2020 Ferri's CLINICAL ADVISOR

FRED F. FERRI, M.D., F.A.C.P.
Clinical Professor
Department of Medicine
The Warren Alpert Medical School
Brown University
Providence, Rhode Island

ELSEVIER

FERRI'S CLINICAL ADVISOR 2020 ISBN: 978-0-323-67254-2

Notices

Practitioners and researchers must always rely on their own experience and knowledge in evaluating and using any information, methods, compounds or experiments described herein. Because of rapid advances in the medical sciences, in particular, independent verification of diagnoses and drug dosages should be made. To the fullest extent of the law, no responsibility is assumed by Elsevier, authors, editors or contributors for any injury and/or damage to persons or property as a matter of products liability, negligence or otherwise, or from any use or operation of any methods, products, instructions, or ideas contained in the material herein.

ISBN: 978-0-323-67254-2

Senior Content Strategist: Sarah Barth
Content Development Specialist: Mary Hegeler
Publishing Services Manager: Catherine Jackson
Senior Project Manager: Kate Mannix
Design Direction: Bridget Hoette

Printed in the United States

Last digit is the print number: 9 8 7 6 5 4 3 2 1

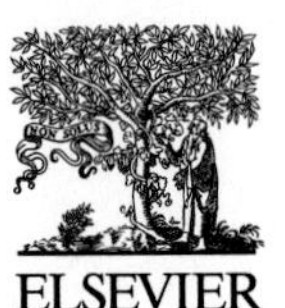

1600 John F. Kennedy Blvd.
Ste 1800
Philadelphia, PA 19103-2899

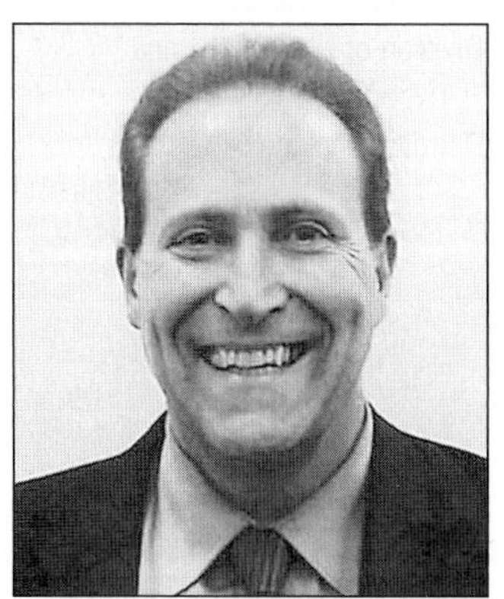

FRED F. FERRI, M.D., F.A.C.P.
Clinical Professor
Department of Medicine
The Warren Alpert Medical School
Brown University
Providence, Rhode Island

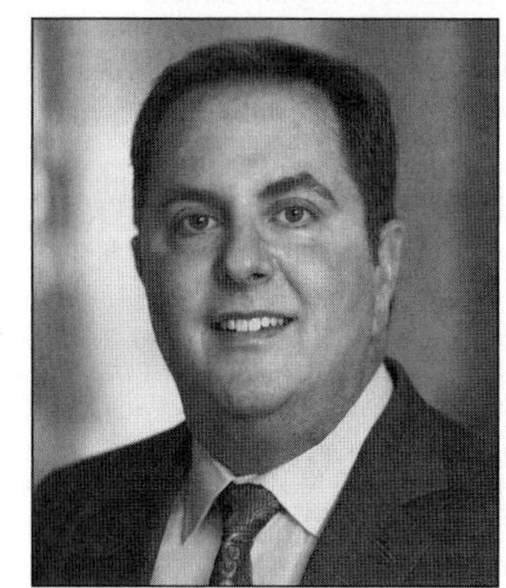

JOSEPH S. KASS, M.D., J.D., F.A.A.N.
Associate Dean of Student Affairs
Professor of Neurology, Psychiatry, and Medical Ethics
Director, Alzheimer's Disease and Memory Disorders Center
Baylor College of Medicine;
Chief of Neurology
Director of Comprehensive Stroke Program
Ben Taub General Hospital
Houston, Texas

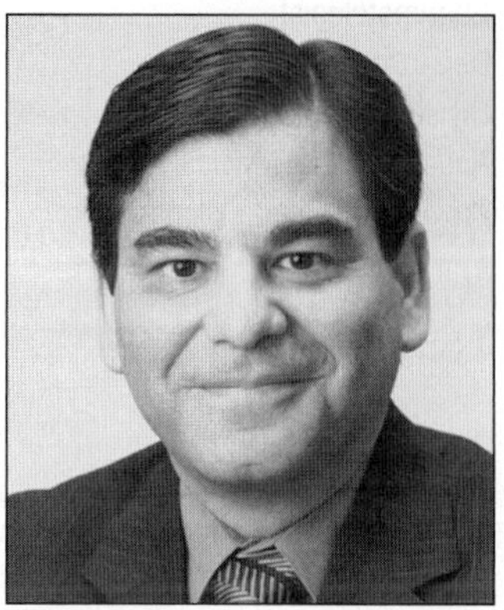

GLENN G. FORT, M.D., M.P.H., F.A.C.P., F.I.D.S.A.
Clinical Associate Professor of Medicine
The Warren Alpert Medical School
Brown University;
Chief, Infectious Diseases
Our Lady of Fatima Hospital and Landmark Medical Center
Providence, Rhode Island

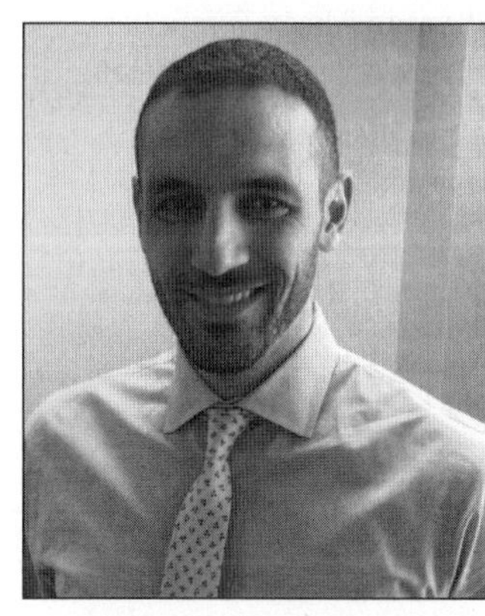

SAMAAN RAFEQ, M.D., F.C.C.P.
Clinical Associate Professor of Medicine and Cardiothoracic Surgery
New York University School of Medicine;
Director, Interventional Pulmonary Fellowship
Associate Director, Interventional Pulmonary Section
NYU Langone Health
New York, New York

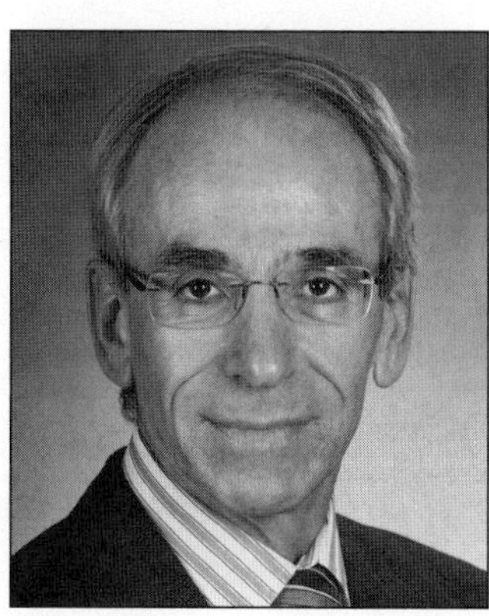

RICHARD J. GOLDBERG, M.D., M.S.
Psychiatrist-in-Chief
Rhode Island Hospital
The Miriam Hospital;
Professor
Department of Psychiatry and Human Behavior
The Warren Alpert Medical School
Brown University
Providence, Rhode Island

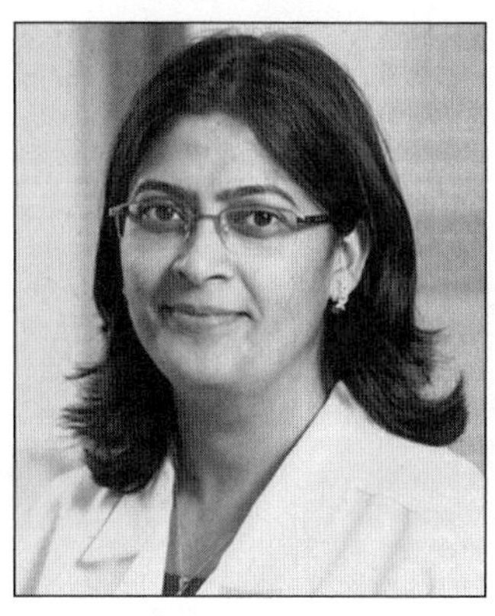

BHARTI RATHORE, M.D.
Program Director, Hematology/Oncology Fellowship
Roger Williams Medical Center
Providence, Rhode Island;
Assistant Professor of Medicine
Boston University School of Medicine
Boston, Massachusetts

Section Editors

ANTHONY SCISCIONE, D.O.
Professor
Department of Obstetrics and Gynecology
Jefferson Medical College
Philadelphia, Pennsylvania;
Residency Program Director
Director of Maternal-Fetal Medicine
Department of Obstetrics and Gynecology
Christiana Care Health System
Newark, Delaware

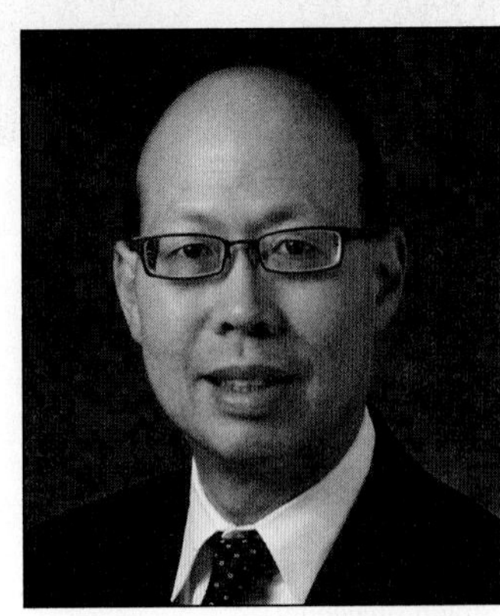

JERRY YEE, M.D.
Clinical Professor of Medicine
Department of Internal Medicine
Wayne State University School of Medicine;
Division Head
Henry Ford Hospital
Division of Nephrology and Hypertension
Detroit, Michigan

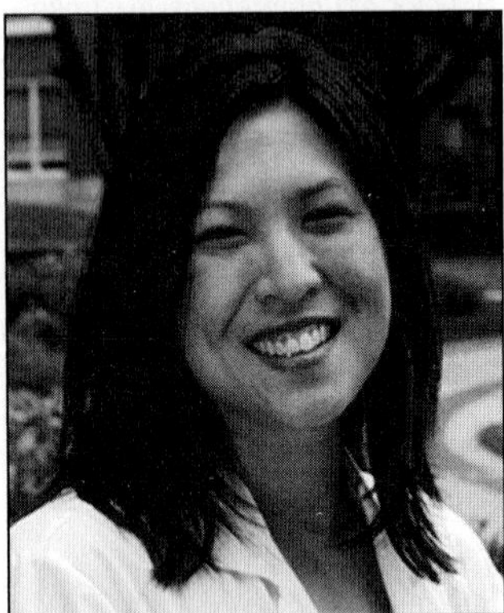

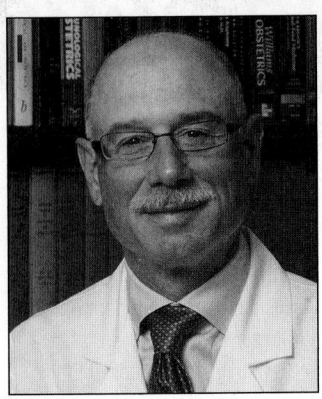

IRIS L. TONG, M.D.
Associate Professor
Department of Medicine
The Warren Alpert Medical School
Brown University;
Attending Physician
Women's Primary Care
Women's Medicine Collaborative
Providence, Rhode Island

BERNARD ZIMMERMANN, M.D.
Associate Professor Emeritus
Department of Medicine
Boston University
Boston, Massachusetts;
Rheumatologist
Department of Medicine
Division of Rheumatology
Roger Williams Medical Center
Providence, Rhode Island

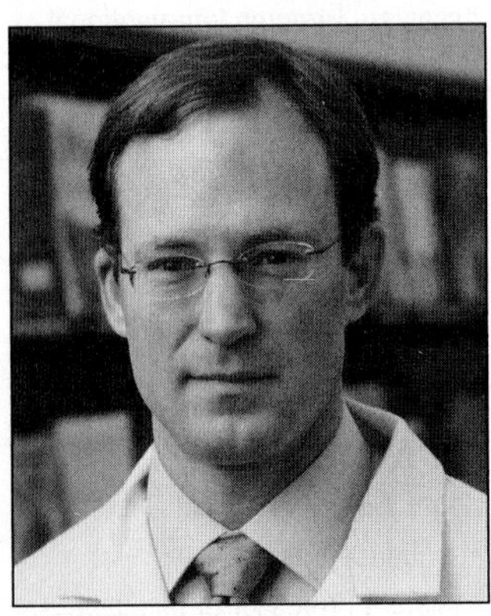

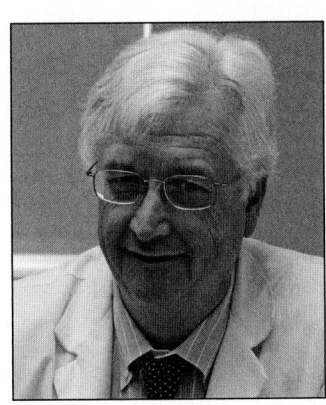

JOHN WYLIE, M.D., F.A.C.C.
Director, Cardiac Electrophysiology
Steward Health Care System
Assistant Professor of Medicine
Tufts University School of Medicine
Boston, Massachusetts

ALEXANDRA ABRAMS-DOWNEY, M.D.
Professor, Department of Medicine
Icahn School of Medicine at Mount Sinai
New York, New York

MAXWELL AFARI, M.D.
Advanced Heart Failure and Transplant Cardiology Fellow
Massachusetts General Hospital
Harvard Medical School
Boston, Massachusetts

SANDEEP AGARWAL, M.D.
Associate Professor of Medicine
Division of Nephrology and Hypertension
Drexel University College of Medicine
Philadelphia, Pennsylvania

MONZR M. AL MALKI, M.D.
Assistant Professor
Hematology and Hematopoietic Cell Transplantation
City of Hope National Medical Center
Duarte, California

BAHA AL-ABID, M.D.
Fellow
Division of Nephrology and Hypertension
Department of Internal Medicine
Henry Ford Hospital
Detroit, Michigan

TANYA ALI, M.D.
Clinical Assistant Professor of Medicine
Department of Medicine
Warren Alpert Medical School of Brown University
Providence, Rhode Island

STEPHANIE MICHELLE ALLEN, M.S.
Baylor College of Medicine
Houston, Texas

ROWENA ALMEIDA, M.D.

IHAB ALOMARI, M.D.
Interventional Cardiologist
Assistant Professor of Medicine
University of California, Irvine
Orange, California

RASHA B. ALQADI, M.D.
Rheumatologist
Providence Sacred Heart Medical Center and Children's Hospital
Spokane, Washington

JORDAN R. ANDERSON, D.O.
Rhode Island Hospital
Departments of Neurology and Psychiatry
Providence, Rhode Island

MARIA ANDRIEVSKAYA, M.D.
Nephrology Fellow
Henry Ford Hospital
Detroit, Michigan

KATHRYN TAYLOR ANILOWSKI, M.S., P.T., C.L.T.-L.A.N.A.
Physical Therapist
Kinder Touch Lymphedema Center
Saratoga Springs, New York

ANNGENE ANTHONY, M.D., M.P.H., F.A.A.F.P.
Teaching Faculty
Mountainside Family Medicine
Residency Program
Verona, New Jersey

JOE AOUN, M.D.
Internal Medicine Resident
Steward St Elizabeth's Medical Center
Tufts University School of Medicine
Brighton, Massachusetts

COSBY G. ARNOLD, M.D., M.P.H.
Emergency Medicine Resident
University of Tennessee Health Science Center
Memphis, Tennessee

ZUHAL ARZOMAND, M.D.
Rheumatology Fellow
Rhode Island Hospital
Warren Alpert Medical School of Brown University
Providence, Rhode Island

DANIEL K. ASIEDU, M.D., PH.D., F.A.C.P.
Staff Physician
Coastal Medical, Inc.
Lincoln, Rhode Island

SUDEEP K. AULAKH, M.D., F.A.C.P., F.R.C.P.C.
Director Ambulatory Education
Baystate Internal Medicine Residency
Assistant Professor
UMASS Medical School - Baystate
Baystate Health
Springfield, Massachusetts

MICHAEL AUSTIN, D.O.
United States Navy

RUPALI AVASARE, M.D.
Assistant Professor of Medicine
Oregon Health & Science University
Portland, Oregon

SARAH AZIZ, M.D.
Rowan University School of Osteopathic Medicine
Stratford, New Jersey

Contributors

TANIA B. BABAR, M.D.
Assistant Professor
West Virginia University School of Medicine, Charleston Division
Charleston, West Virginia

EMELIA ARGYROPOULOS BACHMAN, M.D.
Director of Fertility Preservation
Reproductive Associates of Delaware
Department of Obstetrics and Gynecology
Christiana Hospital
Newark, Delaware

BENJAMIN BAKER, M.D.
Emergency Medicine Assistant Professor
University of Tennessee Health Sciences Center
Memphis, Tennessee

BRIANNA R. BAKOW, M.D.
Department of Medicine
Warren Alpert Medical School of Brown University
Providence, Rhode Island

T. CAROLINE BANK, M.D.
Christiana Care Health System
Wilmington, Delaware

TRACE BARRETT, M.D.
Cardiology Fellow
Department of Medicine
University of Vermont
Burlington, Vermont

AILIN BARSEGHIAN, M.D.
Assistant Professor of Cardiology
University of California, Irvine
Orange, California

CRAIG L. BASMAN, M.D.
Department of Cardiovascular Medicine
Lenox Hill Hospital – Northwell Health
New York, New York

LEE BAUMGARTEN, M.D.
Vattikuti Urology Institute
Henry Ford Health System
Detroit, Michigan

DEANNA BENNER, A.P.R.N., C.R.N.P.
Women's Health Nurse Practitioner
Christiana Care Health System
Newark, Delaware

ARNALDO A. BERGES, M.D.
Director, Division of Inpatient Psychiatry
Rhode Island Hospital
Assistant Clinical Professor
Warren Alpert Medical School of Brown University
Providence, Rhode Island

VICKY H. BHAGAT, M.D., M.P.H.
Gastroenterology Fellow
Robert Wood Johnson University Hospital
New Brunswick, New Jersey

HARIKRASHNA B. BHATT, M.D.
Assistant Professor of Medicine
Department of Medicine
Warren Alpert Medical School of Brown University
Chief of Endocrinology
Providence VA Medical Center
Providence, Rhode Island

DANISH BHATTI, M.D.
Assistant Professor
Department of Neurological Sciences
University of Nebraska Medical Center
Omaha, Nebraska

COURTNEY CLARK BILODEAU, M.D., F.A.C.P.
Assistant Professor
Internal Medicine – Obstetric Medicine
Warren Alpert Medical School of Brown University
Attending Physician
Women's Medicine Collaborative
Providence, Rhode Island

STEFANI BISSONETTE, M.D.
Obstetrics and Gynecology Resident Physician
Christiana Care Health System
Newark, Delaware

GHAMAR BITAR, M.D.
Obstetrics and Gynecology
Christiana Care Health System
Newark, Delaware

CRAIG BLAKENEY, M.D.
Clinical Assistant Professor
Department of Emergency Medicine
Memphis, Tennessee

CHRISTOPHER P. BLOMBERG, D.O.
Cardiovascular Medicine
Southern Maine Health Care / Maine Health
Biddeford, Maine

TRAVIS D. BLOOD, M.D.
University Orthopedics
Warren Alpert Medical School of Brown University
Providence, Rhode Island

STEVEN L. BOKSHAN, M.D.
Orthopedics Resident
Warren Alpert Medical School of Brown University
Providence, Rhode Island

ALEX BORCHERT, M.D.
Vattikuti Urology Institute
Henry Ford Health System
Detroit, Michigan

MARK ELIOT BOROWSKY, M.D.
Division Director, Gynecologic Oncology
Christiana Care Health System
Newark, Delaware

ALEXANDRA BOSKE, M.D.
Director of Inpatient Neurology
Stroke Program Director
Saint David's Round Rock Medical Center
Round Rock, Texas

butors

HER CHOE, B.S.
Tennessee Health Science Center
nessee

CHOLANKERIL, M.D.
patology
Tennessee Health Science Center
nessee

CHOLANKERIL, M.D.
rsity School of Medicine
s Medical Center
hode Island

RK, M.D., M.P.H.
dicine Fellow
Medical School of Brown University
Hospital
hode Island

YNE, M.D.
Assistant Professor
Medical School of Brown University
f Emergency Medicine
hode Island

EN, M.D.
fessor
f Medicine
ephrology
ersity William Beaumont School of Medicine
ichigan

EN, PHARM.D.
fessor of Pharmacy
Rhode Island
de Island

REE CONGRETE, M.D.
dent
cine, Department of Medicine
th's Medical Center
achusetts

COPELIN II, M.D., M.H.A.
cine
rsity School of Medicine
s Medical Center
hode Island

RL CORLEY III, M.D.
ledicine Resident Physician
Tennessee Health Science Center
nessee

CRAINE, M.S.ED., C.C.C.-S.L.P.
uage Pathologist
ren's Hospital
ce, Rhode Island

CRAMER, M.D.
sician
f Obstetrics and Gynecology
re Health System
ware

CRISTOFARO, M.D.
fessor of Medicine
Medical School of Brown University
hode Island

JOANNE SZCZYGIEL CUNHA, M.D.
Assistant Professor of Medicine
Division of Rheumatology
Warren Alpert Medical School of Brown University
Department of Medicine, Division of Rheumatology
University Medicine Foundation
Rhode Island Hospital
Providence, Rhode Island

KARLENE CUNNINGHAM, PH.D.
Clinical Assistant Professor
Department of Psychiatry and Behavioral Medicine
Brody School of Medicine, East Carolina University
Greenville, North Carolina

ALICIA J. CURTIN, PH.D
Assistant Professor
Division of Geriatrics
Warren Alpert Medical School of Brown University
Providence, Rhode Island

GANARY DABIRI, M.D., PH.D.
Department of Medicine
Division of Dermatology
Roger Williams Medical Center
Boston University School of Medicine
Providence, Rhode Island

LYNN DADO, M.D.
Internal Medicine
Providence, Rhode Island

DEEPAN S. DALAL, M.D., M.P.H.
Assistant Professor of Medicine
Warren Alpert Medical School of Brown University
Rheumatologist
Department of Medicine, Division of Rheumatology
Rhode Island Hospital
Providence, Rhode Island

KRISTIN DALPHON, P.A.
Physician Assistant
New York University School of Medicine
New York, New York

KRISTY L. DALRYMPLE, PH.D.
Director of Adult Psychology
Rhode Island and The Miriam Hospitals
Associate Professor, Clinician Educator
Warren Alpert Medical School of Brown University
Providence, Rhode Island

GERARD H. DALY, M.D., M.S.
Division of Cardiology
Saint Elizabeth's Medical Center
Tufts University School of Medicine
Boston, Massachusetts

SHIVANG U. DANAK, M.D.
St. George's University
Detroit, Michigan

RITUPARNA DAS, M.D.
Assistant Professor of Neurology
Baylor College of Medicine
Houston, Texas

LYNN A. BOWLBY, M.D.
Associate Professor of Medicine
Duke University Medical Center
Durham, North Carolina

AMANDA BOX, M.D., M.S.
Emergency Medicine Resident
University of Tennessee Health Science Center
Memphis, Tennessee

ROB W. BRADSHER III, M.D.
Program Director, Internal Medicine
University of Tennessee Health Science Center
Memphis, Tennessee

MARK F. BRADY, M.D., M.P.H., M.M.S.
University of Tennessee Health Science Center
Memphis, Tennessee

KEITH BRENNAN, M.D.
Geriatric Medicine
Stony Brook University
Stony Brook, New York

GAVIN BROWN, M.D.
General Neurologist
Laureate Medical Group at Northside Hospital
Atlanta, Georgia

JENNIFER BUCKLEY, M.D.
Clinical Instructor of Family Medicine
Warren Alpert Medical School of Brown University
Providence, Rhode Island;
Family Medicine
Memorial Hospital of Rhode Island
Pawtucket, Rhode Island;
Family Medicine
Kent Memorial Hospital
Warwick, Rhode Island

ALEXANDRA BUFFIE, M.D.
Graduate Medical Resident
Obstetrics and Gynecology
University of Pittsburgh
Pittsburgh, Pennsylvania

D. BRANDON BURTIS, D.O.
Assistant Professor, Neurology
University of Florida
Gainesville, Florida

CLAUDIA RODRIGUEZ CABRERA, M.D.
Department of Medicine
Universidad Tecnológica de Santiago
Department of Medicine
Hospital Regional Universitario de José María Cabral y Báez
Santiago, Dominican Republic

KATE CAHILL, M.D.
Assistant Professor of Medicine, Clinician Educator
Warren Alpert Medical School of Brown University
Providence, Rhode Island

ANDREW CARAGANIS, M.D.
Internal Medicine
Boston University School of Medicine
Roger Williams Medical Center
Providence, Rhode Island

MATTHEW CARSON, D.P.M.
Podiatrist
Providence, Rhode Island

JORGE J. CASTILLO, M.D.
Division of Hematologic Malignancies
Dana-Farber Cancer Institute
Harvard Medical School
Boston, Massachusetts

ANDREEA M. CATANA, M.D.
Instructor in Medicine, Gastroenterology and
Harvard Medical School
Boston, Massachusetts

CAROLINA S. CEREZO, M.D., F.A.
Medical Director
Division of Pediatric Gastroenterology, Nutri
Hasbro Children's / Rhode Island Hospital
Associate Professor
Department of Pediatrics
Warren Alpert Medical School of Brown Uni
Providence, Rhode Island

JOSHUA CHALKELY, M.S., D.O.
Department of Neurology
University of Kentucky Medical Center
Lexington, Kentucky

PAUL D. CHAMBERLAIN, M.D.
Department of Neurology
Baylor College of Medicine
Houston, Texas

PHILIP A. CHAN, M.D., M.S.
Associate Professor of Medicine
Warren Alpert Medical School of Brown
Providence, Rhode Island

ARLENE CHAPMAN, M.D.
Professor of Medicine
Director, Section of Nephrology
Department of Medicine
University of Chicago
Chicago, Illinois

HANNAH CHAUDRY, M.D.
Warren Alpert Medical School of Brow
Providence, Rhode Island

ANJULIKA CHAWLA, M.D.
Associate Medical Director
Bluebird Bio
Providence, Rhode Island

VICKY CHENG, M.D.
Warren Alpert Medical School of Bro
Providence, Rhode Island

SARAH L. CHISHOLM, M.D.
Resident Physician
Department of Obstetrics and Gynec
University of Colorado Hospital
Denver, Colorado

CHANDRIKA CHITTURI, M.
Fellow, Division of Nephrology and
Henry Ford Hospital
Detroit, Michigan

KATIA DASILVA, B.A.
Research Assistant
Department of Orthopedics
Warren Alpert Medical School of Brown University
Providence, Rhode Island

MANUEL F. DASILVA, M.D.
Assistant Professor of Orthopedics
Director of Medical Student Education
Warren Alpert Medical School of Brown University
Attending Physician in Orthopedics
Rhode Island Hospital
Providence, Rhode Island

CATHERINE D'AVANZATO, PH.D.
Psychologist
Rhode Island Hospital
Clinical Assistant Professor
Warren Alpert Medical School of Brown University
Providence, Rhode Island

AMADEO J. DE LUCA-WESTRATE, M.D.
Battalion Surgeon
3d Battalion, 7th Marine Regiment
MCAGCC
Twentynine Palms, California

STEVEN F. DEFRODA, M.D., M.ENG.
Warren Alpert Medical School of Brown University
Department of Orthopaedic Surgery
Providence, Rhode Island

ALEXANDRA DEGENHARDT, M.D., M.M.SC.
Director, Multiple Sclerosis Center
Pen Bay Medical Center
Rockport, Maine

ASHWINI U. DHOKTE, M.D.
Resident Physician
Christiana Care Hospital
Newark, Delaware

JOSEPH A. DIAZ, M.D., M.P.H.
Associate Dean for Diversity and Multicultural Affairs
Associate Professor of Medicine
Associate Professor of Medical Science
Warren Alpert Medical School of Brown University
Providence, Rhode Island

PRATIMA DIBBA, M.D., M.B.A.
Nutrition Fellow
Memorial Sloan Kettering Cancer Center
Cornell University
New York, New York

THOMAS H. DOHLMAN, M.D.
Cornea Service
Massachusetts Eye and Ear Infirmary
Harvard Medical School
Boston, Massachusetts

DAVID J. DOMENICHINI, M.D.
Clinical Instructor
Endocrinology and Metabolism
Hartford Hospital
University of Connecticut Health Center
West Hartford, Connecticut

KATHLEEN DOO, M.D.
Sleep Medicine Fellow
New York University
New York, New York

AMANDA C. DORAN, M.D., PH.D.
Cardiology Fellow
Department of Medicine, Division of Cardiology
Columbia University
New York, New York

JOHN DUDLEY, M.D., M.P.H.
PGY-3 Internal Medicine
Brown University
Providence, Rhode Island

ANDREW P. DUKER, M.D.
Associate Professor, Movement Disorders Division
Director, Department of Neurology and Rehabilitation Medicine
University of Cincinnati College of Medicine
Cincinnati, Ohio

SHASHANK DWIVEDI, M.D.
Orthopaedic Surgery Resident
Rhode Island Hospital / Warren Alpert Medical School of Brown University
Providence, Rhode Island

CHRISTINE EISENHOWER, PHARM.D
Clinical Assistant Professor
Pharmacy Practice
University of Rhode Island College of Pharmacy
Kingston, Rhode Island

GREGORY ELIA, M.D.
Orthopaedic Surgery Resident
Department of Orthopaedics, Warren Alpert Medical School of Brown University
Providence, Rhode Island

PAMELA ELLSWORTH, M.D.
Chief, Division of Pediatric Urology
Nemours Children's Hospital
Orlando, Florida

BRYAN ENGLAND, M.D.
Assistant Professor of Emergency Medicine
University of Tennessee Health Science Center
Memphis, Tennessee

ALAN EPSTEIN, M.D.
Roger Williams Medical Center
Providence, Rhode Island

AHARON EREZ, M.D.
Clinical Electrophysiology Fellow
Saint Elizabeth's Medical Center
Brighton, Massachusetts

PATRICIO SEBASTIAN ESPINOSA, M.D., M.P.H.
Associate Professor
Department of Neurology
Department of Clinical Biomedical Science
Charles E. Schmidt College of Medicine at Florida Atlantic University
Boca Raton, Florida

DANYELLE EVANS, M.D.
Baylor College of Medicine
Houston, Texas

Contributors

MARK D. FABER, M.D.
Senior Staff Physician
Division of Nephrology
Henry Ford Hospital
Detroit, Michigan

VALERIA FABRE, M.D.
Clinical Instructor, Medicine
Warren Alpert Medical School of Brown University;
Providence, Rhode Island,
Medicine, Memorial Hospital of Rhode Island
Pawtucket, Rhode Island

MATTHEW J. FAGAN, M.D., F.A.C.O.G.
Attending Physician
Director of Undergraduate Medical Education
Obstetrics and Gynecology
Christiana Care Health System
Newark, Delaware

TIMOTHY W. FARRELL, M.D., A.G.S.F.
Associate Professor of Medicine
Adjunct Associate Professor of Family Medicine
Director, University of Utah Health Interprofessional Education Program
Physician Investigator
VA Salt Lake City Geriatric Research, Education, and Clinical Center
University of Utah School of Medicine
Salt Lake City, Utah

MARIAM FAYEK, M.D.
Clinical Assistant Professor
Department of Medicine
Attending Physician
Warren Alpert Medical School of Brown University
Center for Women's Gastrointestinal Health
Women and Infants Hospital
Providence, Rhode Island

JASON D. FERREIRA, M.D.
Gastroenterologist
University Gastroenterology, LLC
Providence, Rhode Island

FRED F. FERRI, M.D., F.A.C.P.
Clinical Professor
Department of Medicine
Warren Alpert Medical School of Brown University
Providence, Rhode Island

HEATHER FERRI, D.O.
Department of Medicine
Warren Alpert Medical School of Brown University
Rhode Island Hospital
Providence, Rhode Island

BARRY FINE, M.D., PH.D
Assistant Professor of Medicine
Division of Cardiology
Columbia University Vagelos College of Physicians and Surgeons
New York, New York

STACI A. FISCHER, M.D.
Field Representative
Clinical Learning Environment Review program
Accreditation Council for Graduate Medical Education
Chicago, Illinois

TAMARA G. FONG, M.D., PH.D.
Assistant Professor of Neurology
Harvard Medical School
Staff Neurologist
Beth Israel Deaconess Medical Center
Assistant Scientist
Aging Brain Center, Institute for Aging Research, Hebrew SeniorLife
Boston, Massachusetts

YANEVE FONGE, M.D.
Resident Physician
Christiana Care Health Network
Newark, Delaware

MICHELLE FORCIER, M.D., M.P.H.
Professor, Pediatrics
Warren Alpert Medical School of Brown University
Providence, Rhode Island

FRANK G. FORT, M.D., F.A.C.S., R.PH.S.
Medical Director
Capital Region Vein Centre
Schenectady, New York

GLENN G. FORT, M.D., M.P.H., F.A.C.P., F.I.D.S.A.
Clinical Associate Professor of Medicine
Warren Alpert Medical School of Brown University
Chief, Infectious Diseases
Our Lady of Fatima Hospital and Landmark Medical Center
Providence, Rhode Island

JUSTIN F. FRASER, M.D.
Assistant Professor of Cerebrovascular, Endovascular, and Skull Base Surgery
Department of Neurosurgery
University of Kentucky
Lexington, Kentucky

MICHAEL FRIEDMAN, M.D.
Clinical Associate Professor
Department of Psychiatry and Human Behavior
Clinical Associate Professor
Department of Neurology
Warren Alpert Medical School of Brown University
Providence, Rhode Island

DANIEL R. FRISCH, M.D.
Jefferson University Sidney Kimmel Medical College
Philadelphia, Pennsylvania

ANTHONY GALLO, M.D.
Director of ECT Service
Rhode Island Hospital
Clinical Assistant Professor
Warren Alpert Medical School of Brown University
Providence, Rhode Island

KRISHNA GANNAMRAJ, D.O.
Resident Physician
Department of Internal Medicine
University of Tennessee Health Science Center
Memphis, Tennessee

EDITH GARNEAU, M.D., M.S.
Associate Program Director
Rheumatology Program
Roger Williams Medical Center
Providence, Rhode Island

PAUL GEORGE, M.D., M.H.P.E.
Professor of Family Medicine and Medical Science
Associate Dean for Medical Education
Warren Alpert Medical School of Brown University
Providence, Rhode Island

MOSTAFA GHANIM, M.D.
Internal Medicine Resident Steward
Saint Elizabeth's Medical Center
Tufts University School of Medicine
Brighton, Massachusetts

ROXANA GHASHGHAEI, M.D.

IRENE M. GHOBRIAL, M.D.
Professor of Medicine
Medical Oncology
Dana Farber Cancer Institute
Boston, Massachusetts

KATARZYNA GILEK-SEIBERT, M.D., RH.M.U.S.
Program Director, Rheumatology Fellowship
Director, Division of Rheumatology
Adjunct Assistant Professor of Medicine
Warren Alpert Medical School of Brown University
Roger Williams Medical Center
Providence, Rhode Island

RICHARD GILLERMAN, M.D., PH.D.
Clinical Assistant Professor of Surgery
Warren Alpert Medical School of Brown University
Providence, Rhode Island

DIMITRI GITELMAKER, M.D.
Internal Medicine Resident
Roger Williams Medical Center
Boston University School of Medicine
Providence, Rhode Island

CHARIS GN, M.D.
Rheumatology Fellow
Rhode Island Hospital
Warren Alpert Medical School of Brown University
Providence, Rhode Island

RICHARD J. GOLDBERG, M.D., M.S.
Psychiatrist-in-Chief
Rhode Island Hospital and The Miriam Hospital
Professor
Department of Psychiatry and Human Behavior
Warren Alpert Medical School of Brown University
Providence, Rhode Island

ALLA GOLDBURT, M.D.
Assistant Clinical Professor
Family Medicine
Warren Alpert Medical School of Brown University
Providence, Rhode Island

DANIELLE GOLDFARB, M.D.
Neurologist / Psychiatrist
Banner Alzheimer's Institute
Phoenix, Arizona

JESSE GOLDMAN, M.D., F.A.S.H.
Professor of Medicine
Drexel University College of Medicine
Philadelphia, Pennsylvania

COREY GOLDSMITH, M.D.
Assistant Professor of Neurology
Baylor College of Medicine
Houston, Texas

MAHESWARA SATYA GANGADHARA RAO GOLLA, M.D.
Saint Elizabeth's Medical Center
Brighton, Massachusetts

CAROLINE GOLSKI, M.D.
General Psychiatry Resident
Warren Alpert Medical School of Brown University
Providence, Rhode Island

HELEN B. GOMEZ, M.D.
Resident Physician
Christiana Care Health System
Newark, Delaware

NATHANIEL P. GOODRICH, M.D.
University of Nebraska College of Medicine
Department of Pediatrics
Children's Hospital & Medical Center
Omaha, Nebraska

MICHAEL P. GOOLD, M.D.
Camp Pendleton Naval Hospital
Camp Pendleton, California

PAUL GORDON, M.D.
Clinical Assistant Professor of Medicine
Division of Cardiology
Warren Alpert Medical School of Brown University
Providence, Rhode Island

JOHN A. GRAY, M.D., PH.D.
Assistant Professor
Department of Neurology
Center for Neuroscience
University of California, Davis
Davis, California

ALISON GRAZIOLI, M.D.
Assistant Professor of Medicine
University of Maryland School of Medicine
Baltimore, Maryland

NADIA GRILLER, M.D.
Gastroenterology
University of Toronto
Toronto, Ontario, Canada

SIMON GRINGUT, M.D.
Cardiac Electrophysiology Fellow
Yale New Haven Hospital
New Haven, Connecticut

LAUREN GROCOTT, B.A.
Clinical Research Assistant
Rhode Island Hospital
Providence, Rhode Island

STEPHEN L. GRUPKE, M.D., M.S.
Assistant Professor
Department of Neurosurgery
University of Kentucky
Lexington, Kentucky

Contributors

PATAN GULTAWATVICHAI, M.D.
Assistant Professor of Medicine
Hematology-Oncology
University of Massachusetts Medical School
Worcester, Massachusetts

PRIYA SARIN GUPTA, M.D., M.P.H.
Adolescent Medicine Fellow
Division of General Pediatrics and Adolescent Medicine
Department of Pediatrics
Johns Hopkins Hospital
Baltimore, Maryland

NAWAZ K.A. HACK, M.D.
Assistant Professor of Neurology
F. Edward Hébert School of Medicine
Uniformed Services University of the Health Sciences
Bethesda, Maryland

DENISA L. HAGAU, M.D., F.A.C.C.
Non-invasive Cardiologist
Mercy Medical Center North Iowa
Mason City, Iowa

MOTI HAIM, M.D.
Director, Cardiac Electrophysiology and Pacing
Cardiology Department
Soroka Medical Center
Ben Gurion University of the Negev
Beer-Sheva, Israel

LEO HAN, M.D., M.P.H.
Assistant Professor
Obstetrics and Gynecology
Oregon Health and Science University
Portland, Oregon

SAJEEV HANDA, M.D., S.F.H.M.
Chief, Hospital Medicine
Lifespan Physician Group
Rhode Island / Miriam & Newport Hospitals
Clinical Assistant Professor of Medicine and Neurology
Warren Alpert Medical School of Brown University
Providence, Rhode Island

M. OWAIS HANIF, M.D.
Hahnemann Hospital
Philadelphia, Pennsylvania

NIKOLAS HARBORD, M.D.
Division Chief
Nephrology & Hypertension
Mount Sinai Beth Israel
Assistant Professor
Icahn School of Medicine
New York, New York

ERICA HARDY, M.D., M.M.S.
Division of Infectious Diseases
Warren Alpert Medical School of Brown University
Women and Infants Hospital
Providence, Rhode Island

COLIN J. HARRINGTON, M.D.
Director of CL Psychiatry and Neuropsychiatry Education
Director of Psychosomatic Medicine Fellowship
Co-Director of CNS-Psychiatry Clerkship
Rhode Island Hospital / Warren Alpert Medical School of Brown University
Providence, Rhode Island

ANDREW PAUL HARRIS, M.D.
Orthopedic Surgery Trauma Fellow
Department of Orthopedic Surgery
Warren Alpert Medical School of Brown University
Providence, Rhode Island

LEONARD JEFFERSON HARRIS JR., M.D.
Clinical Affiliate Instructor
Methodist University Hospital
University of Tennessee Emergency Department
Memphis, Tennessee

TAYLOR HARRISON, M.D.
Assistant Professor of Neurology
Department of Neurology
Emory University
Atlanta, Georgia

DON HAYES JR., M.D., M.S., M.ED.
Professor
Departments of Pediatrics, Internal Medicine, Surgery, Epidemiology
The Ohio State University
Columbus, Ohio

DWAYNE R. HEITMILLER, M.D., F.A.P.M.
Attending Physician
Consultation-Liaison Division
Abbott Northwestern Hospital
Minneapolis, Minnesota

DYLAN HENDY, D.O.
Emergency Medicine Attending
Naval Medical Center Camp Pendleton
Camp Pendleton, California Position

RUTH HENNEBERY, M.D.
Obstetrics and Gynecology Resident
Christiana Care Health System
Newark, Delaware

MARGARET R. HINES, M.D.
FPMRS Fellow
Texas A&M College of Medicine
Scott & White Medical Center
Temple, Texas

BRIAN HOCHMAN, D.P.M.
Crystal Falls Foot and Ankle Specialists
Leander, Texas

MATTHEW K. HOFFMAN, M.D., M.P.H., F.A.C.O.G.
Chairman, Department of Obstetrics/Gynecology
Christiana Care Health System
Newark, Delaware

PAMELA E. HOFFMAN, M.D.
Assistant Director
Hasbro Psychiatric Emergency Services
Assistant Professor, Clinician Educator
Department of Psychiatry and Human Behavior
Warren Alpert Medical School of Brown University
Providence, Rhode Island

R. SCOTT HOFFMAN, M.D.
Ophthalmology
Doctors Eye Institute
Assistant Clinical Professor
Department of Ophthalmology
University of Louisville
Louisville, Kentucky

DAWN HOGAN, M.D.
Clinical Assistant Professor of Family Medicine
Warren Alpert Medical School of Brown University
Providence, Rhode Island

N. WILSON HOLLAND, M.D.
Associate Professor of Medicine
Division of Geriatrics and Gerontology
Emory University School of Medicine
Acting Designated Learning Officer
Atlanta Veterans Administration Medical Center
Atlanta, Georgia

SIRI M. HOLTON, M.D.
Obstetrics and Gynecology Resident
Christiana Care Health System
Newark, Delaware

ANNE L. HUME, PHARM.D.
Professor of Pharmacy
University of Rhode Island
Kingston, Rhode Island

DONNY V. HUYNH, M.D.
Staff Physician
McLeod Oncology and Hematology at Seacoast
Little River, South Carolina

TERRI Q. HUYNH, M.D.
Faculty Physician
Department of Obstetrics & Gynecology
Division of Minimally Invasive Gynecologic Surgery
Christiana Care Health System
Newark, Delaware

SARAH HYDER, M.D.

DINA A. IBRAHIM, M.D.
Kent Hospital
Warren Alpert Medical School of Brown University
Providence, Rhode Island

CAITLIN INGRAHAM, M.D.
Christiana Care Health System
Newark, Delaware

LOUIS INSALACO, M.D.
Otolaryngology Resident
Boston University School of Medicine
Boston, Massachusetts

CHRISTOPHER D. JACKSON, M.D.
Chief Resident of Quality and Safety
Internal Medicine
Veterans Affairs Medical Center
University of Tennessee Health Science Center
Memphis, Tennessee

AMIT K. JAIN, M.D.
Cardiovascular Disease Fellow
University of California, Irvine
Orange, California

VANITA B.D. JAIN, M.D.
Clinical Assistant Professor
Christiana Care Health Systems
Thomas Jefferson University
Newark, Delaware

ROBERT H. JANIGIAN, M.D.
Clinical Assistant Professor of Surgery
Warren Alpert Medical School of Brown University
Providence, Rhode Island

NOELLE MARIE JAVIER, M.D.
Assistant Professor of Medicine
Brookdale Department of Geriatrics and Palliative Care
Icahn School of Medicine at Mount Sinai
New York, New York

STEPHANIE JEAN, M.D.

XIBEI JIA, M.D.
Fellow, Female Pelvic Medicine and Reconstructive Surgery
Hahnemann University Hospital
Drexel University College of Medicine
Philadelphia, Pennsylvania

CHRISTINA M. JOHNSON, M.D.
Division of Minimally Invasive Gynecologic Surgery
Department of Obstetrics and Gynecology
Christiana Care Health Systems
Newark, Delaware

COURTNY JOHNSON, D.P.M., M.S.H.S.
Podiatry Resident
Boston University
Boston, Massachusetts

MICHAEL P. JOHNSON, M.D.
Associate Professor of Medicine
Warren Alpert Medical School of Brown University
Providence, Rhode Island

ANGAD JOLLY, M.D.
Baylor College of Medicine
Houston, Texas

KIMBERLY JONES, M.D.
Associate Professor of Child Neurology
Department of Neurology
University of Kentucky
Lexington, Kentucky

SHYAM JOSHI, M.D.
Assistant Professor of Medicine
Oregon Health Sciences University
Portland, Oregon

SIDDHARTH KAPOOR, M.D.
Assistant Professor of Neurology
Director, Headache Medicine
Program Director, Fellowship in Headache Medicine
Department of Neurology
University of Kentucky College of Medicine
Lexington, Kentucky

JAN M. KARCZEWSKI, M.D.
Rheumatology Fellow
Roger Williams Medical Center
Providence, Rhode Island

VANJI KARTHIKEYAN, M.D.
Senior Staff Physician
Henry Ford Hospital
Detroit, Michigan

Contributors

JOSEPH S. KASS, M.D., J.D., F.A.A.N.
Associate Dean of Student Affairs
Professor of Neurology, Psychiatry, and Medical Ethics
Director, Alzheimer's Disease and Memory Disorders Center
Baylor College of Medicine;
Chief of Neurology
Director of Comprehensive Stroke Program
Ben Taub General Hospital
Houston, Texas

EMILY R. KATZ, M.D.
Associate Professor (Clinician Educator)
Department of Psychiatry and Human Behavior
Department of Pediatrics
Warren Alpert Medical School of Brown University;
Director, Child and Adolescent Psychiatry Consultation-Liaison Service
Hasbro Children's Hospital
Providence, Rhode Island

ALI KAZIM, M.D.
Chief of Psychiatry
Phoenix VA Health Care System
Clinical Professor Psychiatry
University of Arizona Medical College
Phoenix, Arizona

SUDAD KAZZAZ, M.D.
Baylor College of Medicine
Houston, Texas

SACHIN KEDAR, M.B.B.S., M.D.
Associate Professor
Neurological Sciences; Ophthalmology and Visual Sciences
University of Nebraska Medical School
Truhlsen Eye Institute
Omaha, Nebraska

PAUL S. KELLERMAN, M.D.
Professor of Medicine
Oakland University William Beaumont School of Medicine
Section Head, Nephrology
Auburn Hills, Michigan

A. BASIT KHAN, B.A.
Baylor College of Medicine
Houston, Texas

MOHAMMAD KHAN, M.D.
Hospitalist
Westerly Hospital
Westerly, Rhode Island

BYUNG KIM, M.D.
Department of Hematology Oncology
Harold Alfond Center for Cancer Care
Augusta, Maine

BRANDI KIMBLE, D.P.M.
Podiatrist
Coolidge, Arizona

ROBERT M. KIRCHNER, M.D.
Fellow, Cardiology
Warren Alpert Medical School of Brown University
Providence, Rhode Island

DIANE KOCOVSKY, A.P.R.N.
Nurse Practitioner
Children's Hospital & Medical Center
Omaha, Nebraska

ROBERT KOHN, M.D.
Department of Psychiatry and Human Behavior
Warren Alpert Medical School of Brown University
Providence, Rhode Island

ERNA MILUNKA KOJIC, M.D.
Professor, Division of Infectious Diseases
Icahn School of Medicine at Mount Sinai
New York, New York

ARAVIND RAO KOKKIRALA, M.D., F.A.C.C.
Warren Alpert Medical School of Brown University
Providence, Rhode Island

YUVAL KONSTANTINO, M.D.
Cardiology
Clinical Cardiac Electrophysiology
Soroka University Medical Center
Beer-Sheva, Israel

NELSON KOPYT, D.O.
Chief of Nephrology
Lehigh Valley Hospital
Allentown, Pennsylvania;
Clinical Professor of Medicine
Morsani College of Medicine
Tampa, Florida

LINDSAY KOSINSKI, M.D.
Resident Physician
Warren Alpert Medical School of Brown University
Rhode Island Hospital
Providence, Rhode Island

KATHERINE KOSTROUN, B.S.
Medical Student
Baylor College of Medicine
Houston, Texas

IOANNIS KOULOURIDIS, M.D., M.S.
Tufts University School of Medicine
Saint Elizabeth's Medical Center
Department of Medicine
Division of Cardiology
Boston, Massachusetts

TIMOTHY R. KREIDER, M.D., PH.D.
Assistant Professor
Department of Psychiatry
Donald and Barbara Zucker School of Medicine at Hofstra/Northwell
Hempstead, New York

PRASHANTH KRISHNAMOHAN, M.B.B.S., M.D.
Neurocritical Care
Stanford University
Palo Alto, California

LALATHAKSHA KUMBAR, M.D.
Section Head, Interventional Nephrology
Division of Nephrology and Hypertension
Henry Ford Hospital
Detroit, Michigan

DAVID I. KURSS, M.D., F.A.C.O.G., N.C.M.P
Clinical Assistant Professor
SUNY at Buffalo School of Medicine
Buffalo, New York

SEBASTIAN G. KURZ, M.D.
Associate Professor
Department of Internal Medicine
Division of Pulmonary, Critical Care and Sleep Medicine
Mount Sinai Hospital
New York, New York

PETER LACAMERA, M.D.
Assistant Professor of Medicine
Tufts University School of Medicine
Boston, Massachusetts

ANN S. LACASCE, M.D., M.M.SC.
Associate Professor of Medicine
Medical Oncology
Harvard Medical School
Boston, Massachusetts

ASHLEY LAKIN, D.O., M.A.
Assistant Professor of Family Medicine (Clinical)
Warren Alpert Medical School of Brown University
Providence, Rhode Island

UYEN T. LAM, M.D.
Noninvasive Cardiology
Saint Elizabeth's Medical Center
Boston, Massachusetts

JHENETTE LAUDER, M.D.
Obstetrics/Gynecology Resident
Christiana Care Health Services
Newark, Delaware

NYKIA LEACH, B.A.
Clinical Research Assistant
Rhode Island Hospital
Providence, Rhode Island

DAVID A. LEAVITT, M.D.
Associate Director of Endourology
Director of Laser Surgery
Vattikuti Urology Institute
Detroit, Michigan

KACHIU C. LEE, M.D., M.P.H.
Department of Dermatology
Warren Alpert Medical School at Brown University
Providence, Rhode Island

NICHOLAS J. LEMME, M.D.
Resident Physician
Department of Orthopedics
Warren Alpert Medical School at Brown University
Rhode Island Hospital
Providence, Rhode Island

BETH LEOPOLD, M.D.
Obstetrics/Gynecology Resident
Christiana Care Health System
Newark, Delaware

JIAN LI, M.D., PH.D.
Senior Staff Physician
Henry Ford Hospital
Detroit, Michigan

NEILL Y. LI, M.D.
Department of Orthopaedic Surgery
Warren Alpert Medical School of Brown University
Providence, Rhode Island

DONITA DILLON LIGHTNER, M.D.
Assistant Professor of Pediatric Neurology
Department of Neurology
University of Kentucky
Lexington, Kentucky

PATRICIA W. LO, M.D.
Orange Coast Women's Medical Group
Laguna Hills, California

KITO LORD, M.D., M.B.A.
Assistant Professor
Department of Emergency Medicine
University of Tennessee Health Science Center
Memphis, Tennessee

ELIZABETH A. LOWENHAUPT, M.D.
Associate Professor (Clinician Educator)
Department of Psychiatry and Human Behavior
Warren Alpert Medical School of Brown University
Providence, Rhode Island

RANDY L. LUCIANO, M.D., PH.D.
Assistant Professor of Medicine
Yale University School of Medicine
New Haven, Connecticut

DAVID J. LUCIER JR., M.D., M.B.A., M.P.H., C.P.P.S.
Director of Quality Improvement and Patient Safety, Hospital Medicine
Attending Physician, Hospital Medicine
Massachusetts General Hospital
Boston, Massachusetts

MICHELLE C. MACIAG, M.D.
Boston Children's Hospital
Department of Immunology
Boston, Massachusetts

SUSANNA R. MAGEE, M.D., M.P.H.
Assistant Professor
Department of Family Medicine
Warren Alpert Medical School of Brown University
Providence, Rhode Island

MARTA MAJCZAK, M.D.
Attending Psychiatrist
Bradley Hospital
Riverside, Rhode Island

SHEFALI MAJMUDAR, D.O.
Rheumatologist
Miramar, Florida

GRETCHEN MAKAI, M.D.
Christiana Care Health System
Department of Obstetrics and Gynecology
Newark, Delaware

PIEUSHA MALHOTRA, M.D., M.P.H.
Assistant Professor
Division of Rheumatology
Rutgers New Jersey School of Medicine
Newark, New Jersey

EISHITA MANJREKAR, PH.D
Postdoctoral Fellow
Rhode Island Hospital
Warren Alpert Medical School of Brown University
Providence, Rhode Island

ABIGAIL K. MANSFIELD, PH.D.
Assistant Professor
Warren Alpert Medical School of Brown University
Providence, Rhode Island

STEPHEN MARCACCIO, M.D.
Orthopedic Surgery Resident
Rhode Island Hospital
Warren Alpert Medical School of Brown University
Providence, Rhode Island

MICHAEL C. MARIORENZI, M.S., M.D.
Resident Physician
Department of Orthopedic Surgery
Warren Alpert Medical School of Brown University
Providence, Rhode Island

KELLY L. MATSON, PHARM.D., B.C.P.P.S.
Clinical Professor
Department of Pharmacy Practice
University of Rhode Island
Kingston, Rhode Island

MAITREYI MAZUMDAR, M.D., M.P.H., M.SC.
Assistant Professor of Neurology
Harvard Medical School
Staff Physician
Department of Neurology
Boston's Children's Hospital
Boston, Massachusetts

NADINE MBUYI, M.D.
Assistant Professor of Medicine
Division of Rheumatology
The George Washington University School of Medicine and Health Sciences
Washington, DC

RUSSELL J. MCCULLOH, M.D.
Associate Professor
Pediatrics and Internal Medicine
University of Nebraska Medical Center, Children's Hospital & Medical Center
Omaha, Nebraska

CHRISTOPHER MCDONALD, M.D.
Orthopedic Surgery Resident
Rhode Island Hospital
Warren Alpert Medical School of Brown University
Providence, Rhode Island

BARBARA MCGUIRK, M.D.
Director of Surgery
Reproductive Associates of Delaware
Newark, Delaware

RACHEL MEEKS, M.D.
Aviation Combat Element Surgeon
Marine Medium Tiltrotor Squadron 164
Marine Aircraft Group 39, 3rd Marine Aircraft Wing
Camp Pendleton, California

AKANKSHA MEHTA, M.D., M.S.
Assistant Professor of Urology
Director of Undergraduate Medical Education
Emory University School of Medicine
Atlanta, Georgia

JORGE MERCADO, M.D.
Assistant Professor of Medicine
Assistant Chief of Pulmonary & Critical Care Medicine
Director of Pulmonary Section
NYU Langone Health
Brooklyn, New York

JENNIFER B. MERRIMAN, M.D.
Attending Physician
Delaware Center for Maternal & Fetal Medicine
Christiana Care Medical Center
Newark, Delaware

RORY MERRITT, M.D.
Teaching Fellow
Assistant Dean of Medicine
Warren Alpert Medical School of Brown University
Department of Emergency Medicine
Providence, Rhode Island

ROBIN METCALFE-KLAW, M.D.
Obstetrics and Gynecology
Christiana Care Health Network
Newark, Delaware

GAETANE MICHAUD, M.D.
Professor of Medicine and Cardiothoracic Surgery
NYU Langone Health
New York, New York

TARO MINAMI, M.D.
Associate Professor of Medicine, Clinician Educator
Warren Alpert Medical School of Brown University
Providence, Rhode Island

HASSAN M. MINHAS, M.D.
Clinical Assistant Professor
Department of Law and Psychiatry
Yale University
New Haven, Connecticut;
Medical Director, Outpatient Autism Services
Hospital for Special Care
New Britain, Connecticut

JARED D. MINKEL, PH.D.
Assistant Professor, Psychiatry & Human Behavior
Warren Alpert Medical School of Brown University
Providence, Rhode Island

FARHAN A. MIRZA, M.D.
Neurosurgery Resident
University of Kentucky
Lexington, Kentucky

THERESA A. MORGAN, PH.D.
Clinical Assistant Professor, Psychiatry and Human Behavior
Warren Alpert Medical School of Brown University
Providence, Rhode Island

ALEEM I. MUGHAL, M.D.
Cardiac Electrophysiologist
Heart Center of North Texas
Fort Worth, Texas

SHIVA KUMAR R. MUKKAMALLA, M.D., M.P.H.
Hematology / Medical Oncology Attending
Presbyterian Medical Group, Rust Medical Center
Rio Rancho, New Mexico

VIVEK MURTHY, M.D.
Assistant Professor of Medicine
Albert Einstein College of Medicine
Montefiore Medical Center
Bronx, New York

ALEISHA NABOWER, M.D.
Assistant Professor, Pediatrics
University of Nebraska Medical Center
Children's Hospital & Medical Center
Omaha, Nebraska

CATHERINE E. NAJEM, M.D.
Section of Rheumatology
Lewis Katz School of Medicine at Temple University
Philadelphia, Pennsylvania

BILAL H. NAQVI, M.D.
Hematologist / Oncologist
Marshfield Clinic Regional Cancer Center
Eau Claire, Wisconsin

HUSSAIN MOHAMMAD H. NASERI, M.D.
Hematology / Oncology Physician
Ohio Valley Medical Center
Wheeling, West Virginia

UZMA NASIR, M.D.
Assistant Professor, Clinical Anesthesia and Pain Management
SUNY at Stony Brook University Hospital, VA Hospital
Northport, New York

SHAW NATAN, M.D.
Cardiac Electrophysiologist
Saint Elizabeth Medical Center
Brighton, Massachusetts

ADRIENNE B. NEITHARDT, M.D.
Reproductive Associates of Delaware
Newark, Delaware

DANIEL C. NEUBAUER, M.D.
Surgery Resident
Department of General Surgery
Naval Medical Center San Diego
San Diego, California

MARISSA NORBERTO, PHARM.D. CANDIDATE
University of Rhode Island
Kingston, Rhode Island

MELISSA NOTHNAGLE, M.D., M.SC.
Naval Medical Center San Diego
San Diego, California

JAMES E. NOVAK, M.D., PH.D.
Division of Nephrology and Hypertension
Henry Ford Hospital
Detroit, Michigan

CHLOE MANDER NUNNELEY, M.D.
Baylor College of Medicine
Houston, Texas

GAIL M. O'BRIEN, M.D.
Physician, Internal Medicine / Obesity Medicine
Lahey Hospital Primary Care
Burlington, Massachusetts

RYAN M. O'DONNELL, M.D.
Orthopedic Surgery Resident
Warren Alpert Medical School of Brown University
Rhode Island Hospital
Providence, Rhode Island

ADAM J. OLSZEWSKI, M.D.
Assistant Professor of Medicine
Warren Alpert Medical School of Brown University
Providence, Rhode Island

LINDSAY M. ORCHOWSKI, PH.D.
Associate Professor (Research)
Department of Psychiatry and Human Behavior
Warren Alpert Medical School of Brown University
Providence, Rhode Island

THOMAS J. OSWALD, M.D.
Department of Emergency Medicine
University of Tennessee Health Science Center
Memphis, Tennessee

PAOLO G. PACE, M.A.SC., M.D.
Resident Physician, Internal Medicine
Roger Williams Medical Center
Providence, Rhode Island

CHRIS PAN, M.D., M.B.A., M.S.
Assistant Clinical Professor
Associated Fellowship Program Director
University of California, Irvine
Orange, California

LISA PAPPAS-TAFFER, M.D.
Assistant Professor of Dermatology
University of Pennsylvania
Philadelphia, Pennsylvania

YUVRAJSINH J. PARMAR, M.D.
Department of Cardiovascular Medicine
Lenox Hill Hospital – Northwell Health
New York, New York

BIRJU B. PATEL, M.D.
Assistant Professor of Medicine
Department of Medicine
Division of Geriatrics and Gerontology
Emory University School of Medicine
Atlanta Veterans Affairs Medical Center
Atlanta, Georgia

DEVAN PATEL, M.D.
Resident Physician
Warren Alpert Medical School of Brown University
Rhode Island Hospital
Providence, Rhode Island

NIMA R. PATEL, M.D., M.S.
Assistant Residency Director
Division of Minimally Invasive Gynecologic Surgery
Department of Obstetrics & Gynecology
Christiana Care Health Systems
Newark, Delaware

PRANAV M. PATEL, M.D., F.A.C.C., F.A.H.A., F.S.C.A.I.
Professor of Medicine and Biomedical Engineering
Chief, Division of Cardiology
University of California, Irvine
Orange, California

SAAGAR N. PATEL, B.A., B.S.
Baylor College of Medicine
Houston, Texas

SHYAM A. PATEL, M.D.
Resident Physician
Warren Alpert Medical School of Brown University
Rhode Island Hospital
Providence, Rhode Island

CYRIL PATRA, M.P.H.
M.D. Candidate
St. George's University
Grenada, West Indies

BRETT PATRICK, M.D.
University of Tennessee Health Science Center
Memphis, Tennessee

GRACE REBECCA PAUL, M.B.B.S., M.D.
Assistant Professor of Pediatrics
Division of Pulmonary and Sleep Medicine
Nationwide Children's Hospital
Columbus, Ohio

KATHARINE A. PHILLIPS, M.D.
Professor of Psychiatry
DeWitt Wallace Senior Scholar
Weill Cornell Medical College
Attending Psychiatrist
New York-Presbyterian Hospital
New York, New York;
Adjunct Professor of Psychiatry and Human Behavior
Warren Alpert Medical School of Brown University
Providence, Rhode Island

TONI PICERNO, D.O.
Mayo Clinic
Rochester, Minnesota

CHRISTOPHER PICKETT, M.D.
Associate Professor of Medicine
University of Connecticut
Farmington, Connecticut

WENDY A. PLANTE, PH.D.
Staff Psychologist/Director of Outpatient Services
Division of Child and Adolescent Psychiatry
Hasbro Children's Hospital / Rhode Island Hospital
Clinical Associate Professor of Psychiatry and Human Behavior
Warren Alpert Medical School of Brown University
Providence, Rhode Island

KEVIN V. PLUMLEY, M.D., M.P.H.
Roger Williams Medical Center
Providence, Rhode Island

MICHAEL POHLEN, M.D.
Baylor College of Medicine
Houston, Texas

SHARON S. HARTMAN POLENSEK, M.D., PH.D.
Assistant Professor of Neurology
Center for Dizziness and Balance Disorders
Emory University
Atlanta, Georgia

DONN POSNER, PH.D.
Adjunct Clinical Associate Professor
Psychiatry and Behavioral Sciences
Stanford University School of Medicine
Palo Alto Veterans Institute for Research
Veterans Affairs Palo Alto Health Care System
Palo Alto, California

ROHINI PRASHAR, M.D.
Senior Staff Physician
Henry Ford Hospital
Detroit, Michigan

AMANDA PRESSMAN, M.D.
Assistant Professor
Department of Medicine
Warren Alpert Medical School of Brown University
Providence, Rhode Island

KITTICHAI PROMRAT, M.D.
Assistant Professor
Division of Gastroenterology
Department of Medicine
Warren Alpert Medical School of Brown University
Providence, Rhode Island

IMRANA QAWI, M.D.
Assistant Professor, Medicine
Pulmonary / Critical Care
Tufts Medical Center
Boston, Massachusetts

SAMAAN RAFEQ, M.D., F.C.C.P.
Clinical Associate Professor of Medicine and Cardiothoracic Surgery
New York University School of Medicine
Director, Interventional Pulmonary Fellowship
Associate Director, Interventional Pulmonary Section
NYU Langone Health
New York, New York

THARANI RAJESWARAN, M.D.
Warren Alpert Medical School of Brown University
Providence, Rhode Island

TARAK S. RAMBHATLA, M.D.

NEHA RANA, M.D.
Fellow, Female Pelvic Medicine and Reconstructive Surgery
Drexel University College of Medicine
Philadelphia, Pennsylvania

GINA RANIERI, D.O.
Obstetrics/Gynecology Resident
Christiana Care Health System
Wilmington, Delaware

MEGHANA RAO, M.D.
Department of Cardiology
Warren Alpert Medical School of Brown University
Providence, Rhode Island

BHARTI RATHORE, M.D.
Program Director, Hematology/Oncology Fellowship
Roger Williams Medical Center
Providence, Rhode Island;
Assistant Professor of Medicine
Boston University School of Medicine
Boston, Massachusetts

RITESH RATHORE, M.D.
Associate Professor
Boston University School of Medicine
Director, Hematology/Oncology
Roger Williams Medical Center
Providence, Rhode Island

NEHA P. RAUKAR, M.D., M.S.
Associate Professor, Emergency Medicine
Warren Alpert Medical School of Brown University
Providence, Rhode Island

JOHN L. REAGAN, M.D.
Assistant Professor of Medicine
Warren Alpert Medical School of Brown University
Providence, Rhode Island

BHARATHI V. REDDY, M.D.
Associate Professor of Medicine
University of Chicago
Chicago, Illinois

CHAKRAVARTHY REDDY, M.D.
Associate Professor
Pulmonary and Critical Care
University of Utah
Salt Lake City, Utah

SNIGDHA T. REDDY, M.D.
Senior Staff Physician
Division of Nephrology and Hypertension
Henry Ford Medical Center-Columbus
Novi, Michigan

ANTHONY M. REGINATO, PH.D., M.D.
Director, Division of Rheumatology
Warren Alpert Medical School of Brown University
Providence, Rhode Island

JAMES P. REICHART, M.D.
Associate Program Director, Nephrology Fellowship
Lehigh Valley Health Network
Allentown, Pennsylvania

DANIEL BRIAN CARLIN REID, M.D., M.P.H.
Resident Physician
Warren Alpert Medical School of Brown University
Rhode Island Hospital
Providence, Rhode Island

VICTOR I. REUS, M.D.
Distinguished Professor of Psychiatry
UCSF School of Medicine
UCSF Weill Institute for Neurosciences
Langley Porter Psychiatric Institute
San Francisco, California

CANDICE REYES, M.D., RH.M.S.U.S.
Associate Clinical Professor of Medicine
Division of Rheumatology, Department of Medicine
University of California, San Francisco
Fresno, California

MELISSA RICCI, D.P.M., M.B.S.
Podiatrist
Saugus, Massachusetts

HARLAN G. RICH, M.D., F.A.C.P., A.G.A.F.
Associate Professor of Medicine and Medical Science
Warren Alpert Medical School of Brown University
Director of Endoscopy
Rhode Island Hospital
Clinical Director of the Division of Gastroenterology
Brown Medicine/Brown Physicians, Inc.
Providence, Rhode Island

ROCCO J. RICHARDS, M.D.
Roger Williams Medical Center
Department of Internal Medicine
Boston University School of Medicine
Boston, Massachusetts

NATHAN RIDDELL, M.D.
Cardiology Fellow
Saint Elizabeth's Medical Center
Brighton, Massachusetts

GIULIA RIGHI, PH.D.
Staff Psychologist
E. P. Bradley Hospital
East Providence, Rhode Island;
Assistant Professor (Research)
Warren Alpert Medical School of Brown University
Providence, Rhode Island

DAVID O. RILEY, M.D.
Resident Physician
Warren Alpert Medical School of Brown University
Providence, Rhode Island

ALVARO M. RIVERA, M.D.
Internal Medicine
Roger Williams Medical Center
Providence, Rhode Island

NICOLE A. ROBERTS, M.D.
Assistant Professor
University of South Florida
Tampa, Florida

TODD F. ROBERTS, M.D., F.R.C.P.(C.)
Medical Director, Leukemia, Blood and Marrow Transplant Program
Medical Director, Immunotherapy Program
Roger Williams Medical Center
Providence, Rhode Island

JAFET OJEDA RODRIGUEZ, M.D.
Flight Surgeon
United States Air Force
Las Vegas, Nevada

EMILY ROSENFELD, M.D., M.P.H.
Obstetrics/Gynecology Resident
Christiana Care Health Systems
Newark, Delaware

ASHLEY N. ROSSI, M.D.
Internal Medicine Residency Program
Warren Alpert Medical School of Brown University
Rhode Island Hospital
Providence, Rhode Island

JULIE L. ROTH, M.D.
Assistant Professor, Neurology
Warren Alpert Medical School of Brown University
Providence, Rhode Island

STEVEN ROUGAS, M.D., M.S., F.A.C.E.P.
Director, Doctoring Program
Assistant Professor of Emergency Medicine and Medical Science
Warren Alpert Medical School of Brown University
Providence, Rhode Island

BRETON ROUSSEL, M.D.
Resident Physician
General Internal Medicine
Warren Alpert Medical School of Brown University
Providence, Rhode Island

AMITY RUBEOR, D.O., C.A.Q.S.M.
Assistant Professor
Department of Family Medicine
Warren Alpert Medical School of Brown University
University
Providence, Rhode Island

KELLY RUHSTALLER, M.D.
Christiana Care Health Systems
Newark, Delaware

JAVERYAH SAFI, M.D.
Clinical Associate
Department of Pulmonary and Critical Care Medicine
Tufts University
Boston, Massachusetts

EMILY SAKS, M.D., M.S.C.E.
Adjunct Clinical Assistant Professor of Obstetrics and Gynecology
Drexel University College of Medicine
Philadelphia Pennsylvania;
Attending Physician
Center for Urogynecology and Pelvic Surgery
Christiana Care Health System
Newark, Delaware

RADHIKA SAMPAT, D.O.
Instructor
Department of Neurology, Neuromuscular Division
Emory University School of Medicine
Atlanta, Georgia

SONIA R. SAMTANI, M.D.
Interventional Cardiology Fellow
University of California, Irvine
Orange, California

HEMANT K. SATPATHY, M.D.
Fellow, Division of Maternal Fetal Medicine
Department of Obstetrics and Gynecology
Emory University
Atlanta, Georgia

RUBY K. SATPATHY, M.D.
Fellow, Cardiology
Department of Internal Medicine
Creighton University
Omaha, Nebraska

SYEDA M. SAYEED, M.D.
Attending Physician
Department of Rheumatology
South Coast Health
Fall River, Massachusetts

DAPHNE SCARAMANGAS-PLUMLEY, M.D.
Rheumatologist
Attune Health
Cedars-Sinai Medical Center
Los Angeles, California

PAUL J. SCHEEL JR., M.D.
Nephrologist
CEO, Washington University Physicians
Associate Vice Chancellor of Clinical Affairs
Washington University in St. Louis
Barnes-Jewish Hospital
St. Louis, Missouri

BRADLEY SCHLUSSEL, M.D.
Rheumatology Fellow
Roger Williams Medical Center
Boston University School of Medicine
Providence, Rhode Island

HEIKO SCHMITT, M.D., PH.D.
Associate Professor of Medicine
Department of Cardiology
Co-director, Cardiac Electrophysiology
Director Anticoagulation Clinic
UConn Health
Farmington, Connecticut

ANTHONY SCISCIONE, D.O.
Professor, Department of Obstetrics and Gynecology
Jefferson Medical College
Philadelphia, Pennsylvania;
Residency Program Director
Director of Maternal-Fetal Medicine
Department of Obstetrics and Gynecology
Christiana Care Health System
Newark, Delaware

CHRISTINA D. SCULLY, M.D.
Consultation Liaison Psychiatry Attending
Rhode Island Hospital
Providence, Rhode Island

PETER J. SELL, D.O.
Associate Professor
Department of Pediatrics
University of Massachusetts Medical School
Worcester, Massachusetts

STEVEN M. SEPE, M.D., PH.D.
Chair, Department of Medicine
Roger Williams Medical Center;
Clinical Professor of Medicine
Assistant Dean of Clinical Affairs
Boston University School of Medicine
Boston, Massachusetts

HESHAM SHABAN, M.D.
Division of Nephrology
Henry Ford Hospital
Detroit, Michigan

KALPIT N. SHAH, M.D.
Warren Alpert Medical School of Brown University
Department of Orthopaedic Surgery
Providence, Rhode Island

SANJEEV R. SHAH, M.D.
Assistant Clinical Professor of Medicine
University of Pennsylvania
Philadelphia, Pennsylvania

SHIVANI SHAH, M.D.
Obstetrician/Gynecologist
Geisinger Health System
Wilkes-Barre, Pennsylvania

JESSICA E. SHILL, M.D.
Senior Staff Physician
Division of Endocrinology, Diabetes and Bone and Mineral Disorders
Henry Ford Health System
Clinical Associate Professor of Medicine
Wayne State University School of Medicine
Detroit, Michigan

ALEXANDRA SHINGINA, M.D.C.M.
Gastroenterology
University of Toronto
Toronto, Ontario, Canada

PHILIP A. SHLOSSMAN, M.D.
Associate Director Maternal and Fetal Medicine
Christiana Hospital
Newark, Delaware

ASHA SHRESTHA, M.D.
Rheumatology
St. Joseph Hospital
Bangor, Maine

ELIZABETH SHY, M.D.
Clinical Instructor
Department of Obstetrics and Gynecology
Christiana Care Health System
Newark, Delaware

MARK SIGMAN, M.D.
Professor of Surgery (Urology)
Professor of Pathology and Laboratory Medicine
Warren Alpert Medical School of Brown University
Providence, Rhode Island

JAMES SIMON, M.D.
Assistant Professor
Lerner College of Medicine
Cleveland, Ohio

HARINDER P. SINGH, M.D.
Clinical Associate
Department of Pulmonary and Critical Care Medicine
St. Elizabeth Medical Center, Tufts University
Boston, Massachusetts

DIVYA SINGHAL, M.D.
Medical Director, Oklahoma City VAMC Residents' Longitudinal Clinic
Vice Chair, Women's Issues in Neurology, American Academy of Neurology
Assistant Professor of Neurology,
University of Oklahoma
Epileptologist, Department of Neurology / Rehabilitation Services
Oklahoma City, Oklahoma

IRINA A. SKYLAR-SCOTT, M.D.
Resident Physician
Department of Neurology
Harvard Medical School
Boston, Massachusetts

JOHN SLADKY, M.D.
Staff Neurologist
Associate Program Director
Wilford Hall Medical Center
San Antonio, Texas

BRETT SLINGSBY, M.D.
Child Abuse Pediatrician
Lawrence A. Aubin Sr. Child Protection Center
Assistant Professor of Pediatrics
Warren Alpert Medical School of Brown University
Providence, Rhode Island

JEANETTE G. SMITH, M.D.
Assistant Professor
Department of Medicine
Warren Alpert Medical School of Brown University
Providence, Rhode Island

JONATHAN H. SMITH, M.D.
Assistant Professor of Neurology
University of Kentucky
Lexington, Kentucky

U. SHIVRAJ SOHUR, M.D., PH.D
Assistant Professor of Neurology
Harvard Medical School
Boston, Massachusetts

VIVEK SOI, M.D.
Senior Staff Physician
Henry Ford Hospital
Detroit, Michigan

REBECCA SOINSKI, M.D.
Rheumatologist
Women's Medicine Collaborative
Providence, Rhode Island

MARIA E. SOLER, M.D., M.P.H., M.B.A.
Director, Education Division and OB Triage
Department of Obstetrics/Gynecology
Christiana Care Health System
Newark, Delaware

SANDEEP SOMAN, M.D.
Division of Nephrology
Henry Ford Hospital
Detroit, Michigan

AKSHAY SOOD, M.D.
Vattikuti Urology Institute
Henry Ford Hospital Health System
Detroit, Michigan

C. JOHN SPERATI, M.D., M.H.S.
Associate Professor of Medicine
Johns Hopkins University School of Medicine
Division of Nephrology
Baltimore, Maryland

JOHANNES STEINER, M.D.
Assistant Professor
Division of Cardiology
University of Vermont
Burlington, Vermont

PHILIP STOCKWELL, M.D.
Assistant Professor of Medicine
Warren Alpert Medical School of Brown University
Providence, Rhode Island;
Lifespan Cardiovascular Institute
East Providence, Rhode Island

LARA STONE, D.P.M.
Podiatrist
University of Vermont Medical Center
Assistant Professor
University of Vermont
Burlington, Vermont

PADMAJA SUDHAKAR, M.B.B.S.
Assistant Professor
Department of Neurology
University of Kentucky
Lexington, Kentucky

ARUN SWAMINATHAN, M.B.B.S.
Neurology Resident
University of Kentucky College of Medicine
University of Kentucky Hospital
Lexington, Kentucky

JOSEPH SWEENEY, M.D., F.A.C.P., F.R.C.PATH.
Professor, Laboratory Medicine and Pathology
Warren Alpert Medical School of Brown University
Providence, Rhode Island

WAJIH A. SYED, M.D.
Cardiologist
Kaiser Permanente
Roseville, California

MAHER TABBA, M.D., F.A.C.P., F.C.C.P.
Associate Professor of Medicine and Surgery
Department of Pulmonary & Critical Care Medicine and Sleep Disorders
Tufts Medical Center
Boston, Massachusetts

DOMINICK TAMMARO, M.D.
Associate Professor of Medicine
Warren Alpert Medical School of Brown University
Rhode Island Hospital
Providence, Rhode Island

MICHELE TARTAGLIA, D.O., F.A.C.O.O.G., C.S.
Faculty Attending Physician
Department of Obstetrics & Gynecology
Christiana Care Health System
Newark, Delaware

ALAN TAYLOR, M.D.
Assistant Professor of Emergency Medicine
University of Tennessee Health Science Center
Memphis, Tennessee

TAHIR TELLIOGLU, M.D.
Assistant Professor of Psychiatry and Human Behavior
Warren Alpert Medical School of Brown University
Medical Codirector, Lifespan Recovery Center
Providence, Rhode Island

JIGISHA P. THAKKAR, M.D.
Chief Resident
Department of Neurology
University of Kentucky
Lexington, Kentucky

ANTHONY G. THOMAS, D.O., F.A.C.P.
Assistant Clinical Professor of Medicine
Warren Alpert Medical School of Brown University
Lifespan Cancer Institute / The Miriam Hospital
Providence, Rhode Island

ANDREW P. THOME JR., M.D.
Orthopedic Surgery Resident
Warren Alpert Medical School of Brown University
Rhode Island Hospital
Providence, Rhode Island

ERIN TIBBETTS, PHARM.D.
Clinical Pharmacist
Boston Children's Hospital
Boston, Massachusetts

ALEXANDRA MEYER TIEN, M.D.
Clinical Assistant Professor of Family Medicine
Warren Alpert Medical School of Brown University
Providence, Rhode Island

DAVID ROBBINS TIEN, M.D.
Clinical Associate Professor of Surgery (Ophthalmology)
Warren Alpert Medical School of Brown University
Providence, Rhode Island

HELEN VALERIE TOMA, M.D., M.S.P.H.
Obstetrics/Gynecology Resident
Christiana Care Health System
Newark, Delaware

IRIS L. TONG, M.D.
Associate Professor, Department of Medicine
Warren Alpert Medical School of Brown University
Attending Physician, Women's Primary Care
Women's Medicine Collaborative
Providence, Rhode Island

STEVEN P. TREON, M.D.
Director, Bing Center for Waldenström's Macroglobulinemia
Dana Farber Cancer Institute
Boston, Massachusetts

HIRSH D. TRIVEDI, M.D.
Gastroenterology and Hepatology Fellow
Department of Medicine
Beth Israel Deaconess Medical Center
Harvard Medical School
Boston, Massachusetts

MARGARET TRYFOROS, M.D.
Assistant Professor of Family Medicine (Clinical)
Warren Alpert Medical School of Brown University
Providence, Rhode Island

HISASHI TSUKADA, M.D., PH.D.
Instructor in Surgery
Harvard Medical School
Boston, Massachusetts

JOSEPH R. TUCCI, M.D., F.A.C.P., F.A.C.E.
Professor of Medicine
Boston University School of Medicine
Director, Division of Endocrinology
Roger Williams Medical Center
Providence, Rhode Island

MELISSA H. TUKEY, M.D., M.S.
Department of Pulmonary and Critical Care
Kaiser Oakland Medical Center
Oakland, California

CHRISTOPHER TUOHY, M.D., M.P.H.
Warren Alpert Medical School of Brown University
Providence, Rhode Island

JUNIOR UDUMAN, M.D.
Medical Director, Acute Dialysis
Division of Nephrology and Hypertension
Henry Ford Hospital
Detroit, Michigan

SEAN H. UITERWYK, M.D.
Clinical Assistant Professor, Community and Family Medicine
Geisel School of Medicine at Dartmouth
Hanover, New Hampshire

NICOLE J. ULLRICH, M.D., PH.D.
Associate Professor of Neurology
Harvard Medical School
Director of Neurologic Neuro-oncology
Boston Children's Hospital
Boston, Massachusetts

KAUSIK UMANATH, M.D., M.S.
Assistant Professor of Medicine
Section Head, Clinical Research
Division of Nephrology and Hypertension
Henry Ford Hospital
Detroit, Michigan

BABAK VAKILI, M.D.
Director, Center for Urogynecology and Pelvic Surgery
Christiana Care Health System
Newark, Delaware

EMILY VAN KIRK, M.D.
Internal Medicine Resident
Department of Medicine
Roger Williams Medical Center
Providence, Rhode Island

DANNY H. VANVALKINBURGH, M.D.
Emergency Medicine Assistant Professor
University of Tennessee Health Science Center
Memphis, Tennessee

JENNIFER E. VAUGHAN, M.D.
Fellow, Department of Neurology and Rehabilitation Medicine
University of Cincinnati College of Medicine
Cincinnati, Ohio

ROBERT VAZQUEZ, M.D.
Warren Alpert Medical School of Brown University
Providence, Rhode Island

EMIL STEFAN VUTESCU, M.D.
Orthopedics Resident
Warren Alpert Medical School at Brown University
Rhode Island Hospital
Providence, Rhode Island

BRENT T. WAGNER, M.D.
Professor of Medicine
University of New Mexico Health Sciences Center
Director, Kidney Institute of New Mexico
Albuquerque, New Mexico

J. RICHARD WALKER III, M.D., M.S.
Interim Chair of Emergency Medicine
University of Tennessee Health Science Center
Memphis, Tennessee

RAY WALTHER, M.D.
Assistant Professor, Emergency Medicine
University of Tennessee Health Science Center
Memphis, Tennessee

JOZAL WAROICH, M.D.
Department of Medicine
Warren Alpert Medical School of Brown University
Providence, Rhode Island

RYAN WATSON, M.D.
Cardiology Fellow
Jefferson Heart Institute
Philadelphia, Pennsylvania

EMMA H. WEISS, B.B.A.
Baylor College of Medicine
Houston, Texas

MAX WEISS, M.D.
Cardiology Fellow
Jefferson Heart Institute
Philadelphia, Pennsylvania

MARY-BETH WELESKO, M.S., A.P.R.N.-B.C., W.C.C.
Nurse Practitioner
Division of Geriatrics and Palliative Medicine
Care New England Medical Group
Pawtucket, Rhode Island

DENNIS M. WEPPNER, M.D.
Associate Professor of Clinical Gynecology/Obstetrics
SUNY at Buffalo
Buffalo, New York

ADRIENNE WERTH, M.D.
Resident Physician
Christiana Care Health System
Newark, Delaware

MATTHEW J. WHITE, D.O.
Rheumatology Fellow
Roger Williams Medical Center
Providence, Rhode Island

ESTELLE H. WHITNEY, M.D.
Clinical Instructor
Christiana Care Health Systems
Newark, Delaware

MATTHEW P. WICKLUND, M.D.
Professor, Department of Neurology
Penn State College of Medicine;
Vice-Chair for Education
Department of Neurology
Milton S. Hershey Medical Center
Hershey, Pennsylvania

JEFFREY P. WINCZE, PH.D.
Department of Psychiatry
Rhode Island Hospital
Providence, Rhode Island

JOHN P. WINCZE, PH.D.
Clinical Professor Emeritus
Department of Psychiatry and Human Behavior
Warren Alpert Medical School of Brown University
Providence, Rhode Island

MARLENE FISHMAN WOLPERT, M.P.H., C.I.C., F.A.P.I.C.
Director, Infection Prevention and Control
Our Lady of Fatima Hospital
North Providence, Rhode Island

TZU-CHING (TEDDY) WU, M.D., M.P.H.
Assistant Professor of Neurology
University of Texas Medical School at Houston
Director of Telemedicine
Mischer Neuroscience Institute
Houston, Texas

MANIDA WUNGJIRANIRUN, M.D.
Gastroenterology Fellow
Warren Alpert Medical School of Brown University
Providence, Rhode Island

JOHN WYLIE, M.D., F.A.C.C.
Director, Cardiac Electrophysiology
Steward Health Care System
Assistant Professor of Medicine
Tufts University School of Medicine
Boston, Massachusetts

NICOLE B. YANG, M.D.
Rheumatology Fellow
Brigham and Women's Hospital
Boston, Massachusetts

JERRY YEE, M.D.
Clinical Professor of Medicine
Department of Internal Medicine
Wayne State University School of Medicine
Division Head, Henry Ford Hospital
Division of Nephrology and Hypertension
Detroit, Michigan

GEMINI YESODHARAN, M.D.
Internal Medicine Resident, Steward
Saint Elizabeth's Medical Center
Tufts University School of Medicine
Brighton, Massachusetts

AGUSTIN G. YIP, M.D., PH.D.
Associate Medical Director, Short Term Unit
McLean Hospital
Belmont, Massachusetts

JOHN Q. YOUNG, M.D., M.P.P., PH.D.
Professor and Vice Chair for Education
Department of Psychiatry
Donald and Barbara Zucker School of Medicine at Hofstra/Northwell
Hempstead, New York

ELIZABETH ZADZIELSKI, M.D., M.B.A., N.C.M.P.
Education Faculty
Department of Obstetrics and Gynecology
Christiana Care Health System
Newark, Delaware

FARIHA ZAHEER, M.D.
Assistant Professor of Neurology
Baylor College of Medicine
Michael. E. DeBakey VA Medical Center
Houston, Texas

TALIA ZENLEA, M.D.
Assistant Professor of Medicine
University of Toronto;
Division of Gastroenterology
Women's College Hospital
Toronto, Ontario, Canada

MARK ZIMMERMAN, M.D.
Director, Outpatient Psychiatry and Partial Hospital Program
Rhode Island Hospital
Professor, Department of Psychiatry and Human Behavior
Warren Alpert Medical School of Brown University
Providence, Rhode Island

BERNARD ZIMMERMANN, M.D.
Associate Professor Emeritus
Department of Medicine
Boston University
Boston, Massachusetts;
Rheumatologist
Department of Medicine
Division of Rheumatology
Roger Williams Medical Center
Providence, Rhode Island

ALINE N. ZOUK, M.D.
Fellow
New York University School of Medicine
New York, New York

To my sons, Dr. Vito F. Ferri and Dr. Christopher A. Ferri, and my daughter-in-law, Dr. Heather A. Ferri, for their help and constant support, and to my wife, Christina, for her patience during manuscript preparation. A special thanks to all the readers who have personally commented on the merits of this book and through their suggestions have helped make this product a bestseller in the medical field.

Fred F. Ferri, M.D., F.A.C.P.
Clinical Professor
Department of Medicine
The Warren Alpert Medical School
Brown University
Providence, Rhode Island

This book is intended to be a clear and concise reference for physicians and allied health professionals. Its user-friendly format is designed to provide a fast and efficient way to identify important clinical information and to offer practical guidance in patient management. The book is divided into five sections and an appendix, each with emphasis on clinical information.

The tremendous success of the previous editions and the enthusiastic comments from numerous colleagues have brought about several positive changes over time. Each section has been significantly expanded from prior editions, bringing the total number of medical topics covered in this book to more than 1200. Hundreds of new illustrations, tables, and boxes have been added to this edition to enhance recollection of clinically important facts. The expedited claims submission and reimbursement ICD-10CM codes are included in all topics.

Section I describes in detail 964 medical disorders and diseases—including 27 new topics this edition—each of which is arranged alphabetically and presented in outline format for ease of retrieval. Topics with an accompanying algorithm are identified with an ALG icon. Similarly, those topics with an accompanying online Patient Teaching Guide (PTG) are identified with a PTG symbol. Throughout the text, key quick-access information is consistently highlighted, with clinical photographs to further illustrate selected medical conditions, and relevant ICD-10CM codes listed. Most references focus on current peer-reviewed journal articles rather than outdated textbooks and old review articles. Evidence-based medicine data are offered with relevant topics.

Topics in **Section I** use the following structured approach:

1. Basic Information (Definition, Synonyms, ICD-10CM Codes, Epidemiology & Demographics, Physical Findings & Clinical Presentation, Etiology)
2. Diagnosis (Differential Diagnosis, Workup, Laboratory Tests, Imaging Studies)
3. Treatment (Nonpharmacologic Therapy, Acute General Rx, Chronic Rx, Disposition, Referral)
4. Pearls & Considerations (Comments, Suggested Readings)
5. Evidence-Based Data and References

Section II includes the differential diagnosis, etiology, and classification of signs and symptoms. It is a practical section that allows the user investigating a physical complaint or abnormal laboratory value to follow a "workup" leading to a diagnosis. The physician can then easily look up the presumptive diagnosis in Section I for information specific to that illness.

Section III includes more than 150 clinical algorithms to guide and expedite the patient's workup and therapy. For the 2020 edition, we have continued to update algorithms and colorize online versions for improved readability. Physicians describe this section as particularly valuable in today's managed-care environment.

Section IV includes normal laboratory values and interpretation of results of commonly ordered laboratory tests. New illustrations and tables have been added for this edition. By providing interpretation of abnormal results, this section facilitates the diagnosis of medical disorders and further adds to the comprehensive "one-stop" nature of our text.

Section V focuses on preventive medicine. Information in this section includes screening recommendations for major diseases and disorders, patient counseling, and immunization and chemoprophylaxis recommendations.

The **Appendix** is divided into six major sections. Appendix I contains extensive information on complementary and alternative medicine (CAM). With this material, we hope to lessen the current scarcity of exposure of allopathic and osteopathic physicians to the diversity of CAM therapies. Appendix II focuses on nutrition, with an emphasis on dietary supplements, vitamins, and minerals. Appendix III deals with diagnosis and treatment of acute poisoning. Appendix IV is a guide on impairment and disability evaluation. Appendix V focuses on the protection of travelers. Appendix VI is new for the 2020 edition and introduces Physician Quality Reporting System (PQRS) measures.

As clinicians, we all realize the importance of patient education and the need for clear communication with our patients. To that end, practical patient instruction sheets, organized alphabetically and covering the majority of topics in this book, are available in the online version of *Ferri's Clinical Advisor* and can be easily customized and printed from any computer. These guides are valuable tools for improving physician-patient communication, patient satisfaction and, ultimately, quality of care.

I believe that we have produced a state-of-the-art information system with significant differences from existing texts. The information offered in all five sections and patient education guides could be sold separately based on their content, yet are available under a single cover, offering the reader tremendous value. I hope that the *Clinical Advisor*'s user-friendly approach, numerous unique features, and yearly updates will make this book a valuable medical reference, not only to primary care physicians but also to physicians in other specialties, medical students, and allied health professionals.

Fred F. Ferri, M.D., F.A.C.P.
Clinical Professor
Department of Medicine
The Warren Alpert Medical School
Brown University
Providence, Rhode Island

Note: Comments from readers are always appreciated and can be forwarded directly to Dr. Ferri at fred_ferri@brown.edu.

EVALUATION OF EVIDENCE

Ferri's Clinical Advisor evaluates all evidence based on a rating system published by the American Academy of Family Physicians. Each summary statement is accorded one of three levels to indicate the strength of the supporting evidence:

Level A
- Systematic reviews of randomized controlled trials, including meta-analyses
- Good-quality randomized controlled trials

Level B
- Good-quality nonrandomized clinical trials
- Systematic reviews not in Level A
- Lower-quality randomized controlled trials not in Level A
- Other types of study: case-control studies, clinical cohort studies, cross-sectional studies, retrospective studies, and uncontrolled studies

Level C
- Evidence-based consensus statements and expert guidelines

SOURCES OF EVIDENCE

Evidence is summarized principally from three critically evaluated, very highly regarded sources:

- **Cochrane Systematic Reviews** are respected throughout the world as one of the most rigorous searches of medical journals for randomized controlled trials. They provide highly structured systematic reviews, with evidence included or excluded on the basis of explicit quality-related criteria, and they often use meta-analyses to increase the power of the findings of numerous studies.
- ***Clinical Evidence*** is produced by the BMJ Publishing Group. It provides synopses of the best currently available evidence on the treatment and prevention of many clinical conditions, based on searches and appraisals of the available literature.
- **The National Guideline Clearinghouse™** is a comprehensive database of evidence-based clinical practice guidelines and related documents produced by the Agency for Healthcare Research and Quality in partnership with the American Medical Association and the American Association of Health Plans.

In addition, where evidence exists that has not yet been critically reviewed in one of the three sites mentioned previously, the evidence is summarized briefly, categorized, and fully referenced. Guidelines are also sourced from government and professional bodies.

Ferri's Clinical Advisor 2020—How to Use This Book

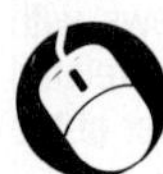 Mouse icon: Indicates content with additional references, figures, or tables available at ExpertConsult.com.

PTG icon: Indicates an accompanying Patient Teaching Guide available at ExpertConsult.com. Many additional PTGs are available online that are not linked to a topic in Section I.

ALG icon: Indicates a topic with an accompanying algorithm.

EBM icon: Indicates relevant evidence-based medicine data available at ExpertConsult.com.

SECTION I Diseases and Disorders

Additional Topics Available at ExpertConsult.com

SECTION II **Differential Diagnosis**

Detailed Contents

SECTION III Clinical Algorithms

Additional Clinical Algorithms Available at ExpertConsult.com

SECTION IV Laboratory Tests and Interpretation of Results

Detailed Contents

SECTION V Clinical Practice Guidelines

APPENDIX I Complementary and Alternative Medicine

APPENDIX II Nutrition

APPENDIX III Acute Poisoning

APPENDIX IV Impairment and Disability Issues

APPENDIX V Protection of Travelers

APPENDIX VI Physician Quality Reporting System (PQRS) Measures, Available at ExpertConsult.com

APPENDIX VII Patient Teaching Guides, Available at ExpertConsult.com

Additional PTGs Available at ExpertConsult.com Not Linked to Topics in Section I

Diseases and Disorders

BASIC INFORMATION

DEFINITION

An abdominal aortic aneurysm (AAA) is a focal full-thickness dilation of the abdominal aortic artery to at least 1.5 times the diameter measured at the level of the renal arteries, or exceeding the normal diameter of the abdominal aorta by 50%. The normal diameter at the renal arteries is 2 cm (range 1.4-3.0 cm), and a diameter 3 cm or larger is generally considered aneurysmal.

ICD-10CM CODES

I71.4 Abdominal aortic aneurysm, without rupture
I71.3 Abdominal aortic aneurysm, ruptured

EPIDEMIOLOGY & DEMOGRAPHICS

- Approximately 15,000 deaths/yr in the United States are attributed to AAA.
- AAA is predominantly a disease of older adults, affecting men more than women (4:1).
- The prevalence rate ranges from 4% to 9% in men in developed countries.
- Clinically important AAAs ≥4 cm are present in 1% of men between age 55 and 64; and the prevalence rate increases by 2% to 4% per decade thereafter.
- The peak incidence is among men approximately 70 yr old.
- The frequency is much higher in smokers than in nonsmokers (8:1); and the risk decreases with smoking cessation.
- Risk factors for AAA are similar to those for other atherosclerotic cardiovascular diseases. They include age, Caucasian race, smoking, male gender, family history, hypertension, hyperlipidemia, peripheral vascular disease, and aneurysm of other large vessels.
- AAA is two to four times more common in first-degree male relatives of known AAA patients.
- A decreased risk of AAA is associated with female gender, non-Caucasian race, and diabetes.
- Rupture of the AAA occurs in 1% to 3% of men age 65 or older.
  1. Rupture is the 10th leading cause of death in men older than age 55.
  2. Mortality from rupture is 70% to 95%.
  3. Risk factors for rupture include cardiac or renal transplants, severe obstructive lung disease, uncontrolled blood pressure, female sex, and ongoing tobacco use.
- A recent decline in incidence and prevalence of AAA and related mortality has been attributed to reductions in tobacco use.

ETIOLOGY

- Exact etiology is unknown and is likely multifactorial.
  1. Degenerative:
     a. Alterations in vascular wall biology leading to a loss of vascular structural proteins and wall strength.
     b. The most common association is atherosclerosis. It is uncertain whether atherosclerosis causes or results from AAAs.
     c. Tobacco use: >90% of people who develop an AAA have smoked at some point in their lives.
  2. Inherited: Familial clusters are common. High familial prevalence rate is notable in male individuals. The nature of the genetic disorder is unclear but may be linked to alpha-1-antitrypsin deficiency or X-linked mutation. Connective tissue disorders, such as Marfan syndrome and Ehlers-Danlos syndrome, have also been strongly associated with AAA.
  3. Inflammatory: AAA is a progressive inflammatory disease of the artery walls. Activated B lymphocytes promote AAA by producing immunoglobulins, cytokines, and matrix metalloproteinases (MMPs), resulting in the activation of macrophages, mast cells (MCs), and complement pathways that lead to the degradation of collagen and matrix proteins and to aortic wall remodeling.
  4. Infection, mycotic: Syphilis, *Salmonella.*

NATURAL HISTORY

- AAAs tend to develop in the infrarenal aorta and to expand, on average, at a rate of 0.3 to 0.4 cm per yr.
- The risk of aneurysmal rupture is largely influenced by aneurysm size, rate of expansion, and sex. Other factors associated with increased risk for rupture include continued smoking, uncontrolled hypertension, and increased wall stress.
- Higher tension in the abdominal aorta (together with histopathologic changes such as accumulation of foam cells, cholesterol crystals, and matrix metalloproteinases) renders the abdominal aortic wall more susceptible to dilation and subsequent rupture.
- The 5-yr rupture rate of asymptomatic AAAs is 25% to 40% for aneurysms >5.0 cm in diameter, 1% to 7% for AAAs 4.0 to 5.0 cm, and nearly 0% for AAAs <4.0 cm. The likelihood that an aneurysm will rupture is increased in aneurysms with a diameter >5.5 cm; this size also demonstrates a faster rate of expansion (>0.5 cm over 6 months) and is more likely to be found in those who continue to smoke and in females.
- Mortality rate after rupture can be as high as 90% because most patients do not reach the hospital in time for surgical repair. Of those who reach the hospital, the mortality rate is still 50%, compared with the 1% to 4% mortality rate for elective repair of a nonruptured AAA. The U.S. Preventive Services Task Force (USPSTF) also concludes that the current evidence is insufficient to assess the balance of benefits and harms of screening for AAA in women aged 65 to 75 who ever smoked and recommends against routine screening in women who never smoked (most recent update in June 2014).

SCREENING AND MONITORING

- The USPSTF recommends one-time screening for AAA by ultrasonography in men ages 65 to 75 who have a history of smoking, and in those 60 yr of age or older with a history of AAA in a parent or sibling. These populations have been shown to have a higher prevalence of AAA, and selectively screening this group has been shown to decrease AAA-specific mortality.
- The USPSTF has found little benefit in repeat screening in men with a negative ultrasound and has determined that men over the age of 75 are unlikely to benefit from screening. It was also concluded that the current evidence is insufficient to assess the balance of the harms and benefits of screening for AAA in women ages 65 to 75 who have ever smoked.
- Monitoring by ultrasound or CT scan should be performed every 6 to 12 months for patients with AAAs measuring 4.0 to 5.4 cm in diameter and by ultrasound every 2 yr for those with AAAs measuring <4 cm.

PHYSICAL FINDINGS & CLINICAL PRESENTATION

- Most aneurysms are asymptomatic and incidentally discovered on imaging studies; however, symptomatic aneurysms are at an increased risk for rupture.
- Physical examination has a sensitivity of 76% for detecting AAAs >5 cm and only 29% for AAAs 3.0-3.9 cm. The accuracy of the physical examination is markedly diminished by obese body habitus.
- Symptomatic patients may present with abdominal, back, flank, or groin pain.
- A pulsatile epigastric mass that may or may not be tender may be present.
- Abdominal pain radiating to the back, flank, and groin.
- Abdominal bruits can be present in case of renal or visceral arterial stenosis.
- Common iliac arteries can be aneurysmal and palpable in the lower abdominal quadrants. In addition, prominent femoral and popliteal pulses warrant an abdominal ultrasound and lower extremity ultrasound.
- Early satiety, nausea, and vomiting may be caused by compression of adjacent bowel.
- Venous thrombosis or insufficiency may occur from iliocaval venous compression.
- Thromboembolization can cause lower extremity pain and discoloration.
- Ureteral obstruction and hydronephrosis can cause flank and groin pain and lead to obstructive renal failure.
- Rupture classically presents as a triad of abdominal or back pain, hypotension, and a pulsatile abdominal mass in 50% of patients.
- Acute blood loss may lead to myocardial infarction; arteriovenous fistulas may present as heart failure; aortoenteric fistulas may present as hematemesis or melena associated with abdominal and back pain.

DIAGNOSIS

DIFFERENTIAL DIAGNOSIS

Almost 75% of patients with AAA are asymptomatic, and the condition is discovered on routine examination or serendipitously when ordering studies for other symptoms. Diagnosis of AAA should be considered in the differential of the following symptoms: Abdominal pain, back pain, and/or pulsatile abdominal mass.

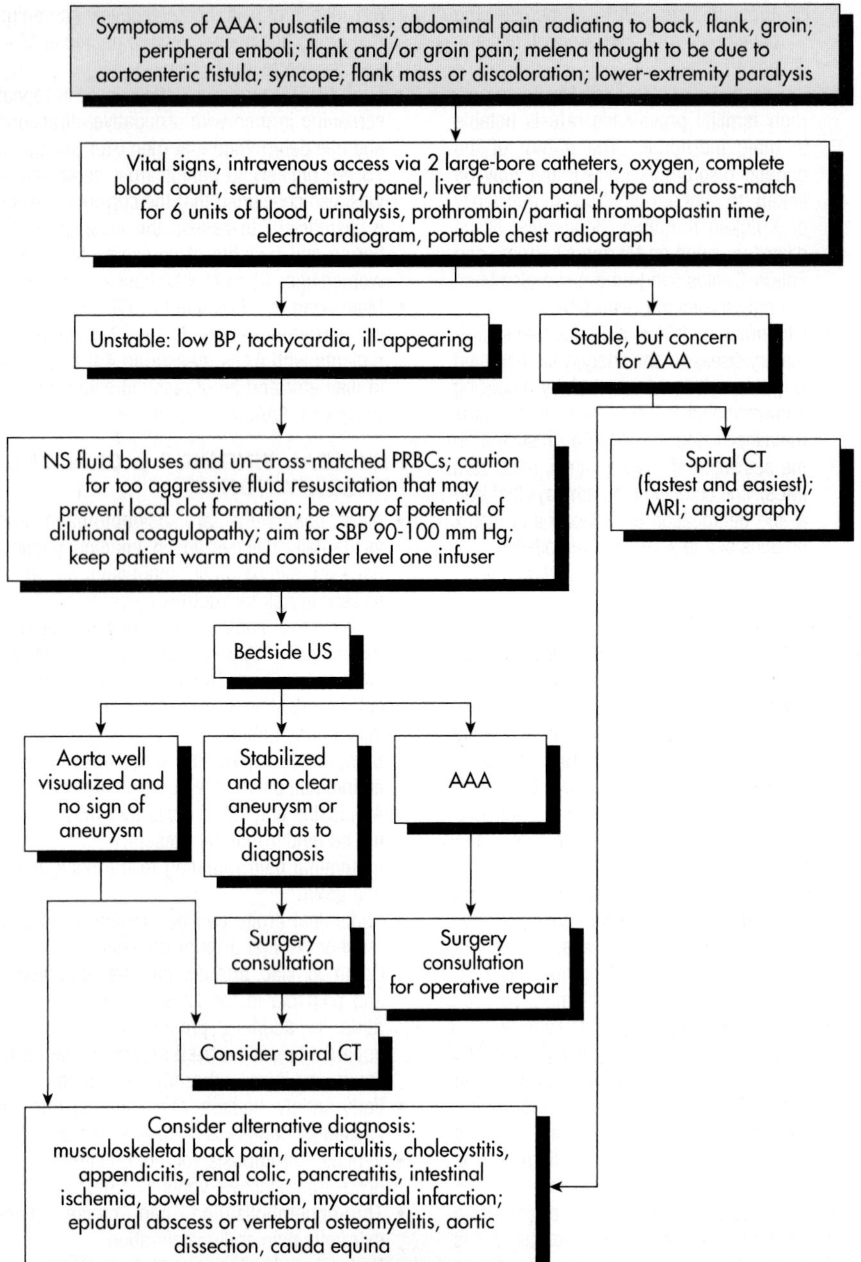
Symptoms of AAA: pulsatile mass; abdominal pain radiating to back, flank, groin; peripheral emboli; flank and/or groin pain; melena thought to be due to aortoenteric fistula; syncope; flank mass or discoloration; lower-extremity paralysis
Vital signs, intravenous access via 2 large-bore catheters, oxygen, complete blood count, serum chemistry panel, liver function panel, type and cross-match for 6 units of blood, urinalysis, prothrombin/partial thromboplastin time, electrocardiogram, portable chest radiograph
Unstable: low BP, tachycardia, ill-appearing
Stable, but concern for AAA
NS fluid boluses and un–cross-matched PRBCs; caution for too aggressive fluid resuscitation that may prevent local clot formation; be wary of potential of dilutional coagulopathy; aim for SBP 90-100 mm Hg; keep patient warm and consider level one infuser
Spiral CT (fastest and easiest); MRI; angiography
Bedside US
Aorta well visualized and no sign of aneurysm
Stabilized and no clear aneurysm or doubt as to diagnosis
AAA
Surgery consultation
Surgery consultation for operative repair
Consider spiral CT
Consider alternative diagnosis: musculoskeletal back pain, diverticulitis, cholecystitis, appendicitis, renal colic, pancreatitis, intestinal ischemia, bowel obstruction, myocardial infarction; epidural abscess or vertebral osteomyelitis, aortic dissection, cauda equina

FIG. 1 Algorithm for the diagnosis and treatment of abdominal aortic aneurysms *(AAAs)*. *BP*, Blood pressure; *CT*, computed tomography; *MRI*, magnetic resonance imaging; *NS*, normal saline; *PRBCs*, packed red blood cells; *SBP*, systolic blood pressure; *US*, ultrasonography. (From Adams JG et al: *Emergency medicine, clinical essentials*, ed 2, Philadelphia, 2013, Elsevier.)

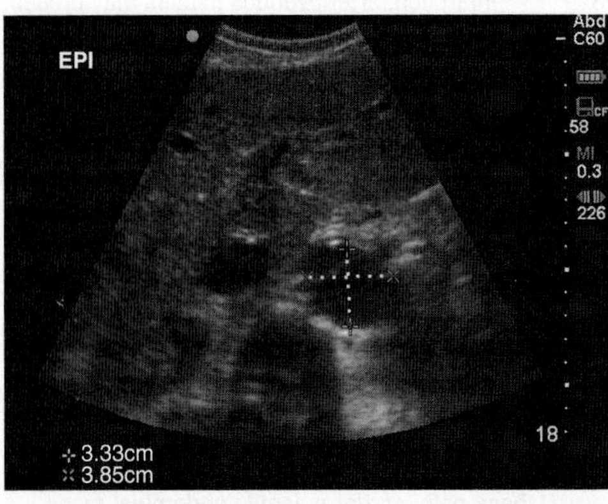
EPI
Abd
C60
.58
MI
0.3
226
18
3.33cm
3.85cm

FIG. 2 Transverse image of an abdominal aortic aneurysm. Note the measurements of 3.33 × 3.85 cm. The inferior vena cava is seen to the patient's right of the aorta, and the vertebral body is seen below the two vessels. Note also that there appears to be an echogenic flap within the aorta, possibly representing an aortic dissection. (From Adams JG, et al.: *Emergency medicine, clinical essentials*, ed 2, Philadelphia, 2013, Elsevier.)

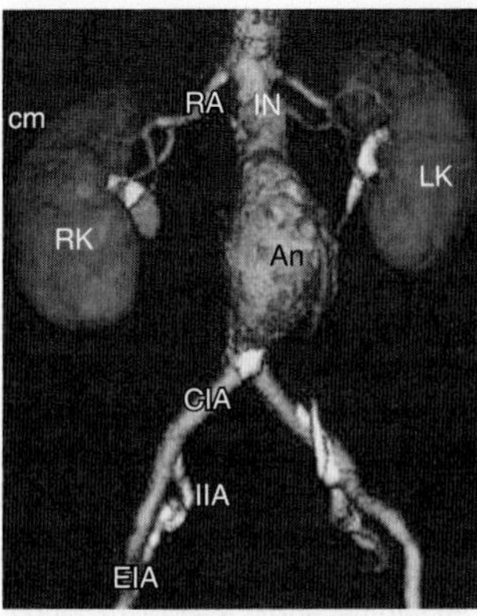
cm
RA
IN
LK
RK
An
CIA
IIA
EIA

FIG. 3 Three-dimensional computed tomography image illustrates the presence of an infrarenal abdominal aortic aneurysm. *An*, Aneurysm; *CIA*, common iliac artery; *EIA*, external iliac artery; *IIA*, internal iliac artery; *IN*, infrarenal neck; *LK*, left kidney; *RA*, renal artery; *RK*, right kidney. (From Townsend CM, et al. [eds]: *Sabiston textbook of surgery*, ed 17, Philadelphia, 2004, Saunders.)

LABORATORY TESTS

Not routinely indicated. For suspected infected or inflammatory aneurysms, WBC, ESR/CRP, and blood cultures can be considered. An elevated D-dimer may indicate a thrombus within the aneurysm. Fig. 1 describes an algorithm for the diagnosis and treatment of abdominal aortic aneurysms.

IMAGING STUDIES

- Abdominal ultrasound (Fig. 2) has nearly 100% sensitivity and specificity in identifying an aneurysm and estimating the size to within 0.3 to 0.4 cm. It is not accurate in estimating the extension to the renal arteries or the iliac arteries.
- Computed tomography (CT) (Fig. 3) scan is recommended for preoperative aneurysm imaging and estimates the size of the AAA to within 0.3 mm. There are no false-negative results, and the scan can localize the extent to renal vessels with more precision than ultrasound. It is the imaging modality of choice for symptomatic AAA. Intravenous contrast is not required to establish a diagnosis of ruptured AAA. CT can also detect the integrity of the wall (Fig. 4) and exclude rupture.
- Magnetic resonance angiography (MRA) may also be used and is at least as accurate as CT.
- Plain radiographs may show the outline of an aneurysm in calcified aortas. This is an insensitive test for diagnosing AAA.
- Diagnostic aortography has essentially been replaced by other noninvasive imaging modalities such as CT or MR angiography. Intraoperative angiography is still used for determining treatment options and post-procedure efficacy (Fig. 5).
- Endovascular aneurysm repair (EVAR) needs a close and lifelong imaging surveillance for a timely detection of possible complications, including endoleaks, graft migration, fractures, and enlargement of aneurysm sac size with eventual rupture. Contrast-enhanced

computed tomography (CTA) is considered the gold standard in EVAR follow-up (Fig. 6), but it is accompanied with radiation burden and renal injury because of the use of contrast media. In the past 2 decades, several studies have shown the role of contrast-enhanced ultrasonography (CEUS) in post-EVAR surveillance, with very good diagnostic performance, absence of renal impairment, and no radiation, accompanied by low costs, in comparison with CTA. In numerous prospective studies and meta-analyses, the detection and characterization of endoleaks with CEUS is comparable to that of CTA imaging.

Rx TREATMENT

NONPHARMACOLOGIC THERAPY

- Despite lack of data substantiating reduction in expansion rate through treatment of cardiac risk factors, nonpharmacologic treatment continues to focus on risk factor modification (most importantly smoking cessation, diet, and exercise).
- Serial studies have shown that expansion rates are faster in current smokers than in former smokers. Patients with known AAA or a family history of aneurysms should be advised to stop smoking and be offered smoking cessation interventions.
- Definitive treatment depends on the size of the aneurysm (see "Chronic Rx").

ACUTE GENERAL Rx

- Acute symptomatic or ruptured AAA can be treated with open surgical or endovascular aneurysm repair (EVAR). The choice is determined by anatomic considerations, operative risks, and availability of regular patient follow-up for EVAR.
- Emergent open repair has been the traditional method of treatment. However, multiple trials including Impact of Managed Pharmaceutical care on Resource utilization and Outcomes in Veterans affairs medical centers (IMPROVE) study have shown lower mortality and shorter hospital stay with EVAR. More centers are increasingly using endovascular repair for patients who fit certain anatomic and physiologic criteria.

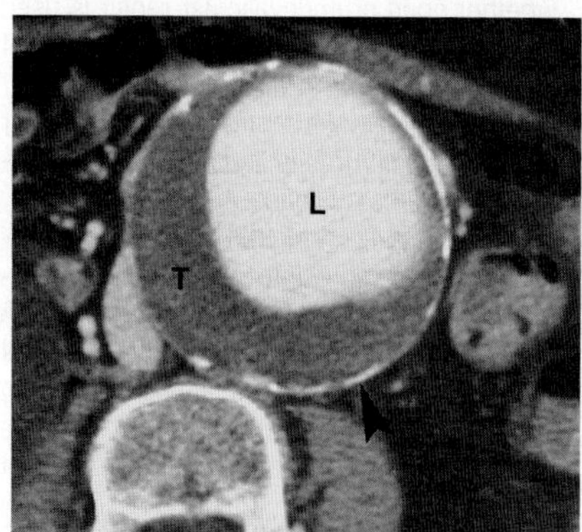

FIG. 4 Aneurysm of the abdominal aorta. A large aortic aneurysm is evident. The aorta exceeds 5 cm in diameter. A large amount of thrombus *(T)* partially surrounds the contrast-enhanced patent lumen *(L)*. Note the atherosclerotic calcification (*arrowhead*) in the wall of the aneurysm.

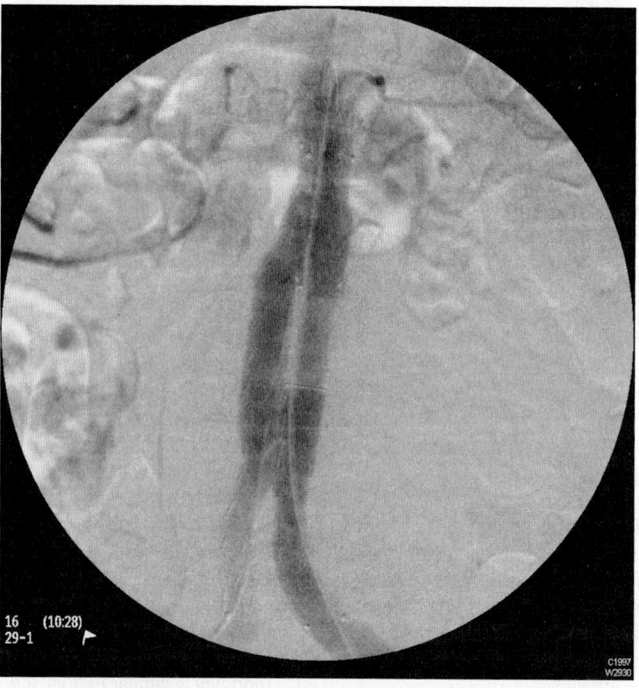

FIG. 6 Completion digital subtraction angiogram following endovascular aneurysm repair. (From Fillit HM: *Brocklehurst's textbook of geriatric medicine and gerontology*, ed 8, Philadlphia, 2017, Elsevier.)

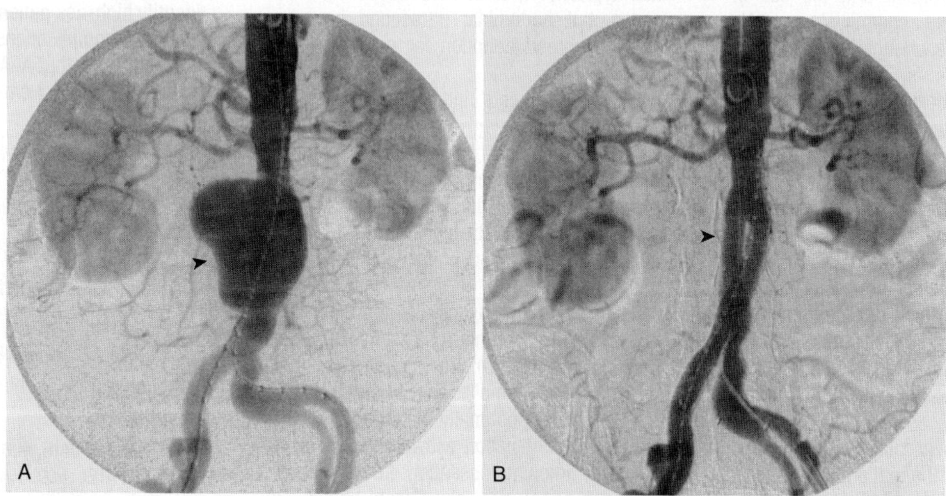

FIG. 5 A, Conventional catheter angiography with bilateral marked catheters in place demonstrates a large, lobulated, infrarenal aortic aneurysm (*arrowhead*) with a 4-cm proximal neck suitable for endovascular repair. **B,** An image after endovascular repair demonstrates complete exclusion of the aneurysm (*arrowhead*) with no endoleak and preservation of the renal and hypogastric arteries. (Soto JA, Lucey BC: *Emergency radiology: the requisites*, ed 2, Philadelphia, 2017, Elsevier.)

- However, a recent Cochrane meta-analysis involving pooled data for four trials comparing EVAR versus open repair for ruptured abdominal aortic aneurysm failed to show a difference in 30-day mortality between EVAR versus open repair. There was a higher incidence of reintervention for patients undergoing EVAR, although interventions to deal with procedural complications were generally less invasive and involved catheter-based approaches.
- The major limitations for EVAR include anatomical issues such as tortuosity or small caliber iliac arteries and inability to follow up patients to exclude late failure of stent-grafts and development of endoleaks.

CHRONIC Rx

- Blood pressure and fasting lipids should be monitored and controlled as recommended for patients with atherosclerotic disease. Statins are associated with decreased mortality after successful AAA repair, and are recommended for those with known AAA to reduce the progression of atherosclerosis and overall cardiovascular risk.
- The most commonly used predictor of rupture is the maximum diameter of the AAA.
- Monitoring by ultrasound or CT scan should be performed every 6 to 12 months for patients with AAAs measuring 4.0 to 5.4 cm in diameter and by ultrasound every 2 yr for those with AAAs measuring 3 to 4 cm and every 5 yr for those with AAAs between 2.6 and 2.9 cm.
- Long-term beta-blocker therapy has slowed the rate of aortic dilation and decreased the incidence of aortic complications in patients with Marfan's syndrome. Several studies have also suggested that beta-blocker therapy may reduce the rate of expansion and risk of rupture; however, conclusive evidence is lacking.
- A recent multicenter study of 5362 patients with AAA found no significant association between AAA progression and the use of statins, beta-blockers, angiotensin-converting enzyme inhibitors, or angiotensin II receptor blockers.
- Antibiotics such as doxycycline and roxithromycin have been shown to limit the expansion of small AAAs.
- Surgical repair to eliminate the risk for rupture should be performed for patients with infrarenal or juxtarenal AAA of approximately 5.5 cm or larger in diameter. All patients who are symptomatic should undergo repair, regardless of size. Timing of repair in symptomatic unruptured AAA is still under debate.
- There is no clear advantage to early repair (open or endovascular) for small AAAs (less than 5.5 cm).
- Percutaneous, endovascular, stent-anchored grafts placed with the patient under local anesthesia have provided an alternative approach for patients with favorable anatomy. In patients who have undergone endovascular repair, long-term surveillance is required to assess for an endoleak, stent migration, change in aneurysm size, and need for re-intervention.
- Fenestrated endovascular repair is an alternative to open repair in the management of juxtarenal aortic aneurysms (JRAs) and short-neck abdominal aortic aneurysms. Contemporary literature shows that it is a safe and efficacious treatment, particularly for those deemed surgically high risk. Growing experience and innovation of stent-grafts are essential for the advancement of fenestrated grafting.
- Randomized trials have shown that endovascular repair of AAA is associated with a significantly lower operative mortality than open surgical repair but it has increased rates of graft-related complications and reintervention, and is more costly. There are no differences between endovascular repair and open surgical repair in total mortality or aneurysm-related mortality at 7 yr.
- Compared with open aneurysm repair, EVAR is associated with better health-related quality of life up to 12 months postoperatively for unruptured aneurysms.
- Most recent meta-analysis concludes that EVAR has lower rates of 30-day mortality, 30-day MI, and length of hospital stay in both elective and emergency AAA repair. However, there were no differences in death rates between treatment groups at 4 yr postprocedure.
- Based on current data, less than 2% of endovascular repairs require open conversion, and approximately half of all early endoleaks resolve spontaneously within a period of 30 days.
- Open repair still represents a valuable solution for many patients with failed EVAR with relatively low mortality rates when performed electively.
- Perioperative mortality is significantly less for EVAR compared with open repair (1.8% vs. 4.3%), whereas overall cumulative long-term mortality is similar (9.3 vs. 8.9 deaths) based upon the data obtained from the EVAR-1 trial.
- Surveillance for endovascular AAA repair has typically involved use of periodic CT scans, but abdominal ultrasound is gaining widespread adoption for postprocedure monitoring.
- In high-risk patients undergoing AAA repair, specifically those with coronary artery disease or those with more than one clinical risk factor based on the American Heart Association (AHA) guidelines, preoperative administration of beta-blockers titrated to a goal heart rate of 60 have been shown to decrease incidence of death from cardiac causes or nonfatal myocardial infarctions.
- Patients with chronic obstructive pulmonary disease (COPD) are at higher risk for major clinical complications, particularly if the COPD is suboptimally managed or if it is present in conjunction with cardiac or renal disease. Smoking cessation for 2 months before surgery has also been shown to decrease pulmonary morbidity.
- Renal dysfunction is a strong predictor of mortality, showing up to as high as 41% mortality in those with impaired renal function compared with 6% in those without renal dysfunction.

REFERRAL

- Vascular surgical referral should be made in asymptomatic patients with AAAs that are approximately 4.5 cm.
- In patients with an expansion rate of 0.6-0.8 cm/yr, it is reasonable to offer repair, although small studies have shown that using expansion as a criterion for surgical referral is of unclear benefit.
- It is important to optimize any comorbid conditions before surgical referral.

PEARLS & CONSIDERATIONS

- Repairing asymptomatic AAAs smaller than 5.5 cm has not been shown to improve survival because the risk of rupture is lower than the risk of surgery.
- The results from multiple trials to date demonstrate no advantage to immediate repair for small AAA (4.0-5.5 cm), regardless of whether open or endovascular repair is used and, at least for open repair, regardless of patient age and AAA diameter. Thus, neither immediate open nor immediate endovascular repair of small AAAs is supported by the currently available evidence.
- Five-yr survival remains poor after elective AAA repair despite advances in short-term outcomes and is associated with AAA diameter and patient age at the time of surgery. Research in this field should attempt to improve the life expectancy of patients with repaired AAA and to optimize patient selection.

COMMENTS

- Most AAAs are infrarenal.
- Surgical risk is increased in patients with coexisting coronary artery disease, pulmonary disease, or chronic renal failure. Evaluation for ischemia and aggressive perioperative hemodynamic monitoring help identify high-risk patients and decrease postoperative complications.
- It is estimated that AAAs at <5 cm expand at a rate of 0.3 to 0.4 cm/yr.

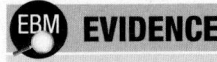

EVIDENCE

Available at ExpertConsult.com

SUGGESTED READINGS

Available at ExpertConsult.com

RELATED CONTENT

Abdominal Aortic Aneurysm (AAA) (Patient Information)

AUTHOR: **AMIT K. JAIN, M.D.,** and
PRANAV M. PATEL, M.D., F.A.C.C., F.A.H.A., F.S.C.A.I.

BASIC INFORMATION

DEFINITION

Abruptio placentae is the separation of placenta from the uterine wall before delivery of the fetus. The condition occurs in approximately 1% of pregnancies. There are three classes of abruption based on maternal and fetal status, including an assessment of uterine contractions, quantity of bleeding, fetal heart rate monitoring, and abnormal coagulation studies (fibrinogen, prothrombin time, partial thromboplastin time).

- Grade I: Mild vaginal bleeding, uterine irritability, stable vital signs, reassuring fetal heart rate, normal coagulation profile (fibrinogen 450 mg/dl). Approximately half of abruptions are grade I.
- Grade II: Moderate vaginal bleeding, hypertonic uterine contractions, orthostatic blood pressure measurements, unfavorable fetal status, fibrinogen 150 to 250 mg. Approximately a quarter of abruptions are grade II.
- Grade III: Severe bleeding (may be concealed), hypertonic uterine contractions, overt signs of hypovolemic shock, fetal death, thrombocytopenia, fibrinogen <150 mg/dl. Approximately a quarter of abruptions are grade III.

SYNONYM

Premature separation of placenta

ICD-10CM CODES	
O45.8X9	Other premature separation of placenta, unspecified trimester
O45.8X1	Other premature separation of placenta, first trimester
O45.8X2	Other premature separation of placenta, second trimester
O45.8X3	Other premature separation of placenta, third trimester
O45.91	Premature separation of placenta, unspecified, first trimester
O45.92	Premature separation of placenta, unspecified, second trimester
O45.93	Premature separation of placenta, unspecified, third trimester

EPIDEMIOLOGY & DEMOGRAPHICS

INCIDENCE (IN U.S.): 9.6 per 1000 births; 80% occur before the onset of labor.

RISK FACTORS: Hypertension (greatest association), trauma, polyhydramnios, multifetal gestation, smoking, use of cocaine, chorioamnionitis, preterm premature rupture of membranes. Table 1 summarizes placental abruption risk factors.

RECURRENCE RATE: 5% to 17%, some studies showing a 5- to 10-fold increase in risk; with two prior episodes, 25%.

PHYSICAL FINDINGS & CLINICAL PRESENTATION

- Triad of uterine bleeding (concealed or per vagina), hypertonic uterine contractions or signs of preterm labor, and evidence of fetal compromise exists.
- More than 80% of cases have external bleeding; 20% of cases have no bleeding but have indirect evidence of abruption, such as failed tocolysis for preterm labor.
- Tetanic uterine contractions are found in only 17%.

ETIOLOGY

- Primary etiology: Unknown
- Hypertension: Found in 40% to 50% of grade III abruptions
- Rapid decompression of uterine cavity, as can occur in polyhydramnios or multifetal gestation
- Blunt external trauma (motor vehicle accident, spousal abuse)

DIAGNOSIS

DIFFERENTIAL DIAGNOSIS

- Placenta previa
- Cervical or vaginal trauma
- Labor
- Cervical cancer
- Rupture of membranes
- The differential diagnosis of vaginal bleeding in pregnancy is described in Section III

TABLE 1 Placental Abruption Risk Factors

Increasing parity or maternal age
Cigarette smoking
Cocaine abuse
Trauma
Maternal hypertension
Preterm premature rupture of membranes
Rapid uterine decompression associated with multiple gestation and polyhydramnios
Inherited or acquired thrombophilia
Uterine malformations or fibroids
Placental abnormalities or ischemia
Prior abruption

From Gabbe SG: *Obstetrics*, ed 6, Philadelphia, 2012, Saunders.

WORKUP

- Placental abruption is primarily a clinical diagnosis that is supported by laboratory, radiographic (Fig. 1), and pathologic studies.
- Initial assessment should evaluate for the source of bleeding, ruling out placenta previa that may contraindicate any type of vaginal examination (e.g., pelvic speculum examination).
- Continuous fetal heart monitoring is indicated for all viable gestations (60% incidence of fetal distress in labor); may show early signs of maternal hypovolemia (late decelerations or fetal tachycardia) before overt maternal vital sign changes.
- Actual amount of blood loss is often greater than initially perceived because of the possibility of concealed retroplacental bleeding and apparent "normal" vital signs. The relative hypervolemia of pregnancy initially protects the patient until late in the course of bleeding, when abrupt and sudden cardiovascular collapse can occur.

LABORATORY TESTS

- Baseline serum hemoglobin helps quantify blood loss and establish baseline values for serial comparisons during expectant management.
- Coagulation profile: Platelets, fibrinogen, prothrombin, and partial thromboplastin time. Diffuse intravascular coagulation can develop with severe abruption. If fibrinogen is <150 mg/dl, estimated blood loss is approximately 2000 ml; if fibrinogen is <100 mg/dl, consider fresh frozen plasma to prevent further bleeding.
- Type and antibody screen is important to identify Rh-negative patients who need Rh immune globulin.

IMAGING STUDIES

Ultrasound should include fetal presentation and status, amniotic fluid volume, placental location,

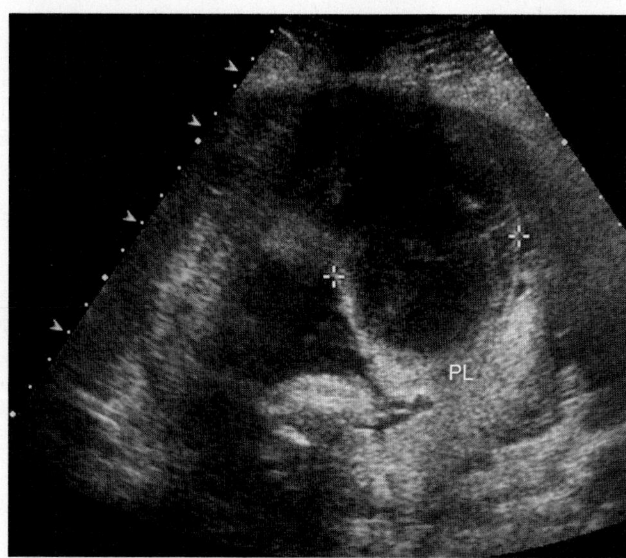

FIG. 1 Placental abruption. Transabdominal sonogram of the placenta *(PL)* with a hematoma *(calipers)* lifting the placenta away from the uterine wall. (From Rumack CM et al [eds]: *Diagnostic ultrasound*, ed 4, Philadelphia, 2011, Mosby.)

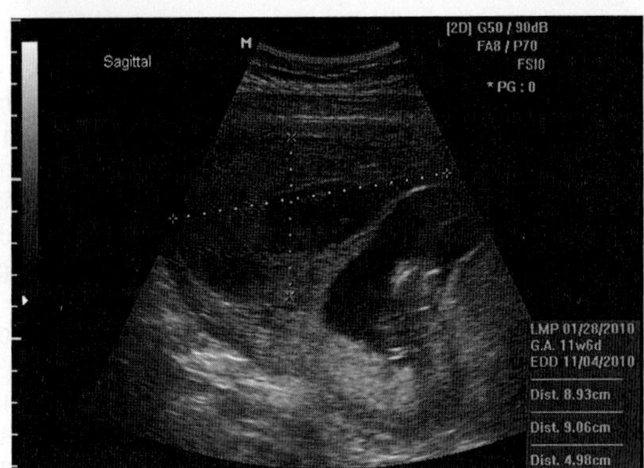

FIG. 2 Ultrasonic image of a subchorionic abruption. (Courtesy K. Francois; from Gabbe SG: *Obstetrics,* ed 6, Philadelphia, 2012, Saunders.)

as well as any evidence of hematoma (retroplacental, subchorionic, or preplacental) (Fig. 2).

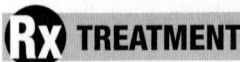

TREATMENT

ACUTE GENERAL Rx

- Stabilization of the mother is the first priority.
- Treatment depends on gestational age of the fetus, severity of the abruption, and maternal status.
- Initial assessment for signs of maternal hemodynamic compromise or hemorrhagic shock; large-bore intravenous access, with crystalloid fluid resuscitation using a replacement of 3 ml lactated Ringer's solution for every 1 ml estimated blood loss.
- Indwelling Foley catheter to monitor urine output and maternal volume status, with a goal of 30 ml/hr urine output.
- Assess fetal status and gestational age by sonogram and continuous fetal heart rate monitoring.
- Because of the unpredictable nature of abruptions, cross-matched blood should be made available during the initial resuscitation period.

CHRONIC Rx

- In the term fetus, delivery is indicated.
- In the preterm fetus, consider betamethasone 12.5 mg IM q24h for two doses and then delivery, depending on the severity of the abruption and the likelihood of fetal complications from preterm birth.
- Cesarean section should be reserved for cases of fetal distress or for standard obstetric indications. While cesarean delivery may be needed to stabilize the fetal and/or maternal status, the mother's coagulation status may complicate the procedure and availability of blood products may be critical.
- In cases of maternal stability and fetal prematurity, expectant management can occur in the setting of close follow-up, including regular evaluation of fetal growth and reassuring antenatal testing.

DISPOSITION

Because of the unpredictable nature of abruptions, expectant management should occur only under controlled circumstances.

REFERRAL

Abruptio placentae places mother and fetus in a high-risk situation and should be managed by a qualified obstetrician in a facility with capability for neonatal and maternal resuscitation, for supporting a preterm infant if delivery is indicated at an early gestational age, and for performing emergency cesarean sections.

RELATED CONTENT

Abruptio Placentae (Patient Information)
Premature Labor (Related Key Topic)
Vaginal Bleeding During Pregnancy (Related Key Topic)

AUTHOR: **KELLY RUHSTALLER, M.D.**

BASIC INFORMATION

DEFINITION

Absence seizures are a type of generalized seizure characterized by brief episodes of staring with impairment of consciousness (absence). They usually last no more than 20 to 30 sec. The onset and the end of the seizures are sudden. Usually the patients are not aware of them and resume the activity they were performing before the seizure. The electroencephalogram signature of absence seizures consists of a generalized 3-Hz spike and slow wave discharges.

SYNONYMS

Childhood absence epilepsy
Seizures, absence

ICD-10CM CODE

G40.309 Generalized idiopathic epilepsy and epileptic syndromes, not intractable, without status epilepticus

EPIDEMIOLOGY & DEMOGRAPHICS

INCIDENCE: 1 to 10 cases per 100,000 population.
PEAK INCIDENCE: 6 to 7 yr.
PREVALENCE: Represents up to 18% of all pediatric epilepsy syndromes.
PREDOMINANT SEX AND AGE: More common in girls than in boys, absences typically begin between 4 and 8 yr.

PHYSICAL FINDINGS & CLINICAL PRESENTATION

- Patients with absence seizures usually have normal physical and neurologic examinations.
- During the seizures, the patients are unresponsive and can have motor phenomena (automatisms, eye blinks, mouth and hand movements).
- Absence seizures are not associated with postictal confusion.
- They may be triggered by hyperventilation associated with activity.
- Tonic clonic seizures are not usually a feature of this syndrome. If the patient also experiences tonic clonic seizures, other etiologies should be investigated, such as juvenile absence epilepsy, juvenile myoclonic epilepsy, complex partial seizures, etc.

ETIOLOGY

Genetic

DIAGNOSIS

DIFFERENTIAL DIAGNOSIS

- Juvenile absence epilepsy
- Juvenile myoclonic epilepsy
- Complex partial seizures
- Focal seizures with altered consciousness (Table E1)
- Nonepileptic spells comprised of staring

WORKUP

- EEG with hyperventilation and photic stimulation is crucial in the diagnosis.
- Ambulatory EEG and video EEG are recommended for patients with diagnostic uncertainty.

LABORATORY TESTS

No specific studies needed

IMAGING STUDIES

- MRI of the brain should be performed in all epilepsy patients, especially if the EEG does not show the typical characteristic of absence seizures (3-Hz spike and slow wave discharges).
- CT scans of the head should be avoided in children due to unnecessary exposure to radiation and low yield of the test except when MRI cannot be obtained.

TREATMENT

The medication of choice based on the best current evidence available is ethosuximide, followed by valproic acid and lamotrigine.

NONPHARMACOLOGIC THERAPY

Not applicable

GENERAL Rx

- Ethosuximide: Initial dose: 10 mg/kg/day; then after 7 days, 20 mg/kg
- Divalproex sodium (Depakote): Initial dose: 5 to 10 mg/kg/day (divided bid), maximum dose: 60 mg/kg/day
- Lamotrigine (Lamictal): Dose for patients on no other antiepileptic drugs. Wk 1 and 2: 0.3 mg/kg/day. Wk 3 and 4: 0.6 mg/kg/day. Wk 5 onward: Increase every 1 to 2 wk by 0.6 mg/kg/day. Maintenance: 4.5 to 7.5 mg/kg/day. Warning: Should be used with caution due to the potential for toxicity and Stevens-Johnson syndrome. Patients on other antiepileptic drugs can also have severe adverse reactions (e.g., valproate can cause increased levels of lamotrigine, and lamotrigine must be titrated much more slowly in patients on valproate therapy).

CHRONIC Rx

- Children with recurrent seizures require chronic treatment.
- If children are seizure-free for a period of 1 to 2 yr, a trial on no medications should be considered; children typically outgrow childhood absence seizures.

COMPLEMENTARY & ALTERNATIVE MEDICINE

Not applicable

DISPOSITION

- Response to treatment is excellent.
- Absence seizures tend to remit in teenage yr.
- Epilepsy can be considered as resolved once 10 yr have elapsed since the last event, including 5 yr free from medications.

REFERRAL

Patients with epilepsy and seizures should be referred for a consultation by a neurologist, preferably one specializing in epilepsy.

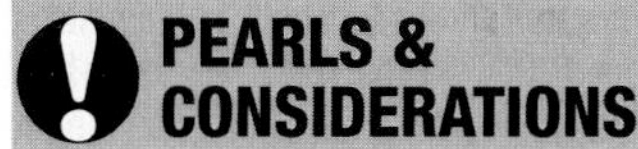

PEARLS & CONSIDERATIONS

COMMENTS

- Absence seizures can be present in other epilepsy syndromes.
- Valproate should be avoided in girls and women with childbearing potential due to the risk of teratogenicity.
- Carbamazepine and phenytoin should be avoided in the treatment of absence seizures, since these medications may worsen seizures and could provoke absence status epilepticus.
- All women of childbearing age taking antiepileptic drugs should take folic acid supplementation (1-4 mg/day) for the prevention of neural tube defects.

PREVENTION

Sleep deprivation and alcohol consumption should be avoided.

PATIENT & FAMILY EDUCATION

- Patients with ongoing seizures are forbidden to drive; check state regulations and laws regarding driving and epilepsy.

SUGGESTED READING

Available at ExpertConsult.com

RELATED CONTENT

Absence Seizures (Patient Information)

AUTHOR: **PATRICIO SEBASTIAN ESPINOSA, M.D., M.P.H.**

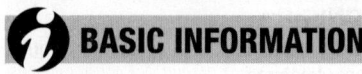

BASIC INFORMATION

DEFINITION

Acetaminophen (APAP) poisoning is a disorder caused by excessive intake of APAP and is manifested by jaundice, nausea, vomiting, and potential death from hepatic necrosis if not treated appropriately.

SYNONYM

Paracetamol poisoning

ICD-10CM CODES

T39.1	Poisoning by 4-aminophenol derivatives, accidental
X60	Intentional self-poisoning by 4-aminophenol derivatives

EPIDEMIOLOGY & DEMOGRAPHICS

- APAP is one of the most widely prescribed antipyretics and analgesics in the U.S. Potentially toxic ingestions, both intentional and unintentional, exceed 100,000 cases annually in the U.S.
- APAP toxicity is the number one cause of acute liver failure in the U.S.
- Death rate is approximately one in 1000 persons. Nearly 50% of exposures occur in children ≤6 yr.
- Hepatic necrosis is most likely to occur in people who are (1) chronically malnourished, (2) regularly abusing alcohol, and (3) using other potentially hepatotoxic medications.

PHYSICAL FINDINGS & CLINICAL PRESENTATION

- The physical examination may vary depending on the amount of time since ingestion.
- Phase I (0 to 24 hr): Initial symptoms may be mild or absent and may consist of anorexia, diaphoresis, malaise, nausea, vomiting, lethargy, and a subclinical rise in transaminase levels.
- Phase II (24 to 72 hr): Right upper quadrant pain, vomiting, somnolence, tachycardia, jaundice, hypotension, and continued increase in transaminases.
- Phase III (72 to 96 hr): Hepatic necrosis with abdominal pain, jaundice, hepatic encephalopathy, coagulopathy, hypoglycemia, renal failure, fatality from multi-organ failure.
- Phase IV (4 days to 2 wk): Complete resolution of symptoms and resolution of organ failure.
- Table E1 summarizes the four phases/stages of acetaminophen poisoning.

ETIOLOGY

- The amount of APAP necessary for hepatic toxicity varies with the patient's body size and hepatic function. It is recommended that APAP intake should not exceed 4 g for adults and 90 mg/kg in children within a 24-hr period.
- A standardized nomogram is used to determine potential hepatic toxicity by knowing the APAP plasma level and the number of hours after ingestion. See the APAP ingestion algorithm (Fig. E1).

Dx DIAGNOSIS

DIFFERENTIAL DIAGNOSIS

- Liver disease from alcohol abuse or viral hepatitis
- Ingestion of other hepatotoxic substances
- Bacterial/viral gastroenteritis

WORKUP

Initial workup is aimed at confirming APAP overdose with plasma APAP level and assessment of hepatic damage. A careful history should elicit the time of APAP ingestion, amount, preparation (e.g., extended release), and possible coingestants (see "Laboratory Tests").

LABORATORY TESTS

- Initial laboratory evaluation should include an initial plasma APAP level with a second level drawn approximately 4 hr after the initial ingestion. Subsequent levels can be obtained every 2 to 4 hr until the levels stabilize or decline. Levels starting from 4 hrs post-ingestion should be plotted on the Rumack-Matthew nomogram (see acetaminophen ingestion algorithm [Fig. E1] to calculate potential hepatic toxicity). The nomogram cannot be used with patients who present >24 hr after ingestion, took extended-release preparations, had chronic ingestions, or when the time of ingestion is unknown.
- Transaminases (AST, ALT), serum glucose, bilirubin level, lipase level, prothrombin time (INR), blood urea nitrogen, creatinine, EKG, and urinalysis should be initially obtained on all patients.
- Serum and urine toxicology screens for other potential toxic substances is also recommended on admission. Screening for infectious hepatitis should also be considered.
- Urine for β-hCG should be obtained from all women of childbearing age.

Rx TREATMENT

NONPHARMACOLOGIC THERAPY

Consultation with a Poison Control Center is recommended for patients who have ingested a large amount of APAP and/or other toxic substances. A single toxic dose of APAP usually exceeds 7 g or 150 mg/kg in adults.

ACUTE GENERAL Rx

- Hepatotoxicity is defined as any increase in alanine aminotransferase (ALT) or aspartate aminotransferase (AST) >1000 IU/L, and hepatic failure manifests as hepatotoxicity with hepatic encephalopathy. For those who cannot be risk stratified using the nomogram, the American College of Emergency Physicians recommends that *N*-acetylcysteine be administered without delay to those >12 yr and >8 hr after ingestion at presentation. This would include anyone with an ingestion of APAP over many days with an APAP level <20 μg/ml (with or without ALT elevation) or anyone with undetectable APAP levels with an elevated ALT and a history of excessive APAP intake.
- Administer activated charcoal 1g/kg PO if the patient is seen within 1 hr of ingestion or the clinician suspects polysubstance ingestion that delays gastric emptying.
- Determine blood levels 4 hr after ingestion; if in the toxic range based on the Rumack-Matthew nomogram, start *N*-acetylcysteine (NAC) either IV (Acetadote) or PO (Mucomyst). Acetylcysteine IV loading dose is 150 mg/kg ×1 diluted in 200 ml D5W over 15 to 60 min. Maintenance dose is 50 mg/kg diluted in 500 ml D5W over 4 hr, followed by 100 mg/kg diluted in 1000 ml D5W over 16 hr. The dose does not require adjustment for renal or hepatic impairment or for dialysis. Total administration time is 21 hours.
- Oral administration is 140 mg/kg PO as a loading dose, followed after 4 hr by 70 mg/kg PO q4h for a total of 18 doses. *N*-acetylcysteine therapy should be started within 24 hr of APAP overdose. Total administration time is 72 hours.
- Advantages of IV administration include more reliable absorption, fewer doses, and shorter duration of treatment. Disadvantages include cost and lower hepatic concentrations from first-pass flow as compared to oral acetylcysteine.
- Monitor APAP level; use Rumack-Matthew nomogram to trend hepatic toxicity. Repeat AST/ALT and APAP levels after 12 to 14 hr of IV acetylcysteine infusion and continue infusion longer than 16 hr if transaminases are elevated, if APAP concentration is still measurable, or if coagulopathy exists (INR >1.5-2.0). Patients with severe, irreversible liver failure may need to continue NAC until liver transplantation is available.
- Provide adequate IV hydration (e.g., D_5½NS at 150 ml/hr).
- Patients on IV *N*-acetylcysteine with liver failure require frequent monitoring of vital signs, oxygen saturation by pulse oximetry, and frequent blood draws. Frequent reassessment for hypoglycemia and infection is also essential.
- If APAP level is nontoxic, *N*-acetylcysteine therapy may be discontinued.

DISPOSITION

All patients with confirmed APAP poisoning will require admission, usually to an intensive care unit. Most patients (90%) will recover fully without persistent hepatic abnormalities. Hepatic failure is particularly unusual in children <6 yr.

REFERRAL

Psychiatric referral is recommended after intentional ingestions.

RELATED CONTENT

Acetaminophen Overdose (Patient Information)

AUTHOR: **STEVEN ROUGAS, M.D., M.S., F.A.C.E.P.**

BASIC INFORMATION

DEFINITION

Achalasia is a motility disorder of the esophagus classically characterized by incomplete relaxation of the lower esophageal sphincter (LES) and aperistalsis of the esophageal smooth muscle. The result is functional obstruction of the esophagus.

SYNONYMS

Achalasia and cardiospasm
Achalasia (of cardia)
Aperistalsis of esophagus
Megaesophagus
Esophageal achalasia
Esophageal cardiospasm

ICD-10CM CODE
K22.0 Achalasia of cardia

EPIDEMIOLOGY & DEMOGRAPHICS

- Annual incidence is approximately 0.5-1.0 in 100,000 persons.
- Prevalence is <10 per 100,000 persons.
- Although the onset of symptoms may occur at any age, incidence is typically bimodal, 20 to 40 yr, then after 60 yr, with greater incidence in the older group.
- Men and women are affected equally.

PHYSICAL FINDINGS & CLINICAL PRESENTATION

Symptoms:

- Dysphagia (most commonly with both solids and liquids)
- Difficulty belching
- Regurgitation
- Chest pain and/or heartburn
- Globus
- Frequent hiccups
- Vomiting of undigested food
- Symptoms of aspiration such as nocturnal cough; possible dyspnea and pneumonia
- Weight loss
- The Eckardt symptom score (assessing dysphagia, regurgitation, retrosternal pain, and weight loss), a fairly reliable and valid measure of achalasia severity, may be used to assess response to therapy

Physical findings:

- Focal lung examination abnormalities and wheezing are also possible.

ETIOLOGY

- Etiology is poorly understood.
- Loss of intrinsic inhibitory neurons in the myenteric plexus in the LES and smooth muscle portion of the esophagus as well as depletion of networks of interstitial cells of Cajal of the LES result in the loss of inhibitory neurotransmitters nitric oxide and vasoactive intestinal polypeptide and unopposed excitatory activity, leading to incomplete relaxation of the LES and loss of esophageal peristalsis.
- Loss of myenteric nerve fibers is associated with lymphocytic and eosinophilic infiltrates, capillaritis, plexitis, venulitis, nerve hypertrophy, and fibrosis.
- This disorder may be caused by autoimmune degeneration of the esophageal myenteric plexus in association with several HLA class II DQ antigens. Antimyenteric plexus and other antineural autoantibodies have also been described. Patients with achalasia are more likely to have other autoimmune diseases.
- Abnormal immune reactions to neurotropic viruses, such as varicella zoster, measles, and particularly herpes simplex type 1, have been implicated. A host T cell–mediated response may lead to neuronal injury; this has been suggested as the cause of types I and II achalasia (see "Imaging Studies" section).
- Achalasia is also seen in the rare autosomal recessive disorder, Allgrove syndrome (achalasia, alacrima, autonomic disturbance, and acetylcholine insensitivity), which has been linked to a gene mutation on chromosome 12q13. Neurons in this syndrome may be susceptible to oxidative injury.
- Recent studies suggest that type III achalasia (see "Imaging Studies" section) is associated with myenteric inflammation but not neuronal loss and that downregulation of nitric oxide synthase expression and increased cholinergic sensitivity are cytokine-mediated.

DIAGNOSIS

DIFFERENTIAL DIAGNOSIS

- Primary achalasia:
  1. Idiopathic
- Secondary achalasia:
  1. Chagas disease
  2. Vagal injury or surgery, including fundoplication
  3. Achalasia-like esophageal dilation has been described after laparoscopic gastric banding
- Pseudoachalasia (diseases that may mimic achalasia):
  1. Esophageal cancer
  2. Infiltrating gastric cancer
  3. Oat cell and bronchogenic lung cancer
  4. Lymphoma
  5. Amyloidosis
  6. Paraneoplastic syndrome
- Angina
- Bulimia
- Anorexia nervosa
- Gastric bezoar
- Gastritis
- Peptic ulcer disease
- Postvagotomy dysmotility
- Esophageal disease (Table 1):
  1. Gastroesophageal reflux disease
  2. Sarcoidosis
  3. Amyloidosis
  4. Esophageal stricture
  5. Esophageal webs and rings
  6. Scleroderma
  7. Barrett's esophagus
  8. Esophagitis
  9. Diffuse esophageal spasm

WORKUP

- Physical examination and laboratory analyses to rule out other causes (Fig. 1, Table 2) and assess complications
- Imaging studies, manometry, and endoscopy (may be supportive or complementary)

LABORATORY TESTS

- Assessment of nutritional status
- Complete blood count, ECG, stress test if diagnosis is in doubt
- Serologic assays for *Trypanosoma cruzi* (Chagas disease) in appropriate individuals

IMAGING STUDIES

Barium swallow with fluoroscopy (particularly a timed barium esophagogram) may demonstrate:

- Uncoordinated or absent esophageal contractions (loss of peristalsis)
- An acutely tapered contrast column ("bird's beak"; Fig. E2)

TABLE 1 Esophageal Motor Disorders

	Achalasia	Scleroderma	Diffuse Esophageal Spasm
Symptoms	Dysphagia Regurgitation of nonacidic material	Gastroesophageal reflux disease Dysphagia	Substernal chest pain (angina-like) Dysphagia with pain
Radiographic appearance	Dilated, fluid-filled esophagus Distal *bird-beak* stricture	Aperistaltic esophagus Free reflux Peptic stricture	Simultaneous noncoordinated contractions
Manometric findings			
Lower esophageal sphincter	High resting pressure Incomplete or abnormal relaxation with swallow	Low resting pressure	Normal pressure
Body	Low-amplitude, simultaneous contractions after swallowing	Low-amplitude peristaltic contractions or no peristalsis	Some peristalsis Diffuse and simultaneous nonperistaltic contractions, occasionally high amplitude

From Andreoli TE et al: *Andreoli and Carpenter's Cecil essentials of medicine*, ed 8, Philadelphia, 2010, Saunders.

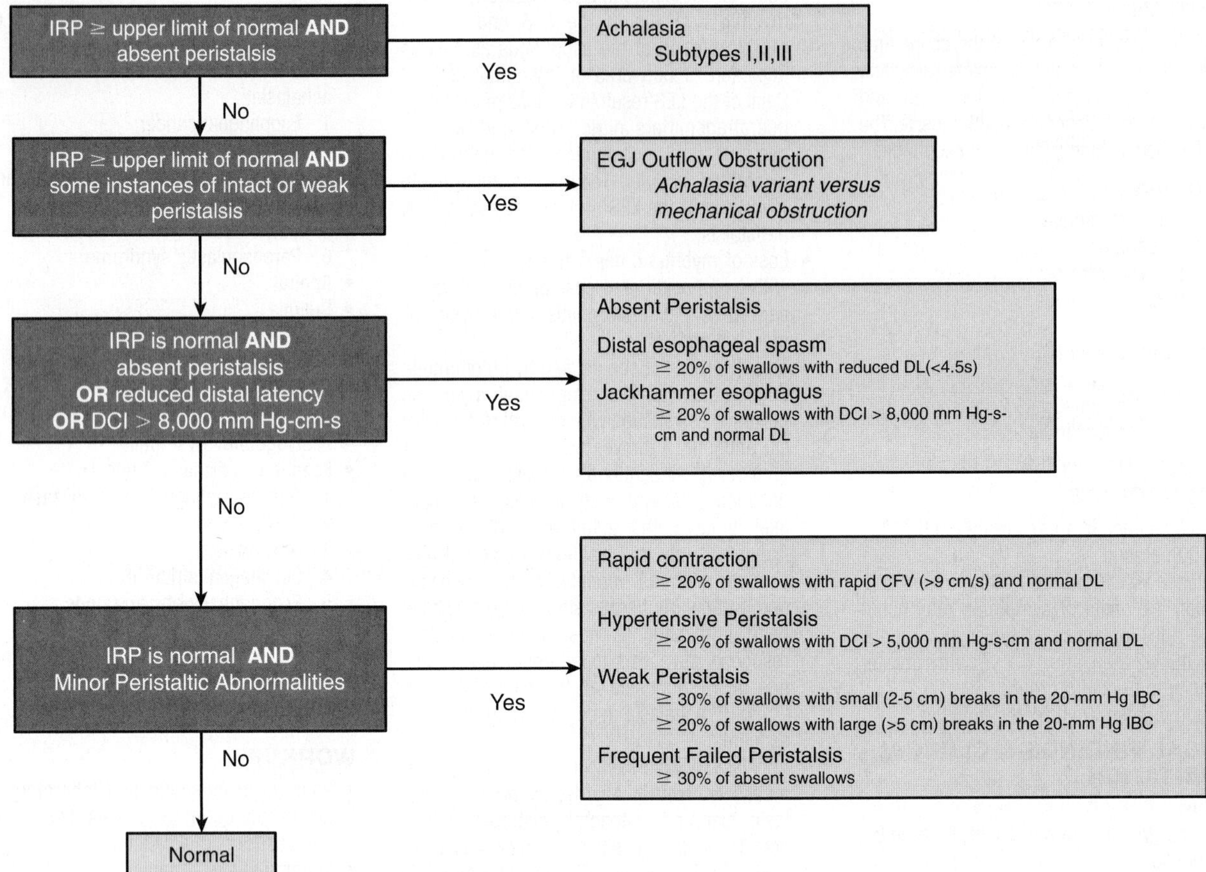

FIG. 1 Algorithm for applying the Chicago Classification of esophageal motor disorders. *CFV*, contractile front velocity; *DCI*, distal contractile interval; *DL*, distal latency; *EGJ*, esophagogastric junction; *IBC*, isobar contour; *IRP*, integrated relaxation pressure (see Table 2 for more details). (From Feldman M, et al.: *Sleisenger and Fortran's gastrointestinal and liver disease*, ed 10, Philadelphia, 2016, Elsevier.)

TABLE 2 Chicago Classification of Esophageal Motility Disorders

Diagnosis	Diagnostic Criteria
Achalasia	
Type I	100% failed peristalsis, mean IRP >10 mm Hg
Type II	No esophageal contraction and panesophageal pressurization with ≥20% of swallows; mean IRP >10 mm Hg
Type III	Premature contractions with ≥20% of swallows, mean IRP ≥17 mm Hg
EGJ outflow obstruction	Mean IRP ≥15 mm Hg; mix of normal, weak, rapid, hypertensive, failed peristalsis or panesophageal pressurization
Motility Disorders	(Patterns not observed in normal individuals)
Distal esophageal spasm	Mean IRP <17 mm Hg, ≥20% premature contractions
Hypercontractile esophagus (jackhammer esophagus)	At least one swallow DCI >8000 mm Hg·s·cm
Absent peristalsis	Mean IRP ≤10 mm Hg, 100% failed peristalsis
Peristaltic Abnormality	(Defined by exceeding statistical limits of normal)
Weak peristalsis	Mean IRP <15 mm Hg and ≥20% swallows with large breaks (≥5 cm) or ≥30% with small breaks (2-5 cm) in the 20-mm Hg isobaric contour Or DCI of 150-450 mm Hg·s·cm in ≥30% test swallows
Frequent failed peristalsis	>30%, but <100% of swallows with failed peristalsis
Rapid peristalsis	Rapid contraction with ≥20% of swallows, DL >4.5 s
Hypertensive peristalsis (nutcracker esophagus)	Mean DCI >5000 mm Hg·s·cm, but not meeting criteria for hypercontractile esophagus
Normal	Not achieving any of the above diagnostic criteria

DCI, Distal contractile interval; *DL*, distal latency; *EGJ*, esophagogastric junction; *IRP*, integrated relaxation pressure.
From Feldman M, Friedman LS, Brandt LJ: *Sleisenger and Fortran's gastrointestinal and liver disease*, ed 10, Philadelphia, 2016, Saunders.

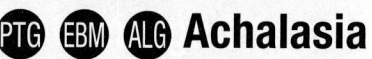

- Dilation of the distal esophagus (smooth muscle portion)
- Esophageal air-fluid level with evidence of poor esophageal emptying
- Late-stage changes include tortuosity, angulation, dilated megaesophagus, retained food, and secretions

Manometry is considered the "gold standard" test to confirm the diagnosis.

- In classic achalasia (type I achalasia), conventional manometric abnormalities are as follows: low-amplitude disorganized contractions/aperistalsis, incomplete or absent LES relaxation (with residual pressure >10 mm Hg) after swallow, and high resting LES pressure.
- A subset of patients with "vigorous achalasia" may have high-amplitude, long-duration, simultaneous esophageal contractions. This term is now thought to be imprecise because of a newer classification of the disease.
- High-resolution manometry (HRM), or high-resolution esophageal pressure topography (HREPT), has defined subsets of patients with achalasia who may have different responses to medical or surgical therapies. Unlike type I achalasia, type II achalasia shows panesophageal pressurization to greater than 30 mm Hg with ≥20% of test swallows, and type III achalasia shows spastic, lumen-obliterating contractions of the distal esophagus with ≥20% of swallows. This technique uses the integrated relaxation pressure (IRP) >15 mm Hg to define better the failure of esophagogastric junction relaxation. HRM also utilizes the distal contraction integral (DCI) to define hypercontractile vs. weak swallows vs. failed peristalsis. The distal latency (DL) defines premature contractions, seen with diffuse esophageal spasm and type III achalasia.
- HREPT has also defined an achalasia variant described as esophagogastric junction outflow obstruction, where the IRP is >15 mm Hg, but peristalsis is present.
- Direct visualization by endoscopy, including careful visualization of the esophagogastric junction and cardia, should be performed to exclude other causes of dysphagia, including "functional esophagogastric junction obstruction," strictures, secondary causes of achalasia (including infiltrating cancers), and pseudoachalasia.
- Functional luminal imaging probe (FLIP) technology is a new technique that may help demonstrate both impaired LES relaxation and response to therapy.

Rx TREATMENT

NONPHARMACOLOGIC THERAPY

- The goals of therapy are to decrease LES pressure to relieve the functional obstruction, relieve symptoms, and prevent progression to a dilated esophagus, sometimes referred to as a megaesophagus. Treatment does not improve esophageal peristalsis. Achalasia is treatable but incurable.
- Pneumatic dilation (PD) to disrupt the LES muscle fibers may benefit 65% to 90% of patients. Multiple sessions may be required, and most protocols use a graded dilation approach, starting with a 30-mm balloon, and repeating if required with a 35-mm or 40-mm balloon. Some studies suggest this may be more effective in females, older patients, and particularly HRM type II patients. Esophageal rupture or perforation is a rare complication (2% to 4%) that may be managed conservatively in some stable patients with a small perforation.
- Surgical: Laparoscopic, or less commonly, open Heller esophagomyotomy (HM) is effective (90%). Approximately 35% of patients undergoing surgery will develop reflux disease. As a result, some surgeons will perform a "loose" or partial antireflux repair (fundoplication) as part of the surgical procedure. Some studies suggest this may be more effective in men and younger patients. An observational study has suggested that those who have had prior endoscopic treatment before myotomy may not do as well as those who have a primary myotomy.
- A large European study suggested that in experienced hands, patients may expect similar medium-term outcomes from myotomy and balloon dilation. A meta-analysis suggests better long-term durability of myotomy. Balloon dilation may be the more cost-effective treatment. A small percentage (20 to 30%) of patients undergoing either therapy may require re-treatment within 5 to 7 yr.
- Endoscopic submucosal myotomy (per-oral endoscopic myotomy [POEM]) has a high success rate comparable to laparoscopic HM (particularly in HRM type III patients in whom a longer myotomy, tailored to the length of the diseased segment, improves outcome), few adverse events (which can include pneumomediastinum, pneumothorax, pneumoperitoneum, pleural effusion, pneumonia, and bleeding), and exceedingly rare mortality. Because no antireflux procedure is performed, there is a modest risk (up to 53%) of developing pathologic reflux. It should only be performed at high-volume centers.
- FLIP and timed barium esophagogram may help determine response to therapy.
- Esophagectomy has been performed in patients with end-stage achalasia with a dilated, often sigmoid-shaped or megaesophagus, who have failed myotomy or pneumatic dilation.

GENERAL Rx

- Medications may be useful for short-term symptom relief and in patients with refractory chest pain. They should only be considered in patients unable to receive, or who are scheduled for, more definitive procedures. LES pressure may be lowered by up to 50% through sublingual use of long-acting nitrates (e.g., isosorbide dinitrate 5 to 20 mg) or calcium channel blockers (e.g., nifedipine 10 to 30 mg). Side effects are common and duration of relief tends to be short. Sildenafil was shown to be effective in a few small, short-term studies, but it is generally not recommended.
- Botulinum toxin injection will benefit up to 85% of patients by inhibiting acetylcholine release from cholinergic nerve endings, blocking the unopposed cholinergic stimulation of the LES, but having no impact on the myogenic tone. Up to half of these patients will require repeat injections by 6 months. A few studies have suggested that repeated injections may have diminished efficacy and can lead to fibrosis, which may complicate subsequent attempts at surgical therapy.
- Many patients will require proton pump inhibitor therapy for gastroesophageal reflux after effective disruption of the LES.

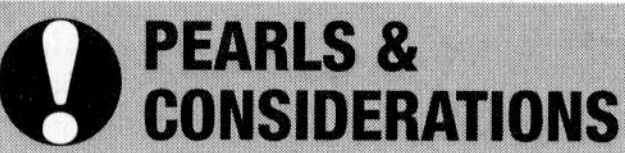

PEARLS & CONSIDERATIONS

COMMENTS

- Medication has a limited role in treatment.
- Botulinum toxin is transiently effective in improving symptoms.
- Pneumatic dilation, surgical myotomy, and POEM provide more durable long-term responses and are the treatment of choice for most patients. Botulinum toxin should be considered primarily in patients too elderly or ill to be considered for these other therapies.
- Patients with achalasia may be at long-term risk of squamous cell carcinoma of the esophagus and non–reflux-associated esophagitis. Treated patients may be at long-term risk for reflux esophagitis, Barrett's esophagus, and adenocarcinoma. Endoscopic surveillance is not routinely recommended in these patients.

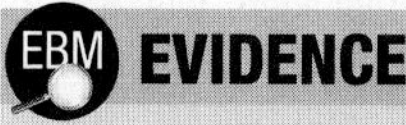

EBM EVIDENCE

Available at ExpertConsult.com

SUGGESTED READINGS

Available at ExpertConsult.com

RELATED CONTENT

Achalasia (Patient Information)
Dysphagia (Related Key Topic)

AUTHOR: **HARLAN G. RICH, M.D., F.A.C.P., A.G.A.F.**

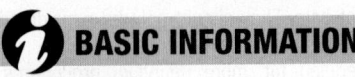

BASIC INFORMATION

DEFINITION

Acne vulgaris is a chronic disorder of the pilosebaceous apparatus caused by abnormal desquamation of follicular epithelium leading to obstruction of the pilosebaceous canal, resulting in inflammation and subsequent formation of papules, pustules, nodules, comedones, and scarring. Based on their appearance, the acne lesions can be divided into inflammatory (presence of papules, pustules, and nodules) or noninflammatory (open and closed comedones) For inflammatory acne, lesions can be classified as papulopustular, nodular, or both. The American Academy of Dermatology classification scheme for acne denotes the following three levels:

1. Mild acne: characterized by the presence of comedones (Figs. E1 and E2) (noninflammatory lesions), few papules and pustules (generally <10), but no nodules.
2. Moderate acne: presence of several to many papules and pustules (10 to 40) along with comedones (10 to 40). The presence of >40 papules and pustules along with larger, deeper nodular inflamed lesions (Figs. E3 and E4) (up to five) denotes moderately severe acne.
3. Severe acne: presence of numerous or extensive papules and pustules as well as many nodular lesions (Fig. E5).

SYNONYM

Acne

ICD-10CM CODES

L70.0 Acne vulgaris
L70.1 Acne conglobata
L70.2 Acne varioliformis
L70.3 Acne tropica
L70.4 Infantile acne
L70.5 Acne excoriee des jeunes filles
L70.8 Other acne
L70.9 Acne, unspecified
L73.0 Acne keloid

EPIDEMIOLOGY & DEMOGRAPHICS

- Acne is the most common skin disease in the U.S.
- It is most common in teenagers, with 85% of all teenagers being affected to some degree.
- Highest incidence between ages of 15 and 18 yr in both genders.
- Involution of the disease usually occurs before age 25 yr, but 12% of women and 3% of men will continue to have clinical acne until the mid-40s.

PHYSICAL FINDINGS & CLINICAL PRESENTATION

- Open comedones (blackheads), closed comedones (whiteheads)
- Greasiness (oily skin)
- Presence of scars from prior acne cysts
- Various stages of development and severity may be present concomitantly
- Common distribution of acne: face, back, and upper chest
- Inflammatory papules, pustules, and ectatic pores

ETIOLOGY

- Acne vulgaris is exclusively a follicular disease, with the principal abnormality being comedone formation.
- Overactivity of the sebaceous glands and blockage in the ducts. The obstruction leads to the formation of comedones, which can become inflamed because of overgrowth of *Propionibacterium acnes.*
- Exacerbated by environmental factors (hot, humid, tropical climate), medications (e.g., iodine in cough mixtures, hair greases), industrial exposure to halogenated hydrocarbons.
- Mechanical or frictional forces can aggravate existing acne (e.g., excessive washing by some patients to help rid them of their blackheads or oiliness).

Dx DIAGNOSIS

DIFFERENTIAL DIAGNOSIS

- Gram-negative folliculitis
- Staphylococcal pyoderma
- Acne rosacea
- Drug eruption
- Sebaceous hyperplasia
- Angiofibromas, basal cell carcinomas, osteoma cutis
- Occupational exposures to oils or grease
- Steroid acne
- Hidradenitis suppurativa
- Perioral dermatitis
- Pseudofolliculitis barbae
- Miliaria
- Seborrheic dermatitis

WORKUP

History and physical examination:

- Inquire about previous treatment
- Careful drug history (including all OTC products)
- Family history, history of cyclic menstrual flares
- History of use of cosmetics and cleansers
- Oral contraceptive use
- Use of medications that may worsen acne such as corticosteroids, anabolic steroids, lithium, neuroleptics, cyclosporine
- Consider the possibility of hyperandrogenic state in all women (hirsutism, irregular menses, androgenic alopecia) or children (seborrhea, acanthosis nigricans, onset of acne between ages 1 and 7 yr and no obvious external factors)

LABORATORY TESTS

- Laboratory evaluation is generally not helpful. Patients who are candidates for therapy with isotretinoin should have baseline liver enzymes, cholesterol, and triglycerides checked because this medication may result in elevation of lipids and liver enzymes.
- A negative serum pregnancy test or two negative urine pregnancy tests should also be obtained in females 1 wk before initiation of isotretinoin; it is also imperative to maintain effective contraception during and 1 mo after therapy with isotretinoin ends because of its teratogenic effects. Pregnancy status should be rechecked at monthly visits.
- If hyperandrogenism is suspected in female patients, levels of dehydroepiandrosterone sulfate (DHEAS), testosterone (total and free), and androstenedione should be measured. For women with regular menstrual cycles, serum androgen measurements generally are not necessary.

Rx TREATMENT

NONPHARMACOLOGIC THERAPY

- Blue light (ClearLight therapy system) can be used for treatment of moderate inflammatory acne vulgaris. Light in the violet/blue range can cause bacterial death by a photoreaction in which porphyrins react with oxygen to generate reactive oxygen species, which damage the cell membranes of *P. acnes.* Treatment usually consists of 15-min exposures twice weekly for 4 wk. Phototherapy may be effective for short-term treatment of acne, but long-term efficacy and how it compares with conventional acne therapy is unclear.
- Diet: In obese patients, dietary counseling is recommended. A high-glycemic diet may worsen acne, although the strength of its influence is controversial.

ACUTE GENERAL Rx

Treatment generally varies with the type of lesions (comedones, papules, pustules, cystic lesions) and the severity of acne. Table 1 summarizes an acne treatment algorithm. First-line treatment for mild acne vulgaris includes benzoyl peroxide, a topical retinoid, or a combination of topical medications, including topical antibiotics. Use of topical treatments for 6 to 8 weeks is required to judge their efficacy. Table 2 describes prescription topical therapies for acne.

- Comedones (noninflammatory acne) can be treated with retinoids or retinoid analogs. Topical retinoids are comedolytic and work by normalizing follicular keratinization. Commonly available agents are Adapalene (Differin, 0.1% gel or cream, applied once or twice daily), tazarotene (Tazorac 0.1% cream or gel applied daily), tretinoin (Retin-A 0.1% cream or 0.025 gel applied once daily), tretinoin microsphere (Retin-A Micro, 0.1% gel, applied at bedtime). Tretinoin is inactivated by ultraviolet light and oxidized by benzoyl peroxide; therefore it should only be applied at night and not used concomitantly with benzoyl peroxide.
- Tretinoin is pregnancy category C and tazarotene is pregnancy category X. Salicylic acid preparations (e.g., Neutrogena 2% wash) have keratolytic and antiinflammatory properties and are also useful in the treatment of comedones. Large, open comedones (blackheads) should be expressed.
- Patients should be reevaluated after 4 to 6 wk. Benzoyl peroxide gel (2.5% or 5%) may be added if the comedones become inflamed or form pustules. The most common adverse effects are dryness, erythema, and peeling. Topical antibiotics (erythromycin, clindamycin lotions or pads) can also be used in patients with significant inflammation. They reduce *P. acnes* in the pilosebaceous follicle and have

TABLE 1 Acne Treatment Algorithm

Therapy	Severity (Lesion Type): Mild (Comedonal)	Mild (Inflammatory/Mixed)	Moderate (Inflammatory/Mixed)	Severe (Inflammatory/Mixed)	Severe (Nodular/Scarring)
*Initial therapy options**,†	Topical retinoid BP Salicylic acid cleanser	BP/retinoid combo BP/antibiotic combo Antibiotic/retinoid combo + BP	BP/retinoid combo BP/antibiotic combo ± topical retinoid Antibiotic/retinoid combo + BP ± oral antibiotic	BP/retinoid combo + oral antibiotic BP/antibiotic combo + topical retinoid + oral antibiotic Antibiotic/retinoid combo + BP + oral antibiotic	Isotretinoin
*Alternative therapy options**,†,‡	Add BP or retinoid if not already prescribed BP/antibiotic combo BP/retinoid combo Antibiotic/retinoid combo	Substitute another combo product Add missing component (i.e., topical retinoid, BP, topical antibiotic) Change type, strength, or formulation of topical retinoid	Substitute another combo product Add missing component (i.e., topical retinoid, BP, topical antibiotic, oral antibiotic) Change type, strength, or formulation of topical retinoid Consider hormonal therapy for females Consider oral isotretinoin	Consider changing oral antibiotic Consider isotretinoin Consider hormonal therapy for females	Consider hormonal therapy for females
Maintenance therapy	Topical retinoid or BP/retinoid combo	Topical retinoid or BP/retinoid combo	Topical retinoid or BP/retinoid combo	Topical retinoid or BP/retinoid combo	Topical retinoid or BP/retinoid combo

BP, benzoyl peroxide.
*If combination products not available to patient, consider substitution of individual components as separate prescriptions.
†Topical dapsone may be considered in place of topical antibiotic.
‡If needed as determined by physician assessment and patient satisfaction.
Modified from Zaenglein AL, Thiboutot DM: Expert committee recommendations for acne management, *Pediatrics* 118(3):1188–99, 2006; Thiboutot D, Gollnick H, Bettoli V, et al: New insights into the management of acne: an update from the Global Alliance to Improve Outcomes in Acne Group, *J Am Acad Dermatol* 60:S1–50, 2009; Eichenfield LF, Krakowski AC, Piggott C, et al: Evidence-based recommendations for the diagnosis and treatment of pediatric acne, *Pediatrics* 131(3):S163–86, 2013; Thiboutot DM, Gollnick HP: Treatment considerations for inflammatory acne: clinical evidence for adapalene 0.1% in combination therapies, *J Drugs Dermatol* 5(8):785–94, 2006; Gollnick H, Cunliffe W, Berson D, et al: Management of acne: a report from a Global Alliance to Improve Outcomes in Acne, *J Am Acad Dermatol* 49(Suppl. 1):S1–37, 2003.

some antiinflammatory effects. The combination of 5% benzoyl peroxide and 3% erythromycin (Benzamycin) or 1% clindamycin with 5% benzoyl peroxide (BenzaClin) is highly effective in patients who have a mixture of comedonal and inflammatory acne lesions.

- Fixed-dose combinations of clindamycin phosphate 1.2% and tretinoin 0.025% are available (Veltin gel, Ziana) and are more effective than either product used alone; however, they are much more expensive than the individual generic components.
- Pustular acne can be treated with tretinoin and benzoyl peroxide gel applied on alternate evenings; drying agents (sulfacetamide-sulfa lotions [Novacet, Sulfacet]) are also effective when used in combination with benzoyl peroxide; oral antibiotics (doxycycline 100 mg qd or erythromycin 1 g qd given in 2 to 3 divided doses) are effective in patients with moderate to severe pustular acne. Patients not responding well to these antibiotics can be switched to minocycline 50 to 100 mg bid. Table 3 summarizes oral antibiotics for acne vulgaris.
- Patients with nodular cystic acne and those with moderate to severe inflammatory acne unresponsive to topical drugs can be treated with systemic agents: antibiotics (erythromycin, tetracycline, doxycycline, minocycline), isotretinoin (available on a restricted basis), or oral contraceptives. Periodic intralesional triamcinolone (Kenalog) injections by a dermatologist are also effective. The possibility of endocrinopathy should be considered in patients responding poorly to therapy.
- Isotretinoin is the most effective drug available for treatment of severe nodulocystic acne. It is indicated for acne resistant to antibiotic therapy and severe acne. It inhibits *P. acne's* colonization by reducing sebum production and has antiinflammatory and keratolytic effects. It is available only on a restricted basis. Dosage is 0.5 to 1 mg/kg/day in 2 divided doses (maximum of 2 mg/kg/day); duration of therapy is generally 20 wk for a cumulative dose ≥120 mg/kg for severe cystic acne. Before using this medication patients should undergo baseline laboratory evaluation (see "Laboratory Tests"). This drug is absolutely contraindicated during pregnancy because of its teratogenicity. It should be used with caution in patients with history of depression. Physicians, distributors, pharmacies, and patients must register in the iPLEDGE program (http://www.ipledgeprogram.com) before using isotretinoin.
- Azelaic acid is a bacteriostatic dicarboxylic acid used to normalize keratinization and reduce inflammation. It can be used in pregnant women.
- Oral contraceptives reduce androgen levels and therefore sebum production. They represent a useful adjunctive therapy for all types of acne in women and adolescent girls. Commonly used agents are norgestimate/ethinyl estradiol (Ortho Tri-Cyclen) and drospirenone/ethinyl estradiol (Yasmin).

REFERRAL

Referral for intralesional injection and dermabrasion should be considered in patients with severe acne unresponsive to conventional therapy. Table 4 summarizes alternative treatments for acne vulgaris.

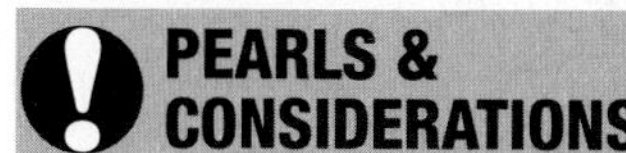

PEARLS & CONSIDERATIONS

- Gram-negative folliculitis should be suspected if inflammatory acne worsens after several months of oral antibiotic therapy.
- Acne may worsen during the first 3 to 4 wk of retinoid therapy before improving.

COMMENTS

Indications for systemic therapy of acne are:

- Painful deep papules or nodules
- Extensive lesions
- Active acne with severe scarring or hyperpigmentation
- Patient's morale

Patients should be educated that in most cases acne can be controlled but not cured and that at least 4 to 6 wk of initial therapy should be required before significant improvement is noted.

SUGGESTED READINGS

Available at ExpertConsult.com

RELATED CONTENT

Acne (Patient Information)

AUTHOR: **FRED F. FERRI, M.D.**

TABLE 2 Prescription Topical Therapies for Acne Vulgaris

Drug	Brand*	Formulation
Antibiotics		
Clindamycin	Cleocin T	1% solution, gel, pledgets, lotion
	ClindaMax	1% lotion
	Clindets	1% pledgets
	Clindagel	1% gel
	Evoclin	1% foam
Clindamycin/BP†	BenzaClin	1% (5% BP) gel
	Duac	1% (5% BP) gel
	Acanya	1.2% (2.5% BP) gel
	Onexton	1.2% (3.75% BP) gel
Dapsone	Aczone	5% gel
Erythromycin	Emgel, Erygel	2% gel
	Eryderm, Erymax, T-Stat	2% solution
	Staticin	1.5% solution
	Akne-Mycin	2% ointment
	Theramycin Z	2% solution + ZA
Erythromycin/BP†	Benzamycin	3% (5% BP) gel, pak
Sulfacetamide	Klaron	10% lotion
	Plexion	10% (5% sulfur) cloths, wash
	Clenia	10% (5% sulfur) cream, wash
	Rosula	10% (4% sulfur) wash
Azelaic acid	Azelex	20% cream
Retinoids		
Adapalene	Differin	0.1% cream, gel, lotion
		0.3% gel
Adapalene/BP†	Epiduo	0.1% (2.5% BP) gel
Tazarotene	Tazorac	0.05, 0.1% cream
		0.05, 0.1% gel
	Fabior	0.1% foam
Tretinoin	Retin-A	0.025, 0.05, 0.1% cream
		0.01, 0.025% gel
	Retin-A Micro	0.04, 0.1% gel
	Avita	0.025% cream, gel
	Atralin	0.05% gel
Tretinoin/Clindamycin†	Ziana	0.025% (1.2% clindamycin) gel
	Veltin	0.025% (1.2% clindamycin) gel

BP, Benzoyl peroxide; *ZA*, zinc acetate.
*Listed are examples; this list is not exhaustive. Many of these preparations have generic alternatives.
†Combination therapy product.
From Paller AS, Mancini AJ: *Hurwitz clinical pediatric dermatology: a textbook of skin disorders of childhood and adolescence*, ed 5, Philadelphia, 2016, Elsevier.

TABLE 3 Oral Antibiotics for Acne Vulgaris

Drug	Usual Dosage*	Comments/Side-Effects
Commonly used		
Tetracycline	250-500 mg	Dental staining <9 yr
		Dairy products decrease absorption
		GI upset, photosensitivity, teratogenic, PTC, VVC, IBD
Minocycline	50-100 mg	Dental staining <9 yr
	55, 65, 80, 105, 115 mg ER (1 mg/kg once daily)	Dairy products decrease absorption
		Vertigo (lower incidence with ER preparation), GI upset, blue-gray skin pigmentation, severe drug reactions with hepatitis/pneumonitis, lupus-like reactions, SJS, teratogenic, hepatitis, PTC, VVC, IBD
Doxycycline	50-100 mg	Dental staining <9 yr
	75, 100, 150 mg ER, once daily	Dairy products decrease absorption
	20 mg ("subantimicrobial dose")	Photosensitivity, photoonycholysis, GI upset (rare), teratogenic, PTC, VVC, IBD
Erythromycin	250-500 mg	GI upset (common), VVC, drug–drug interactions, prolongation of the QT interval; no longer recommended by most experts given increased resistance
Less commonly used		
Trimethoprim-sulfamethoxazole	80/400 mg, 160/800 mg	Severe drug reactions, SJS, bone marrow suppression, hepatitis, GI upset, VVC, fixed drug eruption; routine use for acne strongly discouraged
Clindamycin	75-150 mg	Pseudomembranous colitis, GI upset, drug reactions, VVC
Cephalexin	250-500 mg	GI upset, drug reactions, VVC

ER, Extended release formulation; *GI*, gastrointestinal; *IBD*, inflammatory bowel disease; *PTC*, pseudotumor cerebri; *SJS*, Stevens–Johnson syndrome; *VVC*, vulvovaginal candidiasis.
*Usually given twice daily for acne unless otherwise noted in table.
From Paller AS, Mancini AJ: *Hurwitz clinical pediatric dermatology: a textbook of skin disorders of childhood and adolescence*, ed 5, Philadelphia, 2016, Elsevier.

TABLE 4 Alternative Treatments for Acne Vulgaris

Treatment	Comment
Comedone extraction	Performed with comedone extractor
Injections	Intralesional triamcinolone injected into large cysts or nodules
Light therapy	Blue light (may photoinactivate *P. acnes*)
	Red light (may have antiinflammatory effect)
	Combination blue-red light
	Intensed pulse light (IPL)
	Photodynamic therapy (PDT)
Laser therapy	KTP, pulsed dye laser (rarely used)
	Resurfacing laser (including both nonablative and ablative resurfacing lasers); useful for acne scarring
Dermabrasion/dermasanding	Useful for acne scarring
Collagen injection	Useful for acne scarring
Chemical peels	Useful for acne scarring and hyperpigmentation
Punch grafts/tissue augmentation	Useful for acne scarring
Trichloroacetic acid	Useful for atrophic acne scars
Radiation therapy	Outdated modality

KTP, Potassium titanyl phosphate.
From Paller AS, Mancini AJ: *Hurwitz clinical pediatric dermatology: a textbook of skin disorders of childhood and adolescence*, ed 5, Philadelphia, 2016, Elsevier.

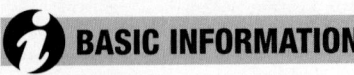

BASIC INFORMATION

DEFINITION

Acoustic neuroma is a benign proliferation of the Schwann cells that cover the vestibular branch of the eighth cranial nerve (CN VIII). Symptoms are commonly a result of compression of the acoustic branch of CN VIII, the facial nerve (CN VII), and the trigeminal nerve (CN V). The glossopharyngeal nerve (CN IX) and vagus nerve (CN X) are less commonly involved. In extreme cases, compression of the brain stem may lead to obstruction of cerebrospinal fluid (CSF) outflow and elevated intracranial pressure (ICP).

SYNONYM

Vestibular schwannoma

ICD-10CM CODE

D33.3 Benign neoplasm of cranial nerves

EPIDEMIOLOGY & DEMOGRAPHICS

Overall incidence is approximately 1.2 in 100,000 person-yr with a higher incidence in patients with neurofibromatosis type 2 (NF2). The prevalence is 2 in 10,000 people. The tumor most commonly presents in the fifth and sixth decades.

PHYSICAL FINDINGS & CLINICAL PRESENTATION

- Most frequently unilateral hearing loss and/or tinnitus. Also balance problems, vertigo, facial pain (trigeminal neuralgia) and weakness, difficulty swallowing, fullness or pain of the involved ear. Headache may occur.
- With elevated ICP, patients may also have vomiting, fever, and visual changes.
- Hearing loss is the most common presenting complaint and is usually high frequency.

ETIOLOGY

The etiology is incompletely understood, but long-term exposure to acoustic trauma has been implicated. Bilateral acoustic neuromas may be inherited in an autosomal-dominant manner as part of NF2. This disease is associated with a defect on chromosome 22q1. Childhood exposure to low-dose radiation for benign head and neck conditions may increase risk for acoustic neuromas. There is inconclusive evidence to link chronic exposure to radiofrequency radiation from cellular telephone use and the risk for developing brain tumors.

DIAGNOSIS

DIFFERENTIAL DIAGNOSIS

- Benign positional vertigo
- Menière disease
- Trigeminal neuralgia
- Cerebellar disease
- Normal-pressure hydrocephalus
- Presbycusis
- Glomus tumors
- Vertebrobasilar insufficiency
- Ototoxicity from medications
- Other tumors:
  1. Meningioma, glioma
  2. Facial nerve schwannoma
  3. Cavernous hemangioma
  4. Metastatic tumors

WORKUP

- A detailed neurologic examination with special attention to the cranial nerves is crucial.
- Rinne and Weber tests help determine conductive or sensorineural hearing loss.
- Common office balance tests (i.e., Romberg, Dix-Hallpike) are typically normal.
- Otoscopic evaluation may help rule out other causes of hearing loss.

LABORATORY TESTS

- Audiometry is useful, often showing asymmetric, sensorineural, high-frequency hearing loss.
- CSF protein may be elevated.

IMAGING STUDIES

- MRI with gadolinium (Fig. 1) is the preferred test. It can detect tumors as small as 2 mm in diameter.
- High-resolution CT scan with and without contrast can detect tumors 1 cm in diameter or larger.
- Treatment decisions should be based on the size of the tumor, rate of growth (older patients tend to have slower-growing tumors), degree of neurologic deficit, desire to preserve hearing, life expectancy, age of the patient, and surgical risk. A combination of treatments can also be used.

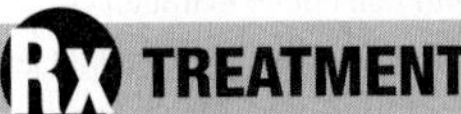

TREATMENT

NONPHARMACOLOGIC THERAPY

- Surgery is the definitive treatment. Choice of approach (middle cranial fossa, translabyrinthine, or retromastoid suboccipital) may vary depending on the size of the tumor, amount of residual hearing desired, and degree of surgical risk that can be tolerated. Partial resection is sometimes undertaken to minimize the risk of injury to nearby structures. Intraoperative facial nerve monitoring is recommended.
- Radiation therapy (stereotactic radiotherapy, stereotactic radiosurgery, or proton beam radiotherapy) is useful for tumors <3 cm in diameter or for those in whom surgery is not an option. Radiotherapy after partial resection has also been used to minimize complications.
- Age alone is not a contraindication to surgery.

GENERAL Rx

- Bevacizumab, an antivascular endothelial growth factor (VEGF) monoclonal antibody, has been shown to improve hearing and reduce the volume of growing acoustic neuromas in some neurofibromatosis type 2 patients.
- Observation with MRI every 6 to 12 mo may be appropriate for frail patients with small tumors, but risk of unrecoverable hearing loss may increase if surgery is delayed. Also, progressive hearing loss may occur despite absence of growth on subsequent imaging.

DISPOSITION

Hearing can be preserved at near-preoperative levels in more than two thirds of patients with small- to medium-sized tumors. Occurrence of secondary radiation-related tumors following radiosurgery is rare. There are no standard posttreatment follow-up recommendations. Therefore, an individualized approach to follow-up imaging and audiometry is recommended.

REFERRAL

Prompt referral to an otolaryngologist or neurosurgeon who is facile with all three surgical approaches is recommended.

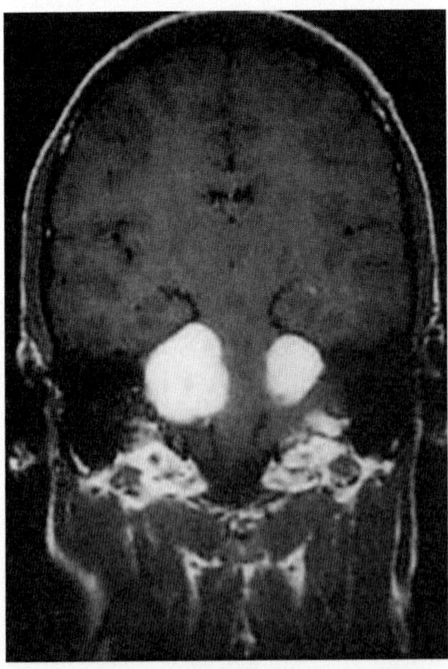

FIG. 1 MRI with enhancement shows bilateral acoustic neuromas. Coronal view. (From Kanski JJ, Bowling B: *Clinical ophthalmology, a systematic approach*, ed 7, Philadelphia, 2011, Saunders.)

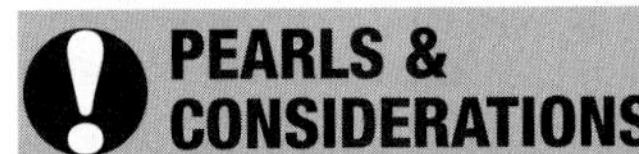

PEARLS & CONSIDERATIONS

COMMENTS

- Presents most commonly as unilateral, sensorineural hearing loss.
- Treatment outcomes are excellent, with surgical cure rates greater than 95%.
- Of those who are managed with observation only, approximately half have continued enlargement, and approximately one fifth eventually have a surgical intervention.

PATIENT/FAMILY EDUCATION

Acoustic Neuroma Association: https://www.anausa.org/

SUGGESTED READINGS

Available at ExpertConsult.com

RELATED CONTENT

Acoustic Neuroma (Patient Information)
Tinnitus (Related Key Topic)

AUTHOR: **COURTNEY CLARK BILODEAU, M.D., F.A.C.P.**

BASIC INFORMATION

DEFINITION

Acquired immunodeficiency syndrome (AIDS) is a disorder caused by infection with the human immunodeficiency virus (HIV) and marked by progressive deterioration of the cellular immune system, leading to secondary (opportunistic) infections and/or malignancies.

SYNONYM

AIDS

ICD-10CM CODE

B20 Human immunodeficiency virus [HIV] disease

EPIDEMIOLOGY & DEMOGRAPHICS

INCIDENCE (IN U.S.):

- The estimated number of persons diagnosed with AIDS in the U.S. is approximately 18,000/yr.
- There is a disproportionate number of new AIDS cases among Black/African Americans and Latino/Hispanic Americans compared with White Americans.
- The majority of all new AIDS diagnoses are among gay, bisexual, or other men who have sex with men (MSM).

PREVALENCE (IN U.S.): The cumulative number of AIDS diagnoses in the U.S. exceeds 1.2 million.

PREDOMINANT SEX: Men constitute approximately 75% of incident AIDS diagnoses in the U.S.; more than half of AIDS diagnoses occur in MSM.

PREDOMINANT AGE: The predominant age group diagnosed with AIDS is 25 to 54 yr of age.

PEAK INCIDENCE: Ages 25 to 94 yr

GENETICS:

- Familial disposition: Although there is no proven genetic predisposition, individuals with deletions in the *CCR5* gene are immune from HIV infection with macrophage tropic virus (the predominant virus in sexual transmission) and may progress to AIDS more slowly.
- Congenital infection:
  1. HIV is transmittable from an infected mother to the fetus in utero in as many as 30% of pregnancies if untreated.
  2. No specific congenital malformations associated with infection; low birth weight and spontaneous abortion are possible.

PHYSICAL FINDINGS & CLINICAL PRESENTATION

- Nonspecific findings: Fever, weight loss, anorexia.
- Specific syndromes:
  1. Seen in association with opportunistic infections and malignancies, so-called indicator diseases; these include:
     a. Opportunistic infections:
        (1) Disseminated strongyloidiasis
        (2) Disseminated toxoplasmosis, cryptococcosis, histoplasmosis, cytomegalovirus (CMV), herpes simplex, or mycobacterial disease (most common is mycobacterium avium complex)
        (3) *Candida* esophagitis or bronchopulmonary disease
        (4) Chronic cryptosporidiosis diarrhea
        (5) *Pneumocystis jiroveci* pneumonia (PJP)
        (6) Extensive pulmonary and extrapulmonary tuberculosis
        (7) Recurrent pneumonia or other bacterial infections
        (8) Progressive multifocal leukoencephalopathy (PML)
     b. AIDS-related neoplasms:
        (1) Kaposi's sarcoma
        (2) Primary brain lymphoma
        (3) Invasive cervical carcinoma
        (4) High-grade B cell non-Hodgkin's lymphoma, Burkitt's lymphoma, undifferentiated non-Hodgkin's lymphoma, or immunoblastic lymphoma
  2. Most common:
     a. Respiratory infections (*Pneumocystis jiroveci* [formerly known as *Pneumocystis carinii*] pneumonia, TB, bacterial pneumonia, fungal infection)
     b. CNS infections (toxoplasmosis, TB)
     c. GI (cryptosporidiosis, isosporiasis, CMV); Sections II and III describe organisms associated with diarrhea in patients with AIDS
     d. Eye infections (CMV, toxoplasmosis)
     e. Kaposi's sarcoma (cutaneous or visceral) or lymphoma (nodal or extranodal)
- Possibly asymptomatic.
- Diagnosis of AIDS if the CD4 cell count is <200 or <14% of total lymphocyte in the presence of proven HIV infection, even in the absence of other infections.
- The various manifestations of HIV infection are described in Section II.

ETIOLOGY

- Caused by infection with HIV-1 or HIV-2 (less common).
- HIV is transmitted by sexual contact, needle-sharing (during IV drug use), transfusion of contaminated blood or blood products, and from infected mother to fetus or neonate.

Dx DIAGNOSIS

DIFFERENTIAL DIAGNOSIS

- Other wasting illnesses mimicking the nonspecific features of AIDS:
  1. TB
  2. Neoplasms
  3. Disseminated fungal infection
  4. Malabsorption syndromes
  5. Depression
- Other disorders associated with dementia or demyelination producing encephalopathy, myelopathy, or neuropathy.

WORKUP

Prompt evaluation of respiratory, CNS, and GI complaints

LABORATORY TESTS

- HIV antibody testing. See "Human Immunodeficiency Virus" topic for the updated surveillance case definition for HIV infection.
- T-lymphocyte subset analysis: performed to determine the degree of immunodeficiency (i.e., CD4 cell count).
- Viral load assay: to plan long-term antiviral therapy and to follow progression and success of treatment (i.e., HIV RNA PCR).
- CSF examination: for meningitis (if indicated).
- Serologic tests for syphilis, hepatitis A, hepatitis B, hepatitis C, and toxoplasmosis.
- Testing for other sexually transmitted diseases, such as gonorrhea and chlamydia.
- Genotypic resistance testing: used to assess for primary resistance in naïve patients and secondary resistance in patients failing a regimen.
- Eye exam: to evaluate for CMV retinitis in patients with CD4 counts <50 cells/mm^3.
- Cryptococcal antigen: part of the evaluation in AIDS patients with CD4 counts <100 cells/mm^3 who have fever, diffuse pneumonia, or evidence of meningitis.
- Evaluation for infection with mycobacterium (TB or MAI) including a tuberculin skin test (TST) or interferon-gamma release assay (IGRA), sputum cultures, chest radiograph, and blood cultures for acid-fast bacteria, depending on clinical presentation.

IMAGING STUDIES

- MRI or CT of head for encephalopathy or focal CNS complications (e.g., toxoplasmosis [Fig. E1], lymphoma)
- Chest radiography or CT to aid in the diagnosis of *Pneumocystis jiroveci* (*P. carinii*) pneumonia, TB, or bacterial pneumonia.

Rx TREATMENT

The most important aspect in management of AIDS due to HIV infection is the timely initiation of antiretroviral therapy (see section on HIV treatment).

NONPHARMACOLOGIC THERAPY

- Maintain adequate caloric intake.
- Encourage good oral hygiene and regular dental care.

- Avoid high-risk behaviors that increase the risk of other potential pathogens—use condoms, avoid sharing needles, etc.
- Update vaccines—particularly the pneumococcal and hepatitis A/B vaccine along with annual influenza vaccines.
- Avoid administration of any live attenuated vaccines that may be a risk to these immunocompromised patients (e.g., MMR, varicella). (See Section V for immunization schedules for HIV-infected children.)
- When feasible, avoid activities that might increase risk of exposure to opportunistic infections (e.g., cleaning out a cat litter box [toxoplasmosis], getting scratched by a cat [*Bartonella* infections], exposure to pet reptiles [salmonellosis], traveling to developing countries [cryptosporidiosis, tuberculosis], eating undercooked foods and drinking from unsafe water supplies, etc.). A description of enteropathogens causing infections in HIV-infected patients is provided in Table 1.

TABLE 1 Organisms That Cause Gastrointestinal Tract Infections in Patients with HIV/AIDS

Organisms	
Esophagus	*Candida albicans*[a]
	Cytomegalovirus[a]
	Herpes simplex virus[a]
Hepatobiliary	Cytomegalovirus
	Cryptosporidium[a]
	Hepatotropic viruses
	Mycobacterium avium complex[a]
Small intestine	*Campylobacter* species
	Cytomegalovirus[a]
	Cryptosporidium[a]
	Giardia lamblia[a]
	Isospora belli[a]
	Mycobacterium avium complex[a]
	Microsporidia[a] (*Enterocytozoon bieneusi* and *Encephalitozoon intestinalis*)
	Salmonella species[a]
	Enteroaggregative *E. coli*
	Strongyloides stercoralis
Large intestine	*Campylobacter* species
	Clostridium difficile
	Cytomegalovirus[a]
	Entamoeba histolytica
	Herpes simplex virus[a]
	Salmonella species[a]
	Enteroaggregative *E. coli*
	Shigella species

[a]Diseases of the gastrointestinal tract that fulfill the Centers for Disease Control and Prevention surveillance case definition of AIDS.

Cherry JD, et al: *Feigin and Cherry's pediatric infectious diseases*, ed 8, Philadelphia, 2019, Elsevier.

ACUTE GENERAL Rx

Acute management of opportunistic infections is summarized in Table 2 and reviewed elsewhere in this text under specific AIDS-related disorders. For management of AIDS-related malignancies, please refer to the specific malignancy elsewhere in this text.

CHRONIC Rx

For all HIV-infected patients, particularly those meeting the case definition of AIDS:

- Preventive therapy for *Pneumocystis jiroveci* pneumonia and *Mycobacterium avium* (see specific chapters elsewhere in this text). With the advent of modern antiretroviral therapy, many patients have experienced substantial restoration of cellular immune function. Preventive therapy for *Pneumocystis jiroveci* and *Mycobacterium avium* complex as well as suppressive therapy for CMV and cryptococcal infection can be safely stopped if the CD4 cell count rises above 200 for at least 6 months.
- Based on the Department of Health and Human Services (DHHS) Guidelines, active antiretroviral therapy (ART) should be started regardless of CD4 cell count. Individuals with CD4 cell counts <350 and especially CD4 cell counts <200 should be strongly encouraged to start ART in a timely fashion.
- ART usually includes three-drug combinations of:
  1. Nucleoside reverse transcriptase inhibitors (NRTI): Tenofovir disoproxil fumarate (TDF), tenofovir alafenamide fumarate (TAF), lamivudine (3TC), emtricitabine (FTC), and abacavir (ABC)
  2. Protease inhibitors (PI): Atazanavir or darunavir
  3. Nonnucleoside reverse transcriptase inhibitors (NNRTI): Nevirapine, efavirenz (EFV), etravirine, and rilpivirine
  4. Integrase inhibitors: Raltegravir, elvitegravir, bictegravir, and dolutegravir.
  5. Others: Maraviroc and enfuvirtide

The protease inhibitors ritonavir or cobicistat should be used in combination with other protease inhibitors to obtain more sustained drug levels. Usual initial dosing regimens include two NRTIs and an NNRTI or PI or integrase inhibitor. Currently, integrase inhibitors are recommended as first-line drugs because of tolerability. Examples of initial regimens recommended by the guidelines:

1. Dolutegravir/abacavir/lamivudine (in patients who are HLA-B*5701 NEGATIVE)
2. Dolutegravir plus tenofovir/emtricitabine*
3. Elvitegravir/cobicistat/tenofovir/emtricitabine
4. Bictegravir/emtricitabine/tenofovir
5. Raltegravir plus tenofovir/emtricitabine
6. Darunavir/ritonavir plus tenofovir/emtricitabine

Previous first-line drugs, including efavirenz/tenofovir/emtricitabine and rilpivirine/tenofovir/emtricitabine, are now considered alternative regimens.

All these drugs have unique and class-specific side effects and require careful and expert follow-up to achieve optimal antiviral effects, ensure compliance, and maintain efficacy. Antiviral response should be monitored by baseline HIV viral load and CD4 count and repeat measurement at 2 weeks and 4 weeks into treatment and then periodically (every 3-6 months) to ensure viral suppression.

- The approach to a patient with CNS signs and symptoms is described in Fig. E2 and Fig. E3 describes the management of CNS mass lesions.
- Genotypic resistance testing is strongly encouraged for all patients initiating treatment and for any patient failing antiretroviral therapy. Poor adherence to therapy, however, often underlies virologic failure.

DISPOSITION

The outlook for AIDS has changed radically since the advent of ART therapy from an essentially fatal disease to a chronic medical illness compatible with long-term survival and remarkably good quality of life. Patients should be aggressively treated for severe illnesses as outcomes following ICU admissions remain good. This is accomplished through expert and continuous follow-up, use of ART, and careful detail to compliance to medications and lifestyle modification.

*Tenofovir-based formulations can include tenofovir disoproxil fumarate (TDF) or tenofovir alafenamide (TAF).

TABLE 2 Treatment of AIDS-Associated Opportunistic Infections

Opportunistic Infection	Preferred Therapy	Alternative Therapy	Other Comments
PJP	• Patients who develop PJP despite TMP-SMX prophylaxis can usually be treated with standard doses of TMP-SMX. • Duration of PJP treatment: 21 days • *For Moderate to Severe PJP:* • TMP-SMX: (TMP 15-20 mg and SMX 75-100 mg/kg/day) IV given q6h or q8h, may switch to PO after clinical improvement. • *For Mild to Moderate PJP:* • TMP-SMX: (TMP 15-20 mg and SMX 75-100 mg/kg/day), given PO in 3 divided doses, *or* • TMP-SMX: (160 mg/800 mg or DS) 2 tablets PO tid. • *Secondary Prophylaxis, after completion of PJP treatment:* • TMP-SMX DS: 1 tablet PO daily *or* • TMP-SMX (80 mg/400 mg or SS): 1 tablet PO daily	*For Moderate to Severe PJP:* • Pentamidine 4 mg/kg IV daily infused over ≥60 minutes; can reduce dose to 3 mg/kg IV daily because of toxicities, *or* • Primaquine 30 mg (base) PO daily + (clindamycin 600 mg q6h IV or 900 mg IV q8h) or (clindamycin 300 mg PO q6h or 450 mg PO q8h). • *For Mild to Moderate PJP:* • Dapsone 100 mg PO daily + TMP 5 mg/kg PO tid, *or* • Primaquine 30 mg (base) PO daily + (clindamycin 300 mg PO q6h or 450 mg PO q8h), or • Atovaquone 750 mg PO bid with food. • *Secondary Prophylaxis, after completion of PJP treatment:* • TMP-SMX DS: 1 tablet PO tiw, *or* • Dapsone 100 mg PO daily, *or* • Dapsone 50 mg PO daily + (pyrimethamine 50 mg + leucovorin 25 mg) PO weekly, *or* • (Dapsone 200 mg + pyrimethamine 75 mg + leucovorin 25 mg) PO weekly, *or* • Aerosolized pentamidine 300 mg monthly via Respirgard II nebulizer, *or* • Atovaquone 1500 mg PO daily, *or* • (Atovaquone 1500 mg + pyrimethamine 25 mg + leucovorin 10 mg) PO daily.	*Indications for Adjunctive Corticosteroids:* • Pa_{O_2} <70 mm Hg at room air, *or* • Alveolar-arterial O_2 gradient >35 mm Hg • *Prednisone Doses (beginning as early as possible and within 72 hours of PJP therapy):* • Days 1-5: 40 mg PO bid • Days 6-10: 40 mg PO daily • Days 11-21: 20 mg PO daily • IV methylprednisolone can be administered as 75% of prednisone dose. • Benefit of corticosteroid if started after 72 hours of treatment is unknown, but some clinicians will use it for moderate-to-severe PJP. • Whenever possible, patients should be tested for G6PD before use of dapsone or primaquine. Alternative therapy should be used in patients found to have G6PD deficiency. • Patients who are receiving pyrimethamine/sulfadiazine for treatment or suppression of toxoplasmosis do not require additional PJP prophylaxis. • If TMP-SMX is discontinued because of a mild adverse reaction, reinstitution should be considered after the reaction resolves. The dose can be increased gradually (desensitization) or be reduced, or the frequency can be modified. • TMP-SMX should be permanently discontinued in patients with possible or definite Stevens–Johnson syndrome or toxic epidermal necrosis.
Toxoplasma gondii encephalitis	*Treatment of Acute Infection:* • Pyrimethamine 200 mg PO 1 time, followed by weight-based therapy: • If <60 kg, pyrimethamine 50 mg PO once daily + sulfadiazine 1000 mg PO q6h + leucovorin 10-25 mg PO once daily. • If ≥60 kg, pyrimethamine 75 mg PO once daily + sulfadiazine 1500 mg PO q6h + leucovorin 10-25 mg PO once daily. • Leucovorin dose can be increased to 50 mg daily or bid. • *Duration for Acute Therapy:* • At least 6 weeks; longer duration if clinical or radiologic disease is extensive or response is incomplete at 6 weeks • *Chronic Maintenance Therapy:* • Pyrimethamine 25-50 mg PO daily + sulfadiazine 2000-4000 mg PO daily (in 2-4 divided doses) + leucovorin 10-25 mg PO daily (AI)	*Treatment of Acute Infection:* • Pyrimethamine (leucovorin)* + clindamycin 600 mg IV or PO q6h *or* • TMP-SMX (TMP 5 mg/kg and SMX 25 mg/kg) IV or PO bid, *or* • Atovaquone 1500 mg PO bid with food + pyrimethamine (leucovorin), *or* • Atovaquone 1500 mg PO bid with food + sulfadiazine 1000-1500 mg PO q6h (weight-based dosing, as in preferred therapy) *or* • Atovaquone 1500 mg PO bid with food, *or* • Pyrimethamine (leucovorin)* + azithromycin 900-1200 mg PO daily. • *Chronic Maintenance Therapy:* • Clindamycin 600 mg PO q8h + (pyrimethamine 25-50 mg + leucovorin 10-25 mg) PO daily *or* • TMP-SMX DS 1 tablet bid, *or* • Atovaquone 750-1500 mg PO bid + (pyrimethamine 25 mg + leucovorin 10 mg) PO daily, *or* • Atovaquone 750-1500 mg PO bid + sulfadiazine 2000-4000 mg PO daily (in 2-4 divided doses), *or* • Atovaquone 750-1500 mg PO bid with food • *Pyrimethamine and leucovorin doses are the same as for preferred therapy.	• Adjunctive corticosteroids (e.g., dexamethasone) should only be administered when clinically indicated to treat mass effect associated with focal lesions or associated edema; discontinue as soon as clinically feasible. • Anticonvulsants should be administered to patients with a history of seizures and continued through acute treatment but should not be used as seizure prophylaxis. • If clindamycin is used in place of sulfadiazine, additional therapy must be added to prevent PCP.

Continued

TABLE 2 Treatment of AIDS-Associated Opportunistic Infections—cont'd

Opportunistic Infection	Preferred Therapy	Alternative Therapy	Other Comments
Mycobacterium tuberculosis disease (TB)	• After collecting specimen for culture and molecular diagnostic tests, empiric TB treatment should be started in individuals with clinical and radiographic presentation suggestive of TB. *Initial Phase (2 months, given daily, 5-7 times/week by DOT):* • INH + [RIF or RFB] + PZA + EMB *Continuation Phase:* • INH + (RIF or RFB) daily (5-7 times/week) *Total Duration of Therapy (for drug-susceptible TB):* • Pulmonary TB: 6 months • Pulmonary TB and culture-positive after 2 months of TB treatment: 9 months • Extrapulmonary TB with CNS infection: 9-12 months • Extrapulmonary TB with bone or joint involvement: 6 to 9 months • Extrapulmonary TB in other sites: 6 months • Total duration of therapy should be based on number of doses received, not on calendar time.	*Treatment for Drug-Resistant TB* • *Resistant to INH:* • (RIF or RFB) + EMB + PZA + (moxifloxacin or levofloxacin) for 2 months; followed by (RIF or RFB) + EMB + (moxifloxacin or levofloxacin) for 7 months. • *Resistant to Rifamycins ± Other Drugs:* • Regimen and duration of treatment should be individualized based on resistance pattern, clinical and microbiologic responses, and in close consultation with experienced specialists.	• Adjunctive corticosteroid improves survival for TB meningitis and pericarditis. See text for drug, dose, and duration recommendations. • RIF *is not recommended* for patients receiving HIV PI because of its induction of PI metabolism. • RFB is a less potent CYP3A4 inducer than RIF and is preferred in patients receiving PIs. • Once-weekly rifapentine can result in development of rifamycin resistance in HIV-infected patients and *is not recommended.* • Therapeutic drug monitoring should be considered in patients receiving rifamycin and interacting ART. • Paradoxical IRIS that is not severe can be treated with NSAIDs without a change in TB or HIV therapy. • For severe IRIS reaction, consider prednisone and taper over 4 weeks based on clinical symptoms. For example: • *If receiving RIF:* prednisone 1.5 mg/kg/day for 2 weeks, then 0.75 mg/kg/day for 2 weeks • *If receiving RFB:* Prednisone 1.0 mg/kg/day for 2 weeks, then 0.5 mg/kg/day for 2 weeks • A more gradual tapering schedule over a few months may be necessary for some patients.
Disseminated MAC disease	*At Least 2 Drugs as Initial Therapy with:* • Clarithromycin 500 mg PO bid + ethambutol 15 mg/kg PO daily, *or* • azithromycin 500-600 mg + ethambutol 15 mg/kg PO daily if drug interaction or intolerance precludes the use of clarithromycin *Duration:* • At least 12 months of therapy, can discontinue if no signs and symptoms of MAC disease and sustained (>6 months) CD4 count >100 cells/μl in response to ART	• Addition of a third or fourth drug should be considered for patients with advanced immunosuppression (CD4 counts <50 cells/μl), high mycobacterial loads (>2 log CFU/ml of blood), or in the absence of effective ART. *Third or Fourth Drug Options May Include:* • RFB 300 mg PO daily (dosage adjustment may be necessary based on drug interactions), or • Amikacin 10-15 mg/kg IV daily, or • Streptomycin 1 g IV or IM daily, or • Moxifloxacin 400 mg PO daily or levofloxacin 500 mg PO daily	• Testing of susceptibility to clarithromycin and azithromycin is recommended. • NSAIDs can be used for patients who experience moderate to severe symptoms attributed to IRIS. • If IRIS symptoms persist, short-term (4-8 weeks) systemic corticosteroids (equivalent to 20-40 mg prednisone) can be used.
Bacterial respiratory diseases *(with focus on pneumonia)*	Empiric antibiotic therapy should be initiated promptly for patients presenting with clinical and radiographic evidence consistent with bacterial pneumonia. The recommendations listed are suggested empiric therapy. The regimen should be modified as needed once microbiologic results are available. *Empiric Outpatient Therapy:* • A PO β-lactam + a PO macrolide (azithromycin or clarithromycin) • *Preferred β-lactams*: High-dose amoxicillin or amoxicillin/clavulanate • *Alternative β-lactams*: Cefpodoxime or cefuroxime, *or* • *For penicillin-allergic patients:* Levofloxacin 750 mg PO once daily, or moxifloxacin 400 mg PO once daily	*Empiric Outpatient Therapy:* • A PO β-lactam + PO doxycycline • *Preferred β-lactams*: High-dose amoxicillin or amoxicillin/clavulanate • *Alternative β-lactams*: Cefpodoxime or cefuroxime • *Empiric Therapy for Non-ICU Hospitalized Patients:* • An IV β-lactam + doxycycline	• Fluoroquinolones should be used with caution in patients in whom TB is suspected but is not being treated. • Empiric therapy with a macrolide alone is not routinely recommended because of increasing pneumococcal resistance. • Patients receiving a macrolide for MAC prophylaxis should not receive macrolide monotherapy for empiric treatment of bacterial pneumonia.

TABLE 2 Treatment of AIDS-Associated Opportunistic Infections—cont'd

Opportunistic Infection	Preferred Therapy	Alternative Therapy	Other Comments
	• *Duration:* 7-10 days (a minimum of 5 days). Patients should be afebrile for 48-72 hours and clinically stable before stopping antibiotics. *Empiric Therapy for Non-ICU Hospitalized Patients:* • An IV β-lactam + a macrolide (azithromycin or clarithromycin) • *Preferred β-lactams:* ceftriaxone, cefotaxime, *or* ampicillin-sulbactam • *For penicillin-allergic patients:* • Levofloxacin, 750 mg IV once daily, *or* moxifloxacin, 400 mg IV once daily *Empiric Therapy for ICU Patients:* • An IV β-lactam + IV azithromycin, *or* • An IV β-lactam + (levofloxacin 750 mg IV once daily or moxifloxacin 400 mg IV once daily) • *Preferred β-lactams:* ceftriaxone, cefotaxime, or ampicillin-sulbactam *Empiric Therapy for Patients at Risk of* Pseudomonas *Pneumonia:* • An IV antipneumococcal, antipseudomonal β-lactam + ciprofloxacin 400 mg IV q8-12h or levofloxacin 750 mg IV once daily • *Preferred β-lactams:* piperacillin-tazobactam, cefepime, imipenem, or meropenem • *Empiric Therapy for Patients at Risk for Methicillin-Resistant* Staphylococcus aureus *Pneumonia:* • Add vancomycin IV or linezolid (IV or PO) to the baseline regimen. • Addition of clindamycin to vancomycin (but not to linezolid) can be considered for severe necrotizing pneumonia to minimize bacterial toxin production.	• *Empiric Therapy for ICU Patients:* • *For penicillin-allergic patients:* Aztreonam IV + (levofloxacin 750 mg IV once daily or moxifloxacin 400 mg IV once daily) *Empiric Therapy for Patients at Risk of Pseudomonas Pneumonia:* • An IV antipneumococcal, antipseudomonal β-lactam + an aminoglycoside + azithromycin, *or* • above β-lactam + an aminoglycoside + (levofloxacin 750 mg IV once daily or moxifloxacin 400 mg IV once daily), *or* • *For penicillin-allergic patients:* Replace the β-lactam with aztreonam	• For patients begun on IV antibiotic therapy, switching to PO should be considered when they are clinically improved and able to tolerate oral medications. • Chemoprophylaxis can be considered for patients with frequent recurrences of serious bacterial pneumonia. • Clinicians should be cautious about using antibiotics to prevent recurrences because of the potential for developing drug resistance and drug toxicities.
Bacterial enteric infections *Empiric therapy pending definitive diagnosis*	• Diagnostic fecal specimens should be obtained before initiation of empiric antibiotic therapy. • Empiric antibiotic therapy is indicated for patients with advanced HIV (CD4 count <200 cells/μl or concomitant AIDS-defining illnesses), with clinically severe diarrhea (>6 stools/day), and/or accompanying fever or chills. *Empiric Therapy:* • Ciprofloxacin 500-750 mg PO (or 400 mg IV) q12h. • Therapy should be adjusted based on the results of diagnostic workup. • For patients with chronic diarrhea (>14 days) without severe clinical signs, empiric antibiotics therapy is not necessary; can withhold treatment until a diagnosis is made.	*Empiric Therapy:* • Ceftriaxone 1 g IV q24h, *or* • Cefotaxime 1 g IV q8h	• Hospitalization with IV antibiotics should be considered in patients with marked nausea, vomiting, diarrhea, electrolyte abnormalities, acidosis, and blood pressure instability. • Oral or IV rehydration if indicated. • Antimotility agents should be avoided if there is concern about inflammatory diarrhea, including *Clostridium difficile*–associated diarrhea. • If no clinical response after 5-7 days, consider follow-up stool culture with antibiotic susceptibility testing or alternative diagnostic tests (e.g., toxin assays, molecular testing), alternative diagnosis, or antibiotic resistance.
Salmonellosis	All HIV-infected patients with salmonellosis should be treated because of high risk of bacteremia. • Ciprofloxacin 500-750 mg PO (or 400 mg IV) q12h, if susceptible *Duration of Therapy:* • *For gastroenteritis without bacteremia:* • If CD4 count ≥200 cells/μl: 7-14 days • If CD4 count <200 cells/μl: 2-6 weeks *For gastroenteritis with bacteremia:* • If CD4 count ≥200/μl: 14 days; longer duration if bacteremia persists or if the infection is complicated (e.g., if metastatic foci of infection are present) • If CD4 count <200 cells/μl: 2-6 weeks *Secondary Prophylaxis Should Be Considered for:* • Patients with recurrent *Salmonella* gastroenteritis ± bacteremia, *or* • Patients with CD4 <200 cells/μl with severe diarrhea	• Levofloxacin 750 mg (PO or IV) q24h, *or* • Moxifloxacin 400 mg (PO or IV) q24h, *or* • TMP, 160 mg-SMX 800 mg (PO or IV) q12h, *or* • Ceftriaxone 1 g IV q24h, *or* • Cefotaxime 1 g IV q8h	• Oral or IV rehydration if indicated. • Antimotility agents should be avoided. • The role of long-term secondary prophylaxis in patients with recurrent *Salmonella* bacteremia is not well established. Must weigh benefit against risks of long-term antibiotic exposure. • Effective ART may reduce the frequency, severity, and recurrence of *Salmonella* infections.

Continued

TABLE 2 Treatment of AIDS-Associated Opportunistic Infections—cont'd

Opportunistic Infection	Preferred Therapy	Alternative Therapy	Other Comments
Mucocutaneous candidiasis	*For Oropharyngeal Candidiasis; Initial Episodes (for 7-14 days):* • *Oral therapy* • Fluconazole 100 mg PO daily, *or* • *Topical therapy* • Clotrimazole troches, 10 mg PO 5 times daily, *or* • Miconazole mucoadhesive buccal 50-mg tablet—apply to mucosal surface over the canine fossa once daily (do not swallow, chew, or crush). *For Esophageal Candidiasis (for 14-21 days):* • Fluconazole 100 mg (up to 400 mg) PO or IV daily, *or* • Itraconazole oral solution 200 mg PO daily. *For Uncomplicated Vulvovaginal Candidiasis:* • Oral fluconazole 150 mg for 1 dose, *or* • Topical azoles (clotrimazole, butoconazole, miconazole, tioconazole, or terconazole) for 3-7 days. *For Severe or Recurrent Vulvovaginal Candidiasis:* • Fluconazole 100-200 mg PO daily for ≥7 days, *or* • Topical antifungal ≥7 days	*For Oropharyngeal Candidiasis; Initial Episodes (for 7-14 days):* • *Oral therapy* • Itraconazole oral solution 200 mg PO daily, *or* • Posaconazole oral solution 400 mg PO bid for 1 day, then 400 mg daily • *Topical therapy* • Nystatin suspension 4-6 ml qid or 1-2 flavored pastilles 4-5 times daily. *For Esophageal Candidiasis (for 14-21 days):* • Voriconazole 200 mg PO or IV bid, *or* • Posaconazole 400 mg PO bid, *or* • Anidulafungin 100 mg IV 1 time, then 50 mg IV daily, *or* • Caspofungin 50 mg IV daily, *or* • Micafungin 150 mg IV daily, *or* • Amphotericin B deoxycholate 0.6 mg/kg IV daily, *or* • Lipid formulation of amphotericin B 3-4 mg/kg IV daily. *For Uncomplicated Vulvovaginal Candidiasis:* • Itraconazole oral solution 200 mg PO daily for 3-7 days	• Chronic or prolonged use of azoles may promote development of resistance. • Higher relapse rate for esophageal candidiasis is seen with echinocandins than with fluconazole use. • Suppressive therapy is usually not recommended unless patients have frequent or severe recurrences. If Decision Is to Use Suppressive Therapy: • *Oropharyngeal Candidiasis:* • Fluconazole 100 mg PO daily or tiw • Itraconazole oral solution 200 mg PO daily • *Esophageal Candidiasis:* • Fluconazole 100-200 mg PO daily • Posaconazole 400 mg PO bid *Vulvovaginal Candidiasis:* • Fluconazole 150 mg PO once weekly
Cryptococcosis	*Cryptococcal Meningitis* • *Induction Therapy (for at least 2 weeks, followed by consolidation therapy):* • Liposomal amphotericin B 3-4 mg/kg IV daily + flucytosine 25 mg/kg PO qid. (NOTE: Flucytosine dose should be adjusted in patients with renal dysfunction.) • *Consolidation Therapy (for at least 8 weeks followed by maintenance therapy):* • Fluconazole 400 mg PO (or IV) daily. • *Maintenance therapy:* • Fluconazole 200 mg PO daily for at least 12 months. *For Non-CNS, Extrapulmonary Cryptococcosis and Diffuse Pulmonary Disease:* • Treatment same as for cryptococcal meningitis. *Non-CNS Cryptococcosis with Mild to Moderate Symptoms and Focal Pulmonary Infiltrates:* • Fluconazole, 400 mg PO daily for 12 months.	*Cryptococcal Meningitis* • *Induction Therapy (for at least 2 weeks, followed by consolidation therapy):* • Amphotericin B deoxycholate 0.7 mg/kg IV daily + flucytosine 25 mg/kg PO qid, *or* • Amphotericin B lipid complex 5 mg/kg IV daily + flucytosine 25 mg/kg PO qid, *or* • Liposomal amphotericin B 3-4 mg/kg IV daily + fluconazole 800 mg PO or IV daily, *or* • Amphotericin B deoxycholate 0.7 mg/kg IV daily + fluconazole 800 mg PO or IV daily, *or* • Fluconazole 400-800 mg PO or IV daily + flucytosine 25 mg/kg PO qid, *or* • Fluconazole 1200 mg PO or IV daily • *Consolidation Therapy (for at least 8 weeks followed by maintenance therapy):* • Itraconazole 200 mg PO bid for 8 weeks—less effective than fluconazole • *Maintenance therapy:* • No alternative therapy recommendation	• Addition of flucytosine to amphotericin B has been associated with more rapid sterilization of CSF and decreased risk for subsequent relapse. • Patients receiving flucytosine should have either blood levels monitored (peak level 2 hours after dose should be 30-80 μg/ml) or close monitoring of blood counts for development of cytopenia. Dosage should be adjusted in patients with renal insufficiency. • Opening pressure should always be measured when an LP is performed. Repeated LPs or CSF shunting are essential to effectively manage increased intracranial pressure. • Corticosteroids and mannitol are ineffective in reducing intracranial pressure and are *not* recommended. • Some specialists recommend a brief course of corticosteroid for management of severe IRIS symptoms.
Histoplasmosis	*Moderately Severe to Severe Disseminated Disease Induction Therapy (for at least 2 weeks or until clinically improved):* • Liposomal amphotericin B 3 mg/kg IV daily. • *Maintenance Therapy:* • Itraconazole 200 mg PO tid for 3 days, then 200 mg PO bid. *Less Severe Disseminated Disease* • *Induction and Maintenance Therapy:* • Itraconazole 200 mg PO tid for 3 days, then 200 mg PO bid. • *Duration of Therapy:* • At least 12 months. *Meningitis* • *Induction Therapy (4-6 weeks):* • Liposomal amphotericin B 5 mg/kg/day. • *Maintenance Therapy:* • Itraconazole 200 mg PO bid to tid for ≥1 yr and until resolution of abnormal CSF findings. • *Long-Term Suppression Therapy:*	*Moderately Severe to Severe Disseminated Disease Induction Therapy (for at least 2 weeks or until clinically improved):* • Amphotericin B lipid complex 3 mg/kg IV daily, *or* • Amphotericin B cholesteryl sulfate complete 3 mg/kg IV daily • *Alternatives to Itraconazole for Maintenance Therapy or Treatment of Less Severe Disease:* • Voriconazole 400 mg PO bid for 1 day, then 200 mg bid, *or* • Posaconazole 400 mg PO bid • Fluconazole 800 mg PO daily *Meningitis* • No alternative therapy recommendation • *Long-Term Suppression Therapy:* • Fluconazole 400 mg PO daily	• Itraconazole, posaconazole, and voriconazole may have significant interactions with certain ARV agents. These interactions are complex and can be bidirectional. • Therapeutic drug monitoring and dosage adjustment may be necessary to ensure triazole antifungal and ARV efficacy and to reduce concentration-related toxicities. • Random serum concentration of itraconazole + hydroxyitraconazole should be >1 μg/ml. • Clinical experience with voriconazole or posaconazole in the treatment of histoplasmosis is limited. • Acute pulmonary histoplasmosis in HIV-infected patients with CD4 counts >300 cells/μl should be managed as nonimmunocompromised host.

TABLE 2 Treatment of AIDS-Associated Opportunistic Infections—cont'd

Opportunistic Infection	Preferred Therapy	Alternative Therapy	Other Comments
	• *For patients with severe disseminated or CNS infection after completion of at least 12 months of therapy; and those who relapse despite appropriate therapy* • Itraconazole 200 mg PO daily.		
Coccidioidomycosis	*Clinically Mild Infections (e.g., focal pneumonia):* • Fluconazole 400 mg PO daily or • Itraconazole 200 mg PO bid. *Severe, Nonmeningeal Infection (diffuse pulmonary infection or severely ill patients with extrathoracic, disseminated disease):* • Amphotericin B deoxycholate 0.7-1.0 mg/kg IV daily • Lipid formulation amphotericin B 4-6 mg/kg IV daily • Duration of therapy: continue until clinical improvement, then switch to an azole. *Meningeal Infections:* • Fluconazole 400-800 mg IV or PO daily. • *Chronic Suppressive Therapy:* • Fluconazole 400 mg PO daily, *or* • Itraconazole 200 mg PO bid	*Mild Infections (focal pneumonia) for patients who failed to respond to fluconazole or itraconazole:* • Posaconazole 200 mg PO bid, *or* • Voriconazole 200 mg PO bid. *Severe, Nonmeningeal Infection (diffuse pulmonary infection or severely ill patients with extrathoracic, disseminated disease):* • Some specialists will add a triazole (fluconazole or itraconazole, with itraconazole preferred for bone disease) 400 mg per day to amphotericin B therapy and continue triazole once amphotericin B is stopped. *Meningeal Infections:* • Itraconazole 200 mg PO tid for 3 days, then 200 mg PO bid, *or* • Posaconazole 200 mg PO bid, *or* • Voriconazole 200-400 mg PO bid, *or* • Intrathecal amphotericin B deoxycholate, when triazole antifungals are ineffective. • *Chronic suppressive therapy:* • Posaconazole 200 mg PO bid, *or* • Voriconazole 200 mg PO bid	• Some patients with meningitis may develop hydrocephalus and require CSF shunting. • Therapy should be continued indefinitely in patients with diffuse pulmonary or disseminated diseases because relapse can occur in 25%-33% of HIV-negative patients. It can also occur in HIV-infected patients with CD4 counts >250 cells/μL. • Therapy should be lifelong in patients with meningeal infections because relapse occurs in 80% of HIV-infected patients after discontinuation of triazole therapy. • Itraconazole, posaconazole, and voriconazole may have significant interactions with certain ARV agents. These interactions are complex and can be bidirectional. Therapeutic drug monitoring and dosage adjustment may be necessary to ensure triazole antifungal and antiretroviral efficacy and to reduce concentration-related toxicities. • Intrathecal amphotericin B should be given only in consultation with a specialist and should be administered by an individual with experience with the technique.
Aspergillosis, invasive	*Preferred Therapy:* • Voriconazole 6 mg/kg IV q12h for 1 day, then 4 mg/kg IV q12h, followed by voriconazole 200 mg PO q12h after clinical improvement • *Duration of Therapy:* • Until CD4 cell count >200 cells/μl and the infection appears to be resolved	*Alternative Therapy:* • Lipid formulation of amphotericin B 5 mg/kg IV daily, *or* • Amphotericin B deoxycholate 1 mg/kg IV daily, *or* • Caspofungin 70 mg IV 1 time, then 50 mg IV daily, *or* • Micafungin 100-150 mg IV daily, *or* • Anidulafungin 200 mg IV 1 time, then 100 mg IV daily, *or* • Posaconazole 200 mg PO qid, then, after condition improved, 400 mg PO bid.	• Potential for significant pharmacokinetic interactions between certain ARV agents and voriconazole; they should be used cautiously in these situations. Consider therapeutic drug monitoring and dosage adjustment if necessary.
CMV disease	*CMV Retinitis Induction Therapy for Immediate Sight-Threatening Lesions (adjacent to the optic nerve or fovea)* • Consult ophthalmologist; ganciclovir implant no longer available: • Ganciclovir 5 mg/kg IV q12h for 14-21 days followed by Valganciclovir 900 mg PO bid *For Small Peripheral Lesions:* • Valganciclovir 900 mg PO bid for 14-21 days • One dose of intravitreal ganciclovir can be administered immediately after diagnosis until steady-state plasma ganciclovir concentration is achieved with oral valganciclovir • *Chronic Maintenance (secondary prophylaxis):* • Valganciclovir 900 mg PO daily (for small peripheral lesion). *CMV Esophagitis or Colitis:* • Ganciclovir 5 mg/kg IV q12h; may switch to valganciclovir 900 mg PO q12h once patient can tolerate oral therapy	*CMV Retinitis Induction Therapy:* • Ganciclovir 5 mg/kg IV q12h for 14-21 days, *or* • Foscarnet 90 mg/kg IV q12h or 60 mg q8h for 14-21 days, *or* • Cidofovir 5 mg/kg/week IV for 2 weeks; saline hydration before and after therapy and probenecid, 2 g PO 3 hours before dose, followed by 1 g PO 2 hours and 8 hours after the dose (total of 4 g). (Note: This regimen should be avoided in patients with sulfa allergy because of cross-hypersensitivity with probenecid.) • *Chronic Maintenance (secondary prophylaxis):* • Ganciclovir 5 mg/kg IV 5-7 times weekly, *or*	• The choice of therapy for CMV retinitis should be individualized, based on location and severity of the lesions, level of immunosuppression, and other factors (e.g., concomitant medications and ability to adhere to treatment). • The choice of chronic maintenance therapy (route of administration and drug choices) should be made in consultation with an ophthalmologist. Considerations should include the anatomic location of the retinal lesion, vision in the contralateral eye, the patients' immunologic and virologic status, and response to ART.

Continued

TABLE 2 Treatment of AIDS-Associated Opportunistic Infections—cont'd

Opportunistic Infection	Preferred Therapy	Alternative Therapy	Other Comments
	• Duration: 21-42 days or until symptoms have resolved. • Maintenance therapy is usually not necessary but should be considered after relapses. *Well-Documented, Histologically Confirmed CMV Pneumonia:* • Experience for treating CMV pneumonitis in HIV patients is limited. Use of IV ganciclovir or IV foscarnet is reasonable (doses same as for CMV retinitis). • The optimal duration of therapy and the role of oral valganciclovir have not been established. *CMV Neurologic Disease* • Note: Treatment should be initiated promptly. • Ganciclovir 5 mg/kg IV q12h + (foscarnet 90 mg/kg IV q12h or 60 mg/kg IV q8h) to stabilize disease and maximize response; continue until symptomatic improvement and resolution of neurologic symptoms. • The optimal duration of therapy and the role of oral valganciclovir have not been established.	• Foscarnet 90-120 mg/kg IV once daily, *or* • Cidofovir 5 mg/kg IV every other week with saline hydration and probenecid as above. *CMV Esophagitis or Colitis:* • Foscarnet 90 mg/kg IV q12h or 60 mg/kg q8h for patients with treatment-limiting toxicities to ganciclovir or with ganciclovir resistance, *or* • Valganciclovir 900 mg PO q12h in milder disease and if able to tolerate PO therapy, *or* • For mild cases, if ART can be initiated without delay, consider withholding CMV therapy. • Duration: 21-42 days or until symptoms have resolved	• Patients with CMV retinitis who discontinue maintenance therapy should undergo regular eye examinations for early detection of relapse IRU—optimally every 3 months and then annually after immune reconstitution. • IRU may develop in the setting of immune reconstitution. *Treatment of IRU:* • Periocular corticosteroid or short courses of systemic steroid. • Initial therapy in patients with CMV retinitis, esophagitis, colitis, and pneumonitis should include initiation or optimization of ART.
HSV disease	*Orolabial Lesions (for 5-10 days):* • Valacyclovir 1 g PO bid *or* • Famciclovir 500 mg PO bid *or* • Acyclovir 400 mg PO tid. *Initial or Recurrent Genital HSV (for 5-14 days):* • Valacyclovir 1 g PO bid, *or* • Famciclovir 500 mg PO bid, *or* • Acyclovir 400 mg PO tid *Severe Mucocutaneous HSV:* • Initial therapy acyclovir 5 mg/kg IV q8h • After lesions begin to regress, change to PO therapy as previously. Continue until lesions are completely healed. • *Chronic Suppressive Therapy for Patients with Severe Recurrences of Genital Herpes or for Patients Who Want to Minimize Frequency of Recurrences:* • Valacyclovir 500 mg PO bid • Famciclovir 500 mg PO bid • Acyclovir 400 mg PO bid • Continue indefinitely regardless of CD4 cell count.	*For Acyclovir-Resistant HSV* • *Preferred Therapy:* • Foscarnet 80-120 mg/kg/day IV in 2-3 divided doses until clinical response. • *Alternative Therapy* • IV cidofovir (dosage as in CMV retinitis), *or* • Topical trifluridine, *or* • Topical cidofovir, *or* • Topical imiquimod • *Duration of Therapy:* • 21-28 days or longer	• Patients with HSV infections can be treated with episodic therapy when symptomatic lesions occur, or with daily suppressive therapy to prevent recurrences. • Topical formulations of trifluridine and cidofovir are not commercially available. • Extemporaneous compounding of topical products can be prepared using trifluridine ophthalmic solution and the IV formulation of cidofovir.
VZV disease	*Primary Varicella Infection (Chickenpox):* • *Uncomplicated Cases (for 5-7 days):* • Valacyclovir 1 g PO tid *or* • Famciclovir 500 mg PO tid. • *Severe or Complicated Cases:* • Acyclovir 10-15 mg/kg IV q8h for 7-10 days. • May switch to oral valacyclovir, famciclovir, or acyclovir after defervescence if no evidence of visceral involvement. *Herpes Zoster (Shingles) Acute Localized Dermatomal:* • For 7-10 days; consider longer duration if lesions are slow to resolve. • Valacyclovir 1 g PO tid *or* • Famciclovir 500 mg tid. *Extensive Cutaneous Lesion or Visceral Involvement:* • Acyclovir 10-15 mg/kg IV q8h until clinical improvement is evident. • May switch to PO therapy (valacyclovir, famciclovir, or acyclovir) after clinical improvement (i.e., when no new vesicle formation or improvement of signs and symptoms of visceral VZV), to complete a 10- to 14-day course.	*Primary Varicella Infection (Chickenpox):* • *Uncomplicated Cases (for 5-7 days):* • Acyclovir 800 mg PO 5 times/day *Herpes Zoster (Shingles)* • *Acute Localized Dermatomal:* • For 7-10 days; consider longer duration if lesions are slow to resolve. • Acyclovir 800 mg PO 5 times/day	• In managing VZV retinitis: Consultation with an ophthalmologist experienced in management of VZV retinitis is strongly recommended. • Duration of therapy for VZV retinitis is not well defined and should be determined based on clinical, virologic, immunologic, and ophthalmologic responses. • Optimization of ART is recommended for serious and difficult-to-treat VZV infections (e.g., retinitis, encephalitis).

TABLE 2 Treatment of AIDS-Associated Opportunistic Infections—cont'd

Opportunistic Infection	Preferred Therapy	Alternative Therapy	Other Comments
	Progressive Outer Retinal Necrosis: • Ganciclovir 5 mg/kg + foscarnet 90 mg/kg IV q12h + ganciclovir 2 mg/0.05 ml ± foscarnet 1.2 mg/0.05 ml intravitreal injection twice weekly *or* • Initiate or optimize ART. *Acute Retinal Necrosis:* • Acyclovir 10 mg/kg IV q8h for 10-14 days, followed by valacyclovir 1 g PO tid for 6 weeks.		
Progressive multifocal leukoencephalopathy (JC virus infections)	• There is no specific antiviral therapy for JC virus infection. The main treatment approach is to reverse the immunosuppression caused by HIV. • Initiate ART immediately in ART-naïve patients. • Optimize ART in patients who develop PML in phase of HIV viremia on ART.	None.	• Corticosteroids may be used for PML-IRIS characterized by contrast enhancement, edema, or mass effect and with clinical deterioration.

ART, antiretroviral therapy; *ARV,* antiretroviral; bid, twice a day; *CD4,* CD4 T lymphocyte cell; *CFU,* colony-forming unit; *CMV,* cytomegalovirus; *CNS,* central nervous system; *CSF,* cerebrospinal fluid; *CYP3A4,* cytochrome P-450 3A4; *DOT,* directly observed therapy; *DS,* double strength; *EMB,* ethambutol; *G6PD,* glucose-6-phosphate dehydrogenase; *GI,* gastrointestinal; *HSV,* herpes simplex virus; *ICU,* intensive care unit; *IM,* intramuscular; *INH,* isoniazid; *IRIS,* immune reconstitution inflammatory syndrome; *IV,* intravenous; *LP,* lumbar puncture; *MAC, Mycobacterium avium* complex; *mm Hg,* millimeters of mercury; *NSAID,* nonsteroidal anti-inflammatory drugs; *PCP, Pneumocystis* pneumonia; *PI,* protease inhibitor; *PML,* progressive multifocal leukoencephalopathy; *PO,* oral; *PZA,* pyrazinamide; *qid,* four times a day; *RFB,* rifabutin; *RIF,* rifampin; *SS,* single strength; *tid,* three times daily; *tiw,* three times weekly; *TMP-SMX,* trimethoprim-sulfamethoxazole; *VZV,* varicella zoster virus.

Quality of Evidence for the Recommendation:

I: One or more randomized trials with clinical outcomes and/or validated laboratory endpoints

II: One or more well-designed, nonrandomized trials or observational cohort studies with long-term clinical outcomes

III: Expert opinion

REFERRAL

All patients with AIDS should be referred to a physician knowledgeable and experienced in the management of the disease and its complications.

RELATED CONTENT

Acquired Immunodeficiency Syndrome (AIDS) (Patient Information)
Candidiasis, Cutaneous (Related Key Topic)
Candidiasis, Invasive (Related Key Topic)
Cryptosporidium Infection (Related Key Topic)
Cytomegalovirus Infection (Related Key Topic)
Herpes Simplex (Related Key Topic)
Histoplasmosis (Related Key Topic)
HIV Cognitive Dysfunction (Related Key Topic)
Human Immunodeficiency Virus (Related Key Topic)
Kaposi Sarcoma (Related Key Topic)
Pneumonia, *pneumocystis jiroveci (carinii)* (Related Key Topic)
Progressive Multifocal Leukoencephalopathy (Related Key Topic)
Toxoplasmosis (Related Key Topic)
Tuberculosis (Related Key Topic)

AUTHOR: **PHILIP A. CHAN, M.D., M.S.**

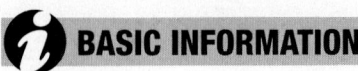

BASIC INFORMATION

DEFINITION

Acute bronchitis is a self-limited inflammation of trachea and bronchi.

SYNONYM

Chest cold

ICD-10CM CODE
J20.9 Acute bronchitis, unspecified

EPIDEMIOLOGY & DEMOGRAPHICS

- Highest incidence in smokers, older adults, and young children and during winter months.
- In the U.S. there are nearly 30 million ambulatory visits annually for cough, leading to more than 12 million diagnoses of "bronchitis."
- Acute lower respiratory tract infection is the most common condition treated in primary care.

PHYSICAL FINDINGS & CLINICAL PRESENTATION

- In most cases, acute bronchitis begins with signs and symptoms typical of the common cold syndrome (nasal congestion, sore throat), followed shortly by the onset of cough
- Cough, usually worse in the morning, often productive; mainly caused by transient bronchial hyperresponsiveness
- Low-grade fever
- Substernal discomfort worsened by coughing
- Postnasal drip, pharyngeal injection
- Rhonchi that may clear after cough, occasional wheezing
- Various host factors (age, immune status, smoking, underlying medical conditions) can influence illness severity and clinical presentation
- In mild cases, the illness lasts only 7 to 10 days, whereas in others, cough may persist for up to 3 weeks or longer

ETIOLOGY

- Viral infections are the leading cause of bronchitis (rhinovirus, influenza virus, adenovirus, respiratory syncytial virus)
- Atypical organisms *(Mycoplasma, Chlamydia pneumoniae)*
- Bacterial infections *(Bordetella pertussis, Haemophilus influenzae, Moraxella, Streptococcus pneumoniae)*
- Table 1 summarizes viral and bacterial causes of acute bronchitis

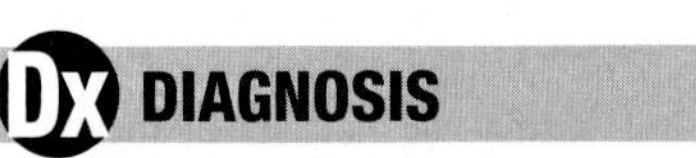

DIAGNOSIS

DIFFERENTIAL DIAGNOSIS

- Pneumonia
- Asthma
- Sinusitis
- Bronchiolitis
- Aspiration
- Cystic fibrosis
- Pharyngitis
- Cough secondary to medications
- Neoplasm (elderly patients)
- Influenza
- Allergic aspergillosis
- Gastroesophageal reflux disease
- Congestive heart failure (in elderly patients)
- Bronchogenic neoplasm

WORKUP

Seldom necessary (e.g., to rule out pneumonia, neoplasm)

LABORATORY TESTS

Laboratory tests are generally not necessary.

IMAGING STUDIES

Chest x-ray is usually reserved for patients with suspected pneumonia, influenza, or underlying chronic obstructive pulmonary disease (COPD) and no improvement with therapy.

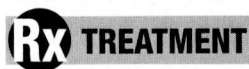

TREATMENT

NONPHARMACOLOGIC THERAPY

- Avoidance of tobacco and other pulmonary irritants
- Increased fluid intake
- Use of vaporizer to increase room humidity

TABLE 1 Viral and Bacterial Causes of Acute Bronchitis

Pathogen	Seasonality	Comments
Influenza viruses	Winter	Local epidemics last 6-8 wk during which clinical illness of cough and fever has high predictive value; laboratory diagnosis readily available; early neuraminidase inhibitor therapy effective
Rhinoviruses	Fall and spring	Most frequent cause of common cold syndrome; immunity is serotype specific
Coronaviruses	Winter to spring	Cause common cold syndrome; newer strains are difficult to culture and require RT-PCR for diagnosis
Adenoviruses	Yr round, winter epidemics	High attack rates in closed populations such as persons living in military barracks or college dormitories; serotype-specific immunity
Respiratory syncytial virus (RSV)	Late fall to early spring	Attack rates approach 75% in neonates, 3%-5% in adults; associated with wheezing in all age groups; rapid antigen test accurate in children but requires culture or RT-PCR to diagnose in adults
Human metapneumovirus (hMPV)	Winter to early spring	Associated with wheezing in adults and in infants; difficult to isolate in tissue culture and often requires RT-PCR
Parainfluenza viruses	Fall to winter	Similar to RSV and hMPV, parainfluenza viruses primarily pediatric pathogens but can cause severe acute disease in some adults
Measles virus	Yr round	Can cause respiratory disease in malnourished children; illness causes transient immune suppression
Mycoplasma pneumoniae	Yr round, fall outbreaks	Long incubation period (10-21 days) results in staggered epidemic pattern in families; nonproductive persistent cough typical; diagnosed by IgM serology; treated with macrolide, quinolone, or tetracycline antibiotics
Chlamydia pneumoniae	Yr round	Associated with sinusitis; diagnosis by RT-PCR not readily available
Bordetella pertussis	Yr round	Severe illness in nonimmunized children; illness milder in partially immune adults; can be associated with prolonged cough; adults often reservoir for epidemics; early therapy with antibiotics can reduce spread

RT-PCR, Reverse-transcriptase polymerase chain reaction.
From Bennett JE, Dolin R, Blaser MJ: *Mandell, Douglas, and Bennett's principles and practice of infectious diseases,* ed 8, Philadelphia, 2015, Saunders.

ACUTE GENERAL Rx

- Therapy is generally symptomatic and directed at relief of cough and wheezing.
- Inhaled bronchodilators (e.g., albuterol, metaproterenol) PRN for 1 to 2 wk in patients with wheezing or troublesome cough. Inhaled albuterol has been proven effective in reducing the duration of cough in adults with uncomplicated acute bronchitis.
- Cough suppression with dextromethorphan and guaifenesin is commonly recommended; addition of codeine for cough suppression if cough is severe and is significantly interrupting patient's sleep pattern.
- Use of antibiotics (TMP-SMX, amoxicillin, doxycycline, cefuroxime) for acute bronchitis is generally not indicated; should be considered only in patients with concomitant COPD and purulent sputum or in patients with suspected pertussis. In the few cases of acute bronchitis caused by *B. pertussis* or atypical bacteria such as *C. pneumoniae* or *Mycoplasma pneumoniae,* early use of macrolide antibiotics is reasonable.
- Antibiotics are overused in patients with acute bronchitis (70% to 90% of office visits for acute bronchitis result in treatment with antibiotics); this practice pattern is contributing to increases in resistant organisms.
- Trials have shown that there are no significant differences in patients receiving antibiotics compared with those receiving placebo in overall clinical improvements or limitations in work or other activities. There was a significant increase in adverse effects in the antibiotic group, particularly gastrointestinal symptoms.[1]

CHRONIC Rx

Avoidance of tobacco and other pulmonary irritants

DISPOSITION

- Complete recovery within 7 to 10 days in most patients.
- Patients should be informed to expect to have a cough for 10 to 14 days after the visit.

REFERRAL

For pulmonary function testing only in patients with recurrent bronchitis and suspected underlying pulmonary disease

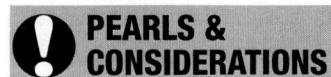

PEARLS & CONSIDERATIONS

COMMENTS

- Patients are more likely to receive prescriptions for antibiotics from mid- or late-career physicians with high patient volumes and from physicians who were trained outside of Canada or the U.S.[2] Intervention studies reveal that patient and physician education are effective in reducing the use of antibiotic therapy. No offer or delayed offer of antibiotics for acute uncomplicated lower respiratory tract infection is acceptable, is associated with little difference in symptom resolution, and is likely to reduce antibiotic use and beliefs in the effectiveness of antibiotics.
- It is helpful to refer to acute bronchitis as a "chest cold." Patients should be informed that antibiotics are probably not going to be beneficial and may result in significant side effects.

SUGGESTED READINGS

Available at ExpertConsult.com.

RELATED CONTENT

Acute Bronchitis (Patient Information)

AUTHOR: **FRED F. FERRI, M.D.**

[1] Smith SM, Smucny J, Fahey T: Antibiotics for acute bronchitis, *JAMA* 312:2678, 2014.

[2] Silverman M et al: Antibiotic prescribing for nonbacterial acute upper respiratory infections in elderly persons. *Ann Intern Med* 166:765–774, 2017.

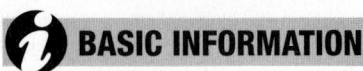

BASIC INFORMATION

Acute coronary syndrome (ACS) represents a spectrum of clinical disorders that includes unstable angina (UA), non–ST-elevation myocardial infarction (NSTEMI), and ST-elevation myocardial infarction (STEMI). Although the severity of disease will vary between the three subsets of ACS, they share a common clinical presentation and pathophysiology. This syndrome is typically caused by atherosclerotic coronary artery disease (CAD). In this spectrum, UA and NSTEMI are represented electrocardiographically by the absence of ST-segment elevation in the appropriate clinical setting (i.e., chest discomfort). NSTEMI is represented by the addition of positive cardiac biomarkers. STEMI is characterized by ST-segment elevation or presumed new left bundle branch block on electrocardiogram (ECG) in the appropriate clinical setting. ACS should be thought of as a continuous spectrum as UA will often progress to a myocardial infarction if left untreated (Table 1). Because of this continuum, the 2014 American College of Cardiology/American Heart Association (ACC/AHA) guidelines have grouped UA and NSTEMI into a single category called non–ST-elevation ACS (NSTE-ACS).

SYNONYMS

Unstable angina
NSTEMI
STEMI
Acute myocardial infarction

ICD-10CM CODES	
I20.0	Unstable angina
I21.0-I21.3	ST elevation (STEMI)
I21.4	Non-ST elevation (NSTEMI) myocardial infarction
I24.9	Acute ischemic heart disease, unspecified

EPIDEMIOLOGY & DEMOGRAPHICS

INCIDENCE: In the U.S., cardiovascular disease accounts for approximately 801,000 deaths each yr. The estimated annual incidence of heart attack in the U.S. is 580,000 new attacks and 210,000 recurrent attacks. Approximately 70% of myocardial infarctions are listed as NSTEMI, with the remainder being listed as STEMI. Patients with NSTE-ACS have more cardiac and noncardiac comorbidities than patients with STEMI. The underlying etiology, atherosclerotic CAD, is the number one cause of mortality.

PREDOMINANT SEX AND AGE: In evaluating chest pain, male gender and older age are important clinical factors that can identify ACS as a potential cause. In a 2005-2011 study sponsored by National Heart, Lung, and Blood Institute, the average age-adjusted first MI or fatal coronary heart disease rates per 1000 population in patients age 35 to 84 yr of age were 3.7 for white men, 5.9 for black men, 2.1 for white women, and 4.0 for black women. As noted in this study, heart disease affects African Americans disproportionately, with more than 39,000 deaths from heart disease in 2013. Heart disease is the number one killer of women. It takes more lives than all forms of cancer combined.

RISK FACTORS: Hypertension, diabetes mellitus, dyslipidemia, tobacco use, and family history of premature CAD (CAD in a male first-degree relative younger than 55 yr or a female younger than 65 yr) are all associated risk factors for CAD. Refer to the topic "Angina Pectoris" for an extensive list of risk factors. Presence of these risk factors causes damage to the vascular endothelium and progression of atherosclerotic coronary artery plaques.

PHYSICAL FINDINGS & CLINICAL PRESENTATION

- Symptoms often, but not always, include chest discomfort described as a pressure that may radiate to the shoulders, neck, jaw, or back. Typical angina is substernal in location, brought on by emotional or physical stress, and relieved with rest and/or nitroglycerin. The pain and discomfort associated with an ACS event is often diffuse rather than localized. It is often associated with diaphoresis.
- Women, diabetics, the elderly, and postoperative patients often have an atypical presentation for ACS.
- Unstable angina has three typical presentations:
  1. Rest angina: Angina occurring at rest and prolonged usually for longer than 20 minutes.
  2. New-onset angina: New-onset angina of at least Canadian Cardiovascular Society (CCS) class III symptoms (Table 2).
  3. Increasing angina: Previously diagnosed angina that has become distinctly more frequent, longer in duration, or lower in threshold (i.e., increased by ≥1 CCS class to at least CCS class III severity).
- "Anginal equivalents" may include dyspnea, nausea, vomiting, and fatigue.
- ECG for NSTE-ACS may reveal ST-segment depression and/or T-wave inversion. ECG for definition of STEMI will reveal at least 1-mm ST-segment elevation in two contiguous leads or new left bundle branch block in the appropriate clinical presentation.
- Physical exam findings alone are insufficient for the diagnosis of ACS. It is, however, important to assess the patient's hemodynamic stability and volume status. The patient may be diaphoretic and tachycardic. Signs of heart failure may be present, which include elevated jugular venous pressure (JVP), presence of an S3 gallop, and peripheral edema. The degree of heart failure with MI can be represented by the Killip classification, with the greater the Killip classification, the greater the mortality noted:
  1. Killip Class 1 is no heart failure.
  2. Killip Class 2 includes individuals with rales, elevated JVP, and S3 on exam.
  3. Killip Class 3 includes individuals with frank pulmonary edema.
  4. Killip Class 4 describes individuals in cardiogenic shock or hypotension with evidence of vasoconstriction noted.

ETIOLOGY

Atherosclerotic CAD is the underlying etiology. The hallmark of ACS is the vulnerable atherosclerotic plaque, which typically has a thin fibrous cap and a large lipid core. This vulnerable plaque ultimately ruptures, which leads to platelet activation and aggregation, leading to thrombus formation. STEMI typically results from complete thrombotic occlusion of a coronary artery, whereas NSTE-ACS often has partial occlusion. Angiographically, it is often the intermediate coronary artery lesions (30% to 50% diameter vessel stenosis) that lead to subtotal or total vessel occlusion in two thirds of STEMI cases.

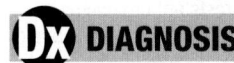

DIAGNOSIS

DIFFERENTIAL DIAGNOSIS

Chest pain mimicking ACS may be the result of various underlying disorders, some of which are also accompanied by ECG changes and/or cardiac biomarker release. Examples include acute pulmonary embolism, acute aortic dissection, pericarditis, myocarditis, costochondritis, pneumonia, tension pneumothorax, perforating ulcer, or Boerhaave syndrome. Refer to topics "Angina Pectoris," "Coronary Artery Disease," and "Myocardial Infarction" for extensive differential diagnoses of chest pain.

WORKUP

Focused history and physical exam, 12-lead ECG, cardiac biomarkers, and chest radiograph (CXR). Initial biomarkers may not be positive early in the disease process. Often serial biomarkers are drawn every 6 to 8 hours for a total of three sets for the purposes of ruling out myocardial infarction (MI), or until peak to

TABLE 1 Acute Coronary Syndromes

	Spectrum of Acute Coronary Syndrome		
	Unstable Angina	**NSTEMI**	**STEMI**
Chest discomfort	1	1	1
Cardiac biomarkers	2	1	1
ECG changes	TWI and/or ST depression	TWI and/or ST depression	ST elevation or presumed new left bundle branch block
Pathophysiology	Partial/transient thrombotic occlusion	Partial/transient thrombotic occlusion	Complete thrombotic occlusion

NSTEMI, Non–ST-segment elevation myocardial infarction; *STEMI*, ST-segment myocardial infarction; *TWI*, T-wave inversion; *ECG*, electrocardiogram.

TABLE 2 Grading of Angina Pectoris According to CCS Classification

Class	Description of Stage
I	"Ordinary physical activity does not cause ... angina," such as walking or climbing stairs. Angina occurs with strenuous, rapid, or prolonged exertion at work or recreation.
II	"Slight limitation of ordinary activity." Angina occurs on walking or climbing stairs rapidly; walking uphill; walking or stair climbing after meals; in cold, in wind, or under emotional stress; or only during the few hours after awakening. Angina occurs on walking 0.2 blocks on the level and climbing 0.1 flight of ordinary stairs at a normal pace and under normal conditions.
III	"Marked limitations of ordinary physical activity." Angina occurs on walking 1 to 2 blocks on the level and climbing 1 flight of stairs under normal conditions and at a normal pace.
IV	"Inability to carry on any physical activity without discomfort—anginal symptoms may be present at rest."

Adapted with permission from Campeau L. Grading of angina pectoris (letter), *Circulation* 54:522–523, 1976. © 1976, American Heart Association, Inc.

From: Braunwald E, et al.: ACC/AHA guidelines for the management of patients with unstable angina and non–ST-segment elevation myocardial infarction. A report of the American College of Cardiology/American Heart Association Task Force on Practice Guidelines (Committee on the Management of Patients With Unstable Angina), *J Am Coll Cardiol* 36:970-1062, 2000.

determine the severity of an established MI. Echocardiogram may reveal new regional wall motion abnormalities or newly depressed LV function or aneurysm formation. Fig. 1 summarizes the evaluation of patients for acute coronary syndrome.

LABORATORY TESTS

- Biomarkers play an important role in the early detection and diagnosis of acute coronary syndrome (ACS). While troponin is essential to the diagnosis of acute myocardial infarction, other markers have demonstrated utility in the setting of acute chest pain and ACS. CK-MB and myoglobin are two traditional markers that are frequently used in combination with troponin and will be elevated in the setting of NSTEMI or STEMI. See Fig. E2, *A* for timing of release of each biomarker. Troponin I is the most sensitive biomarker for cardiac myocyte damage and also predicts 42-day mortality in ACS. Troponin I is considered the gold standard biomarker for diagnosis of myocardial infarction (Fig. E2, *B*).
- Creatinine kinase-myocardial band (CK-MB) is the cardiac specific isoform of creatinine kinase (CK) and is found in high concentrations in the myocardium. After an acute myocardial injury, CK-MB levels peak within 4-6 hours. This delayed rise of CK-MB limits its early diagnostic utility for ACS. However, after approximately 8 hours the negative predictive value of CK-MB reaches 95%, providing valuable information for clinicians attempting to rule out myocardial infarction with serial sampling.
- CK-MB is especially useful when assessing a patient for possible re-infarction. Its shorter half-life leads to normal values within 24-48 hours after an event. Troponin, on the other hand, is often elevated up to 2 weeks following an acute myocardial infarction and will not be as reliable. In these situations, CK-MB is the biomarker of choice and can aid in diagnosis of re-infarction.
- In addition to its utility in diagnosing re-infarction, CK-MB appears to have prognostic value in ACS. CK-MB positivity was found to be predictive of increased all-cause mortality in patients presenting with NSTEMI regardless of their troponin status.
- Meanwhile, other biomarkers also have significant prognostic value. Testing for B-type natriuretic peptide (BNP) has a class IIb recommendation in the 2014 NSTE-ACS guidelines for use as a prognostic tool in patients presenting with an MI. BNP >80 portends a high risk of death at initial presentation of a STEMI.

RISK MODELS AND RISK SCORES

Risk models and scores such as TIMI (see "Risk Assessment" in "Myocardial Infarction" topic), PURSUIT, and GRACE based on clinical, ECG, and laboratory data at presentation help to discriminate patients at high risk versus low risk for short- and intermediate-term adverse outcomes (Fig. E2, *C*).

IMAGING STUDIES

- A CXR to assist in evaluating for volume status and for other possible causes of chest discomfort.
- In patients for whom ECG and cardiac biomarkers are nondiagnostic but the suspicion for ACS is high given the history, an echocardiogram may be helpful to assess left ventricular (LV) function and regional wall motion abnormalities.
- Coronary CT angiography can be performed in patients with possible ACS, a normal 12-lead EKG result, negative troponin results, and no history of coronary artery disease (Class IIa).
- Cardiac stress testing (treadmill ECG, imaging stress studies using echocardiography or nuclear modalities) may further help to diagnose and risk stratify these patients. (See "Coronary Artery Disease" in Section I.)
- Coronary angiogram/cardiac catheterization will reveal coronary artery luminal irregularities/stenotic lesions. In patients with ACS who undergo coronary angiography, approximately 25% will have one vessel disease, 25% will have two vessel disease, 25% will have three vessel disease, 10% will have left main disease, and 15% will have coronary stenosis of <50% or normal coronaries.

Rx TREATMENT

The overall goal for patients with NSTE-ACS is to relieve myocardial ischemia and to prevent recurrent cardiovascular events. Antithrombotic therapy is needed to reduce thrombus burden, prevent further thrombosis, and improve coronary artery flow. Revascularization is needed to prevent further events and improve flow within the coronary artery lumen. For patients with STEMI, the goal is immediate reperfusion therapy, whether it is chemical (i.e., thrombolysis) or mechanical (i.e., percutaneous coronary intervention [PCI]), and time from onset of ischemia to revascularization is an important prognostic factor. STEMI patients presenting to a hospital with PCI capability should be treated with primary PCI within 90 minutes of first medical contact (Figs. 3 and 4). At non–PCI-capable hospitals where the first medical contact to balloon time is more than 120 minutes, thrombolytic therapy should be given if no contraindications are present; thrombolytics should not be administered 24 hours after initial diagnosis of STEMI. Absolute contraindications to thrombolytic therapy include the following: history of hemorrhagic cerebrovascular accident (CVA), history of CVA, dementia or central nervous system damage within the past yr, head trauma or brain surgery within the past 6 months, or intracranial neoplasm. Other contraindications include suspected aortic dissection, internal bleeding within the past 6 weeks, active bleeding or known bleeding disorder, and traumatic CPR within the past 3 weeks.

NONPHARMACOLOGIC THERAPY

- STEMI is a medical emergency and requires immediate reperfusion therapy; the best outcomes are seen in cardiac catheterization with primary PCI. Guidelines call for a goal door-to-balloon time of ≤90 minutes.
- Patients with NSTE-ACS should be risk stratified in conjunction with the cardiology consult service. Risk scores such as the TIMI and GRACE scores can be used to decide between an early invasive strategy and an ischemia-guided strategy. Overall, an early invasive strategy is associated with better outcomes in patients with higher risk (i.e., TIMI score >3 or GRACE >140) and involves cardiac catheterization followed by revascularization with PCI or coronary artery bypass grafting (CABG) within 4 to 24 hours of presentation. An ischemia-guided strategy involves aggressive medical management and revascularization only if ischemia recurs or is documented on noninvasive testing. This should only be reserved for selected patients with low-risk scores (TIMI score 0-2). The early invasive strategy can be further stratified by timing:
  1. Immediate (within 2 hours): Patients with refractory or recurrent angina despite optimal initial treatment, signs or symptoms of heart failure, new or worsening mitral regurgitation, hemodynamic instability, sustained ventricular tachycardia or ventricular fibrillation

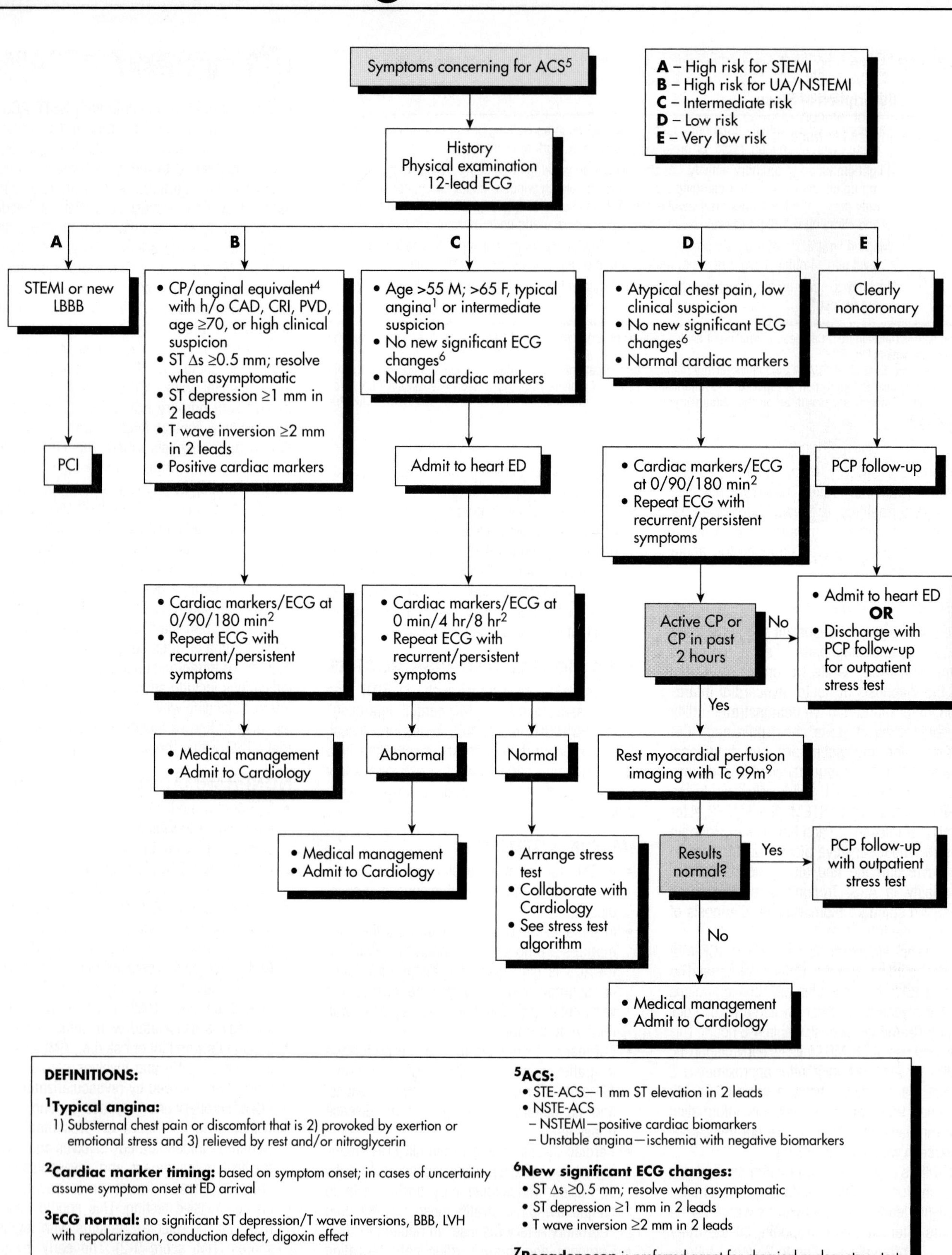

FIG. 1 Evaluation of patients for acute coronary syndrome *(ACS).* *CAD,* Coronary artery disease; *CP,* chest pain; *CRI,* chronic renal insufficiency; *ECG,* electrocardiogram; *ED,* emergency department; *h/o,* history of; *LBBB,* left bundle branch block; *NSTE,* non–ST-segment elevation; *NSTEMI,* non–ST-segment elevation myocardial infarction; *PCP,* primary care physician; *PVD,* peripheral vascular disease; *STE,* ST-segment elevation; *STEMI,* ST-segment elevation myocardial infarction; *UA,* unstable angina. (From Adams JG, et al.: *Emergency medicine, clinical essentials,* ed 2, Philadelphia, 2013, Elsevier.)

2. Early (within 24 hours): No characteristics from the immediate category but new ST-segment depression, a GRACE risk score >140 or temporal change in troponin
3. Delayed invasive: None of the immediate or early characteristics but renal insufficiency, left ventricular ejection fraction of <40%, early post-infarct angina, history of PCI within the past 6 months, prior coronary artery bypass graft, GRACE risk score of 109-140, or TIMI score of 2 or more

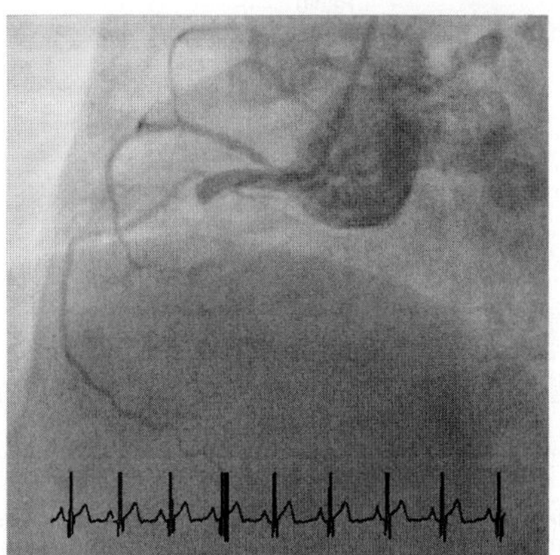

FIG. 3 Right coronary artery totally occluded proximally during ST-elevation mycardial infarction.

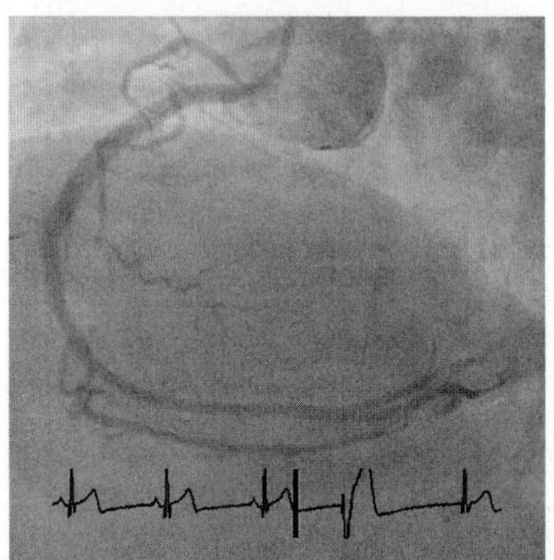

FIG. 4 Right coronary artery after successful percutaneous coronary artery stenting during ST-elevation myocardial infarction.

- Continuous ECG monitoring is recommended for all ACS patients. Supplemental oxygen should be administered to patients with arterial oxygen saturation of less than 90%, respiratory distress, or other high-risk features of hypoxemia. Finger pulse oximetry should be utilized to assess arterial oxygen saturation.

ACUTE GENERAL Rx

- All patients with ACS should receive full-dose non–enteric-coated chewable aspirin of 162 to 325 mg to establish a high blood level for its antiplatelet effects. Thereafter, daily dose of 81 are prescribed and continued indefinitely.
- Antithrombotic therapy is critical in treating the underlying pathophysiology of ACS. This consists of administering antiplatelet and anticoagulant agents.
- Antiplatelet agents (Table 3) inhibit platelet activation and aggregation. Aspirin is a cyclooxygenase inhibitor that blocks platelet aggregation and should be administered to all ACS patients without contraindications.
- Clopidogrel is a thienopyridine agent that inhibits platelet activation and aggregation. It should be administered in all ACS patients, with the timing dependent on the clinical scenario and management strategy. It requires a loading dose of 300 to 600 mg followed by 75 mg daily. It should be discontinued at least 5 days before CABG. If a patient is unable to take aspirin in the setting of hypersensitivity or major gastrointestinal intolerance, a loading dose of clopidogrel followed by daily maintenance should be started. Other antiplatelet agents that can be substituted instead of clopidogrel include prasugrel, ticlopidine, and ticagrelor. However, maintenance doses of aspirin above 100 mg reduce the effectiveness of ticagrelor and should be avoided after an initial dose; ticagrelor should be used with aspirin 75 to 100 mg per day. Because of a more rapid and consistent onset of action, reversibility, and a reduction in death from vascular causes, MI, or stroke, ticagrelor is preferred over clopidogrel in patients with NSTE-ACS. Prasugrel is not recommended in ACS patients with stroke or transient ischemic attack (TIA), or those patients managed with fibrinolysis because of an increased risk of bleeding complications. Cangrelor is a newer IV ADP-P2Y12 receptor antagonist that may be used initially as a load in the emergency department before an invasive strategy, given its initial action and quick platelet recovery time. As a rule, all ACS patients should have two antiplatelet agents initiated and should be continued up to 12 months regardless of ischemia-guided vs invasive strategy.
- GP IIB/IIIa inhibitors (Table 4) may be considered as an intravenous antiplatelet therapy in addition to aspirin for medium- or high-risk patients with NSTE-ACS in whom an invasive strategy is planned (Class IIb). Eptifibatide and tirofiban are preferred agents over abciximab for NSTE-ACS patients; however, for STEMI patients undergoing primary PCI, IV abciximab has the same Class IIa indication as tirofiban and eptifibatide.
- Anticoagulant agents should be administered to all ACS patients. Options include either unfractionated heparin (UFH), or low-molecular-weight heparin (enoxaparin), or factor Xa inhibitors such as fondaparinux, or direct thrombin inhibitors such as bivalirudin (Table 5).
- In the most recent guidelines, enoxaparin and UFH have both received Class I recommendations for use among ACS patients managed conservatively or invasively.
- For STEMI, fondaparinux can be used for anticoagulation. It has been shown to decrease bleeding complications as compared with either UFH or LMWH. However, it has a long half-life (15 hours), and thrombosis on catheters has been noted when using only

TABLE 3 Pharmacologic Characteristics of Oral Antiplatelet Drugs Commonly Used in the Management of Acute Coronary Syndromes

		ADP Receptor Antagonists		
Characteristic	**Aspirin**	**Clopidogrel**	**Prasugrel**	**Ticagrelor**
Class	COX inhibitor	Thienopyridine (second generation)	Thienopyridine (third generation)	Cyclopentyl triazolopyrimidine
Target	COX-1	P2Y12	P2Y12	P2Y12
Dose	162—325-mg loading dose; 75—325mg/day maintenance dose	300—600-mg loading dose; 75mg/day maintenance dose	60-mg loading dose; 10mg/day maintenance dose	180-mg loading dose; 90 mg bid maintenance dose
Prodrug	No	Yes	Yes	No
Time to effect[a]	<1 hour	4 – 6 hours[b]	<1 hour	<1 hour
Drug half-life	20 mmin	Minutes	Minutes	12 hours
Reversible	No	No	No	Yes

ADP, Adenosine diphosphate; bid, twice daily; *COX,* cyclooxygenase.
[a]After loading dose
[b]Increased antithrombotic benefit was seen after the first hour in patients enrolled in the COMMIT trial who did not receive a loading dose, but maximum effect is not seen until after 4-6 hours.
From Hoffman R, et al.: *Hematology, basic principles and practice*, ed 7, Philadelphia, 2018, Elsevier.

TABLE 4 Pharmacologic Characteristics of Intravenous Antiplatelet Drugs Used in the Management of Acute Coronary Syndrome

	GP IIb/IIIa inhibitors			ADP Receptor Antagonists
Characteristic	**Abciximab**	**Eprifibatide**	**Tirofiban**	**Cangrelor**
Class	Fab fragment	Nonpeptide	Cyclic heptapeptide	Nonthienopyridine
Onset	Rapid	Rapid	Rapid	Rapid
Drug half-life	10-30 min	2 hours	2.5 hours	3-6 min
Reversibility of platelet inhibition	Slow	Rapid	Rapid	Rapid
Excretion	Unknown	40%-70% renal	50% renal	Dephosphorylation

From Hoffman R, et al.: *Hematology, basic principles and practice,* ed 7, Philadelphia, 2018, Elsevier.

TABLE 5 Pharmacologic Characteristics of Parenteral Anticoagulants Commonly Used in the Management of Patients with Acute Coronary Syndromes

	Unfractionated Heparin	Enoxaparin	Bivalirudin	Fondaparinux
Route of administration	IV	SC (first dose IV[a])	IV	SC (first dose IV[a])
Frequency of dosing	Continuous IV infusion	Twice daily; once daily if CrCl <30 ml/min	Continuous IV infusion	Once-daily injection
Clearance	Primarily nonrenal	Renal	Renal, proteolytic cleavage	Renal
Use in ACS patients with moderate renal impairment	Yes	Yes (dose reduction)	Yes (dose reduction)	Yes[b]
Use in ACS patients undergoing dialysis	Yes	No experience	Yes (dose reduction)	No experience[c]
Routine laboratory monitoring	Yes	No	No[d]	No
Dose	Adjust dose according to the results of the aPTT	Fixed weight adjusted	Fixed weight adjusted	Fixed
Accumulation in renal failure	No	Yes	Yes	Yes
Nonanticoagulant side effects	Allergy, HIT	HIT (rare)	—	—
Nonbleeding contraindications	Allergy, immune HIT	Allergy, immune HIT	Allergy	Allergy
Antidote	Protamine sulfate	Protamine sulfate partially reverses	No	No

ACS, Acute coronary syndromes; *aPTT,* activated partial thromboplastin time; *CrCl,* creatinine clearance; *HIT,* heparin-induced thrombocytopenia; *IV,* intravenous; *SC,* subcutaneous.
[a]The first dose of enoxaparin was given by the intravenous route in the TIMI-11B (Thrombolysis In Myocardial Infarction 11B) and EXTRACT-TIMI 25 (Enoxaparin and Thrombolysis Reperfusion for Acute Myocardial Infarction Treatment, Thrombolysis in Myocardial Infarction 25) studies. The first dose of fondaparinux was given by the intravenous route in the OASIS-6 (Optimal Antiplatelet Strategy for InterventionS 6) trial.
[b]Acute coronary syndrome patients with creatinine up to 265 μmol/L were eligible for inclusion in the OASIS-5 and -6 trials (equivalent to an estimated creatinine clearance of 15-20 ml/min in a 70-kg patient who is 70 yr of age).
[c]Fondaparinux is contraindicated in patients with venous thromboembolism who have severe renal impairment.
[d]Monitoring and dose adjustment required in patients with creatinine clearance below 30 ml/min.
From Hoffman R, et al.: *Hematology, basic principles and practice,* ed 7, Philadelphia, 2018, Elsevier.

fondaparinux in the cath lab; therefore, it is not recommended as a sole anticoagulation during primary PCI.

- Bivalirudin is a reversible direct thrombin inhibitor and may be considered as an alternative to UFH and GP IIb/IIIa inhibitors in patients with STEMI (HORIZONS AMI trial) who are undergoing primary PCI (PPCI). When bivalirudin was compared to UFH plus a glycoprotein IIb/IIIa inhibitor in patients with STEMI and PCI, less bleeding and a short- and long-term reduction in cardiac events and overall mortality was observed. With bivalirudin, there is no risk of heparin-induced thrombocytopenia, less bleeding is observed, and the anticoagulant effect can be monitored during intervention by the activated clotting time. Similar results were reported in the use of bivalirudin alone in patients with UA/NSTEMI in the ACUITY trial when compared to enoxaparin/UFH with GP IIb/IIIa arms.
- Beta-blocker therapy reduces ischemia by decreasing myocardial oxygen demand and oral therapy should be initiated within 24 hours of onset of ACS unless signs or symptoms of heart failure and shock are present or arrhythmias preclude its use. Oral administration, titrated to a heart rate of 50-60 beats/min, is preferred. Intravenous beta-blockers can be administered to STEMI patients who are hypertensive or have ongoing ischemia; they should be avoided if the patients have any of the following:
  1. Signs of heart failure,
  2. Evidence of a low output state,
  3. Increased risk for cardiogenic shock, or
  4. Other relative contraindications to beta-blockade (PR interval >0.24 second, second- or third-degree heart block, active asthma, or reactive airway disease).
- Nitroglycerin is a vasodilator that should be administered to relieve chest discomfort in all ACS patients. It can be administered sublingually at first, up to 3 doses, followed by intravenous administration if symptoms persist. In the setting of an inferior STEMI, it is necessary to rule out a right ventricular (RV) infarct with a right-sided ECG before the administration of nitroglycerin. This is because RV infarcts are preload dependent

and nitroglycerin decreases preload through venodilation, which leads to hypotension in this setting. This can be corrected by discontinuing nitroglycerin and starting bolus intravenous fluids. Nitroglycerin provides no mortality benefit in ACS patients.

- Oxygen should be administered to patients with shortness of breath, signs of acute heart failure, cardiogenic shock, or an arterial oxyhemoglobin saturation of less than 90%. The 2014 ACC/AHA guidelines report no demonstrated benefit for routine use of supplemental oxygen in normoxic patients with NSTE-ACS; rather, emerging data suggest that routine use of oxygen can lead to adverse effects such as increased coronary vascular resistance, reduced coronary blood flow, and increased mortality rate.
- The 2014 ACC/AHA Guidelines for unstable NSTE-ACS have downgraded the recommendation for morphine use for uncontrolled ischemic chest discomfort from a Class IIa to a Class IIb recommendation due to reports linked to increased adverse events.
- Calcium channel blockers (nondihydropyridine) may be used in patients with persisting or recurrent symptoms, despite treatment with beta-blockers and nitroglycerin. They work by causing coronary vasodilation and decreasing myocardial oxygen demand. They are useful when beta-blockers are contraindicated and in patients with Prinzmetal variant angina. Calcium channel blockers should not be used in cases of severe LV dysfunction, pulmonary edema, increased risk for cardiogenic shock or advanced heart blocks.
- Patients routinely taking nonsteroidal antiinflammatory drugs (NSAIDs) (except for aspirin), both nonselective as well as COX-2 selective agents, before ACS should discontinue those agents at the time of presentation because of the increased risks of mortality, reinfarction, hypertension, heart failure, and myocardial rupture associated with their use.
- Angiotensin-converting enzyme (ACE) inhibitors may be added and should be used within 24 hours of onset of ACS in all patients with depressed LV function (ejection fraction [EF] <40%) or pulmonary vascular congestion. Angiotensin receptor blockers (ARBs) should be used in patients who are ACE inhibitor intolerant.
- Refer to topic "Cocaine Overdose" for treatment of cocaine-related ACS.

CHRONIC Rx

- Post-ACS medical therapy involves aspirin, statin, beta-blocker, and a second anti-platelet agent such as clopidogrel, ticagrelor, or prasugrel.
- In patients already on an oral anticoagulant for another diagnosis such as atrial fibrillation, the duration of triple therapy should be minimized. Strategies aimed at minimizing the risk of bleeding in patients treated with triple therapy (dual antiplatelet therapy and an oral anticoagulant) are summarized in Table 6. The WOEST trial showed that using clopidogrel along with an oral anticoagulant but without aspirin resulted in a significant reduction in bleeding complications with those patients on a triple therapy of oral anticoagulant, aspirin, and clopidogrel. It is a class IIB recommendation in those patients with atrial fibrillation and a CHADS-VASC score of 2 or greater after coronary revascularization to consider using clopidogrel concurrently with oral anticoagulant (Table 7) but without aspirin.
- Lipid lowering with statins has been evaluated in trials such as the MIRACL study, in which high-dose atorvastatin 80 mg reduced death, MI, and cardiac events at 16 weeks when administered early, within 24-96 hours after an ACS. The A-Z trial and PROVE IT-TIMI 22 trials demonstrated benefit of early high-intensity statin therapy with LDL targets <70 mg/dl in ACS.
- ACE inhibitors may be added to treat hypertension and should be used in all patients with depressed LV function (EF <40%) or pulmonary vascular congestion. ARBs should be used in patients who are ACE inhibitor intolerant.
- An aldosterone blocker should be used in post-MI patients without significant renal dysfunction or hyperkalemia who have an ejection fraction of less than 40% and are already on therapeutic doses of an ACE inhibitor and a beta-blocker.
- Cardiac rehabilitation and a monitored exercise program should be recommended at the time of discharge.
- Aggressive risk factor management, including smoking cessation, weight loss, diet and exercise, diabetes control, and so on, for secondary prevention of future events is crucial.

REFERRAL

- All ACS patients should be cared for in conjunction with the cardiology consult service.
- When appropriate, referral to a cardiac surgeon may be necessary for CABG.
- At time of discharge, patients should be considered for cardiac rehabilitation referral.

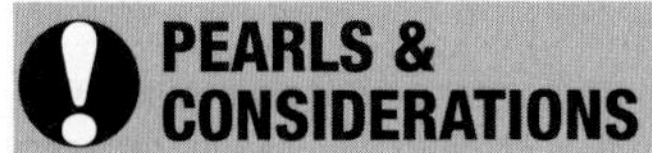

PEARLS & CONSIDERATIONS

COMMENTS

- ACS is common and a leading cause of mortality in the United States.
- The diagnosis hinges on the basics—history and physical, ECG, biomarkers, and CXR.
- Remember the potentially fatal non-ACS causes of chest discomfort, which include acute pulmonary embolism and acute ascending aortic dissection.
- STEMI patients presenting to a hospital with PCI capability should be treated with primary PCI within 90 minutes of first medical contact.

TABLE 6 Strategies Aimed at Minimizing the Risk of Bleeding in Patients Treated with Triple Therapy (Dual Antiplatelet Therapy and an Oral Anticoagulant)

Proposed Approach	Rationale
Aspirin maintenance dose ≤100 mg/day	Higher aspirin maintenance doses increase bleeding, and there is no evidence that they improve efficacy.
PPI with a preference for agents that interfere less with CYP 2C19 (e.g., pantoprazole)	Much of the excess bleeding is from the GI tract. The use of acid-suppressive agents that interfere less with CYP 2C19 minimizes the potential for a negative interaction with clopidogrel.
Preference for a non–vitamin K antagonist oral anticoagulant	Dabigatran 110 mg twice daily and apixaban 2.5 or 5.0 mg twice daily are associated with lower rates of bleeding than warfarin.
For warfarin, use a target INR of 2–2.5	Some evidence that a restricted target INR range reduces the risk of bleeding.
Manage warfarin in a specialized anticoagulation clinic	Compared with usual care, specialist clinics achieve a higher TTR of the INR.
Minimize duration of triple therapy	The risk of bleeding is highest during the first 30 days but remains elevated with long-term treatment.
Avoid NSAIDs	NSAIDs are a common cause of upper GI bleeding.
Avoid prasugrel and ticagrelor	Prasugrel and ticagrelor cannot be recommended because they are more potent than clopidogrel and cause more bleeding.

CYP, Cytochrome P450; *GI*, gastrointestinal; *INR*, international normalized ratio; *NSAID*, nonsteroidal antiinflammatory drug; *PPI*, proton pump inhibitor; *TTR*, time in therapeutic range.
From Hoffman R, et al.: *Hematology, basic principles and practice*, ed 7, Philadelphia, 2018, Elsevier.

TABLE 7 Pharmacological Characteristics of Warfarin and New Oral Anticoagulants Evaluated in Phase III Trials for the Long-Term Management of Acute Coronary Syndromes

Characteristic	Warfarin	Rivaroxaban	Apixaban
Target	VKORC1	Factor Xa	Factor Xa
Prodrug	No	No	No
Bioavailability (%)	100	80	60
Dosing	Variable, once daily	Fixed, 2.5 or 5 mg twice daily[a]	Fixed, 5 mg twice daily (2.5 mg twice daily in selected patients)
Half-life	Mean: 40 hours (range: 20–60 hours)	7–11 hours	12 hours
Renal clearance (%)	Nil	66[b]	25
Routine coagulation monitoring	Yes (INR)	No	No
Drug interactions	Multiple	Potent inhibitors of CYP3A4 and P-gp[c]	Potent inhibitors of CYP3A4 and P-gp c
Antidote	Yes (vitamin K, PCC, FFP)	No[d]	No[d]
Approved for ACS management	Yes	Yes, in Europe	No

ACS, Acute coronary syndromes; *CYP-3A4,* cytochrome P450 3A4; *FFP,* fresh frozen plasma; *fXa,* activated factor X; *INR,* international normalized ratio; *PCC,* prothrombin complex concentrates; *P-gp,* P-glycoprotein; *VKORC1,* C1 subunit of vitamin K epoxide reductase.
[a]A once-daily regimen was tested in atrial fibrillation.
[b]Half of renally cleared rivaroxaban is cleared as unchanged drug and half as inactive metabolites.
[c]Potent inhibitors of both CYP3A4 and P-glycoprotein include azole antifungals (e.g., ketoconazole, itraconazole, voriconazole, posaconazole) and protease inhibitors, such as ritonavir. Potent inhibitors of CYP3A4 include azole antifungals, macrolide antibiotics (e.g., clarithromycin), and protease inhibitors (e.g., atanazavir).
[d]Andexanet alfa is being developed as an antidote for rivaroxaban and apixaban.
Strategies Aimed at Minimizing the Risk of Bleeding in Patients Treated with Triple Therapy (Dual Antiplatelet Therapy and an Oral Anticoagulant)
From Hoffman R, et al.: *Hematology, basic principles and practice,* ed 7, Philadelphia, 2018, Elsevier.

- STEMI patients presenting to a hospital without PCI capability and who cannot be transferred to a PCI center and undergo PCI within 90 minutes of first medical contact should be treated with fibrinolytic therapy within 30 minutes of hospital presentation unless fibrinolytic therapy is contraindicated.
- Refer to topics "Angina Pectoris" and "Myocardial Infarction" for additional discussion of this subject matter.

PREVENTION

Primary prevention of ACS is based on recognizing the major risk factors for CAD:

- Patients should be counseled to end all tobacco use by developing a plan for quitting that may include pharmacotherapy or a referral to a smoking cessation program.
- Patients with blood pressure ≥130/80 mm Hg should be treated, as tolerated, with blood pressure medication, treating initially with β-blockers and/or ACE inhibitors, with addition of other drugs as needed to achieve goal blood pressure.
- All patients should be counseled regarding the need for lifestyle modification: weight control; increased physical activity; alcohol moderation; sodium reduction; and emphasis on increased consumption of fresh fruits, vegetables, and low-fat dairy products.
- It may also be reasonable to add omega 3 fatty acids from fish or fish oil capsules for cardiovascular disease reduction.
- Patients should be encouraged to perform 30-60 minutes of moderate intensity aerobic activity for a minimum of 5 days a week.
- Body mass index and waist circumference should be assessed at every visit and patients should be encouraged to maintain/achieve a body mass index between 18.5 and 24.9 kg/m^2.
- Patients with diabetes mellitus should maintain strict control of their glucose and A1C, under the care of their primary care physician or endocrinologist. Metformin is first line pharmacotherapy. Target HbA1c of ≤7% may be considered.
- Patients with cardiovascular disease should have an annual influenza vaccination.
- For patients with recent myocardial infarction or coronary artery bypass surgery, it is beneficial to screen for depression.
- All eligible patients should be referred to a comprehensive cardiac rehabilitation program.
- Patients with depressed LV function (ejection fraction <35%) at least 40 days after an acute MI benefit from an implantable cardioverter defibrillator (ICD) for the prevention of sudden cardiac death.

SUGGESTED READINGS

Available at ExpertConsult.com

RELATED CONTENT

Acute Coronary Syndrome (Patient Information)
Angina Pectoris (Related Key Topic)
Coronary Artery Disease (Related Key Topic)
Myocardial Infarction (Related Key Topic)
Hypertension (Related Key Topic)

AUTHORS: **ROXANA GHASHGHAEI, M.D.,** and **PRANAV M. PATEL, M.D., F.A.C.C., F.A.H.A., F.S.C.A.I.**

BASIC INFORMATION

DEFINITION

Acute glomerulonephritis (GN) is inflammation of the glomeruli, usually caused by deposition of immunoglobulins or their components and/or complement proteins, that leads to hematuria and/or albuminuria. If untreated, chronic glomerular inflammation may lead to chronic scarring and progressive kidney disease.

SYNONYMS

Acute nephritic syndrome
Glomerulonephritis, acute GN

ICD-10CM CODES

N00.0	Acute nephritic syndrome with minor glomerular abnormality
N00.1	Acute nephritic syndrome with focal and segmental glomerular lesions
N00.2	Acute nephritic syndrome with diffuse membranous glomerulonephritis
N00.3	Acute nephritic syndrome with diffuse mesangial proliferative glomerulonephritis
N00.4	Acute nephritic syndrome with diffuse endocapillary proliferative glomerulonephritis
N00.5	Acute nephritic syndrome with diffuse mesangiocapillary glomerulonephritis
N00.6	Acute nephritic syndrome with dense deposit disease
N00.7	Acute nephritic syndrome with diffuse crescentic glomerulonephritis
N00.8	Acute nephritic syndrome with other morphologic changes
N00.9	Acute nephritic syndrome with unspecified morphologic changes

EPIDEMIOLOGY & DEMOGRAPHICS

- Incidence rates of primary glomerulonephritis vary between 0.2/100,000 per yr and 2.5/100,000 per yr.
- Immunoglobulin A (IgA) nephropathy (Berger's disease) is the most common glomerulonephritis worldwide.
- Glomerulonephritis accounts for 23% of end-stage renal disease cases worldwide.
- Glomerulonephritis affects adults and children.

PHYSICAL FINDINGS & CLINICAL PRESENTATION

- Acute onset of hypertension.
- Dark, "tea-colored" urine.
- Edema (peripheral, periorbital, or pulmonary).
- Fatigue.
- Concurrent pulmonary hemorrhage and rapidly progressive decline in kidney function may indicate antineutrophil cytoplasmic antibody (ANCA) vasculitis or antiglomerular basement membrane (GBM) disease.
- Joint pains, oral ulcers, and malar rash are frequently seen with systemic lupus erythematosus (SLE).
- Palpable purpura may be found in patients with systemic vasculitis such as Henoch-Schönlein purpura, ANCA-associated vasculitis, SLE, or cryoglobulinemia.
- A recent history of endocarditis, or cellulitis or pharyngitis preceding urinary abnormalities may indicate infection-related glomerulonephritis.
- Hepatitis C virus infection may cause membranoproliferative glomerulonephritis (MPGN) with or without cryoglobulinemia.
- Concurrent upper respiratory tract infection (synpharyngitic infection) and gross hematuria may indicate IgA nephropathy.
- Table 1 summarizes the clinical and laboratory features in the different causes of rapidly progressive glomerulonephritis.

ETIOLOGY

Acute glomerulonephritis (GN) may occur as a renal-limited disease or a systemic disorder. A description of target antigens is included in Table 2.

In the past decade, the knowledge of the pathogeneses of several acute GNs has greatly expanded. IgA nephropathy is thought to be caused by a multi-hit process that involves under-galactosylated IgA1, development of antiglycan antibodies, and deposition of immune complexes in the kidney. Post-streptococcal GN is now part of infection-related glomerulonephritis, a broader category that includes IgA-dominant staphylococcus-associated GN. C3 glomerulopathy, composed of C3 glomerulonephritis and dense deposit disease, is caused by dysregulation of the alternative complement pathway. The alternative complement pathway is now implicated in several different GNs, including IgA nephropathy and ANCA-associated vasculitis, which may have treatment implications in the future.

DIAGNOSIS

DIFFERENTIAL DIAGNOSIS FOR HEMATURIA AND/OR PROTEINURIA, IN ADDITION TO ACUTE GLOMERULONEPHRITIS

- Urinary tract infection
- Nephrolithiasis
- Urothelial malignancy
- Polycystic kidney disease
- Acute interstitial nephritis
- Acute tubular necrosis
- Nephrotic syndrome
- Hereditary nephritis (Alport syndrome and thin basement membrane)
- Diabetic nephropathy

WORKUP

Initial evaluation of suspected glomerulonephritis consists of laboratory testing.

LABORATORY TESTS

- Urinalysis, with albuminuria (majority of proteinuria in glomerulonephritis is albuminuria) and hematuria (dysmorphic erythrocytes and red cell casts).
- Blood urea nitrogen and serum creatinine to estimate glomerular filtration rate (GFR).
- 24-hour urine collection for total protein excretion (includes albumin plus tubular proteins) and creatinine clearance to document degree of renal dysfunction. Random urine (spot specimen) protein-to-creatinine ratio instead of a 24-hour collection is also acceptable. Proteinuria primarily, in acute glomerulonephritis typically ranges from 500 mg/day to 3 gram/day, but nephrotic-range proteinuria (>3.5 g/day) may be present.
- Streptococcal tests (Streptozyme), antistreptolysin O (ASO) quantitative titer (highest in 3 to 5 weeks). The ASO titer is not related to severity of kidney disease, duration, or prognosis.
- Additional serologic testing, including ANA, ds-DNA, C3, C4, rheumatoid factor, cryoglobulins, hepatitis B and C viral serologies, ANCA (MPO and PR3), anti-GBM antibodies, serum and urine protein electrophoresis with immunofixation, and serum free light chains analysis.
- Hematocrit and platelet count are decreased during thrombotic microangiopathies.
- Blood cultures are indicated in all febrile patients.

IMAGING STUDIES

- Chest x-rays may demonstrate in ANCA-associated vasculitis and anti-GBM disease (Goodpasture syndrome).
- Renal ultrasound to exclude structural causes of hematuria and proteinuria. A kidney size of <9 cm in length is suggestive of extensive scarring and low likelihood of reversibility.
- Echocardiogram in patients with new cardiac murmurs or positive blood cultures to rule-out endocarditis and pericardial effusion.
- Kidney biopsy with light, electron, and immunofluorescence microscopy to establish diagnosis.
- Biopsy of other affected organs if systemic vasculitis is suspected.

TREATMENT

NONPHARMACOLOGIC THERAPY

- Low-salt diet if edema or hypertension is present.
- Avoidance of high-potassium foods if patient is hyperkalemic.

ACUTE GENERAL Rx

- Diuretics in patients with significant edema or hypertension.
- Correction of electrolyte abnormalities (hypocalcemia, hyperkalemia) and acidosis.
- High-dose steroids for rapidly progressive glomerulonephritis.
- Additional immunosuppressive treatment with alkylating agents, calcineurin inhibitors, or biologic agents may be necessary depending on the underlying disease.
- Treatment of streptococcal infection with penicillin (or erythromycin in penicillin-allergic patients). Hemodialysis in patients with diuretic-resistant volume overload, hyperkalemia, uremic symptoms, and

Acute Glomerulonephritis (AGN) PTG

TABLE 1 Clinical and Laboratory Features in the Different Causes of Rapidly Progressive Glomerulonephritis

Disease	Typical Clinical Features	Serologic Findings	Complement Levels	Immune Deposits in Glomerulus on Renal Biopsy
Vasculitis				Few/pauci-immune
Granulomatosis with polyangiitis (Wegener granulomatosis)	Prodrome of nasal stuffiness, blocked ears, arthralgia; then onset of hemoptysis, purpura, peripheral neuropathy	C-ANCA	Normal or increased	
Microscopic polyangiitis	Similar to granulomatosis with polyangiitis (Wegener granulomatosis) or affecting the kidneys only (renal-limited) or overlap with polyarteritis nodosa	P-ANCA	Normal or increased	
Anti-GBM disease	Macroscopic hematuria and hemoptysis	Anti-GBM antibodies	Normal or increased	Linear staining for IgG and C3
SLE (diffuse proliferative, WHO class IV)	Previous history of SLE, marked hematuria and proteinuria, hypertension "telescoping" urinary sediment	ANA, anti–dsDNA antibodies	Low C3, low C4	Granular immune deposits
IgA disease	Persistent microscopic hematuria with episodes of synpharyngitic macroscopic hematuria, with proteinuria, hypertension	IgA (increased in about half of cases)	Normal or increased	
Poststreptococcal glomerulonephritis	At 1 to 3 weeks after streptococcal pharyngitis or impetigo, macroscopic hematuria, edema, hypertension, oliguria	ASO, anti-DNase B antibodies	Low C3, normal C4	

ANA, Antinuclear antibodies; *anti-DNase B,* anti-deoxyribonuclease B; *anti–dsDNA,* anti–double-stranded DNA; *ASO,* antistreptolysin O; *C-ANCA,* cytoplasmic antineutrophil cytoplasmic antibodies; *GBM,* glomerular basement membrane; *IgA,* immunoglobulin A; *IgG,* immunoglobin G; *P-ANCA,* perinuclear antineutrophil cytoplasmic antibodies; *SLE,* systemic lupus erythematosus; *WHO,* World Health Organization.

Ronco C, et al.: *Critical care nephrology,* ed 3, Philadelphia, 2019, Elsevier.

TABLE 2 Antigens Identified in Glomerulonephritis

Poststreptococcal GN	Streptococcal pyrogenic exotoxin B, plasmin receptor
Anti-GBM disease	α3 type IV collagen (likely induced by molecular mimicry)
IgA nephropathy	Immune complex of anti-glycan antibodies and complement components
Membranous nephropathy	Phospholipase A_2 receptor (idiopathic), neutral endopeptidase in podocyte (congenital), HBeAg (hepatitis associated)
Staphylococcus aureus–associated GN	*Staphylococcus* superantigens induce polyclonal response; not necessarily antigen in glomeruli
Membranoproliferative GN	HCV and HBsAg in hepatitis-associated MPGN
ANCA-associated vasculitis	Proteinase 3 (C-ANCA) and myeloperoxidase (P-ANCA) in neutrophils; antibodies to lysosome-associated membrane protein 2 (LAMP2) on endothelial cells (likely induced by molecular mimicry to fimbriated bacterial antigens)

ANCA, Antineutrophil cytoplasmic antibody; *GBM,* glomerular basement membrane; *GN,* glomerulonephritis; *HBeAg,* hepatitis B virus early antigen; *HBsAg,* hepatitis B surface antigen; *HCV,* hepatitis C virus; *IgA,* immunoglobulin A; *MPGN,* membranoproliferative glomerulonephritis.

Adapted from Floege J, et al.: *Comprehensive clinical nephrology,* ed 4, Philadelphia, 2010, Saunders.

encephalopathy. Plasma exchange therapy for antibody removal for diffuse alveolar hemorrhage or rapidly progressive glomerulonephritis.

CHRONIC Rx

- Periodic monitoring of blood pressure, urinalysis, serum creatinine and blood urea nitrogen, serum albumin, and random urine protein-to-creatinine ratio
- Angiotensin–converting-enzyme (ACE) inhibitors or angiotensin receptor II blockers (ARBs) to reduce proteinuria
- Lipid management with statins and fibrates as indicated
- Monitor for side effects related to immunosuppression such as infection, leukopenia and anemia, osteoporosis or osteopenia, gastrointestinal ulcers, high blood pressure, and tumors
- Routine health maintenance with vaccinations for influenza and pneumococcus, age-appropriate vaccinations, and age-appropriate malignancy screening. Live vaccines are contraindicated in patients on immunosuppression

DISPOSITION

- Prognosis is generally correlated to initial serum creatinine and degree of renal fibrosis on biopsy.
- In general, prognosis is worse in patients with heavy albuminuria/proteinuria, low GFR at presentation, severe hypertension, and kidney biopsy-proven crescentic glomerulonephritis.
- Recovery of kidney function occurs within 8 to 12 weeks in 95% of patients with poststreptococcal glomerulonephritis.

REFERRAL

- Nephrology consultation for all patients with suspected glomerulonephritis. Urgent consultation is recommended if hyperkalemia, acidosis, or azotemia is present.

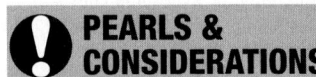

PEARLS & CONSIDERATIONS

COMMENTS

- Diagnosis of acute GN is established by kidney biopsy. Biopsy is indicated when the histologic diagnosis will alter the treatment plan, especially with systemic illnesses, significant proteinuria (>500 mg to 1 g per day), or increasing serum creatinine. A search for systemic illness, including infections, autoimmune disease, and malignancy is needed with careful history, physical examination, and serologic tests. Some patients with suspected glomerulonephritis will not require a kidney biopsy because of the success of supportive therapies (e.g., infection-related GN).
- Nephrology consultation should be obtained before initiating immunosuppressive therapy. ACE inhibitor or ARB therapy is essential for proteinuria reduction, unless there is contraindication. Spironolactone has been added to ACE inhibitor treatment for greater proteinuria reduction.
- Periodic monitoring for side effects of immunosuppressive drugs and complications of corticosteroids is necessary.
- Monitor lipids and treat persistent hyperlipidemia.

SUGGESTED READINGS

Available at ExpertConsult.com

RELATED CONTENT

Glomerulonephritis (Patient Information)
Acute Kidney Injury (Related Key Topic)

AUTHOR: **RUPALI AVASARE, M.D.**

BASIC INFORMATION

DEFINITION

Acute kidney injury (AKI) is defined as a rapid impairment in kidney function that results in retention of products in the blood normally excreted by the kidneys. The decline in kidney function can result in volume overload and dysregulation of acid-base status and electrolytes. Current consensus criteria for diagnosis of AKI requires an increase in serum creatinine of 0.3 mg/dl within 48 hours or 1.5 times baseline serum creatinine, and/or a decline in urine in output to <0.5 ml/kg/hour. AKI is further graded by severity as described in Table 1.

SYNONYMS

AKI
Acute renal failure (ARF)
Acute renal insufficiency syndrome
Acute kidney failure

ICD-10CM CODES

N17.9 Acute kidney failure, unspecified
N17.0 Acute kidney failure with tubular necrosis
N17.1 Acute kidney failure with acute cortical necrosis
N17.2 Acute kidney failure with medullary necrosis
N17.8 Other acute kidney failure
N99.0 Postprocedural (acute) (chronic) kidney failure
O90.4 Postpartum acute kidney failure

EPIDEMIOLOGY & DEMOGRAPHICS

- Using consensus criteria, an estimated 20% of hospitalized patients and nearly 60% of intensive care unit patients develop AKI.
- AKI occurs in 20% of patients with moderate sepsis and in >50% of patients with septic shock and positive blood cultures.
- Greater than 40% of hospital-associated AKI is iatrogenic.
- AKI in hospitalized patients is associated with increased hospital length-of-stay and cost.
- Most common cause of AKI in hospitalized patients is intrinsic kidney failure caused by acute tubular necrosis (ATN) and prerenal azotemia.
- Key risk factors for AKI include older age, preexisting chronic kidney disease, diabetes mellitus, and preexisting proteinuria.

PHYSICAL FINDINGS & CLINICAL PRESENTATION

- Early or mild AKI may be asymptomatic
- Frequent presenting symptoms include weakness, anorexia, generalized malaise, and nausea
- Oliguria is defined as <400 to 500 ml of urine per 24 hours
- Patients may develop nonoliguric or anuric kidney injury
- Physical examination should focus on evaluation of volume status
- Findings vary with duration and rapidity of onset of renal failure and underlying cause of AKI
- Peripheral edema from volume overload, heart failure, liver failure, or nephrotic syndrome
- Pulmonary edema
- Arrhythmias from electrolyte imbalances and metabolic acidosis
- Neurologic findings include altered mental status, delirium, lethargy, myoclonus, seizures, and flapping tremor (asterixis)
- Pruritus, uremic odor
- Flank pain
- Painless hematuria may be seen with glomerulonephritis, whereas painful hematuria is more consistent with obstructive uropathy
- Fasciculations, myoclonus, muscle cramps
- Pericardial effusion and/or pericardial rub
- Fever, skin rash, and arthralgia can be seen with systemic vasculitis
- Classic triad of fever, rash, and eosinophilia in the setting of AKI suggests allergic interstitial nephritis (AIN) and occurs in only 30% of cases. When considering AIN as the cause of AKI, a careful review of medications is required

ETIOLOGY

- **Prerenal:** Inadequate renal perfusion caused by hypovolemia, congestive heart failure (impaired cardiac output), cirrhosis (fluid third-spacing), sepsis (vasodilation), abdominal compartment syndrome, or other. Sixty percent of community-acquired cases of AKI are from prerenal conditions.
- **Postrenal:** Bladder outlet obstruction (prostatic enlargement, urethral fibrosis), ureteral obstruction (stones, bladder masses, retroperitoneal fibrosis, ureteral fibrosis), or renal vein occlusion. With two functioning kidneys, bilateral obstruction is usually required to cause significant AKI. Postrenal causes of AKI account for 5% to 15% of community-acquired AKI.
- **Intrinsic renal:** ATN, glomerulonephritis, AIN. Common causes of ATN include ischemia (e.g., hypotension or shock, postcardiac bypass, or aorta surgery), rhabdomyolysis, sepsis, drug toxicity (e.g., aminoglycosides, amphotericin, cisplatin), and iodinated radiocontrast nephropathy. Contrast-induced nephropathy is the third-most common cause of new-onset AKI in hospitalized patients. AIN can develop after exposure to a variety of medications, most commonly nonsteroidal antiinflammatory drugs, antibiotics, and proton pump inhibitors.
- Causes of AKI are listed in Table 2.
- Nearly one third of cases of AKI may be prevented or mitigated by appropriate intervention.

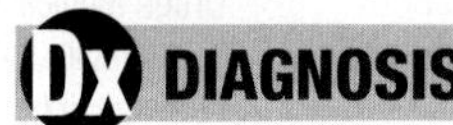

DIAGNOSIS

Table 3 summarizes useful clinical features, urinary findings, and confirmatory tests in the differential diagnosis of AKI.

DIFFERENTIAL DIAGNOSIS

Refer to "Etiology." Diagnostic tests to distinguish prerenal and renal AKI are described in Table 4. A diagnostic approach to patients with suspected AKI is shown in Fig. 1.

LABORATORY TESTS

- Elevated serum creatinine: Rate of rise is approximately 0.5 to 2 mg/dl per day in complete kidney failure.
- Standard estimating equations for glomerular filtration rate (GFR) require steady-state creatinine levels and are not recommended to estimate GFR during AKI.
- Elevated blood urea nitrogen (BUN): BUN-to-creatinine ratio is commonly >20:1 in prerenal azotemia, postrenal azotemia, and acute glomerulonephritis.
- BUN-to-creatinine ratio is <20:1 in acute interstitial nephritis and ATN.
- Hyperkalemia, hyperphosphatemia, and metabolic acidosis are common.
- Hypocalcemia and hyponatremia or hypernatremia may occur, depending on underlying etiology.
- Urinalysis is the initial step of diagnostic evaluation. Prerenal and postrenal AKI are typically characterized by a normal urinalysis. Conversely, abnormal findings should prompt further work-up for specific intrinsic causes of AKI that may require urgent intervention. Hematuria and proteinuria imply

TABLE 1 Kidney Disease: Improving Global Outcomes (KDIGO) Criteria for Diagnosis of Acute Kidney Injury

AKI Definition and Staging		
Stage	**Serum Creatinine Criteria**	**Urine Output Criteria**
1	$\Delta S_{Cr} \geq 0.3$ mg/dl (30 μmol/L) or $S_{Cr} \geq 1.5$, $<2.0 \times$ baseline*	UO <0.5 ml/kg per hour × 6-12 h
2	$S_{Cr} >2.0$, $<3.0 \times$ baseline	UO <0.5 ml/kg per hour > 12 h
3	$S_{Cr} >3.0 \times$ baseline or $S_{Cr} \geq 4.0$ mg/dl with an acute rise ≥ 0.5 mg/dl (50 μmol/L) or on renal replacement therapy	UO <0.3 ml/kg per hour × 24 h or anuria × 12 h

SCr, serum creatinine; *UO,* urinary output.
*To fulfill AKI criteria, a SCr rise of ≥0.3 mg/dl must occur within 48 hours; or increase to ≥1.5 times baseline SCr is known or presumed to have occurred within previous 7 days.
Adapted from KDIGO Clinical Practice Guideline for Acute Kidney Injury, 2012.

TABLE 2 Etiologies of Acute Kidney Injury

Prerenal Causes (Decreased Renal Blood Flow)	Intrinsic Renal Causes	Postrenal Causes
Hypovolemia Renal losses (diuretics, osmotic agents, polyuria) Gastrointestinal losses (vomiting, diarrhea) Cutaneous losses (burns, exfoliative syndromes) Hemorrhage Pancreatitis **Decreased Cardiac Output** Congestive heart failure Pulmonary embolism Acute myocardial infarction Severe valvular heart disease Abdominal compartment syndrome Renal artery obstruction (stenosis, embolism, thrombosis, dissection) **Systemic Vasodilation** Sepsis Anaphylaxis Anesthetics Drug overdose **Afferent Arteriolar Vasoconstriction** Hypercalcemia Drugs (NSAIDs, amphotericin B, calcineurin inhibitors, norepinephrine, radiocontrast agents, aminoglycosides) Hepatorenal syndrome Efferent arteriolar vasodilation (angiotensin converting enzyme inhibitors, aldosterone receptor blockers)	**Vascular: Large and Small Vessels** Trauma Renal vein obstruction (thrombosis, ventilation with high-level PEEP, abdominal compartment syndrome) Microangiopathy (thrombotic thrombocytopenic purpura, hemolytic-uremic syndrome, disseminated intravascular coagulation, preeclampsia) Malignant hypertension Scleroderma renal crisis Transplant rejection Atheroembolic disease **Glomerular** Antiglomerular basement membrane disease (Goodpasture syndrome) Antineutrophil cytoplasmic antibody-associated glomerulonephritis (Wegener granulomatosis) Immune complex glomerulonephritis, systemic lupus erythematosus, postinfectious cryoglobulinemia, primary membranoproliferative glomerulonephritis **Tubular** Ischemic Cytotoxic Heme pigment (rhabdomyolysis, intravascular hemolysis) Crystals (tumor lysis syndrome, seizures, ethylene glycol poisoning, vitamin C megadose, acyclovir, indinavir, methotrexate) Drugs (aminoglycosides, lithium, amphotericin B, pentamidine, cisplatin, ifosfamide, radiocontrast agents), synthetic cannabinoid use **Interstitial** Drugs (penicillins, cephalosporins, NSAIDs, proton pump inhibitors, allopurinol, rifampin, indinavir, mesalamine, sulfonamides, trimethoprim) Infection (pyelonephritis, viral infection) **Systemic Disease** Sjögren syndrome, sarcoidosis, systemic lupus erythematosus, lymphoma, leukemia, tubulonephritis, uveitis	**Ureteral Obstruction** Calculus Tumor (intrinsic or extrinsic) Fibrosis Ligation during pelvic surgery **Bladder Neck Obstruction** Benign prostatic hypertrophy Prostate cancer Neurogenic bladder Tricyclic antidepressants Ganglionic blockers Bladder tumor Calculus Hemorrhage/clot **Urethral Obstruction** Strictures Tumor Phimosis Renal calcinosis Obstructed urinary catheter, ureteral stent, or ileal conduit Pelvic trauma, retroperitoneal hematoma

NSAIDs, Nonsteroidal antiinflammatory drugs; *PEEP,* positive end-expiratory pressure.
Modified from Cameron JL, Cameron AM: *Current surgical therapy,* ed 10, Philadelphia, 2011, Saunders.

glomerulonephritis, heavy (>3+) proteinuria is associated with nephrotic syndrome, and leukocyturia may signify AIN. Microscopic examination of urine sediment may facilitate diagnosis: granular casts in ATN, dysmorphic red blood cells or red blood cell casts in acute glomerulonephritis, and white blood cell casts in AIN.

- In oliguric patients, obtain urine sodium and creatinine concentrations for determination of fractional excretion of sodium [FE_{Na} = 100% × ($U_{Na} \times P_{Cr}$)/($P_{Na} \times U_{Cr}$)]. FE_{Na} <1% is seen in prerenal AKI and >1% in intrinsic AKI. FE_{Na} may be falsely elevated in patients taking diuretics or falsely low in several intrinsic renal conditions, including acute glomerulonephritis, contrast-induced nephropathy, and rhabdomyolysis.
- Fractional excretion of urea (FE_{Urea}) may be used to assess renal dysfunction in AKI. FE_{Urea} is calculated as [FE_{Urea} = 100% × ($U_{Urea} \times P_{Cr}$) / ($P_{Urea} \times U_{Cr}$)]. FE_{Urea} <35% suggests prerenal acute kidney injury, and FE_{Urea} >50% indicates intrinsic AKI. FE_{Urea} is more useful than FE_{Na} during diuretic therapy.
- Urinary osmolarity is 250 to 300 mOsm/kg in ATN (isosthenuria), <400 mOsm/kg in postrenal azotemia, and >500 mOsm/kg in prerenal azotemia and acute glomerulonephritis.
- Blood cultures for suspected sepsis.
- In suspected glomerulonephritis (GN) (e.g., hematuria plus proteinuria, suggestive systemic clinical picture), additional serologic testing may be warranted. Abnormal liver function tests and elevated inflammatory markers are nonspecific. Immune complex deposition disorders (e.g., infectious GN, lupus nephritis, cryoglobulinemic vasculitis) are characterized by decreased complement (C3, C4) levels. Specific testing may include antinuclear antibodies (lupus), antineutrophil cytoplasmic antibodies (ANCA-associated vasculitis), anti-glomerular basement membrane antibodies (Goodpasture syndrome), and cryoglobulins. Kidney biopsy is frequently required for diagnostic confirmation.
- Creatinine kinase level is indicated if rhabdomyolysis is suspected; positive blood reaction on a urine dipstick with few or no red blood cells by microscopy may indicate myoglobinuria from rhabdomyolysis, but this finding is not invariable.
- Serum free light chain analysis, serum and urine protein electrophoresis, and serum and urine immunofixation electrophoresis for suspected multiple myeloma or other plasma cell dyscrasias. Myeloma can cause AKI via a variety of mechanisms, including tubular precipitation of light chains (cast nephropathy), hypercalcemia, and amyloidosis, among others.
- Kidney biopsy may be indicated in patients with intrinsic kidney failure when considering specific therapy. The major reasons for renal biopsy are for the differential diagnosis of nephrotic syndrome, distinguishing lupus vasculitis from other vasculitides, and lupus membranous nephropathy from idiopathic membranous nephropathy, confirmation of hereditary nephropathies based on ultrastructure, diagnosis of rapidly progressive glomerulonephritis, distinguishing AIN from ATN, and separation of primary glomerulonephritides. In addition to establishing a diagnosis, biopsy may determine renal prognosis and guide direction of management. Severe interstitial fibrosis is associated with poor renal outcomes.
- Biomarkers of kidney injury have been explored for earlier diagnosis of AKI or to separate intrinsic from prerenal causes. Candidate markers include cystatin C, neutrophil gelatinase-associated lipocalin (NGAL), kidney-injury molecule 1 (KIM-1), and liver fatty acid binding protein (LFABP).
- In 2014, tissue inhibitor of metalloproteinases and insulin-like growth-factor binding protein 7 (TIMP2*IGFBP7) became the first biomarker for AKI risk prediction approved in the U.S. However, there remains little published experience with this test, and the clinical role remains undefined.

TABLE 3 Useful Clinical Features, Urinary Findings, and Confirmatory Tests in the Differential Diagnosis of Acute Kidney Injury

Cause of Acute Kidney Injury	Some Suggestive Clinical Features	Typical Urinalysis Results	Some Confirmatory Tests
Prerenal azotemia	Evidence of true volume depletion (thirst, postural or absolute hypotension and tachycardia, low jugular venous pressure, dry mucous membranes and axillae, weight loss, fluid output greater than input) or decreased effective circulatory volume (e.g., heart failure, liver failure), treatment with NSAID, diuretic, or ACE inhibitor/ARB	Hyaline casts FE_{Na} <1% U_{Na} <10 mmol/L SG >1.018	Occasionally requires invasive hemodynamic monitoring; rapid resolution of AKI with restoration of renal perfusion
Diseases Involving Large Renal Vessels			
Renal artery thrombosis	History of atrial fibrillation or recent myocardial infarction, nausea, vomiting, flank or abdominal pain	Mild proteinuria Occasionally RBCs	Elevated LDH level with normal transaminase levels, renal arteriogram, MAG3 renal scan, MRA*
Atheroembolism	Usually age >50 yr, recent manipulation of aorta, retinal plaques, subcutaneous nodules, palpable purpura, livedo reticularis	Often normal Eosinophiluria Rarely casts	Eosinophilia, hypocomplementemia, skin biopsy, renal biopsy
Renal vein thrombosis	Evidence of nephrotic syndrome or pulmonary embolism, flank pain	Proteinuria, hematuria	Inferior venacavogram, Doppler flow studies, MRV*
Diseases of Small Renal Vessels and Glomeruli			
Glomerulonephritis or vasculitis	Compatible clinical history (e.g., recent infection), sinusitis, lung hemorrhage, rash or skin ulcers, arthralgias, hypertension, edema	RBC or granular casts, RBCs, white blood cells, proteinuria	Low complement levels; positive antineutrophil cytoplasmic antibodies, anti-glomerular basement membrane antibodies, anti-streptolysin O antibodies, anti-DNase, cryoglobulins; renal biopsy
HUS/TTP	Compatible clinical history (e.g., recent gastrointestinal infection, cyclosporine, anovulants), pallor, ecchymoses, neurologic findings	May be normal, RBCs, mild proteinuria, rarely RBC or granular casts	Anemia, thrombocytopenia, schistocytes on peripheral blood smear, low haptoglobin level, increased LDH, renal biopsy
Malignant hypertension	Severe hypertension with headaches, cardiac failure, retinopathy, neurologic dysfunction, papilledema	May be normal, RBCs, mild proteinuria, rarely RBC casts	LVH by echocardiography or ECG, resolution of AKI with BP control
Ischemic or Nephrotoxic Acute Tubular Necrosis			
Ischemia	Recent hemorrhage, hypotension, surgery often in combination with vasoactive medication (e.g., ACE inhibitor, NSAID)	Muddy-brown granular or tubular epithelial cell casts FE_{Na} >1%, U_{Na} >20 mmol/L SG ≈ 1.010	Clinical assessment and urinalysis usually inform diagnosis
Exogenous toxin	Recent contrast medium-enhanced procedure; nephrotoxic medications; certain chemotherapeutic agents often with coexistent volume depletion, sepsis, or chronic kidney disease	Muddy-brown granular or tubular epithelial cell casts FE_{Na} >1%, U_{Na} >20 mmol/L SG ≈ 1.010	Clinical assessment and urinalysis usually inform diagnosis
Endogenous toxin	History suggestive of rhabdomyolysis (coma, seizures, drug abuse, trauma)	Urine supernatant tests positive for heme in absence of RBCs	Hyperkalemia, hyperphosphatemia, hypocalcemia, increased CK, myoglobin
	History suggestive of hemolysis (recent blood transfusion)	Urine supernatant pink and tests positive for heme in absence of RBCs	Hyperkalemia, hyperphosphatemia, hypocalcemia, hyperuricemia, and free circulating hemoglobin
	History suggestive of tumor lysis (recent chemotherapy), myeloma (bone pain), or ethylene glycol ingestion	Urate crystals, dipstick-negative proteinuria, oxalate crystals, respectively	Hyperuricemia, hyperkalemia, hyperphosphatemia (for tumor lysis); circulating or urinary monoclonal protein (for myeloma); toxicology screen, acidosis, osmolal gap (for ethylene glycol)
Diseases of the Tubulointerstitium			
Allergic interstitial nephritis	Recent ingestion of drug and fever, rash, loin pain, or arthralgias	White blood cell casts, white blood cells (frequently eosinophiluria), RBCs, rarely RBC casts, proteinuria (occasionally nephritic)	Systemic eosinophilia, renal biopsy
Acute bilateral pyelonephritis	Fever, flank pain and tenderness, toxic state	Leukocytes, occasionally white blood cell casts, RBCs, bacteria	Urine and blood cultures
Postrenal AKI	Abdominal and flank pain, palpable bladder	Frequently normal, hematuria if stones, prostatic hypertrophy	Plain abdominal radiography, renal ultrasonography, postvoid residual bladder volume, computed tomography, retrograde or antegrade pyelography

ACE, Angiotensin-converting enzyme; *AKI,* acute kidney injury; *ARB,* angiotensin receptor blocker; *BP,* blood pressure; *CK,* creatine kinase; *DNase,* deoxyribonuclease; *ECG,* electrocardiography; *FE_{Na},* fractional excretion of sodium; *HUS,* hemolytic uremic syndrome; *LDH,* lactate dehydrogenase; *LVH,* left ventricular hypertrophy; *MAG3,* mercaptoacetyltriglycine; *MRA,* magnetic resonance angiography; *MRV,* magnetic resonance venography; *NSAID,* nonsteroidal antiinflammatory drug; *RBC,* red blood cell; *SG,* specific gravity; *TTP,* thrombotic thrombocytopenic purpura; *U_{Na},* urinary sodium concentration.

*Contrast-enhanced MRA and MRV should be used with extreme caution in patients with AKI.

From Skorecki K, Chertow GM, Marsden PA, et al.: *Brenner & Rector's the kidney*, ed 10, Philadelphia, 2016, Elsevier.

TABLE 4 Diagnostic Tests to Distinguish between Prerenal and Renal Acute Kidney Injury

Index	Prerenal Causes	Renal Causes
FENa	<1%	>2%
Urine sodium	<10 mmol/L	>40 mmol/L
Urine/plasma osmolality	>1.5	1 to 1.5
Renal failure index	<1	>2
BUN/creatinine ratio	>20	<10

BUN, Blood urea nitrogen; *FENa,* fractional excretion of sodium. Calculation of FENa: (Urine sodium × Plasma creatinine)/(Plasma sodium × Serum creatinine) × 100. Renal failure index: (Urine sodium × Urine creatinine)/Plasma creatinine.
From Cameron JL, Cameron AM: *Current surgical therapy,* ed 10, Philadelphia, 2011, Saunders.

IMAGING STUDIES

- ECG for arrhythmia detection, especially in hyperkalemia: peaked T waves in precordial leads, widening QRS interval, and/or bradycardia with AV nodal blockade
- Chest radiograph to detect signs of congestive heart failure and pulmonary renal syndromes, which frequently present with alveolar hemorrhage (Goodpasture syndrome, ANCA-associated vasculitis)
- Kidney ultrasonography to determine kidney sizes (distinguishes acute from chronic kidney disease), presence of obstruction, and renal vascular status (Doppler study)
- Bladder scan to assess post-void residual urine when urinary obstruction is suspected
- Computed tomography (CT) with radiocontrast administration is typically avoided in AKI. However, unenhanced CT scans may identify obstructing ureteral stones

Rx TREATMENT

Management of AKI depends on the underlying etiology. Some conditions (e.g., glomerulonephritis) require specific therapy, but the general focus of treatment for established AKI is supportive care and limiting additional injury. Fig. 2 illustrates an algorithm for management of AKI.

NONPHARMACOLOGIC THERAPY

- Withdraw nephrotoxic medications.
- Evaluate volume status and correct hypovolemia. Goal of therapy is to increase cardiac output and improve tissue perfusion.
- Among patients in intensive care units, utilize hemodynamic tools to avoid excessive fluid administration in patients who are non-volume responsive.
- Dietary modification: (1) energy prescription of 29 to 36 Kcal/kg per day, (2) potassium restriction (60 mEq per day), (3) sodium restriction (90 mEq per day), (4) phosphorus restriction (800 mg per day), and (5) protein supplementation of 0.6 to 1.4 g/kg per day depending on requirement for dialysis.
- Daily weight to monitor for fluid retention (in addition to intake and output measurement).
- Modification of drug dosages or schedules of renally excreted medications. Dosing should consider the trajectory of renal function (during evolving and recovering AKI) and may require additional adjustments in patients who require dialysis.

ACUTE GENERAL Rx

- Correct electrolyte abnormalities and metabolic acidosis.
- Administer loop diuretics for volume overload.
- Administer vasopressors or vasodilators, when appropriate, to optimize cardiac output in congestive heart failure.

Specific treatment is variable and dependent on etiology of AKI:

- Prerenal: IV volume expansion with isotonic solutions in hypovolemic patients or those with shock.
- Intrinsic kidney failure: Discontinue all potential nephrotoxins and treat condition(s) causing kidney failure. In severe AIN cases, consider a trial of corticosteroids. For acute noninfectious glomerulonephritis, high-dose pulse corticosteroids are first-line therapy, typically in conjunction with other immunomodulatory therapy and plasma exchange, depending on the clinical scenario.
- Postrenal: Eliminate cause of obstruction. Immediate bladder catheter insertion for suspected bladder outlet obstruction. Percutaneous nephrostomy tubes or ureteral stents may be required for upper tract obstruction.
- Hyperkalemia-related ECG changes: IV (intravenous) calcium if electrocardiographic changes present; IV insulin and/or glucose to shift potassium into cells; and IV bicarbonate therapy when metabolic acidosis is present to shift potassium into cells. These three treatments are temporary, and definitive therapy requires potassium removal via the gastrointestinal tract (potassium-binding agents or cathartics) or urinary tract by diuretics or dialytic therapy.

Dialysis in AKI:

- General indications for initiation of dialysis during AKI.
  1. Uremic symptoms (encephalopathy, pericarditis)
  2. Extracellular fluid volume overload refractory to medical management
  3. Severe acid-base imbalance refractory to medical management
  4. Significant electrolyte derangement (e.g., hyperkalemia, hyponatremia) refractory to medical management
- Among critically ill patients, dialysis may be warranted even in the absence of the previous indications. Optimal timing of initiation of dialysis remains controversial and is not solely dependent on previous metabolic parameters. Ongoing clinical trials may help answer whether early dialysis is beneficial in AKI.
- Intermittent hemodialysis (IHD) and continuous renal replacement therapy (CRRT) have similar outcomes for patients with AKI. However, CRRT is associated with greater hemodynamic stability and fluid removal compared to conventional IHD. CRRT is the preferred modality in critically ill patients with hemodynamic instability.

ADJUNCTIVE Rx

- Monitoring of renal function parameters and electrolytes.
- Renally excreted drugs are adjusted according to creatinine clearance or glomerular filtration rate to prevent further kidney damage or other medication-related toxicities.
- Prevent further renal insult with appropriate volume expansion, particularly before contrast administration, and avoid nephrotoxic agents. Volume expansion with isotonic solutions is more effective than hydration with hypotonic solutions. Isotonic saline or bicarbonate-containing solutions are effective, with or without concomitant N-acetylcysteine prophylaxis, which has shown conflicting results regarding its ability to reduce the risk of iodinated radiocontrast-induced nephropathy.
- Renal function recovery (ability to discontinue dialysis) varies from 50% to 75% in AKI survivors. Preexisting CKD, longer duration of dialysis dependence, congestive heart failure, and older age are negative prognostic factors for renal function recovery.
- Overall mortality rate in AKI is nearly 25% and approaches 50% to 60% in patients who require acute dialysis.
- The combination of AKI and sepsis is associated with a mortality rate as high as 70%.

PEARLS & CONSIDERATIONS

- Patients with AKI are susceptible to infections and sepsis.
- In patients with community-acquired AKI, it is important to obtain a thorough medication history, including nonprescription medications or supplements.
- AKI survivors are at risk for development of CKD, and follow-up with monitoring of kidney function is essential even after apparent renal recovery.

SUGGESTED READINGS

Available at ExpertConsult.com

RELATED CONTENT

Acute Renal Failure (Patient Information)
Chronic Kidney Disease (Related Key Topic)

AUTHOR: **JUNIOR UDUMAN, M.D.**

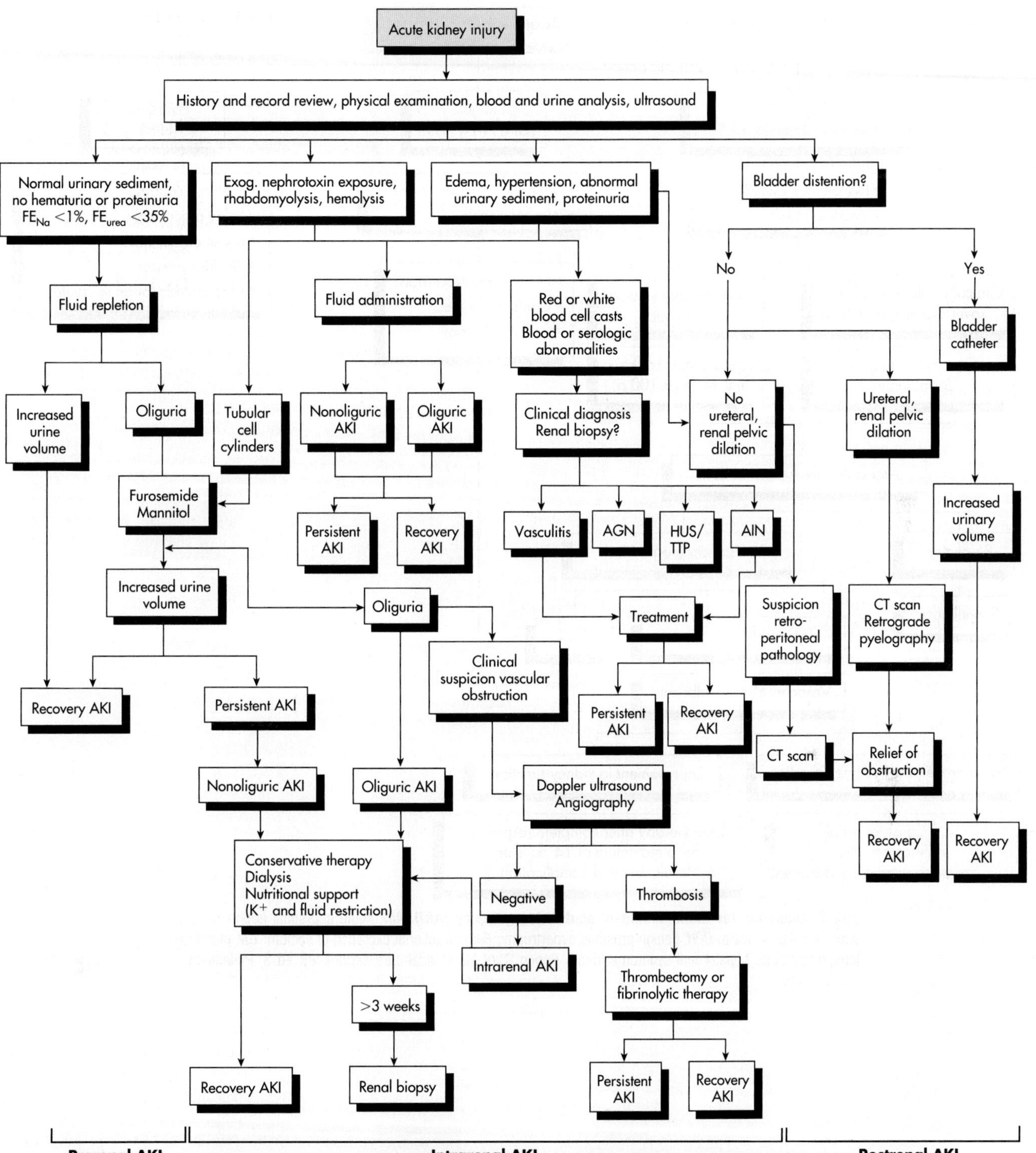

FIG. 1 Diagnostic approach to patients with suspected acute kidney injury *(AKI).* *AGN,* Acute glomerulonephritis; *AIN,* acute interstitial nephritis; *CT,* computed tomography; *Exog.,* exogenous; *HUS/TTP,* hemolytic-uremic syndrome/thrombotic thrombocytopenic purpura. (From Floege J, et al.: *Comprehensive clinical nephrology,* ed 4, Philadelphia, 2010, Saunders.)

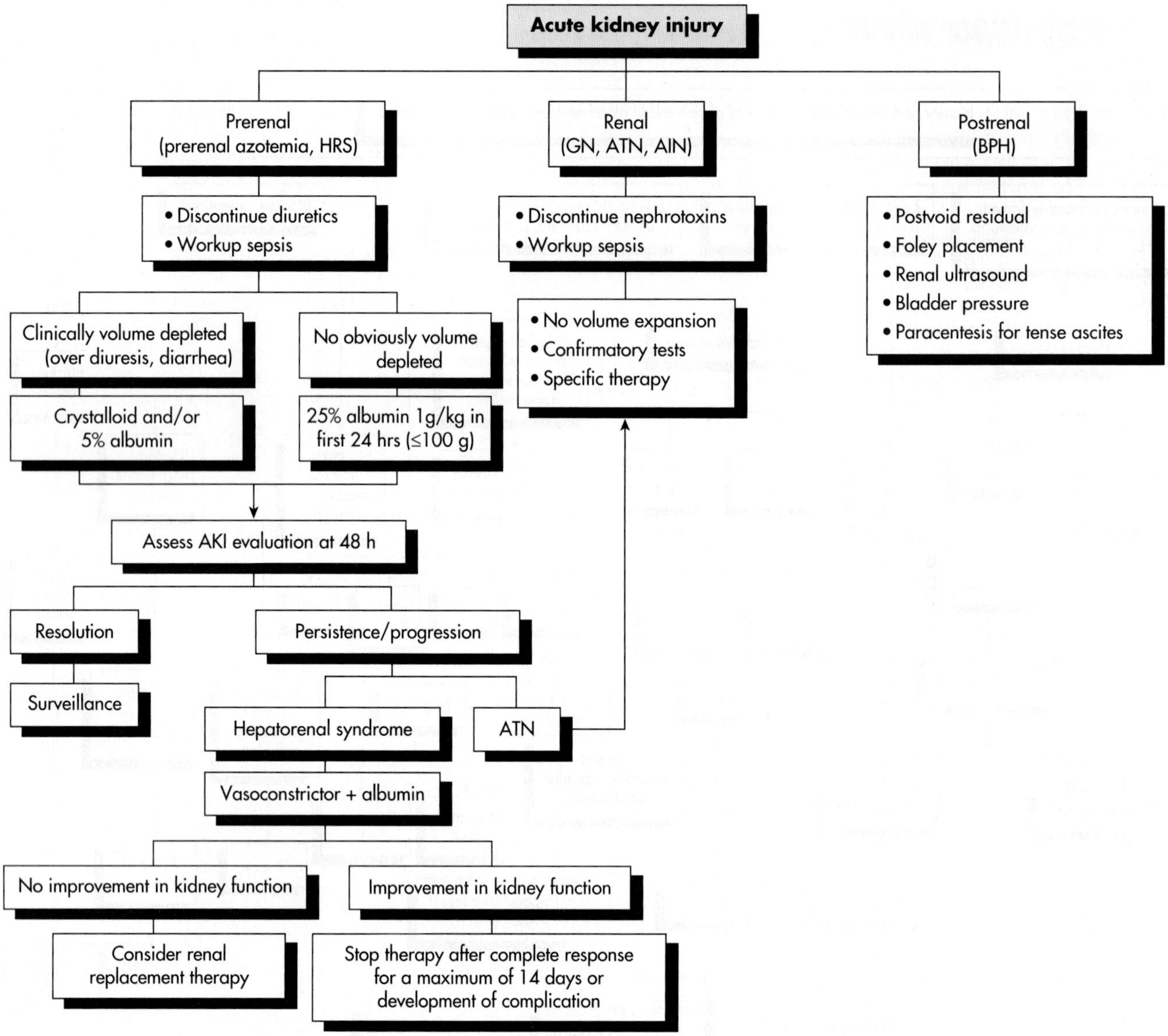

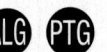

Acute kidney injury

- Prerenal (prerenal azotemia, HRS)
  - • Discontinue diuretics • Workup sepsis
    - Clinically volume depleted (over diuresis, diarrhea)
      - Crystalloid and/or 5% albumin
    - No obviously volume depleted
      - 25% albumin 1g/kg in first 24 hrs (≤100 g)
    - Assess AKI evaluation at 48 h
      - Resolution
        - Surveillance
      - Persistence/progression
        - Hepatorenal syndrome
          - Vasoconstrictor + albumin
            - No improvement in kidney function
              - Consider renal replacement therapy
            - Improvement in kidney function
              - Stop therapy after complete response for a maximum of 14 days or development of complication
        - ATN (→ No volume expansion, Confirmatory tests, Specific therapy)
- Renal (GN, ATN, AIN)
  - • Discontinue nephrotoxins • Workup sepsis
    - • No volume expansion • Confirmatory tests • Specific therapy
- Postrenal (BPH)
  - • Postvoid residual • Foley placement • Renal ultrasound • Bladder pressure • Paracentesis for tense ascites

FIG. 2 Algorithm for management of acute kidney injury *(AKI).* *AIN,* Acute interstitial nephritis; *ATN,* acute tubular necrosis; *BPH,* benign prostatic hypertrophy; *FeNa,* fractional excretion of sodium; *GN,* glomerulonephritis; *HRS,* hepatorenal syndrome. (From Ronco C, et al.: *Critical care nephrology,* ed 3, Philadelphia, 2019, Elsevier.)

BASIC INFORMATION

DEFINITION

Acute liver failure (ALF) is defined as rapid development (<26 wk) of severe hepatic injury, coagulation abnormalities (international normalized ratio [INR] >1.5), and encephalopathy in a patient without preexisting liver disease, in the absence of acute alcoholic hepatitis. However, ALF can also be diagnosed in patients with preexisting Wilson disease, vertically acquired hepatitis B, and autoimmune hepatitis, provided that diagnosis of these conditions was made within the preceding 26 weeks. Box 1 summarizes classifications of acute liver failure.

SYNONYMS

Fulminant hepatic failure
Fulminant hepatitis
Fulminant hepatic necrosis
Acute hepatic necrosis
Acute and subacute necrosis of liver
ALF

ICD-10CM CODES

K72	Hepatic failure, not elsewhere classified
K72.0	Acute and subacute hepatic failure
K72.00	Acute and subacute hepatic failure without coma
K72.01	Acute and subacute hepatic failure with coma

EPIDEMIOLOGY & DEMOGRAPHICS

INCIDENCE (IN U.S.): Affects approximately 2000 people/yr

PREDOMINANT SEX AND AGE: Seen more in women (90% of cases), average age 38 yr

RISK FACTORS:
- Intentional or inadvertent drug overdose
- Risk factors for viral hepatitis:
  - Intravenous drug use
  - Occupational exposure to blood or body fluids
  - Blood transfusions
  - Hemodialysis
  - Intranasal cocaine use
  - Imprisonment
  - Travel to endemic hepatitis areas
- Previous alcohol use
- Hepatotoxic medications
- Critical illness

PHYSICAL FINDINGS & CLINICAL PRESENTATION

- By definition, **symptoms** of ALF must include some degree of encephalopathy (see Table 1) but otherwise are nonspecific, such as fatigue, lethargy, anorexia, and nausea/vomiting. Pruritus, jaundice, and abdominal pain may be present.
- **Physical examination findings** may include jaundice, asterixis, hepatomegaly, decreased hepatic mass on percussion, and ascites. Multisystem organ failure can ensue. In rare cases, cerebral edema and increased intracranial pressure can occur, with abnormal pupillary exam findings, hypertension, bradycardia, respiratory depression (Cushing's triad), seizures, and loss of brain stem reflexes.
- Vesicular skin lesions are suggestive of herpes simplex virus (HSV).
- Family history of unexplained liver disease/cirrhosis should prompt ocular exam to look for Kayser-Fleischer rings (copper rings around the iris seen in Wilson disease).

BOX 1 Classifications of Acute Liver Failure

Trey and Davidson
Fulminant hepatic failure: Development of HE within 8 weeks of onset of symptoms

British Classification
Acute liver failure (includes only patients with encephalopathy)

Subclassification Depending on the Interval between the Onset of Jaundice and HE
- Hyperacute liver failure: 0 to 7 days
- Acute liver failure: 8 to 28 days
- Subacute liver failure: 29 to 72 days
- Late-onset acute liver failure: 56 to 182 days

French Classification
Acute hepatic failure: A rapidly developing impairment of liver function
Severe acute hepatic failure: Prothrombin time or factor V concentration below 50% of normal with or without HE

Subclassification
- Fulminant hepatic failure: HE within 2 weeks of onset of jaundice
- Subfulminant hepatic failure: HE between 3 and 12 weeks of onset of jaundice

International Association for the Study of Acute Liver Failure
Acute liver failure (occurrence of HE within 4 weeks after onset of symptoms)

Subclassification
- Acute liver failure—hyperacute: Within 10 days
- Acute liver failure—fulminant: 10 to 30 days
- Acute liver failure—not otherwise specified
- Subacute liver failure (development of ascites and/or HE from 5 to 24 weeks after onset of symptoms)

HE, Hepatic encephalopathy.
From Vincent JL, Abraham E, Moore FA et al: *Textbook of critical care*, ed 7, Philadelphia, 2017, Elsevier.

ETIOLOGY

- Common causes in the Western world include:
  1. Acetaminophen toxicity (46%)
  2. Indeterminate (14%)
  3. Idiosyncratic drug reaction (12%)
  4. Viral hepatitis (A, B) (10%)

  Rarer causes include alcoholic hepatitis, autoimmune hepatitis, Wilson disease, ischemic hepatopathy, Budd-Chiari syndrome, acute fatty liver of pregnancy, venoocclusive disease, toxin ingestion (e.g., mushroom poisoning *[Amanita phalloides]*), sepsis, infiltrative malignancy (breast cancer, lymphoma, myeloma, melanoma, small cell lung cancer), and other viruses (adenovirus, hepatitis E, HSV). Box 2 summarizes an etiologic classification of liver failure.

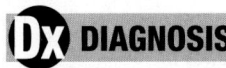

DIAGNOSIS

DIFFERENTIAL DIAGNOSIS

- Severe acute hepatitis, also known as acute liver injury (including alcoholic hepatitis): jaundice and coagulopathy without encephalopathy
- Acute on chronic liver failure (in patients with liver disease duration >26 weeks)
- Cirrhosis (includes decompensated cirrhosis)
- Hepatocellular carcinoma

WORKUP (BOX 3)

- Fig. 1 describes an algorithm for evaluation of acute liver failure.
- Clinical history is critical and should include medication use (6-month history of prescriptions, over-the-counter medications, herbal supplements), alcohol use, recreational drug use, prior symptoms of jaundice, onset of symptoms, history of suicide attempts, recent travel to endemic areas of viral hepatitis, and family history of liver failure/disease.
- Grading of hepatic encephalopathy should be performed (Table 1). Perform an asterixis maneuver, consider psychometric tests (i.e., number connection test) to detect subtle degree of encephalopathy.
- Laboratory evaluation: complete blood count, liver function tests (LFTs) including prothrombin time and INR, chemistry panel (sodium,

TABLE 1 Grades of Encephalopathy

Grade	Description
I	Changes in behavior with minimal change in level of consciousness (mild confusion, slurred speech, sleep difficulties)
II	Gross disorientation, drowsiness, possibly asterixis, inappropriate behavior
III	Marked confusion, incoherent speech, sleeping most of the time but arousable to vocal stimuli
IV	Comatose, unresponsiveness to pain, decorticate or decerebrate posturing

BOX 2 Etiologic Classification of Acute Liver Failure

Acetaminophen Toxicity
Idiosyncratic Drug Injury

Infrequent Agents
Isoniazid
Valproate
Halothane
Phenytoin
Sulfonamide
Propylthiouracil
Amiodarone
Disulfiram
Dapsone
Bromfenac
Troglitazone
Zidovudine
Lamivudine
Lamotrigine
Gatifloxacin
Methotrexate

Miscellaneous Agents
Ecstasy
Cocaine
Phencyclidine

Rare Agents
Carbamazepine
Ofloxacin
Ketoconazole
Lisinopril
Nicotinic acid
Labetalol
Etoposide
Imipramine
Interferon alfa
Flutamide
Tolcapone
Nefazodone
Oral contraceptives

Combination Agents with Enhanced Hepatotoxicity
Alcohol-acetaminophen
Trimethoprim-sulfamethoxazole
Rifampicin-isoniazid
Amoxicillin-clavulanic acid

Viral Hepatitides
Hepatitis A, B, C, D, E, G
Human herpesvirus
Cytomegalovirus
Epstein-Barr virus
Herpes simplex virus
Varicella zoster virus
Paramyxovirus
Parvovirus B19
Adenovirus
Togavirus
Parvovirus
SEN virus
TT virus
Yellow fever virus

Toxins
CCl_4
Amanita phalloides
Yellow phosphorus
Herbal products

Vascular
Ischemic
Veno-occlusive disease
Budd-Chiari syndrome
Malignant infiltration
Non-Hodgkin's lymphoma

Miscellaneous
Wilson disease
Autoimmune hepatitis
Acute fatty liver of pregnancy
Reye syndrome

CCl_4, carbon tetrachloride.
From Vincent JL, Abraham E, Moore FA et al: *Textbook of critical care,* ed 7, Philadelphia, 2017, Elsevier.

BOX 3 Investigations in Fulminant Hepatic Failure

Baseline essential investigations
Biochemistry
- Bilirubin, transaminases
- Alkaline phosphatase
- Albumin
- Urea and electrolytes
- Creatinine
- Calcium, phosphate
- Ammonia
- Acid-base, lactate
- Glucose

Hematology
- Full blood count, platelets
- PT, PTT
- Factors V or VII
- Blood group cross-match

Septic screen
Omitting lumbar puncture
- Radiology
- Chest radiograph
- Abdominal ultrasound
- Head CT scan or MRI

Neurophysiology
- Electroencephalogram

Diagnostic investigations
Serum
- Acetaminophen levels
- Cu, ceruloplasmin (>3 yr)
- Autoantibodies
- Immunoglobulins
- Amino acids
- Lactate
- Pyruvate
- Hepatitis A, B, C, E
- EBV, CMV, HSV viral loads
- Other viruses

Urine
- Toxic metabolites
- Amino acids, succinylacetone
- Organic acids
- Reducing sugars

CMV, Cytomegalovirus; *CT,* computed tomography; *EBV,* Epstein-Barr virus; *HSV,* herpes simplex virus; *PT,* prothrombin time; *PTT,* partial thromboplastin time.
From Fuhrman BP, Zimmerman JJ: *Fuhrman and Zimmerman's pediatric critical care,* ed 4, Philadelphia, 2011, Mosby.

potassium, chloride, bicarbonate, BUN, creatinine, glucose, magnesium, phosphate, calcium), arterial blood gas, arterial lactate, blood type and screen, acetaminophen level, ethanol level, toxicology screen, viral hepatitis serologies (hepatitis A IgM, hepatitis B surface antigen, anti-hepatitis B core IgM, anti-hepatitis C antibody [gM and IgG]), hepatitis C viral load (HCV RNA), anti-hepatitis E IgM and IgG, HSV-1 IgM and HSV PCR, EBV DNA PCR, CMV DNA PCR, anti-hepatitis D IgM and IgG, hepatitis D viral load (HDV RNA), ceruloplasmin level (as well as serum copper and 24-hour urine copper if high suspicion), pregnancy test, arterial ammonia level, autoimmune markers (ANA, ASMA, total IgG levels), HIV-1, HIV-2, amylase, lipase.

- Imaging: abdominal ultrasound with Doppler (hard to diagnose cirrhosis because liver may appear nodular in ALF due to massive necrosis), consider cross-sectional imaging of the liver (triphasic CT, MRCP, or MR with gadolinium), CT/MRI of the head.
- Prompt liver biopsy (via transjugular approach to decrease risk of bleeding) should be performed in cases in which:
  1. The etiology is unknown after the initial workup; *or*
  2. Etiology is thought to be secondary to autoimmune hepatitis, malignancy, or HSV

LABORATORY TESTS

- Patients with ALF typically have a prolonged prothrombin time (INR >1.5), elevated transaminases, elevated bilirubin, and may have a low platelet count (<150,000).
- Other possible lab findings can include an elevated BUN/creatinine (studies show 30% to 50% also have acute kidney injury), hypoglycemia (impairment of gluconeogenesis), hypophosphatemia, hypomagnesemia, hypokalemia, metabolic acidosis or respiratory alkalosis, elevated LDH, and elevated ammonia.

IMAGING STUDIES

- Abdominal ultrasound with Doppler should be ordered to evaluate for Budd-Chiari syndrome, portal hypertension, hepatic congestion, and hepatic steatosis.
- CT or MRI scan of the head should be considered to ensure no other causes for altered mental status.

COMPLICATIONS

Complications or progression of liver failure may result in cerebral edema due to increased intracranial pressure (in up to 40% of patients), high-output cardiac failure, hypoglycemia, lactic acidosis, acute respiratory distress syndrome, upper gastrointestinal hemorrhage (in 1.5% of patients), infectious disease from impaired leukocyte function (in nearly 80% patients), acute kidney injury, and pancreatitis (particularly in acetaminophen-induced ALF). Hypotension can occur due to decreased oral intake as well as extravasation of fluid into extravascular space.

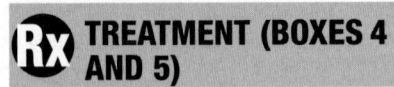

Rx TREATMENT (BOXES 4 AND 5)

NONPHARMACOLOGIC THERAPY

- Initial treatment should focus on the patient's mental status.
  1. Grade I/II encephalopathy may be managed on a medical ward (neuro vital signs q4h).
  2. Grade III and IV encephalopathy should be managed in ICU (elevate head of the bed to 30 degrees).

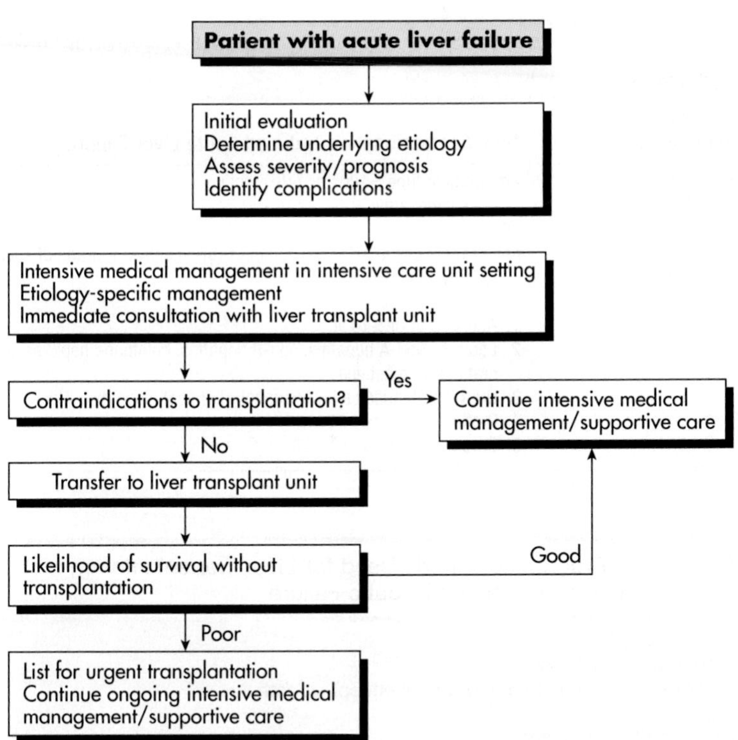

FIG. 1 Management of acute liver failure. (From Tally NJ: *Gastroenterology and hepatology,* Philadelphia, 2008, Churchill Livingston.)

3. Decrease stimulation (quiet room, no audible monitor alarms).
4. Avoid sedatives and opioids.

- A liver specialist should be notified urgently, and arrangements should be made for imminent transfer to a transplant center.
- Nutritional support should be initiated early. A daily intake goal of 60 g of protein is recommended to prevent catabolism of protein stores.
- Fluid support should be initiated if patient is not tolerating oral intake, or signs of hypoperfusion are present. Crystalloid solutions (normal saline in hypotensive patients, ½ normal saline + 75 mEq/L $NaCO_3$ in acidotic patients, normal saline + dextrose in hypoglycemic patients) can be used.

MONITORING

- Neuro exam q4h.
- Patients with suspected acetaminophen toxicity should have LFTs monitored every 12 hr. Otherwise, LFTs can be monitored daily.
- Chemistry panels and PT/INR should be monitored every 8 to 12 hr. Correction of coagulopathy should be avoided because it can interfere with assessment of liver function. In the setting of life-threatening bleeding, fresh frozen plasma (FFP) and recombinant factor VIIa can be considered.
- Glucose finger sticks should be checked every 4 hr initially to evaluate for hypoglycemia. If hypoglycemia is detected, dextrose should be added to crystalloid solution.
- Because of the increased risk of infection, daily urine, sputum, and blood cultures should be checked in the absence of signs or symptoms of infection.

PHARMACOLOGIC TREATMENT

- If acetaminophen is the known or suspected cause, an IV acetylcysteine protocol must be initiated. *N*-acetylcysteine is not harmful and dramatically alters the course in acetaminophen toxicity, so there should be a low threshold to start, particularly in young patients or those with no known cause of ALF.
    - The 20-hr protocol is:
        1. Initial loading dose of 150 mg/kg IV given over 60 min followed by;
        2. 12.5 mg/kg IV/hr over 4 hr followed by;
        3. 6.25 mg/kg IV/hr for 16 hr.
- A repeat acetaminophen level and ALT should be checked at hour 18 of NAC treatment. If either the acetaminophen level or the ALT is elevated, the 16-hour portion of treatment (6.25 mg/kg) should be extended and another ALT, INR, or acetaminophen level should be checked every 12 hr. The acetylcysteine can be stopped once the acetaminophen level is undetectable, INR <2, or ALT is shown to be either normal or decreasing. Additional information on acetaminophen overdose is available in the topic "Acetaminophen Poisoning."
- *N*-acetylcysteine therapy outside of acetaminophen poisoning has been investigated and may be beneficial; however, its routine use is not currently recommended by practice guidelines but is center specific.
- Patients should be placed on stress ulcer prophylaxis given the risk of gastrointestinal bleeding.
- Antibiotics should be started immediately if infection is suspected. Sources usually include respiratory, urinary, and blood; there is no evidence for empiric antibiotic treatment. Antifungals should be initiated if no initial improvement with antibiotics occurs.

BOX 4 Management of Fulminant Hepatic Failure

No sedation except for procedures
Minimal handling
Enteric precautions until infection ruled out
Monitor:
- Heart and respiratory rate
- Arterial BP, CVP
- Core/toe temperature
- Neurologic observations
- Gastric pH (>5.0)
- Blood glucose (>4 mmol/L)
- Acid-base
- Electrolytes
- PT, PTT

Fluid balance
- 75% maintenance
- Dextrose 10% to 50% (provide 6 to 10 mg/kg/min)
- Sodium (0.5 to 1 mmol/L)
- Potassium (2 to 4 mmol/L)

Maintain circulating volume with colloid/FFP
Coagulation support only if required
Drugs
- Vitamin K
- H_2 antagonist
- Antacids
- Lactulose
- *N*-acetylcysteine for acetaminophen toxicity
- Broad-spectrum antibiotics
- Antifungals

Nutrition
- Enteral feeding (1 to 2 g protein/kg/day)
- PN if ventilated

BP, Blood pressure; *CVP,* central venous pressure; *FFP,* fresh frozen plasma; *PN,* parenteral nutrition; *PT,* prothrombin time; *PTT,* partial thromboplastin time.
From Fuhrman BP, Zimmerman JJ: *Fuhrman and Zimmerman's pediatric critical care,* ed 4, Philadelphia, 2011, Mosby.

- Norepinephrine is the initial vasopressor of choice; vasopressin can be added as a second pressor. Persistent hypotension despite fluid resuscitation and pressor support should prompt concern for adrenal insufficiency.
- Lactulose is not routinely recommended for encephalopathy treatment; neomycin should be avoided due to concerns of nephrotoxicity.

PROGNOSIS

- Overall mortality from ALF is 30% to 40% and improved significantly over the last 20 yr.
- Transplant-free survival in ALF in the setting of acetaminophen, hepatitis A, shock liver, and pregnancy-related disease is >50%; for all other causes of ALF, transplant-free survival is <25%.
- Multiple models have been developed to predict spontaneous recovery in ALF patients (King's College criteria, Clichy criteria, MELD score, APACHE II score).
- The King's College criteria form the basis of the model most commonly used for prognostication (Table 2).

BOX 5 Hepatic Replacement Therapeutic Options Available to Patients with Fulminant Hepatic Failure

Liver Transplantation
- Cadaveric transplantation
- Whole liver
- Reduced-size liver
- Split liver
- Auxiliary partial liver
- Orthotopic position
- Heterotopic position
- Auxiliary whole liver
- Living-related transplantation
- Left lateral segment
- Left lobe
- Extended left lobe
- Right lobe

Artificial Liver Assist Devices
- Non–cell-based systems
- Charcoal hemoperfusion
- High-volume plasmapheresis
- Continuous high-frequency hemodiafiltration
- Molecular adsorbent recirculating system (MARS)
- Cell-based systems (bioartificial liver assist devices)
- Primary porcine hepatocytes
- Human hepatoblastoma cells
- Extracorporeal liver assist device (ELAD)

Hepatocyte Transplantation

From Vincent JL, Abraham E, Moore FA et al: *Textbook of critical care,* ed 6, Philadelphia, 2011, Saunders.

- Transplantation.
  1. Contraindications to listing include: medical history of psychiatric illness severe enough to affect patients' survival or likelihood of compliance with medications, active sepsis, severe medical comorbidities, increasing dependence on ventilator/inotropic support, acute substance abuse, previous episodes of self-harm (>5 episodes), refractory mental illness.
  2. Mortality on waiting list is 25%; 1-yr and 5-yr survival is 66% and 70%, respectively.
  3. Various prognostic criteria used for liver transplantation in patients with fulminant hepatic failure are summarized in Box 6.

TABLE 2 King's College Hospital Criteria for Liver Transplantation in Acute Liver Failure

Acetaminophen-Induced Acute Liver Failure	Non–Acetaminophen-Induced Acute Liver Failure
Arterial pH <7.3 (irrespective of grade of encephalopathy)	Prothrombin time >100 sec (irrespective of grade of encephalopathy
OR	*OR*
Grade III or IV encephalopathy *and* Prothrombin time >100 sec *and* Serum creatinine >3.4 mg/dl	Any of three of the following variables (irrespective of grade of encephalopathy): 1. Age <10 yr or >40 yr 2. Etiology: Non-A hepatitis, non-B hepatitis, halothane hepatitis, idiosyncratic drug reactions 3. Duration of jaundice before onset of encephalopathy >7 days 4. Prothrombin time >50 sec 5. Serum bilirubin >18 mg/dl

Sec; seconds.

BOX 6 Various Prognostic Criteria Used for Liver Transplantation in Patients with Fulminant Hepatic Failure

King's College Criteria

Acetaminophen Overdose
- Arterial pH <7.3 (irrespective of grade of encephalopathy)
- *or*
- PT >100 sec (INR >6.5) *and*
- Serum creatinine >3.4 mg/dl (>300 μmol/L) *and*
- Patients with grade III and IV hepatic encephalopathy

Non–Acetaminophen-Induced Liver Injury

Acute form (delayed jaundice-encephalopathy <7 days):
- PT >100 sec (INR >6.5) (irrespective of grade of encephalopathy) or any three of the following variables:
- Aged <10 or >40 yr
- Non-A, non-B hepatitis, halothane hepatitis, idiosyncratic drug reactions
- Subacute form: Delayed encephalopathy >7 days
- Serum bilirubin 17.4 mg/dl (300 μmol/L)
- PT >50 sec

Clichy Criteria
- Grade III or IV encephalopathy
  and
- Factor V <20% in patients <30 yr
  or
- Factor V <30% in patients >30 yr

Serum Gc Globulin Levels

Decreasing Gc levels due to dying hepatocytes

Serum α-Fetoprotein Levels

Serial increase from day 1 to day 3 has been correlated with survival

Liver Biopsy

70% necrosis is discriminant of 90% mortality

Gc, Plasma group-specific component protein; INR, international normalized ratio; PT, prothrombin time.
From Vincent JL, Abraham E, Moore FA et al: *Textbook of critical care,* ed 7, Philadelphia, 2017, Elsevier.

PEARLS & CONSIDERATIONS

- ALF is severe hepatic injury (as evidenced by elevated liver enzymes) with INR >1.5 and hepatic encephalopathy from a disease process that started <26 wk before presentation in a patient with no prior history of liver disease.
- Close to half of ALF is caused by drug ingestion, usually acetaminophen.
- Given the potential rapidity of deterioration, referral must be made as soon as possible to a liver transplant center.
- There should be a low threshold to start *N*-acetylcysteine.
- Do not correct coagulopathy unless life-threatening bleeding occurs or it is recommended by the liver transplant hepatologist.

SUGGESTED READINGS

Available at ExpertConsult.com

RELATED CONTENT

Acetaminophen Poisoning (Related Key Topic)
Ascites (Related Key Topic)
Encephalopathy (Related Key Topic)
Hepatopulmonary Syndrome (Related Key Topic)
Hepatorenal Syndrome (Related Key Topic)

AUTHORS: **TALIA ZENLEA, M.D.,** and **ALEXANDRA SHINGINA, M.D.C.M.**

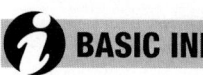

BASIC INFORMATION

DEFINITION

Acute lower gastrointestinal bleeding is defined as sudden colonic blood loss.

SYNONYMS

Acute colonic bleeding
Gastrointestinal hemorrhage
Melena
Hematochezia

ICD-10CM CODES

K92.2	Gastrointestinal hemorrhage, unspecified
K92.1	Melena
K62.5	Hemorrhage of rectum and anus

EPIDEMIOLOGY & DEMOGRAPHICS

INCIDENCE:

- Annual incidence in U.S. of lower gastrointestinal (GI) bleeding is 72/100,000.
- Annual incidence in U.S. of hospitalization is 36/100,000 (about half of that for upper GI bleeding).

PEAK INCIDENCE: The rate of lower GI bleeding, including that necessitating hospitalization, is higher in the elderly.

PREDOMINANT SEX AND AGE: 24.2/100,000 in males versus 17.2/100,000 in females. This increases 200-fold by the ninth decade of life

RISK FACTORS: Risk factors include NSAID use, aspirin use, alcohol abuse, GI malignancy, atrial fibrillation, coagulopathies, prior GI bleed, cirrhosis, constipation, congenital malformations, radiation exposure, recent infectious illness, recent travel, abdominal aortic aneurysm (AAA) repair, and inflammatory bowel disease.

PHYSICAL FINDINGS & CLINICAL PRESENTATION

- Attention should be paid in the history to details suggesting the location and etiology of the bleed. For instance, weight loss and abdominal pain suggest inflammatory bowel disease; recent AAA repair, especially with history of a sentinel bleed, raises suspicion for aortoenteric fistula; a history of cirrhosis suggests bleeding from portal hypertension, e.g., varices. Bright red blood is typically from a brisk upper GI bleed, distal colon, or anorectal disease. Melena arises from the upper GI tract, small bowel, or proximal colon. Take a detailed medication history, noting NSAIDs or other drugs that may cause or mimic GI bleeding as well as beta blockers that may mask tachycardia in the setting of significant blood loss.
- The clinician should first and foremost check vital signs, including orthostatics, if stable. Perform ABCs as indicated. Check for pallor and signs of volume depletion, such as delayed capillary refill and skin tenting. Observe for stigmata of liver disease, such as telangiectasias and jaundice. Auscultate for bowel sounds. Absence of bowel sounds may indicate perforation. Palpate the abdomen for pain, masses, and hepatosplenomegaly. Rectal exam should be performed, noting the presence of blood, rate of bleeding, masses, fissures, hemorrhoids, tenderness, and skin changes. If no gross bleed is seen, perform hemoccult testing. Ensure that the bleeding is, in fact, gastrointestinal, excluding hematuria, vaginal bleeding, and wounds.

ETIOLOGY

Diverticulosis is the most common cause of lower GI bleeding at 30%. Internal hemorrhoids are the second most common cause. 15% of lower GI bleeds are due to upper GI bleeding.

Dx DIAGNOSIS

DIFFERENTIAL DIAGNOSIS

- Upper GI bleed
- Diverticulosis
- Diverticulitis
- Ischemic colitis
- Postpolypectomy bleeding
- Vascular ectasias (angiodysplasia, arteriovenous malformation)
- Anal fissure
- Rectal ulcer
- Colonic polyps
- Advanced neoplasms
- Hemorrhoids
- Intussusception
- Coagulopathies
- Infectious colitis (*E. coli, Shigella, Salmonella, Giardia*)
- Autoimmune (hemolytic uremic syndrome)
- Radiation colitis or proctitis
- Aortoenteric fistula
- Vasculitis
- Inflammatory (ulcerative colitis, Crohn's disease)
- Colonic varices
- Drugs (iron, NSAIDs)
- Foreign body

WORK-UP

Establish large-bore intravenous access. If the patient has significant hematochezia without hematemesis, consider performing nasogastric lavage to evaluate for upper GI bleeding. An algorithm for the management of severe hematochezia is illustrated in Fig. 1.

LABORATORY TESTS

- Complete blood count may reveal anemia and/or thrombocytopenia. The hematocrit and hemoglobin should generally be trended every 4 to 6 hours to document the status of the bleed.
- Order a comprehensive metabolic panel to evaluate the following: elevated blood urea nitrogen, which indicates reabsorption of red blood cells; elevated creatinine, which indicates poor renal perfusion; liver function tests, which could reveal liver disease that is exacerbating bleeding.
- International normalized ratio, especially if patient is taking warfarin.
- Partial thromboplastin time, especially if the patient is on heparin.
- Type and screen/cross in anticipation of the need for blood products.
- Stool studies, including white blood cell count, gram stain, culture, and pathogen-specific testing to identify infectious etiologies.

IMAGING STUDIES

- Computed tomography (CT) angiography can potentially identify the location of the bleed as well as abnormal vasculature.
- Perform a tagged red blood cell scan if source is not identified on CT angiography.
- CT scan of the abdomen and pelvis may identify malignancy as the source of bleeding.
- If free air is suspected from perforation, an abdominal or chest plain film should be ordered immediately. An abdominal plain film can also identify radiopaque foreign bodies.
- Abdominal ultrasound if intussusception is suspected.
- Meckel (technetium-99) scan if Meckel's diverticulum is suspected.

Rx TREATMENT

Begin crystalloid bolus to maintain a systolic blood pressure of at least 100 mm Hg. Transfuse for hemoglobin and hematocrit of 7 and 21, respectively, or less. If the patient has coronary artery disease or multiple medical comorbidities and is older than 65 yr, the goal hemoglobin and hematocrit are 8 and 24, respectively. Platelets should be maintained above 50,000 mm and international normalized ratio 1.5 or less.

NONPHARMACOLOGIC THERAPY

- Colonoscopy defines the colonic anatomy, can identify the source of bleeding, and allows for potential therapy.
- Endoscopy can be performed if the source of the bleed is suspected to be proximal to the ligament of Treitz.
- Anoscopy can be performed for bleeding internal hemorrhoids or other anorectal disorders.
- Balloon tamponade of esophageal or anorectal bleeds.
- Perform surgery if the source of the bleed cannot be otherwise identified, for aortoenteric fistula, or if air enema for intussusception is unsuccessful.
- Interventional radiology for embolization.
- Ablation.

ACUTE GENERAL Rx

Proton pump inhibitor, histamine 2 blocker if suspecting UGI blood with rapid transit

CHRONIC Rx

Avoid NSAIDs and alcohol. Treat the underlying cause of the bleed, e.g., coagulopathy, portal hypertension, etc. Most patients are prescribed

 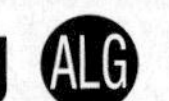

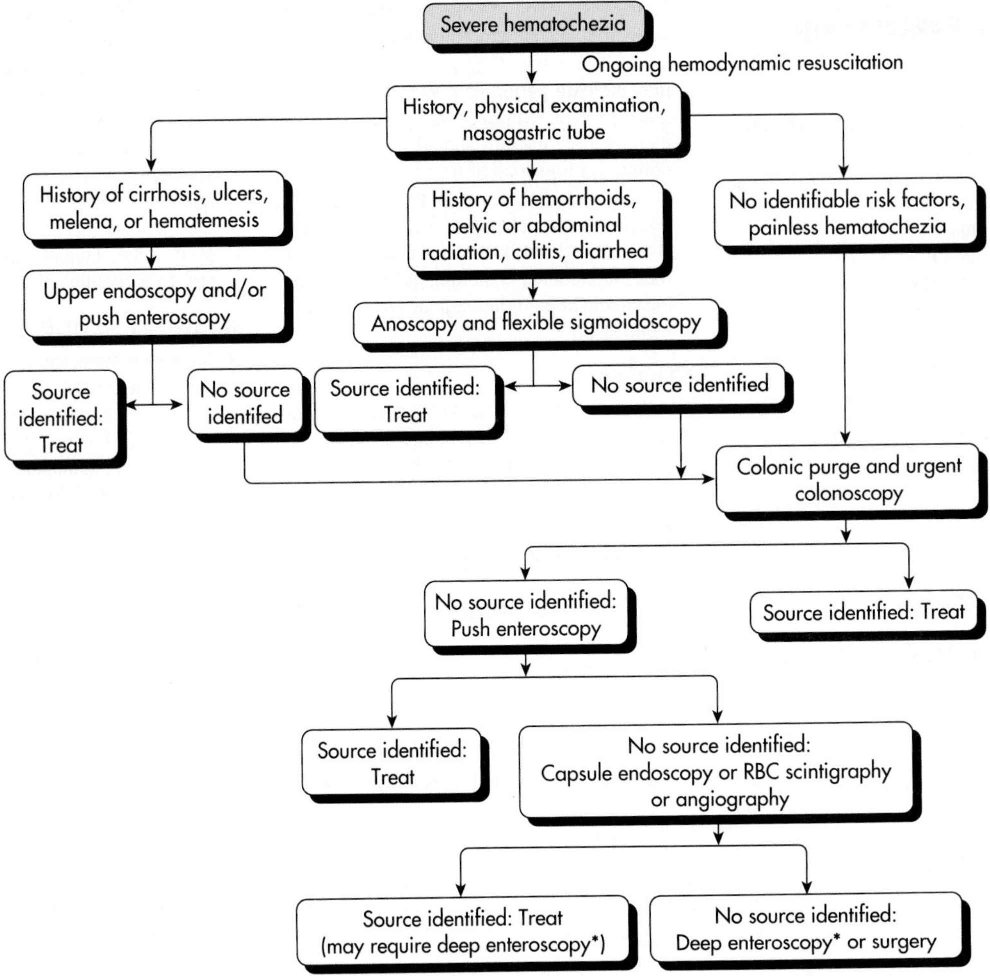

FIG. 1 Algorithm for the management of severe hematochezia modified according to patient's history. *Deep enteroscopy includes double-balloon enteroscopy, single-balloon enteroscopy, and spiral enteroscopy. *RBC,* red blood cell. (From Feldman M, et al.: *Sleisenger and Fortran's gastrointestinal liver disease*, ed 10, Philadelphia, 2016, Elsevier.)

daily proton pump inhibitors. Fiber, stool softeners, and analgesic creams may alleviate development and/or symptoms of hemorrhoids.

DISPOSITION

Most cases of acute lower GI bleeding will resolve spontaneously. Therefore, if the patient is hemodynamically stable without symptomatic anemia or brisk bleeding, he or she may follow up with his or her primary care physician or a gastroenterologist. However, patients with shock or other hemodynamic compromise, severe bleeding, or significant comorbidities should be admitted to the intensive care unit. These patients are at high risk for acute decompensation and as such require close monitoring and aggressive resuscitation; furthermore, they will require urgent diagnosis and intervention to stop the bleeding. Clinical factors predictive of severe colonic bleeding include aspirin use, at least two comorbid illnesses, pulse greater than 100 beats/minute, and systolic blood pressure <115 mm Hg. The overall mortality rate from colonic bleeding is 2.4% to 3.9%. Independent predictors of in-hospital mortality are age over 70 yr, intestinal ischemia, and two or more comorbidities.

REFERRAL

Patients should be referred to gastroenterology for follow-up.

SUGGESTED READINGS

Available at ExpertConsult.com

RELATED CONTENT

Bleeding, Gastrointestinal (Algorithm)
Colorectal Cancer (Related Key Topic)
Diverticular Disease (Related Key Topic)
Meckel Diverticulum (Related Key Topic)

AUTHORS: **AMANDA BOX, M.D., M.S.,** and **J. RICHARD WALKER III, M.D., M.S.**

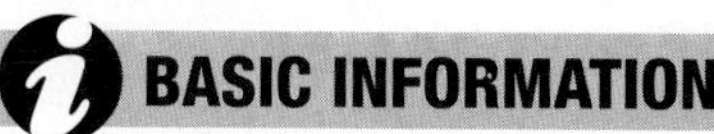

BASIC INFORMATION

DEFINITION

Acute lymphoblastic leukemia (ALL) is a malignancy of precursor B or T lymphocytes (lymphoblasts) characterized by uncontrolled proliferation of malignant lymphocytic cells with replacement of normal bone marrow elements and bone marrow failure. Lymphoblastic lymphoma is diagnosed when the disease presents in extramedullary sites (most commonly as mediastinal mass in T cell disease) *and* less than 25% of the bone marrow is involved.

SYNONYMS

Acute lymphocytic leukemia
Acute lymphoblastic leukemia
ALL

ICD-10CM CODES

C91.00	Acute lymphoblastic leukemia not having achieved remission
C91.01	Acute lymphoblastic leukemia, in remission
C91.02	Acute lymphoblastic leukemia, in relapse

EPIDEMIOLOGY & DEMOGRAPHICS

- ALL is primarily a disease of children (peak incidence occurring at 3-5 yrs of age).
- Overall incidence is 4.5 cases per 100,000 persons per yr; 60% are under age 20. It is the most common malignancy of childhood. (SEER database accessed 11/26/15)
- Incidence varies according to race and ethnic group: 14.8 cases per million for blacks, 35.6 cases per million for whites, and 40.9 cases per million for Hispanics.
- Male:female ratio is 55% to 45%.

PHYSICAL FINDINGS & CLINICAL PRESENTATION

- Findings consistent with bone marrow failure and peripheral cytopenias—pallor, bruising, petechiae.
- Lymphadenopathy or hepatosplenomegaly.
- Fever (disease related or infectious), bone pain, weakness, weight loss, mental status changes, and neurologic findings associated with central nervous system (CNS) involvement (if present).
- T cell lymphoblastic lymphoma is usually associated with a mediastinal mass.
- Table 1 summarizes the clinical presentation of acute lymphoblastic leukemia.

ETIOLOGY

- Most cases are sporadic without established risk factors.
- Ionizing radiation exposure appears to be a risk factor.
- Down's syndrome (trisomy 21) is associated with an approximately 3% risk of developing leukemia by age 30, predominantly ALL. ALL may be seen with other hereditary premalignancy syndromes (e.g., ataxia-telangiectasia)

DIAGNOSIS

DIFFERENTIAL DIAGNOSIS

Disorders associated with lymphocytosis (lymphocytes >5000/mcl):

- Adults: Chronic lymphocytic leukemia, mantle cell lymphoma, marginal zone lymphoma, hairy cell leukemia.
- Adolescents/young adults: Infectious mononucleosis syndromes due to Epstein-Barr virus or cytomegalovirus, among others, may present with lymphocyte abnormalities with appearance suggestive of leukemic blasts.
- Disorders associated with circulating blasts or blastlike cells such as acute myeloid leukemia, prolymphocytic leukemia, blastoid mantle cell lymphoma, and Burkitt's lymphoma (mature B cell leukemia/lymphoma).
- Lymphoblastic lymphoma.
- Aplastic anemia; ALL may present without circulating leukemia cells and with only manifestations of bone marrow failure.

WORKUP

- Identification of circulating abnormal cell population by flow cytometry. CD19 identifies most precursor B cells. Immature leukemic blasts should have *absence* of surface immunoglobulin and will usually express CD34 and stain positive for terminal deoxynucleotidyltransferase (TdT). Cytoplasmic CD3 and CD7 establish immature T cell lineage in most cases. Aberrant myeloid markers (CD13, CD33) can be seen.
- Cytochemical stains are sometimes easier to perform and may be available sooner but are less specific. ALL blasts should be negative for myeloperoxidase and esterase stains.
- Bone marrow examination (Fig. E1).
- Genetic studies define important treatment categories, of which the most important is Philadelphia chromosome positive (Ph+) vs. Philadelphia chromosome negative (Ph–) disease, as these are treated differently. Ph status can be determined rapidly by polymerase chain reaction (PCR) or fluorescence *in situ* hybridization (FISH) and should be available within 24 to 48 hours of diagnosis. The WHO classification recognizes genetic variants of ALL as distinct syndromes (Table 2), and the clinical significance of common abnormalities is outlined in Table 3.
- Genetic profiling for "Ph-like" ALL (genetic profile similar to Ph+ disease, but no BCR/ABL abnormality) or IKZF1 (IKAROS) mutations may provide additional prognostic information, but may not be uniformly available. Ph-like ALL may respond to tyrosine kinase inhibitor therapy and may behave more like Ph+ ALL.
- Lumbar puncture is usually done at diagnosis, if practical, to assess for CNS involvement and to initiate CNS prophylactic therapy.

LABORATORY TESTS

- Complete blood count reveals normochromic, normocytic anemia, thrombocytopenia.
- Peripheral smear will usually reveal lymphoblasts, but in some cases only the marrow is involved.
- Initial blood work should also include assessment for basic organ function (creatinine, bilirubin), blood glucose (glucocorticoids are part of therapy), and spontaneous tumor lysis syndrome (K+, Ca++, PO_4++, uric acid).
- Coagulation studies (full disseminated intravascular coagulation [DIC] screen) prior to lumbar puncture.
- Studies appropriate to identifying and risk-stratifying leukemia as outlined previously.

IMAGING STUDIES

- Chest x-ray to evaluate fever and for the presence of mediastinal mass.
- CT for symptomatic complaints. Be cautious about contrast dye exposure in patients with evidence of spontaneous tumor lysis syndrome to avoid further renal injury.

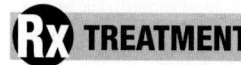

TREATMENT

ACUTE GENERAL Rx

- Survival of children with ALL has improved from 10% to 90% in the last 40 yrs and is a major success story of modern medical science and research. Adults have fared less

TABLE 1 Clinical Presentation of Acute Lymphoblastic Leukemia

Symptoms/ Signs	Etiology	Management
Fever	Disease or infection	Always conduct fever work up and provide broad antimicrobial coverage until infectious etiology is ruled out
Fatigue, pallor	Anemia (ALL infiltrating bone marrow)	Packed red blood cell transfusion (slow if anemia is severe, avoid in hyperleukocytosis)
Petechiae, bruising, bleeding	Thrombocytopenia (ALL infiltrating bone marrow)	Transfuse with platelets
Pain	Leukemia infiltrating bones/ joints, or expanding marrow cavity	Establish diagnosis and start chemotherapy
Respiratory distress/ superior vena cava syndrome	Mediastinal mass	Avoid sedation in presence of tracheal compression. Establish diagnosis as soon as possible and start chemotherapy

ALL, Acute lymphoblastic leukemia.
From Hoffman R, et al.: *Hematology, basic principles and practice*, ed 7, Philadelphia, 2018, Elsevier.

TABLE 2 WHO Classification of Precursor Lymphoid Neoplasms

B-lymphoblastic leukemia/lymphoma, not otherwise specified
B-lymphoblastic leukemia/lymphoma with recurrent cytogenetic abnormalities:
- B-lymphoblastic leukemia/lymphoma with t(9;22)(q34;q11.2); *BCR-ABL1*
- B-lymphoblastic leukemia/lymphoma with t(v*;11q23) *MLL* rearranged.
- B-lymphoblastic leukemia/lymphoma with t(12;21)(p13;q22); *TEL-AML1 (ETV6-RUNX1)*
- B-lymphoblastic leukemia/lymphoma with hyperdiploidy
- B-lymphoblastic leukemia/lymphoma with hypodiploidy
- B-lymphoblastic leukemia/lymphoma with t(5;14)(q32;q32); *IL3-IGH*
- B-lymphoblastic leukemia/lymphoma with t(1;19)(q23;p13.3); *EZA-PBX1 (TCF3-PBX-1)*

T-lymphoblastic leukemia/lymphoma
Provisional entities:
- B-lymphoblastic leukemia/lymphoma BCR/ABL1 like
- B lymphoblastic leukemia/lymphoma with iAMP21

Early T cell precursor lymphoblastic leukemia/lymphoma

*v**, Variable gene partners.

TABLE 3 More Common Recurrent Cytogenetic Abnormalities in B-Lymphoblastic Leukemia/Lymphoma

Abnormality	Clinical Relevance
t(9;22)(q34;q11.2); *BCR-ABL1*	Incidence approximately 3% in children, 25% in adults, rising with age; requires therapy with tyrosine kinase inhibitors.
t(v*;11q23) *MLL* rearranged.	Most common variant is t(4;11); often presents with very high WBC; confers worse prognosis; rare in adults; common in infant leukemia.
t(12;21)(p13;q22); *TEL-AML1*	Common in children (20%-30%); rare in adults; confers improved prognosis.
Hyperdiploidy	Seen in about 25% of children, less in adults; confers favorable prognosis.
Hypodiploidy	Uncommon; confers worse prognosis.
t(5;14)(q32;q32); *IL3-IGH*	Rare; commonly associated with eosinophilia; T cell disease, ? neutral prognostically
t(1;19)(q23;p13.3);	Incidence approximately 5%; intermediate/favorable in children, intermediate/poor in adults.

*v**, Variable gene partners. Many of these disorders also have distinct immunophenotypes by flow cytometry. Additional molecular abnormalities of recently defined relevance include mutations of IKZF1, which encodes a lymphoid transcription factor IKAROS, is associated with high relapse rates and gene expression profile similar to BCR-ABL1 translocated disease. Gene expression profiling has identified a subgroup of "Philadelphia chromosome-like" ALL with a gene expression similar to BCR-ABL1 translocation associated disease, which confers worse prognosis, but which may identify new opportunities for targeted therapies.

well, but cure rates have also improved to about 60% to 70% in standard-risk patients in recent trials. Adults in particular have benefited from tyrosine kinase inhibitor therapy for Ph+ ALL, since this disease is more common in adults and may represent 50% or more of disease in patients over 50.

- **Hyperleukocytic leukemia** (WBC >100,000/mcl) is uncommon in ALL and lymphocyte counts of 100,000 may be well tolerated. Prednisone and vincristine usually offer rapid cytoreduction and leukapheresis is rarely (but sometimes) required.
- **Tumor lysis syndrome** is common in ALL and was seen in 23% of patients in one large series. It is sometimes spontaneous—i.e., present before therapy is given—and is a potential cause of early death. Tumor lysis syndrome is caused by release of intracellular potassium, phosphate, and nucleic acids. The nucleic acids adenosine and guanosine are eventually metabolized to uric acid. Elevated potassium may cause cardiac dysrhythmia and death. Elevated uric acid may cause renal failure through renal urate crystal deposition and possibly other mechanisms. Elevated phosphates cause renal calcium phosphate deposition and kidney injury while also lowering serum calcium, which can cause cardiac dysrhythmia and spasms. Therapy is directed mainly at maintaining renal function through vigorous hydration (3 liters normal saline per day if practical, alkalinization *not* recommended); "forced diuresis" if necessary to maintain urine output at 2 ml/kg/h; and dialysis if necessary to control K^+, phosphates, or fluid balance. Allopurinol, up to 800 mg/day for adults, 300 to 450 mg/m²/day for children, is given routinely. Rasburicase is a recombinant urate oxidase that rapidly lowers uric acid levels. The dose is 0.2 mg/kg, and one dose is usually enough. Rasburicase should be avoided in patients with G6PD deficiency. Phosphate binders are of uncertain value but are usually given. Asymptomatic hypocalcemia is not treated to avoid increasing calcium phosphate deposition. Definitions of laboratory and clinical tumor lysis and defined risk categories are outlined in Table 4.
- Numerous protocols have been used for Ph-ALL, and the specific protocol is likely to be determined by institution/physician familiarity and access to clinical trials, among other factors.
- In the 1990s and early 2000s, it was noted that adolescents and young adult (AYA) patients had better outcomes on pediatric trials than on adult trials. Consequently, this group (currently defined as ages 15-39) is now often (especially younger AYAs) treated on pediatric protocols by pediatric services or on adult "pediatric inspired" protocols.
- Therapy for Ph-negative ALL generally has four components:
  1. Induction therapy, typically with corticosteroids, cyclophosphamide (some regimens), vincristine, an anthracycline (doxorubicin or daunorubicin usually), and asparaginase. The CD20 directed antibody rituximab has shown benefit in patients with greater than 20% CD20 expression on their blast cells.
  2. Consolidation therapy is high-dose chemotherapy aimed at preventing relapse after remission and commonly consists of cytarabine and methotrexate in combination with other agents.
  3. Maintenance therapy is low-intensity outpatient therapy that is continued for 2 to 3 yrs after completion of consolidation. Prednisone, monthly vincristine, methotrexate, and oral 6-mercaptopurine (POMP regimen) are commonly used.
  4. CNS prophylaxis is universal and is usually done with intrathecal therapy (methotrexate alone or in combination with cytarabine and hydrocortisone) administered by lumbar puncture or an Ommaya reservoir. Due to increased toxicity, cranial radiotherapy is reserved for patients with high-risk features, such as active CNS disease at diagnosis.
- Allogeneic bone marrow transplant in first remission of ALL is controversial because of improving results with current nontransplant therapies. It is usually recommended for patients in whom the likelihood of cure is considered less than 50% to 60% with chemotherapy alone, depending on age and donor availability. Autologous bone marrow transplant is rarely used in Ph-ALL. In 2008, the final results of the MRC/UKALL XII/ECOG E2993 study were published. This study evaluated the relative safety and efficacy of chemotherapy, and autologous and allogeneic transplant after first CR in Ph- patients. This was a randomized trial of 1826 patients with newly diagnosed ALL. Patients who had a matched related donor were offered an allogeneic transplant. Patients without a donor were further randomized to an autologous transplant or chemotherapy and maintenance. The key conclusions of this study were:
  1. Allogeneic transplant in first complete remission is associated with lower relapse rates versus autologous transplant or chemotherapy/maintenance therapy alone in Ph- patients.
  2. Allogeneic transplant in first complete remission improved overall survival in standard risk patients. There was a lower risk of relapse in both standard and high-risk patients. There was high treat-

TABLE 4 Tumor Lysis Syndrome

Laboratory Tumor Lysis Syndrome[a]
Uric acid: ≥8 mg/dl or 476 μmol/L
Potassium: ≥6.0 mmol/L
Phosphorus: ≥4.5 mg/dl or 1.5 mmol/L (adults), ≥6.5 mg/dl or 2.1 mmol (children)
- Calcium: Corrected[b] Ca^{++} <7.0 mg/dl or 1.75 mmol/L or ionized Ca^{++} <1.12 mg/dl or 0.3 mmol/L, or 25% increase from baseline uric acid, potassium, phosphorus; 25% decrease for calcium.

Clinical Tumor Lysis Syndrome
Acute kidney injury
- Rise in serum creatinine ≥0.3 mg/dl (26.5 μmol/L).
- Any creatinine >1.5 age-appropriate upper limit normal if no baseline available.
- Oliguria defined as urine output <0.5 ml/kg/hr for 6 hours.

Cardiac arrhythmia
Seizure
Symptomatic hypocalcemia (e.g., neuromuscular irritability such as tetany)

[a]Laboratory tumor lysis syndrome present if two or more abnormalities are present within 3 days before or 7 days after therapy.
[b]Corrected calcium is measured calcium (mg/dl) + 0.8 x (4 – measured albumin g/dl).
From Arber DA et al: The 2016 revision to the World Health Organization classification of myeloid neoplasms and acute leukemia, *Blood* 127:2391-2405, 2016.

TABLE 5 Risk Factors for Treatment Failure in Recent ALL Trials

t(v*;11q23) *MLL* rearranged.
Hypodiploidy
Minimal residual disease after remission or consolidation*
Philadelphia chromosome-like genomic signature (in Ph- ALL)†
Early precursor T (ETP) ALL (absent CD1a, CD8, weak CD5, myeloid or stem cell antigen expression).

*Measured variously after induction or consolidation therapy.
†Standardized testing for this is still in development, but it may have important treatment implications. Note also that many historic risk factors (e.g., T cell vs B cell disease) have not been independent risk factors in current trials.
Roberts KG, et al.: Targetable kinase-activating lesions in Ph-like acute lymphoblastic leukemia, *N Engl J Med* 371(11):1005-1015, 2014.

ment-related mortality in high-risk older patients. The increased mortality offsets the benefit of lower relapse risk for the patient group.
- The findings did not support autologous transplant as replacement therapy in any ALL group.
- Risk factors for treatment failure in recent protocols are outlined in Table 5. Prognostic factors in ALL are summarized in Tables 6 and 7.
- Therapy of Ph+ ALL consists of a tyrosine kinase inhibitor—imatinib, dasatinib, nilotinib, ponatinib have been used—with chemotherapy.
  1. 2-yr survival rates are reported at 50% to 65%, with various regimens.
  2. Low-intensity induction chemotherapy with dasatinib and prednisone or imatinib, vincristine, and prednisone have resulted in remission rates of 100% and 98% and may allow for less toxicity and hospitalization at diagnosis.
  3. Allogeneic bone marrow transplant is commonly used as consolidative therapy if available but has become more controversial. Maintenance therapy with tyrosine kinase inhibitor is usually given after BMT or non-BMT therapy.
- Therapy of relapsed disease:
  1. Allogeneic bone marrow transplant is offered for relapsed disease, but relapse after BMT is common, and long-term cure rates have been low at about 20%.
  2. In 2017, the FDA approved three new therapies for relapsed ALL: Chimeric antigen receptor T-cell (CAR-T) therapy, a form of targeted immunotherapy, yielded a remission rate of 90% in pediatric and young adult (under age 26 yrs) patients with relapsed B cell ALL. Chimeric antigen T-cells are created by harvesting the patient's T cells, then transfecting them with lentivirus vector that inserts DNA expressing an anti-CD19 domain (the target antigen on B cells) coupled to a T cell receptor. The T cells expressing the chimeric anti-CD 19/T-cell receptor specifically target CD1-expressing B cells. The CAR-T cell population is then expanded ex vivo and reinfused to the patient. About 70% of remissions were durable at 6 months. The main side effect is cytokine release syndrome (CRS) associated with "vascular leak," hypotension, respiratory and renal insufficiency, and coagulapathy. CRS is treated with tocilizumab and anti-IL6 receptor blocking antibody. CAR-T cells for ALL have been given the generic designation tisagenlecleucel (trade name "Kymriah"). It currently costs $475,000 and is available at centers certified for its use.
  3. Blinatumomab is a bispecific antibody that binds CD19 and CD3, redirecting T cells to leukemia cells. It was FDA-approved for relapsed ALL, including Ph+ ALL, in adults and children. Blinatumomab is administered as a continuous infusion for 4 weeks (9 μg/day week 1, 28 μg/day thereafter), with maintenance therapy for 4 weeks every 12 weeks. In a large phase III trial, the remission rate was 44% (vs. 25% with chemotherapy), a small number durable. In a smaller phase II trial for Ph+ ALL, the remission rate was 36%. A small number of blinatumomab responses have been durable. Blinatumomab can also be associated with cytokine release syndrome.
- Inotuzumab ozogamicin (IO) is an antibody drug conjugate, in which chemotherapeutic agent calicheamicin is bound to an anti-CD22 antibody. In a large phase III trial, the remission rate was 81% vs. 33% for standard chemotherapy, with a median duration of 4.6 months. Approximately 40% of IO patients were successfully bridged to transplant vs. 10% with chemotherapy. A small number of responses were durable.
- Survivorship
  1. Survivors of childhood and adult ALL are increasingly being seen in primary care practices; as of 2006 there were estimated >50,000 survivors, likely increasing by about 2000+ per yr.
  2. Long-term complications of ALL therapy include secondary malignancy from chemotherapy (usually in first 5-10 yrs) or from radiation (if given, no plateau in risk, congestive heart failure from anthracycline therapy (often manifesting 20-30 yrs after treatment), osteopenia and avascular necrosis from glucocorticoid therapy, obesity, and neurocognitive defects. Key recommendations include the following:
     a. Echocardiography every 3 to 5 yrs for asymptomatic congestive heart failure, more often if anthracycline exposure was >250 to 300 mg/m2, since asymptomatic congestive heart failure may warrant therapy. This may show up decades after therapy.
     b. Screening for malignancy and endocrinopathies in pertinent radiation fields.
     c. Attention to the increased risk of obesity and metabolic derangement in survivors.
     d. Recent reviews (see references) summarizing current recommendations and guidelines are accessible online (www.survivorshipguidelines.org/pdf/LTFUGuidelines_40.pdf, http://www.sign.ac.uk/pdf/sign132.pdf).

SUGGESTED READINGS

Available at ExpertConsult.com

RELATED CONTENT

Acute Lymphocytic Leukemia (ALL) (Patient Information)
Tumor Lysis Syndrome (Related Key Topic)

AUTHOR: **TODD F. ROBERTS, M.D., F.R.C.P.(C.)**

TABLE 6 Prognostic Factors in Acute Lymphoblastic Leukemia

Factor	Prognosis	Clinical Application
Age		
<1 yr	MLL+ (70%-80% infants) poor outcome; MLL− same outcome as older children	MLL− do well on standard ALL therapy Potential role for FLT3 inhibitors, proteasome inhibitors, histone deacetylase inhibitors, and hypomethylating agents for MLL+
1–9 yrs	Lower (standard) risk	ALL biology may change risk
>9 yrs	Higher risk	ALL biology may change risk
WBC		
$<50 \times 10^9/L$	Lower (standard) risk	ALL biology may change risk
$\geq 50 \times 10^9/L$	Higher risk	ALL biology may change risk
CNS		
CNS3	Higher risk of CNS and bone marrow relapse	Therapy intensification
CNS2 Traumatic lumbar puncture with blasts	Higher risk of CNS relapse	CNS directed therapy intensification
Testicular	Higher risk	Therapy intensification
Immunophenotype		
T cell	Higher risk	Poor outcome abolished with current therapy
pre-B (cIgM+)	Standard risk	Poor outcome abolished with current therapy
Early pre-B	Standard risk	Genetics may change risk
Early T-cell precursor	Adverse prognosis	Ongoing studies exploring targeted therapies
Ploidy		
>50 (DI >1.16)	Low risk	Good response to antimetabolites
<44	Higher risk	Therapy intensification
Genetic Alterations		
t(9;22)/*BCR-ABL1*	Higher risk	ABL TKI
t(4;11)/*MLL-AF4*	Higher risk	Potential role for FLT3 inhibitors, proteasome inhibitors, histone deacetylase inhibitors, and hypomethylating agents
t(1;19)/*E2A-PBX1*	Higher risk of CNS relapse	Improved outcome with current therapy
t(12;21)/*ETV6-RUNX1*	Low risk	
IKZF1	Poor prognosis. Present in 80% Ph+ and also in Ph-like ALL	Potential role for tyrosine kinase, JAK inhibitors
NUP214-ABL1	High risk	Potential benefits from TKI
CRLF2	In half of Ph-like cases, associated with Hispanic/Latino, poor outcome	Potential role for JAK inhibitors
CREBBP	Associated with drug resistance and relapse	Potential benefit from histone deacetylase inhibitors
MRD		
Day 15 <0.01%	Excellent outcome	No benefit from 2nd delayed intensification
Slow early responders	Higher MRD = higher risk of relapse	Benefit from augmented delayed intensification
End of induction >1%	Dismal prognosis	Transplantation in first CR
4 months after diagnosis >0.01%	Dismal outcome	Transplantation in first CR

ALL, Acute lymphoblastic leukemia; *CNS,* central nervous system; *CR,* complete remission; *DI,* DNA index; *JAK,* Janus kinase; *MRD,* minimal residual disease; *TKI,* tyrosine kinase inhibitor; *WBC,* white blood cell.
From Hoffman R, et al.: *Hematology, basic principles and practice*, ed 7, Philadelphia, 2018, Elsevier.

TABLE 7 Markers for Poor Prognosis in Adult Acute Lymphoblastic Leukemia

Established Risk Factors	
Age	>60 yrs
Presenting WBC count	>30,000/μL (B-cell ALL); >100,000/μL (T-cell ALL)
Immunophenotype	Pro-B cell; early T cell[a]
Cytogenetics	t(4;11)(q21;q23) and other *MLL* rearrangements t(9;22)(q34;q11.2) – Philadelphia chromosome Hypodiploidy (<44 chromosomes) Complex (>5 abnormalities)
Therapy response	Time to complete remission >4 weeks
MRD	≥0.01% at 3–6 months after initiation of therapy[b]
Emerging Risk Factors	
Immunophenotype	CD20
Molecular	BAALC FUS ERG IKZF1[c] Ph-like ALL

[a]Initial report characterizing ETP ALL showed a poor outcome. However, subsequent studies have shown variable association with response to therapy.
[b]Different studies have used different time points for MRD assessment.
[c]Focal deletions in IKZF1 are present in up to 70% of Ph-like ALL. However, IKZF1 deletions are associated with adverse outcome irrespective of association with Ph-like phenotype.
From Hoffman R, et al.: *Hematology, basic principles and practice*, ed 7, Philadelphia, 2018, Elsevier.
ALL, Acute lymphoblastic leukemia; *ETP,* early T-cell precursor; *MRD,* minimal residual disease; *Ph,* Philadelphia chromosome; *WBC,* white blood cell.

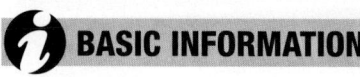

BASIC INFORMATION

DEFINITION

Acute mesenteric ischemia (AMI) is the sudden onset of intestinal hypoperfusion to all or part of the small bowel caused by emboli, arterial or venous thrombosis, or vasoconstriction from low-flow states.

SYNONYMS

AMI
Mesenteric ischemia, acute

ICD-10CM CODE

K55.0 Acute vascular disorders of intestine

EPIDEMIOLOGY & DEMOGRAPHICS

INCIDENCE:

- AMI accounts for 0.1% of hospital admissions.
- The incidence appears to be increasing. Factors for this include increased awareness among clinicians, the aging of the population, and improved intensive care, leading to longer survival of sicker patients. The mortality rate is 60% to 85%.

PREDOMINANT SEX AND AGE:

- AMI caused by arterial embolism or thrombosis occurs more frequently in the elderly.
- AMI due to mesenteric venous thrombosis often presents in younger age groups.

GENETICS: No specific genetic predisposition but may be related to underlying factors such as cardiac disease, atherosclerosis, and hypercoagulable states.

RISK FACTORS:

- Advanced age, atherosclerosis, low cardiac output (especially atrial fibrillation), severe cardiac valvular disease, intraabdominal malignancy.
- In the subgroup of cases caused by venous thrombosis, risk factors include hypercoagulable states, portal hypertension, abdominal infection, blunt trauma, pancreatitis, and portal malignancy.
- Additional risk factors for AMI caused by nonocclusive mesenteric ischemia include recent cardiac or aortic surgery, dialysis, hypovolemia, and vasoconstrictive medications (including illicit drugs such as cocaine).
- Table 1 summarizes risk factors for ischemic bowel disease.
- AMI may occur rarely in patients with no identifiable risk factors.

PHYSICAL FINDINGS & CLINICAL PRESENTATION

- The classic presentation is rapid onset of severe periumbilical pain "out of proportion to physical examination findings." An epigastric bruit may be present in some patients. Generally, patients with mesenteric venous thrombosis tend to present with a less abrupt onset of abdominal pain than those with acute arterial occlusion.
- Nausea and vomiting are commonly associated.
- Initial abdominal examination may be normal, with no rebound or guarding, or may include minimal distention or stool positive for occult blood.
- Later in the course the patient may present with gross distention, absence of bowel sounds, and peritoneal signs. In the elderly, mental status changes may occur.

ETIOLOGY

The pathophysiology of the four different causes of acute mesenteric ischemia are summarized in Table 2. Causes and approximate frequencies of acute mesenteric ischemia are summarized in Table 3. The pathophysiologic mechanisms that cause AMI include:

- Mesenteric arterial embolism (40% to 50% of cases of AMI): Typically from the left atrium, left ventricle, or cardiac valves. The superior mesenteric artery is most commonly affected.
- Mesenteric arterial thrombosis: Often in patients with prior progressive atherosclerotic stenoses, with superimposed abdominal trauma or infection. Thrombotic occlusion of previously stenotic mesenteric vessels accounts for 20% to 35% of cases of AMI.
- Mesenteric venous thrombosis may occur in the setting of hypercoagulable states (acquired or inherited), blunt trauma, abdominal infection, portal hypertension, pancreatitis, and portal malignancy.
- Nonocclusive mesenteric ischemia is caused by reduced intestinal perfusion, as seen with hypotension, hypovolemia, vasoconstricting drugs, and hemodialysis.
- Dissection or inflammation of the mesenteric artery accounts for less than 5% of cases of AMI.

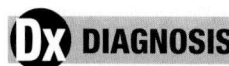

DIAGNOSIS

DIFFERENTIAL DIAGNOSIS

Initially include other causes of abdominal pain of acute onset, including perforated peptic ulcer and early appendicitis, as well as the varied causes of peritonitis.

TABLE 1 Risk Factors for Ischemic Bowel Diseases*

Risk Factor	Arterial Thrombosis	Embolus	Mesenteric Vein Thrombosis	Nonobstructive Mesenteric Ischemia
Advanced age	+	+	+	+
Atherosclerosis	+			
Aortic dissection	+			
Low cardiac output	+	+		+
Congestive heart failure				+
Shock				+
Severe dehydration	+		+	
Cardiac arrhythmias, especially atrial fibrillation		+		+
Severe cardiac valvular disease		+		
Recent myocardial infarction	+			+
Intraabdominal malignancy			+	
Abdominal trauma			+	
Intraabdominal infection			+	
Intraabdominal inflammatory conditions			+	
Parasitic infection (ascariasis)			+	
Hypercoagulable states (venous thrombosis)			+	
Sickle cell anemia			+	
Recent cardiac surgery	+	+		+
Recent abdominal surgery			+	
Vascular aortic prosthetic grafts proximal to the superior mesenteric artery		+		
Hemodialysis				+
Vasculitis	+		+	
Pregnancy			+	
Decompression sickness			+	
Blast lung caused by systemic air embolism		+		
Drugs that cause constriction				
• Digitalis				+
• Cocaine				+
• Amphetamines				+
• Pseudoephedrine				+
• Vasopressin			+†	+
Estrogen therapy			+	

*A plus sign (+) indicates that the factor is a risk for the disease subtype.
†Especially table after sclerotherapy.
From Adams JG et al: *Emergency medicine, clinical essentials,* ed 2, Philadelphia, 2013, Elsevier.

TABLE 2 Pathophysiology of the Four Different Causes of Acute Mesenteric Ischemia (AMI)

Cause	Pathophysiology
Embolism	• Often in patients with atrial fibrillation • Emboli lodge 3–10 cm distal to origin of SMA, often past branching of middle colic artery • Proximal midjejunum is spared
Thrombosis	• Typically these patients have a history of symptomatic stenosis of mesenteric arteries • Any clinical scenario that leads to low flow or hypotension can result in acute-on-chronic arterial thrombosis • Affects the orifice of the SMA • Flush occlusion of the SMA and the entire middle gut is involved during the initial presentation
Nonocclusive	• Low flow state resulting from any type of shock or the use of vasoconstrictors • The entire bowel may be involved
Mesenteric venous thrombosis	• Thrombosis of the veins draining the intestines; SMV, IMV, splenic and portal veins among hypercoagulable patients with cancer or hypercoagulable state • Decreased venous outflow, bowel edema, distension, and decreased mesenteric perfusion

IMV, Inferior mesenteric vein; *SMA*, superior mesenteric artery.
Modified from Cameron JL, Cameron AM: *Current surgical therapy*, ed 12, Philadelphia, 2017, Elsevier.

TABLE 3 Causes and Approximate Frequencies of Acute Mesenteric Ischemia

Cause	Frequency (%)
SMA thrombosis	54–68
SMA embolus	26–32
Nonocclusive mesenteric ischemia	10
Mesenteric venous thrombosis	5
Focal segmental ischemia of the small intestine	5

SMA, Superior mesenteric artery.
From Feldman M, Friedman LS, Brandt LJ: *Sleisenger and Fordtran's gastrointestinal and liver disease*, ed 10, Philadelphia, 2016, Elsevier.

WORKUP

- Early diagnosis is key. Treatment success is related to the duration of symptoms prior to diagnosis.
- Consider early laparotomy for diagnosis in cases with a high index of suspicion when imaging is not readily available.

LABORATORY TESTS

- Laboratory test results are nonspecific, especially early in the course. Elevated lactic acid, leukocytosis, acidosis, and elevated hematocrit from hemoconcentration can occur later in the course, often after progression to bowel necrosis has occurred, hence are not useful for early diagnosis.
- When a hypercoagulable state is suspected, workup may include proteins C and S, antithrombin III, and factor V Leiden. This will likely not affect the diagnosis of AMI but may help guide long-term therapy.
- Amylase levels may be elevated in up to 50% of individuals with intestinal ischemia; phosphate levels may be elevated in up to 80% of affected individuals.
- Normal D-dimer testing may help rule out AMI. Elevated levels are nonspecific.

IMAGING STUDIES

- Biphasic contrast-enhanced computed tomography (CT) is the preferred diagnostic mode. It is more easily available and has similar sensitivity to angiography, the prior gold standard test. Computed tomographic angiography (CTA) has 95% to 100% accuracy for the diagnosis of visceral ischemic syndromes and is also useful in detecting potential sources of emboli and other pathologic processes.
- Plain CT findings are nonspecific and more often found late in the course. Portal venous gas or intramural gas may be seen after the development of gangrene (Fig. 3). In many cases, CT findings remain nonspecific even at advanced stages.
- MR angiography (MRA) may be more useful in cases of mesenteric vein thrombosis causing AMI. It has also been found useful in monitoring the progress of patients with superior mesenteric venous thrombosis who are treated nonsurgically. MRA, however, takes longer than CTA to perform and can overestimate the degree of stenosis.
- Angiography may be considered if the diagnosis remains unclear after CT or MR imaging.
- Plain films are normal 25% of the time in early stages. Suggestive findings may include ileus (Fig. 4), bowel wall thickening, or intramural gas. Free air under the diaphragm may support early surgical intervention prior to further radiologic evaluation.
- Doppler ultrasound evaluation of intestinal blood flow is often limited by the presence of air-filled loops of bowel and is not an appropriate part of the diagnostic workup if AMI is the leading working diagnosis.

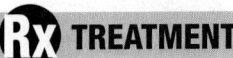

TREATMENT

- The goal of treatment is to restore blood flow to ischemic bowel as rapidly as possible before the occurrence of infarction.
- Treatment varies depending on etiology.

ACUTE GENERAL Rx

- Initial management should include hemodynamic monitoring and support, correction of acidosis, pain control (using parenteral opioids), administration of broad-spectrum antibiotics, and gastric decompression by nasogastric tube.
- Vasoconstricting agents should be avoided.
- In the absence of active bleeding, the use of systemic anticoagulation is usually indicated. The optimal timing of initiation is unclear.

NONPHARMACOLOGIC THERAPY

- Signs of peritonitis mandate early laparotomy and resection of infarcted bowel.
- Specific management will depend on patient status and most likely etiology of the ischemia.
- When workup is positive for major superior mesenteric artery (SMA) embolus, embolectomy is considered standard treatment in the absence of peritoneal signs. Depending on the location and degree of occlusion of the embolus, surgical revascularization, intraarterial infusion of thrombolytics or vasodilators, or systemic anticoagulation may be considered.
- In cases of SMA thrombosis, emergency surgical revascularization is the treatment of choice; stent placement may be a viable alternative.
- Angiography is needed to diagnose nonocclusive mesenteric ischemia before infarct and should be followed up by intraarterial vasodilator infusion. This approach has been shown to reduce mortality rate significantly. Underlying risk factors for reduced blood flow should be assessed and mitigated.
- In patients with mesenteric vein thrombosis, treatment depends on the presence or absence of peritoneal signs. Laparotomy and resection of infarcted bowel is indicated in more advanced cases. If there are no peritoneal signs, immediate anticoagulant therapy with heparin, and ultimately warfarin, may be adequate treatment.
- In general, percutaneous treatment with lytic therapy, balloon angioplasty, or stenting may be limited by the frequent presence of nonviable bowel, which would require laparotomy despite success with percutaneous treatment.
- A "second look" procedure is indicated in most patients, 24 to 48 hours after initial revascularization.

CHRONIC Rx

- In the subgroup of patients with mesenteric venous thrombosis, prevention of further thrombosis is indicated. The optimal duration of anticoagulation is unclear.
- Patients who receive endovascular treatment should be managed with 1 to 3 months of

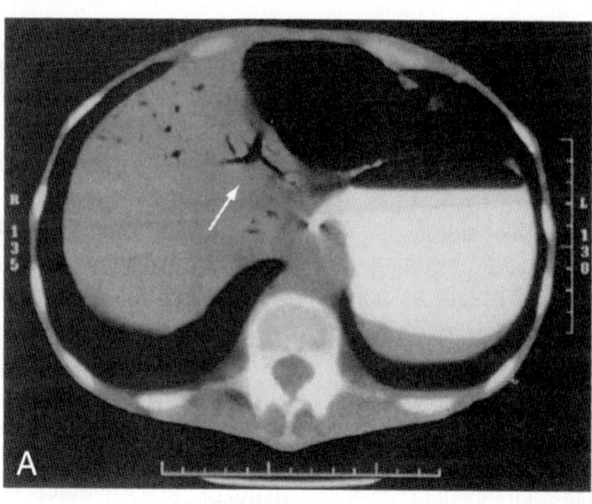

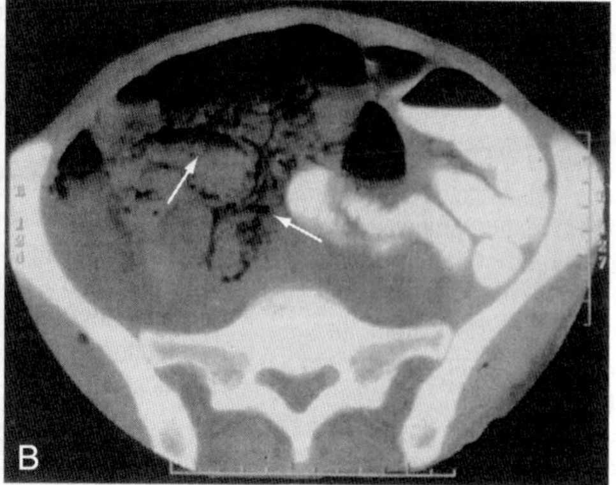

FIG. 3 CT of a patient with acute mesenteric ischemia showing gas *(arrow)* in the portal veins **(A)** and gas *(arrows)* in the wall of the intestine as well as the mesentery and its vessels **(B)** Pneumatosis intestinalis (linearis) is a late sign of ischemic injury, connotes bowel necrosis, and mandates explorative laparotomy. (From Feldman M, Friedman LS, Brandt LJ: *Sleisenger and Fordtran's gastrointestinal and liver disease*, ed 10, Philadelphia, 2016, Elsevier.)

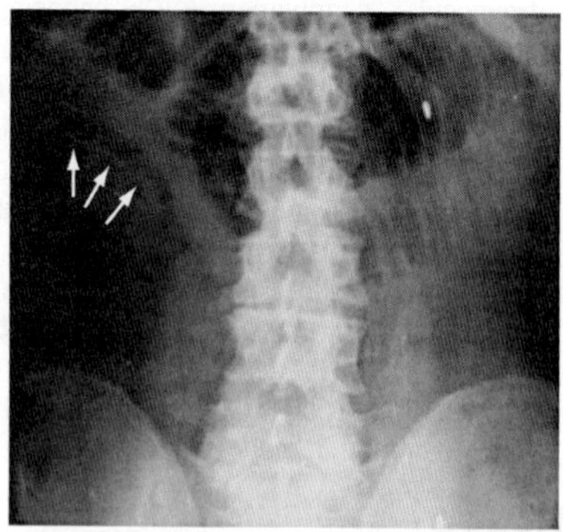

FIG. 4 Plain film of the abdomen showing an ileus and a formless fixed loop of small intestine (arrows) in a patient with acute mesenteric ischemia from a superior mesenteric artery embolus. (From Feldman M, Friedman LS, Brandt LJ: *Sleisenger and Fordtran's gastrointestinal and liver disease*, ed 10, Philadelphia, 2016, Elsevier.)

clopidogrel; additionally, periodic surveillance for restenosis with duplex ultrasound or CTA is indicated.

DISPOSITION

- Prognosis is best in AMI due to mesenteric venous thrombosis and after surgical treatment for acute arterial embolism. It remains poor in cases of arterial thrombosis and nonocclusive ischemia.
- With delayed diagnosis, intestinal infarction—resulting in perforation or gangrenous bowel, sepsis, shock, and death—is typical.

REFERRAL

- Early surgical consultation should be considered. There should be no delay with peritoneal signs.
- Surgery may be warranted for diagnostic purposes.

PEARLS & CONSIDERATIONS

COMMENTS

- The diagnosis of AMI should be considered in any patient with acute onset of abdominal pain out of proportion to physical findings, particularly in at-risk patients.
- Early diagnosis, before intestinal infarction occurs, is critical and correlates with improved survival rates.
- The use of endovascular procedures for AMI is becoming more common and may be most appropriate for patients with ischemia that is not severe and for those who have severe coexisting conditions that place them at high risk for complications and death associated with open surgery.

PREVENTION

Prevention of underlying factors, most notably atherosclerotic disease (smoking cessation, management of hypertension, and use of statins) is indicated for primary prevention as well as prevention of recurrence.

SUGGESTED READINGS

Available at ExpertConsult.com

RELATED CONTENT

Mesenteric Venous Thrombosis (Related Key Topic)

AUTHOR: **PAUL GEORGE, M.D., M.H.P.E**

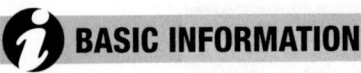

BASIC INFORMATION

DEFINITION

Acute myelogenous leukemia (AML) is a malignancy of hematopoietic progenitor cells that would normally give rise to mature granulocytes. Strictly speaking, AML is a subset of acute nonlymphocytic leukemia (ANLL), a designation that broadly distinguishes these diseases from the biologically distinct leukemias of lymphocytic origin. ANLL includes leukemias involving the spectrum of myeloid stem cells, including precursors of granulocytes, monocytes, erythrocytes, and megakaryocytes. Acute promyelocytic leukemia is a distinct leukemia syndrome that is part of the ANLL spectrum, but that has very different treatment implications. ANLL is characterized by maturation failure of myeloid progenitors, excessive numbers of immature progenitors ("blasts"), and various degrees of bone marrow failure (neutropenia, thrombocytopenia, anemia).

SYNONYMS

Acute nonlymphocytic leukemia (ANLL)
Acute myeloid leukemia (AML)

ICD-10CM CODES

C92.60	Acute myeloid leukemia with 11q23-abnormality not having achieved remission
C92.61	Acute myeloid leukemia with 11q23-abnormality in remission
C92.62	Acute myeloid leukemia with 11q23-abnormality in relapse
C92.90	Myeloid leukemia, unspecified, not having achieved remission
C92.91	Myeloid leukemia, unspecified in remission
C92.92	Myeloid leukemia, unspecified in relapse
C92.A0	Acute myeloid leukemia with multilineage dysplasia, not having achieved remission
C92.A1	Acute myeloid leukemia with multilineage dysplasia, in remission
C92.A2	Acute myeloid leukemia with multilineage dysplasia, in relapse
C92.Z0	Other myeloid leukemia not having achieved remission
C92.Z1	Other myeloid leukemia, in remission
C92.Z2	Other myeloid leukemia, in relapse
C92.00	Acute myeloblastic leukemia, not having achieved remission
C92.01	Acute myeloblastic leukemia, in remission
C92.02	Acute myeloblastic leukemia, in relapse

EPIDEMIOLOGY & DEMOGRAPHICS

- AML incidence rises with age:
  1. Incidence 20 to 55 yr old: 1 to 3/100,000 persons/yr.
  2. Incidence 65 to 80 yr old: 11 to 20/100,000 persons/yr.
- Annual incidence is 4 cases/100,000 persons/yr.
- Males slightly >females; European ancestry slightly >African ancestry.

PHYSICAL FINDINGS & CLINICAL PRESENTATION

Symptoms/exam findings:

- Complications of bone marrow failure:
  1. Thrombocytopenia-associated bleeding
  2. Fatigue and shortness of breath associated with anemia
  3. Infection associated with neutropenia
- Complications of leukocytosis (hyperleukocytic leukemia, WBC >100,000/mcl):
  1. Retinal hemorrhage with visual symptoms
  2. Headache and intracranial bleeding
  3. Respiratory symptoms from pulmonary involvement
- Systemic symptoms:
  1. Fatigue, fever (usually infectious, rarely tumor), bone pain (more common in ALL)
- Hemorrhagic complications of disseminated intravascular coagulation (DIC), especially with acute promyelocytic leukemia (APML).
- Physical exam will reflect consequences of cytopenias (bruising from thrombocytopenia, pallor from anemia). Enlarged lymph nodes and enlarged liver and spleen are rare. Exam is often normal.
- Rarely disease will present as skin lesions (leukemia cutis) or mass lesions (granulocytic sarcoma).
- Gum hypertrophy and organ/skin involvement is more common in monocytic leukemia.

ETIOLOGY

- Environmental/exposure related: Benzene (best documented), organic solvents (including gasoline), cigarette smoking (≥20 pack-yr 1.34 relative risk), obesity, best documented in women
- Hereditary disorders: Numerous, including Fanconi anemia, Bloom syndrome, Schwachman Diamond syndrome, Diamond Blackfan anemia, among others
- Therapy related:
  1. Alkylator (e.g., melphalan, busulfan, cisplatin) related: Typical latency 5 to 7 yrs, associated with chromosome 5 and 7 abnormalities
  2. Topoisomerase II inhibitor (e.g. etoposide, doxorubicin): Typical latency 1 to 3 yrs, associated with 11q23 (mixed lineage leukemia [MLL] gene) rearrangements
- Radiation exposures (therapeutic—generally low risk), occupational
- Antecedent hematologic disorders: Myelodysplasia, myeloproliferative disorders, aplastic anemia

DIAGNOSIS

DIFFERENTIAL DIAGNOSIS

- Disorders that can present with circulating blasts or cells with blastlike appearance:
  1. Acute myeloid leukemia/acute lymphocytic leukemia
  2. Myelodysplasia (up to 20% circulating blasts, if ≥20% = AML)
  3. Primary myelofibrosis
  4. Chronic myeloid leukemia
  5. Blastoid variant of mantle cell lymphoma
  6. Prolymphocytic leukemia
  7. Blastic plasmacytoid dendritic cell neoplasm
  8. Atypical lymphocytes of Epstein-Barr and cytomegalovirus infection may have blastlike appearance

WORKUP

The diagnostic workup consists of a morphologic assessment, immunophenotyping by flow cytometry, assessment of karyotype, and a panel of gene mutations (Fig. 1).

LABORATORY TESTS

- Complete blood counts and blood smear evaluation. Note that morphologic evaluation of blasts may suggest myeloid or lymphoid origin, but flow cytometry or cytochemistries (often faster) are needed to confirm. Auer rods are seen in blasts of myeloid origin.
- LDH is commonly elevated. Other biochemistries to assess organ function (creatinine, liver enzymes) and spontaneous tumor lysis syndrome (uric acid, potassium, phosphate, calcium).
- Coagulation studies to assess DIC. DIC is always present in APML, but can be present in ***all*** forms of acute leukemia, especially acute monocytic leukemia.
- HLA typing for possible bone marrow transplant and platelet support.
- Cytochemical stains:
  1. Myeloperoxidase can be performed in minutes, + in myeloid origin leukemia.
  2. Alpha naphthyl acetate esterase ("nonspecific esterase") stains mainly monocytic cells.
- Flow cytometry on blood and/or bone marrow (see Table E1).
- Cytogenetic studies, ideally on bone marrow, but can be done on peripheral blood. Fluorescence in situ hybridization (FISH) is often used as an adjunct to conventional chromosome analysis.
- Molecular studies to further stratify risk and prognosis, which may affect treatment choices (see Tables E2, 3, and 4). Directing this workup should be done with combined hematology and laboratory expertise and typically will consist of studies for fms-related tyrosine kinase gene (FLT3) mutations, nucleophosmin gene (NPM) mutations, and CCAAT/enhancer binding protein α gene (CEBPA) mutations. Wider molecular panels are increasingly common because of the increasing numbers of potential markers and the potential availability of targeted therapies for FLT3 mutated disease and those with isocitrate dehydrogenase mutations, among others. TP53 mutation, mutated RUNX1, and mutated ASXL1 have recently been added to the NCCN poor-risk category for AML in 2018.
- Formal diagnosis of acute nonlymphocytic leukemia is established if the marrow or peripheral blood blast percentage is ≥20%, unless t(8;21), inv(16), t(16;16) or t(15;17)

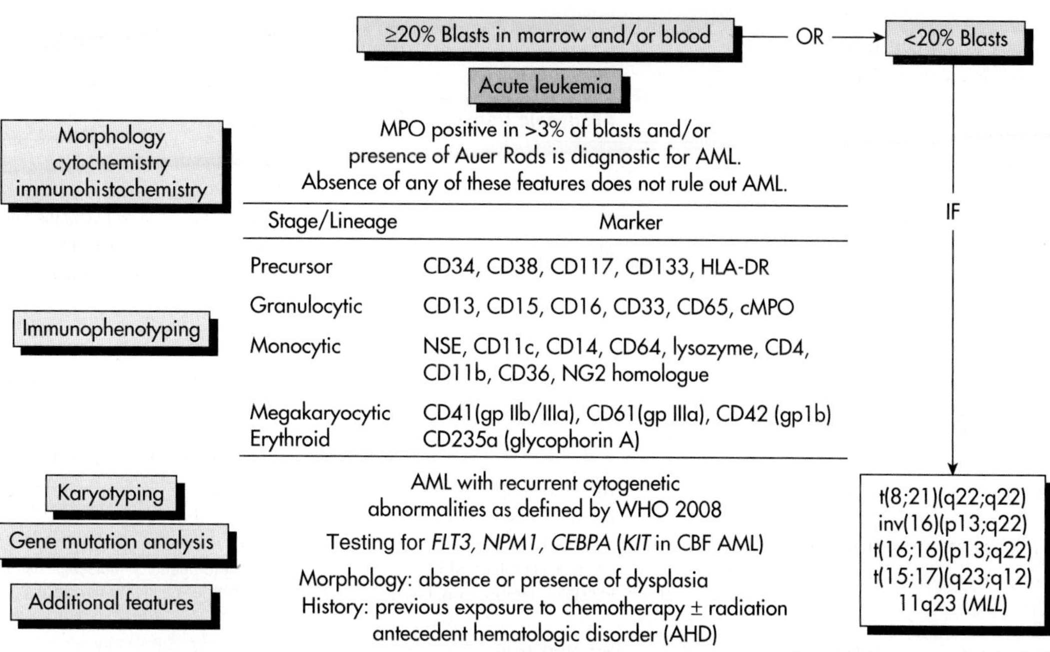

FIG. 1 Workup of acute myeloid leukemia. The diagnostic workup consists of a morphologic assessment, immunophenotyping by flow cytometry, assessment of the karyotype, and a panel of gene mutations. Whereas morphologic assessment by itself is often not sufficient to render a diagnosis, flow cytometry will confirm the lineage assignment (myeloid vs. lymphoid) and stage of differentiation in more than 95% of cases. In the remainder, either no lineage-specific antigens are expressed (acute undifferentiated leukemia) or antigens of more than one lineage are present (mixed-phenotype acute leukemia). In the latter scenario, antigens of several lineages can be found on one (biphenotypic) or separate populations of blasts (bilineal). Karyotyping and gene mutation analysis may add diagnostic information in morphologically ambiguous situations but is otherwise of more interest in determining prognosis. Additional information (exposure to previous chemotherapy and/or radiation therapy, history of an antecedent hematologic disorder, dysplasia) forms the basis for the 2008 revision of the WHO classification of AML. *AHD*, Antecedent hematologic disorder; *AML*, acute myeloid leukemia; *ANLL*, acute nonlymphocytic leukemia; *CBF*, core-binding factor; *MPO*, myeloperoxidase; *WHO*, World Health Organization. (From Hoffman R, et al.: *Hematology, basic principles and practice*, ed 7, Philadelphia, 2018, Elsevier.)

TABLE 3 European LeukemiaNet AML Risk Classification

Genetic Group	Subsets
Favorable	t(8;21)(q22;q22); *RUNX1-RUNX1T1*
	inv(16)(p13.1q22) or t(16;16)(p13.1;q22); *CBFB-MYH11*
	Mutated *NPM1* without *FLT3*-ITD (normal karyotype)
	Mutated *CEBPA* (normal karyotype)
Intermediate-I[a]	Mutated *NPM1* and *FLT3*-ITD (normal karyotype)
	Wild-type *NPM1* and *FLT3*-ITD (normal karyotype)
	Wild-type *NPM1* without *FLT3*-ITD (normal karyotype)
Intermediate-II	t(9;11)(p22;q23); *MLLT3-MLL*
	Cytogenetic abnormalities not classified as favorable or adverse[b]
Adverse	inv(3)(q21q26.2) or t(3;3)(q21;q26.2); *RPN1-EVI1*
	t(6;9)(p23;q34); *DEK-NUP214*
	t(v;11)(v;q23); *MLL* rearranged
	−5 or del(5q); −7; abnl(17p); complex karyotype[c]

[a]Includes all AMLs with normal karyotype except for those included in the favorable subgroup; most of these cases are associated with poor prognosis.
[b]For most abnormalities, adequate numbers have not been studied to draw firm conclusions regarding their prognostic significance.
[c]Three or more chromosome abnormalities in the absence of one of the WHO designated recurring translocations or inversions, that is, t(15;17), t(8;21), inv(16) or t(16;16), t(9;11), t(v;11)(v;q23), t(6;9), inv(3), or t(3;3).
From Hoffman R, et al.: *Hematology, basic principles and practice*, ed 7, Philadelphia, 2018, Elsevier.

are present, in which case the percentage of blasts may be lower.

1. Myeloperoxidase (MPO) staining of 3% of blasts establishes myeloid lineage, but MPO may be negative in some AML cases diagnosed by flow cytometry.
2. Specific criteria exist for diagnosing other forms of ANLL, mainly to distinguish it from myelodysplasia. The WHO AML classification is outlined in Table 5.
3. Bone marrow findings are described in Fig. E2.

IMAGING STUDIES

- Imaging studies are typically directed to evaluating specific complaints.
- Echocardiogram or multigated acquisition scan is usually performed to verify that cardiac function is adequate to tolerate anthracycline (usually daunorubicin) therapy, with left ventricular ejection fraction (LVEF) of >50% typically considered acceptable.

Rx TREATMENT

ACUTE GENERAL Rx

- The general approach to AML is summarized in Fig. 3. Therapy of AML typically has three components:
  1. Immediate therapy to correct metabolic, infectious, or hyperleukocytic emergencies (if needed). Therapy for AML is always urgent but not always an emergency. However, treatment for APML should be considered a medical emergency to prevent catastrophic bleeding.
  2. Induction therapy, which is therapy of active disease intended to obtain remission and restore normal bone marrow function. Remission is defined as blasts <5% in the bone marrow, absolute neutrophils (ANC) of >1000/mcl, platelets >100,000/mcl, and transfusion indepen-

TABLE 4 Allogeneic Transplantation Guidelines for Adult Acute Myeloid Leukemia Based on Commonly Assessed Cytogenetic and Molecular Markers

AML Category	Prognostic Impact	Allogeneic Transplantation	Notes
AML-CR1: Younger Adults			
Good-risk disease			
APL	Favorable	No	APL is treatable by chemotherapy.
CBF-AML *without mKIT*	Favorable	No	t(8;21) AML with high WBC count at diagnosis may have worse prognosis.
CBF-AML *with mKIT*	Intermediate	Possible: MRD, MUD Uncertain: MMUD, UCB, haplo	
Intermediate-Risk Disease			
CN-AML *with CEBPA*	Favorable	No	Benefit likely restricted to *DM-CEBPA*
CN-AML *with mutant NPM1 but not FLT-3-ITD*	Favorable	Possible: MRD	Emerging data suggests allogeneic HSCT benefit for this category, with reduced relapse and improved DFS in patients >40 yrs.
CN-AML *with FLT-3-ITD*	Unfavorable[a]	Yes: MRD, MUD Possible[b]: MMUD, UCB, haplo	Unfavorable risk may be restricted to AML *with FLT-3-ITD allelic ratio >0.51*
Other intermediate-risk disease	Intermediate or Unfavorable	Yes: MRD Likely acceptable[a]: MUD Possible[b]: MMUD, UCB, haplo	Likely considerable underlying clinical heterogeneity. Molecular risk profiling may further delineate risk in this category.
Poor-Risk Disease			
Monosomal karyotype *absent*	Unfavorable	Yes: MRD, MUD Likely acceptable[b]: MMUD, UCB, haplo	
Monosomal karyotype *present*	Very unfavorable	Yes: MRD, MUD. Acceptable[b]: MMUD, UCB, haplo	
Abnormal 17(p)	Very unfavorable	Yes: MRD, MUD Acceptable[b]: MMUD, UCB, haplo	
AML-CR1: older adults	Unfavorable	Yes: MRD, MUD Likely acceptable[b]: MMUD, UCB, haplo	
AML-CR1: t-AML, AML/MDS	Unfavorable	Yes: MRD, MUD Acceptable[b]: MMUD, UCB, haplo	Molecular risk profiling may supersede clinical classification of secondary AML, especially in older patients.
AML-CR2	Very unfavorable	Yes: MRD, MUD Acceptable[b]: MMUD, UCB, haplo	
AML not in remission	Very unfavorable	Yes: MRD, MUD Uncertain: MMUD, UCB, haplo	For selected patients: good performance status, little comorbidity, lower leukemic burden; CIBMTR risk score may be useful.

[a]If no sibling donor available.
[b]If no timely matched donor available.
AML, Acute myeloid leukemia; *APL*, acute promyelocytic leukemia; *CBF*, core binding factor; *CIBMTR*, Center for International Blood and Marrow Transplant Research; *CN*, cytogenetically normal; *CR1*, first complete remission; *CR2*, second complete remission; *haplo*, haploidentical; *MDS*, myelodysplastic syndrome; *MMUD*, mismatched unrelated donor; *MRD*, matched related donor; *MUD*, matched unrelated donor; *t-AML*, therapy-related AML; *UCB*, umbilical cord blood; *WBC*, white blood cell.
From Hoffman R, et al.: *Hematology, basic principles and practice*, ed 7, Philadelphia, 2018, Elsevier.

dence. Complete remission with incomplete marrow recovery (CRi) indicates absence of leukemic blasts in the marrow but persistent cytopenias.

3. Consolidation therapy, typically some form of intensive chemotherapy or stem cell transplant therapy intended to prevent relapse.
4. Hyperleukocytic symptoms are typically seen with WBC >100,000/ml. Leukapheresis requires catheter placement and pheresis but spares tumor lysis. Rapid cytoreduction with chemotherapy (hydroxyurea 3-6 g orally or cytarabine) is often adequate and easier but risks tumor lysis. Optimal management is therefore individualized.
5. Tumor lysis syndrome (TLS) is associated with a rise in uric acid, potassium, and serum phosphate, the last causing a reciprocal fall in calcium. The metabolic changes may result in renal failure, cardiac dysrhythmias, muscle spasms (due to low calcium), seizures, and death (a more detailed discussion is in the section on acute lymphocytic leukemia).
6. The mainstays of therapy for AML are medications dating from the 1970s—daunorubicin and cytarabine—with few medications having meaningful impact on therapy in the last four decades. In 2017, the U.S. FDA approved four new agents, including three targeted agents, for treatment of AML. The role of these agents and their relation to standard therapy is outlined below.
7. Induction chemotherapy typically consists of daunorubicin 60 or 90 mg/m^2 IV for 3 days and cytarabine (Ara-C) 100 or 200 mg/m^2/day as continuous infusion for 7 days ("7+3"). Success rates are 60% to 80% and have been better in recent trials. Other agents that are used include etoposide, idarubicin, fludarabine, and cladribine. Bone marrow examination is usually performed at day 14 of therapy to assess the response.
8. Gemtuzumab ozogamicin (GO, Mylotarg) is an antibody-drug conjugate binding an anti-CD33 antibody to the chemotherapeutic agent calicheamicin that was approved in 2017 for therapy of newly diagnosed CD33+ AML. In newly diagnosed AML, the use of low-dose GO when added to standard 7+3 induction had a success rate of 81%, with 2-yr relapse-free survival improving from 22.7% to 50.3% compared with standard therapy alone. The benefit was seen in favorable and intermediate-risk patients.
9. Midostaurin was also approved in 2017 for treatment of newly diagnosed AML with mutations in the fms-related tyrosine kinase 3 *(FLT3)* gene in combination with standard induction therapy. Four-yr overall survival was 51.4% in FLT3-positive patients receiving midostaurin vs. 44.3% in the placebo arm, with improved durability of remissions in patients achieving remission. The optimal use of these therapies requires rapid access

TABLE 5 Classification of Acute Myeloid Leukemia According to the Revised World Health Organization Classification (2016)

Category	Subtype/Definition*
AML with recurrent cytogenetic abnormalities	t(8;21)(q22;q22); RUNX1-RUNX1T1† inv(16)(p13.1q22); CBFB-MYH11† t(16;16)(p13.1q22); CBFB-MYH11† t(15;17)(q22;q12); PML-RARA† (= acute promyelocytic leukemia) t(9;11)(p22;q23); MLLT3-KMT2A t(6;9)(p23;q34); DEK-NUP214 inv(3)(q21q26.2); GATA2, MECOM t(3;3)(q21;q26.2); RPN1-EVI1 t(1;22)(p13q13); RBM15-MKL1 (megakaryoblastic) with mutated NPM1 with biallelic mutations of CEBPA
AML with MDS-related changes	Morphologic features of MDS, or prior history of MDS or MDS/MPN, or MDS-related karyotype, and none of the recurrent genetic abnormalities above
Therapy-related myeloid neoplasms	Late complications of cytotoxic chemotherapy (alkylating agents, topoisomerase II inhibitors) and/or ionizing radiation therapy†
AML, not otherwise specified	AML with minimal differentiation AML without maturation AML with maturation Acute myelomonocytic leukemia Acute monoblastic/monocytic leukemia Pure erythroid leukemia Acute megakaryoblastic leukemia Acute basophilic leukemia Acute panmyelosis with myelofibrosis
Myeloid sarcoma	
Myeloid proliferations related to Down syndrome	Transient abnormal myelopoiesis Myeloid leukemia associated with Down syndrome
Blastic plasmacytoid dendritic cell neoplasm	
Acute leukemia of ambiguous lineage	Acute undifferentiated leukemia Mixed-phenotype acute leukemia with: t(9;22)(q34;q11.2); BCR-ABL1 t(v;11q23); KMT2A rearranged Mixed-phenotype acute leukemia, B/myeloid, NOS Mixed-phenotype acute leukemia, T/myeloid, NOS
Provisional entities	AML with mutated NPM1 AML with mutated CEBPA NK-cell lymphoblastic leukemia/lymphoma

AML, Acute myeloid leukemia; *MDS*, myelodysplastic syndrome; *MPN*, myeloproliferative neoplasm; *NK*, natural killer; *NOS*, not otherwise specified.

*Diagnosis of AML regardless of percentage of blasts.

†Excluded are patients with AML who have transformed from MPN.

For AML with recurrent genetic abnormalities, specific genes rearranged follow the chromosome rearrangement. In 2016, the MLL gene has been renamed KMT2A.

to genetic data at the time of diagnosis. Also approved in 2017 was CPX-351, a liposomal formulation of cytarabine and daunorubicin encapsulated in a 5:1 ratio, for patients with AML related to previous therapy (t-AML) or with AML with myelodysplasia-related change (AML-MRC). In a trial of t-AML and AML evolving from myelodysplasia or with WHO-defined myelodysplasia-related cytogenetic changes in patients ages 60 to 75 yr, CPX-351 improved survival to 9.56 months vs. 5.95 months with standard 7+3 induction.

10 Gilteritinib was FDA approved in 2018 for treatment of adult patients who have relapsed or refractory acute myeloid leukemia with a FLT3 mutation. Approval was based on an interim analysis of a trial, which included 138 adult patients with relapsed or refractory AML having a FLT3 ITD, D835, or I836 mutation. Gilteritinib was given orally at a dose of 120 mg daily until unacceptable toxicity or lack of clinical benefit. After a median follow-up of 4.6 months, 21% of patients achieved complete remission (CR) or CR with partial hematologic recovery (CRh).

- Consolidation therapy is controversial. For patients managed with chemotherapy, cytarabine 3 g/m^2 for six doses is commonly used (day 1, 3, 5), but intermediate doses (1000-1500 mg/m^2) for six doses appear equally effective and less toxic. Doses above 1000 mg/m^2 are poorly tolerated in patients over 60 yr because of cerebellar toxicity. Renal insufficiency also increases the risk of cerebellar toxicity from Ara-C, which can be severe.
  1. For favorable risk disease, consolidation with chemotherapy alone with two to four cycles of intermediate/high-dose cytarabine is typically given, with long-term survival of 60% to 70%.
  2. For intermediate-risk and unfavorable-risk disease, first-remission allogeneic stem cell marrow transplant is often

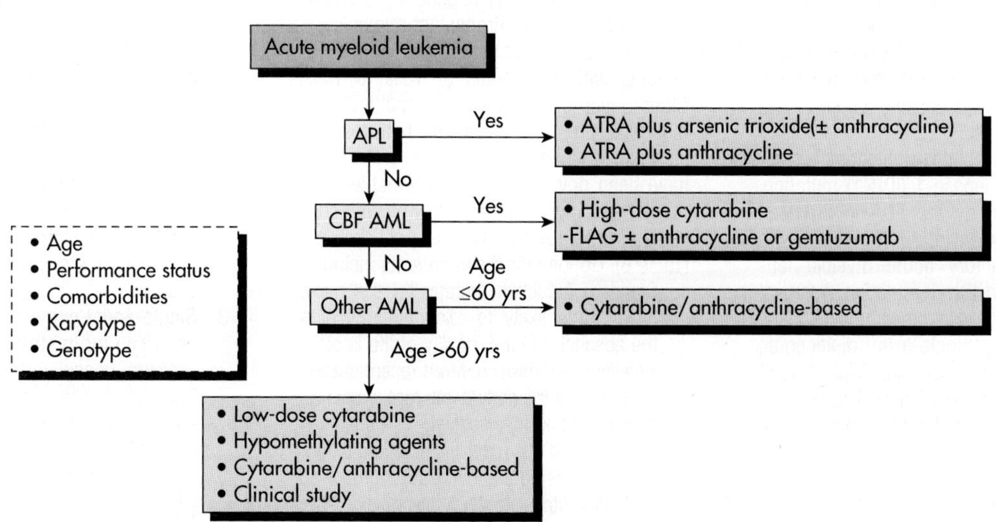

FIG. 3 General approach to acute myeloid leukemia therapy. *AML*, Acute myeloid leukemia; *APL*, acute promyelocytic leukemia; *ATRA*, all-trans retinoic acid; *CBF*, core binding factor; *FLAG*, fludarabine, cytarabine (ara-C), and granulocyte colony-stimulating factor. (From Hoffman R, et al.: *Hematology, basic principles and practice*, ed 7, Philadelphia, 2018, Elsevier.)

recommended if a donor is available. If not, chemotherapy consolidation chemotherapy is offered, although the optimal therapy and schedule, especially for unfavorable disease, is uncertain.

3. In the trial of GO as initial therapy, GO was also used in consolidation with high-dose cytarabine and daunorubicin.
4. The role of autologous bone marrow transplant is controversial, with some evidence of decreased relapse rates after chemotherapy but no clear benefit in overall survival.
5. Allogeneic bone marrow transplant is offered to patients with relapsed disease if a second remission can be obtained in good risk patients. It is offered to high-risk and intermediate-risk patients in first remission if a donor is available. In 2018, most patients will be able to find a donor from either a matched related donor, matched unrelated donor, mismatched unrelated donor, haploidentical donor, or cord blood donor. The Center for International Blood and Marrow Transplant Research (CIBMTR) has published data for 12,309 patients receiving an HLA-matched sibling transplant and 15,632 patients receiving a matched unrelated donor for AML between 2002 and 2012. Their disease status at the time of transplant and the donor type were found to be the best predictors of post-transplant survival. The 3-yr probabilities of survival after HLA-matched sibling transplant in this cohort was 58% ±1%, 50% ± 1%, and 24% ± 1% for patients with early, intermediate, and advanced disease, respectively. The probabilities of survival after an unrelated donor transplant were 49% ± 1%, 47% ± 1%, and 22% ± 1% for patient with early, intermediate, and advanced disease, respectively.
6. Enasidenib, a selective inhibitor of mutated isocitrate dehydrogenase 2 (IDH-2), was approved by the FDA in 2017 for relapsed or refractory AML with IDH-2 mutations. IDH-2 mutations are found in about 12% of AML patients. At a dose of 100 mg orally, the response rate was 40.3%, with 19.3% achieving remission, some durable. Differentiation syndrome can be seen with enasidenib, similar to therapy for APML.
7. Ivosidenib, a selective inhibitor of isocitrate dehydrogenase-1 (IDH-1) mutation, was approved by the FDA in 2018 as the first treatment of adult patients with relapsed/refractory acute myeloid leukemia with an IDH-1 mutation. Approval was based on results from a phase 1, open-label, single-arm, multicenter, dose-escalation, expansion trial of adult patients in this population. The primary end point was combined complete remission and complete remission with partial hematologic improvement; the combined rate was 32.8%, and the median duration of remission was 8.2 months.
8. Relapses after bone marrow transplant can sometimes be managed with donor lymphocyte infusions, adjustment of immune suppression, and chemotherapy (often low intensity). In general, outcomes are poor with posttransplant relapses.

TABLE 6 Prognostic Models in Older Patients with Acute Myeloid Leukemia

Study	Outcome	Unfavorable Characteristics
Study Alliance Leukemia	Survival Disease-free survival	CD34 expression >10% WBC >20 × 10^9/L Age >65 yr LDH >700 U/L NPM1 status wild-type[a]
UK Medical Research Council	Survival	Adverse cytogenetic group Elevated WBC[b] Poor performance status[b] Older age[b] Secondary AML
Acute Leukemia French Association	Survival	High-risk cytogenetics ± Age ≥75 yr Performance status ≥2 WBC ≥50 × 10^9/L
MD Anderson Cancer Center	Remission rate Induction mortality Survival	Age ≥75 yr Secondary AML[c] AHD duration ≥6[c] (12) months Treatment outside LAFR Unfavorable cytogenetics WBC ≥25 × 10^9/L[c] Hemoglobin ≤8 g/dl[c] Creatinine >1.3 mg/dl Performance status >2 LDH >600 U/L[d]
Hematopoietic Cell Transplantation Comorbidity Index	Early mortality Survival	Dyspnea Coronary artery disease, CHF, MI, or EF <50% Chronic hepatitis, elevation of bilirubin and/or transaminases Cirrhosis Elevations of creatinine, dialysis, renal transplant Secondary AML Depression/anxiety requiring therapy Continued use of antimicrobial therapy after day 0 BMI >35 kg/m^2

[a]Favorable and high-risk groups were defined solely by cytogenetic aberrations. Above factors served to further divide the intermediate risk group into good intermediate versus adverse intermediate.
[b]As continuous variables.
[c]Only significant for prediction of remission.
[d]Only significant for prediction of survival.
AHD, Antecedent hematologic disorder; *BMI,* body mass index; *CHF,* congestive heart failure; *EF,* ejection fraction; *LAFR,* laminar air flow room (isolation floor); *LDH,* lactate dehydrogenase; *MI,* myocardial infarction; *WBC,* white blood cell count.
From Hoffman R, et al.: *Hematology, basic principles and practice*, ed 7, Philadelphia, 2018, Elsevier.

- Treatment of older patients (>60 yr) is problematic, with cure rates of 10% to 15%. Older patients do worse because they are more likely to have high-risk features and less likely to tolerate therapy. Several models have been devised to identify variables that predict which patients may do well with conventional therapy versus those who will not (Table 6). Options for these patients include:
  1. Standard induction therapy is reasonable for patients likely to tolerate it. Even in the absence of cure, quality of life is often excellent in remission. More recent studies suggest that the early death rate (within 30 days of diagnosis) was lower for patients in their 70s and 80s receiving standard induction. There is no standardized approach to evaluating fitness for therapy; one algorithm is at www.aml-score.org/.
  2. Hypomethylating agents—decitabine and azacytidine—may be considered in patients unlikely to tolerate induction therapy. Azacytidine (75 mg/m^2 daily for 7 days every 28 days) and decitabine (20 mg/m^2 for 5 days every 28 days) are considered in older patients who are not considered appropriate for induction chemotherapy. Both are outpatient regimens, and decitabine especially is very well tolerated. Recent data with azacytidine suggest benefit in about 20% to 30% lasting 14 to 16 mo in responders, with equivalent results in low blast count (20%-30% in the bone marrow) vs. higher blast count disease.
  3. Single-agent gemtuzumab ozogamicin is an option for treatment of CD33+ AML in patients considered unfit for induction. The benefit compared to best supportive care (BSC) was mainly seen in patients with CD33 expression of greater than 80% and favorable/intermediate cytogenetics (1 yr survival 22% and 37% respectively, BSC <10%), with no benefit in patients with high-risk cytogenetics.
  4. Low-dose cytarabine 20 mg/m^2 twice daily or 40 mg/m^2 daily for 10 days sub-

cutaneously) has shown survival benefit over hydroxyurea in low-/intermediate-risk patients.

5. In November 2018, the FDA granted the accelerated approval to venetoclax (a bcl-2 protein inhibitor) in combination with azacitidine or decitabine or low-dose cytarabine for the treatment of newly diagnosed acute myeloid leukemia in adults who are age 75 yrs or older, or who have comorbidities that preclude use of intensive induction chemotherapy. The recommended venetoclax dose depends upon the combination regimen and is described in prescribing information of venetoclax.
6. In November 2018 the FDA approved glasdegib (a small molecule inhibitor of Sonic hedgehog pathway) in combination with low-dose cytarabine (LDAC), for newly diagnosed acute myeloid leukemia in patients who are 75 yrs old or older or who have comorbidities that preclude intensive induction chemotherapy. Approval was based upon a multicenter, open-label, randomized study that randomized eligible patients 2:1 to receive glasdegib, 100 mg daily, with LDAC 20 mg subcutaneously twice daily on days 1 to 10 of a 28-day cycle or LDAC alone in 28-day cycles until disease progression or unacceptable toxicity. Efficacy was established based on an improvement in overall survival, 8.3 months for LDAC + glasdegib versus 4.3 months for LDAC alone. HR of 0.46 (95% CI: 0.30, 0.71; p=0.0002).
7. Oral hydroxyurea dosed to counts and cytopenias.
8. Best supportive care.
9. Reduced-intensity allogeneic stem cell transplant is an option for patients in remission after standard therapy. A recent meta-analysis of studies including 749 patients over 60 receiving RIT identified a 3-yr relapse-free survival of 35%.

- **Acute Promyelocytic Leukemia** (APML) APML is a distinct leukemia syndrome with very different treatment implications. Cure rates greater than 95% have been seen in current protocols in the absence of high-risk features. It is associated with t(15;17), which translocates the *PML* gene to retinoic acid receptor α (PML-RARa). Uncommon variants are t(11;17) and t(5;17). Risk groups for relapse were defined in studies using retinoic acid and chemotherapy. Patients with presenting WBC >10,000/mcl were considered high risk, patients with WBC <10,000 and platelets >40,000 were considered low risk, and all others were considered intermediate risk. In current protocols, high-risk patients receive some form of intensified therapy.
- APML is a medical emergency because of the high risk of bleeding complications.
  1. All patients with APML have DIC, caused by overexpression of annexin II, (which increases generation of plasmin, degrading fibrin), elastases (which degrade fibrinogen and fibrinolytic inhibitors), and increased endothelial tissue plasminogen activator release.
  2. Early death due to hemorrhage is seen in 5% to 17% of newly diagnosed APML patients, usually intracranial or pulmonary. Risk factors include elevated WBC, increased age, and elevated creatinine.
  3. Retinoic acid rapidly stabilizes the coagulopathy of APML; consideration should be given to starting this immediately for suspected cases.
  4. Cryoprecipitate (usual dose 10 bags) to raise the fibrinogen level to 150 mg/dl and platelet transfusion to raise the count to >50,000//mcl should be given as needed.
  5. Unfractionated heparin may paradoxically stop bleeding in APML by inhibiting DIC, but is rarely used in the retinoic acid treatment era.
- Diagnosis of APML.
  1. Rapid diagnosis is essential due to treatment implications.
  2. Diagnosis by classic APML blast morphology and clinical syndrome (especially DIC with low fibrinogen) is sufficient to justify starting treatment with retinoic acid pending confirmation with molecular studies. Immediate therapy with retinoic acid will rapidly stabilize the coagulopathy and help prevent catastrophic bleeding.
  3. Polymerase chain reaction for PML/RARa.
  4. FISH for t(15;17) or variants.
  5. Flow cytometry is typically distinct with lack of HLA-DR and CD34; CD13, CD33 and CD64 are usually positive.
- Therapy of APML.
  1. Emergency measures to stabilize coagulopathy as outlined previously.
  2. Patients with WBC ≤10,000 (low/intermediate risk) are treated with retinoic acid and arsenic trioxide ("differentiation therapy").
  3. Therapy of high-risk patients is less well standardized but has included intensification with cytarabine, anthracyclines, and gemtuzumab ozogamicin. A recent trial using arsenic and retinoic acid with GO demonstrated 100% 4-yr survival in high-risk patients after 30 days, emphasizing the importance of preventing early deaths in APML.
  4. Maintenance therapy for 2 yrs is given in some APML protocols.
  5. Patients with high-risk disease receive central nervous system prophylaxis with intrathecal chemotherapy.
  6. Treatment of relapsed disease typically consists of autologous bone marrow transplant after obtaining second remission.
- Differentiation syndrome (DS) is a potentially fatal complication of therapy with retinoic acid and arsenic trioxide. It is associated with fever, interstitial pulmonary infiltrates, peripheral edema, pleural and pericardial effusions and renal failure; it is commonly associated with rising WBC seen in patients on differentiation therapy.
  1. Therapy for suspected differentiation syndrome is dexamethasone 10 mg/m^2 every 12 hr. Cytoreductive therapy (hydroxyurea, idarubicin) and stopping retinoic acid and arsenic are appropriate for inadequate response to dexamethasone.
  2. Prophylaxis for differentiation syndrome with dexamethasone 2.5 mg/m^2 every 12 hr has been suggested for WBC >5000 or creatinine >1.4 mg/dl. Hydroxyurea is used to keep the WBC below 10,000/mcl in some protocols.

PEARLS & CONSIDERATIONS

- The diagnosis of acute myeloid leukemia or variants is often, but not always, a medical emergency requiring rapid clinical and laboratory assessment by appropriate expertise.
- APML is a distinct clinical entity that has a high cure rate with current protocols, but which requires intensive supportive care at the time of diagnosis.

RELATED CONTENT

Acute Myelogenous Leukemia (Patient Information)

SUGGESTED READINGS

Available at ExpertConsult.com

AUTHOR: **TODD F. ROBERTS, M.D., F.R.C.P.(C.)**

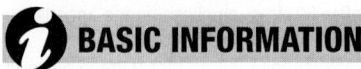

BASIC INFORMATION

DEFINITION

Acute pelvic pain in women is defined as pain in either the pelvis or the bilateral lower quadrants of the abdomen that has been present less than 3 months and is usually sudden in onset.

SYNONYMS

Acute lower abdominal pain
Acute suprapubic pain

ICD-10CM CODE
R10.2 Pelvic and perineal pain/acute female pelvic pain/pelvic pain, acute

EPIDEMIOLOGY & DEMOGRAPHICS

- Acute pelvic pain occurs in women of all ages.

PEAK INCIDENCE: Women of reproductive age report the greatest amount of acute pelvic pain.

PREVALENCE: Acute pelvic pain is a very broad term with multiple etiologies, thus not lending itself to a single calculable prevalence. However, the prevalence of some of the most documented common causes in the U.S. include PID (2,500,000 women with a personal history in the U.S. as of 2015), ovarian torsion (2.7% of emergent gynecologic surgeries each yr), ectopic pregnancy (0.6% to 2.1% of all pregnancies), and appendicitis (6.7% lifetime risk in women).

PREDOMINANT SEX AND AGE: Women of reproductive age report the greatest amount of acute pelvic pain.

PHYSICAL FINDINGS & CLINICAL PRESENTATION

- The history and physical examination are key to narrowing the diagnosis when a patient presents with acute pelvic pain.
- Standard thorough history-taking techniques should be employed, and the patient should be asked about location, onset, severity, radiation, exacerbating and alleviating factors, as well as the quality of the pain.
- Associated symptoms such as nausea, vomiting, anorexia, vaginal discharge, dyspareunia, dysuria, hematuria, urinary frequency, fever, recent upper respiratory infection (URI) symptoms, cyclic midcycle pelvic pain, or any missed or irregular menses should also be inquired about.
- A thorough sexual history should also be taken, including form of birth control used. Patients should also be asked about any history of ovarian cysts, uterine fibroids, recent pregnancies, or other pelvic infections.
- Physical exam is focused on the abdominal and pelvic exam.
- The pelvic exam includes vaginal speculum exam as well as bimanual and rectovaginal pelvic exam. During the speculum exam the patient is evaluated for any active vaginal bleeding, any vaginal or cervical discharge, and for any vulvar or vaginal lesions and masses.
- Testing for gonorrhea and chlamydia via nucleic acid probe should be collected.
- The bimanual and rectovaginal exams help elucidate the size and contour of the uterus, the presence of any adnexal masses or tenderness, and whether the patient has cervical motion tenderness.

ETIOLOGY

Etiologies of acute pelvic pain are varied and depend on the age and pregnancy status of the patient. Please see differential diagnosis for further information.

DIAGNOSIS

DIFFERENTIAL DIAGNOSIS

GYNECOLOGIC CAUSES:
- Pelvic inflammatory disease
- Ruptured ovarian cyst
- Adnexal mass (most pain from ovarian cysts >4 to 5 cm in size and hemorrhagic in nature)
- Ovarian torsion
- Degenerating or torsed uterine fibroid
- Mittelschmerz
- Tubo-ovarian abscess
- Endometriosis
- Dysmenorrhea
- Hematometra/Hematocolpos

EARLY PREGNANCY/POSTPARTUM-RELATED CAUSES:
- Miscarriage
- Ectopic pregnancy
- Postpartum endometritis

NONOBSTETRIC OR GYNECOLOGIC CAUSES:
- Appendicitis
- Urinary tract infection
- Nephrolithiasis
- Diverticulitis
- Colitis
- Bowel obstruction
- Mesenteric lymphadenitis
- Inflammatory bowel disease
- Meckel Diverticulum
- Constipation
- Hernia
- Gastroenteritis
- Musculoskeletal dysfunction
- Trauma

WORKUP

The workup of acute pelvic pain begins with a thorough history and physical exam, then targeted imaging and laboratory studies are ordered to further the diagnosis.

LABORATORY TESTS

- Pregnancy testing via urine or serum
- Rh typing if pregnancy test is positive
- Urinalysis
- Testing for vaginal infections including gonorrhea and chlamydia via direct nucleic acid probe
- Complete blood count (CBC)
- Erythrocyte sedimentation rate (ESR)
- First and foremost, one must determine the pregnancy status of the patient. The most common pregnancy-related causes of acute pelvic pain are ectopic pregnancy (approximately 1 in 7000 spontaneously conceived pregnancies and 1 in 100 pregnancies conceived via artificial reproduction) and spontaneous or threatened miscarriage. In both of these cases, the Rh status of the patient must be determined and RhoGAM administered if she is Rh negative
- Urinalysis will assist with the diagnosis of both acute cystitis and nephrolithiasis and urine culture should be ordered as well when appropriate. Nucleic acid probes for gonorrhea and chlamydia are very sensitive and specific tests and should be collected on any patient with pelvic pain. CBC and ESR can be utilized in the patient with suspected gastrointestinal disease, appendicitis, and pelvic infection of any kind to help determine the severity of disease

IMAGING STUDIES

- Pelvic ultrasound is the primary imaging modality for acute pelvic pain in women that is suspected to be of gynecologic origin. Ultrasound can be used to diagnose intrauterine and ectopic pregnancy (Fig. 1), uterine fibroids, adnexal masses, nephrolithiasis, and even appendicitis, thus assisting with the diagnosis of the vast majority of the differential diagnosis of acute pelvic pain in women. However, there are limitations to the test, such as the level of expertise of the individual sonographer and patient body habitus interfering with the quality of the images.
- In the case of the patient with nonfocal symptoms or an inconclusive ultrasound, computed tomography (CT) of the abdomen and pelvis can be performed. CT is highly useful in the patient with early pelvic inflammatory disease (PID) or tubo-ovarian abscess, as well as in the nonpregnant patient with appendicitis or other gastrointestinal pathology not seen on ultrasound.
- Magnetic resonance imaging (MRI) also plays a role when CT is unable to discern whether a mass in the pelvis is of uterine or adnexal origin such as with a degenerating fibroid or when one must further characterize an ovarian mass. MRI is also extremely helpful in the pregnant patient who presents with many signs and symptoms of appendicitis but has an inconclusive ultrasound result. Pediatric patients are also excellent candidates for MRI when ultrasound is inconclusive. Lower levels of ionizing radiation and its excellent diagnostic capabilities make it a very useful test in this population.

TREATMENT

NONPHARMACOLOGIC THERAPY

- The underlying cause of acute pelvic pain cannot always be diagnosed with history, exam, laboratory, and imaging studies alone. In many cases, diagnostic laparoscopy is

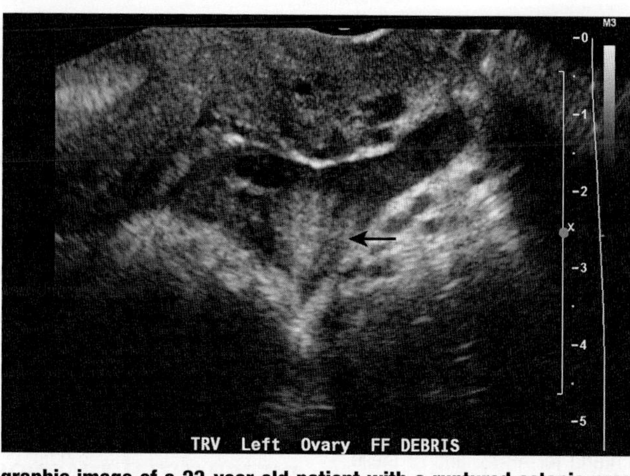

FIG. 1 A sonographic image of a 23-year-old patient with a ruptured ectopic pregnancy. The free fluid containing echogenic debris representing blood is seen in the cul-de-sac *(arrow)*. (From Soto JA, Lucey BC: *Emergency radiology, the requisites,* ed 2, Philadelphia, 2017, Elsevier.)

necessary to complete the diagnosis. In fact, even when the diagnosis seems sure, laparoscopy can reveal an entirely different finding as was illustrated in one study where just over half of women clinically diagnosed with appendicitis actually had the disease.

- The practitioner should not hesitate to take the patient with unstable vital signs and suspected intraabdominal bleeding or findings suggestive of ruptured appendix to the operating room. When one's clinical suspicion is quite high for such diagnoses, laboratory data and imaging studies should be forgone to expedite getting the patient the surgical interventions she needs.

ACUTE GENERAL Rx

The initial treatment of the woman with acute pelvic pain must be tailored to the underlying cause. However, as the workup is in progress, her pain must be managed. Although narcotic pain medications are sometimes initially necessary to control pain, NSAIDs are the traditional first line pharmacotherapy for the patient with pelvic pain of an inflammatory nature. Such medications are highly useful in cases of endometriosis, dysmenorrhea, nonsurgical cases of ovarian masses and ruptured ovarian cysts, spontaneous miscarriage, nephrolithiasis, musculoskeletal dysfunction, and PID/tubo-ovarian abscess. Heat and ice can also be employed as needed for additional symptomatic relief in the appropriate patient.

CHRONIC Rx

Once a diagnosis is made, treatment is based on the underlying cause of the pain. Most patients are managed on a combination of NSAID and narcotic pain medications for a short course until the pathology has resolved or after any surgical interventions. Antibiotic therapy is routinely included in the case of an infectious cause.

REFERRAL

Patients with pain lasting greater than 3 to 6 months should be seen by a specialist in the appropriate field—gynecology, gastroenterology, general surgery, or musculoskeletal medicine—for further workup and management of their now chronic pelvic pain. Referral should also be considered when the underlying cause of pain cannot be found.

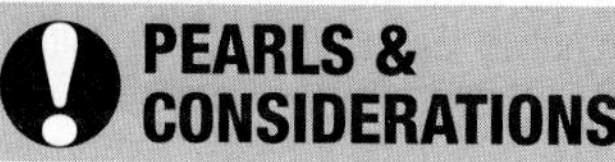

PEARLS & CONSIDERATIONS

A solid knowledge of the differential diagnosis of acute pelvic pain in women and a thorough history and physical examination will lead the practitioner to the underlying cause in the vast majority of cases. But all women who present with acute pelvic pain MUST have a pregnancy test as a part of their initial workup. If imaging is needed, pelvic ultrasound is an excellent tool and should be utilized first before CT and MRI in most cases.

SUGGESTED READINGS

Available at ExpertConsult.com

RELATED CONTENT

Appendicitis (Related Key Topic)
Diverticular Disease (Diverticulosis, Diverticulitis, Diverticular Dysmenorrhea) (Related Key Topic)
Ectopic Pregnancy (Related Key Topic)
Endometriosis (Related Key Topic)
Endometritis (Related Key Topic)
Inflammatory Bowel Disease (Related Key Topic)
Pelvic Inflammatory Disease (Related Key Topic)
Spontaneous Abortion (Related Key Topic)
Urinary Tract Infection (Related Key Topic)
Urolithiasis (Nephrolithiasis) (Related Key Topic)
Uterine Fibroids (Related Key Topic)

AUTHOR: **MICHELE TARTAGLIA, D.O., F.A.C.O.O.G., C.S.**

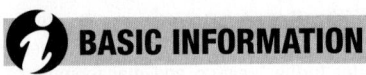

BASIC INFORMATION

DEFINITION

Acute respiratory distress syndrome (ARDS) is a form of noncardiogenic pulmonary edema that results from acute damage to the alveoli. It is characterized by acute diffuse infiltrative lung lesions with resulting interstitial and alveolar edema, severe hypoxemia, and respiratory failure. The cardinal feature of ARDS, refractory hypoxemia, is caused by formation of protein-rich alveolar edema after damage to the integrity of the lung's alveolar-capillary barrier.

The definition of ARDS based on the American–European Consensus Conference (AECC) from 1994 included the following components:

1. The syndrome must present acutely
2. A ratio of Pa_{O_2} to Fi_{O_2} ≤200 regardless of the level of positive end expiratory pressure (PEEP)
3. The detection of bilateral pulmonary infiltrates on frontal chest radiograph
4. Absence of congestive heart failure (pulmonary artery wedge pressure [PAWP] ≤18 mm Hg or no clinical evidence of elevated left atrial pressure on the basis of chest radiograph or other clinical data)

The Berlin definition of ARDS adopted in 2011 addresses some of the limitations of the AECC definition and establishes the following criteria for ARDS:

- Timing: Within 1 week of a known clinical insult or new or worsening respiratory symptoms
- Chest imaging (chest x-ray or computed tomography [CT] scan): Bilateral opacities, not fully explained by effusions, lobar/lung collapse, or nodules
- Origin of edema: Respiratory failure not fully explained by cardiac failure or fluid overload. Need objective assessment (e.g., echocardiography) to exclude hydrostatic edema if no risk factor present
- Oxygenation (if altitude is higher than 1000 m, the correction factor should be calculated as follows: [Pa_{O_2}/Fi_{O_2} × {barometric pressure/760}]
- Mild: 200 mm Hg < Pa_{O_2}/Fi_{O_2} ≤300 mm Hg with PEEP or CPAP ≥5 cm H_2O (this may be delivered noninvasively in the mild ARDS group)
- Moderate: 100 mm Hg < Pa_{O_2}/Fi_{O_2} ≤200 mm Hg with PEEP or CPAP ≥5 cm H_2O
- Severe: Pa_{O_2}/Fi_{O_2} ≤100 mm Hg with PEEP or CPAP ≥5 cm H_2O

SYNONYMS

ARDS
Adult respiratory distress syndrome

ICD-10CM CODE

J80 Acute respiratory distress syndrome

EPIDEMIOLOGY & DEMOGRAPHICS

- More than 150,000 ARDS cases/yr in the U.S. 7.1% of all patients admitted to an intensive care unit (ICU) and 16.1% of all patients on mechanical ventilation develop ARDS.
- An international study of 50 countries revealed that 10% of those admitted to an ICU fulfilled criteria for ARDS, and of these, 93% developed it within 48 hours of admission. The study reinforced the notion that ARDS is underrecognized.
- Black, Hispanic, and other patients belonging to racial minorities in the United States were observed to exhibit significantly higher in-hospital sepsis-related respiratory failure and associated mortality.

PHYSICAL FINDINGS & CLINICAL PRESENTATION

- Signs and symptoms
  1. Dyspnea
  2. Chest discomfort
  3. Cough
  4. Anxiety
- Physical examination
  1. Tachypnea
  2. Tachycardia
  3. Hypertension
  4. Paradoxical breathing and use of accessory muscles
  5. Coarse crepitations or crackles of both lungs
  6. Fever may be present if infection is the underlying etiology

ETIOLOGY

- Sepsis (>40% of cases)
- Aspiration: Near-drowning, aspiration of gastric contents (>30% of cases)
- Trauma (>20% of cases)
- Pneumonia (aspiration of gastric contents and sepsis together account for more than 85% of cases of ARDS in recent clinical trials)
- Multiple transfusions, blood products
- Drugs (e.g., overdose of morphine, methadone, heroin; reaction to nitrofurantoin)
- Noxious inhalation (e.g., chlorine gas, high O_2 concentration)
- Post-resuscitation
- Cardiopulmonary bypass
- Burns
- Pancreatitis
- A history of chronic alcohol abuse significantly increases the risk of developing ARDS in critically ill patients.
- Table 1 describes risk factors associated with development of ARDS.

TABLE 1 Risk Factors Associated with Development of Acute Lung Injury and Acute Respiratory Distress Syndrome

Direct Lung Injury	Indirect Lung Injury
Pneumonia	Sepsis
Aspiration of gastric contents	Multiple trauma
Pulmonary contusion	Cardiopulmonary bypass
Fat, amniotic fluid, or air emboli	Drug overdose
Near-drowning	Acute pancreatitis
Inhalational injury	Transfusion of blood products
Reperfusion pulmonary edema	

From Vincent JL, et al.: *Textbook of critical care*, ed 6, Philadelphia, 2011, Saunders.

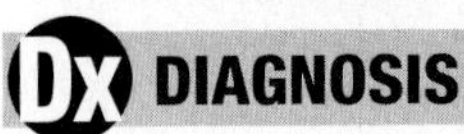

DIAGNOSIS

DIFFERENTIAL DIAGNOSIS

- Congestive heart failure
- Interstitial lung disease (acute interstitial pneumonia, nonspecific interstitial pneumonia [NSIP], cryptogenic organizing pneumonia [COP], acute eosinophilic pneumonia, hypersensitivity pneumonia, pulmonary alveolar proteinosis)
- Connective tissue diseases, such as polymyositis
- Diffuse alveolar hemorrhage
- Lymphangitic carcinomatosis from T-cell or B-cell lymphomas
- Drug-induced lung diseases (amiodarone, bleomycin)

WORKUP

The search for an underlying cause should focus on treatable causes (e.g., infections such as sepsis or pneumonia)

- Arterial blood gases (ABGs)
- Hemodynamic monitoring
- Bronchoalveolar lavage (selected patients)

LABORATORY TESTS

- ABGs:
  1. Initially: Varying degrees of hypoxemia, generally resistant to supplemental oxygen
  2. Respiratory alkalosis, decreased Pc_{O_2}
  3. Widened alveolar-arterial gradient
  4. Hypercapnia as the disease progresses
- Bronchoalveolar lavage:
  1. The most prominent finding is an increased number of polymorphonucleocytes.
  2. The presence of eosinophilia has therapeutic implications because these patients respond to corticosteroids.
- Blood and urine cultures
- Blood work:
  1. Increased or reduced white blood cell count with left shift if concomitant infectious process
  2. Normal or mildly elevated B-type natriuretic peptide level
  3. Increased lactate level if concomitant sepsis or septic shock

IMAGING STUDIES

Chest radiograph (Fig. 1).

- The initial chest radiograph might be normal in the initial hours after the precipitating event.

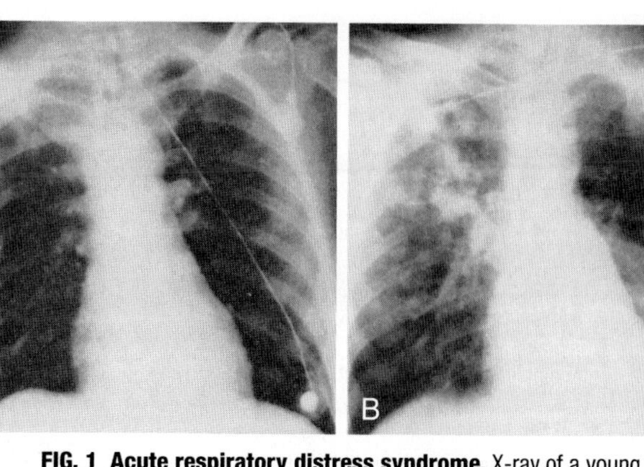

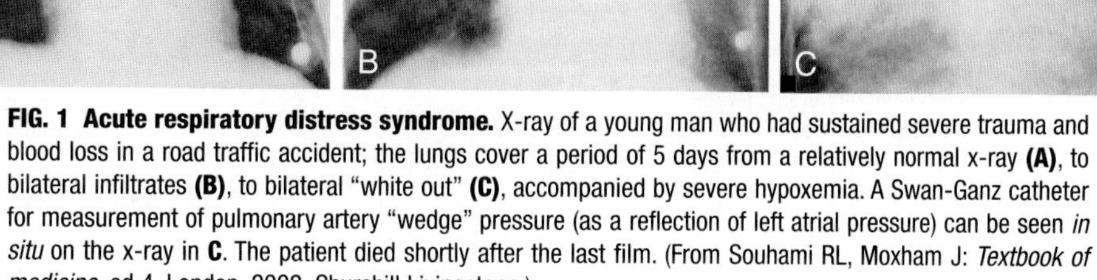

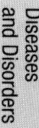

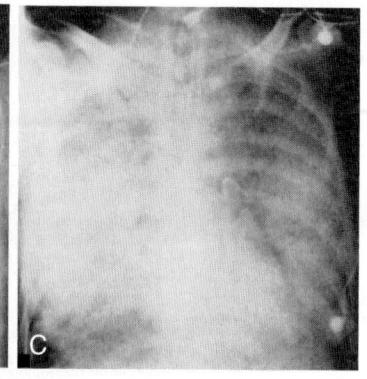

FIG. 1 Acute respiratory distress syndrome. X-ray of a young man who had sustained severe trauma and blood loss in a road traffic accident; the lungs cover a period of 5 days from a relatively normal x-ray **(A)**, to bilateral infiltrates **(B)**, to bilateral "white out" **(C)**, accompanied by severe hypoxemia. A Swan-Ganz catheter for measurement of pulmonary artery "wedge" pressure (as a reflection of left atrial pressure) can be seen *in situ* on the x-ray in **C**. The patient died shortly after the last film. (From Souhami RL, Moxham J: *Textbook of medicine*, ed 4, London, 2002, Churchill Livingstone.)

- Bilateral interstitial infiltrates are usually seen within 24 hr; they often are more prominent in the bases and periphery.
- CT scan of chest: Bilateral diffuse, dense consolidations with air bronchograms.

Rx TREATMENT

NONPHARMACOLOGIC THERAPY

Treatment of ARDS is supportive.

Hemodynamic monitoring:

- Can be used for the initial evaluation of ARDS (in ruling out cardiogenic pulmonary edema) and its subsequent management. However, a pulmonary catheter is not indicated in the routine management of ARDS and trials have shown that clinical management involving the early use of pulmonary artery catheters in patients with ARDS did not significantly affect mortality and morbidity rates and may result in more complications as compared with a central venous catheter.
- Although no dynamic profile is diagnostic of ARDS, the presence of pulmonary edema, a high cardiac output, and a low pulmonary capillary wedge pressure (PCWP) is characteristic of ARDS.
- It is important to remember that partially treated intravascular volume overload and flash pulmonary edema can have the hemodynamic features of ARDS; filling pressures can also be elevated by increased intrathoracic pressures or with fluid administration; cardiac function can be depressed by acidosis, hypoxemia, or other factors associated with sepsis.

Ventilatory support:

- Noninvasive positive-pressure ventilation (NIPPV) (i.e., BiPAP) should only be used in selected cases in patients with hypoxic respiratory failure. A recent randomized control study showed that high-flow oxygen by nasal cannula reduced ventilator-free days and mortality compared with NIPPV in patients with hypoxemic respiratory failure without hypercapnia. Either modality should not delay intubation and mechanical ventilation initiation in patients with rapidly progressing clinical deterioration.
- Mechanical ventilation is generally necessary to maintain adequate gas exchange (Table 2). General recommendations for ventilator settings in ARDS are described in Table 3. A low tidal volume and low plateau pressure ventilator strategy are recommended to avoid ventilator-induced injury. Assist-control is generally preferred initially with the following ventilator settings:
  1. Fio_2 1.0 (until a lower value can be used to achieve adequate oxygenation). When possible, minimize oxygen toxicity by maintaining Fio_2 at <60%.
- Tidal volume: Set initial tidal volume at 6 ml/kg of predicted body weight (PBW). Tidal volumes are reduced from 6 ml/kg of PBW to a minimum of 4 ml/kg if plateau airway pressures exceed 30 cm of water. The concept of using PBW is based on the fact that lung size depends most strongly on height and sex; PBW normalizes the tidal volume to lung size. Aim to maintain plateau pressure (Pplat) at <30 mm Hg.
- PEEP 5 cm H_2O or greater (to increase lung volume and keep alveoli open). PEEP should be applied in small increments of 3 to 5 cm H_2O (see Table 2) to achieve acceptable arterial saturation (>0.9) with nontoxic Fio_2 values (<0.6) and acceptable airway plateau pressures (<30 to 35 cm H_2O). It is important to remember that an increase in PEEP may lower cardiac output and, despite improvement in Pao_2, may actually have a negative effect on tissue oxygenation (the major determinants of tissue oxygenation are hemoglobin, percent saturation, and cardiac output). The optimal level of PEEP remains unestablished. Although higher levels of PEEP may help prevent life-threatening hypoxemia and be associated with lower hospital mortality in patients meeting criteria for ARDS, such benefit is unlikely in patients with less severe lung injury (pa02/Fi02 >200) and a strategy of treating such patients with high PEEP levels may be harmful. In fact, a new study published in 2017 demonstrated that the open lung approach increases mortality in patients with moderate to severe ARDS.
- Inspiratory flow: 60 L/min.
- Ventilatory rate: High ventilatory rates of up to 35 breaths/min are often necessary in patients with ARDS to achieve the desired minute ventilation because of their increased physiologic dead space and smaller lung volumes. Patients must be monitored for excessive intrathoracic gas trapping (auto-PEEP or intrinsic PEEP) that can depress cardiac output.
- Permissive hypercapnia: To maintain a low plateau pressure, a low tidal volume is frequently required, leading to a reduced minute ventilation and hypoventilation with consequently a respiratory acidosis (elevated PCO_2 and reduced pH). Most patients (excluding patients with cerebral edema, acute coronary syndrome, seizures, cardiac arrhythmias, and so on) can tolerate a low pH without major consequences. Bicarbonate replacement is suggested when the pH falls to below 7.20.
- Sedation: Gamma-aminobutyric acid (GABA) receptor agonists (including propofol and benzodiazepines) have traditionally been the most commonly administered sedative drugs for ICU patients. Recent trials indicate that the alpha-2 agonist dexmedetomidine (Precedex) may have distinct advantages. At comparable sedation levels, dexmedetomidine-treated patients spent less time on ventilator, experienced less delirium, and developed less tachycardia and hypertension. The most notable adverse effect of dexmedetomidine was bradycardia. Preliminary trials involving early administration of the neuromuscular blocking agent cisatracurium in patients with severe ARDS have shown improvement in the adjusted 90-day survival and increase in the time off the ventilator without increase in muscle weakness. However, patients who receive continuous infusions of sedatives generally need to be on mechanical ventilation longer than those who receive intermittent dosing. Paralysis of

TABLE 2 Ventilator Management of Patients with ARDS

Calculate Predicted Body Weight (PBW)	• Males: PBW (kg) = 50 + 2.3 [(height in inches) − 60] *or* 50 + 0.91 [(height in cm) − 152.4] • Females: IBW (kg) = 45.5 + 2.3 [(height in inches) − 60] *or* 45.5 + 0.91 [(height in cm) − 152.4]
Ventilator Mode	• Volume assist/control until weaning
Tidal Volume (Vt)	• Initial Vt: 6 ml/kg predicted body weight • Measure inspiratory plateau pressure (Pplat, 0.5 sec inspiratory pause) every 4 hours *and* after each change in positive end-expiratory pressure (PEEP) or Vt. • If Pplat is >30 cm H_2O, decrease Vt to 5 or 4 ml/kg. • If Pplat is <25 cm H_2O and Vt <6 ml/kg PBW, increase Vt by 1 ml/kg PBW
Respiratory Rate (RR)	• With initial change in Vt, adjust RR to maintain minute ventilation. • Make subsequent adjustments to RR to maintain pH 7.30-7.45, but do not exceed RR = 35/min and do not increase set rate if $Paco_2$ is <25 mm Hg.
I:E Ratio	• Acceptable range, 1:1-1:3 (no inverse ratio)
Fio_2, PEEP, and Arterial Oxygenation	• Maintain Pao_2 = 55-80 mm Hg or Spo_2 = 88%-95% using the following PEEP/Fio_2 combinations: Fio_2: 0.3-0.4 / 0.4 / 0.5 / 0.6 / 0.7 / 0.8 / 0.9 / 1 PEEP: 5-8 / 8-14 / 8-16 / 10-20 / 10-20 / 14-22 / 16-22 / 18-25
Acidosis Management	1. If pH is <7.30, increase RR until pH is ≥7.30 or RR = 35/min. 2. If pH remains <7.30 with RR = 35, consider bicarbonate infusion. 3. If pH is <7.15, Vt may be increased (Pplat may exceed 30 cm H_2O).
Alkalosis Management	• If pH is >7.45 and patient is not triggering ventilator, decrease set RR but not below 6/min.
Fluid Management	• Once patients are out of shock, adopt a conservative fluid management strategy. • Use diuretics or fluids to target a central venous pressure (CVP) of <4 or a pulmonary artery occlusion pressure (PAOP) of <8.
Liberation from Mechanical Ventilation	• Daily interruption of sedation • Daily screen for spontaneous breathing trial (SBT) • SBT when all of the following criteria are present: (a) Fio_2 <0.40 and PEEP <8 cm H_2O (b) Not receiving neuromuscular blocking agents (c) Patient is awake and following commands (d) Systolic arterial pressure >90 mm Hg without vasopressor support (e) Tracheal secretions are minimal, and the patient has a good cough and gag reflex
Spontaneous Breathing Trial	• Place patient on 5 mm Hg pressure support with 5 mm Hg PEEP *or* T-piece. • Monitor heart rate, RR, oxygen saturation for 30-90 minutes. • Extubate if there are no signs of distress (tachycardia, tachypnea, agitation, hypoxia, diaphoresis).

FiO_2, Fraction of inspired oxygen; *IBW*, ideal body weight; *$PaCO_2$*, partial pressure of carbon dioxide in the arterial blood; *PaO_2*, partial pressure of oxygen in arterial blood; *SpO_2*, saturation of arterial blood with oxygen as measured by pulse oximetry.
From Vincent JL, et al,: *Textbook of critical care*, ed 7, Philadelphia, 2017, Elsevier.

TABLE 3 Recommendations for Ventilator Settings in ARDS

Conventional Mechanical Ventilation		
Mode		Volume- or pressure-controlled "Airway pressure release ventilation" preferred when preservation of spontaneous ventilation is desired
Tidal volume	6-10 ml/kg	Permissive hypercapnia (increase <5 mm Hg/h) $PaCO_2$ 65-85 mm Hg well tolerated unless increased ICP Arterial pH >7.15
End-inspiratory plateau pressure	<30 cm H_2O	Above this limit, increased risks of barotrauma and air leaks
Positive end-expiratory pressure	10-15 cm H_2O	Lower PEEP levels, if heterogeneous lung injury Higher PEEP levels, if diffuse lung injury Consider early prone positioning (6-12 h)
Respiratory rate	20-60 beats/min	Adjusted to age; higher than normal may limit hypercapnia
Inspiratory/expiratory ratio	1:2 to 1:1	Check for inadvertent PEEP
FiO_2	<60%-80%	Depends on how the diseased lung may be recruited PaO_2 40-60 mm Hg, SpO_2 85%-95%
High-Frequency Oscillatory Ventilation		
Amplitude pressure	30-50 cm H_2O	To achieve visible chest vibrations
Mean airway pressure	15-30 cm H_2O	To achieve adequate chest recruitment (7 to 9 ribs)
Respiratory rate	3-10 Hz	Decrease to increase tidal volume (usually not measured)
Inspiratory/expiratory ratio	1:3 to 1:1	1:1 more appropriate in diffuse lung injury
FiO_2	<60%-80%	Depends on whether the lung may be recruited

FiO_2, Fraction of inspired oxygen; *ICP*, intracranial pressure; *PaO_2*, partial pressure of oxygen in arterial blood; *PEEP*, positive end-expiratory pressure; *$SpO2$*, saturation of arterial blood with oxygen as measured by pulse oximetry.
From Fuhrman BP, et al,: *Pediatric critical care*, ed 4, Philadelphia, 2011, Saunders.

patients with neuromuscular blockade (NMB) to facilitate controlled ventilation is associated with protracted mechanical ventilation and postparalysis weakness. It should ideally be conducted for a brief period, and limited to patients with severe ARDS. Daily interruption of sedation (daily awakening) in mechanically ventilated patients is safe and is associated with a shorter length of mechanical ventilation.

ACUTE GENERAL Rx

Identify and treat precipitating conditions:

- Blood and urine cultures and trial of antibiotics in presumed sepsis (routine administration of antibiotics in all cases of ARDS is not recommended).
- Prompt repair of bone fractures in patients with major trauma.
- Crystalloid resuscitation in pancreatitis.
- Fluid management: In most patients with ARDS, fluid restriction is associated with better outcomes than a liberal fluid policy. Optimal fluid and hemodynamic management of patients with ARDS should be patient specific; in general, administration of crystalloids is recommended if a downward trend in PCWP is associated with diminished cardiac index, resulting in prerenal azotemia, oliguria, and relative tachycardia.
- Positioning the patient: Changes in position can improve oxygenation by improving the distribution of perfusion to ventilated lung regions; repositioning (lateral decubitus positioning) should be attempted in patients with hypoxemia that is not responsive to other medical interventions. Placing patients with moderate and severe hypoxemia in a prone position may improve their oxygenation. A meta-analysis that included the recent trials by Guerin et al have shown that in patients with severe ARDS, early application of prolonged (over 16 hours/day) prone-positioning sessions significantly decreases 28-day and 90-day mortality.
- Corticosteroids: Routine use of corticosteroids in ARDS is not recommended; corticosteroids may be beneficial in patients with many eosinophils in the bronchoalveolar lavage fluid or in patients with severe pneumonia. Systemic infections should be ruled out or adequately treated before administration of corticosteroids. Use of methylprednisolone has not been shown to increase the rate of infectious complications but is associated with a higher rate of neuromuscular weakness. In addition, starting methylprednisolone therapy more than 2 wk after the onset of ARDS may increase the risk of death.
- Nutritional support: Nutritional support, preferably administered by the enteral route, is necessary to maintain adequate colloid oncotic pressure and intravascular volume. The use of antioxidants and dietary oil supplements is still equivocal and cannot be recommended at this time.
- Tracheostomy: Tracheostomy is warranted in patients requiring >2 wk of mechanical ventilation; discussion regarding tracheostomy should begin with patient (if alert and oriented) and/or family members/legal guardian after 5 to 7 days of ventilatory support. Early tracheostomy (within 4 days of admission to critical care) does not limit mortality and results in many unneeded procedures (Young et al, 2013).
- Some form of deep vein thrombosis prophylaxis is indicated in all patients with ARDS.
- Stress ulcer prophylaxis with sucralfate suspension (by nasogastric tube), or proton pump inhibitors (PO or IV) or H_2 blockers (PO or IV). Should be reserved for seriously ill patients who are at high risk for this complication.
- The use of surfactant remains controversial. Patients who receive surfactant have a greater improvement in gas exchange in the initial 24-hour period than patients who receive standard therapy alone; however, the use of exogenous surfactant does not improve survival.

DISPOSITION

- Patients who survive ARDS are at risk of diminished functional capacity, mental illness, and decreased quality of life. Prognosis for ARDS varies with the underlying cause. Prognosis is worse in patients with chronic liver disease, non-pulmonary organ dysfunction, sepsis, and advanced age. ARDS survivors are at high risk for incident joblessness and substantial loss of wages, and 58% of those returning to work received disability.
- Elevated values of dead space fraction ($[Paco_2 > 2\ Peco_2]/Paco_2$; normal is <0.3) is associated with an increased risk of death.
- In ARDS, the percentage of potentially recruitable lung is variable and associated with the response to PEEP.
- Overall mortality rate varies between 32% and 45%. Most deaths are attributable to sepsis or multiorgan dysfunction rather than primary respiratory causes.
- Recent trials have shown that as compared with the current standard of care, a ventilator strategy using esophageal measures to estimate the transpulmonary pressure significantly improves oxygenation and compliance. Further trials will determine if this approach should be widely adapted.
- Strategies for treatment of life-threatening refractory hypoxemia (prone positioning, inhaled nitric acid, extracorporeal membrane oxygenation [ECMO], high-frequency oscillatory ventilation, recruitment maneuvers) may improve oxygenation, but their impact on mortality remains unproven. Use of ECMO in combination with lung-protective ventilation was found to be beneficial as a treatment strategy early in the course of ARDS related to H1N1 infection. Extracorporeal gas exchange may allow the use of low tidal volumes and lower levels of inspired oxygen and use of higher PEEP if desired. ECMO is costly and labor-intensive. The role and proper use of ECMO for patients with ARDS have not been clearly defined.
- General indications for venovenous ECMO in severe cases of ARDS are:
  1. Severe hypoxemia (e.g., ratio of PaO_2 to FiO_2 <80 despite the application of high levels of PEEP [typically 15 to 20 cm H_2O]) for at least 6 hr in patients with potentially reversible respiratory failure
  2. Uncompensated hypercapnia with acidemia (pH <7.15) despite the best accepted standard of care for management with a ventilator
  3. Excessively high end inspiratory plateau pressure (>35 to 45 cm H_2O, according to the patient's body size) despite the best accepted standard of care for management with a ventilator

REFERRAL

Surgical referral for tracheostomy (see "Acute General Rx").

SUGGESTED READINGS

Available at ExpertConsult.com

RELATED CONTENT

Acute Respiratory Distress Syndrome (ARDS) (Patient Information)

AUTHOR: **JORGE MERCADO, M.D.**

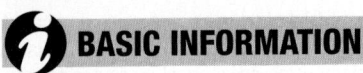

BASIC INFORMATION

DEFINITION

Respiratory failure is a condition in which the respiratory system fails in one or both of its gas exchanging functions (oxygenation and carbon dioxide elimination). Traditionally, there are two types of acute respiratory failure: type I (hypoxic) and type II (hypercapnic). Other sources have defined a type III and a type IV; type III is respiratory failure related to atelectasis, and type IV is related to hypoperfusion of respiratory muscles in patients with shock. Type I is described in detail in another chapter (see ARDS). This chapter focuses on type II respiratory failure. Table 1 summarizes the classification of Acute Respiratory Failure.

Type II Respiratory failure is defined as an elevation in arterial carbon dioxide tension, greater than 45 mm Hg. This is directly proportional to the rate of CO_2 production and inversely proportional to the rate of CO_2 elimination by the lungs. Both hypoxemia and hypercapnia can occur at the same time, depending on the location of the underlying disorder and mechanism.

Respiratory failure can be acute (ARF) or chronic. The acute presentation occurs within minutes to hours, whereas the chronic form develops over days or longer.

SYNONYMS

Respiratory insufficiency
Hypercarbic respiratory failure
Hypoxemic respiratory failure
ARF

ICD-10CM CODES

J96.00 Acute respiratory failure
J96.01 Acute respiratory failure with hypoxia
J96.02 Acute respiratory failure with hypercapnia
J96.90 Respiratory failure, unspecified
J96.91 Respiratory failure, unspecified with hypoxia
J96.92 Respiratory failure, unspecified with hypercapnia

EPIDEMIOLOGY & DEMOGRAPHICS

- An estimated 1.9 million patients discharged from acute care hospitals nationwide meet study criteria for ARF.
- The winter months seem to be where upper and lower respiratory infections are more prevalent, and therefore when there will be a peak incidence of acute respiratory failure cases.
- Comorbid conditions, including chronic disorders of the cardiac, pulmonary, neurologic, renal, hepatic systems, and the patient's advanced age elevate the risk of mortality.

PHYSICAL FINDINGS & CLINICAL PRESENTATION

- Decreased level of consciousness
- Increased cerebral blood flow, with increased intracranial pressure
- Decreased myocardial contractility
- Decreased diaphragmatic function
- Shift of the oxyhemoglobin dissociation curve to the right
- Physical signs:
  1. Dyspnea
  2. Somnolence
  3. Headaches
  4. Confusion
  5. Asterixis
  6. Coma

ETIOLOGY

See Tables 2 and 3.

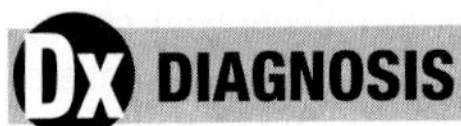

DIAGNOSIS

Diagnosis is made clinically according to physical findings, and it is confirmed by arterial blood gases. Table 4 summarizes common clues obtained from the history and physical examination.

DIFFERENTIAL DIAGNOSIS

See Table 2.

WORKUP

- After supportive therapy is initiated, a careful search for the underlying cause of the respiratory failure is critical, as this may have important implications on its ultimate therapy.

LABORATORY TESTS

- Arterial blood gas (Fig. 1), showing elevated CO_2 level
- Basal metabolic panel, showing elevated bicarbonate level

IMAGING STUDIES

- Chest imaging studies include:
  1. Chest x-ray
  2. CT scan of the chest (with angiography when suspecting pulmonary embolism)
  3. Chest ultrasound

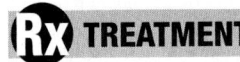

TREATMENT

The treatment of respiratory failure is initially supportive, aiming to determine first the acuity and/or severity of the presentation. Correction of the hypoxemia, hypercapnia, and management of the underlying etiology of the condition are essential to its treatment.

NONPHARMACOLOGIC THERAPY

- Treat the hypoxemia with oxygen support, which may require pressure support in the way of non-invasive ventilation (Bi-PAP) or mechanical ventilation, for the more severe cases.
- Treat hypercapnia with ventilatory support, non-invasive or invasively. The decision for either can be difficult and it is mainly based on clinical presentation, severity of symptoms, comorbidities, and level of acid base derangement, as well as mental status.

TABLE 1 Classification of Acute Respiratory Failure

	Type I	Type II	Type III	Type IV
MECHANISM OF HYPOXEMIA	Low FiO_2 ventilation/perfusion (V/Q) mismatch Shunting Reduced diffusing capacity	Hypoventilation	Shunting Hypoventilation V/Q mismatch	Hypoperfusion or inadequate oxygenation of peripheral tissues
LOCATION OF PATHOLOGICAL PROCESS	Inhaled air composition Alveolar-capillary unit Oxygen-carrying capacity of blood	Airway Central nervous system (CNS) Neuromuscular system Chest wall	Alveolar-capillary unit collapse with regional hypoventilation	Cardiovascular system Peripheral tissues
CLINICAL SYNDROMES	Cardiogenic pulmonary edema Acute respiratory distress syndrome Pneumonia Interstitial lung disease Pulmonary embolism Pulmonary hypertension Atelectasis Alveolar hemorrhage Carbon monoxide poisoning Anatomic shunts	Chronic obstructive pulmonary disease Asthma CNS depression (intoxication) CNS trauma or injury Neuromuscular disorders Skeletal disorders Obesity-hypoventilation syndrome	Thoracic or upper abdominal surgery or trauma Inadequate postoperative analgesia Pleural tumor or inflammation Trapped lung Subdiaphragmatic tumor or inflammation Obesity	Septic (distributive) shock Hypovolemic shock Cardiogenic shock Compromised cellular oxidation Hypermetabolic states

FiO_2, Fraction of inspired oxygen.
Modified from Jean-Louis V: *Intensive care medicine: annual update 2008*, Berlin Heidelberg, 2008, Springer-Verlag.

TABLE 2 Differential Diagnosis of Potential Causes of Acute Respiratory Failure

Central nervous system	Spinal cord, nerves, muscle	Chest wall, thoracic cage	Increased dead space
Medications (anesthetics and/or opioids) Alveolar hypoventilation Trauma Meningoencephalitis Localized tumors or vascular abnormalities of the medulla Strokes affecting medullary control centers Severe alkalosis	Medications Trauma Myasthenia gravis Guillain-Barre Syndrome Electrolyte abnormalities	Trauma Kyphoscoliosis Flail chest Pleural disease Scleroderma Morbid obesity Ascites Severe ileus	Obstructive airways disorders Upper: Acute epiglottitis, foreign body aspiration, tracheal tumor Lower: COPD, asthma, cystic fibrosis

COPD, Chronic obstructive pulmonary disease.

- Contraindications to non-invasive ventilation include respiratory arrest, hemodynamic or cardiac instability, or inability to protect the airway.
- Monitoring carbon dioxide levels has not been standardized, but a change in symptoms and or worsening in mental status can prompt a repeat in blood gas analysis.
- Worsening blood gas levels can be remediated with changes in the pressures on the non-invasive ventilator or by switching to a mechanical ventilator.

ACUTE GENERAL Rx

Ventilatory support, either invasive (mechanical ventilation) or non-invasive

TABLE 3 Pathophysiological Mechanisms That Lead to Hypoxia and Respiratory Insufficiency

Extrapulmonary processes including chest wall and skeletal abnormalities (hypoxic hypoxia)	Deficiency of oxygen in inspired air (high altitude, suffocation) Hypoactive hypoventilation (central nervous system trauma, drug toxicities, and neuromuscular and skeletal disorders) Upper airway obstruction leading to hypoventilation (trauma and angioedema)
Pulmonary etiologies (hypoxic hypoxia)	Hypoventilation caused by increased airway resistance (chronic obstructive pulmonary disease and asthma) Abnormal alveolar ventilation-perfusion ratio (pulmonary embolism, pneumonia, aspiration, and emphysema) Diminished diffusing capacity via the alveolar-capillary membrane (interstitial lung disease and pulmonary vascular disease) Pulmonary shunting (atelectasis, pneumonia, hepatopulmonary syndrome, and arteriovenous malformations)
Cardiac right-to-left shunts; e.g., atrial septal defect (hypoxic hypoxia)	—
Inadequate capacity of blood to transport oxygen (anemic hypoxia)	Anemia Hemoglobinopathies (methemoglobinemia and carbon monoxide poisoning)
Inadequate oxygen transport due to a circulatory defect (static hypoxia)	General circulatory deficiency or collapse (shock or cardiac failure) Localized circulatory deficiency (peripheral, cerebral, and coronary vessels)
Abnormal tissue capability for using oxygen (histotoxic hypoxia)	Late-stage irreversible shock Poisoning of cellular oxidation enzymes (cyanide or arsenic toxicity and heavy ethanol intoxication) Diminished cellular metabolic capacity for using oxygen (severe vitamin deficiencies; e.g., beri-beri)

Vincent JL, et al.: *Textbook of critical care*, ed 7, Philadelphia, 2017, Elsevier.

TABLE 4 Common Clues Obtained from the History, Symptoms, and Clinical Examination Findings That Can Help in the Initial Diagnostic Workup and Management of Acute Respiratory Failure

History and Symptoms	Signs on Physical Examination	Diagnosis
Cough, sputum, secretions	Rales or wheezing	Pneumonia, chronic obstructive pulmonary disease (COPD) exacerbation, bronchiectasis
Sudden onset of shortness of breath	Normal auscultation and percussion, possible signs of leg swelling to suggest deep vein thrombosis	Pulmonary embolism
History of heavy smoking	Wheezing, rhonchi	Emphysema, chronic bronchitis
Orthopnea, chest pain, paroxysmal nocturnal dyspnea	Arrhythmia, peripheral edema, jugular venous distention, peripheral hypoperfusion	Congestive heart failure or acute coronary syndrome
Trauma, aspiration, blood transfusions	Diffuse crackles	Acute respiratory distress syndrome
History of allergies, wheezing or airway disease	Wheezing	Asthma, COPD
Exposure to heavy metals, handling of animals, dust or other significant environmental exposures	"Velcro" rales, clubbing	Chronic interstitial lung disease
Choking, aspiration, vomiting, dental procedures	Inspiratory stridor, poor air entry	Foreign body
Drug abuse	Constricted or dilated pupils, altered mental status, skin marks, perforated nasal septum, hypersalivation, decreased respiratory frequency	Central nervous system depression, intoxication
Exposure to a new drug/chemical or foods known to be allergenic	Swollen oral mucosa and tongue; stridor or wheezing	Angioedema, anaphylaxis
Progressive muscle weakness or immobility	Sensory abnormalities	Neuromuscular disorders
Trauma, procedures, inhalational injury	Absent breath sounds unilaterally, hypertympanic, tracheal deviation	Pneumothorax
Trauma, procedures	Absent breath sounds, dull on percussion, tracheal deviation	Hemothorax

Vincent JL, et al.: *Textbook of critical care*, ed 7, Philadelphia, 2017, Elsevier.

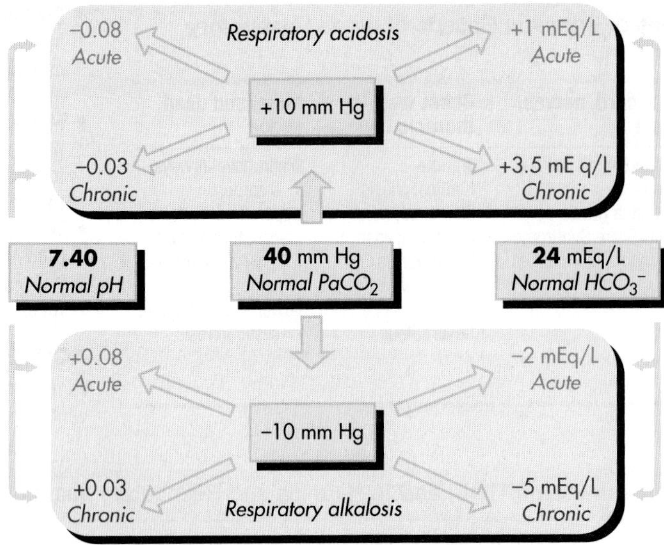

FIG. 1 Interpretation of an arterial blood gas in the setting of respiratory failure. (From Vincent JL, et al.: *Textbook of critical care,* ed 7, Philadelphia, 2017, Elsevier.)

CHRONIC Rx

- Some patients require chronic ventilatory support, such as obesity hypoventilation syndrome patients (alveolar hypoventilation), neuromuscular disease patients (ALS), or those with chronic obstructive pulmonary disease.
- In these cases, the noninvasive form of ventilation is used during sleep.

REFERRAL

Pulmonologist

SUGGESTED READING

Available at ExpertConsult.com

RELATED CONTENT

Acute Respiratory Distress Syndrome (Related key topic)
Pulmonary Edema (Related key topic)
Chronic Obstructive Pulmonary Disease (Related key topic)
Asthma (Related key topic)
Interstitial Lung Disease (Related key topic)
Pneumonia (Related key topic)
Pulmonary Embolism (Related key topic)
Carbon Monoxide Poisoning (Related key topic)

AUTHOR: **JORGE MERCADO, M.D.**

BASIC INFORMATION

DEFINITION

The acute inability to urinate when the bladder is full. This is often, but not always, painful, and the distended bladder may be palpable and percussable. This is distinct from chronic urinary retention, in which patients can still void, but chronically retain a significant volume of urine in the bladder after voiding. Chronic urinary retention is not painful.

SYNONYMS

Acute urinary retention (AUR)
Urinary retention
Retaining urine

ICD-10CM CODES	
R33	Retention of urine
R33.8	Other retention of urine
R33.9	Retention of urine, unspecified

EPIDEMIOLOGY & DEMOGRAPHICS

INCIDENCE: Urinary retention is one of the most common urologic emergencies. This problem typically occurs in aging men, especially men older than 60 yr. However, it may occur in any age group, and in either sex. Over a 5-yr period, AUR will occur in 10% of men older than 70 yrs and in one third of men older than 80 yrs. There is a near-linear increase in age-specific incidence for men ages 40 to 80 yrs.

PREVALENCE: Estimates are 40/100,000 in males and 3/100,000 in females. Prevalence has increased with longer-than-average lifespans.

GENETICS: None known.

PHYSICAL FINDINGS & CLINICAL PRESENTATION

- Acute inability to pass urine or only passing very small amounts of urine.
- Pain and/or pressure in the lower abdomen and suprapubic region is typical. Low back pain may also occur; however, pain may be absent, especially in older patients, patients with underlying neurologic disorders, and cases of chronic urinary retention.
- Palpable and/or percussable bladder may be noted.
- Suprapubic or bladder tenderness with deep palpation may be elicited.
- Increased urge to urinate with bladder palpation.
- Rarely, flank pain and costovertebral angle tenderness can exist if high bladder pressures are transmitted to the ureters and kidney.
- Increased severity of lower urinary tract symptoms (LUTS) is associated with increased risk of AUR. Patients may complain of worsening LUTS prior to episode, including increased urinary urgency, incontinence, nocturia, stranguria, hesitancy, and intermittency. These symptoms usually develop between 1 day and a few weeks prior to AUR.
- Patients with cognitive deficits or inability to communicate may present with restlessness, discomfort, worsened confusion, or delirium.
- Acute kidney injury, electrolyte abnormalities, nausea, and lower extremity edema may be present with delayed presentation.

ETIOLOGY

- Acute urinary retention may be spontaneous or precipitated by a triggering event. Spontaneous AUR may arise from the natural progression of bladder outlet obstruction, more commonly from benign prostatic hyperplasia (BPH), and less commonly from pelvic masses and urethral stricture disease. Conversely, precipitated AUR episodes have an identifiable triggering event, such as acute trauma, surgical procedures (e.g., spinal, orthopedic, and urologic), medications (e.g., over-the-counter [OTC] antihistamines and sympathomimetic agents commonly found in cough medications, anticholinergic drugs), excessive fluid intake (e.g., alcohol), urinary tract infection, central nervous system insults (e.g., strokes, hemorrhage, spinal cord injuries), and severe constipation. There is overlap between spontaneous and precipitated AUR, particularly when triggering events are superimposed on underlying obstructive risk factors.
- Urinary retention generally result from one of three categories: (1) Increased bladder outflow obstruction, as seen in BPH, urethral stricture disease, extrinsic compression from malignancy, constipation, and in gross hematuria where large clots can obstruct the urethra or bladder neck; (2) Disruption of detrusor muscle innervation as with diabetic neuropathy, spinal cord injury, progressive neurologic pathologies, and bladder contractile dysfunction and decompensation, secondary to prolonged outlet obstruction; (3) Bladder overdistension can also lead to impaired contractility, and may result from general anesthesia, epidural anesthesia, or anticholinergic use.
- Often multifactorial in older patients, with an underlying obstructive risk factor and acute precipitant.
- In women, obstructive factors can include benign tumors (especially fibroids); malignant tumors of pelvic, urethral, or vaginal origin; urethral strictures and urethral meatal stenosis; postpartum vulvar edema; and labial fusion. Pelvic organ prolapse, including cystocele, rectocele, and uterine prolapse, can also lead to urinary retention.
- Infection including prostatitis, urethritis, cystitis, genital herpes, and herpes zoster may also produce AUR.
- AUR is common in the postoperative period when patients are less mobile, constipated, and after opioid medications have been administered.

DIAGNOSIS

DIFFERENTIAL DIAGNOSIS

- AUR is typically self-evident to the cognitively intact patient and the treating physician.
- Chronic urinary retention.
- Pelvic masses, fluid collections, uterine fibroids, pregnancies, or ascites may be confused for a full bladder, particularly when using bedside ultrasonic bladder capacity measuring instruments.

WORKUP

- History should focus on urologic symptoms: dysuria, hematuria, baseline voiding symptoms (caliber of stream, nocturia, sensation of incomplete emptying, double-voiding, incontinence, hesitancy), past episodes of retention, surgical history (both urologic and other surgical procedures, especially if recent), and urologic cancer
- History should also include a complete list of prescribed and over-the-counter medications, and recent medication changes
- Review of symptoms should include presence of fever, back pain, neurologic symptoms, and rash
- Rectal exam for masses, fecal impaction, perineal and perianal sensation, prostate size, and sphincter tone
- Genitourinary exam in men, with special attention for meatal stenosis and phimosis or paraphimosis
- Pelvic exam in women with vigilance for any pelvic organ prolapse(s)
- Neurologic exam, with particular evaluation for saddle anesthesia and pelvic sensory or motor deficits, to rule out an underlying neurologic cause

LABORATORY TESTS

- Electrolytes, BUN, and serum creatinine
- Urinalysis and culture, obtained via bladder or suprapubic catheterization
- Prostate-specific antigen testing is not helpful in AUR and may be falsely elevated after catheter placement. This test should not be routinely checked in the acute setting.

IMAGING STUDIES

- Bladder ultrasound or a bedside post-void residual urine scan ("bladder scan") can be diagnostic. Ascites, pelvic fluid collections, body habitus, and presence of surgical implants (e.g., reservoirs for inflatable penile prostheses or artificial urinary sphincters) may confound accurate volume measurement.
- Abdominal ultrasound or computed tomography (CT) may be helpful if there is suspicion of a pelvic mass.
- CT (Fig. 1) can be helpful when high volumes are measured by a bedside bladder scan, but low volumes are returned upon bladder catheterization.
- MRI should be obtained when a spinal cord problem is suspected.
- Renal ultrasound or abdominopelvic CT may be obtained if there is associated renal impairment and hydronephrosis is suspected.
- Evaluation of bladder function. Urodynamic testing may be considered after initial management, particularly in females with no evidence of anatomic obstruction, or patients with long-standing obstruction and/or other neurologic conditions that affect bladder contractility.
- X-rays are of limited utility in evaluating AUR, but may show underlying constipation.

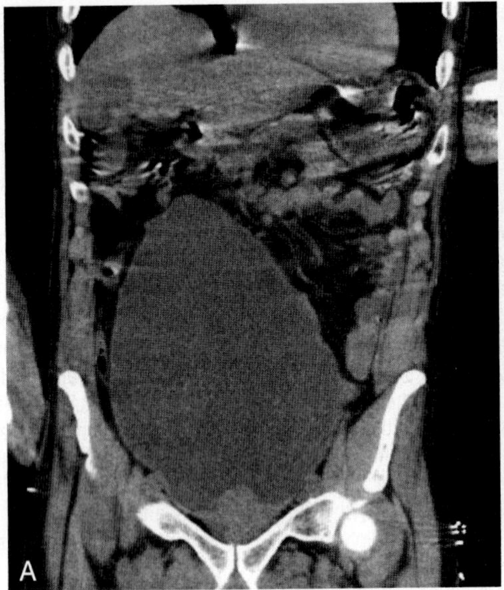

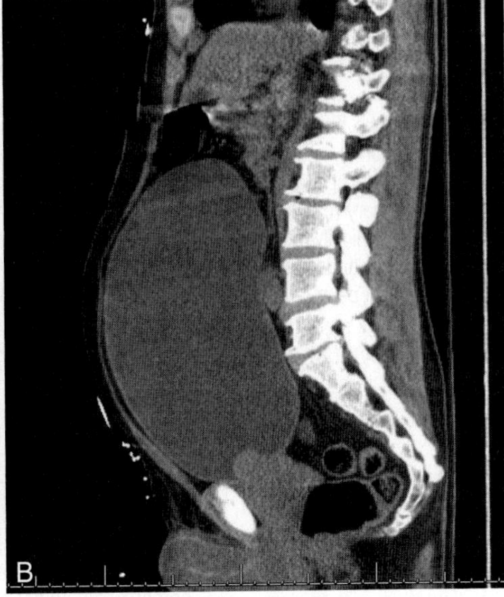

FIG. 1 Large volume urinary retention. Computed tomography images of coronal view **(A)** and sagittal view **(B)** of considerably distended bladder. The bladder extends to the mid-abdomen and well over the pubic bone. More than 2 L of urine was drained.

Rx TREATMENT

ACUTE GENERAL Rx

- Prompt bladder decompression and drainage is the initial management of AUR, generally by indwelling urethral catheterization. Coude-tip catheters (angled-tip catheters) can facilitate catheter placement in men with large prostates. Clean intermittent catheterization (CIC) is an option for patients with sufficient dexterity, vision, and motivation.
- Urological consultation is advised after recent genitourinary surgery, history of urethral stricture disease, or history of difficult catheterizations.
- When urethral catheterization is not possible or contraindicated, suprapubic catheter placement is required.
- Monitor for post-decompression hematuria that usually develops shortly after bladder drainage with small vessel injury of the overstretched bladder wall.
- Monitor for post-obstructive diuresis, produced by mixed osmotic and saline diuresis from urea and salt retention during the period of obstruction.
- Avoid and/or discontinue medications that precipitate AUR (e.g., narcotics, anticholinergics, antihistamines).

CHRONIC Rx

- A voiding trial is reasonable 5 to 7 days after relief of obstruction in most patients.
- α-blockers are effective for treatment of BPH symptoms in males. These agents increase the success rate of early catheter removal, and should be initiated, unless contraindicated. There is limited evidence to suggest benefit in females.
- Discontinue medications that increase the risk of AUR.
- Correct constipation and increase patient mobility.
- Inability to void after 5 to 7 days of catheterization mandates urologic consultation, with more intensive evaluation of AUR, including possible cystoscopic evaluation and/or urodynamic studies.
- Patients unable to void after a voiding trial can either initiate CIC, often 2 to 3 times a day, or have the urinary bladder catheter replaced.

DISPOSITION

- Home disposition when close follow-up is feasible, and progressive kidney injury and post-obstructive diuresis are absent
- Hospital admission if sepsis; complicated urinary tract infection; acute kidney injury; severe post-obstructive diuresis; hyperkalemia; acidemia or azotemia; or if AUR is from malignancy, hematuria, or spinal cord compression

REFERRAL

- Urologist if initial bladder catheterization are unsuccessful, or in surgical scenarios of radical prostatectomy, transurethral resection of prostate, urethral stricture surgery, and other bladder/prostate surgeries
- Urologic referral for recurrent AUR in men
- Gynecologic referral is mandatory if a pelvic mass is determined as etiology of AUR in females

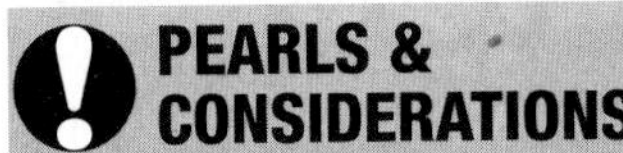

PEARLS & CONSIDERATIONS

- AUR is often painful.
- Rapid bladder drainage is of paramount importance.
- Monitor for postobstructive diuresis and correct electrolyte abnormalities.
- Request urological advice or referral for AUR.

PREVENTION

Patients with BPH should be cautious regarding medications that may precipitate AUR, including antihistamines, sympathomimetics, sedatives, and anticholinergics. On a chronic basis, 5-α reductase inhibitors (e.g., finasteride, dutasteride) can reduce the risk of AUR in men with BPH and large prostates.

SUGGESTED READINGS

Available at ExpertConsult.com

RELATED CONTENT

Benign Prostatic Hyperplasia (Related Key Topic)

AUTHORS: **ALEX BORCHERT, M.D.,** and **DAVID A. LEAVITT, M.D.**

BASIC INFORMATION

DEFINITION

Adrenal insufficiency is characterized by inadequate secretion of corticosteroids resulting from partial or complete destruction of the adrenal glands (primary adrenal failure). Inadequate secretion of cortisol from the adrenals due to critical illness and pituitary insufficiency is known as secondary cortisol deficiency.

SYNONYMS

Primary adrenocortical insufficiency
Addison disease

ICD-10CM CODES

E27.1	Primary adrenocortical insufficiency
E27.2	Addisonian crisis
E27.40	Unspecified adrenocortical insufficiency
E27.49	Other adrenocortical insufficiency
E27.3	Drug-induced adrenocortical insufficiency
E23.3	Hypopituitarism

EPIDEMIOLOGY & DEMOGRAPHICS

PREVALENCE: 10 to 15 per 100,000 persons
PREDOMINANT SEX: Female:male ratio of 2:1

PHYSICAL FINDINGS & CLINICAL PRESENTATION

- Adrenal insufficiency may present insidiously with nonspecific symptoms. A high index of suspicion is required for diagnosis. About half of patients may present acutely with adrenal crises. Table 1 summarizes the clinical features of primary adrenal insufficiency.
- Hyperpigmentation of skin (Figs. E1 and E2) and mucous membranes is a cardinal sign of adrenal insufficiency: more prominent in palmar creases, buccal mucosa, pressure points (elbows, knees, knuckles), perianal mucosa, and around areolas of nipples
- Hypotension, postural dizziness
- Generalized weakness, chronic fatigue, malaise, anorexia
- Amenorrhea and loss of axillary hair in females

ETIOLOGY

- Autoimmune destruction of the adrenal glands (80% of cases)
- Tuberculosis (TB) (7% to 20% of cases)
- Carcinomatous destruction of the adrenal glands, lymphoma
- Adrenal hemorrhage (anticoagulants, trauma, coagulopathies, pregnancy, sepsis)
- Adrenal infarction (antiphospholipid syndrome, arteritis, thrombosis)
- AIDS (adrenal insufficiency develops in 30% of patients with AIDS, often cytomegalovirus [CMV] adrenalitis)
- Genetic causes: Autoimmune polyglandular syndromes (APS) types 1 and 2, X-linked adrenoleukodystrophy, congenital adrenal hyperplasia
- Other: Sarcoidosis, amyloidosis, hemochromatosis, Wegener's granulomatosis, postoperative, fungal infections (candidiasis, histoplasmosis)

TABLE 1 Clinical Features of Primary Adrenal Insufficiency

Feature	Frequency (%)
Symptoms	
Weakness, tiredness, fatigue	100
Anorexia	100
Gastrointestinal symptoms	92
Nausea	86
Vomiting	75
Constipation	33
Abdominal pain	31
Diarrhea	16
Salt craving	16
Postural dizziness	12
Muscle or joint pains	13
Signs	
Weight loss	100
Hyperpigmentation	94
Hypotension (<110 mm Hg systolic)	88-94
Vitiligo	10-20
Auricular calcification	5
Laboratory Findings	
Electrolyte disturbances	92
Hyponatremia	88
Hyperkalemia	64
Hypercalcemia	6
Azotemia	55
Anemia	40
Eosinophilia	17

From Melmed S, Polonsky KS, Larsen PR, Kronenberg HM: *Williams textbook of endocrinology*, ed 12, Philadelphia, 2011, Saunders.

Dx DIAGNOSIS

DIFFERENTIAL DIAGNOSIS

Sepsis, hypovolemic shock, acute abdomen, apathetic hyperthyroidism in the elderly, myopathies, gastrointestinal malignancy, major depression, anorexia nervosa, hemochromatosis, salt-losing nephritis, chronic infection

WORKUP

- An early morning (8 am) serum cortisol <3 mcg/dl (82.8 mmol/L) is consistent with cortisol deficiency.
- If the the cortisol level is 3-15 mcg/dl, the diagnosis can be confirmed with the rapid adrenocorticotropic hormone (ACTH) test:
  1. Give 250 mcg ACTH (Sinachten, tetracosatrin) by IV push and measure cortisol levels at 0, 30, and 60 min.
  2. An increase in serum cortisol level to peak concentration >500 nmol/L (18 mcg/dl) indicates a normal response. Cortisol level ≤18 mcg/dl at 30 or 60 min is suggestive of adrenal insufficiency.
  3. Measure plasma ACTH. A high ACTH level (>200 pg/ml [44 pmol/L]) confirms primary adrenal insufficiency.
- Critical illness-related corticosteroid insufficiency (e.g., in sepsis) is best established with the 1-mcg ACTH stimulation test in which cortisol levels are measured at baseline and 30 min after administration of ACTH. A level <25 mcg/dl (690 nmol/L) or an increment over baseline of <9 mcg (250 nmol/L) represents an inadequate adrenal response.
- Secondary adrenocortical insufficiency (caused by pituitary dysfunction) can be distinguished from primary adrenal insufficiency by the following:
  1. Normal or low plasma ACTH level after rapid ACTH
  2. Absence of hyperpigmentation
  3. No significant impairment of aldosterone secretion (because aldosterone secretion is under control of the renin-angiotensin system)
  4. Additional evidence of hypopituitarism (e.g., hypogonadism, hypothyroidism)

LABORATORY TESTS

- Hyponatremia, hyperkalemia
- Decreased glucose
- Increased BUN/creatinine ratio (prerenal azotemia)

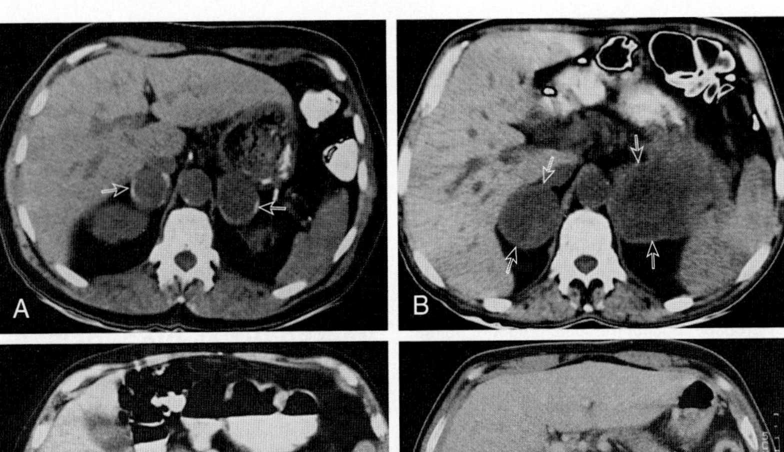

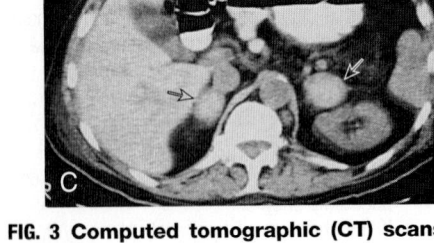

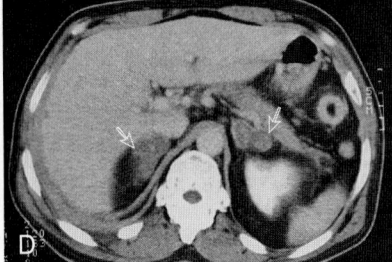

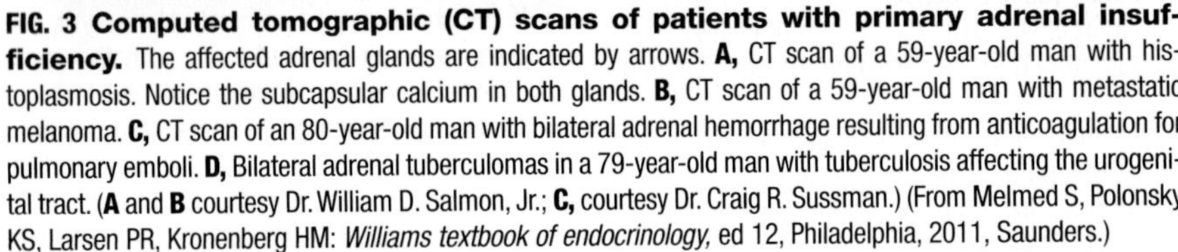
FIG. 3 Computed tomographic (CT) scans of patients with primary adrenal insufficiency. The affected adrenal glands are indicated by arrows. **A,** CT scan of a 59-year-old man with histoplasmosis. Notice the subcapsular calcium in both glands. **B,** CT scan of a 59-year-old man with metastatic melanoma. **C,** CT scan of an 80-year-old man with bilateral adrenal hemorrhage resulting from anticoagulation for pulmonary emboli. **D,** Bilateral adrenal tuberculomas in a 79-year-old man with tuberculosis affecting the urogenital tract. (**A** and **B** courtesy Dr. William D. Salmon, Jr.; **C,** courtesy Dr. Craig R. Sussman.) (From Melmed S, Polonsky KS, Larsen PR, Kronenberg HM: *Williams textbook of endocrinology,* ed 12, Philadelphia, 2011, Saunders.)

- Mild normocytic, normochromic anemia, neutropenia, lymphocytosis, eosinophilia (significant dehydration may mask hyponatremia and anemia), hypercalcemia, metabolic acidosis
- A morning cortisol level >500 mmol/L (18 mcg/dl) generally excludes the diagnosis whereas a level <165 mmol/L (6 mcg/dl) is suggestive of Addison disease and a level <3 mcg/dl requires further evaluation (see "Workup")
- Additional evaluation may include 21-hydroxylase antibodies present in 90% of autoimmune adrenalitis cases. If negative, obtain CT scan of adrenal glands
- PPD or QuantiFERON Gold test to rule out TB

IMAGING STUDIES

- Imaging is not necessary for diagnosis but may help identify potential causes.
- Abdominal CT scan (Fig. 3): Small adrenal glands generally indicate either idiopathic atrophy or longstanding TB, whereas enlarged glands are suggestive of early TB or potentially treatable diseases.
- Chest radiograph may reveal a small heart (Fig. E4).
- Abdominal radiograph: Adrenal calcifications may be noted if the adrenocortical insufficiency is secondary to TB or fungal infection.

Rx TREATMENT

NONPHARMACOLOGIC THERAPY

- Perform periodic monitoring of serum electrolytes, vital signs, and body weight; liberal sodium intake is suggested.
- Periodic measurement of bone density may be helpful in identifying patients at risk for the development of osteoporosis.
- Patients should carry a MedicAlert bracelet and an emergency pack containing hydrocortisone 100-mg ampule, syringe, and needle.
- Patients and partners should be educated on how to give IM injection in case of vomiting or coma.

ACUTE GENERAL Rx

- Addisonian crisis is an acute complication of adrenal insufficiency characterized by circulatory collapse, dehydration, nausea, vomiting, hypoglycemia, and hyperkalemia.
    1. Draw plasma cortisol level; do not delay therapy while waiting for confirming laboratory results.
    2. Administer hydrocortisone 100 mg IV immediately, followed by 100 to 200 mg of hydrocortisone every 24 hours divided into 3 or 4 doses; if patient shows good clinical response, gradually taper dosage and change to oral maintenance dose (usually prednisone 7.5 mg/day).
    3. Provide adequate volume replacement with D_5NS solution until hypotension, dehydration, and hypoglycemia are completely corrected. Large volumes (2 to 3 L) under continuous cardiac monitoring may be necessary in the first 2 to 3 hr to correct the volume deficit and hypoglycemia and to avoid further hyponatremia.
- Identify and correct any precipitating factor (e.g., sepsis, hemorrhage).

CHRONIC Rx

- Give hydrocortisone 15 to 20 mg PO every morning and 5 to 10 mg in late afternoon or prednisone 5 mg in morning and 2.5 mg hs.
- Give oral fludrocortisone 0.05 mg/day to 0.20 mg/day. This mineralocorticoid is necessary if the patient has primary adrenocortical insufficiency. The dose is adjusted based on the serum sodium level and the presence of postural hypotension or marked orthostasis.
- Instruct patients to increase glucocorticoid replacement in times of stress and to receive parenteral glucocorticoids if diarrhea or vomiting occurs. Typical supplementation varies from 25 mg PO qd of hydrocortisone for minor medical and surgical stress to 50 to 100 mg IV hydrocortisone q8h for sepsis-induced hypotension or shock.
- The administration of dehydroepiandrosterone (DHEA) is controversial due to lack of robust data. It is not indicated in men but may be considered in women with primary adrenal failure. A dose of 50 mg PO qd may improve well-being and sexuality in women with adrenal insufficiency.
- Patients with concomitant hypothyroidism should be treated with glucocorticoids first before correcting hypothyroidism because correction of thyroid hormone deficiency will accelerate cortisol clearance and can precipitate adrenal crisis.

SUGGESTED READINGS

Available at ExpertConsult.com

RELATED CONTENT

Addison Disease (Patient Information)

AUTHOR: **FRED F. FERRI, M.D.**

BASIC INFORMATION

DEFINITION

Moderate drinking has been defined as two standard drinks (e.g., 12 oz of beer) per day and one drink per day for women and persons older than 65 yr. Although not generally included under the alcoholism topic, hazardous or at-risk drinking should also be considered. For men, *at-risk drinking* is defined as more than 14 drinks/wk or more than 4 drinks/occasion. For women, at-risk drinking is defined as approximately half that given for men.

The American Psychiatric Association defines diagnostic criteria for *alcohol withdrawal* as follows:

A. Cessation of (or reduction in) alcohol use that has been heavy and prolonged.

B. Two (or more) of the following, developing within several hours to a few days after criterion A:

1. Autonomic hyperactivity (e.g., sweating or pulse rate >100 beats/min)
2. Increased hand tremor
3. Insomnia
4. Nausea and vomiting
5. Transient visual, tactile, or auditory hallucinations or illusions
6. Psychomotor agitation
7. Anxiety
8. Grand mal seizures

C. The symptoms in criterion B cause clinically significant distress or impairment in social, occupational, or other important areas of functioning.

The symptoms are not attributable to a general medical condition and are not better accounted for by another mental disorder.

SYNONYMS

Alcohol dependence syndrome
Substance abuse
Alcohol withdrawal syndrome
Alcoholism

ICD-10CM CODES

F10	Mental and behavioral disorders due to use of alcohol
F10.1	Mental and behavioral disorders due to use of alcohol: harmful use
F10.2	Mental and behavioral disorders due to use of alcohol: dependence syndrome
F10.3	Mental and behavioral disorders due to use of alcohol: withdrawal state
F10.4	Mental and behavioral disorders due to use of alcohol: withdrawal state with delirium
F10.5	Mental and behavioral disorders due to use of alcohol: psychotic disorder
F10.6	Mental and behavioral disorders due to use of alcohol: amnesic syndrome

EPIDEMIOLOGY & DEMOGRAPHICS

INCIDENCE (IN U.S.):

- The clinical history suggests alcohol problems in 15% to 20% of patients in primary care and hospitalized patients. In the U.S., alcohol abuse generates nearly $223 billion in annual economic costs. An estimated 14% of adults in the U.S. have alcohol dependence. Alcohol accounts for 6.8% of age-standardized deaths in men and 2.2% in women.
- 20% achieve abstinence without help; 70% achieve sobriety for 1 yr.

PREVALENCE (IN U.S.): 7% of population ≥18 yr

PREDOMINANT SEX:

- Lifetime risk for males 8% to 10%
- Lifetime risk for females 3% to 5%

PEAK INCIDENCE: 20 to 40 yr. The most common age range for initial treatment of alcohol dependence is 35 to 45 yr. However, the peak period for meeting alcohol dependence criteria is ≥10 yrs earlier.

GENETICS: More common with a family history of alcoholism and in patients of Irish, Scandinavian, and Native American descent

PHYSICAL FINDINGS & CLINICAL PRESENTATION

- Recurring minor trauma
- Gastrointestinal bleeding from gastritis and/or varices
- Pancreatitis (acute and chronic)
- Liver disease
- Odor of alcohol on breath
- Tremulousness
- Tachycardia
- Peripheral neuropathy
- Recent memory loss

ETIOLOGY

- Social and genetic factors important
- Risk factors:
  1. Broken homes
  2. Unemployment
  3. Divorce
  4. Recurrent depression
  5. Addiction to another substance, including tobacco
  6. Working long hours (≥55 hours/week)

DIAGNOSIS

WORKUP

- The USPSTF recommends that clinicians screen adults 18 yrs and older for alcohol misuse and provide persons engaged in risky or hazardous drinking with brief behavioral counseling interventions to reduce alcohol misuse. Several screening tests (CAGE [Table 1], TWEAK, CRAFFT, AUDIT-C [Table 2]) are available. The four-item CAGE (feeling need to **C**ut down, **A**nnoyed by criticism, **G**uilty about drinking, and need for an **E**ye-opener in the morning) is the most popular screening test in primary care. A positive response should lead to further questioning. The sensitivity of the CAGE ranges from 43% to 94% and its specificity ranges from 70% to 97%. The five-item TWEAK scale (**T**olerance, **W**orry, **E**ye-openers, **A**mnesia, [**K**] cut down) and the TACE questionnaire (**T**olerance, **A**nnoyance, **C**ut down, **E**ye-opener) are designed to screen pregnant women for alcohol misuse. They detect lower levels of alcohol consumption that may pose risks during pregnancy. The CRAFFT questionnaire (riding in **C**ar with someone who was drinking, using alcohol to **R**elax, using alcohol while **A**lone, **F**orgetfulness, criticism from **F**riends and **F**amily, **T**rouble) is useful as a screening tool for adolescents. Its sensitivity is 92% and specificity 64% for alcohol abuse. Single-question screening about alcohol consumption in a day ("When was the last time you had more than X drinks in a day?" [where X is 5 for men and 4 for women]) with the threshold set at "in the past 3 months" is 85% sensitive and 70% specific in men and 82% and 70% in women for unhealthy alcohol use. The 3-question AUDIT-C is a shorter form of the 10-item AUDIT, and the questions center on the quantity and frequency of alcohol use. It asks how often someone has had a drink containing alcohol, how many standard drinks containing alcohol one consumes on a typical day when one is drinking, and how often one has six or more drinks on one occasion. Scoring ranges from 0 to 4 on each question with a total score range of 0 to 12. A total score of 3 or higher for women and 4 or higher for men indicates alcohol use disorder and need for further assessment. Its sensitivity ranges from 85% in Hispanic women to 95% in white men.
- Laboratory evaluation (see below).

LABORATORY TESTS

Lab tests alone do not accurately detect alcohol problems but can help identify medical complications related to alcohol use, such as pancreatitis or cirrhosis.

TABLE 1 CAGE Questionnaire for Alcohol Problems Screening[a]

C	Have you felt the need to **C**ut down on your drinking?
A	Have people **A**nnoyed you by criticizing your drinking?
G	Have you ever felt bad or **G**uilty about your drinking?
E	Have you had a drink first thing in the morning to steady your nerves or to get rid of a hangover (i.e., an "**E**ye opener")?

From Stern TA, et al.: Massachusetts General Hospital handbook of general hospital psychiatry, ed 7, Philadelphia, 2018, Elsevier.

TABLE 2 AUDIT-C Questionnaire for Alcohol Problems Screening[a]

Question	Score
How often did you have a drink containing alcohol in the past year?	Never (0 points) Monthly or less (1 point) 2–4 times per month (2 points) 2–3 times per week (3 points) >4 times per week (4 points)

[a]AUDIT-C is scored 0–12, with score >4 (men) and >3 (women) considered positive for problematic drinking.

From Stern TA, et al.: Massachusetts General Hospital handbook of general hospital psychiatry, ed 7, Philadelphia, 2018, Elsevier.

- Gamma-glutamyltransferase (GGTP), generally elevated
- Liver transaminases (alanine aminotransferase [ALT], aspartate aminotransferase [AST]), often elevated, may be normal or low in advanced liver disease.
- Low albumin level, hypophosphatemia, hypomagnesemia from malnutrition
- Complete blood count (CBC) reveals elevated mean corpuscular volume from toxic effect of alcohol on erythrocyte development in nutritional deficiencies.
- Stool for occult blood may be positive as a result of gastritis or variceal bleeding.
- RBC folate, vitamin B_{12} level, vitamin B_6, vitamin B_1 level

IMAGING STUDIES

Indicated only with a history of trauma. CT or ultrasound of abdomen may reveal fatty liver or cirrhosis in advanced stages.

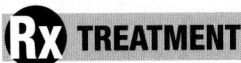

TREATMENT

NONPHARMACOLOGIC THERAPY

- Twelve-step facilitation, cognitive behavioral therapy, and motivational enhancement therapy improve the chances of recovery in patients with alcohol abuse and dependence.
- Depression, if present, should be treated at same time alcohol is withdrawn.

ACUTE GENERAL Rx

Alcohol withdrawal syndrome (AWS) occurs when a person stops ingesting alcohol after prolonged consumption. It can result in four possible clinical patterns depending on the severity of the patient's alcohol abuse and the time from the patient's previous alcohol ingestion. Blood ethanol level decreases by ~20 mg/dl/hr in a normal person. Although discussed separately, these withdrawal states blend together in real life. Table 3 summarizes medications for the treatment of alcohol dependence. The cornerstone of treatment for alcohol withdrawal syndrome is the use of benzodiazepines.

- **Tremulous state** (early alcohol withdrawal, "impending DTs," "shakes," "jitters").
  1. Time interval: usually occurs 6 to 8 hr after the last drink or 12 to 48 hr after reduction of alcohol intake; becomes most pronounced at 24 to 36 hr.
  2. Manifestation: tremors, mild agitation, insomnia, tachycardia; symptoms are relieved by alcohol.
  3. Detoxification can be in the outpatient (ambulatory) or inpatient setting. Candidates for outpatient detoxification should have a reasonable support system (e.g., reliable contact person) who can monitor progress and lack of any significant comorbid conditions (e.g., suicide risk, seizure disorder, coexisting benzodiazepine dependence, prior unsuccessful outpatient detoxification, pregnancy, cirrhosis) or risk factors for severe withdrawal (age >40 yr, drinking >100 g of ethanol daily [e.g., 1 pint of liquor or eight 12-oz cans of beer, random blood alcohol concentration >200 mg/dl]).
  4. Inpatient treatment:
     a. Admit to medical floor (private room); monitor vital signs q4h; institute seizure precautions; maintain adequate sedation.
     b. Administer lorazepam as follows:
        (1) Day 1: 2 mg PO q4h while awake and not lethargic.
        (2) Day 2: 1 mg PO q4h while awake and not lethargic.
        (3) Day 3: 0.5 mg PO q4h while awake and not lethargic.
        (4) NOTE: Hold sedation for lethargy or abnormal vital or neurologic signs. The preceding doses are only guidelines; it is best to titrate the dose case by case.
     c. In patients with mild to moderate withdrawal and without history of seizures, individualized benzodiazepine administration (rather than a fixed-dose regimen) results in lower benzodiazepine administration and avoids unnecessary sedation. The Clinical Institute Withdrawal Assessment Scale for Alcohol, Revised (CIWA-Ar) scale (Box 1) can be used to measure the severity of alcohol withdrawal. It consists of 10 items: nausea; tremor; autonomic hyperactivity; anxiety;

TABLE 3 Medications for the Treatment of Alcohol Dependence*

Medication	Dose and Route	Frequency	Effects	Major Common Adverse Effects
Alcohol Withdrawal				
			Benzodiazepines†	
Chlordiazepoxide*	25-100 mg, PO/IV/IM†	Every 4-6 hr	Decreased severity of withdrawal; stabilization of vital signs; prevention of seizures and delirium tremens	Confusion, oversedation, respiratory depression
Diazepam‡	5-10 mg, PO/IV/IM†	Every 6-8 hr		
Oxazepam‡	15-30 mg, PO†	Every 6-8 hr		
Lorazepam‡	1-4 mg, PO/IV/IM†	Every 4-8 hr		
			β-Blockers	
Atenolol	25-50 mg, PO	Once a day	Improvement in vital signs	Bradycardia, hypotension
Propranolol	10-40 mg, PO	Every 6-8 hr	Reduction in craving	
			α-Agonists	
Clonidine	0.1-0.2 mg, PO	Every 6 hr	Decreased withdrawal symptoms	Hypotension, fatigue
			Antiepileptics	
Carbamazepine	200 mg, PO	Every 6-8 hr	Decreased severity of withdrawal; prevention of seizures	Dizziness, fatigue, red blood cell abnormalities
			Prevention of Relapse	
Disulfiram‡	125-500 mg, PO	Daily	Decreased alcohol use among those who relapse	Disulfiram-alcohol reaction, rash, drowsiness, peripheral neuropathy
Naltrexone‡	50 mg, PO	Daily	Increased abstinence, decreased drinking days	Nausea, abdominal pain, myalgias-arthralgias
	380 mg, IM	Every 4 wk		
Acamprosate‡	666 mg, PO	Three times a day	Increased abstinence	Diarrhea

*Most commonly used medications listed.
†Currently approved by U.S. Food and Drug Administration for the indication noted.
‡Dose and routes given for standard fixed-dose regimens, which include dose tapers over time.
From Goldman L, Schafer AI: *Goldman's Cecil medicine,* ed 24, Philadelphia, 2012, Saunders.

agitation; tactile, visual, and auditory disturbances; headache; and disorientation. Each item is assigned a score from 0 to 7. For example, in the "agitation" category 0 indicates normal activity, and 7 indicates that the patient constantly thrashes about. For the category of "tremor," 0 indicates that tremor is not present and 7 that tremor is severe, even with arms not extended. The maximum total score is 67. Patients with mild AWS symptoms (CIWA-Ar score <8) can be monitored on an outpatient basis. Benzodiazepines are beneficial for most patients with a CIWA-AR score ≥8 and are strongly recommended in patients with substantial withdrawal symptoms (CIWA-Ar score >12). Patients with CIWA-Ar score of ≥15 should be admitted to detox unit. In-patient treatment is also recommended for patients with history of withdrawal seizures and for those with suicidal ideation and significant comorbidities.

d. Beta-adrenergic blockers: Beta-blockers are useful for controlling blood pressure and tachyarrhythmias. However, they do not prevent progression to more serious symptoms of withdrawal and, if used, should not be administered alone but in conjunction with benzodiazepines. Beta-blockers should be avoided in patients with contraindications to their use (e.g., bronchospasm, bradycardia, or severe congestive heart failure). Centrally acting alpha-adrenergic agonists such as clonidine ameliorate symptoms in patients with mild to moderate withdrawal but do not reduce delirium or seizures.
e. Vitamin replacement: Thiamine 100 mg IV or IM for at least 5 days plus oral multivitamins. The IV administration of glucose can precipitate Wernicke's encephalopathy in alcoholics with thiamine deficiency; therefore thiamine administration should precede IV dextrose.
f. Hydration PO or IV (high-caloric solution): If IV, glucose with Na+, K+, Mg2+, and phosphate replacement prn.
g. Laboratory studies:
   (1) CBC, platelet count, INR.
   (2) Electrolytes, glucose, blood urea nitrogen, creatinine.
   (3) GGTP, ALT, AST.
   (4) Phosphorus and magnesium.
   (5) Serum vitamin B_{12} and folic acid (if megaloblastic features in blood smear).
h. Diagnostic imaging: Generally not necessary; if subdural hematoma is suspected (evidence of trauma, persistent lethargy), a CT scan should be ordered.
i. Social rehabilitation: Group therapy such as Alcoholics Anonymous; identification and treatment of social and family problems should be initiated during the patient's hospital stay.

- **Alcoholic hallucinosis:**
  1. Manifestations: Hallucinations usually are auditory, but hallucinations occasionally are visual, tactile, or olfactory; usually there is no clouding of sensorium as in delirium (clinical presentation may be mistaken for an acute schizophrenic episode). Disordered perceptions become most pronounced after 24 to 36 hr of abstinence.
  2. Treatment: Same as for DTs (see "Withdrawal seizures").
- **Withdrawal seizures ("rum fits"):**
  1. Time interval: Usually occurs 7 to 30 hr after cessation of drinking, with a peak incidence between 13 and 24 hr.
  2. Manifestations: Generalized convulsions with loss of consciousness; focal signs are usually absent; consider further investigation with CT scan of head and electroencephalography if clearly indicated (e.g., presence of focal neurologic deficits, prolonged postictal confusion state). In addition, in a febrile patient who is having a seizure or altered mental state, a lumbar puncture is necessary.
  3. Treatment:
     a. Diazepam 2.5 mg/min IV until seizure is controlled (check for respiratory depression or hypotension) may be

BOX 1 Alcohol Withdrawal Assessment Scoring Guidelines (Revised Clinical Institute Withdrawal Assessment for Alcohol Scale)

Nausea and Vomiting (0-7)
0, none; 1, mild nausea with no vomiting; 4, intermittent nausea; 7, constant nausea, frequent dry heaves and vomiting

Tremor (0-7)
0, no tremor; 1, not visible, but can be felt fingertip to fingertip; 4, moderate, with patient's arms extended; 7, severe, even with arms not extended

Paroxysmal Sweats (0-7)
0, no sweats; 1, barely perceptible sweating, palms moist; 4, beads of sweat obvious on forehead; 7, drenching sweats

Anxiety (0-7)
0, no anxiety, patient at ease; 1, mildly anxious; 4, moderately anxious or guarded, so anxiety is inferred; 7, equivalent to acute panic states seen in severe delirium or acute schizophrenic reactions

Agitation (0-7)
0, normal activity; 1, somewhat more than normal activity; 4, moderately fidgety and restless; 7, pacing back and forth during, or constantly thrashing about

Tactile Disturbances (0-7)
Ask, "Have you experienced any itching, pins and needles sensation, burning or numbness, or a feeling of bugs crawling on or under your skin?"
0, none; 1, very mild itching, pins and needles, burning, or numbness; 2, mild itching, pins and needles, burning, or numbness; 3, moderate itching, pins and needles, burning, or numbness; 4, moderately severe tactile hallucinations; 5, severe hallucinations; 6, extremely severe hallucinations; 7, continuous hallucinations

Auditory Disturbances (0-7)
Ask, "Are you more aware of sounds around you? Are they harsh? Do they startle you? Do you hear anything that disturbs you or that you know isn't there?"
0, not present; 1, very mild harshness or ability to startle; 2, mild harshness or ability to startle; 3, moderate harshness or ability to startle; 4, moderate hallucinations; 5, severe hallucinations; 6, extremely severe hallucinations; 7, continuous hallucinations

Visual Disturbances (0-7)
Ask, "Does the light appear to be too bright? Is its color different than normal? Does it hurt your eyes? Are you seeing anything that disturbs you?"
0, not present; 1, very mild sensitivity to light; 2, mild sensitivity; 3, moderate sensitivity; 4, moderate hallucinations; 5, severe hallucinations; 6, extremely severe hallucinations; 7, continuous hallucinations

Headache (0-7)
0, not present; 1, very mild; 2, mild; 3, moderate; 4, moderately severe; 5, severe; 6, very severe; 7, extremely severe

Orientation and Clouding of Sensorium (0-4)
Ask, "What day is this? Where are you? Who am I?"
0, oriented; 1, cannot do serial additions or is uncertain about date; 2, disoriented to date by no more than 2 calendar days; 3, disoriented to date by more than 2 calendar days; 4, disoriented to place and/or person

Total Score
0 to 9: absent or minimal withdrawal
10 to 19: mild to moderate withdrawal
More than 20: severe withdrawal

From Sullivan JT, Sykora K, Schneiderman J, et al.: Assessment of alcohol withdrawal: the revised clinical institute withdrawal assessment for alcohol scale (CIWA-Ar). *Br J Addict* 84:1353-1357, 1989.

beneficial for prolonged seizure activity; IV lorazepam 1 to 2 mg q2h can be used in place of diazepam. Withdrawal seizures generally are self-limited and treatment is not required; the use of phenytoin or other anticonvulsants for short-term treatment of alcohol withdrawal seizures is not recommended.

b. Thiamine 100 mg IV, followed by IV dextrose, should also be administered.

c. Electrolyte imbalances (increased Mg^{2+}, decreased K^+, increased or decreased Na^+, decreased PO_4^{3-}) that may exacerbate seizures should be corrected.

- **DTs:**
  1. Time interval: Variable; usually occurs within 1 wk after reduction or cessation of heavy alcohol intake and persists for 1 to 3 days. Peak incidence is 72 hr and 96 hr after the cessation of alcohol consumption.
  2. Manifestations: Profound confusion, tremors, vivid visual and tactile hallucinations, autonomic hyperactivity; this is the most serious clinical presentation of alcohol withdrawal (mortality rate is approximately 15% in untreated patients).
  3. Treatment:
     a. Admission to a detoxification unit where patient can be observed closely.
     b. Vital signs q30min (neurologic signs, if necessary).
     c. Use of lateral decubitus or prone position if restraints are necessary.
     d. NPO: Nasogastric tube for abdominal distention may be necessary but should not be routinely used.
     e. Laboratory studies: Same as for early alcohol withdrawal.
     f. Vigorous hydration (4 to 6 L/day): IV with glucose (Na^+, K^+, $PO_4^{3}-$ and Mg^{2+} replacement [if patient has hypophosphatemia or hypomagnesemia]).
     g. Vitamins: Thiamine 100 mg IV qd. The initial dose of thiamine should precede the administration of IV dextrose; multivitamins (may be added to the hydrating solution).
     h. Sedation: Control of agitation should be achieved with rapid-acting sedative-hypnotic agents in adequate doses to maintain light somnolence for the duration of delirium.
        (1) Initially: Lorazepam 2 to 5 mg IM/IV repeated prn.
        (2) Maintenance (individualized dosage): Chlordiazepoxide, 50 to 100 mg PO q4-6h, lorazepam 2 mg PO q4h, or diazepam 5 to 10 mg PO tid; withhold doses or decrease subsequent doses if signs of oversedation are apparent.
        (3) Midazolam is also effective for managing DTs. Its rapid onset (sedation within 2 to 4 min of IV injection) and short duration of action (approximately 30 min) make it an ideal agent for titration in continuous infusion.
     i. Treatment of seizures (as previously described).
     j. Diagnosis and treatment of concomitant medical, surgical, or psychiatric conditions.

CHRONIC Rx

- See "Referral."
- Pharmacotherapies for alcoholism include:
  1. Acamprosate is a synthetic compound with a chemical structure similar to the neurotransmitter gamma-aminobutyric acid and the amino acid neuromodulator taurine. Its mechanism of action is not completely understood. It is indicated for the maintenance of abstinence from alcohol in patients with alcohol dependence who are abstinent at treatment initiation. It should be used only as part of a comprehensive psychosocial treatment program. It does not cause a disulfiram-like reaction as a result of ethanol ingestion. Dose is two 333-mg tablets tid. Treatment should be initiated as soon as possible after the period of alcohol withdrawal, when the patient has achieved abstinence, and should be maintained if the patient relapses. Avoid acamprosate if severe renal impairment is present.
  2. The long-acting opiate antagonist naltrexone inhibits the rewarding effects of alcohol. The starting dose is 25 mg/day, increased to 50 mg PO qd after 1 wk. An extended-release, once-monthly injection of naltrexone is also available and can be used along with psychosocial support to maintain alcohol abstinence. In patients with opioid dependence, naltrexone can precipitate acute withdrawal syndrome and should not be used at least 7 days from last opioid use. There are no established guidelines on the appropriate length of naltrexone treatment for alcohol dependence. One study recommends at least 3 mo of treatment. Avoid naltrexone if acute hepatitis, hepatic failure, or ongoing opioid use is present.
  3. Topiramate or gabapentin can be offered to patients with moderate to severe alcohol use disorder who have a goal of abstinence or reducing alcohol use.
  4. Disulfiram (Antabuse): Dosage is 500 mg max qd for 1 to 2 wk, then 125 to 500 mg qd. It interferes with the metabolism of alcohol by inhibiting aldehyde dehydrogenase, causing an accumulation of acetaldehyde. It produces unpleasant symptoms (nausea, flushing, elevated blood pressure, headache, weakness) when alcohol is ingested. It is an older drug that is now rarely used.
  5. Avoid pharmacological treatments in pregnant or breastfeeding women.

DISPOSITION

See "Referral."

REFERRAL

- To Alcoholics Anonymous or Adult Children of Alcoholics
- Family members to Al-Anon or Al-A-Teen
- Many cities have Salvation Army Adult Rehabilitation centers; all patients accepted, regardless of ability to pay

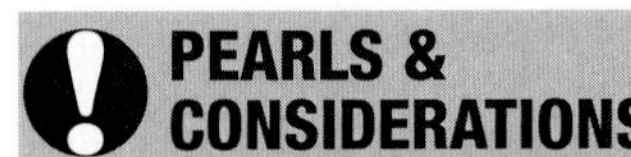

PEARLS & CONSIDERATIONS

COMMENTS

- Relative indications for inpatient alcohol detoxification are as follows: history of DTs or withdrawal seizures, severe withdrawal symptoms, concomitant psychiatric or medical illness, pregnancy, multiple previous detoxifications, recent high levels of alcohol consumption, and lack of reliable support network.
- Detoxification is not a stand-alone treatment but should serve as a bridge to a formal treatment program for alcohol dependence.
- The cure rate for alcoholism is highly disappointing, regardless of the modality. Only those who want to be helped will be helped. An effective strategy for the primary care physician is a prominently displayed sign in the office that states, "If you think you consume too many alcoholic beverages, please discuss it with me." Those who do open up the discussion can be given the facts in a nonjudgmental way and often can be helped. All too often problem drinkers lie on the questionnaire until they face a life-threatening health issue—and even then denial often reigns supreme.
- In a recent clinical trial, patients receiving medical management with naltrexone (100 mg/day), combined behavioral intervention (CBI), or both fared better on drinking outcomes, whereas acamprosate showed no evidence of efficacy, with or without CBI. No combination produced better efficacy than naltrexone or CBI alone in the presence of medical management.

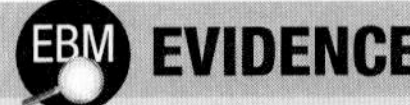

EVIDENCE

Available at ExpertConsult.com

SUGGESTED READINGS

Available at ExpertConsult.com

RELATED CONTENT

Alcohol Abuse (Patient Information)
Abuse, Drug (Related Key Topic)
Alcoholic Hepatitis (Related Key Topic)
Substance Use Disorder (Related Key Topic)
Wernicke Syndrome (Related Key Topic)

AUTHOR: **FRED F. FERRI, M.D.**

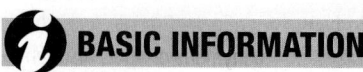

BASIC INFORMATION

DEFINITION

Alcoholic hepatitis (AH) is a severe, progressive, inflammatory, and cholestatic liver disease occurring in patients with long-term ethanol abuse.

SYNONYM

AH

ICD-10CM CODES

K70.10	Alcoholic hepatitis without ascites
K70.9	Alcoholic liver disease, unspecified

EPIDEMIOLOGY & DEMOGRAPHICS

- Approximately 2 million people in the U.S. (about 1% of the population) are affected by alcoholic liver disease.
- Alcoholic hepatitis accounts for 0.8% of all admissions in the U.S.
- Typical presentation age: 40 to 50 yr. Majority occurs before age 60.
- Patients with alcoholic hepatitis typically drink more than 100 g of alcohol daily for two or more decades.

PREVALENCE: Approximately 25% to 30%

PREDOMINANT SEX AND AGE: The majority of patients are males. Males are two times as likely as women to abuse alcohol. However, women develop alcoholic hepatitis after a shorter time and smaller amount of alcoholic exposure than men.

GENETICS: No genetic predilection for any one race. In the U.S., however, there is increased incidence in minority groups.

RISK FACTORS: Drinking multiple alcohol types, drinking alcohol between meal times, poor nutrition, female gender, obesity, Hispanic ethnicity, long-term ingestion of >10 to 20 g/day of alcohol in women and >20 to 40 g/day in men

PHYSICAL FINDINGS & CLINICAL PRESENTATION

Common presenting symptoms include:

- Rapid onset of jaundice
- Right upper quadrant pain
- Nausea/vomiting
- Malaise
- Low-grade fever
- Anorexia
- Abdominal distention/pain (due to ascites)
- Weight loss or malnourishment
- Proximal muscle wasting and weakness
- Complications of liver impairment (GI bleed; confusion, lethargy, ascites)

Findings on physical examination include:

- Jaundice and ascites
- Hepatomegaly, with tender liver on palpation
- Fever (first exclude other causes of fever, such as spontaneous bacterial peritonitis, urinary tract infection [UTI], pneumonia)
- Asterixis (a flapping tremor)
- Splenomegaly
- Tachycardia
- Hypotension
- Peripheral edema
- Abdominal distention with shifting dullness (ascites)
- Hepatic bruit
- With coexistent cirrhosis, look for:
  1. Gynecomastia
  2. Proximal muscles wasting
  3. Spider angiomata
  4. Altered hair distribution

Dx DIAGNOSIS

DIFFERENTIAL DIAGNOSIS

- Hepatitis B
- Hepatitis C
- Nonalcoholic steatohepatitis (NASH)
- Chronic pancreatitis
- Drug-induced liver injury
- Hemochromatosis
- Cholangitis

WORKUP

- A thorough and detailed history is needed.
- Relevant questions may include:
  1. When patient started drinking
  2. Number of times patient drinks per day
  3. How many yrs of regular/daily drinking
  4. Types of alcohol
  5. Home or bar drinking
  6. Rehabilitation for drinking
  7. Social problems (e.g., arrest for public intoxication or driving under the influence, marital discord due to alcoholism)

LABORATORY TESTS

- Elevated transaminase (aspartate aminotransferase [AST] >45 U/L but <300 U/L; AST: alanine aminotransferase [ALT] ratio ≥2.0) but some patients may not have elevations in ALT, AST in early phases
- S-bilirubin >2 mg/dl
- Increased prothrombin time [PT]/international normalized ratio [INR]
- Elevated gamma glutamyltransferase (GGT)
- Carbohydrate-deficient transferrin (CDT) is a reliable marker for chronic alcoholism
- Elevated C-reactive protein
- Electrolyte disorder (hypokalemia, hypomagnesemia, low zinc, hypophosphatemia)
- Hypoalbuminemia
- Hyperferritinemia
- CBC (may reveal leukocytosis with bandemia or anemia or thrombocytopenia); mean corpuscular volume (MCV) may be elevated
- Screening tests to rule out other conditions include checking:
  1. Hepatitis B surface antigen (HBsAg), hepatitis B core antibody (HB_cAb) (IgM), hepatitis A antibody (IgM)
  2. Anti–hepatitis C antibody, hepatitis C ribonucleic acid (RNA)
  3. Ferritin-transferrin saturation
  4. Alpha-fetoprotein
  5. Alkaline phosphatase
- The severity of AH can be calculated with the Maddrey Discriminant Function (MDF) score, which is calculated as follows:

$$MDF = 4.6 \times \text{prothrombin time} - \text{control prothrombin time} + \text{total bilirubin (mg/dl)}$$

IMAGING STUDIES

Ultrasonography is the preferred imaging study. The earliest histologic change in alcoholic liver disease is macrovesicular steatosis.

LIVER BIOPSY

- Liver biopsy is rarely needed.
- Useful to:
  1. Confirm the diagnosis.
  2. Evaluate the effect of coexisting disease.
  3. Rule out cirrhosis.
  4. Exclude other diagnoses (especially other causes of liver diseases, biliary obstruction, Budd-Chiari syndrome).
- Typical histologic findings include:
  1. Micro- or macrovesicular steatosis
  2. Hepatocyte injury (ballooning degeneration and focal hepatocyte necrosis)
  3. Mallory-Denk bodies (characteristic of alcoholic hepatitis)
  4. Perivenular fibrosis
  5. Portal and lobular inflammation with neutrophils or lymphocyte infiltration

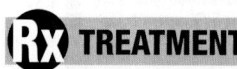

Rx TREATMENT

An algorithm for the management of patients with alcoholic hepatitis is described in Fig. 1. Treatment can be divided into three main components:

1. Lifestyle modifications
2. Nutritional support
3. Pharmacologic therapy

LIFESTYLE MODIFICATIONS

- Abstinence from alcohol (this improves both short- and long-term survival). Fig. 2 describes the effect of subsequent alcohol intake on 5-yr survival in patients with alcoholic hepatitis
- Smoking cessation (to decrease oxidative stress)
- Treatment of substance abuse

NUTRITIONAL SUPPORT

- Good nutrition is an essential part of treatment because many patients with alcoholic hepatitis are usually in a catabolic state.
- Nutritional support includes:
  1. Liberal vitamin supplementation (especially thiamine, folic acid, vitamin K)
  2. Mineral supplementation (**but not iron**)
  3. Calorie counting is essential. A high calorie intake (1.2 to 1.4 times the normal resting intake) may be required.
  4. Protein intake of 1.2 to 1.5 g/kg of ideal body weight per day will provide adequate support. **Exception: In patients with severe encephalopathy, protein restriction may be required.**
  5. Fluid management

PHARMACOLOGIC THERAPY

Severe alcoholic hepatitis may require treatment. Severity can be assessed by calculating the Model for End-Stage Liver Disease (MELD) score or Maddrey's discriminant function (MDF) score or the Glasgow score.

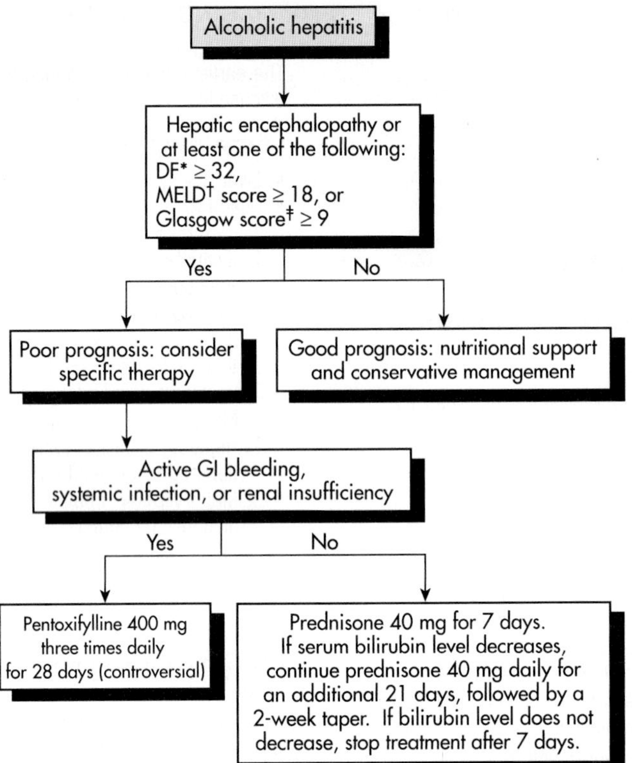

FIG. 1 Algorithm for the management of patients with alcoholic hepatitis. *The DF is calculated as follows: 4.6 (prothrombin time of patient − prothrombin time of control) + serum bilirubin level (in mg/dl). †The Model for End-Stage Liver Disease score is based on the serum bilirubin level, INR, and serum creatinine level. ‡The Glasgow alcoholic hepatitis score is based on the patient's age, white blood cell count, blood urea nitrogen level, ratio of prothrombin time to a control value, and serum bilirubin level. *DF*, Discriminant function. Online calculators for these various models are available at http://www.lillemodel.com. (Modified from Feldman M, et al.: *Sleisenger and Fordtran's gastrointestinal and liver disease*, ed 10, Philadelphia, 2016, Elsevier.)

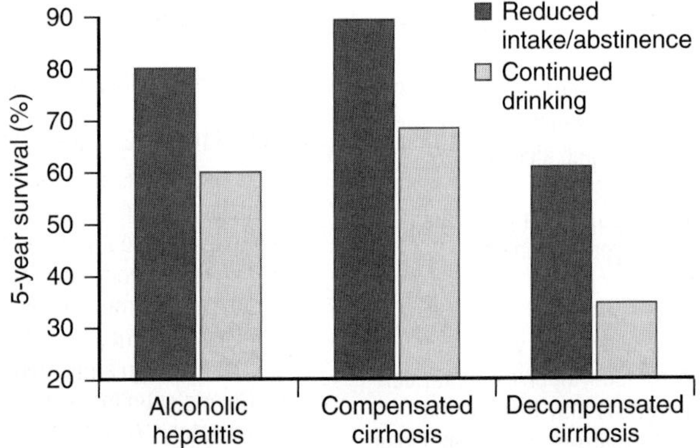

FIG. 2 Effect of subsequent alcohol intake on 5-year survival in patients with alcoholic hepatitis and cirrhosis. (From Day CP: Liver disorder part 1 of 2, *Medicine* 35(1):22–25, 2007.)

- An MDF score ≥32 indicates significant or severe alcoholic hepatitis (30-day mortality of 50%).
- MELD score can easily be calculated (visit http://www.unos.org/resources/meldpeldcalculator.asp?index=98). This score predicts short-term survival in patients with cirrhosis. A score >20 predicts increased short-term mortality.
- Glasgow score: contains four variables (BUN, PT, WBC count, and bilirubin). A score ≥9 indicates increased mortality.

Indications for hospitalization include:

- MDF ≥32
- MELD >20
- Glasgow score >8
- Hepatic encephalopathy

Patients with severe alcoholic hepatitis may be treated with glucocorticosteroids (prednisolone 40 mg/day for 28 days with a 2-wk taper). Glucocorticosteroids reduce hepatic injury, suppress inflammation, and promote liver regeneration. However, not all studies have demonstrated consistent therapeutic benefits for steroids, even in high-risk patients. Prednisolone should be discontinued if bilirubin does not decrease by day 17. An alternative agent for patients with contraindications to corticosteroids is pentoxifylline. Pentoxifylline is not effective in patients who do not respond to prednisone, and data supporting its use is weak.

LIVER TRANSPLANTATION

- Usually reserved for patients with end-stage liver disease. Patients whose hepatitis is not responding to medical therapy have a 6-month survival rate of approximately 30%. Since most hepatitis deaths occur within 2 months, early liver transplantation is attractive and associated with higher than 80% survival at 3 yrs.
- Patients with alcoholic hepatitis must be sober for at least 6 mo before they can be eligible for consideration for liver transplantation. However, transplantation candidates should not be based solely on 6 mo abstinence, and other factors, such as social support and need for rehabilitation, should be considered.

REFERRAL

Severe acute alcoholic hepatitis may require intensive care unit (ICU) care and referral to different subspecialists:

- GI/hepatology (for patients with evidence of GI hemorrhage)
- Nutritional services
- Nephrology (for acute renal failure, hepatorenal syndrome)
- Neurology (for change in mental status, seizures)
- Infectious disease (for fever/leukocytosis)

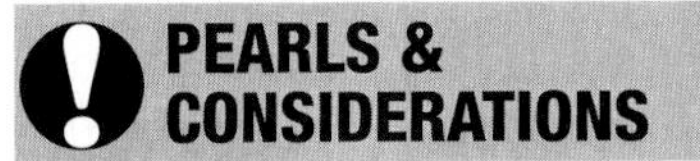

PEARLS & CONSIDERATIONS

COMMENTS

- Referral to substance abuse treatment programs may be helpful.
  1. Stress to patients that there are limited long-term drug treatments for alcoholic hepatitis.
  2. Maintaining good general nutrition is important.
  3. Advise patient about the risk of taking certain medications, especially acetaminophen.
- Periodic follow-up to monitor patient's response to check basic metabolic panel (BMP) and liver function tests (LFTs).
- Encourage alcohol abstinence. Abstinence improves long-term survival.
- If patient develops liver cirrhosis, check serum alpha-fetoprotein every 6 mo and liver ultrasound annually to rule out hepatocellular carcinoma.
- Vaccinate patient against hepatitis A and B viruses, pneumococci, influenza A virus, and routine adult vaccinations, if appropriate.

SUGGESTED READINGS

Available at ExpertConsult.com

RELATED CONTENT

Alcoholic Hepatitis (Patient Information)

AUTHOR: **DANIEL K. ASIEDU, M.D., PH.D., F.A.C.P.**

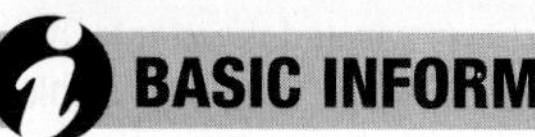

BASIC INFORMATION

DEFINITION

Primary hyperaldosteronism is a clinical syndrome characterized by hypertension, hypokalemia, and excessive aldosterone secretion with either a low (suppressed) plasma renin activity (PRA) or low direct renin concentration (DRC).

SYNONYMS

Hyperaldosteronism
Primary aldosteronism
Conn syndrome

ICD-10CM CODES

E26.0 Primary hyperaldosteronism
E26.1 Secondary hyperaldosteronism
E26.8 Other hyperaldosteronism
E26.9 Hyperaldosteronism, unspecified

EPIDEMIOLOGY & DEMOGRAPHICS

INCIDENCE: 5% to 10% of patients with hypertension

PREVALENCE: More common in females

PHYSICAL FINDINGS & CLINICAL PRESENTATION

- Generally asymptomatic
- If significant hypokalemia is present, muscle cramping, weakness, and paresthesias may occur
- Hypertension
- Polyuria, polydipsia

ETIOLOGY

- Aldosterone-producing adenoma (40%–60%)
- Idiopathic hyperaldosteronism (>30%)
- Glucocorticoid-suppressible hyperaldosteronism (<1%)
- Aldosterone-producing carcinoma (<1%)

Dx DIAGNOSIS

DIFFERENTIAL DIAGNOSIS

- Diuretic use
- Hypokalemia from vomiting, diarrhea
- Renovascular hypertension
- Other endocrine neoplasm (pheochromocytoma, deoxycorticosterone-producing tumor, renin-secreting tumor)

WORKUP

Fig. 1 provides guidance on when to consider testing for primary aldosteronism. Fig. 2 describes a diagnostic approach to patients with suspected primary aldosteronism. CT, MRI, and adrenal vein sampling (AVS) are used to distinguish unilateral from bilateral increased aldosterone secretion. This distinction will dictate treatment options since unilateral primary aldosteronism is treated by surgical resection rather than medically.

LABORATORY TESTS

Routine laboratory tests can be suggestive but are not diagnostic of primary aldosteronism. Common abnormalities are:

When to consider testing for primary aldosteronism:
- Hypertension and hypokalemia
- Resistant hypertension
- Adrenal incidentaloma and hypertension
- Onset of hypertension at a young age (<20 y)
- Severe hypertension (≥160 mm Hg systolic or ≥100 mm Hg diastolic)
- Whenever considering secondary hypertension

↓

Morning blood sample in seated ambulant patient
- Plasma aldosterone concentration (PAC)
- Plasma renin activity (PRA) or PRC

↓

↑ PAC (≥15 ng/dL)
↓ PRA (<1.0 ng/mL per hour) or
↓ PRC (<lower limit of detection for the assay)
and
PAC/PRA ratio ≥20 ng/dL per ng/mL per hour

↓

Investigate for primary aldosteronism

FIG. 1 Algorithm provides guidance on when to consider testing for primary aldosteronism and use of the ratio of plasma aldosterone concentration *(PAC)* to plasma renin activity *(PRA)* as a case-detection tool. *PRC,* Plasma renin concentration. (Melmed S, Polonsky KS, Larsen PR, Kronenberg HM: *Williams textbook of endocrinology,* ed 12, Philadelphia, 2011, Saunders.)

- Spontaneous hypokalemia or severe hypokalemia while receiving conventional doses of diuretics
- Possible alkalosis and hypernatremia

IMAGING STUDIES

- Adrenal CT scans (Fig. E3) or MRI may be used to localize neoplasm.
- Adrenal scanning with iodocholesterol (NP-59) or 6-beta-iodomethyl-19-norcholesterol after dexamethasone suppression. The uptake of tracer is increased in those with aldosteronoma and absent in those with bilateral idiopathic adrenal hyperplasia and adrenal carcinoma.

Rx TREATMENT

NONPHARMACOLOGIC THERAPY

Regular blood pressure monitoring and low-sodium diet, tobacco avoidance, maintenance of ideal body weight, and regular exercise

ACUTE GENERAL Rx

- Control of blood pressure and hypokalemia with spironolactone, eplerenone, or amiloride
- Surgery (unilateral adrenalectomy) for aldosterone-producing adenoma (APA)

CHRONIC Rx

Chronic medical therapy with spironolactone, eplerenone, or amiloride to control blood pressure and hypokalemia is necessary in all patients with bilateral idiopathic adrenal hyperplasia. Eplerenone causes less gynecomastia in men and menstrual irregularities in women because of greater mineralocorticoid receptor selectivity, but is more expensive than spironolactone or amiloride.

DISPOSITION

Unilateral adrenalectomy normalizes hypertension and hypokalemia in 70% of patients with APA after 1 yr. After 5 yrs, 50% of patients remain normotensive.

REFERRAL

Surgical referral for unilateral adrenalectomy after confirmation of unilateral APA or carcinoma

PEARLS & CONSIDERATIONS

- Frequent monitoring of blood pressure and electrolytes postoperatively is necessary because normalization of blood pressure after unilateral adrenalectomy may take up to 4 months.
- With increased use of DRC assays in lieu of PRA assays, caution must be taken during interpretation of results because of different units used for each assay. The aldosterone to DRC ratio is not as widely validated as the plasma aldosterone concentration (PAC)-to-PRA ratio. A PAC-to-DRC ratio of >62 in patients with PAC levels >200 ng/l has been recently established as a reliable screening method for primary hyperaldosteronism from APAs.
- A recent cohort study revealed that suppression of renin and higher aldosterone concentrations in the context of renin suppression are associated with an increased risk for hypertension and possibly also with increased mineralocorticoid receptor activity. These readings suggest a clinically relevant spectrum of subclinical primary

 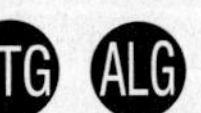

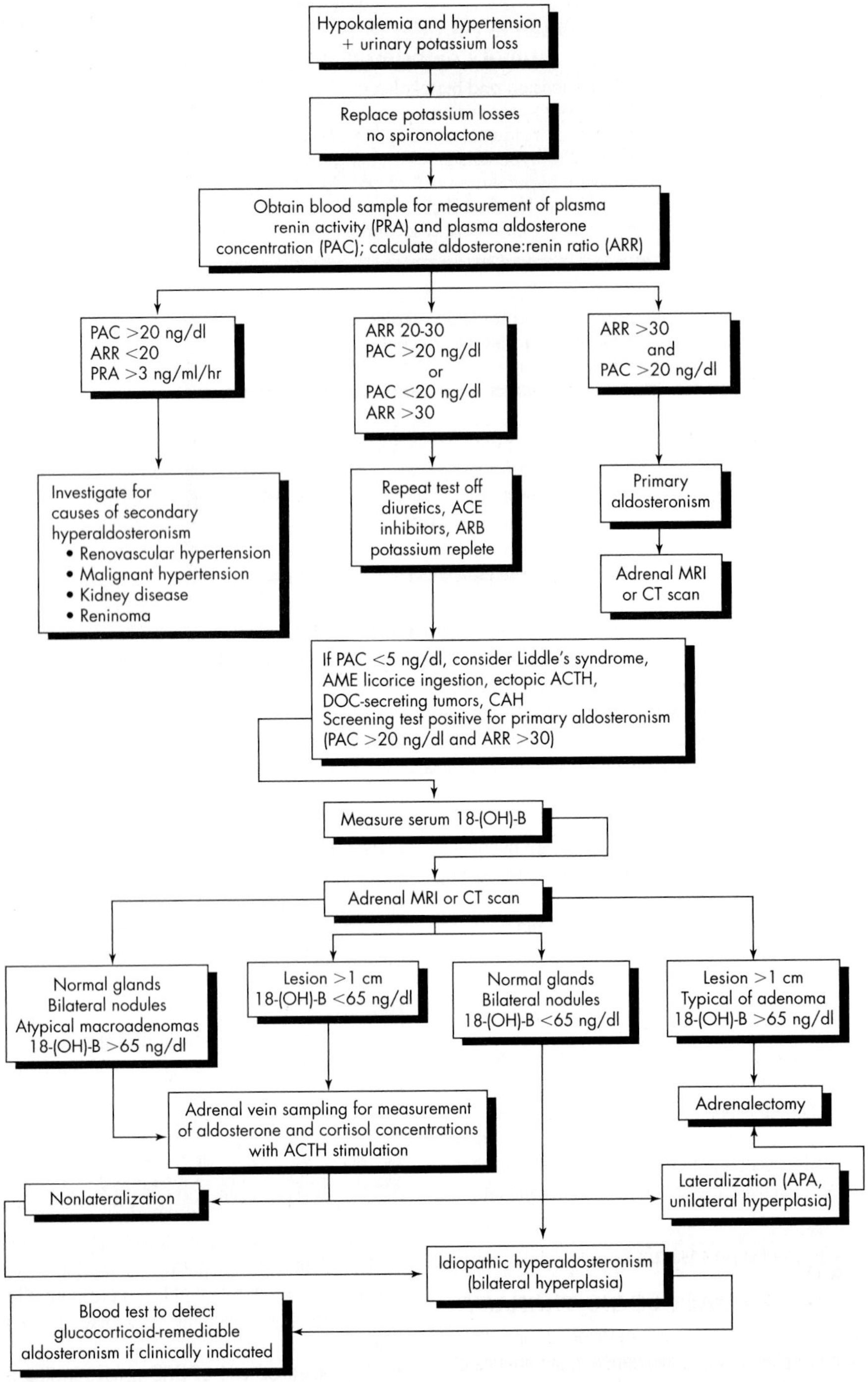

Hypokalemia and hypertension + urinary potassium loss

Replace potassium losses no spironolactone

Obtain blood sample for measurement of plasma renin activity (PRA) and plasma aldosterone concentration (PAC); calculate aldosterone:renin ratio (ARR)

PAC >20 ng/dl
ARR <20
PRA >3 ng/ml/hr

ARR 20-30
PAC >20 ng/dl
or
PAC <20 ng/dl
ARR >30

ARR >30
and
PAC >20 ng/dl

Investigate for causes of secondary hyperaldosteronism
- Renovascular hypertension
- Malignant hypertension
- Kidney disease
- Reninoma

Repeat test off diuretics, ACE inhibitors, ARB potassium replete

Primary aldosteronism

Adrenal MRI or CT scan

If PAC <5 ng/dl, consider Liddle's syndrome, AME licorice ingestion, ectopic ACTH, DOC-secreting tumors, CAH
Screening test positive for primary aldosteronism (PAC >20 ng/dl and ARR >30)

Measure serum 18-(OH)-B

Adrenal MRI or CT scan

Normal glands
Bilateral nodules
Atypical macroadenomas
18-(OH)-B >65 ng/dl

Lesion >1 cm
18-(OH)-B <65 ng/dl

Normal glands
Bilateral nodules
18-(OH)-B <65 ng/dl

Lesion >1 cm
Typical of adenoma
18-(OH)-B >65 ng/dl

Adrenal vein sampling for measurement of aldosterone and cortisol concentrations with ACTH stimulation

Adrenalectomy

Nonlateralization

Lateralization (APA, unilateral hyperplasia)

Idiopathic hyperaldosteronism (bilateral hyperplasia)

Blood test to detect glucocorticoid-remediable aldosteronism if clinically indicated

FIG. 2 Diagnostic approach to patients with suspected primary aldosteronism. Cortisol concentration ratio in an adrenal vein four times greater than that in the other adrenal vein and/or an aldosterone/cortisol concentration ratio from the vein of the unaffected adrenal that is less than the ratio in the vena cava. Urinary loss of potassium can be documented by measuring potassium excretion in a 24-hour urine collection; excretion of more than 30 mEq per day in the presence of hypokalemia indicates potassium wasting. An alternative and simpler approach is to obtain a random sample of urine to calculate the fractional excretion of potassium. A fractional excretion exceeding 10% when hypokalemia is present indicates potassium wasting. *AME,* Syndrome of apparent mineralocorticoid excess; *APA,* aldosterone-producing adenoma; *CAH,* congenital adrenal hyperplasia; *CT,* computed tomography; *DOC,* deoxycorticosterone; *ectopic ACTH,* production of corticotrophin by a tumor outside the pituitary gland; *serum 18-(OH)-B,* serum concentration of 18-hydroxycorticosterone. (From Runge MS, Greganti MA: *Netter's internal medicine,* Philadelphia, 2008, Saunders.)

aldosteronism (renin-independent aldosteronism) in patients with normal blood pressure.[1]

SUGGESTED READINGS

Available at ExpertConsult.com

RELATED CONTENT

Aldosteronism (Patient Information)

AUTHOR: **KAUSIK UMANATH, M.D., M.S.**

[1] Brown JM, et al.: The spectrum of subclinical primary aldosteronism and incident hypertension, *Ann Int Med* 167:630–641, 2017.

BASIC INFORMATION

DEFINITION

Allergic rhinitis is an immunoglobulin E (IgE)-mediated hypersensitivity response to nasally inhaled allergens that involves mucosal inflammation driven by type 2 helper T (Th2) cells that causes sneezing, rhinorrhea, nasal pruritus, and congestion. It may be seasonal or perennial.

SYNONYMS

Hay fever
IgE-mediated rhinitis
Seasonal allergic rhinitis
SAR

ICD-10CM CODES

J30.1	Allergic rhinitis due to pollen
J30.2	Other seasonal allergic rhinitis
J30.3	Other allergic rhinitis
J30.4	Allergic rhinitis, unspecified

EPIDEMIOLOGY & DEMOGRAPHICS

- Allergic rhinitis affects approximately 10% to 20% of the U.S. population and 40% of children.
- Mean age of onset is 8 to 12 yrs.
- The prevalence of allergic rhinitis in patients presenting to their primary care provider with nasal symptoms is estimated to be 30% to 60%.

PHYSICAL FINDINGS & CLINICAL PRESENTATION

- Pale or violaceous mucosa of the turbinates caused by venous engorgement (this can distinguish it from erythema present in viral rhinitis)
- Nasal polyps
- Lymphoid hyperplasia in the posterior oropharynx with cobblestone appearance
- Erythema of the throat, conjunctival and scleral injection
- Clear nasal discharge
- Clinical presentation: Usually consists of sneezing, nasal congestion, cough, postnasal drip, loss of or alteration of smell, and sensation of plugged ears

ETIOLOGY

- Pollens in the springtime, ragweed in fall, grasses in the summer
- Dust, mites, animal allergens
- Smoke or any irritants
- Perfumes, detergents, soaps
- Emotion, changes in atmospheric pressure or temperature

DIAGNOSIS

DIFFERENTIAL DIAGNOSIS

- Infections (sinusitis; viral, bacterial, or fungal rhinitis)
- Rhinitis medicamentosa (cocaine, sympathomimetic nasal drops)
- Vasomotor rhinitis (e.g., secondary to air pollutants)
- Septal obstruction (e.g., deviated septum), nasal polyps, nasal neoplasms
- Systemic diseases (e.g., Wegener granulomatosis, hypothyroidism [rare])

WORKUP

- The initial strategy should be to determine whether patients should undergo diagnostic testing or receive empirical treatment.
- Workup is often unnecessary if the diagnosis is apparent. A detailed medical history is useful in identifying the culprit allergen.
- Selected patients with allergic rhinitis that is not controlled with standard therapy may benefit from allergy testing to target allergen avoidance measures or guide immunotherapy. Allergy testing can be performed using skin testing or radioallergosorbent (RAST) testing. Immunoglobulin E (IgE) testing using newest-generation assays is also an excellent tool for diagnosing the cause of symptoms related to rhinitis. Allergy testing with skin or blood testing is most useful as confirmatory tests when the patient's history is compatible with an IgE-mediated reaction and should generally be reserved for ambiguous or complicated cases.
- Examination of nasal smears for the presence of neutrophils to rule out infectious causes and the presence of eosinophils (suggestive of allergy) may be useful in selected patients.
- Peripheral blood eosinophil counts are not useful in allergy diagnosis.

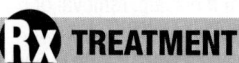

TREATMENT

NONPHARMACOLOGIC THERAPY

- Maintain allergen-free environment by covering mattresses and pillows with allergen-proof casings, eliminating carpeting, eliminating animal products, and removing dust-collecting fixtures.
- Use of air purifiers and dust filters is helpful.
- Maintain humidity in the environment below 50% to prevent dust mites and mold.
- Use air conditioners, especially in the bedroom.
- Remove pets from homes of patients with suspected sensitivity to animal allergens.
- Use of acupuncture to treat seasonal allergic rhinitis is controversial. A recent trial showed that acupuncture led to statistically significant improvement in disease-specific quality of life and antihistamine use measures after 8 weeks of treatment compared with sham acupuncture and with rescue medication alone.

ACUTE GENERAL Rx

- Determine if the patient is troubled by swollen turbinates (best treated with decongestants) or blockages secondary to mucus (effectively treated by antihistamines).
- Topical nasal steroids are very effective and are preferred by many as first-line treatment for allergic rhinitis in persons 12 and older. Patients should be instructed on proper use and informed that improvement might not occur for at least 1 wk after initiation of therapy. Commonly available inhalers follow.
  1. Beclomethasone dipropionate: One to two sprays in each nostril bid
  2. Fluticasone: Initially two sprays in each nostril qd or one spray in each nostril bid, decreasing to one spray in each nostril qd based on response
  3. Flunisolide: Initially two sprays in each nostril bid
  4. Budesonide: Two sprays in each nostril bid or four sprays in each nostril qam
  5. For treatment of moderate to severe seasonal allergic rhinitis in persons aged 12 or older, the best initial treatment is a combination of intranasal corticosteroid and an infranasal antihistamine
  6. Azelastine is an antihistamine nasal spray effective for seasonal allergic rhinitis. Olopatadine is an intranasal H1-antihistamine alternative to azelastine in mild to moderate seasonal allergic rhinitis
- Most oral first-generation antihistamines can cause considerable sedation and anticholinergic symptoms. The second-generation antihistamines (loratadine, fexofenadine, cetirizine, levocetirizine, desloratadine) are preferred because they do not have any significant anticholinergic or sedative effects.
- Montelukast, a leukotriene receptor antagonist commonly used for asthma, is also effective for allergic rhinitis. Usual adult dose is 10 mg qd.

CHRONIC Rx

- Cromolyn sodium: One spray to each nostril three to four times daily can be used for prophylaxis (mast cell stabilizer).
- Immunotherapy is generally reserved for patients responding poorly to the above treatments. Traditionally, immunotherapy consisted of subcutaneous injections of gradually increased doses of allergens. Recently, the FDA has approved several allergen extracts (Oralair, Grastek, Ragwitek, Odactra) for sublingual administration as immunotherapy.

DISPOSITION

Most patients experience significant relief with avoidance of allergens and proper use of medications.

REFERRAL

Allergy testing in patients with severe symptoms who are unresponsive to therapy or when the diagnosis is uncertain

SUGGESTED READINGS

Available at ExpertConsult.com

RELATED CONTENT

Allergic Rhinitis (Patient Information)

AUTHOR: **FRED F. FERRI, M.D.**

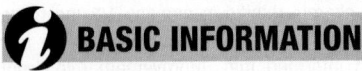

BASIC INFORMATION

DEFINITION

Alopecia is the term used to describe involuntary hair loss, typically on the scalp but can occur anywhere over the body. *Nonscarring alopecia* is hair loss without clinically apparent scarring, inflammation, or skin atrophy. *Scarring alopecia* is characterized by permanent hair loss accompanied by tissue destruction in the form of scarring, inflammation, and/or skin atrophy.

SYNONYMS

Hair loss
Balding

ICD-10CM CODES

L63	Alopecia aerata
L63.0	Alopecia (capitis) totalis
L64	Androgenic alopecia
L64.0	Drug-induced androgenic alopecia
L64.8	Other androgenic alopecia
L64.9	Androgenic alopecia, unspecified
L65	Other nonscarring hair loss
L66	Cicatricial alopecia
L65.9	Nonscarring hair loss, unspecified
L63.8	Other alopecia areata
L65.0	Telogen effluvium

EPIDEMIOLOGY & DEMOGRAPHICS

INCIDENCE: Depends on etiology, for example:
- Alopecia areata affects 1% of the U.S. population by age 50 yr. There is a higher incidence at a younger age and both sexes are affected equally.
- Androgenetic alopecia affects males > females with 50% of Caucasian men affected by age 50 yr. Less common in Asians and African-American men, and often has later onset. By age 70, 40% of females are affected, with incidence increasing after menopause.

GENETICS: Depends on etiology, for example:
- Androgenetic alopecia is polygenic with variable penetrance and can be inherited from one or both parents.
- Certain scarring alopecias are more predominant in people with coarser hair.

ETIOLOGY

NONSCARRING:
- Failure of follicle production
- Hair shaft abnormality
- Pattern hair loss, i.e., androgenetic alopecia
- Hair breakage, i.e., trichotillomania, traction alopecia, cosmetic overprocessing
- Problem with cycling (excess shedding), i.e., telogen effluvium, anagen effluvium, loose chemotherapy anagen syndrome, alopecia areata, syphilis

SCARRING:
- Infectious: Tinea capitis with inflammation (kerion), bacterial folliculitis as in dissecting folliculitis and folliculitis decalvans
- Neoplasm: Alopecia mucinosa in cutaneous T-cell lymphoma or alopecia neoplastica due to metastatic carcinoma (breast cancer)
- Autoimmune: Chronic cutaneous lupus erythematosus
- Congenital

CLINICAL FEATURES

HISTORY: A careful history must be taken and should include time course for hair loss, the pattern of hair loss, any recent change in life situation/stresses, any associated medical conditions, new medications, any family history of hair loss, diet, hair care practices, and other skin/nail symptoms.

PHYSICAL EXAMINATION:
- General: Patient's emotional response to hair loss
- Hair/skin:
  1. Hair thinning/loss
  2. May have fine downy hairs also referred to as vellus hairs
  3. Skin may show changes consistent with inflammation, infection, and/or atrophy
  4. Women may show virilization (e.g., hirsutism)
  5. Exclamation-point hairs can be seen in alopecia areata
  6. Broken hairs of different length may be seen in traumatic alopecia
  7. Hairs that crack or crumble with palpation most often signify shaft damage due to overprocessing

Dx DIAGNOSIS

WORKUP

- Pull test—No shower for 24 hr, 60 hairs are gently pulled from the scalp, removal of 6 or more hairs is considered positive result and indicates telogen effluvium (active shedding). Look for telogen bulbs on recovered hairs to differentiate from breaking (blunt ends).
- Punch biopsy—Mandatory when suspecting scarring alopecia. Send two punches: one for vertical and one for horizontal sectioning for histopathologic analysis, preferably by a dermatopathologist.
- Trichogram—Quantifies hair loss. Pull 25 to 50 hairs and measure proportion of anagen to catagen and telogen hairs under light microscopy: 10% to 20% telogen hairs is normal, whereas >35% is highly suspicious for telogen effluvium.
- Fig. E1 describes the evaluation and treatment of alopecia in females.

LABORATORY TESTS

Initiate laboratory studies if not clear based on clinical presentation:
- CBC—Rule out Fe deficiency
- Total Fe/ferritin—Rule out subclinical Fe deficiency
- TSH—Rule out underlying thyroid disease
- ANA—Screen for autoimmune disease
- RPR—Rule out cutaneous syphilis if history suggestive of increased risk

DIFFERENTIAL DIAGNOSIS

NONSCARRING:
- *Telogen effluvium:* This type of alopecia is usually diffuse thinning that follows significant life stress (death of loved one, high fever, severe infection, crash dieting) or change in hormones (postpartum, change in or cessation of oral contraceptives). Patient often presents with a bag of hair that has fallen out. This is caused by a large number of anagen (growing) hairs entering telogen (dying phase) simultaneously. Telogen effluvium is more common in women.
- *Androgenetic alopecia:* Gradual thinning of hair and a trend toward finer hair, which in men has a typical pattern of receding anterior bitemporal hairline resulting in an M-shaped pattern and hair loss at the vertex (Fig. 2) and in women has a typical pattern of thinning along vertex with or without frontotemporal thinning. This type of thinning is due to a combination of genetic predisposition and androgenic conversion of hair follicles into vellus-like follicles. Widening of the central hair part is often seen, leading to scalp visibility (Fig. 3). This female pattern of more diffuse hair loss is seen in 20% to 30% of adolescent males.

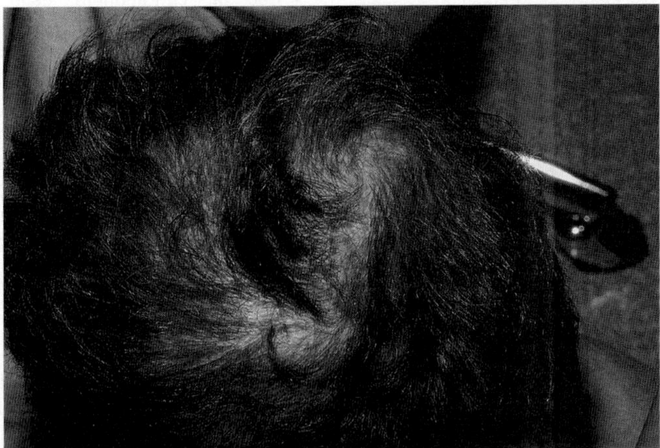

FIG. 2 Androgenetic alopecia. The scalp hair is thinned progressively but most notably between the frontal region of the scalp and the vertex. (From Paller AS, Mancini AJ: *Hurwitz clinical pediatric dermatology, a textbook of skin disorders of childhood and adolescence*, ed 5, Philadelphia, 2016, Elsevier.)

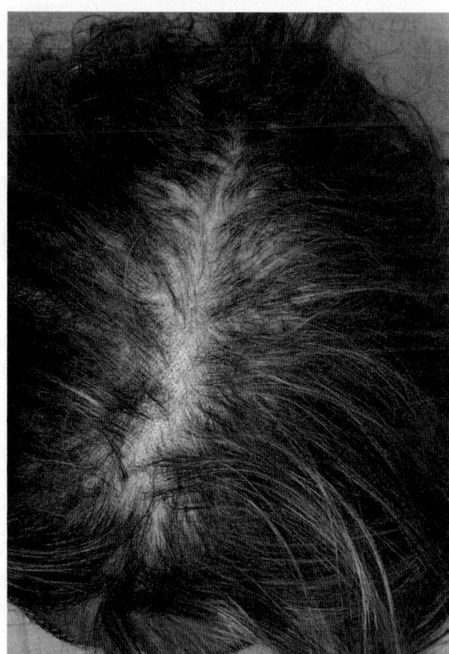

FIG. 3 Androgenetic alopecia. Widening of the central hair part is often seen, leading to scalp visibility. (From Paller AS, Mancini AJ: *Hurwitz clinical pediatric dermatology, a textbook of skin disorders of childhood and adolescence*, ed 5, Philadelphia, 2016, Elsevier.)

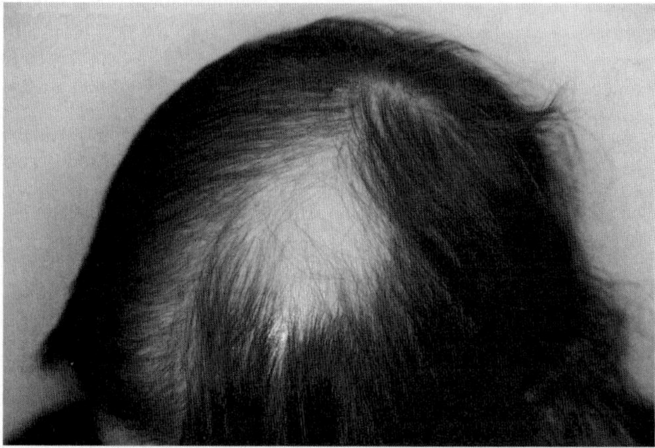

FIG. 4 Alopecia areata: patchy hair loss. The alopecic area is devoid of hairs, and the scalp does not present inflammatory changes. (From Goldman L, Schafer AI: *Goldman's Cecil medicine,* ed 24, Philadelphia, 2012, Saunders.)

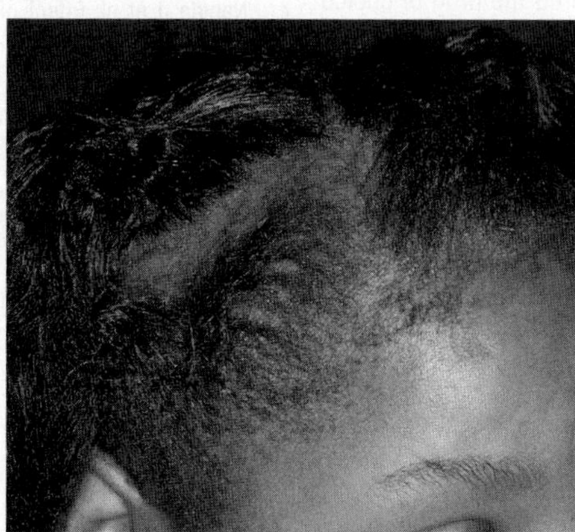

FIG. 5 Traction alopecia. Hair loss can be seen at the margins where hair is pulled most tightly through use of barrettes. (From Paller AS, Mancini AJ: *Hurwitz clinical pediatric dermatology, a textbook of skin disorders of childhood and adolescence*, ed 5, Philadelphia, 2016, Elsevier.)

- *Alopecia areata:* Patches of acute hair loss (Fig. 4), typically 2 to 5 cm in diameter, with normal-appearing skin, black dots (cadaver hairs, point noir) from hair that breaks before reaching the skin's surface, and occasional "exclamation point hairs," which are evidence of hairs breaking off as they are pushed from the follicle. Fingernails may show fine pitting. On biopsy, lymphocytes surround the hair bulb and resemble a "swarm of bees," evidence of the autoimmune etiology. Patients often have positive family history. AA Universalis (AAU)—generalized loss of body hair AA Totalis (AAT)—complete loss of scalp hair
- *Tinea:* This type of hair loss is evident in round patches, possibly with scarring, erythema, and lymphadenopathy. This is the most common type of hair loss in children. Diagnosis can be made by scraping the erythematous edge and placing the scraping with KOH under a microscope to check for hyphae. Wood's lamp only fluoresces if tinea is caused by *Microsporum* spp.; however, the most common (in the U.S.) *Trichophyton* spp. does not fluoresce. If a kerion (severe alopecia associated with bogginess) is present, it may cause scarring.
- *Traumatic alopecia (traction alopecia):* This type of hair loss is in a pattern consistent with breaking off of hairs due to traction (hair pulling) (Fig. 5) or chemical or heating agents (hair straightening or permanent). Etiology usually becomes apparent with careful history taking and visualizing the pattern of hair loss. In trichotillomania (Fig. 6), the alopecia area has an irregular shape, scalp excoriations may present, and hairs are broken at different lengths.

SCARRING:

- *Lichen planus:* The hair loss associated with LP is typically associated with scaling and atrophy of pruritic, painful skin underlying the hair loss. This hair loss is more common in middle-aged women. While there are numerous variations in clinical presentation, the general clinical picture is one of a chronic inflammatory condition of the skin, nails, mucous membranes, and/or hair. The typical skin lesions are flat topped, violaceous lesions with white lines (Wickham's striae), while the typical oral lesions are milky white.
- *Chronic cutaneous (discoid) lupus erythematosus:* This type of hair loss frequently is evident in well-demarcated, erythematous plaques in chronically sun-exposed areas of skin. Lesions exhibit hypopigmentations or hyperpigmentations, atrophy, erythema, and scaling. It may be present concurrently with SLE or be the first presenting symptom of SLE, but in most cases it is a purely cutaneous condition.
- *Tinea with kerion:* A kerion represents an exuberant delayed-type hypersensitivity reaction to the tinea capitis, resulting in one (or many) inflamed boggy plaque(s) on the scalp depending on the severity of the infection.

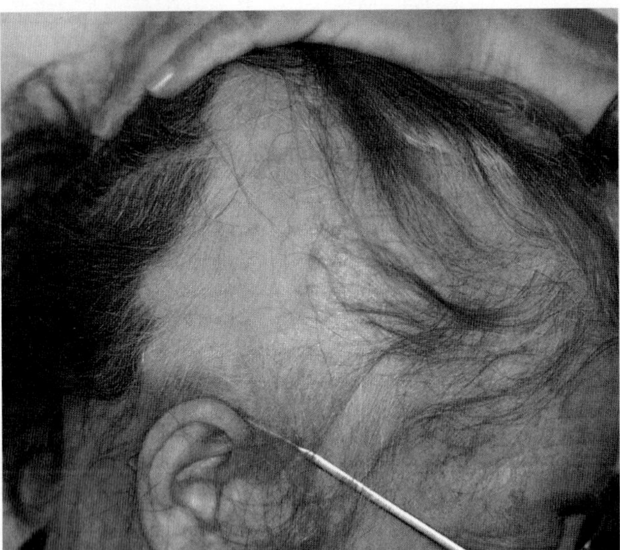

FIG. 6 Trichotillomania: patchy hair loss. The alopecic area has an irregular shape and present hairs are broken at different lengths. Also note scalp excoriations. (From Goldman L, Schafer AI: *Goldman's Cecil medicine,* ed 24, Philadelphia, 2012, Saunders.)

Rx TREATMENT

- *Telogen effluvium:* Stop offending stress/medication and in 3 to 4 months anagen recurs. Hair density should be normalized by 12 months. Multiple medications have been shown to be an inciting factor and one should consider stopping them (these include, but are not limited to, enalapril, colchicine, levodopa, metoprolol, propranolol, oral contraceptives, and lithium). Full regrowth is expected in most cases.
- *Androgenetic alopecia:* For men, the most likely first-line treatment is oral finasteride (type II 5α-reductase inhibitor) which leads to lower levels of dihydrotestosterone. This leads to hair regrowth in about 6 months, but with cessation, hair returns to pattern of loss within 6 to 9 months. Topical minoxidil has shown similar results to finasteride and can be useful in partially restoring lost hair in both men and women. Dutasteride (off-label) has been shown to be superior to finasteride in a randomized trial but requires higher doses than that used for BPH. Discontinuation of minoxidil will result in loss of regrown hair often over several months. Other options include surgical intervention with hair transplantation or hair flaps, camouflaging agents, the use of a hairpiece, or low-level light therapy. In women with elevated androgens, antiandrogens such as spironolactone, flutamide, and cimetidine may be considered.
- *Alopecia areata (AA):* Spontaneous remission occurs in patchy AA, but less commonly in AAT or AAU. Glucocorticoids (GCs) are the mainstay of treatment but have little effect on the long-term outcome of hair loss—topical GC for small patches, intralesional injection of high-potency GC, and even systemic steroids can all be temporarily effective but at the cost of glucocorticoid exposure. Induction of allergic contact dermatitis using short-contact anthralin therapy or squaric acid sensitization can be effective but tends to have significant local discomfort, thereby limiting its use. Photochemotherapy has shown some beneficial outcomes, although there is a high relapse rate after discontinuation.
- *Tinea capitis:* To effectively treat tinea capitis, oral antifungal agents must be used. Griseofulvin is considered the drug of choice in the U.S., and the recommended time course is 6 weeks to several months. Other oral agents to consider include terbinafine, itraconazole, fluconazole, and ketoconazole. If there is a kerion (area of boggy, purulent inflammation underlying the area of hair loss), the patient is at increased risk for scarring alopecia due to bacterial superinfection, and a short course of oral steroids and oral antibiotic must be considered.
- *Traumatic alopecia (traction alopecia):* First priority is stopping inciting activity/agent, ideally leading to gradual resolution of hair loss and hair regrowth.
- *Lichen planus:* Associated hair loss is often permanent; however, for symptomatic control of itching and pain, topical or oral glucocorticoids may be considered.
- *Chronic cutaneous discoid erythematosus:* The best prevention is sun protection, with SPF lotion. Treatment options center around the cautious use of topical or intralesional glucocorticoids. Hydroxychloroquine and retinoids are also used with caution.
- *Chemotherapy-induced alopecia:* Scalp cooling devices may be effective in reducing chemotherapy-induced alopecia. In a recent trial among women with stage I to II breast cancer receiving chemotherapy with taxane, anthracycline, or both, those who underwent scalp cooling were significantly more likely to have less than 50% hair loss after the fourth chemotherapy cycle compared with those who received no scalp cooling.[1]

REFERRAL

Dermatology

PATIENT/FAMILY EDUCATION

Alopecia areata: www.naaf.org

SUGGESTED READINGS

Available at ExpertConsult.com

RELATED CONTENT

Alopecia (Patient Information)

AUTHOR: **FRED F. FERRI, M.D.**

[1] Nangia J et al: Effect of a scalp cooling device on alopecia in women undergoing chemotherapy for breast cancer. The SCALP randomized clinical trial, *JAMA* 317(6):596–605, 2017.

BASIC INFORMATION

DEFINITION

Dementia is a syndrome characterized by progressive loss of previously acquired cognitive skills including memory, language, insight, and judgment. Alzheimer's disease (AD) is thought to account for the majority (50% to 75%) of all cases of dementia.

ICD-10CM CODES

G30.0	Alzheimer's disease with early onset
G30.1	Alzheimer's disease with late onset
G30.8	Other Alzheimer's disease
G30.9	Alzheimer's disease, unspecified

EPIDEMIOLOGY & DEMOGRAPHICS

INCIDENCE: Risk doubles every 5 yrs after the age of 65; above the age of 85, the annual incidence is about 10%.

PREVALENCE: Currently an estimated 5.4 million Americans have AD; 3% of the population between the ages of 65 and 74, 17% between 75 and 84, and 32% at 85 yr and older.

PREDOMINANT SEX: Female greater than male

PHYSICAL FINDINGS & CLINICAL PRESENTATION

- Spouse or other family member, usually not the patient, notes insidious memory impairment.
- Patients have difficulties learning and retaining new information and handling complex tasks (e.g., balancing the checkbook) and have impairments in reasoning, judgment, spatial ability, and orientation (e.g., difficulty driving, getting lost away from home).
- Behavioral changes, such as mood changes and apathy, may accompany memory impairment. In later stages, patients may develop agitation and psychosis.
- Atypical presentations include early and severe behavioral changes, focal findings on examination, parkinsonism, hallucinations, falls, or onset of symptoms younger than the age of 65.

DIAGNOSIS

Diagnosis of AD is evolving with the development of biomarkers that indicate AD pathology such as brain amyloidosis and pathological tau accumulation. Although not yet commonly used in the clinic, the integration of biomarkers into the diagnosis of AD does transform the diagnosis into one that can be established definitively while the patient is still alive. Diagnosis is commonly made based on clinical history, a thorough physical and neurologic examination, and use of reliable and valid diagnostic criteria (i.e., DSM or NINDCS-ADRDA) such as the following:

- Loss of memory and one or more additional cognitive abilities (aphasia, apraxia, agnosia, or other disturbance in executive functioning)
- Impairment in social or occupational functioning that represents a decline from a previous level of functioning and results in significant disability
- Deficits that do not occur exclusively during the course of delirium
- Insidious onset and gradual progression of symptoms
- Cognitive loss documented by neuropsychologic tests
- No physical signs, neuroimaging, or laboratory evidence of other diseases that can cause dementia (i.e., metabolic abnormalities, medication or toxin effects, infection, stroke, Parkinson's disease, subdural hematoma, or tumors)
- Red flags for an AD diagnosis are summarized in Box 1.

The National Institute on Aging (NIA) and the Alzheimer's Association (AA) recommended new diagnostic criteria and guidelines for AD in 2011 (Tables 1 and 2). The NIA-AA criteria differ from prior DSM or NINDCS-ADRDA criteria in the following ways: (1) they recommend AD be considered a disease well before the onset of symptoms by incorporating the biomarkers in diagnosis; and (2) they define three distinct stages of AD: (1) *preclinical* AD, in which there is measurable biologic evidence of AD pathology but no symptoms; (2) *mild cognitive impairment* (MCI) due to AD, in which the patient experiences mild memory loss but no functional impairment at home or work plus biomarker evidence of AD; and (3) *dementia* due to AD, in which the patient experiences cognitive decline causing functional impairment plus biomarker evidence of AD.

DIFFERENTIAL DIAGNOSIS

- Other neurodegenerative dementia: Frontotemporal dementia (see Table 3), dementia with Lewy bodies, corticobasal syndrome, progressive supranuclear palsy
- Cancer (brain tumor, meningeal neoplasia)
- Infection (HIV-associated dementia, neurosyphilis, progressive multifocal leukoencephalopathy [PML])
- Toxic/metabolic (EtOH, hypothyroidism, vitamin B12 deficiency, mercury exposure, drug effects)
- Organ failure (dialysis dementia, Wilson's disease)
- Vascular disorder (vascular dementia due to multiple strokes, severe small vessel changes, chronic vasculitis, or chronic subdural hematoma)
- Subject memory loss
- Depression (pseudodementia)

WORKUP

HISTORY & GENERAL PHYSICAL EXAMINATION:

- Medication lists should always be reviewed for drugs or home remedies that may cause mental status changes, especially anticholinergic medications, benzodiazepines, barbiturates, and neuroleptics.
- Patients should be screened for depression, because it can sometimes mimic dementia but also often occurs as a coexisting condition and should be treated.
- On examination, look for signs of metabolic disturbance, presence of psychiatric features, or focal neurologic deficits.

MENTAL STATUS TESTING: Brief mental status testing can be done easily and quickly in the office. Commonly used cognitive tests to detect dementia include the Folstein Mini-Mental State Examination (MMSE), the Mini-Cog test, and the Addenbrooke's Cognitive Examination-Revised (ACE-R) test. For detecting mild cognitive impairment and dementia, the Montreal Cognitive Assessment (MoCA, http://www.mocatest.org/) is a highly sensitive 30-point test that takes approximately 10 minutes to administer. Cognitive domains tested include visual-spatial, attention, verbal recall, language, abstraction, and orientation. A score of 25 points or less (26 points if the patient has less than 12 yrs of education) indicates cognitive impairment. The test is available in over 35 languages and dialects, and multiple forms in English allow for repeated assessments over time. A summary of commonly used tests may be found in Table 4.

Mental status testing should include tests that assess the following cognitive functions:

- Orientation: Ask the patient to give the day, date, month, yr, and place and to name the current president.

BOX 1 Red Flags for an Alzheimer's Disease Diagnosis

- Age younger than 65 yr
- Fluctuating level of consciousness (consider toxic-metabolic encephalopathy, Lewy body dementia)
- Behavioral, emotional, or personality disturbances overshadowing cognitive impairment (consider frontotemporal dementia, HIV dementia)
- Rapidly (6-12 months) progressive development (consider Creutzfeldt–Jakob disease, paraneoplastic limbic encephalitis, HIV dementia, frontotemporal dementia)
- Presence of physical abnormalities:
  1. Gait impairment (consider vascular dementia, HIV dementia, NPH)
  2. Lateralized signs, e.g., hemiparesis, spasticity, other corticospinal tract signs (consider vascular dementia)
  3. Movement disorders
  4. Myoclonus (consider Creutzfeldt–Jakob disease, paraneoplastic encephalitis)
  5. Rigidity, bradykinesia (parkinsonism) (consider dementia with Lewy bodies and Parkinson's disease)

Modified from Kaufman DM, Geyer HL, Milstein MJ: *Kaufman's clinical neurology for psychiatrists,* ed 8, Philadelphia, 2017, Elsevier.

TABLE 1 New Diagnostic Criteria

Criteria for Probable Alzheimer's Disease	DSM-5 2013	Research Criteria NINCDS–ADRDA 2007	NIA-AA 2011
Insidious onset	X	X	X
Onset over months to yrs		X	X
Progressive decline	X	X	X
Deficits are not explained by delirium or other medical or psychiatric conditions	X	X	X
Social/occupational impairment	X		X
Presence of episodic memory deficit	X	X	
Cognitive deficits in at least two domains	X		X
Neuropsychological testing required for diagnosis?	Preferably	X	Only if routine history and mental status testing are inconclusive
Abnormal PET or MRI scan		Supportive feature*	For research purposes
Genetic markers?	X Required only if there is evidence of multiple causes and no clear evidence of progression and decline in memory and another cognitive domain	Supportive feature*	For research purposes
Abnormal cerebrospinal fluid marker required?		Supportive feature*	For research purposes

DSM-5, Diagnostic and Statistical Manual of Mental Disorders, fifth edition; *MRI,* magnetic resonance imaging; *NIA-AA,* National Institute on Aging–Alzheimer's Association; *NINCDS-ADRDA,* National Institute of Neurological and Communicative Disorders and Stroke–Alzheimer's Disease and Related Disorders Association; *PET,* positron emission tomography.
*At least one supportive feature is required for diagnosis of probable AD.
Fillit HM: *Brocklehurst's textbook of geriatric medicine and gerontology,* ed 8, Philadelphia, 2017, Elsevier.

TABLE 2 National Institute on Aging–Alzheimer's Association Criteria for Alzheimer's Disease (AD)

I. Core Clinical Criteria

- Interferes with work or usual activities *and*
- Represents a decline from previous level of functioning *and*
- Not explained by delirium of psychiatric disorder.
- Documented cognitive impairment by history taking and objective cognitive assessment (bedside mental status examination or neuropsychological testing).
- A minimum of two of the following domains should be impaired:
  1. Impairment in acquisition and recall of new information (symptoms—repetitive questions and/or conversations, misplaced belongings, forgetting appointments, getting lost)
  2. Impairment in reasoning of complex tasks, poor judgment (symptoms—poor safety assessment, poor financial management, poor decision making, inability to plan complex activities)
  3. Impairment in visuospatial abilities (symptoms—inability to recognizes faces or objects or finding objects in plain view, despite good visual acuity; inability to operate simple tools; inability to orient clothing to the body)
  4. Impaired language functions (speaking, reading, writing; symptoms—difficulty thinking of common words while speaking, hesitation; speech, spelling, writing errors)
  5. Changes in personality, behavior, or comportment (symptoms—uncharacteristic mood fluctuations, e.g., agitation, poor motivation, apathy, social withdrawal, decreased interest in previous activities, loss of empathy, compulsions and/or obsessions, social impairment)

II. Probable AD Dementia (meets core criteria plus the following)

- Insidious onset (gradual over months to yrs)
- Clear history of worsening cognition *and*
- Initial and most prominent cognitive deficits fall into two categories (all must include cognitive dysfunction in at least one other domain).
  1. Amnestic—most common presentation; impairment in learning and recall of recent information
  2. Nonamnestic
     a. Language presentation—most prominent in word finding
     b. Visuospatial presentation—most prominent in spatial cognition (object agnosia, face recognition, simultanagnosia, alexia)
     c. Executive dysfunction—impaired reasoning, judgment, problem solving.
- Should not be applied if substantial cerebrovascular disease or core features of dementia with Lewy bodies (other than dementia) are present; features consistent with behavioral variant of frontotemporal dementia, primary progressive aphasia (semantic, nonfluent, or agrammatic variants), or evidence of other neurologic disease or medical comorbidity that could affect cognition
- Increased certainty if there is documented decline based on subsequent evaluations and in persons who have evidence of causative genetic mutations

III. Probable AD With Evidence of AD Pathophysiologic Process

- High probability of AD pathology if both of the following are present:
  1. β-Amyloid level is low in the cerebrospinal fluid (CSF) or there is a positive positron emission tomography (PET) scan
  2. Neuronal injury is proven with high CSF tau levels, decreased fluorodeoxyglucose-PET uptake in the temporoparietal cortex, or disproportionate atrophy in the mediobasolateral temporal lobe and medial parietal cortex on a structural MRI scan.
- Intermediate probability of AD pathology if only one of the two criteria above are met (and the other is absent or negative)

IV. Possible AD Dementia (meets core clinical criteria but has the following features)

- Atypical course—sudden onset of cognitive impairment, insufficient historical details of objective cognitive decline or progressive decline
- Causally mixed presentation—evidence of cerebrovascular disease; features of dementia with Lewy bodies (other than dementia); evidence of other neurologic disease, medical comorbidity, or pharmaceutical use that could have a substantial effect on cognition

TABLE 2 National Institute on Aging–Alzheimer's Association Criteria for Alzheimer Disease (AD)—cont'd

V. Possible AD with Evidence of AD Pathophysiologic Process

- High probability of AD pathology if both of the following are present:
  1. β-Amyloid level is low in the CSF or there is a positive PET scan
  2. Neuronal injury is proven with high CSF tau levels, decreased fluorodeoxyglucose-PET uptake in the temporoparietal cortex, or disproportionate atrophy in the medio-basolateral temporal lobe and medial parietal cortex on a structural MRI scan
- Uninformative unless the above criteria are met
- May also be a second pathophysiologic condition present to explain why the patient does not meet AD criteria (e.g., concomitant dementia with Lewy bodies)

VI. Pathophysiologically Proven AD Dementia

- Clinical and cognitive criteria for AD are satisfied *and* neuropathologic criteria demonstrate presence of AD pathology

VI. Dementia Unlikely to Be Due to AD

- Does not meet clinical criteria for AD dementia *or*
- Regardless of meeting clinical criteria for probable or possible AD dementia, there is sufficient evidence for an alternative diagnosis (e.g., HIV dementia, Huntington disease).
- Regardless of meeting clinical criteria for possible AD dementia, both β-amyloid and neuronal injury biomarkers are negative.

Adapted from McKhann GM, Knopman DS, Chertkow H: The diagnosis of dementia due to Alzheimer's disease: recommendations from the National Institute on Aging-Alzheimer's Association workgroups on diagnostic guidelines for Alzheimer's disease, *Alzheimers Dement* 7:263–269, 2011; Albert MS, DeKosky ST, Dickson D: The diagnosis of mild cognitive impairment due to Alzheimer's disease: recommendations from the National Institute on Aging-Alzheimer's Association workgroups on diagnostic guidelines for Alzheimer's disease, *Alzheimers Dement* 7:270–279, 2011; and Sperling RA, Aisen PS, Beckett LA: Toward defining the preclinical stages of Alzheimer's disease: recommendations from the National Institute on Aging-Alzheimer's Association workgroups on diagnostic guidelines for Alzheimer's disease, *Alzheimers Dement* 7:280–292, 2011.

TABLE 3 Features Distinguishing Alzheimer's Disease and Frontotemporal Dementia

Feature	Alzheimer's Disease	Frontotemporal Dementia
Age at onset (yr)	>65	53 (mean)
Memory impairments	Early, pronounced	Subtle, at least initially, with preserved visual-spatial ability
Behavior abnormalities	None until middle or late stage	Early and prominent perseverative and compulsive behavior; hyperorality; impaired executive ability
Language impairment	Except for anomia, none until late stage	Paraphasias, anomia, decreased fluency
CT/MRI appearance	General atrophy, but especially parietal and temporal lobes	Frontal and temporal lobe atrophy
Histologic marker	Aβ accumulation	Tau accumulation

CT, Computed tomography; *MRI,* magnetic resonance imaging.
From Kaufman DM, Geyer HL, Milstein MJ: *Kaufman's clinical neurology for psychiatrists,* ed 8, Philadelphia, 2017, Elsevier.

TABLE 4 Commonly Used Neuropsychological Tests

Domains to Be Assessed	Tests Used With Age-Corrected and/or Education Norms for Adults Older Than 65 Yr
Premorbid ability	• North American Reading Test (NART) • Vocabulary (WAIS-IV)
Verbal memory	• Rey Auditory Verbal Learning Test (RAVLT) • California Verbal Learning Test (CVLT) • Logical Memory Test (from WMS-IV) • CERAD Word List Test
Visual memory	• Visual Reproduction (from WMS-IV) • Rey Complex Figure Drawing Test (RCFT)
Simple attention	• Digit Span (from WAIS-IV) • Trail-Making Part A
Language	• Animal Naming Test (ANT) • Controlled Oral Word Association Test (COWAT) • Boston Naming Test (BNT)
Executive function	• Trail-Making Part B • Wisconsin Card Sort Test (WCST) • Stroop • Similarities (from WAIS-IV)
Visuospatial	• Coding (from WAIS-IV) • Rey Complex Figure Test (RCFT) • Clock Drawing Test
Motor	• Grooved Pegboard Test • Finger Tapping Test
Mood	• Geriatric Depression Scale (GDS) • Hamilton Depression Rating Scale (HDRS) • Beck Anxiety Inventory (BAI)

WAIS-IV, Wechsler Adult Intelligence Scale, fourth edition; *WMS-IV,* Wechsler Memory Scale, fourth edition.
Fillit HM: *Brocklehurst's textbook of geriatric medicine and gerontology,* ed 8, Philadelphia, 2017, Elsevier.

- Attention: Ask the patient to recite the months of the yr forward and in reverse.
- Verbal recall: Ask the patient to remember three items; test for recall after a 1- and 5-min delay.
- Language: Ask the patient to write and then read a sentence; have the patient name both common and less common objects.
- Visual-spatial: Ask the patient to draw a clock and to set the hands of the clock at 11:10.

Patients with AD typically have trouble with verbal recall plus visuospatial or language deficits. Attention is usually preserved until the late stages of AD, so consider alternate diagnoses in patients who perform poorly on tests of attention. A summary of the pattern of cognitive deficits associated with different dementias and depression may be found in Table 5.

LABORATORY TESTS (TABLE 6)

- CBC
- Serum electrolytes
- Glucose
- BUN/creatinine
- Liver and thyroid function tests
- Serum vitamin B_{12}
- Syphilis serology (RPR), if supported by clinical history
- HIV screening as appropriate
- Lumbar puncture if history or signs of cancer, infectious process, or unusual clinical presentation (e.g., rapid progression of symptoms)
- EEG if there is history of seizures, episodic confusion, rapid clinical decline, or suspicion of Creutzfeldt-Jakob disease
- Apolipoprotein E genotyping, measurement of CSF tau and amyloid, and functional imaging including positron emission tomography (PET), single-photon emission computed tomography (SPECT), or amyloid PET imaging using florbetapir (Amyvid) are not yet routinely indicated

TABLE 5 Patterns of Cognitive Impairment by Domain and Dementia

	Episodic Memory	Attention	Language	Executive	Visuospatial	Behavioral Symptoms
Alzheimer's disease	(I)	Simple (P) Divided (I)	Phonemic (P) Semantic (I) Naming (I)	(I)	Simple (P) Complex (I)	Early apathy, late psychotic symptoms
Mild cognitive impairment—amnestic	Immediate and Delayed recall (I); Recognition (I)	Simple (P) Divided (P)	(P)	(P)	(P)	(P)
Vascular dementia	Immediate and Delayed recall (V) Recognition (P)	Simple (P) Divided (I)	(I)	(I)	(P)	Depression
Behavioral variant FTLD	(V)	Simple (P) Divided (I)	(I)	(I)	(P)	Disinhibition, apathy, hyperorality, inappropriate social interaction
Semantic variant PPA	(P)	(P)	(I) Comprehension (I) Fluency	(P)	(P) (I) Visual agnosia	(P)
Nonfluent variant PPA	(P)	(P)	(I) Fluency (P) Comprehension, (I) Expressive speech	(P)	(P)	(P)
Parkinson disease dementia	(V) Immediate and Delayed recall (P) recognition	(I)	(P)	(I)	(I)	Depression, possible hallucinations, psychomotor slowing
Dementia with Lewy bodies	(V) Immediate and Delayed recall (P) Recognition	(V)	(V)	(I)	(I)	Hallucinations, delusions
Depression	(V) Immediate and Delayed recall (P) Recognition +	(V)	(V) Fluency (P) Naming	I/V	(P)	Psychomotor slowing, apathy

FTLD, Frontotemporal lobar degeneration; *I,* impaired; *P,* preserved; *PPA,* primary progressive aphasia; *V,* variable.

Fillit HM: *Brocklehurst's textbook of geriatric medicine and gerontology*, ed 8, Philadelphia, 2017, Elsevier.

TABLE 6 Laboratory Evaluation of Patients With Dementia

Type of Study	Examples
Basic studies, excluding reversible with specific indication from history for causes of dementia or examination	• Complete blood count (CBC) • Chemistry or metabolic panel (SM-17) • Thyroid function tests (thyroid-stimulating hormone [TSH]) • Vitamin B $_{12}$, folate levels • Computed tomography (CT) or magnetic resonance imaging (MRI) • HIV testing • Sedimentation rate • Hemoglobin A1C (Hb A1C) • Urinalysis • Chest x-ray • Urine or plasma for drugs or heavy metals
Adjuvant studies to aid diagnosis	
Other tests as indicated by history or physical or neurologic examination	• Single-photon emission computed tomography (SPECT) • Positron emission tomography (PET) • Lumbar puncture with cerebrospinal fluid for β-amyloid

Fillit HM: *Brocklehurst's textbook of geriatric medicine and gerontology*, ed 8, Philadelphia, 2017, Elsevier.

- Brain biopsy is usually reserved for diagnoses such as prion disease and cerebral vasculitis. Generally performed postmortem

IMAGING STUDIES

- CT scan or MRI to rule out hydrocephalus, cerebrovascular disease, and mass lesions, including subdural hematoma and to look for typical patterns of atrophy such as hippocampal atrophy
- Florbetapir-PET imaging of the brain correlates with the presence and density of beta-amyloid with high sensitivity and specificity of plaque detection, but it is not covered by most payers. Amyloid scans are not part of routine clinical practice but can be considered on a case-by-case basis. PET scans with tracers detecting tau are available as part of research protocols, correlate with the presence of neurofibrillary tangles, but are not yet FDA approved for clinical use.

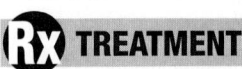

TREATMENT

NONPHARMACOLOGIC THERAPY

- Patient safety, including risks associated with impaired driving, wandering behavior, leaving stoves unattended, and accidents, must be addressed with the patient and family early and appropriate measures implemented.
- Wandering, hoarding or hiding objects, repetitive questioning, withdrawal, and social inappropriateness often respond to behavioral therapies.
- Cognitive stimulation programs are beneficial for maintenance of cognitive function and improved self-reported quality of life in patients with mild to moderate Alzheimer's disease.

ACUTE GENERAL Rx

None

CHRONIC Rx

- Symptomatic treatment of memory disturbance (Table 7):
  1. Cholinesterase inhibitors (ChEIs): Donepezil (Aricept), galantamine (Razadyne), and rivastigmine (Exelon)
     a. FDA approved for the treatment of mild to moderate AD with the exception of donepezil, which is approved for mild, moderate, and severe dementia. Common side effects including nausea, diarrhea, and anorexia may be bothersome enough to require a slower escalation of dosage or switching to another agent. The rivastigmine patch has lower rates of gastrointestinal side effects than rivastigmine. Table 8 summarizes some instruments used to monitor clinical response of AD to pharmacologic therapy.
  2. NMDA receptor antagonist: Memantine (Namenda)
     a. FDA approved for the treatment of moderate to severe AD. Common side effects include constipation, dizziness, or headache. Memantine is contraindicated in patients with renal insufficiency or history of seizures.
- Symptomatic treatment of neuropsychiatric and behavioral disturbances (Table 9).
- Depression, agitation, delusions, or hallucinations may respond to medications.

TABLE 7 Symptomatic Treatment of Memory Disturbance

	Initial Dose	Target Dose
Donepezil	5 mg qd for 4-6 weeks	10 mg qd
Rivastigmine	1.5 mg bid with food, increase by 1.5 mg bid weekly	3-6 mg bid
Galantamine	4 mg bid with food, increase by 4 mg bid every 4 weeks	8-12 mg bid
Memantine	5 mg qd, increase by 5 mg weekly	10 mg bid

TABLE 8 Instruments Used to Monitor Clinical Response of Alzheimer's Disease (AD) to Pharmacologic Therapy

Mini-Mental State Examination
- Global measure of cognition widely used by physicians and third-party caregivers
- Assesses orientation, registration, recall, language, and attention
- Uses a 30-point scale
- Requires ≈5-10 min to complete
- Sensitivity, 80% to 90%; specificity, 80%
- Administered by psychometricians, nurses, and physicians
- AD typically advances by 3 points/yr

Clock Drawing
- Global measure of cognition widely used by physicians
- Multiple scoring systems with proven validity; sensitivity, 59%; specificity, 90%
- Assesses multiple cognitive domains in a single test
- 1-2 min to complete
- Minimal training to administer

Geriatric Depression Scale
- Evaluates depressive symptoms in patients
- Requires 5 min to complete
- Very useful in assessing depression in new patients and in follow-up
- Minimal training to administer
- Ease of administration has led to rapid spread in its use.

Fillit HM: *Brocklehurst's textbook of geriatric medicine and gerontology*, ed 8, Philadelphia, 2017, Elsevier.

DISPOSITION & REFERRAL

- Patients with complex or atypical presentations or challenging management issues should be referred to a neurologist or another specialist with expertise in dementia.
- Approximately 1 in 8 hospitalized patients with AD who develop delirium will have at least one adverse outcome (e.g., institutionalization, cognitive decline, death) associated with delirium.
- Family education and support may help reduce need for skilled nursing facility and reduce caregiver stress, depression, and burnout.

PEARLS & CONSIDERATIONS

The physician should make a thorough search for the treatable causes of dementia. Current American Academy of Neurology practice parameters recommend:
- Treat cognitive symptoms of AD with ChEIs.
- Treat agitation, psychosis, and depression.
- Encourage caregivers to participate in educational programs and support groups.

COMMENTS

- Ginkgo biloba is marketed widely as effective in delaying cognitive impairment; however, trials have shown that it is not effective in reducing the incidence of Alzheimer's dementia or dementia overall.
- Higher midlife fitness levels seem to be associated with lower hazards of developing all-cause dementia later in life independent of cerebrovascular disease. Exercise also may slow the rate of functional deterioration in mild AD.
- Antipsychotics should be used with extreme caution in treating dementia-related psychosis. All antipsychotics carry a warning from the FDA stating that the medication is not approved for dementia-related psychosis because elderly patients on either conventional or atypical antipsychotics experience an increased risk of death due to cardiovascular or infectious causes.

TABLE 9 Treatment of Behavioral and Neuropsychiatric Symptoms

	Initial Dose	Maximum Dose
Atypical Antipsychotics		
Olanzapine	2.5 mg qd to bid, may increase by 2.5 mg as needed	7.5 mg bid
Quetiapine	25 mg bid, may increase by 25 mg every 2 days	250 mg tid
Antidepressants		
Sertraline	25-50 mg qd, may increase by 25 mg every week	200 mg qd
Escitalopram	10 mg qd, may increase after 1 week to 20 mg qd	10 mg qd

- Lower plasma beta-amyloid 42/40 is associated with greater cognitive decline among elderly persons without dementia over 9 yr, and this association is stronger among those with low measures of cognitive reserve.
- Apolipoprotein E (APOE) is the main cholesterol-carrying molecule in the brain, and it exists in three allelic variants: E2, E3, and E4. The E3 allele is most common and has a neutral influence on developing AD, whereas the E2 allele, the rarest allele, may be protective against AD. The E4 alleles are well-established heterozygotes at approximately 3 times AD risk factor. However, neither E4 heterozygosity or homozygosity is required or sufficient to cause AD. Among Caucasians, E4 heterozygosity increases the risk of developing AD approximately threefold, whereas E4 homozygosity increases AD risk by approximately 15 times compared to the E3/E3 baseline. The APOE E4 allele is also associated with an earlier age of onset of AD. Because the benefits of genetic testing are often modest, and the tests themselves are often imprecise in identifying risk, the test is generally discouraged. Recent trials, however, reveal that the disclosure of *APOE* genotyping results to adult children of patients with AD did not result in significant short-term psychological risks. Test-related distress was reduced among those who learned that they were *APOE4* negative. Persons with high levels of emotional distress before undergoing genetic testing are more likely to have emotional difficulties after disclosure.

For additional information for patients, families, and clinicians, contact the following organizations:

- Alzheimer's Association (www.alz.org; 800-272-3900)
- Alzheimer's Disease Education and Referral Center (http://www.nia.nih.gov/Alzheimers; 800-438-4380)

AUTHORS: **TAMARA G. FONG, M.D., PH.D., IRINA A. SKYLAR-SCOTT, M.D.,** and **JOSEPH S. KASS, M.D., J.D.**

SUGGESTED READINGS

Available at ExpertConsult.com

RELATED CONTENT

Alzheimer's Disease (Patient Information)
Dementia with Lewy Bodies (Related Key Topic)
Mild Cognitive Impairment (Related Key Topic)

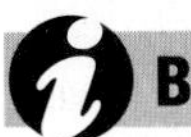

BASIC INFORMATION

DEFINITION

Amaurosis fugax is a temporary loss of monocular vision caused by transient retinal ischemia.

ICD-10CM CODE
G45.3 Amaurosis fugax

EPIDEMIOLOGY & DEMOGRAPHICS

INCIDENCE (IN U.S.): An uncommon but important presentation of carotid artery disease
PEAK INCIDENCE: Approximately 55 yr

PHYSICAL FINDINGS & CLINICAL PRESENTATION

- Onset is sudden, typically lasting seconds to minutes, and often accompanied by scotomas such as a shade or curtain being pulled over the front of the eye (usually downward).
- Vision loss can be complete, hemianopic, or quadrantic.
- Acute stage: Cholesterol emboli may be seen in retinal artery (*Hollenhorst plaque*); carotid bruits or other evidence of generalized atherosclerosis.
- If embolus is cardiac in origin, atrial fibrillation is often present.

ETIOLOGY

- Usually embolic from the internal carotid artery or the heart
- Giant cell arteritis causing inflammation of retinal arteries
- Hyperviscosity syndromes, such as sickle cell disease, which causes ischemia in the vascular territory of the ophthalmic artery
- Hypercoagulable states
- Reversible cerebral vasoconstriction syndrome

Dx DIAGNOSIS

DIFFERENTIAL DIAGNOSIS

- Retinal migraine: In contrast to amaurosis, the onset of visual loss develops more slowly, usually over 15 to 20 min.
- Transient visual obscurations occur in the setting of papilledema; intermittent rises in intracranial pressure briefly compromise optic disc perfusion and cause transient visual loss lasting 1 to 2 seconds. The episodes may be binocular. If the visual loss persists at the time of evaluation (i.e., vision has not yet recovered), then the differential diagnosis should be broadened to include:
    1. Anterior ischemic optic neuropathy: Arteritic (classically GCA) or nonarteritic
    2. Central retinal vein occlusion

WORKUP

- Workup should focus on embolic sources, but GCA should always be considered.
- Careful examination of retina; embolus may be visible and confirm the diagnosis (Fig. 1).
- Auscultation of arteries for carotid bruits.
- Examination of all pulses and for temporal artery tenderness.
- Inquire about symptoms of GCA (scalp tenderness, headache, fever, jaw claudication).
- Examine for signs of hemispheric stroke resulting from intracranial atherosclerosis (contralateral limb and facial weakness or sensory loss, aphasia, etc.).

LABORATORY TESTS

- Complete blood count with erythrocyte sedimentation rate and C-reactive protein.
- Serum chemistries, including lipid profile.
- Cardiac enzymes and ECG.
- Hypercoagulable workup is discretionary based on younger age and history.

IMAGING STUDIES

- CT or MR angiography of head and neck preferred to examine carotid and intracranial vasculature. Carotid doppler if contraindication to MR or CT angiography.
- MRI of the brain with diffusion-weighted imaging to look for infarcts, especially those presenting with focal neurologic disturbances.
- Transthoracic echocardiography is indicated to screen for sources of emboli in patients with evidence of heart disease and in patients without an evident source for transient neurologic deficit. Transesophageal echocardiography is more sensitive for detecting cardiac sources of emboli (ventricular mural thrombus, atrial appendage, patent foramen ovale, aortic arch).
- Extended monitoring for atrial fibrillation if carotid stenosis not found to be etiology.

Rx TREATMENT

NONPHARMACOLOGIC THERAPY

- Diet (decrease saturated fatty acids and high-cholesterol foods)
- Exercise
- Cessation of tobacco use

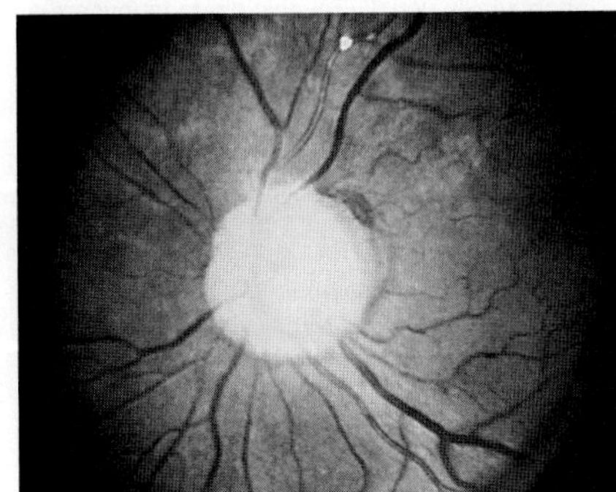

FIG. 1 A cholesterol crystal embolus lodged at an arterial bifurcation. (From Stein JH [ed]: *Internal medicine*, ed 5, St Louis, 1998, Mosby.)

ACUTE GENERAL Rx

- Investigate as an emergency.
- Aspirin
- If GCA is suspected, start prednisone and refer for temporal artery biopsy within 48 hr (see "Giant Cell Arteritis" in Section I).

CHRONIC Rx

- Reduce risks by carotid endarterectomy if stenosis >50%. Carotid stenting may be performed in high-risk surgical candidates.
- Manage vascular risk factors such as hypertension, hyperlipidemia (statin therapy), diabetes, smoking cessation, etc.
- Antiplatelet therapy due to arterial atherosclerosis and postcarotid intervention; anticoagulation if etiology is atrial fibrillation.

DISPOSITION

Among patients with >50% carotid stenosis who do not undergo carotid endarterectomy, those who present with transient monocular blindness have an approximate 10% risk of stroke within 3 yrs compared with an approximate 20% risk in patients who present with a hemispheric transient ischemic attack (TIA).

REFERRAL

- As with any TIA, emergent inpatient workup in a hospital that is a certified stroke center, if possible.
- If significant carotid stenosis, consider either carotid endarterectomy or carotid stenting for the following:
    1. Ipsilateral high-grade (≥70%) stenosis, but consider for ipsilateral stenosis of 50% to 69%.
    2. Multiple TIAs despite medical therapy in the setting of high-grade or ulcerative disease

PEARLS & CONSIDERATIONS

- Cholesterol emboli in retinal arteries on funduscopy confirm the diagnosis.
- Recognize that transient visual loss has multiple other causes.
- Refer to emergent evaluation like any other transient ischemic attack.

RELATED CONTENT

Amaurosis Fugax (Patient Information)
Carotid Stenosis (Related Key Topic)
Giant Cell Arteritis (Related Key Topic)
Transient Ischemic Attack (Related Key Topic)

AUTHORS: **JOSEPH S. KASS, M.D., J.D**, and **TZU-CHING (TEDDY) WU, M.D., M.P.H.**

BASIC INFORMATION

DEFINITION

Anaphylaxis is a severe allergic reaction that is rapid in onset and life-threatening. It is characterized by respiratory, cardiovascular, gastrointestinal, and cutaneous manifestations, as well as vasodilatory hemodynamic changes in response to a particular allergen. Anaphylactoid reaction is an entity closely related to anaphylaxis and is caused by release of mast cells and basophil mediators triggered by non–immunoglobulin E (IgE)-mediated events.

SYNONYM

Anaphylactoid reaction

ICD-10CM CODES

T78.2	Anaphylactic shock, unspecified, initial encounter
T78.00XA	Anaphylactic reaction due to unspecified food, initial encounter
T80.52XA	Anaphylactic reaction due to vaccination, initial encounter
T50.904A	Poisoning by unspecified drugs, medicaments, and biologic substances, undetermined, initial encounter
T63.94XA	Toxic effect of contact with unspecified venomous animal, undetermined, initial encounter

EPIDEMIOLOGY & DEMOGRAPHICS

INCIDENCE: The incidence of anaphylaxis in the U.S. is 50 to 2000 episodes per 100,000 persons. Lifetime prevalence is 0.05% to 2%, with a mortality rate of 1%. Anaphylaxis rates are 0.0004% for food, 0.7% to 10% for penicillin, 0.22% to 1% for contrast media, and 0.5% to 5% after insect stings. Annual mortality is 500 to 1000 persons/yr in the U.S.

PHYSICAL FINDINGS & CLINICAL PRESENTATION

- Urticaria, pruritus, skin flushing, angioedema (Table E1)
- Dyspnea, cough, wheezing, shortness of breath
- Nausea, vomiting, diarrhea, difficulty swallowing
- Hypotension, tachycardia, weakness, dizziness, malaise, vascular collapse (Table E2)

ETIOLOGY

Anaphylaxis results from a sudden systematic release of histamine and other inflammatory mediators from basophils and mast cells. This causes swelling of the mucus membranes and the urticarial rash on the skin. Virtually any substance may induce anaphylaxis.

- Foods and food additives: Peanuts, tree nuts, eggs, shellfish, fish, cow's milk, fruits, soy
- Medications: Antibiotics (especially penicillins and sulfa), insulin, allergen extracts, opiates, vaccines, NSAIDs, contrast media, streptokinase
- Environmental exposures: Bee or wasp sting, snake venom, fire ant venom
- Blood products: Plasma, immunoglobulin, cryoprecipitate, whole blood
- Latex

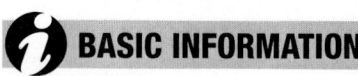

DIAGNOSIS

DIFFERENTIAL DIAGNOSIS

- Endocrine disorders (carcinoid, pheochromocytoma)
- Globus hystericus, anxiety disorder
- Systemic mastocytosis
- Pulmonary embolism, serum sickness, vasovagal reactions
- Severe asthma (the key clinical difference is the abrupt onset of symptoms in anaphylaxis versus a history of progressive worsening of symptoms)
- Septic shock or other form of vasodilatory shock
- Airway foreign body

WORKUP

Workup is aimed at ruling out other conditions that may mimic anaphylaxis.

LABORATORY TESTS

- Laboratory evaluation is generally not helpful because anaphylaxis is typically a clinical diagnosis.
- Arterial blood gas (ABG) analysis may be useful to help differentiate between pulmonary embolism, status asthmaticus, and foreign body aspiration.
- Elevated serum and urine histamine levels and serum tryptase levels can be useful for diagnosis of anaphylaxis, but these tests are not commonly available in the emergency setting.

IMAGING STUDIES

- Generally not helpful.
- Chest radiography for evaluation of foreign body aspiration or pulmonary pathology is indicated in patients with acute respiratory compromise.
- Consider ECG in all patients with sudden loss of consciousness or reports of chest pain or dyspnea and in any elderly patient. ECG in anaphylaxis usually reveals sinus tachycardia.

Rx TREATMENT

NONPHARMACOLOGIC THERAPY

- Establish and protect airway. Provide supplemental O_2 if indicated.
- Intravenous (IV) access should be rapidly established, and IV fluids (i.e., normal saline) should be administered.
- Cardiac monitoring is recommended.

ACUTE GENERAL Rx

- Epinephrine should be rapidly administered as an intramuscular (IM) injection at a dose of 0.3 mg of aqueous epinephrine for adults and children >30 kg. Epinephrine 0.15 mg should be given for children <30 kg (1:1000 concentration). Intramuscular administration is preferred because it provides more reliable and quicker rise to effective plasma levels. The dose may be repeated after approximately 5 to 15 min if symptoms persist.
- Adjunct therapies include H_1 and H_2 receptor antagonists such as diphenhydramine 25 to 50 mg IV or IM (or PO in mild cases) and famotidine 20 to 40 mg IV (or PO in mild cases). Although useful to improve cutaneous erythema and pruritus, H_1 antagonists are not as effective as epinephrine, since onset of action is 1 to 2 hours and they are not effective in reversing upper airway obstruction or improving hypotension.
- Corticosteroids are not useful in the acute episode because of their slow onset of action; however, they should be administered in most cases to prevent prolonged or recurrent anaphylaxis. Commonly used agents are prednisone, methylprednisolone 40 to 250 mg IV in adults (1 to 2 mg/kg in children), or dexamethasone.
- Aerosolized β-agonists (e.g., albuterol, 2.5 mg, repeat prn 20 min) are useful to control bronchospasm.
- Vasopressor therapy with epinephrine (1:10,000), or dopamine is indicated in patients with refractory hypotension/cardiovascular collapse after crystalloid resuscitation.
- Table E3 summarizes drugs and other agents used in anaphylaxis therapy.

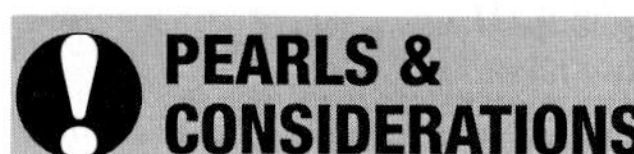

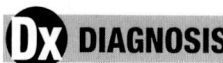

PEARLS & CONSIDERATIONS

COMMENTS

- Patient education regarding the nature of the illness and preventive measures is recommended. A documented history of previous anaphylactic episodes or known triggers is the most reliable method of identifying individuals at risk.
- Prescription for a prefilled epinephrine syringe (EpiPen or EpiPen Jr.) should be given, and the patient should be instructed on the use of this emergency kit, and to carry it with them at all times. School-aged children should keep an additional EpiPen at school with the appropriate staff.
- Patients should also be advised to carry or wear a MedicAlert ID describing substances that have caused anaphylaxis.
- Avoidance of radiologic contrast is also recommended in those who have had a prior reaction. However, pretreatment regimens with methylprednisolone, diphenhydramine, or n-acetylcysteine exist for those who have had contrast reactions in the past.
- Venom immunotherapy immediately after a sting is effective and recommended for up to 5 yr after the anaphylactic incident.

SUGGESTED READINGS

Available at ExpertConsult.com

AUTHOR: **STEVEN ROUGAS, M.D., M.S., FACEP**

BASIC INFORMATION

DEFINITION

Autoimmune hemolytic anemia (AIHA) is anemia secondary to premature clearance of red blood cells (RBCs) caused by binding of autoantibodies and/or complement to RBCs. Primary AIHA comprises approximately 50% of cases, whereas secondary AIHA is usually associated with diseases or drugs. The classification of the hemolytic anemias is described in Table 1.

SYNONYMS

Autoimmune hemolytic anemia
Cold agglutinin disease
Drug-induced hemolytic anemia
Warm autoimmune hemolytic anemia

ICD-10CM CODES

D59.0 Drug-induced autoimmune hemolytic anemia
D59.1 Other autoimmune hemolytic anemias

EPIDEMIOLOGY & DEMOGRAPHICS

The annual incidence is 1–3 cases per 100,000 persons, with 10% mortality; most common in women <50 yr.

PHYSICAL FINDINGS & CLINICAL PRESENTATION

- Most common presentation is dyspnea and fatigue.
- Pallor, jaundice may be present.
- Tachycardia with a flow murmur may be present if anemia is pronounced.
- Patients with intravascular hemolysis may present with dark urine and back pain.
- The presence of hepatomegaly and/or lymphadenopathy suggests an underlying lymphoproliferative disorder or malignancy; splenomegaly may indicate hypersplenism as a cause of hemolysis.

TABLE 1 Classification of the Hemolytic Anemias

Acquired

Environmental factors
- Antibody: Immunohemolytic anemias
- Mechanical trauma: TTP, HUS, heart valve
- Toxins, infectious agents: Malaria, etc.

Membrane defects
- Paroxysmal nocturnal hemoglobinuria
- Spur cell anemia
- Hereditary spherocytosis, etc.

Congenital

Defects of cell interior
- Hemoglobinopathies: Sickle cell, thalassemia
- Enzymopathies: G6PD deficiency, etc.

G6PD, Glucose-6-phosphate dehydrogenase; *HUS,* hemolytic-uremic syndrome; *TTP,* thrombotic thrombocytopenic purpura.
From Goldman L, Schafer AI: *Goldman's Cecil medicine,* ed 24, Philadelphia, 2012, Saunders.

ETIOLOGY

- Warm antibody mediated: IgG only (often idiopathic or associated with leukemia, lymphoma (Table 2), thymoma, myeloma, viral infections (Table 3), babesiosis, and collagen-vascular disease)
- Cold antibody mediated: IgM and complement in majority of cases (often idiopathic; at times associated with infections, lymphoma, or cold agglutinin disease)
- Il-33 may have a role in promoting increasing RBC autoantibodies in AIHA
- Drug induced (Table 4): Three major mechanisms:
  1. Antibody directed against Rh complex (e.g., methyldopa)
  2. Antibody directed against RBC-drug complex (hapten induced; e.g., penicillin)
  3. Antibody directed against complex formed by drug and plasma proteins; the drug-plasma protein-antibody complex causes destruction of RBCs (innocent bystander; e.g., quinidine)

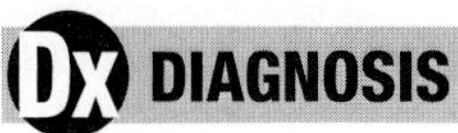

DIAGNOSIS

DIFFERENTIAL DIAGNOSIS

- Hemolytic anemia caused by membrane defects (acquired: paroxysmal nocturnal hemoglobinuria, spur cell anemia, Wilson disease; inherited: spherocytosis, elliptosis), hemoglobinopathies, and enzyme deficiencies (G6PD, pyruvate kinase)
- Non–immune mediated (microangiopathic hemolytic anemias, hypersplenism, cardiac valve prosthesis, giant cavernous hemangiomas, march hemoglobinuria, physical agents, infections, heavy metals, certain drugs [nitrofurantoin, sulfonamides, ribavirin])
- Chronic lymphocytic leukemia (CLL) can be a cause of direct antiglobulin test (DAT) positivity (15% of CLL cases) without AIHA. In a series of patients treated with fludarabine and cyclophosphamide, only 30% of patients with DAT+ disease developed AIHA after therapy; conversely, 85% of patients with AIHA were previously positive for DAT

TABLE 2 Secondary Autoimmune Hemolytic Anemia in Malignancies

Malignancy	Prevalence	WAIHAs	CAIHAs
MGUS	Very low	None	All
All NHL	0.23%–2.6%		
CLL	4.3%–9%	90%	10%
SMZL	10%	2/3	1/3
LPL	3%–5%	None	Most
Angioimmunoblastic T-cell lymphoma	13%	One third	Two thirds
Hodgkin lymphoma	0.19%–1.7%	All	None
Ovarian teratoma	Very low	All	None
Solid tumors	Very low	Two thirds	One third

CAIHAs, Cold antibody autoimmune hemolytic anemias; *CLL,* chronic lymphocytic leukemia; *LPL,* lymphoplasmacytic lymphoma; *MGUS,* monoclonal gammopathy with unknown significance; *NHL,* non-Hodgkin's lymphoma; *SMZL,* splenic marginal zone lymphoma; *WAIHAs,* warm antibody autoimmune hemolytic anemias.
From Hoffman R, et al.: *Hematology, basic principles and practice,* ed 7, Philadelphia, 2018, Elsevier.

TABLE 3 Autoimmune Hemolytic Anemia after Infections

	Infection	WAIHA	CAIHA (Specificities)
Respiratory tract infections (unspecified)	—	—	+ (DL)/PCH
Viral infections (specific)	EBV	+/–	+ (anti-i)
	CMV	+	+/– (anti-i)
	Parvovirus (B19)	+ (often with PRCA)	+/– (DL)
	Varicella	+/–	+ (anti-Pr, anti-I, anti-DL)
	Rubella	—	+ (anti-Pr1) Monotypic IgM
	HIV	+	+ (anti-I, anti-i, anti-Pr)
Bacterial infections (specific)	Mycoplasma	+/–	+ (anti-I, anti-Pr)
	Brucellosis	+/–	+ (anti-I)
	Haemophilus influenzae		+ (DL)
Parasitic infections (specific)	Visceral leishmaniosis	+	—

—, Not reported; +, predominant type of autoimmune hemolytic anemia; +/–, single or few cases reported; *CAIHA,* cold antibody autoimmune hemolytic anemia; *CMV,* cytomegalovirus; *DL,* Donath–Landsteiner antibody; *EBV,* Epstein-Barr virus; *IgM,* immunoglobulin M; *PCH,* paroxysmal cold hemoglobinuria; *PRCA,* pure red blood cell aplasia; *WAIHA,* warm antibody autoimmune hemolytic anemia.
From Hoffman R, et al.: *Hematology, basic principles and practice,* ed 7, Philadelphia, 2018, Elsevier.

TABLE 4 Drug-Induced Autoimmune Hemolytic Anemia

Drug	Risk Factors	AIHA Onset	Type of AIHA	Response to Treatment	Diseases Treated
Methyldopa	Not known	Delayed	WAIHA	Resolution after withdrawal	Hypertension
IFN-α	Pretherapeutic positive DAT	Delayed (8–11 months)	WAIHA	Resolution spontaneous or after steroids	Hepatitis C; hematologic malignancies
Efazulimab	Not known	Many months	WAIHA	Resolution after withdrawal	Arthritis (rare)
Etanercept	Not known	Delayed	CAIHA	Resolution after rituximab	Rheumatoid arthritis (rare)
Fludarabine Cladribine Pentostatin	CLL Pretherapeutic positive DAT result	Early (median, 3–4 cycle) or delayed	WAIHA Mixed AIHA	Half of AIHA resolve after steroids	CLL Lymphomas[a] AML[a]
Bendamustin	CLL	No or only very low risk of AIHA			CLL Lymphomas
Chlorambucil	CLL	Delayed onset	WAIHA		CLL
Eculizumab	Patients with incomplete response	After treatment	CAIHA		PNH
Lenalidomide		During treatment	WAIHA	Resolution after withdrawal	One case treated for lymphoma
Checkpoint inhibitors (anti-CTLA4, anti-PD1/PD1L		During treatment	WAIHA		Solid tumors, Hodgkin lymphoma

[a]No or very low risk.
AIHA, Autoimmune hemolytic anemia; *AML,* acute myeloid leukemia; *CAIHA,* cold autoimmune hemolytic anemia; *CLL,* chronic lymphocytic leukemia; *DAT,* direct antiglobulin test; *IFN,* interferon; *PNH,* paroxysmal nocturnal hemoglobinuria; *WAIHA,* warm autoimmune hemolytic anemia.
From Hoffman R, et al.: *Hematology, basic principles and practice*, ed 7, Philadelphia, 2018, Elsevier.

TABLE 5 Positive Direct Antiglobulin Test Findings, Characteristic Features of Autoantibody in Autoimmune Hemolytic Anemia

	Warm AIHA	CHAD	Mixed-AIHA	PCH	IgA AIHA
DAT	IgG or IgG + C3 or IgG + C3 + IgM	C3 or C3 + IgM	IgG + C3 + IgM	C3	Neg with polyspecific reagent Pos with anti-IgA
Antibody characteristic					
1) Antibody subclass	IgG	IgM	IgG + IgM	IgG	IgA
1) Specificity	Apparent Rh specificity (common)	I, i, Pr		P	
1) Thermal reactivity (in vitro)	Optimal at 37°C by IAT	0-30°C by saline agglutination	Combined	0-24°C, biphasic in nature	
1) Antibody titer at 4°C	Not applicable	≥256	Usually <64 but can be >256	Usually <32	
Autoagglutination	No	Common	Common	Less common	No

AIHA, Autoimmune hemolytic anemia; *C,* complement; *CHAD,* cold hemagglutinin disease; *DAT,* direct antiglobulin test; *IAT,* indirect antiglobulin test; *Ig,* immunoglobulin; *Neg,* negative; *Pos,* positive.
The determination of autospecificity is not required for diagnosis of CHAD, but confirmation of high thermal amplitude (i.e., cold autoagglutinin reacting at or above 30°C) is essential.
From Bain BJ, Bates I, Laffan MA: *Dacie and Lewis practical haematology*, ed 12, Philadelphia, 2017, Elsevier.

WORKUP

Evaluation consists primarily of laboratory evaluation to confirm hemolysis and exclude other causes of the anemia. Although most cases of AIHA are idiopathic, potential causes should always be sought.

LABORATORY TESTS

- The basic features of hemolytic anemia are reticulocytosis (if no concurrent bone marrow suppression), low haptoglobin levels, elevated indirect bilirubin, and elevated LDH.
- Initial laboratory tests: Complete blood count (anemia), reticulocyte count (elevated), liver function studies (elevated indirect bilirubin, LDH), evaluation of peripheral smear (Fig. E1).
- A direct antiglobulin test (DAT, Coombs test) is initially performed with a polyspecific antibody to detect IgG or complement C3d bound to RBCs. If the DAT is positive, the diagnosis of autoimmune hemolytic anemia (AIHA) is confirmed. A positive direct Coombs test indicates presence of antibodies or complement on the surface of RBCs; positive indirect Coombs test implies presence of anti-RBC antibodies freely circulating in the patient's serum. Positive DAT findings and characteristic features of autoantibody in AIHA are summarized in Table 5. Typical serologic features of the different types of drug-induced hemolytic anemia of immunologic origin are summarized in Table 6.
- If the DAT is positive with IgG alone or with IgG + C3d, the AIHA is most likely due to warm antibody (WAIHA), whereas if the DAT is positive with C3d only, it is most likely caused by a cold antibody (CAIHA).
- Hepatitis serology, antinuclear antibody.
- Urinary tests may reveal hemosiderinuria or hemoglobinuria (documenting intravascular hemolysis).

IMAGING STUDIES

- Chest x-ray
- CT scans of chest, abdomen, and pelvis should be considered if underlying lymphoproliferative disorder is suspected

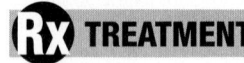

NONPHARMACOLOGIC THERAPY

- Discontinuation of any potentially offending drugs
- Plasmapheresis and exchange transfusion for severe life-threatening cases only
- Avoid cold exposure in patients with cold antibody

TABLE 6 Serologic Features of the Different Types of Drug-Induced Hemolytic Anemia of Immunologic Origin

Mechanism	Prototype drug	DAT	IAT		
Drug-dependent antibody			No drug	Serum + drug	Eluate + drug
C′ activation	Quin(id)ine	C′*	Neg	C′*	Neg
No C′ activation	Penicillin	IgG	Neg	IgG	IgG
Autoantibody	α-Methyldopa	IgG	IgG	NA	NA

C′, Complement; *IgG,* immunoglobulin G; *NA,* not applicable; *Neg,* negative.
*Occasionally also IgG.
From Bain BJ, Bates I, Laffan MA: *Dacie and Lewis practical haematology,* ed 12, Philadelphia, 2017, Elsevier.

TABLE 7 Treatment Options for Primary and Secondary Warm Autoimmune Hemolytic Anemia and Cold Autoimmune Hemolytic Anemia

Disease or Condition	First Line	Second Line	Beyond Second Line	Last Resort
Primary AIHA	Steroids (trituximab)	Splenectomy Rituximab	Azathioprine, MMF, cyclosporine, cyclophosphamide	High-dose cyclophosphamide, alemtuzumab
B- and T-cell NHL	Steroids	Chemotherapy +/− rituximab (splenectomy in SMZL)	Other anti-CD23 antibodies/ ibrutinib	
Hodgkin's lymphoma	Steroids	Chemotherapy		
Solid tumors	Steroids Surgery			
Ovarian dermoid cyst	Ovariectomy			
SLE	Steroids	Azathioprine	MMF	Rituximab Autologous SCT
Ulcerative colitis	Steroids	Azathioprine		Total colectomy
CVID	Steroids + IgG replacement			
ALPD	Steroids	MMF	Sirolimus	
Wiskott-Aldrich syndrome	Steroids	Allogeneic SCT		
Allogeneic SCT	Steroids	Rituximab*	Splenectomy T-cells infusion	
Organ transplantation	Reduction of immune suppression, steroids			
Drug induced	Withdrawal	Steroids		
Primary CAD	Protection from cold exposure	Rituximab Chlorambucil	Fludarabine + rituximab	Eculizumab,† bortezomib†
PCH	Supportive treatment (postinfectious)	Rituximab* (chronic)		

AIHA, Autoimmune hemolytic anemia; *ALPD,* autoimmune lymphoproliferative disorders; *CAD,* cold agglutinin disease; *CVID,* common variable immune deficiency; *IgG,* immunoglobulin G; *MMF,* mycophenolate mofetil; *NHL,* non-Hodgkin lymphoma; *PCH,* paroxysmal cold hemoglobinuria; *SCT,* stem cell transplantation; *SLE,* systemic lupus erythematosus; *SMZL,* splenic marginal zone lymphoma.
*Early second-line treatment because of known poor response to steroids.
†Off-label use in single cases.
From Hoffman R: *Hematology, basic principles and practice,* ed 7, Philadelphia, 2018, Saunders.

ACUTE GENERAL Rx

- Prednisone 1 to 2 mg/kg/day in divided doses initially in warm antibody AIHA. Corticosteroids are generally ineffective in cold antibody AIHA. In cold agglutinin disease treatment, modalities consist of cold avoidance, therapy of underlying lymphoproliferative disorder, and use of rituximab and plasmapheresis in severe cases.
- Splenectomy is indicated in patients responding inadequately to corticosteroids when RBC sequestration studies indicate splenic sequestration.
- Immunosuppressive drugs and/or immunoglobulins only after both corticosteroids and splenectomy (unless surgery is contraindicated) have failed to produce an adequate remission.
- Danazol, typically used in conjunction with corticosteroids (may be useful in warm antibody AIHA).
- Immunosuppressive drugs (azathioprine, cyclophosphamide) may be useful in warm antibody AIHA but are indicated only after both corticosteroids and splenectomy (unless surgery is contraindicated) have failed to produce an adequate remission.
- Table 7 summarizes treatment options for primary and secondary warm autoimmune hemolytic anemia and cold autoimmune hemolytic anemia. Second-line treatment options after steroids are described in Table 8.

DISPOSITION

Prognosis is generally good unless anemia is associated with underlying disorder with a poor prognosis (e.g., leukemia, myeloma).

REFERRAL

- Hematology referral in all cases of AIHA
- Surgical referral for splenectomy in refractory cases

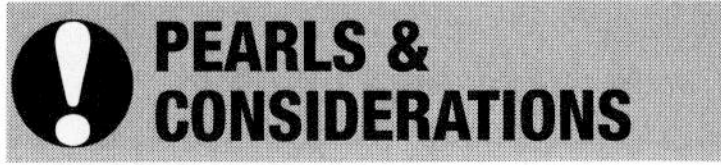

PEARLS & CONSIDERATIONS

COMMENTS

- The direct antiglobulin test demonstrates the presence of antibodies or complement on the surface of RBCs and is the hallmark of autoimmune hemolysis.
- Warm AIHA is often associated with autoimmune diseases, whereas cold AIHA often follows viral infections (e.g., mononucleosis) and *Mycoplasma pneumoniae* infections.
- HIV can induce both warm and cold AIHA.

TABLE 8 Second-Line Treatment Options after Steroids

Treatment	Dosing and Application	Side Effects	Precautions
Splenectomy (acute)	Preferentially laparoscopic	Infections, thrombosis	Postoperative thromboprophylaxis
Splenectomy (long term)	—	Infections Venous thrombosis	Vaccination, patient information
Rituximab	375 mg/m^2 on days 1,8, 15, and 22 IV	Infusional reactions Infections	Premedication with antihistamines (and steroids)
Danazol	200–400/day PO	Hepatotoxicity	None
Cyclophosphamide	PO or IV Dose adjusted to neutrophil count	Neutropenia Mutagenesis	Neutrophil count monitoring, bladder protection after high doses
Azathioprine	2.0–3.mg/kg/day PO Dose adjusted to neutrophil count	Neutropenia	Neutrophil count monitoring; avoid interaction with other drugs (e.g., allopurinol)
MFF	1–2 × 1 g/day PO	Gastrointestinal	
Cyclosporine	PO Dose adjusted to blood levels of CyA Target level, 200–400 ng/ml	Nephrotoxicity Gum hyperplasia	Monitoring of CyA levels and creatinine
Alemtuzumab	SC (variable doses)	Neutropenia	Antiinfectious prophylaxis
Complement inhibition with eculizumab, TNT009		Infections	Vaccination

CyA, Cyclosporine A; *IV,* intravenous; *MMF,* mycophenolate mofetil; *PO,* oral; *SC,* subcutaneous.
From Hoffman R, et al.: *Hematology, basic principles and practice*, ed 7, Philadelphia, 2018, Elsevier.

- Hemolytic anemia is a common autoimmune complication of hematopoietic stem cell transplantation occurring in up to 6% of patients as a late complication (median 202 days); it presents as either warm or cold AIHA.

SUGGESTED READINGS

Available at ExpertConsult.com

AUTHOR: **BHARTI RATHORE, M.D.**

BASIC INFORMATION

DEFINITION

Inflammatory anemia also known as "anemia of chronic disease" (ACD) is a disorder of iron homeostasis (Table 1) promoted by hepcidin-25 in response to an inflammatory condition.

SYNONYMS

Inflammatory anemia
Anemia of chronic disease
ACD

ICD-10CM CODES

D63.8 Anemia in chronic diseases classified elsewhere
D63.0 Anemia in neoplastic disease
D64.8 Anemia, unspecified

EPIDEMIOLOGY & DEMOGRAPHICS

PREVALENCE:

- Second-most prevalent anemia after iron deficiency anemia
  1. Around 11% of men and 10% of women ages 65 to 85 yr
  2. >20% of adults older than 85 yr

Pathophysiology (Fig. 1)

Iron is carried in the bloodstream shelled by a hollow protein called transferrin (<0.2% of total iron body content) or at the core of hemoglobin in RBCs (60% of total iron body content). It is mainly stored (15%–30% of total iron body content) inside the liver, spleen, and skeletal muscle as ferritin and in lysosomes as hemosiderin. The rest of the iron body content is trapped in myoglobin in skeletal muscle and cytochromes in mitochondria. In clinical practice, ferritin is a surrogate for iron stores, and total iron binding capacity (TIBC) is a surrogate for transferrin and the carrying capacity of iron.

Cells involved in the response to inflammatory insults cause the release of cytokines, such as IL-6, which stimulates hepatic release of hepcidin. Hepcidin is a circulating protein that blocks ferroportin, an iron channel responsible for the exit of iron from enterocytes (and thus gastrointestinal absorption) and macrophages (which accumulate iron from engulfed senescent blood cells). IL-1 and TNF-alpha stimulate IFN-gamma release by marrow stromal cells, which in turn suppress the erythroid response to erythropoietin (EPO). In chronic kidney disease, ACD is a consequence of decreased production of EPO and decreased renal clearance of hepcidin. The low availability of serum iron causes iron deficiency in the bone marrow compartment and decreased reticulocyte levels.

TABLE 1 Suspected Causes of Anemia of Chronic Disease

Shortened erythrocyte survival
Block in reuse of iron by erythrocyte
Direct inhibition of erythropoiesis
Relative deficiency of erythropoietin

From Hoffman R et al: *Hematology, basic principles and practice*, ed 7, Philadelphia, 2018, Elsevier.

CLINICAL PRESENTATION

- Besides fatigue, shortness of breath, and generalized weakness from the anemia itself, it is important to consider other complaints if the underlying diagnosis is unknown, such as weight loss (malignancy, chronic infections, connective tissue diseases), anorexia, nausea, paresthesias, pleuritic chest pain, weight gain (CKD), diarrhea, bloody stools, abdominal pain, oral ulcers (IBD), and fevers (HIV, chronic infections).
- Physical findings may include pallor, lymphadenopathy, stigmatas of connective tissue diseases (malar rash, sclerodactyly), palpable or visible masses, and localized findings for infection or malignancy.

DIAGNOSIS

Isolated ACD:

- CBC with differential: Normocytic, normochromic, moderate (Hb rarely <8 g/dl) anemia
- Hypoproliferative anemia (low reticulocyte index; corrected reticulocyte count <2%)

Iron studies:

- Low iron concentration as in IDA (iron deficiency anemia)
- Normal/high ferritin (>35 mg/dl) in ACD as it is an acute phase reactant (Fig. 2)
- Low/normal TIBC (as opposed to IDA) and low transferrin saturation (as in IDA)
- Normal soluble transferrin receptor (sTfR, high in IDA)

Combined ACD/IDA:

- If normal to high ferritin, sTfR/log ferritin ratio <1 defines isolated ACD, and ratio >2 defines combined IDA/ACD

ETIOLOGY

- Malignancy
- CKD (patients with CKD stage IV [GFR<30 ml/min] should be screened for ACD)
- CHF (ACD is the main cause of anemia in CHF patients)
- Chronic infections
- Anemia of critical illness (develops within days)
- Connective tissue diseases

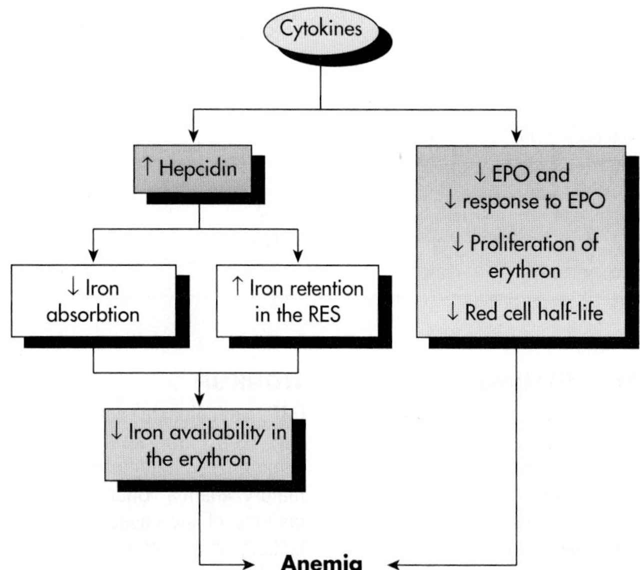

FIG. 1 Pathophysiologic factors associated with the development of anemia of chronic disease. *EPO,* Erythropoietin; *RES,* reticuloendothelial system. (From Hoffman R, et al.: *Hematology, basic principles and practice*, ed 7, Philadelphia, 2018, Elsevier.)

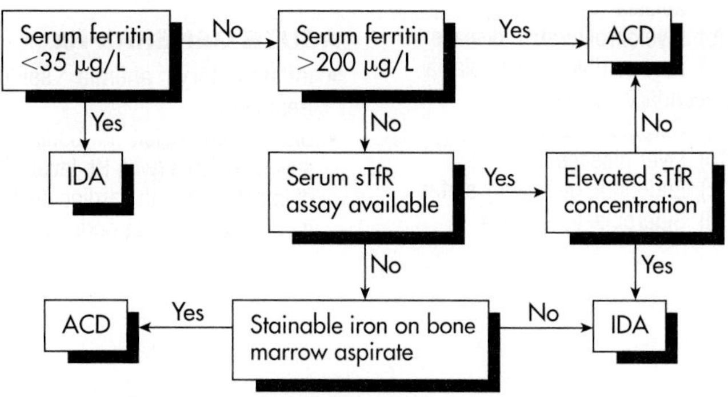

FIG. 2 Differential diagnosis of anemia with low serum iron. *ACD,* Anemia of chronic disease; *IDA,* iron deficiency anemia; *sTfR,* soluble transferrin receptor.

TABLE 2 Laboratory Features in Microcytic Hypochromic Anemias

	Serum Iron	Serum TIBC	% Saturation	MARROW % Sideroblasts	MARROW Iron Stores	Serum Ferritin	ZPP	Hb A_2	Hb F
Iron deficiency	↓	↑	↓	↓	↓	↓	↑	N-↓	N
β-Thalassemia trait	N (↑)	N	N	N	N-↑	N-↑	N	↑	N-↑
ACD	↓	N-↓	↓	↓	N-↑	N-↑	↑	N	N
Sideroblastic anemia	↑	↓	↑	↑	↑	↑	↑ (↓)	N	N-↑

ACD, Anemia of chronic disease; *N,* normal; *TIBC,* total iron-binding capacity; *ZPP,* zinc protoporphyrins; ↓, decreased; ↑, increased.
McPherson RA, Pincus MR: *Henry's clinical diagnosis and management by laboratory methods,* ed 23, Philadelphia, 2017, Elsevier.

TABLE 3 Laboratory Characteristics of ACD, IDA, and IDA With Inflammation

	Anemia of Chronic Disease (ACD)	Iron Deficiency Anemia (IDA)	IDA with Inflammation
Mean corpuscular volume (MCV)	72–100 fL	<85 fL	<100 fL
Mean corpuscular hemoglobin concentration (MCHC)	<36 g/dl	<32 g/dl	<32 g/dl
Serum iron	Decreased	Decreased	Decreased
Serum total iron-binding capacity (TIBC)	Typical below mid-normal range	Elevated	Less than upper limit of normal range
Transferrin saturation*	2%–20%	<15% (usually <10%)	<15%
Serum ferritin	>35 μg/L	<35 μg/L	>35 μg/L, <200μg/L
Serum soluble transferrin receptor concentration (sTfR)	Normal (may be increased if serum ferritin >200 μg/L)	Increased	Increased
TfR index (sTfR/log ferritin)	<1	>2	>2
Hepcidin	High	Low	Normal
Stainable iron in bone marrow	Present	Absent	Absent

*Serum iron/TIBC * 100.

DIFFERENTIAL DIAGNOSIS

- Liver injury (increases ferritin)
  1. Iron deficiency anemia
     a. Other causes of normocytic anemia or microcytic anemia (Table 2)
     b. Red blood cell loss or destruction
        (1) Acute blood loss
        (2) Hypersplenism
        (3) Hemolysis
     c. Decreased red blood cell production
        (1) Primary causes:
           (a) Bone marrow hypoplasia or aplasia
           (b) Myeloproliferative disease
           (c) Pure red blood cell aplasia
        (2) Secondary causes
           (a) Chronic renal failure
           (b) Liver disease
           (c) Endocrine deficiency states
           (d) Sideroblastic anemia

WORKUP

CBC, reticulocyte count, peripheral smear (Fig. E3, A), iron level, ferritin, TIBC. Table 3 summarizes characteristic findings in inflammatory anemia. Characteristic bone marrow findings of increased iron stores in stromal histiocytes and impaired erythroid iron incorporation are shown in Fig. E4.

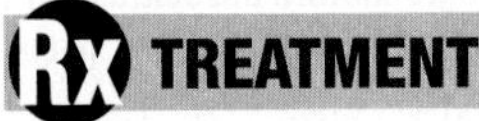

TREATMENT

Treat the underlying disorder/disease.

ACUTE GENERAL Rx

- Inflammatory anemia seldom requires treatment.
- Blood transfusion is usually reserved for severe anemia (with Hb level <7 g/dl or <8 g/dl in patients with cardiac disease) especially if complicated with ongoing bleeding.

CHRONIC Rx

- Erythropoiesis-stimulating agents (ESA) (epoetin alfa and darbepoetin alfa) are FDA approved for use in patients with anemia resulting from:
  1. Chronic kidney disease
  2. Chemotherapy
  3. Zidovudine therapy

A 1998 study, the Normal Hematocrit Cardiac Trial (NHCT), showed a nonsignificant increase in the combined endpoint death and nonfatal MI in patients with goal hematocrit of 33% versus 27%. Subsequent studies (CHOIR, CREATE, and TREAT) showed that higher doses and higher hematocrit targets were associated with increased cardiovascular events.

ESA dose should be individualized for each patient, and the lowest sufficient dose to reduce blood transfusions should be used. A hemoglobin target of approximately 10 g% is widely acceptable. Iron deficiency should be ruled out before ESA is started. After starting ESA therapy, ASH/ASCO guidelines recommend periodic monitoring of iron status. When there is no or suboptimal response to oral therapy, parenteral iron therapy should be considered before concluding that a patient is nonresponsive to iron therapy.

The most promising agents on the hepcidin–ferroportin axis are hypoxia-induced factor modulators. HIF is a transcription factor that promotes expression of erythropoietin. HIF is upregulated by inhibition of PHD. Clinical trials of vadadustat, an oral hypoxia-inducible factor, in patients with anemia of kidney disease have demonstrated efficacy in achieving a hemoglobin of 11 g/dl or an increase of 1.2 g/dl. Also, mean hemoglobin levels were maintained in patients with CKD who were previously receiving ESA.

SUGGESTED READINGS

Available at ExpertConsult.com

AUTHOR: **BHARTI RATHORE, M.D.**

BASIC INFORMATION

DEFINITION

Anemia is defined as a hemoglobin level 2 standard deviations below normal for age and sex. Iron deficiency anemia is anemia resulting from inadequate iron supplementation or excessive blood loss.

ICD-10CM CODES

D50.9	Iron deficiency anemia, unspecified
099.019	Anemia complicating pregnancy, unspecified trimester
D50.0	Iron deficiency anemia secondary to blood loss (chronic)
D50.8	Other iron deficiency anemias

EPIDEMIOLOGY & DEMOGRAPHICS

- Dietary iron deficiency occurs often in infants as a result of unsupplemented milk diets. It is also commonly seen in women during their reproductive years, as a result of heavy menstrual periods, and during pregnancy (increased demand).
- Iron deficiency is the most common nutritional deficiency worldwide.
- The prevalence of iron deficiency is greatest among toddlers ages 1 to 2 yr (7%) from inadequate intake and female individuals ages 12 to 49 yr (9% to 16%) from menstrual losses.
- The prevalence of iron deficiency is 2% in adult men, 9% to 12% in non-Hispanic white women, and 20% in black and Mexican American women.
- GI cancer is diagnosed in 10% of elderly patients with iron deficiency anemia.

PHYSICAL FINDINGS & CLINICAL PRESENTATION

- Most patients have normal examination results.
- Skin pallor and conjunctival pallor may be present.
- Signs and symptoms specific for iron deficiency are koilonychias, pica, pagophagia, blue sclera, glossitis, and angular stomatitis (Fig. 1).
- Patients with severe anemia can have palpitations, headache, weakness, dizziness, and easy fatigability.

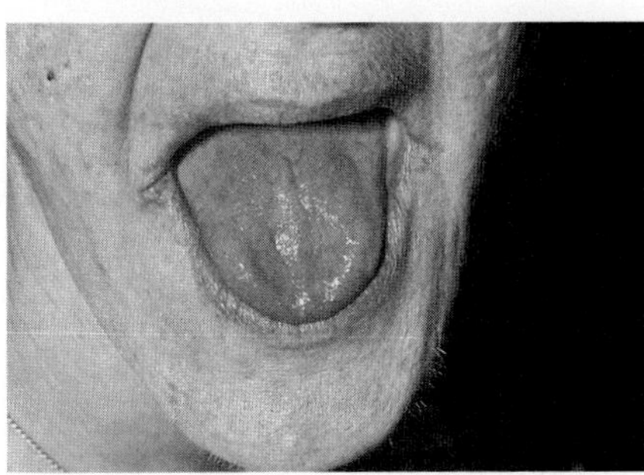

FIG. 1 Iron deficiency. (From White GM, Cox NH [eds]: *Diseases of the skin, a color atlas and text,* ed 2, St Louis, 2006, Mosby.)

ETIOLOGY

- Blood loss from GI or menstrual bleeding (genitourinary blood loss less often the cause)
- Dietary iron deficiency (rare in adults)
- Poor iron absorption in patients with gastric or small-bowel surgery
- Repeated phlebotomy
- Increased requirements (e.g., during pregnancy)
- Other: Traumatic hemolysis (abnormally functioning cardiac valves), idiopathic pulmonary hemosiderosis (iron sequestration in pulmonary macrophages), paroxysmal nocturnal hemoglobinuria (intravascular hemolysis)
- The most common cause worldwide is hookworm infection

DIAGNOSIS

DIFFERENTIAL DIAGNOSIS

- Anemia of chronic disease
- Sideroblastic anemia
- Thalassemia trait
- Lead poisoning

WORKUP

Diagnostic workup consists primarily of laboratory evaluation. Table 1 describes laboratory studies differentiating the most common microcytic anemias. Most patients with iron deficiency anemia are asymptomatic in the early stages. With progressive anemia, the major symptoms are fatigue, dizziness, exertional dyspnea, pagophagia (ice eating), and pica. Patient history may also suggest GI blood loss (melena, hematochezia, hemoptysis).

LABORATORY TESTS

- Laboratory results vary with the stage of deficiency.
- Absent iron marrow stores and decreased serum ferritin are the initial abnormalities.
- Decreased serum iron and increased total iron-binding capacity (TIBC) are the next abnormalities.
- Hypochromic microcytic anemia is present with significant iron deficiency.
- Peripheral smear in patients with iron deficiency generally reveals microcytic hypochromic red blood cells (Fig. 2) with a wide area of central pallor, anisocytosis, and poikilocytosis when severe.
- Laboratory abnormalities consistent with iron deficiency are low serum ferritin level, increased RBC distribution width with values generally >15, low mean corpuscular volume, low mean corpuscular hemoglobin, increased TIBC, and low serum iron.
- In patients diagnosed with iron deficiency anemia, a GI workup including an upper endoscopy and colonoscopy is recommended to look for source of iron loss.

TREATMENT

The goal of therapy is to supply sufficient iron to correct the low hemoglobin and replenish iron stores.

NONPHARMACOLOGIC THERAPY

Patients should be instructed to consume foods that contain large amounts of iron, such as liver, red meat, and legumes.

ACUTE GENERAL Rx

- Iron supplementation will result in reticulocytosis and will generally increase hemoglobin levels by 0.5 to 1 g per wk.
- Treatment consists of ferrous sulfate 325 mg PO daily for 3 to 6 mo. Doses higher than 325 mg/day are poorly tolerated. Calcium supplements can decrease iron absorption; therefore, these medications should be staggered. Supplemental vitamin C can increase oral absorption.
- Parenteral iron therapy is reserved for patients with poor tolerance, noncompliance with oral preparations, or malabsorption.
- Transfusion of packed RBCs is indicated in patients with severe symptomatic anemia.

CHRONIC Rx

Patients should be instructed to continue their iron supplements for at least 6 mo or longer to correct depleted body iron stores.

TABLE 1 Laboratory Studies Differentiating the Most Common Microcytic Anemias

Study	Iron Deficiency Anemia	α or β Thalassemia	Anemia of Chronic Disease
Hemoglobin	Decreased	Decreased	Decreased
MCV	Decreased	Decreased	Normal-decreased
RDW	Increased	Normal	Normal-increased
RBC	Decreased	Normal-increased	Normal-decreased
Serum ferritin	Decreased	Normal	Increased
Total Fe binding capacity	Increased	Normal	Decreased
Transferrin saturation	Decreased	Normal	Decreased
FEP	Increased	Normal	Increased
Transferrin receptor	Increased	Normal	Increased
Reticulocyte hemoglobin concentration	Decreased	Normal	Normal-decreased

Fe, Ferritin; *FEP,* free erythrocyte protoporphyrin; *MCV,* mean corpuscular volume; *RBC,* red blood cell; *RDW,* red cell distribution width.
From Kliegman RM et al: *Nelson textbook of pediatrics,* ed 19, Philadelphia, 2011, Saunders.

 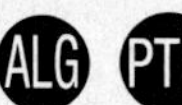

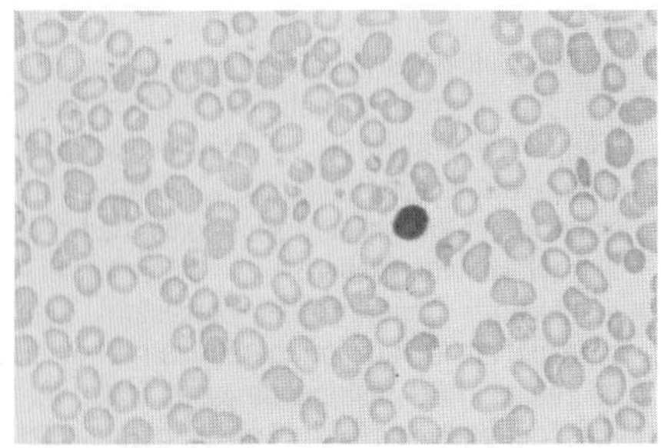

FIG. 2 Iron deficiency anemia. Many of these red blood cells are microcytic (smaller than the nucleus of the normal lymphocyte near the center of the field) and hypochromic (with central areas of pallor that exceed half the diameter of the cells). (From Goldman L, Schafer AI: *Goldman's Cecil medicine,* ed 24, Philadelphia, 2012, Saunders.)

DISPOSITION

- Most patients respond rapidly to iron supplementation with improvement in CBC and general well-being (Table 2). GI side effects from oral iron therapy are common and may require decreased dosage to once every other day or to change to parenteral iron.
- A differential diagnosis of microcytic anemia that fails to respond to oral iron is described in Table 3.

REFERRAL

GI referral for evaluation of GI malignancy is recommended in all patients with iron deficiency and suspected GI blood loss.

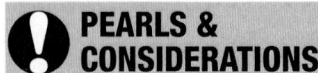

PEARLS & CONSIDERATIONS

COMMENTS

- Iron deficiency may impair aerobic performance and worsen symptoms in patients with heart failure. Treatment with IV iron in patients with chronic heart failure and iron deficiency has been shown to improve symptoms, quality of life, and functional capacity.
- If the diagnosis of iron deficiency anemia is made, locating the suspected site of iron loss is mandatory.

TABLE 2 Responses to Iron Therapy in Iron Deficiency Anemia

Time after Iron Administration	Response
12-24 hr	Replacement of intracellular iron enzymes; subjective improvement; decreased irritability; increased appetite
36-48 hr	Initial bone marrow response; erythroid hyperplasia
48-72 hr	Reticulocytosis, peaking at 5-7 days
4-30 days	Increase in hemoglobin level
1-3 mo	Repletion of stores

From Kliegman RM et al: *Nelson textbook of pediatrics,* ed 19, Philadelphia, 2011, Saunders.

TABLE 3 Differential Diagnosis of Microcytic Anemia That Fails to Respond to Oral Iron

Poor compliance (true intolerance of iron is uncommon)
Incorrect dose or medication
Malabsorption of administered iron
Ongoing blood loss including gastrointestinal, menstrual, and pulmonary
Concurrent infection or inflammatory disorder inhibiting the response to iron
Concurrent vitamin B_{12} or folate deficiency
Diagnosis other than iron deficiency

- Thalassemiass
- Hemoglobin C and E disorders
- Anemia of chronic disease
- Lead poisoning
- Sickle thalassemias, hemoglobin SC disease
- Rare microcytic anemias

From Kliegman RM et al: *Nelson textbook of pediatrics,* ed 19, Philadelphia, 2011, Saunders.

RELATED CONTENT

Algorithm for Diagnosis of Anemias (Algorithm in Section III)
Iron Deficiency Anemia (Patient Information)
Anemia (Patient Information)

AUTHOR: **FRED F. FERRI, M.D.**

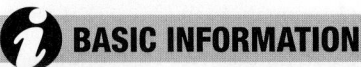

BASIC INFORMATION

DEFINITION

Pernicious anemia (PA) is an autoimmune disease resulting from antibodies against gastric intrinsic factor and gastric parietal cells.

SYNONYMS

Megaloblastic anemia resulting from vitamin B_{12} deficiency
Addison-Biermer anemia

ICD-10CM CODES

D51.0	Vitamin B_{12} deficiency anemia due to intrinsic factor deficiency
D51.8	Other vitamin B_{12} deficiency anemias
D51.9	Vitamin B_{12} deficiency anemia, unspecified
D51.1	Vitamin B_{12} deficiency anemia due to selective vitamin B_{12} malabsorption with proteinuria

EPIDEMIOLOGY & DEMOGRAPHICS

- Increased incidence in females and older adults (40-70 yr)
- More frequent in patients of northern European ancestry
- The overall prevalence of undiagnosed PA after age 60 yr is 1.9%
- Prevalence is highest in women (2.7%), particularly in black women (4.3%)
- Associated with other autoimmune diseases (e.g., type 1 diabetes mellitus, Graves disease, Addison disease), along with possible *Helicobacter pylori* association

PHYSICAL FINDINGS & CLINICAL PRESENTATION

- Mucosal pallor and/or glossitis
- Angular cheilosis
- Mild jaundice (representative of intramedullary hemolysis of megaloblastic cells); "lemon yellow" skin due to pallor and jaundice
- Peripheral sensory neuropathy with paresthesias initially and absent reflexes in advanced disease
- Delirium or dementia
- Worsening weakness and possible subacute combined degeneration of spinal cord (Fig. E1)
- Loss of proprioception and an unsteady gait
- Gastrointestinal symptoms including anorexia, pyrosis, nausea, and vomiting
- Possible splenomegaly and mild hepatomegaly

ETIOLOGY

- Parietal cell antibodies are present in >70% of patients, while intrinsic factor antibodies are noted in >50% of patients
- Atrophic gastric mucosa (Fig. E2) with achlorhydria
- Inborn errors of cobalamin-cofactor synthesis are rare. Fig. E3 illustrates the components and mechanism of cobalamin absorption. An etiopathophysiologic classification of cobalamin deficiency is described in Section II.

DIAGNOSIS

DIFFERENTIAL DIAGNOSIS

- Nutritional vitamin B_{12} deficiency
- Malabsorption (e.g., celiac disease)
- Chronic alcoholism (multifactorial)
- Chronic gastritis related to *H. pylori* infection
- Folic acid deficiency
- Myelodysplasia
- Thyroid abnormalities
- Atrophic gastritis
- Paraproteinemias

WORKUP

- The clinical presentation of PA varies with the stage. Initially, patients may be asymptomatic. In advanced stages patients may have impaired memory, depression, gait disturbances, paresthesias, and generalized weakness.
- Investigation consists primarily of laboratory evaluation. Table 1 describes a step-wise approach to the diagnosis of cobalamin and folate deficiency.
- Endoscopy and biopsy for atrophic gastritis may be performed in selected cases.
- Diagnosis is crucial because failure to treat may result in irreversible neurologic deficits.

LABORATORY TESTS

- Complete blood count generally reveals macrocytic anemia, thrombocytopenia, and mild leukopenia with hypersegmented neutrophils (Fig. E4).
- Mean corpuscular volume (MCV) is significantly elevated in advanced stages.
- Reticulocyte count is low to normal.
- False low serum cobalamin levels can occur in patients who are pregnant or taking oral contraceptives, have multiple myeloma, have transcobalamin I (TCI) deficiency, have severe folic acid deficiency, or are taking large doses of ascorbic acid. False high normal levels in patients with cobalamin deficiency can occur in several conditions including hepatomas, severe liver disease, or monoblastic leukemias (Table 2).
- The absence of anemia or macrocytosis does not exclude the diagnosis of cobalamin deficiency. Anemia is absent in 20% of patients with cobalamin deficiency, and macrocytosis is absent in >30% of patients at the time of diagnosis. Macrocytosis can be masked by concurrent iron deficiency, anemia of chronic disease, or thalassemia trait.
- Laboratory tests used for detecting cobalamin deficiency in patients with normal vitamin B_{12} levels include serum and urinary methylmalonic acid (MMA) level (elevated), total homocysteine level (elevated), and intrinsic factor antibody (positive). Cobalamin is a cofactor for the enzymes L-methylmalonyl coenzyme A mutase and methionine synthase. Inadequate levels of cobalamin will thus result in increased MMA and homocysteine levels. Plasma MMA levels can also be used to differentiate cobalamin deficiency from folate deficiency because patients with folate deficiency have normal or mild elevations of MMA levels
- An increased concentration of plasma MMA does not predict clinical manifestations of vitamin B_{12} deficiency and should not be used as the only marker for diagnosis of B_{12} deficiency

TABLE 1 Stepwise Approach to the Diagnosis of Cobalamin and Folate Deficiency

Megaloblastic Anemia or Neurologic-Psychiatric Manifestations Consistent with Cobalamin Deficiency *Plus* Test Results on Serum Cobalamin and Serum Folate

Cobalamin* (pg/ml)	Folate† (ng/ml)	Provisional Diagnosis	Proceed With Metabolites?‡
>300	>4	Cobalamin or folate deficiency is unlikely	No
<200	>4	Consistent with cobalamin deficiency	No
200-300	>4	Rule out cobalamin deficiency	Yes
>300	<2	Consistent with folate deficiency	No
<200	<2	Consistent with (1) combined cobalamin plus folate deficiency or (2) isolated folate deficiency	Yes
>300	2-4	Consistent with (1) folate deficiency or (2) an anemia unrelated to vitamin deficiency	Yes

Test Results on Metabolites: Serum Methylmalonic Acid and Total Homocysteine

Methylmalonic Acid (Normal, 70-270 nM)	Total Homocysteine (Normal, 5-14 μM)	Diagnosis
Increased	Increased	Cobalamin deficiency confirmed; folate deficiency still possible (i.e., combined cobalamin plus folate deficiency possible)
Normal	Increased	Folate deficiency is likely
Normal	Normal	Cobalamin and folate deficiency is excluded

*Serum cobalamin levels: Abnormally low, less than 200 pg/ml; clinically relevant low-normal range, 200 to 300 pg/ml.
†Serum folate levels: Abnormally low, less than 2 ng/ml; clinically relevant low-normal range, 2 to 4 ng/ml.
‡Any frozen-over sample from serum folate/cobalamin determination can be subjected to metabolite tests.
From Hoffman R et al: *Hematology, basic principles and practice,* ed 7, Philadelphia, 2018, Saunders.

 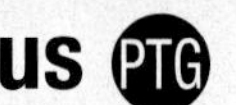

TABLE 2 Serum Cobalamin: False-Positive and False-Negative Test Results

Falsely Low Serum Cobalamin in the Absence of True Cobalamin Deficiency

- Folate deficiency (one-third of patients)
- Multiple myeloma
- TCI deficiency
- Megadose vitamin C therapy
- Pregnancy
- Oral contraceptives

Falsely Raised Cobalamin Levels in the Presence of a True Deficiency*

- Cobalamin binders (TCI and II) increased (e.g., myeloproliferative states, hepatomas, and fibrolamellar hepatic tumors)
- TCII-producing macrophages are activated (e.g., autoimmune diseases, monoblastic leukemias and lymphomas)
- Release of cobalamin from hepatocytes (e.g., active liver disease)
- High serum anti-IF antibody titer

IF, Intrinsic factor; *TC,* transcobalamin.

*Although a low serum cobalamin level is not synonymous with cobalamin deficiency, 5% of patients with true cobalamin deficiency have low-normal cobalamin levels, a potentially serious problem because the patient's underlying cobalamin deficiency will progress if uncorrected.

From Hoffman R et al: *Hematology, basic principles and practice,* ed 6, Philadelphia, 2013, Saunders, 2013.

- Additional laboratory abnormalities can include elevated lactate dehydrogenase, direct hyperbilirubinemia, and decreased haptoglobin.
- Bone marrow aspirate is not necessary to diagnose cobalamin deficiency. It may show giant C-shaped neutrophil bands and megaloblastic normoblasts (Fig. E5).
- Schilling test: No longer used. It was historically used to identify the locus of cobalamin malabsorption and the cause of cobalamin deficiency.

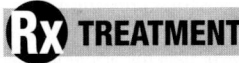

TREATMENT

NONPHARMACOLOGIC THERAPY

Avoid folic acid supplementation without proper vitamin B_{12} supplementation. Folic acid supplementation alone may result in hematologic remission in patients with vitamin B_{12} deficiency but will not treat or prevent neurologic manifestations.

ACUTE GENERAL Rx

Traditional therapy of cobalamin deficiency consists of intramuscular (IM) or deep subcutaneous (SC) injections of vitamin B_{12} 1000 mcg/day for 1 week, followed by 1000 mcg/month, indefinitely. Monitor response and increase dosing if serum B_{12} levels decline.

CHRONIC Rx

- Parenteral vitamin B_{12} 1000 mcg/month or intranasal cyanocobalamin 500 mcg/week for the remainder of life.
- In patients who have no nervous system involvement, intranasal cyanocobalamin may be used in place of parenteral cyanocobalamin after hematologic parameters have returned to normal range. The initial dose of intranasal cyanocobalamin is 1 spray (500 mcg) in one nostril once per week. Nasal cyanocobalamin is expensive.
- Oral cobalamin (1000-2000 mcg/day) is also being effective in mild cases of pernicious anemia because approximately 1% of an oral dose is absorbed by passive diffusion, a pathway that does not require intrinsic factor. Cost for 1 month of therapy is approximately $5. Consider returning to IM vitamin B_{12} supplementation if decline recurs.

DISPOSITION

Anemia generally resolves with appropriate cobalamin replacement therapy. Neurologic deficits, on the other hand, may be corrected only if treated early on.

REFERRAL

Gastroenterology referral for endoscopy on diagnosis of PA followed by periodic surveillance endoscopies to rule out gastric adenocarcinoma or carcinoid tumors.

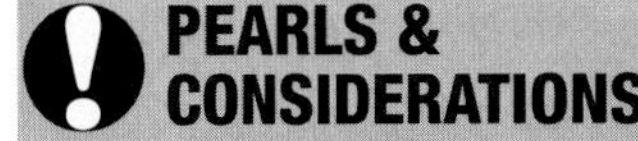

PEARLS & CONSIDERATIONS

COMMENTS

- Early manifestations of negative cobalamin balance are increased serum methylmalonic acid and total homocysteine levels. This occurs when the total cobalamin in serum is still in the low-normal range.

TABLE 3 Causes of Megaloblastosis Not Responding to Therapy With Cobalamin or Folate

Wrong Diagnosis

Combined folate and cobalamin deficiencies being treated with only one vitamin

Associated iron deficiency

Associated hemoglobinopathy (e.g., sickle cell disease, thalassemia)

Associated anemia of chronic disease

Associated hypothyroidism

From Hoffman R et al: *Hematology, basic principles and practice,* ed 7, Philadelphia, 2018, Elsevier.

- Vitamin B_{12} deficiency that is allowed to progress for longer than 3 months may produce permanent degenerative lesions of the spinal cord (e.g., subacute combined degeneration of spinal cord).
- Vitamin B_{12} deficiency may suppress signs of polycythemia vera; treatment of B_{12} deficiency may unmask this disorder.
- Blunted or impeded therapeutic response to vitamin B_{12} may be due to concurrent iron or folic acid deficiency, uremia, infections, or use of drugs with bone marrow suppressant properties. Causes of megaloblastosis not responding to therapy with cobalamin or folate are summarized in Table 3.
- Drugs that interfere with B_{12} absorption include metformin, colchicine, neomycin, and aminosalicylic acid.
- Patients must understand that cobalamin replacement therapy is lifelong.
- Self-injection of vitamin B_{12} may be taught in selected patients. Cost of monthly injections is less than $10.
- Patients who have had bariatric surgery should receive 1 mg of oral vitamin B_{12} per day indefinitely.

SUGGESTED READINGS

Available at ExpertConsult.com

RELATED CONTENT

Pernicious Anemia (Patient Information)

AUTHOR: **SHIVA KUMAR R. MUKKAMALLA, M.D., M.P.H.**

BASIC INFORMATION

DEFINITION

Angina pectoris is a term used to describe a clinical syndrome, typically characterized by chest, jaw, shoulder, back or arm discomfort that is caused by myocardial ischemia. This is most commonly related to atheromatous plaque in one or more than one large epicardial coronary artery; however, myocardial ischemia may occur in the absence of obstructive coronary artery disease (CAD), such as uncontrolled hypertension, microvascular disease, valvular heart disease, hypertrophic cardiomyopathy, coronary spasm, or endothelial dysfunction. Any situation that causes an imbalance in myocardial oxygen supply and demand can cause an angina syndrome. Angina can be classified as follows:

- Chronic stable angina, stable ischemic heart disease (SIHD), or chronic coronary artery disease:
  1. Predictable. Usually follows a precipitating event (e.g., climbing stairs, sexual intercourse, a heavy meal, emotional stress, cold weather).
  2. Generally has the same severity as previous attacks; relieved by rest or by the customary dose of sublingual nitroglycerin.
  3. Caused by a fixed coronary artery obstruction secondary to atherosclerosis. The presence of one or more obstructions in major coronary arteries is likely; the severity of stenosis is usually >70%.
- Unstable (rest, recent onset, crescendo angina; will be reviewed under Acute Coronary Syndrome):
  1. Rest angina: Angina occurring at rest and usually prolonged >20 min, occurring within 1 week of presentation
  2. Recent onset. Angina of at least CCS Class III severity occurring less than 2 months after the onset of the symptoms
  3. Crescendo angina: Previously diagnosed angina that is distinctly more frequent, longer in duration, or lower in threshold (i.e., increased by >1 CCS class within 2 months of initial presentation to at least CCS Class III severity)
- Prinzmetal variant:
  1. Occurs at rest, common after cold exposure.
  2. Cyclical in nature.
  3. EKG finding of episodic ST-segment elevations.
  4. Caused by coronary artery spasm with or without superimposed CAD.
  5. Patients are more likely to develop ventricular arrhythmias.
- Microvascular angina (syndrome X):
  1. Refers to patients with angina symptoms, positive exercise test, normal coronary angiograms and no coronary spasm. Defective endothelium-dependent dilation in the coronary microcirculation contributes to the altered regulation of myocardial perfusion and the ischemic manifestations in these patients.
  2. Patients with chest pain and normal or nonobstructive coronary angiograms are predominantly women, and many have a prognosis that is not as benign as commonly thought (2% risk of death or myocardial infarction [MI] at 30 days of follow-up).
- Refractory angina:
  1. Refers to patients whom, despite optimal medical therapy with at least maximal doses, or as tolerated of 2 antianginal medications, in addition to aspirin, aggressive risk factor modification, such as smoking cessation, adequate control of hypertension, diabetes, and hyperlipidemia, still have both angina and objective evidence of ischemia.
- Other:
  1. Angina due to aortic stenosis and idiopathic hypertrophic subaortic stenosis, cocaine-induced coronary vasoconstriction.

FUNCTIONAL CLASSIFICATION

Stable angina should be classified using a grading system. The most commonly adopted is that of the Canadian Cardiovascular Society (CCS):

- Class I: Ordinary physical activity, such as walking or climbing stairs, does not cause angina. Angina occurs with strenuous, rapid, or prolonged exertion at work or recreation.
- Class II: Slight limitation of ordinary activity. Angina occurs on walking or climbing stairs rapidly; walking uphill; walking or stair climbing after meals, in cold, in wind, or under emotional stress; or only during the few hours after awakening. Angina occurs on walking more than two level blocks and climbing more than one flight of ordinary stairs at a normal pace and in normal conditions.
- Class III: Marked limitations of ordinary physical activity. Angina occurs on walking one to two level blocks and climbing one flight of stairs in normal conditions and at a normal pace.
- Class IV: Inability to carry on any physical activity without discomfort; anginal symptoms may be present at rest.

ICD-10CM CODES

I20.8	Other forms of angina pectoris
I20.9	Angina pectoris, unspecified
I20.1	Angina pectoris with documented spasm
I25.110	Atherosclerotic heart disease of native coronary artery with unstable angina pectoris
I25.111	Atherosclerotic heart disease of native coronary artery with angina pectoris with documented spasm
I25.118	Atherosclerotic heart disease of native coronary artery with other forms of angina pectoris
I25.119	Atherosclerotic heart disease of native coronary artery with unspecified angina pectoris
I25.700	Atherosclerosis of coronary artery bypass graft(s), unspecified, with unstable angina pectoris
I25.790	Atherosclerosis of other coronary artery bypass graft(s) with unstable angina pectoris
I25.791	Atherosclerosis of other coronary artery bypass graft(s) with angina pectoris with documented spasm
I25.798	Atherosclerosis of other coronary artery bypass graft(s) with other forms of angina pectoris
I25.799	Atherosclerosis of other coronary artery bypass graft(s) with unspecified angina pectoris

EPIDEMIOLOGY & DEMOGRAPHICS

- It is estimated that 1 in 3 adults in the United States (about 81 million) has some form of cardiovascular disease. Based on the NHANES survey 2007-2010, an estimated 15.4 million have coronary heart disease of which 7.8 million have angina.
- Angina is most common in middle-aged and elderly men. Among persons 60 to 79 yrs of age, approximately 25% of men and 16% of women have coronary heart disease, and these figures rise to 37% and 23% among men and women >80 yrs of age, respectively.
- The incidence of coronary heart disease and angina in women after menopause is similar to that of men.
- Although the survival rate has steadily improved over time, SIHD remains the number one cause of death in men and women (27% of deaths).
- The initial manifestation of ischemic heart disease is angina pectoris in 50%, and about 50% of patients presenting to the hospital with acute coronary syndrome have preceding angina.
- Two older population-based studies from Olmstead County, MN, and Framingham, MA, showed annual rate of myocardial infarction in patients with symptomatic angina of 3 to 3.5%/yr.
- Within 12 months of initial diagnosis, 10% to 20% of patients with diagnosis of stable angina progress to MI or unstable angina.

PHYSICAL FINDINGS & CLINICAL PRESENTATION

- The assessment of chest pain should include quality, location, severity, and duration of pain; radiation; associated symptoms; provocative factors; and alleviating factors. Anginal pain can be described as "squeezing," "griplike," "suffocating," and "heavy," but it is rarely sharp or stabbing and typically does not vary with position or respiration. The classic Levine's sign is placing a clenched fist over the precordium to describe the pain. Many patients do not, however, describe angina as frank pain but as tightness, pressure, or discomfort. Other patients, in particular women and older adults, can present with atypical symptoms such as nausea, vomiting, midepigastric discomfort, sharp (atypical) chest pain, dizziness, or syncope.

- Ischemic pain of more than 20 minutes' duration should raise concern for possible acute coronary syndrome.
- Women are more likely than men to report atypical chest pain or discomfort (65% reported on Women's Ischemic Syndrome Evaluation [WISE] study).
- Elderly and diabetics may report symptoms other than chest pain, such as dyspnea, fatigue, or diaphoresis.

ETIOLOGY

RISK FACTORS:

- Advanced age.
- Male sex.
- Genetic predisposition, family history of premature coronary artery disease (CAD) in first-degree relatives (men younger than 55 yrs of age, and women younger than 65 yrs of age).
- Smoking (risk of first MI is increased by near threefold).
- Hypertension.
- Hyperlipidemia.
- Impaired glucose tolerance or diabetes mellitus.
- History of stroke or peripheral arterial disease.
- Chronic kidney disease (CKD).
- Metabolic syndrome.
- Physical inactivity.
- Obesity (body mass index >30% over ideal). A higher body mass index during childhood is also associated with an increased risk of coronary heart disease (CHD) in adulthood.
- Entities that cause increased oxygen demand include hyperthermia (particularly if accompanied by volume contraction), hyperthyroidism, and cocaine or methamphetamine abuse.
- Cocaine is used by >5 million Americans regularly and is responsible for >64,000 emergency department (ED) evaluations yearly to rule out myocardial ischemia. Cocaine causes sympathomimetic toxicity and not only increases myocardial oxygen demand but also induces coronary vasospasm and can cause infarction in young patients. Long-term cocaine use can cause premature development of SIHD.
- Severe uncontrolled hypertension causes increased myocardial oxygen demand and decreased subendocardial perfusion that increases LV wall tension. Hypertrophic cardiomyopathy and aortic stenosis can induce even more severe LV hypertrophy and resultant wall tension.
- Other causes of increased myocardial oxygen demand are ventricular or supraventricular tachycardias. Ambulatory monitoring may be required to diagnose these.
- Entities that limit myocardial oxygen supply such as anemia may cause angina when the hemoglobin drops to <9 g/dl, and ST-T-wave changes (depression or inversion) can occur at levels <7 g/dl.
- Hypoxemia resulting from pulmonary disease (e.g., pneumonia, asthma, chronic obstructive pulmonary disease, pulmonary hypertension, interstitial fibrosis, or obstructive sleep apnea) can also precipitate angina.
- Polycythemia, leukemia, thrombocytosis, and hypergammaglobulinemia.
- Oral contraceptive and HRT use.
- Coronary artery calcium is associated with an increased risk of MI.
- Long-term use of nonsteroidal antiinflammatory drugs (NSAIDs).
- Exposure to air pollution from traffic (dilute diesel exhaust) promotes myocardial ischemia and is associated with adverse cardiovascular events.
- Low serum folate levels required for conversion of homocysteine to methionine are associated with an increased risk of fatal CHD. Hyperhomocysteinemia has a toxic effect on vascular endothelium and interferes with proliferation of arterial wall smooth muscle cells. Elevated plasma homocysteine level is a strong and independent risk factor for CHD events, especially in patients with type 2 diabetes mellitus.
- Elevated levels of highly sensitive C-reactive protein (hs-CRP, cardio CRP). Diseases associated with systemic inflammation can lead to accelerated atherosclerosis.
- Depression.
- Vasculitis.
- Elevated levels of lipoprotein-associated phospholipase A_2.
- Elevated fibrinogen levels.
- Low level of red blood cell glutathione peroxidase-1 activity.
- Radiation therapy.

Dx DIAGNOSIS

DIFFERENTIAL DIAGNOSIS

- **Nonischemic Cardiovascular:** Aortic dissection, pericarditis
- **Pulmonary:** Pulmonary embolism, pneumothorax, pneumonia, pleuritis
- **Gastrointestinal:** Esophageal, esophagitis, spasm, reflux, biliary colic, cholecystitis, choledocholithiasis, cholangitis, peptic ulcer, pancreatitis
- **Chest Wall:** Costochondritis, fibrositis, rib fracture, sternoclavicular arthritis, herpes zoster (before the rash)
- **Psychiatric:** Anxiety disorders, hyperventilation, panic disorder, primary anxiety, affective disorders (i.e., depression), somatoform disorders, thought disorders (i.e., fixed delusions)

WORKUP

- In patients with chest pain, the probability of CAD should be estimated on the basis of patient age, sex, cardiovascular risk factors, and pain characteristics.
- The most important diagnostic element is the history. Chest pain or left arm pain or discomfort occurring with exertion and relieved by rest in a patient with cardiovascular risk factors is consistent with a high likelihood of CAD.
- In assessing the likelihood of underlying SIHD it is helpful to classify the chest pain as typical angina, atypical angina, and/or noncardiac chest pain.
- Typical angina, (definite) will have the following three features: (1) Substernal chest discomfort with a characteristic quality and duration, (2) provoked by exertion or emotional stress, and (3) relieved by rest and/or sublingual nitroglycerin (NTG).
- Atypical angina, (probable) will have two of the above listed three features.
- Noncardiac chest pain will have one or none of the previously listed features.
- Physical examination may be completely normal in many patients; however, certain findings may be helpful in the assessment of the patient with suspected SIHD. Some findings may identify consequences of ischemia or possible causes of the anginal syndrome other than CAD. The presence of hypertension, arcus senilis, xanthelasma, carotid or peripheral bruits, and a prominent S4 are all physical signs that could raise concern for the presence of CAD. A murmur of mitral regurgitation may be a marker of an ischemic cardiomyopathy or transient ischemia. A murmur suggestive of hypertrophic cardiomyopathy or aortic stenosis may suggest a cause of angina other than CAD.
- The ultimate goal for an SIHD patient's evaluation is to identify high-risk coronary artery disease patients with minimal use of resources. In general, four common steps would help a clinician to assess high feature of SIHD. Those are 1) CAD risk assessment based on various classical risk factors, 2) Functional capacity and stress test result, 3) LV and RV function, and 4) Coronary anatomy. Every patient does not need each of the modalities. One should classify stable angina without history of CAD patients to low, intermediate, and high pretest probability or likelihood for CAD after assessment of comorbidities. Consider functional capacity and stress test (ETT, ETT-MIBI, or Stress echo) for low and intermediate pretest probability patients. Exercise testing (Fig. 1) is preferred to pharmacologic stress tests when possible. Functional capacity and stress test results categorize SIHD patients based on their risk of annual mortality. Patients with an estimated annual mortality of <1% classify as low risk, 1-3% are considered as intermediate risk, and >3% annual mortality belongs to high-risk patient population (please see "Coronary Artery Disease chapter").

LABORATORY TESTS

- Screen for hypertension, diabetes, and hyperlipidemia per routine guidelines.
- Electrocardiogram should be obtained during pain and when the patient is free of any discomfort. A normal resting electrocardiogram is not unusual in patients with SIHD; in patients who present with chest pain, 1% to 6% who have an acute MI will have a normal or nondiagnostic electrocardiogram.
- Chest x-ray PA and lateral, if symptoms suggestive of heart failure, pericardial disease, aortic aneurysm/dissection.
- Cardio-CRP (hs-CRP): Its elevation is a relatively moderate predictor of CHD, and it adds prognostic information to that conveyed by the Framingham risk score.

EXERCISE TESTING AND IMAGING STUDIES (PLEASE SEE "CORONARY ARTERY DISEASE CHAPTER," FIG. 1)

- Exercise testing is used for diagnosis as well as prognosis of SIHD. If the patient is physically capable to perform at least moderate physical exercise, exercise stress testing (Fig. 1) is useful because of the important prognostic information obtained from exercise performance and the hemodynamic response. Patients who have an intermediate likelihood of CAD, as patients in a low-risk or high-likelihood category are more likely to have a false-positive or false-negative result, respectively. Risk assessment is also indicated in patients with SIHD who are being considered for revascularization of known coronary stenosis of unclear physiological significance.
- Stress echocardiography or stress testing with myocardial perfusion imaging may be employed when baseline electrocardiographic abnormalities are present that render the electrocardiographic response to exercise uninterpretable, such as >1 mm ST segment depression, LBBB, preexcitation, paced ventricular rhythm, digoxin treatment with ST segment changes. Stress echocardiography has the advantage of higher specificity and a lower cost. Stress radionuclide perfusion imaging has a higher sensitivity, particularly for single-vessel coronary disease, and has a higher technical success rate. When the patient is unable to exercise adequately, pharmacologic stress testing (i.e., dobutamine, adenosine, regadenoson) may be used with these imaging modalities.

STRESS TEST ALGORITHM

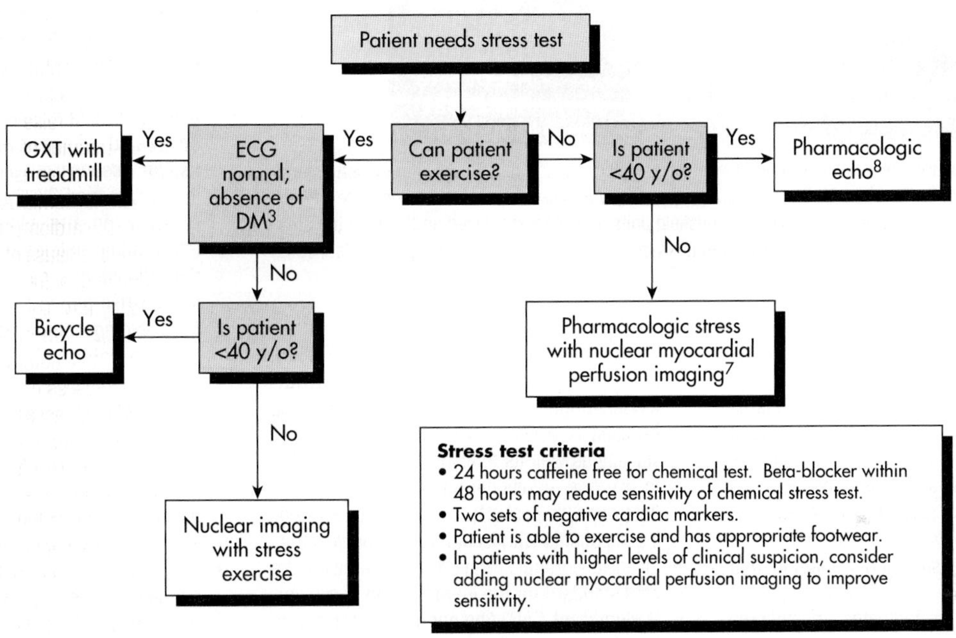
Patient needs stress test
Can patient exercise?
Yes
ECG normal; absence of DM[3]
Yes
GXT with treadmill
No
Is patient <40 y/o?
Yes
Bicycle echo
No
Nuclear imaging with stress exercise
No
Is patient <40 y/o?
Yes
Pharmacologic echo[8]
No
Pharmacologic stress with nuclear myocardial perfusion imaging[7]
Stress test criteria
• 24 hours caffeine free for chemical test. Beta-blocker within 48 hours may reduce sensitivity of chemical stress test.
• Two sets of negative cardiac markers.
• Patient is able to exercise and has appropriate footwear.
• In patients with higher levels of clinical suspicion, consider adding nuclear myocardial perfusion imaging to improve sensitivity.

DEFINITIONS:

[1]Typical angina:
1) Substernal chest pain or discomfort that is 2) provoked by exertion or emotional stress and 3) relieved by rest and/or nitroglycerin

[2]Cardiac marker timing: based on symptom onset; in cases of uncertainty assume symptom onset at ED arrival

[3]ECG normal: no significant ST depression/T wave inversions, BBB, LVH with repolarization, conduction defect, digoxin effect

[4]Anginal equivalent:
- Any symptoms that the physician feels may represent ACS
- Exertional dyspnea—most common anginal equivalent symptom

[5]ACS:
- STE-ACS—1 mm ST elevation in 2 leads
- NSTE-ACS
  - NSTEMI—positive cardiac biomarkers
  - Unstable angina—ischemia with negative biomarkers

[6]New significant ECG changes:
- ST Δs ≥ 0.5 mm; resolve when asymptomatic
- ST depression ≥1 mm in 2 leads
- T wave inversion ≥2 mm in 2 leads

[7]Regadenoson is preferred agent for chemical nuclear stress test. Technitium Tc 99m tetrofosmin is the preferred tracer.

FIG. 1 Stress test algorithm. *ACS*, Acute coronary syndrome; *BBB*, bundle branch block; *DM*, diabetes mellitus; *ECG*, electrocardiogram; echo, echocardiography; *ED*, emergency department; *GTX*, graded exercise test; *LVH*, left ventricular hypertrophy; *NSTE*, non–ST-segment elevation; *NSTEMI*, NSTE myocardial infarction; *STE*, ST-segment elevation; *y/o*, years old. (From Adams JG, et al.: *Emergency medicine: clinical essentials,* ed 2, Philadelphia, 2013, Saunders.)

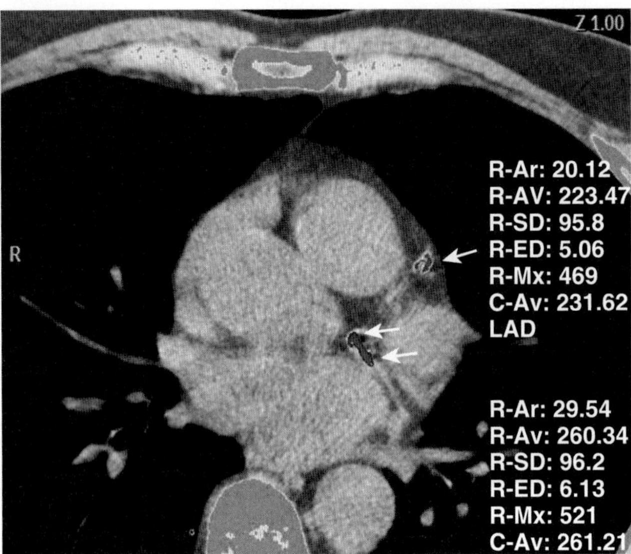

FIG. 2 Example of coronary artery calcium scoring in which calcified foci are identified within the left anterior descending (*orange; single arrow*) and left circumflex (*pink outlined in blue; double arrow*) coronary arteries. The region's area *(R-Ar)* and its average density in Hounsfield units *(R-Av)* are displayed and used in the area-density calcium scoring calculation. (From Bonow RO et al: *Heart disease*, ed 9, Philadelphia, 2012, Saunders.)

- A good predictor of risk for a patient with stable angina is the Duke treadmill score, which incorporates the patient's functional status (METS or time in minutes during the Bruce protocol), ST-segment depression in millimeters, and an angina index (yes or no). Patients with favorable Duke scores (>5) have a 5-yr survival rate of >97%; this is independent of other factors such as coronary anatomy and LV function.
- Echocardiography is indicated in patients with murmurs suggestive of aortic stenosis, hypertrophic cardiomyopathy, mitral regurgitation, mitral valve prolapse, previous MI, pathological Q waves, complex ventricular arrhythmias, heart failure, hypertension, diabetes, and abnormal EKG.
- Cardiac computed tomography (CCTA; Fig. 2) is useful for the detection of subclinical CAD in asymptomatic patients with an intermediate Framingham 10-yr risk estimate of 10% to 20%. Detects and quantifies coronary calcium and evaluates the lumen and wall of the coronary artery. CCTA can be useful as a first-line test for risk assessment in patients with SIHD who are unable to exercise to an adequate workload regardless of interpretability of ECG. Also can be used when a functional test has an indeterminate result and to assess bypass graft patency or patency of previous stents >3 mm diameter. CCTA CT cost and radiation exposure are limiting factors to recommending widespread routine use of this marker.
- Coronary artery calcium (CAC) score is a strong predictor of incidence of CAD and provides predictive information in patients with low to intermediate pretest probability of CAD beyond that provided by standard risk factors. A score below 100 indicates low risk, and a score above 400 high risk.
- Cardiac magnetic resonance imaging (CMRA), in addition to its use for diagnosis of arrhythmogenic right ventricular dysplasia, can also be used to assess myocardial perfusion and viability as well as function in patients unable to exercise. Additional studies are needed to determine the cost effectiveness of these studies in patients with ischemic cardiomyopathy.
- Invasive coronary angiography remains the gold standard for the identification of clinically significant CAD. Angiography is performed to define the location and extent of coronary disease; indicated in selected patients who are candidates for coronary revascularization (either coronary artery bypass graft [CABG] surgery or angioplasty).

Rx TREATMENT

FIVE FUNDAMENTAL OVERLAPPING STRATEGIES ARE RECOMMENDED

- Patient education: Support active participation of patients in the decision-making process of their treatment.
- Management of comorbid conditions that contribute or worsen SIHD.
- Aggressive modification of preventable risk factors such as smoking cessation, weight reduction in obese patients, regular aerobic exercise program (at least 30 to 60 min/day for 5 days a week), correction of folate deficiency, reduced intake of saturated fats (to <7% of total calories) and trans fatty acids (to <1% of total calories), low-sodium diet (<2 g/day), and teaching importance of medication adherence. Whole grains as the main form of carbohydrates, an abundance of fruits and vegetables, and adequate omega-3 fatty acids are optimal for prevention of SIHD.
- Evidence-based pharmacologic management to improve quality of life and survival.
- Use appropriate revascularization procedures to improve survival and long-term outcomes in selected patients.

PHARMACOLOGIC THERAPY (PLEASE SEE "CORONARY ARTERY DISEASE CHAPTER")

Treatment can be classified based on medications that prevent MI and death.

- Aspirin reduces cardiovascular mortality and morbidity rates by 20% to 25% among patients with CAD. Appropriate dose is 75 to 162 mg/day in the absence of contraindications. It inhibits the enzyme cyclooxygenase and synthesis of thromboxane A2 and reduces the risk of adverse cardiovascular events by 33% in patients with unstable angina. Patients intolerant to aspirin can be treated with clopidogrel or can undergo aspirin desensitization. Clopidogrel irreversibly blocks the P2Y12 adenosine diphosphate receptor on the platelet surface, thereby interrupting platelet activation and aggregation. Clopidogrel can be combined with ASA in high-risk patients with SIHD with low risk for bleeding complications or can be given alone in patients that are aspirin intolerant. Dose is 75 mg/day.
- Ticagrelor, the newest CTPT inhibitor (P2Y12 antagonist), in the PEGASUS-TIMI-54 reduced the risk of death, cardiovascular MI, or stroke in patients after 1 yr of MI. However, it is associated with an increased risk of bleeding when compared to placebo.
- Dipyridamole is not recommended as an antiplatelet therapy for the treatment of patients with SIHD.
- Beta-adrenergic blockers, which prevent MI and death, are first-line therapy in the management of angina pectoris. They achieve their major antianginal effect by decreasing myocardial oxygen demand in reducing heart rate and systolic blood pressure product, AV nodal conduction, and myocardial contractility, in this manner contributing to a reduction in angina onset, with improvement in the ischemic threshold during exercise and during the usual daily activities. Absent contraindications, they should be regarded as initial therapy for stable angina for all patients. Their dose should generally be adjusted to reduce the resting heart rate to 55 to 60 beats/min. Despite the difference among the available beta-blockers, they all seem to be equally efficacious in SIHD. Beta-blockers recommended for at least 2-3 yr after MI, and lifelong for patients with LV ejection fraction of <40% with heart failure or prior MI.
- Nitrates cause venodilation and relaxation of vascular smooth muscle; the decreased venous return from venodilation decreases diastolic ventricular wall tension (preload) and thereby reduces mechanical activity (and myocardial oxygen consumption) during systole. Relaxation of vascular smooth muscle increases coronary blood flow and reduces

systemic pressure. Dilatation of the arterial wall will not be affected by plaque, but independent of an intact endothelium, leads to reduced resistance across the obstructed lumen. Nitroglycerin contributes to coronary blood flow redistribution by augmenting collateral flow and lowering ventricular diastolic pressure from areas of normal perfusion to ischemic zones. Nitroglycerin also has demonstrated antithrombotic and antiplatelet effects. Sublingual nitroglycerin or nitroglycerin spray should be prescribed to all patients with SIHD for immediate angina relief. Tolerance to nitrates can be minimized by avoiding sustained blood levels with a daily nitrate-free period (e.g., omission of bedtime dose of oral isosorbide dinitrate or 12 hr on/12 hr off transdermal nitroglycerin therapy). Nitrates are relatively contraindicated in patients with hypertrophic obstructive cardiomyopathy, and should also be avoided in patients with severe aortic stenosis. Nitrates should not be used within 24 hr of sildenafil (Viagra) or vardenafil (Levitra) or within 48 hr of tadalafil (Cialis) because of the potential for hypotension.

- Calcium channel blockers are antiischemic medications that have no proven mortality benefit in SIHD. They improve myocardial oxygen supply by decreasing coronary vascular resistance and augmenting epicardial conduit vessel and systemic arterial blood flow. Myocardial demand is decreased by a reduction in myocardial contractility, systemic vascular resistance, and arterial pressure. They are first-line treatment when beta-blockers are contraindicated. They play a major role in preventing and terminating myocardial ischemia induced by coronary artery spasm. They are particularly effective in treating microvascular angina. All classes of calcium channel blockers reduce anginal episodes, increase exercise duration, and reduce use of sublingual nitroglycerin in patients with effort-induced angina. Short-acting calcium channel blockers should be avoided. Calcium channel blockers (particularly non-dihydropyridine) should generally also be avoided in patients with CHF secondary to systolic dysfunction due to its negative inotropic effect.
- Ranolazine, which has been tested in four different studies with a total of 1737 patients (MARISA, CARISA, RAN080, and ERICA), inhibits the late inward sodium current, indirectly reducing the sodium-dependent calcium current during ischemic conditions and leading to improvement in ventricular diastolic tension and oxygen consumption. It seems to increase the efficiency of energy production in the heart, maintaining cardiac function. Its antianginal and antiischemic effects do not depend on reductions in heart rate or blood pressure. It is indicated for treatment of chronic angina that is inadequately controlled with other antianginals. It represents a new class of drugs known as metabolic modulators and can be useful when prescribed as substitute for beta-blockers or in combination with them for relief of symptoms when initial treatment with beta-blockers is not successful or is contraindicated. Side effects include prolongation of QT interval. Low doses of diltiazem and verapamil should be used with ranolazine. The extended-release preparation reduces the frequency of angina, improves exercise performance, and delays the development of exercise-induced angina and ST-segment depression.
- Angiotensin-converting enzyme (ACE) inhibition through changes in the physiologic balance between angiotensin II and bradykinin could contribute to the reductions in LV and vascular hypertrophy, atherosclerosis progression, plaque rupture, and thrombosis; the favorable changes in cardiac hemodynamics; and the improved myocardial oxygen supply/demand. It has been shown to be effective in reducing cardiovascular death, MI, and stroke in patients who are at risk for or who had vascular disease. They are indicated in patients with hypertension, diabetes, LVEF <40%, and CKD. Angiotensin receptor blockers (ARBs) can be given to patients with SIHD who are intolerant to ACEI and qualify for them.
- Use of high-intensity statin drugs is recommended in all patients with CAD. Among patients who have recently had an acute coronary syndrome, an intensive lipid-lowering statin regimen to reduce LDL cholesterol to <70 mg/dl is a reasonable treatment objective. Statins also decrease the level of the inflammatory marker hs-CRP independently of the magnitude of change in lipid parameters. Recently, the FDA approved two PCSK9 (Proprotein convertase subtilisin/kexin type 9) inhibitors (Alirocumab and Evolocumab) for heterozygous familial hypercholesterolemia in those who maximally tolerated statins or patients with clinical atherosclerotic cardiovascular disease who require lowering of LDL levels.
- Influenza vaccine is recommended for patients with SIHD on annual basis to prevent all-cause mortality, morbidity, and hospitalization caused by the exacerbation of underlying medical conditions produced by influenza.

NEW MODALITIES FOR THE TREATMENT OF CHRONIC STABLE ANGINA PECTORIS

- Although a significant amount of progress has been made in the management of CAD with percutaneous coronary intervention (PCI) and CABG, many patients with the condition require additional therapeutic modalities for relief of symptoms and improvement in quality of life. This group of patients includes those with diffuse CAD who are not suitable for revascularization, patients with previous multiple PCIs or CABG limiting the chances for further revascularization, the lack of vascular conduits for CABG, severe left ventricular systolic dysfunction in patients with previous CABG or PCI, and comorbidities that would render the patients at high risk for revascularization.
- The following pharmacologic agents have been used for the management of stable angina in combination with the standard protocol of nitrates, beta-blockers, calcium channel blockers, and ranolazine: high-dose statin therapy, trimetazidine, perhexiline, nicorandil, allopurinol, ivabradine, fasudil, and testosterone.
- Other, nonpharmacologic modalities that are highly experimental include stem cell therapy, therapeutic angiogenesis, and mechanical therapies like external counterpulsation, spinal cord stimulation, transmyocardial laser revascularization, and coronary sinus reducing device.
- In TACT (Trial to Assess Chelation Therapy), Ethylenediaminetetraacetic acid (EDTA) intravenous infusion resulted significant decrease in total mortality, recurrent MI, stroke, coronary revascularization, or hospitalization for angina. Thus chelation therapy was upgraded from Class III (not recommended) to Class IIb in the 2014 SIHD guidelines. Allopurinol, a xanthine oxidase inhibitor, was shown to reduce myocardial oxygen demand per unit of cardiac output in patients with heart failure in a small crossover study of 65 patients given 600 mg of allopurinol daily for 6 weeks. Allopurinol increased the median time to ST depression from 232 seconds at baseline to 393 seconds. Further and larger studies are necessary to recommend allopurinol as an adjunctive therapy for stable angina.
- Testosterone improves endothelial dysfunction and may be an effective antiangina agent. However, given the potential side effects, additional trials are necessary to recommend testosterone as an adjunctive drug for chronic angina.

The value of enhanced external counterpulsation, or EECP, was assessed with the MUST-EECP trial, which randomly assigned 139 outpatients with angina, documented CAD, and a positive stress test to 35 hours of active EECP. The results indicated the following regarding EECP: (1) was well tolerated; (2) exercise duration increased in both groups; (3) active EECP patients had a significant increase in time to 1-mm ST-segment depression, while there was no change in the inactive group; (4) more patients undergoing active EECP had a decrease in angina episodes, and fewer had an increase in angina symptoms compared with the active group. These data corroborate similar data from multicenter registries. The American Heart Association, American College of Cardiology, Society for Cardiovascular Angiography and Interventions, American Thoracic Society, and Society of Thoracic Surgeons focused update states that EECP may be considered for relief of refractory angina.

The following treatments have NOT been shown to be beneficial in reducing cardiovascular risk or improving clinical outcomes: estrogen therapy, vitamin C, vitamin E, and beta-carotene supplementation; treatment of elevated homocysteine with folate or vitamins B_6 and B_{12}; chelation therapy; garlic; coenzyme Q10; selenium; and chromium.

REFERRAL

Revascularization:

- Revascularization methods should be formulated taking into consideration improved survival or improved symptoms. Revascularization includes either percutaneous coronary intervention (balloon angioplasty and stenting) or CABG. However, note that although the role of PCI is unquestionable in the presence of an acute myocardial infarction, its role is not so clear in stable CAD. The utilization of PCI for stable CAD was reduced by 51.7% from 2007 to 2011, and hospitals with higher volumes of PCI had the largest reduction of these procedures.
- **To improve survival**:
  1. Perform CABG for patients with significant (>50% diameter stenosis) left main coronary artery stenosis, more than 70% diameter stenosis in proximal left anterior descending artery (LAD), or more than 70% diameter stenosis in three major epicardial vessels, >70% diameter stenosis in two major coronary arteries with severe or extensive myocardial ischemia, and in patients with mild to moderate LV systolic dysfunction (EF 35% to 50%) and significant multivessel CAD. Left internal mammary artery (LIMA) graft improves survival when used to bypass a proximal LAD artery stenosis. CABG is recommended in preference to PCI to improve survival in patients with multivessel CAD and diabetes, particularly if a LIMA graft to LAD is used.
  2. PCI is reasonable as an alternative to CABG in selected stable patients (low or intermediate SYNTAX score and[or] high STS score) with unprotected left main CAD, low risk of PCI procedural complications, and a high likelihood of good long-term outcome *and* clinical characteristics that predict a significantly increased risk of adverse surgical outcomes (e.g., STS-predicted risk of operative mortality >5).
- **To improve symptoms:**
  1. CABG or PCI to improve symptoms is beneficial in patients with one or more significant (>70% diameter) coronary artery stenosis amenable to revascularization and unacceptable angina despite maximal medical treatment, or in whom increasing medical therapy cannot be implemented because of medication contraindications, adverse effects, or patient preferences. In 2017, ORBITA trial showed no significant improvement in angina score after PCI for optimally treated stable angina patients. However, 85% of study patients in placebo group underwent PCI within 6 weeks after ORBITA trial completed.
  2. Hybrid coronary revascularization: LIMA-to-LAD artery grafting and of >1 non-LAD coronary artery can be used in patients who have an unfavorable aorta, have poor target vessels for CABG, have unsuitable graft conduits, or have unfavorable LAD for PCI.
- Compared with percutaneous coronary intervention (PCI), CABG is more effective in relieving angina and leads to fewer repeated revascularizations but has a higher risk for procedural stroke. Survival to 10 yrs is similar for both procedures.
- Angioplasty and coronary stents (Fig. E3).
- PCI has an established place in treating angina but is not superior to intensive medical therapy to prevent MI and death in symptomatic or asymptomatic patients. Patients selected for PCI should also be candidates for CABG. Approximately 80% of patients show immediate benefit after PCI. The development of coronary stents has increased the number of patients who can be treated in the cardiac laboratory. Cardiac stents (Fig. E4) are currently used in nearly 95% of all patients with PCI lesions. The rate of restenosis is reduced by placing a stent electively in primary atheromatous lesions. The major limitations of stenting are subacute thrombosis, restenosis within the stent, bleeding complications when antiplatelets are used after stenting, and higher cost. The combination of aspirin and P2Y12 antagonists is effective in preventing coronary stent thrombosis and the duration of therapy depends on whether bare metal stents (BMS) or drug-eluting stents (DES) are used. Duration of dual antiplatelet therapy can be as short as 4 weeks for BMS, but 6 to 12 months of therapy is generally required for DES. This difference in duration is due to the lack of endothelium proliferation in DES initially. New drug-eluting stents with thin struts releasing Limus-family analogs from durable polymers have lowered the risk of stent thrombosis compared with early-generation stents releasing sirolimus or paclitaxel. Current evidence supports the use of drug-eluting stents in most clinical settings without safety concerns (unless there are contraindications to use of dual antiplatelet therapy).

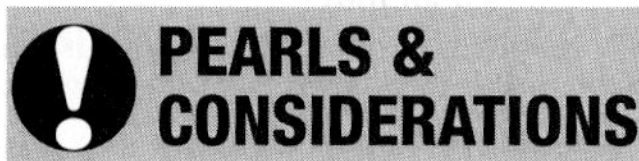

PEARLS & CONSIDERATIONS

COMMENTS

- Although nitrate responsiveness is usually an integral part of a diagnostic strategy for SIHD, recent reports question its value and conclude that in a general population admitted for chest pain, relief of pain after nitroglycerin treatment does not predict active CAD and should not be used to guide diagnosis in the acute care setting.
- CABG is associated with higher long-term survival rates and lower rates of repeat revascularization than PCI and stenting; however, patients often prefer stenting because it is less invasive, involves a shorter hospital stay, and has a lower in-hospital mortality rate.

SUGGESTED READINGS

Available at: ExpertConsult.com

RELATED CONTENT

Angina (Patient Information)
Unstable Angina (Patient Information)
Acute Coronary Syndrome (Related Key Topic)
Coronary Artery Disease (Related Key Topic)
Myocardial Infarction (Related Key Topic)

AUTHOR: **MAHESWARA SATYA GANGADHARA RAO GOLLA, M.D.**

BASIC INFORMATION

DEFINITION

- The mucocutaneous swelling caused by the release of vasoactive mediators is called urticaria and angioedema.
- Urticaria causes edema of the superficial dermis.
- Angioedema involves the deep layers of the dermis and the subcutaneous tissue.

SYNONYMS

Angioneurotic edema
HAE (hereditary angioedema)

ICD-10CM CODES
T78.3 Angioedema
D84.1 Angioedema, hereditary

EPIDEMIOLOGY & DEMOGRAPHICS

INCIDENCE: 100 to 3000/100,000 persons (for urticaria and angioedema)

LIFETIME PREVALENCE: Approximately 20% of the population experiences urticaria and/or angioedema at some time during life. The prevalence of hereditary angioedema is 1 case per 50,000 persons.

DEMOGRAPHICS:

- Race: Slightly more common among African Americans.
- Sex: More occurrences in women than men.
- Angioedema commonly occurs after adolescence in the third decade of life.
- Angioedema can occur together with urticaria (40%) or alone (20%); the remaining 40% have urticaria alone.

PHYSICAL FINDINGS & CLINICAL PRESENTATION

- Angioedema may be acute or chronic.
  1. Acute angioedema is defined as symptoms lasting 6 wk.
  2. Chronic angioedema is defined as symptoms lasting >6 wk.
- Urticaria is commonly known as "hives" and is:
  1. Pruritic
  2. Palpable and well demarcated
  3. Erythematous
  4. Millimeters to centimeters in size
  5. Multiple in number
  6. Fades within 12 to 24 hr
  7. Reappears at other sites
- Angioedema is characterized by the following:
  1. Nonpruritic
  2. Burning
  3. Not well demarcated
  4. Involves eyelids, lips (Fig. 1), tongue, and extremities
  5. Can involve the upper airway, causing respiratory distress
  6. Can involve the gastrointestinal tract, leading to cyclic abdominal pain, nausea, vomiting, and diarrhea
  7. Resolves slowly

ETIOLOGY

- Angioedema, with or without urticaria, is classified as acquired (allergic or idiopathic) or hereditary.
- Angioedema is primarily caused by mast cell activation and degranulation with release of vasoactive mediators (e.g., histamine, serotonin, bradykinins), resulting in postcapillary venule inflammation, vascular leakage, and edema in the deep layers of the dermis and subcutaneous tissue.
- Pathologically, angioedema has both immunologic- and nonimmunologic-mediated mechanisms (Fig. 2).
  1. Immunoglobulin E–mediated angioedema may result from antigen exposure (e.g., foods [milk, eggs, peanuts, shellfish, tomatoes, chocolate, sulfites] or drugs [penicillin, aspirin, nonsteroidal antiinflammatory drugs, phenytoin, sulfonamides, recombinant tissue plasminogen activator]).
  2. Complement-mediated angioedema involving immune complex mechanisms can also lead to mast cell activation that manifests as serum sickness.
  3. Hereditary angioedema is an autosomal-dominant disease caused by a deficiency of or mutation in C1 esterase inhibitor (C1-INH). C1-INH is a protease inhibitor normally present in high concentrations in the plasma. C1-INH serves many functions, one of which is to inhibit plasma kallikrein, a protease that cleaves kininogen and releases bradykinin. Deficient C1-INH activity results in excess concentration of kininogen and the subsequent release of kinin mediators.
  4. Acquired angioedema is usually associated with other diseases, most commonly B-cell lymphoproliferative disorders, but may also result from the formation of autoantibodies directed against C1 inhibitor protein.
  5. Other causes of angioedema include infection (e.g., herpes simplex, hepatitis B, Coxsackie A and B, *Streptococcus, Candida, Ascaris,* and *Strongyloides*), insect bites and stings, stress, physical factors (e.g., cold, exercise, pressure, and vibration), connective tissue diseases (e.g., systemic lupus erythematosus, Henoch-Schönlein purpura), and idiopathic causes. Angiotensin-converting enzyme (ACE) inhibitors can increase kinin activity and lead to angioedema.

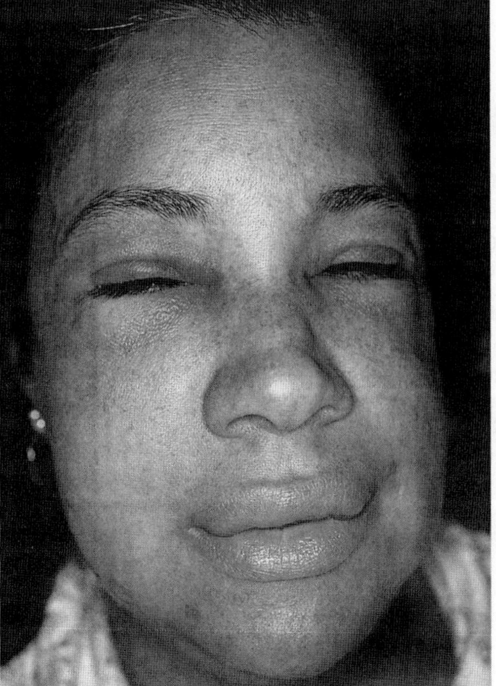

FIG. 1 Angioedema. The swelling is deeper than wheals and may affect mucosal surfaces. Note the swelling of the lips and periorbital region and the lack of erythema. (From Bolognia J, et al.: *Dermatology,* ed 4, London, 2018, Elsevier Limited.)

DIAGNOSIS

A detailed history and physical examination usually establish the diagnosis of angioedema. Extensive laboratory testing is of limited value.

DIFFERENTIAL DIAGNOSIS

- Cellulitis
- Arthropod bite
- Hypothyroidism
- Contact dermatitis
- Atopic dermatitis
- Mastocytosis
- Granulomatous cheilitis
- Bullous pemphigoid
- Urticaria pigmentosa
- Anaphylaxis
- Erythema multiforme
- Epiglottitis
- Peritonsillar abscess

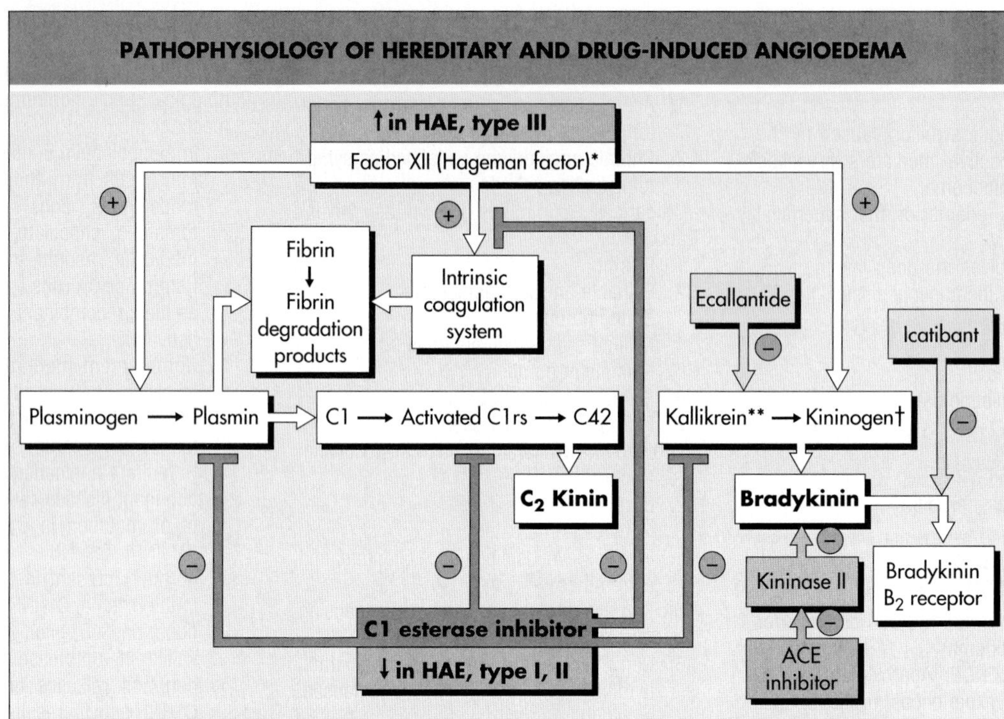

FIG. 2 Pathophysiology of hereditary and drug-induced angioedema. Angiotensin-converting enzyme (ACE) inhibitor-induced urticaria is believed to result from the inhibition of endogenous kininase and a subsequent increase in bradykinin. Icatibant and ecallantide have been approved for the emergency treatment of hereditary angioedema *(HAE)* as alternatives to C1 esterase inhibitor (C1-INH) concentrate (derived from human plasma) or recombinant C1-INH (derived from milk of transgenic rabbits). Icatibant, a decapeptide, is a specific bradykinin B2 receptor antagonist. Ecallantide, a 60-amino acid recombinant protein, selectively inhibits kallikrein. Off label, icatibant has been used to treat ACE inhibitor-induced angioedema. Two forms of C1-INH, one of which is administered intravenously and the other subcutaneously, are approved for prevention of attacks. At the time of writing, twice-monthly administration of lanadelumab, a human monoclonal antibody that inhibits plasma kallikrein, is under investigation for prevention of attacks. *The active form of factor XII (Hageman factor) is XIIa. **Kallikrein is formed from prekallikrein. †High-molecular-weight. (From Bolognia J, et al.: *Dermatology,* ed 4, London, 2018, Elsevier Limited.)

WORKUP

- An extensive workup searching for the cause of angioedema is often unrevealing (90%).
- Workup, including diagnostic blood tests and allergy testing, is performed according to results of the history and physical examination. Fig. 3 illustrates an algorithm for the diagnosis of angioedema.

LABORATORY TESTS

- Complete blood count, erythrocyte sedimentation rate, and urinalysis are sometimes helpful as part of the initial evaluation.
- Stools for ova and parasites.
- Serology testing.
- C4 levels are usually reduced in acquired and hereditary angioedema (occurring without urticaria). If C4 levels are low, C1-INH levels and activity should be obtained. There are isolated reports of hereditary angioedema with normal C4 levels but reduced C1-INH levels.
- Skin and radioallergosorbent testing may be done if food allergies are suspected.
- Skin biopsy is usually done in patients with chronic angioedema refractory to corticosteroid treatment.

Rx TREATMENT

NONPHARMACOLOGIC THERAPY

- Eliminate the offending agent
- Avoid triggering factors (e.g., cold, stress)
- Cold compresses to affected areas

ACUTE GENERAL Rx

- Acute life-threatening angioedema involving the larynx is treated with:
  1. Epinephrine 0.3 mg in a solution of 1:1000 given SC
  2. Diphenhydramine 25 to 50 mg IV or IM
  3. Cimetidine 300 mg IV or ranitidine 50 mg IV
  4. Methylprednisolone 125 mg IV
- Mainstay therapy in nonhereditary angioedema is H_1 antihistamines:
  1. Diphenhydramine 25 to 50 mg q6h
  2. Chlorpheniramine 4 mg q6h
  3. Hydroxyzine 10 to 25 mg q6h
  4. Cetirizine 5 to 10 mg qd
  5. Loratadine 10 mg qd
  6. Fexofenadine 60 mg qd
- H_2 antihistamines can be added to H_1 antihistamines:
  1. Ranitidine 150 mg bid
  2. Cimetidine 400 mg bid
  3. Famotidine 20 mg bid
- Tricyclic antidepressants:
  1. Doxepin 25 to 50 mg qd
- Corticosteroids are rarely required for symptomatic relief of acute angioedema.
- Antihistamines are probably ineffective in acute hereditary angioedema.
- Purified plasma-derived C1-INH replacement therapy is effective and safe in treating acute attacks of hereditary angioedema caused by C1 inhibitor deficiency. Cost is a limiting factor. Acute attacks can be managed with plasma-derived or recombinant preparations of C1 inhibitor, with ecallantide, a specific plasma kallikrein inhibitor, or with the use of the B2 bradykinin-receptor antagonist icatibant.

CHRONIC Rx

- Chronic angioedema is treated as described under "Acute General Rx." Corticosteroids are used more often in chronic nonhereditary angioedema.

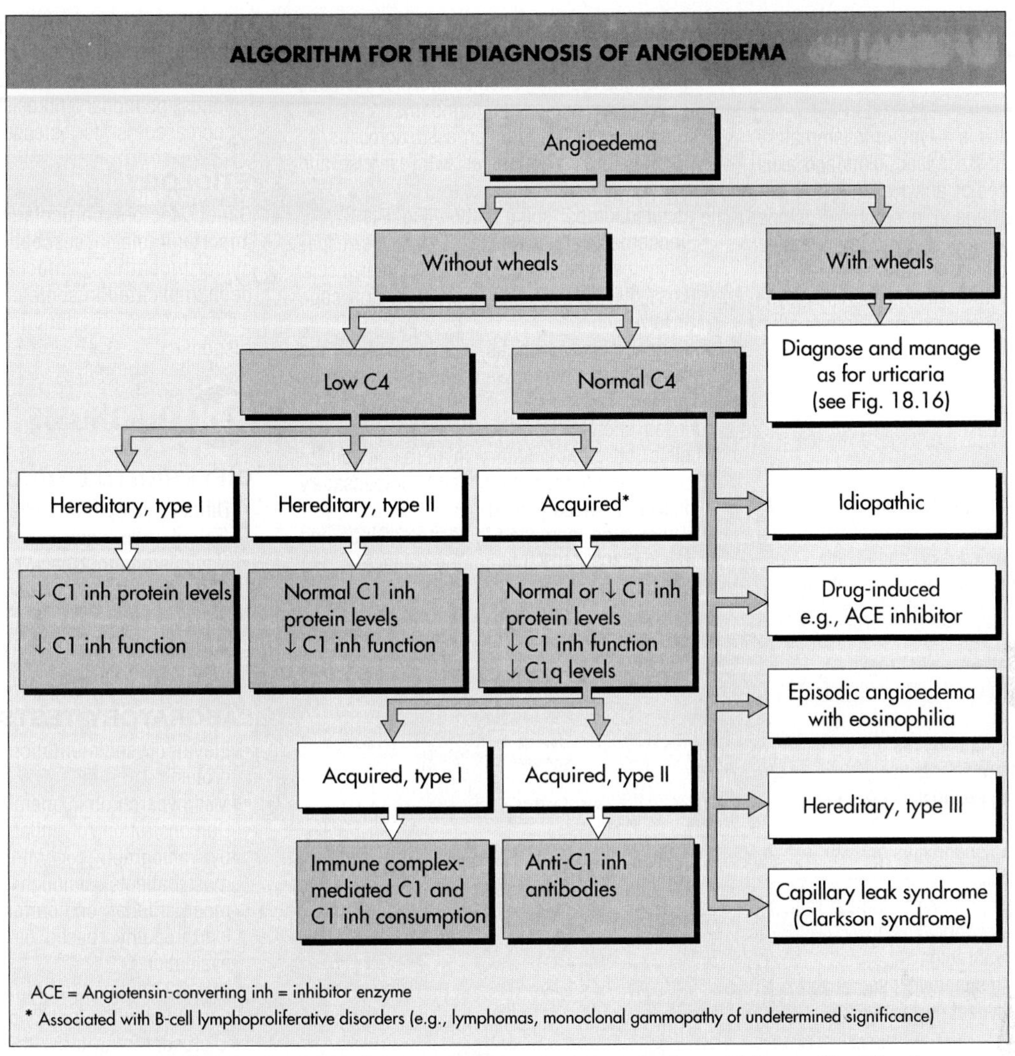

FIG. 3 Algorithm for the diagnosis of angioedema. Episodic angioedema with hypereosinophilia, along with weight gain and fever, is known as Gleich syndrome. (From Bolognia J, et al.: *Dermatology,* ed 4, London, 2018, Elsevier Limited.)

- Prednisone 1 mg/kg/day for 5 days and then tapered over a period of weeks.
- Androgens (danazol, stanozolol, oxandrolone, methyltestosterone) and antifibrinolytic agents can be used for the treatment of chronic hereditary angioedema, which does not respond to antihistamines or corticosteroids but these agents are associated with many adverse effects.
- Long-term prophylaxis with intravenous plasma-derived C1 inhibitors (Cinryze, Berinert) are safe and effective and may be used in patients who have frequent or severe attacks. Cost can be a limiting factor. A twice-weekly subcutaneous formulation (Haegarda/CSL830, CSL Behring) is approved by the FDA to treat type I and type II hereditary angioedema. Icatibant is a bradykinin-receptor antagonist effective in hereditary angioedema. Lanadelumab is a kallikrein inhibitor shown in preliminary studies to reduce attack frequency, although it is not yet FDA approved.

DISPOSITION

- Antihistamines achieve symptomatic relief in more than 80% of patients with nonhereditary acute angioedema.
- In chronic nonhereditary angioedema, corticosteroids are given in addition to antihistamines.
- A small percentage of people will have recurrence of symptoms after steroid treatment.
- Chronic angioedema can last for months and even yrs.

REFERRAL

Consultation with dermatologist and allergist is recommended in patients with chronic angioedema, hereditary angioedema, and recurring angioedema.

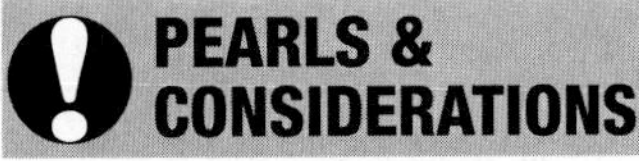

PEARLS & CONSIDERATIONS

ACE inhibitors can cause angioedema up to many months after initiation. There are multiple case reports and case series of angiotensin receptor blocker (ARB)–induced angioedema, although the risk is substantially less than that of ACE inhibitors. (Incidence rates per 1000 person-yrs are 4.38 cases for ACE inhibitors, 1.66 cases for ARBs.) The incidence rate is also very high for the direct renin inhibitor aliskiren (4.67).

COMMENTS

- Identifying a cause for angioedema in patients is often difficult and met with frustration.
- Chronic angioedema, unlike acute angioedema, is rarely caused by an allergic reaction.

SUGGESTED READINGS

Available at: ExpertConsult.com

RELATED CONTENT

Angioedema (Patient Information)

AUTHOR: **FRED F. FERRI, M.D.**

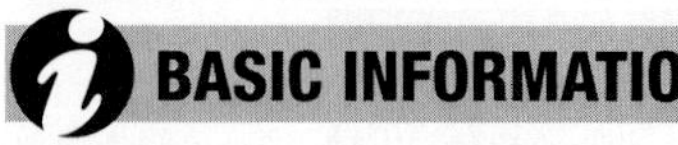

BASIC INFORMATION

DEFINITION

Ankylosing spondylitis is a type of inflammatory arthritis involving the sacroiliac joints and axial skeleton characterized by ankylosis and enthesitis (inflammation at tendon insertions). It is one of a family of overlapping syndromes called seronegative spondyloarthropathies (SpA) that includes reactive arthritis (formerly Reiter syndrome), psoriatic spondylitis, and enteropathic arthritis (Table 1).

SYNONYM

Marie-Strümpell disease

ICD-10CM CODES

M45.9	Ankylosing spondylitis of unspecified sites in spine
M08.1	Juvenile ankylosing spondylitis
M45.0	Ankylosing spondylitis of multiple sites in spine
M45.1	Ankylosing spondylitis of occipito-atlanto-axial region
M45.2	Ankylosing spondylitis of cervical region
M45.3	Ankylosing spondylitis of cervicothoracic region
M45.4	Ankylosing spondylitis of thoracic region
M45.5	Ankylosing spondylitis of thoracolumbar region
M45.6	Ankylosing spondylitis lumbar region
M45.7	Ankylosing spondylitis of lumbosacral region
M45.8	Ankylosing spondylitis sacral and sacrococcygeal region

EPIDEMIOLOGY & DEMOGRAPHICS

PREVALENCE: Between 0.1% and 1% of the population. Varies with prevalence of HLA-B27. Much higher in those with positive family history of spondyloarthropathy.

PREDOMINANT AGE AT ONSET: 15 to 35 yr

PREDOMINANT SEX: Male:female ratio 2 to 3:1

PHYSICAL FINDINGS & CLINICAL PRESENTATION

- Prolonged morning back stiffness of insidious onset lasting more than 3 months
- Bilateral sacroiliac tenderness (sacroiliitis)
- Back pain often improves with exercise and is worse with rest
- Limited lumbar spine motion (Fig. E1)
- Tenderness at tendon insertion sites, especially the Achilles tendons and plantar fascia
- Loss of chest expansion reflecting rib cage involvement
- Peripheral joint arthritis, usually involving the large joints of the lower extremities, may be present
- In advanced cases the typical posture consists of compensatory hyperextension of neck, fixed flexion of hips, and compensatory flexion of knees (Fig. 2)
- There is an increased incidence of iritis and uveitis (30%-40% lifetime prevalence)

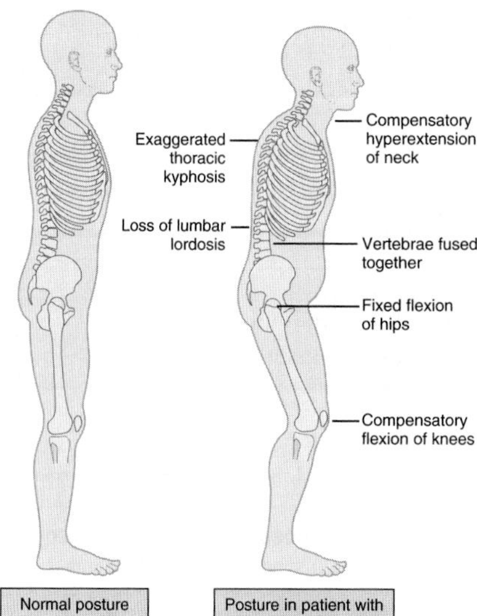

FIG. 2 Ankylosing spondylitis. Typical posture in advanced cases compared with normal posture. (From Ballinger A: *Kumar & Clark's essentials of clinical medicine,* ed 6, Edinburgh, 2012, Saunders.)

TABLE 1 Comparison of Ankylosing Spondylitis and Related Disorders

Feature	Ankylosing Spondylitis	Psoriatic Arthritis	Reactive Arthritis	Enteropathic Arthropathy
Gender (male:female)	2-3:1	1:1	1:1	1:1
Age at onset	<40 yr	35-55 yr	20-40 yr	Any age
Sacroiliitis or spondylitis (%)	100	~20	~40	<20
Symmetry of sacroiliitis	Symmetrical	Asymmetrical	Asymmetrical	Symmetrical
Peripheral arthritis (%)	~25	95	90	5-20
Distribution	Axial and lower limbs	Variable	Lower limbs	Variable
HLA-B27 positivity (%)	85-95	25-60*	30-70	7-70†
Uveitis	0-40	~20	~50	<15

HLA-B27, Human leukocyte antigen B27.
*60% when spondylitis is present.
†70% when spondylitis is present.
From Hochberg M, et al.: *Rheumatology,* ed 7, Elsevier, 2019, Table 121.2.

- Other extraskeletal manifestations include effects on the cardiovascular system (aortic insufficiency and cardiovascular disease) and lungs (pulmonary fibrosis). There is also an increased risk for osteoporosis

ETIOLOGY

Genetic factors, particularly *HLA-B27,* play an important role in susceptibility to the spondyloarthropathies. Infectious triggers have been implicated in some cases. Tumor necrosis factor is important in the inflammatory response.

Dx DIAGNOSIS

DIFFERENTIAL DIAGNOSIS

- Diffuse idiopathic skeletal hyperostosis (Forestier disease)
- Noninflammatory back pain (a clinical algorithm for the evaluation of back pain is described in Section III)
- Table 1 compares ankylosing spondylitis and related disorders

LABORATORY TESTS

- Elevated sedimentation rate, C-reactive protein
- Mild hyperchromic anemia
- Demonstration of inflammatory sacroiliitis by radiography or MRI is diagnostic for most patients, although some patients may meet criteria for "preradiographic spondyloarthropathy" based on compelling clinical evaluation
- HLA-B27 antigen is not useful in the evaluation of noninflammatory back pain because it is present in up to 8% to 10% of the normal population

IMAGING STUDIES

- Classic features are those of bilateral sacroiliitis on radiographs of the pelvis.
- Vertebral bodies lose anterior concave shape and become square.
- With progression, calcification of the annulus fibrosus and paravertebral ligaments develops, giving rise to the so-called *bamboo spine* and a "trolley track" appearance (Fig. 3).
- MRI (Fig. E4) may be useful in detecting early inflammatory lesions and is especially helpful when the history is suggestive but radiographs are equivocal.

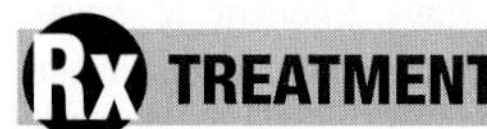

TREATMENT

NONPHARMACOLOGIC THERAPY

- Exercises primarily to maintain flexibility and aerobic activity are important.
- Postural training:
    1. Patients must be instructed on spinal extension exercises to avoid fusion in a flexed position.
    2. Sleeping should be in the supine position on a firm mattress; pillows should not be placed under the head or knees.

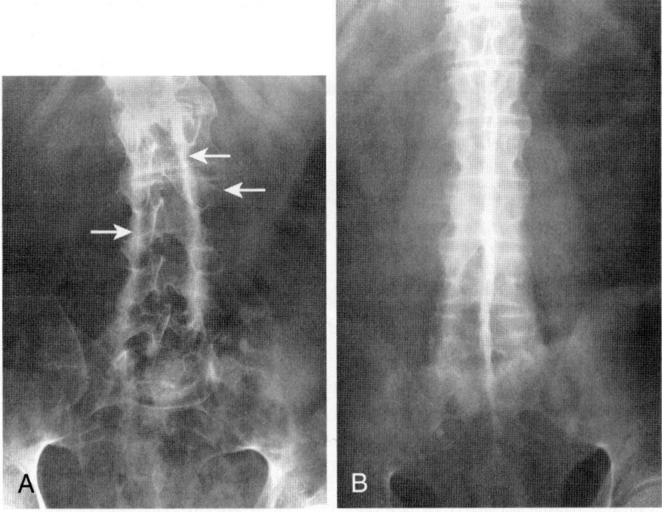

FIG. 3 Ankylosing spondylitis. A, Fusion of the facet joints and ossification of the adjacent soft tissue have produced a "trolley track" appearance *(arrows).* The sacroiliac joints are fused, and syndesmophytes are present. **B,** In another patient, there is a prominent fusion of the interspinous ligaments producing a "saber sheath" appearance. (From Harris ED: *Kelley's textbook of rheumatology,* ed 7, Philadelphia, 2005, Saunders.)

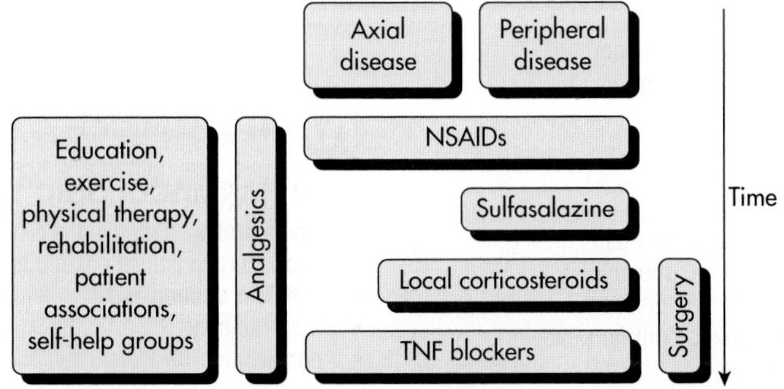

FIG. 5 ASAS/EULAR recommendations for the management of AS. *AS,* ankylosing spondylitis; *ASAS,* The Assessment of SpondyloArthritis international Society; *EULAR,* The European League Against Rheumatism; *TNF,* tumor necrosis factor. (From van der Linden et al: Ankylosing Spondylitis. In Firestein G, et al. (eds): *Kelley & Firestein's textbook of rheumatology,* ed 10, Philadelphia, 2017, Elsevier, Table 75-3, pp 1271.)

PHARMACOLOGIC THERAPY

- NSAIDs: Patients with ankylosing spondylitis should be prescribed full-dose continuous NSAID therapy. There is anecdotal evidence suggesting that indomethacin may be more effective than other NSAIDs, but other NSAIDs are efficacious and may be better tolerated. One study suggested that continuous NSAID therapy may retard the radiographic progression of ankylosing spondylitis, but conflicting data have been published.
- Sulfasalazine may be efficacious in some patients, especially for peripheral arthritis.
- Tumor necrosis factor (TNF) antagonists such as etanercept, infliximab, and adalimumab have been shown to be very effective for relieving symptoms of spinal inflammatory arthritis in numerous controlled studies. Anti-TNF therapy should be recommended for patients whose symptoms are not completely controlled with NSAIDs, and it sometimes results in dramatic improvement in symptoms, range of motion of the spine, and quality of life for these patients. There is evidence suggesting that anti-TNF therapy slows the radiographic progression of the disease.
- Secukinumab, an anti-interleukin-17A monoclonal antibody, has been approved for treatment of ankylosing spondylitis, but its role has yet to be defined.
- Fig. 5 shows American College of Rheumatology (ACR)/The European League Against Rheumatism (EULAR) recommendations for management.

DISPOSITION

Most patients have a normal life span but many suffer significant disability from loss of spinal mobility.

REFERRAL

All patients with seronegative spondyloarthropathy should be referred to a rheumatologist for consideration of anti-TNF therapy.

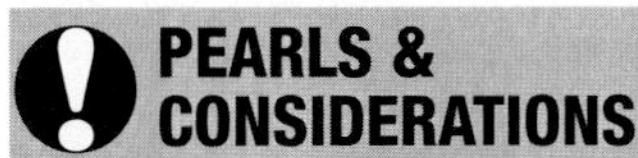

PEARLS & CONSIDERATIONS

A family history of seronegative spondyloarthropathy increases the specificity of testing for HLA-B27. Surgical osteotomy may benefit selected patients with severe spinal deformity. Recent data suggest that men with AS have increased risk of vascular mortality.

SUGGESTED READINGS

Available at ExpertConsult.com

RELATED CONTENT

Ankylosing Spondylitis (Patient Information)

AUTHOR: **BERNARD ZIMMERMANN, M.D.**

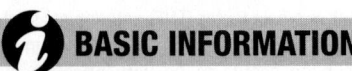

DEFINITION

Abnormal narrowing of the anal canal. Anorectal strictures can be classified based on severity and location (Table 1).

SYNONYMS

Anal stenosis
Küss disease

ICD-10CM CODE

K62.4 Stenosis of anus and rectum

EPIDEMIOLOGY & DEMOGRAPHICS

INCIDENCE: 5%-10% of post-radical hemorrhoidectomy surgeries
RISK FACTORS: Previous anorectal surgery, inflammatory bowel disease, prior radiation

PHYSICAL FINDINGS & CLINICAL PRESENTATION

- History
  1. Most common symptom is pain with defecation
  2. Patients also may report bleeding, narrowing of stools, constipation, fecal incontinence, tenesmus, and urgency
  3. Important to ask about past surgeries, specifically anorectal and any Crohn disease or perianal trauma
- Physical Exam
  1. Visual inspection of the anus which may demonstrate skin tags or chronic fissures
  2. Digital rectal exam which will demonstrate a narrowed anal canal that is difficult to pass a lubricated finger through
  3. In severe cases, exam under anesthesia may be required

ETIOLOGY

- Congenital malformation
- Fibrosis of anoderm or distal rectal mucosa due to a surgical procedure
  1. Hemorrhoidectomy
  2. Low anterior resection
  3. Ileal pouch-anal anastomosis
  4. Anopexy
  5. Excision of perianal skin lesion
- Anal canal muscle hypertrophy
- Anal canal muscle spasm (anismus) secondary to anal fissure
- Neoplasia
  1. Bowen's disease
  2. Paget's disease
  3. Anal squamous cell carcinoma
  4. Rectal adenocarcinoma
  5. Condyloma acuminata

TABLE 1 Classification of Anorectal Stricture

Severity	Location
Mild: Stricture present, but allows passage of well-lubricated finger or medium Hill-Ferguson retractor	**Low:** At least 0.5 cm distal to the dentate line
Moderate: Passage of well-lubricated finger or medium Hill-Ferguson retractor only with forceful dilation	**Middle:** 0.5 cm on either side of the dentate line
Severe: No passage of well-lubricated finger or medium Hill-Ferguson retractor	**High:** At least 0.5 cm proximal to the dentate line

Adapted from Liberman H, Thorson AG. How I do it. Anal stenosis. *Am J Surg* 179:325-329, 2000. In Cameron JL, Cameron AM: *Current surgical therapy,* ed 12, Philadelphia, 2017, Elsevier.

- Inflammation
  1. Anal fissure
  2. Crohn's disease
  3. Tuberculosis
  4. Actinomycosis
  5. Lymphogranuloma venereum
  6. Chronic suppuration
- Trauma
  1. Radiation therapy
  2. Perineal burns
  3. Hot water enemas
  4. Ibuprofen suppositories
  5. Chronic laxative abuse
- Sexually transmitted disease
- Box 1 summarizes common causes of anorectal strictures

DIAGNOSIS

DIFFERENTIAL DIAGNOSIS

- Anorectal stricture/stenosis
- Neoplasm
- Inflammatory bowel disease
- Trauma

WORKUP

- Hydration, fiber supplementation, and stool softeners should be started in all patients regardless of ultimate etiology.
- Suspicious lesions should be biopsied.

LABORATORY TESTS

None

IMAGING STUDIES

None

BOX 1 Cause of Anorectal Stricture

Surgical Procedures
Hemorrhoidectomy
Low anterior resection
Ileal pouch-anal anastomosis
Anopexy
Excision of perianal skin lesions

Neoplastic
Bowen disease
Paget disease
Anal squamous cell carcinoma
Rectal adenocarcinoma
Condyloma acuminata

Inflammatory
Anal fistula
Crohn disease
Tuberculosis
Actinomycosis
Lymphogranuloma venereum

Trauma
Radiation therapy
Perineal burns
Hot water enemas
Ibuprofen suppositories
Chronic laxative abuse

From Cameron JL, Cameron AM: *Current surgical therapy,* ed 12, Philadelphia, 2017, Elsevier.

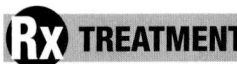

NONPHARMACOLOGIC THERAPY

- Manual dilation started in the clinic or operating room and is continued on an outpatient basis
- Resection of neoplasm
- Stricturoplasty
- Anoplasty

CHRONIC Rx

For mild disease, stool softeners, fiber supplementation, and dietary modification are all that is necessary.

COMPLEMENTARY AND ALTERNATIVE MEDICINE

None

DISPOSITION

Mild strictures can be treated on an outpatient basis in clinic; moderate to severe strictures require colorectal surgical evaluation.

REFERRAL

Referral is indicated when there is concern for neoplasm, patient fails conservative medical management, or if the provider is unable to pass a lubricated finger into the rectum.

AUTHORS: **DANIEL C. NEUBAUER, M.D,** and **MARK F. BRADY, M.D., M.P.H., M.M.S.**

BASIC INFORMATION

DEFINITION

Anorexia nervosa is a psychiatric disorder characterized by abnormal eating behavior, severe self-induced weight loss, and a specific psychopathology (see "Workup").

ICD-10CM CODES

F50.00	Anorexia nervosa, unspecified
F50.01	Restricting type
F50.02	Binge-eating/purging type

EPIDEMIOLOGY & DEMOGRAPHICS

INCIDENCE/PREVALENCE (IN U.S.):

- Anorexia nervosa occurs in 0.2% to 1.3% of the general population, with an annual incidence of 5 to 10 cases per 100,000 persons.
- Participation in activities that promote thinness (athletics, modeling) is associated with a higher incidence of anorexia nervosa.

PREDOMINANT SEX: Female/male ratio is 9:1. Approximately 0.5% to 1% of women between the ages of 15 and 30 yr have anorexia nervosa.

PREDOMINANT AGE: Adolescence to young adulthood is the predominant age. Mean age of onset is 17 yr. Approximately 0.5% to 1% of college-aged women have anorexia nervosa.

PHYSICAL FINDINGS & CLINICAL PRESENTATION

Eating disorders can affect every organ system. Primary care physicians must be skilled at recognizing this disorder because patients with mild cases usually present with nonspecific symptoms such as asthenia, cold intolerance, lack of energy, or dizziness. Children and adolescents are at particular risk due to their active phase of growth and development. The physical examination may be normal in the early stages or in mild cases. Patients with moderate to severe anorexia have the following physical characteristics:

- Patient is emaciated and bundled in clothing.
- Skin is dry and has excessive growth of lanugo. Skin may also be yellow-tinged from carotenodermia.
- Brittle nails, thinning scalp hair are present.
- Bradycardia, hypotension, hypothermia, and bradypnea are common.
- Female fat distribution pattern is no longer evident.
- Axillary and pubic hair is preserved.
- Peripheral edema may be present.

ETIOLOGY

- Etiology is unknown, but probably multifactorial (sociocultural, psychological, familial, and genetic factors).
- A history of sexual abuse has been reported in as many as 50% of patients with anorexia nervosa.
- Psychological factors: Anorexics often have an incompletely developed personal identity. They struggle to maintain a sense of control over their environment, they usually have a low self-esteem, and they lack the sense that they are valued and loved for themselves.

DIAGNOSIS

DIFFERENTIAL DIAGNOSIS

- Other eating disorders (bulimia nervosa, binge eating disorder [Table 1])
- Substance abuse
- Depression with loss of appetite
- Obsessive compulsive disorder
- Schizophrenia
- Conversion disorder
- Occult carcinoma, lymphoma
- Endocrine disorders: Addison disease, diabetes mellitus, hypothyroidism or hyperthyroidism, panhypopituitarism
- Gastrointestinal disorders: Celiac disease, Crohn disease, intestinal parasitosis
- Infectious disorders: AIDS, tuberculosis
- A clinical algorithm for the evaluation of anorexia is described in Section III

WORKUP

- A diagnosis can be made by using the following *DSM-5* diagnostic criteria for anorexia nervosa.
  1. Restriction of energy intake relative to requirements, leading to a significantly low body weight in the context of age, sex, developmental trajectory, and physical health. Significantly low weight is defined as a weight that is less than minimally normal or, for children or adolescents, less than that minimally expected.
  2. Intense fear of gaining weight or becoming fat, or persistent behavior that interferes with weight gain, even though at a significantly low weight.
  3. Disturbance in the way in which one's body or shape is experienced, undue influence of body weight or shape on self-evaluation, or persistent lack of recognition of the seriousness of the current low body weight.
- Specify type:
  1. *Restricting type:* During the last 3 mo, the individual has not engaged in recurrent episodes of binge eating or purging behavior (i.e., self-induced vomiting or the misuse of laxatives, diuretics, or enemas). This subtype describes presentations in which weight loss is accomplished primarily through dieting, fasting, and/or excessive exercise.
  2. *Binge-eating/purging type:* During the last 3 mo, the individual has engaged in recurrent episodes of binge eating or purging behavior (i.e., self-induced vomiting or the misuse of laxatives, diuretics, or enemas).
- Severity level: See "Acute General Rx" section

The SCOFF questionnaire is a screening tool for eating disorders used in England. It consists of the following five questions:

1. Do you make yourself ***s***ick because you feel full?
2. Have you lost ***c***ontrol over how much you eat?
3. Have you lost more than ***o***ne stone (approximately 6 kg) recently?
4. Do you believe yourself to be ***f***at when others say you are thin?
5. Does ***f***ood dominate your life?

A positive response to two or more questions has a reported sensitivity of 100% for anorexia and bulimia and an overall specificity of 87.5%.

In college-aged women a positive response to any of the following screening questions also warrants further evaluation:

1. How many diets have you been on in the past year?
2. Do you think you should be dieting?
3. Are you dissatisfied with your body size?
4. Does your weight affect the way you think about yourself?

Baseline ECG should be performed on all patients with anorexia nervosa. Routine monitoring of patients with prolonged QT interval is necessary; sudden death in these patients is often caused by ventricular arrhythmias related to QT interval prolongation.

A dual-energy x-ray absorptiometry (DEXA) scan to screen for osteopenia should be considered after 6 mo of amenorrhea in patients suspected of anorexia nervosa.

TABLE 1 Diagnostic Features of Eating Disorders

Anorexia nervosa	Body weight willfully maintained below normal level Abnormal perception of body morphology Intense fear of weight gain Amenorrhea
Bulimia nervosa	Large uncontrolled eating binges at least twice weekly Inappropriate compensatory behavior (e.g., vomiting, purging)
Binge eating disorder	Large uncontrolled eating binges at least twice weekly No regular inappropriate compensatory disorders Marked distress about binges

Modified and updated from Besser CM, Thorner MO: *Comprehensive clinical endocrinology,* ed 3, St Louis, 2002, Mosby.

LABORATORY TESTS

- In mild cases, laboratory findings may be completely normal.
- Endocrine abnormalities:
  1. Decreased follicle-stimulating hormone, luteinizing hormone, T_4, T_3, estrogens, urinary 17-OH steroids, estrone, and estradiol
  2. Normal free T_4, thyroid-stimulating hormone
  3. Increased cortisol, growth hormone, rT_3, T_3RU
  4. Absence of cyclic surge of luteinizing hormone

- Leukopenia, thrombocytopenia, anemia, reduced erythrocyte sedimentation rate, reduced complement levels, and reduced CD4 and CD8 cells may be present.
- Metabolic alkalosis, hypocalcemia, hypokalemia, hypomagnesemia, hypercholesterolemia, and hypophosphatemia may be present.
- Increased plasma b-carotene levels are useful to distinguish these patients from others on starvation diets.

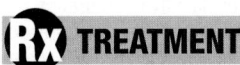

TREATMENT

NONPHARMACOLOGIC THERAPY

- A multidisciplinary approach with psychological, medical, and nutritional support is necessary.
- A goal weight should be set and the patient should be initially monitored at least once a week in the office setting. The target weight is 100% of ideal BW for teenagers and 90% to 100% for older patients.
- Weight gain should be gradual (1 to 3 lb/wk) to prevent gastric dilation. Begin with 800 to 1200 kcal in frequent small meals (to avoid bloating sensation), then increase calories to 1500 to 3000 depending on height and age.
- Add, as necessary, vitamin and mineral supplements.
- In severe cases, total parenteral nutrition must be used (starting at 800 to 1200 kcal/day).
- Electrolyte levels should be strictly monitored.
- Mealtime should be a time for social interaction, not confrontation.
- Postprandially, sedentary activities are recommended. The patient's access to a bathroom should be monitored to prevent purging.

ACUTE GENERAL Rx

- Criteria to decide on the appropriate initial course of treatment for patients with anorexia nervosa are usually based on the presence of complications, percentage of ideal BW, and severity of body image distortion. According to *DSM-5*,[1] the minimum level of severity is based, for adults, on current body mass index (BMI; see below) or, for children and adolescents, on BMI percentile. The level of severity may be increased to reflect clinical symptoms, the degree of functional disability, and need for supervision.
  Mild: BMI ≥ 17 kg/m^2
  Moderate: BMI 16-16.99 kg/m^2
  Severe: BMI 15-15.99 kg/m^2
  Extreme: BMI <15 kg/m^2
- Outpatient treatment is adequate for most patients.
- Indications for inpatient-level care are described under "Referral" section and summarized in Table 2.
- Medically stable patients who are within 85% of ideal BW can be followed up by the primary care physician at 3- or 4-wk intervals, which can be lengthened as the patient improves.

[1] American Psychiatric Association: Desk Reference to the Diagnostic Criteria from DSM-5, Arlington, VA, 2013, American Psychiatric Association.

- Pharmacologic treatment generally has no role in anorexia nervosa unless major depression or another psychiatric disorder is present. SSRIs can be used to alleviate the depressed mood and moderate obsessive-compulsive behavior in some individuals.

CHRONIC Rx

- Psychotherapy continued for years and focused specifically on self-image, family and peer interactions, and relapse prevention is an integral part of a successful recovery.
- Family therapy is also recommended, especially in younger patients.

DISPOSITION

- The long-term prognosis is generally poor and marked by recurrent exacerbations. The percentage of patients with anorexia nervosa who fully recover is modest. Most patients continue to have a distorted body image, disordered eating habits, and psychic difficulties.
- Most patients with anorexia nervosa will recover menses within 6 mo of reaching 90% of their ideal BW. It is important to note that patients with anorexia nervosa can become pregnant despite amenorrhea.
- Mortality rates vary from 5% to 20% and are six times that of peers without anorexia. Frequent causes of death are electrolyte abnormalities, starvation, or suicide.
- Factors that predict improved outcome in patients with eating disorders include early age at diagnosis, brief interval before initiation of treatment, good parent-child

TABLE 2 Clinical Signs and Criteria Warranting Inpatient-Level Care to Stabilize or Treat an Eating Disorder

Domain	General Symptom[a]	Example[b]
Weight	Substantially low weight for height and age Rapidly falling weight	<75% to 85% expected body weight for height and age
Behavioral	Acute food or water refusal Episodes of bingeing and purging of very high and/or escalating frequency Compensatory behaviors likely to result in acute and severe medical complications	Bingeing and/or vomiting multiple times per day resulting in social or occupational impairment and/or serious medical complications; inappropriate withholding of insulin
Other medical compromise	Abnormal vital signs reflecting nutritional compromise Severe medical complications	Severe hematemesis Severe neutropenia and/or thrombocytopenia Severe hypokalemia Uncontrolled type I diabetes Syncope
Psychiatric comorbidity and risk of self-harm	Substantial risk of self-harm or suicide Comorbid psychiatric illness resulting in safety risk or seriously undermining treatment Inability to adhere to treatment plan that will sustain minimal level of safety	Comorbid substance use escalating in the setting of treatment for the eating disorder
Treatment-related	Lack of clinically meaningful progress in an outpatient setting resulting in social or occupational impairment or medical risk Necessity of close supervision to maintain symptom control Previously agreed-on criterion for hospitalization based on patient history	An adolescent's low weight poses risk for decreased peak bone mass or short stature Sustained or persistent inability to eat without supervision or to abstain from intractable purging after food intake Reaching a threshold weight at which the patient repeatedly has rapidly deteriorated

[a]These criteria may be sufficient but do not necessarily need to be present to indicate inpatient care.
[b]Weight, vital signs, metabolic, and other parameters for hospitalization are best interpreted in the context of the patient's overall health, medical and psychiatric history, support systems, and engagement in treatment.
Stern TA et al: *Massachusetts General Hospital handbook of general hospital psychiatry,* ed 7, Philadelphia, 2018, Elsevier.

relationships, and having other healthy relationships with friends or therapists.
- A prolonged QT interval is a marker for risk of sudden death.

REFERRAL

Hospitalization should be considered in the following situations:
- Severe dehydration or electrolyte imbalance
- ECG abnormalities (prolonged QT interval, arrhythmias)
- Significant physiologic instability (hypotension, orthostatic changes)
- Intractable vomiting, purging, or bingeing
- Suicidal thoughts
- Weight loss exceeding 30% of ideal BW and unresponsiveness to outpatient treatment
- Rapidly progressing weight loss (>2 lb in a week)
- Failure to progress in nutritional rehabilitation in outpatient treatment

SUGGESTED READING

Available at ExpertConsult.com

RELATED CONTENT

Anorexia Nervosa (Patient Information)
Binge-Eating Disorder (Related Key Topic)
Bulimia Nervosa (Related Key Topic)

AUTHOR: **FRED F. FERRI, M.D.**

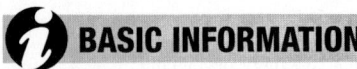

BASIC INFORMATION

DEFINITION

Antiphospholipid antibody syndrome (APS), the most common acquired thrombophilia, is characterized by clinical features of arterial or venous thrombosis and/or pregnancy morbidity *and* the persistence of at least one type of antiphospholipid autoantibody (aPL). aPLs are antibodies directed against anionic phospholipids and phospholipid-binding protein cofactors. These autoantibodies lead to stimulation of procoagulant factors and inhibition of the fibrinolytic system. MTOR pathway upregulation, toll-like receptor signaling, and activation of vascular endothelium, monocytes, neutrophils, platelets, complement, pro-inflammatory cytokines, and various coagulation and fibrinolytic pathway targets have all been shown to play a role in this process.

Three types of aPLs have been characterized:

- Anticardiolipin antibodies (detected in approximately 23% to 44% of patients)
- Lupus anticoagulants (detected in approximately 34% of patients)
- Anti-β2-glycoprotein-I antibodies (detected in approximately 20% of patients)

APS can be primary or secondary to a rheumatic disease, with the most common being systemic lupus erythematosus (SLE). APS can affect all organ systems and includes venous and arterial thrombosis, recurrent fetal losses, and cytopenias, including thrombocytopenia and microangiopathic hemolytic anemia.

SYNONYM

Antiphospholipid syndrome

ICD-10CM CODE
D68.61 Antiphospholipid syndrome

EPIDEMIOLOGY & DEMOGRAPHICS

PREVALENCE:

- Up to 5% of healthy individuals without a history of thrombosis have positive aPLs.
- Approximately 10% of patients with a deep venous thrombosis have aPLs.
- Nearly 20% of women under 50 who have a cerebrovascular accident (CVA) test positive for aPLs.
- 10% to 15% of women with recurrent miscarriages have aPLs.
- aPLs without APS can be seen in patients with certain medications, infections, malignancies, and autoimmune conditions.

PREDOMINANT AGE: Young to middle-aged adults

RISK FACTORS:

- Underlying SLE and collagen-vascular diseases; other autoimmune disorders, including rheumatoid arthritis, Sjögren's syndrome, Behçet's syndrome, primary immune thrombocytopenia (also known as idiopathic thrombocytopenic purpura), AIDS.
- Most individuals are otherwise healthy and have no underlying medical condition.
- Thrombotic risk is increased by the presence of other etiologies of systemic hypercoagulability, including oral contraceptives, pregnancy, smoking, prolonged immobilization, genetic thrombophilia, malignancy, and hyperlipidemia.

PROGNOSIS:

- 91% survival at 10 yr.
- 71% success rate in pregnancy with recommended therapies; prematurity and intrauterine growth restriction are common complications.

GENETICS: Some APS-positive families exist, and human leukocyte antigen (HLA) studies have suggested associations with HLA DR7, DR4, and Dqw7+Drw53.

TABLE 1 Other Features Suggesting the Presence of Antiphospholipid Antibodies

Clinical
Livedo reticularis
Thrombocytopenia (usually 50,000-100,000 platelets/mm^3)
Autoimmune hemolytic anemia
Cardiac valve disease (vegetations or thickening)
Multiple sclerosis–like syndrome, chorea, or other myelopathy

From Firestein GS, et al.: *Kelley's textbook of rheumatology*, ed 9, Philadelphia, 2013, Saunders.

PHYSICAL FINDINGS & CLINICAL PRESENTATION

No pathognomonic findings on examination; Table 1 summarizes other features suggesting the presence of antiphospholipid antibodies, including abnormal findings consistent with ischemia or infarction.

- Thrombosis (Fig. 1):
  1. Patients with APS are at risk for both venous and arterial thromboses. Venous thromboses are more common, occurring as the initial manifestation of APS in approximately 30% of APS patients. Of all patients with deep venous thrombosis, approximately 10% have aPL. The most common site for deep vein thrombosis is the calf, but thromboses may also occur in the renal, hepatic, axillary, subclavian, vena cava, and retinal veins. The most common site of arterial thrombosis is the cerebral vessels, followed by the coronary, renal, mesenteric, and bypass arteries. Recurrent thrombosis is common with APS.

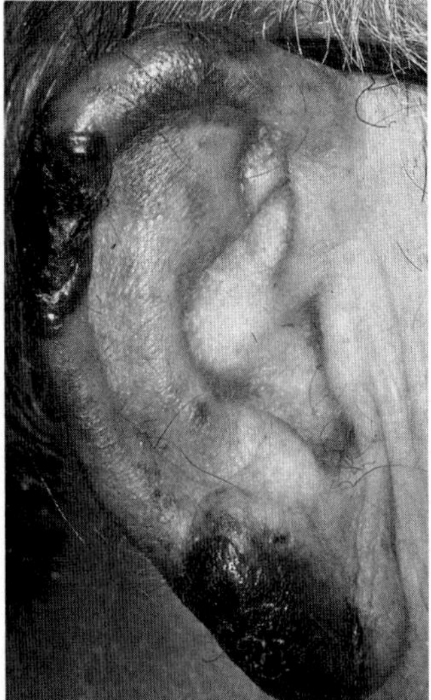

FIG. 1 Cutaneous thrombosis in antiphospholipid antibody syndrome. (From James WD, et al.: *Andrews' diseases of the skin*, ed 12, Philadelphia, 2016, Saunders.)

- Commonly involved organ systems include:
  1. Central nervous system: Stroke, transient ischemic attack, migraine, multi-infarct dementia, epilepsy, movement disorders, transverse myelopathy, depression, Guillain-Barré syndrome.
  2. Pulmonary: Pulmonary embolism and infarction; pulmonary hypertension; acute respiratory distress syndrome; intra-alveolar pulmonary hemorrhage (a postpartum syndrome characterized by fever, pleuritic chest pain, dyspnea, and patchy infiltrates with pleural effusion on chest radiograph).
  3. Cardiology: Libman-Sacks endocarditis, intracardiac thrombosis, coronary artery disease, myocardial infarction, valvulopathy, left ventricular diastolic dysfunction.
  4. Gastrointestinal: Abdominal pain, gastrointestinal bleed secondary to ischemia, splenic or pancreatic infarction, hepatic vein thrombosis, Budd-Chiari syndrome.
  5. Renal: Proteinuria, acute renal failure, hypertension, renal infarct, renal artery or vein thrombosis, post-partum hemolytic uremic syndrome.
  6. Hematology: Thrombocytopenia, hemolytic anemia.
  7. Endocrine: Addison disease secondary to adrenal hemorrhage and, less frequently, thrombosis.
  8. Cutaneous: Livedo reticularis, cutaneous necrosis, skin ulcerations, phlegmasia cerulea dolens, gangrene of digits (Fig. 2).
  9. Obstetric: Recurrent spontaneous abortion, premature delivery, or fetal growth restriction.
- **Catastrophic APS** (CAPS) (Table 2): CAPS is a rapidly progressive multi-organ thrombotic disease. Approximately 1% of APS is CAPS; approximately 45% of CAPS do not present as APS initially. CAPS is associated with a high mortality rate (50%). To make the diagnosis of catastrophic APS, four criteria must be satisfied:
  1. Evidence of involvement of three or more organs, systems, and/or tissues. The most common symptoms are abdominal pain, dyspnea, neurologic symptoms, chest pain, and skin rash.
  2. Development of manifestations simultaneously or in ≤1 week.
  3. Confirmation by histopathology of small-vessel occlusion in at least one organ or tissue.
  4. Laboratory confirmation of the presence of aPL.

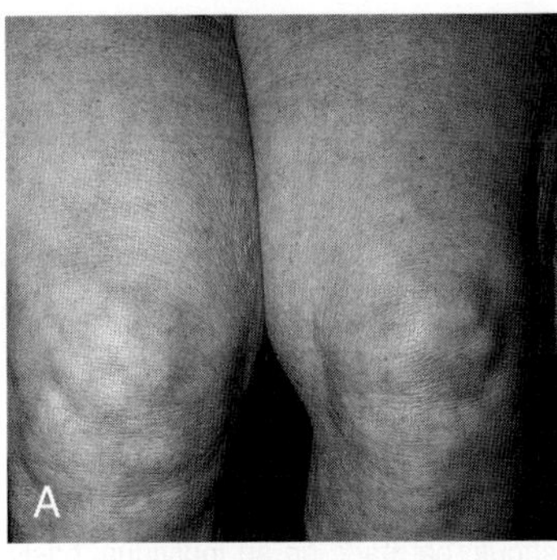
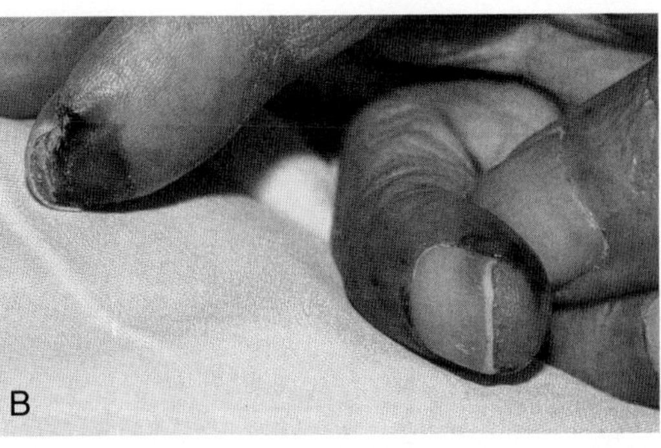

FIG. 2 Antiphospholipid syndrome. The clinical presentations of this disorder are protean and include those shown here. **A,** Broad bands of livedo around the knees in a patient with anticardiolipin antibodies. Physiologic livedo has a finer patterning and less obvious lesions. **B,** Digital infarcts, a nonspecific feature of several vascular occlusion disorders. (From White GM, Cox NH [eds]: *Diseases of the skin, a color atlas and text,* ed 2, St Louis, 2006, Mosby.)

TABLE 2 Differential Diagnosis of Catastrophic Antiphospholipid Syndrome (CAPS)

Laboratory Abnormalities	CAPS	TTP	DIC
Microangiopathic hemolytic anemia	–	+	+
Thrombocytopenia	+	+	+
Fibrinogen/FDP	Normal/Normal	Normal/Increased	Decreased/Increased
Anticardiolipin antibody	+	–	–
Lupus anticoagulant	+	–	–

DIC, Disseminated intravascular coagulation; *FDP,* fibrin degradation products; *TTP,* time to progression.

TABLE 3 Proposed Pathogenic Mechanisms of Antiphospholipid Syndrome

I. aPL-mediated promotion of tissue factor expression
  A. Direct injury and subsequent anti-β2 GPI binding on endothelial cells
  B. Signaling via annexin A2/TLR4/apoER2 inducing proadhesive prothrombotic phenotype
  C. Induction of adhesion molecules and tissue factor on endothelial cells and cytokine release
II. Activation of platelets and monocytes by aPL antibodies
  A. Activation of platelets: via apoER2′, GPIbα, and/or β2 GPI-platelet factor 4 interaction
  B. Interference of β2 GPI in regulating vWF-mediated platelet adhesion
  C. Activation of monocytes: results in increased tissue factor, VEGF, cytokine expression
  D. Activation of monocytes causes mitochondrial dysfunction and oxidative stress
III. Inhibition of endogenous anticoagulant and fibrinolytic mechanisms
  A. Disruption of the annexin A5 anticoagulant shield
  B. Interference with fibrinolysis via annexin A2, β2 GPI cofactor activity, autoactivation of XIIa, direct inhibition of plasmin and increase of PAI-1
  C. Inhibition of the protein C pathway: decreased activation of protein C, barrier of APC proteolysis of factor Va and VIIIa, prevention of protein C and EPCR binding
  D. Interference with tissue factor pathway inhibitor
IV. aPL-mediated activation of complement
  A. Antibodies against β2 GP–HLA-DR7 complexes on cell surfaces trigger complement-mediated cytotoxicity
V. Direct activation of trophoblasts and endometrial cells by aPL antibodies
  A. Abnormal trophoblast proliferation, migration and invasiveness, increased trophoblast apoptosis, and reduced secretion of HCG and adhesion molecules
  B. Disruption in the differentiation of decidual endometrial cells
  C. Disruption of maternal spiral artery transformation and maturation
VI. Other mechanisms
  A. mTORC pathway–mediated vasculopathy
  B. Release in procoagulant microparticles by endothelial cells and platelets

APC, activated protein C; *aPL,* antiphospholipid; *apoER2,* apolipoprotein E receptor 2; *EPCR,* endothelial cell protein C receptor; *β2 GPI,* β2 -glycoprotein I; *HCG,* human chorionic gonadotropin; *HLA,* human leukocyte antigen; *mTORC,* mammalian target of rapamycin complex; *PAI-1,* plasminogen activator inhibitor 1; *TLR,* Toll-like receptor; *VEGF,* vascular endothelial growth factor; *vWF,* von Willebrand factor

Hoffman R, et al.: *Hematology, basic principles and practice*, ed 7, Philadelphia, 2018, Elsevier.

ETIOLOGY

- Endothelial cells are activated by aPLs causing upregulation of adhesion and procoagulant molecules such as tissue factor and von Willebrand factor.
- Table 3 summarizes proposed pathogenic mechanisms of antiphospholipid syndrome.
- Monocyte activation by aPLs yields expression of inflammatory cytokines and additional tissue factor, contributing to the procoagulant state.
- Neutrophil activation by aPLs via complement is proposed to cause the release of neutrophil extracellular traps leading to increased thrombin.
- aPL binding to glycoprotein 1b and ApoE receptor 2 causes platelet activation and increased platelet adhesion.
- aPL binding decreases activation of antithrombin and protein C, while also reducing the ability of activated protein C to inactivate coagulation factors V and VIII.
- aPL binding to annexin A2 (tissue plasminogen activator receptor) contributes to the prothrombotic state seen in APS.
- The mammalian target of rapamycin complex (mTORC) has been shown to be involved in endothelial activation and in regulating expression of tissue factor and IL-8 in monocytes.
- Toll-like receptors 4 and 7 and triggering of the innate immune system are involved in endothelial activation and the development of the prothrombotic state.
- Autoantibodies against other antigens, such as phosphatidylserine, phosphatidyl ethanolamine, and other complexes have been identified in APS patients, but their clinical significance has yet to be elucidated.

Dx DIAGNOSIS

DIFFERENTIAL DIAGNOSIS

Other hypercoagulable states (inherited or acquired):

- Inherited: ATIII, protein C and protein S deficiencies, factor V Leiden, prothrombin gene mutation
- Acquired: Heparin-induced thrombocytopenia, myeloproliferative syndromes, malignancy
- Alternate causes of recurrent pregnancy loss should also be considered (e.g., anatomic or chromosomal abnormalities)

WORKUP

Diagnostic criteria of APS include at least one clinical criterion and at least one laboratory criterion.

- Clinical:
  1. Venous, arterial, or small vessel thrombosis *or*
  2. Morbidity with pregnancy, defined as:
     a. Unexplained fetal death at ≥10 weeks' gestation *or*
     b. ≥1 premature births before 34 weeks' gestation secondary to eclampsia, preeclampsia, or severe placental insufficiency *or*
     c. ≥3 unexplained spontaneous abortions before 10 weeks' gestation.

TABLE 4 Assays Used to Confirm Diagnosis of Antiphospholipid Syndrome

Assay	Methodology
"Criteria" aPL Assays	
aCL	ELISA
Anti-β2-GPI	ELISA
LAC	Clotting/functional assays
"Noncriteria" aPL Assays	
Assays to detect antibodies to other phospholipids (i.e., phosphatidylserine, phosphatidylinositol, phosphatidic acid, phosphatidylglycerol, phosphatidylethanolamine, phosphatidylcholine)	ELISA
Annexin A5 resistance assay	Clotting/mechanistic assay
Assays to detect antibodies to prothrombin or prothrombin/phosphatidylserine	ELISA
Assays to detect antibodies to clotting proteins (i.e., protein C, protein S)	ELISA

aCL, Anticardiolipin; *aPL,* antiphospholipid antibody; *ELISA,* enzyme-linked immunosorbent assay; *β2 GPI,* β2 -glycoprotein I; *LAC,* lupus anticoagulant.
From Hochberg MC, et al.: *Rheumatology*, ed 5, St Louis, 2011, Mosby.

- Laboratory (see Table 4):
  1. Lupus anticoagulant present in plasma on two or more occasions at least 12 weeks apart, *or*
  2. Anticardiolipin antibody, IgG or IgM present in serum or plasma at >40 MPL, GPL, or >99th percentile on two or more occasions at least 12 weeks apart, *or*
  3. Anti-β2-glycoprotein-I antibodies present in serum or plasma at >99th percentile on two or more occasions at least 12 weeks apart
- Screening tests:
  1. Partial thromboplastin time (PTT): Elevated, activated partial thromboplastin time prolongation indicating either the presence of a clotting factor deficiency, or the presence of an inhibitor such as a lupus anticoagulant.
  2. Mixing study: Elevated. Normal plasma is incubated with the patient's plasma. In cases of clotting factor deficiencies the PTT will correct. If an inhibitor is present as in the case with APS, the PTT will not correct.
  3. Dilute Russell viper venom time: Elevated. Laboratory clotting requires the addition of phospholipids and calcium to plasma samples. Antiphospholipid antibodies bind the phospholipids in the test tube, thereby preventing clot formation. The addition of Russell viper venom to plasma results in immediate activation of Factor X (common pathway). Therefore, it will not be prolonged in intrinsic or extrinsic factor deficiencies but will be prolonged in the presence of an antiphospholipid antibody.
  4. The Lupus Anticoagulant screen is the addition of Russell viper venom to plasma. In the Lupus Anticoagulant confirmatory testing, massive doses of phospholipids are added to saturate the antiphospholipid antibody, thereby correcting the prolonged PTT.
- Initial testing for presence of aPL:
  1. Anticardiolipin (aCL) ELISA antibodies (IgG or IgM), *or*
  2. Lupus anticoagulant activity found, *or*
  3. Anti-beta2-glycoprotein (anti-β2GPI) ELISA antibodies (IgG or IgM).
- Confirmatory aPL testing: Repeat testing after 12 weeks is required to confirm the persistence of a positive aCL, anti-β2GPI, or LA test because transient aPL elevations can occur.

LABORATORY TESTS

Diagnostic evaluation of aPLs is indicated in:
- Patient with underlying SLE or collagen-vascular disease with thrombosis.
- Patient with recurrent, familial, or juvenile deep vein thrombosis (DVT) or thrombosis in an unusual location (mesenteric or cerebral).
- One or more unexplained thrombotic events. Do not test those at low risk, e.g., elderly patients with other thrombotic risk factors.
- One or more specific pregnancy events.
- Unexplained thrombocytopenia or microangiopathic hemolytic anemia.
- Patients with an unexplained elevation in PTT, or less commonly, in PT/INR.

Rx TREATMENT

ACUTE Rx

- Initial anticoagulation with heparin or low-molecular-weight heparin (LMWH), before transitioning to a vitamin K antagonist (VKA) such as warfarin, is recommended. DOACs are not recommended due to lack of data demonstrating clinical safety in patients with APS.
- Standard intensity (INR 2.0-3.0) anticoagulation with warfarin is preferred in venous thrombosis, as prior randomized trials failed to show a decrease in recurrent thromboses with high-intensity anticoagulation (INR 3.0-4.0). Task-force reports have not reached a consensus regarding intensity of anticoagulation in secondary thromboprophylaxis of arterial events.
- Unfractionated heparin (UFH) is preferred if quick reversibility is needed.

PRIMARY PREVENTION

- Although other cardiovascular risk factors, such as hypertension and hyperlipidemia, should be controlled, aspirin use for primary prevention remains controversial.
- Adding low-dose warfarin to aspirin for primary prevention seems to confer no benefit.
- Hydroxychloroquine may be useful in those patients with SLE and aPL; it has been shown to reduce the incidence of thrombotic complications in this population.
- Modifiable risk factors for thrombosis, such as smoking and immobility, should also be addressed when possible.
- For pregnant women with a positive test for aPL antibodies without a history of DVT or pregnancy morbidity, decision to treat with low-dose subcutaneous UFH or LMWH and/or low-dose aspirin, or to manage with surveillance should be made on an individual basis as there is no clear consensus data.

SECONDARY PREVENTION

- For men and nonpregnant women, long-term anticoagulation with warfarin, or with UFH or LMWH if warfarin is contraindicated, should be used.
- Modifiable risk factors for thrombosis should be reduced when possible.
- For pregnant women with previously diagnosed APS:
  1. Warfarin should be discontinued before pregnancy due to its teratogenic effects.
  2. Aspirin 81 mg in combination with subcutaneous UFH or LMWH is recommended to improve pregnancy outcomes in women with APS and pregnancy morbidity but without thrombosis.
  3. For pregnant women with APS and prior thrombosis, UFH or LMWH should be used.
  4. Pregnant patients taking LMWH should be transitioned to unfractionated heparin before delivery for ease of reversibility.
  5. Hypertension and hyperlipidemia, if present, should be controlled.

FOR CATASTROPHIC ANTIPHOSPHOLIPID ANTIBODY SYNDROME (CAPS)

- The combination of anticoagulation with heparin products, high-dose corticosteroids, and supportive care, including debriding necrotic tissue and treating underlying infections is the mainstay of therapy.
- Patients may be transitioned to oral anticoagulation with warfarin once clinically stable.
- Plasma exchange with or without IVIG has been shown to improve mortality; however, the decision to use IVIG should be made on an individual basis (e.g., avoid in patients in whom anticoagulation has been discontinued).
- Eculizumab (monoclonal antibody against complement protein C5) and rituximab (monoclonal antibody against CD20) have been used successfully in refractory cases.
- Immunosuppressant therapy with cyclophosphamide should be considered in patients with CAPS and SLE as it has been demonstrated to decrease mortality in this group.

CHRONIC Rx

- Anticoagulation with VKAs, such as warfarin, remains the standard of care.
- Duration of treatment is unknown and should be determined on an individual basis.

However, in the absence of any contraindication to anticoagulation, indefinite therapy is recommended, as the lifelong recurrence rate reached nearly 30% in some studies.
- Immunosuppressive agents such as corticosteroids and cyclophosphamide have not been shown to be effective for chronic treatment of APS.
- Limited data suggest that hydroxychloroquine may be effective in patients with APS and SLE, although efficacy in primary APS remains unproven.
- Recurrent thrombosis can occur even in the setting of "therapeutic" anticoagulation, and multiple assays have been studied to monitor the adequacy of anticoagulation in APS.
- In cases of recurrent thrombosis, hydroxychloroquine and statins (antiinflammatory and antithrombotic activity) may be considered as adjuvant therapies.

DISPOSITION

- APS patients have a 20% to 70% risk for recurrent thrombosis. Positivity in more than one aPL assay is associated with increased thrombotic risk.
- Initial arterial thrombosis tends to be followed by arterial events, and initial venous thrombosis tends to be followed by venous events.
- Incidence of developing catastrophic APS is approximately 1.0% among APS patients.

REFERRAL

Referrals to hematology, rheumatology, and/or obstetric medicine should be placed when diagnosis is made.

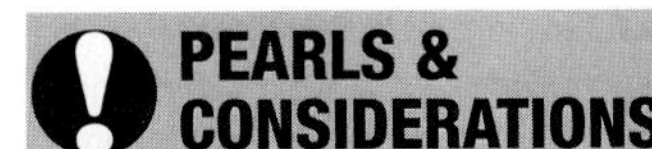

PEARLS & CONSIDERATIONS

COMMENTS

Cerebral features of SLE may be more related to thrombosis than inflammation and may respond better to anticoagulants than immunosuppression.

False-positive lupus anticoagulant (LAC) tests have been reported in patients taking direct oral anticoagulants and heparin. For this reason, thrombophilia testing should be delayed until 2 to 4 weeks after completion of anticoagulation.

PREVENTION

Prophylaxis for asymptomatic patients with positive aPL tests without previous thrombosis:
- No routine prophylaxis is recommended.
- Questionable whether low-dose aspirin is effective.
- Antithrombotic prophylaxis for major surgery, prolonged immobilization, and pregnancy.
- Avoid combination oral contraceptive pills in women with positive aPL tests.

SUGGESTED READINGS

Available at ExpertConsult.com

RELATED CONTENT

Antiphospholipid Antibody Syndrome (Patient Information)
Deep Vein Thrombosis (Related Key Topic)
Hypercoagulable States (Related Key Topic)
Pulmonary Embolism (Related Key Topic)

AUTHORS: **JOZAL WAROICH, M.D.,** and **JOHN L. REAGAN, M.D.**

BASIC INFORMATION

DEFINITION

Generalized anxiety disorder (GAD) is most likely to present in combination with other psychiatric and medical conditions. Individuals with GAD commonly present with excessive and disproportionately high levels of anxiety, fear, or worry for most days over at least a 6-mo period in a number of areas. The worrying must be greater than would be expected given the situation, and it must cause significant interference in functioning. The subjective anxiety must be accompanied by at least three somatic symptoms in adults and one in children (e.g., restlessness, irritability, sleep disturbance, muscle tension, difficulty concentrating, or fatigue). GAD cannot be diagnosed if it occurs only in the context of an active mood disorder, such as depression, or if the anxiety is better explained by another active anxiety disorder, such as PTSD or panic disorder.

SYNONYMS

Anxiety neurosis (former name for a subset of anxiety disorders)
Chronic anxiety
GAD

ICD-10CM CODE

F41.1 Generalized anxiety disorderDSM-5: 300.02

EPIDEMIOLOGY & DEMOGRAPHICS

INCIDENCE (IN U.S.): 6% to 9% per yr in adult primary care clinics; 1-yr incident rate per 100 person-yr of 1.12

PEAK INCIDENCE: Peak incidence tends to occur later relative to other anxiety disorders, such as phobias; cumulative incidence of 4.3% by age 34 in a German community sample

PREVALENCE (IN U.S.):

- In general population: Lifetime morbid risk of 9%; 12-month prevalence of 2.9%
- In primary care setting: 3% (the most common anxiety disorder in this setting)

PREDOMINANT SEX: Women are more frequently affected (2:1 ratio) but may present for treatment less often (3:2 female/male).

PREDOMINANT AGE:

- 30% report onset before age 11
- 50% have onset before age 18
- Median age of onset: 30 yr

GENETICS: Concordance rates in dizygotic twins and monozygotic twins are not different (0% to 5%)

PHYSICAL FINDINGS & CLINICAL PRESENTATION

- Report of being "anxious" all of their lives
- Excessive worry, usually regarding family, finances, work, or health
- Sleep disturbance, particularly early insomnia
- Muscle tension (typically in the muscles of neck and shoulders) or headache
- Difficulty concentrating
- Daytime fatigue
- GI symptoms compatible with IBS (one third of patients)
- Physical symptoms are the usual reason for seeking medical attention
- Comorbid psychiatric illness (e.g., dysthymia or major depression) and substance abuse (e.g., alcohol abuse) are frequent

ETIOLOGY

- Hypotheses include models based on neurotransmitters (catecholamines, indolamines) and developmental psychology (e.g., behavioral inhibition, neuroticism, and harm avoidance)
- Prevalence increased with a family history, increase in stress, history of physical or emotional trauma, and medical illness

DIAGNOSIS

DIFFERENTIAL DIAGNOSIS

- Wide range of psychiatric and medical conditions:
  1. Cardiovascular and pulmonary disease, such as cardiac arrhythmias or COPD
  2. Hyperthyroidism, hypoglycemia
  3. Substance abuse (e.g., cocaine, amphetamines, and PCP) or withdrawal (e.g., alcohol or benzodiazepines)
  4. Other anxiety disorders (e.g., social anxiety disorder), mood disorder
  5. Intrusive thoughts in obsessive-compulsive disorder or illness anxiety disorder

WORKUP

- Screening tests may enhance detection. A screening tool often used in primary care is the GAD-2. It asks, "During the past month, have you been bothered a lot by: (1) Nerves or feeling anxious or on edge? (2) Worrying about a lot of different things?" The response to each question is given a score of 0 (not at all), 1 (several days), 2 (more than half of the days), 3 (nearly every day). A score of ≥3 has a sensitivity of 86% and a specificity of 83% for detecting GAD. A simple 7-item in-office case finding instrument, the GAD-7, includes additional questions to assess symptom severity and can be used to monitor symptoms.
- Physical examination: Additional laboratory and radiologic workup depending on presenting symptoms.
- Iatrogenic cause should be suspected if anxiety follows recent changes in medication.

TREATMENT

NONPHARMACOLOGIC THERAPY

- Cognitive-behavioral therapy
- Acceptance and commitment therapy
- Relaxation training
- Biofeedback
- Psychodynamic psychotherapy

PHARMACOLOGIC THERAPY

- SSRIs/SNRIs
- Azapirones (e.g., buspirone)
- Benzodiazepines (less favored)

ACUTE GENERAL Rx

- Acute treatment is rarely indicated because GAD is a chronic condition.
- If patients are in acute distress, the possibility of another cause, including another anxiety disorder such as panic disorder, should be considered.
- Caution in prescribing benzodiazepines because of the propensity for misuse and dependence. If used, the patient should be educated about the options and the risks.

CHRONIC Rx

- SSRIs and SNRIs (e.g., venlafaxine and duloxetine) are effective typical first-line treatment. Particularly useful if comorbid depression present.
- Buspirone can be effective with minimal potential for tolerance or abuse. May be less effective in patients with previous benzodiazepine exposure and may require a high-dose titration.
- Benzodiazepines can be effective under close supervision; however, they have fallen out of favor as a first-line treatment given their potential for functional impairment, abuse, and dependence.
- Sedating antidepressants, such as mirtazapine, may also be useful for initial insomnia secondary to anxious ruminations.

DISPOSITION

- GAD is chronic with periodic exacerbations.
- Treatment is given to reduce level of symptoms and improve functioning. Suicide risk is higher than in the general population.

REFERRAL

- For refractory symptoms
- For comorbid psychiatric conditions

SUGGESTED READINGS

Available at ExpertConsult.com

RELATED CONTENT

Anxiety (Patient Information)
Panic Disorder (Related Key Topic)
Social Anxiety Disorder (Related Key Topic)

AUTHOR: **KRISTY L. DALRYMPLE, PH.D.**

BASIC INFORMATION

DEFINITION

Aortic dissection is part of a spectrum of aortic pathologies (acute aortic syndromes) that includes intramural hematomas and penetrating atherosclerotic ulcers. Aortic dissection occurs when blood passes through an intimal tear, separating the intima from the medial layers and creating a false lumen. Intramural hematoma (IMH) occurs when the vasa vasorum ruptures within the medial wall. IMH does not involve an intimal tearing unless a dissection develops. Seventeen percent of IMH will transform into aortic dissection. Penetrating atherosclerotic ulcers, which occur in the setting of extensive aortic atherosclerosis and hypertension, destroy the aortic intima and dissect into the aortic media. Rupture of atherosclerotic plaques with subsequent blood entry into the median wall forms a pseudoaneurysm. Fig. 1 illustrates acute aortic syndromes.

SYNONYMS

Dissecting aortic aneurysm
Acute aortic syndrome
AAS

ICD-10CM CODES
I71.00 Dissection of unspecified site of aorta
I71.01 Dissection of thoracic aorta
I71.02 Dissection of abdominal aorta
I71.03 Dissection of thoracoabdominal aorta

EPIDEMIOLOGY & DEMOGRAPHICS

INCIDENCE: 3.5 to 6.0 per 100,000 person-yr

More frequent in winter as compared to other seasons, although no clear reason has been identified

PREDOMINANT SEX AND AGE: Males (65%) females (35%), ages 60 to 80 yr; mean = 63 yr

RISK FACTORS:

- Hypertension (found in up to 77% of patients with aortic dissection)
- Atherosclerosis (found in up to 27% of patients with aortic dissection)
- Preexisting aortic aneurysm (found in up to 16% of patients with aortic dissection)
- Age (60-80 yr)
- Family history of aortic aneurysms/dissection
- History of cardiac surgery, aortic valve replacement, intraaortic catheterization
- Disorders of collagen (Marfan syndrome, Ehlers-Danlos syndrome)
- Vascular inflammation (giant cell arteritis, Takayasu arteritis, rheumatoid arthritis, syphilitic aortitis)
- Aortic coarctation, bicuspid aortic valve
- Turner syndrome
- Cocaine abuse (usually within 12 hours of last use of cocaine)
- Trauma
- Table 1 summarizes genetically triggered conditions associated with aortic dissection

CLASSIFICATION

Aortic dissection is generally classified according to anatomic location (Fig. 2). Table 2 summarizes classification schemes of acute aortic dissection.

- Stanford (more commonly used classification system): Type A ascending aorta (proximal), type B descending aorta (distal)
- DeBakey: Type I ascending and descending aorta, type II ascending aorta, type III descending aorta
- Aortic dissection can also be classified by acuity of presentation: hyperacute (<24 hours), acute (2 to 7 days), subacute (8 to 30 days), and chronic (>30 days). The overall survival rate is inversely related to time of presentation, with the highest survival rate in the hyperacute group and the lowest survival rate in the chronic group

PHYSICAL FINDINGS & CLINICAL PRESENTATION

- Sudden onset of severe sharp, tearing, or ripping chest pain. However, painless dissection occurs in approximately 6.4% of cases
- Anterior chest pain (79% type A, 63% type B)
- Back pain, abdominal pain (43% type A, 64% type B)
- Syncope (19% type A, 3% type B), generally secondary to cardiac tamponade or stroke.
- Congestive heart failure (CHF)
- May present with hypertension (28% for type A, 66% in type B dissection), although 25% present with hypotension (systolic blood pressure <100 mm Hg), which can indicate bleeding, cardiac tamponade, or severe aortic regurgitation
- Pulse and blood pressure differentials (>20 mm Hg between arms) in 19% to 31% of cases caused by partial compression of subclavian arteries
- Aortic regurgitation in 18% to 50% of cases of proximal dissection, often with diastolic decrescendo murmur
- Myocardial ischemia caused by coronary artery occlusion, most commonly involving the right coronary artery
- Stroke in 5% to 10% of patients (secondary to dissection into or decreased blood flow to the carotids)
- Mesenteric ischemia occurs in 3% to 5% of cases, with external compression, flap prolapse, or involvement of arterial ostia
- Horner syndrome (ptosis, miosis, anhidrosis)
- Vocal cord paralysis or hoarse voice (caused by compression of the left recurrent laryngeal nerve)

ETIOLOGY

Genetics, in addition to other risk factors listed previously, contribute to the development of aortic dissection.

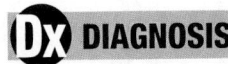

DIAGNOSIS

DIFFERENTIAL DIAGNOSIS

- Known as the great imitator: Pulmonary embolism, acute coronary syndrome, aortic stenosis/insufficiency, nondissecting aneurysm, pericarditis, cholecystitis, peptic ulcer disease, pancreatitis, musculoskeletal pain.
- Consider aortic dissection in patients with unexplained stroke, chest pain, syncope, acute-onset CHF, abdominal pain, back pain, and malperfusion of extremities or internal organs. Acute aortic syndromes may be associated with nonspecific signs and symptoms; a high clinical index of suspicion is necessary to detect the disease early in its course.
- In an emergency situation, a rapid yet comprehensive workup is crucial to reduce diagnostic time delay. This should include clinical assessment, laboratory data (D-dimer and troponin), chest x-ray, electrocardiogram (ECG), and aortic imaging in the appropriate patient.

LABORATORY TESTS

- ECG: Helpful to rule out MI, although dissection can lead to coronary ischemia.
- D-dimer has a 100% negative predictive value in dissection, but lacks specificity in the setting of acute aortic dissection. However, a negative D-dimer does not rule out intramural hematoma or penetrating aortic ulcer.

Aortic dissection
Aortic intramural hematoma
A
B
Penetrating atherosclerotic ulcer
C

FIG. 1 Acute aortic syndromes. A, Classic aortic dissection. **B,** Aortic intramural hematoma. **C,** Penetrating atherosclerotic ulcer. (From Mann DL, et al.: *Braunwald's heart disease,* ed 10, Philadelphia, 2015, Elsevier.)

TABLE 1 Genetically Triggered Conditions Associated With Aortic Dissection

Marfan syndrome (MFS)	Autosomal dominant disorder of connective tissue caused by *FBN1* mutation; incidence of 1 in ≈5000 individuals; multisystem manifestations, including ectopia lentis; mitral valve prolapse, aortic root aneurysm, aortic dissection; skeletal features (pectus deformities, scoliosis, arachnodactyly, hyperflexibility, tall stature, elongated fingers and toes); dural ectasia; spontaneous pneumothorax
Loeys-Dietz syndrome (LDS)	Autosomal dominant disorder caused by mutations in *TGFBR1* and *TGFBR2*, associated with aneurysms and dissections involving the aorta and branch vessels, often at relatively small diameters and young age; manifestations include craniofacial features (hypertelorism, craniosynostosis, cleft palate, bifid or broad uvula), bluish sclera, arterial tortuosity, velvety and hyperlucent skin, easily visible veins, clubfeet, skeletal abnormalities; phenotypes may vary, including those with more pronounced craniofacial features and those with more cutaneous features; ectopia lentis has not been described in LDS; mutations in *TGFB2* lead to a syndrome with an overlap in clinical features of LDS and MFS
Familial thoracic aortic aneurysm (FTAA) syndromes	Autosomal dominant disorders with variable expression and penetrance leading to thoracic aortic aneurysms (TAAs) and dissections at variable ages in families; *ACTA2* mutations occur in 10-15% of cases of FTAA and are associated with bicuspid aortic valve (BAV) disease, cerebral aneurysms, livedo reticularis, iris flocculi, PDA, moyamoya, and premature coronary artery disease; gene mutations causing familial thoracic aortic aneurysm and dissection (TAAD) include *ACTA2, TGFBR1, TGFBR2, FBN1, MYH11, MYLK, TGFB2, SMAD3*
Vascular Ehlers-Danlos syndrome (vEDS)	Autosomal dominant disorder of collagen synthesis caused by a gene mutation in *COL3A1* leading to rupture and dissection of the aorta (usually the descending and abdominal aorta) and branch vessels; manifestations include flexible digits, hyperlucent skin with visible veins, varicose veins, typical facial appearance, and spontaneous rupture of the uterus or bowel
Bicuspid aortic valve (BAV)	Congenital condition affecting ≈1% of the population, familial in ≈9% of cases; often associated with dilation of the ascending aorta and carries increased risk for aortic dissection; gene mutations include *NOTCH1* and loci at 15q, 18q, 5q, and 13q; may be associated with FTAA
Turner syndrome (TS)	Genetic disorder affecting 1 in 2000 live-born girls and caused by complete or partial loss of the second sex chromosome (XO, Xp); women with TS often have BAV and aortic coarctation; associated with ascending aortic dilation for body size and increased risk for aortic dissection, especially when associated with BAV, hypertension, and coarctation
Aneurysms-osteoarthritis syndrome	Autosomal dominant genetic disorder resulting from mutations in the *SMAD3* gene and associated with premature osteoarthritis, osteochondritis dissecans, skeletal features, aortic aneurysms, branch vessel aneurysms, and arterial tortuosity; overlap with LDS phenotype

From Mann DL, et al.: *Braunwald's heart disease*, ed 10, Philadelphia, 2015, Elsevier.

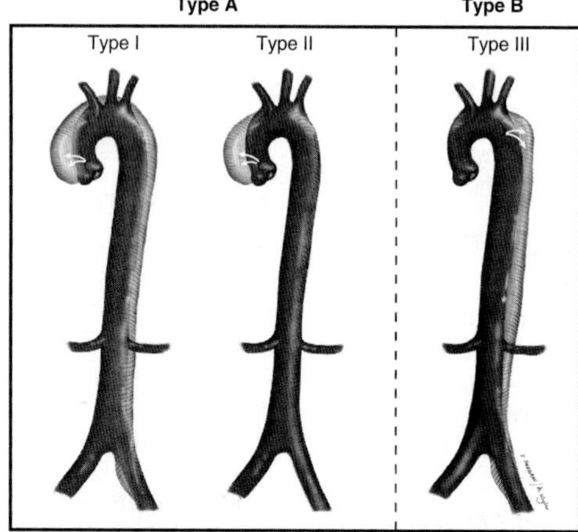

FIG. 2 Classification schemes of acute aortic dissection. (From Mann DL, et al.: *Braunwald's heart disease*, ed 10, Philadelphia, 2015, Elsevier.)

TABLE 2 Classification Schemes of Acute Aortic Dissection

DeBakey Classification	
Type I	Originates in the ascending aorta and extends at least to the aortic arch and often to the descending aorta (and beyond)
Type II	Originates in the ascending aorta and confined to this segment
Type III	Originates in the descending aorta, usually just distal to the left subclavian artery, and extends distally
Stanford Classification	
Type A	Dissections involving the ascending aorta (with or without extension into the descending aorta)
Type B	Dissections not involving the ascending aorta

From Mann DL, et al.: *Braunwald's heart disease*, ed 10, Philadelphia, 2015, Elsevier.

- Three biomarkers with different diagnostic windows can be used in the diagnosis of aortic dissection:
  1. Smooth muscle myosin heavy chain protein (released from damaged medial smooth muscle) can be used to detect proximal aortic dissections (91% sensitivity and 93% specificity). Myosin heavy chains will peak within 3 hr of dissection and clear within 24 hr of aortic injury.
  2. CK-BB isoenzyme also peaks within 6 hr of dissection.
  3. Calponin, a smooth muscle troponin counterpart, increases in aortic dissection with a wider diagnostic window when compared to smooth muscle myosin heavy chain and CK-BB.
  4. C-reactive protein, fibrinogen, soluble ST2, and soluble elastin fragments are under investigation.

IMAGING STUDIES

- Multidetector CT (Figs. 3 and 4) is considered the gold standard, but its use may be limited in patients with renal failure as it involves the use of intravenous contrast.
- Transesophageal echocardiography (TEE), multidetector CT, and MRI are all highly sensitive (98%-100%) and specific (95%-98%). Test of choice depends on clinical circumstances and hospital availability.
- TEE is study of choice in unstable patients with type A dissection but is operator dependent.
- MRI has high sensitivity and specificity but limited availability; not suitable for unstable patients; contraindicated with pacemakers, metal devices.
- With medium or high pretest probability, a second diagnostic test should be done if the first is negative.
- Coronary computed tomographic angiography (CTA) may be an alternative and useful diagnostic study when

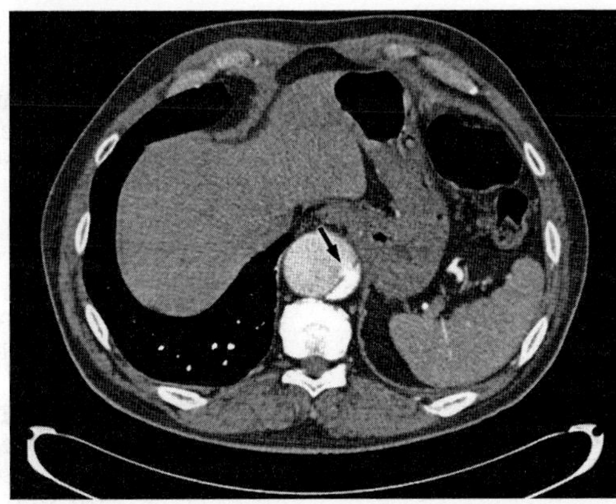

FIG. 3 Contrast-enhanced computed tomography scan of an aortic dissection demonstrating a fenestration in the intimal flap *(arrow)* with contrast material flowing from the small, densely opacified true lumen into the less opacified and larger false lumen of the aorta. (From Mann DL, et al.: *Braunwald's heart disease,* ed 10, Philadelphia, 2015, Elsevier.)

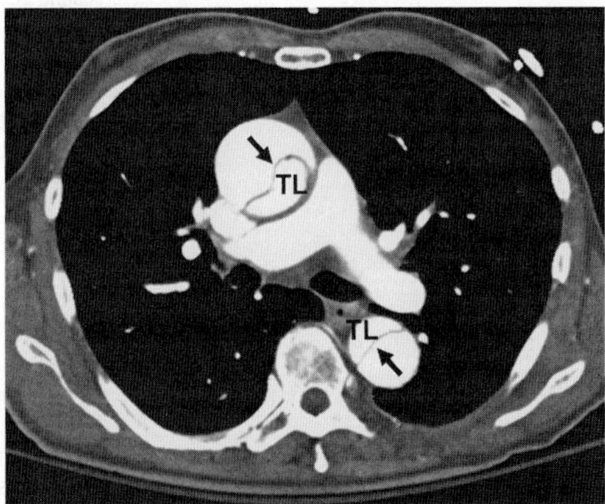

FIG. 4 Contrast-enhanced computed tomography scan demonstrating acute type A aortic dissection with enlargement of the ascending aorta and intimal flaps *(arrows)* in the ascending and descending aorta. Both the true lumen *(TL)* and the false lumen are opacified with contrast material in this example. (From Mann DL, et al.: *Braunwald's heart disease,* ed 10, Philadelphia, 2015, Elsevier.)

evaluating for pulmonary embolism, acute coronary syndrome, and aortic dissection.

- Aortography rarely done, as less sensitive than TEE, CT, or MRI.
- Chest radiograph may show widened mediastinum (52% in type A dissections and 39% in type B dissections) and displacement of aortic intimal calcium. It is normal in 29% to 36% of patients with aortic dissection.
- Although the diagnostic sensitivity of transthoracic echocardiography is suboptimal (31% to 55%), it is useful in assessing potential high-risk features or complications, such as pericardial effusion, and making other potential diagnoses. A negative transthoracic echocardiography, however, does not exclude aortic dissection.

Rx TREATMENT

- Urgent surgical consultation should be obtained for all thoracic aortic dissection regardless of anatomic location.
- Proximal dissections (acute type A) require emergent surgery to prevent rupture or pericardial effusion.
- Distal dissections (Stanford type B) are usually treated medically unless distal organ involvement or impending rupture occurs.
    1. Surgical intervention for distal dissections is reserved for patients who have a complicated course, including occlusion of a major aortic branch, propagation of the dissection, enlarging aneurysm, and evidence of aortic rupture.
    2. Thoracic endovascular aortic repair (TEVAR) is a less invasive option for complicated type B aortic dissections and is associated with lower short- and midterm mortality than medical therapy.
    3. For acute type B dissections, in-hospital mortality in patients managed surgically has been reported to be 33.9% versus those managed with endovascular treatment at 10.6%.
    4. Independent predictors of complication and mortality in distal dissections include periaortic hematoma and descending aortic diameter >5.5 cm, partial false lumen thrombosis, primary tear >10 mm, one entry tear, and false lumen >22 mm.
    5. There is ongoing debate about a possible beneficial role of TEVAR for uncomplicated type B dissections. Data suggest that 30% of uncomplicated type B dissections will progress to an aneurysm.

ACUTE GENERAL Rx

- Admit to ICU for monitoring.
- Target systolic blood pressure 100 to 120 mm Hg or as low as tolerated; heart rate <60 beats/min to reduce aortic wall stress. Treatment with beta-blockers has been associated with improved survival in all patients with acute aortic dissections.
- IV beta-blockers are cornerstones of treatment, but multiple medications may be needed.
    1. Propranolol 1 mg every 3 to 5 min, metoprolol 5 mg IV every 5 min, or labetalol 20 mg IV, then 20 to 80 mg every 10 min, followed by nitroprusside 0.3 to 10 mcg/kg/min.
    2. Vasodilators should not be used without beta-blockade as they can induce reflex sympathetic stimulation and increase aortic shear stress.
    3. IV calcium channel blockers with negative inotropy (i.e., verapamil, diltiazem) may be used if beta-blockers are contraindicated.
- Pain control, often with morphine.

CHRONIC Rx

- Chronic aortic dissection (>2 wk) managed with aggressive blood pressure control; target <120/80 mm Hg in most patients
- Statin therapy to reduce low-density lipoprotein <70 mg/dl
- Tobacco cessation
- Minimize strenuous physical activity such as heavy lifting
- Serial imaging of the aorta, with multidetector CT or MRI should be performed at presentation, at 1, 3, 6, and 12 months given the higher risk of instability early on, followed by yearly clinical and imaging follow-up
- As stated above, endovascular repair should be considered in complicated chronic type B dissections, i.e., when the aortic diameter exceeds 5.5 cm, when there is uncontrolled pain or blood pressure, or when there is rapid growth of the dissecting aneurysm (>4 mm per yr)

DISPOSITION

- 90% mortality rate within 2 weeks for an untreated type A dissection.
- Proximal dissection is a surgical emergency. Time is critical; mortality rate is 1% to 3% per hour, approaching 70% after 48 hours.

TABLE 3 Suggested Imaging Surveillance of Asymptomatic Thoracic Aortic Aneurysms*

Initial Discovery of Aneurysm	Repeated Imaging at 6 Months to Document Stability
Degenerative aneurysm†	
3.5-4.4 cm	Annual imaging
4.5-5.4 cm	Annual to biannual imaging
MFS, BAV with TAA, and familial TAA	
3.5-4.4 cm	Annual imaging
4.5-5.0 cm	Biannual imaging
LDS‡	
<4 cm	At least annual imaging
>4 cm	Biannual imaging

*For aneurysms growing rapidly, more frequent imaging is recommended. Management of TAA must take into account the family history, age, body size, sex, rate of aneurysm growth, and underlying disease.

†For relatively small degenerative aneurysms found by imaging to be stable from year to year, imaging may be performed every 2-3 years. (Hiratzka et al)

‡Some recommend surgery for aortic root dimensions larger than 4 cm in adults with LDS, whereas the American College of Cardiology/American Heart Association guidelines for thoracic aortic disease recommend prophylactic surgery at 4.2 cm by TEE and 4.4 to 4.6 cm by CT or MRI. (Hiratzka et al)

BAV, Bicuspid aortic valve; *LDS,* Loeys-Dietz syndrome; *MFS,* Marfan syndrome; *TAA,* thoracic aortic aneurysm.

(Hiratzka LF et al: 2010 ACCF/AHA/AATS/ACR/ASA/SCA/SCAI/SIR/STS/SVM guidelines for the diagnosis and management of patients with thoracic aortic disease: a report of the American College of Cardiology Foundation/American Heart Association Task Force on Practice Guidelines, American Association for Thoracic Surgery, American College of Radiology, American Stroke Association, Society of Cardiovascular Anesthesiologists, Society for Cardiovascular Angiography and Interventions, Society of Interventional Radiology, Society of Thoracic Surgeons, and Society for Vascular Medicine, *Circulation* 121:e266, 2010.)

From Mann DL, et al.: *Braunwald's heart disease,* ed 10, Philadelphia, 2015, Elsevier.

- Overall, in-hospital mortality rate is 22% with proximal dissections (27% treated surgically and 56% treated medically) and 10% to 17% with distal dissections.
- Table 3 summarizes suggested imaging surveillance of asymptomatic thoracic aortic aneurysms.

REFERRAL

For ICU management and surgical intervention

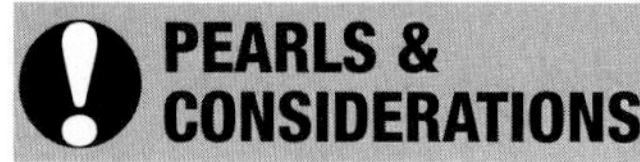

PEARLS & CONSIDERATIONS

- Blood pressure control is essential; beta-blocker is first-line medication.
- Proximal dissection is a surgical emergency.
- Cardiac tamponade is not uncommon in patients with acute type A aortic dissection. Syncope, altered mental status, and a widened mediastinum on chest radiograph on presentation suggest tamponade, which warrants urgent operative therapy.
- Surgery for acute type A aortic dissection in patients ≥70 years old can be performed with acceptable outcomes.

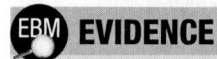

EVIDENCE

Available at ExpertConsult.com

SUGGESTED READINGS

Available at ExpertConsult.com

RELATED CONTENT

Aortic Dissection (Patient Information)

AUTHORS: **MOHAMMAD KHAN, M.D.,** and **PHILIP STOCKWELL, M.D.**

BASIC INFORMATION

DEFINITION

Aortic regurgitation (AR) is retrograde blood flow into the left ventricle from the aorta as a result of an incompetent aortic valve.

Stages of chronic aortic regurgitation:

Stage A = at risk of AR (e.g., bicuspid AV, AV sclerosis) but no aortic regurgitation.

Stage B = progressive AR with mild and moderate aortic regurgitation.

Stage C = asymptomatic severe AR.

Stage D = symptomatic severe AR.

SYNONYMS

Aortic insufficiency
AI
AR

ICD-10CM CODES

I35.1	Nonrheumatic aortic (valve) insufficiency
I35.2	Nonrheumatic aortic (valve) stenosis with insufficiency
Q23.1	Congenital insufficiency of aortic valve

EPIDEMIOLOGY & DEMOGRAPHICS

- Prevalence ranges from 4.9% to 10% and increases with age.
- The most common cause of isolated severe AR is aortic root dilation.
- Infectious endocarditis is the most frequent cause of acute AR.

PHYSICAL FINDINGS & CLINICAL PRESENTATION

The clinical presentation varies depending on whether aortic insufficiency is acute or chronic. Chronic aortic insufficiency is well tolerated (except when secondary to infective endocarditis), and the patients remain asymptomatic for years. Common manifestations after significant deterioration of left ventricular function are dyspnea on exertion, syncope, chest pain, and congestive heart failure (CHF). The stages of chronic AR are summarized in Table 1. Acute aortic insufficiency manifests primarily with hypotension caused by a sudden fall in cardiac output and resultant cardiogenic shock. In addition, a rapid rise in left ventricular diastolic pressure results in a further decrease in coronary blood flow.

Physical findings in chronic aortic insufficiency include the following:

- Widened pulse pressure (markedly increased systolic blood pressure, decreased diastolic blood pressure). Fig. E1 illustrates characteristics of AR murmur.
- Findings associated with the widened pulse pressure:
  1. Bounding pulses, "water hammer," or collapsing pulse (***Corrigan* pulse**) can be palpated at the wrist or on the femoral artery and is caused by rapid rise and sudden collapse of the arterial pressure during late systole.
  2. Head "bobbing" with each systole (***de Musset* sign**).
  3. "Pistol shot femorals" (***Traube* sign**) is a term used to describe a loud sound over the femoral artery.
  4. Capillary pulsations (***Quincke* sign**) may occur at the base of the nail beds.
- A to-and-fro Duroziez double intermittent femoral murmur may be heard over femoral arteries with slight compression with the edge of the stethoscope.
- Popliteal systolic pressure is increased more than 20 mm Hg over brachial systolic pressure (***Hill* sign**) with a 40 to 60 mm difference representing moderate AR and >60 mm difference severe AR.
- Other findings associated with AR, which are more of historical than practical interest, include:
  1. ***Mueller* sign**—Systolic pulsations of the uvula.
  2. ***Becker* sign**—Visible pulsations of the retinal arteries and pupils.
  3. ***Mayne* sign**—More than a 15 mm Hg decrease in diastolic blood pressure with arm elevation from the value obtained with the arm in the standard position.
  4. ***Rosenbach* sign**—Systolic pulsations of the liver.
  5. ***Gerhard* sign**—Systolic pulsations of the spleen.
- Cardiac auscultation reveals:
  1. Displacement of cardiac impulse downward and to the patient's left.
  2. S_3 heard over the apex.
  3. Decrescendo, blowing diastolic murmur heard along left sternal border.
  4. Low-pitched apical diastolic rumble (***Austin-Flint murmur***)—the precise etiology of the murmur is uncertain, but it is generally believed to be related to increased velocity of mitral inflow consequent to the AR.
  5. Early systolic ejection sound and systolic ejection murmur.

In patients with acute aortic insufficiency both the wide pulse pressure and the large stroke volume are absent. A short, blowing diastolic murmur may be the only finding on physical examination.

ETIOLOGY

- Leaflet abnormalities:
  1. Infective endocarditis
  2. Rheumatic fibrosis (most common cause in developing countries)
  3. Trauma with valvular rupture
  4. Congenital bicuspid aortic valve (most common cause in the United States)
  5. Myxomatous degeneration
  6. Fenfluramine, dexfenfluramine, pergolide, cabergoline
  7. Ankylosing spondylitis
- Aortic root or ascending aorta abnormalities:
  1. Annuloaortic ectasia
  2. Ehlers-Danlos syndrome
  3. Marfan's syndrome
  4. Trauma: Ankylosing spondylitis
  5. Syphilitic aortitis
  6. Systemic hypertension
  7. Aortic dissection
- Postprocedural aortic regurgitation, usually due to a paravalvular leak, occurs in 10% to 20% of patients undergoing transcatheter aortic valve replacement. Patients with more than mild aortic regurgitation after transcatheter aortic valve replacement have worse outcomes than those without aortic regurgitation.

Dx DIAGNOSIS

DIFFERENTIAL DIAGNOSIS

- Patent ductus arteriosus, pulmonary regurgitation, and other valvular abnormalities.
- The differential diagnosis of cardiac murmurs is described in Sections II and III.

WORKUP

- Echocardiogram, chest radiograph, electrocardiogram (ECG), cardiac magnetic resonance imaging, and cardiac catheterization (selected patients).
- Medical history and physical examination focused on the following clinical manifestations:
  1. Dyspnea on exertion
  2. Syncope
  3. Chest pain
  4. CHF

IMAGING STUDIES

- Chest radiography:
  1. Left ventricular hypertrophy (LVH) (chronic AR)
  2. Aortic dilation
  3. Normal cardiac silhouette with pulmonary edema: Possible in patients with acute AR
- ECG: LVH.
- Echocardiography (Fig. E2) is the main imaging modality to diagnose AR and assess left ventricular size and function. Quantification of the severity of regurgitation can be made either qualitatively by Doppler vena contracta width (severe if >0.6 cm) or quantitatively by effective regurgitant orifice area (severe if >0.30 cm^2) and/or regurgitant volume (severe if >60 ml per/beat).
- Cardiac magnetic resonance is indicated (class 1) in patients with moderate or severe AR and suboptimal echocardiographic images for the assessment of AR severity as well as LV systolic function and volumes.
- Cardiac catheterization is indicated in selected patients to assess the degree of left ventricular dysfunction, to assess the degree of AR when echocardiographic parameters are inconclusive, and to determine if there is coexistent coronary artery disease.
- Serial evaluation of the size and morphology of the aortic sinuses and ascending aorta by echocardiography, CMR, or CT angiography is recommended in patients with a bicuspid aortic valve and an aortic diameter greater than 4.0 cm, with the examination interval determined by the degree and rate of progression of aortic dilation and by family

TABLE 1 Stages of Chronic Aortic Regurgitation

Stage	Definition	Valve Anatomy	Valve Hemodynamics	Hemodynamic Consequences	Symptoms
A	**At risk of AR**	Bicuspid aortic valve (or other congenital valve anomaly) Aortic valve sclerosis Diseases of the aortic sinuses or ascending aorta History of rheumatic fever or known rheumatic heart disease IE	AR severity none or trace	None	None
B	**Progressive AR**	Mild to moderate calcification of a trileaflet valve bicuspid aortic valve (or other congenital valve anomaly) Dilated aortic sinuses Rheumatic valve changes Previous IE	***Mild AR:*** Jet width <25% of LVOT vena contracta <0.3 cm RVol <30 mlml/beat RF <30% ERO <0.10 cm^2 Angiography grade 1+ ***Moderate AR:*** Jet width 25%–64% of LVOT Vena contracta 0.3–0.6 cm RVol 30–59 ml/beat RF 30%–49% ERO 0.10–0.29 cm^2 Angiography grade 2+	Normal LV systolic function Normal LV volume or mild LV dilation	None
C	**Asymptomatic severe AR**	Calcific aortic valve disease Bicuspid valve (or other congenital abnormality) Dilated aortic sinuses or ascending aorta Rheumatic valve changes IE with abnormal leaflet closure or perforation	***Severe AR:*** Jet width ≥65% of LVOT Vena contracta >0.6 cm Holodiastolic flow reversal in the proximal abdominal aorta RVol ≥60 ml/beat RF ≥50% ERO ≥0.3 cm^2 Angiography grade 3+ to 4+ In addition, diagnosis of chronic severe AR requires evidence of LV dilation	*C1:* Normal LVEF (≥50%) and mild-to-moderate LV dilation (LVESD ≤50 mm) *C2:* Abnormal LV systolic function with depressed LVEF (<50%) or severe LV dilation (LVESD >50 mm or indexed LVESD >25 mm/m^2)	None; exercise testing is reasonable to confirm symptom status
D	**Symptomatic severe AR**	Calcific valve disease Bicuspid valve (or other congenital abnormality) Dilated aortic sinuses or ascending aorta Rheumatic valve changes Previous IE with abnormal leaflet closure or perforation	***Severe AR:*** Doppler jet width ≥65% of LVOT Vena contracta >0.6 cm Holodiastolic flow reversal in the proximal abdominal aorta RVol ≥60 ml/beat RF ≥50% ERO ≥0.3 cm^2 Angiography grade 3+ to 4+ In addition, diagnosis of chronic severe AR requires evidence of LV dilation	Symptomatic severe AR may occur with normal systolic function (LVEF ≥50%), mild-to-moderate LV dysfunction (LVEF 40%–50%), or severe LV dysfunction (LVEF <40%) Moderate-to-severe LV dilation is present	Exertional dyspnea or angina, or more severe HF symptoms

AR, Aortic regurgitation; *ERO,* effective regurgitant orifice; *HF,* heart failure; *IE,* infective endocarditis; *LV,* left ventricle; *LVEF,* left ventricular ejection fraction; *LVESD,* left ventricular end-systolic dimension; *LVOT,* left ventricular outflow tract; *RF,* regurgitant fraction; *RVol,* regurgitant volume.
From Nishimura RA, Otto CM, Bonow RO, et al.: 2014 AHA/ACCF guideline for the management of patients with valvular heart disease: a report of the American College of Cardiology Foundation/American Heart Association Task Force on Practice Guidelines. *J Am Coll Cardiol* 63:e57, 2014. In Mann DL, Zipes DP, Libby P, Bonow RO: *Braunwald's Heart Disease,* ed 10, Philadelphia, 2015, Elsevier.

history. In patients with an aortic diameter greater than 4.5 cm, this evaluation should be performed annually (Class 1).

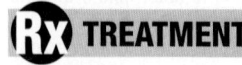

TREATMENT

NONPHASECTIONAMACOLOGIC THERAPY

- Avoidance of competitive sports and heavy weight lifting if the AR is severe and associated with aortic root dilation.
- Salt restriction.
- In 2007, the American Heart Association (AHA) guidelines for prevention of infectious endocarditis were revised; and routine antibiotic prophylaxis to undergo dental or other invasive procedures is no longer recommended, unless the patient has a prior history of endocarditis.

MEDICAL

ACUTE GENERAL RX:

- Afterload reduction: Angiotensin-converting enzyme (ACE) inhibitors and vasodilators (i.e., nitroprusside) in acute AR; diuretics for pulmonary edema.
- Avoid beta-blockers that can prolong diastole.
- Emergent surgical referral for cardiogenic shock.

CHRONIC RX:

- Long-term vasodilator therapy with ACE inhibitors or nifedipine in patients who have concomitant hypertension. In one 1994 study (Scognamiglio et al) nifedipine delayed the need for aortic valve surgery compared to digoxin, but in a second randomized trial (Evangelista et al) comparing placebo to

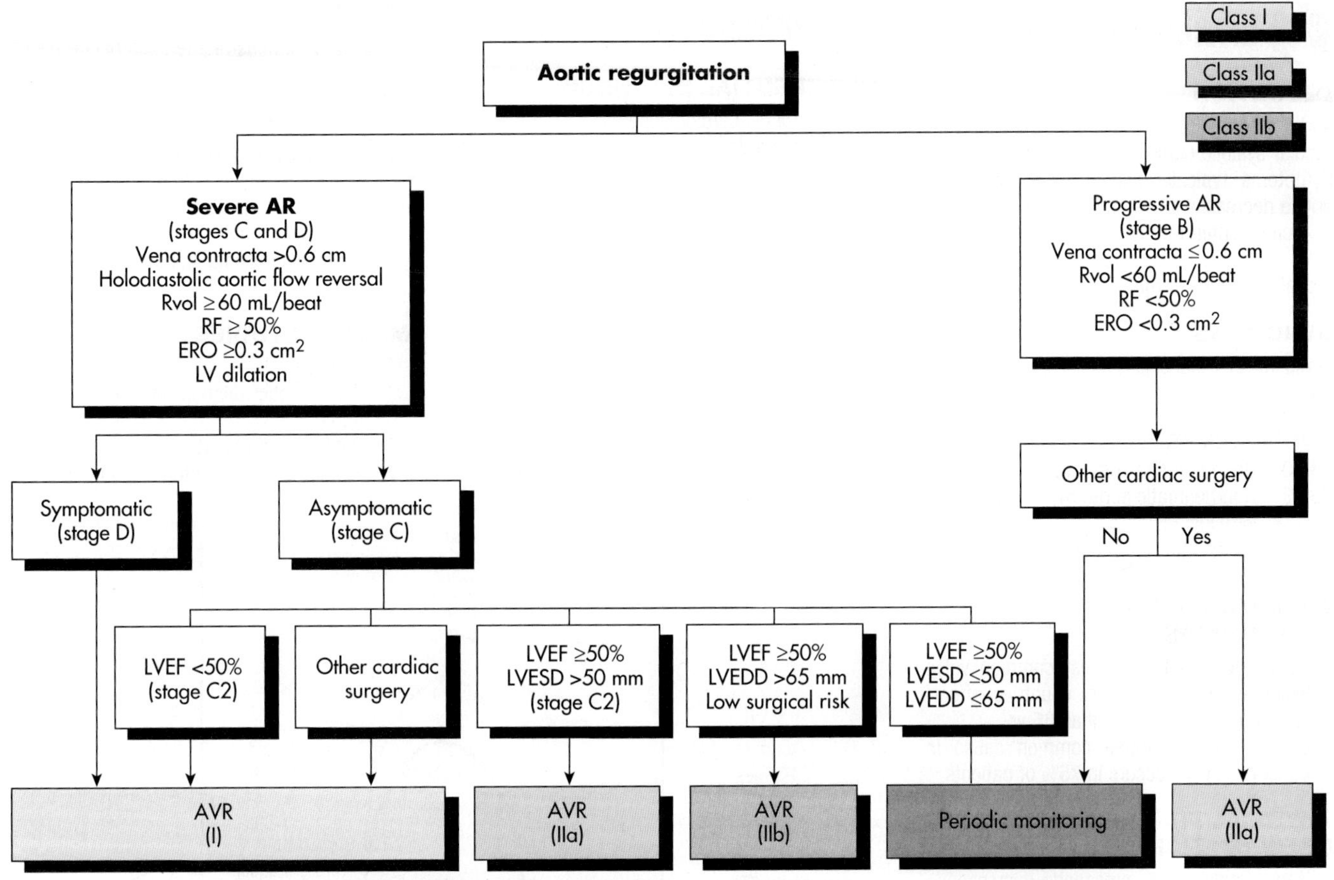

FIG. 3 Management strategy for patients with chronic severe AR. *AR,* Aortic regurgitation; *AVR,* aortic valve replacement (valve repair may be appropriate in selected patients); *ERO,* effective regurgitant orifice; *LV,* left ventricle; *LVEDD,* left ventricular end-diastolic dimension; *LVEF,* left ventricular ejection fraction; *LVESD,* left ventricular end-systolic dimension; *RF,* regurgitant fraction; *RVol,* regurgitant volume. (From Nishimura RA, Otto CM, Bonow RO, et al.: 2014 AHA/ACCF guideline for the management of patients with valvular heart disease: a report of the American College of Cardiology Foundation/American Heart Association Task Force on Practice Guidelines. *J Am Coll Cardiol* 63:e57: 2014. In Mann DL, Zipes DP, Libby P, Bonow RO: *Braunwald's heart disease,* ed 10, Philadelphia, 2015, Elsevier.)

nifedipine and enalapril, there was no reduction in need for aortic valve surgery when followed up to 7 yr. Therefore there is no current definitive indication of medical therapy with afterload reduction for aortic regurgitation other than hypertension control.

- Beta-blockers in combination with ACE inhibitors are reasonable in patients with symptomatic severe AR or LV dysfunction when surgery cannot be performed because of concomitant comorbidities. In a retrospective cohort study of 756 patients with chronic AR, beta-blocker therapy was associated with decreased mortality. Patients treated with beta-blockers were more likely to be taking ACE inhibitors and dihydropyridine calcium channel blockers as well (53% vs. 40%). In the same study, patients treated with beta-blockers and undergoing AVR were also noted to have a mortality benefit.
- Diuretics and sodium restriction for CHF.
- Comparable efficacy of losartan and atenolol was shown in curbing aortic root dilatation growth in children and young adults (6 mo–25 yr) with Marfan's syndrome with similar outcomes of aortic regurgitation severity, surgery, aortic dissection, and death at 3 yr.
- Fig. 3 describes a management strategy for patients with chronic severe AR.

SURGICAL RESERVED FOR: REFERRAL

Reserved for:

- Patients with acute severe AR (i.e., infective endocarditis) and cardiogenic shock.
- Symptomatic patients with severe AR regardless of LV systolic function (class I).
- Patients with hemodynamically stable severe AR undergoing CABG or surgery on the aorta or other heart valves.
- Evidence of systolic dysfunction with left ventricular ejection fraction of less than 50%.
- Asymptomatic patients with severe AR and left ventricular ejection fraction >50%, but with left ventricular dilation:
  1. Echocardiographic end-systolic dimension >50 mm (Class IIa level of evidence) *or;*
  2. Echocardiographic end-diastolic dimension >65 mm with low surgical risk (Class IIb).

SUGGESTED READINGS

Available at ExpertConsult.com

RELATED CONTENT

Aortic Insufficiency (Patient Information)

AUTHOR: **DENISA HAGAU, M.D., F.A.C.C.**

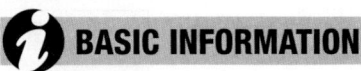

BASIC INFORMATION

DEFINITION

Aortic stenosis (AS) is obstruction to left ventricular systolic outflow across the aortic valve. Symptoms typically appear when the valve orifice decreases to <1 cm^2 (normal orifice is 3 to 4 cm^2). Criteria for severe AS include a valve area <1.0 cm^2, a mean gradient >40 mm Hg, or a peak gradient >4 m/s.

SYNONYMS

Aortic valvular stenosis
AS

ICD-10CM CODES

I35.0	Nonrheumatic aortic (valve) stenosis
I35.2	Nonrheumatic aortic (valve) stenosis with insufficiency
Q23.0	Congenital stenosis of aortic valve

EPIDEMIOLOGY & DEMOGRAPHICS

- Aortic stenosis is the most common valve lesion in adults in Western countries, affecting 3% of persons older than 65 yr.
- Calcific stenosis (most common cause in patients >70 yr) occurs in 75% of patients.

PHYSICAL FINDINGS & CLINICAL PRESENTATION

- Harsh midsystolic, crescendo-decrescendo murmur (Fig. 1) best heard at base of heart and radiating into neck vessels; often associated with a thrill or ejection click; may also be heard well at the apex.
- Signs of severe AS include absent or diminished intensity of the second heart sound and/or late rising carotid upstroke with delayed amplitude (pulsus parvus et tardus), presence of S4, and a reverse splitting of the second heart sound.
- Classic symptoms include angina, syncope, and heart failure.
- Table 1 summarizes the stages of valvular aortic stenosis.
- Acquired von Willebrand disease is seen in approximately 20% of severe AS, which can lead to GI bleeding from angiodysplasia (Heyde syndrome) that resolves after aortic valve replacement.

ETIOLOGY

- Idiopathic calcification of the aortic valve (most common cause, presents at ages 60 to 80)
- Progressive stenosis of congenital bicuspid valve (found in 1% to 2% of the population, presents at ages 40 to 60)
- Rheumatic heart disease
- Less common causes include congenital (major cause of AS in patients <30 yr), radiation, and obstructive vegetations (endocarditis)
- Genetic variation in the LPA locus, mediated by Lp(2) levels, is associated with aortic valve calcification across multiple ethnic groups and with incidental clinical aortic stenosis

Dx DIAGNOSIS

DIFFERENTIAL DIAGNOSIS

- Hypertrophic cardiomyopathy
- Mitral regurgitation
- Ventricular septal defect
- Aortic sclerosis. Aortic stenosis is distinguished from aortic sclerosis by the degree of valve impairment. In aortic sclerosis, the valve leaflets are abnormally thickened but obstruction to outflow is absent or minimal
- Subvalvular membrane or supravalvular AS
- Stages of valvular AS
  1. Stage A = at risk of AS
  2. Stage B = progressive AS (formerly known as mild and moderate AS)
  3. Stage C = asymptomatic severe AS
  4. Stage D = symptomatic severe AS

WORKUP

- ECG: May demonstrate left ventricular hypertrophy and/or left atrial abnormality
- Chest radiograph: May demonstrate cardiomegaly. Poststenotic dilation of the ascending aorta may also be evident
- Echocardiography (see "Imaging Studies")
- Cardiac catheterization in selected patients (see "Imaging Studies")
- Dobutamine challenge (for low-gradient, low-flow AS)

IMAGING STUDIES

- Chest x-ray:
  1. Poststenotic dilation of the ascending aorta
  2. Calcification of aortic cusps
  3. Rounding of left ventricle (LV) apex

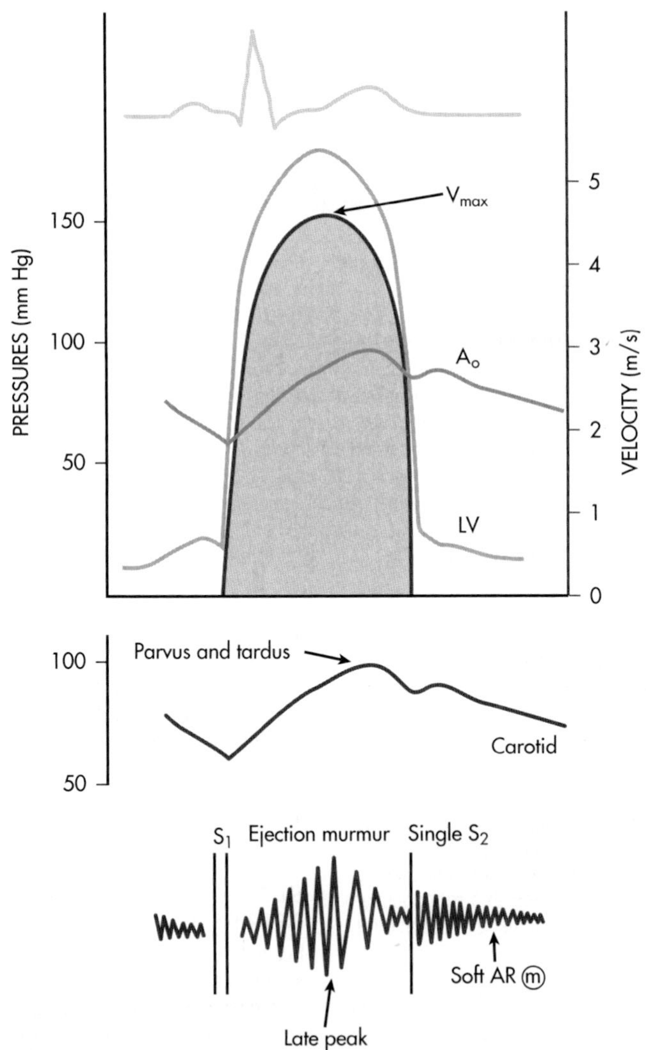

FIG. 1 Relationship between left ventricle (LV) and aortic (Ao) pressures and the Doppler aortic stenosis velocity curve (*in red*). The pressure difference between the LV and aorta in systole is four times the velocity squared (the Bernoulli equation). Thus, a maximum velocity (Vmax) of 4.3 m/sec corresponds to a maximum LV to Ao pressure difference of 74 mm Hg and a mean systolic gradient of 44 mm Hg. On physical examination, the slow rate of rise and delayed peak in the carotid pulse (or parvus and tardus) matches the contour of the aortic pressure waveform. The murmur corresponds to the Doppler velocity curve with a harsh crescendo-decrescendo late-peaking systolic murmur, best heard at the aortic region (upper right sternal border). Often, a soft, high-pitched diastolic decrescendo murmur of aortic regurgitation also is appreciated. (From Bonow, et al. [eds]: *Braunwald's heart disease,* ed 9, Philadelphia, 2012, Saunders.)

TABLE 1 Stages of Valvular Aortic Stenosis

Stage	Definition	Valve Anatomy	Valve Hemodynamics	Hemodynamic Consequences	Symptoms
A	**At risk of AS**	Bicuspid aortic valve (or other congenital valve anomaly) Aortic valve sclerosis	Aortic Vmax <2 m/sec	None	None
B	**Progressive AS**	Mild to moderate leaflet calcification of a bicuspid or trileaflet valve with some reduction in systolic motion or rheumatic valve changes with commissural fusion	***Mild AS:*** Aortic Vmax 2.0–2.9 m/sec or mean ΔP <20 mm Hg ***Moderate AS:*** Aortic Vmax 3.0–3.9 m/sec or mean ΔP 20–39 mm Hg	Early LV diastolic dysfunction may be present Normal LVEF	None
C	**Asymptomatic severe AS**				
C1	Asymptomatic severe AS	Severe leaflet calcification or congenital stenosis with severely reduced leaflet opening	***Severe AS:*** Aortic Vmax ≥4 m/sec or mean ΔP ≥40 mm Hg AVA typically is ≤1 cm^2 (or AVAi ≤0.6 cm^2/m^2) Very severe AS is an aortic Vmax ≥5 m/sec, or mean ΔP ≥ 60 mm Hg	LV diastolic dysfunction Mild LV hypertrophy Normal LVEF	None; exercise testing is reasonable to confirm symptom status
C2	Asymptomatic severe AS with LV dysfunction	Severe leaflet calcification or congenital stenosis with severely reduced leaflet opening	Aortic Vmax ≥4 m/sec or mean ΔP ≥40 mm Hg AVA typically is ≤1 cm^2 (or AVAi ≤0.6 cm^2/m^2)	LVEF <50%	None
D	**Symptomatic severe AS**				
D1	Symptomatic severe high-gradient AS	Severe leaflet calcification or congenital stenosis with severely reduced leaflet opening	***Severe AS:*** Aortic Vmax ≥4 m/sec, or mean ΔP ≥40 mm Hg AVA typically is ≤1 cm^2 (or AVAi ≤0.6 cm^2/m^2), but may be larger with mixed AS/AR	LV diastolic dysfunction LV hypertrophy Pulmonary hypertension may be present	Exertional dyspnea or decreased exercise tolerance Exertional angina Exertional syncope or presyncope
D2	Symptomatic severe low-flow/low-gradient AS with reduced LVEF	Severe leaflet calcification with severely reduced leaflet motion	AVA ≤1 cm^2 with resting aortic Vmax <4 m/sec, or mean ΔP <40 mm Hg Dobutamine stress echo shows AVA ≤1 cm^2 with Vmax ≥4 m/sec at any flow rate	LV diastolic dysfunction LV hypertrophy LVEF <50%	HF, angina, syncope or presyncope
D3	Symptomatic severe low-gradient AS with normal LVEF or paradoxical low-flow severe AS	Severe leaflet calcification with severely reduced leaflet motion	AVA ≤1 cm^2 with aortic Vmax <4 m/sec, or mean ΔP <40 mm Hg AVAi ≤0.6 cm^2/m^2 Stroke volume index <35 ml/m^2 Measured when the patient is normotensive (systolic BP <140 mm Hg)	Increased LV relative wall thickness Small LV chamber with low-stroke volume. Restrictive diastolic filling LVEF ≥50%	HF, angina, syncope or presyncope

AR, Aortic regurgitation; *AS,* aortic stenosis; *AVA,* aortic valve area; *AVAi,* aortic valve area indexed to body surface area; *BP,* blood pressure; *HF,* heart failure; *LV,* left ventricle; *LVEF,* left ventricular ejection fraction; *ΔP,* pressure gradient; *Vmax,* maximum aortic velocity.

From Nishimura RA, et al.: 2014 AHA/ACCF guideline for the management of patients with valvular heart disease: a report of the American College of Cardiology Foundation/American Heart Association Task Force on Practice Guidelines. In Mann DL, et al. (eds): *Braunwald's heart disease*, ed 10, Philadelphia, 2015, Elsevier.

- ECG:
  1. Left ventricular hypertrophy (found in 80% of patients)
  2. Left atrial enlargement
  3. Atrial fibrillation (in late disease)
- Doppler echocardiography: Thickening of the left ventricular wall; allows calculation of both aortic valve area and estimation of pressure gradients to determine severity of AS. (Fig. 2)
- Cardiac catheterization: Indicated in symptomatic patients awaiting aortic valve replacement (AVR) in order to detect coexisting coronary artery stenosis that may need bypass at the same time as aortic valve replacement; also indicated in symptomatic patients when noninvasive tests are inconclusive or when there is a discrepancy between noninvasive tests and clinical findings regarding severity of AS because it confirms the diagnosis and the estimates of the severity of the valvular stenosis by directly measuring the gradient across the valve, allowing calculation of the valve area
- A CT with contrast for imaging the aorta may be needed for annular sizing, aortic measurements, etc., if a transcatheter aortic valve replacement (TAVR) is planned

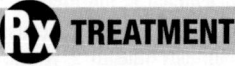

Rx TREATMENT

NONPHARMACOLOGIC THERAPY

- Strenuous activity should be avoided in patients with moderate to severe AS
- Sodium restriction if CHF is present

 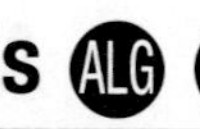

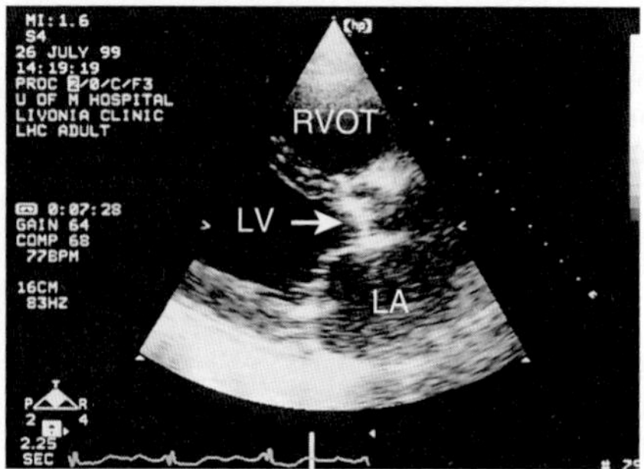

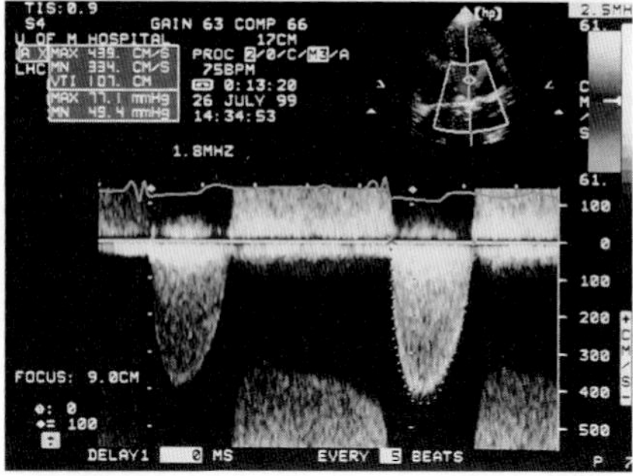

FIG. 2 Echocardiogram recorded in a patient with severe aortic stenosis. The *top panel* is a parasternal long-axis view recorded in systole. Left ventricular function is diminished. The aortic valve is markedly thickened and partially calcified. Its motion is markedly reduced, and in systole it appears that the valve occludes the orifice *(arrow)*. The *lower panel* is a continuous-wave Doppler recorded from the apex of the left ventricle along a line aimed through the stenotic aortic valve. Note the aortic stenosis signal below the zero crossing line. The peak velocity is 430 cm/sec, which corresponds to a maximum gradient of 77 mm Hg and a mean gradient of 49.4 mm Hg. *LA,* Left atrium; *LV,* left ventricle; *RVOT,* right ventricular outflow tract. (From Zipes DP, et al. [eds]: *Braunwald's heart disease,* ed 7, Philadelphia, 2005, Saunders.)

GENERAL Rx

MEDICAL:

- Once symptomatic, AS is a surgical disease. Fig. 3 summarizes a treatment strategy for patients with severe AS.
- Optimize loading conditions by keeping a normal volume status (gentle diuresis for volume overload as preload dependent) and controlling hypertension (HTN) but avoid vasodilators (nitrates); maintain sinus rhythm.
- In 2007, the AHA guidelines for prevention of infectious endocarditis were revised and routine antibiotic prophylaxis to undergo dental or other invasive procedures is no longer recommended, unless the patient has prior endocarditis.

SURGICAL:

- Surgical valve replacement is the treatment of choice in symptomatic patients because there is a 50% mortality rate at 2 yr with medical therapy alone. Valve replacement is a Class I indication for patients with (a) symptomatic severe AS, (b) asymptomatic severe AS with LV ejection fraction (EF) <50%, and (c) severe AS undergoing CABG or surgery on the aorta or other heart valves. Valve replacement is a class 2a indication for patients with (a) asymptomatic severe AS and abnormal blood pressure response (decrease in systolic blood pressure) or decreased exercise tolerance during exercise; (b) asymptomatic patients with very severe AS (peak velocity >5 m/s or mean pressure gradient >60 mm Hg) with low surgical risk; (c) low flow-low gradient (with low ejection fraction <50%) with a positive low-dose dobutamine stress echo; (d) symptomatic patients with low-flow/low gradient severe AS with a **normal LVEF** ≥50%, a valve area ≤1.0 cm^2, and a stroke volume index <35 ml/m^2; and (e) patients with moderate AS who are undergoing cardiac surgery for other indications. Patients with asymptomatic severe AS with rapid disease progression and low surgical risk are a class 2b indication for valve replacement surgery.
- Percutaneous aortic balloon valvuloplasty serves best as palliative therapy in severely symptomatic patients who are not surgical candidates and as a bridge to surgery in hemodynamically unstable adult patients. It is not an option in patients who are good candidates for surgical valve replacement because restenosis occurs in most adult patients at 6 months.
- For patients in whom TAVR or high-risk surgical AVR is being considered, a heart valve team approach is a class I recommendation.
- TAVR is recommended (class I) in patients who have a prohibitive surgical risk and are predicted to survive >12 months after TAVR.
- TAVR is reasonable alternative to surgical aortic valve replacement (SAVR) for symptomatic patients with severe AS and **intermediate surgical risk** (class IIa**).** If transfemoral TAVR is not feasible, SAVR is the recommended approach (grade 1B).
- Valve-in-valve TAVR is reasonable (class IIa) for patients with significant symptoms from bioprosthetic aortic valve regurgitation or stenosis at high risk for reoperation and with anticipated improvement in hemodynamics.
- Percutaneous heart valve replacement is a catheter-based technology that allows for implantation of a prosthetic valve without open heart surgery and sometimes without the need for general anesthesia, decreasing recovery time and hospital stay. TAVR has been shown to reduce mortality by 20% in patients with severe AS and coexisting conditions that exclude them as candidates for surgical replacement of the aortic valve. In a large meta-analysis of **high-risk patients** with severe AS who were candidates for surgery, transfemoral TAVR (but not transthoracic TAVR) was associated with lower mortality at 2 yr. The surgical group had double the incidence of new-onset atrial fibrillation and major bleeding, but the TAVR group had a higher rate of paravalvular regurgitation, major stroke, and vascular complications. In **intermediate-risk patients**, transfemoral TAVR was also associated with lower mortality rates, and nontransfemoral TAVR was similar to surgical aortic valve replacement with respect to death or disabling stroke rates, as demonstrated by the same large meta-analysis of four randomized trials. The notable differences were that TAVR resulted in larger aortic valve areas and had a lower rate of acute kidney injury, severe bleeding, and new-onset atrial fibrillation, whereas surgery resulted in fewer major vascular complications and less paravalvular aortic regurgitation. For **low-risk patients,** the guidelines still recommend surgical aortic valve replacement. However, the NOTION trial showed that patients randomized to either TAVR or SAVR had similar event rates at 1 yr. Limitations of this study included small size and younger patients enrolled subsequently. The trial population was not fully reflective of the population of low-surgical-risk patients with severe symptomatic AS. Other randomized trials are in progress.

Possible predictors of stroke following TAVR were evaluated by a large systematic review and meta-analysis involving 64 studies including 72,318 patients that looked at rates of stroke at 30 days following TAVR. They concluded that female gender, chronic kidney disease, new atrial fibrillation following TAVR, and lower site experience were associated with increased risk of stroke post TAVR.

There also appears to be a risk of early thrombosis after transcatheter aortic valve implantation as demonstrated by a large multicenter study involving 460 patients. There was a 7% incidence of valve thrombosis after Sapien XT or Sapien 3 TAVR, suggesting that warfarin therapy reconsideration may be warranted.

DISPOSITION

- The presence of even mild symptoms is an indicator of poor survival for patients with AS. The average duration of symptoms before death is angina, 5 yr; syncope, 3 yr; CHF, 2 yr.
- Approximately 75% of patients with symptomatic AS will die within 3 yr of symptom onset unless the aortic valve is replaced.

REFERRAL

- Surgical referral for valve replacement in all symptomatic AS patients. There are studies that are examining the presence of moderate or severe valvular calcification, together with a rapid increase in aortic jet velocity and elevated BNP, to identify patients with a very poor prognosis who should be considered for early valve replacement rather than have surgery delayed until symptoms develop. Additionally, patients with severe AS who are asymptomatic should be considered for exercise stress test to see if they are truly without symptoms (low exercise tolerance) or if the BP drops with exercise, both which would be indications for surgical referral. Surgical mortality rate for valve replacement is 3% to 5%; however, it varies with patient's age (>8% in patients >75 yr).

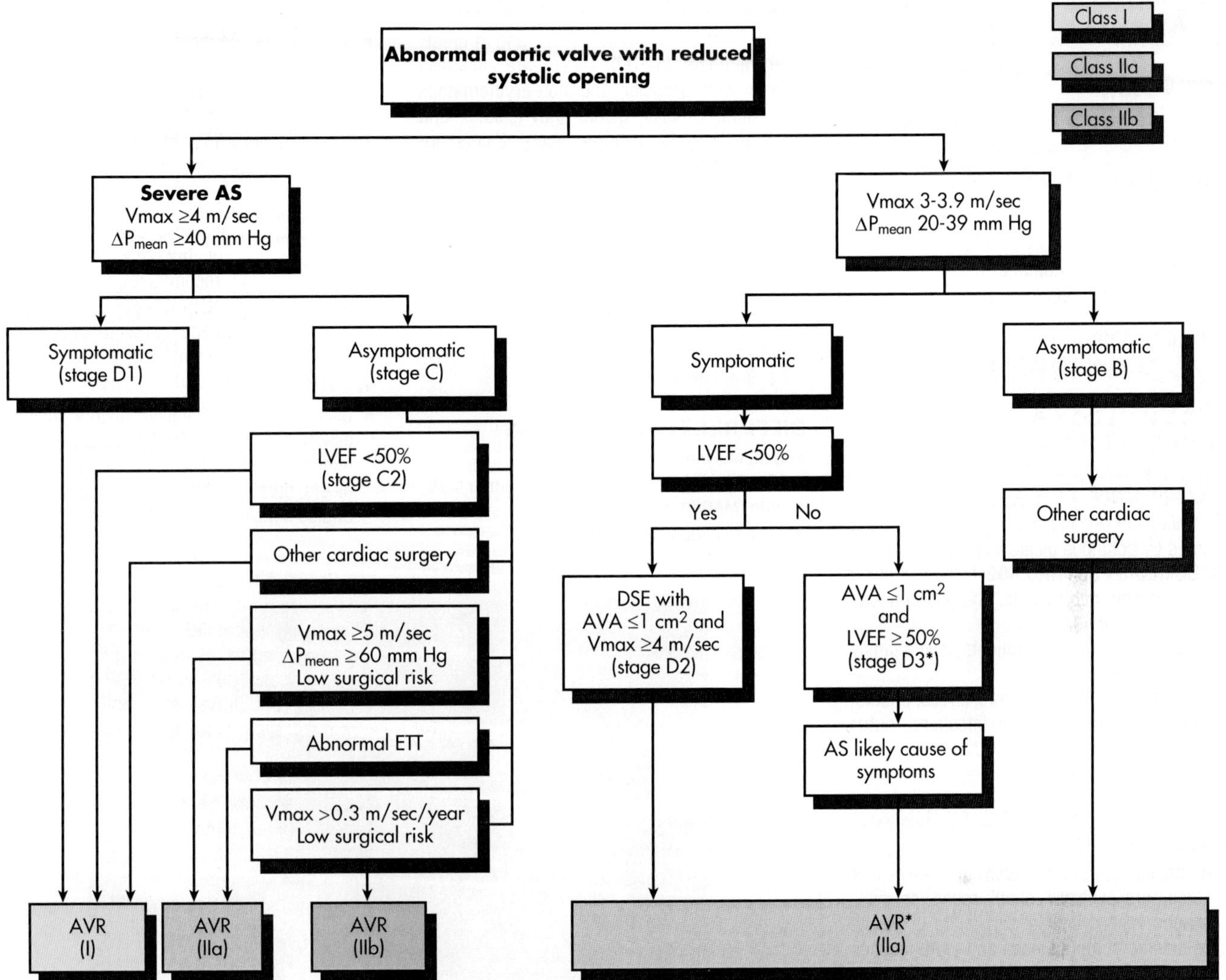

FIG. 3 Management strategy for patients with severe AS. Periodic monitoring is indicated for all patients in whom AVR, by either a surgical or a transcatheter approach, is not yet indicated, including those with asymptomatic AS (stage D or C) and those with low-gradient AS (stage D2 or D3) who do not meet criteria for intervention.*AVR should be considered with stage D3 AS only if valve obstruction is the most likely cause of symptoms, stroke volume index is <35 ml/m^2, indexed AVA is ≤0.6 cm^2/m^2, and data are recorded when the patient is normotensive (systolic BP <140 mm Hg). *AS,* Aortic stenosis; *AVA,* aortic valve area; *AVR,* aortic valve replacement; *BP,* blood pressure; *DSE,* dobutamine stress echocardiography; *ETT,* exercise treadmill test; *LVEF,* left ventricular ejection fraction; ΔP_{mean}, mean pressure gradient; *Vmax,* maximum velocity. (From Nishimura RA et al: 2014 AHA/ACCF guideline for the management of patients with valvular heart disease: a report of the American College of Cardiology Foundation/American Heart Association Task Force on Practice Guidelines. In Mann DL, et al. [eds]: *Braunwald's heart disease*, ed 10, Philadelphia, 2015, Elsevier.)

- In asymptomatic patients, Doppler echocardiography is recommended every 6 to 12 months for severe aortic stenosis, every 1 to 2 yr for moderate disease, and every 3 to 5 yr for mild disease.
- Referral to cardiology should be considered in patient with low-flow, low-gradient (low ejection fraction) symptomatic aortic stenosis for further work-up (dobutamine stress echo).
- Balloon valvuloplasty is useful in infants and children or poor surgical candidates who do not have calcified valve apparatus; it can be done as an intermediate procedure to stabilize high-risk patients before surgery.
- Patients who are considered high risk for cardiac surgery or have contraindications (porcelain aorta) should be referred to a center with a transcatheter program for TAVR evaluation.
- Role of palliative care:
  1. If life expectancy with aortic valve replacement (SAVR or TAVR) is <1 yr **or** the patient's quality of life is unlikely to improve after aortic valve replacement (due to coexisting significant comorbidities), palliative care consultation is extremely valuable as it focuses on shared decision making as well as improving quality of life without interruption of conservative medical therapy.

SUGGESTED READINGS

Available at ExpertConsult.com

RELATED CONTENT

Aortic Stenosis (Patient Information)

AUTHOR: **DENISA HAGAU, M.D., FACC**

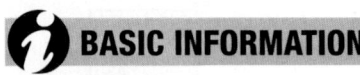

BASIC INFORMATION

DEFINITION

Small painful ulcers predominantly of the oral mucosa

SYNONYMS

Aphthae
Canker sores
Recurrent aphthous stomatitis (RAS)
Recurrent oral aphthae

ICD-10CM CODE

K12.0 Recurrent oral aphthae

EPIDEMIOLOGY & DEMOGRAPHICS

INCIDENCE: Unknown
PEAK INCIDENCE: Adolescence
PREVALENCE: One in five individuals have been affected by aphthous ulcers in their lifetime.
PREDOMINANT SEX AND AGE: Most commonly affects women, adolescents, and young adults under the age of 40.
GENETICS: Up to 40% of patients have a family history of aphthous ulcers.
RISK FACTORS: Genetic factors, stress, trauma, tobacco, viral and bacterial infections, nutritional deficiencies, endocrine and immune disturbances

PHYSICAL FINDINGS & CLINICAL PRESENTATION

- Aphthous ulcers, also referred to as canker sores, are typically small round or oval-shaped lesions with a gray-white or yellow pseudomembranous base and erythematous halo (Fig. 1). Aphthous ulcers can affect any age group. However, they generally appear in childhood and subside by the third decade. The exact cause of aphthous ulcers is poorly understood, but multiple factors may play a role in their occurrence including but not limited to trauma, nutritional deficiencies, viral and bacterial infections, medications, food hypersensitivities, hormonal or endocrine changes, and tobacco use. In the absences of systemic disease and in cases where aphthae reoccur, it is termed Recurrent Aphthous Stomatitis (RAS).
- **Recurrent Aphthous Stomatitis** has three subtypes including minor RAS (up to 80% of cases), major RAS (10% of cases), and herpetiform RAS (10%).
- **Minor RAS:** Classification of Minor RAS depends on the number and size of the ulcers. Generally 1-5 superficial aphthae <10 mm in size and localized to the lips, cheeks, tongue, and floor of the mouth. Lesions tend to self-resolve in 4-14 days and leave no scarring.
- **Major RAS:** These lesions are similar in appearance to Minor RAS except that their size, number, and location increase. Generally, they are >10 mm in diameter, deeper, extend to the gingiva and pharyngeal mucosa, last for weeks to months, and have a higher risk for scarring.
- **Herpetiform RAS:** Herpetiform lesions are often smaller, 1-3 mm, deeper, and in greater numbers (5-100). Ulcers are generally gray with irregular and non-erythematous borders. Smaller ulcers may cluster and coalesce to form larger ulcers. Ulcers are generally very painful and involve the floor of the mouth and ventral surface of the tongue, resolve within 14 days, and generally leave no visible scar.

ETIOLOGY

Both hereditary and environmental causes.

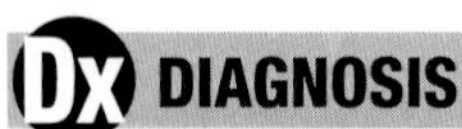

DIAGNOSIS

DIFFERENTIAL DIAGNOSIS

- Behçet syndrome
- Mouth and genital ulcers with inflamed cartilage (MAGIC) syndrome
- Systemic lupus erythematosus
- Gluten-sensitive enteropathy
- Inflammatory bowel disease
- Human immunodeficiency virus infection
- Herpes simplex virus
- Cyclic neutropenia
- Periodic fever with aphthous stomatitis, pharyngitis, and adenitis (PFAPA)
- Hyperimmunoglobulin D syndrome
- Agranulocytosis
- Autoimmune bullous disease
- Oral erosive lichen planus
- Drug-induced mucosal ulcers
- Table 1 summarizes the etiologies and differential diagnosis of recurrent aphthae.

WORKUP

- Clinical history: Detailed history including associated illness, family history, the frequency of ulceration, number and size of ulcers, duration of the outbreak, and location of ulcers including non-oral lesions.

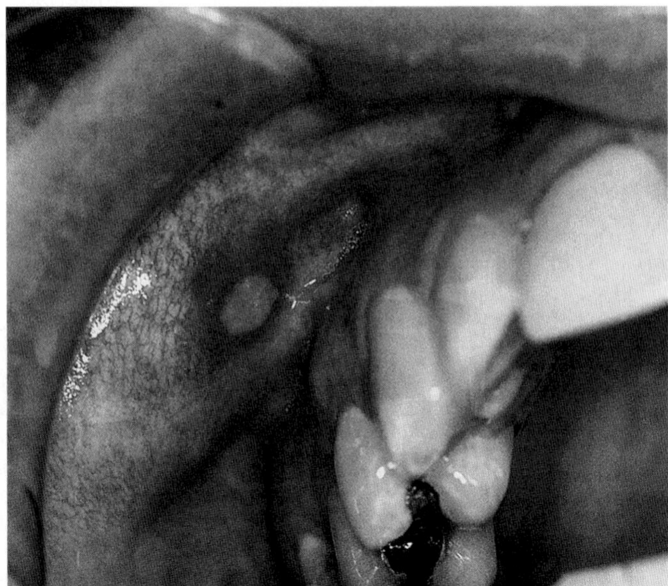

FIG. 1 Recurrent aphthous stomatitis. Minor aphthous ulcer. Shallow, creamy-white ulceration surrounded by an intensely red halo and located on non-keratinized mucosa, representing a classic presentation. (From Bolognia J et al: *Dermatology*, ed 4, Philadelphia, 2018, Elsevier.)

TABLE 1 Recurrent Aphthae—Etiologies and Differential Diagnosis

Etiologies

- Idiopathic (immune-mediated)
- Related to an underlying systemic disorder: Inflammatory bowel disease, systemic lupus erythematosus, HIV infection, Behçet disease, reactive arthritis *, cyclic neutropenia, PFAPA (*p*eriodic *f*ever, *a*phthous stomatitis, *p*haryngitis, and *a*denitis) syndrome, certain hereditary periodic fever syndromes (e.g., HIDS, NOMID)
- Possibly related to an underlying nutritional disorder (controversial): Vitamin B12 , folate, or iron deficiency

Differential Diagnosis

- Recurrent erosions and ulcerations due to an inflammatory disorder, e.g., erythema multiforme, fixed drug eruption, contact stomatitis: Less pain at onset, less peripheral erythema
- Recurrent herpes simplex viral infection: Only involves keratinized mucosa (hard palate, attached gingiva) in immunocompetent hosts.
- Trauma: Less pain at onset, less peripheral erythema, more ragged edges

HIDS, hyperimmunoglobulinemia D with periodic fever syndrome; *HIV,* human immunodeficiency virus; *NOMID,* neonatal-onset multisystem inflammatory disease.
*Previously referred to as Reiter disease.
Modified from Bolognia J et al: *Dermatology*, ed 4, Philadelphia, 2018, Elsevier.

TABLE 2 Recurrent Aphthous Stomatitis (RAS) Subtypes

	Minor Ras	Major Ras	Herpetiform Ras
DESCRIPTION	Round or oval lesions with gray, white, or yellow bases and erythematous border	Round or oval lesions with gray, white, or yellow bases and erythematous border	Small, deep ulcers, may cluster and coalesce to form larger irregular shaped ulcers
LOCATION	Lips, cheeks, tongue, the floor of mouth	Lips, pharynx	Lips, cheeks, tongue, the floor of mouth
SIZE OF ULCERS	<10 mm	>10 mm	1–3 mm
NUMBER OF ULCERS	1–5	1–10	10–100
DURATION	4–14 days; without scarring	>4 weeks; possible scarring	<4 weeks; without scarring

TABLE 3 Therapeutic Ladder for Complex Aphthosis

Key to evidence-based support: (1) prospective controlled trial; (2) retrospective study or large case series; (3) small case series or individual case reports.

Local therapy (agents may be used in combination)

Local anesthetics (2)
Superpotent topical corticosteroids (1*/2) or corticosteroid inhalers (2)
Intralesional corticosteroids (2)
Topical tacrolimus (3)

Systemic therapy

Colchicine (1†/2)
Dapsone (1†/2)
Combination of colchicine and dapsone (2)
Thalidomide (1)

*Clobetasol propionate in an adhesive denture paste.
†In patients with Behçet disease.
Adapted from Letsinger JA et al: *J Am Acad Dermatol* 52:500–8, 2005, with permission. In Bolognia J et al: *Dermatology*, ed 4, Philadelphia, 2018, Elsevier.

- Physical examination: Aphthous ulcers are well-circumscribed small round or oval-shaped lesions with gray-white or yellow pseudomembranous bases with an erythematous halo. RAS may be further broken down into its subtypes as outlined in Table 2.
- RAS is generally a clinical diagnosis; however, if RAS is persistent, then further laboratory testing may be considered.
- Biopsy: Typically not required; however, in more severe or persistent cases a biopsy may aid in ruling out other mucosal pathologies.

LABORATORY TESTS

If RAS is severe, persistent, or occurs at a later age of onset, it is reasonable to investigate further for other potential causes. Screening with hemoglobin, complete blood count, inflammatory markers including erythrocyte sedimentation rate and C-reactive protein, and nutritional deficiencies including serum B12, folate, and iron.

IMAGING STUDIES

None

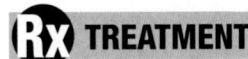

TREATMENT

The exact cause of aphthous ulcers and RAS is still unknown, and the first-line treatment modalities are aimed at supportive care and speeding up healing time. Treatment is based on low-quality studies, and there are no curative pharmacological treatments. If aphthae are secondary to an underlying disease, then treatment of the primary disease may reduce the duration of the aphthae. Treatment is a stepwise approach (Table 3) and includes good oral hygiene, avoiding trauma (e.g., biting lips or cheeks, oral hardware including braces) and known drug or food triggers, topical anesthetics, topical corticosteroids, topical antimicrobials, and systemic medications.

ACUTE GENERAL Rx

- Topical anesthetics: Can be used before eating for temporary relief
  1. 2% viscous lidocaine applied directly or used as swish and spit
  2. Diphenhydramine liquid (12.5 mg/5 ml) use 5 ml as swish and spit
- Topical corticosteroids: First-line treatment for mild to moderate RAS
  3. Dexamethasone elixir (0.5 mg / 5 ml) take 5 ml, swish for 5 minutes before spitting it out. Repeat three to four times daily
- Topical antimicrobial: Not typically necessary in mild cases but may be beneficial in preventing secondary infection in more severe cases or cases involving other immunosuppressive medications
  1. Chlorhexidine 0.12% mouth rinse use 15 ml as swish and spit twice daily
  2. Nystatin suspension swish and swallow four times daily

CHRONIC Rx

Oral options may be tried in patients reporting no benefit with topical treatment alone or in case of severe RAS.

- Oral prednisone 20 mg to 40 mg daily for 4-7 days is typically the first-line treatment of acute severe RAS.
- Montelukast 10 mg daily may be a safe alternative when severe RAS is not well controlled with oral corticosteroids.

COMPLEMENTARY & ALTERNATIVE MEDICINE

- Ascorbic acid 2000 mg/day as an adjunct to topical therapy in managing minor RAS.
- Zinc 50 mg/day may also be beneficial in wound healing.

NONPHARMACOLOGIC THERAPY

Laser therapy or chemical cauterization have been cited as an adjunct to the above therapies to help reduce acute pain; however, their ability to prevent recurrent episodes of aphthae is still unknown.

DISPOSITION

Although a painful condition, aphthous ulcers and RAS are generally self-resolving with an average healing time of 2 weeks and excellent prognosis. Consider an alternative etiology if the patient exhibits systemic symptoms or has other pertinent past medical history.

REFERRAL

Referral to a specialist if an alternative diagnosis is more likely. Severe or persistent cases of RAS may be referred to dermatology.

PREVENTION

Practice good oral hygiene.

PATIENT/FAMILY EDUCATION

Educate patients and parents of pediatric patients on pain control with the use of topical anesthetics before eating or drinking to prevent dehydration. Topical pain control is also beneficial before performing basic dental hygiene. Avoid citrus juices and spicy or salty foods. Return precautions including worsening pain, the spread of ulcers, especially beyond oral mucocutaneous membranes, fever, decreased fluid intake, or other systemic symptoms.

AUTHOR: **DYLAN HENDY, D.O.**

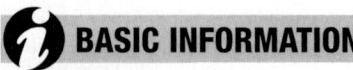

BASIC INFORMATION

DEFINITION

Appendicitis is the acute inflammation of the vermiform appendix.

ICD-10CM CODES

K35.2 Acute appendicitis with generalized peritonitis
K35.3 Acute appendicitis with localized peritonitis
K35.80 Unspecified acute appendicitis
K35.89 Other acute appendicitis
K36 Other appendicitis
K37 Unspecified appendicitis

EPIDEMIOLOGY & DEMOGRAPHICS

- Appendicitis occurs in 10% of the population, most commonly between the ages of 10 and 30 yr. Median age is 22 yr. Lifetime risk is 7% to 14%.
- Approximately 300,000 appendectomies are performed in the U.S. each yr.
- It is the most common abdominal surgical emergency.
- Incidence of appendicitis has declined over the past 30 yr.
- Male/female ratio is 3:2 until mid-20s; it equalizes after age 30 yr.

PHYSICAL FINDINGS & CLINICAL PRESENTATION

- In children with abdominal pain, fever is the single most useful sign associated with appendicitis. Vomiting, rectal tenderness, and rebound tenderness along with fever are more indicative of appendicitis in children than in adults.
- Abdominal pain: Initially the pain may be epigastric or periumbilical in nearly 50% of patients; it subsequently localizes to the right lower quadrant within 12 to 18 hr. Pain can be found in back or right flank if appendix is retrocecal or in other abdominal locations if there is malrotation of the appendix.
- Pain with right thigh extension *(psoas sign)*, low-grade fever: Temperature may be >38° C if there is appendiceal perforation.
- Pain with internal rotation of the flexed right thigh *(obturator sign)* is present.
- Right lower quadrant (RLQ) pain on palpation of the left lower quadrant (LLQ) *(Rovsing sign):* Physical examination may reveal right-sided tenderness in patients with pelvic appendix.
- Point of maximum tenderness is in the RLQ *(McBurney point)*.
- Nausea, vomiting, tachycardia, cutaneous hyperesthesias at the level of T12 can be present.

ETIOLOGY

Obstruction of the appendiceal lumen with subsequent vascular congestion, inflammation, and edema; common causes of obstruction are:

- Fecaliths: 30% to 35% of cases (most common in adults)
- Foreign body: 4% (fruit seeds, pinworms, tapeworms, roundworms, calculi)
- Inflammation: 50% to 60% of cases (submucosal lymphoid hyperplasia [most common etiology in children, teens])
- Neoplasms: 1% (carcinoids, metastatic disease, carcinoma)

Dx DIAGNOSIS

DIFFERENTIAL DIAGNOSIS

- Intestinal: Regional cecal enteritis, incarcerated hernia, cecal diverticulitis, intestinal obstruction, perforated ulcer, perforated cecum, Meckel diverticulitis
- Reproductive: Ectopic pregnancy, ovarian cyst, torsion of ovarian cyst, salpingitis, tubo-ovarian abscess, mittelschmerz, endometriosis, seminal vesiculitis
- Renal: Renal and ureteral calculi, neoplasms, pyelonephritis
- Vascular: Leaking aortic aneurysm
- Psoas abscess
- Trauma
- Cholecystitis
- Mesenteric adenitis
- Table 1 summarizes the differential diagnosis of appendicitis

WORKUP

Patients with RLQ pain, nausea, vomiting, anorexia, and RLQ rebound tenderness should undergo prompt clinical and laboratory evaluation. Imaging studies are generally not necessary in typical appendicitis and generally reserved for patients with an equivocal likelihood of appendicitis. They are useful when the diagnosis is uncertain. Laparoscopy may be useful as both a diagnostic and a therapeutic modality.

LABORATORY TESTS

- Complete blood count with differential reveals leukocytosis with a left shift in 90% of patients with appendicitis. Total white blood cell (WBC) count is generally lower than 20,000/mm^3.

TABLE 1 Differential Diagnosis of Appendicitis

Diagnosis	Findings That Help Differentiate Entity from Appendicitis
Bacterial or viral enteritis	Nausea, vomiting, and diarrhea are severe; pain usually develops after vomiting.
Epiploic appendagitis	Focal abdominal pain and tenderness without migration or progression of the pain; patients have a paucity of other GI symptoms such as anorexia or nausea. Laboratory findings are usually normal.
Mesenteric adenitis	Duration of symptoms is longer; fever is uncommon; RLQ physical findings are less marked; WBC count is usually normal.
Pyelonephritis	Pain is more likely to be felt in the right flank; high fever and rigors are common; marked pyuria or bacteriuria and urinary symptoms are present; abdominal rigidity is less marked.
Renal colic	Pain radiates to the right groin; significant hematuria; character of the pain is clearly colicky.
Acute pancreatitis	Pain and vomiting are more severe; tenderness is less well localized; serum amylase and lipase levels are elevated.
Crohn disease	History of recurrent similar attacks; diarrhea is more common; palpable mass is more common; extraintestinal manifestations may have occurred or be present.
Cholecystitis	History of prior attacks is common; pain and tenderness are greater; radiation of pain is to the right shoulder; nausea is more marked; liver biochemical tests are more likely to be abnormal.
Meckel diverticulitis	Nearly impossible to distinguish preoperatively from appendicitis.
Cecal diverticulitis	Difficult to distinguish preoperatively from appendicitis; symptoms are milder and of longer duration; CT is helpful; patients are usually older.
Sigmoid diverticulitis	Usually occurs in older patients; changes in bowel habits are more common; radiation of the pain is to the suprapubic area, not RLQ; fever and WBC count are higher.
Small bowel obstruction	History of abdominal surgery; pain is colicky; vomiting and distention are more marked; RLQ localization is uncommon.
Ectopic pregnancy	History of menstrual irregularities; characteristic progression of symptoms is absent; syncope; positive pregnancy test.
Ruptured ovarian cyst	Occurs in the middle of the menstrual cycle; pain is of sudden onset; nausea and vomiting are less common; WBC count is normal.
Ovarian torsion	Vomiting is more marked and occurs at the same time as the pain; progression of symptoms is absent; abdominal or pelvic mass often is palpable.
Acute salpingitis or tubo-ovarian abscess	Longer duration of symptoms; pain begins in the lower abdomen; often there is a history of STDs; vaginal discharge and marked cervical tenderness often are present.

RLQ, Right lower quadrant; *STD,* sexually transmitted disease.
From Feldman M, et al.: *Sleisenger and Fordtran's gastrointestinal and liver disease*, ed 10, Philadelphia, 2016, Elsevier.

Higher counts may be indicative of perforation. Less than 4% have a normal WBC and differential. A WBC count <10,000/mm^3 decreases the likelihood of appendicitis. Low hemoglobin and hematocrit levels in an older patient should raise suspicion for GI tract carcinoma.
- Microscopic hematuria and pyuria may occur in <20% of patients.
- HCG to rule out pregnancy in females of reproductive age.

IMAGING STUDIES

- Multidetector computed tomography (Fig. 1) is a useful test for routine evaluation of suspected appendicitis in adults. CT of the abdomen/pelvis without contrast has a sensitivity of >90% and an accuracy >94% for acute appendicitis. A distended appendix, periappendiceal inflammation, and a thickened appendiceal wall are indicative of appendicitis. Table 2 describes CT findings of appendicitis. In children and young adults, exposure to CT radiation is of particular concern. Trials with low-dose CT (116 mGy cm) have shown that low-dose CT is not inferior to standard-dose CT (521 mGy cm) with respect to negative (unnecessary) appendectomy rates in young adults with suspected appendicitis.
- Ultrasonography (Fig. 2) has a sensitivity of 75% to 90% for the diagnosis of acute appendicitis, although it is highly operator dependent and difficult in patients with large body habitus. Ultrasound is useful, especially in pregnancy and in younger women when diagnosis is unclear. Normal ultrasonographic findings should not deter surgery if the history and physical examination are indicative of appendicitis.
- MRI of the abdomen and pelvis can also be used to accurately diagnose acute appendicitis in pregnant patients (100% sensitivity, 93.6% specificity) without exposure to ionizing radiation.

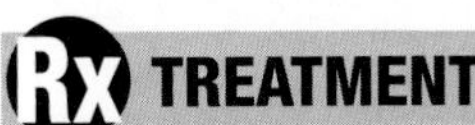

TREATMENT

NONPHARMACOLOGIC THERAPY

- Nothing by mouth
- Do not administer analgesics until the diagnosis is made

ACUTE GENERAL Rx

- Urgent appendectomy (laparoscopic or open), correction of fluid and electrolyte imbalance with vigorous IV hydration, and electrolyte replacement
- IV antibiotic prophylaxis to cover gram-negative bacilli and anaerobes (ampicillin/sulbactam 3 g IV q6h or piperacillin/tazobactam 4.5 g IV q8h in adults)

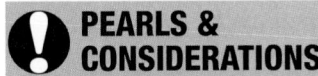

PEARLS & CONSIDERATIONS

COMMENTS

- Perforation is common (20% in adult patients). Indicators of perforation are pain lasting >24 hr, leukocytosis >20,000/mm^3, temperature >102° F, palpable abdominal mass, and peritoneal findings.
- In general, prognosis is excellent. Mortality rate is <1% in young adults without complications; however, it exceeds 10% in elderly patients with ruptured appendix.
- In approximately 20% of patients who undergo exploratory laparotomy because of suspected appendicitis, the appendix is normal.
- An increasing amount of evidence supports the use of antibiotics instead of surgery for treating patients with uncomplicated appendicitis. A trial assessing the feasibility of nonoperative management for uncomplicated acute appendicitis in children using either IV piperacillin-tazobactam or ciprofloxacin metronidazole therapy for at least 24 hours followed by oral antibiotics for 10 days revealed that 90% of children managed nonoperatively had no progression within 30 days.[1] Another trial among patients with CT-proven, uncomplicated appendicitis revealed that antibiotic treatment did not meet the prescribed criterion for noninferiority compared with appendectomy. Most patients randomized to antibiotic treatment for uncomplicated appendicitis did not require appendectomy during the 1-yr

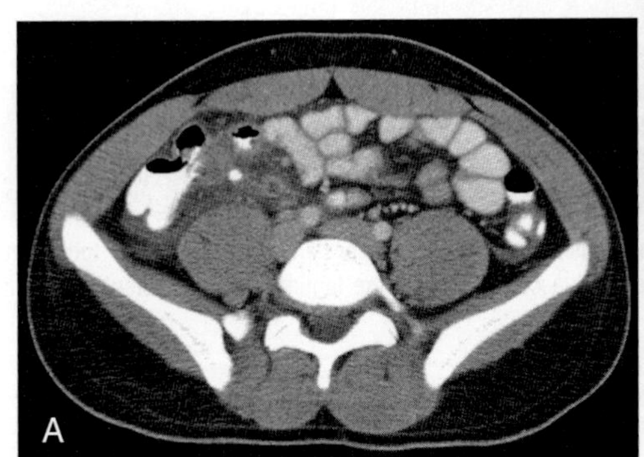

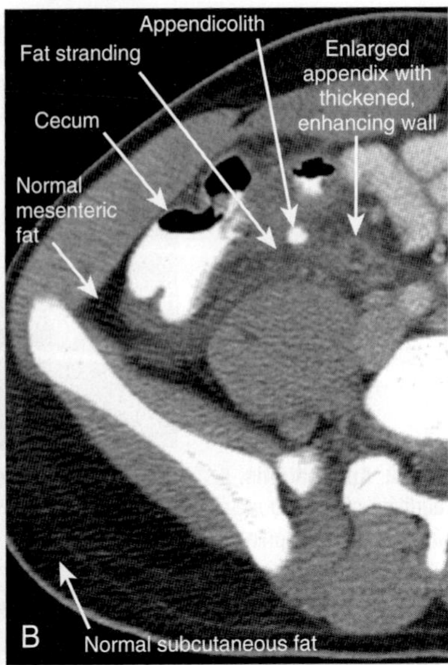

FIG. 1 Appendicitis, computed tomography (CT) with intravenous and oral contrast. This CT demonstrates classic findings of appendicitis in an 18-year-old male with right lower quadrant pain, as seen with CT with IV and oral contrast. Studies suggest that CT without contrast has similar sensitivity and specificity. An enlarged appendix is seen near the cecum as a right lower quadrant tubular structure in short-axis cross section, giving it a circular appearance. The surrounding fat shows stranding, a smoky appearance indicating inflammation (compare with normal mesenteric and subcutaneous fat, which is nearly black). The appendiceal wall shows enhancement, a brightening after administration of IV contrast. This slice also shows an appendicolith, an occasional finding of appendicitis. It does not appear to be within the appendix in this slice, because the appendix bends in and out of the plane of this slice. An appendicolith usually appears as a calcified (white) rounded structure, visible without any contrast. **A,** Axial CT image. **B,** Close-up. (From Broder JS: *Diagnostic imaging for the emergency physician,* Philadelphia, 2011, Saunders.)

TABLE 2 Computed Tomography Findings of Appendicitis: SCALPEL Mnemonic

Term	Description
Stranding	Fat stranding suggests regional inflammation, possibly because of appendicitis.
Cecum	The appendix originates from the cecum, which should be identified first to help localize the appendix. The cecum may show wall thickening, suggesting appendicitis.
Air	Air outside of the lumen of the appendix is pathologic and suggests perforation. Air within the appendiceal wall is also abnormal.
Large	The normal appendix is <6 mm; an enlarged appendix >6 mm suggests appendicitis. Wall thickening >1 mm also suggests appendicitis.
Phlegmon	Inflammatory changes surrounding the appendix suggest a perforated appendix. A heterogeneous collection called a phlegmon may be seen. If the appendix has ruptured, a pericecal phlegmon may be the only remaining evidence, because the appendix itself may not be seen.
Enhancement	The wall of an abnormal appendix enhances with IV contrast and appears brighter than the normal bowel or the normal psoas muscle.
Lith	An appendicolith is a calcified stone sometimes found in the lumen of an inflamed appendix.

From Broder JS: *Diagnostic imaging for the emergency physician,* Philadelphia, 2011, Saunders.

[1] Minneci PC, et al.: Feasibility of a nonoperative management strategy for uncomplicated acute appendicitis in children, *J Am Coll Surg* 219:272-279, 2014.

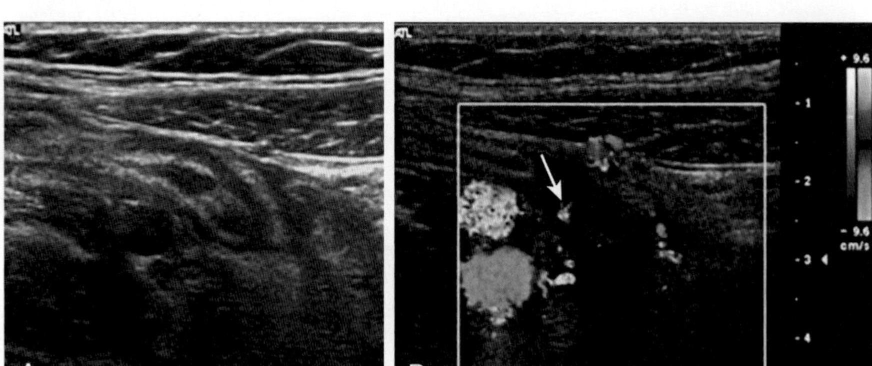

FIG. 2 Appendicitis. A, Transabdominal ultrasound using a linear transducer demonstrates a thick, tubular, noncompressible structure. **B,** Same imaging method with addition of color Doppler ultrasound shows increased vascularity within the luminal wall consistent with inflammation *(arrow).* (From Fielding JR, et al.: *Gynecologic imaging,* Philadelphia, 2011, Saunders.)

follow-up period, and those who required appendectomy did not experience significant complications.[2] A 5-yr follow-up of antibiotic therapy for uncomplicated acute appendicitis in the APPAC randomized clinical trial revealed that among patients who were initially treated with antibiotics for uncomplicated acute appendicitis, the likelihood of late recurrence within 5 yr was 39.1%.[4] It remains to be determined whether the benefits of potentially avoiding an operation with antibiotics-first approach are outweighed by the burden to the patient related to future appendicitis episodes, more days of antibiotic therapy, lingering symptoms, and uncertainty that may affect quality of life.[3]

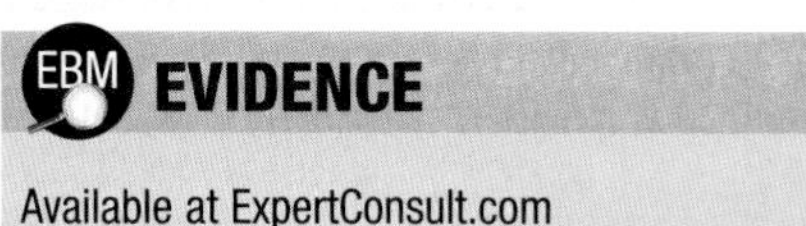

EVIDENCE

Available at ExpertConsult.com

SUGGESTED READINGS

Available at ExpertConsult.com

RELATED CONTENT

Appendicitis (Patient Information)

AUTHOR: **FRED F. FERRI, M.D.**

[2] Salminen P, et al.: Antibiotic therapy vs appendectomy for treatment of uncomplicated acute appendicitis, the APPAC Randomized trial, *JAMA* 313(23):2340-2348, 2015.

[3] Flum DR: Acute appendicitis—appendectomy or the “antibiotics first” strategy, *N Engl J Med* 372:1937-43, 2015.

[4] Salminen P, et al.: Five-year follow-up of antibiotic therapy for uncomplicated acute appendicitis in the APPAC randomized clinical trial, JAMA 320(12):1259–1265, 2018.

BASIC INFORMATION

DEFINITION

Arrhythmogenic right ventricular dysplasia (ARVD) is a cardiomyopathy characterized by replacement of the normal myocardium with fibrofatty tissue, mainly of the right ventricle but also occasionally with involvement of the left ventricle. It is defined clinically by palpitations and syncope and potentially life-threatening ventricular arrhythmias.

SYNONYMS

Arrhythmogenic right ventricular cardiomyopathy
ARVC

ICD-10CM CODE
I42.8 Arrhythmogenic ventricular dysplasia

EPIDEMIOLOGY & DEMOGRAPHICS

PREVALENCE: 1:2000–5000 persons. It is one of the leading causes of arrhythmic cardiac arrest in young people and athletes.

PREDOMINANT SEX AND AGE: Mean age, 31 yr (range, 12 to 50 yr), predominantly male

RISK FACTORS: Family history of ARVD (present in nearly 50% of affected patients)

GENETICS:
- Autosomal dominant (most common) with variable penetrance and polymorphic phenotypic expression
- Autosomal recessive (rarely, e.g., Naxos disease)
- Several different gene mutations in desmosomal proteins
- Gene mutations can be identified in 50% of affected individuals

PHYSICAL FINDINGS & CLINICAL PRESENTATION

- ARVD can present with palpitations, syncope, and chest discomfort and less commonly sudden cardiac arrest and signs of right ventricular failure such as dyspnea, edema, and fatigue. Patients may be clinically asymptomatic for many yrs.
- Cardiac arrest after physical exertion may be the initial presentation.
- Physical examination will be normal in most patients. Widely split S2 is an important diagnostic clue.

ETIOLOGY

ARVD is characterized by progressive replacement of mainly the right ventricular myocardium with fibrofatty tissue after apoptotic myocardial cell death caused by mutations of desmosomal protein.

DIAGNOSIS

- A major criterion equals 2 points; a minor criterion equals 1 point. The diagnosis of ARVD is considered definite if the patient has 4 points and probable with 3 points. See Table 1 for diagnostic criteria.

DIFFERENTIAL DIAGNOSIS

- Cardiomyopathy with involvement of the right ventricle
- Uhl's anomaly: Rare anomaly that presents mainly in childhood with signs and symptoms of right heart failure and characterized by a paper-thin right ventricle resulting from death of the myocytes throughout the right ventricle
- Idiopathic RV tachycardia
- Sarcoidosis
- Right ventricular infarction

WORKUP

- Initial workup includes history with focus on sudden death in the family, resting ECG, 24-Holter ECG, signal-averaged ECG, and imaging studies with echocardiography and MRI.
- ECG will have diagnostic findings in 50% to 90% of patients with ARVD, including T-wave inversions in anterior precordial leads V_1-V_6, epsilon waves, and a QRS duration longer than 110 ms in V1 or >40 ms longer in V1 than v6. (Fig. 1).
- Ventricular tachycardia (VT) with left bundle branch block pattern and frequent PVCs (>500 in 24 h) might be detected by 24-hr Holter monitoring.
- An abnormal signal-averaged ECG is a minor diagnostic criteria.
- Echocardiography will show right ventricular dilation with regional wall motion abnormalities, aneurysms, and depressed RV function that varies with the severity of the disease.
- MRI (Fig. 2) is a noninvasive method to detect structural abnormalities (fibrofatty changes) and regional dysfunction. Cardiac MRI (CMR) is the most sensitive method to detect ARVD, but it has high false-positive rates. Cardiac CT angiogram (Fig. E3) will reveal thinning and aneurysmal dilation of the RV anterior wall and outflow tract.

If the routine tests are not conclusive, endomyocardial biopsy and electrophysiologic testing can be considered. However, biopsies and radionuclide ventriculography are rarely performed in the U.S.

TREATMENT

No curative treatment is available. The treatment goal is focused on preventing sudden cardiac death, symptomatic treatment of right heart failure, and pharmacologic and invasive treatment of arrhythmias. Therapy with cardio-selective beta-blockers is recommended. Family members with a negative phenotype (either healthy gene carriers or those with an unknown genotype) do not need any specific treatment other than sports restriction; however, lifelong clinical assessment with the use of noninvasive tests at least every 2 yr is warranted.[1]

NONPHARMACOLOGIC THERAPY

- Avoidance of activity that may trigger ventricular tachycardia and may lead to disease progression.
- ICD implantation needs to be considered in patients who have the definite diagnosis of ARVD. Patients with unexplained syncope, advanced disease, documented ventricular arrhythmias, or a family history of sudden cardiac death or who have been resuscitated from cardiac arrest are at high risk. A subcutaneous ICD might be an alternative option instead of transvenous implantation.
- Radiofrequency catheter ablation is used in cases of refractory VT or frequent tachycardia after defibrillator placement.
- Cardiac transplantation.
- Fig. 4 describes a management algorithm for ARVD.

PHARMACOLOGIC TREATMENT

Antiarrhythmic therapy with sotalol (first-line treatment) or amiodarone, often in combination with beta-blockers, is used for tachycardia suppression.

REFERRAL

- Early cardiology and electrophysiology referral
- Consider referring for genetic counseling

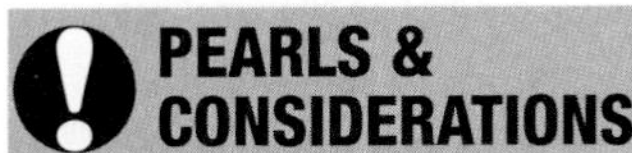

PEARLS & CONSIDERATIONS

PREVENTION

All first-degree relatives should be tested if ARVD is confirmed. Sports activity increases the risk of sudden cardiac death among adolescents and young adults with ARVC. The estimated overall mortality ranges from 0.08% to 3.6% per yr.

SUGGESTED READINGS
Available at ExpertConsult.com

AUTHOR: **HEIKO SCHMITT, M.D., PH.D.**

[1] Corrado D et al: Arrhythmogenic right ventricular cardiomyopathy, *N Engl J Med* 376:61–72, 2017.

TABLE 1 Global or Regional Dysfunction and Structural Alterations

Major

2D echo criteria

Regional RV akinesia, dyskinesia, or aneurysm and one of the following measured at end diastole

PLAX RVOT ≥32 mm or

PSAX RVOT ≥36

Fractional area change ≤33%

MRI criteria

Regional RV akinesia or dyskinesia or dyssynchronous RV contraction and one of the following

Ratio of RV end-diastolic volume to BSA >100, <110 ml/m^2 (male) or >100 ml/m^2

RV ejection fraction >40% ≤45%

RV angiography criteria

Regional RV akinesia, dyskinesia, or aneurysm

Minor

2D echo criteria

Regional RV akinesia or dyskinesia or dyssynchronous RV contraction and one of the following measured at end diastole

PLAX RVOT ≥29 <32 mm or

PSAX RVOT ≥32 <36

Fractional area change >33% ≤40%

MRI criteria

Regional RV akinesia or dyskinesia or dyssynchronous RV contraction and one of the following

Ratio of RV end-diastolic volume to BSA ≥110 ml/m^2 (male) or ≥100 ml/m^2

RV ejection fraction ≤40%

Tissue characterization of wall

Major

Residual myocytes <60% by morphometric analysis (or <50% if estimated) with fibrous replacement of the RV free wall myocardium in >1 sample, with or without fatty replacement of tissue on endomyocardial biopsy

Minor

Residual myocytes 60%-75% by morphometric analysis (or 50%-65% if estimated), with fibrous replacement of the RV free wall myocardium in >1 sample with or without fatty replacement of tissue on endomyocardial biopsy

Repolarization abnormalities

Major

Inverted T waves in right precordial leads (V1, V2, and V3) or beyond in individuals >14 y of age (in the absence of complete RBBB QRS ≥120 ms)

Minor

Inverted T waves in V1 and V2 in individuals >14 y of age (in the absence of complete RBBB) or in V4, V5, and V6

Inverted T waves in leads V1, V2, V3, and V4 in individuals >14 y of age in the presence of a complete RBBB

Depolarization or conduction abnormalities

Major

Epsilon wave (reproducible low-amplitude signals between end of QRS complex to onset of T wave) in the right precordial leads (V1-V3)

Minor

Late potentials by SAECG in ≥1 of 3 parameters in the absence of a QRSd of ≥110 ms on standard ECG

Filtered QRS ≥114 ms

Duration of terminal QRS <40 mV ≥38 ms

Root-mean-square voltage of terminal 40 ms ≤20 μV

Terminal activation duration ≥55 ms measured from the nadir of the end of the QRS, including R', in V1, V2, or V3 in absence of complete RBBB

Arrhythmias

Major

Nonsustained or sustained VT of LBBB morph with superior axis

Minor

Nonsustained or sustained VT of RVOT configuration, LBBB morph with inferior axis or of unknown axis

>500 PVCs per 24 h (Holter)

Family history

Major

ARVD/C in first-degree relative who meets Task Force criteria

ARVD/C confirmed pathologically at autopsy or surgery in first-degree relative

Identification of pathogenic mutation categorized as associated or probably associated with ARVD/C in the patient under evaluation

Minor

History of ARVD/C in first-degree relative in whom it is not possible to determine whether the family member meets Task Force criteria

Premature sudden death (<35 y of age) caused by suspected ARVD/C in a first-degree relative

ARVD/C confirmed pathologically or by current Task Force criteria in second-degree relative

A major criterion equals 2 points, a minor criterion 1 point. The diagnosis of arrhythmogenic right ventricular dysplasia (ARVD) is considered definite if the patient has 4 points and probable with 3 points. *BSA,* body surface area; *MRI,* magnetic resonance imaging; *PLAX,* parasternal long axis; *PSAX,* parasternal short axis; *RBBB,* right bundle branch block; *RV,* right ventricle; *RVOT,* right ventricular outflow tract; *SAECG,* signal-averaged electrocardiogram; *2D,* two dimensional; *VT,* ventricular tachycardia.

From Marcus IM: Diagnosis of arrhythmogenic right ventricular cardiomyopathy/dysplasia proposed modification of the Task Force criteria. *Circulation* 121:1533-1541, 2010

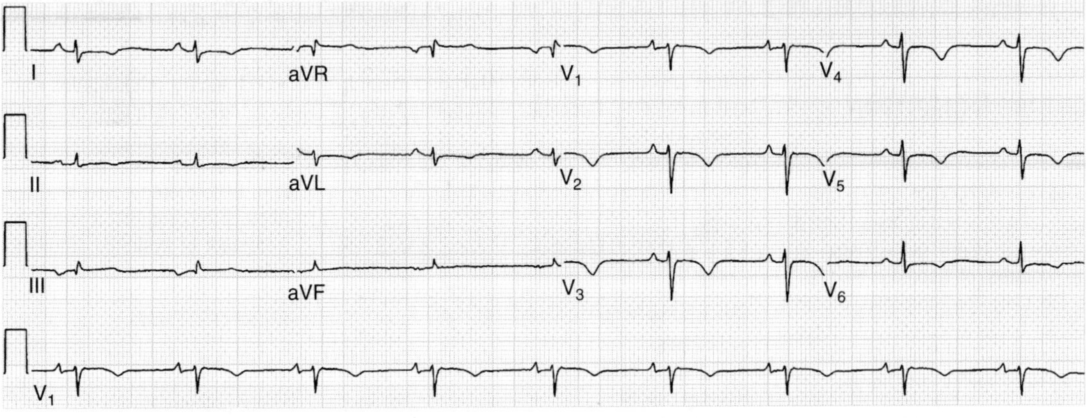

FIG. 1 Arrhythmogenic right ventricular cardiomyopathy—Epsilon wave. This 12-lead ECG tracing with lead Vfn11 rhythm strip **(A)** shows sinus rhythm with T-wave inversion over the right precordial leads. In addition, there is an epsilon wave (small deflection at the end of the QRS complex), evident in lead V^1 **(B)**, which is characteristic of arrhythmogenic right ventricular cardiomyopathy. (From Olshansky B, Chung MK, Pogwizd SM et al: *Arrhythmia essentials*, ed 2, Philadelphia, 2017, Elsevier.)

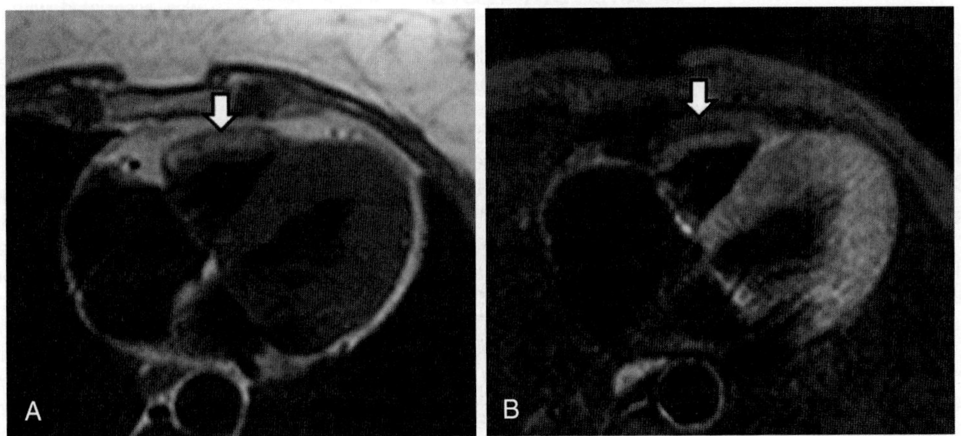

FIG. 2 Arrhythmogenic right ventricular cardiomyopathy. Spin-echo cardiovascular magnetic resonance without **(A)** and with **(B),** a fat-suppression prepulse. There is bright signal in the free wall of the right ventricle that suppresses with fat suppression *(arrows).* (From Sellke FW, del Nido PJ, Swanson SJ et al: *Sabiston & Spencer surgery of the chest*, ed 9, Philadelphia, 2016, Elsevier.)

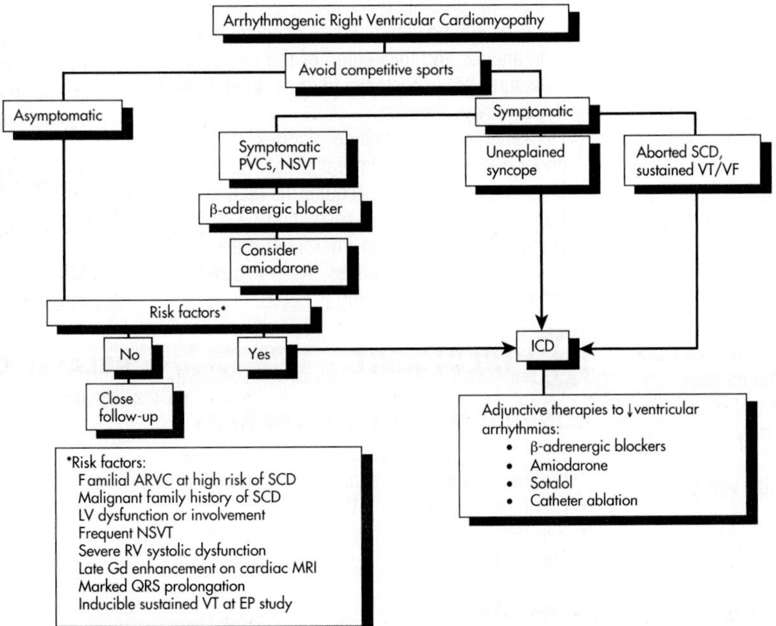

FIG. 4 Arrhythmogenic right ventricular cardiomyopathy. *ARVC,* Arrhythmogenic right ventricular cardiomyopathy; *EP,* electrophysiology; *Gd,* gadolinium; *ICD,* implantable cardiodefibrillator; *NSVT,* nonsustained ventricular tachycardia; *PVCs,* premature ventricular contractions; *SCD,* sequential compression device; *VF,* ventricular fibrillation; *VT,* ventricular tachycardia. (From Olshansky B, Chung MK, Pogwizd SM et al: *Arrhythmia essentials*, ed 2, Philadelphia, 2017, Elsevier.)

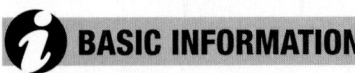

DEFINITION

Asbestosis is a slow, progressive diffuse interstitial fibrosis as a consequence of dose-related inhalation exposure to fibers of asbestos in miners, millers, workers of asbestos textiles, and insulators. Clinically, the lung involvement is characterized by bilateral diffuse interstitial fibrosis, more pronounced in the lower lobes, and pleural thickening, leading to shortness of breath and dry cough.

Asbestos exposure can lead to the spectrum of pulmonary pathology, including pulmonary fibrosis; asbestos-related pleural plaque (ARPD), both focal and diffuse; and malignancies (small cell carcinoma, non–small cell carcinoma, or mesothelioma).

ICD-10CM CODE

J61 Pneumoconiosis due to asbestos and other mineral fibers

EPIDEMIOLOGY & DEMOGRAPHICS

- Five to 10 new cases per 100,000 persons per yr in the U.S.
- Prolonged interval (20 to 30 yr) between exposures to inhaled fibers and clinical manifestations of disease.
- Most common in workers over age 40 yr involved in the primary extraction of asbestos from rock deposits and in those involved in the fabrication and installation of products containing asbestos (e.g., naval shipyards in World War II; installation of floor tiles, ceiling tiles, acoustic ceiling coverings, wall insulation, and pipe coverings in public buildings).
- Smokers and heavy drinkers have the greatest risk of developing this disease.

PHYSICAL FINDINGS & CLINICAL PRESENTATION

- Insidious onset of shortness of breath and dry cough with exertion is usually the first sign of asbestosis.
- Dyspnea becomes more severe as the disease advances; with time, progressively less exertion is tolerated.
- Cough is frequent and usually paroxysmal, dry, and nonproductive. Hemoptysis is rare but reported.
- Scant mucoid sputum may accompany the cough in the later stages of the disease.
- Fine end-respiratory crackles (rales, crepitations) are heard more predominantly in the lung bases.
- Digital clubbing, edema, jugular venous distention are present.
- Advanced cases may have signs of right heart failure.

ETIOLOGY/PATHOGENESIS

Inhalation of asbestos fibers. The pathogenesis of pulmonary interstitial inflammation and fibrosis is related to immune mechanisms. Asbestosis is known to be associated with positive serum antinuclear antibody (ANA) and rheumatoid factor (RF). Recently, an important role of interleukin-1beta (IL-1beta) in the pathogenesis of asbestosis, and its systemic autoimmune manifestations have been reported.

Dx DIAGNOSIS

DIFFERENTIAL DIAGNOSIS

- Silicosis
- Siderosis, other pneumonoconioses
- Lung cancer
- Atelectasis

WORKUP

Documentation of exposure history, diagnostic imaging, pulmonary function testing

LABORATORY TESTS

- Generally not helpful
- Possible mild elevation of erythrocyte sedimentation rate (ESR), positive antinuclear antibody (ANA), and rheumatoid factor (RF) (these tests are nonspecific and do not correlate with disease severity or activity)
- Pulmonary function testing: With decreased vital capacity (VC), decreased total lung capacity (TLC), decreased carbon monoxide gas transfer (DLco)
- FEV1 might be reduced in concomitant smokers
- Arterial blood gases: Hypoxemia, hypercarbia in advanced stages

IMAGING STUDIES

- Chest radiograph (Fig. E1):
  1. Small, irregular shadows in lower lung zones.
  2. The imaging findings vary from benign pleural disease (including discrete plaques, pleural calcification, diffuse pleural thickening with blunting of costophrenic angles, and thickening of the interlobar fissure) to asbestosis (diffuse interstitial pulmonary fibrosis.
- Thickened pleura, calcified plaques (present under diaphragm and lateral chest wall).
- CT scan of chest (Fig. E2) confirms diagnosis. Typical findings on high-resolution CT of the chest include increased interstitial markings found mainly at the bases. As the disease progresses, honeycombing is noted.

Rx TREATMENT

NONPHARMACOLOGIC THERAPY

- Smoking cessation, proper nutrition, exercise program to maximize available lung function
- Home oxygen therapy PRN
- Removal of patient from further asbestos fiber exposure

GENERAL Rx

- Prompt identification and treatment of respiratory infections
- Supplemental oxygen on a PRN basis
- Annual influenza vaccination, pneumococcal vaccination every 6 yr
- Pulmonary rehabilitation can be considered in advanced cases for improved cardiopulmonary capacity

Some new data are coming out targeting IL-1 beta therapy on the progression of lung fibrosis that suggest a new perspective for the treatment of systemic autoimmune features of asbestosis and, possibly, of lung involvement.[1]

DISPOSITION

- There is no specific treatment for asbestosis.
- Death is usually from respiratory failure from cor pulmonale.
- Diffuse pleural thickening and asbestosis are associated with increased risks of malignant peritoneal mesothelioma beyond the risk calculated to be associated with the degree of asbestos exposure.[2]
- None of the benign pleural diseases or ARPD was associated with an increased risk of malignant pleural mesothelioma.
- Asbestos increases the risk for development of lung cancer regardless of smoking status. In patients with diffuse parenchymal disease secondary to asbestos, the risk of lung cancer is nearly 40 times higher than in those with no history of smoking.
- Asbestos exposure without asbestosis and smoking increases the risk of lung cancer. The joint effect of asbestos and smoking is additive and depends in part on the presence of asbestosis. Asbestos workers who stop smoking experience a dramatic decline in lung cancer risk, which approaches that of nonsmokers after 30 yr.
- Low-dose chest CT scanning offers an excellent opportunity to detect early-stage lung cancers in asbestos-exposed workers.
- Computed tomography is more sensitive than radiography, computed tomography without contrast generally suffices for evaluation, and PET scan (fluorodeoxyglucose-positron emission tomography) may have utility in patients with mesothelioma.
- Survival in patients after development of mesothelioma is 4 to 6 yr.

EVIDENCE

Available at ExpertConsult.com

SUGGESTED READINGS

Available at ExpertConsult.com

RELATED CONTENT

Asbestosis (Patient Information)

AUTHOR: **IMRANA QAWI, M.D.**

[1] Niccoli L, et al.: Systemic autoimmune disease in asbestosis rapidly responding to anti-interleukin-1beta antibody canakinumab: a case report, *BMC Musculoskelet Disord* 14(16):146, 2015.

[2] Reid A, et al.: The additional risk of malignant mesothelioma in former workers and residents of Wittenoom with benign pleural disease or asbestosis, *Occup Environ Med* 62:665-669, 2005.

BASIC INFORMATION

DEFINITION

Ascariasis is a parasitic infection caused by the nematode *Ascaris lumbricoides.* The majority of those infected are asymptomatic; however, clinical disease may arise from pulmonary hypersensitivity, intestinal obstruction, and secondary complications.

SYNONYMS

Round worms
Worms

ICD-10CM CODES	
B77.9	Ascariasis, unspecified
B77.81	Ascariasis pneumonia
B77.0	Ascariasis with intestinal complications
B77.89	Ascariasis with other complications

EPIDEMIOLOGY & DEMOGRAPHICS

INCIDENCE (IN U.S.):

- Unknown. Worldwide, *A. lumbricoides* is the most common helminthic infection of humans, infecting as many as 1 billion or more persons. 71% of persons at risk for infection live in Asia and the Western Pacific.
- Three times the infection rates found in blacks as in whites.

PEAK INCIDENCE: Unknown

PREVALENCE (IN U.S.): Estimated at 4 million, the majority of which live in the rural southeastern part of the country; ascariasis is associated with poor sanitation

PREDOMINANT SEX: Both sexes probably equally affected, with a possible slight female preponderance

PREDOMINANT AGE: Most common in children from ages 2 to 10 years old and decreases after age 15; infections tend to cluster in families

NEONATAL INFECTION: Probable transmission, though not specifically studied

PHYSICAL FINDINGS & CLINICAL PRESENTATION

- Most people infected with *Ascaris* are asymptomatic
- Occurs approximately 9 to 12 days after ingestion of eggs (corresponding to the larval migration through the lungs)
- Nonproductive cough
- Substernal chest discomfort
- Fever
- In patients with large worm burdens, especially children, intestinal obstruction associated with perforation, volvulus, and intussusception
- Migration of worms into the biliary tree giving clinical appearance of biliary colic and pancreatitis as well as acute appendicitis with movement into that appendage
- Rarely, infection with *A. lumbricoides* producing interstitial nephritis and acute renal failure
- In endemic areas in Asia and Africa, malabsorption of dietary proteins and vitamins as a consequence of chronic worm intestinal carriage; 1 billion people worldwide are infected with this nematode

ETIOLOGY

- Transmission is usually hand to mouth, but eggs may be ingested via transported vegetables grown in contaminated soil
- Eggs are hatched in the small intestine, with larvae penetrating intestinal mucosa and migrating via the circulation to the lungs
- Larval forms proceed through the alveoli, ascend the bronchial tree, and return to the intestines after swallowing, where they mature into adult worms
- Estimated time until the female adult worm begins producing eggs is 2 to 3 mo
- Eggs are passed out of the intestines with feces and can survive for years in warm, moist, shaded soil
- Within human host, adult worm life span is 1 to 2 yr

DIAGNOSIS

DIFFERENTIAL DIAGNOSIS

- Radiologic manifestations and eosinophilia to be distinguished from drug hypersensitivity and Löffler's syndrome
- Table E1 compares features of major intestinal nematodes

LABORATORY TESTS

- Examination of the stool for *Ascaris* ova (Fig. E1)
- Expectoration or fecal passage of adult worm
- Adult male worms: 10 to 30 cm long; adult female worms: larger than male, up to 40 cm
- Eosinophilia: Most prominent early in the infection and subsides as the adult worm infestation established in the intestines; usually in 5% to 12% range but can be up to 50%
- Serology: Patients develop IgG antibodies, but they cross react with antigens from other helminths and are not protective; thus serology is used more for epidemiologic purposes than for individual diagnosis

IMAGING STUDIES

- Chest x-ray to reveal bilateral oval or round infiltrates of varying size (Löffler syndrome); NOTE: Infiltrates are transient and eventually resolve.
- Plain films of the abdomen and contrast studies to reveal worm masses in loops of bowel.
- Ultrasonography and endoscopic retrograde cholangiopancreatography (ERCP) to identify worms in the pancreaticobiliary tract.
- CT scan with oral contrast can also assist in the detection of GI foreign bodies such as parasites.

TREATMENT

NONPHARMACOLOGIC THERAPY

Aggressive IV hydration, especially in children with fever, severe vomiting, and resultant dehydration

ACUTE GENERAL Rx

- All infected patients, including asymptomatic ones, should be treated.
  1. Albendazole: 400 mg PO × 3 days is the first-line agent. Single-dose albendazole is used in mass treatment campaigns.
  2. Mebendazole 100 mg PO bid y × 3 days.
- Cure rate with these agents is 95% to 100%, but they are contraindicated in pregnancy.
- Side effects: GI discomfort, headache, and rarely leukopenia
- Alternative agent or for use in pregnancy: Pyrantel pamoate (Antiminth)
  1. Given at a dose of 11 mg/kg PO (maximum dose of 1 g/day)
  2. Considered safe for use in pregnant women
- Other alternative agents:
  1. Ivermectin: 150 to 200 mcg/kg orally once
  2. Nitazoxanide: Ages 2 to 3 yrs: 100 mg/5 ml BID × 3 days, and ages 4 to 11 yrs: 200 mg/10 ml BID × 3 days. Cure rates in heavy worm burden are only 50% to 80%
  3. Piperazine citrate: No longer first-line agent due to toxicity but still used in cases of intestinal or biliary obstruction, as drug paralyzes the worm, helping its expulsion. Dose: 50 to 75 mg/kg once daily up to maximum of 3.5 g for 2 days
  4. Levamisole: 2.5 mg/kg once orally is recommended by the WHO as alternative therapy, but not available in the U.S.
- Complete obstruction should be managed surgically.

DISPOSITION

Overall prognosis is good. Patients should be reevaluated in 2 to 3 months. Reinfection is common.

REFERRAL

- To gastroenterologist in cases of visualized pancreaticobiliary tract or appendiceal obstruction
- To surgeon in cases of complete obstruction or suspected secondary complication (e.g., perforation or volvulus)

PEARLS & CONSIDERATIONS

COMMENTS

- Hepatic abscess, containing both viable and dead worms, complicating *Ascaris*-induced biliary duct disease has been documented.
- Given the known transmission of the parasite, routine hand washing with soap and proper disposal of human waste would significantly decrease the prevalence of this disease.
- Other protective measures to avoid ingestion of worm eggs
  1. Peel or cook food.
  2. Boil drinking water.
  3. Do not place small children directly on soil.

SUGGESTED READINGS

Available at ExpertConsult.com

RELATED CONTENT

Ascariasis (Patient Information)

AUTHOR: **GLENN G. FORT, M.D., M.P.H.**

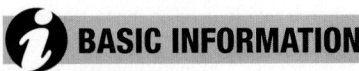

BASIC INFORMATION

DEFINITION

Ascites refers to a pathologic accumulation of fluid in the peritoneal cavity, most commonly caused by liver cirrhosis.

SYNONYMS

Fluid in peritoneal cavity
Hydroperitoneum
Hydroperitonia
Hydrops abdominis

ICD-10CM CODES	
R18	Ascites
C78.6	Malignant ascites
K70.11	Alcoholic hepatitis with ascites
K70.31	Alcoholic cirrhosis of liver with ascites
K71.51	Toxic liver disease with chronic active hepatitis with ascites
R18.8	Other ascites

EPIDEMIOLOGY & DEMOGRAPHICS

Ascites is the most common complication of cirrhosis and signifies decompensation of chronic liver disease. Ascites occurs in 50% of individuals with cirrhosis within ten years of diagnosis. Cirrhosis is the cause of 85% of cases of ascites. Other causes include intraperitoneal malignancy, heart failure, tuberculosis, pancreatitis, nephrotic syndrome, and Budd-Chiari syndrome.

CLINICAL PRESENTATION

- Important information to elicit within history:
  1. History of viral hepatitis
  2. Alcoholism
  3. Intravenous drug use, intranasal cocaine use
  4. Sexual history (i.e., men who have sex with men)
  5. History of transfusions, tattoos, piercings, imprisonment
  6. Symptoms suggestive of peritoneal malignancy (e.g., weight loss, pain, palpable masses, rectal/vaginal bleeding)
  7. Other liver disease symptoms (e.g., increasing abdominal girth, jaundice, pruritus, confusion, pedal edema)
  8. Cardiac symptoms (e.g., pedal edema, shortness of breath, orthopnea, chest pains)
- Important physical exam findings:
  1. Protuberant abdomen (Fig. E1)
  2. Bulging flanks (can be present in obesity)
  3. Flank dullness to percussion
  4. Fluid wave on abdominal exam
  5. Lower extremity edema
  6. Shifting dullness on abdominal exam
  7. Physical signs associated with liver cirrhosis: Spider angiomas, jaundice, loss of body hair, skeletal muscle wasting (sarcopenia), Dupuytren's contracture, bruising, palmar erythema, gynecomastia, testicular atrophy, rectal varices, and caput medusae

ETIOLOGY

Pathophysiology of ascites (Fig. E2): Increased hepatic resistance to portal flow leads to portal hypertension. The splanchnic vessels respond by increased secretion of nitric oxide, causing splanchnic artery vasodilation. Early in the disease increased plasma volume and increased cardiac output compensate for this vasodilation. However, as disease progresses the effective arterial blood volume decreases, causing sodium and fluid retention through activation of the renin-angiotensin system. The change in capillary pressure causes increased permeability and retention of fluid in the abdomen.

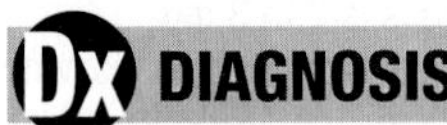

DIAGNOSIS

DIFFERENTIAL DIAGNOSIS

- Chronic parenchymal liver disease, leading to portal hypertension
- Noncirrhotic portal hypertension (e.g., portal vein clot)
- Peritoneal carcinomatosis
- Cardiac disease (e.g., heart failure, constrictive pericarditis)
- Hepatic venous outflow obstruction (e.g., Budd-Chiari syndrome, IVC webs)
- Peritoneal tuberculosis
- Nephrotic syndrome
- Pancreatitis

LABORATORY TESTS

- Initial evaluation should always include:
  1. Diagnostic paracentesis. Laboratory tests on this fluid should include a cell count, cytology, albumin, total protein, culture, and Gram stain. A serum-ascites albumin gradient (SAAG) should be calculated in all patients. The SAAG is measured by subtracting the level of albumin in the ascitic fluid from a concurrent serum albumin measurement: SAAG = serum albumin – ascites albumin.
     a. If the SAAG is greater than 1.1, the cause of ascites can be attributed to portal hypertension.
     b. If SAAG is less than 1.1, a non-portal hypertension etiology of ascites must be sought. Optional tests on paracentesis fluid include amylase, LDH, acid-fast bacilli, and glucose levels.
     c. Causes of ascites in the normal or diseased peritoneum by SAAG are summarized in Table 1.
     d. Fig. 3 illustrates an algorithm for the approach to the differential diagnosis of ascites.
  2. AST, ALT, total and direct bilirubin, albumin, alkaline phosphatase, GGTP.
  3. CBC, coagulation studies.
  4. Electrolytes, BUN, creatinine.

IMAGING STUDIES

- Abdominal ultrasound (Fig. 4) is the most sensitive measure for detecting ascitic fluid; a CT or MRI scan is a viable alternative. Doppler studies of portal and hepatic veins should be added to rule out vascular etiology.

TABLE 1 Causes of Ascites in the Normal or Diseased Peritoneum by Serum-to-Ascites Albumin Gradient (SAAG)

Normal Peritoneum	
Portal Hypertension (SAAG >1.1 G/dl)	**Hypoalbuminemia (SAAG <1.1 g/dl)**
Hepatic congestion	Nephrotic syndrome
Congestive heart failure	Protein-losing enteropathy
Constrictive pericarditis	Severe malnutrition with anasarca
Tricuspid insufficiency	
Budd-Chiari syndrome	
Liver Disease	**Miscellaneous Conditions (SAAG <1.1 g/dl)**
Cirrhosis	Chylous ascites
Alcoholic hepatitis	Pancreatic ascites
Fulminant hepatic failure	Bile ascites
Massive hepatic metastases	Nephrogenic ascites
	Urine ascites
	Ovarian disease
Diseased Peritoneum (SAAG <1.1 g/dl)	
Infections	**Other Rare Conditions**
Bacterial peritonitis	Familial Mediterranean fever
Tuberculous peritonitis	Vasculitis
Fungal peritonitis	Granulomatous peritonitis
HIV-associated peritonitis	Eosinophilic peritonitis
Malignant Conditions	
Peritoneal carcinomatosis	
Primary mesothelioma	
Pseudomyxoma peritonei	
Hepatocellular carcinoma	

From Vincent JL et al: *Textbook of critical care*, ed 7, Philadelphia, 2017, Elsevier.

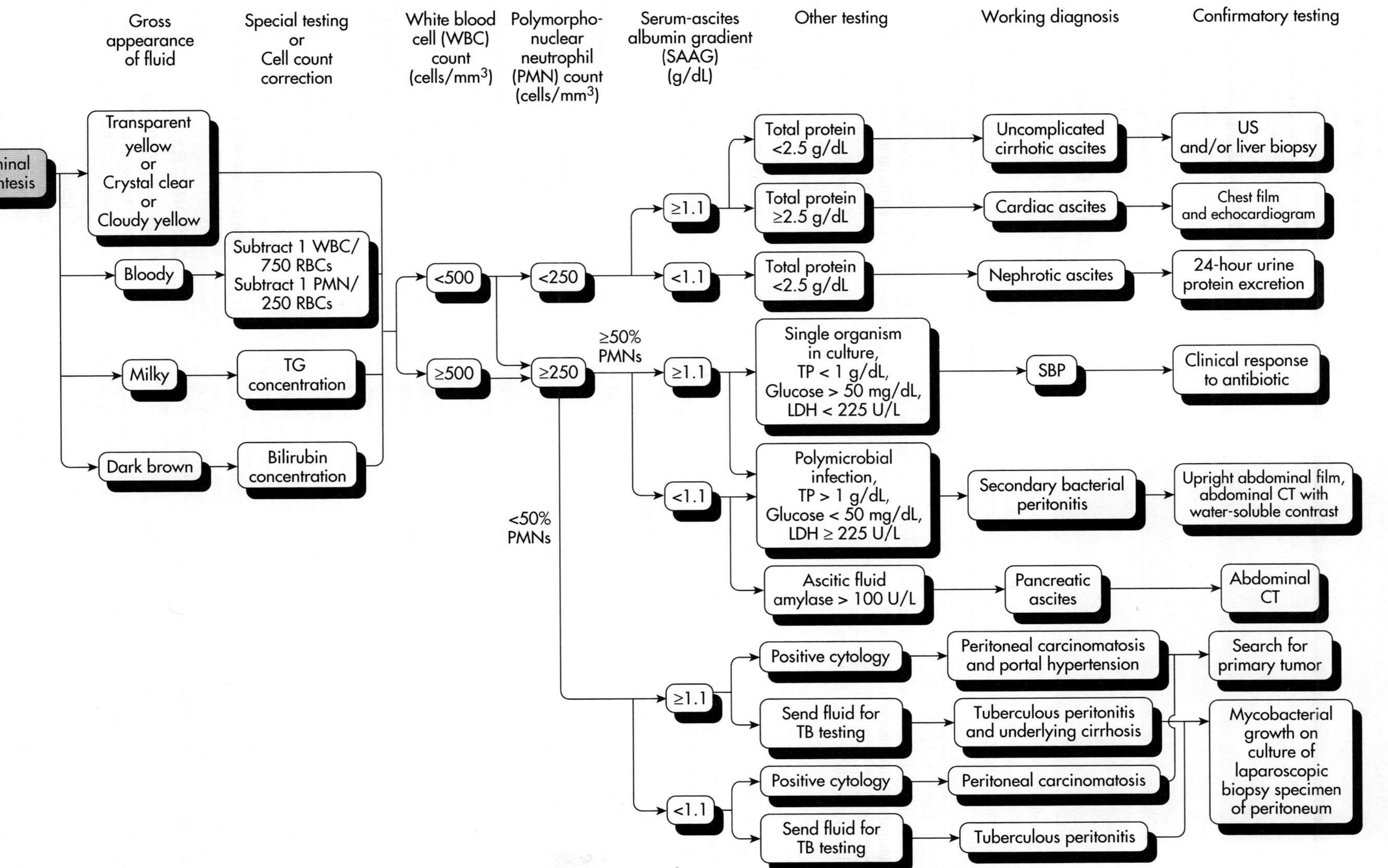

FIG. 3 Algorithm for the approach to the differential diagnosis of ascites. *LDH*, Lactic dehydrogenase; *PMN*, polymorphonuclear neutrophil; *RBC*, red blood cell; *TP*, total protein. (From Feldman M et al: *Sleisenger and Fordtran's gastrointestinal and liver disease*, ed 10, Philadelphia, 2016, Elsevier.)

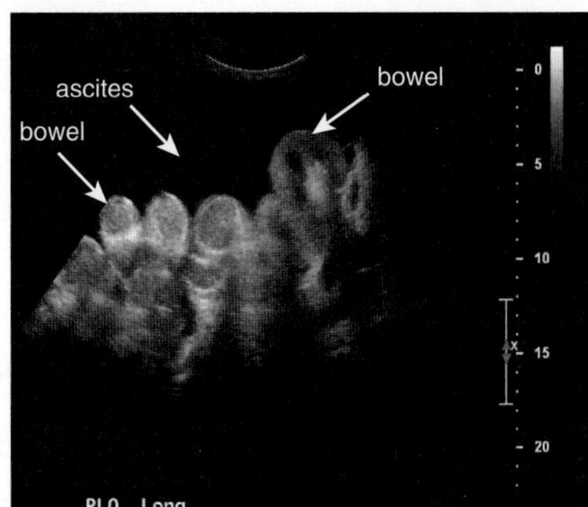

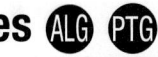

FIG. 4 Ascites, ultrasound. Ultrasound is useful for detection of ascites. Simple fluids such as ascites are excellent sound transmission media, reflecting almost no sound waves. As a consequence, they appear quite hypoechoic *(black)* on ultrasound. This view of the right lower quadrant shows loops of bowel surrounded by fluid. During the ultrasound, the bowel loops would be seen to undergo peristalsis and drift back and forth in the ascitic fluid with patient movement. Ultrasound cannot distinguish the composition of the fluid; ascites, liquid blood, liquid bile, urine, and infectious fluids have a similar appearance, with a few exceptions. Blood may coagulate and form septations within the fluid collection. Infectious fluids also frequently form loculated fluid collections that may be recognized on ultrasound, although the exact composition cannot be determined. *RLQ,* Right lower quadrant. (From Broder JS: *Diagnostic imaging for the emergency physician,* Philadelphia, 2011, Saunders.)

TABLE 2 Primary Medical Therapy and Adjunctive Medications Used to Increase the Efficacy of Primary Therapy in the Treatment of Ascites

Class	Medication	Dosing	Relevant Action	Notes
Diuretics	Spironolactone	400 mg + daily*	Aldosterone receptor antagonist	Primary therapy
	Furosemide	160 mg + daily*	Inhibits Na-K-2Cl symporter	Primary therapy
	Mannitol	20%*	Osmotic diuresis	Give dose just prior to furosemide and spironolactone
Vasoconstrictors	Octreotide	300 mcg bid*	Splanchnic vasoconstriction, inhibits RAAS	Also used in combination with midodrine to treat hepatorenal syndrome; given for first 5 days following variceal bleeding to decrease recurrence
	Midodrine	7.5 mg tid*	Inhibits RAAS	Also used in combination with octreotide and albumin to treat hepatorenal syndrome
α2-Agonist	Clonidine	0.075 mg bid*	Inhibits sympathetic outflow, inhibits RAAS	Increases sensitivity to spironolactone
Colloid	Albumin	25 g*	Increased oncotic pressure	Also utilized with large-volume paracentesis and in the treatment of hepatorenal syndrome
Aquaretics	None are FDA approved	N/A	Vasopressin receptor antagonist	May also treat hyponatremia

*The above doses have been derived from various studies and may not be suitable for all patients. Titration is always recommended. *RAAS,* Renin-angiotensin-aldosterone system. From Cameron JL, Cameron AM: *Current surgical therapy,* ed 10, Philadelphia, 2011, Saunders.

- Endoscopy of the upper GI tract to evaluate for esophageal varices if ascites is secondary to portal hypertension.

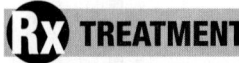

TREATMENT

NONPHARMACOLOGIC THERAPY

- Sodium-restricted diet (<2 g/day)
- Fluid restriction to 1 L/day in patients with severe hyponatremia (sodium <130 mEq/L)
- Counsel on avoiding NSAIDs and discontinuation of ACE inhibitors

ACUTE GENERAL Rx

- Patients with moderate-volume ascites causing only moderate discomfort may be treated on an outpatient basis with the following diuretic regimen:
  1. Spironolactone: Start at 50 to 100 mg/day and titrate up to 400 mg day every 3 to 4 days, can be used alone or
  2. With furosemide: Start at 40 mg/day and titrate up to 160mg/day maximum. Monitor renal function and sodium levels carefully for signs of prerenal azotemia (in patients without edema. Goal weight loss is 300 to 500 g/day; in patients with edema, goal weight loss is 800 to 1000 g/day). Furosemide alone is not recommended.
- Patients with large-volume ascites causing marked discomfort or decrease in activities of daily living may also be treated as outpatients if there are no complications. There are two options for treatment in these patients:
  1. Large-volume paracentesis or
  2. Diuretic therapy until loss of fluid is noted (maximum spironolactone 400 mg daily and furosemide 160 mg daily).
     a. No difference in long-term mortality rate was found; however, paracentesis is faster, more effective, and associated with fewer adverse effects.
     b. Patients receiving large-volume paracentesis should receive albumin replacement therapy at the dose of 7 to 9 g/L of fluid removed if more than 4 to 5 L are taken out. Patients with renal dysfunction or hyponatremia should receive albumin effusion for lower volumes as well.
- Table 2 summarizes primary medical therapy and adjunctive medications used to increase the efficacy of primary therapy in the treatment of ascites.

CHRONIC Rx

- Five to ten percent of patients with large-volume ascites will be refractory to high-dose diuretic treatment. Treatment strategies include repeated large-volume paracentesis with infusion of albumin every 2 to 4 weeks or placement of a transjugular intrahepatic portosystemic shunt (TIPS).
- TIPS evaluation should include echocardiogram, assessment for hepatic encephalopathy, and characterization of liver impairment. The possibility of transplant center referral should be considered at this time.

TABLE 3 Management of Refractory Ascites

Definitions	Ascites that is not eliminated even with maximum diuretic therapy
	Ascites that is not eliminated because maximum dosages of diuretics cannot be attained, given the development of diuretic-induced complications
Recommended therapy	Total paracentesis + IV albumin (7-9 g/L of ascites removed)
	If <5 L of ascites is removed, a synthetic plasma volume expander may be used instead of albumin
	Continue with salt restriction and diuretic therapy as tolerated
Alternative therapy	TIPS for patients who require frequent paracenteses (every 1-2 weeks) and whose CTP score is ≤11
Peritoneovenous shunt for patients who are not candidates for TIPS or transplant	

CTP, Child-Turcotte-Pugh; *IV,* intravenous; *TIPS,* transjugular intrahepatic portosystemic shunt.
Data from Garcia-Tsao G, Lim JK; Members of the Veterans Affairs Hepatitis C Resource Center Program: Management and treatment of patients with cirrhosis and portal hypertension: recommendations from the Department of Veterans Affairs Hepatitis C Resource Center Program and the National Hepatitis C Program, *Am J Gastroenterol,* 104:1802-1829, 2009.
From Vincent JL et al: *Textbook of critical care,* ed 7, Philadelphia, 2017, Elsevier.

- Patients known to have ascites should receive a diagnostic tap if they develop any signs of subacute bacterial peritonitis (SBP) or on any admission to the hospital even in the absence of these signs.
- Primary prophylaxis for SBP is recommended in patients with ascitic fluid protein <1.5 g/dl along with impaired renal function (creatinine ≥1.2, BUN ≥25 or Na ≤130) or liver failure (Child score ≥9 and bilirubin ≥3).
- Secondary prophylaxis should be instituted in all patients who were diagnosed with SBP in the form of a daily fluoroquinolone , ciprofloxacin or norfloxacin.
- Patients with known ascites who develop gastrointestinal bleeding should receive intravenous ceftriaxone for 7 days to prevent bacterial infections.
- Table 3 summarizes the management of refractory ascites. Tolvaptan is reported to be effective in treating refractory ascites, although no effect on prognosis has been reported. A treatment approach to patients with malignant ascites is described in Fig. E5.

DISPOSITION

Monitor closely for worsening liver function and development of spontaneous bacterial peritonitis (SBP).

REFERRAL

Referral to gastroenterology

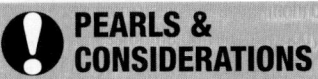

PEARLS & CONSIDERATIONS

COMMENTS

- Prevalence of SBP in patients with ascites ranges between 10% and 30%.
  1. Presence of at least 250 neutrophils per cubic millimeter of ascitic fluid is diagnostic.
  2. Gram-negative bacteria such as *E. coli* are the most common isolates.
  3. Third-generation cephalosporins are the treatment of choice.
  4. By 1 year, 70% of patients have recurrence of SBP and may be prophylaxed with ciprofloxacin 750 mg PO once/wk.

PREVENTION

Prevention of liver cirrhosis through avoidance of long-term use of alcohol, immunization against hepatitis A and B, and treatment of hepatitis C

SUGGESTED READINGS

Available at ExpertConsult.com

RELATED CONTENT

Ascites (Patient Information)
Cirrhosis (Related Key Topic)

AUTHORS: **TALIA ZENLEA, M.D.,** and **PAUL GEORGE, M.D, M.H.P.E.**

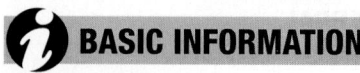

BASIC INFORMATION

DEFINITION

Aspergillosis refers to several forms of a broad range of illnesses caused by infection with *Aspergillus* species. Fig. 1 illustrates the spectrum of *Aspergillus* infection.

ICD-10CM CODES	
B44.0	Invasive pulmonary aspergillosis
B44.1	Other pulmonary aspergillosis
B44.2	Tonsillar aspergillosis
B44.7	Disseminated aspergillosis
B44.81	Allergic bronchopulmonary aspergillosis
B44.89	Other forms of aspergillosis
B44.9	Aspergillosis, unspecified

EPIDEMIOLOGY & DEMOGRAPHICS

INCIDENCE & PREVALENCE:

- *Aspergillus* species are ubiquitous in the environment internationally and occur as a mold found in soil.
- Cause a variety of illness from hypersensitivity pneumonitis to disseminated overwhelming infection in immunosuppressed patients.
- Frequently cultured from hospital wards from unfiltered outside air circulating through open windows as well as water sources.
- Reach the patient by airborne conidia (spores) that are small enough (2.5 to 3 μm) to reach the alveoli on inhalation.
- Can invade the nose, paranasal sinuses, external ear, or traumatized skin.

RISK FACTORS:

- The clinical syndrome depends on the underlying lung architecture, the host's immune response, and the degree of inoculum.
- Incidence of invasive aspergillosis is increasing with advances in the treatment of life-threatening diseases, such as aggressive chemotherapy or bone marrow and organ transplantation. It also can rarely occur in normal hosts, especially associated with influenza A. Liver and lung transplant recipients are at highest risk for pulmonary disease. Genetic deficiency of the soluble-pattern-recognition receptor known as long pentraxin 3 (PTX3) affects the antifungal capacity of neutrophils and may contribute to the risk of invasive aspergillosis in patients treated with hematopoietic stem-cell transplantation (HSCT).
- Patients with AIDS and a CD4 count <50/mm^3 have an increased susceptibility to invasive aspergillosis, but it is otherwise uncommon in patients with HIV.
- Pandemic influenza A (H1N1) infection may predispose immunocompromised patients to invasive aspergillosis.
- Patients with chronic granulomatous disease are at higher risk for infections with *Aspergillus* species.

ETIOLOGY

- *A. fumigatus* is the usual cause.
- *A. flavus* is the second most important species, particularly in invasive disease of immunosuppressed patients and in lesions beginning in the nose and paranasal sinuses. *A. niger* can also cause invasive human infection.

ALLERGIC ASPERGILLOSIS:

- Is a hypersensitivity pneumonitis.
- Presents as cough, dyspnea, fever, chills, and malaise typically 4 to 8 hr after exposure.
- Repeated attacks can lead to granulomatous disease and pulmonary fibrosis.

ALLERGIC BRONCHOPULMONARY ASPERGILLOSIS (ABPA):

- Symptoms occur most commonly in atopic individuals during the third and fourth decades of life.
- Hypersensitivity reaction to *Aspergillus* fungal antigens present in the bronchial tree.
- Results from an initial type I (immediate hypersensitivity) and type III reactions (immune complexes).
- Underdiagnosed pulmonary disorder in patients with asthma and cystic fibrosis (reported prevalence in asthmatic patients varies from 6% to 28% and in cystic fibrosis 6% to 25%).

ASPERGILLOMAS ("FUNGUS BALLS"):

- In the absence of invasion or significant immune response, *Aspergillus* can colonize a preexisting cavity, causing pulmonary aspergilloma.
- Forms masses of tangled hyphal elements, fibrin, and mucus.
- Patients typically have a history of chronic lung disease, tuberculosis, sarcoidosis, or emphysema.
- Manifests commonly as hemoptysis.
- Many are asymptomatic.

INVASIVE ASPERGILLOSIS:

- Patients with prolonged and profound granulocytopenia or impaired phagocytic function are predisposed to rapidly progressive *Aspergillus* pneumonia.
- Typically a necrotizing bronchopneumonia, ranging from small areas of infiltrate to intensive bilateral hemorrhagic infarction.
- Most common presentation: Unremitting fever and a new pulmonary infiltrate despite broad-spectrum antibiotic therapy in an immunosuppressed patient.
- Dyspnea and nonproductive cough are common; sudden pleuritic pain and tachycardia, sometimes with a pleural rub, may mimic pulmonary embolism; hemoptysis is uncommon.
- Chest radiograph (CXR) may reveal patchy bronchopneumonic, nodular densities, consolidation, or cavitation. High-resolution CT scan is more sensitive and specific than CXR in neutropenic patients.
- Immunocompromised patients: Invasive pulmonary *Aspergillus* (IPA) generally is acute and evolves over days to weeks; less commonly, patients with normal or only mild abnormalities of the immune system may develop a more chronic, slowly progressive form of IPA.

EXTRAPULMONARY DISSEMINATION:

- Cerebral infarction from hematogenous dissemination may occur in immunosuppressed individuals.
- Abscess formation from direct extension or invasive disease in the sinuses.
- Esophageal or gastrointestinal ulcerations may occur in the immunosuppressed host.
- Fatal perforation of the viscus or bowel infarction may occur.
- Necrotizing skin ulcers (Fig. 2).
- Osteomyelitis.
- Endocarditis in patients who have recently undergone open heart surgery.
- Infection of an implantable cardioverter-defibrillator has been reported.

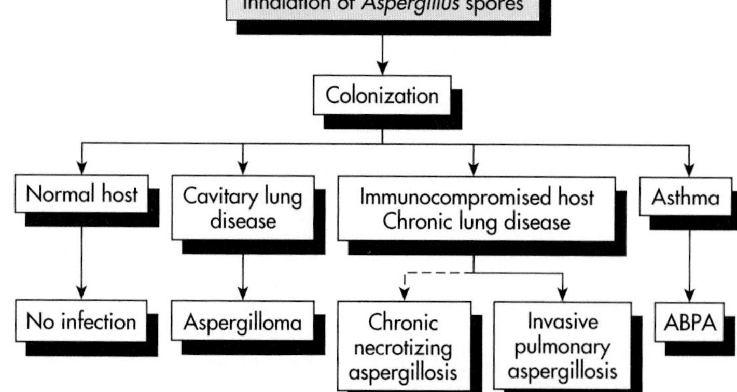

FIG. 1 The spectrum of *Aspergillus* infection. *ABPA,* Allergic bronchopulmonary aspergillosis. (From Sellke FW, del Nido PJ, Swanson SJ: *Sabiston & Spencer surgery of the chest,* ed 9, Philadelphia, 2016, Elsevier.)

DIAGNOSIS

DIFFERENTIAL DIAGNOSIS

- Tuberculosis
- Cystic fibrosis
- Carcinoma of the lung
- Eosinophilic pneumonia
- Bronchiectasis
- Sarcoidosis
- Lung abscess

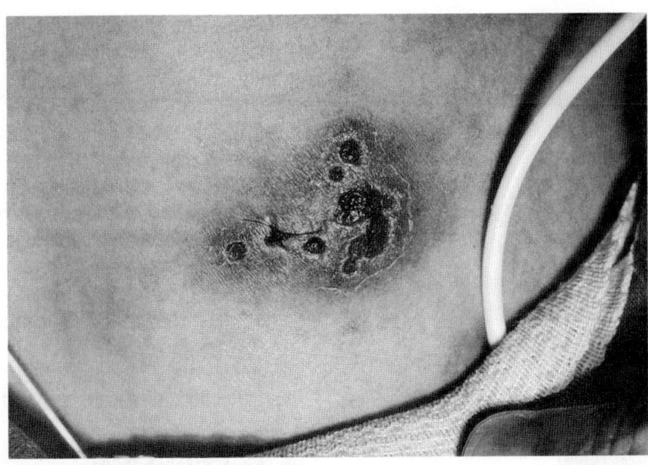

FIG. 2 Cutaneous aspergillosis. Erythematous plaque with necrosis and eschar formation in a young female with immunosuppression and disseminated *Aspergillus fumigatus* infection. (From Paller AS, Mancini, AJ: *Hurwitz clinical pediatric dermatology, a textbook of skin disorders of childhood and adolescence*, ed 5, Philadelphia, 2016, Elsevier.)

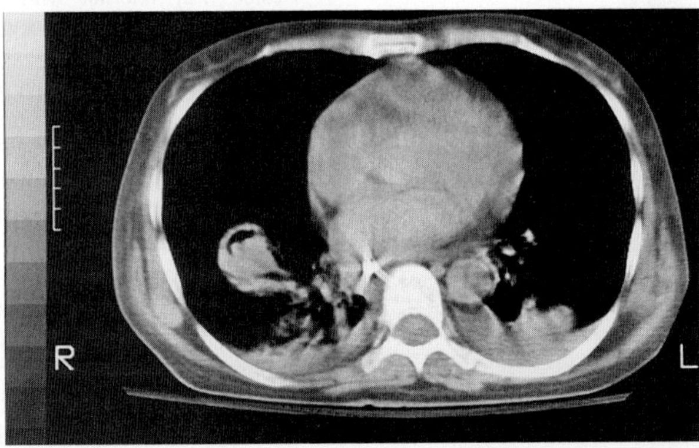

FIG. 3 Computed tomography scan demonstrating an aspergilloma involving the right lower lobe. (From Sellke FW, del Nido PJ, Swanson SJ: *Sabiston & Spencer surgery of the chest*, ed 9, Philadelphia, 2016, Elsevier.)

WORKUP

Physical examination and laboratory data

LABORATORY TESTS

ABPA:

- Peripheral blood eosinophilia and an elevated total serum immunoglobulin E (IgE) level.
- Skin test with *Aspergillus* antigenic extract is usually positive but nonspecific.
- *Aspergillus* serum precipitating antibody is present in 70% to 100% of cases.
- Sputum cultures may be positive for *Aspergillus* spp. but are nonspecific.

ASPERGILLOMAS:

- Sputum culture
- Serum precipitating antibody

Invasive aspergillosis: Definitive diagnosis requires the demonstration of tissue invasion (i.e., septate, acute angle branching hyphae) or a positive culture from the tissue obtained by an invasive procedure such as transbronchial biopsy.

- Sputum and nasal cultures: In high-risk patients a positive culture is strongly suggestive of invasive aspergillosis.
- Serology: The *Platelia Aspergillus* ELISA assay detects a circulating fungal antigen, galactomannan. Galactomannan is a polysaccharide contained in the cell wall of *Aspergillus*. Its presence in serum or other body fluids is indicative of invasive infection, and it is recommended as an accurate marker for diagnosis in certain patient subpopulations (hematologic malignancy and hematopoietic stem cell transplantation). The β-D glucan assay can also be used to detect early infection, but is not specific for *Aspergillus* species.[a]
- Blood cultures: Usually negative.
- Lung biopsy is necessary for definitive diagnosis.
- Biopsy and culture of extrapulmonary lesions.
- Polymerase chain reaction assays may be employed, but their results should be interpreted in conjunction with other diagnostic tests and the clinical context.

[a] False-negative results occur in patients who are receiving antifungal agents other than fluconazole. The sensitivity of the galactomannan assay for invasive pulmonary aspergillosis is higher in bronchoalveolar lavage fluid than in serum. In patients with risk factors and radiologic findings suggestive of invasive aspergillosis, a positive galactomannan confirms the diagnosis of probable invasive pulmonary aspergillosis.

IMAGING STUDIES

ABPA:

- CXRs show a variety of abnormalities, from small, patchy, fleeting infiltrates (commonly in the upper lobes) to lobar consolidation or cavitation.
- A majority of patients eventually develop central bronchiectasis.

ASPERGILLOMAS: CXR or CT scans usually show the characteristic intracavity mass (Figs. 3 and 4) partially surrounded by a crescent of air ("halo sign").

INVASIVE ASPERGILLOSIS: CXR and CT scanning may also reveal cavity formation and the halo sign. Air bronchograms typically disappear as they are filled with hemorrhagic fluid.

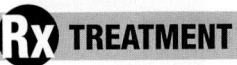

Rx TREATMENT

ACUTE GENERAL Rx

ABPA:

- Prednisone (0.5 to 1 mg/kg PO) until the CXR has cleared, followed by alternate-day therapy at 0.5 mg/kg PO (3 to 6 mo).
- If a patient is corticosteroid dependent, prophylaxis for the prevention of *Pneumocystis jiroveci* infection and maintenance of bone mineralization should be considered.
- Bronchodilators and physiotherapy.
- Serial CXR and serum IgE is useful in guiding treatment.
- Itraconazole 200 mg PO bid for 4 to 6 mo, then taper over 4 to 6 mo may be considered as a steroid-sparing agent or if steroids are ineffective.

ASPERGILLOMAS:

- Controversial and problematic; the optimal treatment strategy is unknown.
- Up to 10% of aspergillomas may resolve clinically without overt pharmacologic or surgical intervention.
- Observation for asymptomatic patients.
- Surgical resection/arterial embolization for those patients with severe hemoptysis or life-threatening hemorrhage.
- For those patients at risk for marked hemoptysis with inadequate pulmonary reserve, consider itraconazole 200 to 400 mg/day PO.

INVASIVE ASPERGILLOSIS (IA):

- Voriconazole 6 mg/kg IV/PO bid on day 1 followed by 4 mg/kg IV/PO bid. Voriconazole serum concentrations need to be monitored to achieve a target range of 1.0 to 5.5 mg/L (trough on day 4).
- Isavuconazonium sulfate (prodrug of Isavuconazole) 372 mg IV/PO tid for six doses and then 372 mg IV/PO daily.

  Alternative Treatment:
- Amphotericin B lipid complex (ABLC) 5 mg/kg IV daily.
- Liposomal amphotericin B (L-AMB) 3 to 5 mg/kg IV daily.
- Posaconazole 200 delayed-release tabs 300 mg PO for two doses, then 300 mg PO daily or posaconazole suspension 200 mgs qid, then 400 mg po bid after stabilization of disease or posaconazole 300 mg IV over 90 minutes bid for one day, then 300 mg IV daily.
- Because azoles and echinocandins target different cellular sites, combination therapy

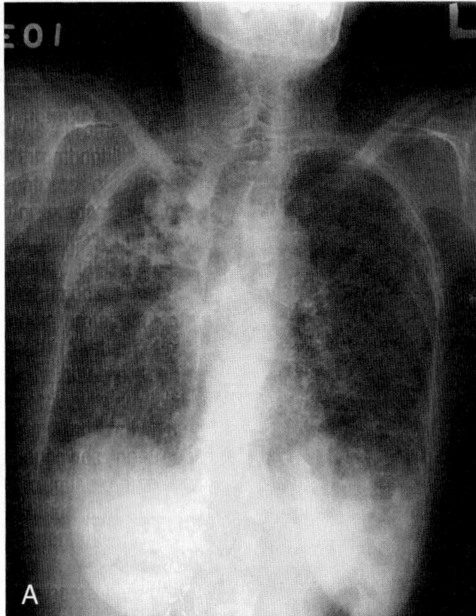

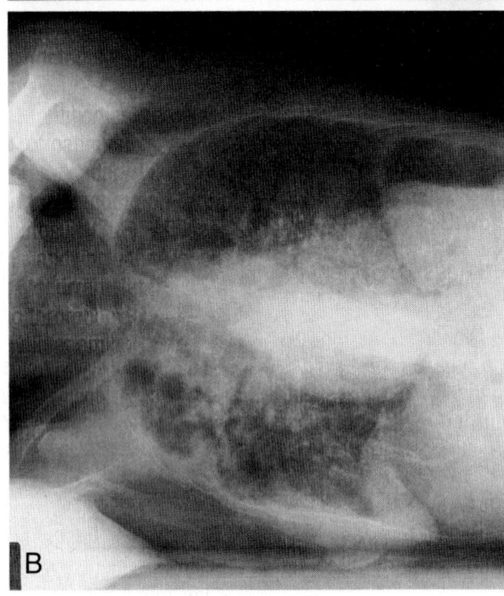

FIG. 4 Posteroanterior **(A)** and decubitus **(B)** chest radiographs demonstrating an aspergilloma within a right upper lobe cavity. The fungus ball "moves" with change in patient position. (From Sellke FW, del Nido PJ, Swanson SJ: *Sabiston & Spencer surgery of the chest*, ed 9, Philadelphia, 2016, Elsevier.)

may have additive activity against *Aspergillus* species. Although still under investigation, some bone marrow transplant units use caspofungin and voriconazole as the preferred initial treatment, especially in patients receiving high-dose corticosteroids. Recent trials (Marr et al, 2015) have shown that compared with voriconazole monotherapy, combination therapy with anidulafungin, and echinocandin antifungal drug that blocks the synthesis of (13)β-D glucan led to higher survival in subgroups of patients with IA.

REFERRAL

To an infectious diseases specialist

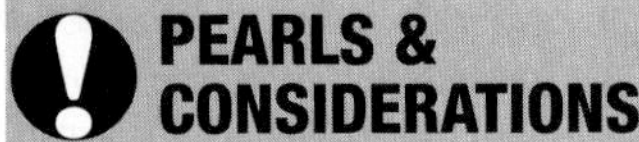

PEARLS & CONSIDERATIONS

- Unlike fluconazole, the potential for drug-drug interactions with voriconazole is high. Azoles may interact with drugs used for chemotherapy by increasing toxicity and/or by reducing efficacy.
- Azole resistance has appeared in *Aspergillus fumigatus*; the main resistance mechanism is a point mutation of CYP51A, the gene coding for 14 alpha-sterol demethylase, the target enzyme of antifungal drugs. Global prevalence of azole resistance in *Aspergillus* is estimated to be approximately 3% to 6%.
- Agitation of hospital buildings by renovations or repairs may increase the incidence of *Aspergillus* infections in immunosuppressed individuals.
- Echinocandins should never be used as primary treatment of aspergillosis.
- *Aspergillus* and *Nocardia* species may co-infect.
- Use of antifungal agents in combination is discussed in Box 1.

SUGGESTED READINGS

Available at ExpertConsult.com

RELATED CONTENT

Aspergillosis (Patient Information)

AUTHOR: **SAJEEV HANDA, M.D., S.F.H.M.**

BOX 1 Use of Antifungal Agents in Combination.

The development of new antifungal drugs gives the clinician more options for prophylaxis and therapy than in previous years. There is an overall level of simplicity to the drug choices once their mechanisms of action are understood. The polyenes, including amphotericin products and the topical agent nystatin, attach onto ergosterol in the fungal cell membrane and are considered fungicidal, because cytoplasm leaks out, and individual cells die. The azoles, including fluconazole, itraconazole, voriconazole, and posaconazole, prevent the formation of new ergosterol. Azoles are considered fungistatic, because removal of the drug permits cell regrowth. Theoretically, use of an azole together with a polyene may have an overall static effect for an established infection as the ergosterol target for the fungicidal polyene is depleted. However, this combination may have advantages in terms of enhanced spectrum of activity. The echinocandins, including caspofungin, micafungin, and anidulafungin, prevent interaction of the catalytic and regulatory subunits of the β-glucan synthesis enzyme, so less β-glucan is formed for the cell wall. The scaffolding for the fungal cell wall is not maintained, and a dividing cell may burst open when trying to extend the new cell wall over daughter cells. The echinocandins are considered fungicidal for yeasts but fungistatic for molds, because drug activity is concentrated at only the tips of the extending hyphae with little effect on less metabolically active subapical compartments of the fungus. Combination therapy may have the most effect when a cell wall agent (an echinocandin) is used together with a cell membrane agent (a polyene or an azole). There is no role for three-drug therapy (an echinocandin, a polyene, and an azole). Aside from cases of cryptococcal meningitis, in which the importance of combination therapy is well established, the benefits of frontline use of combination antifungal for molds remain controversial, although active investigation continues in clinical trials. The value of combination regimens as salvage therapy for refractory mold infections remains uncertain.

From Hoffman R, et al.: *Hematology, basic principles and practice*, ed 7, Philadelphia, 2018, Elsevier.

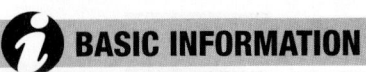

BASIC INFORMATION

DEFINITION

Aspiration pneumonia is a vague term that refers to pulmonary abnormalities following abnormal entry of endogenous or exogenous substances in the lower airways. It is generally classified as:

- Aspiration (chemical pneumonitis)
- Primary bacterial aspiration pneumonia
- Secondary bacterial infection of chemical pneumonitis

SYNONYM

Pneumonia, aspiration

ICD-10CM CODE
J69.0 Pneumonitis due to inhalation of food and vomit

EPIDEMIOLOGY & DEMOGRAPHICS

INCIDENCE (IN U.S.):

- 20% to 35% of all pneumonias
- 5% to 15% of all community-acquired pneumonias

PEAK INCIDENCE: Elderly patients in hospitals or nursing homes
PREVALENCE (IN U.S.): Unknown (unreliable data)
PREDOMINANT SEX: Males and females affected equally
PREDOMINANT AGE: Elderly

PHYSICAL FINDINGS & CLINICAL PRESENTATION

- Shortness of breath, tachypnea, cough, sputum, fever after vomiting, or difficulty swallowing
- Rales, rhonchi, often diffusely throughout lung

ETIOLOGY

Complex interaction of etiologies, ranging from chemical (often acid) pneumonitis after aspiration of sterile gastric contents (generally not requiring antibiotic treatment) to bacterial aspiration. Risk factors for aspiration pneumonia include vomiting, decreased consciousness, poor dentition and GERD. Table 1 summarizes risk factors for aspiration pneumonia.

COMMUNITY-ACQUIRED ASPIRATION PNEUMONIA:

- Generally results from predominantly anaerobic mouth bacteria (anaerobic and microaerophilic streptococci, fusobacteria, gram-positive anaerobic non–spore-forming rods), *Bacteroides* species (*melaninogenicus, intermedius, oralis, ureolyticus*), *Haemophilus influenzae,* and *Streptococcus pneumoniae*
- Rarely caused by *Bacteroides fragilis* (of uncertain validity in published studies) or *Eikenella corrodens*
- High-risk groups: The elderly; alcoholics; IV drug users; patients who are obtunded; stroke victims; and those with esophageal disorders, seizures, poor dentition, or recent dental manipulations

HOSPITAL-ACQUIRED ASPIRATION PNEUMONIA:

- Often occurs among elderly patients and others with diminished gag reflex; those with nasogastric tubes, intestinal obstruction, or ventilator support; and especially those exposed to contaminated nebulizers or unsterile suctioning.
- High-risk groups: Seriously ill hospitalized patients (especially patients with coma, acidosis, alcoholism, uremia, diabetes mellitus, nasogastric intubation, or recent antimicrobial therapy, who are frequently colonized with aerobic gram-negative rods); patients undergoing anesthesia; those with strokes, dementia, or swallowing disorders; the elderly; and those receiving antacids or H_2 blockers, or proton pump inhibitors (but not sucralfate).
- Hypoxic patients receiving concentrated O_2 have diminished ciliary activity, encouraging aspiration.
- Causative organisms:
  1. Anaerobes listed above, although in many studies gram-negative aerobes (60%) and gram-positive aerobes (20%) predominate.
  2. *E. coli, P. aeruginosa, S. aureus* including MRSA, *Klebsiella, Enterobacter, Serratia, Proteus* spp., *H. influenzae, S. pneumoniae, Legionella,* and *Acinetobacter* spp. (sporadic pneumonias) in two thirds of cases.
  3. Fungi, including *Candida albicans,* in <1%.

DIAGNOSIS

DIFFERENTIAL DIAGNOSIS

- Other necrotizing or cavitary pneumonias (especially tuberculosis, gram-negative pneumonias)
- See "Pulmonary Tuberculosis"

WORKUP

- Chest x-ray
- Complete blood count (CBC), blood cultures
- Sputum Gram stain and culture
- Consideration of tracheal aspirate

LABORATORY TESTS

- CBC: Leukocytosis often present
- Sputum Gram stain
  1. Often useful when carefully prepared immediately after obtaining suctioned or expectorated specimen, examined by experienced observer
  2. Only specimens with multiple white blood cells and rare or absent epithelial cells should be examined
  3. Unlike nonaspiration pneumonias (e.g., pneumococcal), multiple organisms may be present
  4. Long, slender rods suggest anaerobes
  5. Sputum from pneumonia caused by acid aspiration may be devoid of organisms
  6. Cultures should be interpreted in light of morphology of visualized organisms

IMAGING STUDIES

- Chest x-ray often reveals bilateral, diffuse, patchy infiltrates and posterior segment upper lobes (Fig. 1). Chemical pneumonitis typically affects the most dependent regions of the lungs.
- Aspiration pneumonia of several days' or longer duration may reveal necrosis (especially community-acquired anaerobic pneumonias) and even cavitation with air-fluid levels, indicating lung abscess.

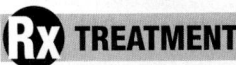

TREATMENT

NONPHARMACOLOGIC THERAPY

- Airway management to prevent repeated aspiration
- Ventilatory support if necessary
- Rehabilitative management: Physical, pulmonary, and dysphagia therapy combined with appropriate nutrition can reduce length of stay and mortality

ACUTE GENERAL Rx

Acute aspiration of acidic gastric contents without bacteria may not require antibiotic therapy; consult infectious disease or pulmonary expert.

- Community-acquired anaerobic aspiration pneumonia: Clindamycin (600 mg IV twice daily followed by 300 mg q6h orally). Intravenous penicillin G (1 to 2 million U q4 to 6h) can also still be used. Alternative oral agents include amoxicillin-clavulanate (875 mg orally twice daily), amoxicillin plus metronidazole or oral moxifloxacin (400 mg orally once daily). Do not use metronidazole alone, as this is associated with high failure rates.

TABLE 1 Risk Factors for Dysphagia and Aspiration Pneumonia

Cerebrovascular disease
Ischemic stroke
Hemorrhagic stroke
Subarachnoid hemorrhage
Degenerative neurologic disease
Alzheimer's disease
Multi-infarct dementia
Parkinson's disease
Amyotrophic lateral sclerosis (motor neuron disease)
Multiple sclerosis
Head and neck cancer
Oropharyngeal malignancy
Oral cavity malignancy
Esophageal malignancy
Other
Scleroderma
Diabetic gastroparesis
Reflux esophagitis
Presbyesophagus
Achalasia

From Vincent JL et al: *Textbook of critical care,* ed 7, Philadelphia, 2017, Elsevier.

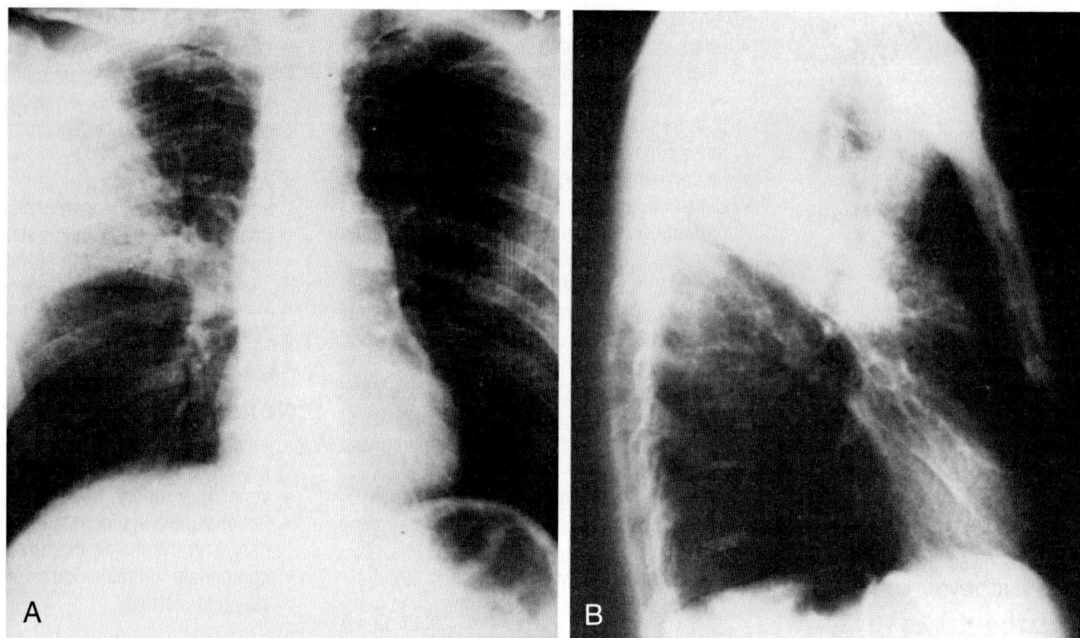

FIG. 1 Anaerobic necrotizing pneumonia following aspiration of oropharyngeal secretions. Multiple, small (<2 cm) radiolucencies are seen throughout the posterior segment of the right upper lobe on the posteroanterior **(A)** and lateral **(B)** projections. (From Mason RJ et al: *Murray & Nadel's textbook of respiratory medicine*, ed 5, Philadelphia, 2010, Saunders.)

- Nursing home aspirations: Levofloxacin 500 to 750 mg qd or piperacillin-tazobactam 3.375 g q6h or cefepime 2 g q8h ± vancomycin if MRSA suspected or known.
- Hospital-acquired aspiration pneumonia:
  1. Piperacillin-tazobactam 3.375 g IV q6h, or meropenem 1 g IV q 8h ± vancomycin IV to cover MRSA. Alternative agents are ceftriaxone 2 g IV q24h plus metronidazole 500 mg IV q8h.
  2. Knowledge of resident flora in the microenvironment of the aspiration within the hospital is crucial to intelligent antibiotic selection; consult infection control nurses or hospital epidemiologist.
  3. Confirmed *Pseudomonas* pneumonia should be treated with antipseudomonal beta-lactam agent (piperacillin/tazobactam, cefepime, meropenem) plus an aminoglycoside until antimicrobial sensitivities confirm that less toxic agents may replace the aminoglycoside.
  4. Do not use metronidazole alone for anaerobes.

DISPOSITION

Repeat chest x-ray in 6 to 8 wk in most patients.

REFERRAL

For consultation with infectious disease and/or pulmonary experts for patients with respiratory distress, hypoxia, ventilatory support, pneumonia in more than one lobe, or necrosis or cavitation on x-ray examination or for those not responding to antibiotic therapy within 2 to 3 days.

SUGGESTED READINGS

Available at ExpertConsult.com

RELATED CONTENT

Aspiration Pneumonia (Patient Information)

AUTHOR: **GLENN G. FORT, M.D., M.P.H.**

BASIC INFORMATION

DEFINITION

The National Asthma Education and Prevention Program (NAEPP) guidelines define asthma as "a chronic inflammatory disease of the airways in which many cells and cellular elements play a role: in particular mast cells, neutrophils, eosinophils, T lymphocytes, macrophages, and epithelial cells. In susceptible individuals, this inflammation causes recurrent episodes of coughing (particularly at night or early in the morning), wheezing, breathlessness, and chest tightness. The episodes are usually associated with widespread but variable airflow obstruction that is reversible either spontaneously or as a result of treatment." **Status asthmaticus,** or acute severe asthma, is a refractory state that does not respond to standard therapy such as inhaled beta-agonists or subcutaneous epinephrine. It may persist for several hours.

SYNONYMS

Bronchospasm
Reactive airway disease
Asthmatic bronchitis

ICD-10CM CODES

J45.20	Mild intermittent asthma, uncomplicated
J45.21	Mild intermittent asthma with (acute) exacerbation
J45.22	Mild intermittent asthma with status asthmaticus
J45.30	Mild persistent asthma, uncomplicated
J45.31	Mild persistent asthma with (acute) exacerbation
J45.32	Mild persistent asthma with status asthmaticus
J45.40	Moderate persistent asthma, uncomplicated
J45.41	Moderate persistent asthma with (acute) exacerbation
J45.42	Moderate persistent asthma with status asthmaticus
J45.50	Severe persistent asthma, uncomplicated
J45.51	Severe persistent asthma with (acute) exacerbation
J45.52	Severe persistent asthma with status asthmaticus
J45.901	Unspecified asthma with (acute) exacerbation
J45.902	Unspecified asthma with status asthmaticus
J45.909	Unspecified asthma, uncomplicated
J45.991	Cough variant asthma
J45.998	Other asthma

EPIDEMIOLOGY & DEMOGRAPHICS

- Asthma has been diagnosed in 7.5% of the population in the United States, and its prevalence is steadily rising. among patients older than 65 years, blacks, women, and persons below the poverty level.
- It accounts for around 440,000 hospitalizations and 1.8 million emergency department visits yearly in the United States.
- It is more common in children, but the gap is closing because of a rapid increase in adult-onset asthma (9.5% of children vs. 8.2% of adults).
- 50% to 80% of children with asthma develop symptoms before 5 yr of age. Early childhood risk factors for asthma are described in Table 1.
- The overall asthma mortality rate in the United States has slightly improved to 11 per 1 million persons.
- Seniors have a high level of mortality from their asthma.

PHYSICAL FINDINGS & CLINICAL PRESENTATION

Physical examination varies with the stage and severity of asthma and may reveal normal lung examination results in many patients. However, some degree of wheezing and prolonged expiratory phases of respiration are seen with persistent or acute disease. Physical examination during status asthmaticus may reveal:

- Tachycardia and tachypnea
- Use of accessory respiratory muscles
- Pulsus paradoxus (inspiratory decline in systolic blood pressure >10 mm Hg)
- Absence of wheezing (silent chest) or decreased wheezing can indicate worsening obstruction
- Mental status changes: Generally secondary to hypoxia and hypercapnia and constitute an indication for urgent intubation
- Paradoxic abdominal and diaphragmatic movement on inspiration (detected by palpation over the upper part of the abdomen in a semirecumbent position) indicates diaphragmatic fatigue, another sign of impending respiratory crisis
- The following abnormalities in vital signs are indicative of severe asthma:
  1. Pulsus paradoxus >18 mm Hg
  2. Respiratory rate >30 breaths/min
  3. Tachycardia with heart rate >120 beats/min

TABLE 1 Early Childhood Risk Factors for Persistent Asthma

Parental asthma
Allergy:
- Atopic dermatitis (eczema)
- Allergic rhinitis
- Food allergy
- Inhalant allergen sensitization
- Food allergen sensitization

Severe lower respiratory tract infection:
- Pneumonia
- Bronchiolitis requiring hospitalization

Wheezing apart from colds
Male gender
Low birthweight
Environmental tobacco smoke exposure
Possible use of acetaminophen (paracetamol)
Exposure to chlorinated swimming pools
Reduced lung function at birth

From Kliegman RM et al: *Nelson textbook of pediatrics,* ed 19, Philadelphia, 2011, Saunders.

ETIOLOGY

- The pathophysiology of asthma involves a complex interaction among various environmental and genetic factors.
- Allergic (extrinsic) asthma is triggered by various aeroallergens or nonspecific (e.g., dust, cigarette smoke, fumes, cold air, exercise) exposures in patients who are prone to develop Ig E antibodies in response to various exposures.
- A recent study of a prebirth cohort observed that maternal intake of foods commonly considered allergenic (peanut and milk) was associated with a decrease in allergy and asthma in the offspring. No dietary changes during pregnancy are therefore recommended for prevention of allergies or asthma.
- A recent trial revealed that supplementation with n-3 long-chain polyunsaturated fatty acids (LCPUFAs, fish oil-derived fatty acids) in the third trimester of pregnancy reduced the absolute risk of persistent wheeze or asthma and infections of the lower respiratory tract in offspring by approximately 7 percentage points, or one third.[1]
- Nonallergic (intrinsic) asthma commonly manifests as adult-onset asthma in response to respiratory tract infection or psychological stress.
- Occupation exposure to certain organic or nonorganic agents can trigger asthma.
- Evidence suggests that dampness and mold contribute to the risk of developing asthma and that remediation of these in homes reduces asthma symptoms and medication use in adults.
- Exercise-induced asthma is seen most frequently in adolescents and manifests with bronchospasm after beginning of exercise and improves with discontinuation of exercise.
- Drug-induced asthma is associated with use of NSAIDs, β-blockers, sulfites, and certain foods and beverages.
- There is a strong association of the *ADAM 33* gene with asthma and bronchial hyperresponsiveness. Experimental, genetic, and clinical studies support an important role for Th2 immune pathways in the pathogenesis of severe asthma. Th2 cells are stimulated by dendritic cells to produce IL-5, IL-13, and IL-4, the latter driving IgE synthesis. This group is characterized by eosinophilia, and IL-5 is felt to be the most specific cytokine in eosinophil regulatory pathways.

Dx DIAGNOSIS

DIFFERENTIAL DIAGNOSIS

- Postinfectious bronchitis
- Rhinitis with postnasal drip
- COPD
- GERD
- Pneumonia and other upper respiratory infections
- Foreign body aspiration (most frequent in younger patients)
- Anxiety disorder
- Diffuse interstitial lung disease
- Hypersensitivity pneumonitis

[1] Bisgaard H et al: Fish oil-derived fatty acids in pregnancy and wheeze and asthma in offspring, *N Engl J Med* 375:2530-2539, 2016.

- CHF
- Pulmonary embolism (in adult and elderly patients)

WORKUP

- Diagnosis of asthma requires documentation of airway obstruction and some degree of reversibility of the obstruction, if and when patient can participate.
- For symptomatic adults and children age >5 yr who can perform spirometry, pre- and postbronchodilator spirometry is the recommended test of choice.
- Airflow reversibility is defined as increase in forced expiratory volume in 1 sec (FEV_1 by at least 12% increase and 200 ml) after inhaling a short bronchodilator.
- The degree of reversibility measured by spirometry correlates with airway inflammation, and patients with a high degree of reversibility have a greater risk of irreversible airflow obstruction in subsequent years.
- For children age<5 yr, spirometry is generally not feasible. Young children with asthma symptoms should be treated as having suspected asthma after alternative diagnoses are ruled out.
- Negative spirometry results do not rule out asthma. Patients with high clinical suspicion should undergo bronchial challenge test using methacholine or other specific agents.
- The clinician should evaluate for environmental causes (e.g., house dust mites, indoor pets) and exposure to other allergens such as tobacco smoke. The degree of reversibility measured by spirometry correlates with airway inflammation, and patients with a high degree of reversibility have a greater risk of irreversible airflow obstruction in subsequent years.
- In the absence of spirometry testing, variability of peak flow measurements by a handheld device can be used to diagnose asthma.
- Fig. E1 describes an algorithm for diagnosing asthma.

After diagnosis, the severity of asthma should be classified during the initial assessment before initiating therapy. Patients are divided into four groups based on the severity of their asthma symptoms and number of exacerbations (see Table 2).

- Once therapy is initiated, the emphasis for clinical management should gear toward achievement of asthma control. The level of asthma control should be used to guide decisions either to maintain or adjust therapy.
- Schedule visits at 2- to 6-wk intervals for patients who are just starting therapy or who require a step up in therapy to achieve or regain asthma control. Schedule visits at 6- to 12-mo intervals, after asthma control is achieved, to monitor whether asthma control is maintained. The interval will depend on factors such as the duration of asthma control or the level of treatment required. Consider scheduling visits at 3-mo intervals if step-down therapy is anticipated.

LABORATORY TESTS

Laboratory tests are usually not necessary and the results can be normal if obtained during a stable period.

- Arterial blood gases (ABGs) can be used during acute bronchospasm in staging the severity of an asthmatic attack:
  1. Mild: Decreased Pa_{O_2} and Pa_{CO_2}, increased pH
  2. Moderate: Decreased Pa_{O_2}, normal Pa_{CO_2}, normal pH
  3. Severe: Marked decreased Pa_{O_2}, increased Pa_{CO_2}, and decreased pH
- Complete blood count: Leukocytosis with left shift may indicate the existence of bacterial infection. Elevated eosinophils point toward allergic component of asthma.
- Spirometry is recommended at the initial assessment and at least every 1 to 2 yr after treatment is initiated and when the symptoms and peak expiratory flow have stabilized. Spirometry as a monitoring measure may be performed more frequently, if indicated, based on severity of symptoms and the disease's lack of response to treatment.
- Peak expiratory flow rate (PEFR) can be used to assess severity of an acute exacerbation episode. Value should be compared with individual's personal best number (see asthma action plan).
- Serum IgE levels help guide treatment for patients with severe persistent asthma, and they also help monitor response to treatment in the same group.

TABLE 2 Classifying Asthma Severity and Initiating Treatment in Youths ≥12 Yr and Adults (Assessing severity and initiating treatment for patients who are not currently taking long-term control medications)

		CLASSIFICATION OF ASTHMA SEVERITY (≥12 YR)			
			PERSISTENT		
Components of Severity		**Intermittent**	**Mild**	**Moderate**	**Severe**
Impairment Normal FEV_1/FVC: yr85% yr80% yr75% yr70%	Symptoms	≤2 days/wk	>2 days/wk but not daily	Daily	Throughout the day
	Nighttime awakenings	≤2x/mo	3-4x/mo	>1x/wk but not nightly	Often 7x/wk
	Short-acting $beta_2$-agonist use for symptom control (not prevention of EIB)	≤2 days/wk	>2 days/wk but not daily, and not more than 1x on any day	Daily	Several times per day
	Interference with normal activity	None	Minor limitation	Some limitation	Extremely limited
	Lung function	Normal FEV_1 between exacerbations FEV_1>80% predicted FEV_1/FVC normal	FEV_1>80% predicted FEV_1/FVC normal	FEV_1>60% but <80% predicted FEV_1/FVC reduced 5%	FEV_1<60% predicted FEV_1/FVC reduced>5%
Risk	Exacerbations requiring oral systemic corticosteroids	0-1 per yr	≥2 per yr		
		Consider severity and interval since last exacerbation. Frequency and severity may fluctuate over time for patients in any severity category. Relative annual risk of exacerbations may be related to FEV_1.			
Recommended Step for Initiating Therapy		Step 1	Step 2	Step 3 and consider short course of oral systemic corticosteroids	Step 4 or 5
		In 2-6 wk, evaluate level of asthma control that is achieved and adjust therapy accordingly.			

The stepwise approach is meant to assist, not replace, the clinical decision-making required to meet individual patient needs.

Level of severity is determined by assessment of both impairment and risk. Assess impairment domain by patient's/caregiver's recall of previous 2-4 wk and spirometry. Assign severity to the most severe category in which any feature occurs.

At present, there are inadequate data to correspond frequencies of exacerbations with different levels of asthma severity. In general, more frequent and intense exacerbations (e.g., requiring urgent, unscheduled care, hospitalization, or ICU admission) indicate greater underlying disease severity. For treatment purposes, patients who had ≥2 exacerbations requiring oral systemic corticosteroids in the past year may be considered the same as patients who have persistent asthma, even in the absence of impairment levels consistent with persistent asthma.

To access the complete *Expert Panel Report 3: Guidelines for the Diagnosis and Management of Asthma,* go to www.nhlbi.nih.gov/guidelines/asthma/asthgdln.pdf.

EIB, Exercise-induced bronchospasm; *FEV_1,* forced expiratory volume in 1 second; *FVC,* forced vital capacity; *ICU,* intensive care unit.

From National Asthma Education and Prevention Program: *Expert panel report 3: guidelines for diagnosis and management of asthma,* National Institutes of Health, National Heart, Lung, and Blood Institute, August 2007, NIH publication 08-4051.

- Specific allergy testing may be helpful in a subgroup of patients.

IMAGING STUDIES

- Chest x-ray: Usually normal, may show evidence of thoracic hyperinflation (e.g., flattening of the diaphragm, increased volume over the retrosternal air space).
- ECG: Tachycardia, nonspecific ST-T wave changes are common during an asthma attack; may also show cor pulmonale, right bundle branch block, right axial deviation, counterclockwise rotation.

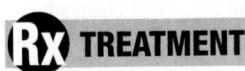

TREATMENT

NONPHARMACOLOGIC THERAPY

- Avoidance of triggering factors (e.g., salicylates, sulfites), environmental or occupational triggers
- Encouragement of regular exercise (e.g., swimming)
- Patient education regarding warning signs of an attack and proper use of medications (e.g., correct use of inhalers)
- Assess asthma control with use of validated questionnaires

GENERAL Rx

The 2007 NAEPP guidelines (see Tables 2 to 10) provide treatment options by age groups: 0 to 4 yr, 5 to 11 yr, and >12 yr. A step-up approach is described based on the severity of symptoms.

An approach to home management of acute asthma is described in Fig. E2. Short-acting beta-selective adrenergic agonists (SABAs) administered by inhalation is the most effective therapy for quick relief of asthmatic symptoms. They are recommended for use only as needed for relief of symptoms or before anticipated exposure to known triggers such as exercise. They should not be use as a single agent except for intermittent asthma symptoms. When symptoms become more frequent or more severe, step-up treatment with maintenance inhalers is recommended (see Table 4). Inhaled steroid is the mainstay of treatment for maintenance therapy. Other treatment options include long-acting beta-agonist (LABA), combination of inhaled steroids and LABA, leukotriene receptor antagonist (LTRA), cromolyn, zileuton, and theophylline. Oral corticosteroids are reserved as a last resort for maintenance therapy for recalcitrant cases. Various studies have showed some degree of benefit when adding LAMA to ICS + LABA in moderate to severe asthma. There are several corticosteroid/LABA combination inhalers available (fluticasone/salmeterol [Advair], budesonide/formoterol [Symbicort], mometasone/formoterol [Dulera], and ICS/LABA fluticasone furoate 200 mcg and vilanterol 25 mcg inhalation powder [Breo Ellipta]) on the market. None of these combinations is indicated for the initial treatment of asthma or for acute therapy of asthma symptoms. There is no evidence that one product is more effective than the others. A large study investigating the safety of LABA and ICS combination inhalers confirmed their long-term safety and demonstrated a reduced risk of exacerbations and improved lung function, when compared with an equivalent dose of ICS alone.

IMMUNOLOGIC TARGETS

Omalizumab, an anti-IgE monoclonal antibody, is indicated for the treatment of moderate and severe persistent asthma with elevated IgE level,

TABLE 3 Assessing Asthma Control and Adjusting Therapy in Youths ≥12 Yr and Adults

		CLASSIFICATION OF ASTHMA CONTROL (≥12 YR)		
	COMPONENTS OF CONTROL	**Well Controlled**	**Not Well Controlled**	**Very Poorly Controlled**
Impairment	Symptoms	≤2 days/wk	>2 days/wk	Throughout the day
	Nighttime awakenings	≤2×/mo	1-3x/wk	≥4/wk
	Interference with normal activity	None	Some limitation	Extremely limited
	Short-acting $beta_2$-agonist use for symptom control (not prevention of EIB)	≤2 days/wk	>2 days/wk	Several times per day
	FEV_1 or peak flow	>80% predicted/personal best	60%-80% predicted/personal best	<60% predicted/personal best
	Validated questionnaires			
	ATAQ	0	1-2	3-4
	ACQ	≤0.75*	≥1.5	N/A
	ACT™	≥20	16-19	≤15
Risk	Exacerbations requiring oral systemic corticosteroids	0-1 per yr	≥2 per yr	
		Consider severity and interval since last exacerbation		
	Progressive loss of lung function	Evaluation requires long-term follow-up care		
	Treatment-related adverse effects	Medication side effects can vary in intensity from none to very troublesome and worrisome. The level of intensity does not correlate to specific levels of control but should be considered in the overall assessment of risk.		
Recommended Action for Treatment		Maintain current step. Regular follow-up every 1-6 mo to maintain control. Consider step down if well controlled for at least 3 mo.	Step up 1 step and reevaluate in 2-6 wk. For side effects, consider alternative treatment options.	Consider short course of oral systemic corticosteroids. Step up 1-2 steps. Reevaluate in 2 wk. For side effects, consider alternative treatment options.

The stepwise approach is meant to assist, not replace, the clinical decision-making required to meet individual patient needs.
The level of control is based on the most severe impairment or risk category. Assess impairment domain by patient's recall of previous 2-4 wk and by spirometry or peak flow measures.
Symptom assessment for longer periods should reflect a global assessment, such as inquiring whether the patient's asthma is better or worse since the last visit.
At present, there are inadequate data to correspond frequencies of exacerbations with different levels of asthma control. In general, more frequent and intense exacerbations (e.g., requiring urgent, unscheduled care, hospitalization, or ICU admission) indicate poorer disease control. For treatment purposes, patients who had ≥2 exacerbations requiring oral systemic corticosteroids in the past year may be considered the same as patients who have not-well-controlled asthma, even in the absence of impairment levels consistent with not-well-controlled asthma.
Validated questionnaires for the impairment domain (the questionnaires do not assess lung function or the risk domain):
- ATAQ = Asthma Therapy Assessment Questionnaire
- ACQ = Asthma Control Questionnaire (user package may be obtained at www.qoltech.co.uk or juniper@qoltech.co.uk)
- ACT = Asthma Control Test™
- Minimal Important Difference: 1.0 for the ATAQ; 0.5 for the ACQ; not determined for the ACT

Before step up in therapy:
- Review adherence to medication, inhaler technique, environmental control, and comorbid conditions
- If an alternative treatment option was used in a step, discontinue and use the preferred treatment for that step

EIB, Exercise-induced bronchospasm; *FEV_1*, forced expiratory volume in 1 second; *ICU*, intensive care unit.
The Asthma Control Test is a trademark of QualityMetric Incorporated.
*ACQ values of 0.76-1.4 are indeterminate regarding well-controlled asthma.
From National Asthma Education and Prevention Program: *Expert panel report 3: guidelines for diagnosis and management of asthma*, National Institutes of Health, National Heart, Lung, and Blood Institute, August 2007, NIH publication 08-4051.

which is refractory to other treatment noted earlier. It is administered subcutaneously every 2 or 4 wk. This medicine is expensive ($10,000 to $30,000/yr). Patients should be closely monitored in the first month because omalizumab can result in allergic reactions (anaphylaxis) in 1 to 2 patients/1000. The NIH guidelines recommend considering omalizumab only after consultation with an asthma specialist.

Dupilumab is a human monoclonal antibody to IL-4 and IL-13 recommended in patients with persistent exacerbations despite multimodal therapy. In patients with persistent, moderate to severe asthma and elevated eosinophil levels who use inhaled glucocorticoids and LABAs, therapy with dupilumab, as compared with placebo, is associated with fewer asthma exacerbations when LABAs and inhaled glucocorticoids are withdrawn, with improved lung function and reduced levels of Th2-associated inflammatory markers.

Mepolizumab (Nucala), an anti-interleukin-5 treatment, is approved by the FDA as an add-on for patients aged ≥12 yr with severe eosinophilic asthma that is uncontrolled on Step 4 treatment. Mepolizumab is a monoclonal antibody to IL-5 that has been shown to reduce exacerbations in patients with severe asthma who have blood eosinophil counts of 150/μL or greater. Mepolizumab is administered subcutaneously into the upper arm, thigh, or abdomen, 100 mg every 4 weeks. Hypersensitivity reactions have been reported with mepolizumab. In addition, herpes zoster infections have led to the recommendation of the administration of the varicella zoster vaccine to adults ages 50 or older 4 weeks prior to initiation of mepolizumab (unless they are at risk for disseminated zoster).

Reslizumab, another anti-IL-5 monoclonal antibody, has a similar indication for eosinophilic asthma and uses a higher eosinophil cutoff (400) based on a greater predictive value for sputum eosinophilia. Benralizumab, a monoclonal anti-IL5 receptor alpha antibody, is an additional FDA-approved add-on treatment to consider for patients 12 years or older with persistent severe eosinophilic asthma. It is administered as a subcutaneous injection every 4 weeks for the first 3 doses then every 8 weeks after that. Hypersensitivity reactions are more common than other anti-IL-5 antibodies and occur in about 3% of patients. Other adverse events include headache and pharyngitis.

Anti-IL-13: IL-13 promotes IgE production by B cells, generation of eosinophil chemoattractants, and contractility of airway smooth muscle cells and is therefore of interest as a potential target for asthma therapy. Preliminary clinical studies, however, have not documented a benefit to anti-IL-13 monoclonal antibodies such as lebrikizumab and tralokinumab.

TABLE 4 Stepwise Approach for Managing Asthma in Youths ≥12 Yr and Adults

Intermittent Asthma	**Persistent Asthma: Daily Medication** Consult with asthma specialist if step 4 care or higher is required. Consider consultation at step 3.					↑
Step 1	**Step 2**	**Step 3**	**Step 4**	**Step 5**	**Step 6**	Step up if needed (first, check adherence, environmental control, and comorbid conditions)
Preferred: SABA prn	*Preferred:* Low-dose ICS *Alternative:* Cromolyn, LTRA, nedocromil, or theophylline	*Preferred:* Low-dose ICS + LABA OR Medium-dose ICS *Alternative:* Low-dose ICS + either LTRA, theophylline, or zileuton	*Preferred:* Medium-dose ICS + LABA *Alternative:* Medium-dose ICS + either LTRA, theophylline, or zileuton	*Preferred:* High-dose ICS + LABA AND Consider omalizumab for patients who have allergies	*Preferred:* High-dose ICS + LABA + oral corticosteroid AND Consider omalizumab for patients who have allergies	**Assess control**
Each step: Patient education, environmental control, and management of comorbidities Steps 2-4: Consider subcutaneous allergen immunotherapy for patients who have allergic asthma						Step down if possible (and asthma is well controlled at least 3 months)
Quick-Relief Medication for All Patients • SABA as needed for symptoms. Intensity of treatment depends on severity of symptoms: up to 3 treatments at 20-minute intervals as needed. Short course of oral systemic corticosteroids may be needed. • Use of SABA >2 days a week for symptom relief (not prevention of EIB) generally indicates inadequate control and the need to step up treatment.						↓

The stepwise approach is meant to assist, not replace, the clinical decision-making required to meet individual patient needs.

If alternative treatment is used and response is inadequate, discontinue it and use the preferred treatment before stepping up.

Zileuton is a less desirable alternative due to limited studies as adjunctive therapy and the need to monitor liver function. Theophylline requires monitoring of serum concentration levels. In step 6, before oral systemic corticosteroids are introduced, a trial of high-dose ICS + LABA + either LTRA, theophylline, or zileuton may be considered, although this approach has not been studied in clinical trials.

Steps 1, 2, and 3 preferred therapies are based on Evidence A; step 3 alternative therapy is based on Evidence A for LTRA, Evidence B for theophylline, and Evidence D for zileuton. Step 5 preferred therapy is based on Evidence B. Step 6 preferred therapy is based on (EPR-2 1997) and Evidence B for omalizumab.

Immunotherapy for steps 2-4 is based on Evidence B for house-dust mites, animal danders, and pollens; evidence is weak or lacking for molds and cockroaches. Evidence is strongest for immunotherapy with single allergens. The role of allergy in asthma is greater in children than in adults.

Clinicians who administer immunotherapy or omalizumab should be prepared and equipped to identify and treat anaphylaxis that may occur.

This information is directly abstracted from the 2007 NAEPP *Expert Panel Report 3: Guidelines for the Diagnosis and Management of Asthma* and is not intended to promote or endorse any of the listed products.

To access the complete *Expert Panel Report 3: Guidelines for the Diagnosis and Management of Asthma,* go to www.nhlbi.nih.gov/guidelines/asthma/asthgdln.pdf.

EIB, Exercise-induced bronchospasm; *ICS,* inhaled corticosteroid; *LABA,* inhaled long-acting beta$_2$-agonist; *LTRA,* leukotriene receptor antagonist; *SABA,* inhaled short-acting beta$_2$-agonist.

From National Asthma Education and Prevention Program: *Expert panel report 3: guidelines for diagnosis and management of asthma,* National Institutes of Health, National Heart, Lung, and Blood Institute, August 2007, NIH publication 08-4051.

TABLE 5 Classifying Asthma Severity and Initiating Treatment in Children 5-11 Yr (Assessing severity and initiating treatment in children who are not currently taking long-term control medications)

Components of Severity		CLASSIFICATION OF ASTHMA SEVERITY (5-11 YR OF AGE)			
			PERSISTENT		
		Intermittent	Mild	Moderate	Severe
Impairment	Symptoms	≤2 days/wk	>2 days/wk but not daily	Daily	Throughout the day
	Nighttime awakenings	≤23/mo	3-4×/mo	>1×/wk but not nightly	Often 7×/wk
	Short-acting beta$_2$-agonist use for symptom control (not prevention of EIB)	≤2 days/wk	>2 days/wk but not daily	Daily	Several times per day
	Interference with normal activity	None	Minor limitation	Some limitation	Extremely limited
	Lung function	Normal FEV$_1$ between exacerbations			
		FEV$_1$>80% predicted	FEV$_1$ = >80% predicted	FEV$_1$ 60%-80% predicted	FEV$_1$ <60% predicted
		FEV$_1$/FVC>85%	FEV$_1$/FVC>80%	FEV$_1$/FVC 75%-80%	FEV$_1$/FVC <75%
Risk	Exacerbations requiring oral systemic corticosteroids	0-1 per yr	≥2 per yr		
		Consider severity and interval since last exacerbation. Frequency and severity may fluctuate over time for patients in any severity category.			
		Relative annual risk of exacerbations may be related to FEV$_1$.			
Recommended Step for Initiating Therapy		Step 1	Step 2	Step 3, medium-dose ICS option	Step 3, medium-dose ICS option, or Step 4
				and consider short course of oral systemic corticosteroids	
		In 2-6 wk, evaluate level of asthma control that is achieved and adjust therapy accordingly.			

The stepwise approach is meant to assist, not replace, the clinical decision-making required to meet individual patient needs.

Level of severity is determined by both impairment and risk. Assess impairment domain by patient's/caregiver's recall of previous 2-4 wk and spirometry. Assign severity to the most severe category in which any feature occurs.

At present, there are inadequate data to correspond frequencies of exacerbations with different levels of asthma severity. In general, more frequent and intense exacerbations (e.g., requiring urgent, unscheduled care, hospitalization, or ICU admission) indicate greater underlying disease severity. For treatment purposes, patients who had ≥2 exacerbations requiring oral systemic corticosteroids in the past year may be considered the same as patients who have persistent asthma, even in the absence of impairment levels consistent with persistent asthma.

EIB, Exercise-induced bronchospasm; *FEV$_1$*, forced expiratory volume in 1 second; *FVC*, forced vital capacity; *ICU*, intensive care unit.

From National Asthma Education and Prevention Program: *Expert panel report 3: guidelines for diagnosis and management of asthma*, National Institutes of Health, National Heart, Lung, and Blood Institute, August 2007, NIH publication 08-4051.

TABLE 6 Assessing Asthma Control and Adjusting Therapy in Children 5-11 Yr

Components of Control		CLASSIFICATION OF ASTHMA CONTROL (5-11 YR OF AGE)		
		Well Controlled	Not Well Controlled	Very Poorly Controlled
Impairment	Symptoms	≤2 days/wk but not more than once on each day	>2 days/wk or multiple times on ≤2 days/wk	Throughout the day
	Nighttime awakenings	≤1×/mo	≥2×/mo	≥2×/wk
	Interference with normal activity	None	Some limitation	Extremely limited
	Short-acting beta$_2$-agonist use for symptom control (not prevention of EIB)	≤2 days/wk	>2 days/wk	Several times per day
	Lung function			
	FEV$_1$ or peak flow	>80% predicted/personal best	60%-80% predicted/personal best	<60% predicted/personal best
	FEV$_1$/FVC	>80% predicted	75%-80%	<75% predicted
Risk	Exacerbations requiring oral systemic corticosteroids	0-1 per yr	≥2 per yr	
		Consider severity and interval since last exacerbation		
	Reduction in lung growth	Evaluation requires long-term follow-up care		
	Treatment-related adverse effects	Medication side effects can vary in intensity from none to very troublesome and worrisome. The level of intensity does not correlate to specific levels of control but should be considered in the overall assessment of risk.		
Recommended Action for Treatment		Maintain current step. Regular follow-up every 1-6 mo. Consider step down if well controlled for at least 3 mo.	Step up 1 step and reevaluate in 2-6 wk. For side effects, consider alternative treatment options.	Consider short course of oral systemic corticosteroids. Step up 1-2 steps. Reevaluate in 2 wk. For side effects, consider alternative treatment options.

The stepwise approach is meant to assist, not replace, the clinical decision-making required to meet individual patient needs.

The level of control is based on the most severe impairment or risk category. Assess impairment domain by patient's/caregiver's recall of previous 2-4 wk and by spirometry or peak flow measures. Symptom assessment for longer periods should reflect a global assessment such as inquiring whether the patient's asthma is better or worse since the last visit.

At present, there are inadequate data to correspond frequencies of exacerbations with different levels of asthma control. In general, more frequent and intense exacerbations (e.g., requiring urgent, unscheduled care, hospitalization, or ICU admission) indicate poorer disease control. For treatment purposes, patients who had ≥2 exacerbations requiring oral systemic corticosteroids in the past year may be considered the same as patients who have persistent asthma, even in the absence of impairment levels consistent with persistent asthma.

Before step up in therapy:

- Review adherence to medications, inhaler technique, environmental control, and comorbid conditions.
- If an alternative treatment option was used in a step, discontinue it and use preferred treatment for that step.

EIB, Exercise-induced bronchospasm; *FEV$_1$*, forced expiratory volume in 1 second; *FVC*, forced vital capacity; *ICU*, intensive care unit.

From National Asthma Education and Prevention Program: *Expert panel report 3: guidelines for diagnosis and management of asthma*, National Institutes of Health, National Heart, Lung, and Blood Institute, August 2007, NIH publication 08-4051.

TABLE 7 Stepwise Approach for Managing Asthma in Children 5-11 Yr

Intermittent Asthma	**Persistent Asthma: Daily Medication** Consult with asthma specialist if step 4 care or higher is required. Consider consultation at step 3.					↑
Step 1 *Preferred:* SABA prn	**Step 2** *Preferred:* Low-dose ICS *Alternative:* Cromolyn, LTRA, nedocromil, or theophylline	**Step 3** *Preferred:* Low-dose ICS + either LABA, LTRA, or theophylline OR Medium-dose ICS	**Step 4** *Preferred:* Medium-dose ICS + LABA *Alternative:* Medium-dose ICS + either LTRA or theophylline	**Step 5** *Preferred:* High-dose ICS + LABA *Alternative:* High-dose ICS + either LTRA or theophylline	**Step 6** *Preferred:* High-dose ICS + LABA + oral corticosteroid *Alternative:* High-dose ICS + either LTRA or theophylline + oral systemic corticosteroid	Step up if needed (first, check adherence, inhaler technique, environmental control, and comorbid conditions) **Assess control** Step down if possible (and asthma is well controlled at least 3 months)
Each step: Patient education, environmental control, and management of comorbidities Steps 2-4: Consider subcutaneous allergen immunotherapy for patients who have allergic asthma						
Quick-Relief Medication for All Patients • SABA as needed for symptoms. Intensity of treatment depends on severity of symptoms: up to 3 treatments at 20-minute intervals as needed. Short course of oral systemic corticosteroids may be needed. • Caution: Increasing use of SABA or use >2 days a week for symptom relief (not prevention of EIB) generally indicates inadequate control and the need to step up treatment.						↓

The stepwise approach is meant to assist, not replace, the clinical decision-making required to meet individual patient needs.
If alternative treatment is used and response is inadequate, discontinue it and use the preferred treatment before stepping up.
Theophylline is a less desirable alternative due to the need to monitor serum concentration levels.
Step 1 and step 2 medications are based on Evidence A. Step 3 ICS 1 adjunctive therapy and ICS are based on Evidence B for efficacy of each treatment and extrapolation from comparator trials in older children and adults—comparator trials are not available for this age group; steps 4-6 are based on expert opinion and extrapolation from studies in older children and adults. Immunotherapy for steps 2-4 is based on Evidence B for house-dust mites, animal danders, and pollens; evidence is weak or lacking for molds and cockroaches. Evidence is strongest for immunotherapy with single allergens. The role of allergy in asthma is greater in children than in adults. Clinicians who administer immunotherapy should be prepared and equipped to identify and treat anaphylaxis that may occur.
This information is directly abstracted from the 2007 NAEPP *Expert Panel Report 3: Guidelines for the Diagnosis and Management of Asthma* and is not intended to promote or endorse any of the listed products.
EIB, Exercise-induced bronchoconstriction; *ICS*, inhaled corticosteroid; *LABA*, inhaled long-acting $beta_2$-agonist; *LTRA*, leukotriene receptor antagonist; *SABA*, inhaled short-acting $beta_2$-agonist.
From National Asthma Education and Prevention Program: *Expert panel report 3: guidelines for diagnosis and management of asthma*, National Institutes of Health, National Heart, Lung, and Blood Institute, August 2007, NIH publication 08-4051.

BRONCHIAL THERMOPLASTY

Selected patients with severe persistent asthma who have failed medical treatment may benefit from bronchial thermoplasty. This requires the insertion of a catheter via bronchoscopy and use of radiofrequency heat to reduce bronchial smooth muscle. Long-term follow-up data showed persistent reduction in asthma exacerbation and fewer ED visits over a period of 5 years. FDA labeling is for "severe persistent asthma inadequately controlled on ICS + LABA."

OTHER MEDICATIONS

Tiotropium (Spiriva) has been used for decades as first-line treatment for COPD. This LAMA is now approved for a second indication for the treatment of asthma and is included in the most recent (2018) Global Initiative for Asthma (GINA) guidelines as a possible add-on at step 4. A systematic review including over 7000 patients demonstrated the use of LAMA compared with placebo as an add-on to inhaled corticosteroids was associated with lower risk of exacerbation. Adding LAMA to a dual LABA-ICS regimen was not shown to reduce exacerbation rates but can improve lung function.

Azithromycin: The AZISAST Trial randomized 109 patients on high-dose ICS/LABA (step 4 or 5 per GINA guidelines) to maintenance therapy with azithromycin or placebo. Overall, there was no benefit seen with azithromycin therapy with regard to any of the outcomes tested. However, subgroup analysis showed that patients with noneosinophilic asthma had fewer exacerbations. More data are needed, but this result suggests azithromycin may be an effective option for the neutrophilic/Th-1 phenotype (COPD is also neutrophilic).

Immunosuppressants such as methotrexate can decrease long-term steroid requirements; however, they have significant side effects, and there is no evidence of persistent therapeutic effect after discontinuing them.

TREATMENT OF SEVERE ASTHMA (ETS/ETA GUIDELINES)

- The American Thoracic Society (ATS) classification of "severe asthma" refers to patients who require high-dose inhaled or near-continuous oral glucocorticoid treatment to maintain asthma control.
- In patients who do not achieve adequate control with the combination of a high-dose inhaled glucocorticoid and LABA, an additional controller medication such as an antileukotriene agent is recommended (tiotropium or theophylline).
- For patients with atopic severe asthma who have a serum IgE level of 30 to 700 IU/ml and documented sensitivity to a perennial allergen, recommend adding omalizumab.
- For patients with severe asthma, frequent exacerbations, and an eosinophilic phenotype despite guideline-based therapy, consider add-on therapy with one of the anti-interleukin (IL)-5 antibodies, mepolizumab, reslizumab, or benralizumab.

TABLE 8 Classifying Asthma Severity and Initiating Treatment in Children 0-4 Yr (Assessing severity and initiating treatment in children who are not currently taking long-term control medications)

Components of Severity		CLASSIFICATION OF ASTHMA SEVERITY (0-4 YR OF AGE)			
		Intermittent	PERSISTENT: Mild	Moderate	Severe
Impairment	Symptoms	≤2 days/wk	>2 days/wk but not daily	Daily	Throughout the day
	Nighttime awakenings	0	1-2×/mo	3-4×/mo	>1×/wk
	Short-acting beta$_2$-agonist use for symptom control (not prevention of EIB)	≤2 days/wk	>2 days/wk but not daily	Daily	Several times per day
	Interference with normal activity	None	Minor limitation	Some limitation	Extremely limited
Risk	Exacerbations requiring oral systemic corticosteroids	0-1 per yr	≥2 exacerbations in 6 mo requiring oral systemic corticosteroids, or ≥4 wheezing episodes/1 yr lasting >1 day AND risk factors for persistent asthma.		
		Consider severity and interval since last exacerbation. Frequency and severity may fluctuate over time. Exacerbations of any severity may occur in patients in any severity category.			
Recommended Step for Initiating Therapy		Step 1	Step 2	Step 3 and consider short course of oral systemic corticosteroids	
		In 2-6 wk, depending on severity, evaluate level of asthma control that is achieved. If no clear benefit is observed in 4-6 wk, consider adjusting therapy or alternative diagnoses.			

The stepwise approach is meant to assist, not replace, the clinical decision-making required to meet individual patient needs.
Level of severity is determined by assessment of both impairment and risk. Assess impairment domain by patient's/caregiver's recall of previous 2-4 wk. Symptom assessment for longer periods should reflect a global assessment such as inquiring whether the patient's asthma is better or worse since the last visit. Assign severity to the most severe category in which any feature occurs.
At present, there are inadequate data to correspond frequencies of exacerbations with different levels of asthma severity. For treatment purposes, patients who had ≥2 exacerbations requiring oral systemic corticosteroids in the past six months, or ≥4 wheezing episodes in the past year, and who have risk factors for persistent asthma may be considered the same as patients who have persistent asthma, even in the absence of impairment levels consistent with persistent asthma.
To access the complete *Expert Panel Report 3: Guidelines for the Diagnosis and Management of Asthma*, go to www.nhlbi.nih.gov/guidelines/asthma/asthgdln.pdf.
EIB, Exercise-induced bronchospasm.
From National Asthma Education and Prevention Program: *Expert panel report 3: guidelines for diagnosis and management of asthma,* National Institutes of Health, National Heart, Lung, and Blood Institute, August 2007, NIH publication 08-4051.

TABLE 9 Assessing Asthma Control and Adjusting Therapy in Children 0-4 Yr of Age

Components of Control		CLASSIFICATION OF ASTHMA CONTROL (0-4 YR OF AGE): Well Controlled	Not Well Controlled	Very Poorly Controlled
Impairment	Symptoms	≤2 days/wk	>2 days/wk	Throughout the day
	Nighttime awakenings	≤13/mo	>1×/mo	>1×/wk
	Interference with normal activity	None	Some limitation	Extremely limited
	Short-acting beta$_2$-agonist use for symptom control (not prevention of EIB)	≤2 days/wk	>2 days/wk	Several times per day
Risk	Exacerbations requiring oral systemic corticosteroids	0-1 per yr	2-3 per yr	>3 per yr
	Treatment-related adverse effects	Medication side effects can vary in intensity from none to very troublesome and worrisome. The level of intensity does not correlate to specific levels of control but should be considered in the overall assessment of risk.		
Recommended Action for Treatment		Maintain current step. Regular follow-up every 1-6 mo. Consider step down if well controlled for at least 3 mo.	Step up 1 step. Reevaluate in 2-6 wk. If no clear benefit in 4-6 wk, consider alternative diagnoses or adjusting therapy. For side effects, consider alternative treatment options.	Consider short course of oral systemic corticosteroids. Step up 1-2 steps. Reevaluate in 2 wk. If no clear benefit in 4-6 wk, consider alternative diagnoses or adjusting therapy. For side effects, consider alternative treatment options.

The stepwise approach is meant to assist, not replace, the clinical decision-making required to meet individual patient needs.
The level of control is based on the most severe impairment or risk category. Assess impairment domain by caregiver's recall of previous 2-4 wk. Symptom assessment for longer periods should reflect a global assessment such as inquiring whether the patient's asthma is better or worse since the last visit.
At present, there are inadequate data to correspond frequencies of exacerbations with different levels of asthma control. In general, more frequent and intense exacerbations (e.g., requiring urgent, unscheduled care, hospitalization, or ICU admission) indicate poorer disease control. For treatment purposes, patients who had ≥2 exacerbations requiring oral systemic corticosteroids in the past year may be considered the same as patients who have not-well-controlled asthma, even in the absence of impairment levels consistent with not-well-controlled asthma.
Before step up in therapy:
- Review adherence to medications, inhaler technique, and environmental control.
- If an alternative treatment option was used in a step, discontinue it and use preferred treatment for that step.

EIB, Exercise-induced bronchospasm; *ICU,* intensive care unit.
From National Asthma Education and Prevention Program: *Expert panel report 3: guidelines for diagnosis and management of asthma,* National Institutes of Health, National Heart, Lung, and Blood Institute, August 2007, NIH publication 08-4051.

TABLE 10 Stepwise Approach for Managing Asthma in Children 0-4 Yr

Intermittent Asthma	**Persistent Asthma: Daily Medication** Consult with asthma specialist if step 3 care or higher is required. Consider consultation at step 2.					
Step 1 *Preferred:* SABA prn	**Step 2** *Preferred:* Low-dose ICS *Alternative:* Cromolyn or montelukast	**Step 3** *Preferred:* Medium-dose ICS	**Step 4** *Preferred:* Medium-dose ICS + either LABA or montelukast	**Step 5** *Preferred:* High-dose ICS + either LABA or montelukast	**Step 6** *Preferred:* High-dose ICS + either LABA or montelukast Oral systemic corticosteroid	↑ Step up if needed (first, check adherence, inhaler technique, and environmental control) **Assess control** Step down if possible (and asthma is well controlled at least 3 months) ↓
Patient Education and Environmental Control at Each Step						
Quick-Relief Medication for All Patients • SABA as needed for symptoms. Intensity of treatment depends on severity of symptoms. • With viral respiratory infection: SABA q 4-6 hours up to 24 hours (longer with physician consult). Consider short course of oral systemic corticosteroids if exacerbation is severe or patient has history of previous severe exacerbations. • Caution: Frequent use of SABA may indicate the need to step up treatment. See text for recommendations on initiating daily long-term-control therapy.						

The stepwise approach is meant to assist, not replace, the clinical decision-making required to meet individual patient needs. If alternative treatment is used and response is inadequate, discontinue it and use the preferred treatment before stepping up.

If clear benefit is not observed within 4-6 wk and patient/family medication technique and adherence are satisfactory, consider adjusting therapy or alternative diagnosis.

Studies on children 0-4 yr are limited. Step 2 preferred therapy is based on Evidence A. All other recommendations are based on expert opinion and extrapolation from studies in other children.

This information is directly abstracted from the 2007 NAEPP *Expert Panel Report 3: Guidelines for the Diagnosis and Management of Asthma* and is not intended to promote or endorse any of the listed products.

ICS, Inhaled corticosteroid; *LABA*, inhaled long-acting beta$_2$-agonist; *SABA*, inhaled short-acting beta$_2$-agonist.

From National Asthma Education and Prevention Program: *Expert panel report 3: guidelines for diagnosis and management of asthma*, National Institutes of Health, National Heart, Lung, and Blood Institute, August 2007, NIH publication 08-4051.

- Bronchial thermoplasty is approved for use in selected adults with severe asthma that is not well controlled with inhaled glucocorticoids and LABAs.
- Potential alternative and experimental therapies include immunomodulatory therapy and macrolide antibiotics.[a]
- In the future, treatments tailored to asthma phenotypes may improve asthma outcomes.

Treatment of status asthmaticus is as follows:

- Oxygen generally started at 2 to 4 L/min by nasal cannula or Venti-Mask at 40% Fio_2; further adjustments are made according to oxygen saturations.
- Bronchodilators: Initiate treatment with high-dose SABA plus ipratropium bromide administered by means of a nebulizer every 20 min. Use of a metered-dose inhaler with valved holding chamber may be acceptable for patients with mild-to-moderate exacerbations.
- Albuterol nebulizer solution (0.63 mg/3 ml, 1.25 mg/3 ml, 2.5 mg/3 ml, or 5.0 mg/ml): 2.5 to 5 mg every 20 min over the first hr, then 2.5-10 mg every 1-4 hr as needed or 10-15 mg/hr continuously. Other useful medications are levalbuterol nebulizer solution (0.31 mg/3 ml, 0.63 mg/3 ml, 1.25 mg/3 ml) and ipratropium nebulizer solution (0.25/ml [0.025%]).
- Corticosteroids:
  1. Early administration is advised, particularly in patients using steroids at home.
  2. Patients may be started on systemic corticosteroids; methylprednisolone, prednisone, or prednisolone may be used. Dose range is from 40-80 mg/day in one or two divided doses, generally given until peak expiratory flow reaches 70% of predicted value.
  3. Generally for corticosteroid courses <1 week there is no need to taper the dose.
- IV hydration: Judicious use is necessary to avoid congestive heart failure in elderly patients. Aggressive IV hydration is not recommended.
- IV antibiotics are indicated when there is suspicion of bacterial infection (e.g., infiltrate on chest radiograph, fever, or leukocytosis).
- Intubation and mechanical ventilation are indicated when previous measures fail to produce significant improvement. Fig. 3 illustrates an approach to acute life-threatening asthma. Table 11 summarizes treatment of life-threatening asthma.
- Discharge home from the emergency department is appropriate if the FEV_1 or PEF after treatment is 70% or greater of the personal best or predicted value and if there is sustained improvement in lung function and symptoms for at least 1 hr.

[a] Recent trials (AMAZES) in patients who have symptomatic asthma despite inhaled maintenance therapy have shown that azithromycin 500 mg 3 times/week reduced exacerbations and improved quality of life.

REFERRAL

Box 1 describes indications for referral to an asthma specialist.

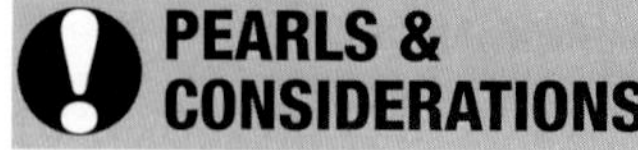

PEARLS & CONSIDERATIONS

COMMENTS

- The differentiation of asthma from COPD can be challenging. A history of atopy and intermittent, reactive symptoms points toward a diagnosis of asthma, whereas smoking and advanced age are more indicative of COPD. Spirometry is useful in distinguishing asthma from COPD.
- In all asthma patients it is important to treat or prevent comorbid conditions (e.g., rhinosinusitis, vocal cord dysfunction, gastroesophageal reflux disease). However, despite the presumed association between asthma and GERD, trials of PPIs in patients with poorly controlled asthma did not reveal any beneficial effects.

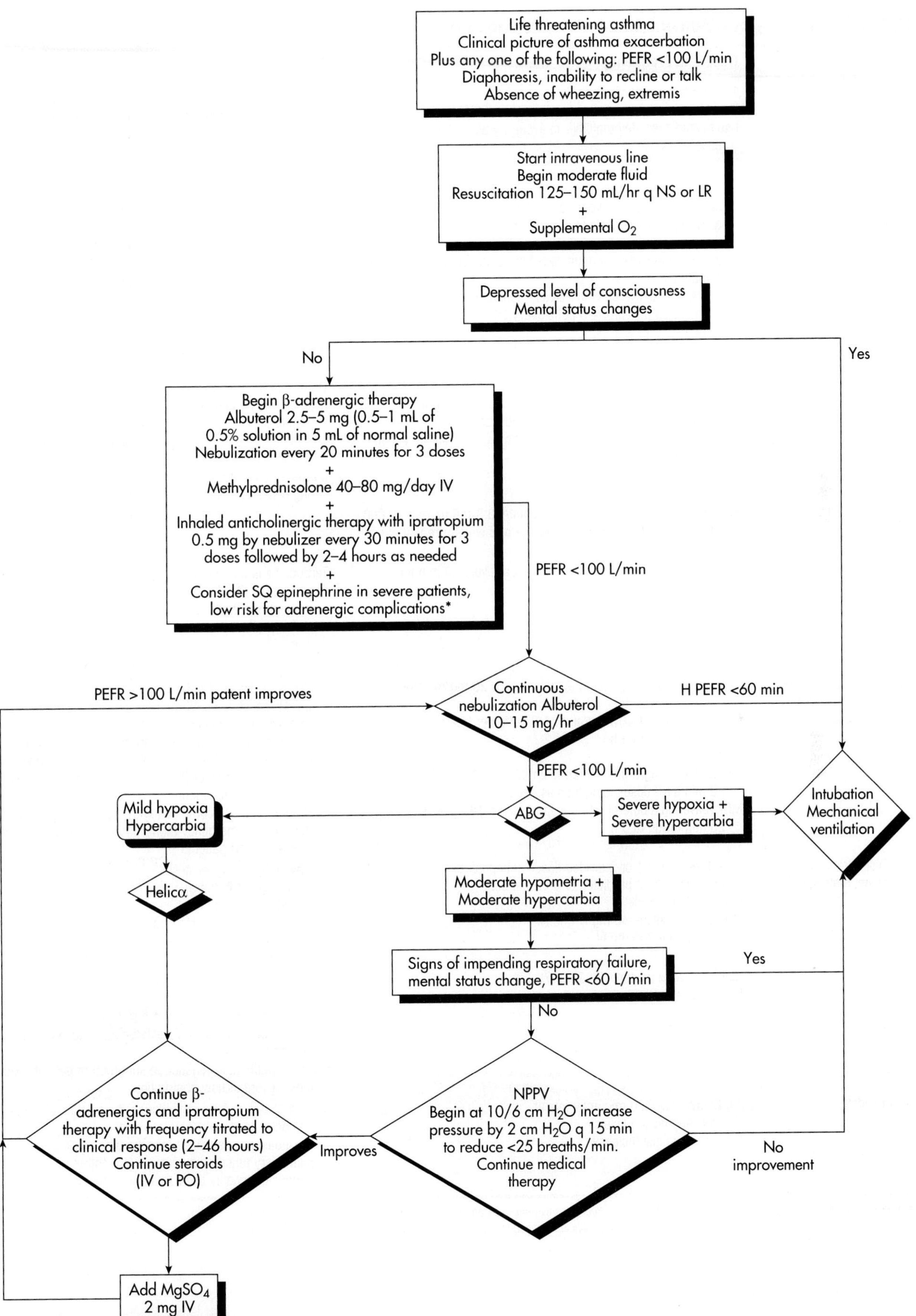

Life threatening asthma
Clinical picture of asthma exacerbation
Plus any one of the following: PEFR <100 L/min
Diaphoresis, inability to recline or talk
Absence of wheezing, extremis
Start intravenous line
Begin moderate fluid
Resuscitation 125–150 mL/hr q NS or LR
+
Supplemental O_2
Depressed level of consciousness
Mental status changes
No
Yes
Begin β-adrenergic therapy
Albuterol 2.5–5 mg (0.5–1 mL of 0.5% solution in 5 mL of normal saline)
Nebulization every 20 minutes for 3 doses
+
Methylprednisolone 40–80 mg/day IV
+
Inhaled anticholinergic therapy with ipratropium 0.5 mg by nebulizer every 30 minutes for 3 doses followed by 2–4 hours as needed
+
Consider SQ epinephrine in severe patients, low risk for adrenergic complications*
PEFR <100 L/min
PEFR >100 L/min patent improves
Continuous nebulization Albuterol 10–15 mg/hr
H PEFR <60 min
PEFR <100 L/min
Mild hypoxia
Hypercarbia
ABG
Severe hypoxia +
Severe hypercarbia
Intubation
Mechanical
ventilation
Helicα
Moderate hypometria +
Moderate hypercarbia
Signs of impending respiratory failure, mental status change, PEFR <60 L/min
Yes
No
Continue β-adrenergics and ipratropium therapy with frequency titrated to clinical response (2–46 hours)
Continue steroids
(IV or PO)
Improves
NPPV
Begin at 10/6 cm H_2O increase pressure by 2 cm H_2O q 15 min to reduce <25 breaths/min.
Continue medical therapy
No
improvement
Add $MgSO_4$
2 mg IV

FIG. 3 Approach to acute life-threatening asthma. *Check for hypokalemia and treat. *ABG*, arterial blood gas; *LR*, lactated Ringer's solution; *NPPV*, noninvasive positive-pressure ventilation; *NS*, normal saline; *PEFR*, peak expiratory flow rate. (From Parrillo JE, Dellinger RP: *Critical care medicine, principles of diagnosis and management in the adult*, ed 4, Philadelphia, 2014, Elsevier.)

TABLE 11 Summary of Treatment for Life-Threatening Asthma

Treatment	Dose and Frequency	Comments
Oxygen	1-3 L/min by nasal cannula Goal is to maintain oxygen saturation (Spo_2) >92% Use heated cascade humidifier to avoid dry air–induced bronchoconstriction	Transient drop in O_2 tension with beta-adrenergic therapy Avoid hyperoxia (may be associated with hypercarbia)
Bronchodilators		
Beta$_2$-selective agonists: Albuterol or salbutamol, levalbuterol	*Albuterol*: 2.5-5 mg (0.5-1 ml of 0.5% solution in 5 ml of normal saline) by nebulizer every 20 min for 3 doses total (for optimal delivery, dilute aerosols to a minimum of 3 ml at gas flow of 6-8 L/min), followed by 2.5-10 mg q1-4h as needed, or 10-15 mg/h continuously; titration based on response and severity of symptoms *Albuterol MDI*, delivered with a spacer (each spacer dose takes 1-2 min; 90 μg/puff), 4-8 puffs every 20 min for 4 h, then q4h as needed *Albuterol*: 5-7.5 mg by jet nebulizer (each treatment takes 15-20 min) *Levalbuterol* (0.63 mg/3 ml and 1.25 mg/3 ml nebulizer): 1.25-2.5 mg every 20 min for 3 doses total, then 1.25-5 mg q1-4h as needed, or 5-7.5 mg/h continuous nebulization *Levalbuterol MDI* (45 μg/puff): 4-8 puffs every 20 min for 4 h, followed by q1-4h as needed	Beta$_2$-selective agonists are the cornerstone of therapy Continuous nebulization used for a majority of severely ill patients In study of continuous vs. intermittent therapy in severe exacerbations (excluding life-threatening asthma), no difference noted in pulmonary function improvement or need for hospitalization Lower frequency of side effects with continuous treatment Watch for hypokalemia, tremors, tachycardia, and lactic acidosis Oral or parenteral route: Loss of beta$_2$-selectivity MDI: 4 puffs of albuterol (0.36 mg) = 2.5 mg of albuterol nebulization Levalbuterol 0.63 mg = racemic albuterol 1.25 mg for efficacy and side effects *Intubated patients*: Nebulizers are less efficient in delivering doses to lower airways (6-10%) than MDIs (11%)
Epinephrine	*Subcutaneous epinephrine* dose for adults: 0.3-0.5 ml of a 1:1000 dilution (1 mg/ml), depending on age and weight; repeat every 20 min for 3 doses total	
Terbutaline	*Subcutaneous terbutaline*, 0.25 mg; repeat every 20 min for 3 doses total	Terbutaline is the parenteral agent of choice in pregnancy For refractory life-threatening asthma: Intravenous epinephrine (high risk for cardiac events, infarction, and arrhythmias) or racemic epinephrine may be considered
Anticholinergics		
Ipratropium (for acute severe asthma warranting visit to emergency department)	*Ipratropium bromide*: 0.5 mg by nebulizer (0.25 mg/ml) every 20 min for 3 doses, then q2-4h as needed *Ipratropium MDI* (0.018 mg/puff): 4-8 puffs per treatment every 20 min for up to 3 h *Combinations*: Albuterol (2.5 mg/3 ml) + ipratropium (0.5 mg/3 ml): 3 ml every 20 min for 3 doses total, then as needed MDI delivering albuterol 90 μg + ipratropium 18 μg: 8 puffs every 20 min for up to 3 h	Ipratropium: Onset of action is slow (20 min), peak effectiveness at 60-90 min, no systemic side effects, improved lung function and reduced recovery time Use a handheld mouthpiece nebulizer (contamination of the ocular area with precipitation of narrow-angle glaucoma may occur if facemask is used for delivery of anticholinergic agent) Ipratropium may be combined with nebulized albuterol dose in the emergency room; no proven benefit shown in hospitalized patients
Corticosteroids: Prednisone, prednisolone, methylprednisolone	40-80 mg/day in 1 or 2 divided doses until peak expiratory flow reaches 70% of predicted or personal best FEV_1 or PEFR <50%[16] Methylprednisolone 40 mg IV q6h OR Hydrocortisone 200 mg IV	No advantage of higher doses No advantage of IV therapy over oral if absorption and gut transit are not impaired Total steroid course: 3-10 days, <1 week; no need to taper steroids Inhaled steroids can be started at any time
Heliox	Helium-oxygen mixture (80-20 or 70-30) Routine use cannot be recommended at this time	Improves O_2 and aerosolized medication delivery to distal lung Decreases flow turbulence and resistance Lower gas density facilitates exhalation, reduces air trapping and intrinsic PEEP Improves pulmonary function in subgroup of patients with most severe airflow obstruction
Magnesium sulfate	2 g IV given over 20 min; may repeat Monitor magnesium levels Avoid in renal insufficiency	Bronchodilatation from inhibition of the calcium channel and decreased acetylcholine release IV and inhaled or nebulized magnesium sulfate improves pulmonary function in acute severe asthma IV magnesium widely used as adjunct therapy

FEV_1, forced expiratory flow in 1 second; *MDI*, metered-dose inhaler; *PEEP*, positive end-expiratory pressure; *PEFR*, peak expiratory flow rate.
From Parrillo JE, Dellinger RP: *Critical care medicine, principles of diagnosis and management in the adult*, ed 4, Philadelphia, 2014, Elsevier.

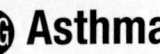

- Inhaled low-dose corticosteroids are the single most effective therapy for adult patients with asthma who require more than an occasional use of SABAs to control their asthma.
- Stepping down inhaled corticosteroids after asthma is well controlled now has level A evidence.
- Leukotriene modifiers/receptor agonists represent a reasonable alternative in adults unable or unwilling to use corticosteroids; however, these agents are less effective than monotherapy with inhaled corticosteroids.
- Use of LABAs alone without use of a long-term asthma medication, such as an inhaled corticosteroid, is contraindicated. LABAs should also not be used in patients whose asthma is adequately controlled on low- or medium-dose inhaled corticosteroids. Continued use of LABAs may cause down-regulation of the beta-2 receptor with loss of the bronchoprotective effect from rescue therapy with a SABA.
- Patients who remain symptomatic despite inhaled corticosteroids benefit from the addition of LABAs. Trials in patients with poorly controlled asthma despite the use of inhaled glucocorticoids and LABAs have shown that the addition of tiotropium, a long-acting anticholinergic bronchodilator approved for treatment of COPD, increased the time to the first severe exacerbation and provided modest sustained bronchodilation.
- Therapy with systemic corticosteroids accelerates the resolution of acute asthma and reduces the risk of relapse. There is no evidence that doses >50-100 mg prednisone equivalent are beneficial.
- In patients with allergies and elevated serum immunoglobulin (Ig) E levels, use of anti-IgE therapy is beneficial.
- Bronchial thermoplasty should be considered in selective patients with severe persistent asthma with recurrent exacerbations or ED visits. Biologic modifiers of the Th2 immune pathways (neutralizing monoclonal antibodies, receptor antagonists, soluble receptors) are potential options for the development of new treatments of severe asthma. Adjunct therapies for bronchospasm are summarized in Table 12.
- The response to treatment for asthma is characterized by wide individual variability. A functional glucocorticoid-induced transcript 1 gene (*GLCCI1*) variant is associated with substantial decrements in the response to inhaled glucocorticoids in patients with asthma. Another potential cause of the variability in response to treatment is heterogeneity in the role of interleukin-13 expression in the clinical asthma phenotype. Patients with asthma who have a certain biochemical signature are more likely to respond to an anti–interleukin-13 monoclonal antibody than those without such a signature. Identification of genetic variants can eventually lead to personalized asthma treatment. Failure of pharmacologic treatment is often due to uncontrolled comorbid conditions (tobacco, allergic rhinitis, pollutants), poor inhaler technique, or lack of adherence to prescribed medication.

BOX 1 Possible Indications for Referral to an Asthma Specialist

- Severe, acute asthma that has caused loss of consciousness, hypoxia, respiratory failure, convulsions, or near death
- Poorly controlled asthma as indicated by admission to a hospital, frequent need for emergency care, need for oral corticosteroids, absence from school or work, disruption of sleep, interference with quality of life
- Severe, persistent asthma requiring step 4 care (consider for patients who require step 3 care)
- Patient <3 yr who requires step 3 or 4 care (consider for patient <3 yr who requires step 2 care)
- Requirement for continuous oral corticosteroids or high-dose inhaled corticosteroids or more than two short courses of oral corticosteroids within 1 yr
- Need for additional diagnostic testing such as allergy skin testing, rhinoscopy, provocative challenge, complete pulmonary function testing, bronchoscopy
- Consideration for immunotherapy
- Need for additional education regarding asthma, complications of asthma and treatment of asthma, problems with adherence to management recommendations, or allergen avoidance
- Uncertainty of diagnosis
- Complications of asthma, including sinusitis, nasal polyposis, aspergillosis, severe rhinitis, vocal cord dysfunction, gastroesophageal reflux

Modified from National Asthma Education and Prevention Program, National Heart, Lung, and Blood Institute: *Expert Panel Report 2: guidelines for the diagnosis and management of asthma,* Bethesda, MD, 1997, National Institutes of Health, NIH publication No 97-4051.

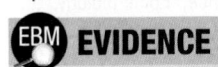

EVIDENCE

Available at ExpertConsult.com

SUGGESTED READINGS

Available at ExpertConsult.com

RELATED CONTENT

Asthma (Patient Information)

Asthma-COPD Overlap Syndrome (Related Key Topic)

AUTHORS: **KRISTIN DALPHON, P.A.,** and **SAMAAN RAFEQ, M.D.**

TABLE 12 Adjunct Therapies for Bronchospasm

Nontraditional Therapy for Severe Bronchospasm	Comments
Intravenous $beta_2$-agonists	No data show any benefit in adding IV agent to nebulization Avoid IV isoproterenol owing to danger of myocardial toxicity
Oral or IV leukotriene receptor antagonists (LTRAs): Montelukast 10 mg oral daily, zafirlukast	Rapid bronchodilation in impending respiratory failure Improves pulmonary function within 10 min Oral LTRAs can be added as an adjunct in severe asthma
Noninvasive positive-pressure ventilation (NPPV)	NPPV reduces the need for endotracheal intubation in severe asthma exacerbation
Inhaled nitric oxide (NO) (adding 15 ppm to the inspiratory circuit)	Rapid improvement in ventilated patients with asthma refractory to medical treatment
Omalizumab (anti-IgE antibody)	Role in acute asthma is unstudied Improves asthma control in allergic asthmatics
General anesthetic agents: Isoflurane or halothane anesthesia IV thiopental, IV propofol, IV ketamine	Propofol relaxes the smooth muscles in arteries and veins and has bronchodilator effect
Plasma exchange (during pregnancy)	Case reports of adjunct therapies; used as salvage therapy for life-threatening asthma
Pumpless extracorporeal carbon dioxide removal	
Extracorporeal life support (ECLS)	
Glucagon	Rapid smooth muscle relaxant, short half-life; small study report
Nebulized DNase (dornase 2.5 mg via tracheal tube)	Case report of use in pregnant patient with rapid improvement
Bronchial lavage	Anecdotal reports: Exacerbates auto-PEEP, decreases oxygenation

IgE, immunoglobulin E; *IV,* intravenous; *PEEP,* positive end-expiratory pressure.
From Parrillo JE, Dellinger RP: *Critical care medicine, principles of diagnosis and management in the adult,* ed 4, Philadelphia, 2014, Elsevier.

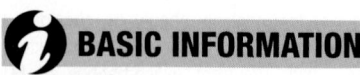

BASIC INFORMATION

DEFINITION

Astrocytoma is a type of neuroepithelial tumor that arises from astrocytes, which are glial precursor cells. The distinction of different grades of astrocytoma provides important clinical prognostic information. According to the World Health Organization (WHO) classification astrocytoma is classified as below based on the histopathology:

- Grade I: Pilocytic astrocytoma
- Grade II: Diffuse astrocytoma
- Grade III: Anaplastic astrocytoma
- Grade IV: Glioblastoma
- Grades III and IV are considered high-grade astrocytomas (HGAs) or malignant.

SYNONYM

Astroglial neoplasms

ICD-10CM CODE
C71.9 Malignant neoplasm of brain, unspecified

EPIDEMIOLOGY & DEMOGRAPHICS

According to Surveillance, Epidemiology, and End Results (SEER) registry, the incidence of primary CNS tumor is 6.4 cases per 100,000 persons per yr with age-adjusted death rate of 4.4 per 100,000. According to the Central Brain Tumor Registry of the United States (CBTRUS) astrocytomas constitute about 10% of the central nervous system neoplasms.

ETIOLOGY

- No agent has been definitely implicated in the causation of CNS tumors, and risk factors can be identified only in minority of patients. Farmers and petrochemical workers have been shown to have a higher incidence of primary brain tumors. Exposure to ionizing radiation is a known risk factor for a small percentage of astrocytomas.
- Different hereditary syndromes are associated with increased risk and high frequency of astrocytoma.
  1. Neurofibromatosis type 1 is associated with increased frequency of astrocytoma.
  2. Li-Fraumeni syndrome (germ line mutation in one of p53 allele) is associated with increased frequency of malignant gliomas.

GENE AND CHROMOSOMAL ALTERATIONS IN ASTROCYTOMA:

- Alteration in p53, a tumor suppressor encoded by the *TP53* gene on chromosome 17p, plays a key role in the development of at least one third of all grades of astrocytoma. In addition, in high-grade astrocytomas, p53 function may be deregulated by alteration of other genes, including amplification of MDM2 or MDM4 and 9p deletions that result in loss of the p14 product of the *CDKN2A* gene.
- Recently mutations of isocitrate dehydrogenase 1 gene (*IDH1*) have been shown to occur in a large fraction of grade II and grade III astrocytomas as well as in other gliomas. Antibodies specific to mutant IDH1 protein are used reliably for glioma diagnosis on routine tissue sections. IDH-mutated tumors have a better prognosis compared to those with IDH-wild type status.

PHYSICAL FINDINGS & CLINICAL PRESENTATION

The presenting symptoms of astrocytoma depend, in part, on the location of the lesion and its rate of growth. Astrocytomas classically present with any one or more of the following features:

- Headache (less frequent)
- New-onset partial or generalized seizures (>50%)
- Nausea and vomiting
- Focal neurologic deficit (cranial nerve palsy, hemiplegia, ataxia)
- Change in mental status
- Papilledema (rare)

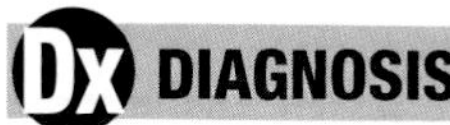

DIAGNOSIS

A provisional diagnosis of astrocytoma is made on clinical grounds and radiographic imaging studies. Tissue pathology is needed to establish the diagnosis and to grade the astrocytoma.

DIFFERENTIAL DIAGNOSIS

The differential diagnosis is vast and includes any cause of headache, seizures, change in mental status, and focal neurologic deficits.

WORKUP

- The imaging modality of choice is contrast enhanced MRI which can demonstrate anatomy and pathological process in detail. CT scanning is reserved for patients who are unable or unwilling to get MRI. Biopsy with histological confirmation is required to establish a diagnosis of astrocytoma.
- Stereotactic biopsy under CT or MRI guidance has been reserved for tumors that are deeply seated, multicentric tumors or diffuse nonfocal tumors where surgical resection is not practical. Major objectives of surgical resection are to maximally remove the tumor bulk, reduce tumor-associated mass effect and elevated intracranial pressure and provide tissue for pathological analysis. The surgical resection is carried out in a manner that minimizes the risk to neurological functioning. Surgery can also rapidly reduce the tumor bulk with potential benefits in terms of mass effect, edema, and hydrocephalus.

LABORATORY TESTS

There are no diagnostic or supportive blood tests for astrocytoma.

IMAGING STUDIES

MRI (Fig. 1) is the diagnostic imaging study of choice. MRI with contrast and magnetic resonance angiography are used to locate the margins of the tumor, distinguish vascular masses from tumors, detect low-grade astrocytomas (LGAs) not seen by CT scan, and provide clear views of the posterior fossa.

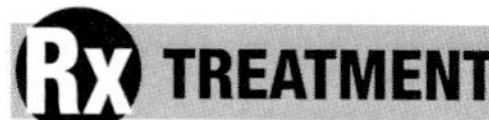

TREATMENT

ACUTE GENERAL Rx

- Corticosteroids (usually dexamethasone) need to be started immediately preoperatively in all primary CNS tumors unless CNS lymphoma is being suspected. Corticosteroids reduce cerebral edema and thus minimize secondary brain injury from cerebral retraction. Corticosteroids needs to be continued in the immediate postoperative period and tapered as quickly as possible. If there is increased intracranial pressure and impending herniation, patient should be started on IV mannitol, and mechanical ventilation with hyperventilation should be considered if there is depressed consciousness.
- The use of preoperative prophylactic anticonvulsants is less commonly indicated. The practice pattern in the U.S. seems to indicate its widespread use.

STAGE-SPECIFIC Rx

- Grade I astrocytoma are usually indolent and circumscribed tumors. Complete surgical

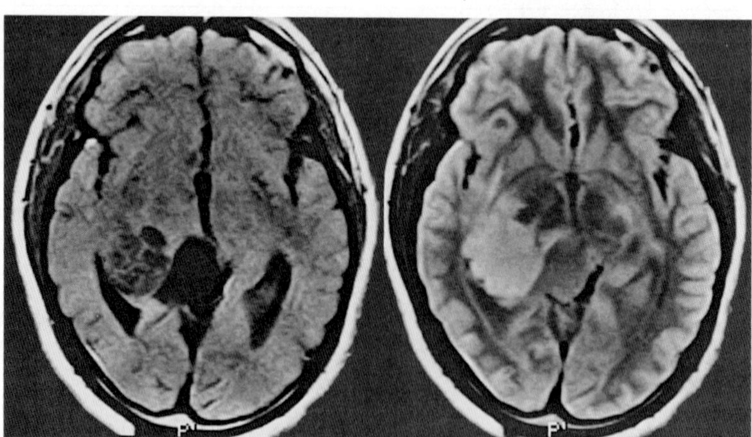

FIG. 1 Magnetic resonance image of a low-grade astrocytoma, demonstrating a hypointense right temporal lesion without contrast enhancement on T1 and hyperintense signal on T2. (From Goetz CG, Pappert EJ: *Textbook of clinical neurology,* Philadelphia, 1999, Saunders.)

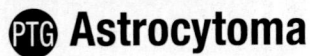

resection is the mainstay of therapy whenever feasible and is curative for these tumors. If complete surgical resection is not feasible due to location of tumor such as when the tumor is in optic pathway, hypothalamus, and in deep midline structures, asymptomatic patients can be observed in these cases until maximally safe resection is feasible upon progression. Unfortunately, despite aggressive near-total resection, delayed recurrence and eventual malignant transformation are common.

- In grade II astrocytoma, the extent of postoperative residual disease is an important variable for time to first relapse. The role and timing of postoperative radiotherapy, in particular, is controversial. Observation with imaging is a reasonable option in patients who are young (<40) and had a gross tumor resection. In patients who have undergone subtotal resection and who are >40 yr of age postoperative radiotherapy is recommended. Radiotherapy in this setting has been shown to improve progression-free survival (PFS) without improvement in overall survival.
- In Grade III anaplastic astrocytoma, surgical resection has shown to prolong survival but almost all of these tumors are characterized by postoperative residual disease. So, postoperative radiotherapy is routinely used adjunctively. Recent randomized clinical trials have established a survival benefit with the use of concurrent chemoradiotherapy compared with radiation alone.
- In Grade IV glioblastoma, surgical resection has been shown to improve median survival. Multiple randomized trials have demonstrated survival benefit with use of chemotherapy concurrent with radiotherapy following surgery. Use of further adjunct temozolomide chemotherapy has been shown to improve the median survival in patients with glioblastoma in randomized clinical trials. Unfortunately, even with chemotherapy and radiation therapy, the 2-yr survival in these patients is only 16%.

TREATMENT OF RECURRENT DISEASE

- For Grade 1 astrocytoma, re-resection should be considered. For patients who have tumors that are not amenable to resection, chemotherapy or radiotherapy can improve recurrence-free survival, although role of chemotherapy in adults remain controversial.
- For Grade 2 astrocytoma, radiation therapy can be considered in the relapsed setting if not given in the adjuvant setting. Data on use of chemotherapy in low-grade gliomas in adults is sparse. Although the results are encouraging, number of patients treated in these studies is small and there were a lot of methodological flaws in the studies. For recurrent Grade III anaplastic astrocytoma treated with radiation therapy in the past (Fig. 2), there is a role for chemotherapy. Nitrosoureas-based regimen and temozolomide (alkylating agent) have shown efficacy in this setting.
- Various targeted therapies are currently being studied in patients with recurrent glioblastoma. Irinotecan with bevacizumab or bevacizumab alone have been studied in a phase 2 trial, and a response rate of 38% and 28% respectively was reported in that study. Median survival was 8.7 months and 9.2 months respectively. The PD-1 checkpoint inhibitors are currently being evaluated and have shown promising early results in relapsed patients.
- In the case of both recurrent and newly diagnosed glioblastoma, the use of tumor-treatment fields (TTF) devices in conjunction with the use of temozolomide chemotherapy has demonstrated a survival benefit and is approved by the FDA.

PROGNOSIS

- Grade 1 astrocytoma has a good prognosis and is usually cured with surgical resection.
- Grade 2 astrocytoma has a median survival of about 7.5 yr with treatment.
- Grade 3 anaplastic astrocytoma has a median survival of approximately 5 yr. The patients with 1p and 19q co deletion have superior survival compared to patients without deletion.
- Median survival of glioblastoma is approximately 14 months.

REFERRAL

A multidisciplinary consultation with a neurosurgeon, radiation oncologist, and neurooncologist is required to assist in the diagnostic workup and to provide immediate and follow-up treatment.

SUGGESTED READINGS

Available at ExpertConsult.com

RELATED CONTENT

Astrocytoma (Patient Information)
Brain Cancer (Patient Information)
Brain Neoplasm, Benign (Related Key Topic)
Brain Neoplasm, Glioblastoma (Related Key Topic)

AUTHOR: **BHARTI RATHORE, M.D.**

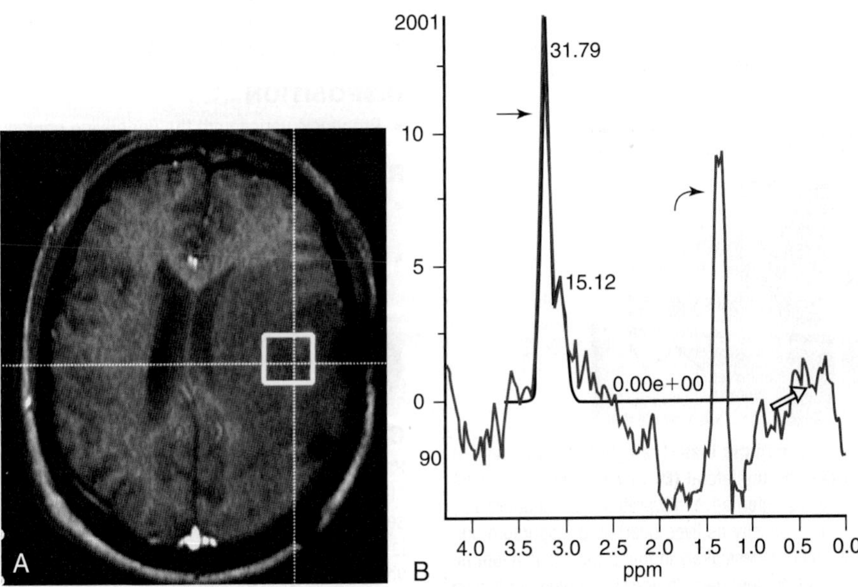

FIG. 2 Recurrent high-grade astrocytoma. Study performed after radiation therapy (not shown) showed increased edema and mass effect; differential diagnosis included recurrent tumor and radiation necrosis. **A,** Axial MRI scan shows volume of tissue *(box)* selected for spectroscopy. **B,** Proton spectroscopy reveals increase in choline peak *(arrow),* decrease in *N*-acetyl aspartate peak *(curved arrow),* and appearance of a lactate peak *(open arrow).* This appearance is consistent with recurrent tumor, which was verified with repeat surgery and biopsy. (From Vincent JL, et al.: *Textbook of critical care,* ed 6, Philadelphia, 2011, Saunders.)

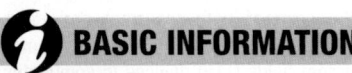

BASIC INFORMATION

DEFINITION

Atelectasis describes collapse of lung with some degree of volume loss. There are two major types of atelectasis. Obstructive atelectasis is the most common type due to reabsorption of gas from alveoli when communication between alveoli and the trachea is obstructed. Nonobstructive atelectasis is usually due to loss of contact between parietal and visceral pleura, compression (pleural effusion), or loss of surfactant.

ICD-10CM CODE
J98.11 Atelectasis

EPIDEMIOLOGY & DEMOGRAPHICS

- Postoperative patients and patients with lung or chest wall injury are at increased risk of atelectasis.
- Asbestos exposure increases risk for an entity called "rounded atelectasis."
- Occurs frequently in patients receiving mechanical ventilation.
- There is no known racial or sexual predilection for atelectasis.
- Dependent regions of the lung are more prone to atelectasis.

PHYSICAL FINDINGS & CLINICAL PRESENTATION

- Decreased or absent breath sounds
- Abnormal chest percussion
- Cough, dyspnea, decreased vocal fremitus, and vocal resonance
- Diminished chest expansion, tachypnea, tachycardia

ETIOLOGY

- Trauma caused by shear force generated by repetitive expansion and collapse during positive-pressure ventilation (e.g., mechanical ventilation)
- Airway obstruction (e.g., endobronchial tumor, a lymph node, foreign bodies, mucus plug)
- Extrinsic bronchial compression (e.g., neoplasms, aneurysms of ascending aorta, enlarged left atrium)
- Pleural disease (e.g., pleural effusion, mesothelioma, rounded atelectasis, pneumothorax)
- Alveolar injury (e.g., toxic fumes, aspiration of gastric contents, infections, ARDS)
- Chest wall abnormalities (e.g., trauma, scoliosis, rib fracture, obesity)
- Impaired respiratory mechanics or decreased cough response (e.g., pain, postanesthetic effect, abdominal distention, neuromuscular disease)

DIAGNOSIS

DIFFERENTIAL DIAGNOSIS

- Neoplasm (Bronchogenic carcinoma must be excluded)
- Pneumonia
- Pleural effusion
- Abnormalities of brachiocephalic vein and the left pulmonary ligament

WORKUP

- Chest x-ray (Fig. 1)
- Thoracic ultrasonography
- CT scan (Prone positioning CT scan with improvement or reduction in atelectasis may be used to differentiate from other etiology.)
- Fiberoptic bronchoscopy (selected patients)

IMAGING STUDIES

- Chest radiograph suggests the diagnosis but fails to confirm the diagnosis in many cases.
- Ultrasonography helps differentiate atelectasis from effusion or consolidation.
- CT scan is useful in patients with suspected endobronchial neoplasm or extrinsic bronchial compression.
- Prone images help differentiate true consolidation from dependent atelectasis.

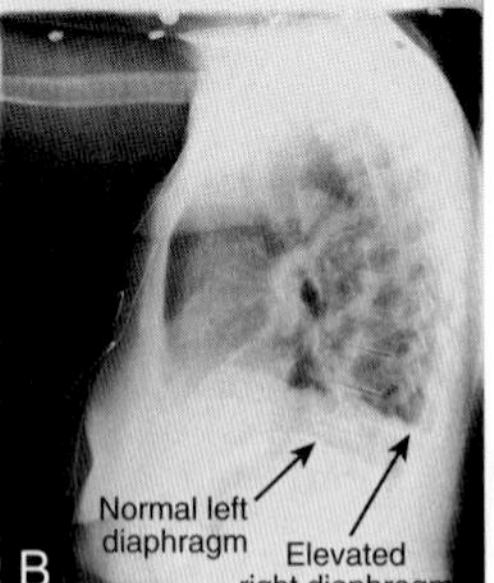

FIG. 1 Atelectasis with elevated diaphragm: an example of volume loss. The right hemidiaphragm in this patient appears elevated on both the posterior-anterior **(A)** and the lateral **(B)** views. Is this the correct interpretation of the x-ray, and if so, what is the cause? Consider the alternative interpretations. A subpulmonic pleural effusion would appear similar, as it would have the same density as liver, heart, and diaphragm and would layer over the diaphragm with the patient upright. This appears less likely in that a meniscus might be seen along the lateral chest wall with a pleural effusion but is not present here. In addition, a pleural effusion occupies space and might be expected to push the heart to the left, whereas in this case the heart may be slightly deviated to the right. Atelectasis of the lower right lung would result in volume loss, pulling the heart and hemidiaphragm into the space normally occupied by lung. This is consistent with the observed features. An infiltrate in this location could explain the x-ray findings but appears less likely for similar reasons to those cited for effusion. Some simple maneuvers could narrow the differential diagnosis. Chest ultrasound, decubitus x-ray views, or CT could identify an effusion. (From Broder JS: *Diagnostic imaging for the emergency physician*, Philadelphia, 2011, Saunders.)

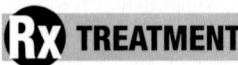

TREATMENT

NONPHARMACOLOGIC THERAPY

- Deep breathing, mobilization of the patient
- Incentive spirometry
- Handheld PEEP devices (e.g., PEEP valve, Acapella)
- Tracheal suctioning in select patients (e.g., mechanical ventilation and tracheostomy)
- Humidification
- Therapies for improving cough and clearance of secretions from airways (chest physiotherapy, chest wall percussion, and postural drainage)
- Fiberoptic bronchoscopy (selected patients) might be helpful with mucous plug, removal of foreign body, or evaluation of endobronchial and peribronchial lesions

ACUTE GENERAL Rx

- Positive-pressure breathing (continuous positive airway pressure by face mask, positive end-expiratory pressure for patients on mechanical ventilation)
- Use of mucolytic agents (e.g., acetylcysteine [Mucomyst])
- Recombinant human DNase (dornase alpha) in patients with cystic fibrosis
- Bronchodilator therapy in selected patients
- Pain control in postoperative and trauma cases
- Pleural drainages in cases of large effusions, hemothorax, or empyema

CHRONIC Rx

- Chest physiotherapy
- Humidification of inspired air
- Frequent nasotracheal suctioning

DISPOSITION

- Prognosis varies with the underlying etiology

REFERRAL

- Bronchoscopy for removal of foreign body or plugs unresponsive to conservative treatment
- Surgical referral for removal of obstructing neoplasm

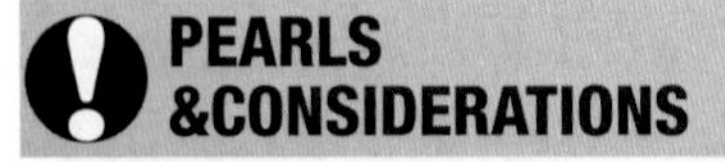

PEARLS & CONSIDERATIONS

COMMENTS

Patients should be educated that frequent changes of position are helpful in clearing secretions. Sitting the patient upright in a chair is recommended to increase both volume and vital capacity relative to the supine position. Adequate pain control is paramount after surgical intervention or rib fractures.

RELATED CONTENT

Atelectasis (Patient Information)

AUTHORS: **HARINDER P. SINGH, M.D.,** and **SAMAAN RAFEQ, M.D.**

BASIC INFORMATION

DEFINITION

Atopic dermatitis is a genetically determined eczematous eruption that is pruritic, symmetric, and associated with personal family history of allergic manifestations (atopy). Box 1 summarizes criteria for atopic dermatitis. Modified criteria for children with atopic dermatitis are described in Box 2.

SYNONYMS

Eczema
Atopic neurodermatitis
Atopic eczema

ICD-10CM CODES
L20.9 Atopic dermatitis, unspecified
L20.89 Other atopic dermatitis

EPIDEMIOLOGY & DEMOGRAPHICS

- Incidence is between 5 and 25 cases/1000 persons.
- Highest incidence is among children (10% to 20%). It accounts for 4% of acute care pediatric visits. It affects 1% to 3% of the adult population.
- Onset of disease before age 5 yr in 85% of patients.
- More than 50% of children with generalized atopic dermatitis develop asthma and allergic rhinitis by age 13 yr.
- Concordance in monozygotic twins is 77%.

PHYSICAL FINDINGS & CLINICAL PRESENTATION

- Atopic dermatitis presentation can be subdivided into three phases:
  1. Acute: Vesicular, crusting, weeping eruption.
  2. Subacute: Dry, scaly, erythematous papules and plaques.
  3. Chronic: Lichenification from repeated scratching.
- The lesions are typically on the neck, face, upper trunk, and bends of elbows and knees (symmetric on flexural surfaces of extremities) (Figs. 1 and E2). Atopic dermatitis lesions are usually discrete but vaguely delineated, scaly, and erythematous.
- There is dryness, thickening of the involved areas, discoloration, blistering, and oozing.
- Papular lesions are frequently found in the antecubital and popliteal fossae.
- In children, red scaling plaques are often confined to the cheeks and the perioral and perinasal areas.
- ***Hertoghe sign:*** Loss of the outer eyebrow from chronic rubbing (Fig. 1, B).
- Constant scratching may result in areas of hypopigmentation or hyperpigmentation (more common in blacks).
- In adults, redness and scaling in the dorsal aspect of the hands or about the fingers are the most common expression of atopic dermatitis; oozing and crusting may be present.
- Secondary skin infections may be present (*Staphylococcus aureus,* dermatophytosis, herpes simplex).

ETIOLOGY

Unknown; elevated T-lymphocyte activation, defective cell immunity, and B-cell IgE overproduction may play a significant role.

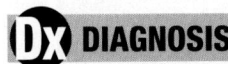

DIAGNOSIS

DIFFERENTIAL DIAGNOSIS

- Scabies
- Psoriasis
- Dermatitis herpetiform
- Contact dermatitis
- Photosensitivity
- Seborrheic dermatitis
- Candidiasis, tinea
- Lichen simplex chronicus
- Other: Xerosis, impetigo, Wiskott-Aldrich syndrome, PKU, ichthyosis, HIV dermatitis, nonnummular eczema, histiocytosis X, malignancies (T-cell lymphoma/mycosis fungoides, Letterer-Siwe disease), graft-versus-host disease, metabolic and nutritional deficiencies (zinc, niacin, pyridoxine deficiencies)

BOX 1 Criteria for Atopic Dermatitis

Major criteria
Must have three of the following:
- Pruritus
- Typical morphology and distribution
  - Flexural lichenification in adults
  - Facial and extensor involvement in infancy
- Chronic or chronically relapsing dermatitis
- Personal or family history of atopic disease (e.g., asthma, allergic rhinitis, atopic dermatitis)

Minor criteria
Must also have three of the following:
1. Xerosis
2. Ichthyosis or hyperlinear palms or keratosis pilaris
3. IgE reactivity (immediate skin test reactivity, RAST test positive)
4. Elevated serum IgE
5. Early age of onset
6. Tendency for cutaneous infections (especially *Staphylococcus aureus* and HSV)
7. Tendency to nonspecific hand/foot dermatitis
8. Nipple eczema
9. Cheilitis
10. Recurrent conjunctivitis
11. Dennie-Morgan infraorbital fold
12. Keratoconus
13. Anterior subcapsular cataracts
14. Orbital darkening
15. Facial pallor or facial erythema
16. Pityriasis alba
17. Itch when sweating
18. Intolerance to wool and lipid solvents
19. Perifollicular accentuation
20. Food hypersensitivity
21. Course influenced by environmental or emotional factors
22. White dermatographism or delayed blanch to cholinergic agents

HSV, Herpes simplex virus; *IgE,* immunoglobulin E; *RAST,* radioallergosorbent assay.
From James WD et al: *Andrews' diseases of the skin*, ed 12, Philadelphia, 2016, Saunders.

BOX 2 Modified Criteria for Children With Atopic Dermatitis

Essential features
1. Pruritus
2. Eczema
   - Typical morphology and age-specific pattern
   - Chronic or relapsing history

Important features
1. Early age at onset
2. Atopy
3. Personal or family history
4. IgE reactivity
5. Xerosis

Associated features
1. Atypical vascular responses (e.g., facial pallor, white dermatographism)
2. Keratosis pilaris, ichthyosis, or hyperlinear palms
3. Orbital or periorbital changes
4. Other regional findings (e.g., perioral changes, periauricular lesions)
5. Perifollicular accentuation, lichenification, or prurigo lesions

IgE, Immunoglobulin E.
From James WD et al: *Andrews' diseases of the skin*, ed 12, Philadelphia, 2016, Saunders.

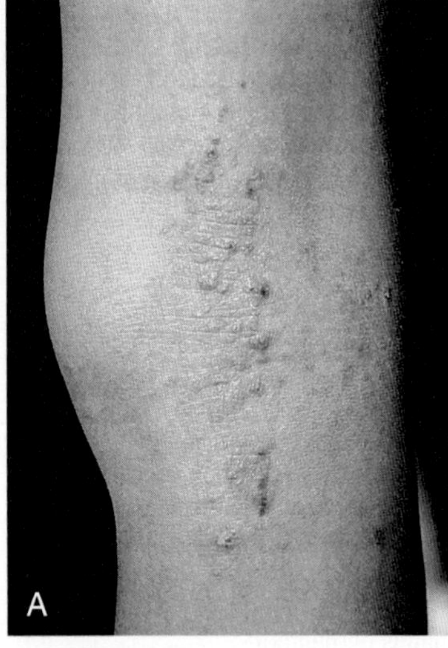

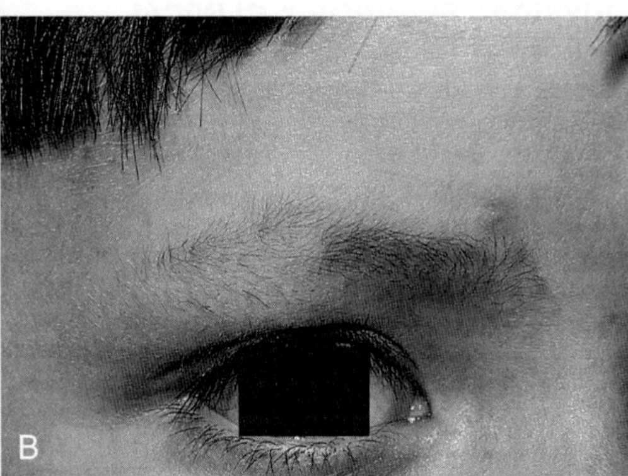

FIG. 1 **A,** Flexural atopic dermatitis with lichenification. Many of the skin changes are secondary to scratching. Linear lichenification, as shown here, and excoriations are typical. **B,** Hertoghe sign: loss of the outer eyebrow may occur in the atopic patient as a result of chronic rubbing. (From White GM, Cox NH, [eds]: *Diseases of the skin, a color atlas and text,* ed 2, St Louis, 2006, Mosby.)

WORKUP

Diagnosis is based on the presence of three of the following major features and three minor features.

MAJOR FEATURES:

- Pruritus
- Personal or family history of atopy: Asthma, allergic rhinitis, atopic dermatitis
- Facial and extensor involvement in infants and children
- Flexural lichenification in adults

MINOR FEATURES:

- Elevated IgE
- Eczema-perifollicular accentuation
- Recurrent conjunctivitis
- Ichthyosis
- Nipple dermatitis
- Wool intolerance
- Cutaneous S. *aureus* infections or herpes simplex infections
- Food intolerance
- Hand dermatitis (nonallergic irritant)
- Facial pallor, facial erythema
- Cheilitis
- White dermographism
- Early age of onset (after 2 mo of age)

LABORATORY TESTS

- Lab tests are generally not helpful.
- Elevated IgE levels are found in 80% to 90% of atopic dermatitis.
- Consider skin biopsy only in cases unresponsive to treatment.

Rx TREATMENT

NONPHARMACOLOGIC THERAPY

- Clip nails to decrease abrasion of skin
- Avoidance of triggering factors:
  1. Sudden temperature changes, sweating, low humidity in the winter
  2. Contact with irritating substance (e.g., wool, cosmetics, some soaps and detergents, tobacco)
  3. Foods that provoke exacerbations (e.g., eggs, peanuts, fish, soy, wheat, milk)
  4. Stressful situations
  5. Allergens and dust
  6. Excessive hand washing
- Phototherapy in moderation may be effective in resistant cases.

GENERAL Rx

- Emollients can be used to prevent dryness. Severely affected skin can be optimally hydrated by occlusion in addition to application of emollients.
- Low-potency topical corticosteroids (e.g., 1% to 2.5% hydrocortisone) may be helpful and are generally considered first-line therapy. Use intermediate-potency steroids (e.g., triamcinolone, fluocinolone) for more severe cases and limit potent corticosteroids (e.g., betamethasone, desoximetasone, clobetasol) to severe cases. Table 1 summarizes relative potencies of topical corticosteroids.
- Crisaborole 2% ointment is a phosphodiesterase type-4 (PDE4) inhibitor modestly effective for short-term treatment of mild to moderate atopic dermatitis.
- Oral antihistamines (e.g., hydroxyzine, diphenhydramine) are effective in controlling pruritus and inducing sedation, restful sleep, and prevention of scratching during sleep. Doxepin and other tricyclic antidepressants also have antihistamine effect, induce sleep, and reduce pruritus.
- The topical immunomodulators pimecrolimus and tacrolimus are especially useful for treatment of the face and intertriginous sites, where steroid-induced atrophy may occur. However, due to concerns about carcinogenic potential, the FDA recommends limiting their use for short periods in patients who are intolerant or unresponsive to other treatments. Pimecrolimus cream 1% is applied bid and has antiinflammatory effects secondary to blockage of activated T-cell cytokine production. Tacrolimus ointment (0.03% or 0.1%) applied bid is a macrolide that suppresses humoral and cell-mediated immune responses.
- Oral prednisone, IM triamcinolone, Goeckerman regimen, PUVA are generally reserved for severe cases.
- Cyclosporine, azathioprine, mycophenolate, and interferon gamma are sometimes tried for recalcitrant disease in adults by physicians who specialize in severe inflammatory skin conditions.
- The human monoclonal antibody dupilumab is effective in adults with moderate to severe atopic dermatitis that have not responded to topical therapies. It can be used with or without corticosteroids. It is injected subcutaneously. Cost is a limiting factor.
- Table 2 summarizes the management of atopic dermatitis.

DISPOSITION

- Resolution occurs in approximately 70% of patients by adulthood.
- Most patients have a course characterized by remissions and intermittent flares.

SUGGESTED READINGS

Available at ExpertConsult.com

RELATED CONTENT

Dermatitis (Patient Information)
Eczema (Patient Information)

AUTHOR: **FRED F. FERRI, M.D.**

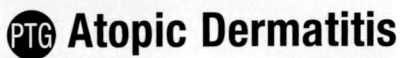

TABLE 1 Relative Potencies of Topical Corticosteroids (From Most Potent to Weakest)

Class	Drug	Dosage Form(s)	Strength (%)
I. Very high potency			
	Augmented betamethasone dipropionate	Ointment	0.05
	Clobetasol propionate	Cream, ointment, foam	0.05
	Diflorasone diacetate	Ointment	0.05
	Halobetasol propionate	Cream, ointment	0.05
II. High potency			
	Amcinonide	Cream, lotion, ointment	0.1
	Augmented betamethasone dipropionate	Cream	0.05
	Betamethasone dipropionate	Cream, ointment, foam, solution	0.05
	Desoximetasone	Cream, ointment	0.25
	Desoximetasone	Gel	0.05
	Diflorasone diacetate	Cream	0.05
	Fluocinonide	Cream, ointment, gel, solution	0.05
	Halcinonide	Cream, ointment	0.1
	Mometasone furoate	Ointment	0.1
	Triamcinolone acetonide	Cream, ointment	0.5
III-IV. Medium potency			
	Betamethasone valerate	Cream, ointment, lotion, foam	0.1
	Clocortolone pivalate	Cream	0.1
	Desoximetasone	Cream	0.05
	Fluocinolone acetonide	Cream, ointment	0.025
	Flurandrenolide	Cream, ointment	0.05
	Fluticasone propionate	Cream	0.05
	Fluticasone propionate	Ointment	0.005
	Mometasone furoate	Cream	0.1
	Triamcinolone acetonide	Cream, ointment	0.1
V. Lower-medium potency			
	Hydrocortisone butyrate	Cream, ointment, solution	0.1
	Hydrocortisone probutate	Cream	0.1
	Hydrocortisone valerate	Cream, ointment	0.2
	Prednicarbate	Cream	0.1
VI. Low potency			
	Alclometasone dipropionate	Cream, ointment	0.05
	Desonide	Cream, gel, foam, ointment	0.05
	Fluocinolone acetonide	Cream, solution, oil	0.01
VII. Lowest potency			
	Dexamethasone	Cream	0.1
	Hydrocortisone	Cream, ointment, lotion, solution	0.25, 0.5, 1
	Hydrocortisone acetate	Cream, ointment	0.5-1

From Paller AS, Mancini, AJ: *Hurwitz clinical pediatric dermatology, a textbook of skin disorders of childhood and adolescence,* ed 5, 2016, Elsevier.

TABLE 2 Management of Mild, Moderate, and Severe Forms of Atopic Dermatitis

Mild	Moderate	Severe
Bathing and barrier repair* Avoidance of irritant and allergic triggers Intermittent, short-term use of class VI or VII topical steroids ± topical calcineurin inhibitors Treatment of superinfection	Bathing and barrier repair* Avoidance of irritant and allergic triggers Intermittent, short-term use of class III–V topical steroids ± topical calcineurin inhibitors Treatment of superinfection Oral antihistamines	Bathing and barrier repair* Avoidance of irritant and allergic triggers Class II topical steroids for flares; class III–V topical steroids ± tacrolimus ointment for maintenance Treatment of superinfection Oral antihistamines Systemic antiinflammatory agents, ultraviolet light therapy

*Barrier repair may be accomplished by application of effective emollients or from barrier-repair agents.
From Paller AS, Mancini, AJ: *Hurwitz clinical pediatric dermatology, a textbook of skin disorders of childhood and adolescence,* ed 5, 2016, Elsevier.

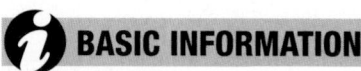

DEFINITION

Atrial fibrillation (AF) is a supraventricular tachyarrhythmia characterized by disorganized and rapid atrial activation and uncoordinated atrial contraction. AF occurs when structural and/or electrophysiologic abnormalities alter atrial tissue to promote abnormal impulse formation and/or propagation. The ventricular rate is dependent on the conduction properties of the atrioventricular (AV) node, which can be influenced by vagal/sympathetic tone, medications, or disease of the AV node.

Multiple classification schemes have been used in the past to characterize AF. The current classification scheme (divided into three major types) used by the American College of Cardiology (ACC)/American Heart Association (AHA) guideline committee is as follows:

- Paroxysmal AF—more than one episode of AF that terminate spontaneously or with intervention within 7 days
- Persistent AF—episodes of AF that last longer than 7 days
  1. Early-persistent AF—AF that has been continuous for longer than 7 days but fewer than 3 months
  2. Long-standing persistent AF—AF that has persisted for longer than 1 yr, either because cardioversion has failed or because cardioversion has not been attempted
- Permanent AF: When patient and physician decide to stop pursuing restoring sinus rhythm
- In addition to the previous AF categories, which are mainly defined by episode timing and termination, the ACC/AHA/European Society of Cardiology (ESC) guidelines describe additional AF categories in terms of other characteristics of the patient:
  1. Lone atrial fibrillation (LAF)—generally refers to AF in younger patients without clinical or echocardiographic evidence of cardiopulmonary disease, diabetes, or hypertension
  2. Nonvalvular AF—absence of rheumatic mitral valve disease, a mechanical or bioprosthetic heart valve, or mitral valve repair
  3. Secondary AF—occurs in the setting of a primary condition that may be the cause of the AF, such as acute myocardial infarction, cardiac surgery, pericarditis, myocarditis, hyperthyroidism, pulmonary embolism, pneumonia, or other acute disease. It is considered separately because AF is less likely to recur once the precipitating condition has resolved
  4. Silent AF—asymptomatic AF diagnosed by an ECG or rhythm strip

SYNONYMS

AF
PAF
AFib

ICD-10CM CODES

I48.0 Paroxysmal atrial fibrillation
I48.1 Persistent atrial fibrillation
I48.2 Chronic atrial fibrillation
I48.91 Unspecified atrial fibrillation

EPIDEMIOLOGY & DEMOGRAPHICS

- The prevalence of AF increases with age, from 2% in adults <65 yr to 9% of those >65 yr.
- AF affects over 3 million people in the United States. AF is uncommon in infants and children and, when present, almost always occurs in association with structural heart disease.
- The incidence of AF is significantly higher in men than in women in all age groups (1.1% versus 0.8%). AF appears to be more common in whites than in blacks, who may have lower awareness of the disease.
- Stroke due to thromboembolism is the most common and dreaded complication of AF. The rate of ischemic stroke in patients with non-rheumatic AF averages 5% a yr, which is somewhere between two and seven times the rate of stroke in patients without AF. The risk of stroke is not due solely to AF; changes in the endothelium and elevated markers of inflammation that may contribute to thrombosis are found in patients with AF, regardless of their rhythm at the time. The attributable risk of stroke from AF is estimated to be 1.5% for those aged 50 to 59 yr, and it approaches 36% for those aged 80 to 89 yr.
- Table 1 summarizes the thromboembolic risk score.

PHYSICAL FINDINGS & CLINICAL PRESENTATION

Clinical presentation is variable:

- Palpitations, dizziness, or lightheadedness
- Fatigue, weakness, or impaired exercise tolerance
- Angina
- Dyspnea
- Some patients are asymptomatic
- Cardiac auscultation revealing irregularly irregular rhythm
- Thromboembolic phenomenon such as stroke

TABLE 1 Thromboembolic Risk Score

CHA_2DS_2-VASc Risk factors	Score
Congestive heart failure	1
Hypertension	1
Age ≥ 75	2
Diabetes	1
Previous stroke, TIA, or thromboembolism	2
Vascular disease	1
Age 65–75	1
Female	1

European Society of Cardiology (ESC), American Heart Association (AHA), and American College of Cardiology (ACC) Guidelines recommend to use CHA2DS2-VASc Score to assess the risk of stroke in patients with atrial fibrillation. ESC Guidelines recommend patients with risk factor(s) ≥1 to receive effective stroke prevention therapy. Antithrombotic therapy is not recommended in patients with AF (irrespective of gender) who are aged <65 and with lone AF as they have very low absolute event rates. AHA/ACC Guidelines recommend oral anticoagulation for patients with CHA2DS2-VASc ≥2; for patients with nonvalvular AF and a CHA_2DS_2-VASc score of 1, no antithrombotic therapy or treatment with an oral anticoagulant or aspirin may be considered.

CHA2DS2-VASc, congestive heart failure, hypertension, age, diabetes, stroke/TIA, and vascular disease; *TIA,* transient ischemic attack.

Ronco C et al: *Critical care nephrology,* ed 3, Philadelphia, 2019, Elsevier.

ETIOLOGY

- The most frequent change in AF is the loss of atrial muscle mass and atrial fibrosis
- Fibrillation is presumed to be caused by multiple wandering wavelets, usually originating from the pulmonary veins. Both reentrant and focal mechanisms have been proposed
- Vascular causes: Hypertensive heart disease
- Valvular heart disease
- Pulmonary causes: Pulmonary embolism, chronic obstructive pulmonary disease, obstructive sleep apnea, carbon monoxide poisoning
- Structural cardiac disease: Hypertrophic cardiomyopathy, congestive heart failure, coronary artery disease, myocardial infarction, congenital heart disease (especially those that lead to atrial enlargement such as atrial septal defect)
- Pericarditis and myocarditis
- Arrhythmias: Atrial tachycardias and atrial flutters have been associated with atrial fibrillation, as has Wolff-Parkinson-White syndrome
- Endocrine: Thyrotoxicosis, hyperthyroidism or subclinical hyperthyroidism, pheochromocytoma, obesity
- Surgery: Both cardiac and noncardiac
- Electrolytes: Hypokalemia, hypomagnesemia
- Systemic stress: Fever, anemia, hypoxia, sepsis, infections (e.g., pneumonia)
- Medications/toxins: Digitalis, adenosine, theophylline, amphetamines, cocaine, antihistamines, alcohol abuse and/or withdrawal, caffeine, steroidal antiinflammatory drugs (SAIDs), nonsteroidal antiinflammatory drugs (NSAIDs)
- Frequency of vigorous exercise is associated with an increased risk of developing AF in young men and joggers
- Porphyrias have been associated with autonomic dysfunction and increased risk of AF
- Patients with metabolic syndrome, excessive vitamin D intake, or excessive niacin intake have a higher risk of AF

Dx DIAGNOSIS

DIFFERENTIAL DIAGNOSIS

- Multifocal atrial tachycardia
- Atrial flutter
- Frequent atrial premature beats
- Atrial tachycardia
- AV nodal reentry tachycardia (AVNRT)
- Wolff-Parkinson-White syndrome

WORKUP

The evaluation of atrial fibrillation involves diagnosis, determination of the etiology, and classification of the arrhythmia. A minimal evaluation includes a history and physical examination, ECG, transthoracic echocardiogram, and case-specific laboratory work to rule out secondary AF.

LABORATORY TESTS

- Thyroid-stimulating hormone, free T_4
- Serum electrolytes
- Toxicity screen
- CBC count (looking for anemia, infection)
- Renal and hepatic function tests
- D-dimer/CT scan of chest pulmonary embolism protocol (if the patient has risk factors to merit a pulmonary embolism workup)

IMAGING STUDIES

- ECG (Fig. 1)
- Absence of P waves
- Fibrillatory or f waves at the isoelectric baseline with varying amplitude, morphology, and intervals
- Irregular ventricular rate
- Echocardiography to rule out structural heart disease (evaluate ventricular size, thickness, and function, atrial size, pericardial disease, and valve function)
- Chest radiography (if pulmonary disease or CHF is suspected)
- Transesophageal echocardiography (TEE): Helpful to evaluate for left atrial thrombus (particularly in the left atrium appendage) to guide cardioversion or ablation (if thrombus is seen, cardioversion should be delayed)
- CT and MRI: In patients with a positive D-dimer result, chest CT angiogram may be necessary to rule out pulmonary embolus. 3D imaging technologies (CT scan or MRI) are often helpful to evaluate atrial anatomy if AF ablation is planned
- 6-minute walk test or exercise test: 6-minute walk or exercise testing can help assess the adequacy of rate control. Exercise testing can also exclude ischemia prior to treatment of patients with class Ic antiarrhythmic drugs and can be used to reproduce exercise-induced AF
- Sleep study (if sleep apnea is suspected)
- Holter monitor or event recorder if the diagnosis of AF is in question and to assess AF burden
- Electrophysiologic study: When initiation of AF is secondary to a supraventricular tachycardia, such as AVNRT or Wolff-Parkinson-White syndrome

Rx TREATMENT

ACUTE TREATMENT

ACUTE GENERAL RX: New-onset AF:

- If the patient is hemodynamically unstable (hypotension, congestive heart failure, or angina), perform synchronized cardioversion after immediate conscious sedation with a rapid short-acting sedative (e.g., midazolam). The likelihood of cardioversion-related clinical thromboembolism is low in patients with AF lasting <48 hr. Patients with AF lasting >2 days have a 5% to 7% risk for clinical thromboembolism if cardioversion is not preceded by several weeks of anticoagulation therapy. However, if transesophageal echocardiography reveals no atrial thrombus, cardioversion may be performed safely after therapeutic anticoagulation has been achieved. Alternatively, patients can be safely anticoagulated for approximately 1 month and then undergo cardioversion without transesophageal echocardiogram. Anticoagulant therapy should be continued for at least 1 month after cardioversion to minimize the incidence of adverse thromboembolic events. It can be stopped after 1 month as long as AF has not recurred if the patient is deemed low risk of stroke using the CHA_2DS_2VASc scoring system (Table 1).
- If the patient is hemodynamically stable, a rate-control strategy is typically pursued initially.
- Treatment options for rate control include the following:
  1. Diltiazem 0.25 mg/kg (maximum of 25 mg) given intravenously (IV) over 2 min followed by a second dose of 0.35 mg/kg (maximum of 25 mg) 15 min later if the rate is not slowed to <100 beats/min. May then follow with IV infusion 10 mg/hr (range, 5-15 mg/h) to achieve a resting heart rate of <100 beats/min. Onset of action after IV administration is usually within 3 min, with peak effect most often occurring within 10 min. After the ventricular rate is slowed, the patient can be changed to oral diltiazem 60 to 90 mg q4 to 6h. High doses of calcium channel blockers can exacerbate heart failure and thus should be used with caution in patients presenting with symptoms of heart failure or depressed ejection fraction.
  2. Verapamil 2.5 to 5 mg IV initially, then 5 to 10 mg IV 10 min later if the rate is still not slowed to <100 beats/min. After the ventricular rate is slowed, the patient can be changed to oral verapamil 80 to 120 mg q6 to 8h. Main concern is hypotension and heart failure with this medication, and it should not be used in patients with CHF.
  3. Esmolol and metoprolol are beta-blockers available in IV preparations that can be used. High doses of β-blockers can have negative inotropic effects in heart failure and should be used with caution.
  4. Digoxin is not a potent AV nodal blocking agent and has a potential for toxicity and therefore cannot be relied on for acute control of the ventricular response, but it may be used in conjunction with beta-blockers and calcium channel blockers. It may be a useful adjunct to a beta-blocker in the hypotensive or heart failure patient, which is not infrequent. When used, give 0.5 mg IV loading dose (slow) and then 0.25 mg IV 6 hr later. A third dose may be

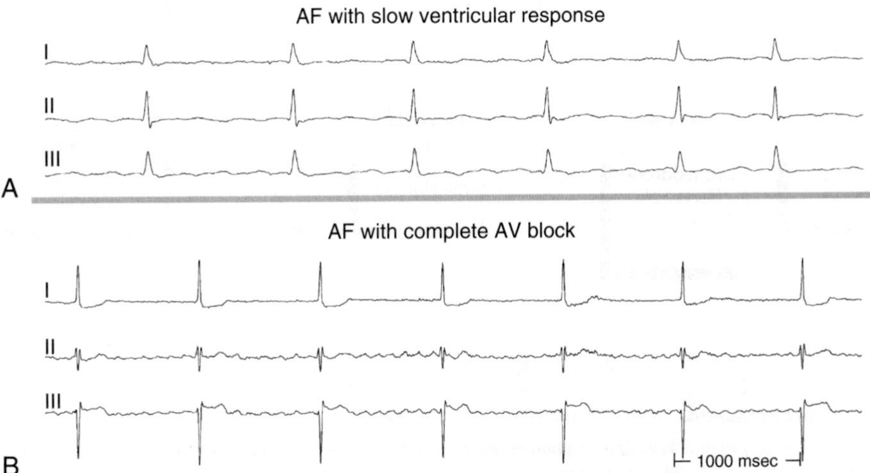

FIG. 1 Atrial fibrillation (AF) with slow ventricular rate. A, The ventricular rhythm is irregular, indicating that it is the result of conducted atrial beats. **B,** The ventricular rhythm is regular, consistent with the presence of complete atrioventricular *(AV)* block and a regular junctional escape rhythm. (From Issa Z, et al.: *Clinical arrhythmology and electrophysiology*, ed 2, Philadelphia, 2012, Saunders Elsevier.)

needed after 6 to 8 hr; the daily dose varies from 0.125 to 0.25 mg (decrease dosage in patients with renal insufficiency and elderly patients) depending on the heart rate and signs or symptoms of digoxin toxicity. Toxicity is manifested by GI and visual complaints, atrial tachyarrhythmias, heart block, and ventricular tachycardia.

5. Amiodarone has a class IIa recommendation from the ACC/AHA/ESC for use as a rate-controlling agent for patients who are intolerant of or unresponsive to other agents, such as patients with heart failure who may otherwise not tolerate diltiazem or metoprolol. Caution should be exercised in those who are not receiving anticoagulation because amiodarone can promote cardioversion, thereby posing a thromboembolic risk.

- AV nodal blocking agents, particularly calcium channel blockers and digoxin, should be avoided in patients with Wolff-Parkinson-White syndrome and AF because, by blocking the AV node, AF impulses may be transmitted exclusively down the accessory pathway, which can result in ventricular fibrillation. If this happens, the patient will require immediate defibrillation. Procainamide, flecainide, or amiodarone can be used instead if Wolff-Parkinson-White syndrome is suspected.
- In the acute setting, pharmacologic cardioversion (e.g., ibutilide, dofetilide) is less commonly used than electrical cardioversion. A major disadvantage with pharmacologic cardioversion is the risk of development of ventricular tachycardia and other serious arrhythmias, especially due to acute prolongation of the QT interval.

CHRONIC THERAPY

- Avoidance of alcohol in patients with suspected excessive alcohol use.
- Treatment of underlying source or cause, if any found.
- Treatment of modifiable risk factors such as obstructive sleep apnea, hypertension, and obesity have been shown to decrease AF burden in patients.
- Per the Atrial Fibrillation Follow-up Investigation of Rhythm Management (AFFIRM) and Rate Control versus Electrical Cardioversion (RACE) trials, either rate control or rhythm control strategies show no difference in composite cardiovascular end points of death, CHF, bleeding, drug side effects, or thromboembolism. Both approaches have similar outcomes as long as appropriate anticoagulation is maintained based on the individual's stroke risk.
- For patients without symptomatic AF, a rate-control strategy with calcium channel blockers, beta-blockers, or digoxin is a reasonable option. The RACE 2 trial indicates that a lenient rate control strategy, with a target resting heart rate of <110 beats/min, is noninferior to a strict control strategy, with a target resting heart rate of <80 beats/min and an exercise heart rate of <110 beats/min. Most recent ACC/AHA guidelines, however, recommend targeting a HR <80 beats/min over a target of <110 beats/min.
- In patients with symptomatic AF, younger patients, or those with difficult to control heart rate, an attempt should be made to maintain sinus rhythm with antiarrhythmic agents. Options of antiarrhythmic agents include amiodarone, dronedarone, (paroxysmal atrial fibrillation only without heart failure), dofetilide, flecainide, propafenone (contraindicated with structural heart disease), or sotalol. The decision of which strategy to follow should be best made in consultation with a cardiologist. Use of dronedarone should be avoided in patients with persistent or permanent atrial fibrillation because of worsened cardiovascular outcomes, especially in those with concomitant symptomatic heart failure (see Fig. 2 for a proposed algorithm to guide maintenance of sinus rhythm).

NONPHARMACOLOGIC THERAPY

- Catheter ablation of AF has become a common procedure for symptomatic drug-refractory or drug-intolerant patients. Sinus rhythm can be maintained long term in the majority of patients with paroxysmal atrial fibrillation (PAF) by circumferential pulmonary vein ablation performed in experienced centers. Established centers have reported success rates of 70% to 85% in patients with paroxysmal AF, but up to 50% of patients may require more than one ablation to achieve success. Complication rates are 4.5% in the largest international survey of hospitals performing this procedure. Success with persistent AF is much lower, with long-term success rates of 40% to 50% in many studies, and such patients often require more than one procedure. The most common

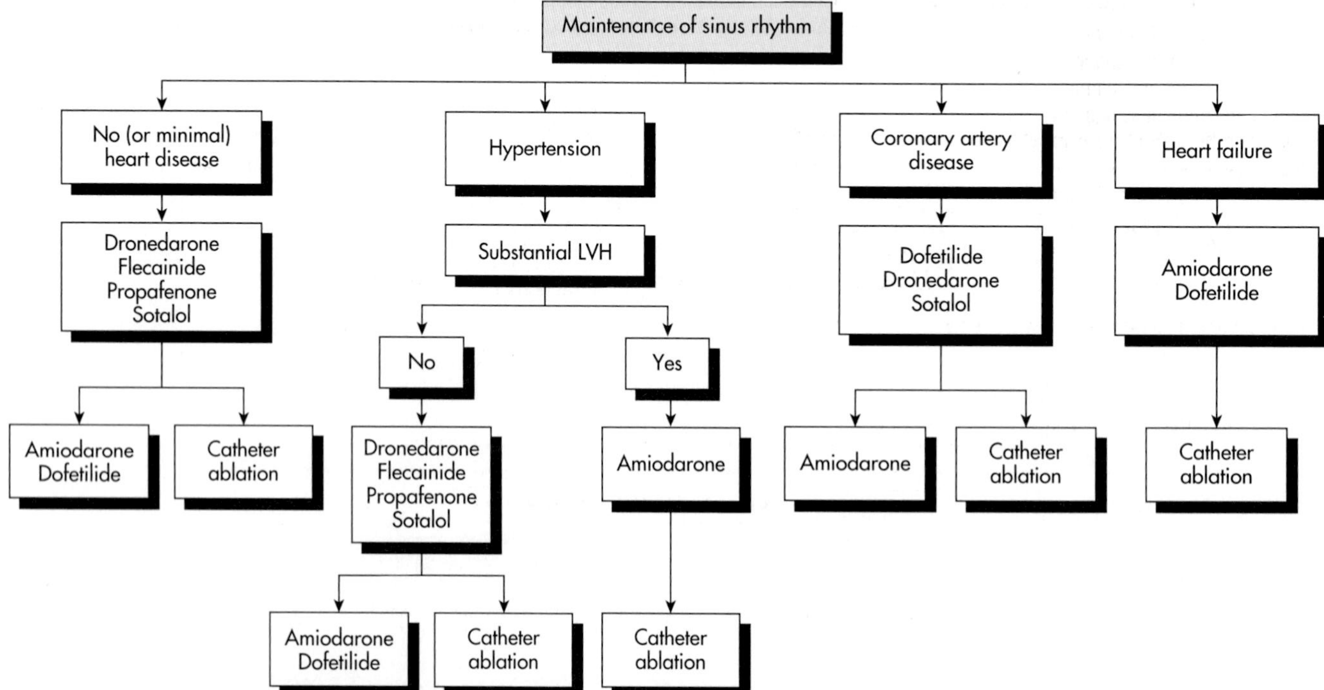

FIG. 2 Therapy to maintain sinus rhythm in patients with recurrent paroxysmal or persistent atrial fibrillation. Drugs are listed alphabetically and not in order of suggested use. The seriousness of heart disease progresses from left to right, and selection of therapy in patients with multiple conditions depends on the most serious condition present. *LVH,* Left ventricular hypertrophy. (From Wann LS, et al.: 2011 ACCF/AHA/HRS Focused update on the management of patients with atrial fibrillation [updating the 2006 guideline]: a report of the American College of Cardiology Foundation/American Heart Association Task Force on Practice Guidelines, *J Am Coll Cardiol* 57[2]:223-242, 2011.)

techniques used to isolate the pulmonary veins are radiofrequency ablation and cryoballoon ablation, which have shown similar results for patients with PAF.

- Pulmonary vein isolation is being increasingly used to treat AF in patients with heart failure. Trials have shown that pulmonary vein isolation is superior to AV node ablation with biventricular pacing in patients with heart failure who have drug-refractory AF.
- AV nodal ablation with permanent pacemaker implantation may become necessary in some patients in whom rate and rhythm are difficult to control despite drugs and cardioversion, although it is generally used as a therapy of last resort.
- The Cox-Maze III surgical procedure, with its modifications creating electrical barriers to the macroreentrant circuits that are believed to underlie AF, is being performed with good results in some medical centers (preservation of sinus rhythm in 70% to 95% of patients without the use of long-term antiarrhythmic medication). Success rates are higher in paroxysmal than in persistent or permanent atrial fibrillation. Surgical ablation is often used for patients undergoing aortic or mitral valve surgery. As a stand-alone procedure, it is a Class IIb recommendation per ACC/AHA Guidelines in 2017. Some centers perform surgical pulmonary vein isolation similar to this procedure using a mini-thoracotomy or video thorascopic "Mini-Maze" approach. Another surgical method is a pericardioscopic approach that allows extensive posterior wall ablation and, when combined with catheter ablation in a "hybrid" approach, has shown promising results for patients with persistent AF.
- It is important to understand that ablation therapy will not eliminate the need to take anticoagulant drugs. Even after ablation, patients with AF face increased risk of thromboembolic events and most electrophysiologists suggest lifelong anticoagulation for patients with elevated stroke risk score. Due to the increasing success rate of ablation, catheter-based therapy is considered the first-line treatment for paroxysmal AF patients intolerant or refectory to one medication or IIa for persistent patients in the ACC/AHA AF Ablation Guidelines in 2017. It remains a IIb indication for patients in long-standing persistent atrial fibrillation.

STROKE PREVENTION

- The decision whether to pursue long-term anticoagulation must be made in light of the patient's risk for a cardioembolic event versus risk for a bleeding event. In nonvalvular AF, CHA2DS2-VASc has superseded the CHADS2 scoring system (C = congestive heart failure; H = hypertension; A = age [>75 yr is 2 points]; D = diabetes; S = stroke, transient ischemic attack, or thromboembolic disease [2 points]; V = vascular disease, A = age 65-74 yr; and Sc = sex category, with females getting 1 extra point). Patients with a CHA2DS2-VASc score of 0 are considered low risk, 1 to 2 are considered moderate risk, and >2 are considered high risk. Per guidelines, patients with a score of 0 do not merit anticoagulation. Patients with a score of 1 can be treated at the discretion of the physician with either aspirin or an oral anticoagulant (warfarin or a novel oral anticoagulant). Anticoagulation with either warfarin or a novel oral anticoagulant is recommended for all patients with a CHADS2VASC score of 2 or above. The available direct-acting oral anticoagulants (DOACs) are at least as effective and as safe as warfarin for patients with nonvalvular AF.
- Increasing amounts of evidence now show that aspirin likely does not protect a person from stroke in AF and has recently been dropped from most of the ACC/AHA and European Atrial Fibrillation guidelines. Target INR for patients with a CHADS-VASc score of >1 is 2 to 3 and should be diligently monitored to avoid risk of stroke versus bleeding. Patients with hypertrophic cardiomyopathy or thyrotoxicosis with AF also have a high risk of stroke and should be anticoagulated irrespective of their CHADS-VASc score.
- Alternatives to warfarin now include several factor Xa inhibitors (Table 2) and a direct thrombin inhibitor.
  1. Dabigatran is a direct thrombin inhibitor indicated to reduce the risk of stroke and systemic embolism in patients with nonvalvular atrial fibrillation. In the RE-LY trial of 18,113 patients with mean CHADS2 score of 2.1, dabigatran 110 mg bid was noninferior to warfarin, and 150 mg bid was superior to warfarin in prevention of thromboembolic events. Bleeding risk was similar to that of warfarin for both doses. Idarucizumab has been approved as a dabigatran reversal agent. Onset is immediate, and it provides full reversal for at least 24 hours in most patients.
  2. Factor Xa inhibitors (apixaban, rivaroxaban, edoxaban) are also effective in reducing stroke and systemic embolism in patients with atrial fibrillation. The Apixaban for Reduction in Stroke and Other Thromboembolic Events in Atrial Fibrillation (ARISTOTLE) trial in patients at high risk for stroke (mean CHADS2 score 2.1) using apixaban, the Rivaroxaban Once Daily Oral Direct Factor Xa Inhibition Compared with Vitamin K Antagonism for Prevention of Stroke and Embolism Trial in Atrial Fibrillation (ROCKET AF) trial using rivaroxaban in patients with CHADS2 score 3.5, and the Effective Anticoagulation with Factor Xa Next Generation in Atrial Fibrillation (ENGAGE-AF) trial using edoxaban in patients with a CHADS2 score of at least 2, showed that these anticoagulants reduce the risk of stroke, systemic embolism, and serious bleeding compared with warfarin. Rivaroxaban showed noninferior efficacy to warfarin in prevention of thromboembolism. Apixaban showed superior stroke reduction, reduced bleeding events, and an overall mortality benefit when compared with warfarin. Edoxaban showed noninferiority to warfarin with respect to stroke and systemic embolism prevention, with lower rates of bleeding and death from cardiovascular causes, but benefit was limited to patients with moderately impaired renal function. Rivaroxaban and edoxaban are dosed once a day, and apixaban is dosed twice a day. A factor Xa reversal agent, andexanet alfa, has received FDA approval as a reversal for the anticoagulant effect of these agents.
- The decision to anticoagulate should be made irrespective of whether the atrial fibrillation is paroxysmal, persistent, or permanent.
- For patients in whom anticoagulation with warfarin or other anticoagulants is contraindicated due to high bleeding risk (Table 3),

TABLE 2 Comparison of the Features of the Direct Oral Anticoagulants

	Dabigatran	Rivaroxaban	Apixaban	Edoxaban
Target	Thrombin (IIa)	Factor Xa	Factor Xa	Factor Xa
Active Drug	No	Yes	Yes	Yes
Onset Time (h)	0.5-2	2-4	3-4	1-3
Half Life (h)	12-17	5-13	~12	9-11
Renal Excretion (%)	80	33	27	50
Reversal Agent	Idarucizumab 5 g IV bolus	PCC	PCC	PCC

IV, Intravenous; *PCC,* prothrombin complex concentrate.
Hoffman R, et al.: *Hematology, basic principles and practice,* ed 7, Philadelphia, 2018, Elsevier.

TABLE 3 Bleeding Risk Score

HAS-BLED Risk factors	Score
Hypertension	1
Abnormal liver function	1
Abnormal renal function	1
Stroke	1
Bleeding	1
Labile INRs	1
Elderly (age >65)	1
Drugs	1
Alcohol	1

HAS-BLED is the most validated bleeding score for patients with AF in whom antithrombotic therapy is indicated. When HAS-BLED score ≥3, caution and regular review are appropriate, as well as efforts to correct the potentially reversible risk factors for bleeding.
INRs, International normalized ratio.
Ronco C, et al.: *Critical care nephrology,* ed 3, Philadelphia, 2019, Elsevier.

left atrial appendage exclusion is an alternative. Several methods can be used, including the Lariat procedure and the AtriClip, but these are still considered unproven for stroke prevention in AF. The Watchman device is a left atrial appendage occlusion device and is the only device approved by the FDA for stroke prevention specifically for patients with AF that require anticoagulation but have an appropriate reason to seek an alternative. Patients with surgical ligation of the left atrial appendages still require anticoagulation due to lack of clinical trials showing a stroke risk reduction and inconsistent techniques.

- Perioperative bridging anticoagulation in patients with AF: Current guidelines advise perioperative continuation of warfarin in low-risk patients (CHADS2 score 0 to 2) and bridging anticoagulation in those at highest risk of thromboembolism (CHADS2 score 5 to 6). The recent Bridging Anticoagulation in Patients who Require Temporary Interruption of Warfarin Therapy for an Elective Invasive Procedure or Surgery (BRIDGE) Study found that for patients who require procedure-related warfarin interruption, forgoing bridging anticoagulation was noninferior to perioperative bridging with low molecular weight heparin and decrease the risk of major bleeding. Based on this study, a no-bridging strategy is appropriate for lower-risk AF and minor procedures but in high-risk patients having major surgery the answer remains debatable.

PROGNOSIS

- AF is associated with a 1.5- to 1.9-fold higher risk of death, which is in part due to the strong association between AF and thromboembolic events.
- AF is also independently associated with an increased risk of incident myocardial infarction, especially in women and blacks.
- Development of AF predicts heart failure and is associated with a worse New York Heart Association Heart Failure classification. AF may also worsen heart failure in individuals who are dependent on the atrial component of the cardiac output.
- AF in the setting of acute myocardial infarction was associated with a 40% increase in mortality compared to patients in sinus rhythm.

DISPOSITION

Factors associated with maintenance of sinus rhythm after cardioversion include:

- Left atrium diameter <60 mm
- Absence of mitral valve disease
- Short duration of AF

REFERRAL

Refer to a cardiologist those patients in whom antiarrhythmic therapy or catheter-based/surgical intervention is being considered.

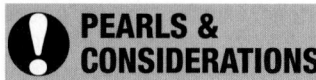

PEARLS & CONSIDERATIONS

COMMENTS

The number of patients anticoagulated in the United States is approximately half the amount that should be anticoagulated for AF, resulting in a large burden of stroke. The exact burden of AF needed to trigger the need for anticoagulation is not known, though recent pacemaker trials have suggested that as little as 6 min confers significant stroke risk. Reversal agents for the new class of anticoagulation are now available: idarucizumab for reversal of dabigatran; andexanet alfa for reversal of apixaban and rivaroxaban (pending FDA approval).

The American Academy of Family Physicians and the American College of Physicians provide the following recommendations for the management of newly detected AF:

- Rate control with chronic anticoagulation is the recommended strategy for the majority of asymptomatic patients with chronic AF. Rhythm control has not been shown to be superior to rate control (with chronic anticoagulation) in reducing morbidity and mortality, and may be inferior in some patient subgroups to rate control. Rhythm control is appropriate when based on other special considerations, such as patient symptoms, exercise tolerance, and patient preference.
- Patients with AF should receive chronic anticoagulation, unless they are at low risk for stroke as stated earlier or have specific contraindications.
- For patients with AF, the following drugs are recommended for their demonstrated efficacy in rate control during exercise and while at rest: atenolol, metoprolol, diltiazem, and verapamil (drugs listed alphabetically by class). Digoxin is effective only for rate control at rest and, therefore, should be used only as a second-line agent for rate control in AF.
- For patients who elect to undergo acute cardioversion to achieve sinus rhythm in AF, both direct-current cardioversion and pharmacologic conversion are appropriate options in an otherwise healthy patient.
- Both transesophageal echocardiography with short-term prior anticoagulation followed by early acute cardioversion (in absence of intracardiac thrombus) with postcardioversion anticoagulation vs. delayed cardioversion with preanticoagulation and postanticoagulation are appropriate management strategies for patients who elect to undergo cardioversion.
- Among patients with paroxysmal AF without previous antiarrhythmic drug treatment, ablation compared with antiarrhythmic drugs resulted in a lower rate of recurrent atrial tachyarrhythmias at 2 yr. However, recurrence was frequent in both groups.
- Among patients with atrial fibrillation who undergo packed cell volume, the risk of bleeding is lower among those who receive dual therapy with dabigatran and a $P2Y_{12}$ inhibitor (clopidogrel or ticagrelor) than among those who receive triple therapy with warfarin, a $P2Y_{12}$ inhibitor, and aspirin. Dual therapy has been shown to be noninferior to triple therapy with respect to the risk of thromboembolic events.[1]

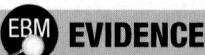

EVIDENCE

Available at ExpertConsult.com

SUGGESTED READINGS

Available at ExpertConsult.com

RELATED CONTENT

Atrial Fibrillation (Patient Information)

AUTHOR: **TANIA B. BABAR, M.D.**

[1] Cannon CP, et al.: Dual antithrombotic therapy with dabigatran after PCV in atrial fibrillation, *N Engl J Med* 377:1513-1524, 2017.

BASIC INFORMATION

DEFINITION

Typical atrial flutter is the term commonly applied to the atrial macroreentrant circuit that circulates around the tricuspid annulus in the right atrium. The critical isthmus of the circuit is the tissue between the inferior vena cava and the tricuspid annulus, and a more precise name for this arrhythmia is *cavotricuspid isthmus-dependent atrial flutter*, or CTI flutter. Because of its anatomic and physiologic stability, the result is regular atrial depolarizations, typically at a rate of 250 to 350 beats/min. Regular, macroreentrant atrial arrhythmias at this rate that do not use the CTI are referred to as *atypical atrial flutter*. Because of the circuit's stability, conduction through the atrioventricular node (AVN) is often predictable at a common mathematical denominator. For example, when the flutter rate is 300 beats/min, 2:1 conduction results in a ventricular rate of 150 beats/min. By extension, 3:1 conduction results in a ventricular rate of 100 beats/min, 4:1 in a rate of 75 beats/min, and 5:1 in a rate of 60 beats/min. If the regular atrial impulses conduct at a variable rate through the AVN, the result may be an irregular QRS pattern.

ICD-10CM CODES	
I48.3	Typical atrial flutter
I48.4	Atypical atrial flutter
I48.92	Unspecified atrial flutter

EPIDEMIOLOGY & DEMOGRAPHICS

- Atrial flutter is the second most common atrial tachyarrhythmia after atrial fibrillation, with an estimated 200,000 new cases annually in the United States.
- Atrial flutter is common in patients with congestive heart failure, COPD, or during the first week after open-heart surgery.
- Atrial flutter occurs more frequently with advancing age (5/10,0000 age <50 vs 587/100,000 age >80 yr) and 2.5 times more frequently in men than in women.
- Patients taking antiarrhythmics for chronic suppression of atrial fibrillation may convert to atrial flutter.
- Atrial flutter is typically seen in patients with underlying structural heart disease and is uncommon in children or young adults.
- More than 50% of patients with atrial flutter will develop atrial fibrillation in 3 yr, and more than 80% will develop atrial fibrillation within 5 yr. This is important when considering treatment options for atrial flutter.

CLASSIFICATION

Historically, the Wells classification designated atrial flutter as type I and type II. However, it is now recognized that tachycardias satisfying either of the definitions for type I or type II can be caused by reentrant circuits or by rapid focal atrial tachycardia, and this classification is infrequently used. Designating atrial flutter based on whether or not it is CTI dependent is more useful because of the management (i.e., ablation) options. Type I CTI-dependent atrial flutter, also known as common atrial flutter or typical atrial flutter, has an atrial rate of 240 to 350 beats/min. The reentrant loop circles the right atrium, passing through the CTI, a body of fibrous tissue in the lower atrium between the inferior vena cava and the tricuspid valve. CTI flutter can revolve around the tricuspid annulus in either direction (counterclockwise or clockwise) when viewing the tricuspid annulus *en face*.

- Counterclockwise atrial flutter is the more common type (~75%). The flutter waves are "sawtooth" and negative on the surface ECG leads II, III, and aVF; positive in V1; and negative in V6. (Fig. 1)
- Clockwise atrial flutter is less common (~25%): The reentry loop cycles in the opposite direction; thus, the flutter waves are upright in leads II, III, and aVF; negative in V1; and positive in V6. (Fig. 2)

Atypical atrial flutter is defined by absence of CTI dependence and may occur in patients with prior cardiac surgery, congenital heart disease, or prior radiofrequency ablation (especially left atrial ablation for atrial fibrillation) or may be idiopathic. One ECG feature is the lack of discordance between the inferior leads (leads II, III, and aVF) and V1. Flutter circuits in the left atrium often have upright flutter waves in all precordial leads.

PHYSICAL FINDINGS & CLINICAL PRESENTATION

- Palpitations
- Dizziness, lightheadedness, syncope, or near syncope
- Angina
- Congestive heart failure
- Embolic phenomena from intracardiac thrombus

ETIOLOGY

- Age-related degenerative changes
- Rheumatic heart disease
- Congenital heart disease
- Left ventricular dysfunction or congestive heart failure
- Acute myocardial infarction (rarely)
- Thyrotoxicosis
- Pulmonary embolism
- Mitral valve disease
- Cardiac surgery
- Chronic obstructive pulmonary disease
- Obesity
- Pericarditis
- Pulmonary hypertension
- Antiarrhythmic therapy use in patients with atrial fibrillation

DIAGNOSIS

DIFFERENTIAL DIAGNOSIS

- Atrial fibrillation
- Atrial tachycardia
- Supraventricular tachycardia:
  1. Atrioventricular node reentry
  2. Orthodromic reciprocating tachycardia (using a concealed bypass tract)
  3. Junctional ectopic tachycardia
  4. Wolff-Parkinson-White syndrome
- Sinus tachycardia

WORKUP

- ECG
- Laboratory evaluation
- Assessment of CHA_2DS_2-VaSc score

LABORATORY TESTS

- Thyroid function studies
- Serum electrolytes, including renal and hepatic tests (anticipating antiarrhythmic therapy use)

IMAGING STUDIES

- ECG:
  1. Absence of P waves.
  2. Regular, "sawtooth," or "F" (flutter)" wave pattern without an isoelectric baseline in leads II, III, and aVF (seen most commonly with counterclockwise typical CTI-flutter).
  3. There is rarely 1:1 atrioventricular (AV) conduction in atrial flutter (unless pre-excitation is present). Rather, AV conduction is usually in a 2:1 (Fig. 1), 3:1, or 4:1 fashion, with corresponding usual ventricular rates of 150, 100, or 75 beats/min, respectively (assuming an atrial rate of 300 beats/min). With high vagal tone or AV block, ventricular rates may be slow in atrial flutter.
- Echocardiography (for new diagnoses) to evaluate for structural heart disease (ventricular size, thickness, and function; atrial size, and valve function).
- Transesophageal echocardiography: Consider in patients with associated structural or functional heart disease to ascertain the presence of intracardiac thrombi, in the absence of an appropriate duration of anticoagulation.
- Holter monitoring or event recorder to assess for paroxysmal atrial flutter or rate control or to identify the arrhythmia if symptoms are nonspecific or to identify triggering events.
- Electrophysiologic studies: Required for a precise diagnosis, for mapping pathway, and for ablation.

TREATMENT

NONPHARMACOLOGIC THERAPY

- Vagal maneuvers (e.g., the Valsalva maneuver or carotid sinus massage) may transiently slow the ventricular rate (by increasing AV block) and may make flutter waves more evident. Adenosine may be similarly helpful for diagnostic purposes, allowing the unmasking of the atrial rhythm in the absence of ventricular activity. Maneuvers that affect AV conduction would be unlikely to terminate atrial flutter.
- Direct current cardioversion is the treatment of choice for acute management of atrial flutter associated with hemodynamic

instability or debilitating symptoms such as angina, congestive heart failure, or hypotension. Electrical cardioversion may be successful with energies as low as 25 joules, but because 100 joules is virtually always successful, this may be a reasonable initial shock strength. If the electrical shock results in atrial fibrillation, a second shock at a higher energy level is used to restore normal sinus rhythm. Sedation of a conscious patient is highly recommended before cardioversion is performed. The use of external defibrillators with biphasic waveforms decreases the amount of energy required for cardioversion and improves cardioversion success rate. Patients should be therapeutically anticoagulated for at least a month or longer depending on their stroke risk (CHA_2DS_2-VASc score; Table 1).

- Overdrive pacing in the atrium may also terminate atrial flutter. This method is especially useful in patients who have recently undergone cardiac surgery and still have temporary atrial pacing wires and in patients who have an implanted pacemaker or defibrillator with an atrial lead.
- Radiofrequency ablation to interrupt the atrial flutter is highly effective for patients with chronic or recurring atrial flutter and is generally considered first-line therapy in those with recurrent episodes of atrial flutter and may be offered for a first-ever episode of atrial flutter. It has been shown to improve health-related quality of life. Despite successful ablation of atrial flutter, however, the risk of future atrial fibrillation remains.

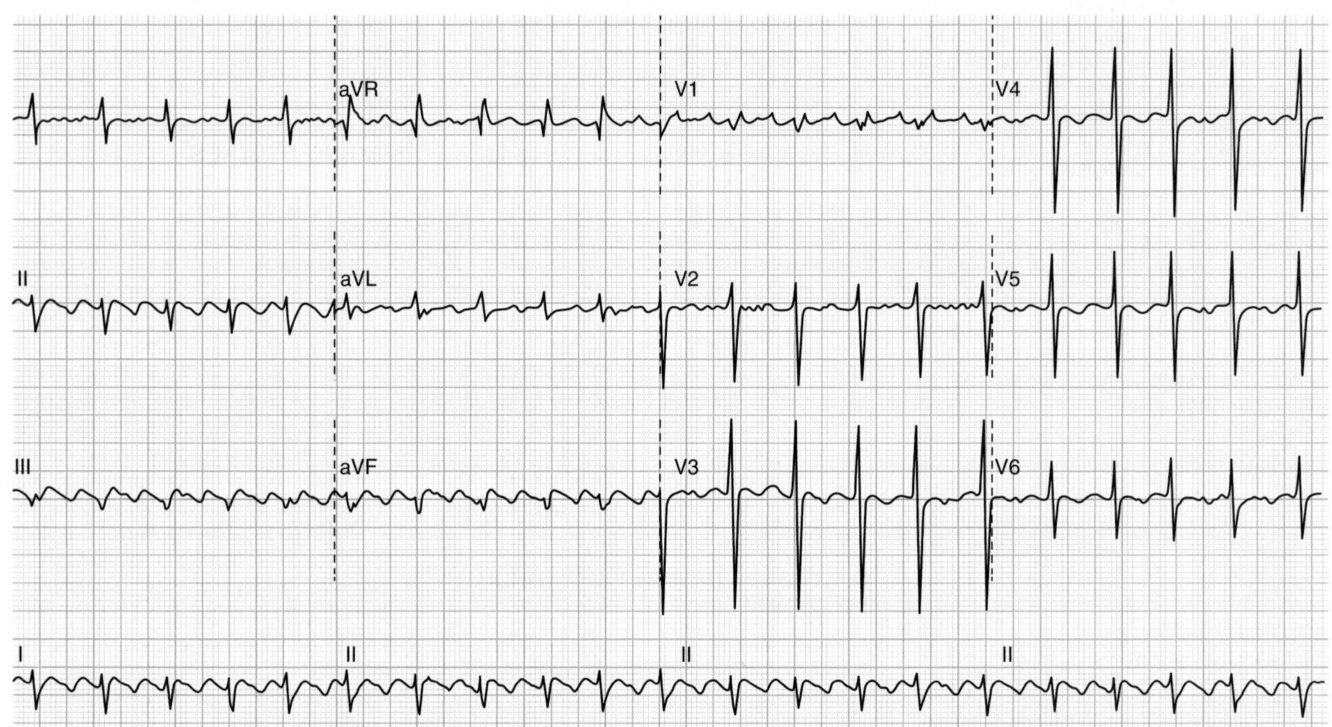

FIG. 1 Counterclockwise atrial flutter with 2:1 AV conduction. Note the negative flutter waves in leads II, III and F, positive in V1 and negative in V6. The second flutter wave can be seen overlying the QRS in the inferior leads and at the end of the QRS in lead V1.

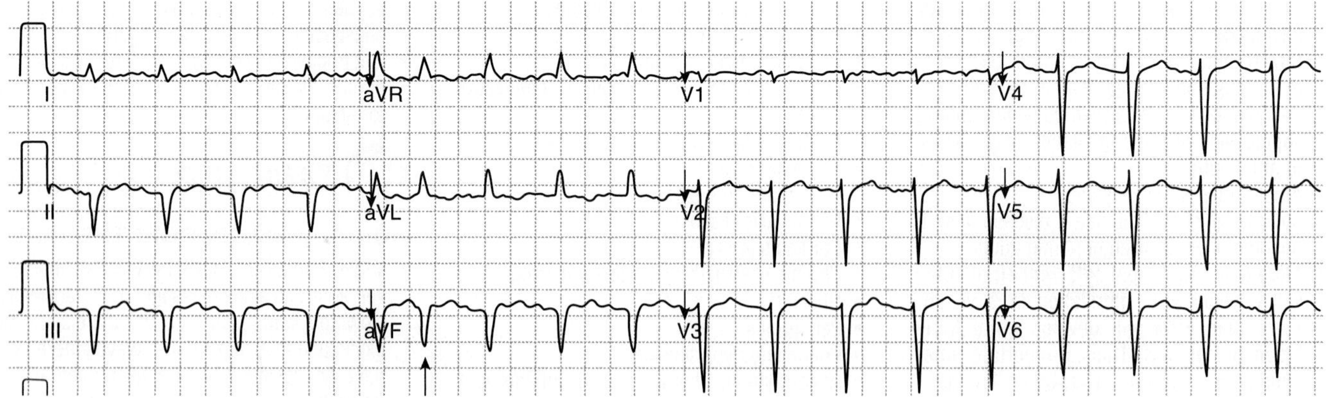

FIG. 2 Clockwise atrial flutter with predominant 2:1 AV conduction. Note the positive flutter waves in leads II, III and F, negative in V1 and positive in V6. The overall ventricular rate is slower than in figure 1 due to a slow flutter rate of approximately 200 bpm. One beat is conducted 1:1 *(arrow)*.

ACUTE Rx

- Treatment choices are based on clinical circumstances. Fig. 3 describes an acute treatment of atrial flutter algorithm. Table 2 summarizes atrial flutter therapy.
- If the patient is unstable, proceed directly to electrical cardioversion.
- In the hemodynamically stable patient, proceed with rate control or rhythm control strategy.
- AV blocking agents such as calcium channel blockers, beta-blockers, and digitalis (second-line treatment) may all be used for rate control. Atrial flutter may spontaneously convert to normal sinus rhythm with this strategy.
- In general, atrial flutter is more difficult to rate-control than atrial fibrillation.
- The rate of recurrence of atrial flutter with cardioversion alone is difficult to determine because most published data combine atrial flutter with atrial fibrillation. However, the recurrence rate is substantial, perhaps 50% at 1 yr.
- Intravenous ibutilide is a first-line medication for pharmacologic cardioversion of atrial flutter in patients with normal systolic function and QT intervals. The success rate is approximately 60%, and it is more effective than procainamide, sotalol, or amiodarone.

TABLE 1 CHA_2DS_2-VASc Risk Score for Prediction of Stroke Risk in Atrial Fibrillation

Risk Factor	Points
CHF/LV dysfunction	1
Hypertension	1
Age ≥75 yr	2
Diabetes mellitus	1
Stroke/TIA/embolism	2
Vascular disease	1
Age 64-74 yr	1
Sex category (female)	1
Maximum score	9

CHF, congestive heart failure; *LV*, left ventricular; *TIA*, transient ischemic attack.

CHRONIC Rx

- Few data exist to decide on the choice of rate control versus rhythm control in patients with atrial flutter. However, rate control may be difficult in atrial flutter, and ablation success exceeds 90%. Although ablation results in more durable freedom from atrial flutter recurrence, there are several pharmacologic options to help maintain sinus rhythm after cardioversion of atrial flutter, such as dofetilide, amiodarone, flecainide, propafenone, or sotalol. The choice of antiarrhythmic therapy is, in part, dictated by the presence or absence of underlying structural heart disease.
- Elective outpatient cardioversion or ablation can be performed either immediately preceded by TEE to evaluate the left atrium and the left atrial appendage for thrombus or after a period of at least 3 weeks of documented therapeutic anticoagulation before cardioversion. At least 4 weeks of anticoagulation should be administered after cardioversion, if not longer, depending on the overall thromboembolic risk of the patient as determined by the CHA_2DS_2-VASc score.

DISPOSITION

More than 85% of patients convert to regular sinus rhythm after cardioversion. Ablation success rates exceed 90%.

REFERRAL

Refer patients who are considered for rhythm control of atrial flutter to cardiologists, especially patients who are candidates for radiofrequency ablation.

PEARLS & CONSIDERATIONS

COMMENTS

- The surface ECG is the best tool for recognizing atrial flutter and distinguishing atrial flutter from atrial fibrillation.
- Ablation for typical atrial flutter is highly effective, straightforward, and relatively safe. It should be considered for patients with recurrent episodes and even for a first-ever episode.
- Patients with atrial flutter carry a significant risk for subsequent development of atrial fibrillation.
- Anticoagulation should be considered for all patients whose CHA_2DS_2-VaSc score is ≥2. Anticoagulation is generally not recommended in patients with a CHA_2DS_2-VaSc score of zero. For patients with a CHA_2DS_2-VaSc score of 1, low-dose aspirin or oral anticoagulants (warfarin, dabigatran, rivaroxaban, apixaban, or edoxaban) are appropriate options.
- Although anticoagulation recommendations for atrial flutter are identical to those for atrial fibrillation, studies suggest that the absolute risk of stroke is lower from atrial flutter than from fibrillation.

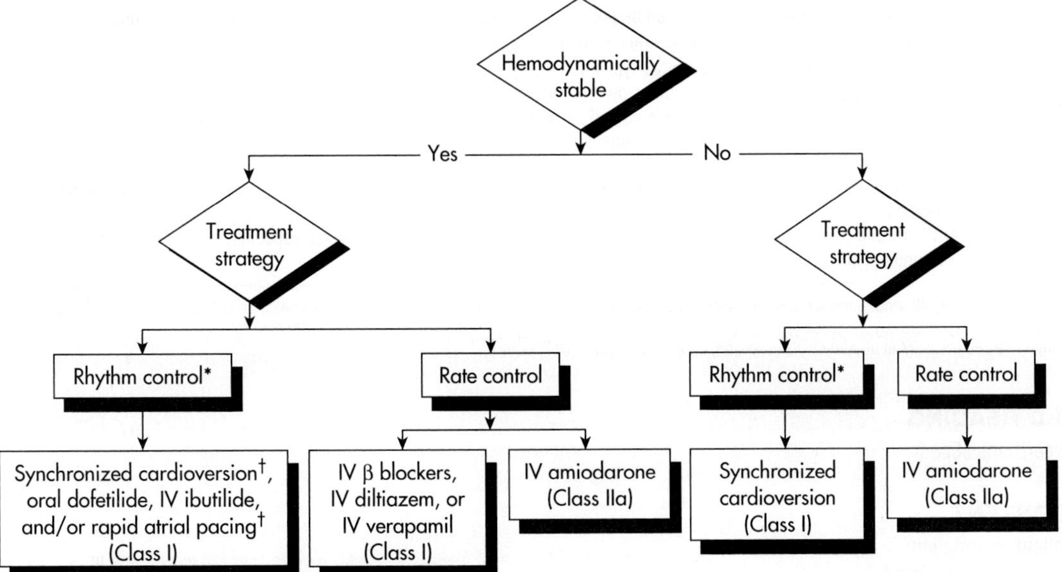

FIG. 3 Acute treatment of atrial flutter. *Anticoagulation as per guideline is mandatory. †For rhythms that break or recur spontaneously, synchronized cardioversion, or rapid atrial pacing is not appropriate. *IV*, Intravenous. (Reproduced with permission from Page RL et al: 2015 ACC/AHA/HRS Guideline for the management of adult patients with supraventricular tachycardia, *JACC* 67(13):e27-e115, 2016. In Olshansky B, Chung MK, Pogwizd SM et al: *Arrhythmia essentials*, ed 2, Philadelphia, 2017, Elsevier.)

TABLE 2 Atrial Flutter Therapy

Acute therapy for poorly tolerated AFL or continuous rapid ventricular rate	• If prolonged (i.e., >48 to 72 h), anticoagulation with heparin followed by therapeutic warfarin or NOAC as cardioversion may be associated with thromboembolic risk. Anticoagulation guidelines for cardioversion are the same as for atrial fibrillation and may indicate need for a TEE for prolonged episodes. Adenosine and carotid massage can be used to help to diagnose AFL masquerading as sinus rhythm. • **First line:** DCC under anesthesia with anticoagulation as necessary. Consider the length of the episode. • **Second line:** Ibutilide or procainamide may be attempted for conversion prior to DCC attempts. Ibutilide may be 70% effective if AFL has been present for <48 h, although often this is not known with certainty. Procainamide may help maintain sinus rhythm. • **Alternate:** Rapid atrial pacing (esophageal, epicardial, or endocardial, depending on the situation). To pace terminate, pace for 10 to 15 s at a rate of 10% to 20% faster than rate of flutter. If ineffective, burst pace 10 bpm faster at a time for 10 to 15 s at a time until conversion to AF or sinus rhythm. Adding procainamide may help pace termination efficacy; however, it may speed AV conduction if the ventricular response is not adequately controlled with AV nodal blocker drugs (see Chronic prevention, below); 20% to 30% will pace to AF and 10% to 20% will have no effect from pacing, depending on patient selection for the procedure. When AF occurs, it is usually short lived and terminates spontaneously within 24 h. If persistent, DCC can be attempted with or without antiarrhythmic drugs. Rapid AFL (atrial rate >350) and atrial fib/flutter usually cannot be pace terminated. However, slower AFL (rate <350) of any flutter wave morphology can often be pace terminated. • Oral drug loading alone to terminate AFL is rarely useful. • If recurrent episodes, use class IC or III antiarrhythmic drugs until steady state is achieved, then attempt cardioversion. These drugs (particularly 1C drugs) may stabilize the flutter circuit. It may also create another form of AFL—"IC" AFL—from AF. Ablation remains first-line therapy, especially if AFL is isthmus dependent. • Consider ablation for all persistent, refractory, or symptomatic AFL. However, despite AFL ablation, AF may occur, especially in individuals with underlying structural heart disease. • AV nodal ablation, although not preferable, could be considered when ventricular rate control cannot be achieved and flutter cannot be ablated, or if symptomatic, refractory, and/or if associated with tachycardia-induced cardiomyopathy. This option may be considered in cases where individuals have multiple forms of nonablatable AFL or AF and especially for those who do have non-isthmus-dependent AFL.
Chronic prevention	• If structural heart disease without CHF: sotalol (initiate in the hospital), dofetilide, amiodarone. • If structural heart disease with CHF: amiodarone, dofetilide. • If no structural heart disease: propafenone, flecainide, sotalol, dofetilide, or amiodarone, but propafenone or flecainide may need concomitant AV nodal blocking drugs to prevent 1:1 conduction. • If class I or III drugs are used, first control the ventricular response rate with an AV nodal blocking drug. Otherwise, the vagolytic effects of class IA drugs can enhance AV nodal conduction, and both 1A and 1C drugs can lead to AFL with 1:1 AV conduction. • Drug therapy alone for pure AFL flutter is usually not effective. • Consider radiofrequency catheter ablation early; it has become first-line therapy.
Nonresponders with severe symptoms	• If type I AFL, radiofrequency ablation of the right atrial isthmus. • Atypical AFL is more difficult to ablate and depends on the location of reentrant circuit. Success rates are lower than that for typical AFL. It is more difficult when there is congenital heart disease, valve disease, or prior surgery in which significant areas of scar are present. • Ventricular rate control, antiarrhythmic drugs, or AV node ablation (less preferable) can be performed for atypical, nonablatable AFL. • If AV node ablation and pacing is performed and AFL is intermittent, mode-switching function should be programmed "ON."
MI	• If hemodynamic intolerance or ongoing refractory myocardial ischemia, emergent cardioversion. AFL may increase MVO_2 due to rapid ventricular rate, causing further ischemia, diastolic dysfunction, and pulmonary congestion and edema. • If recurrent, IV amiodarone or procainamide. • Consider temporary antitachycardia pacing if recurrent and poorly tolerated.
Preoperative	• For cardiac surgery, convert AFL to NSR if adequate anticoagulation has been achieved, or ensure that ventricular response is well controlled. • If surgery is elective and AFL is chronic, antiarrhythmic drugs or catheter ablation may be considered. However, anticoagulation should be continued at least 3 wk after conversion of longer-term (>48 h) AFL prior to elective surgery. • For more urgent surgery in which anticoagulation cannot be used, consider rate control without cardioversion. • For short-duration (<48 h) AFL, DCC can be performed (may consider heparin prior to DCC with surgical consultation as to risk).
Postoperative	• AFL occurs in 10%-20% of all patients after cardiac surgery; it typically occurs with AF. Incidence peaks at days 2-3. It is more common in older patients. It rarely occurs after other types of surgery. The AFL may resolve spontaneously; however, the rhythm can increase the length of hospital stay, exacerbate heart failure, slow the recovery process, and cause symptoms. • Control rate with β-adrenergic blocker if no CHF or bronchospastic disease and good LVEF (> 40%). Diltiazem is often successful as a second-line drug, but use with caution in patients with poor LVEF. Digoxin for rate control is less effective but may be considered, particularly in patients with poor LV function. • IV amiodarone may be useful for persistent and poorly tolerated AFL; amiodarone or other antiarrhythmic drugs may be helpful for recurrent episodes. • DCC or atrial pace termination (if atrial pacing leads are present) is often successful, especially when employed early after the AFL onset. • Discontinue inotropic drugs, if possible.

AF, Atrial fibrillation; *AFL,* atrial flutter; *AV,* atrioventricular; *CHF,* congestive heart failure; *DCC,* direct current cardioversion; *IV,* intravenous; *LV,* left ventricle; *LVEF,* left ventricular ejection fraction; *MI,* myocardial infarction; *MVO_2,* myocardial oxygen consumption; *NOAC,* non-vitamin K oral anticoagulants; *TEE,* transesophageal echocardiography.
From Olshansky B, Chung MK, Pogwizd SM et al: *Arrhythmia essentials,* ed 2, Philadelphia, 2017, Elsevier.

SUGGESTED READING

Available at ExpertConsult.com

RELATED CONTENT

Atrial Flutter (Patient Information)
Atrial Fibrillation (Related Key Topic)

AUTHOR: **DANIEL R. FRISCH, M.D.**

BASIC INFORMATION

DEFINITION

An atrial septal defect (ASD) is a true deficiency in the interatrial septum that allows blood flow between the atria. It should be distinguished from patent foramen ovale (PFO), which is a defect caused by a failure of the septum primum to fuse to the superior limb of the septum secundum at the edge of the fossa ovalis in postnatal life, leaving a flaplike communication between the two atria. PFO occurs in approximately 20%-25% of the normal adult population. Fig. 1 illustrates the physiology of ASD. There are several forms of ASD (Fig. 2):

- Primum: This type of ASD occurs when there is failure of normal fusion of anterior and posterior endocardial cushions with the septum primum, with resultant deficiency in the inferior portion of the septum primum. The defect frequently coexists with abnormalities of the atrioventricular valves, commonly resulting in a cleft anterior mitral leaflet and left ventricular outflow obstruction.
- Secundum: The most common form of ASD; it represents a true deficiency in the septum primum or a septum secundum, or both. This defect most often occurs in the region of the fossa ovalis.
- Sinus venosus defect: This defect is located at the junction of the right atrium and either the superior vena cava or inferior vena cava. In a sinus venosus defect, the wall separating the pulmonary veins and the right atrium is deficient, causing a left-to-right shunt. Most commonly this defect involves the right upper pulmonary vein, which is still anatomically connected to the left atrium but is deficient anteriorly and thus drains anomalously into the right atrium. Less commonly, the right lower pulmonary vein is involved. The left pulmonary veins can also go into a vertical vein that drains into the innominate vein and to the superior vena cava.
- Coronary sinus septal defect (unroofed coronary sinus): This defect results when the wall separating the coronary sinus from the left atrium is deficient, causing a left-to-right shunt. This defect is often associated with a persistent left superior vena cava.
- Iatrogenic atrial septal defect (iASD) is an increasingly common complication after electrophysiological and structural interventional procedures that require transseptal puncture.

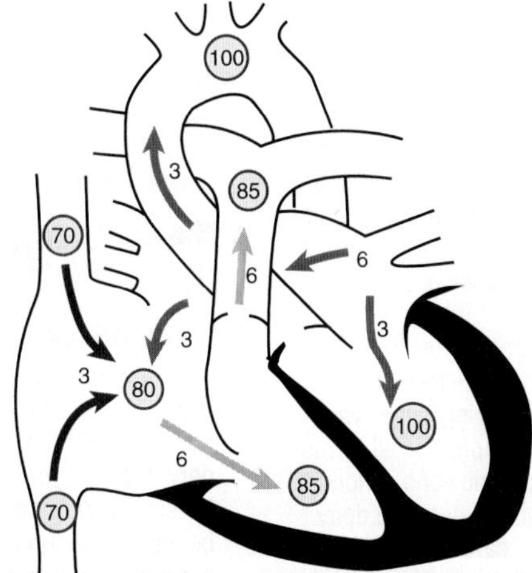

FIG. 1 Physiology of atrial septal defect (ASD). Circled numbers represent oxygen saturation values. The numbers next to the arrows represent volumes of blood flow (in L/min/m^2). This illustration shows a hypothetical patient with a pulmonary-to-systemic blood flow ratio (Qp/Qs) of 2:1. Desaturated blood enters the right atrium from the venae cavae at a volume of 3 L/min/m^2 and mixes with an additional 3 L of fully saturated blood shunting left to right across the ASD; the result is an increase in oxygen saturation in the right atrium. Six liters of blood flow through the tricuspid valve and cause a mid-diastolic flow rumble. Oxygen saturation may be slightly higher in the RV because of incomplete mixing at the atrial level. The full 6 L flows across the RV outflow tract and causes a systolic ejection flow murmur. Six liters return to the left atrium, with 3 L shunting left to right across the defect and 3 L crossing the mitral valve to be ejected by the left ventricle into the ascending aorta (normal cardiac output). (From Kliegman RM et al: *Nelson textbook of pediatrics,* ed 19, Philadelphia, 2011, Saunders.)

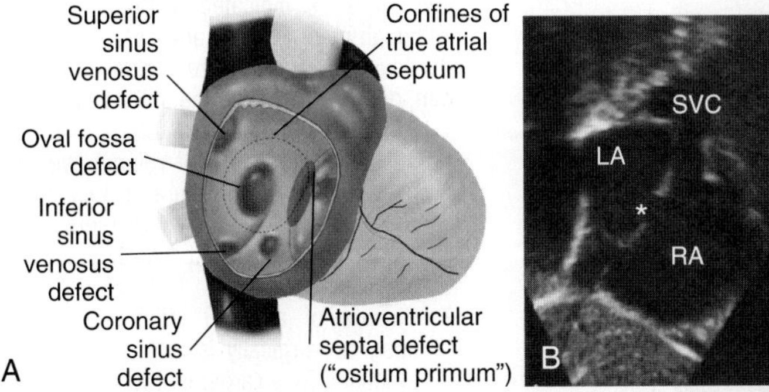

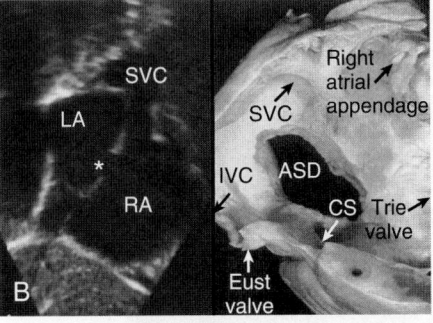

FIG. 2 A, Schematic diagram outlining the different types of interatrial shunting that can be encountered. Note that only the central defect is suitable for device closure. **B,** Subcostal right anterior oblique view of a secundum atrial septal defect *(ASD) (asterisk)* that is suitable for device closure. The right panel is a specimen as seen in a similar view, outlining the landmarks of defect. *CS,* Coronary sinus; *IVC,* inferior vena cava; *LA,* left atrium; *RA,* right atrium; *SVC,* superior vena cava. (From Zipes DP et al [eds]: *Braunwald's heart disease,* ed 7, Philadelphia, 2005, Saunders.)

SYNONYMS

ASD
Interatrial septal defect

ICD-10CM CODES

Q21.1 Atrial septal defect
I23.1 Atrial septal defect as current complication following acute myocardial infarction

EPIDEMIOLOGY & DEMOGRAPHICS

- Secundum, 75%; primum, 15%-20%; sinus venosus, 5%-10%; coronary sinus, <1%
- Incidence is greater in females and in patients with Down syndrome
- Accounts for 8% to 10% of congenital heart abnormalities
- Prevalence is 1.6 per 1000 live births
- Holt-Oram syndrome is an autosomal dominant disorder that involves skeletal anomalies, such as absent radial bones in both arms, as well as ASD (generally secundum) and cardiac conduction disease, such as atrioventricular (AV) blocks.
- Association with other genetic syndromes (e.g., Noonan syndrome, Treacher Collins syndrome, and the thrombocytopenia-absent radii syndrome) has been described for secundum defects. Down syndrome (trisomy 21) is strongly associated with AV canal defects, but these patients also have an increased frequency of secundum defects.
- ASDs may occur as an isolated defect or as part of other congenital cardiac syndromes such as Ebstein anomaly, Lutembacher syndrome, or fetal alcohol syndrome.

CLINICAL PRESENTATION

- Small ASDs or PFOs may close spontaneously during infancy. The majority of ASDs are small and do not cause any symptoms during infancy. These patients are usually diagnosed by the presence of a cardiac murmur during routine physical examination. Infants with large ASDs may presents with heart failure, recurrent respiratory infections, and failure to thrive.
- Exertional fatigue and dyspnea are usually the main presenting symptoms.

- On rare occasions, young adults may present with ischemic stroke caused by paradoxical embolism through the ASD or PFO.
- Platypnea-orthodeoxia (characterized by dyspnea and deoxygenation when changing from a recumbent position to sitting or standing).
- Patients with ASDs caused by congenital syndromes may present with clinical features to the underlying syndrome.
- Atrial arrhythmias such as atrial fibrillation and/or flutter are significantly increased in patients with ASDs, with the estimated incidence of 10% for untreated patients under age 40 yr.

CLINICAL FEATURES

- Cyanosis and clubbing (when abnormal right ventricular [RV] compliance has led to right-to-left shunting)
- Increased jugular venous pressure (with RV failure). Jugular venous pressure may also be a direct reflection of left atrial pressure if there is a significant ASD.
- Prominent RV impulse
- Visible and palpable pulmonary artery pulsations
- Wide fixed splitting of S_2
- An accentuated pulmonic component of S_2 if there is pulmonary hypertension
- Pansystolic murmur best heard at apex secondary to mitral regurgitation (ostium primum defect)
- Ejection systolic flow murmur (pulmonary valve flow murmur) (Fig. E3)
- Diastolic rumble (atrioventricular valve flow murmur)

Dx DIAGNOSIS

DIFFERENTIAL DIAGNOSIS

- Primary pulmonary hypertension
- Pulmonary stenosis
- Rheumatic heart disease
- Mitral valve prolapse
- Cor pulmonale
- Anomalous pulmonary venous connection

WORKUP

- ECG:
  1. Ostium primum defect: Extreme left axis deviation, incomplete or total right bundle branch block, prolongation of PR interval
  2. Sinus venosus defect: Right axis deviation, abnormal P axis (suggesting an absent or deficient sinus node)
  3. Ostium secundum defect: Right axis deviation, incomplete or total right bundle branch block, right atrial enlargement

IMAGING STUDIES

- Chest x-ray: Cardiomegaly, right heart enlargement, increased pulmonary vascular pattern
- Echocardiography (Fig. 4): Transthoracic echocardiography has a high degree of sensitivity for diagnosing secundum and primum ASDs. Echocardiography with saline bubble contrast and Doppler flow studies may demonstrate the size of the defect, the direction of shunting, right heart volume overload, and elevated pulmonary artery pressures. It should be noted that sinus venosus defects are frequently missed.
- Transesophageal echocardiography: It is much more sensitive than transthoracic echocardiography in identifying sinus venosus defects, and can be helpful for all forms of ASD when the transthoracic echo is nondiagnostic. It is also useful to determine defect size, proximity to other cardiac structures, and sizes of rims when determining suitability for device closure and is therefore used in the catheterization laboratory to assist with these issues. In cases of sinus venosus defect, it can be useful to locate anomalous pulmonary venous return.
- Cardiac catheterization: Invasive cardiac catheterization generally is not necessary for the diagnosis of ASDs since noninvasive modalities can generally identify and quantify the defect. Left heart catheterization is generally only useful when the coronary arteries need to be assessed before surgery. When performed, right heart catheterization will reveal a "step-up" in arterial oxygen saturation in the right atrium compared with the superior vena cava. This may not be the case in patients with partial anomalous pulmonary venous return associated with the sinus venosus type of ASD. Right heart catheterization can also aid in assessing shunt severity and the severity of pulmonary hypertension, and it can help to assess pulmonary vascular resistance (PVR) as well as pulmonary artery vasoreactivity in response to vasodilators.
- Cardiac MRI and CT: May be useful if echocardiography is not diagnostic; MRI is the gold standard for assessing RV size and function, and it can determine whether the right-sided chambers are, in fact, enlarged. MRI is also useful to assess anomalous pulmonary venous return and persistent left superior vena cava. Cardiac CT can offer similar information.

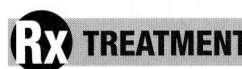

Rx TREATMENT

NONPHARMACOLOGIC THERAPY

- Asymptomatic patients with small defects with shunts with a pulmonary to systemic flow ratio (Qp/Qs) of <1.5:1 without pulmonary artery hypertension (PAH) and normal RV size require no medical therapy and may be observed. Routine assessment of these patients includes assessment of symptoms, arrhythmias, and embolic events and serial echocardiography.
- A repeat echocardiogram should be obtained every 2 to 3 yr to assess RV size and function and pulmonary pressure; with increasing age, the degree of left-to-right shunting may increase due to progressive noncompliance of the left ventricle with age-related acquired heart disease.

GENERAL Rx

- Children and infants: Closure of ASD before age 10 yr is indicated if Qp/Qs is >2:1 (although many experts advocate closure for Qp/Qs >1.5:1), if ASD size is significantly >5 mm, or if there is evidence of RV dilation.
  1. Small ASDs with a diameter of <5 mm and no evidence of RV volume overload do not impact the natural history of the individual and thus may not require closure unless associated with paradoxic embolism.
  2. Closure of an ASD either percutaneously or surgically is indicated for right atrial and RV enlargement with or without symptoms.
  3. A sinus venosus, coronary sinus, or primum ASD should be repaired surgically rather than by percutaneous closure.
  4. Surgical closure of secundum ASD is appropriate when concomitant surgical

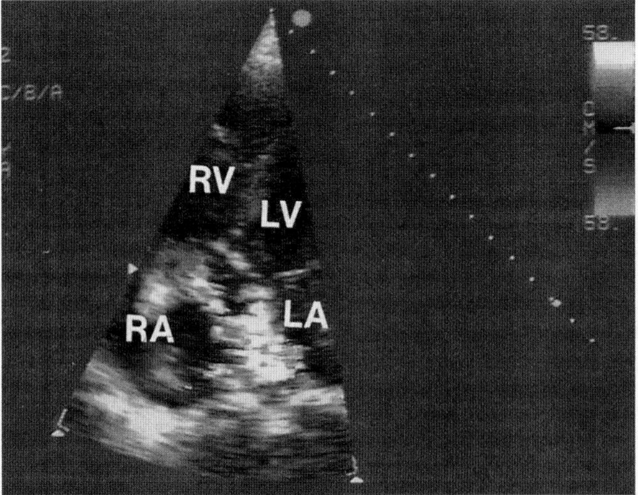

FIG. 4 Color flow Doppler apical four-chamber view showing blood flow from the left atrium *(LA)* to the right atrium *(RA)* through a moderately sized atrial septal defect. *LV,* Left ventricle; *RV,* right ventricle. (From Forbes CD, Jackson WF: *Color atlas and text of clinical medicine,* ed 3, London, 2003, Mosby.)

repair/replacement of associated defects is needed or when the anatomy of the defect precludes the use of a percutaneous device.

- Adults: Closure of an ASD, either percutaneously or surgically, may be considered in the presence of net left-to-right shunting with Qp/Qs >1.5:1, right-sided chamber enlargement, symptoms, pulmonary hypertension with pulmonary artery pressure less than two-thirds systemic levels, PVR less than two-thirds systemic vascular resistance, or when pulmonary hypertension is responsive to either acute or chronic pulmonary vasodilator therapy. These patients must be treated in conjunction with providers who have expertise in the management of adult congenital heart disease and pulmonary hypertension.
- Patients with severe irreversible PAH and no evidence of a left-to-right shunt should not undergo ASD closure.
- Closure of an ASD, either percutaneously or surgically, is reasonable in the presence of:
  1. Paradoxic embolism (Class 2a indication).
  2. Documented orthodeoxia-platypnea (Class 2a indication).
- The majority of iASD close spontaneously. However, if high risk features are present such as large iASD (>8 mm), large shunt, right to left shunting, patients with predisposition to thromboembolism or right ventricular dysfunction, then one should consider ASD closure.
- Percutaneous catheter device closure is possible in many patients with secundum ASDs (if stretched diameter is <41 mm with adequate rims), with >95% success rate in appropriate candidates. The procedure is guided by fluoroscopy and transesophageal echocardiography. A combination of low-dose aspirin and clopidogrel is usually prescribed for 3-6 months after the procedure to prevent thrombus formation. Early complications include device thrombus formation, atrial arrhythmias, erosion, and device dislodgement. Potential mid- and long-term complications include late device erosion into the aortic root or pericardium, atrial dysrhythmias, and infective endocarditis. In one study the long-term outcomes of device closure using the Amplatzer Septal Occluder (ASO) were excellent as evidenced by no deaths and minimal complication in 151 patients followed for 6.5 yr after ASD closure. In October 2013 the FDA began alerting health care providers and patients that in very rare instances, tissue surrounding the Amplatzer ASO can erode and result in life-threatening emergencies that require immediate surgery, especially when the rim adjacent to the aortic root is <5 mm. Based on published estimates, these events occur in approximately 1 to 3 of every 1000 patients implanted with the Amplatzer device. Close clinical follow- up and an echocardiogram is recommended predischarge, at 1 wk, at 6 mo, and at 12 mo after implant.
- Percutaneous closure is contraindicated in those with sinus venosus, primum, or unroofed coronary sinus defects. In addition, it is not suitable for secundum defects with unsuitable anatomy (too large; too close to coronary sinus, AV valves, or pulmonary veins; or inadequate rims), presence of sepsis, bleeding disorder, or intracardiac thrombi.
- In adult patients undergoing surgical closure, the surgical mortality should be <1%. Surgical closure is generally accomplished with a pericardial or Dacron patch, and it can usually be performed through a minimally invasive approach with or without robotic system assistance. Surgical closure of ASD improves function status, exercise capacity, and patient survival; however, it does not prevent atrial fibrillation or stroke, especially if patients are operated on after age 40. Concomitant maze procedure may be considered for intermittent or chronic atrial fibrillation in adults with ASDs who are undergoing surgical repair.

DISPOSITION

- Mortality rate is elevated in patients with large ASDs if left untreated, with complications such as RV failure, arrhythmias, paradoxic embolism, and PAH leading to right-to-left shunting (Eisenmenger syndrome).
- Patients with small shunts (<1.5:1) have a normal life expectancy.
- A reduction in size or spontaneous closure is more likely in younger patients with small defects (<10 mm in diameter).
- Basic assessment for adult congenital heart disease patients should include systemic arterial oximetry, an ECG, chest radiograph, transthoracic echocardiography, and blood tests for full blood count and coagulation screen.
- Intracardiac shunts are considered moderate risk for preoperative evaluation for noncardiac procedure. High-risk features include severe systolic dysfunction (ejection fraction <35%), severe pulmonary hypertension whether primary or secondary, cyanotic heart disease, or severe left-side outlet obstruction.
- Annual clinical follow-up is recommended for patients postoperatively if their ASD was repaired as an adult to monitor for PAH, atrial arrhythmias, RV or left ventricular dysfunction, and coexisting valvular lesions.
- Preoperative atrial fibrillation is a risk factor for immediate postoperative and long-term atrial fibrillation. Patients with a repaired ASD still have an increased risk for development of atrial fibrillation that directly correlates with the age at which the defect is corrected (later correction poses greater risk).
  1. After closure, anticipated benefits include improved functional status and exercise capacity, improved survival after closure as a child, improved quality of life, prevention of right heart failure, and prevention of PAH.
  2. Potential mid- to long-term complications after ASD closure in adulthood include tachyarrhythmias (atrial fibrillation or atrial flutter), bradyarrhythmias (sinus node dysfunction or heart block), stroke (greater risk in older patients), residual ASDs (because of patch dehiscence or incomplete closure by device), right heart failure or PAH (risk is correlated with the size of the original defect and inversely related to age at time of closure), mitral valve regurgitation or subaortic stenosis (in patients with primum ASDs), device migration/erosion, and pulmonary venous congestion (uncommon).
  3. Pregnancy is usually well tolerated in women with ASDs. Follow-up during pregnancy is recommended because of small risk for paradoxic embolus, stroke, arrhythmia, and heart failure. If known, ASDs should be closed before pregnancy is indicated. The sole contraindication to pregnancy in women with an ASD is severe PAH.
  4. Scuba diving is generally contraindicated in patients with unrepaired ASDs because of the risk of paradoxical emboli. In addition, high-altitude climbing should be avoided because it can cause oxygen desaturation from right-to-left shunting in these patients.
- In regard to infective endocarditis prophylaxis for dental procedures:
  1. Prophylaxis is not indicated for an unrepaired ASD.
  2. Prophylaxis is indicated for a repaired ASD or any congenital heart disease with prosthetic material as part of the repair during the first 6 mo after the repair.
  3. Prophylaxis is indicated for a repaired ASD or any congenital heart defect in the presence of residual defects at the site or adjacent to the site of a prosthetic patch or prosthetic device (both of which inhibit endothelialization).

The estrogen-containing oral contraceptive pill is not recommended in acute congenital heart disease patients at risk of thromboembolism, such as those with cyanosis related to an intracardiac shunt, atrial fibrillation, severe PAH, or Fontan repair.

SUGGESTED READINGS

Available at ExpertConsult.com

RELATED CONTENT

Atrial Septal Defect (ASD) (Patient Information)

AUTHORS: **CRAIG L. BASMAN, M.D.** and **TARAK S. RAMBHATLA, M.D.**

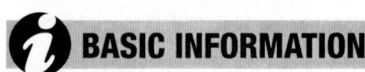

BASIC INFORMATION

DEFINITION

Atrioventricular (AV) dissociation is defined as a lack of association between the atria and the ventricles or independent function of the atria and ventricles. This simple definition will serve as a reminder that AV dissociation should be considered an umbrella rather than a diagnosis. AV dissociation may occur in the setting of bradycardic rhythms (Fig. 1 and Fig. 2) (complete heart block [Fig. 3], as well as tachycardic rhythms [ventricular tachycardia, atrial rhythm with associated accelerated junctional rhythm or AV nodal reentrant tachycardia]).

SYNONYMS

Third-degree AV block
CHB
Complete AV block

ICD-10CM CODE

I44.2 Atrioventricular block, complete

EPIDEMIOLOGY & DEMOGRAPHICS

The prevalence is the sum of the diagnoses that are characterized by AV dissociation.

PHYSICAL FINDINGS & CLINICAL PRESENTATION

Physical examination findings may be normal unless the arrhythmia is causing hemodynamic compromise. If the right atrium contracts against a closed tricuspid valve during ventricular systole, Cannon A waves may be seen in the jugular vein. Patients may present with the following clinical manifestations:

- Dizziness, palpitations
- Syncope or presyncope (caused by reduced cardiac output)
- Fatigue, impaired exercise tolerance
- Mental status changes
- Congestive heart failure
- Angina pectoris
- Some patients may be asymptomatic

ETIOLOGY

- Slow rate of firing from sinus node
- Inappropriately fast pacemaker from the ventricle
- Iatrogenic: Anesthesia, inotrope infusion, ventricular pacing, radiofrequency ablation of slow pathway, digoxin toxicity
- Sinus node disease, ischemia, hyperkalemia, overactive vagal drive
- Complete heart block: Progressive fibrosis of the His-Purkinje system, medications, Lyme disease

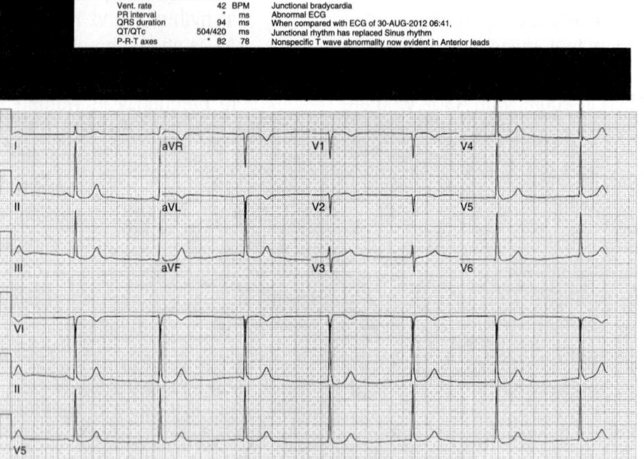
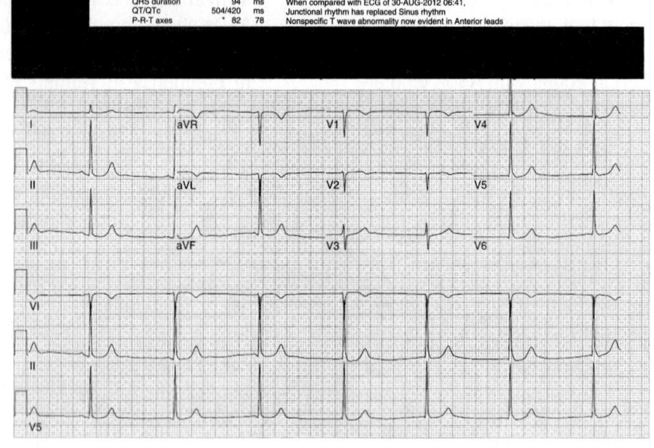

FIG. 1 An electrocardiogram was obtained at the primary care practitioner's office. Computer interpretation indicated junctional bradycardia at a rate of 42 beats per minute. While the rate was regular, not every QRS complex was preceded by a P wave. There were no acute ST- or T-wave changes consistent with ischemia. (From Singh GD et al: Food for thought: atrioventricular dissociation, *Am J Med* 126(12):1050–1053, 2013.)

AV Dissociation

Atrial rate > Ventricular Rate
Complete Heart Block

Reversible
Treat underlying etiology
Withdraw offending agent
TP if needed

Irreversible
PPM

Ventricular rate > Atrial rate

Atrial rate slows:
Isorhythmic AV dissociation
--PPM seldomly warranted
--TP if needed

Junctional (or ventricular) rate accelerates:
Accelerated junctional rhythm or ventricular tachycardia

For both:
Treat underlying etiology

FIG. 2 This flow chart demonstrates the relationship between atrioventricular dissociation due to complete heart block vs. atrioventricular dissociation from a ventricular rate that is greater than the atrial rate. *AV*, atrioventricular; *PPM*, permanent pacemaker; *TP*, temporary pacemaker. (From Singh GD et al: Food for thought: atrioventricular dissociation, *Am J Med* 126(12):1050–1053, 2013.)

Dx DIAGNOSIS

DIFFERENTIAL DIAGNOSIS

- The differential diagnosis should be targeted toward the diagnoses that include AV dissociation.
- NOTE: The atrium does not need to be faster than the ventricular rate in AV dissociation, as is the case in the definition of complete heart block.
  1. Isorhythmic AV dissociation: Atrial and ventricular rates are the same but dissociated.
  2. Interference dissociation: Similar atrial and ventricular rates but conduction occurs sometimes.

WORKUP

- Workup such as routine laboratory studies, cardiac biomarkers, and cardiac imaging should be dictated by the clinical circumstances.
  1. Laboratory studies: Particular attention to electrolyte abnormalities (potassium) and digoxin level
  2. Lyme antibody titer in the case of complete heart block, particularly in the Northeastern U.S.

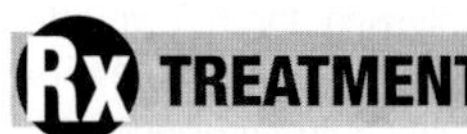

Rx TREATMENT

ACUTE GENERAL Rx

- Initial treatment should focus on the hemodynamic stability and symptoms of the patient.
- Bradycardic rhythms:
  1. If necessary (i.e., symptoms or hemodynamic compromise), a temporary pacemaker is the most reliable therapy.
  2. Hold AV-nodal blocking agents.
  3. Chronotropic medications: Atropine, dopamine, dobutamine, or isoproterenol may be used as second-line agents while preparing for a temporary pacemaker.

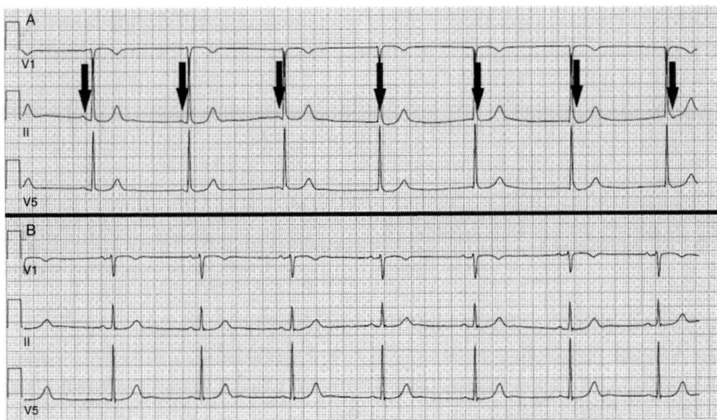

FIG. 3 A, In the initial rhythm strip—also shown in Fig. 1—solid black arrows indicate atrial complexes initiated by the sinus node. Note that for each beat, the sinus impulse is progressively closer to the QRS complex, then becomes obscured within the QRS complex, and finally is seen beginning to emerge on the downstroke of the R wave in the last 3 QRS complexes. The junctional pacemaker, at 42 beats per minute, is slightly faster than the atrial rate of 41 beats per minute. **B,** Another echocardiogram was performed after the patient was treated for dyspepsia. The rhythm strip shows sinus bradycardia with a rate of 45 beats per minute. (From Singh GD et al: Food for thought: atrioventricular dissociation, *Am J Med* 126(12):1050–1053, 2013.)

- Tachycardic rhythms (ventricular tachycardia):
  1. In the setting of hemodynamic compromise, cardioversion is the first-line therapy
  2. IV antiarrhythmic drugs: Amiodarone or lidocaine to suppress the arrhythmia
  3. Treatment of the underlying cause of ventricular tachycardia: Coronary angiogram if ischemia vs electrophysiology (EP) study +/− ablation

REFERRAL

All patients with AV dissociation should be referred to a cardiologist for diagnostic evaluation of the rhythm.

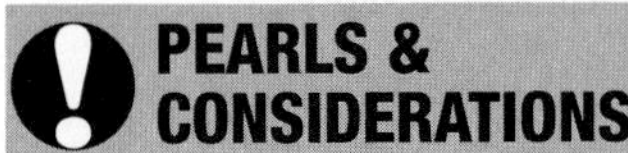

PEARLS & CONSIDERATIONS

COMMENTS

- Recall that AV dissociation is merely an umbrella that includes multiple diagnoses, including both bradycardic and tachycardic arrhythmias.
- Specific considerations regarding etiology, treatment, and disposition should be directed toward the rhythm that has caused AV dissociation.

AUTHOR: **ALEEM MUGHAL, M.D.**

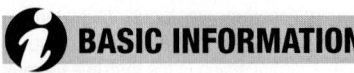

DEFINITION

Attention deficit hyperactivity disorder (ADHD) is a chronic disorder of attention and/or hyperactivity-impulsivity. Symptoms must be present before 12 yr of age, last at least 6 mo, and cause functional impairment in multiple settings. The diagnostic keys for ADHD are described in Table 1.

SYNONYMS

Hyperactivity
Hyperkinetic disorder
Attention deficit disorder (ADD)
ADHD

ICD-10CM CODES

F90.0	Attention-deficit hyperactivity disorder, predominantly inattentive type
F90.1	Attention-deficit hyperactivity disorder, predominantly hyperactive type
F90.2	Attention-deficit hyperactivity disorder, combined type
F90.8	Attention-deficit hyperactivity disorder, other type
F90.9	Attention-deficit hyperactivity disorder, unspecified type

DSM-5 CODES
314.00, 314.01

EPIDEMIOLOGY & DEMOGRAPHICS

PEAK INCIDENCE: Diagnosis is usually first made in school-aged children (6 to 9 yr).

PREVALENCE: Five percent to 10% of school-aged children (most prevalent neurodevelopmental disorder among children) and 2% to 5% of adults. Children from families with low socioeconomic status and children with public insurance are diagnosed with ADHD at higher rates than their peers.

PREDOMINANT SEX: Among children, male predominance with ratio of 2:1 to 4:1. Among adults, ratio is closer to 1:1 (sex difference may reflect referral bias).

PREDOMINANT AGE: Some symptoms must occur before age 12 yr. Symptoms (especially motoric hyperactivity) tend to diminish with age. Up to 70% continue to meet criteria in adolescence, and an estimated 40% to 65% have some symptoms in adulthood.

GENETICS: Strong polygenetic component. First-degree relatives of ADHD patients have 5 times greater risk of ADHD relative to controls. Studies suggest potential involvement of several genes, including those associated with serotonin and glutamate transporters as well as dopamine metabolism in addition to neuronal development.

RISK FACTORS: Possible risk factors include in utero tobacco/drug exposure or hypoxia, low birth weight, prematurity, pregnancy, lead exposure (though most children with elevated lead levels do not develop ADHD), head trauma in young children, family dysfunction, low socioeconomic status. Evidence supports possible association between dietary factors (e.g., refined sugar, food additives) and ADHD in a small percentage of patients. A causal link between environmental toxins and ADHD has not been clearly established.

TABLE 1 Diagnostic Keys for Attention Deficit Hyperactivity Disorder

1. Inattention
   a. Careless mistakes in schoolwork, work, or other activities
   b. Seems not to listen when spoken to directly
   c. Poor follow-through on schoolwork or chores
   d. Difficulty organizing
   e. Easily distracted by extraneous stimuli and is forgetful
2. Hyperactivity
   a. Trouble sitting still
   b. May act as if "driven by a motor"
   c. May talk excessively
3. Impulsivity
   a. Trouble holding back in class
   b. Trouble taking turns
   c. Interrupts

PHYSICAL FINDINGS & CLINICAL PRESENTATION

- Three types:
  1. Predominantly inattentive: Difficulty organizing, planning, remembering, concentrating, starting/completing tasks; symptoms may not be present during preferred activities.
  2. Predominantly hyperactive-impulsive: Edgy/restless, talkative, disruptive/intrusive, disinhibited, impatient.
  3. Combined.
- Usually diagnosed in elementary school when achievement is compromised and behavioral problems are not tolerated. Children with academic underproductivity, problems with peer and family relations, or discipline issues are often referred for evaluation. Of the more than 4 million children in the U.S. who have ADHD, most have comorbid conditions (see the following) and nearly half use special education and mental health services.
- Up to 50% may have associated disorders such as psychiatric diagnoses (oppositional defiant disorder, conduct disorder, depression, anxiety, eating disorders), learning disabilities, or substance abuse.
- In adults, motoric hyperactivity is less common, but restlessness, edginess, and difficulty relaxing are often seen. Disorganization and difficulty completing tasks are other common complaints.

ETIOLOGY

Strongest evidence exists for genetic inheritance. Other theories include abnormal metabolism of brain catecholamines, structural brain abnormalities, reduced activation in the basal ganglia and anterior frontal lobe, as well as environmental factors (see earlier).

Dx DIAGNOSIS

DIFFERENTIAL DIAGNOSIS

- Medical: Visual/hearing impairment, seizure disorder, head injury, sleep disorder, medication interactions, mental retardation intellectual disability, specific learning disorder, autism spectrum disorder/development delay, thyroid abnormalities, lead toxicity, movement disorders.
- Psychiatric: Depression, bipolar disorder, disruptive mood, dysregulation disorder, anxiety, obsessive-compulsive disorder, oppositional defiant disorder, intermittent explosive disorder, conduct disorder, posttraumatic stress disorder, reactive attachment disorder, and substance abuse.
- Psychosocial: Mismatch of learning environment with ability, family dysfunction, abuse/neglect.

WORKUP

- Clinical interview should include assessment of symptoms and impact on work/school and relationships; developmental history; personal and family psychiatric history, including substance abuse; social history, including family dysfunction; medical history.
- Physical examination should be performed to investigate medical causes for symptoms, coexisting conditions, and contraindications to treatment. Special focus should be paid to evaluation of dysmorphic features; neurologic examination, including assessment for neurocutaneous findings; and assessment of hearing and vision.
- Information from collateral sources (parents, partners, teachers) is crucial to diagnosis. Many patients will not display symptoms during an office visit and may underreport or overreport symptoms.
- Self-rating scales and standardized symptom-specific questionnaires from collateral sources can help diagnose and assess response to treatment. The use of ADHD-specific rating scales over broadband behavioral scale is associated with improved sensitivity and specificity.
- Laboratory or imaging studies should be undertaken only if indicated by history or physical examination.
- The FDA has approved a quantitative EEG test to aid in the diagnosis of ADHD in children, but sufficient evidence to support its routine use is lacking.
- Ancillary testing (e.g., IQ/achievement testing, language evaluation, and mental health assessment) may be indicated based on clinical findings and may require referral.

Rx TREATMENT

NONPHARMACOLOGIC THERAPY

- The majority of studies comparing the efficacy of pharmacologic vs nonpharmacologic interventions demonstrate the superiority of pharmacologic treatments.
- Studies on combined treatments have not shown significant improvements in core ADHD symptoms when behavioral treatments are added to stimulant medications. However, improvements in related areas of concern such as parent-child relations, aggressiveness, teacher-rated social skills, and reaching achievement have been seen in combined treatment groups.

- Prevailing opinion favors a multimodal approach in which nonpharmacologic behavioral therapies including parent-child behavioral therapy and social skills training can be used to target comorbid conditions or behaviors that have not responded to medication.
- Behavioral therapy alone is often considered when children are under 6 yr, symptoms and impairment are mild, if parents are opposed to or patients cannot tolerate medications, or if there is uncertainty or disagreement about the diagnosis (e.g., between parents and teachers).
- Educational interventions are recommended, particularly in the setting of learning disabilities. Children with ADHD are entitled to reasonable educational accommodations under a 504 Plan or the Individuals with Disabilities Education Act.
- Behavioral interventions (e.g., goal setting and rewards systems) show short-term efficacy and are endorsed by most national organizations. Time management and organizational skills appear useful. Social skills training may also be useful.
- Psychotherapy such as cognitive therapy, play therapy, or insight-oriented therapy are unlikely to be useful in addressing the core symptoms of ADHD. However, it may be beneficial in treating comorbid psychiatric conditions.
- Preliminary research concentrating on improving diagnosis, treatment outcomes, and medication compliance using eHealth (telemedicine, mobile apps, text reminders) have been promising.
- Elimination diets are not routinely recommended.
- Many support and advocacy groups provide education and other resources (e.g., Children and Adolescents with ADHD, National ADD Association, American Academy of Child and Adolescent Psychiatry).

ACUTE GENERAL Rx

- Most studies on treatment of ADHD are performed in children; limited data available on adults.
- Mainstay of treatment is stimulant medications. Second-line therapies include antidepressants and alpha-agonists. Table 2 summarizes FDA-approved treatments for ADHD.
- Stimulants:
  1. Release or block uptake of dopamine and norepinephrine.
  2. Include short- and long-acting methylphenidate, dextroamphetamine, and dextroamphetamine/amphetamine combinations (mixed amphetamine salts). A methylphenidate patch (Daytrana) is available, as is a pro-drug form of dextroamphetamine, lisdexamfetamine (Vyvanse), which is designed to limit the abuse potential. A long-acting oral suspension of methylphenidate (Quillivant XR), a long-acting chewable tablet of methylphenidate (QuilliChew ER), a long-acting orally disintegrating tablet of mixed amphetamine preparation (Adzenys XR-ODT), and a long-acting liquid amphetamine preparation (Dyanavel XR) are also available.
  3. All stimulants equally effective; however, not all patients improve with stimulants. Patients who do not respond well to one stimulant may respond to another.
  4. Do not cause euphoria or lead to addiction when taken as directed.
  5. Improve cognition, inattention, impulsiveness/hyperactivity, and driving skills. Limited impact on academic performance, learning, and emotional problems.
  6. Side effects are usually mild, reversible, and dose dependent, including anorexia, weight loss, sleep disturbances, increased heart rate and blood pressure, irritability, moodiness, headache, onset or worsening

TABLE 2 FDA-Approved Treatments for Attention Deficit Hyperactivity Disorder

Generic Name	Brand Name	Formulations and Strengths	Duration of Behavioral Effect (h)	Comments
Amphetamines				
D-amphetamine	Dexedrine	Tablets: 5, 10 mg	3–6	
	Dexedrine Spansule	Spansules: 5, 10, 15 mg		
	ProCentra	Oral solution: 5 mg/5 ml		
Mixed amphetamine/ dextroamphetamine	Adderall	Tablets: 5, 7.5, 10, 12.5, 15, 20, 30 mg	4–6	
	Adderall XR	Capsules: 5, 10, 15, 20, 25, 30 mg	8–10	Capsule with 1 : 1 ratio of IR to DR beads
	Evekeo	Tablets: 5, 10 mg	10	Racemic amphetamine sulfate, 1 : 1 D-amphetamine and L-amphetamine
	Dyanavel	Oral suspension: 2.5 mg/ml	8–13	Shake the bottle before administering the dose
Lisdexamfetamine dimesylate	Vyvanse	Capsules: 20, 30, 40, 50, 60, 70 mg	8–12	Inactive prodrug in which L-lysine is chemically bonded to D-amphetamine
Methylphenidates				
Methylphenidate	Ritalin	Tablets: 5, 10, 20 mg	3–4	
	Methylin	Tablets, chewable: 2.5, 5, 10 mg	3–4	
		Oral solution: 5 mg/5 ml, 10 mg/5 ml (500 ml)	3–4	
	Ritalin LA	Capsules: 10, 20, 30, 40 mg	8–9	Capsule with 1 : 1 ratio of IR beads to DR beads
	Metadate ER	Tablets: 10, 20 mg	5–8	
	Metadate CD	Capsules: 10, 20, 30 mg	8–9	Capsule with 3 : 7 ratio of IR beads to DR beads
	Concerta	Tablets: 18, 27, 36, 54 mg	8–12	Ascending profile, OROS technology
	Daytrana	Transdermal patch: 10, 15, 20, 30 mg/9 h	9	Delivery rate of 1.1, 1.6, 2.2, 3.3 mg/h for the patches, respectively, based on 9-h wear times in patients ages 6–12 yr
	Quillivant XR	Oral suspension: 25 mg/ 5 ml	8–12	Shake the bottle before administering the dose
	QuilliChew ER	Chewable tablets: 20, 30, 40 mg	8	
	Aptensio XR	Capsules: 10, 15, 20, 30, 40, 50, 60 mg	9–12	May be swallowed or opened and contents mixed into food.
Dexmethylphenidate	Focalin	Tablets: 2.5, 5, 10 mg		*d-threo*-enantiomer of methylphenidate, twice as potent as racemic methylphenidate
	Focalin XR	Capsules: 5, 10, 20 mg		

DR, Delayed-release; *IR*, immediate-release; *OROS*, osmotic-controlled release oral delivery system.
From Stern TA, et al.: *Massachusetts General Hospital handbook of general hospital psychiatry*, ed 7, Philadelphia, 2018, Elsevier.

of motor tics, reduction of growth velocity (but not adult height). Do not worsen seizures in patients on adequate anticonvulsant therapy. Rebound of symptoms can occur with withdrawal of medication.

7. Stimulants have generally been associated with cardiovascular events and death. Patients should be carefully evaluated for cardiovascular disease before beginning therapy and be periodically monitored, including blood pressure checks, while they are treated. However, despite concerns regarding cardiovascular risk, these medications are generally safe. Recent studies have shown that among young and middle-aged adults, current or new use of ADHD medications, compared with nonuse or remote use, is not associated with an increased risk of serious cardiovascular events. Routine, pre-treatment screening with ECGs is not currently recommended by the American Academy of Pediatrics or the American Academy of Child and Adolescent Psychiatry.

- Atomoxetine (Strattera):
  1. Selective norepinephrine reuptake inhibitor.
  2. Generally felt to be less effective than stimulants, but a useful alternative in patients who have not tolerated or responded to stimulants or in the setting of patient or family substance abuse.
  3. Efficacy and safety of use beyond 2 yr of treatment have not been studied. There have been reports of behavioral abnormalities and increased suicidality in children and adolescents.
  4. Side effects: Gastrointestinal upset, sleep disturbance, decreased appetite, dizziness, sexual side effects in men. Cardiovascular side effects have also been reported.
  5. There have been rare reports of severe liver injury in adults and children.
- Antidepressants (bupropion, imipramine, desipramine, nortriptyline):
  1. May be useful in patients with coexisting psychiatric disorders.
  2. Studies comparing efficacy versus stimulants are inconclusive.
  3. Side effects: Arrhythmias, anticholinergic effects, lowering of seizure threshold.
- Alpha-2-adrenergic agonists (clonidine, guanfacine):
  1. Appear to be less effective than stimulants, but may be particularly useful as an adjunctive treatment to stimulants, particularly in patients with a partial stimulant response or who experience side effects such as sleep disturbance or concurrent symptoms of overarousal, irritability, or aggression.
  2. Extended-release formulations of guanfacine (Intuniv) and clonidine (Kapvay) have been approved by the FDA for treatment of ADHD in children ages 6 to 17 yr. A transdermal clonidine patch is also available.
  3. Potential side effects include sedation, fatigue, headache, bradycardia, hypotension, and depression.
- Use of medications, particularly stimulants (which are monitored under the Controlled Substance Act), requires frequent monitoring.

DISPOSITION

- Although symptoms may change over time, for many patients ADHD represents a chronic condition that requires lifelong management.
- Patients are at higher risk for academic underachievement, lower socioeconomic status, work and relationship difficulties, high-risk behavior, and psychiatric comorbidities.

REFERRAL

- Diagnosis complicated by difficult-to-treat comorbid psychiatric conditions, developmental disorders, or mental retardation
- Lack of adequate response to stimulants/atomoxetine/alpha-adrenergic agents

PEARLS & CONSIDERATIONS

- The World Health Organization's Adult Self-Report Scale (ASRS) v1.1 has good sensitivity and adaptability to the primary care setting.
- Among adults with persistent ADHD symptoms treated with medication, trials have shown that the use of cognitive behavioral therapy compared with relaxation with educational support resulted in improved ADHD symptoms, which were maintained at 12 mo.
- ADHD has been associated with criminal behavior in some studies. Data analysis has shown that among patients with ADHD, rates of criminality are lower during periods when they receive ADHD medication.
- Recommendations for the diagnosis and management of ADHD have been published by the Centers for Disease Control and Prevention (www.cdc.gov/ncbddd/adhd/guidelines.html).

SUGGESTED READINGS

Available at ExpertConsult.com

RELATED CONTENT

Attention Deficit Hyperactivity Disorder (ADHD) (Patient Information)

AUTHORS: **PAMELA E. HOFFMAN, M.D,** and **EMILY R. KATZ, M.D.**

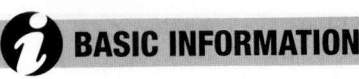

DEFINITION

Autism spectrum disorder (ASD) encompasses a continuum of developmental disabilities characterized by marked social impairment. Box 1 describes the diagnostic keys and case determination criteria under DSM-5. There is usually impairment in several additional domains integral to social functioning, including communication, language, and social interactions. Repetitive/stereotyped behaviors and interests as well as sensory issues (i.e., hypersensitivity, hyposensitivity) also are prominent. Comorbid intellectual disability, neurological and medical problems, and an increased risk of psychiatric disorders are frequently present in ASD. Both core and associated features can vary dramatically among individuals. In addition, timing of onset can differ, as about one quarter of children with ASD are noted to lose skills after developing normally for as long as 2 yr, whereas others present with delays across most developmental domains within the first yr of life. The diagnosis of ASD can accurately be made by 3 yr of age. However, gender and cognitive, linguistic, and adaptive functioning impact ASD presentation and can affect age of diagnosis. DSM-5 criteria no longer differentiate separate disorders. Instead, an overarching diagnosis of ASD is given; severity levels (1, 2, or 3) have been introduced to identify the magnitude of social and behavioral impairment and the support required to ensure the safety and well-being of the individual. Specifiers have been added to capture associated features (e.g., intellectual disability, language impairment, medical or genetic conditions, and catatonia).

SYNONYMS

ASD
Autism
Autistic disorder
Early infantile autism
Childhood autism
Kanner autism
Asperger disorder
Pervasive developmental disorder
PDD NOS

ICD-10CM CODES
F84.0 Autism spectrum disorder
DSM-5 CODES
299.00 Autism spectrum disorder

EPIDEMIOLOGY & DEMOGRAPHICS

INCIDENCE (IN U.S.): Autism spectrum disorder afflicts approximately 1% of children in the United States.

PEAK INCIDENCE: Before age 3 yr

PREVALENCE: 1:68 (1:42 for boys, 1:189 for girls). It is unclear whether the increase in prevalence reflects an expansion of the diagnosis to include subthreshold cases, increased awareness of the disorder, improvement in diagnostic accuracy, changes in public policy related to service eligibility, or a true increase in the frequency of autism spectrum disorder.

PREDOMINANT SEX AND AGE: Male/female ratio of 2-5:1. Lifelong.

GENETICS:

- Autism spectrum disorder is highly inheritable with a heritability index of 82% to 90%.
- The concordance rate for ASD varies across studies and ranges from 36% to 95% for monozygotic twins; the concordance rate is estimated between 20% and 40% for dizygotic twins and between 10% and 20% for non-twin siblings.
- Copy number variants (CVNs) account for 10% to 20% of autism spectrum disorder cases, but each CNV is rare (no more than 1% of cases). Rare chromosomal abnormalities account for about 10% of cases, but each type is rare (no more than 1% of cases).
- Common genetic variants acting in an additive manner account for approximately 35% of cases. Research has identified approximately 1000 gene mutations as being possibly contributory, but only about 20 of them have been associated with ASD with "high confidence."
- In the remaining cases, ASD is suggested to arise from a combination of unknown genetic variations, environmental influences, and epigenetic factors.

RISK FACTORS:
Prenatal and perinatal risk factors identified include hypoxia-related obstetric complications, use of valproic acid during pregnancy, use of thalidomide during pregnancy, advanced parental age, multiple birth, prematurity, congenital sensory deficits, and significant exposure to air pollutions (during pregnancy and in the postnatal period). However, it is not established whether these are causal factors.

PHYSICAL FINDINGS & CLINICAL PRESENTATION

- Common triad of marked impairment in social interactions (poor social-emotional reciprocity), impaired and atypical verbal and nonverbal communication, and repetitive and unusual behavior or play.
- Marked impairment in the understanding and use of both verbal and nonverbal communication, including unchanging facial expression and lack of gestures during interactions.
- Stereotypic behavior (i.e., hand flapping, body rocking) or language (i.e., echolalia, palilalia).
- Perceptual hypersensitivity (i.e., auditory, tactile, olfactory, gustatory) and avoidance of novel stimuli; or perceptual hyposensitivity (e.g., abnormally high threshold for pain).
- Brain abnormalities have been identified at anatomical and functional levels; abnormalities are detected as early as the first yr of

BOX 1 Autism Spectrum Disorder Case Determination Criteria Under DSM-5

DSM-5 behavioral criteria	
A. Persistent deficits in social communication and social interaction	A1: Deficits in social emotional reciprocity A2. Deficits in nonverbal communicative behaviors A3. Deficits in developing, maintaining, and understanding relationships
B. Restricted, repetitive patterns of behavior, interests, or activities, currently or by history	B1: Stereotyped or repetitive motor movements, use of objects or speech B2. Insistence on sameness, inflexible adherence to routines, or ritualized patterns of verbal or nonverbal behavior B3. Highly restricted interests that are abnormal in intensity or focus B4. Hyper- or hyporeactivity to sensory input or unusual interest in sensory aspects of the environment
Historical PDD diagnosis	Any ASD diagnosis documented in a comprehensive evaluation, including a DSM-IV diagnosis of autistic disorder, Asperger disorder, or pervasive developmental disorder–not otherwise specified (PDD-NOS)
DSM-5 case determination	All three behavioral criteria coded under part A, and at least two behavioral criteria coded under part B OR Any ASD diagnosis documented in a comprehensive evaluation, whether based on DSM-IV-TR or DSM-5 diagnostic criteria Note: A child might be disqualified from meeting the DSM-5 surveillance case definition for ASD if, based on the clinical judgment of one or more reviewers, there is insufficient or conflicting information in support of ASD, sufficient information to rule out ASD, or if one or more other diagnosed conditions better account for the child's symptoms.

DSM-IV, *Diagnostic and Statistical Manual of Mental Disorders, Fourth Edition*; DSM-IV-TR, *Diagnostic and Statistical Manual of Mental Disorders, Fourth Edition, Text Revision*; DSM-5, *Diagnostic and Statistical Manual of Mental Disorders, Fifth Edition*; *PDD*, pervasive developmental disorder.

Baio J, et al.: Prevalence of autism spectrum disorder among children aged 8 years — Autism and Developmental Disabilities Monitoring Network, 11 Sites, United States, 2014. *MMWR Surveill Summ* 67(No. SS-6):1-23, 2018. DOI: https://dx.doi.org/10.15585/mmwr.ss6706a1.

BOX 2 Red Flags for Social Communication Development

Prompt evaluation should occur for any of the following: **No vocalizations by 6 months:** *A parent should be able to have a reciprocal "conversation" by this age, consisting of at least several volleys back and forth.* **No polysyllabic consonant babbling by 12 months:** *At least some of these vocalizations should be directed at someone with communicative intent.* **No gestures by 12 months:** *The earliest gesture an infant learns is to raise his/her arms to request to be picked up, usually once sitting independently. Pointing should be with an isolated index finger, not the whole hand, and should be used "to request" or "to show," not just pointing at pictures in a book or pointing to have an adult label items. Any use of hand-over-hand by the child (e.g., putting a parent's hand on the cabinet door where the cookies are kept or using the parent's hand to point at pictures in a book) is a hallmark of ASD.* **No spontaneous (not echoed) single words by 16 months other than mama or dada:** *Spontaneous words must be beyond those used to simply label items and must be used by the child to communicate, to request, to show, or to share.* **No spontaneous (not echoed) phrases by 24 months or sentences by 36 months:** *Spontaneous phrases and sentences must be used by the child to communicate, to request, to show, or to share.* **Any loss of social communication abilities, including babbling, single words, phrases, response to name, social engagement, or gestures:** *If a parent reports their infant has decreased or stopped any social communication milestones, this is usually the hallmark of the onset of regression.*

Swaiman KF, et al.: *Swaiman's pediatric neurology, principles and practice*, ed 6, Philadelphia, 2017, Elsevier.

life and are accompanied by atypical brain maturation trajectories.
- No biomarkers have been identified.

ETIOLOGY

- Majority of cases are not associated with a comorbid medical condition
- High prevalence of comorbid seizure disorder (25%) and/or intellectual disability (up to 75%)
- Sometimes present in the context of medical conditions (e.g., encephalitis, cytomegalovirus, toxoplasmosis, phenylketonuria [PKU], fragile X syndrome, tuberous sclerosis complex, neurofibromatosis)
- Numerous studies have shown **no** association between immunizations (specifically MMR vaccine) or thimerosal-containing vaccines (i.e., DPT) and autism spectrum disorder

Dx DIAGNOSIS

DIFFERENTIAL DIAGNOSIS

- Several genetic syndromes manifest with a phenotype similar to ASD (e.g., 22q11.2 deletion syndrome, Angelman syndrome, Aicardi syndrome, Cornelia de Lange syndrome, Christianson syndrome, fragile X syndrome, Landau-Kleffner syndrome, Klinefelter syndrome, neurofibromatosis, Prader-Willi syndrome, Rett syndrome, tuberous sclerosis complex, Williams syndrome).
- Several psychiatric or neurodevelopmental disorders present with symptoms similar to ASD (e.g., Tourette syndrome, selective mutism, social phobia, obsessive/compulsive disorder, expressive language disorder, mixed receptive-expressive language disorder, stereotypic movement disorder, intellectual disability). Differences are notable in onset of symptoms and developmental trajectories.
- Social (pragmatic) communication disorder, introduced in DSM-5 and characterized by significant difficulties with verbal and nonverbal communication.
- Childhood-onset schizophrenia: Follows period of normal development.
- Attachment disorders (reactive attachment disorder, disinhibited social engagement disorder); individuals with these disorders can present with language delays, cognitive delays, social difficulties, and stereotypies. Differences are notable before 5 yr of age.

WORKUP

- Rule out underlying medical condition, including genetic syndromes.
- "Red flags" for critical delays in social communication development should be recognized or queried and should initiate evaluation for an ASD (Box 2). Validated autism spectrum disorder–specific screening tools are available for children age ≥18 mo. All children should be screened specifically for autism spectrum disorder at 18 and 24 mo. General developmental screening tools are currently used in children 9 to 18 mo.
- Gold standard assessment includes detailed developmental and family history, assessment of developmental/intellectual functioning, assessment of ASD symptomatology, and assessment of adaptive behaviors.
- Additional workup may include assessment of language functioning, neuropsychological functioning, and psychiatric presentation.

LABORATORY TESTS

- PKU screen (usually done at birth in the United States)
- Lead exposure screening
- Audiology testing for young children with autism spectrum disorder; school-based hearing screening may be sufficient in older children with autism spectrum disorders and without significant language or learning deficits
- Karyotype, chromosome microarray analysis, and DNA testing for fragile X syndrome in both boys and girls, as well as for different de novo copy number variants or mutations in specific genes associated with the disorder

IMAGING STUDIES

- EEG to diagnose coexisting seizure disorder if seizures are suspected or if language regression is present (i.e., Landau-Kleffner syndrome)
- Brain MRI if tuberous sclerosis complex or Aicardi syndrome (callosal agenesis) is suspected

Rx TREATMENT

NONPHARMACOLOGIC THERAPY

- Consistent behavioral training program in both the home and school environments.
- A number of treatment programs have been developed; many are based on applied behavioral analysis (ABA) (e.g., Discrete Trial Training); others combine ABA procedures with social-emotional development (e.g., Pivotal Response Training, Floortime, Early Start Denver Model).
- Special educational program focused on language and communication skills, social and life skills development (e.g., TEACCH).
- Cognitive Behavioral Therapy (CBT) has proven effective to ameliorate symptoms of anxiety in higher functioning individuals with ASD.
- Highly structured home environment.
- Education for families and teachers; the Autism Speaks™ website may be helpful in this regard: http://www.autismspeaks.org/about_us.php.

ACUTE GENERAL Rx

- Obsessive or ritualistic behaviors: Selective serotonin reuptake inhibitors (SSRIs), atypical antipsychotics, valproic acid
- Aggression, irritability, self-injury: Atypical antipsychotic agents (e.g., risperidone), anticonvulsant mood stabilizers, SSRIs, beta-blockers, opiate antagonist (self-injury only)
- Hyperactivity, impulsivity, inattention: Stimulants, α-2 adrenergic agonists, atypical antipsychotics
- Anxiety: SSRIs, buspirone, mirtazapine
- Mood lability: Valproic acid, carbamazepine, lithium, aripiprazole
- Depression: SSRIs, mirtazapine
- Only risperidone and aripiprazole are FDA-approved for the management of symptoms associated with ASD
- Medications used to decrease specific symptoms associated with Autism Spectrum Disorder are summarized in Table 1

CHRONIC Rx

- Extended use of medications for acute management of comorbid psychiatric disorder
- Use of medications for comorbid medical conditions, including sleep problems and gastrointestinal problems
- Pharmacotherapy is palliative, not curative, of autism spectrum disorder

COMPLEMENTARY AND ALTERNATIVE MEDICINE (CAM)

- Preliminary evidence is available for effectiveness of melatonin in ameliorating sleep problems.

TABLE 1 Medications Used to Decrease Specific Symptoms Associated with Autism Spectrum Disorder *

Drug	Dose	Age†	N	Efficacy	Side Effects
Neuroleptic Agents					
Risperidone	0.25-2.5 mg/d <20 kg 0.5-2.5 mg/d 20-45 kg 0.5-3.5 mg/d >45 kg Mean = 2.4 mg/d	5-17	101	Decreased tantrums, aggression, self-injury, hyperactivity	Weight gain; increased appetite; transient sedation
Risperidone	1.2-2.9 mg/d child Mean = 2.0 mg/d 2.4-5.3 mg/d adult Mean = 3.6 mg/d	8-56	36	Decreased irritability, hyperactivity	Increased appetite; weight gain; sedation
Risperidone	0.125–0.175 vs. 1.25-1.75 vs. placebo	5-17	96	Higher dose improves global function and irritability	Somnolence sedation increased appetite
Risperidone	0.01-0.06 mg/kg/d Mean = 1.17 mg/d	5-12	79	Decreased irritability, hyperactivity, noncompliance, conduct problems	Weight gain; transient somnolence; mildly increased heart rate and blood pressure
Risperidone	0.5-1.5 mg/d Mean = 1.14 mg/d	2.5-6	24	Minimal improvement in global autism severity scores	Weight gain; increased prolactin levels
Risperidone	1.0-10.0 mg/d	18-43	n =?	Reduced repetitive behavior, aggression, self-injury, property destruction	Transient sedation
Aripiprazole	5 mg/d, 10 mg/d, or 15 mg/d	6-17	218	Reduced irritability, hyperactivity, stereotypy at all doses	Sedation, EPS, weight gain
Aripiprazole	2-15 mg/d	6-17	98	Reduced irritability, hyperactivity, stereotypy, inappropriate speech; global improvement	Decreased prolactin level, weight gain, EPS
Aripiprazole	2-15 mg/d Continuation active tx vs. placebo	6-17	85	No difference in time to relapse	
Opiate Antagonists					
Naltrexone	1.0 mg/kg/d	3-8	41	No improvement over placebo in behavior and learning; improved hyperactivity	None greater than placebo
Naltrexone	1.0 mg/kg/d 2 weeks only	3-8	24	No improvement in communication skills	Transient sedation
Naltrexone	40 mg/d Single dose	3-7	23	Decreased hyperactivity, improved attention	Not reported
Naltrexone	1 mg/kg/dose	3-7	23	Decreased hyperactivity and improved attention by teacher, but not parent, report	No side effects
Serotonin Reuptake Inhibitors					
Fluvoxamine	Mean dose = 276.7 mg/d	18-53	n = 30	Reduced repetitive thoughts and behavior, and aggression; improved social communication	Transient nausea and sedation
Buspirone	2.5 mg or 5 mg/d	2-6	166	Improvement in repetitive behaviors not total ADOS	
Clomipramine	5-10 mg/d	8-17	34	No improvement executive function	Diarrhea, headache, fatigue
Fluoxetine	4.8-20 mg/d Mean = 10.6 mg/d; 0.38 mg/kg/d	5-17	39	Modest reduction in repetitive behaviors, but no improvement in global functioning	Agitation requiring dose reduction
Citalopram	2.5-20 mg/d Mean = 16.5 mg/d	5-17	149	No improvement in repetitive behavior or global functioning	Increased energy, inattention, impulsivity, hyperactivity, stereotypy, diarrhea, insomnia, dry skin
Stimulants					
Methylphenidate	0.125, 0.25, or 0.5 t.i.d. mg/kg/day	5-14	72	Reduced inattention, distractibility, hyperactivity, and impulsivity	Irritability, decreased appetite, difficulty falling asleep, emotional outbursts
Methylphenidate	0.25, 0.5 mg/kg/dose	5-13	33	Positive efforts on social behavior	None discussed
Methylphenidate	10-40 LA AM, 2.5-10 mg afternoon	7-13	24	Decreased hyperactive and impulsive behavior	Loss of appetite, insomnia
Atomoxetine	20-100 mg/d Mean = 44.2 mg/d	5-15	16	Reduced hyperactivity, impulsivity, social withdrawal	Transient nausea and fatigue
Antiseizure Drugs					
Lamotrigine	Mean = 5.0 mg/kg/d	3-11	28	No improvement greater than placebo in disruptive behavior and autism symptoms	Aggression, insomnia, echolalia
Levetiracetam	20-30 mg/kg/d	5-17	20	No improvement in disruptive behavior or irritability	Aggression, agitation
Divalproex sodium	500-1500 mg/d	5-17	13	Reduction in compulsive-type repetitive behavior	Irritability, weight gain, aggression
Divalproex sodium	125 mg QD titrated up to 500 bid	5-17	27	Reduction in irritability	Irritability
Bumetanide	0.5mg bid	3-11	60	Improved autistic behaviors and global function	Diarrhea, increased irritability

ADOS, Autism Diagnostic Observation Schedule; *EPS*, extrapyramidal symptoms; *LA AM*, L-alpha-acetylmethadol; *QD*, every day; *t.i.d.*, three times per day; *tx*, treatment.
*Includes only double-blind, randomized, placebo-controlled trials.
†Age in years.
Swaiman KF, et al.: *Swaiman's pediatric neurology, principles and practice*, ed 6, Philadelphia, 2017, Elsevier.

- Very limited rigorous evidence is available on the effectiveness of CAM, including nutritional interventions.

DISPOSITION

- Most children will require some degree of assistance as adults.
- DSM-5 identifies 3 severity levels based on social communication and restricted, repetitive behaviors: Level 1 (requiring support), Level 2 (requiring substantial support), and Level 3 (requiring very substantial support).
- With early diagnosis and proper treatment/support, the prognosis for children without language and intellectual impairment is fair to very good despite lifelong symptoms.
- Poorer outcomes include a lack of joint attention by age 4 yr, a lack of functional speech by age 5 yr, intellectual disability, seizures, comorbid medical or psychiatric syndromes, and a pervasive lack of social relatedness.
- Best outcomes are associated with early identification and treatment, the development of oral communication skills, and the cognitive and behavioral capacity for inclusion in regular education settings with typically developing peers.

REFERRAL

Assistance may be needed in diagnosis (child psychiatrist, clinical psychologist, geneticist, pediatric neurologist, developmental pediatrician), symptom management (speech language pathologist, occupational therapist, clinical psychologist), parental teaching (clinical psychologist, psychiatric social worker), and intervention with the school system (educational advocate, attorney).

PEARLS & CONSIDERATIONS

- There is no scientific evidence of a relation between childhood vaccination and the development of autism spectrum disorder.
- Evidence suggests that a disproportionate number of children with autism spectrum disorder suffer from a variety of medical problems including sleep difficulties, gastrointestinal problems, and oral health problems.
- Psychiatric comorbidities are very prominent across the life span, with estimated prevalence ranging from 30% to 70%.
- The new U.S. Preventive Services Task Force (USPSTF) recommendation on screening for autism spectrum disorder (ASD) in young children concludes that the current evidence is insufficient to assess the balance of benefits and harms of screening for ASD in young children for whom no concerns of ASD have been raised by their parents or a clinician.
- A recent trial has shown that daily intranasal oxytocin improves social behavior in kids with ASD whose baseline endogenous blood oxytocin levels are low.[1]

SUGGESTED READINGS

Available at ExpertConsult.com

RELATED CONTENT

Autism (Patient Information)

AUTHOR: **GIULIA RIGHI, PH.D.**

[1] Parker KJ, et al.: Intranasal oxytocin treatment for social deficits and biomarkers of response in children with autism. *Proc Natl Acad Sci USA* 114:8119, 2017.

BASIC INFORMATION

DEFINITION

Autoimmune hepatitis (AIH) is a chronic inflammatory condition of the liver characterized by elevated serum globulin levels (IgG), presence of circulating autoantibodies, interface hepatitis on histology, and plasma cell rich infiltrate. Three types have been described:

- Type 1, or "classic," autoimmune hepatitis is the most predominant form in the U.S. and worldwide (80%) and has a bimodal age distribution with peaks between 10 and 20 and 45 and 70 years of age. Patients are positive for antinuclear antibodies (ANA) and/or antismooth muscle antibodies (ASMA) and have specific associated HLA haplotypes: DR3, DR4, DR13. Usually excellent treatment response, but variable relapse rates after drug withdrawal; usually need for long-term maintenance therapy.
- Type 2, up to 10% of AIH cases, primarily affects young children between 2 and 14 years of age, and is characterized by the presence of antibodies to liver/kidney microsomes (anti-LKM-1) or liver cytosol 1. Patients have associated HLA haplotypes: DR3 and DR7. This form is generally more advanced at presentation and is more difficult to treat; need for long-term maintenance therapy is very common.
- Type 3, up to 10% of AIH cases, only SLA/LP positive, otherwise very similar to AIH-1. Often Ro52-antibody positive. Lifelong immunosuppression in most, if not all patients.

SYNONYMS

Autoimmune chronic active hepatitis
AIH
Chronic active hepatitis
Lupoid hepatitis
Plasma cell hepatitis

ICD-10CM CODES

K75.4 Autoimmune hepatitis
K73.2 Chronic active hepatitis, not elsewhere classified

EPIDEMIOLOGY & DEMOGRAPHICS

- Annual incidence (estimated): 0.2 to 2.0 cases per 100,000, similar to PBC, more common than PSC.
- Point prevalence (estimated): 16.9 per 100,000.
- Type 1: Age of onset has a bimodal distribution with peaks between 10 and 20 and 45 and 70 yr.
- Type 2: More common in young children 2-14 years of age.
- Female/male ratio is 3.6:1; type 1 has an 80% female predominance, whereas type 2 has a 90% female predominance.
- Approximately 100,000 to 200,000 persons affected in the U.S.
- Accounts for 4% to 6% of liver transplants in the U.S.
- Associated with HLA-DRB1*0301 and HLA-DRB1*0401 alleles.

CLINICAL PRESENTATION

- Varies from intermittent asymptomatic elevations of liver enzymes to advanced cirrhosis. One third of adults and one half of child patients with AIH have cirrhosis at presentation. AIH can also present initially as a fulminant hepatitis.
- Symptoms may include fatigue, anorexia, nausea, abdominal pain, pruritus, and arthralgia.
- Autoimmune findings may include arthritis, xerostomia, keratoconjunctivitis, cutaneous vasculitis, and erythema nodosum.
- Patients with advanced disease can show hepatosplenomegaly, ascites, peripheral edema, abnormal bleeding, and jaundice.

ETIOLOGY

- Exact etiology is unknown; liver histology demonstrates cell-mediated immune attack against hepatocytes.
- Presence of a variety of autoantibodies suggests an autoimmune mechanism.
- There are likely two components involved: genetic predisposition and an inciting environmental trigger.
- Potential triggering agents such as viruses (hepatitis A, B, C) or drugs (minocycline, nitrofurantoin, biological agents, TNF-blockade) likely possess some homology similar to liver-specific antigens.

Dx DIAGNOSIS

- A simplified diagnostic criteria for routine clinical practice has been developed by the International Autoimmune Hepatitis Group (see Table 1).
- Histology: Lymphoplasmacytic infiltrate invading the hepatocyte boundary surrounding the portal triad (limiting plate). Also, a periportal infiltrate may be seen (interface hepatitis).
- The European Association for the Study of the Liver guidelines require liver biopsy as part of the diagnostic evaluation.
- The American Association for the Study of Liver Disease (AASLD) approach is to obtain a liver biopsy if the diagnosis is unclear or to assess disease activity prior to initiating treatment.

DIFFERENTIAL DIAGNOSIS

- Acute viral hepatitis (A, B, C, D, E, cytomegalovirus, Epstein-Barr, herpes)
- Chronic viral hepatitis (B, C)
- Toxic hepatitis (alcohol, drugs)
- Primary biliary cirrhosis
- Primary sclerosing cholangitis
- Hemochromatosis
- Nonalcoholic steatohepatitis
- Systemic lupus erythematosus
- Wilson's disease
- Alpha-1 antitrypsin deficiency

WORKUP

- History and physical examination with attention to the presence of autoimmune abnormalities such as autoimmune thyroiditis, Graves disease, inflammatory bowel disease, celiac sprue, and rheumatoid arthritis. Fig. 1 illustrates a diagnostic algorithm for autoimmune hepatitis.
- Liver function tests and serum gamma-globulins.
- Tests for autoantibodies: ANA, ASMA, anti-LKM.
- Liver biopsy for establishing diagnosis and disease severity.

LABORATORY TESTS

- Aminotransferases generally elevated and may fluctuate
- Bilirubin and alkaline phosphatase moderately elevated or normal
- Elevation of gamma globulin (>2.0 g/dl [20 g/L]) and immunoglobulin G
- Circulating autoantibodies (Table E2) often present:
  1. Rheumatoid factor
  2. ANA
     a. Present in two thirds of patients
     b. Typical pattern is homogeneous or speckled
     c. Titer does not correlate with the stage, activity, or prognosis
  3. Anti-SMA
     a. Present in 87% of patients
     b. Titer does not correlate with course or prognosis
  4. Anti-LKM antibodies
     a. Typically found in patients who are ANA negative and SMA negative
     b. Characterizes type 2 AIH
     c. Present in pediatric population and up to 20% of adults in Europe; also present in patients with drug-induced hepatitis

TABLE 1 Simplified Diagnostic Criteria for Autoimmune Hepatitis

Variable	Cutoff	Points	Cutoff	Points
ANA or SMA	≥1:40	1	≥1:80	2
LKM			≥1:40	2
SLA			Positive	2
IgG	≥ULN	1	≥1.1 × ULN	2
Histology	Compatible with AIH	1	Typical of AIH	2
Absence of viral hepatitis			Yes	2

Maximum number of points for all antibodies = 2, total = 8. Probable AIH ≥6 points, definite AIH ≥7 points. 88% sensitivity and 97% specificity. *AIH*, Autoimmune hepatitis; *ANA*, antinuclear antibody; *IgG*, immunoglobulin G; *LKM*, liver/kidney microsomes; *SLA*, soluble liver antigen; *SMA*, smooth muscle antibody; *ULN*, upper limit of normal.

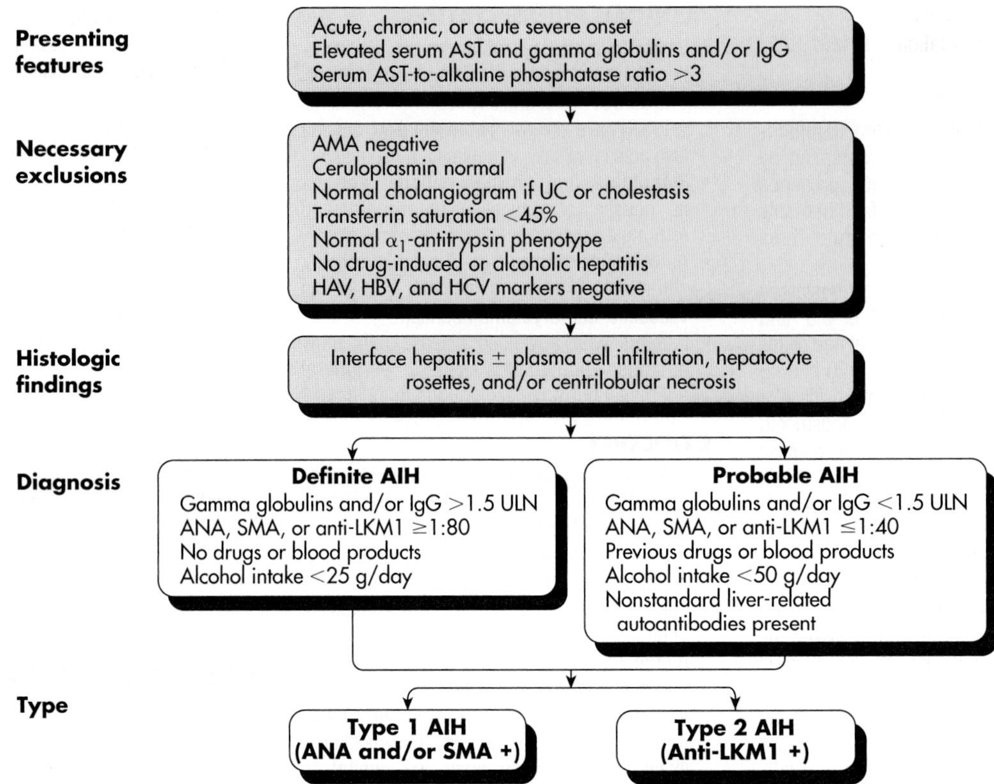

FIG. 1 Diagnostic algorithm for autoimmune hepatitis (AIH). The diagnosis requires predominant elevation of the serum AST level and exclusion of other hepatic diseases (especially PBC, PSC, Wilson disease, hemochromatosis, α1-antitrypsin deficiency, drug-induced or alcoholic hepatitis, and viral hepatitis). Antimitochondrial antibodies (AMA) should be absent; cholangiography should be negative in patients with concurrent UC or cholestasis; and the serologic markers of HAV, HBV, and HCV should be negative. Interface hepatitis should be present on histologic examination, and laboratory manifestations of immune reactivity should be evident by abnormal elevation of the serum gamma globulin and/or immunoglobulin G (IgG) level and the presence of antinuclear antibodies (ANA), smooth muscle antibodies (SMA), or antibodies to liver kidney microsome type 1 (anti-LKM1). The degree of immune reactivity and the presence of confounding etiologic factors, such as alcohol and drug or blood product exposure, distinguish definite from probable AIH. Classification as type 1 AIH or type 2 AIH is based on the type of autoantibodies that predominate in the disease. *AST*, Aspartate aminotransferase; *HAV*, Hepatitis A virus; *HBV*, hepatitis B virus; *HCV*, hepatitis C virus; *ULN*, upper limit of normal. (From Feldman M, Friedman LS, Brandt LJ: *Sleisenger and Fortran's gastrointestinal and liver disease*, ed 10, Philadelphia, 2016, Elsevier.)

5. Autoantibodies against soluble liver antigen and liver-pancreas antigen (anti-SLA/LP)
   a. Present in 10% to 30% of patients
   b. Associated with higher rate of relapse after corticosteroid therapy
   c. Several studies suggest that patients with anti-SLA/LP have a more severe course

Serum p-ANCA levels are useful for diagnosis of the 10% to 15% of patients with negative ASMA, negative ANA, and low gamma globulin levels

- Hypoalbuminemia and prolonged prothrombin time with advanced disease
- There is a well-described overlap syndrome with primary biliary cirrhosis (7%), primary sclerosing cholangitis (6%), and autoimmune cholangitis (11%). In patients who do not respond to therapy after 3 months, consider cholangiographic studies to evaluate for primary sclerosing cholangitis

IMAGING STUDIES

- Ultrasound of liver and biliary tree to rule out obstruction or hepatic mass.
- Cirrhosis secondary to AIH is a risk factor for development of hepatocellular carcinoma (although less so than viral hepatitis). Patients with cirrhosis should get ultrasonography and AFP every 6 months.

Rx TREATMENT

NONPHARMACOLOGIC THERAPY

- Avoid alcohol and hepatotoxic medications.
- Liver transplantation is an option for end-stage disease or fulminant hepatic failure.

PHARMACOLOGIC THERAPY

- Initial treatment:
  1. Predniso(lo)ne 0.5 to 1 mg/kg/day followed by addition of azathioprine when bilirubin levels are <6 mg/dl, ideally 2 wk after initiation of steroid treatment. Initial dose 50 mg/day, increase depending on toxicity and response up to 1-2 mg/kg. A combination of oral budesonide (6-9 mg/day) and azathioprine (1-2 mg/kg/day) can be used to induce and maintain remission in patients with non-cirrhotic AIH, with a lower rate of steroid-specific side effects. Treatment of AIH should be response-guided, and regimens should be individualized. Steroids are contraindicated in brittle diabetes mellitus, uncontrolled hypertension, prior steroid intolerance, severe osteopenia, and psychosis. Azathioprine is contraindicated by thiopurine S-methyltransferase (TPMT) deficiency, leukopenia, or thrombocytopenia. Budesonide is contraindicated in cirrhosis because portal systemic shunting and abnormal hepatic metabolism prevent complete hepatic first-pass extraction, reducing therapeutic efficacy and causing systemic steroid side effects.
  2. Combination therapy allows lower prednisone doses, fewer steroid side effects, and faster normalization of LFTs.
- The primary goal of therapy in AIH is to achieve remission. The 2010 AASLD Practice Guideline (2010 PG) redefined remission to require: normal levels of AST, ALT (optimally <19 U/L in women and <30 U/L in men), total bilirubin, gamma-globulin or IgG and absence of inflammatory activity on liver biopsy. Secondary goals of therapy are the prevention of progression of fibrosis to cirrhosis and reversion of cirrhosis to a lower stage of fibrosis, which has been documented.
- Indications for treatment:
  1. Serum aminotransferases >10 times the upper limit of normal
  2. Serum aminotransferases >5 times the upper limit of normal, with serum gamma-globulin level twice the upper limit of normal
  3. Histologic features of bridging necrosis

4. Symptomatic disease: Incapacitating symptoms such as fatigue and arthralgia
- Relative indications:
  1. Asymptomatic patients with elevated liver enzymes or limited histological activity
- Treatment not indicated:
  1. Inactive cirrhosis
- Evaluation of treatment response:
  1. Goals are the absence of symptoms, normalization of liver function tests, and absence of inflammatory activity on liver biopsy. Generally, this is a steroid-responsive condition, but up to 20% do not respond.
  2. Patients whose transaminase levels normalize may continue to have ongoing active hepatitis involving inflammation and fibrosis.
  3. Histologic improvement may lag behind clinical and laboratory improvement by as much as 6 mo. Because of this, repeat liver biopsy should be considered after normalization of transaminase levels. A review of AIH studies between 1972 and 2013 shows that hepatic fibrosis improves in 53% to 57% of cases and that progressive fibrosis is slowed or prevented in 79% of patients.
  4. After initial remission is achieved, one may consider tapering medications. Steroid withdrawal should be done only if liver function tests normalize and histologic quiescence is achieved. About 50% to 86% of patients will relapse after this and require long-term maintenance medications.
  5. Complete normalization on biopsy is associated with a 15% to 20% risk of relapse, whereas persistent interface hepatitis is associated with a 90% risk of relapse. Do not attempt multiple treatment withdrawals. The risk of developing cirrhosis with single relapse is 9.5%, whereas multiple relapses are associated with 37.5% risk of developing cirrhosis. The patient with sustained remission has a risk of cirrhosis of 4.5%.
  6. Suboptimal response: A failure to adequate response should lead to a reconsideration of the diagnosis or re-evaluation of adherence to treatment. In patients with suboptimal response despite reconfirmation of diagnosis and adherence, doses of prednisolone and azathioprine should be increased, or alternative medications should be used. Patients with acute severe AIH should be treated with high doses of intravenous corticosteroids (>1 mg/kg) as early as possible. Lack of improvement within 7 days should lead to consideration of emergency liver transplantation.

DISPOSITION

- Long-term treatment may be necessary for sustained remission in individuals who continuously relapse and in partial responders.
- Sixty-five percent of patients achieve remission by 18 months; 80% achieve remission by 3 years.
- Approximately 10% to 15% of patients do not respond to conventional therapy. The risk factors for nonresponse include presence of underlying cirrhosis, younger age, or longer duration of disease, HLA-B8 or DR3. High-dose therapy can achieve remission in 70%: Prednisone 60 mg or dual therapy with prednisone 30 mg and AZA 150 mg. Other alternatives such as mycophenolate, the calcineurin inhibitors (CNIs), tacrolimus (TAC) and cyclosporine (CSA), sirolimus (SIR), everolimus (EVR), rituximab, and infliximab, have been used successfully. However, none of the alternative therapies has been studied in multicenter, randomized, controlled trials.
- Orthotopic liver transplantation (OLT) is a life-saving option for AIH patients with acute liver failure, decompensated cirrhosis, or HCC. Allograft and patient survival are excellent; however, AIH recurs in the allograft in a minority (25% probability in first 5 years, 50% in 10 years).

REFERRAL

Patients with advanced cirrhosis or who progress to end-stage liver disease are candidates for liver transplantation and should be referred to appropriate medical centers that provide liver transplantation services.

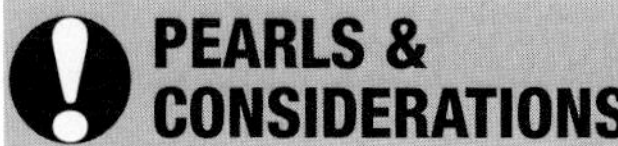

PEARLS & CONSIDERATIONS

COMMENTS

- ANA and SMA are observed together in 60% of cases. Serum titers >1:40 suggest autoimmune hepatitis.
- A variety of autoimmune conditions can be seen in association with autoimmune hepatitis, including thyroiditis, Graves disease, ulcerative colitis, rheumatoid arthritis, uveitis, pernicious anemia, Sjögren's syndrome, mixed connective tissue disease, CREST syndrome, and vitiligo.
- Variant forms of autoimmune hepatitis (overlap syndrome) have clinical and serologic findings of autoimmune hepatitis plus features of other forms of chronic liver disease such as primary biliary cirrhosis (PBC) or primary sclerosing cholangitis (PSC).

PREVENTION

None

PATIENT & FAMILY EDUCATION

- American Liver Foundation (ALF): Phone: 800-GO-LIVER (465-4837); Internet: www.liverfoundation.org
- National Digestive Diseases Information clearinghouse: http://digestive.niddk.nih.gov/ddiseases/pubs/autoimmunehep

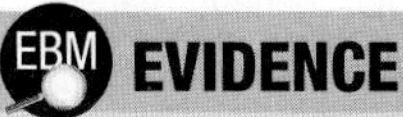

EVIDENCE

Available at ExpertConsult.com

SUGGESTED READINGS

Available at ExpertConsult.com

RELATED CONTENT

Autoimmune Hepatitis (Patient Information).

AUTHORS: **ANDREEA M. CATANA, M.D,** and **KITTICHAI PROMRAT, M.D.**

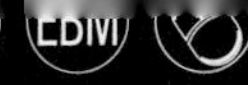

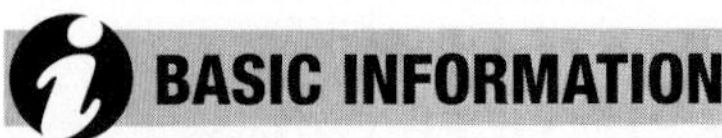

BASIC INFORMATION

DEFINITION

Autosomal dominant polycystic kidney disease (ADPKD) is a systemic inherited disorder due to mutations of either the *PKD1* or *PKD2* gene. These mutations lead to multiple cyst formations and growth in multiple organs including the kidneys, liver, and pancreas. ADPKD is also associated with multiple gastrointestinal and cardiovascular abnormalities. It is the most common inherited kidney disease, and its prevalence is greater than Huntington disease, hemophilia, sickle cell disease, cystic fibrosis, myotonic dystrophy, and Down syndrome combined.

SYNONYMS

Adult polycystic kidney disease
Polycystic kidney disease
ADPKD

ICD-10CM CODES

Q61.3	Polycystic kidney, unspecified
Q61.2	Polycystic kidney, adult type
Q61.19	Other polycystic kidney, infantile type
Z82.71	Family history of polycystic kidney

EPIDEMIOLOGY & DEMOGRAPHICS

- Most common, single, genetic cause of chronic kidney disease (CKD).
- Mendelian dominant disorder: Each child of an affected parent has a 50% chance of inheriting the mutated gene.
- Affects all ethnic groups equally worldwide.
- Approximately 85 percent of ADPKD individuals have a mutation on chromosome 16 (*PKD1* locus), and 15% have a mutation located on chromosome 4 in the *PKD2* gene. A growing number of the ADPKD population have mutations in the glucosidase, alpha, neutral AB form (*GANAB*) gene located on chromosome 11q12.3.
- The disease has 100% penetrance and does not skip generations.

INCIDENCE:

- Between 1 in 400 and 1000 live births in the U.S.

GENETICS: ADPKD is caused by a mutation in the *PKD1* gene, located on the short arm of chromosome 16, which lies next to the tuberous sclerosis complex 2 gene (*TSC2*). The gene encoding polycystin-1 (PC1) plays a vital role in cell-cell and cell-matrix interactions, and primary ciliary function. Mutations in *PKD1* lead to an alteration in the differentiation of epithelial cells and the abnormal phenotypic expressions characteristic of ADPKD. ADPKD is less commonly caused by a mutation in the *PKD2* gene located on chromosome 4. *PKD2* encodes the protein polycystin-2 (PC2), which is involved in intracellular calcium signaling. *PKD2* patients typically have milder disease with later onset of end-stage renal disease (ESRD), death, and hypertension. Polycystins 1 and 2 form a single functional complex through interactions of their intracellular carboxy termini. Consequently, a mutation of either *PKD1* or *PKD2* results in a similar phenotype.

ADPKD is also caused by mutations in the *GANAB* gene in up to 3% of ADPKD patients. This gene is located on chromosome 11q12.3 and is expressed in kidney and liver. *GANAB* encodes the catalytic subunit of glucosidase II (GIIα). GII is thought to play an important role in PC1 maturation. Cystogenesis is likely caused by defects in protein maturation and cell surface localization of polycystin 1 and polycystin 2. Usually patients with ADPKD who have mutations in *GANAB* have mild PKD and mild to severe polycystic liver disease.

CLINICAL PRESENTATION

ADPKD-related symptoms reflect kidney cyst burden and extrarenal involvement, including polycystic liver disease and vascular complications (Fig. 1). Total kidney volume (TKV) and cyst volume in ADPKD increase exponentially over time in patients with ADPKD.

RENAL MANIFESTATIONS

Many patients with ADPKD are asymptomatic. The diagnosis is established by either the identification of an afflicted family member, asymptomatic screening (approximately 40%), or renal imaging performed for another reason. Patients may present with gross hematuria, flank mass/pain, polyuria/nocturia, fever due to a kidney or lower urinary tract infection, nephrolithiasis, or blood pressure elevation. All of these complications are manifested through increased cyst burden or TKV.

Gross hematuria occurs in 35% to 50% of patients with ADPKD and is associated with increased TKV. Hematuria is also caused by rupture of a cyst into the collecting system or secondary to nephrolithiasis. Nephrolithiasis occurs in approximately 27% of ADPKD patients, due in part to low levels of urinary citrate. Kidney stones may present as flank pain or hematuria, commonly microscopic. Polyuria and nocturia reflect impaired urinary concentrating ability, whereas increased thirst indicates elevated circulating vasopressin levels. Proteinuria is not a common feature of ADPKD and is usually less than 1 gram per day. However, the presence of microalbuminuria is correlated with increased TKV and more severe kidney disease.

Urinary tract infections are common in patients with PKD, but do not appear to be more common than in the general population. Renal cyst infections are specific to ADPKD, and patients typically present with localized flank pain, fevers, and nausea and vomiting, similar to pyelonephritis. Acute flank pain can be caused by a kidney stone, kidney, or liver cyst rupture or hemorrhage. Chronic pain is typically due to enlarged kidneys, either unilaterally or bilaterally.

CARDIAC MANIFESTATIONS

Hypertension occurs in 60% of patients with ADPKD prior to any substantial decline in kidney function and appears earlier in males than in females. Hypertension in ADPKD is due to

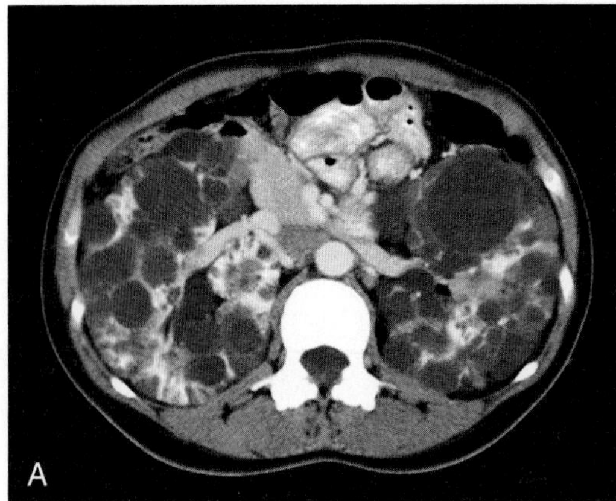

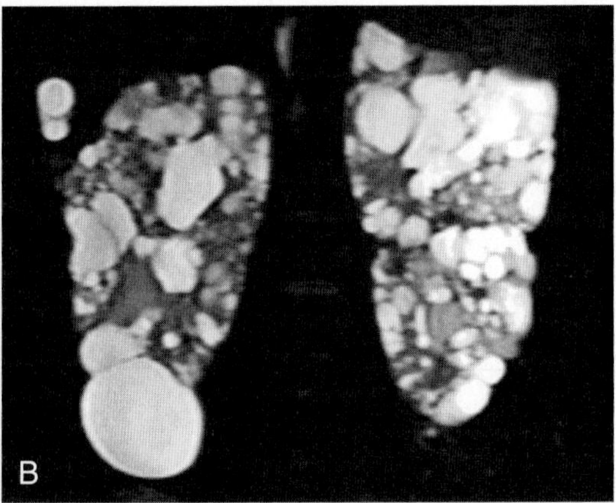

FIG. 1 A, Axial contrast-enhanced computed tomography (CT) image and **B,** coronal T2-weighted single-shot fast spin echo magnetic resonance imaging (MRI) in a 39-year-old woman with autosomal polycystic kidney disease. Contrast administration is necessary to differentiate the cystic tissue from preserved parenchyma and detect small cysts using CT, but it is not necessary using MRI. (From Chebib FT, et al.: Autosomal dominant polycystic kidney disease: core curriculum 2016, *Am J Kidney Dis* 67(5):792-810, 2016.)

upregulation of renin-angiotensin-aldosterone system (RAAS). Hypertension is a predictor of worse renal outcome and is associated with cardiovascular morbidity and mortality. Cardiac valvular abnormalities occur in 25% to 30% of patients and include mitral valve prolapse and aortic regurgitation.

EXTRARENAL MANIFESTATIONS

- The prevalence of intracranial aneurysms (ICA) in ADPKD is approximately 5% and increases to as high as 20% in patients with a first-degree relative with a known intracranial aneurysm rupture.
- Rupture of an ICA is a serious complication of PKD and may produce significant permanent morbidity or death. Routine screening for ICA is recommended for patients with a family history of ICA or intracerebral bleed or for patients with warning symptoms such as a sentinel headache.
- In addition to kidney cysts, cysts can develop in the liver, pancreas, and seminal vesicles. Hepatic cysts are common and occur in up to ~85% of ADPKD patients by the age of 30 yr. Hepatic cysts represent the most common extrarenal manifestation of ADPKD. Liver cystic disease is typically asymptomatic and develops slightly later than kidney cysts in ADPKD. However, hepatic cysts can cause serious complications including pain, infection, bleeding, and biliary obstruction. Liver cysts continue to grow and expand after patients reach ESRD.
- Colonic diverticula and abdominal or inguinal hernias occur more frequently in ADPKD patients.
- Seminal vesical cysts have been reported to occur in up to 40% of men with ADPKD but are not associated with changes in fertility.
- Patients with ADPKD may be at an increased risk of developing liver, colon, and kidney cancer. However, there is sparse evidence upon which to recommend any change in current cancer-screening guidelines for patients with PKD.

NATURAL HISTORY

- Patients with *PKD1* mutations have more rapid disease progression than patients with *PKD2* mutations. The median age of onset of ESRD is 54 yr in *PKD1* patients and 74 yr in PKD2 patients.
- Other clinical risk factors associated with progressive kidney disease in ADPKD include male sex, onset of hypertension before 35 yr of age, early onset of gross hematuria, proteinuria or microalbuminuria, increased urinary sodium excretion, and increased low-density lipoprotein cholesterol levels. All of these risk factors are mediated through cyst burden or TKV.
- Data from the Consortium of Radiologic Imaging studies of Polycystic Kidney Disease (CRISP) indicate that a decline in renal blood flow and increases in TKV and cyst volume are strong predictors of future renal functional decline and progression to CKD stage 3. Baseline height-adjusted TKV (htTKV) of 600 ml/m predicts the risk of developing stage 3 CKD within 8 yr. Patients with ADPKD can be classified into Mayo Clinic imaging categories 1A-1E based on htTKV limits for their ages. This classification helps physicians identify patients with severe disease. Patients in classes 1A and 1B are at a low risk for renal function decline. Patients in classes 1C–1E are at a high risk for progressive disease.

Dx DIAGNOSIS

Ultrasound of the kidneys is the most commonly used imaging modality for screening and diagnosis and is inexpensive, readily available, noninvasive, and free of radiation. CT and MRI are also used, but typically in the setting of acute complications. CT scans (Fig. E2) and MRI are more sensitive than ultrasound with cyst detection at <1 cm in size.

The following diagnostic criteria are used for diagnosis of ADPKD in asymptomatic individuals at risk for development of ADPKD (i.e., those with positive family history of ADPKD):

1. Individuals 15 to 39 yr of age: At least three unilateral or bilateral kidney cysts
2. Individuals 40 to 59 yr of age: At least two cysts in each kidney
3. Individuals older than 60 yr of age: At least four cysts in each kidney

With no family history of ADPKD, there is no definitive number of cysts and/or cyst location that provides an unequivocal diagnosis. The diagnosis is strongly suspected when multiple and bilateral kidney cysts are present along with hepatic cysts. Genetic testing can be done to diagnose ADPKD when imaging results are equivocal and definitive diagnosis is required in a young individual such as a potential living donor.

DIFFERENTIAL DIAGNOSIS

- Multiple benign simple cysts
- Autosomal-recessive PKD
- Familial juvenile nephronophthisis
- Medullary cystic or UMOD (uromodulin) disease
- Medullary sponge kidney
- Tuberous sclerosis
- von Hippel-Lindau syndrome
- Acquired cystic kidney disease

LABORATORY TESTS

- Hemoglobin and hematocrit may be elevated because of increased erythropoietin production but are typically similar to levels in other patients with CKD.
- Urinalysis can show microscopic hematuria and proteinuria (seldom >1 gram per day).
- With decreased kidney function, blood urea nitrogen and creatinine are elevated.
- Platelet counts can be mildly reduced in patients with extensive polycystic liver disease.
- Metabolic acidosis, hyperparathyroidism, and hyperphosphatemia are all associated with CKD in ADPKD.

Rx TREATMENT

NONPHARMACOLOGIC THERAPY

Dietary intervention should be prescribed to all patients with ADPKD.

- Restriction of dietary salt (<2 gram sodium per day) and calories is recommended. Post hoc analysis of the HALT-PKD trial in which all patients were instructed to follow a sodium-restricted diet (2.4 gram per day) showed that the urine sodium excretion is associated with kidney growth and more rapid renal function decline. The HALT Progression of Polycystic Kidney Disease (HALT-PKD) trials were two simultaneously conducted multicenter clinical studies that examined the benefits of renin-angiotensin-aldosterone system (RAAS) blockade on progression of cystic disease and decrease of kidney function in ADPKD.
- Cyclic adenosine monophosphate (cAMP) contributes to cyst formation and growth in ADPKD. Vasopressin stimulates the production of cAMP. Increasing water intake to greater than 3 L per day can suppress vasopressin. Increasing water intake is recommended in all ADPKD patients with preserved renal function. However, serum sodium should be monitored carefully in patients with advanced renal dysfunction as these persons are prone to developing hyponatremia.

CHRONIC GENERAL Rx

- Data from the HALT-PKD trial showed that in young individuals with preserved kidney function, strict BP control of <110/75 mm Hg was associated with slower increase in TKV, reduced urinary albumin excretion, and a greater reduction of left ventricular mass index.
- For all ADPKD patients, the goal BP is <130/80 mm Hg. For young, healthy patients with ADPKD and with intact kidney function, the goal BP target can be <110/75 mm Hg.
- ACE inhibitors or angiotensin receptor blockers are the first drug of choice for treatment of hypertension.
- Hyperlipidemia should be aggressively treated with LDL-cholesterol targets <80 mg/dl.
- Pravastatin was found to have a beneficial effect on htTKV, LVMI, and urinary albumin excretion in a randomized, double-blind placebo-controlled phase II trial involving 91 children and young adults with ADPKD. A 23% change in htTKV was observed in the pravastatin group compared to 31% in the placebo group.
- Statin therapy did not produce benefit in a post hoc analysis of the HALT-PKD trials. However, this study was not randomized, different statin drugs and doses were used, and only a small number of statin users were in that study. Use of statins in the management of patients with ADPKD is a personal physician choice. A larger randomized study is needed to study the effect of statins on cyst growth.

- Patients who progress to ESRD require renal replacement therapy. Peritoneal dialysis or hemodialysis can be used as a bridge to kidney transplantation.
- Pretransplant unilateral or bilateral nephrectomy is recommended only in selected patients with recurrent infections, renal cell carcinoma, and significant kidney enlargement causing limitation of daily activities and malnutrition.

ACUTE GENERAL Rx

- The treatment of gross hematuria is typically supportive with bed rest, hydration, and analgesics. Antihypertensive medications should be stopped during this time.
- Extracorporeal shock wave lithotripsy (ESWL) has been used in patients with small obstructing kidney stones (<2 cm diameter) in the renal pelvis or calyces. Percutaneous nephrolithotomy is another potential option.
- Infections are treated with antibiotics that penetrate cysts, such as fluoroquinolones, trimethoprim/sulfamethoxazole, vancomycin, and chloramphenicol.
- New therapies impacting cyst growth.
- Tolvaptan.
- In a phase 3, double-blind, placebo-controlled, randomized trial (TEMPO 3:4 trial) involving 1,450 patients with PKD and preserved kidney function, the vasopressin-receptor 2 antagonist, tolvaptan, significantly decreased kidney volume and slowed the decline in kidney function. The benefits of tolvaptan on TKV rate of increase and decline of kidney function is greater in patients with increased albuminuria. The benefits of tolvaptan on TKV were seen across chronic kidney disease stages 1–3.
- The effect of tolvaptan on delaying renal function decline was maintained for additional 2 yr in an extension study TEMPO 4:4 trial, where all TEMPO 3:4 participants were offered treatment with tolvaptan for additional 2 yr.
- A second Tolvaptan trial (REPRISE) was conducted examining the safety and efficacy of tolvaptan in patients with more advanced ADPKD. This was a 12-month phase 3, randomized withdrawal, multicenter, placebo-controlled, double-blind trial; 1,370 patients with eGFRs between 25 to 65 ml/min per 1.73 m^2 were included in this trial. Tolvaptan treatments compared to placebo. Those receiving placebo lost 3.61 ml/min per 1.73 m^2 per yr. Tolvaptan-treated patients demonstrated an eGFR decline of 2.34 ml/min/1.73 m^2/yr, a difference of 1.27ml/min/1.73m^2 per yr which was statistically significant. The beneficial effect of tolvaptan on renal function decline was seen in all subgroups (<55 yr of age, men and women, and patients with stage 3a, 3b, and stage 4 CKD). This beneficial effect was not observed in patients older than 55 yr of age. However, firm conclusions cannot be made in this subgroup due to relatively smaller numbers.
- Based on these studies, the FDA approved tolvaptan for treatment of ADPKD in adult patients at risk for rapidly progressing ADPKD on April 24, 2018.
- Aquaretic side effects are commonly observed with tolvaptan. Patients have polyuria, nocturia, pollakiuria (abnormally frequent urination), and polydipsia. Post-hoc analysis of TEMPO 3:4 and TEMPO 4:4 trials reveals that the aquaretic effects are more pronounced early after drug initiation and in patients with better kidney function. Appropriate hydration is essential to prevent thirst, dehydration, and hypernatremia.
- Another important adverse event associated with tolvaptan is liver toxicity. Two patients in the TEMPO 3:4 trial and 1 patient in the TEMPO 4:4 trial developed serious drug-induced liver injury meeting Hy's law criteria: alanine aminotransferase (ALT) >3 times the upper limit of normal, bilirubin >2 the upper limit of normal. In the REPRISE trial, liver adverse effects were higher in the tolvaptan group compared to the placebo (5.6% vs. 1.2%). However, no participant met the Hy's law criteria.
- Because of the risks of serious liver injury, tolvaptan is available only through a restricted distribution program under a Risk Evaluation and Mitigation Strategy (REMS). Under this program, liver function testing is done before initiation of treatment and at monthly intervals after initiation of treatment weekly for the first 2 weeks, monthly for the first 18 months, and then every 6 months, thereafter. A status form must be completed every 3 months for the first 18 months and then every 6 months.
- Patients with Mayo class 1C–1E levels of cyst burden (faster rates of cyst growth) are considered to have rapidly progressive disease and should be considered for treatment with tolvaptan.
- Other therapies impacting cyst growth:
- A small trial involving the somatostatin analogue, octreotide long-acting repeatable depot, showed that there was significantly less increase in TKV in the octreotide group compared to placebo.
- In a phase 2, randomized, double-blind, placebo-controlled study, the oral src/bcr-abl tyrosine kinase inhibitor, bosutinib, reduced kidney growth in patients with ADPKD and preserved renal function. However, side effects of the medication (diarrhea, rash, and pancreatitis) and acute declines in kidney function have limited development of this agent.
- Two randomized, double-blind trials involving mammalian target of rapamycin inhibitors, sirolimus and everolimus, did not show any effect on renal function in these patients. The shorter duration of these trials and inadequate dosing of the medications may have affected the outcome.

REFERRAL

Patients with ADPKD should be referred at time of diagnosis to a nephrologist for ongoing care. Urology can also be consulted in patients with nephrolithiasis for recurrent episodes of gross hematuria or consideration for nephrectomy before transplantation.

Genetic counseling should be offered if patients plan to start a family or are considering having their children screened. Individuals at risk for ADPKD should undergo pretest and posttest counseling if they are found to have ADPKD.

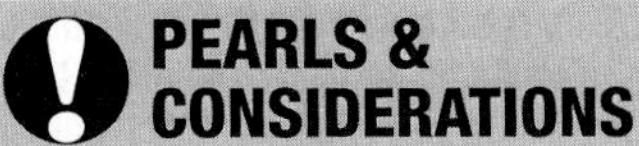

PEARLS & CONSIDERATIONS

- ADPKD is the most common, single, genetic cause of chronic kidney disease.
- TKV is a strong predictor of future renal function decline.
- Increasing water intake to >3 L per day is recommended in patients with ADPKD and preserved renal function.
- Strict blood pressure control is recommended in all patients with ADPKD.

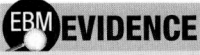

EVIDENCE

Available at ExpertConsult.com

SUGGESTED READINGS

Available at ExpertConsult.com

RELATED CONTENT

Polycystic Kidney Disease (Patient Information)

AUTHORS: **BHARATHI REDDY, M.D.,** and **ARLENE CHAPMAN, M.D.**

BASIC INFORMATION

DEFINITION

Cerebral arteriovenous malformations (AVMs) are congenital vascular lesions that are characterized by blood flow from high-pressure arterial vessels directly into thin-walled veins without passing through an intervening capillary/venule system (Fig. 1).

SYNONYMS

Arteriovenous malformations of the brain
AVM
Brain AVM

ICD-10CM CODE
Q28.2 Arteriovenous malformations of cerebral vessels

EPIDEMIOLOGY & DEMOGRAPHICS

INCIDENCE:

- Detection rates in large prospective studies range from 1.1 to 1.4 per 100,000 person-yr.
- Incidence of hemorrhage, the most common and often most clinically dangerous presentation, is estimated to be 2% to 4% per yr.

PREVALENCE: Estimated about 1.3 per 100,000

PREDOMINANT SEX AND AGE:

- There is a slight male preponderance; studies of varying populations show 1.04:1 to 1.2:1 male:female ratio.
- Peak age at time of hemorrhage occurrence is about 20 yr, but it can occur in younger and older patients.

GENETICS:

- Cerebral AVMs are sporadic in most cases.
- AVMs are present in about 20% of cases of Osler-Weber-Rendu syndrome (also known as hereditary hemorrhagic telangiectasia [HHT]), an autosomal dominant disorder that results in abnormal blood vessel formation in the skin, lungs, liver, brain, and other organs.

RISK FACTORS:

- Male sex and presence of HHT are risk factors for AVM.
- The risk of hemorrhage is increased with prior hemorrhage, presence of a single draining vein, and diffuse nidus morphology.

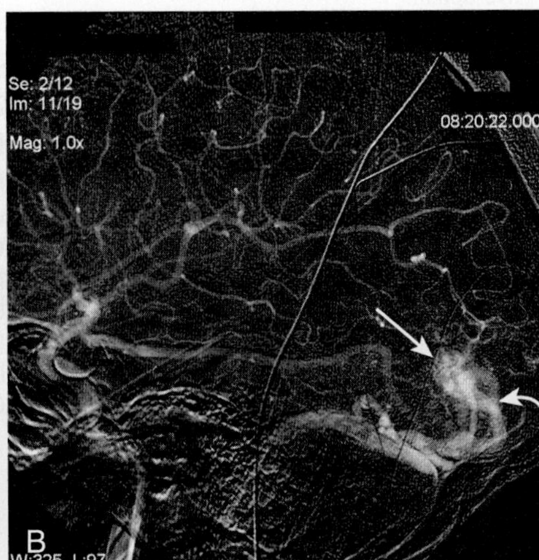

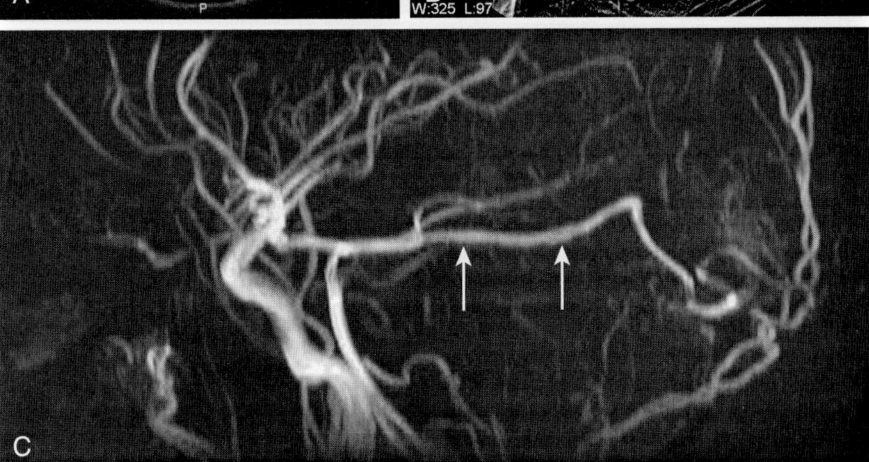

FIG. 1 A 14-year-old child with a left occipital arteriovenous malformation (AVM). A, MRI shows multiple flow voids in the left occipital lobe *(arrow).* **B,** Lateral view from catheter angiogram confirms the presence of an AVM *(arrow)* and early draining veins *(curved arrow).* **C,** Lateral maximum intensity projection image from an MR angiogram shows an enlarged posterior cerebral artery branch *(arrows),* which feeds the tangle of abnormal vessels. (From Fuhrman BP et al: *Pediatric critical care,* ed 4, Philadelphia, 2011, Saunders.)

PHYSICAL FINDINGS & CLINICAL PRESENTATION

- The most common presentation is hemorrhage; symptoms vary based on location and magnitude of hemorrhage.
- Patients may present with seizures or neurologic deficits related to mass effect of the AVM nidus.
- Headache and pulsatile tinnitus may be present.
- In infants, AVM may present as cyanotic heart failure, macrocephaly, or hydrocephalus.
- A bruit may be auscultated through the scalp or orbit.
- AVMs may also present with associated intracranial aneurysms that occur on distant, unrelated vessels, on a proximal artery that feeds the aneurysm (flow-related aneurysm), or within the AVM nidus itself (intranidal aneurysm). Patients may present with a subarachnoid hemorrhage related to the aneurysm rather than to the AVM.

ETIOLOGY

In most cases, AVMs are congenital abnormalities caused by failure of formation of a capillary bed between embryonic arterial and venous vascular plexuses during the first trimester of gestation; however, de novo sporadic AVMs have been reported.

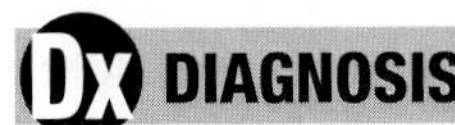

DIAGNOSIS

DIFFERENTIAL DIAGNOSIS

The differential diagnosis of cerebral AVMs includes other vascular lesions such as cavernous malformations, dural arteriovenous fistulas, and intracranial aneurysms. Table E1 compares vascular malformations, and Table E2 describes major differences between hemangiomas and vascular malformations.

LABORATORY TESTS

- CBC and BMP with renal function panel prior to contrast dye administration with CT angiography/cerebral angiogram.
- PT/INR/PTT should be drawn and corrected in the case of bleeding diathesis.

IMAGING STUDIES

- In the acute setting, a CT scan of the head to check for hemorrhage and a CT angiogram of the head for characterization of the lesion may be helpful (although calcification may be present and potentially pose as small acute blood).
- MRI of the brain delineates the nidus and its relationship to surrounding soft tissue structures better than a CT scan; however, in the setting of an acute hemorrhage these details will be obscured.
- Four-vessel cerebral angiogram (arteriogram) is the best study to evaluate AVM. Angiography in multiple projections helps identify the number and location of feeding and draining vessels for treatment planning (Fig. 2). High-resolution images of the nidus may also reveal other irregularities such as

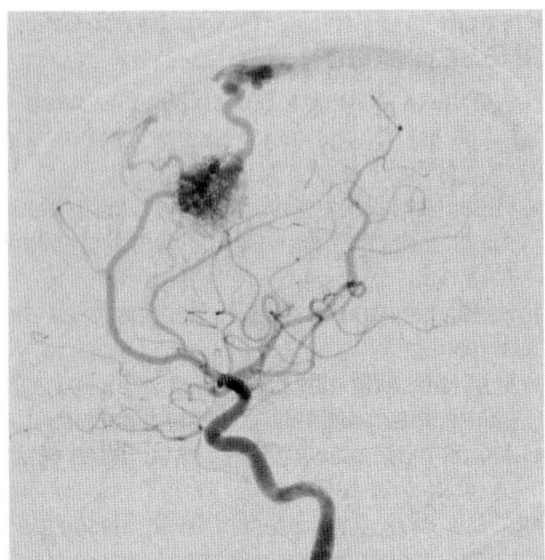

FIG. 2 Arteriovenous malformation of the frontal lobe. The anterior cerebral artery provides primary arterial supply with venous drainage superficially into the superior sagittal sinus.

aneurysms that often arise given the abnormal histology of the vessel walls and the high-pressure blood flow traversing them.

Rx TREATMENT

Pharmacologic management of seizures with antiepilepsy drugs and of headaches with oral analgesics can provide symptomatic relief.

NONPHARMACOLOGIC THERAPY

- Nonemergent outpatient setting: Cerebral angiogram provides characterization of the lesion. Based on angiographic characteristics, the Spetzler-Martin AVM grading system may be used to help guide treatment. In general, grade 5 AVMs are considered unresectable; they are not treated because the risks of treatment likely outweigh the risk of hemorrhage. Current tools for the treatment of AVMs include surgical resection, radiosurgery, and endovascular embolization (with liquid glues or embolic agents).
- Surgical resection: In low-grade lesions by an experienced neurosurgeon yields a high cure rate (~95% in published studies). Resection should include removal of all of the nidus of the AVM; failure to remove the complete nidus may increase the risk of recurrence. An increasing Spetzler-Martin grading scale increases risk of neurologic complications. Intraoperative imaging techniques such as indocyanine-green in-field angiography and conventional digital subtraction angiography are used to verify complete resection.
- Radiosurgery: Alternative definitive treatment for AVMs. Traditionally employed to treat AVMs in eloquent areas (e.g., brainstem); stereotactic radiosurgery is increasingly used for higher Spetzler-Martin grade AVM. Reported rates of confirmed radiographic obliteration after AVM radiosurgery range from 47% to 90%.
- Endovascular embolization involves transarterial superselective blockage of the AVM. It has become an important adjunctive tool. Currently recommended and approved for use before resection, preoperative embolization can reduce arterial flow and pressure within the AVM, assisting in speed and safety of surgical resection. In addition, embolization may often be used to treat intranidal or flow-related aneurysms in coordination with either resection or radiosurgery. Embolization alone in obliterating an AVM is not routinely recommended.
- Treatment decisions should take into consideration the morbidity associated with the treatment modality versus the risk of future hemorrhage or neurologic deterioration. Disability stemming from intractable seizures or severe headaches may make invasive definitive treatment a more attractive option.
- Acute cerebral hemorrhage: In the case of an acute hemorrhage, airway and breathing must be maintained, with intubation if necessary. Acute neurosurgical intervention for clot evacuation may be warranted. Microsurgical resection of the AVM may or may not be feasible in the acute setting and is controversial.

DISPOSITION

Whether the patient is receiving elective treatment of a known lesion or presenting with an acute hemorrhage, the patient should receive care in a progressive or intensive care unit with experience dealing with cerebrovascular disease. Once the patient is stabilized, appropriate rehabilitation should be arranged.

REFERRAL

- Cerebral AVMs should be managed by a qualified neurosurgeon.
- Referral to radiation medicine for adjuvant radiosurgery should be made when indicated.
- Referral to an interventional radiologist for endovascular treatment may be warranted.
- Treatment in a primary stroke center or other specialized center that offers all treatment modalities is recommended.

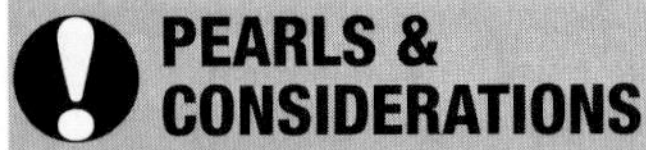

PEARLS & CONSIDERATIONS

COMMENTS

- No two AVMs are exactly the same; individualization of treatment decisions is the mainstay. Additionally, many AVMs could be effectively treated through one of several modalities or a combination thereof. Factors such as patient age, overall health status, radiographic characteristics, route of surgical access, and potential morbidities of each treatment modality are vital variables in consideration for treatment. The advisability of intervention for unruptured AVMs remains controversial. In a recent randomized trial comparing medical management with specific interventions to obliterate AVMs (neurosurgery, embolization, radiotherapy, or a combination) the rates of neurological disability were higher in the intervention group than with conservative treatment.[1]
- The annual risk of hemorrhage from a cerebral AVM is approximately 3%, but depending on the clinical and anatomical features of the malformations, the risk may be as low as 1% or as high as 33%. The risk of bleeding is increased if the patient has had previous episodes of bleeding, if there is a berry aneurysm on an artery feeding the AVM, and if there is a restriction of venous drainage from the AVM.[2]

PATIENT/FAMILY EDUCATION

If a patient with a known AVM suffers from acute-onset neurologic deficits or stroke-like symptoms, emergency medical attention is warranted for potential hemorrhage. Presence of AVMs, cerebral or otherwise, in family members should be disclosed to the patient's primary care physician because the presence of a genetic condition predisposing to cerebral AVMs should be considered.

SUGGESTED READINGS

Available at ExpertConsult.com

AUTHOR(S): **STEPHEN L. GRUPKE, M.D., M.S.,** and **JUSTIN F. FRASER, M.D.**

[1] Mohr JP et al: Medical management with or without interventional therapy for unruptured brain arteriovenous malformations (ARUBA): a multicentre non-blinded, randomized trial, *Lancet* 383:614–621, 2014.

[2] Solomon RA, Connolly ES: Arteriovenous malformations of the brain. *N Engl J Med* 376:1859–1866, 2017.

BASIC INFORMATION

DEFINITION

Avascular necrosis (AVN) is ischemic death of bone due to insufficient blood supply. It is not a specific disease entity but a final common pathway to several disorders that impair blood supply to the femoral head and other locations.

SYNONYMS

AVN
Osteonecrosis
Aseptic necrosis

ICD-10CM CODES

M87	Idiopathic aseptic necrosis of bone
M87.1	Osteonecrosis due to drugs
M87.2	Osteonecrosis due to previous trauma
M87.3	Other secondary osteonecrosis
M87.9	Osteonecrosis, unspecified

EPIDEMIOLOGY & DEMOGRAPHICS

- 15,000 new cases per yr in the United States. It is most commonly associated with the hip and accounts for 10% of total hip replacements in the United States
- Usually occurs in middle age and is more frequent in males than females
- Associated conditions:
  1. Corticosteroid treatment: 35%
  2. Alcohol abuse: 22%
  3. Idiopathic and other: 43%
  4. Hemoglobinopathies, pancreatitis, chronic renal failure, SLE, chemotherapy, decompression sickness
- Common sites involved
  1. Femoral head
  2. Femoral condyle
  3. Humeral head
  4. Navicular and lunate wrist bones
  5. Talus

PHYSICAL FINDINGS & CLINICAL PRESENTATION

- May be asymptomatic in early stages
- Pain in the involved area exacerbated by movement or weight bearing in later stages
- Decreased range of motion as the disease progresses
- Functional limitation

ETIOLOGY

Final common pathway of conditions that lead to impairment of the blood supply to the involved bone. Trauma disrupting the blood supply is the most common cause of AVN. Arterial factors are considered the most common cause of AVN. Table 1 describes proposed mechanism of disease of common conditions associated with osteonecrosis.

STAGING

Table 2 describes the Modified Steinberg Staging System for osteonecrosis.

Stages:

- Stage 0
  1. Asymptomatic
  2. Normal imaging
  3. Histologic findings only (i.e., silent osteonecrosis)
- Stage 1
  1. Asymptomatic or symptomatic
  2. Normal radiographs and CT scan
  3. Abnormal bone scan or MRI
- Stage 2
  1. Abnormal radiographs or CT scan, including linear sclerosis, focal bead mineralization, cysts; however, the overall architecture of the involved bone is normal
- Stage 3
  1. Early evidence of mechanical bone failure (subchondral fracture), but the overall shape of the bone is still intact
- Stage 4
  1. Flattening or collapse of the bone
- Stage 5
  1. Joint space narrowing
- Stage 6
  1. Extensive joint destruction

TABLE 2 Modified Steinberg Staging System for Osteonecrosis

Stage	Radiographic Appearance	Reversible
I	Normal radiographs, but abnormal bone scan or magnetic resonance image	Yes
II	Lucent and sclerotic changes	Yes
III	Subchondral fracture without flattening	No
IV	Subchondral fracture with flattening or segmental depression of femoral head	No
V	Joint space narrowing or acetabular changes	No
VI	Advanced degenerative changes	No

From Firestein GS et al: *Kelly's textbook of rheumatology*, ed 9, Philadelphia, 2013, Saunders.

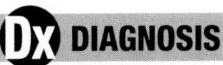

DIAGNOSIS

DIFFERENTIAL DIAGNOSIS

- None in late stages
- Early: Any condition causing focal musculoskeletal pain, including arthritis, bursitis, tendinitis, myopathy, neoplastic bone and joint diseases, traumatic injuries, pathologic fractures

WORKUP

Fig. 1 describes a diagnostic algorithm for osteonecrosis.

IMAGING STUDIES (FIG. 2)

- MRI: The most sensitive technology to diagnose early aseptic necrosis. The first sign is a margin of low signal. An inner border of high signal associated with a low-signal line is specific for aseptic necrosis ("double line sign"). Sensitivity is 75% to 100%.
- Radiography: Insensitive early in the course. The earliest changes include diffuse osteopenia, areas of radiolucency with sclerotic border, and linear sclerosis. Later, a subchondral lucency (crescent sign) indicates subchondral fracture. More advanced cases reveal flattening, collapsed bone, and abnormal bone contour. In late disease, osteoarthritic changes are seen.

TABLE 1 Proposed Mechanism of Disease of Common Conditions Associated with Osteonecrosis

	Mechanism of Osteonecrosis							
Associated Condition	Apoptosis	Osteoblast/ Osteoclast Homeostasis	Lipid Abnormalities	Coagulation Abnormalities	Oxidative Stress	Parathyroid/ Calcium Imbalance	Vascular Plugging	Vasoactive Substances
Corticosteroids	X	X	X	X	X			X
Bisphosphonates	X	X	X					
Alcohol abuse	X	X	X	X	X			
Trauma	X	X						X
Renal transplantation	X	X		X		X		
Dialysis						X		
Sickle cell disease							X	

From Firestein GS et al: *Kelley's textbook of rheumatology*, ed 9, Philadelphia, 2013, Saunders.

 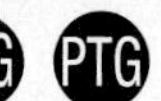

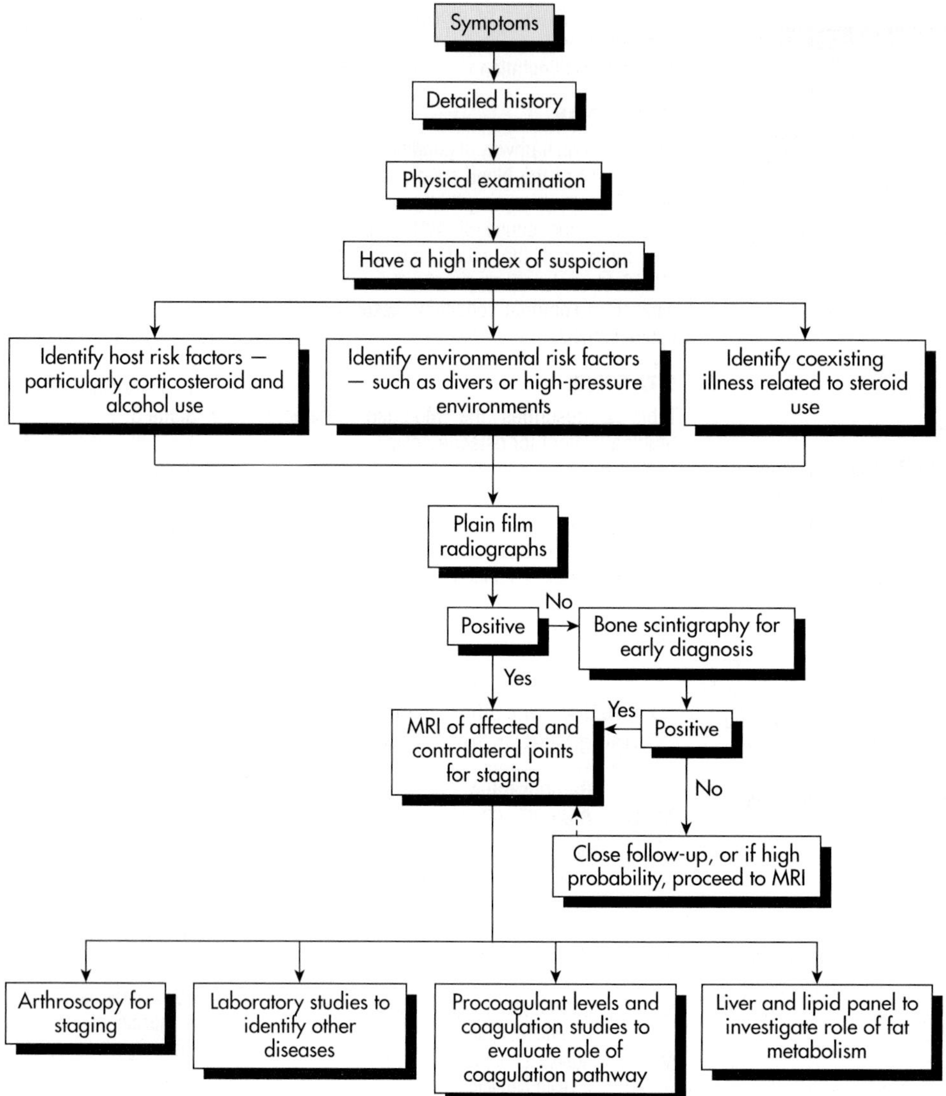

FIG. 1 Diagnostic algorithm for osteonecrosis. *MRI*, Magnetic resonance image. (From Firestein GS et al: *Kelley's textbook of rheumatology*, ed 9, Philadelphia, 2013, Saunders.)

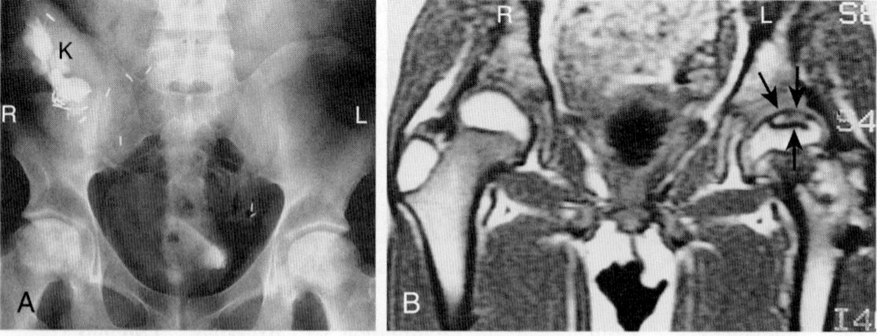

FIG. 2 Aseptic necrosis of the hips. A, Aseptic necrosis can occur from a number of causes, including trauma and steroid use. In this patient, an anteroposterior view of the pelvis shows a transplanted kidney *(K)* in the right iliac fossa. Use of steroids has caused this patient to have bilateral aseptic necrosis. The femoral heads are somewhat flattened, irregular, and increased in density. **B,** Aseptic necrosis in a different patient is demonstrated on an MRI scan as an area of decreased signal *(arrows)* in the left femoral head. This is the most sensitive method for detection of early aseptic necrosis. (From Mettler FA [ed]: *Primary care radiology,* Philadelphia, 2000, Saunders.)

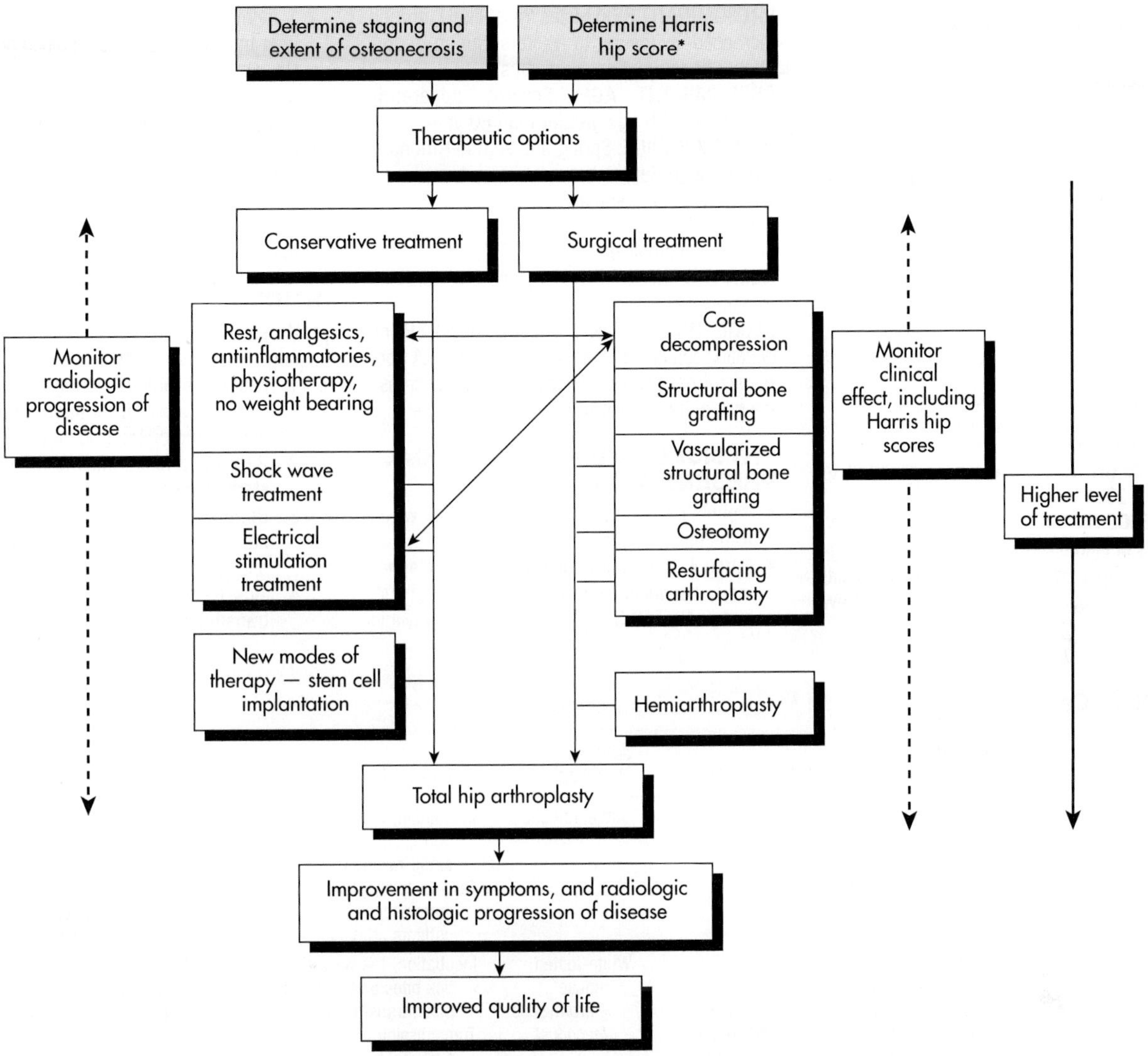

Determine staging and extent of osteonecrosis

Determine Harris hip score*

Therapeutic options

Conservative treatment

Surgical treatment

Monitor radiologic progression of disease

Rest, analgesics, antiinflammatories, physiotherapy, no weight bearing

Shock wave treatment

Electrical stimulation treatment

New modes of therapy — stem cell implantation

Core decompression

Structural bone grafting

Vascularized structural bone grafting

Osteotomy

Resurfacing arthroplasty

Hemiarthroplasty

Monitor clinical effect, including Harris hip scores

Higher level of treatment

Total hip arthroplasty

Improvement in symptoms, and radiologic and histologic progression of disease

Improved quality of life

FIG. 3 Treatment algorithm for osteonecrosis. *www.ncbi.nlm.nih.gov/pubmed/22588745. (From Firestein GS et al: *Kelley's textbook of rheumatology*, ed 9, Philadelphia, 2013, Saunders.)

- Bone scan:
  1. Early: "Cold" area
  2. Later: Increased radionuclide uptake as a result of remodeling
  3. Sensitivity in early disease is only 70% and specificity is poor
- CT scan: May reveal central necrosis and area of collapse before those are visible on radiographs.

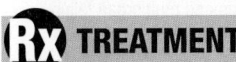

TREATMENT

PREVENTION

- Manage etiologic conditions
- Minimize corticosteroid use

NONPHARMACOLOGIC THERAPY

- Core decompression: Effectiveness 35% to 95% in early phases
- Bone grafting
- Osteotomies
- Joint replacement

ACUTE GENERAL Rx

- Decrease weight bearing of affected area.
- Pulsing electromagnetic fields applied externally (still experimental).
- Peripheral vasodilators (e.g., dihydroergotamine) (unproven).
- Late-stage AVN is most often treated by total joint arthroplasty.
- A treatment algorithm for osteonecrosis is described in Fig. 3.

PROGNOSIS

- When diagnosed at an early stage treatment is appropriate in all cases because 85% to 90% can be expected to progress to a more advanced stage.
- Contralateral joint involvement is common (30% to 70%).

RELATED CONTENT

Avascular Necrosis (Patient Information)

AUTHOR: **FRED F. FERRI, M.D.**

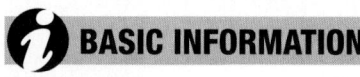

BASIC INFORMATION

DEFINITION

Babesiosis is a tick-transmitted protozoan disease of animals, caused by intraerythrocytic parasites of the genus *Babesia.* Humans are incidentally infected, resulting in a nonspecific febrile illness. The disease can be severe in immunocompromised hosts.

ICD-10CM CODE
B60.0 Babesiosis

EPIDEMIOLOGY & DEMOGRAPHICS

INCIDENCE (IN U.S.): 1744 cases reported to the CDC in 2014

PREVALENCE (IN U.S.):

- In areas of high endemicity, seropositivity ranging from 9% (Rhode Island) to 21% (Connecticut)
- Highest number of reported cases in New York

PREDOMINANT SEX: Males (most likely through increased exposure to vectors during recreational or occupational activities)

PREDOMINANT AGE: Severity apparently increasing with age greater than 60 yr

PEAK INCIDENCE: Spring and summer months, May through September

GENETICS: None known

CONGENITAL INFECTION: Definite evidence of vertical transmission

NEONATAL INFECTION: Many cases of perinatal transmission

BLOOD TRANSFUSION: Many instances. Blood donation screening for antibodies to and DNA from *B. microti* has been shown to significantly decrease the risk of transfusion-transmitted babesiosis

PHYSICAL FINDINGS & CLINICAL PRESENTATION

- Incubation period 1 to 4 wk, or 6 to 9 wk in transfusion-associated disease
- Gradual onset of irregular fever, chills, diaphoresis, headache, myalgia, arthralgia, fatigue, and dark urine. Symptoms usually begin within 1 month after tick bite and within 6 months after transfusion of infected blood products
- On physical examination: Petechiae, frank or mild hepatosplenomegaly, and jaundice. Most patients have a normal physical exam.
- Infection with *B. divergens* (Europe) producing a more severe illness with a rapid onset of symptoms and increasing parasitemia progressing to massive intravascular hemolysis and renal failure

ETIOLOGY

- Vector: Deer tick, *Ixodes scapularis* (also known as *I. dammini*)
  1. Feeds on rodents during the spring and summer while in its larval and nymphal stages and on deer as an adult
  2. Requires a blood meal to mature to each stage, hence human infection
  3. During the warmer months in endemic areas, humans are readily infected while engaging in outdoor activities
  4. Tick must attach for 36 to 72 hours to transmit infection

TABLE 1 Causal Agents and Clinical Manifestations of Babesiosis

Babesia Species	Geographic Distribution	Tick Vectors	Animal Reservoirs	Epidemiology	Clinical Manifestations
B. divergens	United Kingdom, Western Europe, Eastern Europe, Sweden, Russia; not reported in United States	*Ixodes ricinus*	Cattle, reindeer	Incubation, 1-4 wk. Occurs during summer months in cattle-raising regions Targets splenectomized or immunocompromised patients primarily	Fulminant course with high case-fatality rate Fever, rigors, headache, myalgia, jaundice, hemoglobinuria, hemolytic anemia, acute renal failure, multiorgan failure
B. microti	Parallels the U.S. Northeast endemic regions for *Borrelia burgdorferi*, especially the islands off New York, Massachusetts, Connecticut, and Rhode Island and focal areas in Connecticut, New Jersey, Wisconsin, and Minnesota	Deer ticks: *Ixodes dammini* and *Ixodes scapularis*	White-footed mouse *(Peromyscus leucopus)*	Incubation, 1-4 wk after tick bites or 4-9 wk after blood transfusions Transmission primarily by nymphal ticks Targets older, not necessarily immunocompromised patients, particularly severe in those immunocompromised by HIV infection, advanced age, coinfections with *B. burgdorferi* Seasonality parallels tick nymph activity; 80% of cases occur from May to August	Often asymptomatic in young, healthy patients Self-limited influenza-like febrile illness with onset of anorexia, malaise, and lethargy followed in 1 wk by high fever, diaphoresis, myalgias; mild splenomegaly and rarely hepatomegaly Later hemolysis, hemolytic anemia, thrombocytopenia, jaundice, acute renal failure, especially in the splenectomized, older adults, or the immunocompromised Complications include ARDS and DIC Case-fatality rate, 5%
MO-1 (a relative or subspecies of *B. divergens*)	Rural Missouri and Kentucky	*Ixodes dentatus* (rabbit tick)	Rabbits, birds	Incubation, 1-4 wk after tick bites Spring to autumn seasonality Targets the splenectomized, like *B. divergens*	Same as above—often asymptomatic, except in the splenectomized, who will develop high parasitemias and multiorgan failure
WA-1 (a relative or subspecies of *B. gibsoni*)	Rural Washington State	Ixodid ticks, including *Ixodes dentatus*	Unknown—wild canids and ungulates suspected	Incubation, 1-4 wk Targets the splenectomized, older adults, immunocompromised, premature infants May be transmitted by blood transfusion	Same as above—often asymptomatic, except in the splenectomized, who will develop high parasitemias and multiorgan failure
CA-1, CA-2, etc. subspecies (relatives or subspecies of mule deer and bighorn sheep *Babesia* species)	U.S. Pacific coast, primarily rural and semirural areas of California	Ixodid ticks	Unknown—mule deer and bighorn sheep suspected	Incubation, 1-4 wk Targets the splenectomized, elderly, immunocompromised, and premature infants	Same as above—often asymptomatic, except in the splenectomized, who will develop high parasitemias and multiorgan failure

ARDS, Acute respiratory distress syndrome; *DIC,* disseminated intravascular coagulation.
From Bennett JE, Dolin R, Blaser MJ: Mandell, Douglas, and Bennett's principles and practice of infectious diseases, ed 8, Philadelphia, 2015, Saunders.

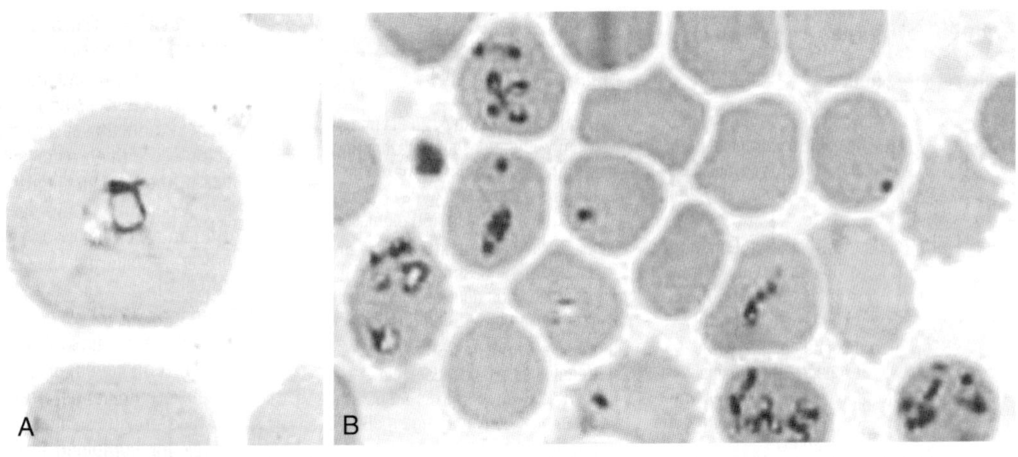

FIG. 1 Babesia Parasites. Human infection with species of piroplasm transmitted by the bite of the tick *Ixodes ricinus* infected from cattle is a rare occurrence. Infection in normal people with this piroplasm may give rise to a self-limiting fever and parasitemia, as in the case of infection with the rodent parasite *Babesia microti* on the northeastern seaboard of the United States via the tick *Ixodes scapularis* (A). Heavy red-cell infection may develop, however, in splenectomized patients, leading to fatal hemolytic anemia. This patient died as a result of an infection acquired from the cattle parasite *Babesia divergens* in Scotland (B). Other species of *Babesia* that occasionally infect humans, for example, the WA1, CA1, and MO1 isolates from the United States, are distinguished by molecular means. (Hoffman R, et al.: *Hematology, basic principles and practice*, ed 7, Philadelphia, 2018, Elsevier.)

- *B. microti* and *B. divergens* account for most human infections. Table 1 compares causal agents and clinical manifestations of babesiosis.
- In the U.S., cases caused by *B. microti* are acquired on offshore islands of the northeastern coast, including Nantucket Island, Cape Cod, and Martha's Vineyard in Massachusetts; Block Island in Rhode Island; and Long Island, Fire Island, and Shelter Island in New York; as well as the nearby mainland including Connecticut, Rhode Island, Massachusetts, and New Jersey.
- Sporadic cases reported from California, Georgia, Maryland, Minnesota, Virginia, Wisconsin, and most recently the WA-1 strain from Washington State and the MO-1 strain from Missouri.
- *B. divergens* is implicated in human disease in Europe, where the disease remains rare and predominantly associated with asplenia.
- Majority of cases are asymptomatic.
- May be transmissible by transfusion, through red cell-contaminated platelets and erythrocytes.
- Mixed infections (*B. microti* and *Borrelia burgdorferi,* the causative agent of Lyme disease) are estimated to occur in 30% (Rhode Island and Connecticut) to 60% (New York) of cases.

Dx DIAGNOSIS

DIFFERENTIAL DIAGNOSIS

- Malaria
- Amebiasis
- Ehrlichiosis
- Hepatic abscess
- Leptospirosis
- Salmonellosis, including typhoid fever
- Acute viral hepatitis
- Hemorrhagic fevers
- Subacute bacterial endocarditis

WORKUP

Should be suspected in any febrile patient living or traveling in an endemic area, irrespective of exposure history to ticks or tick bites, especially if asplenic. The hallmark of babesiosis is hemolysis with resulting anemia. Elevated liver enzymes, thrombocytopenia, and acute kidney injury may occur.

LABORATORY TESTS

- The preferred method for diagnosing babesiosis is PCR using whole blood specimens.
- Babesial DNA by polymerase chain reaction (PCR) has comparable sensitivity and specificity to microscopic analysis of thin blood smears. PCR is more sensitive than smears at the onset of infection when parasite load may be minimal.
- Diagnosis achieved serologically by indirect immunofluorescence assay (IFA) is specific for *B. microti.*
    1. Assay is hampered by the inability to distinguish between exposed patients and those who are actively infected.
    2. IGG titer of ≥1:64 is indicative of seropositivity, whereas one ≥1:1024 is considered diagnostic of acute infection. IGM titer of 1:64 is considered indicative of acute infection.
    3. Immunoglobulin M indirect immunofluorescent-antibody test may be highly sensitive and specific for diagnosis. IGM titer of 1:64 is considered indicative of acute infection.
- CBC to reveal mild to moderate thrombocytopenia and anemia. The WBC count may be normal, elevated, or low. Abnormally elevated serum chemistries, including creatinine, liver function profile, lactate dehydrogenase, and indirect and total bilirubin levels; haptoglobin is low.
- Urinalysis to reveal proteinuria and hemoglobinuria.
- Examination of Giemsa- or Wright-stained thin blood films for intraerythrocytic parasites (Fig. 1):
    1. In its classic, though infrequently seen, form a "tetrad" or "Maltese cross" composed of four daughter cells attached by cytoplasmic strands is observed.
    2. More commonly, smaller forms composed of a single chromatin dot are eccentrically located within bluish cytoplasm.
    3. Parasitized erythrocytes may be multiply infected but not enlarged.
    4. Extra-erythrocytic forms may be seen.

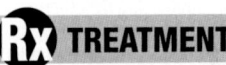

Rx TREATMENT

NONPHARMACOLOGIC THERAPY

Supportive care with adequate hydration

ACUTE GENERAL Rx

- In patients with intact spleens: Predominantly asymptomatic or if symptomatic, generally self-limited
- Therapy may be offered to any symptomatic patient. Table 2 summarizes treatment recommendations.
- Therapy is mandatory for the severely ill patient, especially if asplenic, elderly, or immunosuppressed. Combination of atovaquone 750 mg q12h and azithromycin 500 mg on day 1 and 250 mg per day thereafter for 7 to 10 days appears to be as effective as a regimen of clindamycin and quinine with fewer adverse reactions. This is the preferred regimen for mild disease.
- Combination of quinine sulfate 650 mg PO tid plus clindamycin 600 mg PO tid (600 mg parenterally qid) taken for 7 to 10 days. Severely ill patients are hospitalized and treated with clindamycin and quinine.
- Exchange transfusions in addition to antimicrobial therapy: Successful treatment for severe infections in asplenic patients associated with high levels of *B. microti* or *B. divergens* parasitemia. Exchange transfusion is recommended for patients with >10% parasitemia, but may be considered for any severely ill patient.

TABLE 2 Treatment of Human Babesiosis

Organism	Severity	Adults	Children
*Babesia microti**	Mild†	Atovaquone 750 mg q12h PO plus azithromycin 500 mg PO on day 1 and 250 mg/day PO from day 2 on	Atovaquone 20 mg/kg q12h PO (maximum 750 mg/dose) plus azithromycin 10 mg/kg PO on day 1 (maximum 500 mg/dose) and 5 mg/kg/day PO from day 2 on (maximum 250 mg/dose)
	Severe‡,§	Clindamycin 300-600 mg q6h IV or 600 mg q8h PO plus quinine 650 mg q8h PO	Clindamycin 7-10 mg/kg q6-8h IV or 7-10 mg/kg q6-8h PO (maximum 600 mg/dose) plus quinine 8 mg/kg q8h PO (maximum 650 mg/dose)
*Babesia divergens**		Immediate complete RBC exchange transfusion plus clindamycin 600 mg q6-8h IV plus quinine 650 mg q8h PO	Immediate complete RBC exchange transfusion plus clindamycin 7-10 mg/kg q6-8h IV (maximum 600 mg/dose) plus quinine 8 mg/kg q8h PO (maximum 650 mg/dose)

Note: Monitor patients on quinine with electrocardiography; monitor quinine serum levels in the setting of hepatic or renal disease.
IV, intravenously; *PO,* orally; *RBC,* red blood cell.
*Treatment for 7 to 10 days, but duration may vary.
†Atovaquone (750 mg twice daily) combined with higher doses of azithromycin (600 to 1000 mg/day) has been used in immunocompromised patients. With this regimen, symptoms and parasitemia resolve faster.
‡Consider partial or complete RBC exchange transfusion in cases of high-grade parasitemia (≥10%), severe anemia (<10 g/dl), or pulmonary, renal, or hepatic compromise. Even when parasitemia is less than 10%, consider exchange transfusion if acute respiratory distress syndrome or syndrome resembling a systemic inflammatory response syndrome is present.
§In asplenic individuals and in immunocompromised patients, persistent or relapsing babesiosis should be treated for at least 6 wk, including 2 wk during which parasites are no longer detected.
From Bennet, et al.: *Principles and practice of infectious diseases*, ed 8, Philadelphia, 2015, Elsevier.

- Relapsed and immunocompromised patients may require a longer duration of therapy.

DISPOSITION

Prognosis is usually good and fatal outcomes are rare.

REFERRAL

- For prompt consultation with an infectious disease specialist if the diagnosis is acutely suspected, especially in the asplenic, elderly, or immunocompromised patient
- For hospitalization for the severely ill patient who may require exchange transfusions in addition to antibiotic therapy

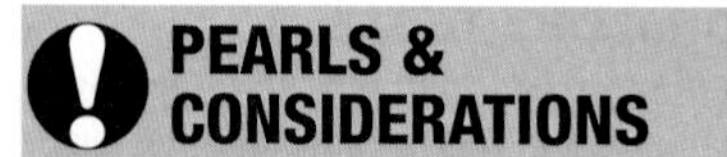

PEARLS & CONSIDERATIONS

COMMENTS

- Prevention of babesiosis in asplenic or immunocompromised hosts is best achieved by avoidance of areas where the vector is endemic, especially May through September.
- If residence or travel in endemic areas is unavoidable, advise patients to perform daily cutaneous self-examination, wear light-colored clothing (to facilitate removal of ticks), tuck pants into socks, and apply tick repellent (diethyltoluamide and dimethyl phthalate) to skin or clothing.
- Advise a daily inspection for ticks in family pets (e.g., cats and dogs).
- Infection with *B. divergens,* especially in the asplenic patient, is often fatal.
- Concurrent cases of babesiosis and Lyme disease, anaplasma, *Borrelia miyamotoi*, and Powassan virus have been documented—check for combined infection in severely ill patients.
- A combination of clindamycin and quinine has been successfully used to treat babesiosis during the third trimester of pregnancy without incurring apparent adverse effect on the fetus.
- In 2011 the CDC added babesiosis to the list of nationally notifiable diseases.

SUGGESTED READINGS

Available at ExpertConsult.com

RELATED CONTENT

Babesiosis (Patient Information)

Tick avoidance is paramount in prevention of babesiosis.

AUTHOR: **PATRICIA CRISTOFARO, M.D.**

BASIC INFORMATION

DEFINITION

Barrett esophagus occurs when the squamocolumnar junction is displaced ≥1 cm proximal to the gastroesophageal junction and the squamous lining of the lower esophagus is replaced by metaplastic columnar epithelium, which predisposes to the development of esophageal adenocarcinoma. While cardia-type epithelium has been shown to predispose to esophageal cancer, the presence of intestinalized epithelium is still considered essential for the diagnosis. Recent data show that the absolute annual risk for esophageal carcinoma in Barrett esophagus is 0.12%, which is much lower than the assumed risk of 0.5% that is the basis for current surveillance guidelines.

SYNONYMS

Barrett esophagus
Esophagus, Barrett
Esophagus, columnar-lined
Ulcer, Barrett

ICD-10CM CODES

K22.70	Barrett esophagus without dysplasia
K22.710	Barrett esophagus with low grade dysplasia
K22.711	Barrett esophagus with high grade dysplasia
K22.719	Barrett esophagus with dysplasia, unspecified

EPIDEMIOLOGY & DEMOGRAPHICS

- Male/female ratio of 4:1.
- Mean age of onset is 40 yr, with a mean age range of diagnosis of 55 to 60 yr.
- Occurs more frequently in white and Hispanic individuals than in African American individuals, with a ratio of 10 to 20:1.
- Mean prevalence of 5% to 15% in patients undergoing endoscopy (EGD) for symptoms of gastroesophageal reflux disease (GERD).
- Independent risk factors include chronic reflux (>5 yr), hiatal hernia, age >50 yr, male gender, white ethnicity, smoking history, and intraabdominal obesity. A family history with at least one first-degree relative with Barrett esophagus or adenocarcinoma of the esophagus may also be a risk factor.
- It is estimated that 5.6% of adults in the United States have Barrett esophagus. Prevalence rate in asymptomatic cohorts ranges from 5% to 25%.

PHYSICAL FINDINGS & CLINICAL PRESENTATION

SYMPTOMS:

- Chronic heartburn
- Dysphagia with solid food
- May be an incidental finding on EGD in patients without reflux symptoms
- Less frequent: Chest pain, hematemesis, melena
- Patients may be asymptomatic.

PHYSICAL FINDINGS:

- Nonspecific; can be completely normal
- Epigastric tenderness on palpation

ETIOLOGY

- Metaplasia is thought to result from reepithelialization of esophageal tissue injured as a result of chronic GERD.
- Patients with Barrett esophagus tend to have more severe esophageal motility disturbances (decreased lower esophageal sphincter pressure, ineffective peristalsis) and greater esophageal acid exposure on 24-hour pH monitoring. Table 1 lists some physiologic abnormalities that have been reported in Barrett patients and suggests how these abnormalities may contribute to GERD severity.
- Bile salts in the presence of acid may produce oxidative stress, induce reactive oxygen species, and alter transcriptional factor activity, all of which may induce the formation of Barrett epithelium, DNA damage, and dysplastic progression.
- Familial clustering of GERD and Barrett esophagus suggests a genetic predisposition, but no gene has yet been identified. Early data suggest that patients who develop Barrett are genetically predisposed to a severe inflammatory response to GERD. Candidate susceptibility loci include *CRTC1*, *BARX1*, and *FOXP1*.
- Progression from metaplasia to carcinoma is associated with changes in gene structure and expression, including the caudal-related homeobox family of transcription factors (*CDX1* and *CDX2*), the embryonic transcription factor SOX2, and the tumor suppressors p16 *(CDKN2A)* and *TP53*.

DIAGNOSIS

DIFFERENTIAL DIAGNOSIS

- GERD, uncomplicated
- Erosive esophagitis
- Gastritis
- Peptic ulcer disease
- Angina
- Malignancy
- Stricture or Schatzki ring

WORKUP

- The American Gastroenterological Association Medical Position Panel gave a weak recommendation for screening patients with multiple risk factors, including age over 50, male sex, white race, chronic GERD, hiatal hernia, elevated body mass index, and intraabdominal distribution of body fat. An international consensus group suggested screening men over 60 with GERD symptoms for more than 10 yr. An American College of Gastroenterology (ACG) Clinical Guideline suggested screening men with >5 yr and/or frequent symptoms of GERD and two or more risk factors including age >50, Caucasian race, presence of central obesity, current or past history of smoking, and a confirmed family history of Barrett or esophageal adenocarcinoma. General population screening is not currently recommended. Although screening has become standard of practice in some communities, the effectiveness of screening using current techniques is controversial because it may not improve mortality rates from adenocarcinoma.
- EGD with biopsy is necessary for diagnosis. Ideally, this should be done via high-resolution white-light endoscopy with at least four biopsies for every 2-cm segment. If erosive esophagitis is present, patients should be treated to heal esophagitis with repeat endoscopy and biopsies 8-12 wk later to determine if underlying Barrett esophagus is present.
- Unsedated transnasal endoscopy and an esophageal cytology device (*Cytosponge®*) may be acceptable alternatives to conventional endoscopy. Wireless esophageal capsule endoscopy may detect Barrett esophagus but with too low a sensitivity and specificity to be recommended. Imaging studies are not useful.
- Diagnosis requires the presence of metaplastic columnar epithelium at least 1 cm proximal to the gastroesophageal junction (Figs. 1 and E2). Longer-segment (≥3 cm) Barrett esophagus is more readily diagnosed. Barrett esophagus may be described using the Prague criteria, documenting the circumferential and maximal length via a C and M score. The Paris classification may be used to

TABLE 1 Proposed Physiologic Abnormalities Contributing to Gastroesophageal Reflux Disease in Patients with Barrett Esophagus

Abnormality	Potential Consequences
Extreme hypotension of the lower esophageal sphincter	Gastroesophageal reflux
Ineffective esophageal motility	Defective clearance of refluxed material
Gastric acid hypersecretion	Reflux of highly acidic gastric juice
Duodenogastric reflux	Esophageal injury caused by reflux of bile acids and pancreatic enzymes
Decreased salivary secretion of EGF	Delayed healing of reflux-damaged esophageal mucosa
Decreased esophageal pain sensitivity to refluxed caustic material	Failure to initiate therapy

EGF, Epidermal growth factor.
From Feldman M, et al.: *Sleisenger and Fordtran's gastrointestinal and liver disease*, ed 10, Philadelphia, 2016, Saunders.

 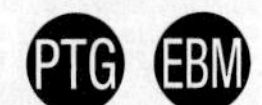

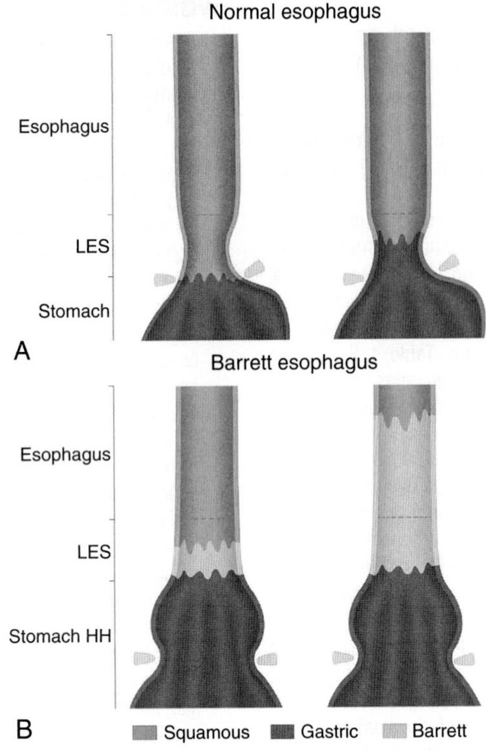

FIG. 1 Anatomic landmarks of the normal LES region (A) and of Barrett esophagus (B). Note that gastric mucosa is very common and normal in the LES region and that in Barrett esophagus, the squamocolumnar junction is not only proximally displaced within the tubular esophagus, but that the intervening mucosa is composed of intestinalized Barrett metaplastic epithelium. *HH,* Hiatal hernia; *LES,* lower esophageal sphincter. (From Silverburg SG: *Principles of practice of surgical pathology and cytopathology,* ed 4, New York, 2006, Churchill Livingstone.)

report associated visible lesions. At least two expert gastrointestinal pathologists should concur if any grade of dysplasia is diagnosed.

- Intestinal metaplasia of the gastric cardia is not Barrett esophagus and does not have the same risk for malignancy.
- Biomarkers and advanced imaging techniques such as chromoendoscopy, narrow band imaging, autofluorescence imaging, white light postprocessing algorithms, confocal laser endomicroscopy, and optical coherence tomography (recently incorporated into volumetric laser endomicroscopy) are being evaluated to assist with diagnosis and to better understand progression of disease, prediction of response to therapy, or prognosis.
- Screening for *Helicobacter pylori* infection in patients with GERD and Barrett esophagus is not recommended.

Rx TREATMENT

The goal is to control GERD symptoms and maintain healed mucosa.

NONPHARMACOLOGIC THERAPY

Nonpharmacologic therapy includes lifestyle modifications; elevating head of bed; and avoiding chocolate, tobacco, caffeine, mints, and certain drugs (see "Gastroesophageal Reflux Disease").

ACUTE GENERAL Rx

- Proton pump inhibitors are the most effective treatment for GERD. Therapy should be titrated to control symptoms and/or to promote healing of endoscopic signs of disease.
- If patient is asymptomatic and incidentally found to have Barrett esophagus, once-daily proton pump inhibitors should be prescribed, as they may reduce the risk of neoplastic progression.

CHRONIC Rx

- Chronic acid suppression is recommended to control symptoms, maintain healing, and reduce neoplastic progression. For patients with Barrett esophagus, the benefits of the use of proton-pump inhibitors is thought to outweigh the potential risks.
- Antireflux surgery may be considered for management of GERD and associated sequelae, but it has not been proven to be superior to medical therapy. Patients continue to require endoscopic surveillance of their esophagus.
- When GERD is controlled by either medical or surgical therapy, ablation of metaplastic epithelium usually leads to replacement by normal squamous epithelium. Because only a minority of patients with Barrett esophagus progress to high-grade dysplasia or carcinoma, endoscopic eradication therapy is not recommended for the general population of patients with nondysplastic Barrett esophagus.
- Endoscopic eradication therapy is becoming the treatment of choice for low-grade dysplasia and is the treatment of choice for high-grade dysplasia. Radiofrequency ablation or photodynamic therapy, combined with endoscopic mucosal resection (EMR) or endoscopic submucosal dissection (ESD) of visible mucosal irregularities, should be performed in conjunction with aggressive surveillance and eradication of all remaining Barrett epithelium. Endoscopic therapy is preferred over surgical treatment in properly staged individuals. These therapies may even be considered for patients with focal intramucosal carcinoma, if properly staged (T1SM1 or lower). Cryotherapy is being evaluated for the complete eradication of both dysplasia and intestinal metaplasia and reduced risk for disease progression. All these options run the risk for residual or buried metaplasia. Ultimate goals of therapy include both complete eradication of dysplasia (CE-D) and complete eradication of intestinal metaplasia (CE-IM). Even with CE-IM, recurrence has been documented in 5% to 39.5% of patients. Modalities for endoscopic treatment of Barrett esophagus are summarized in Table 2.
- Surgical resection is definitive therapy and may be offered for multifocal high-grade dysplasia, carcinoma that has extended into the submucosa (T1 SM2 or 3), or patients with poorly differentiated carcinomas or with evidence of lymphovascular invasion. Mortality appears to be lower with experienced surgeons operating in high-volume centers.
- Patients with cardiovascular risk factors may be considered for low-dose aspirin therapy for chemoprevention of esophageal adenocarcinoma. NSAIDs or NSAIDs combined with statins are potentially effective at reducing the risk of esophageal adenocarcinoma but are not currently recommended for use because of the risk of adverse effects.

DISPOSITION

- The relative risk of developing esophageal adenocarcinoma for a patient with Barrett esophagus, as compared with the general population, is 11.3, a substantial drop from the relative risk of 30 or 40 estimated in earlier reports. The risk is greater in men and in patients with longer (≥8 cm) columnar-lined segments.
- The risk of progression to esophageal adenocarcinoma from untreated Barrett with low-grade dysplasia is 0.5% per yr, and with high-grade dysplasia ranges from 6% to 19% per yr.
- Frequency of monitoring is controversial. No prospective studies have proven that endoscopic surveillance is cost effective or increases life expectancy. Although some studies have suggested that close adherence to surveillance protocols is associated with higher rates of detection of dysplasia and cancer, a recent case-control study showed no reduction in mortality.
- Patients with Barrett esophagus currently undergo surveillance EGD and systematic four-quadrant biopsy ("Seattle protocol") at intervals determined by the presence and grade of dysplasia. All mucosal abnormalities should undergo biopsy.

TABLE 2 Modalities for Endoscopic Treatment of Barrett Esophagus

Modality	HGD Resolved	BE Resolved	Recurrence Rate	Subsquamous BE Rate	Stricture Rate	Complication Rate	Advantages	Disadvantages
APC	67%-98.6%	38%-98%	33%-68% low power	25%-45% low power 0-30% high power	4%-10%	24% low power 40%-60% high power	Noncontact, technically simple	Requires several treatment sessions
MPEC	–	25%-88%	7%	7%	2%	41%-43%	Noncontact, technically simple, relatively inexpensive, readily available	Requires several treatment sessions
PDT	77%-88%	13%	5%-11%	2%-24%	4.8%-53%	4.8%-53%	Easy to perform; only FDA-approved ablation method for treatment of precancerous lesions in BE	Photosensitivity, relatively high stricture rate
EMR	59%-97%	53%	4%-30%	–	3%-30%	12%-60%	Histologic assessment; Complete removal of circumferential short-segment BE; 1-2 sessions	Difficulty treating long-segment BE

APC, Argon plasma coagulation; *BE,* Barrett esophagus; *EMR,* endoscopic mucosal resection; *FDA,* U.S. Food and Drug Administration; *HGD,* high-grade dysplasia; *MPEC,* multipolar electrocoagulation; *PDT,* photodynamic therapy.
From Cameron JL, Cameron AM: *Current surgical therapy*, ed 12, Philadelphia, 2017, Elsevier.

1. Patients without dysplasia should have follow-up every 3 to 5 yr. Patients with low-grade dysplasia should have aggressive antisecretory (proton pump inhibitor) therapy, repeat endoscopy within 2 to 6 mo, and endoscopic ablation therapy or extensive mucosal sampling every 12 mo or until dysplasia is no longer present. They then revert to a 3- to 5-yr interval.
2. Patients with high-grade dysplasia should have expert confirmation and extensive mucosal sampling. High-grade dysplasia with visible mucosal irregularities should be removed by EMR or ESD, followed by mucosal ablation. Consider intensive surveillance every 3 mo for at least a year; the optimal timing and duration of surveillance over the long term is unknown. Indefinite dysplasia requires aggressive medical therapy and close follow-up and resampling. Endoscopic treatment is preferred over intensive surveillance in patients with high-grade dysplasia.

- Patients should be treated aggressively for GERD before surveillance.

REFERRAL

- Consider EGD with biopsy in male or selected female patients with multiple risk factors who have not had previous EGD.
- Refer patients with GERD for evaluation if "red flag" symptoms are present (dysphagia, odynophagia, weight loss, vomiting, early satiety, GI bleeding, iron deficiency).
- Refer patients with biopsy-proved Barrett esophagus for surveillance.
- For those with low-grade or high-grade dysplasia, refer for ablative therapy with EMR or ESD if appropriate, followed by intensive surveillance. Esophageal resection may be considered.

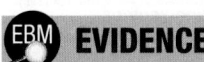

Available at ExpertConsult.com

SUGGESTED READINGS

Available at ExpertConsult.com

RELATED CONTENT

Barrett Esophagus (Patient Information)
Esophageal Tumors (Related Key Topic)
Gastroesophageal Reflux Disease (Related Key Topic)

AUTHOR: **HARLAN G. RICH, M.D., FACP, AGAF.**

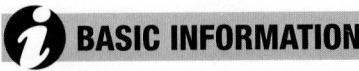

BASIC INFORMATION

DEFINITION

Basal cell carcinoma (BCC) is a malignant tumor of the skin arising from basal cells of the lower epidermis and adnexal structures. It may be classified as one of six types: nodular, superficial, pigmented, cystic, sclerosing or morpheaform, and nevoid. The most common type is nodular (21%); the least common is morpheaform (1%). A mixed pattern is present in approximately 40% of cases. BCC advances by direct expansion and destroys normal tissue.

SYNONYMS

BCC

ICD-10CM CODES

C44.01	Basal cell carcinoma of skin of lip
C44.111	Basal cell carcinoma of skin of unspecified eyelid, including canthus
C44.112	Basal cell carcinoma of skin of right eyelid, including canthus
C44.119	Basal cell carcinoma of skin of left eyelid, including canthus
C44.211	Basal cell carcinoma of skin of unspecified ear and external auricular canal
C44.212	Basal cell carcinoma of skin of right ear and external auricular canal
C44.219	Basal cell carcinoma of skin of left ear and external auricular canal
C44.310	Basal cell carcinoma of skin of unspecified parts of face
C44.311	Basal cell carcinoma of skin of nose
C44.319	Basal cell carcinoma of skin of other parts of face
C44.41	Basal cell carcinoma of skin of scalp and neck
C44.510	Basal cell carcinoma of anal skin
C44.511	Basal cell carcinoma of skin of breast
C44.519	Basal cell carcinoma of skin of other part of trunk
C44.611	Basal cell carcinoma of skin of unspecified upper limb, including shoulder
C44.612	Basal cell carcinoma of skin of right upper limb, including shoulder
C44.619	Basal cell carcinoma of skin of left upper limb, including shoulder
C44.711	Basal cell carcinoma of skin of unspecified lower limb, including hip
C44.712	Basal cell carcinoma of skin of right lower limb, including hip
C44.719	Basal cell carcinoma of skin of left lower limb, including hip
C44.81	Basal cell carcinoma of overlapping sites of skin
C44.91	Basal cell carcinoma of skin, unspecified

EPIDEMIOLOGY & DEMOGRAPHICS

- Most common cutaneous neoplasm
- 85% of cases appear on the head and neck region
- Most common site: Nose (30%)
- Annual incidence is nearly 2 million cases
- Increased incidence in men and over age 40
- Risk factors: Fair skin, increased sun exposure, use of tanning salons with ultraviolet A or B radiation, history of irradiation (e.g., Hodgkin's disease), personal or family history of skin cancer, impaired immune system

PHYSICAL FINDINGS & CLINICAL PRESENTATION

Variable with the histologic type:

- Nodular: Dome-shaped (Fig. 1), painless lesion that may become multilobular and frequently ulcerates (rodent ulcer) (Fig. 2); prominent telangiectatic vessels are noted on the surface. Border is translucent, elevated, pearly white (Fig. 3). Some nodular BCCs may contain pigmentation (Fig. 4), giving an appearance similar to a melanoma.
- Superficial: Circumscribed, scaling, black appearance with a thin, raised, pearly-white border; a crust and erosions may be present. Occurs most frequently on the trunk and extremities.
- Cystic: Dome-shaped, blue-gray cystic nodules, appearing clinically similar to eccrine and apocrine hidrocystomas (Fig. 5).
- Morpheaform: Flat or slightly raised yellowish or white appearance (similar to localized scleroderma); appearance similar to scars; surface has a waxy consistency.

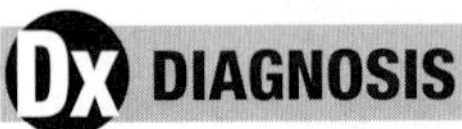

DIAGNOSIS

DIFFERENTIAL DIAGNOSIS

- Keratoacanthoma
- Melanoma (pigmented BCC)
- Xeroderma pigmentosa
- Basal cell nevus syndrome

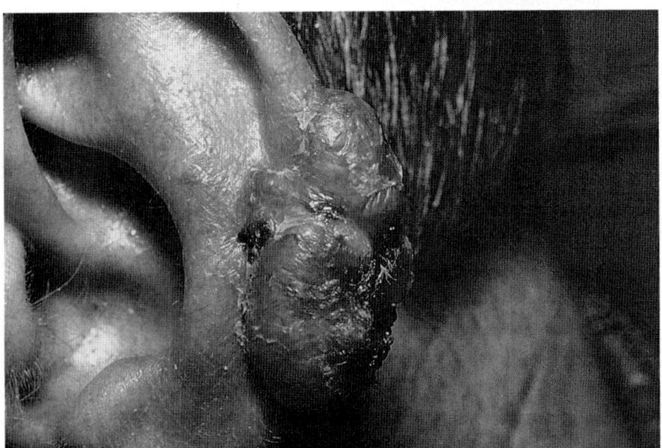

FIG. 1 Basal cell carcinoma, nodular type. (From James WD, Berger TG, Elston DM et al: *Andrews' diseases of the skin*, ed 12, Philadelphia, 2016, Elsevier.)

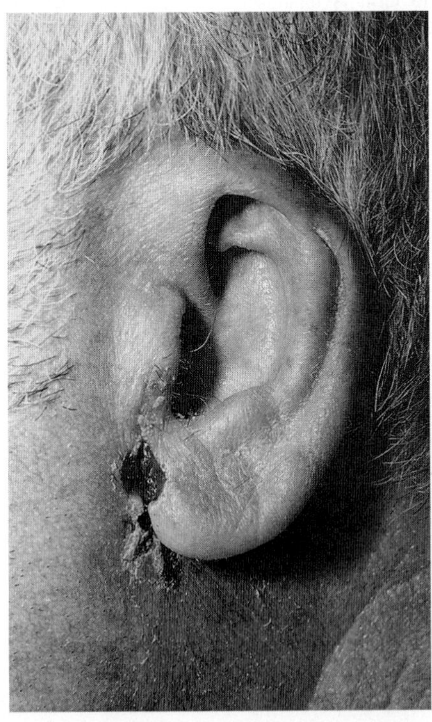

FIG. 2 Basal cell carcinoma, rodent ulcer. (From James WD, Berger TG, Elston DM et al: *Andrews' diseases of the skin*, ed 12, Philadelphia, 2016, Elsevier.)

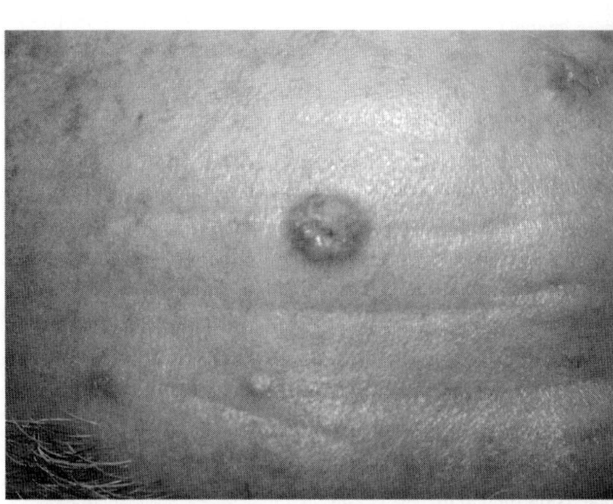

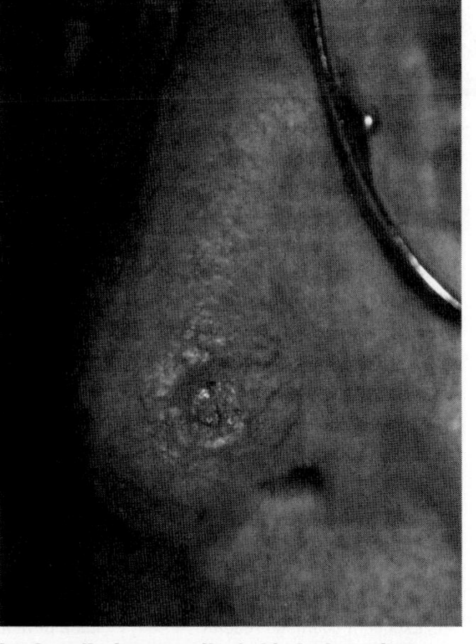

FIG. 3 Basal cell cancer typically is seen as a pearly, raised, well-circumscribed skin lesion, often on the face, sometimes with ulceration and associated telangiectasias. (From Cameron JL, Cameron AM: *Current surgical therapy*, ed 12, Philadelphia, 2017, Elsevier.)

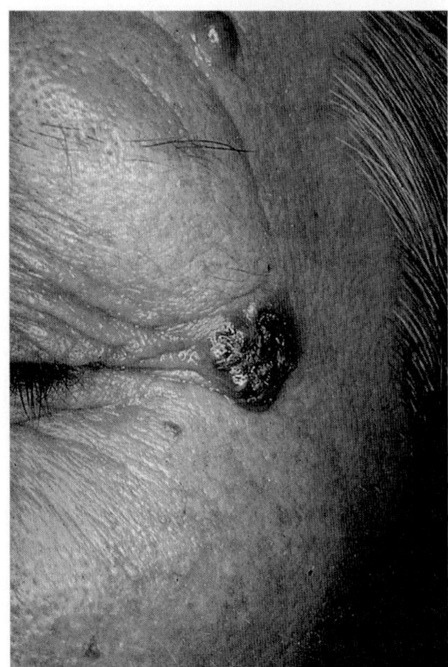

FIG. 4 Basal cell carcinoma, pigmented. (From James WD, Berger TG, Elston DM et al: *Andrews' diseases of the skin*, ed 12, Philadelphia, 2016, Elsevier.)

- Molluscum contagiosum
- Sebaceous hyperplasia
- Psoriasis

WORKUP

Biopsy to confirm diagnosis

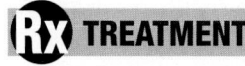

TREATMENT

Variable with tumor size, location, and cell type:

- Excision surgery: Preferred method for large tumors with well-defined borders on the legs, cheeks, forehead, and trunk.

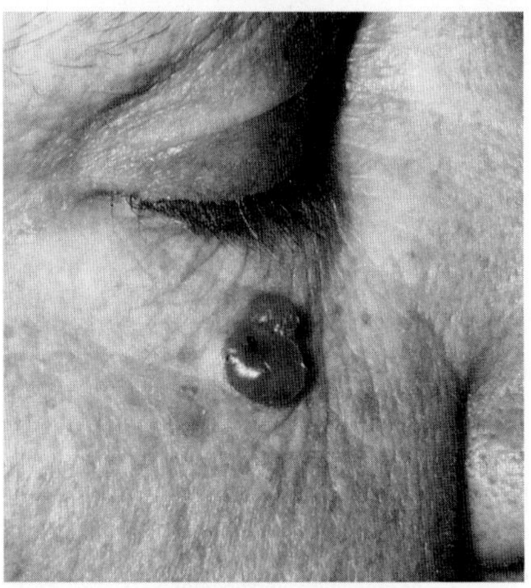

FIG. 5 Basal cell carcinoma, cystic. (From James WD, Berger TG, Elston DM et al: *Andrews' diseases of the skin*, ed 12, Philadelphia, 2016, Elsevier.)

- Mohs micrographic surgery: Preferred for lesions in high-risk areas (e.g., nose, eyelid), very large primary tumors, recurrent BCCs, and tumors with poorly defined clinical margins.
- Electrodesiccation and curettage: Useful for small (>6 mm) nodular BCCs.
- Cryosurgery with liquid nitrogen: Useful in BCCs of the superficial and nodular types with clearly definable margins; no clear advantages over the other forms of therapy; generally reserved for uncomplicated tumors.
- Radiation therapy: Generally used for BCCs in areas requiring preservation of normal surrounding tissues for cosmetic reasons (e.g., around lips); also useful in patients who cannot tolerate surgical procedures or for large lesions and surgical failures.
- Imiquimod 5% cream can be used for treatment of small, superficial BCCs of the trunk and extremities. Efficacy rate is approximately 80%. Its main advantage is lack of scarring, which must be weighed against higher cure rates with surgical intervention.
- Vismodegib and sonidegib are orally active hedgehog pathway inhibitors FDA approved for metastatic BCC, recurrent basal cell carcinoma post-surgery, and locally advanced BCC in patients who are not candidates for surgery or radiation.
- Table 1 summarizes advantages and disadvantages of BCC treatment options.

DISPOSITION

- More than 90% of patients are cured; however, periodic evaluation for at least 5 yr is necessary because of increased risk of recurrence of another BCC (<40% risk within 5 yr of treatment).
- A lesion is considered low risk if it is >1.5 cm in diameter, is nodular or cystic, is not in a difficult-to-treat area (H zone of face), and has not been previously treated.
- Nodular and superficial BCCs are the least aggressive.
- Morpheaform lesions have the highest incidence of positive tumor margins (<30%) and the greatest recurrence rate.

PREVENTION

Oral nicotinamide, a form of vitamin B_3 available without prescription (500 mg bid), has been reported to prevent development of new nonmelanoma skin cancer in high-risk patients.

SUGGESTED READINGS

Available at ExpertConsult.com

RELATED CONTENT

Basal Cell Skin Cancer (Patient Information)
Actinic Keratosis (Related Key Topic)
Melanoma (Related Key Topic)
Squamous Cell Carcinoma (Related Key Topic)

AUTHOR: **FRED F. FERRI, M.D.**

TABLE 1 Advantages and Disadvantages of Basal Cell Carcinoma Treatment Options

Modality	Advantages	Disadvantages
Mohs micrographic surgery	Complete margin analysis Well tolerated by elderly Gold standard treatment	Cost Longer procedure (stages)
Conventional surgical excision	Well tolerated by elderly	Cost Lack of complete margin analysis
Electrodesiccation and curettage	Shorter procedure Does not require return visit Patients can avoid surgery	Lack of histologic confirmation of malignancy removal Not appropriate for lesions with extension into deep dermis
Cryosurgery	Patients can avoid surgery	Higher recurrence rates than surgery Lack of histologic confirmation of malignancy removal Recurrent carcinoma could be extensive (can be obscured by fibrous scar tissue) Hypertrophic scarring Postinflammatory pigment changes
Imiquimod	Patient self-administration Excellent cosmetic results	Local skin reactions Lack of histologic confirmation of malignancy removal Cost
Photodynamic therapy	Excellent cosmetic outcome	Higher recurrence rates than with surgery Lack of histologic confirmation of malignancy removal
5-FU	Patient self-administration	Higher recurrence rates than with surgery
Radiation therapy	Good option in patients who are not surgical candidates	Cost Higher recurrence rates than with surgery Scars tend to worsen with time Can require 15-30 visits Side effects are considerable
Vismodegib	Approved for metastatic BCC and locally advanced BCC that has recurred following surgery; option in patients who are not surgical or radiation therapy candidates	Cost
Observation	Patients can avoid surgery Cost	No standard as to length of time for which it is appropriate to monitor patients clinically More dangerous neoplasms may be missed (such as Merkel cell carcinoma or amelanotic melanoma)

BCC, Basal cell carcinoma; *5-FU*, 5-fluorouracil.

From Wiznia LE, Federman DG: Treatment of basal cell carcinoma in the elderly: what nondermatologists need to know, *Am J Med* 129:655–660, 2016.

BASIC INFORMATION

DEFINITION

A bedbug's bite is a wound caused by the penetration of the bedbug mouthpiece into the skin as the insect feeds on blood from vessels or extravasated blood from the damaged surrounding tissue. The saliva of the bedbug contains pharmacologically active substances responsible for a spectrum of undesirable skin reactions depending on the individual. The bugs typically feed during times when an individual is at rest and may feed without being detected. Typically feedings take 5 to 10 minutes.

SYNONYMS

Insect bite
Bedbug *Cimex lectularius* bite

ICD-10CM CODE

T00.9 Multiple superficial (insect bite) injuries, unspecified

EPIDEMIOLOGY & DEMOGRAPHICS

- Traditionally, bedbugs were considered more common in poorer areas, but they are now increasingly found in areas of frequent travel.
- Bedbug infestations may spread among multifamily and institutional facilities with shared walls and are consequently difficult to eradicate.
- Reports of bedbug infestations have increased dramatically in the U.S., as well as worldwide, likely because of the decreased use of pesticides and increased international travel.
- Bedbugs are attracted to carbon dioxide gas and warm bodies.
- Bedbugs do not have a preference for specific age groups, ethnicity, or sex.
- Persons at higher risk include those who have recently stayed overnight in a hotel, dorm room, hospital, or new home.
- Studies have shown increased sensitivity of cutaneous reaction in previous bite victims.

PHYSICAL FINDINGS AND CLINICAL PRESENTATION

- Bites typically occur at night on exposed areas of skin, most often the face, neck, arms, and legs.
- The bites are painless and so do not awaken the individual.
- Onset of signs and symptoms of bites can be immediately on awakening or up to 10 days after the bite.
- Firm, purpuric or erythematous macules, urticaria, papules (Fig. 1), or bullae may be present. Bites are often inflammatory and pruritic, although bedbug-naive individuals may be asymptomatic to their first bites.
- Bite may have a central hemorrhagic punctum.
- Victim may observe a linear series often consisting of three bites ("breakfast, lunch, and dinner").
- Bites are typically pruritic.
- The size, degree of itching, and propensity toward vesiculation all increase with repeated bedbug bites.
- Fig. 2 illustrates symptoms and behaviors resulting from bed bug bites.

ETIOLOGY

- The *Cimex lectularius* species, also known as the common bedbug (Fig. 3), have flat, oval bodies and retroverted mouth parts used for taking blood meals. It feeds on mammals and birds. *Cimex hemipterus* is a tropical species that bites mostly humans, and hybrid species of the two insects exist. Both generally feed nocturnally on the blood of sleeping humans. They hide in beds, the floor, or furniture crevices during the day and emerge at night. They go through a larva stage (Fig. 4) and have a life span from 4 months up to 1 yr. The adult bedbug is wingless and about 5 to 7 mm in length. It has a modified mouthpart for piercing and sucking that usually leaves a bite mark of papular urticarial presentation to exposed areas of skin. Bedbugs have weak appendages for latching on to their hosts and are not usually transported from person to person.
- The saliva of the bedbug contains nitrophorin that enables vasodilation, an anticoagulant that interferes with production of coagulation factor Xa, a salivary apyrase that inhibits platelet aggregation, and an anesthetic. Consequently, the host often does not feel the bite until the effects have worn off.

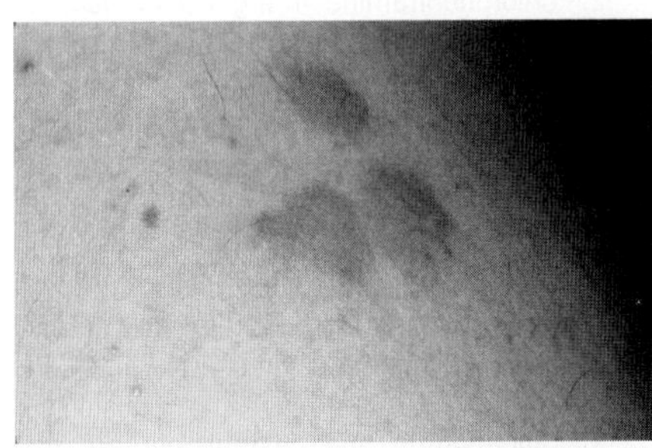

FIG. 1 Pruritic papules after bedbug bites. (From Kliegman RM et al: *Nelson textbook of pediatrics*, ed 19, Philadelphia, 2011, Saunders.)

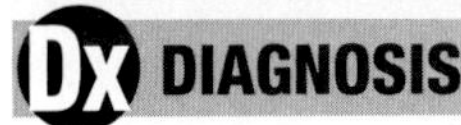

DIAGNOSIS

DIFFERENTIAL DIAGNOSIS

Scabies, flea and mite bites, vesicular disorders, delusional parasitosis, dermatitis herpetiformis, pemphigus herpetiformis, ecthyma, drug eruptions

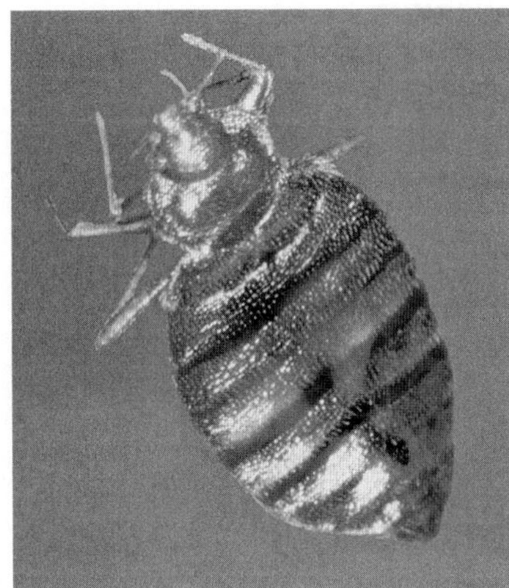

FIG. 3 Bedbug. (From James WD et al: *Andrews' diseases of the skin*, ed 12, Philadelphia, 2016, Saunders.)

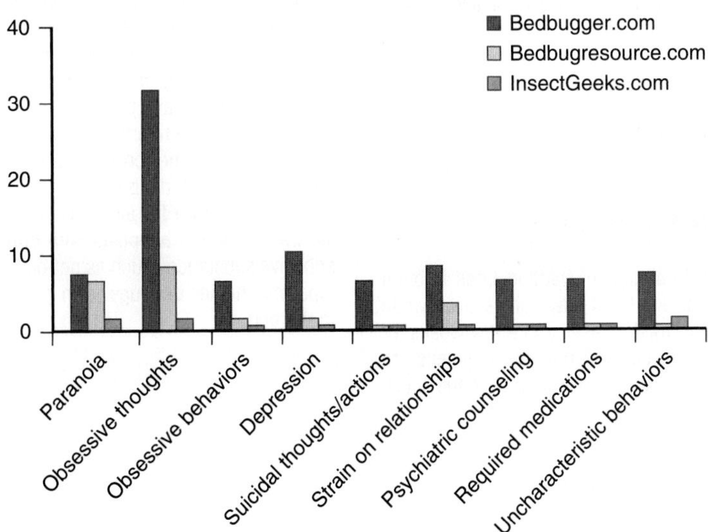

FIG. 2 Distribution of symptoms in 135 Internet reports describing effects of bed bug bites. (From Goddard J, de Shazo R: Psychological effects of bed bug attacks *(Cimex lectularius L.), Am J Med* 125:101-103, 2012.)

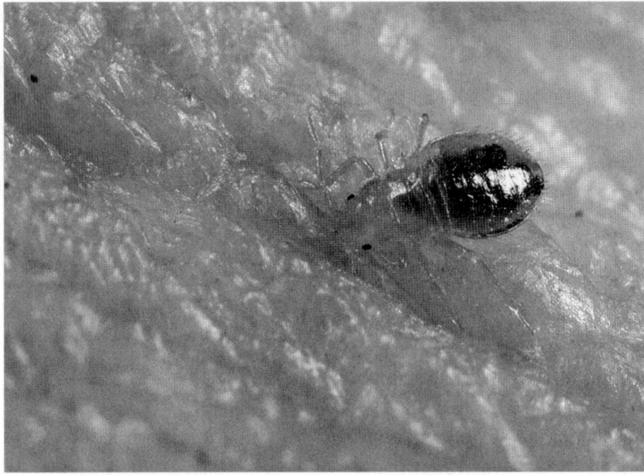

FIG. 4 Bedbug—second-stage larva. (From Habif TP: *Clinical dermatology: a color guide to diagnosis and therapy*, ed 6, Philadelphia, 2016, Elsevier.)

WORKUP

- Workup begins with history and physical for clinical symptoms and environmental findings suggestive of insect bites.
- Victims should carefully scrutinize the bedroom for signs of bedbug infestation. One may encounter fecal smears or flecks of blood on bed linens, inside furniture cracks and crevices, and behind peeling wallpaper. Bedbugs may travel as far as 20 feet for a meal. Densely infested rooms may also have a distinctive, pungent, soda syrup–like odor.

LABORATORY TESTS

- No specific tests recommended except for identification of the insect.
- The histology of bedbug bites is similar to other insect bites. Perivascular infiltrate of lymphocytes, histiocytes, eosinophils, and mast cells is seen within the upper dermis. One may also observe collagen bundles with interstitial eosinophils, dermal edema, and extravasated erythrocytes.
- Hypersensitivity to bedbug salivary proteins may be tested via intradermal allergy skin testing.
- Skin biopsy results are nonspecific and are not helpful in making the diagnosis.

IMAGING STUDIES

None

Rx TREATMENT

- Specific treatment of bedbug bites is often not necessary. Bites may self-resolve within a week for milder cases and a few weeks for more severe cases. Treatment regimens are based on resolving symptoms of the bites, mainly pruritus.
- To prevent infection, avoid scratching the area.
- Topical glucocorticoids or systemic antihistamines are appropriate in patients with severe pruritus from the bedbug bite.
  1. Triamcinolone cream 0.1%; apply thin film to affected areas bid.
  2. Chlorpheniramine 4 mg PO at bedtime (adults), 2 mg PO at bedtime (children).
- Insecticides may be effective in eradicating the bedbug, but growing resistance has been seen and multi-insecticide therapy is recommended.
  1. Use permethrin spray for clothing and bedsheets or bed nets.
  2. Diethyltoluamide (DEET): Be wary of toxic levels in children when used at high concentrations.
  3. Deltamethrin and chlorfenapyr are two common insecticides used.
  4. Please consult a pest control professional for safe eradication.

NONPHARMACOLOGIC THERAPY

Vacuuming is effective in removing bedbugs but does not remove the eggs. Wash bedsheets and clothing in hot water with detergent with at least 20 minutes in a dryer. Bedbugs have a high thermal death point of 45° C and also may survive at temperatures as low as 7° C. Some companies perform a treatment in which the room is heated above 50° C, which is a lethal temperature for all stages of a bedbug's life cycle. Coating bedposts with antifriction or adhesive substances such as petrolatum or duct tape may hinder bedbugs from gaining access to the bed.

ACUTE GENERAL Rx

Immunologic response is dependent on immunocompetence and individual sensitivity to the salivary components of the bedbug bite. Often, patients with papular urticaria have IgG antibodies to specific bedbug proteins. IgE antibodies may also mediate bullae formation. Anaphylaxis and death from bites is rare but documented in literature.

DISPOSITION

Patient may resume normal activity and lifestyle. Travelers should inspect their clothing and suitcases before returning home.

BEDBUGS AS POTENTIAL VECTORS

The bedbug has been studied extensively as a potential vector for human pathogens such as HIV, hepatitis B, hepatitis C, and Chagas' disease. To date, there is no evidence of transmission from an infected bedbug to a human.

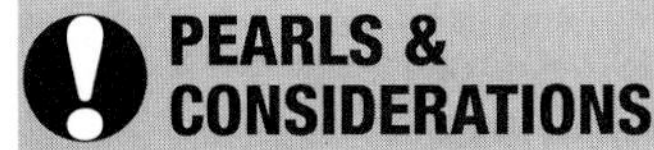

PEARLS & CONSIDERATIONS

COMMENTS

- Bedbugs are an increasing source of anguish and frustration for humans, and clinicians should evaluate for signs of stress and depression.
- A combination of chemical and physical intervention is often necessary for complete eradication. All hiding areas must be carefully inspected and cleaned. Treatment may include pesticides, laundering, heat, freezing, vacuuming, and hiring a professional service to eradicate bedbugs.

SUGGESTED READINGS

Available at ExpertConsult.com

RELATED CONTENT

Bedbugs (Patient Information)
Bites and Stings, Insect (Related Key Topic)

AUTHOR: **FRED F. FERRI, M.D.**

BASIC INFORMATION

DEFINITION

Acute peripheral facial nerve (cranial nerve VII) palsy

SYNONYMS

Idiopathic facial paralysis
Facial nerve palsy

ICD-10CM CODE

G51.0 Bell palsy

EPIDEMIOLOGY & DEMOGRAPHICS

INCIDENCE: 20-30 cases per 100,000
PEAK INCIDENCE: Patients less than 70 yr old and pregnant females, especially during the third trimester and first postpartum week.
PREDOMINANT SEX AND AGE: Sexes are equally affected. The median age is 40.
RISK FACTORS: Diabetes and pregnancy

PHYSICAL FINDINGS & CLINICAL PRESENTATION

- Patients present with acute or subacute (hours to days) onset of unilateral facial paralysis with maximal weakness at 3 wk. Clinical findings are dependent on the location of facial nerve injury and involvement of associated branches (Fig. 1). One third of patients demonstrate incomplete paralysis, and the remaining two thirds have complete paralysis. Recovery usually occurs within the first 6 mo.
- Patients may also present with variable involvement of taste over the anterior two thirds of the tongue and/or altered secretion of the lacrimal and salivary glands.

ETIOLOGY

Most cases of Bell palsy are thought to be secondary to either a viral inflammatory or immune injury. Herpes simplex virus is thought to be the most common viral pathogen followed by herpes zoster. Other infectious causes include Epstein-Barr virus, cytomegalovirus, adenovirus, rubella, and mumps.

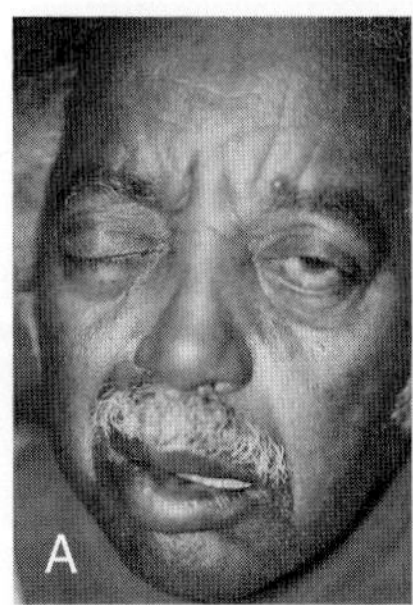

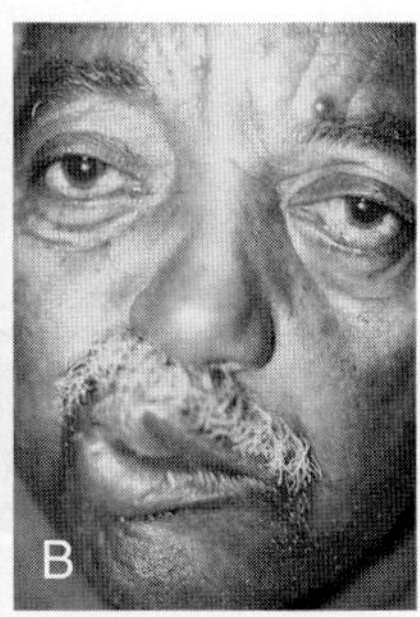

FIG. 1 A patient with a lesion of the facial nerve. A, The patient has difficulty in closing his left eye, and the left corner of his mouth droops. **B,** The latter defect is especially evident when the patient attempts to purse his lips. (From Haines DE: *Fundamental neuroscience for basic and clinical applications,* ed 3, Philadelphia, 2006, Churchill Livingstone.)

Dx DIAGNOSIS

DIFFERENTIAL DIAGNOSIS

- Cortical stroke: Forehead and periorbital muscles are spared in stroke patients because of bilateral innervation of the upper face.
- Brainstem stroke: Ipsilateral weakness in the upper and lower muscles of facial expression due to a stroke affecting the nucleus or fascicle of the seventh nerve.
- Lyme disease: Facial nerve palsy is the most common cranial neuropathy associated with Lyme disease. In Lyme meningitis, facial nerve palsy may be unilateral or bilateral.
- HIV.
- Ramsay Hunt syndrome: Facial nerve paralysis associated with ipsilateral zoster oticus.
- Parotid gland tumors.
- Trauma/temporal bone fracture.
- Meningeal processes:
  1. Infectious: Lyme disease, HIV, syphilis, leprosy, tuberculosis meningitis, fungal meningitis.
  2. Inflammatory: Sarcoidosis, Sjögren syndrome, and Guillain-Barré syndrome and its variants.
  3. Leptomeningeal carcinomatosis or lymphomatosis: Breast cancer, lung cancer, and lymphoma are most common.
- Möbius syndrome.
- Melkersson-Rosenthal syndrome.

WORKUP

- Bell palsy is a clinical diagnosis.
- Additional workup may be necessary in patients with an uncertain diagnosis, complete seventh nerve injury, evidence of neurologic dysfunction in addition to seventh nerve injury, and lack of recovery.

LABORATORY TESTS

Laboratory tests are not typically recommended. However, if the diagnosis of Bell palsy is in question (e.g., bilateral facial nerve palsy, concern for a secondary etiology), then it is reasonable to pursue the following tests:

- Lyme antibody followed by Western blot for positive cases for confirmation. Consider lumbar puncture for CSF analysis for Lyme serologies
- ACE level
- Glycosylated hemoglobin (HgA1C)
- HIV
- RPR and VDRL in CSF
- ESR

ELECTRODIAGNOSTIC TESTING

Electrodiagnostic testing may be performed 2 wk after the onset of symptoms to assess the integrity of a motor unit and the degree of nerve damage. Facial motor response remains normal for the first 3 days following an injury and then rapidly decreases depending on the severity of the lesion. A facial motor study may be performed at 10 days and compared to the contralateral side. A motor response that is 10% the amplitude of the unaffected side on electrodiagnostic testing corresponds with 90% motor axon degeneration. One study found that patient recovery was poor when this critical value was reached.

IMAGING STUDIES

Imaging studies are not usually indicated.

- Brain MRI is indicated in certain cases, such as an upper motor neuron pattern (able to wrinkle forehead) where the temporalis branch of the facial nerve is spared.
- Brain MRI with gadolinium is indicated either when other cranial nerve palsies are present or when a meningeal process is suspected.
- CT temporal bone is indicated in cases of either trauma or complete facial paralysis in which the surgeon is considering decompression.

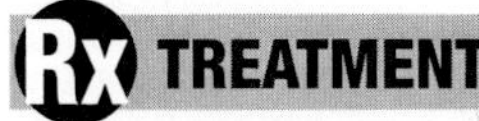

Rx TREATMENT

NONPHARMACOLOGIC THERAPY

- Reassurance that most patients will have a full recovery and that the patient did not sustain a stroke.
- Eye patch to prevent corneal drying/abrasion and subsequent ulceration. Patients may protect their eyes with Lacri-Lube at night and artificial tears during the day.
- Acupuncture with needle manipulation and strong stimulation has been shown to improve recovery after Bell palsy when compared to acupuncture without needle manipulation.[1]

ACUTE GENERAL Rx

- Corticosteroids started within 72 hr will expedite speed and rate of recovery in most patients. Antiviral therapy alone has no benefit.
  1. Two high-quality randomized trials assessed efficacy of early (<72 hr) treatment with glucocorticoids alone, antiviral therapy alone, and combination therapy in the treatment of Bell palsy. Glucocorticoids alone were effective, while antiviral therapy showed no benefit when given either alone or with concomitant glucocorticoid therapy.
  2. The largest study compared groups receiving the following treatments: (a) 60 mg prednisolone daily, (b) 1000 mg valacyclovir three times daily for 1 wk, (c) combination therapy, and (d) placebo. All interventions were administered within 72 hr of presentation.
  3. Time to recovery, determined at a 1-yr follow-up appointment, was shortest in the group treated with prednisolone

[1] Xu SB et al: Effectiveness of strengthened stimulation during acupuncture for the treatment of Bell palsy: a randomized controlled trial, *CMAJ* 185:473–479, 2013.

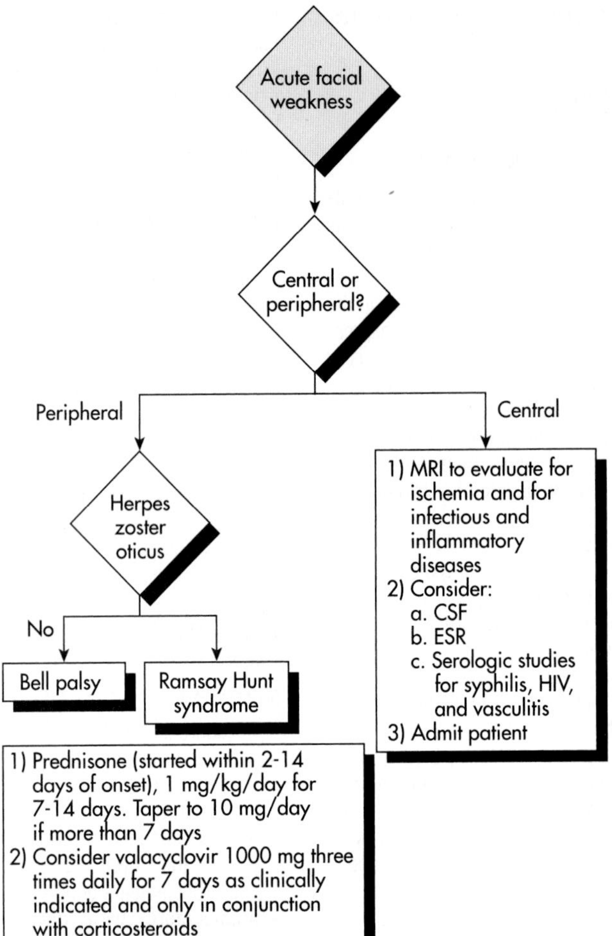

FIG. 2 Algorithm outlining the treatment of patients with Bell palsy. *CSF,* Cerebrospinal fluid; *ESR,* erythrocyte sedimentation rate; *HIV,* human immunodeficiency virus; *MRI,* magnetic resonance imaging. (Modified from Adams JG et al: *Emergency medicine, clinical essentials,* ed 2, St Louis, 2013, Elsevier.)

monotherapy. The efficacy of valacyclovir monotherapy did not differ from placebo, and no added benefit was seen with combination therapy.

- Treatment guidelines recommend prednisone 60 to 80 mg daily for 1 wk.
  1. Despite the lack of strong clinical evidence, some authors still recommend treatment with valacyclovir (1000 mg 3 times daily for 1 wk) in severe cases (i.e., level IV or greater on the House-Brackmann grading system).
- Surgical decompression is not currently recommended.
  1. The 2001 American Academy of Neurology Practice Parameter concluded there was insufficient evidence to make any recommendation regarding surgical decompression for Bell palsy.
  2. This conclusion was further substantiated by a 2011 Cochrane systematic review, which looked at two additional studies, again citing insufficient evidence regarding surgical decompression for Bell palsy.
- Fig. 2 describes an algorithm for the treatment of patients with Bell palsy.

CHRONIC Rx

Botulinum toxin may be used in cases of hemifacial spasm that may follow recovery from Bell palsy.

DISPOSITION

- Between 70% and 90% of patients with Bell palsy have a complete recovery within a few weeks.
- 85% show recovery after 3 wk. Prognosis is favorable if recovery is seen during this timeframe.

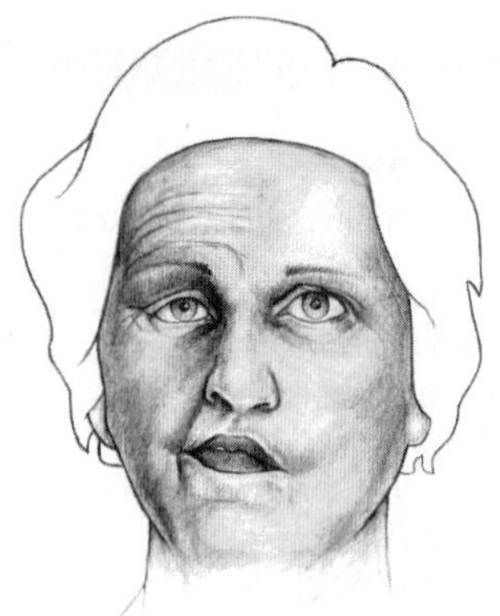

FIG. 3 Bell palsy. The patient with Bell palsy (facial nerve palsy) will demonstrate an unwrinkled forehead, widely opened eyes (with weakness of eyelid closure), flattening of the nasolabial fold, and a droop of the corner of the mouth. (From Remmel KS et al: *Handbook of symptom-oriented neurology,* ed 3, St Louis, 2002, Mosby.)

- 13% have slight sequelae, and 16% have residual weakness, synkinesis, or contracture.
- Recurrence rate is 7%, and the average time to recurrence is 10 yr.

REFERRAL

- Neurologist if clinical diagnosis is in question.
- Ophthalmologist if concern for corneal abrasion or ulceration.

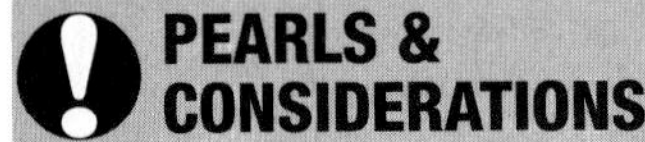

PEARLS & CONSIDERATIONS

COMMENTS

- Assess wrinkling of forehead (Fig. 3). If present on affected side, ensure that the facial weakness is not central.
- Assess for strength of eye closure. A patient with Bell palsy will have difficulty with ipsilateral eye closure, whereas a patient with a central lesion with have equal eye closure strength bilaterally.
- Assess for other cranial nerve deficits or long-tract signs because brainstem fascicular lesions of the seventh nerve can show peripheral facial pattern of weakness.

SUGGESTED READINGS

Available at ExpertConsult.com

RELATED CONTENT

Bell Palsy (Facial Palsy) (Patient Information)

AUTHORS: **ALEXANDRA BUFFIE, M.D., JOSEPH S. KASS, M.D., J.D.,** and **JOHN SLADKY, M.D.**

BASIC INFORMATION

DEFINITION

Benign paroxysmal positional vertigo (BPPV) is a labyrinthine disorder and is the most common cause of vertigo. It is characterized by paroxysms of brief spinning sensation accompanied by nystagmus that usually lasts less than a minute. These paroxysms are generally induced by changes in head position with respect to gravity.

SYNONYM

BPPV

ICD-10 CM CODES
H81.1 Benign paroxysmal vertigo

EPIDEMIOLOGY & DEMOGRAPHICS

Higher prevalence seen in elderly and women.

INCIDENCE: Incidence increases with advancing age. Unrecognized BPPV can be found in about 10% of certain geriatric populations, and there is a cumulative incidence of nearly 10% by age 80 yr.

PREVALENCE: Lifetime prevalence is 2.4%. Reported prevalence is 10.7 and 64 cases per 100,000 population. BPPV is by far the most common type of vertigo.

PREDOMINANT SEX AND AGE: Female (2:1 to 3:1 ratio); peak onset: 50-60 yr.

GENETICS: Unknown

RISK FACTORS: Head trauma, inner ear surgery, viral labyrinthitis, Ménière disease, migraine. The majority are idiopathic.

PHYSICAL FINDINGS & CLINICAL PRESENTATION

- Brief paroxysms of vertigo and nystagmus with certain head positions are seen in 70%.
- Episodes are typically triggered by head position changes such as while getting in or out of bed, rolling over in bed, forward head tilt, or bending forward.
- Episodes are brief, usually lasting 30 to 40 seconds but can recur for several days or months.
- Usually no hearing abnormalities are present.
- Direction of nystagmus depends on the canal affected with reversal of direction being seen while sitting up, and fatigability with repeated testing.
- Rarely persistent vertigo and disequilibrium may be seen.

POSTERIOR SEMICIRCULAR CANAL (PSC)

While posterior, horizontal or superior semicircular canal can be affected as isolated or in different combinations, PSC involvement is commonest (60%-90%) and will be discussed in the following sections. Nystagmus is up-beating and torsional and can be elicited by the Dix-Hallpike maneuver.

DIX-HALLPIKE MANEUVER: With head turned to one side at an angle of 45 degrees, patient is moved from sitting to supine position with head hanging below the end of the table at an angle of 15-20 degrees. The posterior semicircular canal comes into the sagittal plane and the free floating otolith debris moves down and away from the ampulla. An up-beating and torsional nystagmus will be seen with the top poles of the eye beating towards the lower ear.

HORIZONTAL SEMICIRCULAR CANAL

Involvement may be underestimated as it may remit spontaneously. It produces either geotropic nystagmus beating towards the ground or apogeotropic nystagmus beating towards the ceiling when the head is turned to either side in the supine position. The nystagmus beats stronger towards the affected ear.

HEAD ROLL TEST FOR THE RIGHT HORIZONTAL SEMICIRCULAR CANAL (INDUCING GEOTROPIC NYSTAGMUS): Patient is moved from sitting to supine position, then head is rolled 90 degrees to the left. The otolithic debris moves away from the cupula of horizontal semicircular canal, a left beating geotropic nystagmus (towards the ground) is seen. Next the head is turned 90 degrees to the right—a right-beating stronger geotropic nystagmus is seen as otolithic debris moves towards the cupula of the right horizontal semicircular canal.

SUPINE HEAD ROLL TEST FOR THE RIGHT HORIZONTAL SEMICIRCULAR CANAL (INDUCING APOGEOTROPIC NYSTAGMUS): Patient is moved from sitting to supine position, then head is rolled 90 degrees to the left. This induces deflection of the cupula of the right horizontal semicircular canal due to otolithic debris near or attached to the cupula. A strong, right-beating apogeotropic nystagmus (towards the ceiling) is induced. Next, the head is turned 90 degrees in the opposite direction. Now the right horizontal semicircular canal cupula is deflected in the opposite direction and a weak, left-beating apogeotropic nystagmus results.

ANTERIOR SEMICIRCULAR CANAL

Involvement is rare as it is located uppermost in the labyrinth and so otolithic debris is unlikely to become trapped. A downbeat and torsional nystagmus where the top poles of the eye beat towards the lower ear is seen. Evaluating for central lesions is a must in these cases.

ETIOLOGY

The fundamental pathologic process is believed to be the movement of otolithic debris in the endolymph of the inner ear. The debris may be present in the cupula (cupulolithiasis) or free floating within the semicircular canal near the cupula (canalithiasis). Static head position changes with respect to gravity, causing the debris to move within the semicircular canal and creating a false sense of rotation.

Dx DIAGNOSIS

Elicitation of a typical nystagmus with Dix-Hallpike is the standard for diagnosing posterior canal BPPV. However, 25% of symptomatic patients may not exhibit nystagmus. Appropriate referral to a neurologist or neuro-otologist should be considered in these cases.

Fig. E1 shows a diagnostic algorithm for vertigo and dizziness.

DIFFERENTIAL DIAGNOSIS

- Vestibular neuritis
- Vestibular migraine
- Ménière disease
- Stroke
- Box 1 lists causes of vertigo with and without hearing loss.
- Table 1 describes the differential diagnosis of true vertigo.

WORKUP

None; BPPV is a clinical diagnosis.

IMAGING STUDIES

- To be obtained only when stroke remains high in the differential diagnosis

Rx TREATMENT

- BPPV usually resolves without treatment in 2 to 4 weeks. Recurrences are common in the first yr, and long-term recurrence rates range from 30% to 50%.
- Nausea and vomiting may be treated symptomatically with medications.
- Canalith repositioning maneuvers (Epley and Semont maneuvers for the posterior canal) are effective. They are designed to "flush" otolithic debris out of the semicircular canals into the vestibule where they are resorbed. Epley maneuver for BPPV of the posterior canal is recommended as standard of care by the American Academy of Neurology and American Academy of Otolaryngology-Head and Neck Surgery. When patients do not respond, it may be related to the technique,

BOX 1 Causes of Vertigo with and without Hearing Loss

Hearing Loss
Conductive
- Otitis media with effusion
- Chronic suppurative otitis media or cholesteatoma should be considered

Sensorineural
- Perilymphatic fistula
- Tumor
- Ménière disease
- Migraine headache
- Genetic syndromes
- Temporal bone fracture
- Vestibular concussion

No Hearing Loss
Acute Vertigo
- Perilymphatic fistula
- Benign positional vertigo
- Seizure
- Labyrinthitis

Recurrent or Chronic Vertigo
- Acoustic neuroma
- Multiple sclerosis

From Marx JA et al: *Rosen's emergency medicine: concepts and clinical practice*, ed 7, Philadelphia, 2010, Elsevier.

TABLE 1 Differential Diagnosis of Patients with True Vertigo

Cause	History	Associated Symptoms	Physical
Peripheral			
1. Benign paroxysmal positional vertigo	Short-lived, positional, fatigable episodes	Nausea, vomiting	Single position can precipitate vertigo. Horizontorotary nystagmus often can be induced at bedside.
2. Labyrinthitis			
• Serous	Mild to severe positional symptoms. Usually coexisting or antecedent infection of ear, nose, throat, or meninges	Mild to severe hearing loss can occur	Usually nontoxic patient with minimal fever elevation
• Acute suppurative	Coexisting acute exudative infection of the inner ear. Severe symptoms	Usually severe hearing loss, nausea, vomiting	Febrile patient showing signs of toxicity. Acute otitis media
• Toxic	Gradually progressive symptoms: Patients on medication causing toxicity	Hearing loss that may become rapid and severe, nausea and vomiting	Hearing loss. Ataxia common feature in chronic phase
3. Ménière disease	Recurrent episodes of severe rotational vertigo usually lasting hours. Onset usually abrupt. Attacks may occur in clusters. Long symptom-free remissions	Nausea, vomiting, tinnitus, hearing loss	Positional nystagmus not present
4. Vestibular neuronitis	Sudden onset of severe vertigo, increasing in intensity for hours, then gradually subsiding over several days. Mild positional vertigo often lasts weeks to months. Sometimes history of infection or toxic exposure that precedes initial attack. Highest incidence is found in third and fifth decades	Nausea, vomiting. Auditory symptoms do not occur	Spontaneous nystagmus toward the involved ear may be present.
5. Acoustic neuroma	Gradual onset and increase in symptoms. Neurologic signs in later stages. Most occur in women between 30 and 60	Hearing loss, tinnitus. True ataxia and neurologic signs as tumor enlarges	Unilateral decreased hearing. True truncal ataxia and other neurologic signs when tumor enlarges. May have diminution or absence of corneal reflex. Eighth cranial nerve deficit may be present
Central			
1. Vascular disorders			
• Vertebrobasilar insufficiency	Should be considered in any patient of advanced age with isolated new-onset vertigo without an obvious cause. More likely with history of atherosclerosis. Initial episode usually seconds to minutes	Often headache. Usually neurologic symptoms including dysarthria, ataxia, weakness, numbness, double vision. Tinnitus and deafness uncommon	Neurologic deficits usually present, but initially neurologic examination can be normal.
• Cerebellar hemorrhage	Sudden onset of severe symptoms	Headache, vomiting, ataxia	Signs of toxicity. Dysmetria, true ataxia. Ipsilateral sixth cranial nerve palsy may be present.
• Occlusion of posterior inferior cerebellar artery (Wallenberg syndrome)	Vertigo associated with significant neurologic complaints	Nausea, vomiting, loss of pain and temperature sensation, ataxia, hoarseness	Loss of pain and temperature sensation on the side of the face ipsilateral to the lesion and on the opposite side of the body, paralysis of the palate, pharynx, and larynx. Horner syndrome (ipsilateral ptosis, miosis, and decreased facial sweating)
• Subclavian steal syndrome	Classic picture is syncopal attacks during exercise, but most cases present with more subtle symptoms.	Arm fatigue, cramps, mild lightheadedness may be only other symptoms than vertigo	Diminished or absent radial pulses in affected side or systolic blood pressure differentials between the two areas occur in most patients.
2. Head trauma	Symptoms begin with or shortly after head trauma. Positional symptoms most common type after trauma. Self-limited symptoms that can persist weeks to months	Usually mild nausea	Occasionally, basilar skull fracture
3. Neck trauma	Usual onset 7-10 days after whiplash injury. Symptoms may last weeks to months. Episodes seconds to minutes when turning head	Neck pain	Neck tenderness, pain on movement, and positional nystagmus and vertigo when head is turned to side of the whiplash
4. Vertebrobasilar migraine	Vertigo almost always followed by headache. Patient has usually had similar episodes in past. Most patients have a family history of migraine. Syndrome usually begins in adolescence	Dysarthria, ataxia, visual disturbances, or paresthesias usually precede headache	No residual neurologic or otologic signs are present after attack.

TABLE 1 Differential Diagnosis of Patients with True Vertigo—Cont'd

Cause	History	Associated Symptoms	Physical
5. Multiple sclerosis	Vertigo presenting symptoms in 7%-10% and appears in the course of the disease in a third. Onset may be severe and suggest labyrinth disease. Disease onset usually between ages 20 and 40. Often history of other attacks with varying neurologic signs or symptoms	Nausea and vomiting, which may be severe	May have horizontal, rotary, or vertical nystagmus. Nystagmus may persist after the vertiginous symptoms have subsided. Bilateral internuclear ophthalmoplegia and ataxic eye movements suggest multiple sclerosis.
6. Temporal lobe epilepsy	Can be initial or prominent symptom in some patients with the disorder	Memory impairment, hallucinations, trancelike states, seizures	May have aphasia or convulsions
7. Hypoglycemia	Should be considered in diabetics and any other patient with unexplained symptoms	Sweating, anxiety	Tachycardia, mental status change may be present.

From Marx JA et al: *Rosen's emergency medicine: concepts and clinical practice*, ed 7, Philadelphia, 2010, Elsevier.

or they may be refractory. There is no clear consensus on how many times the maneuver should be performed at a single visit. Many prefer to do it two or three times if nystagmus is still present with the second maneuver. Other maneuvers such as Barbecue, Vannucchi, and Gufoni are used to reposition debris in the horizontal semicircular canal and will not be discussed here.

EPLEY MANEUVER:

- Head is turned 90 degrees towards unaffected side. The head and trunk are then turned an additional 90 degrees in the same direction, so that the patient lies on the unaffected side with head pointing towards the floor. The otolithic debris moves in the same direction, producing a brief nystagmus. The patient is then moved to a sitting position, which allows the debris to fall out of the canal into the utricle through the common crus.
- Each position should be maintained for 30 seconds or until the nystagmus or vertigo resolves. Sometimes nystagmus in the opposite direction is seen. It is prudent for patients to sit still in the upright position for about 15 minutes and then to walk cautiously.

NONPHARMACOLOGIC THERAPY

Transection of the ampullary nerve (singular nerve) and plugging of the involved canal are rarely performed for intractable and treatment-resistant cases.

ACUTE GENERAL Rx

Canalith repositioning

CHRONIC Rx

If multiple treatments are needed, patients should be instructed to perform the maneuvers at home.

REFERRAL

To a neuro-otologist, otolaryngologist, neurologist

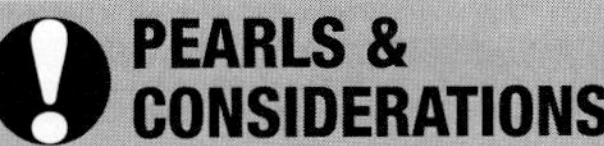

PEARLS & CONSIDERATIONS

- BPPV is a benign and self-limiting condition but can be disabling.
- Diagnosis is clinical and canalith repositioning maneuvers are effective.

PATIENT/FAMILY EDUCATION

- Reassurance
- Fall precautions

RELATED CONTENT

Ménière Disease (Related Key Topic)
Vestibular Neuritis (Related Key Topic)

SUGGESTED READING

Available at ExpertConsult.com

AUTHORS: **PADMAJA SUDHAKAR, M.B.B.S.,** and **SACHIN KEDAR, M.B.B.S., M.D.**

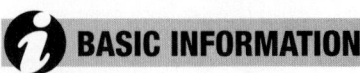

BASIC INFORMATION

DEFINITION

Benign prostatic hyperplasia (BPH) is the benign growth of the prostate, generally originating in the periureteral and transition zones, with subsequent obstructive and irritative voiding symptoms. Histologically, BPH refers to the proliferation of smooth muscle, epithelium, and stromal cells within the transition zone of the prostate that surrounds the proximal urethra.

SYNONYMS

Benign prostatic hypertrophy
BPH
Prostatic hypertrophy

ICD-10CM CODES

N40.0 Enlarged prostate without lower urinary tract symptoms
N40.1 Enlarged prostate with lower urinary tract symptoms
N40.2 Nodular prostate without lower urinary tract symptoms
N40.3 Nodular prostate with lower urinary tract symptoms

EPIDEMIOLOGY & DEMOGRAPHICS

- 80% of men have evidence of BPH by age 80 yr.
- Medical and surgical intervention for problems caused by BPH is required in <20% of males by age 75 yr.
- Transurethral resection of the prostate (TURP) is the tenth most common operative procedure (<400,000/yr in U.S.).
- 10% to 30% of men with BPH have occult prostate cancer.

PHYSICAL FINDINGS & CLINICAL PRESENTATION

- Digital rectal examination (DRE) reveals enlargement of the prostate.
- Focal enlargement may be indicative of malignancy.
- There is poor correlation between size of prostate and symptoms (BPH may be asymptomatic if it does not encroach on the urethral lumen).
- Most patients with BPH report difficulty in initiating urination (hesitancy), decrease in caliber and force of stream, incomplete emptying of bladder often resulting in double voiding (need to urinate again a few minutes after voiding), postvoid "dribbling," and nocturia.

ETIOLOGY

Multifactorial (Fig. E1); a functioning testicle is necessary for development of BPH (as evidenced by the absence in males who were castrated before puberty).

Dx DIAGNOSIS

DIFFERENTIAL DIAGNOSIS

- Prostatitis
- Prostate cancer
- Strictures (urethral)
- Medications interfering with the muscle fibers in the prostate and also with bladder function:
  1. Opiates: Impaired autonomic function
  2. Decongestants: Increased sphincter tone
  3. Antihistamines: Decreased parasympathetic tone
  4. Tricyclic antidepressants: Anticholinergic effects
- Neurogenic bladder
- Bladder cancer

WORKUP

Symptom assessment (use of American Urological Association [AUA] Symptom Index for BPH [Table 1]), laboratory tests, and imaging studies. Fig. E2 describes a diagnostic approach to patients with BPH.

LABORATORY TESTS

- Prostate-specific antigen (PSA): Protease secreted by epithelial cells of the prostate; elevated in 30% to 50% of patients with BPH. Testing for PSA increases detection rate for prostate cancer and tends to detect cancer at an earlier stage. However, the PSA test does not discriminate well between patients with symptomatic BPH and those with prostate cancer, particularly if the cancer is pathologically localized and curable. The test may also trigger additional evaluation, including ultrasound biopsy of the prostate. Asymptomatic men with PSA levels >2 ng/ml do not need annual testing. According to the AUA, PSA testing and DRE should be offered to any asymptomatic man <50 yr with a life expectancy of 10 yr. PSA testing can also be offered at an earlier age in men at higher risk of prostatic cancer (e.g., first-degree relatives with prostate cancer; African American race).
- Measurement of "free" PSA is useful to assess the probability of prostate cancer in patients with normal DRE and total PSA between 4 and 10 ng/ml. In these patients the global risk of prostate cancer is 25%. However, if the free PSA is >25%, the risk of prostate cancer decreases to 8%, whereas if the free PSA is <10%, the risk of cancer increases to 56%. Free PSA is also useful to evaluate the aggressiveness of prostate cancer. A low free PSA percentage generally

TABLE 1 International Prostate Symptom Score (I-PSS)

	Score						
Symptom	**Not at All**	**Less Than 1 Time in 5**	**Less Than Half the Time**	**About Half the Time**	**More Than Half the Time**	**Almost Always**	**Total Score**
Incomplete emptying: Over the past month, how often have you had a sensation of not emptying your bladder completely after you finished urinating?	0	1	2	3	4	5	
Frequency: Over the past month, how often have you had to urinate again <2 hr after you finished urinating?	0	1	2	3	4	5	
Intermittency: Over the past month, how often have you found you stopped and started again several times when you urinated?	0	1	2	3	4	5	
Urgency: Over the past month, how often have you found it difficult to postpone urination?	0	1	2	3	4	5	
Weak stream: Over the past month, how often have you had a weak urinary stream?	0	1	2	3	4	5	
Straining: Over the past month, how often have you had to push or strain to begin urination?	0	1	2	3	4	5	
	None	1 Time	2 Times	3 Times	4 Times	5 or More Times	
Nocturia: Over the past month, how many times did you most typically get up to urinate from the time you went to bed at night until the time you got up in the morning?	0	1	2	3	4	5	
Total I-PSS score =							

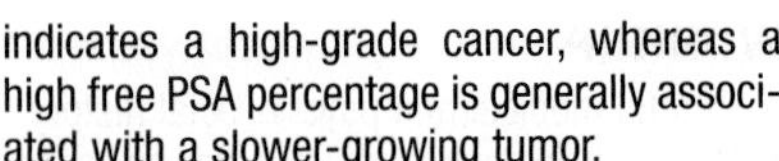

indicates a high-grade cancer, whereas a high free PSA percentage is generally associated with a slower-growing tumor.

- Elevated measurement of prostate cancer gene 3 (*PCA3*) in urine specimens collected after digital exam is helpful in deciding about prostate biopsy in men with elevated PSA (increased *PCA3* = increased likelihood of prostate cancer).
- Urinalysis, urine culture, and sensitivity to rule out infection (if suspected).
- Blood urea nitrogen and creatinine to rule out postrenal insufficiency.

IMAGING STUDIES

- Transrectal ultrasound may be indicated in patients with palpable nodules or significant elevation of PSA. It is also useful to estimate prostate size. BPH may also be evident in suprapubic ultrasound and MRI.
- Uroflowmetry may be used to determine relative impact of obstruction on urine flow. Urethral pressure profile is useful to predict prostatic hypertrophy within the urethral lumen.
- Pressure flow studies, although invasive, are particularly helpful in patients whose history and/or examination suggest primary bladder dysfunction as a cause of symptoms of prostatism. They are also useful in patients for whom a distinction between prostatic obstruction and impaired detrusor contractility may affect the choice of therapy. However, pressure flow studies may not be useful in the workup of the usual patient with symptoms of prostatism.
- Postvoid residual urine measurement has not been proved useful in predicting the need for or response to treatment; it may be useful in monitoring the course of the disease in patients who elect nonsurgical treatment.
- Urethral cystoscopy is an option during later evaluation if invasive treatment is being planned.

Rx TREATMENT

NONPHARMACOLOGIC THERAPY

- Avoidance of caffeine or any other foods that may exacerbate symptoms
- Avoidance of medications that may exacerbate symptoms (e.g., most cold and allergy remedies)

GENERAL Rx

- Asymptomatic patients with prostate enlargement caused by BPH generally do not require treatment. Patients with mild to moderate symptoms are candidates for pharmacologic treatment (see the following). For patients who have specific complications from BPH, prostate surgery is usually the most appropriate form of treatment. However, surgery may result in significant complications (e.g., incontinence, infection).
- Alpha-blockers (e.g., tamsulosin, alfuzosin, doxazosin, prazosin, terazosin) relax smooth muscle of the bladder neck and prostate and can increase peak urinary flow rate. They have no effect on the size of the prostate. Alpha-1 blockers are useful in symptomatic patients to relieve symptoms of obstruction by causing relaxation of smooth muscle tone in the prostatic capsule, urethra, and bladder neck.
- Hormonal manipulation with finasteride, a 5-alpha-reductase inhibitor that blocks conversion of testosterone to dihydrotestosterone, can reduce the size of the prostate. Usual dose is 5 mg qd. Treatment requires ≥6 mo for maximal effect.
- Dutasteride is also a 5-alpha-reductase inhibitor useful to decrease prostate size and improve urinary flow. In addition to inhibiting the isoform of 5-alpha-reductase located in the prostate, the medication inhibits a second isoform and reduces dihydrotestosterone formation in the skin and liver. Usual dose is 0.5 mg qd.
- Tadalafil 2.5 to 5 mg qd has been FDA-approved to treat patients with signs and symptoms of BPH and patients with both ED and signs and symptoms of BPH. Tadalafil can potentiate the hypotensive effect of alpha-blockers and should not be used in combination with alpha-blockers.
- The dietary supplement saw palmetto is commonly used for relief of symptoms of BPH. Recent trials using 160 mg of saw palmetto bid did not improve symptoms of BPH. This contrasts with the positive findings of many previous studies. Trials with higher dose-ranging protocols are currently in progress.
- TURP is the most commonly used surgical procedure for BPH. It is recommended for patients unresponsive to medical therapy who have renal insufficiency, recurrent UTIs, bladder stones, or gross hematuria. Transurethral incision of the prostate (TUIP), a procedure almost equivalent in efficacy, is limited to patients whose estimated resection tissue weight would be 30 g or less. TUIP can be performed in an ambulatory setting or during a 1-day hospitalization. Open prostatectomy is typically performed on patients with very large prostates. A prostatic urethral lift implant (UroLift) is now available for BPH. It is placed transurethrally at the site of obstruction to open the urethra by compressing the obstructing prostatic lobes and holding them permanently retracted with suture-based implants.
- Laser therapy for BPH is a less invasive alternative to TURP; YAG laser enucleation has minimal effect on potency, libido, or patient satisfaction with his sex life and is associated with retrograde ejaculation. However, recent studies indicate that at least in the initial 7 mo after surgery, TURP is moderately more effective than laser therapy in relieving symptoms of BPH.
- Transurethral needle ablation with radiofrequency to remove periurethral prostate tissue is being increasingly used in patients with prostate volume >60 ml and moderate symptoms. It has a low morbidity rate, but treatment failure is approximately 25% at 5 yr and <80% at 10 yr.
- Balloon dilation of the prostatic urethra is less effective than surgery for relieving symptoms but is associated with fewer complications. It is a reasonable treatment option for patients with smaller prostates and no middle lobe enlargement.
- Surgery need not be the treatment of last resort for most patients; that is, patients need not undergo other treatments for BPH before they can have surgery. However, recommending surgery on the grounds that a patient's surgical risk will "only increase with age" is generally inappropriate.

DISPOSITION

With appropriate therapy, symptoms improve or stabilize in <70% of patients with BPH.

REFERRAL

Urology referral for patients with severe or intolerable symptoms and for any patient suspected of having prostate cancer (10%-30% of men with BPH)

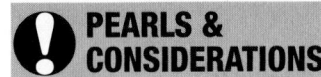

PEARLS & CONSIDERATIONS

COMMENTS

- Emerging technologies for treating BPH, including prostatic artery embolization, transurethral holmium laser enucleation, transurethral electrovaporization, and transurethral microwave thermotherapy of the prostate, appear promising; however, long-term effectiveness has not yet been demonstrated.
- The increase in the use of pharmacologic management has resulted in <30% reduction in the total number of TURP procedures.
- Combined drug therapy for BPH with an alpha-blocker and a 5-alpha-reductase inhibitor is superior to monotherapy with either agent. After 1 yr of combination therapy, withdrawal of the alpha-blocker will usually not exacerbate symptoms.

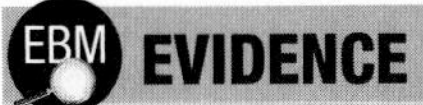

EVIDENCE

Available at ExpertConsult.com

SUGGESTED READINGS

Available at ExpertConsult.com

RELATED CONTENT

Enlarged Prostate (Patient Information)

AUTHOR: **FRED F. FERRI, M.D.**

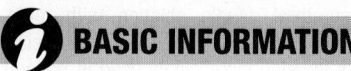

BASIC INFORMATION

DEFINITION

Binge eating disorder (BED) is characterized by recurrent binge eating episodes, during which an abnormally large amount of food is consumed in a short period of time, accompanied by a sense of loss of control. At least 3 of the following features need to be present in a binge eating episode:

1. Consuming food faster than normal
2. Consuming food until uncomfortably full
3. Consuming large amounts of food when not hungry
4. Consuming food alone due to embarrassment
5. Feeling disgusted, depressed, or guilty after eating a large amount of food

In order to meet criteria for BED, individuals must engage in binge eating episodes at least once per week for 3 months, feel significant distress with regard to their binge eating behaviors, and not utilize compensatory behaviors (e.g., induced vomiting, laxative misuse, overexercising) seen in other eating disorders like bulimia nervosa.

SYNONYMS

Compulsive overeating
BED

ICD-10CM CODES
F50.81 Binge eating disorder
DSM-5 CODES
307.51

EPIDEMIOLOGY & DEMOGRAPHICS

INCIDENCE: To our knowledge, no incidence studies on BED yet exist.

PREVALENCE (IN US): Approximately 2% lifetime prevalence in adult community samples was found (women 3.5%; men 2.0%). BED was found to be the most common eating disorder in males—the female-to-male ratio being more balanced (about 3:2) compared with other eating disorders (about 9:1). Lower lifetime prevalence rates among 13- to 18-yr-old adolescents (girls 2.3%; boys 0.8%) were found. The 12-month prevalence among adult women and men is 1.6% and 0.8%, respectively.

PREDOMINANT AGE (IN US): Higher prevalence rates in females (1.75:1) were found among adults.

GENETICS:

- BED appears to aggregate in families and have a significant genetic component
- Family studies report odds ratios between 1.9 and 2.2 for the risk of BED in a relative of a proband with BED compared with relatives of controls
- Twin studies of BED have reported heritability estimates ranging from 41% to 57% for varying definitions of this disorder

RISK FACTORS:

- Mental health concerns and psychopathology (mood disorders, anxiety disorders, personality disorders, conduct problems, negative affectivity, substance abuse)
- Temperament and coping style (e.g., high avoidance motivation, low distress tolerance, low extraversion, and self-directedness)
- Severe childhood obesity
- Experience of bullying/weight-related stigmas
- Lifestyle disruptions and deprivation
- Family weight and eating concerns (family dieting, family history of bulimia nervosa, family overeating)
- Quality of parenting (family discord, maternal/paternal problem parenting, parental separation/absence/death)
- Sexual and physical abuse

PHYSICAL FINDINGS & CLINICAL PRESENTATION

- Although not necessary for a diagnosis, individuals presenting with BED are often overweight or obese
- BED is highly comorbid with other forms of psychopathology, especially mood and anxiety disorders. Individuals seeking treatment with acute symptoms of other disorders might not initially report binging episodes, which underscores the importance of thorough initial assessment
- Males with BED are more likely to underreport symptoms
- Among individuals with BED, men tend to have significantly higher BMI, whereas women tend to have significantly higher eating-disorder psychopathology
- Disordered eating symptoms can improve or worsen over time, and diagnostic labels might transition from BED to other eating disorders over time
- There is potential for higher suicide risk among individuals with BED, possibly because of comorbid psychopathology, and suicidal ideation/intent should be monitored
- General difficulty to cope with negative emotions and avoidance of aversive experiences/feelings might be apparent
- Significant shame and self-conscious emotions regarding bingeing behaviors might be present, often resulting in underreporting of binge-eating behaviors

ETIOLOGY

Research suggests that individual factors (e.g., genetic, biologic, temperamental), environmental factors (e.g., family environment, external sources of stress), and their interactions each contribute.

Dx DIAGNOSIS

DIFFERENTIAL DIAGNOSIS

- Important to establish the presence of objective binge eating episodes versus subjective binge eating episodes and nonbinge forms of overeating.
- Important to establish that binge eating episodes are not associated with the recurrent use of inappropriate compensatory behaviors (e.g., purging, overexercising).
- Important to establish that binge eating episodes do not occur exclusively during the course of anorexia nervosa, bulimia nervosa, or avoidant/restrictive food intake disorder.

WORKUP

- Careful medical and psychosocial history
- Physical examination reveals no specific diagnostic signs of BED
- Mental status examination

LABORATORY TESTS

No laboratory tests are diagnostic. However, given that BED is frequently associated with overweight and obesity, tests examining associated medical problems (e.g., Type II diabetes, high triglycerides) might benefit an individual's overall treatment plan.

IMAGING STUDIES

Neuroimaging studies suggest there are corticostriatal circuitry alterations in BED similar to those observed in substance abuse, including altered function of prefrontal, insular, and orbitofrontal cortices and the striatum. Imaging is not recommended as part of routine evaluation.

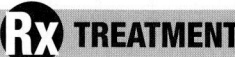

TREATMENT

NONPHARMACOLOGIC THERAPY

- The primary goal of therapeutic approaches to BED is reduction and/or elimination of binge eating episodes and the associated symptoms of distress.
- Variations of cognitive behavior therapy (CBT) and interpersonal psychotherapy (IPT) remain the most established treatments for BED.
- Growing literature on other psychotherapeutic approaches to BED has also yielded empirical support for dialectical behavior therapy (DBT) and mindfulness-based therapies.
- Combining different interventions at the same time does not add significant advantages. Planning sequential treatments, with more specific interventions for nonresponders, seems to be a more promising strategy.
- Behavioral weight loss (BWL) and self-help interventions evidenced some efficacy in patients with lower psychopathological features. Moreover, BWL approaches have not fared as well as CBT and IPT approaches in ameliorating disordered eating patterns.
- Morbidly obese patients with BED might be well-served by weight loss (bariatric) surgery, which has been found to be associated with sustained, substantial weight loss, as well as reduction in binge eating episodes.
- Preliminary findings regarding electronically delivered psychotherapeutic interventions (e.g., Internet-based CBT) for BED have yielded some empirical support.
- One of the limitations of extant literature is the predominant inclusion of female participants in RCTs.

ACUTE GENERAL Rx

- The pharmacotherapy literature on treating BED in the short-term has focused on achieving the following objectives: Reducing the frequency of binge eating episodes, reducing weight, and improving associated psychopathology (e.g., depression/anxiety symptoms).

- Preliminary support for specific medications within the classes of antidepressants, anticonvulsants, and antiobesity agents has been found for treating symptoms associated with BED.
- Antidepressants are thought to influence treatment outcomes by addressing the mood and anxiety symptoms that often co-occur with BED. Anticonvulsants have been examined in the treatment of BED because of their success in treating other impulse control disorders. Antiobesity agents have been used to address the overweight and obesity that usually accompanies BED.
- Lisdexamfetamine dimesylate (Vyvanse) is the only medication that has been approved by the Food and Drug Administration (FDA) for the treatment of BED. Two studies found that participants taking the medication experienced a decrease in the number of binge-eating days per week and had fewer obsessive-compulsive binge eating behaviors compared with those on placebo. Longer-term maintenance studies examining the treatment of BED have not yet been published.
- Exploratory work using substance use treatment agents to address BED symptoms is currently under way.
- The existing literature on pharmacotherapy approaches to BED has several limitations, including short duration of RCTs and lack of adequately sized RCTs.

CHRONIC Rx

The long-term treatment of BED using pharmacotherapy has not as yet been systematically investigated.

COMPLEMENTARY & ALTERNATIVE MEDICINE

One study found that hour-long, weekly yoga sessions were associated with reductions in binge eating, BMI, and hip and waist measurements, and an increase in physical activity. More follow-up research is needed in this area.

DISPOSITION

- Data on the long-term outcome of BED, including mortality, are scarce.
- Most outcome data on BED are derived from RCTs. In studies on the outcome of binge eating disorder with a follow-up duration over 3 yr, remission rates in the samples treated with psychotherapy ranged from 19% to 65% across the studies.
- Prospective longitudinal studies with adolescents have found that girls with BED had a twofold risk of becoming overweight or obese, or developing high depressive symptoms compared with nondisordered girls. Among boys, weekly binges predicted drug use as well.
- Various factors may affect treatment response to BED. For instance, higher frequency of binges, increased comorbid psychopathology, and decreased social/family support have been found to be associated with worse treatment outcomes.

REFERRAL

- Referral to mental health specialists: For diagnosis and symptom management (using psychotherapy, pharmacotherapy)
- Referral to nutrition, exercise specialist and/or bariatric surgeon: If patient with BED is morbidly obese and has associated medical problems

PEARLS & CONSIDERATIONS

COMMENTS

- Individuals with BED who are overweight or obese and are interested in weight loss, should also be encouraged to engage in treatment for disordered eating. Although the psychological treatments for BED do not produce substantial weight loss, the elimination of binge eating protects against future weight gain.
- If possible, including family in treatment can be helpful for building social and environmental supports, especially for adolescent and young adult clients.

PREVENTION

There are no known ways to prevent BED (or other eating disorders). However, research suggests that involving education on weight stigma, healthy eating, and body confidence in interventions among school children might ameliorate future body dissatisfaction and disordered eating.

PATIENT/FAMILY EDUCATION

- National Education Disorders Association (NEDA, https://www.nationaleatingdisorders.org/) provides patient, family, and professional information on eating disorders including BED.
- Binge Eating Disorder Association (BEDA, http://bedaonline.com/) provides patient and professional information on BED.
- Additional, local and/or online support groups for BED are common and should be investigated.

SUGGESTED READINGS

Available at ExpertConsult.com

RELATED TOPICS

Anorexia Nervosa (Related Key Topic)
Bulimia Nervosa (Related Key Topic)

AUTHORS: **EISHITA MANJREKAR, PH.D.**, and **MARK ZIMMERMAN, M.D.**

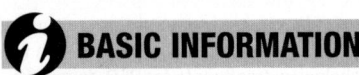

DEFINITION

Bipolar disorder is an episodic, recurrent, and frequently progressive condition in which the afflicted individual experiences at least one episode of mania, characterized by at least 1 wk of continuous symptoms of elevated, expansive, or irritable mood, in association with three or more of the following symptoms (four if irritability is the presenting mood):

- Decreased need for sleep
- Grandiosity or inflated self-esteem
- Pressured speech
- Flight of ideas or subjective sense of racing thoughts
- Distractibility
- Increased level of goal-directed activity
- Problematic behavior with a high potential for painful consequences

Most individuals with bipolar disorder also experience one or more episodes of major depression over their lifetimes or have symptoms of a depressive episode commingled with those of mania (mixed episode). Hypomanic episodes may also occur.

SYNONYMS

Manic-depression
Cycloid psychosis

ICD-10CM CODES

F42.0	Bipolar affective disorder, current episode hypomanic
F31.1	Bipolar affective disorder, current episode manic without psychotic symptoms
F31.2	Bipolar affective disorder, current episode manic with psychotic symptoms
F31.3	Bipolar affective disorder, current episode mild or moderate depression
F31.4	Bipolar affective disorder, current episode severe depression without psychotic symptoms
F31.5	Bipolar affective disorder, current episode severe depression with psychotic symptoms
F31.6	Bipolar affective disorder, current episode mixed
F31.8	Bipolar II disorder

DSM-5 CODES

296.41-296.80	(Depends on specific diagnosis)

EPIDEMIOLOGY & DEMOGRAPHICS

INCIDENCE: 0.016% to 0.021%

PREVALENCE (IN U.S.): 0.4% to 1.6% (lifetime); bipolar spectrum disorders: 2.8%; approximately 25% attempt suicide, and suicide deaths occur 20x more frequently than in the general population

PREDOMINANT SEX: Equal distribution among male and female

PREDOMINANT AGE: Lifelong condition with age of onset 14 to 30 yr

PEAK INCIDENCE: Onset in 20s

GENETICS:

- Concordance rates for monozygotic twins: 0.7 to 0.8; for dizygotic twins: 0.2
- Risk of affective disorder in offspring with one affected parent with bipolar disorder: 27% to 29%; with two affected parents: 50% to 74%
- Heritability estimate of 0.85
- No specific causal mutations have been identified, but cross-disorder studies indicate an overlap with genes associated with a risk for autism or schizophrenia. Genome-wide association analyses and exome sequencing have suggested a role for *CACNA1C, ANK3, TRANK1, ODZ4, ZNF 804A,* and *KDM5B,* among others, and have implicated ion channelopathies, immune and neuronal signaling, and histone methylation in pathogenesis of bipolar disorder. It is hypothesized that heritability derives from the additive effect of a number of common risk alleles in association with a few higher-risk deleterious variants

PHYSICAL FINDINGS & CLINICAL PRESENTATION

- Mania associated with:
  1. Psychomotor activation that is usually goal directed but not necessarily productive
  2. Increase in goal-directed activity and excessive involvement in activities leading to unexpected adverse outcomes
  3. Elevated, euphoric, and frequently labile mood
  4. Decreased need for sleep
  5. Flight of ideas with rapid, loud, pressured speech
- Psychosis often occurs (75%), with delusions, hallucinations, and/or formal thought disorder
- Depressive episodes resembling major depressive disorder (see "Depression, Major"), although usually of shorter duration and more frequent; atypical features (hypersomnia, prominent anxiety, weight gain) may be present
- Mixed states, characterized by activation, irritability, and dysphoria, also possible.

KEY DIAGNOSTIC CRITERIA DISTINGUISHING BIPOLAR I DISORDER FROM BIPOLAR II DISORDER:

[1]**Manic episode (Bipolar I Disorder)**

- Distinct period during which there is an abnormally and persistently elevated, expansive, or irritable mood and abnormally and persistently increased goal-directed activity or energy lasting at least 1 wk (or less if hospitalization is required)
- Must be accompanied by at least three of the following symptoms (four if mood is only irritable): Inflated self-esteem or grandiosity, decreased need for sleep, pressured speech, racing thoughts, distractibility, increased involvement in goal-directed activity or psychomotor agitation, excessive involvement in pleasurable activities with a high potential for painful consequences
- Symptoms do not meet criteria for a mixed episode
- Disturbance must be sufficiently severe to cause marked impairment in social or occupational functioning or to require hospitalization, or it is characterized by the presence of psychotic features
- Symptoms not due to direct physiologic effect of medication, general medication condition, or substance abuse, although if they persist after a direct condition is addressed, a primary bipolar condition should be considered

Hypomanic episode (Bipolar II Disorder)

- Distinct period during which there is an abnormally and persistently elevated, expansive, or irritable mood and abnormally and persistently elevated activity or energy lasting at least 4 consecutive days
- Must be accompanied by at least three of the following symptoms (four if mood is only irritable): Inflated self-esteem or grandiosity, decreased need for sleep, pressured speech, racing thoughts, distractibility, increased involvement in goal-directed activity or psychomotor agitation, excessive involvement in pleasurable activities with a high potential for painful consequences
- Hypomanic episodes must be clearly different from the person's usual nondepressed mood, and there must be a clear change in functioning that is not characteristic of the person's usual functioning; consider using checklist (HCL-32) for accuracy
- Changes in mood and functioning must be observable by others. In contrast to a manic episode, a hypomanic episode is not severe enough to cause marked impairment in social or occupational functioning or to require hospitalization, and there are no psychotic features
- Symptoms not due to direct physiologic effect of medication, general medication condition, or substance abuse

ETIOLOGY

Hypotheses:

- Abnormalities of GABAA and G protein–coupled receptor and membrane function, calcium dysregulation
- Alteration of cAMP, MAP kinase, protein kinase C, arachidonic acid cascade, and glycogen synthase kinase-3 signal transduction pathways; mitochondrial dysfunction
- Alteration in cell survival pathways, glial and neuronal death and loss of neuroplasticity; proposed biomarkers include BDNF and measures of inflammation, oxidative stress, and endothelial function

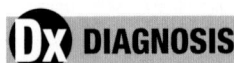

DIFFERENTIAL DIAGNOSIS

- Secondary manias caused by medical disorders (e.g., hyperthyroidism, AIDS, early dementia, stroke, Cushing syndrome) or pharmacologic treatment (e.g., steroids, stimulants)

---

[1] Criteria are from the American Psychiatric Association: *Diagnostic and statistical manual of mental disorders, fifth edition,* Washington, DC, 2013, American Psychiatric Association.

- First onset of mania after age 50 yr suggestive of secondary mania
- Less severe, and possibly distinct, conditions of bipolar type II and cyclothymia
- Comorbid substance abuse or dependency occurs in 60% to 75% of patients and may confound diagnosis and treatment
- Presentation can be confused with schizophrenia or paranoid psychosis

WORKUP

- History
- Physical examination
- Mental status examination
- Mood Disorder Questionnaire (MDQ); Composite International Diagnostic Interview (CIDI) (3.0)

LABORATORY TESTS

Because of high rate of secondary manias, initial evaluation to confirm health of all major organ systems (routine chemistries, complete blood count, urinalysis, sedimentation rate)

IMAGING STUDIES

- Consider brain imaging if late onset or if neurologic examination is abnormal.
- Neuroimaging may show evidence of ventricular enlargement or increased white matter hyperintensities; decrements in prefrontal and temporal lobe cortical thickness also reported. Corresponding changes in neurocognition, including changes in executive function, verbal memory, and processing speed, may occur.

Rx TREATMENT

NONPHARMACOLOGIC THERAPY

- Cognitive-behavioral and family-focused psychoeducational psychotherapy to help patients cope with consequences of the disease, improve adherence with medications, and identify possible environmental triggers; consider life charting
- Bright light therapy in the northern latitudes in individuals exhibiting a seasonal pattern of winter depression
- Lifestyle "regularization"; interpersonal and social rhythm therapy; integrated care management for chronic conditions
- Many smartphone mobile apps for bipolar disorder are available to provide information, help monitor symptoms, and deliver interventions

ACUTE GENERAL Rx

- First-line agents for acute mania and mixed states: Lithium 1500 to 1800 mg/day (0.8 to 1.2 mEq/L), valproate 1000 to 1500 mg/day (50 to 125 ng/ml), carbamazepine 600 to 800 mg/day (4 to 12 micrograms/ml), oxcarbazepine 900 to 2400 mg/day, olanzapine 10 to 20 mg/day, risperidone 2 to 4 mg/day, quetiapine 350 to 800 mg/day, ziprasidone 80 to 120 mg/day, asenapine 10 to 20 mg/day, or aripiprazole 10 to 30 mg/day. Treatment-resistant cases may respond to varying combinations of these agents or to the addition of clozapine.
- Useful adjuncts to acute treatment of mania: Benzodiazepines: lorazepam 1 to 2 mg q4h, clonazepam 1 to 2 mg q4h.
- Traditional antidepressants can induce manic episodes and exacerbate mania in mixed episodes and may be less effective than in treatment of unipolar depression.
- First-line options for bipolar depression include lithium, lurasidone, quetiapine, lamotrigine, and olanzapine/fluoxetine combination. Bupropion may have a lower risk for triggering mania, and MAOIs or ECT may be efficacious in treatment-resistant cases. Off-label agents with possible efficacy include modafinil, pramipexole, and intravenous ketamine.

CHRONIC Rx

- Goal of long-term treatment: Prevention of relapse or episode recurrence
- Best agents for prophylaxis of mania: Lithium, quetiapine, aripiprazole, and olanzapine (valproate, carbamazepine/oxcarbazepine possibly beneficial)
- Best agents for prophylaxis of depression: Lamotrigine and lithium
- Risk/benefit of atypical antipsychotics versus traditional mood stabilizers in maintenance unclear
- Long-term use of antidepressants: Frequently destabilizes patient and leads to more frequent relapses; depression outweighs mania as the most debilitating dimension over the life span; bipolar disorder accounts for 7% of all disease-related disability-adjusted life yrs

DISPOSITION

- Course is variable.
- More than 90% of patients having a single manic episode are likely to experience others.
- Uncontrolled manic or depressive episodes can lead to additional episodes.
- Lithium, in comparison to other mood stabilizers or atypical antipsychotic agents, has been shown to specifically decrease suicidal risk.
- Socioeconomic consequences of both mania and depression can be severe and disabling.
- Mortality rate from all causes is 15× that of the general population.

REFERRAL

- If use of antidepressant contemplated or in cases of pediatric bipolar disorder
- If patient is severely manic, rapid cycling, pregnant, or suicidal or is in a bipolar, mixed episode

PEARLS & CONSIDERATIONS

COMMENTS

- All patients presenting with depression should be asked about past personal and family history of mania and hypomania; 70% of bipolar patients have previously been misdiagnosed. Onset before age 25, postpartum onset, and poor prior response to antidepressants are additional clues.
- Prompt recognition of the earliest signs of mania in a given individual (e.g., decreased need for sleep, increased rate of speech) allows earlier intervention and a better likelihood of preventing a full episode.
- Bipolar disorder in children frequently manifests as episodic behavioral disinhibition, affective lability, and temper dysregulation, but current consensus indicates that the condition is overdiagnosed in this age group. Disruptive mood dysregulation disorder (DMDD) describes children who exhibit persistent irritability and severe temper outbursts on a frequent basis (at least three times/wk for a yr or more).
- Rapid cycling (greater than three episodes/yr) and mixed states are associated with a poorer prognosis, including a longer course, more treatment resistance, more substance use comorbidity, and increased suicidal risk.
- Patients treated with atypical antipsychotic agents should be carefully monitored for development of metabolic syndrome. Independent of medication effect, there is a higher prevalence of metabolic syndrome and abdominal obesity in those with bipolar disorder.
- Despite some variation in prevalence, the severity, impact, and patterns of comorbidity of bipolar disorder are similar in different countries in world health surveys.
- Bipolar disorder often co-occurs with anxiety disorders and attention deficit hyperactivity disorder (ADHD), making attribution of specific symptoms difficult.
- Patients receiving anticonvulsants or antidepressants should be monitored for a possible increase in suicidal thoughts or behavior.
- There is preliminary evidence that nutraceutical agents like omega-3 fatty acids and *N*-acetyl cysteine (NAC) may have efficacy in the treatment of bipolar disorder.
- Multiple studies show a correlation between bipolar disorder and heightened creativity.

PATIENT/FAMILY EDUCATION

Information available at www.NMHA.org/ and www.dbsalliance.org/.

SUGGESTED READINGS

Available at ExpertConsult.com

RELATED CONTENT

Bipolar Disorder (Patient Information)
Depression, Major (Related Key Topic)

AUTHOR: **VICTOR I. REUS, M.D.**

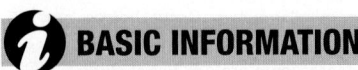

BASIC INFORMATION

DEFINITION

A bite wound can be animal or human, accidental, or intentional.

ICD-10CM CODES

T14.1	Open wound of unspecified body region
T01.9	Multiple open wounds, unspecified
S31.000A	Unspecified open wound of lower back and pelvis without penetration into retroperitoneum, initial encounter
S41.159A	Open bite of unspecified upper arm, initial encounter

EPIDEMIOLOGY & DEMOGRAPHICS

- Bite wounds account for 1% of emergency department visits, and about 2% of patients need hospitalization.
- More than 1 million bites occur in human beings annually in the U.S.
- Dog bites account for 85% to 90% of all bites and result in 10 to 20 fatalities yearly in the U.S.; most dog bite victims are children. Cat bites account for 10% to 20%. The animal typically is owned by the victim.
- Infection rates are highest for cat bites (30%-50%), followed by human bites (15%-30%) and dog bites (5%).
- The extremities are involved in 75% of bites.

PHYSICAL FINDINGS & CLINICAL PRESENTATION

- The appearance of the bite wound is variable (e.g., puncture wound, tear, avulsion).
- Cellulitis, lymphangitis, and focal adenopathy may be present in infected bite wounds.
- Patient may have fever and chills.

ETIOLOGY

- Increased risk of infection: Human and cat bites, closed-fist injuries, wounds involving joints, puncture wounds, face and lip bites, bites with skull penetration, bites in immunocompromised hosts
- Mixed aerobes and anaerobes typically compose the bacteria in bite wounds. Most frequent infecting organisms:
  1. *Pasteurella* spp.: Responsible for majority of infections within 24 hr of dog *(P. canis)* and cat *(P. multocida, P. septica)* bites
  2. *Capnocytophaga canimorsus* (formerly DF-2 bacillus): A gram-negative organism responsible for late infection, usually after dog bites
  3. Gram-negative organisms *(Pseudomonas, Haemophilus)*: Often found in human bites
  4. *Streptococcus* spp., *Staphylococcus aureus*
  5. *Eikenella corrodens* in human bites

Dx DIAGNOSIS

DIFFERENTIAL DIAGNOSIS

- Bite from a rabid animal (often the attack is unprovoked)
- Factitious injury

WORKUP

- Determination of the time elapsed since the patient was bitten, status of rabies immunization of the animal, and underlying medical conditions that might predispose the patient to infection (e.g., DM, immunodeficiency)
- Documentation of bite site, notification of appropriate authorities (e.g., police department, animal officer)
- Box 1 summarizes management procedures for bite wounds

LABORATORY TESTS

- Generally not necessary
- Hct if there has been significant blood loss
- Wound cultures (aerobic and anaerobic) if there is evidence of sepsis or victim is immunocompromised; cultures should be obtained before irrigation of the wound but after superficial cleaning

IMAGING STUDIES

Radiographs are indicated when bony penetration is suspected or if there is suspicion of fracture or significant trauma; they are also useful for detecting foreign bodies (when suspected).

BOX 1 Management Procedures for Bite Wounds

Obtain history from patient
- Situation leading to injury
- Place of occurrence
- Patient allergies
- Other medications (potential interactions)

Perform evaluation of patient
- Nerve function
- Tendon function
- Vascular integrity
- Range of motion
- Potential bone and joint involvement

Diagram or photograph wound
Mark leading edge of cellulitis
Culture wound (if infected)
Irrigate wound (do not irrigate puncture wounds)
Debride wound cautiously
Obtain diagnostic imaging for penetrating injuries overlying bones or joints, if fracture suspected or foreign body suspected
Drain abscesses
Operative debridement (for removal of devitalized tissue and for severe bites, as indicated)
Administer antimicrobial agents (prophylactic therapy, 3-5 days; longer duration for established infection)
Elevate injured area
Close the wound (see text)
Immobilize wound area (3 days for hands)
Have the patient exercise the injured area (if previously immobilized)
Administer tetanus toxoid
Submit health department report (if required)

Cherry JD et al: *Feigin and Cherry's textbook of pediatric infectious diseases,* ed 8, Philadelphia, 2019, Elsevier.

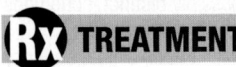

TREATMENT

NONPHARMACOLOGIC THERAPY

- Local care with debridement, vigorous cleansing, and saline irrigation of the wound; debridement of devitalized tissue
- High-pressure irrigation to clean bite wound and ensure removal of contaminants (e.g., use saline solution with a 30- to 35-ml syringe equipped with a 20-gauge needle or catheter with tip of syringe placed 2 to 3 cm above the wound)
- Avoid blunt probing of wounds (increased risk of infection)
- If the animal is suspected to be rabid: Infiltrate wound edges with 1% procaine hydrochloride, swab wound surface vigorously with cotton swabs and 1% benzalkonium solution or other soap, and rinse wound with normal saline

ACUTE GENERAL Rx

- Avoid suturing of hand wounds and any wounds that appear infected.
- Clenched fist injuries that develop after a punch to another's mouth usually require hospitalization, IV antibiotics, and evaluation by a hand specialist.
- Puncture wounds should be left open.
- Give antirabies therapy and tetanus immune globulin (250-500 units IM in limb contralateral to toxoid) and toxoid (adult or child older than 5 yr: 0.5 ml DT given IM, child <5 yr 0.5 ml DPT IM) as needed.
- Use empiric antibiotic therapy in high-risk wounds (e.g., cat bite, hand bites, face bites, genital area bites, bites with joint or bone penetration, human bites, immunocompromised host): Amoxicillin-clavulanate 875 to 1000 mg bid for 7 days or cefuroxime 500 mg bid for 7 days.
- In hospitalized patients, IV antibiotics of choice are cefoxitin 1 to 2 g q6h, ampicillin-sulbactam 1.5 to 3 g q6h, ticarcillin-clavulanate 3 g q6h, cefoxitin 2 g IV q8h, or ceftriaxone 1 to 2 g q24h.
- Penicillin allergy: Animal bite (doxycycline or moxifloxacin or trimethoprim/sulfamethoxazole with either clindamycin or metronidazole); human bite (moxifloxacin plus clindamycin, trimethoprim/sulfamethoxazole plus metronidazole).
- Prophylactic therapy for persons bitten by others with HIV and hepatitis B (see Section V).
- Table 1 summarizes the treatment of mammalian bites. The comparative in vitro antimicrobial activity of selected oral antimicrobial agents against common bite wound pathogens is summarized in Table 2.

DISPOSITION

- Prognosis is favorable with proper treatment.
- Important prognostic factors are type and depth of wound, which compartments are

TABLE 1 Treatment of Mammalian Bites

Type	Wound Care	Antibiotic PR	Tetanus PR	Rabies PR	HIV PR	Hepatitis PR
Human	High-pressure irrigation of the wound with normal saline or dilute (<1%) povidone-iodine solution; débride devitalized tissue or ragged edges	Amoxicillin-clavulanate, second-generation cephalosporin with anaerobic activity, penicillin plus dicloxacillin, clindamycin plus ciprofloxacin or trimethoprim-sulfamethoxazole	Tetanus immunoglobulin (250 units IM) and tetanus toxoid (0.5 mg IM) if never had a tetanus vaccine or have not had 3 doses of tetanus toxoid; tetanus toxoid (0.5 mg IM) if >5 yr since previous tetanus booster	None	ART therapy started within the first 48-72 hr and continued for 28 days or bite source tested HIV negative; refer to the hospital for the specific drugs used in ART therapy	HBIG (0.06 ml/kg IM); HBV given at separate site from HBIG
Cat	High-pressure irrigation of the wound with normal saline or dilute (<1%) povidone-iodine solution; débride devitalized tissue or ragged edges	Amoxicillin-clavulanate, second-generation cephalosporin with anaerobic activity, penicillin plus a first-generation cephalosporin, clindamycin plus a fluoroquinolone or trimethoprim-sulfamethoxazole	Tetanus immune globulin (250 units IM) and tetanus toxoid (0.5 mg IM) if never had a tetanus vaccine or have not had 3 doses of tetanus toxoid; tetanus toxoid (0.5 mg IM) if >5 yr since previous tetanus booster	HRIG (20 IU/kg) injected IM and/or around the bite site; rabies vaccine (1 ml IM) given in the deltoid in adults and in the thigh in children, on days 0, 3, 7, 14, and 28	None	None
Dog	High-pressure irrigation of the wound with normal saline or dilute (<1%) povidone-iodine solution; débride devitalized tissue or ragged edges	Amoxicillin-clavulanate, second-generation cephalosporin with anaerobic activity, penicillin plus a first-generation cephalosporin, clindamycin plus a fluoroquinolone or trimethoprim-sulfamethoxazole	Tetanus immune globulin (250 units IM) and tetanus toxoid (0.5 mg IM) if never had a tetanus vaccine or have not had 3 doses of tetanus toxoid; tetanus toxoid (0.5 mg IM) if >5 yr since previous tetanus booster	HRIG (20 IU/kg) injected IM and/or around the bite site; rabies vaccine (1 ml IM) given in the deltoid in adults and in the thigh in children, on days 0, 3, 7, 14, and 28	None	None

ART, Antiretroviral therapy; *HBIG,* hepatitis B immune globulin; *HBV,* hepatitis B vaccine; *HIV,* human immunodeficiency virus; *HRIG,* human rabies immune globulin; *IM,* intramuscularly; *PR,* prophylaxis.
From Adams JG et al: *Emergency medicine: clinical essentials,* ed 2, Philadelphia, 2013, Elsevier.

TABLE 2 Comparative in Vitro Antimicrobial Activity of Selected Oral Antimicrobial Agents Against Common Bite Wound Pathogens

Staphylococcus aureus[a]	Eikenella corrodens	Streptococcus	Haemophilus	Pasteurella	Anaerobes	
Amoxicillin	–	+	v	v	v	v
Amoxicillin–clavulanic acid	v	+	+	+	+	+
Cephalexin	v	–	v	–	v	–
Cefaclor	v	–	v	v	v	–
Cefuroxime	v	v	v	v	v	–
Meropenem	v	+	+	+	+	+
Dicloxacillin	v	–	v	–	–	–
Erythromycin	v	–	v	–	v	–
Azithromycin	v	v	v	–	v	v
Clarithromycin	v	v	v	–	v	–
Trimethoprim-sulfamethoxazole	+	+	v	+	+	–
Moxifloxacin	+	+	+	+	+	+
Clindamycin	+	–	+	–	–	+

+, Active; –, poorly active or inactive; *v,* variable.
[a]Methicillin-resistant *S. aureus* can be a pathogen in bite wounds.
Cherry JD et al: *Feigin and Cherry's textbook of pediatric infectious diseases,* ed 8, Philadelphia, 2019, Elsevier.

BOX 2 Advice for Avoiding the Bites and Attacks of Common Pets*

Dogs
- Do not leave a young child alone with a dog.
- Never approach or try to pet an unfamiliar dog, especially if it is tied up or confined.
- Always ask the dog's owners if you can pet the dog.
- Do not lean over a dog or pet it directly on the head.
- Do not kiss a dog.
- Avoid quick or sudden movements that may startle a dog.
- Never pet or step over a sleeping dog.
- Never try to take a bone or toy away from a dog (other than your own dog).
- Know the appearance of an angry dog: barking, growling, snarling with teeth showing, ears laid flat, legs stiff, tail up, and hair on the back standing up.
- Never step between two fighting dogs; if you need to separate them, use a bucket of water or a hose.
- Do not approach a female dog that is nursing her pups.
- Teach injury prevention advice to children from an early age.

Cats
- Be aware that some cats do not like prolonged petting.
- Know warning signs of an impending bite: twitching of the tail, restlessness, and "intention" bites (i.e., the cat moves to bite but does not bite).

Ferrets
- Do not sell or adopt a ferret that is known to bite.
- Do not push your fingers through the wires of a ferret cage.
- Reach for a ferret from the side with the palm upward rather than from above.
- Do not handle food and then handle young ferrets without washing your hands first.
- Do not poke a ferret or pull on its tail or ears.
- Never leave a ferret alone with a child or infant.
- If a ferret bites and locks on very tightly, pour cold and fast-running water over its face.

From Auerbach P: *Wilderness medicine, expert consult,* premium edition—enhanced online features and print, Philadelphia, 2012, Elsevier.

entered, and pathogenicity of inoculated bacteria.
- Punctures that are difficult to irrigate adequately, carnivore bites over vital structures (arteries, nerves, joints), and tissue crushing that cannot be debrided have a worse prognosis.
- In general, human bites have a higher complication and infection rate than do animal bites.
- Nearly 50% of the anaerobic gram-negative bacilli isolated from human bite wounds may be penicillin resistant and beta-lactamase positive.

PREVENTION

Box 2 provides advice for avoiding the bites and attacks of common pets.

REFERRAL

- Hospitalization and IV antibiotic therapy for infected human bites; bites with injury to joints, nerves, or tendons; or any animal bites unresponsive to oral therapy.
- Human bites with tendon involvement should go to operating room for washout.
- In the outpatient setting, bite wounds should be reevaluated within 48 hr to assess for signs of infection.

SUGGESTED READING

Available at ExpertConsult.com

RELATED CONTENT

Animal and Human Bites (Patient Information)

AUTHOR: **FRED F. FERRI, M.D.**

BASIC INFORMATION

DEFINITION

There are two major classes of arthropods: insects and Arachnida. This chapter focuses on the class Arachnida. Arachnid bites consist of bites caused by:

- Spiders
- Scorpions
- Ticks

ICD-10CM CODES

T63.301	Toxic effect of unspecified spider venom, accidental (unintentional), initial encounter
T63.2	Toxic effect of venom of scorpion, accidental (unintentional), initial encounter
E906	Bite of nonvenomous arthropod; insect bite NOS

EPIDEMIOLOGY & DEMOGRAPHICS

- Spiders—ubiquitous; only three types potentially significantly harmful:
  1. Sydney funnel web spider—Australia
  2. Black widow (Fig. E1)—worldwide (excluding Alaska)
  3 Brown recluse (Fig. E2)—most common (South Central U.S.)
- Scorpions—various warm climates: Africa, Central South America, Middle East, India; Texas, New Mexico, California, and Nevada in the U.S.
- Ticks—woodlands

PHYSICAL FINDINGS & CLINICAL PRESENTATION

Spiders:

- Sydney funnel web—atracotoxin toxin
  1. Piloerection, muscle spasms leading to tachycardia, hypertension, increased intracranial pressure, coma
- Black widow—females toxic
  1. Initial reaction: Local swelling, redness (two fang marks) leading to local piloerection, edema, urticaria, diaphoresis, lymphangitis
  2. Pain in limb leading to rest of body (chest pain, abdominal pain), compartment syndrome
- Brown recluse
  1. Minor sting or burn
  2. Wound may become pruritic and red with a blanched center with vesicle (Fig. E3). Can necrose, especially in fatty areas (Fig. E4). Leaves eschar, which sloughs and leaves ulcer; can take months to heal
  3. Systemic symptoms: Headache, fever, chills, gastrointestinal upset, hemolysis, renal tubular necrosis, disseminated intravascular coagulation possible

Scorpions:

- Sting leading to sympathetic and parasympathetic stimulation: Hypertension, bradycardia, vasoconstriction, pulmonary edema, reduced coronary blood flow, priapism, inhibition of insulin
- Also possible: Tachycardia, arrhythmia, vasodilation, bronchial relaxation, excessive salivation, vomiting, sweating, bronchoconstriction, pancreatitis
- Clinically significant scorpion envenomation by Centruroides sculpturatus produces a severe neuromotor syndrome and respiratory insufficiency that often requires ICU admission

Ticks: U.S., Europe, Asia

- Very small (<1 mm). Must be attached >36 hr to transmit disease
- Lyme disease—most common (see "Lyme Disease"). Caused by the bacterium *Borrelia burgdorferi* and is transmitted to humans through the *Ixodes scapularis* tick
  1. Early localized (days): Erythema migrans in 60% to 80% of cases
  2. Early disseminated (weeks): Mild to moderate constitutional symptoms, secondary skin lesions, fever, adenopathy, facial palsy, peripheral neuropathy, lymphocytic meningitis, meningoencephalitis, cardiac manifestations (heart block)
  3. Late (months to yrs): Chronic arthritis, dermatitis, neuropathy, keratitis
- Babesiosis (see "Babesiosis")
- Ehrlichiosis/anaplasmosis (see "Ehrlichiosis and Anaplasmosis")

Dx DIAGNOSIS

DIFFERENTIAL DIAGNOSIS

- Cellulitis
- Urticaria

Other tick-borne illnesses:

- Babesiosis
- Tick-borne relapsing fever/*Borrelia miyamotoi*
- Tularemia
- Rocky Mountain spotted fever
- Ehrlichiosis/anaplasmosis
- Colorado tick fever
- Tick paralysis, Powassan disease
- Community-acquired cutaneous methicillin-resistant *Staphylococcus aureus*

WORKUP

Physical examination: Thorough skin examination may reveal fang marks, attached ticks, black eschar.

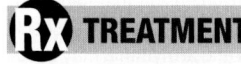

TREATMENT

ACUTE GENERAL Rx

Spiders:

- Sydney funnel web
  1 Pressure, immediate immobilization, supportive care, antivenin
- Black widow
  1. Treatment based on severity of symptoms; bite is rarely fatal
  2. All should receive oxygen, IV, cardiac monitor, tetanus prophylaxis
  3. Symptomatic/supportive therapy
  4. 10% calcium gluconate for muscle cramps (controversial)
  5. Antivenin only for more severe reactions; it carries a risk of anaphylaxis
     a. Dose: One vial in 100 ml 0.9% saline over 20 to 30 min
     b. Skin test before use
     c. Give antihistamines with use
- Brown recluse
  1. Pain management, tetanus, supportive treatment
  2. No consensus regarding best treatment; some evidence for hyperbaric oxygen

Scorpions:

- Fluids, supportive care, species-specific antivenin (equine based, risk of serum sickness) is controversial.
- IV administration of scorpion-specific F(ab')2 antivenin has been reported effective in resolving the clinical syndrome within 4 hours and reducing the need for concomitant sedation with midazolam and reducing the levels of circulating unbound venom.

Ticks:

- Prophylactic: Tick >36 hr: Single dose of doxycycline 200 mg
- Early localized disease
  1. Duration of antibiotics: 10 to 21 days
  2. Doxycycline preferred in patients with possible concurrent ehrlichiosis
  3. Treatment of choice in children: Amoxicillin for 14 days
- Early disseminated: Treatment depends on manifestation
- Late disease: May require longer-term or IV therapy; controversial for neurologic disease (see "Lyme Disease")

DISPOSITION

- For patients with systemic reactions, send home with emergency epinephrine kit.
- If severe or anaphylactic reaction, admit and observe for 48 hr for cardiac, renal, or neurologic problems.

REFERRAL

For patients with systemic reactions, refer to allergist for immunotherapy; 95% to 98% effective in preventing anaphylaxis.

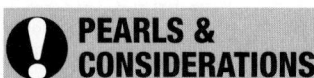

PEARLS & CONSIDERATIONS

Actual spider bites rare; need witnessed bite. Patient should bring spider if possible for confirmation. Bites usually occur in settings of unusually close contact with spider. Bedbugs becoming more prevalent; repeated exposure increases severity of reaction.

SUGGESTED READINGS

Available at ExpertConsult.com

RELATED CONTENT

Bites and Stings (Patient Information)
Bites and Stings, Insect (Related Key Topic)

AUTHOR: **GAIL M. O'BRIEN, M.D.**

BASIC INFORMATION

DEFINITION

Most stinging insects belong to the Hymenoptera order and include the winged: honey bees, hornets, bumblebees, sweat bees, wasps (including yellow jackets), and the unwinged: harvester ants, fire ants, and the Africanized honey bee ("killer bee"). Thousands of species can sting. Wasps cause 70% of all reactions to stings. Spiders, which are arachnids, not insects, are another cause of bites (Fig. 1) (see "Bites and Stings, Arachnids"). The venom of the Hymenoptera order contains vasoactive and proinflammatory mediators that can cause local reactions. A small number of those stung can develop a systemic hypersensitivity reaction. The usual local effect of a sting is intense pain, immediate erythema, edema, and pruritus from the injecting venom. Allergic reactions can be either local or generalized. Generalized reactions can lead to anaphylactic shock. This is a rapid-onset event and can cause death. The majority of reactions occur within the first 6 hr after the sting or bite, but a delayed reaction may occur up to 24 hr after the sting. Delayed reactions are rare and include serum sickness (fever, malaise, urticaria, and arthralgias). A biphasic reaction can occur.

SYNONYM

Venom allergy

ICD-10CM CODES

T63.444	Toxic effect of venom of bees, undetermined, initial encounter
T63.464	Toxic effect of venom of wasps, undetermined, initial encounter
T63.424	Toxic effect of venom of ants, undetermined, initial encounter

EPIDEMIOLOGY & DEMOGRAPHICS

PREVALENCE (OF BEE STINGS AND INSECT BITES):

- Unknown prevalence, very underreported.
- Account for 2.3% of ED visits; 5% to 7.5% of the population is hypersensitive, with large local or systemic reactions to the venom of one or more stinging insects.
- Insect bites are the most common cause of anaphylaxis reactions and account for 20% of all anaphylaxis-related deaths.
- Most anaphylactic reactions occur during summer months in those most likely to be exposed, including children, males, and outdoor workers. There are no tests to predict reaction accurately; the reaction to a prior sting is still the best predictor. Anaphylaxis can occur after a number of uneventful stings.
- Approximately half of fatal reactions occur without prior allergic response.
- Bites by fire ants are less likely to cause systemic disease.
- Spider bites are rare; only a few of the thousands of spider species cause a reaction in humans. Observation and collection of the spider inflicting the bite is necessary (see Bites and Stings, Arachnids).

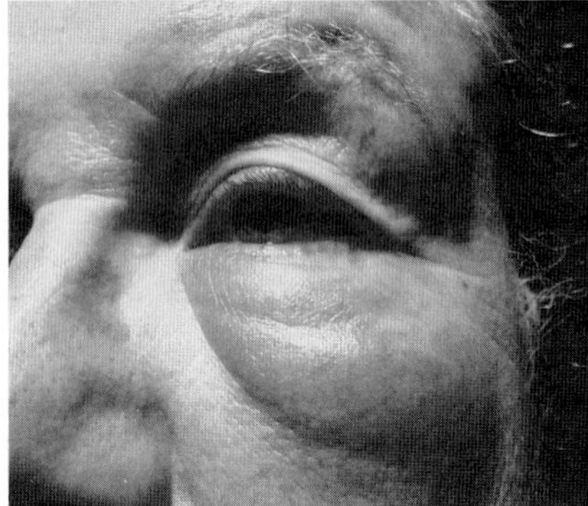

FIG. 1 Spider bite to lower eyelid. (From Swartz MH: *Textbook of physical diagnosis*, ed 7, Philadelphia, 2014, Elsevier.)

INCIDENCE (IN U.S.): Forty to 100 people die each yr from insect sting anaphylaxis; anaphylaxis occurs most often within 10 to 30 min of a sting. Delayed reactions are rare, occurring only in <0.3% of stings.

PHYSICAL FINDINGS & CLINICAL PRESENTATION

- Stings:
  1. Local reactions:
     a. Cutaneous: The skin is the most common site of a local allergic reaction. Manifestations include flushing, urticaria, pruritus, and angioedema. Local reactions may last several days.
  2. Systemic reactions:
     a. Local swelling greater than 10 cm is associated with increased risk of a systemic reaction with repeat exposure.
     b. Respiratory: This is the leading cause of anaphylactic death. Anaphylaxis as defined by consensus of the NIH 2006 is a severe life-threatening hypersensitivity reaction. Symptoms of upper or lower airway obstruction including hoarseness, choking, throat tightness or tingling that may progress to stridor, laryngeal edema, laryngospasm, and bronchoconstriction.
     c. Cardiovascular: Cardiac manifestations are the second leading cause of death from anaphylaxis; the most common reaction is hypotension that can progress to profound hypovolemic shock. Tachycardia and arrhythmia may occur. Myocardial infarction is rare.
     d. General symptoms: Abdominal pain, nausea, vomiting, lightheadedness, and diarrhea.

Fire ant bites:
- Initial wheal and flare response
- Subsequent development of circularly arrayed blisters within 24 hr (Fig. E2)
- Blisters may develop the appearance of pustules, but they are not infected

Flea bites:
- Classic linear configuration (Fig. 3)
- Multiple excoriated, clustered red papules (Fig. 4)

ETIOLOGY

Stings:
- Most systemic reactions to insect stings are classic immunoglobulin E (IgE)–mediated reactions. Anaphylaxis can be the presenting sign of indolent mastocytosis.
- Reactions occur in previously sensitized patients who have produced high titers of IgE antibody to insect venom antigens.
- Sensitization to wasp venom can occur after a single sting but is more common after a few stings.
- Sensitization to bee venom occurs mainly in people who have been stung frequently by bees.

Bites:
- Fire ant venom contains proteins toxic to the skin.

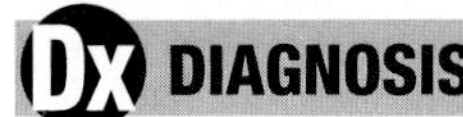

DIAGNOSIS

DIFFERENTIAL DIAGNOSIS

- Stings: Cellulitis, bites, rash
- Bites: Stings, cellulitis

WORKUP

The history is essential for accurate diagnosis including timing of sting or bite and type of insect (bee, wasp, spider, or ant) if known.

LABORATORY TESTS (FOR HYPERSENSITIVITY REACTION)

- Skin test: Either skin prick test or intradermal method with fire ant or hymenoptera venom
- Venom skin tests and occasionally radioallergosorbent tests (RAST) to provide additional information, only for those with history of a systemic reaction
- Venom-specific IgE tests
- Basophil activation tests and mast cell mediator testing are being developed to identify those with allergy and predict those who will have more severe reactions
- Measuring baseline serum tryptase can identify patients as high risk for anaphylaxis and those with mastocytosis

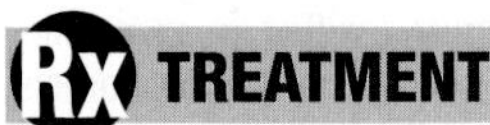

TREATMENT

ACUTE GENERAL Rx

Sting:
- Local Poison Control Center can be contacted.
- Removal of the stinger most easily performed with a flat tool such as a credit card within 30 seconds of the sting, followed by cleansing and application of ice.
- Venom may all be released within 20 seconds of bite or sting.
- Avoid squeezing, which may push venom out of the venom sac and into the tissue.
- Supportive care with oral antihistamines, nonsteroidal antiinflammatory medications/pain medications, topical corticosteroids for 5 to 7 days, and cold compresses for limited reactions.
- Large local reactions (LLR>10 cm) may benefit from oral steroids. 50 mg/day prednisone

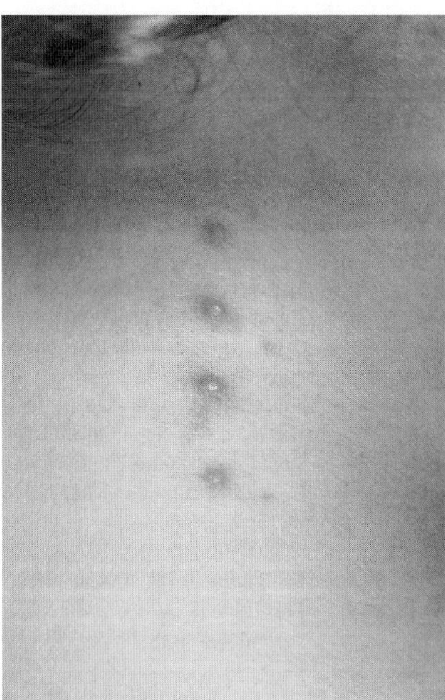

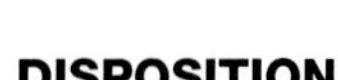

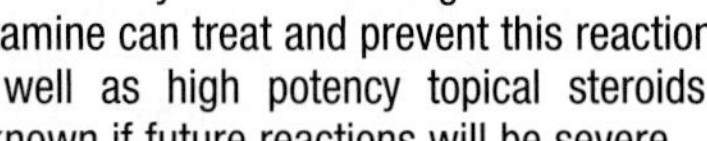

FIG. 3 Flea bites. The classic linear configuration of flea bites (the breakfast, lunch, and dinner sign) caused by the tendency of fleas to jump and crawl rather than fly. (From Paller AS, Mancini AJ: *Hurwitz clinical pediatric dermatology, a textbook of skin disorders of childhood and adolescence*, ed 5, Philadelphia, 2016, Elsevier.)

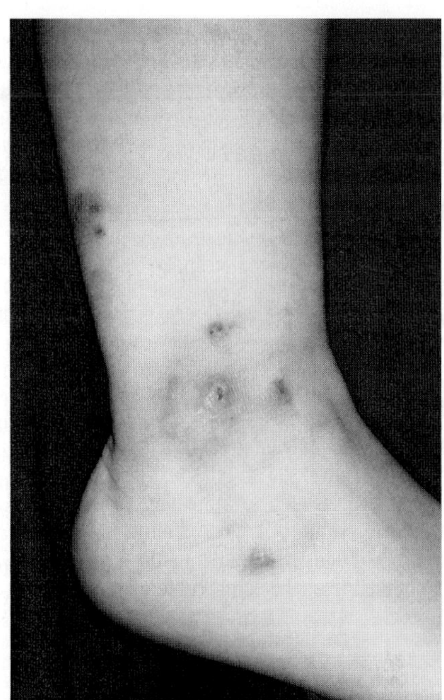

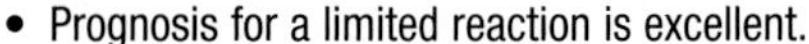

FIG. 4 Flea bites. Multiple excoriated, clustered red papules. (From Paller AS, Mancini AJ: *Hurwitz clinical pediatric dermatology, a textbook of skin disorders of childhood and adolescence*, ed 5, Philadelphia, 2016, Elsevier.)

for 5 to 7 days. Oral second-generation antihistamine can treat and prevent this reaction as well as high potency topical steroids. Unknown if future reactions will be severe.
- Patients with previous reactions or multiple stings to the mouth or neck should be evaluated in an emergency department.
- Unusual reactions to multiple stings include cerebrovascular accident or acute kidney injury due to many causes, including hypotension or direct toxicity from venom.
- Systemic reactions = Anaphylaxis: Treat quickly with intramuscular epinephrine (no contraindication for use). Increased risk of death if epinephrine delayed. The patient should be supine with 0.30 mg IM in anterior/lateral thigh. Patient should be observed for 4 to 8 hours. Adults with preexisting CV disease are at greater risk.
  1. H1- and H2-blockers, oxygen, IV glucocorticoids, beta-agonists, pressors, and IV fluids may also be beneficial for anaphylaxis. No data that glucocorticoids improve clinical outcomes.
  2. Patients should be given 2 units of self-injectable epinephrine pens for home use and referral to allergy indicated after a systemic reaction. Patients should be transported to ED if epinephrine is used, due to 20% risk of recurrence of symptoms.
- Tetanus not needed.

Bite:
- Supportive care—wash with soap and water
- Application of ice or cooling. Calamine lotion may be helpful
- Surveillance for secondary cellulitis—more common with yellow jacket bites

DISPOSITION

Sting:
- Prognosis for a limited reaction is excellent.
- Subsequent anaphylaxis may occur in up to 65% of patients stung again with history of prior systemic reaction. Large local reaction does not predict a systemic reaction.
- There is no evidence that the next sting will necessarily cause a more severe reaction. Variable outcome is due to the patient's age, comorbidities, time elapsed since prior exposure, dose of venom injected, and site of sting.
- Watch for secondary cellulitis.
- Patients who have a history of a severe systemic reaction should:
  1. Be educated to avoid stinging insects.
  2. Carry 2 syringes preloaded with epinephrine for self-administration.
  3. Undergo testing for serum levels of venom-specific IgE.
  4. Be referred to allergist for venom immunotherapy (VIT), which reduces chance of serious allergic reaction from 60% to <5%. VIT is typically needed for 3 to 5 yr.
  5. Carry medical identification for stinging insect hypersensitivity.
  6. Have a baseline tryptase level checked if an anaphylactic reaction to a sting has been experienced in the past to evaluate the possibility of an underlying mast cell disorder. Patients with levels >20 ng/ml need further evaluation. VIT may benefit those with mastocytosis and wasp venom allergy.

Bite:
- Prognosis for fire ant bite is excellent.
- Large lesions from brown recluse spider bites may take months to heal.
- Watch for secondary cellulitis.

REFERRAL

- Consider referral to an allergist for venom immunotherapy (VIT). All patients with severe systemic reactions should be referred for testing and, if positive, should receive VIT for 5 yr.
- Risk of subsequent anaphylaxis with immunotherapy falls to <5%.
- VIT for 5 yr induces long-term protection in most patients.

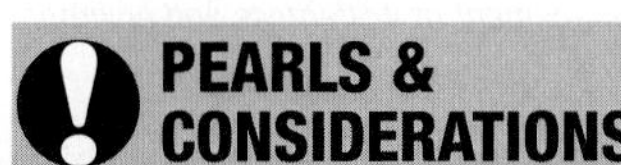

PEARLS & CONSIDERATIONS

Hypersensitivity to stings is common. Reactions range from local nonallergic reaction to venom to life-threatening systemic reaction with anaphylaxis. This could indicate underlying mast cell disorder; tryptase level is indicated. Venom-specific immunotherapy is highly effective in decreasing subsequent anaphylaxis. Although venom immunotherapy is currently indicated only for systemic reactions, investigation is under way to assess efficacy for prevention of large local reactions, which can result in significant morbidity.

SUGGESTED READINGS

Available at ExpertConsult.com

RELATED CONTENT

Bites and Stings (Patient Information)
Bites and Stings, Arachnids (Related Key Topic)

AUTHOR: **LYNN A. BOWLBY, M.D.**

BASIC INFORMATION

DEFINITION

Injury resulting from a snake biting a human.

ICD-10CM CODES

T63.0	Toxic effect of snake venom
T63.001A	Toxic effect of unspecified snake venom, accidental (unintentional), initial encounter

EPIDEMIOLOGY & DEMOGRAPHICS

- The CDC reports that, between 1950 and 2010, there were on average 5000 snakebites per yr, which correlates to 1.56 bites per 100,000 people. In the U.S. alone, there are 5 cases of snake bites resulting in death per yr. Data from the National Electronic Injury Surveillance System reveals that the number of snakebites (including from non-venomous snakes) to be close to 9200 on average per yr over the period 2001–2010, with more than 2800 venomous bites per yr.
- The highest incidence is reported in southern states, with Texas and Florida reporting the highest incidence.
  1. Snakebites peak during the warmer months of April through November.
  2. Worldwide, farm workers have the highest incidence of snakebites, whereas in the U.S., most snakebites result from intentional provocation of wild snakes or in the setting of handling captive snakes.
  3. In the US, 13.9% of bites occurred predominantly in landscapers, snake handlers, and outdoor professionals, with 76% of the envenomations involving the upper extremity.
  4. The sex ratio (male:female) is 2.7.
  5. Incidence peaks in those between 10-14 yr of age and then steadily decreases in adults to about 2 bites per 100,000. Alcohol use and drug intoxication are implicated in many snakebites. The risk of death is highest in children, the elderly, and in those with delayed presentation to care.
  6. Exotic, nonnative pets also account for 1% to 2% of snake envenomations.
- In the U.S., at least one species of poisonous snake (Fig. 1) has been identified in every state, with the exception of Alaska, Hawaii, and Maine. Table 1 summarizes medically important snake families.
- The Viperidae family includes the Crotalinae subfamily which is the only subfamily native to North America. These are commonly referred to as crotalids or pit vipers and include rattlesnakes, copperheads, and cottonmouths (water moccasins).
  1. Crotalids are responsible for 98% of snake envenomations in the U.S.
  2. Crotalids are characterized by a prominent, diamond-shaped head, a heat-sensing pit between the eye and nostril, long retractable fangs, and, in the case of rattlesnakes, the telltale rattler.
  3. Crotalid bites are typically very painful. Their venom contains a hemotoxin, a neurotoxin, a cardiotoxin, and necrotizing factors leading to direct tissue damage and necrosis. Dry bites (when envenomation does not occur) make up approximately 3-25% of pit viper bites.
- The Elapidae family includes mambas, cobras, and coral snakes.
  1. Coral snakes are the only member of the Elapidae family found in the U.S.
  2. Coral snakes are much less common than crotalids, are innately less aggressive, and represent only 2% of reported snakebites in the U.S.

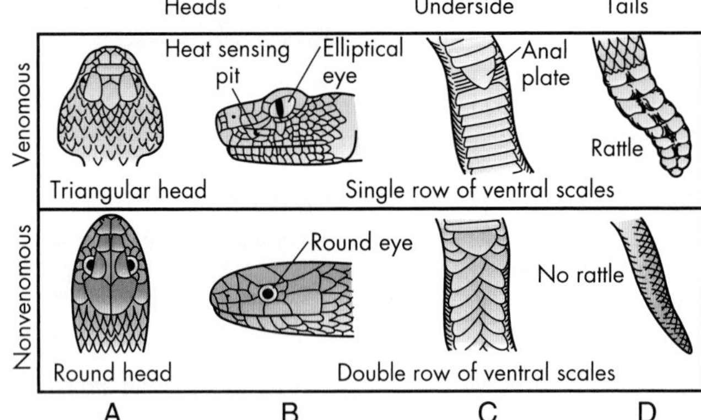

FIG. 1 Comparison of pit vipers and nonvenomous snakes. Rattle in **D** *(top)* applies to rattlesnakes only. (**A** to **D,** From Sullivan JB et al: North American venomous reptile bites. In Auerbach PS [ed]: *Wilderness medicine: management of wilderness and environmental emergencies,* ed 7, Philadelphia, 2015, Elsevier.)

TABLE 1 Medically Important Snake Families

Family	Venomous?	Location	Examples	Toxin Effects/Other Comments
Colubridae	Some species	Most parts of the world	Garter snakes (*Thamnophis* spp.), king snakes, and milk snakes (*Lampropeltis* spp.)	Largest family of snakes; most are considered harmless to humans; a few species are dangerously toxic (e.g., African boomslang [*Dispholidus typus*])
Boidae	None	Most parts of the world	*Boa* sp., *Python* sp.	Constrictors; unsupervised children should not be allowed access to large constrictors
Viperidae				
Subfamily Crotalinae (pit vipers)	All	Americas, Asia	Rattlesnakes (*Crotalus* spp.), cottonmouths, and copperheads (*Agkistrodon* spp.), Lancehead pit vipers (*Bothrops* spp.)	Heat-sensing "pit" between each eye and nostril
Subfamily Viperinae (true vipers)	All	Europe, Africa, Middle East, Asia	Puff adder (*Bitis arietans*), Gaboon viper (*Bitis gabonica*)	No heat-sensing pits
Elapidae	All	Americas, Africa, Middle East, Asia	Cobras (*Naja* spp.), mambas (*Dendroaspis* spp.), kraits (*Bungarus* spp.), coral snakes (*Micrurus* spp.), and the venomous snakes of Australia	Highly variable venom effects—some largely neurotoxic, others causing severe local tissue damage
Hydrophiidae	All	Warm waters of the Pacific Ocean, Indian Ocean, and Oceania (none in the Atlantic Ocean)	Sea snakes including the pelagic sea snake (*Pelamis platurus*)	Neurotoxins and myotoxins; rarely bite humans unless provoked

From Kliegman RM et al: *Nelson textbook of pediatrics,* ed 19, Philadelphia, 2011, Saunders.

3. Elapids have smaller heads and shorter fangs, and they are identified by vibrant bands of yellow, red, and black. The popular saying "Red on yellow, kill a fellow; red on black, venom lack" is used to distinguish between venomous and nonvenomous snakes in the U.S. Caution should be used when applying this axiom internationally, as some coral snakes within South America display red-on-black coloring and are in fact venomous.
4. Because of their shorter fangs, elapids rely on a longer bite time to inject their venom. Less than 40% of coral bites result in envenomation.
5. The elapid venom competitively blocks the acetylcholine receptor leading to a delayed onset of systemic symptoms. The venom lacks proteolytic enzymes so there is minimal soft tissue destruction. In the last 40 yr, there has only been 1 fatality from a coral snake bite, and this was because the patient did not seek treatment.

- The degree of envenomation correlates to the size of the snake, with envenomation from larger snakes producing significantly worse local and systemic symptoms than bites from smaller animals.

PHYSICAL FINDINGS & CLINICAL PRESENTATION

The effects of envenomation vary by the type of snake but may include local tissue injury, coagulopathy, neurotoxicity, and cardiovascular instability, as well as renal failure. Crotalids typically cause severe local effects as well as hematologic symptoms including primary consumptive coagulopathies and, less commonly, neurologic complications. The exception is the Mojave rattlesnake bite, in which case local tissue destruction following envenomation is minimal, but severe neurologic symptoms can occur up to 12 hours after the bite. This is similar to elapid bites, which cause less localized tissue damage but have more severe and often delayed neurotoxic manifestations.

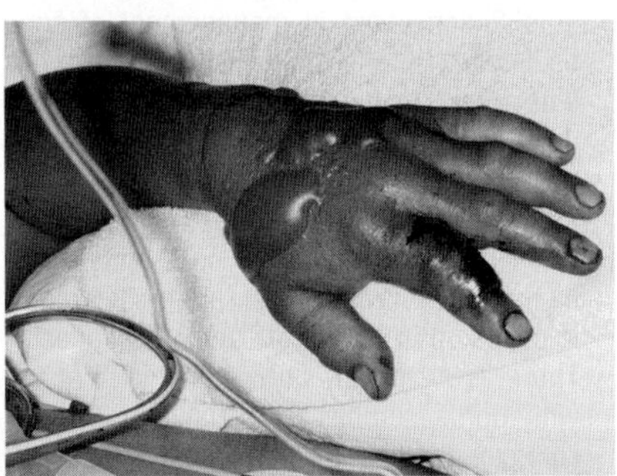

FIG. 2 Southern Pacific rattlesnake *(Crotalus helleri)* bite wounds. (Courtesy Sean Bush, M.D.)

CROTALINAE (PIT VIPERS): Local signs and symptoms:

- Intense pain within 5 minutes.
- Localized edema within 30 minutes.
- Erythema, ecchymosis, and serous/hemorrhagic bullae can develop over hours (Fig. 2).
- Compartment syndrome is rare but can develop around the site of the bite from significant amounts of soft tissue swelling and subcutaneous tissue fluid accumulation.
- If edema or erythema does not occur within 8 hours of a confirmed crotalid snakebite, it is assumed envenomation did not occur ("dry bite"). Roughly 25% of crotalid bites are "dry bites."

Systemic manifestations:

- Nonspecific: Nausea, vomiting, diarrhea, light-headedness, weakness, diaphoresis, chills
- Coagulopathy: Epistaxis, bleeding from gums, internal hemorrhage
- Neurotoxicity: Perioral paresthesias, metallic taste, tingling of fingers or toes (especially with rattlesnake bites), localized/generalized fasciculations, mental status change
- Nephrotoxicity: Secondary to rhabdomyolysis
- Increased vascular permeability: Severe hypotension, tachycardia, respiratory distress

ELAPIDAE (CORAL SNAKES): Local signs and symptoms:

- Absent or minimal local effects, such as mild pain, swelling, or paresthesias at site of bite.

Systemic manifestations:

- May be delayed for up to 12 hours.
- Nonspecific: Nausea, vomiting, abdominal pain, dizziness.
- Neurotoxic: Cranial neuropathies typically appear first, including ptosis, ophthalmoplegia, dysphagia, drooling, and mydriasis with absent or prolonged pupillary light reflex. Descending paralysis and respiratory failure (due to diaphragmatic weakness) can be delayed many hours.

Dx DIAGNOSIS

DIFFERENTIAL DIAGNOSIS

- Bite: Nonvenomous snakebite, "dry bite," scorpion bite, insect bite, cellulitis, laceration, puncture wound, necrotizing fasciitis
- Descending paralysis: Myasthenia gravis, botulism, shellfish poisoning
- Rhabdomyolysis: Crush injury, prolonged immobilization, marked exercise, hyperthermia, metabolic myopathies, drugs or toxins, infections, electrolyte disorders
- Coagulopathy: Sepsis, multiple trauma, obstetrical complications, malignancy

WORKUP

- Stabilize and resuscitate unstable patients.
- Initial evaluation of the bite (see details below):
  1. Complete physical and neurologic examination.
  2. Obtain past medical history, including any history of allergic reaction to horse serum, sheep serum, or papaya in those previously treated for snakebite (see antivenom treatment). Patients with allergies to papain, chymopapain, or other papaya extracts may be at risk of an allergic reaction to crotalid antivenom.
- Labs and imaging (see details below).
- Determine need for antivenom (see the following and Table 2).
- Call Poison Control Hotline: 1-800-222-1222.
- Call local zoo when treating patients with envenomations from exotic pets or nonnative snakes.
- Serially reassess, including serial neurologic exams, all cases of suspected envenomation for 8 hours, longer if clinical status deteriorates.

LABORATORY TESTS

- CBC with peripheral smear, electrolytes, BUN, creatinine, PT, INR, PTT, fibrinogen, d-dimer, creatine kinase, liver function tests (LFTs), sedimentation rate (ESR), arterial blood gas (ABG), type and crossmatch, urinalysis, and electrocardiogram (ECG).
- Repeat labs every 4 to 6 hours to monitor trend.

IMAGING STUDIES

- Consider chest x-ray in cases of severe envenomation or in patients over 40 yr old with underlying cardiopulmonary disease to rule out pulmonary edema.
- Plain films of bite site for retained fangs (poor sensitivity). Bedside ultrasound is another option to rule out a retained foreign body in the setting of a snakebite (negative predictive value of 96%).
- Computed tomography (CT) of head if concern for intracranial hemorrhage or if any cognitive/neurologic deficit is appreciated on exam.
- CT abdomen or focused assessment with sonography in trauma (FAST) if concern for intraabdominal bleeding exists or if patient complains of abdominal pain or distention.

TABLE 2 Indications for Snake Antivenom Administration

Evidence of Systemic Toxicity:	
Hemodynamic or respiratory instability	Hypotension, respiratory distress
Hemotoxicity	Clinically significant bleeding or abnormal coagulation studies
Neurotoxicity	Any evidence of toxicity: Usually beginning with cranial nerve abnormalities and progressing to descending paralysis including the diaphragm
Evidence of local toxicity	*Progressive* soft tissue swelling

From Kliegman RM et al: *Nelson textbook of pediatrics,* ed 19, Philadelphia, 2011, Saunders.

Rx TREATMENT

ACUTE GENERAL Rx

IN THE FIELD:

- There is no field first aid that will significantly treat the envenomation; therefore, the most important intervention is to transport the patient quickly to the nearest medical facility.

- Remove any constricting items including rings, watches, jewelry, or tight clothing.
- The affected part should be kept at the level of the heart. Keep the joint in a functional position to minimize disability should the limb or joint become severely swollen or immobile.
- Do *not* apply a tourniquet, incise wound, apply mechanical or oral suction, attempt electrotherapy, or apply ice. These interventions have not been shown to provide any benefit and have the potential to cause further harm, including tissue damage, infection, and caregiver envenomation.
- A loose tourniquet, applied to occlude only lymphatic drainage and loosened every 60-90 seconds, can be applied for 10 minutes if the patient was bitten by a coral snake or other species with neurotoxic venom and the patient is exhibiting neurologic symptoms or there is a prolonged transport time. A properly applied pressure bandage should produce a pressure of 40 to 70 mm Hg and 55 to 70 mm Hg in the upper and lower extremity, respectively.
- Avoid alcohol, stimulants (caffeine), or agents that can suppress mental status.
- Do *not* pick up a dead snake, as the strike reflexes remain intact and can still envenomate.
- When possible, a picture can be taken from a safe distance for later classification of the snake.

IN THE HOSPITAL:

- Assess airway, breathing, and circulation and intervene as needed. Patients with neurotoxic envenomation from elapids or Mojave rattlesnakes can develop respiratory failure (from diaphragmatic paralysis) and may require intubation. Be cautious and repeat the examination as neurotoxic symptoms may be delayed for many hours.
- Place on monitor, obtain vital signs, place 2 large-bore IVs and give crystalloid.
- Unstable patients should be given antivenom immediately. Administration should not be delayed for wound care of the bite.
- If patient is stable, obtain a history, including the time of bite and description of snake.
- Inspect bite site for fang marks and local tissue injury. Clean bite site and remove any retained fangs. Bite may appear like two distinct puncture wounds or small scratches.
- Mark leading edge of erythema and edema, and obtain circumferential measurements every 15 minutes to assess for progression.
- Obtain initial labs and repeat every 4 to 6 hours.
- Determine need for antivenom and begin preparation. It can take up to 1 hour to reconstitute antivenom, so this process should be started as early as possible.
- Contact Poison Control at 1-800-222-1222, which will connect you to your local poison control center. They will provide guidance for treatment and use of antivenom, and also track snakebite incidence.
- Immunize against tetanus if no booster within the past 5 yr. If never immunized, give immunoglobulin as well as toxoid.
- Prophylactic antibiotics are not recommended. Antibiotics should be given only if purulence or other signs of infection are identified, at which time the patient should be given broad-spectrum antibiotics that cover gram-negative bacteria (i.e., ampicillin-sulbactam or quinolone derivatives).
- Aggressive pain control with opioids. Avoid NSAIDs, as they increase risk of bleeding, platelet dysfunction, and nephrotoxicity.

ANTIVENOM TREATMENT

CROTALID (RATTLESNAKE, COPPERHEAD, COTTONMOUTH) ENVENOMATIONS:

- CroFab (Crotalinae polyvalent ovine immune Fab), made from sheep serum, is the antivenom commercially available in the U.S. for crotalid envenomations.
- Indications for antivenom administration include swelling, pain, and/or ecchymosis extending beyond area immediately adjacent to bite, any progression of local symptoms (≥2 cm of erythema spread), any systemic symptoms, any development of coagulation lab abnormalities, or abnormal bleeding.
- Patients with crotalid envenomation who have minimal or nonprogressive symptoms should *not* be given CroFab and instead should be monitored for 8 to 12 hours.
- Dosing:
  1. For moderate symptoms, reconstitute 4 to 6 vials of antivenom (CroFab). Each vial should be mixed in 25 ml of normal saline. The 4 to 6 reconstituted vials should then be mixed in 250 ml normal saline and infused over 60 minutes. Infuse the first 25 ml slowly over the first 10 minutes to monitor for allergic reaction.
  2. For patients with shock or serious active bleeding, give an initial dose of 8 to 12 vials.
  3. If no improvement after first round (defined as progression of local symptoms, persistent systemic symptoms, derangement of laboratory values, or continued bleeding), repeat the initial dose of antivenom.
  4. Between 4 and 18 vials of antivenom may be necessary to control initial symptoms.
- After initial control of symptom progression, give maintenance dose of 2 vials every 6 hours for 3 doses to prevent recurrent toxicity.
- Hematologic labs (fibrinogen, platelet levels, and coagulation studies) should be repeated within an hour of antivenom administration.
- The manufacturer of CroFab maintains a 24/7 hotline: 877-377-3784.
- A new Crotalinae antivenom, Anavip, was approved by the FDA in May 2015, with anticipated availability in October 2018. Anavip is an equine antivenom that has venom specific $F(ab')_2$ fragments of immunoglobulin G (IgG), as opposed to two separate Fab fragments, increasing the half-life in the blood and leading to greater binding and therefore greater elimination of the venom. Because of the longer half-life, dosing with Anavip also eliminates the need for repeat outpatient antivenom dosing, as is required with CroFab. There is a low risk of adverse reactions and serum sickness because, similar to CroFab, these antivenoms lack the Fc component of the IgG.

ELAPID (CORAL SNAKE) ENVENOMATIONS:

- In the U.S., production of coral snake antivenom by Pfizer/Wyeth was discontinued in 2003, and only one lot of antivenom still exists (Lot #L67530). The antivenom's expiration date was extended to January 31, 2018. The use of expired antivenom may be considered in a patient with life-threatening symptoms but should only be administered in conjunction with Poison Control and/or a medical toxicologist. If coral snake antivenom is not available, providers may consider contacting their local zoo to determine whether a provisional antivenom is available. Small-animal studies support the use of Mexican Coral Snake, Australian Tiger Snake, or anti-coral antivenom for neutralization of North American coral snake venom. Many zoos caring for wild snake species stock these specific antivenoms. It is important to note that the effectiveness of these particular antivenoms in human snakebites by the North American coral snake has not been studied. If considering administering alternate antivenom, the provider should contact Poison Control to help orchestrate acquisition. Clinical trials for a new coral snake antivenom have started; however, only 7 of the required 55 patients that are necessary for FDA approval have been recruited.
- A potent, safe, sheep-based antivenom for elapid bites exists and is being used internationally but is not yet approved in the U.S. The University of Arizona is currently sponsoring a clinical trial evaluating the use of a new F(ab')2 antivenom in management of coral snakebites in the U.S. The results of this study have not yet been published.
- In the U.S., only symptomatic patients with confirmed coral snake bites should receive antivenom. The initial dose is 3 to 5 vials given by slow intravenous push, although a higher dose may be necessary in children or in envenomations from large coral snakes.
- There is a high risk of allergic reaction with horse serum-based elapid antivenom so epinephrine, diphenhydramine, IV corticosteroids, and albuterol should be readily available prior to giving antivenom.

NONNATIVE OR EXOTIC SNAKE ENVENOMATIONS: Contact the Poison Control Center or your local zoo, as zoos with exotic snakes are required to maintain a supply of snake-specific antivenom on their premises.

DISPOSITION

- All patients who are given antivenom must be admitted and monitored in an ICU for further observation and supportive care. Patients should be observed for a minimum of 18 to 24 hours after initial control of symptom

progression, and they are safe for discharge when symptom progression has resolved and laboratory values have normalized.
- Victims of crotalid envenomations with minimal to no toxicity and normal serial lab values should be observed for 8 to 12 hours.
- Children, the elderly, those with significant comorbidities, and patients who sustain bites to the legs, face, or neck may require observation for 24 hours.
- Suspected Mojave rattlesnake bites should be observed 12 to 24 hours as their venom predominantly causes neurotoxicity and symptoms may be delayed (similar to elapids).
- Asymptomatic patients with coral snakebites should be observed for 12 to 24 hours because neurotoxicity may be delayed.

FOLLOW-UP:
- All patients who receive antivenom should have repeat labs at 2 to 3 days and 5 to 7 days after the last administered antivenom dose to evaluate for delayed hematologic complications or serum sickness.
- Return for worsening, nondependent swelling, abnormal bleeding, or signs of serum sickness, which include fatigue, rash, or arthralgias.
- Patients should adhere to bleeding precautions (no contact sports, dental extractions, elective surgery, etc.) for 2 weeks.

REFERRAL

Refer to a medical facility with an ICU for administration of antivenom. The approach to snakebites should be multidisciplinary and should include medical toxicology or other physician snakebite specialists, as well as hematology or nephrology if needed. All snakebites should be reported to Poison Control and the local health department for surveillance.

PEARLS & CONSIDERATIONS

OTHER CONSIDERATIONS
- Frequent assessment and clinical judgment is essential in the treatment of snakebites, as patients do not have a uniform response to envenomation and treatment.
- Dosage of antivenom is based on typical envenomation rather than age or weight, so the dose is the same for children and adults.
- Antivenom is most effective when given within 4 hours of the bite and least effective if delayed beyond 12 hours. Systemic symptoms (coagulopathy, CNS effects, etc.) respond better to treatment than do local symptoms (erythema/edema, bullae, etc.).
- Antivenom is not contraindicated in pregnancy. There have been no adverse reactions to mother or to fetus reported secondary to antivenom treatment. The potential coagulopathy associated with envenomation may place the fetus at higher risk for placental abruption, so prompt treatment with antivenom is prudent. Pregnant victims of snakebites who are treated with antivenom have a significantly lower rate of miscarriage when compared with those who did not receive antivenom.
- Although local wound effects can be severe, wound management should not take precedence over antivenom administration. Some studies suggest that even in the case of compartment syndrome, antivenom may be more effective than fasciotomy, although both may be necessary.

COMPLICATIONS
- Hypersensitivity reactions and serum sickness can occur following antivenom administration. These reactions are much more common with equine-derived antivenom than with ovine-derived antivenom. CroFab derived from sheep serum should be used preferentially over equine serum if available, given the decreased risk for adverse reaction. Elapid antivenom is derived from horse serum, so the risk for allergic reaction and anaphylaxis remains high.
- Anaphylaxis to antivenom can occur within 30 minutes and should be treated by immediately stopping the infusion and managing the symptoms. Epinephrine, diphenhydramine, and hydrocortisone should be administered as needed. If the anaphylaxis is well-controlled and the envenomation is severe, the antivenom infusion can then be resumed.
- In patients with a known hypersensitivity to antivenom, prophylactic epinephrine has been found to reduce the rate of adverse effects.
- Delayed or recurrent hematologic complications are common and can manifest up to 2 weeks post treatment. Most bleeding is self-limited but can rarely be severe, necessitating close follow-up and occasionally repeat doses of antivenom.
- Serum sickness occurs 7 to 14 days after antivenom administration and is characterized by fever, rash, arthralgias, and lymphadenopathy. It can be treated with prednisone 60 mg PO daily, tapered over 7 to 10 days.

SUGGESTED READINGS

Available at ExpertConsult.com

RELATED CONTENT

Snakebites (Patient Information)

AUTHOR: **NEHA P. RAUKAR, M.D., M.S.**

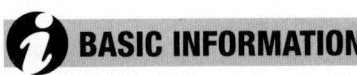

DEFINITION

Bladder cancer is a field change disease in which the entire urothelium from the renal pelvis to the urethra is susceptible to malignant transformation. The disease stages include non-muscle-invasive bladder cancer, muscle-invasive bladder cancer, and metastatic urothelial carcinoma. The three types of bladder cancer are transitional cell carcinoma, squamous cell carcinoma, and adenocarcinoma.

ICD-10CM CODES

C67.9	Malignant neoplasm of bladder, unspecified
C79.11	Secondary malignant neoplasm of bladder
D09.0	Carcinoma in situ of bladder
D30.3	Benign neoplasm of bladder
D41.4	Neoplasm of uncertain behavior of bladder
D49.4	Neoplasm of unspecified behavior of bladder

EPIDEMIOLOGY & DEMOGRAPHICS

In 2018, an estimated 81,190 new cases and 17,240 deaths in the U.S. will be attributed to bladder cancer. It is the sixth commonest malignancy in the U.S., with a median age of diagnosis of 73 years.

PREDOMINANT SEX: It is 3 to 4 times more common in men than in women; lifetime risks are 1 in 26 for men and 1 in 88 for women.

RISK FACTORS:

Smoking:

- More than half of bladder cancers are related to smoking.
- Smoking risk is based on consumption; there is a two- to three-fold increase for subjects smoking >10 cigarettes per day.
- Smokers of low-tar and low-nicotine cigarettes have a lower risk when compared with higher tar and nicotine cigarettes.
- Those who smoke unfiltered cigarettes have a 50% increased risk of bladder cancer compared with those who smoke filtered cigarettes.
- Pipe smokers have a lower risk of bladder cancer compared with cigarette smokers.
- Cigars, snuff, and chewing tobacco, although implicated in nonurologic cancers, are not thought to influence bladder cancer risk.

Diet:

- Diets rich in beef, pork, and animal fat increase risk of bladder cancer.
- Beer consumption has been linked to bladder cancer development as a result of the presence of nitrosamines in the beer. Drinking coffee is not thought to contribute to bladder cancer risk.
- Medications: Long-term (>1 yr) use of pioglitazone and rosiglitazone.

PEAK INCIDENCE: Incidence increases with age: Higher after age 60 yr, uncommon in those younger than 40 yr.

GENETICS: It is thought to be multifactorial in etiology, involving both genetic and environmental interactions. Overall, approximately 20% to 25% of the male population in the U.S. with bladder cancer is estimated to have the disease as a result of occupational exposure.

DISTRIBUTION: In North America, transitional cell carcinomas (TCC) account for 93%, squamous cell carcinomas account for 6%, and adenocarcinomas account for 1% of bladder cancers.

PATHOGENESIS: Two pathways exist for bladder cancer (TCC):

1. Papillary superficial disease occasionally leading to invasive cancer (75%)
2. Carcinoma in situ (CIS) and solid invasive cancer with high risk of disease progression (25%)

Two distinct forms of "superficial cancer" exist:

1. T_a: Papillary low-grade tumor with a high rate of recurrence; disease progression occurs in 5%.
2. T_1: Higher-grade papillary tumor that infiltrates the lamina propria; often associated with flat CIS that may involve the urothelium diffusely. Disease progression occurs in 30% to 50%. This is subdivided into:
   a. T_{1a}: Penetration up to the muscularis mucosa; disease progression in 5%.
   b. T_{1b}: Penetration through the muscularis mucosa; disease progression in 53%.

Flat CIS:

- Entirely different and separate pathway of cancer development whose mechanism is manifested by dysplasia, which leads to the occurrence of poorly differentiated malignant cells that replace or undermine the normal urothelium and extend along the plane of the bladder wall. It penetrates the basement membrane and lamina propria in 20% to 30% of cases and is associated with the development of solid tumor growth. A p53 defect occurs in 50% of these cases.

At presentation, 50% to 51%% of cancers are in situ, 34% to 35%% are localized to the bladder, 17% are regionally spread to the lymph nodes, and 4% to 5% present with distant metastases. Eighty percent of superficial TCC recur, with up to 30% progressing to a higher stage or grade. Younger patients most commonly develop low-grade papillary noninvasive TCC and are less likely to have recurrences when compared with older patients with similar lesions. Involvement of the upper tracts with tumor occurs in 25% to 50% of cases (see Tables E1 and E2).

MOLECULAR EPIDEMIOLOGY: TCC is usually a field change disease with tumors arising at different times and sites in the urothelium, suggesting a polyclonal etiology of bladder cancer. Non-muscle-invasive bladder cancer (NMIBC) and muscle-invasive bladder cancer (MIBC) are genetically different. NMIBC is characterized by a high frequency of mutations in the *FGFR3* oncogene, leading to constitutive activation of the RAS/MAPK pathway. In MIBC, mutations in the *TP53* gene prevail. In general, mutations in *FGFR3* and *TP53* are mutually exclusive, suggesting that NMIBC and MIBC develop along different oncogenetic pathways. However, these mutations often occur simultaneously in stage pT_1 tumors that invade the connective tissue layer underlying the urothelium. Recently, somatic mutations in the *PIK3CA* oncogene, which encodes the catalytic subunit p110α of class-IA PI3 kinase, were described in 13% to 27% of bladder tumors. https://meetinglibrary.asco.org/record/116712/edbook These mutations often coincided with *FGFR3* mutations. Mutations in the *RAS* oncogenes (*HRAS*, *KRAS*, and *NRAS*) have also been found in 13% of bladder tumors and in all stages and grades; they are mutually exclusive with *FGFR3* mutations.

PHYSICAL FINDINGS & CLINICAL PRESENTATION

- Gross, painless hematuria
- Microhematuria
- Frequency, urgency, occasional dysuria
- With locally invasive to distant metastatic disease, the presentation can include:
  1. Abdominal pain
  2. Flank pain
  3. Lymphedema
  4. Renal failure
  5. Anorexia
  6. Bone pain

ETIOLOGY

Bladder cancer is a potentially preventable disease associated with specific etiologic factors:

- Cigarette smoking is associated with 45% to 65% of cases. The risk of developing a TCC is two to four times higher in smokers than in nonsmokers, and that risk persists for many years, being equal to nonsmokers only after 12 to 15 yr of smoking abstinence. Smoking is associated with higher histologic grade and stage, increase in the numbers of tumors, and increased size
- Occupational exposures: Dye workers, textile workers, tire and rubber workers, petroleum workers
- Chemical exposure: O-toluidine, 2-naphthylamine, benzidine, 4-amino-biphenyl, and nitrosamines
- Exposure to herpes papilloma virus type 16

Squamous carcinomas are associated with:

- Schistosomiasis
- Urinary calculi
- Indwelling catheters
- Bladder diverticula

Miscellaneous causes:

- Phenacetin abuse
- Cyclophosphamide
- Pelvic irradiation
- Tuberculosis

Adenocarcinomas are associated with:

- Exstrophy
- Endometriosis
- Neurogenic bladder
- Urachal abnormalities
- As a secondary site for distant metastases from other organs (e.g., colon cancer)

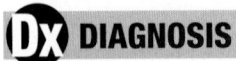

- History and physical examination.
- Urinalysis.

- Cystoscopy with bladder barbotage and biopsy. Fluorescence cystoscopy offers improvement in the detection of flat neoplastic lesions such as carcinoma in situ.
- Transurethral resection of bladder tumor (TURBT).
- There is insufficient evidence to determine whether a decrease in mortality rate from bladder cancer occurs with hematuria testing, urinary cytology, or a variety of other tests on exfoliated urinary cells or other substances.
- In addition to urinary cytology and bladder barbotage, BTA, NMP22, and fibrin degradation products have been approved by the FDA as bladder cancer tumor markers. No marker has general, widespread acceptance because the results are affected by the presence of stents, recent urologic manipulation, stones, infection, bowel interposition, and prostatitis, creating false-positive results.
- Urinary biomarkers: Six urinary biomarkers have been approved by the FDA for diagnosis on surveillance of bladder cancer.
    1. Quantitative nuclear matrix protein 22 (Alere NMP22)
    2. Qualitative NMP22 (BladderChek)
    3. Qualitative bladder tumor antigen (BTA stat)
    4. Quantitative BTA (BTA TRAK)
    5. Fluorescence in situ hybridization (FISH)
    6. Fluorescent immunohistochemistry (ImmunoCyt)
- Generally, urinary biomarkers miss a substantial proportion of patients with bladder cancer and are subject to false-positive results in others. Accuracy is poor for low-stage and low-grade tumors.[1]

DIFFERENTIAL DIAGNOSIS

- Urinary tract infection
- Frequency-urgency syndrome
- Interstitial cystitis
- Stone disease
- Endometriosis
- Neurogenic bladder

LABORATORY TESTS

- Urine cytology.
- Urine telomerase: Telomerase activity in voided urine or bladder washings determined by the telomeric repeat amplification protocol (TRAP) assay. This test has been reported to accurately detect the presence of bladder tumors in men. It represents a potentially useful noninvasive diagnostic innovation for bladder cancer detection in high-risk groups such as habitual smokers or in symptomatic patients.

RADIOLOGIC TESTS

- Renal ultrasound, retrograde pyelography, CT scan, and MRI.
- One or a combination of studies can be used. In the absence of skeletal symptoms, bone scan is not recommended.

[1] Chou R, et al.: Urinary biomarkers for diagnosis of bladder cancer: a systematic review and meta-analysis, *Ann Intern Med* 163:922-931, 2015.

Rx TREATMENT

NONPHARMACOLOGIC THERAPY

- The goal of any resection should be the visual eradication of any tumor burden and the assurance of an adequate depth of resection
- Initially, transurethral resection of bladder tumor (TURBT). Using cutting current, a loop electrode is used to resect the tumor inclusive of muscularis propria (Fig. E1). Histologically, bladder tumors frequently exhibit growth beyond the visible edge, and, as such, resection should include an approximate 2-cm margin of normal-appearing tissue. Wide resection of tumors will ensure completeness, whether the tumor has a broad base or a tentacular growth pattern (Fig. E2)
- Loop biopsy of the prostatic urethra if high-grade TCC is suspected
- If superficial disease, follow-up protocol with repeat TURBT and/or the use of intravesical agents is recommended
- For advanced bladder cancer, radical cystectomy with urethrectomy (unless orthotopic diversion is planned), and either ileal loop conduit or orthotopic diversion

BLADDER PRESERVATION APPROACHES: After cystectomy for muscle-invasive disease, 50% or more of the patients will develop metastases. Most patients develop metastases at distant sites; a third relapse locally. Bladder preservation management is offered in individuals who refuse surgery or who might not be suitable radical cystectomy patients. Bladder-sparing protocols include extensive TURBT or partial cystectomy with external-beam or interstitial radiotherapy and systemic chemotherapy. Radiotherapy as a single treatment modality is not effective. The best predictor of successful bladder preservation is a complete response after the combination of initial TURBT and neoadjuvant chemotherapy with stages T_2 to T_{3a}.

INDICATIONS FOR PARTIAL CYSTECTOMY:

- Tumor within a bladder diverticulum
- Solitary, primary, and muscle-invasive or high-grade lesion of a region of the bladder that allows complete excision with adequate surgical margins
- Inability to adequately resect tumor by TURBT alone because of size or location
- Tumor overlying a ureteral orifice requiring ureteral reimplantation
- Biopsy of a radiation-induced ulceration
- Palliation of severe local symptoms
- Patient refusal of urinary diversion
- Poor-risk patient who is not a diversion candidate

CONTRAINDICATIONS:

- Multiple tumors
- CIS
- Cellular atypia on biopsy
- Prostatic invasion
- Invasion of the trigone
- Inability to achieve adequate surgical margins
- Prior radiotherapy
- Inability to maintain adequate bladder volume after resection
- Evidence of extravesical tumor extension
- Poor surgical risk

ACUTE GENERAL Rx

INDICATIONS FOR INTRAVESICAL CHEMOTHERAPY:

- High-grade tumor
- Tumor size <5 cm
- Multiple tumors
- Presence of CIS
- Positive urinary cytologic findings after a resection
- Incomplete tumor resection

Intravesical agents: Thiotepa, doxorubicin, mitomycin C, AD-32, BCG, interferon, bropirimine, Epodyl, interleukin-2, and keyhole-limpet hemocyanin. Photodynamic therapy with hematoporphyrin derivatives has also been used.

INDICATIONS FOR CYSTECTOMY:

- Large tumors not amenable to complete TURBT
- High-grade tumor
- Multiple tumors with frequent recurrences
- Diffuse CIS not responsive to intravesical chemotherapy
- Prostatic urethra involvement
- Irritative bladder symptoms with upper tract deterioration
- Muscle-invasive disease
- Disease outside the bladder

SYSTEMIC CHEMOTHERAPY: Used as neoadjuvant and adjuvant therapy for systemic disease. The most effective regimens include MVAC (cisplatin, methotrexate, vinblastine, doxorubicin), GC (gemcitabine, cisplatin), and CMV (cyclophosphamide, methotrexate, vinblastine). Other agents include ifosfamide, paclitaxel, and mitomycin C. Combination chemotherapy can provide palliation and modest survival benefit.

IMMUNOTHERAPY: The use of checkpoint inhibitors has now been demonstrated to improve overall survival in relapsed metastatic bladder cancer after failure of first-line chemotherapy regimens. Available agents include the PD-1 inhibitors (nivolumab, pembrolizumab) and PDL-1 inhibitors (atezolizumab, durvalumab).

RADIOTHERAPY: Conflicting reports suggest that superficial bladder cancer is more sensitive to radiotherapy. Only 20% to 30% of patients with invasive bladder cancer can be cured by external-beam radiation therapy alone. It is used in combination with surgery or with systemic agents to treat bladder cancer primarily in patients who are not surgical candidates or who refuse surgery. Combination chemotherapy (cisplatin) given concurrently with radiotherapy has shown significant improved locoregional control of bladder cancer in bladder-preservation strategies.

CHRONIC Rx

FOLLOW-UP RECOMMENDATIONS FOR SUPERFICIAL BLADDER CANCER:

- Cystoscopy, bladder barbotage, and bimanual examination every 3 mo for 2 yr, then every 6 mo for 2 yr, and annually thereafter.
- Upper tract studies are based on the risk of upper tract tumor development, generally every 2 to 5 yr.

BOX 1 American Urological Association Guideline Recommendations

For all index patients
- Standard: Physicians should discuss with the patient the treatment options and the benefits and harms, including side effects, of intravesical treatment.

For a patient who presents with an abnormal growth on the urothelium but who has not yet been diagnosed with bladder cancer
- Standard: If the patient does not have an established histologic diagnosis, a biopsy should be obtained for pathologic analysis.
- Standard: Under most circumstances, complete eradication of all visible tumors should be performed.
- Standard: If bladder cancer is confirmed, periodic surveillance cystoscopy should be performed.
- Option: An initial single dose of intravesical chemotherapy may be administered immediately postoperatively.

For a patient with small volume, low-grade Ta bladder cancer
- Recommendation: An initial single dose of intravesical chemotherapy may be administered immediately postoperatively.

For a patient with multifocal and/or large volume, histologically confirmed, low-grade Ta or a patient with recurrent low-grade Ta bladder cancer
- Recommendation: An induction course of intravesical therapy with bacillus Calmette-Guérin or mitomycin C is recommended for the treatment of these patients with the goal of preventing or delaying recurrence.
- Option: Maintenance bacillus Calmette-Guérin or mitomycin C may be considered.

For a patient with initial histologically confirmed high-grade Ta, T1, and/or carcinoma in situ bladder cancer
- Standard: For patients with lamina propria invasion (T1) but without muscularis propria in the specimen, repeat resection should be performed prior to additional intravesical therapy.
- Recommendation: An induction course of bacillus Calmette-Guérin followed by maintenance therapy is recommended for treatment of these patients.
- Option: Cystectomy should be considered for initial therapy in select patients.

For a patient with high-grade Ta, T1, and/or carcinoma in situ bladder cancer that has recurred after prior intravesical therapy
- Standard: For patients with lamina propria invasion (T1) but without muscularis propria in the specimen, repeat resection should be performed prior to additional intravesical therapy.
- Recommendation: Cystectomy should be considered as a therapeutic alternative for these patients.
- Option: Further intravesical therapy may be considered for these patients.

FOLLOW-UP RECOMMENDATIONS FOR ADVANCED DISEASE: Bladder preservation:
- Cystoscopy, barbotage, bimanual examination, biopsy (when indicated), every 3 mo for 2 yr, then every 6 mo for 2 yr, yearly thereafter
- CT scan of abdomen and pelvis every 6 mo for 2 yr in addition to chest x-ray examination, liver function testing, and serum creatinine

Cystectomy with ileal loop/orthotopic bladder:
- Neobladder endoscopy and IVP yearly
- CT scan of abdomen and pelvis every 6 mo for 2 yr in addition to chest x-ray examination, liver function tests, and serum creatinine
- Loopogram every 6 mo for 2 yr, then annually

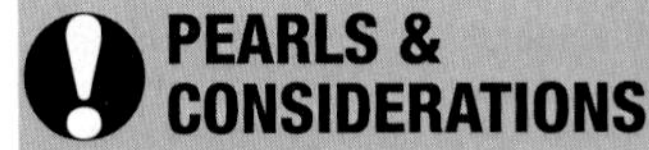

PEARLS & CONSIDERATIONS

COMMENTS
- Useful prognostic parameters for bladder tumor recurrence and subsequent progression are tumor grade, tumor depth, multifocal tumors, frequency of recurrence, tumor size, CIS, lymphatic invasion, papillary or solid tumor configuration.
- Currently, the incidence of occupational bladder cancer seems to be increasing faster in women than in men. Workers with aromatic amine exposure have the highest incidence, whereas those exposed to polycyclic aromatic hydrocarbons and heavy metals have the greatest mortality.
- The 5-year survival for bladder cancer is 76%; it ranges from 96% for in situ, 70% for localized, 35% for regional, and 5% for distant cancers.
- Box 1 describes the American Urological Association Guideline Recommendations for bladder cancer.

SUGGESTED READINGS
Available at ExpertConsult.com

RELATED CONTENT
Bladder Cancer (Patient Information)

AUTHOR: **BHARTI RATHORE, M.D.**

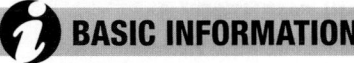

BASIC INFORMATION

DEFINITION

The International Continence Society defines bladder pain syndrome, otherwise known as interstitial cystitis (IC), as a clinical syndrome consisting of suprapubic pain related to bladder filling and accompanied by other symptoms, such as increased daytime and nighttime frequency in the absence of proven infection or other obvious pathology. The American Urological Association defines interstitial cystitis/bladder pain syndrome (IC/BPS) as an unpleasant sensation perceived to be related to the urinary bladder that is associated with lower urinary tract symptoms >6 weeks' duration, in the absence of infection or other unidentifiable causes.

SYNONYMS

Interstitial cystitis
Interstitial cystitis/bladder pain syndrome (IC/BPS)
Painful bladder syndrome
Tic douloureux of bladder

ICD-10CM CODES

N30.1	Interstitial cystitis (chronic)
N30.9	Cystitis, unspecified
N30.10	Interstitial cystitis (chronic) without hematuria
N30.11	Interstitial cystitis (chronic) with hematuria

EPIDEMIOLOGY & DEMOGRAPHICS

INCIDENCE: 21 cases per 100,000 women and four cases per 100,000 men annually

PREVALENCE:

- 197 per 100,000 women and 41 per 100,000 men in the U.S.
- Because the disease is substantially underdiagnosed, it may actually affect one in five women and one in 20 men.
- More than 81% of women diagnosed with chronic pelvic pain and up to 84% of men initially diagnosed with chronic prostatitis actually have IC.
- More than 90% of patients diagnosed with overactive bladder who do not respond to anticholinergics are subsequently diagnosed with IC.

PREDOMINANT SEX AND AGE:

- White women constitute 95% of patients with IC.
- Female/male ratio of 5 to 10:1.
- Most prevalent in fourth and fifth decades of life.

PHYSICAL FINDINGS & CLINICAL PRESENTATION

- Urinary urgency, frequency (>8 in daytime), nocturia (>2 at night), and suprapubic pain are the most common symptoms.
- Suprapubic pain is worse with bladder filling or urinating and relieved after emptying.
- Dyspareunia.
- Symptoms lasting longer than 6 mo.
- Intensity of symptoms waxes and wanes.
- Insidious onset and worsens to the final stage within 5 to 15 yr.
- Exercise, stress, sexual activity, ejaculation, certain foods with high potassium and acids (beer, spices, bananas, tomatoes, chocolate, strawberries, artificial sweeteners, oranges, cranberries, caffeine), menstruation, prolonged sitting, and activation of allergies exacerbate the symptoms.
- Often associated with irritable bowel syndrome, migraine, endometriosis, skin sensitivities, multiple drug allergies, other allergies, vulvodynia, fibromyalgia, chronic fatigue syndrome, systemic lupus erythematosus, and mood disorders.
- Dysphoric mood.
- Lower abdominal tenderness.
- Tender prostate in digital rectal examination.
- Levator ani tenderness in female.
- Tenderness of anterior vaginal wall/bladder neck in female.

ETIOLOGY

Unknown. Fig. 1 illustrates a hypothesis for etiologic cascade of painful bladder syndrome/interstitial cystitis.

DIAGNOSIS

DIFFERENTIAL DIAGNOSIS

- Chronic pelvic pain
- Overactive bladder
- Recurrent urinary tract infection
- Endometriosis
- Pelvic adhesions
- Vulvar vestibulitis
- Vulvodynia
- Urethral pain syndrome
- Chronic nonbacterial prostatitis
- Frequent vaginitis
- Benign prostatic hyperplasia

WORKUP

- IC can be considered a diagnosis of exclusion when no known cause of painful bladder can be identified.
- There is no definite diagnostic test.
- Validated questionnaires such as Pelvic Pain and Urgency/Frequency scale (PUF), O'Leary-Sant symptoms and problem index, and Wisconsin IC scale. PUF is the most commonly used.

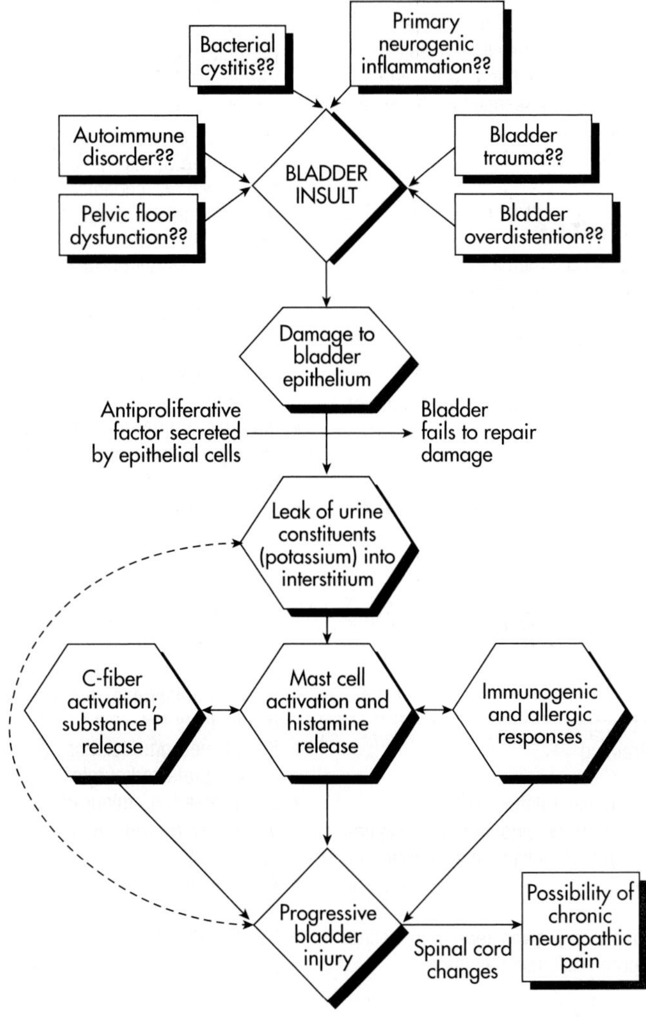

FIG. 1 Hypothesis for etiologic cascade of painful bladder syndrome/interstitial cystitis. (From Wein AJ: Painful bladder syndrome/interstitial cystitis and related disorders. In Wein AJ et al [eds]: *Campbell-Walsh urology*, ed 11, Philadelphia, 2007, Elsevier.)

- Voiding diary shows low-volume (<100 ml) and high-frequency voiding pattern.
- National Institute of Diabetes and Diseases of the Kidney diagnostic criteria misses 60% of IC patients and is not clinically used anymore.
- Anesthetic bladder challenge: With this test the symptoms dissipate on instillation of an anesthetic cocktail into the bladder.
- Cystoscopy and hydrodistention under general anesthesia may show terminal hematuria (Fig. E2), glomerulation, Hunner's ulcers (Fig. E3), and small bladder capacity of less than 350 ml. Cystoscopy and/or urodynamic testing should be considered when the diagnosis is in doubt, but the tests are not necessary to confirm an IC/BPS diagnosis in uncomplicated cases.
- Bladder biopsy is not essential for diagnosis of IC.
- Parson's potassium sensitivity test (PST).
- Urodynamics are unnecessary in diagnosis of IC.

LABORATORY TESTS

- Urine analysis and culture.
- Urine cytology should be performed if microscopic or gross hematuria is present, or with other risk factors such as smoking, age >40 yr, and other bladder cancer risk factors.
- Culture of sexually transmitted diseases if clinically indicated. Nonbacteriuric patients with pyuria should be screened for *Chlamydia.*
- Urine biomarkers (e.g., antiproliferative factor) are promising but not ready for clinical use.

IMAGING STUDIES

CT or ultrasound of abdomen and pelvis may be considered to rule out other pathology.

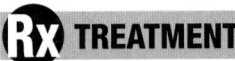

TREATMENT

- There is no consensus for optimal management.
- There is no cure for this disease.

NONPHARMACOLOGIC THERAPY

- Avoidance of activities associated with flare-ups
- Avoidance of smoking
- Dietary restriction, avoiding common irritants (e.g., coffee, citrus fruits)
- Physical therapy
- Exercise
- Behavioral therapy
- Bladder retraining
- Biofeedback
- Warm sitz bath, ice, heating pad
- Thiele massage (transrectal and transvaginal manual therapy of pelvic floor muscle) in presence of pelvic floor muscle tenderness and spasm
- Hydrodistention only gives temporary relief, so it is not commonly used anymore

ACUTE AND CHRONIC Rx

- A course of empiric antibiotics if not tried yet. Long-term oral antibiotics are not recommended.
- Oral therapy is tried first.
- Pentosan polysulfate sodium (Elmiron) is the only FDA-approved and most effective oral therapy.
- Most treatment takes 3 to 6 mo before maximum benefit is seen.
- Adjunct oral therapy includes tricyclic antidepressants (amitriptyline), cimetidine, antihistaminics (hydroxyzine, montelukast), neuroleptics (gabapentin, topiramate), analgesics (NSAIDs, opioid analgesics), and occasionally antimuscarinics.
- Oral therapies can be used in combination.
- Antihistaminics are preferred for patients with an allergy history or those who show mast cells in bladder biopsy.
- Oral prednisone is used in presence of Hunner's ulcers.
- Other drugs rarely used for IC are cyclosporin A, interleukin-10, imatinib, methotrexate, suplatast, misoprostol, and quercetin.
- Growth factor inhibitors, gene therapy, RDP 58, and vitamin B_3 analogue (BXL 628) may represent future therapies.
- Intravesical treatment is used when oral medications fail, for acute flare-ups, or before the oral medications take full effect.
- Dimethyl sulfoxide (DMSO), heparin, lidocaine, hyaluronic acid, capsaicin, botulinum toxin A, chondroitin sulfate, steroids, and Elmiron are drugs used for intravesical treatment.
- DMSO is the only FDA-approved intravesical treatment.
- DMSO is used less often now because of its side effects, specifically a garlic-like odor or taste on breath or skin that lasts 72 hr after treatment.
- Intravesical therapy typically involves mixture of heparin or Elmiron with lidocaine and sodium bicarbonate.
- Silver nitrate and clorpactin have fallen out of favor.

SURGERY

- Major surgical intervention is not the mainstay of treatment.
- Patients whose condition is extreme and who are miserable may consider surgery if medications fail.
- Sacral neuromodulation (InterStim) is the current preferred surgical intervention.
- Laser ablation, fulguration, or resection is offered when Hunner's ulcers are seen in cystoscopy.
- Augmentation cystoplasty is not recommended.
- Cystourethrectomy with urinary diversion is rarely done.

COMPLEMENTARY & ALTERNATIVE MEDICINE

- Transcutaneous electric nerve stimulation
- Intravaginal electric nerve stimulation
- Acupuncture
- Urinary chelating agents such as Polycitra-K crystals, Urocit-K
- Prelief, an over-the-counter food additive
- Herbal remedies such as Algnot Plus, CystoProtek, Cysta-Q, aloe vera

DISPOSITION

Voiding diary and symptom questionnaire are helpful to monitor response to treatment.

REFERRAL

- Urologist
- Pain specialist
- Physical therapist

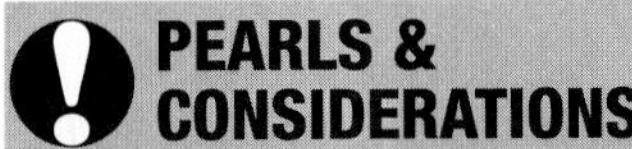

PEARLS & CONSIDERATIONS

COMMENTS

- On average, these patients see five physicians and endure irritating voiding symptoms for 5 yr before the disease is identified.
- Besides symptom questionnaire and urine analysis, all other diagnostic tests are optional.
- PST is well tolerated.
- Negative cystoscopy does not rule out IC.

PREVENTION

Early identification and timely intervention improve patient outcome.

PATIENT & FAMILY EDUCATION

- IC support groups
- Interstitial Cystitis Association
- Interstitial Cystitis Network

SUGGESTED READINGS

Available at ExpertConsult.com

AUTHOR: **FRED F. FERRI, M.D.**

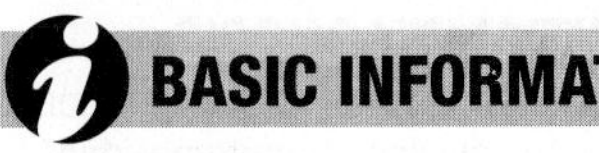

BASIC INFORMATION

DEFINITION

Blepharospasm (BSP) is a movement disorder characterized by hyperactivity of the orbicularis oculi and other muscles around the eyes.

SYNONYMS

BSP
Orbicularis oculi spasms
Focal dystonia

ICD 10-CM CODE

G24.5 Blepharospasm

EPIDEMIOLOGY & DEMOGRAPHICS

INCIDENCE: Not applicable
PEAK INCIDENCE: Not applicable
PREVALENCE: Prevalence is between 20 and 133 cases per million depending on geographic area.
PREDOMINANT SEX AND AGE: Female preference, peak age at onset between the fifth and seventh decade.
GENETICS: Predominantly a sporadic disorder, however 25% of patients have one or more family members affected by dystonia. No specific genetic association specific to BSP is known.
RISK FACTORS: Risk of primary BSP increases with diseases of the anterior segment of the eye and preceding head trauma. Risk of secondary BSP increases with focal lesions in multiple brain regions, comorbid Parkinson's disease, tardive dyskinesia, or conditions associated with eyelid weakness such as facial palsy and myasthenia.

PHYSICAL FINDINGS & CLINICAL PRESENTATION

- Motor manifestations include orbicularis oculi (OO) spasms (Fig. 1), apraxia of eyelid opening, increased blinking rate, and dystonia at other body sites (most commonly oromandibular and cervical regions).
- OO spasms are stereotyped, bilateral, and synchronous. Spasms may be brief or sustained, and may induce narrowing or closure of the eyelids.
- Apraxia of eyelid opening is transient failure to voluntarily reopen the eyes without an apparent spasm of the OO muscle and despite sustained frontalis muscle contraction.
- Nonmotor manifestations include the presence of a so-called "sensory trick" (certain actions involving gentle stimulation to the face alleviate symptoms and allow patients with BSP to keep eyes open, e.g., light touch to certain areas of the face, wearing tinted lenses, talking, singing, or chewing/eating); other sensory symptoms (burning sensation and grittiness in the eye, dry eye, and photophobia); psychiatric disturbances (depression and obsessive/compulsive symptoms); sleep abnormalities, and cognitive dysfunction.

ETIOLOGY

- Primary BSP is predominantly sporadic, although up to 25% of patients have one or more family members with dystonia. Several genes are associated with adult-onset dystonia, though none have been associated with pure BSP.
- Secondary BSP is associated with several different focal lesions of the brain (thalamus, basal ganglia, lower brain stem, cerebellum, midbrain, and cortex) or may be associated with other movement disorders including PD, TD, facial palsy, or myasthenia.
- A proposed mechanism involves loss of striatal dopamine leading to reduced tonic inhibition of trigeminal reflex circuits combined with weakening of lid closure by the OO muscle. This leads to an adaptive increase in activity of trigeminal sensory-motor blink circuits.

DIAGNOSIS

DIFFERENTIAL DIAGNOSIS

- Pure apraxia of eyelid opening, a common feature of lesions of the nondominant parietal lobe (among other regions)
- Bell's palsy (unilateral facial weakness involving both the upper and lower face due to lower-motor-neuron facial nerve palsy; etiology may be viral, inflammatory, autoimmune, or ischemic)
- Eyelid myokymia (typically unilateral, spontaneous, fine fascicular contractions of the lower orbicularis oculi without atrophy or weakness)
- Hemifacial spasm (brief clonic movements of OO typically spreading to other facial regions, often associated with chronic irritation of the facial nerve or nucleus)
- Dry eye, or conjunctivitis/kerratitis with frequent blinking
- Myasthenia gravis with eyelid ptosis

WORK-UP

BSP is a clinical diagnosis that relies on thorough neuropsychiatric and ophthalmologic evaluation.

LABORATORY TESTS

No tests are diagnostic. However, certain findings on electromyography (evaluation of blink reflex excitability recovery curve) present in dystonia and BSP, but not in psychogenic BSP, may reinforce clinical suspicion.

IMAGING STUDIES

Standard brain imaging has not consistently demonstrated clinical utility for BSP.

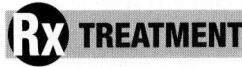

TREATMENT

ACUTE GENERAL Rx

- Botulinum neurotoxin type A is first-line treatment for BSP. Side effects such as transient ptosis, blurred vision, and diplopia are uncommon and tend to improve spontaneously within weeks.
- Modest improvement has come with anticholinergics (e.g., trihexyphenidyl), benzodiazepines, baclofen, and tetrabenazine. However, side effects may be too problematic.

CHRONIC Rx

Long-term efficacy of Botulinum neurotoxin type A treatment in BSP has been documented. However, this has not led to significant improvements upon quality of life, indicating non-motor manifestations of BSP require individual attention. More literature is needed in this regard.

REFERRAL

Movement disorder specialist consultation is common.

AUTHOR: **JORDAN R. ANDERSON, D.O.**

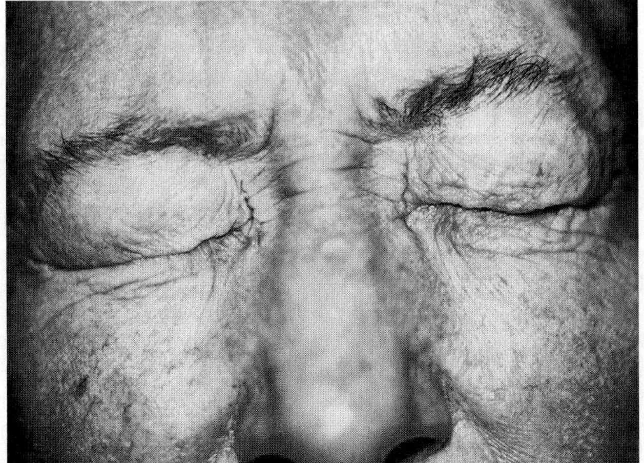

FIG. 1 Essential blepharospasm. (From Bowling B: *Kanski's clinical ophthalmology, a systemic approach*, ed 8, 2016, Philadelphia, Elsevier.)

BASIC INFORMATION

DEFINITION

Body dysmorphic disorder (BDD) is classified as an obsessive-compulsive and related disorder. It is characterized by preoccupation with one or more perceived defects or flaws in physical appearance that are not observable or appear only slight to others, as well as repetitive behaviors (e.g., excessive grooming, mirror checking, skin picking, reassurance seeking) in response to the appearance concerns. The preoccupations cause clinically significant distress or impairment in social, occupational, or other important areas of functioning (usually both). The appearance preoccupations are not better explained by concerns with body fat or weight in a person whose symptoms meet diagnostic criteria for an eating disorder.

SYNONYMS

Dysmorphophobia
BDD

ICD-10CM CODES
F45.22 Body dysmorphic disorder
DSM-5 CODES
300.50

EPIDEMIOLOGY & DEMOGRAPHICS

- Affects 1.7% to 2.9% of the general population (in nationwide epidemiologic studies)
- Prevalence among general cosmetic surgery patients is 13%–15%
- Weighted prevalence in rhinoplasty surgery settings is 20.1%
- Weighted prevalence among dermatology outpatients is 11.3%
- Slightly higher prevalence among females (but not in cosmetic surgery or dermatology settings)
- Onset most commonly in early adolescence (two thirds have onset before age 18)

PHYSICAL FINDINGS & CLINICAL PRESENTATION

- Excessive preoccupation (obsession) with one or more perceived defects in appearance that are not observable or appear only slight to others. Patients believe they look abnormal, ugly, unattractive, or deformed, whereas in reality they look normal. Any part of the body may be a focus of concern; skin (e.g., perceived acne or scarring), hair (e.g., perceived thinning or excessive body or facial hair), and nose (e.g., size or shape) concerns are most common. Muscle dysmorphia is a form of BDD that occurs primarily in men and focuses on excessive concern that one's body build is too small or is insufficiently muscular. Most patients are preoccupied with multiple body areas.
- The body areas with which the patient is concerned appear physically normal; if a physical defect is present, it is slight, and the patient's reaction to it is excessive.
- Most patients have poor insight (i.e., are mostly convinced) or absent insight (i.e., delusional beliefs; are completely convinced) regarding the accuracy of their beliefs about the appearance of the perceived defects.
- At some point during the course of the disorder, all patients engage in repetitive behaviors such as frequent mirror checking, excessive grooming, skin picking to try to fix perceived skin flaws, reassurance seeking, and repeatedly measuring or feeling the perceived defect. The intent of these behaviors is to check, try to improve, or gain reassurance about the appearance of the perceived flaws. Nearly all patients attempt to camouflage or hide the perceived defects—e.g., with makeup, a hat, hair, or body position.
- Nearly all experience impairment in psychosocial functioning and quality of life as a result of their appearance concerns; impairment is usually substantial.
- Suicidal ideation, suicide attempts, and completed suicide appear common.
- Commonly co-occurring mental disorders are major depressive disorder, substance use disorders (including abuse of anabolic androgenic steroids in muscle dysmorphia), social anxiety disorder, obsessive-compulsive disorder (OCD), and personality disorder.

ETIOLOGY

Likely multifactorial, with both genetic and environmental risk factors (e.g., teasing). Has shared genetic vulnerability with obsessive-compulsive disorder plus BDD-specific genetic influences. Neuropsychological and fMRI studies indicate abnormalities in visual processing consisting of excessive focus on details rather than on larger global and configural elements of visual stimuli (with some similarities to anorexia nervosa). Information processing deficits and biases also characterize BDD, which may also play a role in the disorder's development and/or maintenance.

DIAGNOSIS

Psychiatric interview
Ask:

1. Are you very worried about your appearance in any way? *OR:* Are you unhappy with how you look?
2. Does this concern with your appearance preoccupy you? If you add up all the time you spend each day thinking about your appearance, how much time would you estimate it takes (at least an hour a day)?
3. How much distress does this concern cause you?
4. What effect does this concern have on your life?
5. Is there anything you feel an urge to do over and over again in response to your appearance concerns? (Give examples, such as mirror checking, comparing with others, skin picking to remove perceived skin flaws)
6. Determine that the perceived appearance defects are actually nonexistent or only slight

DIFFERENTIAL DIAGNOSIS

- Often undiagnosed because of patient's reluctance to divulge symptoms due to shame and fear of being misunderstood (e.g., considered vain)
- OCD
- Eating disorder
- Social anxiety disorder
- Major depressive disorder

WORKUP

Clinical evaluation focused on BDD symptoms and associated impairment in functioning.

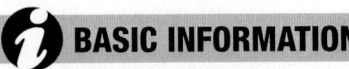

TREATMENT

NONPHARMACOLOGIC THERAPY

- CBT, with a focus on cognitive restructuring, exposure, perceptual retraining, and response (ritual) prevention; CBT must be specifically tailored to BDD's unique symptoms.
- Do not try to talk patients out of their concern; it is ineffective.
- Avoid cosmetic procedures; a majority of patients with BDD receive them, but such treatments do not appear effective for BDD. Dissatisfied patients may sue or even become violent toward the treating clinician.

CHRONIC Rx

- SRIs are medication of choice both acutely and chronically; high doses (similar to those for OCD) often needed.
- Other agents (e.g., neuroleptics, tricyclic antidepressants other than clomipramine) do not appear as beneficial, although limited evidence suggests that atypical neuroleptics and buspirone may be helpful as SRI augmentation agents.
- CBT tailored specifically to BDD is recommended, with an SRI if BDD symptoms are moderate to severe, the patient is suicidal because of BDD symptoms, or comorbidity is present that may benefit from an SRI.
- Support groups if available.
- More intensive BDD-focused treatment (e.g., intensive outpatient, residential treatment) if outpatient care is insufficient.

DISPOSITION

- Untreated BDD tends to be chronic and can lead to social isolation; school dropout; loss of employment; major depression; abuse of drugs or alcohol; unnecessary surgery, dermatologic treatment, or other cosmetic treatment; and suicide.
- With correct diagnosis and treatment, a majority improve.

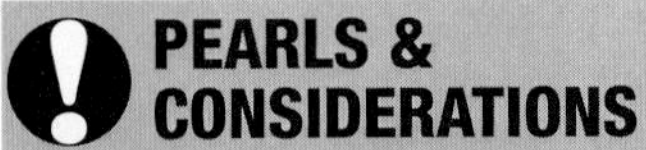

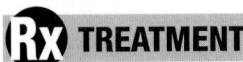

PEARLS & CONSIDERATIONS

- In clinical settings, approximately three quarters have lifetime co-occurring major depressive disorder; suicidal ideation is common.
- Reassurance that the patient looks normal is rarely helpful.

- Patients often have an unrealistic expectation of improvement with plastic surgery, dermatologic treatment, and other cosmetic procedures; these treatments do not appear to be effective.
- All patients should be screened and monitored for suicidality.

PATIENT/FAMILY EDUCATION

- Family support and encouragement of appropriate treatment is important.
- Phillips KA: *Understanding Body Dysmorphic Disorder: An Essential Guide.* Oxford University Press, 2009.
- www.KatharinePhillipsMD.com
- https://bdd.iocdf.org/

RELATED CONTENT

Body Dysmorphic Disorder (Patient Information)
Obsessive Compulsive Disorder (Related Key Topic)

AUTHOR: **KATHARINE A. PHILLIPS, M.D.**

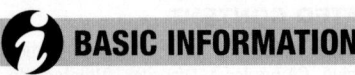

BASIC INFORMATION

DEFINITION

Primary malignant bone tumors are invasive and anaplastic and have the ability to metastasize. These neoplasms can arise from the marrow (myeloma), but may also develop from bone, cartilage, fat, and fibrous tissues. Leukemia and lymphoma are excluded from this discussion.

FIBROSARCOMA AND LIPOSARCOMA: They are extremely rare and similar to tumors arising in soft tissue.

OSTEOSARCOMA: A rare primary malignant tumor of bone characterized by malignant tumor cells that produce osteoid or bone. Several variants have been described: parosteal sarcoma, periosteal sarcoma, multicentric, and telangiectatic forms.

CHONDROSARCOMA: A malignant cartilage tumor that may develop primarily or secondarily from transformation of a benign osteocartilaginous exostosis or enchondroma.

EWING SARCOMA: A malignant tumor of the bone or soft tissues characterized by the presence of small, round, blue cells on immunohistochemical evaluation.

MULTIPLE MYELOMA: A neoplastic proliferation of plasma cells in the bone marrow.

SYNONYMS

Multiple myeloma:
1. Plasma cell myeloma
2. Plasmacytoma

ICD-10CM CODES

C41.9	Malignant neoplasm of bone and articular cartilage, unspecified
C40.00	Malignant neoplasm of scapula and long bones of unspecified upper limb
C40.01	Malignant neoplasm of scapula and long bones of right upper limb
C40.02	Malignant neoplasm of scapula and long bones of left upper limb
C40.10	Malignant neoplasm of short bones of unspecified upper limb
C40.11	Malignant neoplasm of short bones of right upper limb
C40.12	Malignant neoplasm of short bones of left upper limb
C40.20	Malignant neoplasm of long bones of unspecified lower limb
C40.21	Malignant neoplasm of long bones of right lower limb
C40.22	Malignant neoplasm of long bones of left lower limb
C40.30	Malignant neoplasm of short bones of unspecified lower limb
C40.31	Malignant neoplasm of short bones of right lower limb
C40.32	Malignant neoplasm of short bones of left lower limb
C40.80	Malignant neoplasm of overlapping sites of bone and articular cartilage of unspecified limb
C40.81	Malignant neoplasm of overlapping sites of bone and articular cartilage of right limb
C40.82	Malignant neoplasm of overlapping sites of bone and articular cartilage of left limb
C40.90	Malignant neoplasm of unspecified bones and articular cartilage of unspecified limb
C40.91	Malignant neoplasm of unspecified bones and articular cartilage of right limb
C40.92	Malignant neoplasm of unspecified bones and articular cartilage of left limb
C41.0	Malignant neoplasm of bones of skull and face
C41.4	Malignant neoplasm of pelvic bones, sacrum and coccyx
C41.9	Malignant neoplasm of bone and articular cartilage, unspecified

EPIDEMIOLOGY & DEMOGRAPHICS

Table 1 summarizes incidence, in decreasing order, of lesions that may present as a primary bone tumor.

MULTIPLE MYELOMA:
- The most common tumor in bone
- Age at onset: Usually >40 yr
- Male/female ratio of 2:1

OSTEOGENIC SARCOMA:
- Average age at onset: 10 to 20 yr
- Males afflicted more often than females
- Parosteal sarcoma in older patients

CHONDROSARCOMA:
- Age at onset: 40 to 60 yr
- Male/female ratio of 2:1

EWING SARCOMA: Age at onset: 10 to 15 yr

PHYSICAL FINDINGS & CLINICAL PRESENTATION

MULTIPLE MYELOMA:
- May present as a systemic process or, less commonly, as a "solitary" extramedullary lesion
- Early manifestations: Anorexia, weight loss, and bone pain; majority of cases present initially with back pain that often leads to the detection of a destructive skeletal lesion
- Other organ systems eventually become involved, resulting in more bone pain, anemia, renal insufficiency, and/or bacterial infections, usually as a result of the dysproteinemia typical of this disorder
- Possible secondary amyloidosis, leading to cardiac failure or nephrotic syndrome

OSTEOSARCOMA:
- Most originating in the metaphysis
- 50% to 60% around the knee
- Possible pain and swelling, but otherwise healthy patient
- Osteosarcoma in conjunction with Paget's disease, manifested primarily as a sudden increase in bone pain

CHONDROSARCOMA:
- Tumor most commonly involving the pelvis, upper femur, and shoulder girdle
- Painful swelling

EWING SARCOMA:
- Painful soft tissue mass often present
- Possibly increased local heat
- Midshaft of a long bone usually affected (in contrast to other tumors)
- Weight loss, fever, and lethargy

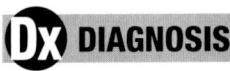

DIAGNOSIS

DIFFERENTIAL DIAGNOSIS

- Osteomyelitis
- Metastatic bone disease

LABORATORY TESTS

- Slightly elevated alkaline phosphatase in osteosarcoma

TABLE 1 Incidence, in Decreasing Order, of Lesions That May Present as a Primary Bone Tumor

Lesion	Incidence of All Tumors (%)[†,‡]
Osteosarcoma	17
Chondrosarcoma	11
Enchondroma*	6
Fibrous dysplasia*	6
Giant cell tumor	6
Nonossifying fibroma/fibrous cortical defect*	5
Ewing sarcoma	5
Malignant fibrous histiocytoma/fibrosarcoma	5
Osteochondroma*	4
Aneurysmal bone cyst	4
Metastasis	4
Osteomyelitis	4
Solitary bone cyst	3
Osteoid osteoma	3
Langerhans cell histiocytosis (eosinophilic granuloma)	3
Chondroblastoma	2
Others	12

*Lesions are often asymptomatic and therefore much more frequent than the table suggests.
†Benign tumors and tumor-like lesions in general are underreported in these frequency distributions.
‡Data are based on 6873 tumors on file in the Netherlands Committee on Bone Tumors.
Pope TL, Bloem HL et al: *Musculoskeletal imaging*, ed 2, Philadelphia, 2015, Elsevier.

TABLE 2 Systemic Approach in Diagnosing Osseous Tumors or Tumor-Like Lesions

1. Categorize the radiograph (normal, variant, tumor-like lesion, tumor).
2. Determine the prevalence of lesions in relation to the age of the patient.
3. Determine the prevalence of lesions in the affected bone.
4. Is the lesion solitary, or are there multiple lesions?
5. Determine the prevalence of osseous lesions in the affected part of the bone.
6. Analyze the radiograph in detail.
7. Analyze additional information (MR, CT, clinical and laboratory data, and so on).
8. Perform a biopsy, if needed, based on the comprehensive imaging findings.

From Pope TL, Bloem HL et al: *Musculoskeletal imaging*, ed 2, Philadelphia, 2015, Elsevier.

- In Ewing sarcoma: Reflective of systemic reaction; includes anemia, an increase in white blood cell count, and an elevated sedimentation rate
- In multiple myeloma:
  1. Bence Jones protein in the urine
  2. Anemia and elevated erythrocyte sedimentation rate
  3. Characteristic dysproteinemia on serum protein electrophoresis showing a monoclonal spike
  4. Elevated quantitative immunoglobulins, beta-2 microglobulin, and elevated kappa:lambda ratio upon serum-free light chain assay
  5. Rouleaux formation in the peripheral blood smear
  6. Often presence of hypercalcemia
  7. Elevated serum lactate dehydrogenase (LDH)

IMAGING STUDIES

- Table 2 summarizes a systemic approach in diagnosing osseous tumors or tumor-like lesions.
- Classic osteogenic sarcoma penetrates the cortex early in many cases.
  1. A blastic (dense), lytic (lucent), or mixed response may be seen in the affected bone (Fig. 1).

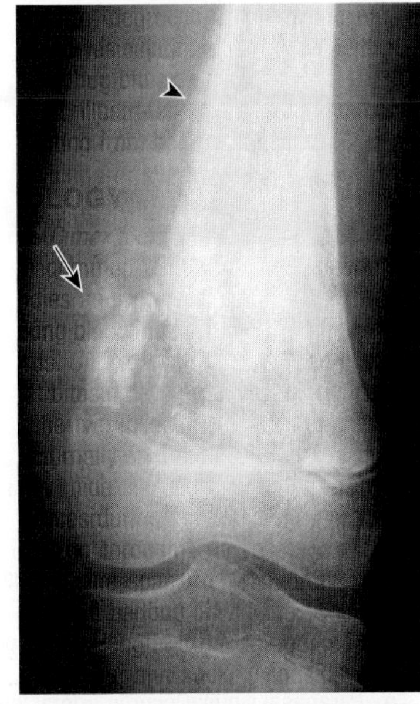

FIG. 1 Conventional central osteosarcoma. AP radiograph of the distal femur showing a classic osteosarcoma with mixed lytic and sclerotic areas, tumor bone formation in the extraosseous mass *(arrow)*, and a proximal Codman's triangle *(arrowhead)*. (From Adam A et al: *Grainger & Allison's diagnostic radiology,* ed 5, Philadelphia, 2008, Churchill Livingstone.)

  2. An aggressive perpendicular sunburst pattern may be present as a result of periosteal reaction, and peripheral Codman's triangles are often noted.
  3. Margins of the tumor are poorly defined.
- Speckled calcifications in a destructive radiolucent lesion are usually suggestive of chondrosarcoma.
- Ewing sarcoma is characterized radiographically by mottled, irregular destructive changes with periosteal new bone formation. The latter may be multilayered, producing the typical "onion skin" appearance.
- Typical x-ray finding in multiple myeloma is the "punched out" lesion with sharply demarcated edges.
  1. Multiple lesions are usual.
  2. Diffuse osteoporosis may be the only finding in many cases.
  3. Pathologic fractures are common.
- In multiple myeloma, MRI scans or PET are routinely utilized for the purposes of staging extent of disease and also for monitoring for response and/or disease progression.

Rx TREATMENT

The evaluation and treatment of malignant bone tumors are complicated. Diagnostic studies and treatment should be supervised by an orthopedic cancer specialist and oncologist.

DISPOSITION

- In the past 20 yr, dramatic improvements have been made in the treatment protocols for osteosarcoma with the use of adjuvant multidrug regimens and limb-sparing surgery.
- Prognosis of multiple myeloma has markedly improved with introduction of several newer therapies, including proteasome inhibitors, immunomodulatory drugs, histone deacetylase inhibitors, and monoclonal antibodies. Additionally, immunotherapy approaches with checkpoint inhibitors are under investigation with promising initial results.
- Prognosis for Ewing sarcoma has improved with a combination of chemotherapy, local resection, and radiation therapy.
- Chondrosarcomas are not sensitive to chemotherapy or radiation, and prognosis depends on the grade of the tumor and the ability to obtain an adequate resection.

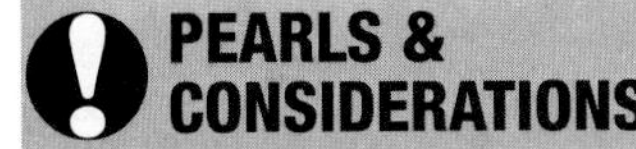

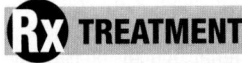

PEARLS & CONSIDERATIONS

Early diagnosis is important because most bone tumors are initially localized and have not metastasized at the time of initial presentation. In multiple myeloma, early utilization of autologous stem cell transplantation confers a survival benefit in eligible patients.

RELATED CONTENT

Multiple Myeloma (Related Key Topic)
Sarcoma (Related Key Topic)

AUTHOR: **BHARTI RATHORE, M.D.**

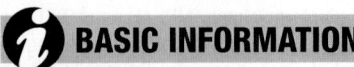

BASIC INFORMATION

DEFINITION

A brain abscess is a focal intracerebral infection that can arise as a complication of a bacterial, mycobacterial, fungal, or parasitic infection, or as a sequelae after surgery or trauma.

ICD-10CM CODE
G06.0 Intracranial abscess and granuloma

EPIDEMIOLOGY & DEMOGRAPHICS

INCIDENCE: Uncommon (reported incidence 0.4 to 0.9 cases per 100,000 population; occurs about 2% as commonly as brain tumors)
PEAK INCIDENCE: Preadolescence and middle age (and depends on predisposing condition); increased rates in the immunocompromised host
PREDOMINANT AGE: Occurs at any age
PREDOMINANT SEX: Men affected more than women (ratio 2:1 to 3:1)

PHYSICAL FINDINGS & CLINICAL PRESENTATION

- Classic triad: Fever, headache, and focal neurologic deficit (present in approximately 20% of cases).
- Clinical presentation is often due to the manifestations of the space-occupying lesion rather than to signs of systemic infection.
- Fever is present in only 32% to 79% of patients.
- Headache is usually localized to the side of the abscess; onset can be gradual or severe; present in an average of 70% to 75% of cases.
- Focal neurologic findings (e.g., seizures, hemiparesis, aphasia, ataxia) depend on the location of the abscess and are seen in 23% to 66% of cases.
- Papilledema is present in 9% to 51% of cases.
- Presence of adjacent infections (dental abscess, otitis media, sinusitis, or postneurosurgical infection) may be a clue to the underlying diagnosis and should be sought in any suspected case.
- Time course from symptom onset to presentation ranges from hours in fulminant cases to more than 1 month; 75% present in the first 2 weeks.
- The nonspecific presentation of a brain abscess warrants that clinicians maintain a high index of suspicion. Table 1 describes common initial features of brain abscess.

ETIOLOGY

- Brain abscesses are classified based on the likely portal of entry and can arise from:
  1. Contiguous infection (e.g., dental abscess, otitis media, sinusitis, or post neurosurgical infection)
  2. Hematogenous spread from a remote site (e.g., endocarditis, bacteremia), which typically causes multiple lesions

TABLE 1 Brain Abscess: Initial Features in 123 Cases

Headache	55%
Disturbed consciousness	48%
Fever	58%
Nuchal rigidity	29%
Nausea, vomiting	32%
Seizures	19%
Visual disturbance	15%
Dysarthria	20%
Hemiparesis	48%
Sepsis	17%

From Goldman L, Schafer AI: *Goldman's Cecil medicine*, ed 24, Philadelphia, 2012, Saunders.

- Likely source of abscess and common organisms involved:
  1. Contiguous focus or primary infection (55% of all brain abscesses):
     a. Paranasal sinus: Occur in frontal lobe; streptococci (especially microaerophilic and anaerobic streptococci), *Bacteroides*, *Haemophilus*, and *Fusobacterium* spp.
     b. Otitis media/mastoiditis: Occur in temporal lobe and cerebellum; aerobic and anaerobic streptococci, *Enterobacteriaceae*, *Bacteroides*, and *Pseudomonas* spp.
     c. Dental infection: Occur in frontal lobe; mixed *Fusobacterium*, *Bacteroides*, and *Streptococcus* spp. (especially *S. viridans* and anaerobic streptococci)
     d. Penetrating head injury: Site of abscess depends on site of wound; *Staphylococcus aureus*, aerobic streptococci, *Clostridium* spp., *Enterobacteriaceae*
     e. Postoperative: *Staphylococcus epidermidis* and *S. aureus, Enterobacteriaceae,* and *Pseudomonas aeruginosa*
  2. Hematogenous spread from a distant site of infection (25% of all brain abscesses): Abscesses most commonly multiple, especially in middle cerebral artery distribution; infecting organism(s) depend on source
     a. Congenital heart disease: Streptococci, *Haemophilus* spp.
     b. Endocarditis: *S. aureus*, viridans streptococci
     c. Urinary tract: Enterobacteriaceae, Pseudomonadaceae
     d. Intraabdominal: Streptococci, *Enterobacteriaceae*, anaerobes
     e. Lung: streptococci, *Actinomyces* spp., *Fusobacterium* spp.
     f. Immunocompromised host: *Toxoplasma* spp., *Enterobacteriaceae*, *Nocardia* spp., listeriosisi, other fungi, tuberculosis
        (1) Fungi are responsible for up to 90% of cerebral abscesses in solid organ transplant recipients
  3. Cryptogenic (unknown source): 20% of all brain abscesses

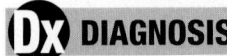

DIAGNOSIS

DIFFERENTIAL DIAGNOSIS

- Other parameningeal infections: Subdural empyema, epidural abscess, thrombophlebitis of the major dural venous sinuses and cortical veins
- Embolic strokes in patients with bacterial endocarditis
- Mycotic aneurysms with leakage
- Acute hemorrhagic leukoencephalitis
- Parasitic infections: Toxoplasmosis, echinococcosis, cysticercosis
- Metastatic or primary brain tumors
- Cerebral infarction
- CNS vasculitis
- Chronic subdural hematoma

WORKUP

Physical examination, laboratory tests, and imaging studies

LABORATORY TESTS

- White blood cell counts are elevated in 60% of patients.
- Erythrocyte sedimentation rate is usually elevated but may be normal.
- Lumbar puncture is contraindicated because of the potential for increased intracranial pressure and the risk for herniation due to the space-occupying abscess. Lumbar puncture may be helpful only in those with suspicion for meningitis or abscess rupture into the ventricular system; however, the risk of herniation must be considered.
- The yield of gram stain and culture of material aspirated at time of surgical drainage is very high.
- Cultures of contiguous sites of infection should be considered (e.g., paranasal sinus, otitis, skin site abscess from a neurosurgical procedure). These sites of infection may need surgical drainage in order to control the infection.
- Blood cultures and cerebrospinal fluid cultures may identify the causative organism in up to 25% of patients.
- Based on the appearance of lesions on imaging, then antitoxoplasma IgG antibodies from the blood and anticysticercal antibodies in the CSF can aid in the diagnosis of CNS toxoplasma and neurocysticercosis infections, respectively.

IMAGING STUDIES

- CT scan with contrast enhancement or MRI with gadolinium can be used to detect brain abscess. CT is rapid and available in most medical settings. An MRI with gadolinium (Fig. E1) is able to provide more detailed images in order to differentiate between abscess and tumor or other mass.
- CT scan (Fig. 2) with intravenous contrast enhancement is still an excellent test (sensitivity 95%-99%).
- Serial CT or MRI scanning is recommended to follow the response to therapy.

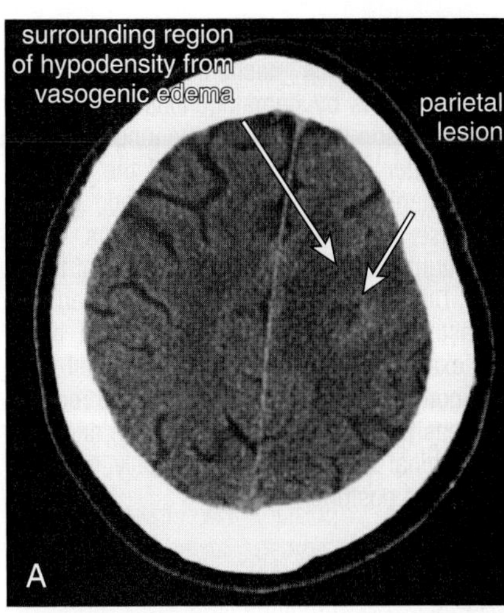

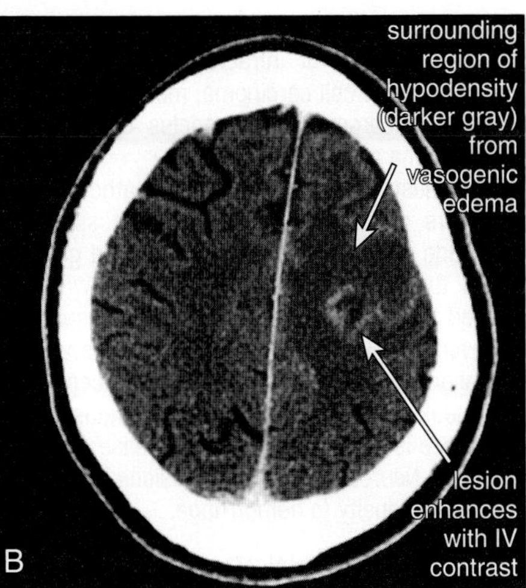

FIG. 2 Brain abscess. This 48-year-old male presented with status epilepticus. Computed tomography (CT) of the brain showed a parietal mass, which at brain biopsy was found to be an abscess. Cultures grew mixed gram-positive and gram-negative organisms and anaerobes. The patient was subsequently found to be human immunodeficiency virus positive. **A,** Noncontrast head CT, brain windows. **B,** CT with intravenous (IV) contrast moments later, brain windows. Abscesses and other infectious, inflammatory, or neoplastic lesions typically have surrounding hypodense regions representing vasogenic edema. When IV contrast is administered **(B),** the lesion may enhance peripherally, often referred to as ring enhancement. (From Broder JS: *Diagnostic imaging for the emergency physician*, Philadelphia, 2011, Saunders.)

Rx TREATMENT

ACUTE GENERAL Rx

- Effective treatment involves a combination of empiric antibiotic therapy and timely excision or aspiration of the abscess.
- If evidence of edema or mass effect, treatment of elevated intracranial pressure is paramount.
  1. Hyperventilation of mechanically ventilated patient.
  2. Dexamethasone initially in a dosage of 10 mg IV followed by 4 mg IV q6h until symptoms of cerebral edema subside. Steroids should be discontinued as soon as possible.
  3. Mannitol 0.25 to 1 g/kg IV over 20 to 30 min q6 to 8h; maximum of 6 g/kg in 24 hr.
- Medical therapy is never a substitute for surgical intervention to relieve increased intracranial pressure. Neurologic deterioration usually mandates surgical intervention.
- Steroids should be limited to patients with severe cerebral edema or midline shift.

MEDICAL Rx

If abscess <2.5 cm and patient is neurologically stable and conscious, may start antibiotics and observe. Empiric antibiotic therapy guided by:

- Abscess location
- Suspicion of primary source
- Presence of single or multiple abscesses
- Patient's underlying medical conditions (e.g., HIV, immunocompromised)

  Selection of empiric antibiotic therapy:
- Primary infection or contiguous source:
  1. Otitis media/mastoiditis, sinusitis: Third-generation cephalosporin (cefotaxime 2 g q4h IV or ceftriaxone 2 g q12h IV) plus metronidazole 15 mg/kg IV as a loading dose, then 7.5 mg/kg q8h IV, not to exceed 4 g per day
  2. Dental infection: Penicillin G (20 million to 24 million units per day IV in six divided doses) plus metronidazole (dose as above)
  3. Head trauma: Third- or fourth-generation cephalosporin (cefotaxime 2 g IV q4h or ceftriaxone 2 g IV q12h or cefepime 2 g IV q8h) plus vancomycin (30 mg/kg IV in two divided doses adjusted for renal function)
  4. Postoperative neurosurgery: Vancomycin (dose as above) plus ceftazidime (2 g IV q8h) or cefepime (2 g IV q8h), or meropenem (1 g IV q8h). Replace vancomycin with nafcillin (2g IV q4h) if susceptibility testing reveals methicillin-sensitive *Staphylococcus aureus*
- Hematogenous spread (congenital heart disease, endocarditis, urinary tract, lung, intraabdominal): Vancomycin (empiric therapy, dose as above) or nafcillin (if susceptibility testing reveals methicillin-sensitive *S. aureus*, dose as above) plus metronidazole plus third-generation cephalosporin (cefotaxime 2 g IV q4h or ceftriaxone 2 g IV q12h). Antibiotic therapy can be adjusted based on the etiology of the underlying infection, if known. Depending on the source, many experts advocate for anaerobic coverage, even with no documentation given suboptimal sensitivity of current techniques
- HIV infected or immunocompromised patient: Metronidazole plus a third-generation cephalosporin, antifungal, or antiparasitic agent. Duration of antibiotic therapy is guided by the clinical course and by whether the abscess was surgically aspirated or excised; it is usually prolonged. Most recommend parenteral treatment for at least 4 to 8 weeks, with serial neuroimaging to ensure adequate resolution. (Imaging weekly could be considered for first 2 weeks of therapy, then every 2 weeks until resolution.) Surgical therapy may be required for clinical failure (i.e., increasing size of abscess on imaging despite antibiotic therapy).

SURGICAL Rx

- Three indications for surgical intervention:
  1. Collect specimens for culture and sensitivity
  2. Reduce mass effect
  3. Clinical failure with antibiotic therapy alone
- Stereotactic biopsy or aspirate of the abscess if surgically feasible
- Essential to selection of targeted antimicrobial coverage
- Timing and choice of surgery depend on:
  1. Primary infection source
  2. Number and location of the abscesses
  3. Whether the procedure is diagnostic or therapeutic
  4. Neurologic status of the patient

DISPOSITION

- Prompt diagnostic consideration, early institution of appropriate antimicrobial therapy, and advanced neuroradiologic imaging have reduced the mortality rate from brain abscesses from 40% to 80% in the preantibiotic era to 10% to 20% at present.
- Morbidity is usually manifest as persistent neurologic sequelae (seizures, intellectual or behavioral impairment, motor deficits).

REFERRAL

Consultation with infectious disease and neurosurgery

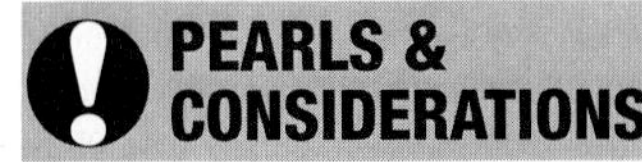

PEARLS & CONSIDERATIONS

COMMENTS

- It is important to maintain a high index of suspicion because a brain abscess often presents with nonspecific symptoms.
- Rapid imaging and early institution of appropriate antimicrobial therapy improve patient morbidity and mortality.
- Neurosurgical consultation is mandatory.

PREVENTION

Because brain abscesses arise from either contiguous infections or hematogenously from a remote site, early and appropriate treatment of predisposing infections is paramount to prevent brain abscess.

SUGGESTED READINGS

Available at ExpertConsult.com

RELATED CONTENT

Brain Abscess (Patient Information)

AUTHOR: **ERICA HARDY, M.D., M.M.S.**

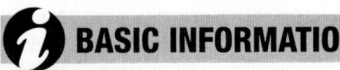

BASIC INFORMATION

DEFINITION

Brain metastases result from a spread of cancers originating in other organs to the brain and are devastating complications of cancer. Brain metastases are the most common intracranial tumors in adults and account for more than one half of brain tumors.

ICD-10CM CODES

C80.0	Disseminated malignant neoplasm, unspecified
C80.9	Malignant neoplasm, unspecified
C79.89	Secondary malignant neoplasm of other specified sites

EPIDEMIOLOGY & DEMOGRAPHICS

INCIDENCE:

- Accurate data on the incidence of metastatic brain disease are not available. Population studies based on review of epidemiological data show an overall incidence of 8.3 to 14.3 per 100,000 population per yr. However, these studies underestimate the true incidence of brain metastases because they rely on historical data from times when diagnostic imaging was poor. Autopsy-based studies are thought to show higher incidence of brain metastases because they identify asymptomatic brain metastases. However, autopsy-based data are now more than 20 yr old. Ultimately, the incidence of metastatic brain malignancy is rising, likely due to improved detection and better control of extracerebral disease.
- In the U.S., an estimated 98,000 to 170,000 new cases occur each yr, representing 24% to 45% of all cancer patients. The incidence is higher in autopsy series, where 20% of patients with systemic disease have brain metastases.

PREDOMINANT SEX AND AGE:

- In patients with systemic malignancies, brain metastases occur in 10% to 30% of adults and 6% to 10% of children. Of these, about 60% of patients are between the ages of 50 and 70 yr.
- There is no definite gender predilection. Some data indicate that metastatic brain malignancy has a higher incidence in men because men have a higher incidence of primary lung cancer.

RISK FACTORS

- In adults, the cumulative incidence (CI) of metastases to the brain depends on the type of primary cancer as follows: lung cancer (16%-20% CI), renal cell carcinoma (7%-10% CI), melanoma (7% CI), breast cancer (5% CI), and colorectal cancers (1%-2% CI). Lymphoma is also known to metastasize to the brain. These metastatic lesions may or may not be present at the patient's initial presentation. The majority of patients with metastases to the brain have greater than one metastasis. The cancers with the highest association of intracranial hemorrhage include renal cell carcinoma, melanoma, and the less common malignancies of thyroid carcinoma and choriocarcinoma.
- The most common primary pediatric solid tumors associated with metastatic spread include sarcomas, neuroblastoma, and germ cell tumors. Leukemias are well known to seed the CNS. Metastatic disease is usually never seen when a child first presents with malignancy, with the occasional exception of leukemia. For solid tumors, metastatic disease is seen at the time of disease recurrence. Neuroblastoma CNS lesions have a high propensity to hemorrhage.

PHYSICAL FINDINGS & CLINICAL PRESENTATION

- Clinical presentations vary depending on where the lesion is located. Brain metastases should be suspected in any cancer patient developing acute neurologic signs or symptoms. Neurologic symptoms, however, are common in patients with systemic cancer. In an analysis of more than 800 patients with neurologic symptoms, brain metastases were found in only 16%.
- Symptoms:
  1. Headache occurs in 40% to 50% of patients with brain metastases. Frequency is higher with metastases located in the posterior fossa, which may result in obstructive hydrocephalus. The headache can be accompanied by nausea, vomiting, focal neurologic signs, and postural variation.
  2. Focal neurologic signs/symptoms are the presenting symptom in 20% to 40% of patients. Hemiparesis is the most frequent complaint. However, the specific neurologic dysfunction depends on the location of the brain metastasis.
  3. Cognitive dysfunction, including memory problems or mood or personality changes, is the presenting problem in 30% to 45% of patients.
  4. Seizures are the presenting symptom for 10% to 20% of patients with metastatic brain tumors and indicate supratentorial metastases.
  5. Acute stroke secondary to hemorrhage into a metastasis, hypercoagulability, or local vascular invasion occurs in 5% to 10% of patients.

ETIOLOGY

The most common mechanism of metastasis to the brain is by hematogenous spread. The most common location is at the junction of the gray matter and white matter of the cerebral hemispheres (almost 80%). The blood vessels decrease in diameter in these regions, which is thought to act like a trap for clumps of tumor cells. Different tumor types have a tendency to metastasize to different regions of the brain. For example, metastases of small cell lung carcinoma are equally distributed in all regions, whereas pelvic (prostate and uterine) and gastrointestinal tumors more commonly metastasize to the posterior fossa.

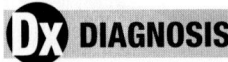

DIAGNOSIS

DIFFERENTIAL DIAGNOSIS

- Primary brain tumor
- Infection: Bacterial abscess or fungal disease
- Progressive multifocal leukoencephalopathy
- Demyelinating disease: Multiple sclerosis, post-infectious encephalomyelitis
- Cerebral infarction or bleeding
- Effects of treatment, such as radiation necrosis

LABORATORY TESTS

- Routine laboratory studies are not typically helpful.
- Lumbar puncture is generally contraindicated due to increased intracranial pressure and risk of herniation.
- Brain biopsy is necessary in some cases for a definitive diagnosis, particularly in the case of unknown primary tumor. Illustrating this situation is a study of cancer patients with solitary brain lesions that were presumed to be metastatic disease; in about 10% of study participants, the lesions were proved to be a different pathology.

IMAGING STUDIES

- MRI (Fig. 1) with and without contrast is the imaging study of choice. Important features on MRI suggesting brain metastases include: presence of multiple lesions, localization at the junction of the gray and white matter, circumscribed margins, or large amounts of vasogenic edema. CT of the head with contrast (Fig. 2) can be used when MRI is contraindicated.
- MR spectroscopy and PET are useful to differentiate tumor from either other space-occupying lesions or radiation necrosis.

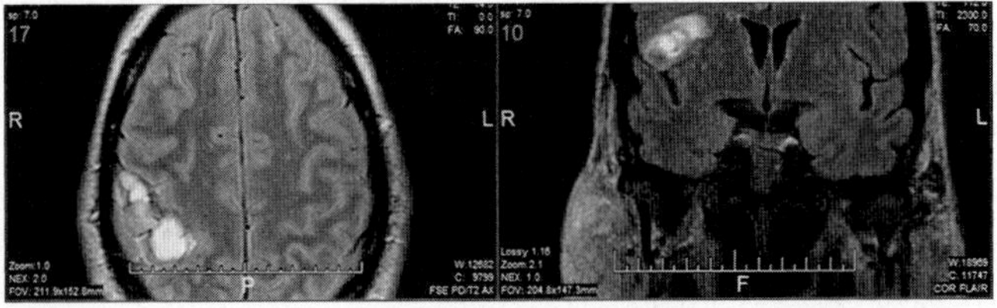

FIG. 1 Brain magnetic resonance imaging (axial and coronal fluid-attenuated inversion recovery sequences) showing hemorrhagic metastatic deposition in the inferior right frontoparietal lobe (lobulated high signal focus) in a 40-year-old woman with metastatic choriocarcinoma to the brain. (From Fielding JR, et al.: *Gynecologic imaging,* Philadelphia, 2011, Saunders.)

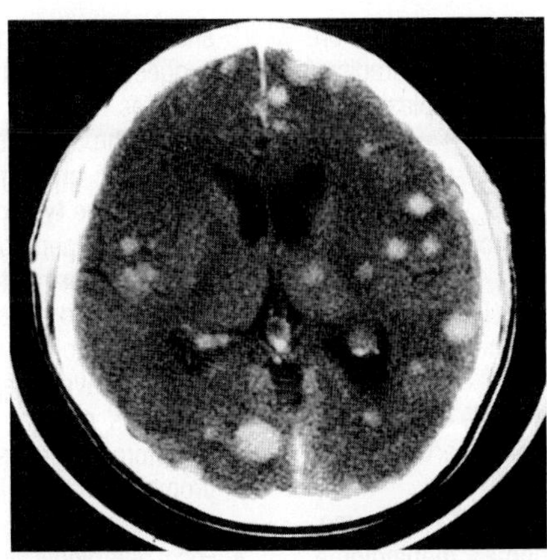

FIG. 2 Intracranial metastatic disease. Axial contrast-enhanced CT scan of head reveals multiple enhancing nodules throughout gray and white matter structures consistent with metastatic disease. (From Vincent JL, et al. [eds]: *Textbook of critical care*, ed 6, Philadelphia, 2011, Saunders.)

- Newer experimental imaging studies, such as receptor-targeted and ligand-based molecular imaging, are on the horizon.
- In about 80% of patients, brain metastases develop after the diagnosis of systemic cancer. In the remaining patients, brain metastases are diagnosed either simultaneously or before the primary tumor is found. In patients without a known primary tumor, the lung should be the primary focus of evaluation. Other frequent primary cancer types include melanoma, colon cancer, and breast cancer. PET scan may be useful in these patients to help identify either the primary tumor or other sites of metastatic disease, which may be more amenable to biopsy.

Rx TREATMENT

- Management of patients with brain metastases is influenced by the overall prognosis and may include treatments targeted at the metastases, management and prevention of complications (seizures, edema), and treatment of systemic malignancy.
- In patients considered to have a favorable prognosis (i.e., one to three metastases, good Karnofsky performance score, and controlled or absent systemic disease), treatment focuses on surgical resection and stereotactic radiation either to eradicate or control the brain metastases. Whole-brain radiation (WBRT) is widely used but has significant side effects. A study through the European Organisation for Research and Treatment of Cancer (EORTC), along with prior randomized studies, has shown the addition of WBRT did not improve overall survival but seemed to reduce the rates of disease relapse. A meta-analysis of five randomized controlled trials found that WBRT decreased the relative risk of intracranial disease progression at 1 yr by 53% but did not improve survival. Additionally, the individuals who did not receive WBRT after stereotactic radiosurgery or surgery had better quality-of-life scores. Unfortunately, few patients with metastatic disease are able to meet inclusion criteria for such studies.
- In patients with poor prognosis, treatment focuses on symptom control and WBRT.

ACUTE GENERAL Rx

- Steroids are used to reduce peritumoral edema and intracranial pressure.
- Antiepileptics are started for patients who present with seizures. Prophylactic treatment for seizures is not indicated in patients without a prior history of seizure.
- Anticoagulants are sometimes used to prevent venous thromboembolic disease but should be used with caution in patients with brain metastases that are at increased risk of hemorrhage.

CHRONIC Rx

- Radiation therapy has become the mainstay of treatment for brain metastases, including whole brain radiation therapy and stereotactic radiosurgery (SRS).
- For highly chemosensitive tumors, chemotherapy has been integrated into the primary management of patients with disseminated disease.
- For other tumors (e.g., small cell and non–small cell lung cancers, breast cancer, melanoma) systemic chemotherapy or molecularly targeted agents may be of palliative value when surgery, whole brain radiation therapy, and SRS have failed or are inappropriate. In most cases, two to three agents in combination are used in conjunction with whole brain radiation therapy. A phase II trial has shown combination treatment of lapatinib, an epidermal growth factor receptor inhibitor (EGFR-inhibitor), and capecitabine, an antimetabolite prodrug that is converted to 5-fluorouracil, as active for first-line treatment of *HER2*-positive breast brain metastases. Another phase II trial showed sagopilone (low-molecular-weight epothilone B analogue) as showing modest activity in patients with metastatic breast cancer. Additionally, dabrafenib, a tyrosine kinase inhibitor of BRAF, had some activity and an acceptable safety profile for metastatic melanoma with $BRAF^{V600E}$ mutations. Ipilimumab, a monoclonal antibody against cytotoxic T-lymphocyte antigen 4, was used for patients with metastatic melanoma and showed an improved median overall survival of 7 months in clinically asymptomatic lesions and 3.7 months in patients with neurologic symptoms. There are also other reports of its efficacy.

DISPOSITION

- The median survival of patients who receive supportive care and are treated with corticosteroids only is approximately 1 to 2 months.
- Key prognostic factors are performance status, extent of systemic disease, and age. Most favorable outcome is found in patients with Karnofsky performance score ≥70, age younger than 70 yr, no systemic disease or local control of primary tumor without extracranial metastases, and female gender. In this group, median survival is estimated at 7.1 months.

REFERRAL

Treatment involves a multispecialty team. Consultations from oncology, neurosurgery, neurology, radiation oncology, psychiatry, and physical therapy are all warranted.

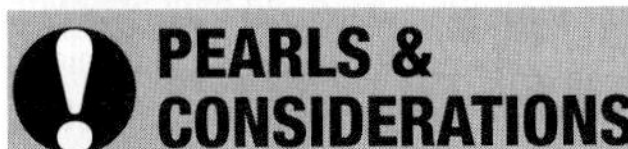

PEARLS & CONSIDERATIONS

COMMENTS

- Brain metastases are the most common intracranial tumors in adults, accounting for more than half of all brain tumors.
- Lung cancer, melanoma, renal cell carcinoma, and breast cancer are the most common primary tumors that metastasize to the brain.
- MRI of the brain with and without contrast is the most reliable imaging study.
- Treatment depends upon the patient's overall prognosis.

PATIENT/FAMILY EDUCATION

- American Brain Tumor Association (http://www.abta.org)
- National Brain Tumor Society (http://www.braintumor.org)

SUGGESTED READINGS

Available at ExpertConsult.com

RELATED CONTENT

Brain Cancer (Patient Information)

AUTHORS: **A. BASIT KHAN, B.A., JOSEPH S. KASS, M.D., J.D.,** and **NICOLE J. ULLRICH, M.D., PH.D.**

B

Diseases and Disorders

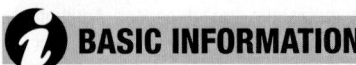

DEFINITION

Brain neoplasms are a diverse group of primary (nonmetastatic) tumors arising from one of many different cell types within the central nervous system (CNS). Specific tumor subtypes and prognosis depend on the tumor cell of origin and pattern of growth. The diffuse low-grade gliomas (LGGs) include World Health Organization Grade II astrocytomas, oligodendrogliomas, and oligoastrocytomas.

SYNONYMS

Low-grade glioma (LGG)
Glioneuronal tumor
Meningioma
Primary brain tumor

ICD-10CM CODE
D33.2 Benign neoplasm of brain, unspecified

EPIDEMIOLOGY & DEMOGRAPHICS

INCIDENCE: U.S. incidence rate of a new brain tumor is approximately 6.4/100,000 persons per yr for all primary brain tumors (Table 1). One third of these are considered malignant and the remainder benign or borderline malignant. The incidence rate in children aged 0 to 19 yr is lower (5.6 per 100,000 children). Primary brain neoplasms account for ~2% of all cancers, with a disproportionate share of cancer morbidity and mortality. It is the most common cause of cancer death in children up to 15 yr.

PEAK INCIDENCE: Depends on histology, though highest peak at ~age 50 yr.

PREDOMINANT SEX AND AGE: Slight male predominance of malignant brain tumors (8.0 vs. 5.5/100,000 person/yr). Men account for slightly less than half of cases of both benign and malignant brain tumors, as meningiomas have a higher incidence in women.

GENETICS: Most primary CNS neoplasms are sporadic; 5% are associated with hereditary syndromes that predispose to neoplasia. The most common of these include:

- Li-Fraumeni syndrome: *p53* mutation on chromosome 17q13, gliomas
- Von Hippel-Lindau: VHL, chromosome 3p25, hemangioblastoma
- Tuberous sclerosis: TSC1/TSC2 (chromosome 9q34/16p13), subependymal giant cell astrocytoma
- Neurofibromatosis type 1: NF1, chromosome 17q11, neurofibroma, optic nerve glioma, low-grade glioma
- Neurofibromatosis type 2: NF2, chromosome 22q12, schwannoma, meningioma, ependymoma
- Retinoblastoma: pRB, chromosome 13q, retinoblastoma
- Gorlin syndrome: PTCH, chromosome 9q31, desmoplastic medulloblastoma
- Hereditary nonpolyposis colorectal cancer (HNPCC): Mismatch repair deficiency, high-grade gliomas

RISK FACTORS: Exposure to ionizing radiation has been implicated in meningiomas, gliomas, and nerve sheath tumors. No convincing evidence has shown a link with trauma, occupation, cellular phone use, diet, or electromagnetic fields.

PHYSICAL FINDINGS & CLINICAL PRESENTATION

- In general, the location, size, and rate of growth will determine the symptoms and signs of a brain tumor.
- Headache is common and is the worst symptom in nearly half of all patients. The headaches are usually dull, constant pain that is often worse at night. Symptoms of increased intracranial pressure may also be present, including nausea and vomiting, and may worsen with changes in body position that increase thoracic pressure (coughing, sneezing, Valsalva maneuver). Papilledema is suggestive of obstructive hydrocephalus.
- Seizures occur in 33% of patients and are among the most common symptoms, particularly with brain metastases and low-grade gliomas. The type of seizure and clinical presentation depend on the location of the brain tumor. Tumor-related seizures are typically repetitive and have similar presentation patterns. It is thought that patients with seizures typically have smaller tumors at the time of diagnosis compared with those with other symptoms, because the onset of seizures prompts an imaging study, leading to an earlier diagnosis.
- Focal neurologic signs and symptoms, including muscle weakness, sensory changes, or visual disturbances are also quite frequent. In addition, cognitive dysfunction, accompanied by changes in memory or personality change, may be recounted, often in retrospect.

ETIOLOGY

Most cases are idiopathic, though specific chromosomal abnormalities have been implicated in some tumor types.

Dx DIAGNOSIS

- Diagnosis is typically based on clinical presentation and imaging characteristics. Specifically, neuroimaging is critical for preoperative planning and tumor etiology.
- Tumors are best seen on brain MRI with and without contrast; calcifications are sometimes present.
- Benign and low-grade tumors, typically in the glioma family, are heterogeneous and are generally seen as an infiltrating hemispheric lesion.

LABORATORY TESTS

- Ultimately, only histologic examination can provide the exact diagnosis. Additional features such as proliferative index, immunohistochemical stains, and electron microscopy can also be used to aid in diagnosis.
- The current classification schema for gliomas is based on pathologic and microscopic criteria. Tumor histology/histologic diagnosis (World Health Organization [WHO] grading system), includes number of mitoses, capillary endothelial proliferation, and necrosis. However, even tumors with benign histology can cause significant morbidity due to their location and effect on surrounding structures.
- Genetic analysis of tumors is rapidly becoming important for genetic classification, stratification of treatments, and predicting outcome. Different subtypes of gliomas have distinct gene-expression profiles, which can be distinguished from one another and from normal tissue; these differences typically involve pathways of cell proliferation, energy metabolism, and signal transduction. In adults, global expression profiling identified differences in 360 genes between low-grade and high-grade tumors.

TABLE 1 Frequency of Primary Central Nervous System Tumors

Children (0-14 Yr)		Adults (≥15 Yr)	
Type	**Percentage**	**Type**	**Percentage**
Glioblastoma	20	Glioblastoma	50
Astrocytoma	21	Astrocytoma	10
Ependymoma	7	Ependymoma	2
Oligodendroglioma	1	Oligodendroglioma	3
Medulloblastoma	24	Medulloblastoma	2
Neuroblastoma	3	Neurilemmoma	2
Neurilemmoma	1	Pituitary adenoma	4
Craniopharyngioma	5	Craniopharyngioma	1
Meningioma	5	Meningioma	17
Teratoma	2	Pinealoma	1
Pinealoma	2	Hemangioma	2
Hemangioma	3	Sarcoma	1
Sarcoma	1	Others	5
Others	5	Total	100
Total	100		

From Goetz CG, Pappert EJ: *Textbook of clinical neurology*, Philadelphia, 1999, Saunders.

DIFFERENTIAL DIAGNOSIS

- Stroke/cerebral hemorrhage
- Abscess/parasitic cyst
- Demyelinating disease: Multiple sclerosis, postinfectious encephalomyelitis
- Metastatic tumors
- Primary CNS lymphoma

WORKUP

Neuroimaging studies and pathologic sampling are the most important diagnostic modalities in evaluation of brain tumors and may be critical for preoperative planning.

IMAGING STUDIES

- MRI with gadolinium enhancement is highly sensitive and permits visualization of the tumor with relation to the surrounding tissue. Specifically, enhancing tumor can be distinguished from surrounding edema. Low-grade tumors often present as an infiltrating lesion without mass effect. MRI is superior to CT scanning for evaluating the meninges, subarachnoid space, and posterior fossa, and for defining relation to major intracranial vessels, although CT scanning is useful if calcification or hemorrhage is suspected (Fig. E1). Fig. E2 shows the appearance of astrocytoma in imaging studies.
- Magnetic resonance spectroscopy is increasingly being used as a diagnostic tool to help differentiate intracranial tumors from other intracranial processes using different chemical markers. For example, *N*-acetylaspartate is often decreased in brain tumors, whereas choline, a component of cell membranes, is often increased in brain tumors because of high cellular turnover.
- PET scan is helpful to distinguish neoplastic lesions (with high rate of metabolism) from other lesions such as demyelination or radiation necrosis (with a much lower metabolic rate). Such lesions take up greater amounts of glucose than surrounding tissues or tumors with slower metabolic rates. May be useful to help map functional areas of the brain before surgery or radiation.
- Functional MRI is now used as an adjunct in perioperative planning for patients whose lesion is in vital regions, such as those responsible for speech, language, and motor control.

Rx TREATMENT

NONPHARMACOLOGIC THERAPY

- Maximal surgical removal or debulking is the initial treatment of choice and provides tissue for diagnosis and molecular characterization. Maximal safe resection is often favored with a trend toward improved survival with this approach.
- Biopsy alone is performed if the tumor is located in eloquent regions of brain or is inaccessible; this is essential for histopathologic diagnosis. Biopsy can be performed under CT or MRI guidance using stereotactic localization.
- If the tumor is benign (e.g., meningioma, acoustic neuroma), often no further therapy is required.

ACUTE GENERAL Rx

Antiseizure medications have been used perioperatively and to control seizures resulting from focal lesions. Prophylactic use of anticonvulsants is not typically recommended without clear history of seizures.

CHRONIC Rx

- Chemotherapy (combination or single agent) may be used before, during, or after surgery and radiation therapy. In children, chemotherapy is often used to delay radiation therapy. A recent trial in patients with grade 2 glioma who were younger than 40 yr of age and had undergone subtotal tumor resection or who were 40 yr of age or older, progression-free survival and overall survival were longer among those who received combination chemotherapy in addition to radiation therapy than among those who received radiation therapy alone.[1]
- Radiation is useful for certain types of tumors and is often used if there is residual tumor after surgery; conventional radiation uses external beams over a period of weeks, whereas stereotactic radiosurgery delivers a single, high dose of radiation to a well-defined area (usually <1 cm). Long-term effects of radiation therapy include radiation necrosis (particularly of white matter), blood vessel hyalinization, and secondary tumors (usually meningiomas, sarcomas, and malignant astrocytomas). Radiosensitizers may help increase the therapeutic effect of radiation therapy.
- Experimental therapies are continually in development and target molecular characterization of tumors and small molecule blockers of signal transduction cascades involved in tumor growth. Some of these therapies involve antisense molecules, biologic agents, immunotherapies, or angiogenesis inhibitors. Intratumoral drug infusions and convection-enhanced delivery of novel agents are currently under study.

[1] Buckner JC et al: Radiation plus procarbazine, CCNU, and vincristine in low-grade glioma, *N Engl J Med* 374:1344–1355, 2016.

DISPOSITION

In general, younger age, high performance status, and lower pathologic grade have more favorable prognosis. For all histologic subtypes of brain tumors, pediatric and young adult patients have a better survival rate.

REFERRAL

- All cases warrant evaluation by an oncologist and neurosurgeon.
- Patients should be evaluated for physical and occupational therapy.
- Children should undergo neuropsychologic evaluations and screening for learning disabilities.

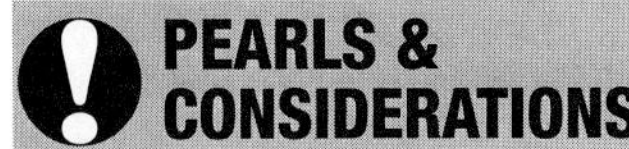

COMMENTS

In general, younger age, high performance status, and lower pathologic grade have more favorable prognosis. For all histologic subtypes of brain tumors, pediatric and young adult patients have a better survival.

PATIENT/FAMILY EDUCATION

American Brain Tumor Association (http://www.abta.org)
National Brain Tumor Society (http://www.braintumor.org)
Pediatric Low Grade Astrocytoma (PLGA) (http://fightplga.org)

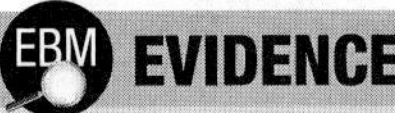

Available at ExpertConsult.com

SUGGESTED READINGS

Available at ExpertConsult.com

RELATED CONTENT

Brain Cancer (Patient Information)
Astrocytoma (Related Key Topic)
Meningioma (Related Key Topic)

AUTHORS: **EMMA H. WEISS, B.B.A., NICOLE J. ULLRICH, M.D., PH.D.,** and **JOSEPH S. KASS, M.D., J.D.**

DEFINITION

Glioblastoma (GBM) is the most aggressive diffuse glioma of astrocytic lineage and corresponds to grade IV in the World Health Organization's (WHO) classification system. GBM is the most common brain and central nervous system (CNS) malignancy, accounting for 45.2% of malignant primary brain and CNS tumors, 54% of all gliomas, and 16% of all primary brain and CNS tumors.

GBM represents a molecularly heterogeneous disease with numerous subclassifications. GBMs comprise primary and secondary subtypes that evolve through different genetic pathways, affect patients at different ages, and have differences in outcomes. Primary (*de novo*) GBMs account for 80% of GBMs and occur in older patients (mean age 62 yr). Secondary GBMs develop from lower-grade astrocytomas or oligodendrogliomas and occur in younger patients (mean age 45 yr).

ICD-10CM CODE

C71.9 Malignant neoplasm of brain, unspecified

EPIDEMIOLOGY & DEMOGRAPHICS

INCIDENCE: Based on the 2014 CBTRUS report, the average annual age-adjusted incidence rate (IR) of GBM is 3.19/100,000 population.

PREDOMINANT SEX AND AGE: GBM is primarily diagnosed at older ages, with the median age of diagnosis at 64 yr. It is uncommon in children, accounting for ~3% of all brain and CNS tumors reported among infants to 19-yr-olds. A higher incidence of GBM has been reported in men compared with women; the incidence rate is 1.6 times higher in males [3.97 versus 2.53]. Whites have the highest incidence rates for GBM compared with any other race in the U.S.

RISK FACTORS: Many genetic and environmental factors have been studied in GBM, but no risk factor that accounts for a large proportion of GBM has been identified. Like many cancers, the causes are sporadic. Factors associated with GBM risk are prior therapeutic radiation, decreased susceptibility to allergy, immune factors and immune genes, and some single nucleotide polymorphisms (SNPs) detected by genome-wide association studies (GWAS). There is no substantial evidence of GBM association with lifestyle characteristics such as cigarette smoking, alcohol consumption, drugs, or dietary exposure to N-nitroso compounds (cured or smoked meat or fish). Inconsistent and non-definitive results have been published regarding the risk of glioma with use of mobile phones.

PHYSICAL FINDINGS & CLINICAL PRESENTATION

Patients present with a variety of symptoms, including headache, seizures, symptoms of increased intracranial pressure, and cognitive disturbances.

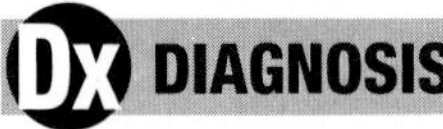

DIAGNOSIS

IMAGING STUDIES

Initial workup includes imaging studies. Brain MRI with and without contrast is the study of choice, and demonstrates a contrast-enhancing tumor. Functional MRI is now used as an adjunct modality in perioperative planning for patients whose lesion is in vital regions (eloquent regions), such as those responsible for speech, language, and motor control. Pathologically, GBM is a high-grade astrocytoma characterized by hypercellularity, mitotic activity, nuclear atypia, pseudopalisading necrosis, and microvascular proliferation. Various molecular markers have been identified distinguishing GBM from other lower grade astrocytomas, as well as differentiating primary and secondary subtypes of GBM.

Rx TREATMENT

- GBM is an aggressive neoplasm with a median survival of 3 months if untreated.
- Combined modality therapy with surgery, RT, and chemotherapy has significantly improved survival of GBM patients. Treatment is complex and initially consists of maximal-safe surgical resection followed by RT with concurrent temozolomide (TMZ) chemotherapy followed by six cycles of maintenance TMZ with tumor-treating fields.
- Surgical intervention has decompressive and cytoreductive effects, and there is increasing evidence of a significant survival advantage with complete resection.
- Various emerging treatment modalities under investigation seem promising, including immunotherapy. Regression of glioblastoma after chimeric antigen receptor T-cell therapy has been reported (see Brown CE et al, in Suggested Readings). Intratumoral infusion of recombinant nonpathogenic polio-rhinovirus chimera (PVSRIPO) has improved survival rate in advanced stage glioblastoma (see Desjardins et al in Suggested Readings).
- Symptomatic treatment includes corticosteroids to reduce cerebral edema, antiepileptic drugs for seizures, and painkillers for headache.

REFERRAL

Treatment involves a multidisciplinary team approach including oncology, neurosurgery, neurology, and radiation oncology.

PROGNOSIS

Survival: GBM has a poor prognosis with a low relative survival estimate; only a few patients reach long-term survival status of 2.5 yr, and less than 5% of patients survive 5 yr post-diagnosis. The relative survival for the first yr after diagnosis is 35%, falls in the second yr post-diagnosis to 13.7%, and continues to fall thereafter. Median survival of GBM post-diagnosis is 15 months following standard therapy. Several variables affect the prognosis of GBM patients, including age, preoperative performance status, tumor location, preoperative imaging characteristics of the tumor, and the extent of resection.

Prognostic molecular markers in GBM: All GBMs are WHO grade IV but exhibit significant genetic heterogeneity. Tumor subtypes, based on genetic alterations, exist within this larger homogeneous histologic category and carry prognostic significance. These markers include methylation status of the gene promoter for O^6-methylguanine-DNA methyltransferase (MGMT), isocitrate dehydrogenase enzyme 1/2 (IDH1/2) mutation, epidermal growth factor receptor (EGFR) overexpression and amplification, tumor protein (TP53) mutation, ATRX mutation and genetic losses of chromosomes.

- Primary GBMs show EGFR overexpression, phosphatase and tensin homolog gene (*PTEN*) mutations, and loss of heterozygosity (LOH) 10q, p16 deletions; less frequently shown are mouse double-minute 2 (MDM2) amplification, high frequency of telomerase reverse transcriptase (hTERT) promoter mutations, and absence of IDH1 mutation.
- The hallmark of secondary GBMs is TP53, alpha thalassemia/mental retardation syndrome X-linked (ATRX) and IDH1 mutations; additionally, they show LOH 10q.
- The MGMT promoter is methylated in approximately 50% of newly diagnosed GBMs. MGMT methylation is more common in secondary than primary GBM (75% versus 36%, respectively) and has prognostic and predictive significance of better overall survival in patients with GBM, irrespective of treatment choices.
- IDH1/2 mutations are far more common in grades II and III astrocytomas and oligodendrogliomas compared with GBMs, and more than 90% of the mutations involve IDH1. IDH1/2 mutations are a selective molecular marker of secondary GBMs, help distinguish them from primary GBMs, and are a marker of more favorable prognosis in high-grade gliomas.
- In GBMs, EGFR signaling promotes cell division, tumor invasiveness, and resistance to radiation therapy (RT) and chemotherapy. About 40% of all GBMs have EGFR amplification, and it is more common in primary as compared with secondary GBMs.
- Mutation of the *TP53* gene has been found in 60% to 70% of secondary GBMs and 25% to 30% of primary GBMs, and it occurs more frequently in younger patients. Studies of *TP53* mutations as a prognostic marker have not been definitive.
- *ATRX* is frequently mutated in grade II-III astrocytomas (71%), oligoastrocytomas (68%), and secondary GBMs (57%), but is infrequent in primary (4%) and pediatric GBMs (20%) as well as pure oligodendroglial tumors (14%). In a prospective cohort of patients with astrocytic tumors, those harboring *ATRX* loss had a significantly better prognosis than the ones that expressed *ATRX* and had IDH mutation.
- *TERT* mutation is one of the most frequent genetic alterations in primary adult GBMs and is significantly higher in these tumors as compared with secondary adult or any pediatric GBMs. GBMs with *TERT* mutation have a shorter survival than those without *TERT* mutations. However, when adjusted for GBM subtype (primary and secondary), they do not have a significant impact on survival.

SUGGESTED READINGS

Available at ExpertConsult.com

AUTHOR: **JIGISHA P. THAKKAR, M.D.**

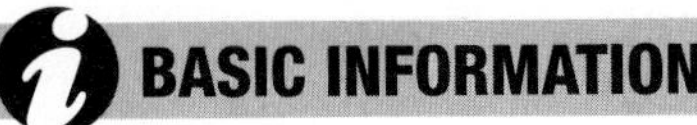

BASIC INFORMATION

DEFINITION

Breast abscess is an acute inflammatory process resulting in the formation of a collection of purulent material in breast tissue. Typically there is painful erythematous mass formation in the breast, occasionally draining through the overlying skin or nipple duct.

SYNONYMS

Subareolar abscess
Lactational or puerperal abscess

ICD-10CM CODES

091.111	Abscess of breast associated with pregnancy, first trimester
091.112	Abscess of breast associated with pregnancy, second trimester
091.113	Abscess of breast associated with pregnancy, third trimester
091.119	Abscess of breast associated with pregnancy, unspecified trimester
091.12	Abscess of breast associated with the puerperium
091.13	Abscess of breast associated with lactation

EPIDEMIOLOGY & DEMOGRAPHICS

INCIDENCE: 10% to 30% of all breast abscesses are lactational; acute mastitis occurs in 10% of nursing mothers, with one in 15 of these women developing abscess. A recent Cochrane review, however, found that as many as 30% of nursing mothers may have evidence of mastitis. Smoking and diabetes may be risk factors for nonpuerperal mastitis with abscess. More recently, nipple piercing may also be associated with infection.

PHYSICAL FINDINGS & CLINICAL PRESENTATION

Painful erythematous induration involving breast and leading to fluctuant abscess

ETIOLOGY

- Lactational abscess: Milk stasis and bacterial infection leading to mastitis and then abscess, with *Staphylococcus aureus* the most common causative agent
- Subareolar abscess:
  1. Central ducts involved, with obstructive nipple duct changes leading to bacterial infection
  2. Cultured organisms mixed, including anaerobes, staphylococci, streptococci, and others

DIAGNOSIS

DIFFERENTIAL DIAGNOSIS

- Inflammatory carcinoma
- Advanced carcinoma with erythema, edema, and/or ulceration
- Tuberculous abscess (rare in the United States)
- Hidradenitis of breast skin
- Sebaceous cyst with infection

WORKUP

- Clinical examination. Fig. 1 illustrates the various areas where breast abscesses can develop.
- If abscess suspected, referral to surgeon for incision, drainage, and biopsy.

LABORATORY TESTS

- Perform culture and sensitivity test of abscess contents.
- If mammogram or ultrasound is required but prevented by discomfort, perform after treatment and subsequent resolution of abscess.

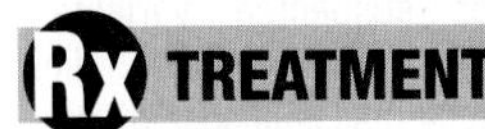

TREATMENT

NONPHARMACOLOGIC THERAPY

- Established abscess: Incision and drainage
- Biopsy of abscess cavity wall to exclude carcinoma

ACUTE GENERAL Rx

- Antibiotics: Generally staphylococci in lactational abscess. Recommended initial antibiotic therapy is nafcillin or oxacillin 2 g q4h IV or cefazolin 1 g q8h IV for 10 to 14 days. Alternative includes vancomycin 1 g IV q12h.
- If acute mastitis is identified and treated early without the development of an abscess, resolution without drainage is possible.
- Subareolar abscess: Broad-spectrum antibiotic treatment (e.g., cephalexin 500 mg PO qid or cefazolin 1 g q8h IV for 10 to 14 days for more severe infection) and drainage (Fig. 1) are needed to control acute phase. If abscess is odoriferous, consider anaerobes as most likely etiology and add metronidazole 500 mg PO/IV tid.

CHRONIC Rx

Further surgical treatment for recurrences or fistula

DISPOSITION

- Lactational abscess: Possible to continue breastfeeding without risk of infection to the infant
- Subareolar abscess:
  1. High risk for recurrence or complication of fistula formation
  2. Patient informed and referred to General Surgery for evaluation and treatment

REFERRAL

- If abscess drainage required.
- If subareolar abscess involved, refer to surgery.

SUGGESTED READING

Available at ExpertConsult.com

RELATED CONTENT

Breast Abscess (Patient Information)
Breast Cancer (Related Key Topic)
Mastodynia (Related Key Topic)

AUTHOR: **ANTHONY SCISCIONE, D.O.**

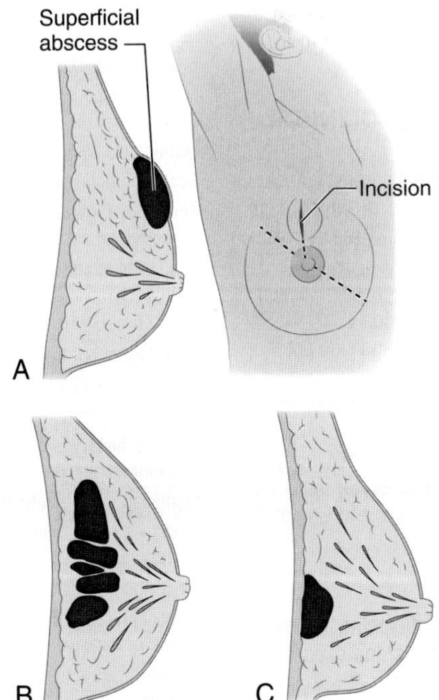

FIG. 1 A, A superficial breast abscess may be drained with a linear incision that radiates from the nipple. **B** and **C,** Diagrams of intramammary abscess **(B)** and retromammary abscess **(C)**. Both require drainage under general anesthesia. The abscess itself may not be fully appreciated if it is deep seated, and the mistaken diagnosis of cellulitis may be made. (Redrawn from Wolcott MW: *Ferguson's surgery of the ambulatory patient*, 5th ed. Philadelphia, JB Lippincott, 1974. Reprinted with permission.)

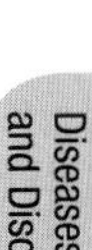

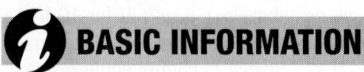

BASIC INFORMATION

DEFINITION

Breast cancer refers to both in situ and invasive carcinoma of the breast. Breast cancer can be of either ductal or lobular types.

SYNONYM

Carcinoma of the breast

ICD-10CM CODES

C50.911	Malignant neoplasm of unspecified site of right female breast
C50.912	Malignant neoplasm of unspecified site of left female breast
C50.919	Malignant neoplasm of unspecified site of unspecified female breast
C50.921	Malignant neoplasm of unspecified site of right male breast
C50.922	Malignant neoplasm of unspecified site of left male breast
C50.929	Malignant neoplasm of unspecified site of unspecified male breast

EPIDEMIOLOGY & DEMOGRAPHICS

- In the U.S., there will be an estimated 268,670 new patients and an estimated 41,400 deaths in 2018.
- The most common form of breast cancer is hormone-receptor positive; its incidence has increased particularly among young women. Breast cancer is nearly exclusively the disease of women, with only 1% of breast cancers occurring in males.
- Table 1 enumerates risk factors for breast cancer.
- Genetically defined group of women with *BRCA-1* or *BRCA-2* genes identified to carry lifetime risk as high as 85%.

PHYSICAL FINDINGS & CLINICAL PRESENTATION

- Increasing number of small breast cancers are found by mammograms in which case patients are usually completely free of symptoms or physical findings.
- Palpable lump or mass which can be self-detected or physician-detected.
- Skin and/or nipple retraction and skin edema, erythema, ulcer, satellite nodule.
- Nodal enlargement in axilla and supraclavicular areas.
- Nipple discharge may be serous or bloody.
- Generalized symptoms and signs, including fatigue, weight loss, jaundice, and anorexia, may be present in metastatic cases.

ETIOLOGY

- The precise mechanism of carcinogenesis is not understood. Endogenous and exogenous estrogen exposure is key to the development of receptor-positive breast cancer.
- Breast cancer is no longer perceived as a single disease. Molecular classification based on gene expression profiling has shown breast cancer to be of the following types:
  1. Luminal A type: Endocrine responsive with favorable prognosis.
  2. Luminal B type: Endocrine responsive with less favorable prognosis.
  3. Normal type: Resemble normal epithelium and prognosis similar to luminal B type.
  4. *HER-2* amplified type: *HER-2* gene amplification.
  5. Basal type: Hormone receptor and *HER-2* negative cancers with poor prognosis.
- Approximately 10% of all women with breast cancer have a germline mutation of *BRCA-1, BRCA-2, P53*, or other mutations.
- Possibly interaction of ovarian estrogen, nonovarian estrogen, estrogens of exogenous origin with breast tissue of varied carcinogenic susceptibility to develop cancer.
- Other known or suspected variables: Childbearing, breastfeeding practice, diet, physical activity, body mass, alcohol intake.

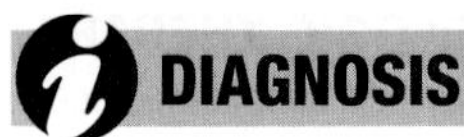

DIAGNOSIS

DIFFERENTIAL DIAGNOSIS

The following nonmalignant breast lesions can simulate breast cancer on both physical and mammogram examinations:

- Fibrocystic changes
- Fibroadenoma
- Hamartoma

TABLE 1 Risk Factors for Breast Cancer

Risk Factor	Relative Risk
Any benign breast disease	1.5
Postmenopausal hormone replacement	1.5
Menarche at <12 yr	1.1-1.9
Moderate alcohol intake (2-3 drinks/day)	1.1-1.9
Menopause at >55 yr	1.1-1.9
Increased bone density	1.1-1.9
Sedentary lifestyle and lack of exercise	1.1-1.9
Proliferative breast disease without atypia	2
Age at first birth >30 yr or nulliparous	2-4
First-degree relative with breast cancer	2-4
Postmenopausal obesity	2-4
Upper socioeconomic class	2-4
Personal history of endometrial or ovarian cancer	2-4
Significant radiation to chest	2-4
Increased breast density on mammogram	2-4
Older age	>4
Personal history of breast cancer (in situ or invasive)	>4
Proliferative breast disease with atypia	>4
Two first-degree relatives with breast cancer	5
Atypical hyperplasia and first-degree relative with breast cancer	10

From Goldman L, Schafer AI: *Goldman's Cecil medicine*, ed 24, Philadelphia, 2012, Saunders.

WORKUP

- Initial workup:
  1. Mass assessment by medical professional.
  2. Diagnostic mammogram followed by breast ultrasound for suspicious lesions.
  3. MRI (Fig. 1) may detect suspicious lesions better than mammography alone in women with dense breasts or inherited predisposition to breast cancer.
- Diagnosis:
  1. Positive aspiration cytology on a clinically and mammographically suspicious mass is highly accurate, but it requires open biopsy confirmation.
  2. Stereotactic, ultrasound-guided core-needle biopsy procedures are accurate and have low complication rates. Indications for stereotactic core biopsy are summarized in Box 1. Box 2 describes contraindications to stereotactic core biopsy.
  3. Excisional surgical biopsy establishes diagnosis.
- Breast radiologic evaluation and an algorithm for breast cancer screening and evaluation are described in Section III. The differential diagnosis of breast lumps is described in Section II.

STAGING

Table 2 describes the pathologic staging of breast cancer.

IMAGING STUDIES

Mammograms (Figs. E2 and E3): 30% to 50% of breast cancers are detected by screening mammograms as a spiculated mass, a mass with or without microcalcifications, or a cluster of microcalcifications. MRI is a modality that is particularly useful in patients with breast implants and when there is a strong family history of breast cancer. MRI is also better for assessing the response to neoadjuvant chemotherapy and is useful in identifying the primary tumor in patients who present with axillary adenopathy.

Rx TREATMENT

NONPHARMACOLOGIC THERAPY

- These approaches include various types of surgical resection and reconstruction as well as adjuvant radiotherapy.
- For early breast cancer, the primary therapy is typically surgical. The choice is between modified radical mastectomy and breast-conserving treatment, which consists of lumpectomy, axillary staging with sentinel node biopsy, or axillary dissection.
- Table 3 compares ductal versus lobular carcinoma in situ. Adjuvant treatment guidelines for patients with early-stage invasive breast cancer are described in Table 4.
- Among patients with limited sentinel lymph nodes (SLN) who are treated with breast conservation and systemic therapy, sentinel lymph node dissection (SLND) alone compared with axillary lymph node dissection (ALND) did not result in inferior survival.

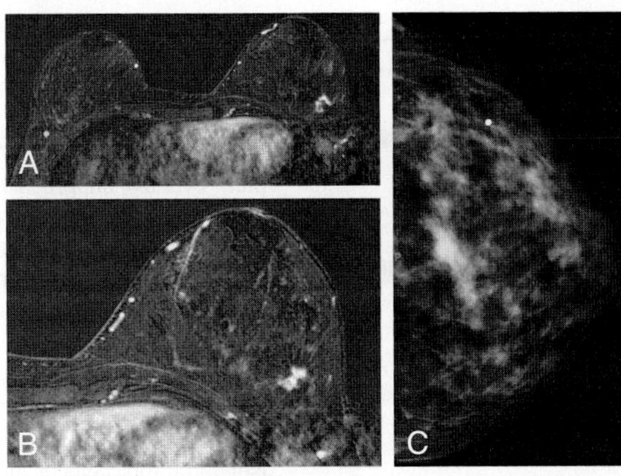

FIG. 1 A 42-year-old woman with *BRCA2* mutation. Magnetic resonance imaging (MRI) screening showed a 1.2-cm invasive ductal cancer in the lower outer left breast seen only on MRI (**A** and **B**) and subsequently on second-look ultrasound. **C,** The mammogram showed only dense breast tissue. (From Cameron JL, Cameron AM: *Current surgical therapy*, ed 12, Philadelphia, 2017, Elsevier.)

BOX 1 Indications for Stereotactic Core Biopsy

- Certain probably benign lesions, BI-RADS 3, depending on clinical suspicion, patient or physician preference, or when short-term follow-up is not practical
- Lesions suspicious, BI-RADS 4
- Lesions highly suspicious, BI-RADS 5
- New suspicious microcalcifications, developing asymmetries, or architectural distortions
- Nonpalpable asymmetry, focal asymmetry, or solid mass on mammogram not seen on ultrasound
- Mammographic lesions corresponding to suspicious areas of enhancement on MRI

BI-RADS, Breast Imaging-Reporting and Data System; *MRI,* magnetic resonance imaging.
From Cameron JL, Cameron AM: *Current surgical therapy*, ed 12, Philadelphia, 2017, Elsevier.

BOX 2 Contraindications to Stereotactic Core Biopsy

- Patient unable to lie prone or cooperate
- Patient's weight
- Lesion location near nipple, too superficial to skin, or too posterior to chest wall
- Lesion mammographically occult
- Patient has severe kyphosis or movement disorders
- Lack of breast tissue thickness for adequate compression

From Cameron JL, Cameron AM: *Current surgical therapy*, ed 12, Philadelphia, 2017, Elsevier.

- DCIS: Local breast-conserving therapy (lumpectomy plus radiation therapy) or mastectomy followed by endocrine therapy in estrogen receptor-positive cases.
- Invasive breast cancer: Mastectomy or lumpectomy, along with sentinel lymph node evaluation followed by radiation therapy for large tumors.
- Invasive breast cancer may require adjuvant endocrine therapy and chemotherapy. Endocrine therapy is recommended alone or after chemotherapy in patients with hormone-receptor positive tumors. Breast cancer intrinsic subtypes are summarized in Table 5. Treatment according to breast cancer subtypes is described in Table 6. Adjuvant hormone therapy with anti-estrogen drugs reduces disease recurrence and mortality in women with breast cancer. Aromatase inhibitors (anastrozole, letrozole, fulvestrant) decrease the agonist effect of estrogen by inhibiting estrogen synthesis and have become preferred first-line hormonal treatment agents over the selective estrogen receptor modulator tamoxifen.
- Standard *adjuvant chemotherapy* regimens in current use in the U.S. include second-generation regimens such as AC (cyclophosphamide plus doxorubicin) and FEC (5-fluorouracil, epirubicin, cyclophosphamide). Third-generation regimens such as AC-T (doxorubicin and cyclophosphamide followed by a taxane) and TC (docetaxel and cyclophosphamide) are also in routine use. A recent meta-analysis has demonstrated equivalence of anthracycline and platinum-containing regimens, with the sequential AC-T regimen likely to be the most effective regimen regardless of hormone receptor status. Fig. E4 illustrates considerations for adjuvant chemotherapy in breast cancer.
- *Neoadjuvant chemotherapy* (same regimens as used in the adjuvant setting) results in pathologic complete responses in significant number of cases, causes downstaging, provides an assessment of chemosensitivity, and provides no deleterious effect on survival.
- The benefit of adjuvant chemotherapy or hormone therapy can be assessed by commercially available *multigene assays* (OncotypeDx, Mammaprint) that have demonstrated utility in determining prognostic and predictive benefit with both hormonal therapy and chemotherapy in breast cancer. Recently published results from the prospective TAILORx trial support the routine use of multigene assays so as to identify intermediate-risk score patients in which chemotherapy can be safely omitted.
- *Metastatic breast cancer* is approached based on the extent of bone-only or visceral disease sites as well as the rate of symptomatic progression. Typically, bone-only metastatic disease is approached with upfront, sequential hormonal therapy. The combination of mTOR inhibitors (everolimus) or CDK4/CDK6 inhibitors (palbociclib, ribociclib) with aromatase inhibitors has been associated with improved overall survival. Patients with progressive bone disease or those with visceral disease are treated with typically single-agent chemotherapy and occasionally with combination chemotherapy regimens. The chemotherapy agents are the same as those used in early stages of disease. Sequential chemotherapy with different classes of chemotherapy agents are usually used to provide palliation with improvement in survival and symptoms.
- In patients with metastatic *HER2/neu-positive* breast cancer, the addition of the monoclonal antibody pertuzumab to the standard regimen of trastuzumab and docetaxel significantly improves the median overall survival by 16 months without increasing cardiac toxicity.

CHRONIC Rx

Follow-up after treatment of early breast cancer stages includes:

- Regular clinical evaluations as delineated by medical oncologist or surgeon.
- Annual mammograms and breast MRI as indicated.
- Laboratory tests as indicated.
- Tumor markers and CT scans for surveillance are not recommended.
- Patient instruction in monthly breast self-examination.
- Prognosis after curative therapy: Depends on size of tumor, extent of nodal metastasis, and pathologic grade of tumor.
- Systemic adjuvant therapy: Improves prognosis significantly. Women who take tamoxifen for 10 yr lower their recurrence risk by 25% and their dying of breast cancer risk by 27% compared with those who took it for just 5 yr. Adjuvant therapy with an aromatase inhibitor improves survival outcomes, compared with tamoxifen, in postmenopausal women with

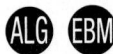

TABLE 2 Pathological Staging of Breast Cancer

T_X	Primary tumor cannot be assessed
T_0	No evidence of primary tumor
T_{is}	Carcinoma in situ
T_{is} (DCIS)	Ductal carcinoma in situ
T_{is} (LCIS)	Lobular carcinoma in situ
T_{is} (Paget)	Paget disease of the nipple NOT associated with invasive carcinoma and/or carcinoma in situ (DCIS and/or LCIS) in the underlying breast parenchyma. Carcinomas in the breast parenchyma associated with Paget disease are categorized based on the size and characteristics of the parenchymal disease, although the presence of Paget disease should still be noted
T_1	Tumor ≤ 20 mm in greatest dimension
T_{1mi}	Tumor ≤ 1 mm in greatest dimension
T_{1a}	Tumor >1 mm but ≤ 5 mm in greatest dimension
T_{1b}	Tumor >5 mm but ≤ 10 mm in greatest dimension
T_{1c}	Tumor >10 mm but ≤ 20 mm in greatest dimension
T_2	Tumor >20 mm but ≤ 50 mm in greatest dimension
T_3	Tumor >50 mm in greatest dimension
T_4	Tumor of any size with direct extension to the chest wall and/or to the skin (ulceration or skin nodules)
T_{4a}	Extension to chest wall, not including only pectoralis muscle adherence/invasion
T_{4b}	Ulceration and/or ipsilateral satellite nodules and/or edema (including peau d'orange) of the skin, which do not meet the criteria for inflammatory carcinoma
T_{4c}	Both T4a and T4b
T_{4d}	Inflammatory carcinoma
N_X	Regional lymph nodes cannot be assessed (e.g., previously removed)
N_0	No regional lymph node metastasis
N_1	Metastasis to movable ipsilateral level I, II axillary lymph node(s)
N_2	Metastases in ipsilateral level I, II axillary lymph nodes that are clinically fixed or matted or in clinically detected* ipsilateral internal mammary nodes in the *absence* of clinically evident axillary lymph node metastasis
N_{2a}	Metastases in ipsilateral level I, II axillary lymph nodes fixed to one another (matted) or to other structures
N_{2b}	Metastases only in clinically detected* ipsilateral internal mammary nodes and in the *absence* of clinically evident level I, II axillary lymph node metastases
N_3	Metastases in ipsilateral infraclavicular (level III axillary) lymph node(s), with or without level I, II axillary node involvement, or in clinically detected* ipsilateral internal mammary lymph node(s) and in the *presence* of clinically evident level I, II axillary lymph node metastasis; or metastasis in ipsilateral supraclavicular lymph node(s), with or without axillary or internal mammary lymph node involvement
N_{3a}	Metastasis in ipsilateral infraclavicular lymph node(s)
N_{3b}	Metastasis in ipsilateral internal mammary lymph node(s) and axillary lymph node(s)
N_{3c}	Metastasis in ipsilateral supraclavicular lymph node(s
M_0	No clinical or radiographic evidence of distant metastasis
$cM_{0(i+)}$	No clinical or radiographic evidence of distant metastases, but deposits of molecularly or microscopically detected tumor cells in circulating blood, bone marrow, or other nonregional nodal tissue that are no larger than 0.2 mm in a patient without symptoms or signs of metastases
M_1	Distant detectable metastases as determined by classic clinical and radiographic means and/or histologically proven >0.2 mm
G_X	Grade cannot be assessed
G_1	Low combined histologic grade (favorable)
G_2	Intermediate combined histologic grade (moderately favorable)
G_3	High combined histologic grade (unfavorable)

Stage Groupings in Breast Cancer

Stage	T	N	M
0	T_{is}	N_0	M_0
I_A	T_1	N_0	M_0
I_B	T_0-T_1	N_{1mi}	M_0
II_A	T_0-T_1	N_1	M_0
	T_2	N_0	M_0
II_B	T_2	N_1	M_0
	T_3	N_0	M_0
III_A	T_0-T_2	N_2	M_0
	T_3	N_1-N_2	M_0
III_B	T_4	N_0-N_2	M_0
III_C	Any T	N_3	M_0
IV	Any T	Any N	M_1

From Goldman L, Schafer AI: Goldman's Cecil medicine, ed 24, Philadelphia, 2012, Saunders. (AJCC 8th ed., 2018)

hormone receptor–positive breast cancer. Recent trials have shown that in premenopausal women with hormone receptor–positive early breast cancer, adjuvant treatment with the aromatase inhibitor exemestane plus ovarian suppression, compared with tamoxifen plus ovarian suppression, significantly reduced recurrence.

- Isolated tumor cells or micrometastases in regional lymph nodes are associated with a reduced 5-yr rate of disease-free survival among women with favorable early-stage breast cancer who do not receive adjuvant therapy. Survival is improved in patients with isolated tumor cells or micrometastases who received adjuvant therapy.
- Retrospective analyses suggest that occult lymph-node metastases are an important prognostic factor for disease recurrence or survival among patients with breast cancer; however, recent trials indicate that the magnitude of the difference in outcome at 5 yr is small (1.2 percentage points). These data do not favor a clinical benefit of additional evaluation (including immunohistochemical analysis) of initially negative sentinel nodes in patients with breast cancer.
- The addition of zoledronic acid to adjuvant endocrine therapy improves disease-free survival in premenopausal patients with estrogen-responsive early breast cancer.

REFERRAL

Referral to a multidisciplinary team consisting of a breast surgeon, reconstructive surgeon, medical oncologist, and radiation oncologist is necessary as soon as breast cancer is suspected.

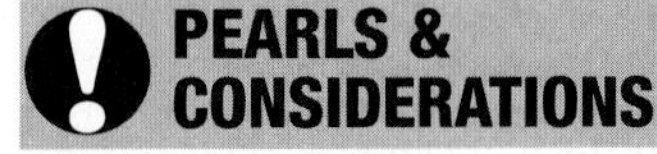

PEARLS & CONSIDERATIONS

BREAST CANCER IN PREGNANCY AND LACTATION

- Frequency in women 40 yr or younger reported to be 15%
- May carry worse prognosis because disease discovery delayed by engorged and nodular breast changes and/or because disease progression more rapid in pregnancy
- Survival rates similar to those for nonpregnant early-stage patients in same age group
- Expedient workup recommended, including mammography and sonography
- Choice of mastectomy or lumpectomy with axillary dissection for treatment
- Adjuvant chemotherapy delayed until third trimester or after delivery
- Irradiation to breast after lumpectomy delayed until after delivery

DUCTAL CARCINOMA IN SITU (DCIS, INTRADUCTAL CARCINOMA) (SEE TABLE 3)

- Discovered by mammogram as cluster of microcalcifications and/or density
- Presents less often as a palpable mass or nipple discharge

TABLE 3 Carcinoma In Situ: Lobular Versus Ductal

Feature	Lobular Carcinoma In Situ	Ductal Carcinoma In Situ
Age	Younger	Older
Palpable mass	No	Uncommon
Mammographic appearance	Not detected on mammography	Microcalcifications, mass
Immunophenotype	E-cadherin negative	E-cadherin positive
Usual manifestation	Incidental finding on breast biopsy	Microcalcifications on mammography or breast mass
Bilateral involvement	Common	Uncertain
Risk and site of subsequent breast cancer	25% risk for invasive breast cancer in either breast over remaining lifespan	At site of initial lesion; 0.5% risk/yr of invasive breast cancer in opposite breast
Prevention	Consider tamoxifen or raloxifene	Consider tamoxifen or raloxifene if estrogen-receptor positive
Treatment	Yearly mammography and breast examination	Lumpectomy ± radiation; mastectomy for large or multifocal lesions

From Goldman L, Schafer AI: *Goldman's Cecil medicine*, ed 24, Philadelphia, 2012, Saunders.

TABLE 4 Adjuvant Treatment Guidelines for Patients with Early-Stage Invasive Breast Cancer

Patient Group	Treatment
Hormone Receptor-Positive and HER-2 Positive Breast Cancer	
<0.5 cm	Consider adjuvant endocrine therapy
0.6-1 cm	Adjuvant endocrine therapy Consider adjuvant chemotherapy and trastuzumab
>1 cm	Adjuvant endocrine therapy Adjuvant chemotherapy and trastuzumab
Node positive	Adjuvant endocrine therapy Adjuvant chemotherapy with pertuzumab and trastuzumab
Hormone Receptor-Positive and HER-2 Negative Breast Cancer	
<0.5 cm	No adjuvant therapy
>0.5 cm	Adjuvant hormonal therapy Consider adjuvant chemotherapy based on 21-gene recurrence score
Node-positive	Adjuvant hormonal therapy + adjuvant chemotherapy
Hormone Receptor-Negative and HER-2 Positive Breast Cancer	
<0.5 cm	Consider adjuvant chemotherapy and trastuzumab
0.6-1 cm	Consider adjuvant chemotherapy and trastuzumab
>1 cm	Adjuvant chemotherapy and trastuzumab
Node positive	Adjuvant endocrine therapy Adjuvant chemotherapy with pertuzumab and trastuzumab
Hormone Receptor-Negative and HER-2 Negative Breast Cancer	
≤0.5 cm	No adjuvant therapy
0.6-1.0 cm	Consider adjuvant chemotherapy
>1 cm or node positive	Adjuvant chemotherapy

HER2, human epidermal growth factor receptor 2.
Modified from National Comprehensive Cancer Network Guidelines. Available at www.nccn.org.

- Before mammogram screening, DCIS accounted for 1% of all breast cancers
- Now 15% to 20% or even higher proportion have DCIS
- Treated with lumpectomy with cure rates 98% to 99%
- Higher-risk cases require breast radiation and adjuvant hormone therapy
- Mastectomy possibly required with multifocal and/or high-grade DCIS

INFLAMMATORY CARCINOMA

- Rare, rapidly progressive and often lethal form of breast cancer
- Presents as erythematous and edematous breast resembling mastitis
- Biopsy required, including that of the skin
- Treatment with upfront combination chemotherapy followed by surgery and radiotherapy
- Prognosis once dismal; now 5-yr disease-free survival approaches 50% (Fig. E5)

COMMENTS

- The U.S. Preventive Services Task Force (USPSTF) now recommends against automatic "routine" screening of younger women (age range 40 to 49). The task force recommends biennial screening mammography for all middle-aged women (age range 50 to 74). It also states that current evidence is insufficient to assess the benefits and harms of screening mammography in older women (aged 75 and older). The task force also discourages women from performing breast self-examination. Several other U.S. organizations, such as the American Congress of Obstetricians and Gynecologists, however, still recommend annual screening beginning at age 40 yr.
- The American Cancer Society guidelines for breast cancer screening are summarized in the following:
  1. Women with an *average risk* of breast cancer should undergo regular screening mammography as below:
     a. Women should have the opportunity to begin annual screening between the ages of 40 and 44 yr. (Qualified recommendation)
     b. Women aged 45 to 54 yr should be screened annually. (Qualified recommendation)
     c. Women 55 yr and older should transition to biennial screening or have the opportunity to continue screening annually. (Qualified recommendation)
  2. Women should continue screening mammography as long as their overall health is good and they have a life expectancy of 10 yr or longer. (Qualified recommendation)
  3. Women who are at *high risk* for breast cancer based on certain factors should get an MRI and a mammogram every yr, typically starting at age 30 yr. This includes women who:
     a. Have a lifetime risk of breast cancer of about 20% to 25% or greater, according to risk assessment tools that are based mainly on family history.
     b. Have a known *BRCA1* or *BRCA2* gene mutation (based on genetic testing).
     c. Have a first-degree relative (parent, brother, sister, or child) with a *BRCA1* or *BRCA2* gene mutation and have not had genetic testing themselves.
     d. Had radiation therapy to the chest between the ages of 10 and 30 yr.
     e. Have Li-Fraumeni syndrome, Cowden syndrome, or Bannayan-Riley-Ruvalcaba syndrome, or have first-degree relatives with one of these syndromes.
- Physicians should be familiar with the risks and benefits of various competing recommendations in order to better counsel patients.
- Breast radiologic evaluation, evaluation of nipple discharge, and evaluation of palpable mass are described in Section III.

TABLE 5 Breast Cancer Intrinsic Subtypes

Subtype	Characteristics	Markers
Luminal A	Low grade High ER ~40% of all breast cancer Good prognosis	ER+, PR+, HER2– Low Ki-67 (<14%)
Luminal B	Higher grade Lower ER ~20% of all breast cancer Poorer prognosis than luminal A	ER+, PR+/–, HER2+/– High Ki-67 (>14%)
HER2-enriched	High grade Often node positive *P53* mutations ~10%-15% of all breast cancer	ER–, PR–, HER2+
Basal-like	High proliferation *BRCA* dysfunction ~15%-20% of all breast cancer Poor prognosis	ER–, PR–, HER2– CK5/6 Or EGFR+

CK, Cytokeratin; *EGFR*, epidermal growth factor receptor; *ER*, estrogen receptor; *HER2*, human epidermal growth factor receptor 2; *PR*, progesterone receptor.
From Cameron JL, Cameron AM: *Current surgical therapy*, ed 12, Philadelphia, 2017, Elsevier.

TABLE 6 Treatment According to Breast Cancer Subtype

Subtype	Treatment Response and Prognosis
Luminal A	Respond to endocrine therapy • Premenopausal: SERMs (tamoxifen) • Postmenopausal: AIs (exemestane, anastrozole, letrozole)
Luminal B	Response to endocrine therapy lower Response to chemotherapy greater than luminal A
HER2-enriched	Respond to anti-HER2 agents (trastuzumab, pertuzumab, lapatinib)
Basal-like	No response to endocrine therapy or anti-HER2 agents Chemotherapy only treatment outside of a clinical trial

AIs, Aromatase inhibitors; *HER2*, human epidermal growth factor receptor 2; *SERMs*, selective estrogen receptor modulators.
From Cameron JL, Cameron AM: *Current surgical therapy*, ed 12, Philadelphia, 2017, Elsevier.

BOX 3 Counseling Points for Women with Average Risk Interested in Contralateral Prophylactic Mastectomy (CPM)

- There is a low annual contralateral breast cancer risk in women with average risk factors.
- Risk of contralateral breast cancer is decreasing with use of adjuvant therapy.
- Removing the contralateral breast does not decrease the risk for developing distant metastases.
- Breast cancer does not commonly metastasize from one breast to the other.
- CPM does not improve breast cancer–specific survival.
- CPM does not decrease local recurrence.
- Contralateral breast cancers tend to be at a lower stage than the initial primary cancer.
- CPM increases the surgical complication risk.
- Choice of CPM may influence reconstruction options.
- There are alternatives to CPM, including chemoprevention and surveillance.

From Cameron JL, Cameron AM: *Current surgical therapy*, ed 12, Philadelphia, 2017, Elsevier.

- Exposure of the heart to ionizing radiation during breast cancer radiotherapy increases risk of ischemic heart disease. The increased rate of ischemic heart disease begins within a few yrs of exposure and continues for at least 20 yr. The increase is proportional to the mean radiation dose to the heart.

RISK REDUCTION STRATEGIES

- Prophylactic bilateral mastectomy reduces the risk for invasive breast cancer by >90%.
- Counseling points for women with average risk interested in contralateral prophylactic mastectomy (CPM) are summarized in Box 3.
- Selective estrogen receptor modulators (SERM) reduce the incidence of hormone receptor-positive invasive breast cancer by 50%.
- Ovarian failure is a common toxic effect of chemotherapy. Administration of the gonadotropin-releasing hormone (GnRH) agonist Goserelin appears to protect against ovarian failure, reducing the risk of early menopause and improving prospects for fertility.

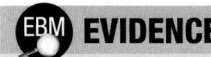

EVIDENCE

Available at ExpertConsult.com

SUGGESTED READINGS

Available at ExpertConsult.com

RELATED CONTENT

Breast Cancer (Patient Information)
Breast Cancer: For Men (Patient Information)
Breast Abscess (Related Key Topic)
Fibrocystic Breast Disease (Related Key Topic)

AUTHOR: **BHARTI RATHORE, M.D.**

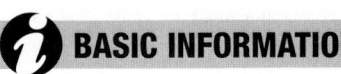

BASIC INFORMATION

DEFINITION

Bronchiectasis is an irreversible pathologic dilatation of the bronchi or bronchioles resulting from a variety of causes through an interplay of host factors (either anatomic or immune defense abnormality), respiratory pathogens, and environmental factors. Radiographically, it is often divided into cylindrical, varicose, and cystic varieties, although these variants have no significant etiologic or prognostic relevance.

ICD-10CM CODES

J47.0 Bronchiectasis with acute lower respiratory infection
J47.1 Bronchiectasis with (acute) exacerbation
J47.9 Bronchiectasis, uncomplicated
Q33.4 Congenital bronchiectasis

EPIDEMIOLOGY & DEMOGRAPHICS

- The exact prevalence of bronchiectasis is unknown.
- Cystic fibrosis is responsible for nearly 50% of all cases of bronchiectasis.
- Acquired primary bronchiectasis is uncommon because of rapid diagnosis of pulmonary infections and frequent use of antibiotics.
- Effective childhood immunizations have led to a significant decrease in the incidence of bronchiectasis resulting from pertussis.
- Declining incidence of pulmonary tuberculosis has also resulted in a decline in bronchiectasis without apparent causes.
- In developed countries, an increasing proportion of patients with an identifiable cause of bronchiectasis is being seen.
- Data on morbidity and mortality from bronchiectasis are limited because patients with the highest morbidity typically are not adequately represented in randomized controlled studies.

PHYSICAL FINDINGS & CLINICAL PRESENTATION

- Moist crackles at lung bases
- Chronic cough, typically with expectoration of large amount of purulent sputum
- Fever, night sweats, generalized malaise, weight loss
- Hemoptysis
- Halitosis, skin pallor
- Clubbing (infrequent)

ETIOLOGY

- Cystic fibrosis
- Lung infections (pneumonia, lung abscess, TB, nontubercular mycobacterial infections, fungal infections, viral infections)
- Impaired host defense (panhypogammaglobulinemia, primary ciliary dyskinesia/Kartagener's syndrome, AIDS, chemotherapy)
- Localized airway obstruction (congenital structural defects, foreign bodies, neoplasms)
- Inflammation (inflammatory pneumonitis, granulomatous lung disease, allergic aspergillosis)
- Rheumatoid arthritis, ulcerative colitis, and so on
- Congenital disorders such as tracheobronchomegaly (Mounier Kuhn syndrome), cartilage deficiency (Williams-Campbell syndrome)

Dx DIAGNOSIS

DIFFERENTIAL DIAGNOSIS

- TB
- Asthma
- Chronic bronchitis or chronic rhinosinusitis
- Interstitial fibrosis
- Chronic lung abscess
- Foreign body aspiration
- Cystic fibrosis
- Lung carcinoma
- GERD

LABORATORY TESTS

- Sputum for Gram stain, culture and sensitivity, and acid-fast bacteria
- Complete blood count with differential (leukocytosis with left shift, anemia)
- Serum protein electrophoresis to evaluate for hypogammaglobulinemia
- Antibody test for aspergillosis
- Testing for allergic bronchopulmonary aspergillosis
- Serum immunoglobulins (total IgG, IgA, IgM)
- Sweat test in patients with suspected cystic fibrosis
- Pulmonary function tests: Mild to moderate airflow obstruction
- Serum anti-Pseudomonas aeruginosa (PA) IgG antibody testing is highly accurate to detect chronic PA colonization in bronchiectasis patients

IMAGING STUDIES

- Chest radiograph: Hyperinflation, crowded lung markings, small cystic spaces at the base of the lungs.
- High-resolution CT scan of the chest (Fig. E1) has become the best tool to detect cystic lesions and exclude underlying obstruction from neoplasm with a sensitivity and specificity exceeding 90%. The CT study should be a noncontrast study with the use of 1- to 1.5-mm window every 1 cm with acquisition time of 1 sec. Typical findings on CT include enlarged internal bronchial diameter, bronchi appearing larger than accompanying artery, lack of tapering of an airway toward periphery, ballooned cysts at the end of bronchus, and varicose constrictions along airways.
- Bronchoscopy may be helpful to evaluate hemoptysis, rule out obstructive lesions, remove mucus plugs, and also obtain microbiologic data on respiratory pathogens.
- Table 1 summarizes diagnostic studies for the classification and management of patients with bronchiectasis.

Rx TREATMENT

NONPHARMACOLOGIC THERAPY

- Postural drainage (reclining prone on a bed with the head down on the side) and chest percussion with use of inflatable vests/high-frequency chest wall oscillation or mechanical vibrators applied to the chest may enhance removal of respiratory secretions.
- Adequate hydration.
- Supplemental oxygen for hypoxemia.
- Inhaled hypertonic saline in conjunction with chest physiotherapy improves airway clearance.

ACUTE GENERAL Rx

- Antibiotic therapy is based on the results of sputum, Gram stain, and culture and sensitivity; in patients with inadequate or inconclusive results, empiric therapy with amoxicillin/clavulanate 500 to 875 mg q12h, TMP-SMX q12h, doxycycline 100 mg bid, a fluoroquinolone, or cefuroxime 250 mg bid for 14-21 days is recommended.
- There is strong consideration for intravenous antibiotics in patients who require hospitalizations for acute exacerbation with signs of respiratory distress.
- Bronchodilators are useful in patients with demonstrable airflow obstruction.

CHRONIC Rx

- Avoidance of tobacco.
- Maintenance of proper nutrition and hydration.
- Prompt identification and treatment of infections.
- Pneumococcal vaccination and annual influenza vaccination.
- In patients with cystic fibrosis, using rhDNase and aerosolized antipseudomonal antibiotics should be considered. This should not be offered to patients with non-cystic fibrosis related bronchiectasis.
- Specific immunoglobulin replacement in patients with selective immunoglobulin deficiency.
- Adults with bronchiectasis with a new isolation of P. aeruginosa should be offered eradication antibiotic treatment. This should not be offered to adults with bronchiectasis following new isolation of pathogens other than P. aeruginosa.
- Inhaled corticosteroids should not be offered to adults with isolated bronchiectasis. However, the diagnosis of bronchiectasis should not affect the use of inhaled corticosteroid in patients with comorbid asthma of chronic obstructive pulmonary disease.
- Long-term antibiotics should be offered for adults with bronchiectasis who have three or more exacerbations per yr.
- Long-term mucoactive treatment (≥3 months) should be considered in patients who have difficulty in expectorating sputum and poor quality of life and where standard airway clearance techniques such as chest physiotherapy have failed to control symptoms.
- Bronchodilators should be used before physiotherapy, including inhaled mucoactive drugs, as well as before inhaled antibiotics, as this increases tolerability and optimizes delivery of medications in diseased areas of the lungs.

DISPOSITION

- Prognosis is variable with severity of the disease and underlying etiology of bronchiectasis.

TABLE 1 Diagnostic Studies for the Classification and Management of Patients with Bronchiectasis

Test	Comments
Routine, Universal Studies	
Computed tomography lung scan (CTLS)	If bronchiectasis (BXSIS) is suspected, CTLS is the definitive test. Thin-section, high-resolution images may help detect subtle airway dilation before bronchial walls are grossly thickened. Contrast is generally not helpful and may, in fact, compromise the overall resolution of the study. CTLS may also identify esophageal abnormalities.
Pulmonary function tests (PFTs)	For patients with significant bronchiectasis, comprehensive PFTs, including spirometry, bronchodilator responsiveness, lung volumes, and diffusion capacity, are important studies that aid in management and prognosis. PFTs may also provide useful hints regarding predisposing conditions.
Complete blood count	Anemia may reflect effects of chronic infection or blood loss (consider inflammatory bowel disorders). Leukocytosis may mark severity of infection. Eosinophilia may suggest ABPA/M.
ESR, C-reactive protein	Nonspecific markers of inflammation; very high levels may suggest underlying connective tissue disease or vasculitis.
Routine sputum culture	Antibiotic therapy in bronchiectasis should generally be directed against specific pathogens and guided by in vitro susceptibility. The presence of mucoid strains of *Pseudomonas aeruginosa* and *Staphylococcus aureus* may raise suspicions for CF. *Stenotrophomonas maltophilia, Alcaligenes xylosoxidans*, and *Burkholderia cepacia* are gram-negative bacilli that may prove problematic pathogens in patients with long-standing bronchiectasis. Isolation of *B. cepacia* and *Helicobacter pylori* requires special laboratory techniques.
Mycobacterial sputum culture	Environmental mycobacteria such as *Mycobacterium avium* complex, *M. chelonae*, and *M. abscessus* appear to be increasingly common in contemporary bronchiectasis. May be commensal but often are pathogenic.
Fungal sputum culture	In patients with an asthmatic component, the presence of *Aspergillus* species (or other molds including Pseudallescheria or penicillium) may be suggestive of etiology.
CT scan of sinuses	Many patients with bronchiectasis also suffer chronic rhinosinusitis. The presence of extensive sinus involvement suggests possible CF, immunoglobulin deficiencies, or ciliary disorders. Also, optimal management often entails aggressive sinus care.
Specific, Directed Studies	
Sweat chloride, CF genotyping, and nasal potential differences	For bronchiectasis patients with bilateral disease, recurrent sinusitis, and no other identified risk factor, mild variants of CF appear to be relatively common. Sweat chloride is regarded as the primary screening test for CF, but a considerable portion of adults with CF have borderline or normal results. Nasal potential difference may be useful for identifying CF in equivocal cases.
Alpha$_1$-antitrypsin (AAT) levels and phenotype	AAT anomalies appear to be a substantial risk factor for bronchiectasis, especially with white females. Abnormal proteinase inhibitor (Pi) phenotypes, even heterozygous patterns such as MS, appear to confer risk even with normal levels of AAT. Repletion of AAT may enhance resistance to lower respiratory tract infections.
Immunoglobulin (Ig) levels	Deficiencies of IgG or IgA may promote bronchiectasis; IgG subclass deficiencies may also be a factor. Elevated levels of IgE may suggest ABPA/M or Job's syndrome. Hyper-IgM may be associated, as well, with chronic infections.
Ciliary morphology or function	For individuals with suggestive stories, a nasal ciliated epithelium biopsy with transmission electron microscopy may identify primary ciliary dyskinesia. Other studies including ex vivo ciliary activity, the saccharine test, or spermatozoa analysis may aid in this diagnosis.
Nasal nitric oxide (NNO) levels	Patients with documented PCD have significantly lower levels of NNO than normal or patients with CF. Although not universally available, such testing may prove highly useful in identifying PCD. Paradoxically, exhaled NO levels have been elevated in bronchiectasis of diverse etiologies except CF.
Barium swallow (BaS)	The BaS may detect disturbed deglutition, esophageal diverticula, obstructing lesions (tumors or strictures), hypomotility, achalasia, hiatal hernias, or lower esophageal sphincter (LES) incompetence with reflux. The absence of reflux on a BaS, however, does not exclude this problem (see pH probe).
pH probe	For patients suspected of gastroesophageal reflux, an 18- to 24-hour study with a transnasal pH probe may identify, quantitate, and characterize reflux. Medications that inhibit acid production must be stopped before such tests.
Esophageal manometry	For patients being considered for surgical repair of the LES, manometry should be performed to determine that the esophagus generates sufficient pressure to propel food and liquids through the tightened sphincter.
Tailored hypopharyngography (TH)	TH is useful in detecting abnormalities of the initial phase of swallowing, deglutition. Persons particularly prone to problems include those with prior strokes, Parkinson's disease, bulbar disorders including postpolio syndrome, and those with prior laryngeal or pharyngeal surgery. Note that some patients have gross aspiration without clinical manifestations (choking, coughing); this may occur in individuals with none of the above risk factors.
Less Common, Exotic Studies	
Collagen vascular disease (CVD) serologies	Various CVDs may contribute to the risk for bronchiectasis, including RA, ankylosing spondylitis, and systemic lupus erythematosus. Thus, for patients with compatible histories or physical findings, assays for rheumatoid factor, HLA-B27, and ANA may provide insight into predisposing conditions. CVD serologies may also suggest the diagnosis of Sjögren's syndrome, particularly SSA/Ro and/or SSB/La.
Schirmer's test	For patients with histories suggestive of "sicca syndrome" (dry eyes, dry mouth, oral ulcers), a positive Schirmer's test may indicate the presence of either primary or secondary (associated with a CVD) Sjögren's syndrome.

ABPA/M, Allergic bronchopulmonary aspergillosis/other mycoses; *ANA*, antinuclear antibody; *CF*, cystic fibrosis; *ESR*, erythrocyte sedimentation rate; *HLA*, human leukocyte antigen; *MS*, multiple sclerosis; *NO*, nitric oxide; *PCD*, primary ciliary dyskinesia; *RA*, rheumatoid arthritis.
From Mason, RJ: *Murray & Nadel's textbook of respiratory medicine*, ed 5, Philadelphia, 2010, Saunders.

- In overlap syndrome of bronchiectasis with rheumatoid arthritis, worse outcomes occurred compared with other bronchiectasis etiologies.

REFERRAL

- Surgical referral for partial lung resection in patients with localized, severe disease unresponsive to medical therapy or in patients with massive hemoptysis. Surgical resection of localized bronchiectasis is safe and improves quality of life.
- Lung transplantation for bronchiectasis accounts for about 2% to 3% of all lung transplant candidates (*The Registry of the International Society for Heart and Lung Transplantation*).

SUGGESTED READINGS

Available at ExpertConsult.com

RELATED CONTENT

Bronchiectasis (Patient Information)

AUTHORS: **ALINE N ZOUK, M.D.**, and **SAMAAN RAFEQ, M.D.**

BASIC INFORMATION

DEFINITION

Brugada syndrome (BRS) is an inherited disorder involving cardiac sodium channels characterized by typical electrocardiographic abnormalities. Patients with a Brugada pattern on ECG and symptoms such as palpitations, syncope, or sudden death are deemed to have BRS. BRS predisposes one to sudden cardiac death (SCD) secondary to polymorphic ventricular tachycardia (PVT)/ventricular fibrillation (VF) in the absence of structural heart disease.

SYNONYM

Sudden unexpected nocturnal death syndrome (SUNDS)

ICD-10CM CODES
I49.9 Cardiac arrhythmia, unspecified
I47.2 Ventricular tachycardia

EPIDEMIOLOGY & DEMOGRAPHICS

INCIDENCE: The incidence ranges from 1 to 5:10,000 people in Europe and 12:10,000 in Southeast Asia.

PREVALENCE: It comprises 4% of SCD and 20% of SCD in structurally normal hearts. Although found in every population, the prevalence is much higher in Asian and Southeast Asian countries; in fact in some Southeast Asian countries, such as Laos and Thailand, it may be the most common form of natural death in younger males.

PREDOMINANT SEX AND AGE: BRS is more common in males (58% to 80% of patients). Mean age at presentation is 40 to 45.

GENETICS: The disease is autosomal dominant with variable expression (Table 1).

- *SCN5A,* the gene that encodes for the alpha subunit of the cardiac sodium channel, accounts for about 20% to 30% of cases of BRS.
- *SCN10a,* the gene that encodes the Nav1.8 subunit of the sodium channel, has been found in 17% of BRS patients, making it the second most common known mutation.
- Known genetic abnormalities are only found in half of patients; thus the impact of genetic testing is limited. When available, it may be useful in identifying silent carriers.
- In all genotypes, the basic abnormality is either a decrease in the inward sodium or calcium current or an increase in the outward potassium current.

RISK FACTORS: First-degree relatives with sudden death or known BRS

PHYSICAL FINDINGS & CLINICAL PRESENTATION

- Physical exam is usually benign.
- Classic ECG finding is a pattern of atypical right bundle branch block (RBBB) with persistent ST elevation of cove-like morphology and T-wave inversion in the anterior leads (V_1-V_2).
- Often an incidental finding diagnosed from a typical ECG pattern.
- Palpitations.
- Nocturnal agonal respirations.
- Syncope.
- Sudden cardiac arrest (SCA)/SCD secondary to rapid PVT that frequently degenerates into VF more often at night.
- Fig. 1 illustrates Brugada ECG patterns. Type 1 is the most common and characteristic (Fig. 2).
- Type 1 ECG pattern is defined as an elevated ST segment ≥2 mm that descends in a coved pattern to an inverted T wave. This finding can be transient and may be provoked (sodium channel blockers, vagal maneuvers, increased alpha-adrenergic tone, beta-blockers, tricyclic or tetracyclic antidepressants, fever, hypokalemia, hyperkalemia, hypercalcemia, and alcohol and cocaine toxicity).
- Type 2 ECG pattern (Fig. 3) is not diagnostic of BRS but may be suggestive and warrant further testing. This pattern is a "saddle back" ST-T wave morphology with an upright or biphasic T wave. Type 2 (formerly known as types 2 and 3) can change to a type 1 pattern with the triggers noted above. Table 2 describes drugs used to unmask Brugada ECG pattern.

ETIOLOGY

Autosomal dominant inheritance with variable penetration.

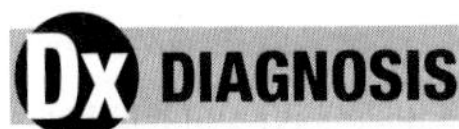

DIAGNOSIS

Diagnosis is made by the presence of a type 1 ECG *and* symptoms.

- ST segment elevation with type 1 morphology ≥2 mm in one or more right-sided leads (V_1-V_2), occurring either spontaneously or after provocative drug testing
- Type 2 ECG that converts into type 1 following sodium channel blocker (procainamide/flecainide/ajmaline) challenge (Fig. 2)

TABLE 1 Molecular Basis of the Brugada Syndrome

Disease	Gene	Protein	Ionic Current	Function	Inheritance
BRS type 1	*SCN5A*	$Na_v1.5$	Subunit alpha I_{Na}	Loss	Autosomal dominant
BRS type 2	*GPD1L*	G3PD1L	Interaction subunit alpha I_{Na}	Loss	Autosomal dominant
BRS type 3	*CACNA1C*	$Ca_v1.2$	Subunit alpha I_{CaL}	Loss	Autosomal dominant
BRS type 4	*CACNB2B*	$Ca_v\beta_2$	Subunit beta I_{CaL}	Loss	Autosomal dominant
BRS type 5	*SCN1B*	$Na_v\beta_1/\beta_{1b}$	Subunit beta I_{Na}	Loss	Autosomal dominant
BRS type 6	*KCNE3*	MiRP2	Subunit beta I_{Ks}/I_{to}	Gain	Autosomal dominant
BRS type 7	*SCN3B*	$Na_v\beta_3$	Subunit beta I_{Na}	Loss	Autosomal dominant

From Issa ZF, et al.: *Clinical arrhythmology and electrophysiology: a companion to Braunwald's heart disease*, ed 2, Philadelphia, 2012, Saunders.

Brugada Syndrome - Diagnosis
ECG changes may be variable:
3 types (I — III) based on the ST, T wave morphology in right precordial leads (V1 — V3)
May be unmasked by Na+ channel blockers (proc., flec., etc)
Brugada syndrome DIAGNOSED with:
• Type 1 ECG: ≥2 mm coved STE in ≥1 V1-V2 leads positioned in the 2nd, 3rd, or 4th intercostal space (spontaneous or induced)
OR
• Type 2 (saddleback STE) or type 3 (≤1mm STE) ECG when a provocative drug (IV class 1 Na ch blocker AAD) induces a Type 1 ECG
Type 1 ECG
Type 2 (saddleback STE)
Type 3 (≤1mm STE)
Type 1 ECG

FIG. 1 Brugada ECG patterns. A type 1 ECG pattern supports diagnosis of Brugada syndrome. Brugada syndrome can be considered for type 2 or 3 ECG patterns if ECG pattern converts to a type 1 pattern after challenge with a sodium channel blocker. (From Olshansky B, et al.: *Arrhythmia essentials*, ed 2, Philadelphia, 2017, Elsevier.)

DIFFERENTIAL DIAGNOSIS

A number of diseases can lead to a BRS-like abnormality on the surface ECG, including the following:

- Atypical RBBB
- Early repolarization
- Acute pericarditis
- Acute myocardial infarction or ischemia
- Pulmonary embolism
- Various central and autonomic system abnormalities
- Duchenne's muscular dystrophy
- Electrolyte abnormalities such as hyperkalemia and hypercalcemia
- Arrhythmogenic right ventricular cardiomyopathy
- Pectus excavatum

WORKUP

- Clinical history with special emphasis on syncope, palpitations, nocturnal agonal respirations, and family history.
- Echocardiography to rule out structural heart disease. While no structural heart disease is usually apparent, there are some recent reports indicating mild abnormalities in the right ventricle (RV) and left ventricle (LV).
- MRI, especially to rule out ARVC (arrhythmogenic right ventricular cardiomyopathy).
- Electrophysiology study. No consensus exists on the value of arrhythmia induction in predicting future clinical events in individual patients. However, findings such as HV (His ventricular) conduction interval >60 ms and VERP (ventricular effective refractory period) <200 ms during electrophysiology study can help in supporting a diagnosis. Repeated trials have failed to show a predictive power of electrophysiology study, and although it still exists as a IIb recommendation in the most recent consensus statement, a recent meta-analysis has suggested it may have some utility, its use in risk stratification remains controversial.
- Laboratory tests are unhelpful. Genetic testing may be helpful for prognosis and family evaluation, but it is not necessary for diagnostic purposes.
- First-degree relatives should obtain ECG and be evaluated for symptoms.
- The following are considered indicators of high risk in an asymptomatic patient:
  1. Spontaneous type 1 ECG at baseline.
  2. Presence of fragmented QRS on ECG.
  3. RVERP (right ventricular effective refractory period) <200 ms on EPS.
  4. Male sex.
  5. Spontaneous atrial fibrillation.

  Note that family history of sudden death is not considered a high-risk feature in BRS.

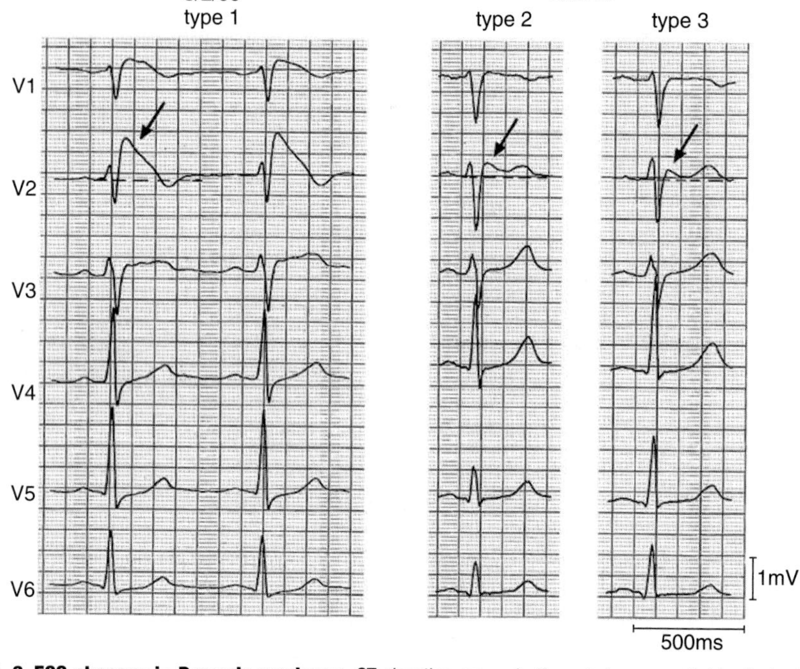

FIG. 2 ECG changes in Brugada syndrome. ST elevation occurs in the anterior precordial leads, leads V1 and V2. Type 1 (coved) ECGs with 1 mV of ST elevation have the most prognostic significance. (From Strickberger SA, et al.: AHA/ACCF scientific statement on the evaluation of syncope, *J Am Coll Cardiol* 47:473–484, 2006.)

Rx TREATMENT

NONPHARMACOLOGIC THERAPY

- The only effective strategy that prevents sudden cardiac death in BRS is implantable cardioverter-defibrillator (ICD). Currently there are no class I recommendations for primary prevention because clinical events are extremely rare, even in high-risk patients. Fig. 4 depicts the algorithm for clinical decision making regarding recommendation of an ICD.
- Definitive candidates for ICD (class I) are patients who survived SCD or have had sustained VT (secondary prevention).
- ICD can be useful (class IIa) for patients who have type 1 ECG pattern in the absence of class IC drug test associated with history of syncope.
- ICD may be considered (class IIb) if there is inducible VF on electrophysiologic (EP) study, but the literature on EP study in patients with BRS does not support this practice.

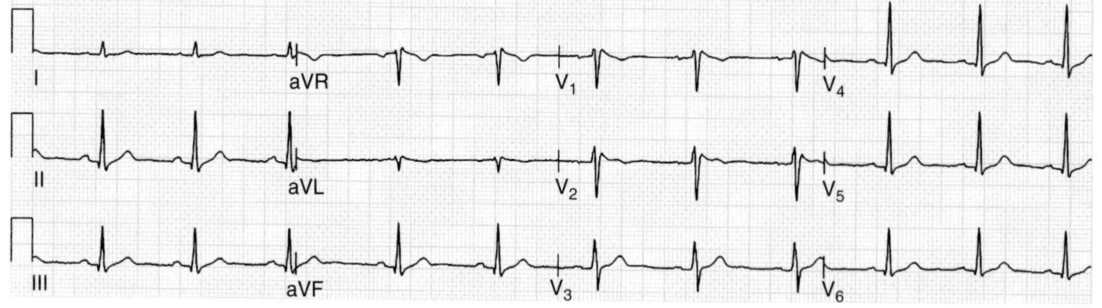

FIG. 3 Type II Brugada pattern ECG. This 12-lead ECG shows a type II Brugada pattern in leads V_1 and V_2. Whereas a type I ECG pattern supports a diagnosis of Brugada syndrome, Brugada syndrome can be considered for type 2 or 3 ECG patterns (see Fig. 1) if the ECG pattern converts to a type 1 pattern after challenge with a sodium channel blocker. *aVF*, Augemented vector foot; *aVL*, augmented vector left; *aVR*, augmented vector right. (From Olshansky B, Chung MK, Pogwizd SM, et al.: *Arrhythmia essentials*, ed 2, Philadelphia, 2017, Elsevier.)

TABLE 2 Drugs Used to Unmask Brugada ECG Pattern

Drug	Dose
Ajmaline	1-mg/kg IV infusion over 5 min
Flecainide	2-mg/kg IV infusion over 10 min, maximum 150 mg; or 400 mg PO
Procainamide	10-mg/kg IV infusion over 10 min
Pilsicainide	1-mg/kg IV infusion over 10 min

- Patients with spontaneous type 1 ECG without syncope or inducible VF on EP study or asymptomatic patients with drug-induced type 1 ECG pattern are considered a lower risk group for SCD, and ICD is not indicated in these patients.
- Radiofrequency catheter ablation of the RV epicardium may be performed for patients with recurrent ventricular arrhythmias and may eliminate the Brugada ECG phenotype. It has also been associated with very low recurrence of arrhythmia in small studies. This has become an accepted therapy for patients with ICD shocks and requires referral to specialized centers.

ACUTE GENERAL RX:

- Isoproterenol (class IIa) may be used for electrical storm.
- Quinidine, which blocks both Ito and IKr currents in the RV epicardium, is used in patients with a history of multiple appropriate ICD shocks, as well as for electrical storms and treatment of supraventricular tachycardia (SVT) in these patients. It is also useful in cases where the patient refuses an ICD implant or when an ICD implant is contraindicated.

REFERRAL

Consultation with cardiology is strongly recommended if BRS is suspected.

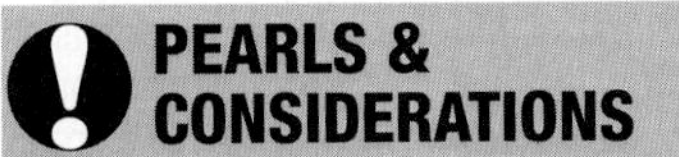

PEARLS & CONSIDERATIONS

COMMENTS

- The clinical manifestations, such as syncope and SCD, are rare in the pediatric group, but fever can acutely predispose to cardiac arrest. Mean age of presentation is 40 to 45 years.
- Cardiac events may occur during sleep, at rest, or after a large meal.
- BRS patients should be advised to avoid all drugs that may induce a type 1 ECG pattern and/or be known to trigger ventricular arrhythmias and avoid unnecessary use of drugs (a drug that is not yet identified as potentially dangerous for these patients does not make its use safe). For up-to-date information on this matter, a full list can be found at www.brugadadrugs.org.
- Fever may induce the appearance of a type 1 BRS ECG pattern and may trigger episodes of PVT/VF in BRS patients. In the case of fever, close ECG monitoring is appropriate in combination with lowering of the body temperature.
- The classic ECG changes in BRS can be transient with patients having normal ECGs in between highly abnormal ones.
- The appearance of syncope, seizures, or nocturnal agonal respiration must lead to prompt medical evaluation.
- Family screening for BRS in first-degree relatives is strongly recommended.
- Although participation in sports is not strictly prohibited, competitive training can lead to development of strong vagal tone and subsequent higher risk of clinical events. Hence, participation in sports at a competitive or professional level is not advised.
- Once diagnosed initially by an ECG pattern, all patients must be followed up on a regular basis by an electrophysiologist.

PREVENTION

Identification of patients with BRS, risk stratification, and appropriate screening of family members are paramount to the prevention of SCD. Patients with known BRS should have fevers aggressively treated with antipyretics and avoid drugs associated with drugs that induce a type 1 pattern.

PATIENT/FAMILY EDUCATION

Immediate family members should be notified and be screened for BRS.

SUGGESTED READINGS

Available at ExpertConsult.com

AUTHOR: **JOHN WYLIE, M.D.**

Prior cardiac arrest or sustained VT?
Yes
ICD recommended
No
Spontaneous type I ECG and hx of syncope judged to be caused by vent arrhythmias?
Yes
ICD can be useful
No
Inducible VF on EP study?
Yes
ICD may be considered
No *or* No EP study
Asymptomatic with drug-induced type I ECG and family history of SCD?
Yes
ICD is not indicated
Class I
Class IIa
Class IIb
Class III

FIG. 4 Consensus recommendations for ICDs in patients diagnosed with Brugada syndrome. (*hx*, History; *ICD*, implantable cardioverter-defibrillator; *SCD*, sequential compression device; *VF*, ventricular fibrillation; *VT*, ventricular tachycardia. Priori SG, et al.: HRS/EHRA/APHRS expert consensus statement on the diagnosis and management of patients with inherited primary arrhythmia syndromes, *Heart Rhythm* 10:1932–1963, 2013.)

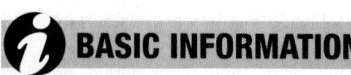

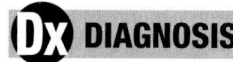

BASIC INFORMATION

DEFINITION

Budd-Chiari syndrome (BCS) is a rare disorder defined by the obstruction of hepatic venous outflow anywhere from the small hepatic veins to the junction of the inferior vena cava (IVC) and the right atrium. Primary BCS is defined by endoluminal obstruction as seen in thromboses, phlebitis, or webs. Secondary BCS occurs when the obstruction is caused by compression or invasion by a lesion originating outside of the veins (tumor, abscess, cyst, etc.). It can also be a postoperative complication of orthotopic liver transplantation (OLT).

SYNONYMS

BCS
Hepatic vein thrombosis
Obliterative endophlebitis of the hepatic veins
IVC thrombosis
Chiari-Budd syndrome
Budd syndrome
Chiari disease
Rokitansky disease

ICD-10CM CODE

I82.0 Budd-Chiari syndrome

EPIDEMIOLOGY & DEMOGRAPHICS

INCIDENCE: Males: 2.0/1 million persons per yr
Females: 2.2/1 million persons per yr

PREDOMINANT SEX: In Western countries, women are more commonly affected (approximately 2/3 of cases).

In Asia, men are slightly more affected (approximately 1.5/1).

PREDOMINANT AGE: In Western countries, presentation is usually in the third and fourth decades of life, with the median age being 35-50 yr.

In Asia, presentation is usually at a median age of 36 yr.

PHYSICAL FINDINGS & CLINICAL PRESENTATION

Clinical presentation and characteristics vary with geography. The classic presentation of Budd-Chiari syndrome includes hepatomegaly, ascites, and right upper quadrant pain. In Africa and South Asia, intravascular webs are more often associated with IVC thrombosis with a stronger association with subsequent liver cirrhosis and hepatocellular carcinoma. In the U.S., BCS is more commonly associated with primary myeloproliferative disorders and underlying hypercoagulable states. Underlying factors that contribute to BCS can be identified in more than 80% of cases; multiple causative factors are identified in up to 50% of cases.

- Clinical manifestations can be caused by complete or partial occlusion of any or all of the three major hepatic veins or the inferior vena cava.
- Presentation is variable according to the degree, location, acuity of obstruction, and presence of collateral circulation:
  1. Fulminant/acute (25%): Severe right upper quadrant abdominal pain, fever, nausea, vomiting, mild jaundice, hepatomegaly, transudative and intractable ascites, marked elevation in serum aminotransferases (AST/ALT >5 times the upper limit of normal), elevation of alkaline phosphatase to 300–400 IU/L, serum-ascites albumin gradient ≥ 1.1 with total protein >2.5 g/dl, coagulopathy (usually international normalized ratio [INR] >1.5), variceal bleeding, encephalopathy within 8 wk of onset of jaundice, renal failure. Biopsy, if performed, would reveal hepatic necrosis. Early recognition and treatment are essential for survival; a slow decrease in ALT is associated with poor survival.
  2. Subacute/chronic (60%): Vague abdominal discomfort, gradual progression to caudate lobe hypertrophy with atrophy of the rest of the liver, portal hypertension with or without cirrhosis and its sequelae, transudative ascites, lower-extremity edema, esophageal varices, splenomegaly, coagulopathy, mild to moderate elevation in aminotransferases, bilirubin and alkaline phosphatase, hepatorenal syndrome, hepatopulmonary syndrome, and rarely, encephalopathy; biopsy, if performed, could reveal minimal hepatic necrosis.
  3. Asymptomatic (up to 20%): Usually discovered incidentally by abnormal liver function tests or imaging attained for other reasons.

ETIOLOGY: APPROXIMATELY 80-87% OF PATIENTS HAVE ONE PROTHROMBOTIC RISK FACTOR, AND APPROXIMATELY 50% HAVE MULTIPLE

- Primary myeloproliferative diseases: Up to 53% of BCS patients have a primary myeloproliferative disease and polycythemia vera is responsible for 10% to 40% of these cases.
  1. Essential thrombocythemia and idiopathic myelofibrosis are less common causes.
  2. *JAK2* mutations are implicated in cases of idiopathic BCS (identified in 25%-60% of cases).
- Hypercoagulable states (inherited and acquired) often coexist with other causes.
  1. Anticardiolipin antibodies (up to 25%).
  2. Hyperhomocysteinemia (22%).
  3. Paroxysmal nocturnal hemoglobinuria (5%-19%).
  4. Factor V Leiden (25%).
  5. Factor II gene mutation (5%).
- Protein C, protein S, and antithrombin III deficiency are difficult to interpret because the presence of liver disease may confound results. However, they account for 4.0%, 3.0%, and 3.0% of BCS, respectively.
- Heterozygosity for *G20210A* prothrombin gene mutation, methylenetetrahydrofolate reductase (MTHFR) mutation, Tet methylcytosine dioxygenase 2 mutation, and calreticulin mutation may be seen in BCS.
- Pregnancy and oral contraceptive pills are also predisposing factors to develop BCS.
- Malignancy causing external compression or invasion of vascular structures (up to 10% of cases).
  1. Most commonly due to hepatocellular carcinoma but also can be due to neoplasms of the kidney, adrenal gland, pancreas, stomach, lung and sarcomas of the right atrium, inferior vena cava, and hepatic veins.
- Rare but reported: Sickle cell anemia, infections with liver abscess, hydatid cyst (echinococcosis), schistosomiasis, sarcoidosis, Behçet's disease, membranous webs of IVC or hepatic veins (more common in Africa and South Asia, can be congenital or acquired secondary to underlying myeloproliferative disorder), abdominal trauma, liver torsion, granulomatous venulitis, ulcerative colitis, celiac disease, systemic lupus erythematous, minimal change nephrotic syndrome, neurofibromatosis, α-1 antitrypsin deficiency, hypereosinophilic syndrome, idiopathic (10%-25%).

Dx DIAGNOSIS

DIFFERENTIAL DIAGNOSIS

- Hepatitis from ischemia, viral infection, toxin, alcohol
- Cholecystitis
- Hepatic veno-occlusive disease (sinusoidal obstruction syndrome)
- Congestive hepatopathy, also known as *cardiac cirrhosis*, from tricuspid regurgitation, right atrial myxoma, constrictive pericarditis
- Cirrhosis from any etiology

LABORATORY TESTS

- Assessment of liver injury and function: Serum aminotransferases, alkaline phosphatase, prothrombin time (PT), albumin, bilirubin.
- Exclusion of another form of liver disease: Viral hepatitis panel, autoantibodies (antinuclear antibody, anti–smooth muscle antibody, anti-mitochondrial antibody), iron studies, ceruloplasmin, and α-1 antitrypsin.
- Ascites protein content ≥2.5 g/dl and serum ascites albumin gradient >1.1 g/dl are suggestive of transudative ascites from BCS or cardiac ascites.
- Evaluation for underlying myeloproliferative disorder and hypercoagulable state: CBC, bone marrow biopsy, tests for hypercoagulable states (Factor V Leiden, prothrombin gene *G20210A* mutation, protein C, protein S, antithrombin deficiencies, antiphospholipid syndrome, and paroxysmal nocturnal hemoglobinuria). Protein C, protein S, and antithrombin deficiencies may be difficult to interpret in the setting of liver dysfunction, but levels <20% of normal are suggestive of a true deficiency; thrombophilia screening for the JAK2 V617F mutation, hyperhomocysteinemia, and MTHFR C677T mutation may be useful if no other cause for myeloproliferative disorders or hypercoagulable states are identified.

IMAGING STUDIES

- Diagnosis of BCS is made by radiographic imaging.
- Doppler ultrasonography is the first-line test. Diagnostic sensitivity and specificity are 85% to 90%. Findings include large hepatic vein with an absent flow signal, or with reversed or turbulent flow; large intrahepatic or subcapsular collateral vessels; enlarged, stenotic, thickened, or tortuous hepatic veins; spiderweb pattern near hepatic vein ostia and associated absent flow in that region; caudate lobe hypertrophy (as the caudate lobe has an alternate blood supply through anastomoses); flattened or absent hepatic venous waveform without fluttering; hyperechoic cord replacing a normal vein.
- MRI with gadolinium contrast is the second-line test. It is superior to contrast-enhanced CT (Fig. E1) with a sensitivity and specificity of approximately 90%, and it is preferred in younger patients due to the lack of radiation. Findings include obstructed hepatic veins or IVC, large intrahepatic or subcapsular collaterals, and caudate lobe hypertrophy. MRI is beneficial to visualize the entire length of the IVC and distinguish between acute, subacute, and chronic BCS. Three-dimensional contrast-enhanced magnetic resonance angiography (MRA, see Fig. 2) rivals hepatic venography in sensitivity.
- Contrast-enhanced CT may reveal similar findings as Doppler ultrasound as well as delayed or absent filling of the hepatic veins, parenchymal opacification of the liver, narrowing and/or compression of the inferior vena cava, and caudate lobe hypertrophy. Contrast enhancement localizes more centrally than peripherally and has a patchy and flea-bitten appearance. The use of CT is limited given that in almost 50% of patients, the test is indeterminate or a false-positive. Ultrasonography is more accurate than CT for detecting lesions in the hepatic veins and IVC.
- CT image reconstruction of vasculature is becoming more available.
- Venography: Although it is the the gold standard, it is not essential for diagnosis, and it should be performed when other noninvasive imaging tests are nondiagnostic in the setting of strong clinical suspicion for BCS. Measurement of pressure gradients can help predict success of percutaneous or surgical shunt intervention. Confirms the pathognomonic web pattern caused by collateral venous flow.
- Liver biopsy: Not necessary to diagnose BCS but may be helpful in patients with cirrhosis in whom the diagnosis remains uncertain and is critical for differentiating from hepatic veno-occlusive disease or congestive hepatopathy. Findings include hepatic congestion, hepatocyte necrosis and fibrosis in centrilobular areas, and compensatory nodular regenerative hyperplasia with progression to fibrosis and cirrhosis. In advanced BCS, infarction caused by concomitant thrombosis of the intrahepatic, extrahepatic, and portal veins may be seen. There are conflicting studies regarding the association of histologic findings and prognosis.

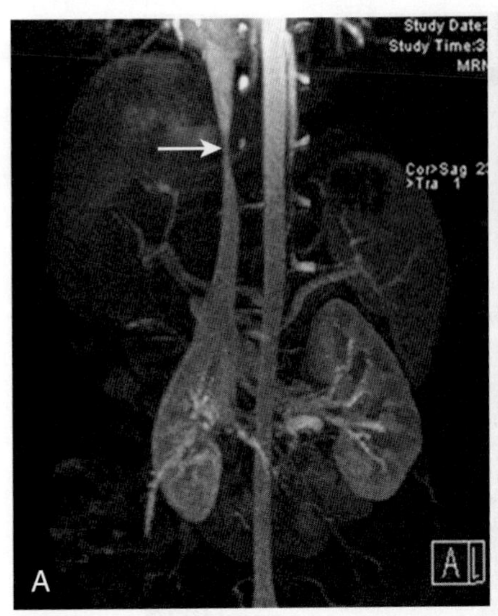

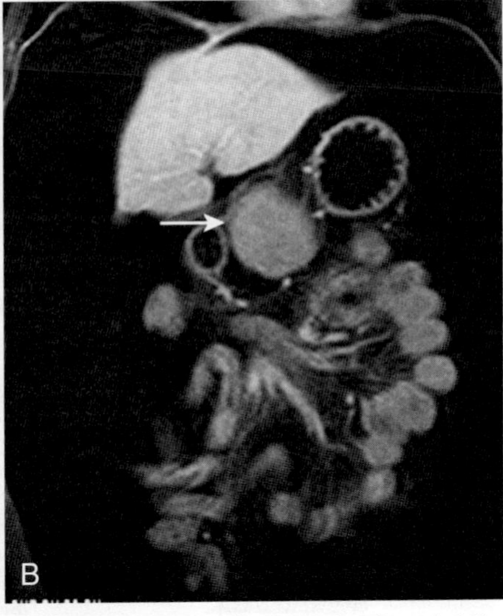

FIG. 2 Magnetic resonance venogram. A, Intravenous cholangiography (IVC) obstruction *(arrow)* at the level of the caudate. **B,** Hypertrophic caudate lobe *(arrow)*. (From Cameron JL, Cameron AM: *Current surgical therapy,* ed 10, Philadelphia, 2011, Saunders.)

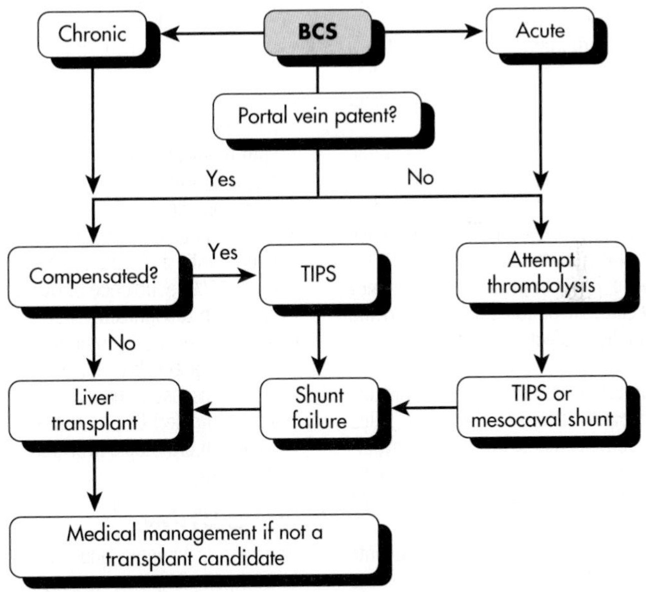

FIG. 3 Treatment algorithm for patients with Budd-Chiari syndrome (BCS). *TIPS,* Transjugular intrahepatic portosystemic shunt. (From Cameron JL, Cameron AM: *Current surgical therapy,* ed 12, Philadelphia, 2017, Elsevier.)

Rx TREATMENT

NONPHARMACOLOGIC THERAPY

- Goal of therapy is decompression of hepatic congestion.
- In general, therapeutic procedures should be introduced by order of increasing invasiveness based on response/failure to therapy rather than disease severity. Fig. 3 illustrates a treatment algorithm for patients with Budd-Chiari syndrome.
- Hypercoagulable states should be investigated in all patients.

ACUTE GENERAL RX:

- Anticoagulation, first with low-molecular-weight heparin (LMWH), followed by warfarin, even in the absence of an underlying hypercoagulable disorder. Recent research also suggests that using direct-acting oral anticoagulants in BCS is safe and effective.
- In situ thrombolysis: Can be successful when performed in patients with recently thrombosed veins (within 2-3 weeks after symptom onset) that are well defined on venography. Mature clots are nonresponsive to thrombolysis, and bleeding risk is high if portal hypertension has developed.

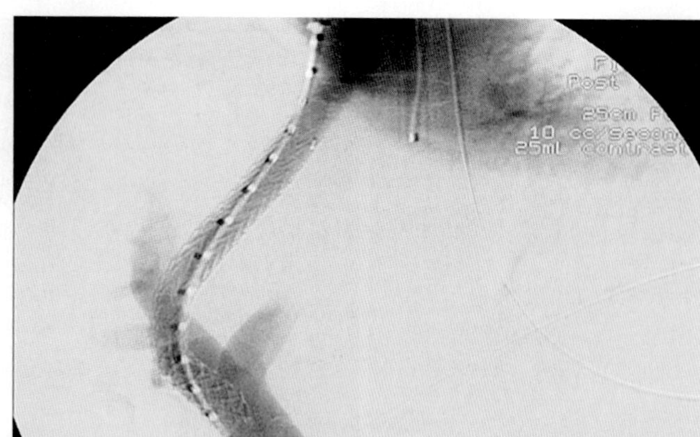

FIG. 4 Transjugular intrahepatic portosystemic shunt extending from the right portal vein into the right atrium. (From Cameron JL, Cameron AM: *Current surgical therapy*, ed 12, Philadelphia, 2017, Elsevier.)

- Balloon angioplasty: Complicated by 50% restenosis rate within 2 yr; effective when membranous webs or short segment hepatic vein stenosis are the etiology.
- Stenting: May improve long-term patency rates to 90%, but if placed above the intrahepatic IVC, may complicate future liver transplantation.
- Transjugular intrahepatic portosystemic shunt (TIPS) (Fig. 4): Indicated with diffuse hepatic vein thrombosis, refractory ascites, recurrent variceal bleeding and progressive liver failure. Polytetrafluoroethylene (ePTFE)-coated stents have improved TIPS-patency rates, especially in patients with underlying hypercoagulable defects with a 76% 10-yr survival rate.
- Surgical portal systemic shunts: Indicated when angioplasty and stenting have failed and when complications from portal hypertension are also present. This option is no longer common practice and provides no survival benefit.
- Liver transplant may be indicated in patients with cirrhosis or fulminant hepatic failure and in patients who fail to respond to TIPS; 10-yr survival is reported to range between 69% and 84%.
- Supportive measures.

CHRONIC Rx

- Lifelong anticoagulation: Warfarin therapy, with a target INR of 2 to 3 or low-molecular-weight heparin, lessens, but does not completely prevent, recurrence. Anticoagulation should be continued permanently unless the patient has an adverse event to anticoagulation, the obstruction is because of an anatomic cause that has been corrected, or anticoagulation is contraindicated.
- In patients with an underlying myeloproliferative disorder, first-line treatment is with hydroxyurea and aspirin.
- Treat liver dysfunction and complications related to portal hypertension such as ascites and variceal bleeding.
- Invasive interventions should be reserved for symptomatic patients who do not improve with medical therapy.
- Manage shunt thrombosis; which is a common complication.
- Liver transplantation is another treatment option with a 71-89% survival rate at 5 yr; up to 27% recurrence of BCS after transplant has been recognized.
- Monitor for development of hepatocellular carcinoma and transformation of myeloproliferative disease in patients with long-standing, well-controlled BCS and post-transplant lymphoma in orthotopic liver transplantation (OLT) recipients.

DISPOSITION

Prognosis is variable and depends on multiple factors, including time to recognition and treatment, etiology, acuity, the type of intervention, and the condition of the patient at the time of treatment. Overall mortality rates are decreasing with the use of anticoagulation and early diagnosis of asymptomatic cases. Given numerous therapeutic options, the survival rate is 90%, 83%, and 72% at 1, 5, and 10 yr from diagnosis.

- A prognostic index called the *Rotterdam BCS Index* has been described: 1.27 × Encephalopathy + 1.04 × Ascites + 0.72 × PT + 0.004 × Bilirubin.
  1. Encephalopathy and ascites are scored as 1 for present or 0 as absent, and PT is scored as greater (1) or less than (0) an INR of 2.3.
  2. An index of <1.1 correlates to low risk (5-yr survival rate, 89%), 1.1 to 1.5 with intermediate risk (5-yr survival rate, 74%), and >1.5 with high risk (5-yr survival rate, 42%).
- There is also the *BCS-TIPS PI score*, which is a prognostic index for survival 1 yr after TIPS: age (yr) × 0.08 + bilirubin × 0.16 + INR × 0.63.
  1. Seven is the most specific discriminative factor, with those scoring above 7 necessitating emergent OLT as the first line treatment.

REFERRAL

Fulminant presentations should immediately be referred to a center capable of liver transplantation. All cases benefit from referral to a hepatologist, a hematologist, an interventional radiologist, and a surgeon specializing in hepatobiliary disease.

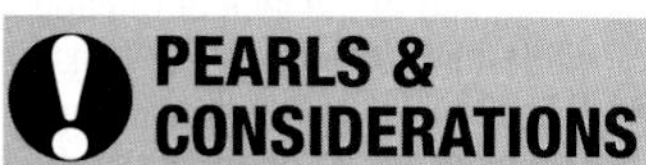

PEARLS & CONSIDERATIONS

COMMENTS

- Look for one or more underlying causes, especially hypercoagulable or hematologic disorders, and malignancies or space-occupying lesions that may compress or invade the hepatic outflow tract.
- Myeloproliferative disorders are most common.
- Diagnosis relies on imaging; beginning with Doppler ultrasound.
- Treatment with anticoagulation comes first; followed by invasive interventions as needed. Prophylaxis of portal hypertension can reduce the risk of major bleeding associated with anticoagulation therapy.
- Referral for liver transplantation may be necessary.
- Prognostic indices can assist in management and estimate survival rates.

PREVENTION

In the setting of known risk factors, such as a hypercoagulable state or myeloproliferative disorder, any additional risks, such as smoking or oral contraceptive therapy, should be avoided.

SUGGESTED READINGS

Available at ExpertConsult.com

RELATED CONTENT

Budd-Chiari Syndrome (Patient Information)
Hypercoagulable States (Related Key Topic)

AUTHORS: **JEANETTE G. SMITH, M.D.**, and **DINA IBRAHIM, M.D.**

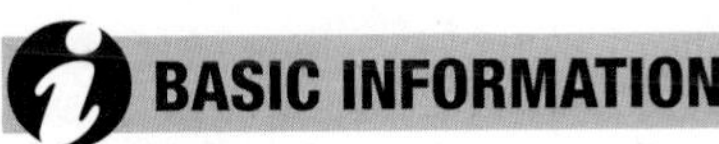

BASIC INFORMATION

DEFINITION

Bulimia nervosa is a prolonged illness characterized by a specific psychopathology. According to the *Diagnostic and Statistical Manual of Mental Disorders,* 5th edition, bulimia nervosa can be diagnosed by: (A) recurrent episodes of binge eating. An episode of binge eating is characterized by both of the following:

1. Eating, in a discrete period of time, an amount of food that is definitely larger than what most individuals would eat in a similar period of time under similar circumstances.
2. A sense of lack of control over eating during the episode.

(B) Recurrent inappropriate compensators/behaviors in order to prevent weight gain, such as self-induced vomiting; misuse of laxatives, diuretics, or other medications; fasting; or excessive exercise. (C) The binge eating and inappropriate compensatory behaviors both occur, on average, at least once a week for 3 mo. (D) Self-evaluation is unduly influenced by body shape and weight. (E) The disturbance does not occur exclusively during episodes of anorexia nervosa.

ICD-10CM CODE
F50.2 Bulimia nervosa

EPIDEMIOLOGY & DEMOGRAPHICS

INCIDENCE/PREVALENCE: Affects 1% to 3% of female adolescents and young adults
PREDOMINANT SEX: Female/male ratio of 10:1
PREDOMINANT AGE: Adolescence to young adulthood; mean age of onset: 17 yr

PHYSICAL FINDINGS & CLINICAL PRESENTATION

- Parotid and salivary gland swelling
- Scars on the back of the hand and knuckles (Russell sign) from rubbing against the upper incisors when inducing vomiting
- Eroded enamel, particularly on the lingual surface of the upper teeth; pyorrhea and other gum disorders possible
- Petechial hemorrhages of the cornea, soft palate, or face possibly noted after vomiting
- Loss of gag reflex, well-developed abdominal musculature
- Often no emaciation; normal physical examination possible

ETIOLOGY

- Etiology is unknown but likely multifactorial (sociocultural, psychological, familial factors).
- Bulimia is much more common in Western societies, where there is a strong cultural pressure to be slender.
- According to the American Psychiatric Association, patients with eating disorders display a broad range of symptoms that occur along a continuum between those of anorexia nervosa and bulimia.

Dx DIAGNOSIS

DIFFERENTIAL DIAGNOSIS

- Schizophrenia
- Gastrointestinal disorders
- Neurologic disorders (seizures, Kleine-Levin syndrome, Klüver-Bucy syndrome)
- Brain neoplasms
- Psychogenic vomiting

WORKUP

- The following questions are useful to screen patients for bulimia:
    1. "Are you satisfied with your eating habits?"
    2. "Do you ever eat in secret?"
- Answering "no" to the first question and/or "yes" to the second question has 100% sensitivity and 90% specificity for bulimia. The SCOFF questionnaire can also be used as a screening tool for eating disorders (see "Anorexia Nervosa").
- According to the DSM-5, the level of severity is based on the frequency of inappropriate compensatory behaviors and may be increased to reflect other symptoms and degree of functional disability, as noted below:
    1. Mild: An average of 1 to 3 episodes of inappropriate compensatory behaviors per week
    2. Moderate: An average of 4 to 7 episodes of inappropriate compensatory behaviors per week
    3. Severe: An average of 8 to 13 episodes of inappropriate compensatory behaviors per week
    4. Extreme: An average of ≥14 inappropriate compensatory behaviors per week
- Table 1 describes eating and weight control habits commonly found in children and adolescents with an eating disorder.

LABORATORY TESTS

- Electrolyte abnormalities from vomiting (hypokalemia and metabolic alkalosis) or diarrhea from laxative abuse (hypokalemia and hyperchloremic metabolic acidosis)
- Hyponatremia, hypocalcemia, hypomagnesemia (caused by laxative abuse)
- Elevated cortisol, decreased luteinizing hormone, decreased follicle-stimulating hormone

Rx TREATMENT

NONPHARMACOLOGIC THERAPY

- Cognitive behavioral therapy, particularly interpersonal therapy to control abnormal behaviors
- Use of food diaries, nutritional counseling, and planning meals at least 1 day in advance are useful measures to counter abnormal eating behaviors
- Correction of electrolyte abnormalities

ACUTE GENERAL Rx

- Selective serotonin reuptake inhibitors are generally considered to be the safest medication option in these patients. They are useful in severely depressed patients and in those who do not benefit from cognitive behavioral therapy.
- Prompt recognition and treatment of complications:
    1. Ipecac cardiotoxicity from laxative abuse
    2. Electrolyte abnormalities (see "Laboratory Tests")
    3. Esophagitis and Mallory-Weiss tears; esophageal rupture from repeated vomiting
    4. Aspiration pneumonia and pneumomediastinum
    5. Menstrual irregularities (including amenorrhea)
    6. Gastrointestinal abnormalities: Acute gastric dilation, pancreatitis, abdominal pain, constipation

CHRONIC Rx

- Psychotherapy continued for yrs and focused specifically on self-image and family and peer interactions is an integral part of successful recovery.
- Family therapy is also recommended, especially in younger patients.

DISPOSITION

Course is variable and marked by frequent recurrence of exacerbations.

REFERRAL

- In addition to the primary care physician, the multidisciplinary team should include a dietician, a psychiatrist, and a family therapist.
- Hospitalization should be considered for patients with severe electrolyte abnormalities or those with suicidal thoughts.

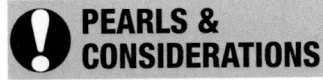

PEARLS & CONSIDERATIONS

COMMENTS

- Bulimia has a close association with depression, bipolar disorder, obsessive-compulsive disorder, alcoholism, and substance abuse.
- Bulimia should be considered in all patients (especially adolescents) with unexplained hypokalemia and metabolic alkalosis.

RELATED CONTENT

Bulimia (Patient Information)
Anorexia Nervosa (Related Key Topic)
Binge-Eating Disorder (Related Key Topic)

AUTHOR: **FRED F. FERRI, M.D.**

TABLE 1 Eating and Weight Control Habits Commonly Found in Children and Adolescents with an Eating Disorder

	Prominent Features		Clinical Comments Regarding Eating Disorder Habits	
Habit	**Anorexia Nervosa**	**Bulimia Nervosa**	**Anorexia Nervosa**	**Bulimia Nervosa**
Overall intake	Inadequate energy (calories), although volume of food and beverages may be high due to very low caloric density of intake due to "diet" and nonfat choices	Variable, but calories normal to high; intake in binges often "forbidden" food or drink that differs from intake at meals	Consistent inadequate caloric intake leading to wasting of the body	Inconsistent balance of intake, exercise, and vomiting, but severe caloric restriction is short-lived
Food	Counts and limits calories, especially from fat; emphasis on "healthy food choices" with reduced caloric density Monotonous, limited "good" food choices, often leading to vegetarian or vegan diet Strong feelings of guilt after eating more than planned leads to exercise and renewed dieting	Aware of calories and fat, but less regimented in avoidance than AN Frequent dieting interspersed with overeating, often triggered by depression, isolation, or anger	Obsessive-compulsive attention to nutritional data on food labels and may have "logical" reasons for food choices in highly regimented pattern, such as sports participation or family history of lipid disorder	Choices less structured, with more frequent diets
Beverages	Water or other low- or no-calorie drinks; nonfat milk	Variable, diet soda common; may drink alcohol to excess	Fluids often restricted to avoid weight gain	Fluids ingested to aid vomiting or replace losses
Meals	Consistent schedule and structure to meal plan Reduced or eliminated caloric content, often starting with breakfast, then lunch, then dinner Volume can increase with fresh fruits, vegetables, and salads as primary food sources	Meals less regimented and planned than in AN; more likely impulsive and unregulated, often eliminated following a binge-purge episode	Rigid adherence to "rules" governing eating leads to sense of control, confidence, and mastery	Elimination of a meal following a binge-purge only reinforces the drive for binge later in the day
Snacks	Reduced or eliminated from meal plan	Often avoided in meal plans, but then impulsively eaten	Snack foods removed early because "unhealthy"	Snack "comfort foods" can trigger a binge
Dieting	Initial habit that becomes progressively restrictive, although often appearing superficially "healthy" Beliefs and "rules" about the patient's idiosyncratic nutritional requirements and response to foods are strongly held	Initial dieting gives way to chaotic eating, often interpreted by the patient as evidence of being "weak" or "lazy"	Distinguishing between healthy meal planning with reduced calories and dieting in ED may be difficult	Dieting tends to be impulsive and short-lived, with "diets" often resulting in unintended weight gain
Binge eating	None in restrictive subtype, but an essential feature in binge-purge subtype	Essential feature, often secretive Shame and guilt prominent afterward	Often "subjective" (more than planned but not large)	Relieves emotional distress, may be planned
Exercise	Characteristically obsessive-compulsive, ritualistic, and progressive May excel in dance, long-distance running	Less predictable May be athletic, or may avoid exercise entirely	May be difficult to distinguish active thin vs. ED	Males often use exercise as means of "purging"
Vomiting	Characteristic of binge-purge subtype May chew then spit out, rather than swallow, food as a variant	Most common habit intended to reduce effects of overeating Can occur after meal as well as a binge	Physiologic and emotional instability prominent	Strongly "addictive" and self-punishing, but does not eliminate calories ingested—many still absorbed
Laxatives	If used, generally to relieve constipation in restrictive subtype, but as a cathartic in binge-purge subtype	Second most common habit used to reduce or avoid weight gain, often used in increasing doses for cathartic effect	Physiologic and emotional instability prominent	Strongly "addictive," self-punishing, but ineffective means to reduce weight (calories are absorbed in the small intestine, but laxatives work in the colon)
Diet pills	Very rare, if used; more common in binge-purge subtype	Used to either reduce appetite or increase metabolism	Use of diet pills implies inability to control eating	Control over eating may be sought by any means

AN, Anorexia nervosa; *BN,* bulimia nervosa; *ED,* eating disorder.
From Kliegman RM et al: *Nelson textbook of pediatrics,* ed 19, Philadelphia, 2011, Saunders.

BASIC INFORMATION

DEFINITION

- Delayed conduction in the His-Purkinje system that meets criteria for right bundle branch block (RBBB), left bundle branch block (LBBB), or hemifascicular block. The latter can be either left anterior fascicular block (LAFB) or left posterior fascicular block (LPFB). Bifascicular block is a combination of RBBB and either LAFB or LPFB. All of these are categories of bundle branch block. Any delayed conduction that does not meet these criteria is not considered bundle branch block but rather categorized as intraventricular conduction delay (IVCD) [see separate topic]. Repolarization abnormalities may be seen in multiple leads with LBBB and in leads V1-V3 in RBBB. These include T wave inversions and ST segment depression in the opposite direction from the QRS complex. Fig. 1 illustrates a diagrammatic representation of fascicular blocks in the left ventricle. Tables 1 and 2 summarize common diagnostic criteria for fascicular blocks and bundle branch blocks.
- The bundle branch block can be persistent or intermittent. The latter is most commonly rate-related, during tachycardia or acute shortening of the R-R interval, and usually RBBB. Bradycardia dependent aberrancy can also be seen. Alternating bundle branch block between RBBB and LBBB is a sign of conduction system disease and will often progress to complete heart block.

SYNONYMS

- Fascicular block
- Aberrancy
- Conduction disturbance
- Conduction delay
- Conduction defect

ICD 10-CM CODES

Bundle branch block (fascicular block):

I45.2	Bilateral (bifascicular)
I44.7	Left
I44.60	Hemiblock (hemifascicular block)
I44.4	Anterior
I44.5	Posterior
I44.7	Incomplete
I45.10	Right

EPIDEMIOLOGY & DEMOGRAPHICS

INCIDENCE: The cumulative incidence of any type of bundle branch block increases with age (1.5% at age 50, 18% at age 80)

PEAK INCIDENCE: Cumulative incidence of 18% at age 80 for any type of bundle branch block

PREVALENCE:

- Complete LBBB: 0.4% men age 50, 5.7% men age 80, 1.1% women age 50-80
- Complete RBBB: 0.2% men before age 30, 0.8% men age 50, 1.3% men age 80, 1.3% women age 50-80, 2.3% in men and women age 60
- Incomplete RBBB: 13.5% age 20, 3.4% age 50

PREDOMINANT SEX AND AGE: More common in men, incidence increases with age

GENETICS: Most cases of bundle branch block are not hereditary. The Brugada syndrome is an autosomal dominant genetic disorder with pseudo-RBBB but is not a true bundle branch block (see section on Brugada Syndrome). The hereditary bundle branch defect is an autosomal dominant genetic disease that has been described in Lebanon and was mapped to the long arm of chromosome 19.

RISK FACTORS: Male gender, elder age, structural heart disease, cardiomyopathy, hypertension

PHYSICAL FINDINGS & CLINICAL PRESENTATION

- RBBB can cause wide splitting of the second heart sound (S_2). Either LBBB or RBBB can cause continuous splitting of S_2 during respiration.
- Isolated bundle branch block does not cause symptoms. Nevertheless, it is usually a result of heart disease, either in the conduction system or the surrounding cardiac tissues, and its existence can aggravate the clinical picture of the causal entity.
- In patients with heart failure, the presence of LBBB can cause ventricular dyssynchrony and worsen heart failure. LBBB or RBBB, when coexistent with coronary artery disease, diabetes, or heart failure, are markers for increased mortality.
- RBBB can be seen in pulmonary hypertension or acute pulmonary embolism, generally in entities that increase the right ventricular afterload. The presence of bundle branch block can be associated with other conduction defects such as second or third degree AV block.

ETIOLOGY

- Bundle branch block can be a result of disease in the His-Purkinje conduction system but can also result from disease or fibrosis surrounding the conduction system (i.e., myocardial infarction), antiarrhythmic drugs, or hyperkalemia. Selected causes of bundle branch block are the following: intracardiac catheter manipulation, myocardial ischemia or infarction, myocarditis, cardiomyopathy, and Lenegre's or Lev's disease.

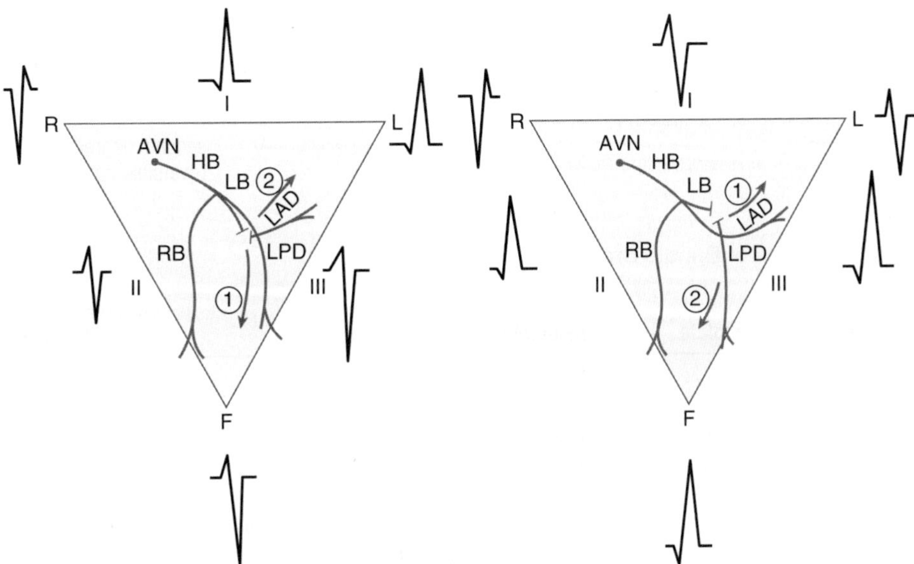

FIG. 1 Diagrammatic representation of fascicular blocks in the left ventricle. *Left,* Interruption of the left anterior fascicle or division (here labeled LAD) results in an initial inferior (1) followed by a dominant superior (2) direction of activation. *Right,* Interruption of the left posterior fascicle or division (here labeled LPD) results in an initial superior (1) followed by a dominant inferior (2) direction of activation. *AVN,* atrioventricular node; *HB,* His bundle; *LB,* left bundle; *RB,* right bundle. (Courtesy Dr. C. Fisch.) (From Mann DL et al: *Braunwald's heart disease,* ed 10, Philadelphia, 2015, Elsevier.)

RBBB in particular is associated with pulmonary hypertension and pulmonary embolism, whereas LBBB can be caused by an anterior myocardial infarction.

- Rate-related branch block in normal hearts is usually seen in tachycardia or in atrial fibrillation where a long R-R interval is followed by a shorter one. This is due to Ashman's phenomenon, where a long cycle length interval causes prolongation in the refractory period resulting in bundle branch block on the subsequent early beat. This is a common property of all cardiac tissues but more evident in the conduction system. The rate-related bundle block is usually RBBB since the right bundle has a longer refractory period than the left bundle for the same heart rate. Another phenomenon is bradycardia-dependent aberrancy. This may be due to automaticity in a bundle branch block during diastole leading to BBB on a subsequent beat. Other explanations include vagal tone inhibition or phase 4 block. In phase 4 block, the cells have depleted sodium reserves resulting in low resting membrane potentials that impose difficulty in cell excitability resulting in conduction block.

Dx DIAGNOSIS

DIFFERENTIAL DIAGNOSIS (TABLE 3)

- An accessory pathway can cause an appearance of RBBB or LBBB. If lead V1 is placed higher than the fourth intercostal space or more right than the parasternal area, the EKG can resemble incomplete RBBB.
- An inferior myocardial infarction can resemble left anterior fascicular block, but in the inferior myocardial infarction, the inferior leads (II, III, aVF) will have qR instead of QS morphology. Left posterior fascicular block can resemble lateral myocardial infarction, right ventricular hypertrophy, dextrocardia, or lateral accessory pathway. Accelerated idioventricular rhythm can resemble LBBB or RBBB, depending on the origin of the ventricular pacemaker site.

WORK-UP

- Resting, ambulatory, and exercise electrocardiogram
- Investigation of coexistent comorbidities such as heart failure, myocardial infarction, and cardiomyopathies
- Acute LBBB should prompt investigation for anterior myocardial infarction (Fig. 2) whereas acute RBBB for pulmonary hypertension, or pulmonary embolism (Fig. 3)
- Figures 2 and 3 illustrate diagnostic evaluations for bundle branch block.

LABORATORY TEST(S)

- Standard laboratory testing appropriate for age, gender, and metabolic abnormalities.
- Electrolyte abnormalities and especially hyperkalemia should be excluded.

IMAGING STUDIES

Electrocardiogram (Figs. 4 and 5)

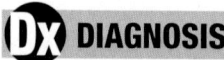

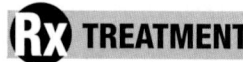

Rx TREATMENT

- Treat the underlying cause (Tables 4 and 5).
- In asymptomatic patients with an isolated bundle branch block, no therapy is required.

NONPHARMACOLOGIC THERAPY

Cardiac resynchronization therapy (CRT) with biventricular or His-bundle devices can benefit selected patients with LBBB and depressed EF, if heart failure is present. Permanent pacemaker is appropriate for patients with cardiac syncope or coexisting third degree, or Mobitz type II second degree AV block, when not due to a reversible cause.

TABLE 1 Common Diagnostic Criteria for Fascicular Blocks

Left Anterior Fascicular Block
Frontal plane mean QRS axis between −45 and −90 degrees qR pattern in lead aVL
QRS duration <120 msec
Time to peak R wave in aVL ≥45 msec

Left Posterior Fascicular Block
Frontal plane mean QRS axis between +90 and +180 degrees rS pattern in leads I and aVL with qR patterns in leads III and aVF
QRS duration <120 msec
Exclusion of other factors causing right axis deviation (e.g., right ventricular overload patterns, lateral infarction)

From Mann DL, et al: *Braunwald's heart disease*, ed 10, Philadelphia, 2015, Elsevier.

TABLE 2 Common Diagnostic Criteria for Bundle Branch Blocks

Complete Left Bundle Branch Block
QRS duration ≥120 msec
Broad, notched, or slurred R waves in leads I, aVL, V_5, and V_6
Small or absent initial r waves in right precordial leads (V_1 and V_2) followed by deep S waves
Absent septal q waves in leads I, V_5, and V_6
Prolonged time to peak R wave (>60 msec) in V_5 and V_6

Complete Right Bundle Branch Block
QRS duration ≥120 msec rsr′, rsR′, or rSR′, patterns in leads V_1 and V_2
S waves in leads I and V_6 ≥40 msec wide
Normal time to peak R wave in leads V_5 and V_6 but >50 msec in V_1

From Mann DL, et al: *Braunwald's heart disease*, ed 10, Philadelphia, 2015, Elsevier.

TABLE 3 Differential Diagnosis of Bundle Branch Block

	Incomplete	Complete	Incomplete	Complete	Left Anterior Fascicular Block	Left Posterior Fascicular Block
QRS Axis	Normal	Normal	Normal or left	Normal or left	Left and >−45°	Right and >+90°
QRS Duration	<120 msec	>120 msec	<120 msec	>130 msec	<120 msec	<120 msec
I	qRs	Deep S	No q wave	Tall R wave, no q wave, no S wave	Positive QRS	rS
aVL	qRs	Deep S		Tall R wave, no q wave, no S wave	qR	rS
II, III, aVF					rS	qR
Precordial Leads	rSR' in V1-V2, qRs in V5-V6	RsR' in V1-V2, deep S in V5-V6	No q wave in V5-V6	QS or rS in V1-V2, tall R wave and no q wave or S wave in V5-V6	Poor R wave progression in V1-V3	
aVR	rsR'				Often tall R wave	

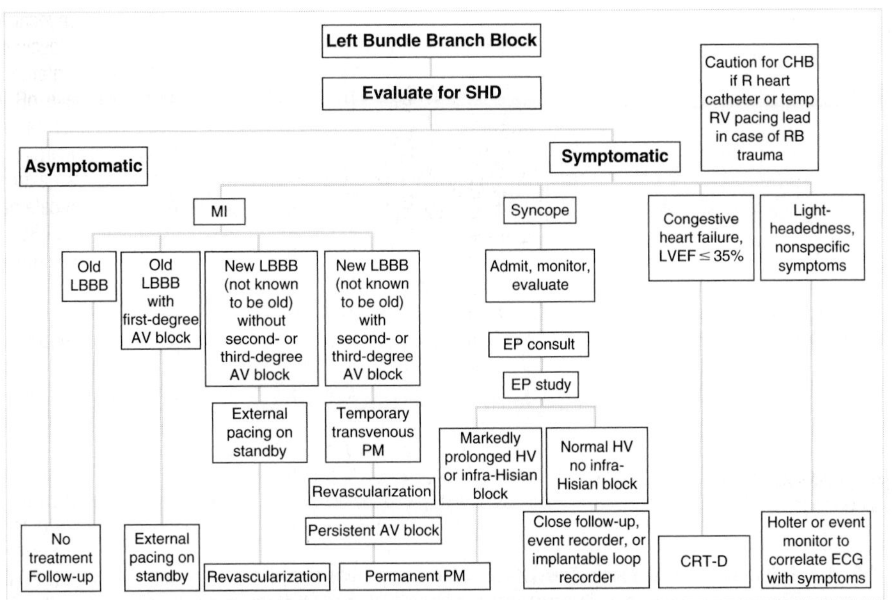

FIG. 2 Left bundle branch block. *CHB*, Complete heart block; *LBBB*, left bundle branch block; *LVEF*, left ventricular ejection fraction; *MI*, myocardial infarction; *PM*, pacemaker; *SHD*, structural heart disease (no overt evidence of myocardial, valvular, congenital, or coronary heart disease). (From Olshansky B, Chung MK, Pogwizd SM, Goldschlager N: *Arrhythmia essentials*, ed 2, Philadelphia, 2017, Elsevier.)

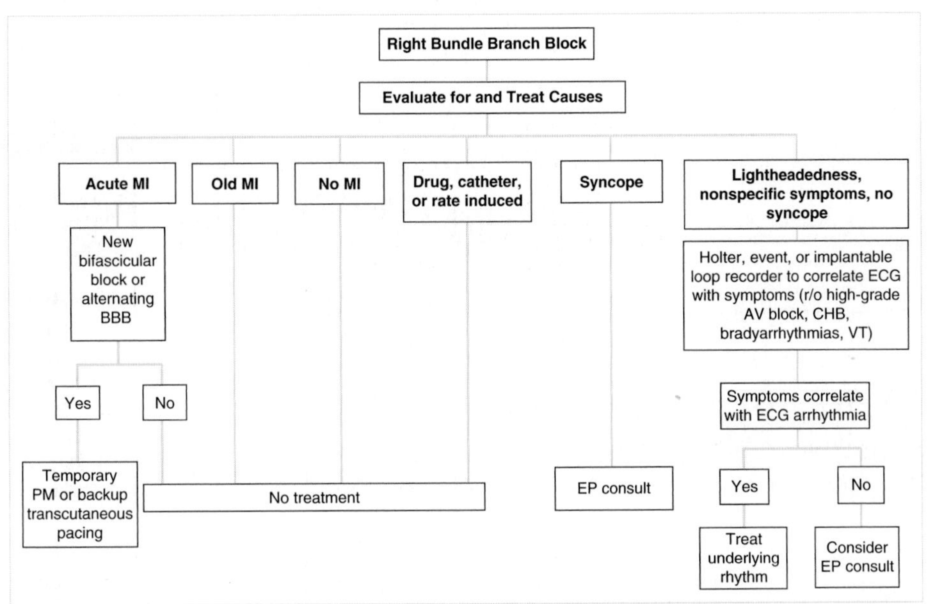

FIG. 3 Right bundle branch block. *BBB*, Bundle branch block; *CHB*, complete heart block; *EP*, electrophysiology, *MI*, myocardial infarction; *PM*, pacemaker; *VT*, ventricular tachycardia. (From Olshansky B, Chung MK, Pogwizd SM, Goldschlager N: *Arrhythmia essentials*, ed 2, Philadelphia, 2017, Elsevier.)

ACUTE GENERAL Rx

In acutely established bundle branch block, investigate the cause. In acute LBBB, anterior myocardial infarction should be investigated whereas in acute RBBB investigation should target pulmonary embolism.

CHRONIC Rx

Optimization of potential coexisting comorbidities such as coronary artery disease, heart failure, hyperkalemia, diabetes

DISPOSITION

There is no specific disposition plan for isolated bundle branch block. Entities such as myocardial ischemia or infarction, myocarditis, and cardiomyopathy should be investigated prior to disposition in a new bundle branch block with associated symptoms. Pulmonary embolism should also be investigated in a new RBBB with suspecting symptoms.

REFERRAL

In selected patients at risk for sudden cardiac death such as Brugada syndrome, or in cases of new bundle branch block associated with acute symptoms, referral is indicated.

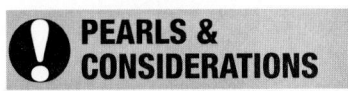

PEARLS & CONSIDERATIONS

COMMENTS

Acute LBBB can be caused by anterior myocardial infarction. Acute RBBB can be due to pulmonary embolism. Bundle branch block is a normal variant, especially in young individuals.

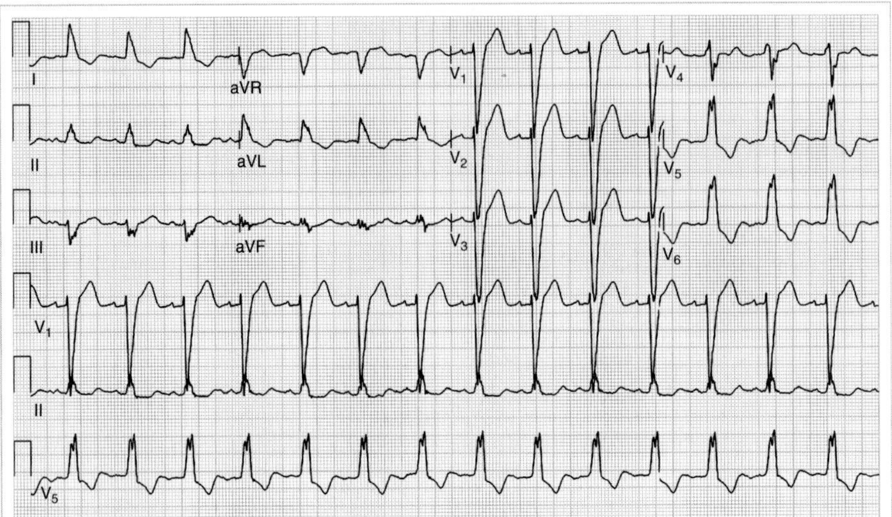

FIG. 4 Left bundle branch block. This 12-lead ECG shows LBBB that is characterized by a wide (>0.12 seconds) QRS complex; broad monophasic R waves in leads V_5, V_6, and I that are commonly slurred or notched; rS or QS complexes in the right precordial leads; and secondary ST- and T-wave changes that are opposite in direction to the major QRS deflections. The mean frontal plane QRS axis is normal, but left-axis deviation may be present. (From Olshansky B, Chung MK, Pogwizd SM, Goldschlager N: *Arrhythmia essentials*, ed 2, Philadelphia, 2017, Elsevier.)

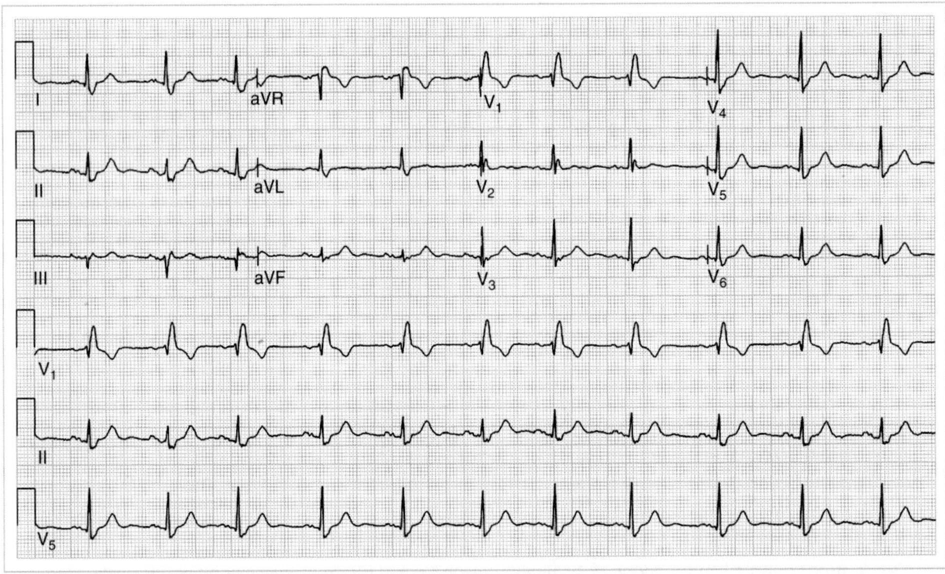

FIG. 5 Right bundle branch block. This 12-lead ECG shows RBBB that is characterized by a wide (≥0.12 seconds) QRS complex; a secondary R wave (R′) in V_1 and V_2 (rsR′ or rSR′) with R′ usually taller than the initial R wave; a wide, slurred S wave in leads V_5, V_6, and I; and secondary ST- and T-wave changes that are opposite in direction to the terminal QRS deflections over the right precordial leads. The mean frontal plane QRS axis is normal. (From Olshansky B, Chung MK, Pogwizd SM, Goldschlager N: *Arrhythmia essentials*, ed 2, Philadelphia, 2017, Elsevier.)

History and physical exam are needed to identify associated cardiac abnormalities. In patients with heart failure, and depressed ejection fraction, cardiac resynchronization is beneficial in the presence of LBBB but not in the presence of RBBB.

PREVENTION

Modification of associated comorbidities such as optimization of heart failure, coronary artery disease, hypertension, and diabetes.

PATIENT/FAMILY EDUCATION

Bundle branch block is a problem in the heart's electrical system. There are several types, but clinically the most important is the left bundle branch block in which one of the two main "wires" in the heart is not functioning correctly. As a result, the heart's pumping chambers are squeezing out of sync and can worsen the heart's ability to pump in people with heart failure. It is more common in older adults and people with serious heart disease.

TABLE 4 Left Bundle Branch Block Management

Setting	Therapy
Asymptomatic normal LV function	• No therapy—rule out structural heart disease, ischemic heart disease. • Requires long-term follow-up. • If instrumentation of the right ventricle is planned, be ready to temporarily pace (preferably externally or via a temporary pacemaker wire) if transient traumatic RBBB with resultant complete AVB is induced. • Trauma to the right bundle can last from minutes to more than 24 hours.
Symptomatic (syncope, lightheadedness)	• Admit, monitor, and evaluate for structural heart disease. • If syncope occurs, EP consultation and possible EP testing is indicated. • If HV interval is 100 ms or more or if infra-Hisian block is provoked with atrial pacing at rates of <160 bpm with or without procainamide challenge, implant a permanent pacemaker.
Symptomatic (CHF)	• LVEF is 35% or less, NYHA class II, III or IV heart failure symptoms are present with LBBB with QRS duration of more than 130 ms: CRT-D ICD implantation is indicated and may improve LV function and heart failure symptoms, and reduce the risk of sudden death.
MI	• New (or not known to be old) LBBB: revascularization with direct PTCA with or without stent. • Temporary pacemaker if second-degree or third-degree AVB is present. • New onset LBBB indicates extensive myocardial ischemia or infarction and can be associated with a poorer prognosis. • Have external (transcutaneous) pacing on standby if no AVB is present.
Preoperative	• No therapy is required if the patient is asymptomatic, whether or not coronary artery disease or systolic dysfunction is known to be present. • Cardiac workup (stress test, echocardiogram) to exclude structural heart disease if symptomatic. • LBBB is not per se an indication for treadmill testing. If stress testing is performed, imaging must accompany the test if the aim is to document the presence of obstructive coronary artery disease; imaging is not required if the aim of the stress test is the assessment of effort tolerance.
Postoperative	• No therapy if asymptomatic. • Common after aortic valve replacement (usually persistent) and after CABG (transient due to cardioplegia).
Alternating LBBB and RBBB	• Alternating BBB may be due to trifascicular disease (see trifascicular block). • Because of the high rate of progression to CHB, permanent pacemaker implantation is advised. • Alternating BBB may also be seen as a digitalis toxic rhythm, although in current practice this occurs only rarely.

AVB, Atrioventricular block; *BBB*, bundle branch block; *CABG*, coronary artery bypass graft; *CHB*, complete atrioventricular block; *CHF*, congestive heart failure; *CRT-D*, cardiac resynchronization and defibrillation therapy; *EP*, electrophysiology; *HV*, histoventricular; *ICD*, implantable cardioverter defibrillator; *LBBB*, left bundle branch block; *LV*, left ventricular; *LVEF*, left ventricular ejection fraction; *MI*, myocardial infarction; *NYHA*, New York Heart Association; *PTCA*, percutaneous transluminal coronary angioplasty; *RBBB*, right bundle branch block.
From Olshansky B, Chung MK, Pogwizd SM, Goldschlager N: *Arrhythmia essentials*, ed 2, Philadelphia, 2017, Elsevier.

TABLE 5 Right Bundle Branch Block Management

Setting	Therapy
Outpatient asymptomatic	• No therapy. • May occur with instrumentation of the right ventricle (e.g., Swan-Ganz catheter) and trauma to the right bundle. • Can last up to 24 h.
Symptomatic (syncope)	• Admit the patient with RBBB who has syncope. • If symptoms of syncope occur (may be related to AVB or VT), attempt to correlate symptoms with rhythm by Holter or event monitoring. • Evaluate for underlying structural cardiac disease. • Consider EP testing to assess AV conduction and the presence of inducible VT (present in up to 30% of symptomatic RBBB patients) if the patient is syncopal.
MI	• Isolated RBBB: No therapy. • RBBB with LAFB or LPFB (that is new or not known to be old) or alternating BBB: • Temporary pacemaker • Alternatively, placement of a transcutaneous pacing system • RBBB occurs in 3% to 7% of MIs, often with LAFB, and usually because of anterior or anteroseptal infarction. • The combination is less common in the current era of early revascularization via percutaneous techniques.
Preoperative	• No therapy—temporary pacemaker not required. • Perform cardiac evaluation to exclude other cardiovascular disease.
Postoperative	• No treatment. • Most common conduction disturbance in this setting.
Alternating LBBB and RBBB	• Permanent pacemaker if not due to reversible cause.

AV, Atrioventricular; *AVB*, atrioventricular block; *BBB*, bundle branch block; *EP*, electrophysiology; *LAFB*, left anterior fascicular block; *LBBB*, left bundle branch block; *LPFB*, left posterior fascicular block; *MI*, myocardial infarction; *RBBB*, right bundle branch block; *VT*, ventricular tachycardia.
From Olshansky B, Chung MK, Pogwizd SM, Goldschlager N: *Arrhythmia essentials*, ed 2, Philadelphia, 2017, Elsevier.

RELATED CONTENT

Intraventricular Conduction Delay (Related Key Topic)
Atrioventricular Block (Related Key Topic)
Brugada Syndrome (Related Key Topic)
Myocardial Infarction (Related Key Topic)
Heart Failure (Related Key Topic)
Pulmonary Embolism (Related Key Topic)

AUTHORS: **IOANNIS KOULOURIDIS, M.D., M.S.,** and **JOHN WYLIE, M.D., F.A.C.C.**

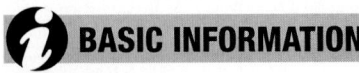

BASIC INFORMATION

DEFINITION

- Cutaneous burns can be classified by type of injury (e.g., thermal vs. chemical), burn depth (e.g., 1st, 2nd, 3rd degree), extent of burn (total burn surface area [TBSA]), and burn severity (e.g., minor vs. major). Types of burn injury include thermal (flames, scalds, hot contactants), chemical, electrical, and radiation burns. This chapter will focus on thermal and electrical burns.
- Burns can affect skin and respiratory, ocular, oral, and genital mucosa.

SYNONYMS

Thermal injury
Chemical injury
Electrical injury
Radiation injury

ICD-10CM CODES

T29.0 Burns of multiple regions, unspecified degree
T30.0 Burn of unspecified body region, unspecified degree
T30.1 Burn of first degree, body region unspecified
T30.2 Burn of second degree, body region unspecified
T30.3 Burn of third degree, body region unspecified
T31.0 Burns involving less than 10% of body surface
T31.1 Burns involving 10-19% of body surface
T31.2 Burns involving 20-29% of body surface
T31.3 Burns involving 30-39% of body surface
T31.4 Burns involving 40-49% of body surface
T31.5 Burns involving 50-59% of body surface

EPIDEMIOLOGY & DEMOGRAPHICS

PREVALENCE (IN U.S.):

- More than 1.2 million individuals experience burns in the U.S., and burn injuries account for approximately 500,000 emergency department visits, with 9% (45,000) requiring hospitalization and 0.8% (4000) resulting in death annually.
- Of thermal injury, scald burn from liquid is most common—followed by flame, flash burn, and then contact burn.

PREDOMINANT AGE & SEX: Children ages 2-4 yr have the greatest frequency of burns (most commonly scald burns), with male adolescent and young adults ages 17 to 25 with second greatest frequency (most commonly from flammable liquids).

PHYSICAL FINDINGS & CLINICAL PRESENTATION

- It is important to note that burns occur unevenly—often with various depths (Table 1).
- 1st-degree (superficial) burns—penetrate epidermis only (minimal barrier loss)
    1. Very painful, intact, erythematous skin with minimal to no edema and no blistering.
- 2nd-degree (partial-thickness) burns—epidermis and part of dermis is affected.
    1. Moist, very painful skin with edema and blistering/blebs
    2. Superficial partial-thickness burns—cherry red with two-point discrimination intact, incredibly painful
    3. Deep partial-thickness burns—mottled white and cherry red; only the sensation of pressure is intact in these areas
- 3rd-degree (full-thickness) burns—entire epidermis and dermis are affected, with destruction of hair follicles and sweat glands.
    1. The skin is dry, charred, pale, painless, and leathery. Charred vessels may be visible beneath, little or no pain, and hair pulls out easily.

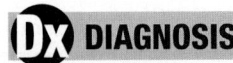

DIAGNOSIS

CLASSIFICATION

- Burns are classified by (1) depth of injury, (2) extent of injury, and (3) severity, according to the American Burn Association.
- Depth of injury (see Table 1):
    1. Indicates how the wound will heal and whether grafting will be needed.
- Extent of TBSA:
    1. The TBSA is best classified by using age-specific burn charts and the "rule of nines" (Fig. 1).
    2. For scattered burns, utilizing patient's palm including fingers to equate 1% body surface area can be helpful.
    3. TBSA indicates how aggressively the patient will need to be resuscitated.
- Severity—determined by burn depth, TBSA, age, location, type of injury, and presence/absence of coexisting conditions. Severity classification helps triage patients to outpatient, inpatient, or burn unit care (see Table 2).
    1. Minor burns—outpatient management.
    2. Moderate burns—admission to hospital with experience managing burns or burn center referral.
    3. Major burns—referral to burn center.

LABORATORY STUDIES (MODERATE OR MAJOR BURNS)

- CBC, electrolytes, BUN, creatinine, glucose, liver function tests, venous blood gas, blood coagulation, and type and screen in anticipation of blood transfusion
- *If smoke inhalation expected:* Serial ABG carboxyhemoglobin and continuous ECG
- *If electrical burn or if concern for rhabdomyolysis:* Urinalysis, urine myoglobin, and CPK levels
- *If severe lactic acidosis:* Consider checking cyanide level

IMAGING STUDIES

- If smoke inhalation suspected: Chest radiograph and bronchoscopy
- If high-voltage electrical burn: Cardiac monitoring first 24 hours

TABLE 1 Categorization of Burn by Depth

Burn Type	Histologic Depth	Clinical Presentation	Treatment	Healing Time/Prognosis
1st degree	Epidermis	Erythematous but intact skin, no blisters, pain may range in severity	Topical salves, cold compresses, NSAIDs for pain control	2-5 days with no scarring
Superficial 2nd degree (partial thickness)	Papillary dermis	Erythematous with superficial blisters, intense pain	Topical antimicrobials with gauze dressing or biosynthetic dressing (if widespread), pain control	5-21 days with no grafting
Deep 2nd degree (partial thickness)	Reticular dermis	Erythematous with superficial/deep blisters, range of pain depending on nerve involvement	Same	21-35 days with no infection; if infected, converts to full-thickness burn
3rd degree (full thickness)	Through dermis to subcutaneous tissue. Can involve fascia, muscle and bone.	White or black, possible eschar, may or may not be painful depending on nerve damage	Usually requires grafting, may require resuscitation depending on TBSA affected, pain control	Large areas require grafting, but small areas may heal from the edges after weeks

From Kliegman RM et al: *Nelson textbook of pediatrics,* ed 19, Philadelphia, 2011, Saunders; and Kessides MC, Skelsey MK: Management of acute partial-thickness burns, *Cutis* 86:249-257, 2010.

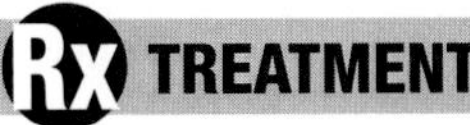

TREATMENT

DIFFERENTIAL DIAGNOSIS

Cultural practices leading to burn-like lesions in distinctive patterns (e.g., cupping, coining, moxibustion), cellulitis, Stevens-Johnson syndrome/toxic epidermolytic necrolysis

ACUTE GENERAL Rx

MINOR BURNS (1ST DEGREE BURNS AND 2ND/3RD DEGREE BURNS OF LIMITED TBSA):

- Outpatient management—"6 Cs"
  1. Clothing: Remove hot or burned clothing.
  2. Cooling: Cool (approximately 54° F) for 10 to 30 minutes (under faucet or compress) to reduce edema/pain by conducting heat away from skin. Not recommended with extensive burns due to theoretical risk of hypothermia and shock. No ice packs.
  3. Cleaning: Wash gently with mild alcohol-free soap, then normal saline daily. Remove all old ointment and any loose skin. Blot dry. No evidence supports vigorous cleansing with antiseptic solutions. Embedded materials should be removed by copious irrigation using a large-gauge syringe.
  4. Chemoprophylaxis: Tetanus immunization (all deep 2nd and 3rd degree burns). Routine skin cultures are NOT recommended except when wound infection suspected, and prophylactic systemic antibiotics are NOT recommended. All 2nd and 3rd degree burns are treated with a topical antimicrobial agent. This may include silver sulfadiazine, bacitracin, bismuth-impregnated vaseline gauze, or silver-impregnated synthetic dressings.
  5. Covering: All 2nd and 3rd degree burns should be covered with sterile dressing. If financial resources are limited, instead of gauze, can purchase cotton gloves, T-shirts, or similar at discount stores, wash, and reuse.
  6. Comfort: Analgesics (Tylenol and NSAIDs—alone or in combination with opioids) around the clock are recommended. Additional "rescue" analgesics before dressing changes and physical activity recommended.

MODERATE AND MAJOR BURNS (2ND/3RD DEGREE BURNS OF EXTENSIVE TBSA):

- Patients with moderate/major burns (Fig. 1) should be admitted to the hospital or referred to a burn center. Indications for hospitalization for burns are described in Table 2
- Resuscitation (in addition to previous)
  1. Assessment of ABCs: Establish airway and assess breathing (inspect for inhalation injury and intubate for suspected airway edema, often seen 12 to 24 hours later); O_2; establish circulation (place two large-bore peripheral IV lines, ECG)
  2. IV fluid resuscitation—Parkland formula (Ringer's lactate at 2 to 4 ml/kg per % TBSA per 24 hours with half the calculated fluid given in the first 8 hours is an effective modality in severe burns (Fig. 2)
  3. Baseline neurologic and vascular assessment
  4. Foley catheter and NG tube (20% of patients develop an ileus)—urine output 30 ml/hr (Fig. 3)
  5. Optimize nutritional support: Mayes equations to calculate energy requirements after burn (Box 1)
- Frequent reassessment in the first 24 to 72 hours, as wound depth can change significantly
- The four phases of burn care, with physiologic changes and objectives, are described in Table 3. Box 2 describes the modified Brooke resuscitation formula

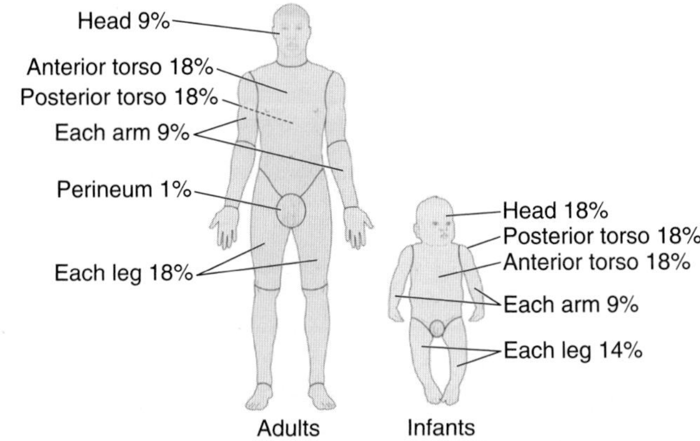

FIG. 1 The "rule of nines" for estimating second-degree and third-degree burns. Because infants have significantly larger heads and smaller legs than do adults, different rules must be used in evaluating these patients. A simple, practical rule is that the palm of the patient's hand, with fingers, equals 1% of the total body area. (From Ferri F: *Practical guide to the care of the medical patient*, ed 9, St Louis, 2014, Elsevier.)

BURN WOUND CARE BY BURN DEPTH Rx

GENERAL:

- Vigilant wound care with dressings to prevent evaporation and minimize threat of wound colonization and infection of nonintact skin
- Daily activity necessary to maintain function of burned extremity, decrease pain and swelling, and promote healing
- 1st-degree burns (skin intact):
  1. *Dressing:* None required (except to protect from injury); topical antibacterial agents NOT recommended
  2. *Other:* Emollients, cool compresses (avoid ice), if pruritic, trial of antihistamines
  3. *Prognosis:* Heals within 1 week without scarring. May heal with pigmentary changes (limit by sunscreen and sun avoidance of area for 1 yr)

TABLE 2 Classification of Burns by Severity and Indications for Hospitalization or Burn Center Referral

Criteria	Minor Burn	Moderate Burn	Major Burn
Total body surface area (%)	• All 1st degree burns <10% adults <5% children or elderly • <2% for 3rd degree	• 2nd degree burns 10%-20% adults 5%-10% in children or elderly • 2%-5% 3rd degree	• All 1st degree burns >20% adults >10% children and elderly • >5% 3rd degree
Type of burn injury		• Low-voltage burn • Suspected inhalation injury	• High-voltage burn • Chemical burn • Known
Location		Circumferential burn	• Clinically significant burn to face, eyes, ears, genitalia, over joints
Coexisting conditions		• Concomitant medical problem predisposing to infection (e.g., diabetes, sickle cell anemia)	• Significant associated injuries (e.g., fracture, other major trauma)
	Outpatient management	Inpatient management—consider referral to burn center*	Referral to burn center

*Per the American Burn Association (ABA), any partial-thickness burn >10% total body surface area or any factors listed in moderate or major burn category warrant referral to burn center. Additional factors per the ABA include burned children in a hospital without qualified personnel or equipment for the care of children and burn injury in a patient who will require special social, emotional, or rehabilitative intervention (including suspected child abuse).

Modified from Singer AJ, Dagum AB: Current management of acute cutaneous wounds, *N Engl J Med* 359 (10):1037-1046, 2008; www.ameriburn.org.

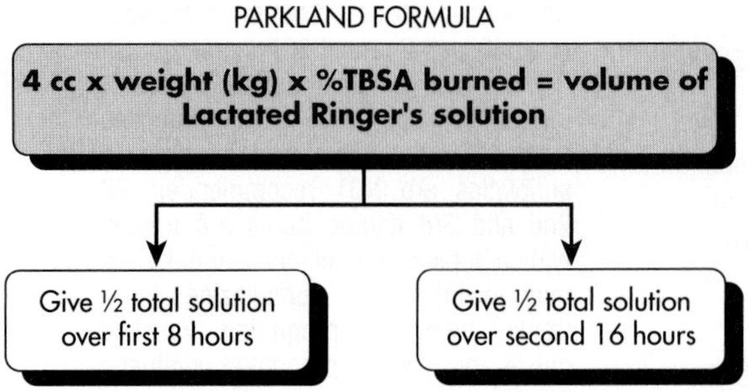

PARKLAND FORMULA

4 cc x weight (kg) x %TBSA burned = volume of Lactated Ringer's solution

Give ½ total solution over first 8 hours

Give ½ total solution over second 16 hours

FIG. 2 Parkland formula. *TBSA*, Total body surface area. (From Cameron JL, Cameron AM: *Current surgical therapy*, ed 12, Philadelphia, 2017, Elsevier.)

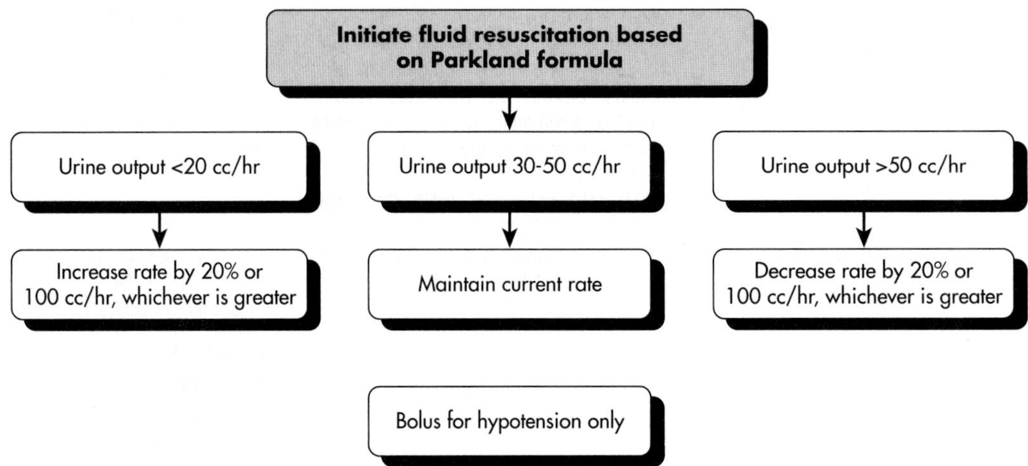
Initiate fluid resuscitation based on Parkland formula
Urine output <20 cc/hr
Urine output 30-50 cc/hr
Urine output >50 cc/hr
Increase rate by 20% or 100 cc/hr, whichever is greater
Maintain current rate
Decrease rate by 20% or 100 cc/hr, whichever is greater
Bolus for hypotension only

FIG. 3 Proposed resuscitation protocol. (From Cameron JL, Cameron AM: *Current surgical therapy*, ed 12, Philadelphia, 2017, Elsevier.)

BOX 1 Mayes Equations to Calculate Energy Requirement after a Burn

Mayes equation for a 5- to 10-yr-old burn patient with injury <50% TBSA:

$$818 + 37.4\,(\text{weightinkilograms}) + 9.3 \times \text{TBSAburn}$$

Mayes equation for a 5.5-yr-old patient with a 45% TBSA scald burn weighing 20 kg:

$$818 + 37.4\,(20\text{kg}) + 9.3 \times 45\text{TBSAscald}$$

$$818 + 748 + 481.5 = 2047.5\text{calories/day}$$

From Fuhrman BP et al: *Pediatric critical care,* ed 4, Philadelphia, 2011, Saunders.

TABLE 3 The Four Phases of Burn Care, with Physiologic Changes and Objectives

Phase and Timing	Physiologic Changes	Objectives
1: Initial evaluation and resuscitation, 0 to 72 hr	Massive capillary leak and burn shock	Accurate fluid resuscitation and thorough evaluation
2: Initial wound excision and biologic closure, days 1-7	Hyperdynamic and catabolic state with high risk of infection	Accurately identify and remove all full-thickness wounds and achieve biologic closure
3: Definitive wound closure, day 7 to week 6	Continued catabolic state and risk of nonwound septic events	Replace temporary with definitive covers and close small complex wounds
4: Rehabilitation, reconstruction, and reintegration, day 1 through discharge	Waning catabolic state and recovering strength	Initially to maintain range of motion and reduce edema; subsequently to strengthen and facilitate return to home, work, school

From Vincent JL et al: *Textbook of critical care,* ed 6, Philadelphia, 2011, Saunders.

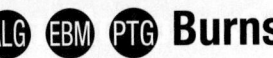

B

Diseases and Disorders

I

BOX 2 Modified Brooke Resuscitation Formula

0-24 Hours

Adults and Children >10 kg

- Lactated Ringer's: 2 to 4 ml/kg/% burn/24 hr (first half in first 8 hr)
- Colloid: None

Children <10 kg

- Lactated Ringer's: 2 to 3 ml/kg/% burn/24 hr (first half in first 8 hr)
- Lactated Ringer's with 5% dextrose: 4 ml/kg/hr
- Colloid: None

24-48 Hours

All Patients

- Crystalloid: To maintain urine output. If silver nitrate is used, sodium leaching will mandate continued isotonic crystalloid. If other topical is used, free water requirement is significant. Serum sodium should be monitored closely. Nutritional support should begin, ideally by the enteral route.
- Colloid: (5% albumin in lactated Ringer's):
    - 0% to 30% burn: None
    - 30% to 50% burn: 0.3 ml/kg/% burn/24 hr
    - 50% to 70% burn: 0.4 ml/kg/% burn/24 hr
    - >70% burn: 0.5 ml/kg/% burn/24 hr. Note: The Modified Brooke formula is a common consensus formula that is only useful in individual patients if adjusted to physiologic endpoints. Like all resuscitative formulas, it is a helpful starting point, but optimal-quality resuscitation requires the bedside presence of a physician capable of regularly evaluating resuscitation endpoints.

From Vincent JL et al: *Textbook of critical care,* ed 6, Philadelphia, 2011, Saunders.

- 2nd degree (superficial partial-thickness) burns without adherent exudate or eschar:
    1. *Blisters:* Sharp debridement of ruptured blisters; leave intact blisters. Quicker healing and reduced infections when intact blisters are not disturbed. Consider unroofing blisters that show no sign of resorption over several weeks or contain cloudy fluid
    2. *Dressing:* Topical antimicrobial ointment (e.g., bactroban) or A&D ointment with nonadherent dressing twice a day. Alternate: Biosynthetic dressing (alginates, hydrofibers, or foam dressings)—many with silver as antimicrobial (absorb exudates, maintain moist environment, require fewer dressing changes, which reduces pain/anxiety)
    3. *Prognosis:* Heals with minimal scarring in 10 to 14 days. May heal with pigmentary changes (reduced with sunscreen and sun avoidance of area × 1 yr)
- 2nd degree (deep partial-thickness) burns with adherent exudates; localized 3rd degree burns; cellulitic wounds:
    1. *Dressing:* Silver sulfadiazine 1%: Broader spectrum, better penetration of necrotic tissue than bactroban, but inhibits epithelialization and promotes hypertrophic scarring in studies. Must stop use once exudates and eschar have separated from wound. Alternative: Enzymatic debrider (e.g., Santyl or Accuzyme)—chemically debrides devitalized tissue without harming healthy tissue
    2. *Referral:* Burn specialist for consultation regarding need for excision and grafting
    3. *Prognosis:* Deep 2nd degree burns heal with significant scarring, often take 3 to 4 weeks to heal. If infected, convert to 3rd degree burns. 3rd degree burns typically require skin graft, but small areas may heal from edges after weeks

DISPOSITION/FOLLOW-UP CARE

- Outpatient: Evaluate next day to assess level of injury, level of pain, and ability to manage dressing changes on own. If insufficient, daily evaluation until complete wound epithelialization recommended. Epithelialization: Tiny islands of epithelialization throughout wound. If no epithelialization after 2 weeks, or subsequent evaluation reveals 3rd degree burn, referral to burn surgeon recommended. Box E3 describes common complications in burn patients.
- Following re-epithelialization, visits every 4 to 6 weeks to monitor for hypertrophic scar formation (early referral to burn/scar specialist if occurs).
- Mortality rates higher in patients >60 yr of age, with burns >40% TBSA, or with inhalation injury. Long-term risk of developing squamous cell carcinoma of the skin within burn injury. Long-term skin monitoring necessary.

REFERRAL

Consultation of burn specialist or burn center referral per Table 2.

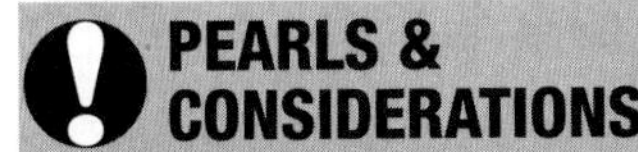

COMMENTS

- In circumferential skin burns, look for compartment syndrome of limbs (e.g., tightening, progressive deterioration of peripheral motor and sensory exam findings, severe pain, and loss of arterial Doppler signals). Escharotomy may be necessary.
- If child abuse is suspected, social services at the hospital or child protective services must be contacted.
- Fig. E4 describes an algorithm for the treatment of chemical burns.

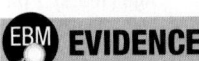

Available at ExpertConsult.com

SUGGESTED READINGS

Available at ExpertConsult.com

RELATED CONTENT

Burns (Patient Information)
Electrical and Lightning Injury (Related Key Topic)

AUTHOR: **LISA K. PAPPAS-TAFFER, M.D.**

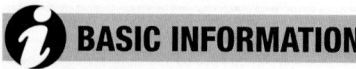

BASIC INFORMATION

DEFINITION

Carcinoma of unknown primary (CUP) refers to a diverse group of malignancies for which the anatomic site of origin cannot be determined despite extensive investigations.

SYNONYMS

Cancer NOS
Cancer unspecified site
Malignancy unspecified site
CUP

ICD-10CM CODE
C80.1 Malignant (primary) neoplasm, unspecified

EPIDEMIOLOGY & DEMOGRAPHICS

- CUP accounts for about 4% of all cancers, and the annual incidence in the United States is 7-12 cases per 100,000 persons.
- It is the seventh most frequent common cause of cancer and the fourth most common cause of cancer death. It predominantly occurs in adults and is more common in males.
- In the United States, an estimated 31,810 new cases are expected in 2018. CUP incidence rates have been decreasing since the early 1980s, 3.6 % per yr in the last two decades.
- Most cases of CUP are carcinomas, which are divided into adenocarcinomas (90%), squamous cell carcinomas (5%), and undifferentiated carcinomas (5%).
- There is a variable rate of mutations detected in CUP (18%-30%). The tumor suppressor gene *p-53* has overexpression rates (40%-50%) or mutation rates (25%-40%) that are comparable to that seen in other solid tumors. The evaluation of VEGF-A (vascular endothelial growth factor-A, angiogenesis factor) and matrix metalloproteinases (enzymes that degrade stroma) showed that these are universally expressed and active angiogenesis is present in CUP.

PHYSICAL FINDINGS & CLINICAL PRESENTATION

- Physical findings can be variable and include generalized and organ-specific findings.
- General findings can include cachexia, pallor, edema, icterus, edema, skin rash, muscle wasting among others.
- Organ-specific findings are related to the dysfunction of the underlying organ(s) involved with CUP.
- The clinical course is often highlighted by a short presentation history, with symptoms and signs associated with metastatic sites, early dissemination, aggressive clinical course, and occasionally an unpredictable metastatic pattern.
- Multiple organs are involved at diagnosis in up to half of patients.
- The clinicopathologic subsets comprising CUP are shown in Table 1.

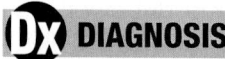

DIAGNOSIS

WORKUP

- Comprehensive medical history
- Complete physical examination with particular attention to skin, lymph node sites, organ enlargement, and testes; also rectal examination and pelvic examination (in women) (Table 2)
- Histopathology review of biopsy specimens

LABORATORY TESTS

- Complete blood count.
- Comprehensive chemistry panel.
- Urine analysis.
- Stool for occult blood.
- Tumor markers (in selected cases): Prostate-specific antigen (PSA), β-human chorionic gonadotrophin, α-fetoprotein.
- Adequate tissue biopsy with immunohistochemical (IHC) staining is done to guide broad diagnostic category assignments—carcinoma, melanoma, sarcoma, or lymphoma.
- Subtyping with IHC panels helps further classifying into adenocarcinoma, squamous carcinoma, germ cell tumor, neuroendocrine, thyroid, hepatocellular, or renal origin.
- Stepwise approach for IHC derived diagnosis of likely site of origin are depicted in Table 3.
- In up to 25% cases, a single site of origin can be narrowed down by IHC staining (e.g., TTF-1 positive and CK-1 positive lung cancer profile).
- Molecular diagnosis is carried out by commercially available multi-gene assays that utilize micro-array or polymerase chain reaction assays and can assist in finalizing diagnosis in up to 80% to 90% of cases in which initial IHC staining has been inconclusive.

IMAGING STUDIES

- CT scans of the chest, abdomen, and pelvis; also CT of the neck in case of neck lymphadenopathy
- For selected cases
  1. PET scan
  2. Mammography and/or breast MRI
  3. Testicular ultrasonography

Rx TREATMENT

- CUP patients often require early supportive care for their advanced cancer; also there is elevated psychosocial distress with the uncertainties of diagnosis and treatment options. Anxiety and depression are more common in CUP patients compared to patients with known primaries.
- Treatment is based according to the most likely site of origin for the cancer, with systemic chemotherapy typically being the mainstay of therapy.
- Next-generation gene sequencing and in situ hybridization techniques in a large study of 1806 CUP cases were able to identify potential biomarkers predictive of therapeutic efficacy in 96% of cases. Additionally, biomarkers associated with a potential lack of benefit were identified in numerous cases, which could further refine the management of patients with CUP.
- In another study of 442 patients with CUP, the use of targeted clinical-grade, next-generation sequencing resulted in the detection of alterations in circulating tumor DNA in 80% of patients. Among the patients harboring characterized alterations, distinct genomic profiles were observed in the majority of cases exhibited potentially targetable alterations with currently available biologic therapies.

TABLE 1 Clinicopathologic Subsets of Patients with CUP

	Median Age (Years)	Sex of Patients (M/F)	Histopathology
Lymph nodes			
Mediastinal retroperitoneal	<50	70%/30%	UDF or PDF
Axillary	52	0%/100%	Adenocarcinoma (WDF, MDF, or PDF)
Cervical	57-60	80%/20%	SCC
Inguinal	58	50%/50%	UDF, SCC, mixed SCC and adenocarcinoma
Peritoneal cavity			
Primary peritoneal in women	55-65	0%/100%	Adenocarcinoma (serous papillary)
Ascites of other unknown origin	–	–	Adenocarcinoma (MDF or PDF; mucin; with or without signet ring cells)
Neuroendocrine tumors	63	60%/40%	PDF with neuroendocrine features; low-grade neuroendocrine cancers; small-cell anaplastic cancers
Liver (mainly) or other organs, or both	62	61%/39%	Adenocarcinoma (MDF or PDF)
Lungs			
Pulmonary metastases	–	–	Adenocarcinoma (WDF, MDF, or PDF)
Pleural effusions	–	–	Adenocarcinoma (MDF or PDF)
Bones (one or more)	–	–	Adenocarcinoma (WDF, MDF, or PDF)
Brain (one or more)	51-55	M>F	Adenocarcinoma (WDF, UDF, or PDF); SCC

CUP, Cancer of unknown primary; *F,* Women; *M,* men; *MDF,* moderately differentiated; *PDF,* poorly differentiated; *SCC,* squamous cell carcinoma; *UDF,* undifferentiated; *WDF,* well differentiated.
From Pavlidis N, Pentheroudakis G: Cancer of unknown primary site, *Lancet* 379(9824):1428–1435, 2012.

TABLE 2 Recommended Evaluation Following Initial Light Microscopic Diagnosis

Diagnosis	Clinical Evaluation*	Special Pathologic Studies
Adenocarcinoma (or poorly differentiated adenocarcinoma)	PET CT of chest, abdomen; men: serum psa; women: mammogram; additional directed radiologic or endoscopic studies to evaluate abnormal symptoms, signs, laboratory values	Men: PSA stain; women: estrogen and progesterone receptor stains (if clinical features suggest metastatic breast cancer)
Poorly differentiated carcinoma	PET CT of chest, abdomen; serum hCG, AFP; additional directed radiologic or endoscopic studies to evaluate abnormal symptoms, signs, laboratory values	Immunoperoxidase staining; electron microscopy (if immunoperoxidase stains indeterminate)
Squamous carcinoma, cervical nodes	PET direct laryngoscopy with visualization; biopsy of nasopharynx, pharynx, hypopharynx, larynx; fiberoptic bronchoscopy (if laryngoscopy is negative)	—
Squamous carcinoma, inguinal nodes	PET complete examination of perineal area (including pelvic examination); anoscopy cystoscopy	—

AFP, α-Fetoprotein; *CT*, computed tomography; *hCG*, human chorionic gonadotropin; *PET*, positron emission tomography; *PSA*, prostate-specific antigen.
*In addition to a history, physical examination, complete blood cell counts, chemistry profile, and chest radiograph.
From Goldman L, Schafer AI: *Goldman's Cecil medicine,* ed 25, Philadelphia, 2016, Saunders.

TABLE 3 Immunohistochemical Approaches for Diagnosis of CUP

	Diagnosis
Step One	
AE1 or AE3 pan-cytokeratin	Carcinoma
Common leukocyte antigen	Lymphoma
S100; HMB-45	Melanoma
S100; vimentin	Sarcoma
Step Two	
CK7 or CK20; PSA	Adenocarcinoma
PLAP; OCT4; AFP; human chorionic gonadotropin	Germ cell tumors
Hepatocyte paraffin1; canalicular pCEA, CD10, or CD13	Hepatocellular carcinoma
RCC; CD10	Renal cell carcinoma
TTF1; thyroglobulin	Thyroid carcinoma
Chromogranin; synaptophysin, PGP9.5; CD56	Neuroendocrine carcinoma
CK5 or CK6; p63	Squamous cell carcinoma
Step Three	
PSA; PAP	Prostate
TTF1	Lung
GCDFP-15; mammaglobin; ER	Breast
CDX2; CK20	Colon
CDX2 (intestinal epithelium); CK20; CK7	Pancreas or biliary
ER; CA-125; mesothelin; WT1	Ovary

Step one detects broad type of cancer. Step two detects subtype. Step three detects origin of adenocarcinoma. Positive results with any of these stains indicates a tumor is present, but without absolute certainty.
AFP, α-Fetoprotein; *CA-125*, cancer antigen 125; *ER*, estrogen receptor; *GCDFP-15*, gross cystic disease fluid protein 15; *OCT4*, octamer-binding transcription factor 4; *PAP*, prostatic acid phosphatase; *pCEA*, polyclonal carcinoembryonic antigen; *PLAP*, placental alkaline phosphatase; *PSA*, prostate-specific antigen; *RCC*, renal cell carcinoma antigen *TTF-1*, thyroid transcription factor 1; *WT1*, Wilms' tumor 1.
From Pavlidis N, Pentheroudakis G: Cancer of unknown primary site, *Lancet* 379(9824):1428-1435, 2012.

TABLE 4 Prognostic Classification of CUP Patients

Favorable Subset
Women with papillary adenocarcinoma of the peritoneal cavity
Women with adenocarcinoma involving the axillary lymph nodes
Poorly differentiated carcinoma with midline distribution
Poorly differentiated neuroendocrine carcinoma
Squamous cell carcinoma involving cervical lymph nodes
Adenocarcinoma with a colon-cancer profile (CK20+, CK7−, CDX2+)
Men with blastic bone metastases and elevated prostate-specific antigen (adenocarcinoma)
Isolated inguinal adenopathy (squamous carcinoma)
Patients with one small, potentially resectable tumor
Unfavorable Subset
Adenocarcinoma metastatic to the liver or other organs
Nonpapillary malignant ascites (adenocarcinoma)
Multiple cerebral metastases (adenocarcinoma or squamous carcinoma)
Several lung or pleural metastases (adenocarcinoma)
Multiple metastatic lytic bone disease (adenocarcinoma)
Squamous cell carcinoma of the abdominopelvic cavity

From Pavlidis N, Pentheroudakis G: Cancer of unknown primary site, *Lancet* 379(9824):1428-1435, 2012.

- Favorable and unfavorable CUP subsets are shown in Table 4.
- ***Favorable CUP:***
  1. Women with peritoneal adenocarcinoma when treated as advanced ovarian cancer with surgical cytoreduction and adjuvant systemic chemotherapy can have median survivals in the 36-month range.
  2. Patients with a midline tumor characteristically treated as germ cell tumors have median survivals of 12 months.
  3. Patients with poorly differentiated neuroendocrine cancers are treated with combination platinum-containing chemotherapy and median survivals are in the 15-month range.
  4. Women with axillary nodal adenocarcinoma are approached as breast cancers with treatment plans incorporating axillary and breast surgery followed by adjuvant chemotherapy, hormone therapy and radiotherapy; survival rates are comparable to similarly staged breast cancers.
  5. Patients with metastatic squamous neck nodal cancer are treated as head–neck cancers with chemoradiotherapy and/or neck dissection.
  6. Patients with a colon adenocarcinoma profile are treated with systemic regimens as in metastatic colorectal cancers with median survivals in the 24-month range.
  7. Men with blastic bone metastases and elevated prostate specific antigen are treated with initial androgen deprivation therapy and later on with systemic chemotherapy.
- ***Unfavorable CUP:***
  1. Account for 75% to 80% of all CUP patients.
  2. The most common presentation is advanced visceral disease, often with liver metastases; median survivals with systemic platinum and taxane-containing chemotherapy are typically in the range of 6 to 7 months.

DISPOSITION

Newer clinical practice guidelines recommend that gene panel testing be routinely undertaken to support diagnosis based on the findings of genomic mutations and to select a therapeutic drug that is likely to be effective.

SUGGESTED READINGS

Available at ExpertConsult.com

AUTHOR: **RITESH RATHORE, M.D.**

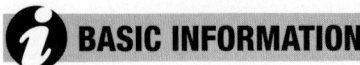

BASIC INFORMATION

DEFINITION

Infection caused by the species of the genus *Candida.* All the different *Candida* species can cause disease, but infections caused by *Candida albicans* are the most common. *Candida* species are ubiquitous and are the most common fungal pathogens affecting mankind. Cutaneous candidiasis comprises superficial *Candida* infections of the skin and mucosal membranes.

Cutaneous candidiasis can be classified into two subgroups: cutaneous candidiasis syndromes and chronic mucocutaneous syndromes. Cutaneous candidiasis syndromes include:

- Generalized cutaneous candidiasis
- Intertrigo
- *Candida* folliculitis
- Paronychia/onychomycosis
- Perianal candidiasis
- Erosio interdigitalis blastomycetica
- Balanitis

Chronic mucocutaneous syndromes include:

- Oropharyngeal candidiasis
- Esophageal candidiasis
- Vulvovaginal candidiasis
- GI candidiasis (gastric/intestines/perianal)
- *Candida* cystitis

SYNONYMS

Yeast infection
Candidosis
Moniliasis
Oidiomycosis

ICD-10CM CODES

B37.2	Candidiasis of skin and nail
B37.8	Candidiasis, unspecified
B37.89	Other sites of candidiasis

EPIDEMIOLOGY & DEMOGRAPHICS

- *Candida* species: It is the most common fungal infection in immunocompromised people.
- Most females (75%) experience an episode of vulvovaginal candidiasis in their lifetime.

INCIDENCE: Estimated to be 50 cases per 100,000 persons

PREVALENCE: Colonizes more than 50% of U.S. population

PREDOMINANT SEX AND AGE:

- Female > male
- No predominant age, but neonates and the elderly (adults >65 yr) are susceptible to *Candida* colonization and to getting mucocutaneous candidiasis.

RISK FACTORS: Risk factors that allow *Candida* infection include:

- Age >65 yr
- Females in the third trimester
- Defects in the mucocutaneous barrier (e.g., wounds, burns, ulcerations)
- Decreased/defective granulocytes/monocytes
- Diseases of white blood cells (e.g., chronic granulomatous disease)
- Complement deficiency
- Certain diseases associated with cell-mediated immunity (e.g., HIV, DM)
- Use of certain medications (e.g., broad-spectrum antibiotics, high doses of corticosteroids)
- Increased skin pH due to panty liners and occlusive attire
- **Chronic mucocutaneous candidiasis** (CMC) is characterized by susceptibility to *Candida* infection of skin, nails (Fig. 1), and mucous membranes. Patients with recessive CMC and autoimmunity have mutations in the autoimmune regulator *AIRE.* Mutations in the CC domain of *STAT1* underlie autosomal-dominant CMC and lead to defective Th1 and Th17 responses, which may explain the increased susceptibility to fungal infections (van de Veerdonk et al).

Anatomical sites predisposed to *Candida* infection include:

- Axilla
- Beneath the breast, abdominal fold, intertriginous areas
- Periungual creases
- Inguinal creases
- Back and buttocks of bedridden persons

PHYSICAL FINDINGS & CLINICAL PRESENTATION

There are several clinical presentations of cutaneous candidiasis. A few are presented here.

- **Cutaneous candidiasis**
  1. Presents as erythematous, sometimes shiny with flakes and fluid lesions at the edge of the redness (satellite pustules). It is itchy and the skin becomes inflamed. Pustules may be present in candidiasis of the scrotal and perineal skin
- **Gastrointestinal tract candidiasis**
  1. Oropharyngeal candidiasis
     a. Usually seen in diabetics, after exposure to inhaled steroids, broad-spectrum antibiotics, chemotherapy, radiation to head and neck, and in immunosuppressed individuals (e.g., patients with a history of HIV infection). It is also seen in some patients who wear dentures Symptoms include:
        (1) White, thick patches on the oral mucosa (Fig. 2), tongue, palate, or oropharynx or under dentures
        (2) Dysphagia, mouth soreness, and pain on eating and swallowing
        (3) Tongue burning
  2. Physical examination shows:
     a. Erythema of the buccal mucosa
     b. White patches on buccal cavity surfaces (described previously)
     c. Transverse fissuring
  3. Esophageal candidiasis:
     a. Most common in patients with:
        (1) Hematologic cancers
        (2) HIV/AIDS
     b. History of oropharyngeal candidiasis Symptoms include:
        (1) Odynophagia (pain on swallowing), hallmark of the disease
        (2) Dysphagia
        (3) Epigastric pain
        (4) Retrosternal pain
     c. Physical examination shows:
        (1) Affects mainly the distal one third of the esophagus. Endoscopy shows areas of the erythema and edema; scattered white patches or ulcers
  4. Perianal candidiasis:
     a. Skin maceration
     b. Itching
     c. Frequently extends to the perineum

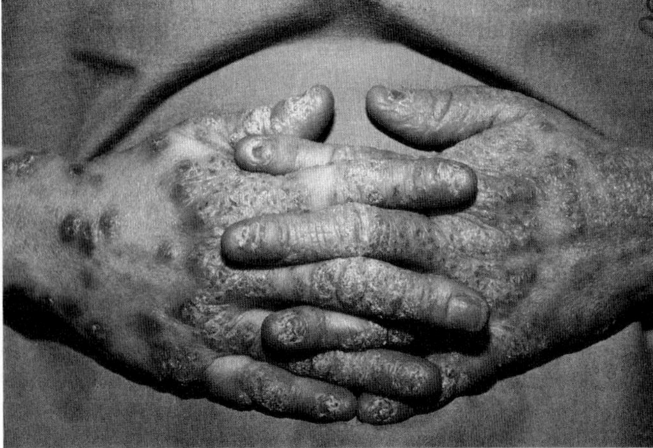

FIG. 1 Hand and nail involvement in chronic mucocutaneous candidiasis. (From James WD et al: *Andrews' diseases of skin,* ed 12, Philadelphia, 2016, Saunders.)

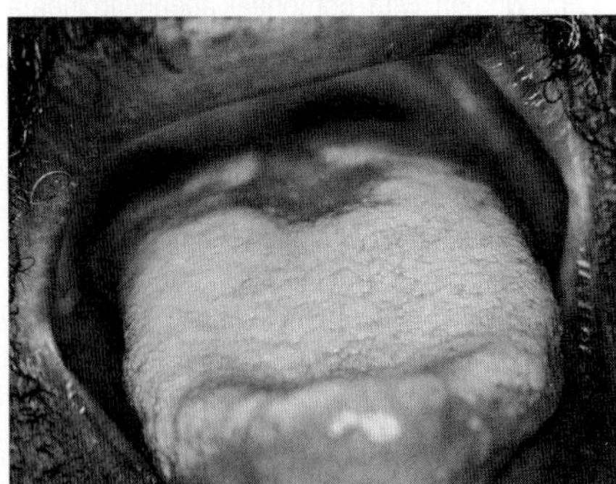

FIG. 2 Oral candidiasis. (From Swartz, MH: *Textbook of physical diagnosis,* ed 7, Philadelphia, 2014, Elsevier.)

- **Paronychia/onychomycosis**
  1. Fungal infection of the nail and surrounding tissues
  2. Associated with diabetes mellitus and immersion of hands or feet in water
  3. History: Pain and redness around and beneath the nail and nail bed
  4. Physical exam: Inflammation around the toe nail. There may also be nail thickening and discoloration (dystrophic nails). Nail loss may also occur
- **Respiratory tract candidiasis**
  1. Usually seen in hospitalized patients
  2. About 25% of outpatients have their respiratory tract colonized by *Candida* species
- **Genitourinary tract candidiasis**
  1. Vulvovaginal candidiasis
     a. Commonest form of mucosal candidiasis
     b. Risk factors include increased estrogen level (e.g., contraceptive pill), steroid or antibiotic use, diabetes, HIV infection, IUD, and diaphragm use
     c. It causes itching, curdy white discharge, and occasionally dysuria, dyspareunia, and vaginal irritation
     d. On examination the mucosa may be inflamed with vulvar and vaginal erythema, and vaginal discharge, classically described as white and curdy
     e. Painful erythema or itchy penile inflammation may occur in male sexual partners of affected females
  2. *Candida* balanitis
     a. Usually acquired through sexual contact with a partner who has vulvovaginal candidiasis
     b. Symptoms include penile pruritus and white patches on penis. There could be severe burning and itching. Infection could also spread to the perineum
     c. Physical exam: Dry, erythematous, and scaly patches on penis and sometimes on the thighs, scrotum, and buttocks
- **Others**
  1. Erosio interdigitalis blastomycetica: Denudating/macerating area commonly seen in third web space
  2. Mastitis: Injured nipples in lactating women can lead to infections, including candida infections
  3. *Candida* folliculitis: Pustulous nodules in hairy areas
  4. Intertrigo: This occurs in folds of the skin and creases (Fig. 3). It is characterized by erosions, exudation, oozing, and maceration

ETIOLOGY

The most common cause of cutaneous candidiasis is *Candida albicans.*

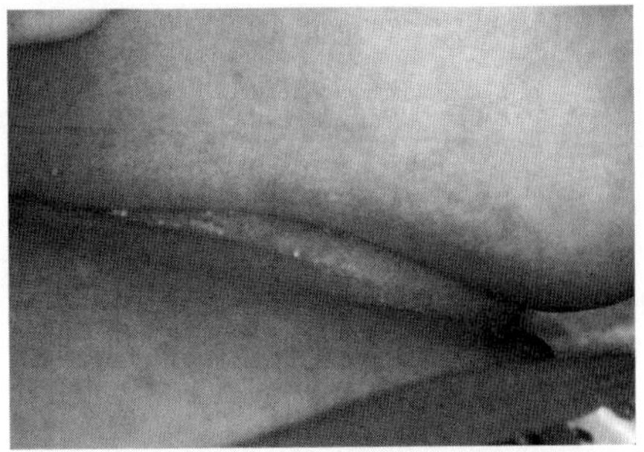

FIG. 3 Intertriginous candidiasis of the neck. (From Kliegman RM et al: *Nelson textbook of pediatrics,* ed 19, Philadelphia, 2011, Saunders.)

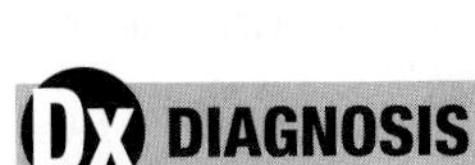

DIAGNOSIS

DIFFERENTIAL DIAGNOSIS

Intertrigo
Seborrheic dermatitis
Psoriasis

WORKUP

Mucocutaneous and cutaneous candidiasis

- Obtain scrapings from the skin, oral, and vaginal mucosa or nails.
- The presence of hyphae/pseudohyphae or budding yeast cells on wet smear, as well as confirmation by culture, is the recommended procedure to diagnose cutaneous candidiasis.
- KOH smears are helpful.

Respiratory candidiasis

- Sputum gram stain: Shows yeast cells
- Sputum cultures
- Lung biopsy: Establishes the diagnosis

Gastrointestinal candidiasis

- Upper endoscopy with or without biopsy (Fig. 4)

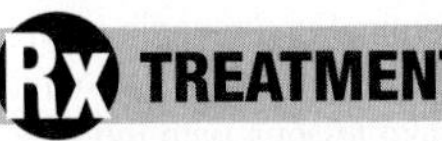

TREATMENT

PHARMACOLOGIC THERAPY

- Cutaneous candidiasis
  1. Decrease/prevent moisture in area
  2. Apply antifungal agents (nystatin powder or cream with an azole or ciclopirox [e.g., clotrimazole, econazole, miconazole])
- Gastrointestinal candidiasis
  1. Oropharyngeal candidiasis
     a. Treat with either
        (1) Oral topical antifungal agent (e.g., nystatin swish and swallow) OR
        (2) Systemic oral azoles (e.g., fluconazole)
  2. In HIV-positive patients, use high doses of fluconazole (100-200 mg PO qd for 7-14 days), itraconazole, or posaconazole
- *Candida* esophagitis
  1. Treat with systemic fluconazole for 2 to 3 wk
  2. Treat with IV fluconazole if patient is unable to take oral medication

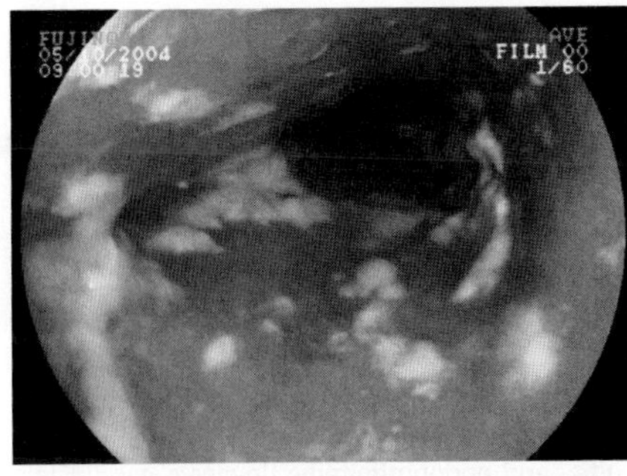

FIG. 4 Endoscopic appearance of esophageal candidiasis. (Courtesy Dr. B. Rembacken, Leeds, U.K.)

- Genitourinary tract candidiasis
  1. Vulvovaginal candidiasis: Treatment options for acute cases include:
     a. A single dose of oral fluconazole (fluconazole 150 mg PO × 1 dose) OR
     b. Topical antifungal agent
  2. For chronic or recurrent cases, treat with fluconazole 150 mg qod × 3 doses and then 150 mg/wk for 6 mo
- Chronic mucocutaneous candidiasis
  1. Treatment with azoles is effective (e.g., fluconazole 100-400 mg daily)
  2. When patient improves, follow with maintenance treatment with same azole for life

FOLLOW-UP CARE

Mucocutaneous candidiasis

- Patient should be instructed to call or follow up if symptoms persist, recur, or worsen.
- For recurrent infections:
  1. Check HIV antibodies.
  2. Check FBS, HbA_{1c}.
  3. Rule out hematologic malignancy or solid organ malignancy.
  4. Refer to infectious disease specialist if no etiology is found.

PREVENTION

- Maintaining dry environment (e.g., by wearing cotton underwear)
- Decreased use of antibiotic
- No douching

SUGGESTED READING

Available at ExpertConsult.com

RELATED CONTENT

Candidiasis (Patient Information)

AUTHOR: **DANIEL K. ASIEDU, M.D., PH.D., F.A.C.P.**

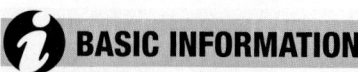

BASIC INFORMATION

DEFINITION

Severe and invasive diseases are caused by *Candida* infection. The most common pathogen is *C. albicans*. Invasive candidiasis embodies a variety of diseases caused by hematogenous spread of *Candida* to multiple viscera (e.g., kidney, brain, heart). These diseases include candidemia, disseminated candidiasis, meningitis, and endophthalmitis. Invasive candidiasis is a significant cause of morbidity and mortality for certain groups of patients.

SYNONYM

Systemic candidiasis

ICD-10CM CODES

B37.89	Other sites of candidiasis
B37.1	Pulmonary candidiasis
B37.2	Candidiasis of skin and nail
B37.5	Candidal meningitis
B37.6	Candidal endocarditis
B37.7	Candidal sepsis
B37.9	Candidiasis unspecified

EPIDEMIOLOGY & DEMOGRAPHICS

INCIDENCE: Invasive candidiasis is the most common fungal disease among hospitalized patients in the developed world. It is an important nosocomial infection. It affects over 250,000 people worldwide each yr and causes more than 50,000 deaths.

In the U.S., *Candida* species cause 8% to 10% of nosocomial bloodstream infections (fourth most common bloodstream infection). *C. albicans* is the most common cause of candidemia, but other non-*albicans* species have been implicated in recent yrs. These include *C. glabrata, C. parapsilosis, C. tropicalis,* and *C. krusei.* Incidence rates of candidemia are between 2 and 14 cases/100,000 persons.

PREVALENCE: No data available

PREDOMINANT SEX AND AGE: Equal between males and females; all ages are susceptible.

RISK FACTORS: Prolonged hospitalization and ICU stay, use of broad-spectrum antibiotics, prolonged indwelling of catheters (especially central venous catheters), acute and chronic renal failure, surgery requiring general anesthesia, cancer (e.g., solid neoplasms), transplantation (bone marrow or solid organ), recent chemotherapy/radiation therapy, use of immunosuppressive drugs, parenteral alimentation, use of internal prosthetic devices, organ transplant, hemodialysis, mechanical, surgical procedures

PHYSICAL FINDINGS & CLINICAL PRESENTATION

- History
  1. Fever unresponsive to broad-spectrum antibiotics
  2. History of prolonged indwelling IV catheter
  3. A personal history of any of the risk factors listed earlier
- Physical findings (general)
  1. Fever
  2. Hypotension
  3. Generalized malaise
  4. Tachycardia
  5. Change in mental status
  6. Signs of multiorgan system failure
- Specific diseases
  1. Candidemia
     a. A positive blood culture is the gold standard for the diagnosis of candidemia. Obtain blood cultures in patients suspected to have candidemia. *Candida* species must be isolated from at least one blood culture
     b. Most common manifestation of invasive candidiasis
     c. Physical exam may include fever, macronodular skin lesions, septic shock, *Candida* endophthalmitis
  2. Disseminated candidiasis
     a. Seen in patients with neutropenia
     b. Associated with multiple deep-organ infections or failure
     c. Blood culture negative
     d. Fever not responding to broad-spectrum antibiotics
     e. Physical exam: Discrete erythematous or palpable rash, sepsis/septic shock
  3. Endophthalmitis
     a. Iatrogenic/accidental or traumatic fungal infection of the eye (exogenous) or hematogenous seeding of the eye (endogenous)
     b. Starts as choroidal lesion, progresses to vitreitis and endophthalmitis and eventually blindness
     c. Physical exam shows fever. An early funduscopic exam by an ophthalmologist should be performed in all patients with candidemia. Funduscopic examination may show large and off-white cotton ball–like lesions with indistinct borders. Patients usually present with decreased visual acuity and occasional pain
  4. *Candida* infection of the CNS
     a. Exogenous and endogenous forms
     b. Usually invades the meninges
     c. Commonly found in long-term ICU patients
     d. May present as meningitis, mycotic aneurysms, change in mental status
     e. Physical examination reveals fever, neck rigidity, confusion, headache, and coma
  5. Candidal musculoskeletal infections
     a. Candida infect the skeletal system, especially the joints as a result of trauma, joint injections, and other surgical interventions, such as IV drug use (hematogenous seeding)
     b. Previously uncommon; now relatively common probably due to increased frequency of candidemia and disseminated candidiasis
     c. Knee and vertebral column (especially lumbosacral vertebral disks and vertebral bodies) are involved
     d. Physical exam is usually unremarkable but may show tenderness over involved area, fever, erythema, bone deformity, weight loss, and sometimes a draining fistulous tract
  6. Candidal infections of the heart
     a. Usually found in patients with artificial heart valves, IV drug users, and patients with an indwelling central venous catheter
     b. May present as infective endocarditis, myocarditis, or pericarditis
     c. Physical examination reveals fever, hypotension, tachycardia, new or changing murmur, and signs and symptoms of heart failure
  7. Hepatosplenic candidiasis (chronic systemic candidiasis)
     a. Seen in patients with hematologic malignancy and neutropenia; usually develops during recovery from a neutropenic state (normally after undergoing myeloablative chemotherapy)
     b. On examination, patients have low-grade fever, right upper quadrant pain, palpable/tender liver, splenomegaly, and rarely jaundice
  8. *Candida* peritonitis
     a. Associated with GI surgery: Perforations, acute necrotizing pancreatitis, peritoneal dialysis
     b. Clinical manifestations include fever, chills, abdominal pain; nausea, vomiting, constipation
     c. Physical examination reveals abdominal distention, abdominal pain, absent bowel sounds
  9. Other forms of invasive candidiasis
     a. *Candida* splenic abscess
     b. *Candida* cholecystitis
     c. Renal candidiasis
     d. Mediastinitis
     e. Empyema
     f. Pneumonia (rare)

ETIOLOGY

- Several species of *Candida* exist in nature
- Medically significant include:
  1. *C. albicans:* Together with *C. glabrata,* they account for 70% to 80% of *Candida* in invasive candidiasis.
  2. *C. glabrata:* Together with *C. albicans,* they account for 70% to 80% of *Candida* in invasive candidiasis.
  3. *C. parapsilosis:* Associated with indwelling vascular catheters and prosthetic devices
  4. *C. tropicalis:* Especially in leukemic patients
  5. *C. krusei:* Resistant to fluconazole and ketoconazole

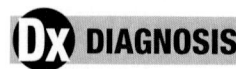

DIAGNOSIS

DIFFERENTIAL DIAGNOSIS

- Sepsis (bacterial)
- Septic shock
- Cryptococcosis
- Aspergillosis

WORKUP

LABORATORY TESTS:

- Laboratory studies are nonspecific. It is often necessary to perform several diagnostic tests to achieve maximum accuracy.
- High index of suspicion is needed.
- Candidemia/disseminated candidiasis: Candidemia represents the tip of the iceberg with respect to the more invasive forms of candidiasis. Central lines often contribute to the propagation of candidemia. From the blood, infection can spread to almost any organ.
    1. Blood cultures are the mainstay of diagnosis. They are helpful but have low positive yield. Only 40% to 60% of patients with infection have positive culture. Candida in a blood culture is NOT a contamination, and the source of the infection should be sought.
    2. Diagnosis can also be made from normally sterile sites. Specific species identification is necessary since only 10% of known *Candida* species produce disease in humans.
    3. The T2 magnetic resonance assay of whole blood can be performed on blood samples even after initiation of antifungal therapy.
    4. Serum (1,3) beta-D-glucan detection assay: High specificity and high positive predictive value. It can also be used for diagnosing invasive candidiasis when blood cultures are negative.
- Hepatosplenic candidiasis (focal):
    1. Elevated serum alkaline phosphatase.

IMAGING STUDIES:

- Imaging studies are generally not required or useful.
- Ultrasound is useful for diagnosing hepatosplenic abscess. "Bull's eye or target lesions" are observed in the liver and spleen.
- CT scanning may be used to diagnose hepatosplenic candidiasis, as well as intraabdominal/renal abscesses.
- ECHO is useful to rule in or rule out *Candida* endocarditis.

Rx TREATMENT

- To successfully treat invasive *Candida* infection, it is important to start antifungal medication as early as possible. A small delay (approximately 12-24 hr) in starting treatment may result in a significantly excessive mortality rate.
    1. Do not dismiss *Candida* spp. as a contaminant when it is isolated in blood cultures or other sterile sites.
    2. Before treatment, also consider removal of an intravenous catheter.
- Antifungals available include:
    1. Azoles (e.g., fluconazole, posaconazole, itraconazole, voriconazole). They inhibit the synthesis of ergosterol, a fungal cell component.
    2. Echinocandins (e.g., caspofungin, micafungin, anidulafungin). These are glucan synthesis inhibitors. Glucan is an important component of fungal cell walls. Most studies have provided reasonable support for echinocandins as treatment of choice for the majority of patients with invasive candidiasis.
    3. Polyenes (e.g., amphotericin B, lipid formulation of amphotericin, nystatin). Broad spectrum. Their mechanism of action is to increase cytoplasmic permeability.
    4. Antimetabolites (e.g., flucytosine). Flucytosine is deaminated to 5-fluorouracil in fungal cell. 5-Fluorouracil inhibits RNA and protein synthesis.

TREATMENT PLANS

CANDIDEMIA:

- Treatment depends on whether the patient is neutropenic or not.
    1. Nonneutropenic adult patients: Drug of choice is fluconazole; 800 mg as loading dose then 400 mg/day for at least 2 wk after clinical improvement or negative blood culture. Amphotericin B is equally efficacious.
    2. Neutropenic adult patients: An echinocandin is the drug of choice (e.g., caspofungin) 70 mg IV loading dose then 50 mg/day IV or micafungin 100 mg/day IV or anidulafungin 200 mg IV loading dose then 100 mg IV all for at least 2 wk after clear blood culture and after clinical improvement.

DISSEMINATED CANDIDIASIS: Fluconazole is the drug of choice.

DISSEMINATED CANDIDIASIS WITH END-ORGAN INFECTION:

- Treatment is the same as for candidemia of nonneutropenic patients. In most cases, therapy is prolonged for at least 4 to 6 wk.
- The echinocandins are the first-line therapy.

OSTEOMYELITIS OR SEPTIC ARTHRITIS:

- Fluconazole 400 mg IV or PO *or*
- Lipid-based amphotericin B 3 to 5 mg/kg qd

ENDOCARDITIS:

- Caspofungin 50 to 150 mg/day *or*
- Micafungin 100 to 150 mg/day *or*
- Anidulafungin 100 to 200 mg/day

MYOCARDITIS:

- Lipid-based amphotericin B 3 to 5 mg/kg daily *or*
- Fluconazole 400 to 800 mg daily IV or PO

ESOPHAGITIS:

- Fluconazole 200 to 400 mg/day *or*
- Caspofungin 50 mg IV daily

PERICARDITIS:

- Lipid-based amphotericin B 3 to 5 mg/kg daily *or*
- Fluconazole 400 to 800 mg PO qd IV or PO

SURGICAL CARE: Include:

- Drainage
- Removal of any foreign bodies
- Surgical debridement
- Organ-specific care (e.g., valve replacement for endocarditis, splenectomy for splenic abscess, or vitrectomy for fungal endophthalmitis)

DISPOSITION

- Several factors affect prognosis: Infection site, degree of immune suppression, and how quickly diagnosis and therapy are initiated
- Overall mortality rate: 30% to 40%

REFERRAL

- Always involve an infectious disease specialist.
- Referral to specialist will depend on the organ involved. For example:
    1. Endocarditis will require a cardiothoracic surgeon.
    2. Endophthalmitis will require an ophthalmologist.

FOLLOW-UP CARE

- Prolonged periods, mainly in the hospital, of antifungal treatment may be necessary.
- Closely monitor patients on amphotericin B because of the high incidence of side effects. Check basic metabolic panel, magnesium, and CBC at least twice a week.

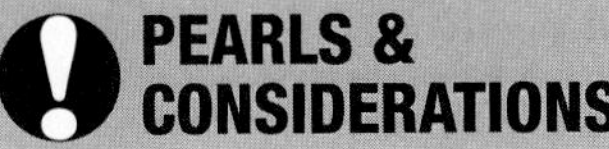

PEARLS & CONSIDERATIONS

PREVENTION

Basic preventive measures are similar to those used for nosocomial infections. This includes:

- Maximizing hand hygiene recommendations:
    1. Hand washing.
    2. Using alcohol/chlorhexidine solution.
- Adhering strictly to recommendations for placement and care of central lines and catheters.
- Judicious use of antimicrobials
    1. Notes on *C. auris*:
        a. CDC issued warnings in 2016 about the emergence of *C. auris*, a multidrug-resistant *Candida* species.
        b. It has caused invasive health care–associated infections in many countries and has high mortality rates.
        c. Initial treatment is with echinocandin. Patient should be closely followed with cultures.
        d. Special infection control precautions should be followed for patients infected with or colonized by *C. auris*.

PROPHYLAXIS

Antifungal prophylaxis should be limited to patients in whom it has proved beneficial: patients with gastrointestinal anastomotic leakage, patients undergoing transplantation of the pancreas or small bowel, selected patients undergoing liver transplantation who are at high risk for candidiasis, and extremely low-birth-weight neonates in settings with a high incidence of neonatal candidiasis.

PATIENT/FAMILY EDUCATION

- Inform them about the risk factors for invasive candidiasis.
- Inform them of the seriousness of the disease and the associated high morbidity/mortality rates, thus requiring aggressive treatment.
- Side effects and toxicities associated with treatment.

SUGGESTED READINGS

Available at ExpertConsult.com

RELATED CONTENT

Candidiasis (Patient Information)
Candidiasis, Cutaneous (Related Key Topic)

AUTHOR: **DANIEL K. ASIEDU, M.D., PH.D., F.A.C.P.**

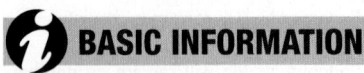

DEFINITION

Carbon monoxide (CO) is a colorless, odorless, tasteless, nonirritating gas. When inhaled, it produces toxicity by causing cellular hypoxia and damage.

ICD-10CM CODES

T68	Toxic effect of carbon monoxide
T58.01	Toxic effect of carbon monoxide from motor vehicle exhaust, accidental (unintentional), initial encounter

EPIDEMIOLOGY & DEMOGRAPHICS

- A leading cause of accidental and intentional poisoning in the U.S.
- Can occur because of acute toxicity or chronic exposure.
- CO poisoning is seen more frequently during the fall and winter months in cold climates. Frequently seen after storm-related power outages, mostly due to the use of portable gasoline-powered electrical generators.
- Most fatal cases of CO poisoning occur in the home.

PHYSICAL FINDINGS & CLINICAL PRESENTATION

- Depends on the severity and duration of exposure. The brain and heart are most sensitive to CO poisoning. Table 1 summarizes carboxyhemoglobin concentration and related symptoms.
- Presentation is often nonspecific and may be mistaken for a flulike illness.
- Severity of poisoning does not correlate with carboxyhemoglobin (COHb) levels.
- Mild to moderate poisoning may present with headache, malaise, dizziness, nausea, dyspnea, difficulty concentrating, confusion, and blurred vision. Patients may have tachypnea and tachycardia.
- Severe poisoning may present with hypotension, arrhythmias, myocardial ischemia, pulmonary edema, lethargy, ataxia, loss of consciousness, seizure, coma, or, rarely, cherry-red skin.
- Delayed neurologic sequelae may develop days to weeks after apparent recovery from acute poisoning. Patients may present with neurologic or psychiatric symptoms (cognitive deficits, memory loss, personality changes, movement disorders, Parkinson's, psychosis, neurologic deficits).

ETIOLOGY

- CO results from the incomplete combustion of carbon-containing compounds. CO poisoning occurs from inhaling smoke from fires, motor vehicle/motor boat exhaust, or the burning of fuel (oil, wood, coal, gasoline, natural gas) in poorly functioning or improperly ventilated devices (heating systems, stoves/grills, portable generators, etc.). Methylene chloride (paint stripper) fumes are converted to CO by the liver.
- CO toxicity results from tissue hypoxia and direct CO-mediated damage at the cellular level. This may explain why COHb levels alone are not predictive of clinical toxicity. The mechanisms of CO toxicity are not completely understood.
- CO impairs oxygen delivery. CO reversibly binds hemoglobin with an affinity 250 times greater than oxygen, displacing oxygen from hemoglobin and decreasing the oxygen-carrying capacity of blood. By binding to hemoglobin, CO changes the structure of the hemoglobin molecule and decreases oxygen release to tissue.
- CO may also interfere with peripheral oxygen utilization by binding to other heme-containing proteins including cytochromes and myoglobin. Cellular respiration may be depressed by inhibition of mitochondrial function.
- Neurologic toxicity is not explained by hypoxia alone and is related to the complex intracellular actions of CO. CO precipitates an inflammatory cascade that results in oxidative damage and brain lipid peroxidation.

Dx DIAGNOSIS

DIFFERENTIAL DIAGNOSIS

- Viral syndromes
- Cyanide, hydrogen sulfide
- Methemoglobinemia
- Amphetamines and derivatives
- Cocaine, phencyclidine (PCP)
- Cyclic antidepressants
- Phenothiazines
- Theophylline

WORKUP

History (duration and source of CO exposure, loss of consciousness), physical examination (detailed neurologic examination), laboratory and imaging tests

LABORATORY TESTS

- COHb level (measured by CO-oximetry on arterial or venous blood). COHb level >3% in nonsmokers confirms exposure. Heavy smokers may have baseline levels up to 10%-15%. Levels may be low if the patient has already received supplemental oxygen or if delays occur between exposure and testing.
- NOTE: Pulse oximetry and arterial blood gas (ABG) may be falsely normal because neither measures oxygen saturation of hemoglobin directly. Pulse oximetry is inaccurate because of the similar absorption characteristics of oxyhemoglobin and COHb. An ABG is inaccurate because it measures oxygen dissolved in plasma (which is not affected by CO) and then calculates oxygen saturation of hemoglobin.

TABLE 1 Treatment Strategies for Acute Smoke Inhalation

Current	Under Investigation
Rescue victim from source	Activated protein C
High-flow 100% O_2	Antiinflammatory drugs • Methylprednisolone • Phenytoin
Body check	Nitric oxide synthase inhibitors
Intravenous access	Antioxidants • Gamma-tocopherol • 21-aminosteroid
± Intubation	Endothelin-I-receptor antagonist tezosentan
If upper airway edema: • Nebulized adrenaline • Nebulized corticosteroids	P-selectin blockade
If bronchospasm: • Nebulized $alpha_2$-agonists	Nebulized deferoxamine-pentastarch complex
If elevated COHb: • High-flow 100% O2 • Hyperbaric oxygen	Mechanical ventilation • High-frequency percussive ventilation • Airway pressure release ventilation • Volumetric diffuse ventilator
If cyanide intoxication: • Amyl nitrate • Sodium thiosulfate • Hydroxocobalamin (Cyanokit)	Extracorporeal membrane oxygenation
Mechanical ventilation, Low tidal volume	Arteriovenous carbon dioxide removal
Nebulized heparin	Pulmonary decontamination with nebulized amphoteric chelating agents
Nebulized *N*-acetylcysteine	

From Parrillo JE, Dellinger RP: *Critical care medicine, principles of diagnosis and management in the adult,* ed 4, Philadelphia, 2014, Elsevier.

TABLE 2 Carboxyhemoglobin Concentration and Related Symptoms

COHb [in %]	Symptoms
<20	Slight headache and dilation of peripheral blood vessels
21-40	Severe headache and pulsating in temporal blood vessels, vertigo, dizziness, nausea and vomiting, circulatory collapse
41-60	Symptoms as above, syncope, tachycardia, hyperventilation, intermittent seizures, cyanosis, coma, shock, Cheyne-Stokes respiration
61-80	Coma, intermittent seizures, impaired heart and lung function, weak pulses, slow breathing, death within hours
>81	Death occurs within minutes

From Parrillo JE, Dellinger RP: *Critical care medicine, principles of diagnosis and management in the adult,* ed 4, Philadelphia, 2014, Elsevier.

TABLE 3 Half-Life of COHb

Oxygen Concentration	Half-Life
21% (room air)	4-5 hr
100% (mask or endotracheal)	60-90 min
100% (hyperbaric molecular oxygen)	20-30 min

From Fuhrman BP et al: *Pediatric critical care,* ed 4, Philadelphia, 2011, Saunders.

- Electrolytes, glucose, BUN, creatinine, cardiac biomarkers, ABG (lactic acidosis and rhabdomyolysis may develop), CBC (polycythemia from hypoxia in chronic CO poisoning).
- ECG (ischemia, arrhythmia).
- Pregnancy test (fetus at high risk).
- Consider toxicology screen.
- Table 2 summarizes treatment strategies for acute smoke inhalation.

IMAGING STUDIES

- Chest x-ray (noncardiogenic edema)
- Brain CT, MRI if neurologic abnormalities are present, to exclude other causes

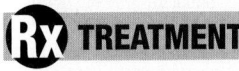

TREATMENT

ACUTE GENERAL Rx

- Remove from site of CO exposure.
- Ensure adequate airway.
- Continuous ECG monitor.
- Fetal monitoring if pregnant.
- 100% oxygen by nonrebreather mask or endotracheal tube (decreases half-life of COHb from 4 to 6 hr to 60 to 90 min) until COHb level is <5% and patient is asymptomatic. Table 3 describes the half-life of COHb.
- Hyperbaric oxygen (2.5 to 3 atm).
    1. Questionable beneficial effect over normobaric oxygen. Disparate findings in various studies: Some suggest hyperbaric oxygen treatment reduces the incidence of neurologic sequelae, and others have found it worsens neurologic outcomes compared to normobaric oxygen treatment. A large retrospective study suggests it may decrease short-term and long-term mortality, especially in individuals <20 yr old and those with acute respiratory failure. Multiple sessions were associated with lower mortality than a single session.
    2. Decreases half-life of COHb to 20 to 30 min; increases amount of oxygen dissolved in plasma. It also reduces CO binding to other heme-containing proteins.
    3. Consider for:
        a. Severe intoxication (COHb >25%, history of loss of consciousness, neurologic symptoms or signs, cardiovascular compromise, severe metabolic acidosis).
        b. Pregnant women with COHb >20% or signs of fetal distress. CO elimination is slower in fetus than mother, fetal Hgb has greater affinity for CO than adult Hgb.
        c. Should be instituted quickly if deemed necessary.
- Consider concomitant poisoning with other toxic/irritant gases that may be present in smoke (e.g., cyanide) or thermal injury to airway. Toxic effects of CO and cyanide are synergistic.
- Identify source of exposure and determine if poisoning was accidental.

DISPOSITION

- Patients with mild accidental poisoning can be treated in an ambulatory setting. Those with moderate/severe poisoning or coexisting illness require hospitalization.
- About 35% of patients with moderate to severe poisoning have cardiac dysfunction (arrhythmia, LV systolic dysfunction, ischemia).
- Survivors of severe poisoning are at 14% to 40% risk for neurologic sequelae.
    1. Deficits are usually apparent within 3 wk of poisoning but may present months later.
    2. Risk of developing sequelae is greater if patient lost consciousness during acute poisoning and with older age.
    3. Brain MRI and functional CT may reveal changes; damage is seen most often in the globus pallidus and deep white matter.
    4. Recovery may occur over months to yrs.
- Severe CO poisoning is associated with increased long-term morbidity and mortality.
- High risk of fetal demise.

REFERRAL

- American Association of Poison Control Centers: 1-800-222-1222
- Hyperbaric unit; accredited facilities are listed on the Undersea & Hyperbaric Medical Society website (www.uhms.org)
- Psychiatric evaluation if intentional poisoning

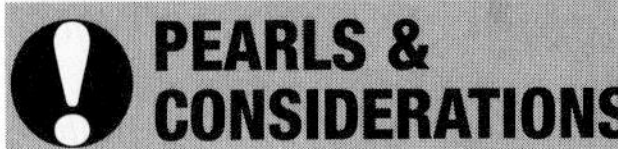

PEARLS & CONSIDERATIONS

- Hookah smoking is increasingly being recognized as a cause of CO poisoning, especially among young adults.
- Severity of poisoning and prognosis do not correlate with COHb levels because hypoxia represents only a component of CO's toxic effect. New therapies to address CO toxicity are being proposed.
- Neuropsychometric testing is an objective measure of cognitive function but is not universally used.
- Imaging techniques and biomarkers to define severity of CO poisoning, early prediction of CNS damage and prognosis are being studied, but are not ready for application.
- Pulse CO-oximetry measurement of CO saturation has limited clinical use.
- Treatment with hydroxocobalamin (for cyanide toxicity) may make subsequent COHb testing unreliable.
- Contact local fire department to assess environment and identify source of CO.

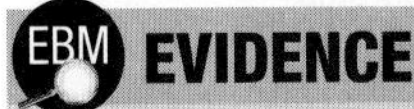

EVIDENCE

Available at ExpertConsult.com

SUGGESTED READINGS

Available at ExpertConsult.com

RELATED CONTENT

Carbon Monoxide Poisoning (Patient Information)

AUTHOR: **SUDEEP K. AULAKH, M.D., F.A.C.P., F.R.C.P.C.**

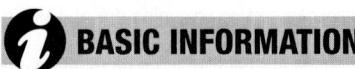

BASIC INFORMATION

DEFINITION

Cardiac tamponade is a life-threatening condition where an accumulation of fluid within the pericardial sac causes equal elevation of atrial, end diastolic pressures in the ventricles, and pericardial pressures, as well as an exaggerated inspiratory decrease in arterial systolic pressure (pulsus paradoxus) along with arterial hypotension.

ICD-10CM CODE
I31.4 Cardiac tamponade

PHYSICAL FINDINGS & CLINICAL PRESENTATION

- Tachypnea/dyspnea
- Chest pain may be present
- Beck triad
  1. Absolute or relative hypotension
  2. Elevated jugular venous pressure (with prominent *x* descent and blunted *y* descent)
  3. Muffled heart sounds
- Tachycardia (except in uremia or hypothyroid patients)
- Pulsus paradoxus (decrease in systolic arterial pressure of 10 mm Hg or more during normal inspiration while in normal sinus rhythm)
- Pericardial friction rub may be heard in patients with cardiac tamponade due to inflammatory pericarditis.
- Reduced or absent apical cardiac impulse
- Signs of varying degrees of shock (diaphoresis, cool extremities, peripheral cyanosis, and depressed sensorium)

ETIOLOGY

- Acute (rapidly accumulating pericardial effusion leading to cardiac tamponade): Does not need a large amount of effusion to cause tamponade; rather, it is the rapidity of fluid accumulation that leads to clinical tamponade. Clinical presentation typically resembles that of cardiogenic shock requiring urgent reduction of pericardial pressure. Causes for acute cardiac tamponade include:
  1. Penetrating trauma
  2. Aortic dissection (more commonly in Type A)
  3. Postinfarction myocardial rupture and/or hemorrhagic pericarditis
  4. Iatrogenic (central line and pacemaker insertions, cardiac ablation, post–coronary bypass surgery or post–percutaneous coronary intervention)
- Subacute or chronic: Occurs over days to weeks, and the effusion is usually large; causes include the following:
  1. Malignancy (e.g., lung, breast, lymphoma)
  2. Viral pericarditis (e.g., Coxsackie, human immunodeficiency virus, enterovirus, HSV 6, parvovirus, etc.)
  3. Bacterial, fungal, or tuberculous pericarditis
  4. Uremia
  5. Hypothyroidism/myxedema (rare)
  6. Collagen vascular disease (e.g., lupus, rheumatoid arthritis, scleroderma)
  7. Radiation
  8. Post–myocardial infarction or post–cardiac ablation inflammation
  9. Idiopathic
- Regional cardiac tamponade occurs when the localized or loculated hematoma compresses only selected cardiac chambers

Dx DIAGNOSIS

Cardiac tamponade is a clinical diagnosis made at the bedside from history and physical examination. The echocardiogram will help confirm or reject the clinical diagnosis. Tamponade can be confirmed invasively by the measurement of elevated intrapericardial pressures with an intrapericardial catheter and right-sided heart catheterization. Typical findings are diastolic equalization of pressures, usually ranging from 10 to 30 mm Hg (diastolic pulmonary artery pressure = right ventricular diastolic pressure = right atrial pressure = intrapericardial pressure), and lowering of the intrapericardial pressure with fluid drainage. Thereafter, the underlying etiology must be determined with specific laboratory work (see "Laboratory Tests").

DIFFERENTIAL DIAGNOSIS

Other conditions that can also lead to elevated jugular venous pressure, decreased systemic pressure, and pulsus paradoxus include:

- Chronic obstructive pulmonary disease and asthma exacerbations
- Constrictive pericarditis (Table 1)
- Effusive-constrictive pericarditis
- Restrictive cardiomyopathy
- Right ventricular infarction
- Pulmonary embolism
- Chronic biventricular heart failure

LABORATORY TESTS

- Electrolytes, blood urea nitrogen, creatinine, erythrocyte sedimentation rate, thyroid function tests, antinuclear antibody, rheumatoid factor, PPD, blood cultures, viral titers, and pericardial fluid analysis including cytology and cultures
- Possible 12-lead ECG findings:
  1. Sinus tachycardia
  2. PR depression and/or diffuse ST elevations if acute pericarditis is present
  3. Electrical alternans (beat to beat alternations in the QRS complex heights) (Fig. E1)
  4. Low QRS voltage in patients with a pericardial effusion may be a specific manifestation of cardiac tamponade, not of the effusion (QRS complex <0.5 mV in the limb leads and <1.0 mV in precordial leads)

IMAGING STUDIES

- Chest radiograph (enlarged cardiac silhouette with clear lung fields) (Fig. 2)
- Chest CT (may overestimate size of the effusion) (Fig. 3)
- Cardiac MRI (as an adjunct to echocardiography)
- Echocardiogram findings (Fig. 4):
  1. Pericardial effusion
  2. Right atrial inversion for greater than one third of systole has a sensitivity of 94% and a specificity of 100% for the diagnosis of tamponade
  3. Diastolic collapse of the right ventricle (early diastole) is pathognomonic and very specific
  4. >25% mitral and >50% tricuspid valve inflow variation on the first beat of inspiration and expiration, respectively
  5. Plethoric inferior vena cava (IVC dilation and <50% decrease in the diameter of the IVC during inspiration)
  6. Left atrial collapse (high specificity)
- Cardiac catheterization as discussed earlier will see equalization of intracardiac diastolic pressures and increase of right-sided

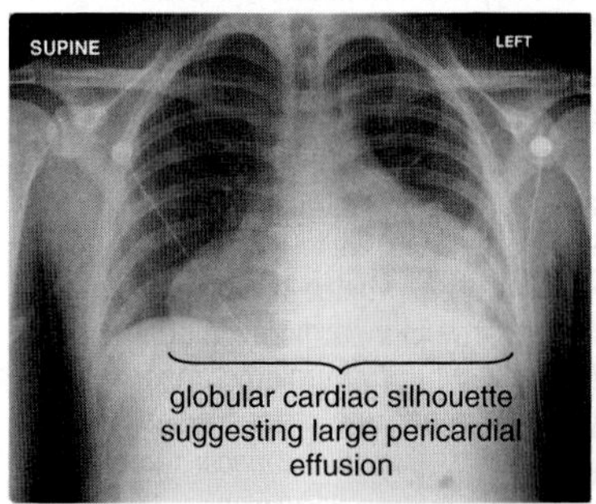

FIG. 2 Massive pericardial effusion and tamponade. This 23-year-old male has a history of aortic valve replacement for infective endocarditis. He presented with increased chest pain and dyspnea. His chest x-ray shows a globular cardiac silhouette, suggesting a large pericardial effusion. The lung fields and right costophrenic angle appear clear, although the left costophrenic angle is hidden behind the heart and cannot be assessed. The patient underwent chest computed tomography to evaluate his aorta, as he complained of severe interscapular pain as well (see Fig. 3). (From Broder JS: *Diagnostic imaging for the emergency physician,* Philadelphia, 2011, Saunders.)

TABLE 1 Hemodynamics in Cardiac Tamponade and Constrictive Pericarditis

	Tamponade	Constriction
Paradoxical pulse	Usually present	Present in ~1/3
Equal left- and right-sided filling pressures	Present	Present
Systemic venous wave morphology	Absent *y* descent	Prominent *y* descent (M or W shape)
Inspiratory change in systemic venous pressure	Decrease (normal)	Increase or no change (Kussmaul sign)
"Square root" sign in ventricular pressure	Absent	Present

From Fuhrman BP et al: *Pediatric critical care,* ed 4, Philadelphia, 2011, Saunders.

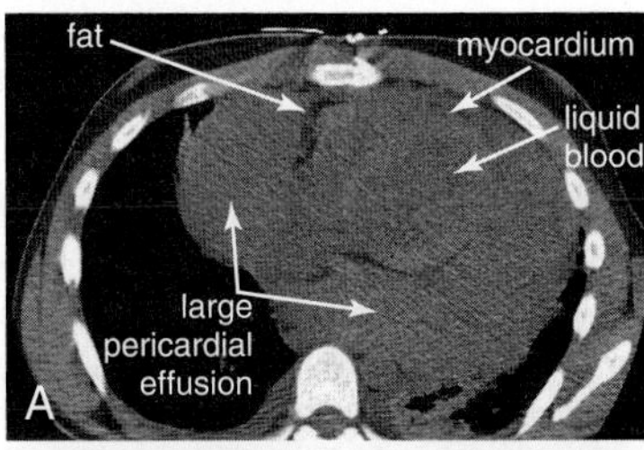

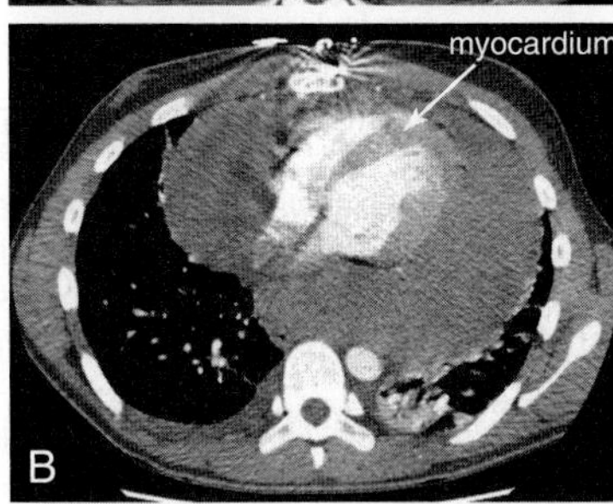

FIG. 3 Massive pericardial effusion. Same patient as Fig. 2. The patient underwent chest computed tomography (CT) without **(A)** and then with **(B)** intravenous contrast to evaluate his aorta, which was normal. However, the CT confirmed a massive pericardial effusion surrounding a normal-appearing heart. Without contrast, note that fluid blood within the chambers of the heart has a slightly lower density than the pericardial effusion, which has a density more similar to that of myocardium. When contrast is administered, the ventricular chambers fill completely, and the myocardium enhances and becomes somewhat brighter than the surrounding pericardial effusion. The heart itself is outlined by a thin stripe of fat, which appears nearly black on soft tissue windows. The patient developed hypotension, suggesting cardiac tamponade, and pericardial window was performed for drainage of the effusion. In the operating room, the effusion was found to be coagulated blood. (From Broder JS: *Diagnostic imaging for the emergency physician,* Philadelphia, 2011, Saunders.)

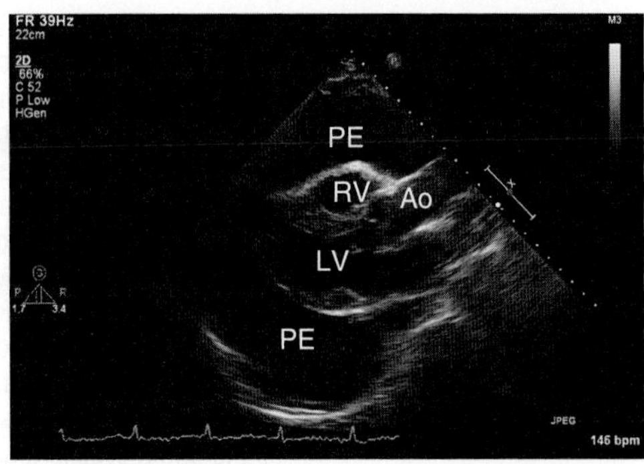

FIG. 4 Two-dimensional echocardiogram of a large, circumferential pericardial effusion *(PE).* *Ao,* Aorta; *LV,* left ventricle; *RV,* right ventricle. (From Kabbani SS, LeWinter M: Cardiac constriction and restriction. In Crawford MH, DiMarco JP [eds]: *Cardiology,* St Louis, 2001, Mosby.)

pressures and reduction of left-sided pressures, which subsequently causes pulsus paradoxus (the pathognomonic finding on physical examination)

Rx TREATMENT

NONPHARMACOLOGIC THERAPY

- Cardiac tamponade should be treated emergently with removal of the pericardial fluid.
- Avoid drugs that reduce preload (e.g., nitrates, diuretics).
- Large pericardial effusions without hemodynamic compromise (tamponade) can be managed conservatively with careful monitoring, IV fluids, treatment of the underlying cause, clinical follow-up, and frequent serial surveillance echocardiography.

ACUTE GENERAL Rx

- Aggressive intravascular volume expansion (saline or blood).
- Emergency pericardial fluid removal by pericardiocentesis or surgical pericardiotomy by way of the subxiphoid pericardial window.
- Pericardiocentesis should be performed under fluoroscopic or echocardiographic guidance when available.
- Pericardiocentesis is an absolute contraindication if the etiology of the pericardial effusion is aortic dissection, wherein emergent surgical management is indicated.
- Inotropic or vasopressor support if above measures cannot be performed immediately.

CHRONIC Rx

- Depends on etiology. Patients with inflammatory causes of pericarditis leading to effusion should be treated with an extended course of colchicine.
- Pericardiocentesis with draining catheter: The catheter can be left inside the pericardium to allow continued drainage for 24 to 48 hr. If residual fluid still persists with hemodynamic compromise, surgical drainage should be considered. In the absence of hemodynamic compromise or significant residual fluid, discontinuation of the draining catheter can be done with periodic postprocedure echocardiographic monitoring for reaccumulation (e.g., 24 hr, 7 days, 30 days, 3 mo, 6 mo, 12 mo) depending on the etiology and the rate of reaccumulation.
- Other surgical drainage procedures include:
    1. Subxiphoid pericardiotomy drainage.
    2. Pericardial window; draining the pericardial fluid into the left hemithorax.
    3. Limited pericardiectomy.
    4. Complete pericardiectomy, especially in patients with effusive-constrictive pericarditis, bacterial pericarditis, or tuberculous pericarditis. (see "Pearls & Considerations").

DISPOSITION

The prognosis of cardiac tamponade depends on the underlying cause.

REFERRAL

- Emergent cardiology consultation along with thorough echocardiographic exam should be made if cardiac tamponade is suspected.
- Cardiothoracic surgery or interventional cardiology consultation should also be considered if pericardial drainage is indicated.

PEARLS & CONSIDERATIONS

- Cardiac tamponade should always be considered during pulseless electrical activity arrest and may require emergent pericardiocentesis at the bedside.
- Evaluation for pulsus paradoxus should always be performed during normal respiration because deep inspiration may render a false-positive finding.
- Strong consideration should be given to performing early pericardiocentesis in patients who have pericardial effusion associated with bacterial pneumonia or empyema because the incidence of bacterial pericarditis is especially high in this clinical situation and the subsequent development of cardiac tamponade and severe chronic constrictive pericarditis are ominous complications.
- Pericardiocentesis is an absolute contraindication if the etiology of the pericardial effusion is due to aortic dissection extending into the pericardial sac.
- As little as 100 ml of fluid can lead to acute cardiac tamponade if the rate of accumulation is rapid, whereas with gradual accumulation, the pericardial sac can hold up to 5 L of fluid before tamponade occurs.
- With effusions that are small, organized, and/or loculated, needle aspiration should generally be avoided. An exception is acute cardiac tamponade complicating a cardiac procedure (e.g., percutaneous coronary intervention) with anticoagulation. In this setting, the effusion is often small, but pericardial pressure rises very quickly, resulting in hemodynamic compromise.

SUGGESTED READINGS

Available at ExpertConsult.com

RELATED CONTENT

Cardiac Tamponade (Patient Information)
Pericarditis (Related Key Topic)

AUTHORS: **ROBERT VAZQUEZ, M.D.,** and **ARAVIND RAO KOKKIRALA, M.D. FACC.**

DEFINITION

Cardiomyopathy, chemical-induced (CMc), is a change in cardiac structure and/or function caused by chemical compounds. Many chemicals, including environmental substances, prescription drugs, and illicit drugs, are associated with cardiomyopathy (CM). These include (but are not limited to) alcohol, cocaine, amphetamines, chloroquine, anabolic steroids, anthracyclines, 5-fluorouracil (5-FU), zidovudine, tyrosine kinase inhibitors, and trastuzumab.

SYNONYMS

Alcoholic cardiomyopathy (ACM)
Cocaine-induced CM
Anabolic steroid-induced CM
Anthracycline-induced CM
Chemotherapy-induced CM
CMc

ICD-10CM CODE
I42.7 Cardiomyopathy due to drug and external agent

EPIDEMIOLOGY & DEMOGRAPHICS

- ACM occurs in about 5% to 10% of alcoholics and accounts for 21% to 36% of dilated cardiomyopathy in high-income countries. Most patients in whom alcoholic cardiomyopathy develops have been drinking more than 80 to 90 g of ethanol per day for more than 5 yr.
- The risk of doxorubicin-induced cardiotoxicity is dose dependent: 3% to 5% with 400 mg/m^2, 7% to 26% at 550 mg/m^{22}, and 18% to 48% at 700 mg/m^2.
- The addition of trastuzumab to an anthracycline-based chemotherapy regimen markedly increases the incidence of heart failure (28% vs. 1.7%-21% with trastuzumab alone). The incidence can be significantly reduced by introducing a drug-free interval between the agents. Long-term follow-up data regarding trastuzumab cardiotoxicity are favorable, as the cardiotoxic effects generally manifest during treatment and are reversible.
- Other chemotherapeutic agents known to cause cardiomyopathy include idarubicin (>90 mg/m^2, 5%-18%), epirubicin (>900 mg/m^2, 0.9%-11.4%), docetaxel (2.3%-13%), cyclophosphamide (7%-28%), bortezomib (2%-5%), sunitinib (2.7%-19%), 5-fluorouracil [5-FU] (6%-7%), and carfilzomib (11%-25%). Table 1 summarizes chemotherapeutic agents implicated in clinical syndromes of cardiotoxicity.

PREDOMINANT SEX AND AGE: The prevalence of ACM appears to be similar among alcoholic men and women, with women developing left ventricular (LV) dysfunction at a lower ethanol dose than men. Significant racial differences exist, with blacks having higher mortality rates than non-Hispanic whites. Anthracycline- and trastuzumab-induced cardiomyopathy is more common in those aged >50 yr.

GENETICS:

- In patients with ACM, the deletion (DD) genotype of angiotensin-converting-enzyme (ACE) is more common than insertion (II) and deletion, insertion (DI) genotypes. The underlying mechanism involves direct toxicity of ethanol to the myocardium through uncoupling of adenosine triphosphate.
- Anthracycline-induced CM is linked to an increase in cardiac oxidative stress via the pathways of mitochondrial nitric oxide synthesis, and nicotinamide adenine dinucleotide phosphate reduction.
- One study suggests that polymorphisms in the carbonyl reductase genes could be related to anthracycline-induced CM.

RISK FACTORS:

- Consumption of more than 80 to 100 g/day of alcohol for more than 10 yr significantly increases the risk of ACM.
- The occurrence of chronic anthracycline-induced CM is correlated to cumulative dose, age, preexisting heart disease, concomitant chemotherapy, and history of mediastinal radiation therapy. Children are more susceptible to anthracycline-induced CM.
- Additional risk factors for anthracycline-induced CM include radiation therapy involving the cardiac silhouette as well as use of trastuzumab.
- Infusional dosing may reduce the risk for cardiotoxicity compared to bolus regimens.

PHYSICAL FINDINGS & CLINICAL PRESENTATION

The majority of clinical characteristics of CMc are similar to dilated cardiomyopathy of other etiologies. Symptoms may be insidious or acute in onset.

- Acute anthracycline-induced CM can start at any time after the first dose and may present with arrhythmias (most commonly supraventricular tachycardia), LV dysfunction, or pericardial disease. Typically the first manifestation of anthracycline-induced cardiotoxicity is subtle diastolic dysfunction noted on tissue Doppler. The subacute and chronic symptoms may occur 3 months to 10 yr after the last dose. Patients usually present with heart failure. More recently, mortality has improved as a result of medical treatment with ACE inhibitors and beta-blockers. In fact, recent trials, including the OVERCOME trial, have demonstrated a benefit in preemptively treating low-cardiac-risk patients undergoing anthracycline therapy with beta-blockers and ACE-inhibitors to prevent the development of CM.
- Cardiac symptoms after 5-FU treatment include angina (most common), myocardial infarction, arrhythmia, acute pulmonary edema, cardiac arrest, and pericarditis. The mechanism of angina and myocardial infarction is coronary vasospasm and endothelial injury. The overall incidence of angina is approximately 10%.
- ACM typically occurs after yrs of heavy drinking. Concurrent cirrhosis may be present. The presentation is typically heart failure with or without arrhythmia. Atrial fibrillation is the most common arrhythmia associated with chronic alcohol abuse and can also be seen with acute intoxication (holiday heart syndrome).
- Patients with cocaine-induced CM may present with adrenergic symptoms (palpitations, pallor, diaphoresis, and anxiety), hypertension, angina, atrial and ventricular arrhythmias, and heart failure.
- Anabolic steroids can cause LV hypertrophy and dilation, and lead to heart failure, arrhythmia, myocardial infarction, hypertension, and sudden death.

ETIOLOGY

- The underlying mechanism of chemotherapy-induced cardiotoxicity is not well established. Several pathways have been proposed, including an increase in oxidative stress, free radical production, apoptosis, disturbance of DNA, RNA and protein synthesis, and vasospasm.
- Nutritional deficiencies, such as thiamine deficiency, also play a role in ACM.
- Table 2 describes mechanisms of ethanol-induced myocardial injury. Table 3 summarizes the effects of light-to-moderate and heavier alcohol intake on cardiovascular risk factors and outcomes.

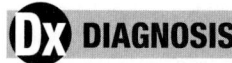

DIAGNOSIS

DIFFERENTIAL DIAGNOSIS

- Infectious cardiomyopathy: Viral, HIV related, Lyme disease, Chagas disease
- Ischemic cardiomyopathy
- Dilated cardiomyopathy, related to valvular disease or hypertension
- Cirrhotic cardiomyopathy
- Tachycardia-induced cardiomyopathy
- Stress-related (takotsubo) cardiomyopathy
- Peripartum cardiomyopathy
- Genetic causes of dilated cardiomyopathy

WORKUP

- Chemical exposure history.
- Electrocardiogram, serum electrolytes, renal function, and hepatic function.
- Serum troponin and brain natriuretic peptide (BNP) levels.
- Transthoracic echocardiogram for the evaluation of heart structure and function.
- Rule out the diagnosis of coronary artery disease by coronary angiography.
- Cardiac magnetic resonance (CMR) imaging can be used to evaluate for myocardial scar and fibrosis.

LABORATORY TESTS

- There are no specific diagnostic tests to help differentiate CMc from other forms of CM, but the following laboratory tests are generally helpful; serum electrolytes, renal function, hepatic function, thyroid-stimulating hormone, iron profile, and inflammatory markers.
- Recent studies have suggested that early elevation of troponin levels, BNP, and myeloperoxidase following chemotherapy may be a predictor of future development of cardiomyopathy.

TABLE 1 Chemotherapeutic Agents Implicated in Clinical Syndromes of Cardiotoxicity

Agent	Frequency of Cardiotoxicity*	Comments
Left Ventricular Dysfunction–Heart Failure		
Chemotherapeutics		
Anthracyclines		
Doxorubicin	+++	Highly dose-dependent
Epirubicin	+	Risk factors include age (old and young), prior mediastinal radiation, history of heart disease, decreased ejection fraction; drop in ejection fraction on drug therapy, female sex (for children), and other agents (especially trastuzumab)
Idarubicin	++	Risk decreased by liposomal encapsulation or dexrazoxane
Alkylating agents		
Cyclophosphamide	+++	Primarily seen with high-dose "conditioning" regimens
Ifosfamide	+++	Risk factors are previous mediastinal irradiation and anthracycline drug therapy Also can have myocarditis, pericarditis, myocardial necrosis
Taxanes		
Paclitaxel	+/++	Also employed in paclitaxel-eluting stent
Docetaxel	+	
Proteasome inhibitor		
Bortezomib	+/++	Moderately high rates of HF seen in trials (5%), but rates only minimally higher than in patients receiving dexamethasone
Targeted Therapeutics		
Monoclonal antibodies		
Trastuzumab	++	Not common as single agent Increased risk with anthracyclines, paclitaxel, cyclophosphamide
Pertuzumab	+/++	Targets HER2 Rates of LV dysfunction as high as ~25% in one series
Bevacizumab	+/++	Targets VEGF-A (ligand for VEGFRs) and serves as a trap, preventing interaction with its receptor HF can be seen in setting of severe hypertension, which occurs in 10%-25% of patients, depending on dose; anthracyclines may increase HF risk
Tyrosine kinase inhibitors		
Imatinib, nilotinib	+	Can cause severe fluid retention with peripheral edema, pleural and pericardial effusion not secondary to LV dysfunction
Dasatinib	++	Same as above regarding fluid retention Can cause severe pulmonary hypertension; mechanism unclear
Sunitinib	+++	LV dysfunction common; hypertension likely plays role
Sorafenib	++	Rate of cardiotoxicity not clear as of yet
Ischemic Syndromes		
Fluorouracil, capecitabine	++	ACS; patients with CAD at increased risk Recurs with rechallenge; multiple mechanisms proposed; etiology remains unknown
Cisplatin, carboplatin	+	ACS caused by vasospasm or vascular injury Hypertension common; thromboembolism more common (see below)
Interferon-α	+	Risk of ischemia increased in patients with CAD; hypertension common
Paclitaxel	+	Myocardial ischemia in 1%-5%; serious ischemic cardiac events not common
Docetaxel	+	Limited data, but rate probably ~1%
Bevacizumab	++	Arterial thrombotic events including MI and stroke
Vinca alkaloids	+	~1% risk of cardiac events; ischemia possibly caused by coronary spasm
Sorafenib	+/++	~2.5% risk of ACS
ErlotinibNilotinib	+/++	Limited data, but rate ~2% Concern over possible increase in peripheral vascular events
Hypertension		
Cisplatin	++++	
Bevacizumab	++++	Extremely common with all anti-VEGF therapeutics to date
Sunitinib	++++	Intrinsic in mechanism of action of these agents
Sorafenib	+++	
Venous Thrombosis		
Cisplatin	+++	Deep vein thrombosis or pulmonary embolism in 8.5%; most occur early in treatment Additional risk factors for deep vein thrombosis often present
Thalidomide	++++	Uncommon with monotherapy, but risk rises with concurrent chemotherapy
Lenalidomide	+++	See comments for thalidomide
Erlotinib	++	Rate with erlotinib plus gemcitabine ~2% over that with gemcitabine alone

*Relative frequency of cardiotoxicity is scored as follows: + = ≤1%; ++ = 1% to 5%; +++ = 6% to 10%; ++++ = >10%.
ACS, acute coronary syndrome; *CAD,* coronary artery disease; *HER2,* human epidermal growth factor receptor 2; *HF,* heart failure; *LV,* left ventricular; *MI,* myocardial infarction; *VEGF,* vascular endothelial cell growth factor; *VEGFR,* vascular endothelial cell growth factor receptor.
From Mann DL, et al.: *Braunwald's heart disease,* ed 10, Philadelphia, 2015, Elsevier.

TABLE 2 Mechanisms of Ethanol-Induced Myocardial Injury

Direct Toxic Effects
- Uncoupling of the excitation/contraction system
- Reduced calcium sequestration in the sarcoplasmic reticulum
- Inhibition of the sarcolemmal adenosine triphosphate–dependent Na^+/K^+ pump
- Reduction in the mitochondrial respiratory ratio
- Altered substrate uptake
- Increased interstitial/extracellular protein synthesis

Toxic Effect of Metabolites
- Acetaldehyde
- Ethyl esters

Nutritional or Trace Metal Deficiencies
- Thiamine
- Selenium

Electrolyte Disturbances
- Hypomagnesemia
- Hypokalemia
- Hypophosphatemia

Toxic Additives
- Cobalt
- Lead
- Arsenic

K, Potassium; *Na*, sodium. From Mann DL, Zipes DP, Libby P, Bonow RO: *Braunwald's heart disease*, ed 10, Philadelphia, 2015, Elsevier.

TABLE 3 Qualitative Effects of Light-to-Moderate and Heavier Alcohol Intake on Cardiovascular Risk Factors and Outcomes

Cardiovascular Risk Factors and Outcomes	Light-to-Moderate Alcohol Intake (<2 Drinks per Day)	Heavier Alcohol Intake (>2 Drinks per Day)
Blood pressure	↔	↑↑
HDL cholesterol	↑↑	↑↑↑
Triglycerides	↑	↑↑
LDL cholesterol	↔ or ↓	↑
Platelet aggregability/coagulability	↓	↓↓
Systemic inflammation	↓	↑
Congestive heart failure	↓	↑↑
Coronary artery disease (angina, nonfatal MI)	↓↓	↓
Atrial fibrillation	↔	↑↑
Stroke	↓	↑↑
Sudden cardiac death	↓↓	↑

HDL, High-density lipoprotein; *LDL*, low-density lipoprotein; *MI*, myocardial infarction. From Mann DL, Zipes DP, Libby P, Bonow RO: *Braunwald's heart disease*, ed 10, Philadelphia, 2015, Elsevier.

IMAGING STUDIES

- ECG

  Nonspecific findings of a cardiomyopathy may be present, including sinus tachycardia, nonspecific ST-T wave changes, decreased QRS voltage, interventricular conduction delay or bundle branch block, and QT interval abnormalities. In 5-FU toxicity, significant ST segment deviations may present.
- Echocardiogram
  1. Asymptomatic alcoholics may present with mild LV hypertrophy, diastolic dysfunction, LV dilation, and decrease in left ventricular ejection fraction (LVEF).
  2. Baseline LVEF should be performed before initiation of anthracycline-based chemotherapy, preferably with an echocardiogram or MUGA scan (multigated acquisition).
     a. Anthracycline-based chemotherapy should generally be avoided for patients with an LVEF ≤40, or LVEF >40 but <50 with prior heart failure.
     b. Total doxorubicin dose should be limited to 450 mg/m^2.
     c. If baseline LVEF is ≥55%, then subsequent evaluation should be at the end of treatment if the doxorubicin dose is <200 mg/m^2 or serially at 200, 300, 350, and 400 mg/m^2 for higher doses. Doxorubicin therapy should be discontinued if there is a >15% absolute drop in LVEF, decease in LVEF to ≤40%, or symptomatic congestive heart failure with an LVEF <50. There has been no direct causal link between anthracyclines and the development of heart failure with a preserved ejection fraction.
     d. Peak systolic global longitudinal strain imaging (GLS) is an emerging echocardiographic measurement. A 10% to 15% early decrease in GLS by speckle tracking echocardiography during treatment seems to be the most useful parameter for the early detection of cardiotoxicity. Echocardiographic strain and strain rate imaging are sensitive, noninvasive methods for assessment of myocardial function.
- Radionuclide imaging (Fig. 1).
  1. If baseline LVEF is <50% with no prior history of heart failure, the cardiac risks vs. oncological benefits should be discussed with the patient, cardiologist, and oncologist before initiating therapy. Cardio-protective agents such as ACE inhibitors and beta-blockers should be initiated and serial LVEF measurements done after each dose.
  2. Even after chemotherapy, periodic screening with echocardiography and/or biomarkers should be considered for up to 10 yr for those with high cumulative anthracycline doses or a history of reversible LV dysfunction during treatment.

Rx TREATMENT

Prevention
- Noninvasive assessment of LV function before, during, and after anthracycline-containing chemotherapy with echocardiography or MUGA scan.
- To reduce the risk of doxorubicin cardiotoxicity, the lifetime cumulative dosage should be limited to <450 mg/m^2 in adults.
- Other approaches include the use of infusion rather than bolus dosing, liposomal encapsulated doxorubicin, less cardiotoxic analogs of doxorubicin such as epirubicin, and coadministration of protective agents such as dexrazoxane.
- 5-FU treatment should be terminated if cardiac symptoms develop. Readministration is not recommended.

ACUTE GENERAL Rx

- Treat decompensated heart failure with diuresis and inotropes if there is a low cardiac output state.
- For angina in acute cocaine intoxication or induced by 5-FU, benzodiazepines, nitrites, and calcium channel blockers are first-line therapy. If ECG provides evidence of acute myocardial infarction, patients should proceed to emergent cardiac catheterization and coronary angiography.

CHRONIC Rx

- Dexrazoxane is an ethylenediaminetetraacetic acid-like chelator that acts by binding to iron, which prevents anthracycline cardiotoxicity. Cardio-oncology experts suggest a 10:1 ratio of dexrazoxane to anthracycline, given 15 to 30 minutes before doxorubicin

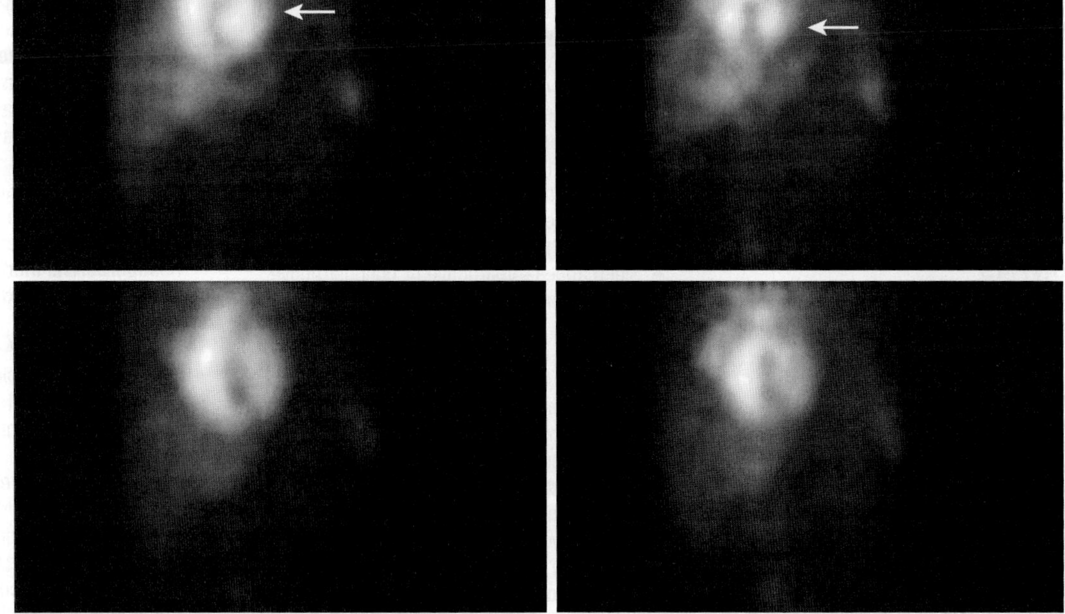

FIG. 1 Technetium-99m-pertechnetate multigated acquisition scans in a 47-year-old woman with breast cancer treated with doxorubicin. The top scan was taken before initiation of doxorubicin and cyclophosphamide therapy in September 2009. The left ventricular ejection fraction *(LVEF)* (left ventricular end-diastolic counts minus left ventricular end-systolic counts/left ventricular end-diastolic counts 100) was calculated at 60%. The bottom scan was taken in March 2010 after treatment with a total doxorubicin dose of 451 mg/m^2. Left ventricular ejection fraction was calculated at 28%. Left ventricle (*white arrows*) during end-diastole and end-systole. (From Figueredo VM: Chemical cardiomyopathies: the negative effects of medications and nonprescribed drugs on the heart, *Am J Med* 124:480-488, 2011.)

administration. However, its routine use is not currently recommended in adults except in cases of a cumulative doxorubicin dose of 300 mg/m^2 or greater with an ongoing indication to receive doxorubicin-based chemotherapy.

- Those developing anthracycline-induced CM generally should not be rechallenged with the drug, as the cardiac damage is usually irreversible due to cell death.
- Beta-blocker: Carvedilol and nebivolol have been shown to have protective effects on LV systolic function during anthracycline therapy. Larger trials with metoprolol have shown no benefit.
- The following ACE inhibitors and angiotensin receptor blocker (ARB) have been shown to protect against anthracycline cardiotoxicity: enalapril, ramipril, and telmisartan. Results from the PRADA trial suggest that use of the ARB candesartan mitigates anthracycline-induced decline in LVEF.
- There is growing interest in the use of statins for primary prevention of anthracycline-mediated cardiotoxicity based on their antioxidant and anti-inflammatory properties, although a cardioprotective effect has not been established.
- Thiamine, folic acid, and multivitamins are adjunctive treatments for ACM. Abstinence can usually reverse the cardiomyopathy.

DISPOSITION

Prognosis depends on the dosage of chemicals and the severity of LV dysfunction.

REFERRAL

Close follow-up with a cardiooncologist.

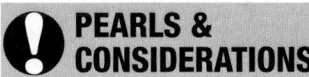

PEARLS & CONSIDERATIONS

The presentation of chemotherapy-induced cardiac toxicity ranges from an asymptomatic decline in LVEF to overt heart failure. The incidence is dose-dependent in the case of anthracyclines and may manifest up to 10 yr after the initial exposure. Therefore, regular clinical follow-up with echocardiographic surveillance is advised.

SUGGESTED READINGS

Available at ExpertConsult.com

AUTHORS: **HANNAH CHAUDRY, M.D.**, and **ARAVIND RAO KOKKIRALA, M.D. FACC.**

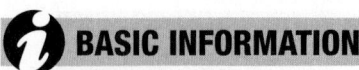

BASIC INFORMATION

DEFINITION

Dilated cardiomyopathy describes a group of diseases involving the myocardium and characterized by myocardial dysfunction that is not wholly the result of hypertension, coronary atherosclerosis, valvular dysfunction, congenital, or other structural heart disease. As a result, the heart is enlarged and the ventricles are dilated with impaired systolic function.

SYNONYMS

Congestive cardiomyopathy
Idiopathic cardiomyopathy

ICD-10CM CODES	
B33.24	Viral cardiomyopathy
I11.0	Hypertensive heart disease with heart failure
I42.0	Dilated cardiomyopathy (includes congestive cardiomyopathy)
I42.9	Cardiomyopathy, unspecified (includes cardiomyopathy [primary] [secondary] NOS)
I43	Cardiomyopathy in diseases classified elsewhere
I50.20 to I50.9	(Unspecified, acute, chronic, or acute on chronic) + (systolic, diastolic, or combined) (congestive) heart failure
O90.3	Peripartum cardiomyopathy

EPIDEMIOLOGY & DEMOGRAPHICS

- The estimated prevalence of dilated cardiomyopathy in the general adult population is approximately 1:2500. The incidence is approximately 4 to 8 per 100,000 persons per yr.
- The incidence of dilated cardiomyopathy is greatest in middle age and among men.
- African Americans have a threefold increased risk for developing DCM, irrespective of comorbidities or socioeconomic factors, compared with whites.
- It is the most common cardiomyopathy and accounts for 25% of cases of congestive heart failure.

PHYSICAL FINDINGS & CLINICAL PRESENTATION

The patient will present with common symptoms of congestive heart failure, which may be of insidious or sudden onset. The patient may also be asymptomatic and the diagnosis made by the unexpected finding of cardiomegaly on a chest x-ray. The history should focus also on information that could help determine the etiology. Classical signs of heart failure may be absent. When present, findings are indistinguishable from other heart failure syndromes, including:

- Increased jugular venous pressure
- Narrow pulse pressure
- Pulmonary rales, hepatomegaly, peripheral edema
- S3, S4
- Mitral regurgitation, tricuspid regurgitation (less common)

ETIOLOGY

In approximate order of occurrence:

- Idiopathic (often a viral infection that cannot be confirmed)
- Infections (viral [human herpesvirus 6, influenza, echovirus, cytomegalovirus, Coxsackie B, adenovirus, parvovirus, HIV], rickettsial, mycobacterial, toxoplasmosis, trichinosis, Chagas' disease)
- Alcoholism (15% to 40% of all cases in Western countries)
- Uncontrolled tachyarrhythmia ("tachycardia-mediated")
- Sleep apnea–obstructive or nonobstructive
- Cirrhotic–not necessarily alcohol-induced
- End-stage renal disease–related
- Nutritional deficiencies–selenium, L-carnitine, thiamine
- Peripartum (greatest risk from last trimester of pregnancy to 6 months postpartum)
- Chemotherapeutic (anthracycline, doxorubicin, daunorubicin) or pharmacologic agents (antiretrovirals, phenothiazines) (see "Cardiomyopathy, Chemical-Induced")
- Substance abuse (cocaine, heroin, organic solvents "glue-sniffer's heart")
- Postmyocarditis
- Toxins (cobalt, lead, phosphorus, carbon monoxide, mercury) Collagen-vascular disease (systemic lupus, rheumatoid arthritis, polyarteritis, dermatomyositis, sarcoidosis)
- Heredofamilial neuromuscular disease (e.g., muscular dystrophy)
- Excess hormones (acromegaly, osteogenesis imperfecta, myxedema, thyrotoxicosis, diabetes)
- Hematologic (e.g., sickle cell anemia, hemochromatosis, hypereosinophilia)
- Stress-induced (i.e., takotsubo or broken heart syndrome)
- LV noncompaction
- TTN truncating mutations (mutations in TTN, the gene encoding the sarcomere protein titin) are a common cause of dilated cardiomyopathy, occurring in approximately 25% of familial cases of idiopathic dilated cardiomyopathy and in 18% of sporadic cases

Dx DIAGNOSIS

Dilated cardiomyopathy is a diagnosis of exclusion, made after ruling out other potential causes of myocardial dysfunction.

DIFFERENTIAL DIAGNOSIS

- Coronary atherosclerosis, that is, left ventricular dysfunction secondary to ischemia and/or myocardial infarction
- Valvular dysfunction (especially aortic and mitral regurgitation)
- Other cardiomyopathies (restrictive, hypertrophic)
- Pulmonary disease (embolism, obstructive, restrictive)
- Pericardial abnormalities (constrictive pericarditis, tamponade)
- Hypothyroidism/myxedema
- Athlete's heart

WORKUP

- Medical history: Emphasis on symptoms of dyspnea, orthopnea, paroxysmal nocturnal dyspnea, weight gain, palpitations, fatigue, or signs of systemic and pulmonary embolism, substance abuse history, possible toxin exposures (especially occupational)
- Physical exam (see "Physical Findings & Clinical Presentation")
- Testing (see "Laboratory Tests" and "Imaging Studies" for more detail): Laboratory, chest x-ray, ECG, echocardiogram, cardiac catheterization; myocardial biopsy is not routinely recommended, unless acute myocarditis requiring immunosuppressive therapy is considered (e.g., giant cell myocarditis)

LABORATORY TESTS

- Chemistries/metabolites (deficiencies), renal function tests (renal dysfunction)
- Cardiac biomarkers (elevation of cardiac troponin or BNP)
  1. Persistently increased cardiac troponin T levels are a marker of poor outcome in cardiomyopathy patients
- Endocrine (particularly thyroid)
- Iron studies (hemochromatosis, deficiency)
- Rheumatologic and inflammatory (ANA, ESR, CRP)
- Others as indicated (HIV, Lyme, neurohormonal)

IMAGING STUDIES

Chest x-ray:

- Cardiac silhouette enlargement (particularly left ventricle)
- Pulmonary vascular redistribution and congestion (Kerley B lines, cephalization of vasculature), pleural effusion (may appear as unilateral, most often on the right side)

ECG:

- ECG findings are typically nonspecific, and sinus tachycardia is usually a reflection of underlying heart failure. Large voltage in precordial leads and low voltage in limb leads may be seen in advanced disease.
- Intraventricular conduction defects and left bundle branch block
- Arrhythmias (atrial fibrillation, premature ventricular or atrial contractions, ventricular tachycardia)

Echocardiogram (Fig. E1):

- Low ejection fraction with global hypokinesis
- Four-chamber enlargement (LV enlargement usually predominates)
- Mitral or tricuspid regurgitation ("secondary" regurgitation from tethering due to incomplete leaflet closure caused by ventricular dilation)

Cardiac catheterization:

- On initial presentation to exclude obstructive epicardial coronary artery disease

Cardiac magnetic resonance imaging (CMRI):

- Particularly if infiltrative or inflammatory etiology suspected

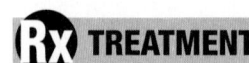

Rx TREATMENT

NONPHARMACOLOGIC THERAPY

- Treatment of underlying disease (systemic lupus, alcoholism)
- Dietary sodium restriction (<2 g/day)

- Exercise training has been shown to be associated with reduced risk for hospitalization and death in patients with history of heart failure in limited trials; enrollment in a formal cardiac rehabilitation program may be beneficial in improving patient's functional status

ACUTE GENERAL Rx

- Identify and treat the etiology of the acute exacerbation, when able. A helpful mnemonic is FAILURE: failure to take medications, anemia/arrhythmia, ischemia/infection/infarction, lifestyle (dietary indiscretion), upregulation of cardiac output (hyperthyroidism or pregnancy), renal failure, embolus (pulmonary).
- Diuretics are indicated for all patients with current symptoms or history of heart failure and reduced left ventricular ejection fraction (LVEF) with evidence of volume overload (see "Physical Findings and Clinical Presentation") to improve symptoms. It is important to note that diuretics have not been shown to improve mortality rates.
- Patients with associated coronary atherosclerosis (angina, ECG changes, reversible defects on myocardial perfusion imaging) may benefit from percutaneous or surgical revascularization.

CHRONIC Rx

- Diuretics and digoxin as noted in "Acute General Rx."
- ACE inhibitors (and angiotensin receptor blockers) have been shown to have favorable effects on ventricular remodeling in patients with cardiomyopathy and a demonstrable mortality benefit in these patients. They also reduce afterload and improve cardiac output. Therefore, they are recommended in all patients with reduced LV systolic function (EF ≤40%), regardless of symptoms unless specific contraindications exist.
- Beta-blockers work by inhibiting the adverse effects of the sympathetic nervous system in patients with ventricular systolic dysfunction (EF ≤40%). Only carvedilol, long-acting metoprolol succinate, and bisoprolol have shown a mortality benefit in patients with LV systolic dysfunction. Unless specifically contraindicated, they should be started after the acute exacerbation has resolved and titrated to the maximum tolerated dose.
- Aldosterone antagonists (spironolactone and eplerenone) have shown mortality benefit along with a decreased rate of hospitalization for heart failure in patients with symptomatic heart failure and reduced LV systolic function (EF ≤35%). They should be used following label guidelines and with close monitoring of renal function and potassium.
- Hydralazine/nitrates improve both morbidity and mortality, and should be considered in the following populations: African Americans with persistent NYHA class III or IV heart failure with an EF <40%, on optimal medical therapy (beta blocker and ACE or ARB); or for those unable to take ACE inhibitors or ARBs due to intolerance, hypotension, or renal insufficiency.
- Digoxin has no mortality benefit but has been shown to improve patients' quality of life in appropriately selected patients.
- The angiotensin receptor-neprilysin inhibitor sacubitril/valsartan (LCZ696 or Entresto™) in place of an ACE inhibitor or angiotensin receptor blocker and on top of optimal medical therapy in patients with class II-IV heart failure and an EF of 40% or less was found to significantly reduce multiple heart failure end points, including death, hospitalizations, and CV death in comparison to enalapril. This medication was approved in the U.S. in 2015.
- Ivabradine was FDA approved in 2015 for patients with stable, symptomatic chronic heart failure with left ventricular ejection fraction ≤35% who are in sinus rhythm with resting heart rates ≥70 beats/min and either of the following: (1) are on maximally tolerated doses of beta-blockers or (2) have a contraindication to beta-blocker use. It acts by blocking the hyperpolarization-activated cyclic nucleotide-gated (HCN) channel responsible for the cardiac pacemaker I_f current, which regulates heart rate.

DISPOSITION

- Annual mortality rate is 20% in patients with moderate heart failure, and it exceeds 50% in patients with severe heart failure. Once symptomatic, hospitalizations are frequent and readmission rates are high (>50% at 3 mo). A multispecialty treatment approach (e.g., primary care, cardiology, nutrition, cardiac rehabilitation) is recommended.
- Factors associated with an adverse outcome in dilated cardiomyopathy are described in Table 1.

REFERRAL

- Implantation of a cardiac defibrillator for primary prevention of sudden cardiac death can be considered for patients with LVEF <35% on optimal medical therapy regardless of symptom status. Emerging data have called into question the benefit of ICD implantation in patients with nonischemic heart failure (the DANISH Study), although these findings have not yet made it into the guidelines.
- Patients with LVEF <35%, left bundle branch block on ECG (QRS ≥0.13 sec), and persistent heart failure symptoms may benefit from cardiac resynchronization therapy via a biventricular pacemaker.
- Consider heart transplantation for relatively young patients (there is no precise age threshold) free of other significant comorbid conditions who are unresponsive to medical therapy. Dilated cardiomyopathy is the reason for 45% of all heart transplantations in the U.S.

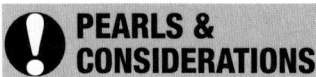

COMMENTS

- Patients should be encouraged to restrict or eliminate alcohol and reduce sodium intake (<2 g daily).
- Patients may benefit from daily weight checks as a means of early detection of volume overload and decompensated heart failure.
- Vulnerability to cardiomyopathy among chronic alcohol abusers is partially genetic and related to the presence of the ACE DD genotype.
- Idiopathic dilated cardiomyopathy is often familial, and apparently healthy relatives may have latent, early, or undiagnosed disease. Echocardiographic evaluation of family members is recommended.
- Incorporation of sequencing approaches that detect TTN truncations into genetic testing for dilated cardiomyopathy may substantially increase test sensitivity and allow earlier diagnosis of dilated cardiomyopathy.

SUGGESTED READINGS

Available at ExpertConsult.com

RELATED CONTENT

Dilated Cardiomyopathy (Patient Information)
Cardiomyopathy, Chemical Induced (Related Key Topic)

AUTHOR: **CHRISTOPHER P. BLOMBERG, D.O.**

TABLE 1 Factors Associated with an Adverse Outcome in Dilated Cardiomyopathy

Clinical	Noninvasive	Invasive
NYHA Class III/IV	Low LV ejection fraction	High LV filling pressures
Increasing age	Marked LV dilation	
Low exercise peak oxygen consumption	Low LV mass	
Marked intraventricular conduction delay	≥Moderate mitral regurgitation	
Complex ventricular arrhythmias	Abnormal diastolic function	
Abnormal signal-averaged ECG	Abnormal contractile reserve	
Evidence of excessive sympathetic stimulation	Right ventricular dilation or dysfunction	
Protodiastolic gallop (S_3)		
Elevated serum BNP		
Elevated uric acid		
Decreased serum sodium		

BNP, Brain natriuretic peptide; *ECG*, electrocardiogram; *LV*, left ventricular; *NYHA*, New York Heart Association.
From Hare JM: The dilated, restrictive, and infiltrative cardiomyopathies. In Bonow RO et al, (eds): *Braunwald's heart disease—a textbook of cardiovascular medicine,* ed 9, St Louis, 2011, Saunders.

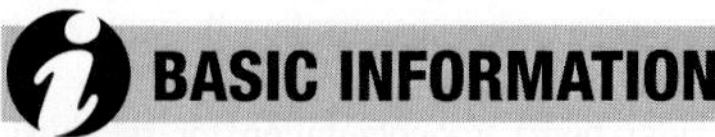

BASIC INFORMATION

DEFINITION

Hypertrophic cardiomyopathy (HCM) is most commonly an autosomal dominant myocardial disorder characterized by disorganized myocyte architecture and marked thickening (hypertrophy) of the left ventricular wall (≥15 mm), without dilation, not explained by another cardiac or systemic disorder. The interventricular septum is the most common site of enlargement, though hypertrophy may involve other focal regions or may be concentric. HCM may result in hemodynamically significant obstruction within the left ventricular outflow tract (LVOT) and/or impairment of the diastolic function of the left ventricle. However, about one third of patients have no obstruction at rest or with provocation.

SYNONYMS

HCM
Hypertrophic cardiomyopathy
Idiopathic hypertrophic subaortic stenosis (IHSS)
Hypertrophic obstructive cardiomyopathy (HOCM)
Hypertrophic nonobstructive cardiomyopathy
Asymmetric septal hypertrophy (ASH)
Familial hypertrophic cardiomyopathy

ICD-10CM CODES

I42.1	Obstructive hypertrophic cardiomyopathy (Includes hypertrophic subaortic stenosis)
I42.2	Other hypertrophic cardiomyopathy (Includes nonobstructive hypertrophic cardiomyopathy)
I42.8	Other cardiomyopathies
I42.9	Cardiomyopathy, unspecified (includes cardiomyopathy [primary] [secondary] NOS)

EPIDEMIOLOGY & DEMOGRAPHICS

- Prevalence in the general population in the U.S., China, and Japan is estimated to be between 1/500 to 1/200 (the most common genetically transmitted cardiovascular disease).
- HCM is the most common cause of sudden cardiac death in young athletes (more commonly among blacks).
- There is equal prevalence in men and women (probably underdiagnosed in women).
- It occurs across ethnicities, perhaps underdiagnosed among blacks.
- Mortality rate is approximately 1%/yr, as high as to 2%/yr in children.
- The most common form of the disease is familial (60%-70% of cases), and it follows an autosomal dominant inheritance pattern with variable expression.
- Spontaneous mutations can also occur, accounting for approximately 20% of cases. It is otherwise indistinguishable from the familial form.
- A variant form seen in the elderly (5%-10% of cases) has a better prognosis, and it is not typically associated with sudden cardiac death.
- The familial form is usually diagnosed in young patients. It is most often caused by a mutation in one of the contractile protein genes of the cardiac sarcomere. See "Etiology" for more details.
- Nonsarcomeric genetic mutations that cause storage disease (e.g., Fabry disease) have a very similar clinical presentation.
- Apical HCM is a variant more common among Asians: As many as 41% of Chinese HCM and 15% of Japanese HCM patients. Clinically there is no LVOT obstruction.

PHYSICAL FINDINGS & CLINICAL PRESENTATION

Patients may have subtle symptoms of progressive congestive heart failure (CHF). At the time of diagnosis, most patients are asymptomatic, referred and diagnosed based on family history. HCM may be suspected on the basis of abnormalities found on physical examination. Classic findings include:

- Harsh, systolic, crescendo–decrescendo murmur at the left sternal border or apex. The murmur increases with maneuvers that decrease venous return or LV size (Valsalva, standing), and decreases with those that increase venous return or afterload (squatting, hand grip, post-Valsalva release).
- Paradoxical splitting of S2 (if left ventricular obstruction is present).
- S4 may be present.
- Double or triple LV apical impulse ("triple ripple": Atrial contraction, early rapid ejection, and late slow ejection).
- Pulsus bisferiens (double pulsation on palpation of the carotid pulse).

Increased obstruction can occur with:

- Drugs: Digitalis, β-adrenergic stimulators (isoproterenol, dopamine, epinephrine), nitroglycerin, vasodilators, diuretics, alcohol, inhalation of amyl nitrate
- Hypovolemia
- Tachycardia
- Valsalva maneuver
- Standing position

Decreased obstruction is seen with:

- Drugs: β-adrenergic blockers, calcium channel blockers, disopyramide, α-adrenergic stimulators
- Volume expansion
- Bradycardia
- Hand-grip exercise
- Squatting position
- Release phase of the Valsalva maneuver

Clinical manifestations are as follows:

- Syncope or presyncope (usually seen with exercise)
- Angina
- Palpitations
- Sudden cardiac death
- Heart failure (typically with advanced stages): Dyspnea on exertion, orthopnea, edema, increased jugular venous pressure, paroxysmal nocturnal dyspnea

ETIOLOGY

- Genetic: Autosomal dominant trait with variable penetrance caused by mutations in multiple genes encoding proteins of the cardiac sarcomere and calcium regulation. To date, >1400 mutations have been identified among at least 13 genes, with variable phenotypes, expressivity, and penetrance. The most vigorous evidence indicates that 8 genes are known to definitively cause HCM: beta myosin heavy chain, myosin binding protein C, troponin T, troponin I, tropomyosin alpha-1 chain, actin, regulatory light chain, and essential light chain. HCM may be caused by a single mutation in one of two alleles; however, 5% of patients have at least two mutations. Sarcomeric protein gene mutations account for up to 60% of cases of HCM.
- Metabolic: Most are autosomal recessive, but some are X-linked. Most commonly, they are due to Anderson-Fabry disease (a lysosomal storage disease). Other metabolic etiologies include the glycogen storage diseases Pompe and Danon, AMP-kinase (PRKAG2), and carnitine disorders.
- Mitochondrial: These comprise autosomal dominant, autosomal recessive, X-linked, and maternally inherited traits. Most frequently, they are due to mutations in the respiratory chain protein complexes. The age of onset and severity of involvement are variable.
- Neuromuscular: These are most commonly associated with Friedreich's ataxia, but they are also associated with FHLI.
- Malformation syndromes: These etiologies include Noonan, LEOPARD, Costello, and cardiofasciocutaneous.
- Amyloidosis: These include familial ATTR, wild-type TTR (senile), and amyloid light-chain (AL) amyloidosis.
- Drug-induced: Tacrolimus, hydroxychloroquine, and steroids.
- Sporadic occurrence.

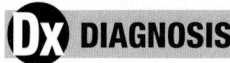

DIAGNOSIS

DIFFERENTIAL DIAGNOSIS

- Hypertensive heart disease
- Aortic stenosis
- Subaortic stenosis
- Athlete's heart
- Volume depletion

WORKUP

- Medical history: Unexplained clinical manifestations and/or family history of sudden death.
- Physical exam: See "Physical Findings & Clinical Presentation."
- Genetic counseling with or without testing.
- ECG is abnormal in 75% to 95% of patients, although there are no pathognomonic findings. Typical findings include:
  1. LV hypertrophy (abnormally tall R waves in the precordial leads) in up to 80% of patients (Fig. E1).
  2. Abnormal Q waves in lateral and inferior leads.
  3. T wave inversions (associated with the apical hypertrophy predominant variant).

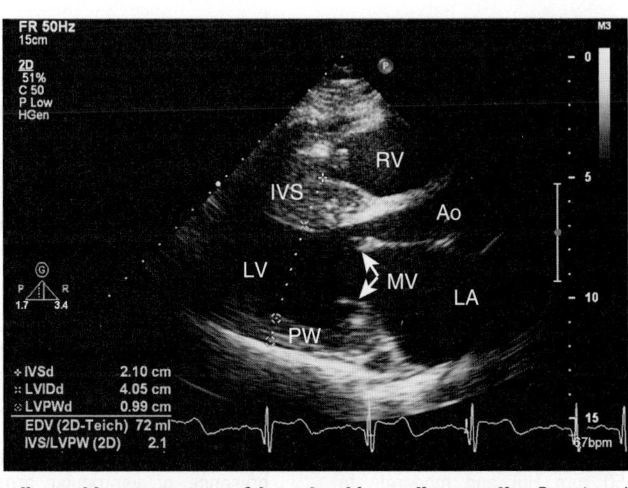

FIG. 2 Echocardiographic appearance of hypertrophic cardiomyopathy. Parasternal long-axis view from a patient with hypertrophic cardiomyopathy demonstrating asymmetrical septal hypertrophy. The interventricular septum (marked by *arrow*) measures 2.1 cm; the posterior wall measures 0.99 cm. *Ao*, Aorta; *IVS*, interventricular septum; *LA*, left atrium; *LV*, left ventricle; *MV*, mitral valve; *PW*, posterior wall; *RV*, right ventricle. (From Issa Z, et al.: *Clinical arrhythmology and electrophysiology*, ed 2, Philadelphia, 2012, Saunders.)

- Echocardiography (Fig. 2) is usually diagnostic as the majority of patients have significant LV hypertrophy (See "Imaging Studies" for details) and should be repeated every 12 to 24 months or as clinically needed.
- 24-hour Holter monitor to screen for potentially lethal ventricular arrhythmias (principal cause of syncope or sudden death in obstructive cardiomyopathy) should be performed at the initial diagnosis and in patients that subsequently develop palpitations, lightheadedness, or syncope. The presence of these arrhythmias identifies patients who are candidates for ICD therapy.
- In the absence of significant LVOT obstruction, exercise testing is indicated at diagnosis and annually thereafter to evaluate for symptoms and response to exercise. A drop in systolic blood pressure by at least 20 mm Hg or failure to augment by at least 20 mm Hg with exercise are markers of poor prognosis and are indicators for referral for myotomy/myomectomy. Cardiopulmonary exercise testing can provide objective evidence for worsening diseases, but need only be performed every 2 to 3 yr.
- Biomarkers of myocardial fibrosis in HCM include BNP and high-sensitivity cardiac troponin T and I. Other labs include CBC, BMP, LFTs, TSH, SPEP, UPEP, Kappa/Lambda.
- Screening for sarcomere protein gene mutations in family members of patients with HCM can identify a broad subgroup of patients with increased propensity toward long-term impairment of left ventricular function and adverse outcome, irrespective of the myofilament (thick, intermediate, or thin) involvement.
- In individuals with pathogenic mutations who do not express the HCM phenotype, it is recommended to perform serial electrocardiogram (ECG), transthoracic echocardiogram (TTE), and clinical assessment at periodic intervals (12 to 18 months in children and adolescents and about every 5 yr in adults), based on the patient's age and change in clinical status.
- Endomyocardial biopsy may be helpful to rule out diseases other than HCM if a diagnosis remains inconclusive after extensive testing.

IMAGING STUDIES

- Chest x-ray may be normal or show cardiomegaly.
- Two-dimensional echocardiography is used to establish the diagnosis and assess the severity of obstruction when present. LV wall thickness will usually be ≥15 mm (although some may be genetically positive but phenotype negative), and most patients (up to 95%) will have asymmetric (ratio of septum thickness to left ventricular wall thickness >1.3:1) LV wall hypertrophy. Symmetric LV hypertrophy is less common. The septum is most often affected, followed by the left ventricular midcavity and apex. In addition, 25% to 30% of patients will manifest systolic anterior motion (SAM) of the anterior leaflet of the mitral valve, causing obstruction of the LVOT and mitral regurgitation. Two-dimensional strain imaging echocardiography is useful for differentiation of HCM and cardiac amyloidosis from other causes of ventricular wall thickening. Up to 80% of HCM patients will also have diastolic dysfunction as evidenced by pulsed mitral valve inflow pattern and tissue Doppler.
- Cardiac MRI or cardiac CT may be of diagnostic value when echocardiographic studies are technically inadequate. MRI is also useful in identifying unusual segmental hypertrophy undetectable by standard echocardiography and can detect myocardial replacement fibrosis (an independent predictor of adverse cardiac outcomes and ventricular arrhythmias) using late gadolinium enhancement. CMR evaluation may be considered every 5 yr or every 2 to 3 yr in patients with progressive disease.

Rx TREATMENT

NONPHARMACOLOGIC THERAPY

- Avoid volume depletion: HCM patients experience decrease in stroke volume and consequent increase in left ventricular outflow gradient with exercise. This may lead to hypotension, dizziness, and syncope.
- Exercise restriction: The risk of sudden cardiac death is increased by exercise in HCM patients. Participation in competitive sports and intense physical activity should be avoided. As a part of a healthy lifestyle, low-intensity aerobic exercise is reasonable.
- Avoidance of alcohol: Alcohol use (even in small amounts) may result in increased obstruction of the left ventricular outflow tract. Other stimulants such as cocaine and other sympathomimetic recreational drugs should also be avoided.

GENERAL Rx

- Therapy for HCM is directed at blocking the effect of catecholamines and avoiding vasodilator or diuretic agents that can exacerbate the dynamic left ventricular outflow tract obstruction.
- Beta-blockers' beneficial effects on symptoms (principally dyspnea and chest pain) and exercise tolerance appear to be largely a result of a decrease in the heart rate with consequent prolongation of diastole and increased passive ventricular filling. By reducing the inotropic response, beta-blockers may also reduce myocardial oxygen demand and decrease the outflow gradient during exercise, when sympathetic tone is increased.
- Nondihydropyridine calcium channel blockers (e.g., verapamil is the preferred agent, diltiazem) can also decrease left ventricular outflow obstruction through a mechanism similar to beta-blockers. However, they are mainly second-line agents used in patients who cannot tolerate beta-blockers as they also theoretically have vasodilatory properties that may worsen severe outflow tract gradients.
- Disopyramide is an antiarrhythmic that is also a negative inotrope, resulting in further decrease in outflow gradient. It is sometimes used in combination with beta-blockers.
- Prophylactic antibiotics before dental, GI, and genitourinary procedures are no longer recommended according to the 2007 American Heart Association (AHA) guidelines.
- Avoid use of digitalis, intravenous inotropes, dihydropyridine calcium channel blockers (e.g., nifedipine, amlodipine), nitrates, and vasodilators.
- Diuretics, angiotensin-converting enzyme inhibitors, and angiotensin receptor blockers should be used with caution.
- Intravenous phenylephrine (or another pure vasoconstricting agent) is recommended for the treatment of acute hypotension in patients with obstructive HCM who do not respond to fluid administration.

- Implantable cardiac defibrillators (ICDs) are a safe and effective therapy in HCM patients prone to ventricular arrhythmias. In their practice guidelines, the major cardiology societies (AHA/ACC/HRS) give a strong recommendation (Class I) for ICD implantation in all patients with HCM who have had an episode of sustained ventricular tachycardia or fibrillation. In addition, they endorse the prophylactic placement of an ICD (Class IIa recommendation) for patients with one or more of the major risk factors for sudden cardiac death (outlined in "Disposition").
- Dual-chamber pacing may provide symptomatic relief of symptoms attributable to LVOT obstruction and refractory to medical therapy.
- HCM patients are at an increased risk of atrial fibrillation (AF) as well as systemic thromboembolization. AF occurs in over 20% of the HCM population. AF is an important source of symptoms, morbidity, and mortality and correlates to a worse prognosis. AF therapy is indicated independent of CHA2DS2-VASc score and should aim for thromboembolic risk mitigation with a vitamin K antagonist (unless contraindicated) and symptom alleviation via rhythm (generally preferred due to poor tolerance of AF with HCM) or rate control. If a vitamin K antagonist cannot be used in a patient (due to inability to maintain a therapeutic INR, inability to adequately perform INR monitoring, or other side effects), the 2014 ESC HCM (Class Ib) and 2014 ACC/AHA/HRS AF (Class Ic) guidelines recommend the use of direct thrombin or factor Xa inhibitors, even though there is no data on their use in patients with HCM.

DISPOSITION

HCM is not a static disease. Some adults may experience subtle regression in wall thickness, whereas others (~5%-10%) paradoxically evolve into an end-stage cardiomyopathy resembling dilated cardiomyopathy, characterized by cavity enlargement, left ventricular wall thinning, and systolic dysfunction. Patients with HCM are at increased risk for sudden death, especially if the onset of symptoms began during childhood. Severe left ventricular outflow obstruction at rest is also a strong, independent predictor of severe symptoms of heart failure and death. ICD implantation for primary prevention should be considered if patients (particularly the young) have any of the following high-risk features:

- Personal history of sudden cardiac death or out of hospital cardiac arrest (major risk factor)
- Spontaneous sustained ventricular tachycardia or ventricular fibrillation (major risk factor)
- Family history of premature death in a first-degree relative possibly caused by HCM
- Unexplained syncope
- Nonsustained ventricular tachycardia during Holter monitoring
- Substantial septal hypertrophy (>30 mm)
- Abnormal blood pressure response during exercise
- Increased delayed gadolinium enhancement on cardiac magnetic resonance imaging is suggested in some recent studies as a marker of increased SCD risk

The European Society of Cardiology sponsors a HCM Risk-SCD calculator that is useful in estimating the 5-yr risk of sudden cardiac death in appropriate populations using the aforementioned data points and can help guide recommendations for placement of an ICD (http://www.doc2do.com/hcm/webHCM.html).

REFERRAL

- Surgical treatment (septal myectomy involving resection of the basal septum) is now the gold standard for relieving outflow tract obstruction in patients with large outflow gradient (≥50 mm Hg) and moderate to severe symptoms unresponsive to medical therapy. The risk for sudden death from arrhythmias is not altered by surgery. When this operation is performed by experienced surgeons in tertiary referral centers, the operative mortality rate is <1%, and many patients are able to achieve near-normal exercise capacity after surgery. Mitral valvuloplasty or plication in combination with myectomy may be necessary in <5% of patients. Risks of surgery include AV nodal block, ventricular septal defect, and aortic regurgitation (AR).
- Alcohol septal ablation is a nonsurgical alternative to reduce the size of the interventricular septum. This can be done in patients with HCM refractory to pharmacologic treatment, particularly in those who are not candidates for myectomy due to high surgical risk or patient preference. This technique involves the injection of ethanol in a septal perforator branch of the left anterior descending coronary artery (Fig. E3), producing a controlled myocardial infarction of the interventricular septum, and thereby reducing septal mass and consequently the left ventricular outflow tract gradient. This method may lead to improvement in both subjective and objective measures of exercise capacity, but results are not as effective as surgery because they are associated with a high incidence of heart block, requiring permanent pacing in approximately one fourth of patients, and/or recurrence of obstruction and symptoms. This should be done only at centers with experienced operators.
- Refractory end-stage HF symptoms can be treated with LVAD, BiVAD, or heart transplant.

PEARLS & CONSIDERATIONS

COMMENTS

- Clinical screening of first-degree relatives with two-dimensional echocardiography and ECG is indicated. Starting at the age of 12, periodic screening at 12- to 18-month intervals is recommended for children of patients with HCM and in competitive athletes. Periodic screening of first-degree adult family members not in competitive athletics is recommended at 5-yr intervals because hypertrophy may not be detected until the sixth decade of life. Genetic testing is not indicated in relatives of index patients who do not have a definite pathogenic mutation.
- Genetic counseling and screening (Fig. 4) is recommended in first-degree relatives of patients with HCM. Genetic screening of first-degree relatives can refine or eliminate the need for periodic clinical screening. At least 13 genes are known to cause HCM, among them: cardiac myosin binding protein-C, beta-myosin heavy chain, troponin T, troponin I, alpha tropomyosin, actin regulatory light chain, and essential light chain. Clinical predictors of positive genotype, such as the presence of ventricular arrhythmias, age at diagnosis, degree of left ventricular wall hypertrophy, and family history of HCM, may aid in patient selection for genetic testing and increase the yield of cardiac sarcomere gene screening. Currently a mutation can be identified in 40% to 60% of all cases, sporadic or familial.
- All HCM patients who wish to become pregnant should be given prenatal counseling about the risk of transmission (about 50%) to their offspring and should be followed at a tertiary care center that specializes in high-risk pregnancies. Most patients with HCM tolerate pregnancy well due to the higher circulating blood volume.
- The mortality rate in HCM is approximately 1% to 2% per yr.
- About one third of HCM patients will not have a resting or labile outflow gradient (i.e., nonobstructive form of HCM), but it is important to note that lethal ventricular arrhythmias can occur in the absence of obstruction or symptoms.
- Myocardial fibrosis is a hallmark of hypertrophic cardiomyopathy. Biomarkers of collagen metabolism such as serum C-terminal propeptide of type I procollagen (PICP) are significantly higher in mutation carriers without left ventricular hypertrophy and in subjects with overt hypertrophic cardiomyopathy than in controls, indicating that a probiotic state precedes the development of hypertrophy of fibrosis identifiable with cardiac MRI.

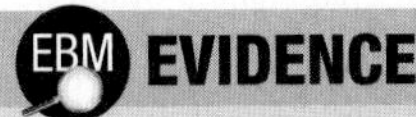

EVIDENCE

Available at ExpertConsult.com

SUGGESTED READINGS

Available at ExpertConsult.com

RELATED CONTENT

Hypertrophic Cardiomyopathy (Patient Information)

AUTHOR: **CHRISTOPHER P. BLOMBERG, D.O.**

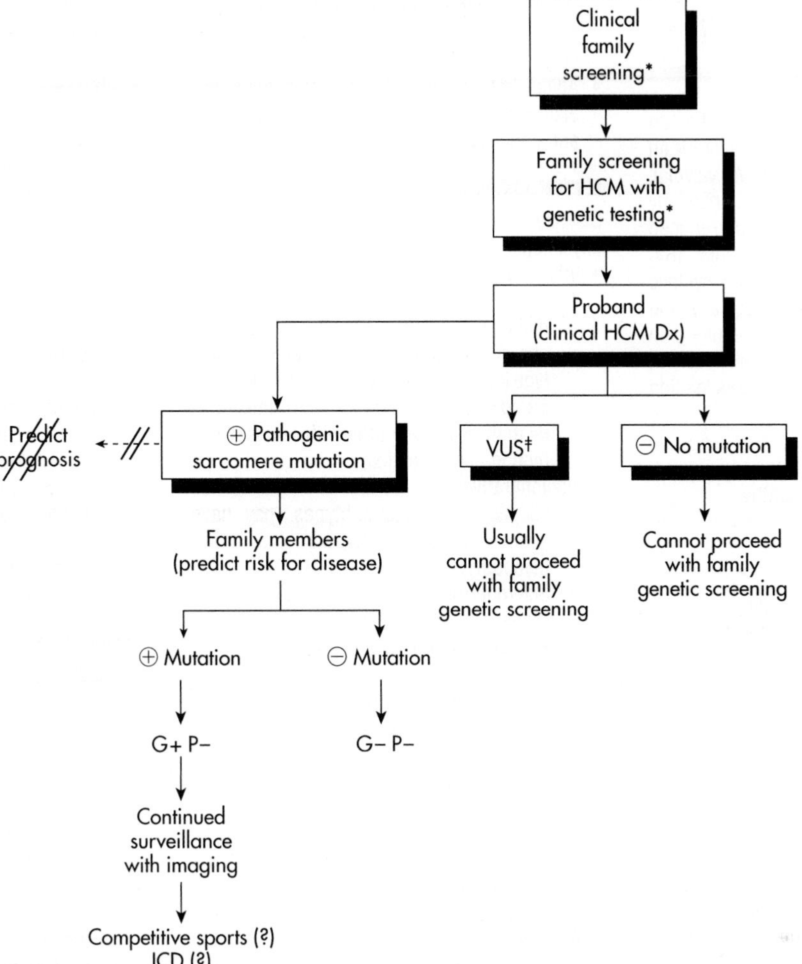

FIG. 4 Role of genetic testing in family screening strategies in hypertrophic cardiomyopathy (HCM). Some form of family screening for HCM in family members of the proband is universally recommended. The preferred first option (*) for clinical testing family members is usually with cardiac imaging and electrocardiography to identify phenotype-positive relatives. The predominant role for genetic testing in this setting is to identify those family members who are at risk for developing disease who do not have left ventricular (LV) hypertrophy. This strategy is initiated by successfully genotyping the proband with a clinically expressed HCM phenotype. Failure to identify the causative mutation in the proband is an indeterminate result that provides no useful information and precludes predictive testing in family members. The likelihood of obtaining a positive test result in the proband is less than 50%, insofar as all genes causing HCM have not yet been identified. Furthermore, many of the detected mutations will not be judged to be pathogenic, thereby eliminating substantially more than 50% of families from the option of genotyping for identification of relatives at risk for HCM. Accordingly, the genetic test results in the proband will be actionable in terms of family screening in only a minority of cases. *Dx*, diagnosis; *G+ P–*, genotype-positive, phenotype-negative; *G– P–*, genotype-negative, phenotype-negative; *ICD*, implantable cardioverter-defibrillator; *VUS*, variant of uncertain significance. (Modified from Maron BJ, Maron MS, Semsarian C: Genetics of hypertrophic cardiomyopathy after 20 years: clinical perspectives, *J Am Coll Cardiol* 60:705, 2012. In Mann DL, Zipes DP, Libby P, Bonow RO: *Braunwald's heart disease*, ed 10, Philadelphia, 2015. Elsevier.)

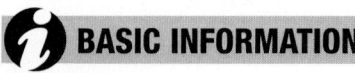

BASIC INFORMATION

DEFINITION

Restrictive cardiomyopathy refers to either an idiopathic or a systemic myocardial disorder (in the absence of ischemic, hypertensive, valvular, or congenital heart disease) characterized by restrictive filling (Fig. E1), normal or reduced left ventricular (LV) and right ventricular (RV) volumes, and normal or near normal systolic LV and RV function. Pathophysiologically, the heart muscle is abnormally stiff, resulting in decreased compliance, abnormal relaxation in diastole, and increased filling pressures leading to enlarged left atria.

SYNONYMS

Idiopathic restrictive cardiomyopathy
Infiltrative cardiomyopathy

ICD-10CM CODES

D86.XX	Sarcoidosis-related codes
E83.11X	Hemochromatosis-related codes
E85.X	Amyloidosis-related codes
I42.5	Other restrictive cardiomyopathy
I42.8	Other cardiomyopathies
I43.1	Cardiomyopathy in metabolic diseases
I42.9	Cardiomyopathy, unspecified

EPIDEMIOLOGY & DEMOGRAPHICS

- A relatively uncommon cardiomyopathy, accounting for 5% of all primary myocardial diseases.
- Most frequently caused by amyloidosis or myocardial fibrosis (following open heart surgery, transplantation or radiation).
- Patients classified as having "idiopathic" restrictive cardiomyopathy may have mutations in the gene for cardiac troponin I, and restrictive cardiomyopathy may represent an overlap with hypertrophic cardiomyopathy in many familial cases.

PHYSICAL FINDINGS & CLINICAL PRESENTATION

Restrictive cardiomyopathy presents with symptoms of progressive left-sided and right-sided heart failure:

- Fatigue, weakness (caused by low output as patients are unable to augment cardiac output by increasing heart rate without compromising ventricular filling).
- Progressively worsening exercise intolerance and dyspnea.
- Anginal chest pain can be seen (particularly in patients with amyloidosis) from myocardial compression of small coronaries.
- Palpitations (atrial fibrillation is common), dizziness or syncope (from orthostasis, heart block, or malignant arrhythmia).
- Edema, ascites, hepatomegaly, distended neck veins (from elevated right heart pressures).
- Kussmaul sign may be present (rise, or failure to fall, of the jugular veins on inspiration).
- On auscultation: Murmurs of mitral or tricuspid regurgitation may be heard; an S3 may be present.
- Apical impulse may be palpable (can help distinguish it from constrictive pericarditis) and nondisplaced.

ETIOLOGY

Disease may be classified according to pathophysiologic processes:

- Infiltrative:
  1. Amyloidosis (most common overall): The main types include AA, AL, Aß (ß amyloid), and ATTR (transthyretin-mutated or wild type [commonly known as senile systemic])
  2. Sarcoidosis (more commonly causing a dilated cardiomyopathy with regional wall motion abnormalities)
- Noninfiltrative:
  1. Idiopathic (familial subtypes may have genetic overlap with hypertrophic cardiomyopathy)
  2. Scleroderma
  3. Diabetic cardiomyopathy
  4. Pseudoxanthoma elasticum
- Storage diseases:
  1. Hemochromatosis (more commonly associated with a dilated cardiomyopathy)
  2. Glycogen or other storage diseases (Gaucher, Hurler, Fabry—all rare)
- Endomyocardial:
  1. Endomyocardial fibrosis
  2. Hypereosinophilic syndrome (Loeffler's syndrome)
- Carcinoid heart disease
- Radiation
- Metastatic cancers
- Drug related (anthracyclines, serotonin, ergotamine, busulfan, methysergide)

DIAGNOSIS

The diagnosis of idiopathic or primary restrictive cardiomyopathy is rare and is a diagnosis of exclusion.

DIFFERENTIAL DIAGNOSIS

- Constrictive pericarditis (see Table E1)
- Valvular dysfunction (especially aortic stenosis)
- Hypertrophic cardiomyopathy
- Hypertensive heart disease

WORKUP

- Complete blood count with differential (to identify eosinophilia), iron studies, serum renal function studies, chest x-ray, ECG, echocardiogram.
- Right and left heart catheterization, magnetic resonance imaging, and computed tomography (in select cases).
- Aspiration biopsy of subcutaneous fat to detect amyloidosis.
- Endomyocardial biopsy if diagnostic confirmation needed.
- Brain natriuretic peptide (BNP) serum levels (>400 pg/ml): There is data suggesting that BNP levels are markedly elevated in restrictive cardiomyopathy but near normal in constrictive pericarditis, most likely resulting from the lack of myocardial stretching in constriction that is required for BNP release.
- Genetic testing.

IMAGING STUDIES

- Chest x-ray:
  1. Ranges from normal cardiomediastinal silhouette to moderate cardiomegaly (primarily because of biatrial enlargement).
  2. Evidence of heart failure may be present.
  3. Presence of pericardial calcification favors alternative diagnosis of constrictive pericarditis.
- ECG:
  1. Nonspecific ST-T wave abnormalities are the most common finding. Voltage may be low in infiltrative etiologies such as amyloidosis.
  2. Frequent atrial and ventricular ectopy are often present. Atrial fibrillation may be present.
  3. High-degree atrioventricular block, intraventricular conduction delay may be seen in advanced cases.
- Echocardiogram (Fig. 2):
  1. Biatrial enlargement almost always present.
  2. Wall thickness depends on etiology; often thickened in infiltrative disease.

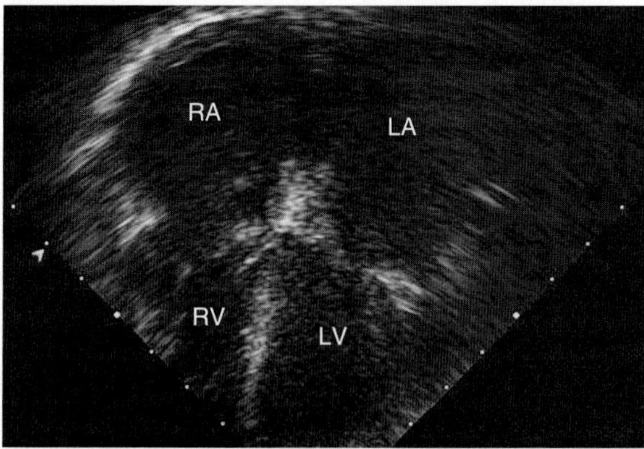

FIG. 2 Echocardiogram of a patient with restrictive cardiomyopathy. The optical four-chamber view shows the markedly enlarged right and left atria, compared to the normal-sized left and right ventricular chambers. *LA,* Left atrium; *LV,* left ventricle; *RA,* right atrium; *RV,* right ventricle. (From Kliegman RM et al: *Nelson textbook of pediatrics,* ed 19, Philadelphia, 2011, Saunders.)

3. Myocardial appearance may be altered (speckled pattern suggestive of infiltration).
4. Ventricular chamber sizes and systolic function are often normal or reduced.
5. Echo Doppler shows evidence of diastolic dysfunction. Tissue Doppler demonstrates low mitral annular velocities.

- Cardiac catheterization:
  1. Characteristic hemodynamic findings are a dip and plateau, or square-root sign, in the left ventricular tracing where a deep and rapid decline in ventricular pressure at the onset of diastole is immediately followed by rapid rise and plateau in early diastolic phase.
  2. To distinguish restrictive cardiomyopathy from constrictive processes (Fig. 3):
     a. Constrictive: Usually involves both ventricles and leads to equalization of diastolic pressures between all four cardiac chambers to within 5 mm Hg. There is discordance in RV and LV pressures generated during inspiration, which is due to increased ventricular interdependence and decreased left atrial filling (caused by a decreased gradient in inspiration between the pulmonary veins, which are outside the constrictive process and the left atrium).
     b. Restrictive cardiomyopathy: Impairs the left ventricle more than the right, often with left-sided end-diastolic pressures of 5 mm Hg greater than the right. The presence of increased pulmonary arterial systolic pressures is also suggestive of restrictive disease. Simultaneous RV and LV pressure tracings demonstrate concordant patterns during the respiratory cycle.
- Cardiac computed tomographic scan may be helpful to identify a thickened and calcified pericardium, consistent with constrictive pericarditis.
- Cardiac magnetic resonance imaging (CMRI) may also be useful to distinguish restrictive cardiomyopathy from constrictive pericarditis (thickness of the pericardium greater than 4 mm in the latter). CMRI is particularly helpful in the diagnosis of the amyloid or sarcoid variants and may have value in other variants as well. Late gadolinium enhancement can be seen with infiltrative diseases.

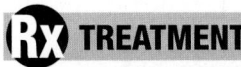

TREATMENT

NONPHARMACOLOGIC THERAPY

Congestive symptoms may respond to dietary sodium restriction (<2 g/day).

ACUTE GENERAL Rx

Treatment of volume overload and heart failure symptoms with diuretic therapy.

CHRONIC Rx

- Treatment involves management of the underlying disease if it exists:
  1. Hemochromatosis may respond to repeated phlebotomy and iron chelators to decrease iron deposition in the heart.
  2. Sarcoidosis may respond to corticosteroid therapy.
  3. Primary amyloidosis may respond to chemotherapy (high-dose melphalan with autologous stem cell therapy or bortezomib-based regimens). ATTR may be treated with liver transplant or other promising novel therapeutic agents that are currently being tested in clinical trials.
  4. Eosinophilic cardiomyopathy may respond to corticosteroid and cytotoxic drugs.
  5. There is no effective therapy for other causes of restrictive cardiomyopathy.
- Overall, the goal of treatment is to reduce symptoms by decreasing filling pressures while preserving cardiac output. Since there is currently no drug available to specifically act on myocardial relaxation, therapy centers on low-dose diuretics to lower the preload.
- Beta-blockers or calcium channel blockers have not been demonstrated to improve symptoms or alter the course of disease. Must be careful not to decrease HR too far, as this will affect cardiac output (CO = HR × stroke volume).
- ACE inhibitors (or angiotensin receptor blockers [ARBs]) and vasodilators should be avoided in patients with amyloidosis as they are poorly tolerated. Even small doses can trigger profound hypotension (probably due to associated autonomic neuropathy). Adequate preload is necessary for LV filling and ultimately cardiac output.
- Atrial fibrillation is common and patients with it or with a history of embolization should be anticoagulated. Tachycardia (of any cause) is poorly tolerated and a common cause of decompensation. Rate control is of paramount importance. Cardioversion in case of rapid atrial fibrillation should be considered. Of note, digoxin should be used with caution as it is potentially arrhythmogenic (particularly in patients with amyloidosis).
- Fibrosis of the cardiac conduction system may result in complete heart block presenting as dizziness or syncope (especially in amyloidosis) and pacemaker implantation may be required. The course of restrictive cardiomyopathy is variable and depends on the underlying etiology. Death usually results from heart failure or arrhythmias, and interventions aimed at addressing these are recommended.
  1. For the amyloid variant, an implantable cardiac defibrillator offers little prophylactic benefit beyond the ability to pace because the cause of sudden cardiac death is usually electromechanical disassociation.

DISPOSITION

Prognosis varies with the etiology of the cardiomyopathy but is poor overall as disease is rarely detected before advanced stages.

REFERRAL

Cardiac transplantation can be considered in patients with refractory symptoms and idiopathic or familial restrictive cardiomyopathies.

SUGGESTED READINGS

Available at ExpertConsult.com

RELATED CONTENT

Restrictive Cardiomyopathy (Patient Information)

AUTHOR: **NATHAN RIDDELL, M.D.**

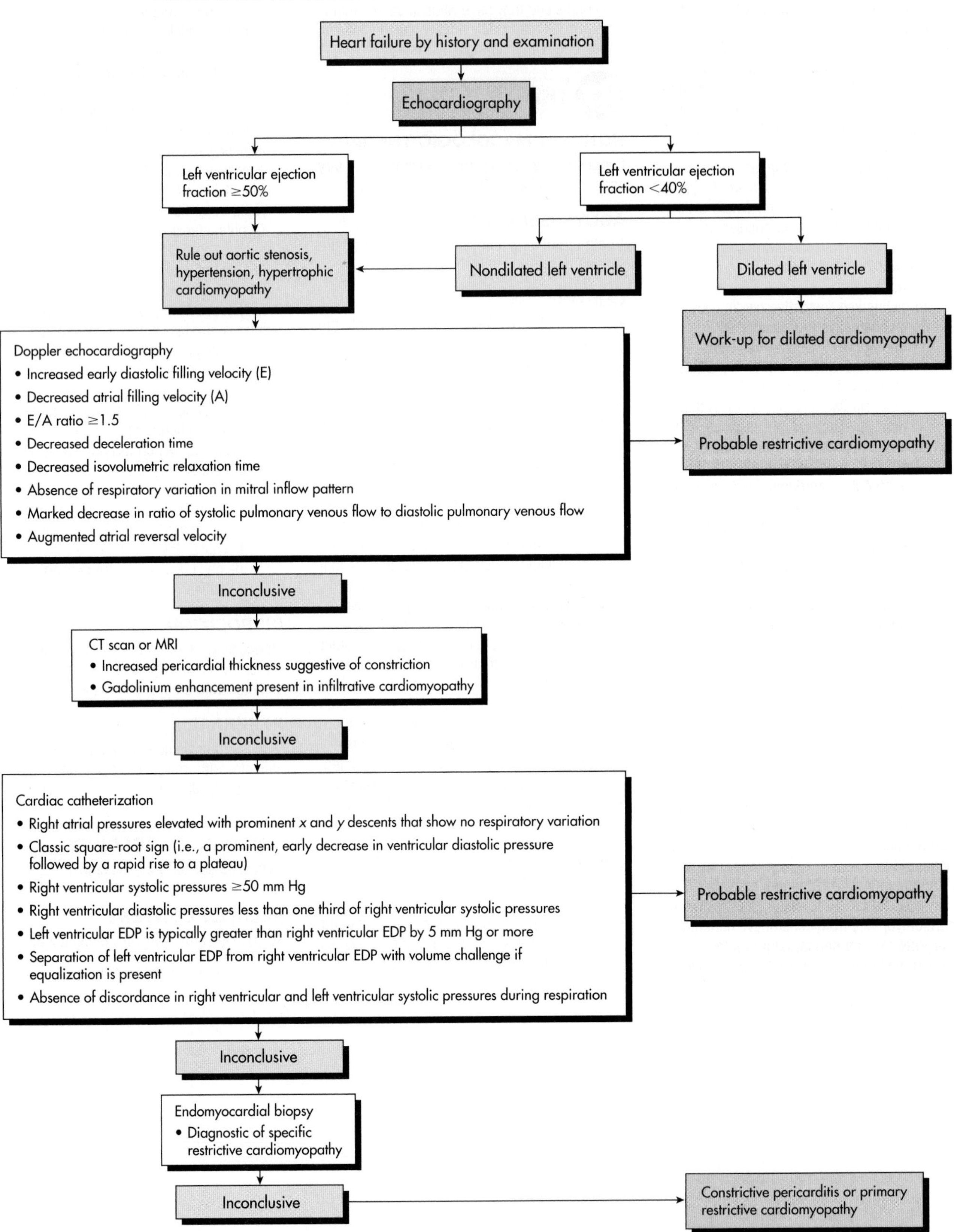

FIG. 3 Differentiation of restrictive cardiomyopathy from constrictive pericarditis. *CT*, Computed tomography; *MRI*, magnetic resonance imaging; *EDP*, end-diastolic pressure. (From Pereira NL, Dec GW: Restrictive and infiltrative cardiomyopathies. In Crawford MH et al: *Cardiology*, Philadelphia, 2010, Elsevier.)

BASIC INFORMATION

DEFINITION

Light-headedness, dizziness, presyncope, or syncope in a patient with carotid sinus hypersensitivity is defined as carotid sinus syndrome (CSS). Carotid sinus hypersensitivity is the exaggerated response to carotid stimulation resulting in bradycardia, hypotension, or both. CSS is often considered a variant of neurocardiogenic syncope. The 2013 European Guidelines (ESC) defines CSS as syncope with reproduction of symptoms during carotid sinus massage of 10-second duration. There are two components of CSS: cardioinhibitory and vasodepressor.

SYNONYMS

Carotid sinus syncope
CSS
Carotid sinus hypersensitivity

ICD-10CM CODES

G90.01	Carotid sinus syncope
R55	Syncope and collapse

EPIDEMIOLOGY & DEMOGRAPHICS

- Carotid sinus hypersensitivity accounts for 1% of syncopal episodes (Fig. 1).
- Carotid sinus hypersensitivity is frequently associated with atherosclerosis and diabetes mellitus.
- Incidence increases with age, with an average age of onset at 61 to 74 yr. Fig. 2 illustrates age distribution of the patients with carotid sinus syndrome.
- Men are affected more often than women (2:1).
- CSS is rarely found in patients younger than 50 yr.

MECHANISM

- The carotid sinus is located in the internal carotid artery.
- There is a reflex loop between the mechanoreceptors of the carotid sinus and the vagal nucleus in the midbrain.
- There is an exaggerated cardioinhibitory and vasodepressor reaction caused by decreased sympathetic and increased parasympathetic outflow to the heart and vasculature, respectively.

PHYSICAL FINDINGS & CLINICAL PRESENTATION

- Often associated with sudden neck movements, especially rotation, neck palpation, shaving, or tight-fitting collars, but can occur in the absence of clear provocation.
- Mild form has symptoms such as fatigue, lightheadedness, nausea, warmth, pallor, or diaphoresis.
- More severe form of the condition has sudden abrupt loss of consciousness without prodrome.

Properly performed carotid sinus massage (CSM) at the bedside is diagnostic. The European Society of Cardiology recommends carotid sinus massage as part of the exam in patients with syncope of unknown etiology and age over 40. This maneuver can elicit three types of responses in patients with carotid sinus hypersensitivity (see "Diagnosis").

- CSM should be performed with the patient in the supine and upright positions while monitoring the patient's blood pressure by cuff and heart rate by ECG.
- CSM should be performed on both the right and left sides but on only one carotid artery at a time.
- Vigorous pressure is applied over the carotid artery, directed posterior to compress the artery against the spinous process of the vertebrae, at the level of the cricoid cartilage for 10 to 30 seconds. Repeat on the opposite side if no effect is produced.
- Contraindications to CSM include the presence of carotid artery bruits, documented carotid artery stenosis >70%, history of stroke or transient ischemic attack <3 mo, history of myocardial infarction <6 mo, history of serious ventricular arrhythmia, or prior carotid endarterectomy.
- Complications of CSM are rare (0.1%-1%) and may include transient visual disturbance, transient paresis, tachyarrhythmias, or bradyarrhythmias.
- False-positive results with carotid sinus massage may be relatively common in the elderly population. Thus alternative explanations for syncope should be investigated prior to attribution of symptoms to carotid sinus hypersensitivity.

ETIOLOGY

- Idiopathic
- Head and neck tumors (e.g., thyroid)
- Significant lymphadenopathy
- Carotid body tumors
- Prior neck surgery

DIAGNOSIS

- The diagnosis of CSS is made in a patient with a history of syncope when carotid sinus hypersensitivity is demonstrated by CSM and no other cause of syncope is identified.
- CSM can elicit three types of responses diagnostic of carotid sinus hypersensitivity:
  1. Cardioinhibitory type: CSM producing (1) asystole for at least 3 sec in the absence of symptoms or (2) reproduction of symptoms occurring with a decline in heart rate of 30% to 40% or asystole of up to 2 sec in duration. Symptoms should not recur when CSM is repeated after atropine infusion.
  2. Vasodepressor type: CSM producing (1) a decrease in systolic blood pressure of 50 mm Hg in the absence of symptoms or 30 mm Hg in the presence of neurologic symptoms; (2) no evidence of asystole; or (3) neurologic symptoms that persist after infusion of atropine.
  3. Mixed type: CSM producing both types of responses.

DIFFERENTIAL DIAGNOSIS

All causes of syncope

WORKUP

- Evaluation for structural heart disease and other arrhythmias.
- Exclude other causes of syncope or presyncope: Detailed history, physical examination including orthostatic vital signs, ECG.
- Evaluation for vasovagal syncope which may include tilt table testing.

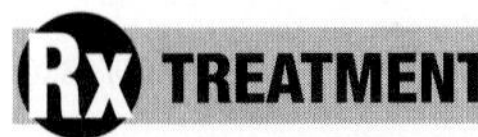

TREATMENT

NONPHARMACOLOGIC THERAPY

Reassurance and education are important. Avoid applying neck pressure from tight collars, shaving, or rapid head turning.

ACUTE GENERAL Rx

Treatment will vary according to the type of carotid hypersensitivity response and symptoms present (see "Chronic Rx").

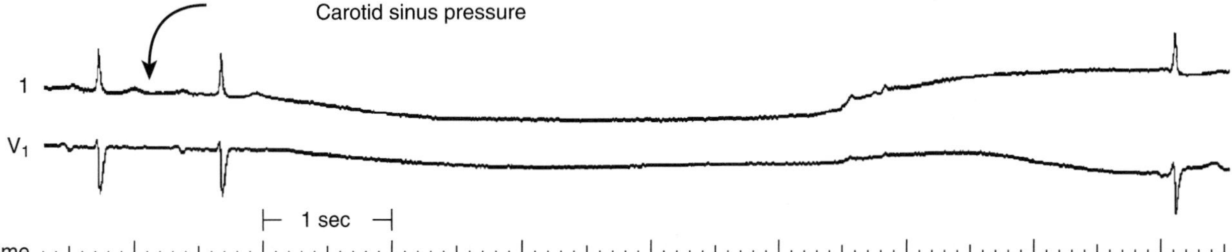

FIG. 1 Carotid sinus hypersensitivity. Two surface ECG leads are shown during carotid sinus pressure, as indicated. The PR interval is prolonged and followed by a 7.5-second sinus pause ended by a P wave and probable junctional escape complex. The patient was nearly syncopal during this period. (From Issa ZF et al: *Clinical arrhythmology and electrophysiology: a companion to Braunwald's heart disease*, ed 2, Philadelphia, 2012, Saunders.)

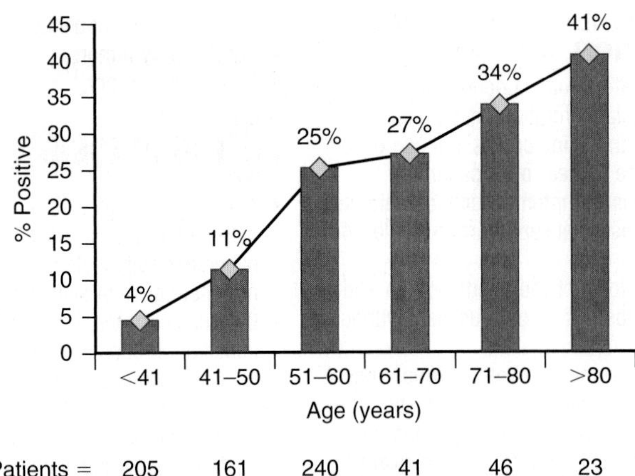

FIG. 2 Age distribution of patients with carotid sinus syndrome. (From Puggioni E et al: Results and complications of the carotid sinus massage performed according to the "method of symptoms," *Am J Cardiol* 89:599–601, 2002.)

CHRONIC Rx

Therapy is divided into three classes: medical, surgical (carotid denervation), and cardiac pacing.

- Surgical therapy has been largely abandoned except in cases of compressing tumors or masses responsible for CSS.
- For infrequent and mildly symptomatic carotid sinus hypersensitivity of either the cardioinhibitory or vasodepressor type, treatment is generally not necessary.
- Cardiac pacing is indicated in patients with recurrent syncope in whom CSM induces ventricular asystole of more than 6 seconds and accompanied by syncope. Dual chamber pacing is recommended as there is evidence that single-chamber pacing worsens syncope recurrence.

Permanent pacing is not indicated for carotid sinus hypersensitivity with no, or only vague, symptoms.

For symptomatic patients with a vasodepressor response to CSM:

- No medical treatment is proven to be effective
- Drugs, such as vasodilators, that would worsen the response should be discontinued or reduced if feasible
- Permissive hypertension
- Increased fluids (≥2 L) and salt intake (>6 g/day)
- Sympathomimetics: Midodrine, titrate from 2.5 to 10 mg tid based on BP and therapeutic response (major side effect in urinary retention in elderly males)
- Serotonin-specific reuptake inhibitors
- Fludrocortisone
- Elastic knee-high or thigh-high stockings
- Carotid sinus denervation

For symptomatic patients with CSS with a mixed response to CSM:

- Combination of dual-chamber permanent pacemaker and agents used to treat vasodepressor response

DISPOSITION

- Up to 50% of the patients have recurrent symptoms.
- No increased mortality rate in patients with idiopathic CSS compared with the general population.

REFERRAL

Cardiology referral is indicated if pacemaker placement is being considered.

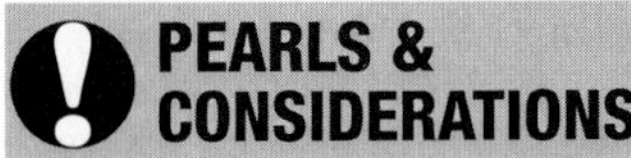

- The most common type of CSS is cardioinhibitory, followed by mixed and vasodepressor responses.
- Driving restrictions in the 2009 ESC syncope update and 2006 AHA/ACCF consensus document on syncope are stratified according to whether patients have mild or severe syncope.
- Mild carotid sinus syndrome is defined as infrequent mild symptoms (without syncope), with clear precipitating causes (usually standing), warning signs, and infrequent occurrence. For patients with mild sinus hypersensitivity, no driving restrictions are recommended for private or commercial driving.
- Severe carotid sinus syndrome is marked by syncope without warning occurring in any position, without precipitating causes and frequent occurrences. For patients with severe hypersensitivity, all driving is prohibited. If symptoms are controlled, driving is permitted 1 to 6 months after, based on the modality of treatment.

COMMENTS

Prognosis depends on the underlying cause.

RELATED CONTENT

Syncope (Patient Information)
Orthostatic Hypotension (Related Key Topic)
Syncope (Related Key Topic)

AUTHOR: **BARRY FINE, M.D., PH.D.**

BASIC INFORMATION

DEFINITION

Carotid stenosis is narrowing of the carotid arterial lumen, typically as a result of atherosclerosis.

SYNONYMS

Atherosclerotic disease of the carotid artery

ICD-10CM CODES

I65.29	Occlusion and stenosis of unspecified carotid artery
I65.21	Occlusion and stenosis of right carotid artery
I65.22	Occlusion and stenosis of left carotid artery
I65.23	Occlusion and stenosis of bilateral carotid arteries

EPIDEMIOLOGY & DEMOGRAPHICS

INCIDENCE: 2.2 to 8/1000 persons per yr

PREVALENCE: 11 to 77/100,000 persons; it is estimated that 5/1000 persons aged 50 to 60 yr and 100/1000 persons >80 yr have carotid stenosis >50%. (*Note:* The incidence of carotid stenosis is unknown as screening is not routine. However, the incidence of transient ischemic attack [TIA], a common presenting symptom of carotid stenosis, is well known.)

PREDOMINANT SEX AND AGE: Male/female ratio of 2:1; more common in whites than African Americans and Asians

PEAK INCIDENCE: Peak incidence is between 50 and 60 yr.

GENETICS: Multifactorial; twin studies (monozygotic versus dizygotic) suggest a familial influence.

RISK FACTORS: Hypertension, dyslipidemia, diabetes mellitus, and smoking are the four major risk factors.

PHYSICAL FINDINGS & CLINICAL PRESENTATION

Patients with carotid stenosis are often asymptomatic, but many either have a carotid bruit or experience a TIA.

- Carotid bruit: The presence of a carotid bruit is a better indicator of generalized atherosclerosis and is thus a better predictor of ischemic heart disease than future stroke.
- TIA: Carotid stenosis is classically heralded by ipsilateral transient monocular blindness (amaurosis fugax), contralateral numbness or weakness, contralateral homonymous hemianopsia, or aphasia.

ETIOLOGY

- Atherosclerosis (most common by far)
- Aneurysm
- Arteritis
- Carotid dissection
- Fibromuscular dysplasia
- Post-radiation necrosis
- Vasospasm

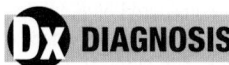

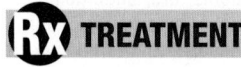

DIAGNOSIS

DIFFERENTIAL DIAGNOSIS

Aneurysm, arteritis, and carotid dissection

WORKUP

Systematic history, examination, and diagnostic studies to assess for carotid stenosis and other risk factors of TIA and stroke.

LABORATORY TESTS

CBC, basic metabolic panel, fasting lipid profile, PT/international normalized ratio, APTT, HgA1C

IMAGING STUDIES

- Four imaging modalities are available for the evaluation of carotid stenosis (Table 1).
- Patients who have neurologic sequelae suggestive of carotid stenosis should be screened via carotid duplex. If carotid stenosis is suspected on carotid duplex, but inconclusive, magnetic resonance angiography, computed tomography angiography, or conventional angiography should be obtained to confirm the degree of stenosis (Fig. 1).
- Screening of asymptomatic patients without any risk factors for atherosclerosis is not routinely recommended.
- When required, carotid duplex is considered the imaging modality of choice for screening.
- Screening with carotid duplex may be considered in asymptomatic patients with carotid bruit, in those with multiple risk factors for atherosclerosis, or those with known atherosclerotic disease at other sites such as coronary artery disease, peripheral arterial disease, or abdominal aortic aneurysms.
- Patients identified to have >50% stenosis on carotid duplex may be re-imaged annually to assess progression.

TREATMENT

ACUTE GENERAL Rx

- General medical therapy should be aimed at risk factor reduction. The major risk factors for carotid stenosis are hypertension, diabetes mellitus, dyslipidemia, and smoking (see "Stroke, Secondary Prevention").
- Antiplatelet therapy: Three antiplatelet options are available for patients with carotid stenosis: ASA, ASA plus dipyridamole, or clopidogrel.

NONPHARMACOLOGIC THERAPY

Carotid endarterectomy (CEA) and carotid angioplasty and stenting (CAS) are the two

TABLE 1 Imaging Modalities for Carotid Stenosis

Imaging Modality	Benefit	Drawback
Cerebral angiography	• Gold standard • Assesses plaque morphology • Assesses presence of collaterals	• Invasive • High cost • 4% incidence rate of complications • 1% incidence rate of serious complications or death
Carotid duplex	• Sensitive in detecting high-grade stenosis (>70%) • Less invasive • Lower cost	• Can be limited by body habitus • Technician dependent • Overestimates degree of stenosis
Magnetic resonance angiography (MRA)	• Sensitive in detecting high-grade stenosis (>70%) • Less operator dependent	• Overestimates degree of stenosis • Cannot be performed in patients who are critically ill, unable to tolerate supine positioning, have pacemaker or other ferromagnetic hardware, or are claustrophobic* • Expensive • Takes much longer to obtain compared with other modalities
Computed tomography angiography (CTA)	• Sensitive for high-grade stenosis	• Contraindicated in patients with serum creatinine concentration >1.5 mg/dl

*One study revealed that ~17% of patients are unable to tolerate MRA secondary to claustrophobia or are unable to lie still for procedure.

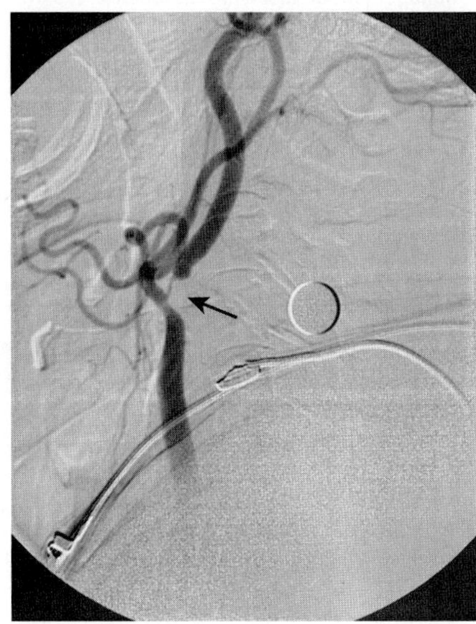

FIG. 1 Conventional angiography demonstrating severe stenosis of the internal carotid artery at the bifurcation.

nonpharmacologic options available. The decision on which revascularization procedure to favor is dependent upon the presence or absence of symptoms, degree of stenosis, medical comorbidities, operative risk of the patient, and experience and outcomes data of the proceduralist.

In a trial involving asymptomatic patients with severe carotid stenosis who were not at high risk for surgical complications, stenting was noninferior to endarterectomy with regard to the rate of the primary composite end point at 1 yr. In analyses that included up to 5 yr of follow-up, there were no significant differences between the study groups in the rates of nonprocedure-related stroke, all stroke, and survival.[1]

ASYMPTOMATIC CAROTID STENOSIS

The benefit of surgical revascularization of the carotids (CEA or CAS) in asymptomatic patients is not well established. In the U.S., more than 90% of carotid artery interventions are performed in asymptomatic patients, even though evidence suggests that up to 90% of these patients are undergoing an ultimately unnecessary and potentially harmful procedure. In contrast, the percentage of interventions performed for asymptomatic stenosis is approximately 60% in Germany and Italy, 15% in Canada and Australia, and 0% in Denmark.[2]

According to the most recent guidelines, revascularization procedures may be considered in asymptomatic patients with >70% stenosis if the anticipated perioperative risk is low, but surgery should only be recommended after considering their medical comorbidities and life expectancy, and after discussing the risks and benefits in detail with the patients. It is important to note that trials of CEA for asymptomatic carotid stenosis were performed prior to the era of aggressive medical management of vascular risk factors. Recently launched studies of asymptomatic carotid stenosis versus aggressive contemporary medical management will answer lingering questions from older studies.

[1] Rosenfield K, Matsumura JS, Chaturvedi S, et al., for the ACT I Investigators: Randomized trial of stent versus surgery for asymptomatic carotid stenosis, *N Engl J Med* 374:1011–1020, 2016.

[2] Spence DJ, Naylor AR: Endarterectomy, stenting, or neither for asymptomatic carotid artery stenosis, *N Engl J Med* 374:1087–1088, 2016.

SYMPTOMATIC CAROTID STENOSIS

In patients who have suffered a non-disabling ischemic stroke or TIA in the preceding 6 months, surgical revascularization by CEA is recommended if the degree of stenosis is >70% by noninvasive imaging or >50% by catheter angiogram and if the anticipated rate of perioperative stroke or mortality is <6%.

All patients undergoing CEA should be started on aspirin (ASA; 81 or 325 mg daily) before surgery and this should be continued indefinitely.

CAS can be an alternative to CEA in select patients considered to be at high surgical risk or with unfavorable neck anatomy for surgery.

CEA is preferred over CAS in older patients.

For patients undergoing CAS, dual antiplatelet therapy is recommended for a minimum of 30 days.

When feasible, early revascularization within 14 days after incident event should be undertaken unless there are definite contraindications. For patients undergoing early intervention, CEA is associated with lower periprocedural complication rate than CAS.

Surgical revascularization is not recommended in <50% stenosis, total occlusion, or in patients with major disabling strokes.

In patients who are considered high surgical risk for either CEA or CAS, the role of medical therapy alone compared with surgical revascularization is not well established.

DISPOSITION

Disposition and prognosis depend on several variables (Table 2): the degree of stenosis, the presence of symptoms, medication compliance, and the type of intervention (if any).

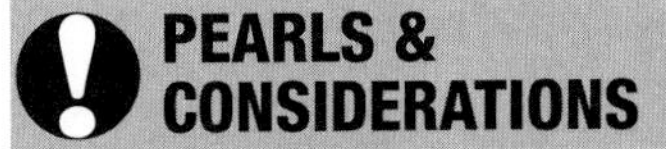

PEARLS & CONSIDERATIONS

The results of ongoing studies concerning the best treatment of patients with carotid artery stenosis may result in guideline changes.

SPECIAL CONSIDERATION

Some studies have shown that in patients with bilateral hemodynamically significant stenosis (>70%), blood pressure reduction resulted in worsened outcomes for stroke. These patients would likely be candidates for CEA.

Carotid artery occlusion (100% blockage), for which there is no routine treatment, was reexamined in the national Carotid Occlusion Surgery Study (www.cosstrial.org). Recently published results from the COSS trial demonstrate that superficial temporal artery to middle cerebral artery anastomosis does not provide an overall benefit for ipsilateral 2-yr stroke recurrence when compared to medical therapy alone.

PREVENTION

Prevention of carotid stenosis should include pursuit of a healthy lifestyle and management of risk factors for atherosclerosis.

PATIENT/FAMILY EDUCATION

Patients should be counseled to pursue a healthy lifestyle including exercise and smoking cessation. In addition, patients should take an active role in controlling blood pressure and blood glucose. Further educational materials can be found online at: www.strokecenter.org/education.

SUGGESTED READINGS

Available at ExpertConsult.com

RELATED CONTENT

Carotid Stenosis (Patient Information)
Transient Ischemic Attack (Related Key Topic)

AUTHORS: **SAAGAR N. PATEL, B.A., B.S., JOSEPH S. KASS, M.D., J.D.,** and **PRASHANTH KRISHNAMOHAN, M.B.B.S., M.D.**

TABLE 2 Carotid Stenosis Management

Degree of Carotid Stenosis	<50%	50%-69%	70%-99%
Asymptomatic	• Medical management	• Medical management • Inconclusive evidence base to favor surgical treatment. May be considered in select patients with >60% stenosis.*	• Medical management • CEA in highly selected patients*
Symptomatic	• Medical management	• CEA • CAS can be an alternative	• CEA • CAS can be an alternative

CAS, Carotid artery stenting; *CEA,* carotid endarterectomy.
*CEA can be considered in asymptomatic patients with >70% stenosis if the anticipated rate of perioperative complications (stroke, myocardial infarction, and death) is low, their life expectancy is greater than 5 years, and the risks and benefits (including medical comorbidities) have been discussed thoroughly with the patients and their families

BASIC INFORMATION

DEFINITION

Carpal tunnel syndrome (CTS) is a compression neuropathy of the median nerve as it passes under the transverse carpal ligament at the wrist (Figs. E1 and E2). It is the most common entrapment neuropathy.

SYNONYM

CTS

ICD-10CM CODES	
G56.0	Carpal tunnel syndrome, unspecified upper limb
G56.01	Carpal tunnel syndrome, right upper limb
G56.02	Carpal tunnel syndrome, left upper limb

EPIDEMIOLOGY & DEMOGRAPHICS

INCIDENCE: 3.8% of the general population (the most common entrapment neuropathy)
PREVALENT AGE: 30 to 60 yr
PREVALENT SEX: Females are affected two to five times as often as males.

PHYSICAL FINDINGS & CLINICAL PRESENTATION

- Pain, paresthesia in 1st, 2nd, 3rd, and lateral half of 4th fingers, worse at night.
- ***Tinel sign*** at wrist (Fig. 3): Tapping lightly over the median nerve on the volar surface of the wrist produces a tingling sensation radiating from the wrist to the hand.
- ***Phalen sign*** (Fig. 4): Reproduction of symptoms after 1 min of gentle, unforced wrist flexion.
- Carpal compression test: Direct pressure over the patient's carpal tunnel for 30 sec elicits symptoms.

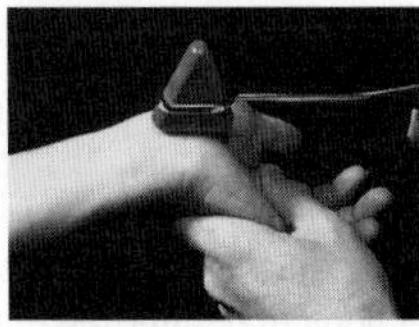

FIG. 3 Tinel sign. The wrist is held in extension while gentle percussion is performed over and just proximal to the transverse carpal ligament. (From Hochberg MC, et al.: *Rheumatology,* ed 5, St Louis, 2011, Mosby.)

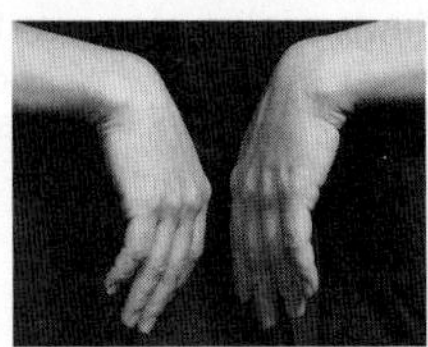

FIG. 4 Phalen (wrist flexion) test. With the wrists held in unforced flexion for 30 to 60 seconds, a positive test reproduces or worsens the patient's symptoms. (From Hochberg MC, et al.: *Rheumatology,* ed 5, St Louis, 2011, Mosby.)

- Thenar atrophy in long-standing cases with weakness of thumb abduction and opposition.
- Findings may be bilateral in up to 65% of patients.

ETIOLOGY

- Idiopathic in most cases—caused by increased intracarpal tunnel pressure
- Commonly associated with diabetes, obesity, female gender, advancing age, pregnancy, hypothyroidism, rheumatologic disorders, autoimmune disorders, and trauma
- Specific occupations with repetitive strain or job-related mechanical overuse

DIAGNOSIS

DIFFERENTIAL DIAGNOSIS

- Cervical radiculopathy
- Chronic tendinitis
- Pronator teres syndrome
- Anterior interosseous syndrome
- Complex regional pain syndrome
- Brachial plexopathy, thoracic outlet syndrome
- Polyneuropathy
- Other entrapment neuropathies
- Traumatic wrist injuries
- Vascular disorders (Raynaud syndrome)
- Cervical myelopathy

IMAGING STUDIES

Carpal tunnel syndrome is a clinical diagnosis, but imaging may assist workup in uncertain situations. Accumulating evidence suggests that diagnostic ultrasound may be almost as sensitive as nerve conduction velocity tests and may help identify the structural cause of nerve compression. X-ray or MRI may be helpful in ruling out other conditions.

ELECTRODIAGNOSTIC STUDIES

Nerve conduction velocity tests (NCS) demonstrate impaired sensory conduction across the carpal tunnel and may help guide treatment based on the severity of median nerve compression. Electromyography may show active denervation muscle potentials. Specificity of NCS and electromyography for CTS is >95%, and sensitivity is >85%.

TREATMENT

ACUTE GENERAL Rx

- Activity modification and ergonomic changes (desk, keyboard).
- Nocturnal wrist splint has been shown to be effective.
- No evidence for effectiveness of NSAIDs.
- Corticosteroid injection of carpal canal on ulnar side of palmaris longus tendon proximal to wrist crease (Figs. E5 and E6): Can be done with palpation guidance or under ultrasound guidance. In different clinical studies, injections have increased patient satisfaction and improved clinical symptoms, albeit temporarily.
- Low-dose oral corticosteroids are optional but usually not effective.
- Short-term benefit from ultrasound therapy (physical therapy modality).
- Carpal tunnel release if no response from nonoperative treatment.

DISPOSITION

Clinical course may have remissions and exacerbations. Some may progress from intermittent to persistent sensory complaints (numbness, tingling, paresthesia) and then to motor symptoms. In pregnancy, symptoms usually resolve spontaneously weeks after delivery.

REFERRAL

Surgical referral is needed if conservative treatment fails. Surgery (sectioning of transverse carpal ligament) is performed by open, endoscopic, or minimal incision techniques, with good long-term results. Carpal tunnel release is one of the most common surgeries performed, with approximately 400,000 conducted per yr.

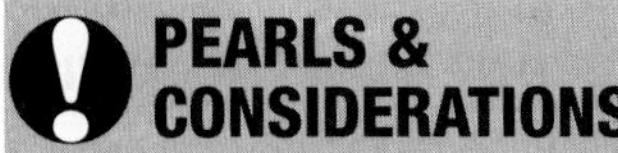

PEARLS & CONSIDERATIONS

- The sensory changes of carpal tunnel syndrome spare the thenar eminence. This distinctive pattern occurs because the palmar sensory cutaneous branch of the median nerve arises proximal to the wrist, passing superficial to the tunnel.
- Role of repetitive hand or wrist use and workplace factors in the development of carpal tunnel syndrome remains controversial.
- Recent trials from the Mayo Clinic using ultrasound-guided perineural injection therapy (PIT) using 5% dextrose (D_5W) have shown promising results in patients with mild-to-moderate CTS.[1]

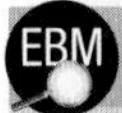

EVIDENCE

Available at ExpertConsult.com

SUGGESTED READINGS

Available at ExpertConsult.com

RELATED CONTENT

Carpal Tunnel Syndrome (Patient Information)

AUTHORS: **MANUEL F. DASILVA, M.D.,** and **KATIA A. DASILVA, B.A.**

[1] Wu YT et al: Six-month efficacy of perneural dextrose for carpal tunnel syndrome: a prospective, randomized, double-blind, controlled trial, *Mayo Clin Proc* 92(8):1179–1189, 2017.

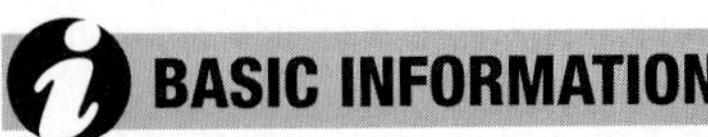

BASIC INFORMATION

DEFINITION

Cat-scratch disease (CSD) is an infectious disease consisting of gradually enlarging regional lymphadenopathy occurring after contact with a feline. Atypical presentations are characterized by a variety of neurologic manifestations as well as granulomatous involvement of the eye, liver, spleen, and bone. The disease is usually self-limiting, and recovery is complete; however, patients with atypical presentations, especially if immunocompromised, may suffer significant morbidity and mortality.

SYNONYMS

CSD
Cat-scratch fever
Benign inoculation lymphoreticulosis
Nonbacterial regional lymphadenitis

ICD-10CM CODES
A28.1 Cat-scratch disease

EPIDEMIOLOGY & DEMOGRAPHICS

PREVALENCE: Unknown

INCIDENCE (IN U.S.):

- 9 to 10 cases per 100,000 persons per yr (22,000 cases per yr)
- Majority of reported cases occur in persons <21 yr

PEAK INCIDENCE: August through January

PHYSICAL FINDINGS & CLINICAL PRESENTATION

- Classic, most common finding: Regional lymphadenopathy occurring within 2 wk of a scratch or contact with felines; usually a new kitten in the household
- Tender, swollen lymph nodes most commonly found in the head and neck (Fig. E1), followed by the axilla and the epitrochlear, inguinal, and femoral areas
- Erythematous overlying skin, showing signs of suppuration from involved lymph nodes
- On careful examination, evidence of cutaneous inoculation in the form of a nonpruritic, slightly tender pustule or papule
- Fever in most patients
- Malaise and headache in fewer than a third of patients
- Atypical presentations in fewer than 15% of cases
  1. Usually in association with lymphadenopathy and a low-grade or frank fever (>101 °F, >38.3 °C)
  2. Include granulomatous involvement of the conjunctiva (Parinaud's oculoglandular syndrome) and focal masses in the liver, spleen, and mesenteric nodes
- CNS involvement: Neuroretinitis, encephalopathy, encephalitis, transverse myelitis, seizure activity, and coma
- Osteomyelitis in adults and children
- Can be a cause of culture-negative endocarditis
- In HIV-infected and other immunocompromised patients, *Bartonella henselae* is the cause of bacillary angiomatous and peliosis hepatis

ETIOLOGY

- Major cause: *Bartonella henselae*, possibly *Afipia felis* and *Bartonella clarridgeiae*
- Mode of transmission: Predominantly by direct inoculation through the scratch, bite, or lick of a cat, especially a kitten
- Also can be transmitted by flea bite (with the flea obtaining the bacteria from a bacteremic cat); rarely after exposure to a dog, probably secondary to flea bites
- Approximately 2 wk after introduction of the bacteria into the host, regional lymphatic tissues displaying granulomatous infiltration associated with gradual hypertrophy
- Possible dissemination to distant sites (e.g., liver, spleen, and bone), usually characterized by focal masses or discrete parenchymal lesions

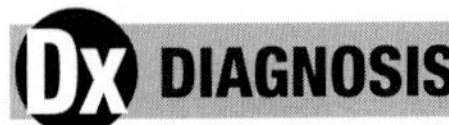

DIAGNOSIS

DIFFERENTIAL DIAGNOSIS

Granulomas of this syndrome must be differentiated from those associated with:

- Tularemia
- Tuberculosis or other mycobacterial infections
- Brucellosis
- Sarcoidosis
- Sporotrichosis or other fungal diseases
- Toxoplasmosis
- Lymphogranuloma venereum
- Benign and malignant tumors such as lymphoma

WORKUP

Diagnosis should be considered in patients who present with a predominant complaint of gradually enlarging regional (focal) lymphadenopathy, often with fever and a recent history of having contact with a cat. A primary ulcer at the site of the cat scratch may or may not be present at the time lymphadenopathy becomes manifest.

LABORATORY TESTS

- Serologies: An IFA or EIA *Bartonella* serology (titer ≥1:64) is diagnostic. A PCR assay on tissue or blood is also available.
- Lymph node biopsy: Granulomatous inflammation consistent with CSD.
- Warthin-Starry silver stain on biopsy can identify the bacteria.
- Histopathologically, Warthin-Starry silver stain has been used to identify the bacillus.
- Culture: *B. henselae* is a fastidious, slow-growing, gram-negative rod that requires specific culture techniques for tissue or blood.
- Routine laboratory findings:
  1. Mild leukocytosis or leukopenia.
  2. Infrequent eosinophilia.
  3. Elevated ESR or CRP.
- Abnormalities of bilirubin excretion and elevated hepatic transaminases are usually secondary to hepatic obstruction by granuloma, mass, or lymph node.
- In patients with neurologic manifestations, lumbar puncture usually reveals normal CSF, although there may be a mild pleocytosis and modest elevation in protein.
- CSD skin test is no longer used for clinical purposes.

Rx TREATMENT

NONPHARMACOLOGIC THERAPY

- Warm compresses to the affected nodes
- In cases of encephalitis or coma: Supportive care

ACUTE GENERAL Rx

- This disease is typically self-limited and generally resolves within 2 to 6 months. Most studies show no additional benefit from antibiotic therapy.
- It would be prudent to treat severely ill patients, especially if immunocompromised, with antibiotic therapy, because these patients tend to suffer dissemination of infection and increased morbidity.
- *Bartonella* is usually sensitive to a 5-day course of azithromycin (500 mg on day 1 followed by 250 mg for 4 days for weight >45.5 kg; 10 mg/kg on day 1 followed by 5 mg/kg for 4 days for weight <45.5 kg) or alternatively tetracycline, sulfa, and the quinolones can be used for 7 to 10 days.
- Hepatosplenic disease, neuroretinitis, and endocarditis require longer courses of therapy.
- Antipyretics and NSAIDs may also be used for lymphadenitis.

DISPOSITION

Overall prognosis is good.

REFERRAL

- For diagnostic aspiration or excision in presence of regional lymphadenopathy, bone lesions, and mesenteric lymph nodes and organs
- Infectious diseases specialist for organ involvement including endocarditis
- To ophthalmologist for ocular granulomas

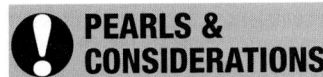

PEARLS & CONSIDERATIONS

COMMENTS

- A presentation of this syndrome, especially in patients with HIV infection or impaired cellular immunity, may be fever of unknown origin.
- Hepatic and splenic granulomas, coronary valve infections may offer few physical clues to diagnosis, emphasizing the need for a complete history.
- CSD should be considered in the differential diagnosis of school-aged children presenting with status epilepticus.
- Chronically immunocompromised patients considering the acquisition of a young feline should be made aware of the possible risk of infection.
- No signs of illness may be apparent in bacteremic kittens.

SUGGESTED READINGS
Available at ExpertConsult.com

RELATED CONTENT

Cat-Scratch Disease (Patient Information)

AUTHOR: **GLENN G. FORT, M.D., M.P.H.**

BASIC INFORMATION

DEFINITION

Cavernous sinus thrombosis (CST) is a late complication of either facial or paranasal sinus infection, resulting in thrombosis of the cavernous sinus and inflammation of its surrounding anatomic structures, including cranial nerves III, IV, V (ophthalmic and maxillary branch), and VI, and the internal carotid artery.

SYNONYMS

CST
Intracranial venous sinus thrombosis or thrombophlebitis
Dural sinus thrombosis

ICD-10CM CODE

G08 Intracranial and intraspinal phlebitis and thrombophlebitis

EPIDEMIOLOGY & DEMOGRAPHICS

- CST is rare in the post-antibiotic era.
- Before antibiotics the mortality rate was 80% to 100%.
- With antibiotics and early diagnosis, mortality rates have fallen to ~20%.
- Reported morbidity rates have also declined from between 50% and 70% to about 20% to 30% with advances in imaging modalities and aggressive medical care.

PHYSICAL FINDINGS & CLINICAL PRESENTATION

- Can be either an acute and fulminant disease or an indolent and subacute presentation.
- Septic cases of CST commonly present with high-grade fever (picket fence pattern) and signs of sepsis.
- Headache, although not specific, is the most common presenting symptom and may precede fever and periorbital edema by several days. Elderly patients, however, may only demonstrate alteration in mental status without antecedent headache. The triad of unilateral or bilateral progressive chemosis, periorbital edema, and proptosis with headache is a classical presentation in patients with CST. These signs and symptoms are related to the anatomic structures affected within the cavernous sinus, notably cranial nerves III to VI, as well as impaired venous drainage from the orbit and eye.

Other common signs and symptoms include:

- Ptosis.
- Cranial nerve palsies (III, IV, V1, V2, VI).
    1. Ophthalmoplegia caused by involvement of cranial nerves III, IV, and VI is present in most cases. Sixth nerve palsy can occur early in some cases of septic CST, especially when originating from the sphenoid sinus owing to its anatomic proximity.
    2. Hypoesthesia or hyperesthesia of the ophthalmic and maxillary branch of the fifth nerve is common. Periorbital sensory loss and impaired corneal reflex may be noted.
- Papilledema, retinal hemorrhages, and decreased visual acuity progressing to blindness may occur from venous congestion within the retina.
- Pupil may be dilated and sluggishly reactive.
- Headache with nuchal rigidity and changes in mental status may occur if the infection spreads intracranially to the meninges and brain parenchyma.
- Infection can spread to the contralateral cavernous sinus through the intercavernous sinuses within 24 to 48 hours of initial presentation.
- Patients may also develop signs and symptoms of pituitary insufficiency.

ETIOLOGY

- CST most commonly results from contiguous spread of an infection from either the sinuses (sphenoid, ethmoid, or frontal) or the medial third of the face (areas around the eyes and nose that drain to the ophthalmic vein). Nasal furuncles are the most common facial infection to produce this complication. Less-common primary sites of infection include dental abscess, tonsils, soft palate, middle ear, or orbit (orbital cellulitis).
- CST also can result from hematogenous spread of infection to the cavernous sinus by the superior and inferior ophthalmic veins or through the lateral and sigmoid sinuses. Depending on the pressure gradients, infection can spread in a retrograde direction because the dural sinuses are valveless.
- *Staphylococcus aureus* is the most commonly identified pathogen, found in 60% to 70% of the cases.
- *Streptococcus* is the second leading cause.
- Gram-negative rods and anaerobes may also lead to CST.
- Rarely, *Aspergillus fumigatus* and mucormycosis cause CST.
- Risk factors for dural sinus thrombosis include venous hypercoagulable disorders, infections (see previous), trauma, malignancies, systemic inflammatory disorders, pregnancy, and dehydration.

DIAGNOSIS

- The diagnosis of CST is made by clinical suspicion and confirmed by appropriate imaging studies.
- Proptosis, ptosis, chemosis, and cranial nerve palsy beginning in one eye and progressing to the other eye establish the diagnosis.

DIFFERENTIAL DIAGNOSIS

- Orbital or periorbital cellulitis.
- Internal carotid artery aneurysm or fistula.
- Cerebrovascular disease.
- Migraine headache.
- Allergic blepharitis.
- Thyroid ophthalmopathy.
- Orbital neoplasm.
- Meningitis.
- Epidural and subdural infections.
- Epidural and subdural hematoma.
- Subarachnoid hemorrhage.
- Acute angle-closure glaucoma.
- Trauma.

WORKUP

CST is a clinical diagnosis, with laboratory tests and imaging studies confirming the clinical impression.

LABORATORY TESTS

- Complete blood count, erythrocyte sedimentation rate, blood cultures, and sinus cultures help establish and identify an infectious primary source. Metabolic panel to look for electrolyte imbalances in cases of suspected pituitary involvement (DI/SIADH).
- Lumbar puncture (LP) helps to distinguish CST from more localized processes (e.g., sinusitis, orbital cellulitis). LP reveals inflammatory cells in 75% of cases. In half of these cases, the cerebrospinal fluid profile is typical for a parameningeal focus (high white blood cells with polymorphonuclear and/or mononuclear cells, normal glucose, normal protein, culture negative), and in one third may be similar to that of bacterial meningitis.

IMAGING STUDIES

- MRI with gadolinium, including magnetic resonance angiography and magnetic resonance venogram (Fig. 1), is more sensitive than CT scan and is the imaging study of choice to diagnose CST. Findings may include deformity of the internal carotid artery within the cavernous sinus and an obvious signal hyperintensity within thrombosed vascular sinuses.
- Noncontrast CT scan of the head and orbits may demonstrate increased density in the region of the cavernous sinus but has relatively low sensitivity. Contrast-enhanced CT scan may reveal underlying sinusitis, thickening of the superior ophthalmic vein, and irregular filling defects within the cavernous sinus; however, findings may be normal early in the disease course.

TREATMENT

NONPHARMACOLOGIC THERAPY

Recognizing the primary source of infection (i.e., facial cellulitis, middle ear, and sinus infections) and treating the primary source expeditiously is the best way to prevent CST.

ACUTE GENERAL Rx

- Appropriate therapy should take into account the primary source of infection as well as possible associated complications such as brain abscess, meningitis, or subdural empyema.
- Broad-spectrum intravenous antibiotics are used as empiric therapy until a definite pathogen is found. Treatment should include vancomycin to cover hospital or community-acquired methicillin-resistant *Staphylococcus aureus* or resistant *Streptococcus pneumoniae* plus a third- or fourth-generation cephalosporin:
    1. Vancomycin (1 g q12h with normal renal function) plus either ceftriaxone (2 g q12h) or cefepime (2 g q8 to 12h).

 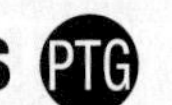

2. Metronidazole 500 mg IV q6h should be added if anaerobic bacterial infection is suspected (dental or sinus infection).

- Most experts recommend anticoagulation with heparin after the diagnosis is confirmed, unless surgical intervention is planned, or there is evidence of an expanding hematoma. Spontaneous intracranial hemorrhage should first be ruled out before initiating heparin therapy. Early heparinization has been suggested in patients with unilateral CST to prevent clot propagation. Coumadin therapy should be avoided in the acute phase of the illness, but should ultimately be instituted to achieve an INR of 2 to 3 and continued until the infection, symptoms, and signs of CST have either resolved or significantly improved. Anticoagulation with warfarin is generally continued for a minimum of 3 to 6 months. Retrospective case reports and case series have demonstrated a favorable outcome in terms of decreased mortality and morbidity in the anticoagulated patients.
- Steroid therapy is also controversial but may prove helpful in reducing cranial nerve dysfunction or when progression to pituitary insufficiency occurs. Corticosteroids should only be instituted after appropriate antibiotic coverage. Dexamethasone 10 mg q6h is the treatment of choice.
- Emergent surgical drainage with sphenoidotomy is indicated if the primary site of infection is believed to be the sphenoid sinus.

CHRONIC Rx

- Patients with CST are usually treated with prolonged courses (3 to 4 weeks) of IV antibiotics. If there is evidence of complications such as intracranial suppuration, 6 to 8 weeks of total therapy may be warranted.
- All patients should be monitored for signs of complicated infection, continued sepsis, or septic emboli while antibiotic therapy is being administered. Relapse of septic CST can occur after an initial improvement weeks after stopping antibiotic treatment.

DISPOSITION

- CST can be a life-threatening, rapidly progressive infectious disease with high morbidity and mortality rates (30%) despite antibiotic use. Morbidity and mortality rates are increased in cases of sphenoid sinus infection.
- Complications of untreated CST include extension of thrombus to other dural sinuses, carotid thrombosis with concomitant strokes, subdural empyema, brain abscess, or meningitis. Septic embolization may also occur to the lungs, resulting in acute respiratory distress syndrome, pulmonary abscess, empyema, and pneumothorax.
- Thirty percent of treated patients develop long-term sequelae, including cranial nerve palsies, blindness, pituitary insufficiency, and hemiparesis.

REFERRAL

If suspected, CST should be considered a medical emergency. Depending on source of infection, appropriate consultation should be made (i.e., ear-nose-throat, ophthalmology, and infectious disease).

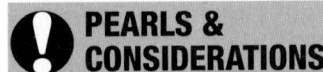

PEARLS & CONSIDERATIONS

COMMENTS

CST is a medical emergency and should be suspected with progressing chemosis, proptosis, and cranial neuropathy in a patient with headaches with or without fever.

The anatomy of the cavernous sinus explains the clinical findings: The cavernous sinus lies just above and lateral to the sphenoid sinus and drains the middle portion of the face by the superior and inferior ophthalmic veins; cranial nerves III, IV, V, and VI pass alongside or through the cavernous sinus.

SUGGESTED READINGS

Available at ExpertConsult.com

RELATED CONTENT

Cavernous Sinus Thrombosis (Patient Information)

AUTHORS: **DANYELLE EVANS, M.D., JOSEPH S. KASS, M.D.J.D,** and **PRASHANTH KRISHNAMOHAN, M.B.B.S., M.D.**

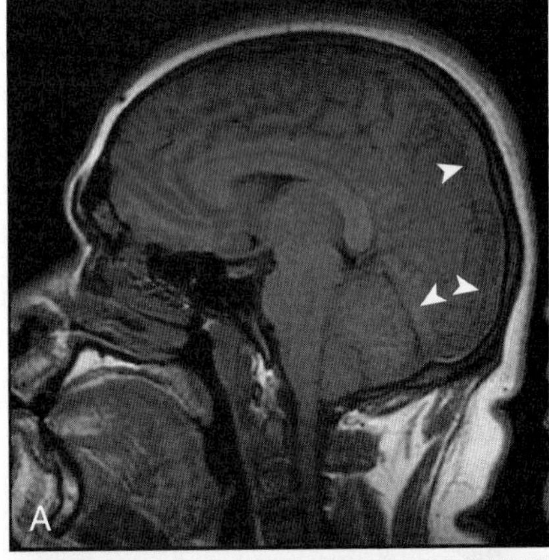

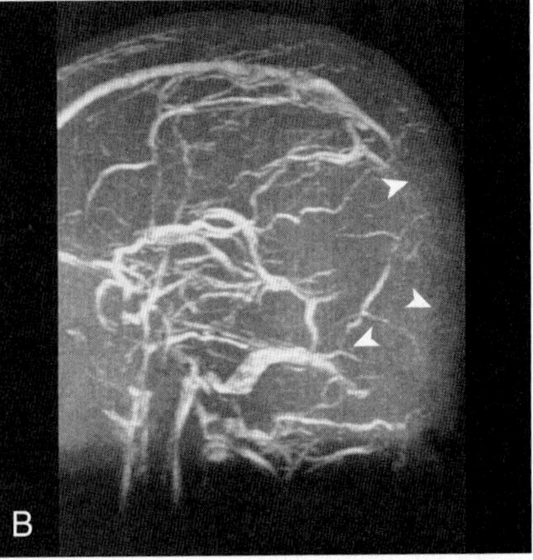

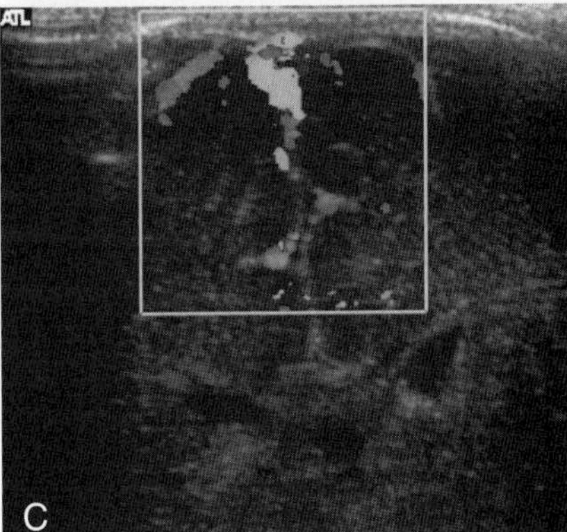

FIG. 1 Superior sagittal sinus (SSS) thrombosis on magnetic resonance venogram (MRV). Sagittal T1 magnetic resonance imaging **(A)** shows intermediate signal intensity in sagittal and straight sinuses *(arrowheads).* No flow is seen on MRV **(B)** in these vessels *(arrowheads),* which is consistent with thrombosis. Color Doppler evacuation **(C)** of the SSS in another 6-mo-old patient with suspected thrombosis demonstrated a patent SSS with normal draining cortical veins. (From Fuhrman BP, et al.: *Pediatric critical care,* ed 4, Philadelphia, 2011, Saunders.)

BASIC INFORMATION

DEFINITION

Celiac disease is a chronic autoimmune disease characterized by malabsorption and diarrhea precipitated by ingestion of food products containing gluten. Gluten is a protein complex found in wheat, rye, and barley.

SYNONYMS

Gluten-sensitive enteropathy
Celiac sprue
Nontropical sprue

ICD-10CM CODE

K90.0 Celiac disease

EPIDEMIOLOGY & DEMOGRAPHICS

- The prevalence of celiac disease is 0.5% to 1% in the general population in North America and Western Europe and 5% in high-risk groups such as first-degree relatives of persons with the disease. The prevalence of celiac disease in the U.S. has increased fourfold over the past three decades, but the trend is flattening. The decline in undiagnosed celiac disease may reflect greater public and professional attention to gluten-related issues. Worldwide celiac disease affects 0.6% to 1% of the population. Celiac disease is significantly more common in persons with type 1 DM and is associated with greater risk of retinopathy and nephropathy in this population.
- Incidence is highest during infancy and the first 36 mo of life (after introduction of foods containing gluten), in the third decade (frequently associated with pregnancy and severe anemia during pregnancy), and in the seventh decade.
- There is a slight female predominance.
- The average age of diagnosis is in the fifth decade of life.
- The risk for celiac disease is 5% to 10% in newborn children of parents with the disease and nearly 20% in siblings.
- It is estimated that only 10% to 15% of persons with celiac disease in the U.S. have been diagnosed.

PHYSICAL FINDINGS & CLINICAL PRESENTATION

- Physical examination may be entirely within normal limits.
- Weight loss, dyspepsia, short stature, and failure to thrive may be noted in children and infants.
- Weight loss, fatigue, and diarrhea are common in adults.
- Abdominal pain, nausea, and vomiting are unusual.
- Pallor as a result of iron-deficiency anemia is common.
- Atypical forms of the disease are being increasingly recognized and include osteoporosis, short stature, anemia, infertility, and neurologic problems. Manifestations of calcium deficiency, such as tetany and seizures, are rare and can be exacerbated by coexistent magnesium deficiency.
- Angular cheilitis, aphthous ulcers, atopic dermatitis, and dermatitis herpetiformis are frequently associated with celiac disease.
- Table 1 summarizes the clinical spectrum of celiac disease.
- Table 2 summarizes extraintestinal manifestations of celiac disease.
- Disorders associated with celiac disease are summarized in Box 1.

ETIOLOGY

- Celiac sprue is considered an autoimmune-type disease, with tissue transglutaminase (tTG) suggested as a major autoantigen. It results from an inappropriate T-cell–mediated immune response against ingested gluten in genetically predisposed individuals who carry either *HLA-DQ2* or *HLA-DQ8* genes. There is sensitivity to gliadin, a protein fraction of gluten found in wheat, rye, and barley. In patients with celiac disease, immune responses to gliadin fractions promote an inflammatory reaction, mainly in the upper small intestine, manifested by infiltration of the lamina propria and the epithelium with chronic inflammatory cells and villous atrophy. The susceptibility to celiac disease may also be related to other environmental factors such as bacterial microbiome and reovirus infection). Table 3 summarizes biomarkers in the diagnosis of celiac disease and monitoring compliance to gluten-free diet.
- Seroconversion to celiac autoimmunity may occur at any time.
- Timing of introduction of gluten into the infant diet is associated with the appearance of celiac disease in children at risk. Children initially exposed to gluten in the first 3 mo of life have a fivefold increased risk. Current recommendations are to delay introduction of gluten into the diet of a genetically susceptible infant until 4 to 6 mo of age while the mother continues to breastfeed.

DIAGNOSIS

Diagnostic criteria for celiac disease require at least four out of five or three out of four if the *HLA* genotype is not performed:

1. Typical symptoms of celiac disease
2. Positivity of serum celiac disease Ig A class autoantibodies at high titer
3. *HLA-DQ2* or *HLA-DQ8* genotypes
4. Celiac enteropathy at the small intestinal biopsy
5. Response to gluten-free diet

DIFFERENTIAL DIAGNOSIS

- Inflammatory bowel disease
- Laxative abuse
- Intestinal parasitic infestations
- Lactose intolerance
- Other: Irritable bowel syndrome, tropical sprue, chronic pancreatitis, Zollinger-Ellison syndrome, cystic fibrosis (children), lymphoma, eosinophilic gastroenteritis, short bowel syndrome, Whipple's disease
- Intestinal lymphoma, tuberculosis, radiation enteritis, HIV enteropathy

LABORATORY TESTS

- IgA anti-tTG antibody by enzyme-linked immunosorbent assay (tissue transglutaminase [tTG] test) is the best screening serologic test for celiac disease. IgA antiendomysial antibodies (EMA) test is also a good screening test for celiac disease but is best used as a confirmatory test in cases of borderline positive results. In patients with IgA deficiency, the IgG DPG test (deamidated gliadin peptides) can be used for diagnosis. Screening of close relatives is initially done with PCR testing for *HLA DQ2* or *HLA DQ8*. Those that are positive should then have serum tTG IgA screening. All diagnostic serologic testing for celiac disease should be performed before a gluten-free diet is initiated. Table 4 summarizes the sensitivity, specificity, and positive and negative predictive values of serologic tests for untreated celiac disease.
- CBC, ferritin level: Iron-deficiency anemia (microcytic anemia, low ferritin level) may be present.
- Celiac disease can lead to malabsorption: Screen for vitamin B_{12} level, folate level, vitamin D level, serum calcium, albumin, magnesium; vitamin B_{12} deficiency, vitamin D deficiency, hypomagnesemia, and hypocalcemia are not uncommon in celiac disease.
- Biopsy of the small bowel, considered the gold standard, has been questioned as a reliable and conclusive test in all cases. It may be reasonable in children with significant elevations of tTG levels (>100 U) to first try a gluten-free

TABLE 1 Clinical Spectrum of Celiac Disease

Symptomatic
Frank malabsorption symptoms: Chronic diarrhea, failure to thrive, weight loss
Extraintestinal manifestations: Anemia, fatigue, hypertransaminasemia, neurologic disorders, short stature, dental enamel defects, arthralgia, aphthous stomatitis
Silent
No apparent symptoms in spite of histologic evidence of villous atrophy
In most cases identified by serologic screening in at-risk groups (see Laboratory Tests)
Latent
Subjects who have a normal histology, but at some other time, before or after, have shown a gluten-dependent enteropathy
Potential
Subjects with positive celiac disease serology but without evidence of altered jejunal histology
It might or might not be symptomatic

From Kliegman RM, et al.: *Nelson textbook of pediatrics,* ed 19, Philadelphia, 2011, Saunders.

TABLE 2 Extraintestinal Manifestations of Celiac Disease

Manifestation	Probable Cause(s)
Cutaneous	
Ecchymoses and petechiae	Vitamin K deficiency; rarely, thrombocytopenia
Edema	Hypoproteinemia
Dermatitis herpetiformis	Epidermal (type 3) tTG autoimmunity
Follicular hyperkeratosis and dermatitis	Vitamin A malabsorption, vitamin B complex malabsorption
Endocrinologic	
Amenorrhea, infertility, impotence	Malnutrition, hypothalamic-pituitary dysfunction, immune dysfunction
Secondary hyperparathyroidism	Calcium and/or vitamin D malabsorption with hypocalcemia
Hematologic	
Anemia	Iron, folate, vitamin B_{12}, or pyridoxine deficiency
Hemorrhage	Vitamin K deficiency; rarely, thrombocytopenia due to folate deficiency
Thrombocytosis, Howell-Jolly bodies	Hyposplenism
Hepatic	
Elevated liver biochemical test levels Autoimmune hepatitis	Lymphocytic hepatitis Autoimmunity
Muscular	
Atrophy	Malnutrition due to malabsorption
Tetany	Calcium, vitamin D, and/or magnesium malabsorption
Weakness	Generalized muscle atrophy, hypokalemia
Neurologic	
Peripheral neuropathy	Deficiencies of vitamin B_{12} and thiamine; immune-based neurologic dysfunction
Ataxia	Cerebellar and posterior column damage
Demyelinating central nervous system lesions	Immune-based neurologic dysfunction
Seizures	Unknown
Skeletal	
Osteopenia, osteomalacia, and osteoporosis	Malabsorption of calcium and vitamin D, secondary hyperparathyroidism, chronic inflammation
Osteoarthropathy	Unknown
Pathologic fractures	Osteopenia and osteoporosis

tTG, Tissue transglutaminase.
From Feldman M, Friedman LS, Brandt LJ: *Sleisenger and Fortran's gastrointestinal and liver disease*, ed 10, Philadelphia, 2016, Elsevier.

BOX 1 Disorders Associated with Celiac Disease

Definite Association
Bird-fancier's lung
Dermatitis herpetiformis
Diabetes mellitus type 1
Down syndrome
Epilepsy with cerebral calcification
Fibrosing alveolitis
Hypothyroidism or hyperthyroidism
IBD
IgA mesangial nephropathy
Idiopathic pulmonary hemosiderosis
Immunoglobulin (Ig)A deficiency
Microscopic colitis
Recurrent pericarditis
RA
Sarcoidosis

Negative Association
Diabetes mellitus type 2

Possible Association
Addison disease
Autoimmune hemolytic anemia
Autoimmune liver diseases
Cavitary lung disease
Congenital heart disease
Cystic fibrosis
Immune thrombocytopenic purpura
Iridocyclitis or choroiditis
Macroamylasemia
Myasthenia gravis
Polymyositis
Schizophrenia
Sjögren's syndrome
Systemic and cutaneous vasculitides
SLE

Modified from Mulder CJ, Tytgat GN: Coeliac disease and related disorders, *Neth J Med* 31:286–299, 1987. In Feldman M, Friedman LS, Brandt LJ: *Sleisenger and Fortran's gastrointestinal and liver disease*, ed 10, Philadelphia, 2016, Elsevier.

diet and consider biopsy in those who do not improve with diet. Repeat small-bowel biopsies are no longer required to show healing when there is a clear response to a gluten-free diet.
- The HLA-DQ2 allele is identified in >90% of patients with celiac disease, and HLA-DQ8 is identified in most of the remaining patients. These genes occur in only 30% to 40% of the general population. Their greatest diagnostic value is in their negative predictive value, making them useful when negative in ruling out the disease.

IMAGING STUDIES

- Consider bone density in newly diagnosed adult patients.
- Capsule endoscopy can be used to evaluate mucosa of the small intestine, especially if future innovations will allow mucosal biopsy.

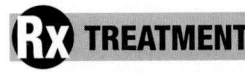

TREATMENT

NONPHARMACOLOGIC THERAPY

Patients should be instructed on a gluten-free diet (avoidance of wheat, rye, and barley). Safe grains (gluten-free) include rice, corn, oats, buckwheat, millet, amaranth, quinoa, sorghum, and teff (an Ethiopian cereal grain). The lowest amount of daily gluten that causes damage to the celiac intestinal mucosa is 10-15 mg/day. One slice of bread contains 1.6 g of gluten. Principles of initial dietary therapy for patients with celiac disease are summarized in Box 2.

GENERAL Rx

- Correct nutritional deficiencies with iron, folic acid, calcium, vitamin D, and vitamin B_{12} as needed.
- Prednisone 20 to 60 mg qd gradually tapered is useful in refractory cases.
- Lifelong gluten-free diet is necessary. A referral to a nutritionist experienced in celiac disease and gluten-free diet is recommended at initial diagnosis.

DISPOSITION

- Prognosis is good with adherence to a gluten-free diet. Rapid improvement is usually seen within a few days of treatment. Healing of the intestinal damage typically occurs within 6 to 24 mo after initiation of the diet. Lack of response to gluten-free diet occurs in 5% of patients and is due to unintentional ingestion of gluten or presence of coexisting GI disorders such as IBD, lactose or other carbohydrate intolerance, and pancreatic insufficiency.
- Serial antigliadin or antiendomysial antibody tests can be used to monitor the patient's adherence to a gluten-free diet.
- Repeat small-bowel biopsy after treatment generally reveals significant improvement. It is also useful to evaluate for increased risk of small-bowel T-cell lymphoma in these patients, especially untreated patients. Some experts recommend a repeat biopsy only in selected patients who have an unsatisfactory response to a strict gluten-free diet; however, recent data (Lebwohl et al) show that the risk for lymphoproliferative malignancy (LPM) is affected by the results of follow-up intestinal biopsy performed to document mucosal healing. Increased risk for LPM in CD is associated with the follow-up biopsy results, with a higher risk among patients with persistent villous atrophy. Follow-up biopsy may effectively stratify patients with CD by risk for subsequent LPM.

TABLE 3 Biomarkers in the Diagnosis of Celiac Disease and Monitoring Compliance to Gluten-Free Diet

Biomarker	Method	Comments
Antireticulin antibodies—IgG/IgA	IFA (rat kidney)	Lack optimal sensitivity and specificity for routine diagnostic use
Total IgA	Quantitative nephelometry	Useful in ruling out IgA deficiency; specific IgG antibodies need to be tested in IgA-deficient individuals
Antigliadin antibodies—IgG/IgA	Quantitative EIA	Low sensitivity and specificity; useful in monitoring dietary compliance
Antideaminated gliadin antibodies—IgG/IgA	Quantitative EIA	Inferior performance relative to other diagnostic assays
Antiendomysial antibodies—IgG/IgA	IFA (rhesus monkey esophagus; human umbilical cord)	High sensitivity and specificity in CD; observer bias limits usefulness
Antitissue glutaminase—IgG/IgA	Quantitative EIA	Assays using purified human or recombinant human tTG are more sensitive than those using guinea pig tTG; useful in both diagnosis and monitoring dietary compliance
HLA-DQ2/HLA-DQ8	PCR-based assays	High negative predictive value; not affected by dietary gluten; found in ≈30% of general population

IgA, Immunoglobulin A; *IgG,* immunoglobulin G; *PCR,*; *tTG,* tissue transglutaminase.
From McPherson RA, Pincus MR: *Henry's clinical diagnosis and management by laboratory methods,* ed 23, Philadelphia, 2017, Elsevier.

TABLE 4 Sensitivity, Specificity, and Positive and Negative Predictive Values of Serologic Tests for Untreated Celiac Disease

Serologic Test	Sensitivity* (%)	Specificity* (%)	Positive Predictive Value (%)	Negative Predictive Value (%)
Immunoglobulin A Tissue Transglutaminase				
Endomysial antibody by indirect immunofluorescence assay	85-98	97-100	98-100	80-95
Guinea pig tTG ELISA	95-98	94-95	91-95	96-98
Human tTG ELISA	95-100	97-100	80-95	100
Antigliadin Antibodies (AGAs)				
IgA	75-90	82-95	28-100	65-100
IgG	69-85	73-90	20-95	41-88

AGA, Antigliadin antibodies; *ELISA,* enzyme-linked immunosorbent assay; *Ig,* immunoglobulin; *tTG,* tissue transglutaminase.
*Wide variations in test sensitivity and specificity rates are reported among different laboratories. (Stern M: Comparative evaluation of serologic tests for celiac disease: a European initiative toward standardization, *J Pediatr Gastroenterol Nutr* 31:513–519, 2000.)
From Feldman M, Friedman LS, Brandt LJ: *Sleisenger and Fortran's gastrointestinal and liver disease,* ed 10, Philadelphia, 2016, Elsevier.

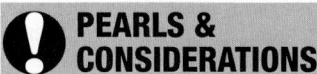

PEARLS & CONSIDERATIONS

COMMENTS

- The presence of dermatitis herpetiformis is pathognomonic for celiac disease.
- In close relatives, repeated serum tTG IgA testing may be useful in those with positive *HLA-DQ2* or *HLA-DQ8* tests because celiac disease may not manifest until later in life, and initial negative results do not preclude the possibility of future onset of celiac disease.
- Celiac disease should be considered in patients with unexplained metabolic bone disease, osteoporosis, transaminasemia, or hypocalcemia, because gastrointestinal symptoms are absent or mild. Clinicians should also consider testing children and young adults for celiac disease if unexplained weight loss, abdominal pain or distention, or chronic diarrhea is present.
- Screening for celiac disease is recommended in first-degree relatives. It should also be considered in patients with type 1 diabetes mellitus and in those with certain autoimmune disorders such as primary biliary cirrhosis, primary sclerosing cholangitis, autoimmune hepatitis, IBD, thyroid disease (hypothyroidism occurs in up to 15% of patients with celiac disease), SLE, RA, and Sjögren's syndrome due to increased risk of celiac disease in these populations. Screening persons with Down syndrome or Turner syndrome has also been recommended.
- The prevalence of celiac disease in patients with dyspepsia is twice that of the general population. Screening for celiac disease should be considered in all patients with persistent dyspepsia.

BOX 2 Principles of Initial Dietary Therapy for Patients with Celiac Disease.

Avoid all foods containing wheat, rye, and barley gluten (pure oats usually safe).
Avoid malt unless clearly labeled as derived from corn.
Use only rice, corn, maize, buckwheat, millet, amaranth, quinoa, sorghum, potato or potato starch, soybean, tapioca, and teff, bean, and nut flours.
Wheat starch and products containing wheat starch should only be used if they contain less than 20 ppm gluten and are marked "gluten free."
Read all labels and study ingredients of processed foods.
Beware of gluten in medications, supplements, food additives, emulsifiers, or stabilizers.
Limit milk and milk products initially if there is evidence of lactose intolerance.
Avoid all beers, lagers, ales, and stouts (unless labeled gluten free).
Wine, most liqueurs, ciders, and spirits, including whiskey and brandy, are allowed.

ppm, Parts per million.
Modified from Trier JS: Celiac sprue and refractory sprue. In Feldman M, Scharschmidt BF, Sleisenger MH [eds]: *Gastrointestinal and liver disease,* ed 6, Philadelphia, 1997, WB Saunders, p 1557; In Feldman M et al: *Sleisenger and Fortran's gastrointestinal and liver disease,* ed 10, Philadelphia, 2016, Elsevier.

- Patients with celiac disease have an overall risk of cancer that is almost twice that of the general population. The risk of adenocarcinoma of the small intestine is increased manifold compared with the risk in the general population. Celiac disease is also associated with an increased risk for non-Hodgkin's lymphoma, especially of T-cell type and primarily localized in the gut. Lymphoma is 4 to 40 times more common, and death from lymphoma is 11 to 70 times more common in patients with celiac disease.
- Patients with celiac disease who have followed a gluten-free diet for prolonged periods may not experience relapse of symptoms for several months after gluten is reintroduced.

Trials involving randomized feeding intervention in infants at high risk for celiac disease have shown that as compared to placebo, the introduction of small quantities of gluten at 16 to 24 weeks of age did not reduce the risk of celiac disease by 3 yr of age.

SUGGESTED READINGS

Available at ExpertConsult.com

RELATED CONTENT

Celiac Disease (Patient Information)
Dermatitis Herpetiformis (Related Key Topic)
Malabsorption (Related Key Topic)

AUTHOR: **FRED F. FERRI, M.D.**

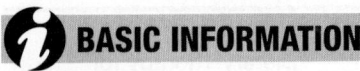

DEFINITION

Cellulitis is an infection of the deep dermis and subcutaneous tissues characterized by erythema, warmth, and tenderness of the involved area. Diagnosis is made on the basis of history and physical examination.

SYNONYMS

Erysipelas (cellulitis generally caused by group A β-hemolytic streptococci [GABHS])
SSSIs (skin and skin structure infections)
ABSSSIs (acute bacterial skin and skin structure infections)

ICD-10CM CODES

H05.011	Cellulitis of right orbit
H05.012	Cellulitis of left orbit
H05.013	Cellulitis of bilateral orbits
H05.019	Cellulitis of unspecified orbit
H60.10	Cellulitis of external ear, unspecified ear
H60.11	Cellulitis of right external ear
H60.12	Cellulitis of left external ear
H60.13	Cellulitis of external ear, bilateral
K12.2	Cellulitis and abscess of mouth
L03.011	Cellulitis of right finger
L03.012	Cellulitis of left finger
L03.019	Cellulitis of unspecified finger
L03.031	Cellulitis of right toe
L03.032	Cellulitis of left toe
L03.039	Cellulitis of unspecified toe
L03.111	Cellulitis of right axilla
L03.112	Cellulitis of left axilla
L03.113	Cellulitis of right upper limb
L03.114	Cellulitis of left upper limb
L03.115	Cellulitis of right lower limb
L03.116	Cellulitis of left lower limb
L03.119	Cellulitis of unspecified part of limb
L03.211	Cellulitis of face
L03.221	Cellulitis of neck
L03.311	Cellulitis of abdominal wall
L03.312	Cellulitis of back [any part except buttock]
L03.313	Cellulitis of chest wall
L03.314	Cellulitis of groin
L03.315	Cellulitis of perineum
L03.316	Cellulitis of umbilicus
L03.317	Cellulitis of buttock
L03.319	Cellulitis of trunk, unspecified
L03.811	Cellulitis of head [any part, except face]
L03.818	Cellulitis of other sites
L03.90	Cellulitis, unspecified

EPIDEMIOLOGY & DEMOGRAPHICS

- Occurs most frequently in diabetics, immunocompromised hosts, and patients with venous and lymphatic compromise.
- Frequently found near skin breaks (trauma, surgical wounds [surgical site infections develop in 2% to 5% of all surgical procedures], ulcerations, tinea infections). Edema, animal or human bites, subadjacent osteomyelitis, and bacteremia are potential sources of cellulitis.
- Skin and soft-tissue infections account for >14 million outpatient visits per yr and $3.7 billion in ambulatory care costs. They also are responsible for more than 650,000 admissions in the U.S./yr.

PHYSICAL FINDINGS & CLINICAL PRESENTATION

Variable with the causative organism:

- Erysipelas (Fig. E1): Superficial-spreading, warm, erythematous lesion distinguished by indurated, elevated margin; lymphatic involvement, vesicle formation common.
- Staphylococcal cellulitis: Area involved is erythematous, hot, and swollen; differentiated from erysipelas by nonelevated, poorly demarcated margin; local tenderness and regional adenopathy are common; up to 85% of cases occur on the legs and feet.
- *Haemophilus influenzae* cellulitis: Area involved is a blue-red/purple-red color; occurs mainly in children; generally involves the face in children and the neck or upper chest in adults.
- *Vibrio vulnificus:* Larger hemorrhagic bullae, cellulitis, lymphadenitis, myositis; often found in critically ill patients in septic shock.
- Table 1 describes anatomic variants of or predispositions to cellulitis. Typically, nonpurulent cellulitis is caused by β-hemolytic streptococci, whereas cellulitis with purulent drainage is caused by MRSA.

ETIOLOGY

- Any disruption of the skin barrier provides a portal for pathogens to enter the skin and soft tissues.
- Group A β-hemolytic streptococci (may follow a streptococcal infection of the upper respiratory tract). β-hemolytic streptococci are implicated in most cases of nontraumatic cellulitis.
- Staphylococcal cellulitis: Diabetics, athletes, men who have sex with men, people living in public housing, and incarcerated men are at greater risk for methicillin-resistant *Staphylococcus aureus* (MRSA) infection. A community-acquired MRSA strain, USA 300, is replacing nosocomial strains of MRSA in hospitals.
- IV drug use: MRSA, *Pseudomonas aeruginosa.*
- *V. vulnificus:* Higher incidence in patients with liver disease (75%) and in immunocompromised hosts. *V. vulnificus* infection is the leading cause of death related to seafood consumption in the U.S.
- *Erysipelothrix rhusiopathiae:* Common in people handling poultry, fish, or meat.
- *Aeromonas hydrophila:* Generally occurs in contaminated open wounds in fresh water.
- Fungi *(Cryptococcus neoformans):* In immunocompromised granulopenic patients.
- Gram-negative rods *(Serratia, Enterobacter, Proteus, Pseudomonas):* May be present in immunocompromised or granulopenic patients.
- Hot tub exposure: *P. aeruginosa*; fish tank exposure: *Mycobacterium marinum.*
- Bites: Human *(Eikenella corrodens),* dog *(Pasteurella multocida, C. canimorsus),* cat *(P. multocida),* rat *(Streptobacillus moniliformis).*

Dx DIAGNOSIS

DIFFERENTIAL DIAGNOSIS

- Necrotizing fasciitis (reddish-purple discoloration of skin, rapid increase in size, woody induration and pale appearance rather than erythema, violaceous bullae, pain out of proportion to appearance, sepsis)
- Deep vein thrombosis
- Peripheral vascular insufficiency (venous stasis dermatitis)
- Paget disease of the breast
- Thrombophlebitis
- Acute gout
- Psoriasis
- *Candida* intertrigo
- Pseudogout
- Osteomyelitis
- Insect bite
- Fixed drug eruption
- Lymphedema
- Contact dermatitis
- Olecranon bursa infection
- Herpetic whitlow, early herpes zoster (before blisters)
- Erythema migrans (Lyme disease)
- Rare: *Vaccinia* vaccination, Kawasaki disease, pyoderma gangrenosum, Sweet syndrome, carcinoma erysipeloides, anaerobic myonecrosis, erythromelalgia, eosinophilic cellulitis (Well's syndrome), familial Mediterranean fever

LABORATORY TESTS

- Laboratory testing is generally not required for the evaluation of cellulitis and uncomplicated soft tissue infections in the absence of comorbidities
- CBC with differential: Leukocytosis may be present but is a non-specific finding
- Gram stain, culture (aerobic and anaerobic):
  1. Aspirated material from:
     a. Advancing edge of cellulitis
     b. Any vesicles
  2. Swab of any drainage material
  3. Punch biopsy (in selected patients)
- Blood cultures in hospitalized patients, patients with cellulitis superimposed on lymphedema, patients with buccal or periorbital cellulitis, and patients suspected of having a salt- or fresh-water source of infection. Bacteremia uncommon in cellulitis (positive blood cultures in 4% of patients)
- Anti-streptolysin O (ASLO) titer (in suspected streptococcal disease)

The cause of cellulitis remains unidentified in most patients. Patients with recurrent lower-extremity cellulitis should be inspected for tinea pedis. If found, it should be treated.

IMAGING STUDIES

- Imaging is generally not necessary but may be helpful in suspected purulent soft tissue infections and osteomyelitis.

TABLE 1 Anatomic Variants of or Predispositions to Cellulitis

Anatomic Variant or Predisposition	Location	Likely Bacterial Cause
Periorbital cellulitis	Periorbital	*Staphylococcus aureus, Streptococcus pneumoniae,* group A streptococci
Buccal cellulitis	Cheek	*Haemophilus influenzae* type b
Cellulitis complicating body piercing	Ear, nose, umbilicus	*S. aureus,* group A streptococci
After mastectomy (with axillary node dissection)	Ipsilateral upper extremity	Non–group A β-hemolytic streptococci
After lumpectomy (with limited axillary node dissection, breast irradiation)	Ipsilateral breast	Non–group A β-hemolytic streptococci
After saphenous vein harvest for coronary artery bypass	Ipsilateral leg	Group A or non–group A β-hemolytic streptococci
After radical pelvic surgery, radiation therapy	Vulva, inguinal areas, legs	Group B and group G streptococci
After liposuction	Thigh, abdominal wall	Group A streptococci, peptostreptococci
Postoperative (very early) wound infection	Abdomen, chest, hip	Group A streptococci
Injection drug use ("skin popping")	Extremities, neck	*S. aureus,* streptococci (groups A, C, F, G)*
Perianal cellulitis	Perineum	Group A streptococcus

*Other bacteria to consider based on isolation from skin or abscesses in this setting include *Enterococcus faecalis,* viridans group streptococci, coagulase-negative staphylococci, anaerobes (including *Bacteroides* and *Clostridium* spp.), and Enterobacteriaceae.

From Bennett JE, Dolin R, Blaser MJ: *Mandell, Douglas, and Bennett's principles and practice of infectious diseases,* ed 8, Philadelphia, 2015, Saunders

- CT or MRI in patients with suspected necrotizing fasciitis (deep-seated infection of the subcutaneous tissue that results in the progressive destruction of fascia and fat).

TREATMENT

NONPHARMACOLOGIC THERAPY

Immobilization and elevation of the involved limb. Cool sterile saline dressings to remove purulence from any open lesion. Support stockings in patients with peripheral edema.

ACUTE GENERAL Rx

Treatment should initially cover *Streptococcus* and methicillin-sensitive *S. aureus* and should be expanded for MRSA in patients with risk factors (e.g., IV drug users, residents of long-term care facilities, athletes, children, men who have sex with men, prisoners).

Erysipelas:
- PO: dicloxacillin 500 mg PO q6h or cephalexin 500 mg qid
- IV: cefazolin 1 g q6 to 8h or nafcillin 1.0 or 1.5 g IV q4 to 6h

NOTE: Use vancomycin 1 g IV q12h in patients allergic to penicillin.

Staphylococcal cellulitis:
- PO: dicloxacillin 250 to 500 mg qid
- IV: nafcillin 1 to 2 g q4 to 6h
- Cephalosporins (cephalexin 500 mg qid) also provide adequate antistaphylococcal coverage, except for MRSA.
- Trimethoprim-sulfamethoxazole (160 mg/800 mg 1 PO bid) may be appropriate in outpatient mild MRSA infections. Use vancomycin 1.0 to 2.0 g IV qd or linezolid 0.6 g IV q12h in patients with moderate/severe MRSA. Daptomycin (Cubicin), a cyclic lipopeptide, can be used as an alternative to vancomycin for complicated skin and skin structure infections. Usual dose is 4 mg/kg IV given over 30 min every 24 hr. Telavancin is a new glycopeptide derivative of vancomycin effective for gram-positive skin and skin structure infections, including those caused by MRSA. Tedizolid is an oxazolidinone effective in ABSSSI as an alternative to linezolid. Ceftaroline fosamil (Teflaro) is a newer IV cephalosporin also effective against MRSA. Dalbavancin and tedizolid are two new drugs FDA-approved for skin and skin structure infections, including those caused by MRSA.

***H. influenzae* cellulitis:**
- PO: cefixime or cefuroxime
- IV: cefuroxime or ceftriaxone

Vibrio vulnificus:
- Doxycycline 100 mg IV bid + ceftazidime 2 g IV q8h or IV ciprofloxacin 400 mg bid. Mild cases treated with oral antibiotics (doxycycline 100 mg bid + ciprofloxacin 750 mg bid).
- IV support and admission into intensive care unit (mortality rate >50% in septic shock).

E. rhusiopathiae:
- Penicillin

A. hydrophila:
- Aminoglycosides
- Chloramphenicol
- Complicated skin and skin structure infections in hospitalized patients can be treated with daptomycin (Cubicin) 4 mg/kg IV q24h

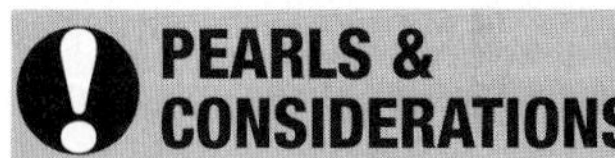

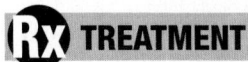

PEARLS & CONSIDERATIONS

- 16.6% of acute cellulitis cases are unresponsive to initial treatment mainly due to inappropriate antibiotic selection and dosing (weight-based dosing is preferred).
- Prophylactic antibiotics (e.g., dicloxacillin 500 mg bid or erythromycin 250 mg bid) are controversial but can be considered with patients with ≥4 episodes of cellulitis despite optimized control of risk factors. Recurrent cellulitis with no identifiable cause occurs in 22% of cases despite antibiotic prophylaxis.
- In patients with uncomplicated cellulitis in the outpatient setting, adding trimethoprim-sulfamethoxazole to cephalexin for MRSA coverage is unnecessary and does not increase the likelihood of clinical cure.

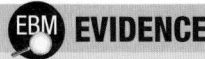

EVIDENCE

Available at ExpertConsult.com

SUGGESTED READINGS

Available at ExpertConsult.com

RELATED CONTENT

Cellulitis (Patient Information)
Erysipelas (Related Key Topic)
Necrotizing Fasciitis (Related Key Topic)

AUTHOR: **FRED F. FERRI, M.D.**

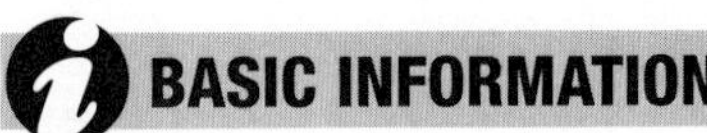

BASIC INFORMATION

DEFINITION

Cervical cancer is the penetration of the basement membrane and infiltration of the stroma of the uterine cervix by malignant cells.

ICD-10CM CODES

C53.8	Malignant neoplasm of overlapping sites of cervix uteri
C53.9	Malignant neoplasm of cervix uteri, unspecified
D06.7	Carcinoma in situ of other parts of cervix
D06.9	Carcinoma in situ of cervix, unspecified

EPIDEMIOLOGY & DEMOGRAPHICS

INCIDENCE: According to the World Health Organization, cervical cancer is the fourth most common malignancy in women. It is reported that nearly 9 out of 10 women who died of cervical cancer were in an underdeveloped region of the world.

PREDOMINANCE: Higher incidence rates occur in developing countries. Among the U.S. population, Hispanics have a higher incidence than African Americans, who likewise have a higher incidence than Caucasians.

RISK FACTORS: Infection with high-risk human papillomavirus (HPV; types 16 and 18 are the most oncogenic with 31, 33, 35, 45, 52, and 58 also labeled high risk). Smoking, early age of coitarche, multiple sexual partners, immunocompromised state, nonbarrier methods of birth control, and multiparity are also risk factors.

PHYSICAL FINDINGS & CLINICAL PRESENTATION

- Unusual vaginal bleeding, particularly postcoital (Fig. 1)
- Vaginal discharge and/or odor
- Pelvic pain in early stage disease, back pain, or disrupted urination or defecation in later stages
- Advanced cases may present with lower-extremity edema or renal failure
- In early stages, there may be little or no obvious cervical lesion; more advanced cases may have large, bulky, friable lesions encompassing majority of vagina

ETIOLOGY

- Infection with high-risk HPV types is a necessary, although not sufficient, cause of almost all cases of cervical cancer. Persistent HPV infection leads to precancerous changes of cervix (cervical intraepithelial neoplasia [CIN]). CIN can progress to invasive cervical cancer.
- Both squamous cell and adenocarcinoma of cervix are associated with HPV infection (Table 1).
- More than 40 HPV types can infect the cervix. Most cases are believed to be linked to presence of HPV 16, 18, 31, 35, 39, 45, 51, 52, 56, 58, 59, and 68 by interaction of E6 and E7 oncoprotein on *p53* gene product.

DIAGNOSIS

DIFFERENTIAL DIAGNOSIS

- Cervical polyp or prolapsed uterine fibroid
- Neoplasia metastatic from a separate primary neoplasia
- Box 1 summarizes benign mimics of cervical adenocarcinoma
- Categories of squamous carcinoma are described in Box 2
- Table 2 summarizes the differential diagnosis of squamous intraepithelial lesions

WORKUP

- Thorough history and physical examination.
- Pelvic examination with careful rectovaginal examination.
- Table 3 summarizes the clinical evaluation of patients with newly diagnosed cervical cancer.
- Compared with Pap testing, HPV testing has greater sensitivity for detection of CIN. Addition of HPV test for high-risk types to Pap test to screen women in mid-30s for cervical cancer reduces incidence of grade 2 or 3 CIN or cancer detected by subsequent screening examinations.
- Colposcopy with directed biopsy and endocervical curettage.
- FIGO staging described in Table 4.

LABORATORY TESTS

- Complete blood count, chemistry profile
- SCC antigen in research setting
- Carcinoembryonic antigen

IMAGING STUDIES

- Chest x-ray
- Depending on stage, may need CT scan, MRI (Fig. 2), PET/CT
- Table 3, intravenous pyelogram

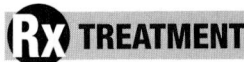

TREATMENT

NONPHARMACOLOGIC THERAPY

- FIGO stage IA: Cone biopsy or simple hysterectomy
- FIGO stage IB or IIA: Type III radical hysterectomy and pelvic lymphadenectomy or pelvic radiation therapy. Minimally invasive radical hysterectomy is associated with shorter overall survival than open surgery among women with stage IA2 or IB2 cervical carcinoma (Melamed A et al, in Suggested Reading N Engl J Med 379:1905, 2018.)
- Advanced or bulky disease: Multimodality therapy (radiation, chemotherapy, and/or surgery); platinum use before radiation therapy

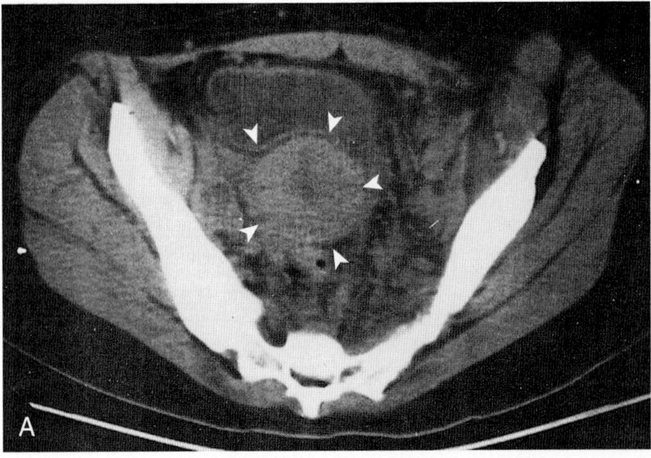

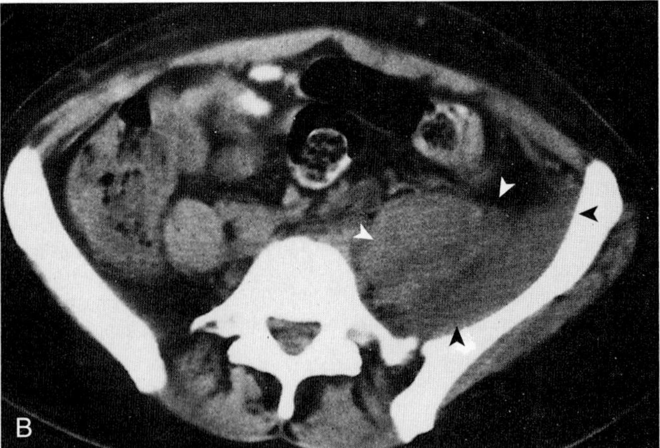

FIG. 1 Stage IIIb cervical carcinoma. A 27-year-old woman presented with increased vaginal bleeding, left leg swelling, and abdominal pain. Examination revealed a large, fixed pelvic mass. Computed tomography scan evaluation **(A)** confirms the mass *(arrowheads)* and **(B)** shows extension into the left psoas and iliacus muscles *(arrowheads)*. She also had hydronephrosis. Pathologic examination showed an adenosquamous carcinoma. (Skarin AT: *Atlas of diagnostic oncology*, ed 4, Philadelphia, 2010, Mosby.)

C

TABLE 1 Descriptive Categories of Low-Grade Squamous Intraepithelial Lesion and High-Grade Squamous Intraepithelial Lesion

	Descriptors	Human Papillomavirus	p16 Immunostaining
LSIL	CIN1, flat condyloma, mild dysplasia	HR (70%)	Usually diffuse
	Exophytic condyloma	LR	Negative or patchy
	Immature condyloma (papillary immature metaplasia)	LR	Negative or patchy
	Immature flat metaplastic LSIL	HR	Usually diffuse
HSIL	CIN2 or moderate dysplasia	HR (45% type 16)	Diffuse
	CIN3 or severe dysplasia/carcinoma in situ	HR (60% type 16)	Diffuse
	Keratinizing SIL	HR	Diffuse
	HSIL with immature metaplastic phenotype	HR	Diffuse
	Papillary carcinoma in situ	HR	Diffuse
	Adenosquamous carcinoma in situ	HR	Diffuse

CIN, Cervical intraepithelial lesion; *HR*, high risk; *HSIL*, high-grade squamous intraepithelial lesion; *LR*, low risk; *LSIL*, low-grade squamous intraepithelial lesion; *SIL*, squamous intraepithelial lesion.
Crum CP et al: *Diagnostic gynecologic and obstetric pathology*, ed 3, Philadelphia, 2018, Elsevier.

BOX 1 Benign Mimics of Cervical Adenocarcinoma

1. Deep nabothian cysts, florid deep glands
2. Tunnel clusters
3. Endocervical gland hyperplasias
   a. Lobular hyperplasia
   b. Diffuse laminar hyperplasia
4. Adenomyoma of the endocervical type
5. Endocervicosis, florid cystic endosalpingiosis
6. Müllerian papilloma
7. Microglandular hyperplasia
8. Mesonephric hyperplasia
9. Ectopic prostate
10. Deep tubal metaplasia

Crum CP et al: *Diagnostic gynecologic and obstetric pathology*, ed 3, Philadelphia, 2018, Elsevier.

BOX 2 Categories of Squamous Carcinoma

Squamous cell carcinoma
Large cell keratinizing (well-differentiated)
Large cell nonkeratinizing (moderately differentiated)
Small cell nonkeratinizing (poorly differentiated)
Lymphoepithelial-like carcinoma
Spindle cell (sarcomatoid) carcinoma
Verrucopapillary carcinomas
Papillary (squamo-transitional) carcinoma
Verrucous carcinoma (rare)[a]
Condylomatous carcinoma[a]
Basaloid carcinomas[b]

[a] In young women, an extensive (giant) condyloma must be excluded.
[b] May be associated with adenoid basal and adenoid cystic carcinomas, as well as carcinosarcomas.
Crum CP et al: *Diagnostic gynecologic and obstetric pathology*, ed 3, Philadelphia, 2018, Elsevier.

TABLE 2 Differential Diagnosis of Squamous Intraepithelial Lesions

Category	Mimic	Distinguishing Features
LSIL	Mucosal polyp (vaginal)	Minimal acanthosis, no koilocytosis
	Reactive epithelial changes	Mild superficial karyomegaly, occasional binucleated intermediate cells
	Postmenopausal changes	Superficial cell karyomegaly, cytoplasmic halos
HSIL	Immature reactive/repair	Basal hyperchromasia, uniform nuclear spacing and nuclear contour, nucleoli
	Immature metaplasia	Uniform maturation, minimal surface hyperchromasia
	Atrophy	No mitoses, uniform chromasia, nuclear density
	Atypical atrophy	Enlarged nuclei, uncommon
	Implantation site	Uniform and wide nuclear spacing, bizarre nuclei
	Endometrial histiocytes	Small indented nuclei, granular cytoplasm, lack of polarity

HSIL, High-grade squamous intraepithelial lesion; *LSIL*, low-grade squamous intraepithelial lesion.
Crum CP et al: *Diagnostic gynecologic and obstetric pathology*, ed 3, Philadelphia, 2018, Elsevier.

ACUTE GENERAL Rx

- Table 4 summarizes treatment according to tumor stage. Fig. 3 describes a treatment algorithm for invasive cervical cancer.

Chemotherapy is cisplatin-based. In advanced cases, cervical cancer may present with massive and acute vaginal bleeding requiring volume and blood replacement, vaginal packing or other hemostatic modalities, and/or high-dose local radiotherapy.

CHRONIC Rx

- Physical examination with Pap smear every 3 mo for 2 yr, every 6 mo for 3 to 5 yr, annually thereafter. Table 5 summarizes a proposed schedule for interval evaluation of cervical cancer after radiotherapy or surgery in asymptomatic patients
- Chest x-ray annually (optional)
- Other imaging done only as clinically indicated
- Localized pelvic recurrence may be treated and cured with pelvic exenteration

DISPOSITION

Five-yr survival varies by stage:

- Stage I: 90% to 95%
- Stage II: 40% to 80%
- Stage III: <60%
- Stage IV: <15%

Early detection by Pap smear is imperative for long-term improvements in survival.

REFERRAL

Gynecologic oncologist for all invasive disease

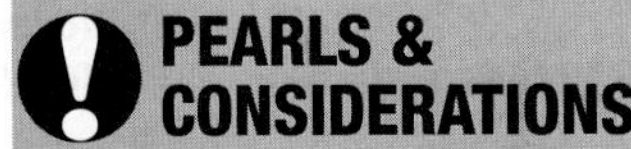

PEARLS & CONSIDERATIONS

- HPV vaccination is indicated in males and females age 9 to 26 yr for the prevention of cervical cancer caused by HPV types 6, 11, 16, and 18. HPV vaccination is over 90% effective in preventing infection and cervical cancer. There are now HPV vaccines that are effective against nine strains of high-risk HPV.
- Available evidence supports discontinuation of cervical cancer screening among women aged 65 yr or older who have had adequate screening and are not otherwise at high risk.
- Updated recommendations from the American College of Physicians on screening for cervical cancer in average-risk women are as follows.[1]
- Women should be screened with cervical cytology every 3 yr beginning at age 21 until age 30.
- After age 30, women can be screened with cytology and HPV testing every 5 yr.

[1] Sawaya GF et al: Cervical cancer screening in average-risk women: best practice advice from the Cervical Guidelines Committee of the American College of Physicians, *Ann Intern Med* 162(12):851–859, 2015.

TABLE 3 Clinical Evaluation of Patients with Newly Diagnosed Cervical Cancer

History	Review of Systems	General Physical Examination
Risk factors (STDs, smoking, OCPs, HIV), prior abnormal Pap tests, previous dysplasia, and treatment	Abnormal vaginal bleeding or discharge, pelvic pain, flank pain, sciatica, hematuria, rectal bleeding, anorexia, weight loss, bone pain	Peripheral lymphadenopathy
Evaluation	Common procedures (FIGO)	Alternative procedures
Invasive cancer	Cervical biopsy	Histologic diagnosis required
	Endocervical curettage	
	Cervical conization	
Tumor size; involvement of the vagina, bladder, rectum and parametria	Pelvic examination under anesthesia	MRI of pelvis preferred over CT
Anemia	Complete blood count	—
Renal failure	Serum chemistries	—
Hematuria	Urinalysis	—
Bladder involvement	Cystoscopy with biopsy and urine cytology	CT, MRI pelvis
Rectal infiltration	Proctoscopy with biopsy	CT, MRI pelvis; barium enema
Hydronephrosis	IVP	Renal ultrasonography; CT abdomen
Pulmonary metastases	Chest radiography	CT chest; PET scan
Retroperitoneal lymphadenopathy	—	lymphangiogram, CT, MRI, PET scan

CT, Computed tomography; *FIGO,* Federation of International Gynecologists and Obstetricians; *HIV,* human immunodeficiency virus; *IVP,* intravenous pyelography; *MRI,* magnetic resonance imaging; *OCP,* oral contraceptive pill; *PET,* positron emission tomography; *STD,* sexually transmitted disease.
From Disaia PJ et al: *Clinical gynecologic oncology,* ed 9, Philadelphia, 2017, Elsevier.

TABLE 4 FIGO Staging of Cervical Cancer

Stage	Invasion	Prognosis: 5-yr Survival	Treatment
I_{A1}	Depth of invasion ≤3 mm and width ≤7 mm (includes early stromal invasion of ≤1 mm)	84% to 90% if tumor <3 cm; 85% will have negative pelvic nodes, and 95% of these patients will be "cured"	Local excision; if margins of cone clear (i.e., no residual tumor or CIN), then conization is adequate, with no need for pelvic lymphadenectomy
I_{A2}	Depth of invasion between 3 and 5 mm (i.e., 3.1-5 mm) and width up to 7 mm	66% if tumor >3 cm	Simple hysterectomy and pelvic lymphadenectomy
I_{B1}	Tumor confined to cervix and diameter <4 cm		Radical hysterectomy or radiotherapy
I_{B2}	Tumor confined to cervix and diameter >4 cm		Radical hysterectomy or radiotherapy
II_A	Upper third of the vagina	62%	Radical hysterectomy or radiotherapy
II_B	Upper two thirds of the vagina plus parametrial disease		Radiotherapy ± chemotherapy
III_A	Lower third of the vagina	40%	Radiotherapy ± chemotherapy
III_B	Pelvic sidewall and/or hydronephrosis		Radiotherapy ± chemotherapy
IV_A	Bladder, rectum	15%	Radiotherapy ± chemotherapy
IV_B	Beyond pelvis		Radiotherapy ± chemotherapy

CIN, cervical intraepithelial neoplasia; FIGO, Federation of International Gynecologists and Obstetricians. From Drife J, Magowan B: *Clinical obstetrics and gynecology,* Philadelphia, 2004, Saunders.

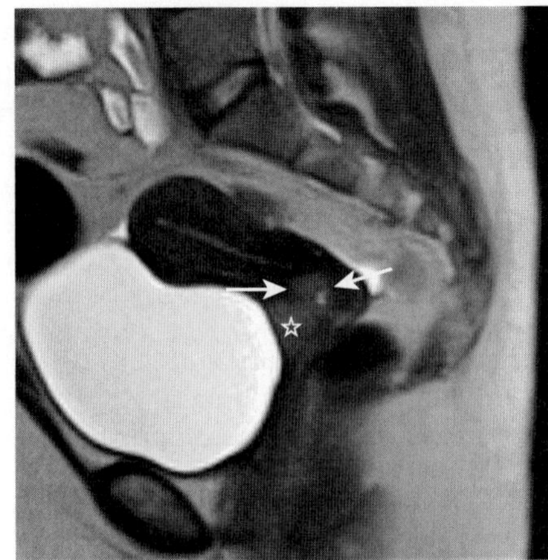

FIG. 2 Cervical carcinoma. T2-weighted sagittal image through the cervix shows an intermediate signal mass *(arrows)* disrupting the normally intense low signal ring of the cervical stroma with areas of high signal. The mass infiltrates the upper vagina *(star).* (From Fielding JR et al: *Gynecologic imaging,* Philadelphia, 2011, Saunders.)

- Before age 21, women should not be scanned, unless HIV positive. If HIV positive, they should enter screening within 1 yr of coitarche.
- Before age 30, women should not be screened with HPV testing.
- At age 65, screening can stop in women with three consecutive negative cytology results or two consecutive negative cytology results combined with a negative HPV test within the last 10 yr (with the most recent test within 5 yr).
- Women without a cervix should not be screened.

SUGGESTED READINGS

Available at ExpertConsult.com

RELATED CONTENT

Cervical Cancer (Patient Information)
Cervical Dysplasia (Related Key Topic)

AUTHOR: **BETH LEOPOLD, M.D.**

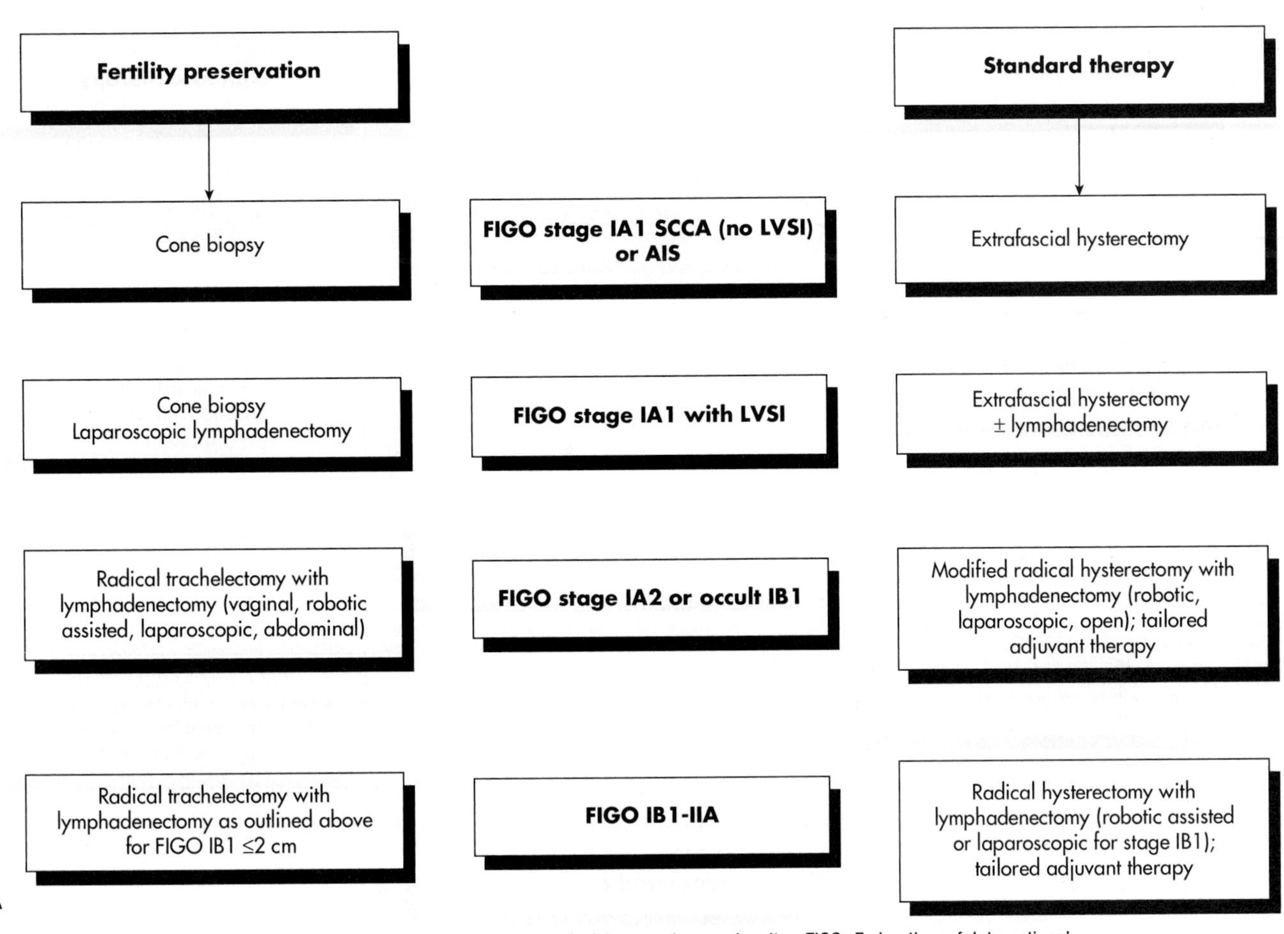

FIG. 3 A and **B,** Algorithm for therapy. *AIS,* Adenocarcinoma *in situ; FIGO,* Federation of International Gynecologists and Obstetricians; *GOG,* gynecologic oncology group; *HDR,* high-dose rate; *LVSI,* lymphovascular space invasion, *SCCA,* squamous cell carcinoma associated antigen. (From Disaia PJ et al: *Clinical gynecologic oncology*, ed 9, Philadelphia, 2017, Elsevier.)

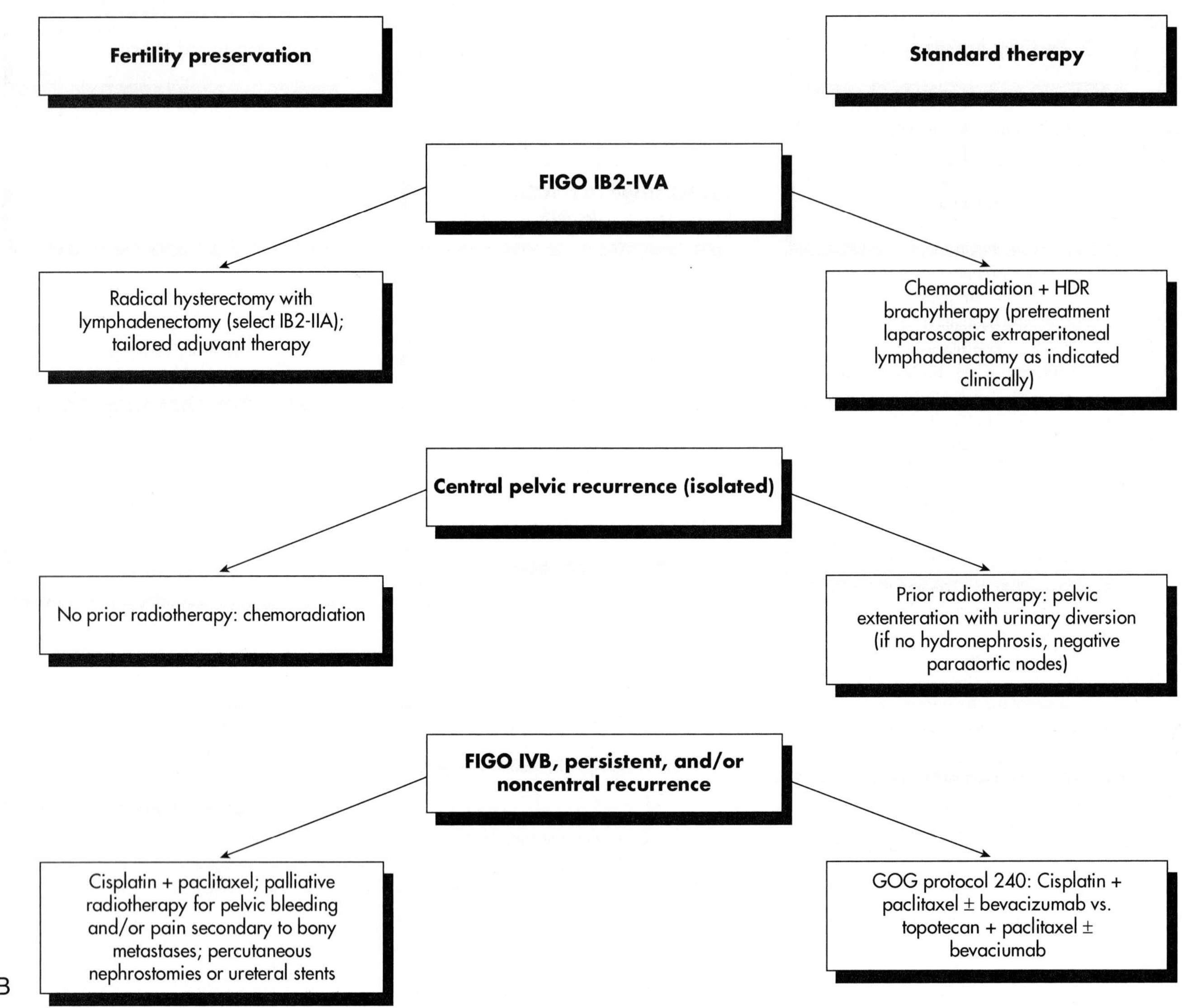

FIG. 3, cont'd

TABLE 5 Proposed Schedule for Interval Evaluation of Cervical Cancer after Radiotherapy or Surgery (Asymptomatic Patient*)

Year	Frequency	Examination
1	3 mo	Pelvic examination, Pap smear
	6 mo	Chest radiography, CBC, BUN, creatinine
	1 yr	IVP or CT scan with contrast
2	4 mo	Pelvic examination, Pap smear
	1 yr	Chest radiography, CBC, BUN, creatinine, IVP or CT scan with contrast
3-5	6 mo	Pelvic examination, Pap smear

BUN, Blood urea nitrogen; *CBC,* complete blood count; *CT,* computed tomography; *IVP,* intravenous pyelogram; *Pap,* Papanicolaou.
*Symptomatic patients should have appropriate examination where indicated.
From Disaia PJ et al: *Clinical gynecologic oncology,* ed 9, Philadelphia, 2017, Elsevier.

BASIC INFORMATION

DEFINITION

Cervical dysplasia refers to atypical development of immature squamous epithelium that does not penetrate the basement epithelial membrane. Characteristics include increased cellularity, nuclear abnormalities, and increased nuclear/cytoplasmic ratio. A progressive loss of squamous differentiation exists beginning adjacent to the basement membrane and progressing to the most advanced stage (severe dysplasia), which encompasses the complete squamous epithelial layer thickness. The revised 2001 Bethesda System terminology was used in a National Institutes of Health consensus conference, sponsored by the American Society for Colposcopy and Cervical Pathology (ASCCP) and its partner professional organizations in 2006. The conference updated therapeutic options for women based on studies such as the **A**SC-US (atypical squamous cells of undetermined significance)/**L**SIL (low-grade squamous intraepithelial lesions) **T**riage **S**tudy (ALTS) that appeared after revision of the Bethesda classification. Fig. 1 provides a comparison of grading systems for cervical squamous dysplasia.

In 2012, the American Cancer Society (ACS), ASCCP, and American Society for Clinical Pathology (ASCP) published a new set of recommendations for lifetime assessment and early diagnosis of cervical dysplasia and cancer. The recommendations attempted to reduce the number of lifetime assessments, thereby reducing the possible morbidity associated with excess testing and also optimizing the co-evaluation with Pap smear and HPV testing.

UPDATED SCREENING PROTOCOL:

- Women younger than 21 yr of age should not have any screening, unless HIV positive. If HIV positive, screening should start within 1 yr of coitarche.
- Women 21-29 yr of age should have testing every 3 yr with only cytology. With negative cytology or HPV-negative ASC-US, patients can repeat every 3 yr. For HPV-positive ASC-US or cytology with LG-SIL, follow-up is as per the 2006 guidelines (essentially a colposcopic examination as the initial step with follow-up steps depending on the findings).
- Women between the ages of 30 and 65 yr should have co-testing every 5 yr with both Pap cytology and HPV testing. Alternatively, it is also acceptable to perform cytology alone, but then the testing interval should be every 3 yr. With negative cytology or HPV-negative ASC-US, patients can repeat with co-testing every 5 yr. For HPV-positive ASC-US or cytology with LG-SIL, follow-up is as per the 2006 guidelines, as previously documented. For patients with positive HPV but negative cytology, the patient can repeat testing 12 months later with co-testing; patients can also specifically test for HPV 16 or HPV 16/18 genotypes and, if positive, should be referred for colposcopy. Patients with positive HPV but negative 16 and/or 18 should be retested in 12 months with co-testing.

Women older than the age of 65 yr and those with a history of hysterectomy (including removal of cervix) should no longer be tested unless they had previous diagnosis of cervical intraepithelial neoplasia (CIN) 2 or more severe; these women should be tested for at least 20 yr. Women who have been vaccinated for HPV should still use age-specific recommendations for screening.

BETHESDA 2001 UPDATED CLASSIFICATION: The Bethesda 2001 System was the result of a yr-long iterative process held to update the original 1991 system and to broaden participation in the consensus process, clarify reporting of abnormalities, and incorporate data that had been collected since the initial system was created.

The reporting system includes the following areas:

- *Specimen adequacy:* The system defines the specimen as either satisfactory for evaluation or unsatisfactory and then specifies the reason for inadequacy if necessary.
- *General categorization (optional):* This serves to triage the specimen into normal finding (negative for intraepithelial lesion or malignancy) or identifies it as an "epithelial abnormality." The descriptions are meant to be mutually exclusive.
- *Interpretation/result:* Makes a distinction between "interpretation" and "diagnosis" of the specimen so that the interpretation may be incorporated into the overall clinical context for the particular patient being evaluated.
- *Negative for intraepithelial lesion or malignancy:* In this screening test, no intraepithelial lesion or malignancy is identified. Non-neoplastic findings such as organisms or reactive cellular findings may be specified but are still considered to be a negative result.
- Epithelial cell abnormalities:
  1. Squamous cell:
     a. Atypical squamous cell (ASC) of undetermined significance (ASC-US) emphasizing the unusual but still possible association with underlying CIN II/III and extremely rare possibility of squamous cell carcinoma.
     b. ASC cannot exclude high-grade squamous intraepithelial lesion (HSIL) (ASC-H), suggesting a risk for CIN II/III that is intermediate between ASC-US and HSIL.
     c. Low-grade squamous intraepithelial lesion (LSIL) suggests a transient viral infection with a greater likelihood for regression, more likely to encompass human papillomavirus (HPV) infection and CIN I histologically.
     d. HSIL suggestive of a more persistent viral infection and with a greater risk for progressive disease, more likely to encompass CIN II/III and carcinoma in situ (CIS) histologically.
     e. Squamous cell carcinoma.
  2. Glandular cell:
     a. Atypical glandular cells (should specify endocervical, endometrial, or not otherwise specified).
     b. Atypical glandular cell, favor neoplasia (should specify endocervical or not otherwise specified).
     c. Endocervical adenocarcinoma in situ (AIS).

Histological features	Traditional system	WHO system	British Society for Cervical Cytology	Bethesda system
Atypical squamous cells not meeting the criteria for dysplasia	Mild atypia	Mild atypia	Borderline nuclear abnormality	Atypical squamous cells (ASC)
Koilocytes plus mild atypia	HPV infection	HPV infection	HPV plus borderline change	Low-grade squamous intraepithelial lesion (SIL)
Dysplasia limited to lower third of epithelium	Mild dysplasia	CIN 1	Mild dyskaryosis (low-grade dyskaryosis)	Low-grade SIL
Dysplasia limited to lower two-thirds of epithelium	Moderate dysplasia	CIN 2	Moderate dyskaryosis (high-grade dyskaryosis)	High-grade SIL
Dysplasia extending into upper third of epithelium	Severe dysplasia	CIN 3	Severe dyskaryosis (high-grade dyskaryosis)	High-grade SIL
Dysplasia of full thickness of epithelium	Carcinoma in situ	CIN 3	Severe dyskaryosis (high-grade dyskaryosis)	High-grade SIL

FIG. 1 Comparison of grading systems. *CIN,* Cervical intraepithelial neoplasia; *HPV,* human papillomavirus. (From Young B et al: Female reproductive system. In *Wheater's basic pathology,* Philadelphia, 2011, Elsevier, pp. 216–315.)

- ■ Adenocarcinoma.

3. Other: Endometrial cells in a woman ≥>40 yr of age. Because menopausal status is sometimes uncertain, age was chosen to discriminate women who might, with the findings of endometrial cells on cytology, warrant further evaluation with endometrial sampling.

KEY POINTS:
- The cytologic distinctions of low grade (LSIL) and high grade (HSIL) do not necessarily equate to the histologic classifications CIN I and CIN II/III.
- The 2006 conference noted that one cytologic abnormality can have different histologic risk in different women and highlights "special populations" such as adolescent and young women, and those women who are pregnant. In young women, spontaneous HPV clearance rates are exceptionally high. The testing recommendations essentially removed the possibility of testing women younger than 21 yr of age.
- DNA testing for high-risk HPV types is incorporated into the evaluation and treatment algorithms for women with cytologic cervical abnormalities.

Histologically, a two-tiered system is developed in this guideline that distinguishes between the lower-risk CIN I and higher-risk CIN II/III diagnoses.

ICD-10CM CODES

N87.9	Dysplasia of cervix uteri, unspecified
R87.610	Atypical squamous cells of undetermined significance on cytologic smear of cervix (ASC-US)
R87.611	Atypical squamous cells cannot exclude high grade squamous intraepithelial lesion on cytologic smear of cervix (ASC-H)
R87.612	Low grade squamous intraepithelial lesion on cytologic smear of cervix (LGSIL)
R87.613	High grade squamous intraepithelial lesion on cytologic smear of cervix (HGSIL)
R87.614	Cytologic evidence of malignancy on smear of cervix
R87.615	Unsatisfactory cytologic smear of cervix
R87.618	Other abnormal cytological findings on specimens from cervix uteri
R87.619	Unspecified abnormal cytological findings in specimens from cervix uteri
Z12.4	Encounter for screening for malignant neoplasm of cervix

EPIDEMIOLOGY & DEMOGRAPHICS

PREDOMINANT AGE:
- Dysplasia: Peak age, 26 yr (3600 cases/100,000 persons)
- CIS: Peak age, 32 yr (1100 cases/100,000 persons)
- Invasive cancer: Peak age <60 yr (800 cases/100,000 persons)

PEAK INCIDENCE:
- Age 35 yr
- Abnormal Pap smear rate revealing dysplasia approximates 2% to 5% depending on population risk factors and false-negative rate variance
- False-negative rate approaching 40%
- Average age-adjusted incidence of severe dysplasia is 35 cases/100,000 persons
- Approximately half of the cases of new cervical cancer had never been screened, and another 10% had not been screened in more than 5 yr. Many of these women come from underserved or underresourced communities. The single biggest impact in reducing the morbidity and mortality from cervical cancer would come from appropriately addressing these health disparities

PHYSICAL FINDINGS & CLINICAL PRESENTATION

- Cervical lesions associated with dysplasia often are not visible to the naked eye; therefore, physical findings are best viewed by colposcopy of a 3% acetic acid–prepared cervix or lugols solution
- Patients evaluated by colposcopy are identified by abnormal cervical cytology screening from Pap smear screening
- Colposcopic findings:
  1. Leukoplakia (white lesion seen by the unaided eye that may represent condyloma, dysplasia, or cancer)
  2. Acetowhite epithelium with or without associated punctation, mosaicism, abnormal vessels
  3. Abnormal transformation zone (abnormal iodine uptake, "cuffed" gland openings)
- Studies have looked at the benefit of taking random biopsies at time of colposcopy and have shown that there may be increased detection of CIN II or greater if biopsies are taken at random rather than only directed toward abnormal appearing lesions

ETIOLOGY

- Strongly associated and initiated by oncogenic HPV infection (high-risk HPV types are 16, 18, 31, 33, 35, 45, 51, 52, 56, and 58; low-risk HPV types are 6, 11, 42, 43, and 44)
- Risk factors:
  1. HPV
  2. Any heterosexual coitus
  3. Coitus during puberty (transformation-zone metaplasia peak)
  4. Diethylstilbestrol exposure
  5. Multiple sexual partners
  6. Lack of prior Pap smear screening
  7. History of STD
  8. Other genital tract neoplasia
  9. HIV
  10. Tuberculosis
  11. Substance abuse
  12. "High-risk" male partner (HPV)
  13. Low socioeconomic status
  14. Early first pregnancy
  15. Tobacco use

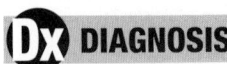

Dx DIAGNOSIS

DIFFERENTIAL DIAGNOSIS

- Metaplasia
- Hyperkeratosis
- Condyloma
- Microinvasive carcinoma
- Glandular epithelial abnormalities
- Vulvar intraepithelial neoplasm
- Vaginal intraepithelial neoplasm
- Metastatic tumor involvement of the cervix

WORKUP

- Periodic history and physical examination (including cytologic screening) depending on age, risk factors, and history of preinvasive cervical lesions
- Consider screening for sexually transmitted disease (gonorrhea, *Chlamydia,* herpes, HIV, HPV)
- Abnormal cytology (HSIL/LSIL, initial ASC/ASC-US/ASC-H in high-risk patients, recurrent in low-risk/postmenopausal patients) and grossly evident suspicious lesions; refer for colposcopy and possible directed biopsy/endocervical curettage (ECC; examination should include cervix, vagina, vulva, and anus)
- For glandular cell abnormalities (AGCs): Refer for colposcopy and possible directed biopsy/ECC, and consider endometrial sampling
- In pregnancy: Abnormal cytology followed by colposcopy in the first trimester and at 28 to 32 wk; only high-grade lesions suspicious for carcinoma biopsied; ECC is contraindicated

LABORATORY TESTS

- Gonorrhea, chlamydia NAATs to rule out STD
- Pap cytology screening (requires appropriate sampling, preparation, cytologist interpretation, and reporting)
- Colposcopy and directed biopsy, ECC for indications (see "Workup")
- HPV DNA typing if identified abnormal cytology
- As compared with Pap testing, HPV testing has greater sensitivity for the detection of intraepithelial neoplasia

IMAGING STUDIES

- Cervicography
- Computer-enhanced Pap cytology screening (e.g., PAPNET)

MANAGEMENT

Refer to the literature for a more comprehensive approach. The following treatment paradigms in Table 1 give a general outline for care.

DISPOSITION

- Because of the large number of women in high-risk groups, the prevalence of HPV, and the high false-negative Pap smear rate, routine Pap smear screening should be strongly encouraged for all women, especially those with a history of cervical dysplasia. The

TABLE 1 Summary of Recommendations

Population	Recommended Screening Method	Management of Screen Results	Comments
<21 yr	No screening		
21-29 yr	Cytology alone every 3 yr	HPV-positive ASC-US or cytology of LSIL or more severe: Refer to ASCCP Guidelines Cytology Negative or HPV-Negative ASC-US; Rescreen with cytology in 3 yr	
30-65 yr	HPV and cytology "co-testing" every 5 yr (preferred)	HPV-positive ASC-US or cytology of LSIL or more severe: Refer to ASCCP guidelines	Screening by HPV testing alone is not recommended for most clinical settings.
		HPV positive, cytology negative: Option 1: Y 12-month follow-up with co-testing	
		Option 2: Y test for HPV16 or HPV16/18 genotypes. If HPV16 or HPV16/18 positive, refer to colposcopy. If HPV16 or HPV16/18 negative, 12-mo follow-up with co-testing	
		Co-test negative or HPV-negative ASC-US: Rescreen with co-testing in 5 yr	
	Cytology alone every 3 yr (acceptable)	HPV-positive ASC-US or cytology of LSIL or more severe: Refer to ASCCP guidelines	
		Cytology negative or HPV-negative ASC-US: Rescreen with cytology in 3 yr	
>65 yr	No screening following adequate negative prior screening		Women with a history of CIN2 or a more severe diagnosis should continue routine screening for at least 20 yr
After hysterectomy	No screening		Applies to women without a cervix and without a history of CIN2 or a more severe diagnosis in the past 20 yr or cervical cancer ever.
HPV vaccinated	Follow age-specific recommendations (same as unvaccinated women)		

ASCCP, American Society for Colposcopy and Cervical Pathology; *ASC-US,* atypical squamous cells of undetermined significance; *CIN,* cervical intraepithelial neoplasia; *HPV,* human papillomavirus; *LSIL,* low-grade squamous intraepithelial lesions.

Modified from Saslow D et al: American Cancer Society, American Society for Colposcopy and Cervical Pathology, and American Society for Clinical Pathology screening guidelines for the prevention and early detection of cervical cancer, *J Low Gen Tract Dis* 16(3):175–204, 2012.

addition of an HPV test to the Pap test reduces the incidence of CIN II or III, or cancer detected by subsequent screening.

- Success rates for treatment approach 80% to 90%.
- Detection of persistence of recurrence requires careful follow-up.
- Cervical treatment possibly results in infertility (cervical stenosis or incompetence), which requires careful consideration and discretion for use of LEEP and cone biopsy.
- Appropriate counseling and informed consent are needed when considering any form of management of cervical dysplasia.

REFERRAL

- Patients with abnormal Pap cytology should be referred to a provider, likely a trained obstetrician/gynecologist, who can appropriately treat the patient in an age-specific manner and also perform a colposcopy if indicated as part of the new recommendations. Given the morbidity associated with both underevaluating and treating as well as reacting excessively to cytologic findings, a provider who is intimately familiar with ASCCP guidelines should be sought.
- If treatment is required, patient should be referred to a gynecologist or gynecologic oncologist skilled in the diagnosis and treatment of preinvasive cervical disease.

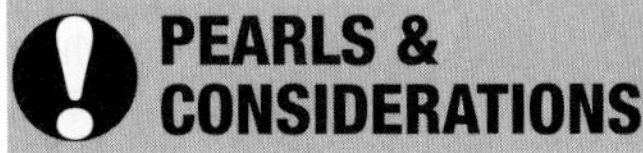

PEARLS & CONSIDERATIONS

COMMENTS

- Testing for human papillomavirus by Hybrid capture 2 DNA test will identify 91% of the small proportion of women with post-treatment residual or recurrent disease, but 30% of all women who are tested will test positive and need colposcopy.
- HPV vaccination is recommended for males and females from ages 9 to 26.

SUGGESTED READINGS

Available at ExpertConsult.com

RELATED CONTENT

Cervical Dysplasia (Patient Information)
Pap Smear Abnormalities (Patient Information)
Cervical Cancer (Related Key Topic)
Cervical Polyps (Related Key Topic)

AUTHOR: **BETH LEOPOLD, M.D.**

BASIC INFORMATION

DEFINITION

Cervicitis is an inflammation of the uterine cervix, primarily affecting the columnar epithelial cells of the endocervical glands. Acute cervicitis results from direct infection of the cervix secondary to a uterine or vaginal infection—most commonly chlamydia or gonorrhea—whereas chronic cervicitis is due to an exposure to a local irritation.

SYNONYMS

Endocervicitis
Ectocervicitis
Mucopurulent cervicitis

ICD-10CM CODES

N72	Inflammatory disease of cervix uteri
A54.03	Gonococcal cervicitis, unspecified
A74.89	Other chlamydial diseases
A60.03	Herpesviral cervicitis
086.11	Cervicitis following delivery

EPIDEMIOLOGY & DEMOGRAPHICS

The published prevalence of cervicitis varies greatly, ranging from 8% to as high as 40% of women attending sexually transmitted disease (STD) clinics. Cervicitis is most common in women aged 15 to 24 but it can occur in any sexually active woman. Women who have had sex without condoms or sex with multiple partners are at increased risk of developing cervicitis as well as other STDs.

PHYSICAL FINDINGS & CLINICAL PRESENTATION

Cervicitis is usually asymptomatic or associated with mild symptoms. Patients may complain of copious purulent or mucopurulent vaginal discharge, pelvic pain, postcoital or intermenstrual bleeding, vulvovaginal irritation, or dyspareunia.

The CDC emphasizes that the two diagnostic signs of cervicitis are either mucopurulent discharge or sustained cervical bleeding with gentle trauma. On physical exam, the cervix can be erythematous and tender on palpation. The cervix may also bleed easily when obtaining cultures or a Pap smear. Yellow discharge will be seen on a Q-tip inserted into the cervix.

INFECTIOUS ETIOLOGY

- *Chlamydia trachomatis*
- *Neisseria gonorrhoeae*
- *Trichomonas vaginalis*
- Herpes simplex
- Human papillomavirus
- *M. genitalium*
- Bacterial vaginosis

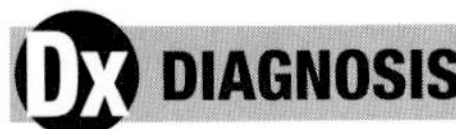

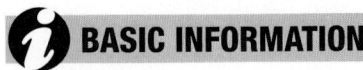

DIAGNOSIS

The diagnosis of acute cervicitis is clinical and based upon the presence of purulent or mucopurulent cervical exudate and/or cervical friability—bleeding induced by gently touching the area with a swab.

DIFFERENTIAL DIAGNOSIS

- Carcinoma of the cervix
- Cervical erosion (from tampons or other intravaginal devices)
- Cervical metaplasia
- Cervical ectropion
- Cervical and vaginal irritation due to chemicals or hormonal imbalance

WORKUP

If cervicitis is suspected, testing for infectious causes should be performed and pelvic inflammatory disease (PID) should be excluded.

LABORATORY TESTS

- A finding of leucorrhea (>10 WBC per high-power field on microscopic examination of vaginal fluid) has been associated with chlamydial and gonococcal infection of the cervix.
- Nucleic acid amplification tests (NAAT) should be used for diagnosing *C. trachomatis* and *N. gonorrhoeae* in women with cervicitis; this testing can be performed on vaginal, cervical, or urinary samples.
- Use a wet mount to look for evidence of bacterial vaginitis (BV) and trichomonads, but because the sensitivity of microscopy to detect *T. vaginalis* is relatively low (~50%), symptomatic women with cervicitis and negative microscopy for BV and trichomonads should receive further testing with NAAT or culture if there is concern for resistant infection.
- HIV testing is recommended in all patients with supposed cervicitis.
- Although HSV-2 infection has been associated with cervicitis, the utility of specific testing (i.e., culture or serologic testing) for HSV-2 in this setting is not recommended unless there are clinical findings suggestive of herpes infection.

Rx TREATMENT

NONPHARMACOLOGIC THERAPY

- The patient's history of hygiene habits, which may increase her risk for cervicitis, should be obtained including history of douching, tampon usage, and other potential chemical exposures to vaginal irritants.
- Uncomplicated cervicitis is typically treated as an outpatient.
- Safe sex should be recommended including monogamous relationships and the consistent use of condoms (male and female).
- Sexual partners should be offered treatment in all cases of STD infection proven by culture.

ACUTE GENERAL Rx

Because *Chlamydia* and *N. gonorrhoeae* cause 50% of cases of infectious cervicitis, if either of these infections is suspected, then treatment should be initiated without waiting for the test results. Administer ceftriaxone 250 mg IM single dose followed by azithromycin 1 g single dose or doxycycline 100 mg PO bid for 7 days. If the patient is pregnant, treat with azithromycin 1 g single dose instead of using doxycycline, which is contraindicated in pregnant or nursing mothers. If *Trichomonas* is the etiologic agent, treat with metronidazole or tinidazole 2 g single dose, which is curative in 95% of cases. An alternative treatment option is metronidazole 500 mg twice daily for 7 days. Alcohol should be avoided during the treatment course.

For herpes infection, treat with acyclovir, valacyclovir, or famciclovir.

M. genitalium might be considered for cases of clinically significant cervicitis that persist after azithromycin or doxycycline therapy in which reexposure to an infected partner or medical nonadherence is unlikely. If *M. genitalium* infection is confirmed, treatment is with moxifloxacin.

DISPOSITION

Bacterial cervicitis responds well to antibiotics. Possible complications to watch for include subsequent PID and infertility (found in 5%-10% of patients with increasing rates with repeat episodes of PID). Repeat cervical cultures are recommended after treatment in pregnancy or if there is concern of treatment failure. Screening for reinfection is recommended within 3 months. Condoms should be recommended and sexual relations should be resumed after negative cultures for both partners.

REFERRAL

If subsequent PID develops, attempt outpatient therapy and consider hospital admission for IV antibiotics for severe or specialty cases as outlined in the CDC guidelines.

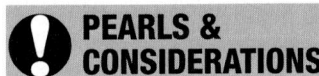

PEARLS & CONSIDERATIONS

COMMENTS

- Management of sex partners of women tested for cervicitis should be appropriate for the identified or suspected STD.
- Repeat testing 3 to 6 months after treatment is recommended for all women diagnosed with chlamydia or gonorrhea, and all sex partners in the preceding 60 days should be evaluated and treated for the STDs for which the index patient received treatment.

SUGGESTED READING

Available at ExpertConsult.com

RELATED CONTENT

Cervicitis (Patient Information)
Chlamydia Genital Infections (Related Key Topic)
Gonorrhea (Related Key Topic)
Nongonococcal Urethritis (Related Key Topic)

AUTHOR: **HELEN B. GOMEZ, M.D.**

BASIC INFORMATION

DEFINITION

Painless localized granulomatous nodule caused by obstruction and inflammation of the glands of Zeis or the meibomian glands of the eyelid.

SYNONYMS

Meibomian gland lipogranuloma
Meibomian cyst

ICD-10CM CODES

H00.1	Chalazion
H00.11	Right upper eyelid
H00.12	Right lower eyelid
H00.13	Right eye, unspecified eyelid
H00.14	Left upper eyelid
H00.15	Left lower eyelid
H00.16	Left eye, unspecified eyelid
H00.19	Unspecified eye, unspecified eyelid

EPIDEMIOLOGY & DEMOGRAPHICS

INCIDENCE: Relatively common condition, although U.S. and worldwide incidence are unknown.
PEAK INCIDENCE: Most common in adults age 30 to 50
PREVALENCE: Unknown
PREDOMINANT SEX AND AGE: Affects men and women equally
GENETICS: Not applicable

RISK FACTORS:

- Consider demodicidosis in patients with recurrent chalazia
- Consider low serum vitamin A

PHYSICAL FINDINGS & CLINICAL PRESENTATION

- Painless localized nodule on the eyelid (Fig. 1)
- Lesion will be firm and rubbery. Can see mild erythema
- Can be visualized on the external eyelid or internal eyelid
- Tend to present for longer than 2 weeks compared to styes, which usually have a shorter course
- Typically, benign and self-limited lesion. If persistent or recurrent, a chalazion should be evaluated for malignancy

ETIOLOGY

- Granulomatous lesions that forms after obstruction of the sebaceous glands of Zeis or Meibomian glands
- Can develop from a hordeolum after the infection and inflammation have resolved

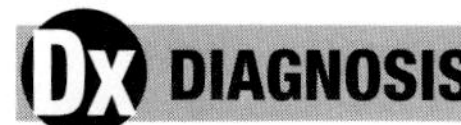

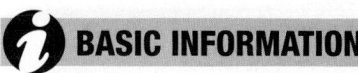

DIAGNOSIS

DIFFERENTIAL DIAGNOSIS

- Hordeola (stye)
- Xanthalasma
- Molluscum contagiosum
- Seborrheic keratosis

Recurrent or persistent lesions:

- Basal cell carcinoma
- Sebaceous cell carcinoma
- Meibomian gland carcinoma

WORKUP

Diagnosed based on clinical appearance

LABORATORY TESTS

None

IMAGING STUDIES

None

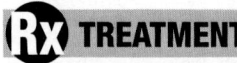

TREATMENT

- A small chalazion will often resolve without intervention within a few weeks.
- Conservative management including warm compresses placed on the affected eyelid four times a day for 15-minute intervals can successfully expedite drainage of the nodule. Most chalazia will resolve within a month with conservative treatment.
- Persistent lesions may require intralesional triamcinolone acetonide injections or surgical incision and curettage by an ophthalmologist. Intralesional corticosteroid (ILS) injections are the preferred procedure for children, patients with allergies to local anesthesia, if the chalazia is located close to the lacrimal duct, or if the operating physician is not an ophthalmologist. Incision and curettage is recommended for patients with infected chalazia.

ACUTE GENERAL Rx

- None
- Chalazion are not an infectious process so antibiotics are not indicated

CHRONIC Rx

None

DISPOSITION

Excellent patient prognosis. Small chalazia can be discharged home with instructions for conservative management. Large, recurrent, or persistent lesions may require an ophthalmology referral.

REFERRAL

Refer to ophthalmology for ILS injections or surgical intervention if indicated and evaluation of recurrent or persistent eyelid lesions.

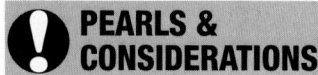

PEARLS & CONSIDERATIONS

COMMENTS

- A chalazion is a painless firm eyelid nodule.
- A chalazion is not an infectious process so antibiotics are not indicated.

PREVENTION

No specific strategy for prevention

SUGGESTED READINGS

Available at ExpertConsult.com

RELATED CONTENT

Hordeolum (Stye)

AUTHORS: **RACHEL MEEKS, M.D.,** and **MARK F. BRADY, M.D., M.P.H., M.M.S.**

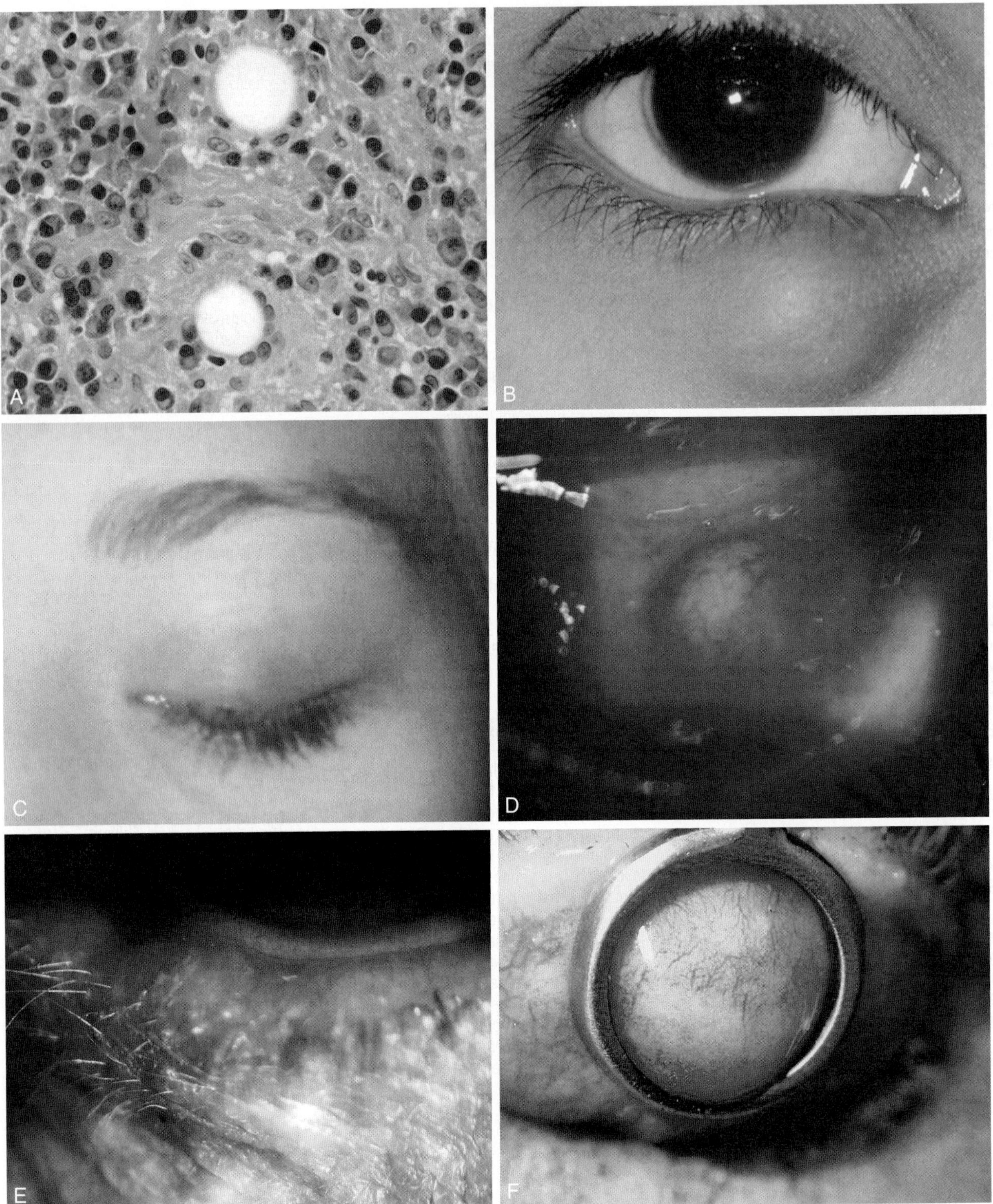

FIG. 1 Chalazion. A, Histopathology shows a lipogranuloma; the large pale cells are epithelioid cells and the well-demarcated empty space contained fat dissolved out during processing. **B,** Uninflamed chalazion. **C,** Acutely inflamed lesion. **D,** Conjunctival granuloma. **E,** Marginal chalazion. **F,** Conjunctival view of chalazion clamp in place prior to incision and curettage. (A, Courtesy of J Harry and G Misson, from Harry J, Misson G: *Clinical ophthalmic pathology: principles of diseases of the eye and associated structures*, Boston, 2001, Butterworth-Heinemann; F, from Nerad J, Carter K, Alford M: *Rapid diagnosis in ophthalmology: oculoplastic and reconstructive surgery*, St Louis, 2008, Mosby.) (From Bowling B: *Kanski's clinical ophthalmology, a systemic approach*, ed 8, Philadelphia, 2016, Elsevier.)

BASIC INFORMATION

DEFINITION

Chemotherapy-induced nausea and vomiting (CINV) refers to adverse emetic effects associated with the use of drugs used to treat cancer. There are five recognized subtypes:

- Acute-phase CINV: Nausea and vomiting start within minutes to hours after receiving chemotherapy.
- Delayed-phase CINV: Nausea and vomiting begin or return 24 hours or more after receiving chemotherapy.
- Breakthrough CINV: Occurring despite appropriate prophylactic treatment.
- Anticipatory CINV: Symptoms begin before receiving therapy as a conditioned response in patients who have developed significant nausea and vomiting during previous chemotherapy.
- Refractory CINV: Recurring in subsequent cycles of therapy, excluding anticipatory CINV.

SYNONYMS

Drug-induced nausea and vomiting
Chemotherapy-induced emesis
CINV

ICD-10CM CODES

R11.2	Nausea with vomiting, unspecified
R11.0	Nausea
R11.10	Vomiting, unspecified
Z51.11	Encounter for antineoplastic chemotherapy

EPIDEMIOLOGY & DEMOGRAPHICS

- The patient's risk for development of nausea and vomiting is most strongly dependent on the emetogenicity of the chemotherapy agent(s) being used.
- Emetogenicity is classified into four categories: highly emetic (>90%), moderately emetic (>30%–90%), low emetic (10%–30%), and minimally emetic (0%–10%).
- With certain chemotherapy regimens, CINV will occur in the majority of patients. However, patients' tolerance may vary, and symptoms may occur in as low as 10% of patients.
- Symptoms may be dose dependent (the higher the dose, the greater the risk for symptoms).
- CINV is more likely to affect female and younger patients.
- Patients expecting CINV before receiving therapy (anticipatory emesis) are at greater risk of experiencing symptoms.
- Patients with a history of alcohol consumption are at lower risk.
- Patients with a history of motion sickness are at greater risk.

INCIDENCE: The highest incidence of CINV is before or during the first cycle of chemotherapy.

GENETICS: Some rapid metabolizers of certain 5-HT3 receptor antagonists and polymorphisms in the 5-HT3 receptor confer greater risk for CINV.

RISK FACTORS:

- Previous history of CINV
- History of motion sickness or vestibular dysfunction
- Higher levels of anxiety
- History of alcohol use decreases risk

PHYSICAL FINDINGS & CLINICAL PRESENTATION

- Symptoms may include anxiety and lightheadedness.
- The most common physical findings are increased pulse rate and abnormal blood pressure (elevated if the person is highly anxious, reduced if the patient is dehydrated).
- Symptoms such as diarrhea, fever, headache, and abdominal pain may suggest an alternative diagnosis; physical examination findings such as increased blood pressure, abdominal tenderness, or focal neurologic deficits may suggest symptoms caused by cancer progression or other acute illness such as infection.

PATHOPHYSIOLOGY

CINV is likely the result of chemotherapy acting in two places: directly in the gastrointestinal tract and in the vomiting center of the brain. In both areas, nausea and vomiting are mediated by the actions of certain neurotransmitters, with serotonin, dopamine, and neurokinin-1 being the most important.

DIAGNOSIS

DIFFERENTIAL DIAGNOSIS

- The two main considerations are progression of cancer and infection
- Intestinal/gastric: Obstruction or partial obstruction of the digestive tract from tumor
- Neurologic: Metastases to the brain causing vomiting; metastatic infiltration of nerves affecting the digestive tract
- Infectious: Acute bacterial, viral, or parasitic infections of the digestive tract causing symptoms (can be associated with diarrhea or pain)
- Renal: Dehydration leading to acute kidney injury and failure, causing worsening of nausea and vomiting

WORKUP

No workup is indicated if patient's symptoms and onset of nausea and vomiting fit the usual presentation for CINV. If other symptoms or unexpected physical examination findings are present, then other causes need to be ruled out. A combination of blood work and imaging may be helpful.

LABORATORY TESTS

- If the onset of symptoms is not typical for CINV, then blood tests such as a CBC, liver function tests, electrolytes, and kidney function tests may be indicated.
- Stool studies looking for infections from viruses, bacteria, or parasites may be ordered if diarrhea is also present.

IMAGING STUDIES

- Abdominal radiographs may be ordered to look for obstruction of the digestive tract but will not provide any information about tumor progression.
- Abdominal CT scan may provide more detailed information about local cancer progression/invasion in the proximity of the digestive tract and whether obstruction of the digestive tract is present.
- CNS imaging with CT scan or magnetic resonance imaging (MRI) of the brain may provide information about possible metastases.

TREATMENT

- Choice and duration of antiemetic use are dependent on the chemotherapy regimen used.
- For chemotherapy agents with high emetogenic potential, the use of multidrug antiemetic regimens has proven to be highly effective in symptom prevention.
- The most common treatment combination includes a serotonin-receptor antagonist (ondansetron, granisetron, dolasetron, or palonosetron), a corticosteroid (methylprednisolone or dexamethasone), and a neurokinin-1 receptor antagonist (aprepitant, rolapitant, or fosaprepitant).
- A fixed-dose combination of oral palonosetron and netupitant (NK-1 receptor antagonist) is now available.
- Many other adjunct drugs are available, such as olanzapine, prochlorperazine, metoclopramide, haloperidol, and marinol; comparatively, they are less effective and have greater potential for adverse effects.
- Benzodiazepines (usually lorazepam) may help in patients with significant anxiety levels that lead to anticipatory CINV.
- Patients with uncontrolled symptoms may require hospitalization for supportive care including intravenous medications and fluids.

NONPHARMACOLOGIC THERAPY

For those patients with a significant anxiety component to their CINV, cognitive behavioral therapy may help.

DISPOSITION

Although CINV is one of the most feared complications of cancer therapy, its treatment has been revolutionized in the last 20 yr, with most patients achieving adequate symptom control.

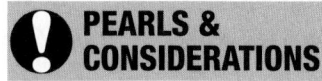

PEARLS & CONSIDERATIONS

COMMENTS

- Aggressive symptom control in the acute phase of CINV is the key initial therapeutic approach. Prevention of the acute phase has led to much improved control of the delayed phase and has greatly decreased the incidence of anticipatory CINV.
- Prevention of symptoms is much easier to achieve than controlling or treating active symptoms.

SUGGESTED READINGS

Available at ExpertConsult.com

AUTHOR: **BYUNG KIM, M.D.**

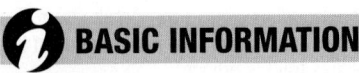

BASIC INFORMATION

DEFINITION

Genital infection with *Chlamydia trachomatis* (CT) is the most prevalent sexually transmitted disease in the U.S. Chlamydia infection can result in cervicitis, acute urethral syndrome, endometritis, pelvic inflammatory disease, ectopic pregnancy, infertility, and chronic pelvic pain in women (see "Pelvic Inflammatory Disease"). In men, CT infection may cause mucopurulent discharge, urethritis, epididymitis, and prostatitis. Newborns born via an infected birth canal are at risk for conjunctivitis and pneumonia. A majority of the men and women affected with CT are asymptomatic. Thus, screening tests play a very important role in detection of this infection to initiate treatment, impede disease sequelae, and prevent further transmissions.

ICD-10CM CODES

A56.2	Chlamydial infection of genitourinary tract, unspecified
A56	Other sexually transmitted chlamydial diseases
A56.0	Chlamydial infection of lower genitourinary tract
A56.00	Chlamydial infection of lower genitourinary tract, unspecified
A56.01	Chlamydial cystitis and urethritis
A56.02	Chlamydia vulvovaginitis
A56.09	Other chlamydial infection of lower genitourinary tract
A56.1	Chlamydial infection of pelviperitoneum and other genitourinary organs
A56.19	Other chlamydial genitourinary infection
A56.2	Chlamydial infection of genitourinary tract, unspecified
A56.3	Chlamydial infection of anus and rectum
A56.4	Chlamydial infection of pharynx
A56.8	Sexually transmitted chlamydial infection of other sites

EPIDEMIOLOGY & DEMOGRAPHICS

- *C. trachomatis* is the most commonly reported sexually transmitted disease in the U.S., with more than 1.4 million cases reported annually to the Centers for Disease Control and Prevention. However, it is thought that this number is an underestimate, since many cases of CT infection are asymptomatic and potentially can remain undiagnosed.
- Age is a strong predictor for risk of CT infection. Individuals less than 25 yr old are the largest age group affected by *C. trachomatis.* Chlamydia infections are 10 times more prevalent than gonococcal infections in young women between the ages of 18 and 26 yr.
- Chlamydia conjunctivitis occurs in 18% to 44% of infants, and chlamydial pneumonia occurs in 3% to 16% of infants who are delivered by mothers with untreated CT infection at the time of delivery.
- Pelvic inflammatory disease develops in 10% to 15% of women with untreated CT infections.
- Untreated CT increases a person's risk of acquiring HIV.
- In men, 15% to 55% of nongonococcal urethritis cases are caused by C. trachomatis.
- Table 1 summarizes clinical characteristics of common *C. trachomatis* infections.

PHYSICAL FINDINGS & CLINICAL PRESENTATION

Clinical manifestations in symptomatic women affected with *C. trachomatis* are vaginal discharge or irregular vaginal bleeding. Purulent discharge or cervicitis may be visualized on speculum exam. Easily induced endocervical bleeding can be noted on exam and is caused by inflammation of endocervical columnar epithelium. Untreated infection can ascend the reproductive tract, causing pelvic inflammatory disease. Clinical signs of pelvic inflammatory disease are cervical, uterine, or adnexal tenderness on exam. Complications of pelvic disease are ectopic pregnancy, infertility, and chronic pelvic pain.

Most men are asymptomatic, but when they do experience symptoms, it is usually dysuria or a mucopurulent penile discharge. A complication that can arise from CT infection in men is epididymitis, which manifests as unilateral testicular pain, hydrocele, or swelling of the epididymis. An untreated CT infection can also cause prostatitis in men. Prostatitis may present as urinary dysfunction, pain with ejaculation, and pelvic pain.

Chlamydial conjunctivitis can be experienced by both men and women and is the result of conjunctiva exposed to infected genital secretions. CT infection can also cause proctitis or infection of the rectum in men and women. This usually presents with rectal pain, discharge, or bleeding. CT infection of the throat is usually asymptomatic in both men and women and not a usual cause of pharyngitis. Less frequent manifestations of CT infection may include perihepatitis (Fitz-Hugh–Curtis syndrome) or reactive arthritis (Reiter's syndrome).

ETIOLOGY

- *C. trachomatis* consists of 15 serotypes
- Obligate, intracellular bacteria

Dx DIAGNOSIS

DIFFERENTIAL DIAGNOSIS

Differential diagnosis depends on presenting symptoms. Some of the common differentials are listed in the following:

- Candidiasis
- Conjunctivitis
- Ectopic pregnancy
- Endometriosis
- Gonorrhea
- Mycoplasma infection
- Pelvic inflammatory disease
- Trichomonas
- Urethritis
- Urinary tract infection

WORKUP

- Individuals with signs and symptoms mentioned previously should be screened for CT infection. Since the majority of CT infections are asymptomatic, routine screening should be offered to individuals at risk for CT infection. Annual screening of all sexually active women less than 25 yr and women at any age at risk for sexually transmitted diseases is recommended. Risk factors include a new sexual partner, more than one sexual partner, individuals not in a mutually monogamous relationship, a previous or concurrent sexually transmitted disease, or working in the sex industry for profit. Screening interval is determined by any new risk for exposure since the last negative screening. The CDC recommends CT screening for all pregnant women under the age of 25 and for any pregnant woman over the age of 25 who is at increased risk for acquiring CT. These same pregnant women should be screened again during the third trimester.

LABORATORY TESTS

- Nucleic acid amplification tests (NAATs) are the gold standard for diagnosis because of their high sensitivity and specificity for the detection of CT infection. The FDA has approved these tests for male and female urine collection and for provider-collected endocervical, vaginal, and male urethral specimens.
- Rectal and pharyngeal collection site specimens may be taken from individuals who engage in receptive anal and oral intercourse, but these collection sites are not FDA approved.
- For best results, urine collection should be completed with a first-void urine sample.
- Self-collected vaginal swab samples for women have the same sensitivity and specificity as provider-collected samples.
- The same specimen can be used to test for chlamydia and gonorrhea.
- Sexual partners of a person testing positive for CT infection should be treated if they had sexual contact with that individual within 60 days prior to onset of symptoms or CT diagnosis.
- Microscopy should not be used for chlamydia diagnosis; however, greater than 10 white blood cells per high-power field with a mucopurulent discharge can be a presumptive diagnosis.

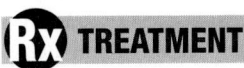

Rx TREATMENT

ACUTE GENERAL Rx

Nongonococcal urethritis, urethritis, cervicitis, conjunctivitis (except for lymphogranuloma venereum):

- Azithromycin 1 g PO × single dose therapy *or*
- Doxycycline 100 mg PO bid for 7 days

Infection in pregnancy:

- Azithromycin 1 gm PO single-dose therapy

Alternatives:

- Erythromycin 500 mg PO qid for 7 days *or*
- Erythromycin ethylsuccinate 800 mg PO qid for 7 days

TABLE 1 Clinical Characteristics of Common *Chlamydia trachomatis* Infections

	Infection	Symptoms and Signs	Presumptive Diagnosis	Definitive Diagnosis	Treatment
Men	Nongonococcal urethritis	Urethral discharge, dysuria	Urethral leukocytosis; no gonococci seen	Urine or urethral NAAT	Azithromycin, 1 g PO (single dose) *or* Doxycycline, 100 mg PO bid, for 7 days
	Epididymitis	Unilateral epididymal tenderness, swelling; pain; fever, presence of NGU	Urine or urethral NAAT	Urethral leukocytosis; pyuria on urinalysis	STI likely: Ceftriaxone 250 mg IM plus doxycycline, 100 mg PO bid, for 10 days *History of insertive anal intercourse:* Ceftriaxone, 250 mg IM, plus levofloxacin, 500 mg bid for 10 days
	Proctitis (non-LGV)	Rectal pain, discharge and bleeding; history of receptive anal intercourse	≥1 PMN/OIF on rectal Gram stain; no gonococci seen	Urine or urethral NAAT; rectal culture or NAAT	Doxycycline, 100 mg PO bid, for 7 days
	LGV	Painful, tender inguinal lymphadenopathy, fever	"Groove sign"	Urine, urethral, lymph node or rectal NAAT; rectal or lymph node culture; LGV-specific testing if available	Doxycycline, 100 mg PO bid, for 21 days
	LGV proctitis	Rectal pain, discharge, and bleeding in MSM; absence of inguinal lymphadenopathy	≥1 PMN/OIF on rectal Gram stain; no gonococci seen	Urine, urethral, or rectal NAAT; rectal culture; LGV-specific testing if available	Doxycycline, 100 mg PO bid, for 21 days
	Conjunctivitis	Ocular pain, redness, discharge; simultaneous genital infection	Gram stain of conjunctival swab negative for bacterial pathogens; PMNs on smear	Rectal culture or NAAT; NAAT of conjunctivae	Azithromycin, 1 g PO (single dose) *or* Doxycycline, 100 mg PO bid, for 7 days
Women	Cervicitis	Mucopurulent cervical discharge; ectopy, easily induced bleeding	≥20 PMN/OIF on cervical Gram stain	Urine or cervical NAAT	Azithromycin, 1 g PO (single dose) *or* Doxycycline, 100 mg PO bid, for 7 days
	Urethritis	Dysuria, frequency; no hematuria	Pyuria on UA; negative urine Gram stain and culture	Urine, cervical, or urethral NAAT	Azithromycin, 1 g PO (single dose) *or* Doxycycline, 100 mg PO bid for 7 days
	Pelvic inflammatory disease	Lower abdominal pain, adnexal pain, cervical motion tenderness	Evidence of mucopurulent cervicitis	Urine or cervical NAAT	Outpatient: Ceftriaxone 250 mg IM as a single dose, plus doxycycline 100 mg PO bid for 14 days, with or without metronidazole, 500 mg PO bid for 14 days
Adults	Conjunctivitis	Ocular pain, redness, discharge; simultaneous genital infection	Gram stain of conjunctival swab negative for bacterial pathogens; PMNs on smear	DFA or NAAT on conjunctival swab	Azithromycin, 1 g PO (single dose) *or* Doxycycline, 100 mg PO bid for 7 days
Newborns	Conjunctivitis	Ocular pain, redness, discharge; simultaneous genital infection	Gram stain of conjunctival swab negative for bacterial pathogens; PMNs on smear	DFA or NAAT on conjunctival swab; vagina, rectum, pharynx also often positive	Erythromycin base 50 mg/kg/day, orally divided into four doses daily for 14 days; evaluate and treat parents as well
	Pneumonia	Staccato cough, tachypnea, hyperinflation	Diffuse interstitial infiltrate, eosinophilia	Nasopharyngeal NAATs or culture; MIF serology (IgM)	Erythromycin base 50 mg/kg/day, orally divided into four doses daily for 14 days; evaluate and treat parents as well

DFA, Direct fluorescent antibody; *IgM*, immunoglobulin M; *LGV*, lymphogranuloma venereum; *MIF*, microimmunofluorescence; *MSM*, men who have sex with men; *NAAT*, nucleic acid amplification test; *NGU*, nongonococcal urethritis; *OIF*, oil immersion field; *PMN*, polymorphonuclear neutrophil; *STI*, sexually transmitted infection; *UA*, urinalysis.
From Bennett JE, Dolin R, Blaser MJ. *Mandell, Douglas, and Bennett's principles and practice of infectious diseases*, ed 8, Philadelphia, 2015, Saunders.

NOTE: Azithromycin (Pregnancy Risk Category B) is generally considered safe and effective during pregnancy and with lactation. Erythromycin base (Pregnancy Risk Category B) is an acceptable alternate agent for treatment of CT infection in pregnancy. Doxycycline is contraindicated in pregnancy. Erythromycin estolate is contraindicated in pregnancy because of drug-related hepatotoxicity.

FOLLOW-UP:

- Observed single-dose therapy should be offered to individuals for whom compliance is a concern.
- To minimize disease transmission to partners, affected persons should be advised to refrain from sexual intercourse for 7 days after single-dose therapy, until completion of 7-day therapy, or until resolution of symptoms.
- To prevent reinfection, affected individuals should refrain from sexual intercourse until all of their partners have been treated.
- Test of cure to detect treatment failure is not needed.
- Re-collection by NAAT method in less than 3 weeks from treatment can yield a false-positive result due to the sensitivity of this testing method.
- Both men and women treated for chlamydia should be retested at approximately 3 months after treatment to screen for reinfection. If patients do not return to clinical settings within 3 months, rescreen the patient at the next presentation for clinical care.
- Pregnant women with chlamydia trachomatis infection should have a test of cure 3 to 4 weeks after treatment and should then be retested within 3 months.

Refer partners for evaluation and treatment.

RECURRENT AND PERSISTENT URETHRITIS: Retreat noncompliant patients with the above regimens. If patient was initially compliant, recommended regimens: metronidazole 2 g PO in single dose plus erythromycin base 500 mg PO qid for 7 days or erythromycin ethylsuccinate 800 mg PO qid for 7 days.

REFERRAL

Refer to infectious disease specialist if persistent infection or gynecologist if salpingitis is suspected.

SUGGESTED READINGS

Available at ExpertConsult.com

RELATED CONTENT

Cervicitis (Related Key Topic)
Gonococcal Urethritis (Related Key Topic)
Gonorrhea (Related Key Topic)
Nongonococcal Urethritis (Related Key Topic)
Pelvic Inflammatory Disease (Related Key Topic)

AUTHOR: **DEANNA L. BENNER, A.P.R.N., C.R.N.P.**

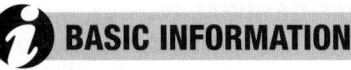

BASIC INFORMATION

DEFINITION

Cholangitis refers to an inflammation and/or infection of the hepatic and common bile ducts associated with obstruction of the common bile duct.

SYNONYMS

Biliary sepsis
Ascending cholangitis
Suppurative cholangitis

ICD-10CM CODE

K83.0 Cholangitis

EPIDEMIOLOGY & DEMOGRAPHICS

INCIDENCE (IN U.S.): Complicates approximately 1% of cases of cholelithiasis
PEAK INCIDENCE: Seventh decade
PREVALENCE (IN U.S.): 2 cases/1000 hospital admissions
PREDOMINANT SEX:

- Females, for cholangitis secondary to gallstones
- Males, for cholangitis secondary to malignant obstruction and HIV infection

PREDOMINANT AGE: Seventh decade and older; unusual <50 yr of age

PHYSICAL FINDINGS & CLINICAL PRESENTATION

- Usually acute onset of fever, abdominal pain (RUQ), and jaundice (Charcot's triad)
- All signs and symptoms in only 50% to 85% of patients
- Often, dark coloration of the urine resulting from bilirubinuria
- Complications:
  1. Bacteremia (50%) and septic shock
  2. Hepatic abscess and pancreatitis

ETIOLOGY

Obstruction of the common bile duct causing rapid proliferation of bacteria in the biliary tree

- Most common cause of common bile duct obstruction: stones, usually migrated from the gallbladder
- Other causes: Prior biliary tract surgery with secondary stenosis, tumor (usually arising from the pancreas or biliary tree), and parasitic infections from Ascaris lumbricoides or Fasciola hepatica
- Iatrogenic after contamination of an obstructed biliary tree by endoscopic retrograde cholangiopancreatoscopy (ERCP) or percutaneous transhepatic cholangiography (PTC)
- Primary sclerosing cholangitis (PSC)
- HIV-associated sclerosing cholangitis: Associated with infection by CMV, *Cryptosporidium,* Microsporida, and *Mycobacterium avium* complex

DIAGNOSIS

DIFFERENTIAL DIAGNOSIS

- Biliary colic
- Acute cholecystitis
- Liver abscess
- Peptic ulcer disease (PUD)
- Pancreatitis
- Intestinal obstruction
- Right kidney stone
- Hepatitis
- Pyelonephritis

WORKUP

- Blood cultures
- CBC
- Liver function tests

LABORATORY TESTS

- Usually, elevated WBC count with a predominance of polymorphonuclear forms
- Elevated alkaline phosphatase and bilirubin in chronic obstruction
- Elevated transaminases in acute obstruction
- Positive blood cultures in 50% of cases, typically with enteric gram-negative aerobes (e.g., *Escherichia coli, Klebsiella pneumoniae),* enterococci, or anaerobes

IMAGING STUDIES

- Ultrasound:
  1 Allows visualization of the gallbladder and bile ducts to differentiate extrahepatic obstruction from intrahepatic cholestasis
  2 Insensitive but specific for visualization of common duct stones
- CT scan:
  1. Less accurate for gallstones
  2. More sensitive than ultrasound for visualization of the distal part of the common bile duct
  3. Also allows better definition of neoplasm
- ERCP:
  1. Confirms obstruction and its level
  2. Allows collection of specimens for culture and cytology
  3. Indicated for diagnosis if ultrasound and CT scan are inconclusive
  4. May be indicated in therapy (see "Treatment")

TREATMENT

NONPHARMACOLOGIC THERAPY

Biliary decompression:

- May be urgent in severely ill patients or those unresponsive to medical therapy within 12 to 24 hr
- May also be performed semielectively in patients who respond
- Options:
  1. ERCP with or without sphincterotomy or placement of a draining stent
  2. Percutaneous transhepatic biliary drainage for the acutely ill patient who is a poor surgical candidate
  3. Recently, endoscopic ultrasound–guided biliary drainage has been proven as an alternative to percutaneous transhepatic biliary drainage in specialized centers when ERCP fails or is not available
  4. Surgical exploration of the common bile duct

ACUTE GENERAL Rx

- Nothing by mouth
- Intravenous hydration
- Broad-spectrum antibiotics directed at gram-negative enteric organisms, anaerobes, and enterococcus such as carbapenems (meropenem: 1 g q8h or imipenem: 500 mg IV q6h if life threatening), piperacillin/tazobactam: 3.375 or 4.5 g IV q6h, or ampicillin-sulbactam, or ticarcillin-clavulanate; if infection is nosocomial, post-ERCP, or the patient is in shock, broaden antibiotic coverage

CHRONIC Rx

Repeated decompression may be necessary, particularly when obstruction is related to neoplasm.

DISPOSITION

Excellent prognosis if obstruction is amenable to definitive surgical therapy; otherwise relapses are common.

REFERRAL

- To biliary endoscopist if obstruction is from stones or a stent needs to be placed
- To interventional radiologist if external drainage is necessary
- To a general surgeon in all other cases
- To an infectious disease specialist if blood cultures are positive or the patient is in shock or otherwise severely ill

PEARLS & CONSIDERATIONS

- Cholangitis is a life-threatening form of intra-abdominal sepsis, though it may appear to be rather innocuous at its onset.
- Antibiotics alone will not resolve cholangitis in the presence of biliary obstruction, because high intrabiliary pressures prevent antibiotic delivery. Decompression and drainage of the biliary tract to alleviate the obstruction with antimicrobial therapy is the therapy of choice.

SUGGESTED READING

Available at ExpertConsult.com

AUTHORS: **GLENN G. FORT, M.D., M.P.H.,** and **TANYA ALI, M.D.**

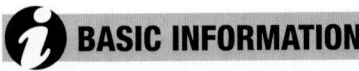

BASIC INFORMATION

DEFINITION
Cholecystitis is acute or chronic inflammation of the gallbladder generally caused by gallstones (>95% of cases).

SYNONYM
Gallbladder attack

ICD-10CM CODES
K81.9 Acute cholecystitis
K80.00 Calculus of gallbladder with acute cholecystitis without obstruction
K81.9 Cholecystitis, unspecified

EPIDEMIOLOGY & DEMOGRAPHICS
- Acute cholecystitis occurs most commonly in women during the fifth and sixth decades. Approximately 120,000 cholecystectomies are performed for acute cholecystitis annually in the U.S.
- The incidence of gallstones is 0.6% in the general population and much higher in certain ethnic groups (>75% of Native Americans by age 60 yr). Most patients with gallstones are asymptomatic. Of such patients, biliary colic develops in 1% to 4% annually.

PHYSICAL FINDINGS & CLINICAL PRESENTATION
- Pain and tenderness in the right hypochondrium or epigastrium; pain possibly radiating to the infrascapular region
- Palpation of the right upper quadrant (RUQ) eliciting marked tenderness and stoppage of inspired breath ***(Murphy sign)***
- Guarding
- Fever (33%)
- Jaundice (25% to 50% of patients)
- Palpable gallbladder (20% of cases)
- Nausea and vomiting (>70% of patients)
- Fever and chills (>25% of patients)
- Medical history often revealing ingestion of large, fatty meals before onset of pain in the epigastrium and RUQ

ETIOLOGY
- Gallstones (>95% of cases)
- Ischemic damage to the gallbladder, critically ill patient (acalculous cholecystitis)
- Infectious agents, especially in patients with AIDS (cytomegalovirus, *Cryptosporidium*)
- Strictures of the bile duct
- Neoplasms, primary or metastatic
- Risk factors for cholelithiasis include age, obesity, female sex, rapid weight loss, ethnicity/race (Native American), use of contraceptives, pregnancy, diabetes mellitus, hemolysis, total parenteral nutrition, biliary parasites

Dx DIAGNOSIS

DIFFERENTIAL DIAGNOSIS
- Hepatic: Hepatitis, abscess, hepatic congestion, neoplasm, trauma
- Biliary: Neoplasm, stricture, sphincter of Oddi dysfunction
- Gastric: Pelvic ulcer disease, neoplasm, alcoholic gastritis, hiatal hernia, non-ulcer dyspepsia
- Pancreatic: Pancreatitis, neoplasm, stone in the pancreatic duct or ampulla
- Renal: Calculi, infection, inflammation, neoplasm, ruptured kidney
- Pulmonary: Pneumonia, pulmonary infarction, right-sided pleurisy
- Intestinal: Retrocecal appendicitis, intestinal obstruction, high fecal impaction, irritable bowel syndrome (IBS), inflammatory bowel disease (IBD)
- Cardiac: Myocardial ischemia (particularly involving the inferior wall), pericarditis
- Cutaneous: Herpes zoster
- Trauma
- Fitz-Hugh–Curtis syndrome (perihepatitis), ruptured ectopic pregnancy
- Subphrenic abscess
- Dissecting aneurysm
- Nerve root irritation caused by osteoarthritis of the spine

WORKUP
Workup consists of detailed history and physical examination coupled with laboratory evaluation and imaging studies. No single clinical finding or laboratory test is sufficient to establish or exclude cholecystitis without further testing.

LABORATORY TESTS
- Leukocytosis (12,000 to 20,000) is present in >70% of patients.
- Elevated alkaline phosphatase, ALT, AST, bilirubin; bilirubin elevation >4 mg/dl is unusual and suggests presence of choledocholithiasis.
- Elevated amylase may be present (consider pancreatitis if serum amylase elevation exceeds 500 U).

IMAGING STUDIES
- Ultrasound of the gallbladder (Fig. E1) is the preferred initial test; it will demonstrate the presence of stones and also dilated gallbladder with thickened wall and surrounding edema in patients with acute cholecystitis.
- Nuclear imaging (HIDA scan) (Fig. E2) is useful for diagnosis of cholecystitis when sonogram is inconclusive: Sensitivity and specificity exceed 90% for acute cholecystitis. This test is only reliable when bilirubin is <5 mg/dl. A positive test result (absence of gallbladder filling within 60 min after the administration of tracer) will demonstrate obstruction of the cystic or common hepatic duct; the test will not demonstrate the presence of stones.
- CT scan of abdomen is useful in cases of suspected abscess, neoplasm, or pancreatitis.
- Plain radiograph of the abdomen generally is not useful because <25% of stones are radiopaque.

Rx TREATMENT

NONPHARMACOLOGIC THERAPY
Provide IV hydration; withhold oral feedings.

ACUTE GENERAL Rx
- Laparoscopic (percutaneous) cholecystectomy (PC) is considered the treatment of choice for most patients. The rate of conversion to open cholecystectomy is higher when laparoscopic cholecystectomy (CCY) is performed for acute cholecystitis rather than for uncomplicated cholelithiasis; conservative management with IV fluids and antibiotics (ampicillin-sulbactam 3 g IV q6h or piperacillin-tazobactam 4.5 g IV q8h) may be justified in some high-risk patients to convert an emergency procedure into an elective one with a lower mortality rate.
- Endoscopic retrograde cholangiopancreatography with sphincterectomy and stone extraction can be performed in conjunction with laparoscopic cholecystectomy for patients with choledochal lithiasis; approximately 7% to 15% of patients with cholelithiasis also have stones in the common bile duct.

DISPOSITION
- Prognosis is good; elective laparoscopic cholecystectomy can be performed as outpatient procedure.
- Hospital stay (when necessary) varies from overnight with laparoscopic cholecystectomy to 4 to 7 days with open cholecystectomy.
- Complication rate is approximately 1% (hemorrhage and bile leak) for laparoscopic cholecystectomy and <0.5% (infection) with open cholecystectomy.

REFERRAL
Surgical referral in all patients with acute cholecystitis

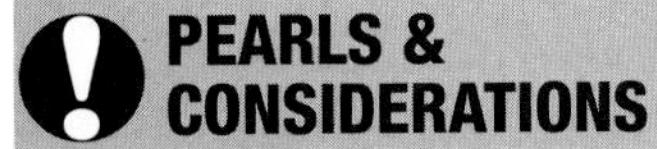

PEARLS & CONSIDERATIONS

COMMENTS
- Patients should be instructed that stones may recur in bile ducts.
- Gallbladder aspiration, in which all fluid visualized by ultrasound is aspirated, represents a nonsurgical treatment when patients who are at high operative risk develop acute cholecystitis. Salvage cholecystectomy is reserved for nonresponders.

SUGGESTED READINGS
Available at ExpertConsult.com

RELATED CONTENT
Gallbladder Attack (Cholecystitis) (Patient Information)
Choledocholithiasis (Related Key Topic)
Cholelithiasis (Related Key Topic)
Cholangitis (Related Key Topic)
Functional Gallbladder Disorder (Related Key Topic)

AUTHOR: **FRED F. FERRI, M.D.**

DEFINITION

Choledocholithiasis is a derivation from the Greek words of *choli* (bile), *docheion* (container), and *lithos* (stone) and refers to the presence of gallstones within the common bile duct (CBD).

SYNONYM

Common bile duct stone(s)

ICD-10CM CODE
K80.50 Calculus of bile duct

EPIDEMIOLOGY & DEMOGRAPHICS

- While the exact incidence and prevalence are unknown, an estimated 10% to 20% of patients are found to have choledocholithiasis at the time of cholecystectomy.
- Passage of gallstones into the CBD occurs in approximately 10% to 15% of those with cholelithiasis, and the incidence is known to increase with age. Approximately 95% of those with choledocholithiasis will also have cholelithiasis.
- Risk factors for gallstone formation include nonmodifiable factors such age, female sex, family history, ethnic background, and genetic predilection, while modifiable factors are centripetal obesity and metabolic syndrome, rapid weight loss, ileal Crohn's disease, cirrhosis, total parenteral nutrition, and medications such as estrogen replacement therapy.

PHYSICAL FINDINGS & CLINICAL PRESENTATION

- Uncomplicated choledocholithiasis presents with biliary colic; it is classically described as intense and constant pain in the right upper quadrant or epigastric region, associated with nausea and vomiting.
- Occasionally patients may remain asymptomatic, but resolution of pain more often reflects passage of stone into the bowel.
- Physical examination demonstrates right upper quadrant or epigastric tenderness and occasionally jaundice.
- Courvoisier's sign for a palpable gallbladder is more typically associated with malignant obstruction of the CBD, but it has been reported with choledocholithiasis.
- Other clinical findings of fever (Charcot's triad), hypotension, and altered mental status (Reynolds' pentad) are found only when choledocholithiasis is complicated by acute cholangitis.
- Choledocholithiasis can also be complicated by acute pancreatitis.

ETIOLOGY

- The majority of cases are due to passage of cholesterol stones from the gallbladder into the common bile duct.
- De novo formation of choledocholithiasis (primary choledocholithiasis) is uncommon but is seen among those with increased propensity for pigment stone formation due to chronic recurrent pyogenic cholangitis from trematodes, congenital biliary duct anomalies, dilated or strictured ducts or *MDR3* gene defects causing impairments in biliary phospholipid secretions, or biliary stasis such as from cystic fibrosis.
- Brown pigment stones comprise the majority of pigment stones in the bile duct, often found proximal to biliary stricture and associated with cholangitis.

Dx DIAGNOSIS

DIFFERENTIAL DIAGNOSIS

- Biliary pain
- Acute cholecystitis
- Sphincter of Oddi dysfunction
- Functional gallbladder disorder
- Malignant obstruction
- Choledochal cyst
- Papillary stenosis
- AIDS-associated cholangiopathy

WORKUP

- The constellation of symptomatic cholelithiasis with elevated liver enzymes should prompt a transabdominal ultrasound (US) of the right upper quadrant to evaluate for a stone in the CBD, which is the most reliable predictor of choledocholithiasis.
- Elevated liver enzymes are 94% sensitive in detecting choledocholithiasis.
- Clinical predictors may be utilized to risk-stratify patients and to inform the next step in management. For instance, strong predictors for high-risk choledocholithiasis are a CBD stone or dilated CBD seen on transabdominal US, clinical or biochemical evidence of cholangitis, and elevated bilirubin (>1.8 mg/dl).
- See Fig. 1 for the ASGE guideline for a proposed risk stratification model.

LABORATORY TESTS

- Elevations in serum alanine aminotransferase (ALT) and aspartate aminotransferase (AST) reflect early biliary obstruction, followed by a disproportionate increase in serum bilirubin, alkaline phosphatase (ALP), and gamma-glutamyl transpeptidase (GGT), which are independent predictors of a CBD stone.
- Elevation in ALP is rapid and precedes the rise in bilirubin level, the latter being proportional to the degree of obstruction.
- An isolated and transient increase in alanine transaminase or amylase reflects passage of the gallstone.
- In addition, patients with choledocholithiasis complicated by acute pancreatitis and cholangitis have elevated serum amylase or lipase (>3 times upper limit of normal) and leukocytosis, respectively.

IMAGING STUDIES

- Ultrasound of the gallbladder has a relatively poor sensitivity (22%-55%) for stone detection but is relied on for CBD dilation, which is associated with choledocholithiasis.
- The finding of CBD dilation >8 mm (sensitivity 77%-87%, negative predictive value 95%-96%) with an intact gallbladder is indicative of biliary obstruction. Multiple small gallbladder stones (<5 mm) portend a fourfold higher risk of passage of stones into the CBD.
- Other imaging modalities such as helical CT (Fig. 2), magnetic resonance cholangiopancreatography, CT cholangiography, and endoscopic ultrasound have improved performance characteristics for CBD stone detection; however, their use as first-line diagnostic tools is contingent on diagnostic uncertainty, patient factors, and availability.
- Magnetic resonance cholangiopancreatography should be considered in intermediate-risk patients or in those with prior cholecystectomy.
- High-risk patients should proceed directly to endoscopic retrograde cholangiopancreatography (ERCP) for diagnosis and treatment.

Rx TREATMENT

ACUTE GENERAL Rx

- Presence of choledocholithiasis warrants treatment.
- The mainstay is removal of CBD stones via ERCP and papillotomy either before or at the time of laparoscopic or open cholecystectomy.
- Failure of ERCP to clear the biliary duct warrants biliary stenting for drainage as a temporary measure in the event of acute cholangitis.
- ERCP without subsequent cholecystectomy may be performed in select high-risk patients, but 10% of these patients will require a subsequent cholecystectomy for recurrence.

CHRONIC Rx

- Patients with recurrent choledocholithiasis from cholesterol gallstones after cholecystectomy might be considered for chronic treatment with ursodeoxycholic acid to facilitate reduction of cholesterol saturation of bile.

REFERRAL

- Gastroenterology
- General surgery

SUGGESTED READINGS

Available at ExpertConsult.com

RELATED CONTENT

Cholangiocarcinoma (Related Key Topic)
Cholelithiasis (Related Key Topic)
Cholecystitis (Related Key Topic)

AUTHORS: **ROWENA ALMEIDA, M.D.,** and **TALIA ZENLEA, M.D.**

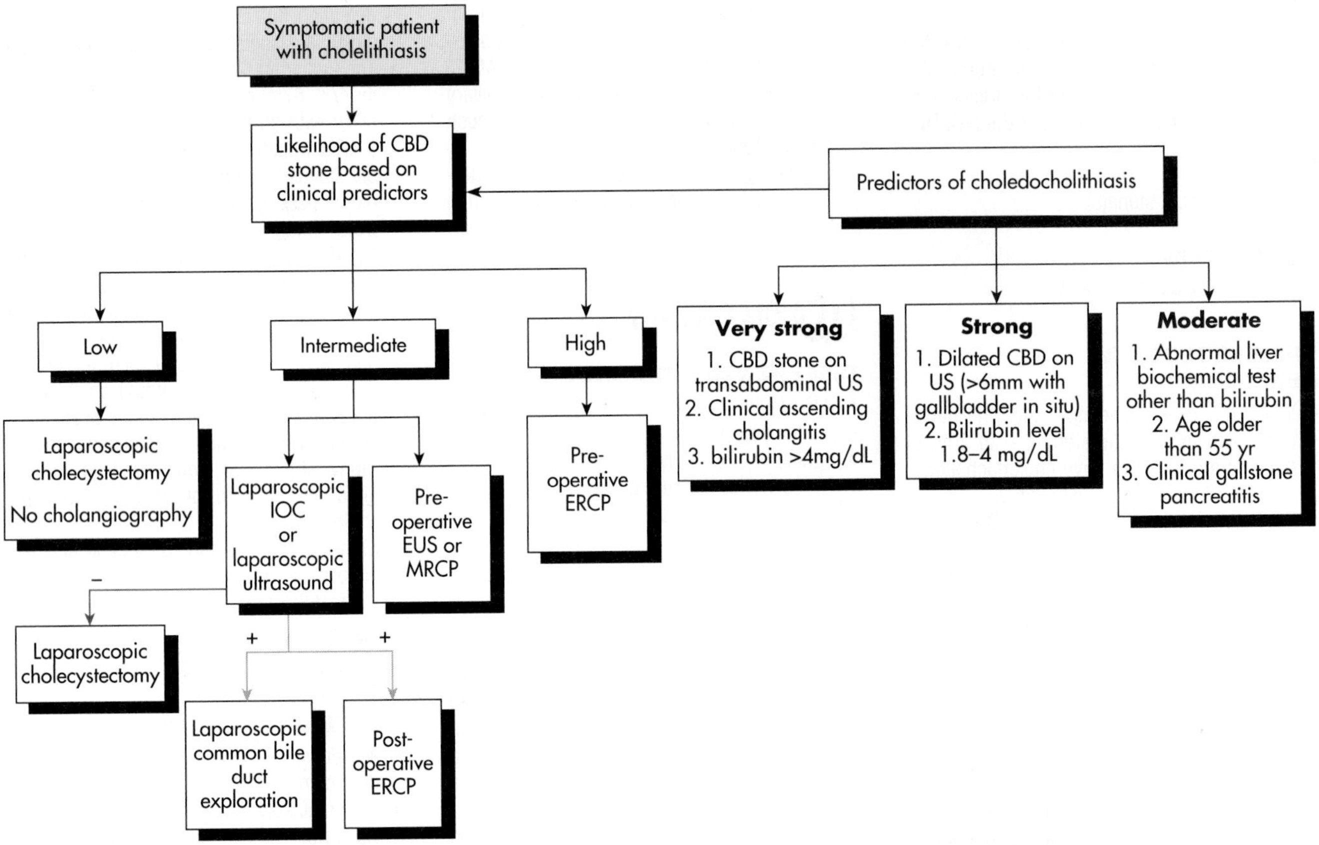

- Symptomatic patient with cholelithiasis
  - Likelihood of CBD stone based on clinical predictors ← Predictors of choledocholithiasis
    - Low
      - Laparoscopic cholecystectomy
        No cholangiography
    - Intermediate
      - Laparoscopic IOC or laparoscopic ultrasound
        - −: Laparoscopic cholecystectomy
        - +: Laparoscopic common bile duct exploration
        - +: Post-operative ERCP
      - Pre-operative EUS or MRCP
    - High
      - Pre-operative ERCP

- Predictors of choledocholithiasis
  - **Very strong**
    1. CBD stone on transabdominal US
    2. Clinical ascending cholangitis
    3. bilirubin >4mg/dL
  - **Strong**
    1. Dilated CBD on US (>6mm with gallbladder in situ)
    2. Bilirubin level 1.8–4 mg/dL
  - **Moderate**
    1. Abnormal liver biochemical test other than bilirubin
    2. Age older than 55 yr
    3. Clinical gallstone pancreatitis

FIG. 1 Algorithm for the management of patients with symptomatic cholelithiasis. (From Feldman M, et al.: *Sleisenger and Fordtran's gastrointestinal and liver disease*, ed 10, Philadelphia, 2016, Elsevier.)

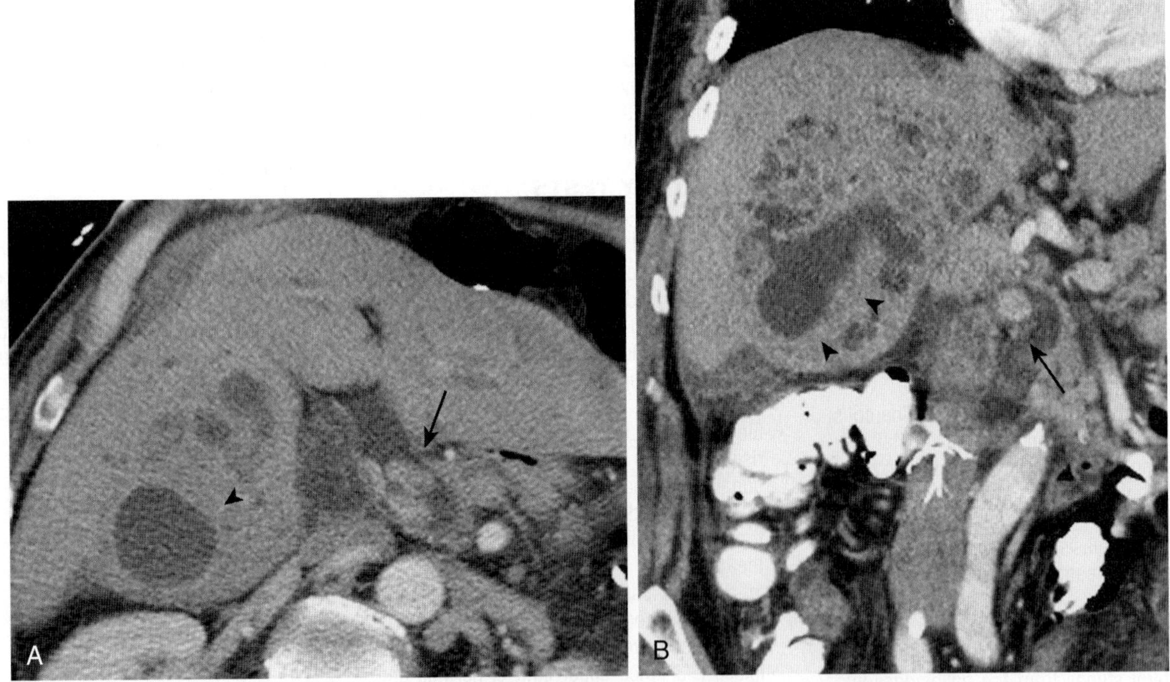

FIG. 2 A 70-year-old man with choledocholithiasis and a hepatic abscess. Axial **(A)** and coronal **(B)** portal venous phase computed tomography images demonstrate large bile duct stones *(arrows)* with a focal intrahepatic fluid collection *(arrowheads)* consistent with the patient's known pyogenic abscess. (From Soto JA, Lucey BC: *Emergency radiology: the requisites*, ed 2, Philadelphia, 2017, Elsevier.)

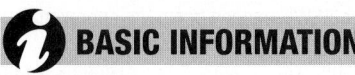

DEFINITION

Cholelithiasis is the presence of stones in the gallbladder

SYNONYM

Gallstones

ICD-10CM CODES

K80.80 Other cholelithiasis without obstruction
K80.81 Other cholelithiasis with obstruction
K91.86 Retained cholelithiasis following cholecystectomy

EPIDEMIOLOGY & DEMOGRAPHICS

- Gallstone disease can be found in 12% of the U.S. population. Of these, 2% to 3% (500,000 to 600,000) are treated with cholecystectomies each yr.
- Annual medical expenditures for gallbladder surgeries in the U.S. exceed $5 billion.
- Incidence of gallbladder disease increases with age. Highest incidence is in the fifth and sixth decades. Predisposing factors for gallstones are female sex, pregnancy, age >40 yr, family history of gallstones, obesity, ileal disease, oral contraceptives, diabetes mellitus, rapid weight loss, estrogen replacement therapy.
- Patients with gallstones have a 20% chance of developing biliary colic or its complications at the end of a 20-yr period. Significant predictors of gallstone-related events are large stone (>10 mm), presence of multiple stones, and female sex.

PHYSICAL FINDINGS & CLINICAL PRESENTATION

- Physical examination is entirely normal unless patient is having biliary colic; 80% of gallstones are asymptomatic.
- Typical symptoms of obstruction of the cystic duct include intermittent, severe, cramping pain affecting the right upper quadrant.
- Pain occurs mostly at night and may radiate to the back or right shoulder. It can last from a few minutes to several hours.
- Symptoms of gallstone disease and its complications are described in Table 1.

ETIOLOGY

- 75% of gallstones contain cholesterol and are usually associated with obesity, female sex, and diabetes mellitus; mixed stones are most common (80%); pure cholesterol stones account for only 10% of stones and are the result of biliary supersaturation due to cholesterol secretion into the gallbladder and accelerated cholesterol nucleation and crystallization.
- 25% of gallstones are pigment stones (bilirubin, calcium, and variable organic material) associated with hemolysis and cirrhosis. These tend to be black-pigmented stones that are refractory to medical therapy.
- 50% of mixed-type stones are radiopaque.

Dx DIAGNOSIS

DIFFERENTIAL DIAGNOSIS

- Peptic ulcer disease
- Gastroesophageal reflux disease
- Irritable bowel disease
- Pancreatitis
- Neoplasms
- Nonnuclear dyspepsia
- Inferior wall myocardial infarction
- Hepatic abscess

LABORATORY TESTS

Generally normal unless patient has biliary obstruction (elevated alkaline phosphatase, bilirubin).

IMAGING STUDIES

- Ultrasound of the gallbladder (Fig. E1) will detect small stones and biliary sludge (sensitivity, 95%; specificity, 90%); the presence of dilated gallbladder with thickened wall is suggestive of acute cholecystitis.
- Nuclear imaging (HIDA scan) can confirm acute cholecystitis (>90% accuracy) if gallbladder does not visualize within 4 hr of injection and the radioisotope is excreted in the common bile duct.
- Common bile duct stones can be detected noninvasively by magnetic resonance cholangiopancreatography or invasively by endoscopic retrograde cholangiopancreatography (ERCP) and intraoperative cholangiography.

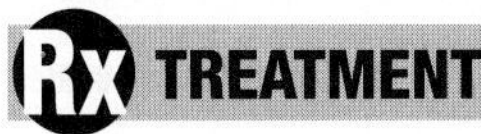

NONPHARMACOLOGIC THERAPY

Lifestyle changes (avoidance of diets high in polyunsaturated fats, weight loss in obese patients; however, avoid rapid weight loss)

ACUTE GENERAL Rx

- The management of gallstones is affected by the clinical presentation.
- Asymptomatic patients do not require therapeutic intervention. Proposed criteria for prophylactic cholecystectomy are described in Table 2.
- Surgical intervention is generally the ideal approach for symptomatic patients. Laparoscopic cholecystectomy is preferred over open cholecystectomy because of the shorter recovery period and lower mortality rate.

TABLE 1 Symptoms of Gallstone Disease and Its Complications

Disease	Pathophysiology	Symptoms
Biliary colic	Transient gallstone impaction at the cystic duct or ampulla of Vater	Intermittent RUQ pain associated with nausea or vomiting. Pain in the epigastrium or radiating to the right scapular tip. Episodes last 30 min to several hours with days or months between episodes.
Acute cholecystitis	Inflammation of the gallbladder caused by obstruction of the cystic duct. May occur in the presence or absence of bacterial superinfection	Patients appear ill and cannot take deep breaths. They have constant pain that lasts 30-60 min and worsens with movement. Persistent common bile duct impaction usually promotes vomiting. Physical examination demonstrates RUQ tenderness with voluntary guarding and a positive Murphy sign (arrest of inspiration during deep palpation over the gallbladder).
Emphysematous cholecystitis	Infection with gas-producing bacteria such as *Escherichia coli, Clostridium perfringens*, and anaerobic streptococci	Symptoms are similar to those with acute cholecystitis. Gas may be seen on abdominal plain films or CT. Male diabetics are most commonly affected.
Chronic cholecystitis	Persistent inflammation and fibrosis of the gallbladder with poor motor and absorptive function	Patients are usually asymptomatic but may report multiple previous attacks of colic. Porcelain gallbladder develops from chronic inflammation and may progress to carcinoma.
Acalculous cholecystitis	Probably related to biliary stasis in the setting of critical illness and altered gastrointestinal motility	Seen in patients with traumatic injuries, burns, and critical illness, as well as in those receiving total parenteral nutrition. The mortality for this disorder is twice as high as that for acute calculous cholecystitis.
Gallbladder perforation	Stones erode through an inflamed and necrotic gallbladder wall. Stones may travel into the peritoneal cavity or cause adhesions between nearby structures. Bile peritonitis may develop	More than half of patients with gallbladder perforation have fever and a palpable RUQ mass. Mortality in these patients is 30%.

CT, Computed tomography; *RUQ*, right upper quadrant.
From Adams JG et al: *Emergency medicine, clinical essentials*, ed 2, Philadelphia, 2013, Elsevier.

Between 5% and 26% of patients undergoing elective laparoscopic cholecystectomy will require conversion to an open procedure. Most common reason is the inability to clearly identify the biliary anatomy.

- Laparoscopic cholecystectomy after endoscopic sphincterectomy is recommended for patients with common bile duct stones and residual gallbladder stones. Where possible, single-stage laparoscopic treatments with removal of duct stones and cholecystectomy during the same procedure are preferable. Percutaneous cholecystectomy is an alternative for patients who are critically ill with gallbladder empyema and sepsis.
- Patients who are not appropriate candidates for surgery because of coexisting illness or patients who refuse surgery can be treated with oral bile salts: ursodiol or chenodiol. Candidates for oral bile salts are patients with cholesterol stones (radiolucent, noncalcified stones), with a diameter of ≤15 mm and having three or fewer stones. Candidates for medical therapy must have a functioning gallbladder and must have absence of calcifications on CT scans.
- Extracorporeal shock wave lithotripsy (ESWL) is another form of medical therapy. It can be used in patients with stone diameter of ≤3 cm and having three or fewer stones.

TABLE 2 Proposed Criteria for Prophylactic Cholecystectomy

Life expectancy >20 yr
Calculi >2 cm in diameter
Calculi >3 mm and patent cystic duct
Radiopaque calculi
Gallbladder polyps >15 mm
Nonfunctioning or calcified gallbladder ("porcelain" gallbladder)
Women <60 yr
Patients in areas with high prevalence of gallbladder cancer

From Cameron JL, Cameron AM: *Current surgical therapy,* ed 10, Philadelphia, 2011, Saunders.

DISPOSITION

- Complicated gallstone events develop in 8% of patients with incidentally discovered gallstones after 17 yr (Shabanzadeh DM et al in Suggested Readings: *Gastroenterology* 150:156, 2016).
- After ESWL, stones recur in approximately 20% of patients after 4 yr.
- Patients with at least one gallstone <5 mm in diameter have a greater than fourfold increased risk of presenting with acute biliary pancreatitis. A policy of watchful waiting in such cases is generally warranted.
- A potential serious complication of gallstones is acute cholangitis. ERCP and endoscopic sphincterectomy followed by interval laparoscopic cholecystectomy are effective in acute cholangitis.
- Uncommon complications of gallstone disease are summarized in Table 3.

SUGGESTED READINGS

Available at ExpertConsult.com

RELATED CONTENT

Gallstones (Patient Information)
Cholecystitis (Related Key Topic)
Choledocholithiasis (Related Key Topic)

AUTHOR: **FRED F. FERRI, M.D.**

TABLE 3 Uncommon Complications of Gallstone Disease

Complication	Pathogenesis	Clinical Features	Diagnosis/Treatment
Emphysematous cholecystitis	Secondary infection of the gallbladder wall with gas-forming organisms (*Clostridium welchii, Escherichia coli,* and anaerobic streptococci) More common in older adult diabetic men; can occur without stones	Symptoms and signs similar to those of severe acute cholecystitis	Plain abdominal films may show gas in the gallbladder fossa US and CT are sensitive for confirming gas Treatment is with IV antibiotics, including anaerobic coverage, and early cholecystectomy High morbidity and mortality rates
Cholecystoenteric fistula	Erosion of a (usually large) stone through the gallbladder wall into the adjacent bowel, most often the duodenum, followed in frequency by the hepatic flexure, stomach, and jejunum	Symptoms and signs similar to those of acute cholecystitis, although sometimes a fistula may be clinically silent Stones >25 mm, especially in older adult women, may produce a bowel obstruction, or "gallstone ileus"; the terminal ileum is the most common site of obstruction Gastric outlet obstruction (Bouveret syndrome) may occur rarely	Plain abdominal films may show gas in the biliary tree and/or a small bowel obstruction in gallstone ileus, as well as a stone in the RLQ if the stone is calcified Contrast upper GI series may demonstrate the fistula A fistula from a solitary stone that passes may close spontaneously Cholecystectomy and bowel closure are curative Gallstone ileus requires emergency laparotomy; the diagnosis is often delayed, with a resulting mortality rate of ≈20%
Mirizzi syndrome	An impacted stone in the gallbladder neck or cystic duct, with extrinsic compression of the common hepatic duct from accompanying inflammation or fistula	Jaundice and RUQ pain	ERCP demonstrates dilated intrahepatic ducts and extrinsic compression of the common hepatic duct and possible fistula Preoperative diagnosis is important to guide surgery and minimize the risk of BD injury
Porcelain gallbladder	Intramural calcification of the gallbladder wall, usually in association with stones	No symptoms attributable to the calcified wall per se, but carcinoma of the gallbladder is a late complication in ≈20%	Plain abdominal films or CT show intramural calcification of the gallbladder wall Prophylactic cholecystectomy is indicated to prevent carcinoma

BD, bile duct; *CT,* computed tomography; *ERCP,* endoscopic retrograde cholangiopancreatography; *GI,* gastrointestinal; *IV,* intravenous; *RLQ,* right lower quadrant; *RUQ,* right upper quadrant *US,* ultrasound.
From Feldman M, et al: *Sleisenger and Fortran's gastrointestinal and liver disease,* ed 10, Philadelphia, 2016, Elsevier.

BASIC INFORMATION

DEFINITION

Chronic fatigue syndrome (CFS), also known as myalgic encephalomyelitis/chronic fatigue syndrome (ME/CFS) and Systemic Exertion Intolerance Disease (SEID), is characterized by at least three of the following symptoms, present concurrently for at least 6 mo:

- Impaired memory or concentration (cognitive impairment)
- Sore throat
- Tender cervical or axillary lymph nodes
- Muscle pain
- Multijoint pain
- New headaches
- Unrefreshing sleep
- Postexertion malaise for longer than 24 hr
- Orthostatic intolerance

There are currently several sets of clinical criteria to define ME/CFS, yet there is no consensus regarding which set of criteria best identifies patients with this condition. In 2015, the Institute of Medicine (IOM) recommended renaming ME/CSF "Systemic Exertion Intolerance Disease (SEID)." Their definition requires that patients have: 1. Substantial reduction or impairment in the ability to engage in premorbid levels of activities persisting for >6 months and associated with new-onset fatigue not alleviated by rest; 2. Postexertional fatigue; 3. Unrefreshing sleep; and 4. Presence of cognitive impairment and/or orthostatic intolerance.

SYNONYMS

Systemic exertion intolerance disease (SEID)
Yuppie flu
CFS
Chronic Epstein-Barr syndrome
Myalgic encephalomyelitis/chronic fatigue syndrome (ME/CFS)
Neurasthenia

ICD-10CM CODES

R53.82	Chronic fatigue, unspecified
F45.8	Other somatoform disorders

EPIDEMIOLOGY & DEMOGRAPHICS

PREVALENCE IN U.S: Prevalence rates of CFS in the U.S. range from 0.3% to 2.5%. It is estimated that 800,000 to 2.5 million Americans have CFS.

PREDOMINANT AGE: Young adulthood and middle age

PREDOMINANT SEX: Females affected more often than males

ECONOMICS: The estimated annual cost of lost productivity is estimated to be between $17 billion and $24 billion annually.

PHYSICAL FINDINGS & CLINICAL PRESENTATION

- There are no physical findings specific for CFS.
- The physical examination may be useful to identify fibromyalgia and other rheumatologic conditions that may coexist with CFS.

ETIOLOGY

- The etiology of CFS is unknown. The pathophysiologic dysregulation of the thalamus, hypothalamus, and amygdala is believed by some to be a potential cause of SEID.
- Some theorize that a viral illness may trigger certain immune responses that lead to the various symptoms. Most patients often report the onset of their symptoms with a flulike illness.
- The presence of numerous psychiatric comorbidities in CFS have led some experts to question the existence of any organic etiology.

Dx DIAGNOSIS

DIFFERENTIAL DIAGNOSIS

- Psychosocial depression, dysthymia, anxiety-related disorders, and other psychiatric diseases
- Sleep apnea
- Infectious diseases (subacute bacterial endocarditis, Lyme disease, fungal diseases, mononucleosis, HIV, chronic hepatitis B or C, tuberculosis [TB], chronic parasitic infections)
- Autoimmune diseases: Systemic lupus erythematosus, myasthenia gravis, multiple sclerosis, thyroiditis, rheumatoid arthritis
- Endocrine abnormalities: Hypothyroidism, hypopituitarism, adrenal insufficiency, Cushing's syndrome, diabetes mellitus, hyperparathyroidism, pregnancy, reactive hypoglycemia
- Occult malignant disease
- Substance abuse
- Systemic disorders: Chronic renal failure, chronic obstructive pulmonary disease, cardiovascular disease, anemia, electrolyte abnormalities, liver disease
- Other: Inadequate rest, sleep apnea, narcolepsy, fibromyalgia, sarcoidosis, medications, toxic agent exposure, Wegener granulomatosis, vitamin deficiency

LABORATORY TESTS

- No specific laboratory tests exist for diagnosing CFS. Initial laboratory tests are useful to exclude other conditions that may mimic or may be associated with CFS.
    1. Screening laboratory tests: CBC, ESR, ALT, total protein, albumin, globulin, alkaline phosphatase, calcium, phosphorus, glucose, BUN, creatinine, electrolytes, TSH, and urinalysis are useful.
    2. Serologic tests for Epstein-Barr virus, *Candida albicans,* human herpesvirus 6, and other studies for immune cellular abnormalities are not useful; these tests are expensive and generally not recommended.
- Other tests may be indicated depending on the history and physical examination (e.g., ANA, RF in patients presenting with joint complaints or abnormalities on physical examination, Lyme titer in areas where Lyme disease is endemic).

IMAGING STUDIES

Generally not recommended unless history and physical examination indicate specific abnormalities (e.g., chest radiography in any patient suspected of TB or sarcoidosis)

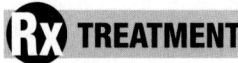

TREATMENT

NONPHARMACOLOGIC THERAPY

- Patients should be reassured that the illness is not fatal and that most patients improve over time.
- An initially supervised exercise program to preserve and increase strength is beneficial for most patients and can improve symptoms.
- Cognitive-behavioral therapy trials have shown positive effects on fatigue levels, work, depression/anxiety, and social adjustment.

GENERAL Rx

Therapy is generally palliative. The following medications may be helpful; however, evidence is conflicting:

- Antidepressants: The choice of antidepressant varies with the desired side effects. Patients with difficulty sleeping or fibromyalgia-like symptoms may benefit from low-dose trazodone 50 mg hs. When sedation is not desirable, low-dose SSRIs (fluoxetine 20 mg qd) often help alleviate fatigue and associated symptoms.
- NSAIDs can be used to relieve muscle and joint pain and headaches.

"Alternative" medications (herbs, multivitamins, nutritional supplements) are very popular with many CFS patients but are generally not very helpful.

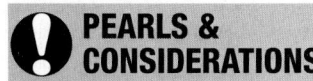

PEARLS & CONSIDERATIONS

COMMENTS

- In CFS the symptoms are serious enough to reduce daily activities by >50% in the absence of any other medically identifiable disorders.
- The suicide rate is nearly sevenfold higher in people with CFS.
- Moderate to complete recovery at 1 yr occurs in 22% to 60% of patients with CFS.

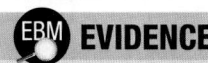

EVIDENCE

Available at ExpertConsult.com

SUGGESTED READINGS

Available at ExpertConsult.com

RELATED CONTENT

Evaluation of Fatigue (Algorithm, Section III)
Chronic Fatigue Syndrome (Patient Information)

AUTHOR: **FRED F. FERRI, M.D.**

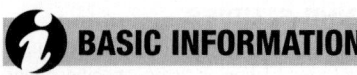

BASIC INFORMATION

DEFINITION

Chronic kidney disease (CKD) is diagnosed when there is evidence for more than 3 months of **kidney damage** (urine albumin >30 mg/g creatinine, hematuria, or parenchymal abnormalities) and/or **decreased kidney function** (glomerular filtration rate, GFR <60 ml/min per 1.73 m^2). CKD is characterized by accumulation of metabolic waste products in blood, electrolyte abnormalities, mineral and bone disorders, and anemia. The manifestations of CKD are summarized in Table 1.

SYNONYMS

CKD
Chronic renal failure
CRF
Chronic renal insufficiency
CRI

ICD-10CM CODES

N18.1	Chronic kidney disease, stage 1
N18.2	Chronic kidney disease, stage 2
N18.3	Chronic kidney disease, stage 3
N18.4	Chronic kidney disease, stage 4
N18.5	Chronic kidney disease, stage 5
N18.6	End-stage renal disease
N18.9	Chronic kidney disease, unspecified

EPIDEMIOLOGY & DEMOGRAPHICS

- The overall prevalence of CKD (Stages 1–5) in the United States (U.S.) adult general population was 14.8% in 2011–2014. CKD Stage 3 (6.6%) was the most prevalent.
- Incidence of end-stage renal disease (ESRD) is 7% to 9% per yr in the U.S., primarily due to diabetes mellitus and hypertension, the leading risk factors for CKD. Annually, 3 in 10,000 persons develop ESRD, and more than 100,000 patients begin dialysis annually.
- By 2015, there were 703,243 prevalent cases of ESRD with an annual average cost per patient of approximately $88,000 for hemodialysis.
- Kidney transplantation is the best option for kidney replacement therapy, but many patients are not eligible for transplantation.

PHYSICAL FINDINGS & CLINICAL PRESENTATION

- Skin pallor, ecchymosis
- Sleep disorder
- Hypertension
- Edema, leg cramps, restless legs, peripheral neuropathy
- Emotional lability, depression, decreased cognitive function
- Clinical presentation varies with the degree of kidney disease and its underlying etiology. Common symptoms are generalized fatigue, nausea, anorexia, pruritus, sleep disturbances, smell and taste disturbances, hiccoughs, and seizures

ETIOLOGY

- Diabetes (43.2%), hypertension (23%), chronic glomerulonephritis (12.3%)
- Failed kidney transplant
- Polycystic kidney disease (2.9%)
- Interstitial nephritis (e.g., drug hypersensitivity, analgesic nephropathy)
- Obstructive nephropathies (e.g., nephrolithiasis, prostatic disease)
- Vascular diseases (renal artery stenosis, hypertensive nephrosclerosis)
- Autoimmune diseases

TABLE 1 Pathophysiology of Chronic Kidney Disease

Manifestation	Mechanisms
Accumulation of nitrogenous waste products	Decrease in glomerular filtration rate
Acidosis	Decreased ammonia synthesis Impaired bicarbonate reabsorption Decreased net acid excretion
Sodium retention	Excessive renin production Oliguria
Sodium wasting	Solute diuresis Tubular damage
Urinary concentrating defect	Solute diuresis Tubular damage
Hyperkalemia	Decrease in glomerular filtration rate Metabolic acidosis Excessive potassium intake Hyporeninemic hypoaldosteronism
Renal osteodystrophy	Impaired renal production of 1,25-dihydroxycholecalciferol Hyperphosphatemia Hypocalcemia Secondary hyperparathyroidism
Growth retardation	Inadequate caloric intake Renal osteodystrophy Metabolic acidosis Anemia Growth hormone resistance
Anemia	Decreased erythropoietin production Iron deficiency Folate deficiency Vitamin B_{12} deficiency Decreased erythrocyte survival
Bleeding tendency	Defective platelet function
Infection	Defective granulocyte function Impaired cellular immune functions Indwelling dialysis catheters
Neurologic symptoms (fatigue, poor concentration, headache, drowsiness, memory loss, seizures, peripheral neuropathy)	Uremic factor(s) Aluminum toxicity Hypertension
Gastrointestinal symptoms (feeding intolerance, abdominal pain)	Gastroesophageal reflux Decreased gastrointestinal motility
Hypertension	Volume overload Excessive renin production
Hyperlipidemia	Decreased plasma lipoprotein lipase activity
Pericarditis, cardiomyopathy	Uremic factor(s) Hypertension Fluid overload
Glucose intolerance	Tissue insulin resistance

From Kliegman RM et al: *Nelson textbook of pediatrics*, ed 19, Philadelphia, 2011, Saunders.

Dx DIAGNOSIS

Although GFR is considered the best overall index of kidney function, it is not the only measure of kidney health. The qualifying criterion for use of estimated glomerular filtration rate (eGFR) equations is that kidney disease must be present for 3 mo. Therefore, the serum creatinine must be repeated and trended to establish a diagnosis of CKD in individuals who must also be in a steady state of creatinine generation or production. Although staging systems for CKD based on eGFR have limitations, they have proven useful in many clinical settings and are now embedded into guidelines developed for CKD management.

WORKUP

- Laboratory evaluation and imaging studies can identify reversible causes of acute GFR decline (e.g., volume depletion, urinary tract obstruction, heart failure).
- Ultrasound evaluation of the kidneys often reveals small kidneys (<9 cm sagittal length) with increased echogenicity.

- Kidney biopsy is generally not considered when kidneys are small or CKD is advanced.
- Fig. E1 provides a summary of a practical approach to the detection and management of chronic kidney disease.

LABORATORY TESTS

- Elevated blood urea nitrogen (BUN), creatinine, and low GFR are the best overall indicators of kidney function. GFR is estimated by multivariable (creatinine, age, sex, and race) prediction equations normalized to body surface area. GFR calculators are available online (http://www.kidney.org/kls/professionals/gfr_calculator.cfm). The Modification of Diet in Renal Disease (MDRD) equation has been in common use in clinical laboratories until recently, but has been replaced by the Chronic Kidney Disease Epidemiology Collaboration (CKD-EPI) equation, which more accurately categorizes the risk of mortality and progression to ESRD.
- Urinalysis may reveal proteinuria, hematuria, or formed elements such as casts.
- Serum chemistries: Elevated BUN and creatinine, hyperkalemia, hyperuricemia, hypocalcemia, hyperphosphatemia, hyperglycemia, and decreased serum bicarbonate concentration.
- Urinary protein excretion. A urine total protein-to-creatinine ratio >1000 mg/g generally indicates glomerular disease.
- Special studies: Serum and urine immunoelectrophoresis (multiple myeloma), antinuclear antibody (i.e., systemic lupus erythematosus).
- Cystatin C measurement or direct glomerular filtration clearance methods may confirm CKD in situations when serum creatinine–based GFR equations are less accurate (e.g., HIV, malnutrition) or more precise measurement is desired (e.g., kidney transplant organ donation).

IMAGING STUDIES

- Ultrasound of kidneys for size measurements and to rule out obstruction.
- Plain radiographs of the aorta and extremities ordered for other reasons may reveal vascular and extraskeletal calcification.

CLASSIFICATION

The 2012 Kidney Disease: International Global Outcomes classifies CKD by CGA categories: Cause (etiology), GFR (G1 to G5), and Albuminuria (A1 to A3) by urine albumin-to-creatinine ratio (Table 2). This format is recommended when documenting and/or discussing CKD. Table 3 depicts how CKD prognosis worsens with either increasing levels of albuminuria or declining GFR.

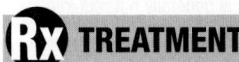

TREATMENT

Management varies according to stage (Table 4).

NONPHARMACOLOGIC THERAPY

- Kidney Disease: Improving Global Outcomes (KDIGO) has recommended that protein intake should be lowered to 0.8 g/kg per day in adults with CKD and GFR below 30 ml/min per 1.73 m^2, whereas high protein intake (>1.3 g/kg per day) should be avoided in adults with CKD at risk of progression. Table 5 describes nutritional recommendations in CKD. Referral to a dietitian for nutritional therapy for patients with GFR <50 ml/min per 1.73 m^2 is recommended and is a Medicare-covered service.
- Dietary restriction of sodium (~100 mmol/day), potassium (≤60 mmol/day), and phosphorus (<800 mg/day).
- Blood pressure: Target blood pressure of ≤140/90 mm Hg if CKD (diabetic and nondiabetic) and urine albumin excretion ≤30 mg/24 hr. If CKD (diabetic and nondiabetic) and albumin excretion >30 mg/24 hr are present, consider a target blood pressure ≤130/80 mm Hg.
- Adjust medication doses for reduced GFR.
- Restrict fluid intake if significant edema is present or hyponatremia (serum Na <130 mEq/L) is present.
- Resistance exercise training can preserve lean body mass, improve nutritional status, and muscle function in patients with moderate CKD.
- Avoid iodinated radiocontrast agents. Prophylactic volume expansion with sodium chloride or sodium bicarbonate before dye exposure is equally effective.
- Smoking cessation.
- Prompt referral to a nephrologist is helpful. Late evaluation of patients with CKD is associated with greater burden and severity of comorbid disease and complications and increased mortality. Suggested criteria for nephrology referral are described in Table 6.
- Referral for kidney transplantation in selected patients.

GENERAL Rx

Angiotensin–converting-enzyme inhibitors (ACEIs) and angiotensin II receptor blockers (ARBs) reduce proteinuria and slow progression of CKD, especially in hypertensive diabetic patients. The combination of ACEI and ARB is not recommended due to increased risks of hyperkalemia, hypotension, and acute kidney injury. Increases of serum creatinine of up to 25%–30% greater than baseline within 3 months of initiating ACEI or ARB therapy may be acceptable.

- Addition of chlorthalidone to CKD patients with difficult-to-treat hypertension may reduce blood pressure and proteinuria. Successful blood pressure–lowering is associated with weight loss. Loop diuretic therapy may be associated with complications of hypokalemia.
- Initiation of dialysis:
  1. Urgent indications: Uremic pericarditis, neuropathy, neuromuscular abnormalities (e.g., "foot drop"), heart failure, hyperkalemia, and seizures.
  2. Other indications: GFR 10 to 15 ml/min; progressive anorexia, weight loss, disordered sleep, pruritus, uncontrolled fluid gain with hypertension and signs of heart failure.
  3. General indications for initiation of dialysis are summarized in Table 7. Suggested steps for resolving conflict in the shared decision-making process regarding dialysis initiation are described (Fig. E2). Early initiation of dialysis when the GFR is 10 to 15 ml/min per 1.73 m^2 does not enhance survival compared with a symptom-driven strategy for initiation of dialysis at eGFR <8 to 10 ml/min per 1.73 m^2.
- Erythropoiesis-stimulating agents (ESAs), including epoetins alfa and beta, pegylated erythropoietin, and darbepoetin alfa, are administered to reduce transfusions in anemic CKD patients. A target hemoglobin of 9

TABLE 2 Criteria for Definition of Chronic Kidney Disease

Kidney damage for ≥3 months, as defined by structural or functional abnormalities of the kidney, with or without decreased GFR, that can lead to decreased GFR, manifest by either:
- Pathologic abnormalities
- Markers of kidney damage, including abnormalities in the composition of blood or urine, or abnormalities in imaging tests
- GFR <60 ml/min per 1.73 m^2 for ≥3 months, with or without kidney damage

GFR, Glomerular filtration rate.
From Floege J et al: *Comprehensive clinical nephrology*, ed 5, Philadelphia, 2015, Saunders.

TABLE 3 Classification of Chronic Kidney Disease Based on GFR

CKD Stage	Definition
1	Normal or increased GFR; some evidence of kidney damage reflected by microalbuminuria, proteinuria, and hematuria as well as radiologic or histologic changes
2	Mild decrease in GFR (89 to 60 ml/min per 1.73 m^2) with some evidence of kidney damage reflected by albuminuria, proteinuria, and hematuria as well as radiologic or histologic changes
3	GFR 59 to 30 ml/min per 1.73 m^2
3A	GFR 59 to 45 ml/min per 1.73 m^2
3B	GFR 44 to 30 ml/min per 1.73 m^2
4	GFR 29 to 15 ml/min per 1.73 m^2
5	GFR <15 ml/min per 1.73 m^2; when renal replacement therapy in the form of dialysis or transplantation must be considered to sustain life

Classification and prognosis of chronic kidney disease from 2012 KDIGO guidelines.
CKD, Chronic kidney disease; *GFR*, glomerular filtration rate; *KDIGO*, Kidney Disease: Improving Global Outcomes.
From Floege J et al: *Comprehensive clinical nephrology*, ed 5, Philadelphia, 2010, Saunders.

to 11 g/dl is reasonable to maintain quality-of-life, while avoiding premature and excessive ESA use. Higher hemoglobin values have been associated with adverse cardiovascular events. Iron sufficiency defined as transferrin saturation >20% and ferritin >100 ng/ml, must be present before initiating ESA therapy.

- Optimal diuretic therapy should be prescribed for edema or cardiopulmonary congestion.
- ACEIs or ARBs retard progression of CKD and lower blood pressure, but may reduce GFR and renal potassium excretion.

TABLE 4 Management Plan for Patients with Chronic Kidney Disease, According to Stage

Stage & GFR	Action	Clinical Testing	Treatment Considerations
1 **>90** **ml/min per 1.73 m^2**	Establish risk or etiology of CKD Diagnose and treat CVD risk factors and comorbid conditions	***eGFR**: Every* 12 mo **UA** with microscopic evaluation **UPC** if non-diabetic: *Every* 12 mo **UACR** if diabetic: *Every* 12 mo	**Consult** Nephrology if ***eGFR*** declines by ≥4 ml/min per yr **BP:** <130/80 mm Hg **Proteinuria:** UPC <0.2; UACR <30 mg/g with ACEI or ARB
2 **60-89** **ml/min per 1.73 m^2**	Estimate CKD progression rate Diagnose and treat CVD risk factors and comorbid conditions	***eGFR**: Every* 6-12 mo **CBC,** reticulocyte ct, TSAT, ferritin if Hb 10-12 g/dl: every 12 mo Annual Ca/P/PTH/25(OH)D evaluations **UACR** or **UPC:** *Every* 6-12 mo	**Avoid** nephrotoxins **Treat** Hypertension **Hb:** 10-12 g/dl, TSAT >20%, and ferritin >100 ng/ml **UACR:** <30 mg/g or UPC <0.2 with ACEI or ARB
3A **45-59** **ml/min per 1.73 m^2** **3B** **30-44** **ml/min per 1.73 m^2**	Estimate CKD progression rate Diagnose and treat CVD risk factors and comorbid conditions Kidney imaging study (e.g., US or CT) Consider Nephrology Consultation	**BP** monitoring**:** *Every* 3-6 mo ***eGFR**: Every* 6 months, if stable every 12 mo **CBC:** Hb <10 g/dl *every* 1-3 mo until Hb 9-12 g/dl; then *every* 3-6 mo **TSAT** and ferritin if Hb <13 g/dl (males) or 12 g/dl (females) and after therapy Baseline Ca/P/PTH/Alk Phos/25(OH)D Ca/P/PTH/Alk Phos, depending on baseline and CKD progression **25(OH)D,** depending on baseline and response to treatment **UPC or UACR:** *Every* 6-12 mo	**Avoid** nephrotoxins **Treat** Hypertension **Hb:** 9-12 g/dl, TSAT >20%, ferritin >100 ng/ml with p.o. and/or *iv* iron and/or erythropoiesis stimulating agent **Ca & P:** To normal range with P-binders **25(OH)D:** ≥30 ng/ml with vitamin D2/D3 **iPTH:** 130-600 pg/ml with calcitriol or vitamin D analogs if iPTH progressively increases **NaHCO3:** 22-26 mEq/L and titrate $NaHCO_3$ therapy **UPC:** <0.2 or UACR <30 mg/g with ACEI or ARB
4 **15-29 ml/min per 1.73 m^2**	Transition of management and care to Nephrology Initiate decisions regarding kidney replacement therapy, vascular access, and kidney transplant Diagnose and treat CVD risk factors and comorbid conditions Adjust drug dosing for CKD stage	**BP** monitoring**:** *Every* 3 mo ***eGFR**: Every* 3 mo **CBC,** TSAT, ferritin**:** *Every* 3-6 mo Baseline Ca/P/PTH/Alk Phos/25(OH)D; then repeat levels *every* 6-12 mo **UPC or UACR:** *Every* 3-6 mo	**ALL OF THE ABOVE PLUS** **CKD**-specific education: Kidney replacement therapy modality Immunizations: TIV, PPV-23, and HBV Reinforce dietary prescription Protect dominant (handwriting) arm Vascular access surgery evaluation

ACEI, Angiotensin-converting enzyme inhibitors; *ARB,* angiotensin-receptor blockers; *BP,* blood pressure; *CKD,* chronic kidney disease; *CT,* computed tomography; *ct,* count; *CVD,* cardiovascular disease; *eGFR,* estimated glomerular filtration rate; *HBV,* hepatitis B virus; *TSAT,* transferrin saturation; *UA,* urine analysis; *UACR,* urine albumin to creatinine ratio; *UPC,* urine protein test; *US,* ultrasonography.
CKD Stage 5 (GFR <15 ml/min per 1.73 m^2) patients require management by a nephrologist.
From Inker LA, Astor BC, Fox CH et al: *Am J Kidney Dis* 63(5);713–735, 2014.

TABLE 5 Nutritional Recommendations in Renal Disease

Daily Intake	Predialysis CKD	Hemodialysis	Peritoneal Dialysis
Protein (g/kg ideal BW) (see KDOQI for estimation of adjusted edema-free body weight)	0.6-1.0 Level depends on the view of the nephrologist 1.0 for nephrotic syndrome	1.1-1.2 This is a broad recommendation as protein intake would be individualized for the patient's nutritional status, serum phosphate levels, and dialysis adequacy	1.0-1.3
Energy (kcal/kg BW)	35 (<60 yr) 30-35 (>60 yr)	35 (<60 yr) 30-35 (>60 yr)	35 including dialysate calories (<60 yr) 30-35 including dialysate calories (<60 yr)
Sodium (mmol)	<100 (more if salt wasting)	<100	<100
Potassium	Reduce if hyperkalemic If hyperkalemic, advice will take the form of decreasing certain foods (e.g., some fruits and vegetables) and giving information about cooking methods	Reduce if hyperkalemic	Reduce if hyperkalemic; potassium restriction is generally not required
Phosphorus	Reduce; level dependent on protein intake Advice will take the form of reducing certain foods (e.g., dairy, offal, some shellfish) and giving information about the timing of binders with high-phosphorus meals and snacks		
Calcium	In CKD stages 3-5, total intake of elemental calcium (including dietary calcium) should not exceed 2000 mg/day	Total intake of elemental calcium (including dietary calcium) should not exceed 2000 mg/day	Total intake of elemental calcium (including dietary calcium) should not exceed 2000 mg/day

Recommendations are for typical patients but should always be individualized based on clinical, biochemical, and anthropometric indices. *BW,* Body weight; *CKD,* chronic kidney disease; *CRF,* chronic renal failure; *KDOQI,* Kidney Disease Outcomes Quality Initiative.
From Floege J et al: *Comprehensive clinical nephrology,* ed 5, Philadelphia, 2015, Saunders.

TABLE 6 Suggested Criteria for Referral of Patients with Chronic Kidney Disease to a Nephrologist

	NICE 2008	KDIGO 2012
Advanced CKD	Stage 4 and 5 CKD	Category G4 and G5 CKD
Proteinuria	High proteinuria: ACR ≥70 mg/mmol unless known to be caused by diabetes and appropriately treated	Consistent proteinuria: ACR ≥ 300 mg/g (≥30 mg/mmol)
Hematuria	Proteinuria (ACR ≥30 mg/mmol) together with hematuria	Urinary red cell casts, RBCs >20 per high-power field sustained; not readily explained
Progression of CKD	Rapidly declining eGFR: >5 ml/min per 1.73 m^2 in 1 yr >10 ml/min per 1.73 m^2 in 5 yr	Progression of CKD: Sustained decline in eGFR >5 ml/min per 1.73 m^2 in 1 yr Drop in GFR category with a ≥25% drop in eGFR from baseline
Uncontrolled hypertension	Hypertension that remains poorly controlled despite the use of at least four antihypertensive drugs at therapeutic doses	CKD and hypertension refractory to treatment with four or more antihypertensive agents
Hereditary kidney disease	Known or suspected rare or genetic causes of CKD	Hereditary kidney disease
Other conditions	Suspected renal artery stenosis	Recurrent or extensive nephrolithiasis Persistent abnormalities of serum potassium

ACR, Albumin-creatinine ratio; *eGFR*, estimated glomerular filtration rate; *KDIGO*, Kidney Disease: Improving Global Outcomes; *NICE*, National Institute for Health and Care Excellence; *PTH*, parathyroid hormone; *RBC*, red blood cell.

Data from: KDIGO 2012 clinical practice guideline for the evaluation and management of chronic kidney disease, *Kidney Int Suppl* 3:1–150, 2013; and National Institute for Health and Care Excellence: Chronic kidney disease: Early identification and management of chronic kidney disease in adults in primary and secondary care. http://publications.nice.org.uk/chronic-kidney-disease-cg73.

From Floege J et al: *Comprehensive clinical nephrology,* ed 5, Philadelphia, 2015, Saunders.

TABLE 7 When to Initiate Dialysis

Indications for early start on dialysis

- Intractable fluid overload
- Intractable hyperkalemia
- Malnutrition due to uremia
- Uremic neurologic dysfunction
- Uremic serositis
- Functional deterioration otherwise unexplained

Uremic cognitive dysfunction can affect learning

Therefore, home-based self-dialysis may need to start earlier than center-assisted dialysis.

Start of dialysis may be delayed if patient is

asymptomatic, awaiting imminent kidney transplant, awaiting imminent placement of permanent HD or PD access, or, after appropriate education, has chosen conservative therapy.

If start of dialysis is delayed,

patient should be reevaluated regularly to see if dialysis has become necessary.

Patients who choose PD

should not be required to have HD access placed, but venous sites for possible future HD access in arms should be preserved since HD may be required in the future.

Incremental start on PD may be considered if there is significant residual renal function.

Nephrologists should consider conservative (non-dialysis) treatment of kidney failure an integral part of their clinical practice.

HD, Hemodialysis; *PD*, peritoneal dialysis.

Modified from NKF KDOQI Clinical Practice Guideline for initiation of dialysis. http://www.kidney.org/professional/Kdoqi/guideline_upHD_PD_VA/pd_rec1.htm.

From Floege J et al: *Comprehensive clinical nephrology*, ed 5, Philadelphia, 2015, Saunders.

- Treat metabolic acidosis with oral sodium bicarbonate to attain a serum HCO_3 level of 22 to 26 mEq/L.
- Statin or a combination of statin and ezetimibe is recommended in adults aged ≥50 yr with eGFRs <60 ml/min per 1.73 m^2. Lipid management focuses on absolute risk for coronary events, and there are no target cholesterol levels.
- Therapy of mineral and bone disease in CKD is geared toward normalizing serum phosphorus concentration. Calcitriol and vitamin D analogs should be reserved for patients at CKD stages 4–5 and for those with severe and progressive hyperparathyroidism.
- Dietary phosphate restriction is recommended for nearly all CKD patients. For additional management of hyperphosphatemia, phosphate-binder therapy is recommended. Calcium-based phosphate binders, although inexpensive, should be restricted if total serum calcium is >10.2 mg/dl. Sevelamer carbonate and lanthanum carbonate are effective as phosphate binders but are more expensive. Two iron-based phosphate-binding agents, sucroferric oxyhydroxide and ferric citrate, have recently been approved by the FDA.
- Annual influenza vaccination for all adults with eGFRs <30 ml/min per 1.73 m^2. Those at high risk for pneumococcal infection should receive vaccination with polyvalent pneumococcal vaccine unless contraindicated. In addition, those at high risk of progression of CKD with eGFR <30 ml/min per 1.73 m^2 should undergo hepatitis B virus immunization to ensure seroconversion.

TABLE 8 Continuing Assessment of the Chronic Kidney Disease Patient

Kidney Function

Has kidney function declined?
Has kidney function declined at the predicted rate?
If not, are there exacerbating factors?
Should dialysis be started?
Are there life-threatening complications?
Pericarditis
Fluid overload
Resistant hypertension
Hyperkalemia
Uncompensated metabolic acidosis
Should access be created or transplantation planned?

Supportive Treatment

Can salt, potassium, and fluid balance be improved by diet or diuretics?
Is the phosphate controlled?
Is the dose of vitamin D compound appropriate?
Should erythropoietin (EPO) be prescribed?
Are nutritional supplements needed?
Does the patient need counseling?

Questions to be posed in evaluation of the patient.

From Floege J et al: *Comprehensive clinical nephrology,* ed 5, Philadelphia, 2010, Saunders.

- General considerations in the continuing assessment of the CKD patient as discussed previously are summarized in Table 8.

DISPOSITION

- Prognosis is related to CKD stage and burden of comorbid illness. Late referral of patients to a nephrologist is associated with greater morbidity and mortality. Despite recommendations for early referral, nearly two thirds of CKD patients are referred late.
- *Choosing Wisely* is an initiative of the American Board of Internal Medicine Foundation that aims to promote conversations between clinicians and patients by helping patients choose care that is supported by evidence and aims at avoiding wasteful or unnecessary medical tests, treatments, and procedures. The five American Society of Nephrology initiatives are summarized in Table E9.
- Genetic susceptibility for CKD is prominent in African Americans. Apolipoprotein E2 allele status predicts CKD progression, independent of diabetes, race, lipid, and non-lipid factors.
- Kidney transplantation in selected patients improves survival. Currently, the 2-yr kidney graft survival rate for living related donor transplantations is >80%, and the 2-yr graft survival rate for cadaveric donor transplantation is nearly 70%.
- Principles underlying withdrawal from dialysis treatment are described in Table E10.

SUGGESTED READINGS

Available at ExpertConsult.com

AUTHOR: **SNIGDHA T. REDDY, M.D.**

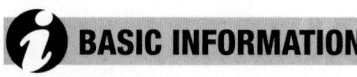

BASIC INFORMATION

DEFINITION

Chronic lymphocytic leukemia (CLL) is a lymphoproliferative disorder characterized by proliferation and accumulation of mature-appearing neoplastic B-cells.

SYNONYM

CLL

ICD-10-CM CODES

C91.10 Chronic lymphocytic leukemia of B-cell type not having achieved remission
C91.11 Chronic lymphocytic leukemia of B-cell type in remission
C91.12 Chronic lymphocytic leukemia of B-cell type in relapse

EPIDEMIOLOGY & DEMOGRAPHICS

- Most frequent form of leukemia in Western countries (20,940 new cases and 4510 deaths annually in the U.S.). Incidence rate is 5 per 100,000 person-yr, increasing to 17 cases per 100,000 at age 65. It is more common in patients with a family history of CLL or other lymphoid malignancy.
- Generally occurs in older patients: Median age at diagnosis in the U.S. is 70 yr.
- Male/female ratio of 2:1.
- CLL accounts for 1% of all cancers and 11% of all hematologic neoplasms.
- May be preceded by monoclonal B-cell lymphocytosis—a premalignant, asymptomatic condition with less than 5000 /mm^3 CLL-like cells circulating in the blood.

PHYSICAL FINDINGS & CLINICAL PRESENTATION

- At presentation most patients are asymptomatic. Many cases are diagnosed on the basis of incidentally discovered lymphocytosis.
- Symptoms include fatigue, recurrent infections (pneumonia, herpes zoster), enlarging lymph nodes.
- B symptoms (fever, weight loss, and drenching night sweats) occur in 10% of patients at presentation.
- Small diffuse lymphadenopathy and splenomegaly are typical findings on clinical examination, but they are absent in a majority of patients at diagnosis.
- A minority of CLL patients (<10%) may develop autoimmune hemolytic anemia or immune thrombocytopenia at diagnosis or during the course of the disease.
- At a rate of 1% per yr, CLL may undergo a histologic transformation into an aggressive lymphoma (Richter's transformation), characterized by a rapidly growing nodal mass, elevated LDH, and constitutional symptoms.

ETIOLOGY

Remains largely unknown. Accumulation of genetic defects causing resistance to apoptosis and chronic stimulation of the B-cell receptor by autoantigens or undefined microorganisms have been implicated.

Dx DIAGNOSIS

- The diagnosis of CLL requires presence of >5000/mm^3 clonal B-cells, for >3 months, with a characteristic immunophenotype on flow cytometry, which is essential for diagnosis.
- CLL cells are typically positive for CD5, CD19, CD23 and weakly positive for CD20, while they are negative for CD10, Cyclin D1, and CD103. In some cases, molecular studies for CLL-specific chromosomal alterations (deletion of chromosome 13q, 11q, 17p or trisomy 12) may be helpful.
- Table 1 describes the evaluation of CLL patients at diagnosis.

DIFFERENTIAL DIAGNOSIS

- Few acute infections with lymphocytosis (mononucleosis, pertussis).
- Other lymphoproliferative disorders that involve blood (can be distinguished using flow cytometry): Follicular lymphoma, mantle cell lymphoma, splenic marginal zone lymphoma, prolymphocytic leukemia, adult T-cell lymphoma/leukemia, hairy cell leukemia (Table 2).
- Acute lymphocytic leukemia can be differentiated by presence of lymphoblasts rather than mature lymphocytes.
- Persistent polyclonal B-cell lymphocytosis: A rare, benign condition affecting (predominantly female) middle-aged smokers.

LABORATORY TESTS

- Complete blood count demonstrates lymphocytosis with mature lymphocytes and characteristic "smudge cells" on the peripheral smear (Fig. 1); anemia and thrombocytopenia may be present in more advanced cases.
- Bone marrow examination is **not** indicated in most cases, except when differentiation between autoimmune cytopenias and marrow infiltration by CLL is difficult.
- Hypogammaglobulinemia and elevated lactate dehydrogenase may be present at the time of diagnosis.
- Cytogenetic evaluation (using fluorescent *in-situ* hybridization, FISH) is essential for prognostic assessment and optimal treatment selection.
- Other prognostic markers include: Mutational status of the immunoglobulin heavy chain variable region (*IGHV*, unmutated gene with >98% homology indicates poor prognosis), presence of CD38 or ZAP-70 (also associated with poor prognosis). Additional mutation analysis is gaining importance for identifying patients with worse prognosis (mutations in *TP53, NOTCH1, SF3B1,* and *BIRC3* genes).

TABLE 1 Evaluation of Chronic Lymphocytic Leukemia Patients at Diagnosis

History
- B symptom and fatigue assessment
- Infectious history assessment
- Occupational assessment for chemical exposure
- Familial history of CLL and lymphoproliferative disorders
- Preventive interventions for infections and secondary cancers

Physical Examination

Laboratory Assessment
- CBC with differential
- Morphology assessment of lymphocytes
- Chemistry, LFT enzymes, LDH
- Flow cytometry assessment to confirm immunophenotype of CLL
- Serum immunoglobulins
- Serum β_2M levels
- Interphase cytogenetics for del(17p13.1), del(11q22.3), del(13q14), del(6q21), and trisomy 12
- IGHV mutational analysis
- Stimulated metaphase karyotype (if available)

Selected Tests Under Certain Circumstances
- DAT, haptoglobin, reticulocyte count if anemia present
- CT scan if unexplained abdominal pain or enlargement present
- PET scan or biopsy (or both) if large nodal mass present
- BM aspirate and biopsy if cytopenias present
- Familial counseling if first-degree relative with CLL

Teaching
- Varicella zoster identification instruction
- Skin cancer identification
- Disease education (Leukemia and Lymphoma Society)

B symptoms, Fever, night sweats, weight loss; *BM,* bone marrow; β_2M, beta-2 microglobulin; *CBC,* complete blood count; *CLL,* chronic lymphocytic leukemia; *CT,* computed tomography; *DAT,* direct antiglobulin test; *IGHV,* immunoglobulin heavy chain variable region; *LDH,* lactate dehydrogenase; *LFT,* liver function test; *PET,* positron emission tomography.
From Hoffman R et al: *Hematology, basic principles and practice*, ed 7, Philadelphia, 2018, Elsevier.

STAGING

Staging reflects the clinical burden of disease and aids assessment of prognosis and treatment decision making. The historical staging systems by Rai and Binet remain in clinical use. They use **only** physical examination and the CBC (i.e., no scans). The modified Rai system distinguishes three risk groups:

- Low risk (lymphocytosis alone, or Stage 0)
- Intermediate risk (presence of lymphadenopathy, hepatomegaly or splenomegaly, formerly Stage I/II)
- High risk (presence of anemia with hemoglobin <11 g/dl, or thrombocytopenia with platelet count <100,000/mm³, formerly stage III/IV)

The Binet system divides CLL into three stages:

- Stage A: Involvement of <3 nodal areas (counting separately cervical, axillary, or inguinal lymph nodes, spleen, and liver)
- Stage B: Three or more areas involved
- Stage C: Presence of anemia (hemoglobin <10 g/dl) or thrombocytopenia (<100,000/mm³), independent of the areas involved

Prognosis in CLL can be determined using the CLL-International Prognostic Index (CLL-IPI), which includes five factors: 17p/*TP53* status, *IGVH* mutational status, serum beta-2-microglobulin, Rai/Binet stage (0/A versus others), and age >65 yr. Overall 5-yr survival varies from 93% for the low-risk group to 23% for the very high-risk group (Table 3).

TABLE 2 Diseases That Can Mimic Chronic Lymphocytic Leukemia

- Follicular lymphoma
- Mantle cell lymphoma
- Marginal zone lymphoma
- Hairy cell leukemia
- Acute lymphoblastic leukemia
- T-cell prolymphocytic leukemia
- Large granular natural killer or T-cell leukemia

From Hoffman R et al: *Hematology, basic principles and practice*, ed 7, Philadelphia, 2018, Elsevier.

IMAGING STUDIES

Imaging studies (CT or PET/CT scans) are not necessary for asymptomatic patients at diagnosis. They are obtained in case of clinical concerns for bulky internal adenopathy, Richter's transformation, or prior to starting chemotherapy.

Rx TREATMENT

- At present, there is no standard curative therapy for CLL, so treatment is only instituted for progressive or symptomatic disease (Table 4) with a goal of symptom relief and prolongation of life.
- "Watchful waiting" (i.e., observation without therapy) is the optimal strategy for all early-stage, asymptomatic patients outside of clinical trials because early chemotherapy provides no survival or quality-of-life benefit.
- Treatment with the Bruton tyrosine kinase (BTK) inhibitor ibrutinib or with immunochemotherapy is the standard of care for patients with symptoms related to disease, bulky adenopathy, rapidly increasing lymphocyte count, or progressive cytopenias (except for autoimmune cytopenias, which can be treated without chemotherapy).

ACUTE GENERAL Rx

- The initial chemotherapy is chosen depending on the patient's age, comorbidities, and CLL cytogenetics (Fig. 2).
- BTK inhibitor ibrutinib is the most effective first-line treatment strategy in every studied setting, demonstrating improved survival against aggressive immunochemotherapy in younger/fit patients, or against less intensive approaches in older patients. Its downsides include lack of complete remissions and need for long-term daily drug therapy. Combinations of ibrutinib with venetoclax are currently studied to achieve deep complete remissions that would allow discontinuation of therapy.
- Ibrutinib is typically prescribed at the dose of 420 mg daily and is associated with diarrhea, increased risk of hypertension, atrial fibrillation (10%), and occasional bleeding (particularly with concurrent anticoagulants).
- Immunochemotherapy with fludarabine, cyclophosphamide, and rituximab (FCR) results in complete remission in 72% of patients, with about 30% remaining in remission after 12 yr of follow-up. It may be considered for fit patients younger than 65 yr with unmutated *IGVH*, but is associated with high rates of toxicity.
- Immunochemotherapy with bendamustine and rituximab or with chlorambucil and obinutuzumab is an option for older patients, and provides at least a partial remission for most patients, with median progression-free survival of about 2 to 4 yr.
- CLL with deletion 17p or *TP53* mutation does not respond well to standard immunochemotherapy, and BTK inhibitors are the standard approach.
- Recurrent CLL is often characterized by acquired deletion or mutation of the *TP53* gene and can also be treated with a variety of salvage regimens:
  1. Ibrutinib for patients who did not receive it as first line of treatment;
  2. Venetoclax, an oral BCL2 inhibitor, in combination with rituximab or alone; venetoclax is characterized by a high response rate (79%) and risk of tumor lysis, requiring extremely careful dosing and monitoring in the first days of therapy;
  3. Idelalisib, an oral PI3K inhibitor;
  4. Anti-CD20 monoclonal antibodies: Ofatumumab, obinutuzumab, rituximab, alone or in combination with chemotherapy: Purine analogues (fludarabine, pentostatin), alkylating agents (bendamustine, cyclophosphamide, CHOP-like combinations);
  5. Alemtuzumab (anti-CD52 monoclonal antibody);
  6. High-dose methylprednisolone;
  7. Palliative radiation therapy to bulky lymph nodes or spleen.
- Allogeneic bone marrow transplantation is occasionally used for younger patients with recurrent, refractory, or ultra-high cytogenetic risk disease, but is associated with high rates of transplant-related mortality.

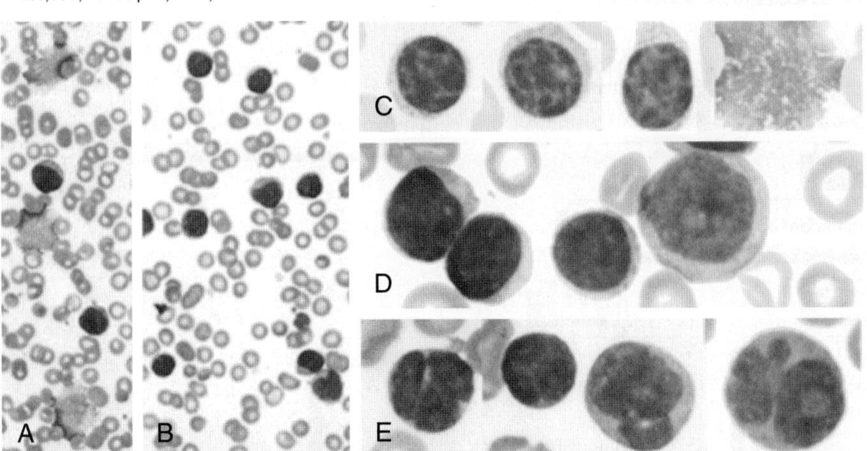

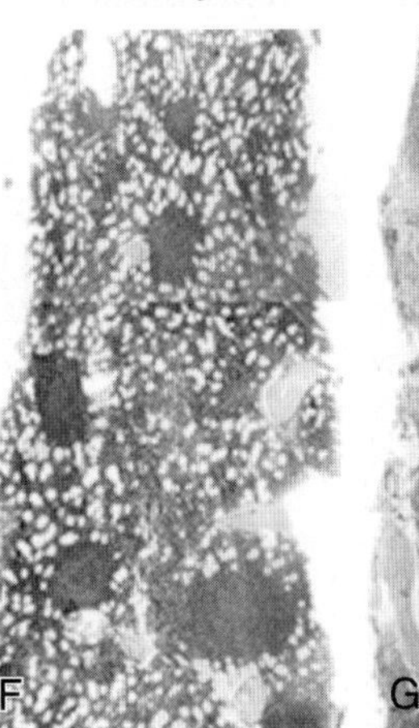

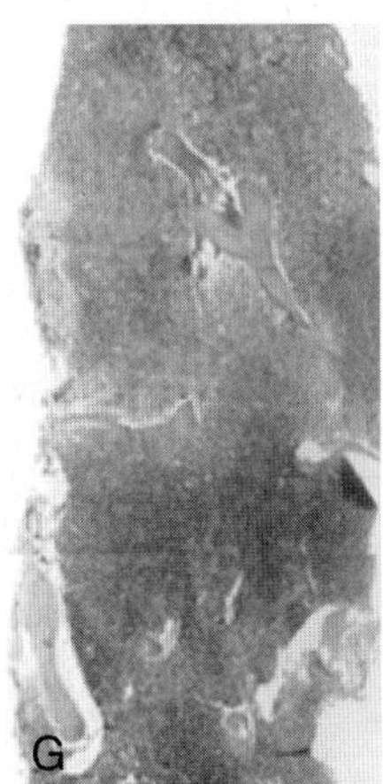

FIG. 1 Microscopic images of chronic lymphocytic leukemia. Peripheral blood smear **(A-E)** typically shows mature lymphocytes slightly larger than the red cells a with small amount of cytoplasm and smudge cells **(A)**. Bone marrow biopsy **(F, G)** shows hypercellularity with infiltration by the leukemic cells.

CHRONIC Rx

Treatment of systemic complications:

- Tumor lysis syndrome may occur during initial or subsequent chemotherapy but is extremely unlikely without chemotherapy in CLL, even with high lymphocyte counts.
- CLL patients are at increased risk of solid tumors and should adhere to age-appropriate screening modalities; skin cancers, including melanoma, are particularly common.
- Hypogammaglobulinemia is frequent in CLL and may cause recurrent infections, particularly pneumonias. Immunoglobulin supplementation (250 mg/kg IV every 4 wk) may prevent infections but has no effect on the course of CLL.
- Patients after chemoimmunotherapy are at risk for, and often ultimately succumb to, opportunistic infections. Herpes zoster and *Pneumocystis jiroveci* prophylaxis is used during and after some chemoimmunotherapy regimens.
- Novel targeted agents are associated with specific adverse effects during prolonged therapy. Ibrutinib may cause atrial fibrillation, chronic diarrhea, and hemorrhage and must be held before surgical procedures. Idelalisib may cause severe hepatitis and pneumonitis. Venetoclax may cause tumor lysis syndrome and neutropenia.
- Autoimmune hemolytic anemia, thrombocytopenia, and (rare) neutropenia may be treated with steroids, immunoglobulin, or immune suppression without cytotoxic chemotherapy.
- CLL is a contraindication to administration of live vaccines (varicella zoster, mumps/measles/rubella, yellow fever, intranasal influenza). Patients should adhere to the recommended schedule of immunization against *Pneumococcus* and influenza.

TABLE 3 Prognosis of Patients With CLL at the Time of Diagnosis, Stratified by the CLL-International Prognostic Index.

Number of high risk factors	Risk group	Percent of patients	Median time to first chemotherapy	Overall survival at 5 years
0-1	Low	38%	5-10 yr	93%
2-3	Intermediate	34%	4-5 yr	79%
4-6	High	23%	1-3 yr	63%
7-10	Very high	5%	<1 yr	23%

Risk factors include age >65 years (1 point), stage Rai I-IV or Binet B-C (1 point), unmutated *IGVH* (2 points), beta-2-microglobulin >3.5 mg/L (2 points), or deletion 17p/*TP53* mutation (4 points). *CLL,* Chronic lymphocytic leukemia.

TABLE 4 Modified Indications for Treatment of Chronic Lymphocytic Leukemia

- Grade 2 or greater fatigue limiting life activities
- B symptoms persisting for ≥2 weeks
- Lymph nodes >10 cm or progressively enlarging lymph nodes causing symptoms
- Spleen or liver with progressive enlargement or causing symptoms
- Anemia (hemoglobin <11 g/dl) referable to CLL
- Thrombocytopenia (platelets $<100 \times 10^{12}$/L) referable to CLL or ITP poorly responsive to traditional therapy
- Severe paraneoplastic (e.g., insect hypersensitivity, vasculitis, myositis) process related to CLL not responsive to traditional therapies

B symptoms, Fever, night sweats, weight loss; *CLL,* chronic lymphocytic leukemia; *ITP,* idiopathic thrombocytopenic purpura.
From Hoffman R et al: *Hematology, basic principles and practice,* ed 7, Philadelphia, 2018, Elsevier.

DISPOSITION

Most patients die due to infectious complications of therapy for refractory disease after several lines of treatment. Histologic transformation to an aggressive lymphoma is also associated with high mortality. Palliative treatment should be offered to patients who are no longer benefiting from aggressive therapy to avoid pervasive and futile treatment with distressing complications.

SUGGESTED READINGS

Available at ExpertConsult.com

RELATED CONTENT

Chronic Lymphocytic Leukemia (Patient Information)

AUTHOR: **ADAM J. OLSZEWSKI, M.D.**

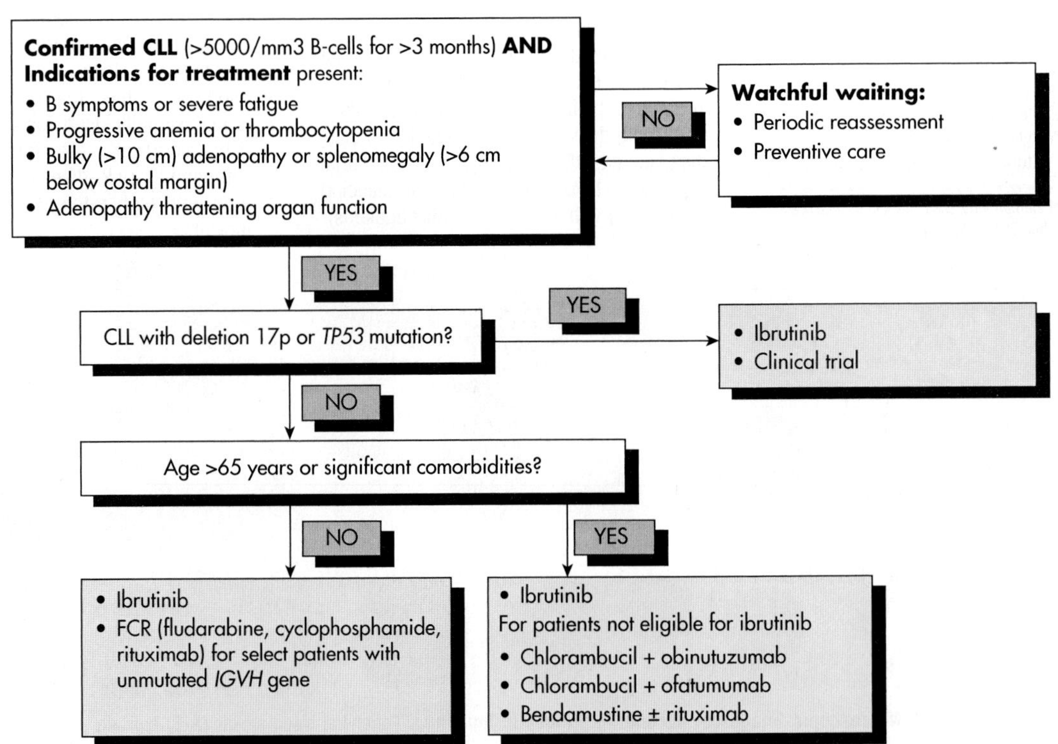

FIG. 2 Initial treatment approach in chronic lymphocytic leukemia. *CLL,* Chronic lymphocytic leukemia.(Courtesy of Adam J. Olszewski, M.D.)

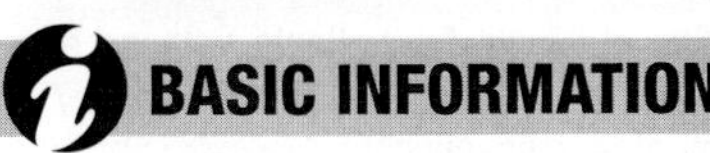

BASIC INFORMATION

DEFINITION

Chronic myelogenous leukemia (CML) is a malignant clonal stem disease characterized by the Philadelphia chromosome, an acquired cytogenetic abnormality arising out of the reciprocal translocation of long arms of the *ABL* and *BCR* genes on chromosomes 9 and 22. The resultant *BCR:ABL* fusion oncogene is associated with the development of abnormal myeloid proliferation and accumulation of immature granulocytes. The initial chronic phase (CP-CML) is marked by a myeloproliferative picture lasting months to yrs, which evolves into an advanced phase (AP-CML) characterized by poor response to therapy, worsening anemia, or thrombocytopenia; finally this phase then evolves into a terminal blast phase (BP-CML) resulting in acute leukemia (70% myeloid and approximately 30% lymphoid subtype). The WHO criteria for accelerated and blast phases of CML are described in Table 1.

SYNONYMS

CML
Chronic granulocytic leukemia
Chronic myeloid leukemia

ICD-10CM CODES

C92.10 Chronic myeloid leukemia, BCR/ABL-positive, not having achieved remission
C92.11 Chronic myeloid leukemia, BCR/ABL-positive, in remission
C92.12 Chronic myeloid leukemia, BCR/ABL-positive, in relapse

EPIDEMIOLOGY & DEMOGRAPHICS

- The median age for CML presentation is usually in the mid-50 yr range. It accounts for 15% to 20% of adult leukemias.
- Incidence is 1 to 1.5 cases per 100,000 people annually.
- In 2018, nearly 8430 new cases and more than 1090 deaths are estimated to occur in the U.S.

PHYSICAL FINDINGS & CLINICAL PRESENTATION

- Up to 50% patients are asymptomatic, with diagnosis based on abnormal blood counts.
- In chronic phase, symptomatic patients can have fatigue, weight loss, early satiety, and left abdomen pain. Examination can reveal splenomegaly. Occasionally, a very high WBC count may lead to hyperviscosity-related symptoms.
- Patients in accelerated phase are usually symptomatic with fevers, sweats, weight loss, abdomen pain, and progressive splenomegaly.
- Patients in blast phase in addition can have bone pain; symptoms of anemia, infectious complications, and bleeding are also present.

ETIOLOGY

The etiology of CML is unclear, though radiation exposure has been linked in its development.

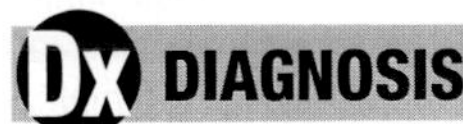

DIAGNOSIS

DIFFERENTIAL DIAGNOSIS

- Splenic lymphoma
- Myeloproliferative syndrome
- Chronic neutrophilic leukemia
- Essential thrombocythemia

LABORATORY TESTS

- CBC showing left-shifted myeloid cells, with the presence of precursor polymorphonuclear cells, basophils, and eosinophils; can be accompanied by thrombocytosis and anemia.
- Bone marrow biopsy demonstrates hypercellularity with granulocytic hyperplasia, increased ratio of myeloid cells to erythroid cells, and increased megakaryocytes (Fig. E1).
- Bone marrow cytogenetics demonstrated the 9:22 translocation (Philadelphia chromosome) in >95% of patients (Fig. 2).

TABLE 67.1 Who Criteria for Accelerated and Blast Phases of Chronic Myeloid Leukemia

Accelerated phase	Diagnosis can be made if one or more of the following is present:
	Blasts 10% to 19% of peripheral blood white cells or bone marrow cells
	Peripheral blood basophils at least 20%
	Persistent thrombocytopenia ($<100 \times 10^9$/L) unrelated to therapy, or persistent thrombocytosis ($>100 \times 10^9$/L) unresponsive to therapy
	Increasing spleen size and increasing WBC count unresponsive to therapy
	Cytogenic evidence of clonal evolution (i.e., the appearance of an additional genetic abnormality that was not present in the initial specimen at the time of diagnosis of CP CML)
	Megakaryocytic proliferation in sizable sheets and clusters, associated with marked reticulin or collagen fibrosis, and/or severe granulocytic dysplasia, should be considered as suggestive of AP CML. (These findings have not yet been analyzed in large clinical studies; thus, it is not clear whether they are independent criteria for AP. They often occur simultaneously with one or more of the other features listed.)
Blast crisis	Diagnosis can be made if one or more of the following is present:
	Blasts 20% or more of peripheral WBCs or bone marrow cells
	Extramedullary blast proliferation
	Large foci or clusters of blasts in bone marrow biopsy

AP, Accelerated phase; *CML,* chronic myeloid leukemia; *CP,* chronic phase; *WBC,* white blood cell.
Hoffman R et al. *Hematology: Basic Principles and Practice,* 7 ed, Philadelphia, 2018, Elsevier.

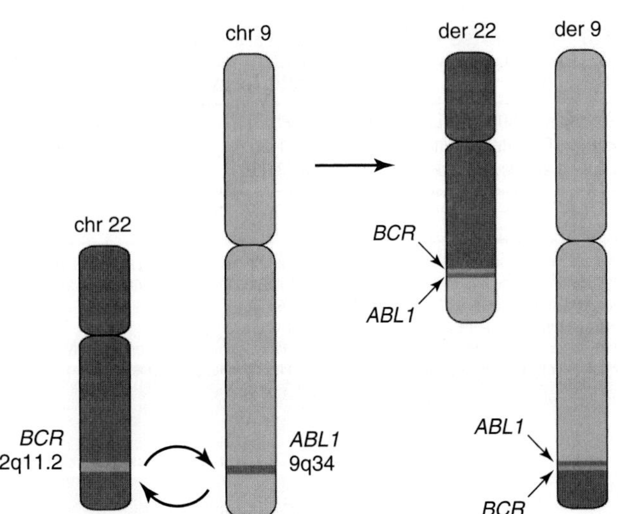

FIG. 2 The Philadelphia chromosome, der(22q), results from the reciprocal translocation of a portion of the *ABL1* gene on chromosome 9 at band q34 to the region of the *BCR* gene on chromosome 22 at band q11.2. In turn, a portion of *BCR* is translocated to chromosome 9 to the region of *ABL1*. In 5% to 10% of patients with chronic myelogenous leukemia, cryptic or complex rearrangements result in a *BCR-ABL1* fusion gene, even though no Philadelphia chromosome is detected cytogenetically. (From Jaffe ES et al: *Hematopathology,* Philadelphia, 2011, Saunders.)

- Leukocyte alkaline phosphatase is markedly decreased (unlike other myeloproliferative disorders).
- *BCR-ABL* fusion transcripts can be measured using quantitative RT-PCR technology using either peripheral blood or bone marrow; serial peripheral blood monitoring of transcript level is utilized at 3-month intervals to determine molecular remission status.

RISK STRATIFICATION

- Chronic phase CML patients can be stratified into low-, intermediate-, or high-risk criteria using the Sokal or Hasford criteria; more recently, the EUTOS score has been validated as an effective tool used to stratify patients into low- or high-risk categories.
- Patients developing secondary mutations have variable response to second- or third-line therapies; the T315I mutation is typically associated with resistance and is treated with allogeneic stem cell transplantation (SCT).

IMAGING STUDIES

Ultrasound or CT scan of abdomen can be done.

Rx TREATMENT

Treatment with a potential to either cure CML or prolong long-term survival should be used according to the phase of the disease.

- Chronic phase: The therapeutic approach involves the use of either a first-generation (imatinib) or second-generation (dasatinib, nilotinib, or bosutinib) oral tyrosine kinase inhibitor (TKI). The decision to select a particular TKI is based on patient comorbidities, age, and often formulary restrictions. The large majority of patients obtain hematologic and cytogenetic remissions; major molecular remissions are observed in 25%-60% cases. Patients who lose their initial response, develop secondary mutations, or develop intolerance to therapy can be treated with newer third-generation TKIs (bosutinib, ponatinib). Omacetaxine, a protein synthesis inhibitor, is also effective in patients who have previously received TKI therapy.
- Second-generation TKIs (dasatinib, nilotinib, or bosutinib) are preferred for patients with an intermediate- or high-risk Sokal or Hasford score, especially for young women whose goal is to achieve a deep and rapid molecular response and eventual drug discontinuation of TKI therapy for fertility purposes.
- During therapy for chronic phase CML, treatment efficacy is monitored by the use of serial RT-PCR to measure peripheral blood *BCR-ABL* transcripts every 3 to 6 months.
- Accelerated phase: Patients are initially treated with second-generation TKIs but ultimately require allogeneic SCT.
- Blast phase: Patients are initially treated with conventional induction chemotherapy as per the type of evolved acute leukemia and then subsequently undergo allogeneic SCT.
- Symptomatic hyperleukocytosis is treated with leukapheresis and hydroxyurea; allopurinol should be started to prevent urate nephropathy after the rapid lysis of the leukemia cells.

DISPOSITION

- Response definition and monitoring are summarized in Table 2.
- Median survival for patients with chronic phase CML undergoing therapy with current TKIs is estimated to last 25+ yr.
- Median survivals for patients with accelerated and blast phase CML are 5 yr and 7 to 11 months, respectively.
- Discontinuing oral TKI therapy in chronic phase CML patients who have achieved deep molecular remissions is associated with molecular relapses in up to half the cases; as such, indefinite therapy is preferred in all cases.

REFERRAL

To hematology physician.

PEARLS

- Chronic-phase CML patients should be risk-stratified at diagnosis to define prognosis upfront; patients achieving complete cytogenetic remission or major molecular remission by 12 months have consistently superior long-term outcomes.
- Regular monitoring of molecular response using peripheral blood RT-PCR for BCR:ABL transcript levels is done every 3 to 6 months for disease monitoring.
- Allogeneic stem cell transplantation is a useful modality for advanced CML patients and chronic phase CML patients who develop resistance to standard TKI therapy.

SUGGESTED READINGS

Available at ExpertConsult.com

RELATED CONTENT

Chronic Myelogenous Leukemia (Patient Information)

AUTHOR: **RITESH RATHORE, M.D.**

TABLE 67.2 Response Definition and Monitoring

Hematologic Response	Cytogenetic Response	Molecular Response
Complete: platelet count <450 × 10^9/L; WBC count <10 × 10^9/L; differential without immature granulocytes and with less than 5% basophils; nonpalpable spleen	Complete: Ph^+ 0 Major: Ph^+ 1-35% Minor: Ph^+ 36-65% Minimal: Ph^+ 66-95% None: Ph^+ <95%	Complete: *BCR-ABL* transcripts nonquantifiable and nondetectable[a] Major: ≤0.10%

BCR-ABL to control gene ratio according to the proposed international scale for measuring molecular response, with a standardized "baseline", as established in the IRIS trial, taken to represent 100% on the international scale, and a 3-log reduction from the standardized baseline (major molecular response) fixed at 0.10%.

[a]Qualified by the limit of sensitivity of the polymerase chain reaction assay employed.

ABL, Abelson leukemia virus; *BCR,* breakpoint cluster region; *Ph+,* Philadelphia chromosome positive; *WBC,* white blood cell.

Hoffman R et al. *Hematology: Basic Principles and Practice,* 7 ed, Philadelphia, 2018, Elsevier.

BASIC INFORMATION

DEFINITION

Chronic obstructive pulmonary disease (COPD) is an inflammatory respiratory disease usually caused by exposure to tobacco smoke. It is characterized by the presence of airflow limitation that is not fully reversible. The pathophysiology of COPD is related to enhanced inflammatory response to noxious particles and gases, chronic airway irritation, mucus production, and pulmonary scarring and changes in pulmonary vasculature.

Acute exacerbations and comorbidities contribute to the overall severity and prognosis of the disease in individual patients.

Traditionally, COPD was described as encompassing *emphysema*, characterized by loss of lung elasticity and destruction of lung parenchyma with enlargement of air spaces, and *chronic bronchitis*, characterized by obstruction of small airways and productive cough >3 months for more than 2 successive yrs. These terms are no longer included in the formal definition of COPD, although they are still used clinically. Although emphysema and chronic bronchitis are commonly associated with COPD, neither is required to make the diagnosis.

An overlap syndrome known as ACOS (asthma-COPD overlap syndrome), characterized by persistent airflow limitation with several features associated with asthma and several features associated with COPD, has been gaining recognition and may have treatment and mortality implications (Global Initiative for Chronic Obstructive Lung Disease (GOLD) and Global Initiative for Asthma (GINA) consensus statement).

SYNONYMS

COPD
Emphysema
Chronic bronchitis

ICD-10CM CODES

J42 Chronic bronchitis, unspecified chronic bronchitis type
J44.9 Chronic obstructive pulmonary disease, unspecified COPD type
J44.0 Chronic obstructive pulmonary disease with acute lower respiratory infection
J44.1 Chronic obstructive pulmonary disease with acute exacerbation
J43.0 Unilateral emphysema
J43.1 Panlobular emphysema
J43.2 Centrilobular emphysema
J43.8 Other emphysema
J43.9 Pulmonary emphysema, unspecified emphysema type

EPIDEMIOLOGY & DEMOGRAPHICS

- COPD affects 14% of U.S. adults aged 40 to 79 yr.
- Between 10% and 20% of COPD in the U.S. is due to occupational or other exposure to chemical vapors, irritants, and fumes; 80% to 90% is due to cigarette smoking.
- COPD is the third leading cause of death in the U.S.
- Highest incidence is in males >40 yr.
- 16 million office visits, 500,000 hospitalizations, 120,000 deaths annually, and >$18 billion in direct health care costs annually can be attributed to COPD.
- Patients with COPD living in isolated rural areas of the U.S. are at greater risk for COPD exacerbation-related mortality than those living in urban areas, independent of hospital rurality and volume.

PHYSICAL FINDINGS & CLINICAL PRESENTATION

- Patients with COPD have historically been classically subdivided in two major groups based on their phenotype:
  1. *Blue bloaters* are patients with chronic bronchitis; the name is derived from the bluish tinge of the skin (as a result of chronic hypoxemia and hypercapnia) and from the frequent presence of peripheral edema (from cor pulmonale); chronic cough with production of large amounts of sputum is characteristic.
  2. *Pink puffers* are patients with emphysema; they have a cachectic appearance but pink skin color (adequate oxygen saturation); shortness of breath is manifested by pursed-lip breathing and use of accessory muscles of respiration.
- COPD may present with combinations of the following signs and symptoms:
  1. Cyanosis, chronic cough (usually productive but may be intermittent and may be unproductive), tachypnea, tachycardia.
  2. Dyspnea (persistent, progressive), pursed-lip breathing with use of accessory muscles for respiration, decreased breath sounds, wheezing.
  3. Chronic sputum production.
  4. Chest wall abnormalities (hyperinflation, "barrel chest," protruding abdomen).
  5. Flattening of diaphragm.
- Systemic manifestations and comorbidities of COPD are described in Table 1.
- Acute exacerbation of COPD is mainly a clinical diagnosis and generally manifests with worsening dyspnea, increase in sputum purulence, and increase in sputum volume. Respiratory symptom status, however, is not a reliable indicator of the presence of airflow obstruction. Individuals with normal spirometry values may report respiratory symptoms, whereas individuals who have severe to very severe airflow obstruction by spirometry may report no symptoms. Individuals with sedentary lifestyles may underestimate their symptoms and careful history taking is important to elicit symptoms suggestive of COPD.

TABLE 1 Systemic Manifestations and Comorbidities of COPD

Cardiovascular	Infarction Arrhythmia Congestive heart failure Aortic aneurysm
Hypercoagulability	Stroke Pulmonary embolism Deep vein thrombosis Atrophy
Systemic	Weight loss Osteoporosis Skin wrinkling Anemia Fluid retention
Lung cancer	Depression

From Mason RJ: *Murray & Nadel's textbook of respiratory medicine*, 5th ed, Philadelphia, 2010, Saunders.

ETIOLOGY

- Tobacco exposure
- Occupational exposure to pulmonary toxins (e.g., dust, noxious gases, vapors, fumes, cadmium, coal, silica). The industries with the highest exposure risk are plastics, leather, rubber, and textiles.
- Atmospheric pollution.
- Alpha-1-antitrypsin deficiency (rare; <1% of COPD patients).

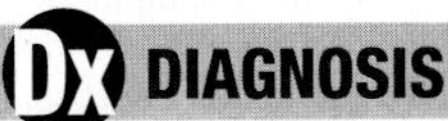

DIAGNOSIS

DIFFERENTIAL DIAGNOSIS

- Heart failure (HF)
- Asthma
- Tuberculosis, other respiratory infections
- Bronchiectasis
- Anemia
- Cystic fibrosis
- Neoplasm
- Pulmonary embolism
- Obliterative bronchiolitis
- Diffuse panbronchiolitis
- Sleep apnea, obstructive
- Hypothyroidism <50% predicted
- Neuromuscular disease

DIAGNOSTIC WORKUP

- Chest x-ray is seldom diagnostic but useful to visualize significant hyperinflation and to exclude alternative diagnosis (e.g., CHF, TB).
- Pulmonary function testing (spirometry). Measurement of airflow limitation (by forced expiratory volume in 1 second [FEV_1]) is recommended to confirm diagnosis and establish prognosis.
- Oxygen saturation and arterial blood gases (useful in selected patients with FEV_1 <50% predicted, with acute exacerbation or hypoxia by pulse oximetry).
- Alpha-1-antitrypsin: All patients with COPD should be screened one time for alpha-1 antitrypsin deficiency.

LABORATORY TESTS

- CBC: Generally not helpful, may reveal leukocytosis with left shift during acute exacerbation and secondary polycythemia in COPD with significant, chronic hypoxia. Recent trials have shown that eosinophilia in COPD patients predicts response to corticosteroids. Eosinophilia may also be found in an acute exacerbation in an asthma-COPD overlap syndrome.
- Sputum may be purulent with bacterial respiratory tract infections. Sputum staining

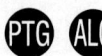

and cultures are usually reserved for cases refractory to antibiotic therapy.

- Arterial blood gases: Normocapnia, mild to moderate hypoxemia may be present. ABGs and pulse oximetry are usually used to determine if a patient is a candidate for long-term oxygen therapy or if hypercapnia is present (ABGs).
- Spirometry pulmonary function testing (PFT) with measurement of forced vital capacity (FVC) and forced expiratory volume in 1 s (FEV_1). Spirometry should be obtained to diagnose airflow obstruction in clinically stable patients with respiratory symptoms. It should not be used to screen for airflow obstruction in individuals without respiratory symptoms. Spirometry reveals that the primary physiologic abnormality in COPD is an accelerated decline in FEV_1 from the normal rate in adults >30 yr of approximately 30 ml/yr to nearly 60 ml/yr. PFT results in COPD reveal abnormal diffusing capacity, increased total lung capacity and/or residual volume, and fixed reduction in FEV_1 in patients with emphysema; normal diffusing capacity and reduced FEV_1 are found in patients with chronic bronchitis. Stage and severity of COPD according to post-bronchodilator spirometry are described in Table 2. It is important to note that FEV_1 does not correlate well with individual patients' severity of dyspnea, exercise limitations, or health status. Evaluation of patients should also focus on symptom control and risk for adverse events in addition to FEV_1.
- Patients with COPD can generally be distinguished from asthmatics by their incomplete response to short-acting beta agonist (change in FEV_1 <200 ml and 12%) and absence of an abnormal bronchoconstrictor response to methacholine or other stimuli. Nearly 40% of patients with COPD will, however, respond to bronchodilators. Similarly, patients without a smoking history but with chronic asthmatic bronchitis may have airflow obstruction that is not completely reversible.

ASSESSMENT

The global initiative for chronic obstructive lung disease (GOLD) assigns patients with COPD into four groups (A, B, C, D) based on (1) the degree of airflow restriction (Table 2), (2) a patient symptom score using one of two symptom questionnaires (CAT or mMRC), or (3) the number of COPD exacerbations in one yr.[1]

IMAGING STUDIES

Chest x-ray:

- Hyperinflation with flattened diaphragm, tenting of the diaphragm at the rib, and increased retrosternal chest space (Fig. 1)
- Decreased vascular markings and bullae in patients with emphysema
- Thickened bronchial markings and enlarged right side of the heart in patients with chronic bronchitis
- Computed tomography: Emphysematous lung, tracheobronchomalacia

Rx TREATMENT

NONPHARMACOLOGIC THERAPY

- Smoking cessation and elimination of air pollutants.
- Vaccination (pneumococcal vaccine and annual influenza vaccine).
- Supplemental oxygen, usually through a face mask/nasal cannula, to ensure oxygen saturation >90% as measured by pulse oximetry. Continuous oxygen therapy should be prescribed for patients with COPD who have arterial partial pressure of oxygen 55 mm Hg or less, or oxygen saturation 88% or less as measured by pulse oximetry. In patients with stable COPD and moderate resting desaturation (SpO2 89 to 93%) or moderate exercise-induced moderate desaturation (during the 6-minute walk test, Spo2 ≥80% for ≥5 minutes and <90% for ≥10 seconds), long-term supplemental oxygen did not improve mortality or time to first hospitalization.
- Pulmonary secretion clearance: Careful nasotracheal suction is indicated only in patients with excessive secretions and an inability to expectorate. Mechanical percussion of the chest as applied by a physical or respiratory therapist is ineffective with acute exacerbations of COPD.
- Pulmonary rehabilitation should be considered in COPD patients who remain symptomatic despite optimal medical management. Medicare will cover up to 36 sessions of pulmonary rehabilitation in COPD patients.
- Weight loss in obese patients.
- Identification of depression in patients newly diagnosed with COPD is important, as it may be associated with decreased adherence to maintenance therapy of COPD (Albrecht JS, et al: *Ann Am Thorac Soc* 13(9):1497-1594, 2016).
- Use of continuous positive airway pressure (CPAP) in patients with COPD and obstructive sleep apnea, as it improves both survival and reduces hospital admissions.

TABLE 2 Stage and Severity of COPD According to Postbronchodilator Spirometry

GOLD Stage and Severity	Definition
I: Mild	FEV_1/FVC <0.70, FEV_1 ≥80% of predicted
II: Moderate	FEV_1/FVC <0.70, 50%≤FEV_1 <80% of predicted
III: Severe	FEV_1/FVC <0.70, 30%≤FEV_1 <50% of predicted
IV: Very severe	FEV_1/FVC <0.70, FEV_1 <30% of predicted or FEV_1 <50% of predicted plus chronic respiratory failure

FEV_1, Forced expiratory volume in 1 sec; *FVC*, forced vital capacity.
Data from the Global Initiative for Chronic Obstructive Lung Disease, 2017 Report.

GENERAL Rx

- Pharmacologic treatment should be administered in a stepwise approach according to the severity of disease and patient's tolerance for specific drugs. When using the GOLD assessment criteria, pulmonary rehabilitation is recommended for patients in groups B, C, and D. Those in group A should receive a

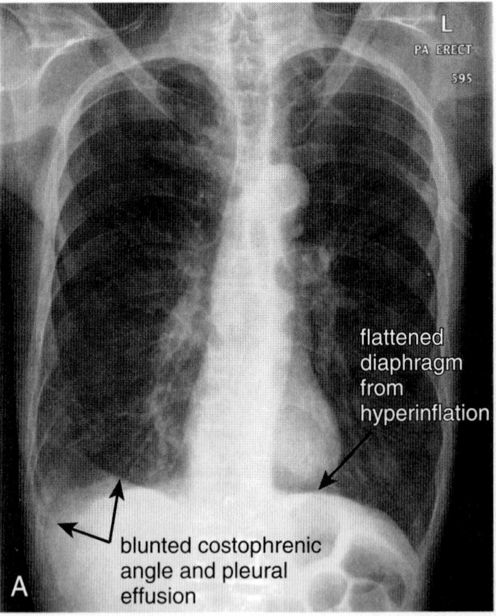

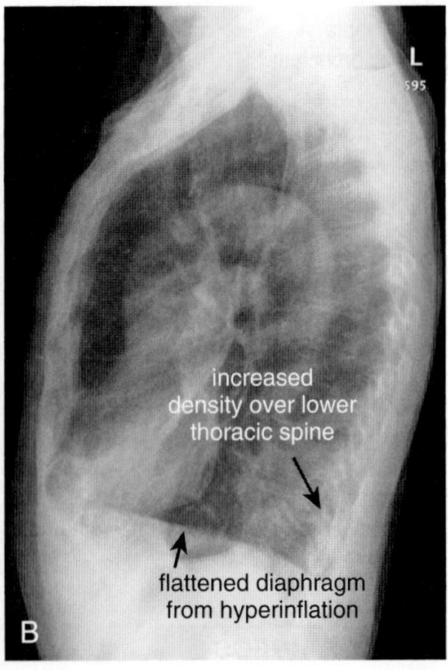

FIG. 1 Chronic obstructive pulmonary disease (COPD). A, Posterior-anterior (PA) upright chest x-ray. **B,** Lateral upright chest x-ray. This 63-year-old man with a history of COPD presented with 2 weeks of worsening cough with yellow sputum and dyspnea. His oxygen saturation was 87% in the emergency room. He has evidence of hyperinflation with flat diaphragms (particularly evident on the lateral x-ray, **(B)**. The patient also has a blunted right costophrenic angle with an apparent effusion and increased densities in both the right and the left lung base **(A)**. The lateral x-ray also shows increased density overlying the inferior thoracic spine, an abnormal spine sign. (From Broder JS: *Diagnostic imaging for the emergency physician*, Philadelphia, 2011, Saunders.)

[1] Lee H, Kim J, Tagmazyan K: Treatment of stable chronic obstructive pulmonary disease: the GOLD guidelines, *Am Fam Physician* 88(10):655-663, 2013.

short-acting or long-acting anticholinergic or β_2-agonist for mild intermittent symptoms. For patients in group B, long-acting anticholinergics or long-acting β_2-agonists should be added, and both if symptoms persist on one drug. Patients in group C or D are at high risk of exacerbations and should receive a long-acting anticholinergic or a combination of either an inhaled corticosteroid and a long-acting β_2-agonist or a long-acting anticholinergic and long-acting bronchodilator if symptoms persist. Patients in group D are more complicated and require individual management, multiple drugs, and consideration of roflumilast and azithromycin.

1. Bronchodilators improve symptoms, quality of life, and exercise tolerance and decrease incidence of exacerbations. Inhaled bronchodilators *should be offered* for stable COPD patients with respiratory symptoms and FEV_1 between 60% and 80% of predicted. Long-acting bronchodilators are *recommended* for stable COPD patients with respiratory symptoms and FEV_1 <60% of predicted. Recent guidelines from ACP, ACCP, ATS, and ERS recommend that clinicians prescribe monotherapy using either long-acting inhaled anticholinergics or long-acting inhaled β-agonists for symptomatic patients with COPD and FEV_1 <60% of predicted. Clinicians should base the choice of specific monotherapy on patient preference, cost, and adverse effect profile. Long-acting inhaled bronchodilators are superior to short-acting bronchodilators when taken as needed.
2. Short-acting β_2-agonists (e.g., albuterol metered-dose inhaler 1 to 2 puffs q4 to 6h prn) or short-acting anticholinergic agents (e.g., ipratropium inhaler 2 puffs qid) are acceptable in patients with mild, variable symptoms. Anticholinergics (antimuscarinic agents) are also effective and are available in combination with albuterol (e.g., Combivent). Long-acting inhaled agents are preferred in patients with mild to moderate or continuous symptoms. Tiotropium is an excellent long-acting bronchodilator. It is very effective for long-term, once-a-day use. It has been shown to be superior to salmeterol, an inhaled long-acting β-agonist (LABA) in patients with moderate to severe COPD and may possibly slow the rate of decline in FEV1. Some recent trials, however, have shown higher hospitalization rates and mortality with tiotropium compared to LABAs. Indacaterol, umeclidinium, olodaterol, and vilanterol are other available LABAs for long-term maintenance treatment of bronchospasm associated with COPD. Indacaterol provides the convenience of once-daily dosing. Aclidinium, unlike tiotropium, is another long-acting anticholinergic that is predominantly renally excreted and can be used safely in renal impairment. Olodaterol is also for once-a-day use. As with other LABAs, these medications should not be used with other sympathomimetic drugs, medications that can prolong the QT interval, or beta-blockers. LABAs and long-acting antimuscarinic agents (LAMAs) in different combinations are now available on the market. Although LAMAs and LABAs perform equally well for symptom control, LAMAs are generally preferred for symptom control.
3. Addition of inhaled steroids (fluticasone, budesonide, triamcinolone) is used to reduce exacerbations in patients with moderate to severe COPD. Inhaled steroids are reserved for patients with either ≥2 exacerbations annually or FEV_1 <50% of predicted. The role of inhaled corticosteroids (ICS) in COPD is controversial. Although some trials have demonstrated mild improvement in patients' symptoms and decreased frequency of exacerbations, most pulmonologists believe that these drugs are ineffective in most patients with COPD but should be considered for patients with moderate to severe airflow limitation who have persistent symptoms despite optimal bronchodilator therapy. ICS therapy does not affect 1-yr all-cause mortality among patients with COPD and is associated with a higher risk of pneumonia.
4. Roflumilast is a selective oral PDE4 inhibitor useful to reduce the risk of COPD exacerbations in patients with severe COPD associated with chronic bronchitis and a history of exacerbations. It is not a bronchodilator and is not indicated for the relief of acute bronchospasm.
5. Recent guidelines from ACP (American College of Physicians), ACCP (American College of Chest Physicians), ATS (American Thoracic Society), and ERS (European Respiratory Society) suggest that clinicians may administer combination inhaled therapies for symptomatic patients with stable COPD and FEV_1 <60% predicted. They also recommend that clinicians should prescribe pulmonary rehabilitation for symptomatic patients with an FEV_1 <50% predicted and continuous oxygen therapy in patients with COPD who have resting hypoxemia (PaO_2 <55 mm Hg or SpO_2 <88%).
6. Chronic antibiotic therapy: Chronic antibiotic therapy, specifically macrolide such as azithromycin, should be considered in patients with frequent acute exacerbations of COPD despite optimal therapy with bronchodilators and antiinflammatory agents.
7. Systemic glucocorticoid therapy: Chronic systemic glucocorticoid therapy is generally not recommended even in severe COPD due to associated increase in mortality and morbidity.
8. Triple therapy (two long-acting bronchodilators and an inhaled corticosteroid): A double-blind, parallel group, RCT (TRINITY) reported that treatment with extrafine fixed triple therapy reduced rates of moderate-to-severe exacerbation and improved baseline FEV_1 at 52 weeks as compared with tiotropium in patients with symptomatic COPD, FEV1 <50%, and a history of exacerbations. Another double-blind RCT (FULFIL) reported similar benefits of single-inhaler triple therapy compared with ICS/LABA therapy in patients with advanced COPD.

- Acute exacerbation of COPD (increase in sputum volume and purulence, worsening dyspnea) can be treated with:
  1. Aerosolized β_2-agonists (e.g., metaproterenol nebulizer solution 5% 0.3 ml or albuterol nebulized 5% solution 2.5 to 5 mg).
  2. Anticholinergic agents, which have equivalent efficacy to inhaled beta-adrenergic agonists. Inhalant solution of ipratropium bromide 0.5 mg can be administered every 4 to 8 hr.
  3. Short courses of systemic corticosteroids have been shown to improve spirometric and clinical outcomes. Treatment failure occurs less often in patients who receive low-dose steroids than in those receiving high-dose parenteral steroids. Oral prednisone 40 mg/day for 5 to 14 days is generally effective. Courses of treatment that are extended for >14 days confer no added benefit and increase the risk of adverse events. Trials have shown that in patients with acute COPD exacerbations, systemic glucocorticoid treatment for 5 days is not inferior to treatment for 14 days.
  4. Use of noninvasive positive pressure ventilation (NIPPV) decreases the risk of endotracheal intubation and decreases intensive care unit admission rates. Contraindications to its use are uncooperative patient, decreased level of consciousness, hemodynamic instability, inadequate mask fit, and severe respiratory acidosis. Increased airway pressure can be delivered by using inspiratory positive airway pressure, continuous positive airway pressure, or bilevel positive airway pressure, which combines the other modalities. When using NIPPV, the nasal mask is usually tolerated the best; however, patients must be instructed to keep their mouths closed while breathing with the nasal apparatus. Oxygen can be delivered at 10 to 15 L/min and started in spontaneous ventilation mode with an initial expiratory positive airway pressure setting of 3 to 5 cm H_2O and an inspiratory positive airway pressure setting of up to 10 cm H_2O. Adjustments in these settings should be made in 2-cm H_2O increments. It is important to monitor patients with frequent vital signs measurements, arterial blood gases, or pulse oximetry. Intubation and mechanical ventilation may be necessary if previous measures fail to provide improvement.
  5. IV aminophylline administration is controversial and generally not recommended. When used in patients with refractory symptoms, serum levels should be closely monitored (keep level 8 to 12 mcg/ml) to minimize risks of tachyarrhythmias.
- Approximately 50% of COPD exacerbations are caused by bacterial infection. Antibiotics are indicated in suspected bacterial respiratory infection (e.g., increased purulence and volume of phlegm).

 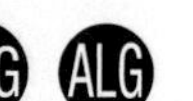

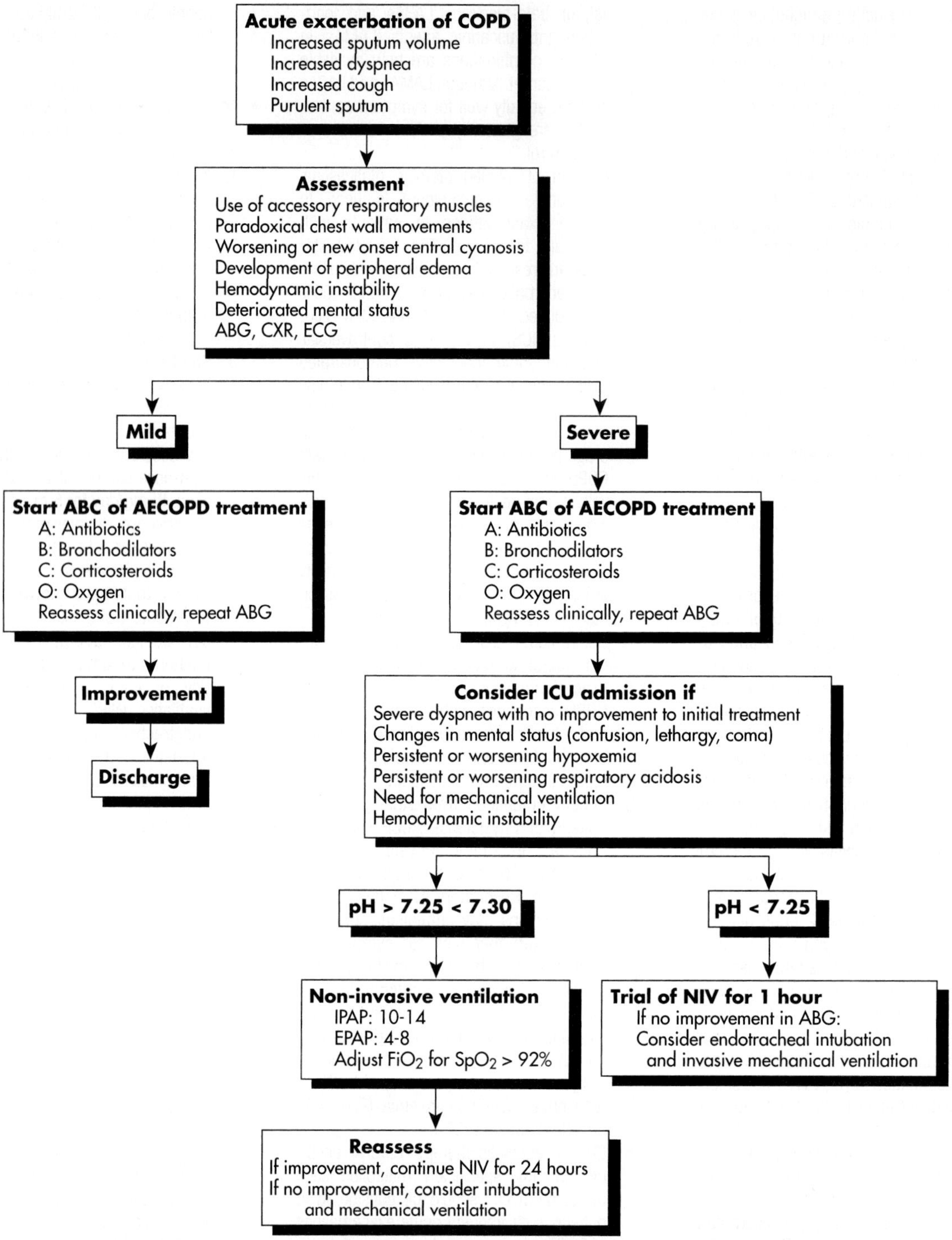

Acute exacerbation of COPD
Increased sputum volume
Increased dyspnea
Increased cough
Purulent sputum

↓

Assessment
Use of accessory respiratory muscles
Paradoxical chest wall movements
Worsening or new onset central cyanosis
Development of peripheral edema
Hemodynamic instability
Deteriorated mental status
ABG, CXR, ECG

Mild

↓

Start ABC of AECOPD treatment
A: Antibiotics
B: Bronchodilators
C: Corticosteroids
O: Oxygen
Reassess clinically, repeat ABG

↓

Improvement

↓

Discharge

Severe

↓

Start ABC of AECOPD treatment
A: Antibiotics
B: Bronchodilators
C: Corticosteroids
O: Oxygen
Reassess clinically, repeat ABG

↓

Consider ICU admission if
Severe dyspnea with no improvement to initial treatment
Changes in mental status (confusion, lethargy, coma)
Persistent or worsening hypoxemia
Persistent or worsening respiratory acidosis
Need for mechanical ventilation
Hemodynamic instability

pH > 7.25 < 7.30

↓

Non-invasive ventilation
IPAP: 10-14
EPAP: 4-8
Adjust FiO_2 for SpO_2 > 92%

↓

Reassess
If improvement, continue NIV for 24 hours
If no improvement, consider intubation and mechanical ventilation

pH < 7.25

↓

Trial of NIV for 1 hour
If no improvement in ABG:
Consider endotracheal intubation and invasive mechanical ventilation

FIG. 2 Management of acute exacerbations of chronic obstructive pulmonary disease. *ABG*, Arterial blood gas; *AECOPD*, acute exacerbation of chronic obstructive pulmonary disease; *CXR*, chest x-ray; *ECG*, electrocardiogram; *EPAP*, expiratory positive airway pressure; *FiO_2*, fraction of inspired oxygen; *ICU*, intensive care unit; *IPAP*, inspiratory positive airway pressure; *NIV*, noninvasive ventilation; *SpO_2*, the saturation of arterial blood with oxygen as measured by pulse oximetry.(From Parrillo JE, Dellinger RP: *Critical care medicine, principles of diagnosis and management in the adult*, ed 4, Philadelphia, 2014, Elsevier.)

1. *Haemophilus influenzae* and *Streptococcus pneumoniae* are frequent causes of acute bronchitis.
2. Oral antibiotics of choice are azithromycin, levofloxacin, amoxicillin-clavulanate, trimethoprim-sulfamethoxazole, doxycycline, and cefuroxime.
3. The two best predictors of potential benefit from antibiotics are purulent sputum and C-reactive protein (CRP) level >40 mg/L.
4. Procalcitonin-based protocols to trigger antibiotic use are associated with significantly decreased antibiotic use without affecting clinical outcomes such hospital length of stay, treatment failure, and mortality.

- Guaifenesin may improve cough symptoms and mucus clearance; however, mucolytic medications are generally ineffective. Their benefits may be greatest in patients with more advanced disease.
- Fig. 2 illustrates the management of acute exacerbations of COPD. Guideline recommendations for hospital management of COPD exacerbations are described in Table 3. Indications for invasive mechanical ventilation are described in Box 1.

TABLE 3 Guideline Recommendations for Hospital Management of COPD Exacerbations

	Global Initiative for Chronic Obstructive Lung Disease*	American Thoracic Society/ European Respiratory Society†	National Institute for Clinical Excellence‡
Date of statement	2017	2017	2010
Diagnostic testing	Chest radiograph, oximetry, ABGs, ECG. Other testing as warranted by clinical indication.	Chest radiograph, oxygen saturation, ABGs, ECG, sputum Gram stain and culture.	Chest radiograph, ABG, ECG, complete blood count, sputum smear and culture, blood cultures if febrile.
Bronchodilator therapy	Inhaled short-acting β_2-agonist is recommended. Consider ipratropium if inadequate clinical response. Methylxanthamines are not recommended due to increased side effect profiles.	Inhaled short-acting β_2-agonist and/ or ipratropium with spacer or nebulizer, as needed.	Administer inhaled drugs by nebulizer or handheld inhaler. Specific agents and dosing regimens not specified. Consider theophylline if inadequate response to inhaled bronchodilators.
Antibiotics	Recommended if (1) increases in dyspnea, sputum volume, and sputum purulence all are present; (2) increase in sputum purulence along with increase in either dyspnea or sputum volume; or (3) need for assisted ventilation. See original document for complex treatment algorithm.	Base choice on local bacterial resistance patterns. Consider amoxicillin/clavulanate or respiratory fluoroquinolones. If *Pseudomonas* species and/or other Enterobacteriaceae are suspected, consider combination therapy.	Administer only if history of purulent sputum. Initiate with an aminopenicillin, a macrolide, or a tetracycline, taking into account local bacterial resistance patterns. Adjust therapy according to sputum and blood cultures.
Systemic corticosteroids	Daily prednisolone 30-40 mg (or its equivalent) orally for not more than 5-7 days.	Daily prednisone 30-40 mg orally for 10-14 days. Equivalent dose intravenously if unable to tolerate oral intake. Consider inhaled corticosteroids.	Daily prednisolone 30 mg (or its equivalent) orally for 7-14 days.
Supplemental oxygen	Maintain oxygen saturation >90%. Monitor ABGs for hypercapnia and acidosis.	Maintain oxygen saturation >90%. Monitor ABGs for hypercapnia and acidosis.	Maintain oxygen saturation within the individualized target range. Monitor ABGs.
Assisted ventilation	Indications for NPPV include severe dyspnea, acidosis (pH ≤7.35) and/or hypercapnia (PCO_2 >45 mm Hg), and respiratory rate >25 breaths/min. Contraindications to NPPV include respiratory arrest, hemodynamic instability, impaired mental status, copious bronchial secretions, and extreme obesity. Intubate if contraindication to NPPV or failure of NPPV (worsening ABGs or clinical status). Consider likelihood of recovery and patient's wishes and expectations before intubation.	Consider with pH <7.35 and PCO_2 >45-60 mm Hg and respiratory rate >24 breaths/min. Institute NPPV in a controlled environment, unless there are contraindications (e.g., respiratory arrest, hemodynamic instability, impaired mental status, copious bronchial secretions, and extreme obesity). Intubate if contraindication to NPPV or failure of NPPV (worsening ABGs or clinical status).	NPPV treatment of choice for persistent hypercapnic respiratory failure. Consider functional status, body mass index, home oxygen, comorbidities, prior ICU admissions, age, and FEV_1 when assessing suitability for intubation and ventilation.

ABGs, Arterial blood gases; *ECG,* electrocardiogram; *FEV_1,* forced expiratory volume in 1 sec; *ICU,* intensive care unit; *NPPV,* noninvasive positive pressure ventilation.
*Data from http://www.goldcopd.com.
†Data from MacNee W. Standards for the diagnosis and treatment of patients with COPD: a summary of the ATS/ERS position paper. *Eur Respir J* 23:932-946, 2004.
‡Data from http://www.nice.org.uk.

BOX 1 Indications for Invasive Mechanical Ventilation

Severe dyspnea, with use of accessory muscles and paradoxical abdominal motion
Respiratory frequency >35 breaths/min
Life-threatening hypoxemia (Pao_2 <40 mm Hg or Pao_2/Fio_2 <200 mm Hg)
Severe acidosis (pH <7.25) and hypercapnia ($Paco_2$ >60 mm Hg)
Respiratory arrest
Somnolence, impaired mental status
Cardiovascular complications (hypotension, shock, heart failure)
Other complications: Metabolic abnormalities, sepsis, pneumonia, pulmonary embolism, barotrauma, massive pleural effusion
Noninvasive positive-pressure ventilation failure (or exclusion criteria)
Fio_2, Inspired oxygen fraction; *$Paco_2$*, partial pressure of carbon dioxide in arterial blood; *Pao_2*, partial pressure of oxygen in arterial blood.

From Vincent JL, et al.: *Textbook of critical care*, ed 6, Philadelphia, 2011, Saunders.

- Lung volume reduction surgery has been proposed as a palliative treatment for severe emphysema. Overall it increases the chance of improved exercise capacity but does not confer a survival advantage over medical therapy. It is most beneficial in patients with both predominantly upper-lobe emphysema and low baseline exercise capacity.
- Preliminary trials involving lung volume reduction using bronchoscopic treatment with nitinol coils have shown improved exercise capacity in patients with severe emphysema (Deslee G, et al.: *JAMA* 315[2]:175-184, 2016). Selection criteria for lung volume reduction surgery is described in Table 4. Box 2 summarizes indications and contraindications for lung volume reduction surgery and lung transplantation.
- Endobronchial valve (EBV) placement (Zephyr valve) via bronchoscopy to reduce lung volume with one-way valves that are allowed to leave but not enter a lung segment is now FDA approved since June 2018. (Klooster K, et al.: *NEJM* 373:2325, 2015).
- Single-lung transplantation (Box 2) should be considered a surgical option in patients with end-stage emphysema who have an FEV_1 <25% of predicted normal value after administration of bronchodilator and additional complications such as severe hypoxemia, hypercapnia, and pulmonary hypertension.

DISPOSITION

- After the initial episode of respiratory failure, 5-yr survival is approximately 25%.
- Development of cor pulmonale or hypercapnia and persistent tachycardia are poor prognostic indicators.
- The need for oxygen at rest may be the strongest predictor of mortality in chronic respiratory failure from COPD.

TABLE 4 Selection Criteria for Lung Volume Reduction Surgery

Inclusion Criteria	Exclusion Criteria
General	
Disability despite maximal rehabilitation	Inability to participate in rehabilitation
Cessation of tobacco use >6 mo	Continued use of tobacco
Patient's expectation of goals reasonable	Significant comorbidity Previous pleurodesis or thoracotomy
	Underweight, overweight
Anatomic-Radiographic Evaluation	
Marked emphysema	Bronchiectasis
	Minimal radiographic emphysema
Heterogeneously distributed emphysema	Homogeneously distributed emphysema
Target zones of poorly perfused lung	No target zones
Areas with better preserved lung	No preserved lung tissue
Marked thoracic hyperinflation	Chest wall or thoracic cage abnormalities
Physiologic Evaluation	
Marked airflow obstruction	Minimal to moderate airflow obstruction
Marked hyperinflation	Minimal to moderate thoracic hyperinflation
Alveolar gas exchange	Markedly disordered alveolar gas exchange
DL_{co} <50% (steady state)	DL_{co} <10%
	$Paco_2$ >60 mm Hg
Cardiovascular function	Cardiovascular function
Essentially normal ejection fraction	Mean pulmonary artery pressure >35 mm Hg
	Left ventricular ejection fraction <40%
	Significant coronary artery disease

DL_{co}, Diffusing capacity of the lungs for carbon monoxide; *$Paco_2$*, partial pressure of carbon dioxide in arterial blood. From Sellke FW, et al.: *Sabiston & Spencer surgery of the chest*, ed 9, Philadelphia, 2016, Elsevier.

BOX 2 Indications and Contraindications for Lung Volume Reduction Surgery and Lung Transplantation

Indications Common to Both Procedures
Emphysema with destruction and hyperinflation
Marked impairment (FEV_1 <35% predicted)
Marked restriction in activities of daily living
Failure of maximal medical treatment to correct symptoms

Contraindications to Both Procedures
Abnormal body weight (<70% or >130% of ideal)
Coexisting major medical problems increasing surgical risk
Inability or unwillingness to participate in pulmonary rehabilitation
Unwillingness to accept the risk of morbidity and mortality of surgery
Tobacco use within the past 6 mo
Recent or current diagnosis of malignant disease
Increasing age (>65 yr for transplantation, >70 yr for volume reduction)
Psychological instability, such as depression or anxiety disorder

Discriminating Conditions Favoring Lung Volume Reduction Surgery
Marked thoracic distention
Heterogeneous disease with obvious apical target areas
FEV_1 >20% predicted
Age between 60 and 70 ye

Discriminating Conditions Favoring Lung Transplantation
Diffuse disease without target areas
FEV_1 <20% predicted
Hypercapnia with $Paco_2$ >55 mm Hg
Pulmonary hypertension
Age younger than 60 yr
α_1-Antitrypsin deficiency

FEV_1, Forced expiratory volume in 1 sec. From Sellke FW, et al.: *Sabiston & Spencer surgery of the chest*, ed 9, Philadelphia, 2016, Elsevier.

PEARLS & CONSIDERATIONS

COMMENTS

- All patients with COPD should receive pneumococcal vaccine and yearly influenza vaccine.
- Early antibiotic administration is associated with improved outcomes among patients hospitalized for acute exacerbations of COPD regardless of the risk of treatment failure.
- In assessing the severity of COPD, the FEV_1 is limited by the fact that it does not take into account the systemic manifestations of COPD. The BODE index (body mass index, degree of obstruction, dyspnea, and exercise capacity) has been proposed as a multidimensional scale to better assess the morbidity and mortality associated with COPD. It is better than the FEV_1 alone at predicting the risk of death from any cause and from respiratory causes among patients with COPD. In the BODE index, obstruction is measured by FEV_1 and dyspnea is measured by the modified Medical Research Council (MMRC) dyspnea questionnaire in a 6-minute walk test. A score of 0 on the MMRC indicates that the individual is not troubled with breathlessness except with strenuous exercise, 1 indicates shortness of breath when hurrying or walking up a slight hill, and 2 means the individual walks slower than people of the same age due to breathlessness or has to stop for breath when walking at own pace on level ground. A score of 3 means severe dyspnea because the person has to stop for breath after walking approximately 100 meters or after a few minutes on level ground, and a score of 4 indicates very severe dyspnea and is given when the individual is too breathless to leave the house or is breathless when dressing or undressing.
- Pulmonary artery enlargement as determined by a ratio of the diameter of the pulmonary artery to the diameter of the aorta [PA:A ratio] of >1 detected by CT is associated with severe exacerbations of COPD.
- The average person with COPD has one or two acute exacerbations each yr. Prophylactic use of macrolide antibiotics (azithromycin 250 mg/day) has been shown to decrease the frequency of exacerbations and improve quality of life among selected patients with COPD; however, it leads to hearing decrements in a small percentage of patients and increased prevalence of macrolide-resistant bacteria colonizing the airway and is therefore not recommended.
- Eosinophilic airway inflammation may contribute to COPD exacerbations. Patients with COPD with eosinophilic phenotype may benefit from mepolizumab, a monoclonal antibody directed against interleukin-5.
- Current and former smokers (within 15 yr) with at least a 30-pack-yr history of smoking should be assessed for lung cancer using low-dose computed tomography.

SUGGESTED READINGS

Available at ExpertConsult.com

RELATED CONTENT

Chronic Obstructive Pulmonary Disease (Patient Information)
Emphysema (Patient Information)
Asthma-COPD Overlap Syndrome (Related Key Topic)

AUTHORS: **ALINE N. ZOUK, M.D.,** and **SAMAAN RAFEQ, M.D.**

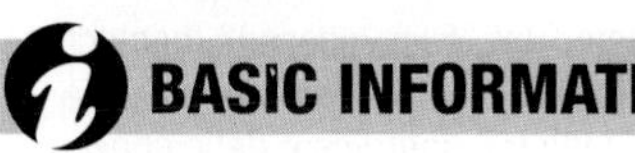

BASIC INFORMATION

DEFINITION

CTE is a neurogenerative disorder often found in athletes, veterans, and those with repeated head injuries. It presents with cognitive, psychiatric, and sometimes motor symptoms.

SYNONYMS

CTE
Traumatic encephalopathy syndrome (clinical diagnosis)
Dementia pugilistica (older term)
Punch drunk syndrome (older term)

ICD 10-CM CODE

G93.49 Other encephalopathy

EPIDEMIOLOGY & DEMOGRAPHICS

PEAK INCIDENCE & PREVALENCE: The incidence and prevalence of CTE are currently unknown. Among 202 deceased former football players, CTE was never pathologically diagnosed in 177 players (87%). Among participants with severe CTE pathology, 89% had behavior, mood symptoms, or both, 95% had cognitive symptoms, and 85% had signs of dementia.[1]

PREDOMINANT SEX AND AGE: CTE may present early (20s to 30s) or later (50s to 60s) in adulthood. The relationship with gender is unknown.

GENETICS: Currently there are no known genetic risk factors that predispose to the development of CTE.

RISK FACTORS: Repetitive head injuries leading to concussions are the strongest risk factor for the development of CTE. Atheletes, veterans, and victims of repetitive head trauma are at highest risk.

PHYSICAL FINDINGS & CLINICAL PRESENTATION

Currently, it is thought that CTE presents in two forms. The first presents early in life (later 20s to 30s), with primarily psychiatric and behavioral manifestations. These may include depression, anxiety, paranoia, impulsivity, explosivity, and aggression. Cognitive problems are more common as the disease progresses. The second form presents later in life (60s), with mainly cognitive impairments and is likely to progress to dementia. Symptoms of this variant include impairment in episodic memory, attention, and executive function. Currently it is thought that CTE progresses in four stages with increasing severity along each stage. Symptoms progress from headaches, attention problems, and depression to explosivity, aggression, dementia, and suicidality as the disease progresses.

Physical findings are not always present in CTE but may include symptoms of parkinsonism and motor dysfunction, such as gait disturbance, tremors, ataxia, and dysarthria. These have been found to be particularly more common in boxers.

Of note, the symptoms of CTE may present similarly to the behavior subtype of frontotemporal dementia (FTD), but the characteristic disinhibition found in FTD is often missing. In addition, TBI patients may also have some symptoms of CTE, but these will present more acutely, whereas CTE develops after multiple yrs of injuries.

ETIOLOGY

CTE is believed to occur due to repetitive head injuries. Definitive diagnosis is made only through autopsy, where neurofibrillary tangles and p-tau aggregates may be found around blood vessels and in deep cortical sulci, amygdala, hopocampus, brainstem, and cerebellum depending on the stage of the disease.

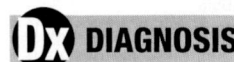

DIAGNOSIS

DIFFERENTIAL DIAGNOSIS

Alzheimer's disease
Frontotemporal dementia
Post-concussion syndrome
Bipolar disorder
Major depressive disorder

WORK-UP

CTE should be suspected in those with a history of repetitive head injuries and the symptoms previously listed. The history and progression of symptoms is of most benefit in the diagnostic process. Neuropsychological testing may be helpful in delineating specific cognitive deficits.

LABORATORY TESTS

Tests including complete blood count, comprehensive metabolic panel, thyroid function tests, HIV, syphilis

IMAGING STUDIES

- MRI may aid in ruling out other causes of dementia.
- The usefulness of advanced imaging such as PET, SPECT, and DTI in CTE is still under investigation.

Rx TREATMENT

NONPHARMACOLOGIC THERAPY

Cognitive behavioral therapy is helpful for depression and anxiety symptoms.

GENERAL Rx

- **SSRIs**, especially sertraline and citalopram, may be effective in treating depression symptoms. Close monitoring for suicidality is recommended in all patients with CTE.
- **Methylphenidate** has been shown to help in alleviating agitation, irritability, and aggressive symptoms.
- **Pain management** to improve quality of life.

COMPLEMENTARY AND ALTERNATIVE MEDICINE

None

DISPOSITION

CTE is chronic and progressive. Emphasis should be placed on improving quality of life through pain management, therapy, and symptom management.

REFERRAL

Patients may benefit from referral to neurology, psychiatry, and psychology.

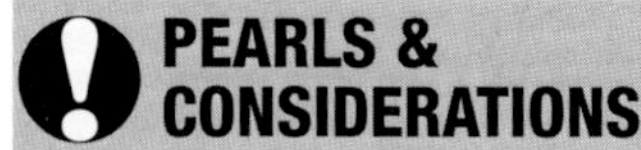

PEARLS & CONSIDERATIONS

COMMENTS

CTE is a slow developing illness. Although it should be considered in patients with repetitive head injuries, it is important to conduct a thorough work-up to rule out psychiatric illnesses and other forms of dementia that may present with similar symptoms.

PREVENTION

For athletes, wearing proper protective equipment as well as using techniques to avoid direct head impacts when playing sports is important. Furthermore, if a concussion is suspected, the player should not be allowed to resume play without further evaluation.

PATIENT/FAMILY EDUCATION

Concussion foundation—CTE resources
https://concussionfoundation.org/CTE-resources
CDC—HEADS UP: For prevention of concussions
https://www.cdc.gov/headsup/index.html

SUGGESTED READINGS

Available at ExpertConsult.com

RELATED CONTENT

Concussion (Related Key Topic)
Postconcussive Syndrome (Related Key Topic)
Depression, Major (Related Key Topic)
Suicide (Related Key Topic)

AUTHORS: **SUDAD KAZZAZ, M.D.,** and **JOSEPH S. KASS, M.D., J.D.**

[1] Mez J et al: Clinicopathological evaluation of chronic traumatic encephalopathy in players of American football, *JAMA* 318(4):360-370, 2017.

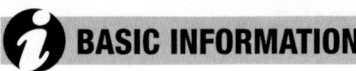

BASIC INFORMATION

DEFINITION

Cirrhosis is defined histologically as the presence of irreversible fibrosis in the liver. It can be classified as micronodular, macronodular, or mixed; however, each form may be seen in the same patient at different stages of the disease, and this classification system has little utility in determining the underlying etiology of cirrhosis. Cirrhosis manifests clinically with portal hypertension, ascites and peripheral edema, hepatic encephalopathy, and variceal bleeding.

ICD-10CM CODES

K70.30	Alcoholic cirrhosis of liver without ascites
K70.31	Alcoholic cirrhosis of liver with ascites
K71.7	Toxic liver disease with fibrosis and cirrhosis of liver
K74.3	Primary biliary cirrhosis
K74.4	Secondary biliary cirrhosis
K74.5	Biliary cirrhosis, unspecified
K74.60	Unspecified cirrhosis of liver
K74.69	Other cirrhosis of liver
P78.81	Congenital cirrhosis (of liver)

EPIDEMIOLOGY & DEMOGRAPHICS

- Cirrhosis was the fourteenth-leading cause of death in the U.S. in 2015 and the thirteenth-leading cause of death globally.
- Alcohol abuse, hepatitis C, and nonalcoholic steatohepatitis are the major causes of cirrhosis in the U.S.
- Economic burden of cirrhosis in the U.S. exceeds $2 billion in direct costs and over $10 billion in indirect costs.

PHYSICAL FINDINGS & CLINICAL PRESENTATION

GENERAL: Fever (spontaneous bacterial peritonitis)

SKIN: Jaundice, palmar erythema, spider angiomata, ecchymosis (thrombocytopenia or coagulation factor deficiency), increased pigmentation (hemochromatosis), xanthomas (primary biliary cirrhosis), diffuse pruritus, and needle tracks (viral hepatitis). Cutaneous lesions often accompany cirrhosis and can be found in >40% of people with chronic alcoholism.

EYES: Kayser-Fleischer rings (corneal copper deposition seen in Wilson disease; best diagnosed with slit lamp examination), scleral icterus

BREATH: Fetor hepaticus (breath has a sweet musty odor found in cirrhosis with hepatic failure)

CHEST: Possible gynecomastia in men

ABDOMEN: Tender or nontender hepatomegaly (congestive hepatomegaly), small, nodular liver (cirrhosis), palpable, nontender gallbladder (neoplastic extrahepatic biliary obstruction), palpable spleen (portal hypertension), dilated superficial periumbilical vein (caput medusae), venous hum auscultated over periumbilical veins (portal hypertension), ascites (portal hypertension, hypoalbuminemia), diffuse abdominal tenderness (spontaneous bacterial peritonitis)

RECTAL EXAMINATION: Hemorrhoids (portal hypertension), guaiac-positive stools (alcoholic gastritis, bleeding esophageal varices, peptic ulcer disease, bleeding hemorrhoids, portal gastropathy)

GENITALIA: Testicular atrophy in males (chronic liver disease, hemochromatosis)

EXTREMITIES: Pedal edema (hypoalbuminemia, anasarca), arthropathy (hemochromatosis), Dupuytren contractures

NEUROLOGIC: Asterixis (hepatic encephalopathy), choreoathetosis, dysarthria (Wilson disease)

ETIOLOGY

- Chronic hepatitis B virus (HBV) and hepatitis C virus (HCV) infection
- Alcoholism
- Nonalcoholic steatohepatitis
- Primary biliary cirrhosis
- Secondary biliary cirrhosis, obstruction of the common bile duct (stone, stricture, pancreatitis, neoplasm, sclerosing cholangitis)
- Autoimmune hepatitis
- Drugs with chronic hepatitis (e.g., acetaminophen, isoniazid, methotrexate, methyldopa)
- Chronic hepatic congestion (e.g., CHF, constrictive pericarditis, tricuspid insufficiency, thrombosis of the hepatic vein, obstruction of the vena cava)
- Hemochromatosis
- Wilson disease
- Alpha-1-antitrypsin deficiency
- Infiltrative diseases (amyloidosis, glycogen storage diseases, hemochromatosis, nonhepatocellular malignancies)
- Nutritional: Jejunoileal bypass
- Others: Parasitic infections (schistosomiasis), idiopathic portal hypertension, congenital hepatic fibrosis, systemic mastocytosis

Dx DIAGNOSIS

WORKUP

In addition to an assessment of liver function, the evaluation of patients with cirrhosis should also include an assessment of renal and circulatory function. Diagnostic workup is aimed primarily at identifying the most likely cause of cirrhosis. The history is extremely important:

- Alcohol abuse: Alcoholic liver disease
- History of hepatitis B or hepatitis C
- Obesity, type 2 diabetes mellitus, hyperlipidemia (nonalcoholic steatohepatitis)
- History of IBD (primary sclerosing cholangitis)
- History of pruritus, hyperlipoproteinemia, and xanthomas in a middle-aged or elderly woman (primary biliary cholangitis)
- Impotence, diabetes mellitus, hyperpigmentation, arthritis (hemochromatosis)
- Neurologic disturbances (Wilson disease, hepatolenticular degeneration)
- Family history of "liver disease" (hemochromatosis [positive family history in 25% of patients], alpha-1-antitrypsin deficiency)
- History of recurrent episodes of right upper quadrant pain (biliary tract disease)
- History of blood transfusions, IV drug abuse (hepatitis C)
- History of repetitive hepatotoxic drug exposure
- Coexistence of other diseases with immune or autoimmune features (immune thrombocytopenic purpura, myasthenia gravis, thyroiditis, autoimmune hepatitis)

Biopsy is the gold standard to diagnosis cirrhosis and is helpful when multiple etiologies are possible that might change management (autoimmune hepatitis, small duct primary sclerosing cholangitis, antimitochondrial antibody-negative primary biliary cholangitis, and infiltrative diseases such as lymphoma, amyloidosis, and granulomatous hepatitis). However, it is generally unnecessary if the clinical picture is highly suggestive of cirrhosis and management would not change. Biopsy can be useful in alcoholics to distinguish between decompensated cirrhosis and cirrhosis with alcoholic hepatitis.

LABORATORY TESTS

- Decreased hemoglobin and hematocrit, elevated mean corpuscular volume (Fig. E1). Increased blood urea nitrogen (BUN) and creatinine (the BUN may also be "normal" or low if the patient has severely diminished liver function)
- Decreased sodium (dilutional hyponatremia), and decreased potassium (as a result of secondary aldosteronism or urinary losses). Evaluation of renal function should also include measurement of urinary sodium and urinary protein from 24-hr urine collection.
- Decreased glucose in a patient with liver disease indicates severe liver damage.
- Other laboratory abnormalities:
  1. Alcoholic hepatitis and cirrhosis: Possible mild elevation of alanine aminotransferase (ALT) and aspartate aminotransferase (AST), usually <500 IU; AST >ALT (ratio >2:3).
  2. Extrahepatic obstruction: Possible moderate elevations of ALT and AST to levels <500 IU.
  3. Viral, toxic, or ischemic hepatitis: Extreme elevations (>500 IU) of ALT and AST.
  4. Transaminases may be normal despite significant liver disease in patients with jejunoileal bypass operations or hemochromatosis or after methotrexate administration.
  5. Alkaline phosphatase elevation can occur with extrahepatic obstruction, primary biliary cholangitis, and primary sclerosing cholangitis.
  6. Serum lactate dehydrogenase is significantly elevated in metastatic disease of the liver; lesser elevations are seen with hepatitis, cirrhosis, extrahepatic obstruction, and congestive hepatomegaly.
  7. Serum gamma-glutamyl transpeptidase is elevated in alcoholic liver disease and

may also be elevated with cholestatic disease (primary biliary cholangitis, primary sclerosing cholangitis).
8. Serum bilirubin may be elevated; urinary bilirubin can be present in hepatitis, hepatocellular jaundice, and biliary obstruction.
9. Serum albumin: Significant liver disease results in hypoalbuminemia. Malnutrition occurs in 20% to 60% of patients with cirrhosis.

- Prothrombin time/INR: Elevation in patients with liver disease indicates severe liver damage and poor prognosis. Table 1 summarizes hemostatic balance in liver disease.
    1. Presence of hepatitis B surface antigen implies acute or chronic hepatitis B.
    2. Presence of antimitochondrial antibody suggests primary biliary cholangitis, chronic hepatitis.
    3. Elevated serum copper, decreased serum ceruloplasmin, and elevated 24-hr urine may be diagnostic of Wilson disease.
    4. Protein immunoelectrophoresis may reveal decreased α-1 globulins (alpha-1-antitrypsin deficiency), increased IgA (alcoholic cirrhosis), increased IgM (primary biliary cirrhosis), increased IgG (chronic hepatitis, cryptogenic cirrhosis).
    5. An elevated serum ferritin and increased iron saturation are suggestive of hemochromatosis.
    6. An elevated blood ammonia suggests hepatocellular dysfunction; serial values, however, are generally not useful in monitoring patients with hepatic encephalopathy because there is poor correlation between blood ammonia level and degree of hepatic encephalopathy.
    7. Serum cholesterol is elevated in cholestatic disorders.
    8. Antinuclear antibodies (ANA) may be found in autoimmune hepatitis.
    9. Alpha fetoprotein: Levels >1000 pg/ml are highly suggestive of hepatocellular carcinoma.
    10. Hepatitis C viral testing identifies patients with chronic hepatitis C infection.
    11. Elevated level of serum globulin (especially gamma-globulins) and positive ANA test may occur with autoimmune hepatitis.
    12. End-stage liver disease is characterized by decreased levels of most procoagulant factors with the notable exceptions of factor VIII and von Willebrand factor, which are elevated. Table 2 summarizes hemostatic indices in liver disease.

IMAGING STUDIES

- Ultrasonography is the procedure of choice. It can identify the size and shape of the liver (generally small and nodular in advanced cirrhosis) and can detect gallstones and dilation of bile ducts. The use of sonography on a periodic basis to screen for hepatocellular carcinoma in patients with cirrhosis should be considered.
- CT scan (Figs. 2 and 3) is useful for detecting mass lesions in liver and pancreas, assessing hepatic fat content, identifying idiopathic hemochromatosis, diagnosing Budd-Chiari syndrome early, assessing dilation of intrahepatic bile ducts, and detecting varices and splenomegaly. However, ultrasound is generally the preferred imaging modality of choice.
- MRI can be used to identify hemangiomas, hepatocellular carcinoma.
- Vibration-controlled transient elastography and magnetic resonance elastography are useful to assess advanced fibrosis. These noninvasive tests are less expensive and safer than biopsy and can be repeated over time to monitor disease progression.
- Technetium-99m sulfur colloid scanning is rarely used but can be useful for diagnosing cirrhosis (there is a shift of colloid uptake to the spleen and bone marrow), identifying hepatic adenomas (cold defect is noted), and diagnosing Budd-Chiari syndrome (there is increased uptake by the caudate lobe).
- Endoscopic retrograde cholangiopancreatography can be used for diagnosing periampullary carcinoma and common duct stones; it is also useful in diagnosing primary sclerosing cholangitis.
- Percutaneous transhepatic cholangiography is useful when evaluating patients with cholestatic jaundice and dilated intrahepatic ducts by ultrasonography; presence of intrahepatic strictures and focal dilation is suggestive of primary sclerosing cholangitis.

TABLE 1 Hemostatic balance in Liver disease

	Hemostatic Balance in Liver Disease	
	Promotes Thrombosis	**Promotes Bleeding**
Primary hemostasis	• Increased vWF • Decreased ADAMTS13	• Thrombocytopenia • Platelet dysfunction
Secondary hemostasis	• Increased factor VIII • Decreased protein C, protein S, antithrombin	• Factor deficiencies: II, V, VII, IX, XI • Vitamin K deficiency • Hypofibrinogenemia • Dysfibrinogenemia
Fibrinolysis	• Reduced plasminogen • Increased PAI-1	• Reduced α2-antiplasmin, TAFI, factor VIII • Increased t-PA

ADAMST13, A disintegrin and metalloproteinase with thrombospondin; *PAI-1,* plasminogen activator inhibitor-1; *TAFI,* thrombin activatable fibrinolysis inhibitor; *t-PA,* tissue plasminogen activator; *vWF,* von Willebrand factor.
From Hoffman R et al: *Hematology, basic principles and practice,* ed 7, Philadelphia, 2018, Elsevier.

TABLE 2 Hemostatic Indices in Liver Disease

Laboratory Changes	PT	PTT	TCT	Fib	Clauss	Plt	Platelet Aggregation	FVII	DD	ELT
Thrombocytopenia	N	N	N	N	N	↓	N	N	N	N
Platelet dysfunction	N	N	N	N	N	N	abnormal	N	N	N
Vitamin K deficiency[a]	↑	↑	N	N	N	N	N	↓	N	N
Factor deficiency	↑	↑	N	N	N	N	N	↓	N	N
Hypofibrinogenemia	N/↑	N/↑	↑	↓	↓	N	N	N	N	N
Dysfibrinogenemia	N/↑	N/↑	↑	N	↓	N	N	N	N	N
Hyperfibrinolysis	N/↑	N/↑	N/↑	N/↓	N/↓	N	N	↓	↑	↓
DIC	N/↑	N/↑	N/↑	↓	↓	↓	N	N/↓	↑	↓

Clauss, Clauss fibrinogen; *DD,* D-dimer; *DIC,* disseminated intravascular coagulation; *ELT,* euglobulin lysis time (measure of fibrinolysis); *Fib,* fibrinogen; *FVII,* factor VII functional assay; *N,* normal; *Plt,* platelet; *PT,* prothrombin time; *PTT,* partial thromboplastin time; *TCT,* thrombin clotting time.
[a]Differentiating between vitamin K deficiency and liver disease can be challenging with conventional laboratory tests. If available, performing a factor II assay with and without Echis venom (factor II biologic and factor II Echis) may be useful. Ecarin is derived from *Echis carinatus* snake venom and can activate prothrombin irrespective of γ-carboxylation. Factor II activity (biologic) is reduced in both vitamin K deficiency and liver disease. In contrast, the factor II Echis is reduced in liver disease but is normal in vitamin K deficiency.
From Hoffman R et al: *Hematology, basic principles and practice,* ed 7, Philadelphia, 2018, Elsevier.

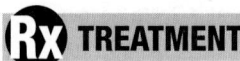

TREATMENT

NONPHARMACOLOGIC THERAPY

- Avoid any hepatotoxins (e.g., ethanol, acetaminophen), improve nutritional status, vaccinate against hepatitis A and B if not already immune.
- Transjugular intrahepatic portosystemic shunt (TIPS) in patients with recurrent variceal hemorrhage despite optical medical therapy (Fig. 4). Early use of TIPS is associated with significant reductions in treatment failure and in mortality in patients with cirrhosis who are hospitalized for acute variceal bleeding and are at high risk for treatment failure.
- Correction of malnutrition: Daily protein intake of 1.0 to 1.5 g per kg of body weight.

GENERAL Rx

- Nonselective beta blockers (nadolol, propranolol) in patients with cirrhosis and variceal hemorrhage, and some without hemorrhage but with high-risk bleeding features. Use with caution in patients with severe alcoholic hepatitis and decompensated cirrhosis with refractory ascites. They should be temporarily discontinued in patients with spontaneous bacterial peritonitis due to increased mortality and hepatorenal syndrome incidence.
- Pruritus due to liver disease may be treated with cholestyramine 4 g/day initially. Dose can be increased to 24 g/day as needed.
- Pain management: Avoid opiates (may precipitate or aggravate hepatic encephalopathy) and NSAIDs (increased risk of gastrointestinal bleeding and renal failure). Low-dose tramadol and lidocaine patches are generally well tolerated.
- Sedatives: Benzodiazepines (lorazepam or oxazepam) may be used for alcohol withdrawal but should be avoided in patients with hepatic encephalopathy. Avoid benzodiazepines with liver metabolites (diazepam, chlordiazepoxide).
- Statins: Can be safely started and continued in patients with hyperlipidemia and/or nonalcoholic fatty liver disease.
- Proton pump inhibitors: Not routinely indicated; their use in patients with cirrhosis is associated with excess risk for spontaneous bacterial peritonitis and hepatic encephalopathy; avoid indiscriminate use of PPIs in patients with cirrhosis.
- Antibiotics: Trimethoprim-sulfamethoxazole or ciprofloxacin/norfloxacin for spontaneous bacterial peritonitis prophylaxis in patients with a history of SBP, an ascites protein

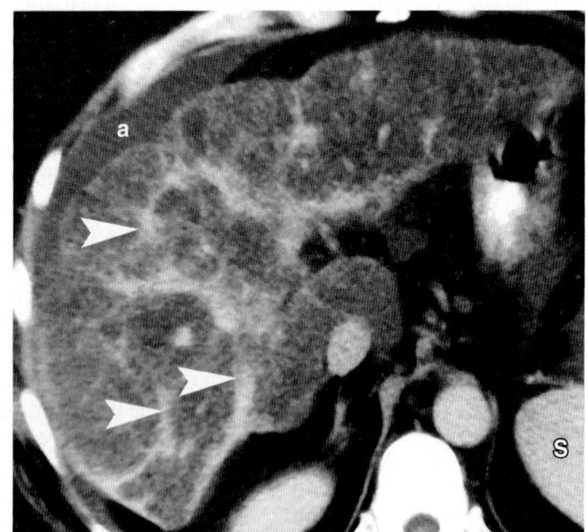

FIG. 2 Advanced cirrhosis with fatty infiltration. Delayed portal venous–phase computed tomography reveals that the liver is misshapen and nodular in contour. Parenchymal density that is significantly lower than that of the spleen *(S)* is indicative of fatty infiltration and continuing liver injury. Prominent scars and bands of fibrosis *(arrowheads)* are seen throughout the liver. Ascites *(a)* is present. (From Webb WR et al: *Fundamentals of body CT*, ed 4, Philadelphia, 2015, Saunders.)

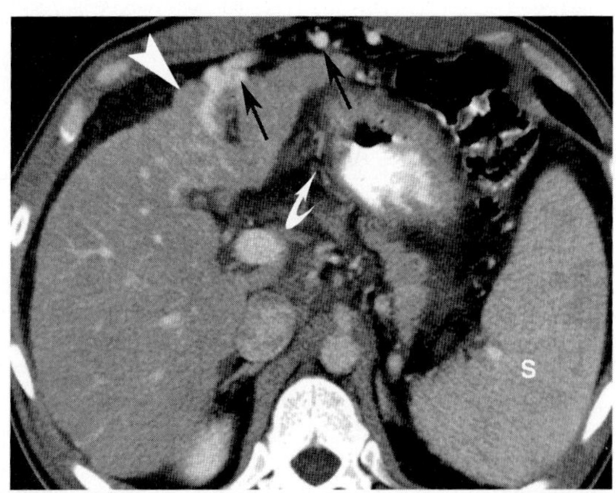

FIG. 3 Cirrhosis with portal hypertension. Postcontrast computed tomography reveals a liver that is nodular in contour *(arrowhead)* with patent enlarged paraumbilical veins (*blue arrows*) and splenomegaly *(S)*, findings indicative of portal hypertension. Mildly enlarged portosystemic collateral vessels (*curved arrow*) are also evident in the gastrohepatic ligament. (From Webb WR et al: *Fundamentals of body CT*, ed 4, Philadelphia, 2015, Saunders.)

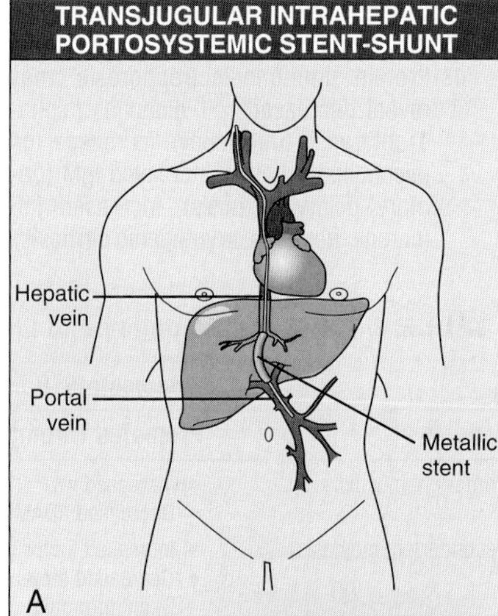

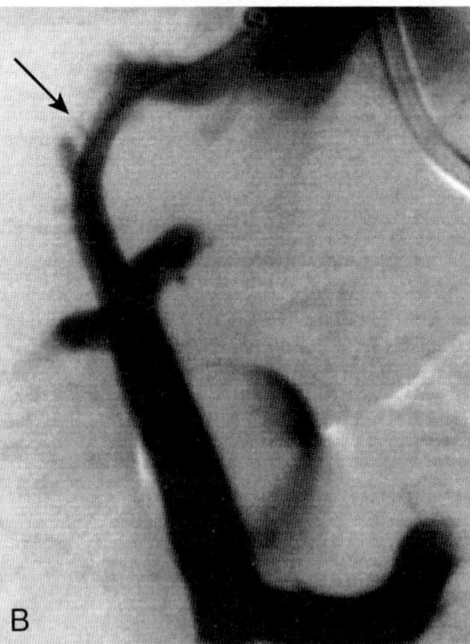

FIG. 4 Transjugular intrahepatic portosystemic stent shunt. A, An intrahepatic track has been created between the right hepatic vein and the right portal vein. **B,** The track is dilated *(arrow)* and stented, creating a shunt as demonstrated on shuntogram. (Courtesy Dr. W. K. Tso, Queen Mary Hospital, Hong Kong.)

concentration less than 1 g/dl, or variceal hemorrhage.
- Liver transplantation may be indicated in otherwise healthy patients (ages <65 yr) with severe cirrhosis and lack of contraindications. Contraindications to liver transplantation are AIDS, most metastatic malignancies, active substance abuse, uncontrolled sepsis, and uncontrolled cardiac or pulmonary disease.
- Treatment of complications of portal hypertension (ascites, esophagogastric varices, hepatic encephalopathy, spontaneous bacterial peritonitis, and hepatorenal syndrome; refer to these individual topics in Section I).
- Box 1 summarizes the management of coagulopathy in liver disease.

TREATMENT BASED ON SPECIFIC CAUSE OF CIRRHOSIS

- Remove excess body iron with phlebotomy and deferoxamine in patients with hemochromatosis.
- Remove copper deposits with D-penicillamine in patients with Wilson disease.
- Long-term ursodiol therapy will slow the progression of primary biliary cirrhosis. It is, however, ineffective in primary sclerosing cholangitis.
- Glucocorticoids (prednisone 20 to 30 mg/day initially or combination therapy or prednisone and azathioprine) are useful in autoimmune hepatitis.
- Antivirals in chronic hepatitis C.

BOX 1 Management of coagulopathy in liver disease

- Actively bleeding patients should be adequately resuscitated. Admission to the intensive care setting may be appropriate.
- Basic coagulation tests should be ordered to identify the cause of bleeding; these include CBC, PT (INR), PTT, thrombin clotting time, fibrinogen, D-Dimer, FDP, and mixing studies. The need for more specialized tests will be dictated by the clinical situation and response to therapy.
- It is important to identify any localized source of bleeding (e.g., varices) amenable to procedural intervention to achieve hemostasis.
- A trial of 5 to 10 mg of vitamin K is reasonable in asymptomatic patients with prolonged PT and PTT but should be used with other therapies in actively bleeding patients.
- In patients with thrombocytopenia platelet transfusions can be used, targeting platelet counts greater than 50 × 109 /L.
- In patients who can tolerate volume, FP 4 to 6 units (1000–1500 ml) given over 1 to 2 hours can be used to replace coagulation factors. Coagulation parameters should be monitored to document effect and determine the timing and need for additional units.
- Dysfibrinogenemia or hypofibrinogenemia should be suspected if coagulation assays do not correct with FP or fibrinogen levels are low, respectively. Replacement can be attempted with 10 to 20 units of cryoprecipitate while following laboratory results.
- Patients who are intravascularly overloaded or who do not respond to FP should be considered for rFVIIa. Low doses of rFVIIa (25–50 μg/kg) are generally used, and repeated doses may be required because of the short rfVIIa half-life of 2 to 3 hours. rFVIIa may be most suitable as a temporizing measure to enable invasive procedures or hemostasis to be achieved by other means. Avoid use in the setting of DIC.

CBC, Complete blood count; *DIC,* disseminated intravascular coagulation; *FDP, FP,* frozen plasma; *INR,* international normalized ratio; *PT,* prothrombin time; *PTT,* partial thromboplastin time; *rFVIIa*, recombinant factor VIIa.
From Hoffman R et al: *Hematology, basic principles and practice,* ed 7, Philadelphia, 2018, Elsevier.

TABLE 3 Child-Pugh Staging Criteria

	CHILD-PUGH SCORE		
Criteria	**1 Point**	**2 Points**	**3 Points**
Total serum bilirubin (mg/dl)	<2	2-3	>3
Serum albumin (g/dl)	>3.5	2.8-3.5	<2.8
INR	<1.70	1.71-2.20	>2.20
Ascites	No ascites	Ascites controlled	Ascites not controlled
Encephalopathy	No encephalopathy	Encephalopathy controlled	Encephalopathy not controlled

	INTERPRETATION OF CHILD-PUGH SCORES		
	Points	**Life Expectancy**	**Perioperative Mortality**
Child Class A	5-6	15-20 yr	10%
Child Class B	7-9	Candidate for liver transplant	30%
Child Class C	10-15	1-3 yr	82%

PROGNOSIS

- Prognosis varies with the etiology of the patient's cirrhosis and whether there is ongoing hepatic injury. Patients with compensated cirrhosis (no associated complications or esophageal varices without bleeding) have a good prognosis with median survival of 12 yr.
- In patients with decompensated cirrhosis, the Model for End-stage Liver Disease with sodium (MELDNa) scoring is useful to predict 3-month mortality and so is the main method of prioritizing patients awaiting liver transplantation. It also has prognostic value following TIPS placement for patients with cirrhosis undergoing nontransplant surgeries. Mortality rate exceeds 80% in patients with hepatorenal syndrome.
- Regression of cirrhosis has been demonstrated after antiviral therapy in some patients with chronic hepatitis C. Regression is associated with decreased disease-related morbidity and improved survival.
- Cirrhosis is associated with an increased risk for hepatocellular carcinoma. However, the risk is low (1% 5-yr cumulative risk in alcoholic cirrhosis).

PEARLS & CONSIDERATIONS

COMMENTS

- Thrombocytopenia and advanced Child-Pugh classes (Table 3) are associated with the presence of varices. These factors are useful to identify cirrhotic patients who benefit most from referral for endoscopic screening for varices.
- A combination of endoscopic and drug therapy reduces overall and variceal rebleeding in cirrhosis more than either therapy alone.
- PPI use, but not H_2RA use, is associated with risk for serious infections in patients with decompensated cirrhosis.

SUGGESTED READINGS

Available at ExpertConsult.com

RELATED CONTENT

Cirrhosis (Patient Information)
Ascites (Related Key Topic)
Esophageal Varices (Related Key Topic)
Hepatic Encephalopathy (Related Ke y Topic)
Hepatopulmonary Syndrome (Related Key Topic)
Hepatorenal Syndrome (Related Key Topic)
Peritonitis, Spontaneous Bacterial (Related Key Topic)
Primary Biliary Cholangitis (Related Key Topic)

AUTHOR: **DAVID J. LUCIER JR., M.D., M.B.A., M.P.H., C.P.P.S**

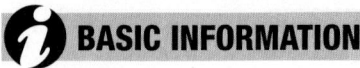

DEFINITION

Claudication refers to reproducible pain, fatigue, or cramping due to vascular origin in a muscle group that is consistently brought on by exertion and is relieved with rest. The pain experienced results from inadequate blood flow to the target muscle group, which is not able to meet increased metabolic demand. Claudication is therefore a supply-and-demand mismatch and is due to peripheral arterial disease (PAD). Intermittent vascular claudication is more common in the lower extremities but can also affect the upper extremities.

SYNONYM

Intermittent claudication

ICD-10CM CODES

I70.211 Atherosclerosis of native arteries of extremities with intermittent claudication, right leg
I70.212 Atherosclerosis of native arteries of extremities with intermittent claudication, left leg
I70.213 Atherosclerosis of native arteries of extremities with intermittent claudication, bilateral legs
I70.219 Atherosclerosis of native arteries of extremities with intermittent claudication, unspecified extremity
I70.311 Atherosclerosis of unspecified type of bypass graft(s) of the extremities with intermittent claudication, right leg
I70.312 Atherosclerosis of unspecified type of bypass graft(s) of the extremities with intermittent claudication, left leg
I70.313 Atherosclerosis of unspecified type of bypass graft(s) of the extremities with intermittent claudication, bilateral legs
I70.319 Atherosclerosis of unspecified type of bypass graft(s) of the extremities with intermittent claudication, unspecified extremity
I70.719 Atherosclerosis of other type of bypass graft(s) of the extremities with intermittent claudication, unspecified extremity

EPIDEMIOLOGY & DEMOGRAPHICS

- Symptomatic claudication in Western countries affects 5% of patients between the ages of 55 and 74.
- Lower-extremity PAD, which includes both symptomatic claudication and asymptomatic disease, is estimated to affect approximately 8.5 million Americans above age 40 yr and 202 million people around the world. This finding demonstrates that a large portion of patients is at risk of developing claudication.
- At-risk patients include:
  1. Patients with exertional leg symptoms
  2. Nonhealing lower-extremity wounds
  3. Asymptomatic patients 50 yr or older with a history of smoking or diabetes
  4. Patients younger than age 50 yr with diabetes and an additional cardiovascular risk factor (smoking, dyslipidemia, hypertension, or homocysteinemia)
  5. All patients age 65 yr or older
- Risk factors associated with development of PAD are similar to coronary atherosclerosis (CAD) and include increasing age, cigarette smoking (odds ratio 2.72), hypertension (odds ratio 1.55), diabetes mellitus (odds ratio 1.88), and hypercholesterolemia (odds ratio 1.19). In addition, patients with chronic kidney disease, metabolic syndrome, and elevated levels of C-reactive protein, lipoprotein(a), and homocysteine are at increased risk. Nontraditional risk factors include race/ethnicity, with African American patients being at higher risk. Hispanics also have similar to slightly higher rates of PAD compared to non-Hispanic whites.
- There is a strong correlation among PAD, CAD, carotid artery stenosis, and generalized cerebrovascular disease. Individuals with known atherosclerotic disease in one vascular bed are likely to have disease in another.
- The American College of Cardiology/American Heart Association (ACC/AHA) guidelines suggested the following distribution of clinical presentation of PAD in patients 50 yr of age or older:
  1. Asymptomatic: 20% to 50%
  2. Atypical leg pain: 40% to 50%
  3. Classic intermittent claudication: 10% to 35%
  4. Critical limb ischemia with threatened limb: 1% to 2%

PHYSICAL FINDINGS & CLINICAL PRESENTATION

- The severity of symptoms varies with degree of PAD, collateral blood supply, and exertional demands.
- Classic symptoms include exertional calf pain, which limits the patient's activity and self-resolves with rest within 10 minutes. Claudication can also typically present in the buttock and hip, thigh, calf, or foot, with one or more of the following signs or symptoms, depending on the level and degree of peripheral stenosis:
  1. Diminished or absent pedal pulses
  2. Bruit over the distal aorta, iliac, or femoral arteries
  3. Pallor of the distal extremities and cool to the touch upon elevation
  4. Rubor with prolonged capillary refill upon dependent positioning
  5. Trophic changes, including hair/nail loss and muscle atrophy
  6. Non-healing ulcers, necrotic tissue, and gangrene
  7. Weakness, numbness, or heaviness in the lower extremities
- True vascular claudication must be distinguished from "pseudoclaudication," which can be caused by severe venous obstruction or insufficiency, chronic compartment syndrome, spinal stenosis, osteoarthritis, and inflammatory muscle diseases. The characteristic features of pseudoclaudication that distinguish it from claudication are summarized in Table 1. Table 2 illustrates the differential diagnosis of intermittent claudication.
- Location of pain usually corresponds to analogous anatomy:
  1. Buttock and hip: Aortic or iliac disease
  2. Thigh: Aorta, iliac, or common femoral artery
  3. Upper two thirds of calf: Superficial femoral artery
  4. Lower one third of calf: Popliteal artery
  5. Foot: Tibial or peroneal artery
- Asymptomatic PAD is typically diagnosed by screening studies (exercise ankle brachial index, lower-extremity ultrasound) or incidentally on physical exam. Patients who are at significant risk for PAD often have multiple comorbidities that can alter their presentation. In the PARTNERS program report, 47% of those with a new diagnosis of PAD had no history of leg symptoms, 47% had atypical symptoms, and only 6% had classic symptoms.
- Symptoms of intermittent claudication classically start distally within a muscle group (below the stenosis) and then ascend with continued activity.
- Rest pain that occurs with leg elevation and is paradoxically relieved by walking may suggest severe PAD.
- Critical limb ischemia may present as tissue ulceration and gangrene, which require prompt intervention.

ETIOLOGY

The primary cause of claudication is peripheral atherosclerosis, resulting in a stenosis that impedes blood flow beyond the level necessary to meet the metabolic demand of limb muscles first with activity and then ultimately at rest.

TABLE 1 Characteristic Features of Pseudoclaudication That Distinguish It from Claudication

	Claudication	Pseudoclaudication
Characteristics	Limb cramping, tightness, fatigue	Similar to claudication with numbness
Location of discomfort	Lower extremity involving buttock, hip, thigh, calf, foot	Similar to claudication
Induced by exercise	Yes	Variable
Reproducible with distance walked	Consistent	Variable
Occurs with standing	No	Yes
Actions which provide relief	Stand	Sit
Time to relief	<5 min	≥30 min

TABLE 2 Differential Diagnosis of Intermittent Claudication

	Intermittent Claudication	Venous Claudication	Neurogenic Claudication
Quality of pain	Cramping	Aching, heaviness, tightness	"Pins and needles" sensation going down the leg, weakness
Onset	Gradual, consistent	Gradual; can, however, be immediate	Can be immediate
Relieved by	Stopping walking	Activity, elevation of leg	Sitting down, stooping, flexion at the waist
Location	Muscle groups (e.g., buttocks, thigh, calf)	Whole leg	Poorly localized, but can affect whole leg
Legs affected	Usually one	Usually one	Often both

From Swartz, MH: *Textbook of physical diagnosis*, ed 7, Philadelphia, 2014, Saunders.

Other etiologies include neuropathy, musculoskeletal or degenerative disease, compartment or entrapment syndrome, vasculitis, and embolic events.

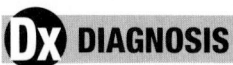

DIAGNOSIS

DIFFERENTIAL DIAGNOSIS

- Spinal stenosis (neurogenic or pseudoclaudication)
- Musculoskeletal disorders: Arthritis or myositis
- Degenerative osteoarthritic joint disease, predominantly of the lumbar spine and hips
- Chronic compartment or popliteal artery entrapment syndrome
- Peripheral neuropathy
- Atheromatous embolization and deep venous thrombosis
- Vasculitis: Thromboangiitis obliterans, Takayasu, or giant cell arteritis
- Symptomatic Baker cyst
- Venous claudication

WORKUP

History and physical findings suggest the diagnosis of claudication and noninvasive studies help confirm the diagnosis.

- Careful physical examinations include:
  1. Measurement of blood pressure in both arms and notation of asymmetry.
  2. Palpation and recording of carotid pulses, upstroke, amplitude, and presence of bruits.
  3. Auscultation and palpation of abdomen for bruits, aortic pulsation, and diameter.
  4. Palpation of brachial, radial, ulnar, femoral, popliteal, dorsalis pedis, and posterior tibial pulses. Pulse intensity should be recorded as follows: 0, absent; 1+, diminished; 2+, normal; 3+, bounding.
  5. Auscultation of femoral arteries for the presence of bruits.
  6. Extremities should be inspected for color, temperature, integrity of the skin, hair loss, and hypertrophic nails.
- Measurement of resting ankle–brachial index (ABI) should be considered first-line test in patients at risk for PAD.
- An ABI is the ratio of highest ankle systolic pressure of each leg to the highest brachial systolic pressure of either arm. A normal ABI is 1.00 to 1.40. A low ABI has been shown to be an independent predictor of mortality.
- The severity of PAD is based on the resting ABI. The absolute value of the ABI is reported to 2 decimal places:
  1. Abnormal: ABI at rest ≤0.90
  2. Borderline: ABI 0.9-0.99
  3. Normal: 1.00-1.40
  4. Noncompressible >1.40
- ABI >1.4 may represent significant PAD caused by heavy calcification. In such cases, measuring a toe–brachial index (TBI) can increase the sensitivity of testing, as highly calcified arteries are incompressible and may have an elevated ABI. A toe–brachial index <0.7 is considered abnormal and diagnostic of PAD.
- Borderline resting ABI (>0.90 and ≤1.40) in patients with exertional leg symptoms should undergo treadmill ABI testing to evaluate for PAD. This can help differentiate claudication from pseudoclaudication. If posttreadmill ABI is normal, alternative causes of leg pain should be considered. If no treadmill is available, the pedal plantarflexion ABI test is a reasonable alternative.
- Progression of PAD is considered to have occurred if a decrease in ABI of 0.15 occurs while the patient is in treatment.
- If a patient has a history concerning for PAD but a normal ABI, and if the clinician is concerned about a potential false-negative finding, performing an exercise stress ABI can potentially demonstrate lower-extremity PAD.
- If after exercise an ABI reading decreases by more than 20% or an ankle pressure decreases by 30 mm Hg, the patient should be considered to have significant PAD.
- Segmental systolic pressures are measured at the level of the thigh, calf, ankle, metatarsal, and toes. Normally, successive segments have <20 mm Hg difference in pressures. If the gradient is >20 mm Hg, a significant stenosis is suspected in the interval vascular segment.

IMAGING STUDIES

- Duplex ultrasound can be used to assess occlusion location, length, and patency of the distal arterial system or prior grafts; it is a good choice for initial imaging and surveillance monitoring after revascularization.
- In patients with prior infra-inguinal venous bypass grafts, the long-term patency should be evaluated at regular intervals using a duplex ultrasound. The 2016 AHA/ACC guidelines recommend routine surveillance approximately 4 to 6 weeks post procedure, 6 and 12 months after graft placement, and then yearly
- Magnetic resonance angiography (MRA) and CT angiography (CTA) are effective for imaging of the aorta and peripheral lower-extremity arteries above the knee. MRA has almost replaced catheter-based angiography, with 90% sensitivity and 97% specificity in identification of hemodynamically significant stenosis in the lower extremities.
- MRA and CTA are useful to define the anatomy and assist in planning percutaneous and surgical revascularization; however, the utility of each is decreased by necessity of gadolinium contrast and non-iodinated contrast agents, respectively.
- CTA of occlusive aortoiliac disease with fractional flow reserve (FFR) has been correlated with invasive angiographic evaluation with FFR and demonstrated, although in a small sample of people the correlation is excellent. One may then surmise that the patients could benefit from noninvasive CTA to plan and evaluate any potential areas of disease amenable to revascularization.
- Angiography (Fig. 1) remains the gold standard for diagnosing PAD, particularly below the knee.

Rx TREATMENT

NONPHARMACOLOGIC THERAPY

- Smoking cessation is of paramount importance. Smokers and former smokers should be asked about tobacco use status on each visit. Assistance and counseling for smoking cessation should be addressed thoroughly.
- Aggressive risk factor modification for hypertension, dyslipidemia, and diabetes mellitus, including diet, weight loss, and lifestyle counseling, is recommended (Fig. 2)
- Supervised exercise training should be performed as a first-line therapy for a minimum of 30 to 45 minutes, in sessions performed at least 3 times per week for a minimum of 12 weeks.
- Supervised exercise training programs under direct supervision in a hospital or outpatient facility and structured exercise are recommended for all patients with PAD. This has been shown to increase maximal walking

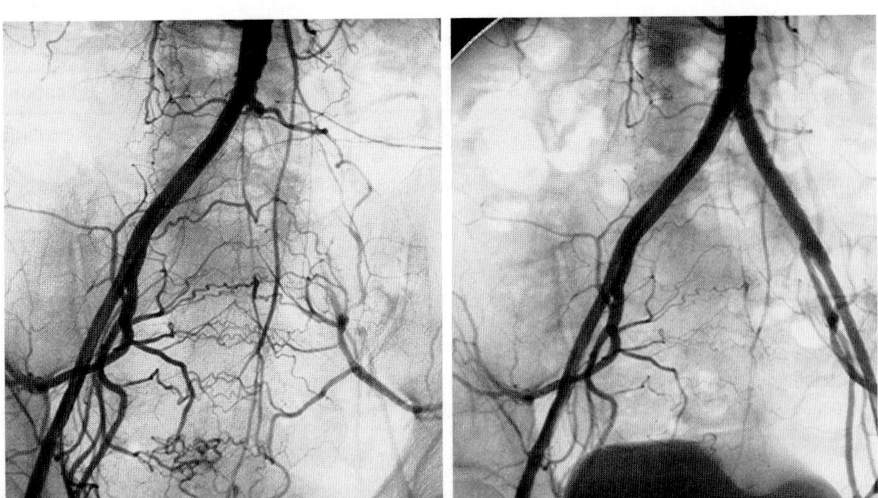

FIG. 1 Angiogram of the distal abdominal aorta and iliac arteries demonstrates an occluded left common iliac artery with extensive collateral circulation from contralateral internal iliac artery *(left panel),* which resolved after successful stent implantation *(right panel).* Images courtesy of Bart Domatch, MD, Radiology Department, University of Texas Southwestern Medical Center, Dallas, Texas. (From Andreoli TE et al: *Andreoli and Carpenter's Cecil essentials of medicine,* ed 8, Philadelphia, 2010, Saunders.)

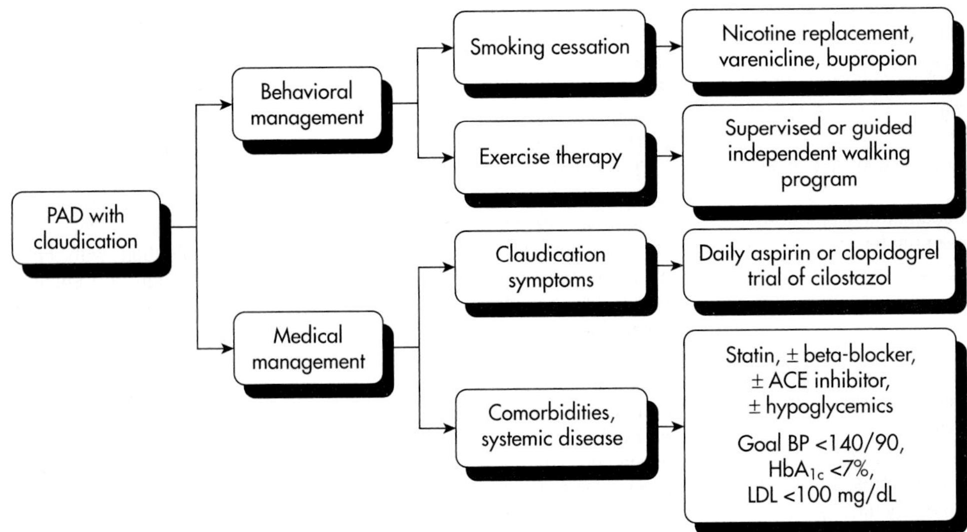

FIG. 2 Algorithm for revascularization in the management of claudication. *ACE,* Angiotensin-converting enzyme; *BP,* blood pressure; *HbA_{1C},* hemoglobin A_{1c}; *LDL,* low-density lipoprotein; *PAD,* peripheral arterial disease. (From Cameron JL, Cameron AM: *Current surgical therapy,* ed 12, Philadelphia, 2017, Elsevier.)

distance, pain-free walking distance, and the 6-minute walking distance. This treatment modality should be attempted prior to revascularization attempts.

- Structured or home-based walking exercise program may be considered as an alternative treatment modality, but it has not been shown to be as efficacious. It can be combined with group-mediated cognitive behavioral intervention that can significantly improve endurance and physical activity for patients unable or unwilling to participate in supervised exercise training.
- Lifestyle therapy in conjunction with exercise can be as or more effective than pharmacologic therapy and in some cases more effective than stent revascularization, as shown by the CLEVER Study.
- Intermittent pneumatic compression may hold promise as an adjunctive therapy.

ACUTE GENERAL Rx

Revascularization by an endovascular or surgical approach is usually reserved for patients with symptoms refractory to medical therapy or those with impending critical limb ischemia.

CHRONIC Rx

- Aspirin 75 to 325 mg daily is standard therapy.
- Thienopyridine medications such as clopidogrel 75 mg daily may be considered as an alternative to aspirin, especially for those intolerant of aspirin.
- Current data do not support combination treatment with aspirin and clopidogrel (CHARISMA trial).
- Asymptomatic patients with PAD (ABI ≤0.90) without claudication symptoms may benefit from the addition of an antiplatelet agent, either ASA or clopidogrel, as there is an increased cardiovascular risk in this subgroup.
- Hydroxymethyl glutaryl (HMG) coenzyme-A reductase inhibitor (statin) medications are indicated for all patients with PAD.
  1. LDL cholesterol level of less than 100 mg/dl is recommended.
  2. A goal LDL cholesterol level of less than 70 mg/dl is recommended for patients with PAD and high risk for coronary atherosclerotic disease.

3. Although new lipid guidelines have been published, the guidelines did not specifically address patients with PAD; therefore, the numerical targets can be considered. In those unable to reach the targets, a reduction in LDL >50% should be approached at a minimum.

- Antihypertensive therapy with beta-adrenergic blocking drugs and/or ACE inhibitors should be administered to all hypertensive patients with PAD to reduce the risk of MI, stroke, congestive heart failure, and cardiovascular death.
  1. In nondiabetics, the target blood pressure is <140 mm Hg systolic over 90 mm Hg diastolic.
  2. In diabetics or patients with chronic renal disease, the target blood pressure is <130 mm Hg systolic over 80 mm Hg diastolic.
  3. Recent hypertension guidelines have raised the targets for some diseases; however, they do not address the higher risk posed by multiple comorbidities.
- Cilostazol 100 mg bid may be used in conjunction with aspirin or clopidogrel. It has been shown to increase walking distance by 50% to 67% in symptomatic patients.
- Among patients with intermittent claudication, a single randomized controlled trial has shown a 24-week treatment with ramipril resulted in significant increases in pain-free and maximum treadmill walking times compared with placebo. Furthermore, the use of ACE inhibitors may be considered in patients with PAD to reduce the risk of cardiovascular events compared with ARBs, as their effect has not been studied.
- Pentoxifylline is not effective for treatment of claudication. In a review of 24 studies with over 3000 participants, results remained unclear, and a randomized control trial showed no difference between pentoxifylline and placebo; thus this is not recommended as a treatment for claudication.
- In patients with type II diabetes, a secondary analysis of the BARI 2D trial showed that an insulin-sensitizing approach (metformin, glitazones) reduces the risk of developing PAD when compared to insulin-providing therapy (glipizide, insulin). These patients also have lower rates of revascularization and amputation.
- Patients who are tobacco smokers should be advised at every visit to quit smoking and offered either varenicline or bupropion along with nicotine replacement therapy in the absence of any contraindications. Patients with PAD should avoid tobacco smoke exposure at work, at home, and in public places.
- Anticoagulation should not be used to reduce the risk of cardiovascular ischemic events in patients with PAD, as there is increased morbidity with no mortality benefit (WAVE trial). Its use to improve patency after bypass is uncertain.
- Novel agents, such as protease-activated receptor-1 (e.g., vorapaxar), added to existing antiplatelet therapy may have some benefit in decreasing acute limb-related ischemic events; however, its association with a risk of moderate to severe bleeding makes its benefits uncertain at this time. There was no cardiovascular benefit demonstrated in symptomatic PAD.
- Fig. 3 summarizes the nonoperative management of claudication.
- Revascularization through either a percutaneous or surgical approach is indicated in patients with refractory rest pain or claudication that is lifestyle limiting. It is also

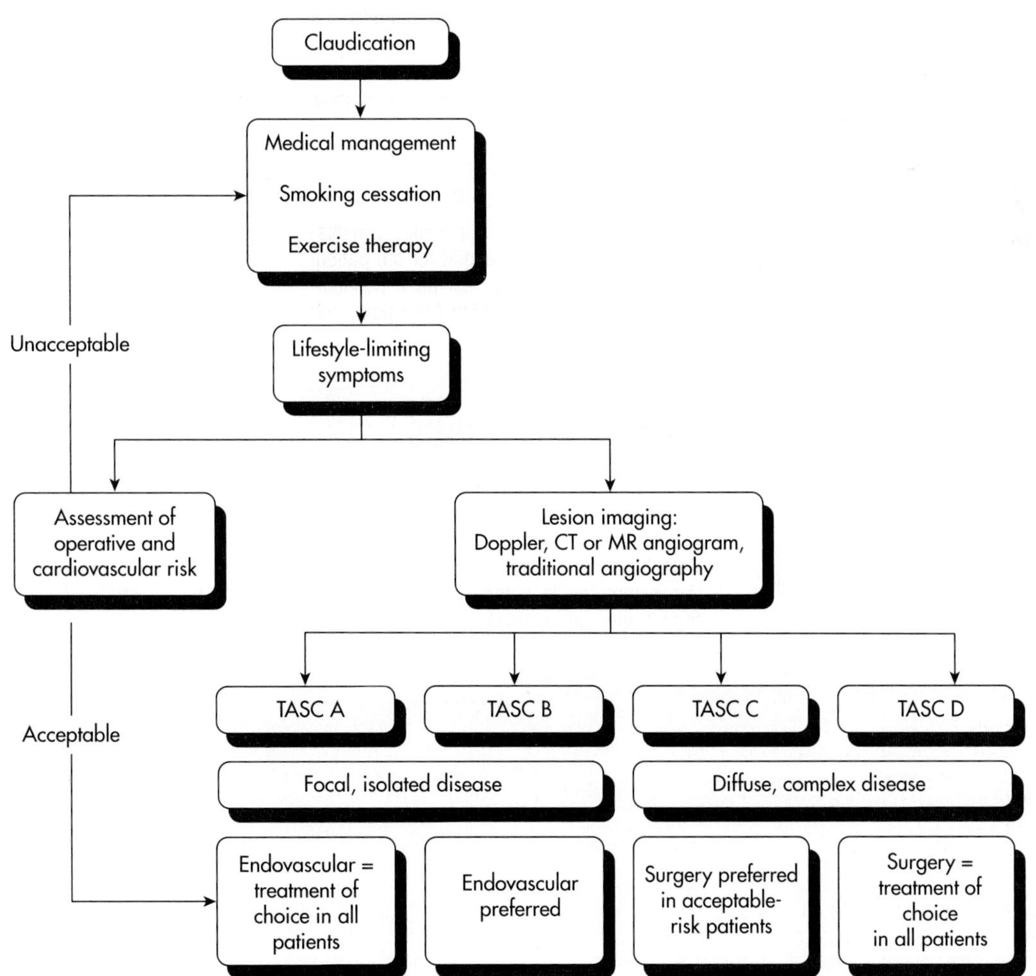

FIG. 3 Nonoperative management of claudication. *CT*, Computed tomographic; *MR*, magnetic resonance; *TASC*, TransAtlantic Inter-Society Consensus class. (From Cameron JL, Cameron AM: *Current surgical therapy*, ed 12, Philadelphia, 2017, Elsevier.)

indicated in those with non-healing ulcers or gangrene and in select patients with functional disability. Before such revascularization, each patient should have:

1. Participated in a supervised exercise training program and been given goal-directed medical therapy
2. Received comprehensive risk factor modification, including smoking cessation and optimal management of comorbidities
3. Significant disability with either the inability to perform normal work or a serious impairment of other activities important to the patient
4. Lower-extremity PAD lesion anatomy amenable to revascularization, defined by a low risk and a high probability of initial and long-term success

- Common procedures include:
  1. Aorto-iliofemoral reconstruction or bypass or infrainguinal bypass (e.g., femoropopliteal, femorotibial).
  2. Percutaneous balloon angioplasty, often with stenting, is primarily used on discrete stenotic lesions in the iliac or femoropopliteal arteries.
  3. Endovascular intervention is recommended as the preferred revascularization technique for iliac and femoropopliteal arterial lesions.
  4. Stenting is effective primary therapy for common and external iliac artery stenosis and occlusions. However, it is not recommended in the femoral, popliteal, or tibial arteries due to a low success rate except to salvage suboptimal balloon dilation.
- Endovascular procedures should not be performed in patients with PAD solely to prevent progression to critical limb ischemia, as reported rates of amputation or progression to critical limb ischemia are <10% to 15% over 5 yr or more, and increased mortality rate associated with claudication is usually the result of cardiovascular events rather than limb-related events.

COMPLEMENTARY & ALTERNATIVE MEDICINE

- A meta-analysis found that over 12 to 24 weeks, *Ginkgo biloba* increased pain-free walking distance by 34 m compared with placebo, although the benefit is not well established according to ACC/AHA guidelines.
- Naftidrofuryl, a serotonin receptor inhibitor, available in Europe and other parts of the world, has shown some efficacy in improving claudication symptoms.
- Estrogen replacement therapy, propionyl-L-carnitine, L-arginine, oral vasodilators, prostaglandins, and chelation therapy are ineffective in the treatment of intermittent claudication.
- B-complex vitamin supplementation to lower homocysteine levels for prevention of cardiovascular events in patients with PAD is not recommended (HOPE-2 trial).
- Acupuncture has shown some improvement in symptom relief and functional capacity in small studies but mainly in neurogenic claudication or mild peripheral arterial disease.

DISPOSITION

- It is unusual for intermittent claudication to progress to ischemic leg or limb loss, especially with aggressive use of conservative treatments, risk factor modification, exercise, and smoking cessation.
- The 5-yr risk for development of ischemic ulceration in patients treated for diabetes and with ABI <0.5 was 30% compared with only 5% in patients without either characteristic.
- A screening duplex ultrasound for abdominal aortic aneurysm (AAA) is recommended for patients with symptomatic PAD.
- All patients with PAD should receive annual influenza vaccination based on observational studies that have demonstrated a reduced cardiovascular event rate.

REFERRAL

Consultation with physicians specializing in vascular medicine is recommended for the patient with threatened limb loss, rest pain, nonhealing ulcers, functional disability from pain, and gangrene.

PEARLS & CONSIDERATIONS

- Approximately 70% of patients with peripheral vascular disease will have concomitant coronary artery disease.
- Beta-blockers may worsen claudication symptoms in some patients, although their underuse is associated with excess cardiovascular death. Patients with intermittent claudication are less likely to receive beta-blocker therapy after a myocardial infarction. Those who do not receive post-MI beta-blockers have at least a threefold higher mortality.
- Patients with peripheral vascular disease may benefit from secondary cardiovascular prevention with clopidogrel versus aspirin more so than other high-risk patients (CAPRIE trial).
- Often, PAD can be asymptomatic or with atypical symptoms, and a thorough history, physical exam, and clinical suspicion based on medical comorbidities may help guide therapy before lifestyle-limiting claudication or limb ischemia develops.

COMMENTS

- Claudication is a marker for generalized atherosclerosis. Patients have a higher risk of death from cardiovascular events than from limb loss. Patients with PAD experience diminished overall quality of life similar to patients with diagnosed coronary artery or cerebrovascular disease.
- The ABI is more closely associated with exercise tolerance and severity of disease in persons with PAD rather than intermittent claudication or other leg symptoms.

SUGGESTED READINGS

Available at ExpertConsult.com

RELATED CONTENT

Poor Circulation (Claudication) (Patient Information)

Peripheral Arterial Disease (PAD) (Related Key Topic)

AUTHORS: **CHRIS PAN, M.D., M.B.A., M.S.,** and **PRANAV M. PATEL, M.D., FACC, FAHA, FSCAI**

C

Diseases and Disorders

BASIC INFORMATION

DEFINITION

Clostridium difficile infection (CDI) is the occurrence of diarrhea and bowel inflammation associated with antibiotic use caused by *C. difficile*, an anaerobic gram-positive, spore-forming, toxin-producing bacillus transmitted through the fecal–oral route. CDI can manifest clinically in several forms ranging from fulminant diarrhea and leukocytosis associated with pseudomembranous colitis, mild to severe acute diarrhea, short-term colonization seen typically in health care facilities, and recurrent CDI within 60 days after initial treatment occurring in 20% to 30% of cases.

SYNONYMS

Antibiotic-induced colitis
Pseudomembranous colitis
CDI

ICD-10CM CODES

A04.7 Enterocolitis due to *Clostridium difficile*

EPIDEMIOLOGY & DEMOGRAPHICS

- Cephalosporins are the most frequent offending agent in CDI because of their high rates of use.
- The antibiotic with the highest incidence is clindamycin (10% incidence of CDI with its use).
- Since 1996, the incidence of CDI has more than doubled. Severity of CDI has also increased due to the emergence of an epidemic virulent strain (NAP1/BI/027). CDI is the most common infectious cause of health-care–associated diarrhea in adults. In 2011, *C. difficile* was responsible for nearly half a million infections and was associated with approximately 29,000 deaths.
- Nosocomial CDI quadruples the cost of hospitalizations and increases annual expenditures by $1.5 billion in the U.S.
- Asymptomatic carriage of *C. difficile* is identified in more than 20% of patients hospitalized without diarrhea.

PHYSICAL FINDINGS & CLINICAL PRESENTATION

- Abdominal tenderness (generalized or lower abdominal)
- Fever
- In patients with prolonged diarrhea, poor skin turgor, dry mucous membranes, and other signs of dehydration may be present

ETIOLOGY

C. difficile colonizes the large intestines and releases 2 protein exotoxins (TcdA and TcdB) that cause colitis. Infection is transmitted by spores that are resistant to antibiotics, heat, and acid. The NAP1 strain is predominant among patients with *C. difficile* infection, whereas asymptomatic patients are more likely to be colonized with other strains. Risk factors for *C. difficile* (the major identifiable agent of antibiotic-induced diarrhea and colitis):

- Administration of antibiotics: Can occur with any antibiotic, but occurs most frequently with clindamycin, ampicillin, cephalosporins, and fluoroquinolone
- Prolonged hospitalization
- Advanced age
- Abdominal surgery
- Underlying disease (malignancy, renal failure, debilitated status)
- Hospitalized, tube-fed patients are at risk for *C. difficile*–associated diarrhea. Clinicians should consider testing for *C. difficile* in tube-fed patients with diarrhea unrelated to the feeding solution.
- PPI and H_2 blocker therapy increases risk of CDI and recurrent CDI. Risk is 1.7-fold higher with PPIs.

Dx DIAGNOSIS

The clinical signs of CDI generally include diarrhea, fever, and abdominal cramps after use of antibiotics. Although a history of recent antibiotic use is common, it is not a requirement for diagnosis.

DIFFERENTIAL DIAGNOSIS

- Gastrointestinal bacterial infections (e.g., *Salmonella, Shigella, Campylobacter, Yersinia*)
- Enteric parasites (e.g., *Cryptosporidium, Entamoeba histolytica*)
- Inflammatory bowel disease
- Celiac sprue
- Irritable bowel syndrome
- Ischemic colitis
- Antibiotic intolerance

WORKUP

- All patients with diarrhea accompanied by current or recent antibiotic use should be tested for *C. difficile* (see later discussion). *C. difficile* stool tests are positive in 3% of outpatients and up to 29% of inpatients without signs of infection. Testing and treatment for CDI is not recommended in asymptomatic individuals.
- Sigmoidoscopy (without cleansing enema) may be necessary when the clinical and laboratory diagnosis is inconclusive and the diarrhea persists.
- In antibiotic-induced pseudomembranous colitis, the sigmoidoscopy often reveals raised white-yellow exudative plaques adherent to the colonic mucosa pseudomembranes. These are seen more commonly in severe CDI.

LABORATORY TESTS

- Stool test for *C. difficile* toxin: Enzyme-linked immunosorbent assay for *C. difficile* toxins A and B. The latter is used most widely in the clinical setting. It has a sensitivity of 85% and a specificity of 100%.
- *C. difficile* toxin can be detected by cytotoxin tissue culture assay (cytotoxin assay, gold standard for identifying *C. difficile* toxin in stool specimen). This test is difficult to perform, and results are not available for 24 to 48 hr.
- Fecal leukocytes (assessed by microscopy or lactoferrin assay) are generally present in stool samples.
- Complete blood count usually reveals leukocytosis. A sudden increase in white blood cells to >30,000/mm^3 may be indicative of fulminant colitis.
- Laboratory indicators of **severe CDI** are leukocyte count >15,000/mm^3, serum creatinine ≥1.5 times baseline level, serum albumin <2.5 g/dl.

IMAGING STUDIES

- Abdominal film (flat plate and upright) is useful in patients with abdominal pain or evidence of obstruction on physical examination.
- CT can demonstrate typical findings of colonic wall thickening, dilatation, and the so-called *accordion sign* (thickened haustral folds and trapped contrast material, ascites, or pericolonic stranding [Fig. 1]).

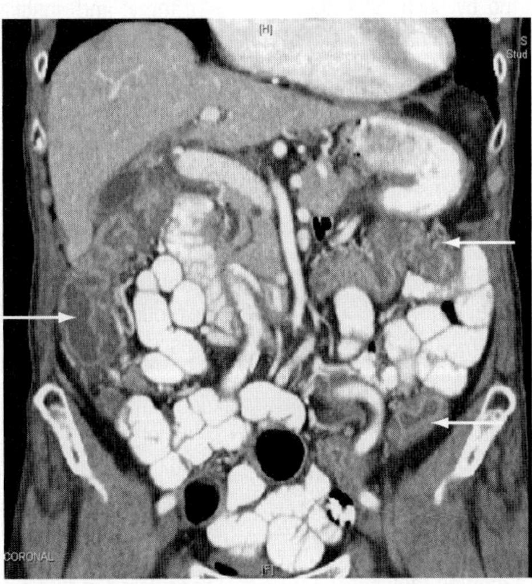

FIG. 1 Computed tomography with oral and intravenous contrast in a patient with *Clostridium difficile* colitis. Typical findings include colonic wall thickening *(arrows)*, dilation, and accordion sign (thickened haustral fold and trapped contrast material, ascites, and pericolonic stranding). (From Vincent JL, et al.: *Textbook of critical care*, ed 7, Philadelphia, 2017, Elsevier.)

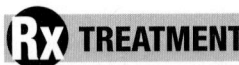

TREATMENT

NONPHARMACOLOGIC THERAPY

- Discontinue offending antibiotic.
- Fluid hydration and correction of electrolyte abnormalities.
- Probiotics to restore natural defense mechanisms may be useful as adjuvant therapy; however, evidence is limited. Probiotic trials have failed to show benefit in preventing *C. difficile*–associated diarrhea.
- Fecal microbiota transplantation (FMT) is an excellent treatment modality for recurrent CDI. It replaces the altered gut flora to allow colonization resistance. Trials have shown that it is more effective than vancomycin and may become standard treatment for recurrent CDI. Recent trials have shown that donor stool administered via colonoscopy are safe and more efficacious than autologous FMT in preventing further CDI episodes.

ACUTE GENERAL Rx

- Vancomycin 125 mg PO qid for 10 days can be used as initial treatment in patients with nonsevere or severe CDI. Patients with fulminant CDI will require 500 mg qid for 10 days.
- Fidaxomicin 200 mg bid for 10 days has shown non-inferiority to vancomycin and a lower rate of CDI recurrence (25% with vancomycin vs. 15% with fidaxomicin); however, its higher cost is a limiting factor. Fidaxomicin can be used for initial treatment of nonsevere or severe CDI or for recurrence of CDI if vancomycin was used for initial treatment.
- Metronidazole 500 mg PO qid for 10 days can be used in patients with mild disease if oral vancomycin or fidaxomicin are not available or contraindicated. A significant rise in clinical failure has been seen with metronidazole over the past decade, especially in patients with the BI/NAP/027 strain.
- When parenteral therapy is necessary (e.g., patient with paralytic ileus), IV metronidazole 500 mg qid can be used. It can also be supplemented with vancomycin 500 mg by nasogastric tube with intermittent clamping or retention enema.
- Fecal microbiota transplantation (FMT): When standard treatment has failed, intestinal microbiota transplantation (IMT) is an effective alternative therapy (eradication rate is 94%). It involves infusing intestinal microorganisms (in a suspension of healthy donor stool) into the intestine of a sick patient via enema, oral capsule, gastroscope/colonoscope, or nasojejunal tube to restore the microbiota. In patients with recurrent C. difficile infection, FMT by oral capsule has been shown to be noninferior to transplantation by colonoscopy for recurrence at 12 weeks. Trials comparing fresh versus frozen fecal microbiota transplantation have shown equal efficacy.
- The human monoclonal antibody bezlotoxumab has been FDA-approved for use with antibacterial drug treatment to reduce recurrence of CDI. Cost is a limiting factor.

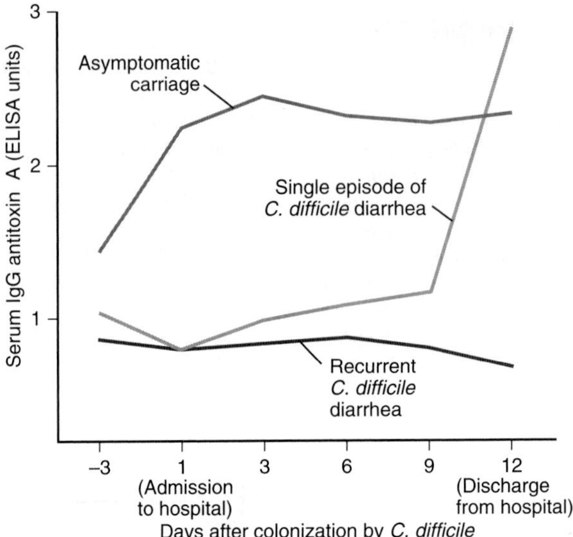

FIG. 2 Serum immunoglobulin G (IgG) antitoxin A antibody response and clinical outcome of infection with *Clostridium difficile*. Patients with nosocomial *C. difficile* diarrhea were studied prospectively, and serum IgG antitoxin A antibody concentrations were measured by enzyme-linked immunosorbent assay (ELISA) at regular intervals. A correlation was observed between the IgG response to toxin A and the clinical outcome of infection. Asymptomatic carriers mounted an early memory immune response to toxin A. By contrast, no significant increase was found in serum IgG antitoxin A of patients who experienced recurrent *C. difficile* diarrhea. In those who had a single episode of diarrhea, IgG antitoxin A levels generally were increased on day 12 of their first episode. Thus, a serum antibody response to toxin A during *C. difficile* infection is associated with protection against symptoms and against recurrent diarrhea. (From Feldman M, et al. [eds]: *Sleisenger and Fordtran's gastrointestinal and liver disease*, ed 10, Philadelphia, 2016, Saunders.)

SURGICAL MANAGEMENT OF CDI

- Indications: CDI unresponsive to medical therapy, fulminant colitis
- Clinical features: Colonic distention, severe abdominal pain/tenderness, systemic inflammatory response syndrome. Diarrhea may be absent because of ileus.
- Surgical approaches:
  1. Traditional (subtotal or total colectomy), high mortality (50%)
  2. Colon-sparing (loop ileostomy with intraoperative colonic lavage using warmed polyethylene glycol solution via the ileostomy and instillations of postoperative vancomycin flushes via the ileostomy); lower mortality compared to traditional approach

CHRONIC Rx

- Judicious future use of antibiotics to prevent recurrences (e.g., avoid prolonged antibiotic therapy).
- Probiotics have been shown mildly effective in reducing the risk for CDI among patients prescribed antibiotics. They should not be used in immunocompromised or severely debilitated patients.
- Alcohol-based hand gels are inadequate for eradication of spores. They are inferior to soap and water for eradication of spores.
- Gastric acid suppression with PPIs increases risk of CDI. Preferential use of H_2RA should be considered in these patients.

DISPOSITION

- Most patients recover completely with appropriate therapy. Fever resolves within 48 hr and diarrhea within 4 to 5 days. Overall mortality rate is 1% to 2.5% but exceeds 10% in untreated patients. CDI recurrence after an initial episode is 20% to 25% regardless of initial treatment with metronidazole or vancomycin. Each recurrence increases risk of repeat episodes (65% chance of recurrence after 3 CDI episodes). Recurrent CDI usually represents relapse rather than reinfection, no matter how long between episodes (Fig. 2). Recurrent episodes are best treated with a prolonged course of oral vancomycin tapered off over several weeks to months.
- Hospital-acquired CDI is independently associated with an increased risk of in-hospital death. All hospitalized patients with CDI should be placed in contact isolation at least until resolution of diarrhea.

SUGGESTED READINGS

Available at ExpertConsult.com

RELATED CONTENT

Clostridium difficile Infection (Patient Information)
Pseudomembranous Colitis (Patient Information)

AUTHOR: **FRED F. FERRI, M.D.**

BASIC INFORMATION

DEFINITION

The term *cluster headache* refers to attacks of severe, unilateral pain that is orbital, supraorbital, temporal, or any combination of these sites, lasting 15 to 180 minutes, and occurring from once every other day to eight times a day over a span of weeks to months. The attacks are associated with one or more ipsilateral signs and symptoms of parasympathetic activation: conjunctival injection, lacrimation (Fig. 1), nasal congestion, rhinorrhea, forehead and facial sweating, miosis, ptosis, or eyelid edema. Most patients are restless or agitated during an attack.

SYNONYMS

Headache, cluster
Ciliary neuralgia
Erythromelalgia of the head
Erythroprosopalgia of Bing
Horton's headache

ICD-10CM CODES	
G44.001	Cluster headache syndrome, unspecified, intractable
G44.009	Cluster headache syndrome, unspecified, not intractable
G44.011	Episodic cluster headache, intractable
G44.019	Episodic cluster headache, not intractable
G44.021	Chronic cluster headache, intractable
G44.029	Chronic cluster headache, not intractable

EPIDEMIOLOGY & DEMOGRAPHICS

INCIDENCE: Estimated to occur in 0.05% to 1% of the population

PREDOMINANT SEX: Occurs in males at least five times more commonly than in females

PREDOMINANT AGE: Peak age of onset between 20 and 40 yr

GENETICS: May be inherited in up to 20% of cases, although uncertainty exists over the mode or modes of inheritance.

PHYSICAL FINDINGS & CLINICAL PRESENTATION

- Many of the attacks are nocturnal and some may be provoked by alcohol ingestion.
- During attack: Conjunctival injection, lacrimation, nasal congestion, rhinorrhea, facial sweating, Horner syndrome.
- In contrast to migraine sufferers, patients are agitated and active during an attack.
- Symptoms associated with an attack remain ipsilateral during the attack but may switch sides from one attack to the next.
- Permanent partial Horner syndrome in 5% of patients; otherwise examination is normal.

ETIOLOGY

Activation of the posterior hypothalamic gray matter resulting in trigeminal activation coupled with parasympathetic activation. The pathophysiology remains controversial.

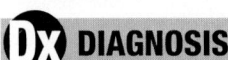

DIAGNOSIS

Per the *International Classification of Headache Disorders, 3rd edition,* the diagnosis of cluster headache requires all of the following:

- At least five attacks of severe or very severe unilateral orbital, supraorbital, and/or temporal pain lasting 15 to 180 minutes.
- Frequency of every other day to eight per day; they may cluster seasonally or at a certain time in a patient's life.
- Headache is accompanied by a sense of restlessness or agitation and/or at least one of the following (ipsilateral):
  1. Conjunctival injection and/or lacrimation
  2. Nasal congestion and/or rhinorrhea
  3. Eyelid edema
  4. Forehead and facial sweating
  5. Forehead and facial flushing
  6. Miosis and/or ptosis
  7. Sensation of fullness in the ear
  8. Restlessness or agitation

A diagnosis of episodic cluster headache requires the above criteria plus attacks that occur in bouts, also called cluster periods. These periods last 1 week to 1 yr and are separated by attack-free intervals lasting at least 1 month.

A diagnosis of chronic cluster headache requires meeting the criteria for cluster headache plus at least 1 yr of attacks without a pain-free interval of at least 1 month.

DIFFERENTIAL DIAGNOSIS

- Migraine
- Trigeminal neuralgia
- Primary stabbing headache
- Temporal arteritis
- Post-herpetic neuralgia
- Venous sinus thrombosis
- Carotid-cavernous fistula or other cavernous sinus lesions
- Other trigeminal autonomic cephalalgias
- Section II describes the differential diagnosis of headaches

WORKUP

Diagnosis is made clinically.

IMAGING STUDIES

- None, unless history or examination suggests focal neurologic deficit or headaches change in character or are of new onset.
- MRI of the brain along with vascular imaging may be necessary to exclude secondary headaches at the time of initial diagnosis.

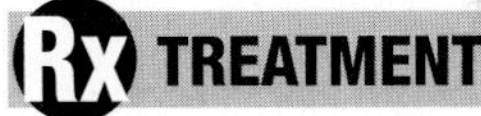

TREATMENT

NONPHARMACOLOGIC THERAPY

Avoidance of alcohol, histamine, nitroglycerin, and tobacco during clusters

ABORTIVE Rx

- Inhalation of 100% oxygen by face mask at a flow rate of 12 L/min or greater for 15 min aborts the attack in 60% to 80% of patients.
- In approximately 75% of patients, subcutaneous or nasal triptans (e.g., sumatriptan, zolmitriptan) will result in freedom from pain within 20 minutes. Only injectable and nasal formulations achieve a response that is rapid enough to be efficacious.
- Cafergot, octreotide, intranasal lidocaine, or dihydroergotamine may abort an attack or prevent one if given just before a predictable episode. An attack typically resolves before oral analgesics can take effect, although indomethacin and other NSAIDs may be effective in prolonged attacks.

PROPHYLAXIS Rx

For patients with episodic cluster headache, prophylactic treatment should be started at the onset of the cluster period and tapered at its end. Patients with chronic cluster headache should be

FIG. 1 This 43-year-old man with cluster headaches suffers from nightly right-sided unrelenting, severe, stabbing unilateral periorbital pain for 45 minutes to 3 hours accompanied by ipsilateral tearing and nasal discharge, along with ptosis and miosis (a partial Horner syndrome). Note that the ptosis prompts compensatory elevation of the eyebrow. (From Kaufman DM, et al.: *Kaufman's clinical neurology for psychiatrists*, ed 8, Philadelphia, 2017, Elsevier.)

started on prophylactic treatment at increasing doses until good control is achieved. Preventative therapy should begin with verapamil. Alternative treatment options are also listed below.

- Verapamil: Start at 240 mg/day; increase up to 960 mg/day as tolerated. Dosing three times per day may be more effective than extended release. First-degree AV block may develop with escalating doses, so ECG should be checked.
- Topiramate: Up to 50 mg bid; can be used as add-on to verapamil.
- Lithium: 200 mg tid with frequent monitoring and adjustment to maintain therapeutic serum level of 0.4 to 1 mEq/L. Equally effective as verapamil, but with more side effects.
- Ergotamine tartrate: 3 to 4 mg/day during clusters.
- Melatonin: 10 mg per night. Evidence is weak and comes from scattered case reports.
- Prednisone: 60 mg PO daily for 1 wk followed by taper; headaches can return during taper.
- Greater and lesser occipital nerve blocks, with the use of local anesthetics including lidocaine and bupivacaine along with steroids like Depo-Medrol, dexamethasone, or triamcinolone, may be used to shorten the duration of the cluster period. Consensus guidelines from the American Headache Society have been published recently.
- There is emerging evidence for benefit of a sphenopalatine ganglion block that may be available at some centers for both treatment and prophylaxis of cluster attacks.

DISPOSITION

Headache-free periods tend to increase with increasing age.

REFERRAL

Refractory cluster headaches may require referral to a headache specialist.

PEARLS & CONSIDERATIONS

COMMENTS

- Cluster headaches are divided into episodic (attacks lasting up to 1 yr with more than 1 month pain-free periods) and chronic (>1 yr without remission). Episodic cluster headache is six times more common than the chronic form.
- Home oxygen therapy is reasonable for cluster headache sufferers.

SUGGESTED READINGS

Available at ExpertConsult.com

RELATED CONTENT

Cluster Headaches (Patient Information)

AUTHORS: **MICHAEL POHLEN, M.D., JOSEPH S. KASS, M.D., J.D., F.A.A.N.** and **SIDDHARTH KAPOOR, M.D.**

BASIC INFORMATION

DEFINITION

Cocaine is an alkaloid derived from the coca plant *Erythroxylum coca,* native to South America, which contains approximately 0.5% to 1% cocaine. The drug produces physiologic and behavioral effects when administered orally, intranasally, intravenously, or by inhalation after smoking. Cocaine has potent pharmacologic effects on dopamine, norepinephrine, and serotonin neurons in the central nervous system (CNS) involving alteration and blockade of cellular membrane transport and prevention of reuptake. Cocaine's second action involves the blockage of voltage-gated sodium ion membrane channels, which is responsible for its anesthetic effect. Table 1 describes the pharmacokinetics of cocaine according to route of administration. The mechanism by which cocaine alters sympathetic tone is illustrated in Fig. 1.

SYNONYMS

Cocaine hydrochloride: Topical solution (FDA approved as a topical anesthetic)

Crack: This is produced when the hydrochloride molecule is removed by ether extraction, which frees the basic cocaine molecule or "free base." Heating does not destroy the free base; rather, it melts at 98° F and vaporizes at higher temperatures, allowing it to be smoked.

Freebase: Aqueous solution of cocaine hydrochloride converted to a more volatile base state by the addition of alkali, thereby extracting the cocaine base in a residue or precipitate.

Street names include Bernice, Blow, C, Carrie, Cecil, Charlie, Coke, Dust, Dynamite, Flake, Gin, Girl, Gold dust, Green gold, Jet, Powder, Star dust, Paradise, Pimp's drug, Snow, Stardust, White girl, Yay, Yayo

Liquid lady: Alcohol + cocaine

Speedball: Heroin + cocaine

Street measures: Git (2-200 mg), snort, line, dose, spoon (approximately 1 g)

ICD-10CM CODES

T40.5 Poisoning, cocaine

F14.20 Cocaine dependence, uncomplicated

EPIDEMIOLOGY & DEMOGRAPHICS

- The 2016 National Survey on Drug Use and Health published by the U.S. Department of Health and Human Services estimates that in 2016 1.9 million people aged 12 or older were current users of cocaine. This includes about 432,000 users of "crack" cocaine. The estimate is similar to those in most years between 2007 and 2015 but was lower than the estimates in 2002 to 2006.
- Table 2 summarizes characteristics of patients with cocaine-induced myocardial infarction.

PHYSICAL FINDINGS & CLINICAL PRESENTATION

PHASE I:

- CNS: Euphoria, agitation, headache, vertigo, twitching, bruxism, unintentional tremor
- Nausea, vomiting, fever, hypertension, tachycardia

PHASE II:

- CNS: Lethargy, hyperreactive deep tendon reflexes, seizures (status epilepticus)
- Sympathetic overdrive: Tachycardia, hypertension, hyperthermia
- Incontinence

PHASE III:

- CNS: Flaccid paralysis, coma, fixed dilated pupils, loss of reflexes
- Pulmonary edema
- Cardiopulmonary arrest

Psychological dependence manifests with habituation, paranoia, and hallucinations (cocaine "bugs").

CNS: Cerebral ischemia and infarction, cerebral arterial spasm, cerebral vasculitis, cerebral vascular thrombosis, subarachnoid hemorrhage, intraparenchymal hemorrhage, seizures, cerebral atrophy, movement disorders, and hyperthermia

Cardiac: Acute myocardial ischemia and infarction (Fig. 2), arrhythmias (Table 3), and sudden death, dilated cardiomyopathy and myocarditis, infective endocarditis, aortic rupture, acceleration of coronary atherosclerosis

Pulmonary: Inhalation injuries (secondary to smoking crack cocaine): Cartilage and nasal septal perforation, oropharyngeal ulcers; immunologically mediated diseases: Hypersensitivity pneumonitis, bronchiolitis obliterans; pulmonary vascular lesions and hemorrhage, pulmonary infarction, pulmonary edema secondary to left ventricular failure, pneumomediastinum, and pneumothorax

TABLE 1 Pharmacokinetics of Cocaine According to Route of Administration

Route of Administration	Onset of Action	Peak Effect	Duration of Action
Inhalation (smoking)	3-5 sec	1-3 min	5-15 min
Intravenous	10-60 sec	3-5 min	20-60 min
Intranasal or other mucosal	1-5 min	15-20 min	60-90 min

From Bonow RO et al: *Heart disease,* ed 9, Philadelphia, 2012, Saunders.

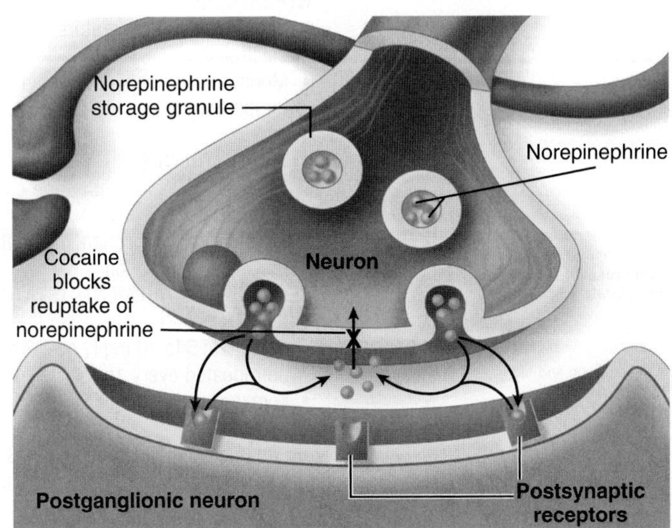

FIG. 1 Mechanism by which cocaine alters sympathetic tone. Cocaine blocks the reuptake of norepinephrine by the preganglionic neuron (X), thereby resulting in excess amounts of this neurotransmitter at postganglionic receptor sites. (From Mann DL et al: *Braunwald's heart disease,* ed 10, Philadelphia, 2015, Elsevier.)

TABLE 2 Characteristics of Patients with Cocaine-Induced Myocardial Infarction

Dose of Cocaine

5-6 lines (150 mg) to as much as 2 g

Serum concentration, 0.01-1.02 mg/L

Frequency of Use

Reported in chronic, recreational, and first-time users

Route of Administration

Occurs with all routes of administration

75% of reported MIs occurred after intranasal use

Age

Mean, 34 (range, 17-71) yr

20% younger than 25 yr

Sex

80%-90% male

Timing

Often within minutes of cocaine use

Reported as late as 5-15 hr after use

MI, Myocardial infarction.

From Mann DL et al: *Braunwald's heart disease,* ed 10, Philadelphia, 2015, Elsevier.

Gastrointestinal: Gastroduodenal ulceration and perforation; intestinal infarction or perforation, colitis
Renal: Acute renal failure secondary to rhabdomyolysis and myoglobinuria; renal infarction; focal segmental glomerulosclerosis
Obstetric: Placental abruption, low infant weight, prematurity, microcephaly
Psychiatric: Anxiety, depression, paranoia, delirium, psychosis, suicide

Adulterants such as levamisole (an immunomodulator) and clenbuterol (a beta-adrenergic agonist) have been found mixed with cocaine. Levamisole can cause agranulocytosis, leukoencephalopathy, and cutaneous vasculitis leading to necrosis of the skin. Clenbuterol may cause tachycardia, hyperglycemia, and hypokalemia.

TABLE 3 Cardiac Dysrhythmias and Conduction Disturbances Reported with Cocaine Use

Sinus tachycardia
Sinus bradycardia
Supraventricular tachycardia
Bundle branch block
Complete heart block
Accelerated idioventricular rhythm
Ventricular tachycardia
Ventricular fibrillation
Asystole
Torsades de pointes
Brugada pattern (right bundle branch block with ST-segment elevation in leads V_1, V_2, and V_3)

From Mann DL et al: *Braunwald's heart disease*, ed 10, Philadelphia, 2015, Elsevier.

ETIOLOGY

Cocaine may be absorbed through different routes with varying degrees of speed:
- Nasal insufflation/snorting: 2.5 min
- Smoking: <30 sec
- Oral: 2 to 5 min
- Mucosal: <20 min
- Intravenous injection: <30 sec

Dx DIAGNOSIS

DIFFERENTIAL DIAGNOSIS

- Methamphetamine ("speed") abuse
- Methylenedioxyamphetamine ("ecstasy") abuse
- Cathinone ("khat") abuse
- Lysergic acid diethylamide (LSD) abuse

WORKUP

Physical examination and laboratory evaluation

LABORATORY TESTS

- Toxicology screen (urine): Cocaine is metabolized within 2 hr by the liver to major metabolites, benzoylecgonine, and ecgonine methyl ester, which are excreted in the urine. Metabolites can be identified in urine within 5 min of IV use and up to 48 hr after oral ingestion.
- Blood: CBC, electrolytes, glucose, BUN, creatinine, calcium
- Arterial blood gas analysis
- ECG
- Serum creatine kinase and troponin concentration

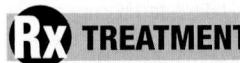

Rx TREATMENT

There is no specific antidote, and at present, no drug therapy is uniquely effective in treating cocaine abuse and dependence. Modifying cocaine's pharmacokinetic properties by sequestering or hydrolyzing it in serum and limiting its access to its sites of action may prove helpful by using a bacterial cocaine esterase, currently investigational. Adulterants (such as levamisole and clenbuterol, discussed earlier), contaminants, and other drugs may be admixed with street cocaine and should be kept in mind with patients presenting with unusual manifestations. Amantadine may provide effective treatment for cocaine-dependent patients with severe cocaine withdrawal symptoms, as well as the other dopamine agonist bromocriptine (1.5 mg PO tid), which may alleviate some of the symptoms of craving associated with acute cocaine withdrawal.

ACUTE GENERAL Rx

Acute cocaine toxicity requires following advanced poisoning treatment and life support. A suspected "body packer" should have an abdominal radiograph to detect the continued presence of cocaine-containing condoms in the intestinal tract. If present, gentle catharsis with charcoal and mineral oil should be performed with ICU admission and monitoring.

SPECIFIC TREATMENT

INHALATION: Wash nasal passages

AGITATION:
- Check STAT glucose
- Diazepam 15 to 20 mg PO or 2 to 10 mg IM or IV for severe agitation

HYPERTHERMIA:
- Check rectal temperature, creatine kinase, electrolytes
- Monitor with continuous rectal probe; bring temperature down to 101° F within 30 to 45 min

RHABDOMYOLYSIS:
- Vigorous hydration with urine output at least 2 ml/kg
- Mannitol or bicarbonate for rhabdomyolysis resistant to hydration

SEIZURE MANAGEMENT (STATUS EPILEPTICUS):
- Diazepam 5 to 10 mg IV over 2 to 3 min; may be repeated every 10 to 15 min.
- Lorazepam 2 to 3 mg IV over 2 to 3 min; may be repeated.
- Phenytoin loading dose 15 to 18 mg/kg IV at a rate not to exceed 25 to 50 mg/min under cardiac monitoring.
- Phenobarbital loading dose 10 to 15 mg/kg IV at a rate of 25 mg/min; an additional 5 mg/kg may be given in 30 to 45 min if seizures are not controlled.

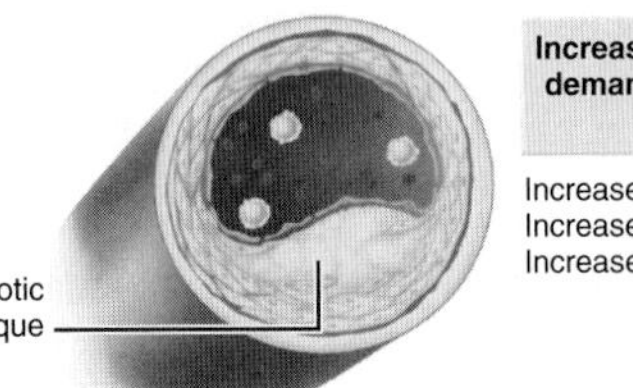

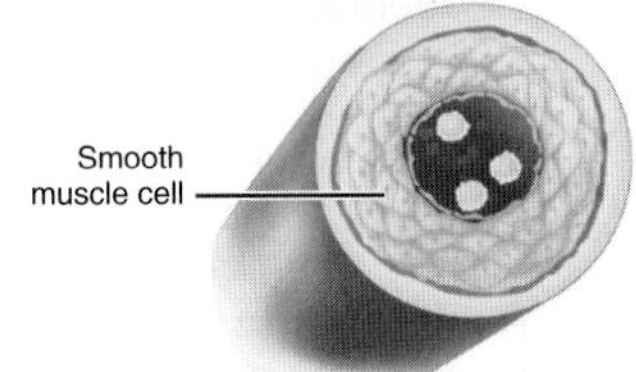

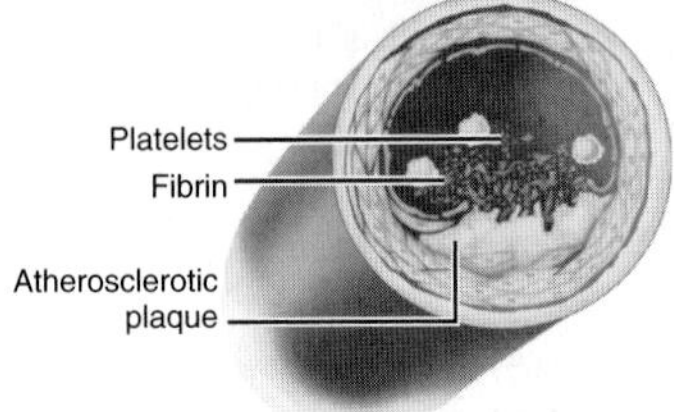

FIG. 2 Mechanisms by which cocaine may induce myocardial ischemia or infarction. Cocaine may induce myocardial ischemia or infarction by increasing the determinants of myocardial oxygen demand in the setting of limited oxygen supply (*top*), thereby causing intense coronary arterial vasoconstriction (*middle*) or inducing accelerated atherosclerosis and thrombosis (*bottom*). (From Mann DL et al: *Braunwald's heart disease*, ed 10, Philadelphia, 2015, Elsevier.)

- For refractory seizures, consider:
  1. Pancuronium 0.1 mg/kg IV
  2. Halothane general anesthesia
  3. Both require EEG monitoring to determine brain seizure activity.

HYPERTENSION: Cocaine-induced hypertension usually responds to benzodiazepines. If this fails:

- Consider arterial line for continuous blood pressure monitoring.
- Avoid the use of calcium channel blockers because they may potentiate the incidence of seizures and death, especially in body packers.
- The use of beta-blockers may exacerbate cocaine-induced vasoconstriction and may cause paradoxical hypertension, worsening patient outcomes.
- Phentolamine (unopposed adrenergic effects) or nitroglycerin may be required.
- If diastolic pressure >120 mm Hg: Hydralazine hydrochloride 25 mg IM or IV; may repeat q1h.
- If hypertension is uncontrolled or hypertensive encephalopathy is present: Sodium nitroprusside initially at 0.5 mg/kg/min not to exceed 10 mg/kg/min.

CHEST PAIN:

- Chest radiograph, ECG, cardiac enzymes
- Benzodiazepines (diazepam 5mg IV or lorazepam 1 mg IV every 5 minutes) for agitation until sedation is achieved
- Acetylsalicylic acid and nitroglycerin for ischemic pain (Aspirin is contraindicated if dissection is suspected.)
- Percutaneous transluminal coronary angioplasty possibly better than thrombolysis for cocaine-associated myocardial infarction
- Phentolamine will reverse cocaine-induced vasoconstriction and may be administered 5 to 10 mg every 5 to 10 minutes
- The use of beta-adrenergic blockers is not generally recommended for reasons highlighted earlier
- If beta-blockers are to be used, this should be preceded by administration of phentolamine to prevent unopposed alpha-adrenergic stimulation. Many authors recommend not using beta-blockers until the cocaine has been systemically eliminated

VENTRICULAR ARRHYTHMIAS (CONSIDERATIONS):

- The Advanced Cardiac Life Support (ACLS) protocol should be followed.
- Antiarrhythmic agents should be used with caution during the early period after cocaine exposure as a result of their proarrhythmic and proconvulsant effects.
- Termination of ventricular arrhythmias may be resistant to lidocaine and even cardioversion.
- In a cardiac arrest situation secondary to cocaine toxicity, vasopressin offers a theoretical advantage over epinephrine as it increases coronary blood flow and myocardial oxygen availability. In the 2015 ACLS update, however, vasopressin was removed from the treatment algorithm, so it may not be readily available.

BOX 1 Complications Associated with Cocaine Use

Cardiovascular
Myocardial ischemia, infarction
Arrhythmias
Aortic dissection, rupture
Hypertension
Atherosclerosis
Cardiomyopathy
Vasculitis

Central Nervous System
Seizures
Cerebral infarction
Transient ischemic attack
Intracranial hemorrhage (intraparenchymal, intraventricular, subarachnoid)
Cerebral vasculitis
Cognitive dysfunction

Pulmonary
Bronchospasm
Barotrauma
Noncardiogenic edema
Pulmonary hypertension

Renal
Renal infarction
Renal failure
Scleroderma renal crisis

Gastrointestinal
Mesenteric ischemia, infarction
Gastrointestinal tract perforations

Metabolic
Hyperthermia
Rhabdomyolysis
Weight loss
Multiple organ failure

Other
Deep venous thrombosis
Skin ischemia
Dystonic reactions

From Parrillo JE, Dellinger RP: *Critical care medicine, principles of diagnosis and management in the adult,* ed 4, Philadelphia, 2014, Elsevier.

DISPOSITION

Although many patients who use cocaine may not require treatment because of the short half-life of the drug, others may require specific treatment for possible cocaine-related complications. Box 1 summarizes complications associated with cocaine use.

REFERRAL

Consider psychotherapy or behavioral therapy once stable. There is some evidence that topiramate 300 mg orally daily added to cognitive behavioral therapy may be beneficial in patients with severe withdrawal symptoms.

PEARLS & CONSIDERATIONS

- Cocaine-induced vasoconstriction may be exacerbated by the use of selective and nonselective beta-adrenergic blocking agents.
- The use of lidocaine in treating ventricular arrhythmias may precipitate seizures and further arrhythmias.
- Clinical trials with the SSRI sertraline 200 mg/day have shown that it may help prevent relapse in individuals with some depression symptoms.

SUGGESTED READINGS

Available at ExpertConsult.com

RELATED CONTENT

Cocaine Abuse and Dependence (Patient Information)
Drug Abuse (Patient Information)
Drug Abuse (Related Key Topic)

AUTHOR: **SAJEEV HANDA, M.D., S.F.H.M.**

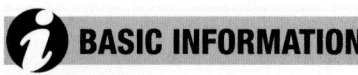

BASIC INFORMATION

DEFINITION

Colorectal cancer (CRC) is a neoplasm arising from the luminal surface of the large bowel; locations include descending colon (40% to 42%), rectosigmoid and rectum (30% to 33%), cecum and ascending colon (25% to 30%), and transverse colon (10% to 13%).

ICD-10CM CODES

C18	Malignant neoplasm of colon
C18.2	Malignant neoplasm of colon, ascending colon
C18.4	Malignant neoplasm of colon, transverse colon
C18.6	Malignant neoplasm of colon, descending colon
C18.7	Malignant neoplasm of colon, sigmoid colon
C19	Malignant neoplasm of rectosigmoid junction

EPIDEMIOLOGY & DEMOGRAPHICS

- Worldwide, CRC accounts for about 1.4 million new cases and 700,000 deaths annually. The highest incidence is in North America, Australasia, Europe, and South Korea.
- CRC is the fourth most common cancer and the second leading cause of cancer deaths in the U.S. (140,250 new cases and 50,630 deaths for 2018). Distant metastatic disease is present in 18% to 22% of patients at time of diagnosis.
- The peak incidence is in the seventh decade of life. The lifetime risk for development of CRC is 1 in 17, with 90% of cases occurring after age 50 yr.
- Risk factors:
  1. Hereditary polyposis syndromes
  2. Familial polyposis (high risk)
  3. Gardner syndrome (high risk)
  4. Turcot syndrome (high risk)
  5. Peutz-Jeghers syndrome (low to moderate risk)
  6. Inflammatory bowel disease (IBD), both ulcerative colitis and Crohn disease
  7. Family history of "cancer family syndrome"
  8. Heredofamilial breast cancer and colon carcinoma
  9. Pelvic irradiation history
  10. First-degree relatives with colorectal carcinoma
  11. Age >50 yr
  12. Dietary factors (diet high in fat or red meat, alcohol use, low vegetable intake)
  13. Hereditary nonpolyposis colon cancer (HNPCC): Autosomal dominant disorder characterized by early age of onset (mean age, 44 yr) and right-sided or proximal colon cancers, synchronous and metachronous colon cancers, mucinous and poorly differentiated colon cancers; accounts for 1% to 5% of all cases of CRC
  14. Previous endometrial or ovarian cancer, particularly when diagnosed at an early age

PHYSICAL FINDINGS & CLINICAL PRESENTATION

- Physical examination may be completely unremarkable.
- Digital rectal examination can detect approximately 50% of rectal cancers.
- Palpable abdominal masses may indicate metastasis or complications of colorectal carcinoma (abscess, intussusception, volvulus).
- Abdominal distention and tenderness are suggestive of colonic obstruction.
- Hepatomegaly is indicative of hepatic metastasis.

ETIOLOGY

CRC can arise through either of two mutational pathways: microsatellite instability or chromosomal instability. Germline genetic mutations are the basis of inherited colon cancer syndromes; an accumulation of somatic mutations in a cell is the basis of sporadic colon cancer. Approximately 15% of CRC lack one or more mismatch repair enzymes (mismatch repair deficient [dMMR]-CRC).

DIAGNOSIS

DIFFERENTIAL DIAGNOSIS

- Diverticular disease
- Strictures or adhesions
- Inflammatory bowel disease (IBD)
- Infectious or inflammatory lesions
- Arteriovenous malformations
- Metastatic carcinoma
- Extrinsic masses (cysts, abscesses)

WORKUP

The clinical presentation of colorectal malignancies may consist of nonspecific symptoms (weight loss, anorexia, malaise) or of specific symptoms related to mass effect or bleeding. It is useful to divide colon cancer symptoms into those usually associated with the right- or left-sided cancers because the clinical presentation can vary with the location.

- Right side of colon:
  1. Anemia (from chronic blood loss).
  2. Abdominal pain may be present, or the patient may be completely asymptomatic.
  3. Rectal bleeding is often missed because blood is mixed with feces.
  4. Obstruction and constipation are unusual because of large lumen and more liquid stools.
- Left side of colon:
  1. Change in bowel habits (constipation, diarrhea, tenesmus, pencil-thin stools).
  2. Rectal bleeding (bright red blood coating the surface of the stool).
  3. Intestinal obstruction is frequent because of small lumen.

CLASSIFICATION AND STAGING

AJCC 8th edition classification for CRC:

A. Confined to the mucosa-submucosa (stage I)
B. Invasion of muscularis propria (stage II)
C. Local node involvement (stage III)
D. Distant metastasis (stage IV)

TNM Classification:

Stage	TNM Classification
I	T_{1-2}, N_0, M_0
II_A	T_3, N_0, M_0
II_B	T_{4a}, N_0, M_0
II_C	T_{4b}, N_0, M_0
III_A	T_{1-2}, N_1, M_0; T_1, N_{2a}, M_0
III_B	T_{3-4a}, N_1, M_0 T_{2-3}, N_{2a}, M_0 T_{1-2}, N_{2b}, M_0
III_C	T_{4a}, N_{2a}, M_0 T_{3-4a}, N_{2b}, M_0 T_{4b}, N_{1-2}, M_0
IV_A	T(any), N(any), M_{1a}
IV_B	T(any), N(any), M_{1b}
IV_C	T(any), N(any), M_{1c}

LABORATORY TESTS

- Positive fecal occult blood test (FOBT): Many primary care physicians use single digital FOBT as their primary screening test for CRC. Single FOBT has low specificity for detecting human hemoglobin, is a poor screening method for CRC (sensitivity, 4.9%), and is inappropriate as the only test because negative results do not decrease the odds of advanced neoplasia. The American College of Gastroenterology recommends fecal immunochemical test (FIT) as a replacement for guaiac-based FOBT for CRC detection. FIT measures intact human globin protein (as opposed to heme) in the stool. It detects more advanced adenomas than FOBT. Fecal DNA testing is a newer screening method that detects colonic cells shed into the fecal stream that possess specific genetic or epigenetic changes. The technique has a reported sensitivity of 97% and a specificity of 90% for CRC stages I-III. In trials involving asymptomatic persons at average risk for colorectal cancer, multitarget stool DNA testing detects significantly more cancers than FIT but has more false-positive results. High cost and rate of false positives are the main obstacles inhibiting broader adoption of fecal DNA testing. Microcytic anemia on CBC may be indicative of chronic blood loss.
- Molecular markers including abnormal DNA from cancerous cells can be detected in stool. FIT combined with stool DNA test (FIT-DNA) has been approved by the FDA for colorectal screening. One study showed that one-time FIT-DNA had a higher sensitivity for detection of colorectal cancer than one-time FIT alone (92.3% vs. 73.8%), but specificity was lower (86.6% vs. 94.9%).[1]
- Circulating methylated SEPT9 DNA: Does not reliably detect precancerous neoplasia. Studies showing mortality benefit are lacking.

[1] Inadomi JM: Screening for colorectal neoplasia, *N Engl J Med* 376:149–156, 2017.

TABLE 1 Colorectal Cancer (CRC) Screening and Surveillance Recommendations*

Indication	Recommendations
Average risk	Beginning at age 50 yr: Colonoscopy every 10 yr; Computed tomographic colonography every 5 yr; Flexible sigmoidoscopy every 5 yr; Double-contrast barium enema every 5 yr; Stool blood testing annually or stool; DNA testing acceptable but not preferred
One or two first-degree relatives with CRC at any age or adenoma at age <60 yr	Colonoscopy every 5 yr beginning at age 40 yr, or 10 yr younger than earliest diagnosis, whichever comes first
Hereditary nonpolyposis CRC	Genetic counseling and screening†Colonoscopy every 1 to 2 yr beginning at age 25 yr and then yearly after age 40 yr‡
Familial adenomatous polyposis and variants	Genetic counseling and testing†Flexible sigmoidoscopy yearly beginning at puberty‡
Personal history of CRC	Colonoscopy within 1 yr of curative resection; repeat at 3 yr and then every 5 yr if normal
Personal history of colorectal adenoma	Colonoscopy every 3 to 5 yr after removal of all index polyps
Inflammatory bowel disease	Colonoscopy every 1 to 2 yr beginning after 8 yr of pancolitis or after 15 yr if only left-sided disease

*Recommendations proposed by the American Cancer Society and U.S. Multi-Society Task Force on Colorectal Cancer; recommendations for average-risk patients also endorsed by the American College of Radiology.
†Whenever possible, affected relatives should be tested first because of potential false-negative results.
‡Screening recommendation for individuals with positive or indeterminate tests as well as for those who refuse genetic testing.
From Andreoli TE, et al.: *Andreoli and Carpenter's Cecil essentials of medicine,* ed 8, Philadelphia, 2010, Saunders.

- Plasma carcinoembryonic antigen (CEA) level is not useful for screening because it can be increased in nonmalignant conditions (smoking, IBD, alcoholic liver disease). A normal CEA result does not exclude the diagnosis of CRC.

IMAGING STUDIES

- Colonoscopy with biopsy (primary assessment tool): The American College of Physicians (ACP) recommends that patients should be offered a colonoscopy beginning at age 50, and it should be repeated every 10 yr in average-risk patients. Screening is recommended in African Americans beginning at age 45 yr. Persons with only one first-degree relative with CRC or advanced adenomas diagnosed at 60 yr or older may be screened as at average risk. The U.S. Preventive Services Task Force guidelines state that screening should not be routinely recommended in persons older than 75 yr, and it should not be recommended at all in persons older than 85 yr. If persons between the ages of 75 and 85 yr have never undergone screening, the decision about screening should be individualized according to health status. The ACP recommends that clinicians stop screening for colorectal cancer in adults over age 75 yr or in adults with a life expectancy of <10 yr. Table 1 describes CRC screening and surveillance recommendations.
- Computed tomography colonoscopy (CTC) virtual colonoscopy (VC) uses helical (spiral) CT scanning to generate a two- or three-dimensional virtual colorectal image (Fig. 1). CTC does not require sedation, but, like optical colonoscopy, it requires some bowel preparation (either bowel cathartics or ingestion of iodinated contrast medium with meals during the 48 hr before CT) and air insufflation. It also involves substantial exposure to radiation. In addition, patients with lesions detected by VC will require traditional colonoscopy. Compared with colonoscopy, CTC sensitivity for detection of polyps >10 mm ranges from 70% to 96%, and specificity ranges from 72% to 96%. CTC has replaced double-contrast barium enema as the radiographic screening alternative when patients decline colonoscopy.
- Capsule endoscopy allows visualization of the colonic mucosa but is not recommended as a screening procedure because its sensitivity for detecting colonic lesions is low compared with colonoscopy.
- CT scanning of the abdomen (Fig. 2), pelvis, and chest assists in preoperative staging.
- PET scanning can display functional information and is accurate in the detection of CRC and its distant metastases. Colonography composed of a combined modality of PET and CT is a newer diagnostic modality that can provide whole-body tumor staging in a single session.

Rx TREATMENT

GENERAL Rx

- Surgical resection is the definitive and curative upfront treatment for stages I-III colon cancers. Selected patients (high-risk stage II, all stage III) are recommended to receive adjuvant chemotherapy.
- The standard chemotherapy regimen for adjuvant therapy of resected CRC is the combination of oxaliplatin with a fluoropyrimidine (5-fluorouracil or capecitabine). Older patients and patients with significant comorbidities are recommended treatment with single-agent fluoropyrimidine therapy.
- Neoadjuvant chemotherapy and radiation therapy is used to downsize and downstage rectal cancers before definitive resection and improves overall survival and local disease control in stage II-III cancers.
- Adjuvant chemotherapy in stage II disease (no nodal involvement) provides an improvement in overall survival by 3% to 4%, with current 5-yr survival rates in the 80% range. Given this modest benefit, current guidelines recommend consideration of adjuvant chemotherapy only in high-risk stage II patients. The magnitude of survival benefit is higher in stage III patients, and combination chemotherapy is associated with 5-yr overall survival in the 70% range with wide variation in the subgroups. More recent data has revealed that low-risk stage III colon cancer patients may have equivalent survival with adjuvant multiagent chemotherapy of 3 months duration.
- The outlook for patients with metastatic and relapsed CRC has improved dramatically in the past few yr. Median overall survival in patients with unresectable metastases is now expected in the 30-month range with modern chemotherapeutic regimens. In patients with limited, resectable metastases in sites such as the liver, the 5-yr median overall survival is in the 50% range.
- Chemotherapy agents used in the metastatic setting include 5-fluorouracil (5-FU), capecitabine, irinotecan, oxaliplatin, and mitomycin. Chemotherapy regimens using a combination of antimetabolite (5-FU or capecitabine) in combination with either oxaliplatin or irinotecan form the backbone of systemic chemotherapy.
- Molecularly targeted therapy against the epidermal growth factor receptor (EGFR) and the angiogenesis pathway are used in combination with the chemotherapy backbone in metastatic CRC. Antiangiogenic agents include monoclonal antibodies bevacizumab, aflibercept, and ramucirumab. Cetuximab and panitumumab are EGFR receptor blockers that are active in metastatic CRC patients whose tumors do not harbor mutated RAS oncogenes.
- The liver is generally the initial and most common site of CRC metastases. Resection of metastases limited to the liver followed by systemic chemotherapy is curative in more than 30% of selected patients. Metasectomy of limited pulmonary metastases can also be considered in selected cases.
- Unresectable multiple liver metastases are often approached by locoregional therapeutic approaches such as transarterial chemoembolization (TACE), selective internal radiation therapy (SIRT) using yttrium-90 brachytherapy, or hepatic arterial infusional chemotherapy.
- The oral multitargeted kinase inhibitor regorafenib and the oral antimetabolite drug TAS-102 provide modest survival benefit in

 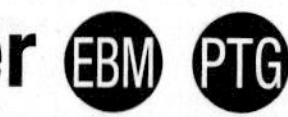

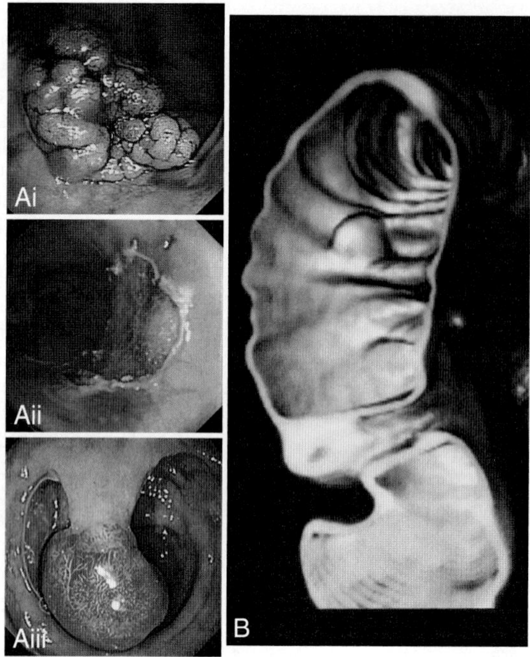

FIG. 1 Colon polyps seen at (Ai–iii) colonoscopy and (B) computed tomography (CT) colonography. Aii is after endoscopic resection of the polyps in Ai. (From Ballinger A: *Kumar & Clark's essentials of medicine*, ed 5, Edinburgh, 2012, Saunders.)

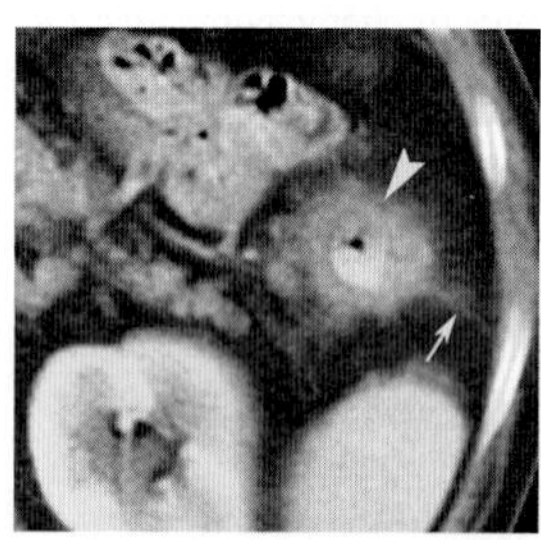

FIG. 2 Colon carcinoma: wall thickening. A carcinoma of the descending colon near the splenic flexure causes thickening of the colon wall (*arrowhead*) and narrowing of the lumen. Stranding densities (*arrow*) extending into the pericolonic fat suggest tumor extension through the bowel wall. (From Webb WR, Brant WE, Major NM: *Fundamentals of body CT*, ed 4, Philadelphia, 2015, Saunders.)

patients who have failed standard chemotherapy approaches.
- In patients with pathologically confirmed microsatellite instability in their cancers, the checkpoint inhibitors (pembrolizumab, nivolumab) are effective options after failure of standard therapies and have been recently approved in this setting.
- Reviews of randomized trials in metastatic CRC have demonstrated that right-sided cancers are associated with shorter overall survival when compared with left-sided cancers.

CHRONIC Rx

Follow-up is indicated with:
- Physician visits with a focus on clinical and disease-related history, directed physical examination, coordination of follow-up, and counseling every 3 to 4 mo for the first 3 yr and then every 6 months for 2 yr.
- Colonoscopy at end of first yr, then after 3 yr, and subsequently every 5 yr.
- Baseline CEA level, if elevated, can be used after surgery as a measure of completeness of tumor resection. It is used to monitor tumor recurrence and is obtained every 3 to 6 mo for up to 5 yr.

DISPOSITION

The 5-yr survival rate varies with the stage of the carcinoma:

TNM Stage	5-yr Survival Rate (%)
I	>90
II_{A-C}	60-85
III_{A-C}	25-65
IV	5-10

- Overall 5-yr disease-free survival rate has increased from 50% to 63% during the past two decades.
- High-frequency microsatellite instability in CRC is independently predictive of a relatively favorable outcome and reduces the likelihood of metastases.
- In patients with high-risk stage II and with stage III CRC, there is improved 5-yr survival among patients treated with adjuvant chemotherapy.
- Expression patterns of microRNA are systemically altered in colon adenocarcinomas. High miR-21 expression is associated with poor survival and poor therapeutic outcome.
- The optimal timing from surgery to initiation of adjuvant chemotherapy is 4 to 8 wk. A longer time to initiation of adjuvant chemotherapy is associated with worse survival rates.
- Regular aspirin use after the diagnosis of CRC has been reported to be associated with lower risk for CRC-specific and overall mortality, especially among individuals with tumors that overexpress cyclooxygenase-2. Regular aspirin use is associated with lower BRAF-wild type colorectal cancer but not with BRAF-mutated cancer risk. All aspirin doses starting with 75 mg daily had similar effects on CRC incidence and mortality.

REFERRAL

- Multidisciplinary referral to colorectal surgery or surgical oncology, medical oncology, radiation oncology

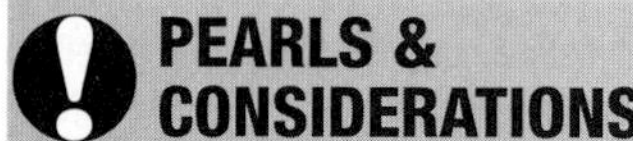

PEARLS & CONSIDERATIONS

COMMENTS

- Metastases of tumor cells to regional lymph nodes is the single most important prognostic factor in patients with colon cancer.
- Decreased fat intake to 30% of total energy intake, increased fiber through fruit and vegetable consumption may reduce CRC risk.
- Chemoprophylaxis with aspirin (81 mg/day) reduces the incidence of colorectal adenomas in persons at risk.
- The National Cancer Institute has published consensus guidelines for universal screening for HNPCC in patients with newly diagnosed CRC. Tumors in mutation carriers of HNPCC typically exhibit microsatellite instability, a characteristic phenotype caused by expansion or contraction of short nucleotide repeat sequences. These guidelines (Bethesda Guidelines) are useful for selective patients for microsatellite instability testing. Screening patients with newly diagnosed CRC for HNPCC is cost effective, especially if the benefits to their immediate relatives are considered.
- The use of either annual or biennial FOBT significantly reduces the incidence of CRC.
- The detection of mutations in the *APC* gene from stool samples is a promising new modality for early detection of colorectal neoplasms.

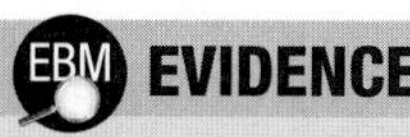

EVIDENCE

Available at ExpertConsult.com

SUGGESTED READINGS

Available at ExpertConsult.com

RELATED CONTENT

Colon Cancer (Patient Information)
Familial Adenomatous Polyposis and Gardner Syndrome (Related Key Topic)
Lynch Syndrome (Related Key Topic)
Peutz-Jeghers Syndrome and Other Polyposis Syndromes (Related Key Topic)

AUTHOR: **RITESH RATHORE, M.D.**

BASIC INFORMATION

DEFINITION

- Concussion is a mild traumatic brain injury manifesting with self-limited symptoms at the less severe end of the brain injury spectrum.
- The fourth International Conference on Concussion (2012) defines concussion as "a complex pathophysiological process affecting the brain, induced by traumatic biomechanical forces," characterized by the following features: (1) caused by a direct blow to the head or blow to the body that transmits an "impulsive" force to the head; (2) results in rapid onset of short-lived neurologic impairment that resolves spontaneously; (3) variable clinical symptoms that may not include loss of consciousness; (4) symptoms that largely reflect a functional disturbance rather than structural injury (thus, no abnormalities are seen on standard structural neuroimaging studies); and (5) symptom resolution that typically follows a sequential course but may be prolonged in a small percentage of cases.

SYNONYM

Mild traumatic brain injury (mTBI)

ICD-10CM CODES

S06.0	Concussion
S06.0X0A	Concussion without loss of consciousness, initial encounter
S06.0X0D	Concussion without loss of consciousness, subsequent encounter
S06.0X0S	Concussion without loss of consciousness, sequela
S06.0X1A	Concussion with loss of consciousness of 30 minutes or less, initial encounter
S06.0X9A	Concussion with loss of consciousness of unspecified duration, initial encounter

EPIDEMIOLOGY & DEMOGRAPHICS

INCIDENCE: 3.8 million sports- and recreation-related concussions occur each yr in the U.S. It is estimated that as many as 50% of concussions go unreported.

PREVALENCE: Each yr, U.S. emergency departments treat an estimated 135,000 sports- and recreation-related TBIs, including concussions, among children ages 5 to 18.

PREDOMINANT SEX AND AGE:

- Children and teens are more likely to get a concussion and take longer to recover than adults.
- Limited studies have shown that in sports that are played by both men and women, women are at more risk of sustaining a concussion. In males the incidence is highest in football, followed by hockey, and in females, soccer. Player contact is the most common cause.

RISK FACTORS:

- Participating in high-impact sports and recreational activities
- Previous history of concussion
- Athletes with a body mass index (BMI) >27 kg/m^2 and those who train <3 hr/wk
- Individuals who sustain a sports-related concussion and continue playing immediately after the injury require nearly twice as much time to recover as those who are removed immediately

PHYSICAL FINDINGS & CLINICAL PRESENTATION

See Table 1.

ETIOLOGY

- Occurs when rotational or angular acceleration forces are applied to the brain, resulting in shear strain of the underlying neural elements, including altered autonomic function and impaired control of cerebral blood flow
- May be associated with a blow to the skull; however, direct impact to the head is not required

TABLE 1 Symptoms and Signs of Concussion

Mental Status Changes
Amnesia
Confusion
Disorientation
Easily distracted
Excessive drowsiness
Feeling dinged, stunned, or foggy
Impaired level of consciousness
Inappropriate play behaviors
Poor concentration and attention
Seeing stars or flashing lights
Slow to answer questions or to follow directions
Physical or Somatic
Ataxia or loss of balance
Blurry vision
Decreased performance or playing ability
Dizziness
Double vision
Fatigue
Headache
Light-headedness
Nausea, vomiting
Poor coordination
Ringing in the ears
Seizures
Slurred, incoherent speech
Vacant stare/glassy-eyed
Vertigo
Behavior or Psychosomatic
Emotional lability
Irritability
Low frustration tolerance
Personality changes
Nervousness, anxiety
Sadness, depressed mood

From Patel DR et al: Sports concussions in adolescents, *Pediatr Clin N Am* 57:652, 2010.

DIAGNOSIS

DIFFERENTIAL DIAGNOSIS

- Migraine
- Cervical strain
- Posttraumatic vestibular injury

WORKUP

- There is no definitive diagnostic test for concussion. Physical exam should include smooth pursuits (examine mons finger horizontally across field of vision), saccades, gaze instability, near point of convergence, accommodation, and balance. Patients with loss of consciousness or post-traumatic convulsive seizures should be transported to the emergency department.
- Sideline assessment:
  1. No athlete with a suspected concussion should return to play that day.
  2. Neurologic assessment using a standardized tool, such as s SCAT-3 (Sports Concussion Assessment Tool), which includes the BESS (Balance Error Scoring System), Maddocks Questions, and SAC (Standardized Assessment of Concussion).
  3. Monitor for deterioration; no athlete should be left alone.
- Office assessment:
  1. History focused on current symptoms. Consider using Postconcussion Symptom Checklist.
  2. Neurologic exam
     a. Gait/balance testing. Consider the Balance Error Scoring System (BESS).
     b. Cerebellar coordination: Finger-to-nose testing (tested on SCAT-3 card).
     c. Convergence of Accommodative Sufficiency.
- Neurocognitive testing:
  1. Computer-based programs, such as ImPACT, ANAM, CogSport
  2. Neuropsychiatric testing administered by a neuropsychologist
- When used in combination, symptom assessment, balance assessment, and neurocognitive testing provide a sensitivity of >90% for the identification of concussion.
- Consider the Buffalo Concussion Treadmill Test, which identifies physiologic dysfunction in concussion, rules out other diagnoses, and can quantify a safe level of activity in concussion recovery.

IMAGING STUDIES

- CT imaging is not universally indicated and should be considered on an individual basis. It is indicated in any athlete with a rapidly changing or focal neurologic exam or with a suspected intracranial bleed.
- Consider following PECARN guidelines.

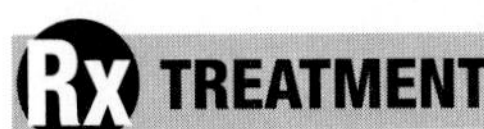

TREATMENT

ACUTE GENERAL Rx

- Removal from game
- Physical rest

TABLE 2 Graduated Return to Play Protocol

Rehabilitation Stage	Functional Exercise at Each Stage of Rehabilitation	Objective of Each Stage
1. No activity	Complete physical and cognitive rest	Recovery
2. Light aerobic exercise	Walking, swimming, or stationary cycling, keeping intensity <70% maximum predicted heart rate. No resistance training	Increase heart rate
3. Sport-specific exercise	Skating drills in ice hockey, running drills in soccer. No head impact activities	Add movement
4. Noncontact training drills	Progression to more complex training drills, e.g., passing drills in football and ice hockey. May start progressive resistance training	Exercise, coordination, and cognitive load
5. Full contact practice	After medical clearance, participate in normal training activities	Restore confidence and assess functional skills by coaching staff
6. Return to play	Normal game play	

From Putukian M: The acute symptoms of sports-related concussion: diagnosis and on-field management, *Clin Sports Med* 30(58), 2011.

1. No return to play until asymptomatic for at least 24 hours.
2. Follow the return-to-play guidelines (Table 2).
3. There is no evidence to support prolonged rest in concussed athletes longer than several weeks (see "Postconcussive Syndrome"). Prolonged inactivity after concussion has been linked to negative health effect. Light aerobic activity that avoids risk for reinjury decreases concussion symptoms, suggesting that low-level physical activity post-concussion might be beneficial.

- Cognitive rest to limit symptoms
  1. Limit screen time to less than 2 hours per day.
  2. Academic accommodations at school. Consider return to school for half-days when tolerating 2 hours of work at home.
  3. Encourage good sleep hygiene.

CHRONIC Rx

See "Postconcussive Syndrome"

DISPOSITION

- Physiologic recovery is slower than symptomatic recovery. Protocols involving a symptom-free waiting period before return to play are warranted. Table 2 summarizes the American Academy of Neurology, American Medical Society for Sports Medicine, and International Conference on Concussion recommendations on returning to play after a concussion.
- If concussion symptoms occur with activity at one level, the athlete should stop the activity, rest until symptoms resolve, and then restart his or her progression at the level that did not elicit symptoms.
- There are no evidence-based guidelines for disqualifying or retiring an athlete from sport after a concussion. Each case should be individually considered.

REFERRAL

Referral to sports-medicine physician, neuropsychology, or concussion center is indicated if there is concern about the timing of return to contact or collision sport. Referral is also indicated in patients with preexisting neurologic disorders such as migraines, depression or anxiety, and in those who have had multiple concussions.

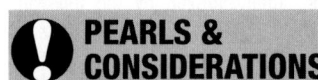

PREVENTION

- Pre-participation evaluations for all athletes
- Pre-participation neurocognitive and balance testing to establish a baseline
- There is currently no evidence to support the use of concussion prevention headbands or mouth guards.
- Spontaneous recovery from acute concussion ranges from 1-2 weeks in adults and up to 4 weeks in adolescents.

PATIENT/FAMILY EDUCATION

Centers for Disease Control and Prevention: www.cdc.gov/TraumaticBrainInjury/causes.html.

SUGGESTED READINGS

Available at ExpertConsult.com

RELATED CONTENT

Concussion (Patient Information)
Traumatic Brain Injury (Related Key Topic)
Post-Concussion Syndrome (Related Key Topic)

AUTHORS: **PETER J. SELL, D.O.,** and **AMITY RUBEOR, D.O., C.A.Q.S.M.**

BASIC INFORMATION

DEFINITION

Condyloma acuminatum, also known as anogenital warts, is a sexually transmitted viral disease of the penis, vulva, vagina, cervix, perineum, and perianal area caused by the human papillomavirus (HPV). More than 100 subtypes of the HPV virus have been identified, yet 90% of genital warts are caused by HPV types 6 or 11.

SYNONYMS

Genital warts
Venereal warts
Anogenital warts

ICD-10CM CODE

A63.0 Anogenital (venereal) warts

EPIDEMIOLOGY & DEMOGRAPHICS

- The estimated prevalence rate of HPV anogenital infection in the U.S. adult population is 10% to 20% among unvaccinated individuals
- Seen mostly in young adults, with peak age of onset of 16 to 25 yr
- A sexually transmitted disease spread by skin-to-skin contact
- Highly contagious, with 75% of sexually active adults in the United States having been infected with at least one genital HPV type at some time
- Virus shed from both macroscopic and microscopic lesions
- Average incubation time is 2 months (range, 1 to 8 months)
- Predisposing conditions: Diabetes, pregnancy, local trauma, and immunosuppression (e.g., transplant recipients, those with HIV infection)

PHYSICAL FINDINGS & CLINICAL PRESENTATION

- Usually found in genital area but can be present elsewhere on the body (larynx, oropharynx, trachea, and extremities)
- Lesions usually in similar positions on both sides of perineum
- Initial lesions are pedunculated, soft papules about 2 to 3 mm in diameter, 10 to 20 mm long; may occur as single papule or in clusters
- Size of lesions varies from pinhead to large cauliflower-like masses (Fig. 1)
- Usually asymptomatic, but if infected can cause pain, odor, or bleeding
- Vulvar condyloma more common than vaginal and cervical
- Four morphologic types: Condylomatous, keratotic, papular, and flat warts
- Intra-anal warts are observed predominantly in persons who have had receptive anal intercourse

ETIOLOGY

- HPV is a group of nonenveloped, double-stranded DNA viruses belonging to the family Papillomaviridae.
- HPV DNA types 6 and 11 usually found in exophytic warts and have no malignant potential. 90% of genital warts are caused by HPV 6 and 11.
- HPV types 16 and 18 usually found in flat warts and are associated with increased risk of malignancy.
- Recurrence associated with persisting viral infection of adjacent normal skin in 25% to 50% of cases.

DIAGNOSIS

DIFFERENTIAL DIAGNOSIS

- Molluscum contagiosum
- Seborrhea keratosis
- Fordyce spots
- Lichen planus
- Lichen nitidus
- Condylomata lata of syphilis
- Malignancy
- Abnormal anatomic variants or skin tags around labia minora and introitus

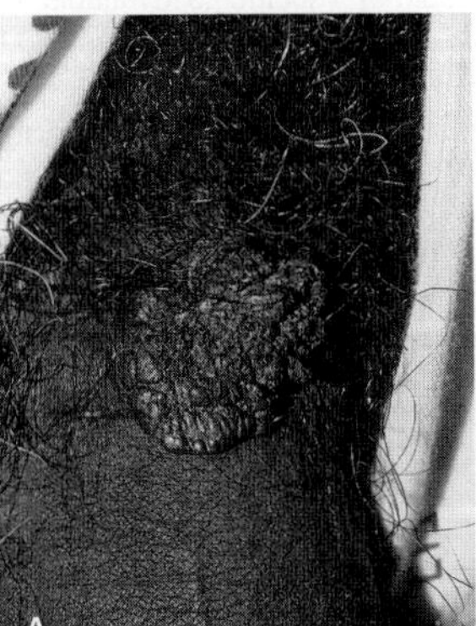

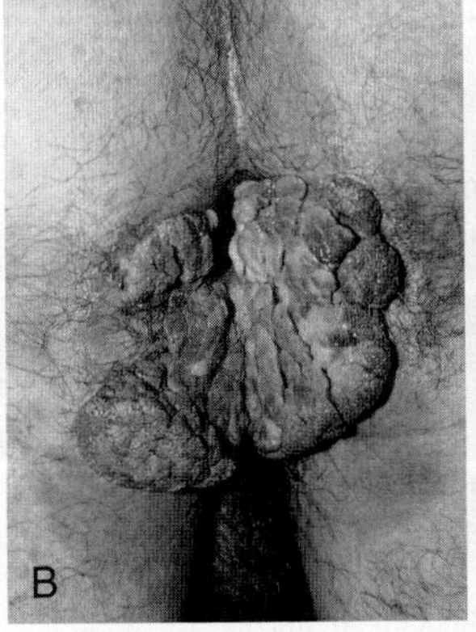

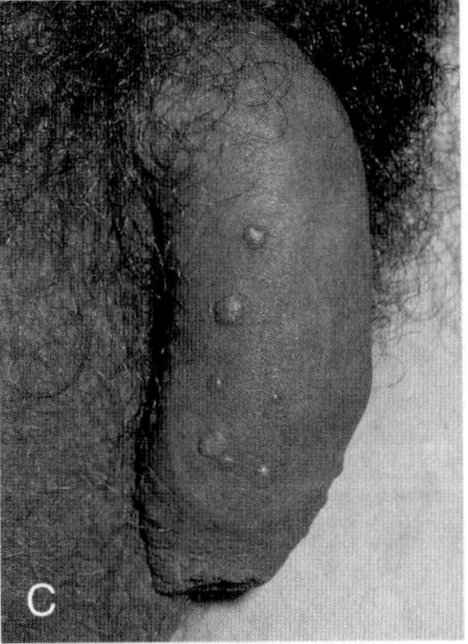

FIG. 1 Condyloma acuminatum. A, Scattered, flesh-colored or hyperpigmented, smooth or verrucous papules or erythematous macules along the shaft of the penis, scrotum, and perianal area are characteristic. The term *bowenoid papulosis* is used when the histologic picture of a lesion resembles Bowen disease. **B,** Perianal condyloma acuminatum. The viral particles causing perianal condyloma may have originated from warts elsewhere on the body and been transmitted via the patient's own hands, or they may have been contracted during anal sex. **C,** Condyloma acuminatum. Multiple lesions on the shaft of the penis. (From White GM, Cox NH [eds]: *Diseases of the skin: a color atlas and text,* ed 2, St Louis, 2006, Mosby.)

- Dysplastic warts
- Table 1 summarizes treatment options for anal warts

WORKUP

- Colposcopic examination of lower genital tract from cervix to perianal skin with 3% to 5% acetic acid
- Biopsy of vulvar lesions that lack the classic appearance of warts and that become ulcerated or do not respond to treatment
- Biopsy of flat, white, or ulcerated cervical lesions

LABORATORY TESTS

- HPV tests are available to detect oncogenic types of HPV infection and are used in the context of cervical cancer screening and management or follow-up of abnormal cervical cytology or histology.
- Cervical cultures for *Neisseria gonorrhoeae* and Chlamydia.
- Serologic test for syphilis.
- HIV testing offered.
- Wet mount or DNA testing for trichomoniasis, *Candida albicans*, and *Gardnerella vaginalis* (if patient has abnormal vaginal discharge).

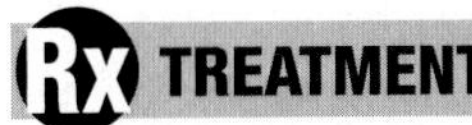

TREATMENT

NONPHARMACOLOGIC THERAPY

- Cryotherapy with liquid nitrogen
- Surgical removal

ACUTE GENERAL Rx

Factors that influence selection of treatment include wart size, wart number, anatomic site of wart, wart morphology, patient preference, cost of treatment, convenience, adverse effects, and provider experience.
Keratolytic agents:

- Podophyllin (Podofilox 0.5% solution or gel)
  1. Acts by poisoning mitotic spindle and causing intense vasospasm
  2. Applied by patient directly to lesion weekly and washed off in 6 hours
  3. Used in minimal vulvar or anal disease
  4. Applied cautiously to nonkeratinized epithelial surfaces
  5. Contraindicated in pregnancy
  6. Discontinued if lesions do not disappear in 6 weeks; switch to other treatment
- Sinecatechins 15% ointment (green tea flavonoid extracts)
  1. Acts by upregulating apoptosis-associated genes
  2. Applied by patient three time daily (0.5 cm strand of ointment to each wart)
  3. Should not be continued longer than 16 weeks
- Trichloroacetic acid (30% to 80% solution)
  1. Acts by destruction of the warty lesions through precipitation of surface proteins
  2. Applied weekly to lesion by a trained clinician
  3. Indicated for vulvar, anal, and vaginal lesions; can be used for cervical lesions

TABLE 1 Treatment Options for Anal Warts

Treatment	Success Rate	Comments
Podophyllin	20%-50%	May need repeat applications Skin irritation can occur Not used in the anal canal Poorly absorbed by keratinized lesions (most chronic warts are keratinized)
Trichloroacetic or dichloroacetic acid	75%	Can be used in the anal canal Care is required to control the size of the slough
Cryotherapy	75%	Can be used in the anal canal Care is required to limit the size of the wound Fumes from the therapy can contain active HPV*
Topical 5-fluorouracil	50%-75%	Probably better used after surgical excision to decrease the frequency of recurrence
Imiquimod	75% in women 33% in men	Cannot be used in the anal canal; works better in women than in men
Surgical excision (usually combined with cautery)	60%-90%	Fumes from the cautery may contain HPV* May need to be done in more than one session to avoid excising or burning excessive anoderm if a thick carpet of lesions is present
Intralesional interferon-α	>70%	Injected into the base of up to 5 warts 3 times a week for 3-8 weeks Approved by the FDA for refractory condyloma
HspE7	Experimental	Promising treatment involving subcutaneous injections Fusion protein that combines immune-stimulating properties and a target antigen from HPV
External-beam radiation therapy	Variable	Reserved for giant cavitating condyloma (Buschke-Löwenstein lesions) Used as a last resort, usually when bleeding or tissue invasion cannot be controlled

*The risk of HPV transmission from such fumes is unknown.
From Feldman M, Friedman LS, Brandt LJ: *Sleisenger and Fortran's gastrointestinal and liver disease*, ed 10, Philadelphia, 2016, Elsevier.

4. Less painful and irritating to normal tissue than podophyllin
- 5-Fluorouracil
  1. Acts by causing necrosis and sloughing of growing tissue
  2. Can be used intravaginally or for vulvar, anal, or urethral lesions
  3. Better tolerated; 3 g (two-thirds of vaginal applicator) applied weekly for 12 weeks
  4. Possible vaginal ulceration and erythema
  5. Patient's vagina examined after four to six applications
  6. 80% cure rate

Physical agents:
- Cryotherapy with liquid nitrogen or cryoprobe
  1. Acts by causing tissue damage by formation of ice crystals, leading to disruption of cell membranes and cell death
  2. Can be used weekly for 3 to 6 weeks
  3. 62% to 79% cure rate
  4. Not suitable for large warts
- Laser therapy
  1. Done by physician with necessary expertise and equipment
  2. Painful; requires anesthesia
- Electrocautery or excision
  1. For recurrent, very large lesions
  2. Local anesthesia needed

Immunotherapy:
- Interferon A
  1. Injected intralesionally at a dose of 3 million U/m2 three times weekly for 8 weeks
  2. Side effects: Fever, chills, malaise, headache
- Imiquimod 5% cream: Immunomodulatory drug that increases the immune response to warts
  1. Applied by patient at night, 3 times per week; wash off after 6 to 10 hours
  2. Usage for 16 weeks maximum
  3. Increases wart clearance after 3 months
- 40% to 77% cure rate
- Interferon, topical: Increases wart clearance at 4 weeks

DISPOSITION

- Most genital warts resolve without therapy.
- Follow-up exam every 6 to 12 months as needed.
- Referral to a specialist experienced in the treatment of anogenital warts (e.g., dermatologist, urologist, or colorectal surgeon) is appropriate for patients who are immunosuppressed or who have treatment-refractory anogenital warts.
- Patients with large, bulky perianal or genital warts that may require extensive surgical removal should be referred to a colorectal surgeon or urologist.

PREVENTION

- Male and female condoms should be used consistently and correctly to lower the risks of acquiring and transmitting HPV. However, because HPV can infect areas not covered by a condom, condoms will not fully protect against HPV.
- New guidelines for the routine vaccination of young adolescents (females and males) ages 9 to 14 are 2 doses of the HPV vaccine given at a 6- to 12-month interval, which offers the same protection as the 3-dose vaccination.
- Young women from ages 15 to 26 should receive 3 doses of the HPV vaccine (the 9vHPV, 4vHPV, and 2vHPV are approved for females).
- Young males from ages 15 to 21 should receive 3 doses of the HPV vaccine. The age limit for male HPV vaccination may be extended up to age 26 (only the 4vHPV and 9vHPV vaccines are approved for males). For men who have sex with men (including young men who identify as gay and bisexual), for young transgender adults, and for young adults who are immunocompromised (secondary to HIV, chronic steroid usage, or prior history of transplant), HPV vaccination is recommended up to age 26. Three-dose HPV vaccination series are administered as IM injections over a 6-month period, with the second and third doses given 1 to 2 and 6 months after the first dose, respectively. The same vaccine type should be used for the entire 3-dosage series.
- 4vHPV (Gardasil) vaccinates against types 6, 11, 16, and 18, which account for 66% of all cervical cancers.
- 2vHPV (Cervarix) vaccinates against types 16 and 18 (licensed for females only).
- 9vHPV (Gardasil 9) vaccine is available for preventing infection against HPV types 6, 11, 16, 18, 31, 33, 45, 52, and 58. It offers protection against five additional types of HPV accounting for 15% of cervical cancers not covered by Gardasil or Cervarix.
- HPV vaccines are not recommended for use in pregnant women.

SUGGESTED READING

Available at ExpertConsult.com

RELATED CONTENT

Genital Warts (Patient Information)
Warts (Related Key Topic)

AUTHOR: **HELEN B. GOMEZ, M.D.**

BASIC INFORMATION

DEFINITION

The term *conjunctivitis* refers to an inflammation of the conjunctiva resulting from a variety of causes, including allergies and bacterial, viral, and chlamydial infections.

SYNONYMS

"Red eye"
Pink eye
Acute conjunctivitis
Subacute conjunctivitis
Chronic conjunctivitis
Purulent conjunctivitis
Pseudomembranous conjunctivitis
Papillary conjunctivitis
Follicular conjunctivitis
Newborn conjunctivitis

ICD-10CM CODES

H10.9	Unspecified conjunctivitis
B30	Viral conjunctivitis
H10.0	Mucopurulent conjunctivitis
H10.1	Acute atopic conjunctivitis
H10.4	Chronic conjunctivitis

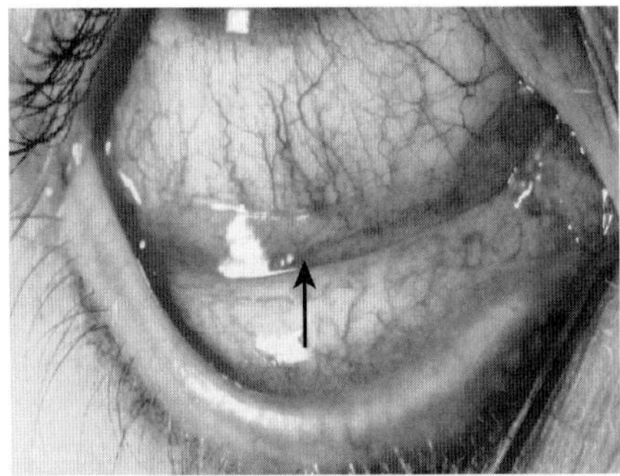

FIG. 1 Allergic conjunctivitis. *Arrow* indicates area of chemosis in the conjunctivitis. (From Adkinson NF Jr et al [eds]: *Middleton's allergy principles and practice,* ed 7, vol 2, Philadelphia, 2008, Mosby.)

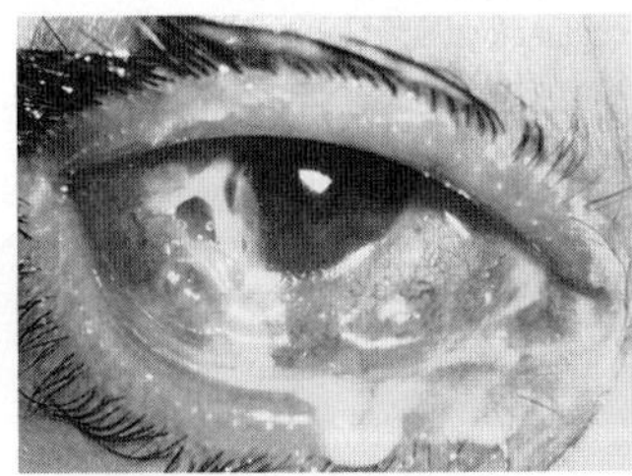

FIG. 2 Bacterial conjunctivitis. Purulent discharge and conjunctiva hyperemia suggest bacterial conjunctivitis. Viral conjunctivitis produces watery discharge, foreign body sensation, preauricular lymphadenopathy, and conjunctival follicles seen on slit lamp examination. (Reproduced with permission from the American Academy of Ophthalmology. From Goldman L, Schafer AI: *Goldman's Cecil medicine,* ed 24, Philadelphia, 2012, Saunders.)

EPIDEMIOLOGY & DEMOGRAPHICS

INCIDENCE (IN U.S.): 1.6% to 12% in *newborns*

PREVALENCE (IN U.S.):

- Allergic conjunctivitis (Fig. 1), the most common form of ocular allergy, is usually associated with allergic rhinitis and may be seasonal or perennial.
- Bacterial or viral conjunctivitis is often seasonal and can be extremely contagious.

PREDOMINANT AGE: Occurs at *any* age. Most cases in adults are due to viral infection. Children are more prone to develop bacterial conjunctivitis than viral forms.

PEAK INCIDENCE: More common in the spring and fall, when *viral* infections and pollens increase.

PHYSICAL FINDINGS & CLINICAL PRESENTATION

- Infection and chemosis of conjunctivae with discharge. Gluing of the eyelids and no itching is more indicative of a bacterial cause (Fig. 2).
- Cornea is clear or can be involved (certain bacteria, such as *Neisseria*, can rapidly develop into corneal infection).
- Vision is often normal but can be blurred. Mucus and watering can cause fluctuating vision.
- Fig. E3 illustrates the difference between papillary and follicular conjunctivitis.

ETIOLOGY

- Bacterial: *Haemophilus influenzae, Streptococcus pneumoniae*, and *Moraxella catarrhalis* in children; *Staphylococcus* species in adults. Gram-negative infections are more common in contact lens wearers. *Gonococcal ophthalmia neonatorum* is caused by *Neisseria gonorrhoeae* acquired by exposure of the neonatal conjunctivae to infected cervicovaginal secretions during delivery.
- Viral: Most common overall cause of infectious conjunctivitis.
- Chlamydial.
- Allergic.
- Traumatic (chemical or toxin exposure).
- Chronic eyelid inflammation (blepharitis).

DIAGNOSIS

DIFFERENTIAL DIAGNOSIS

- Acute glaucoma (fixed pupil with headache may indicate acute angle closure)
- Corneal lesions
- Acute iritis (with pain and photophobia, blurred vision)
- Episcleritis
- Scleritis (more severe pain, local globe tenderness, and no drainage)
- Canalicular obstruction (eye watering, inflammation near the tear punctum)
- Table 1 compares allergic diseases of the eye. Histologic and laboratory manifestations of allergic ocular disease are described in Table 2

WORKUP

- History and physical examination
- Visual acuity and eye examination
- Reports of itching, pain, and visual changes

LABORATORY TESTS

Cultures are useful if not *successfully* treated with antibiotics; initial culture is usually not necessary, since normal conjunctival flora interferes with helpful culture results.

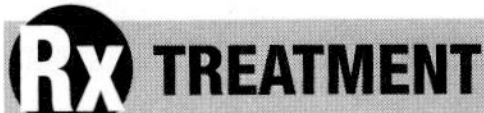

TREATMENT

NONPHARMACOLOGIC THERAPY

- Warm compresses if infective conjunctivitis.
- Cold compresses if irritative or allergic conjunctivitis.
- Contact lenses should be taken out until an infection is completely resolved. Nondisposable lenses should be cleaned thoroughly as recommended by the manufacturer, and a new lens case should be used. Disposable contact lenses should be thrown away.

ACUTE GENERAL Rx

- The majority of cases of bacterial conjunctivitis are self-limiting, and no treatment is necessary in uncomplicated cases.[1] Antibiotic drops (e.g., levofloxacin, ofloxacin, ciprofloxacin, tobramycin, gentamicin ophthalmic solution, 1 or 2 drops q2 to 4h) are indicated for complicated bacterial conjunctivitis, in conjunctivitis caused by gonorrhea or chlamydia, and in bacterial conjunctivitis in contact lens wearers.
- Caution: Be careful with ophthalmic corticosteroid treatment and avoid unless sure of diagnosis; corticosteroids can exacerbate infections and have been associated with increased intraocular pressure and cataract formation.
- An oral antihistamine (e.g., cetirizine, loratadine, desloratadine, or fexofenadine) is effective in relieving itching.
- Mast cell stabilizers (e.g., ketotifen, olopatadine, azelastine bid) are effective for allergic conjunctivitis. Others include Elestat, Optivar, and Patanol.
- Bepotastine, alcaftadine, azelastine, epinastine, and ketotifen are H1-antihistamines and mast cell stabilizers effective for topical treatment of itching associated with allergic conjunctivitis. The topical NSAID ketorolac (0.5%, 1 drop qd) is also useful in allergic conjunctivitis. Table 3 describes topical ophthalmic medications for allergic conjunctivitis.

[1] Azari AA, Barney NP: Conjunctivitis, a systematic review of diagnosis and treatment, *JAMA* 310(16):1721-1729, 2013.

TABLE 1 Allergic Diseases of the Eye

Disease	Clinical Parameters	Signs and Symptoms	Differential Diagnosis
Seasonal allergic conjunctivitis (SAC)	Occurs in sensitized individuals Both females and males affected Bilateral involvement Seasonal allergens Self-limiting	Ocular itching Tearing (watery discharge) Chemosis, redness Often associated with rhinitis Not sight threatening	Infective conjunctivitis Preservative toxicity (any eye drop with preservative) Medicamentosa Dry eye Perennial allergic conjunctivitis Vernal keratoconjunctivitis (VKC) Atopic keratoconjunctivitis (AKC)
Perennial allergic conjunctivitis (PAC)	Occurs in sensitized individuals Both females and males affected Bilateral involvement Year-round allergens Self-limiting	Ocular itching Tearing (watery discharge) Chemosis, redness Often associated with rhinitis Not sight-threatening	Infective conjunctivitis Preservative toxicity Dry eye SAC/AKC/VKC
Atopic keratoconjunctivitis (AKC)	Occurs in sensitized individuals Peak incidence: 20-50 yr of age Both females and males affected Bilateral involvement Seasonal or perennial allergens Atopic dermatitis Chronic symptoms	Severe ocular itching Red, flaking periocular skin Mucoid discharge, photophobia Corneal erosions Scarring of conjunctiva Cataract (anterior subcapsular) Sight threatening	Contact dermatitis Infective conjunctivitis Blepharitis Pemphigoid VKC/SAC/PAC/GPC
Vernal keratoconjunctivitis (VKC)	Occurs in some sensitized individuals Peak incidence: 3-20 yr of age Males predominate (in 3:1 ratio) Bilateral involvement Warm, dry climate Seasonal/perennial allergens Chronic symptoms	Severe ocular itching Severe photophobia Thick, ropy discharge Cobblestone papillae Corneal ulceration and scarring Sight threatening	Infective conjunctivitis Blepharitis AKC/SAC/PAC/GPC
Giant papillary conjunctivitis (GPC)	Sensitization not necessary Both females and males affected Bilateral involvement Prosthetic and contact lens exposure Occurs anytime Chronic symptoms Nonseasonal occurrence	Mild ocular itching Mild mucoid discharge Giant papillae Contact lens intolerance Foreign body sensation Protein buildup on contact lens Not sight threatening	Infective conjunctivitis Preservative toxicity SAC/PAC/AKC/VKC

From Adkinson NF et al: *Middleton's allergy principles and practice*, ed 8, Philadelphia, 2014, Saunders.

TABLE 2 Histopathologic and Laboratory Manifestations of Allergic Ocular Disease

Disease	Histopathologic Features	Laboratory Manifestations
Seasonal/perennial allergic conjunctivitis	Mast cell/eosinophil infiltration in conjunctival epithelium and substantia propria Mast cell activation Upregulation of ICAM-1 on epithelial cells	Increased in tears: Specific IgE antibody Histamine Tryptase TNF-α
Atopic keratoconjunctivitis	Increased mast cells, eosinophils in conjunctival epithelium and substantia propria Epithelial cell/goblet cell hypertrophy Increased CD4/CD8 ratio in conjunctival epithelium and substantia propria Increased collagen	Increased specific IgE antibody in tears Depressed cell-mediated immunity Increased IgE antibody and eosinophils in blood Eosinophils found in conjunctival scrapings
Vernal keratoconjunctivitis	Increased mast cells, eosinophils in conjunctival epithelium and substantia propria Eosinophil major basic protein deposition in conjunctiva CD4^{+} clones from conjunctiva found to have helper function for local production of IgE antibody Increased collagen Increased ICAM-1 on corneal epithelium	Increased specific IgE/IgG antibody in tears Elevated histamine and tryptase in tears Reduced serum histaminase activity Increased serum levels of nerve growth factor and substance P
Giant papillary conjunctivitis	Giant papillae Conjunctival thickening Mast cells in epithelium	No increased histamine in tears Increased tryptase in tears

ICAM-1, Intercellular adhesion molecule 1; *IgE, IgG*, immunoglobulins E and G; *TNF-α*, tumor necrosis factor-α.
From Adkinson NF et al: *Middleton's allergy principles and practice*, ed 8, Philadelphia, 2014, Saunders.

TABLE 3 Topical Ophthalmic Medications for Allergic Conjunctivitis

Generic Drug Name (Trade Name)	Mechanism of Action and Dosing	Cautions and Adverse Events
Azelastine hydrochloride 0.05% (Optivar)	Antihistamine Children ≥3 yr: 1 gtt bid	Not for treatment of contact lens–related irritation; the preservative may be absorbed by soft contact lenses. Wait at least 10 min after administration before inserting soft contact lenses.
Emedastine difumarate 0.05% (Emadine)	Antihistamine Children ≥3 yr: 1 gtt qid	Soft contact lenses should not be worn if the eye is red. Wait at least 10 min after administration before inserting soft contact lenses.
Levocabastine hydrochloride 0.05% (Livostin)	Antihistamine Children ≥12 yr: 1 gtt bid-qid up to 2 wk	Not for use in patients wearing soft contact lenses during treatment.
Pheniramine maleate 0.3% or 0.025%	Antihistamine/vasoconstrictor	Avoid prolonged use (>3 to 4 days) to avoid rebound symptoms. Not for use with contact lenses.
Naphazoline hydrochloride (Naphcon-A, Opcon-A)	Children >6 yr: 1 to 2 gtt qid	
Cromolyn sodium 4% (Crolom, Opticrom)	Mast cell stabilizer Children >4 yr: 1 to 2 gtt q4-6h	Can be used to treat giant papillary conjunctivitis and vernal keratitis. Not for use with contact lenses.
Lodoxamide tromethamine 0.1% (Alomide)	Mast cell stabilizer Children ≥2 yr: 1 to 2 gtt qid up to 3 mo	Can be used to treat vernal keratoconjunctivitis. Not for use in patients wearing soft contact lenses during treatment.
Nedocromil sodium 2% (Alocril)	Mast cell stabilizer Children ≥3 yr: 1 to 2 gtt bid	Avoid wearing contact lenses while exhibiting the signs and symptoms of allergic conjunctivitis.
Pemirolast potassium 0.1% (Alamast)	Mast cell stabilizer Children >3 yr: 1 to 2 gtt qid	Not for treatment of contact lens–related irritation; the preservative may be absorbed by soft contact lenses. Wait at least 10 min after administration before inserting soft contact lenses.
Epinastine hydrochloride 0.05% (Elestat)	Antihistamine/mast cell stabilizer Children ≥3 yr: 1 gtt bid	Contact lenses should be removed before use. Wait at least 15 min after administration before inserting soft contact lenses. Not for the treatment of contact lens irritation.
Ketotifen fumarate 0.025% (Zaditor)	Antihistamine/mast cell stabilizer Children ≥3 yr: 1 gtt bid q8-12h	Not for treatment of contact lens–related irritation; the preservative may be absorbed by soft contact lenses. Wait at least 10 min after administration before inserting soft contact lenses.
Olopatadine hydrochloride 0.1%, 0.2% (Patanol, Pataday)	Antihistamine/mast cell stabilizer Children ≥3 yr: 1 gtt bid (8 hr apart), 1 gtt qid	Not for treatment of contact lens–related irritation; the preservative may be absorbed by soft contact lenses. Wait at least 10 min after administration before inserting soft contact lenses.
Ketorolac tromethamine 0.5% (Acular)	NSAID Children ≥3 yr: 1 gtt qid	Avoid with aspirin or NSAID sensitivity. Use ocular product with caution in patients with complicated ocular surgeries, corneal denervation or epithelial defects, ocular surface diseases (e.g., dry eye syndrome), repeated ocular surgeries within a short period of time, diabetes mellitus, or rheumatoid arthritis; these patients may be at risk for corneal adverse events that may be sight threatening. Do not use while wearing contact lenses.

NSAID, Nonsteroidal antiinflammatory drug.
Modified from Kliegman RM et al: *Nelson textbook of pediatrics,* ed 19, Philadelphia, 2011, Saunders.

- Antihistamine/decongestant combinations such as pheniramine/naphazoline (Visine A), available over the counter, are more effective than either agent alone but have a short duration and can result in rebound vasodilatation with prolonged use. Others include Naphcon-A, Albalon-A, and Opcon-A.

CHRONIC Rx

- Depends on cause.
- If allergic, nonsteroidals such as ketorolac, and bromfenac ophthalmic solution; mast cell stabilizers such as Patanol and Zaditor (ketotifen) are useful for improving ocular itching in patients with allergic conjunctivitis.
- If an infection, use antibiotic drops (see "Acute General Rx").
- Dry eyes need artificial tears, topical cyclosporine, or lacrimal duct plugs when indicated.
- Chronic and recurrent conjunctivitis often occurs with blepharitis. Daily warm compresses and lid scrub treatment may help relieve symptoms.

DISPOSITION

Follow carefully for the first 2 wk to ensure secondary complications do not occur. Otitis media can develop in 25% of children with *H. influenzae* conjunctivitis. Bacterial keratitis occurs in 30/1000 contact lens wearers.

REFERRAL

To ophthalmologist if symptoms are refractory to initial treatment. Indications for urgent referral are severe eye pain or headache, photophobia, decreased vision, and contact lens use.

PEARLS & CONSIDERATIONS

COMMENTS

- Red eyes are not simply conjunctivitis when the patient has significant pain or loss of sight. However, it is usually safe to treat pain-free eyes and the normal-seeing red eye with lid hygiene and topical treatment.
- Use caution with patients wearing soft contact lenses, infants, and the elderly.
- Do not use steroids indiscriminately; use only when the diagnosis is certain.
- Bacterial conjunctivitis is generally self-limiting. More than 60% of persons will improve with placebo within 2 to 5 days.

RELATED CONTENT

Conjunctivitis (Patient Information)

AUTHOR: **R. SCOTT HOFFMAN, M.D.**

BASIC INFORMATION

DEFINITION

Vasculitis is defined by inflammatory leukocytes and subsequent necrosis of blood vessel walls that can eventually lead to tissue ischemia. When vasculitis is associated with a connective tissue disease (CTD), it is defined as a secondary vasculitis. The connective tissue diseases that most commonly cause vasculitis include rheumatoid arthritis (RA), systemic lupus erythematosus (SLE), and Sjögren's syndrome (SS). Vasculitis rarely occurs in the setting of other connective tissue diseases, including systemic sclerosis (SSc), relapsing polychondritis, primary antiphospholipid syndrome, inflammatory myopathies, and mixed connective tissue disease. Vasculitis is typically classified into large, medium, and small vessel vasculitis. When associated with a connective tissue disease, any type of vasculitis can occur; however, small vessel vasculitis is most common.

SYNONYMS

Connective tissue disorder–associated vasculitis
CTD

ICD-10CM CODE
M35.9 Systemic involvement of connective tissue, unspecified

EPIDEMIOLOGY & DEMOGRAPHICS

- Rheumatoid vasculitis: Estimated to occur in 1% to 5% of patients with RA, with no racial or ethnic predominance.
- Lupus-associated vasculitis: Estimates of the prevalence of vasculitis among SLE patients range from 11% to 36%.
- Sjögren's-associated vasculitis: Cutaneous vasculitis occurs in approximately 10% of patients with primary Sjögren's disease.
- Other CTD: Rare, but well described.

PHYSICAL FINDINGS & CLINICAL PRESENTATION

General
- Constitutional symptoms—fatigue, myalgias, weight loss, fever
- Skin manifestations—nail fold lesions (splinter hemorrhages), palpable purpura, leg ulcers, panniculitis, digital gangrene, livedo reticularis, urticaria, Janeway lesions, Osler nodes
- Neurologic manifestations—mononeuritis multiplex, distal symmetric sensorimotor neuropathy, transverse myelitis
- Ocular manifestations—episcleritis, scleritis, ulcerative keratitis.
- Cardiac manifestations—arrhythmias, pericarditis, aortitis
- Gastrointestinal manifestations—pancreatitis, peritonitis, colitis
- Pulmonary manifestations—pneumonitis, alveolar hemorrhage
- Renal manifestations—glomerulonephritis

Note: Any organ may be involved because vasculitis can disrupt the corresponding vasculature (an example would be kidney injury due to destructive inflammation of the renal vasculature).

Most Common Syndromes
- Rheumatoid vasculitis
  1. The most common clinical presentation of rheumatoid vasculitis includes skin lesions and peripheral neuropathy.
  2. Although a diagnosis of RA is needed to develop a secondary vasculitis, occasionally the vasculitic symptoms are the first manifestation of RA.
  3. Most patients with rheumatoid vasculitis have long-standing uncontrolled erosive RA, with rheumatoid nodules and high levels of rheumatoid factor and anti-CCP antibodies.
  4. The diagnosis of rheumatoid vasculitis is usually made by obtaining a biopsy of the clinically involved organ.
- Lupus-associated vasculitis
  1. Skin lesions are the most common manifestation.
  2. The most common types of skin lesions are palpable purpura, petechiae, papulonodular lesions, livedo reticularis, panniculitis, and splinter hemorrhages.
- Sjögren's-associated vasculitis
  1. Vasculitis is one of the most common extraglandular manifestations of Sjögren's syndrome.
  2. The most common skin lesions are palpable purpura, which most often represents a leukocytoclastic vasculitis.
  3. It can be quite difficult to tell the difference between vasculitis secondary to Sjögren's disease and a concomitant primary vasculitis. Sjögren's disease has been associated with several other primary vasculitides, including ANCA-associated vasculitis and polyarteritis nodosa.

ETIOLOGY

The vasculitis usually reflects the pathophysiology of the underlying connective tissue disease.

DIAGNOSIS

DIFFERENTIAL DIAGNOSIS

- Infection
- Hypercoagulable states (TTP, HUS)
- Malignancy (leukemia, lymphoma)
- Primary vasculitides

WORKUP

The diagnosis usually requires multiple modalities, including a full history and physical, as well as laboratory testing, imaging, and sometimes a biopsy of skin or other involved organ. In order to have a connective tissue disease–associated vasculitis, one must meet diagnostic criteria for an underlying connective tissue disease.

LABORATORY TESTS

- ESR/CRP
- CBC with diff. and platelets
- Albumin
- Complement studies
- Blood urea nitrogen and creatinine
- Urinalysis
- ANA, RF, Anti-CCP antibodies
- Double-stranded DNA (dsDNA) (if patient has a history suggesting SLE)
- Antineutrophil cytoplasmic antibodies (ANCA) that include ANCA-specific antibodies (anti-proteinase-3 and anti-myeloperoxidase antibodies)

IMAGING AND OTHER STUDIES

- Imaging may be helpful depending on the clinical manifestations of the disease. For instance, in aortitis or renal artery vasculitis, an angiogram, computed tomography angiography, or magnetic resonance angiography may be useful.
- Biopsy of the affected site may be very useful. Skin, nerve, muscle, and kidney biopsies, depending on the affected organ system, will usually help to arrive at a final diagnosis and rule out vasculitis mimics.

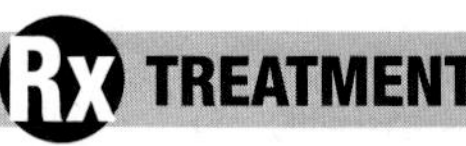

TREATMENT

Initial treatment is aimed at the underlying connective tissue disease. Additional immunosuppressive therapy may be needed depending on the severity of the vasculitis.

CHRONIC Rx

May need extended immunosuppressive therapy to prevent relapse

REFERRAL

Rheumatology

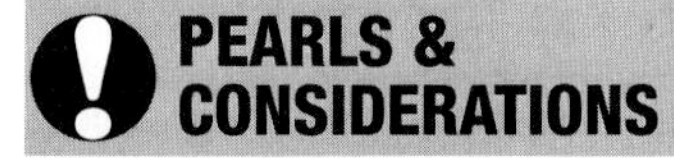

PEARLS & CONSIDERATIONS

COMMENTS

Patients with a history of CTD who present with new cutaneous lesions or systemic symptoms should be evaluated for vasculitis. Conversely, in patients who present with vasculitis, consideration should be given to the possibility of underlying CTD.

It is important not to confuse vasculitis with vasculopathy. The latter is a noninflammatory vascular process that is integral to the pathophysiology of some CTDs, such as SLE and SSc.

RELATED CONTENT

Rheumatoid Arthritis (Related Key Topic)
Sjögren's Syndrome (Related Key Topic)
Systemic Lupus Erythematosus (Related Key Topic)
Vasculitis, Systemic (Related Key Topic)

AUTHOR: **BRADLEY SCHLUSSEL, M.D.**

BASIC INFORMATION

DEFINITION

Decreased stool frequency (fewer than three bowel movements [BM] per week) with complaints of excessive straining, lower abdominal fullness, hard stools, or feeling of incomplete evacuation.

Rome IV criteria (see "Diagnosis") are used to classify patients.

ICD-10CM CODES	
K59.00	Constipation
K59.03	Drug-induced constipation
K59.01	Slow-transit constipation
K59.9	Functional intestinal disorder, unspecified

EPIDEMIOLOGY & DEMOGRAPHICS

PREVALENCE:

- 12% to 19% of adults
- Chronic constipation increases with age
- Approximately 26% of men and 34% of women >65 have constipation

RISK FACTORS: More prevalent in women, non-whites, patients with low income, patients older than 60 yr, patients who perform little physical activity, patients with low education level

PHYSICAL FINDINGS & CLINICAL PRESENTATION

- A thorough history is paramount for evaluation. The duration of constipation, change in bowel movements, medication history, or any other concurrent medical history is important to inform your diagnosis.
- Clinical presentation varies for every patient, as their personal definition of constipation may differ from medical lexicon.
- Constipation can be accompanied by an increased frequency of liquid stools (overflow diarrhea), typically caused by stool impaction.
- Must rule out alarm features such as hematochezia, weight loss of greater than 10 lbs, a family history of colon cancer or inflammatory bowel disease, anemia, positive fecal occult blood tests, or acute onset of constipation.
- Physical examination must include a digital rectal exam.
- Rectal examination will rule out etiologies that can result in constipation. Pain on examination, asymmetric anal opening, impaired sphincter function, masses, strictures, or the presence and character of stool (soft, hard, impacted) can help determine the etiology.
- Clinical clues to an evacuation disorder are summarized in Box 1.

ETIOLOGY

- Characterized as idiopathic vs. secondary causes of constipation
- Secondary causes include neurologic, metabolic, or endocrine disturbances; psychiatric disorders; gastrointestinal (GI) malignancies; and medication-induced constipation.
- Types of anorectal dysfunction causing rectal outlet delay in older people are summarized in Table 1.
- Medication-induced constipation is very common; frequent offenders include:
  1. Anticholinergics
  2. Iron supplements
  3. Antacids
  4. Opiates
  5. Antihypertensive medications (especially calcium channel blockers)
  6. Serotonin antagonists
  7. Ganglionic blockers

DIAGNOSIS

BASED ON ROME IV CRITERIA

- Symptoms present for at least 3 months out of the previous 6 months.
- Loose stools are rarely present without the use of laxatives.
- Criteria for irritable bowel syndrome (IBS) are not met.
- Presence of two or more of the following specific symptoms:
  1. Straining during more than 25% of defecations
  2. Lumpy or hard stools in more than 25% of defecations
  3. Sensation of incomplete evacuation for more than 25% of defecations
  4. Sensation of anorectal obstruction/blockage for more than 25% of defecations
  5. Manual maneuvers to facilitate more than 25% of defecations (e.g., digital evacuation, support of the pelvic floor)
  6. Fewer than three spontaneous bowel movements per week
- See Fig. 1 for an algorithmic approach to the diagnosis of constipation.

DIFFERENTIAL DIAGNOSIS

- First delineate between functional constipation vs. secondary causes.
- Secondary causes of constipation include medications, diabetes, hyperparathyroidism, hypothyroidism, lead poisoning, uremia, Parkinson's disease, multiple sclerosis, scleroderma, lupus, and malignancy.
- Functional constipation must be differentiated from irritable bowel syndrome (IBS), inflammatory bowel disease (IBD), appendicitis, ileus, and Ogilvie syndrome.

WORKUP

- A thorough history should include presence of alarm signs, dietary habits, list of medications, underlying systemic or neurological disorders, and patient's lifestyle/level of activity.
- Physical examination must include a rectal examination to evaluate for hemorrhoids, stool consistency, melena, hematochezia, rectal prolapse, abnormal rectal tone, or rectocele. The sensitivity and specificity

BOX 1 Clinical Clues to an Evacuation Disorder

History

Prolonged straining to expel stool
Assumption of unusual postures on the toilet to facilitate stool expulsion
Support of the perineum, digitation of rectum, or application of pressure to the posterior vaginal wall to facilitate rectal emptying
Inability to expel enema fluid
Constipation after subtotal colectomy for constipation

Rectal Examination (with patient in left lateral position)

Inspection

Anus "pulled" forward during attempts to simulate strain during defecation
Anal verge descends <1 cm or >4 cm (or beyond ischial tuberosities) during attempts to simulate straining at defecation.
The perineum balloons down during straining; rectal mucosa partially prolapses through anal canal.

Palpation

High anal sphincter tone at rest precludes easy entry of the examining finger (in absence of a painful perianal condition [e.g., anal fissure]).
Anal sphincter pressure during voluntary squeeze only minimally higher than anal pressure at rest.
The perineum and examining finger descend <1 cm or >4 cm during simulated straining at defecation.
The puborectalis muscle is tender to palpation through the rectal wall posteriorly, or palpation reproduces pain.
Palpable mucosal prolapse during straining.
"Defect" in anterior wall of the rectum, suggestive of rectocele.

Anorectal Manometry and Balloon Expulsion (with patient in left lateral position)

Elevated resting anal sphincter pressure
Delay in balloon expulsion test (normal values for women <50 yr: 4-75 seconds; normal values for women ≥50 yr of age: 3-15 seconds*

*Noelting J et al: Normal values for high-resolution anorectal manometry in healthy women: effects of age and significance of rectoanal gradient, *Am J Gastroenterol* 107:1530–1536, 2012.
From Feldman M, Friedman LS, Brandt LJ: *Sleisenger and Fordtran's gastrointestinal and liver disease*, ed 10, Philadelphia, 2016, Elsevier.

TABLE 1 Types of Anorectal Dysfunction Causing Rectal Outlet Delay in Older People

	Pathophysiology	Clinical Picture
Rectal dysmotility	Reduced rectal motility and contractions Increased rectal compliance Variable degree of rectal dilation Impaired rectal sensation with blunting of urge to pass stool Over time, increasing rectal distention required to reflexively trigger the defecation mechanism	Rectal hard or soft stool retention on digital examination of which patient may be unaware Chronic rectal distention leads to relaxation of the internal sphincter and fecal soiling One postulated cause is diminished parasympathetic outflow as a result of impaired sacral cord function (e.g., from ischemia or spinal stenosis). May also develop through persistent disregard or suppression of the urge to defecate as a result of dementia, depression, immobility, or painful anorectal conditions
Pelvic floor dyssynergia	Paradoxical contraction or failure to relax the pelvic floor and external anal sphincter muscles during defecation Manometric studies show paradoxical increases in anal canal pressure on straining	Severe and long-standing symptoms of rectal outlet delay Parkinson's disease More common in younger women
Irritable bowel syndrome	Increased rectal tone and reduced compliance Lower pain threshold on distending the rectum during anorectal function tests	Usually constipation-predominant in older people Rome criteria symptoms: Abdominal distention or pain relieved by defecation, passage of mucus, and feeling of incomplete emptying

Fillit HM: *Brocklehurst's textbook of geriatric medicine and gerontology*, ed 8, Philadelphia, 2017, Elsevier.

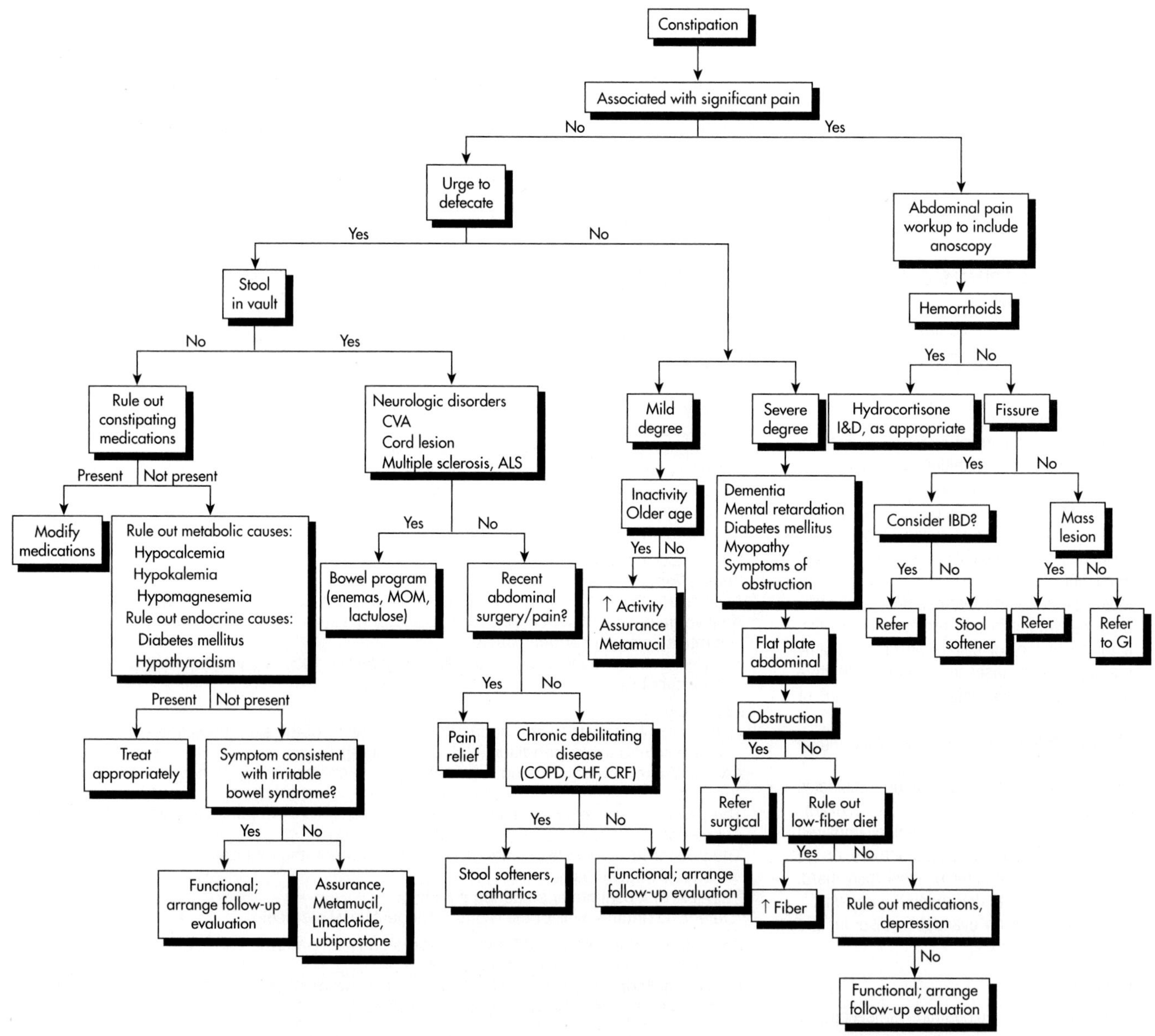

FIG. 1 Algorithmic approach to the diagnosis of constipation. *ALS,* Amyotrophic lateral sclerosis; *CHF,* congestive heart failure; *COPD,* chronic obstructive pulmonary disease; *CRF,* chronic renal failure; *CVA,* cerebrovascular accident; *GI,* gastroenterology; *IBD,* inflammatory bowel disease; *I&D,* incision and drainage; *MOM,* milk of magnesia. (From Marx JA et al: *Rosen's emergency medicine*, ed 8, Philadelphia, 2014, Saunders.)

of a digital rectal exam to diagnose dyssynergic defecation are 75% and 87%, respectively.
- Stool impaction can present as diarrhea and is diagnosed with a digital rectal exam and physical/radiologic findings consistent with increased stool burden.

LABORATORY TESTS

Routine laboratory tests are not required to diagnose constipation. However, patients with alarm signs should get a complete blood cell count, basic metabolic panel, thyroid-stimulating hormone, and fecal occult blood test.

IMAGING STUDIES

- Not required but may help rule out secondary causes.
- Plain film x-rays of the abdomen can be used to diagnose stool retention, which can possibly suggest ileus vs. obstruction vs. possible malignancy.
- If infrequent defecation is the major complaint, colon transit studies (via wireless motility capsule study) and whole-gut transit times can be useful, but they are only indicated in patients with chronic constipation that is refractory to laxatives and other conservative measures.
- Defecography is performed when the anorectum has anatomical and functional changes and is thought to contribute to constipation.
- Motility studies include anorectal manometry, colonic manometry, and balloon expulsion.

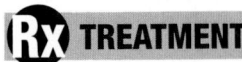

TREATMENT

After a thorough history and physical examination, combined with the absence of alarm signs, it is appropriate to initiate empiric treatment, including patient education, dietary changes, and fiber therapy without further diagnostic workup. If there is no response, then laxative therapy is indicated.

See Box 2 for a general approach to the treatment of constipation.

NONPHARMACOLOGIC THERAPY

- In patients with pelvic floor dysfunction as the major cause of constipation, biofeedback is a behavioral approach that can be used to correct inappropriate contraction of the pelvic floor muscles and external anal sphincter during defecation.
- Manual disimpaction can be a necessary intervention to remove hard stool in the rectal vault; at times this must be done in the operating room (depending on the volume of impacted stool).
- In patients unresponsive to medical therapy and with favorable manometry studies, subtotal colectomy with ileorectal anastomosis may be considered.

ACUTE GENERAL Rx

- Fiber (dietary or supplemental) is the first-line treatment.
- Laxatives, including bulk-forming, osmotic, and stimulant, are the next therapy to utilize.
  1. Bulk-forming laxatives include psyllium, methylcellulose, wheat dextrin, and polycarbophil.
  2. Osmotic laxatives include polyethylene glycol, lactulose, milk of magnesia, and magnesium citrate.
  3. Stimulant laxatives include bisacodyl, senna, and sodium picosulfate.
- Suppositories and/or enemas should be used if oral therapy is ineffective.
- Many agents can be used in combination if no alarm signs are present.
- Bowel preparation in older people is summarized in Table E3.

CHRONIC Rx

- Many of the agents used in acute constipation also have a role in chronic constipation.
- Be wary of the chronic use of stimulant laxatives, as they can cause colonic epithelial dysfunction.
- Less common, but used for chronic constipation, include:
  1. Linaclotide: Guanylate cyclase-c reactor agonist. It stimulates intestinal fluid secretion and transit.
  2. Plecanatide: Guanylate cyclase-c reactor agonist. It stimulates intestinal fluid secretion and transit.
  3. Lubiprostone: Chloride channel activator that enhances chloride-rich intestinal fluid secretion.
  4. Misoprostol: Prostaglandin analog.
  5. Botulinum toxins: In patients with pelvic floor dysfunction with injection into the puborectalis muscle.
  6. Naldemedine: Opioid receptor antagonist useful for opioid-induced constipation.

COMPLEMENTARY & ALTERNATIVE MEDICINE

Acupuncture can be recommended for chronic idiopathic constipation.

DISPOSITION

- Constipation can be treated in outpatient clinic settings with dietary modifications, medications, and follow-up visits.
- Occasionally, constipation must be addressed in the inpatient setting.

BOX 2 General Approach to Treatment of Constipation

For specific agents, dosages, and precautions, see Table 2.

I. Core Program for All Patients
- Adequate intake of fluid and fiber is one key to preventing constipation. Fiber is available primarily from grains and bran cereals. Flatulence, bloating, and cramps are common side effects encountered when bran fiber is introduced.
- Another source of bulk is from synthetic bulk agents (e.g., psyllium). Bulk agents require an adequate amount of fluid intake; otherwise, they may worsen constipation.
- Avoid irritant laxatives as part of a core program, because long-term use may decrease bowel motility. Encourage the patient to exercise and respond promptly to the urge to defecate.

II. Individualized Program-Specific Indications and General Comments
- *Stimulant laxatives (e.g., senna, bisacodyl)*: Many believe that long-term use of these agents leads to dependency and habituation, but this is not substantiated. When used appropriately, these medications are not harmful and are very effective. Senna is probably the first-line choice among this class of laxatives.
- *Osmotic laxatives (e.g., polyethylene glycol [PEG], lactulose, milk of magnesia, magnesium citrate)*: These agents are most commonly used for colonic preparation before bowel procedures. These agents are safe and well tolerated. PEG has been shown to be slightly more effective than lactulose and causes less bloating and flatus.
- *Lubricants and stool softeners*: Oral mineral oil lubricants and stool softeners are particularly helpful in patients who have acute painful perianal lesions. The softening and coating of the stool can make passage much easier and less painful, preventing constipation. Mineral oil is contraindicated in patients with swallowing problems or in those who are particularly debilitated, to prevent aspiration leading to lipid pneumonia.
- *Suppositories and enemas*: These agents may be helpful in patients who tend to have trouble expelling soft stool from the rectum. Glycerin suppositories may have a soothing effect and be helpful in patients with constipation caused by local, painful perianal lesions. Tap-water enemas are helpful when disimpaction is necessary.

From Marx JA et al: *Rosen's emergency medicine*, ed 8, Philadelphia, 2014, Saunders.

TABLE 2 Preparations Used in the Symptomatic Treatment of Constipation

Medication	Maximal Recommended Dose	Onset of Action	Comments
Bulk Laxatives			Indigestible fiber attracts water, which leads to larger, softer fecal mass.
Psyllium (Metamucil)	Titrate up to 20 g	12-72 hr	Natural fiber that undergoes bacterial degradation, which may contribute to bloating and flatus. Should be taken with plenty of water to avoid intestinal obstruction.
Methylcellulose (Citrucel)	Titrate up to 20 g		Semisynthetic cellulose fiber that is relatively resistant to colonic bacterial degradation.
Polycarbophil (Fibercon)	Titrate up to 20 g		Synthetic fiber of polymer of acrylic acid, resistant to bacterial degradation.
Osmotic Laxatives			Draw water into the intestines along osmotic gradient.
Magnesium or Sodium Salts			
Magnesium Hydroxide (Milk of Magnesia)	30-45 ml once daily	1-6 hr	A small percentage of magnesium is absorbed. Use caution in patients. with renal insufficiency and in children.
Magnesium Citrate	150-300 ml as needed	3-6 hr	
Sodium Phosphate (Fleet Phospho-soda)	20-45 ml with 12 oz of water as needed		Hyperphosphatemia may result if patient has renal insufficiency. Commonly used before colonoscopy.
Poorly Absorbed Sugars			
Lactulose	15-30 ml once or twice a day	24-48 hr	Synthetic disaccharide not absorbed by the small intestine. Gas and bloating common.
Sorbitol	15-30 ml once or twice a day		Poorly absorbed by small intestine.
Polyethylene Glycol and Electrolytes (GoLYTELY, MiraLax)	17 g two or three times a day	12-24 hr	Organic polymers that are poorly absorbed and not metabolized by bacteria, thus may cause less bloating and cramping. Can be mixed with noncarbonated beverages.
Stimulant Laxatives			Stimulate intestinal motility or secretion.
Senna (Senokot, Ex-Lax)	8-34 mg daily	6-12 hr	Stimulates secretion and motility of small intestine and colon.
Bisacodyl (Dulcolax, Correctol)	5-10 mg daily		
Stool Softeners			Increase water penetration and soften stool.
Docusate Sodium (Colace)	100 mg twice a day; some use higher doses	24-48 hr	In many studies, no better than placebo. Not recommended as first-line or solo therapy.
Mineral Oil (Fleet Mineral Oil)	5-15 ml orally at night		Provides lubrication for the passage of stool. Long-term use is not recommended. Lipid pneumonia can occur in patients predisposed to aspiration.
Newer Agents			
Lubiprostone (Amitiza)	24 μg once or twice per day	1 hr	A chloride channel activator. FDA-approved for treatment of chronic idiopathic constipation in adults. Adverse effects: Headache, nausea, diarrhea.
Methylnaltrexone (Relistor)	8-12 mg SQ		Used in refractory opioid-induced constipation.
Linaclotide (Linzess)	145 mcg daily 30 min prior to meals	2-6 hr	Peptide agonist of the guanylate cyclase 2C. It increases smooth muscle contractions. Useful in IBS with constipation.
Plecanatide (Trulance)	3 mg once/day	<24 hr	Peptide agonist of the guanylate cyclase 2C. It increases smooth muscle contractions. Useful in IBS with constipation.
Naldemedine (Symproic)	0.2 mg once/day	2 h	Opioid receptor antagonist

FDA, U.S. Food and Drug Administration; *SQ*, subcutaneously.
Modified from Marx JA et al: *Rosen's emergency medicine*, ed 8, Philadelphia, 2014, Saunders.

REFERRAL

- A referral to a gastroenterologist is not typically necessary for routine cases but is essential for refractory patients or those who may need a colonoscopy, sigmoidoscopy, or manometric studies.
- A referral to a surgeon may be required in patients with large volumes of impacted stool (requiring disimpaction under anesthesia), megacolon, megarectum, or chronic slow transit constipation that is nonresponsive to medical treatment.

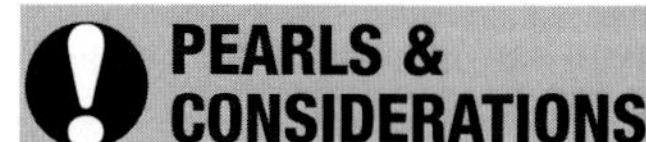

PEARLS & CONSIDERATIONS

- The presence of weight loss, rectal bleeding, or anemia with constipation mandates a colonoscopy or flexible sigmoidoscopy.
- A thorough history and physical examination including digital rectal examination is important in diagnosis and cause of constipation.
- History that includes a survey of the patient's diet, medications, and psychosocial issues is key to the successful treatment of constipation.
- Key components in patient education are summarized in Table E4.

SUGGESTED READINGS

Available at ExpertConsult.com

AUTHORS: **CHRISTOPHER D. JACKSON, M.D.,** and **ROB W. BRADSHER III, M.D.**

BASIC INFORMATION

DEFINITION

Contact dermatitis is an acute or chronic skin inflammation resulting from exposure to substances in the environment. It can be subdivided into "irritant" contact dermatitis (nonimmunologic physical and chemical alteration of the epidermis) and "allergic" contact dermatitis (delayed hypersensitivity reaction).

SYNONYMS

Irritant contact dermatitis
Allergic contact dermatitis

ICD-10CM CODES

L23	Allergic contact dermatitis
L23.0	Allergic contact dermatitis due to metals
L23.1	Allergic contact dermatitis due to adhesives
L23.2	Allergic contact dermatitis due to cosmetics
L23.3	Allergic contact dermatitis due to drugs in contact with skin
L23.4	Allergic contact dermatitis due to dyes
L23.5	Allergic contact dermatitis due to other chemical products
L25.9	Unspecified contact dermatitis, unspecified cause

EPIDEMIOLOGY & DEMOGRAPHICS

- 20% of all cases of dermatitis in children are caused by allergic contact dermatitis.
- Rhus dermatitis (poison ivy, poison oak, and poison sumac) is responsible for most cases of contact dermatitis.
- Frequent causes of irritant contact dermatitis are soaps, detergents, eye drops (Fig. E1), and organic solvents.
- Chemical irritants (e.g., cutting fluids used in machining, solvents) account for most cases of irritant contact dermatitis. Occupational skin diseases are second only to traumatic injuries as the most common types of occupational disease.

PHYSICAL FINDINGS & CLINICAL PRESENTATION

Clinical presentation varies with the responsible agent and affected area of skin.

IRRITANT CONTACT DERMATITIS:

- Mild exposure may result in dryness, erythema, and fissuring of the affected area (e.g., hand involvement in irritant dermatitis caused by exposure to soap [Fig. E2], genital area involvement in irritant dermatitis caused by prolonged exposure to wet diapers).
- Eczematous inflammation may result from chronic exposure.

ALLERGIC CONTACT DERMATITIS:

- Poison ivy dermatitis can present with vesicles and blisters; linear lesions (as a result of dragging of the resins over the surface of the skin by scratching) are a classic presentation.
- The pattern of lesions is asymmetric; itching, burning, and stinging may be present.
- The involved areas are erythematous, warm to touch, swollen, and may be confused with cellulitis.

ETIOLOGY

- Irritant contact dermatitis: Cement (construction workers), rubber, ragweed, malathion (farmers), orange and lemon peels (chefs, bartenders), hair tints, shampoos (beauticians), rubber gloves (medical, surgical personnel)
- Allergic contact dermatitis: Poison ivy, poison oak, poison sumac, rubber (shoe dermatitis), nickel (jewelry), balsam of Peru (hand and face dermatitis), neomycin, formaldehyde (cosmetics)

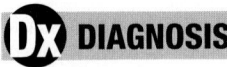

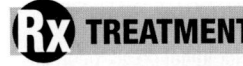

DIAGNOSIS

DIFFERENTIAL DIAGNOSIS

- Impetigo
- Lichen simplex chronicus
- Atopic dermatitis
- Nummular eczema, dyshidrotic eczema
- Seborrheic dermatitis
- Inverse psoriasis, palmoplantar psoriasis
- Scabies
- Tinea pedis

WORKUP

- Medical history: Gradual onset versus rapid onset, number of exposures, clinical presentation, occupational history.
- Physical examination: Contact dermatitis in the neck may be caused by necklaces, perfumes (Fig. E3), aftershave lotion. Involvement of the axillae is often secondary to deodorants, clothing. Face involvement can occur with cosmetics, airborne allergens, aftershave lotion.

LABORATORY TESTS

- Patch testing has a sensitivity and specificity of 70% to 80%. It is useful to confirm the diagnosis of contact dermatitis; it is indicated only when inflammation persists despite appropriate topical therapy and avoidance of suspected causative agent; patch testing should not be used for irritant contact dermatitis because this is a nonimmunologic-mediated inflammatory reaction.
- Dermoscopy and microscopy when suspecting scabies and mites.
- A potassium hydroxide (KOH) preparation may be useful if suspecting tinea or Candida infection.

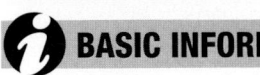

TREATMENT

NONPHARMACOLOGIC THERAPY

Avoidance of suspected allergens (e.g., use of plain petrolatum instead of topical antibiotics for clean wounds)

ACUTE GENERAL Rx

- Removal of the irritant substance by washing the skin with plain water or mild soap within 15 min of exposure is helpful in patients with poison ivy, poison oak, or poison sumac dermatitis.
- Cold or cool water compresses for 20 to 30 min 5 to 6 times a day for the initial 72 hr are effective during the acute blistering stage.
- Topical steroids (clobetasol 0.05%, triamcinolone 0.1%) are effective for acute localized allergic contact dermatitis lesions. Lower-potency topical steroids are preferred on face, anogenital regions, and flexural surfaces to minimize risk of skin atrophy. Oral corticosteroids (e.g., prednisone 20 mg bid for 6 to 10 days) are generally reserved for severe, widespread dermatitis.
- IM steroids (e.g., Kenalog) are used for severe reactions and in patients requiring oral corticosteroids but unable to tolerate PO.
- Oral antihistamines (e.g., hydroxyzine 25 mg q6h) will control pruritus, especially at night; calamine lotion is also useful for pruritus; however, it can lead to excessive drying.
- Colloidal oatmeal (Aveeno) baths can also provide symptomatic relief.
- Patients with mild to moderate erythema may respond to topical steroid gels or creams.
- Patients with shoe allergy should change their socks at least once a day; use of aluminum chloride hexahydrate in a 20% solution (Drysol) qhs will also help control perspiration.
- Use hypoallergenic surgical gloves in patients with rubber and surgical glove allergy.

DISPOSITION

Allergic contact dermatitis generally resolves within 2 to 4 wk if re-exposure to allergen is prevented.

REFERRAL

For patch testing in selected patients, see "Laboratory Tests."

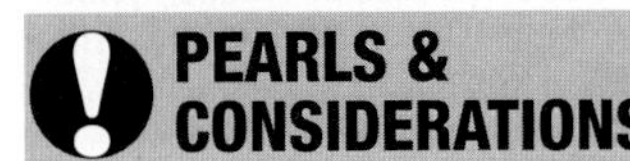

PEARLS & CONSIDERATIONS

COMMENTS

Commercially available corticosteroid dose packs should be avoided, because they generally provide an inadequate amount of medication.

SUGGESTED READINGS

Available at ExpertConsult.com

RELATED CONTENT

Contact Dermatitis (Patient Information)
Poison Ivy Dermatitis (Related Key Topic)

AUTHOR: **FRED F. FERRI, M.D.**

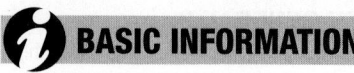

BASIC INFORMATION

DEFINITION

Contraception refers to the various modalities that a sexually active couple uses to prevent pregnancy. These options can be either medical or nonmedical and used by men or women or both. The options are as follows:

- No contraception (unprotected intercourse); failure rate 85% both typical use and perfect use
- Abstinence
  1. 12.4% of unmarried men
  2. 13.2% of unmarried women
  3. More frequently practiced before age 17 yr
  4. No intercourse experienced by 13% of women ages 30 to 34 yr
  5. Failure rate 0%
- Withdrawal
  1. Used in only 2% of sexually active women
  2. Failure rate with perfect use, 4%; with typical use, 19%
- Rhythm method (natural family planning)
  1. Failure rate with perfect use, 1% to 9%; with typical use, 20%
  2. Symptothermal type: Mucus method and ovulation pain combined with basal body temperature
  3. Ovulation (Billings method): Takes into account mucus quality
  4. Basal body temperature method: Uses biphasic temperature chart
  5. Lactation amenorrhea method: Effective in fully breastfeeding women, especially 70 to 100 days after delivery; depends on number of feedings per day
- Barriers
  1. Diaphragm and cervical cap: Failure rate 5% to 9% in nulliparous women, 20% in multiparous women
  2. Female condom: Failure rate with perfect use, 5.1%; with typical use, 12.4%; FDA labeling states 25% failure rate
  3. Male condom: Failure rate with perfect use, 3%; with typical use, 12%
  4. Spermicides (aerosols, foam, jellies, creams, tabs): Failure rate with perfect use, 3%; with typical use, 21%
- Oral contraceptives
  1. Failure rate with perfect use, <<1%; with typical use, 3%
  2. Come in combinations of estrogen/progestin or as progestin only
- Hormonal implants and injectables
  1. Implanon (etonogestrel) implant 2-yr cumulative pregnancy rate 0.05%. Nexplanon is essentially the same as Implanon but with a barium sulfate core for easier radiologic detection and a preloaded applicator to facilitate insertion.
  2. Depo-Provera: Failure rate 0.3% in first yr of use.
  3. Nestorone-releasing single implant: Not yet available.
  4. Jadelle implant: Successor to the Norplant implant, which has been discontinued in the U.S. The Jadelle implant is not available in the U.S.
- Mini pill (progesterone only pill)
  1. Failure rate with typical use, 1.1% to 13.2%
  2. With perfect use, 5 pregnancies per 1000 women
     a. Requires precise timing of daily use for effectiveness
- Emergency postcoital contraception
  1. Decreases pregnancy rate by 75% or more with women treated within 72 hrs of coitus
  2. Progestin-only method: 1.5 mg levonorgestrel single dose or 0.75 mg given 12 hrs apart
  3. Selective progesterone receptor modulator: 30 mg Ulipristal single dose is more effective than levonorgestrel
  4. Copper IUD: Can be inserted up to 5 days after ovulation and results in the lowest pregnancy rate (0.1%)
- IUD (available over the counter in some states)
  1. Progestasert: Failure rate with perfect use, 2%; with typical use, 3%
  2. Copper T (30-A): Failure rate with perfect use, 0.6%; with typical use, 0.8%
  3. Levonorgestrel Intrauterine System (Mirena)
     a. 1-yr failure rate, 0.2%
     b. 5-yr cumulative failure rate, 0.7%
- Skyla, a smaller version of the Mirena, which also releases Levonorgestrel, and is targeted for younger users, was released in 2014. In 2015, the FDA approved Liletta, which also releases levonorgestrel. Liletta is marketed by Medicine 360, a nonprofit pharmaceutical firm, and is intended for use by women with fewer economic resources. Cost, which limits access to long-acting reversible contraceptives for many women, has been cited as a public health problem. Although Liletta has been approved for a 3-yr lifespan, the lower initial cost may allow many more women access to affordable contraception. Kyleena was FDA approved in 2016 for nulliparous and parous women, releases lower dose of levonorgestrel than Mirena, and was approved for 5 yr.
- Female sterilization (tubal ligation): Failure rate with perfect use, 0.2%; with typical use, 3%.
- Male sterilization (vasectomy): Failure rate of 0.1% in first yr.
- Vaginal ring (NuvaRing): Failure rate pearl index 0.77.
- Contraceptive patch (Ortho Evra): Failure rate 0.4% to 0.7%.

SYNONYMS

Birth control
Family planning

ICD-10CM CODES	
Z30.011	Encounter for initial prescription of contraceptive pills
Z30.018	Encounter for initial prescription of other contraceptives
Z30.09	Encounter for other general counseling and advice on contraception
Z30.430	Encounter for insertion of intrauterine contraceptive device
Z30.2	Encounter for sterilization

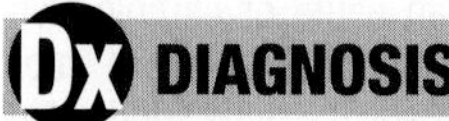

DIAGNOSIS

WORKUP

- Thorough medical history
- Thorough surgical history
- Obstetric history (was fertility desired with conception?)
- Gynecologic history, including:
  1. History of previous sexually transmitted diseases
  2. Number of partners
  3. Previous difficulties with contraception
  4. Frequency of intercourse
- Family history
- Table E1 summarizes when to start using contraceptive methods
- Examinations and tests needed before initiation of contraceptive methods described in Table 2
- Recommendations for routine follow-up after contraceptive initiation summarized in Table E3

LABORATORY TESTS

- Pap smear
- *Chlamydia* and *Gonorrhea* screening when appropriate
- Pregnancy test if suspected pregnancy
- Lipid profile if family history of premature vascular event

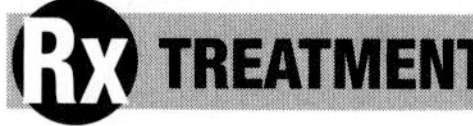

TREATMENT

NONPHARMACOLOGIC THERAPY

- Male condoms
  1. 95% latex (rubber), 5% polyurethane, or natural membrane (lamb's intestine does not block transmission of sexually transmitted infections).
  2. Proper use: Place on an erect penis and leave ½-inch empty space at the tip of the condom; use with non–oil-based lubricants.
  3. Effectiveness increased when used with spermicides.
  4. Main advantage: Condoms are the only method shown to reduce HIV transmission.
- Female condoms
  1. Composed of polyurethane, with one end open and one end closed.
  2. Proper use: Place closed end over cervix, open end hanging out of vagina to cover penis and scrotum.
  3. Highly effective against HIV.
- Spermicides
  1. Types: Nonoxynol, octoxynol.
  2. Forms: Jellies, creams, foams, suppositories, tablets, soluble films.
  3. Proper use: Put in immediately before intercourse; may be used with other barrier methods.

C

TABLE 2 Examinations and Tests Needed before Initiation of Contraceptive Methods

	Contraceptive Method and Class							
Examination or Test	Cu-IUD and LNG-IUD	Implant	Injectable	CHC	POP	Condom	Diaphragm or Cervical Cap	Spermicide
Examination								
Blood pressure	C	C	C	A*	C	C	C	C
Weight (BMI) (weight [kg]/height [m]^2)	—†	—†	—†	—†	—†	C	C	C
Clinical breast examination	C	C	C	C	C	C	C	C
Bimanual examination and cervical inspection	A	C	C	C	C	C	A‡	C
Laboratory Test								
Glucose	C	C	C	C	C	C	C	C
Lipids	C	C	C	C	C	C	C	C
Liver enzymes	C	C	C	C	C	C	C	C
Hemoglobin	C	C	C	C	C	C	C	C
Thrombogenic mutations	C	C	C	C	C	C	C	C
Cervical cytology (Papanicolaou test)	C	C	C	C	C	C	C	C
STD screening with laboratory tests	—¶	C	C	C	C	C	C	C
HIV screening with laboratory tests	C	C	C	C	C	C	C	C

BMI, body mass index; *CHC*, combined hormonal contraceptive; *Cu-IUD*, copper-containing intrauterine device; *HIV*, human immunodeficiency virus; *LNG-IUD*, levonorgestrel-releasing intrauterine device; *POP*, progestin-only pill; *STD*, sexually transmitted disease; *U.S. MEC*, U.S. Medical Eligibility Criteria for Contraceptive Use.

*In instances in which blood pressure cannot be measured by a provider, blood pressure measured in other settings can be reported by the woman to her provider.

†Weight (BMI) measurement is not needed to determine medical eligibility for any methods of contraception because all methods can be used (U.S. MEC 1) or generally can be used (U.S. MEC 2) among obese women. However, measuring weight and calculating BMI at baseline might be helpful for monitoring any changes and counseling women who might be concerned about weight change perceived to be associated with their contraceptive method.

‡A bimanual examination (not cervical inspection) is needed for diaphragm fitting.

¶Most women do not require additional STD screening at the time of IUD insertion. If a woman with risk factors for STDs has not been screened for gonorrhea and chlamydia according to CDC's *STD Treatment Guidelines* (http://www.cdc.gov/std/treatment), screening can be performed at the time of IUD insertion, and insertion should not be delayed. Women with current purulent cervicitis or chlamydial infection or gonococcal infection should not undergo IUD insertion (U.S. MEC 4).

From Curtis KM et al: U.S. selected practice recommendations for contraceptive use, 2016, *MMWR Recomm Rep* 65(4):1–66, 2016.

- Diaphragm and cervical cap
  1. Must be fitted by practitioner, used with contraceptive gels, and refitted with weight gain or loss of 4.5 kg. Must also be refitted after pregnancy.
  2. Diaphragm sizes: 50 to 105 mm; cervical cap sizes 26, 28, and 30 mm.
  3. The correct fit allows the woman to remain ambulatory without feeling the device.
  4. Proper use of diaphragm: Put in immediately before intercourse and keep in for 6 hr after intercourse; must not remain in the vagina for longer than 24 hr.
  5. Proper use of cervical cap: Fit over the cervix exactly; must not remain in place for longer than 48 hr.
- Lactation amenorrhea method
  1. Depends on number of feedings per day; effective as birth control for 6 mo if 15 or more feedings, lasting 10 min each, are accomplished daily. If woman meets criteria (e.g., breastfeeding only source of infant feeding), 0.5% to 2.0% failure rate in the first 6 months after delivery.
  2. Not a common practice in the U.S.
- Withdrawal
  1. Withdrawal of the penis from the vagina before ejaculation.
  2. Depends on self-control, but there is a high typical use failure rate.
- Rhythm method
  1. Depends on awareness of physiology of male and female reproductive tracts.
  2. Sperm viable in vagina for 2 to 7 days.
  3. Ovum lifespan 24 hr.
- Sterilization
  1. Male
     a. Vasectomy to interrupt vas deferens and block passage of sperm to seminal ejaculate.
     b. Scalpel and nonscalpel techniques available.
     c. More easily performed procedure than female sterilization and does not require general anesthesia.
  2. Female
     a. Leading method of birth control in U.S. in women older than 30 yr.
     b. Interrupts fallopian tubes, blocking passage of ovum proximally and sperm distally through tube.
     c. Several types; modified Pomeroy done during cesarean section or interval laparoscopic using clips (Filshie, Hulka) or banding.
     d. Essure-tubal occlusion through hysteroscopic placement of microinserts into the fallopian tubes; current controversy regarding safety and efficacy.

ACUTE GENERAL Rx

- Combination oral contraceptives
  1. Standard administration: Taken daily for 21 days, pill-free interval of 7 days.
  2. Alternative regimen: Extended or continuous administration of active pills.
  3. Less than 50 mcg ethinyl estradiol in most common combination oral contraceptives; progestins most commonly used in combination pills are norethindrone, levonorgestrel, norgestrel, norethindrone acetate, ethynodiol diacetate, norgestimate, or desogestrel; triphasic combination oral contraceptives (give varying doses of progestin and estrogens throughout cycle); monophasic oral contraceptives: Offer same dose of progestin and estrogen throughout cycle, taken daily at same time; estrophasic pill (constant progesterone with variation of estrogen throughout the cycle).
  4. If pill taken with antibiotics, efficacy affected by inadequate gastrointestinal absorption in most cases; only rifampin truly reduces pill's effectiveness.
  5. Increased body weight decreases effectiveness.
  6. Table E4 describes oral contraceptive formulations available in the U.S. Guidelines for use of combination estrogen-progestin contraceptives in women 35 yr of age and older are described in Table E5.

7. Fig. E1 describes recommended actions after late or missed combined oral contraceptives.
8. Recommended actions after vomiting or diarrhea while using combined oral contraceptives are described in Fig. E2.

- Mini pill
  1. Progestin only; taken without a break.
  2. May cause irregular bleeding because of the lack of estrogen effect on the lining of the uterus.
  3. Table E6 provides a summary and recommendations for progestin-only oral contraceptive use.
- Hormonal implants and injectables
  1. Implanon/Nexplanon
     a. Single etonogestrel-secreting device that is inserted underneath the skin.
     b. Among the most effective contraceptive available.
     c. Approved by FDA in 2006 and effective over 3-yr period.
  2. Depo-Provera
     a. Medroxyprogesterone acetate given every 3 mo in IM injection form.
     b. Major side effect: Irregular bleeding.
     c. Fertility return possibly delayed up to 1 yr or longer after last injection.
     d. Table E7 provides a summary and recommendations for depot medroxyprogesterone acetate (DMPA) use.
- Postcoital contraception
  1. Done on emergency basis, usually as a result of noncompliance with birth control or failure of birth control (e.g., condom breakage) at the time of ovulation.
  2. Methods:
     a. Hormonal methods:
        (1) Levonorgestrel is available either as two 0.75 mg tablets taken 12 hr apart (next choice) or as a 1.5 mg tablet taken once (Plan B, one step). It is indicated for emergency contraception to be used within 72 hr after unexpected intercourse. It can be obtained OTC by women >15 yr of age and by prescription by younger patients.
        (2) Ulipristal (ELLA) is a progesterone-receptor agonist/antagonist available by prescription only. It is a 30-mg, single-dose tablet and can be taken up to 5 days after unexpected intercourse.
        (3) Copper IUD insertion within 5 days of coitus.
- IUD
  1. Device inserted into uterus to prevent sperm and ovum from uniting in fallopian tube.
  2. Types available in the U.S.:
     a. ParaGard (Copper T/30-A): A polyethylene T wrapped with a fine copper wire effective for 10 yr.
     b. Mirena Levonorgestrel Intrauterine System: A T-shaped system with a chamber that contains levonorgestrel. Releases 20 mcg/day; is effective for 5 yr.
     c. Skyla: Smaller and lowest dose of levonorgestrel, approved for 3 yr.
     d. Liletta: Cheaper levonorgestrel secreting system, approved for 3 yr.
     e. Kyleena: Another 5-yr levonorgestrel system.
- Vaginal ring (NuvaRing)
  1. Provides daily dose of 120 mcg of etonogestrel and 15 mcg ethinyl estradiol.
  2. Stays in vagina 3 wk and is removed the fourth for a contraceptive-free interval analogous to the placebo pills in oral contraceptive pills.
  3. Increased body weight decreases effectiveness.
  4. Delivers lower total dose of estrogen than the combination oral contraceptive, but may have higher risk of DVT.
  5. Recommended actions after delayed insertion or reinsertion with combined vaginal ring are described in Fig. E3.
- Contraceptive patch
  1. Releases a progestin and estrogen (ethinyl estradiol)
  2. Each patch contains 6 mg norelgestromin and delivers an estimated continuous systemic dose of 150 mcg norelgestromin and 15 mcg of ethinyl estradiol daily
  3. Worn 3 out of 4 wk
  4. Increased body weight decreases effectiveness
  5. Concern for increased risk of thromboembolic events
  6. Ortha Evra brand discontinued; Xulane (generic) available in the U.S.
  7. Recommended actions after delayed application or detachment with combined hormonal patch are described in Fig. E4

CHRONIC Rx

- With all the previously mentioned types of birth control, patient is followed up at least yearly, or as necessary, if problems arise.
- Full history, physical examination, and Pap smear, including cultures when needed, are performed yearly.
- Patients with medical problems are followed up approximately every 6 mo when taking hormonal therapy.

DISPOSITION

- Follow yearly or more frequently according to patient's side effects.
- Tailor birth control to patient according to different needs or side effects present at different times in life. Effective counseling also requires an understanding of a woman's preference and medical risks, benefits, side effects, and contraindications of each contraceptive method.

COMMENTS

- With hormonal contraception, if neurologic or cardiac symptoms arise, stop method immediately, evaluate, and refer to internist when appropriate.
- The effectiveness of long-acting reversible contraception (IUDs and implants) is superior to that of contraceptive pills, patch, or ring and is not altered in adolescents and young women.
- Management of women with bleeding irregularities while using contraception is described in Fig. E5.

SUGGESTED READINGS

Available at ExpertConsult.com

RELATED CONTENT

Contraception (Patient Information)
Emergency Contraception (Related Key Topic)

AUTHOR: **ANTHONY SCISCIONE, D.O.**

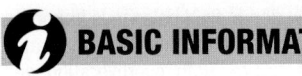

BASIC INFORMATION

DEFINITION

Cor pulmonale is an alteration in the structure and function of the right ventricle (RV) from pulmonary hypertension caused by diseases of the upper or lower airways, lungs, or pulmonary vasculature. It is a state of cardiopulmonary dysfunction that may result from multiple etiologies rather than a specific disease state. Right-sided heart failure resulting from primary disease of the left heart and congenital heart disease are not considered in this disorder.

SYNONYMS

Acute cor pulmonale
Chronic cor pulmonale

ICD-10CM CODES	
I26.0	Pulmonary embolism with acute cor pulmonale
I27.81	Cor pulmonale (chronic)
I26.01	Septic pulmonary embolism with acute cor pulmonale
I26.02	Saddle embolus of pulmonary artery with acute cor pulmonale
I26.09	Other pulmonary embolism with acute cor pulmonale
I26.90	Septic pulmonary embolism without acute cor pulmonale
I26.92	Saddle embolus of pulmonary artery without acute cor pulmonale
I26.99	Other pulmonary embolism without acute cor pulmonale

ETIOLOGY

Acute cor pulmonale is a disorder in which the right ventricle (RV) is dilated and the muscular wall is stretched thin, usually as a result of acute pulmonary embolism or acute respiratory distress syndrome (ARDS). This may present with often life-threatening obstructive shock, or death, but if the patient survives the initial event, they can develop pulmonary hypertension, right ventricular hypertrophy, and subsequent failure. Critical care echocardiography is essential and defines acute cor pulmonale as the presence of RV dilatation along with a paradoxical interventricular septal motion at end systole, suggesting both RV systolic and diastolic overload.

Chronic cor pulmonale is hypertrophy of the right ventricle caused by increased afterload in the pulmonary circuit, i.e., pulmonary hypertension, resulting in either acute or chronic right ventricular failure depending on the time course of the elevation in pulmonary vascular resistance.

Mechanisms leading to pulmonary hypertension and thus predisposing to the development of cor pulmonale include the following:

- Passive pulmonary vascular congestion as a result of "back-filling" due to elevated left ventricular filling pressures.
- Pulmonary vasoconstriction leading to increased RV afterload, often resulting from conditions causing alveolar hypoxia and/or respiratory acidosis (e.g., high-altitude/hypobaric hypoxia, obstructive sleep apnea/obesity-hypoventilation syndrome, chronic obstructive pulmonary disease). In pulmonary arterial hypertension (PAH), pulmonary vasoconstriction may occur in the absence of a primary cause of hypoxemia, due to imbalances between vasoconstrictor and vasodilator expression in the pulmonary circulation.
- Pulmonary vascular endothelial dysfunction also plays a major role in the development of pulmonary hypertension. There is reduction in the production of nitric oxide as well as prostacyclins, resulting in an imbalance of vasoconstriction opposed to dilation.
- Anatomic reduction or remodeling of the pulmonary vascular bed leading to increased RV afterload (e.g., emphysema, interstitial lung disease, pulmonary emboli, pulmonary arterial hypertension).
- Chronic thromboembolic disease.

PHYSICAL FINDINGS & CLINICAL PRESENTATION

No symptoms are specific for cor pulmonale. Typically, the symptoms depend on the underlying disease process. The symptoms are most often a result of right ventricular failure:

- Dyspnea, fatigue, chest pain, or syncope with exertion (from pulmonary hypertension, RV ischemia, and impaired cardiac output)
- Right upper quadrant abdominal pain and anorexia (from passive hepatic congestion)
- Hoarseness (caused by compression of the left recurrent laryngeal nerve by dilation of the main pulmonary artery; known as *Ortner's syndrome*)
- Signs of right ventricular failure: Jugular venous distention, peripheral edema, hepatic congestion, ascites, and a right ventricular third heart sound
- Signs of associated tricuspid regurgitation: Holosystolic murmur heard best along the left parasternal border (augments during inspiration), prominent V-wave on jugular venous pulse, and pulsatile hepatomegaly (in severe tricuspid regurgitation)
- Pulmonary hypertension will increase the intensity of the pulmonic component of S2, which may be narrowly split
- Rarely, cough and hemoptysis

Dx DIAGNOSIS

WORKUP

Search for an underlying pulmonary process resulting in pulmonary hypertension:

- Left ventricular dysfunction should be excluded in initial assessment with an echocardiogram.
- Worldwide, chronic mountain sickness and schistosomiasis are important causes of cor pulmonale.
- Prevalence of cor pulmonale cases attributable to chronic obstructive pulmonary disease (COPD) ranges from 25% to 90%. Workup should include complete pulmonary function tests (PFTs) and chest CT.
- Consideration of obstructive sleep apnea, chronic thromboembolic disease, pulmonary arterial hypertension, and musculoskeletal disease should be given in the absence of parenchymal lung disease.
- A multiple gated acquisition right ventricular ejection fraction (MUGA RVEF) <45% is considered abnormal. However, MUGA scan is largely being replaced by cardiac MRI (CMR), which is the gold standard for RV function and size.

LABORATORY TESTS

- Complete blood count may show erythrocytosis from chronic hypoxia.
- Arterial blood gas levels confirm hypoxemia and acidosis or hypercapnia.
- B-type natriuretic peptide (BNP) may be elevated from RV dilation and/or hypoxia.
- Connective tissue disorder workup to exclude scleroderma, lupus, rheumatoid arthritis.
- HIV testing.

IMAGING STUDIES

- Chest radiograph may show underlying pulmonary disease and evidence of pulmonary hypertension (e.g., enlargement of the pulmonary arteries or right atrium and right ventricular dilation or "pruning" of the peripheral vasculature) (Fig. 1).
- ECG (Fig. 2) may reveal right ventricular hypertrophy with R/S ratio >1 in leads V_1 and R/S ratio <1 in leads V_5,V_6, right atrial enlargement (P-pulmonale), right-axis deviation, or the triad of $S_1Q_3T_3$ indicative of RV strain.
- Echocardiogram to detect right ventricular enlargement and/or hypertrophy and estimate systolic pulmonary artery pressure.
- PFTs, including spirometry, lung volumes, and diffusion capacity, should be performed in all patients to evaluate for restrictive, obstructive, or combined restrictive-obstructive lung disease.
- Perfusion scintigraphy (VQ scan) to rule out chronic thromboembolic pulmonary hypertension (CTEPH)
- Cardiac MRI can accurately measure right ventricular dimensions and function.
- Right-sided heart catheterization measures pulmonary artery pressures and pulmonary vascular resistance. It can also determine response to vasodilators. Importantly, right heart catheterization allows assessment of pulmonary capillary wedge pressure, allowing right heart failure from pulmonary venous hypertension due to left heart disease to be ruled out.
- Chest CT can assess for pulmonary parenchymal disease and embolus in the pulmonary vasculature.

Rx TREATMENT

The treatment of cor pulmonale is directed toward the underlying etiology while also reversing hypoxemia, improving right ventricular contractility, decreasing pulmonary artery vascular resistance, and improving pulmonary hypertension. Table 1 summarizes therapeutic strategies for cor pulmonale.

NONPHARMACOLOGIC THERAPY

- Supplemental oxygen to correct hypoxemia is an important management step in the treatment of cor pulmonale related to hypoxemia. Goal O_2 sat of more than 90% is recommended. Oxygen is the only modality that has demonstrated mortality benefit in patients with group 3 pulmonary hypertension.
- Continuous positive airway pressure is used in patients with obstructive sleep apnea.
- Sodium and fluid restriction in setting of edema from RV failure.
- Low-level aerobic exercise, avoiding heavy physical exercise or isometric exercises that may cause syncope.

ACUTE GENERAL Rx

- Pulmonary embolism is the most common cause of acute cor pulmonale (see "Pulmonary Embolism"). The treatment is anticoagulation, hemodynamic support, and consideration of thrombolytics. Thrombolytics have been reserved for patients with large pulmonary embolism (PE) resulting in hemodynamic instability. Catheter-based thrombectomy or surgical embolectomy are potential salvage therapies in patients who cannot receive anticoagulation or thrombolysis, or whose condition continues to deteriorate despite thrombolytics and anticoagulation.
- Acute cor pulmonale may also be seen in cases of acute respiratory distress syndrome (ARDS), related to hypercapnia/acidosis, hypoxic pulmonary vasoconstriction, and the effects of mechanical ventilation. The treatment is supportive care for ARDS with low tidal volume ventilation. Extracorporeal membrane oxygen support (ECMO) while awaiting lung recovery from ARDS may also be helpful in maintaining blood oxygenation. Venoarterial ECMO can provide hemodynamic support as well as blood oxygenation.
- In patients with preexisting cor pulmonale, acute pulmonary illnesses or hypoxia can increase pulmonary hypertension and worsen right ventricular function. The underlying exacerbating conditions should be treated.
- Careful attention to fluid balance is important in the management of acute decompensated right heart failure. Both overhydration and overdiuresis should be avoided, with careful monitoring of intake and output, electrolytes and creatinine, and hemodynamics.
- Intravenous inotropes may be employed to support right heart contractility in decompensated right heart failure. Dobutamine, milrinone, or epinephrine all have been used in clinical studies with variable success.
- In acutely decompensated right heart failure due to pulmonary arterial hypertension, IV prostanoid medications are the treatment of choice to acutely decrease pulmonary vascular resistance. Oral pulmonary vasodilators may also be added to the IV prostanoids, but should not be initiated as monotherapy in patients with advanced right heart failure from pulmonary arterial hypertension (PAH).

CHRONIC Rx

- The long-term use of oxygen therapy results in decreased clinical right heart failure and improved pulmonary hemodynamics in hypoxic patients.
- Indications for oxygen in chronic obstructive pulmonary disease (COPD) patients include the following:
  1. Resting PaO_2 ≤55 mm Hg on arterial blood gas
  2. Resting PaO 56 to 59 mm Hg if clinical presence of right heart failure with dependent edema, P pulmonale on ECG
  3. Desaturation to SpO_2 ≤88% on oximetry with activity or at night
     - Right ventricular volume overload should be treated with loop diuretics (e.g., furosemide) and potassium-sparing diuretics such as spironolactone.
- Anticoagulation with warfarin has been shown to have some benefit in patients with idiopathic pulmonary arterial hypertension, provided that there are no obvious contraindications to long-term anticoagulation.

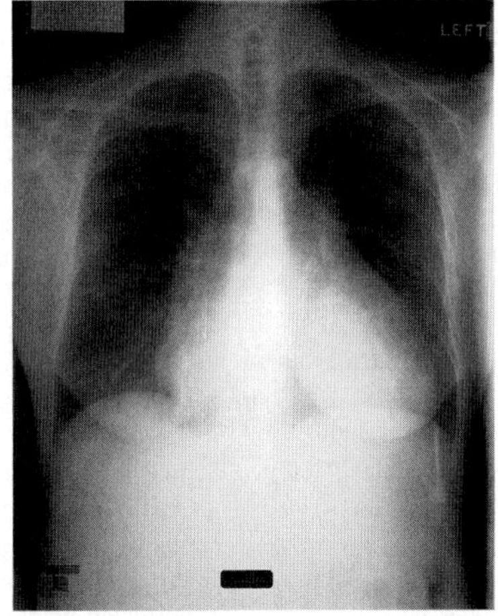

FIG. 1 Chest radiography in a patient with severe intrinsic pulmonary vascular disease demonstrating enlargement of the main pulmonary artery, right ventricle, and right atrium. (From Crawford MH, et al. [eds]: *Cardiology,* ed 2, St Louis, 2004, Mosby.)

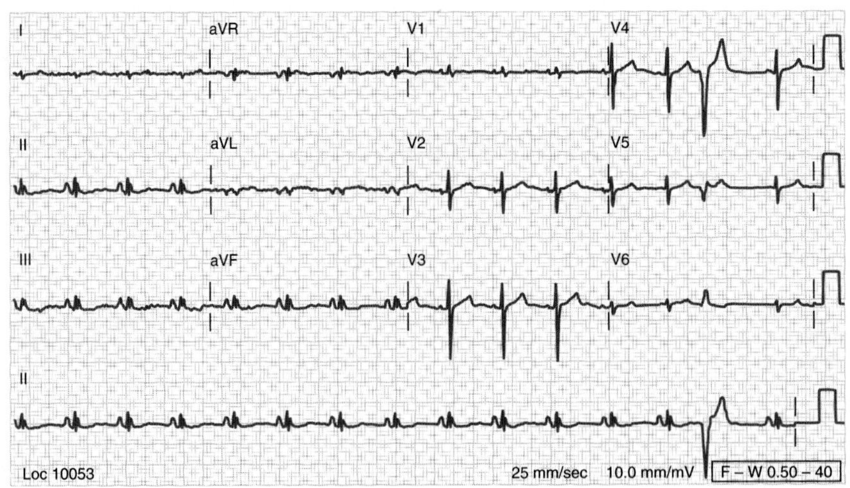

FIG. 2 An electrocardiogram in a patient with chronic cor pulmonale reveals prominent "P pulmonale" and other characteristic features (see text). *aVF,* Augmented vector foot; *aVL,* augmented vector left; *aVR,* augmented vector right. (From Mason RJ: *Murray & Nadel's textbook of respiratory medicine,* ed 5, Philadelphia, 2010, Saunders.)

TABLE 1 Therapeutic Strategies for Cor Pulmonale

Diet and Lifestyle

Smoking cessation
Weight loss
Sodium restriction
Judicious exercise training
Structured rehabilitation and breathing training programs
Avoidance of overexertion
Avoidance of pregnancy
Avoidance of high altitudes

Interventions

Treatment of underlying condition
- COPD (bronchodilators, corticosteroids, antibiotics, oxygen)
- Interstitial lung disease (immunosuppression, oxygen, interferon gamma [investigational])
- Sleep-disordered breathing and alveolar hypoventilation disorders (CPAP, BiPAP, surgery)
- Chronic exposure to high altitudes (return to sea level)
- Chronic thromboembolic disease (anticoagulation, inferior vena cava filters, thromboendarterectomy)

Supplemental oxygen
Pulmonary vasodilators
Anticoagulation
Diuretics
Digitalis glycosides (chronic therapy)
Nonglycoside inotropes (low-dose dobutamine or milrinone in acute severe right heart decompensation with hypoperfusion)
Lung volume reduction surgery
Lung transplantation
Heart-lung transplantation (PAH secondary to complex congenital heart disease)
Percutaneous blade-balloon atrial septostomy (investigational)
- Severe right-sided heart failure
- Recurrent syncope

BiPAP, Bilevel positive airway pressure; *COPD,* chronic obstructive pulmonary disease; *CPAP,* continuous positive airway pressure; *PAH,* pulmonary arterial hypertension.
From Mason RJ: *Murray & Nadel's textbook of respiratory medicine,* ed 5, Philadelphia, 2010, Saunders.

- Digoxin, though controversial, may be employed as an oral inotropic agent to improve right heart contractility and control atrial arrhythmias.
- Selective oral or parenteral pulmonary vasodilators such as oral calcium channel blockers (CCBs), prostanoids, phosphodiesterase inhibitors, and endothelin receptor blockers may be used after a right heart catheterization that establishes pulmonary hypertension. If vasoreactivity is established, CCBs may be used to lower pulmonary vascular resistance. However, if there is no vasoreactivity, prostanoids such as epoprostenol or treprostinil, phosphodiesterase type 5 inhibitors such as sildenafil, or endothelin receptor blockers such as bosentan may be tried. However, such agents have been shown to be beneficial in the treatment of idiopathic PAH, PAH related to connective tissue disease, and PAH due to congenital heart disease. Pulmonary vasodilators are sometimes considered in other forms of PAH when primary disease management strategies have failed to improve right heart failure.
- Pulmonary endarterectomy may be curative in the special case of cor pulmonale due to chronic thromboembolic pulmonary hypertension.
- Atrial septostomy is a salvage option for patients with ongoing decompensated right heart failure from PAH despite pulmonary vasodilators. Such patients should undergo rapid assessment for possible transplantation.
- Lung transplantation or heart-lung transplantation should be considered in the setting of cor pulmonale from lung diseases or from pulmonary vascular disease.

DISPOSITION

Patients with cor pulmonale should have regular assessment of their functional class (e.g., New York Heart Association or World Health Organization [NYHA or WHO] functional class); worse functional class indicates a poorer prognosis. Other poor prognostic features include high right atrial pressure, impaired cardiac output, elevated BNP levels, low systemic blood pressure, and poor exercise tolerance as demonstrated by a 6-minute walk test.

REFERRAL

Patients with pulmonary disease who have progressed to cor pulmonale should be followed up by a pulmonologist and a tertiary care center that specializes in treatment of advanced pulmonary hypertension.

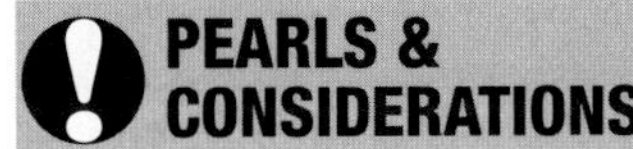

- Identification and treatment of the underlying cause of cor pulmonale is key.
- Prognosis and treatment are related to the underlying cause, whereas the presence of cor pulmonale is merely a marker of the underlying disease severity.
- Right heart catheterization is the gold standard to establish diagnosis and to determine treatment, including response to calcium channel blockers, prostanoids, and endothelin receptor blockers.

COMMENTS

There is increasing interest in selective pulmonary vasodilators to improve right ventricular heart function in patients with cor pulmonale outside of the setting of idiopathic PAH, PAH related to connective tissue disease, and PAH related to congenital heart disease. However, more data on the safety and efficacy of these agents, especially in the setting of hypoxemic lung disease, is needed.

The importance of maintaining or improving right heart function, rather than solely lowering pulmonary pressures, is becoming increasingly apparent in the therapeutic management of patients with pulmonary hypertension and right heart failure.

Long-term survival is related to improved pulmonary artery hemodynamics (lower mean PAP). Improved pulmonary hemodynamics are apparent within the first 6 months of oxygen therapy. Continuous oxygen therapy improves pulmonary hemodynamics with more than 19 hr/day therapy.

SUGGESTED READINGS

Available at ExpertConsult.com

RELATED CONTENT

Pulmonary Embolism (Related Key Topic)
Pulmonary Hypertension (Related Key Topic)

AUTHOR: **WAJIH A. SYED, M.D.**

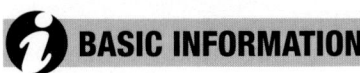

DEFINITION

Coronary artery disease (CAD) is a clinical syndrome that suggests limitation of coronary blood flow to the myocardium as a result of flow-limiting atherosclerotic lesions. Atherosclerosis can be defined as the narrowing of the artery due to plaque formation in the setting of lipid accumulation inside the arterial walls. It is silent in the early stages and characterized by exertional symptoms in later stages as described in the following.

This topic addresses only stable CAD. Acute coronary syndromes (ACS), angina pectoris, and myocardial infarction are addressed as separate topics elsewhere.

SYNONYMS

Atherosclerotic heart disease
CAD
Chronic stable angina
Stable ischemic heart disease
Coronary arteriosclerosis

ICD-10CM CODES	
I25.1	Atherosclerotic heart disease
I25.0	Atherosclerotic cardiovascular disease
I25.10	Atherosclerotic heart disease of native coronary artery without angina pectoris
I25.110	Atherosclerotic heart disease of native coronary artery with unstable angina pectoris
I25.111	Atherosclerotic heart disease of native coronary artery with angina pectoris with documented spasm
I25.118	Atherosclerotic heart disease of native coronary artery with other forms of angina pectoris
I25.119	Atherosclerotic heart disease of native coronary artery with unspecified angina pectoris

EPIDEMIOLOGY & DEMOGRAPHICS

INCIDENCE: For persons who are 40 yr old, the lifetime risk of developing CAD is 49% in men and 32% in women. The risk increases with age in both men and women; however, the incidence in women lags behind that seen in men by approximately 10 yr.

The incidence in premenopausal women is relatively low, with the incidence increasing significantly in postmenopausal women.

The initial presentation in men is more likely to be that of a myocardial infarction, whereas women present initially with angina more frequently.

PREVALENCE: The 2017 Heart Disease and Stroke Statistics update from the American Heart Association estimated that 16.5 million Americans ≥20 yr of age have CAD. There is a slight male predominance at 55%, with incidence increasing with age. CAD prevalence is 7.9% for men and 5.1% for women.

RISK FACTORS: Age, male sex, hypertension, hyperlipidemia, diabetes mellitus, obesity, tobacco use, family history, peripheral vascular disease. Coronary plaque, especially noncalcified plaque, is more prevalent and extensive in HIV-infected men, independent of CAD risk factors.

PHYSICAL FINDINGS & CLINICAL PRESENTATION

- Left anterior chest discomfort often described as squeezing, heavy pressure, burning, and occasionally hot or cold sensations.
- Associated symptoms include fatigue, dyspnea, weakness, lightheadedness, nausea, diaphoresis, altered mental status, and syncope.
- Angina typically lasts 3 to 5 minutes but usually does not last more than 30 minutes.
- Women and diabetics may not present with classic symptoms, but may manifest more frequently with dyspnea or GI complaints.
- Elicited by physical exertion, emotional stress, cold exposure, consumption of heavy meal, smoking.
- Early coronary disease is asymptomatic.
- Stigmata of atherosclerosis may include xanthelasma, tendon xanthomata, and evidence of peripheral vascular disease such as claudication and diminished peripheral pulses.

ETIOLOGY

The development of atherosclerosis occurs over many yrs. The order of events has been well studied. Multiple factors contribute to the pathogenesis, including endothelial dysfunction, dyslipidemia, inflammatory conditions, and smoking. Under such conditions, cholesterol molecules, primarily low-density lipoprotein (LDL), adhere to the intima of the vessel walls and are taken into the intimal layers. LDL is then oxidized, causing cytokine release, which initiates adhesion molecule expression on endothelial layers. Monocytes are then recruited and pass across the endothelium, where they digest the LDL and become "foam cells." Smooth muscle cells then migrate from the media to the intima. This causes further smooth cell proliferation and fibrosis to occur. In later stages, calcification of the matrix also develops. This causes a relatively acellular fibrous capsule to surround a lipid-rich core. This "plaque" then causes narrowing of the vessel lumen, ultimately leading to symptoms related to ischemia.

Dx DIAGNOSIS

DIFFERENTIAL DIAGNOSIS OF ACUTE CHEST PAIN

- Cardiovascular causes
  1. Acute coronary syndrome
  2. Aortic dissection
  3. Pericarditis
  4. Coronary arterial vasospasm
- Pulmonary causes
  1. Pulmonary embolism
  2. Pneumonia
  3. Pleuritis
  4. Pneumothorax
- Gastrointestinal causes
  1. Esophageal spasm
  2. Esophagitis
  3. GERD
- Chest wall causes
  1. Rib fracture
  2. Sternoclavicular arthritis
  3. Herpes zoster
  4. Costochondritis
- Psychiatric causes
  1. Anxiety disorders

WORKUP

See Fig. 1. ACCF/HFA guidelines for stress testing and advanced imaging are summarized in Tables 1 to 3.

LABORATORY TESTS

- Focused metabolic studies to rule out noncardiac causes (BMP, liver function tests)
- Complete blood count can help rule out anemia-related chest discomfort.
- Fasting cholesterol panel is important in assessment of lipid-related risk factors.
- Hemoglobin A1c is important to follow glycemic control.
- High-sensitivity C-reactive protein.

IMAGING STUDIES

- Electrocardiography (ECG) is important for assessing for prior cardiac injury or ischemia.
- Exercise treadmill test (ETT) is the gold standard to assess physiologic cardiac stress response if the patient is able to exercise and has a normal baseline ECG.
- Stress tests combined with imaging is the next best option if ETT cannot be performed due to physical limitation or if baseline ECG is abnormal.
- Echocardiogram to assess left ventricular ejection fraction (LVEF) and the presence of wall motion abnormalities.
- Although not used in the acute setting, a coronary artery calcium (CAC) score can be used to improve CVD risk classification. The CAC is estimated from noncontrast CT (Fig. E2) images. Normal coronary arteries do not have plaques or calcium, and the normal score is 0. A CAC score of 300 or higher, or 75th percentile or higher for age, sex, and ethnicity is considered a high risk. According to the recent ACC/AHA guidelines, CAC is most appropriate among adults with an estimated 10-yr ASCVD risk <7.5% in whom questions remain about whether statin therapy is indicated. A CAC score >75th percentile for age, sex, and ethnicity is considered high risk and would justify revising a patient's risk upward.
- Those with high-risk features (Box 1) should undergo coronary angiography to assess coronary anatomy for revascularization.
- Cardiac computed tomography angiography is an emerging imaging modality that can be considered as an alternative to stress testing.
- Coronary angiography is useful for both diagnostic and therapeutic interventions if there is evidence of significant ischemia

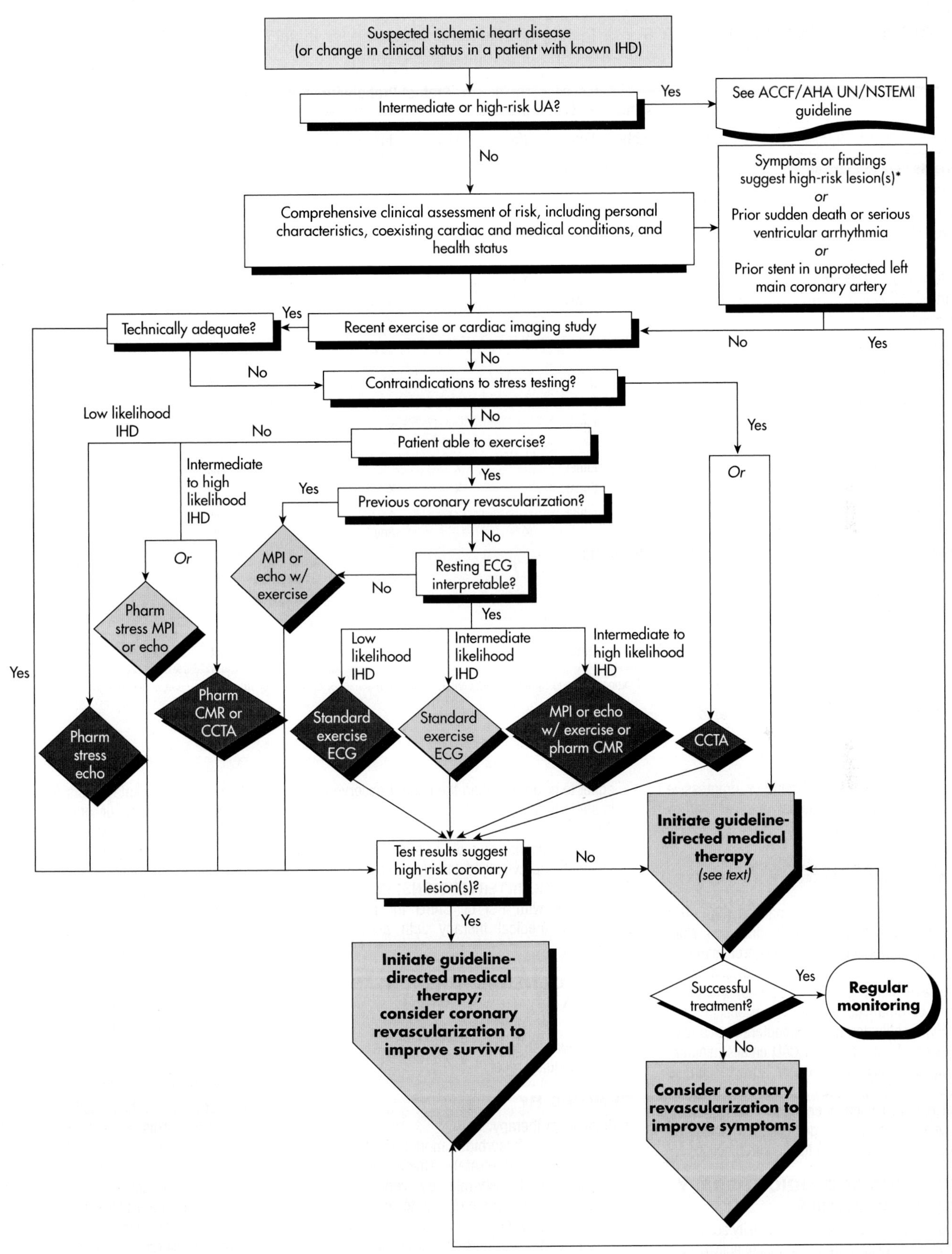

FIG. 1 Diagnosis of patients with suspected ischemic heart disease.
*CCTA is reasonable only for patients with intermediate probability of IHD. *CCTA,* Computed coronary tomography angiography; *CMR,* cardiac magnetic resonance; *ECG,* electrocardiogram; *Echo,* echocardiography; *IHD,* ischemic heart disease; *MI,* myocardial infarction; *MPI,* myocardial perfusion imaging; *Pharm,* pharmacologic; *UA,* unstable angina; *UA/NSTEMI,* unstable angina/non–ST-elevation myocardial infarction. (From 2012 ACCF/AHA/ACP/AATS/PCNA/SCAI/STS Guideline for the Diagnosis and Management of Patients With Stable Ischemic Heart Disease: A report of the American College of Cardiology Foundation/American Heart Association Task Force on Practice Guidelines, and the American College of Physicians, American Association for Thoracic Surgery, Preventive Cardiovascular Nurses Association, Society for Cardiovascular Angiography and Interventions, and Society of Thoracic Surgeons, *J Am Coll Cardiol* 60:e44-e164, 2012.)

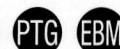

TABLE 1 ACCF/AHA Guidelines for Stress Testing and Advanced Imaging for Initial Diagnosis in Patients With Suspected Stable Ischemic Heart Disease Who Require Noninvasive Testing

Test	Exercise Status		ECG Interpretable		Pretest Probability of Ischemic Heart Disease			Recommendation	Level of Evidence
	Able	Unable	Yes	No	Low	Intermediate	High		
Patients Able to Exercise									
Exercise ECG	X		X			X		I	A
Exercise ECG with MPI or Echo	X			X		X	X	I	B
Exercise ECG	X		X		X			IIa	C
Exercise ECG with MPI or Echo	X		X			X	X	IIa	B
Pharmacologic stress CMR	X			X		X	X	IIa	B
CCTA	X		Either			X		IIb	B
Exercise Echo	X		X			X		IIb	C
Pharmacologic stress with nuclear MPI, Echo, or CMR	X		X			Any		III	C
Exercise stress with MPI	X		X		X			III	C
Patients Unable to Exercise									
Pharmacologic stress with nuclear MPI or Echo		X	Either			X	X	I	B
Pharmacologic stress Echo		X	Either		X			IIa	C
CCTA		X	Either		X	X		IIa	B
Pharmacologic stress CMR		X	Either			X	X	IIa	B
Exercise ECG		X		X		Any		III	C
Other Reasons for Cardiac Computed Tomography Angiography									
Continued symptoms after normal test resultsInconclusive stress test results Unable to undergo stress test	Either		Either			X		IIa	C
CAC	Either		Either		X			IIb	C

CAC, Coronary artery calcium (imaging); *CCTA,* coronary computed tomography angiography; *CMR,* cardiac magnetic resonance; *ECG,* electrocardiography; *Echo,* echocardiography; *MPI,* myocardial perfusion imaging.
From Mann DL et al: *Braunwald's heart disease,* ed 10, Philadelphia, 2015, Elsevier.

by noninvasive assessment or progressive symptoms despite optimal medical therapy (as in the following).

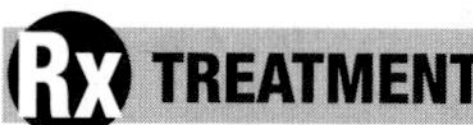 TREATMENT

- See Fig. 3. Table 4 summarizes ACCF/AHA guidelines for risk factor modification. Note that hypertension and cholesterol management guidelines have been revised since release of these CAD guidelines, and these are summarized in the "Hypertension" and "Hypercholesterolemia" chapters in this text.
- Successful treatment of CAD entails minimizing the likelihood of major adverse cardiac events (MACE), which include death, myocardial infarction, need for emergent coronary artery bypass grafting, or target lesion revascularization, while maximizing health and function.

NONPHARMACOLOGIC THERAPY

LIFESTYLE MODIFICATION:

- ≥150 min/wk of moderate-intensity activity or ≥75 min/wk of vigorous-intensity activity or a combination thereof (for adults) as 1 of the 7 components of ideal cardiovascular health.
- Mediterranean diet with a focus on vegetables, fruit, fish, whole grains, and olive oil has proven to reduce cardiovascular events to a degree greater than low-fat diets and equal to or greater than the benefit observed in statin trials.
- Smoking cessation.
- Weight reduction can reduce various risk factors with improved lipid and glycemic control.

THERAPEUTIC INTERVENTIONS: Coronary angiography with PCI or CABG for patients on optimal medical therapy with persistent symptoms.

ACUTE GENERAL Rx FOR STABLE ANGINA

- Rest.
- Sublingual nitroglycerin if rest does not provide adequate relief.

CHRONIC Rx

- Antianginal therapy:
  1. Nitrates (isosorbide mononitrate and isosorbide dinitrate). These medications treat ischemia by venodilation to decrease preload, dilate epicardial coronary arteries, and recruit coronary collaterals. Furthermore, they attenuate platelet aggregation. Although they do not influence survival or decrease cardiovascular death in patients with chronic CAD, they do lower the rate of angina frequency and increase time to ischemic ECG findings on treadmill testing.
  2. Beta-adrenergic antagonists (metoprolol, atenolol, carvedilol, or any other beta-blockers with the exception of those with intrinsic sympathomimetic activity). These medications work to relieve angina by decreasing myocardial oxygen demand by reducing heart rate, blood pressure, and contractility. Drugs should be titrated to a heart rate of 50 to 60 beats/min at rest and ≤100 beats/min with exercise
  3. Calcium channel blockers (CCBs; amlodipine or verapamil). The antianginal efficacy of CCBs is comparable to beta-blockers; however, the efficacy of monotherapy for reducing MI or cardiac death has not been demonstrated.
  4. Ranolazine. This is a selective inhibitor of late sodium influx into myocytes, which leads to decreased myocardial contractility. It can be used in combination with beta-blockers and significantly reduces frequency of angina and increases exercise duration and time to onset of angina (CARISA trial). Although it rarely may cause QT prolongation, it has not been linked to any clinically important arrhythmias.
  5. May benefit from combination therapy of the above.

TABLE 2 ACCF/AHA Guidelines for Stress Testing and Advanced Imaging for Patients With Known Stable Ischemic Heart Disease Who Require Noninvasive Testing for Risk Assessment

Test	Exercise Status		ECG Interpretable		Additional Considerations	Recommendation	Level of Evidence
	Able	Unable	Yes	No			
Patients Able to Exercise							
Exercise ECG	X		X			I	B
Exercise ECG with MPI or Echo	X			X	Abnormalities other than LBBB or ventricular pacing	I	B
Exercise ECG with MPI or Echo	X		X			IIa	B
Pharmacologic stress CMR	X			X		IIa	B
CCTA	X			X		IIb	B
Pharmacologic stress imaging or CCTA	X		X			III	C
Patients Unable to Exercise							
Pharmacologic stress with nuclear MPI or Echo		X	Either			I	B
Pharmacologic stress CMR		X	Either			IIa	B
CCTA		X	Either		Without previous stress test	IIa	C
Regardless of Ability to Exercise							
Pharmacologic stress with nuclear MPI or Echo	Either			X	LBBB present	I	B
Exercise or pharmacologic stress with nuclear MPI, Echo, or CMR	Either		Either		Known coronary stenosis being considered for revascularization	I	B
CCTA	Either		Either		Indeterminate result of functional testing	IIa	C
	Either		Either		Unable to undergo stress imaging	IIb	C
	Either		Either		Alternative to invasive coronary angiography when functional testing indicates moderate to high risk	IIb	C
Multiple stress tests or cardiac imaging at the same time	Either		Either			III	

CMR, Cardiac magnetic resonance; *ECG,* electrocardiography; *Echo,* echocardiography.
From Mann DL et al: *Braunwald's heart disease*, ed 10, Philadelphia, 2015, Elsevier.

TABLE 3 ACCF/AHA Guidelines for Coronary Angiography to Assess Risk in Patients With Known or Suspected Stable Ischemic Heart Disease

Class	Indication	Level of Evidence
I (indicated)	1. Patients with SIHD who have survived sudden cardiac death or potentially life-threatening ventricular arrhythmia should undergo coronary angiography to assess cardiac risk.	B
	2. Patients with SIHD in whom symptoms and signs of heart failure develop should be evaluated to determine whether coronary angiography should be performed for risk assessment.	B
	3. Coronary arteriography is recommended for patients with SIHD whose clinical characteristics and results of noninvasive testing indicate a high likelihood of severe IHD and when the benefits are deemed to exceed risk.	C
IIa (good supportive evidence)	1. Coronary angiography is reasonable to further assess risk in patients with SIHD who have depressed LV function (EF <50%) and moderate-risk criteria on noninvasive testing with demonstrable ischemia.	C
	2. Coronary angiography is reasonable to further assess risk in patients with SIHD and inconclusive prognostic information after noninvasive testing or in patients for whom noninvasive testing is contraindicated or inadequate.	C
	3. Coronary angiography for risk assessment is reasonable for patients with SIHD who have unsatisfactory quality of life because of angina, have preserved LV function (EF >50%), and have intermediate-risk criteria on noninvasive testing.	C
III (no benefit)	1. Coronary angiography for risk assessment is not recommended in patients with SIHD who elect not to undergo revascularization or who are not candidates for revascularization because of comorbid conditions or individual preferences.	B
	2. Coronary angiography is not recommended to further assess risk in patients with SIHD who have preserved LV function (EF >50%) and low-risk criteria on noninvasive testing.	B
	3. Coronary angiography is not recommended to assess risk in patients who are at low risk according to clinical criteria and who have not undergone noninvasive risk testing.	C
	4. Coronary angiography is not recommended to assess risk in asymptomatic patients with no evidence of ischemia on noninvasive testing.	C

EF, Ejection fraction.
From Mann DL et al: *Braunwald's heart disease*, ed 10, Philadelphia, 2015, Elsevier.

BOX 1 Noninvasive Risk Stratification

High risk (>3% annual mortality rate)

1. Severe resting left ventricular dysfunction (LVEF <35%).
2. High-risk treadmill score (≤−11).
3. Severe exercise left ventricular dysfunction (exercise LVEF <35%).
4. Stress-induced large perfusion defect (particularly if anterior).
5. Stress-induced multiple perfusion defects of moderate size.
6. Large, fixed perfusion defect with LV dilation or increased lung uptake (thallium-201).
7. Stress-induced moderate perfusion defect with LV dilation or increased lung uptake (thallium-201).
8. Echocardiographic wall motion abnormality (involving >2 segments) developing at low dose of dobutamine (≤10 mg/kg/min) or at a low heart rate (<120 beats/min).
9. Stress echocardiographic evidence of extensive ischemia.

Intermediate risk (1% to 3% annual mortality rate)

1. Mild/moderate resting left ventricular dysfunction (LVEF 35% to 49%).
2. Intermediate-risk treadmill score (score between −11 and <5).
3. Stress-induced moderate perfusion defect without LV dilation or increased lung intake (thallium-201).
4. Limited stress echocardiographic ischemia with a wall motion abnormality only at doses of dobutamine involving ≤2 segments.

Low risk (<1% annual mortality rate)

1. Low-risk treadmill score (≥5).
2. Normal or small myocardial perfusion defect at rest or with stress.
3. Normal stress echocardiographic wall motion or no change of limited resting wall motion abnormalities during stress.

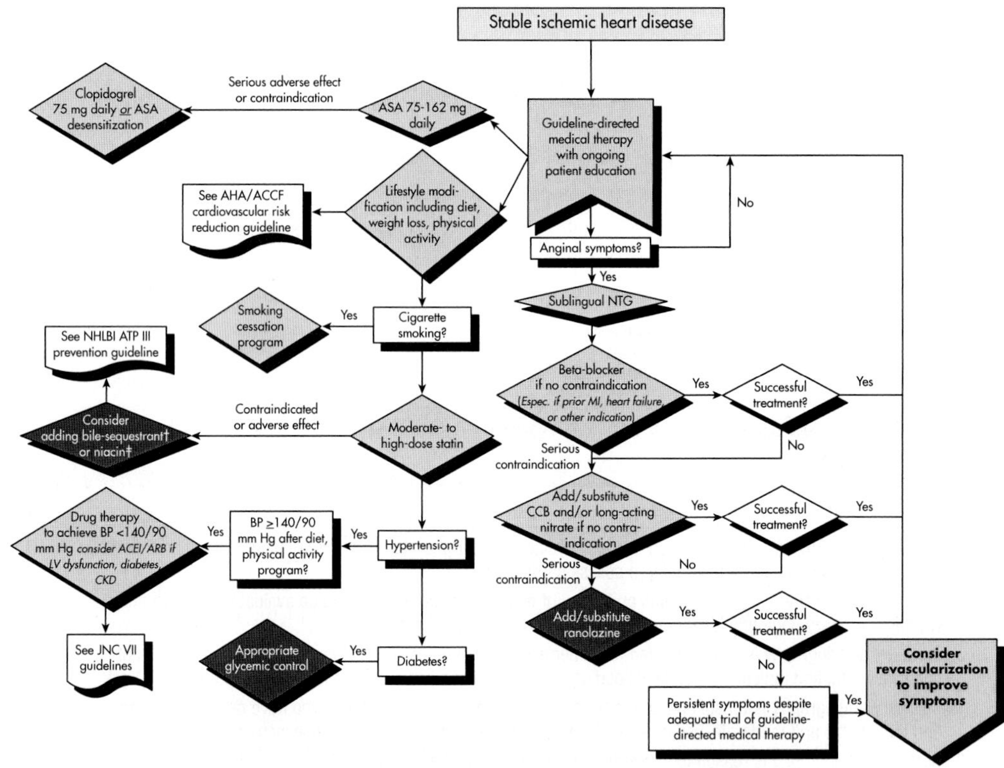

FIG. 3 Algorithm for guideline-directed medical therapy for patients with SIHD.*

*The algorithms do not represent a comprehensive list of recommendations (see text for all recommendations). †The use of bile acid sequestrant is relatively contraindicated when triglycerides are ≥200 mg/dl and is contraindicated when triglycerides are ≥500 mg/dl. ‡Dietary supplement niacin must not be used as a substitute for prescription niacin. *ACCF,* American College of Cardiology Foundation; *ACEI,* angiotensin-converting enzyme inhibitor; *AHA,* American Heart Association; *ARB,* angiotensin-receptor blocker; *ASA,* aspirin; *ATP III,* Adult Treatment Panel 3; *BP,* blood pressure; *CCB,* calcium channel blocker; *CKD,* chronic kidney disease; *HDL-C,* high-density lipoprotein cholesterol; *JNC VII,* Seventh Report of the Joint National Committee on Prevention, Detection, Evaluation, and Treatment of High Blood Pressure; *LDL-C,* low-density lipoprotein cholesterol; *LV,* left ventricular; *MI,* myocardial infarction; *NHLBI,* National Heart, Lung, and Blood Institute; *NTG,* nitroglycerin. (From 2012 ACCF/AHA/ACP/AATS/PCNA/SCAI/STS Guideline for the Diagnosis and Management of Patients With Stable Ischemic Heart Disease: A report of the American College of Cardiology Foundation/American Heart Association Task Force on Practice Guidelines, and the American College of Physicians, American Association for Thoracic Surgery, Preventive Cardiovascular Nurses Association, Society for Cardiovascular Angiography and Interventions, and Society of Thoracic Surgeons, *J Am Coll Cardiol* 60:e44-e164, 2012.)

TABLE 4 ACCF/AHA Guidelines for Risk Factor Modification

Class	Indication	Level of Evidence
Lipid Management		
I (indicated)	1. Lifestyle modifications, including daily physical activity and weight management, are strongly recommended for all patients with SIHD.	B
	2. Dietary therapy for all patients should include reduced intake of saturated fats (to <7% of total calories), trans fatty acids (to <1% of total calories), and cholesterol (to <200 mg/day).	B
	3. In addition to therapeutic lifestyle changes, a moderate or high dose of a statin should be prescribed in the absence of contraindications or documented adverse effects.	A
IIa (good supportive evidence)	For patients who do not tolerate statins, LDL cholesterol–lowering therapy with bile acid sequestrants, niacin, or both is reasonable.	B
Blood Pressure Management		
I (indicated)	1. All patients should be counseled about the need for lifestyle modification: weight control; increased physical activity; alcohol moderation; sodium reduction; and emphasis on increased consumption of fresh fruits, vegetables, and low-fat dairy products.	B
	2. In patients with SIHD and a BP of 140/90 mm Hg or higher, antihypertensive drug therapy should be instituted in addition to or after a trial of lifestyle modifications.	A
	3. The specific medications used for the treatment of high BP should be based on specific patient characteristics and may include ACE inhibitors and/or beta-blocking agents, as well as the addition of other drugs such as thiazide diuretics or calcium channel blocking agents if needed to achieve a goal BP of less than 140/90 mm Hg.	B
Diabetes Management		
IIa (good supportive evidence)	1. For selected individual patients, such as those with a short duration of diabetes mellitus and a long life expectancy, a goal hemoglobin A1c (HbA1c) of 7% or less is reasonable.	B
	2. A goal HbA1c between 7% and 9% is reasonable for certain patients according to age, history of hypoglycemia, presence of microvascular or macrovascular complications, or presence of coexisting medical conditions.	C
IIb (weak supportive evidence)	Initiation of pharmacotherapy interventions to achieve a target HbA1c might be reasonable.	A
III (not indicated)	Therapy with rosiglitazone should not be initiated in patients with SIHD.	C
Physical Activity		
I (indicated)	1. For all patients, clinicians should encourage 30 to 60 minutes of moderate-intensity aerobic activity at least 5 days and preferably 7 days per week, supplemented by an increase in daily lifestyle activities (e.g., walking breaks at work, gardening, household work) to improve cardiorespiratory fitness and move patients out of the least-fit, least-active, high-risk cohort (bottom 20%).	B
	2. For all patients, risk assessment with a physical activity history and/or an exercise test is recommended to guide prognosis and prescription.	B
	3. Medically supervised programs (cardiac rehabilitation) and physician-directed, home-based programs are recommended for at-risk patients at first diagnosis.	A
IIa (good supportive evidence)	It is reasonable for clinicians to recommend complementary resistance training at least 2 days per week.	C
Weight Management		
I (indicated)	1. BMI and/or waist circumference should be assessed at every visit, and clinicians should consistently encourage weight maintenance or reduction through an appropriate balance of lifestyle physical activity, structured exercise, caloric intake, and formal behavioral programs when indicated to maintain or achieve a BMI of between 18.5 and 24.9 kg/m^2 and a waist circumference of less than 102 cm (40 inches) in men and less than 88 cm (35 inches) in women (less for certain racial groups)	B
	2. The initial goal of weight loss therapy should be to reduce body weight by approximately 5% to 10% from baseline. With success, further weight loss can be attempted if indicated.	C
Smoking Cessation		
I (indicated)	Smoking cessation and avoidance of exposure to environmental tobacco smoke at work and home should be encouraged for all patients with SIHD. Follow-up, referral to special programs, and pharmacotherapy are recommended, as is a stepwise strategy for smoking cessation (Ask, Advise, Assess, Assist, Arrange, Avoid).	B
Management of Psychological Factors		
IIa (good supportive evidence)	It is reasonable to consider screening patients with SIHD for depression and to refer or treat when indicated.	B
IIb (weak supportive evidence)	Treatment of depression has not been shown to improve cardiovascular disease outcomes but might be reasonable for its other clinical benefits.	C
Alcohol Consumption		
IIb (weak supportive evidence)	In patients with SIHD who drink alcohol, it might be reasonable for nonpregnant women to have 1 drink (4 oz of wine, 12 oz of beer, or 1 oz of spirits) a day and for men to have 1 or 2 drinks a day unless alcohol is contraindicated (such as in patients with a history of alcohol abuse or dependence or those with liver disease).	C
Exposure to Air Pollution		
IIa (good supportive evidence)	It is reasonable for patients with SIHD to avoid exposure to increased air pollution to reduce their risk for cardiovascular events.	C

BMI, Body mass index.
From Mann DL et al: *Braunwald's heart disease*, ed 10, Philadelphia, 2015, Elsevier.

- Antiplatelet therapy:
  1. Aspirin therapy (81-162 mg/day).
  2. Clopidogrel for those intolerant to aspirin therapy.
  3. Combination of aspirin and clopidogrel does not reduce cardiovascular events in stable CAD (CHARISMA trial).
  4. Newer antiplatelet drugs such as prasugrel and ticagrelor have been studied in ACS but not in stable CAD.
- Statins:
  1. HMG-CoA reductase inhibitors (Statins) (atorvastatin, rosuvastatin) with high-intensity therapy for a target LDL reduction of >50% if safely achieved in high-risk patients; if not a candidate for high-intensity therapy, patient should receive at least moderate-intensity statin therapy that lowers LDL by 30% to 50% as advised by the ATP IV cholesterol guidelines from the 2013 ACC/AHA expert panel.
- PCSK9 inhibitors:
  1. This is a novel class of monoclonal antibodies that inhibit proprotein convertase subtilisin/kexin type 9. In the OSLER trial, PCSK9 inhibition in addition to standard therapy reduced LDL cholesterol by 61%. The rate of cardiovascular events at 1 yr reduced to 0.98% with therapy versus 2.18% in the standard therapy group. In the FOURIER trial, in patients with LDL >70 despite being on high- or moderate-intensity statin therapy, the addition of evolocumab resulted in 1.5% absolute reduction in major adverse cardiovascular events. However, there was no overall or cardiovascular-specific mortality benefit.

TABLE 5 ACCF/AHA Guidelines for Revascularization to Improve Survival Versus Medical Therapy in Patients With Stable Ischemic Heart Disease

Anatomic Setting	Class	Recommendation	Level of Evidence
Unprotected Left Main or Complex Coronary Artery Disease			
CABG and PCI	I	Heart team approach	C
CABG and PCI	IIa	Calculation of STS and SYNTAX Scores	B
Unprotected Left Main			
CABG	I		B
PCI	IIa	For SIHD when both of the following are present: 1. Anatomic conditions associated with a low risk for PCI procedural complications and a high likelihood of a good long-term outcome 2. Clinical characteristics that predict a significantly increased risk for adverse surgical outcomes	B
	IIb	For SIHD when both of the following are present: 1. Anatomic conditions associated with a low to intermediate risk for PCI procedural complications and an intermediate to high likelihood of a good long-term outcome 2. Clinical characteristics that predict increased risk for adverse surgical outcomes (e.g. STS-predicted operative mortality >2%)	B
	III	For SIHD in patients (versus performing CABG) with unfavorable anatomy for PCI and who are good candidates for CABG	B
Three-Vessel Coronary Artery Disease with or without Proximal Left Anterior Descending Coronary Artery Disease			
CABG	I		B
	IIa	It is reasonable to choose CABG over PCI in patients with complex 3-vessel CAD (e.g., SYNTAX score ≥22) who are good candidates for CABG	B
PCI	IIb		B
Two-Vessel Coronary Artery Disease with Proximal Left Anterior Descending Coronary Artery Disease			
CABG	I		B
PCI	IIb		B
Two-Vessel Coronary Artery Disease without Proximal Left Anterior Descending Coronary Artery Disease			
CABG	IIa	With extensive ischemia	B
	IIb	Without extensive ischemia	C
PCI	IIb		B
One-Vessel Proximal Left Anterior Descending Coronary Artery Disease			
CABG	IIa	With LIMA	B
PCI	IIb		B
One-Vessel Coronary Artery Disease without Proximal Left Anterior Descending Coronary Artery Disease			
CABG	III	Harm	B
PCI	III	Harm	B
Left Ventricular Dysfunction			
CABG	IIa	EF of 35% to 50%	B
CABG	IIb	EF <35% without significant left main disease	B
PCI	N/A	Insufficient data	
Survivors of Sudden Cardiac Death with Presumed Ischemia-Mediated Ventricular Tachycardia			
CABG	I		B
PCI	I		C
No Anatomic or Physiologic Criteria for Revascularization			
CABG	III	Harm	B
PCI	III	Harm	B

EF, Ejection fraction; *LIMA,* left internal mammary artery; *N/A,* not applicable; *SYNTAX,* synergy between PCI with taxus and cardiac surgery.
From Mann DL et al: *Braunwald's heart disease*, ed 10, Philadelphia, 2015, Elsevier.

TABLE 6 ACCF/AHA Guidelines for Revascularization to Improve Symptoms in Patients With Significant Anatomic (>50% Left Main or >70% Non–Left Main Coronary Artery Disease) or Physiologic (Fractional Flow Reserve <0.80) Coronary Artery Stenoses

Clinical Setting	Recommendation		Level of Evidence
≥1 significant stenosis amenable to revascularization and unacceptable angina despite GDMT	I	CABG or PCI	A
≥1 significant stenoses and unacceptable angina in whom GDMT cannot be implemented because of medication contraindications, adverse effects, or patient preferences	IIa	CABG or PCI	C
Previous CABG with ≥1 significant stenosis associated with ischemia and unacceptable angina despite GDMT	IIa	PCI	C
	IIb	CABG	C
Complex 3-vessel CAD (e.g., SYNTAX score ≥22) with or without involvement of the proximal LAD artery and a good candidate for CABG	IIa	CABG preferred over PCI	B
Viable ischemic myocardium that is perfused by coronary arteries that are not amenable to grafting	IIb	TMR as an adjunct to CABG	B
No anatomic or physiologic criteria for revascularization	III	CABG or PCI	C

SYNTAX, Synergy between PCI with taxus and cardiac surgery; *TMR,* transmyocardial revascularization.
From Mann DL et al: *Braunwald's heart disease,* ed 10, Philadelphia, 2015, Elsevier.

TABLE 7 ACC/AHA Guidelines for Follow-Up Noninvasive Testing in Patients With Known Stable Ischemic Heart Disease: New, Recurrent, or Worsening Symptoms (Not Consistent With Unstable Angina)

	Exercise Status		ECG Interpretable				
Test	**Able**	**Unable**	**Yes**	**No**	**Additional Considerations**	**Recommendation**	**Level of Evidence**
Patients Able to Exercise							
Exercise ECG	X		X			I	B
Exercise ECG with MPI or Echo	X			X		I	B
Exercise ECG with MPI or echo	X		Either		Previous requirement for imaging or known to be at high risk for multivessel CAD	IIa	B
Pharmacologic stress MPI, Echo, or CMR	X		X			III	C
Patients Unable to Exercise							
Pharmacologic stress with nuclear MPI or Echo		X	Either			I	B
Pharmacologic stress CMR		X	Either			IIa	B
Exercise ECG		X		X		III	C
Regardless of Ability to Exercise							
CCTA	Either		Either		To assess patency of coronary stent or bypass graft ≥3 mm in diameter	IIb	C
	Either		Either		In absence of known moderate or severe calcification and to assess coronary stent <3 mm in diameter	IIb	C
	Either		Either		Known moderate or severe calcification or assessment of stent <3 mm in diameter	III	C

CMR, Cardiac magnetic resonance; *ECG,* electrocardiography; *Echo,* echocardiography.
From Mann DL et al: *Braunwald's heart disease,* ed 10, Philadelphia, 2015, Elsevier.

- ACE-inhibitors (captopril, enalapril, lisinopril) are a class I recommendation for patients with chronic CAD with LV dysfunction LVEF <40% or diabetes and a class II recommendation for CAD patients without these features.

CORONARY ARTERY REVASCULARIZATION

- Patients with symptoms refractory to optimal medical therapy (OMT) as above or those with high clinical, stress testing, or an angiographic risk profile and suitable coronary anatomy may benefit from revascularization with either PCI (percutaneous coronary intervention) or CABG (coronary artery bypass graft) surgery. ACCF/AHA guidelines for revascularization are summarized in Tables 5 and 6.
- ACC/AHA class I indications for CABG surgery in chronic CAD patients include the following:
  1. High grade (>50%) left main CAD
  2. Left main CAD-equivalent anatomy including >70% luminal stenosis in the left anterior descending artery and left circumflex arteries
  3. Three-vessel disease with LVEF <50%
  4. Single- or two-vessel CAD with a large area of viable myocardium at risk
  5. Severe angina despite medical therapy if CABG can be performed with acceptable risk
- PCI has not been shown to reduce long-term rates of MI and death in patients with stable chronic CAD and therefore has no class I indications in this group. PCI is suitable in patients with suitable anatomy with refractory or lifestyle-limiting angina who have failed optimal medical therapy (OMT). Recent trials such as the COURAGE Trial have demonstrated no significant difference between OMT and PCI in overall survival, MI, and ACS over 5 yr in patients with chronic stable CAD. A recent meta-analysis

TABLE 8 ACC/AHA Guidelines for Follow-Up Noninvasive Testing in Patients With Known Stable Ischemic Heart Disease: Asymptomatic or Stable Symptoms

Test	Exercise Status		ECG Interpretable		Pretest Probability of Ischemia	Additional Considerations	Recommendation	Level of Evidence
	Able	Unable	Yes	No				
Exercise or pharmacologic stress with MPI, Echo, or CMR at ≥2-yr intervals		X		X	Previous evidence of silent ischemia or at high risk for recurrent event	Unable to exercise, uninterpretable ECG, or incomplete revascularization	IIa	C
Exercise ECG at ≥1-yr intervals	X		X		Previous silent ischemia or at high risk for recurrent event		IIb	C
Exercise ECG	X		X		No previous silent ischemia and not at high risk for recurrent events		IIb	C
Exercise or pharmacologic stress imaging or CCTA	Either		Either			<5-yr intervals after CABG or <2 yr intervals after PCI	III	C

ECG, Electrocardiography; *CMR,* cardiac magnetic resonance; *Echo,* echocardiography.
From Mann DL et al: *Braunwald's heart disease*, ed 10, Philadelphia, 2015, Elsevier.

demonstrated no objective reduction in death, nonfatal MI, unplanned revascularization, or angina versus medical therapy alone.

- The SYNTAX trial, which used a numerical score based on qualitative plaque features on angiography, showed that surgical revascularization was associated with a lesser risk of stroke and major cardiac events if the SYNTAX score was high (>33).
- The FREEDOM trial showed that in diabetic patients with multivessel disease, CABG is superior to PCI with drug-eluting stents in chronic CAD and should remain the revascularization strategy of choice in this patient population. CABG resulted in lower rates of death and MI but a higher risk of stroke. This is true for patients with either insulin-dependent or non–insulin-dependent DM.

DISPOSITION

CAD is a common chronic condition with which many patients can live for yrs with good symptom control on optimal medical therapy.

REFERRAL

Cardiovascular disease specialist

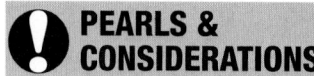

PEARLS & CONSIDERATIONS

COMMENTS

- The transition from stable CAD to unstable angina must be carefully monitored. Symptoms of concern include more frequent episodes of chest pain, exertional dyspnea, chest pain that is less responsive to nitroglycerin, or first episode of chest pain. Regarding unstable angina, please refer to section on acute coronary syndromes.
- ACC/AHA guidelines for follow-up non-invasive testing are summarized in Tables 7 and 8.

EVIDENCE-BASED MEDICINE

Available at ExpertConsult.com

SUGGESTED READINGS

Available at ExpertConsult.com

RELATED CONTENT

Coronary Artery Disease (Patient Information)
Acute Coronary Syndrome (Related Key Topic)
Angina Pectoris (Related Key Topic)
Hypercholesterolemia (Related Key Topic)
Hyperlipoproteinemia, Primary (Related Key Topic)
Myocardial Infarction (Related Key Topic)

AUTHOR: **NATHAN RIDDELL, M.D.**

BASIC INFORMATION

DEFINITION

Crohn disease (CD) is an inflammatory disease of the bowel of unknown etiology, most commonly involving the terminal ileum and manifesting primarily with diarrhea, abdominal pain, fatigue, and weight loss.

SYNONYMS

CD
Regional enteritis
Inflammatory bowel disease (IBD)

ICD-10CM CODES

K50.00	Crohn disease of small intestine without complications
K50.011	Crohn disease of small intestine with rectal bleeding
K50.012	Crohn disease of small intestine with intestinal obstruction
K50.013	Crohn disease of small intestine with fistula
K50.014	Crohn disease of small intestine with abscess
K50.018	Crohn disease of small intestine with other complication
K50.019	Crohn disease of small intestine with unspecified complications
K50.10	Crohn disease of large intestine without complications
K50.111	Crohn disease of large intestine with rectal bleeding
K50.112	Crohn disease of large intestine with intestinal obstruction
K50.113	Crohn disease of large intestine with fistula
K50.114	Crohn disease of large intestine with abscess
K50.118	Crohn disease of large intestine with other complication
K50.119	Crohn disease of large intestine with unspecified complications
K50.80	Crohn disease of both small and large intestine without complications
K50.811	Crohn disease of both small and large intestine with rectal bleeding
K50.812	Crohn disease of both small and large intestine with intestinal obstruction
K50.813	Crohn disease of both small and large intestine with fistula
K50.814	Crohn disease of both small and large intestine with abscess
K50.818	Crohn disease of both small and large intestine with other complication
K50.819	Crohn disease of both small and large intestine with unspecified complications
K50.90	Crohn disease, unspecified, without complications
K50.911	Crohn disease, unspecified, with rectal bleeding
K50.912	Crohn disease, unspecified, with intestinal obstruction
K50.913	Crohn disease, unspecified, with fistula
K50.914	Crohn disease, unspecified, with abscess
K50.918	Crohn disease, unspecified, with other complication
K50.919	Crohn disease, unspecified, with unspecified complications

EPIDEMIOLOGY & DEMOGRAPHICS

PREVALENCE:

- Annual incidence ranges from 3 to 20 cases per 100,000.
- Median age of onset is 30 yr.
- Crohn disease has 2 peaks, the first between age 20 and 30 yr and the second a smaller peak around 50 yr.

PHYSICAL FINDINGS & CLINICAL PRESENTATION

- Physical exam findings vary depending on disease location and severity
- Abdominal tenderness, mass, or distention
- Chronic or nocturnal diarrhea
- Weight loss, fever, night sweats
- Hyperactive bowel sounds in patients with partial obstruction, bloody diarrhea
- Delayed growth and failure of normal development in children
- Perianal and rectal abscesses, multiple sinuses and scarring (Fig. E1), mouth ulcers, cobblestone appearance of oral mucosa (Fig. E2), and atrophic glossitis
- Extraintestinal manifestations (Table E1): Joint swelling and tenderness, hepatosplenomegaly, erythema nodosum, clubbing, tenderness to palpation of the sacroiliac joints
- Symptoms may be intermittent, with varying periods of remission
- Overall 45% to 50% of patients have ileocolonic inflammation, 30% have isolated small bowel disease, 20% have isolated colonic disease, and 5% have isolated upper GI or perianal manifestations

ETIOLOGY

Unknown. Pathophysiologically, Crohn disease involves an immune system dysfunction.

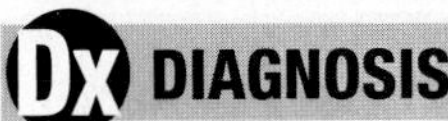

DIAGNOSIS

DIFFERENTIAL DIAGNOSIS

- Ulcerative colitis (see Table 2)
- Infectious diseases (tuberculosis, *Yersinia, Salmonella, Shigella, Campylobacter*)
- Parasitic infections (amebic infection)
- Pseudomembranous colitis
- Ischemic colitis in elderly patients
- Lymphoma
- Colon carcinoma
- Diverticulitis
- Radiation enteritis
- Collagenous colitis
- Fungal infections (*Histoplasma, Actinomyces*)
- Gay bowel syndrome (in homosexual patient)
- Carcinoid tumors
- Celiac sprue
- Mesenteric adenitis

LABORATORY TESTS

- Decreased hemoglobin and hematocrit from chronic blood loss, effect of inflammation on bone marrow, and malabsorption of vitamin B_{12}
- Hypokalemia, hypomagnesemia, hypocalcemia, and low albumin in patients with chronic diarrhea
- Vitamin B_{12} and folate deficiency
- Elevated erythrocyte sedimentation rate and CRP
- Positive anti–*Saccharomyces cerevisiae* antibodies
- Elevated INR (due to vitamin K malabsorption)
- Fecal calprotectin has been reported as useful in screening of patients with suspected IBD. Based on a pretest probability of 32% in adults, an abnormal calprotectin test result increases the posttest probability to 91%, and a normal result reduces the probability of IBD to 3%. False elevations may occur with other gastrointestinal diseases such as bacterial, viral, and protozoal causes of infective diarrhea

TABLE 2 Differentiating Features

	Ulcerative Colitis	Crohn Disease
Site of involvement	Only involves colon Rectum almost always involved	Any area of the gastrointestinal tract Rectum usually spared
Pattern of involvement	Continuous	Skip lesions
Diarrhea	Bloody	Usually nonbloody
Severe abdominal pain	Rare	Frequent
Perianal disease	No	In 30% of patients
Fistula	No	Yes
Endoscopic findings	Erythematous and friable Superficial ulceration	Aphthoid and deep ulcers Cobblestoning
Radiologic findings	Tubular appearance resulting from loss of haustral folds	String sign of terminal ileum RLQ mass, fistulas, abscesses
Histologic features	Mucosa only Crypt abscesses	Transmural crypt abscesses, granulomas (about 30%)
Smoking	Protective	Worsens course
Serology	p-ANCA more common	ASCA more common

ASCA, Anti–*Saccharomyces cerevisiae* antibodies; *p-ANCA,* perinuclear antineutrophil cytoplasmic antibody; *RLQ,* right lower quadrant.
From Andreoli TE et al: *Andreoli and Carpenter's Cecil essentials of medicine,* ed 8, Philadelphia, 2010, Saunders.

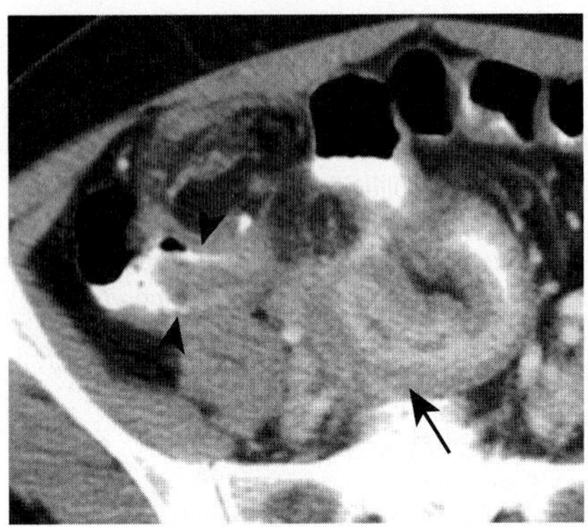

FIG. 4 Crohn disease: fistulas. The ileum (*arrow*) in the right lower quadrant exhibits marked wall thickening and matting of bowel loops caused by inflammation of the mesentery. A double-tract bowel lumen (*arrowheads*) is seen, indicating the formation of an ileo–ileal fistula. (From Webb WR, Brant WE, Major NM: *Fundamentals of body CT*, ed 4, Philadelphia, 2015, Saunders.)

ENDOSCOPIC EVALUATION

Endoscopic features of Crohn disease include asymmetric and discontinued disease, deep longitudinal fissures, cobblestone appearance, and presence of strictures (Fig. E3). Crypt distortion and inflammation are also present. Granulomas may be present.

IMAGING STUDIES

- CT of abdomen may show thickening of the terminal ileum and is helpful in identifying abscesses, fistulas (Fig. 4), and other complications.
- Magnetic resonance enterography (MRe) is superior to other imaging modalities in its ability to distinguish active from chronic fibrotic disease. It is, however, more expensive.
- In 10% to 15% of patients with IBD, a clear distinction between ulcerative colitis and Crohn disease cannot be made. In general, Crohn disease can be distinguished from ulcerative colitis by the presence of transmural involvement and the frequent presence of noncaseating granulomas and lymphoid aggregates on biopsy.

Rx TREATMENT

The medical management of Crohn disease is based on disease activity. According to Hanauer and Sanborn, disease activity can be defined as follows:

- Mild to moderate disease: The patient is ambulatory and able to take oral alimentation. There is no dehydration, high fever, abdominal tenderness, painful mass, obstruction, or weight loss of >10%.
- Moderate to severe disease: Either the patient has not responded to treatment for mild to moderate disease or has more pronounced symptoms, including fever, significant weight loss, abdominal pain or tenderness, intermittent nausea and vomiting, or significant anemia.
- Severe fulminant disease: Either the patient has persistent symptoms despite outpatient steroid therapy or has high fever, persistent vomiting, evidence of intestinal obstruction, rebound tenderness, cachexia, or evidence of an abscess.
- Remission: The patient is asymptomatic or without inflammatory sequelae, including patients responding to acute medical intervention.

NONPHARMACOLOGIC THERAPY

- Nutritional supplementation is needed in patients with advanced disease. Total parenteral nutrition may be necessary in selected patients.
- Low-residue diet is necessary when obstructive symptoms are present.
- If diarrhea is prominent, increased dietary fiber and decreased fat in the diet are sometimes helpful.
- Psychotherapy is useful for situational adjustment crises. A trusting and mutually understanding relationship and referral to self-help groups are very important because of the chronicity of the disease and the relatively young age of the patients.
- Avoid oral feedings during acute exacerbation to decrease colonic activity: a low-roughage diet may be helpful in early relapse.

ACUTE GENERAL Rx

- Corticosteroids are used to induce remission. They have been the mainstay for treating moderate to severe active Crohn disease. Prednisone 40 to 60 mg/day is useful for acute exacerbation. Steroids are usually tapered over approximately 2 to 3 mo. Some patients require a low dose for a prolonged period of maintenance.
- Steroid analogues are locally active corticosteroids that target specific areas of inflammation in the gastrointestinal tract. Budesonide is available as a controlled-release formulation and is approved for mild to moderate active Crohn disease involving the ileum and/or ascending colon. The adult dose is 9 mg qd for a maximum of 8 wk.
- Patients responding to glucocorticoids are transitioned to immunomodulators as their glucocorticoid is tapered.
- Immunosuppressants such as azathioprine or mercaptopurine are used for maintenance of remission. Methotrexate is an alternative agent.
- Metronidazole 500 mg qid may be useful for colonic fistulas and treatment of mild to moderate active Crohn disease. Ciprofloxacin 1 g qd has also been found to be effective in decreasing disease activity.
- TNF inhibitors are agents useful to induce remission and maintain remission in patients with moderate to severe Crohn disease. Infliximab, a chimeric monoclonal antibody targeting tumor necrosis factor-α, is effective in the treatment of enterocutaneous fistulas. This medication can induce clinical improvement in 80% of patients with Crohn disease refractory to other agents. It can be used in combination with other medications such as azathioprine in patients with severe Crohn disease. A PPD test should be done before using this medication. Adalimumab and certolizumab are other TNF inhibitors also effective in inducing remissions and may be useful in adult patients with Crohn disease who cannot tolerate infliximab or have symptoms despite receiving infliximab therapy. Efficacy is better when an anti-TNF is used together with an immunomodulator.
- Natalizumab, a selective adhesion-molecule inhibitor, has been reported to be effective in increasing the rate of remission and response in patients with active Crohn disease. It is effective for patients in whom anti-TNF therapy has been unsuccessful. Prior to using natalizumab, serologic testing should be done for JC virus, which causes multifocal leukoencephalopathy (PML), and if the patient is seronegative, the risk of PML from natalizumab is low. Vedolizumab is another IV integrin receptor antagonist recently FDA approved for moderate to severe Crohn disease patients who have not responded to or cannot tolerate standard treatment. Vedolizumab use is not associated with high risk of PML. Ustekinumab, a monoclonal antibody to the P_40 subunit of interleukin-12 and interleukin-23, has shown efficacy for induction and maintenance therapy for Crohn disease. It has been FDA-approved for moderate to severely active Crohn disease unresponsive to immunomodulators or corticosteroids or a tumor necrosis factor inhibitor.
- Hydrocortisone enema bid or tid is useful for proctitis.
- Most patients who have anemia associated with Crohn disease respond to iron supplementation. Erythropoietin is useful in patients with anemia refractory to treatment with iron and vitamins.

CHRONIC Rx

- Monitor disease activity with symptom review and laboratory evaluation (complete blood count and sedimentation rate).
- Liver tests and vitamin B_{12} levels monitored on a yearly basis.

DISPOSITION

There is no cure for CD, and most patients require at least one surgical resection. One tenth of patients have prolonged remission, three quarters have a chronic intermittent disease course, and one eighth have an unremitting course. Patients with IBD are at increased risk of colon cancer.

REFERRAL

Surgical referral is needed for complications such as abscess formation, obstruction, fistulas, toxic megacolon, refractory disease, or severe hemorrhage. Approximately 40% to 50% of patients will require some type of bowel surgery within the first 5 yr of Crohn disease. A conservative surgical approach is necessary because surgery is not curative. Multiple surgeries may also result in short bowel syndrome.

SUGGESTED READINGS

Available at ExpertConsult.com

RELATED CONTENT

Crohn Disease (Patient Information)

AUTHOR: **FRED F. FERRI, M.D.**

BASIC INFORMATION

DEFINITION

Cryoglobulins are serum immunoglobulins that precipitate when cooled and redissolve when heated. A classification of cryoglobulins is described in Table 1 and Fig. 1. Cryoglobulinemia is a clinical syndrome that results from systemic inflammation caused by cryoglobulin-containing immune complexes. Mixed cryoglobulinemia is a vasculitis of small and medium-sized arteries and veins due to the deposition of complexes of antigen, cryoglobulin, and complement in the vessel walls.

SYNONYMS

Cryoglobulinemic vasculitis
Cryoproteinemia
Mixed cryoglobulinemia
Essential cryoglobulinemia

ICD-10CM CODES
D89.1 Cryoglobulinemia

EPIDEMIOLOGY & DEMOGRAPHICS

PREVALENCE:
- Prevalence of mixed cryoglobulinemia is approximately 1:100,000 and accounts for 85% to 90% of cryoglobulinemic vasculitis cases.
- Approximately 50% of patients with HCV are found to have mixed cryoglobulinemia; only 5% to 10% develop vasculitis.
- Three types: I (monoclonal), II (IgM monoclonal and IgG polyclonal), and III (polyclonal).

PREDOMINANT SEX AND AGE: Female-to-male ratio of 3:1

PREDOMINANT AGE: Mean age reported is 42 to 52 yr.

RISK FACTORS:
- HCV infection
- Connective tissue disorders
- Lymphoproliferative disorders

PHYSICAL FINDINGS & CLINICAL PRESENTATION

- *Meltzer triad* of purpura, arthralgias/myalgia, and weakness is seen in one third of patients.
- Other symptoms include dyspnea, cough, numbness, abdominal pain, acrocyanosis.
- Hypertension, hepatosplenomegaly, Raynaud's phenomenon, and in severe cases, distal necrosis, retiform purpura of lower extremities (Fig. 2), and ulcerations of lower limbs.

ETIOLOGY

- Intravascular deposition of cryoglobulins leading to ischemic insults in territory supplied by vasa nervorum
- Necrotizing vasculitis caused by cryoglobulin precipitation in cooler areas (distal extremities) and kidneys (increased concentration due to ultrafiltration)
- Infections: HCV, mycosis fungoides, HBV, HIV, Epstein-Barr virus, cytomegalovirus, *Treponema pallidum,* Mycobacterium leprae, and in post-streptococcal glomerulonephritis
- Lymphoproliferative disorders: Chronic lymphocytic leukemia, Waldenström's macroglobulinemia, multiple myeloma
- Connective tissue disorders: Rheumatoid arthritis, systemic lupus erythematosus (SLE), scleroderma, Sjögren's syndrome, vasculitis
- Renal diseases including proliferative glomerulonephritis

DIAGNOSIS

DIFFERENTIAL DIAGNOSIS

- Antiphospholipid syndrome
- SLE
- Churg-Strauss syndrome
- Cirrhosis
- Glomerulonephritis
- Goodpasture syndrome
- Hemolytic uremic syndrome
- Hepatitis
- Lymphoma
- Sarcoidosis
- Waldenström's hypergammaglobulinemia

WORKUP

History and physical examination; laboratory tests; imaging tests depending on patients' presentation.

LABORATORY TESTS

- Serum cryoglobulins, rheumatoid factor, serum complement, hepatitis C titer, urinalysis, CBC, ALT, AST, BUN, creatinine.
- Electromyogram/nerve conduction studies may demonstrate axonal changes and distal muscle denervation.
- Sural nerve and skin biopsy.

IMAGING STUDIES

Chest x-ray for pulmonary involvement, CT scan to evaluate for malignancy, and angiography for vasculitis

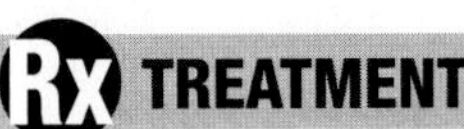

TREATMENT

- Management of type I cryoglobulinemia is directed at treating the underlying disorder.

TABLE 1 Classification of Cryoglobulins

Type	Composition	Associated Disease
I	Monoclonal IgG, IgA, or IgM	Multiple myeloma (IgG, IgM) Chronic lymphocytic leukemia Waldenstrom macroglobulinemia Idiopathic monoclonal gammopathy Lymphoproliferative disorders
II	Polyclonal IgG and monoclonal IgM (with rheumatoid factor activity)	Hepatitis C, hepatitis B, HIV Neoplasms: Chronic lymphocytic leukemia, diffuse lymphoma, B lymphocytic neoplasia
III	Polyclonal IgG and polyclonal IgM	Infections: Viral (hepatitis B and C, Epstein-Barr virus, cytomegalovirus), bacterial (endocarditis, leprosy, poststreptococcal glomerulonephritis), parasitic (schistosomiasis, toxoplasmosis, malaria) Autoimmune disorders: Systemic lupus erythematosus, rheumatoid arthritis Lymphoproliferative disorders Chronic liver disease

IgG, Immunoglobulin G; *IgA,* immunoglobulin A; *IgM,* immunoglobulin M.
From Floege J et al: *Comprehensive clinical nephrology,* ed 4, Philadelphia, 2010, Saunders.

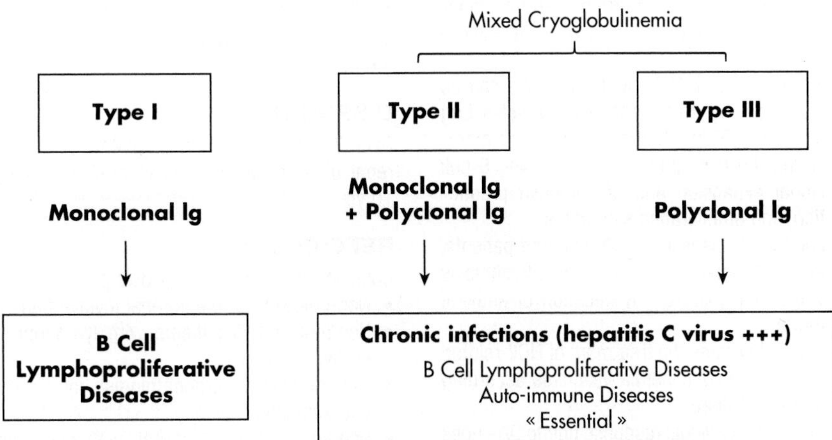

FIG. 1 Cryoglobulin immunotyping and related underlying diseases. *Ig,* Immunoglobulin. (From Cacoub P et al: Cryoglobulinemia vasculitis. *Am J Med* 128[9]:950–955.)

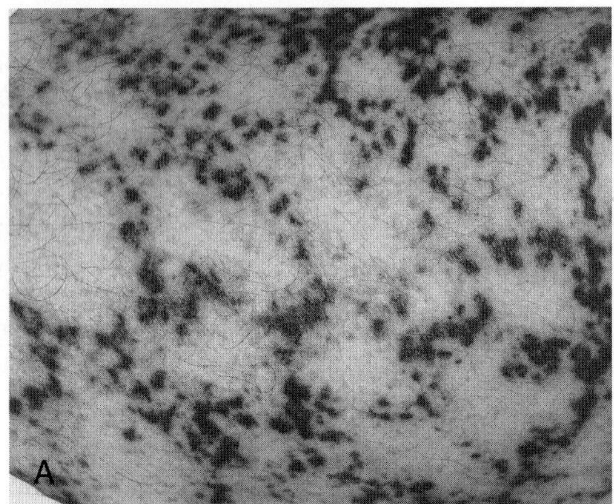

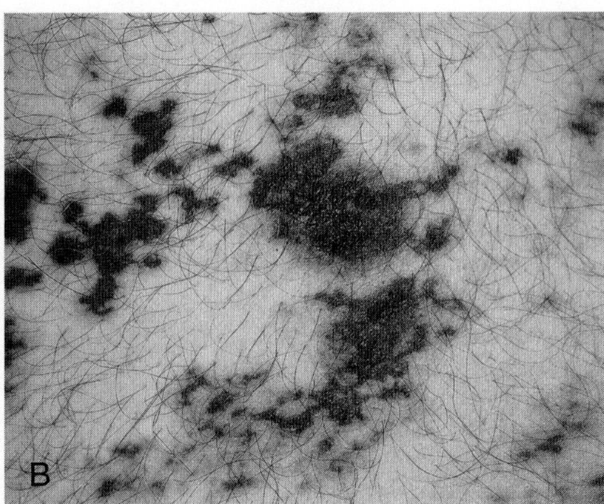

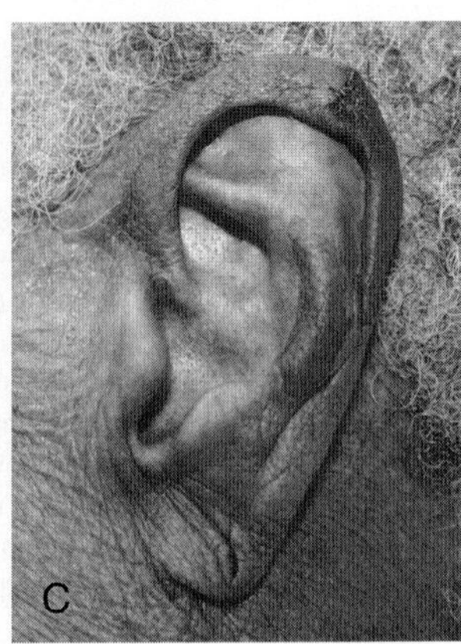

FIG. 2 Type I cryoglobulinemia in two patients with multiple myeloma (IgG type). A, Retiform purpura of the lower extremity. **B**, Areas of necrosis within the areas of retiform purpura. **C**, Purpuric lesions of the antihelix and helix of the ear. (**A, B**, Courtesy, Jean L. Bolognia, MD; **C**, Courtesy, Jonathan Leventhal, MD, In Bolognia J: *Dermatology*, ed 4, Philadelphia, 2018, Elsevier.)

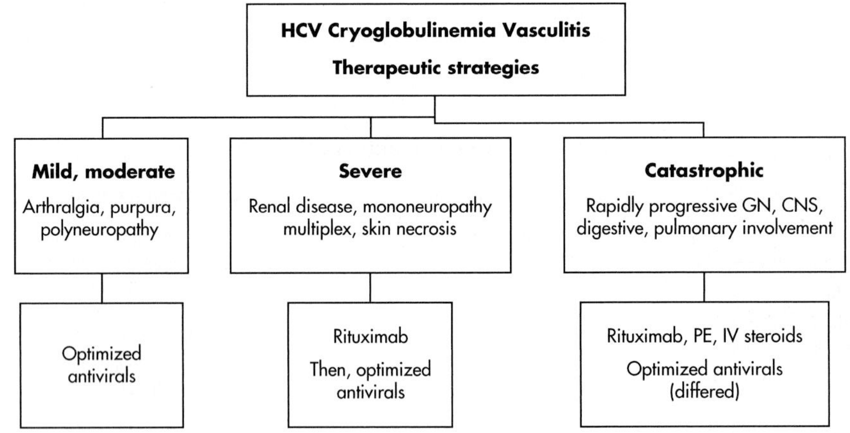

FIG. 3 Treatment of HCV-related mixed cryoglobulinemia vasculitis according to the presentation. *CNS,* Central nervous system; *GN,* glomerulonephritis; *HCV,* hepatitis C virus; *IV,* intravenous; *PE,* pulmonary embolism. (From Cacoub P et al: Cryoglobulinemia vasculitis, *Am J Med* 128[9]:950–955.)

- For noninfectious mixed cryoglobulinemia, treatment is based on disease severity. Low-dose corticosteroids, NSAIDs, and colchicine should be given for mild symptoms. Rituximab, high-dose corticosteroids, cyclophosphamide, and/or plasmapheresis should be given for severe disease.
- In patients with HCV, mild symptoms can be managed by treatment with direct-acting antivirals (DAA). Therapy is aimed at eradicating the HCV infection, suppressing B-cell clonal expansion and cryoglobulin production, and ameliorating symptoms.
- For severe disease in HCV-infected patients, initial immunosuppression with rituximab is warranted, followed by initiation of antiviral therapy.
- Fig. 3 illustrates the treatment of HCV-related mixed cryoglobulinemia vasculitis according to presentation.
- Sustained virologic response due to DAA does not always fully eradicate cryoglobulinemia but can help mitigate its manifestations.

NONPHARMACOLOGIC THERAPY

Avoidance of cold exposure, diabetic food care guidelines

ACUTE GENERAL Rx

NSAIDs in those with general fatigue and arthralgia; see "Treatment" for further management.

DISPOSITION

Overall prognosis is worse with concomitant renal disease. Mean survival rate is ~50% at 10 yr.

REFERRAL

Consider referring to the following:

- Nephrologist if there is renal involvement
- Hematologist in patients with lymphoproliferative disorders
- Gastroenterologist/hepatologist in patients with hepatitis
- Rheumatologist in patients with connective tissue disease cases
- Clinical immunologist in severe cases

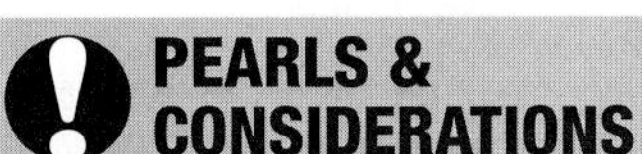

COMMENTS

Always look for underlying cause of cryoglobulinemia.

PREVENTION

Avoidance of cold exposure, avoidance of late complications.

PATIENT/FAMILY EDUCATION

Inform patients about early signs/symptoms of cryoglobulinemia so that treatment can be rendered before the development of complications.

SUGGESTED READINGS

Available at ExpertConsult.com

AUTHOR: **REBECCA SOINSKI, M.D.**

C

Diseases and Disorders

BASIC INFORMATION

DEFINITION

Cryptococcosis is an infection caused by the encapsulated yeast *Cryptococcus spp.*

SYNONYMS

C. *neoformans* infection
C. *gattii* infection
C. *albidus* infection
C. *laurentii* infection

ICD-10CM CODES	
B45.09	Pulmonary cryptococcosis
B45.1	Cerebral cryptococcosis
B45.2	Cutaneous cryptococcosis
B45.3	Osseous cryptococcosis
B45.7	Disseminated cryptococcosis
B45.9	Cryptococcosis, unspecified

EPIDEMIOLOGY & DEMOGRAPHICS

INCIDENCE (IN U.S.):
- 0.8 cases per million persons/yr; *C. neoformans* is an important opportunistic infection in patients with deficits in cell-mediated immunity.
- 2 to 7 per 1000 persons living with AIDS/yr.

PEAK INCIDENCE: 20 to 40 yr (parallel to HIV/AIDS epidemic)
PREDOMINANT SEX: Equal sex distribution when adjusted for HIV status
PREDOMINANT AGE: Less than 2 yr of age; 20 to 40 yr of age
NEONATAL INFECTION: Very uncommon

PHYSICAL FINDINGS & CLINICAL PRESENTATION

- More than 90% present with meningitis (generally subacute); almost all have fever and headache.
- Meningismus, photophobia, mental status changes are seen in approximately 25%.
- Increased intracranial pressure may be present.
- Most common infections outside the CNS:
  1. In the lungs (fever, cough, dyspnea, and typically with lobar consolidation).
  2. In the skin (cellulitis, papular eruption).
  3. In the lymph nodes (lymphadenitis).
  4. Potential involvement of virtually any organ (e.g., prostate and bone).

ETIOLOGY

- There are four *Cryptococcus spp.* that cause disease in humans, although most laboratories are not able to differentiate between species. *C. neoformans* (Table E1) is the cause of a majority of global disease burden, primarily in immunocompromised patients. *C. gattii* infections are much less common and occur more often in normal hosts, with recent outbreaks in the Pacific Northwest. *C. albidus* and *C. laurentii* are even rarer causes of disease.
- Infection originates by inhalation into the respiratory tract followed by dissemination to the CNS in most cases, usually without recognizable lung involvement.
- Almost always in the setting of AIDS (most with CD4 counts <100) or other disorders of cellular immune function, such as organ transplantation.
- Neutropenia alone poses a much lower risk of significant cryptococcal infection.

DIAGNOSIS

DIFFERENTIAL DIAGNOSIS

- Subacute meningitis (caused by *Listeria monocytogenes,* Mycobacterium tuberculosis, *Histoplasma capsulatum,* viruses).
- Intracranial mass lesion (neoplasms, toxoplasmosis, TB).
- Pulmonary involvement confused with *Pneumocystis jiroveci* pneumonia when diffuse or confused with TB or bacterial pneumonia when focal or involving the pleura.
- Skin lesions can take many forms and may be confused with bacterial cellulitis or molluscum contagiosum.

WORKUP

- Lumbar puncture to exclude cryptococcal meningitis, with measurement of opening pressure because CSF opening pressure is elevated in 60% to 80% of HIV patients and may require drainage. In cryptococcal meningitis, CSF reveals lymphocytic pleocytosis (although a paucity of WBCs may be found in CSF of HIV patients).
- CT scan of the head when focal lesion or increased intracranial pressure is suspected.
- Biopsy of enlarged lymph nodes and skin lesions if feasible.

LABORATORY TESTS

- Culture and India ink stain (60% to 80% sensitive in culture-proven cases [Fig. E1]); examination of the CSF in all cases when CNS involvement is suspected.
- Blood and serum cryptococcal antigen assay (>90% sensitivity and specificity in immunocompromised patients; lower sensitivity in immunocompetent patients).
- Culture and histologic examination of biopsy material.
- HIV antibody testing.

IMAGING STUDIES

- CT scan or MRI of the head if focal neurologic involvement or cryptococcoma is suspected.
- Chest x-ray examination to exclude pulmonary involvement.

TREATMENT

ACUTE GENERAL Rx

- Treatment of cryptococcosis consists of three stages: induction, consolidation, and maintenance. Induction therapy for CNS disease (meningitis) was historically initiated with IV amphotericin B deoxycholate (0.7-1.0 mg/kg/day) with flucytosine 100 mg/kg/day PO in four divided doses; however, there is growing clinical evidence for liposomal amphotericin B (3-6 mg/kg/day) plus flucytosine, especially in HIV-infected patients and in those with renal dysfunction. Induction therapy is generally recommended for 2 to 4 weeks and until repeat CSF cultures are negative; it is then recommended to transition to consolidation therapy with fluconazole 400 mg PO q24h for 8 weeks, followed by ongoing fluconazole 200 mg PO q24h maintenance therapy (up to 2 year) to reduce relapse rate. Maintenance therapy is indicated in patients with AIDS until these patients have been receiving antifungal therapy for at least 1 yr and they have responded to antiretroviral therapy (CD4 cell count ≥100/microliter for ≥3 months). In patients without HIV, the duration of maintenance therapy is generally 6 to 12 months. Lifelong antifungal therapy is needed in organ transplant patients.
- Alternative: IV fluconazole combined with flucytosine for initial therapy in patients unable to tolerate amphotericin B.
- If symptomatic increased intracranial pressure, consider multiple therapeutic lumbar taps or intraventricular shunt.
- Data support increased mortality with early initiation of antiretroviral therapy in the setting of cryptococcal meningitis due to immune reconstitution syndrome; therefore, it is generally recommended to wait 2 to 10 weeks after starting cryptococcal therapy prior to starting antiretroviral therapy.
- CSF removal with daily lumbar puncture or insertion of a shunt is beneficial in patients with elevated intracranial pressure.

CHRONIC Rx

- Fluconazole (200-400 mg PO qd) is highly effective in preventing a relapse in HIV-infected patients; development of resistance may occur. Itraconazole is an alternative agent, along with growing evidence for voriconazole and posaconazole use.

DISPOSITION

Without maintenance therapy, relapse rate is >50% among AIDS patients.

REFERRAL

- For consultation with infectious diseases specialist in all cases.
- For neurologic consultation if level of consciousness is depressed or focal lesion is present.

SUGGESTED READINGS

Available at ExpertConsult.com

RELATED CONTENT

Cryptococcosis (Patient Information)

AUTHORS: **PHILIP A. CHAN, M.D., M.S.,** and **GLENN G. FORT, M.D., M.P.H.**

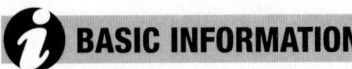

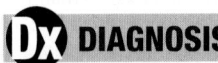

DEFINITION

The intracellular protozoan parasite *Cryptosporidium parvum* is associated with gastrointestinal disease and diarrhea, especially in patients with AIDS or other immunocompromised hosts. It is also associated with sporadic infections and waterborne outbreaks in immunocompetent hosts. Cryptosporidiosis is a notifiable disease in the U.S.

Other species, including *C. hominis, C. felis, C. muris,* and *C. meleagridis,* are now described to be pathogens as well.

SYNONYM

Cryptosporidiosis

ICD-10CM CODE
A07.2 Cryptosporidiosis

EPIDEMIOLOGY & DEMOGRAPHICS

INCIDENCE:

- Approximately 2% in industrial countries, 5% to 10% in developing countries.
- Immunocompromised patients, especially those with HIV/AIDS, are particularly susceptible to infection. 10% to 20% of HIV patients in the United States may excrete cyst.
- Cryptosporidiosis is a leading cause of all waterborne outbreaks in the U.S. An estimated 748,000 cryptosporidiosis cases occur annually, although fewer than 2% are reported. In 2011, more than 9000 cases of cryptosporidiosis were reported in the country. The highest overall reporting rates were observed in the Midwest.[1]

PREVALENCE: Worldwide, especially third-world countries; associated with poor hygiene as a waterborne pathogen.

PREDOMINANT SEX: Male = female.

TRANSMISSION:

- Person-to-person (day care, family members).
- Animal-to-person (pets, farm animals). Fig. 1 describes the life cycle of *Cryptosporidium.*
- Environmental (water-associated outbreaks, including travel associated with swimming in or drinking contaminated water or eating contaminated food).
- May be significant pathogen causing diarrhea in patients with AIDS.

PHYSICAL FINDINGS & CLINICAL PRESENTATION

- Spectrum of illness ranging from asymptomatic to severe enteritis (Table 1). Typical cases in immunocompetent hosts result in self-limited diarrhea, whereas immunocompromised hosts are characterized by profuse, watery, nonbloody diarrhea that may lead to dehydration and weight loss.
- Usually limited to the gastrointestinal tract; however, in individuals with AIDS, the disease may be fulminant and life-threatening (CD4 counts <50).
- Diarrhea, severe abdominal pain (2-28 days).
- Impaired digestion, dehydration.
- Fever, malaise, fatigue, nausea, vomiting.
- Pneumonia if aspirated.

ETIOLOGY

C. hominis, C. parvum, C. felis, C. muris, C. meleagridis.

Dx DIAGNOSIS

Clinical presentation of acute gastrointestinal illness, especially associated with HIV/AIDS or with travel and waterborne outbreaks.

DIFFERENTIAL DIAGNOSIS

- *Campylobacter*
- *Clostridium difficile*
- *Entamoeba histolytica*
- *Giardia lamblia*
- *Salmonella*
- *Shigella*
- Microsporidia
- Cytomegalovirus
- *Mycobacterium avium*

Disease may cause cholecystitis, reactive arthritis, hepatitis, urethritis, pancreatitis, or pneumonia in immunocompromised or HIV-infected patients.

WORKUP

(Table 2)

- Stool evaluation looking for characteristic oocyst by modified acid-fast stain (Fig. 2)
- Direct immunofluorescence using monoclonal antibodies is the gold standard for stool exams
- Rapid antigen detection
- PCR
- HIV antibody testing

Rx TREATMENT

- Handwashing and appropriate decontamination of drinking and recreational water sources.
- May be self-limited in normal host over several weeks. Antidiarrheal agents Pepto-Bismol, Kaopectate, or loperamide may give symptomatic relief.
- Pharmacologic treatment with antibiotics has been largely unsatisfactory in patients with AIDS. Antiviral therapy is the treatment of choice to restore the immune system. Oocyst excretion reduction has been shown with nitazoxanide 500 mg PO bid for 3 days in immunocompetent patients. If treatment fails, consider a trial of paromomycin, metronidazole, azithromycin, or trimethoprim/sulfamethoxazole. However, these medications have not been approved for treatment of *Cryptosporidium.*
- Nitazoxanide elixir has been approved for the treatment of cryptosporidiosis in children ages 1 to 11 yr.
- Biliary cryptosporidiosis can be treated with antiretroviral therapy in the HIV setting.

DISPOSITION

- A self-limited disease in immunocompetent patients with complete recovery over 2 to 3 weeks.
- In patients with AIDS, chronic infection often clears with initiation and maintenance of antiretroviral therapy.
- Chronic arthralgia, headache, malaise, and weakness may persist after infection, even in immunologically normal people.
- If severe and prolonged disease (>30 days), testing for HIV and other immunocompromised states is appropriate, along with a referral to an infectious diseases specialist or gastroenterologist.

REFERRAL

- To an infectious diseases specialist if symptoms persist and/or HIV infection is found
- To a gastroenterologist if chronic malabsorption, or biliary or pancreatic complications occur

PEARLS & CONSIDERATIONS

- Chronic cryptosporidiosis (>30 days of diarrhea from *Cryptosporidium* spp. infection) in a patient with HIV is an AIDS-qualifying opportunistic infection.
- *Cryptosporidium hominis* has a limited host range (humans), whereas *Cryptosporidium parvum* has a wide host range including humans, horses, cattle, other domesticated animals, and wild animals; both species present similarly in humans.

SUGGESTED READING

Available at ExpertConsult.com

AUTHORS: **PHILIP A. CHAN, M.D., M.S.,** and **GLENN G. FORT, M.D., M.P.H.**

[1] Cryptosporidiosis surveillance, United States, 2011-2012. MMWR 64 3 (2015).

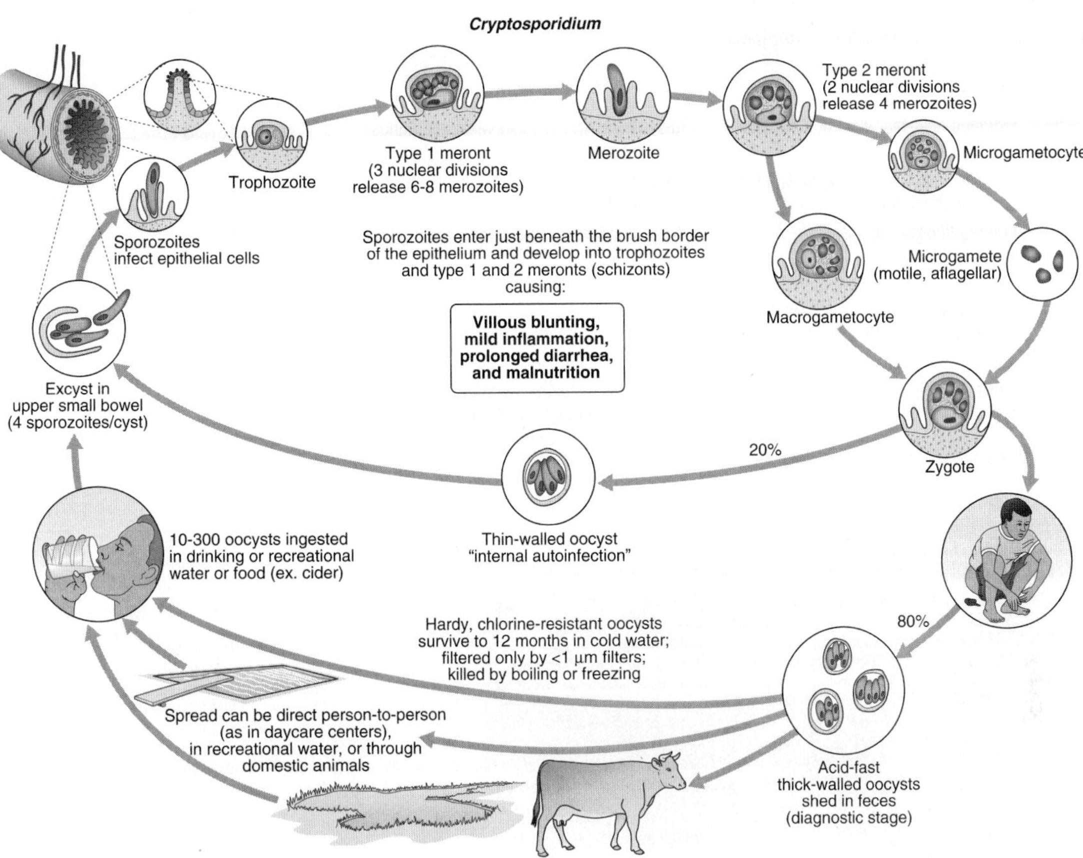

FIG. 1 Life cycle of *Cryptosporidium*. Oocysts are excreted in the feces. After ingestion, the sporozoites are released from the oocysts and attach to and invade intestinal epithelial cells. The cells engulf the parasites into a parasitophorous vacuole, where they enlarge to form the trophozoites; undergo asexual multiplication, forming type 1 meronts; and release the motile merozoites. The type II meronts differentiate into microgamonts and macrogamonts. The microgametes fertilize the macrogametes to form the zygote. The zygotes develop into the oocysts. Two different types of oocysts are produced: the thick-walled, which is commonly excreted from the host, and the thin-walled, which is primarily involved in autoinfection. Oocysts are infective upon excretion, thus permitting direct and immediate fecal-oral transmission. (From Lima AM et al: Cryptosporidiosis. In: Guerrant RL et al [eds]: *Tropical infectious diseases,* ed 3, Philadelphia, 2011, Saunders; Bennett JE et al: *Mandell, Douglas, and Bennett's principles and practice of infectious diseases,* ed 8, Philadelphia, 2005, Saunders.)

TABLE 1 Clinical Manifestation of Cryptosporidiosis

Host	Clinical Manifestations	Comments
Normal host	Acute watery diarrhea	Relapses common Persistent diarrhea common
Children in developing countries	Acute watery diarrhea	Diarrhea more severe in children with malnutrition
	Persistent diarrhea	Persistent diarrhea affecting nutritional status, growth, and intellectual function
Immunocompromised host	Acute watery diarrhea	Transient, self-limited, similar to disease in normal host
	Relapsing diarrhea	Very common
	Persistent or chronic diarrhea	Usually found in patients with low CD4 count or malnutrition
	Cholera-like illness	Voluminous watery diarrhea, only with very low CD4 count
	Extraintestinal involvement	Respiratory tract, biliary tract, and pancreas

From Cherry JD et al: *Feigin and Cherry's pediatric infectious diseases*, ed 8, Philadelphia, 2019, Elsevier.

TABLE 2 Diagnosis of *Cryptosporidium* Infection

Test Type	Method	Comments
Microscopic examination of stools	Modified acid-fast stain of stools	Inexpensive and widely available diagnostic test
	Fluorescent stains (auramine O, auramine-rhodamine)	Faster than other acid-fast stains and may improve sensitivity
	Immunofluorescent assays	More sensitive than acid-fast staining but also more expensive
Antigen-detection assays	Enzyme immunoassay and immunochromatographic tests: Direct and indirect immunofluorescence assay	Good sensitivity (66-100%) and excellent specificity (93-100%), but occasional lots associated with false-positive test results
Molecular methods	Polymerase chain reaction	Increased sensitivity in contrast to microscopic or antigen-detection studies

From Cherry JD et al: *Feigin and Cherry's pediatric infectious diseases*, ed 8, Philadelphia, 2019, Elsevier.

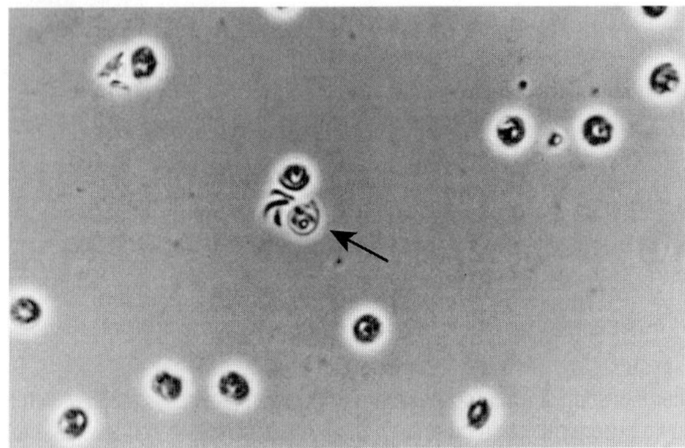

FIG. 2 Human stool-derived *Cryptosporidium* oocysts. Excysting oocyst *(arrow)* is releasing three of its four sporozoites. (Phase-control microscopy ×630.) (From Gorbach SL: *Infectious diseases*, ed 2, Philadelphia, 1998, Saunders.)

BASIC INFORMATION

DEFINITION

- Cushing's syndrome is the occurrence of clinical abnormalities associated with glucocorticoid excess as a result of exaggerated adrenal cortisol production or long-term glucocorticoid therapy.
- Cushing's disease is Cushing's syndrome caused by pituitary adrenocorticotropic hormone (ACTH) excess.

ICD-10CM CODES

E24	Cushing's syndrome
E24.2	Drug-induced Cushing's syndrome
E24.3	Ectopic ACTH syndrome
E24.8	Other Cushing's syndrome
E24.9	Cushing's syndrome, unspecified
E24.9	Pituitary-dependent Cushing's disease

PHYSICAL FINDINGS & CLINICAL PRESENTATION

- Hypertension
- Central obesity with rounding of the facies (moon facies); thin extremities. Fig. 1 illustrates the distribution of adipose tissue in Cushing's syndrome
- Hirsutism, menstrual irregularities, hypogonadism
- Skin fragility, ecchymoses, red-purple abdominal striae (Fig. E2), acne, poor wound healing, hair loss, facial plethora, hyperpigmentation (with ACTH excess). The frequency of individual findings in Cushing's syndrome is summarized in Table 1
- Psychosis, emotional lability, paranoia
- Muscle wasting with proximal myopathy

NOTE: The previous characteristics are not commonly present in Cushing's syndrome caused by ectopic ACTH production. Many of these tumors secrete a biologically inactive ACTH that does not activate adrenal steroid synthesis. These patients may have only weight loss and weakness.

ETIOLOGY

- Iatrogenic from long-term glucocorticoid therapy (common).
- Pituitary ACTH excess (Cushing's disease; 60%).
- Adrenal neoplasms (30%).
- Ectopic ACTH production (neoplasms of lung, pancreas, kidney, thyroid, thymus; 10%).
- Table E2 summarizes the incidence of tumors associated with the ectopic adrenocorticotropic hormone syndrome.
- A classification of causes of Cushing's syndrome is described in Table E3.

Dx DIAGNOSIS

DIFFERENTIAL DIAGNOSIS

- Alcoholic pseudo-Cushing's syndrome (endogenous cortisol overproduction)
- Obesity associated with diabetes mellitus
- Adrenogenital syndrome

WORKUP

- Initial tests include the overnight low-dose dexamethasone suppression test (LDST), 24-hour urine free cortisol (UFC), and late-night (LN) salivary cortisol. The LN and UFC tend to be more convenient.
- Late-night salivary cortisol: A single midnight serum cortisol level (normal diurnal variation leads to a nadir around midnight) >7.5 mcg/dl has been reported as 96% sensitive and 100% specific for the diagnosis of Cushing's syndrome. This test assesses the normal diurnal rhythm of cortisol (lost in Cushing's syndrome) and is not useful in patients who have inconsistent sleep patterns or do shift work. It can also be affected by tobacco use and use of topical corticosteroids.
- In patients with a clinical diagnosis of Cushing's syndrome, the classic initial screening test is the overnight dexamethasone suppression test:
  1. Dexamethasone 1 mg PO given at 11 PM.
  2. Plasma cortisol level measured 9 hr later (8 AM).
  3. Plasma cortisol level <5 mcg/100 ml excludes Cushing's syndrome.
- Serial measurements (two or three consecutive measurements) of 24-hr urinary free cortisol and creatinine (to ensure adequacy of collection) are undertaken if overnight dexamethasone test is suggestive of Cushing's syndrome. Persistent elevated cortisol excretion (>300 mcg/24 hr) indicates Cushing's syndrome.
- The low-dose (2 mg) dexamethasone suppression test is useful to exclude pseudo-Cushing's syndrome if the previous results are equivocal. Corticotropic-releasing hormone (CRH) stimulation after low-dose dexamethasone administration (dexamethasone-CRH test) is also used to distinguish patients with suspected Cushing's syndrome from those who have mildly elevated urinary free cortisol level and equivocal findings.

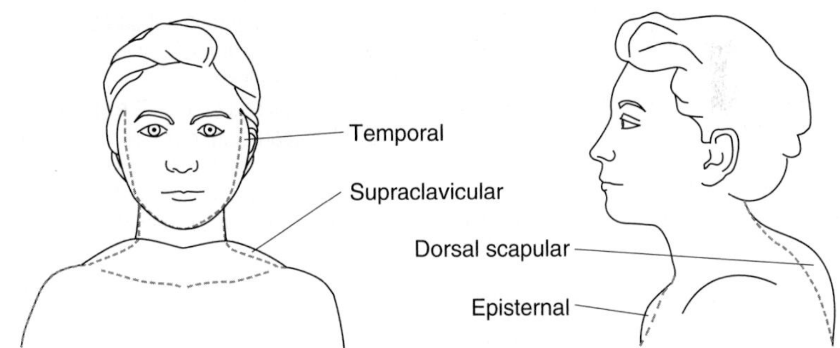

FIG. 1 Distribution of adipose tissue in Cushing's syndrome. Rounding of the cheeks and prominent bitemporal fat produce the characteristic moon facies. Fat also may accumulate bilaterally above the clavicles (supraclavicular collar), in front of the sternum (episternal area, or dewlap), and over the back of the neck (dorsal cervical fat pad, or buffalo hump). In these drawings, the dotted line depicts normal contours of patients without Cushing's syndrome. (From McGee S: *Evidence-based physical diagnosis*, ed 4, Philadelphia, 2018, Elsevier.)

TABLE 1 Cushing's Syndrome—Frequency of Individual Findings

Physical Finding†	Frequency (%)‡
Vital Signs	
Hypertension	64-88
Body Habitus	
Moon facies	67-92
Central obesity	44-97
Buffalo hump	34-75
Skin Findings	
Thin skin	27
Plethora	28-94
Hirsutism, women	48-81
Ecchymoses	23-75
Red or purple striae	46-68
Acne	21-52
Extremity Findings	
Proximal muscle weakness	39-68
Edema	15-66
Other	
Significant depression	12-40

†*Diagnostic standard*: For *Cushing's syndrome*, elevated daily cortisol or corticosteroid metabolites, or both, with loss of circadian rhythm and with abnormal dexamethasone suppression tests.

‡Results are overall mean frequency or, if statistically heterogeneous, the range of values.

From McGee, S: *Evidence-based physical diagnosis*, ed 4, Philadelphia, 2018, Elsevier.

- The high-dose (8 mg) dexamethasone test and measurement of ACTH by radioimmunoassay are useful to determine the etiology of Cushing's syndrome.
  1. ACTH undetectable or decreased and lack of suppression indicate adrenal cause of Cushing's syndrome.
  2. ACTH normal or increased and lack of suppression indicate ectopic ACTH production.
  3. ACTH normal or increased and partial suppression suggest pituitary excess (Cushing's disease).

Bilateral inferior petrosal sinus sampling (BIPSS) can be used to distinguish pituitary Cushing's disease from the ectopic ACTH syndrome.

TABLE 4 Differential Diagnosis of Hormonal Values Seen in Cushing's Syndrome

Cause	Plasma ACTH	Plasma Cortisol (PM)	High-Dose or Overnight Dexamethasone Suppression
Pituitary-dependent	N—slightly ↑	↑	Yes
Adrenal disease	↓—undetectable	↑	No
Ectopic Cushing's*	↑↑↑	↑↑	Usually no
Pseudo-Cushing's	N—slightly ↑	N–↑	Usually yes

ACTH, Adrenocorticotropin; *N*, normal.
*ACTH levels may overlap with values seen in pituitary-dependent disease.
From McPherson RA, Pincus MR (eds): *Henry's clinical diagnosis and management by laboratory methods*, ed 23, St Louis, 2017, Elsevier.

LABORATORY TESTS

- Hypokalemia, hypochloremia, metabolic alkalosis, hyperglycemia, hypercholesterolemia.
- Increased 24-hr urinary free cortisol (>100 mcg/24 hr).
- Table 4 describes the differential diagnosis of hormonal values seen in Cushing's syndrome.
- Fig. 3 describes an algorithm for the evaluation of Cushing's syndrome.

IMAGING STUDIES

- CT scan or MRI of adrenal glands in suspected adrenal Cushing's syndrome (Fig. E4).
- MRI of pituitary gland with gadolinium is the preferred procedure for localizing a pituitary edema in suspected pituitary Cushing's syndrome.
- Additional imaging studies to localize neoplasms of the lung, pancreas, kidney, thyroid, or thymus in patients with ectopic ACTH production.

Rx TREATMENT

GENERAL Rx

The definitive treatment of Cushing's syndrome is surgical removal of the tumor causing excessive production of cortisol:

- Pituitary adenoma: Transsphenoidal microadenomectomy is the therapy of choice in adults. Pituitary irradiation is reserved for patients not cured by transsphenoidal surgery. In children, pituitary irradiation may be considered as initial therapy because 85% of children are cured by radiation. Stereotactic radiotherapy (photon knife or gamma knife) is effective and exposes the surrounding neuronal tissues to less irradiation than does conventional radiotherapy. Total bilateral adrenalectomy is reserved for patients not cured by transsphenoidal surgery or pituitary irradiation.
- Adrenal neoplasm:
  1. Surgical resection of the affected adrenal.
  2. Glucocorticoid replacement for approximately 9 to 12 mo after the surgery to allow time for the contralateral adrenal gland to recover from its prolonged suppression.
  3. In nonsurgical candidates, suppression of adrenal steroid production can be accomplished with ketoconazole. Mifepristone, an antiprogestin, can also be used for control of hyperglycemia secondary to hypercortisolism in adults with endogenous Cushing's syndrome. It should be avoided in women who are or who could become pregnant.
- Bilateral micronodular or macronodular adrenal hyperplasia: Bilateral total adrenalectomy.
- Ectopic ACTH:
  1. Surgical resection of the ACTH-secreting neoplasm
  2. Control of cortisol excess with metyrapone, aminoglutethimide, mifepristone, or ketoconazole
  3. Control of the mineralocorticoid effects of cortisol and 11-deoxycorticosteroid with spironolactone
  4. Bilateral adrenalectomy: A rational approach to patients with indolent, unresectable tumors

DISPOSITION

Prognosis is favorable in patients with surgically amenable disease.

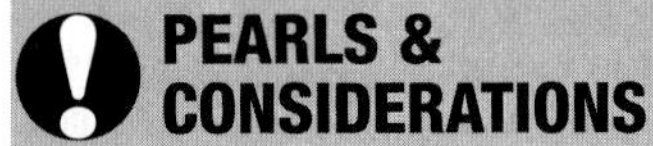

COMMENTS

Screening for multiple endocrine neoplasia type I should be considered in patients with Cushing's disease.

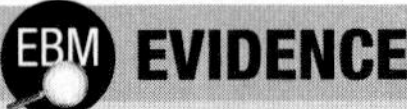

Available at ExpertConsult.com

SUGGESTED READING

Available at ExpertConsult.com

RELATED CONTENT

Cushing's Syndrome (Patient Information)

AUTHOR: **FRED F. FERRI, M.D.**

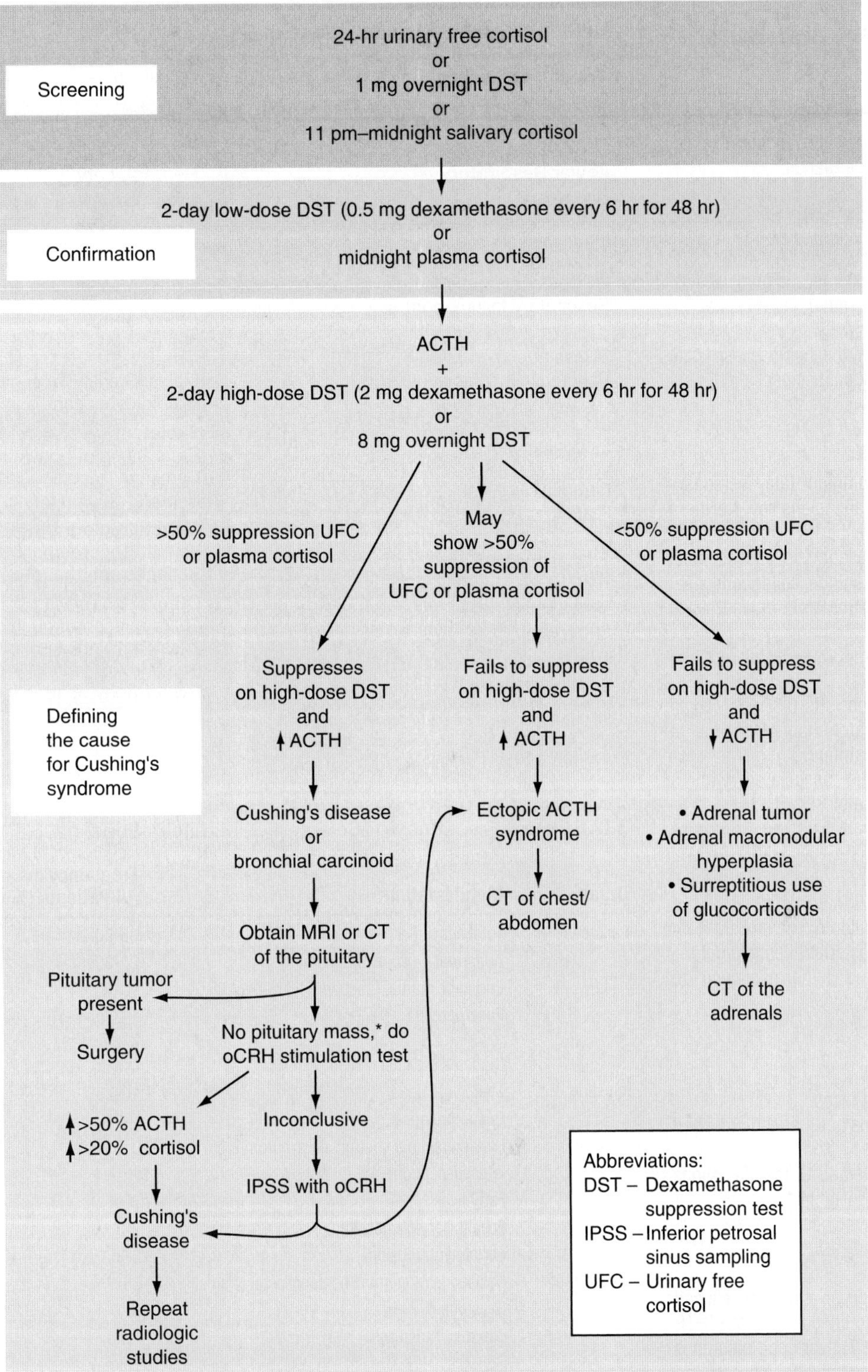

FIG. 3 Algorithm for the evaluation of Cushing's syndrome. All screening tests must be followed by a confirmatory test. If there is no pituitary mass, obtain a chest radiograph and chest CT to rule out bronchial carcinoid before proceeding to IPSS. *ACTH,* Adrenocorticotropin; *CT,* computed tomography; *oCRH,* ovine corticotropin-releasing hormone; *MRI,* magnetic resonance imaging. (From McPherson RA, Pincus MR: *Henry's clinical diagnosis and management by laboratory methods,* ed 23, Philadelphia, 2017, Elsevier.)

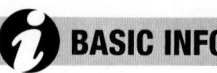

BASIC INFORMATION

DEFINITION

Cystic fibrosis (CF) is an autosomal recessive disorder characterized by dysfunction of chloride channels of exocrine glands.

ICD-10CM CODES

E84.0	Cystic fibrosis with pulmonary manifestations
E84.11	Meconium ileus in cystic fibrosis
E84.19	Cystic fibrosis with other intestinal manifestations
E84.8	Cystic fibrosis with other manifestations
E84.9	Cystic fibrosis, unspecified

EPIDEMIOLOGY & DEMOGRAPHICS

- CF is the most common fatal hereditary disorder among Caucasians of Northern European descent in the U.S. (one case per approximately 3000) and the second most common life-shortening childhood-onset inherited disorder in the U.S., behind sickle cell disease.
- Worldwide it affects 80,000 children and adults.
- Median age at diagnosis is 5.3 mo. Median survival is now greater than 40 yr due to advancements in treatment.
- Carrier screening is associated with a decrease in incidence of CF.

PHYSICAL FINDINGS & CLINICAL PRESENTATION

- Meconium ileus
- Failure to thrive in children
- Increased anterior/posterior chest diameter
- Basilar crackles and hyperresonance to percussion
- Digital clubbing
- Chronic cough
- Abdominal distention
- Greasy, foul-smelling feces
- Clinical manifestations of CF are summarized in Box 1
- The frequency of selected GI manifestations in CF is summarized in Table 1.
- See Box 1.

ETIOLOGY

CF is an autosomal-recessive disease caused by mutations to the gene encoding for the CFTR protein on chromosome 7, over gene mutations organized into six classes have been associated with CF. About half of patients in the U.S. with CF are homozygous for the Phe508del mutation in *CFTR*, and more than 90% have at least one Phe508del allele. These mutations result in abnormalities in chloride transport and thus water flux across the surface of epithelial cells; the resulting abnormally viscous secretions cause obstruction of glands and ducts in various organs and subsequent damage to exocrine tissue (recurrent pneumonia, atelectasis, bronchiectasis, diabetes mellitus, biliary cirrhosis, cholelithiasis, intestinal obstruction, increased risk of gastrointestinal malignancies).

BOX 1 Clinical Manifestations of CF

Upper Respiratory
Sinusitis
Mucous membrane hypertrophy, nasal polyposis

Lower Respiratory
Atelectasis
Emphysema
Infections
Bronchitis, bronchopneumonia, bronchiectasis, lung abscess
Respiratory failure, right-sided heart failure

GI
Bile salt deficiency
Pancreatic insufficiency
GERD
PUD
Meconium ileus
Volvulus
Peritonitis
Ileal atresia
Distal intestinal obstruction syndrome
Fecal masses
Intussusception
Rectal prolapse

Pancreatic
Pancreatitis
Nutritional failure
Diabetes mellitus
Calcification
Maldigestion with steatorrhea and azotorrhea
Vitamin deficiencies

Hepatobiliary
Mucus hypersecretion
Gallstones, atrophic gallbladder
Focal biliary cirrhosis
Portal hypertension ± esophageal varices
Hypersplenism

Reproductive
Females: Increased viscosity of vaginal mucus, decreased fertility
Males: Sterility; absent ductus deferens, epididymis, and seminal vesicles

Skeletal
Retardation of bone age
Demineralization
Hypertrophic pulmonary osteoarthropathy

Ophthalmologic
Venous engorgement
Retinal hemorrhage

Other
Salt depletion through excessive loss of salt through skin
Heat stroke
Hypertrophy of apocrine glands

From Feldman M, Friedman LS, Brandt LJ: *Sleisenger and Fortran's gastrointestinal and liver disease*, ed 10, Philadelphia, 2016, Elsevier.

TABLE 1 Frequency of Selected GI Manifestations in CF*

Organ	Manifestation	Frequency in All Patients (%)	Frequency in Adults (%)
Pancreas	Total achylia	85-90	85-90*
	Abnormal glucose tolerance	20-30	20-30
	Partial or normal function	10-15	10-15
	Pancreatitis	1-2 (all CF) 22 (PS-CF)	2-3
	Diabetes mellitus	4-7	4-7
Intestine	Meconium ileus	10-25	
	Rectal prolapse	1-2	
	Distal intestinal obstruction syndrome	3	18
	Intussusception	1	1-2
Liver	Fatty liver	7	20-60
	Focal biliary cirrhosis	2-3	11-70
	Portal hypertension	2-3	28
Biliary tract	Gallbladder abnormal, nonfunctional, or small	25	5-20
	Gallstones	8	10-25
	Bile duct strictures	1-20	1-20
Esophagus	GERD	Unknown	80

*Frequency may depend on the genotype.
PS-CF, CF with pancreatic sufficiency.
From Feldman M, Friedman LS, Brandt LJ: *Sleisenger and Fortran's gastrointestinal and liver disease*, ed 10, Philadelphia, 2016, Elsevier.

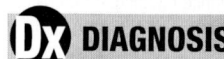

DIAGNOSIS

DIFFERENTIAL DIAGNOSIS

- Immunodeficiency states
- Celiac disease
- Asthma
- Recurrent pneumonia
- Primary ciliary dyskinesia

WORKUP

A diagnosis of CF requires proof of both CFTR dysfunction (i.e., elevated sweat chloride ≥60 mmol/L measured twice, two disease-causing mutations in CFTR from each parental allele, or abnormal nasal potential difference) and one or more phenotypic features consistent with CF (e.g., chronic suppurative obstructive lung disease, pancreatic insufficiency). Table 2

TABLE 2 Diagnostic Criteria for Cystic Fibrosis (CF)

Presence of typical clinical features (respiratory, gastrointestinal, or genitourinary)
OR
A history of CF in a sibling
OR
A positive newborn screening test
PLUS
Laboratory evidence for CFTR (CF transmembrane regulator) dysfunction:
Two elevated sweat chloride concentrations obtained on separate days
OR
Identification of two CF mutations
OR
An abnormal nasal potential difference measurement

From Kliegman RM et al: *Nelson textbook of pediatrics*, ed 19, Philadelphia, 2011, Saunders.

TABLE 4 Sweat Test (Quantitative Pilocarpine Iontophoresis): Indications and Conditions with High Electrolyte Levels

Indications	Conditions with High Sweat Electrolyte Levels
Siblings with CF	CF
Chronic pulmonary symptoms	Ectodermal dysplasia
Persistent cough	Glycogen storage disease, type 1
Recurrent respiratory infection	Adrenal insufficiency
Bronchitis	Familial hypoparathyroidism
Bronchiectasis	Fucosidosis
Lobar atelectasis	Pitressin-resistant diabetes insipidus
Failure to thrive (stunting of growth)	Mucopolysaccharidosis
Rectal prolapse	Familial cholestasis syndrome
Nasal polyposis	Environmental deprivation syndrome
Intestinal obstruction of newborn	Acute respiratory disorders (croup, epiglottitis, viral pneumonia)
Meconium ileus	Chronic respiratory disorders (bronchopulmonary dysplasia)
Jaundice in early infancy	α_1-Antitrypsin deficiency
Cirrhosis in childhood or adolescence	
Portal hypertension	
Adult males with aspermia or azoospermia	
Heat stroke	
Hypoproteinemia	
Hypoprothrombinemia	

From Feldman M et al: *Sleisenger and Fordtran's gastrointestinal and liver disease*, ed 10, Philadelphia, 2016, Elsevier.

TABLE 3 Approach to Diagnosis of Cystic Fibrosis in Adult Patients

Conditions Suggesting the Diagnosis of Cystic Fibrosis in Adults
Recurrent pancreatitis
Male infertility
Chronic sinusitis
Nasal polyposis
Nontuberculous mycobacterial infection
Allergic bronchopulmonary mycosis
Bronchiectasis

Recommended Diagnostic Studies
Sweat electrolyte determination
Extended CFTR mutation analysis
Nasal potential difference
High-resolution CT scan to identify bronchiectasis
CT scan of sinuses for polyposis
Sputum induction or bronchoalveolar lavage to identify bacterial and fungal pathogens

CFTR, Cystic fibrosis transmembrane conductance regulator; *CT*, computed tomography.
From Goldman L, Schafer AI: *Goldman's Cecil medicine*, ed 24, Philadelphia, 2012, Saunders.

describes diagnostic criteria for CF. Conditions suggesting the diagnosis of CF in adults and recommended diagnostic studies are described in Table 3.

LABORATORY TESTS

- Pilocarpine iontophoresis (sweat chloride test): Diagnostic of CF in children if sweat chloride is >60 mmol/L (>80 mmol/L in adults) on two separate tests on consecutive days. Repeat testing may be necessary because not all infants have sufficient quantities of sweat for reliable testing. Indications for sweat test and conditions with associated high electrolyte levels are summarized in Table 4. Table 5 describes conditions associated with false-positive and false-negative sweat test results.
- DNA testing may be useful for confirming the diagnosis and providing genetic information for family members.

TABLE 5 Conditions Associated with False-Positive and False-Negative Sweat Test Results

With False-Positive Results
Eczema (atopic dermatitis)
Ectodermal dysplasia
Malnutrition/failure to thrive/deprivation
Anorexia nervosa
Congenital adrenal hyperplasia
Adrenal insufficiency
Glucose-6-phosphatase deficiency
Mauriac syndrome
Fucosidosis
Familial hypoparathyroidism
Hypothyroidism
Nephrogenic diabetes insipidus
Pseudohypoaldosteronism
Klinefelter's syndrome
Familial cholestasis syndrome
Autonomic dysfunction
Prostaglandin E infusions
Munchausen syndrome by proxy

With False-Negative Results
Dilution
Malnutrition
Edema
Insufficient sweat quantity
Hyponatremia
Cystic fibrosis transmembrane conductance regulator (CFTR) mutations with preserved sweat duct function

From Kliegman RM et al: *Nelson textbook of pediatrics*, ed 19, Philadelphia, 2011, Saunders.

- Sputum culture and sensitivity and Gram stain (frequent bacterial infections with *Staphylococcus aureus* [both MSSA and MRSA], *Pseudomonas aeruginosa* [most common virulent respiratory pathogen], *Stenotrophomonas maltophilia*, and *Burkholderia cepacia*).
- Bronchoalveolar lavage (BAL) may be used to aid in the early diagnosis of pulmonary infection in nonexpectorating patients; however, evidence for its clinical benefit is lacking. Trials have shown that among infants diagnosed with CF, BAL-directed therapy did not result in a lower prevalence of *P. aeruginosa* infection or lower total CF-CT score when compared with standard therapy at age 5 yr.
- Low albumin level, increased 72-hr fecal fat excretion.
- Pulse oximetry or arterial blood gases: Hypoxemia.
- Pulmonary function studies: Decreased total lung capacity, forced vital capacity, pulmonary diffusing capacity.

IMAGING STUDIES

- Chest x-ray (Fig. E1): May reveal focal atelectasis, peribronchial cuffing, bronchiectasis, increased interstitial markings, hyperinflation
- High-resolution chest CT scan: Bronchial wall thickening, cystic lesions, ring shadows (bronchiectasis)

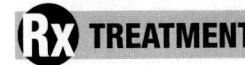

TREATMENT

NONPHARMACOLOGIC THERAPY

- Mucus clearance (i.e., using postural drainage techniques, chest percussion, pneumatic vest, acapella)
- Encouragement of regular exercise and proper nutrition (daily caloric intake of 120%-200% of healthy population)
- Psychosocial evaluation and counseling of patient and family members

ACUTE GENERAL Rx

- Primary goal of CF treatment in regard to pulmonary disease is to maintain lung function as near to normal as possible by controlling respiratory infections and clearing airways of mucus.

- Antibiotic therapy is based on the results of sputum Gram stain and culture and sensitivity. *S. aureus* infections are treated with either cefazolin 1.5 g q6h or nafcillin 2 g 4-6h. MRSA should be treated with vancomycin 45-60 mg/kg/day in 3 divided doses or with linezolid 600 mg q12h. *P. aeruginosa* infections can be treated with piperacillin-tazobactam 4.5 g q6h plus ciprofloxacin 750 mg PO q12h. Treatment of CF exacerbations should be aimed at least at mucoid *P. aeruginosa* and *S. aureus* (i.e., piperacillin-tazobactam and ciprofloxacin). A recent study using azithromycin maintenance in children with CF for 6 mo found less use of additional antibiotics and improvement in some aspects of pulmonary function. Additional studies will be necessary to determine if azithromycin should be used as a primary therapy or rescue treatment. Inhaled antibiotics (aztreonam or tobramycin) can also be used and can achieve high airway concentration with lower systemic side effects. Intermittent administration of inhaled tobramycin has been reported to be beneficial in CF.
- Bronchodilators for patients with airflow obstruction.
- Long-term pancreatic enzyme replacement.
- Alternate-day prednisone (2 mg/kg) possibly beneficial in children with CF (decreased hospitalization rate, improved pulmonary function). Glucocorticoids are used in selected patients during an exacerbation that has characteristics of an acute asthmatic episode (e.g., chest tightness, wheezing, acute symptomatic response to inhaled beta-adrenergic agonists). Routine use of corticosteroids not recommended in adults. Boys with CF who have received alternate-day treatment with prednisone have shown persistent growth impairment after treatment is discontinued.
- Proper nutrition and vitamin supplementation (including fat-soluble vitamins A, D, E, and K).
- The mucolytic recombinant human deoxyribonuclease (DNase [dornase alfa]) 2.5 mg qd or bid given by aerosol for patients ≥6 yr of age with viscid sputum. It lowers the viscosity of sputum. It is useful to improve mucociliary clearance by liquefying difficult-to-clear pulmonary secretions. It is, however, very expensive. It is most beneficial in patients with forced vital capacity values >40% of predicted. Its cost can be decreased by using alternate-day rhDNase therapy.
- Newer treatment modalities act by improving production, intracellular processing, and/or function of the defective CFTR protein. Ivacaftor (a CFTR potentiator) is FDA approved for oral treatment of CF in patients 2 and older with the G551D mutation (5% of patients with CF). It can decrease the frequency of pulmonary exacerbations and improve lung function. Cost is a significant limiting factor. A new combination drug, tezacaftor-ivacaftor, has been reported to work as well or better than ivacaftor for most of the same mutations as were approved for ivacaftor. Tezacaftor-ivacaftor is approved only for patients aged 12 yr and above. Another combination treatment, lumacaftor-ivacaftor, has been FDA-approved for patients aged 12 yr and above who are homozygous for the F508del mutation in the *CFTR* gene. Most recommendations call for the use of tezacaftor-ivacaftor for residual function mutations and F508del homozygotes mutations >12 yr of age. If the patient's genotype is unknown, an FDA-cleared CF mutation test should be used to detect the presence of the F508del mutation on both alleles of the *CFTR* gene. Recent phase 3 trials involving the next-generation cystic fibrosis transmembrane conductance regulator (CFTR) corrector VX-659 in triple combination with tezacaftor and ivacaftor resulted in significant improvements for patients with Phe508del-MF or Phe508del-Phe508del genotypes. Based on these results, VX-659 triple combination regimens have the potential to treat the underlying cause of disease in ~90% of patients with CF.
- Limitations of use: Efficacy and safety have not been established in patients with CF other than those homozygous for the F508del mutation.
- Treatment of impaired glucose tolerance and diabetes mellitus.

CHRONIC Rx

- Pneumococcal and influenza vaccination.
- Chronic treatment with oral antibiotics to control infection is not recommended with two exceptions (see below).
- Azithromycin is recommended for many patients due to its benefits from antiinflammatory and/or antibacterial properties. Should be started on patients ≥6 yr of age with persistent *P. aeruginosa* in airway cultures for inhibition of neutrophil migration and elastase production.
- Chronic treatment with nebulized antibiotics (aztreonam or tobramycin) can be used daily for *P. aeruginosa* colonization.

DISPOSITION

- Bronchiectasis develops early in the course of cystic fibrosis, being detectable in infants as young as 10 wk of age, and is persistent and progressive. Recent data[1] reveal that neutrophil elastase activity in BAL fluid in early life is associated with early bronchiectasis in children with cystic fibrosis.
- More than 50% of children with CF live beyond age 20 yr. During the past 2 decades, survival among patients with late-stage CF has lengthened substantially. Survival has improved at the rate of 1.8% annually during the past decade. This is believed due to increased use of NBH DNase.
- Lung transplantation is the only definitive treatment; 3-yr survival after transplantation exceeds 50%.

[1] Sly PD et al: Risk factors for bronchiectasis in children with cystic fibrosis, *N Engl J Med* 368:1963-1970, 2013.

- Obstructive azoospermia is present in >98% of postpubertal males.
- The SERPINA Z allele is a risk factor for liver disease in CF. Patients who carry the Z allele are at a greater risk of developing severe liver disease with portal hypertension.

REFERRAL

- Lung transplantation is advised in selected patients. Indications for lung transplantation include FEV_1 <30% of predicted, rapidly progressive respiratory deterioration, increasing number of hospital admissions, massive hemoptysis, recurrent pneumothorax, arterial partial pressure of oxygen <55 mm Hg, arterial partial pressure of carbon dioxide >50 mm Hg, multidrug-resistant organisms (although most centers will deny transplant to patients with *Burkholderia* colonization), and wasting. Young female patients should be referred earlier because of overall poorer prognosis. Selected patients must undergo double lung transplant.
- For screening of family members with DNA analysis.

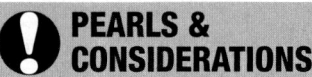

PEARLS & CONSIDERATIONS

COMMENTS

- Clinicians should think of CF in any patient with bronchiectasis plus any of the following: male infertility, recurrent idiopathic pancreatitis, recurrent nasal polyposis.
- Genetic testing for CF should be offered to adults with a positive family history of CF, couples currently planning a pregnancy, and couples seeking prenatal care.
- Inhalation of hypertonic saline (5 ml of 7% sodium chloride qid) has been reported to produce a sustained acceleration of mucus clearance and improved lung function.
- The prevalence of MRSA in the respiratory tract of individuals with CF has increased dramatically over the past decade and is associated with worse survival.

SUGGESTED READINGS

Available at ExpertConsult.com

RELATED CONTENT

Cystic Fibrosis (Patient Information)
Bronchiectasis (Related Key Topic)

AUTHORS: **HARINDER P. SINGH, M.D.,** and **SAMAAN RAFEQ, M.D.**

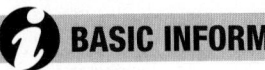

BASIC INFORMATION

DEFINITION

Venous thromboembolism is any thromboembolic event occurring within the venous system. Deep vein thrombosis (DVT) is the development of thrombi in the deep veins of the extremities or pelvis.

SYNONYMS

DVT
Venous thromboembolism (VTE) (VTE includes DVT and pulmonary embolism [PE])
Deep venous thrombosis
VTE

ICD-10CM CODES

I82.401	Acute embolism and thrombosis of unspecified deep veins of right lower extremity
I82.402	Acute embolism and thrombosis of unspecified deep veins of left lower extremity
I82.403	Acute embolism and thrombosis of unspecified deep veins of lower extremity, bilateral
I82.621	Acute embolism and thrombosis of deep veins of right upper extremity
I82.622	Acute embolism and thrombosis of deep veins of left upper extremity
I82.623	Acute embolism and thrombosis of deep veins of upper extremity, bilateral

EPIDEMIOLOGY & DEMOGRAPHICS

- Annual incidence of VTE is 0.1% to 0.27%, affecting up to 5% of the population during their lifetimes.
- The risk of recurrent thromboembolism is higher among men than women.
- In the U.S., there are approximately 900,000 DVT events annually. About 5% to 15% of persons with untreated DVT die from pulmonary embolism.
- Venous thromboembolism occurs in nearly 2 cases per 1000 pregnancies and is a leading cause of maternal mortality and morbidity.

PHYSICAL FINDINGS & CLINICAL PRESENTATION

- Pain and swelling of the affected extremity
- In lower extremity DVT: Leg pain on dorsiflexion of the foot (***Homans* sign**)
- Physical examination may be unremarkable in early DVT

ETIOLOGY

The etiology is often multifactorial (prolonged stasis, coagulation abnormalities, vessel wall trauma). The following are risk factors for DVT:

- Prolonged immobilization (>3 days)
- Postoperative state
- Trauma to pelvis and lower extremities for lower extremity DVT; central line placement for upper extremity DVT
- Birth control pills, high-dose estrogen therapy; conjugated equine estrogen but not esterified estrogen is associated with increased risk of DVT; estrogen plus progestin is associated with doubling the risk of venous thrombosis. The use of bevacizumab is also significantly associated with an increased risk of developing DVT in cancer patients receiving this drug
- Visceral cancer (lung, pancreas, alimentary tract, genitourinary tract)
- Occult cancer is detected in 1 in 20 patients within a year of receiving a diagnosis of unprovoked VTE
- Age >60 yr
- History of thromboembolic disease
- Hematologic disorders (e.g., factor V Leiden mutation [FVL], antithrombin III deficiency, protein C deficiency, protein S deficiency, heparin cofactor II deficiency, sticky platelet syndrome, G20210A prothrombin mutation, lupus anticoagulant, dysfibrinogenemias, anticardiolipin antibody, hyperhomocysteinemia, concurrent homocystinuria, high levels of factors VIII, XI, and single nucleotide polymorphisms [SNPs] such as CYP4V2)
- Pregnancy and early puerperium
- Obesity (BMI >30)
- Congestive heart failure
- Surgery, fracture, or injury involving lower leg or pelvis
- Plaster cast immobilization
- Surgery requiring >30 min of anesthesia
- Gynecologic surgery (particularly gynecologic cancer surgery)
- Recent travel (within 2 wk, lasting ≥2 hr). Every 2 hr spent traveling increases VTE risk by 18%.
- Smoking and abdominal obesity
- Central venous catheter or pacemaker insertion
- Superficial vein thrombosis (10% risk of DVT within 3 mo), varicose veins
- Collagen vascular disease
- Nephrotic syndrome
- Myeloproliferative disorders
- Testosterone therapy
- Long-term exposure to particulate air pollution is also associated with altered coagulation function and DVT risk.
- Varicose veins

DIAGNOSIS

DIFFERENTIAL DIAGNOSIS

- Postphlebitic syndrome
- Superficial thrombophlebitis
- Ruptured Baker cyst
- Cellulitis, lymphangitis, Achilles tendinitis
- Hematoma
- Muscle or soft tissue injury, stress fracture
- Varicose veins, lymphedema
- Arterial insufficiency
- Abscess
- Claudication
- Venous stasis

WORKUP

- The clinical diagnosis of DVT is inaccurate. Pain, tenderness, swelling, or color changes are not specific for DVT.
- Clinical prediction rules can be used to establish pretest probability of DVT. The Wells prediction rules for DVT and for pulmonary embolism are described in Table 1. These rules perform better in younger patients without a history of DVT and in those without comorbidities. In younger patients without associated comorbidities and a low pretest probability using Wells criteria and a negative high-sensitivity D-dimer test, the diagnosis of DVT can be reasonably excluded.
- Compression ultrasonography (CUS; Fig. E1) is preferred as the initial study to diagnose DVT in patients with intermediate to high pretest probability. An initial negative test limited to the proximal leg should be repeated after 5 days (if the clinical suspicion of DVT persists) to exclude DVT that is propagating proximally from the calf. Comprehensive ultrasonography (whole-leg CUS) is a more extensive test that examines the deep veins from the inguinal ligament to the level of the malleolus. Literature reports indicate that it may be safe to withhold anticoagulation after negative results on comprehensive duplex ultrasonography in nonpregnant patients with

TABLE 1 Wells Scoring Scheme for Pre-Test Probability of Deep Vein Thrombosis*

Clinical Feature	Points
Risk Factors	
Active cancer	1
Paralysis, paresis, or recent plaster immobilization of the lower extremities	1
Recently bedridden >3 days or major surgery, within 4 weeks	1
Signs	
Localized tenderness along the distribution of the deep venous system	1
Entire leg swollen	1
Asymmetric calf swelling (>3 cm difference, 10 cm below tibial tuberosity)	1
Asymmetric pitting edema	1
Collateral superficial veins (nonvaricose)	1
Alternative Diagnosis	
Alternative diagnosis as likely or more likely than deep venous thrombosis	−2

*Interpretation of score: High probability if 3 points or more, moderate probability if 1 or 2 points, and low probability if 0 points or less.
From Wells PS, et al.: Value of assessment of pretest probability of deep-vein thrombosis in clinical management. *Lancet*. 350:1795–1798, 1997. In McGee S: *Evidence-based physical diagnosis*, ed 4, Philadelphia, 2018, Elsevier.

a suspected first episode of symptomatic DVT of the leg.

LABORATORY TESTS

- Laboratory tests are not specific for DVT. Baseline prothrombin time (INR), partial thromboplastin time, and platelet count should be obtained on all patients before starting anticoagulation. D-dimer testing is sensitive but not specific for DVT. A negative result (D-dimer <0.5 mcg/ml) can exclude the diagnosis in a patient with low probability of DVT, but a positive result (≥0.5 mcg/ml) mandates additional testing with venous ultrasonography.
- Use of D-dimer assay by ELISA is useful in the management of suspected DVT. The combination of a normal D-dimer study on presentation together with a normal compression venous ultrasound is useful to exclude DVT. DVT can be ruled out in patients who are clinically unlikely to have DVT and who have a negative D-dimer test. Compressive ultrasonography can be safely omitted in such patients.
- Laboratory evaluation of young patients with DVT, patients with recurrent thrombosis without obvious causes, and those with a family history of thrombosis should include protein S (both total and free PS), protein C, fibrinogen, antithrombin III level, lupus anticoagulant, anticardiolipin antibodies, anti-b2 glycoprotein1, factor V Leiden, factor VIII, factor IX, and fasting plasma homocysteine levels. It is important to remember that the lupus anticoagulant assay and antithrombin, protein C, protein S, and dysfibrinogenemia testing cannot be properly interpreted if the patient is already on warfarin, whereas anticardiolipin antibody test, prothrombin G20210A factor VII:C, factor V Leiden, and PT polymorphism can be performed when the patient is on warfarin.

IMAGING STUDIES

- Compression ultrasonography (CUS) is generally preferred as the initial study because it is noninvasive and can be repeated serially (useful to monitor suspected acute DVT); it offers good sensitivity for detecting proximal vein thrombosis (in the popliteal or femoral vein). Its disadvantages are poor visualization of deep iliac and pelvic veins and poor sensitivity in isolated or nonocclusive calf vein thrombi. Whole-leg compression ultrasound can generally exclude proximal and distal DVT in a single evaluation. Withholding anticoagulation following a single negative whole-leg CUS is associated with a relatively low risk of venous thromboembolism (3.5% of inpatients will develop DVT) during a 3-mo follow-up.
- Contrast venography is the gold standard for evaluation of DVT of the lower extremity. It is, however, invasive and painful and rarely used in clinical practice. Additional disadvantages are the increased risk of phlebitis, new thrombosis, renal failure, and hypersensitivity reaction to contrast media; it also gives poor visualization of the deep femoral vein in the thigh and the internal iliac vein and its tributaries.
- Magnetic resonance direct thrombus imaging (MRDTI) is an accurate noninvasive test for diagnosis of DVT. It is particularly useful in suspected DVT patients with leg casts, which prevent CUS, and in pregnant patients with positive D-dimer and negative CUS. Current limitations are its cost and lack of widespread availability.

Rx TREATMENT

NONPHARMACOLOGIC THERAPY

- Gradual resumption of normal activity. Immobility promotes stasis and propagation of DVT. Patients should get up and walk as tolerated. The theoretical risk that ambulation may dislodge thrombi in the legs, precipitating PE, is unfounded.
- Patient education on anticoagulant therapy and associated risks.

ACUTE GENERAL Rx

- Direct oral anticoagulants (DOACs) apixaban or rivaroxaban are prepared as monotherapy for initial treatment of DVT. These new anticoagulants (Table 2) are noninferior to warfarin, do not require periodic lab monitoring, and have a relatively low bleeding risk. They are preferred agents for extended treatment of venous thromboembolism if cost is not a significant issue.
- When apixaban or rivaroxaban are not available or contraindicated, initial treatment of DVT requires therapeutic doses of heparin (low-molecular-weight heparin [LMWH] or unfractionated). LMWH is preferred due to ease of administration, less hemorrhage, and significantly fewer deaths. Unfractionated heparin is recommended in patients with renal insufficiency because LMWH is predominantly excreted in the urine.
- LMWH is generally administered for 5 to 7 days. Recommended dose of enoxaparin is 1 mg/kg q12h SC. Once-daily fondaparinux, a synthetic analogue of heparin, is also as effective and safe as twice-daily enoxaparin in the initial treatment of patients with symptomatic DVT. Once systemic anticoagulation is initiated, vitamin K antagonist warfarin is initiated. Warfarin is titrated to maintain an INR between 2 and 3. After ≥5 days, heparin is stopped and warfarin is continued as monotherapy. Long-term LMWH may be preferable to warfarin in patients with cancer or those whose INR is difficult to control.
- Outpatient treatment of DVT is appropriate for patients without thrombophilic conditions or substantial comorbidity. Exclusions from outpatient treatment of DVT include patients with potential high complication risk (e.g., hemoglobin <7, platelet count <75,000, guaiac-positive stool, recent cerebrovascular accident or noncutaneous surgery, noncompliance).
- Compression stockings are effective in reducing the incidence of postthrombotic syndrome and should be used starting within 1 mo of proximal DVT and continued for at least 1 yr after diagnosis.
- Insertion of an inferior vena cava filter to prevent pulmonary embolism is recommended in patients with contraindications to anticoagulation (e.g., hemorrhagic stroke, active internal bleeding, pregnancy), HIT in a patient with an active VTE/PE, recurrent PE despite adequate anticoagulant therapy, emergent surgery in patient with DVT, presence of free-floating iliofemoral thrombus, lower IVC thrombosis (incipient embolization), and chronic pulmonary (thromboembolic) hypertension with limited pulmonary reserve. Table 3 summarizes indications for IVC filter placement.
- Thrombolytic therapy (streptokinase) can be used in rare cases (unless contraindicated) in patients with extensive iliofemoral venous thrombosis and a low risk of bleeding. There are concerns about hemorrhagic complications related to the large doses of thrombolytics required in systemic thrombolysis for DVT (2% to 10% risk of major hemorrhagic complications).
- Other treatment modalities for DVT include surgical thrombectomy and catheter-directed thrombolysis (CDT). Thromboreduction by surgical thrombectomy is effective but invasive and expensive. CDT is also invasive, carries a bleeding risk, and will generally require ICU admission.

CHRONIC Rx

- The optimal duration of anticoagulant therapy varies with the cause of DVT and the patient's risk factors. The risk of recurrence is low

TABLE 2 Comparison of Dabigatran, Rivaroxaban, Apixaban, and Edoxaban

	Dabigatran	Rivaroxaban	Apixaban	Edoxaban
Target	Thrombin (IIa)	Factor Xa	Factor Xa	Factor Xa
Active drug	No	Yes	Yes	Yes
Onset time (hr)	0.5–2	2–4	3–4	1–3
Half-life (hr)	12–17	5–13	~12	9–11
Renal excretion (%)	80	33	27	50

Hoffman R, et al.: *Hematology, basic principles and practice*, ed 7, Philadelphia, 2017, Elsevier.

TABLE 3 Indications for Inferior Vena Cava Filter Placement

	Indications for IVC Filter Placement	Examples
1.	DVT and contraindication to anticoagulation (A)	Hemorrhage while on anticoagulation
2.	DVT and failure of anticoagulation (A)	Recurrent DVT or PE despite anticoagulation, inability to achieve or maintain adequate anticoagulation
3.	DVT and low cardiopulmonary reserve or high mortality risk from possible PE (R)	Severe pulmonary hypertension, right heart failure, known large right-to-left shunt
4.	Populations with very high risk for PE (R)	Some postbariatric, orthopedic, or neurosurgical patients or multitrauma patients. Patients with expected prolonged immobilization
5.	High risk for life-threatening PE (R)	Large, unstable (free-floating) IVC clot
6.	DVT and high fall risk (R)	
7.	Prophylaxis during catheter-directed thrombolysis of DVT (R)	

There are two absolute indications for IVC filter placement: first, if the patient is at risk for PE (i.e., DVT) but for whatever reason he/she is not a candidate for systemic anticoagulation (i.e., hemorrhage); and second, if the patient developed a PE, new DVT, or an extension of DVT while on proper anticoagulation. There are a number of relative indications for filter placement. They are presented in rows 3 through 7. In every case the decision to place a filter compels careful consideration of the risks and benefits and may require multidisciplinary input. *(A)*, Absolute; *DVT*, deep vein thrombosis; *IVC*, inferior vena cava; *PE*, pulmonary embolism; *(R)*, relative.

From Cameron JL, Cameron AM: *Current surgical therapy*, ed 12, Philadelphia, 2017, Elsevier.

if VTE is provoked by surgery, intermediate if provoked by a nonsurgical risk factor, and high if unprovoked. These risks should determine whether patients with VTE should undergo short-term vs. indefinite treatment.

- Therapy for 3 mo is generally satisfactory in patients with reversible risk factors (low-risk group). A high D-dimer level measured after 3 mo of anticoagulation in patients with unprovoked DVT should favor a longer duration of therapy. The American College of Chest Physicians Guidelines suggests that patients with first unprovoked VTE receive indefinite anticoagulation unless their bleeding risk is high.
- The risk of recurrence in patients with a first unprovoked VTE who have negative D-dimer results is not low enough to justify stopping anticoagulant therapy in men but may be low enough in some cases to justify stopping therapy in women who were taking estrogen at the time of initial VTE.[1]
- Anticoagulation for 6 mo is recommended for patients with idiopathic venous thrombosis or medical risk factors for DVT (intermediate-risk group). About 20% of patients with unprovoked venous thromboembolism have a recurrence within 2 yr after the withdrawal of oral anticoagulant therapy. Use of daily low-dose aspirin after discontinuation of anticoagulant treatment may provide a modest reduction in DVT risk.
- Indefinite anticoagulation is necessary in patients with DVT associated with active cancer; long-term anticoagulation is also indicated in patients with inherited thrombophilia (e.g., deficiency of antithrombin III, protein C or S antibody), high factor VIII levels, antiphospholipid antibody, and those with recurrent episodes of idiopathic DVT (high-risk group). Long-term anticoagulation should also be considered in the presence of comorbidities such as paroxysmal nocturnal hemoglobinuria (PNH), SLE (especially with nephrotic syndrome), some myeloproliferative disorders, IBD, and Cushing's syndrome.

[1]Kearon C, et al.: D-Dimer testing to select patients with a first unprovoked venous thromboembolism who can stop anticoagulant therapy: a cohort study. *Ann Intern Med* 162:27–34, 2015.

- Measurement of D-dimer after withdrawal of oral anticoagulation may be useful to estimate the risk of recurrence in selected patients. In patients with a first unprovoked DVT, positive D-dimer test results after cessation of anticoagulation predict recurrence, regardless of test timing or patient's age. Patients with a first spontaneous DVT and a D-dimer level <250 mg/ml after withdrawal of oral anticoagulation have a low risk of DVT recurrence. Risk is lower in women than in men. In patients who have completed at least 3 mo of anticoagulation for a first episode of unprovoked DVT and after approximately 2 yr of follow-up, a negative D-dimer result is associated with a 3.5% annual risk of recurrent disease, whereas a positive D-dimer result is associated with an 8.9% annual risk for recurrence. Hence, elevated D-dimer levels would be an indication for prolonged therapy (for 1 or 2 more yr at a minimum).
- The presence of residual thrombosis on ultrasonography when anticoagulant therapy is discontinued is also associated with an increased risk for subsequent recurrent DVT; a recent trial showed that tailoring the duration of anticoagulation on the basis of the persistence of residual thrombi on ultrasonography may reduce the rate of recurrent DVT. Additional trials are needed before this approach can be adapted for all patients.
- Patients with DVT and pulmonary embolism are at high risk of recurrence whenever anticoagulation is discontinued; therefore, many experts recommend prolonged anticoagulation in this population group, especially if other risk factors for recurrence are present.

PEARLS & CONSIDERATIONS

COMMENTS

- The prevalence of occult cancer is low among patients with a first unprovoked venous embolism. Routine screening with CT of the abdomen and pelvis does not provide a clinically significant benefit.[2]

[2]Carrier M, Lazo-Langner A, Shivakumar S, et al.: Screening for occult cancer in unprovoked venous thromboembolism, *N Engl J Med* 373:697–704, 2015.

- When using heparin, there is a risk of heparin-induced thrombocytopenia (HIT) (with unfractionated more so than with LMWH). Platelet count should be obtained initially and repeated every 3 days while on heparin.
- ***ISOLATED DEEP VEIN THROMBOSIS OF THE CALF:*** The American College of Chest Physicians Guidelines suggest (1) anticoagulation in patients with severe symptoms or risk factors for proximal extension, and (2) repeat sonogram in 2 weeks in lower risk patients and anticoagulation only in those patients whose DVTs extend proximally.
- ***Prophylaxis of DVT:*** Recommended in all patients at risk (e.g., low-molecular-weight heparin [enoxaparin 30 mg SC bid or fondaparinux 2.5 mg SC daily] after major trauma, postsurgery of hip and knee; enoxaparin 40 mg SC qd post–abdominal surgery in patients with moderate to high DVT risk; gradient elastic stockings alone or in combination with intermittent pneumatic compression [IPC] boots following neurosurgery). Graduated compression stockings (GCSs) are effective for preventing air-travel-related DVT and in reducing the risk of DVT in patients hospitalized for conditions other than stroke. The type of GCSs is also important because proximal DVT occurs more often in patients with stroke who wear below-knee stockings than in those who wear high-length stockings. The new oral anticoagulants (rivaroxaban, apixaban, etc.) are effective for thromboprophylaxis after THR and TKR. However, their clinical benefits over LMWH are marginal. Betrixaban is the first FDA-approved once-daily oral direct factor Xa inhibitor for prophylaxis of VTE in adults hospitalized for an acute medical illness with risk factors for VTE and moderately or severely restricted mobility. Apixaban appears to be as effective as LMWH for thromboprophylaxis in cancer patients but poses similar risk of bleeding and should be used with caution in patients with GI malignancies, thrombocytopenia, or renal impairment.

- ***RECURRENT THROMBOEMBOLISM:*** The risk of recurrent venous thromboembolism in heterozygous carriers of factor V Leiden and a first spontaneous venous thromboembolism is similar to that of noncarriers of factor V Leiden; therefore, heterozygous patients should receive secondary thromboprophylaxis for a similar length of time as patients without factor V Leiden.
- ***POSTTHROMBOTIC SYNDROME:*** Approximately 20% to 50% of patients with DVT develop postthrombotic syndrome characterized by leg edema, pain, venous ectasia, skin induration, and ulceration. Patients with extensive DVT and those with more severe postthrombotic manifestations 1 mo after DVT have poorer long-term outcomes. Recent trials have shown that compression stockings after DVT do not prevent postthrombotic syndrome.
- Exercise following DVT is reasonable because it improves flexibility of the affected leg and does not increase symptoms in patients with postthrombotic syndrome.
- Previously undiagnosed cancer is frequent in patients with newly diagnosed DVT. A cancer screening strategy should be considered in all patients with unprovoked venous thromboembolism.
- ***UPPER EXTREMITY DVT:*** It is less common than lower extremity DVT and is seen more frequently in patients requiring central venous catheters or wires. It confers risk for mortality, recurrent thromboembolic events, and postthrombotic syndrome similar to that of lower extremity DVT. It is classified as primary upper extremity DVT ***(Paget-Schroetter syndrome)***, defined as a thrombus in the axillary and subclavian veins in absence of identifiable thrombosis risk factors. It accounts for 20% of upper extremity DVT cases and may be due to an underlying anatomic abnormality at the thoracic outlet in combination with local hypercoagulability due to venous stretching or perivascular fibrosis from recurrent venous compression. Secondary upper extremity DVT is defined as any DVT related to a predisposing factor (e.g., insertion of central venous catheter, wires, or other devices, malignancy). In patients with secondary upper extremity DVT removal of the catheter is not routinely recommended but is warranted if there is a catheter malfunction or infection, if anticoagulation therapy is contraindicated or has failed, or if the catheter is no longer needed. Anticoagulation therapy in upper extremity DVT consists of use of vitamin K antagonists, except in patients with cancer, for whom LMWH is preferred. Optimal duration of anticoagulation treatment in upper extremity DVT is 3 to 6 mo (including in those in whom a central catheter has been removed).
- ***DVT THERAPY IN PREGNANCY:*** Vitamin K antagonists such as warfarin are contraindicated in pregnancy. Low-molecular-weight heparins are safe and effective. Typical agents used in pregnancy include dalteparin (200 IU per kilogram of body weight daily or 100 IU per kilogram twice daily) or enoxaparin (1.5 mg per kilogram daily or 1 mg per kilogram twice daily).
- ***REVERSAL OF ANTICOAGULATION:*** Vitamin K (1 mg PO or 2 mg IV) can be used to reverse elevated INR (3 to 6) from warfarin when elective or urgent procedures are needed. The administration of vitamin K can take more than 24 hr to fully restore vitamin K dependent coagulation factors II, VII, IX, and X. The American College of Chest Physicians recommends the following guidelines for managing elevated INRs or bleeding in patients receiving vitamin A antagonist therapy:
  1. INR between 4.5 and 10 and no significant bleeding: Omit dose and monitor the next day, routine use of vitamin K is not recommended.
  2. INR >10 and no significant bleeding: Hold vitamin K antagonist, give 5 to 10 mg orally of vitamin K. Monitor the next day and use additional vitamin K if necessary. Resume therapy at lower dose when INR therapeutic.
  3. Serious bleeding at any elevation of INR: Hold vitamin K antagonist and supplement with prothrombin complex concentrates (PCC). Give vitamin K (10 mg by slow IV infusion over 30 min to reduce the risk of anaphylaxis). Vitamin K1 can be repeated every 12 hr. PCC composition in the United States (3-factor PCC) includes clotting factors II, IX, and X but minimal amounts of factor VII (unlike PCC products available outside of the United States [4-factor PCC], which have a significant amount of factor VII). In order to replace the low factor VII, some clinicians in the United States will also give fresh frozen plasma (FFP) in addition to vitamin K and PCC in patients with life-threatening warfarin-related bleeding.
- ***SPECIFIC REVERSAL AGENTS FOR NON–VITAMIN K ANTAGONIST ANTICOAGULANTS:***
  - Idarucizumab, an antibody fragment given at a dose of 5 g IV, has been shown to completely reverse the anticoagulant effect of dabigatran within minutes.
  - The anticoagulant activity of factor Xa inhibitors apixaban, rivaroxaban, and edoxaban can be rapidly reversed with IV administration of andexanet alfa.
  - These reversal agents are very expensive (over $20,000 for each use).

SUGGESTED READINGS

Available at ExpertConsult.com

RELATED CONTENT

Deep Vein Thrombosis (DVT) (Patient Information)
Antiphospholipid Antibody Syndrome (Related Key Topic)
Hypercoagulable State (Related Key Topic)
Postthrombotic Syndrome (Related Key Topic)
Pulmonary Embolism (Related Key Topic)
Upper Extremity Deep Vein Thrombosis (Related Key Topic)

AUTHOR: **FRED F. FERRI, M.D.**

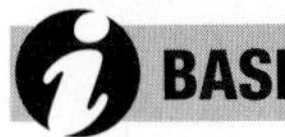

BASIC INFORMATION

DEFINITION

The American Psychiatric Association's *Diagnostic and Statistical Manual*, 5th edition (DSM-5) defines delirium as:

- Disturbance of consciousness with reduced ability to focus, sustain, or shift attention.
- The disturbance develops over a short period of time (usually hours to days) and tends to fluctuate during the course of a day.
- An additional disturbance in cognition (e.g., memory deficit, disorganization, language, visuospatial ability, or perception).
- A change in cognition or development of a perceptual disturbance that is not better accounted for by a preexisting, established, or evolving dementia.
- There is evidence from history, physical exam, or lab findings that the disturbance is caused by medical condition, substance intoxication or withdrawal (i.e., due to a drug of abuse or to a medication), or exposure to a toxin, or is due to multiple etiologies.

SYNONYMS

Acute confusional state
Toxic or metabolic encephalopathy

THEORIES REGARDING PATHOPHYSIOLOGY

- Neuroinflammation, with increased permeability of the blood-brain barrier
- Acetylcholine deficiency
- Other neurotransmitter imbalances, including excesses of norepinephrine, serotonin, and, most important, dopamine

CLASSIFICATION

Hyperactive, hypoactive, and mixed subtype

ICD-10CM CODES

F05	Delirium, not induced by alcohol and other psychoactive substances
F05.9	Delirium, unspecified
F06.0	Organic hallucinosis
F05.8	Other delirium
F05.0	Delirium not superimposed on dementia
F05.1	Delirium superimposed on dementia

EPIDEMIOLOGY & DEMOGRAPHICS

Nearly 30% of older patients experience delirium at some time during the hospital course. In old surgical patients, the risk varies from 10% to 50%. Hypoactive is more common. Delirium is the most common mental disorder in patients with medical illness. Any age, race, or gender can be affected. Pediatric delirium is often missed but remains important because delirium is associated with longer hospital stays, decreased cognitive performance, and increased mortality. Risk factors include extremes of age, severe pain, illicit substance use, surgery, dementia, and kidney or liver failure (Table 1).

PHYSICAL FINDINGS & CLINICAL PRESENTATION

- One of the earliest symptoms is change in level of awareness and ability to focus, sustain, or shift attention. Symptoms may differ both among patients and within one patient. Family members or caregivers report that the patient "isn't acting quite right." Symptoms may include poor attention, sleepiness, agitation, or psychosis.
- Acuteness of presentation helps in differentiating delirium with dementia. Change in cognition, perceptual problems (such as visual, auditory, or somatosensory hallucination usually with lack of insight), memory loss, disorientation, difficulty with speech and language. It is important to ascertain from family member or caregivers the patient's level of functioning before onset of delirium.
- Elderly patients with delirium often do not look sick, but patients with delirium are sick by definition.
- Hyperactive delirium represents only 25% of cases, with the others having hypoactive (quiet) delirium.
- There is often a prodrome phase that later blends into hypoactive delirium or erupts into an agitated confusional state.
- Physical examination should be performed, focusing on signs of infection, dehydration, or chronic disease that may be exacerbated. Vital signs are key. Consider using the Mini-Mental Status Exam or the Montreal Cognitive Assessment.
- Fig. 1 describes an algorithm for evaluation of mental status changes in an older patient.
- Table 2 summarizes delirium assessment tools.

ETIOLOGY

Can be multifactorial; often falls into one of the following categories:

- Drugs: Benzodiazepines are the worst offenders, but other drugs such as narcotics, anticholinergics, beta-blockers, steroids, nonsteroidal antiinflammatory drugs, digoxin, cimetidine can cause delirium; also, withdrawal states such as alcohol withdrawal or benzodiazepine withdrawal can cause delirium
- Infection or inflammation
- Metabolic: Kidney or liver failure, thyroid, adrenal, or glucose dysregulation, anemia, vitamin deficiency such as Wernicke encephalopathy or vitamin B_{12} deficiency, inborn metabolic errors such as porphyrias or Wilson disease
- Stress: Surgery, sleep problems, pain, fever, hypoxia, anesthesia, environmental changes, fecal or urinary retention, burns
- Fluids, electrolytes, nutrition (FEN): Dysregulation of calcium, magnesium, potassium, or sodium; dehydration; volume overload; altered pH
- Brain disorder: CNS infection, head injury, hypertensive encephalopathy

Dx DIAGNOSIS

DIFFERENTIAL DIAGNOSIS

- Primary psychiatric illness
- Focal syndromes
- Dementia
- Sundowning
- Nonconvulsive status epilepticus

Remember, delirium may coexist with any of the above. Table 3 summarizes the differential diagnosis of delirium. Table 4 describes clinical factors that help differentiate delirium and dementia from psychiatric disease.

LABORATORY TESTS

- Complete blood count, electrolytes, liver function tests, ammonia, drug levels (digoxin, lithium)
- Toxicology screen, urinalysis, urine culture
- Thyroid function tests, vitamin B_{12}, and folate levels
- Rapid plasma reagin for syphilis, blood, urine, and spinal fluid culture
- Arterial blood gas
- Lumbar puncture is mandatory when cause of delirium is not obvious

IMAGING STUDIES

- Consider head CT (to look for bleed, trauma, tumor, atrophy, dementia, stroke)
- Chest radiograph (to look for tumor, infection)

TABLE 1 Mnemonic for Risk Factors for Delirium and Agitation

Iwatchdeath	Delirium
Infection	**D**rugs
Withdrawal	**E**lectrolyte and physiologic abnormalities
Acute metabolic	**L**ack of drugs (withdrawal)
Trauma/pain	**I**nfection
Central nervous system pathology	**R**educed sensory input (blindness, deafness)
Hypoxia	**I**ntracranial problems (CVA, meningitis, seizure)
Deficiencies (vitamin B_{12}, thiamine)	**U**rinary retention and fecal impaction
Endocrinopathies (thyroid, adrenal)	**M**yocardial problems (MI, arrhythmia, CHF)
Acute vascular (hypertension, shock)	
Toxins/drugs	
Heavy metals	

CHF, Congestive heart failure; *CVA,* cerebrovascular accident; *MI,* myocardial infarction.
From Vincent JL et al: *Textbook of critical care,* ed 6, Philadelphia, 2011, Saunders.

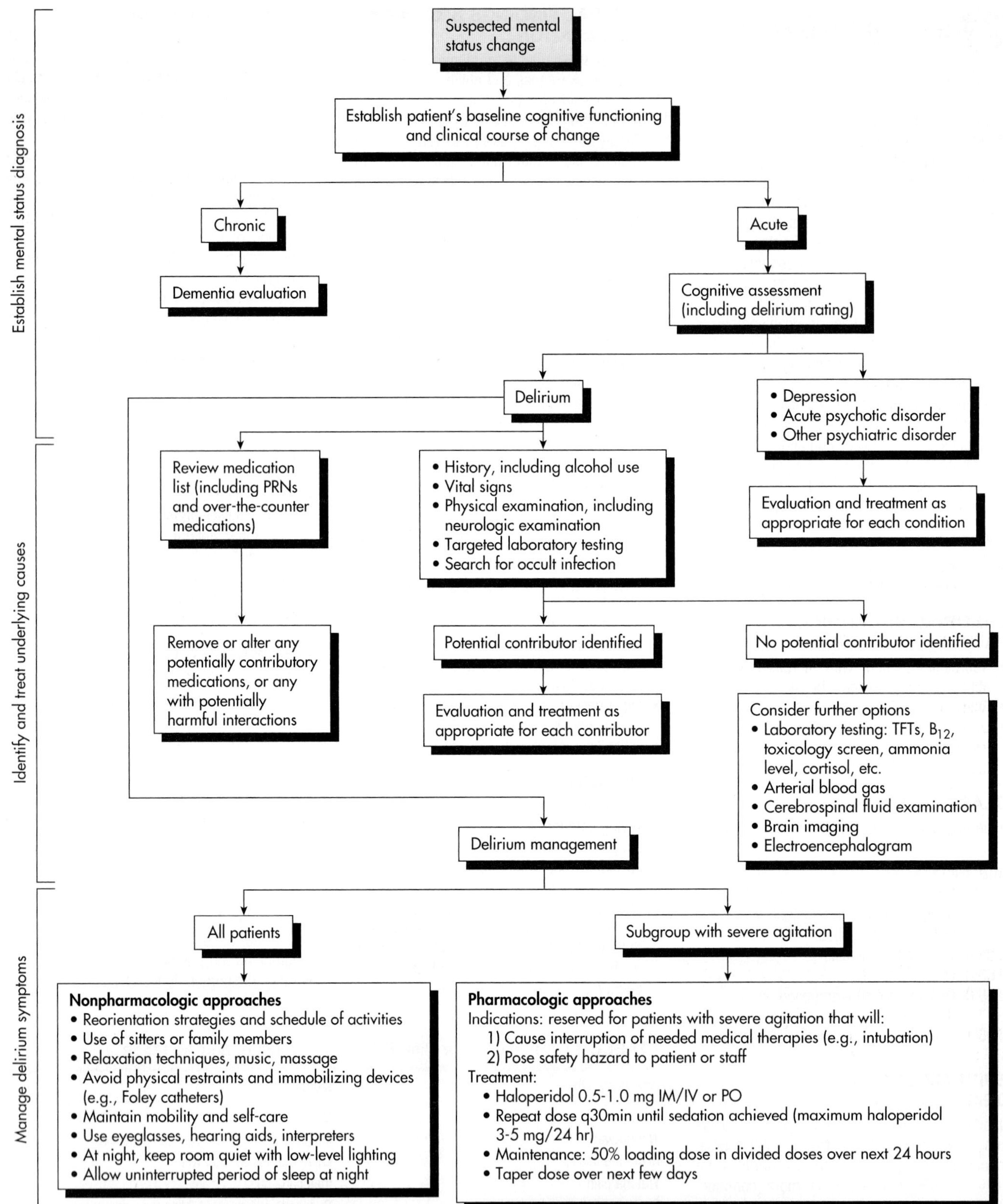

FIG. 1 Algorithm for evaluation of suspected mental status change in an older patient. *IM,* Intramuscular; *NG,* nasogastric; *PO,* by mouth; *PRN,* as needed; *TFTs,* thyroid function tests. (Modified from Goldman L, Ausiello D [eds]: *Cecil textbook of medicine,* ed 24, Philadelphia, 2012, Saunders.)

TABLE 2 Delirium Assessment Tools

Tool	Structure	Notes
Confusion Assessment Method (CAM)	Full scale of 11 items Abbreviated algorithm targeting four cardinal symptoms	Intended for use by nonpsychiatric clinicians
Confusion Assessment Method for the Intensive Care Unit (CAM-ICU)	Algorithm targeting four cardinal symptoms	Designed for use by nursing staff in the ICU
Intensive Care Delirium Screening Checklist (ICDSC)	8-item screening checklist	Bedside screening tool for use by nonpsychiatric physicians or nurses in the ICU
Delirium Rating Scale (DRS)	Full scale of 10 items Abbreviated 7- or 8-item subscales for repeated administration	Provides data for confirmation of diagnosis and measurement of severity
Delirium Rating Scale—Revised–98 (DRS-R-98)	16-item scale that can be divided into a 3-item diagnostic subscale and a 13-item severity subscale	Revision of DRS is better suited to repeat administration
Memorial Delirium Assessment Scale (MDAS)	10-item severity rating scale	Grades severity of delirium once diagnosis has been made
Neecham Confusion Scale	10-item rating scale	Designed for use by nursing staff and primarily validated for use in elderly populations in acute medical or nursing home setting

ICU, Intensive care unit.
Stern TA et al: *Massachusetts General Hospital handbook of general hospital psychiatry,* ed 7, Philadelphia, 2017, Elsevier.

ELECTROENCEPHALOGRAM

To exclude seizure, confirm diagnosis of metabolic encephalopathy

Rx TREATMENT

NONPHARMACOLOGIC THERAPY

- The most important consideration is to keep the patient safe by using a variety of methods, including frequent reorientation.
- A quiet, restful, simplified environment with cues to time and location such as clock or calendar is helpful, as well as consistent staff providing both personal and medical care. If possible, encourage familiar family members and friends to keep the patient company.
- Early mobilization and minimized use of physical restraints (use of physical restraints if necessary to ensure safety).
- Visual and hearing aids for patients with these impairments.

ACUTE GENERAL Rx

- Reverse any treatable cause, such as volume repletion for patients with dehydration, antibiotics for urinary tract infection.
- Pharmacologic treatment with antipsychotic agents should be initiated only when symptoms are severe, dangerous, or cause significant distress to the patient. In general these agents are similarly effective and the choice among them is usually made on the basis of side effects. Haloperidol is the least sedating but has a high risk of extrapyramidal side effects; quetiapine has the least side effects but is highly sedating.
- Haloperidol can be used with caution to control agitation, with doses ranging from 0.25 to 2 mg IM/IV twice daily, repeating the dose every 20 to 30 min until patient has calmed and using lower doses for the elderly.
- Most antipsychotics can prolong the QT interval and increase the risk of torsades de pointes.

TABLE 3 Differential Diagnosis of Delirium

General Cause	Specific Cause
Vascular	Hypertensive encephalopathy Cerebral arteriosclerosis Intracranial hemorrhage or thrombosis Emboli from atrial fibrillation, patent foramen ovale, or endocarditic valve Circulatory collapse (shock) Systemic lupus erythematosus Polyarteritis nodosa Thrombotic thrombocytopenic purpura Hyperviscosity syndrome Sarcoid Posterior reversible encephalopathy syndrome (PRES) Cerebral aneurysm
Infectious	Encephalitis Bacterial or viral meningitis, fungal meningitis (*cryptococcal, coccidioidal, histoplasma*) Sepsis General paresis Brain, epidural, or subdural abscess Malaria Human immunodeficiency virus Lyme disease Typhoid fever Parasitic (*toxoplasma, trichinosis, cysticercosis, echinococcosis*) Behçet's syndrome Mumps
Neoplastic	Space-occupying lesions, such as gliomas, meningiomas, abscesses Paraneoplastic syndromes Carcinomatous meningitis
Degenerative	Dementias Huntington disease Creutzfeldt–Jakob disease Wilson disease
Intoxication	Chronic intoxication or withdrawal effect of drugs, including sedative-hypnotics, opiates, tranquilizers, anticholinergics, dissociative anesthetics, anticonvulsants
Neurophysiologic	Epilepsy Postictal states Complex partial status epilepticus
Traumatic	Intracranial bleeds Postoperative trauma Heat stroke Fat emboli syndrome

Continued

TABLE 3 Differential Diagnosis of Delirium—cont'd

General Cause	Specific Cause
Intraventricular	Normal-pressure hydrocephalus
Vitamin deficiency	Thiamine (Wernicke–Korsakoff syndrome) Niacin (pellagra) B_{12} (pernicious anemia)
Endocrine/metabolic	Diabetic coma and shock Uremia Myxedema Hyperthyroidism Parathyroid dysfunction Hypoglycemia Hepatic or renal failure Porphyria Severe electrolyte or acid/base disturbances Cushing's or Addison syndrome Sleep apnea Carcinoid Whipple disease
Autoimmune	Autoimmune encephalitides Steroid-responsive encephalopathy associated with thyroiditis (SREAT)/ Hashimoto encephalopathy Systemic lupus erythematosus Multiple sclerosis
Poisoning	Heavy metals (lead, manganese, mercury) Carbon monoxide Anticholinergics Other toxins
Anoxia	Hypoxia and anoxia secondary to pulmonary or cardiac failure, anesthesia, anemia
Psychiatric	Depressive pseudodementia, catatonia, Bell mania

Stern TA et al: *Massachusetts General Hospital handbook of general hospital psychiatry,* ed 7, Philadelphia, 2017, Elsevier.

The effect is greatest with IV haloperidol and least with aripiprazole. Aripiprazole is available in tablets, solution, and injection. Starting dose is 1 mg twice a day.

- Risperidone 0.5 mg twice daily (off-label use, non-FDA approved) can also be used with caution with a slow increase to desired dose, not to exceed 1.0 to 2.0 mg.
- Avoid benzodiazepines and meperidine. Drug toxicity accounts for approximately 30% cases of delirium.

CHRONIC Rx

Delirium is not a chronic condition; if assessing a more long-term mental status change, consider other diagnoses.

DISPOSITION

Requires frequent monitoring often necessitating hospital level of care to ensure safety and assess etiology.

REFERRAL

Consider neurologic or psychiatric consultation if not improved in several days or in complicated cases.

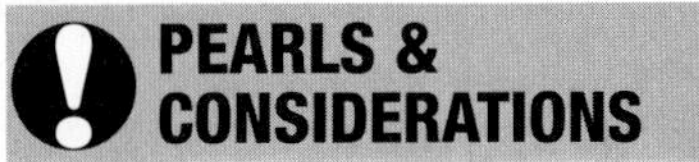

PEARLS & CONSIDERATIONS

COMMENTS

Although benzodiazepines are frequently used in hospitalized patients for sedation and are the mainstay of therapy for alcohol withdrawal, they must be used with caution in the elderly because they can have a paradoxical effect on agitation.

PREVENTION (TABLE 5)

- Avoid polypharmacy as much as possible.
- Optimize chronic medical conditions.
- Provide frequent reorientation and a soothing environment for high-risk patients (e.g., lights on during the day, off at night; open curtains during the day so patient can see the weather).
- In patients over 70 without dementia, regular exercise has been associated with lower risk for developing delirium, and early return to physical activity can improve outcomes in ill patients.

PATIENT & FAMILY EDUCATION

Inform about the above preventive techniques, especially polypharmacy risks.

SUGGESTED READINGS

Available at ExpertConsult.com

RELATED CONTENT

Delirium Tremens (Related Key Topic)

AUTHOR: **FRED F. FERRI, M.D.**

TABLE 4 Clinical Factors That Help Differentiate Delirium and Dementia from Psychiatric Disease

Characteristic	Delirium	Dementia	Psychiatric Illness
Symptoms			
Age at onset	<12 or >40 yr	Usually elderly, >50 yr	13-40 yr
Onset	Acute	Gradual or insidious	Gradual
Symptom course	Rapid, fluctuating	Stable and progressive	Stable
Duration	Days to weeks	Months to years	Months to years
Reversibility	Usually	Rarely	Rarely
History			
Past medical history	Substance abuse, medical illness	Comorbid conditions of aging	Previous psychiatric history
Family history	Unusual	History of dementia	History of psychiatric illness
Physical Examination			
Vital signs	Usually abnormal	Usually normal	Usually normal
Involuntary activity	May have tremors, asterixis, etc.	None unless coexistent disease	None
Mental Status			
Affect	Emotional lability	Flat affect with advanced disease	Flat affect
Orientation	Usually impaired	Impaired with advanced disease	Rarely impaired
Attention	Impaired	Slow to focus	Disorganized
Hallucinations	Primarily visual	Rare	Primarily auditory
Speech	Slow, incoherent, dysarthric	Usually coherent	Usually coherent
Consciousness	Decreased to impaired	Normal (clear)	Alert
Intellectual function	Usually impaired	Impaired	Intact

From Adams JG et al: *Emergency medicine, clinical essentials*, ed 2, Philadelphia, 2013, Elsevier.

TABLE 5 Priorities (Consensus, Evidence-Based, and Speculative) for the Prevention, Management, and Advancement of the Treatment of Delirium

Community-Based Prevention	Hospital-Based Prevention	Hospital-Based Management	Postdischarge Management	Clinical Research Opportunities
Hospital avoidance strategies	Implementation of basic standards (e.g., screening for delirium) Minimization of iatrogenesis*	Implementation of basic standards (e.g., review of medications)*	Responsive, proportionate, and holistic follow-up*	Pragmatic research into optimizing care delivery
Identification and management of frailty	Multicomponent interventions to address frailty† Reorientation† Nutrition† Multidisciplinary care* Physiologic correction† Sensory optimization† Minimization of ward transfers* Avoidance of polypharmacy†	Multicomponent interventions to address frailty* Reorientation* Nutrition* Multidisciplinary care* Physiologic correction* Sensory optimization* Minimization of ward transfers* Reduction of drug burden*	Identification and management of frailty Reduction and cessation of antipsychotics	The interaction between frailty, interventions to ameliorate frailty, and delirium Transference from basic science models to trials of newer therapies Validation of delirium models using advanced imaging
Pleiotropic interventions (e.g., exercise/ nutrition)	Monitor and promote early mobilization†	Monitor and promote early mobilization*	Review of the primary triggers for delirium and other state variables (e.g., mobility)	Delirium, mobility, and response to physical therapy
Early diagnosis and management of dementia	Screening for dementia*	Screening for delirium resolution and residual cognitive impairment	Screening for subsyndromal delirium or dementia*	The interaction between dementia, including non-Alzheimer dementia, and delirium
Education of nursing home facilities and staff	Education of nursing and medical staff*	Education of medical and nursing staff*	Caregiver support and education	The role of education of non-medical staff, families,‡ and general public using multimedia solutions
Integrated geriatric care for planned major surgery	Targeted drug treatments (e.g., melatonin for sleep disturbance)† Family-based screening/ reorientation†	Delirium units Supported early discharge Family-based screening/ reorientation* Management in the nursing home with CGA capability	Adaptive and versatile methods of follow-up such as telemedicine	The role of novel and targeted interventions and models of care supported by assistive technologies
Public health awareness	Audit of care and cycle of care improvement*	Audit of care and cycle of care improvement*	Public health awareness/ NGO engagement	Development of key indicators in the management of delirium

*Consensus role.
†Evidence-based role.
‡Speculative role.
CGA, Comprehensive geriatric assessment; *NGO*, non-governmental organization.
Fillit HM: *Brocklehurst's textbook of geriatric medicine and gerontology*, ed 8, 2017, Elsevier.

BASIC INFORMATION

DEFINITION

Delirium tremens, also known as withdrawal delirium, is overactivity of the central nervous system after cessation of alcohol intake. The time interval is variable; it usually occurs within 1 wk after reduction or cessation of heavy alcohol intake and persists for 1 to 3 days.

SYNONYMS

Withdrawal delirium
Alcohol withdrawal syndrome
DTs
Alcoholic delirium

ICD-10CM CODE

F10.231 Alcohol dependence with withdrawal delirium

EPIDEMIOLOGY & DEMOGRAPHICS

INCIDENCE (IN U.S.): Up to 500,000 cases annually, 3% to 5% of patients who are hospitalized for alcohol withdrawal meet the criteria for withdrawal delirium
PEAK INCIDENCE: 30 yr and older
PREDOMINANT SEX: Male
PEAK AGE: Teenage yrs and older
GENETICS: More common with patients who have relatives who are alcoholics

PHYSICAL FINDINGS & CLINICAL PRESENTATION

- Ethanol withdrawal symptoms usually begin within 8 hours after blood alcohol levels decrease, peak at about 72 hours, and are markedly reduced by days 5 to 7 of abstinence
- Initially: Anxiety, insomnia, tremulousness
- Early: Tachycardia, sweating, anorexia, agitation, headache, gastrointestinal distress
- Late: Seizures, visual hallucinations, delirium

ETIOLOGY

Alcoholism

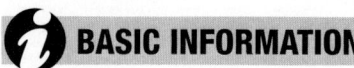

DIAGNOSIS

DIFFERENTIAL DIAGNOSIS

- Coexisting illness
- Trauma
- Drug use

WORKUP

- Frequent rating of symptoms (hallucinations, tremor, sweating, agitation, orientation).
- The Clinical Institute Withdrawal Assessment-Alcohol (CIWA-A) scale can be used to measure the severity of alcohol withdrawal. It consists of the 10 following items:
  1. Nausea
  2. Tremor
  3. Autonomic hyperactivity
  4. Anxiety
  5. Agitation
  6. Tactile disturbances
  7. Visual disturbances
  8. Auditory disturbances
  9. Headache
  10. Disorientation

  The maximum score is 67. Scores <8 indicate mild symptoms; scores 8-15 indicate moderate withdrawal symptoms; and scores >15 indicate severe withdrawal symptoms.

LABORATORY TESTS

- Electrolytes (including magnesium, phosphate)
- Close monitoring of glucose levels
- Drug screen (blood and urine)

IMAGING STUDIES

CT scan of head if there is a history of head trauma.

Rx TREATMENT

NONPHARMACOLOGIC THERAPY

Refer to drug rehabilitation program after patient recovers.

ACUTE GENERAL Rx

- Admission to a detoxification unit where patient can be observed closely.
- Vital signs q30min initially (neurologic signs, if necessary).
- Use of lateral decubitus or prone position if restraints are necessary.
- Nothing by mouth: Nasogastric tube for abdominal distention may be necessary but should not be routinely used.
- Vigorous hydration (4-6 L/day): IV with glucose (Na^+, K^+, PO_4^{-3}, and Mg^{2+} replacement). May be necessary in some patients but commonly there is little support for routine administration of magnesium. Use vigorous hydration with caution in patients with CHF.
- Vitamins: Thiamine 500 mg infused IV over the course of 30 minutes daily for 3 days. The initial dose of thiamine should precede the administration of IV dextrose; multivitamins (may be added to the hydrating solution).
- Sedation (sedation can be achieved using fixed-dose regimen or individualized benzodiazepine administration [see CIWA-Ar score] in "Alcohol-Related Disorders"):
  1. Initially: Lorazepam 8 mg IM/IV every 15 minutes as needed, after the patient has received 16 mg. If delirium is still severe, administer an 8 mg bolus IV, then administer 10 to 30 mg/hr.[1]
  2. Maintenance (individualized dosage): Chlordiazepoxide, 50 to 100 mg PO q4 to 6h, lorazepam 2 mg PO q4h, or diazepam 5 to 10 mg PO tid; withhold doses or decrease subsequent doses if signs of oversedation are apparent.
  3. Midazolam is also effective for managing DTs. Its rapid onset (sedation within 2 to 4 min of IV injection) and short duration of action (approximately 30 min) make it an ideal agent for titration in continuous infusion.
- In addition to benzodiazepines, administer medications such as the antipsychotic agent haloperidol for uncontrolled agitation or hallucinations (0.5-5 mg IV/IM every 30-60 minutes as needed for severe agitation or hallucinations, not to exceed 20 mg).
- Treatment of seizures: Diazepam 2.5 mg/min IV until seizure is controlled (check for respiratory depression or hypotension) may be beneficial for prolonged seizure activity; IV lorazepam 1 to 2 mg q2h can be used in place of diazepam. In general, withdrawal seizures are self-limited and treatment is not required; the use of phenytoin or other anticonvulsants for short-term treatment of alcohol withdrawal seizures is not recommended.
- Diagnosis and treatment of concomitant medical, surgical, or psychiatric conditions.

CHRONIC Rx

Alcoholics Anonymous has the best record in breaking addiction, but the results are still disappointing.

DISPOSITION

Refer to drug rehabilitation program

REFERRAL

If cardiac arrhythmias are prominent or respiratory distress develops.

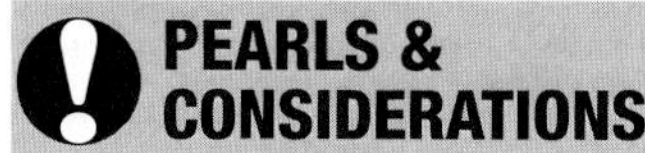

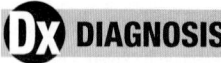

PEARLS & CONSIDERATIONS

COMMENTS

- This is a potentially lethal disease if not carefully treated. Mortality rate is 15% in untreated patients, and approximately 1% to 6% of hospitalized patients who have withdrawal delirium die.

SUGGESTED READING

Available at ExpertConsult.com

RELATED CONTENT

Delirium Tremens (Patient Information)
Alcohol Abuse (Related Key Topic)
Delirium (Related Key Topic)
Wernicke Syndrome (Related Key Topic)

AUTHOR: **FRED F. FERRI, M.D.**

[1] Schuckit MA: Recognition and management of withdrawal delirium (delirium tremens). *N Engl J Med* 371:2109-2113, 2014.

BASIC INFORMATION

DEFINITION

Dementia with Lewy bodies (DLB) is a neurodegenerative dementia occurring concurrently with or within 1 yr (either before or after) of the onset of parkinsonism. DLB also has other core features including fluctuations in attention and alertness and recurrent vivid visual hallucinations. Diagnostic criteria for dementia syndrome associated with Lewy body pathology are described in Box 1. Patients generally respond to cholinesterase inhibitors, are very sensitive to the adverse effects of neuroleptics, and compared with Parkinson's disease patients, are relatively unresponsive to L-dopa.

SYNONYMS

DLB
Lewy body dementia
Diffuse Lewy body disease
Lewy body type senile dementia
Cortical Lewy body disease

ICD-10CM CODE
G31.83 Dementia with Lewy bodies

EPIDEMIOLOGY & DEMOGRAPHICS

INCIDENCE: Accounts for 10% to 15% of all dementias. DLB is the second most common neurodegenerative cause of dementia after Alzheimer's disease.

PEAK INCIDENCE: Affects individuals in their sixth decade or older

PREVALENCE: Estimated 0.7% of individuals older than age 65

PREDOMINANT SEX AND AGE:
- Sex: Male predominance
- Mean age of onset: 75 yr. On average, 10 yr greater for dementia with Lewy bodies (DLB) than Parkinson's disease (PD).

GENETICS:
- Most cases are sporadic with a discordance among monozygotic twins, suggesting that either environmental or other epigenetic factors may play a major role in the incidence of DLB.
- Copy number variation of the alpha-synuclein gene (*SNCA*) has been reported in families with DLB. Rare autosomal dominant variants in *LRRK2* have also been reported. These genes are associated with Parkinson's disease and Parkinson's disease dementia in addition to DLB, suggesting a common molecular etiology with a spectrum of clinical phenotypes.
- The *APOE* ε4 allele has a higher prevalence in DLB than in control individuals, suggesting heightened disease risk conferred by the allele. Conversely, the *APOE* ε2 allele is enriched in control individuals, suggesting a neuroprotective role, or at least the lack of a deleterious effect, for the allele.
- Other factors include glucocerebrosidase genetic mutations, high prevalence of Lewy bodies with presenilin-1 mutations, and polymorphisms of the coding region for the synuclein genes.

RISK FACTORS:
- Male sex
- Advanced age

PHYSICAL FINDINGS & CLINICAL PRESENTATION

- Importance of recognizing DLB relates to its pharmacologic management, including responsiveness to cholinesterase inhibitors, sensitivity to the adverse effects of neuroleptics, and relative unresponsiveness to L-dopa.
- Onset of dementia is insidious, with core features of fluctuations in cognition, attention, and alertness; recurrent vivid visual hallucinations; and extrapyramidal motor symptoms, along with other features either suggestive or supportive of the clinical diagnosis.
- Syncopal events or unexplained episodes of severe alteration in mentation.
- Repeated falls.
- Detailed neuropsychological assessment demonstrates a characteristic profile of impairments in visuoperceptual, attentional, and executive functions, with relative sparing of episodic memory (in contradistinction to Alzheimer's diseases, in which impairment in episodic memory is a hallmark), reflecting a combination of cortical and subcortical damage.

ETIOLOGY

- *SNCA* encodes for a protein normally found at the synapse with a role in vesicle production. In its insoluble form, SNCA aggregates into Lewy bodies found at the cortical and subcortical levels.
- Lewy bodies (Fig. E1) are round, eosinophilic, intracytoplasmic inclusions in the nuclei of neurons.
- Cortical Lewy bodies are found in deep cortical layers of the anterior frontal and temporal lobes, the cingulate gyrus, and insula.
- As in Parkinson's disease, Lewy bodies aggregate in the following structures: substantia nigra, locus ceruleus, raphe nuclei, nucleus basalis of Meynert, and brainstem nuclei.
- Fig. 2 shows the relationships among the subtypes of dementia.

DIAGNOSIS

DIFFERENTIAL DIAGNOSIS

- Diagnosis of DLB when dementia occurs before or concurrently with extrapyramidal features—arbitrarily set as the "1-year rule" vs. Parkinson's disease with dementia, which occurs in the setting of well-established Parkinson's disease.
- Dementia: Alzheimer's disease (AD), vascular dementia, frontotemporal dementia.
- Parkinsonian features: Parkinson's disease dementia, progressive supranuclear palsy (PSP), multisystem atrophy (MSA), corticobasal syndrome (CBS).
- Rapidly progressive form: Creutzfeldt-Jakob disease (CJD). Lack of cerebellar signs and lack of typical MRI may help distinguish DLB from classic CJD (but not variant form of CJD).
- Psychiatric features: Late-onset psychosis or depression with psychotic features.
- Hallucinations with fluctuations in consciousness: Temporal lobe epilepsy (TLE) or delirium due to metabolic derangement.

WORKUP

- Lumbar puncture to rule out underlying chronic infections. Protein 14-3-3 may be present in both DLB and CJD.
- Electroencephalogram (EEG) to rule out potential TLE. However, either DLB or TLE may show nonspecific slowing or periodic complexes.
- MRI of the brain to evaluate for structural causes of dementia and to exclude MRI features of CJD.

LABORATORY TESTS

- Rule out other potential reversible causes for dementia including:
  1. Hormonal dysregulation: Thyroid stimulating hormone, free thyroxine
  2. Vitamin deficiency: Thiamine, cyanocobalamin, folate
  3. Vascular risk factors: Lipid profile, Hgb A_{1c}, homocysteine, syphilis (FTA-ABS), or ApoE genotype

IMAGING STUDIES

- MRI typically shows a relative preservation of the hippocampi and medial temporal lobe volumes (in contrast to AD) but generalized atrophy and white matter changes.

BOX 1 Diagnostic Criteria for the Dementia Syndrome Associated with Lewy Body Pathology

The cognitive disturbance is of insidious onset and is progressive, based on evidence from the history or serial cognitive examination
The presence of at least two of the following:
- Parkinsonism (rigidity, resting tremor, bradykinesia, postural instability, parkinsonian gait disorder)
- Prominent, fully formed visual hallucinations
- Substantial fluctuations in alertness or cognition
- Rapid eye movement sleep behavior disorder
- Severe worsening of parkinsonism by antipsychotic drugs
- The disturbance is not better accounted for by a systemic disease or another brain disease

From Goldman L, Schafer AI: *Goldman's Cecil medicine,* ed 24, Philadelphia, 2012, Saunders.

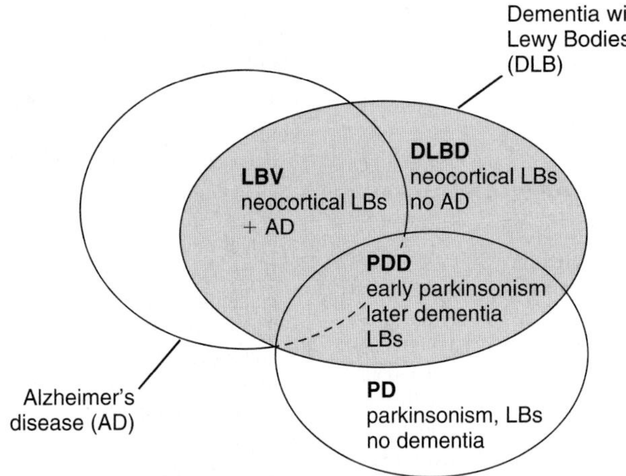

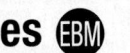

FIG. 2 Relationships among Alzheimer's disease (AD), the three subtypes of dementia with Lewy bodies (DLB), and Parkinson's disease (PD). Parkinsonism refers to the clinical symptoms of PD (hypokinesia, tremor, and muscular rigidity). *DLBD,* Diffuse Lewy body disease; *LBs,* Lewy bodies; *LBV,* Lewy body variant of Alzheimer's disease; *PD,* Parkinson's disease; *PDD,* Parkinson's disease dementia. (From Lewis KA, et al.: Abnormal neurites containing C-terminally truncated α-synuclein are present in Alzheimer's disease without conventional Lewy body pathology, *Am J Pathol* 177(6):3037–3050, 2010.)

- Functional imaging including single photon emission computed tomography (SPECT) may demonstrate hypoperfusion of the occipital region (specific finding but not sensitive).

Rx TREATMENT

Patient and caregiver education on benefits, side effects, and limitations of treatment is very important. Based on the preference of the patient and caregiver, a fine balance between psychosis and parkinsonism features confounds the treatment choices. Caregivers may be encouraged to avoid neuroleptics unless the psychotic features either trouble or endanger the patient. If neuroleptics must be used, typical neuroleptics must be avoided.

NONPHARMACOLOGIC THERAPY

- Social interaction and environmental novelty may improve cognitive dysfunction and psychiatric features often exacerbated by low levels of arousal and attention.
- Behavioral methods, such as avoiding previously exposed environmental triggers known to cause anxiety, agitation, or aggression.
- Physical therapy, mobility aids, and daily exercise.

ACUTE GENERAL Rx

Atypical neuroleptic for disabling, persistent, bothersome (to the patient) psychotic features despite initiation of a cholinesterase inhibitor. A very low dose of an atypical antipsychotic (quetiapine 12.5 mg daily) may be started after patient/caregiver education regarding the sensitivity to neuroleptics. However, neuroleptics do carry a black box warning about the increased mortality risk associated with their use in patients with dementia. Patients and/or caregivers should be informed of this risk and allowed to balance the risk against the perceived benefit.

CHRONIC Rx

- Cholinesterase inhibitors for cognitive and behavioral symptoms. Rivastigmine (6 to 12 mg per day orally or 9.5 mg per day by transdermal patch) has shown in randomized controlled trial (RCT) a significant reduction in anxiety, delusions, and hallucinations, as well as significantly improved performance on neuropsychological testing.
- Antiparkinson medications for disabling parkinsonian features. L-dopa is reported to be more effective with fewer side effects than dopamine agonists. Begin at a low dose of L-dopa (25/100 mg tid), and slowly titrate over several weeks as tolerated and according to response.
- Selective serotonin reuptake inhibitors are commonly used for depression.
- If rapid eye movement (REM) sleep disorder remains disabling (or patient has not responded to an atypical antipsychotic initiated for psychosis), a trial of low-dose clonazepam (0.25-0.5 mg) or melatonin (3 mg) at bedtime remains an option.
- Orthostatic hypotension may be aided by nonpharmacologic therapy such as supportive stockings or pharmacologically by midodrine and/or fludrocortisone.
- Memantine demonstrated an improvement in clinical global measure and remains well tolerated but may worsen hallucinations or delusions.
- Avoid anticholinergics (including tricyclic antidepressants) and benzodiazepines, as they can trigger delirium and worsen symptoms.

DISPOSITION

- Survival resembles the progression of AD, but a minority of cases may have a rapid disease course.
- Progression in cognitive decline, similar to AD, by approximately 10% per yr on cognitive testing.

REFERRAL

DLB requires a multidisciplinary approach including the general practitioner, neurologist, neuropsychologist, and/or neuropsychiatrist.

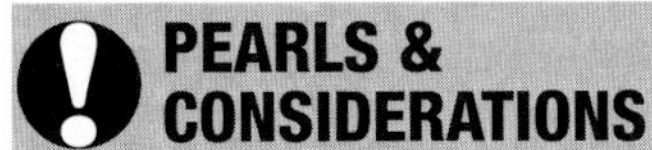

PEARLS & CONSIDERATIONS

COMMENTS

- Clinical presentation helps differentiate DLB from AD. AD presents with early signs of anterograde episodic memory loss without the benefit of cues on neuropsychological testing due to cortical atrophy at the medial temporal lobe region.
- Vascular dementia may also present with evidence of frontal-subcortical features but typically without the core features listed in the criteria above.
- Bed partners may report that individuals with DLB "act out their dreams," sometimes violently, leading to sleeping in separate beds. This history may indicate REM sleep behavior disorder. A history of REM sleep behavior may precede the diagnosis by many yrs. However, REM sleep behavior does not necessarily lead to DLB.

PATIENT/FAMILY EDUCATION

- Visual hallucinations (VH) typically consist of innocuous, well-formed, detailed images of animate figures. These are classically labeled Lilliputian, as the hallucinatory images are often relatively small. Unless VH lead to a potential threat to self or others, avoid antipsychotics due to the sensitivity of neuroleptics. Family/friends are often more alarmed by the VH than the patient with DLB.
- Apathy is a common clinical feature of DLB and mimics changes in mood, including depression, or excessive daytime somnolence. These features are often noticed by family/friends.

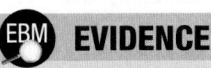

EVIDENCE

Available at ExpertConsult.com

SUGGESTED READINGS

Available at ExpertConsult.com

AUTHORS: **ANGAD JOLLY, M.D,** and **JOSEPH S. KASS, M.D., J.D.**

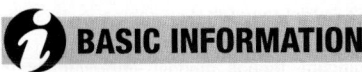

BASIC INFORMATION

DEFINITION

Major depression is an episodic, frequently recurring syndrome. The diagnosis requires that 5 of 9 criteria be present for 2 wk. One of these 9 criteria must be either a persistent depressed mood or pervasive anhedonia (loss of interest or pleasure in all, or almost all, usual interests or activities). Other symptoms include sleep disturbance (insomnia or hypersomnia), appetite loss/gain or weight loss/gain, fatigue, psychomotor retardation or agitation, difficulty concentrating or indecisiveness, feelings of guilt or worthlessness, and recurrent thoughts of death or suicidal ideation.

SYNONYMS

Unipolar affective disorder
Clinical depression
Melancholia
Manic-depressive illness, depressed type
Depressive episode

Codes depend on whether the episode is single or recurrent, and also on clinical severity.

ICD-10CM CODES

F32.9	Depressive episode, unspecified
F33.0	Recurrent depressive episode, current episode mild
F33.1	Recurrent depressive disorder, current episode moderate
F33.2	Recurrent depressive disorder, current episode severe without psychotic symptoms
F33.3	Recurrent depressive disorder, current episode severe with psychotic symptoms
F33.4	Recurrent depressive disorder, currently in remission
F33.9	Recurrent depressive disorder, unspecified

DSM-5 CODES

296.21	Single episode
296.22	Single episode, moderate
296.23	Single episode, severe
296.24	Single episode, with psychotic features
296.31	Recurrent, mild
296.32	Recurrent, moderate
296.33	Recurrent severe
296.34	Recurrent, with psychotic features

EPIDEMIOLOGY & DEMOGRAPHICS

LIFETIME RISK (IN U.S.): 10% of men, 20% of women

PREVALENCE (IN U.S.): Point prevalence in a community sample is 3% of men, 4.5% to 9.3% of women, and 1% of children. Prevalence of 20% to 40% in patients with comorbid medical conditions.

PREDOMINANT SEX: Female/male ratio 2:1

PREDOMINANT AGE: 25 to 44 yr; 5% of adolescents

PEAK INCIDENCE: 30 to 40 yr; 13% of postpartum women

GENETICS:

- Clear evidence of familial predominance.
- Prevalence is 2 to 3 times greater among first-degree relatives.
- Concordance among monozygotic twins approximately 50%.
- Several studies have documented associations between various genes and increased risk for MDD, but there remains no established pattern of inheritance.

PHYSICAL FINDINGS & CLINICAL PRESENTATION

- Clinical evaluation facilitated by organizing the major symptoms into four hallmarks: (1) depressed mood, (2) anhedonia, (3) physical symptoms (sleep disturbance, appetite problem, fatigue, psychomotor changes), and (4) psychological symptoms (difficulty concentrating or indecisiveness, guilt or worthlessness, and suicidal ideation).
- A stressful life event, typically a serious loss, may trigger a depressive episode. DSM-5 recommends that clinical judgment be used to determine if depression in the context of a loss should be diagnosed as a major depressive episode.
- Patients often present with somatic complaints such as pain, fatigue, insomnia, dizziness, headache, or gastrointestinal problems. Somatic complaints may be reported more frequently among certain ethnic groups than depressed mood, increasing risk for underdetection in these groups.
- Comorbid psychiatric disorders are often present. Anxiety disorders are the most common comorbid conditions.
- May be associated with mood-congruent delusional thinking (paranoid and melancholic themes).
- May be associated with active or passive suicidal ideation.
- Serious misconduct may appear in adolescents.
- May be underdiagnosed in elderly patients, with signs and symptoms attributed to normal aging.
- May be underdiagnosed in medically ill patients, with signs and symptoms attributed to medical illness or considered appropriate reaction to medical condition.

ETIOLOGY

- A heterogeneous group of disorders probably arising from various etiologies.
- Genetic and environmental experiences, and their interaction, each contribute.
- Significant psychosocial stressors, including loss and history of childhood abuse or adversity, often trigger depression, particularly for first episodes.
- Numerous biologic correlates have been identified, though none is considered causative or diagnostic. Genes that influence the production and reuptake of serotonin, norepinephrine, dopamine, and glutamate, as well as nerve cell growth in brain regions underlying memory and emotional processing, are of greatest interest. Abnormalities in brain regions underlying executive functioning, emotion regulation, and reward processing, as well as irregularities in functional connectivity have been identified. Irregularities in cortisol responding and inflammation also may play a role.
- Cognitive risk factors include a pessimistic style of explaining negative events, a tendency to ruminate, and biases in processing emotional information and events.

DIAGNOSIS

DIFFERENTIAL DIAGNOSIS

- Anxiety disorders (e.g., social phobia, PTSD, obsessive compulsive disorder), substance abuse, and personality disorders often present with depressive symptoms.
- Important to determine if a depressive episode is part of major depression or part of bipolar disorder.
- Important to distinguish from adjustment disorder. Depression in the context of a stressful life event is diagnosed as major depressive disorder if the symptom criteria are met and adjustment disorder if the symptom criteria are not met. There is no evidence that medication is effective for adjustment disorder.
- Approximately 10% to 15% of depression caused by general medical illnesses, such as Alzheimer's disease, Parkinson's disease, stroke, end-stage renal failure, cardiac disease, HIV infection, and cancer.
- Some medical conditions present as depression (e.g., hypothyroidism, hyperthyroidism, or neurosyphilis).
- Premenstrual dysphoric disorder.
- In elderly, depression often coexists with dementia.

WORKUP

- Careful medical history is required.
- Physical examination reveals no specific diagnostic signs of depression.
- Mental status examination.
- Self-report scales can assist in screening.
- Commonly used validated screening tools include the 15-item Geriatric Depression Scale in the elderly and the Patient Health Questionnaire (PHQ)-2 and PHQ-9. The PHQ-2 has a 97% sensitivity and 67% specificity in adults. If it is positive for depression, the PHQ-9 should be administered. The PHQ-9 has a 61% sensitivity and 94% specificity for depression in adults.

LABORATORY TESTS

- Research is underway to identify biomarkers that may be useful in diagnosis, but as of yet no laboratory studies are diagnostic.
- The following can assist in ruling out other confounding issues:
  1. Routine blood chemistry evaluation
  2. CBC with differential
  3. Thyroid function studies
  4. Vitamin B_{12} levels

IMAGING STUDIES

With unusual presentations (e.g., associated with new-onset severe headache, focal neurologic signs, a cognitive or sensory disturbance), the following may be performed:

- EEG (diffuse slowing indicates metabolic encephalopathy)
- Anatomic brain imaging (CT scan or MRI)

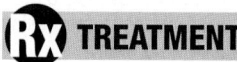

TREATMENT

NONPHARMACOLOGIC THERAPY

- Good evidence that cognitive-behavioral therapy is as effective as antidepressant medication in achieving significant reduction or remission (Table 1).
- Problem solving and interpersonal psychotherapies are comparably efficacious.
- "New wave" cognitive-behavioral therapies (e.g., acceptance and commitment therapy, mindfulness-based CBT) have demonstrated efficacy in numerous studies. It is unclear as of yet whether new-wave versus traditional behavioral therapies differ in mechanisms of action. Individuals not responding adequately to traditional behavioral therapies may benefit.
- Growing evidence indicates that Internet-based CBT and brief therapy interventions integrated into primary care to expand access to therapy are efficacious, with some studies finding comparable efficacy to standard length interventions, but further research is needed.
- By 12 wk or earlier, psychotherapy and medication approaches are equally effective.
- Augmentation of standard depression treatment with CBT to address insomnia (CBT-I) was found to significantly improve response rates.
- Official treatment guidelines recommend that medication be used as the first-line treatment for patients with severe depression, although some studies have found equal efficacy of medication and psychotherapy in the treatment of severe depression.
- Evidence, although mixed, indicates that combined psychotherapy and medication may be more effective than either treatment alone. Various types of evidence-based psychotherapy or augmentation with psychotherapy, including CBT and mindfulness-based behavioral therapy, appear to reduce the risk for future recurrences compared to medication alone in some but not all studies, particularly when medication is discontinued after symptomatic remission.
- Factors, including history of childhood maltreatment, presence of precipitant stressful life events, family psychiatric history, the presence of anhedonia, and depression severity, may affect treatment response and risk of recurrence. Numerous genetic and neurobiologic variables that predict treatment response have been identified, particularly in combination with one another or with clinical characteristics. However, as of yet there are no universally accepted markers that can aid clinicians in matching individuals to particular medications or interventions.

ACUTE GENERAL Rx

- Concurrent medical or psychiatric illnesses, history of prior response, cost, patient preference, and side effects should be considered when selecting initial treatment.
- Antidepressants are helpful in approximately 60% to 70% of cases, though sustained remission rates are lower.
- Selective serotonin reuptake inhibitors (SSRIs) generally are first-line. According to the STAR-D trial, approximately 30% achieve remission with the first prescribed medication after 3 months of treatment. Another 25% to 30% respond to treatment but do not achieve remission. Treatment-refractory patients should be switched to another SSRI or to another class of medication, offered adjunctive medication such as bupropion, or referred for evidence-based counseling. Approximately 25% more patients will achieve remission with this secondary intervention.
- Response to antidepressants for many patients is seen as early as 2 wk, and among patients showing little to no response, the odds of later response decrease the longer patients remain unimproved. Conversely, rapid response to treatment predicted improved outcomes in multiple studies.
- To date no benefit of combining antidepressants as first-line treatment. Also no clear advantage has been identified for switching medications within vs. across different classes, or to switching vs. augmentation. The VAST-D trial found that switching to the antipsychotic aripiprazole resulted in statistically significant, though modest, improvement in remission rates compared with switching or augmenting with an antidepressant, although greater side effects resulted. More research is needed.
- Therapy should be continued for 4 to 9 mo after the full remission of symptoms.
- Electroconvulsive therapy is the most effective means available for the treatment of severe, refractory depression. Transcranial magnetic stimulation has also shown evidence of efficacy though the magnitude of effects is more variable. To date electroconvulsive therapy has shown superior efficacy; research is under way to investigate mechanisms to increase the efficacy of TMS.
- Antipsychotic medication should be added for psychotic depression. Antipsychotic medication has also been shown to be helpful in augmenting antidepressants for nonpsychotic depression, and it may be beneficial for individuals with mixed features, although more research is needed.
- Ketamine found to be rapidly effective in treatment-resistant depression. However, treatment remains experimental, and effects usually do not persist.

TABLE 1 Treatments of Depression

Name of Psychotherapy	Approach
Cognitive psychotherapy	Identify and correct negativistic patterns of thinking.
Interpersonal psychotherapy	Identify and work through role transitions or interpersonal losses, conflicts, or deficits.
Problem-solving therapy	Identify and prioritize situational problems; plan and implement strategies to deal with top-priority problems.
Psychodynamic psychotherapy	Use therapeutic relationship to maximize use of the healthiest defense mechanisms and coping strategies.

From Goldman L et al: *Goldman's Cecil medicine,* ed 24, Philadelphia, 2012, Saunders.

CHRONIC Rx

Long-term treatment, in some cases lifelong, is recommended for multiple depressive episodes, an episode duration longer than 2 yr, a severe episode or significant suicidality, or a strong family history of severe depression or bipolar disorder.

DISPOSITION

- Major depression is often a relapsing and remitting illness.
- Physical symptoms may predict a favorable response to biologic intervention in some but not all studies.
- Additional episodes experienced by >50% after one episode, with each additional episode linked to increased risk for subsequent episodes.
- Without treatment, episodes last an average of 6 to 12 mo; risk of recurrence higher without treatment.
- For many depressed individuals, subthreshold residual symptoms are present between episodes and define the majority of an individual's course of depression. Such symptoms may lead to impairment and warrant prolonged treatment.
- Anxious distress, as defined by the DSM-5 specifier, was found in one recent study to predict greater clinical severity and functional impairment, above and beyond comorbid anxiety disorder diagnoses.

REFERRAL

- If treatment refractory
- If patient suicidal or psychotic
- For suspected bipolar depression

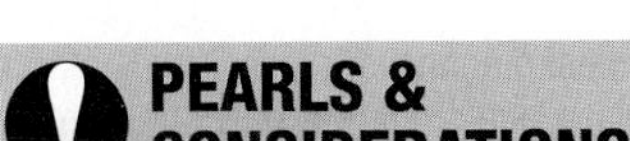

PEARLS & CONSIDERATIONS

COMMENTS

- All threats of suicide should be taken very seriously. Clinicians can use the mnemonic SAL: Is the method specific? Is it available? Is it lethal?
- Rule out bipolar affective disorder before initiating antidepressant medication. Screening scales for bipolar disorder can be helpful in primary care settings to identify patients at increased risk for bipolar disorder, although unclear benefit in mental health settings.
- Many patients and families reluctant to acknowledge depression because of stigma.
- A two-question screener is as effective as longer instruments. A positive answer to either question warrants a full assessment.
  1. Over the past 2 weeks, have you ever felt down, depressed, or hopeless?
  2. Over the past 2 weeks, have you felt little interest or pleasure in doing things?
- Depression screening programs without treatment programs are unlikely to improve depression outcomes.
- Strict monitoring of patients who initiate antidepressant therapy is necessary both for safety and to ensure optimal treatment. Use of self-report scales to measure symptom severity is helpful in monitoring outcome and may result in improved outcomes.

SUGGESTED READING

Available at ExpertConsult.com

RELATED CONTENT

Depression (Patient Information)
Bipolar Disorder (Related Key Topic)

AUTHORS: **MARK ZIMMERMAN, M.D.,** and **CATHERINE D'AVANZATO, PH.D.**

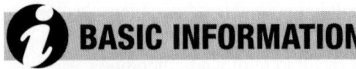

BASIC INFORMATION

DEFINITION

Dermatitis herpetiformis (DH) is an autoimmune blistering disease that is considered to be a cutaneous manifestation of celiac disease (CD). It is associated with gluten-sensitive enteropathy in nearly all cases, although only 20% of patients have gastrointestinal symptoms. 15% to 25% of patients with CD will have DH.

SYNONYMS

DH
Duhring disease

ICD-10CM CODE
L13.0 Dermatitis herpetiformis

EPIDEMIOLOGY & DEMOGRAPHICS

PREVALENCE (IN U.S.): 11 cases per 100,000 persons per yr; prevalence for CD is one in 133 adults

PREDOMINANT SEX: Male predominance (2:1); however, female predominance in children

PREDOMINANT AGE: Fourth decade of life, but can occur at any age

PREDOMINANT RACE: Most common in Caucasians of Northern European ancestry

GENETICS: Both CD and DH have a strong genetic component. 10% to 15% of patients with DH have a first-degree relative with either DH or CD. Specific HLA genes (involved in processing gliadin antigen in genetically susceptible individuals) have also been shown to predispose to developing DH (HLA-DQ2 in 90%, DQ8 in the remaining 10%). However, less than 50% of genetic predisposition is attributed to HLA genes.

PHYSICAL FINDINGS & CLINICAL PRESENTATION

- Classically, the lesions of DH are small, grouped, "herpetiform" vesicles that are distributed symmetrically on extensor surfaces (elbows, knees [Fig. 1], scalp, back, and buttocks). However, due to intense pruritus and scratching, pinpoint erosions and excoriations in the above distribution are often the most prominent findings on examination, with intact vesicles rarely seen.
- Spontaneous improvement with cyclic exacerbations is common.
- Celiac-type enamel defects to permanent teeth, oral vesicles, or palmoplantar purpura have been reported as potential associated findings.

PATHOGENESIS

CD and DH are both autoimmune-mediated by IgA class autoantibodies. Dietary gluten is central to the pathogenesis in both. In genetically predisposed individuals, it is hypothesized that the gluten by-product, gliadin, complexes with tissue transglutaminase (tTG) in the gut, binding as an antigen to HLA-DQ2 on T-cells, creating an immune response that results in anti-tTG IgA antibodies (i.e., antiendomysial antibodies) in the blood. tTG cross-reacts with epidermal TG (eTG). The blood of CD patients with and without skin disease is found to have both skin and gut anti-TG IgA antibodies. Yet, it is thought that the high-affinity IgA against eTG form complexes that are responsible for DH. The deposition of IgA-eTG complexes in the papillary dermis triggers an immunologic cascade resulting in neutrophil recruitment and complement activation.

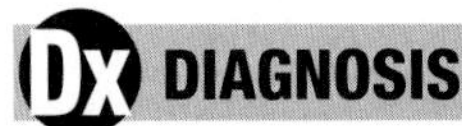

DIAGNOSIS

Physical examination and routine histopathology are often suggestive of DH; however, direct immunofluorescence (DIF) of a perilesional skin biopsy has pathognomonic findings and is the gold standard for diagnosis. Fig. 2 describes an approach to the patient with suspected dermatitis herpetiformis.

DIFFERENTIAL DIAGNOSIS

- Clinically and histologically, the differential diagnosis includes:
  1. Linear IgA dermatosis
  2. Bullous pemphigoid
  3. Bullous lupus

  These diagnoses can be differentiated by DIF on perilesional skin biopsy.
- Other clinical diagnoses to consider:
  1. Scabies (check for interdigital burrows and involvement of genitalia)
  2. Arthropod bite (papular urticaria over exposed areas)
  3. Eczematous dermatitis (ill-defined, weeping erythematous plaques)
  4. Herpes simplex or zoster infection (painful, not symmetric)
  5. Generalized pruritus (no blister history)

WORKUP, LABORATORY TESTS

- Evaluation for gastrointestinal symptoms, family history of DH or CD, and pruritus should be sought in patients with suspected DH.
- **Lesional skin biopsy**: Will demonstrate a neutrophil-rich subepidermal bulla and rule out many conditions.
- **DIF of normal-appearing perilesional skin biopsy**: Will demonstrate pathognomonic IgA deposits localized to the dermal papillae and dermal-epidermal junction in a granular pattern.
- Although circulating antibodies in the blood exist (IgA tissue transglutamase, IgA epidermal transglutaminase, IgA endomysial antibodies), they are not part of the diagnostic work-up due to high false-positive rate for antitissue TG and one third of patients being negative for antiendomysial antibodies. However, they can be helpful in suggesting the diagnosis of DH in cases where linear IgA cannot be excluded on DIF or for monitoring disease activity response to treatment. It is important to check total IgA levels because an IgA-deficient DH patient may have negative serologic results. ELISA testing is also available for these antibodies.

TREATMENT

A gluten-free diet (GFD) and dapsone are considered first-line therapy and are often started in conjunction.

- GFD improves symptoms of both GI and skin disease, with GI responding quicker (skin responds after 2 months). A retrospective study showed remission (2 yr without symptoms) in 12%.
- Dapsone results in improvement of skin manifestations within days but does not treat GI manifestations. Dapsone is typically tapered over time, while lifelong gluten avoidance is often necessary.

One study demonstrated GFD alone was comparable to GFD plus dapsone in the treatment of DH; hence GFD is an essential component in the treatment of DH.

NONPHARMACOLOGIC THERAPY

- First line: GFD
  1. Avoid barley, rye, wheat (can consume rice, corn, and oats).
  2. Consultation with a dietitian is recommended.
  3. Most patients need to follow diet indefinitely; however, cases of spontaneous remission have been reported.
- Second line: Elemental diet (controversial)
  1. Can consider elemental diet (avoidance of whole proteins) in those patients who do

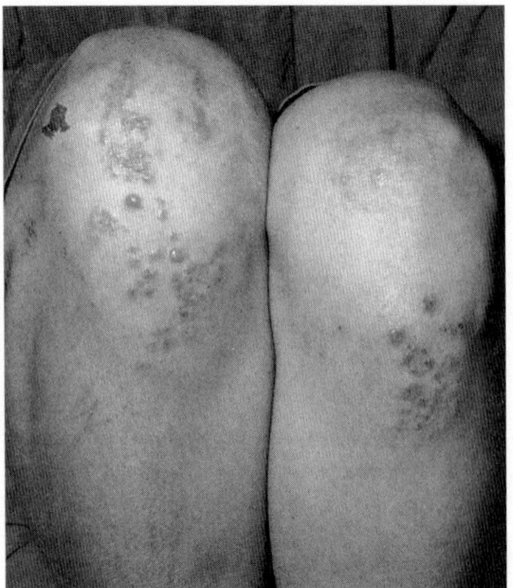

FIG. 1 Dermatitis herpetiformis. (From James WD, et al.: *Andrews' diseases of the skin*, ed 12, Philadelphia, 2016, Elsevier.)

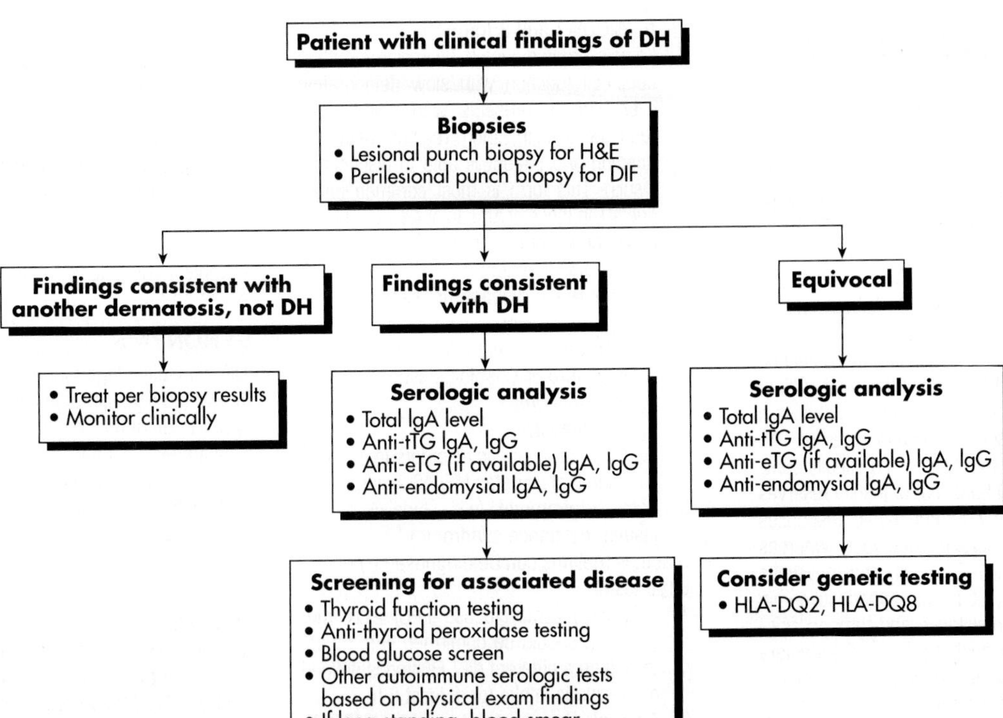

FIG. 2 Approach to the patient with suspected dermatitis herpetiformis. *DH*, Dermatitis herpetiformis; *DIF*, direct immunofluorescence; *eTG*, epidermal transglutaminase; *H&E*, hematoxylin and eosin; *HLA-DQ2*, histocompatibility locus antigen haplotype DQ2; *HLA-DQ8*, histocompatibility locus antigen haplotype DQ8; *Ig*, immunoglobulin; *tIG*, tetanus immune globulin. (From Bolotin D, Petronic-Rosic V: Dermatitis herpetiformis: Part II. Diagnosis, management, and prognosis, *J Am Acad Dermatol* 64(6):1027–1033, 2011.)

not adequately respond to a strict GFD; however, data are limited.

ACUTE GENERAL Rx

- First line: Dapsone
  1. Initial dose 25-50 mg PO daily with gradual increase to an average maintenance dose of 0.5-1 mg/kg daily (often maintenance dose of 100 mg daily).
  2. Clinical monitoring weekly is recommended to optimize dose (optimal dose is when 1-2 new lesions/wk).
  3. Caution: Dapsone may produce hemolysis (especially if G6PD deficiency), agranulocytosis, methemoglobinemia, systemic drug hypersensitivity reaction (DRESS), and a peripheral neuropathy.
  4. Baseline labs: CBC, LFTs, G6PD levels. After the initiation of therapy, monitor CBC every week ×1 month, then every other week ×2 months, monthly ×3 months, then every 3-4 months. Monitor LFTs every 3-4 months.
- Second-line alternatives
  1. Sulfapyridine (500-1500 mg/day) or sulfasalazine (500-1000 mg bid) may be substituted in cases of dapsone intolerance or in the rare case that neuropathy develops.
  2. Case reports of efficacy using topical dapsone 5% twice daily in patients who do not tolerate oral dapsone; also reported to be efficacious as an adjuvant to oral dapsone.
  3. Uncontrolled studies and case reports have suggested efficacy with tetracyclines, nicotinamide, cyclosporine, colchicine, and heparin.
- Symptomatic relief for pruritus
  1. Potent and superpotent topical corticosteroids (atrophy with prolonged use, limit to 14 days per month), nonsedating antihistamines twice daily, sedating antihistamines at bedtime, mentholated lotion

CHRONIC Rx

- As DH is considered to represent the cutaneous manifestations of CD, lifelong avoidance of gluten is typically recommended. Information about educational resources, such as national and local support groups, should be provided (www.celiac.org).
- Patients with DH and CD have an increased risk of developing Hashimoto thyroiditis (50% with thyroid disease), non-Hodgkin's lymphoma, and GI lymphomas. An increased incidence of other autoimmune disorders (type 1 diabetes mellitus, pernicious anemia, Addison disease, vitiligo, systemic lupus erythematosus, rheumatoid arthritis, and Sjögren's syndrome) and osteoporosis have also been reported.
  1. Screening for thyroid disease (TSH, antithyroid peroxidase antibody titers) is typically recommended.
  2. Screening for autoimmune connective tissue diseases should be considered if there are suspicious signs or symptoms.
  3. Routine screening for GI lymphomas is controversial.

REFERRAL

- Dermatologist for skin biopsy and management of cutaneous disease
- Gastroenterologist for evaluation of CD
- Nutritionist to educate patients about gluten-free diet
- National support groups (www.celiac.org) and local support groups

PEARLS & CONSIDERATIONS

- Classic areas involved are those that are exposed if in a "fetal position."
- Lesions may be worsened by iodides and certain NSAIDs; systemic steroids ineffective.
- Location of biopsies is IMPORTANT: False-negative DIF can result if biopsies are taken from lesional skin (should be taken from normal-appearing skin adjacent to lesion) as diagnostic IgA deposits are usually destroyed by the blistering process.
- GFD results in reduced IgA in skin on DIF (with eventual disappearance) and reduced antiendomysial antibodies in the blood. Hence, serologies (e.g., antiendomysial antibodies) can be used to monitor degree of compliance to dietary gluten restriction.
- Some studies have suggested a possible protective effect of GFD against intestinal lymphoma. First-degree relatives do not appear to be at increased risk for GI or systemic lymphomas in the absence of DH or CD.

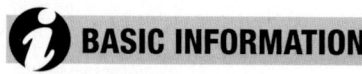

BASIC INFORMATION

DEFINITION

- Diabetes mellitus (DM) refers to a syndrome of hyperglycemia resulting from many different causes (see "Etiology"). It is broadly classified into type 1 (T1DM) and type 2 DM (T2DM). The terms "insulin-dependent" and "non–insulin-dependent" diabetes are obsolete because when a person with type 2 diabetes needs insulin, he or she remains labeled as type 2 and is not reclassified as type 1. Immune-mediated type 1 DM (type 1A) represents 5% to 10% of newly diagnosed diabetics. Table 1 provides a general comparison of the two types of DM. One difference is that type 1 has usually complete or near-total knockout of insulin reserves mediated solely by immunogenic responses from carriers of certain genotypes, whereas type 2 is of polygenetic origin and may have patients who may start with hyperinsulinemia but have insulin resistance and through environmental factors such as diet and sedentary lifestyle leads to an imbalance between glucagon and insulin levels, resulting in combination of causes toward hyperglycemia.
- Recently, however, it has been noted that some type 1 diabetics also may exhibit high levels of glucagon and not all type 1 diabetics have complete islet cell destruction.
- The classification of diabetes also includes:
  1. **LADA**: Latent autoimmune diabetes of adult onset (sometimes called type 1.5 DM). These individuals are typically not insulin dependent initially and are often misclassified as having type 2 DM.
  2. **MODY**: Maturity onset diabetes of youth. These have various genetic expressions and can be classified into various subtypes:
     a. MODY 1, 2, 3, 4, and 5 (with 3 being most prevalent: 70% incidence with HNF-1-alpha [12q24] genetic expression)
     b. MODY 7 and 8 (rare)
  3. Ketosis-prone diabetes: Relapsing/remitting beta cell function with slow deterioration over time. It presents with ketoacidosis requiring insulin, then regains beta cell function and patient is able to discontinue insulin. This form is most common under age 40, in those of African or Afro-Caribbean origin, and in obese or overweight patients.
  4. Secondary diabetes:
     a. Pancreatic disease or resection (e.g., cystic fibrosis)
     b. Chronic excessive corticosteroid exposure or Cushing's syndrome
     c. Glucagonoma
     d. Acromegaly
     e. Other rare genetic disorders (e.g., mitochondrial diabetes MELAS syndrome)
  5. Rare autoimmune (e.g., type A and B insulin resistance syndrome)
- Diabetes mellitus can be diagnosed by one of three tests:
  1. A fasting plasma glucose (FPG) ≥126 mg/dl, which should be confirmed with repeat testing on a different day. Fasting is defined as no caloric intake for at least 8 hr.
  2. An oral glucose tolerance test (OGTT) with a plasma glucose ≥200 mg/dl 2 hr after a 75 g (100 g for pregnant women) glucose load.
  3. A hemoglobin A_{1c} (HbA_{1c}) value ≥6.5%.
- Of these three tests the OGTT has the highest sensitivity. Symptoms of hyperglycemia and a casual (random) plasma glucose ≥200 mg/dl are also indicative of DM. Classic symptoms of hyperglycemia include polyuria, polydipsia, and unexplained weight loss. (At the time of diagnosis as a diabetic, B cell function is at 25% to 30%.)
- Individuals with glucose levels higher than normal but not high enough to meet the criteria for diagnosis of DM are considered to have "prediabetes," the diagnosis of which is made as follows:
  1. A fasting plasma glucose 100 to 125 mg/dl; this is referred to as ***impaired fasting glucose***.
  2. After OGTT, a 2-hr plasma glucose of 140 to 199; this is referred to as ***impaired glucose tolerance***. Patients with impaired glucose tolerance or prediabetes have B-cell function at 50% of normal.
  3. A hemoglobin A_{1c} value of 5.7% to 6.4%.
- Table 2 describes diagnostic categories for DM and at-risk states.

SYNONYMS

IDDM (insulin-dependent diabetes mellitus)
NIDDM (non–insulin-dependent diabetes mellitus)
Type 1 diabetes mellitus (insulin-dependent diabetes mellitus)
Type 2 diabetes mellitus (non–insulin-dependent diabetes mellitus)
LADA (latent autoimmune diabetes of adult)
MODY (mature onset diabetes of youth)

ICD-10CM CODES

E11.5 Type 2 diabetes mellitus with peripheral circulatory complications
E11.7 Type 2 diabetes mellitus with multiple complications
E11.8 Type 2 diabetes mellitus with unspecified complications
E11.9 Type 2 diabetes mellitus without complications
E10.69 Type 1 diabetes mellitus with other specified complication
E10.8 Type 1 diabetes mellitus with unspecified complications
E10.9 Type 1 diabetes mellitus without complications
E11.69 Type 2 diabetes mellitus with other specified complication
E11.8 Type 2 diabetes mellitus with unspecified complications
E11.9 Type 2 diabetes mellitus without complications

TABLE 1 General Comparison of the Two Types of Diabetes Mellitus

	Type 1	Type 2
Previous terminology	Insulin-dependent diabetes mellitus (IDDM), type I, juvenile-onset diabetes	Non–insulin-dependent diabetes mellitus, type II, adult-onset diabetes
Age of onset	Usually <30 yr, particularly childhood and adolescence, but any age	Usually >40 yr, but any age
Genetic predisposition	Moderate; environmental factors required for expression; 35%-50% concordance in monozygotic twins; several candidate genes proposed	Strong; 60%-90% concordance in monozygotic twins; many candidate genes proposed; some genes identified in maturity-onset diabetes of the young
Human leukocyte antigen associations	Linkage to DQA and DQB, influenced by DRB (3 and 4) (DR2 protective)	None known
Other associations	Autoimmune; Graves' disease, Hashimoto's thyroiditis, vitiligo, Addison's disease, pernicious anemia	Heterogeneous group, ongoing subclassification based on identification of specific pathogenic processes and genetic defects
Precipitating and risk factors	Largely unknown; microbial, chemical, dietary, other	Age, obesity (central), sedentary lifestyle, previous gestational diabetes
Findings at diagnosis	85%-90% of patients have one and usually more autoantibodies to ICA512/IA-2/IA-2b, GAD_{65}, insulin (IAA)	Possibly complications (microvascular and macrovascular) caused by significant preceding asymptomatic period
Endogenous insulin levels	Low or absent	Usually present (relative deficiency), early hyperinsulinemia
Insulin resistance	Only with hyperglycemia	Mostly present
Prolonged fast	Hyperglycemia, ketoacidosis	Euglycemia
Stress, withdrawal of insulin	Ketoacidosis	Nonketotic hyperglycemia, occasionally ketoacidosis

GAD, Glutamic acid decarboxylase; *IA-2/IA-2b,* tyrosine phosphatases; *IAA,* insulin autoantibodies; *ICA,* islet cell antibody; *ICA512,* islet cell autoantigen 512 (fragment of IA-2).
From Andreoli TE (ed): *Cecil essentials of medicine,* ed 6, Philadelphia, 2005, Saunders.

TABLE 2 Diagnostic Categories*: Diabetes Mellitus and At-Risk States

Fasting Plasma Glucose Level	2-Hour (75-g) OGTT Result		
	<140 mg/dl	140-199 mg/dl	≥200 mg/dl
<100 mg/dl	Normal	IGT†	DM
100-125 mg/dl	IFG†	IGT† *and* IFG†	DM
≥126 mg/dl	DM	DM	DM
HbA_{1c} Level	**<5.7%**	**5.7-6.4%**	**≥6.5%**
	Normal	High-risk†	DM

DM, Diabetes mellitus; *IFG,* impaired fasting glucose; *IGT,* impaired glucose tolerance; *OGTT,* oral glucose tolerance test.

*These diagnostic categories are based on the combined fasting plasma glucose level and a 2-hour, 75-g oral glucose tolerance test (OGTT) result. Note that a confirmed random plasma glucose level of 200 mg/dl or higher in the appropriate clinical setting is diagnostic of diabetes and precludes the need for further testing.

†May be referred to as prediabetes.

From Goldman L, Schafer AI: *Goldman's Cecil medicine,* ed 24, Philadelphia, 2012, Saunders.

EPIDEMIOLOGY & DEMOGRAPHICS

- DM affects 9% to 10% of the U.S. population. Prevalence rates vary considerably by race/ethnicity. T1DM accounts for approximately 5% of diagnosed diabetes cases and is defined by the presence of one or more autoimmune markers. While incidence of diabetes in adolescents is mostly type 1, the rate of type 2 being diagnosed in adolescents has increased by 1.5 times in certain given areas. This seems to correlate with the epidemic of pediatric obesity.
- Incidence rate increases with age, varying from 2% in persons age 20 to 44 yr to 18% in persons 65 to 74 yr. T2DM can have a long presymptomatic phase, leading to a 4- to 7-yr delay in diagnosis. In the U.S. 1.2 million new cases of diabetes are diagnosed each yr, and 86 million have prediabetes. Currently, 30 million Americans have diabetes; with this current trend, it is predicted that by 2050 1 out of 3 Americans will be diabetic.
- Diabetes accounts for 8% of all legal blindness in the U.S. and is the leading cause of end-stage renal disease (ESRD). Approximately 40% of patients in a given dialysis center are diabetic.
- Patients with diabetes are 2 to 4 times more likely than nondiabetic patients to experience development of cardiovascular disease.

PHYSICAL FINDINGS & CLINICAL PRESENTATION

- Physical examination varies with the presence of complications and may be normal in early stages.
- Diabetic retinopathy:
  1. Nonproliferative (background diabetic retinopathy):
     a. Initially: Microaneurysms, capillary dilation, waxy or hard exudates, dot and flame hemorrhages, arteriovenous shunts
     b. Advanced stage: Microinfarcts with cotton wool exudates, macular edema
  2. Proliferative retinopathy: Characterized by formation of new vessels, vitreous hemorrhages, fibrous scarring, and retinal detachment
- Cataracts and glaucoma occur with increased frequency in patients with diabetes.
- Diabetic macular edema—swelling of the macula leading to loss of sharp vision in this part of the eye. People with this disorder usually already have retinopathy but may present separately as well.
- Diabetic neuropathy:
  1. Distal sensorimotor polyneuropathy:
     a. Symptoms include paresthesia, hyperesthesia, or burning pain involving bilateral distal extremities in a "stocking glove" distribution. This can progress to motor weakness and ataxia.
     b. Physical examination may reveal decreased pinprick sensation, decreased sensation to light touch, decreased vibration sense, and loss of proprioception. Motor disturbances such as decreased deep tendon reflexes and atrophy of interosseous muscles can also be seen.
  2. Autonomic neuropathy:
     a. GI disturbances: Esophageal motility abnormalities, gastroparesis, diarrhea (usually nocturnal)
        (1) Increased gastric emptying seen in type 2
        (2) Decreased gastric emptying seen in type 1
     b. Genitourinary (GU) disturbances: Neurogenic bladder (hesitancy, weak stream, and dribbling), impotence
     c. Cardiovascular (CV) disturbances: Orthostatic hypotension, tachycardia, decreased heart rate variability (HRV). Decreased heart rate variability is associated with increased cardiac mortality, independent of ejection fraction.
  3. Polyradiculopathy: Painful weakness and atrophy in the distribution of ≥1 contiguous nerve roots.
  4. Mononeuropathy involving cranial nerves III, IV, or VI or peripheral nerves can also occur.
- Diabetic nephropathy: Pedal edema, pallor, weakness, uremic appearance
- Nephrotic syndrome: Proteinuria, hypertriglyceridemia, edema
- Nephritis: Progressive degeneration of nephrons focal glomerulosclerosis

  Type IV renal tubular acidosis, hyperkalemic nephropathy, interstitial nephritis, causing hyporeninemic hypoaldosteronism. It is important to keep in mind that NSAIDs, ACE inhibitors, trimethoprim, and heparin can all reduce aldosterone and can cause or exacerbate the condition. 50% of patients on dialysis have diabetes as primary diagnosis; whereas glycemia is important to prevent nephropathy, the most significant contributing factor is hypertension.
- Foot ulcers: Occur in 15% of individuals with diabetes (annual incidence rate 2%) and are the leading causes of hospitalization; they are usually secondary to a combination of factors, including peripheral vascular insufficiency, repeated trauma (unrecognized because of sensory loss), and superimposed infection.
  1. Patient symptoms are usually less than would be expected from clinical findings, due to loss of sensation related to peripheral neuropathy.
  2. Comprehensive foot exams include visual inspection, assessment of pedal pulses, and assessment of protective sensation using a 10-g monofilament to test sensation.
  3. Prevention of foot ulcers in an individual with diabetes includes strict glucose control, patient education, prescription footwear, intensive podiatric care, and evaluation for surgical interventions.
  4. Foot examination should be done annually on all diabetics.
- Neuropathic arthropathy (Charcot joints): Bone or joint deformities from repeated trauma (secondary to peripheral neuropathy; Fig. E1).
- Necrobiosis lipoidica diabeticorum: Plaquelike reddened areas with a central area that fades to white-yellow, found on the anterior surfaces of the legs (Fig. E2); in these areas, the skin becomes very thin and can ulcerate easily.
- Other diabetic skin manifestations with diabetes include:
  1. Sclerodema diabeticorum—thickening of skin and epidermis giving skin a "leatherlike texture"; typically affects type 2, mainly on upper back and neck.
  2. Dermatitis herpetiformis—diffuse petechial rash associated with gluten insensitivity.
  3. Vitiligo: Associated with type 1 and type 2, and affects skin coloration due to autoimmune reaction to pigmentation (at times may be associated with adrenal insufficiency, especially in type 1 patients). Patients should use SPF 30 sunscreen to prevent sunburn.
  4. Acanthosis nigricans—darkening of skin folds in neck and axilla, at times raised and velvety, thought to be associated with insulin resistance; other conditions such as Cushing's and acromegaly can have this as well.
  5. Diabetic dermopathy—appears as shiny round or oval lesions on thin skin of the lower extremity, also known as "shin

spots"; these are usually not painful and do not require treatment.
6. Eruptive xanthomatosis—associated with uncontrolled blood sugars and extremely high triglycerides. There is a high risk for pancreatitis in patients with this finding; treatment is aimed at lowering blood sugars with insulin and fibrates.
7. Digital sclerosis—skin on toes fingers and hands become waxy, thick, and tight, with joint stiffness; treatment is aimed at lowering blood sugars and encouraging use of lotions and moisturizers.
8. Bullosis diabeticorum—rare disorder manifesting with blisters on hands, forearms, toes, and feet, usually painless. Lesions generally heal on their own.

ETIOLOGY

IDIOPATHIC DIABETES: Type 1 DM: Results from autoimmune beta-cell destruction, usually leading to absolute insulin deficiency.
- Hereditary factors:
  1. Islet cell antibodies (found in 90% of patients within the first yr of diagnosis)
  2. Higher incidence of human leukocyte antigen (HLA) types DR3, DR4
  3. 50% concordance rate in identical twins
- Environmental factors: Viral infection (possibly coxsackievirus, mumps virus)

Type 2 DM: Results from insulin resistance and a progressive defect in insulin secretion.
- Hereditary factors: 90% concordance rate in identical twins
- Environmental factors: Obesity, sedentary lifestyle, high carbohydrate content in food

DIABETES SECONDARY TO OTHER FACTORS:
- Hormonal excess: Cushing's syndrome, acromegaly, glucagonoma, pheochromocytoma
- Drugs: Glucocorticoids, diuretics, oral contraceptives
- Insulin receptor unavailability (with or without circulating antibodies)
- Pancreatic disease: Pancreatitis, pancreatectomy, hemochromatosis, cystic fibrosis
- Genetic syndromes: Maturity onset diabetes of the young (MODY, monogenetic diabetes accounting for 2% to 5% of diabetes), familial hyperlipidemias, myotonic dystrophy, lipoatrophy
- Gestational diabetes (GDM): Diabetes diagnosed during pregnancy that is due to pregnancy-related insulin resistance

Dx DIAGNOSIS

DIFFERENTIAL DIAGNOSIS

- Diabetes insipidus
- Stress hyperglycemia
- Diabetes secondary to hormonal excess, drugs, pancreatic disease

LABORATORY TESTS

- Diagnosis of DM is made on the basis of the following tests:
  1. Fasting glucose ≥126 mg/dl on two occasions.
  2. Non-FPG ≥200 mg/dl and symptoms of DM.
  3. OGTT (75 g glucose load for nonpregnant individuals) with 2-hr value >200 mg/dl.
  4. Glycosylated hemoglobin (HbA_{1c}) ≥6.5%. HbA_{1c} level reflects average glycemia over previous 3 months or longer. In known diabetics, this test should be performed at least twice yearly in stable patients and more frequently when therapy changes or patients are not meeting glycemic goals. HbA_{1c} alone does not provide a measure of glycemic variability or hypoglycemia and is affected by the presence of hemoglobin variants, hemolysis, or blood loss.
- Measurement of autoantibodies glutamic acid decarboxylase (GAD65) and tyrosine phosphatase IA-2 are useful in suspected immune mediated type 1 DM (strong association).
- Screening for prediabetes and diabetes in asymptomatic patients (see Table 3):
  1. Should be considered in adults of any age who are overweight (body mass index [BMI] >25 kg/m^2) or obese (BMI >30) and who have one or more additional risk factors for diabetes.
  2. In those who are without these risk factors, testing should begin at age 45 yr.
  3. If screen is normal, repeat testing should be carried out at least at 3-yr intervals.
  4. ADA recommends screening all Asian Americans with BMI 23 or higher every 2 yr.
- Detection and diagnosis of gestational diabetes mellitus (GDM):
  1. Screen for GDM using risk factor analysis and use of an OGTT. Pregnant women who are not known to have diabetes should be screened for gestational diabetes at 24 to 28 weeks' gestation with a "1-step" strategy with 75 g oral glucose tolerance test or a "2-step" approach with a 50-g (nonfasting) screen followed by a 100-g oral glucose tolerance test for those who screen positive. A diagnosis of GDM is made if any of the following levels of plasma glucose are exceeded: ≥92 mg/dl (5.1 mmol/L) when fasting, ≥80 mg/dl (10 mmol/L) at 1 hour, or ≥153 mg/dl (8.5 mmol/L) at 2 hours.
  2. Women with GDM should be screened for diabetes 6 to 12 wk postpartum and should be followed with subsequent screening for the development of diabetes or prediabetes at least every 3 yr. A woman who had GDM during pregnancy has 50% risk of developing diabetes later in life; this is dependent on ethnicity (e.g., Pima Indians, Hispanic, African American).
- Screening for diabetic nephropathy (Fig. E3):
  1. Screening should be done at diagnosis and then yearly for type 2 diabetes and 5 yr after diagnosis then yearly in type 1 diabetes. 18% of type 1 DM may have early kidney changes, and future guidelines may change screening to 1 yr after diagnosis if poorly controlled then annually for both type 1 and type 2.
  2. Screening can be performed using an albumin:creatinine ratio (microalbumin) in a random spot urine collection or by measurement of a 24-hr urine collection for albumin and creatinine clearance. The urine albumin to creatinine ratio (ACR) is independently associated with mortality at all levels of estimated glomerular filtration rate (eGFR) in older adults with diabetes.
  3. The diagnosis of microalbuminuria (ACR 30-299 mg/24 hr) should be based on 2 to 3 elevated levels within a 3- to 6-mo period because there is a marked variability in day-to-day albumin excretion. Patients with overt macroalbuminuria (>300 mg albumin/24 hr or albumin:creatinine ratio >300) should be followed by urine protein:creatinine ratio.
- A fasting serum lipid panel, serum creatinine, and electrolytes should be obtained yearly on all adult patients with diabetes.
- Self-monitoring of blood glucose (SMBG) is crucial for assessing the effectiveness of the management plan. The frequency and timing of SMBG varies with the needs and goals of

TABLE 3 Criteria for Diabetes Screening in Asymptomatic Individuals

1. Testing should be considered in all adults who are overweight (BMI >25 kg/m2*) and have additional risk factors:
   - Physical inactivity
   - A first-degree relative with diabetes
   - High-risk ethnic population (e.g., African American, Hispanic American, Native American, Asian American, Pacific Islander)
   - Delivered a baby weighing more than 9 lb or diagnosed with gestational diabetes mellitus
   - Systemic hypertension (blood pressure >140/90 mm Hg or on antihypertensive therapy)
   - High-density lipoprotein cholesterol level <35 mg/dl or triglyceride level >250 mg/dl
   - Polycystic ovary syndrome
   - Hemoglobin A1c ≥5.7%, impaired glucose tolerance or impaired fasting glucose on prior testing
   - Other clinical conditions associated with insulin resistance (e.g., severe obesity, acanthosis nigricans)
   - History of cardiovascular disease
2. If none of the above criteria are present, screening for diabetes should begin at age 45 yr.
3. If the results are normal, screening should be repeated at least every 3 yr. Depending on initial results and risk status, more frequent testing may need to be considered.

*In some ethnic groups, such as Asians, at-risk body mass index (BMI) may be lower.
Modified from American Diabetes Association, Diagnosis and classification of diabetes mellitus *Diabetes Care* 33(Suppl. 1):S14, 2010. Borrowed from Goldman L, Schafer AI: *Goldman's Cecil medicine*, ed 24, Philadelphia, 2012, Saunders.

each patient. In most patients with type 1 DM and pregnant women taking insulin, SMBG is recommended at least 3 times/day. In patients with type 2 DM not on insulin, recommendations are unclear for SMBG, but testing once or twice/day is acceptable in most patients. Glycemic control is best evaluated when SMBG is combined with HbA_{1c} testing.

- Continuous glucose monitoring (CGM) is now starting to play a more prominent role in reducing the number of fingersticks. Dexcom CGM has been approved by FDA for use by patients to adjust insulin based on CGM readings.
- The use of insulin pump and CGM readings and computer software can adjust insulin automatically (known as the "artificial pancreas").
- CGM can also be used in patients with type 2 on multiple daily injections.
- Limitations of CGM are that it cannot predict accuracy of blood glucose when <70 mg/dl.
- Screening for thyroid dysfunction (TSH level), vitamin B12 deficiency, and celiac disease should be considered in type 1 diabetes due to the increased frequency of other autoimmune diseases in these individuals.
- Consider screening for autoimmune polyendocrine syndromes (APS-2):
    1. APS-2: Most commonly known as Schmidt syndrome, heterogeneous not linked to one gene (HDLA-DQ2, HDLA-DQ8, AND HLA-DR4). Patients can have IDDM, hyperthyroidism, other autoimmune conditions, B_{12} deficiency, and myasthenia.

Rx TREATMENT

- Type 1 diabetes requires immediate initiation of insulin therapy.
- In type 1 diabetes, intensive glycemic control (HbA_{1c} <7) has been shown in randomized controlled trials (RCT) to reduce the risk of microvascular (neuropathy, retinopathy, nephropathy) and macrovascular (cardiovascular events) complications.
- Type 2 DM: The ADA and European Association for the Study of Diabetes recommend lifestyle intervention (diet and exercise) and metformin initiation (unless contraindications exist such as serum creatinine levels ≥1.5 mg/dl in males or ≥1.4 mg/dl in females or patients ≥30 yr of age with reduced renal function as measured by creatinine clearance) at the time of diagnosis of type 2 diabetes. Therapy should then be augmented with additional agents (including early initiation of insulin therapy) to achieve adequate glycemic control.
- In type 2 diabetes, intensive glycemic control (HbA_{1c} <7) has been shown in RCT to reduce the risk of microvascular complications. While intensive glucose control reduced the risk of some cardiovascular disease outcomes (such as nonfatal MI), it did not reduce the risk of cardiovascular death or all-cause mortality and increased the risk of severe hypoglycemia.
- It is important to remember that tight glycemic control may burden patients with complex treatment programs, hypoglycemia, weight gain, and costs. Clinicians should individualize HbA_{1c} targets so that they are reasonable and reflect patients' personal and clinical contexts and their informed values and preferences. A target HbA_{1c} <7 is reasonable for motivated new diabetic patients with long life expectancies, whereas less stringent controls (HbA_{1c} 7.5 or higher) may be reasonable in elderly patients with limited life expectancy and elevated risk of hypoglycemia. The American Geriatrics Society recommends a general goal for glycated hemoglobin in older adults of 7.5% to 8.0%. Higher HbA_{1c} targets (8%-9%) are appropriate for older adults with multiple comorbidities, poor health, and limited life expectancy.[1]

NONPHARMACOLOGIC THERAPY

- Diet: The ADA does not recommend a special diet. However, newly diagnosed diabetics who are overweight or obese should be counseled to lose at least 5% of their body weight. Medical association therapy with a registered dietitian is recommended.
    1. Calories
        a. The patient with diabetes can be started on 15 calories/lb of ideal body weight; this number can be increased to 20 calories/lb for an active person and 25 calories/lb if the patient does heavy physical labor.
        b. The calories should be distributed as 45% to 65% carbohydrates, <30% fat, with saturated fat limited to <7% of total calories, and 10% to 30% protein. Daily cholesterol intake should not exceed 300 mg.
        c. The emphasis should be on complex carbohydrates rather than simple and refined starches, and on polyunsaturated instead of saturated fats in a ratio of 2:1.
    2. Seven food groups
        a. The exchange diet of the ADA includes bread or starches, meat or proteins, vegetables, fruits, fats, milk, and free foods (e.g., black tea, sugar-free gelatin).
        b. The name of each exchange is meant to be all-inclusive (e.g., cereal, muffins, spaghetti, potatoes, rice are in the bread group; meats, fish, eggs, cheese, peanut butter are in the protein group).
        c. The glycemic index compares the increase in blood sugar after the ingestion of simple sugars and complex carbohydrates with the increase that occurs after the absorption of glucose; equal amounts of starches do not give the same increase in plasma glucose (pasta equal in calories to a baked potato causes less of an increase than the potato); thus, it is helpful to know the glycemic index of a particular food product.
        d. Fiber: Insoluble fiber (bran, celery) and soluble globular fiber (pectin in fruit) delay glucose absorption and attenuate the postprandial serum glucose peak.
            (1) They also appear to reduce the increased triglyceride level often present in patients with uncontrolled diabetes. A diet high in fiber should be emphasized (20 to 35 g/day of soluble and insoluble fiber).
            (2) Diet programs: In 2015, a meta-analysis review of all research revealed that weight loss was equal no matter which diet program patients were involved in.
            (3) However, the only data to show evidence-based prevention of diabetes in prediabetics was the "Mediterranean diet."
            (4) The Mediterranean diet also showed a significant decrease in the percentage of established diabetics from needing insulin in the future and significant benefit in reducing cardiovascular events.
    3. Other principles
        a. Modest sodium restriction to 2400 to 3000 mg/day. If hypertension is present, restrict to <2400 mg/day; if nephropathy and hypertension are present, restrict to <2000 mg/day.
        b. Moderation of alcohol intake recommended (≤2 drinks/day in men, ≤1 drink/day in women).
        c. Non-nutritive artificial sweeteners are acceptable in moderate amounts.
            (1) However, it has been shown that artificial sweeteners may actually increase insulin resistance by affecting the action of insulin at receptor level.
- Exercise: Increases the cellular glucose uptake by increasing the number of insulin receptors. The following points must be considered:
    1. Exercise program must be individualized and built up slowly. Consider beginning with 15 min of low-impact aerobic exercise 3 times per wk and increasing the frequency and duration to 30 to 45 min of moderate aerobic activity (50% to 70% of maximum age predicted heart rate) to 3 to 5 days/wk.
        a. In the absence of contraindications, resistance training three times per wk should be encouraged.
    2. Insulin is more rapidly absorbed when injected into a limb that is then exercised, and this can result in hypoglycemia.
    3. Physical activity can result in hypoglycemia if medication dose or carbohydrate consumption is not modified. Ingestion of additional carbohydrates is recommended if pre-exercise glucose levels are <100 mg/dl.

[1] Huang ES, Davis AM: Glycemic control in older adults with diabetes mellitus, *JAMA* 314:1509-1510, 2015.

4. Diabetes prevention program: Low-fat diet with exercise reduced diabetes by 58%. This encompassed diet of 1200 to 1800 kcal/day <30% from fat, exercise unsupervised and supervised, akin to brisk walking >150 min/wk of moderately intensity physical activity.

- Weight loss: To ideal body weight if the patient is overweight. Recent trials have shown that although weight loss has many positive health benefits for people with type 2 DM, such as slower decline in mobility, it does not reduce the number of cardiovascular events.
- Screening for nephropathy, neuropathy, and retinopathy: Annual serum creatinine and urine albumin excretion; initial comprehensive eye examination and at least annually thereafter.
- Diabetes self-management education: Could also address psychosocial issues.
- Self-monitoring of blood glucose should occur three to four times per day for patients using multiple insulin injections or on insulin pump therapy.
- Perform HbA_{1c} at least two times a yr in patients who are meeting treatment goals and who have stable glycemic control.
    1. HbA_{1c} quarterly in patients whose therapy has changed or who are not meeting glycemic goals.
    2. The HbA_{1c} goal for nonpregnant adults in general is <7%.
    3. In the elderly, those with comorbidities, or those at risk for complications from hypoglycemia, a more moderate glycemic target (HbA_{1c} 7-8) may be appropriate.
    4. In elderly patients (>80 yr of age) with average life expectancy of 5 yr, a target HbA_{1c} <8.0 is reasonable. In patients >80 yr with comorbidities and life expectancy of 3 yr, a target HbA_{1c} of <9.0 may be appropriate.

GENERAL Rx

- Type 1 DM: Lifelong insulin therapy is required for persons with type 1 DM. It should consist of basal coverage, prandial coverage, and supplemental insulin for correction of hyperglycemia. Initial total insulin dosing ranges from 0.4 to 1.0 U/kg/day, 50% of which is basal insulin and 50% prandial insulin.
- Type 2 DM: When the previous measures fail to normalize the serum glucose, oral hypoglycemic agents should be added to the regimen in T2DM. Tables 4 and 5 compare therapies for T2DM and classes of antihyperglycemic agents. Treatment options in patient with type 2 diabetes should be tailored to try to target core diabetic defects and apply therapies that lower HbA_{1c} in a weight-neutral or weight-lowering fashion if possible; of course, cost of therapies needs to be considered as well.
- **Metformin:** The primary mechanism of metformin is to decrease hepatic glucose production and improve insulin sensitivity. Because metformin does not produce hypoglycemia when used as a monotherapy, it is preferred initially for most patients. Metformin reduces mean HbA_{1c} level by 1.1%. It is contraindicated in patients with

TABLE 4 Comparison of Therapies for Type 2 Diabetes

Property	Lifestyle	Insulins	Sulfonylureas	Metformin	α-Glucosidase Inhibitors	Glitazones	Glinides	Exenatide	Pramlintide
Target tissue	Muscle or fat	Beta cell supplement	Beta cell	Liver	Gut	Muscle	Beta cell	Various	Brain
ΔHbA_{1c} (%) as (monotherapy)	Variable	1->2	1-2	1-2	0.5-1	0.5-2	Re: 1-2 N: 0.5-1	~1	~0.5
Fasting effect	Good	Excellent	Good	Good	Poor	Good	Re: Moderate N: Poor	Poor	Poor
Postprandial effect	Good	Excellent	Good	Good	Excellent	Good	Re: Good N: Excellent	Excellent	Excellent
Severe hypoglycemia	No	Yes	Yes	No	No	No	Re: Yes N: No	No	No
Dosing interval	Continuous	qd to continuous	qd to tid	bid or tid	bid to qid	P: qd Ro: qd or bid	tid to qid with meals	bid	tid
ΔWeight (lb/yr)	+1	+3	+1 to 3	0 to −6	0 to −10	+1 to 13	+1 to 3	−6 to −12	−3 to −6
ΔInsulin	Variable	Increase	Increase	Modest decrease	Modest decrease	Decrease	Increase	Increase	None
ΔLDL	Minimal decrease	Minimal decrease	None	Decrease	Minimal decrease	Increase	None	None	None
ΔHDL	Minimal increase	None	None	Increase	None	Increase	None	Decrease	None
ΔTG	Minimal decrease	Decrease	None	Decrease	Minimal decrease	P: Decrease Ro: None	None	Decrease	None
Common problem	Recidivism, injury	Hypoglycemia, weight gain	Hypoglycemia, weight gain	Transient GI	Flatulence	Weight gain, edema, anemia	Hypoglycemia	GI	GI
Rare problem	—	—	—	Lactic acidosis	—	Hepatotoxicity?	—	—	—
Contraindications	None	None	Allergy	Renal failure, Liver failure, CHF (>80 yr old)	Intestinal disease	Hepatocellular disease	—	None	None
Cost ($/mo)	0-200	30-450	10-15	30-60	40-80	75-180	70-110	170-200	200-400
Maximum effective dose	—	1-2 U/kg per day	maximum or double starting	1000 mg bid	50 mg tid	P: 45 mg qd Ro: 4 mg bid	Re: 2 mg tid N: 120 mg tid	10 μg bid	120 μg ac

Δ, Change; *ac,* before food; *bid,* twice a day; *CHF,* congestive heart failure; *GI,* gastrointestinal disturbance; *HbA_{1c},* glycosylated hemoglobin; *HDL,* high-density lipoprotein; *LDL,* low-density lipoprotein; *N,* nateglinide; *P,* pioglitazone; *qd,* every day; *qid,* four times a day; *Re,* repaglinide; *Ro,* rosiglitazone; *TG,* triglycerides; *tid,* three times a day.
From Melmed S, Polonsky KS, Larsen PR, Kronenberg HM: *Williams textbook of endocrinology,* ed 12, Philadelphia, 2011, Saunders.

TABLE 5 Classes of Antihyperglycemic Therapy

Class	Representative Agents	Major Action	HbA_{1c} Lowering (%)	Fasting or Prandial Effect	Usual Dosing Frequency (Doses/Day)	Route	Hypoglycemia	Weight Effect	CVD Risk Factor Benefits	Important Contraindications	Daily Cost ($)
Lifestyle	—	Broad	>1	Both	—	—	No	Loss	Yes	—	—
Biguanide	Metformin	Liver sensitizer	>1	Fasting	1-2	Oral	No	Neutral	Modest	Renal or hepatic failure	<$1
Sulfonylurea	Glimepiride, glipizide	Insulin secretagogue	>1	Fasting	1-2	Oral	Yes	Gain	Negligible	—	<<$1
Meglitinide	Repaglinide	Insulin secretagogue	>1	Both	With meals	Oral	Yes	Gain	Negligible	—	~$5
Benzoic acid–derived	Nateglinide	Insulin secretagogue	<1	Prandial	With meals	Oral	Minimal	Minimal	Negligible	—	~$5
Basal insulin	NPH, glargine, detemir	Insulin supplement/ substitute	>1	Fasting	1	SQ	Yes++	Gain++	Lowers TG	—	~$5
Bolus insulin	R, lispro, aspart, glulisine	Insulin supplement/ substitute	>1	Prandial	With meals	SQ	Yes++	Gain++	Lowers TG	—	~$5
Thiazolidinediones	Pioglitazone, rosiglitazone	Peripheral sensitizer	>1	Fasting	1	Oral	No	Gain++	Variable (see text)	Heart or liver failure	~$5
α-Glucosidase inhibitors	Acarbose, miglitol	Slow carbohydrate absorption	<1	Prandial	With meals	Oral	No	Neutral	Negligible	—	~$3
Amylinomimetics	Pramlintide	Broad	<1	Prandial	With meals	SQ	No	Loss	Negligible	—	~$10
GLP1 receptor agonists	Exenatide	Broad	~1	Prandial	2	SQ	No	Loss	Modest with weight loss	Pancreatitis, renal failure	~$9
Long-acting GLP1 receptor agonists	Liraglutide, albiglutide, dulaglutide	Broad	>1	Both	1	SQ	No	Loss	Lowers BP	Pancreatitis, medullary thyroid cancer	~$13
DPP4 inhibitors	Sitagliptin, saxagliptin	Improved insulin/ glucagon secretion	<1	Both	1	Oral	No	Neutral	Negligible	Pancreatitis	~$7
Bile acid sequestrants	Colesevelam	Uncertain	<1	Prandial	1-2	Oral	No	Neutral	Lowers LDL	Hypertriglyceridemia	~$9
$SGIT_2$ inhibitor	Canagliflozin, dapagliflozin, empagliflozin	Decrease renal glucose reabsorption, increase urinary glucose excretion	<1	Both	1	Oral	No	Loss	Negligible	Volume dilution	~$10

BP, Blood pressure; *CVD,* cardiovascular disease; *LDL,* low-density lipoprotein; *$SGLT_2$,* sodium-glucose co-transporter 2; *SQ,* subcutaneous; *TG,* triglyceride.

severe renal insufficiency with an estimated glomerular filtrate rate <30 ml/min, serum creatinine level of 1.5 per dl or greater in men or 1.4 per dl or greater in women, heart failure, or other clinical states of hypoperfusion, and in patients with significant liver disease. Starting metformin in patients with GFR between 30 and 45 ml/min is also not recommended. Renal dosing of metformin is preferred, based on GFR levels rather than creatinine levels.

1. When the HbA_{1c} level is 9% or greater, initial dual-regimen combination therapy should be considered. Clinicians should consider adding either a DPP-4 inhibitor, an SGLT-2 inhibitor, a thiazolidinedione, or sulfonylurea to metformin to improve glycemic control when a dual regimen is considered.

- **DPP-4 inhibitors:** Sitagliptin, saxagliptin, vildagliptin, alogliptin, and linagliptin inhibit the enzyme DPP-4, responsible for inactivation and degradation of glucagon-like peptide-1 (GLP-1) and glucose-dependent insulinotropic polypeptide (GIP). These drugs, known as "DPP-4 inhibitors" or "gliptins," raise blood incretin levels, thereby inhibiting glucagon release and lowering blood glucose levels. When used with metformin, they do not cause hypoglycemia and are preferred over sulfonylureas as second-line agents. Linagliptin does not require a dosage adjustment in renal insufficiency. Cost is a major barrier to their use. Sitagliptin can be used in any degree of kidney disease but needs to be dosed based on GFR and creatinine levels.
- **GLP-1 agonists:** Exenatide, dulaglutide, albiglutide, lixisenatide, and liraglutide are glucagon-like peptide-1 (GLP-1) agonists. They are incretin mimetics that stimulate release of insulin from pancreatic beta cells and can be used as adjunctive therapy for patients with T2DM. GLP-1 agonists are not indicated in T1DM and are contraindicated in patients with severe renal impairment. Cost is a barrier to their use. The difference in a DDP-4 versus a GLP-1 analog is that with the DDP-4, we are enhancing physiologic levels of GLP-1 and GIP, assuming patients have GLP reserve, whereas with a GLP-1 analog, one is administering a pharmacologic dose of GLP-1, which overrides any resistance and restores insulin secretion and glucagon lowering.
- **Sodium-glucose co-transporter 2 ($SGLT_2$) inhibitors** (e.g., canagliflozin [Invokana], dapagliflozin [Farxiga], empagliflozin [Jardiance]) are useful for oral treatment of type 2 DM. By inhibiting $SGLT_2$, these medications decrease glucose reabsorption, increase urinary glucose excretion, and lower blood glucose levels (decrease HbA_{1c} by 0.7%). Empagliflozin has been shown to slow progression of renal disease in type 2 diabetics with cardiovascular disease. Side effects include increased risk of genital mycotic infections, UTIs, and volume depletion. Renal function should be evaluated before starting $SGLT_2$ inhibitors and periodically thereafter. Temporary discontinuation of these meds is recommended in cases of reduced oral intake or fluid loss. Higher cost and limited drug formulary availability are limiting factors.
  1. Recent trials using canagliflozin have also shown cardiovascular and renal benefit, particularly in reversal of microalbuminuria, thus also showing primary and secondary prevention.
  2. These cardiovascular and renal benefits may be a class effect.
  3. However, in these trials there was an unexplained increase in amputations of toes and limbs, which should make one consider using these agents with caution in vasculopathies and patients prone to dehydration.
  4. Canafliglitazone has partial SGLT-1 blocking activity at the intestinal level, but not at renal level, and only at 300-mg dose.
  5. Future therapies will be looking at dual blockade of SGLT-2 and SGLT-1 carriers (not available at this time).
  6. DKA has been seen in some patients using these agents, mostly in off-label use in type 1 patients, but some type 2 patients have exhibited this as well. In type 1 DM patients, it seems to be related to cutting down insulin dosing; in type 2, exact mechanism of action is unknown.
  7. Mycotic infections with UTI are common side effects of these agents. This is especially problematic in patients already at risk for mycotic infections (uncircumcised men and women who are prone to dermatomycosis). Mycotic infections may also be related to poor control of diabetes and may decrease as glycemia is lowered.
- **Sulfonylureas:** Sulfonylureas increase insulin secretion and work best when given before meals. All sulfonylureas are contraindicated in patients who are allergic to sulfa. Use of sulfonylureas confers a greater risk of hypoglycemia than the other agents.
  1. These agents are now being considered to be used as last or later resort or when cost is of major concern for the patient and when other therapies cannot be incorporated or are contraindicated.
- **Acarbose and miglitol:** These agonists inhibit pancreatic amylase and small intestinal glucosidases, thereby delaying carbohydrate absorption in the gut and reducing associated postprandial hyperglycemia. The major side effects are flatulence, diarrhea, and abdominal cramps.
- **The meglitinides nateglinide and repaglinide and the bile acid sequestrant colesevelam** can also be used to lower glucose levels but are expensive and generally poorly tolerated.
- **Pramlintide** is a synthetic analog of human amylin, which is synthesized by pancreatic beta cells and cosecreted with insulin in response to food intake. It suppresses glucagon secretion and slows stomach emptying and can be used as an adjunctive treatment for patients with T1DM or T2DM who inject insulin at mealtime. Nausea is its major side effect. This therapy has been largely replaced with use of GLP-1 analogs.
- **Thiazolidinediones (pioglitazone and rosiglitazone)** increase insulin sensitivity and have been used in the therapy of type 2 diabetes. Serum transaminase levels should be obtained before starting therapy and monitored periodically. Thiazolidinediones, in general, result in moderate weight gain and increase the risk for heart failure and osteoporosis/fractures. Rosiglitazone has an FDA black box warning for heart failure exacerbations and myocardial ischemia. Pioglitazone and rosiglitazone cause increased incidence of bladder cancer. Use thiazolidinediones with caution with calcium channel blockers, especially amlodipine (can cause fluid retention and edema).
- Combination therapy of various hypoglycemic agents is commonly used when dual therapy results in inadequate glycemic control.
- **Insulin** is indicated for the treatment of all T1DM and for T2DM patients whose condition cannot be adequately controlled with diet and oral agents. The American College of Endocrinology and the American Association of Clinical Endocrinologists recommend initiation of insulin therapy in patients with type 2 diabetes and an initial HbA_{1c} level >9%, or if the diabetes is uncontrolled despite optimal oral glycemic therapy. Insulin therapy may be initiated as augmentation, starting at 0.1 to 0.2 unit/kg of body weight, or as replacement, starting at 0.6 to 1.0 unit/kg. Table 6 describes commonly used types of insulin.
  1. The risks of insulin therapy include weight gain, hypoglycemia, and in rare cases, allergic or cutaneous reactions.
  2. Replacement insulin therapy should mimic normal release patterns.
     a. Approximately 50% to 60% of daily insulin can be given as a long-acting insulin (NPH, Ultralente, glargine, detemir) injected once or twice daily.
     b. The remaining 40% to 50% can be short-acting (regular) or rapid-acting (lispro, aspart, glulisine) to cover mealtime carbohydrates and correct increased current glucose levels.
     c. NPH and older basal insulins can be mixed with rapid-acting insulins like Humalog and regular; all newer basal insulins cannot be mixed in one syringe.
     d. Basal-bolus regimens are now preferred on injection of long-acting basal at bedtime or in AM to target fasting glycemia between 80 and 130, and rapid-acting mealtime insulins to target lower postprandial blood glucose <140 mg/dl.
     e. New combinations of basal insulins with GLP-1 analogs are now available:
        (1) Soliqua: Combines glargine insulin and lixisenatide in one pen. Patients taking <30 units start at

TABLE 6 Types of Insulin[a]

Preparation	Brand	Onset (hr)[b]	Peak (hr)	Duration (hr)[c]	Route
Insulin Aspart	NovoLog[d]	<0.25	1-3	3-5	SC, IV, CSII
Insulin Aspart Protamine/Insulin Aspart	NovoLog Mix 70/30[d]	<0.25	1-4	24	SC
Insulin Detemir	Levemir	1-4	None	24	SC
Insulin Glargine	Lantus[d]	1-4	None	≥24	SC
Insulin Degludec	Tresiba	1-9	None	>42	SC
Insulin Glulisine	Apidrad	≤0.25	1	2-4	SC, IV
Insulin Lispro	Humalog[d]	<0.25	1	3.5-4.5	SC
Insulin Lispro Protamine/Insulin Lispro	Humalog Mix 75/25[d]	≤0.25	0.5-1.5	24	SC
	Humalog Mix 50/50[d]	≤0.25	1	16	SC
Insulin Injection Regular (R)	Humulin R[f]	0.5	2-4	6-8	SC, IM, IV
	Novolin N[e]	0.5	2.5-5	8	SC, IM, IV
Insulin Isophane Suspension (NPH)/ Regular Insulin (R)	Humulin 70/30[f]	0.5	2-12	24	SC
	Humulin 50/50[f]	0.5	3-5	24	SC
	Novolin 70/30[e]	0.5	2-12	24	SC
Insulin Isophane Suspension (NPH)	Humulin N[f]	1-2	6-12	18-24	SC
	Novolin N[e]	1.5	4-12	24	SC

CSII, Continuous subcutaneous infusion; *IM*, intramuscularly; *IV*, intravenously; *N*, NPH or isophane suspension; *NPH*, neutral protamine Hagedorn; *SC*, subcutaneous.

[a]Injectable insulins listed are available in a concentration of 100 U/ml; Humulin R, in a concentration of 500 U/ml for subcutaneous (SC) injection. SC injection only is available by prescription from Lilly for insulin-resistant patients who are hospitalized or in need of medical supervision.

[b]Onset for injectable formulations is always for the subcutaneous (SC) route. All times are approximate.

[c]Maximum effect occurs between these times; actual effect may last longer.

[d]Recombinant human insulin analog (using *E. coli*).

[e]Recombinant (using *S. cerevisiae*).

[f]Recombinant (using *E. coli*).

Modified from Melmed S, Polonsky KS, Larsen PR, Kronenberg HM: *Williams textbook of endocrinology*, ed 12, Philadelphia, 2011, Saunders.

15 units and patient taking >30 units start at 30 units and are titrated every 3 to 4 days until fasting blood glucose levels are between 80 and 130 mg/dl. One should not exceed 60 units of glargine insulin.

(2) Xultophy 100/3.6 is degludec insulin and liraglutide combination in one pen. Dosing is based on tresiba dose. Patients start at 16 units and increase by 2 units every 5 to 7 days to target fasting glycemia between 80 and 130 mg/dl, and dose cannot exceed 50 units. The use of this combination may eliminate or reduce prandial insulin needs and limits weight gain caused by insulin.

3. Continuous subcutaneous insulin infusion (CSII, or insulin pump) provides comparable or slightly better control than multiple daily injections. It should be considered for diabetes presenting in childhood or adolescence and during pregnancy. The guidelines for insulin pump therapy from the American Association of Diabetes Educators include "frequent and unpredictable fluctuations in blood glucose" and "patient perceptions that diabetes management impedes the pursuit of personal or professional goals." Use of insulin pumps are today coupled with CGM monitoring and with software in which the computer is making the automatic adjustments to glucose levels, constituting what is referred to as an "artificial pancreas." This allows for fewer fluctuations of glycemia.

- Antiplatelet therapy: Low-dose aspirin (ASA; 81 mg/day) has been proven to lower the risk of subsequent myocardial infarction, stroke, or vascular death in secondary prevention studies. The ADA recommends low-dose aspirin for primary prevention in diabetic patients with one additional cardiovascular risk factor, including age older than 50 yr, cigarette smoking, hypertension, obesity, albuminuria, hyperlipidemia, and family history of coronary artery disease. Clopidogrel can be used in patients with atherosclerotic cardiovascular disease (ASCVD) and a documented aspirin allergy. The ADA does not recommend aspirin therapy in diabetics younger than 50 yr of age at low risk for coronary artery disease.
- Lipid management: Measure fasting lipid profile at least annually in adults.
  1. All patients with diabetes with one or more additional risk factors for cardiovascular disease should be on statin therapy together with lifestyle modification regardless of baseline lipid levels.
  2. Diabetic patients aged 40 to 75 with LDL cholesterol of 70 to 189 mg/dl and without clinical ASCVD should receive at least moderate-intensity statin therapy and consider high-intensity statin therapy if 10-yr ASCVD risk is ≥7.5%.
  3. Ezetimibe can be added to moderate-intensity statin therapy in those who cannot tolerate high-intensity statin therapy.
  4. Combination therapy with statin and fenofibrate is not recommended but may be considered in those with triglyceride levels equal or greater than 204 mg/dl. If triglycerides are not at goal with combination of statin and fibrate, then prescription fish oil is advised if triglyceride levels still exceed 300 mg/dl.
  5. PCK-9 inhibitors may be considered in diabetics with CAD risk when statins are insufficient and in those who cannot tolerate statins, have had cardiovascular events, and cannot achieve A_{1c} to target goal.
- Hypertension: Antihypertensive therapy is recommended to keep systolic blood pressure (BP) <140 and diastolic BP <90 mm Hg. Use of angiotensin-converting enzyme (ACE) inhibitors or angiotensin receptor blockers (ARBs) to decrease albuminuria and for prevention of progression of kidney disease should be considered regardless of presence of hypertension. Combination therapy with an ACE inhibitor and an ARB should be avoided due to increased risk of adverse effects among patients with diabetic nephropathy. In older adults a treatment goal of <130/70 mm Hg is not recommended due to higher mortality and morbidity.
- Bariatric surgery should be considered in adults with BMI >35 kg/m2 and type 2 diabetes, especially if the diabetes is difficult to control with lifestyle and pharmacologic therapy. Five-yr outcome data showed that, among patients with type 2 DM and a BMR of 27 to 43, bariatric surgery plus intensive medical therapy was more effective than intensive medical therapy alone in decreasing, or in some cases resolving, hyperglycemia.[2]
- Treat hypoglycemia in a conscious person with glucose tab or gel 15 to 20 g, and intramuscular injection of glucagon if unconscious. Patient and family members should be instructed on the administration of glucagon for individuals at significant risk for severe hypoglycemia. A sick day management protocol for diabetic patients is described in Box 1.

DISPOSITION

- Diabetic retinopathy occurs in nearly 15% of patients with diabetes after 15 yr of diagnosis and increases 1%/yr after diagnosis. Glycemic, lipid, and blood pressure controls are essential to reduce the risk

[2]Schauer PR, et al.: Bariatric surgery versus intensive medical therapy for diabetes—5-year outcomes, *N Engl J Med* 376(7):641–651, 2017.

BOX 1 Sick Day Management Protocol for Diabetic Patients

Examples of "Sick Day" Scenarios

- Feeling sick or presence of fever for 2 days or longer without getting better
- Vomiting or diarrhea for more than 6 hours

Management

General Measures

- Check blood sugar levels at least every 4 hours, but when values are changing quickly, check more often.
- Check urine or blood ketones.
- Modify usual insulin regimen according to a plan developed by the diabetes physician or team.
- Maintain adequate food and fluid intake. If your appetite is poor, aim for consumption of 50 g of carbohydrate every 3-4 hours. If you are nauseous, high-carbohydrate liquids, such as regular (not diet) soft drinks or juice, or frozen juice bars, sherbet, pudding, creamed soups, or fruit-flavored yogurt usually are tolerated. Broth also is a good alternative.

Taking Medications When You Are Sick

- If you are eating: Continue taking your pills for diabetes or your insulin. Your blood sugar may continue to rise because of your illness.
- If you are nauseous or vomiting or otherwise cannot take your medicines:
- Continue to take your long-acting insulin (Lantus, Levemir, NPH).
- Call your doctor and discuss whether you need to adjust your short- or rapid-acting insulin dose (regular, lispro [Humalog], aspart [Novolog], glulisine [Apidra]) or your other diabetes medicines.

Examples of When to Call Physician or Diabetes Team

- If glucose levels are higher than 240 mg/dl despite taking extra insulin according to a sick day plan
- If you take diabetes pills and blood sugar is still above 240 mg/dl before meals and remains there for more than 24 hours
- If symptoms/signs develop that might signal DKA or dehydration, such as dizziness, trouble breathing, fruity breath, or dry and cracked lips or tongue

DKA, Diabetic ketoacidosis; *NPH*, neutral protamine Hagedorn.

Parrillo JE, Dellinger RP: *Critical care medicine: principles of diagnosis and management in the adult*, ed 4, Philadelphia, 2014, Mosby.

and progression of diabetic retinopathy. An annual comprehensive eye exam by an ophthalmologist or optometrist should begin at the time of diagnosis for those with T2DM and after 5 yr in those with T1DM. Retinal laser photocoagulation and vitrectomy are effective treatment modalities. Prevention is best accomplished by strict glucose and BP control. Early blockade of the renin-angiotensin system has been shown to slow progression of retinopathy in patients with type 1 diabetes.

- The frequency of neuropathy in patients with type 2 diabetes approaches 70% to 80%. It can be subdivided into sensorimotor neuropathy and autonomic neuropathy. Duloxetine, a selective serotonin and norepinephrine reuptake inhibitor, is effective and FDA approved for relief of diabetic peripheral neuropathy. Pregabalin and gabapentin (900 to 3600 mg/day) are also effective for the symptomatic treatment of peripheral neuropathic pain. Topical capsaicin, 5% lidocaine transdermal patches, amitriptyline, and carbamazepine are also modestly effective. Use of high-dose vitamin combination of B_{12}, B_6 with alpha lipoic acid may help with nerve preservation and worsening of neuropathy, but will have no immediate effect on pain.
- Diabetic gastroparesis is most often seen in patients who have had diabetes for at least 10 yr and typically have retinopathy, neuropathy, and nephropathy. Major manifestations are postprandial fullness, nausea, vomiting, and bloating. Pharmacologic therapy involves prokinetic agents (metoclopramide). Endoscopic injection of botulinum toxin into the pylorus and gastric electrical stimulation (using f electrodes placed laparoscopically in the muscle wall of the stomach antrum and connected to a neurostimulator) represent newer approaches to nonpharmacologic therapy.
- Nephropathy: The first sign of renal involvement in patients with DM is most often microalbuminuria, which is classified as incipient nephropathy. Before the current period of intensive glycemic control and blood pressure with ACE inhibitors and angiotensin receptor blockade, it was suggested that 25% to 45% of diabetic patients would develop clinically evident renal disease (proteinuria) and 4% to 17% would progress to end-stage renal disease. In the current era of intensive glycemic and blood pressure control and ACE/ARB use, clinically evident diabetic nephropathy has declined to 9% and end-stage renal disease 2% to 7%. Use of ACE inhibitor or ARB is not recommended in diabetics with normal blood pressure, no microalbuminuria (urine albumin to creatinine ratio less than 30 mg/g creatinine) and normal renal function (eGFR >60 ml/min/1.73m^2).
- Infections are generally more common in patients with diabetes because of multiple factors, such as impaired leukocyte function, decreased tissue perfusion secondary to vascular disease, repeated trauma because of loss of sensation, and urinary retention secondary to neuropathy.
- Prevention/delay of type 2 diabetes: Patients with prediabetes should achieve weight loss of 5% to 10% of body weight and increase physical activity to at least 150 min/wk of moderate activity such as walking. Metformin therapy may be considered in those at high risk, especially if they have hyperglycemia (HbA_{1c} ≥6) despite lifestyle interventions.
- The Mediterranean diet has been shown to prevent type 2 diabetes in patients with prediabetes and can delay the need of insulin use in type 2 diabetes in up to 50% of patients.
- Use of metformin in prediabetics can prevent onset of diabetes in up to 30% of patients, independent of diet.

REFERRAL

- Patients with diabetes should be advised to have annual ophthalmologic examinations. In T1DM, ophthalmologic visits should usually begin 5 yr after diagnosis, whereas T2DM patients should be seen from disease onset.
- Podiatric care can significantly reduce the rate of foot infections and amputations in patients with DM. Noninfected neuropathic foot ulcers require debridement and reduction of pressure.
- Nephrology consultation in all cases of proteinuria, hyperkalemia, uncontrolled BP, and when GFR has decreased to <30 ml/min/1.73 m^2.

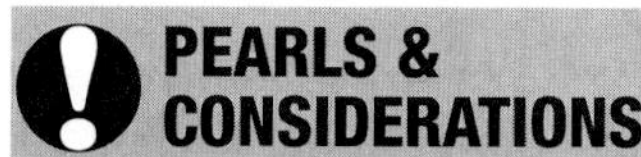

PEARLS & CONSIDERATIONS

COMMENTS

- Because normalization of serum glucose level is the ultimate goal, every patient with diabetes should measure his or her blood glucose with commercially available glucometers unless contraindicated by senility or blindness.
- Continuous glucose monitoring is now commercially available for all types of diabetics on multiple daily injections of insulin. In the near future there will be weekly disposable sensors that can replace fingersticks. The advantage of CGM is that it not only gives a patient a value, but it shows a rate of change at that moment and predicts impending hyperglycemia or hypoglycemia, allowing a patient to react appropriately.
- Underinsured children and those with psychiatric illness are at greater risk for acute complications in T1DM and require frequent monitoring and aggressive risk management with diet, exercise, and periodic laboratory evaluation.
- Significant sustained weight loss using bariatric surgery has been reported as effective in achieving remission of type 2 diabetes in morbidly obese patients. Bariatric surgery may be considered for adults with BMI >35 kg/m2 and T2DM, especially if diabetes or

associated comorbidities are difficult to control with lifestyle and pharmacologic therapy.

- Cigarette smoking predicts incident type 2 diabetes. For a smoker at risk for diabetes, smoking cessation should be coupled with strategies for diabetes prevention and early detection.
- Glycemic control in hospitalized patients: The American College of Physicians (ACP) recommends against using intensive insulin therapy to strictly control blood glucose in non-surgical intensive care unit (SICU)/medical intensive care unit (MICU) in patients with or without DM. The ACP recommends a target blood glucose level of 130 to 180 mg/dl if insulin therapy is used.
- Studies have shown that tight glycemic control in SICU patients can reduce infection rates and ICU stay. This was not seen in MICU patients. However, there is evidence showing that patients using continuous IV insulin infusions to keep tight glycemic control after open heart surgery reduces sternal wound infection rates.
- Now many institutions are incorporating automated log adjustment, such as Glucommander, which reduces workload of staff in maintaining smooth glycemic control.

SUGGESTED READING

Available at ExpertConsult.com

RELATED CONTENT

Diabetes Mellitus type 1 (Patient Information)
Diabetes Mellitus type 2 (Patient Information)
Diabetic Foot (Related Key Topic)
Diabetic Ketoacidosis (Related Key Topic)
Diabetic Polyneuropathy (Related Key Topic)
Diabetic Retinopathy (Related Key Topic)
Gestational Diabetes Mellitus (Related Key Topic)
Hyperosmolar Hyperglycemic Syndrome (Related Key Topic)

AUTHOR: **DAVID J. DOMENICHINI, M.D.**

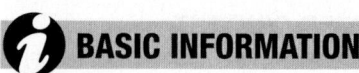

BASIC INFORMATION

DEFINITION

Diabetic foot infections (DFIs) are a common and potentially serious problem in persons with diabetes. They usually arise from either a skin ulceration that occurs secondarily to peripheral neuropathy or in a wound caused by some form of trauma. The infection usually involves one or more bacteria and can spread to contiguous tissues including bone, causing an osteomyelitis.

SYNONYMS

Diabetic foot ulcer
Diabetic foot infection
DFI

ICD-10CM CODES

E10.5	Diabetes mellitus with peripheral circulatory complications
E10.6D	Diabetes mellitus with other specific complications
E11.621	Type 2 diabetes mellitus with foot ulcer

EPIDEMIOLOGY & DEMOGRAPHICS

INCIDENCE: DFIs are the most common cause of hospitalizations for diabetic patients. They account for 20% of all hospital admissions. Nearly one in six patients will die within a yr of their infection.

PEAK INCIDENCE: More common in Hispanics, African Americans, and Native Americans due to increased rates of diabetes in those populations

PREVALENCE: 25 million people in the U.S. have diabetes, of which 19% to 34% will develop a foot ulcer in their lifetime and more than 50% of these will become infected.

PREDOMINANT SEX AND AGE: Females greater than males

RISK FACTORS:
- Diabetes greater than 10 yr
- Poor glucose control
- Peripheral neuropathy: Altered protective sensation and altered pain response
- Diabetic angiopathy: Atherosclerotic obstruction of larger vessels leading to peripheral vascular disease
- Evidence of increased local pressure: Callus or erythema

PHYSICAL FINDINGS & CLINICAL PRESENTATION

- Based on guidelines by Infectious Diseases Society of America, infection is present if obvious purulent drainage and/or the presence of two or more signs of inflammation:
  1. Erythema
  2. Pain
  3. Tenderness
  4. Warmth
  5. Induration
- Systemic signs of infection include:
  1. Anorexia, nausea/vomiting
  2. Fever, chills, night sweats
  3. Change in mental status and recent worsening of glycemic control

An earlier and commonly used classification system was originally proposed by Wagner.

An update to the Wagner system was introduced at the University of Texas (UT), San Antonio, United States. While similar to Wagner in its first three categories, this later system eliminated grades 4 and 5 and added stages A-D for each of the grades. The UT system was the first diabetic foot ulcer classification to be validated. University of Texas system Grade:
- Grade 0: Pre- or postulcerative (Stages A-D)
- Grade 1: Full-thickness ulcer not involving tendon, capsule, or bone (Stage A-D)
- Grade 2: Tendon or capsular involvement without bone palpable (Stage A-D)
- Grade 3: Probes to bone (Stage A-D)
  Stage:
  1. A: Noninfected
  2. B: Infected
  3. C: Ischemic
  4. D: Infected and ischemic
- Etiology: Most diabetic foot infections are polymicrobial (can involve 5-7 different bacteria) and depend on the extent of involvement
  1. Superficial infections are likely due to gram-positive skin bacteria:
     a. *Staphylococcus aureus*, includes methicillin-resistant *S. aureus* (MRSA)
     b. *Streptococcus agalactiae* (group B streptococcus) and *Streptococcus pyogenes* (group A streptococcus)
     c. Coagulase-negative *Staphylococcus*
  2. Infections that are deep, chronically infected, or previously treated are likely to be polymicrobial:
     a. Include above bacteria plus enterococci, gram-negative rods including *Pseudomonas aeruginosa* and anaerobes
     b. With gangrene can expect more anaerobic bacteria such as *Clostridia* and *Bacteroides* species
     c. Patients with multiple admissions can have more resistant bacteria such as ESBL-type resistant gram-negative rod bacteria, MRSA, and *Acinetobacter*

Dx DIAGNOSIS

DIFFERENTIAL DIAGNOSIS

Other inflammatory conditions that can mimic diabetic foot infections include:
- Crystal-associated arthritis such as gout
- Trauma
- Acute Charcot arthropathy from long-standing diabetes
- Venous stasis ulcers
- Deep vein thrombosis

WORKUP

Evaluation of a patient with a DFI involves determining the extent and severity of the infection, identifying the underlying factors that predispose to the infection, and determining the microbiologic etiology.

PHYSICAL EXAMINATION

- Vital signs: Fever, chills, hypotension, tachycardia can be present.
- Detailed wound description: Length, width, and depth of wound, consistency of drainage, character of wound base: Granular fibrous necrotic.
- Determination of osteomyelitis: Highly likely if bone visible. A positive probe test to bone has a sensitivity of 66% and specificity of 85% in diagnosing bone infection.
- Necrotizing infections may present with cutaneous bullae, soft tissue gas, foul odor, and skin discoloration (Fig. E1).
- Severe infections may present with gangrene, tissue necrosis, and evidence of tissue ischemia, all of which may be limb threatening.

LABORATORY TESTS

Important to obtain at baseline and to assess response to therapy:
- Fewer than 50% of patients have an elevated WBC.
- Determine BUN/Cr, acidosis, hemoglobin A_{1C}, and blood sugar.
- Acute phase reactants: Sed rate and CRP are markers for inflammation.
  1. Sed rate >70 increases probability of bone infection.
- Serum prealbumin and albumin are markers for nutritional status and ability to heal.
- An ulcer size larger than 2 cm^2 is indicative of osteomyelitis.
- Gram stains and cultures: Superficial cultures should not be obtained as they may contain colonizing bacteria; instead deep tissue cultures (aerobic and anaerobic) should be obtained.

IMAGING STUDIES

- Plain film x-ray evaluates bones and soft issues and can detect presence of tissue gas, which would represent an emergent situation (Fig. 2).
- Osteomyelitis appears as radiolucencies, periosteal reaction, and destructive changes. Plain films are 67% specific and 60% sensitive for osteomyelitis.
- Bone scan: Indium-111 or technetium-99 can distinguish acute and chronic infections.
- CT and MRI: MRI is the most sensitive and specific test to detect osteomyelitis and abscess formation.

OTHER DIAGNOSTIC TESTS

- Annual noninvasive vascular studies: Ankle brachial index (ABI): <0.90 or >1.30 indicates peripheral arterial disease
- Transcutaneous oxygen (TcPO2) tension measurements: Predictive of wound healing failure at levels below 25 mm Hg

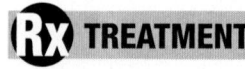

TREATMENT

Empiric antibiotic regimen should be started based on likely pathogens suspected and severity of disease. Wound management and debridement including surgical consultation are important as well.

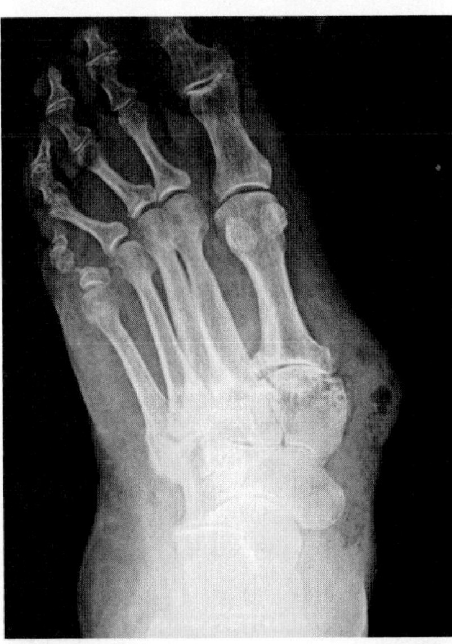

FIG. 2 X-ray. Significant soft tissue swelling in midfoot with numerous gas bubbles seen in the soft tissues

NONPHARMACOLOGIC THERAPY

- Good nutrition will promote wound healing.
- Glycemic control will promote healing.
- Fluid and electrolyte balance will improve healing.

ACUTE GENERAL TREATMENT

WOUND MANAGEMENT:

- Debridement of callus and necrotic tissues by wound care specialist or surgeon and at times may require multiple debridements.
- Wound dressing: To absorb exudates and promote healing. Many products are available but none has been proven superior and include:
  1. Enzymes
  2. Gels
  3. Hydrocolloids
  4. Antiseptics containing iodine or silver salts
  5. Honey
- Relieve pressure on the foot: Casts or special shoes.
- Amputation or revascularization procedures such as angioplasty or bypass grafting may be necessary.

ANTIBIOTIC MANAGEMENT

- Prior to receiving culture results an empiric antibiotic regimen should be started as soon as possible to cover skin bacteria, gram-negative rods, and anaerobes. Options for intravenous therapy include:
  1. Piperacillin-tazobactam: 3.375 g IV q6h with normal kidney function. Will cover gram-negative rods including *Pseudomonas aeruginosa*, streptococci, anaerobes, and *Staphylococcus aureus.* Adjust dose based on CrCl.
  2. Meropenem: 1 g IV q8h with normal kidney function has comparable coverage as piperacillin-tazobactam. Similar agents include imipenem and doripenem.
  3. Third-generation cephalosporin such as cefepime, 2 g IV q8h, or ceftriaxone, 2 g IV qd, have excellent gram-negative coverage, and for anaerobic coverage add metronidazole, 500 mg IV q8h, or clindamycin 900 mg IV q8h. Cefepime will cover *Pseudomonas aeruginosa* but ceftriaxone will not.
  4. For penicillin-allergic patients a combination of ciprofloxacin, 400 mg IV q12h, plus metronidazole or clindamycin is an option. Aztreonam is another option for gram-negative rod coverage, 2 g IV q8h.
  5. If MRSA is suspected, need to add IV vancomycin, 15-20 mg/kg IV q8-12h, depending on age and CrCL and follow trough levels to keep above 15. Other options include daptomycin, 4 mg/kg IV qd, which does not have to be adjusted for CrCL, or linezolid, 400-600 mg IV q12h.
  6. If VRE is suspected, options include tigecycline, 100-mg IV load dose, then 50 mg IV q12h, which also covers MRSA and gram-negative rods but not *Pseudomonas aeruginosa,* or can use daptomycin or linezolid.
  7. If ESBL gram-negative bacteria are suspected, then options include meropenem or ertapenem, 1 g IV qd, or tigecycline.
  8. Once culture results are known can tailor antibiotics to more specific agent.
- Oral antibiotics used for milder infections include amoxicillin-clavulanate, 875 mg PO q12h, which will cover gram-negative rods, streptococci, and anaerobes, or ciprofloxacin plus metronidazole or clindamycin. Bactrim will cover MRSA and MSSA and some gram-negative rods.

The expert panel on diabetic foot infection (DFI) of the International Working Group on the Diabetic Foot conducted a systematic review. Results of comparisons of different antibiotic regimens generally demonstrated that newly introduced antibiotic regimens appeared to be as effective as conventional therapy.

CHRONIC TREATMENT

- Length of therapy: Highly variable depending on the severity of the infection. In general, 2 to 4 weeks of antibiotics is sufficient. If bone infection suspected or documented, may need 4-8 weeks of antibiotics, preferably intravenous via a peripherally inserted central line (PICC line).
- Surgical debridement may also be necessary for several weeks.

COMPLEMENTARY MEDICINE

- Hyperbaric oxygen (HBO): Used as an adjunct to antibiotics, debridement, and revascularization in the therapy of chronic, nonhealing wounds associated with diabetes. Evidence of effectiveness is conflicting, and recent trials have failed to show improvement in clinical outcomes.[1] HBO acts by:
  1. Inducing vasoconstriction and reducing vasogenic edema
  2. Facilitating fibroblast activity, angiogenesis, and wound healing
  3. Killing anaerobic bacteria and augmenting neutrophil bactericidal activity
- Negative pressure wound therapy (wound vac): Controlled, subatmospheric pressure applied to an open wound can accelerate healing and closure.
  1. An open cell foam insert is cut to fit the open wound and then secured under a clear, vapor-permeable, plastic dressing.
  2. Tubing extends from the sponge to a disposable collection canister.
  3. A portable pump applies 125 mm Hg of controlled suction to the system. The subatmospheric pressure (suction) is equally distributed across the open wound and evacuates stagnant fluid from the wound.

DISPOSITION

- Following up on sed rates, CRP, BUN/CR, and levels of vancomycin if that antibiotic used.
- Surgical or wound center care follow-up.
- HBO usually involves multiple sessions over several weeks.
- Wound vac is applied for weeks and requires periodic nursing follow-up.
- The risk of death at 5 yr for a patient with a diabetic foot ulcer is 2 to 5 times as high as the risk for a patient with diabetes without a foot ulcer.

REFERRAL

- Infectious disease consultant for antibiotic management.
- Surgeon or wound care center for surgical treatments.
- Endocrinologist for good diabetes care.
- Vascular surgeon for angioplasty or bypass procedures.

PEARLS & CONSIDERATIONS

- In a meta-analysis of randomized controlled trials on the outcome of DFIs, there was a 22.7% treatment failure rate.
- Patients should be advised to seek prompt medical attention as these infections can progress rapidly to gangrene.

SUGGESTED READINGS

Available at ExpertConsult.com

AUTHORS: **GLENN G. FORT, M.D., M.P.H.,** and **TANYA ALI, M.D.**

[1] Santema KTB et al: Hyperbaric oxygen therapy in the treatment of ischemic lower-extremity ulcers in patients with diabetes: results of the Damocles multicenter randomized clinical trial, *Diabetes Care* 41:112, 2018.

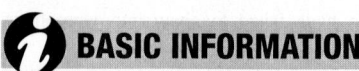

BASIC INFORMATION

DEFINITION

Diabetic ketoacidosis (DKA) is a life-threatening complication of diabetes mellitus (DM). It results from an absolute or relative insulin deficiency, which, when paired with counterregulatory hormone and free fatty acid excess, results in insulin resistance. DKA is characterized by the presence of an anion gap metabolic acidosis, ketonemia, and hyperglycemia.

ICD-10CM CODES

E10.10	Type 2 diabetes mellitus with other specified complication
E10.11	Diabetic ketoacidosis with coma associated with type 1 diabetes mellitus
E08.10	Diabetes mellitus due to underlying condition with ketoacidosis without coma
E08.11	Diabetes mellitus due to underlying condition with ketoacidosis with coma
E13.10	Diabetic ketoacidosis
E13.11	Diabetic ketoacidosis with coma

EPIDEMIOLOGY & DEMOGRAPHICS

DKA is the most common hyperglycemic emergency among patients with type 1 (T1D) and type 2 diabetes (T2D). The reported number of DKA hospitalizations in the United States is >140,000/yr. DKA most commonly occurs in T1D, with one third in T2D. Those with ketosis-prone T2D are especially vulnerable. Overall, DKA prevalence has increased, yet mortality has decreased to <5%, significantly less than from hyperglycemic hyperosmolar syndrome (HHS). Mortality from DKA in children and adolescents is most commonly due to cerebral edema, whereas in adults it is usually related to the precipitating illness (i.e., sepsis, cardiac or CNS ischemia, pneumonia).

PHYSICAL FINDINGS & CLINICAL PRESENTATION

- Polyuria, polydipsia, weight loss, weakness
- Signs of dehydration (tachycardia, hypotension, dry mucous membranes, sunken eyeballs, poor skin turgor)
- Nausea, vomiting, abdominal tenderness, ileus
- Mental obtundation (can range from full alertness to coma)
- Tachypnea with air hunger (Kussmaul respirations)
- Fruity breath (caused by acetone)
- Evidence of precipitating factors (i.e., ischemia or infection)

ETIOLOGY

Hyperglycemia occurs from ineffective insulin concentrations with transient insulin resistance plus increased hepatic gluconeogenesis and glycogenolysis. Increased lipolysis and fatty oxidation result in ketonemia and metabolic acidosis.

DKA can be precipitated by various conditions:

- Infection
- Insulin deficiency (undiagnosed diabetes or medication nonadherence)
- Inflammatory conditions (i.e., acute pancreatitis)
- Ischemia/infarction (i.e., myocardial infarction, bowel ischemia)
- Kidney failure
- Severe extracellular fluid volume depletion
- Drugs (i.e., steroids, thiazides, atypical antipsychotics, SGLT2 inhibitors, alcohol, sympathomimetics including cocaine, immunotherapy for cancer [such as anti-programmed death 1 (PD-1) antibody treatment])

Dx DIAGNOSIS

DIFFERENTIAL DIAGNOSIS

- Hyperosmolar nonketotic state
- Alcoholic/starvation ketoacidosis
- Lactic acidosis
- Acute kidney injury/chronic kidney disease
- Metabolic acidosis caused by exogenous poisons, e.g., methanol, ethylene glycol, paraldehyde
- Salicylate poisoning
- Hypovolemic/septic shock

WORKUP

After initial history is obtained, perform physical examination, including evaluation of airway, breathing, circulation, mental status, volume status, and signs suggestive of precipitating event(s).

LABORATORY TESTS

- Serum glucose level: Generally >250 mg/dl. However, "euglycemic DKA" can occur in 10% of the DKA population (i.e., exogenous insulin injection en route to hospital, use of an SGLT2-inhibitor, food restriction).
- Arterial blood gas (demonstrating metabolic acidosis): Arterial pH <7.30.
- Serum beta hydroxybutyrate and urine ketones: Positive (beta hydroxybutyrate >3 mmol/L, ≥2+ urine ketones).
- Serum electrolytes:
  1. Serum bicarbonate: <15 mEq/L (mild DKA may decline to levels to <18 mEq/L).
  2. Serum potassium: Levels may initially measure as normal or high from extracellular shift with insulin deficiency and hyperosmolality. However, overall total body potassium depletion occurs from urinary losses and vomiting.
  3. Serum sodium: May be low, normal, or high. Hyperglycemia increases plasma osmolality, which attracts intracellular water to the extracellular compartment, decreasing serum sodium. Correct serum sodium by adding 1.6 mEq/L to the measured serum sodium for every 100 mg/dl rise in serum glucose above 100 mg/dl up to 400 mg/dl, then 4 mEq/L for each glucose increment of 100 mg/dl >400 mg/dl.
  4. Serum calcium, magnesium, and phosphorus: May be significantly low and may decrease further with DKA treatment.
  5. Anion gap (AG): Na − (Cl + HCO_3). AG is increased (>10) from elevated ketones.
  6. Blood urea nitrogen (BUN) and creatinine: Generally reveal acute kidney injury.
- Hemoglobin A1c (if not performed in past 3 months).
- Complete blood count with differential: May indicate underlying infection (leukocytosis >25,000/mm^3), inflammatory condition, or hemoconcentration. A leukocytosis of 10,000–15,000/mm^3 is expected from the stress of illness alone.
- Urinalysis, urine/blood cultures: As indicated based on exam findings.
- Pregnancy test: Perform in all female patients of reproductive age.
- Lipase/liver enzymes: Obtain if abdominal pain present. Elevated lipase can occur without underlying pancreatitis.

IMAGING STUDIES

ECG, chest x-ray, and other imaging studies as indicated to evaluate the precipitating cause(s).

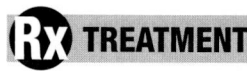

Rx TREATMENT

NONPHARMACOLOGIC THERAPY

- Monitor mental status, vital signs, and urine output hourly until improved.
- Monitor serum glucose hourly and serum electrolytes, BUN, and creatinine every 2–4 hours until DKA resolves.

ACUTE GENERAL Rx (FIG. 1)

FLUID REPLACEMENT Fluid therapy is initiated to expand volume and restore renal perfusion for a usual total body water deficit of 8–10 liters. In the absence of cardiac compromise or end-stage renal disease, infuse 0.9% normal saline (NS) at an initial rate of 1–1.5 L/hr (alternatively, use 15–20 ml/kg per hour) for the first 1–2 hours. Subsequently, fluid choice depends on patient hemodynamics, electrolytes, and urinary output. If corrected serum sodium is normal or high, infuse 0.45% NS at 250–500 ml/hr. If corrected serum sodium is low, continue 0.9% NS at a similar rate. Once serum glucose decreases to 200 mg/dl, add 5% dextrose to the IV fluid. Recommended sodium decline is 0.5 mEq/L per hour and should not surpass 10–12 mEq/L per day. Hyperglycemia (>250 mg/dl) resolves sooner than ketoacidosis (6 versus 12 hours, respectively).

INSULIN ADMINISTRATION Administer initial bolus of IV regular insulin 0.1 units/kg followed by 0.1 units/kg per hour infusion or a continuous infusion of 0.14 units/kg per hour without initial bolus. If serum glucose declines less than 50–75 mg/dl in the first hour, increase insulin infusion rate hourly until a steady glucose decline is seen. Once serum glucose reaches 200 mg/dl and until resolution of DKA, maintain serum glucose between 150 and 200 mg/dl by decreasing insulin infusion to 0.02–0.05 units/kg per hour or giving subcutaneous rapid-acting insulin at 0.1 units/kg every 2 hours.

PROTOCOL FOR MANAGEMENT OF ADULT PATIENTS WITH DKA *

Complete initial evaluation. Check capillary glucose and serum/urine ketones to confirm hyperglycemia and ketonemia/ketonuria. Obtain blood for metabolic profile. Check blood glucose by finger stick every hr. until it is ≤ 200 mg/dl. Get an ECG. Start IV fluids: 1.0 L of 0.9% NaCl per hour.†

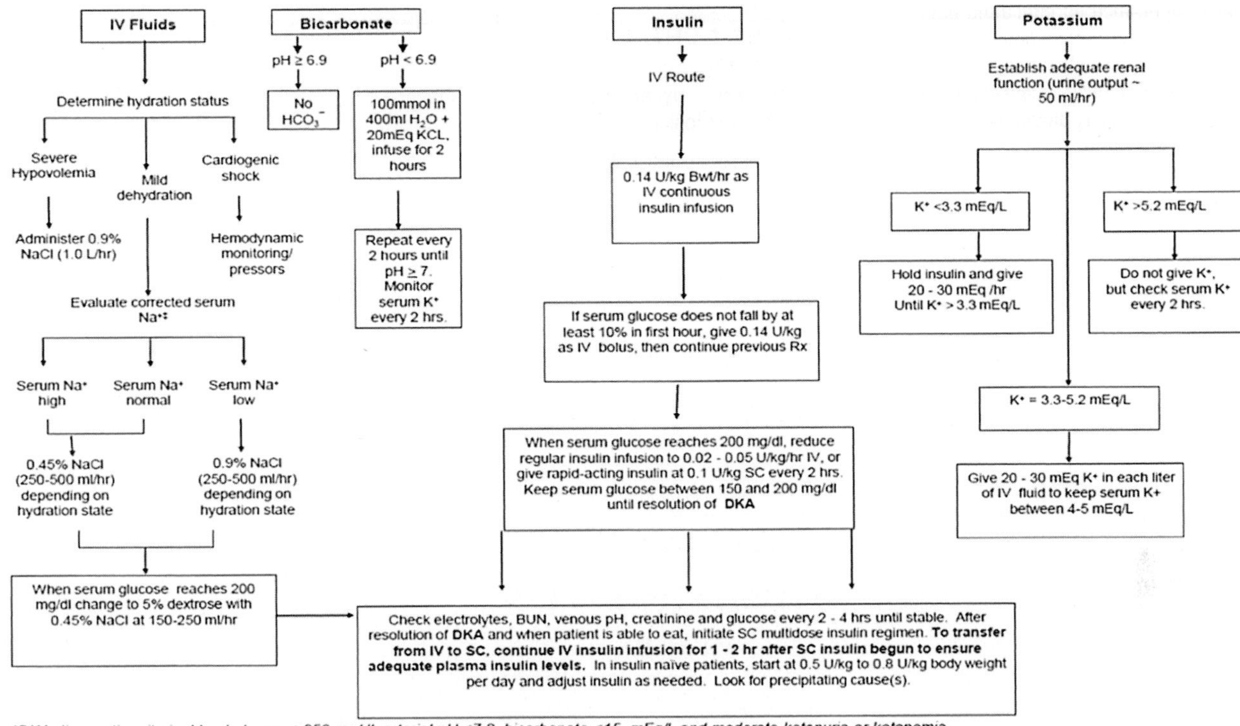

*DKA diagnostic criteria: blood glucose >250 mg/dl, arterial pH <7.3, bicarbonate <15, mEq/l, and moderate ketonuria or ketonemia.
‡ Serum Na should be corrected for hyperglycemia (for each 200 mg/dl glucose, add 1.6 mEq to sodium value for corrected serum value)

Modified from * Kitabchi et al., Diabetes Care 2009

FIG. 1 Management of diabetic ketoacidosis. *BUN,* Blood urea nitrogen; *DKA,* diabetic ketoacidosis; *ECG,* electrocardiogram; *IV,* intravenous; *Rx,* prescription; *SC,* subcutaneous. (From Nyenwe EA, et al.: The evolution of diabetic ketoacidosis: an update of its etiology, pathogenesis, and management, *Metabolism* 65(4):507–521, 2016.)

POTASSIUM REPLACEMENT Insulin therapy shifts potassium intracellularly, frequently causing hypokalemia. If serum potassium at presentation is between 3.3 and 5.2 mEq/L, infuse 20–30 mEq of potassium chloride (KCl) with each liter of IV fluid to maintain serum potassium at 4–5 mEq/L. If serum potassium is <3.3 mEq/L, hold insulin until serum potassium is >3.3 mEq/L and replace potassium by administering KCl infusion at 20–30 mEq/hr. If serum potassium at presentation is >5.2 mEq/L, monitor serum potassium level every 2 hours without replacement.

BICARBONATE REPLACEMENT The use of bicarbonate in DKA is debated. There are numerous adverse effects associated with severe metabolic acidosis (decreased cardiac contractility, cerebral vasodilation). In adult patients with pH <6.9, give 100 mmol (2 ampules) of sodium bicarbonate in 400 ml of sterile water (isotonic solution) with 20 mEq KCl at 200 ml/hr for 2 hours until venous pH is >7.0. If pH is still <7 after infusion, repeat infusion every 2 hours until pH is >7.

PHOSPHATE REPLACEMENT Phosphate replacement is not routinely recommended, yet phosphorus decreases with insulin administration. In patients with cardiac dysfunction, respiratory depression, or anemia, and serum phosphate <1 mg/dl, add 20–30 mEq/L of potassium phosphate to IV fluids to prevent inadequate diaphragm function.

TRANSITION TO SUBCUTANEOUS INSULIN Resolution of DKA occurs when blood glucose is <200 mg/dl and two of the following occur: venous pH >7.3, serum bicarbonate >15, anion gap ≤12. At this point, patients can transition to subcutaneous insulin but may remain on IV insulin if NPO. Overlap subcutaneous long- or intermediate-acting insulin with IV insulin by 2–4 hours to maintain adequate insulin levels and prevent rebound hyperglycemia. In patients with a known history of controlled diabetes, their home insulin regimen may be resumed. In patients with known poorly controlled diabetes, the subcutaneous insulin dose can be determined based on their stable insulin drip requirement. Insulin-naïve patients may be started on basal-bolus insulin therapy, starting with a total daily dose of 0.5–0.8 units/kg (split as half-basal and half-bolus: Administer 1/3 total bolus for each meal). Their stable insulin drip requirement will also help guide initial doses of subcutaneous insulin. Further subcutaneous insulin dose titration will be based on resultant blood glucoses. Resolution of glucotoxicity and the inciting condition(s) will decrease insulin requirements.

DISPOSITION In general, patients with DKA should be admitted to the intensive care unit on an insulin drip. Alert patients who are able to take fluids orally and have mild DKA (plasma glucose >250 mg/dl, arterial pH 7.25–7.3, bicarbonate 15–18 mEq/L with anion gap >10 and alert mental status) occasionally can be treated with rapid-acting insulin analogues under observation and sent home. Timely follow-up with primary care or endocrinology is important, preferably with appointment made before discharge.

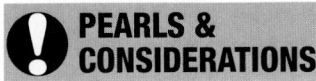

PEARLS & CONSIDERATIONS

COMMENTS

- DKA is the initial presentation of diabetes in 15%–20% of adults and 30%–40% of children. This underscores the importance of educating patients, families, and school administrators regarding early symptoms of diabetes with the aim of earlier diagnosis.
- Address affordability of insulin before discharge. Consider use of NPH and regular insulin for $25/vial at Walmart when needed.
- Proper instructions for insulin storage, dosing, timing of mealtime insulin before meals, preparation of insulin before injection (i.e., resuspend NPH), and use of syringe/vial or pen are paramount.

PREVENTION

Many cases of DKA can be prevented by effective patient education and communication. Place importance on educating patients regarding sick day management to include early communication with provider, continuing insulin during illness, checking ketones, and continuing an easily digestible liquid diet containing carbohydrates.

SUGGESTED READING

Available at ExpertConsult.com

RELATED CONTENT

Diabetes Mellitus (Related Key Topic)
Hyperosmolar Hyperglycemic Syndrome (Related Key Topic)

AUTHOR: **JESSICA E. SHILL, M.D.**

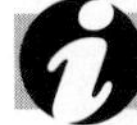

BASIC INFORMATION

DEFINITION

Diabetic polyneuropathy is a distal symmetric polyneuropathy (DSPN) characterized by numbness, tingling, pain, or weakness that affects the nerves in a stocking-and-glove pattern, beginning in the distal extremities. DSPN leads to substantial pain, morbidity, and impaired quality of life. A number of different classification schemes exist for diabetic neuropathy; a common one is outlined in Box 1.

SYNONYMS

Distal symmetric polyneuropathy (DSPN)
Diabetic peripheral neuropathy

ICD-10CM CODES

E11.40	Type 2 diabetes mellitus with neurological complications
E11.40	Type 2 diabetes mellitus with diabetic neuropathy, unspecified
E11.41	Type 2 diabetes mellitus with diabetic mononeuropathy
E11.42	Type 2 diabetes mellitus with diabetic polyneuropathy
E11.43	Type 2 diabetes mellitus with diabetic autonomic (poly)neuropathy
E11.44	Type 2 diabetes mellitus with diabetic amyotrophy
E11.49	Type 2 diabetes mellitus with other diabetic neurological complication

EPIDEMIOLOGY & DEMOGRAPHICS

PREVALENCE: The prevalence of diabetic polyneuropathy varies from 10% to 100% in patients with diabetes mellitus in population-based studies. It is the most common form of peripheral neuropathy in the western world.
RISK FACTORS: Patients with poor glycemic control, diabetic nephropathy, or retinopathy are at increased risk.

PHYSICAL FINDINGS & CLINICAL PRESENTATION

- Patients most commonly experience numbness and tingling, but they may also experience either feelings of tightness or a sensation of heat or cold.
- Pain is common, is often worst at night, and can be burning, aching, shooting, or lancinating in nature.
- Sensory symptoms begin in the feet and may slowly ascend over months to years. Symptoms in the hands do not generally occur until symptoms in the lower extremities have reached the level of the knees. In more severe cases, the symptoms can spread to the trunk and head.
- Neurologic examination reveals early loss of small-fiber modalities resulting in decreased pinprick and temperature sensation and later involvement of large-fiber modalities leading to a reduction in vibratory and proprioceptive sensation. Ankle reflexes are usually reduced or absent, and more proximal reflexes may also become involved as the neuropathy progresses. Strength is usually normal, but there can be some motor involvement leading to mild weakness and atrophy, which is usually limited to intrinsic foot muscles and ankle dorsiflexors.

BOX 1 Clinical Classification of Diabetic Neuropathies

Symmetric
- Diabetic polyneuropathy
- Diabetic autonomic neuropathy
- Painful diabetic neuropathy

Asymmetric
- Diabetic radiculoplexopathy
- Diabetic thoracic radiculoneuropathy
- Mononeuropathies
- Carpal tunnel syndrome
- Ulnar neuropathy at the elbow
- Peroneal neuropathy at fibular head
- Cranial neuropathies

Fillit HM: *Brocklehurst's textbook of geriatric medicine and gerontology*, ed 8, Philadelphia, 2017, Elsevier.

ETIOLOGY

The precise etiology is unknown but most likely involves a complex interaction of metabolic derangements and microvascular insults occurring in the setting of diabetes.

Dx DIAGNOSIS

DIFFERENTIAL DIAGNOSIS

Although diabetes is the leading cause of peripheral neuropathy in developed countries, there are numerous other causes requiring further investigation(s).

WORKUP

- A thorough history and neurologic examination are essential to confirm features consistent with a diabetic polyneuropathy and exclude other features suggesting alternative diagnoses.
- For some patients, neuropathy may be the presenting feature of previously undiagnosed diabetes.
- Electrodiagnostic evaluation to include nerve conduction studies and electromyography can be helpful in confirming the presence, extent, and severity of a neuropathy.
- Patients with DSPN typically have a reduction of amplitudes and slowing of conduction velocities involving sensory and possibly motor nerves in a length-dependent and symmetric fashion.
- Electromyographic examination of distal muscles may reveal fibrillation potentials, positive sharp waves, and large motor unit action potentials, all suggestive of denervation and reinnervation.
- Electrodiagnostic testing may be negative if the neuropathy is limited to small fiber involvement.
- Neither skin biopsy nor nerve biopsy is necessary in the vast majority of cases.
- Fig. 1 describes a diagnosis and treatment algorithm of diabetic autonomic neuropathy.

LABORATORY TESTS

- Fasting blood sugar, hemoglobin A1c, and 2-hour oral glucose tolerance tests should all be considered in patients with peripheral neuropathy without a known history of diabetes.
- A focused laboratory evaluation for other common or potentially treatable causes of neuropathy is also indicated: Complete blood cell count, complete metabolic panel to include electrolytes and liver function tests, erythrocyte sedimentation rate, vitamin B12 and folate levels, thyroid function tests, serum protein electrophoresis with immunofixation.
- Additional laboratory tests can be considered, based on either history or exam findings suggesting other underlying diagnoses, such as antinuclear antibodies, extractable nuclear antigens, ANCAs, rheumatoid factor, HIV, hepatitis B and C, and cryoglobulins.

IMAGING STUDIES

Imaging is not necessary unless there is concern for an alternate or coexisting process based on the history and examination.

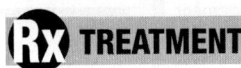

TREATMENT

CHRONIC Rx

- Table 1 summarizes clinical features, diagnosis, and treatment of diabetic autonomic neuropathy.
- Glycemic control: The primary treatment for diabetic polyneuropathy is effective glycemic control, as this may either improve or at least slow progression of the neuropathy.
- Symptomatic management: Another aspect of treatment is the symptomatic management of pain and paresthesias. The American Academy of Neurology, the American Association of Neuromuscular and Electrodiagnostic Medicine, and the American Academy of Physical Medicine and Rehabilitation have together developed an evidence-based guideline for the treatment of painful diabetic neuropathy. Pregabalin, an anticonvulsant, is the only agent in the guideline that has been established as effective for painful diabetic neuropathy. Other probably effective agents are listed in the following:
  1. Topical agents: Lidocaine 5% patch can be applied to painful areas for 12 hours a day, capsaicin 0.075% applied qid.
  2. Anticonvulsants: Gabapentin (100 to 1200 mg tid) and pregabalin (50 to 100 mg tid).
  3. Antidepressants: Amitriptyline (10 to 100 mg qhs), nortriptyline (25 to 150 mg qhs), duloxetine (60 to 120 mg daily), and venlafaxine (75 to 225 mg/day).
  4. Tramadol (50 mg qid as needed) can be a useful adjunctive analgesic.
- Fig. 2 describes a treatment algorithm for neuropathic pain after exclusion of nondiabetic etiologies and stabilization of glycemic control.

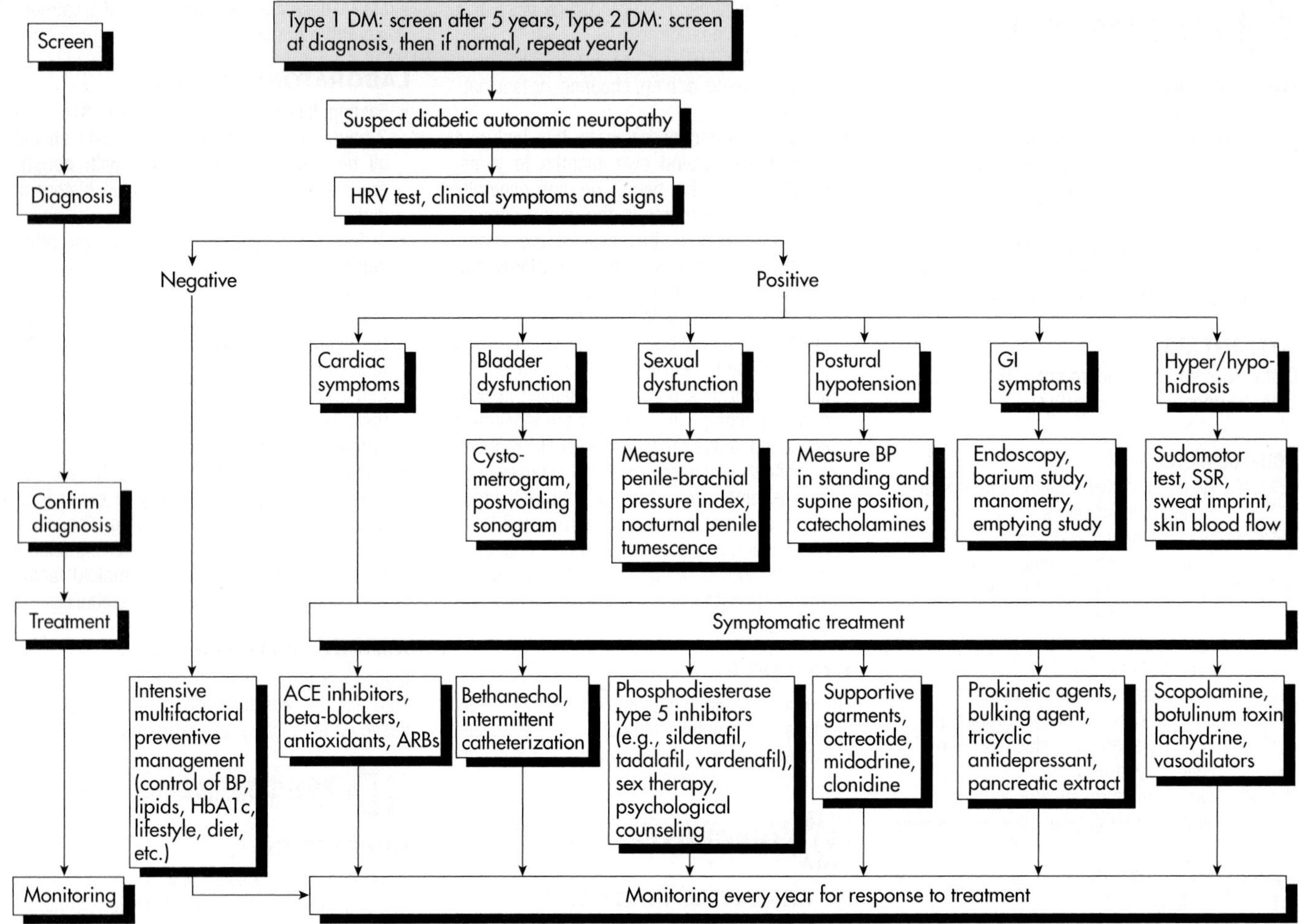

FIG. 1 Diagnosis and treatment algorithm of diabetic autonomic neuropathy. *ACE*, Angiotensin-converting enzyme; *ARBs*, angiotensin receptor blockers; *BP*, blood pressure; *DM*, diabetes mellitus; *GI*, gastrointestinal; *HRV*, heart rate variability; *SSR*, sympathetic skin response. (Modified from Larsen PR et al [eds]: *Williams textbook of endocrinology*, ed 11, Philadelphia, 2008, Saunders.)

DISPOSITION

The distal sensory loss of diabetic polyneuropathy places patients at increased risk of trauma to the extremities, with the potential for ulceration and infection that could ultimately require amputation if not attended to in a timely fashion.

REFERRAL

- A neurologist can assist in the diagnosis and management of diabetic polyneuropathy.
- Patients with diabetic polyneuropathy should also be evaluated at least annually by a podiatrist and ophthalmologist.
- Progression of diabetic polyneuropathy can be minimized by paying close attention to strict glycemic control as well as other risk factors such as hypertension and obesity.

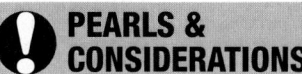

PEARLS & CONSIDERATIONS

COMMENTS

- For many patients, either DSPN or another form of diabetic neuropathy may be the initial presentation of previously undiagnosed diabetes.
- In addition to regular visits with podiatry, patients with diabetic polyneuropathy should be educated on aggressive foot hygiene and the importance of examining their own feet.

PATIENT/FAMILY EDUCATION

The following websites are recommended:

http://patienteducationcenter.org/articles/diabetic-neuropathies/

http://www.mayoclinic.com/health/diabetic-neuropathy/DS01045

SUGGESTED READINGS

Available at ExpertConsult.com

AUTHOR: **DIVYA SINGHAL, M.D.**

TABLE 1 Clinical Features, Diagnosis, and Treatment of Diabetic Autonomic Neuropathy

Symptoms	Tests	Treatments
Cardiac		
Resting tachycardia, exercise intolerance	HRV, MUGA thallium scan, MIBG scan	Graded supervised exercise, ACE inhibitors, β-blockers
Postural hypotension, dizziness, weakness, fatigue, syncope	HRV, supine and standing BP, catecholamines	Mechanical measures, clonidine, midodrine, octreotide, erythropoietin
Gastrointestinal		
Gastroparesis, erratic glucose control	Gastric emptying study, barium study	Frequent small meals, prokinetic agents (metoclopramide, domperidone, erythromycin)
Abdominal pain, early satiety, nausea, vomiting, bloating, belching	Endoscopy, manometry, electrogastrogram	Antibiotics, antiemetics, bulking agents, tricyclic antidepressants, pyloric botulinum toxin, gastric pacing
Constipation	Endoscopy	High-fiber diet, bulking agents, osmotic laxatives, lubricating agents
Diarrhea (often nocturnal alternating with constipation)		Soluble fiber, gluten and lactose restriction, anticholinergic agents, cholestyramine, antibiotics, somatostatin, pancreatic enzyme supplements
Sexual Dysfunction		
Erectile dysfunction	H&P, HRV, penile-brachial pressure index, nocturnal penile tumescence	Sex therapy, psychological counseling, phosphodiesterase inhibitors, PGE_1 injections, devices or prostheses
Vaginal dryness		Vaginal lubricants
Bladder Dysfunction		
Frequency, urgency, nocturia, urinary retention, incontinence	Cystometrogram, postvoid sonography	Bethanechol, intermittent catheterization
Sudomotor Dysfunction		
Anhidrosis, heat intolerance, dry skin, hyperhidrosis	Quantitative sudomotor axon reflex, sweat test, skin blood flow	Emollients and skin lubricants, scopolamine, glycopyrrolate, botulinum toxin, vasodilators
Pupillomotor and Visceral Dysfunction		
Blurred vision, impaired adaptation to ambient light, Argyll-Robertson pupil	Pupillometry, HRV	Care with driving at night
Impaired visceral sensation: silent MI, hypoglycemia unawareness		Recognition of unusual presentation of MI, control of risk factors, control of plasma glucose levels

ACE, acetylcholinesterase; *BP*, blood pressure; *H&P*, history and physical examination; *HRV*, heart rate variability; *MI*, myocardial infarction; *MIBG*, metaiodobenzylguanidine; *MUGA*, multigated angiography; PGE_1, prostaglandin E_1.
From Melmed S, Polonsky KS, Larsen PR, Kronenberg HM: *Williams textbook of endocrinology*, ed 12, Philadelphia, 2011, Saunders.

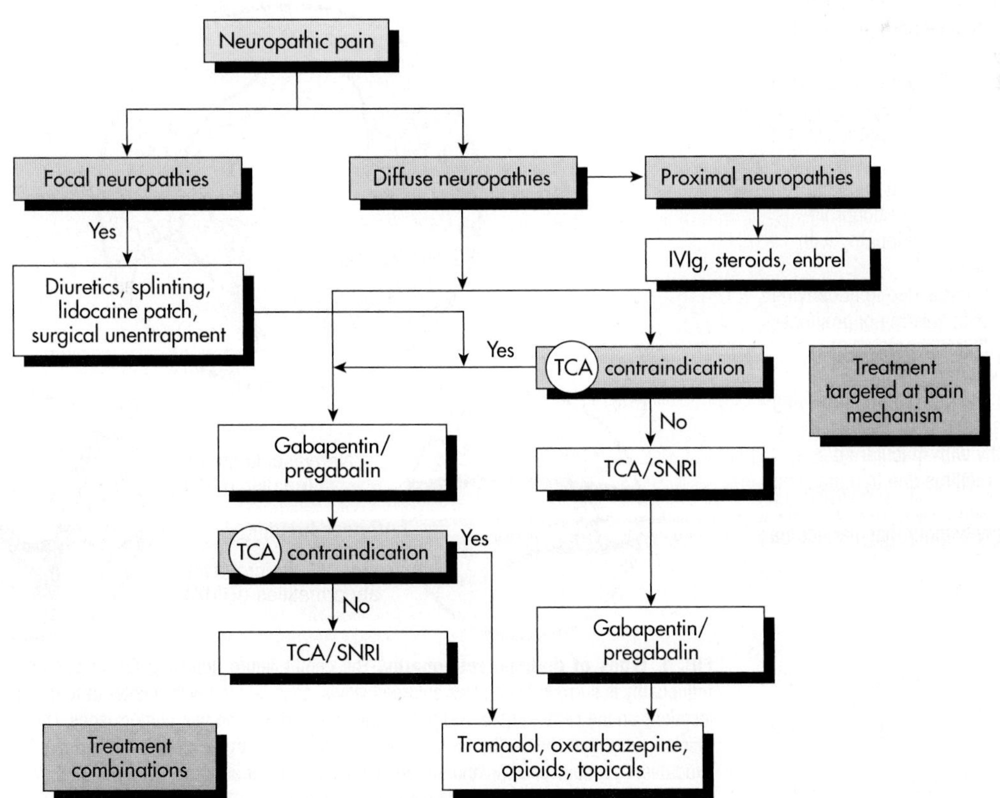

FIG. 2 Treatment algorithm for neuropathic pain after exclusion of nondiabetic etiologies and stabilization of glycemic control. *IVIg*, Intravenous immune globulin; *SNRI*, serotonin-norepinephrine reuptake inhibitors; *TCA*, tricyclic antidepressants. (From Melmed S, Polonsky KS, Larsen PR, Kronenberg HM: *Williams textbook of endocrinology*, ed 12, Philadelphia, 2011, Saunders.)

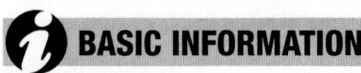

BASIC INFORMATION

DEFINITION

Diabetic retinopathy (Fig. 1) is a microvascular abnormality of the retina resulting in microaneurysms (Fig. E2), retinal hemorrhages, lipid exudates (Fig. E3), macular edema, and neovascular vessel growth (Fig. E4) and can ultimately end in blindness. Diabetic retinopathy can be classified into two stages: nonproliferative (mild, moderate, and severe) and proliferative.

SYNONYMS

Nonproliferative diabetic retinopathy (NPDR)
Proliferative diabetic retinopathy (PDR)
Diabetic macular edema (DME)

ICD-10CM CODES

E08.311	Diabetes mellitus due to underlying condition with unspecified diabetic retinopathy with macular edema
E08.319	Diabetes mellitus due to underlying condition with unspecified diabetic retinopathy without macular edema
E08.321	Diabetes mellitus due to underlying condition with mild nonproliferative diabetic retinopathy with macular edema
E08.329	Diabetes mellitus due to underlying condition with mild nonproliferative diabetic retinopathy without macular edema
E08.331	Diabetes mellitus due to underlying condition with moderate nonproliferative diabetic retinopathy with macular edema
E08.339	Diabetes mellitus due to underlying condition with moderate nonproliferative diabetic retinopathy without macular edema
E08.341	Diabetes mellitus due to underlying condition with severe nonproliferative diabetic retinopathy with macular edema
E08.349	Diabetes mellitus due to underlying condition with severe nonproliferative diabetic retinopathy without macular edema
E08.351	Diabetes mellitus due to underlying condition with proliferative diabetic retinopathy with macular edema
E08.359	Diabetes mellitus due to underlying condition with proliferative diabetic retinopathy without macular edema

EPIDEMIOLOGY & DEMOGRAPHICS

INCIDENCE (IN U.S.):

- After 20 yr of diabetes mellitus, nearly 99% of patients with type 1 and 60% with type 2 disease demonstrate some degree of diabetic retinopathy.
- A leading preventable cause of blindness in the U.S. between the ages of 20 and 74 yr.
- There are approximately 8000 new cases of diabetic retinopathy–induced blindness each yr in the U.S.

PREVALENCE (IN U.S.):

- Prevalence of retinopathy increases with duration of diabetes. Found in 18% of people diagnosed with diabetes for 3- to 4-yr duration and in up to 80% of diabetics with a diagnosis of ≥15 yr.
- In the U.S., the prevalence of diabetic macular edema (the most common cause of vision impairment) is 4%, or approximately 750,000 people.
- CDC data reveal that 4 million Americans were visually impaired due to diabetic retinopathy in 2011.
- The number of Americans with diabetic retinopathy is expected to nearly double, from 7.7 million to 14.6 million between 2010 and 2050. Expected to triple in the Hispanic population.

PREDOMINANT SEX: Males and females affected equally

PREDOMINANT AGE: ≥30 yr

GENETICS:

- The development of diabetes involves the interaction of genetic and nongenetic factors.
- Type 1 has an autoimmune basis, resulting in destruction of beta islet cells and has strong HLA associations.
- Type 2 has genetic predisposition, but the specific genes are not yet well characterized.

PHYSICAL FINDINGS & CLINICAL PRESENTATION

- Microaneurysms
- Hemorrhages
- Cotton-wool spots
- Lipid exudates
- Macular edema
- Neovascularization
- Retinal detachment (in advanced cases)
- Vitreous hemorrhage
- In early cases, patient may not report a visual disturbance

ETIOLOGY

Prolonged hyperglycemia results in basement membrane thickening in retinal capillaries with subsequent loss of pericytes and endothe-

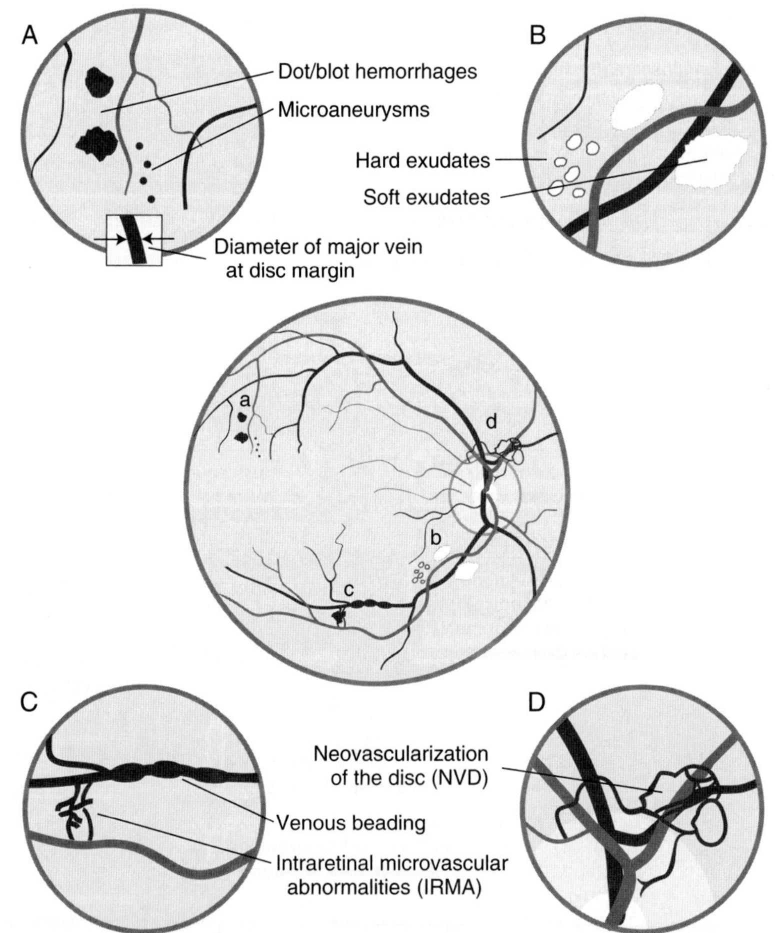

FIG. 1 Types of diabetic retinopathy. The center figure depicting the fundus of a patient with diabetic retinopathy is surrounded by four enlarged views, each labeled with a letter (a to d) corresponding to specific locations on the center figure. **A,** Microaneurysms and dot and blot hemorrhages. The diameter of microaneurysms is less than the width of a major vein at the disc margin (reproduced in square inset). **B,** Hard and soft exudates. **C,** Venous beading and intraretinal microvascular abnormalities (IRMA). **D,** Neovascularization, which may be located within one disc diameter of the optic disc (NVD) or elsewhere (NVE). Although both IRMA and neovascularization represent the formation of new blood vessels, IRMA are confined to the layers of the retina, whereas neovascularization is on the inner surface of the retina or vitreous. (From McGee, S: *Evidence-based physical diagnosis*, ed 4, Philadelphia, 2018, Elsevier.)

lial decompensation resulting in breakdown of the blood–retina barrier and capillary occlusion, ischemia, and serum leakage. This leads to the clinical findings of dot hemorrhages, microaneurysms, lipid exudate, and edema. Upregulation of vascular endothelial growth factor (VEGF) and other cytokines contributes to vascular incompetence and promotes growth of neovascular tissue.

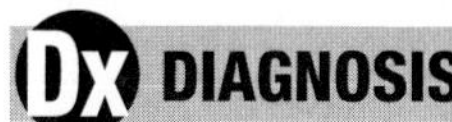

DIAGNOSIS

DIFFERENTIAL DIAGNOSIS

- Branch or central retinal vein occlusion
- Hypertensive retinopathy
- Ocular ischemic syndrome (carotid occlusion)
- Radiation retinopathy
- Retinal macroaneurysm
- Sickle cell retinopathy
- Valsalva retinopathy
- Lupus
- Retinal vasculitis

WORKUP

- Fundus photography
- Optical coherence tomography
- Fluorescein angiogram
- Laboratory workup if indicated based on DDx

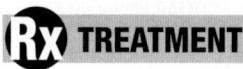

TREATMENT

NONPHARMACOLOGIC THERAPY

- Tight glycemic control remains the cornerstone in the primary prevention of diabetic retinopathy, particularly in type 1 as seen in the Diabetes Control and Complications Trial (DCCT) and less so in type 2 as seen in the United Kingdom Prospective Diabetes Study (UKPDS) and more recently in the Action to Control Cardiovascular Risk in Diabetes Trial (ACCORD). ADA guidelines recommend A1c <7.0.
- Intensive lowering of blood pressure was shown in UKPDS but not ACCORD to reduce progression of diabetic retinopathy. ADA guidelines recommend BP target of <140/90 mm Hg.
- Lipid lowering results in reduction of retinopathy progression (ACCORD Trial).
- Laser treatment (photocoagulation) for proliferative disease or macular edema.
- Table 1 summarizes classification and management of diabetic retinopathy.

ACUTE GENERAL Rx

- Intravitreal pharmacotherapy with anti-VEGF agents (e.g., bevacizumab, ranibizumab, aflibercept) and/or corticosteroids is the standard of care for patients with center-involved diabetic macular edema.
- Laser therapy: Panretinal laser photocoagulation reduces the risk of severe visual loss in patients with proliferative retinopathy.
- Focal laser reduces risk of moderate visual loss by 50% in patients with clinically significant macular edema.
- Vitrectomy for traction retinal detachment or vitreous hemorrhage.

TABLE 1 Abbreviated Early Treatment Diabetic Retinopathy Study (ETDRS) Classification of Diabetic Retinopathy

Category/Description	Management
Nonproliferative diabetic retinopathy (NPDR)	
No DR	Review in 12 months
Very mild NPDR	Review most patients in 12 months
Microaneurysms only	
Mild NPDR	Review range 6-12 months, depending on severity of signs, stability, systemic factors, and patient's personal circumstances
Any or all of: microaneurysms, retinal hemorrhages, exudates, cotton wool spots, up to the level of moderate NPDR. No intraretinal microvascular anomalies (IRMA) or significant beading	
Moderate NPDR	Review in approximately 6 months
• Severe retinal hemorrhages (more than ETDRS standard photograph 2A: about 20 medium to large per quadrant) in 1-3 quadrants or mild IRMA • Significant venous beading can be present in no more than 1 quadrant • Cotton wool spots commonly present	Proliferative diabetic retinopathy (PDR) in up to 26%, high-risk PDR in up to 8% within a yr
Severe NPDR	Review in 4 months
The 4–2–1 rule; one or more of: • Severe hemorrhages in all 4 quadrants • Significant venous beading in 2 or more quadrants • Moderate IRMA in 1 or more quadrants	PDR in up to 50%, high-risk PDR in up to 15% within a yr
Very severe NPDR	Review in 2-3 months
Two or more of the criteria for severe NPDR	High-risk PDR in up to 45% within a yr
Proliferative diabetic retinopathy (PDR)	
Mild–moderate PDR	Treatment considered according to severity of signs, stability, systemic factors, and patient's personal circumstances such as reliability of attendance for review. If not treated, review in up to 2 months
New vessels on the disc (NVD) or new vessels elsewhere (NVE), but extent insufficient to meet the high-risk criteria	
High-risk PDR	Treatment advised (see text)
• New vessels on the disc (NVD) greater than ETDRS standard photograph 10A (about 1⁄3 disc area) • Any NVD with vitreous hemorrhage • NVE greater than ½ disc area with vitreous hemorrhage	Should be performed immediately when possible, and certainly same day if symptomatic presentation with good retinal view

DR, Diabetic retinopathy. From Bowling B: *Kanski's clinical ophthalmology, a systematic approach,* ed 8, Philadelphia, 2016, Elsevier.

CHRONIC Rx

- Monthly anti-VEGF injections until macular edema has resolved with surveillance at regular intervals for additional treatment
- Both ranibizumab (Lucentis) and aflibercept (Eylea) have been FDA-approved for treatment of diabetic retinopathy in patients with macular edema
- Repeated laser treatments may be necessary
- Diet and exercise; good medical control of disease, blood pressure, and cholesterol

DISPOSITION

- Retinal examination should be performed on all routine medical visits. Referral if abnormality seen.
- Routine annual eye examination in all patients with diabetes.
- Prognosis is improved with early diagnosis and treatment.

REFERRAL

Refer to ophthalmologist immediately on finding retinal abnormality to institute early treatment.

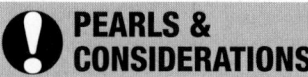

PEARLS & CONSIDERATIONS

COMMENTS

- Early treatment of severe nonproliferative and proliferative retinopathy may minimize complications and visual loss.
- Tight blood sugar control in type 1 patients significantly reduces the probability of developing new-onset retinopathy as well as progression of existing retinopathy.
- Retinopathy is an independent risk marker for cardiovascular disease in patients with type 2 DM.

SUGGESTED READINGS

Available at ExpertConsult.com

RELATED CONTENT

Diabetic Retinopathy (Patient Information)
Diabetes Mellitus (Related Key Topic)

AUTHOR: **ROBERT H. JANIGIAN, M.D.**

Diarrhea, Persistent

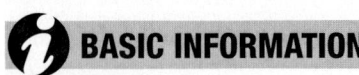

BASIC INFORMATION

DEFINITION

Persistent diarrhea is generally defined as an increase in stool frequency (>3 per day) or loose stool consistency for ≥4 wk. Some clinicians define persistent diarrhea as diarrhea lasting ≥14 days.

SYNONYM

Chronic diarrhea

ICD-10CM CODES

R19.7 Diarrhea, unspecified
K52.9 Noninfective gastroenteritis and colitis, unspecified
K58.0 Irritable bowel syndrome with diarrhea
K59.1 Functional diarrhea
K90.9 Intestinal malabsorption, unspecified

EPIDEMIOLOGY & DEMOGRAPHICS

PREVALENCE:

- Chronic diarrhea affects approximately 3%-5% of the U.S. population.
- According to the World Health Organization, the prevalence of chronic diarrhea in children worldwide ranges from 3% to 20%.

PREDOMINANT SEX & AGE: Dependent on etiology:

- Irritable bowel syndrome (IBS) has a female/male ratio of 2:1, with peak prevalence from 20 to 39 yr of age.
- Celiac disease has a slight female predominance, and incidence is highest during infancy, in the third decade, and in the seventh decade.
- Crohn disease has bimodal incidence with peaks in the third and fifth decades.
- Ulcerative colitis has bimodal incidence first between ages 15 and 40 yr and then between ages 50 and 80 yr.
- Lactose intolerance incidence generally increases with age.
- Microscopic colitis is most common in middle-aged women.

PHYSICAL FINDINGS & CLINICAL PRESENTATION

History:

- Specific symptoms: Loose stools, frequent stools, or urgency
- Fecal incontinence: Present or absent
- Duration
- Onset: Congenital, abrupt (infectious, idiopathic secretory diarrhea), or gradual
- Stool characteristics: Watery, bloody, fatty, malodorous
- Stool volume (watery, voluminous stool suggests disorder of small bowel or proximal colon. Frequent small stools suggest a disorder of left colon or rectum.)
- Abdominal pain: Location, relation to meals or bowel movements (inflammatory bowel disease [IBD], IBS, ischemia)
- Weight loss or fever (malabsorption, malignancy, IBD)
- Medical history: Immunologic, endocrine, neoplastic, human immunodeficiency virus (HIV), diabetes, surgery, radiation
- Travel history: Countries with infectious sources
- Medications: All medications and supplements, especially focusing on new medications, drugs containing magnesium, any antibiotics in the past 6 to 8 weeks; Box 1 summarizes medications and toxins associated with diarrhea
- Dietary history: Recent changes, "sugar-free" foods, fiber intake, raw seafood or shellfish, raw milk, impure drinking water
- Family history: Absorptive defects (lactose intolerance), IBD, celiac disease, IBS, cancer
- Social history: Risk factors for HIV, receptive anal intercourse (infection or proctitis)
- Aggravating and alleviating factors: Relation to meals, diet, stress
- Excessive flatus (carbohydrate malabsorption)
- Nocturnal diarrhea (suggests secretory diarrhea)
- Symptoms suggesting IBS: Abdominal pain associated with altered bowel habits and improvement with defecation; often aggravated by stress

Physical:

- General: Fluid balance, nutrition (dehydration, malnutrition)
- Skin: Flushing (carcinoid syndrome), dermatitis herpetiformis (celiac disease)
- Mouth: Ulcers (Crohn disease)
- Neck: Thyroid mass or nodule (hyperthyroidism, multiple endocrine neoplasia), lymphadenopathy (malignancy or chronic infection)
- Abdomen
  1. Hepatomegaly (endocrine tumor, amyloidosis)
  2. Scars (surgical causes of diarrhea)
  3. Tenderness (inflammation)
  4. Mass, ascites, tenderness (multiple)
- Rectal:
  1. Sphincter weakness (fecal incontinence), anal fistula, fecal impaction

ETIOLOGY

Cause-specific etiology: Secretory, osmotic, steatorrheal, inflammatory, dysmotile, factitial, iatrogenic

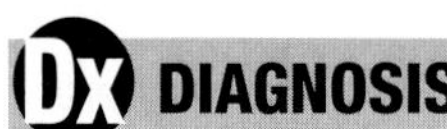

DIAGNOSIS

DIFFERENTIAL DIAGNOSIS

(See Box 2)

- Steatorrheal (fatty) diarrhea
  1. Malabsorption syndromes
     a. Mesenteric ischemia
     b. Mucosal diseases (e.g., celiac disease, Whipple disease)
     c. Small intestinal bacterial overgrowth (SIBO)
     d. Drug-induced enteropathy
  2. Maldigestion
     a. Inadequate luminal bile acid
     b. Pancreatic exocrine insufficiency
     c. Liver disease
     d. Bariatric surgery
- Inflammatory diarrhea (Table 1)
  1. Diverticulitis
  2. IBD (Crohn disease, ulcerative colitis)
  3. Infectious diseases
     a. Bacterial (e.g., tuberculosis, yersiniosis)
     b. Parasitic (e.g., amebiasis, strongyloidiasis)
     c. Pseudomembranous colitis (*C. difficile*)
     d. Ulcerating viral (e.g., cytomegalovirus, herpes simplex virus)
  4. Ischemic colitis
  5. Neoplasia (colon cancer, lymphoma)
  6. Radiation colitis
- Watery diarrhea (Table 2)
  1. Osmotic diarrhea
     a. Carbohydrate malabsorption (e.g., lactose intolerance)
     b. Osmotic laxatives (e.g., magnesium, phosphate, sulfate, sorbitol)
     c. Gluten and FODMAP intolerance
  2. Secretory diarrhea
     a. Bacterial toxins
     b. Congenital syndromes (e.g., congenital chloridorrhea)
     c. Disordered motility
        (1) Diabetic neuropathy
        (2) IBS
        (3) Postsympathectomy
        (4) Postvagotomy
        (5) Diabetic neuropathy
     d. Endocrinopathies
        (1) Addison disease
        (2) Carcinoid syndrome
        (3) Gastrinoma
        (4) Hyperthyroidism
        (5) Mastocytosis
        (6) Medullary carcinoma of the thyroid
        (7) Pheochromocytoma
        (8) Somatostatinoma
        (9) VIPoma

BOX 1 Medications and Toxins Associated with Diarrhea

Acid-reducing agents (e.g., H_2RAs, PPIs)
Antacids (e.g., those that contain magnesium)
Antiarrhythmics (e.g., quinidine)
Antibiotics (most)
Antiinflammatory agents (e.g., 5-aminosalicylates, gold salts, NSAIDs)
Antihypertensives (e.g., β-adrenergic receptor blocking drugs)
Antineoplastic agents (many)
Antiretroviral agents
Colchicine
Heavy metals
Herbal products
Prostaglandin analogs (e.g., misoprostol)
Theophylline
Vitamin and mineral supplements

H_2RA, Histamine-2 receptor agonist; *NSAID,* nonsteroidal antiinflammatory drug; *PPI,* proton pump inhibitor.
From Feldman M, Friedman LS, Brandt LJ: *Sleisenger and Fordtran's gastrointestinal and liver disease*, ed 10, Philadelphia, 2016, Elsevier.

BOX 2 Differential Diagnosis of Diarrhea

Acute Diarrhea
Infection
- Bacteria
- Parasites
- Protozoa
- Viruses

Food allergies
Food poisoning
Medications
Initial presentation of chronic diarrhea

Chronic Diarrhea
Fatty diarrhea
Malabsorption syndromes
- Mesenteric ischemia
- Mucosal diseases (e.g., celiac disease, Whipple disease)
- Short bowel syndrome
- SIBO

Maldigestion
- Inadequate luminal bile acid concentration
- Pancreatic exocrine insufficiency

Inflammatory Diarrhea
Diverticulitis
Infectious diseases
- Invasive bacterial infections (e.g., tuberculosis, yersiniosis)
- Invasive parasitic infections (e.g., amebiasis, strongyloidiasis)
- Pseudomembranous colitis (*Clostridium difficile* infection)
- Ulcerating viral infections (e.g., cytomegalovirus, HSV)

Inflammatory bowel diseases
- Crohn disease
- UC
- Ulcerative jejunoileitis

Ischemic colitis
Neoplasia
- Colon cancer
- Lymphoma

Radiation colitis

Watery Diarrhea
Osmotic diarrhea
- Carbohydrate malabsorption
- Osmotic laxatives (e.g., Mg^{2+}, PO_4^{3-}, SO_4^{2-})

Secretory diarrhea
- Bacterial toxins
- Congenital syndromes (e.g., congenital chloridorrhea)
- Disordered motility, regulation
  - Diabetic autonomic neuropathy
  - IBS
  - Postsympathectomy diarrhea
  - Postvagotomy diarrhea
- Diverticulitis
- Endocrinopathies
  - Addison disease
  - Carcinoid syndrome
  - Gastrinoma
  - Hyperthyroidism
  - Mastocytosis
  - Medullary carcinoma of the thyroid
  - Pheochromocytoma
  - Somatostatinoma
  - VIPoma
- Idiopathic secretory diarrhea
  - Epidemic secretory (Brainerd) diarrhea
  - Sporadic idiopathic secretory diarrhea
- Ileal bile acid malabsorption
- IBD
  - Crohn disease
  - Microscopic colitis
  - Collagenous colitis
  - Lymphocytic colitis
  - UC
- Laxative abuse (stimulant laxatives)
- Medications and toxins (see Box 1)
- Neoplasia
  - Colon carcinoma
  - Lymphoma
  - Villous adenoma in rectum
- Vasculitis

HSV, Herpes simplex virus; *IBD,* inflammatory bowel disease; *IBS,* inflammatory bowel syndrome; *SIBO,* small bacterial overgrowth; *UC,* ulcerative colitis.
From Feldman M, Friedman LS, Brandt LJ: *Sleisenger and Fordtran's gastrointestinal and liver disease*, ed 10, Philadelphia, 2016, Elsevier.

TABLE 1 Clinical Findings That Suggest the Causative Organisms for Some Inflammatory Diarrheas

Finding	Causative Organisms
Hemolytic-uremic syndrome/thrombotic thrombocytopenic purpura	Shiga toxin-producing *Escherichia coli*; most common with *Shigella dysenteriae* among *Shigella* spp., but *S. dysenteriae* is not found in the U.S.
Reactive arthritis*	*Salmonella* spp., *Shigella* spp., *Campylobacter* spp., *Yersinia* spp.
Bone-marrow suppression	*Salmonella* serovars Typhi and Paratyphi
Guillain-Barré syndrome	*Campylobacter jejuni*
Toxic megacolon	*Shigella* spp., *Clostridium difficile, Salmonella* (rarely)
Aortitis/endovascular infection	Nontyphoidal *Salmonellae*
Intestinal hemorrhage/perforation	*Salmonella* serovars Typhi and Paratyphi, TB enteritis
Right lower quadrant tenderness	*Yersinia* spp.
Cellulitis	*Vibrio vulnificus* and *alginolyticus* (see text)
Postinfection IBS	All, including viral gastroenteritis; viruses typically yield less severe postinfection IBS
Small-bowel lymphoproliferative disease	*Campylobacter jejuni*

*Can occur with any enteric pathogen.
From Feldman M, Friedman LS, Brandt LJ: *Sleisenger and Fordtran's gastrointestinal and liver disease*, ed 10, Philadelphia, 2016, Elsevier.

   e. Idiopathic secretory diarrhea
   f. Ileal bile acid malabsorption
   g. IBD (Crohn disease, ulcerative colitis)
   h. Laxative abuse
   i. Medications and toxins
   j. Microscopic colitis (lymphocytic, collagenous)
   k. Neoplasia (colon carcinoma, lymphoma, villous adenoma in rectum)
   l. Vasculitis
3. Factitial causes
   a. Munchausen
   b. Eating disorders
4. Iatrogenic causes
   a. Cholecystectomy
   b. Ileal resection
   c. Bariatric surgery

WORKUP

- Due to the many potential causes of chronic diarrhea, it is impractical to use the same diagnostic tests on every patient.

TABLE 2 Secretory Versus Osmotic Diarrhea

Type of Diarrhea	Causes	Examples
Secretory	Exogenous secretagogues	Enterotoxins (e.g., cholera)
	Endogenous secretagogues	Neuroendocrine tumors (e.g., carcinoid syndrome)
	Absence of ion transporter	Congenital chloridorrhea
	Loss of intestinal surface area	Intestinal resection, diffuse intestinal mucosal disease
	Intestinal ischemia	Diffuse mesenteric atherosclerosis
	Rapid intestinal transit	Intestinal hurry following vagotomy
Osmotic	Ingestion of poorly absorbed agent	Magnesium ingestion
	Reduced nutrient transport	Lactase deficiency

From Feldman M, Friedman LS, Brandt LJ: *Sleisenger and Fordtran's gastrointestinal and liver disease*, ed 10, Philadelphia, 2016, Elsevier.

- Good history and physical examination should be obtained (as mentioned previously), and the workup should be tailored accordingly.
- First determine the type of diarrhea (watery, fatty, or inflammatory) based on the history and physical examination. Further tests may then be obtained to differentiate the diseases in that subtype of diarrhea.
- Basic laboratory testing may include complete blood count (CBC) (anemia, leukocytosis), electrolyte tests, liver function tests, albumin, erythrocyte sedimentation rate (nonspecific), and thyroid stimulating hormone.
- Initial stool studies may include fecal leukocyte and fecal occult blood testing.
- Further lab testing as indicated by clinical suspicion:
  1. IBD: Fecal calprotectin
  2. Diarrhea after hospitalization or recent antibiotics: *Clostridium difficile* stool toxin
  3. Suspected laxative abuse: Stool laxative screen
  4. Malabsorption: Fecal fat, Sudan stain
  5. Celiac panel (tissue transglutaminase immunoglobulin A), especially in patients with iron deficiency anemia on CBC
  6. Watery diarrhea
     a. Fecal osmotic gap: $290 - 2([Na^+] - [K^+])$
        (1) Gap >125 mOsm/kg suggests osmotic diarrhea.
        (2) Gap <50 mOsm/kg suggests secretory diarrhea.
     b. Fecal pH
        (1) pH <5.3 suggests carbohydrate malabsorption (lactose intolerance).

Rx TREATMENT

In most cases, an underlying etiology should be discovered and treated accordingly. However, nonspecific treatment may be used in several situations:

- Volume depletion that requires treatment (or hospitalization) during evaluation
- Specific treatment for a condition fails to adequately treat diarrhea
- No specific treatment is available

NONPHARMACOLOGIC THERAPY

- If etiology can be managed with diet modification (e.g., lactose intolerance or celiac disease), offending substance should be eliminated from diet.
- Reasonable to have trial of reduced dietary lactose and caffeine and monitor for improvement.
- Fiber supplementation (psyllium) can thicken stool consistency; however, it may increase stool output.
- Patients with stool output greater than 1000 g per day often receive IV hydration, but as an alternative, most could be managed with oral rehydration solution (ORS).
- Other therapies would be determined by the specific etiology of persistent diarrhea.

CHRONIC GENERAL Rx

- General principles:
  1. Opiates are the most effective nonspecific antidiarrheal drugs. In general, they should not be used in severe diarrhea due to acute infections, massive intestinal resection, or secretion of endogenous secretagogues.
  2. Less potent opiate agents (loperamide) should be attempted first, but treatment should be escalated to more potent agents if low-potency opiates fail.
  3. Avoid high-potency agents when concerns of narcotic abuse and/or dependence exist.
  4. When prescribed, opiates should be used on a scheduled basis rather than as needed.
- Low-potency opiate antidiarrheals
  1. Diphenoxylate with atropine (Lomotil) 2.5-5 mg 4 times daily
  2. Loperamide (Imodium) 2-4 mg 4 times daily
- More potent opiate antidiarrheals (avoid in alcoholics or history of drug abuse)
  1. Codeine 15-60 mg 4 times daily
  2. Morphine 2-20 mg 4 times daily
  3. Tincture of opium 2-20 drops 4 times daily
- Alpha-2 agonist
  1. Clonidine 0.1-0.3 mg 3 times daily
  2. Utility limited by hypotensive effect. Opiate agents should be attempted first.
- Intraluminal agents
  1. Used to bind toxins and change stool consistency
  2. Usually ineffective as monotherapy in managing chronic diarrhea
  3. Fibers: Psyllium, calcium polycarbophil, methylcellulose
  4. Bismuth: Pepto-Bismol
  5. Clays: Attapulgite, kaolin
  6. Bile acid–binding resins: Cholestyramine, colestipol
- Newer agent
  1. Racecadotril, an antisecretory enkephalinase inhibitor
  2. Not yet available in the U.S.

COMPLEMENTARY & ALTERNATIVE MEDICINE

- There is growing evidence that shows some benefit of probiotics in the treatment of infectious diarrhea, IBS, *Clostridium difficile* disease, and antibiotic-associated diarrhea.

DISPOSITION

Etiology dependent

REFERRAL

Gastroenterology referral is warranted depending on severity of symptoms, need for endoscopic procedures, and/or need for long-term disease management.

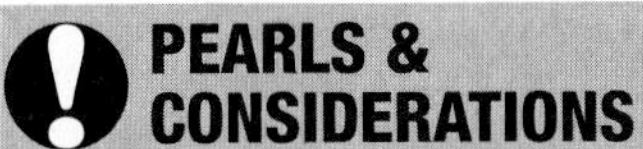

PEARLS & CONSIDERATIONS

COMMENTS

- A good history is crucial in the evaluation of chronic diarrhea. An attempt should be made to classify diarrhea as watery, fatty, or inflammatory.
- Fecal incontinence is often described by patients as diarrhea, and many patients are reluctant to volunteer more information on this subject unless specifically asked.
- IBS is one of the most common causes of chronic diarrhea and requires minimal laboratory studies. Patients should be screened appropriately.
- An underlying etiology of chronic diarrhea should be determined and treated accordingly.

PATIENT/FAMILY EDUCATION

- Disease-specific education

SUGGESTED READINGS

Available at ExpertConsult.com

RELATED CONTENT

Amebiasis (Related Key Topic)
Celiac Disease (Related Key Topic)
Colorectal Cancer (Related Key Topic)
Crohn Disease (Related Key Topic)
Gastroenteritis (Related Key Topic)
Giardiasis (Related Key Topic)
Hyperthyroidism (Related Key Topic)
Incontinence, Bowel, Elderly Patient (Related Key Topic)
Irritable Bowel Syndrome (Related Key Topic)
Lactose Intolerance (Related Key Topic)
Malabsorption (Related Key Topic)
Pancreatitis, Chronic (Related Key Topic)
Paraneoplastic Syndromes (Related Key Topic)
Small Bowel Intestinal Bacterial Overgrowth (SIBO) (Related Key Topic)
Traveler's Diarrhea (Related Key Topic)
Tropical Sprue (Related Key Topic)
Ulcerative Colitis (Related Key Topic)
Whipple Disease (Related Key Topic)

AUTHOR: **JAFET OJEDA RODRIGUEZ, M.D.**

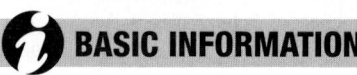

BASIC INFORMATION

DEFINITION

Diffuse idiopathic skeletal hyperostosis (DISH) is a systemic disorder primarily involving the axial skeleton. DISH is characterized by widespread bone proliferation as well as calcification and ossification of soft tissues, including ligaments and their sites of insertion. DISH is known to be associated with certain metabolic abnormalities.

SYNONYMS

Ankylosing hyperostosis
Forestier disease
DISH

ICD-10CM CODES

M48.10	Ankylosing hyperostosis, site unspecified
M48.11	Ankylosing hyperostosis, occipito-atlanto-axial region
M48.12	Ankylosing hyperostosis, cervical region
M48.13	Ankylosing hyperostosis, cervicothoracic region
M48.14	Ankylosing hyperostosis, thoracic region
M48.15	Ankylosing hyperostosis, thoracolumbar region
M48.16	Ankylosing hyperostosis, lumbar region
M48.17	Ankylosing hyperostosis, lumbosacral region
M48.18	Ankylosing hyperostosis, sacral and sacrococcygeal region
M48.19	Ankylosing hyperostosis, multiple sites in spine

EPIDEMIOLOGY & DEMOGRAPHICS

PREVALENCE: The prevalence of DISH varies in different populations. Factors such as age, ethnicity, geography, and clinical setting affect the prevalence of the disease. Studies have shown DISH is more common in developed nations, although this may be secondary to more frequent use of radiologic imaging in these countries. Higher prevalence rates are seen in men, 10% to 25% versus 5% to 15% in women over the age of 50 yr. Rates increase with age, with prevalence reported as high as 35% in men and 26% in women over the age of 70 yr.

PREDOMINANT SEX AND AGE:

- Male predominance with a ratio of 2:1
- Mostly seen in elderly patients, usually after the age of 50 yr

GENETICS: Association with *COL6A1* gene in some populations, which causes ossification of the posterior longitudinal ligament, a condition that is related to DISH

RISK FACTORS:

- Obesity
- Type II diabetes mellitus
- Hyperuricemia
- Dyslipidemia
- Hypertension
- Hyperinsulinemia
- Elevated growth hormone levels
- Elevated insulin-like growth factor (IGF-1)
- Chronic vitamin A toxicity/retinoid use

PHYSICAL FINDINGS & CLINICAL PRESENTATION

Patients with DISH are usually asymptomatic or experience only increased stiffness in the spine or peripheral joints. In the spine, osteophytes can obstruct or impinge on other structures or tissues, causing dysphagia (DISH affecting the cervical spine), myelopathy, quadriplegia, spinal stenosis, and ossification of posterior longitudinal ligament. Spinal ligament calcification and ossification leads to decreased range of motion and a stooped posture as well as an increase in the risk for fractures. Peripheral enthesopathies are usually asymptomatic, but mechanical stresses can injure the entheses and cause pain. In patients with DISH, pronounced hypertrophic changes can be seen affecting certain peripheral joints that are not typically associated with OA, such as the metacarpophalangeal joints, elbows, shoulders, and ankles. Thoracic spinal involvement is common in DISH and not usually seen in OA. Patients with DISH are at increased risk for heterotopic ossification after orthopedic surgery (i.e., hip arthroplasty).

ETIOLOGY

Etiology of DISH is unknown and the cause of excess bone formation is unclear. Chondrocytes located in entheseal areas become activated and cause changes in the adjacent matrix leading to ossification. Local vascular infiltration in these areas promotes ossification as well.

DIAGNOSIS

Diagnosis of DISH is made by radiographic imaging. Bone formation is typically seen in the thoracic spine, and less frequently in the cervical and lumbar spines. Coarse osteophytes that seem to "flow" between adjacent vertebrae are seen on the right side of the thoracic spine, thought to be subsequent to the pressure effect of the left-sided aorta (Figs. 1 and 2). Ossification occurs within the overlying anterior longitudinal ligament, preserving the original bone cortex. The intervertebral disc height is preserved in the involved segments. Peripheral bone formation is seen in entheseal areas, especially around the heels (Achilles tendon and plantar fascia), knees (peripatellar ligaments), and elbows (olecranon). Peripheral new bone formation can be seen as well, with increased distal finger tuft thickening, increased sesamoid bone size, and increased cortical bone thickness. There is no evidence of apophyseal joint ankylosis or sacroiliac involvement.

Resnick and Niwayama criteria: Most frequently used and is based on radiographic findings in the spine:

- Findings of new bone formation/osteophytes bridging four adjoining vertebral bodies or ossification of the anterolateral longitudinal ligament
- Preserved intervertebral disc height
- Absence of degenerative disc disease, sacroiliac joint, or facet joint involvement or changes

Others have proposed different criteria for diagnosis, which include the presence of peripheral enthesopathy. New diagnostic criteria are needed to recognize milder forms of the disease, those affecting other parts of the spine, and those that manifest initially with peripheral enthesopathy.

DIFFERENTIAL DIAGNOSIS

- Ankylosing spondylitis
- Degenerative disc disease
- Acromegaly

WORKUP

Diagnosis of DISH is made with radiologic imaging. Patients with the above risk factors (increased weight, BMI, waist circumference, and systolic blood pressure) are at risk for cardiovascular disease and evaluation for this should be pursued.

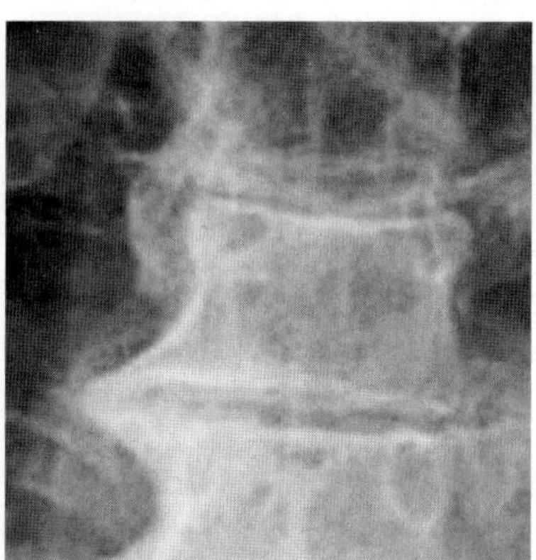

FIG. 1 Large, flowing, right-sided osteophytes of the thoracic spine. (Firestein GS, Budd RC, Gabriel SE, McInnes IB, O'Dell JR: Proliferative bone diseases. In Firestein G, et al. [eds]: *Firestein: Kelley's textbook of rheumatology,* ed 9, Philadelphia, 2013, Elsevier, pp 1680-1691.)

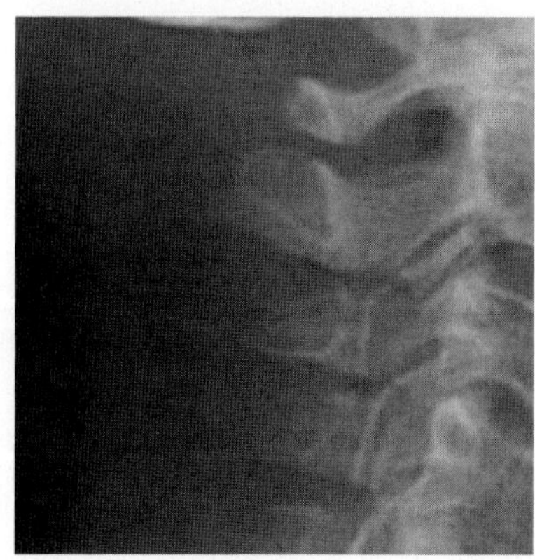

FIG. 2 Severe bulky ossification of the anterior longitudinal ligament of the cervical spine. (Firestein GS, Budd RC, Gabriel SE, McInnes IB, O'Dell JR: Proliferative bone diseases. In Firestein G, et al. [eds]: *Firestein: Kelley's textbook of rheumatology,* ed 9, Philadelphia, 2013, Elsevier, pp 1680-1691.)

LABORATORY TESTS

- Routine biochemical tests and erythrocyte sedimentation rate (ESR) are normal
- Laboratory testing should include evaluation for metabolic syndrome, i.e., fasting glucose or HgbA1c, cholesterol panel, etc.
- Uric acid

IMAGING STUDIES

- Posteroanterior and lateral (Fig. 3) x-ray views of the spine
- Computed tomography (CT) (Fig. 4) or magnetic resonance imaging (MRI) of the spine (not routinely needed unless evaluating for other possible conditions such as spinal stenosis)
- Plain radiographs of symptomatic peripheral joints

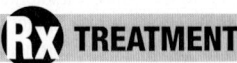

TREATMENT

There is no specific treatment available for DISH.

- Weight management
- Treatment and control of components of metabolic syndrome
- Treat cardiovascular risk factors

NONPHARMACOLOGIC THERAPY

- Physical therapy, light exercise
- Heat
- For peripheral enthesopathy pain, local soft applications such as insoles for plantar spurs or orthotics can be used as well as protective bandages at other sites.
- Surgical intervention rarely necessary, unless complications such as dysphagia from cervical osteophytes or spinal stenosis occurs

ACUTE GENERAL Rx

- Analgesics and nonsteroidal antiinflammatory medications (NSAIDs)
- Local corticosteroid injections

CHRONIC Rx

- Pain management as above
- Prevention of heterotopic ossification after orthopedic surgical procedures: NSAIDs, anti-vitamin K, and irradiation

SUGGESTED READINGS

Available at ExpertConsult.com

RELATED CONTENT

Ankylosing Spondylitis (Related Key Topic)
Osteoarthritis (Related Key Topic)

AUTHOR: **JOANNE SZCZYGIEL CUNHA, M.D.**

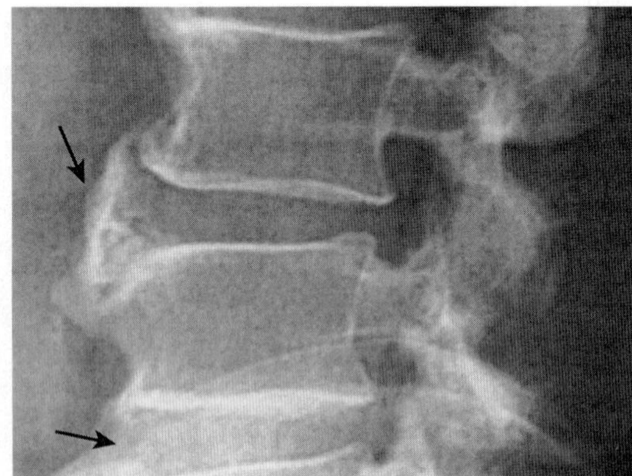

FIG. 3 Diffuse idiopathic skeletal hyperostosis (DISH): lumbar spine. This lateral radiograph of the lumbar spine shows early changes of DISH. Calcifications of the anterior longitudinal spinal ligament *(arrows)* are evident and will eventually evolve into flowing osteophytes extending across multiple spinal levels. (From Firestein GS: *Kelley's textbook of rheumatology*, ed 9, Philadelphia, 2013, Saunders.)

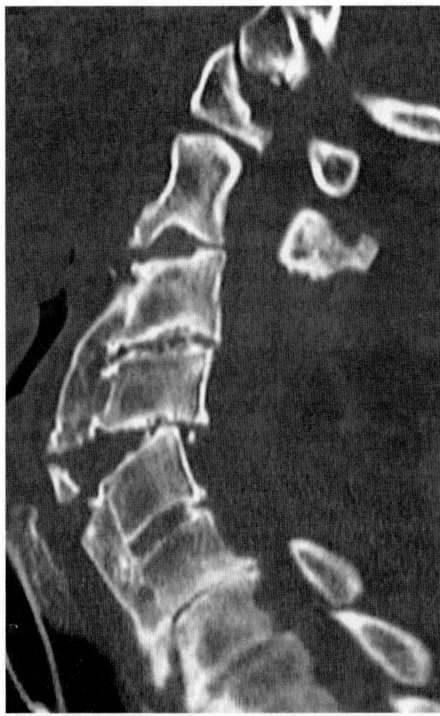

FIG. 4 Sagittal reformatted multidetector computed tomography image showing hyperextension fracture with subluxation through C4 and C5 levels in a patient with massive diffuse idiopathic skeletal hyperostosis. Such injuries may occur after relatively trivial trauma in such patients. (Pope TL, Bloem HL, Beltran J, Morrison WB, Wilson DJ: *Musculoskeletal imaging*, ed 2, Philadelphia, 2014, Saunders.)

BASIC INFORMATION

DEFINITION

Diplopia is the perception of two images of a single object that may be displaced horizontally, vertically, or obliquely. Diplopia may be monocular or binocular. Monocular diplopia is double vision in one eye and persists when the unaffected eye is covered. It is an ophthalmologic problem that results from abnormal light transmission to the retina. Binocular diplopia results from ocular misalignment and resolves when either eye is covered. There are multiple possible causes that can be localized along the visual pathway, from the eye to the brainstem.

SYNONYM

Double vision

ICD-10CM CODE
H53.2 Diplopia

EPIDEMIOLOGY & DEMOGRAPHICS

- Diplopia represents 1.4% of ophthalmologic emergencies.
- The majority of cases are binocular.

GENETICS: Some diseases have a genetic basis, such as Marfan syndrome (dislocation of lens), or to a lesser degree, autoimmune conditions (MG, Graves) that have a possible genetic link.

RISK FACTORS: Risk factors for diplopia include risk factors for vasculopathies (e.g., hypertension, diabetes mellitus, smoking, cerebrovascular accident) or trauma.

PHYSICAL FINDINGS & CLINICAL PRESENTATION

- Monocular diplopia persists when the unaffected eye is covered and, unless caused by a retinal defect, resolves when a pinhole is used.
- Restrictive, mechanical orbitopathy: Gradual onset, sensation of mass effect/discomfort/pain in a single eye, may result from rectus muscle entrapment secondary to orbital blowout fracture, possible fever if infectious, diplopia worse in the morning in Graves myopathy, proptosis, periorbital swelling, edema, palpebral swelling, conjunctival or scleral injection, abrupt restriction of eye movement away from the affected muscle.
- Cranial nerve (CN; III, IV, or VI) palsy: May occur as an isolated nerve palsy as a result of microvascular ischemia, or in combination in the case of cavernous sinus or posterior orbit pathologies.
  1. CN III palsy: Multidirectional diplopia except on lateral gaze toward the affected side
  2. CN IV palsy: Rotational diplopia that worsens looking down and toward the nose; difficulty descending stairs, reading, or watching television in bed
  3. CN VI palsy: Diplopia that worsens on lateral gaze toward the affected side
- Neuroaxial process: Diplopia may occur in isolation or may be accompanied by multiple neurological signs and symptoms; vertical diplopia without vertical skew deviation suggests a brainstem lesion.
- Neuromuscular disorder: Muscle atrophy/weakness, weakness on forced eyelid closure, normal reflexes, and no sensory deficits.

ETIOLOGY

- The etiology of diplopia differs between monocular and binocular diplopia. Monocular diplopia is caused by primary ophthalmologic structural problems in the transmission of light to the retina. Binocular diplopia, when not caused by trauma, is most often a vascular lesion (small-vessel vasculopathy or aneurysmal disease) or occasionally due to endocrinopathy or neuromuscular, neoplastic, or autoimmune sources.
- Table 1 summarizes important causes of diplopia.

DIAGNOSIS

DIFFERENTIAL DIAGNOSIS

- Psychogenic (functional deficit)
- Monocular diplopia:
  - Dry eyes
  - Corneal irregularity
  - Astigmatism
  - Cataract
  - Lens dislocation
  - Retinal wrinkles involving the macula
- Binocular diplopia:
  1. Restrictive, mechanical orbitopathy
     a. Abscess
     b. Trauma
     c. Entrapment
     d. Orbital myositis (may be associated with Wegener granulomatosis, giant cell arteritis, systemic lupus erythematosus, dermatomyositis, sarcoidosis, rheumatoid arthritis, Graves disease, or orbital pseudotumor)
     e. Craniofacial mass
  2. Cranial nerve (III, IV, or VI) palsy
     a. Isolated mononeuropathy of a single nerve
        (1) Demyelination (e.g., multiple sclerosis)
        (2) Hypertensive or diabetic vasculopathy
        (3) Nerve compression (e.g., aneurysm, tumor)
     b. Unilateral palsy of multiple oculomotor nerves
        (1) Infection, mass, or vasculitis affecting cavernous sinus or posterior orbit
  3. Neuroaxial process involving the brainstem
     1. Multiple sclerosis may manifest as a focal brainstem lesion.
     2. A more diffuse but localized brainstem lesion may result from brainstem tumor, brainstem lacunar stroke, basilar artery thrombosis, vertebral artery dissection, ophthalmoplegic migraine, infection, autoimmune disorder (e.g., Miller-Fischer or Guillain-Barré syndrome), Wernicke encephalopathy, meningoencephalitis, or botulism.
- Neuromuscular disorder
  1. Myasthenia gravis
  2. Lambert-Eaton syndrome

WORKUP

- Full neurologic examination with careful attention to the cranial nerves.
- Monocular diplopia: Slit-lamp, funduscopic examination, and ophthalmology referral.
- Diagnostic testing should be guided by clinical judgment as applied to the differential diagnosis. Imaging is the mainstay of the workup and is indicated in most cases of undifferentiated binocular diplopia. Laboratory studies are rarely helpful.
- Fig. 1 describes an algorithm for the diagnostic approach to diplopia.

LABORATORY TESTS

- Thyroid panel may be useful in cases of suspected thyroid disease.
- Lumbar puncture for meningitis or Miller-Fischer syndrome.

IMAGING STUDIES

- Magnetic resonance imaging (MRI) of the orbits with gadolinium is the test of choice in patients with suspected restrictive, mechanical orbitopathy; cavernous sinus; or posterior orbit pathology. Computed tomography (CT) of the head with contrast is a second-line option.
- For an isolated mononeuropathy, MRI of the brain and orbits with gadolinium is preferred. CT angiography (CTA) or magnetic resonance angiography (MRA) should be obtained in cases of suspected aneurysm. MRA should be used with caution when aneurysm is highly suspected because the sensitivity of MRA decreases with aneurysm size less than 5 mm.
- MRI with and without gadolinium is recommended for detection of brainstem lesions. The addition of a diffusion-weighted imaging protocol may be useful when ischemia is suspected.

TREATMENT

- The treatment of diplopia is directed at the underlying disorder.
- Signs of basilar meningoencephalitis: Empiric antibiotics pending CT, lumbar puncture, and confirmation of infection
- Signs of Wernicke encephalopathy: Give thiamine
- Signs of stroke: IV fluid bolus and emergent evaluation for reperfusion therapy

DISPOSITION

Most patients will require hospital admission for further evaluation and treatment. However, a CN III or CN IV palsy from microvascular ischemia typically self-resolves over a few days; these patients can usually be followed on an outpatient basis for spontaneous resolution.

TABLE 1 Important Causes of Diplopia

Diplopia-Causing Entity	Mechanism and Mortality	Distinguishing Features
Tier 1—Critical		
Basilar artery thrombosis	Acute thrombosis of the basilar artery with brainstem ischemia; untreated, mortality 70%-90%	Vertigo, dysarthria, other cranial nerve involvement; risk factors for stroke
Botulism	Toxin inhibits release of acetylcholine (ACh) at cholinergic synapses and presynaptic myoneural junctions; untreated, mortality 60%	Dysarthria, dysphagia, autonomic dysreflexia, pupillary dysfunction
Basilar meningitis	Infection; untreated, mortality close to 100% if bacterial (25%-40% if treated)	Headache, meningismus, fever
Aneurysm	Enlarging aneurysm directly compresses cranial nerve; untreated, rupture risk is 1% per year; mortality 26%-50% per rupture	CN III palsy with pupillary involvement
Tier 2—Emergent		
Vertebral dissection	Dissection causes vertebrobasilar ischemia; acute untreated, mortality 28% (2%-5% if neurologically asymptomatic)	Neck pain, vertigo; risk factors for vertebral dissection
Myasthenia gravis	Autoantibodies develop against ACh nicotinic postsynaptic receptors; untreated, crisis mortality 42% (5% if treated)	Fluctuating muscle weakness, ptosis, and diplopia worsen with activity and improve with rest
Wernicke encephalopathy	Thiamine-dependent metabolic failure and tissue injury; untreated, mortality 20%	Nystagmus, ataxia, altered mental status, and ophthalmoplegia; risk factors and nutritional deficiency
Orbital apex syndrome, cavernous sinus process	Inflammation or infection in the orbital apex or cavernous sinus directly affects oculomotor cranial nerves; acute mortality low unless infectious and complicated by meningitis	A combination of palsies of CN III, IV, or VI, with retroorbital pain, conjunctival injection, and possible periorbital or facial numbness
Tier 3—Urgent		
Brainstem tumor	Tumor involvement at the supranuclear level; acute mortality low (long-term mortality variable)	Skew deviation vertical diplopia, internuclear ophthalmoplegia
Miller-Fisher syndrome	Autoantibodies develop to a cranial nerve ganglioside, GQ1b; acute mortality low if fully differentiated from GBS; mortality 2%-12% if GBS	Ophthalmoplegia, ataxia, areflexia
Multiple sclerosis	Demyelinating lesions; acute mortality low	Internuclear ophthalmoplegia
Thyroid myopathy (Graves disease)	Autoimmune myopathy; acute mortality low with regard to ocular complaints	Proptosis, restriction of elevation and abduction of the eye, signs of Graves disease
Ophthalmoplegic migraine	Inflammatory cranial neuropathy; low mortality—self-limited disease	Ipsilateral headache, CN (usually III) palsy
Ischemic neuropathy	Microvascular ischemia; mortality low—self-limited disease	Isolated CN palsy (pupil-sparing if CN III)
Orbital myositis, pseudotumor	Autoimmune or idiopathic myositis; acute mortality low with regard to ocular complaints	Eye pain, restriction of movement, periorbital edema; exophthalmos and chemosis when more severe
Orbital apex mass	A tumor, infiltration, or mass effect in the orbital apex or cavernous sinus directly compresses oculomotor cranial nerves; acute mortality low	A combination of palsies of CN III, IV, or VI, and possible periorbital or facial numbness, with retroorbital pain, proptosis, signs of venous congestion

CN, Cranial nerve; *GBS*, Guillain-Barré syndrome.
From Marx JA et al: *Rosen's emergency medicine*, ed 8, Philadelphia, 2014, Saunders.

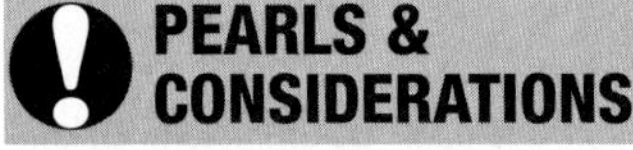

PEARLS & CONSIDERATIONS

- All patients with diplopia merit a thorough neurologic examination.
- Consider potential critical and emergent causes, including infection, stroke, and Wernicke encephalopathy.
- Treat the underlying problem.
- Most patients merit hospital admission.

PREVENTION

No specific prevention has been published, although it stands to reason that preventing the antecedent vascular insults by managing hypertension and diabetes, as well as avoiding tobacco use and trauma, should have an impact on the disease prevalence.

PATIENT/FAMILY EDUCATION

Patients should be counseled to avoid driving or performing tasks that could be considered dangerous with impaired vision until symptoms resolve.

SUGGESTED READINGS

Available at ExpertConsult.com

RELATED CONTENT

Botulism (Related Key Topic)
Giant Cell Arteritis (Related Key Topic)
Granulomatosis With Polyangiitis (Related Key Topic)
Graves Disease (Related Key Topic)
Guillain-Barré Syndrome (Related Key Topic)
Inflammatory Myopathies (Related Key Topic)
Multiple Sclerosis (Related Key Topic)
Myasthenia Gravis (Related Key Topic)
Rheumatoid Arthritis (Related Key Topic)
Sarcoidosis (Related Key Topic)
Systemic Lupus Erythematosus (Related Key Topic)
Wernicke Syndrome (Related Key Topic)

AUTHORS: **COSBY G. ARNOLD, M.D., M.P.H.,** and **BRYAN ENGLAND, M.D.**

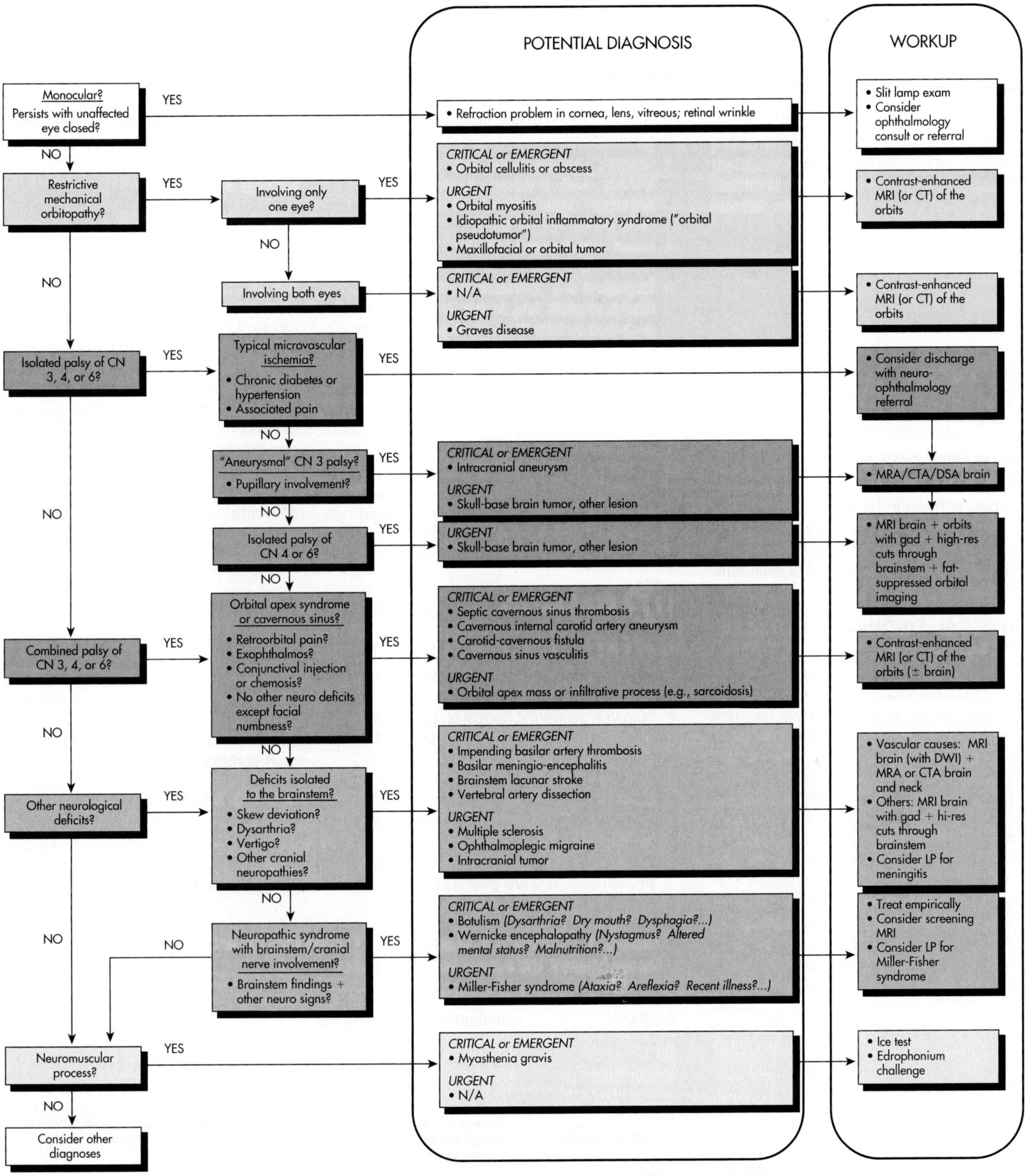

POTENTIAL DIAGNOSIS

WORKUP

Monocular? Persists with unaffected eye closed?
YES → • Refraction problem in cornea, lens, vitreous; retinal wrinkle → • Slit lamp exam • Consider ophthalmology consult or referral
NO ↓

Restrictive mechanical orbitopathy?
YES → Involving only one eye?
YES → CRITICAL or EMERGENT • Orbital cellulitis or abscess URGENT • Orbital myositis • Idiopathic orbital inflammatory syndrome ("orbital pseudotumor") • Maxillofacial or orbital tumor → • Contrast-enhanced MRI (or CT) of the orbits
NO ↓
Involving both eyes → CRITICAL or EMERGENT • N/A URGENT • Graves disease → • Contrast-enhanced MRI (or CT) of the orbits
NO ↓

Isolated palsy of CN 3, 4, or 6?
YES → Typical microvascular ischemia? • Chronic diabetes or hypertension • Associated pain
YES → • Consider discharge with neuro-ophthalmology referral
NO ↓
"Aneurysmal" CN 3 palsy? • Pupillary involvement?
YES → CRITICAL or EMERGENT • Intracranial aneurysm URGENT • Skull-base brain tumor, other lesion → • MRA/CTA/DSA brain
NO ↓
Isolated palsy of CN 4 or 6?
YES → URGENT • Skull-base brain tumor, other lesion → • MRI brain + orbits with gad + high-res cuts through brainstem + fat-suppressed orbital imaging
NO ↓
NO ↓

Combined palsy of CN 3, 4, or 6?
YES → Orbital apex syndrome or cavernous sinus? • Retroorbital pain? • Exophthalmos? • Conjunctival injection or chemosis? • No other neuro deficits except facial numbness?
YES → CRITICAL or EMERGENT • Septic cavernous sinus thrombosis • Cavernous internal carotid artery aneurysm • Carotid-cavernous fistula • Cavernous sinus vasculitis URGENT • Orbital apex mass or infiltrative process (e.g., sarcoidosis) → • Contrast-enhanced MRI (or CT) of the orbits (± brain)
NO ↓
NO ↓

Other neurological deficits?
YES → Deficits isolated to the brainstem? • Skew deviation? • Dysarthria? • Vertigo? • Other cranial neuropathies?
YES → CRITICAL or EMERGENT • Impending basilar artery thrombosis • Basilar meningio-encephalitis • Brainstem lacunar stroke • Vertebral artery dissection URGENT • Multiple sclerosis • Ophthalmoplegic migraine • Intracranial tumor → • Vascular causes: MRI brain (with DWI) + MRA or CTA brain and neck • Others: MRI brain with gad + hi-res cuts through brainstem • Consider LP for meningitis
NO ↓
Neuropathic syndrome with brainstem/cranial nerve involvement? • Brainstem findings + other neuro signs?
YES → CRITICAL or EMERGENT • Botulism *(Dysarthria? Dry mouth? Dysphagia?...)* • Wernicke encephalopathy *(Nystagmus? Altered mental status? Malnutrition?...)* URGENT • Miller-Fisher syndrome *(Ataxia? Areflexia? Recent illness?...)* → • Treat empirically • Consider screening MRI • Consider LP for Miller-Fisher syndrome
NO → Neuromuscular process?
NO ↓

Neuromuscular process?
YES → CRITICAL or EMERGENT • Myasthenia gravis URGENT • N/A → • Ice test • Edrophonium challenge
NO ↓
Consider other diagnoses

FIG. 1 Algorithm for the diagnostic approach to diplopia in the emergency department—a guideline. *CN,* Cranial nerve; *CT,* computed tomography; *CTA,* CT angiogram; *DSA,* digital subtraction angiography (conventional angiography); *DWI,* diffusion-weighted imaging; *gad,* gadolinium; *hi-res,* high-resolution; *LP,* lumbar puncture; *MRA,* magnetic resonance angiography; *MRI,* magnetic resonance imaging. (From Marx JA et al: *Rosen's emergency medicine,* ed 8, Philadelphia, 2014, Saunders.)

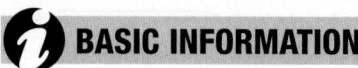

BASIC INFORMATION

DEFINITION

Disseminated intravascular coagulation (DIC) is an acquired thromboembolic disorder characterized by generalized activation of the clotting pathways, which results in the intravascular formation of fibrin and ultimately thrombotic occlusion of small and midsize vessels, followed by end-organ damage.

SYNONYMS

Consumptive coagulopathy
DIC
Defibrination syndrome

ICD-10CM CODE
D65 Disseminated intravascular coagulation [defibrination syndrome]

EPIDEMIOLOGY & DEMOGRAPHICS

DIC can be found in up to 1% of hospitalized patients. There is no predilection for age or gender. More than 50% of cases are associated with gram-negative sepsis or other septicemic infections.

PHYSICAL FINDINGS & CLINICAL PRESENTATION

Both acute and chronic DIC can present with bleeding or thrombosis. Bleeding manifestations are more commonly seen in acute DIC. Risk of bleeding can increase up to fivefold when platelet count is below <50 × 10^9/liter. Sudden exposure to procoagulants may extensively activate a coagulation cascade and platelet consumption. Platelet regeneration from bone marrow and also replacement of coagulation factors from liver synthesis might not be able to keep up with this acute consumptive process. In contrast, chronic DIC more frequently causes thrombotic complications, although PT and PTT values may be normal. Multiple pathways are involved in DIC simultaneously, including (1) thrombin generation due to releasing of tissue factor, (2) suppression of physiologic anticoagulant (e.g., protein C or antithrombin insufficiency), (3) impaired fibrinolytic system characterized by increased level of plasminogen activator inhibitor type 1 (PAI-1), and (4) activation of inflammatory pathways.

With DIC, multiple organs may be involved, including:

- Central nervous system: Altered mental status, transient neurological deficits
- Cardiovascular: Hypotension, tachycardia
- Respiratory: Hypoxia, dyspnea, localized rales, and acute respiratory syndrome
- Gastrointestinal: Intestinal bleeding, bowel infarction
- Genitourinary: Oliguria, anuria, uremia, acidosis, metrorrhagia
- Skin: Wound site bleeding, epistaxis, gingival bleeding, hemorrhagic bullae, petechiae, ecchymosis, purpura

ETIOLOGY

DIC results from the simultaneous formulation of coagulation and fibrinolysis. Its various causes are listed below:

- Infections (e.g., gram-negative sepsis, Rocky Mountain spotted fever, malaria, viral or fungal infection)
- Obstetric complications (e.g., dead fetus, amniotic fluid embolism, toxemia, abruptio placentae, septic abortion, eclampsia, placenta previa, uterine atony)
- Tissue trauma (e.g., burns, hypothermia rewarming)
- Neoplasms (e.g., adenocarcinomas [gastrointestinal, prostate, lung, breast], lymphoproliferative/myeloproliferative, acute promyelocytic leukemia)
- Quinine, cocaine-induced rhabdomyolysis
- Liver failure
- Acute pancreatitis
- Transfusion reactions
- Respiratory distress syndrome
- Toxins (snake bites, amphetamine overdose)
- Other: Systemic lupus erythematosus (SLE), vasculitis, aneurysms, polyarteritis, hemangiomas with thrombocytopenia, and consumptive coagulopathy (Kasabach-Merritt syndrome)

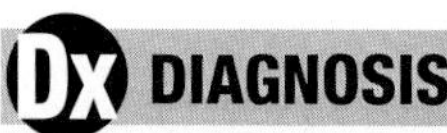

DIAGNOSIS

DIFFERENTIAL DIAGNOSIS

- Hepatic necrosis: Normal or elevated factor VIII concentrations
- Vitamin K deficiency: Normal platelet count
- Hemolytic uremic syndrome: Coagulation assays are usually normal
- Thrombotic thrombocytopenic purpura: Low ADAMTS13 activity
- Renal failure, SLE, sickle cell crisis, dysfibrinogenemias
- HELLP syndrome (**h**emolysis, **e**levated **l**iver function tests, and **l**ow **p**latelets)

WORKUP

Diagnostic workup includes laboratory screening to confirm the diagnosis and exclude conditions noted in the differential diagnosis (Tables 1 and 2, Box 1). Workup is also aimed at distinguishing DIC progression (acute vs. chronic), chief manifestations (thrombotic or hemorrhagic), and extent (localized or systemic).

Specific criteria

LABORATORY TESTS

- Peripheral blood smear generally shows red blood cell fragments (schistocytes) and low platelet counts.
- Coagulation factors are consumed at a rate in excess of the capacity of the liver to synthesize them, and platelets are consumed in excess of the capacity of the bone marrow megakaryocytes to release them. Diagnostic characteristics of DIC are decreased fibrinogen level; thrombocytopenia; and increased prothrombin time (PT), partial thromboplastin time (PTT), TT, fibrin split products, bleeding time, and D-dimer.
- Coagulopathy secondary to DIC must be differentiated from that secondary to liver disease or vitamin K deficiency.
  1. Vitamin K deficiency manifests with prolonged PT and normal PTT, TT, platelet, and fibrinogen level; PTT may be elevated in severe cases.
  2. Patients with liver disease have abnormal PT and PTT; TT and fibrinogen are usually normal unless severe disease is present; platelets are usually normal unless splenomegaly is present.
  3. Factor VIII is low in DIC but is normal in liver disease with coagulopathy.

IMAGING STUDIES

Imaging studies are generally not useful. Chest radiographs may be helpful to exclude infectious processes in patients with pulmonary symptoms such as dyspnea, cough, or hemoptysis.

TABLE 1 Differential Diagnosis of Thrombocytopenia in Suspected Disseminated Intravascular Coagulation

Differential Diagnosis	Additional Diagnostic Clues
DIC	Prolonged aPTT and PT, increased FDP, low levels of antithrombin or protein C
Sepsis without DIC	Positive (blood) cultures, positive sepsis criteria, hemophagocytosis in bone marrow
Massive blood loss	Major bleeding, low hemoglobin, prolonged aPTT and PT
Thrombotic microangiopathy	Schistocytes evident on blood smear, Coombs-negative hemolysis, fever, neurologic symptoms, renal insufficiency, coagulation tests usually normal, ADAMTS13 levels decreased
Heparin-induced thrombocytopenia	Use of heparin, venous or arterial thrombosis, positive HIT test (usually immunoassay for heparin-platelet factor 4 antibodies), increase in platelet count after cessation of heparin; coagulation tests usually normal
Immune thrombocytopenia	Antiplatelet antibodies, normal or increased number of megakaryocytes in bone marrow aspirate, normal levels of TPO (TPO levels are usually normal or slightly increased in ITP); coagulation tests usually normal
Drug-induced thrombocytopenia	Decreased number of megakaryocytes in bone marrow aspirate or detection of drug-induced antiplatelet antibodies, increase in platelet count after cessation of drug; coagulation tests usually normal

ADAMTS13, A disintegrin and metalloproteinase with thrombospondin 13; *aPTT,* activated partial thromboplastin time; *DIC,* disseminated intravascular coagulation; *FDP,* fibrin degradation products; *HIT,* heparin-induced thrombocytopenia; *PT,* prothrombin time; *ITP,* immune thrombocytopenia; *TPO,* thrombopoietin.
Hoffman R et al: *Hematology, basic principles and practice,* ed 7, Philadelphia, 2018, Elsevier.

TABLE 2 Differential Diagnosis of Prolonged aPTT and/or PT in Suspected Disseminated Intravascular Coagulation

Test Result	Cause
PT prolonged, aPTT normal	Factor VII deficiency Mild vitamin K deficiency Mild liver insufficiency Low doses of vitamin K antagonists
PT normal, aPTT prolonged	Factor VIII, IX, or XI deficiency Unfractionated heparin Inhibitory antibody and/or antiphospholipid antibody Factor XII or prekallikrein deficiency
Both PT and aPTT prolonged	Factor X, V, II, or fibrinogen deficiency Severe vitamin K deficiency Vitamin K antagonists Global clotting factor deficiency • Decreased synthesis: Liver failure • Increased loss: Massive bleeding, DIC

aPTT, Activated partial thromboplastin time; *PT,* prothrombin time.
Hoffman R et al: *Hematology, basic principles and practice,* ed 7, Philadelphia, 2018, Elsevier.

BOX 1 Diagnostic Algorithm for the Diagnosis of Overt Disseminated Intravascular Coagulation[a]

- Presence of an underlying disorder known to be associated with disseminated intravascular coagulation (DIC) (Table 2) (no = 0, yes = 2)
- Score global coagulation test results
  - Platelet count (>100 = score 0; <100 = score 1; <50 = score 2)
  - Level of fibrin markers (e.g., D-dimer, fibrin degradation products) (no increase = score 0; moderate increase = score 2; strong increase = score 3)[b]
  - Prolonged prothrombin time (<3 s = score 0; >3 s but <6 s = score 1; >6 s = score 2)
  - Fibrinogen level (>1.0 g/L = score 0; <1.0 g/L = score 1)
- Calculate score
- If ≥5: Compatible with overt DIC; repeat scoring daily if <5: Suggestive (not affirmative) for nonovert DIC; repeat next 1–2 days.

[a] According to the Scientific Standardization Committee of the International Society of Thrombosis and Haemostasis.
[b] Strong increase, greater than 5× upper limit of normal; moderate increase, greater than upper limit of normal but less than 5× upper limit of normal.
Hoffman R et al: *Hematology, basic principles and practice,* ed 7, Philadelphia, 2018, Elsevier.

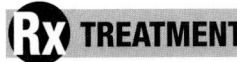

Rx TREATMENT

ACUTE GENERAL Rx

- Correct and eliminate underlying cause (e.g., antimicrobial therapy for infection, removal of necrotic bowel, evacuation of uterus in obstetric emergencies).
- Give replacement therapy with fresh frozen plasma (FFP) and platelets in patients with significant hemorrhage:
  1. FFP 10 to 15 ml/kg can be given with a goal of normalizing international normalized ratio.
  2. Platelet transfusions are given when platelet count is <10,000 (or higher if major bleeding is present).
  3. Cryoprecipitate 1 U/5 kg is reserved for fibrinogen level <100 mg/dl.
  4. Antithrombin treatment may be considered as a supportive therapeutic option in patients with severe DIC. Its modest results and substantial cost are limiting factors.
- Heparin therapy using unfractionated heparin at lower doses than those used in venous thrombosis (300-500 U/hr) may be useful in selected cases in which thrombosis usually predominates, with a view to increase neutralization of thrombin (e.g., in acute promyelocytic leukemia, purpura fulminans, acral ischemia). Low-molecular-weight heparin also may be used in this scenario.
- The mainstays of supportive treatment of DIC are summarized in Box 2.

DISPOSITION

Mortality rate in severe DIC exceeds 75%. Death generally results from progression of the underlying disease and complications such as acute

BOX 2 Mainstays of Supportive Treatment of Disseminated Intravascular Coagulation

Modality	Details	Expectations/Rationale
Treating the underlying disorder	Dependent on the primary diagnosis	Inhibit or block the complicating pathologic mechanism of disseminated intravascular coagulation (DIC) in parallel with the response (if any) of the disorder
Antithrombotic agents	Prophylactic heparin to prevent venous thromboembolic complications (Low-dose) therapeutic heparin in case of confirmed thromboembolism or if clinical picture is dominated by (micro) vascular thrombosis and associated organ failure	Risk of thromboembolism is increased in critically ill patients, trauma patients, or patients with cancer Prevent fibrin formation; tip the balance within the microcirculation toward anticoagulant mechanisms and physiologic fibrinolysis; allow reperfusion of the skin, kidneys, and brain
Transfusion	Infuse platelets, plasma, and fibrinogen (cryoprecipitate) if there is overt bleeding or a high risk of bleeding	Bleeding should diminish and stop over the course of hours Platelet count, coagulation tests, and fibrinogen should return toward normal
Anticoagulant factor concentrates	Recombinant human activated protein C may be effective in sepsis and DIC (24 μg/kg per hour for 4 days); currently withdrawn from the market	Restore anticoagulation in microvascular environment and may have antiinflammatory activity Latest trials were negative.
Fibrinolytic inhibitors	Tranexamic acid (e.g., 500–1000 mg q8–12 h or ε-aminocaproic acid 1000–2000 mg q8–12 h)	May be useful if there is (hyper)fibrinolysis Bleeding ceases, but there is a risk of microvascular thrombosis and renal failure

Hoffman R et al: *Hematology, basic principles and practice,* ed 7, Philadelphia, 2018, Elsevier.

renal failure, intracerebral bleeding, shock, or cardiac tamponade.

REFERRAL

Hematology consultation is recommended in all cases of DIC.

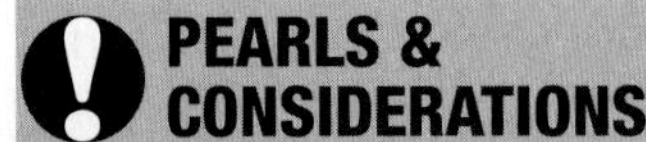

COMMENTS

The treatment of chronic DIC is controversial. Low-dose SC heparin and/or combination antiplatelet agents such as aspirin and dipyridamole may be useful.

SUGGESTED READINGS

Available at ExpertConsult.com

RELATED CONTENT

Disseminated Intravascular Coagulation (Patient Information)

AUTHOR: **PATAN GULTAWATVICHAI, M.D.**

Diverticular Disease (Diverticulosis, Diverticulitis, Diverticular Hemorrhage)

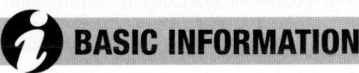

BASIC INFORMATION

DEFINITION

- Colonic diverticula are herniations of mucosa and submucosa (Figs. 1 and 2) through the muscularis. They are generally found along the colon's mesenteric border at the site where the vasa recta penetrates the muscle wall (anatomic weak point).
- *Diverticulosis* is the asymptomatic presence of multiple colonic diverticula.
- *Diverticulitis* is an inflammatory process or localized perforation of diverticulum.

ICD-10CM CODES

K57.30	Diverticulosis of large intestine without perforation or abscess without bleeding
K57.32	Diverticulitis of large intestine without perforation or abscess without bleeding
K57.31	Diverticulosis of large intestine without perforation or abscess with bleeding

EPIDEMIOLOGY & DEMOGRAPHICS

- Incidence of diverticulosis in the general population is 35% to 50%. Prevalence of diverticulosis increases with ages (<10% under age 40 to over 50% in those >85).
- Diverticulosis is more common in Western countries, affecting >30% of people >40 yr and >50% of people >70 yr.
- Approximately 20% of patients with diverticula have an episode of diverticulitis.

PHYSICAL FINDINGS & CLINICAL PRESENTATION

- Physical examination in patients with diverticulosis is generally normal.
- Painful diverticular disease can present with left lower quadrant (LLQ) pain, often relieved by defecation; location of pain may be anywhere in the lower abdomen because of the redundancy of the sigmoid colon.
- Diverticulitis can cause muscle spasm, guarding, and rebound tenderness predominantly affecting the LLQ. Factors associated with diverticulitis are pain localized to left lower quadrant and exacerbated by movement, left-lower-quadrant tenderness on examination, fever 38.5°C or higher, absence of vomiting, age >50 yr, and history of one or more episodes of diverticulitis.

ETIOLOGY

- Diverticular disease is believed to be secondary to low intake of dietary fiber.
- Recent studies indicate a pathogenetic role for inflammation in diverticulitis that may be similar to that of IBS, IBD, or both, based on common histologic findings such as granulomas, infiltrating lymphocytes, TNF, histamine, and matrix metalloproteinases.[1]

[1] Morris AM et al: Sigmoid diverticulitis: a systematic review, *JAMA* 311(3):287-297, 2014.

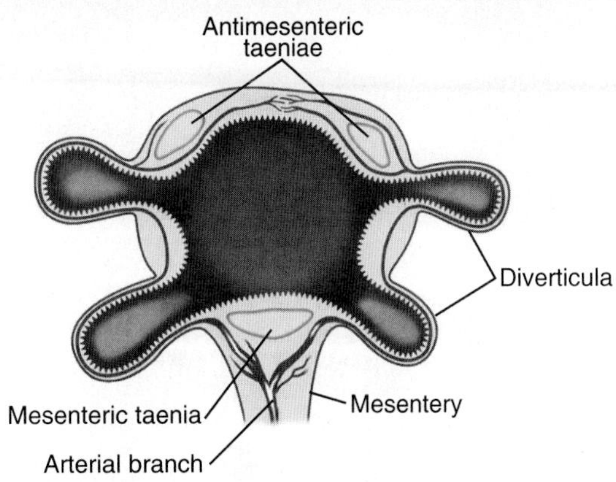

FIG. 1 Diagram showing colonic diverticula and their relationship to the taeniae coli. (From Feldman M et al (eds): *Sleisenger and Fordtran's gastrointestinal and liver disease*, ed 10, Philadelphia, 2016, Saunders.)

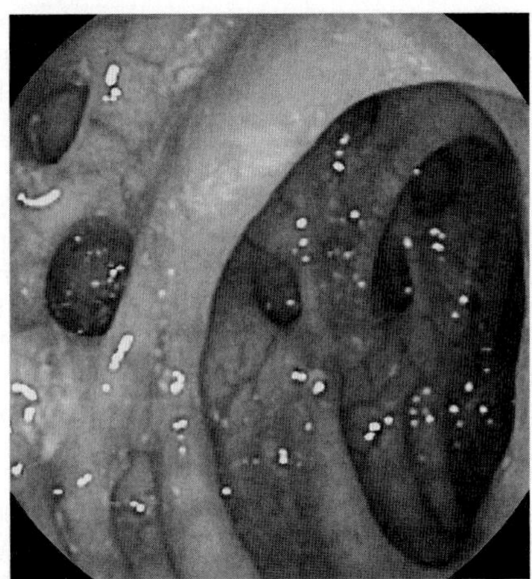

FIG. 2 Colonoscopic view of sigmoid diverticulosis. (From Feldman M et al (eds): *Sleisenger and Fordtran's gastrointestinal and liver disease*, ed 10, Philadelphia, 2016, Saunders.)

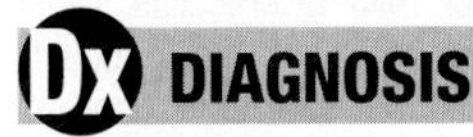

DIAGNOSIS

DIFFERENTIAL DIAGNOSIS

- IBS
- IBD
- Colorectal cancer
- Endometriosis
- Ischemic colitis
- Bowel obstruction/volvulus
- Urinary tract disorders (urolithiasis, hydronephrosis)
- Infections (pseudomembranous colitis, appendicitis, pyelonephritis, PID)
- Lactose intolerance
- Celiac disease
- Epiploic appendagitis
- Gynecologic disorders (ectopic pregnancy, menstrual irregularities, dyspareunia, endometriosis)
- Cholecystitis, biliary disease

LABORATORY TESTS

- WBC count in diverticulitis reveals leukocytosis with left shift.
- Microcytic anemia can be present in patients with chronic bleeding from diverticular disease. MCV may be elevated in acute bleeding secondary to reticulocytosis.
- Urinalysis is useful to exclude urinary causes of pain.
- Pregnancy test is indicated in women of child-bearing age.
- Electrolytes and liver enzymes are useful in ruling out biliary causes of pain.
- CRP levels of 50 mg/L or greater is common in acute diverticulitis.

PROCEDURES: Colonoscopy should be avoided during acute diverticulitis due to the risk of perforation. It can generally be performed after 6 wk to rule out the presence of cancer and IBD.

IMAGING STUDIES

- If clinical features are highly suggestive of diverticulitis, imaging studies are generally not necessary.
- A CT scan of the abdomen (Fig. 3) with IV and luminal contrast is the preferred radiologic examination to diagnose acute diverticulitis. It can also diagnose diverticulosis. It has a sensitivity of 93% to 97% and a specificity approaching 100% for diverticulitis. Typical findings are thickening of the bowel wall, fistulas, or abscess formation. CT may also reveal other disease processes (e.g., appendicitis, tubo ovarian abscess, Crohn's disease) accounting for lower abdominal pain. In the Hinchey classification scheme based on CT results, stages 0 and Ia indicate uncomplicated diverticulitis, whereas stages Ib (pericolic or mesenteric abscess in proximity to the

 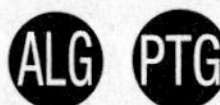

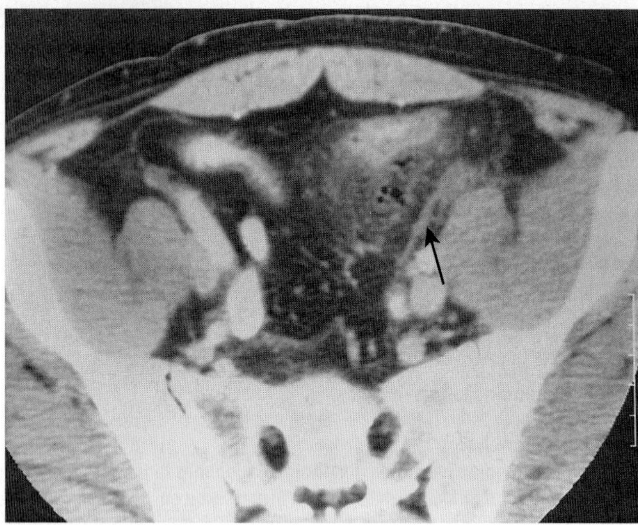

FIG. 3 Sigmoid diverticulitis. Enhanced CT shows haziness associated with extraluminal air in the sigmoid mesocolon due to perforated diverticulitis, also manifested as a thickened sigmoid wall. Thickening at the root of the sigmoid mesocolon is also present *(arrow).* (From Grainger RG et al [eds.]: *Grainger and Allison's diagnostic radiology,* ed 4, Philadelphia, 2001, Churchill Livingstone.)

primary inflammatory process), II (intraabdominal abscess distant from primary inflammatory process or pelvic/retroperitoneal abscess), III (generalized purulent peritonitis), and IV (generalized fecal peritonitis) indicate complicated diverticulitis. Ultrasonography and MRI can also be used. Abdominal ultrasonography has a 90% sensitivity and specificity for acute diverticulitis. MRI is also highly sensitive and specific for acute diverticulitis.
- Evaluation of suspected diverticular bleeding (Fig. 4):
  1. Arteriography if the bleeding is faster than 1 ml/min (advantage: the possible infusion of vasopressin directly into the arteries supplying the bleeding, as well as selective arterial embolization; disadvantages: its cost and invasive nature)
  2. Technetium-99m sulfa colloid
  3. Technetium-99m labeled RBC (can detect bleeding rates as low as 0.12 to 5 ml/min)

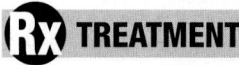

TREATMENT

NONPHARMACOLOGIC THERAPY

- Increase in dietary fiber intake and regular exercise to improve bowel function. However, recent studies have challenged the common view that fiber intake protects against diverticulosis.
- Oral diet of clear liquids is recommended until pain resolves in cases of mild uncomplicated diverticulitis.
- NPO and IV hydration in severe diverticulitis; NG suction if ileus or small bowel obstruction is present.
- Emergent surgery is required for perforation, peritonitis, or uncontrolled sepsis.

ACUTE GENERAL Rx

TREATMENT OF DIVERTICULITIS:

- Mild uncomplicated diverticulitis (75% of cases of diverticulitis): Broad-spectrum PO antibiotics (e.g., ciprofloxacin 750 mg bid or levofloxacin 750 mg bid or trimethoprim/sulfamethoxazole DS bid to cover aerobic component of colonic flora *and* metronidazole 500 mg q6h for anaerobes) and liquid diet for 7 to 10 days are commonly prescribed. Single-agent therapy with amoxicillin-clavulanic acid 875 mg/125 mg PO every 12 hours or moxifloxacin 400 mg PO every hour is also effective. Trials have shown no benefit of IV versus oral antibiotics and similar outcomes when using a 4-day course instead of a 7-day course of antibiotics. Other randomized trials and cohort studies have shown that antibiotics are not as beneficial or necessary as previously thought in cases of mild diverticulitis. Other modalities such as 5-aminosalicylate products and probiotics remain controversial and of unclear benefit.
- Mild- to moderate complicated diverticulitis, in-patient treatment: Single-agent therapy with ertapenem 1 mg IV every 24 hours, ticarcillin-clavulanic acid 200–300 mg/kg per day divided doses every 6 hours, or moxifloxacin 400 mg IV every 24 hours for 4–7 days. Combination therapy of cefazolin (1–2 mg every 8 hours) or levofloxacin (750 mg every 24 hours) plus metronidazole (500 mg every 8 hours) is also effective.
- Severe complicated diverticulitis: NPO and aggressive IV antibiotic therapy
  1. Imipenem-cilastin 500 mg IV q6h *or*
  2. Piperacillin-tazobactam 4.5 g IV q8h *or*
  3. Meropenem 1 g IV q8h *or*
  4. Doripenem 500 mg IV q8h
  5. Cefepime 2 g IV q8h or ciprofloxacin 400 mg IV q12h each in combination with metronidazole 500 mg IV q8h
- Surgical treatment (laparoscopic preferred over open colectomy) consisting of resection of involved areas and reanastomosis (if feasible); otherwise, a diverting colostomy with reanastomosis is performed when infection has been controlled. The need for surgery as well as its optimal timing is unclear, and surgery is no longer considered necessary after a couple of episodes of diverticulitis. Surgery may be considered in patients with:
  1. Repeated episodes of diverticulitis
  2. Poor response to appropriate medical therapy (failure of conservative management)
  3. Abscess or fistula formation
  4. Obstruction
  5. Peritonitis: Colonic resection with a Hartmann pouch is the procedure of choice in critically ill patients with generalized peritonitis
  6. Immunocompromised patients, first episode in young patient (<40 yr old)
  7. Inability to exclude carcinoma (10%-20% of patients diagnosed with diverticulosis on clinical grounds are subsequently found to have carcinoma of the colon)

DIVERTICULAR HEMORRHAGE:

- Bleeding is painless and stops spontaneously in the majority of patients (60%); it is usually caused by erosion of a blood vessel by a fecalith present within the diverticular sac.
- Medical therapy consists of blood replacement and correction of volume and any clotting abnormalities.
- Colonoscopic treatment with epinephrine injections, bipolar coagulation, or both may prevent recurrent bleeding and decrease the need for surgery. Endoclips (Fig. 5) can also be used to stop the bleeding.
- Surgical resection is necessary if bleeding does not stop spontaneously after administration of 4 to 5 U of PRBCs or recurs with severity within a few days; if attempts at localization are unsuccessful, total abdominal colectomy with ileoproctostomy may be indicated (high incidence of rebleeding if segmental resection is performed without adequate localization).

DISPOSITION

- The risk of recurrence among patients with uncomplicated diverticulitis is 32% to 36%. Most patients with diverticulitis respond well to antibiotic management and bowel rest. Up to 30% of patients with diverticulitis will eventually require surgical management.
- Diverticular bleeding can recur in 15% to 20% of patients within 5 yr.

REFERRAL

- GI referral for colonoscopy 4 to 6 wk after resolution of symptoms. In patients who have complications from diverticulitis, colonoscopy is generally not necessary after radiologically proven uncomplicated diverticulitis.
- Surgical referral when considering resection.

SUGGESTED READINGS

Available at ExpertConsult.com

RELATED CONTENT

Diverticular Disease (Patient Information)
Diverticulitis (Patient Information)
Diverticulosis (Patient Information)

AUTHOR: **FRED F. FERRI, M.D.**

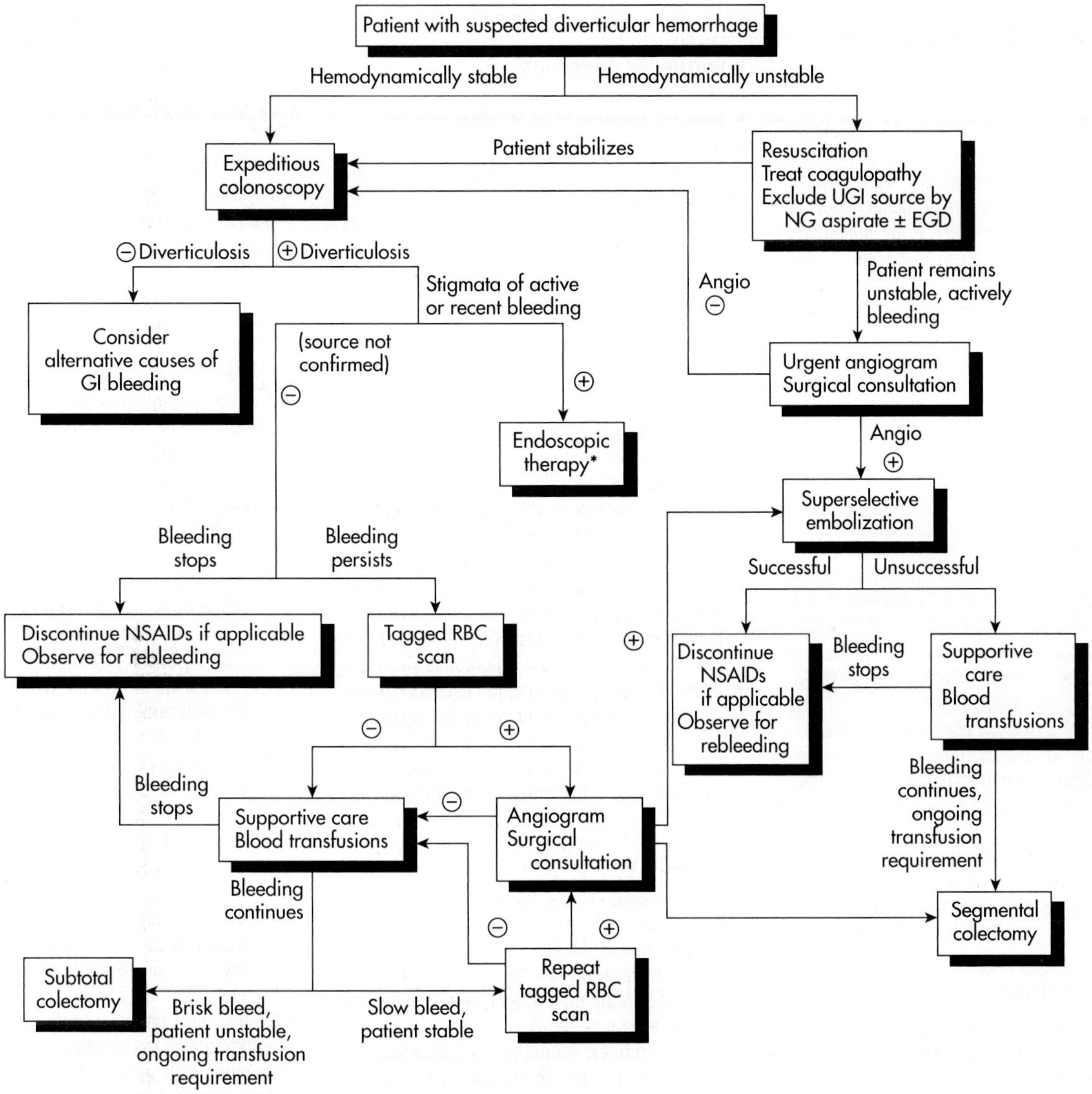

Patient with suspected diverticular hemorrhage

Hemodynamically stable

Hemodynamically unstable

Expeditious colonoscopy

Patient stabilizes

Resuscitation
Treat coagulopathy
Exclude UGI source by NG aspirate ± EGD

⊖ Diverticulosis

⊕ Diverticulosis

Stigmata of active or recent bleeding

Angio ⊖

Patient remains unstable, actively bleeding

Consider alternative causes of GI bleeding

(source not confirmed) ⊖

⊕

Urgent angiogram
Surgical consultation

Endoscopic therapy*

Angio ⊕

Superselective embolization

Bleeding stops

Bleeding persists

Successful

Unsuccessful

Discontinue NSAIDs if applicable
Observe for rebleeding

Tagged RBC scan

⊕

Discontinue NSAIDs if applicable
Observe for rebleeding

Bleeding stops

Supportive care
Blood transfusions

⊖

⊕

Bleeding stops

⊖

Supportive care
Blood transfusions

Angiogram
Surgical consultation

Bleeding continues, ongoing transfusion requirement

Bleeding continues

Segmental colectomy

⊖

⊕

Subtotal colectomy

Brisk bleed, patient unstable, ongoing transfusion requirement

Slow bleed, patient stable

Repeat tagged RBC scan

FIG. 4 Algorithm for the management of patients with suspected diverticular hemorrhage. *Angio*, angiogram; *EGD*, esophagogastroduodenoscopy; *NG*, nasogastric; *NSAID*, nonsteroidal antiinflammatory drugs; *RBC*, red blood cell; *UGI*, upper GI. *Endoscopic therapy may consist of epinephrine injection alone or in combination with other therapies, such as heater probe coagulation, bipolar coagulation, endoclips, fibrin sealant, and band ligation. (From Feldman M et al [eds.]: *Sleisenger and Fordtran's gastrointestinal and liver disease*, ed 10, Philadelphia, 2016, Saunders.)

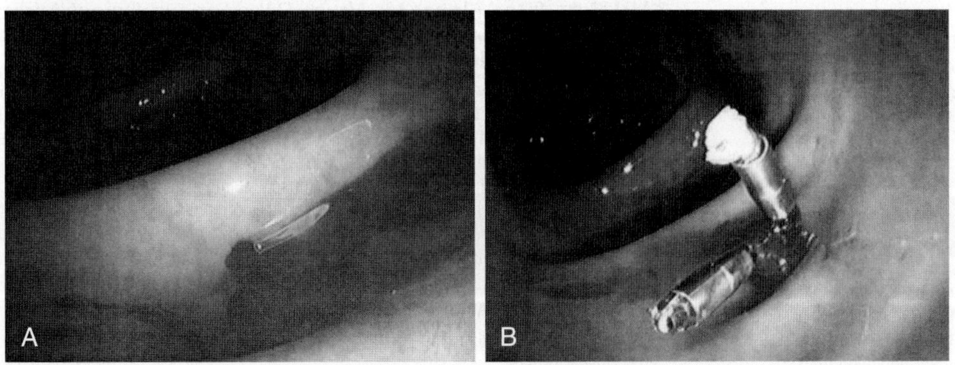

FIG. 5 Colonoscopy in a patient with lower intestinal bleeding from a diverticulum in whom a site of active bleeding was identified **(A)** and treated successfully with placement of two endoclips **(B)**. (Courtesy Janak Shah, MD. San Francisco, CA.) (From Feldman M et al [eds.]: *Sleisenger and Fordtran's gastrointestinal and liver disease*, ed 10, Philadelphia, 2016, Saunders.)

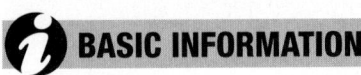

BASIC INFORMATION

DEFINITION

Drug abuse is a recurring pattern of harmful use of a substance despite adverse consequences to work, school, relationships, the legal system, or physical health. This may occur concurrently with or independently from *substance dependence,* in which the impairment or distress is more pervasive and often (though not necessarily) includes physical dependence and withdrawal symptoms (Table 1).

SYNONYMS

Substance use disorder
Substance abuse
Addiction

ICD-10CM CODES

F19.129	Other psychoactive substance abuse, unspecified
F10-F19	Defined by specific substance
Z71.51	Drug abuse counseling and surveillance of drug abuser
Z71.51	Drug abuse counseling and surveillance of drug abuser

The new term *substance use disorder* in the fifth edition of the *Diagnostic and Statistical Manual of Mental Disorders* (DSM-5) combines the categories of substance abuse and substance dependence into a single disorder measured on a continuum from mild to severe.

DSM-5 CODE

Depends on specific drug of abuse

EPIDEMIOLOGY & DEMOGRAPHICS

INCIDENCE (IN U.S.): Alcohol or drug dependence: 5% to 10% of population

PREVALENCE (IN U.S.): Approximately 15% of patients in primary care practice have an at-risk pattern of drug and/or alcohol use; lifetime prevalence of any alcohol use disorder: 30%; prescription drug misuse is on the rise with 5% past-yr prevalence.

PREDOMINANT SEX: Males > females

PREDOMINANT AGE:
- Problematic use of substances may begin in early life (8-10 yr).
- Mean age of onset of problem drinking is approximately 25 yr for men and 30 yr for women.

PEAK INCIDENCE: For most substances: Age 15 to 30 yr

DURATION OF CONDITION:
- Men: Average >20 yr of heavy drinking
- Women: Average 15 yr of heavy drinking
- In general, substance use disorders are chronic and relapsing and often progressive

GENETICS: There is evidence of nonspecific genetic factors. Addiction may result in part from underlying, inherited abnormalities in brain structure that impair behavior control and encourage impulsive behavior.

PHYSICAL FINDINGS & CLINICAL PRESENTATION

- Polysubstance use and comorbidity with psychiatric disorders are common.
- History often reveals recurring behavioral problems, such as relationship, work, or legal problems; violence and traumatic injuries; and anxiety, depression, insomnia, and cognitive and memory dysfunction.
- Repeated requests for early refills of controlled substances and obtaining prescriptions from multiple providers should raise concern for prescription drug abuse (Table 2).
- Physical findings may include injection marks (Fig. 1), nasal lesions or recurrent epistaxis, poor dentition, scars or bruises from falls or trauma, and poor nutritional status; signs/symptoms of intoxication or withdrawal are highly suggestive of substance use disorder.

ETIOLOGY

Several models of addiction have been proposed:
- Disease model: Addiction is a mental illness, which occurs as a result of the impairment of healthy neurochemical or behavioral processes.
- Genetic model: Genetic predisposition is often a factor in dependency and certain addictive behaviors.
- Social model: Person–environment interactions (i.e., socialization, imitation of observable behavior, and the influence of modeling) shape addictive behavior.

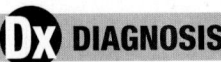

DIAGNOSIS

DIFFERENTIAL DIAGNOSIS

- Psychiatric disorders such as depression, mania, psychosis, and anxiety disorders may coexist or occur as a consequence of substance use.
- Rule out seizure disorder and underlying illness.

WORKUP

- A thorough history is crucial for diagnosis.
- The physician's history-taking style and techniques strongly affect patient's willingness to report use and participate in future treatment activities.
- A structured, nonjudgmental approach is generally preferable:
  1. Ask about quantity and frequency of alcohol or drug use. For example, the National Institute on Alcohol Abuse and Alcoholism (NIAAA) declares that *problem drinking* is defined as more than two drinks per day for men and more than one drink per day for women or anyone older than 65 yr.
  2. Use a short screening instrument such as the CAGE questionnaire ("1. Have you ever felt you need to **C**ut down on your alcohol or drug use? 2. Have people **A**nnoyed you by criticizing your alcohol or drug use? 3. Have you ever felt **G**uilty about alcohol or drug use? 4. Have you ever felt you need to drink first thing in the morning [**E**ye opener] to stop shakiness?").
- Problematic behavior during intoxication or withdrawal is diagnostic.
- Because self-report of substance use and its consequences can be unreliable, obtaining corroborating information, such as from family members, past detoxifications, or drug rehabilitations, is often helpful.

TABLE 1 Key Features of Substance Abuse

1. The substance is often taken in larger amounts over a longer period than intended
2. Unsuccessful efforts to cut down
3. A great deal of time spent obtaining the substance or recovering from its effects
4. Craving
5. Social, occupational, or recreational
6. Recurrent despite hazards
7. Tolerance or withdrawal

Reprinted from Goldman L, Bennett JC (eds): *Cecil textbook of medicine,* ed 22, Philadelphia, 2004, Saunders.

TABLE 2 "Red Flags" for Abuse Behavior and Opioid Addiction

Potential Abuse/Addiction Behaviors*

1. Patient displays an overwhelming focus on opioid issues during clinic visits that occupies a significant proportion of the clinic visit and impedes progress with other pain issues or medical problems.
2. Patient has a pattern of early refills (three or more) or escalating drug use in the absence of acute change or progression of his or her medical condition.
3. Patient generates multiple telephone calls or unscheduled visits to request more opioids, early refills, or problems associated with the opioid prescription that often creates a disturbance of the clinic staff.
4. There is a pattern of prescription problems with reports of medications lost, spilled, or stolen.
5. Patient has supplemental sources of opioids from multiple providers, emergency departments, or illegal sources.

Additional "Red Flag" Abuse Behavior

1. Selling prescribed medications
2. Prescription forgery
3. Stealing another patient's medications
4. Injecting or snorting oral medication
5. Concurrent use of illicit drug(s)
6. Appearing intoxicated or oversedated
7. Insisting on obtaining a specific opioid medication

*Adapted from Chabal criteria for opioid abuse.
From Hochberg MC et al: *Rheumatology,* ed 5, St Louis, 2011, Mosby.

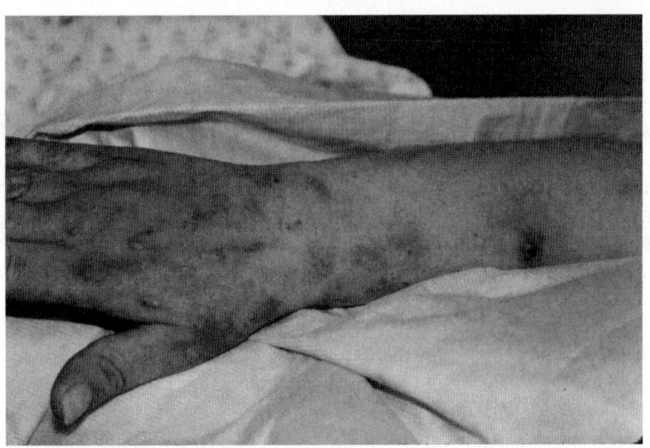

FIG. 1 Tracks secondary to intravenous heroin abuse. (Marx JA et al: *Rosen's emergency medicine*, ed 8, Philadelphia, 2014, Saunders.)

- Adolescent drug abuse detection and treatment is extremely challenging. Stages of adolescent substance use are described in Table 3. An assessment for evaluating the seriousness of adolescent drug abuse is described in Table 4.

LABORATORY TESTS

- Blood alcohol content (BAC) measured on the breath is practical to define intoxication and provides a rough measure of impairment. In general, two standard drinks may cause BAC 0.08% or higher, which is considered legally impaired.
- Obtain toxicology screen in urine or blood samples.
- Biologic markers such as elevated mean corpuscular volume (MCV), γ-glutamyltransferase (GGT), liver function tests (AST and ALT), and carbohydrate deficient transferrin (CDT) may also be used to diagnose and monitor.

TABLE 3 Stages of Adolescent Substance Abuse

Stage	Description
1	Potential for abuse Decreased impulse control Need for immediate gratification Available drugs, alcohol, inhalants Need for peer acceptance
2	Experimentation: learning the euphoria Use of inhalants, tobacco, marijuana, and alcohol with friends Few, if any, consequences Use may increase to weekends regularly Little change in behavior
3	Regular use: seeking the euphoria Use of other drugs, e.g., stimulants, LSD, sedatives Behavioral changes and some consequences Increased frequency of use; use alone Buying or stealing drugs
4	Regular use: preoccupation with the "high" Daily use of drugs Loss of control Multiple consequences and risk-taking Estrangement from family and "straight" friends
5	Burnout: use of drugs to feel normal Polysubstance use/cross-addiction Guilt, withdrawal, shame, remorse, depression Physical and mental deterioration Increased risk-taking, self-destructive, suicidal

LSD, lysergic acid diethylamide.
From Kliegman RM et al: *Nelson textbook of pediatrics,* ed 19, Philadelphia, 2011, Saunders.

IMAGING STUDIES

Not helpful in routine diagnosis and management of substance abuse, but possibly useful in the management of sequelae of substance abuse (e.g., brain imaging to evaluate the alcohol abuse–associated increased risk of subdural hematomas or increased evidence of cerebral atrophy).

Rx TREATMENT

NONPHARMACOLOGIC THERAPY

- First assess readiness for change; if precontemplative or contemplative, counsel about risks of use and benefits of abstinence; a motivational interviewing approach has been shown to be effective.
- Nonpharmacologic strategies have the greatest documented efficacy: Advice, feedback, goal setting, problem solving, and additional contacts for further assistance.
- Opiate contracts, prohibiting a patient from getting early refills or obtaining opiates from multiple prescribers, should be considered for all patients with chronic pain receiving opioid painkillers, especially for patients with a history of substance abuse or medication abuse.
- Relapse prevention facilitated by avoidance of trigger stimuli or by uncoupling trigger stimuli from substance ingestion.
- Self-help and support groups such as Alcoholics Anonymous and Narcotics Anonymous are helpful in achieving and maintaining sobriety.
- Residential or inpatient treatment programs should be a consideration for any individual with continued or escalating use despite outpatient treatment.

ACUTE GENERAL Rx

- Detoxification is an important first step. Its goals are to facilitate withdrawal and reduce

TABLE 4 Assessing the Seriousness of Adolescent Drug Abuse

Variable	0	+1	+2
Age (yr)	>15	<15	
Sex	Male	Female	
Family history of drug abuse		Yes	
Setting of drug use	In group		Alone
Affect before drug use	Happy	Always poor	Sad
School performance	Good, improving		Recently poor
Use before driving	None		Yes
History of accidents	None		Yes
Time of week	Weekend	Weekdays	
Time of day		After school	Before or during school
Type of drug	Marijuana, beer, wine	Hallucinogens, amphetamines	Whiskey, opiates, cocaine, barbiturates

Total score: 0–3, less worrisome; 3–8, serious; 8–18, very serious.
From Kliegman RM et al: *Nelson textbook of pediatrics,* ed 19, Philadelphia, 2011, Saunders.

symptoms, initiate abstinence, and refer the patient to ongoing treatment.

- Benzodiazepines are effective in acute alcohol withdrawal for the management of symptoms as well as the prevention of seizures. One strategy is to give the patient a loading dose of a long-acting benzodiazepine (e.g., 20 mg of diazepam) and then continue the benzodiazepine as scheduled while tapering down the dose gradually. An alternative "symptom-driven" strategy is to follow the patient closely with serial assessments, such as the Clinical Institute Withdrawal Assessment for Alcohol (CIWA) scale, and to dose with 1 to 2 mg of lorazepam as needed to treat withdrawal symptoms.
- The prophylactic administration of thiamine and folic acid (first intravenously or intramuscularly followed by supplemental oral doses) in alcohol withdrawal is recommended before starting any carbohydrate-containing fluids or food to prevent Wernicke-Korsakoff syndrome (alcoholic encephalopathy and psychosis). Magnesium appears to be effective in the treatment of alcohol withdrawal–related cardiac arrhythmias, but not other symptoms of alcohol withdrawal.
- Beta-blockers and clonidine generally should be avoided in alcohol withdrawal; they may mask markers of the severity of the withdrawal (blood pressure and pulse rate).
- Unlike withdrawal from alcohol or benzodiazepines, opioid withdrawal is not life threatening.
- Clonidine alleviates the discomfort of opiate withdrawal. Clonidine tablets, 0.1 mg q4-6h as needed, can be used while monitoring patient's blood pressure. Clonidine transdermal patch, 0.1 mg/24 hr, can be used to treat autonomic hyperactivity symptoms; however, it has a very slow onset and may take 2 to 3 days to achieve therapeutic levels. Antidiarrheals, ibuprofen, and dicyclomine can be used as adjuncts to treat opiate withdrawal symptoms.
- Methadone taper is an effective approach for detoxification in opioid dependence.
- Buprenorphine is a partial μ-opioid receptor agonist that may be used for detoxification and maintenance in treatment of opioid dependence (see dosing in next section).

LONG-TERM Rx

- Naltrexone helps reduce craving for alcohol. Naltrexone 50 mg once daily for 12 wk can be a useful adjunct to substance abuse counseling or rehabilitation programs. Randomized treatment studies are equivocal for long-term outcomes. Naltrexone reduces relapse and the intensity or frequency of any drinking that does occur. It can be hepatotoxic and is contraindicated in opiate users. Intramuscular naltrexone (380 mg monthly) may be considered if adherence is an issue.
- Acamprosate also helps reduce craving for alcohol. Acamprosate 666 mg three times daily may be an effective adjunct to counseling. A recent meta-analysis showed overall benefit with increase in the number of abstinent days.
- Disulfiram provokes acetaldehyde accumulation after alcohol ingestion, producing a toxic state manifested by nausea, headache, flushing, and respiratory distress. Studies have shown limited efficacy mostly due to noncompliance.
- Topiramate may be an alternative treatment for alcoholism. In a 12-wk randomized trial topiramate up to 300 mg daily significantly reduced the number of heavy drinking days.
- Methadone maintenance for opiate addiction is effective and involves once-daily dosing of methadone in a controlled setting via methadone clinics.
- Buprenorphine is as effective as low-dose methadone and may be prescribed by physicians who have completed approved training. For induction, initiate 12 to 24 hr after short-acting opioid use and 24 to 48 hr after long-acting opioid use. Use buprenorphine/naloxone tablets in most patients, since buprenorphine-only tablets have risk of abuse. Maximum first-day dosage is 4 to 8 mg of buprenorphine. Titrate buprenorphine dose up to 12 mg on day 2 for signs of withdrawal. Then adjust dosage in frequent outpatient visits (weekly) to minimum needed for maintenance (up to 32 mg daily).
- Naltrexone (oral or injectable) may also be used for maintenance in opioid dependence treatment, though evidence of effectiveness is limited.
- Always combine pharmacotherapy with counseling. There is good evidence that this combination improves outcome.
- Treatment of comorbid psychiatric disorders improves outcomes.
- Intervention may be used to break through **denial** of a person with a serious addictive disorder to help the person acknowledge that he or she suffers from a disorder and agree to treatment.

DISPOSITION

- Substance abuse is a chronic relapsing illness, so relapses are best approached as part of the course of the illness, as opposed to as treatment failure.
- The goal of treatment is always abstinence, but success of treatment is measured by return of function, increasing duration between relapses, and prevention of sequelae of use.

REFERRAL

Physicians should refer patients who do not make progress on changing substance use patterns to addiction specialists and/or specialized substance abuse programs. Patients with comorbid psychiatric illness should be referred for mental health care.

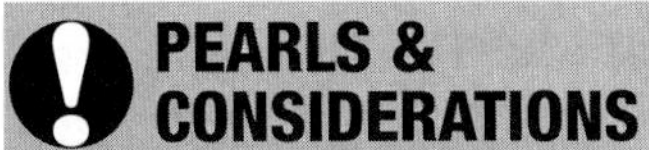

PEARLS & CONSIDERATIONS

- Acute withdrawal from alcohol can become life threatening.
- Withdrawal from opioids can resemble a severe case of the flu.
- A brief intervention (providing information and advising the patient to reduce consumption of alcohol) by the primary care doctor has been demonstrated in randomized trials to reduce drinking in at-risk patients.
- Treatment rates for alcohol use disorders remain low despite available effective treatments.

SUGGESTED READINGS

Available at ExpertConsult.com

RELATED CONTENT

Drug Abuse (Patient Information)
Alcohol Abuse (Related Key Topic)
Opioid Dependence (Related Key Topic)

AUTHOR: **TAHIR TELLIOGLU, M.D.**

BASIC INFORMATION

DEFINITION

Dysfunctional uterine bleeding (DUB) describes abnormal uterine bleeding in the absence of identified causative disease in the pelvis, pregnancy, or medical illness. Specific types of abnormal bleeding include the following (Table 1):

- Menorrhagia: Regular normal intervals, excessive flow and duration
- Metrorrhagia: Irregular intervals
- Menometrorrhagia: Irregular and excessive bleeding during menstruation and between periods
- Oligomenorrhea: Intervals greater than 35 days
- Polymenorrhea: Intervals less than 21 days

These terms, while commonly used in practice, increasingly are felt to be confusing. The term *dysfunctional uterine bleeding* was initially used in 1935 but has never been clearly defined and has been used as both a diagnosis and a symptom. It is generally understood to be a term of exclusion when no other cause of bleeding has been established. In 2011, the FIGO Working Group on Menstrual Disorders released a classification system intended to simplify these definitions. FIGO recommends that the three classifications typically comprising DUB—endometrial dysfunction, ovulatory dysfunction, and coagulopathy—be grouped under the nonstructural causes of abnormal uterine bleeding. However, these new FIGO terms have not yet made their way into common usage.

SYNONYM

DUB

ICD-10CM CODES

N92.5 Other specified irregular menstruation
N92.0 Excessive and frequent menstruation with regular cycle
N91.5 Oligomenorrhea, unspecified
N92.1 Excessive and frequent menstruation with irregular cycle
N94.6 Dysmenorrhea, unspecified

EPIDEMIOLOGY & DEMOGRAPHICS

- Many cases of DUB occur in reproductive extremes of age: the perimenarchal or perimenopausal periods.
- During reproductive age, >80% of abnormal bleeding results from anovulatory DUB.

PHYSICAL FINDINGS & CLINICAL PRESENTATION

- A clinical diagnosis of exclusion
- Thorough physical and pelvic examination to exclude the other causes of abnormal bleeding:
  1. Includes thyroid, breast, liver (e.g., presence or absence of ecchymotic lesions)
  2. Patient habitus: Obese and hirsute (polycystic ovarian disease) or thin (think eating disorders or excessive exercise)
  3. Presence or absence of vulvar, vaginal, or cervical lesions, uterine (fibroid) or ovarian tumors, urethral caruncles or diverticula, hemorrhoids, anal fissures, colorectal lesions
  4. Bimanual pelvic examination: Normal-sized or enlarged uterus, regular or irregular contour

ETIOLOGY

- 90% is caused by anovulation.
- 10% is ovulatory in origin—can be caused by dysfunction of corpus luteum or midcycle (estrogen withdrawal) bleeding.
- Table 2 describes the various causes of abnormal uterine bleeding. The causes of AUB in the fourth and fifth decade are summarized in Table 3.

Dx DIAGNOSIS

DIFFERENTIAL DIAGNOSIS

- PALM–COEIN:
  1. Polyps
  2. Adenomyosis
  3. Leiomyoma
  4. Malignancy/hyperplasia
  5. Coagulopathy
  6. Ovulatory dysfunction
  7. Endometrial
  8. Iatrogenic
  9. Not yet classified
- Anatomic nonuterine causes:
  1. Cervical neoplasia, cervicitis
  2. Vaginal neoplasia, adhesions, trauma, foreign body, atrophic vaginitis, infections, condyloma
  3. Vulvar trauma, infections, neoplasia, condyloma, dystrophy, varices
  4. Urinary tract: Urethral caruncle, diverticulum, hematuria
  5. Gastrointestinal tract: Hemorrhoids, anal fissure, colorectal lesions
- Systemic diseases/effects:
  1. Exogenous hormone intake
  2. Medications
  3. Coagulopathies: von Willebrand's disease, thrombocytopenia, hepatic failure
  4. Endocrinopathies: Thyroid disorder, diabetes mellitus
  5. Renal diseases
- Section II describes a differential diagnosis of vaginal bleeding abnormalities.

WORKUP

- A detailed history and thorough physical examination, including a pelvic examination to exclude causes mentioned above.
- Clinical algorithms for the evaluation of vaginal bleeding are described in Section III, "Bleeding, Vaginal."

TABLE 1 Definitions of Abnormal Uterine Bleeding

Term	Description
Oligomenorrhea	Bleeding at intervals greater than 35 days
Polymenorrhea	Bleeding at intervals less than 21 days
Hypermenorrhea (menorrhagia)	Excessive flow or bleeding with normal intervals
Metrorrhagia	Bleeding between menses
Menometrorrhagia	Excessive flow or duration with periods and between periods
Withdrawal bleeding	Bleeding after the withdrawal of hormones

Crum CP et al: *Diagnostic gynecologic and obstetric pathology,* ed 3, Philadelphia, 2018, Elsevier.

TABLE 2 Causes of Abnormal Uterine Bleeding

Age (Years)	Causes (In Order of Decreasing Frequency)
Prepubertal	Precocious puberty (hypothalamic, pituitary, ovarian)
Adolescence	• Disorders in the hypothalamic-pituitary axis (transient) • Disorders in folliculogenesis (transient) • Sexually transmitted infections, undiscovered pregnancy • Hematologic disorders (von Willebrand factors VII, XI)
Third and fourth decades	• Oral contraceptive pill (OCP) related • Postpregnancy • Benign organic lesions (polyps, leiomyomata, endometritis) • Anovulatory cycle
Fifth decade	• Anovulatory or altered cycle • Benign organic lesions (polyps, adenomyosis, leiomyomata, or endometritis) • Neoplasia
Sixth decade	• Hormone replacement therapy (HRT) • Benign organic lesions (polyps, adenomyosis, leiomyomata, endometritis) • Atrophy • Neoplasia

Crum CP et al: *Diagnostic gynecologic and obstetric pathology,* ed 3, Philadelphia, 2018, Elsevier.

TABLE 3 Causes of Abnormal Uterine Bleeding in the Fourth and Fifth Decades

Cause	Differential Diagnosis
Anovulation	• Endometrial polyp • Basalis
Endometrial polyp	• Basalis/lower uterine segment • Tangentially sectioned functionalis • Atypical polypoid adenomyoma • Adenomyomatous polyp • Intraendometrial leiomyoma • Adenosarcoma
Chronic endometritis	• Late menstrual endometrium • Postpartum/postabortal endometrium • Cervical tissue (plasma cells) • Menstrual endometrium • Lymphoproliferative disorder
Submucosal leiomyoma	• Progestin/tamoxifen therapy • Endometrial polyp • Stromal neoplasm

Crum CP et al: *Diagnostic gynecologic and obstetric pathology,* ed 3, Philadelphia, 2018, Elsevier.

LABORATORY TESTS

- Complete blood count with platelets to evaluate for possible iron-deficiency anemia or thrombocytopenia
- Prothrombin/INR; partial thromboplastin and bleeding time (or PFA-100 assay) if coagulopathy is suspected
- von Willebrand's panel, particularly in women with heavy bleeding since menarche
- Serum or urine human chorionic gonadotropin
- Chemistry profile, including liver function tests
- Thyroid profile
- Pap smear
- Cultures for gonorrhea and *Chlamydia*
- Serum gonadotropins and prolactin
- Serum androgens
- Endometrial biopsy or dilation and curettage, especially in women over 45, with a longstanding history of anovulatory bleeding with fewer than three menstrual cycles per yr or with a high risk of endometrial neoplasia with prolonged unopposed estrogen exposure
- Stool testing for occult blood if source of bleeding is unclear
- Urinalysis for hematuria if source of bleeding is unclear

IMAGING STUDIES

- Pelvic ultrasound, including measurement of endometrial thickness and assessment of myometrial or endometrial defects
- Fluid contrast ultrasound (also called saline sonogram, sonohysterogram, saline infusion sonogram, etc.). Distends the uterine cavity so that "filling defects" of the endometrium can be assessed for possible endometrial polyp, uterine fibroid, or neoplasm
- Hysteroscopy

Rx TREATMENT

NONPHARMACOLOGIC THERAPY

- Increase iron intake in the form of pills and a diet rich in iron to combat anemia.
- Initiate lifestyle changes, including weight loss, exercise, and low-carb diet, if indicated.

ACUTE GENERAL Rx

- Progestational agents:
  1. Progesterone in oil, 100 to 200 mg IM
  2. Medroxyprogesterone acetate, 10 to 20 mg daily for 15 days
  3. Megestrol acetate, 40 to 120 mg daily in divided doses for 15 days
  4. Oral contraceptives: one tablet tid for 5 to 7 days, followed by one tablet low-dose estrogen daily for 21 days; will cause withdrawal bleeding; patient should then be on cyclical medroxyprogesterone or continue on oral contraceptives daily
- Estrogens:
  1. Conjugated estrogen 25 mg IV q4h until bleeding is under control (in cases of severe or life-threatening bleeding); maximum 24 hr
  2. For prolonged bleeding that is not life threatening: Premarin 1.25 mg (Estrace 2 mg) q4h for 24 hr, followed by Provera to bring on withdrawal bleeding; then sequential regimen of estrogen and progestin (Premarin 1.25 mg qd for 24 days, Provera 10 mg for last 10 days) or oral contraceptives

CHRONIC Rx

- Progestational agents:
  1. Medroxyprogesterone acetate 10 mg daily for 12 days, then cyclically to induce monthly withdrawal bleeding
  2. Norethindrone 2.5 to 10 mg qd for 12 days each mo
  3. Depo-Provera 150 mg IM every 3 mo
  4. Oral contraceptives, one tablet qd either cyclically or continuously using only active pills
  5. Levonorgestrel-releasing intrauterine device (Mirena has an FDA indication for heavy menstrual bleeding)
- Letrozole or clomiphene citrate: Patients with anovulatory bleeding who want to become pregnant. Progesterone withdrawal may be counterproductive in patients wishing to start an ovulation induction regimen. Pregnancy rates are lower when patients undergo withdrawal compared to when random ovulation induction start is used. Letrozole is superior to clomiphene citrate in ovulation induction in women with PCOS. Human menopausal gonadotropin (HMG) can be used for women who do not ovulate with oral agents or who have hypothalamic dysfunction.
- Others:
  1. Antiprostaglandins (ibuprofen or naproxen sodium can reduce bleeding by 40%).
  2. Danazol (rarely used due to side-effect profile).
  3. Gonadotropin-releasing hormone (GnRH) analogues; often used to reduce bleeding and ameliorate anemia and in preparation for a surgical procedure.
  4. Tranexamic acid (Lysteda) is an antifibrinolytic agent FDA approved for cyclic heavy menstrual bleeding. Dosage in normal renal function is 3900 mg daily (650 mg tablets, 2 tablets tid) for up to five days during menses.
  5. Endometrial tamponade with Foley catheter.
- Surgical treatment:
  1. D&C and operative hysteroscopy
  2. Endometrial ablation
  3. Uterine artery embolization
  4. Hysterectomy

DISPOSITION

Cyclical treatment on birth control pills or Provera for several cycles, then discontinue pill and watch patient for onset of regular menses. If the patient does not want to conceive, continued cycle management with oral contraceptives is commonly used.

REFERRAL

To gynecologist in case of failure of treatment

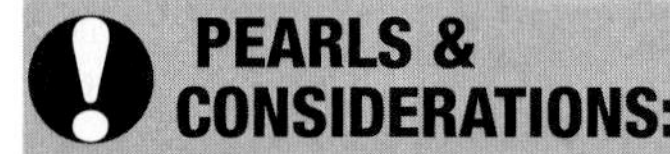

PEARLS & CONSIDERATIONS:

- Always get a pregnancy test.
- If a young patient presents at menarche with bleeding severe enough to warrant emergency evaluation, there is a higher risk of a bleeding disorder, such as von Willebrand's disease.

COMMENTS

Patient education material may be obtained from the American College of Obstetricians and Gynecologists, 409 12th Street SW, Washington, DC 20024-2188; phone 202-638-5577.

SUGGESTED READING

Available at ExpertConsult.com

RELATED CONTENT

Dysfunctional Uterine Bleeding (Patient Information)
Endometrial Cancer (Related Key Topic)
Menorrhagia (Related Key Topic)
Uterine Fibroids (Related Key Topic)

AUTHOR: **NICOLE A. ROBERTS, M.D.**

BASIC INFORMATION

DEFINITION

Dysmenorrhea is painful menstrual cramps of uterine origin. Prevalence is estimated to vary between 45% and 95%. Dysmenorrhea is the most common gynecologic condition in women, regardless of age and nationality.

Types of Dysmenorrhea:

- Primary dysmenorrhea is menstrual pain without organic disease.
- Secondary dysmenorrhea is menstrual pain associated with an identifiable disease.

SYNONYMS

Menstrual cramps
Painful periods

ICD-10CM CODES	
N94.3	Primary dysmenorrhea
N94.5	Secondary dysmenorrhea
N94.6	Dysmenorrhea, unspecified

EPIDEMIOLOGY & DEMOGRAPHICS

- Approximately 50% of menstruating women are affected by dysmenorrhea, with approximately 10% of them having severe dysmenorrhea with incapacitation for 1 to 3 days/mo.
- Dysmenorrhea is most common in the age group from 20 to 24 yr.
- Primary dysmenorrhea may appear 6 to 12 months after ovulatory menstrual cycles begin.
- Secondary dysmenorrhea may occur at any time after menarche, but it may arise in a woman's 30s to 40s due to a causative underlying condition. The woman may also complain of dyspareunia, menorrhagia, intermenstrual bleeding, or postcoital bleeding.

PHYSICAL FINDINGS & CLINICAL PRESENTATION

- Sharp, crampy, midline, lower abdominal pain without a lower quadrant or adnexal component but possible radiation to the lower back and upper thighs
- Unremarkable pelvic examination in nonmenstruating patient
- Accompanying symptoms: Nausea, vomiting, headaches, anxiety, fatigue, diarrhea, fainting, and abdominal bloating
- Cramps usually lasting <24 hr and seldom lasting >2 to 3 days
- Secondary dysmenorrhea: Dyspareunia is a common complaint, and bimanual pelvic-abdominal examination may demonstrate uterine or adnexal tenderness, fixed uterine retroflexion, uterosacral nodularity, a pelvic mass, or an enlarged, irregular uterus

ETIOLOGY

Prostaglandin $F_2\alpha$ is the agent responsible for dysmenorrhea. It stimulates uterine contractions and cervical stenosis (narrowing) and increases vasopressin release. Behavior and psychological factors have also been implicated in the etiology of primary dysmenorrhea. Primary dysmenorrhea only occurs in ovulatory cycles. Secondary dysmenorrhea is usually caused by endometriosis, adenomyosis, leiomyomas and, less commonly, intrauterine device (IUD) use, or congenital or acquired outflow tract obstruction, including cervical stenosis.

Dx DIAGNOSIS

DIFFERENTIAL DIAGNOSIS: SECONDARY DYSMENORRHEA

- Adenomyosis
- Adhesions
- Cervical structures or stenosis
- Congenital malformation of müllerian system
- Ectopic pregnancy
- Endometriosis
- Imperforate hymen
- IUD use
- Leiomyomas
- Ovarian cysts
- Pelvic congestion syndrome
- Pelvic inflammatory disease
- Polyps
- Transverse vaginal septum

WORKUP AND EVALUATION

- Primary dysmenorrhea: Characteristic history, physical examination and ultrasound normal with the absence of an identifiable cause of pelvic pain
- Secondary dysmenorrhea: Physical examination and ultrasound may reveal vaginal/uterine abnormalities, fibroids, adenomyosis, polyps, endometriomas

LABORATORY TESTS

- No specific tests diagnostic for dysmenorrhea
- Elevated white blood cell count in the presence of infection
- Human chorionic gonadotropin to rule out ectopic pregnancy

IMAGING STUDIES

- Ultrasound scan of the pelvis to evaluate the presence of leiomyomas, adenomyosis, ovarian cysts
- Saline ultrasonography to assess the uterine cavity to rule out endometrial polyps or submucosal or intraluminal leiomyomas

Rx TREATMENT

NONPHARMACOLOGIC THERAPY

- Applying heat to the lower abdomen with hot compresses, heating pads, or hot water bottles seems to offer some relief.
- Offer reassurance that this is a treatable condition.

ACUTE GENERAL Rx

- Nonsteroidal antiinflammatory drugs such as ibuprofen 400 to 600 mg q4 to 6h or naproxen sodium 500 mg q12h
- Oral contraceptives cyclically or continuously (taking only active pills), primarily in women with primary dysmenorrhea
- The levonorgestrel-containing IUD is increasingly being used to ameliorate symptoms of dysmenorrhea. Pain improvement has been shown in many cases to be even better than oral contraceptive pills
- Magnesium supplements (research ongoing)
- Thiamine supplements (research ongoing)
- Fish oil supplements (research ongoing)
- Secondary dysmenorrhea: Treatment directed to the specific underlying condition

CHRONIC Rx

Acupuncture and transcutaneous electrical nerve stimulation may be tried. However, there is not enough evidence to support the use of yoga, acupuncture, or massage. In cases in which medical therapy has not worked, laparoscopy or other surgical treatments should be considered depending on the secondary cause of the dysmenorrhea. A directed physical examination looking for gynecologic masses or nodularity should be performed. Nontraditional approaches such as acupuncture have been tried with relief in some patients. The levonorgestrel IUD has been shown to effectively reduce pain in women with primary dysmenorrhea.

DISPOSITION

The majority of patients are satisfactorily treated with good outcomes. Possible chronic complications with primary dysmenorrhea that has not been adequately treated can lead to anxiety and depression. With certain causes of secondary dysmenorrhea, infertility can become a problem.

REFERRAL

If a secondary cause of dysmenorrhea is revealed, refer to the appropriate specialist for further medical or surgical treatment (e.g., gynecologist, urogynecologist, reproductive endocrinologist, pain management center).

RELATED CONTENT

Dysmenorrhea (Patient Information)
Dyspareunia (Related Key Topic)
Endometriosis (Related Key Topic)
Premenstrual Dysphoric Disorder (Related Key Topic)
Premenstrual Syndrome (Related Key Topic)

AUTHOR: **BARBARA MCGUIRK, M.D.**

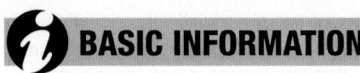

BASIC INFORMATION

DEFINITION

Dyspepsia is a constellation of symptoms referable to the gastroduodenal region of the upper GI tract. *Nonulcerative dyspepsia* is a term used to describe signs and symptoms of persistent or recurrent dyspepsia that have no identifiable organic cause.

SYNONYMS

Nonulcer dyspepsia
Functional dyspepsia
Idiopathic dyspepsia

ICD-10CM CODE
K30 Functional dyspepsia

EPIDEMIOLOGY & DEMOGRAPHICS

Up to 25% of the general population will experience dyspepsia each yr. Of these, 75% will have no evident causative agent.

PHYSICAL FINDINGS & CLINICAL PRESENTATION

Typical clinical presentation is dyspepsia without findings on physical examination to explain the symptoms.

ETIOLOGY

The etiology and pathophysiology are still unclear. Box 1 summarizes causes of dyspepsia. Research is focused on abnormalities of gastric motor function and visceral hypersensitivity, as well as:

- *Helicobacter pylori* infection
- Psychosocial factors—associated with anxiety and depression

RISK FACTORS

Risk factors include the following:

- Genetic predisposition: Homozygous *GNB3* gene
- Dietary habits such as caffeine, alcohol, or smoking
- Medications such as NSAIDs, calcium channel blockers, methylxanthines, alendronate, orlistat, acarbose, and potassium supplements
- Psychological disorders such as anxiety, depression, somatization, or personal history of childhood sexual or physical abuse

Dx DIAGNOSIS

DIFFERENTIAL DIAGNOSIS

Nonulcerative dyspepsia is diagnosed when all other organic causes have been excluded, including:

- Peptic ulcer disease (PUD)
- Gastroesophageal reflux
- Gastric/esophageal/other abdominal cancers
- Biliary tract disease
- Gastroparesis, including diabetic gastroparesis
- Pancreatitis
- Medications (i.e., NSAIDs, erythromycin)
- Metabolic disturbances (i.e., hypercalcemia, heavy metals, or hyperkalemia)
- Ischemic bowel disease
- Systemic disorders (i.e., eosinophilic gastritis, Crohn's disease, sarcoidosis, celiac disease, thyroid disorders)

DIAGNOSIS

The Rome IV criteria lists the following factors, which must be present at least 3 months and first noticed within 6 months of diagnosis:

- At least one of the following:
  1. Postprandial fullness, *or*
  2. Early satiety, *or*
  3. Epigastric pain, *or*
  4. Epigastric burning
  5. *And* no evidence of structural disease likely to explain the symptoms

WORKUP

The American Gastroenterological Association, as well as the Maastricht III and the IV European consensus, suggest the following:

- The pattern of symptoms overlaps considerably for all types of dyspepsia; therefore, the history and physical should focus on finding specific symptoms that help exclude other causes of dyspepsia.
- Endoscopy should be performed only in patients >55 yr old and in younger patients with alarming symptoms (e.g., weight loss, progressive dysphagia, recurrent vomiting, evidence of gastrointestinal bleeding, or family history of cancer) presenting with new-onset dyspepsia. Findings consistent with diagnosis of nonulcerative dyspepsia are not conclusive, no presence of *H. pylori*, no signs of gastroesophageal reflux disease, no mucosal inflammation. NOTE: Patients <55 yr old and without any alarming symptoms can be treated without endoscopy.

LABORATORY TESTS

H. pylori: Laboratory methods include serologic tests,[1] monoclonal stool antigen, or urea breath test.

[1] Serologic testing for *H. pylori* has a low predictive value because colonization is lifelong; it can therefore determine prevalence better than incidence.

BOX 1 Causes of Dyspepsia

Luminal GI Tract
Functional dyspepsia
Chronic gastric volvulus
Chronic gastric or intestinal (mesenteric) ischemia
Food intolerance
Gastric or esophageal neoplasm
Gastric infections (cytomegalovirus, fungus, tuberculosis, syphilis)
Gastroparesis (diabetes mellitus, postvagotomy, scleroderma, chronic intestinal pseudo-obstruction, postviral, idiopathic)
GERD
Infiltrative gastric disorders (Ménétrier disease, Crohn disease, eosinophilic gastroenteritis, sarcoidosis, amyloidosis)
IBS
Parasites (*Giardia lamblia, Strongyloides stercoralis*)
PUD

Systemic Conditions
Adrenal insufficiency
Diabetes mellitus
Heart failure, myocardial ischemia
Intraabdominal malignancy
Pregnancy
Renal insufficiency
Thyroid disease, hyperparathyroidism

Medications
Acarbose
Aspirin and other NSAIDs (including COX-2 selective agents)
Colchicine
Digitalis preparations
Estrogens
Ethanol
Gemfibrozil
Glucocorticoids
Iron
Levodopa
Narcotics
Niacin
Nitrates
Orlistat
Potassium chloride
Quinidine
Sildenafil
Theophylline

Pancreaticobiliary Disorders
Biliary pain: cholelithiasis, choledocholithiasis, sphincter of Oddi dysfunction
Chronic pancreatitis
Pancreatic neoplasms

COX-2, Cyclooxygenase-2; *GERD*, gastroesophageal reflux disease; *IBS*, irritable bowel syndrome; *NSAID*, nonsteroidal antiinflammatory drug; *PUD*, peptic ulcer disease.
From Feldman M et al (eds): *Sleisenger and Fordtran's gastrointestinal and liver disease*, ed 10, Philadelphia, 2016, Elsevier.

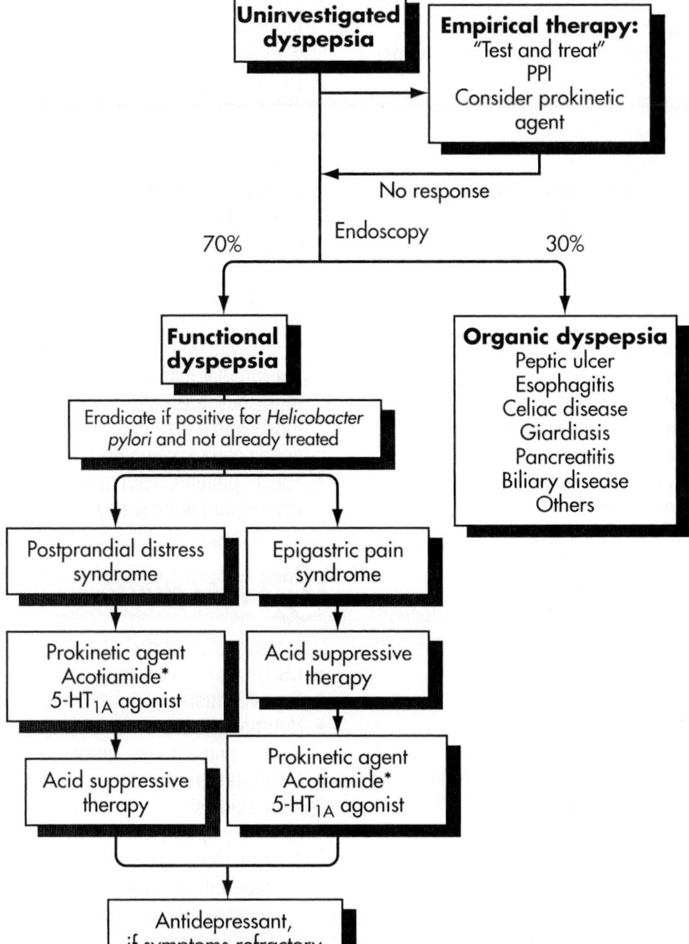

FIG. 1 An algorithm for management of patients with dyspepsia. Patients younger than age 45 to 55 years who do not have alarm features may be treated empirically, whereas all others should be evaluated initially by endoscopy. *5-HT,* 5-hydroxytryptamine; *PPI,* proton pump inhibitor. *Not available in the U.S. (From Feldman M et al [eds]: *Sleisenger and Fordtran's gastrointestinal and liver disease,* ed 10, Philadelphia, 2016, Elsevier.)

Rx TREATMENT

ACUTE GENERAL Rx

PHARMACOLOGIC THERAPY: Primary treatment is usually initiated with proton pump inhibitors (PPIs), which can be started without performing endoscopy, especially if the patient comes from a population with low prevalence of *H. pylori* infection. If symptoms persist, a trial of antidepressants can be started. An algorithm for the management of patients with dyspepsia is described in Fig. 1.

Treatment of accompanying symptoms includes:

Predominant Symptom	Possible Etiology	Medication Recommended
Nausea	Motility dysfunction	Prokinetic agent
Bloating	Motility dysfunction	Simethicone and/or prokinetic agent
Pain	Mucosal disease or *H. pylori* infection	Antibiotic trial
Somatic complaints	Psychosocial	Psychotropic medication trial

Medication categories:

- Antacids (i.e., aluminum hydroxide, calcium carbonate)
- Gas-reducing agents, such as those containing simethicone
- H_2-receptor antagonists (i.e., cimetidine)
- PPIs (i.e., omeprazole)
- Prokinetic agents (i.e., metoclopramide, domperidone)
- Antidepressants (i.e., selective serotonin receptor inhibitors, tricyclics)
- *H. pylori* therapy/antibiotic therapy (various antibiotic regimens, usually 1 PPI) if *H. pylori* present

CHRONIC Rx

Controversy currently exists around the long-term use of PPIs. Due to the high association with psychological factors, patients with functional dyspepsia should undergo psychological intervention, even if there is good response to pharmacotherapeutic approaches.

COMPLEMENTARY & ALTERNATIVE THERAPIES

Peppermint and caraway oil may be helpful, as well as acupuncture; however, no definitive trials have been performed.

REFERRAL

- Referral to gastroenterology if patient has alarming symptoms (such as GI bleeding, dysphagia, odynophagia, unexplained anemia, change in appetite, and weight loss) or when endoscopy is indicated—although controversy exists about the workup of younger patients.
- Referral to cardiology if cardiac etiology suspected.

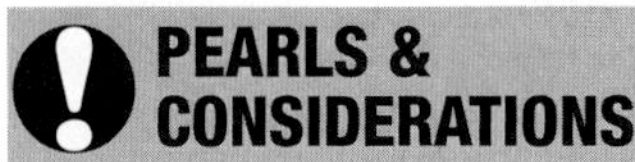

PEARLS & CONSIDERATIONS

PREVENTION

Avoid excessive amounts of caffeine, alcohol, smoking, or long-term use of steroids and NSAIDs.

PATIENT AND FAMILY EDUCATION

http://www.mayoclinic.com/health/stomach-pain/DS00524

SUGGESTED READINGS

Available at ExpertConsult.com

RELATED CONTENT

Approach to the patient with dyspepsia (Algorithm, Section III)

AUTHORS: **ALVARO M. RIVERA, M.D.,** and **NADINE MBUYI, M.D.**

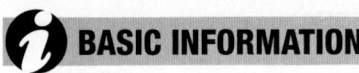

DEFINITION

The term "dysphagia" is derived from the Greek words *dys* (with difficulty) and *phagia* (to eat). It is characterized by abnormal transfer of food from mouth to the stomach, which may involve the oral, pharyngeal, or esophageal stages of swallowing.

ICD-10CM CODES

R13.10	Dysphagia, unspecified
D50.1	Sideropenic dysphagia
I69.091	Dysphagia following nontraumatic subarachnoid hemorrhage
I69.191	Dysphagia following nontraumatic intracerebral hemorrhage
I69.291	Dysphagia following other nontraumatic intracranial hemorrhage
I69.391	Dysphagia following cerebral infarction
I69.891	Dysphagia following other cerebrovascular disease
I69.991	Dysphagia following unspecified cerebrovascular disease
R13.11	Dysphagia, oral phase
R13.12	Dysphagia, oropharyngeal phase
R13.13	Dysphagia, pharyngeal phase
R13.14	Dysphagia, pharyngoesophageal phase
R13.19	Other dysphagia

EPIDEMIOLOGY & DEMOGRAPHICS

- This is seen in 10% of individuals above the age of 50 yr. Its prevalence increases with advancing age.
- Nearly 12% of hospitalized patients have symptoms of dysphagia.
- Up to 30% to 60% of nursing home patients have some form of dysphagia.
- Special populations, including patients with head injury, stroke, or Parkinson's disease, have 30% to 50% prevalence of oropharyngeal dysphagia.

ETIOLOGY

- Oropharyngeal:
  1. Neuromuscular causes:
     a. Stroke
     b. Parkinson's disease
     c. Multiple sclerosis
     d. Myasthenia gravis
     e. Amyotrophic lateral sclerosis
     f. CNS tumors
     g. Muscular dystrophy
     h. Thyroid dysfunction
     i. Polymyositis and dermatomyositis
     j. Sarcoidosis
     k. Cerebral palsy
     l. Head trauma
     m. Metabolic encephalopathy
     n. Dementia
     o. Bell palsy
  2. Structural causes:
     a. Oropharyngeal tumors
     b. Zenker diverticulum
     c. Infection of pharynx or neck (mucositis from *Candida,* herpes, and CMV)
     d. Thyromegaly
     e. Prior surgery or radiotherapy
     f. Osteophytes and other spinal disorders
     g. Proximal esophageal webs
     h. Congenital anomalies (e.g., cleft palate)
     i. Poor dentition
- Esophageal:
  1. Neuromuscular disorders:
     a. Achalasia
     b. Diffuse esophageal spasm
     c. Nutcracker esophagus
     d. Hypertensive lower esophageal sphincter
     e. Ineffective esophageal motility
     f. Scleroderma
     g. Reflex-associated dysmotility
  2. Structural disorder:
     a. Peptic stricture
     b. Esophageal rings and webs
     c. Diverticuli
     d. Carcinoma and benign tumors
     e. Foreign bodies
     f. Vascular compression
     g. Mediastinal masses
     h. Spinal osteophytes
     i. Mucosal injury (from pills, infection, gastroesophageal reflux disease [GERD], etc.)

PATHOGENESIS

The inability to swallow is caused either by a problem in strength or coordination of the muscles required to move material from the mouth to stomach or by a fixed obstruction somewhere between the mouth and the stomach.

CLINICAL FEATURES

Oropharyngeal dysphagia (transfer dysphagia):
- The patient is unable to transfer the food bolus from the mouth to the upper esophagus. Problem arises within 2 seconds of initiating the voluntary phase of swallowing.
- Typical symptoms include drooling, spillage of food, postnasal regurgitation, difficulty in initiation of swallowing, sialorrhea, sensation of food stuck in the neck, coughing or choking during swallowing, the need to swallow repeatedly to clear food or fluid from the pharynx, dysphonia, nasal speech, hoarseness of voice, and dysarthria.
- A thorough physical examination including that of the nervous system, oral cavity, and the head/neck is very important in patients with oropharyngeal dysphagia.

Esophageal dysphagia:
- Problem usually arises several seconds after swallowing.
- Patients often complain of food being stuck in lower substernal area.
- Dysphagia to solids suggests mechanical obstruction whereas dysphagia with liquids or combination of solids and liquids favors a motility disorder.
- Neuromuscular causes result in dysphagia to both solids and liquids. Particularly, patients with achalasia tend to drink a lot of fluids while eating or apply maneuvers such as straightening the back, raising their arms over their heads, or standing to increase intraesophageal pressure to facilitate the emptying of food into the stomach.
- Oftentimes, ingestion of very cold or very hot foods precipitates the dysphagia associated with neuromuscular disorder.
- Delayed regurgitation of food, heartburn, and chest pain are usually present.
- Weight loss is usually associated with malignancy or achalasia.
- Symptoms are intermittent in patients with esophageal dysphagia from benign causes of structural obstruction or diffuse esophageal spasm. However, it is progressive in patients with peptic stricture, esophageal carcinoma, scleroderma, and achalasia.
- In patients with structural obstruction, when the luminal diameter is more than 18 to 20 mm, they are rarely symptomatic, whereas those with a diameter of less than 13 mm are nearly always symptomatic.
- These patients with esophageal dysphagia usually do not have any characteristic physical findings.

Dx DIAGNOSIS

Laboratory evaluation:
- CBC
- Thyroid studies
- Nutritional assessment by checking serum protein and albumin levels
- Other studies based on specific clinical conditions

Special studies:
- Oropharyngeal dysphagia
  1. Videofluoroscopy is the first test often ordered in evaluation of patients with oropharyngeal dysphagia.
  2. Double contrast modified barium swallow study (Fig. E1).
  3. Fiberoptic flexible nasopharyngeal laryngoscopy is mandatory in all cases when a structural lesion, particularly malignancy, is suspected.
  4. Pharyngeal and upper esophageal manometry (Fig. E2) is occasionally of value to predict which patients will have a favorable outcome from cricopharyngeal myotomy or dilation.
  5. Radiography of head and neck when indicated.
- Esophageal dysphagia
  1. Barium esophagography should precede upper endoscopies to identify patients at risk from potential perforation with an endoscopy and to help plan fluoroscopically guided dilation. It is often the first step in evaluating patients with dysphagia, especially if an obstructive lesion is suspected.
  2. EGD.
  3. Esophageal manometry is indicated if no abnormality is identified by barium study or EGD.
  4. Esophageal pH monitoring in patients with suspected reflux disease.
  5. Endoscopic ultrasonography.
  6. Radiograph, CT, and MRI of chest.

DIFFERENTIAL DIAGNOSIS (FIG. 3)

- Globus pharyngeus
- Odynophagia
- Phagophobia
- GERD

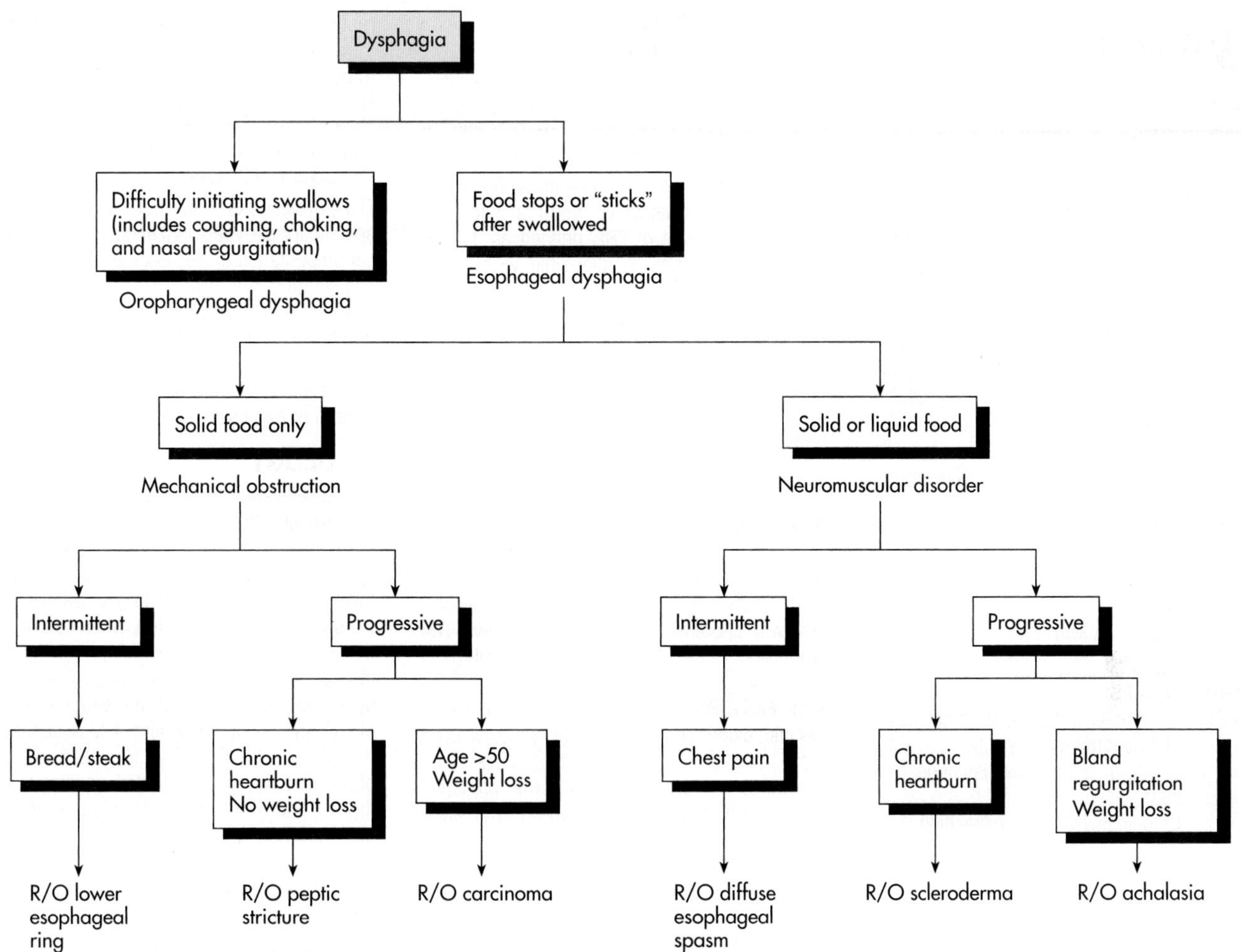

FIG. 3 Differential diagnosis of dysphagia. *RO,* Rule out. (Modified from Andreoli TE [ed]: *Cecil essentials of medicine,* ed 7, Philadelphia, 2008, Saunders.)

Rx TREATMENT

- Treatment should be approached with the help of specialists of multiple disciplines (ENT, head and neck surgeon, radiologist, speech pathologist, physical therapist, dietitian, gastroenterologist, physical medicine and rehabilitation specialist, dentist, neurologist, etc.).
- Goal of therapy is airway protection and maintenance of nutrition.
- Alteration of food consistency, volume, and delivery rate plays a major role.
- The goal of direct therapy is to change swallowing physiology with medical treatment of primary disease, maxillofacial prosthesis, and cricopharyngeal myotomy.
- Indirect therapies include exercise programs for tongue coordination and chewing under the guidance of a speech therapist.
- Maintenance of oral feeding often requires compensatory techniques such as chin-tuck position, rotation of head to the affected side, tilting of head to the strong side, and lying on one's back or on one's side during swallowing.
- Some of the voluntary maneuvers applied include supraglottic swallow, effortful swallow, Mendelson maneuver, Shaker exercise, and the Heimlich maneuver.
- Placement of nasogastric tube, jejunostomy tube, or percutaneous endoscopic gastrotomy (PEG) tube is considered for enteral feeding when other measures fail and the patient remains at significant risk for aspiration or nutrition becomes compromised.
- Treatment of associated GERD should not be forgotten.
- Surgery for chronic aspiration may involve tracheostomy, medialization, laryngeal suspension, laryngeal closure, and/or laryngotracheal separation-diversion.
- Other measures include esophageal dilation removal of foreign body, esophageal resection, chemotherapy, radiotherapy, endoscopic ablation of tumor, photodynamic therapy, esophageal prosthesis/stents, diverticulectomy, intrasphincteric injection of botulinum toxin, surgical myotomy, and others. Smooth muscle relaxants such as nitrates and calcium channel blockers have been used to effectively treat patients with diffuse esophageal spasm and nutcracker esophagus.
- Several scales have been suggested to determine patients' functional outcome. One of them is the "Swallowing Rating Scale."

COMPLICATIONS

- Dehydration
- Malnutrition
- Aspiration pneumonia
- Airway obstruction
- Death resulting from pulmonary complications

PROGNOSIS

- Depends on the etiology.
- Nursing home patients with oropharyngeal dysphagia and a history of aspiration have an approximately 45% mortality rate over 1 yr.
- All patients, especially the elderly, should take their medications with a full glass of water while in upright position well before bedtime.
- Dysphagia should be considered an alarm symptom, indicating the need for immediate evaluation.

PATIENT EDUCATION

Elderly patients with dysphagia should not attribute their symptoms to aging.

SUGGESTED READING

Available at ExpertConsult.com

RELATED CONTENT

Achalasia (Related Key Topic)
Dyspepsia, Nonulcerative (Related Key Topic)
Esophageal Tumors (Related Key Topic)
Gastroesophageal Reflux Disease (Related Key Topic)

AUTHOR: **FRED F. FERRI, M.D.**

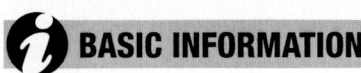

DEFINITION

An early repolarization pattern (ERP) in a QRS complex with a duration <120 ms, a peak J point elevation of ≥0.1 mV in two or more contiguous leads **excluding** leads V_1-V_3, with a notch or slur noted in the end of the QRS complex at the downslope of a prominent R wave (Fig. 1). This notch must be above the baseline T-P segment (Fig. 2). Previously thought to be benign, the pattern has been noted in higher prevalence in patients with idiopathic ventricular fibrillation (VF). Recently it has been cited as a predictor of symptom status in the setting of long QT syndrome, as well as a predictor of arrhythmic events in patients with structural heart disease.

SYNONYMS

Early repolarization syndrome—sudden cardiac arrest in a patient with ERP
J point elevation
Persistent juvenile pattern

ICD-10CM CODES	
R94.310	Abnormalities ECG—Abnormalities of ST segment
R00.9	Unspecified abnormalities of heart beat
I49.9	Cardiac arrhythmia unspecified

EPIDEMIOLOGY & DEMOGRAPHICS

INCIDENCE: The clinical entity "early repolarization pattern" is commonly asymptomatic; therefore, the true incidence of the pattern is difficult to definitively establish. In one comparison of patients with idiopathic ventricular fibrillation (VF) vs. young athletes vs. age-matched controls, the presence of ERP, defined as J point elevation >1.0 mm, in idiopathic VF patients was 31.1% in any lead, 17.8% in inferior leads, 11.1% in leads I and aVL, and 6.7% in leads V_4 to V_6. For comparison, the incidence in age-matched controls was 8.9% in any lead, 6.5% in inferior leads, 0% in leads I and aVL, and 4.9% in leads V_4 to V_6.

PREDOMINANT SEX: J point elevation >1 mm was documented significantly higher in males vs. females.

GENETICS: The mode of transmission and the genetic basis of the syndrome are unclear. An autosomal dominant pattern of inheritance of the *KCNJ8* gene, which has been associated with sporadic cases, has been shown. The prognostic value of the inheritance pattern is not known.

RISK FACTORS: Male sex, younger age, lower systolic blood pressure, higher Sokolow-Lyon index, and lower Cornell voltage have been shown to be associated with the presence of the early repolarization pattern. The early repolarization pattern carries an increased risk for future arrhythmic death. This is considered to be higher in the setting of a downsloping ST segment.

PHYSICAL FINDINGS & CLINICAL PRESENTATION

The physical exam will not show any findings specific for early repolarization. Rather, the clinical presentation is well documented in patients resuscitated from cardiac arrest. This is particularly shown in a pattern in which the early repolarization is seen in the inferior and/or the lateral leads but not in the precordial leads. The pattern has been shown to have an intermittent pattern of expression.

ETIOLOGY

J point elevation is considered to be the electrocardiographic representation of a voltage gradient between different layers from the epicardium to the endocardium. The epicardium has a relatively higher density of transient outward potassium current (I_{TO}), when compared to the endocardium, resulting in a prominent notch in phase I of the action potential. The Brugada syndrome is considered an extreme version of this phenomenon, where a loss of function mutation in the *SCN5A* gene results in loss of phase II in the action potential, causing marked J point and ST segment elevation, allowing for polymorphic ventricular tachycardia.

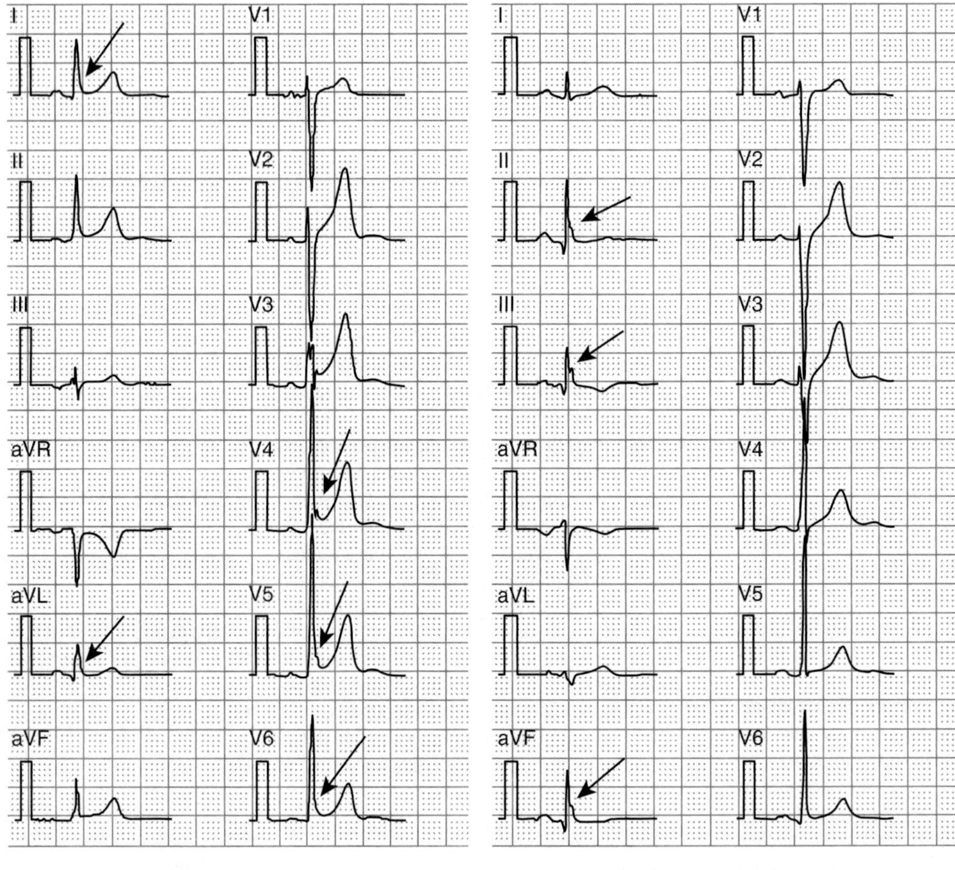

FIG. 1 A, Notching in lead V_4 progressing to slurring in V_6, I, aVL. **B,** Notching in lead III, aVF and slurring in lead II. (From Macfarlane PW et al: The early repolarization pattern: a consensus pattern, *J Am Coll Cardiol* 66:470-477, 2015.)

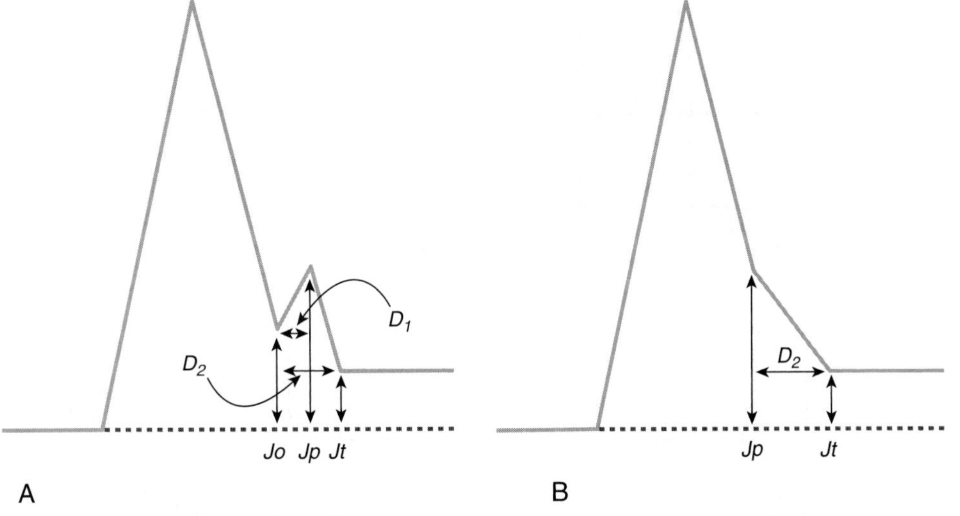

FIG. 2 A, Illustration of the amplitudes J onset (Jo), J peak (Jp), and J termination (Jt) as well as durations D1 and D2 in relation to an end QRS notch, as defined previously. **B,** Illustration of Jp and Jt as well as D2 in relation to an end QRS slur. (From Macfarlane PW et al: The early repolarization pattern: a consensus pattern, *J Am Coll Cardiol* 66:470-477, 2015.)

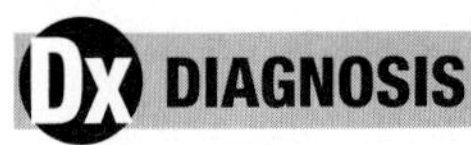

DIAGNOSIS

DIFFERENTIAL DIAGNOSIS

- Benign vs. malignant early repolarization
- Brugada syndrome
- Persistent juvenile pattern

WORKUP

- Primarily guided by the clinical scenario. In a patient where the early repolarization pattern is an incidental finding (Figs. 3 and 4), detailed family history for sudden cardiac death is indicated.
- However, should the pattern be identified in the setting of a cardiac arrest, then the workup would be directed to identification of potentially reversible causes.
  1. Basic metabolic panel
  2. Echocardiogram
  3. Ischemic evaluation—noninvasive stress testing vs. left heart catheterization
  4. Electrophysiology testing
  5. ICD implant for secondary prevention of sudden cardiac death if no reversible cause is identified

LABORATORY TEST

- BMP
- Thyroid function studies

IMAGING STUDIES

Echocardiogram

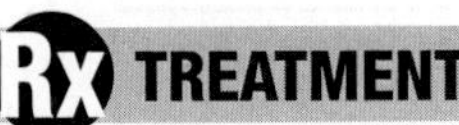

TREATMENT

No treatment is indicated in the case of the early repolarization pattern. In the setting of early repolarization syndrome with sudden cardiac death, the treatment would be that of sudden cardiac death as detailed under "Workup."

REFERRALS

Cardiology referral should be obtained, particularly in the setting of syncope, nonsustained ventricular tachycardia, or cardiac arrest.

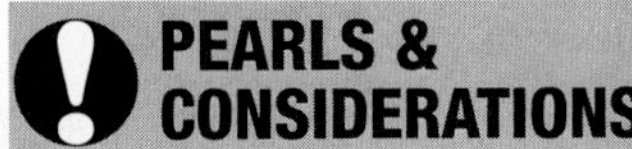

PEARLS & CONSIDERATIONS

COMMENTS

The early repolarization pattern has previously been considered a benign pattern; however, the body of evidence suggests it to be a risk factor for sudden cardiac death. Therefore, all patients with early repolarization, particularly with risk factors or an isolated pattern in the inferior leads, merit a detailed evaluation.

PREVENTION

None

SUGGESTED READINGS

Available at ExpertConsult.com

RELATED CONTENT

Brugada Syndrome (Related Key Topic)
Long QT Syndrome (Related Key Topic)
Ventricular Fibrillation (Related Key Topic)
Ventricular Tachycardia (Related Key Topic)

AUTHOR: **ALEEM I. MUGHAL, M.D.**

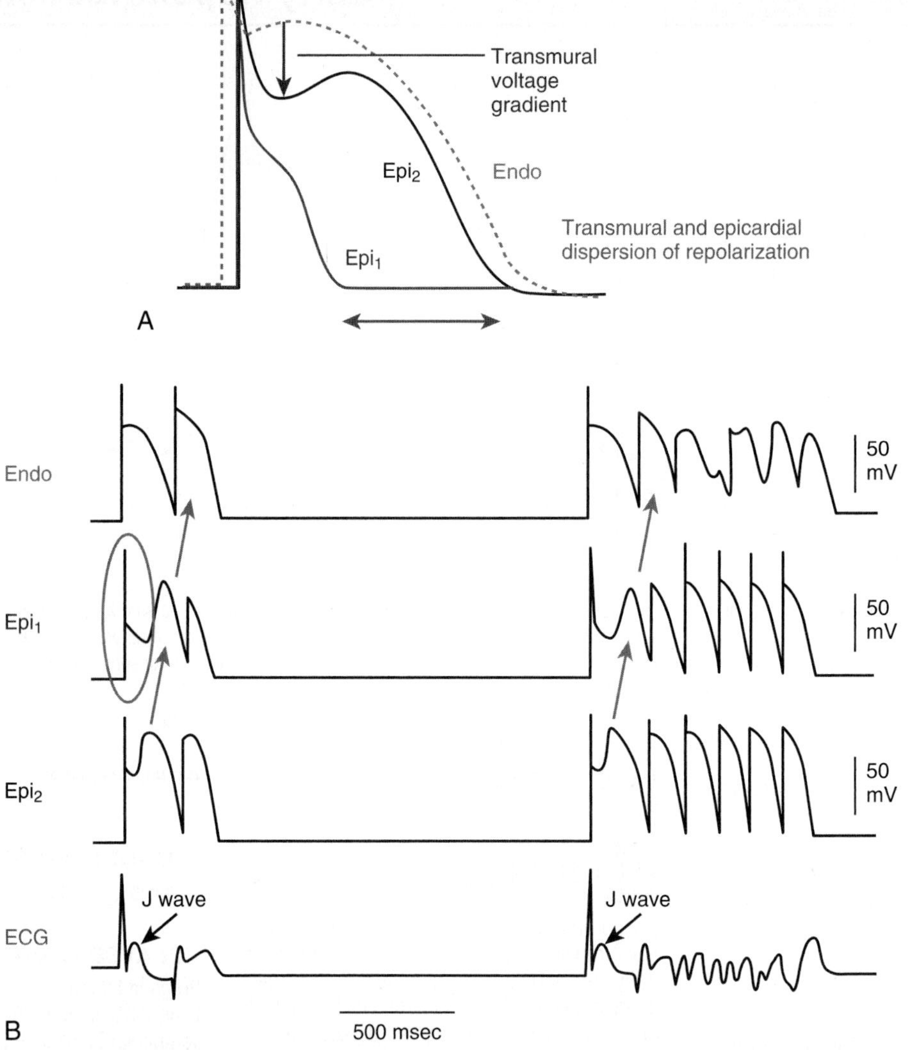

FIG. 3 Potential mechanism for arrhythmogenesis in the Brugada and early repolarization syndromes. A, With enhanced repolarization in regions with prominent transient outward current (I_{to}), all-or-none repolarization can occur, creating a substrate for arrhythmias. **B,** Simultaneous action potentials from two epicardial sites (Epi_1 and Epi_2) and one endocardial site (Endo), and surface ECG. A loss of the action potential dome in Epi_1, but not in Epi_2, leads to apparent propagation of the dome from Epi_2 to Epi_1, inducing reentry. (From Issa ZF, Miller JM: *Clinical arrhythmology and electrophysiology: a companion to Braunwald's heart disease*, ed 2, Philadelphia, 2012, Saunders.)

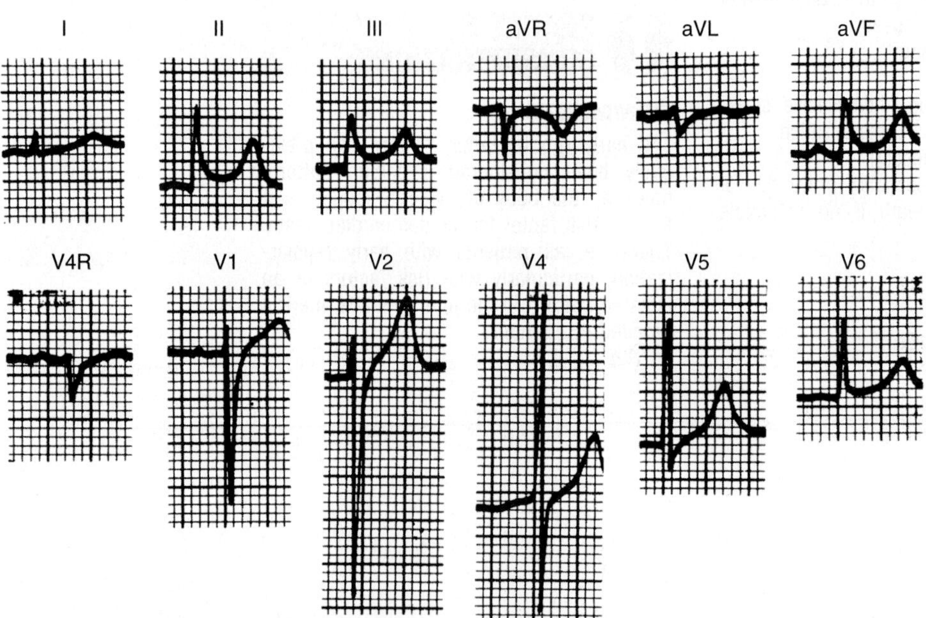

FIG. 4 Tracing from a healthy 16-year-old boy that exhibits early repolarization and J-depression. The ST segment is shifted toward the direction of the T wave and is most marked in II, III, and aVF. J-depression is seen in most of the precordial leads. (From Park MK: *Park's pediatric cardiology for practitioners*, ed 6, Philadelphia, 2014, Saunders.)

BASIC INFORMATION

DEFINITION

Eclampsia is the occurrence of seizures or coma in a woman with signs or symptoms of preeclampsia, occurring at >20 wk of gestation or <48 hr postpartum. Atypical eclampsia occurs at <20 wk of gestation or as much as 23 days postpartum.

SYNONYMS

Toxemia
Seizures of pregnancy

ICD-10CM CODES

015.00	Eclampsia in pregnancy, unspecified trimester
015.02	Eclampsia in pregnancy, second trimester
015.03	Eclampsia in pregnancy, third trimester
015.1	Eclampsia in labor
015.2	Eclampsia in the puerperium
015.9	Eclampsia, unspecified as to time period

EPIDEMIOLOGY & DEMOGRAPHICS

INCIDENCE: One case per 1500 to 3000 pregnancies; 2% to 4% of those with preeclampsia; one large Australian series found 8.6 cases per 10,000 live births.

GENETICS: Increased incidence with a first-degree relative (sister or mother) having had eclampsia.

RISK FACTORS: Multifetal gestation (3.6% in twin gestation), molar pregnancy, nonimmune hydrops fetalis, uncontrolled hypertension, preexisting hypertension, renal disease, systemic lupus, and existing heart disease.

PHYSICAL FINDINGS & CLINICAL PRESENTATION

- Seizure often begins as facial twitching, then spreads to generalized tonic-clonic state, with cessation of respiration followed by a postictal period of amnesia, agitation, and confusion.
- The most common symptoms preceding eclampsia are headache (80%), visual disturbance (45%), and epigastric pain (20%). 17% are completely asymptomatic prior to seizure.
- 40% have severe hypertension, 40% have mild to moderate hypertension, and 20% are normotensive.
- Generalized edema with rapid weight gain (>2 lb/wk) may precede eclampsia.

ETIOLOGY

Common pathway relates to abnormalities in autoregulation of cerebral blood flow. This may involve transient vasospasm, ischemia, cerebral hemorrhage, and edema occurring by a mechanism involving hypertensive encephalopathy, decreased colloid osmotic pressure, and prostaglandin imbalance.

DIAGNOSIS

DIFFERENTIAL DIAGNOSIS

- Preexisting seizure disorder
- Metabolic abnormalities (hypoglycemia, hyponatremia, hypocalcemia)
- Substance abuse
- Head trauma, infection (meningitis, encephalitis)
- Intracerebral bleeding or thrombosis
- Amniotic fluid embolism
- Space-occupying brain lesions or neoplasms
- Pseudoseizure
- Hypertensive encephalopathy
- Venous or arterial thrombosis, arterial embolism
- Posterior reversible encephalopathy syndrome (often seen in eclampsia)
- Vasculitis, angiopathy
- Thrombotic thrombocytopenic purpura

WORKUP

- Rule out other causes of seizures during pregnancy.
- Atypical presentations such as prolonged postictal state; status epilepticus; gestational age <20 wk or >48 hr postpartum; or signs of meningitis, substance abuse, or severe uncontrolled hypertension should prompt a search for other seizure etiologies.

LABORATORY TESTS

- Proteinuria: Severe (49%), mild to moderate (29%), absent (22%).
- HCT: Elevated as a result of hemoconcentration.
- Platelet count: Decreased; LFTs elevated in HELLP syndrome (hemolysis, elevated liver enzymes, and low platelet count).
- BUN and creatinine: Elevated with renal involvement.
- Serum electrolytes, glucose, calcium, toxicology profile: Rule out other causes of seizures.
- ABG: Maternal acidemia and hypoxia.

IMAGING STUDIES

- CT scan or MRI indicated in atypical presentation, suspected intracerebral bleeding, or focal neurologic deficit.
- Over 90% of patients will have findings consistent with posterior reversible encephalopathy syndrome on MRI.
- There are other abnormal findings, including cerebral edema, hemorrhage, and infarction, in 50% of patients.

TREATMENT

ACUTE GENERAL Rx

- Maintain airway, adequate oxygenation, and IV access.
- Fetal resuscitation involving maternal oxygenation, left lateral positioning, and continuous fetal heart rate monitoring is needed.
- Magnesium sulfate is the drug of choice. Give magnesium sulfate 6 g IV load over 20 min, then 2 g/hr maintenance, for treatment and recurrent seizure prophylaxis. Adjust maintenance dose for renal insufficiency. If there is no IV access, may give 10 g IM (5 g to each buttock). If repeated convulsions, may give an additional 2 g IV over 3 to 5 min. Approximately 10% to 15% of patients will have a second seizure after initial loading dose. Clinical signs of progressive Mg^{2+} toxicity, such as loss of reflexes, should also be followed. If magnesium toxicity is suspected, check magnesium level (therapeutic range 4 to 7 mEQ/L). Respiratory and cardiac arrest occur at extremely high magnesium levels. Antidote for toxicity is calcium gluconate 10 ml of 10% solution. Phenytoin has been used as an alternative in patients in whom magnesium sulfate is contraindicated (heart block, myasthenia gravis).
- Give sodium amobarbital 250 mg IV over 3 min for persistent seizures not responsive to magnesium sulfate.
- Treat BP >160 mm Hg systolic or BP >110 mm Hg diastolic with either hydralazine 5-10 mg IV, then 10 mg, then 20 mg every 20 minutes; or labetalol hydrochloride 20, 40, 80 mg IV, escalating the dose every 10 minutes to maximum total dose of 300 mg; or nifedipine 10, 20 mg orally every 20 minutes can be used for acute blood pressure control, if no IV access. If maximum dose of one medication is reached, add an additional medication to reach goal of BP 140-150/90-100 mm Hg.
- Evaluate patient for delivery.

CHRONIC Rx

- The first priority is stabilization of the mother in terms of adequate oxygenation, hemodynamics, and laboratory abnormalities, such as associated coagulopathies.
- Cervical status and gestational age should be assessed. If unfavorable cervix and <30 wk of gestation, consider C-section; otherwise consider induction.
- Give antenatal corticosteroids if 24 to 34-weeks' gestation. Consider antenatal corticosteroids if 34 to 36-6/7 weeks' gestation or 23-0/7 to 24 weeks' gestation.
- Controlled epidural is the anesthesia of choice for labor or C-section.
- Avoid general anesthesia in uncontrolled hypertension to minimize risk of catastrophic cerebral events.
- Continue magnesium sulfate through delivery process and for 24 hr postpartum or for at least 24 hr after the last convulsion.

DISPOSITION

The maternal mortality rate for eclampsia averages 5% to 6%. Morbidity rate is 25%, including placental abruption (10%), disseminated intravascular coagulation, maternal apnea with fetal asphyxia, aspiration pneumonia, pulmonary edema (4%), renal failure, cardiopulmonary arrest, and coma.

There is an increased risk of fetal death, neonatal death, preterm birth, and small-for-gestational-age birth.

In patients with eclampsia, the risk of recurrence of eclampsia in a subsequent pregnancy is about 2% and the risk of preeclampsia is about 25%. The use of low-dose aspirin starting at 12–16 (28) weeks may decrease that risk.

REFERRAL

Because of the potential for serious permanent maternal and fetal sequelae, all cases should be managed by a team approach of obstetrician, maternal and fetal medicine, neonatologist, and intensivist.

SUGGESTED READINGS

Available at ExpertConsult.com

RELATED CONTENT

Eclampsia (Patient Information)
HELLP Syndrome (Related Key Topic)
Preeclampsia (Related Key Topic)

AUTHOR: **PHILIP A. SHLOSSMAN, M.D.**

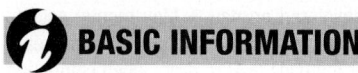

BASIC INFORMATION

DEFINITION

An ectopic pregnancy (EP) occurs when a fertilized ovum implants outside the endometrial cavity.

SYNONYMS

Tubal pregnancy (97%)
Interstitial (cornual) pregnancy (1%-2%)
Ovarian pregnancy (1%-3%)
Abdominal pregnancy (0.03%-1%)
Cervical pregnancy (0.5%)

ICD-10CM CODES

000.0	Abdominal pregnancy
000.1	Tubal ectopic pregnancy
000.2	Ovarian ectopic pregnancy
000.8	Other ectopic pregnancy
000.9	Ectopic pregnancy, unspecified

EPIDEMIOLOGY & DEMOGRAPHICS

- 1.5% to 2% of pregnancies
- 2.7% of maternal deaths

PREVALENCE (IN U.S.): Accounts for up to 18% of women presenting to the emergency room with vaginal bleeding or abdominal pain. Currently over 100,000 reported cases/yr.

RISK FACTORS: Previous EP, previous pelvic infection (pelvic inflammatory disease, tubo-ovarian abscess, salpingitis), previous tubal ligation, previous tuboplasty, intrauterine device use, assisted reproductive techniques, infertility, cigarette use, age >35 yr, multiple lifetime sexual partners, DES exposure in utero

PHYSICAL FINDINGS & CLINICAL PRESENTATION:

- Abdominal tenderness: 95%
- Adnexal tenderness: 87% to 99%
- Peritoneal signs: 71% to 76%
- Amenorrhea or abnormal vaginal bleeding: 75%
- Adnexal mass: 33% to 53%
- Enlarged uterus: 6% to 30%
- Shock: 2% to 17%
- Shoulder pain: 10%
- Tissue passage: 6% to 7%

ETIOLOGY

- Anatomic obstruction to zygote passage
- Abnormalities in tubal motility
- Transperitoneal migration of the zygote

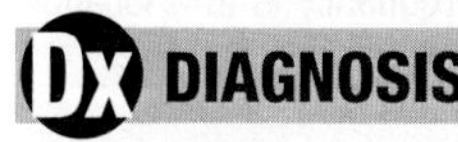

DIAGNOSIS

DIFFERENTIAL DIAGNOSIS

- Corpus luteum cyst
- Rupture or torsion of ovarian cyst
- Threatened or incomplete abortion
- Pelvic inflammatory disease
- Appendicitis
- Gastroenteritis
- Dysfunctional uterine bleeding
- Degenerating uterine fibroids
- Endometriosis

WORKUP

- The classic presentation of EP includes the triad of abnormal vaginal bleeding, pelvic pain, and an adnexal mass. Fig. 1 describes a diagnostic approach to suspected EP. Fig. E2 *(top)* describes potential sites of ectopic implantations. Consider in all women with abdominopelvic pain and a positive pregnancy test.
- Transvaginal ultrasound.
- Quantitative serum human chorionic gonadotropin level.
- Type and screen if presents with vaginal bleeding; give Rhogam if Rh-negative status on initial presentation of vaginal bleeding with positive pregnancy test.
- Laparoscopy in equivocal situations and possibly for treatment.

LABORATORY TESTS

- Quantitative human chorionic gonadotropin (qhCG): Check on initial presentation. qhCG allows one to interpret initial ultrasound. If

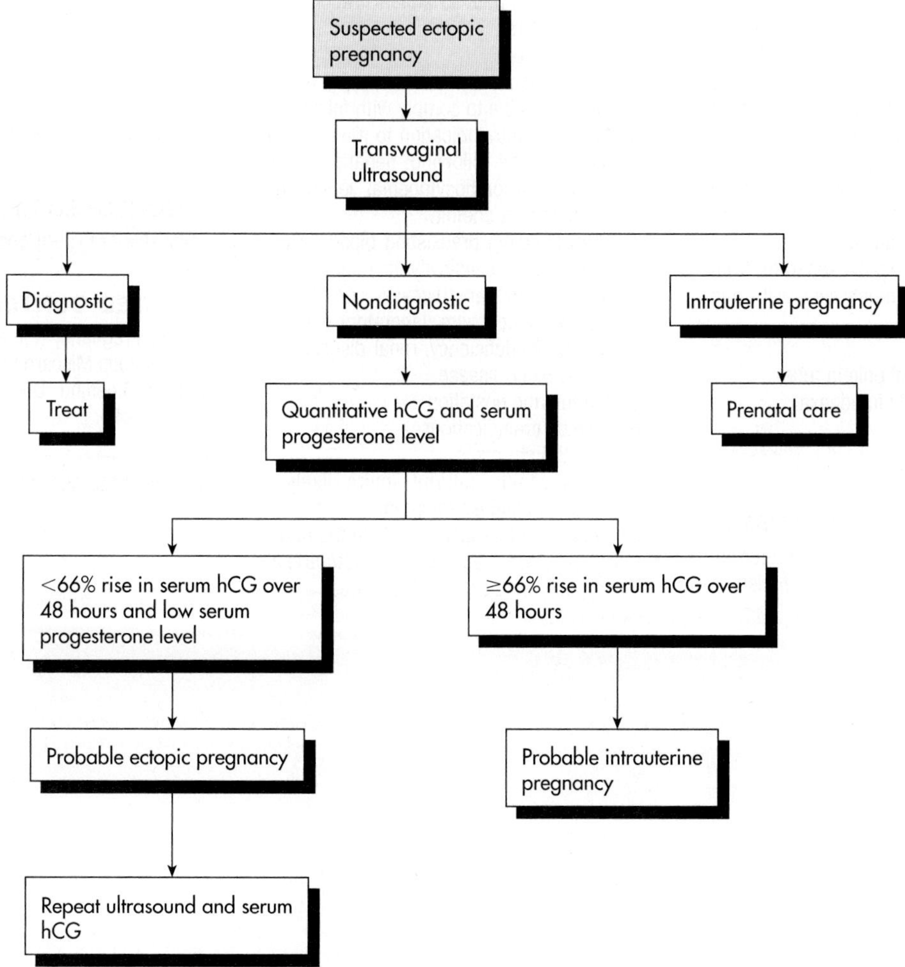

FIG. 1 Ectopic pregnancy. *hCG,* Human chorionic gonadotropin.

qhCG >6000 mIU/ml, should see intrauterine pregnancy (IUP) on abdominal scan; qhCG >1500 mIU/ml for transvaginal scan. The ability to visualize an early pregnancy is dependent on the gestational age and expertise of the ultrasonographer; therefore, some may use up to qhCG >3500 mIU/ml as the discriminatory threshold for transvaginal ultrasonography.

- Approximately 25% to 50% of women with an EP present with a pregnancy of unknown location, meaning that the initial ultrasound does not show a pregnancy in the uterus or the fallopian tube. Therefore, serial measurement of qhCG, typically obtained every 2 days, can help distinguish between an IUP, resolving miscarriage, or EP.
- The expected rate of qhCG increase varies by the initial starting hCG. For an initial hCG level <1500 mIU/ml, the expected rate of increase is 49%, compared to 40% for an initial hCG level between 1500 and 3000 mIU/ml, and a 33% increase for an initial hCG >3000 mIU/ml.
- Dropping hematocrit may be associated with tubal rupture or possible abnormal intrauterine pregnancy.

IMAGING STUDIES

- Ultrasound: Presence of an intrauterine yolk sac makes EP extremely unlikely. However, if the patient used assisted reproductive technologies, a heterotopic pregnancy (an EP with concurrent IUP) is a possibility. A repeat ultrasonographic examination within 7 days after presentation may identify the location of a pregnancy that was not identified on initial ultrasonographic examination.
- Findings on ultrasound in EP include:
  1. Empty uterus (i.e., no yolk sac or fetal pole; a pseudosac in uterus may appear similar to a gestational sac).
  2. Adnexal mass (typically separate from adjacent ovary, commonly seen with "ring of fire" appearance).
  3. Fluid in cul-de-sac.
  4. Yolk sac and/or fetal pole in tube.
  5. Fetal cardiac activity in adnexa.

Rx TREATMENT

NONPHARMACOLOGIC THERAPY

Surgery performed via laparoscopy is preferred; however, laparotomy is appropriate if patient is very unstable or if visualization of the pelvis is poor at the time of laparoscopy.

- Salpingostomy, or resecting EP with conservation of tube, has the potential benefit of higher rates of subsequent IUP; however, recent randomized controlled trials suggest there is no difference in fecundity rate between salpingostomy and salpingectomy. The procedure requires postoperative serial monitoring of qhCG.
- Salpingectomy, or removal of affected fallopian tube, is considered the standard surgical procedure and is preferred in the following circumstances:
  1. Ruptured tube
  2. Future fertility not desired
  3. Recurrent EP in the same tube
  4. Uncontrolled hemorrhage
- Salpingiosis is the direct injection of chemotherapy into the EP by laparoscopy, transvaginal ultrasound, or hysteroscopy. Direct injection of methotrexate, and possibly KCl if there is active cardiac activity, may be performed when the pregnancy is in a location where there is high morbidity, such as the cervix, cesarean section scar, or cornu.

ACUTE GENERAL Rx

- Medical management with methotrexate, a folic acid antagonist, is a safe alternative if the patient is stable. Check the methotrexate safety labs prior to administration (CBC, creatinine, LFTs).
- Contraindications:
  1. Hemodynamically unstable; ruptured EP
  2. Patient unable to comply with follow-up
  3. Medical contraindication to methotrexate including the following: hepatic or renal disease, thrombocytopenia, leukopenia, or significant anemia
  4. Breastfeeding, preexisting blood dyscrasias, known sensitivity to methotrexate, active pulmonary disease, chronic liver disease, alcoholism, laboratory evidence of immunodeficiency, renal disease, and peptic ulcer disease
  5. Intrauterine gestation
- Relative contraindications:
  1. EP >3.5 cm mass
  2. qhCG >5000 mIU/ml (more likely to require multidose regimen)
  3. Presence of cardiac activity in the fetus
- Most common regimen is methotrexate 50 mg/m^2 of body surface area and is administered on day 1. May require second dose or surgical intervention if qhCG increases or plateaus (<15% drop) when comparing values from day 4 and 7.
- Success rate of single-dose protocol approximately 88.1%. Rupture during methotrexate treatment ranges from 7% to 14%.
- Other methotrexate regimens include multidose protocol ± leucovorin rescue.
- Methotrexate side effects include nausea, vomiting, stomatitis, diarrhea, elevated LFTs, abdominal pain, and nephrotoxicity.

CHRONIC Rx

Persistent EP results from residual trophoblastic tissue or secondary implantation after conservative surgery. There is a 5% incidence of persistent EP with conservative treatment.

DISPOSITION

If diagnosed and treated early (before rupture), prognosis is excellent for good recovery. Monitor qhCG weekly until negative. Use reliable contraception until qhCG is negative. With subsequent pregnancies, follow qhCG and perform early ultrasound to confirm IUP. There is a 10% recurrence rate for EP.

REFERRAL

Should obtain gynecologic consultation if EP is suspected.

PEARLS & CONSIDERATIONS

Any patient who presents with vaginal bleeding, abdominal pain, or both with a positive pregnancy test and no prior documented IUP needs to be assessed for ectopic pregnancy.

SUGGESTED READINGS

Available at ExpertConsult.com

RELATED CONTENT

Ectopic Pregnancy (Patient Information)
Spontaneous Miscarriage (Related Key Topic)
Vaginal Bleeding During Pregnancy (Related Key Topic)

AUTHORS: **TERRI Q. HUYNH, M.D,** and **NIMA R. PATEL, M.D., M.S.**

BASIC INFORMATION

DEFINITION

Human monocytic ehrlichiosis (HME) and human granulocytic anaplasmosis (HGA) are tick-borne rickettsial diseases. Ehrlichiosis is the generic name for infections caused by both *Ehrlichia* and *Anaplasma* genera. Table 1 describes the agent, vector, and geographic prevalence of these diseases.

SYNONYMS

Human granulocytic ehrlichiosis (HGE)
Ehrlichiosis
Human monocytic ehrlichiosis (HME)
Human monocytotropic ehrlichiosis
Human granulocytic anaplasmosis (HGA)
Human granulocytotropic ehrlichiosis
Anaplasmosis
Human granulocytropic anaplasmosis
HGE
HGA
HME

ICD-10CM CODES
A77.40 Ehrlichiosis, unspecified
A77.41 Ehrlichiosis chaffeensis [*E. chaffeensis*]
A77.49 Other ehrlichiosis

EPIDEMIOLOGY & DEMOGRAPHICS

INCIDENCE (IN U.S.): Highest overall incidence in Rhode Island (36.5 per 1 million), New York, New Jersey, Connecticut, Wisconsin, Minnesota, and northern California; >3000 cases identified in the United States since 2006.

PREDOMINANT SEX: Males outnumber females by 2 to 1.

PREDOMINANT AGE: Most severe disease 50 to 70 yr

PEAK INCIDENCE: Occurs throughout the year, with peak incidence between May and July and again in September

PHYSICAL FINDINGS & CLINICAL PRESENTATION

- Symptoms of ehrlichiosis typically appear after a median of 9 days (range 5-14 days)
- Most common initial symptoms
  1. Fever (96%)
  2. Chills, rigor
  3. Headache (72%)
  4. Myalgia
- Subsequent symptoms
  1. Anorexia, nausea
  2. Arthralgia
  3. Cough
  4. Confusion (meningoencephalitis in 20% of patients with HME)
  5. Abdominal pain
  6. Rash (erythematous to pustular) <30% in HME, uncommon in HGA
- Complications
  1. Hepatitis
  2. Interstitial pneumonitis; acute respiratory distress syndrome
  3. Renal and respiratory failure
  4. Demyelinating polyneuropathy
  5. Toxic shock–like syndrome
  6. Life-threatening opportunistic infections

ETIOLOGY

- The causative agents are *Ehrlichia chaffeensis* for human monocytic ehrlichiosis (HME) and *Anaplasma phagocytophilum* for human granulocytic anaplasmosis (HGA) and *Ehrlichia ewingii* for human granulocytic ehrlichiosis (HGE)
- Vector
  1. Almost certainly tick-borne, recently confirmed to be rarely transmitted by infected blood (including nosocomial infection). Perinatal and transplant transmission have been documented.
  2. Transmitted by *Ixodes scapularis* in the northeastern states and *Amblyomma americanum* in the south central, southeastern, and mid-Atlantic states. Fig. 1 illustrates the life cycles of human monocytic ehrlichiosis (HME, with *Ehrlichia chaffeensis*) and human granulocytic ehrlichiosis (anaplasmosis).
  3. Tick exposure reported in >90% of patients, with ~60% reporting tick bite.
- Mammalian host: Deer, horses, dogs, white-footed mice, cattle, sheep, goats, bison
- Host inflammatory and immune responses define final spectrum of disease beyond granulocytes, including hepatitis, interstitial pneumonitis, and nephritis with mild azotemia
- Between 6% and 21% of patients with HGE also have serologic evidence of other *Ixodes* spp. tick-borne diseases: Lyme disease or babesiosis
- Recovery is usual outcome; fatality rate of HGE is about 1%
- ICU care required: 7%

DIAGNOSIS

DIFFERENTIAL DIAGNOSIS

- Rocky Mountain spotted fever, Colorado tick fever, Q fever, relapsing fever
- Babesiosis
- Leptospirosis
- Lyme disease
- Tularemia
- Typhoid fever, paratyphoid fever
- Brucellosis
- Viral hepatitis
- Meningococcemia
- Infectious mononucleosis
- Hematologic malignancy
- TTP (thrombotic thrombocytopenic purpura)
- Table 2 describes clinical clues suggesting a diagnosis of a tick-borne illness manifesting as a nonspecific febrile illness

WORKUP

- Acute blood samples for Giemsa-stained smears
- CBC (leukopenia, thrombocytopenia), liver function (elevated), BUN/creatinine
- Acute serum samples for serology. Antibodies are seldom detected at time of acute infection (they usually appear 2-4 weeks following clinical illness).
- Chest radiograph examination
- Bone marrow rarely needed

LABORATORY TESTS

- Polymerase chain reaction (PCR) to facilitate early diagnosis: Detection of *Ehrlichia/Anaplasma* DNA in blood or CSF by PCR (Table E3)
- Giemsa-stained smear demonstrating morulae of the organism within granulocytes or monocytes (sensitivity 20% to 75%) (Fig. E2)
- CBC: Progressive leukopenia and thrombocytopenia with nadir near day 7
- C-reactive protein concentration is generally elevated
- Liver function tests (LFTs): Increase in hepatic transaminases, lactate dehydrogenase, and alkaline phosphatase
- Elevated plasma creatinine concentration may be seen
- Serologic titer (IFA) >80 or fourfold increase in titer to antigen

IMAGING STUDIES

- Chest radiograph examination to show interstitial pneumonitis (unusual)
- MRI of the brain in cases of encephalitis

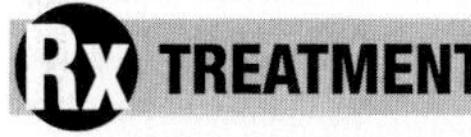

TREATMENT

ACUTE GENERAL Rx

- Immediate therapy to limit extent of acute illness and complication
- Doxycycline: 100 mg twice a day for 7 to 14 days is therapy of choice for adults and children >8 yr (4 mg/kg/day in 2 divided doses)
- Doxycycline is now recommended as well for children aged <8 yr (Redbook 2018)
- Rifampin: 300 mg twice a day for 7 to 10 days can be used in pregnancy and for children <8 yr at 10 mg/kg twice per day
- Most patients defervesce within 24 to 48 hr given appropriate treatment.

PROGNOSIS

Poor prognostic indicators include:

- Advanced age or immunosuppression
- Concomitant chronic illness (such as diabetes mellitus, collagen-vascular disease)
- Lack of diagnosis recognition
- Delayed onset of specific antibiotic therapy
- Concomitant HIV or organ transplant status

DISPOSITION

Repeat CBC every 2 to 4 wk until normal.

REFERRAL

For consultation with infectious diseases specialist in suspected cases

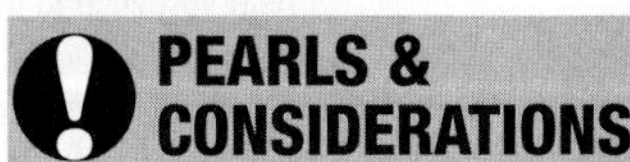

PEARLS & CONSIDERATIONS

- A new pathogenic *Ehrlichia* species, closely related to *E. muris,* has been identified in Minnesota and Wisconsin. Organism-specific PCR and serologic testing can be used for identification.
- Duration of time tick must be attached to produce illness as few as 4 hr

- Delay in antibiotic treatment results in poorer outcome. Antibiotic treatment should be initiated as soon as infection is suspected.

SUGGESTED READINGS

Available at ExpertConsult.com

RELATED CONTENT

Anaplasmosis (Patient Information)

AUTHOR: **PATRICIA CRISTOFARO, M.D.**

TABLE 1 Human Ehrlichioses and Anaplasmosis

	Human Monocytotropic Ehrlichiosis	Human Granulocytotropic Ehrlichiosis	Human Granulocytotropic Anaplasmosis
Former disease nomenclature	Human monocytic ehrlichiosis	Human granulocytic ehrlichiosis	Human granulocytic ehrlichiosis
Causative agent(s)	*Ehrlichia chaffeensis*	*Ehrlichia ewingii, Ehrlichia cani*—one asymptomatic human case reported in Venezuela	*Anaplasma phagocytophilum*
Leukocyte targets	Monocytic cell phagosomes	Neutrophil phagosomes	Granulocyte-neutrophil phagosomes
Tick vectors	*Amblyomma americanum* (lone star ticks)	*Amblyomma americanum* (lone star ticks), *Dermacentor variabilis* (American dog ticks)	*Ixodes persulcatus* complex (American deer ticks)—*I. scapularis, I. ricinus, I. pacificus*
Animal reservoirs	White-tailed deer, coyotes, dogs	White-tailed deer, dogs	Rodents, deer, ruminants, horses
U.S. regional distribution	Southeastern and south central United States	South central United States	Northeastern United States, upper Midwest, northern California
U.S. regional prevalence	2-5 cases/100,000	≤10% of presumed HME cases have *E. ewingii* infections in south central United States	50-60 cases/100,000; high seroprevalence rates in children (>20%) who have had subclinical infections
Seasonal occurrences	April-September, peaking in July	Spring-fall	May-July
Incubation periods (wk)	1-4	1-4	1-4
Modes of transmission	Tick bite, blood product transfusion	Tick bite, blood product transfusion	Tick bite, blood product transfusion, nosocomial
Frequently presenting clinical manifestations	Fever, malaise, headache, myalgias, rash in <40%	Same initial manifestations, but much milder, except in immunocompromised individuals	Fever, malaise, headache, myalgias; rarely rash
Laboratory abnormalities	Leukopenia, thrombocytopenia, transaminitis	Leukopenia, thrombocytopenia, transaminitis	More pronounced and prolonged leukopenia, thrombocytopenia, transaminitis
Potential complications, especially in immunocompromised individuals	Meningoencephalitis, acute renal and respiratory failure, hepatitis, myocarditis	Milder and less likely, except in patients immunocompromised by HIV/AIDS, organ transplantation, prolonged corticosteroid therapy	May be significant in immunocompromised patients with high fevers, seizures, confusion, hemorrhagic diathesis, rhabdomyolysis, shock, acute tubular necrosis, adult respiratory distress syndrome; some specific CNS complications may include eighth nerve palsy, brachial plexopathy, demyelinating polyneuropathy
Case-fatality rate (CFR)	3%, higher in immunocompromised individuals	No deaths reported	0.5%, higher CFR in immunocompromised individuals
Recommended confirmatory diagnostic tests	Wright-stained peripheral blood smears with characteristic intracytoplasmic morulae in monocytes, DNA detection by PCR assay, culture	Wright-stained peripheral blood smears with characteristic intracytoplasmic morulae in neutrophils, DNA detection by PCR	Wright-stained peripheral blood smears with characteristic intracytoplasmic aggregates in neutrophils, DNA detection by PCR assay, increased immunofluorescent antibodies in initial and paired serum samples
Current antibiotic resistance	Fluoroquinolones	Fluoroquinolones	Fluoroquinolones
Currently recommended antibiotic therapy, adults	Doxycycline, 100 mg PO bid, or tetracycline, 250-500 mg PO qid, for minimum of 3 days after defervescence to maximum of 14-21 days	Doxycycline, 100 mg PO bid, or tetracycline, 250-500 mg PO qid, for minimum of 3 days after defervescence to maximum of 14-21 days	Doxycycline, 100 mg PO bid, or tetracycline, 250-500 mg PO qid for minimum of 3 days after defervescence to maximum of 14-21 days
Currently recommended antibiotic therapy, children	Doxycycline, 4.4 mg/kg PO bid, or tetracycline, 25-50 mg/kg PO qid, for minimum of 3 days after defervescence to maximum of 14-21 days	Doxycycline, 4.4 mg/kg PO bid, or tetracycline, 25-50 mg/kg PO qid, for minimum of 3 days after defervescence to maximum of 14-21 days	Doxycycline, 4.4 mg/kg PO bid, or tetracycline, 25-50 mg/kg PO qid, for minimum of 3 days after defervescence to maximum of 14-21 days

bid, Twice daily; *CNS,* central nervous system; *DNA,* deoxyribonucleic acid; *HME,* human monocytotropic ehrlichiosis; *HIV/AIDS,* human immunodeficiency virus infection/acquired immunodeficiency syndrome; *PCR,* polymerase chain reaction; *PO,* by mouth; *qid,* four times a day.
From Bennett JE, et al.: *Mandell, Douglas, and Bennett's principles and practice of infectious diseases,* ed 8, Philadelphia, 2015, Saunders.

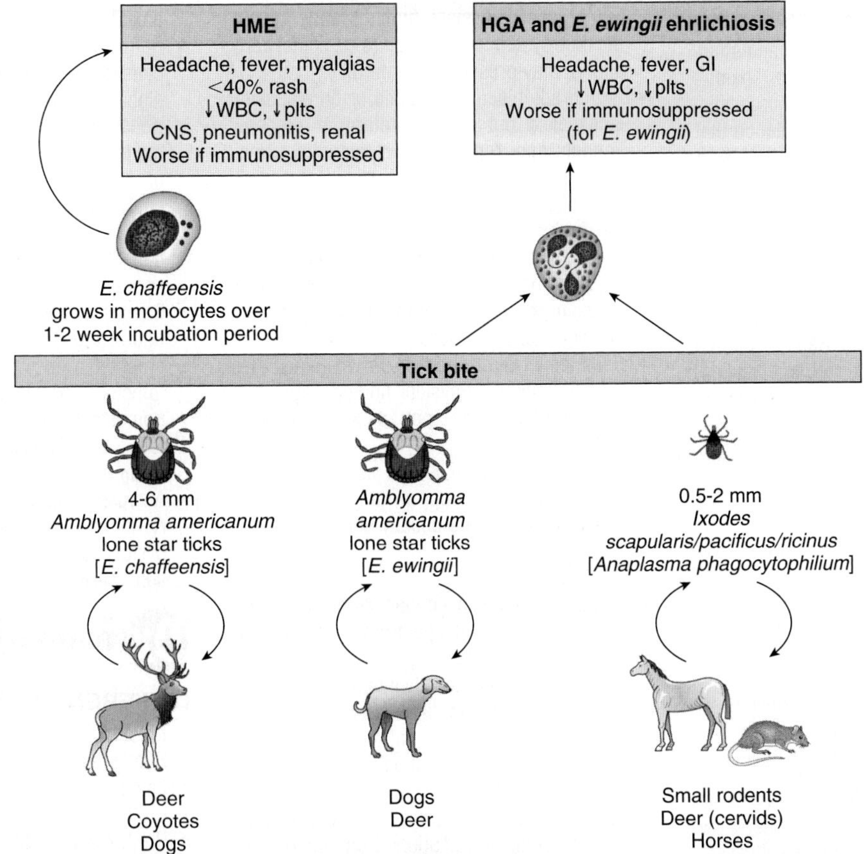

FIG. 1 Life cycles of human monocytic ehrlichiosis (*HME*, with *Ehrlichia chaffeensis*) and human granulocytic ehrlichiosis (anaplasmosis, *HGA* with *Anaplasma phagocytophilum*) or infection with *E. ewingii*. *CNS*, Central nervous system; *GI*, gastrointestinal; *WBC*, white blood cell count. (From Dumler JS: Ehrlichiosis and anaplasmosis. In Guerrant RL, Walker DH, Weller PF (eds): *Tropical infectious diseases: principles, pathogens and practice*, 3rd ed, Philadelphia, 2011, Elsevier, pp. 339-343.)

TABLE 2 Clinical Clues (History, Physical Examination, or Laboratory) Suggesting the Diagnosis of a Tick-Borne Illness Manifesting as a Nonspecific Febrile Illness*

Disease	Clues
Anaplasmosis	Faint rash possible Low white blood cell or platelet count Elevated hepatic transaminases
Babesiosis	Findings of hemolysis History of splenectomy Presence of faint rash, hepatomegaly, or splenomegaly
Lyme disease	Careful skin examination for any rash consistent with erythema migrans Bradycardia from heart block Associated seventh nerve palsy or lymphocytic meningitis
Colorado tick fever	Saddle-back fever curve
Rocky Mountain spotted fever	Maculopapular or petechial rash Normal white blood cell count or low platelet count Hyponatremia Peripheral edema
Relapsing fever	Recurring episodes of fever with afebrile intervals
Tularemia	Acrally located ulcer Regional lymphadenopathy Possible associated pneumonia

*Apart from an epidemiologic context suggesting a tick-borne disease.

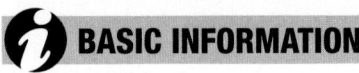

BASIC INFORMATION

DEFINITION

Disorders of ejaculation and orgasm include premature ejaculation, delayed ejaculation, anejaculation, retrograde ejaculation, painful ejaculation, hematospermia, and anorgasmia. Premature ejaculation refers to ejaculation that occurs sooner than desired, either before or shortly after penetration, whereas delayed ejaculation refers to ejaculation that occurs after prolonged sexual stimulation. Anejaculation occurs when semen is not propulsed into the urethra during orgasm, resulting in a dry ejaculate. Retrograde ejaculation is a backward flow of semen into the bladder. Hematospermia is the appearance of blood in the ejaculate. Anorgasmia is the inability to achieve orgasm in a timely manner.

SYNONYMS

Ejaculatory dysfunction
Anejaculation
Aspermia
Dry ejaculate
Failure of emission

ICD-10CM CODES

R36.1	Hematospermia; Bloody ejaculation
F52.4	Premature ejaculation
F52.32	Male orgasmic disorder; Inhibited male orgasm; Anorgasmia
N53.11	Delayed ejaculation; Retarded ejaculation
N53.12	Painful ejaculation
N53.13	Anejaculatory orgasm; Anejaculation
N53.14	Retrograde ejaculation
N53.19	Other ejaculatory dysfunction

EPIDEMIOLOGY & DEMOGRAPHICS

INCIDENCE: Not well understood, due to variability in definitions and reporting.

PEAK INCIDENCE: Not well understood.

PREVALENCE: Premature ejaculation is the most prevalent male sexual complaint, affecting 20% to 30% of men and may be primary (lifelong) or acquired. Delayed ejaculation is the least common, least studied, and least understood of the male sexual dysfunctions.

PREDOMINANT SEX AND AGE: These disorders have been reported among men aged 18 to 70 yr.

GENETICS: No known genetic predisposition.

RISK FACTORS: Men with ejaculatory dysfunction of any type usually indicate higher levels of relationship stress, sexual dissatisfaction, anxiety about sexual performance, and general health issues, compared to sexually functional men.

PHYSICAL FINDINGS & CLINICAL PRESENTATION

- Premature ejaculation: Ejaculation occurs sooner than desired, often within 1 minute of penetration. Physical examination is normal. Up to 30% of patients may report concomitant erectile dysfunction.
- Delayed ejaculation: Ejaculation requires prolonged sexual stimulation, often 30 minutes or longer. Physical examination is normal.
- Anejaculation: No ejaculate is produced during orgasm. Physical findings may reveal nervous system dysfunction (e.g., spinal cord injury); may present with infertility.
- Retrograde ejaculation: Little or no ejaculate is expelled out of the urethra at orgasm. Patients may report cloudy postcoital urine. Physical examination is usually normal; may present with infertility.
- Painful ejaculation: Perineal, scrotal, or testicular pain during or shortly after ejaculation. Physical examination may demonstrate pain on examination of external genitalia, or with digital rectal examination.
- Hematospermia: Reddish-brown ejaculate, usually painless. Physical findings are usually unremarkable; not associated with malignancy.
- Anorgasmia: Patient is not able to achieve orgasm despite appropriate stimulation. Physical findings are usually unremarkable.

ETIOLOGY

- Premature and delayed ejaculation represent opposite ends of the spectrum of ejaculatory disorders. The underlying etiology is complex and multifactorial and includes organic and psychogenic contributions. Box 1 summarizes recommended and optional questions to establish the diagnosis of delayed ejaculation and direct treatment.
- Anejaculation may result from pelvic surgery, trauma, or radiation; from neurologic diseases such as Parkinson's disease, multiple sclerosis, spinal cord injury, or diabetes mellitus; from bilateral ejaculatory duct obstruction; or from psychological stress and anxiety.
- Retrograde ejaculation is most commonly caused by the use of medications (e.g., alpha-blockers) or surgical procedures (e.g., transurethral resection of prostate) that relax the bladder neck, but it can also be the result of retroperitoneal surgery and the previously mentioned neurologic diseases. Box 2 summarizes causes of retrograde ejaculation, delayed ejaculation, anejaculation, and anorgasmia.
- Causes of painful ejaculation may be infectious (e.g., epididymo-orchitis, urethritis, prostatitis), obstructive (e.g., vasectomy, prostatectomy, hernia repair), or psychological.
- Hematospermia may be idiopathic, secondary to prolonged abstinence, or due to infection or inflammation of the genitourinary tract.
- Anorgasmia may be caused by spinal cord injury, hormonal dysfunction, psychological factors, dysfunctional sexual techniques, or medications, particularly serotonin reuptake inhibitors.

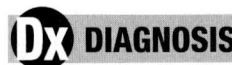

DIAGNOSIS

DIFFERENTIAL DIAGNOSIS

- Erectile dysfunction
- Hypogonadism
- Ejaculatory duct obstruction
- Urethral stricture disease
- Urethritis or sexually transmitted infection

BOX 1 Recommended and Optional Questions to Establish the Diagnosis of Delayed Ejaculation (DE) and Direct Treatment

Recommended Questions for Diagnosis of DE

For Diagnosis

What proportion of the time can you ejaculate during sexual intercourse?
During intercourse, how long after penetration does it take for you to ejaculate?
When you cannot ejaculate during sexual intercourse, how often do you feel that you are close to ejaculation?
If you cannot ejaculate, why do you stop intercourse?
Do you ever feel that you have ejaculated, but fail to release semen?
Do you feel bothered, annoyed, and/or frustrated by your DE?
How often can you ejaculate during masturbation by yourself or with your partner?

Optional Questions

Differentiate Lifelong and Acquired DE

When did you first experience DE?
Have you experienced DE since your first sexual experience on every/almost every attempt and with every partner?

Assess Erectile Function

Is your erection hard enough for penetration?
Do you have difficulty in maintaining your erection during intercourse?
During masturbation, are you able to achieve an erection that is hard enough for penetration?
Do you wake up at night or in the morning with an erection that is hard enough for penetration?

Assess Relationship Impact

How upset is your partner with your DE?
Do you or your partner avoid sexual intercourse?
Is your DE affecting your overall relationship?

Previous Treatment

Have you received any medical or psychological treatment for your DE?

Impact on Quality of Life

Do you feel anxious, depressed, or embarrassed because of your DE?

From Wein AJ et al: *Campbell-Walsh urology*, ed 11, Philadelphia, 2016, Elsevier.

BOX 2 Causes of Retrograde Ejaculation, Delayed Ejaculation, Anejaculation, and Anorgasmia

Degeneration of penile afferent nerves

Psychogenic
Inhibited ejaculation

Congenital
Müllerian duct cyst
Wolffian duct abnormality
Prune belly syndrome

Anatomic Causes
Transurethral resection of prostate
Bladder neck incision

Neurogenic Causes
Diabetic autonomic neuropathy
Multiple sclerosis
Spinal cord injury
Radical prostatectomy
Retroperitoneal lymph node dissection
Proctocolectomy
Bilateral sympathectomy
Abdominal aortic aneurysmectomy
Para-aortic lymphadenectomy

Infectious
Urethritis
Genitourinary tuberculosis
Schistosomiasis

Endocrine
Hypogonadism
Hypothyroidism

Medication
α-Methyldopa
Alpha blockers
Thiazide diuretics
Tricyclic and SSRI antidepressants
Phenothiazine
Alcohol abuse

SSRI, Selective serotonin reuptake inhibitor.

From Wein AJ et al: *Campbell-Walsh urology*, ed 11, Philadelphia, 2016, Elsevier Aging Male.

LABORATORY TESTS

- For a low-volume ejaculate, post-ejaculate urine should be evaluated for the presence of spermatozoa to differentiate failure of emission from retrograde ejaculation.
- Hematuria, in the setting of hematospermia or painful ejaculation, may signal an underlying inflammatory disorder or a malignancy, and it should prompt a complete evaluation.
- A fasting blood glucose test may be considered if diabetes is suspected as a cause of lack of emission or retrograde ejaculation.
- Urinalysis, urine culture, and screening for sexually transmitted diseases, when indicated, can rule out an infectious etiology of painful ejaculation.

IMAGING STUDIES

Transrectal ultrasonography or pelvic MRI can rule out ejaculatory duct obstruction or absence of the seminal vesicles.

Rx TREATMENT

NONPHARMACOLOGIC THERAPY

- Premature ejaculation can improve with psychotherapy and behavioral interventions (e.g., "coronal squeeze" or "start-and-stop" technique) and effective partner communication. These approaches may be more effective when combined with pharmacologic therapy.
- Retrograde ejaculation and anejaculation do not require treatment unless fertility is desired.
- In the setting of retrograde ejaculation, viable sperm can be recovered from the post-ejaculate urine and used for intrauterine insemination or in vitro fertilization.
- Idiopathic hematospermia may be followed expectantly and is usually self-limited to 10 or 15 ejaculations.
- Anorgasmia caused by serotonin reuptake inhibitors usually improves with withdrawal of the medication. Sexual therapy and counseling can improve anorgasmia caused by dysfunctional sexual techniques or psychological issues. Vibratory or electrical stimulation of emission is helpful in selected cases.
- Fig. E1 illustrates an algorithm for the management of delayed ejaculation, anejaculation, and anorgasmia. Drug therapy for delayed ejaculation and anejaculation is summarized in Table E1.

ACUTE GENERAL Rx

- Premature ejaculation: Selective serotonin reuptake inhibitors (SSRI) (e.g., sertraline, fluoxetine) and the tricyclic antidepressant clomipramine can successfully delay ejaculation when taken daily. Dapoxetine, a short-acting SSRI, may be used as an "on-demand" treatment for premature ejaculation (not available in the U.S.). Topical anesthetics such as lidocaine cream and topical sprays have been used with variable success. The use of phosphodiesterase inhibitors (PDE5i) (e.g., sildenafil, vardenafil, tadalafil) with SSRIs may be beneficial in men with concomitant erectile dysfunction and premature ejaculation. Table E2 summarizes drug therapy for premature ejaculation.
- Retrograde ejaculation: Pharmacologic therapy is only effective in patients without an anatomic disturbance of the bladder neck. Sympathomimetic medications (phenylpropanolamine, ephedrine, pseudoephedrine) and imipramine may be useful in converting retrograde ejaculation to antegrade ejaculation.
- Antimicrobial treatment (if indicated), NSAIDs, and muscle relaxants may help decrease discomfort associated with painful ejaculation.
- The use of the pharmacologic therapies listed above for the treatment of various disorders of ejaculation is strictly off label and does not carry FDA approval.
- Fig. E2 illustrates an algorithm for the office management of premature ejaculation.

CHRONIC Rx

Rarely, painful ejaculation due to long-standing obstructive causes may show improvement with surgical intervention (e.g., vasectomy reversal). The pharmacologic therapies listed above can also be used for the chronic treatment of disorders of ejaculation and orgasm.

COMPLEMENTARY AND ALTERNATIVE MEDICINE

- A variety of nutritional supplements and herbs have been used for the treatment of erectile dysfunction, but their benefit for the specific treatment of ejaculation and orgasm disorders is unknown.
- Acupuncture and traditional Chinese medicine may be helpful in treating underlying hormonal imbalances.
- Yoga and meditation can reduce the effects of stress and relieve anxiety about sexual dysfunction.
- Therapeutic massage can decrease stress.

DISPOSITION

Prognosis varies with etiology. Ejaculatory dysfunction attributable to sexual techniques or psychological issues can improve with psychotherapy. Pharmacologic treatment is helpful in treating premature, retrograde, or painful ejaculation.

REFERRAL

All fertility issues and suspected anatomic problems should be referred to a urologist. Professional psychotherapy should be considered for appropriate patients.

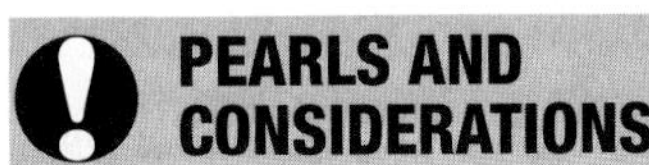

PEARLS AND CONSIDERATIONS

COMMENTS

Ejaculatory and orgasmic disorders are common male sexual dysfunctions and include premature ejaculation, delayed ejaculation, anejaculation, retrograde ejaculation, painful ejaculation, hematospermia, and anorgasmia. Physical exam is usually normal.

PREVENTION

Preventing sexually transmitted infections and treating other inflammatory disorders of the genitourinary tract may be of some benefit in reducing the incidence of these sexual disorders.

PATIENT/FAMILY EDUCATION

These sexual disorders can exert a significant psychological burden on affected men and their partners. A combination of pharmacologic and nonpharmacologic therapies, including a urologic and psychologic evaluation, when indicated, may be helpful in the treatment of these complaints.

SUGGESTED READINGS

Available at ExpertConsult.com

RELATED CONTENT

Erectile Dysfunction (Patient Information)
Premature Ejaculation (Patient Information)
Erectile Dysfunction (Related Key Topic)

AUTHORS: **AKANKSHA MEHTA, M.D., M.S.,** and **MARK SIGMAN, M.D.**

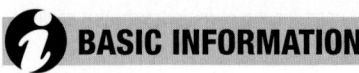

BASIC INFORMATION

DEFINITION

Elder abuse consists of actions that cause harm committed by someone in a trust relationship whether in the community or institutional setting.

- Physical abuse: Inflicting physical pain or injury
- Sexual abuse: Inflicting nonconsensual sexual activity
- Psychological abuse: Inflicting mental anguish, including intimidation, humiliation, or threats
- Financial abuse: Improper use of resources, property, or assets without the person's consent
- Neglect: Abandonment, failure to fulfill a care-taking obligation, including provision of food, safe shelter, physical health and mental health care, or basic custodial care
- Box 1 summarizes definitions of types of abuse, with examples of behavior and effects

SYNONYMS

Battered elder syndrome
Elder mistreatment
Domestic violence in the elderly
Diogenes syndrome
Intimate partner violence (IPV)

Adult abuse, neglect, and maltreatment cover a range of diagnostic codes depending on whether the issue is confirmed or suspected and whether the problem is neglect, physical, psychological, or sexual. The DSM-5 includes these codes under other conditions that may be a focus of clinical attention.

Core Codes:

ICD-10CM CODES

T74 and T76	Abuse, neglect, and other maltreatment
T74.0 and T76.0	Neglect or abandonment
T74.1 and T76.1	Physical abuse
T74.2 and T76.2	Sexual abuse
T74.3 and T76.3	Psychological abuse
T74.9 and T76.9	Unspecified adult maltreatment

DSM-5 CODES

Depends on specific diagnosis

EPIDEMIOLOGY & DEMOGRAPHICS

INCIDENCE: As high as 5,000,000 elders are abused annually in the U.S.

PEAK INCIDENCE: >75 yr; more recent studies now suggest <75 yr

PREVALENCE:

- About 10% of those 60 yr or older have been abused.
- Emotional followed by financial abuse are the most common forms.
- 12-month U.S. prevalence rates: Emotional abuse 9.0% and 4.6%; physical abuse 0.2% and 1.6%; sexual abuse 0.6%; neglect 0.5%; and financial abuse 3.5% and 5.2%.
- Family members reported 21% of nursing home residents were neglected on one or more occasion in the past 12 months, and over 24% had been subjected to physical abuse during their entire stay.
- Among caregivers of patients with dementia in the U.K., one half reported behaving abusively at least some of the time, and one third reported "important" levels of abuse. Verbal abuse was common and physical abuse was rare.
- Elder abuse is associated with increased risk of mortality, with the highest for caregiver neglect, functional impairment, and greater emotional distress, including depression, anxiety, and posttraumatic stress.
- Adult intimate partner violence perpetrators are significantly more likely to have witnessed intimate partner violence as a child than nonperpetrators.
- Older women are more likely than older men to be victims of abuse.

RISK FACTORS (VICTIM):

- Impaired cognition
- Behavioral problems
- Psychiatric illness or psychological problems
- Mental or physical dependence
- Poor physical health or frailty
- Trauma or past abuse
- Shared living situation and premorbid relationship with abuser
- Social isolation and poor social support
- Low household income

RISK FACTORS (PERPETRATOR):

- Relationship conflict with the victim
- Substance abuse, mental illness, particularly depression
- Caregiver burden or stress, being an involuntary caregiver, overwhelmed or resentful

PHYSICAL FINDINGS & CLINICAL PRESENTATION

- Physical abuse with multiple injuries at various stages with implausible descriptions of their origins
- Fear, hypervigilance, or withdrawal
- Evidence of poor nutrition, dehydration, poor hygiene, multiple or neglected pressure ulcers, genital or anal pain, neglected medical conditions, or evidence of restraint use (bruises around wrists or ankles)
- Toxicologic evidence of unprescribed medications
- Poor adherence, frequent no-shows, or little contact with health care system
- Caregiver not allowing interviewing the patient alone

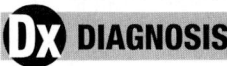

DIAGNOSIS

DIFFERENTIAL DIAGNOSIS

- Dementia
- Depression, substance misuse, posttraumatic stress disorder (PTSD), or other psychiatric disorder
- Malnutrition from intrinsic causes

BOX 1 Definitions of Types of Abuse, with Examples of Behavior and Effects

- **Physical abuse:** Nonaccidental infliction of physical force that results in bodily injury, pain, or impairment
  - *Examples of behavior:* Hitting, slapping, pushing, burning, physical restraint
  - *Examples of effects:* Bruises, fractures, burns, broken teeth, sprains, cuts, hair loss, bleeding from scalp, fear, anxiety, depression
- **Psychological abuse:** The persistent use of threats, humiliation, bullying, swearing and other verbal conduct, and/or of any other form of mental cruelty that results in mental or physical distress
  - *Examples of behavior:* Treating an older person as a child, blaming, swearing, intimidating, name-calling, threatening violence, isolating older person
  - *Examples of effects:* Fear, depression, confusion, loss of sleep, loss of appetite
- **Financial abuse:** Unauthorized and improper use of funds, property, or any resources of an older person
  - *Examples of behavior:* Misappropriating money, valuables, or property; forcing changes to will; denying access to personal funds
  - *Examples of effects:* Loss of money, etc., inability to pay bills, deterioration in health or standard of living, lack of amenities, unusual activity in bank accounts, signatures on documents uncertain, lack of solid arrangements for financial management, eviction or house sale notices
- **Sexual abuse:** Direct or indirect involvement in sexual activity without consent
  - *Examples of behavior:*
    - *Noncontact:* Looking, photography, indecent exposure, harassment, serious teasing or innuendo, pornography
    - *Contact:* Touching breast, genitals, anus, mouth; masturbation of either or both persons; penetration or attempted penetration of vagina, anus, mouth, with or by penis, fingers, other objects
  - *Examples of effects:* Difficulty in walking or sitting, bruises, bleeding, venereal disease, psychological trauma
- **Neglect:** Repeated deprivation of assistance needed by the older person for important activities of daily living
  - *Examples of behavior:* Failure to provide food, shelter, clothing, medical care, hygiene, personal care; inappropriate use of medication or overmedication
  - *Examples of effects:* Malnutrition, pressure ulcers, oversedation, untreated medical problems, depression, confusion

From Fillet HM: *Brocklehurst's textbook of geriatric medicine and gerontology,* ed 8, Philadelphia, 2017, Elsevier.

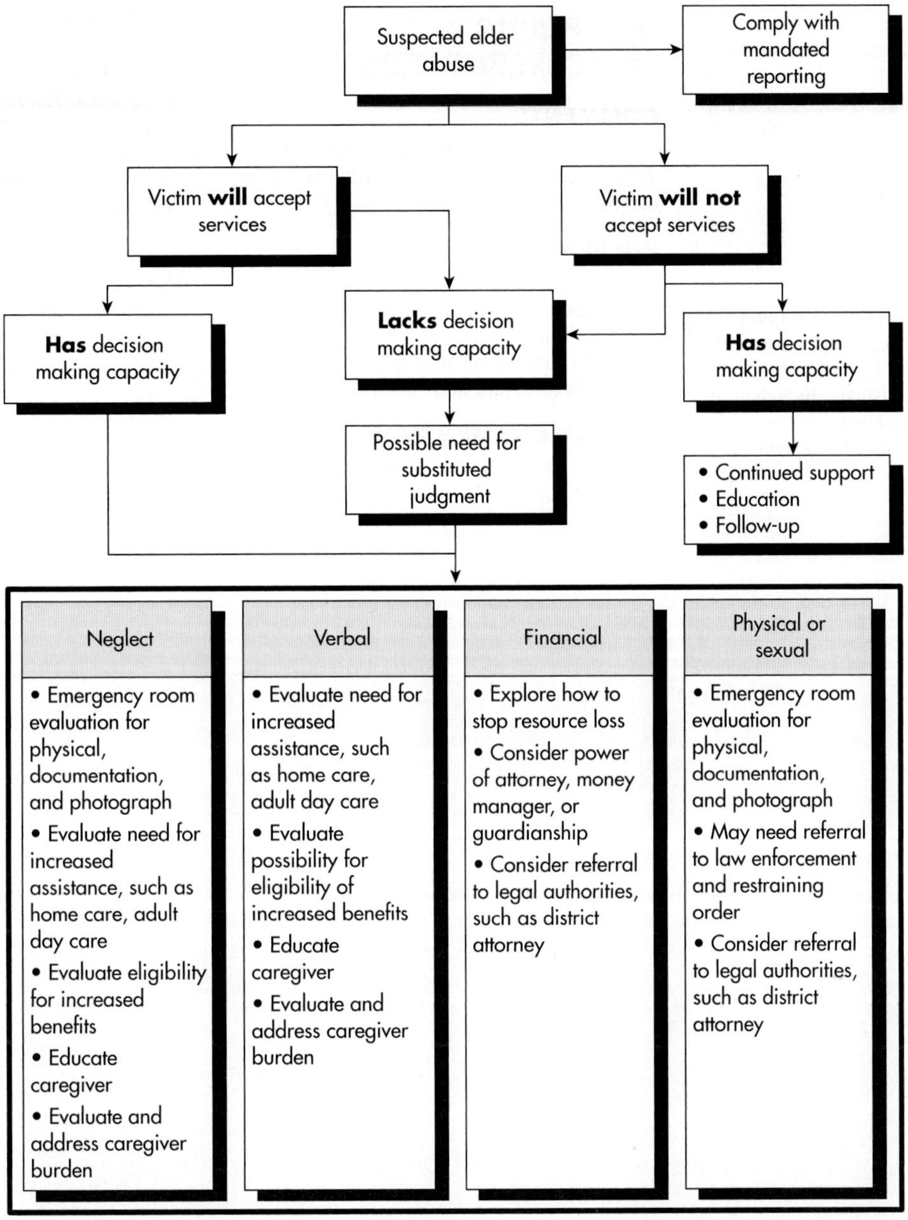

Suspected elder abuse → Comply with mandated reporting

Suspected elder abuse → Victim **will** accept services; Victim **will not** accept services

Victim **will** accept services → **Has** decision making capacity; **Lacks** decision making capacity

Victim **will not** accept services → **Lacks** decision making capacity; **Has** decision making capacity

Lacks decision making capacity → Possible need for substituted judgment

Has decision making capacity (victim will not accept services) →
- Continued support
- Education
- Follow-up

Has decision making capacity (victim will accept services) and Possible need for substituted judgment →

Neglect	Verbal	Financial	Physical or sexual
• Emergency room evaluation for physical, documentation, and photograph • Evaluate need for increased assistance, such as home care, adult day care • Evaluate eligibility for increased benefits • Educate caregiver • Evaluate and address caregiver burden	• Evaluate need for increased assistance, such as home care, adult day care • Evaluate possibility for eligibility of increased benefits • Educate caregiver • Evaluate and address caregiver burden	• Explore how to stop resource loss • Consider power of attorney, money manager, or guardianship • Consider referral to legal authorities, such as district attorney	• Emergency room evaluation for physical, documentation, and photograph • May need referral to law enforcement and restraining order • Consider referral to legal authorities, such as district attorney

FIG. 1 Management of elder abuse. (Adapted from Kohn R, Warner J, Murphy E, Verhoek-Oftedahl W: Elder abuse. In Holzer JC, Kohn R, Recupero PR, Ellison JM [eds]: *Textbook of geriatric forensic psychiatry*, New York, 2018, Oxford University Press.)

- Nonadherence to medical treatment
- Relationship distress
- Falling

WORKUP

- Ask direct specific questions such as:
    1. "Has anyone close to you called you names or put you down recently?"
    2. "Are you afraid of anyone who lives with you or cares for you?"
    3. "Has anyone at home ever hurt you?"
    4. "Has anyone touched you without your consent?"
    5. "Has anyone forced you to do things you didn't want to do?"
    6. "Has anyone taken things or money that belong to you without your OK?"
    7. "Have you signed any documents that you don't understand?"
    8. "Are you often alone?"
    9. "When you need help has anyone ever failed to help you take care of yourself?"
    10. If appropriate, ask, "Have you been abused?"
- Interview patient and alleged perpetrator separately.
- Pelvic examination if sexual abuse suspected.
- Take photographs of physical injuries as legal evidence.

LABORATORY TESTS & IMAGING STUDIES

- Screen for dehydration, malnutrition, and rhabdomyolysis.
- Toxicology screens and therapeutic drug monitoring are sometimes helpful.
- Other tests and radiology according to presentation.

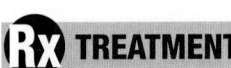

TREATMENT

NONPHARMACOLOGIC THERAPY

- Separate patient and abuser.
- Patient and caregiver may benefit from psychiatric evaluation and treatment for substance abuse, mental illness, or cognitive impairment.
- If appropriate, assess the patient's capacity.
- Fig. 1 describes a management algorithm for elder abuse.

ACUTE GENERAL Rx

- As indicated for injury or pain relief
- As indicated for mental disorders, dementia, or delirium

DISPOSITION

If the patient's level of disability does not allow independent living, institutionalization may be required. Guidelines vary at the state and county levels regarding guardianship and conservatorship requirements.

REFERRAL

- For outpatients, report to local adult protective services agency. Reporting is mandatory in most states.
- Resident-to-resident elder mistreatment (R-REM) in nursing homes is highly prevalent. For nursing home patients, report to regional long-term care ombudsman. Reporting is mandatory under federal law.
- Mental health services may be needed.

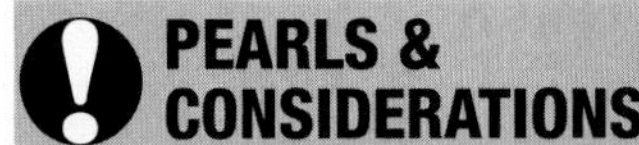

PEARLS & CONSIDERATIONS

COMMENTS

Care should be taken in interacting with the alleged abuser so that access to the victim is not lost.

PREVENTION

- Offer social services (e.g., respite care or homecare) for stressed caregivers.
- Make financial arrangements and arrange durable power of attorney for health care and finances while patient is still cognitively intact.

PATIENT & FAMILY EDUCATION

In the U.S., the elder care help line is 1-800-677-1116.

National Center on Elder Abuse: http://www.ncea.aoa.gov

National Domestic Violence Hotline: 800-799-7233 or 800-799-SAFE

TTY: 800-787-3224

CDC: Violence Prevention www.cdc.gov/violenceprevention/intimatepartnerviolence

SUGGESTED READINGS

Available at ExpertConsult.com

RELATED CONTENT

Elder Abuse (Patient Information)

AUTHOR: **ROBERT KOHN, M.D.**

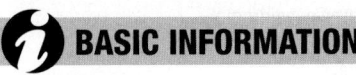

BASIC INFORMATION

DEFINITION

An accumulation of pus in the pleural space, most often caused by bacterial infection.

SYNONYMS

Infected pleuritis
Infected pleural effusion
Purulent pleural effusion

ICD-10CM CODES

J86 Pyothorax
A16.5 Empyema due to tuberculosis

EPIDEMIOLOGY & DEMOGRAPHICS

- Empyema is most commonly a complication of bacterial pneumonia, especially in association with pneumococcal or anaerobic infection (40% to 60% of cases of empyema).
- Occurs as a complication of thoracic surgery ($<20\%$ of cases).
- Penetrating chest trauma (4% to 10% of cases).
- Bronchopleural fistulae resulting from malignancy or lung biopsy.

PHYSICAL FINDINGS & CLINICAL PRESENTATION

- May be abrupt or chronic and insidious depending on the etiologic agent and host factors.
- Typically presents as progressive pleuritic chest pain, persistent fever, and other sustained signs and symptoms of infection.
- In anaerobic empyema, particularly that caused by the actinomycetes, the clinical picture is dominated by systemic symptoms and signs: weight loss, malaise, and low-grade fever.
- A slowly enlarging chest wall mass.
- As a complication of thoracic trauma or surgery, empyema typically results from contamination of blood within the pleural space several days following the event.
- The physical findings of empyema are those of pleural effusion. Decreased breath sounds and dullness to percussion over the involved part of the thorax is typical. Systemic signs include fever, tachycardia, leukocytosis, and warmth and erythema over the involved area.

ETIOLOGY

Infection of the lung parenchyma spreading to pleural space caused by

- *Streptococcus pneumoniae.*
- *Haemophilus influenzae.*
- *Staphylococcus aureus.*
- *Legionella* species.
- *Mycobacterium tuberculosis.*
- *Actinomyces* spp.
- A variety of oral anaerobic bacteria have been cultured in 36% to 37% of empyemas: *Bacteroides fragilis*, *Prevotella* species, *Fusobacterium nucleatum*, and *Peptostreptococcus* are the most common.

Dx DIAGNOSIS

DIFFERENTIAL DIAGNOSIS

- Uninfected parapneumonic effusion
- Lung abscess (see Fig. 1)
- Congestive heart failure
- Malignancy involving the pleura
- Tuberculous pleurisy
- Collagen vascular disease (particularly rheumatoid lung and systemic lupus erythematosus)

LABORATORY TESTS

- Complete blood count; arterial blood gas.
- Blood cultures; pleural fluid cultures.
- Pleural fluid cultures identify pathogens in only 60% of cases.
- Pleural fluid analysis in empyema has the characteristics of an exudate with a ratio of pleural fluid to serum protein >0.5 or pleural fluid to serum LDH >0.6. Characteristically, empyema fluid is grossly purulent with visible organisms on Gram stain with glucose <50 mg/dl and pH <7. These findings justify immediate drainage by chest tube or surgery because of the high risk of loculation and progressive systemic infection.

IMAGING STUDIES

- Chest x-ray (Fig. E2*A*)
- Lateral decubitus view to establish the presence of free fluid in the pleural space
- Computed tomography (Fig. E2*B*) to establish the presence of fluid loculation, underlying mass lesions, and other intrathoracic pathology

Rx TREATMENT

NONPHARMACOLOGIC THERAPY

Prompt drainage by thoracostomy (chest tube) or open thoracotomy. Video-assisted thoracoscopic surgery (VATS) has greatly improved surgical management of empyemas.

ACUTE GENERAL Rx

- Maintenance of drainage until infection controlled.
- Antibiotics directed at suspected or proven bacterial or fungal pathogens. Initial regimens include cefotaxime or ceftriaxone for suspected *S. pneumoniae* or group A *Streptococcus*, nafcillin or oxacillin for suspected methicillin-sensitive *S. aureus*, vancomycin or linezolid for suspected MRSA, ceftriaxone for suspected *H. influenzae*, and clindamycin plus ceftriaxone when suspecting anaerobes. Other agents with excellent anaerobic coverage include carbapenem antibiotics such as meropenem and ertapenem and piperacillin/tazobactam. These agents also have excellent Gram-negative coverage.
- Thoracoscopy or instillation of thrombolytic agents (streptokinase or urokinase) may be considered in refractory, loculated empyema.

CHRONIC Rx

- If thorough drainage cannot be accomplished, open thoracotomy with pleural decortication may be required.
- Lung function should be monitored following completion of therapy.

DISPOSITION

Hospitalization with supplemental oxygen with ventilatory support if necessary

REFERRAL

Consultation by infectious diseases, pulmonary, or thoracic surgery specialists as needed.

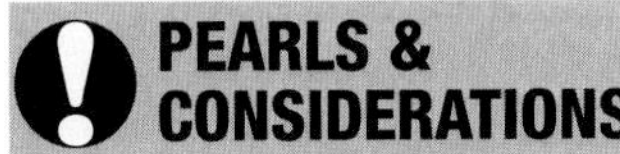

PEARLS & CONSIDERATIONS

COMMENTS

- Empyema caused by actinomycetes may present with erosion through the chest wall and formation of a fistulous tract.
- Nosocomial infection caused by relatively resistant bacterial or fungal pathogens may result in empyema in patients with indwelling thoracostomy tubes.

SUGGESTED READINGS

Available at ExpertConsult.com

AUTHOR: **GLENN G. FORT, M.D., M.P.H.**

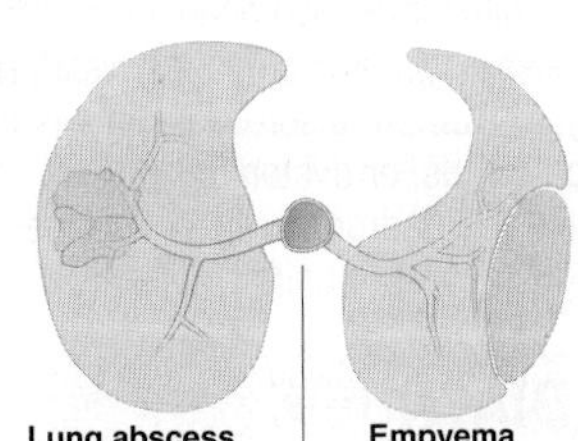

FIG. 1 Empyema versus lung abscess. (From Webb WR, Brant WE, Major NM: *Fundamentals of body CT*, ed 4, Philadelphia, 2015, Saunders.)

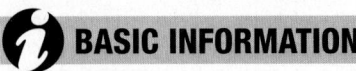

BASIC INFORMATION

DEFINITION

Acute viral encephalitis is an acute febrile syndrome with evidence of meningeal involvement and of derangement of the function of the cerebrum, cerebellum, or brain stem.

SYNONYMS

Arboviral encephalitis
Brain stem encephalitis
Acute necrotizing encephalitis
Rasmussen encephalitis
Encephalitis lethargica

ICD-10CM CODES

A86	Unspecified viral encephalitis
A83.0	Japanese encephalitis
A83.1	Western equine encephalitis
A83.2	Eastern equine encephalitis
A83.3	St Louis encephalitis
A83.4	Australian encephalitis
A83.5	California encephalitis
A83.8	Other mosquito-borne viral encephalitis
A83.9	Mosquito-borne viral encephalitis, unspecified
A84.8	Other tick-borne viral encephalitis
A84.9	Tick-borne viral encephalitis, unspecified
A85.0	Enteroviral encephalitis
A85.1	Adenoviral encephalitis
A85.2	Arthropod-borne viral encephalitis, unspecified
A85.8	Other specified viral encephalitis
A92.31	West Nile virus infection with encephalitis
B00.4	Herpesviral encephalitis
B01.11	Varicella encephalitis and encephalomyelitis
B02.0	Zoster encephalitis
B05.0	Measles complicated by encephalitis
B06.01	Rubella encephalitis
B10.01	Human herpesvirus 6 encephalitis
B10.09	Other human herpesvirus encephalitis
B26.2	Mumps encephalitis
B94.1	Sequelae of viral encephalitis
G04.00	Acute disseminated encephalitis and encephalomyelitis, unspecified
G04.81	Other encephalitis and encephalomyelitis
G04.90	Encephalitis and encephalomyelitis, unspecified
G05.3	Encephalitis and encephalomyelitis in diseases classified elsewhere

EPIDEMIOLOGY & DEMOGRAPHICS

INCIDENCE (IN U.S.): About 20,000 cases/yr are reported to the CDC. In 2016, there were 2149 cases of West Nile virus with 106 deaths. Each year in the U.S. approximately seven patients are hospitalized for encephalitis per 100,000 population.

PEAK INCIDENCE: Any age, but children and older adults are more likely to have significant morbidity

PREVALENCE (IN U.S.):
- Arbovirus infections are transmitted by mosquitoes and thus cause infection when mosquitoes are active, especially summer and fall. Herpes simplex infections can occur at any time.
- Geography also plays a role (Fig. 1): Whereas Eastern equine encephalitis is more likely on the East Coast of U.S., West Nile virus has spread to 48 states. Powassan virus is more common in northern New England and Canada. La Crosse virus is more common in the upper Midwestern and mid-Atlantic and southeastern states.

PREDOMINANT SEX: Male = female
PREDOMINANT AGE: Any age
GENETICS: No specific genetic or congenital predisposition

ETIOLOGY

- Can be caused by a host of viruses (Table E1), with herpes simplex the most common virus identified.
- Arboviruses transmitted by mosquitoes include Eastern equine encephalitis, Western equine encephalitis, St. Louis encephalitis, Venezuelan equine encephalitis, California virus encephalitis, Japanese B encephalitis, La Crosse encephalitis, Murray Valley and West Nile encephalitis. Tick-borne diseases include Russian spring-summer encephalitis, Powassan encephalitis, and other lesser known agents.
- Also implicated: Rabies-causing agents, CMV, Epstein-Barr, varicella-zoster, echo virus, mumps, adenovirus, coxsackie, rubeola, and herpes viruses.
- Meningoencephalitis: Acute retroviral infection from HIV.
- In the U.S., the most commonly identified etiologies are herpes simplex virus, West Nile virus, and the enteroviruses.

PHYSICAL FINDINGS & CLINICAL PRESENTATION

- Initially, fever and evidence of meningeal irritation
- Headache and stiff neck
- Later, development of signs of cortical dysfunction: Lethargy, coma, stupor, weakness, seizures, facial weakness, as well as brainstem findings
- Cerebellar findings: Ataxia, nystagmus, hypotonia, myoclonus, cranial nerve palsies, and abnormal tendon reflexes
- Patients with rabies: Hydrophobia, anxiety, facial numbness, psychosis, coma, or dysarthria
- Rarely, movement disorders, such as chorea, hemiballismus, or dystonia
- Recall of a prodromal viral-like illness (this finding is not at all uniform)

Dx DIAGNOSIS

DIFFERENTIAL DIAGNOSIS

- Bacterial infections: Brain abscess, toxic encephalopathies, TB
- Protozoal infections
- Behçet's disease
- Lupus encephalitis
- Sjögren's syndrome
- Multiple sclerosis
- Syphilis
- Cryptococcus
- Toxoplasmosis
- Brucellosis
- Leukemic or lymphomatous meningitis
- Other metastatic tumors
- Lyme disease
- Cat-scratch disease
- Vogt-Koyanagi-Harada syndrome
- Mollaret's meningitis

WORKUP (BOX 1)

- Lumbar puncture to reveal pleocytosis, usually lymphocytic, although neutrophils may be seen early on
- Usually, elevated CSF protein
- Normal or low CSF glucose
- In herpes simplex encephalitis: RBCs and xanthochromia
- Selected tests on CSF fluid in viral encephalitis are described in Table 2
- EEG changes showing periodic high-voltage sharp waves in the temporal regions and slow wave complexes suggestive of herpes encephalitis (Fig. E2)
- CT scan and MRI (Fig. 3) to reveal edema and hemorrhage in the frontal and temporal lobes
- Temporal lobe involvement suggests herpes simplex encephalitis (Fig. E4)
- Basal ganglia and thalami are areas involved as generally seen in Eastern equine encephalitis
- With West Nile infection, MRI changes have shown changes in basal ganglia, thalami, mesial temporal structures, brain stem, and cerebellum
- Arboviral infections suspected during outbreaks in specific areas
- Rising titers of neutralizing antibodies from the acute to the convalescent stage demonstrated but often not helpful in the acutely ill patient
- Polymerase chain reaction (PCR) that amplifies DNA from the CSF for herpes simplex encephalitis
- Rarely, brain biopsy to assist in the diagnosis; viral culture of cerebral tissue obtained if biopsy done
- Classic herpetic skin lesions suggestive of herpes encephalitis
- In diagnosing arboviral encephalitis:
  1. Presence of antiviral IgM within the first few days of symptomatic disease; detected and quantified by ELISA
  2. Unusual to recover an arbovirus from the blood or CSF

LABORATORY TESTS

- Aside from the lumbar puncture, most other laboratory studies are nonspecific.
- Skin lesions and urine may be cultured for herpes simplex and CMV.

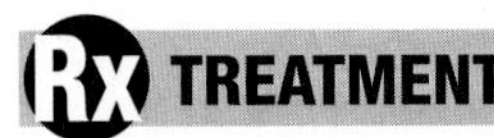

TREATMENT

ACUTE GENERAL Rx

- Supportive care, frequent evaluation, and neurologic examination

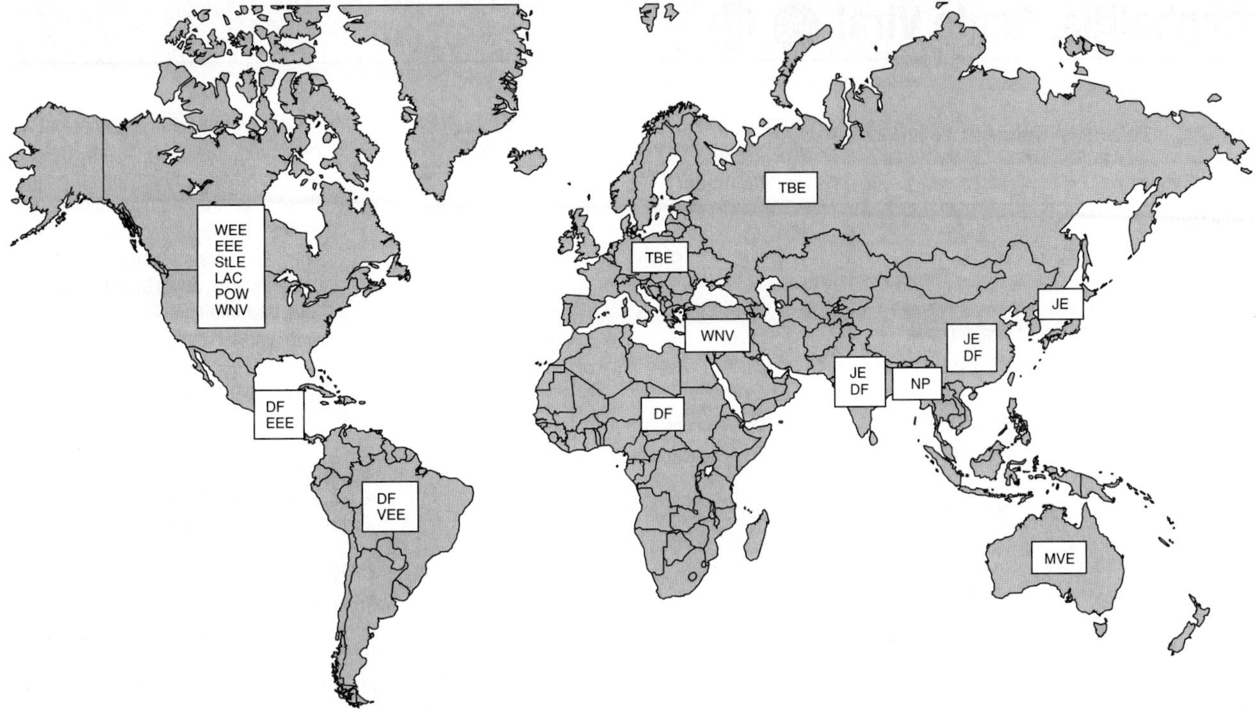

DF: Dengue fever
EEE: Eastern equine encephalitis
JE: Japanese encephalitis
LAC: La Crosse encephalitis
MVE: Murray Valley encephalitis
NP: Nipah encephalitis
POW: Powassan encephalitis
StLE: St. Louis encephalitis
TBE: Tick-borne encephalitis
VEE: Venezuelan equine encephalitis
WEE: Western equine encephalitis
WNV: West Nile encephalitis

FIG. 1 Map showing the worldwide geographic distribution of encephalitis caused by arthropod-borne viruses (the "arboviruses"). (Swaiman KF et al: *Swaiman's pediatric neurology, principles and practice,* ed 6, Philadelphia, 2017, Elsevier.)

BOX 1 Diagnostic Algorithm

All Cases

CSF
- WBC count with differential, RBC count, protein, glucose
- Gram stain and bacterial culture
- Herpes simplex virus–1/2 PCR (if test available, consider HSV CSF IgG and IgM in addition)
- VZV PCR (sensitivity may be low; if test available, consider VZV CSF IgG and IgM in addition)
- Enterovirus PCR

Blood/Serum
- Routine blood culture
- Epstein-Barr virus (EBV) antibodies (if positive for acute infection, check CSF EBV PCR)
- Hold acute serum and collect convalescent serum 10-14 days later for paired antibody testing

Respiratory, Stool
- Enterovirus PCR (respiratory, stool)
- Enterovirus (stool)

Conditional

Host Factors
- Neonate: Herpes simplex virus–2 PCR (CSF), swabs of skin vesicles, mouth, nasopharynx, conjunctivae, and rectum (viral culture)
- ≤3 yr: Parechovirus PCR (CSF and respiratory)
- Immunocompromised: Cytomegalovirus, human herpesvirus–6/7, JC virus, human immunodeficiency virus PCR (CSF)

Season and Exposure
- Summer/fall: West Nile virus (WNV) IgM (CSF, serum), WNV IgG (paired serum), and other appropriate arboviruses as geographically relevant
- Cat (particularly if with seizures and paucicellular CSF): *Bartonella* antibody (serum)
- Animal bite exposure: Rabies test[a]

[a]Contact health department for assistance with testing.
- Rodent exposure: LCM antibody (serum)
- Tick and/or camping exposure: *Rickettsia* spp., antibody (serum), *Anaplasma* phagocytophila antibody (serum)
- Swimming or diving in brackish water: *Naegleria fowleri* (wet mount)[a]
- If history of sexual activity: Herpes simplex virus–2 (CSF PCR)

Signs and Symptoms
- Psychotic component or movement disorder: Anti-NMDAR antibody (CSF and serum), and abdominal ultrasound evaluation for teratoma
- Vesicular rash: Varicella zoster virus PCR (CSF)
- Rapid decompensation (especially with bite history or foreign travel): Rabies test[a]
- Respiratory (during influenza season): Influenza PCR (respiratory)
- Diarrhea and seizure (especially young child): Rotavirus (check stool for antigen), if positive then rotavirus PCR (CSF)

Laboratory Features
- CSF protein >100 mg/dl or CSF glucose less than two-thirds peripheral glucose and/or lymphocytic pleocytosis:
  1. Mycobacterial tuberculosis: Culture (CSF, respiratory), place PPD, and check IGRA, chest radiograph, fungal culture (CSF)
  2. Fungal (specific types depend on geographic residence and/or travel to endemic areas): Culture CSF *and* check antibody and antigen
  3. Balam*uthia mandrillaris:* Contact health department/CDC for assistance with testing
- CSF eosinophilia: *Baylisascaris procyonis* antibody

Travel
- Consider consultation with public health department concerning specific diseases such as arboviruses, rabies, and other diseases

CDC, Centers for Disease Control and Prevention; *CSF,* cerebrospinal fluid; *HSV,* herpes simplex virus; *Ig,* immunoglobulin; *IGRA,* interferon gamma release assay; *LCM,* lymphocytic choriomeningitis; *NMDAR, N*-methyl-D-aspartate receptor; *PCR,* polymerase chain reaction; *PPD,* purified protein derivative; *RBC,* red blood cell; *VZV,* varicella zoster virus.

Cherry JD et al: *Feigin and Cherry's pediatric infectious diseases,* ed 8, Philadelphia, 2019, Elsevier.

TABLE 2 Selected Tests for Viral Encephalitis

Organism/Syndrome	Test	Comment
West Nile Virus		
West Nile encephalitis	IgM in CSF	Diagnostic of CNS invasive disease or acute flaccid paralysis
Herpes Simplex Virus Type 1		
Herpes simplex encephalitis	PCR in CSF	Sensitive and specific in the acute phase
	CSF–serum antibody ratio	Useful 2 weeks to 3 months after onset
Herpes Simplex Virus Type 2		
Neonatal encephalitis	PCR in CSF	Confirmatory, high sensitivity
Relapsing meningitis	PCR in CSF	Sensitive and specific in first 3 days of illness
Varicella-Zoster Virus		
Meningoencephalitis	PCR in CSF	Confirmatory when used with clinical and spinal fluid findings; sensitivity unclear
Epstein-Barr Virus		
EBV encephalitis	PCR in CSF	Suggests CNS invasion by virus
JC virus		
Progressive multifocal leukoencephalopathy	PCR in CSF	Diagnostic but incompletely (70%) sensitive
Cytomegalovirus		
CMV ventriculitis	PCR in CSF	Sensitive and specific

CMV, Cytomegalovirus; *CNS,* central nervous system; *CSF,* cerebrospinal fluid; *EBV,* Epstein-Barr virus; *IgM,* immunoglobulin M; *PCR,* polymerase chain reaction.
From Goldman L, Schafer AI: *Goldman's Cecil medicine,* ed 24, Philadelphia, 2011, Saunders.

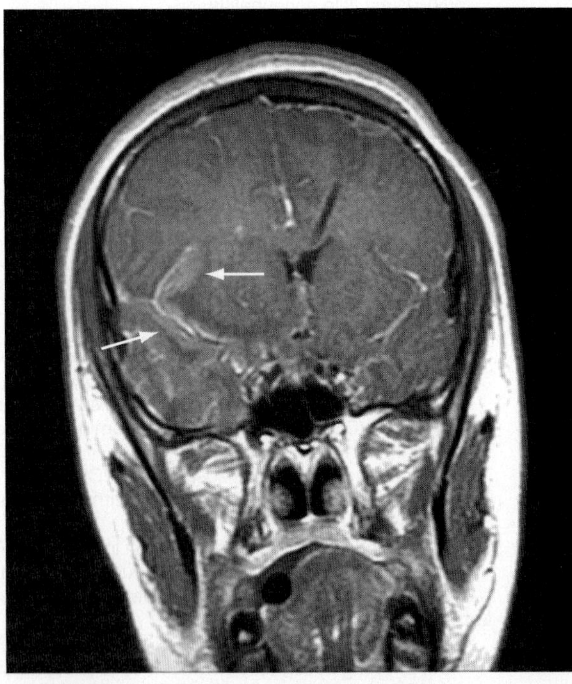

FIG. 3 Gadolinium-enhanced, T1-weighted brain magnetic resonance imaging in a teenager with herpes simplex virus encephalitis. The scan shows gadolinium enhancement in the right insular cortex *(arrows).* (Swaiman KF et al: *Swaiman's pediatric neurology, principles and practice,* ed 6, Philadelphia, 2017, Elsevier.)

- Ventilatory assistance for patients who are moribund or at risk for aspiration
- Avoidance of infusion of hypotonic fluids to minimize the risk of hyponatremia
- For patients who develop seizures: Anticonvulsant therapy and follow-up in a critical care setting
- For comatose patients:
  1. Aggressive care to avoid decubitus ulcers, contractures, and DVT
  2. Close attention to weights, input/output, and serum electrolytes
- Acyclovir 30 mg/kg/day IV total dose divided in q8 hour intervals for 14 days for herpes simplex encephalitis
- Short courses of corticosteroids to control brain edema and prevent herniation
- In patients with suspected rabies:
  1. Human rabies immune globulin (HRIG) should be given at a dose of 20 U/kg.
  2. Active immunization may be stimulated by rabies vaccine, which is grown on a human diploid cell line (HDCV) and has reduced the number of doses needed to five.
  3. If suspect animal is a dog or cat and can be found, observe closely for 10 days to detect rabid behavior; any significant illness in the animal should promptly initiate humane sacrifice of the animal with the brain submitted to local or state health departments for pathology and immunologic testing for rabies. Any wild animal suspected of rabies should be humanely sacrificed, if possible, and submitted for rabies testing immediately.
  4. If signs are seen, animal should be euthanized and its brain examined for signs of rabies.
- No specific pharmacologic therapy for most other viral pathogens

CHRONIC Rx

Some patients may develop permanent neurologic sequelae; these patients will benefit from intensive rehabilitation programs, including physical, occupational, and speech therapy.

DISPOSITION

- Patients with suspected encephalitis of any cause should generally be admitted for initial diagnostic workup and specific treatment (if available).
- Long-term management of patients with significant neurologic sequelae from encephalitis (e.g., memory defects, depression, difficulty with organization of thoughts, movement disorders) may benefit from rehabilitation services, home care, or nursing home placement.

REFERRAL

- To a neurologist for initial workup and management
- To an infectious disease specialist for diagnostic and therapeutic plan
- To a rehabilitation service for long-term evaluation and convalescent services

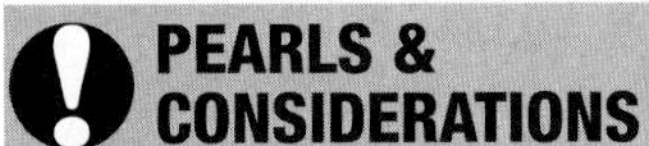

PEARLS & CONSIDERATIONS

- West Nile virus encephalitis occurs primarily in elderly patients >65 yr of age.
- Rabies may occur months after contact with the rabid animal, and the exposure (especially bat rabies) may have been seemingly insignificant and even inapparent.
- Experimental therapies are worthy of consideration for some forms of viral encephalitis (e.g., immune plasma, ribavirin, interferons), and expert consultation should be obtained early on for possible treatment interventions with promising therapies.

SUGGESTED READINGS

Available at ExpertConsult.com

RELATED CONTENT

Herpes Encephalitis (Patient Information)
Rabies (Related Key Topic)
West Nile Virus Infection (Related Key Topic)

AUTHOR: **GLENN G. FORT, M.D., M.P.H.**

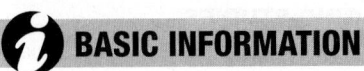

BASIC INFORMATION

DEFINITION

Encephalopathy is a clinical syndrome of global cognitive impairment characterized by impaired arousal, inattention, and disorientation.

SYNONYMS

Acute confusional state
Altered mental status

ICD-10CM CODES

G93.40	Encephalopathy, unspecified
G93.41	Metabolic encephalopathy
G93.49	Other encephalopathy
G92	Toxic encephalopathy
E51.2	Wernicke encephalopathy
G04.30	Acute necrotizing hemorrhagic encephalopathy, unspecified
G04.31	Postinfectious acute necrotizing hemorrhagic encephalopathy
G04.32	Postimmunization acute necrotizing hemorrhagic encephalopathy
G04.39	Other acute necrotizing hemorrhagic encephalopathy
G93.49	Other encephalopathy
I67.4	Hypertensive encephalopathy
I67.83	Posterior reversible encephalopathy syndrome
J10.81	Influenza due to other identified influenza virus with encephalopathy
J11.81	Influenza due to unidentified influenza virus with encephalopathy
P91.60	Hypoxic ischemic encephalopathy [HIE], unspecified
P91.61	Mild hypoxic ischemic encephalopathy [HIE]
P91.62	Moderate hypoxic ischemic encephalopathy [HIE]
P91.63	Severe hypoxic ischemic encephalopathy [HIE]

EPIDEMIOLOGY & DEMOGRAPHICS

POINT PREVALENCE: 1.1% of adults in the general population >55 yr, 10% to 40% of hospitalized elderly, and 60% of nursing home patients >75 yr; 100,000 to 200,000 cases annually with anoxic encephalopathy

RISK FACTORS: Advanced age; cancer; AIDS; terminal illness; bone marrow transplant; postoperative state; poor nutritional status; acute or chronic cardiac, pulmonary, renal, or hepatic dysfunction; history of previous insult to the brain; epilepsy; drug abuse; alcoholism; overtreatment and undertreatment of pain; use of anticholinergics, benzodiazepines, narcotics, barbiturates, and neuroleptics

PHYSICAL FINDINGS & CLINICAL PRESENTATION

- Common to all encephalopathies is a fluctuating level of arousal, poor attention, and disorientation. Table 1 summarizes stages of encephalopathy in chronic liver disease.
- Some patients may appear agitated and others lethargic.
- Delusions (fixed false beliefs) and hallucinations are common.
- Asterixis (negative myoclonus) is common.
- Other physical findings, such as fever, ascites, jaundice, or tachycardia, may vary depending on the underlying cause of encephalopathy.
- Because toxins and metabolic disturbances are common causes of encephalopathy, the history should focus on exposure to toxins, especially medications, and symptoms suggesting a concurrent illness such as a urinary tract infection, pneumonia, sepsis, meningitis, or encephalitis. Clinical events precipitating hepatic encephalopathy in patients with cirrhosis are summarized in Box 1.

ETIOLOGY

The final common pathway of all causes of encephalopathy is widespread neuronal dysfunction from either a structural or functional cause. Many conditions are reversible and carry a good prognosis if treated in a timely manner.

- Organ failure (e.g., hepatic encephalopathy [Fig. 1], hypoxia, hypercapnia, uremia).
- Infection: Systemic (e.g., urinary tract, pneumonia, sepsis) or involving the central nervous system (e.g., meningitis, encephalitis).
- Toxin ingestion or withdrawal: Special consideration should be paid to alcohol, benzodiazepines, anticholinergics, neuroleptics, antibiotics (such as fluoroquinolones), and recreational drugs.
- Metabolic disturbance: Hyperosmolar states, hypernatremia, hyponatremia, hyperglycemia, hypoglycemia, hypercalcemia, hypophosphatemia, acidosis, alkalosis, inborn errors of metabolism.
- Endocrinopathy: Hyperthyroidism, hypothyroidism, Cushing's syndrome, adrenal insufficiency, pituitary failure.
- Neoplasm: Tumors of the central nervous system, primary or metastatic; effects of distant tumors (e.g., paraneoplastic limbic encephalitis).
- Nutritional deficiency, mostly in alcoholics and chronically ill patients, such as vitamin B_1 deficiency (Wernicke encephalopathy).
- Seizures: Postictal state, nonconvulsive status epilepticus, complex partial seizures, absence seizures.
- Trauma: Concussion, contusion, subdural hematoma, epidural hematoma, diffuse axonal injury.
- Vascular: Ischemic and hemorrhagic strokes, vasculitis, venous thrombosis.
- Postanoxic encephalopathy.
- Psychiatric disease: Acute psychosis, depression with psychiatric features.
- Acute demyelinating disease: Acute disseminating encephalomyelitis, tumefactive multiple sclerosis.
- Other autoimmune diseases: Autoimmune encephalitis (associated with antibodies such as anti-NMDA), lupus cerebritis, cerebral vasculitis (primary angiitis of the central nervous system [CNS] of a secondary cerebral vasculitis).
- Other: Hypertensive encephalopathy, postoperative status, sleep deprivation.

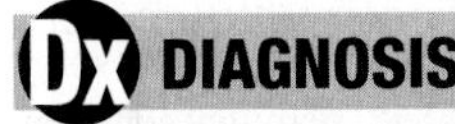

DIAGNOSIS

DIFFERENTIAL DIAGNOSIS

Differential diagnosis for encephalopathy is broad. It is typically helpful to distinguish toxic metabolic causes from primary neurologic causes.

TABLE 1 Stages of Encephalopathy in Chronic Liver Disease (West Haven Criteria)

Stage	Clinical Signs
Stage I	Mental slowness, euphoria or anxiety, shortened attention span, impaired calculating ability
Stage II	Lethargy or apathy, inappropriate behavior, personality change, more obvious problems with calculations
Stage III	Lethargic, somnolent, marked confusion and disorientation, but responds to verbal stimuli
Stage IV	Coma, patient may or may not respond to noxious stimuli

Patients with chronic liver disease rarely, if ever, demonstrate cerebral edema, regardless of the stage of encephalopathy.
From Vincent JL, Abraham E, Moore FA et al: *Textbook of critical care*, ed 7, Philadelphia, 2017, Elsevier.

BOX 1 Clinical Events Precipitating Hepatic Encephalopathy in Patients with Cirrhosis

Gastrointestinal hemorrhage
Infection (including spontaneous bacterial peritonitis)
Sepsis
Dehydration
Imbalance of electrolytes or acid-base
Renal failure
Drugs, toxins, medications (especially sedative-hypnotics or narcotics)
Illicit substances
Alcohol
Dietary indiscretion (excessive protein intake)

From Vincent JL, Abraham E, Moore FA et al: *Textbook of critical care*, ed 7, Philadelphia, 2017, Elsevier.

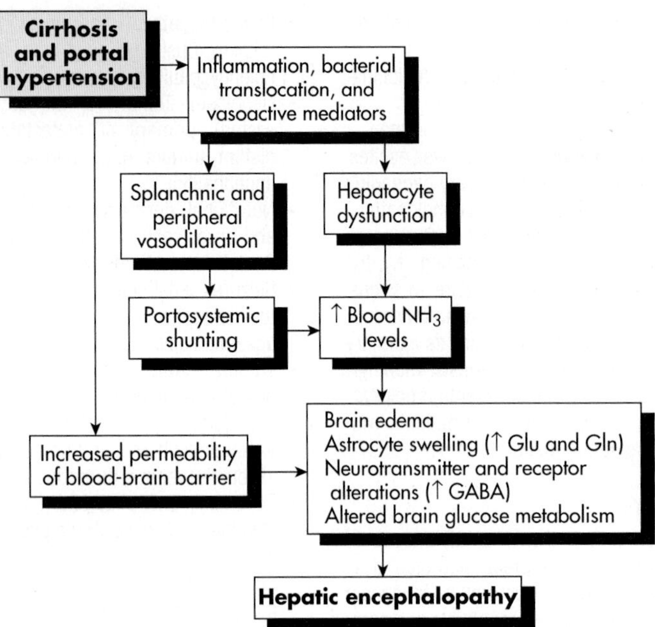

FIG. 1 Proposed pathophysiology of hepatic encephalopathy. *GABA*, gamma-aminobutyric acid; *Gln*, glutamine; *Glu*, glutamate; *NH_3*, ammonia. (From Feldman M et al [eds]: *Sleisenger and Fordtran's gastrointestinal and liver disease*, ed 10, Philadelphia, 2016, Saunders.)

- Dementia: Distinguished from encephalopathy by a history of slowly progressive cognitive decline over time (fluctuating cognitive function is rare except in diffuse Lewy body disease).
- Hypersomnia.
- Aphasia: Distinguished from encephalopathy by virtue of its representing a specific disorder of language rather than a global disturbance of cognitive function.
- Depression.
- Psychosis: Some overlap with encephalopathy because delusions and hallucinations may be common to both.
- Mania.
- Vegetative state from cerebral injury; these patients appear awake (eyes are open) but there is no content to their consciousness.
- Akinetic mutism: These patients do not talk and do not move; there is little fluctuation in their state, and there is no asterixis or other focal deficit.
- Locked-in syndrome: May be distinguished from encephalopathy by the presence of fixed neurologic deficits (e.g., paralysis of all four limbs); however, the patient is aware of his or her environment.

WORKUP

The best tool in the evaluation of encephalopathy is a good history and physical exam, which will help tailor the remainder of the diagnostic workup. Interview family members and other providers to identify preceding events, medication changes, and medical history. Evaluate focal deficits.

LABORATORY TESTS

- General chemistry: Electrolytes, glucose, creatinine, ammonia, blood urea nitrogen, transaminases, amylase, lipase
- Complete blood count
- Drug screen and alcohol level (must order ethylene glycol separately if suspected)
- Lumbar puncture if meningitis, encephalitis, autoimmune process, or subarachnoid hemorrhage with negative imaging is suspected
- HIV testing
- Endocrine testing: Cortisol level, thyroid function test
- Urinalysis and microscopy, urine culture, blood cultures
- Arterial blood gases

IMAGING STUDIES

The following imaging and diagnostic studies may be indicated depending on history and physical examination:

- Chest radiograph to rule out pneumonia
- Head CT to rule out intracranial hemorrhage, hydrocephalus, tumors
- Brain MRI with and without contrast and with diffusion-weighted images for suspected encephalitis, tumors, acute strokes, or acute autoimmune processes
- Magnetic resonance angiography/venography for strokes, arterial dissection, venous thrombosis
- Conventional angiography for CNS vasculitis and aneurysms
- EEG: Evaluate for subclinical status epilepticus

Rx TREATMENT

The encephalopathy itself is a symptom of these underlying problems. In general, it is best to avoid treating the symptom of encephalopathy with antipsychotics or sedatives. The best approach is to treat the underlying toxic or metabolic disturbance.

- Thiamine supplementation.
- Glucose for hypoglycemia.
- Antibiotics in cases of infections (choose an agent with good CNS penetration in cases of primary CNS infections; to prevent exacerbation of underlying problem, ensure also that the agent is not associated with causing encephalopathy, if possible).
- Insulin in hyperglycemic conditions (e.g., diabetic ketoacidosis, hyperosmolar nonketosis, and sepsis).
- Correct electrolyte disturbances properly.
- Treat organ failure and its sequelae; for example, implement appropriate therapy for hyperammonemia and uremia.
- Ensure hemodynamic stability (blood pressure and heart rate).

SUGGESTED READINGS

Available at ExpertConsult.com

RELATED CONTENT

Delirium (Related Key Topic)
Encephalitis, Acute Viral (Related Key Topic)
Hepatic Encephalopathy (Related Key Topic)

AUTHORS: **CHLOE MANDER NUNNELEY, M.D., JOSEPH S. KASS, M.D., J.D.,** and **JOSHUA CHALKELY, M.S., D.O.**

BASIC INFORMATION

DEFINITION

Infective endocarditis is an infection of the endocardial surface of the heart or mural endocardium. Box 1 describes the modified Duke criteria for the diagnosis of infective endocarditis.

ACUTE ENDOCARDITIS: Usually caused by *Staphylococcus aureus, Streptococcus pyogenes, S. pneumoniae,* and *Neisseria* organisms; classic clinical presentation of high fever, positive blood cultures, vascular and immunologic phenomenon

SUBACUTE ENDOCARDITIS: Usually caused by viridans streptococci in the presence of valvular pathology; less toxic, often indolent presentation with lower fevers, night sweats, fatigue

ENDOCARDITIS IN INJECTION DRUG USERS: Often involving *S. aureus* or *Pseudomonas aeruginosa* with variation that may be geographically influenced; tricuspid or multiple valvular involvement; high mortality rate of 50% to 60%

PROSTHETIC VALVE ENDOCARDITIS (EARLY): Usually caused by *S. aureus* (leading cause of PVE) within 2 mo of valve replacement; other organisms include *S. epidermidis,* gram-negative bacilli, diphtheroids, *Candida* organisms

PROSTHETIC VALVE ENDOCARDITIS (LATE): Typically develops >60 days after valvular replacement; involved organisms similar to early prosthetic valve endocarditis, including viridans streptococci, enterococci, and group D streptococci

NOSOCOMIAL ENDOCARDITIS: Secondary to intravenous catheters, TPN lines, pacemakers; coagulase-negative staphylococci, *S. aureus,* and streptococci most common

Non-HACEK gram-negative bacillus endocarditis is not primarily a disease of injection drug users. More than half of all cases are associated with health care contact

SYNONYMS

Bacterial endocarditis
Subacute bacterial endocarditis (SBE)
Endocarditis

ICD-10CM CODES

I33.0 Acute and subacute infective endocarditis
I33.9 Acute endocarditis, unspecified

EPIDEMIOLOGY & DEMOGRAPHICS

INCIDENCE (IN U.S.): 3 to 10 cases/100,000 persons/yr with the incidence rising

PEAK INCIDENCE: Females: Often <35 yr old; males: 45 to 65 yr old

NOSOCOMIAL ENDOCARDITIS: 14% to 28% of cases

PREVALENCE (IN U.S.): 0.3 to 3 cases/1000 hospital admissions. 40,000 to 50,000 new cases a yr in the U.S.

PREDOMINANT SEX: Male < female

PREDOMINANT AGE: 45 to 65 yr

ENDOCARDITIS TRENDS

From 1998 through 2013 the population of patients with prosthetic valve endocarditis increased from 2% to 13.8%, as did cardiac device-related endocarditis, from 1.3% to 4.1%, whereas native valve endocarditis decreased from 74.5% to 68.4%.

PHYSICAL FINDINGS & CLINICAL PRESENTATION

- Clinical manifestations of infective endocarditis are described in Table 1.
- Fever may be variable in presentation; may be high, hectic, or absent.
- Fever, chills, fatigue, and rigors occur in 25% to 80% of patients.
- Heart murmur may be absent in right-sided endocarditis.
- Embolic phenomenon with peripheral manifestations is found in 50% of patients.
- Skin manifestations include petechiae, Osler nodes (Fig. E1), splinter hemorrhages, Janeway lesions (Fig. E2).
- Splenomegaly is more common with subacute course.

BOX 1 Modified Duke Criteria for the Diagnosis of Infective Endocarditis[1]

Major Criteria

Positive blood cultures for infective endocarditis.
Typical microorganism for infective endocarditis from two separate blood cultures in the absence of a primary focus: *Streptococcus viridans, Streptococcus bovis*
HACEK group: *Haemophilus* species, *Actinobacillus actinomycetemcomitans, Cardiobacterium hominis, Eikenella corrodens,* and *Kingella kingae*
Community-acquired *Staphylococcus aureus* or enterococci
Persistently positive blood cultures, defined as recovery of a microorganism consistent with infective endocarditis from blood cultures drawn more than 12 hr apart or all of three or the majority of four or more separate blood cultures, with first and last drawn at least 1 hr apart
Single positive blood culture for *Coxiella burnetii* or antiphase IgG antibody titer >1:800
Evidence for endocardial involvement
TTE (TEE in prosthetic valve) showing oscillating intracardiac mass on a valve or supporting structures, in the path of regurgitant jet or on implanted material, in the absence of an alternative anatomic explanation, *or*
Abscess, *or*
New partial dehiscence of prosthetic valve.

Minor Criteria

Predisposition (e.g., prosthetic valve, intravenous drug use).
Fever: 38° C.
Vascular phenomena.
Immunologic phenomena.
Microbiologic evidence: Positive blood culture but not meeting major criteria.

TEE, Transesophageal echocardiogram; *TTE,* transthoracic echocardiogram.
[1] Adapted from Li JS et al: Proposed modifications to the Duke criteria for the diagnosis of infective endocarditis, *Clin Infect Dis* 30:633-638, 2000.
From Ballinger A: *Kumar & Clark's essentials of clinical medicine,* ed 6, Edinburgh, 2012, Saunders.

TABLE 1 Clinical Manifestations of Infective Endocarditis Myalgia/Arthralgia

Symptoms	Patients Affected (%)	Signs	Patients (%)
Fever	80	Fever	90
Chills	40	Heart murmur	85
Weakness	40	Changing murmur	5-10
Dyspnea	40	New murmur	3-5
Sweats	25	Embolic phenomenon	>50
Anorexia	25	Skin manifestations	18-50
Weight loss	25	Osler nodes	10-23
Malaise	25	Splinter hemorrhages	15
Cough	25	Petechiae	20-40
Skin lesions	20	Janeway lesion	<10
Stroke	20	Splenomegaly	20-57
Nausea/vomiting	20	Septic complications	20
Headache	20	(e.g., pneumonia, meningitis)	
Myalgia/arthralgia	15	Mycotic aneurysms	20
Edema	15	Clubbing	12-52
Chest pain	15	Retinal lesion	2-10
Abdominal pain and delirium/coma	15	Signs of renal failure	10-25
Delirium/coma	10-15		
Hemoptysis	10		
Back pain	10		

From Mandell GL et al: *Principles and practice of infectious diseases,* ed 6, Philadelphia, 2005, Churchill Livingstone.

ETIOLOGY

Staphylococcal infection is now the leading cause of native or prosthetic valve infection. Variation in incidence may occur that is influenced by the patient's risk for developing infection. Risk factors include hemodialysis (8%), IV drug use (10%), mitral regurgitation (43%), aortic regurgitation (26%), and rheumatic heart disease (3.3%).

ACUTE ENDOCARDITIS:
- *Staphylococcus aureus* (MSSA and MRSA)
- *Staphylococcus lugdunensis*
- *Streptococcus pneumoniae*
- Streptococcal species and groups A through G
- *Haemophilus influenzae*

SUBACUTE ENDOCARDITIS:
- Viridans streptococci (alpha-hemolytic)
- *S. bovis*
- Enterococci
- *S. aureus*

ENDOCARDITIS IN INJECTION DRUG USERS:
- *S. aureus*
- *P. aeruginosa*
- *Candida spp.*
- Enterococci

PROSTHETIC VALVE ENDOCARDITIS (EARLY):
- *S. epidermidis*
- *S. aureus*
- Gram-negative bacilli
- Group D streptococci

PROSTHETIC VALVE ENDOCARDITIS (LATE):
- *S. epidermidis*
- Viridans streptococci
- *S. aureus*
- Enterococci and group D streptococci

NOSOCOMIAL ENDOCARDITIS:
- Coagulase-negative staphylococci
- *S. aureus*
- Streptococci: Viridans, group B, enterococcus

HACEK ORGANISMS:
- Fastidious gram-negative bacilli
- *H. parainfluenzae*
- *H. aphrophilus*
- *A. actinomycetemcomitans*
- *Cardiobacterium hominis*
- *Eikenella corrodens*
- *Kingella kingae*

Other unusual pathogens:
- Q fever: *Coxiella burnetti*
- *Bartonella henselae* (etiologic agent of cat scratch disease)
- *Tropheryma whippelii* (Whipple disease)

RISK FACTORS

- Poor dental hygiene
- Long-term hemodialysis
- Diabetes mellitus
- HIV infection
- Mitral valve prolapse

Dx DIAGNOSIS

DIFFERENTIAL DIAGNOSIS

- Brain abscess
- FUO
- Pericarditis
- Meningitis
- Rheumatic fever
- Osteomyelitis
- *Salmonella*
- TB
- Bacteremia
- Pericarditis
- Glomerulonephritis

WORKUP

Physical examination to evaluate for the previous physical findings followed by laboratory testing (see "Laboratory Tests"). Fig. 3 describes a diagnostic evaluation of suspected endocarditis. The modified Duke criteria for diagnosis of endocarditis defines "major criteria" as persistently positive blood cultures of organisms typical of endocarditis or endocardial involvement (new valvular regurgitation or positive echocardiogram). "Minor criteria" are defined as presence of predisposing condition or injection drug use, fever, embolic vascular pneumonia (e.g., glomerulonephritis, rheumatoid factor), or positive blood cultures not meeting major criteria. Definite endocarditis is two major criteria or one major criteria and three minor criteria or five minor criteria or presence of organisms by culture or histologic examination of a vegetation.

LABORATORY TESTS

- Blood cultures: Three sets in first 24 hr. Table 2 describes causes of culture-negative endocarditis.
- More culturing if patient has received prior antibiotic.
- CBC (anemia possibly present, subacute).
- WBC (leukocytosis is higher in acute endocarditis).
- ESR and C-reactive protein (elevated).
- Positive rheumatoid factor (subacute endocarditis).
- Proteinuria, hematuria, RBC casts.
- Serologies or PCR for more unusual pathogens (*B. henselae, C. burnetti, etc.*)

IMAGING STUDIES

- Echocardiogram: Two-dimensional. Transthoracic echocardiography (TTE) (Fig. E4) is noninvasive and more easily available but has less-than-optimal sensitivity (50%-80%) for endocarditis.
- Transesophageal echocardiography (TEE): More sensitive in detecting vegetations and preferred diagnostic modality. It is especially helpful with prosthetic valves or in detecting perivalvular disease (Fig. E5).
- Electrocardiogram: Look for cardiac conduction abnormalities, injury pattern, or evidence of pericarditis—any such new findings are suggestive of myocardial abscess.

Rx TREATMENT

Initial IV antibiotic therapy (before culture results) is aimed at the most likely organism. The American Heart Association has developed guidelines based on the most frequently encountered bacteria. Tables 3 through 7 summarize treatment recommendations.

- **Native valve endocarditis** caused by penicillin-susceptible *S. viridians, S. gallolyticus* (previously called *S. bovis*), and other streptococci (MIC of penicillin ≤0.12 mcg/ml): Pen G 12 to 18 million U IV q24h continuous or divided q4h for 4 weeks **or** ceftriaxone 2 g IV or IM q day for 4 weeks for penicillin-allergic patients. Vancomycin at 30 mg/kg per 24 hr in 2 equally divided doses assuming normal kidney function, for 4 weeks.
- **Native valve endocarditis** caused by strains of viridians streptococci and *S. gallolyticus (S. bovis)* relatively resistant to penicillin (MIC >0.12 mcg/ml): Pen G: 24 million units per 24 hr IV either continuously or in 4 or 6 equally divided doses for 4 weeks **or** ceftriaxone 2 g per 24 hr IV or IM for 4 weeks **plus** gentamicin 3 mg/kg per 24 hr IV or IM in one dose or in 2 to 3 equally divided doses for 2 weeks or monotherapy with vancomycin 30 mg/kg per 24 hr IV in 2 equally divided doses for 4 weeks not to exceed 2 g per 24 hr unless concentrations in serum too low.
- **Native valve endocarditis** due to *Staphylococcus:*
  1. **MSSA:** Nafcillin (or oxacillin) 12 per 24 hr IV in 4 or 6 equally divided doses for 6 weeks **plus** optional addition of gentamicin 3 mg/kg per 24 hr IV or IM in 2 or 3 equally divided doses for 3 to 5 days **or** cefazolin 6 g per 24 hr IV in 3 equally divided doses for 6 weeks, **plus** optional addition of gentamicin 3 mg/kg per 24 hr IV or IM in 2 or 3 equally divided doses for 3 to 5 days. A newer antibiotic daptomycin has an indication for right-sided endocarditis with MSSA at 6 mg/kg IV q24h.
  2. **MRSA:** Vancomycin 30 mg/kg per 24 hr in 2 equally divided doses for 6 weeks; not to exceed 2 g per 24 hr unless concentrations in serum are low.
- For culture-negative native valve endocarditis one of the following regimens is suggested: Ampicillin-sulbactam: 12 g per 24 hr IV in 4 equally divided doses for 4 to 6 weeks **plus** gentamicin 3 mg/kg per 24 hr IV or IM in 3 equally divided doses for 4 to 6 weeks **or** vancomycin 30 mg/kg per 24 hr IV in 2 equally divided doses for 4 to 6 weeks; not to exceed 2 g per 24 hr unless concentrations in serum low **plus** gentamicin 3 mg/kg per 24 hr IV or IM in 3 equally divided doses for 4 to 6 weeks **plus** ciprofloxacin 1000 mg per 24 hr orally or 800 mg per 24 hr IV in 2 equally divided doses for 4 to 6 weeks.
- For treatment of native valve endocarditis due to HACEK organisms: Ceftriaxone 2 g per 24 hr IV or IM in 1 dose for 4 weeks **or** ampicillin-sulbactam 12 g per 24 hr IV in 4 equally divided doses for 4 weeks **or** ciprofloxacin 1000 mg per 24 hr orally or 800 mg per 24 hr IV in 2 equally divided doses for 4 weeks.
- **Patients with prosthetic valves** endocarditis:
- Methicillin-susceptible strains: Nafcillin or oxacillin 12 g per 24 hr IV in 6 equally divided doses for at least 6 weeks **plus** rifampin 900 mg per 24 hr IV or orally in 3 equally divided doses for at least 6 weeks **plus** gentamicin 3 mg/kg IV or IM in 2 or 3 equally divided doses for 2 weeks.

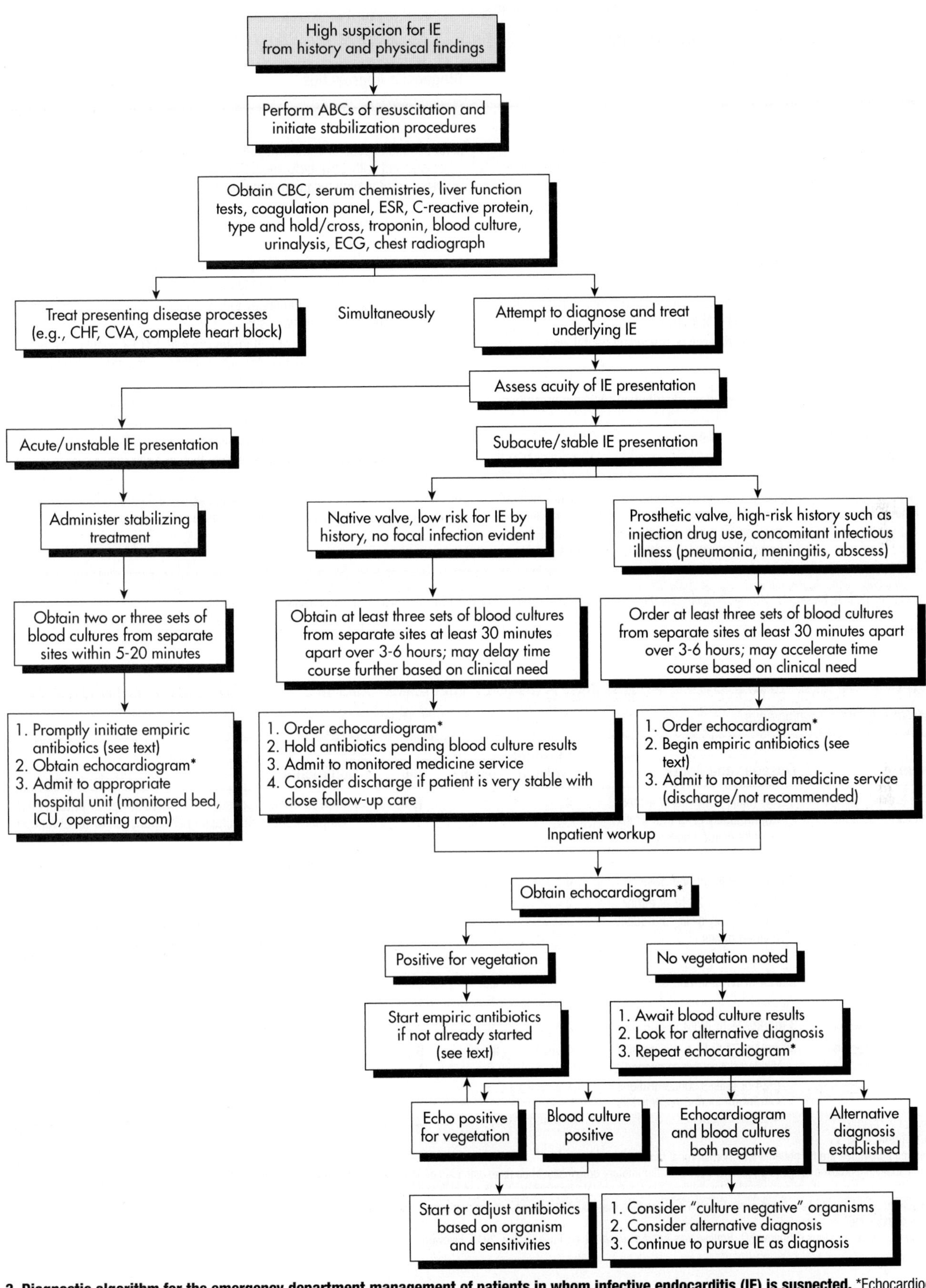

FIG. 3 Diagnostic algorithm for the emergency department management of patients in whom infective endocarditis (IE) is suspected. *Echocardiography can be performed via either the transthoracic (TTE) or transesophageal (TEE) technique. TEE is more invasive but is more sensitive for detecting vegetations and complications of IE, such as perivalvular abscesses; it is recommended for prosthetic valves; for situations in which optimal visualization by TTE will be difficult, such as emphysema and morbid obesity; for high suspicion of IE but normal TTE findings; and for high suspicion of a complication of IE, such as perivalvular abscess. Normal findings with either technique do not exclude IE if clinical suspicion is high. Echocardiograms can be repeated in an attempt to identify problems such as vegetations and abscesses that may not be noted initially. *ABCs*, Airway, breathing, and circulation; *CBC*, complete blood count; *CHF*, congestive heart failure; *CVA*, cerebrovascular accident; *ECG*, electrocardiogram; *ESR*, erythrocyte sedimentation rate; *ICU*, intensive care unit. (From Adams JG et al: *Emergency medicine, clinical essentials*, ed 2, Philadelphia, 2013, Elsevier.)

TABLE 2 Causes of Culture-Negative Endocarditis

Organism	Epidemiology and Exposures	Diagnostic Approaches
Aspergillus and other noncandidal fungi	Prosthetic valve	Lysis-centrifugation technique; also culture and histopathologic examination of any emboli
Bartonella spp.	*B. henselae:* Exposure to cats or cat fleas *B. quintana:* Louse infestation; homelessness, alcohol abuse	Most common cause of culture-negative IE in United States; serologic testing (may cross-react with *Chlamydia* spp.); PCR assay of valve or emboli is best test; lysis-centrifugation technique may be useful
Brucella spp.	Ingestion of unpasteurized milk or dairy products; livestock contact	Blood cultures ultimately become positive in 80% of cases with extended incubation time of 4-6 wk; lysis-centrifugation technique may expedite growth; serologic tests are available
Chlamydia psittaci	Bird exposure	Serologic tests available but exhibit cross-reactivity with *Bartonella;* monoclonal antibody direct stains on tissue may be useful; PCR assay now available
Coxiella burnetii (Q fever)	Global distribution; exposure to unpasteurized milk or agricultural areas	Serologic tests (high titers of antibody to both phase 1 and phase 2 antigens); also PCR assay on blood or valve tissue
HACEK spp.	Periodontal disease or preceding dental work	Although traditionally a cause of culture-negative IE, HACEK species are now routinely isolated from most liquid broth continuous monitoring blood culture systems without prolonged incubation times
Legionella spp.	Contaminated water distribution systems; prosthetic valves	Serology available; periodic subcultures onto buffered charcoal yeast extract medium; lysis-centrifugation technique; PCR assay available
Nutritionally variant streptococci	Slow and indolent course	Supplemented culture media or growth as satellite colonies around *Staphylococcus aureus* streak; antimicrobial susceptibility testing often requires processing specialized microbiology laboratory
Tropheryma whipplei (Whipple's disease)	Typical signs and symptoms include diarrhea, weight loss, arthralgias, abdominal pain, lymphadenopathy, central nervous system involvement; IE may be present without systemic symptoms	Histologic examination of valve with periodic acid–Schiff stain; valve cultures may be done using fibroblast cell lines; PCR assay on vegetation material

HACEK, *Haemophilus* spp., *Aggregatibacter* spp., *Cardiobacterium hominis, Eikenella corrodens,* and *Kingella* spp.; IE, infective endocarditis; PCR, polymerase chain reaction.
From Bennett JE, Dolin R, Blaser MJ: *Mandell, Douglas, and Bennett's principles and practice of infectious diseases*, ed 8, Philadelphia, 2015, Saunders.

TABLE 3 Therapy of Native Valve Endocarditis Caused by Highly Penicillin-Susceptible Viridans Group Streptococci and *Streptococcus gallolyticus*

Regimen	Dosage* and Route	Duration (weeks)	Class	loe	Comments
Aqueous crystalline penicillin G sodium	12-18 million U/24 hr IV either continuously or in four or six equally divided doses	4	IIa	B	Preferred in most patients >65 years of age or patients with impairment of 8th cranial nerve function or renal function
or					
Ceftriaxone sodium	2 g/24 hr IV/IM in one dose	4	IIa	B	
Aqueous crystalline penicillin G sodium	12-18 million U/24 hr IV either continuously or in six equally divided doses	2	IIa	B	2-week regimen not intended for patients with known cardiac or extracardiac abscess or for those with creatinine clearance of <20 ml/min, impaired 8th cranial nerve function, or *Abiotrophia, Granulicatella,* or *Gemella* spp. infection; gentamicin dosage should be adjusted to achieve peak serum concentration of 3-4 μg/ml and trough serum concentration of <1 μg/ml when three divided doses are used; there are no optimal drug concentrations for single daily dosing[‡]
or					
Ceftriaxone sodium	2 g/24 hr IV/IM in one dose	2	IIa	B	
plus					
Gentamicin sulfate[†]	3 mg/kg/24 hr IV/IM in one dose	2			
Vancomycin hydrochloride[‖]	30 mg/kg/24 hr IV in two equally divided doses, not to exceed 2 g/24 hr unless concentrations in serum are inappropriately low	4	IIa	B	Vancomycin recommended only for patients unable to tolerate penicillin or ceftriaxone; vancomycin dosage should be adjusted to a trough concentration range of 10-15 μg/ml

MIC ≤0.12 μg/ml.
*Dosages recommended are for patients with normal renal function.
†Other potentially nephrotoxic drugs (e.g., nonsteroidal antiinflammatory drugs) should be used with caution in patients receiving gentamicin therapy.
‡Data for once-daily dosing of aminoglycosides for children exist, but no data for treatment of IE are available.
§Vancomycin dosages should be infused over at least 1 hr to reduce the risk of histamine-release "red man" syndrome.
LOE, Level of evidence.
From Mann DL, Zipes DP, Libby P, Bonow RO: *Braunwald's heart disease*, ed 10, Philadelphia, 2015, Elsevier.

TABLE 4 Therapy of Native Valve Endocarditis Caused by Strains of Viridans Group Streptococci and *Streptococcus gallolyticus* Relatively Resistant to Penicillin

Regimen	Dosage* and Route	Duration (weeks)	Class	loe	Comments
Aqueous crystalline penicillin G sodium	24 million U/24 hr IV either continuously or in four to six equally divided doses	4	IIa	B	Patients with endocarditis caused by penicillin-resistant (MIC ≥0.5 μg/ml) strains should be treated with regimen recommended for enterococcal
or					
Ceftriaxone sodium	2 g/24 hr IV/IM in one dose	4	IIa	B	
plus					
Gentamicin sulfate†	3 mg/kg/24 hr IV/IM in one dose	2			
Vancomycin hydrochloride‡	30 mg/kg/24 hr IV in two equally divided doses, not to exceed 2 g/24 hr, unless serum concentrations are inappropriately low	4	IIb	C	Vancomycin‡ therapy recommended only for patients unable to tolerate penicillin or ceftriaxone therapy

Minimum inhibitory concentration (MIC) >0.12 μg/ml to <0.5 μg/ml.
*Dosages recommended are for patients with normal renal function.
†See Table 3 for appropriate dosage of gentamicin.
‡See Table 3 for appropriate dosage of vancomycin.
LOE, Level of evidence.
From Mann DL, Zipes DP, Libby P, Bonow RO: *Braunwald's heart disease*, ed 10, Philadelphia, 2015, Elsevier.

TABLE 5 Therapy for Endocarditis of Prosthetic Valves or Other Prosthetic Material Caused by Viridans Group Streptococci and *Streptococcus gallolyticus*

Regimen	Dosage* and Route	Duration (weeks)	Class	loe	Comments
Penicillin-Susceptible Strain (MIC ≤0.12 μg/ml)					
Aqueous crystalline penicillin G sodium	24 million U/24 hr IV either continuously or in four to six equally divided doses	6	IIa	B	Penicillin or ceftriaxone together with gentamicin has not demonstrated cure rates superior to those for monotherapy with penicillin or ceftriaxone for patients with highly susceptible strain; gentamicin should not be administered to patients with creatinine clearance of <30 ml/min.
or					
Ceftriaxone	2 g/24 hr IV/IM in one dose	6	IIa	B	
with or without					
Gentamicin sulfate†	3 mg/kg/24 hr IV/IM in one dose	2			
Vancomycin hydrochloride‡	30 mg/kg per 24 h IV in two equally divided doses	6	IIa	B	Vancomycin therapy recommended only for patients unable to tolerate penicillin or ceftriaxone.
Penicillin–Relatively or Fully Resistant Strain (MIC >0.12 μg/ml)					
Aqueous crystalline penicillin sodium	24 million U/24 hr IV either continuously or in four to six equally divided doses	6	IIa	B	
or					
Ceftriaxone	2 g/24 hr IV/IM in one dose	6	IIa	B	
plus					
Gentamicin sulfate	3 mg/kg/24 hr IV/IM in one dose	6			
Vancomycin hydrochloride	30 mg/kg/24 hr IV in two equally divided doses	6	IIb	C	Vancomycin therapy is recommended only for patients unable to tolerate penicillin or ceftriaxone.

*Dosages recommended are for patients with normal renal function.
†See Table 3 for appropriate dosage of gentamicin.
‡See text and Table 3 for appropriate dosage of vancomycin.
LOE, Level of evidence.
From Mann DL, Zipes DP, Libby P, Bonow RO: *Braunwald's heart disease*, ed 10, Philadelphia, 2015, Elsevier.

TABLE 6 Therapy for Endocarditis Caused by Staphylococci in the Absence of Prosthetic Materials

Regimen	Dosage* and Route	Duration (weeks)	Class	loe	Comments
Oxacillin-Susceptible Strains					
Nafcillin or oxacillin†	12 g/24 hr IV in four to six equally divided doses	6	IIa	B	For complicated right-sided IE and for left-sided IE; for uncomplicated right-sided IE, 2 weeks (see text)
For penicillin-allergic (non-anaphylactoid type) patients:					Consider skin testing for oxacillin-susceptible staphylococci and questionable history of immediate-type hypersensitivity to penicillin
Cefazolin	6 g/24 hr IV in three equally divided doses	6	IIa	B	Cephalosporins should be avoided in patients with anaphylactoid-type hypersensitivity to β-lactams; vancomycin should be used in these cases‡
Oxacillin-Resistant Strains					
Vancomycin‡	30 mg/kg/24 hr IV in two equally divided doses	6	IIa	B	Adjust vancomycin dosage to a trough serum concentration of 10-15 μg/ml (see text for vancomycin alternatives)

*Dosages recommended are for patients with normal renal function.
†Penicillin G 24 million U/24 hr IV in four to six equally divided doses may be used in place of nafcillin or oxacillin if strain is penicillin-susceptible (MIC ≤0.1 μg/ml) and does not produce beta-lactamase.
‡For specific dosing adjustment and issues concerning vancomycin, see Table 3 footnotes.
LOE, Level of evidence.
From Mann DL, Zipes DP, Libby P, Bonow RO: *Braunwald's heart disease*, ed 10, Philadelphia, 2015, Elsevier.

TABLE 7 Therapy for Endocarditis of Prosthetic Valves or Other Prosthetic Material Caused by Staphylococci

Regimen	Dosage* and Route	Duration (weeks)	Class	loe	Comments
Oxacillin-Susceptible Strains					
Nafcillin or oxacillin	12 g/24 hr IV in six equally divided doses	≥6	IIa	B	Penicillin G 24 million U/24 hr IV in four to six equally divided doses may be used in place of nafcillin or oxacillin if strain is penicillin susceptible (MIC ≤ 0.1 μg/ml) and does not produce beta-lactamase; vancomycin should be used in patients with immediate-type hypersensitivity reactions to beta-lactam antibiotics (see Table 3 for dosing guidelines); cefazolin may be substituted for nafcillin or oxacillin in patients with nonimmediate hypersensitivity reactions to penicillins
Plus					
Rifampin	900 mg/24 hr IV/PO in three equally divided doses	≥6			
Plus					
Gentamicin†	3 mg/kg/24 hr IV/IM in two or three equally divided doses	2			
Oxacillin-Resistant Strains					
Vancomycin	30 mg/kg/24 hr in two equally divided doses	≥6	IIa	B	Adjust vancomycin to achieve a trough serum concentration of 10-15 μg/ml (see text for gentamicin alternatives)
plus					
Rifampin	900 mg/24 hr IV/PO in three equally divided doses	≥6			
plus					
Gentamicin	3 mg/kg/24 hr IV/IM in two or three equally divided doses	2			

*Dosages recommended are for patients with normal renal function.
†Gentamicin should be administered in close proximity to vancomycin, nafcillin, or oxacillin dosing.
LOE, Level of evidence.
From Mann DL, Zipes DP, Libby P, Bonow RO: *Braunwald's heart disease*, ed 10, Philadelphia, 2015, Elsevier.

- Methicillin-resistant strains: Vancomycin 30 mg/kg per 24 hr in two equally divided doses for at least 6 weeks **plus** rifampin 900 mg per 24 hr IV or orally in three equally divided doses for at least 6 weeks **plus** gentamicin 3 mg/kg per 24 hr IV or IM in two or three equally divided doses for 2 weeks.

Antibiotic therapy after identification of the organism should be guided by susceptibility testing, preferably by formal testing by MIC (minimum inhibitory concentration).

DISPOSITION

- The patient may need outpatient IV antibiotic therapy, and arrangements need to be made to ensure safe vascular access and continuity of care with outpatient IV therapy team.
- Long-term follow-up is essential after therapy has ended; relapse of endocarditis may occur.
- Prophylaxis with antibiotics will be needed before dental procedures as a previous episode of endocarditis increases the risk of recurrent endocarditis associated with transient bacteremia from dental procedures.

REFERRAL

- To an infectious disease specialist.
- To a cardiologist or a cardiac surgeon if evidence of heart failure, refractory infection, myocardial abscess, valve disruption, or major embolic events occur.
- The timing and indications for surgical intervention to prevent systemic embolism in infective endocarditis remain controversial. Trials have shown that early surgery in patients with infective endocarditis and large vegetations significantly reduced death and embolic events by decreasing the risk of systemic embolism.

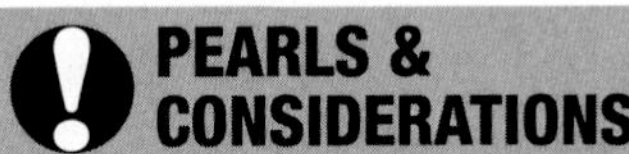

COMMENTS

- For endocarditis prophylaxis refer to Section V.
- In regards to antibiotic prophylaxis before dental procedures in patients with orthopedic implants, the 2013 guidelines from the American Academy of Orthopedic Surgeons (AAOS) and the American Dental Association (ADA) advises clinicians to consider discontinuing the practice of routinely prescribing prophylactic antibiotics for patients with hip and knee prosthetic joint implants undergoing dental procedures.
- *Streptococcus viridians* are a large group of commensal bacteria that are either alpha hemolytic on blood agar plates or nonhemolytic. Common members of this family include *S. mutans*, *S. anginosus*, *S. mitis*, *S. sanguis*, *S. oralis,* and *S. salivarius.* These tend to be oral/dental flora and most highly penicillin susceptible.
- Recent European trials have shown that in patients with endocarditis in the left side of the heart who were in stable condition, changing to oral antibiotic treatment was non-inferior to continued intravenous antibiotic treatment.[1] Additional trials will be necessary before changing current parenteral antibiotic guidelines to include oral antibiotic regimens.

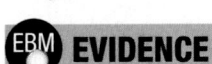

Available at ExpertConsult.com

SUGGESTED READINGS

Available at ExpertConsult.com

RELATED CONTENT

Endocarditis (Patient Information)

AUTHOR: **GLENN G. FORT, M.D., M.P.H.**

[1]Iverson K, et al.: Partial oral versus intravenous antiobiotic treatment of endocarditis, *N Engl J Med* 380:415–424, 2019.

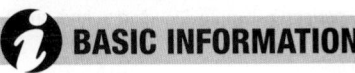

BASIC INFORMATION

DEFINITION

Endometrial carcinoma (EC) is the malignant transformation of endometrial glands with stromal invasion. The changes are typified by irregular nuclear membranes, nuclear atypia, mitotic activity, loss of glandular pattern, loss of intervening stroma, and irregular cell size. The two main histologic subcategories of EC (Table 1), low-grade endometrioid (Type 1) and high-grade endometrioid and nonendometrioid EC (Type 2), show unique molecular aberrations and differing clinical behaviors.

SYNONYMS

Uterine cancer (some forms)
Carcinoma of the endometrium
EC

ICD-10CM CODES
C54.1 Malignant neoplasm of endometrium
C55 Malignant neoplasm of uterus, part unspecified
C54.9 Malignant neoplasm of corpus uteri, unspecified

EPIDEMIOLOGY & DEMOGRAPHICS

INCIDENCE: 25.4 cases per 100,000 persons; approximately 63,000 new cases annually. It is the most common gynecologic malignancy in the U.S. 2.8% of women will be diagnosed in their lifetime

PREDOMINANCE: Median age at diagnosis: 62 yr; only 5% occur in women <40 yr; 5-yr survival >80%

RISK FACTORS: Obesity, diabetes, nulliparity, early menarche and late menopause, unopposed estrogen therapy, tamoxifen use, oligoovulation with chronic unopposed estrogen exposure such as with polycystic ovary syndrome (PCOS), endometrial atypical hyperplasia, endometrial polyps (malignancy is found in 3.6% of endometrial polyps), family history. The relative risk for endometrial cancer is summarized in Table 2.

PHYSICAL FINDINGS & CLINICAL PRESENTATION

- Abnormal uterine bleeding or postmenopausal bleeding in 90%
- Pyometra or hematometra
- Abnormal Pap smear
- Incidental finding at hysterectomy

ETIOLOGY

Endogenous or exogenous chronic unopposed estrogen stimulation of the endometrium

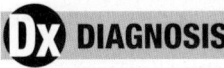

DIAGNOSIS

DIFFERENTIAL DIAGNOSIS

- Endometrial atypical hyperplasia
- Transvaginal sonography
- Other genital tract malignancy
- Uterine polyps
- Atrophic vaginitis
- Granulosa cell tumor
- Fibroid uterus
- Adenomyosis

WORKUP

- Complete history and physical examination
- Endometrial biopsy or dilation and curettage (Table 3)
- Assessment of operative risk
- Staging (Tables 4 and 5)

LABORATORY TESTS

- Complete blood count
- Prothrombin time and partial thromboplastin time if bleeding is heavy
- Chemistry profile including liver function tests
- Consider CA-125 level

IMAGING STUDIES

- Chest x-ray
- CT scan if concern for metastatic disease, and/or pelvic ultrasound (Fig. 1)

TABLE 1 Pathogenetic Subsets of Endometrial Carcinoma

Parameter	Type I	Type II
Age	50s–60s	60s-70s
Obesity	Common	Uncommon
Estrogenic stimuli	Common	Uncommon
Endometrium	Anovulatory	Atrophic
Precursor	Endometrial intraepithelial neoplasia	Presumed EmGD
Transition	Slow	Unknown
Type	Endometrioid	Papillary serous or mixed
Molecular genetics	MSI, *PTEN* mutation; loss of PAX2	p53 mutation, 1p deletions; loss of PAX2
Familial	Hereditary nonpolyposis colonic cancer syndrome	
Spread	Lymph nodes	Peritoneum
Concurrent ovarian	Common	Uncommon
Prognosis	Good	Poor

EmGD, Endometrial glandular dysplasia; *MSI,* microsatellite instability.
Crum CP et al: *Diagnostic gynecologic and obstetric pathology,* ed 3, Philadelphia, 2018, Elsevier.

TABLE 2 Risk Factors for Endometrial Cancer

Factor	Relative Risk
Overweight (lb)	
• 20-50	3.0
• 50+	10.0
Nulliparous	
• Versus one child	2.0
• Versus five children	5.0
Late menopause (>52 vs. 49 yr)	2.4
Diabetes mellitus	2.7
Unopposed estrogen therapy	6.0
Tamoxifen therapy	2.0
Sequential oral contraceptives	7.0
Combination oral contraceptives	0.5
Cowden syndrome (*PTEN* mutation)	Three- to fivefold increased risk
Hereditary nonpolyposis colonic cancer syndrome	40%-60% lifetime risk
Family member with endometrial cancer	3.4

Crum CP et al: *Diagnostic gynecologic and obstetric pathology,* ed 3, Philadelphia, 2018, Elsevier.

TABLE 3 Differential Diagnosis of Endometrial Carcinoma (Curettings)

Parameter	Mimicking	Differential Diagnosis
Gland architecture	Cancer	Telescoping artifact; stromal collapse breakdown; sectioning artifacts
	Benign	Microglandular mucinous carcinoma; surface endometrioid carcinoma
Nuclear atypia	Cancer	Surface or glandular repair; Arias-Stella changes (hormonal therapy); radiation effect
Papillary changes	Cancer	Exfoliation artifact; stromal breakdown with papillary changes; papillary syncytial changes
	Benign	Papillary mucinous carcinoma

Crum CP et al: *Diagnostic gynecologic and obstetric pathology,* ed 3, Philadelphia, 2018, Elsevier.

TABLE 4 Revised FIGO Staging for Endometrial Cancer (Adopted 2009)

Stages*	Characteristic
I	Tumor confined to the corpus uteri
IA	No or less than half myometrial invasion
IB	Invasion equal to or more than half of the myometrium
II	Tumor invades cervical stroma but does not extend beyond the uterus†
III	Local or regional spread of the tumor
III_A	Tumor invades serosa of the corpus uteri or the adnexa‡
III_B	Vaginal or parametrial involvement‡
III_C	Metastases to pelvic or paraaortic lymph nodes‡
III_{C1}	Positive pelvic nodes
III_{C2}	Positive paraaortic lymph nodes with or without positive pelvic lymph nodes
IV	Tumor invades bladder or bowel mucosa, or distant metastasis
IV_A*	Tumor invasion of bladder or bowel mucosa
IV_B	Distant metastases, including intraabdominal or inguinal lymph nodes

*G1, G2, or G3.
†Endocervical glandular involvement only should be considered as stage I and no longer as stage II.
‡Positive cytology has to be reported separately without changing the stage.
FIGO, Fédération Internationale de Gynécologie et d'Obstétrique (International Federation of Gynecology and Obstetrics).
From Lobo RA et al: *Comprehensive gynecology*, ed 7, Philadelphia, 2017, Elsevier.

TABLE 5 Carcinoma of the Corpus Uteri: Patients Treated in 1990-1992: Survival by 1988 FIGO Surgical Stage, *N* = 5562

Stage	5-Year Survival Rate
I_A	90.9%
I_B	88.2%
I_C	81.0%
II	71.6%
III	51.4%
IV	8.9%

FIGO, Fédération Internationale de Gynécologie et d'Obstétrique (International Federation of Gynecology and Obstetrics).
From Lobo RA et al: *Comprehensive gynecology*, ed 7, Philadelphia, 2017, Elsevier.

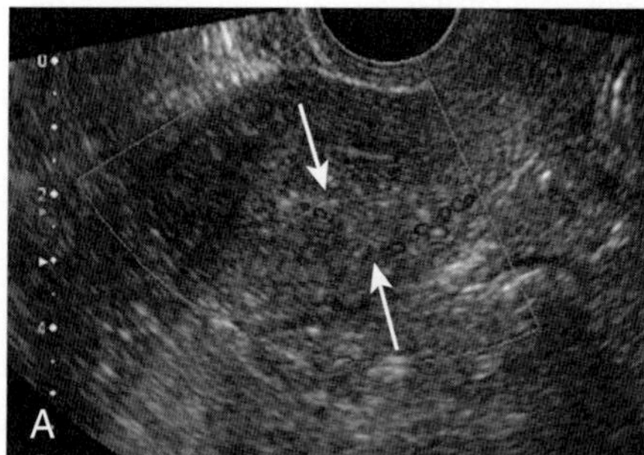

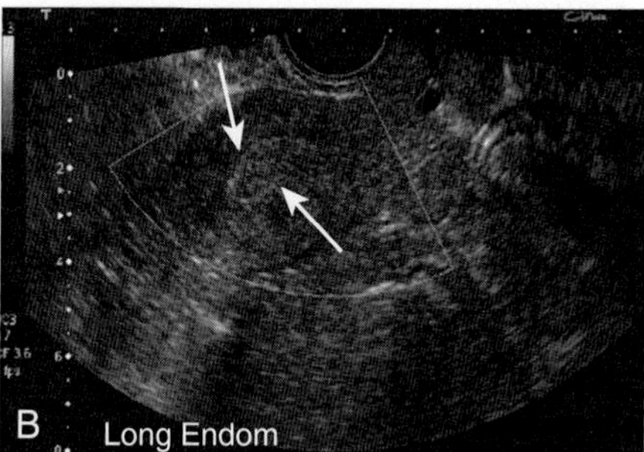

FIG. 1 A 48-year-old woman with endometrial carcinoma. A, Endovaginal ultrasound (US) showing thickened, heterogeneous, cystic, and vascular hyperechoic tissue filling the endometrial cavity *(arrows).* **B,** Second, sagittal US image showing the same *(arrows).* (*Endom*, Endometrium. From Fielding JR et al: *Gynecologic imaging*, Philadelphia, 2011, Saunders.)

- Transvaginal ultrasound (Fig. 2) in postmenopausal women with vaginal bleeding

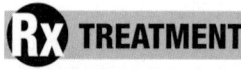

TREATMENT

NONPHARMACOLOGIC THERAPY

- Surgery is the mainstay of treatment, with or without adjuvant radiation and/or chemotherapy, depending on tumor histology, stage, and grade. Laparoscopic surgery for early-stage EC is as safe and effective as laparotomy. Robotic laparoscopy procedures have increased significantly in recent yrs for this indication.
- Surgery generally consists of pelvic washings, total abdominal hysterectomy and bilateral salpingo-oophorectomy, selective pelvic and periaortic lymphadenectomy, and omental biopsy depending on stage, grade, and histology.
- Brachytherapy and/or teletherapy are added in an advanced stage.
- Chemotherapy (carboplatin, paclitaxel) or hormonal therapy (tamoxifen, progestational agents, aromatase inhibitors) may also be used, especially for advanced or recurrent endometrial cancers.
- Hormonal therapy, commonly a levonorgestrel intrauterine device, is an option for some young women with early-stage, low-grade EC who wish to preserve fertility. This choice should be discussed with a gynecologic oncologist.

ACUTE GENERAL Rx

- A thorough workup should be completed before any therapy for EC.
- Surgery hysterectomy with bilateral salpingo-oophorectomy is the treatment of choice.

CHRONIC Rx

- Physical and pelvic examination every 3 mo for 2 yr, then every 6 mo for 2 yr, and annually thereafter with imaging as clinically indicated
- Hormone replacement (combination) a consideration in low-risk patients (stage I or early stage II)

DISPOSITION

- Survival is generally defined by the stage of the disease and histology.
- The majority of cases present early, and the 5-yr survival is generally good (Fig. 3).
- Some histologic types (clear cell, papillary serous) have worse survival rates, as they tend to be more aggressive with higher rates of metastatic disease at the time of diagnosis.

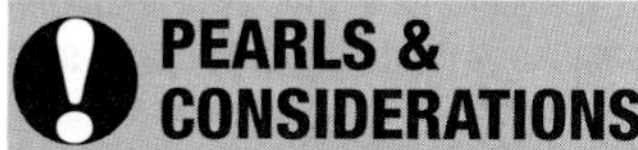

PEARLS & CONSIDERATIONS

Any woman with postmenopausal bleeding or abnormal uterine bleeding with risk factors for endometrial cancer needs evaluation by a gynecologist and either endometrial biopsy and/or pelvic ultrasound. When endometrial cancer is diagnosed, the patient should be cared for by a gynecologic oncologist and undergo surgical staging in a minimally invasive procedure when possible.

SUGGESTED READINGS

Available at ExpertConsult.com

RELATED CONTENT

Endometrial Cancer (Patient Information)
Dysfunctional Uterine Bleeding (Related Key Topic)
Uterine Malignancy (Related Key Topic)

AUTHORS: **TONI PICERNO, D.O.,** and **MARK ELIOT BOROWSKY, M.D.**

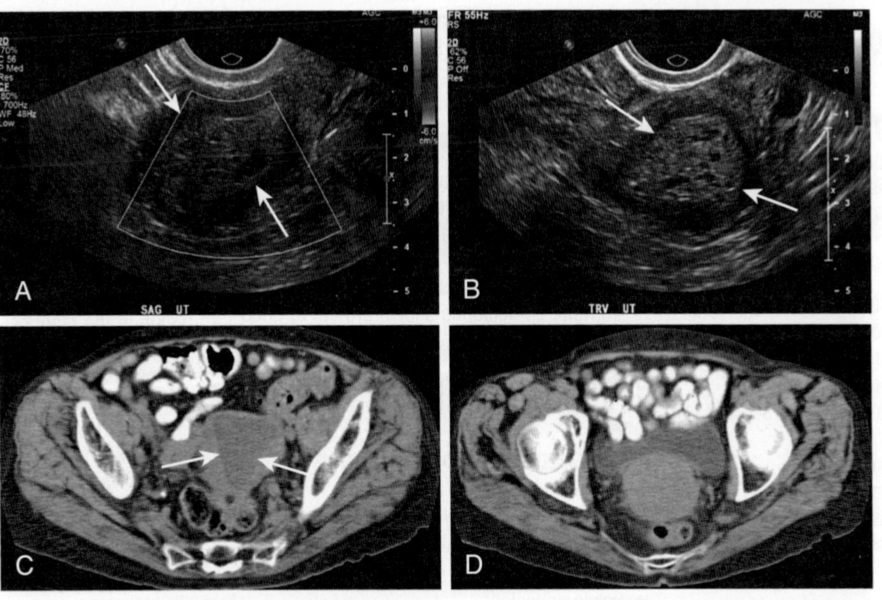

FIG. 2 A 56-year-old woman with endometrial carcinoma. A, Sagittal ultrasound (US) image showing thickened cystic echogenic soft tissue filling the endometrial cavity *(arrows).* **B,** Axial US image showing thickened cystic echogenic soft tissue filling the endometrial cavity *(arrows).* **C,** Non–contrast-enhanced axial computed tomographic (CT) image showing low-attenuation tissue filling the endometrial canal *(arrows)* in a postmenopausal patient. Note fundal thinning. **D,** Non–contrast-enhanced axial CT image showing cervical soft tissue fullness. (From Fielding JR et al: *Gynecologic imaging*, Philadelphia, 2011, Saunders.)

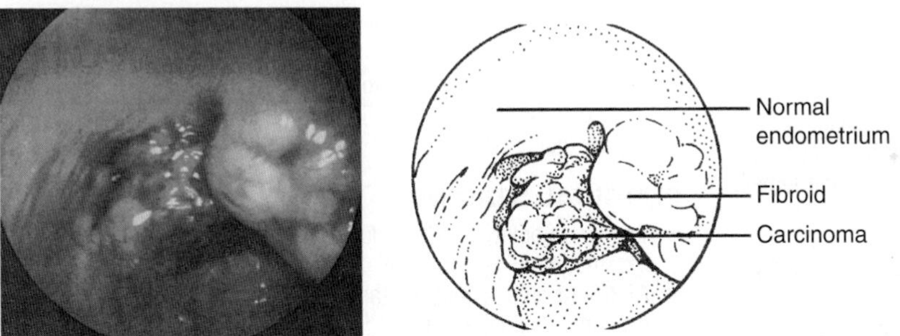

FIG. 3 Stage I endometrial carcinoma. A small carcinoma can be seen adjacent to a uterine fibroid in this hysteroscopy photograph. Occasionally, a tumor this small may be missed on curettage. (From Skarin AT: *Atlas of diagnostic oncology*, ed 4, St Louis, 2010, Mosby.)

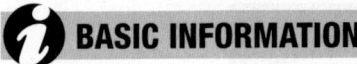

BASIC INFORMATION

DEFINITION

Endometriosis is defined as the presence of functioning endometrial glands and stroma outside the uterine cavity. It is a chronic, estrogen-dependent condition that causes dysmenorrhea and pelvic pain.

ICD-10CM CODES

N80.0	Endometriosis of uterus
N80.1	Endometriosis of ovary
N80.2	Endometriosis of fallopian tube
N80.3	Endometriosis of pelvic peritoneum
N80.4	Endometriosis of rectovaginal septum and vagina
N80.5	Endometriosis of intestine
N80.6	Endometriosis in cutaneous scar
N80.8	Other endometriosis
N80.9	Endometriosis, unspecified

EPIDEMIOLOGY & DEMOGRAPHICS

PREVALENCE:

- Endometriosis affects 10% of reproductive-aged women.
- Women with dysmenorrhea: 40% to 60%.
- Subfertile women: 28% to 50%.
- Incidence peaks at approximately 40 yr.

MOST COMMON AGE AT DIAGNOSIS: 25 to 29 yr.

GENETICS:

- Familial association: If first-degree relative is affected, the patient has a seven- to tenfold increased risk of having the disease.
- Polygenic-multifactorial inheritance pattern.
- 6.9% occurrence rate in first-degree female relatives.

PHYSICAL FINDINGS & CLINICAL PRESENTATION

- Classic triad is dysmenorrhea, dyspareunia, and infertility.
- Presence of pelvic pain does not correlate with the total area of endometriosis (stage of disease), type of lesion, or volume of disease but is correlated with the depth of infiltration.
- Other symptoms include abnormal bleeding (premenstrual spotting, menorrhagia), cyclic abdominal pain, intermittent constipation/diarrhea, dyschezia, dysuria, hematuria, and urinary frequency.
- Rare manifestations: Catamenial hemothorax, bloody pleural effusion, massive ascites occurring during menses.
- Most severe discomfort is associated with lesions >1 cm in depth.
- Bimanual examination may reveal tender uterosacral ligaments, cul-de-sac nodularity, induration of the rectovaginal septum, fixed retroversion of the uterus, adnexal mass, and generalized or localized tenderness.

ETIOLOGY

- Reflux and direct implantation theory: Retrograde menstruation with implantation of viable endometrial cells to surrounding pelvic structures (Sampson theory).
- Coelomic metaplasia theory: Transformation of multipotential cells of the coelomic epithelium into endometrium-like cells.
- Vascular dissemination theory: Transport of endometrial cells to distant sites by the uterine vascular and lymphatic systems.
- Autoimmune disease theory: Disorder of immune surveillance allows growth of endometrial implants.

DIAGNOSIS

DIFFERENTIAL DIAGNOSIS

- Ectopic pregnancy
- Acute appendicitis
- Chronic appendicitis
- Pelvic inflammatory disease (PID)
- Pelvic adhesions
- Hemorrhagic cyst
- Hernia
- Irritable bowel syndrome
- Uterine leiomyomata
- Adenomyosis
- Nerve entrapment syndrome
- Interstitial cystitis

WORKUP

- Thorough history and physical examination including ultrasound.
- Definitive diagnosis of endometriosis can be made only by histologic confirmation during surgery (gold standard).

SURGICAL STAGING

- American Society for Reproductive Medicine classification system for endometriosis (ASRM revised 1996) is the most widely accepted staging system.
- Value: Uniform recording of operative findings.
- Limitations
  1. Not a good predictor of successful pregnancy after treatment.
  2. Does not correlate well with the symptoms of pain, dyspareunia, or infertility.

Stage I	Minimal
Stage II	Mild
Stage III	Moderate
Stage IV	Severe

LABORATORY TESTS

Cancer antigen 125 (CA125): Limited overall value in the diagnosis of endometriosis

- Also elevated in ovarian epithelial neoplasm, myomas, adenomyosis, acute PID, ovarian cysts, pancreatitis, chronic liver disease, menstruation, and pregnancy.
- CA125 value >35 U/ml: Positive predictive value of 0.58 and a negative predictive value of 0.96 for the presence of endometriosis.

IMAGING STUDIES

- Ultrasound: For evaluating adnexal mass; ultrasound characteristics may suggest endometriomas versus other benign or malignant ovarian conditions but persistent solid or cystic-solid ovarian masses require definitive tissue diagnosis with laparoscopy.
- MRI:
  1. Highly accurate in detecting endometriomas.
  2. Limited sensitivity in detecting diffuse pelvic endometriosis, especially if sessile lesions.
- CT scan may show adnexal masses of varying density (Fig. 1).

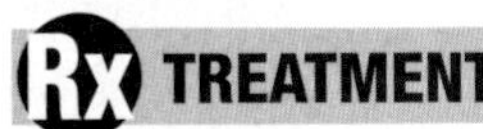

TREATMENT

NONPHARMACOLOGIC THERAPY

Expectant management (observation for 5 to 12 months) for stage I or stage II endometriosis-associated infertility. Evaluation should take place if the couple meets the diagnostic criteria for infertility.

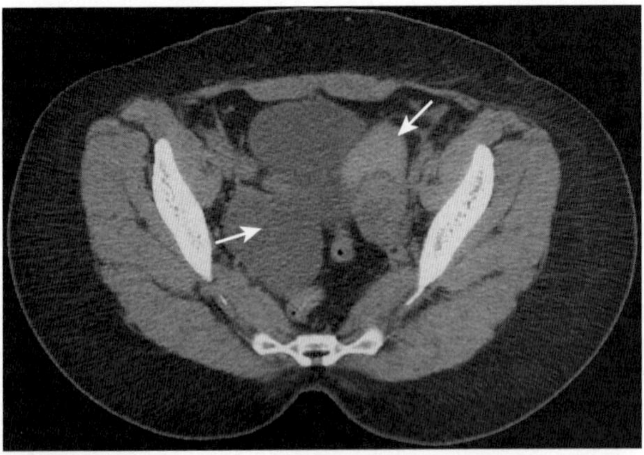

FIG. 1 Computed tomographic scan demonstrates adnexal masses of varying density, subsequently proven to be endometriomas. (From Fielding JR et al: *Gynecologic imaging,* Philadelphia, 2011, Saunders.)

ACUTE GENERAL Rx

Nonsteroidal antiinflammatory drugs for symptomatic relief of dysmenorrhea.

CHRONIC Rx

PHARMACOLOGIC MANAGEMENT: Estrogen-progesterone:
- State of "pseudopregnancy" created by continuous (discarding pill pack when placebo pills remaining and starting active pills from new pill pack) use of combination oral contraceptives for minimum of 6 months and continuing indefinitely.

Progestins:
- Medroxyprogesterone acetate 10 to 30 mg orally qd and occasionally up to 100 mg orally qd.
- Alternatively, 100 mg IM q2wk for four doses, followed by 200 mg IM monthly for 4 mo.
- Comparison with danazol: Progestins cost less, have a more tolerable side-effect profile, and have comparable efficacy with regard to pain relief and so are often the first-line drug. Very little justification for the use of danazol.

Gonadotropin-releasing hormone (GnRH) agonists:
- Induces medical menopause.
- Use usually limited to 6 to 12 months due to hypoestrogenic effects such as osteopenia or osteoporosis but can be given longer in certain circumstances, particularly when paired with estrogen add-back therapy. Referral to specialist strongly advised.
- Elagolix is an oral GnRH antagonist that provides partial to nearly full estrogen suppression. Dosage is 150 mg once daily or 200 mg twice daily. It is effective in improving dysmenorrhea and non-menstrual pain, but is associated with hypoestrogenic side effects (hot flashes, hyperlipidemia, decreased bone density).
- Leuprolide acetate depot 3.75 mg IM monthly or 11.25 mg IM q3mo or nafarelin 400 mcg nasal puffs bid or goserelin 3.6 mg SC monthly.
- Add-back therapy for protection against vasomotor symptoms and bone loss: Norethindrone acetate 5 mg PO qd alone or in combination with conjugated estrogen 0.625 mg orally qd.
- Add-back therapy allows gonadotropin-releasing hormone (GnRH) agonist use to be extended to 1 yr based on limited studies available.

Alternative therapies for inhibition of estrogen action currently under investigation are:
- Aromatase inhibitors: Anastrozole, letrozole
- SERM: Raloxifene
- Agents enhancing cell-mediated immunity are cytokines (interleukin-12 and interferon-α2b)
- Immunomodulators (loxoribine, levamisole)
- Antiinflammatory: Pentoxifylline

SURGICAL MANAGEMENT: Conservative:
- Directed at enhancing fertility or treating pain unresponsive to first-line medical treatment.
- Usually accomplished through laparoscopy.
- Removal or destruction of endometriotic implants by excision, electrocautery, or laser.
- Cystectomy for endometrioma; must remove cyst wall to be effective long-term.
- Laparoscopic uterosacral nerve ablation (LUNA) for midline pain such as dysmenorrhea or dyspareunia (evidence does not support its use).
- Unless pregnancy is desired, patient is usually started on GnRH agonist therapy or continuous OCP immediately after surgery.
- For those desiring pregnancy, surgery alone results in significant increase in fertility.

Definitive:
- Directed at relieving endometriosis-associated pain.
- Total abdominal hysterectomy with bilateral salpingo-oophorectomy and complete excision or ablation of endometriosis.
- Thorough abdominal exploration to ensure removal of all disease.
- Must be prepared to manage possible gastrointestinal and urinary tract endometriosis.
- 90% effective in pain relief; patient must be counseled that pain relief is not guaranteed.
- Estrogen replacement therapy (ERT) to be considered in all women undergoing definitive surgical management; after ERT, recurrence rate is 0% to 5% in women with endometriosis confined to the pelvis but 18% in women with bowel involvement.
- Concern for malignant degeneration exists in implants if unopposed estrogen is used after definitive surgical therapy.

MANAGEMENT OF ENDOMETRIOSIS-ASSOCIATED INFERTILITY: Conservative surgery:
- Yields significantly higher pregnancy rate than does expectant management, in part because of correction of mechanical factors such as adhesions.

Assisted reproductive technologies:
- Can be used to circumvent unknown mechanism of endometriosis-associated infertility.
- Superovulation with clomiphene citrate or human menopausal gonadotropins; clomiphene citrate results in threefold pregnancy rate over expectant management.
- Further improvement with intrauterine insemination combined with superovulation.
- In vitro fertilization if above procedures are unsuccessful.

DISPOSITION

Tends to recur unless definitive surgery is performed, and should be considered a chronic condition.

REFERRAL

To a reproductive endocrinologist for advanced surgical management or infertility management.

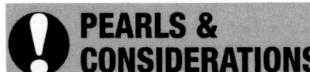

COMMENTS

Patient information can be obtained through the following organizations: Endometriosis Association, 8585 North 76th Place, Milwaukee, WI 53223, 414-355-2200 or 800-992-ENDO; Women's Reproductive Health Network, P.O. Box 30167, Portland, OR 97230-9067 or 503-667-7757.

SUGGESTED READINGS

Available at ExpertConsult.com

RELATED CONTENT

Endometriosis (Patient Information)
Dysmenorrhea (Related Key Topic)
Dyspareunia (Related Key Topic)

AUTHOR: **BARBARA A. MCGUIRK, M.D.**

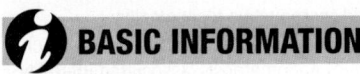

DEFINITION

Enteropathic arthritis (EA) is an inflammatory joint disease associated with inflammatory bowel diseases (IBD) such as Crohn disease (CD), ulcerative colitis (UC), and microscopic colitis. Less frequently, EA is associated with other gastrointestinal disorders, including Whipple disease, celiac disease, and bowel-associated dermatitis-arthritis syndrome related to bypass surgery or intestinal disease. EA is included in the family of spondyloarthropathies (SpA), which have features of peripheral inflammatory arthritis, axial spondylitis and sacroiliitis, enthesitis, dactylitis, uveitis, and rashes. Arthritis is the most common extraintestinal manifestation of IBD.

SYNONYMS

IBD-related spondyloarthropathy
Enteroarthritis
Arthritis associated with gastrointestinal disease

ICD 10-CM CODE(S)

M.07.60	Enteropathic arthropathies, unspecified sites
M.07.69	Enteropathic arthropathies, multiple sites
M.07.68	Enteropathic arthropathies, vertebra
M07.611	Enteropathic arthropathies, right shoulder
M07.612	Enteropathic arthropathies, left shoulder
M07.619	Enteropathic arthropathies, unspecified shoulder
M07.621	Enteropathic arthropathies, right elbow
M07.622	Enteropathic arthropathies, left elbow
M07.629	Enteropathic arthropathies, unspecified elbow
M07.631	Enteropathic arthropathies, right wrist
M07.632	Enteropathic arthropathies, left wrist
M07.639	Enteropathic arthropathies, unspecified wrist
M07.641	Enteropathic arthropathies, right hand
M07.642	Enteropathic arthropathies, left hand
M07.649	Enteropathic arthropathies, unspecified hand
M07.651	Enteropathic arthropathies, right hip
M07.652	Enteropathic arthropathies, left hip
M07.659	Enteropathic arthropathies, unspecified hip
M07.661	Enteropathic arthropathies, right knee
M07.662	Enteropathic arthropathies, left knee
M07.669	Enteropathic arthropathies, unspecified knee
M07.671	Enteropathic arthropathies, right ankle and foot
M07.672	Enteropathic arthropathies, left ankle and foot
M07.679	Enteropathic arthropathies, unspecified ankle and foot
M07.68	Enteropathic arthropathies, vertebrae
M07.69	Enteropathic arthropathies, multiple sites

EPIDEMIOLOGY AND DEMOGRAPHICS

Peripheral arthritis occurs in 5% to 15% of patients with IBD in most studies and is slightly more common in CD than in UC. Spinal involvement occurs in 10% to 20% of cases and may be the only articular manifestation or be accompanied by oligoarthritis.

PREDOMINANT SEX AND AGE: Males and females equally affected. Inflammatory back pain usually presents before the age of 45 yr. Onset of peripheral arthritis is usually between 25 and 45 yr of age.

GENETICS: The presence of HLA-B27 is the strongest association with SpA. Recent genome-wide association studies demonstrated a genetic overlap between IBD and SpA, implicating NOD2 (CARD15) and interleukin 23 receptor (IL23R) as susceptibility genes.

RISK FACTORS:
- Active large bowel disease
- Family history of IBD
- Cigarette smoking
- Genetics
- Complicating intestinal manifestations such as abscesses and perianal disease

PHYSICAL FINDINGS & CLINICAL PRESENTATION

- Two types of joint involvement in IBD: Peripheral and/or axial. Peripheral: Affects peripheral joints, predominantly lower limb joints. Axial: Affects the spine in the form of sacroiliitis with or without spondylitis; can be similar to ankylosing spondylitis or other idiopathic SpA (e.g., psoriatic arthritis, reactive arthritis, undifferentiated SpA).
- Axial involvement is found more commonly in CD than in UC. Axial disease is independent of IBD activity.
- Peripheral arthritis is the most frequent finding in both CD and UC. Peripheral and spinal disease equally affects both sexes (Table 1).
- Type 1 peripheral arthropathy (pauciarticular, less than five joints): Usually acute and self-limited asymmetric inflammatory arthritis; commonly affects large joints of legs such as the knee; occurs early in the course of IBD and commonly parallels the disease activity or flares of IBD.
- Type 2 peripheral arthropathy (polyarticular, five or more joints): Affects mainly the metacarpophalangeal, proximal interphalangeal, knee and ankle joints; bilateral and symmetric; may be migratory. Symptoms may take a more chronic course, independent of IBD activity.
- Type 3 includes patients with both axial and peripheral forms.
- Main complaints are inflammatory back pain, buttock pain, joint pain, and swelling (with prolonged morning stiffness and fatigue); symptoms worse with rest or inactivity and improve with exercise.
- Examination reveals evidence of synovitis, progressive limitation of spinal mobility.
- Periarticular and other extraintestinal manifestations include enthesitis (inflammation of tendon insertion sites into bone such as Achilles or plantar fascia), dactylitis (flexor tenosynovitis of a finger or toe causing sausagelike swelling of digit), uveitis, and psoriasis.
- Uveitis in IBD is more often bilateral and more prone to chronicity.
- Erythema nodosum, pyoderma gangrenosum can be associated with skin lesions in IBD.

ETIOLOGY

In genetically predisposed individuals with intestinal disease, the co-occurrence of joint inflammation provides important support to the theory that dysbiosis in the gut microbiome can link colitis to the development of EA.

TABLE 1 Enteropathic Arthritis

Feature	Peripheral Arthritis	Sacroiliitis, Spondylitis
Crohn Disease		
Frequency in CD	10%-20%	2%-7%
HLA-B27 associated	No	Yes
Pattern	Transient, symmetrical	Chronic
Course	Related to activity of CD	Unrelated to activity of CD
Effect of surgery	Remission of arthritis uncommon	No effect
Effect of anti-TNF therapy	Effective	Effective
Ulcerative Colitis		
Frequency in UC	5%-10%	2%-7%
HLA-B27 associated	No	Yes
Pattern	Transient	Chronic
Course	More common in pancolitis than proctitis; related to activity of UC	Unrelated
Effect of surgery	Remission of arthritis	No effect

CD, Crohn disease; *HLA,* human leukocyte antigen; *TNF,* tumor necrosis factor; *UC,* ulcerative colitis.
From Goldman L, Schafer AI: *Goldman's Cecil Medicine,* ed 24, Philadelphia, 2012, Saunders.

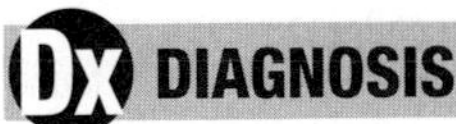

DIFFERENTIAL DIAGNOSIS

- Hypertrophic osteoarthropathy
- Osteonecrosis (avascular necrosis)
- Septic arthritis
- Other idiopathic seronegative spondyloarthropathies (e.g., reactive arthritis, psoriatic arthritis, ankylosing spondylitis)
- Behçet's syndrome
- Rheumatoid arthritis

WORK-UP

Diagnosis mainly relies on clinical features and imaging data. There is no gold standard for diagnosis.

LABORATORY TEST(S)

- Laboratory testing: Markers of inflammation such as sedimentation rate and CRP may reflect underlying disease activity of bowel disease and thus may not be useful to track for EA activity. CBC can reveal leukocytosis, anemia, thrombocytosis suggestive of inflammatory response.
- Synovial fluid is nonspecific; shows mild to marked inflammation: WBC 1500-50,000/mm^3.
- Serologic tests for rheumatoid arthritis are negative (rheumatoid factor, cyclic-citrullinated peptide antibodies), and lupus-related antinuclear antibodies are absent.
- Tests for other intestinal diseases based on clinical suspicion: Whipple diagnosis is based on histology with PAS-positive cells, serology for T. whipplei, and culture; celiac disease IgA anti-tissue transglutaminase and anti-endomysial antibodies along with diagnostic villous atrophy on small bowel biopsy; microscopic colitis diagnosed only through histology from colonoscopy showing collagenous colitis or lymphocytic colitis.

IMAGING STUDIES

- Plain x-ray of the spine and pelvis may appear normal in early disease but with progression may show evidence of sacroiliitis, spondylitis, ankyloses.
- X-ray of peripheral joints may show soft tissue swelling, periostitis, or joint effusion.
- MRI may be used to assess early changes of spondyloarthritis when plain x-rays are negative. MRI is the most sensitive method of detecting sacroiliitis in IBD patients.
- Musculoskeletal ultrasonography is a noninvasive, safe, and easily reproducible means of detecting early pathologic changes in SpA patients. It can identify characteristic features of enthesitis, bone erosions, synovitis, bursitis, and tenosynovitis.

Rx TREATMENT

- Effective treatment of underlying IBD is helpful in controlling the peripheral arthritis. The goal of treatment of EA is reducing inflammation to relieve suffering and prevent joint deformity and disability.
- When IBD and SpA coexist, treatment strategy should also address extraintestinal and extraarticular features such as enthesitis, dactylitis, uveitis, and psoriasis, with need for tailored consideration of certain limited biologic options.
- Avoidance of NSAIDs due to controversial increased risk of exacerbation of intestinal disease.

NONPHARMACOLOGIC THERAPY

Rest, physical therapy, and exercise such as swimming

ACUTE GENERAL Rx

- There has been concern that NSAIDs exacerbate IBD and that NSAID-related adverse events such as ulcers and GI bleeding may mimic IBD flares. COX-2 inhibitors may be preferred to traditional NSAIDs, but similar concerns and cautions apply.
- Intraarticular steroid injections may help treat joint synovitis.
- Systemic steroids can help reduce polyarticular joint and IBD activity but should be used at the lowest effective dose and ideally for only short courses.

CHRONIC Rx

- Immunomodulatory agents such as sulfasalazine, azathioprine, 6-mercaptopurine, methotrexate, and cyclosporine can be used to treat active IBD, peripheral arthritis, and associated skin conditions. Peripheral joint disease responds better to these agents than axial disease. TNF inhibitors, particularly infliximab, adalimumab, and certolizumab, are useful to treat both arthritis (axial or peripheral) and severe, refractory IBD. Golimumab is also in use for refractory IBD and is used for arthritis. Etanercept is effective only to control the arthritis but not the IBD.
- The axial disease associated with IBD is treated as is any SpA. Medications approved for other SpAs, such as ustekinumab (anti-IL12/23) and secukinumab (anti-IL17A), may be effective therapies for EA, although their effectiveness for IBD treatment is not clear.
- The choice of biologic requires the consideration of extra-intestinal features such as uveitis. This condition can be treated with infliximab or adalimumab, both of which also treat the IBD.
- For highly active IBD, particularly UC, colectomy has been found to ameliorate peripheral joint inflammatory disease but does not influence axial involvement.

REFERRAL

Rheumatology and gastroenterology

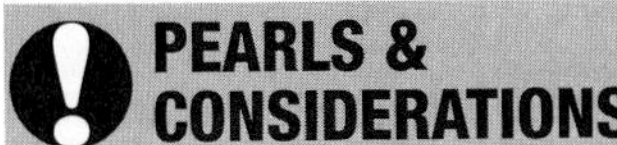

- When a single joint is affected, consider joint aspiration to rule out septic arthritis. Signs of infection may be atypical in those receiving antiinflammatory or immunosuppressive medications.
- Other extra-intestinal manifestations of enteropathic arthritis include skin and mucous membrane involvement, anterior uveitis, Hashimoto's thyroiditis, genitourinary involvement (nephrolithiasis), aortic insufficiency, and cardiac conduction abnormalities. These are often seen in patients with prolonged disease activity and with positive HLA-B 27.
- Pyoderma gangrenosum is the most severe skin manifestation in IBD.

SUGGESTED READINGS

Available at ExpertConsult.com

RELATED TOPICS

Ankylosing Spondylitis (Related Key Topic)
Crohn Disease (Related Key Topic)
Psoriatic Arthritis (Related Key Topic)
Ulcerative Colitis (Related Key Topic)

AUTHOR: **CANDICE REYES, M.D., R.H.M.S.U.S.**

BASIC INFORMATION

DEFINITION

Eosinophilic esophagitis is a chronic, antigen- and immune-mediated disease, which requires three inclusion criteria:

1. Inflammation secondary to eosinophilic infiltration within the esophagus (confirmed with at least 15 eosinophils per high power field (hpf) detected on biopsy of mucosa taken at mid and distal esophagus)
2. Symptoms of esophageal dysfunction
3. Exclusion of proton pump inhibitor–responsive esophageal eosinophilia after response to a proton pump inhibitor (PPI) trial

SYNONYMS

Esophageal eosinophilia
EoE
EE

ICD-10CM CODE

K20.0 Eosinophilic esophagitis

EPIDEMIOLOGY & DEMOGRAPHICS

INCIDENCE (IN U.S.): One to 20 new cases per 100,000 inhabitants per yr, increased from last yr

PEAK INCIDENCE: Older children; in adults, ages 30 to 50

PREVALENCE: Between 13 and 49 cases per 100,000 inhabitants

PREDOMINANT SEX: Male predominance (ratio ~3:1)

PREDOMINANT AGE: Peak of disease activity at age 35 to 39

GENETICS

- Association between thymic stromal lymphopoietin *(TSL)* gene mutation and risk for EoE
- Higher risk in those with homozygous pattern for the mutation
- *TSL* gene found on Yp11.3 chromosome
- Association with polymorphism on eotaxin-3 (CCL-26)

RISK FACTORS/ETIOLOGY: Genetic, host immune, and environmental

PHYSICAL FINDINGS & CLINICAL PRESENTATION

- Adults: Dysphagia to solid foods, food impaction, heartburn, noncardiac chest pain, increased time to consume meals, concurrent allergic disease (asthma, eczema, rhinitis, atopic dermatitis, seasonal/food allergies)
- Children: Vomiting, regurgitation, nausea, epigastric/abdominal pain, chest pain, water brash, globus, decreased appetite, gagging, choking, refusal of food, possible atopy
- Often associated with asthma, rhinitis, dermatitis, and other atopic conditions

Dx DIAGNOSIS

DIFFERENTIAL DIAGNOSIS

- Gastroesophageal reflux disease
- PPI-responsive esophageal eosinophilia (PPI-REE)—see "Acute General Treatment"
- Celiac disease
- Eosinophilic gastroenteritis
- Crohn's disease
- Hypereosinophilic syndrome
- Achalasia
- Vasculitis/pemphigus/connective tissue diseases
- Infectious (fungal/viral)
- Graft-versus-host disease

WORKUP

- EGD with at least two to four biopsies from distal and mid/proximal esophagus after a PPI trial
- Confirmation: Persistence of symptoms *and* ≥15 eosinophils/hpf on pathology (Fig. 1) although esophagus is normal in ~5% to 10% of patients
- Other histological findings can include basal zone hyperplasia, dilated intracellular spaces, and subepithelial fibrosis
- Endoscopic findings can include white mucosal papules, which represent eosinophilic microabscesses, linear furrows, esophageal narrowing with stricture, mucosal tearing, and esophageal trachealization (Fig. 2), esophageal rings, felinization of esophagus. Felinization of the esophagus is a radiologic term used to describe 1 to 2 mm transverse folds found circumferentially along the entire lumen of the esophagus that appear transiently on EGD and barium studies, possibly attributed to thickened and contracted muscularis mucosae

LABORATORY TESTS

- 40% to 50% have elevated peripheral eosinophilia
- 50% to 60% have elevated serum IgE levels

IMAGING STUDIES

Esophagram can reveal rings and strictures.

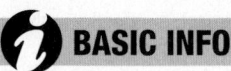

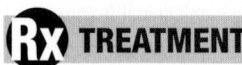

Rx TREATMENT

NONPHARMACOLOGIC THERAPY

- Step-Up (2-4-6) elimination diet (eliminates milk and wheat, then additionally eggs and soy/legumes, then nuts and seafood)
    1. For patients with response, foods can be reintroduced one at a time for 6 weeks
- Dilation if stricture is present and/or patient is refractory to therapy with the goal of creating a tear in the mucosa

ACUTE GENERAL Rx

- An 8-week trial of PPI therapy, which has newly demonstrated antiinflammatory therapy, should be initiated after an initial EGD

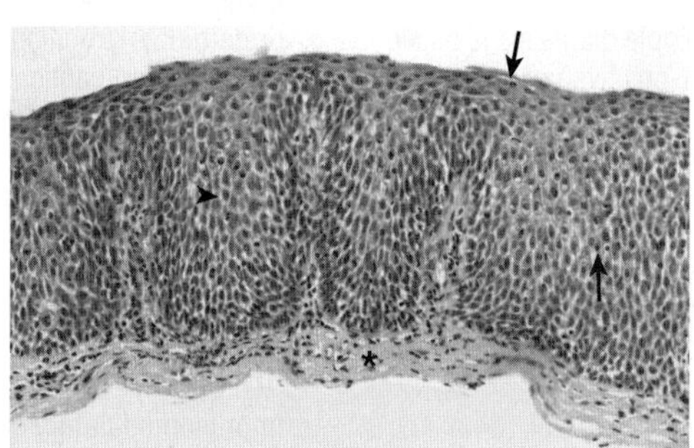

FIG. 1 H&E staining of an esophageal specimen from a patient with eosinophilic esophagitis. *Arrows* point to eosinophils, including some at the surface. *Arrowhead* points to dilated intercellular spaces. *Asterisk* marks the lamina propria, showing inflammation and fibrosis. *Green arrow* points to elongated papillae. There is also marked basal layer hyperplasia, with the basal layer reaching almost to the luminal surface. *H&E,* haematoxylin and eosin. (From Feldman M, Friedman LS, Brandt LJ: *Sleisenger and Fortran's gastrointestinal and liver disease,* ed 10, Philadelphia, 2016, Elsevier.)

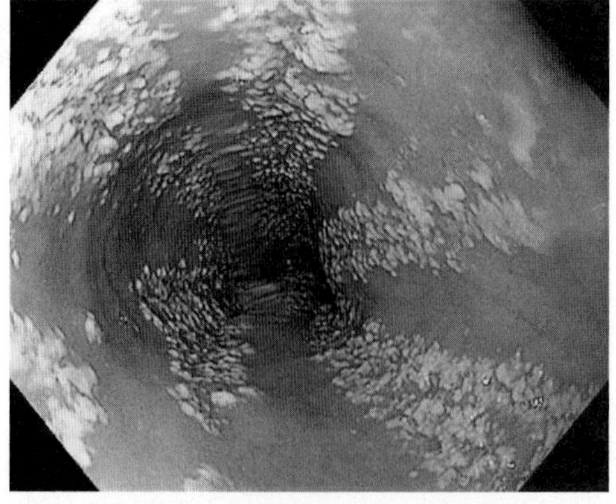

FIG. 2 Endoscopic view of eosinophilic esophagitis with furrowing and exudates. (From Feldman M, Friedman LS, Brandt LJ: *Sleisenger and Fortran's gastrointestinal and liver disease,* ed 10, Philadelphia, 2016, Elsevier.)

with biopsy based on clinical symptoms with subsequent EGD (with biopsies)

1. If eosinophilia persists on biopsy despite PPI use, diagnosis is EoE
2. If eosinophilia is reduced on repeat biopsies, patient is considered to have PPI-REE, not EoE

- An EGD (with biopsies) should be performed initially if a critical stricture is present (e.g., patient presents with food impaction)
- If EoE is confirmed, patient should be tried on aerosolized topical glucocorticoids (fluticasone or budesonide) and/or dietary elimination
  1. Topical steroids shown to be most effective:
     a. Swallowed fluticasone 880 mcg bid
        (1) Delivered by meter-dosed inhaler without a spacer
        (2) Medication is sprayed into the patient's mouth and then swallowed
        (3) Patient should **not** inhale when the medication is being delivered
        (4) Patient should not eat or drink for 30 minutes following administration
     b. Swallowed budesonide 2 mg daily
        (1) Administered using a nebulizer: Patient then instructed to swallow accumulated liquid
        (2) Administered as viscous slurry: Mixing four 0.5 mg/2 ml nebulizer respules with sucralose (10 1-gram packets per 1 mg of budesonide, creating a volume of approximately 8 ml)
        (3) Patient should not eat or drink for 30 min after taking the budesonide suspension.

CHRONIC Rx

- If patient is responsive to PPI therapy, EoE has been excluded and patient can be continued on PPI therapy with surveillance of symptoms.
- If patient is responsive to aerosolized topical steroids and/or dietary modification, continue steroids at lowest dose and/or continue dietary elimination.
- If lack of response to initial therapy:
  1. Assess compliance.
  2. Restrict diet further.
  3. Increase steroid dose or consider alternate steroid.
  4. Switch from dietary modification to steroid therapy and vice versa.
  5. Consider second-line agents or clinical trials.
  6. Reevaluate diagnosis.
- Chronic histologic and symptomatic surveillance is recommended.
- If dysphagia persists, endoscopic dilation is recommended for amelioration of symptoms.

DISPOSITION

Follow-up by gastroenterologist is important to gauge progression or regression of disease.

REFERRAL

Referrals to gastroenterologists, allergists, and dieticians allow for a multidisciplinary approach to diagnosis and management of EoE.

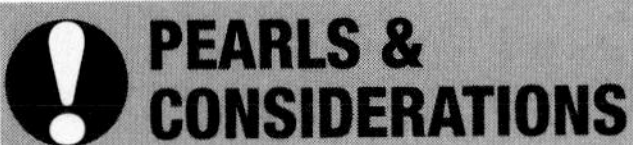

COMMENTS

- EoE can be confused with PPI-REE, and patients should undergo a PPI trial before confirmation of EoE and utilization of topical steroids, step-up elimination diet, or esophageal dilation.
- Endoscopic surveillance of disease with or without symptoms is important.
- While esophageal dilation is the mainstay of therapy in patients with esophageal strictures, narrowing of esophagus, and esophageal rings, dilation will not reduce the risk of recurrence as eosinophilic burden is unaffected.

SUGGESTED READINGS

Available at ExpertConsult.com

RELATED CONTENT

Gastroesophageal Reflux Disease (GERD) (Related Key Topic)

AUTHORS: **PRATIMA DIBBA, M.D., M.B.A.,** and **MARIAM FAYEK, M.D.**

BASIC INFORMATION

DEFINITION

Epidermolysis bullosa (EB) is a rare disorder presenting in adults with the development of blisters on the hands, feet, elbows, knees, and other body regions after mild trauma. It represents a group of genetic disorders characterized by mechanically fragile skin with a propensity to develop blisters and/or erosions. There are four major types: dystrophic (DEB), junctional (JEB), simplex (EBS), and ***Kindler syndrome.*** They differ in the ultrastructural site within which cutaneous blisters form. Kindler syndrome is an extremely rare form characterized by trauma-induced blistering, photosensitivity, progressive poikiloderma, cutaneous atrophy, and mucosal inflammation.

SYNONYMS

EB
Kindler syndrome

ICD 10-CM CODES	
Q81.9	Epidermolysis bullosa, unspecified
L12.30	Acquired epidermolysis bullosa, unspecified
Q81.2	Epidermolysis bullosa dystrophica
Q81.0	Epidermolysis bullosa simplex

EPIDEMIOLOGY & DEMOGRAPHICS

PREVALENCE AND INCIDENCE: The estimated overall prevalence and incidence of EB in the U.S. are 11.1 per 1 million population and 19.6 per 1 million live births, respectively. The approximate prevalences and incidences, respectively, of the major types of EB are as follows: EB simplex, 6.0 and 7.9; junctional EB, 0.5 and 2.7; dominant dystrophic EB, 1.5 and 2.1; and recessive dystrophic EB, 1.4 and 3.0.

PREDOMINANT SEX AND AGE

GENETICS: The most common forms of EB simplex (EBS) are transmitted in an autosomal dominant manner. Table E1 summarizes the various clinical phenotypes and inheritance.

RISK FACTORS

Physical Findings & Clinical Presentation
EB is marked by development of painful blisters on the hands, feet (Fig. E1), elbows, and knees after mild trauma. Extensive blistering (Fig. E2) may occur. EB may also be complicated by atrophic scarring, milia formation, and nail dystrophy. Fig. 3 illustrates helpful cutaneous findings in patients with EB.

Table 2 summarizes major extracutaneous complications of EB.

ETIOLOGY

- This is an inherited disorder (see Table E1).

DIAGNOSIS

DIFFERENTIAL DIAGNOSIS

- Bullous pemphigoid
- Pemphigus vulgaris
- Linear IgA bullous dermatosis
- Porphyria cutanea tarda
- Chemical burn
- Thermal burn
- Blisters due to trauma (friction blisters)
- Cicatricial pemphigoid

WORKUP

An approach to the laboratory diagnosis of EB is illustrated in Fig. 4.

LABORATORY TEST(S)

Skin biopsy and serum for direct and indirect immunofluorescence can detect skin basement membrane–specific autoantibodies.

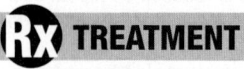

TREATMENT

ACUTE GENERAL RX

- Nutritional support, avoidance of trauma
- Topical antibiotics, sterile dressing
- Dressings frequently used in patients with EB are described in Table 3
- Systemic corticosteroids
- Dapsone
- Azathioprine
- Colchicine
- Cyclosporine

CHRONIC Rx

The management of long-term complications of EB is summarized in Table E4.

REFERRAL

Dermatology in all cases

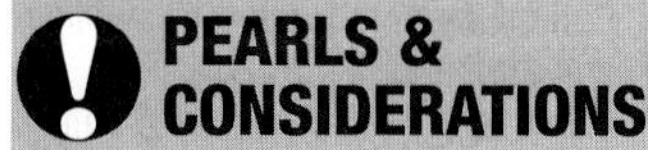

PEARLS & CONSIDERATIONS

COMMENTS

Workup for inflammatory bowel disease and ELISA for type VII collagen-specific autoantibodies should also be considered.

SUGGESTED READINGS

Available at ExpertConsult.com

AUTHOR: **FRED F. FERRI, M.D.**

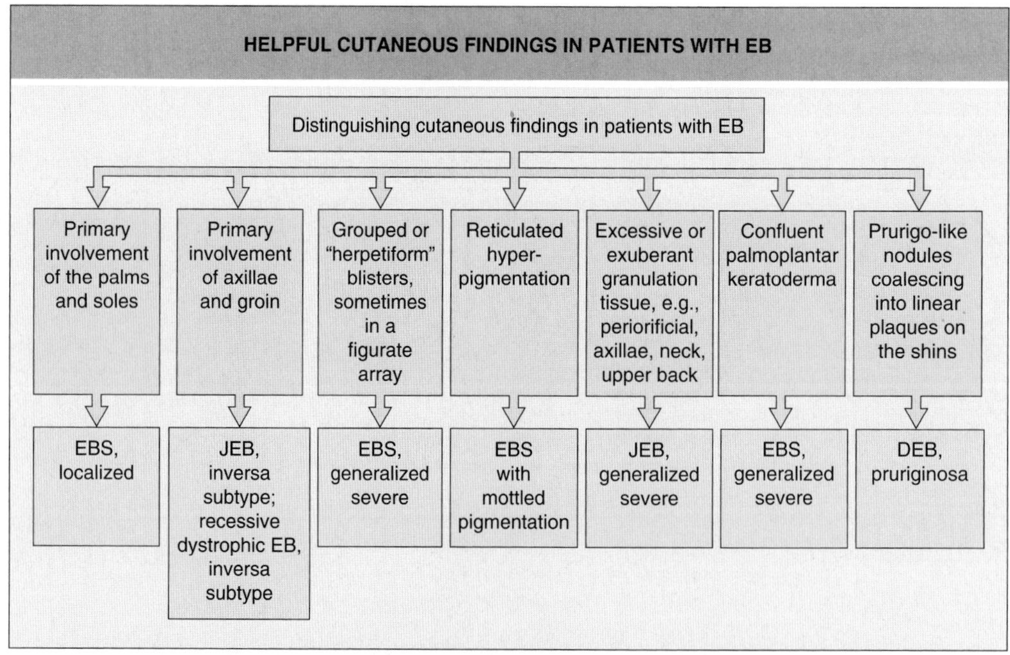

FIG. 3 Helpful cutaneous findings in patients with epidermolysis bullosa *(EB).* *DEB*, dystrophic EB; *EBS*, EB simplex; *JEB*, junctional EB. (From Bolognia J: *Dermatology*, ed 4, Philadelphia, 2018, Elsevier.)

TABLE 2 Major Extracutaneous Complications of Epidermolysis Bullosa (EB)

Complication	EB Subtype(s) Most Commonly Affected	
	≥50% of patients	<50% of patients
Eyes		
Corneal blisters, ulcers, and scarring	RDEB-gen/sev	JEB-gen/sev > RDEB-gen/intermed, RDEB-inv, JEB-gen/intermed
Ectropion formation		JEB-gen/sev; Kindler
Oral cavity and upper airway (excluding blisters)		
Microstomia	RDEB-gen/sev	JEB-gen/sev, RDEB-inv
Enamel hypoplasia	JEB (all subtypes)	
Excessive caries and premature loss of teeth	RDEB gen/sev, JEB-gen/sev	
Tracheolaryngeal stenosis	JEB-gen/sev	JEB-gen/intermed
Gastrointestinal tract		
Esophageal strictures	RDEB-gen/sev, RDEB-inv	RDEB-gen/intermed, Kindler > JEB-gen/sev
Pyloric atresia	JEB-PA, EBS-PA	
Malnutrition/failure to thrive	RDEB-gen/sev, JEB-gen/sev	JEB-gen/intermed
Severe constipation	RDEB-gen/sev	JEB-gen/sev, EBS-gen/sev
GERD	RDEB	JEB, EBS-gen/sev
Colitis		Kindler, RDEB-gen/sev
Genitourinary tract		
Urethral meatal stenosis		RDEB-gen/sev, JEB-gen/sev, Kindler
Chronic renal failure*		RDEB-gen/sev
Hydroureter and hydronephrosis		JEB-PA, JEB-gen/sev
Nephrotic syndrome	JEB-resp/renal	JEB-gen/sev
Heart		
Dilated cardiomyopathy		RDEB-gen/sev > JEB, RDEB-gen/intermed
Musculoskeletal system		
Pseudosyndactyly	RDEB-gen/sev	RDEB-gen/intermed, Kindler
Osteoporosis or osteopenia	RDEB-gen/sev	RDEB-gen/sev, JEB-gen/sev
Muscular dystrophy	EBS-MD	
Bone marrow		
Severe multifactorial anemia	RDEB-gen/sev, JEB-gen/sev	

*Causes include renal amyloidosis and glomerulonephritis.

EBS, EB simplex; *GERD*, gastroesophageal reflux disease; *gen/intermed*, generalized intermediate; *gen/sev*, generalized severe; *inv*, inversa; *JEB*, junctional EB; *MD*, muscular dystrophy; *PA*, pyloric atresia; *RDEB*, recessive dystrophic EB; *resp/renal*, respiratory and renal involvement.

From Bolognia J: *Dermatology*, ed 4, Philadelphia, 2018, Elsevier.

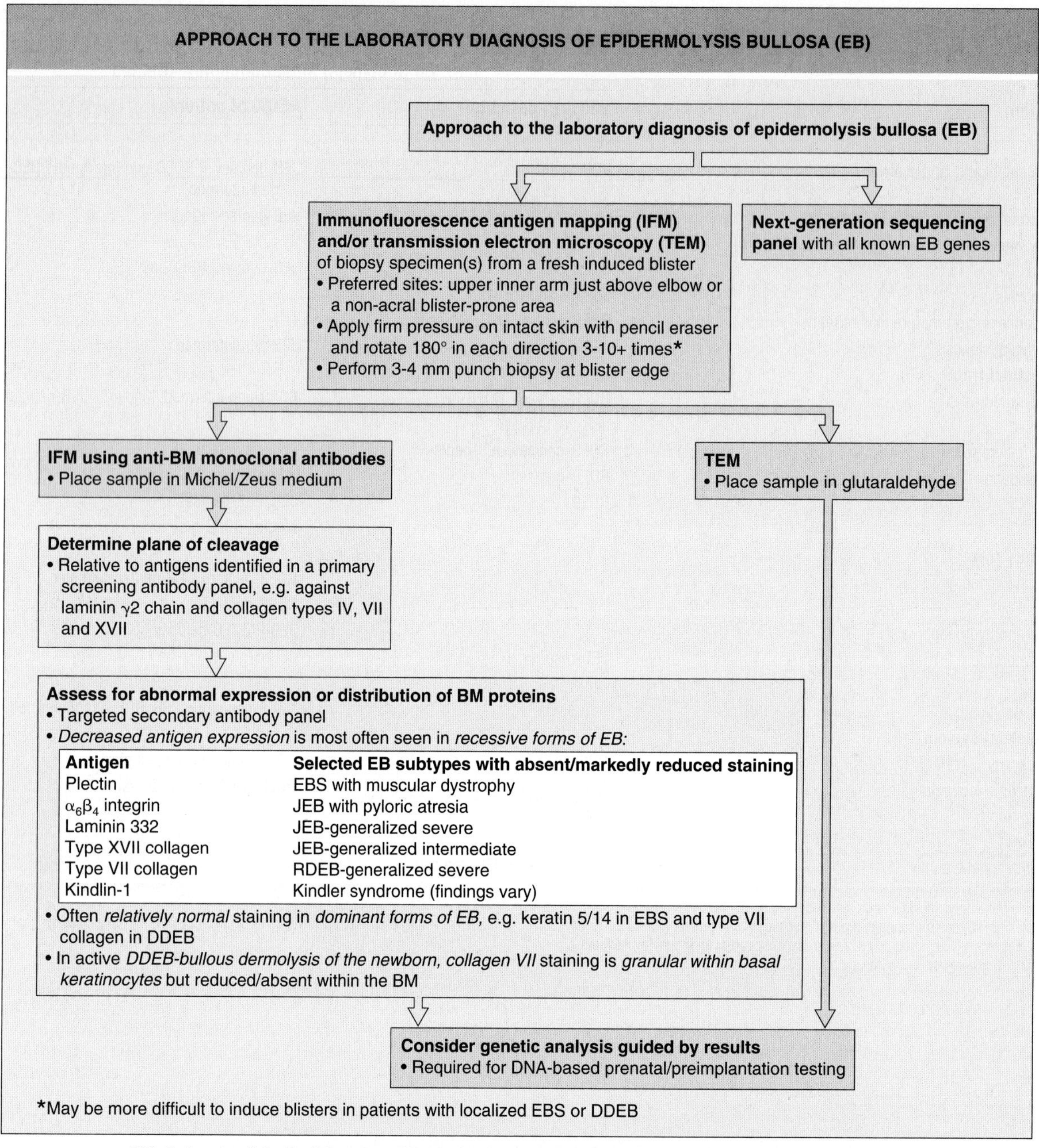

FIG. 4 Approach to the laboratory diagnosis of epidermolysis bullosa *(EB)*. *BM*, basement membrane; *DDEB*, dominant dystrophic EB; *DNA*, deoxyribonucleic acid; *EBS*, EB simplex; *JEB*, junctional EB; *RDEB*, recessive dystrophic EB. (From Bolognia J: *Dermatology*, ed 4, Philadelphia, 2018, Elsevier.)

TABLE 3 Dressings Frequently Used in Patients With Epidermolysis Bullosa (EB)

Dressing type	Use	Examples®,™
Soft silicone dressings ("low-tack")	• Suitable as primary or secondary dressings in many types of EB • May have a foam backing for mechanical protection or to wick exudate away from the wound	Mepitel, Mepilex, Mepilex Transfer, Mepilex Border
Nonadherent lipido-colloid dressings	• Suitable for primary contact	Urgotul
Hydrogel dressings	• Provide moisture to drier wounds to facilitate healing • May provide relief from pain or itch	Flexigel, Curagel, ActiForm Cool
Foam dressings	• Useful to absorb moderate amounts of wound exudate	Mepilex, Allevyn
Absorptive dressings	• Useful to absorb heavy amounts of wound exudate	Eclypse, Sorbion Sana
Silver-containing dressings	• Clinically infected or highly colonized wounds • Avoid prolonged use due to risk of silver absorption	Urgotul SSD, Mepilex AG
Other antimicrobial dressings	• Clinically infected or highly colonized wounds	PolyMem, Cutimed Sorbact, Activon Tulle, Suprasorb X + PHMB

From Bolognia J: *Dermatology*, ed 4, Philadelphia, 2018, Elsevier.

BASIC INFORMATION

DEFINITION

- Epididymitis is an inflammatory reaction of the epididymis caused by either an infectious agent or local trauma. In most cases of acute epididymitis, the testis is also involved (orchitis).
- Epididymitis is considered chronic if lasting ≥6 wk. Chronic epididymitis has been subcategorized into inflammatory chronic epididymitis, obstructive chronic epididymitis, and chronic epididymalgia.

SYNONYMS

Nonspecific bacterial epididymitis
Sexually transmitted epididymitis

ICD-10CM CODES

N45.1	Epididymitis
A54.00	Gonococcal infection of lower genitourinary tract, unspecified

EPIDEMIOLOGY & DEMOGRAPHICS

INCIDENCE (IN U.S.): Cause of >600,000 visits to physicians per yr
PEAK INCIDENCE: Sexually active yrs
PREDOMINANT SEX: Exclusive to males
PREDOMINANT AGE: All ages affected but usually in sexually active men or older males
CONGENITAL: Congenital urologic structural disorders possibly predisposing to infections

PHYSICAL FINDINGS & CLINICAL PRESENTATION

- Tender swelling of the scrotum with erythema, usually unilateral testicular pain and tenderness
- Dysuria and/or urethral discharge
- Fever and signs of systemic illness (less common)
- Pain and redness on scrotal examination
- Hydrocele or even epididymo-orchitis, especially late
- Chronic draining scrotal sinuses with a "beadlike" enlargement of the vas deferens in tuberculous disease

ETIOLOGY

- In young, sexually active men (<35 yr of age), the most common causes of infections are *Neisseria gonorrhoeae* and *Chlamydia trachomatis.*
- In older men (>35 yr of age) or those with underlying urologic disease:
  1. Gram-negative aerobic rods are predominant (i.e., *Escherichia coli*).
  2. Similar organisms are found in men following invasive urologic procedures.
  3. Gram-positive cocci are rarely seen in these groups.
  4. Mycobacteria may also be a cause of epididymitis.
- Acute epididymitis caused by sexually transmitted enteric organisms (e.g., *Escherichia coli*) also occurs among men who are the insertive partner during anal intercourse.
- Young, prepubertal boys may present with epididymitis caused by coliform bacteria; almost always a complication of underlying urologic disease such as reflux.
- In AIDS patients, CMV and *Salmonella* epididymitis have been described. CMV may have a negative urine culture. Toxoplasmosis and *Cryptococcus* should also be considered as a cause of epididymitis in AIDS patients.
- Chronic infectious epididymitis is most frequently seen in conditions associated with granulomatous reaction; mycobacterium tuberculosis is the most common granulomatous disease affecting the epididymis.

Dx DIAGNOSIS

DIFFERENTIAL DIAGNOSIS

- Orchitis
- Testicular torsion, trauma, or tumor
- Epididymal cyst
- Hydrocele
- Varicocele
- Spermatocele
- Testicular torsion should be considered in all cases (Table E1).

WORKUP

- Consideration of a full assessment of the urologic tract in patients with bacterial infection, especially if recurrent
- If discharge is present, cultures and Gram stain smear of urethral exudate. Gram stain should demonstrate ≥5 WBC per oil immersion field.
- In sexually active men: Gonococcal cultures of the throat and rectum possibly of value
- If testicular torsion a consideration: Radionuclear imaging
- Examination of first void uncentrifuged urine for leukocytes if the urethral Gram stain is negative. Positive leukocyte esterase test on first-void urine or microscopic examination of first-void urine sediment will demonstrate ≥10 WBC per high power field. A culture and Gram-stained smear of this urine specimen should be obtained along with nucleic acid amplification testing (NAAT) from urine samples for gonorrhea and chlamydia.
- Imaging with sonogram (Fig. E1)

LABORATORY TESTS

- All suspected cases of acute epididymitis should be tested for *C. trachomatis* and for *N. gonorrhoeae* by NAAT. Urine is the preferred specimen for NAAT testing.
- Urinalysis and urine culture if dysuria is present or if urinary tract infection is suspected
- HIV testing and counseling.
- PPD placed and chest x-ray viewed if TB suspected (rare cases).
- Rarely, biopsy to ensure the diagnosis of tuberculous epididymitis.

Rx TREATMENT

ACUTE GENERAL Rx

- Ice packs and scrotal elevation for relief of pain
- Analgesia with acetaminophen with or without codeine or NSAIDs
- Antibiotics to cover suspected pathogens. Empiric therapy is indicated before laboratory test results are available
- Recommended regimens are ceftriaxone 250 mg IM in a single dose plus doxycycline 100 mg bid for 10 days. For acute epididymitis most likely caused by enteric organisms, treatment options are levofloxacin 500 mg qd × 10 days or ofloxacin 300 mg bid × 10 days. Add ceftriaxone 250 mg IM single dose to levofloxacin or ofloxacin in men who practice insertive anal sex and are suspected to have chlamydia and gonorrhea and enteric organisms
- Best treatment for older men with gram-negative bacteriuria: Ofloxacin 300 mg PO bid for 10 days or levofloxacin 500 mg PO qd for 10 days
- *Pseudomonas* covered by ciprofloxacin PO or IV or cefepime (2 g IV q8h)
- Consider ampicillin-sulbactam, 3rd-generation cephalosporin, ticarcillin-clavulanate, or piperacillin-tazobactam in toxic-appearing patients.
- Surgical aspiration of local abscesses or even open surgical drainage
- Diabetics: Especially prone to develop more extensive scrotal infections, including Fournier gangrene
- Reinforcement of compliance with antibiotics to avoid partial treatment

CHRONIC Rx

- Repair of underlying structural defects is considered especially if infections are severe or recur.
- Surgical repair of reflux in young boys should be undertaken promptly and at a young age when possible.
- Sex partners of patient should be referred for evaluation and treatment.

REFERRAL

- If abscess or chronic structural problems suspected
- If another diagnosis, such as testicular torsion, is suspected

PEARLS & CONSIDERATIONS

- Recurrent epididymitis in sexually active men is usually related to failure to simultaneously treat sexual partners for STDs.
- Recurrent epididymitis in non-sexually active men is generally related to structural-anatomic defects in the genitourinary system or relapsing disease from inadequate initial treatment or antimicrobial resistance.
- Tuberculous epididymitis fails to respond to seemingly adequate antimicrobial therapy even without characteristic radiographic changes on chest films.

RELATED CONTENT

Epididymitis (Patient Information)
Orchidis (Related Key Topic)
Testicular Torsion (Related Key Topic)

AUTHORS: **PHILIP A. CHAN, M.D., M.S.** and **GLENN G. FORT, M.D., M.P.H.**

BASIC INFORMATION

DEFINITION

Epidural abscess is a suppurative infection of the central nervous system localized between the dura mater and the overlying skull or vertebral column. There are two types of epidural abscess: spinal epidural abscess (SEA) and intracranial epidural abscess (IEA), depending on the location within the central nervous system.

SYNONYMS

SEA
Spinal epidural abscess
IEA
Intraspinal abscess

ICD-10CM CODES

G06.2 Extradural and subdural abscess, unspecified

EPIDEMIOLOGY & DEMOGRAPHICS

INCIDENCE: Spinal epidural abscess: 2 to 25 patients per 100,000 admissions; spinal epidural abscess is 9 times more common than intracranial abscess
PEAK INCIDENCE: Median age at onset of spinal epidural abscess: 50 yr old
PREVALENCE: Greatest between 50 and 70 yr of age
PREDOMINANT SEX: More common in men
RISK FACTORS: Bacteremia, secondary to distant infection; epidural catheter placement (0.5%-3% risk), paraspinal injections of glucocorticoids or for pain management, contiguous bone or soft tissue infection, intravenous drug abuse, diabetes, immunosuppressive therapy, HIV

PHYSICAL FINDINGS & CLINICAL PRESENTATION

- Initially nonspecific, such as fever and malaise
- Classic triad: Fever, spinal pain, and neurologic deficits are not common
- More commonly:
  1. Localized and significant back pain is present.
  2. Nerve root pain is present ("shooting" or "electrical" from involved nerve root).
  3. Motor weakness, sensory changes, and even paralysis can occur.
  4. Fever may not be a prominent sign.

ETIOLOGY

- Bacteria enter the epidural space most often secondary to hematogenous spread from foci elsewhere in the body (25%-50% of cases) or by direct extension from nearby infected tissues such as vertebral body or psoas muscle. A local intervention such as injection can also cause infection.
- Hematogenous foci include furuncles, cellulitis, urinary tract infection, pharyngitis, and pneumonia.
- Microbiology:
  1. *Staphylococcus aureus*, including methicillin-resistant S. *aureus* (MRSA), accounts for 50% to 90% of cases.
  2. Aerobic and anaerobic streptococci account for 8% to 17% of cases.
  3. Aerobic gram-negative rods (*Escherichia coli* and *Pseudomonas*) account for 10% to 17% of cases.
  4. Coagulase-negative staphylococci can be seen with spinal procedures.

DIAGNOSIS

DIFFERENTIAL DIAGNOSIS

- Disc and degenerative bone disease
- Metastatic tumors
- Vertebral discitis and osteomyelitis

WORKUP

Includes a combination of physical exam with neurologic evaluation, blood work, and radiographic studies

LABORATORY TESTS

- Blood cultures
- Culture of fluid or pus for bacteria aerobically and anaerobically by CT-guided aspiration if possible. Fungal stain and cultures and AFB stain and culture should also be obtained to exclude more unusual pathogens.
- Erythrocyte sedimentation rate and/or C-reactive protein
- CBC with differential

IMAGING STUDIES

- MRI with gadolinium is the diagnostic test of choice (Fig. E1) and imperative if diagnosis is considered.
- CT is an alternative but not as good as MRI for visualizing spinal cord and epidural space.
- CT myelography can be performed if MRI is not available.

TREATMENT

NONPHARMACOLOGIC THERAPY

- Immediate surgery is required if neurologic deficits occur or the patient worsens with medical therapy.
- CT-guided aspiration of abscess with antimicrobial therapy is an alternative treatment to surgery for patients without neurologic deficits.

ACUTE GENERAL Rx

- Empiric antibiotic regimen should include antibiotics effective against staphylococci (including MRSA), streptococci, and gram-negative rods.
- Examples are vancomycin (30-60 mg/kg daily divided in q12h doses adjusted for creatinine clearance *plus* metronidazole (500 mg IV q8h) *plus* ceftriaxone (2 g IV q12h) or ceftazidime (2 g IV q8h) if *Pseudomonas* is suspected. Meropenem: 1 g IV q8h with vancomycin as an alternative, especially if penicillin allergic
- If cultures reveal methicillin-sensitive S. *aureus*, use nafcillin 2 g IV q4h.

CHRONIC Rx

Antimicrobial therapy tailored to culture results may have to be continued for 4 to 6 weeks depending on whether or not there was surgical or CT-guided drainage. If osteomyelitis is suspected, treat for 6 to 8 weeks.

DISPOSITION

- Mortality rates vary from 5% to 32%. Irreversible paralysis can affect 4% to 22% of patients.
- Complete recovery is more likely if neurologic signs are present less than 24 hours before the start of treatment.
- Final functional capacity may continue to improve for up to 1 yr after the end of treatment.

REFERRAL

- Neurosurgery should be involved early when this diagnosis is considered.
- Refer to an interventional radiologist for possible aspiration.
- An infectious diseases evaluation is needed for antimicrobial therapy.

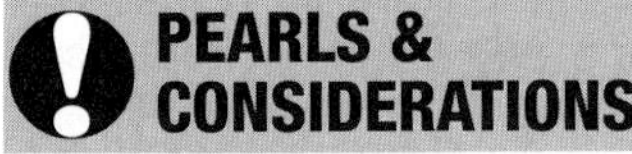

PEARLS & CONSIDERATIONS

COMMENTS

It is important to think of spinal epidural abscess early to permit early treatment and prevent permanent neurologic deficits.

SUGGESTED READINGS

Available at ExpertConsult.com

RELATED CONTENT

Abscess, Brain (Related Key Topic)

AUTHOR: **GLENN G. FORT, M.D., M.P.H.**

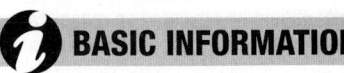

BASIC INFORMATION

DEFINITION

Epidural hematoma (EDH) is the accumulation of blood in the potential space surrounding the brain, between the dura mater and the inner surface of the skull.

SYNONYMS

Extradural hematoma/hemorrhage
EDH

ICD-10CM CODES	
S06.4	Epidural hemorrhage
I62.1	Non-traumatic extradural hemorrhage
S06.4X0A	Epidural hemorrhage without loss of consciousness, initial encounter
S06.4X1A	Epidural hemorrhage with loss of consciousness of 30 minutes or less, initial encounter
S06.4X9A	Epidural hemorrhage with loss of consciousness of unspecified duration, initial encounter

EPIDEMIOLOGY & DEMOGRAPHICS

INCIDENCE: Exact incidence is unknown; however, it is found in 1% to 4% of traumatic head injury cases and 5% to 15% of autopsy series.
PREDOMINANT SEX AND AGE: Male > female
PEAK INCIDENCE: Peak incidence is among adolescents and young adults. It is rarely found in patients older than 50 to 60 yr old.
GENETICS: There is a role for genetics in spontaneous (nontraumatic) EDH caused by coagulopathies and vascular malformations.
RISK FACTORS: Head trauma, especially in cases involving skull fracture

PHYSICAL FINDINGS & CLINICAL PRESENTATION

- History of head trauma is present.
- Signs and symptoms vary depending on severity.
- Symptoms: Altered mental status, nuchal rigidity, headache, vomiting, drowsiness, confusion, aphasia, photophobia, and paralysis.
- Signs: Transient loss of consciousness, followed by a "lucid interval" in 47% of cases, in which the patient is free of any neurologic signs or symptoms. This is followed by clinical deterioration including vomiting, lethargy, confusion, or seizures. Other signs may include focal neurologic deficits such as paralysis of limbs, unequal pupils, and coma. Signs of increased intracranial pressure could be found including the Cushing reflex of hypertension, bradycardia, and respiratory distress. External signs of skull fracture—lacerations, ecchymoses, cerebrospinal fluid (CSF) rhinorrhea or otorrhea—may be observed. Skull fractures can be found in 75% to 95% of EDH patients.
- Coma or stupor with ipsilateral cranial nerve III palsy and contralateral hemiparesis may indicate transtentorial (uncal) herniation.

ETIOLOGY

- Traumatic: Commonly caused by arterial injury (the middle meningeal artery) from a temporal bone fracture (Fig. 1) but may also be injury of the anterior meningeal artery, a dural arteriovenous (AV) fistula at the vertex, or from venous bleeding
- Nontraumatic: Caused by an infection/eroding abscess, coagulopathy, hemorrhagic tumors, vascular malformations, postsurgical procedures, and in special populations (e.g., pregnant women, patients receiving hemodialysis)

DIAGNOSIS

DIFFERENTIAL DIAGNOSIS

In the setting of head trauma: Subdural hematoma, subarachnoid hemorrhage, cerebral contusion, brain laceration, diffuse brain swelling

WORKUP

- Imaging is the mainstay of diagnosis.
- Serial head CT is the test most commonly used due to its simplicity, widespread use, and availability. Typical appearance is a "lens shaped," or "lentiform" hyperdensity (Fig. 2). Box 1 describes CT findings of EDH.
- Note: Head CT is not conclusive in 8% of cases possibly due to severe anemia, early scanning (before blood has time to accumulate), and severe hypotension.
- Brain MRI: More sensitive. Indicated in situations in which there is a strong clinical suspicion but no evidence of EDH on head CT (Fig. 3).
- Angiography: Rarely necessary but may be used to evaluate an underlying vascular lesion.
- Note: Lumbar puncture (LP) is contraindicated in EDH due to risk of brain stem herniation.

LABORATORY TESTS

- Laboratory tests are helpful as adjunct to diagnosis but are not the mainstay of diagnosis or treatment.
- CBC may be helpful to evaluate for anemia, although in an acute onset of bleeding hemoglobin levels can be normal.
- Other tests: Renal functions, electrolytes, liver functions, INR may be helpful depending on the case scenario.

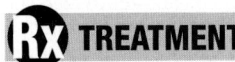

TREATMENT

Acute symptomatic EDH is a neurologic emergency that requires surgical treatment to prevent permanent brain injury.

NONPHARMACOLOGIC THERAPY

- Immediate surgical decompression, ideally within 1 to 2 hr after traumatic event

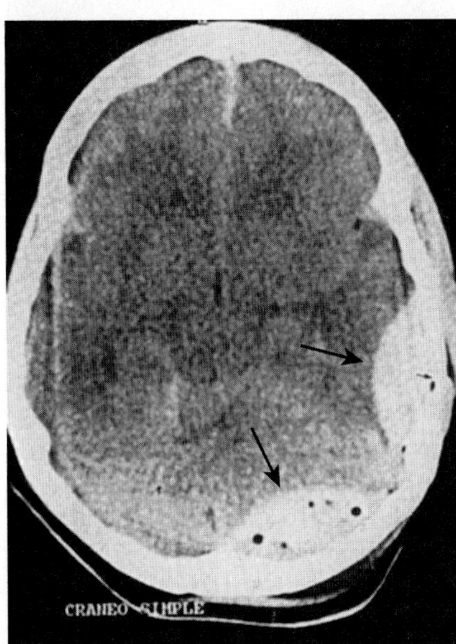

FIG. 2 Head CT showing two epidural hematomas in a 23-year-old involved in a motor vehicle accident. Note air bubbles that are a result of linear fracture in the left temporal bone *(short arrow)*.

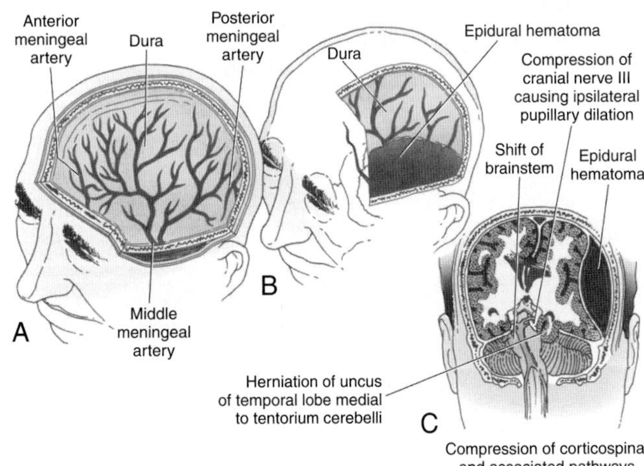

FIG. 1 Epidural hematoma is typically caused by trauma resulting in laceration of the middle meningeal artery. A, The middle meningeal artery. The typical traumatic epidural hematoma is caused by a laceration of this vessel. **B** and **C,** A linear fracture of the squamous portion of the temporal bone has torn the middle meningeal artery, which has resulted in an epidural hematoma. (From Rothrock, JC: Neurosurgery. In Rothrock, JC [ed] *Alexander's care of the patient in surgery*, ed 13, Philadelphia, 2007, Elsevier.)

BOX 1 Computed Tomography (CT) Findings of Epidural Hematoma

- CT appearance: variable white to gray on brain windows
- Location: peripheral to brain, variable but usually temporal region
- Shape: biconvex disc or lens
- Pearl: does not cross suture lines
- White swirl sign means active bleeding
- Significance: may cause mass effect and herniation
- Look for midline shift
- Look for effacement of ventricles and sulci
- Surgical indications: 15-mm thickness or 5-mm midline shift

From Broder JS: *Diagnostic imaging for the emergency physician*, Philadelphia, 2011, Saunders.

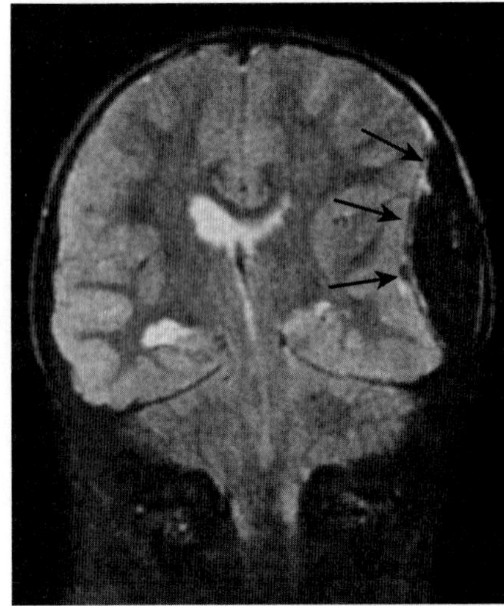

FIG. 3 Epidural hematoma on MRI. Coronal T2-weighted images show hypointense biconvex extraaxial collection in the left temporal region.

- Craniotomy and hematoma evacuation is the treatment of choice. When indicated, identify and ligate the bleeding vessel.
- Burr hole evacuation: This involves drilling a hole in the skull to evacuate the hematoma. It is a lifesaving procedure that is indicated if surgical expertise is limited.

ACUTE GENERAL Rx

- Cardiopulmonary resuscitation and assessment for disability.
- Medical resuscitation maneuvers: Head elevation, hyperventilation, monitoring of vital signs and avoidance of hypotension and hyperthermia, sedation if necessary.
- Medications: Osmotic diuresis with IV mannitol, cerebrosedating medications, antiepileptics may be used to treat or, in some situations, prevent seizures. The patient should also be started on a proton pump inhibitor to decrease risks of developing an upper gastrointestinal bleed.
- Reversing anticoagulation should be weighed in terms of advantages versus disadvantages.
- Note: Glucocorticoid therapy is *not* indicated following head injury and may be related to increased mortality.
- Evaluation for surgery: The best available evidence points toward advantages of decompression procedures. Nonoperative treatment may only be indicated if the patient has no symptoms, no focal neurologic deficit, no coma (Glasgow coma score >8), and EDH volume is less than 30 ml by CT scan, with clot thickness <15 mm and midline shift of less than 5 mm.
- Nonoperative treatment involves close monitoring, hourly neurologic checks, and serial head CT scans.

CHRONIC Rx

- There is a risk of permanent brain damage whether the disorder is treated or not. Most recovery occurs in the first 6 months with some improvement over 2 yr.
- Children have a tendency to recover more quickly.
- Patients should be educated on rehabilitative exercises and to alert medical professionals in the event of new neurologic symptoms.
- Support and encouragement to patient and family should always be provided.

REFERRAL

Neurosurgery should be the first service consulted. If not available, then general surgery needs to be called. Clinical nurse practitioners, pastoral care staff, and social workers to help patients and families are also appropriate.

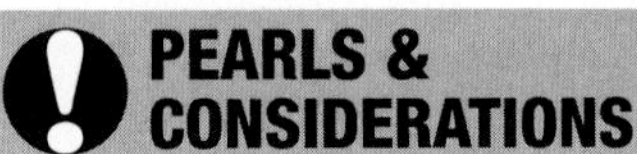

PEARLS & CONSIDERATIONS

- Acute symptomatic EDH is a neurologic emergency. Urgent surgical evacuation is necessary in patients with Glasgow coma score (GCS) less than 9, hematoma greater than 30 ml in volume, or presence of anisocoria.
- EDH should be suspected in any patient with a history of blow to the head leading to a period of loss of consciousness.
- Initial resuscitation is extremely important, but surgery is the mainstay of treatment for acute symptomatic EDH.

PREVENTION

Should be directed toward preventing head trauma: Use of appropriate safety equipment (e.g., helmets, hard hats, safe driving, avoiding diving into unknown depths)

PATIENT/FAMILY EDUCATION

Online head injury support groups are helpful: www.headinjury.com/linktbisup.htm, www.headinjury.com/, www.dailystrengthorg/c/Brain-Injury/support-group.

SUGGESTED READING

Available at ExpertConsult.com

AUTHOR: **FRED F. FERRI, M.D.**

BASIC INFORMATION

DEFINITION

Epiglottitis is a rapidly progressive cellulitis of the epiglottis and adjacent soft tissue structures with the potential to cause abrupt airway obstruction, which can be life-threatening.

SYNONYMS

Supraglottitis
Cherry-red epiglottitis

ICD-10CM CODE

J05.1 Acute epiglottitis

EPIDEMIOLOGY

INCIDENCE (IN U.S.): Due to vaccination against *Haemophilus influenzae* type B, this is a rare infection in children estimated at between 0.6 to 0.8 per 100,000 in one study and for adults at 1.6 per 100,000.

PEAK INCIDENCE: Now highest in children ages 6 to 12

PREDOMINANT SEX: Males

PHYSICAL FINDINGS & CLINICAL PRESENTATION

- Irritability, fever, dysphonia, and dysphagia
- Respiratory distress, with child tending to lean up and forward
- Often, drooling or oral secretions
- Often, presence of tachycardia and tachypnea
- On visualization, edematous and cherry-red epiglottis
- Often, no classic barking cough as seen in croup
- Possibly fulminant course (especially in children), leading to complete airway obstruction

ETIOLOGY

- In children, *Haemophilus influenzae* type b, still most common cause but now rare due to vaccination *Streptococcus pyogenes,* (group A Streptococcus) *Streptococcus pneumoniae, and Staphylococcus aureus* (includes MRSA).
- In adults, *Streptococcus pyogenes* (group A Streptococcus), *H. influenzae* (can be isolated from blood and/or epiglottis [about 26% of cases]).
- Pneumococci, streptococci, and staphylococci are also implicated.
- Role of viruses in epiglottitis unclear.

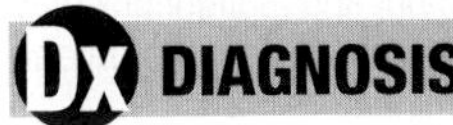

DIAGNOSIS

DIFFERENTIAL DIAGNOSIS

- Croup (Table E1)
- Angioedema
- Retropharyngeal or peritonsillar abscess
- Diphtheria
- Foreign body aspiration
- Lingual tonsillitis
- Bacterial tracheitis

WORKUP

- Cultures of blood and urine.
- Lateral neck radiograph to show an enlarged epiglottis, ballooning of the hypopharynx, and normal subglottic structures (Fig. 1).
  1. Radiographs are of only moderate sensitivity and specificity and take time to perform.
  2. Visualization of the epiglottis may be safer in adults than in children.
- Cultures of the epiglottis.

LABORATORY TESTS

- CBC: May reveal a leukocytosis with a shift to the left.
- Chest radiograph examination: May reveal evidence of pneumonia in close to 25% of cases.
- Cultures of blood, urine, and the epiglottis, as noted previously.

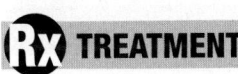

TREATMENT

ACUTE GENERAL Rx

- Maintenance of adequate airway is critical. Fig. E2 describes the optimal assessment and management of upper airway obstruction caused by epiglottitis or severe croup. It is crucial to have a tracheostomy set "at bedside."
- Early placement of an endotracheal or nasotracheal tube in a child is advised.
- Closely follow the adult patient, if no signs of airway obstruction, and defer intubation.
- In children, visualization and intubation are best done in the most controlled environment.
- *H. influenzae* in children is much less common in large part due to the HIB vaccine.

Empiric antibiotics:

1. **In children:** Use cefotaxime 50 mg/kg IV q8h or ceftriaxone 50 mg/kg IV q24h *plus* vancomycin for its coverage of MRSA. If penicillin allergy, use levofloxacin 10 mg/kg IV q24h *plus* clindamycin 7.5 mg/kg IV q6h.
2. **In adults:** Ceftriaxone 2 g IV q24h or cefotaxime *plus* vancomycin.
3. If possible, obtain cultures before initiating antibiotics.
4. If there is an unvaccinated child for *H. influenzae* at home (or in a day care center) who is >4 yr and living with an index case, give close family contacts of the patient (including adults) rifampin 20 mg/kg/day for 4 days (up to 600 mg/day) for prophylaxis.
5. Role of epinephrine or corticosteroids in the management of epiglottitis is not firmly established.

DISPOSITION

Invasive *H. influenzae* infections and epiglottitis are reportable illnesses; this may be particularly important in recognizing an outbreak in a day care center with unvaccinated children.

REFERRAL

- Close cooperation between the pediatrician or internist, anesthesiologist, and otorhinolaryngologist, especially when epiglottis is visualized and when the patient requires endotracheal intubation.
- Best managed in a critical care setting or ICU.

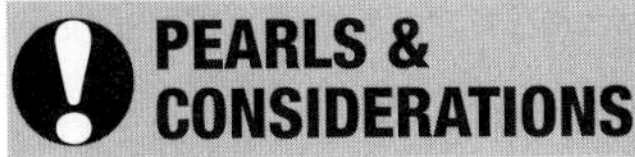

PEARLS & CONSIDERATIONS

The incidence of epiglottitis has diminished markedly since the introduction of the protein conjugate vaccine against *H. influenzae* serotype B into routine childhood immunization.

The mortality rate now in children is about 1% but still remains at about 7% in adults.

SUGGESTED READING

Available at ExpertConsult.com

RELATED CONTENT

Epiglottitis (Patient Information)

AUTHOR: **GLENN G. FORT, M.D., M.P.H.**

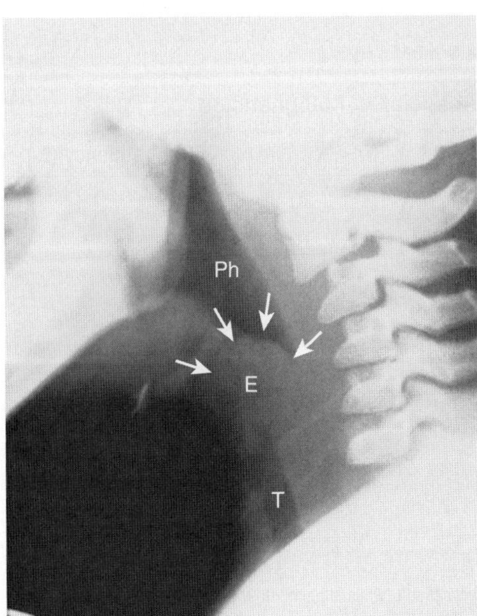

FIG. 1 Epiglottitis. A lateral soft tissue view of the neck shows a ballooned pharynx *(Ph)* with swollen epiglottis *(E)* in the shape of a large thumbprint *(arrows). T,* Trachea. (From Mettler FA [ed]: *Primary care radiology,* Philadelphia, 2000, Saunders.)

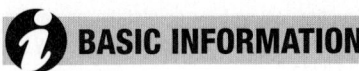

BASIC INFORMATION

DEFINITION

Epstein-Barr virus infection refers to a disease caused by Epstein-Barr virus (EBV), a human herpesvirus.

SYNONYMS

Infectious mononucleosis (IM)
Kissing disease

ICD-10CM CODES

B27.80 Other infectious mononucleosis without complication
B27.81 Other infectious mononucleosis with polyneuropathy
B27.82 Other infectious mononucleosis with meningitis
B27.89 Other infectious mononucleosis with other complication
B27.90 Infectious mononucleosis, unspecified without complication
B27.91 Infectious mononucleosis, unspecified with polyneuropathy
B27.92 Infectious mononucleosis, unspecified with meningitis
B27.99 Infectious mononucleosis, unspecified with other complication

EPIDEMIOLOGY & DEMOGRAPHICS

INCIDENCE (IN U.S.): 5 cases/100,000 persons per yr of IM

PREDOMINANT SEX: Neither, although peak incidence occurs about 2 yr earlier in women

PREDOMINANT AGE:

- Clinical evidence of IM: Occurs most commonly at ages 15 to 24 yr
- EBV infection: Occurs earlier in life in lower socioeconomic groups

PHYSICAL FINDINGS & CLINICAL PRESENTATION

- Most EBV infections either are asymptomatic or cause a nonspecific viral illness.
- Incubation period is 1 to 2 mo, possibly followed by a prodrome of anorexia, low-grade fever, malaise, headache, and chills; after several days, clinical triad of pharyngitis, moderate to high fever, and adenopathy may appear, accompanied by fatigue and malaise.
- Pharyngitis is usually the most severe symptom; white or necrotic exudates are common.
- Symmetrical lymphadenopathy is most prominent in the posterior more than anterior cervical region but may be diffuse.
- Splenomegaly (50% of cases) is possible, most commonly during the second week of illness.
- Maculopapular or morbilliform rash is uncommon but will often occur in patients who receive ampicillin (Fig. 1). Patients may have palatal petechiae, periorbital, or palpebral edema. Mucocutaneous oral hairy leukoplakia (OHL), which is associated with intense EBV replication and the action of EBV-encoded proteins such as latent membrane protein-1, may occur.
- Possible IM presentation: Fever and adenopathy without pharyngitis.
- Nausea, vomiting, and anorexia are frequent in patients with IM, probably reflecting mild hepatitis encountered in 90% of infected individuals.
- Although complications such as spleen rupture, airway obstruction, and malignancy may be severe and fatal, they are uncommon and tend to resolve completely.
- Hematologic involvement includes hemolytic or aplastic anemia, thrombocytopenia, thrombotic thrombocytopenic purpura/hemolytic-uremic syndrome, and disseminated intravascular coagulation (DIC). Pneumonia, myocarditis, pancreatitis, mesenteric adenitis, myositis, and glomerulonephritis may occur as well. Nervous system involvement includes Guillain-Barré syndrome, facial nerve palsy, meningoencephalitis, aseptic meningitis, transfer myelitis, peripheral neuritis, and optic neuritis.
- IM is usually a self-limited illness. Acute symptoms resolve in 1 to 2 wk, but symptoms of malaise and fatigue often persist for months.
- EBV is related to lymphoproliferative syndromes in transplant recipients and in AIDS patients.
- Increasing evidence showing an association between EBV infection and African Burkitt, B-cell, T-cell lymphoma, and nasopharyngeal carcinoma. Table 1 describes EBV-associated malignancies.

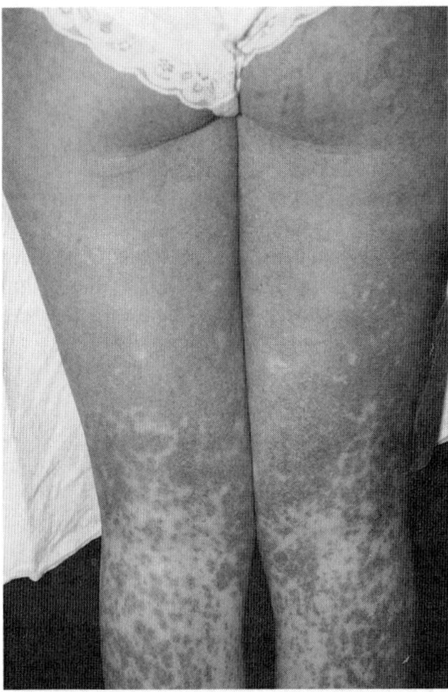

FIG. 1 Patient with infectious mononucleosis and ampicillin-induced rash. Maculopapular rash extends over the trunk and extremities. Rash frequently has a violaceous hue and is often accompanied by pruritus. (Bennett JE et al: *Mandell, Douglas, and Bennett's principles and practice of infectious diseases,* ed 8, Philadelphia, 2015, Saunders.)

ETIOLOGY

- EBV is a ubiquitous virus.
- Infection during childhood is much less likely to cause significant illness.
- Frequency of IM in late adolescence is attributed to the onset of social contact between the sexes.
- Close personal contact is usually necessary for transmission, although EBV is occasionally transmitted by blood transfusion; transfer via saliva while kissing may be responsible for many cases.

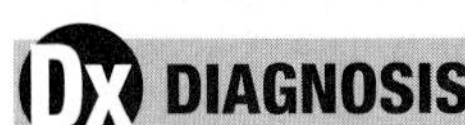

DIAGNOSIS

DIFFERENTIAL DIAGNOSIS

- Heterophile-negative IM caused by cytomegalovirus (CMV)
- Although clinical presentation similar, CMV more frequently follows transfusion
- Bacterial and viral causes of pharyngitis
- Toxoplasmosis
- Acute retroviral syndrome of HIV
- Lymphoma
- Lyme disease

TABLE 1 Epstein-Barr Virus (EBV)–Associated Malignancies

Malignancy	EBV Frequency (%)
Hodgkin's disease	~40
Non-Hodgkin's lymphomas	
Burkitt lymphoma	20-95
Diffuse large B-cell lymphoma and $CD30^+$ $Ki\text{-}1^+$ anaplastic large cell lymphoma	10-35
Lymphomatoid granulomatosis	80-95
T-cell–rich B-cell lymphoma	20
Angioimmunoblastic lymphoma	>80
T-cell, NK-cell, and T/NK-cell lymphomas	30-90
Nasopharyngeal carcinoma	>95
Gastric adenocarcinoma	5-10
Pyothorax-associated lymphoma	>95
Leiomyosarcoma in immunocompromised patients	>95

NK cell, Natural killer cell; *T cell,* T lymphocyte cell.
From Hoffman R et al: *Hematology: basic principles and practice,* ed 5, Philadelphia, 2009, Churchill Livingstone.

TABLE 2 Frequently Determined EBV-Specific Antibodies

Antibody Specificity	Positive in IM (%)	Time of Appearance in IM	Persistence	Comments
Viral Capsid Antigen				
VCA-IgM	100	At clinical presentation	4-8 weeks	Highly sensitive and specific; of major diagnostic utility
VCA-IgG	100	At clinical presentation	Lifelong	Useful for documentation of past EBV infection
Early Antigen				
Anti-D	70	Peaks 3-4 weeks after onset	3-6 months	Correlates with disease severity; seen in NPC patients
Anti-R	Low	2 weeks to several months after onset	2 months to >3 years	Occasionally seen with unusually severe cases; seen in African Burkitt lymphoma patients
EBNA	100	3-4 weeks after onset	Lifelong	Presence excludes primary EBV infection

EBNA, EBV nuclear antigen; *EBV,* Epstein-Barr virus; *Ig,* immunoglobulin; *IM,* infectious mononucleosis; *NPC,* nasopharyngeal carcinoma; *VCA,* viral capsid antigen.
Adapted from Schooley RT: Epstein-Barr virus (infectious mononucleosis). In Mandell GL et al (eds): *Principles and practice of infectious diseases,* Philadelphia, 2010, Churchill Livingstone.

WORKUP

Heterophile antibody and CBC with blood smear. Table 2 describes frequently determined EBV-specific antibodies.

LABORATORY TESTS

- Increased WBC common, with a relative lymphocytosis of more than 50% and neutropenia identified.
- Hallmark of IM: Atypical lymphocytes of more than 10% (not pathognomonic) are found.
- Mild thrombocytopenia is present.
- Falling hematocrit signals the possibility of splenic rupture or immune hemolytic anemia.
- Elevated hepatocellular enzymes and cryoglobulins are found in most cases.
- Heterophile antibody:
  1. As measured by the monospot test, may be positive at presentation or may appear later in the course of illness.
  2. Negative test is repeated in 1 wk if clinical suspicion is high.
  3. A positive test has been reported with primary HIV infection.
- Viral capsid antigen (VCA) IgG and IgM are rarely used for diagnosis, but better value in children because heterophile antibody is negative in most children younger than 8 yr.
- PCR DNA for CMV is the test of choice in transplant recipients who develop lymphoproliferative syndromes.

IMAGING STUDIES

Chest radiograph examination:
- May rarely show infiltrates
- Possible elevated left hemidiaphragm with splenic rupture

Rx TREATMENT

NONPHARMACOLOGIC THERAPY

- Supportive including rest
- Splenectomy if rupture occurs
- Transfusions for severe anemia or thrombocytopenia

ACUTE GENERAL Rx

- Pharmacologic therapy is not indicated in uncomplicated illness.
- Avoid aspirin due to the risk of Reye syndrome.
- Avoid ampicillin and amoxicillin as their use can frequently precipitate a nonallergic rash.
- Use of steroids is suggested in patients who have severe thrombocytopenia, hemolytic anemia, impending airway obstruction resulting from enlarged tonsils, or fulminant liver failure. Prednisone 60 to 80 mg PO qd for 3 days, then tapered over 1 to 2 wk.
- Although it may reduce initial viral shedding, there is little evidence to support the use of antiviral agents such as acyclovir in the management of IM.

CHRONIC Rx

An extremely rare, chronic form of IM with persistent fevers and fatigue has been described and should be differentiated from chronic fatigue syndrome, which is not related to EBV.

DISPOSITION

Eventual resolution of all symptoms

REFERRAL

If more than mild illness

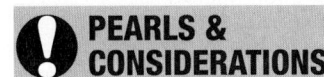

PEARLS & CONSIDERATIONS

COMMENTS

Avoidance of contact sports during the first month of illness because splenic rupture can occur even in the absence of clinically detectable splenomegaly.

RELATED CONTENT

Epstein-Barr Virus Infection (Patient Information)
Mononucleosis (Related Key Topic)

AUTHOR: **MONZR M. AL MALKI, M.D.**

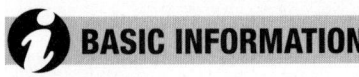

BASIC INFORMATION

DEFINITION

Erectile dysfunction (ED) is the persistent inability to achieve or sustain a penile erection of adequate rigidity to make sexual penetration possible or satisfactory.

SYNONYMS

ED
Impotence
Male erectile disorder
Sexual dysfunction (a nonspecific term)

ICD-10CM CODES

N48.4	Impotence of organic origin
F52.2	Failure of genital response
F52.9	Unspecified sexual dysfunction, not caused by organic disorder or disease
N52.01	Erectile dysfunction due to arterial insufficiency
N52.02	Corporo-venous occlusive erectile dysfunction
N52.03	Combined arterial insufficiency and corporo-venous occlusive erectile dysfunction
N52.1	Erectile dysfunction due to diseases classified elsewhere
N52.2	Drug-induced erectile dysfunction
N52.31	Erectile dysfunction following radical prostatectomy
N52.32	Erectile dysfunction following radical cystectomy
N52.33	Erectile dysfunction following urethral surgery
N52.34	Erectile dysfunction following simple prostatectomy
N52.39	Other post-surgical erectile dysfunction
N52.8	Other male erectile dysfunction
N52.9	Male erectile dysfunction, unspecified

DSM-5:
302.72 Failure of genital response

EPIDEMIOLOGY & DEMOGRAPHICS

PREVALENCE (IN U.S.):

- Increases with age and presence of specific medical comorbidities
- Approximately 8% in the 20s to 30s, 18% in the 50s, 25% in the 60s, 37% in the 70s, 80% in the 80s

PREDOMINANT SEX: By definition, only in males
PREDOMINANT AGE: Increases with age
RISK FACTORS: Age, coronary artery disease, peripheral vascular disease, hypertension, hypogonadism, diabetes mellitus, hypercholesterolemia, prostate surgery, neurologic injury, numerous medications, alcohol, smoking or drug abuse, obesity, obstructive sleep apnea, systemic sclerosis; psychological: performance anxiety.

ETIOLOGY

- A classification of male erectile dysfunction is described in Box 1.
- Most cases involving men older than 50 yr are caused by organic problems related to neurologic, hormonal, or vascular abnormalities or prescription or recreational drugs. In organic ED, nocturnal penile tumescence is generally diminished or absent, and ED is also experienced during private masturbation and across partners.
- Psychogenic ED results from mental stress, depression, a stressful partner relationship, a partner's sexual and mental health problems, and performance anxiety. Performance anxiety is extremely common and is characterized by a focus on the performance outcome of sex (i.e., obtaining and maintaining an erection) rather than a focus on the process and enjoyment of sex. Psychogenic ED is characterized by normal nocturnal penile tumescence and/or erections associated with erotic material or other partners, and by otherwise negative medical test results.
- Vascular disease: History of hypertension (HTN), peripheral vascular disease, ischemic heart disease, diabetes, smoking. In approximately 40% of men >50 yr, the primary cause of ED is related to atherosclerotic disease, diabetes mellitus (DM), neuropathy, or vascular disease.
- Obesity and metabolic syndrome.
- Medication side effects: Antihypertensives such as thiazides and clonidine, guanethidine or methyldopa (consider change to ACE inhibitors and calcium channel blockers with lower reported incidence of ED); antiandrogens such as spironolactone, finasteride, ketoconazole; cimetidine (but not ranitidine or famotidine); antidepressants such as selective serotonin reuptake inhibitors [SSRIs]; and antipsychotics. Table 1 summarizes drug-induced erectile dysfunction and suggested alternatives.

BOX 1 Classification of Male Erectile Dysfunction

Organic
- I. Vasculogenic
  - A. Arteriogenic
  - B. Cavernosal
  - C. Mixed
- II. Neurogenic
- III. Anatomic
- IV. Endocrinologic

Psychogenic
- I. Generalized
  - A. Generalized unresponsiveness
    1. Primary lack of sexual arousability
    2. Aging-related decline in sexual arousability
  - B. Generalized inhibition
    1. Chronic disorder of sexual intimacy
- II. Situational
  - A. Partner-related
    1. Lack of arousability in specific relationship
    2. Lack of arousability owing to sexual object preference
    3. High central inhibition owing to partner conflict or threat
  - B. Performance-related
    1. Associated with other sexual dysfunction (e.g., rapid ejaculation)
    2. Situational performance anxiety (e.g., fear of failure)
  - C. Psychological distress or adjustment related
    1. Associated with negative mood state (e.g., depression) or major life stress (e.g., death of partner)

From Wein AJ, Kavoussi LR, Partin AW et al: *Campbell-Walsh urology*, ed 11, Philadelphia, 2016, Elsevier.

TABLE 1 Drug-Induced Erectile Dysfunction and Suggested Alternatives

Class	Known to Cause Erectile Dysfunction	Suggested Alternatives
Antihypertensives	Thiazide diuretics General β blockers	α-Blockers Calcium channel blockers Specific β-blockers Angiotensin-converting enzyme inhibitors Angiotensin II receptor antagonists
Psychotropics	Antipsychotics Antidepressants Anxiolytics	Newer anxiolytics (bupropion, buspirone)
Antiandrogen	Androgen receptor antagonists Luteinizing hormone–releasing hormone agonists 5α-Reductase inhibitors	
Opiates		
Antiretroviral agents		
Tobacco		Quit smoking
Alcohol	Large amount	Small amount

From Wein AJ, Kavoussi LR, Partin AW et al: *Campbell-Walsh urology*, ed 11, Philadelphia, 2016, Elsevier.

- Excessive alcohol and nicotine use.
- Recreational drugs, including cocaine, heroin, amphetamines, and marijuana. These may increase libido but impair performance.
- Hormonal dysfunction such as testosterone deficiency (decreases libido and erection), hypothyroidism or hyperthyroidism, hyperprolactinemia, and adrenal insufficiency.
- Neurogenic causes including spinal cord lesions, cortical lesions, and peripheral neuropathies.
- Trauma or pelvic surgeries such as radical prostatectomy or cystectomy.

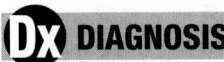

DIAGNOSIS

DIFFERENTIAL DIAGNOSIS

- A useful tool to diagnose/evaluate ED severity is the Sexual Health Inventory for Men (SHIM).
- Distinguish psychogenic and organic contributions to ED.
- Evaluate for underlying etiology of organic ED and comorbid psychiatric condition.

WORKUP

- Clinical history should include time course (abrupt onset may correlate with reversible cause such as medications, psychosocial stress, psychiatric complaint, trauma; nonsustained erection may be secondary to anxiety or vascular steal syndrome), cause (psychogenic vs. organic), and change in libido. Box 2 describes symptoms suggesting neurologic sexual impairment.
- Report of spontaneous nocturnal or morning erections indicate intact neurologic reflexes and penile blood flow.
- Decreased libido may indicate endocrinologic or psychogenic cause.
- If possible, interview partner regarding partner's sexual function, relationship satisfaction, and mental health history.
- Medical and social history should address cardiac disease symptoms and risk factors (HTN, DM, hyperlipidemia, smoking, and substance abuse), pelvic surgery, medications, and mental health. Coronary artery calcium score (CAC) is best indicator of subclinical coronary artery disease.

BOX 2 Symptoms Suggesting Neurologic Sexual Impairment

Continual erectile dysfunction
  Absence of morning erections
  No erection or orgasm during masturbation or sex with different partners
Related somatic complaints
Sensory loss in genitals, pelvis, or legs
Urinary incontinence
Certain neurologic conditions
  Spinal cord injury
  Diabetic neuropathy
  Multiple sclerosis
  Herniated intervertebral disk
Use of many medications

From Kaufman DM, Geyer HL, Milstein MJ: *Kaufman's clinical neurology for psychiatrists*, ed 8, Philadelphia, 2017, Elsevier.

- Physical examination to check blood pressure, visual field defects to evaluate for pituitary tumors; femoral and peripheral pulses, femoral bruits; gynecomastia; neuronal damage (genital sensation, cremasteric reflex); direct penile damage (e.g., plaque formation such as Peyronie's disease); prostate examination; or testicular atrophy and other secondary sexual characteristics. Signs of neurologic sexual impairment are summarized in Box 3.

LABORATORY TESTS

Screen for diabetes mellitus with fasting glucose. Consider lipid panel, thyroid-stimulating hormone, morning serum testosterone (free and total). If decreased testosterone, check prolactin, follicle-stimulating hormone, and luteinizing hormone.

IMAGING STUDIES

Imaging studies are rarely performed except in situations of pelvic trauma or surgery.

OTHER STUDIES

- Nocturnal penile tumescence testing is very specific for distinguishing psychogenic versus organic causes.
- Neurogenic etiologies examined by the cremasteric reflex (inner-thigh touch elicits scrotal contraction), the bulbocavernosus reflex, or the pudendal-evoked response.
- Intracorporeal injection of prostaglandin E_1 to distinguish vascular and nonvascular etiologies (erection is achieved in patients with normal vascular systems). If no erection with direct injection of vasoactive substance, consider duplex ultrasound of penile vasculature.
- In patients without an obvious cause of ED, consider screening for cardiovascular disease prior to starting treatment.

Rx TREATMENT (FIG. 1)

NON-PHARMACOLOGIC THERAPY

- Various psychotherapeutic approaches: Cognitive-behavioral therapy preferred; success rates decrease with advancing age and duration of symptoms.
- Psychosexual therapy is first line for psychogenic ED. Psychosexual therapy may be used as for adjunctive therapy in ED from any cause to address contributing, performance anxiety, social, and relationship issues.
- Performance anxiety is best addressed by sensate focus in which a couple is asked to refrain from sexual penetration but enjoy erotic touching.
- Mechanical vacuum devices (function by drawing blood into corpus cavernosum) are 70% to 90% effective but are difficult to use and subject to noncompliance.
- Incorporate vascular risk factor reduction including counsel on diet, exercise, smoking cessation, ETOH intake and screening/treatment for HTN, insulin resistance, and hypercholesterolemia as appropriate. Trials have shown that lifestyle modification and pharmacotherapy for cardiovascular risk factors are effective in improving sexual function in men with ED.

BOX 3 Signs of Neurologic Sexual Impairment

Signs of spinal cord injury
  Paraparesis or quadriparesis
  Leg spasticity
  Urinary incontinence
Signs of autonomic nervous system injury
  Orthostatic hypotension or lightheadedness
  Anhidrosis in groin and legs
  Urinary incontinence
  Retrograde ejaculation
Signs of peripheral nervous system injury
  Loss of sensation in the genitals, "saddle area," and legs
  Paresis and areflexia in legs
  Scrotal, cremasteric, and anal reflex loss

From Kaufman DM, Geyer HL, Milstein MJ: *Kaufman's clinical neurology for psychiatrists*, ed 8, Philadelphia, 2017, Elsevier.

ACUTE GENERAL Rx

- First-line treatment: In setting of sexual stimulation, four selective phosphodiesterase type 5 (PDE5) inhibitors (Table 2) prolong nitric oxide–induced vasodilation by increase of intracavernosal cyclic guanosine monophosphate levels. Sildenafil (Viagra) and vardenafil (Levitra, Staxyn) can be taken 30 to 60 min before sexual activity, and both are effective for about 4 hr. Avanafil (Stendra) can be taken 15 to 30 min before sexual activity and is effective for about 6 hr. Tadalafil (Cialis) can be taken several hours before sexual activity (although 50% respond within 30 min) and lasts up to 36 hr. All four PDE5 inhibitors have similar efficacy and tolerability, but tadalafil has a longer duration of action and is less affected by high-fat meals and alcohol. Counsel patients to avoid high-fat meals and excessive alcohol when taking PDE5 inhibitors, as they may impede effectiveness.
- With PDE5 inhibitors, avoid concomitant use of nitrates (absolute contraindication), drugs that inhibit or induce cytochrome P450 CYP3A4, and drugs that prolong the QT interval. Caution in men on alpha-adrenergic blocker therapy because of concern for hypotension; start the lowest dose of PDE5 inhibitor. Caution in men who have had myocardial infarction in the past 6 mo, resting hypotension or uncontrolled hypertension, unstable angina, positive exercise stress test or poor exercise tolerance. Counsel on side effects of headache, flushing, dyspepsia, nasal congestion, changes in color perception (including blue vision for sildenafil and vardenafil but not tadalafil), sudden hearing loss, and priapism (rare). Nonarteritic anterior ischemic optic neuropathy is also a rare association with sildenafil and tadalafil. Consider counseling on safe sexual practices when prescribing PDE5 inhibitors.
- Second-line treatment if PDE5 inhibitors fail: Self-injection with intraurethral alprostadil

(prostaglandin E_1 [medicated urethral suppository]) applied into meatus of penis before intercourse; or intracavernosal injections of vasodilators (e.g., papaverine or prostaglandin E_1). Consider combining intraurethral alprostadil with PDE5 inhibitor. Relatively high success with self-injection, but attrition is high (Table E3).
- Second-line treatment alternative: Vacuum constriction pump; has variable satisfaction rate.

CHRONIC Rx

- Psychosexual therapy is helpful as an adjunctive treatment.
- Psychogenic impotence: PDE5 inhibitors are effective in patients with depression because tissues, nerves, hormones, and vasculature are normal. PDE5 inhibitors are also effective as a way of providing positive experiences and building sexual confidence. Full psychological evaluation is recommended before starting treatment.
- For men not responding to other approaches: Surgical implantation of penile prosthesis may be considered. Full psychological evaluation is recommended to evaluate the possibility of unrealistic expectations or partner problems contributing to ED.
- Testosterone therapy in men with low testosterone (i.e., hypogonadal); evaluate for prostate cancer before prescribing testosterone.
- Aerobic exercise may improve ED along with pharmacologic treatment.

DISPOSITION

- Psychogenic-acquired ED will remit spontaneously in 15% to 30% of cases.
- Lifelong ED is usually a chronic and unremitting condition.
- Situational ED may remit with changes in social environment and reducing performance anxiety.

REFERRAL

- Refer if psychotherapy, sexual focused therapy, or invasive organic treatment required
- Refer to urology if PDE5 inhibitors fail or sudden onset occurs after penile trauma

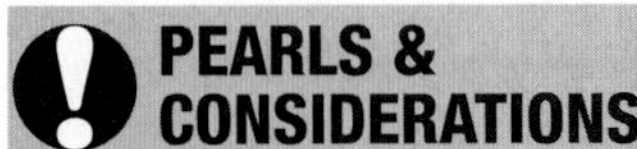

PEARLS & CONSIDERATIONS

- ED is commonly evaluated and treated by primary care physician; refer to urologist if oral therapy fails or surgery is required.
- PDE5 inhibitors are treatment of choice for most causes of ED. Main contraindications are nitrate use and decompensated cardiac disease. Caution in patients on alpha-adrenergic blockers and with blood pressures at extreme ends (significant hypotension or hypertension).
- For optimal response, patients should be appropriately informed of proper use, precautions, and adverse effects of PDE5 inhibitors. Try six to eight times at optimal doses before declaring PDE5 inhibitors a failure. Consider switching among the four PDE5 inhibitors if one fails.
- Men with ED are at increased risk of coronary, cerebrovascular, and peripheral vascular diseases. Screen for cardiovascular risk factors in these patients.

SUGGESTED READINGS

Available at ExpertConsult.com

RELATED CONTENT

Erectile Dysfunction (Patient Information)
Ejaculation and Orgasm Disorders (Related Key Topic)

AUTHOR: **JOHN P. WINCZE, PH.D.**

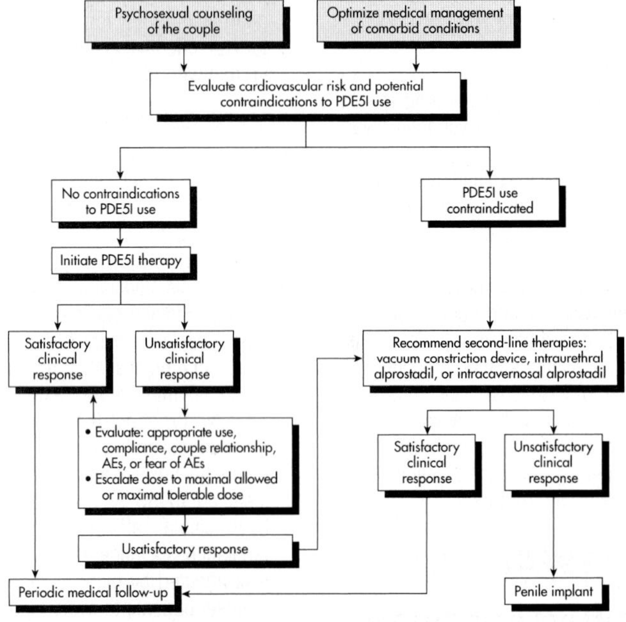

FIG. 1 An algorithmic approach to the treatment of erectile dysfunction in men. *AE,* Adverse effects; *PDE5I,* phosphodiesterase 5 inhibitor. (From Melmed S, Polonsky KS, Larsen PR, Kronenberg HM: *Williams textbook of endocrinology,* ed 12, Philadelphia, 2011, Saunders.)

TABLE 2 Comparison of Four Phosphodiesterase Type 5 Inhibitors Currently Available in the United States

	Sildenafil	Vardenafil	Tadalafil	Avanafil
Cmax (ng/ml)	450	20.9	378	2153
Tmax (hr)	0.8	0.7-0.9	2	0.3-0.5
Onset of action (min)	15-60	15-60	15-120	15-60
Half-life (hr)	3-5	4-5	17.5	3-5
Bioavailability	40%	15%	Not tested	30%
Fatty food	Reduced absorption	Reduced absorption	No effect	Reduced absorption
Recommended dosage	25, 50, 100 mg	5, 10, 20 mg	5, 10, 20 mg	50, 100, 200 mg
Side effects				
Headache, dyspepsia, facial flushing	Yes	Yes	Yes	Yes
Backache, myalgia	Rare	Rare	Yes	Rare
Blurred/blue vision	Yes	Rare	Rare	No
Precaution with antiarrhythmics	No	Yes	No	No
Contraindication with nitrates	Yes	Yes	Yes	Yes

Cmax, Maximal plasma concentration; *half-life,* time required for elimination of one half of the medication from plasma; *Tmax,* time required to attain Cmax.
From Wein AJ, Kavoussi LR, Partin AW et al: *Campbell-Walsh urology,* ed 11, Philadelphia, 2016, Elsevier.

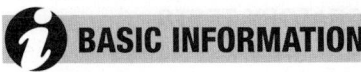

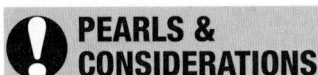

BASIC INFORMATION

DEFINITION

Erysipelas is a type of cellulitis caused by infection of the superficial layers of the skin and cutaneous lymphatics. Erysipelas is characterized by redness, induration, lymphangitis, lymphadenopathy, and a sharply demarcated, raised border.

SYNONYM

St. Anthony's fire

ICD-10CM CODE
A46 Erysipelas

EPIDEMIOLOGY & DEMOGRAPHICS

PREDOMINANT AGE: Occurs most often in the young or old
RISK FACTORS: Patients with impaired lymphatic or venous drainage (mastectomy, saphenous vein harvesting) and immunocompromised patients. Athlete's foot is a common portal of entry.
RECURRENCE RATE: Relatively common

PHYSICAL FINDINGS & CLINICAL PRESENTATION

- Distinctive red, warm, tender skin lesion with induration and a sharply defined, advancing, raised border (Fig. 1).
- Most common sites are lower extremities and face.
- Systemic signs of infection (fever) are often present.
- Vesicles or bullae may develop.
- After several days, lesions may appear ecchymotic.
- After 7 to 10 days, desquamation of affected area may occur.

ETIOLOGY

- Usually group A β-hemolytic streptococci (GABHS)
- Less often group B, C, or G streptococci
- Rarely *Staphylococcus aureus*

COMPLICATIONS

- Abscess
- Necrotizing fasciitis
- Thrombophlebitis
- Gangrene
- Metastatic infection

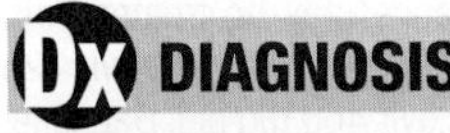

DIAGNOSIS

DIFFERENTIAL DIAGNOSIS

- Other types of cellulitis
- Necrotizing fasciitis
- Deep vein thrombosis
- Stasis dermatitis
- Erythema nodosum
- Contact dermatitis
- Erythema migrans (Lyme disease)
- Insect bite
- Herpes zoster
- Erysipeloid
- Acute gout
- Pseudogout

WORKUP

History, physical examination, and laboratory evaluation

LABORATORY TESTS

Diagnosis is usually made by characteristic clinical setting and appearance.

- Complete blood count: White blood cell count often elevated.

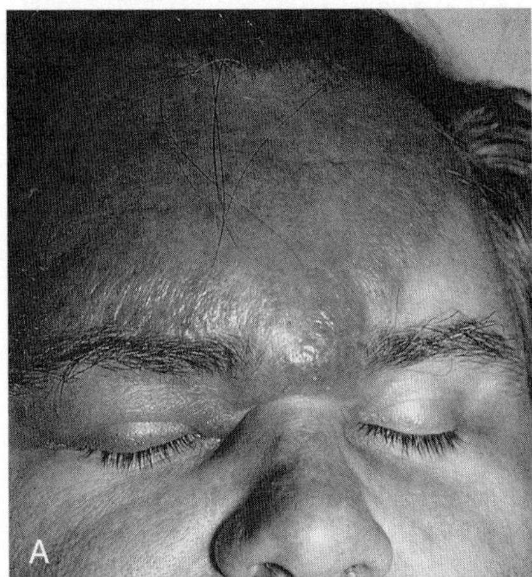

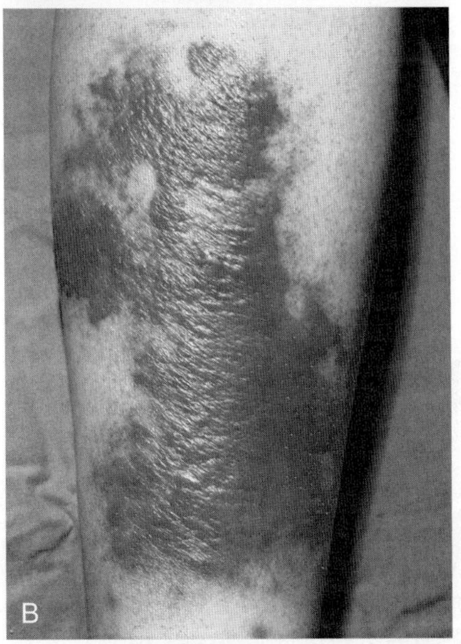

FIG. 1 A and B, Erysipelas. (From James WD, Berger TG, Elston DM et al: *Andrews' diseases of the skin*, ed 12, Philadelphia, 2016, Elsevier.)

- Blood cultures positive in 5% of patients. Septic, or there is a history of animal bites for immersion injury and are not routinely indicated unless the host is immunocompromised.
- Gram stain and culture of any drainage from skin lesions.
- Culture of aspirated fluid from leading edge of skin lesion has low yield.

IMAGING STUDIES

- Not routinely indicated
- Duplex ultrasound for patients suspected of having deep vein thrombosis
- CT scan or MRI for patients with suspected necrotizing fasciitis

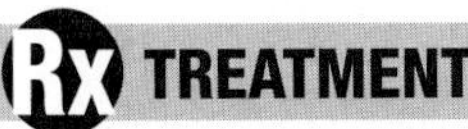

TREATMENT

NONPHARMACOLOGIC THERAPY

- Elevation of the affected limb
- Warm compresses

ACUTE GENERAL Rx

Typical erysipelas of extremity in nondiabetic patient:

- PO: Penicillin V 500 mg q6h. Use clindamycin in patients who are allergic to penicillin.
- IV: Penicillin G (aqueous) 1 to 2 million units q6h. Use vancomycin 15 mg/kg IV q12h in penicillin-allergic patients.

Facial erysipelas (include coverage for *Staphylococcus aureus*):

- PO dicloxacillin 500 mg q6h
- IV nafcillin or oxacillin 2 g q4h
- IV vancomycin 1 g q12h
- Daptomycin 4 mg/kg IV q24h
- Linezolid 600 mg IV q12h

DISPOSITION

Prognosis is good with antibiotic treatment but recurrence is common.

REFERRAL

For surgical debridement for patients with necrotizing fasciitis or for drainage of abscess

PEARLS & CONSIDERATIONS

- Consider early surgical referral when necrotizing fasciitis suspected. Consider skin biopsy when not responding to appropriate antibiotics.
- Look for tinea pedis as portal of entry in erysipelas of lower extremities, and treat if present.

RELATED CONTENT

Erysipelas (Patient Information)
Cellulitis (Related Key Topic)

AUTHOR: **GAIL M. O'BRIEN, M.D.**

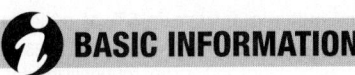

BASIC INFORMATION

DEFINITION

Erythema multiforme is an inflammatory disease characterized by eruption of annular, maculopapular lesions with dark raised, erythematous, or vesiculobullous center surrounded by a pale zone. It is believed to be caused by immune complex formation and subsequent deposition in the skin and mucous membranes. It is considered a hypersensitivity reaction to infection or drugs.

SYNONYM

EM

ICD-10CM CODES
L51.9 Erythema multiforme, unspecified
L51.0 Nonbullous erythema multiforme
L51.8 Other erythema multiforme

EPIDEMIOLOGY & DEMOGRAPHICS

PREDOMINANT AGE: 20 to 40 yr
RISK FACTORS: Often associated with herpes simplex and other infectious agents, drugs, or connective tissue diseases

PHYSICAL FINDINGS & CLINICAL PRESENTATION

- Prodromal symptoms are mild or absent. Itching or burning at the site of eruption may occur.
- Symmetric skin lesions (Fig. E1) with a classic "target" appearance (caused by the centrifugal spread of red maculopapules to circumference of 1 to 3 cm with a purpuric, cyanotic, or vesicular center) are present (Fig. 2). The papules may enlarge into plaques measuring a few centimeters in diameter with a dark or red central portion (Fig. E3). Target lesions may not be apparent for several days and generally heal in 1 to 2 weeks without scarring.
- EM lesions are most common on the face, back of the hands and feet, and extensor aspect of the forearms and legs (EM minor). Trunk involvement can occur in severe cases (EM major).
- Urticarial papules, vesicles, and bullae may also be present and generally indicate EM major.
- EM major bullae and erosions may also be present in the oral cavity. The most common sites are the lips and buccal mucosa.

ETIOLOGY

- Immune complex formation and subsequent deposition in the cutaneous microvasculature may play a role in the pathogenesis of erythema multiforme.
- The majority of cases follow outbreaks of herpes simplex virus 1 and 2.
- *Mycoplasma pneumoniae,* fungal infections, medications (bupropion, sulfonamides, penicillins, nonsteroidal antiinflammatory drugs, barbiturates, phenothiazines, hydantoins).
- In >50% of patients no specific cause is identified.

Dx DIAGNOSIS

DIFFERENTIAL DIAGNOSIS

- Chronic urticaria
- Pityriasis rosea
- Contact dermatitis
- Pemphigus vulgaris
- Lichen planus
- Serum sickness
- Drug eruption
- Granuloma annulare
- Polymorphic light eruption
- Viral exanthema
- Stevens-Johnson syndrome (SJS)
- Toxic epidermal necrolysis (TEN)
- Bullous pemphigoid
- Viral exanthems
- Leukocytoclastic vasculitis
- Lupus erythematosus
- Secondary syphilis

WORKUP

- Medical history with emphasis on drug ingestion.
- Laboratory evaluation in patients with suspected collagen-vascular diseases.
- Skin biopsy when diagnosis is unclear.

LABORATORY TESTS

- Complete blood count with differential, elevated ESR
- Antinuclear antibody
- Serology for *Mycoplasma pneumoniae,* HSV-1, HSV-2
- Biopsy for atypical cases
- Direct immunofluorescence if suspecting bullous diseases

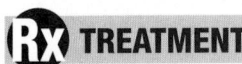

TREATMENT

NONPHARMACOLOGIC THERAPY

- Mild cases generally do not require treatment; lesions resolve spontaneously within 1 mo.
- Potential drug precipitants should be removed.

ACUTE GENERAL Rx

- Treatment of associated diseases (e.g., valacyclovir or famciclovir for herpes simplex, erythromycin for *Mycoplasma* infection).
- Dapsone, antimalarials or azathioprine for severe or resistant cases.
- Prednisone 40 to 80 mg/day for 1 to 3 wk is effective for decreasing inflammation and pain and may be tried in patients with many target lesions; however, the role of systemic steroids remains controversial.
- Levamisole, an immunomodulator, may be effective in the treatment of patients with chronic or recurrent oral lesions (dose is 150 mg/day for 3 consecutive days used alone or in combination with prednisone).
- IV immunoglobulins in severe cases.
- Antimicrobial therapy is indicated if *M. pneumoniae* is the trigger of EM.

DISPOSITION

The rash generally evolves over a 2-wk period and resolves within 3 to 4 wk without scarring. A severe bullous form can occur (see entry for "Stevens-Johnson Syndrome").

REFERRAL

Hospital admission in patients with suspected Stevens-Johnson syndrome

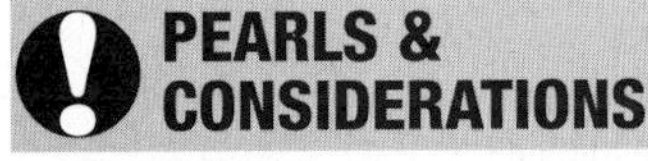

PEARLS & CONSIDERATIONS

COMMENTS

The risk of recurrence of erythema multiforme exceeds 30%. Recurrence may be treated with valacyclovir 500 to 1000 mg/day, famciclovir 125 to 250 mg/day, or acyclovir 400 mg bid. Dapsone, antimalarials, azathioprine, or cyclosporine use is reserved for cases resistant to antivirals.

RELATED CONTENT

Erythema Multiforme (Patient Information)
Stevens-Johnson Syndrome (Related Key Topic)

AUTHOR: **FRED F. FERRI, M.D.**

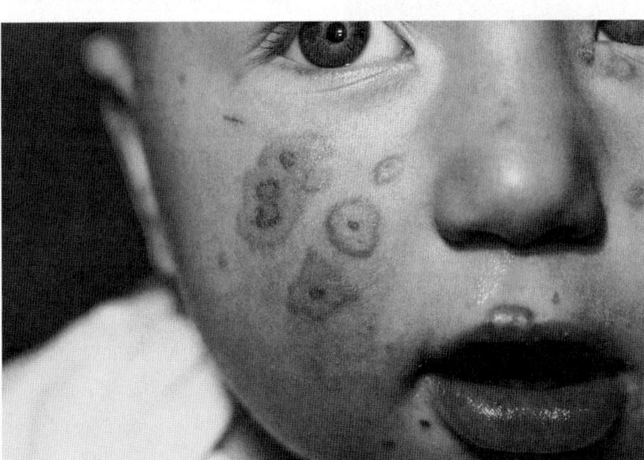

FIG. 2 Erythema multiforme. Classic target lesions and marginated wheals with central vesicles are characteristic. (From Paller AS, Mancini, AJ: *Hurwitz clinical pediatric dermatology: a textbook of skin disorders of childhood and adolescence,* ed 5, Philadelphia, 2016, Elsevier.)

BASIC INFORMATION

DEFINITION

Erythema nodosum (EN) is an acute, tender, erythematous, nodular skin eruption resulting from inflammation of subcutaneous fat, often associated with bruising. It is the most common form of panniculitis.

SYNONYM

EN

ICD-10CM CODE
L52 Erythema nodosum

EPIDEMIOLOGY & DEMOGRAPHICS

INCIDENCE: It is the most common form of panniculitis. Two to three cases/100,000 persons per yr.
PREDOMINANT SEX: Female:male ratio of 3 to 4:1
PREDOMINANT AGE: 25 to 40 yr

PHYSICAL FINDINGS & CLINICAL PRESENTATION

- Prodromal symptoms of fatigue, malaise, upper respiratory infection symptoms may precede eruption by 1 to 2 wk.
- Acute onset of tender nodules typically located on the shins and occasionally seen on the thighs and forearms (Fig. 1).
- The nodules are usually 1/8 to 1 inch in diameter but can be as large as 4 inches; they begin as light red lesions, then become darker and often ecchymotic. The nodules heal within 8 wk without ulceration.
- Associated findings:
  1. Fever (60%)
  2. Lymphadenopathy (<50%)
  3. Arthralgia (64%)
  4. Signs of the underlying illness

ETIOLOGY

Cell-mediated hypersensitivity reaction is seen more frequently in persons with human leukocyte antigen (HLA) B8. The lesion results from an exaggerated interaction between an antigen and cell-mediated immune mechanisms leading to granuloma formation. Up to 55% of cases of EN are idiopathic.
Infections:
- Bacteria
  1. Campylobacter
  2. Streptococcal pharyngitis (28% to 48%)
  3. *Salmonella* enteritis
  4. *Yersinia* enteritis
  5. Psittacosis
  6. *Chlamydia pneumoniae* infection
  7. *Mycoplasma* pneumonia
  8. Meningococcal infection
  9. Gonorrhea
  10. Syphilis
  11. Lymphogranuloma venereum
  12. Tularemia
  13. Cat-scratch disease
  14. Leprosy
  15. Tuberculosis
- Fungi
  1. Histoplasmosis
  2. Coccidioidomycosis
  3. Blastomycosis
  4. Tri*chophyton verrucosum*
- Viruses
  1. Cytomegalovirus
  2. Hepatitis B
  3. Epstein-Barr virus
- Drugs (3% to 10%)
  1. Sulfonylureas
  2. Sulfonamides
  3. Penicillins
  4. Oral contraceptives
  5. Gold salts
  6. Prazosin
  7. Aspirin
  8. Bromides
- Sarcoidosis (11% to 25%)
- Inflammatory bowel disease
- Hodgkin's disease, non-Hodgkin's lymphoma
- Ankylosing spondylosis and reactive arthropathies (e.g., associated with inflammatory bowel disease)
- Behçet's disease
- Löfgren syndrome
- Acute myelogenous leukemia

FIG. 1 Erythema nodosum. Tender, red, oval nodules on the extensor aspect of the legs. Note that several have darkened and resemble bruises. (From Paller AS, Mancini, AJ: *Hurwitz clinical pediatric dermatology: a textbook of skin disorders of childhood and adolescence,* ed 5, 2016, Elsevier.)

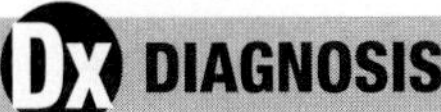

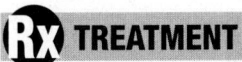

DIAGNOSIS

DIFFERENTIAL DIAGNOSIS

- Insect bites
- Posttraumatic ecchymoses
- Vasculitis
- Weber-Christian disease
- Fat necrosis associated with pancreatitis
- Necrobiosis lipoidica
- Scleroderma
- Lupus panniculitis
- Subcutaneous granuloma

WORKUP

- Physical examination
- Diagnosis of underlying illness by history, physical examination, and laboratory tests as indicated

LABORATORY TESTS

- Erythrocyte sedimentation rate
- Throat culture and antistreptolysin O titer
- PPD
- Others depending on index of suspicion (e.g., stool culture and evaluation for ova and parasites in patients with diarrhea and gastrointestinal symptoms)
- Skin biopsy in doubtful cases:
  1. Early lesion: Inflammation and hemorrhage in subcutaneous tissue
  2. Late lesion: Giant cells and granulomata

IMAGING STUDIES

Chest radiograph to rule out sarcoidosis and tuberculosis

TREATMENT

- The disease is self-limited and treatment is symptomatic. EN nodules develop in pretibial locations and resolve spontaneously over several weeks without scarring or ulceration.
- Treatment of underlying disorders.
- Avoidance of contact irritation of affected areas.
- Nonsteroidal antiinflammatory drugs for pain.
- Systemic steroids (prednisone 1 mg/kg of body weight/day, tapered over several days) may be useful in severe cases if underlying risk of sepsis and malignancy have been excluded.
- Potassium iodide given as tablet 300 mg tid or as a supersaturated solution (five drops three times/day in orange juice) has been reported as effective for symptom control.
- Intralesional corticosteroid injections for persistent lesions.

PROGNOSIS

Typical case:
- Pain for 2 wk
- Resolution within 8 wk

RELATED CONTENT

Erythema Nodosum (Patient Information)
Sarcoidosis (Related Key Topic)

AUTHOR: **FRED F. FERRI, M.D.**

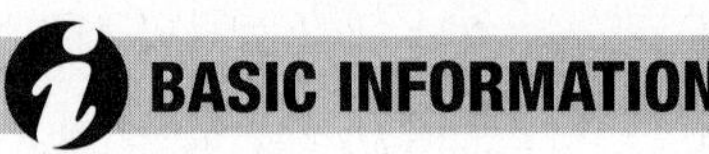

BASIC INFORMATION

DEFINITION

Esophageal tumors include benign and malignant neoplasms of the esophageal mucosa and wall. Carcinomas of the esophageal epithelium, both squamous cell carcinoma and adenocarcinoma (including adenoacanthoma, mucoepidermoid, and adenoid cystic), are the most common tumors of the esophagus. Rare esophageal tumors include both malignant (spindle cell, small cell, sarcoma, lymphoma, melanoma, and choriocarcinoma) and benign neoplasms (leiomyoma, papilloma, and fibrovascular polyps). One can also develop metastatic disease from a cancer that originated in another organ, but this is very rare. Breast cancer, lung cancer, and melanoma would be the most likely culprits. Approximately 15% of esophageal tumors arise in the proximal esophagus, 50% in the middle third of the esophagus, and 35% in the lower third. Tumors involving the esophageal-gastric junction are usually staged and treated as esophageal cancers if the tumor epicenter is no more than 2 cm into the proximal stomach. Tumors in the upper two thirds are usually squamous cell cancers, and tumors in the lower third are usually adenocarcinomas. The incidence of superficial esophageal cancers is increasing. These invade no deeper than the submucosa.

ICD-10CM CODES	
C15.X	Malignant neoplasm of the esophagus (X defines location)
C15.3	Malignant neoplasm of upper third of esophagus
C15.4	Malignant neoplasm of middle third of esophagus
C15.5	Malignant neoplasm of lower third of esophagus
D00.2	Carcinoma of esophagus, in situ

EPIDEMIOLOGY & DEMOGRAPHICS

INCIDENCE: It is the eighth most common cancer worldwide and the seventh leading cause of cancer deaths. Rates are increasing every decade and are highest in the Asian esophageal cancer belt, extending from the Caspian Sea to northern China, with certain high-incidence pockets in Finland, Ireland, southeast Africa, and northwest France. Incidence has increased six-fold since 1975. Foods including cured meats and spicy regional fare likely play a role in certain areas. Rates of squamous cell carcinoma are decreasing while those of adenocarcinomas are dramatically increasing. The causes of squamous cell carcinoma most commonly include tobacco and alcohol abuse. Epithelial dysplasia usually occurs, which progresses to carcinoma in situ. Adenocarcinomas are usually the result of GERD and obesity. The mucosa of the esophagus undergoes intestinal metaplasia. Genetic alterations occur, which perpetuate the cell changes during proliferation.

PREVALENCE: In the U.S., there was an estimated 16,000 new cases and 15,000 deaths are reported yearly, making it the seventh leading cause of death by cancer among men. The majority of cases are diagnosed at an advanced stage (unresectable or metastatic disease).

RACE, AGE, & SEX PREDOMINANCE: In the United States, squamous cell esophageal cancer is more common among blacks than whites, whereas adenocarcinoma is more common in whites than blacks. The overall male/female ratio is 3 to 4:1; the highest male/female ratio is in the Hispanic population. It usually develops in the fifth to seventh decades and is associated with lower socioeconomic status.

GENETICS: Increasing evidence shows that genetics may play a role by increasing susceptibility to esophageal cancer. One well-identified disease associated with esophageal cancer is tylosis (focal non-epidermolytic palmoplantar keratoderma), linked to loss of heterozygosity on chromosome 17q. Familiar clustering of Barrett esophagus and the recent identification of germline mutations in affected sibling pairs support a genetic link to esophageal adenocarcinoma. Also, up to 35% of esophageal adenocarcinomas can have overexpression of HER2, which can lead to the use of targeted therapy (trastuzumab) in the treatment plan.

CLINICAL PRESENTATION

Symptoms and signs:

- Dysphagia (74%): Initially with solid foods, gradually progresses to semisolids and liquids; the latter signs usually indicate incurable disease with tumor involving more than 60% of the esophageal circumference. It may be felt as chest pain.
- Unintentional weight loss: Usually of short duration. Losing >10% of body mass predicts poor outcome.
- Hoarseness: Suggests recurrent laryngeal nerve involvement.
- Odynophagia and halitosis: Unusual symptoms.
- Cervical adenopathy: Usually involving supraclavicular lymph nodes.
- Dry cough: Suggests tracheal involvement.
- Aspiration pneumonia: Caused by fistula between the esophagus and trachea.
- Iron deficiency anemia: Related to chronic GI blood loss.
- Massive hemoptysis or hematemesis from the invasion of vascular structures.
- Advanced disease spreads to lymph nodes, liver, lungs, peritoneum, and pleura.
- Hypercalcemia: Associated with squamous cell carcinoma from secretion of a parathyroid-like tumor peptide.

Clinical findings:

- 50% to 60% of patients present with the inoperative stage of their disease (locally advanced, regional, or metastatic).

ETIOLOGY

The pathogenesis of esophageal cancers is attributable to chronic recurrent oxidative damage from any of the following etiologic agents, which cause inflammation, and esophagitis, increased cell turnover, and, ultimately, initiation of the carcinogenic process.

ETIOLOGIC AGENTS: Squamous cell carcinoma

- Excess alcohol consumption is strongly associated with squamous cell esophageal cancer in the United States; hard liquor is associated with a higher incidence than wine or beer.
- Tobacco and alcohol synergistically increase risk for squamous cell cancer.
- Other ingested carcinogens:
  1. Nitrates (converted to nitrites): South Asia, China.
  2. Smoked opiates: Northern Iran.
  3. Fungal toxins in pickled vegetables.
  4. Betel nut chewing.
- Mucosal damage:
  1. Long-term exposure to extremely hot tea (>70° C 158° F).
  2. Lye ingestion.
- Radiation-induced strictures.
- Achalasia: Incidence of esophageal cancer is seven times greater in this population.
- Host susceptibility as a result of precancerous lesions:
  1. Plummer-Vinson syndrome (Paterson-Kelly): Glossitis with iron deficiency.
  2. Congenital hyperkeratosis and pitting of palms and soles (tylosis).
- Human papillomavirus infection (particularly types 16 and 18) has been variably detected in squamous cell carcinoma of the esophagus, sometimes associated with p53 tumor suppressor gene mutations.
- Questionable relationship with prolonged bisphosphonate use (≥10 prescriptions, or use >3 yrs).
- Possible association with celiac sprue or dietary deficiencies of molybdenum, selenium, zinc, vitamin A.

ADENOCARCINOMA: The incidence of adenocarcinoma is continually rising, whereas that of squamous cell carcinoma is unchanged.

- Smoking increases the risk of developing adenocarcinoma, particularly in patients with Barrett.
- Obesity, hiatal hernia, and diets lacking in fresh fruit and vegetables and high in fat (particularly from red meat and processed foods).
- Chronic GERD leading to Barrett metaplasia and adenocarcinoma via immune cell infiltration and production of inflammatory mediators and reactive oxygen species. The annual rate of transformation from Barrett to adenocarcinoma is <0.5%.
- *H. pylori* infection may reduce the risk of adenocarcinoma.

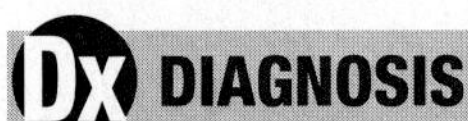

DIAGNOSIS

DIFFERENTIAL DIAGNOSIS

- Achalasia
- Scleroderma of the esophagus
- Diffuse esophageal spasm
- Esophageal rings and webs

LABORATORY TESTS

Complete blood cell count, blood chemistry, and liver enzymes should be obtained at diagnosis. No biomarkers are currently recommended to diagnose, monitor, or predict outcomes. While both the CEA and CA-19-9 can be elevated in patients with esophageal cancer (up to 70%), the sensitivity is low (18 % to 35%) and there is no proven predictive value.

IMAGING STUDIES

Imaging studies are important not only for diagnosis but for accurate staging:

- Esophagogastroduodenoscopy (EGD) (Fig. E1) should be performed initially to visualize smaller tumors, which may be missed by esophagogram, and to allow histopathologic confirmation.
- Endoscopic inspection of the larynx, trachea, and bronchi may identify concomitant cancers of head, neck, and lung ("triple endoscopy").
- Endoscopic ultrasound (EUS) (Fig. E1) appears to be the most accurate method for locoregional staging: To determine the depth of tumor invasion and to assess for and possibly obtain fine needle aspiration biopsies of suspicious lymph nodes.
- PET CT has become the standard of care, along with EUS, for the most accurate staging. These modalities can determine tumor spread for preoperative staging. CT scans of the chest (Fig. E2) and abdomen are more useful for restaging patients after initial therapy.
- Staging laparoscopy may alter treatment plans in 20% to 30% of cases by more accurately staging regional lymph nodes and detecting occult peritoneal metastases.
- Double-contrast esophagogram effectively identifies large esophageal lesions.
    1. In contrast to benign esophageal leiomyomata, which cause narrowing with preservation of normal mucosal pattern, esophageal carcinomas cause ragged ulcerating mucosal changes in association with deeper infiltration.

STAGING

Table 1 describes the TNM staging system for cancer of the esophagus from the American Joint Committee on Cancer Criteria. Fig. 3 illustrates an algorithm for staging thoracic esophageal cancer.

TABLE 1 TNM Staging System for Cancer of the Esophagus (American Joint Committee on Cancer Criteria)

Primary Tumor (T)*	
T_X	Primary tumor cannot be assessed
T_0	No evidence of primary tumor
T_{is}	High-grade dysplasia†
T_1	Tumor invades lamina propria, muscularis mucosae, or submucosa
T_{1a}	Tumor invades lamina propria or muscularis mucosae
T_{1b}	Tumor invades submucosa
T_2	Tumor invades muscularis propria
T_3	Tumor invades adventitia
T_4	Tumor invades adjacent structures
T_{4a}	Resectable tumor invading pleura, pericardium, or diaphragm
T_{4b}	Unresectable tumor invading other adjacent structures, such as aorta, vertebral body, trachea, etc.
Lymph Node (N)‡	
N_X	Regional lymph nodes cannot be assessed
N_0	No regional lymph node metastasis
N_1	Metastasis in 1-2 regional lymph nodes
N_2	Metastasis in 3-6 regional lymph nodes
N_3	Metastasis in 7 or more regional lymph nodes
Distant Metastasis (M)	
M_X	Metastasis cannot be assessed
M_0	No distant metastasis
M_1	Distant metastasis

*(1) At least maximal dimension of the tumor must be recorded and (2) multiple tumors require the T(m) suffix.
†High-grade dysplasia includes all noninvasive neoplastic epithelia that was formerly called carcinoma in situ.
‡Number must be recorded for total number of regional nodes sampled and total number of reported nodes with metastasis.
TNM, tumor, node, metastases.
From Edge S, et al. (eds): AJCC cancer staging manual, ed 7, New York, 2010, Springer.

Rx TREATMENT

TREATMENT OF ALL STAGES OF ESOPHAGEAL CANCER:

Although the histology of esophageal cancer can differ, most studies have combined tissue types in exploring treatment options. The histology develops secondary to differing pathogenesis and causative agents with tumor biology likely playing a role through varying mutations. The likelihood of response and prognosis can differ as well. However, as there is a lack of data on how histology should dictate the treatment approach, we therefore generally attack this cancer in a uniform manner as most studies have suggested the optimum benefit be obtained through a neoadjuvant chemoradiation approach followed by surgery when applicable in up to stage III disease.

COMBINATION THERAPY: CHEMORADIOTHERAPY FOLLOWED BY SURGICAL RESECTION: Induction chemotherapy that occurs before chemoradiation for patients with locally advanced but still possibly resectable disease has been given with good results. However, no studies have shown this being superior to chemoradiation alone. It can, however, provide relief of dysphagia. Standard fractionation 3D-RT is used in chemoradiotherapy.

- Chemotherapy is most often given with concurrent radiotherapy. Chemotherapy acts as a radiosensitizer and makes tumor cells more vulnerable to the effects of ionizing radiation, thus improving tumoricidal effects on cancer. Neoadjuvant chemoradiotherapy followed by surgery is the most common approach for patients with resectable disease but is employed primarily for patients with stage IIA or higher disease. Five-yr survival is improved with neoadjuvant approach (39%) versus surgery alone (16%). Several trials have now shown that preoperative therapy improves survival among patients with potentially curable esophageal or esophagogastric junction cancer. Neoadjuvant chemotherapy alone is another option for locally advanced disease, but results are not as good as with neoadjuvant chemoradiotherapy.
- Chemoradiotherapy followed by surgery should be offered to late stage I ($T_{1b}N_0$ or higher), stage II, and stage III esophageal cancer patients as the current standard of care. In several studies, this approach significantly improved local control, reduced recurrence, and reduced mortality compared with surgery alone in patients with resectable esophageal cancer. Trimodality therapy is the preferred treatment for most esophageal cancers.
- Chemoradiotherapy alone may be offered as the definitive treatment for patients who are not surgical candidates, and some of these patients may be cured.
- Combination chemotherapy using a platinum doublet (platinum agent plus second agent) can achieve significant tumor reduction in 30% to 60% of patients. Cisplatin, oxaliplatin, or carboplatin is usually given with 5-FU (5-fluorouracil) or paclitaxel to obtain the desired tumoricidal effects. Other chemotherapeutic agents with activity in esophageal cancer include irinotecan, epirubicin, and docetaxel.
- Capecitabine in combination with either cisplatin or oxaliplatin is as effective as 5FU in the neoadjuvant or definitive treatment setting.
- Complications of chemoradiotherapy primarily include mucositis, nausea, vomiting, diarrhea, myelosuppression, nephrotoxicity, ototoxicity, neurotoxicity with peripheral neuropathy, esophageal stricture, esophageal rupture, trachea-esophageal fistula (6%), and radiation pneumonitis. These can occur to varying degrees and are certainly more significant in the elderly and those with significant comorbidities.
- Postoperative adjuvant chemoradiotherapy should be offered to node-positive patients who underwent initial surgery alone.

SURGICAL RESECTION:

- Surgical resection of squamous cell carcinoma and adenocarcinoma of the middle esophagus and lower third of the esophagus is an acceptable initial modality for local and resectable disease in the absence of widespread metastases detected by CT-PET and transesophageal ultrasound (T_1 and T_2 tumors). Gastric pull-through or colonic interposition typically is used to provide luminal continuity.
- Endoscopic mucosal resection may replace radical surgical resection in patients with dysplasia and some small early tumors with no lymph node involvement (T_{is} or T_{1a}), but a recent Cochrane review found no studies comparing endoscopic treatment vs. surgery. Endoscopic mucosal resection may be beneficial for patients who are poor surgical candidates. It may be performed in conjunction with ablative therapies, including radiofrequency ablation, thermal ablation techniques,

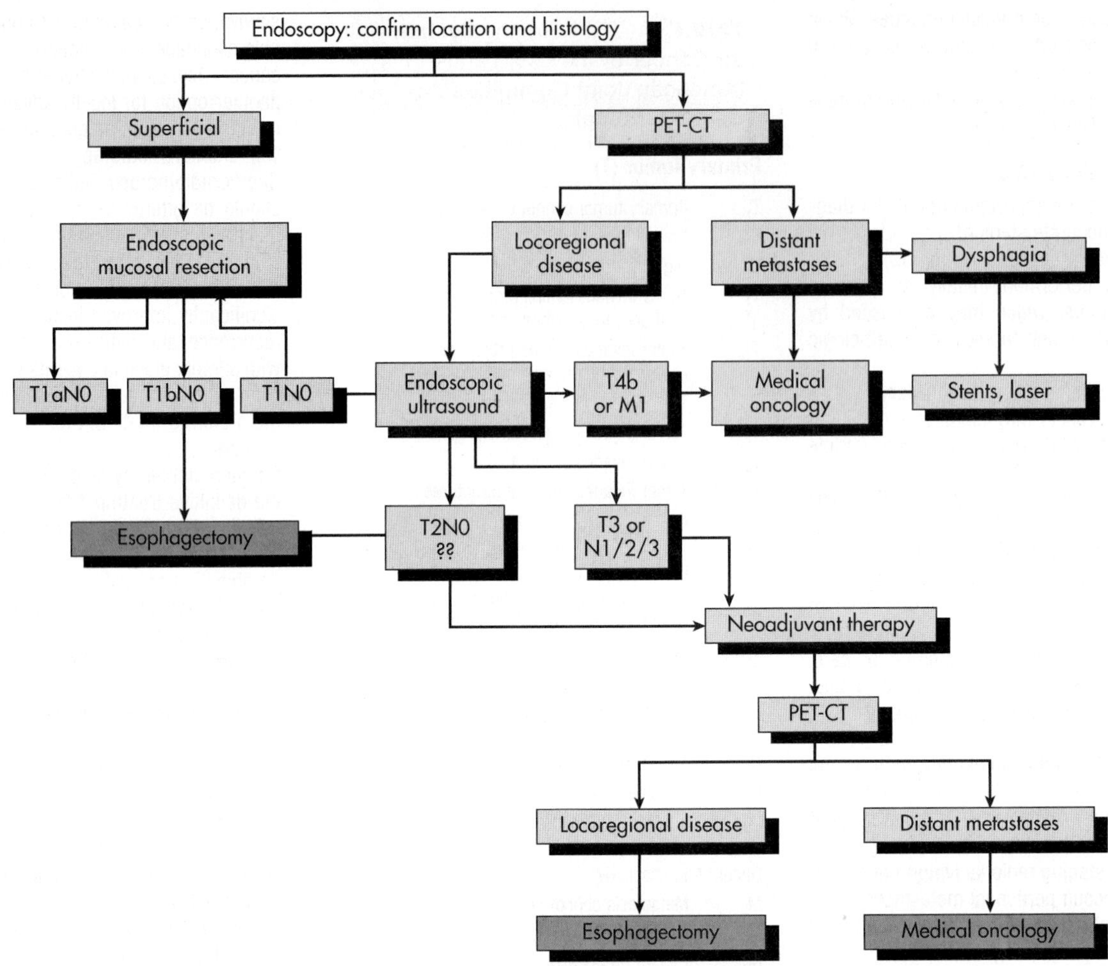

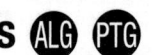

FIG. 3 An algorithm for staging a thoracic esophageal cancer patient. Metastatic disease must always be confirmed by pathologic evaluation of the tissue in question. *PET-CT,* Positron emission tomography–computed tomography. (From Sellke FW, del Nido PJ, Swanson SJ: *Sabiston & Spencer surgery of the chest*, ed 9, Philadelphia, 2016, Elsevier.)

laser ablation, argon plasma coagulation, or photodynamic therapy. Electrocoagulation (electrofulguration) is also being used and may aid in the relief of esophageal blockage.

- Complications of surgery:
  1. Anatomic fistula (usually with colon interposition, subphrenic abscesses).
  2. Respiratory complications.
  3. Cardiovascular complications are most common, including MI, CVA, and PE.
  4. Mortality is lower and clinical outcomes are better at high-volume hospitals and with minimally invasive surgery.
  5. Hybrid minimally invasive esophagectomy has been reported to have a lower incidence of intraoperative and postoperative major complications, specifically pulmonary complications, than open esophagectomy, without compromising overall and disease-free survival over a 3-yr period.[1]

Despite adequate preoperative staging, 25% of patients initially treated with surgical resection will have microscopically positive resection margins and are upstaged at the time of surgery. This has led to the majority of patients receiving neoadjuvant chemoradiotherapy as demonstrated in the CROSS Trial. The median disease-free survival for this group of patients was significantly prolonged as compared with the surgery-alone group. Death from recurrent cancer was decreased by 9% in the neoadjuvant group as well. The benefit of neoadjuvant therapy on survival was consistent regardless of histologic subtype.

PRE-TREATMENT PATIENT PREPARATION

The patient needs to stop smoking and drinking alcohol if at all possible. Before neoadjuvant or definitive chemoradiotherapy, the patient should have placement of an intravenous access device and a feeding tube (J-tube is preferable before surgical resection).

RADIATION THERAPY:

- Squamous cell carcinomas are more radiosensitive. Radiotherapy achieves good local control but is generally only used as monotherapy in a palliative mode for obstructive symptoms in patients with unresectable or advanced cancer or those with multiple comorbidities that limit treatment. It is best used for cervical esophageal tumors, but response rates are best when combined with chemotherapy.
- Radiotherapy in the preoperative/neoadjuvant setting is taken to a total dose of 40-50 Gy. For definitive therapy, the dose range is 50-55 Gy.
- Palliative radiotherapy for bone metastasis is also effective.
- Complications of radiotherapy: Can best be avoided by 3D conformal therapy.
  1. Esophageal stricture, fistula formation, radiation-induced pulmonary fibrosis, and transverse myelitis are the most common.
  2. Radiotherapy-induced cardiomyopathy and skin changes are rare.

IMRT can also be used for the treatment of esophageal cancers. It is associated with a more favorable toxicity profile. Very few studies have been completed to date using chemotherapy with IMRT and is therefore not considered a standard approach at this time for neoadjuvant therapy.

Brachytherapy: This is also an option for patients in a palliative mode. It provides high-dose radiation to a localized area and may prevent the need for a stent in patients with dysphagia. Its use

[1] Mariette C, et al.: Hybrid minimally invasive esophagectomy for esophageal cancer, *N Engl J Med* 380(2):152–162, 2019.

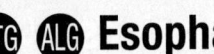

is very limited in prior irradiated tissue for fear of fistula and perforation of the esophagus.

TREATMENT OF UNRESECTABLE, LOCALLY ADVANCED, OR METASTATIC DISEASE

- Combination chemotherapy regimens as a rule have a higher response rate than single-agent therapy. Response rates can be as high as 50% but that does not always translate into prolonged survival.
- Neoadjuvant chemotherapy regimens can also be utilized in locally advanced or metastatic settings. Cisplatin is probably the most active agent, and this combined with 5FU can yield response rates shown in several studies of 20% to 50%. If a taxane is added to this regimen in the metastatic setting, the triple drug regimen can lead to a prolongation in disease progression by about 2 months, which may translate into prolonged survival. However, the patients have to be carefully chosen for this triple drug regimen because of increased toxicity. Other active double regimens can combine cisplatin with irinotecan, etoposide, or gemcitabine. Again, capecitabine can be substituted for 5FU in these regimens.

TARGETED MOLECULAR THERAPY

This is only applicable in adenocarcinoma of the esophagus that has overexpression of HER2. There is no apparent role for this treatment in squamous cell carcinoma.

- Ramucirumab is a recombinant monoclonal IgG1 antibody that is a vascular endothelial growth factor receptor 2 (VEGFR-2) antagonist. It inhibits ligand proliferation and migration of endothelial cells and ultimately inhibits angiogenesis. It is indicated for second-line therapy in conjunction with paclitaxel or as third line as monotherapy.
- Trastuzumab, in combination with cisplatin and 5FU, can be used as first-line therapy for metastatic esophageal cancer in patients with HER-2 overexpressing adenocarcinoma. Approximately 22% of adenocarcinomas will overexpress the type II epidermal growth factor receptor HER2. The overall response rate is 47%.

IMMUNOTHERAPY IN ESOPHAGEAL CANCER

- This involves an immune checkpoint inhibitor that targets PD-1.
- Studies have been done using nivolumab and pembrolizumab with varying response rates of 10-30% in patients who have progressive disease and failed traditional therapy with at least two previous chemotherapy regimens. Currently, only pembrolizumab is approved in the U.S. for treatment of esophageal cancer.

FOLLOW-UP CARE

The majority of recurrences develop within 12 months. Clinical monitoring, lab tests, imaging, and endoscopic evaluation where appropriate (particularly Barrett), are performed for post-operative surveillance, without clear benefit in earlier detection or decreased mortality. For patients who have undergone definitive therapy, it is recommended that endoscopic surveillance be performed every 3 months for the first year, and then annually. Palliative procedures such as repeated endoscopic dilation, endoscopic ablation, endoscopic mucosal resection, photodynamic therapy, brachytherapy, feeding tube insertion, or placement of expandable metal stents or polyvinyl prostheses to bypass tumors have been used for unresectable patients. The morbidity and mortality associated with resection in patients with advanced disease and/or for palliation argues against offering this modality to most of these patients.

SURVIVORSHIP

- Overall 5-yr survival for all stages at presentation is 15% (39% for localized disease, 21% for regional disease, and 4% for distant disease).
- Endoscopic therapy for highly selected stage 0 or stage I patients with disease limited to the submucosa may have 5-yr survival rates of 70% to 90%.
- Surgical resection without neoadjuvant treatment: 5-yr survival rate is 5% to 30%, with higher survival (up to 45% to 50%) in early-stage cancers.
- Radiation therapy without chemotherapy or surgery: 5-yr survival rate of 6% to 20%.
- Chemoradiotherapy without surgery: 5-yr survival up to 30%.
- Combined trimodality treatment: Up to 45% to 50% 5-yr survival rates (all stages of disease treated).
- Patients with metastatic disease have median survivals of less than 1 yr with palliative chemotherapy.

REFERRAL

- To gastroenterologist for endoscopy for patients with dysphagia, odynophagia, or unexplained weight loss, or for palliative care
- To medical oncologist for evaluation of preoperative chemotherapy and care of the metastatic patient
- To radiation oncologist for palliative therapy if tumor is actively bleeding, unresectable, or if obstruction is present
- To hospice if appropriate

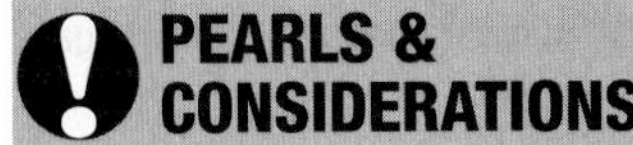

PEARLS & CONSIDERATIONS

COMMENTS

More than 50% of patients with esophageal cancer are diagnosed when the disease is metastatic or unresectable.

PREVENTION

- A diet high in fruits, vegetables, and antioxidants may be associated with lower risk of esophageal cancer.
- Avoid tobacco and excessive alcohol use.
- Avoid ingested toxins known to cause esophageal cancers.
- Aspirin may have a chemopreventive role in Barrett but is only currently recommended for patients with other (e.g., cardiac) indications.
- There is no evidence that vitamins, Chinese herbal regimens, or green tea prevent esophageal cancer.
- Screening the general population is not recommended. If Barrett esophagus is detected, regularly scheduled surveillance endoscopies are necessary, with consideration for radiofrequency or other ablation therapy if dysplasia is detected.

PATIENT/FAMILY EDUCATION

Provide education and support about the likely prognosis because most esophageal cancers are diagnosed at an advanced stage.

SUGGESTED READINGS

Available at ExpertConsult.com

RELATED CONTENT

Esophageal Cancer (Patient Information)
Barrett Esophagus (Related Key Topic)

AUTHOR: **ANTHONY G. THOMAS, D.O., FACP.**

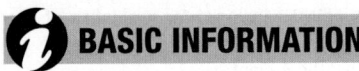

BASIC INFORMATION

DEFINITION

Esophageal varices are dilated submucosal veins that occur in patients with underlying portal hypertension, function as a shunt between the portal venous and systemic venous circulation, and can result in severe upper GI hemorrhage.

ICD-10CM CODES
I85.00 Esophageal varices without bleeding
I85.01 Esophageal varices with bleeding

EPIDEMIOLOGY & DEMOGRAPHICS

INCIDENCE:
- Esophageal varices: 5% to 15% per yr in patients with cirrhosis
- Hemorrhage:
  1. One third of all patients with varices will develop hemorrhage.
  2. Variceal hemorrhage occurs in 25% to 40% of patients with cirrhosis.
  3. The risk of bleeding from varices is approximately 15% at 1 yr.
  4. Survivors of an episode of active bleeding have a 70% risk of recurrent hemorrhage within 1 yr.

PREVALENCE: Approximately 50% of patients with cirrhosis have varices at the time of diagnosis.
RISK FACTORS: Cirrhosis, low platelet count and advanced Child-Pugh class, hepatitis C with advanced fibrosis

PHYSICAL FINDINGS & CLINICAL PRESENTATION

- Often asymptomatic until acute upper GI hemorrhage: Hematemesis, hypovolemia
- No physical findings specific for esophageal varices
- Stigmata of cirrhosis and portal hypertension may be evident: Palmar erythema, telangiectasias, gynecomastia, testicular atrophy, jaundice, caput medusae, lower extremity edema, ascites, splenomegaly, hemorrhoids, asterixis

ETIOLOGY

- Portal hypertension results from obstruction to portal venous outflow, and varices subsequently develop in order to decompress the hypertensive portal vein and return blood to the systemic circulation.
- Varices may appear when portal vein pressures rise above 10 to 12 mm Hg.
- Cirrhosis is the most common cause of portal hypertension.

Dx DIAGNOSIS

DIFFERENTIAL DIAGNOSIS

- Budd-Chiari syndrome, cirrhosis, portal vein thrombosis, schistosomiasis, Wilson's disease
- Other causes of upper GI bleeding: Duodenal or gastric ulcers, gastric cancer, Mallory-Weiss tear

WORKUP

Upper endoscopy, laboratory tests, and imaging

LABORATORY TESTS

- CBC:
  1. Anemia (blood loss, nutritional deficiencies, alcohol myelosuppression)
  2. Thrombocytopenia (hypersplenism, alcohol myelosuppression)
- Renal function panel:
  1. BUN: Often increased in setting of upper GI bleeding
  2. Creatinine: Often elevated by hypovolemia, monitor for hepatorenal syndrome
  3. Sodium: Dilutional hyponatremia
- Heme-positive stools:
- Type and Crossmatch: In preparation for blood transfusion
- INR/PT and PTT: Coagulation factors produced in liver and may be prolonged in liver disease or impairment
- Liver function tests: ALT/AST may be normal in cirrhotic patients due to longstanding fibrosis; elevated alkaline phosphatase and a direct hyperbilirubinemia may be present if cholestatic liver disease is present
- Serum albumin: Severe liver disease results in hypoalbuminemia

IMAGING STUDIES

Invasive:
- Esophagogastroduodenoscopy (EGD) (upper endoscopy):
  1. In all patients with cirrhosis, screen for the presence or absence of varices and determine subsequent risk for variceal hemorrhage.
  2. In patients with small varices (<5 mm) repeat EGD in 2 yr (unless decompensation occurs).
  3. In patients with compensated cirrhosis who do not have varices, screening is repeated every 2 to 3 yr.
  4. In patients with decompensated cirrhosis (ascites, hepatic encephalopathy, variceal hemorrhage, or jaundice), it is repeated every yr or at the time of first decompensation.
  5. Emergently performed if there is evidence of acute upper GI bleeding to diagnose and treat variceal hemorrhage.

Noninvasive:
- Esophagography with barium can diagnose esophageal varices (Fig. E1).
- Capsule endoscopy can also diagnose esophageal varices, although sensitivity is not yet established.
- CT scan (Figs. E1 and E2).

Rx TREATMENT

NONPHARMACOLOGIC THERAPY

- Endoscopic variceal ligation (Fig. E3) is an alternative to nonselective beta-blockers for primary prophylaxis against variceal hemorrhage. It is also used in patients unable to tolerate beta-blockers.
  1. Typically for patients with medium or large varices at highest risk for hemorrhage (Child-Pugh B/C or red wale markings viewed on endoscopy)
  2. Usually two to four sessions
  3. May not be a permanent solution because varices can recur after initial eradication
  4. Associated with significant complications, including hemorrhage from banding-induced ulcerations
     a. Therefore should be performed by endoscopists with expertise in prophylactic banding
     b. First surveillance endoscopy 1-3 mo after obliteration, then every 6 to 12 mo indefinitely

ACUTE GENERAL Rx

- Variceal hemorrhage: Acute hemodynamic resuscitation with packed red blood cell transfusion, correct coagulopathy and thrombocytopenia, airway protection and intubation as necessary, antibiotics (ceftriaxone or norfloxacin) for SBP prophylaxis, octreotide maintained for 2 to 5 days in conjunction with endoscopic therapy
- EGD to treat bleeding esophageal varices by esophageal band ligation or sclerotherapy (Fig. 4)

CHRONIC Rx

Primary prophylaxis (Fig. 5):
- Nonselective beta-blockers such as propranolol (20 mg twice daily), nadolol (40 mg once daily) or carvedilol (6.25 mg twice daily)
  1. Increase as tolerated for goal heart rate of approximately 55 beats/min
  2. Blocks the adrenergic dilatory tone in mesenteric arterioles, resulting in unopposed alpha-adrenergic mediated vasoconstriction and therefore a decrease in portal inflow

Secondary prophylaxis (Fig. E6):
- All patients with compensated cirrhosis who have bled from esophageal varices should receive esophageal band ligation and beta-blockers, unless beta-blockers are contraindicated.
  1. Transjugular intrahepatic portosystemic shunt or surgical shunt may be performed if bleeding from esophageal varices continues or recurs despite this dual therapy.
- For patients with decompensated cirrhosis there is evidence, although limited, against the use of prophylactic beta-blockers due to the risk for increased mortality.

REFERRAL:

Consultation with a gastroenterologist is recommended in all patients with cirrhosis or portal hypertension in order to screen for esophageal varices.

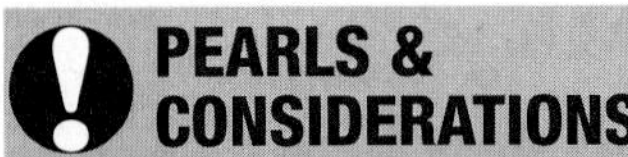

PEARLS & CONSIDERATIONS

Besides variceal size, risk factors for variceal hemorrhage include Child-Pugh class B/C or variceal red wale markings on endoscopy.

RELATED CONTENT

Cirrhosis (Related Key Topic)
Portal Hypertension (Related Key Topic)

AUTHOR: **FRED F. FERRI, M.D.**

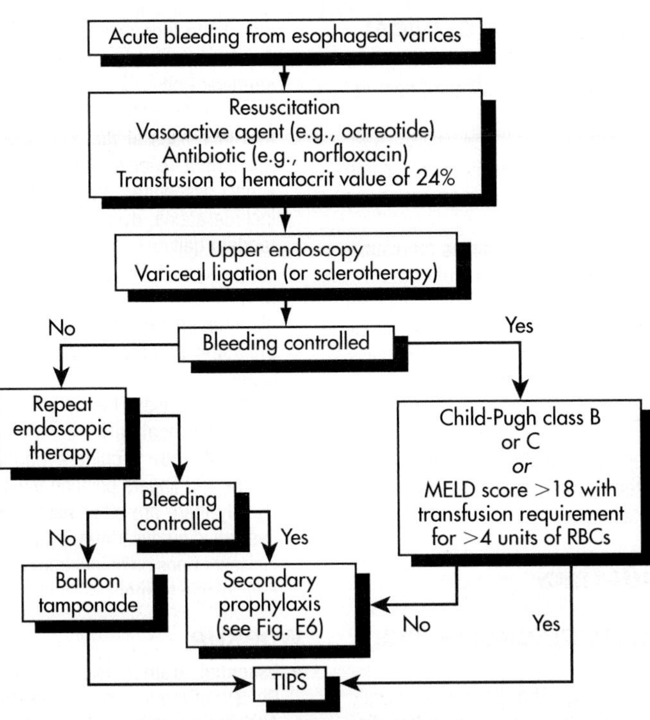

FIG. 4 Algorithm for the management of bleeding esophageal varices. *MELD*, Model end state liver disease; *RBC*, red blood cell; *TIPS*, transjugular intrahepatic portosystemic shunt. (From Feldman M, Friedman LS, Brandt LJ: *Sleisenger and Fordtran's gastrointestinal and liver disease*, ed 10, Philadelphia, 2016, Elsevier.)

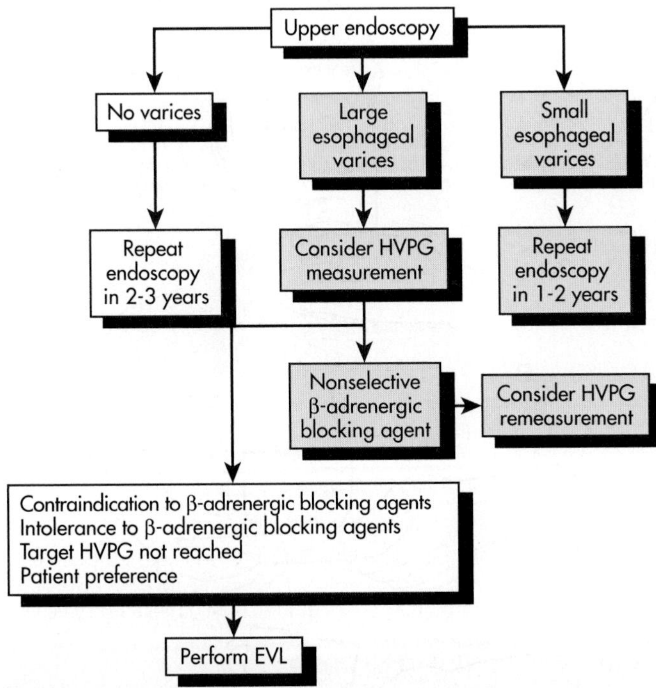

FIG. 5 Algorithm for the primary prophylaxis of esophageal variceal hemorrhage in patients with cirrhosis. The hepatic vein pressure gradient (HVPG) may be measured in patients with large varices before a nonselective β-adrenergic blocking agent is started and remeasured 1 mo after the maximum tolerated dose of the beta-blocker is reached. The goal of treatment is to reduce the HVPG to <12 mm Hg or by ≥20%. *EVL*, Endoscopic variceal ligation. (From Feldman M, Friedman LS, Brandt LJ: *Sleisenger and Fordtran's gastrointestinal and liver disease*, ed 10, Philadelphia, 2016, Elsevier.)

BASIC INFORMATION

DEFINITION

A tremor is an oscillatory movement of a body part. Essential tremor is a predominantly postural and action tremor that is bilateral and tends to progress slowly over the years in the absence of other neurologic abnormalities.

SYNONYMS

Benign essential tremor
Familial tremor

ICD-10CM CODE
G25.0 Essential tremor

EPIDEMIOLOGY & DEMOGRAPHICS

Essential tremor is one of the most prevalent neurologic diseases. It affects nearly 7 million persons in the U.S. It is the most common movement disorder.

PREDOMINANT AGE: Can begin at any age, but incidence increases after age 40 yr. Prevalence is 6% to 9% for those >60 yr of age.

GENETICS: Positive family history is found in 50% of patients. No gender or racial predominance.

PHYSICAL FINDINGS & CLINICAL PRESENTATION

- Tremor (Fig. 1), 4 to 12 Hz, bilateral postural and action tremor of the upper extremities (90%-95%), head (30%), legs (10%-15%), and voice (20%). Typically, it is the same amplitude throughout the action, such as bringing a cup to the mouth.
- No other neurologic abnormalities on examination except difficulty with tandem gait.
- Symptoms worsen under emotional distress with fatigue or use of caffeine or other stimulants and improve with intake of small amounts of alcohol.

ETIOLOGY

Often an inherited disease in an autosomal dominant pattern. Sporadic cases without a family history can occur.

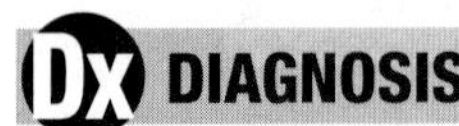

DIAGNOSIS

DIFFERENTIAL DIAGNOSIS (SEE TABLE 1)

- Parkinson's disease: The tremor is usually asymmetric, especially early on in the disease, and is predominantly a resting tremor. Patients with Parkinson's disease will also have increased tone, decreased facial expression, slowness of movement, and shuffling gait.
- Cerebellar tremor: This is an intention tremor that increases at the end of a goal-directed movement (such as finger to nose testing). Other associated neurologic abnormalities include ataxia, dysarthria, and difficulty with tandem gait.
- Drug-induced: Many drugs enhance normal, physiologic tremor. These include caffeine, nicotine, lithium, levothyroxine, β-adrenergic bronchodilators, amiodarone, valproate, and SSRIs.
- Wilson disease: This is often characterized by a wing-beating tremor that is most pronounced with shoulders abducted, elbows flexed, and fingers pointing toward each other. Usually there are other neurologic abnormalities including dysarthria, dystonia, and Kayser-Fleischer rings on ophthalmologic examination.
- Physiologic tremor.

WORKUP

- Essential tremor is a clinical diagnosis. Review of medications is essential.
- All imaging studies (MRI, CT) are unnecessary unless other neurologic abnormalities are present.

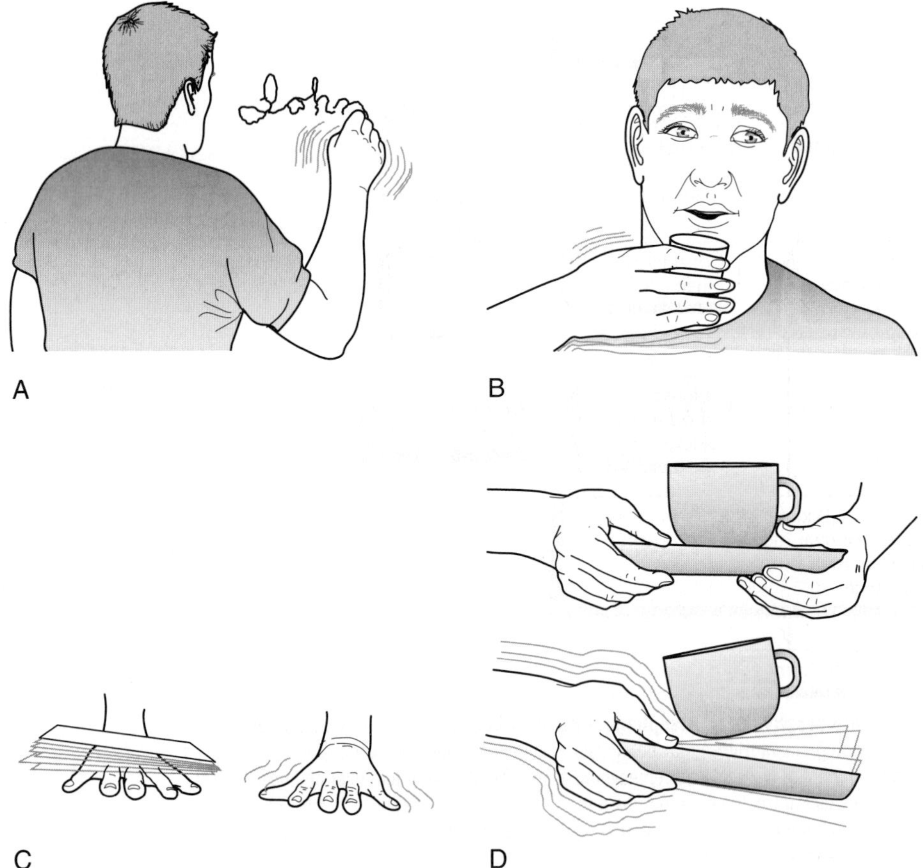

FIG. 1 Physicians elicit this 34-year-old gentleman's essential tremor by having him write his name **(A)**, drink from a filled glass **(B)**, support an envelope on his outstretched and pronated hand **(C)**, or transfer a cup and saucer from one hand to the other **(D)**. When his hands rest in his lap, the tremor completely subsides. Essential tremor is a prime example of an action tremor. (From Kaufman DM et al: *Kaufman's clinical neurology for psychiatrists,* ed 8, Philadelphia, 2017, Elsevier.)

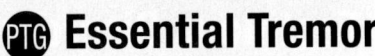

TABLE 1 Overlapping Features of Various Types of Tremor

Feature	Parkinson's Syndrome	Cerebellar Tremor	Essential Tremor
Present at rest	Yes	No	Yes
Increased tone	Yes	No	No
Decreased tone	No	Yes	No
Postural abnormality	Yes	Yes	No
Head involvement	Yes	Yes	Yes
Intentional component	No	Yes	Yes
Incoordination	No	Yes	No

From Remmel KS et al: *Handbook of symptom-oriented neurology*, ed 3, St Louis, 2002, Mosby

- Obtain TSH to rule out hyperthyroidism.
- In patients younger than 40 yr old with other neurologic abnormalities, send ceruloplasmin, serum copper, and 24-hr urine copper to evaluate for Wilson disease.

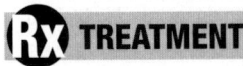

TREATMENT

Treat essential tremor when it is functionally impairing. Treatments are up to 75% effective.

NONPHARMACOLOGIC THERAPY

- Stress management
- Minimization of caffeine use if consumption is correlated with worsened symptoms
- Wrist weights and use of weighted utensils may be helpful in reducing tremor amplitude during feeding. Consumption of small quantities of alcohol at social functions, although relief may be short in duration and may be followed by tremor rebound
- A recent trial using MRI-guided focus ultrasound thalamotomy found it effective in reducing hand tremor in patients with essential tremor. Side effects included sensory and gait disturbances[1]

[1] Elias WJ et al: A randomized trial of focused ultrasound thalamotomy for essential tremor, *N Engl J Med* 375:730-739, 2016.

ACUTE GENERAL Rx

Propranolol (20 to 40 mg) may be used in preparation for specific event.

CHRONIC Rx

First-line agents:

- Propranolol/Inderal LA: Typical starting dose is 30 mg. The usual therapeutic dose is 160 to 320 mg. Although not contraindicated, this medication must be used with caution in those with asthma, depression, cardiac disease, and diabetes. Atenolol or sotalol are also effective.
- Primidone: Typical starting dose is 12.5 to 25 mg qhs. Usual therapeutic dose is between 62.5 and 750 mg daily (assuming side effects are tolerated). Sedation and nausea are common at treatment initiation.
- Topiramate: 25 mg qhs, may titrate up to about 400 mg

Other (second-line) agents:

- Gabapentin: Typical starting dose is 300 mg tid. Usual therapeutic dose is 1200 to 3600 mg daily.
- Pregabalin: Typical starting dose is 50 mg twice a day. Usual therapeutic dose is 150 to 600 mg per day.
- Benzodiazepines (i.e., alprazolam): 0.125 to 3 mg daily.
- Focal botulinum toxin injections.

SURGICAL Rx

Thalamic deep brain stimulation (or possibly thalamotomy) contralateral to side of tremor is reserved for resistant tremor or for patients who do not tolerate drug therapy. Surgical ablation of the neutral intermediate nucleus or the thalamus with use of magnetic resonance-guided focused ultrasound was recently FDA approved.

DISPOSITION

Patients should be reassured that the condition is not associated with other neurologic disabilities; however, it can become quite functionally disabling over time.

REFERRAL

This is a condition that usually can be treated by the primary care physician; however, if patient fails first-line therapies, the patient should be referred to a neurologist for other drug trials and discussion of possible surgical options.

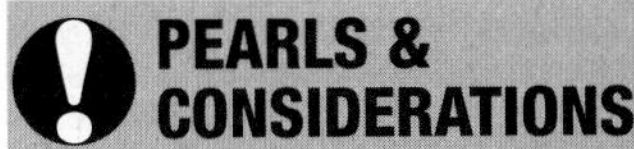

PEARLS & CONSIDERATIONS

- Essential tremor is the most common of all movement disorders.
- In addition to motor dysfunction, essential tremor can cause significant psychological impact on patients in social situations.

SUGGESTED READINGS

Available at ExpertConsult.com

RELATED CONTENT

Essential Tremor (Patient Information)

AUTHORS: **CHLOE MANDER NUNNELEY, M.D., JOSEPH S. KASS, M.D., J.D.,** and **U. SHIVRAJ SOHUR, M.D., PH.D.**

BASIC INFORMATION

DEFINITION

Factitious disorder, according to the DSM-5, occurs when an individual feigns physical or psychological signs or symptoms or induces injury or disease with identified deception. Individuals present to others as ill, impaired, or injured and create signs or symptoms by lying, simulating (e.g., putting drops of blood into a urine sample), or actually creating disease (e.g., injecting bacteria or taking medications). The primary aim is to achieve the patient role, and the behavior persists even in the absence of apparent external rewards such as monetary gain or obtaining narcotics. More is known about factitious physical disorder.

The individual may seek examination and treatment including invasive diagnostic testing or surgery. The term *Munchausen syndrome* is reserved for the most severe variant of factitious physical disorder and is characterized by exaggerated lying (pseudologia fantastica), sociopathy, geographic wandering (peregrinating) from hospital to hospital, and seeking the role of a patient.

SYNONYMS

Munchausen syndrome (severe form of factitious disorder)
Munchausen by proxy (factitious disorder created in another person, usually a child)
Hospital addiction syndrome
Surreptitious illness

ICD-10CM CODE

F68.10 Intentional production or feigning of symptoms or disabilities, either physical or psychological (factitious disorder)

DSM-5 CODE

300.19 Factitious disorder

EPIDEMIOLOGY & DEMOGRAPHICS

INCIDENCE (IN U.S.): Unknown
PEAK INCIDENCE: Approximately 30 to 40 yrs of age
PREVALENCE (IN U.S.): Likely underdiagnosed because of the role of deception, but estimates range between 0.5% and 2%
PREDOMINANT SEX: Variable. With psychological subtype M > F; with predominant physical symptoms F > M by a ratio of 3:1. Munchausen syndrome M > F, and Munchausen by proxy mostly younger females
PREDOMINANT AGE: 30 to 40 yr of age
GENETICS: No genetic predisposition known

PHYSICAL FINDINGS & CLINICAL PRESENTATION

- Patient is inconsistent or intentionally misleading and resistant to allowing providers to obtain outside records.
- Clinical picture is atypical for the natural history of disease (e.g., an infection that does not respond to multiple courses of appropriate antibiotics).
- Tests, consultations, and medical and surgical treatments done to no avail and often contradicting history provided by the patient.
- Presentation may be acute and dramatic and in excess of what might be expected.
- The patient may predict deterioration or report exacerbation just before scheduled discharge.
- Opposition to psychiatric consultation.

ETIOLOGY

- A history of significant childhood illness; traumatic experiences such as having witnessed violence and physical, emotional, or sexual abuse can predispose.
- Personality disorders and psychodynamic factors often play a significant role in the development and maintenance of this disorder.

DIAGNOSIS

This is a diagnosis of exclusion. It requires demonstrating that the individual is taking surreptitious actions to misinterpret, simulate, or cause signs or symptoms of illness or injury in the absence of any obvious external reward. Early diagnosis is helpful to prevent extensive and unnecessary testing, which can cause iatrogenic injury.

There may be direct observation of fabrication, the presence of signs or symptoms that contradict laboratory testing, nonphysiologic response to treatment, physical evidence of fabrication (e.g., syringes at the bedside), recurrent patterns of illness exacerbation, or failure to follow the expected natural history of disease. Box 1 describes clues that increase the likelihood of subtle forms of factitious disease.

DIFFERENTIAL DIAGNOSIS

- Primary medical condition
- Somatic symptoms disorder: Not intentionally produced
- Conversion disorder
- Conditions in which self-injurious behavior is common such as borderline personality disorder. The goal is self-injury and not to attain the sick role
- Malingering: Clear secondary gain (e.g., financial gain or avoidance of unwanted duties)

WORKUP

- Dictated by the presenting complaints. A reasonable index of suspicion when presentation is not consistent with known pathology.
- Methods that have been used to bolster or confirm a suspicion of self-induced or factitious disease are summarized in Box 2.

LABORATORY TESTS

- Laboratory testing often reveals inconsistencies.
- Laboratory abnormalities may reflect the underlying factitious behavior (e.g., hypokalemia in an individual surreptitiously taking furosemide or a clean urine sample obtained by straight catheterization in someone complaining of hematuria).

TREATMENT

NONPHARMACOLOGIC THERAPY

Two approaches may be considered:

- Nonpunitive constructive confrontation by the primary physician and a psychiatrist in collaboration. A supportive stance should be maintained and an offer for ongoing support and follow-up made. Box E3 summarizes consensus opinions on the treatment of factitious disease.
- Avoid overt confrontation with patient but provide him or her with a face-saving way to recover. For example, a therapeutic double bind would involve saying, "There are two possibilities here: one is that you have a medical problem that should respond to the next intervention we do, or two, you have a factitious disorder. The outcome will give us the answer." Features of supportive confrontation are described in Box E4.

Munchausen syndrome is the most severe variant and may be virtually impossible to treat

BOX 1 Clues That Increase the Likelihood of Subtle Forms of Factitious Disease

Predominantly women
Previous experience in the medical field, which provides an unusual grasp of terminology and access to medical supplies
Multiple surgeries, multiple procedures
Inexplicable laboratory test results
Inconsistency and implausibility of certain aspects of the history
Visits to three or more medical centers previously for the same symptoms, or to a nationally known referral center such as the Mayo Clinic or Cleveland Clinic, despite residing far away
History of substance abuse or prior psychiatric disorder
Vagueness in regard to details of past history and/or reluctance to allow release of previous medical records

From Feldman M, Friedman LS, Brandt LJ: *Sleisenger and Fordtran's gastrointestinal and liver disease*, ed 10, Philadelphia, 2016, Elsevier.

BOX 2 Methods That Have Been Used to Bolster or Confirm a Suspicion of Self-Induced or Factitious Disease

Review old medical records and discuss case with previous doctors and family members if appropriate. Identify discrepancies and inconsistencies, and estimate influence of gain derived from the sick role. Inquire about psychosomatic illness, previous psychiatric treatment, suicide attempts, stress in the patient's life, childhood abuse, marital/sexual problems, eating disorders, and so on. The Internet can be used to facilitate such a review. A forensic consultant with access to multiple records can be uniquely helpful in identifying conflicting stories.

Review previous biopsy slides, looking for foreign body material in wounds, melanosis coli, and other clues, as appropriate for the patient's symptoms.

Obtain a psychiatric evaluation to help determine whether the patient has a personality disorder or psychiatric disease, absence of which would argue against factitious disease. Psychiatrists should not attempt initially to discover the underlying unconscious motivation that may have impelled the patient to assume the sick role.

If symptoms and signs may be explained by surreptitious ingestion of medications and poisons, obtain appropriate medication and toxicology screens. Consider obtaining a urine test for diuretics even in the absence of renal or electrolyte disorders. Evaluate results of such screens in light of the sensitivity and specificity of the tests employed.

Test biological fluids collected under direct observation and compare results with fluids collected privately by the patient. For example, compare fecal material obtained at "unprepped" sigmoidoscopy with fecal material submitted by the patient.

Have nursing staff observe the patient to detect tampering behavior.

Search the patient's personal belongings.

Conduct covert videotape surveillance, especially in suspected Munchausen syndrome by proxy.

From Feldman M, Friedman LS, Brandt LJ: *Sleisenger and Fordtran's gastrointestinal and liver disease*, ed 10, Philadelphia, 2016, Elsevier.

except to avoid further invasive and iatrogenic intervention.

ACUTE GENERAL Rx

- Treatment of comorbid psychiatric disorders may be helpful with medications and/or psychotherapy, which may ameliorate the factitious behavior.
- Multidisciplinary staff meetings can be useful to ventilate feelings and develop cohesive treatment plans.

CHRONIC Rx

- Attempt to engage the patient in some form of psychotherapy or at least a harm-reduction strategy.
- Establishment of a central reporting register has been proposed to aid development of evidence-based guidelines.

DISPOSITION

- After being confronted with their behavior, patients may cease factitious behavior, but they may also seek other physicians or hospitals, as in the Munchausen variant.
- Some patients may enter psychotherapy, particularly when they have been given a face-saving approach with avoidance of a humiliating confrontation.

REFERRAL

Always obtain psychiatric referral. Risk management attorneys and hospital ethicists may contribute to challenging decision making in these patients.

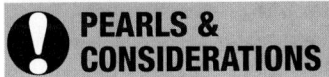

PEARLS & CONSIDERATIONS

- Think of factitious disorders whenever there is an unexplained medical course that continues to repeat itself despite appropriate treatment.
- Patients may have a history of working in the health care field.
- Gratuitous, self-aggrandizing deception may be noted.

SUGGESTED READINGS

Available at ExpertConsult.com

AUTHORS: **CHRISTINA SCULLY, M.D.,** and **DWAYNE R. HEITMILLER, M.D., F.A.P.M.**

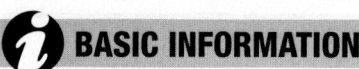

BASIC INFORMATION

DEFINITION

A tumor is defined as "primary fallopian tube" when it is restricted to the fallopian tube or is the most affected site. Recent data show that the fallopian tube may be the site of origin of many high-grade serous carcinomas of the pelvis.

SYNONYMS

Fallopian tube cancers, serous tubal intraepithelial carcinomas

ICD-10CM CODES

C57.00	Malignant neoplasm of unspecified fallopian tube
C57.01	Malignant neoplasm of right fallopian tube
C57.02	Malignant neoplasm of left fallopian tube

EPIDEMIOLOGY & DEMOGRAPHICS

INCIDENCE: Only 0.3% to 1.1% of all gynecologic cancers are fallopian tube primary

PEAK INCIDENCE: Highest incidence in white, non-Hispanic women aged 60 to 79 yr

PREDOMINANT SEX AND AGE: Highest in white women in the fourth to sixth decade

GENETICS: Patients with BRCA mutations have a 0% to 12% incidence of serous tubal intraepithelial carcinomas based on 16 studies. Also, more common in women with hereditary nonpolyposis colorectal cancer. GOG199 looking at 966 high-risk women found the rate of serous tubal intraepithelial carcinomas (STICs) or invasive carcinoma to be 2.6%.

RISK FACTORS:

- Protective factors: Multiparity, pregnancy, oral contraception use
- Age, weight, education level, pelvic inflammatory disease, infertility, hysterectomy, and endometriosis do not seem to be risk factors
- Highest incidence in white, non-Hispanic women aged 60 to 79 yr

PHYSICAL FINDINGS & CLINICAL PRESENTATION

Physical exam findings are similar to those of ovarian and primary peritoneal cancers. Patients can have abdominal bloating, early satiety, abdominal distention, and weight loss. However, many early fallopian tube cancers are detected at time of risk-reducing bilateral salpingo-oophorectomy.

ETIOLOGY

Etiology is unknown at this time. STIC is now thought to be the precursor lesion to high-grade serous carcinomas (HGSC) of the ovary.

DIAGNOSIS

DIFFERENTIAL DIAGNOSIS

- Ovarian cancer
- Primary peritoneal cancer

WORK-UP

LABORATORY TEST(S)

- CBC, BMP
- CA125
- Pathology:
  1. Until recently grossly positive tubal mass was required to assign the tumor origin to the fallopian tube.
  2. Fimbrial carcinoma is unlikely to cause tubal dilation.
  3. More recently the SEE-FIM protocol for pathologic evaluation of fallopian tubes has been used to better evaluate the potential for primary fallopian tube cancers.
  4. SEE-FIM—sectioning and extensively examining the fimbriated end.
  5. Contain TP53 mutations.

IMAGING STUDIES

- Pelvic ultrasonography
- CT abdomen/pelvis

STAGING

See Table 1.

TREATMENT

Approach mirrors treatment for ovarian cancers

NONPHARMACOLOGIC THERAPY

Surgery: Generally, total hysterectomy with removal of both tube and ovaries is the first-line treatment with goal of complete resection of all visible tumors; pelvic and para-aortic lymph node resection is often also performed.

ACUTE GENERAL Rx

Medications to control nausea and vomiting, constipation associated with tumor burden

CHRONIC RX

- Adjuvant chemotherapy:
  1. Usually with platinum-based combination chemotherapy regimens, usually platinum-taxane combination
- Radiotherapy is no longer recommended

DISPOSITION

SURVIVAL

- 5-yr survival is about 65% or higher.
- Stage of disease at time of diagnosis is the most important factor in survival.
- Overall survival is about 30% to 50%.

AUTHOR: **BETH H. LEOPOLD, M.D.**

TABLE 1 International Federation of Gynecology and Obstetrics Staging

- **Stage 0.** Carcinoma in situ (limited to tubal mucosa)
- **Stage I.** Growth limited to the fallopian tubes
  1. **Stage I_A.** Growth limited to one tube with extension into submucosa and/or muscularis, but not penetrating the serosal surface, no ascites. Ascites refer to a build-up of abdominal fluid that may occur as a result of cancer or other illnesses
  2. **Stage I_B.** Growth limited to both tubes with extension into submucosa and/or muscularis but not penetrating the serosal surface, no ascites
  3. **Stage 1_C.** Tumor either stage I_A or I_B with tumor extension through or onto the tubal serosa OR with ascites containing malignant cells OR with positive peritoneal washings. Peritoneal washings are performed by instilling fluid into the abdominal cavity and withdrawing it to assess for the presence of tumor cells in the abdominal cavity
- **Stage II.** Growth involving one or both fallopian tubes with pelvic extension.
  1. **Stage II_A.** Extension and/or metastasis to the uterus and/or ovaries
  2. **Stage II_B.** Extension to other pelvic tissues
  3. **Stage II_C.** Tumor either stage II_A or II_B AND with ascites containing malignant cells OR with positive peritoneal washing
- **Stage III.** Tumor involving one or both fallopian tubes with peritoneal implants outside of the pelvis, involvement of the small bowel, omentum, or liver surface, and/or positive retroperitoneal or inguinal nodes. Peritoneal implants are studs of tumors implanted in the abdominal wall
  1. **Stage III_A.** Tumor grossly limited to the true pelvis with negative nodes, but with histologically confirmed microscopic seeding of abdominal peritoneal surfaces (small bowel, omentum, or liver surface)
  2. **Stage III_B.** Tumor involving one or both tubes with histologically confirmed implants visualized on the abdominal peritoneal surfaces (small bowel, omentum, liver surface), none exceeding 2 cm in diameter. Lymph nodes negative for tumor
  3. **Stage III_C.** Abdominal implants greater than 2 cm in diameter and/or positive retroperitoneal or inguinal nodes
- **Stage IV.** Growth invading one or both fallopian tubes with distant metastases, including parenchymal liver metastases. Parenchymal liver disease refers to cancer inside the liver; it differs from disease on the liver surface, which may qualify as stage III disease. Fluid on the lungs (pleural effusion) may classify as stage IV disease, but only if cancer cells are found to be present in the fluid

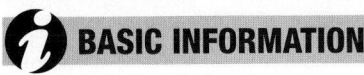

BASIC INFORMATION

DEFINITION

A fall is an "event which results in a person coming to rest inadvertently on the ground and other than a consequence of the following: loss of consciousness, sudden onset of paralysis, or epileptic seizure" (Kellogg International Work Group, *Danish Medical Bulletin,* 34, 1-24).

SYNONYMS

Syncope
Collapse

ICD-10CM CODES

E880-E888.9	Accidental fall
R29.6	Repeated falls

EPIDEMIOLOGY & DEMOGRAPHICS

INCIDENCE:

- Trauma is the fifth leading cause of death in persons >65 yr of age, and falls are responsible for 70% of accidental deaths in persons ≥75 yr.
- The incidence of falls among community-dwelling older adults is 30% to 40%. Two thirds of falls in the community are preventable; 6% to 7% of these falls result in fracture.
- The incidence of falls for nursing home and hospitalized older adults is three times the rate of community-dwelling older adults. Over 50% of nursing home residents fall during their stay.
- 20% to 30% of older adults who fall suffer significant injury leading to immobility, dependence, and an increased risk of early death.

HEALTH CARE COST: In 2006, patients ≥65 had over 2.1 million visits to the ED for injurious falls, which was 10.5% of all ED visits among the elderly and 29.6% of these visits required hospital admission. In those that were admitted, the mean length of stay was 5.5 days with a mean cost of $10,800. The aggregate hospital cost for those requiring admission in 2006 was $6.8 billion. (Source: Healthcare Cost and Utilization Project.)

PREDOMINANT SEX & AGE:

- Fall-related mortality is highest among older white men followed by white women, black men, and black women.
- The incidence rates of falls increase with advancing age.
- Older adults ≥85 yr are 10 to 15 times more likely to have a fracture compared with those aged 60 to 65 yr.

RISK FACTORS: Four groups of risk factors for falls have been identified (Table 1):

- Intrinsic factors inherent in the older adult who falls.
- Extrinsic factors circumstantial to the older adult who falls.
- Falls in nursing homes.
- Situational or the activity in which the older adult is engaged in when a fall occurs.

CLINICAL PRESENTATION

- Older adults who fall may present with minor soft tissue injuries, such as lacerations or bruising, hip fracture, or head trauma; however, most falls are not reported unless an injury has occurred.
- If an older adult presents for medical attention for a fall or reports recurrent falls in the past year or difficulties in walking or balance, a multifactorial fall risk assessment should be completed.
- The multifactorial fall risk assessment should include:
  1. Focused history: A detailed history of events and circumstances surrounding fall, relevant risk factors including review of medications, acute and chronic medical problems (e.g., osteoporosis, urinary incontinence, and cardiovascular disease), and whether the fall was witnessed
  2. Physical examination:
     a. Vital signs including orthostatics.
     b. Cardiovascular examination assessing for arrhythmias, carotid bruits, or new murmurs.
     c. Neurologic examination including vision assessment, evaluation of lower-extremity strength, peripheral nerves, proprioception, and testing of cortical, extrapyramidal, and cerebellar function.
     d. Gait and balance assessment: Multiple screening tools are available for fall risk screening and balance assessment (Tables 2 and 3). "Get up and go test" is a rapid assessment that will quickly tell you if the patient needs rehabilitation and what to work on. (Ask patient to stand from a seated position without use of hands, walk 10 feet forward, turn around, and return to chair and sit).
     e. Musculoskeletal exam with attention to joints of lower extremity, feet, and footwear.
  3. Functional assessment including the older adult's activities of daily living skills, use of adaptive equipment, and fear of falling
  4. Environmental assessment of home safety

TABLE 1 Risk Factors for Falls in the Elderly

Intrinsic

Aging

Age-related decline in vestibular function might lead to loss of balance, dizziness, and falls. Aging of the vision system (e.g., glaucoma, cataracts, retinopathy) may result in decreased visual acuity, inability to discriminate dark/light, and decreased spatial perception.

Cardiac

Cardiac arrhythmias, carotid sinus hypersensitivity, neurocardiogenic syncope

Neurologic

Parkinson's disease, normal pressure hydrocephalus (NPH), sensory neuropathy, dementia/impaired cognition, cervical myelopathy, senile gait disorder, prior stroke (One third of the elderly have abnormal position sense.)

Musculoskeletal

Lower extremity weakness, impaired knee extension and ankle plantar flexion strength contribute to abnormalities in gait velocity and step length, deconditioning, arthritis, foot abnormalities (such as bunions, calluses, or nail abnormalities)

Vascular

Vertebrobasilar insufficiency, postural hypotension, postprandial hypotension

Metabolic

Hypoglycemia, hypothyroidism, hyponatremia

Psychiatric

Depression

Medications

Use of more than four medications may be associated with an increased risk of falls. Medications that may increase fall risk include benzodiazepines, sleeping medications, neuroleptics, antidepressants, anticonvulsants, class I antiarrhythmics, and antihypertensives (Rao, 2005).

Extrinsic

Environmental

Environmental hazards cause >50% of falls in the elderly (cords, furniture, small objects, ill-fitting shoes, slippery surfaces, loose rugs, uneven steps, optical patterns on escalators). Majority occurs with mild-moderate activity (walking, stepping up/down, changing position); 70% occur at home and 10% on stairs (descending > ascending).

Nursing Home Falls

20% have a cardiovascular cause (hypotension: Drug induced, postprandial, postural, or bradycardia)
5% are the result of an acute illness such as PNA, febrile illness, UTI, CHF.
3% are from an overwhelming intrinsic event such as syncope, seizure, stroke, psychoactive drugs.

Situational

Tripping over obstacles, carrying heavy items, descending/ascending stairs, rapid turning, reaching overhead, climbing ladders, ill-fitting shoes, lack of assistive devices

CHF, Congestive heart failure; *PNA,* pneumonia; *UTI,* urinary tract infection.

TABLE 2 Scales Used for Fall Risk Screening and Balance Assessment

Instrument	Items	Setting		
		Community	Acute	Chronic
Multifactorial Reports				
STRATIFY[71]	Five items—history of falls, agitation, visual impairment, frequent toileting, able to stand but needs assistance with moving		X	X
Morse Fall Scale[72]	Six items—history of falls, secondary diagnoses, parenteral therapy, use of ambulation aids, gait, mental status		X	X
FROP-Com[73]	13 risk factors in 26 items—fall and fall injury history, medications, medical conditions, sensory loss, feet, cognitive status, toileting, nutrition, environment, function, behavior, balance, gait; total score, 0 to 60; fall risk high with score >24	X		
Fall risk for residential care[74]	Among persons who can stand without assistance—poor balance or two of three the following: Fall history, nursing home residence, urinary incontinence Among persons who cannot stand without assistance—one of three of the following: fall history, hostel residence, use of nine or more medications			X
Functional Mobility				
Berg Balance test[50,75]	14 tasks scored 0 to 4; total range 0 to 56; fall risk increases as score decreases	X	X	X
Functional reach[76]	Distance reached in inches without moving the feet; fall risk <7 inches	X	X	X
Performance-oriented mobility and balance[77]	Balance subscale score 0 to 16, gait subscale 0 to 12, summary score 0 to 28; summary score <19 indicates high fall risk	X		X
Timed up and go[78]	Time in seconds to rise from a chair, walk 3 m, turn, walk back, and sit down; <10 sec normal; fall risk increases with time >13.5 sec	X		X
Dynamic gait index[51]	Eight walking tasks scored 0 to 3, total score 0 to 24; <18 or 19 indicates fall risk	X		
Functional mobility tests[79]	Time to complete eight step ups (alternate step test) >10 sec, timed sit to stand five times >12 sec, 6-m walk time >6 sec increased fall risk	X		
Physiologic profile assessment[80]	Performance in five domains: Sway, reaction time, strength, proprioception, contrast sensitivity; total score 0 to >3; fall risk increased with score ≥2	X		

FROP-Com, Falls Risk for Older People in the Community; *STRATIFY,* St. Thomas Risk Assessment Tool in Falling elderly inpatients.
From Fillit HM et al: *Brocklehurst's textbook of geriatric medicine and gerontology,* ed 8, Philadelphia, 2017, Elsevier.

TABLE 3 Clinical Assessment Based on Components of Postural Control

Organ System	Impairment	Clinical Evaluation	Potential Cause
Eye	Decreased acuity	Vision chart	Presbyopia, macular degeneration, cataracts
	Reduced visual fields	Confrontation, perimetry	Glaucoma, posterior circulation stroke
	Decreased depth perception	Stereo or depth testing	Monocular vision
	Decreased dark adaptation	Self-report—inability to dilate pupil in low light	Aging, miotic agents for glaucoma
Vestibular apparatus	Otoliths	Ability to detect true vertical, Hallpike maneuver	Benign positional vertigo
	Semicircular canals	Ability to detect position during rotation with eyes closed, nystagmus, visual acuity during head motion	Meniere disease, vestibular hypofunction
Peripheral nerve	Peripheral neuropathy	Light touch, filaments, two-point discrimination, vibratory sense	Diabetes, peripheral vascular disease, vitamin B_{12} deficiency
Circulation	Reduced cerebral perfusion	Low blood pressure, altered level of consciousness, lightheadedness	Medications, arrhythmias, postprandial hypotension
	Orthostatic hypotension	Positional change in blood pressure	Medications, autonomic dysfunction, dehydration
Brain	Reduced attention	Ability to perform dual tasks like timed up and go with cup of water, executive function tasks	Mild cognitive impairment, dementia, medications
	Psychomotor slowing	Timed tapping, timed finger to nose test, trails A test (connect the dots)	Medications, degenerative and vascular brain diseases
	Altered postural reflexes	Absent or slowed righting reflexes	Parkinson's disease, other extrapyramidal and degenerative brain diseases
Muscle	Reduced strength	Manual muscle testing, strength-based functional performance (chair rise, squat)	Generalized—inactivity, sarcopenia, vitamin D deficiency, myopathies
			Focal deficits, spinal cord and peripheral motor nerve conditions
Musculoskeletal pain	Loss of flexibility	Contractures, decreased range of motion	Arthritis, inactivity
	Bone and joint deficits	Weight-bearing pain	Arthritis, fractures, periarticular conditions, foot problems
	Disturbance of spinal cord, roots, nerves	Leg and back pain with activity	Spinal stenosis, radiculopathies, peripheral neuropathies

From Fillit HM et al: *Brocklehurst's textbook of geriatric medicine and gerontology,* ed 8, Philadelphia, 2017, Elsevier.

ETIOLOGY

- Falls are a multifactorial syndrome resulting from the cumulative effects of impaired gait and balance, aging, polypharmacy, depression, cognitive impairment, acute medical illness, or environmental factors (Fig. E1).
- Most falls among community-dwelling older adults are due to environmental factors, whereas falls among nursing home residents are a result of confusion, gait impairment, or postural hypotension.

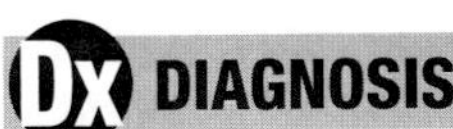

DIAGNOSIS

DIFFERENTIAL DIAGNOSIS

Falls are often a nonspecific symptom of an acute illness (such as delirium, urinary tract infection, acute anemia, or pneumonia) or an exacerbation of a chronic disease (chronic heart failure [CHF] or chronic obstructive pulmonary disease [COPD]). The mnemonic "DELIRIUMS" can be used to assess the differential diagnosis in acute delirium. (**D**rugs, **E**motional [depression], **L**ow PaO_2 [CHF, COPD], **I**nfection, **R**etention [urinary, fecal], **I**ctal status, **U**nder nutrition/hydration, **M**etabolic, **S**ubdural/Sensory [all neurologic causes] workup).

WORKUP

- Older adults presenting with a noninjurious fall need a detailed history and physical exam to identify acute medical illnesses and potential modifiable risk factors. Laboratory and neuroimaging studies may be necessary if the history and physical exam indicate a specific problem. ECG and Holter monitoring may be considered if cardiac arrhythmia is suspected.
- See Fig. E1.

LABORATORY TESTS

CBC, stool guaiac, blood chemistries, thyroid function, liver function, vitamin B_{12} level, folate level, erythrocyte sedimentation rate, vitamin D level, drug levels, and urinalysis depending on physical/historical findings.

IMAGING STUDIES

- CT or MRI of the brain or cervical spine films in the presence of neurologic or gait impairment.
- Chest x-ray if pulmonary pathology (pneumonia, pulmonary edema) is suspected.
- Consider ECG, echocardiography, or Holter monitor if suspicious for structural cardiac abnormality or syncope.

Rx TREATMENT

NONPHARMACOLOGIC THERAPY

- Physical therapy evaluation for gait and balance training, evaluation of appropriate assisted devices (e.g., cane, walker), the use of fall prevention equipment (e.g., low beds, bed alarms).
- Home safety assessment: Studies show that 50% of recurrent fallers fell doing the same activity that caused them to fall the first time. This can be prevented by creating a home safety evaluation checklist (preferably done by family member to improve compliance) or arranging for a home safety inspection by a visiting nurse or occupational therapist.
- Minimization or discontinuation of certain medications associated with falls (psychotropics).
- Customized exercise program to improve strength, gait, and balance.
- Evaluation of proper footwear, hard sole, and low heel height.

ACUTE GENERAL Rx

Hospitalization may be necessary for treatment of hip fracture, subdural hematoma, lacerations, or trauma as well as the treatment of underlying cause of the fall such as infection, metabolic disturbances, cardiovascular (e.g., carotid sinus hypersensitivity, vasovagal syndrome, bradyarrhythmias, and tachyarrhythmias) or neurologic abnormality.

CHRONIC Rx

- Screen and treat for osteoporosis as low bone density increases the risk of hip or other fractures.
- Optimize treatment of chronic illnesses such as CHF, COPD, osteoarthritis, Parkinson's disease, dementia, postural hypotension, and visual problems.
- Vitamin D supplementation of at least 800 IU per day. Epidemiological studies reveal that compared with usual care, short-term intervention with oral nutritional supplementation and dietetic counseling significantly decrease falls in malnourished older adults.
- Table 4 summarizes the management of impairments that contribute to instability and falls.

COMPLEMENTARY & ALTERNATIVE MEDICINE

T'ai chi has been shown to reduce the risk of falls in community-dwelling study participants.

DISPOSITION

Falls increase the older adult's risk of hospitalization, institutionalization, and mortality.

REFERRAL

- Referral may be appropriate to cardiologist, ophthalmologist, neurologist, or podiatrist depending on the presence of a specific condition.
- Consider referral to physical therapist for gait and balance training, evaluation for assisted device, or strengthening program.

PEARLS & CONSIDERATIONS

COMMENTS

- Fear of falling may lead to restriction of activities, social isolation, and dependence.
- Older adults with four or more risk factors have a 78% chance of falling.
- Mortality from falls has increased by 42% over the past decade.

PREVENTION

The U.S. Preventive Services Task Force recommends exercise or physical therapy and vitamin D supplementation to prevent falls in community-dwelling adults aged ≥65 who are at increased risk for falls. It does not recommend automatically performing an in-depth multifactorial risk assessment in conjunction with comprehensive management of identified risks to prevent falls in community-dwelling adults aged 65 or older because the likelihood of benefit is small. In determining whether this service is appropriate in individual cases, patients and clinicians should consider the balance of benefits and harms on the basis of the circumstances of prior falls, comorbid medical conditions, and patient values.

SCREENING

The "get up and go test" is a quick assessment of balance and gait. A more in-depth screening tool for falls is the Tinetti gait and balance assessment, which evaluates normal and adaptive ability to maintain balance when rising from a chair, standing with eyes closed, turning, and receiving a sternal nudge. It also evaluates several components of gait (step height, postural sway, path deviation). The test is scored on the patient's ability to perform specific tasks. Scoring is done on a 3-point scale with a range of 0 to 2. Individual scores are combined to form three measures: an overall gait assessment score (maximum score = 12), an overall balance assessment score (maximum score = 16), and a gait and balance score (maximum score = 28). In general, patients who score below 19 are at high risk for falls, and those who score 19-24 are at risk for falls.

PATIENT/FAMILY EDUCATION

Providing education and information for the patient and caregiver regarding fall prevention strategies in addition to multifactorial risk reduction strategies

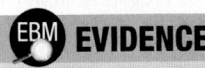

EVIDENCE

Available at ExpertConsult.com

SUGGESTED READINGS

Available at ExpertConsult.com

AUTHORS: **SEAN H. UITERWYK, M.D., ALICIA J. CURTIN, PH.D.,** and **KEITH BRENNAN, M.D.**

TABLE 4 Management of Impairments That Contribute to Instability and Falls

Organ System	Impairment	Medical Management	Restorative Services	Environmental Modifications
Eye	Decreased acuity	Corrective lenses	Low vision rehabilitation	Lighting
	Reduced visual fields	Prisms in spectacles	Low vision rehabilitation, teach to scan using head rotation	
	Loss of depth perception	Cataract removal, if indicated	Teach to use shadows to detect depth	Lighting to accent shadows, contrast
	Poor dark adaptation	Switching to glaucoma medications that do not cause miosis		Lighting
Vestibular system	Benign paroxysmal positional vertigo (BPPV)	Epley maneuver	Vestibular rehabilitation	
	Meniere disease	Cautious use of meclizine, diuretics; rarely, surgery	Vestibular rehabilitation	
Peripheral nerve	Neuropathy	Footwear to protect foot and maximize sensation	Assistive devices for haptic enhancement	Hand holds, railings
Central circulation	Reduced brain perfusion	Treatment varies by cause Arrhythmias—medications to control rate and rhythm, pacemakers Postprandial hypotension—frequent small meals		
	Orthostatic hypotension	Treatment varies by cause Adjust offending medications Autonomic neuropathy—salt loading, fluorinated corticosteroids Dehydration—hydration, reduce diuretic dose	Compression hose, calf muscle contractions	
Brain	Reduced attention	Medication adjustment	Practice dual tasks	
	Psychomotor slowing	Medication adjustment	Practice movement speed	
	Abnormal righting reflexes	Antiparkinsonian medication helps bradykinesia more than balance.	Assistive devices, practice getting up after a fall	Protective clothing
Effector muscle	Weakness	Reduced activity—treat contributing causes (e.g., CHF, anemia, COPD, arthritis)	Strength-training exercises	Raise chair height
		Focal motor deficit due to spinal stenosis—sometimes surgery Myopathy—adjust offending medications, possibly steroids for myositis	Orthotics, exercise, assistive devices	
Musculoskeletal	Decreased range of motion		Active and passive range of motion exercise, orthotics	
Pain	Bone and joint	Analgesics, injections	Physical modalities (e.g., heat, massage, assistive devices, orthoses, adaptive equipment)	Place items within easy reach
	Spinal cord, roots, nerves	Injections, surgery, analgesics	Orthoses, assistive devices	Place items within easy reach

CHF, Congesetive heart failure; *COPD,* chronic obstructive pulmonary disease.
From Fillit HM et al: *Brocklehurst's textbook of geriatric medicine and gerontology,* ed 8, Philadelphia, 2017, Elsevier.

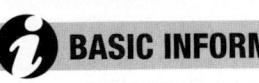

BASIC INFORMATION

DEFINITION

Familial adenomatous polyposis (FAP) is a highly penetrant, autosomal-dominant condition characterized by hundreds of colorectal adenomatous polyps that inevitably progress to cancer (Fig. 1). ***Gardner syndrome*** is a subset of FAP, with prominent extraintestinal manifestations including dental abnormalities, soft tissue lesions, desmoid tumors, and osteomas.

ICD-10CM CODES

D12.5	Benign neoplasm of sigmoid colon
D12.4	Benign neoplasm of descending colon
D12.3	Benign neoplasm of transverse colon
D12.2	Benign neoplasm of ascending colon
D12.6	Benign neoplasm of colon, unspecified

EPIDEMIOLOGY & DEMOGRAPHICS

- FAP occurs in approximately 1 in 10,000 births worldwide.
- FAP accounts for <1% of all colorectal cancers.
- Individuals develop hundreds to thousands of adenomatous colorectal polyps.
- Polyps usually present in adolescence.
- 100% lifetime risk for colorectal cancer; most diagnosed by 40 yr of age.
- Gastric, duodenal, periampullary, and small bowel polyps occur but have lower malignant potential.
- Increased risk for other tumors: Desmoid (15%), duodenal/periampullary (7%), thyroid (2%), brain (1%), childhood hepatoblastoma (1%), nasopharyngeal angiofibroma (benign), pancreatic (2%), adrenal adenoma (10%), and gastric (1%).

PHYSICAL FINDINGS & CLINICAL PRESENTATION

Phenotypic variability is seen in individuals and families with the same mutation. Soft tissue and bone abnormalities may precede intestinal disease. These findings are reported in at least 20% of individuals with FAP.

- Congenital hypertrophy of the retinal pigment epithelium (CHRPE): Benign fundus lesions, usually present at birth
- Dental abnormalities: Supernumerary or unerupted teeth
- Soft tissue lesions: Epidermal or sebaceous cysts, fibromas, lipomas, desmoid tumors (benign, locally invasive, aggressive connective tissue tumor)
- Osteomas (benign bone growths): Skull, mandible, long bone
- Anemia, occult blood in stool, bowel obstruction, weight loss

ETIOLOGY

- FAP is caused by mutations of the tumor suppressor gene adenomatous polyposis coli *(APC)* on chromosome 5q21-q22; more than 1000 disease-causing mutations identified. The site of the mutation often correlates with the extraintestinal findings.
- De novo mutations are responsible for approximately 20% of FAP cases. These may be due to germline mutations or somatic cell mosaicism, which is seen when a new mutation occurs in the APC gene post-fertilization and is present in only a subset of cell types or tissues.

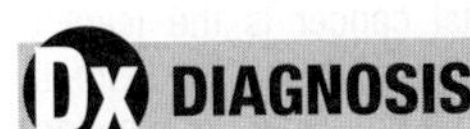

DIAGNOSIS

In individuals with a family history, more than 100 adenomatous colorectal polyps, CHRPE lesions, or positive genetic testing confirms diagnosis. In those without a family history, more than 100 adenomatous colorectal polyps suggest the diagnosis, and genetic testing confirms it. The diagnosis should be considered in individuals with ≥10 adenomatous colorectal polyps or fewer polys in the presence of extraintestinal findings.

DIFFERENTIAL DIAGNOSIS

- Turcot syndrome
- Attenuated FAP (also APC gene mutation, but presents with fewer polyps [<100], at a later age, and has lower cancer risk than FAP [~80% lifetime risk])
- MUTYH-associated polyposis
- Peutz-Jeghers syndrome
- Juvenile polyposis syndrome
- Cowden disease
- Lynch syndrome
- Hereditary mixed polyposis syndrome
- Polymerase proofreading-associated polyposis
- Hyperplastic polyposis
- Table 1 compares various adenomatous polyposis syndromes

WORKUP

History, physical examination, laboratory tests, imaging studies

DIAGNOSTIC SCREENING OPTIONS

GENETIC TESTING: NOTE: Genetic counseling should be performed, and written informed consent obtained before testing. Refer to a specialized center for counseling and evaluation.

- Should be offered to first-degree relatives of affected individuals (with an identified mutation) at age 10 to 12 yr and clinically suspected individuals.
- Able to identify a mutation in approximately 80% of families. To ensure that the family has a detectable mutation, test an affected family member first.
- If positive in the affected individual, the test can differentiate with 100% accuracy affected and unaffected family members. If negative in the affected individual, screening family members will not be useful in determining disease status.
- If no known family history exists, screening the clinically suspected individual is reasonable. A positive test rules in FAP but a negative test does not rule it out.
- Numerous testing techniques available; may require multiple tests to identify the mutation.

SIGMOIDOSCOPY:

- Individuals with a positive genetic test, untested at-risk family members, or patients from families with an unidentified *APC* mutation: Annual flexible sigmoidoscopy or colonoscopy beginning at 10 to 12 yr of age.
- Once adenomatous polyps are detected, patients should undergo colonoscopy and evaluation for colectomy.
- Negative genetic test in patients from families with an identified mutation: Average risk screening.
- Screening with upper endoscopy should begin at age 25 and should include visualization of duodenal papilla. Additional annual screening should include thyroid ultrasound.

CHRPE: Lesions occur in up to 80% of families and are a reliable indicator of affected status in these families.

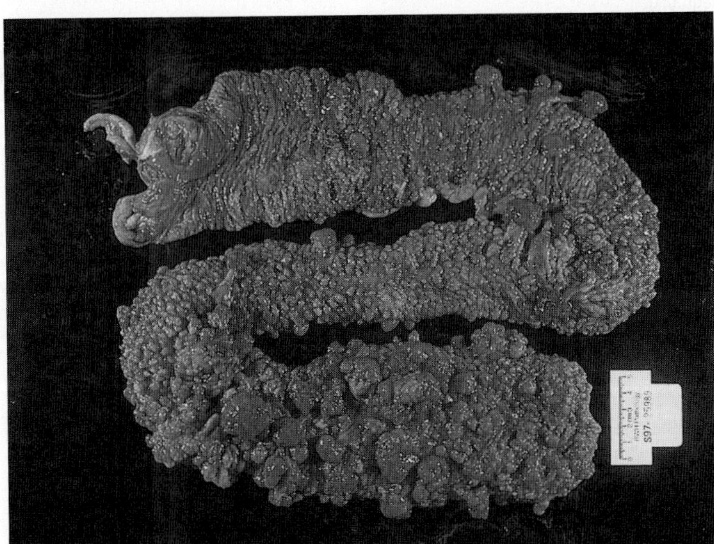

FIG. 1 Familial adenomatous polyposis with innumerable adenomatous polyps, increasing in size and density from proximal (upper left) to distal (lower right). (From Skarin AT: *Atlas of diagnostic oncology*, ed 4, St. Louis, 2010, Mosby.)

TABLE 1 Adenomatous Polyposis Syndromes

Syndrome	Gene Mutation	Polyps	Extraintestinal Abnormalities
Classic FAP	*APC* (usually truncated protein)	Colonic adenomas (thousands) Duodenal, periampullary adenomas Gastric fundic gland polyps Jejunal and ileal adenomas Ileal lymphoid polyps	Mandibular osteomas Dental abnormalities
Gardner variant of FAP	*APC*	Same as FAP	Osteomas (mandible, skull, long bones) CHRPE Desmoid tumors Epidermoid and sebaceous cysts Fibromas, lipomas Thyroid, adrenal tumors
Turcot variant of FAP	*APC* DNA MMR*	Colonic adenomas (sometimes fewer than in classic FAP)	Medulloblastoma Glioblastoma multiforme CHRPE
Attenuated FAP	*APC* 5′ and 3′ regions	Colonic adenomas (<100; proximal colon) Duodenal, periampullary adenomas Gastric fundic gland polyps	Mandibular osteomas (rare)
Familial tooth agenesis	*Axin2* (APC pathway)	Colonic adenomas Hyperplastic polyps	Agenesis of teeth
Bloom's syndrome	*BLM*	Colonic adenomas	Small stature Facial erythema/telangiectasia Male sterility Adenocarcinomas, leukemia, lymphoma
MUTYH polyposis	*MUTYH (MYH)*	Colonic adenomas (5-100) Duodenal polyposis Gastric cancer	CHRPE Osteomas

*May be more appropriately classified under hereditary nonpolyposis colon cancer.
APC, Adenomatous polyposis coli; *CHRPE,* congenital hypertrophy of the retinal pigment epithelium; *FAP,* familial adenomatous polyposis; *MMR,* mismatch repair; *MUTYH* (mutY homolog [*E. coli*]).
From Feldman M, et al. (eds): *Sleisenger and Fordtran's gastrointestinal and liver disease*, ed 10, Philadelphia, 2016, Saunders.

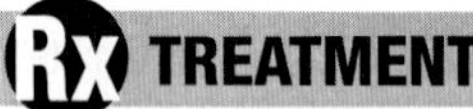

TREATMENT

- Prophylactic colectomy or proctocolectomy: Timing determined by polyp number, size, and degree of dysplasia. Postsurgical endoscopic surveillance annually.
- Screening of remaining GI tract and screening for extraintestinal manifestations continues after colectomy:
  1. Annual physical examination: History, examination (including thyroid), and blood tests
  2. Upper endoscopy to screen for gastric/duodenal polyps: Baseline at age 25 yr (earlier if colon polyps detected) and repeated every 3 months to 4 yr based on findings
  3. Annual thyroid ultrasound
  4. Other possible cancer sites imaged if symptoms occur or if these cancers have occurred in relatives
- Treat soft tissue lesions and osteomas for symptoms or cosmetic concerns. Treat desmoid tumors if they pose a risk to adjacent structures.

DISPOSITION

- 100% chance of colorectal cancer in untreated individuals. Many other neoplasms occur at higher rates.
- Metastatic colorectal cancer is the leading cause of death (58%), followed by desmoid tumors (11%), and duodenal/periampullary adenocarcinoma (8%).

REFERRAL

- Patients should be managed at centers with expertise in FAP, including a gastroenterologist, medical geneticist, and surgeon.
- Genetic counselors can be found at www.nsgc.org.

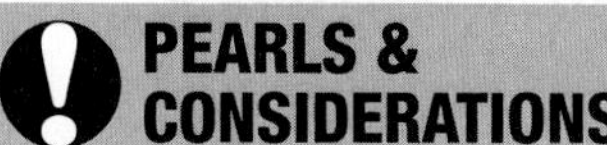

PEARLS & CONSIDERATIONS

- Management should be individualized based on genotype, phenotype, and individual preferences.
- Sulindac (NSAID) and celecoxib (COX-2 inhibitor) can cause duodenal and colorectal polyp regression in individuals with FAP. Preliminary studies with other agents also show polyp regression. Their ability to reduce cancer risk remains unknown; they do not replace colon resection for cancer prevention.
- Desmoid tumors usually present in the 30s, frequently occur in the abdomen, and are difficult to treat with high rates of recurrence. Growth and recurrence are stimulated by surgery.
- Screen children of affected parents (from infancy to age 7 yr) biannually with alpha-fetoprotein level and liver ultrasound to rule out hepatoblastoma.
- Preimplantation and prenatal genetic testing is available.

SUGGESTED READINGS

Available at ExpertConsult.com

RELATED CONTENT

Familial Adenomatous Polyposis and Polyposis Syndromes (Patient Information)
Colorectal Cancer (Related Key Topic)
Lynch Syndrome (Related Key Topic)
Peutz-Jeghers Syndrome (Related Key Topic)

AUTHOR: **SUDEEP K. AULAKH, M.D., F.A.C.P., F.R.C.P.C.**

BASIC INFORMATION

DEFINITION

Acute fatty liver of pregnancy (AFLP) is characterized histologically by microvesicular fatty cytoplasmic infiltration of hepatocytes with minimal hepatocellular necrosis.

SYNONYMS

Acute fatty metamorphosis
Acute yellow atrophy
AFLP
Acute fatty liver of pregnancy

ICD-10CM CODES

026.611	Liver and biliary tract disorders in pregnancy, first trimester
026.612	Liver and biliary tract disorders in pregnancy, second trimester
026.613	Liver and biliary tract disorders in pregnancy, third trimester
026.619	Liver and biliary tract disorders in pregnancy, unspecified trimester

EPIDEMIOLOGY & DEMOGRAPHICS

INCIDENCE:
- Rare: 1 in 10,000 to 1 in 20,000 pregnancies
- Equal frequencies in all races and at all maternal ages

AVERAGE GESTATIONAL AGE: 37 wk (range 28 to 42 wk)
- 20% present postnatally

RISK FACTORS:
- Primiparity
- Multiple gestation
- Male fetus
- History of type II diabetes mellitus
- Preeclampsia

GENETICS: Some with a familial deficiency of long-chain 3-hydroxyacyl-coenzyme A dehydrogenase (LCHAD)

PHYSICAL FINDINGS & CLINICAL PRESENTATION

- Initial manifestations:
  1. Nausea and vomiting (70%)
  2. Pain in right upper quadrant or epigastrium (50% to 80%)
  3. Malaise and anorexia
- Jaundice often in 1 to 2 wk
- Hypoglycemia
- Late manifestations:
  1. Fulminant hepatic failure
  2. Encephalopathy
  3. Renal failure
  4. Pancreatitis
  5. Gastrointestinal and uterine bleeding
  6. Disseminated intravascular coagulation (10%)
  7. Seizures
  8. Coma
- Liver:
  1. Usually small
  2. Normal or enlarged in preeclampsia, eclampsia, HELLP syndrome (hemolysis, elevated liver enzymes, and low platelets), and acute hepatitis
  3. Coexistent preeclampsia in up to 46% of patients

ETIOLOGY

- Fetal LCHAD deficiency results in transplacental passage of excess fetal fatty acids and subsequent accumulation in the maternal liver.
- Postulated that inhibition of mitochondrial oxidation of fatty acids may lead to microvesicular fatty infiltration of liver.
- Fatty metamorphosis of preeclamptic liver disease believed to be of different etiology.

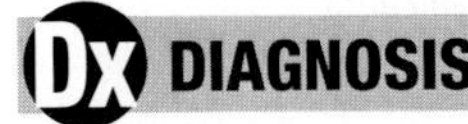

DIAGNOSIS

DIFFERENTIAL DIAGNOSIS

- Acute gastroenteritis
- Preeclampsia or eclampsia with liver involvement
- HELLP syndrome
- Acute viral hepatitis
- Fulminant hepatitis
- Drug-induced hepatitis caused by halothane, phenytoin, methyldopa, isoniazid, hydrochlorothiazide, or tetracycline
- Intrahepatic cholestasis of pregnancy
- Gallbladder disease
- Reye syndrome
- Hemolytic-uremic syndrome
- Budd-Chiari syndrome
- Systemic lupus erythematosus

WORKUP

- A clinical diagnosis is based predominantly on physical and laboratory findings (Swansea criteria).
- Most definitive diagnosis is through liver biopsy with oil red O staining and electron microscopy.
- Liver biopsy is reserved for atypical cases only and only after any existing coagulopathy is corrected with fresh frozen plasma because of concerns for excessive bleeding.

LABORATORY TESTS

Tests to determine the following:
- Hypoglycemia (often profound <60 mg/dl)
- Hyperammonemia
- Elevated aminotransferases (usually <500 U/ml)
- Thrombocytopenia
- Leukocytosis (white blood cell count >15,000)
- Hyperbilirubinemia (usually <10 mg/dl)
- Low albumin
- Hypofibrinogenemia (<300 mg/dl)
- Disseminated intravascular coagulation (DIC) (in 75%)

IMAGING STUDIES

- Ultrasound: Best used to rule out other diseases in the differential diagnosis such as gallbladder disease
- CT scan: Plays minimal role because of a high false-negative rate

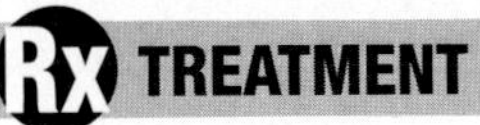

TREATMENT

NONPHARMACOLOGIC THERAPY

- Patient is admitted to intensive care unit for stabilization.
- Fetus is delivered; spontaneous resolution usually follows delivery.
- Mode of delivery is based on obstetric indications and clinical assessment of disease severity.

ACUTE GENERAL Rx

- Decrease in endogenous ammonia through dietary protein restriction; neomycin 6 to 12 g/day PO to decrease presence of ammonia-producing bacteria; magnesium citrate 30 to 50 ml PO or enema to evacuate nitrogenous wastes from colon.
- Administration of IV fluids with glucose to keep glucose levels >60 mg/dl.
- Coagulopathy corrected with fresh frozen plasma.
- Avoidance of drugs metabolized by liver.
- Aggressive avoidance and treatment for nosocomial infections; consideration of prophylactic antibiotics.
- Monitor closely for development of complications such as hepatic encephalopathy, pulmonary edema, DIC, and respiratory arrest.
- Plasma exchange after delivery may result in a lower maternal mortality.

CHRONIC Rx

Orthotopic liver transplantation is the only treatment for irreversible liver failure.

DISPOSITION

- Before 1980, both maternal and fetal mortality rates were approximately 85%.
- Since 2008, maternal mortality rates have been less than 10%.
- Usually rapid return of liver function to normal after delivery.
- Minimal risk of recurrence with future pregnancies.

REFERRAL

- To tertiary health care facility as soon as diagnosis is suspected.
- 20% of infants born to mothers with AFLP have LCHAD; after birth, all infants should be evaluated for the deficiency.

SUGGESTED READINGS

Available at ExpertConsult.com

RELATED CONTENT

Eclampsia (Related Key Topic)
Preeclampsia (Related Key Topic)
HELLP Syndrome (Related Key Topic)

AUTHOR: **KELLY RUHSTALLER, M.D.**

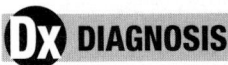

BASIC INFORMATION

DEFINITION

Febrile seizures are seizures that occur in febrile children (fever of at least 100.4° F [38° C]) between the ages of 6 and 60 months in the absence of infection of the central nervous system (CNS), metabolic disturbance, or history of neonatal seizures or a previous unprovoked seizures. Febrile seizures are subdivided into two categories: simple and complex. Simple febrile seizures last <15 min, are generalized (without a focal component), and occur once in a 24-hr period, whereas complex febrile seizures are prolonged (>15 min), show focal neurologic signs, or occur more than once in 24 hr.

SYNONYMS

Febrile convulsions
Seizures, febrile

ICD-10CM CODE
R56.0 Febrile convulsions

EPIDEMIOLOGY & DEMOGRAPHICS

INCIDENCE: Febrile seizures are the most common seizures of childhood. 2% to 5% of children will have a febrile seizure by age 60 mo. Simple febrile seizures represent 65% to 90% of febrile seizures.
PREDOMINANT SEX AND AGE: Slightly more common in boys than girls
PEAK INCIDENCE: 6 to 60 mo
PREVALENCE: Represents up to 18% of all pediatric epilepsy syndromes

PHYSICAL FINDINGS & CLINICAL PRESENTATION

- Children with febrile seizures have normal physical and neurologic examinations.
- Viral illnesses are the predominant cause of febrile seizures.

ETIOLOGY

- Viral infections are a common cause of a fever that triggers febrile seizures.
- Febrile seizures tend to occur in families. Although clear evidence exists for a genetic basis of febrile seizures, the mode of inheritance is unknown.
- Febrile seizures are likely multifactorial with genetic and environmental factors.

DIAGNOSIS

DIFFERENTIAL DIAGNOSIS

- CNS infection (i.e., meningitis)
- Epilepsy

WORKUP

- It is important to first investigate whether an underlying infection exists. Fig. 1 describes guidelines for febrile seizure evaluation.
- In patients with simple self-limited febrile seizures with rapid return to consciousness and a normal neurologic examination, further workup is not routinely recommended.
- In patients with complex febrile seizures, laboratory workup and brain imaging are recommended.
- EEG is not routinely recommended in the evaluation of a neurologically healthy child with simple febrile seizures.

LABORATORY TESTS

- Routine blood workup (CBC with differential, CMP, electrolytes), blood and urine cultures are often performed, but there is no evidence that these tests are necessary for identifying the cause of a simple febrile seizure.
- CSF analysis: Follow lumbar puncture guidelines of the American Academy of Pediatrics.
- Lumbar puncture should be performed in children with febrile seizures and signs and symptoms of meningitis (e.g., neck stiffness, Kernig sign, Brudzinski sign), or if the patient history or examination suggests the presence of meningitis or other intracranial infection.
- In infants 6 to 12 months of age with febrile seizures, lumbar puncture is an option if they have not received the recommended *Haemophilus influenza* type b (Hib) or pneumococcal vaccinations, or if their immunization status is unknown.
- Lumbar puncture is also considered an option in children with febrile seizures pretreated with antibiotics.

IMAGING STUDIES

- MRI of the brain is not required in the routine evaluation of patients with simple febrile seizures.
- Imaging of the brain should be considered in children with complex febrile seizures and in children with focal neurologic deficits.
- CT scans of the head should be avoided in children, if possible, due to exposure to radiation and the relative low yield of the test compared with MRI. CT scans of the head are reserved for neurologic emergencies and are adjusted for weight in children.

TREATMENT

Febrile seizures do not usually require antiepileptic drug treatment.

NONPHARMACOLOGIC THERAPY

Not applicable

GENERAL Rx

Symptomatic treatment of fever

CHRONIC Rx

No chronic treatment for febrile seizures is recommended.

COMPLEMENTARY & ALTERNATIVE MEDICINE

Not applicable

DISPOSITION

- Treatment is not recommended.
- Febrile seizures should stop by age 60 months.
- Risk of recurrence in the first 2 yr after an initial febrile seizure is 15% to 70%.

REFERRAL

Patients with recurrent febrile seizures need to be referred for a consultation by a pediatric neurologist.

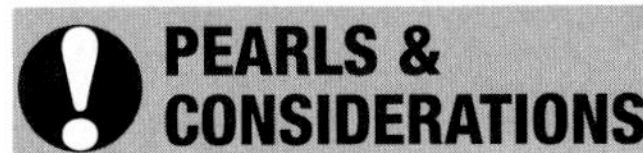

PEARLS & CONSIDERATIONS

COMMENTS

- It is crucial to find out the etiology of the fever and to treat it appropriately.
- Patient with seizures and fever after age 60 mo are not classified as febrile seizures.

PREVENTION

Antipyretics do not reduce the recurrence risk of febrile seizures. However, fever should be treated and worked up independently of the diagnosis of febrile seizures.

PATIENT & FAMILY EDUCATION

- Children with febrile seizures do not need antiepileptic drug treatment.
- Patient education and information can be obtained at the Epilepsy Foundation: www.epilepsyfoundation.org. Parents should be reassured that children without underlying developmental problems will usually not have lasting neurologic effects from febrile seizures.

SUGGESTED READINGS
Available at ExpertConsult.com

RELATED CONTENT

Fever Seizures (Patient Information)

AUTHOR: **PATRICIO SEBASTIAN ESPINOSA, M.D., M.P.H.**

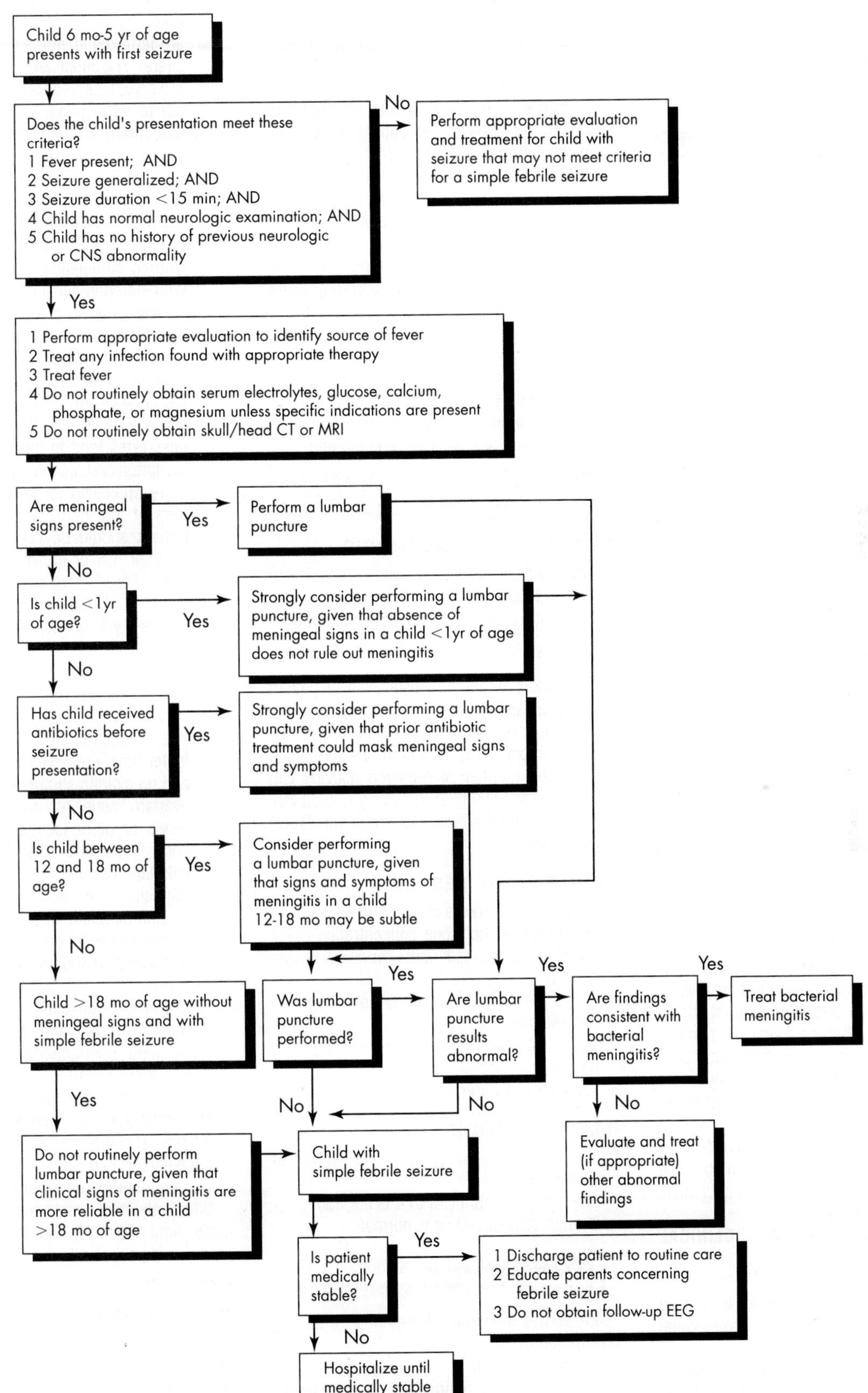

FIG. 1 Guidelines for febrile seizure evaluation. *CNS,* Central nervous system; *CT,* computed tomography; *EEG,* electroencephalogram; *MRI,* magnetic resonance imaging. (From Custer JW, Rau RE: *The Harriet Lane handbook,* ed 18, St Louis, 2009, Mosby.)

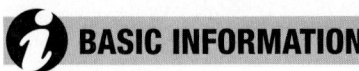

DEFINITION

Fertility preservation is the process of preserving eggs, sperm, or reproductive tissue for future use.

Patients typically seek fertility preservation techniques before undergoing sterilizing therapies for cancer treatment or for elective delay of childbearing.

SYNONYMS

Oncofertility
In vitro fertilization
Cryopreservation

ICD-10CM CODES

Z31.84	Encounter for fertility preservation procedure
Z31.62	Encounter for fertility preservation counseling (before cancer therapy) (before removal of gonads)
Z31.41	Encounter for fertility testing
Z31.9	Other special procreative management

EPIDEMIOLOGY & DEMOGRAPHICS

PREVALENCE: Given the emergence and novelty of fertility preservation techniques, the epidemiology has not been well established. Currently, little is known regarding the perceptions and prevalence of elective fertility preservation. However, there is a growing need for discussions regarding fertility options among cancer patients. In 2006, the American Society of Clinical Oncology published guidelines for oncologists to discuss the possibility of infertility and offer referral for fertility preservation consultation and treatment.

In 2017, nearly 12% of men and women found to have cancer were younger than 45 yr Furthermore, the prevalence of nonsurgical premature menopause in female cancer survivors was 9.1% by age 40, nearly tenfold higher than baseline. Recent literature shows that, among adolescent females with malignancies, 81% of them and 93% of parents were interested in fertility preservation, even if options were described as experimental.

PREDOMINANT SEX AND AGE: Fertility declines with age in both men and women, but the effects of age are more pronounced in women, particularly after age 35.

PHYSICAL FINDINGS & CLINICAL PRESENTATION:

- An increasing proportion of women are choosing to delay childbearing to pursue educational degrees or for professional achievement.
- For women seeking to delayed childbearing, a thorough history and physical should be performed. A thorough reproductive history including previous pregnancies, spontaneous/elective abortions, and pregnancy complications; a gynecologic history including cysts, fibroids, sexually transmitted diseases, and endometriosis also needs to be included.
- A complete assessment of past medical diagnoses, illicit drug use, and family history is indicated. Specifically, age is a determining factor guiding management. The older a woman is at the time of oocyte cryopreservation, the lower the probability of live birth in the future. The highest probability of live birth after oocyte cryopreservation occurs for women ≤35 yr of age, whereas the maximum age for attempting oocyte cryopreservation may be as high as 45 yr.
- For patients undergoing sterilizing therapies, chemotherapy, or radiation, physicians should discuss the risk of treatment-induced infertility and possible interventions to preserve fertility. Ultimately, the optimal preservation approach depends on the type of gonadotoxic treatment (radiation vs. chemotherapy), time available, patient age, cancer type, partner status, costs, and storage.

Dx DIAGNOSIS

DIFFERENTIAL DIAGNOSIS

- Elective delay
- Gonadotoxic treatment with radiation
- Gonadotoxic treatment with chemotherapy

WORKUP

Initial workup requires a discussion of patient goals, ideal family size, and timeline. Physicians should set realistic expectations for their patients' most likely outcome. Factors such as age and number of retrieved oocytes can predict the probability of achieving a live birth. Online calculators are available to guide clinical management.

LABORATORY TEST(S)

Assessment of markers of ovarian reserve:

- Anti-Müllerian hormone concentration (>2.7 ng/ml is associated with improved oocyte quality)
- Day 3 follicle-stimulating hormone (<10–15 mIU/ml is normal)
- Day 3 estradiol concentration (<80 pg/ml is normal)
- Inhibin B (>45 pg/ml is normal)

IMAGING STUDIES

Consider an ultrasound-guided assessment of ovarian reserve:

- Antral follicle count (>3 to 4 is normal)
- Ovarian volume (>3 cc is normal)

Rx TREATMENT

There exist a multitude of methods for fertility preservation:

- Cryopreservation:
  1. Embryo: This method is an established technique for fertility preservation; the percentage of live birth after embryo transfer is similar to the natural fecundity rate of 20% to 30%. Women undergo ovarian stimulation with gonadotropins followed by office oocyte retrieval via needle aspiration under ultrasound guidance. Oocytes are fertilized in vitro with partner or donor sperm. The subsequent embryos that arise are cryopreserved using either slow freezing or vitrification, and stored for future use; there is no time limit for embryo storage. Cryopreserved embryos are not associated with poor obstetrical outcomes. However, for women undergoing chemotherapy, certain time constraints make oocyte retrieve unfeasible. Additionally, ovarian stimulation may not be possible with estrogen-sensitive tumors.
  2. Oocytes: Oocyte cryopreservation is technically more challenging than embryo preservation. Given the increased water content in oocytes, cryopreservation risks ice crystals, excessive osmotic pressure, and electrolyte toxicity. Although the success rates tend to be lower than embryo cryopreservation, harvesting oocytes are more appealing for women without partners at the time of fertility preservation. Patient should be counseled extensively on their risk of transfer success and live birth. Large retrospective cohorts have shown that approximately 5% of thawed oocytes will successfully implant and 4% will result in a live birth in women whose average age was 33.
  3. Ovarian Tissue: This technique remains in its infancy and is currently experimental. The advantages of this technique include faster time, preservation of many oocytes, and no ovarian stimulation necessary. The ovarian tissue can remain either in the pelvis or other locations throughout the body. Retrieval is often invasive, typically with laparoscopy.
- Transposition via oophoropexy: This technique can be useful in patients with planned radiation. The ovary can be removed from the field of radiation and transposed elsewhere in the pelvis.
- Gonadotropin-releasing hormone (GnRH) agonists: This technique is useful in women undergoing chemotherapy. GnRH agonists suppress ovarian function and are speculated to prevent toxic damage to oocytes caused by chemotherapy. This technique remains in its infancy. The efficacy and success have not been established, and this is therefore not the first-line therapy for fertility preservation.

Ultimately, a complete evaluation of patient goals, time available, and cancer type is necessary before selecting a method of fertility preservation.

DISPOSITION

Fertility preservation via cryopreservation of embryos or oocytes is completed in an outpatient setting. GnRH agonist therapy is also managed in an outpatient setting. Harvesting ovarian tissue and transposing via oophoropexy are more invasive procedures, requiring surgical management.

REFERRAL

The American Society of Clinical Oncology and the American Society of Reproductive Medicine recommend early referral to a reproductive endocrine and infertility specialist if fertility is a concern before treatment.

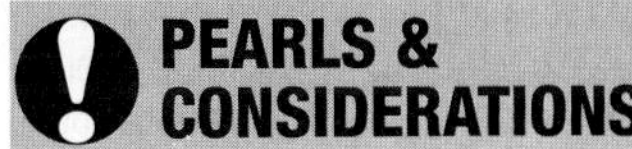

PEARLS & CONSIDERATIONS

COMMENTS

- Two major indications for fertility preservation include prior cancer treatment and elective delay of childbearing.
- Early referral to a reproductive endocrinology and infertility specialist is essential.
- A discussion of patient-centered reproductive goals should be initiated.
- Fertility preservation techniques should be reviewed, and the best option selected for each patient, specific to the situation and reproductive goals.

PATIENT/FAMILY EDUCATION

Fertility Preservation for Cancer Patients: A patient education video sponsored by the American Society of Reproductive Medicine. www.reproductivefacts.org/

Egg Freezing Counseling Tool (EFCT): Predicts likelihood of live birth for elective egg freezing in women. www.mdcalc.com/bwh-egg-freezing-counseling-tool-efct

AUTHOR: **HELEN B. GOMEZ, M.D.**

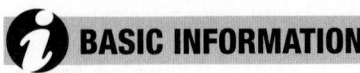

BASIC INFORMATION

DEFINITION

A traveler who returns from a foreign country with a fever or develops a fever within a month of returning.

ICD10-CM CODES

A50 Fever of other and unknown origin
A95 Yellow fever
A90 Dengue fever
A01 Typhoid and paratyphoid fever
B54 Malaria, malarial (fever)
A98.8 Other specified viral hemorrhagic fever

EPIDEMIOLOGY & DEMOGRAPHICS

INCIDENCE: Fever was the chief complaint in 28% of travelers who reported to a travel clinic. Mortality is between 0.2% and 0.5%.

PEAK INCIDENCE: Location and timing of travel influences the incidence of fever.

RISK FACTORS: Morbidity and mortality increased among elderly and young travelers.

PHYSICAL FINDINGS & CLINICAL PRESENTATION

- A detailed history on the trip must be obtained, including areas of travel, activities, sleeping arrangements, pre-trip immunizations, comorbidities, and use of malaria prophylaxis.
- If the incubation period is <21 days, the most common diseases include malaria, typhoid fever, and dengue. Also consider Japanese encephalitis, meningococcemia, plague, typhus, yellow fever, and viral hemorrhagic fevers.
- If incubation period is >21 days, the most common diseases include malaria, tuberculosis (TB), and hepatitis A. Consider acute HIV infection, acute systemic schistosomiasis, borreliosis, other viral hepatitis, and West African trypanosomiasis (Table 1).

Common causes of fever in returning travelers:

- Malaria: Most common cause of fever after travel in endemic areas. Presents with abrupt rigors, relapsing high fevers, diaphoresis, malaise, headaches, myalgias, abdominal pain, nausea, vomiting, diarrhea.
- Enteric fevers (typhoid fever, paratyphoid fever): Clinical syndrome of sustained fever, anorexia, abdominal pain, malaise. Diarrhea usually precedes other symptoms. May see hepatosplenomegaly and rose spots on physical exam. Vaccines are 70% effective. Patient will have traveled to a developing nation. Diagnoses by identification of organism in blood, stool, or urine.
- Dengue fever ("breakbone fever"): Abrupt fever, severe myalgia, headaches with retro-orbital pain, maculopapular blanching rash, petechial fever similar to meningococcus.

Hemorrhagic fevers:

- Yellow fever: Classic presentation of jaundice, black emesis, albuminuria. Patients may also have conjunctival injection, facial flushing, relative bradycardia.
- Ebola: Recent large outbreaks in West Africa with recurring smaller outbreaks. Symptoms of fever, myalgia, and abdominal pain that progress to hemorrhage, shock, and end organ failure.

Fever with CNS involvement:

- Consider malaria, meningococcal meningitis, tuberculosis, rabies.
- Japanese encephalitis: Asian distribution, associated with rural rice fields. High fevers, headache, nuchal rigidity, and seizures.

Chronic fevers: Relapsing or constant fever >3 weeks:

- African trypanosomiasis (African sleeping sickness): Bite from the tsetse fly, painless chancre that grows for 2 to 3 weeks. Fever unresponsive to antimalarials, malaise, wasting, behavioral and neurologic changes, encephalitis, coma occur.
- American trypanosomiasis (Chagas disease): Spread by reduviid bug (kissing or assassin bug). Painful edema at wound near mouth, unilateral periorbital edema, lymphadenopathy for 2 to 4 weeks. Latent phase with nerve destruction causing cardiac and GI manifestations.
- Middle East respiratory syndrome (travel to or near the Arabian Peninsula): Fever, acute respiratory distress syndrome, or pneumonia.

ETIOLOGY

Table 2 summarizes the constellations of exposures and clinical presentations suggestive of particular diagnoses in returning travelers.

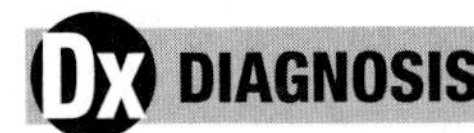

DIAGNOSIS

DIFFERENTIAL DIAGNOSIS

- Malaria
- Dengue
- Hemorrhagic fevers: Yellow fever, Ebola
- Enteric fever: Typhoid, paratyphoid
- Meningococcemia
- TB
- Acute HIV
- Trypanosomiasis
- Viral hepatitis
- Common nontravel causes of fever: Urinary tract infection, upper respiratory tract infections

WORKUP

Must consider travel location, activities, endemic diseases

TABLE 1 Incubation Periods of Common Travel-Related Infections*

Short Incubation (<10 days)	Medium Incubation (10-21 days)	Long Incubation (>21 days)
Malaria	Malaria	Malaria
Arboviruses including dengue, yellow fever, Japanese encephalitis	Flaviviruses: Tick-borne encephalitis and Japanese encephalitis	Schistosomiasis
Hemorrhagic fevers: Lassa, ebola, South American arenaviruses	Hemorrhagic fevers: Lassa, ebola, Crimean-Congo	Tuberculosis
Respiratory viruses including severe acute respiratory syndrome	Acute HIV infection	Acute HIV infection
Typhoid and paratyphoid	Typhoid and paratyphoid	Viral hepatitis
Bacterial enteritis	*Giardia*	Filariasis
Rickettsia: Spotted fever group—Rocky Mountain spotted fever, African tick typhus, Mediterranean spotted fever, scrub typhus, Q fever	*Rickettsia*: Flea-borne, louse-borne, and scrub typhus, Q fever, spotted fevers (rare)	*Rickettsia:* Q fever
Bacterial pneumonia including *Legionella*	Cytomegalovirus	Secondary syphilis
Relapsing fever	*Toxoplasma*	Epstein-Barr virus including mononucleosis
Amebic dysentery	Amebic dysentery	Amebic liver disease
Meningococcemia	Histoplasmosis	Leishmaniasis
Brucella (rarely)	*Brucella*	*Brucella*
Leptospirosis	Leptospirosis	Bartonellosis (chronic)
Fascioliasis	Babesiosis	Babesiosis
Rabies (rarely)	Rabies	Rabies
African trypanosomiasis (acute), East African (rarely)	East African trypanosomiasis (acute)	West African trypanosomiasis (chronic)
	Hepatitis A (rarely)	Cytomegalovirus
	Measles	

*Diseases that commonly have variable incubation periods are shown more than once. However, most diseases may rarely have an atypical incubation period, and this is not shown here.
HIV, Human immunodeficiency virus.
From Bennet et al: *Mandell, Douglas, and Bennett's principles and practice of infectious diseases*, ed 8, Philadelphia, 2015, Elsevier.

TABLE 2 Constellations of Exposures and Clinical Presentations Suggestive of Particular Diagnoses in Returned Travelers*

Exposure Scenario	Distinctive Findings	Diagnosis
Any exposure in any area with documented malaria transmission	Fever with or without any other finding	Malaria
Most tropical countries	Fever and altered mental status	Malaria, meningococcal meningitis, rabies, West Nile virus
Budget travel to India, Nepal, Pakistan, or Bangladesh	Insidious onset, high unremitting fever, toxic patient, paucity of physical findings	Enteric fever due to *Salmonella typhi* or *Salmonella paratyphi*
Freshwater recreational exposure in Africa	Fever, eosinophilia, hepatomegaly, negative malaria smear	Acute schistosomiasis (Katayama fever)
Bitten by *Aedes aegypti* in Central America, Southeast Asia, or the South Pacific	Fever, headache, myalgia, diffuse macular rash, mild to moderate thrombocytopenia	Dengue
Bitten by *A. aegypti* or *Aedes albopictus* in India, Malaysia, Singapore, the Caribbean, or an island in the Indian Ocean	Fever, headache, myalgia, diffuse macular rash, arthralgia, tenosynovitis often followed by chronic polyarthritis after the fever resolves	Chikungunya fever
Hunting or visiting game reserves in southern Africa	Fever, eschar, diffuse petechial rash	African tick typhus due to *Rickettsia africae*
Travel to Southeast Asia	Fever, eschar, diffuse petechial rash	Scrub typhus due to *Orientia tsutsugamushi*
Hiking, biking, swimming, rafting with exposure to fresh surface water	Fever, myalgia, conjunctival suffusion, mild to severe jaundice, variable rash	Leptospirosis
Cruise, elderly traveler	Influenza-like illness	Influenza A or B
Outdoor exposure anywhere in the Americas	Large, single furuncular lesion anywhere on body, with sense of movement inside	Myiasis due to *Dermatobia hominis* (botfly)
Clothing washed or dried out of doors in Africa	Multiple furuncular lesions around clothing contact points with skin	Myiasis due to *Cordylobia anthropophaga* (tumbu fly)
New sexual partner during travel	Fever, rash, mononucleosis-like illness	Acute human immunodeficiency virus infection
Travel to any developing country or to Western Europe	Coryza, conjunctivitis, Koplik spots, rash	Measles
Longer visit to humid areas of Africa, the Americas, or Southeast Asia	Asymptomatic eosinophilia or with periodic cough or wheezing	Strongyloidiasis
Sand fly bite in either New or Old World tropical area	Painless skin ulcer with clean, moist base in exposed area	Cutaneous leishmaniasis
Resort hotel in southern Europe, ± exposure to whirlpool spas	Pneumonia	Legionnaires' disease
Explored a cave in the Americas	Fever, cough, retrosternal chest pain, hilar adenopathy	Histoplasmosis
Ingestion of unpasteurized goat cheese	Chronic fever, fatigue	*Brucella melitensis*
Long trip to West/Central Africa	Afebrile, intensely pruritic, evanescent truncal maculopapular rash	Onchocerciasis
Long trip to West/Central Africa	Migratory localized angioedema or swellings over large joints, eosinophilia	Loiasis
Safari to game parks of East Africa	Fever, nongenital chancre, fine macular rash	East African trypanosomiasis
Travel to Australia	Fever, fatigue, polyarthritis	Ross River virus
Farming areas of India and Southeast Asia	Fever, altered mental status, paralysis	Japanese encephalitis
Forested areas of central and eastern Europe and across Russia	Fever, altered mental status, paralysis	Tick-borne encephalitis
Rodent exposure in West Africa	Fever, sore throat, jaundice, hemorrhagic manifestations	Lassa fever
Ingestion of sushi, ceviche, or raw freshwater fish	Migratory nodules in truncal areas with overlying erythema or mild hemorrhage	Gnathostomiasis
Returning Hajj pilgrim or family contact	Fever, meningitis	Meningococcal meningitis
Ingestion of snails, fish, or shellfish in Asia or Australia	Eosinophilic meningitis	Angiostrongyliasis, gnathostomiasis
Diabetic or compromised host with exposure to moist terrain in Asia or Australia	Fever, sepsis, pneumonia or multifocal abscesses	Melioidosis
Summertime exposure to rodent droppings in Scandinavia	Fever with decreased renal function	Puumala virus
Ingestion of undercooked meat of any animal in any country	Fever, facial edema, myositis, increased creatine phosphokinase, massive eosinophilia, normal erythrocyte sedimentation rate	Trichinosis
Unvaccinated, returning from sub-Saharan Africa or forested areas of Amazonia	Fever, jaundice, proteinuria, hemorrhage	Yellow fever
Exposure to farm animals	Pneumonia, mild hepatitis	Q fever
Possible tick exposure almost anywhere	Fever, headache, rash, conjunctival injection, hepatosplenomegaly	Tick-borne relapsing fever
Poor hygienic conditions with possible body louse exposure in Ethiopia or Sudan	Fever, headache, rash, conjunctival injection, hepatosplenomegaly	Louse-borne relapsing fever

*The table includes illnesses of travelers (listed first) as well as less common diseases with presentations that should suggest the possibility of the appropriate diagnosis. Many diseases have a spectrum of presentation, and the table describes the most common presentations of these diseases. Many diseases have a spectrum of geographic origins, and the table describes the most common exposures seen in daily practice.

From Bennet et al: *Mandell, Douglas, and Bennett's principles and practice of infectious diseases,* ed 8, Philadelphia, 2015, Elsevier.

LABORATORY TESTS

Consider:
- CBC
- Comprehensive metabolic panel
- Prothrombin time/international normalized ratio, partial thromboplastin time
- Urinalysis
- Blood, urine stool cultures
- Cerebrospinal fluid analysis, gram stain, culture
- Rapid HIV screen
- Serial blood smears q8-12h over 2 days
- Specific serology for suspected infections

IMAGING STUDIES

Not usually required, but consider as clinically indicated:
- Chest x-ray
- Upright abdominal x-ray
- CT: Head
- CT: Abdomen and pelvis

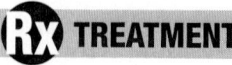

TREATMENT

Pretravel prevention should focus on proper vaccinations and prophylactic antimalarial antibiotics. Post-travel treatment depends on diagnosing or ruling out specific, known causes of fever in the returning traveler. Treatment ranges from supportive care to IV antibiotics, as with malaria and Dengue fever.
- Malaria:
  1. Uncomplicated *Plasmodium falciparum*: Treatment of choice is artemether-lumefantrine (CoArtem) 4 tab bid for 3 days with first 2 doses 8 hr apart
  2. Alternative: Malarone 4 tabs OD for 3 days
  3. Quinine sulfate 650 mg PO q8h for 3 to 7days plus doxycycline 100 mg PO q12h for 7 days
  4. Complicated/severe malaria to non-*P. falciparum* species: Artesunate (from CDC if quinidine fails)
  5. Quinidine gluconate 6.25 mg/kg IV load over 2 hr with 0.0125mg/kg/min continuous infusion PLUS doxycycline 2.2 mg/kg IV q12h for 7 days
- Dengue: Supportive care, pain control
  1. NSAIDs and aspirin contraindicated due to increased bleeding risk
- Typhoid fever: Fluoroquinolone (ciprofloxacin), cephalosporins (cefiximine or ceftraixone), azithromycin. Duration varies based on severity.
- Hemorrhagic viruses: Supportive care
- Meningococcus: Standard bacterial meningitis care

DISPOSITION

- Depending on the specific disease, severity of disease, and possibility of transmission.
- Patients may have outpatient or inpatient medical treatment.
- The most severe cases may need ICU and/or isolation.

REFERRAL

- Infectious disease consult
- Contact the CDC for recommendations pertaining to endemic diseases and treatment
- Some medical treatments and diagnostic testing must be sent from the CDC
- Mandatory reporting of some diseases to CDC

PEARLS & CONSIDERATIONS

COMMENTS

- The differential depends on the geography. Also consider travel to endemic areas, pretrip immunizations, comorbidities, non-travel-related diseases, sleeping arrangements, activities, and immunocompromised status.
- Until demonstrated otherwise, some travel medicine experts recommend assuming that all febrile travelers coming from malaria endemic regions have malaria.

PREVENTION

Check the CDC website and the Yellow Book for pretrip vaccinations.

PATIENT/FAMILY EDUCATION

Visit http://www.CDC.gov for further information.

SUGGESTED READINGS

Available at ExpertConsult.com

RELATED CONTENT

Brucellosis (Related Key Topic)
Dengue Fever (Related Key Topic)
Histoplasmosis (Related Key Topic)
Human Immunodeficiency Virus (Related Key Topic)
Leishmaniasis (Related Key Topic)
Malaria (Related Key Topic)
Measles (Rubeola) (Related Key Topic)
Q Fever (Related Key Topic)
Rabies (Related Key Topic)
Salmonellosis (Related Key Topic)
Trichinosis (Related Key Topic)
West Nile Virus Infection (Related Key Topic)
Yellow Fever (Related Key Topic)
Zika Virus (Related Key Topic)

AUTHORS: **DANNY H. VANVALKINBURGH, M.D.,** and **MARK F. BRADY, M.D., M.P.H., M.M.S.**

BASIC INFORMATION

DEFINITION

Fever of undetermined origin (FUO) was first defined by Petersdorf and Beeson in 1961 as an illness characterized by temperatures >38.3° C (101° F) on several occasions for >3 weeks with an uncertain diagnosis after 1 week of study in the hospital. With the increased availability of outpatient evaluation, the requirement of hospitalization for diagnosis was removed. As of 2017, the widely accepted definition of FUO is:

- Temperature ≥38.3° C (101° F) on at least two occasions
- Duration of illness ≥3 weeks or multiple febrile episodes in ≥3 weeks
- Not immunocompromised
  1. Neutropenic >1 week in last 3 months
  2. Known HIV
  3. Hypogammaglobulinemia
  4. 10 mg prednisone or equivalent for at least 2 weeks

FUO can be classified into classic, nosocomial (health care associated), neutropenic (immune deficient), and HIV-associated. Table 1 provides a summary of definitions and major features of subtypes of FUO.

SYNONYMS

Fever of unknown origin
Pyrexia of unknown origin

ICD-10CM CODE

R50.9 Fever, unspecified

EPIDEMIOLOGY & DEMOGRAPHICS

- Due to advances in medical knowledge and technology, the distribution of causes of FUO has changed.
- Improved imaging and culture techniques have led to decreased diagnosis secondary to malignancy or infection.
- In recent yrs, more FUOs have no identified cause and eluded diagnosis:
  1. In prospective study of 73 immunocompetent patients with FUO, 51% had no identified cause.

CLINICAL PRESENTATION

Significant fever (≥38.3° C [101° F]) that has persisted for longer than an acute self-limiting illness would be expected to and without identified etiology despite reasonable investigations in whatever setting is appropriate.

ETIOLOGY

FUO can be divided into four categories:

- Infectious (17% to 35%)
  1. Localized:
     a. Abscess (intraabdominal, pelvic, renal, dental, intracranial)
     b. Endocarditis (including subacute and culture negative)
     c. Infected peripheral vessels
     d. Osteomyelitis
     e. Urinary tract infection
     f. Sinusitis
     g. *Clostridium difficile* colitis
  1. Generalized:
     a. Bacterial: Typhoid fever, bartonellosis, brucellosis, Q fever
     b. Viral: HIV, CMV, EBV, multicentric Castleman disease
     c. Fungal: Histoplasmosis, blastomycosis, cryptococcosis, coccidioidomycosis
     d. Mycobacterial: Tuberculosis (extrapulmonary, military)
     f. Parasitic: Malaria, toxoplasmosis, visceral leishmaniosis, amoebic abscess
- Non-infectious inflammatory (24% to 36%)
  1. Adult Still disease
  2. Giant cell arteritis, temporal arteritis, polymyalgia rheumatics
  3. Other vasculitides: Polyarteritis nodosa, Takayasu arteritis, granulomatosis with polyangiitis, mixed cryoglobulinemia
  4. Other rheumatologic disorders: Systemic lupus erythematous, rheumatoid arthritis
- Malignancy (10% to 20%)
  1. Lymphoma
  2. Leukemia
  3. Myelodysplastic syndrome
  4. Solid tumors: Renal cell carcinoma, hepatocellular carcinoma, metastatic disease

TABLE 1 Summary of Definitions and Major Features of the Four Subtypes of Fever of Undetermined Origin

Feature	Classic FUO	Health Care–Associated FUO	Immune-Deficient FUO	HIV-Related FUO
Definition	>38.0° C, (100.4° F) >3 wk, >2 visits or 1 wk in hospital	≥38.0° C (100.4° F), >1 wk, not present or incubating on admission	≥38.0° C (100.4° F), >1 wk, negative cultures after 48 hr	≥38.0° C (100.4° F), >3 wk for outpatients, >1 wk for inpatients, HIV infection confirmed
Patient location	Community, clinic, or hospital	Acute care hospital	Hospital or clinic	Community, clinic, or hospital
Leading causes	Cancer, infections, inflammatory conditions, undiagnosed, habitual hyperthermia	Health care–associated infections, postoperative complications, drug fever	Majority due to infections, but cause documented in only 40%-60%	HIV (primary infection), typical and atypical mycobacteria, CMV, lymphomas, toxoplasmosis, cryptococcosis, immune reconstitution inflammatory syndrome (IRIS)
History emphasis	Travel, contacts, animal and insect exposure, medications, immunizations, family history, cardiac valve disorder	Operations and procedures, devices, anatomic considerations, drug treatment	Stage of chemotherapy, drugs administered, underlying immunosuppressive disorder	Drugs, exposures, risk factors, travel, contacts, stage of HIV infection
Examination emphasis	Fundi, oropharynx, temporal artery, abdomen, lymph nodes, spleen, joints, skin, nails, genitalia, rectum or prostate, lower limb deep veins	Wounds, drains, devices, sinuses, urine	Skinfolds, IV sites, lungs, perianal area	Mouth, sinuses, skin, lymph nodes, eyes, lungs, perianal area
Investigation emphasis	Imaging, biopsies, sedimentation rate, skin tests	Imaging, bacterial cultures	CXR, bacterial cultures	Blood and lymphocyte count; serologic tests; CXR; stool examination; biopsies of lung, bone marrow, and liver for cultures and cytologic tests; brain imaging
Management	Observation, outpatient temperature chart, investigations, avoidance of empirical drug treatments	Depends on situation	Antimicrobial treatment protocols	Antiviral and antimicrobial protocols, vaccines, revision of treatment regimens, good nutrition
Time course of disease	Months	Weeks	Days	Weeks to months
Tempo of investigation	Weeks	Days	Hours	Days to weeks

CMV, Cytomegalovirus; *CXR,* chest radiograph; *FUO,* fever of undetermined origin.
Adapted from Mandell GL, Bennett JE, Dolin R (eds): *Mandell, Douglas, and Bennett's principles and practice of infectious diseases,* ed 7, Philadelphia, 2010, Churchill Livingstone. Borrowed from Kliegman RM, et al.: *Nelson textbook of pediatrics,* ed 19, Philadelphia, 2011, Saunders.

- Miscellaneous (3% to 15%)
  1. Drug-induced fever
  2. Inflammatory bowel disease
  3. Sarcoidosis
  4. Pulmonary embolism/deep vein thrombosis
  5. Alcoholic hepatitis
  6. Familial Mediterranean fever
  7. Factitious fever
- No diagnosis in 16% to 39% of cases

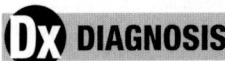

DIAGNOSIS

DIFFERENTIAL DIAGNOSIS

Over 200 possible diagnoses for FUO

WORKUP

- By definition, FUO is a diagnostic challenge. As the list of possible causes is extensive, there is no useful algorithmic approach.
- Accurate history and careful physical examination are essential. Fig. E1 describes an approach to the patient with FUO.
- Laboratory tests and imaging dependent on medical history clues and physical findings.
- When in doubt, perform another complete history and physical examination. Examples of subtle physical findings in patients with FUO are described in Table 2.

MEDICAL HISTORY CLUES

- Duration, accompanying symptoms (rigor, drenching sweats)
  1. Degree of fever, nature of fever curve, apparent toxicity, and response to antipyretic have not be found to be helpful.
- Unintentional weight loss
- Drenching night sweats
- Rash
- Myalgias
- Joint pain
- Unilateral retro-orbital headache or jaw claudication
- History of immunosuppression
- Thromboembolic risk factors (previous episodes, prolonged immobility, oral contraceptive pills recent surgeries)
- Medications
- Sick contacts
- Social history:
  1. Alcohol intake
  2. Occupational exposures
  3. Animal exposures
  4. Insect bites
  5. Sexual exposures
  6. Travel history
- Family history:
  1. Autoimmune disorders
  2. Malignancies
  3. Familial Mediterrenean fever

PHYSICAL FINDINGS

- HEENT (head, ears, eyes, nose, throat): Sinus tenderness, dental abscesses, funduscopic lesions
- Neck: Adenopathy, palpable thyroid
- Lungs: Auscultate for rales
- Heart: Murmur
- Abdomen: Organomegaly
- Rectal: Prostate tenderness
- Pelvic: Cervical motion tenderness, fundal or adnexal masses or pain, inguinal adenopathy
- Extremities: Clubbing, splinter hemorrhages, tenderness or fluctuance at IV access site
- Musculoskeletal: Joint effusions
- Skin: Rashes, wounds

LABORATORY TESTS

- Initial laboratory testing:
  1. Complete blood count with differential
  2. Comprehensive metabolic panel
  3. Inflammatory markers (erythrocyte sedimentation rate [ESR], C-reactive protein)
  4. Urinalysis
  5. Lactate dehydrogenase
  6. Blood cultures
  7. Thyroid-stimulating hormone
  8. HIV antibody testing
- Consider:
  1. HIV viral load
  2. Hepatitis serologies
  3. TB testing (purified protein derivative or interferon gamma release assay)
  4. Testing for endemic fungal infections (based on geographic location and exposure)
  5. Peripheral smear (thick and thin)
  6. Creatine kinase
  7. Ferritin
  8. Antinuclear antibody testing
  9. Rheumatoid factor
  10. Serum protein electrophoresis
  11. Lumbar puncture
  12. Biopsy (based on clinical and laboratory findings)
- May need to repeat tests at regular intervals until diagnosis is established.

IMAGING STUDIES

- Initial:
  1. CXR
  2. Abdominal imaging (CT or US)
- Consider:
  1. Venous duplex imaging
  2. Fluorodeoxyglucose (FDG)-PET
     a. Anatomic localization of focally increased FDG uptake
     b. Consider when initial workup negative and no clear diagnostic clues

Rx TREATMENT

- Therapy should be tailored once etiology of FUO has been established.
- When the cause of FUO remains unknown, empiric treatment with broad spectrum antibiotics should be reserved for patients who are severely ill.

DISPOSITION

- Prognosis is determined primarily by the underlying disease.
- FUO patients who remain undiagnosed after an extensive evaluation generally have a favorable outcome.

REFERRAL

To an infectious disease specialist, hematologist, or rheumatologist if no diagnosis after thoughtful workup.

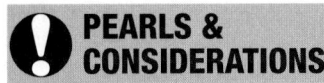

PEARLS & CONSIDERATIONS

COMMENTS

FUO is rarely due to an obscure disease but is more often an atypical presentation of a common illness.

SUGGESTED READINGS

Available at ExpertConsult.com

RELATED CONTENT

Fever of Unknown Origin (Patient Information)

AUTHORS: **ALEXANDRA ABRAMS-DOWNEY, M.D.,** and **ERNA MILUNKA KOJIC, M.D.**

TABLE 2 Examples of Subtle Physical Findings Having Special Significance in Patients with Fever of Undetermined Origin

Body Site	Physical Finding	Diagnosis
Head	Sinus tenderness	Sinusitis
Temporal artery	Nodules, reduced pulsations	Temporal arteritis
Oropharynx	Ulceration	Disseminated histoplasmosis
	Tender tooth	Periapical abscess
Fundi or conjunctivae	Choroid tubercle	Disseminated granulomatosis*
	Petechiae, Roth's spot	Endocarditis
Thyroid	Enlargement, tenderness	Thyroiditis
Heart	Murmur	Infective or marantic endocarditis
Abdomen	Enlarged iliac crest lymph nodes, splenomegaly	Lymphoma, endocarditis, disseminated granulomatosis*
Rectum	Perirectal fluctuance, tenderness	Abscess
	Prostatic tenderness, fluctuance	Abscess
Genitalia	Testicular nodule	Periarteritis nodosa
	Epididymal nodule	Disseminated granulomatosis
Lower extremities	Deep venous tenderness	Thrombosis or thrombophlebitis
Skin and nails	Petechiae, splinter hemorrhages, subcutaneous nodules, clubbing	Vasculitis, endocarditis

*Includes tuberculosis, histoplasmosis, coccidioidomycosis, sarcoidosis, and syphilis.
From Mandell GL et al (eds): *Mandell, Douglas, and Bennett's principles and practice of infectious diseases*, ed 7, Philadelphia, 2010, Churchill Livingstone.

BASIC INFORMATION

DEFINITION

Fibrocystic breast disease (FCD), now called "fibrocystic breast changes" (FBC), includes nonmalignant breast lesions including:

- Microcystic and macrocystic changes
- Fibrosis
- Mild and moderate hyperplasia
- Sclerosing adenosis
- Apocrine metaplasia
- Fibroadenoma
- Papilloma
- Papillomatosis
- Radial scar

SYNONYMS

Cystic changes
Chronic cystic mastitis
Fibrocystic breast changes
FBC
Mammary dysplasia
FCD
Fibrocystic mastopathy
Diffuse cystic mastopathy

Nonmalignant breast lesions can be divided into nonproliferative, proliferative without atypia, and atypical hyperplasia. Nonproliferative lesions such as breasts cysts are considered not to be at increased risk for breast cancer. Patients with proliferative lesions, including ductal hyperplasia, intraductal papillomas, sclerosing adenosis, radial scars, and fibroadenomas, have a small increased risk of progressing to breast cancer.

ICD-10CM CODES

N60.01	Solitary cyst of right breast
N60.02	Solitary cyst of left breast
N60.09	Solitary cyst of unspecified breast
N60.11	Diffuse cystic mastopathy of right breast
N60.12	Diffuse cystic mastopathy of left breast
N60.19	Diffuse cystic mastopathy of unspecified breast
N60.3	Fibrosclerosis

EPIDEMIOLOGY & DEMOGRAPHICS

- FBC affects 30% to 60% of reproductive-age women.
- Most commonly seen in women ages 30 to 50 yr.

PHYSICAL FINDINGS & CLINICAL PRESENTATION

- Lumpy or ropey breast texture
- Nodular areas
- Tenderness of breasts and/or nipples
- Dominant mass more often in the upper outer quadrants
- Symptoms tend to be affected with changes in the menstrual cycle
- Symptoms can be aggravated in postmenopausal women who initiate hormone therapy
- Nipple discharge

ETIOLOGY

- Because it is found in the majority of healthy breasts, it is regarded as a nonpathologic process.
- The relationship of FBC to the menstrual cycle suggests hormonal influence.

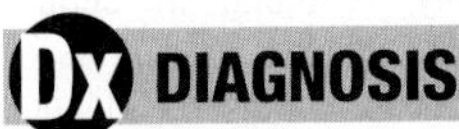

DIAGNOSIS

DIFFERENTIAL DIAGNOSIS

Table 1 differentiates breast masses. Characteristics of breast masses suspect for cancer (90% sensitivity, 40%–60% specificity) are:

- Fixed mass
- Poorly defined mass
- Hard (scirrhous) mass

WORKUP

- Rule out breast carcinoma if breast mass, thickening, discharge, and/or pain are present.
- Perform biopsy of suspected area for histologic confirmation.

IMAGING STUDIES

Mammography and ultrasound studies required:

- For mammographic changes (suspicious densities, microcalcifications, architectural distortion): Careful evaluation, including possibly biopsy to exclude breast cancer.
- Ultrasound study: To evaluate the presence of a solid vs. cystic mass.
- MRI is not recommended for routine evaluation of breast pain or fibrocystic changes.

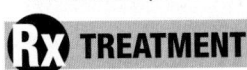

TREATMENT

NONPHARMACOLOGIC THERAPY

Treatment is symptomatic:

- Reassurance.
- Supportive bra.
- OTC pain medications including NSAIDs and Tylenol.
- Reduced intake of methylxanthines (coffee, chocolate), although this is not as effective as previously thought.
- Decreasing vitamin E or salt has not proved to be effective.
- Periodic physician examination to monitor patients with FCD who have pronounced nodular features.
- Aspiration for palpable or symptomatic cysts (NOTE: Cysts often recur; repeat aspiration is not always required unless pain is a problem).

PHARMACOLOGIC TREATMENT

For breast pain:

- Danocrine (Danazol): This is the only FDA-approved drug for breast pain. Moderate success has been reported, but the side effect profile is significant due to androgenic effects.
- Bromocriptine: The medication inhibits prolactin, and its effects are better than a placebo, but side effects such as lightheadedness and gastrointestinal symptoms limit its use.
- Tamoxifen: This has been found to reduce breast pain in 70% of affected women with cyclic breast pain, but the side effects of hot flashes and vaginal dryness interfere with compliance.
- Pharmacology therapy is usually tapered down after 3 to 6 months of treatment.

FOLLOW-UP

- Evaluate carefully to exclude breast cancer; then offer reassurance and periodic reevaluation as required.
- Regular self-examination, annual physician examination.

REFERRAL TO BREAST SURGEON

- For further evaluation and/or biopsy if suspicious changes are associated with FBC (including progression of dominant mass or thickening, persistent or spontaneous nipple discharge, or suspicious mammographic changes or lesions)
- To alleviate anxiety associated with breast symptoms or changes

RELATED CONTENT

Fibrocystic Breast Changes (Patient Information)
Breast Cancer (Related Key Topic)
Mastodynia (Related Key Topic)
Mastitis (Related Key Topic)

TABLE 1 Differentiation of Breast Masses

Characteristic	Cystic Disease	Benign Adenoma	Malignant Tumor
Patient age	25-60 yr	10-55 yr	25-85 yr
Number	One or more	One	One
Shape	Round	Round	Irregular
Consistency	Elastic, soft to hard	Firm	Stony hard
Delimitation	Well delimited	Well delimited	Poorly delimited
Mobility	Mobile	Mobile	Fixed
Tenderness	Present	Absent	Absent
Skin retraction	Absent	Absent	Present

From Swartz, MH: *Textbook of physical diagnosis*, ed 7, Philadelphia, 2014, Saunders.

SUGGESTED READINGS

Available at ExpertConsult.com

AUTHORS: **ESTELLE H. WHITNEY, M.D.,** and **ANTHONY SCISCIONE, D.O.**

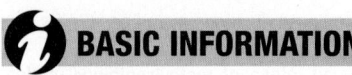

BASIC INFORMATION

DEFINITION

Fibromyalgia (FM) is a syndrome characterized by chronic, widespread musculoskeletal pain without evidence of soft tissue inflammation. Key features include fatigue, sleep disruption, cognitive disturbance, and psychiatric and somatic symptoms. Research suggests that FM is a disorder of pain regulation, which is often classified as a form of central sensitization.

SYNONYMS

"Fibrositis" is a term that is no longer used, because there is no evidence of connective tissue inflammation in FM.

ICD-10CM CODE

M79.7 Fibromyalgia

EPIDEMIOLOGY & DEMOGRAPHICS

Worldwide, the prevalence of FM is estimated to be between 2% and 8%, and it increases with age. In the United States, FM is the most common cause of musculoskeletal pain in women aged 20 to 55 yr. Using the 2010 American College of Rheumatology (ACR) diagnostic criteria for FM, the female:male ratio is approximately 2:1.

PHYSICAL FINDINGS & CLINICAL PRESENTATION

Patients with FM often report the following symptoms:

- Chronic (>3 months) widespread (affecting both sides of the body, above and below the waist, and involving the axial spine) musculoskeletal pain
- Cognitive disturbances
- Fatigue and sleep disturbances (e.g., unrefreshed sleep, easy fatigability)
- Psychiatric symptoms (e.g., anxiety, depression)
- Headache (present in more than half of patients with FM; this includes migraine and tension-type headaches)
- Paresthesias
- Associated disorders: Irritable bowel syndrome, interstitial cystitis/painful bladder syndrome

On physical examination, patients with FM may have tenderness in particular soft tissue locations called tender points (Fig. 1). Examination of tender points requires that the examiner be familiar with the areas to palpate and that they apply enough pressure (4 kg/cm^2 or enough pressure to whiten the nail bed of the fingertips of the examiner).

ETIOLOGY

Although the exact cause of FM is unknown, its etiology is thought to be multifactorial:

- Genetic and environmental factors may play a role. Evidence suggests that both the ascending and descending pain pathways operate abnormally, resulting in central amplification of pain signals. Familial associations of FM provide strongest evidence that reflect both these factors.
- In those predisposed, FM may be precipitated by stressful events such as abuse, injury from accidents, illnesses (including autoimmune disorders), infections, surgical procedures, and psychological stressors.
- Psychosocial, neuroendocrine, hormonal, and sociocultural factors also influence symptom expression.

PATHOGENESIS

Much remains to be discovered about the pathogenesis of FM, even though significant advances have been made in our understanding of this syndrome over the past few decades. Researchers have shown that biochemical, metabolic, and immunoregulatory abnormalities exist in patients with FM. Hence, this condition is now believed to be neurosensory in nature.

- Augmented pain and sensory processing is a hallmark, resulting in diffuse pain, allodynia (pain brought on by nonpainful stimuli), and hyperalgesia (more intense and prolonged pain perception).
- Afflicted persons show altered physiologic responses to painful stimulation at spinal and supraspinal levels.
- Brain neuroimaging studies found differences in brain structure, neurochemical concentrations, and functional brain networks in FM compared with control subjects. PET scans have revealed widespread activation of glial cells in the cortex, particularly in the frontal and parietal lobes.
- Pain augmentation may also result from a loss of tonic inhibition by descending inhibitory pathways from the brain to the spinal cord.

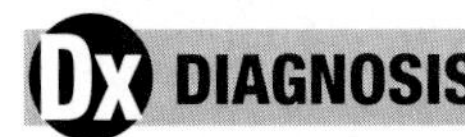

DIAGNOSIS

DIFFERENTIAL DIAGNOSIS

The presence of any of the disorders mentioned below does not necessarily exclude a diagnosis of FM because it may coexist with many conditions:

- Other functional somatic or "central sensitivity" syndromes: Myofascial pain, chronic fatigue syndrome, irritable bowel syndrome, headache/migraines, chronic pelvic and bladder pain disorders, and temporomandibular disorder
- Disorders that can mimic FM and must be ruled out include metabolic (e.g., hypothyroidism), infectious, and neurologic disorders. Arthritis and rheumatic diseases (e.g., rheumatoid arthritis, systemic lupus erythematosus, osteoarthritis, Sjögren syndrome)
- Myalgias and other muscle disease (e.g., inflammatory and metabolic myopathies)
- Mood and anxiety disorders
- Sleep disorders (e.g., sleep apnea, restless leg syndrome)
- Neurologic disorders
- Medications: Statin-induced muscle pain, opioid-induced hyperalgesia

WORK-UP

A thorough history, physical examination, and appropriately selected laboratory or imaging studies can usually differentiate FM from connective tissue or other systemic diseases.

- Chronic (>3 months) widespread pain is the hallmark symptom of FM, but fatigue, tenderness, depression/anxiety, nonrestorative sleep, cognitive difficulties (the so-called "fibrofog"), and functional impairment are other key symptoms.
- The 1990 American College of Rheumatology (ACR) FM Classification Criteria were used for clinical studies:
  1. Chronic, widespread pain in all four quadrants of the body and the axial skeleton.
  2. Pain on digital palpation of at least 11 of 18 tender points (see Fig. 1).
- The 2010 ACR diagnostic criteria for FM do not require a tender point examination; other disorders that would otherwise explain the musculoskeletal pain must be excluded (Table 1).
- A diagnostic screening tool (Fibromyalgia Diagnostic Screen) developed by Arnold and colleagues was found to accurately screen for FM. This tool includes a patient

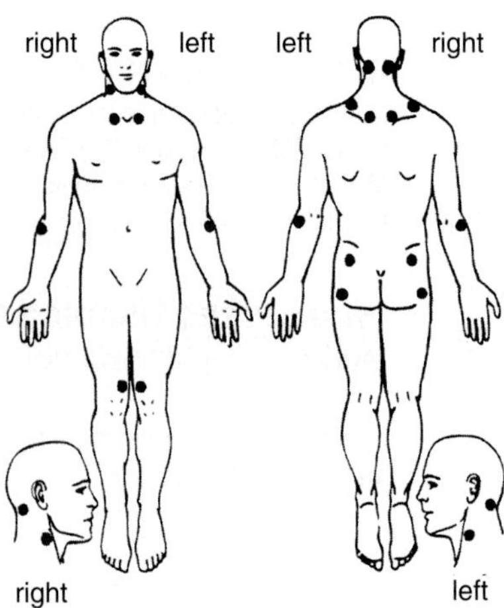

FIG. 1 The sites of the 18 tender points of the 1990 American College of Rheumatology criteria for the classification of fibromyalgia. (From Conn R: *Current diagnosis*, ed 9, Philadelphia, 1997, Saunders.)

TABLE 1 2010 Fibromyalgia Diagnostic Criteria

Criteria

A patient satisfies diagnostic criteria for fibromyalgia if the following three conditions are met:

1. Widespread pain index (WPI) 7 and symptom severity (SS) scale score of 5 or WPI 3–6 and SS scale score of 9.
2. Symptoms have been present at a similar level for at least 3 months.
3. The patient does not have a disorder that would otherwise explain the pain.

Ascertainment

1. WPI: Note the number of areas in which the patient has had pain over the past week. In how many areas has the patient had pain?

Score will be between 0 and 19.

Shoulder girdle, left	Hip (buttock, trochanter), left	Jaw, left	Upper back
Shoulder girdle, right	Hip (buttock, trochanter), right	Jaw, right	Lower back
Upper arm, left	Upper leg, left	Chest	Neck
Upper arm, right	Upper leg, right	Abdomen	
Lower arm, left	Lower leg, left		
Lower arm, right	Lower leg, right		

2. SS scale score:
   Fatigue
   Waking unrefreshed
   Cognitive symptoms

For the each of the three symptoms above, indicate the level of severity over the past week using the following scale:

0, No problem
1, Slight or mild problems, generally mild or intermittent
2, Moderate, considerable problems, often present at a moderate level
3, Severe: Pervasive, continuous, life-disturbing problems

Considering somatic symptoms in general, indicate whether the patient has:*

0, No symptoms
1, Few symptoms
2, A moderate number of symptoms
3, A great deal of symptoms

The SS scale score is the sum of the severity of the three symptoms (fatigue, waking unrefreshed, cognitive symptoms) plus the extent (severity) of somatic symptoms in general. The final score is between 0 and 12.

*Somatic symptoms that might be considered include muscle pain, irritable bowel syndrome, fatigue or tiredness, thinking or remembering problem, muscle weakness, headache, pain or cramps in the abdomen, numbness or tingling, dizziness, insomnia, depression, constipation, pain in the upper abdomen, nausea, nervousness, chest pain, blurred vision, fever, diarrhea, dry mouth, itching, wheezing, Raynaud's phenomenon, hives or welts, ringing in ears, vomiting, heartburn, oral ulcers, loss of or change in taste, seizures, dry eyes, shortness of breath, loss of appetite, rash, sun sensitivity, hearing difficulties, easy bruising, hair loss, frequent urination, painful urination, and bladder spasms.

Adapted from Wolfe F et al: The American College of Rheumatology preliminary diagnostic criteria for fibromyalgia and measurement of symptom severity, *Arthritis Care Res* 62:600–610, 2010.

self-reported questionnaire and an abbreviated physical examination with targeted lab tests.

LABORATORY TESTS

- Selective use of ancillary tests complements the history and physical examination in the diagnosis of FM. Testing should be highly focused on the exclusion of FM mimickers or suspected concurrent diseases.
- Complete blood cell count, routine chemistries, thyroid-stimulating hormone (TSH), 25-hydroxy vitamin D level (low levels can cause muscle pain), vitamin B12 level (low levels can cause fatigue and pain), iron studies (low levels can cause fatigue and depressive symptoms), and magnesium levels (low levels can cause muscle spasms).
- Erythrocyte sedimentation rate (ESR) and C-reactive protein (CRP) are generally normal in FM.
- Routine testing for antinuclear antibody (ANA) and/or rheumatoid factor should be avoided unless history and physical examination suggest an autoimmune disease.

Rx TREATMENT

GENERAL Rx (FIG. E2)

The goal in treating patients with fibromyalgia is to reduce the main symptoms of the syndrome (musculoskeletal pain, fatigue, depression, anxiety, poor sleep).

- Best approach may be combination of drug and nondrug therapies.
- FM can be due to abnormalities in many different neurotransmitter systems; thus, approaches and treatment responses may vary.
- Best evidence for tricyclics (low-dose amitriptyline and cyclobenzaprine), serotonin-norepinephrine reuptake inhibitors (milnacipran and duloxetine), and gabapentinoids (gabapentin and pregabalin).
- Second-tier drug classes include SSRIs.
- "Start low, go slow" approach is best to avoid side effects from medications.
- The only analgesic that has demonstrated efficacy in FM has been tramadol, either alone or in combination with acetaminophen.
- There is no evidence that NSAIDs or corticosteroids are effective in FM.
- Avoid narcotic use. There is concern that opioid use and abuse may aggravate chronic widespread pain.
- Nonpharmacologic: Strong evidence to support exercise (aerobic, strengthening, and stretching exercises, tai-chi, yoga), cognitive behavioral therapy, physical therapy, and patient education (e.g., regarding the disease, importance of good sleep hygiene).

DISPOSITION

- The pain and symptoms of FM can wax and wane, vary in physical location and in intensity day-to-day; many patients continue to have chronic pain and fatigue regardless of therapy.
- Disability rates vary from 10% to 30%.

REFERRAL

Referral to rheumatology, neurology, mental health professionals, physical medicine, and rehabilitation, including physical therapy, may be helpful for a multidisciplinary team approach.

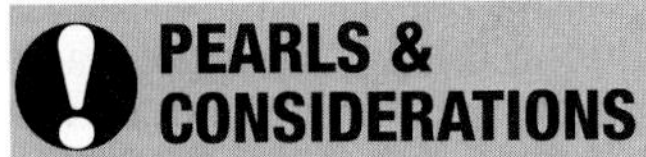

- Fibromyalgia is a neurosensory disorder whereby affected individuals have abnormal central nociceptive processing.
- Diagnosis is based on the presence of chronic musculoskeletal pain in the absence of physical or laboratory evidence of inflammation and in the absence of any other condition that would explain the symptoms.
- Treatment options are varied, but a combination of drug and nondrug options is likely to provide optimal results.
- Myofascial pain syndrome may represent a localized form of FM. It is associated with trigger points (rather than tender points as seen in FM). Some patients with myofascial pain syndrome may progress to FM.

COMMENTS

FM occurs frequently in patients with some rheumatic diseases, such as rheumatoid arthritis, ankylosing spondylitis, and systemic lupus erythematosus, in which prevalence of FM may reach 20%.

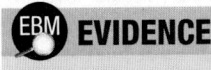

Available at ExpertConsult.com

SUGGESTED READINGS

Available at ExpertConsult.com

RELATED CONTENT

Fibromyalgia (Patient Information)

AUTHOR: **NADINE MBUYI, M.D.**

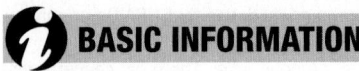

BASIC INFORMATION

DEFINITION

Folliculitis is inflammation of the hair follicle as a result of infection, physical injury, or chemical irritation.

SYNONYM

Sycosis barbae

ICD-10CM CODES

L72.9	Follicular cyst of skin and subcutaneous tissue, unspecified
L73.1	Pseudofolliculitis barbae
L73.8	Other specified follicular disorders
L66.2	Folliculitis decalvans
L66.4	Folliculitis ulerythematosa reticulata
L66.3	Perifolliculitis capitis abscedens

EPIDEMIOLOGY & DEMOGRAPHICS

PREVALENCE: Staphylococcal folliculitis is the most common form of infectious folliculitis; it occurs most commonly in persons with diabetes. Gram-negative folliculitis occurs in patients who have had moderately inflammatory acne for long periods and have been treated with long-term antibiotics such as tetracycline.

PREDOMINANT SEX: Sycosis barbae occurs most frequently in men who have commenced shaving.

PHYSICAL FINDINGS & CLINICAL PRESENTATION

- The lesions generally consist of painful yellow pustules surrounded by erythema; a central hair is present in the pustules. Furuncles with pus may be present.
- Patients with sycosis barbae may initially present with small follicular papules or pustules that increase in size with continued shaving; deep follicular pustules may occur surrounded by erythema and swelling; the upper lip is frequently involved.
- "Hot tub" folliculitis occurs within 1 to 4 days after the use of a hot tub with poor chlorination. It is characterized by papules and pustules (Fig. 1) with surrounding erythema generally affecting the torso, buttocks, and limbs (Fig. 2).

ETIOLOGY

- Staphylococcus infection (e.g., sycosis barbae), *Pseudomonas aeruginosa* ("hot tub" folliculitis)
- Gram-negative folliculitis (*Klebsiella, Enterobacter, Proteus*) associated with antibiotic treatment of acne
- Chronic irritation of the hair follicle (use of cocoa butter or coconut oil, chronic irritation from workplace)
- Initial use of systemic corticosteroid therapy (steroid acne), eosinophilic folliculitis (AIDS patients), *Candida albicans* (immunocompromised patients)
- *Pityrosporum orbiculare*

DIAGNOSIS

DIFFERENTIAL DIAGNOSIS

- Pseudofolliculitis barbae (ingrown hairs)
- Acne vulgaris
- Dermatophyte fungal infections
- Keratosis pilaris
- Cutaneous candidiasis
- Superficial fungal infections
- Miliaris

WORKUP

- Physical examination and medical history (e.g., use of hot tub: "hot tub" folliculitis; adolescent patients who have started shaving: sycosis barbae; use of occlusive topical steroid therapy: *Staphylococcus* folliculitis).
- Gram-negative folliculitis in acne patients on prolonged antibiotic treatment manifests with superficial pustules 3 to 6 mm in diameter flaring out from anterior nares or fluctuant, deep-seated nodules.

LABORATORY TESTS

- Generally not necessary.
- Gram stain is useful to identify the infective organisms in infectious folliculitis and to differentiate infectious folliculitis from noninfectious.

TREATMENT

NONPHARMACOLOGIC THERAPY

- Prevention of chemical or mechanical skin irritation
- Glycemic control in diabetics
- Proper chlorination of hot tubs and spas
- Shaving with a clean razor

ACUTE GENERAL

- Cleansing of the area with chlorhexidine and application of saline compresses to involved area.
- Application of 2% mupirocin ointment or 1% retapamulin ointment for bacterial folliculitis affecting a limited area (e.g., sycosis barbae).
- Treatment of severe cases of *Pseudomonas* folliculitis with ciprofloxacin.
- Treatment of *S. aureus* folliculitis with dicloxacillin 250 mg qd for 10 days.
- Isotretinoin is the treatment of choice in gram-negative folliculitis. Amoxicillin or TMS-SMX can be used when isotretinoin is contraindicated or cannot be tolerated.

CHRONIC Rx

- Chronic nasal or perineal *S. aureus* carriers with frequent folliculitis can be treated with rifampin 300 mg bid for 5 days.
- Mupirocin or retapamulin ointment applied to nares bid is also effective for nasal carriers.

DISPOSITION:

- Most cases of bacterial folliculitis resolve completely with proper treatment.
- Steroid folliculitis responds to discontinuation of steroids.

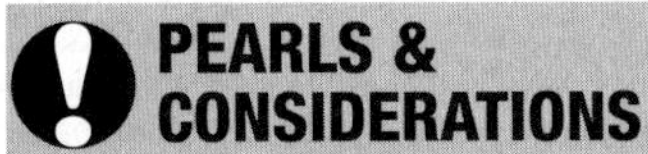

PEARLS & CONSIDERATIONS

COMMENTS

Patients should be instructed in good personal hygiene and avoidance of sharing razors, towels, and washcloths.

RELATED CONTENT

Folliculitis (Patient Information)

AUTHOR: **FRED F. FERRI, M.D.**

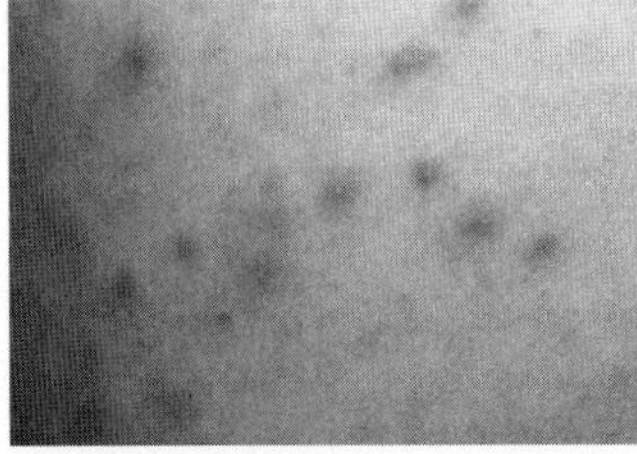

FIG. 1 Papules and pustules in hot tub folliculitis. (From Kliegman RM et al: *Nelson textbook of pediatrics,* ed 19, Philadelphia, 2011, Saunders.)

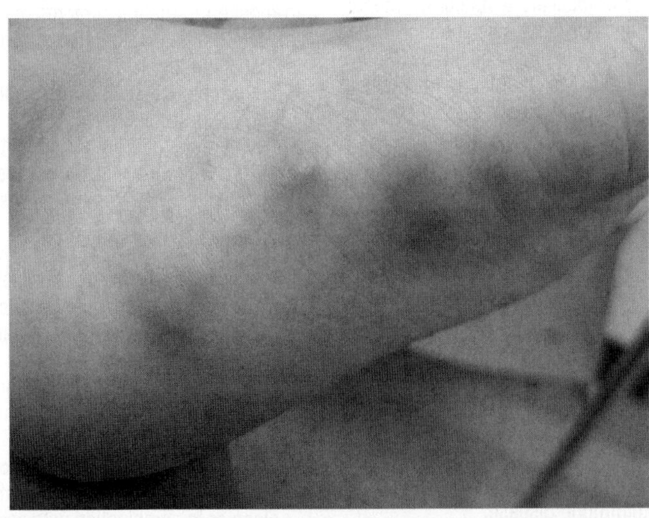

FIG. 2 *Pseudomonas* hot foot syndrome. Tender papules and papulopustules on the plantar aspect of the foot. Culture of a swab from one of the pustules grew *P. aeruginosa*. (Courtesy John J. Van Aalst, M.D. From Paller AS, Mancini AJ: *Hurwitz clinical pediatric dermatology: a textbook of skin disorders of childhood and adolescence,* ed 5, Philadelphia, 2016, Elsevier.)

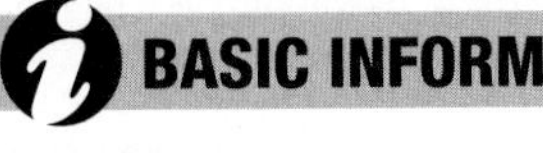

BASIC INFORMATION

DEFINITION

Food allergies are divided into IgE-mediated and immunologically mediated non-IgE reactions. They include a spectrum of disorders that involve adverse immunologic responses to dietary antigens.

ICD-10CM CODES

T78.0	Adverse food reaction (including anaphylactic shock)
T78.1	Other adverse food reactions, not elsewhere classified
L27.2	Dermatitis due to ingested food
Z91.010	Allergy to peanuts
Z91.011	Allergy to milk products
Z91.012	Allergy to eggs
Z91.013	Allergy to seafood
Z91.018	Allergy to other foods
Z91.02	Food additives allergy status

EPIDEMIOLOGY & DEMOGRAPHICS

INCIDENCE: Food allergies have a cumulative incidence of 6% to 8% for the first 3 yr of life.

PREVALENCE:

- Overall prevalence is 1% to 2% in general population, ~3.9% to 8% in children.
- Patient self-reported food allergies have a prevalence of 12% to 13%, demonstrating the importance of objective measures in assessing food allergies.
- Nearly 40% of children with food allergy have a history of severe reactions that, if not treated immediately with proper medication, can lead to hospitalization or even death.[1]
- There is insufficient evidence to conclude a racial predilection (Greenhawt, 2013).

GENETICS: Children with parents or close relatives with allergies may have a tendency to become allergic to foods.

PHYSICAL FINDINGS & CLINICAL PRESENTATION

- IgE-mediated reactions: (within minutes to a few hours): Pruritus, urticaria or angioedema, atopic dermatitis, GI symptoms, conjunctival injection, sneezing, nasal congestion, rhinorrhea, bronchospasm, and anaphylaxis
- Non–IgE-mediated reactions: Food-induced enterocolitis, celiac disease, Crohn disease, dermatitis herpetiformis, and pulmonary reactions such as Heiner syndrome. These illnesses are discussed separately.
- Signs, symptoms, and presentation reflect specific allergic manifestation, but in food allergies there is a reproducible temporal relationship to ingested food allergens.

ETIOLOGY

Failure to establish tolerance to food antigens. IL-33 mediated epithelial permeability and Th2 skewing result in sensitization to food proteins which are presented to primed T cells. Food processing conditions that may affect allergenic activity are described in Table 1.

DIAGNOSIS

- Thorough history (to identify specific food[s], quantity consumed, timing, and nature of reaction) and physical exam should be performed.
- The temporal relationship and reproducibility of the symptoms are most important to establishing the diagnosis.
- A review of ingredient labels may be helpful.
- Confirmatory testing can include skin testing or in vitro testing.
- Skin prick testing (SPT): Positive predictive value <50%, but negative predictive value >95%. Thus a negative skin test effectively rules out an IgE-mediated process.
- In vitro testing: RAST testing: Historically it is less sensitive than skin testing, but sensitivity has improved with cut off points indicating a positive predictive value of 95% for allergies to eggs, milk, peanuts, wheat, and fish.
- Atopy patch test: Used in conjunction with RAST and skin testing in multiallergic children to plan widening the elimination diet. However, it is not recommended in the routine evaluation of food allergies.
- Double-blind, placebo-controlled food challenges are the gold standard test for determining food allergies. These need to be done in a supervised and controlled setting.
- In summary, if the history and lab tests are suggestive of a specific food allergy, that food should be confirmed by SPT, RAST, or food challenge and, once confirmed, eliminated from the diet.

DIFFERENTIAL DIAGNOSIS

- Gastrointestinal disorders
- Irritable bowel syndrome
- Carcinoid syndrome
- Giardiasis
- Structural abnormalities like hiatal hernia, pyloric stenosis, Hirschsprung disease, tracheoesophageal fistula
- Disaccharidase deficiencies: Lactase, sucrase-isomaltase complex, glucose-galactose complex
- Pancreatic insufficiency: Cystic fibrosis
- Gallbladder disease
- Peptic ulcer disease
- Malignancy
- Metabolic disorders
- Galactosemia
- Phenylketonuria
- Pharmacologic-related conditions
- Gustatory rhinitis
- Auriculotemporal syndrome (facial flush from tart food)

TREATMENT

NONPHARMACOLOGIC THERAPY

- Elimination diet should be used in conjunction with nutritional counseling. Fig. 1 illustrates an algorithm for the management of food allergy
- Formula-fed infants: Brief trial of hydrolyzed milk formula as most children with milk allergy–induced skin symptoms will respond to the change of formula. Nonresponders may require amino acid–based formula.
- In older children: Elimination of one to two suspected foods is appropriate for 2 wk or longer and then reintroducing the foods to determine if symptoms recur.

ACUTE GENERAL Rx

- Antihistamines (both H1 and H2 antihistamines), albuterol if wheezing, epinephrine and glucocorticoids in patients with anaphylaxis.
- Patients with documented IgE-mediated reactions should receive and be counseled on the use of epinephrine autoinjector.

NEW TREATMENTS FOR FOOD ALLERGIES

- Oral and sublingual immunotherapy may play a role in management of food allergies, but this is currently under investigation.
- Recombinant vaccines and other immunomodulatory strategies are under development, although monoclonal anti-IgE antibody has shown benefit in adults with peanut allergy.

PEARLS & CONSIDERATIONS

- Eczema that develops in first 6 to 12 mo of life is usually the first manifestation of atopy.
- Egg allergy or sensitization is the strongest recognized predictor of respiratory allergies in children and asthma in adults.
- Consultation with trained dietitian is critical to avoid potentially adverse nutritional consequences in children with multiple food allergies.
- Skin testing is the preferred method for identifying food-specific IgE. RAST is useful if there is chance of severe food reaction causing risk to the patient.
- American Academy of Pediatrics no longer recommends avoiding the influenza and MMR vaccines in patients with severe systemic allergic reactions to egg.

COMMENTS

- Milk allergy usually resolves by age 5. Risk factors for persistence are early cutaneous manifestations following milk ingestion, development of other atopic conditions, and persistence of milk-specific high IgE titers. Soy milk is recommended for these children, keeping in mind that about 15% of these children can develop soy allergy.
- Egg allergy has been thought to resolve in 66% of children by 5 yr of age and in 75% of children by 7 yr of age. Trials have shown that oral immunotherapy can desensitize a high proportion of children with egg allergy and induce sustained unresponsiveness in a clinically significant subset.

[1] Gupta RS et al: The prevalence, severity, and distribution of childhood food allergy in the United States, *Pediatrics* 128(l):e9-e17, 2011.

TABLE 1 Food Processing Conditions That May Affect Allergenic Activity

Processing Stage	Nature of Processing	Impact of Processing on Allergens	Food-Level Evidence	Clinical Implications
Post-harvest treatments	Modified atmosphere for storage of fruit and vegetables	Expression of Bet v 1 homologs is upregulated during storage; levels are higher in fruit stored for 4-5 mo compared with fresh fruit. Expression of LTP allergens is downregulated during storage; levels are higher in fresh fruit and decrease during storage.	Apple	Individuals with birch pollen–related fruit allergies may tolerate freshly picked but not stored fruit. LTP-allergic individuals may experience reverse symptoms, although severity of LTP allergies may completely preclude consumption of problem fruit.
Primary processing	Removal of outer layers by physical or chemical peeling	Loss of allergens such as LTPs located in the outer layers	Peach	Peeling fruits can make them safe for consumption by certain individuals with LTP allergies.
Secondary processing	Fruit purees and fresh juices	Labile Bet v 1 homologs are modified. Prolamin superfamily fruit LTPs retain a native-like structure.	Peach, apple	Individuals with Bet v 1–related fruit allergies usually can consume pureed fruit products. These foods can still trigger reactions in individuals with LTP fruit allergies.
	Preparation of pasteurized, UHT fruit juices and milk	Labile Bet v 1 homologs are modified. Prolamin superfamily fruit LTPs retain a native-like structure. Milk allergens retain much of their native structure.	Peach, apple, milk	Individuals with Bet v 1–related fruit allergies usually can consume UHT-processed fruit products. Processing is insufficient to make UHT juices safe for individuals with LTP fruit allergies. The allergenic potential of UHT milk resembles that of pasteurized and raw milk.
	Boiling	The prolamin superfamily LTPs and 2S albumin retain a native-like structure after boiling, although when seeds are boiled, much of the protein is lost into cooking water. Boiling alters the structure of milk, egg, and fish allergens. Boiling alters the structure of cupin allergens (7S and 11S seed storage proteins) and can render them insoluble.	Maize, wheat, peanut, lentil, fish, milk, egg	Boiling seeds (e.g., peanuts) and milk reduces their allergenicity but does not abolish it. For some foods (e.g., polenta), the extent of cooking affects the residual level of allergenic activity.
	Roasting and frying	Thermostable allergens, notably the prolamin superfamily 2S albumin allergens, retain their native structure and solubility after roasting and frying. Some cupin allergens (7S and 11S seed storage proteins) are altered by roasting and become insoluble. Maillard modification of allergens may take place under these processing conditions	Peanut	The major peanut 2S albumin allergens retain their allergenic activity, explaining why roasted peanuts possess significant allergenic activity. Allergenic activity of the 7S and 11S globulins is retained to some extent after roasting. Maillard modifications may further contribute to the allergenic activity of roasted peanuts.
	Preparation of powdered ingredients, such as celery spice, skimmed milk, and pasteurized egg white powder	Major allergens retain their three-dimensional structure and activity in dry-processed goods. Maillard modifications take place under these processing conditions when residual sugars are present (e.g., lactose in skimmed milk powder).	Celery spice, milk	Powdered food ingredients have allergenic activity similar to unprocessed foods and can promote trigger reactions when included in recipes or through cross-contact in other foods (e.g., residual milk powder in foods otherwise free from milk).
	Deamidation	Acidic conditions are used to treat food ingredients (notably gluten) to improve their food functional properties through deamidation.	Gluten	Induces formation of novel IgE epitopes through glutamine deamidation, which results in individuals reacting to foods prepared with deamidated gluten ingredients who can otherwise safely consume wheat flour–containing foods.

TABLE 1 Food Processing Conditions That May Affect Allergenic Activity—cont'd

Processing Stage	Nature of Processing	Impact of Processing on Allergens	Food-Level Evidence	Clinical Implications
	Hydrolyzed food ingredients	Enzymatic (usually microbial proteases) and chemical treatments are used to hydrolyze protein ingredients to change their functional properties. Ingredients may originate from soy, milk (e.g., caseinates, whey protein), gluten, and other sources.	Milk, egg, gluten	Hydrolysis reduces IgE reactivity but does not abolish it completely, which may in part result from the presence of residual intact protein. Evidence is largely limited to in vitro IgE binding studies and animal models with little direct, in vivo evidence for allergic humans.
	Oil refining	Proteins are removed during the refining process, and residual protein levels in highly refined oils are very low.	Soybean, peanut	In the EU, highly refined soybean oils are considered safe for consumption by individuals with soy allergies. Highly refined peanut oils do not appear to cause adverse reactions in peanut-allergic individuals, but these oils do not have an EU labeling derogation.
Complex foods	Fining agents added to alcoholic beverages	Certain beverages contain residual levels of fining agents based on isinglass, fish gelatin, milk casein, egg albumin, or lysozyme. Fining agents and their residues in beverages usually are highly modified compared with the raw, unprocessed foods.	Beer, wine, and spirits	Individuals with allergies to fish triggered by collagen or egg can react to alcoholic beverages when they are used as fining agents, although this depends on the nature of the individual's allergy and whether fining agents are used in conjunction with other agents, such as bentonite. Reactions to fining agents are rare, and many individuals with egg, milk, or fish allergy can safely consume these beverages.
	Fermented foods	Lactic acid fermentations can cause proteins to unfold and precipitate or form gelled networks due to the reduced pH. Fermentative organisms secrete proteases that can hydrolyze proteins.	Milk, soybean	Although fermented milk and yogurt may retain some allergenic activity, other highly modified foods, such as soy sauce, may have substantially reduced allergenic activity and may not present a hazard to certain allergic patients.
	Baked foods	Food ingredients may be included that are raw or have already been processed (e.g., skimmed milk powder, pasteurized egg white). Complex interactions between different food ingredients coupled with further cooking modify allergens and result in their becoming part of the insoluble food matrix, but data are limited because of the poor solubility of allergens in physiologic buffers.	Milk	Evidence from oral food challenge studies indicates that baking reduces the allergenic activity of milk, and foods with baked milk may be given to children whose infantile cow's milk allergy is beginning to resolve.

EU, European Union; *LTP*, lipid transfer protein; *UHT*, ultrahigh temperature.
From Adkinson NF et al: *Middleton's allergy principles and practice*, ed 8, Philadelphia, 2014, Saunders.

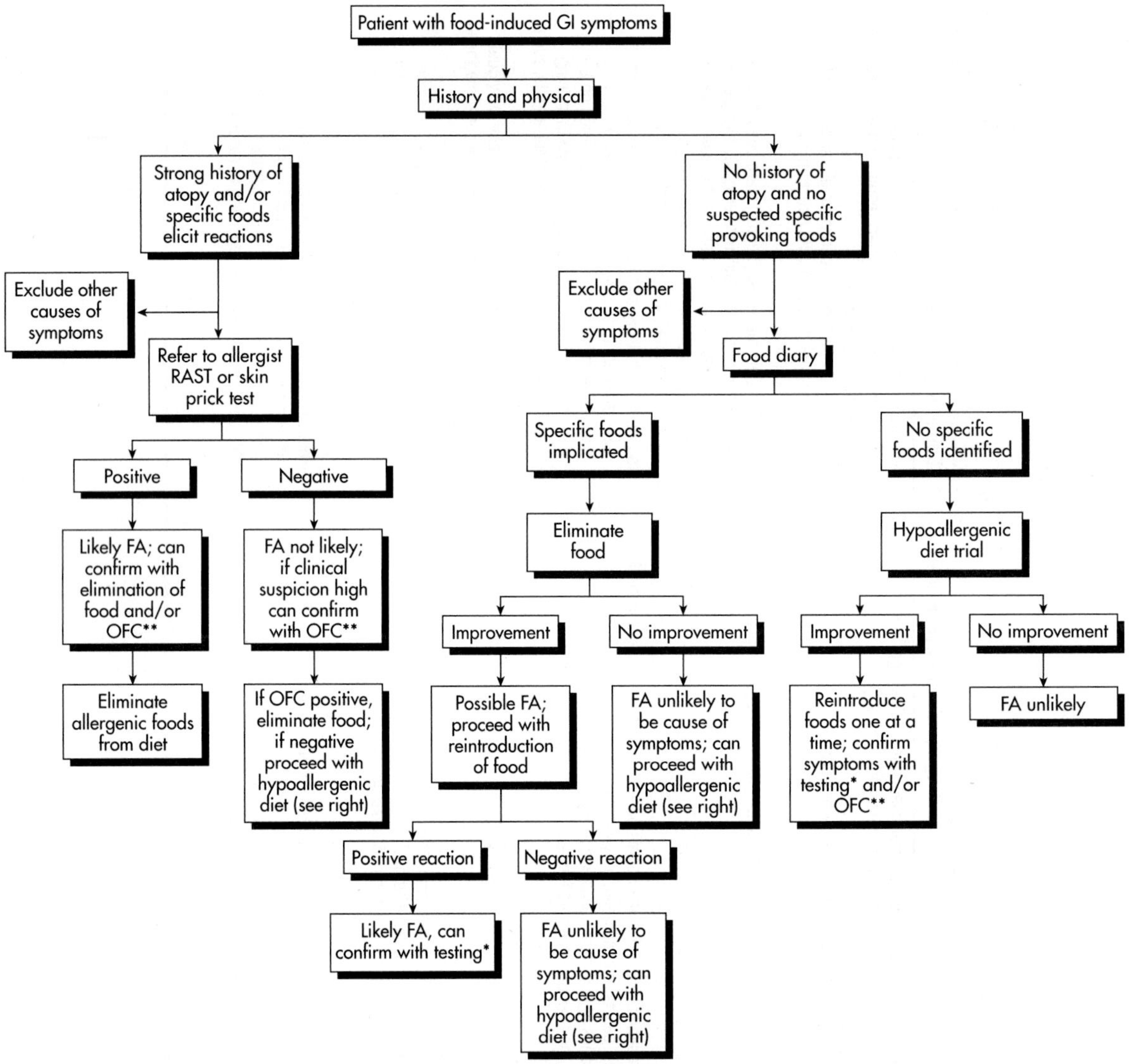

Patient with food-induced GI symptoms

History and physical

- Strong history of atopy and/or specific foods elicit reactions
  - Exclude other causes of symptoms
  - Refer to allergist RAST or skin prick test
    - Positive
      - Likely FA; can confirm with elimination of food and/or OFC**
        - Eliminate allergenic foods from diet
    - Negative
      - FA not likely; if clinical suspicion high can confirm with OFC**
        - If OFC positive, eliminate food; if negative proceed with hypoallergenic diet (see right)
- No history of atopy and no suspected specific provoking foods
  - Exclude other causes of symptoms
  - Food diary
    - Specific foods implicated
      - Eliminate food
        - Improvement
          - Possible FA; proceed with reintroduction of food
            - Positive reaction
              - Likely FA, can confirm with testing*
            - Negative reaction
              - FA unlikely to be cause of symptoms; can proceed with hypoallergenic diet (see right)
        - No improvement
          - FA unlikely to be cause of symptoms; can proceed with hypoallergenic diet (see right)
    - No specific foods identified
      - Hypoallergenic diet trial
        - Improvement
          - Reintroduce foods one at a time; confirm symptoms with testing* and/or OFC**
        - No improvement
          - FA unlikely

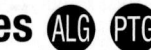

FIG. 1 Algorithm for the management of food allergy *Testing indicates skin-prick testing, radioallergosorbent tests *(RAST)*, IgG_4 assay, and/or patch testing. Note that clinical symptoms must be associated with the food(s) that test positive before the food(s) should be eliminated from the diet. **Oral food challenge *(OFC)* involves reintroducing the food and observing for signs/symptoms of food allergy *(FA)*. Treatment of food allergy involves elimination of the causative food(s) from the diet.

- Wheat allergy found to resolve by 5 yr of age and soybean allergy by 2 yr of age.

PREVENTION

- There is conflicting evidence regarding the protective effect of breastfeeding on food allergies.
- There is no evidence to suggest that exclusive breastfeeding for 6 mo or more is superior to exclusive breastfeeding for 4 to 6 mo in terms of developing food allergies.
- In high-risk infants who are not exclusively breastfed, there is limited evidence to suggest that feeding with hydrolyzed formula compared to cow's milk formula reduces allergies.
- Currently, there is no evidence to support the use of prebiotics and/or probiotics for the prevention of allergic diseases.
- No current evidence exists to support delaying the introduction of solid foods beyond 4 to 6 mo.
- The early introduction of peanuts significantly decreases the frequency of the development of peanut allergy among children at high risk for this allergy and modulated immune responses to peanuts.[2] Early peanut introduction (ages 4-11 months) lowers the risk of developing peanut allergy by 80% compared with peanut introduction after age 5 yr.
- In recent phase 3 trials of oral immunotherapy in children and adolescents who were highly allergic to peanut, treatment with AR101 resulted in higher doses of peanut protein that could be ingested without dose-limiting symptoms.

PATIENT/FAMILY EDUCATION

Information can be found on American Academy of Allergy, Asthma and Immunology (www.aaaai.org), the Food Allergy and Anaphylaxis Network (www.foodallergy.org), and the Anaphylaxis Campaign (www.anaphylaxis.org.uk).

REFERRAL

Patients may be referred to an allergy/immunology specialist when the diagnosis is uncertain or if avoidance measures are not successful.

SUGGESTED READINGS

Available at ExpertConsult.com

RELATED CONTENT

Food Allergies (Patient Information)

AUTHOR: **FRED F. FERRI, M.D.**

[2] Gupta RS et al: The prevalence, severity, and distribution of childhood food allergy in the United States, *Pediatrics* 128(l):e9-e17, 2011.

BASIC INFORMATION

DEFINITION

Food poisoning is an illness caused by ingestion of food contaminated by bacteria and/or bacterial toxins. A foodborne disease outbreak is defined as two or more cases of a similar illness resulting from ingestion of a common food. Table 1 describes pathogenic mechanisms in bacterial foodborne disease.

SYNONYMS

Enterotoxin-poisoning
Epidemic vomiting disease

ICD-10CM CODE

A05.9 Bacterial foodborne intoxication, unspecified

EPIDEMIOLOGY & DEMOGRAPHICS

INCIDENCE (IN U.S.):

- CDC estimates that each yr one in six Americans will experience a foodborne illness.
- Approximately 800 foodborne disease outbreaks are reported in the United States each year, accounting for approximately 15,000 illnesses, 800 hospitalizations, and 20 deaths. Outbreak-associated foodborne illnesses are only a small subset of the estimated 9.4 million foodborne illnesses that occur annually in the U.S.[1]
- Majority of identifiable causes are bacterial, although more than 250 known diseases can be transmitted through food.

PEAK INCIDENCE: Varies with specific organism

- Summer: *Staphylococcus aureus, Salmonella, Shigella* spp.
- Summer and fall: *Clostridium botulinum, Vibrio parahaemolyticus*
- Spring and fall: *Campylobacter jejuni*
- Winter: *Clostridium perfringens, Yersinia enterocolitica*

PREDOMINANT AGE: Varies with specific agent

NEONATAL INFECTION: Rare but severe with *Shigella* and *Salmonella* spp.

PHYSICAL FINDINGS & CLINICAL PRESENTATION

- Any combination of GI symptoms and fever. Orthostatic pulse and blood pressure changes should be noted.
- Specific organisms suspected on the basis of the incubation period and predominant symptoms (Table 2), although a great deal of overlap exists.
  1. Short incubation period (1 to 6 hr): Involve the ingestion of preformed toxin; noninvasive.
     a. *S. aureus:* Nausea, profuse vomiting, and abdominal cramps common; diarrhea possible, but fever uncommon; usually resolves within 24 hr; foods implicated in outbreaks include meats, mayonnaise, and cream pastries.
     b. *B. cereus:* Two forms, a short incubation (emetic) form (characterized by vomiting and abdominal cramps in virtually all patients, diarrhea in one third of patients, fever uncommon) and a long incubation (diarrheal) form; illness usually mild, resolves within 12 hr; unrefrigerated rice most often implicated as vehicle. Other sources include gravy, meats, stews, vanilla, and sauces.
  2. Moderate incubation period (8 to 16 hr): Involves the in vivo production of toxin; noninvasive.
     a. *C. perfringens:* Severe crampy abdominal pain and watery diarrhea common; fever and vomiting unlikely; symptoms usually resolving within 24 hr; outbreaks invariably related to cooked meat or poultry that is allowed to cool without refrigeration; most cases in the fall and winter months. *C. perfringens* is the third most common cause of foodborne illness in the United States.
     b. *B. cereus:* Diarrheal (or long incubation) form most commonly beginning with diarrhea, abdominal cramps, and occasionally vomiting; fever uncommon; usually resolves within 24 hr; the responsible food is usually fried rice.
  3. Long incubation period (>16 hr): Some toxin-mediated, some invasive.
- Toxin-producing organisms include:
  1. *C. botulinum:* Should be considered when a diarrheal illness coincides with or precedes paralysis; severity of illness related to the quantity of toxin ingested; characteristic cranial nerve palsies progressing to a descending paralysis; fever usually absent; usually associated with home-canned foods.
  2. Enterotoxigenic *E. coli* (ETEC): Most common cause of travelers' diarrhea; after 1- to 2-day incubation period, abdominal cramps and copious diarrhea occur; vomiting and fever uncommon; usually resolves after 3 to 4 days; vehicle usually unbottled water or contaminated salad or ice.
  3. Enterohemorrhagic *E. coli* (EHEC): Can cause severe abdominal cramps and watery diarrhea, which may eventually become bloody; bacteria (strain 0157:H7) are noninvasive; no fever; illness may be complicated by hemolytic-uremic syndrome; associated with contaminated beef (especially hamburger), unpasteurized milk or juice. Table 3 summarizes the various strains of diarrheagenic *E. coli.*
  4. *V. cholerae:* Varies from a mild, self-limited illness to life-threatening cholera; diarrhea, nausea, and vomiting, abdominal cramps, and muscle cramps; no fever; severe cases may progress to shock and death within hours of onset; survivors usually have resolution of symptoms in 1 wk; U.S. cases are either imported or result from ingestion of imported food.
- Invasive organisms include:
  1. *Salmonella:* Associated most often with nontyphoidal strains; incubation period generally 12 to 48 hr; nausea, vomiting, diarrhea, and abdominal cramps typical; fever possible; outbreaks of gastroenteritis related to contaminated poultry, meat, and dairy products.
  2. *Shigella:* Asymptomatic infection possible, but some with fever and watery diarrhea that may progress to bloody diarrhea and dysentery; with mild illness, usually self-limited, resolves in a few days; with severe illness, may develop complications; transmission usually from person to person but can occur via contaminated food or water.
  3. *C. jejuni:* The most common foodborne bacterial pathogen; incubation period is about 1 day, then a prodrome of fever, headache, and myalgias; intestinal phase marked by diarrhea associated with fever, malaise, and abdominal pain; diarrhea mild to profuse and bloody; usually resolves in about 7 days, but relapse is possible; associated with undercooked meats and poultry, unpasteurized dairy products, and drinking from freshwater streams.

[1]Dewey-Mattia D et al: Surveillance for foodborne disease outbreaks – United States 2009-2015, *MMWR Surveill Summ* 67(10):1-11, 2018.

TABLE 1 Pathogenic Mechanisms in Bacterial Foodborne Disease

Preformed Toxin	Toxin Production in Vivo	Tissue Invasion	Toxin Production and/or Tissue Invasion
Staphylococcus aureus	*Clostridium perfringens*	*Campylobacter jejuni*	*Vibrio parahaemolyticus*
Bacillus cereus (short incubation)	*B. cereus* (long incubation)	*Salmonella*	*Yersinia enterocolitica*
Clostridium botulinum	*C. botulinum* (infant botulism)	*Shigella*	
	Enterotoxigenic *Escherichia coli*	Invasive *E. coli*	
	Vibrio cholerae 01 or 0139		
	V. cholerae non-01		
	Shiga toxin–producing *E. coli*		

From Mandell GL et al: *Principles and practice of infectious diseases,* ed 6, Philadelphia, 2005, Churchill Livingstone.

TABLE 2 Foodborne Disease Agents and Clinical Presentation

Usual Incubation Periods	Causative Agent	Clinical Illness: Fever	Clinical Illness: Diarrhea	Clinical Illness: Vomiting	Epidemiologic and Laboratory Diagnosis
5 min–6 h (usually <3 h)	Chemical or toxin	Rare	Occasional	Common	Demonstration of toxin or chemical from food or epidemiologic incrimination of food
1–6 h (usually <1 h)	*Staphylococcus aureus* enterotoxin	Rare	Occasional	Profuse	Isolation of organisms in food (>10^5/g)/vomitus/stool; detection of enterotoxin in food
	Bacillus cereus emetic toxin	Rare	Occasional	Profuse	Isolation of organisms in food (>10^5/g)/vomitus/stool
6–24 h	*Clostridium perfringens* enterotoxin	Rare	Typical	Occasional	Isolation of organisms or toxin from food (10^5/g) or stools of ill persons, epidemiologic incrimination of food; detection of enterotoxin in food
	B. cereus enterotoxin	Rare	Typical	Occasional	
12–72 h	*Clostridium botulinum*	Clinical syndrome compatible with botulism	Constipation more common		Isolation of organism or toxin from food (10^5/g) or stools; demonstration of toxin in serum or food
16–96 h	*Shigella*	Common	Typical, often bloody	Occasional	Isolation of organism from clinical specimens from two or more ill persons; isolation of organism from epidemiologically implicated food
	Nontyphoidal *Salmonella*	Common	Typical	Occasional	
	Enteroinvasive *E. coli* (EIEC)	Common	Typical, may be bloody	Occasional	
	Enteropathogenic *E. coli* (EPEC)	Occasional	Typical	Occasional	
	Enterotoxigenic *E. coli* (ETEC)	Rare	Typical	Rare	
	Vibrio parahaemolyticus; V. cholerae enterotoxin	Occasional	Typical	Occasional	
1–3 days	Caliciviruses (noroviruses) Rotavirus	Occasional	Typical	Common	Antigen detection (enzyme immunoassay) in stool; immune electron microscopy of stool; detection of viral RNA in stool or vomitus by PCR
1–10 days	*Yersinia*	Uncommon	Typical, severe abdominal pain	Uncommon	Isolation of organisms from food or clinical specimens of ill persons
2–10 days	*Campylobacter jejuni*	Common	Typical, often bloody	Uncommon	Isolation of organisms from food or clinical specimens of ill persons
1–11 days	*Cryptosporidium*	Occasional	Common	Occasional	Demonstration of oocysts in stool or in small bowel biopsy of ill persons; demonstration of organism in epidemiologically implicated food
	Cyclospora	Occasional	Common	Occasional	Demonstration of parasite in stool or in small bowel biopsy of ill persons; demonstration of organism in epidemiologically implicated food
	Giardia intestinalis	Occasional	Common	Occasional	Demonstration of parasite in stool or in small bowel biopsy of ill persons; demonstration of organism in epidemiologically implicated food
2 days–weeks	*Bacillus anthracis*	Common	Typical	Frequent	Isolation of organism from blood or contaminated meat
1–7 days	*E. coli* O157:H7 and other Shiga toxin–producing *E. coli*	Uncommon	Typical	Frequent	Isolation of organism from food or stool or identification of toxin in stools of ill persons
3–60 days, usually 7–14	*Salmonella typhi*	Common	Diarrhea or constipation	Uncommon	Isolation of organisms from food or clinical specimens of ill persons
7–21 days	*Brucella* spp.	Common	Common	Rare	Isolation of organisms from blood or bone marrow culture of ill persons; fourfold increase in standard agglutination titer overall several weeks or single titer 1:160 in person with compatible clinical syndrome
1–4 wk	*Giardia lamblia*	Rare	Common	Rare	Stool for ova and parasite examination enzyme immunoassay
2 days–8 wk	*Trichinella spiralis*	Common	Common	Common	Serology, muscle biopsy

PCR, Polymerase chain reaction; *RNA*, ribonucleic acid.
From Cherry JD et al: *Feigin and Cherry's Pediatric infectious diseases*, ed 8, Philadelphia, 2019, Elsevier.

4. *Y. enterocolitica* and *Y. pseudotuberculosis:* Infrequent causes of enteritis in the United States; children affected more often than adults; fever, diarrhea, and abdominal pain lasting 1 to 3 wk; some with mesenteric adenitis that mimics acute appendicitis; contaminated food or water is usually responsible.
5. *V. parahaemolyticus:* In the United States, most outbreaks in coastal states or on cruise ships during the summer months; incubation period usually >1 day, followed by explosive watery diarrhea in the majority of cases; nausea, vomiting, abdominal cramps, and headache also common; fever less common; usually resolves by 1 wk; related to ingestion of seafood.
6. Enteroinvasive *E. coli* (EIEC): A rare cause of disease in the United States; high incidence of fever and bloody diarrhea; may resemble bacillary dysentery.
7. *V. vulnificus:* May cause serious, often fatal illness in persons with chronic liver disease; GI symptoms usually absent, but fever, chills, hypotension, and hemorrhagic skin lesions possible; patients with liver disease or at increased risk of developing liver disease should avoid eating raw oysters.

TABLE 3 Diarrheagenic *Escherichia coli*

Strains	Pathogenic Mechanisms	Persons Affected	Clinical Features
DAEC	Diffuse adherence to Hep-2 cells	Children in developing countries	Watery diarrhea (acute) and persistent diarrhea
EAEC	Aggregative adherence to Hep-2 cells	Children in developing countries	Watery diarrhea (acute) and persistent diarrhea
STEC 0157:H7 Non-0157:H7 0104:H4*	Shiga toxins 1 and 2	Children and adults Persons who ingest contaminated food, especially hamburger (outbreaks)	Watery diarrhea Bloody diarrhea (classic)
EIEC	Epithelial cell invasion	Children and adults	Watery diarrhea Dysentery
EPEC Typical Atypical	Attaching and effacing Bundle-forming pilus, attachment and effacement lesions or Atypical adherence pattern	Children	Watery diarrhea (acute) Persistent diarrhea
ETEC	Heat-labile and/or heat-stable toxin Adherence	Children in developing countries; travelers	Watery diarrhea

DAEC, Diffusely adhering *Escherichia coli*; *EAEC,* enteroaggregative *E. coli*; *EIEC,* enteroinvasive *E. coli*; *EPEC,* enteropathogenic *E. coli*; *ETEC,* enterotoxigenic *E. coli*; *STEC,* Shiga toxin–producing *E. coli.*
[a]EAEC that acquired Shiga toxin gene.
From Feldman M, Friedman LS, Brandt LJ: *Sleisenger and Fordtran's gastrointestinal and liver disease*, ed 10, Philadelphia, 2016, Elsevier.

ETIOLOGY

Classically categorized as either inflammatory (invasive) or noninflammatory:

- Noninflammatory: *B. cereus, S. aureus, C. botulinum, C. perfringens, V. cholerae,* enterotoxigenic *E. coli* (ETEC), and enterohemorrhagic *E. coli* (EHEC); toxin-producing organisms that are noninvasive; fecal leukocytes are not seen.
- Inflammatory: *Campylobacter,* enteroinvasive *E. coli* (EIEC), *Salmonella, Shigella, V. parahaemolyticus,* and *Yersinia;* cause disease by invasion of intestinal tissue; fecal leukocytes are seen.

Dx DIAGNOSIS

DIFFERENTIAL DIAGNOSIS

Gastroenteritis caused by viruses (Norwalk, Noro, or rotavirus), parasites *(Amoeba histolytica, Giardia lamblia),* or toxins (ciguatoxins, mushrooms, heavy metals).

LABORATORY TESTS

- Watchful waiting is often the most appropriate option and ancillary testing is usually not necessary.
- In severe or persistent cases stool test for fecal leukocytes may help narrow the differential diagnosis:
    1. Send stool for culture and for ova and parasites.
    2. Send stool for *C. difficile* toxin in patients with current or recent antibiotic use.
    3. Note: Some pathogens are not identified on routine stool culture; laboratory should be advised if *Yersinia, C. botulinum, Vibrio,* or enterohemorrhagic *E. coli* (0157:H7) are suspected.
    4. Finding *B. cereus, C. perfringens,* or *E. coli* in stool is of little value, because these may be part of the normal bowel flora.
    5. Stool cultures are positive in less than 40% of cases.
    6. Newer techniques such as polymerase chain reaction (PCR) testing provide a more rapid and reliable determination of specific pathogens.
- If botulism suspected, send food, serum, and stool for toxin assay.
- Blood cultures should be considered for all febrile patients.
- Consider toxic megacolon (identified on plain abdominal sonography).
- Consider sigmoidoscopy to obtain tissue and histology in hospitalized patients with bloody diarrhea.
- Consider lactoferrin measurement if an inflammatory etiology is suspected.

Rx TREATMENT

NONPHARMACOLOGIC THERAPY

Adequate rehydration is the mainstay of therapy.

ACUTE GENERAL Rx

- Most cases of acute infectious diarrhea are viral and antibiotics are not indicated.
- Gastroenteritis caused by the following bacterial organisms requires no antimicrobial treatment: *B. cereus, S. aureus, C. perfringens, V. parahaemolyticus, Yersinia,* and enterohemorrhagic and enteroinvasive *E. coli.*
- The usual cause of travelers' diarrhea is enterotoxigenic *E. coli.* Although usually a self-limited illness, antibiotics can shorten the course in patients with fever or dysentery.
    1. Azithromycin 1000 mg in a single oral dose or
    2. SMX/TMP one DS tab bid for 3 days or
    3. Ciprofloxacin 500 mg PO bid for 3 days.
- The mainstay of therapy for cholera is fluid replacement. Antibiotics should be given to decrease shedding and duration of illness.
    1. Doxycycline 300 mg in a single dose or 100 mg PO bid for 3 days.
    2. SMX/TMP one DS tab bid for 3 days.
- Treatment is not indicated for *Salmonella* gastroenteritis. Patients who are at high risk of developing bacteremia may be treated for 48 to 72 hr (see "Salmonellosis").
- Although shigellosis tends to be a self-limited illness, antibiotics shorten the course of illness and may limit transmission of the illness (see "Shigellosis").
- Those with moderate or severe *Campylobacter* diarrhea may benefit from treatment.
    1. Azithromycin 500 mg qd for 3 days or
    2. Erythromycin 500 mg PO qid for 5 days or
    3. Ciprofloxacin 500 mg PO bid for 5 days.
- *V. vulnificus* sepsis should be treated with:
    1. Doxycycline 100 mg IV bid for 2 wk.
    2. Ceftazidime 2 g IV q8h for 2 wk.
- For suspected botulism, antitoxin should be administered early (see "Botulism").
- Table 4 summarizes antibiotic therapy for nonsevere infections with common bacterial enteropathogens in immunocompetent adults.

CHRONIC Rx

Patients with *Salmonella* infections may become carriers and may require treatment (see "Salmonellosis").

DISPOSITION

- Most infections are self-limited and do not require therapy.
- In immunocompromised host or patient with underlying disease, serious complications are possible.
- Postinfectious syndromes are important with some infections:

TABLE 4 Antibiotic Therapy for Nonsevere Infections with Common Bacterial Enteropathogens in Immunocompetent Adults

Organism	Recommended Antibiotic(s)	Alternative Antibiotic(s)
***Shigella* Species**		
Shigella infection (non-*dysenteriae*; for *Shigella dysenteriae* type 1, see text)	Ciprofloxacin 500 mg twice daily (or levofloxacin 500 mg daily) × 3 days	Azithromycin 500 mg-1 g daily × 3-5 days TMP/SMX 160 mg/800 mg twice daily, if sensitive, × 3 days
***Salmonella* Species**		
Enterocolitis, uncomplicated	Not usually recommended (see text)	Can consider in areas of high fluoroquinolone quinolone resistance; Azithromycin 1 g daily × 5 days
Typhoid and enteric fevers*	Ciprofloxacin 500 mg twice daily (or ofloxacin 400 mg twice daily) × 7-14 days Ceftriaxone 2-3 g IV daily × 7-14 days	
***Campylobacter* Species**		
Campylobacter jejuni	Not usually required Ciprofloxacin 500 mg twice daily × 3 days	Azithromycin 500 mg-1 g × 3-5 days
Yersinia enterocolitica		
Enterocolitis, uncomplicated	Not usually required	An aminoglycoside (parenteral) Tetracycline 500 mg 4 times daily × 5 days TMP/SMX 160 mg/800 mg twice daily × 5 days Ciprofloxacin 500 mg twice daily × 5 days Doxycycline 100 mg twice daily × 5 days
Escherichia coli†		
Enterotoxigenic	Endemic disease; usually self-limited, supportive care (see text) Travelers' diarrhea: ciprofloxacin 500 mg twice daily × 3 days Rifaximin 200 mg 3 times daily × 3 days	Azithromycin 500 mg-1 g daily × 3-5 days TMP/SMX 160 mg/800 mg twice daily, if sensitive, × 3 days
Shiga toxin–producing	Unclear if antibiotics are effective; may be harmful	
***Vibrio* Species**		
Vibrio cholera	Doxycycline 300 mg × 1 dose	Ciprofloxacin 1 g × 1 dose Azithromycin 1 g × 1 dose Tetracycline 500 mg every 6 hours × 3 days
Vibrio parahaemolyticus	Usually not required; no controlled trials	As for *V. cholerae*

NOTE: All antibiotics are administered orally unless otherwise indicated. Recommendations are given for treatment of mild/moderate infections only. Treatments for complicated infections or severely ill, bacteremic, or immunocompromised patients are not listed above and may differ from treatments for mild disease.
TMP/SMX, Trimethoprim/sulfamethoxazole.
*For severe typhoid fever, consider the addition of glucocorticoids (dexamethasone 3 mg/kg × 1, then 1 mg/kg every 6 hours × 48 hours) to parenteral antimicrobial therapy. Antimicrobial sensitivity testing is required. Fluoroquinolones (e.g., ciprofloxacin) should not be used as empiric therapy in Asia or other areas with high fluoroquinolone resistance.
†Enteropathogenic, enteroaggregative, and diffusely enteroadherent *E. coli* are omitted from this table because these types are defined in research laboratories and are not diagnosed in routine clinical practice. Enteroinvasive *E. coli* presenting as inflammatory diarrhea should be treated empirically as for *Shigella* spp.
From Feldman M, Friedman LS, Brandt LJ: *Sleisenger and Fordtran's gastrointestinal and liver disease*, ed 10, Philadelphia, 2016, Elsevier.

1. Reiter syndrome: *Salmonella, Shigella, Campylobacter, Yersinia* spp.; more common in genetically susceptible host (HLA-B27+).
2. Guillain-Barré syndrome: *Campylobacter* spp.

REFERRAL

If more than a mild illness

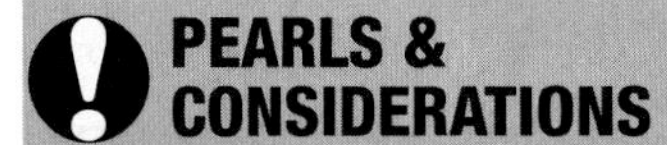

PEARLS & CONSIDERATIONS

COMMENTS

- Grossly underreported and undiagnosed
- All cases to be reported to the local health department
- Table 5 summarizes control and prevention measures of foodborne diseases

SUGGESTED READINGS

Available at ExpertConsult.com

RELATED CONTENT

Bacterial Food Poisoning (Patient Information)
Salmonellosis (Related Key Topic)

AUTHOR: **GLENN G. FORT, M.D., M.P.H.**

TABLE 5 Control and Prevention of Foodborne Diseases

General Recommendations for All Persons

- Thoroughly cook raw food from animal sources, such as beef, pork, poultry, fish, and eggs, to temperatures that eliminate most pathogens.*
- Wash raw fruits and vegetables before eating.
- Keep uncooked meats separate from fruits, vegetables, cooked foods, and ready-to-eat foods.
- Do not thaw meat, poultry, or fish on the counter (instead, thaw in a refrigerator, in cold water, or in a microwave oven).
- Wash hands before, during, and after preparing food and before eating food.
- Wash knives, other utensils, and cutting boards after handling uncooked foods.
- Keep refrigerators set to below 40°F and freezers set to 0°F or lower and verify with a thermometer.
- Refrigerate perishable foods within 2 hr (or within 1 hr if left out at temperatures >90°F).
- Read and follow all cooking and storage instructions on food product packaging. This is especially important for foods prepared in microwave ovens because these ovens heat foods unevenly. Even foods that may appear ready to eat may require thorough cooking.
- Persons with diarrhea or vomiting possibly caused by an infectious agent should not prepare foods for others.
- Keep all animals, including reptiles and amphibians, away from surfaces where foods or drinks are prepared.
- Do not drink unpasteurized (raw) milk or eat foods made from unpasteurized milk. (Exception: Hard cheeses made from raw milk that have been aged >60 days are generally safe to eat.)
- Do not eat home-canned foods that were not known to be adequately heat processed during canning.

Recommendations for Persons at High Risk, Such as Pregnant Women and People With Weakened Immune Systems, in Addition to the Recommendations Listed Above

Measures to Prevent a Variety of Bacterial Infections

- Do not eat uncooked sprouts.
- Do not drink prepackaged juice or juice-containing beverages that have not been processed to reduce or eliminate microbial contamination (e.g., by pasteurization).

Listeriosis Prevention Measures

- Do not eat soft cheeses, such as feta, Brie, and Camembert; blue-veined cheeses; and Mexican-style cheeses, such as queso blanco, queso fresco, and panela, unless the package has a label that clearly states that the cheese is made from pasteurized milk.
- Do not eat refrigerated pâtés or meat spreads. Canned or shelf-stable pâtés and meat spreads are safe to eat.
- Do not eat refrigerated smoked seafood unless it is contained in a cooked dish, such as a casserole. Refrigerated smoked seafood, such as salmon, trout, whitefish, cod, tuna, and mackerel, is most often labeled as "nova-style," "lox," "kippered," "smoked," or "jerky." The fish is found in the refrigerator section or sold at delicatessen counters of grocery stores and delicatessens. Canned or shelf-stable smoked seafood is safe to eat.
- Do not eat hotdogs, luncheon meats, or delicatessen meats unless they are reheated until steaming hot.
- Avoid getting fluid from hotdog packages on other foods, utensils, and food preparation surfaces, and wash hands after handling hot dogs, luncheon meats, and delicatessen meats.

Salmonellosis Prevention Measures

- Choose pasteurized eggs.

Vibriosis, Toxoplasmosis, and Norovirus Prevention Measures

- Do not eat raw or lightly steamed oysters, clams, or other raw shellfish (especially important for patients with liver disease).

More food safety information can be found at www.foodsafety.gov/keep/index.html.

*Poultry: 165°F (73.9°C); ground meats: 160°F (71.1°C); intact cuts of beef, pork, ham, veal, and lamb: 145°F (62.8°C) and allow to rest for at least 3 minutes before eating; fish and shellfish: 145°F (62.8°C); egg dishes: 160°F (71.1°C).

From Bennett JE, Dolin R, Blaser MJ: *Mandell, Douglas, and Bennett's principles and practice of infectious diseases*, ed 8, Philadelphia, 2015, Saunders.

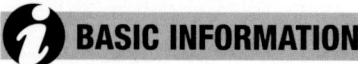

BASIC INFORMATION

DEFINITION

Frostbite represents tissue injury (or death) from freezing and vasoconstriction induced by severe environmental cold exposure.

SYNONYM

Cold-induced tissue injury

ICD-10CM CODES

T35.0	Superficial frostbite involving multiple body regions
T34	Frostbite with tissue necrosis
T345	Frostbite with tissue necrosis of wrist and hand
T34.8	Frostbite with tissue necrosis of ankle and foot
T34.9	Frostbite with tissue necrosis of other and unspecified sites
T35.4	Superficial frostbite involving multiple body regions
T33.9	Superficial frostbite of unspecified sites, initial encounter

EPIDEMIOLOGY & DEMOGRAPHICS

- Environmental factors include windchill factor, temperature, duration of exposure, altitude, and degree of wetness. Hands and feet account for 90% of injuries; nose, cheeks, ears, and male genitalia are also more susceptible.
- Host factors include psychiatric illness and neuroleptic and sedative drugs (especially alcohol, which, in addition to impairing judgment, inhibit shivering and cause cutaneous vasodilation). Other risk factors include immobility, previous frostbite, malnutrition, tobacco use, peripheral neuropathy, peripheral vascular disease, diabetes, exhaustion, and constricting clothing and footwear.

Patients at the extremes of age are at greatest risk, but frostbite is more common in adults ages 30 to 49 yr, and African Americans may be more susceptible than whites.

PHYSICAL FINDINGS & CLINICAL PRESENTATION

- Frostbite may be classified into four degrees of injury severity or, more practically, into *superficial* (corresponding to first and second degree) and *deep* (corresponding to third and fourth degree) groups. In both cases, the degree of frostbite can only be accurately determined after rewarming as initially most frostbite injuries appear similar.
- *Superficial* frostbite involves the skin and subcutaneous tissue. The frozen part is waxy, white (or mottled), and firm but soft and resilient below the surface when gently depressed. After rewarming, there is an initial hyperemia that may be followed by swelling and formation of superficial blisters with clear or milky fluid within 6 to 24 hr. There is no ultimate tissue loss.
- *Deep* frostbite extends into the dermis and may involve muscles, nerves, tendons, or bones. The skin may be hard or wooden, without tissue resilience. Nonblanching cyanosis, hemorrhagic blisters, tissue necrosis (Fig. 1), and gangrene may develop. Affected tissue has a poor prognosis and debridement or amputation is generally required.
- Patients initially feel numbness, prickling, and itching. More severe injury can produce paresthesias and stiffness, with burning or throbbing pain upon thawing.

PATHOPHYSIOLOGY

Two phases of tissue injury:

1. The actual freezing of the tissues, during which cellular damage is caused by the formation of extracellular ice crystals, which cause osmotic shifts, cellular dehydration, cell membrane lysis, and cell death.
2. The reperfusion injury, during which the thawing of damaged endothelial cells releases a cascade of inflammatory mediators (e.g., prostaglandin F, thromboxane A2, bradykinins, histamine), resulting in capillary compression, vascular stasis, progressive ischemic injury, and thrombus formation. These conditions ultimately lead to the destruction of the microcirculation and to cell death.

DIAGNOSIS

DIFFERENTIAL DIAGNOSIS

- Frostnip: A superficial nonfreezing cold injury associated with intense vasoconstriction and characterized by frost forming on the surface of the skin. Transient numbness, tingling, and pallor resolve quickly with warming
- Pernio (chilblains): Self-limited, cold-induced vasculitis associated with purple plaques or nodules, often affecting dorsum of hands and feet; seen with prolonged cold exposure to above-freezing temperatures
- Cold immersion (trench foot): Caused by ischemic injury resulting from sustained, severe vasoconstriction in appendages exposed to wet cold at temperatures above freezing

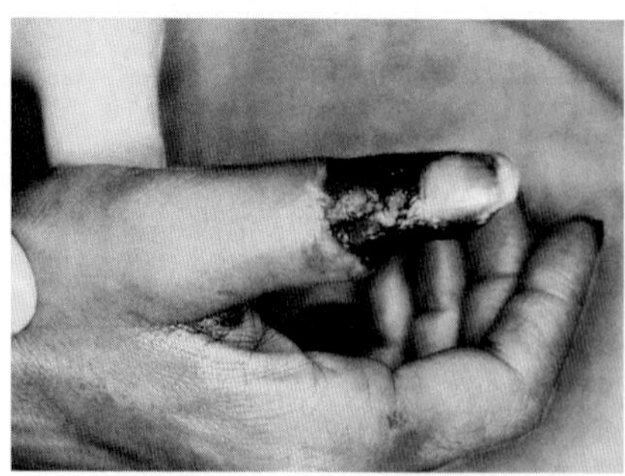

FIG. 1 Third- and fourth-degree frostbite with tissue death. Note demarcation beyond the interphalangeal joint. (From Cameron JL, Cameron AM: *Current surgical therapy,* ed 10, Philadelphia, 2011, Saunders.)

WORKUP

- Laboratory workup is not indicated unless the patient has systemic hypothermia.
- Early presentation (<24 hr from thawing): If there is deep frostbite with potential significant morbidity, perfusion evaluation with angiography (or Tc-99m or MRA) should be done emergently in anticipation of potential thrombolysis treatment.
- Late presentation (>24 hr from thawing): Noninvasive imaging with MRA or multiphase bone scintigraphy (ideally with SPECT/CT) can be used to predict the likely levels of tissue viability for future reconstruction after amputation.

TREATMENT (3 PHASES)

1. FIELD MANAGEMENT

- Prioritize treatment of hypothermia (core body temperature <35° C; 95° F) with systemic and adjunctive rewarming measures if available (e.g., warmed, humidified oxygen, heated IV saline [45° C; 113° F], and warming blankets) before thawing frostbitten extremities.
    1. Shelter patient out of wind and give warm fluids.
- Remove constricting or wet clothing and jewelry from affected digits.
    1. Place cold extremity in a companion's axilla or groin for 10 minutes, then replace dry gloves/boots.
- Insulate, splint, and elevate affected areas if practical to do so.
    1. Never rub or massage the affected area. Avoid dry heat (e.g., fires and heaters).
- Avoid thawing if there is any risk of refreezing and if possible avoid ambulation on thawed lower extremities (unless only distal toes affected).
- Administer pain medication and topical aloe if available.
- Box 1 describes the Alaska State Guidelines for prehospital treatment of frostbite.

2. REWARMING

- Rapid rewarming (with warm water) limits the freezing injury and yields better outcomes than slow rewarming (e.g., moving to a warmer location).
- Rapid rewarming is achieved by immersing the affected area in a circulating warm water bath with or without a mild antibacterial agent (e.g., chlorhexidine or povidone-iodine) maintained at 37° to 39° C for at least 15 to 30 min up to 1 hour, until all tissues are thoroughly rewarmed and pliable with a red-purple color. Active motion during rewarming is advisable; massage is not.
- Administer analgesics during rewarming (ibuprofen and possibly narcotics).

3. POST-THAW TREATMENT

- Tetanus prophylaxis and topical antibiotics if potentially contaminated skin wound.
- Consider systemic antibiotics for patients with significant trauma or signs of infection.

BOX 1 Alaska State Guidelines for Prehospital Treatment of Frostbite

First Responder/Emergency Medical Technician—I, II, III/Paramedic/Small Bush Clinic
Evaluation and Treatment

A. Anticipate, assess, and treat the patient for hypothermia, if present.
B. Assess the frostbitten area carefully because the loss of sensation may cause the patient to be unaware of soft tissue injuries in that area.
C. Obtain a complete set of vital signs and the patient's temperature.
D. Remove jewelry and clothing, if present, from the affected area.
E. Obtain a patient history, including the date of the patient's last tetanus immunization.
F. If there is frostbite distal to a fracture, attempt to align the limb unless there is resistance. Splint the fracture in a manner that does not compromise distal circulation.
G. Determine whether rewarming the frostbitten tissue can be accomplished in a medical facility. If it can, transport the patient while protecting the tissue from further injury from cold or impacts.
H. If the decision is made to rewarm frostbitten tissue in the field, you should prepare a warm water bath in a container large enough to accommodate the frostbitten tissues without them touching the sides or bottom of the container. The temperature of the water bath should be 99° to 102° F (37° to 39° C).
   1. Generally, patients with frostbite do not require opiates for pain relief; they occasionally need non-opiate pain medication or anxiolytics. If possible, consult a physician regarding the administration of oral analgesics, such as acetaminophen, ibuprofen or aspirin. Aspirin or ibuprofen may help improve outcomes by blocking the arachidonic acid pathway.
   2. Immersion injury or frostbite with other associated injuries may produce significant edema and high pain levels. These patients may need opiate pain medications for initial treatment. In this case, advanced life support personnel should administer morphine or other analgesics in accordance with physician-signed standing orders or online medical control.
I. A source of additional warm water must be available.
J. Water should be maintained at approximately at 99° to 102° F (37° to 39° C) and gently circulated around the frostbitten tissue until the distal tip of the frostbitten part becomes flushed.
K. Pain after rewarming usually indicates that viable tissue has been successfully rewarmed.
L. After rewarming, let the frostbitten tissues dry in the warm air. Do **not** towel dry.
M. After thawing, tissues that were deeply frostbitten may develop blisters or appear cyanotic. Blisters should not be broken and must be protected from injury.
N. Pad between affected digits and bandage affected tissues loosely with a soft, sterile dressing. Avoid putting undue pressure on the affected parts.
O. Rewarmed extremities should be kept at a level above the heart, if possible.
P. Protect the rewarmed area from refreezing and other trauma during transport. A frame around the frostbitten area should be constructed to prevent blankets from pressing directly on the injured area.
Q. Do not allow an individual who has frostbitten feet to walk except when the life of the patient or rescuer is in danger. Once frostbitten feet are rewarmed, the patient becomes nonambulatory.

- Debride broken clear vesicles and avoid disrupting intact blisters (especially hemorrhagic ones) unless they interfere with mobility.
- Topical aloe vera (a potent anti-prostaglandin agent) q6h and ibuprofen (a thromboxane inhibitor) 400 to 600 mg bid to tid (or daily aspirin) can be given until wounds are healed or surgery occurs.
- Thrombolytic therapy: If <24 hr from thawing in a patient with severe frostbite and poor prognostic indicators (e.g., cool skin after rewarming, numb, dusky or blue digits, hemorrhagic blisters). First, perfusion evaluation with angiography (or Tc-99m or MRA) is performed to assess for arterial compromise followed by intra-arterial (or intravenous) tPA if perfusion defects are demonstrated and there is no contraindication to thrombolysis. The use of early thrombolytic therapy appears to limit reperfusion injury and reduce subsequent digit amputation significantly. The tissue salvage rate correlates with elapsed time to treatment from time of rewarming.
- Heparin is recommended in addition to tPA to prevent recurrent local thrombosis.
- Vasodilator therapy: Various vasodilators (NTG, pentoxifylline, phenoxybenzamine, nifedipine, reserpine, and buflomedil) have been tried, with the best evidence favoring prostacyclin (or iloprost, which is available in Europe). If iloprost is available, at least one study has shown superior efficacy to tPA, and it is easier to administer, has a better safety profile, fewer contraindications, and can be managed on a general ward.
- Daily dressing changes with dry, sterile, noncompressive, and nonadherent dressings. Splint and elevate hands and feet to reduce edema and separate digits with cotton gauze. Avoid any abrasion to limit risk of infection.
- Whirlpool hydrotherapy: 1 to 2 times per day for 30 minutes with warm water (37°-39° C), with or without an antiseptic solution if severe edema is present, until there is a clear demarcation of necrotic tissues or evidence of tissue healing.
- Gentle, progressive physical therapy after edema resolves.
- Keep site warm, and avoid all vasoconstrictors, including nicotine.
- Dextran, warfarin, sympathectomy, and hyperbaric oxygen are of potential but unproven benefit. In patients treated with thrombolysis, an oral anticoagulant or antiplatelet therapy upon discharge is included in some treatment protocols.

DISPOSITION

A majority of patients have long-term residual symptoms, including cold hypersensitivity, neuropathic pain, sensory deficits, hyperhidrosis, secondary Raynaud's disease, localized osteoporosis, edema, hair or nail deformities, and (rarely) arthritis. Treatment with tricyclics, gabapentin, calcium channel blockers, and careful protection from further cold exposure may be helpful.

REFERRAL

- Hospitalize for hypothermia or deep frostbite; a burn unit is best.
- Surgical decisions regarding amputation should be deferred until demarcation of viable tissue is clear (6 to 12 weeks), unless refractory pain, sepsis, or gangrene occurs.

SUGGESTED READINGS

Available at ExpertConsult.com

RELATED CONTENT

Frostbite (Patient Information)

AUTHOR: **MICHAEL P. JOHNSON, M.D.**

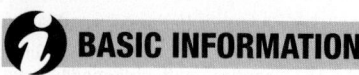

DEFINITION

Biliary pain caused by gallbladder dysmotility in the absence of gallstones, sludge, or microlithiasis. It is a diagnosis of exclusion with no evidence of structural disease seen with normal hepatobiliary and pancreatic laboratory and diagnostic imaging modalities.

SYNONYMS

Biliary dyskinesia
Gallbladder dyskinesia
Gallbladder spasm
Acalculous biliary disease
Chronic acalculous cholecystitis
Chronic acalculous
Gallbladder dysfunction
Cystic duct syndrome

ICD-10CM CODE
K82.9 Disease of gallbladder, unspecified

EPIDEMIOLOGY & DEMOGRAPHICS

INCIDENCE: Biliary dyspepsia has an incidence rate of 1% to 6%.

PREVALENCE: 10% to 45% of total population report dyspepsia.

PREDOMINANT SEX AND AGE: There is a 3:1 female-to-male predominance.

RISK FACTORS

There is no consistent relationship to meals or fatty meal intake.

PHYSICAL FINDINGS & CLINICAL PRESENTATION

These patients present with typical biliary pain that fulfills the Rome III criteria:

- Patients present with sporadic epigastric or right upper quadrant pain lasting for 30 minutes but less than 6 hours.
- Episodes are recurrent and occur in sporadic intervals (but not daily).
- The pain is not relieved by bowel movements.
- The pain is not relieved by postural movements.
- The pain is not relieved by antacids.
- The pain builds up to a steady level.
- The pain is severe enough it impedes daily activities and may even require an emergency department visit.

Dx DIAGNOSIS

DIFFERENTIAL DIAGNOSIS

- Primary gallbladder disorders: Gallstones, cholecystitis
- Pancreatobiliary disorders: Cholelithiasis, choledocholithiasis, pancreatitis, pancreatic neoplasm
- Gastrointestinal disorders: Gastroesophageal reflux disorder, peptic ulcer disease, inflammatory bowel disease, irritable bowel syndrome, gastric or esophageal neoplasm
- Metabolic disorders: Obesity, diabetes mellitus
- Cholecystokinin deficiency: Celiac disease

WORKUP

This is a diagnosis of exclusion in a patient with biliary pain. Patients will have normal blood test results and hepatobiliary and pancreatic enzymes, including AST, ALT, ALP, bilirubin, amylase, and lipase. Imaging, including abdominal ultrasound, is essentially normal without evidence of gallstone or gallbladder sludge pathology.

LABORATORY TESTS

Laboratory tests, including serum AST, ALT, ALP, bilirubin, GGT, amylase, and lipase, are within normal limits.

IMAGING STUDIES

- To exclude gallstone pathology, a transabdominal ultrasound is initial choice for imaging. Transabdominal ultrasound is capable of detecting gallstones up to 3 to 5 mm in size. Patients should fast for at least 8 hours before ultrasound to optimize visualization of the gallbladder.
- If gallstones or gallbladder are not found on ultrasound but still suspected, endoscopic ultrasound (EUS) may be used to detect microlithiasis or gallstones smaller than 3 mm.
- Assessing gallbladder emptying through cholecystokinin (CCK)–stimulated cholescintigraphy is essential in the diagnosis. CCK-stimulated cholescintigraphy allows for the calculation of gallbladder ejection fraction (GBEF). Normal GBEF is >38%. Patients with a GBEF <35% to 40% with reproducible pain on CCK stimulation is suggestive of functional gallbladder disorder.

Rx TREATMENT

In patients with appropriate evaluation for suspected functional gallbladder disorder, surgical management with cholecystectomy is the preferred method of treatment.

NONPHARMACOLOGIC THERAPY

Surgical cholecystectomy is the preferred method of treatment. Studies have shown symptomatic relief in up to 98% of patients postcholecystectomy.

ACUTE GENERAL Rx

- Initial management should include adequate analgesic control for abdominal pain.
- Opioid analgesics should be avoided because they may exacerbate symptoms involved in a hypofunctioning gallbladder.

COMPLEMENTARY AND ALTERNATIVE MEDICINE

Turmeric (Curcuma) has been known to alleviate biliary dyspepsia by stimulating gallbladder contractions.

DISPOSITION

Patients with functional gallbladder disorder are often misdiagnosed. These patients require appropriate evaluation to exclude other hepatobiliary etiology. After they are properly diagnosed, these patients have a favorable prognosis after surgical intervention.

REFERRAL

- Gastroenterology consultation may be considered to rule out microlithiasis via EUS.
- Surgical consultation should be considered for possible cholecystectomy in select patients.

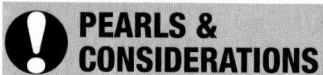

COMMENTS

Functional gallbladder disorder is a diagnosis of exclusion. It is essential that other hepatobiliary pathology be ruled out first. CCK-stimulation scintigraphy showing a reduced GBEF without any other pathology is suggestive of this disorder. Patients fare well with surgical intervention.

RELATED TOPICS

Cholangiocarcinoma (Related Key Topic)
Cholecystitis (Related Key Topic)
Choledocholithiasis (Related Key Topic)
Cholelithiasis (Related Key Topic)

AUTHORS: **ROSANN CHOLANKERIL, M.D.,** and **GEORGE CHOLANKERIL, M.D.**

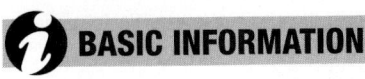

BASIC INFORMATION

DEFINITION

Galactorrhea can be defined as inappropriate lactation (in the absence of pregnancy or postpartum state) as a result of nonphysiologic augmentation of prolactin release.

ICD-10CM CODES

N64.3	Galactorrhea not associated with childbirth
092.6	Galactorrhea in pregnancy

PHYSICAL FINDINGS & CLINICAL PRESENTATION

- Milky discharge from nipples (Fig. 1), usually occurring bilaterally
- Evidence of chest wall irritation from ill-fitting clothing, herpes zoster, or atopic dermatitis may be present
- Visual field defects (bitemporal hemianopsia) may be present with prolactinomas, particularly if large, such as macroadenomas
- Headaches may also occur in cases of large pituitary adenomas
- Evidence of acromegaly, Cushing's syndrome, or hypothyroidism when galactorrhea is caused by these disorders

ETIOLOGY

- Medications (phenothiazines, metoclopramide, selective serotonin reuptake inhibitors, anxiolytics, buspirone, risperidone, atenolol, valproic acid, conjugated estrogen and medroxyprogesterone, methyldopa, verapamil, H_2 receptor blockers [cimetidine], octreotide, danazol, tricyclic antidepressants, isoniazid, amphetamine, reserpine, opiates, sumatriptan, rimantadine, oral contraceptive formulations), after infancy, galactorrhea is often medication induced
- Pituitary tumors (prolactinomas, craniopharyngiomas)
- Hypothyroidism (diminished feedback inhibition increases thyroid-releasing hormone [TRH], which increases prolactin)
- Breast stimulation: Prolonged suckling or during sexual intercourse
- Chest wall irritation from ill-fitting clothing, herpes zoster, atopic dermatitis, burns
- Breast surgery
- Chronic renal failure (decreased prolactin clearance)
- Cushing's syndrome
- Herbs (e.g., fennel, red clover, anise, red raspberry, marshmallow)
- Cocaine
- Cannabis
- Spinal cord surgery or injury, or tumors
- Severe gastroesophageal reflux disease, esophagitis (stimulation of thoracic nerves by the cervical and thoracic ganglia)
- Neonatal ("witch's milk" produced by 2%-5% of neonates because of precipitous drop in maternal estrogen and progesterone postdelivery)
- Cancer: Lymphomas, Hodgkin's disease, bronchogenic carcinoma, renal adenocarcinomas
- Sarcoidosis and other infiltrative disorders
- Tuberculosis affecting pituitary gland
- Pituitary stalk resection
- Multiple sclerosis
- Empty sella syndrome
- Acromegaly
- Increased stress, including major trauma
- Exercise
- Idiopathic, diagnosis of exclusion

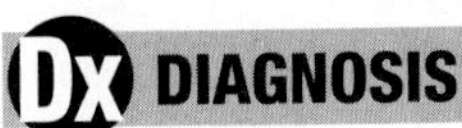

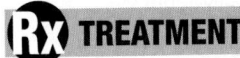

DIAGNOSIS

DIFFERENTIAL DIAGNOSIS

- Intraductal papilloma
- Breast cancer
- Paget disease of breast
- Breast abscess

WORKUP

- Complete history focusing on menstrual irregularity, infertility, previous pregnancies, duration of galactorrhea, medications, visual complaints, fatigue. Age of onset is also significant (e.g., prolactinoma most common between ages 20 and 35 yr; neonatal galactorrhea is usually secondary to transplacental transfer of maternal estrogen)
- Physical examination: Height, weight, vital signs. Evidence of hirsutism, acne, obesity, visual field defects, goiter, neurologic deficits
- Breast examination for presence of nodules, evaluation of discharge (milky versus serosanguineous versus purulent). Inspection of chest wall
- Laboratory testing and imaging studies (see "Laboratory Tests")

LABORATORY TESTS

- β-Human chorionic gonadotropin (HCG) test (positive in pregnancy)
- Prolactin level (elevated, often >200 ng/ml in prolactinoma but may occur at any prolactin level). Confirm with repeat fasting test (avoid exercise and breast stimulation).
- Thyroid-stimulating hormone (TSH) (elevated in hypothyroidism)
- Basic metabolic panel (BMP): Blood urea nitrogen, creatinine (elevated in renal failure), glucose (elevated in Cushing's syndrome)
- Urinalysis (hematuria in renal cell carcinoma)
- Microscopic examination of nipple discharge (scant cellular material, numerous fat globules, can be seen without specific staining)

IMAGING STUDIES

- MRI of brain if prolactin level is elevated, amenorrhea is present, or visual field defects are detected on physical examination.
- High-resolution CT of brain with special coronal cuts through the pituitary region may be helpful in patients with contraindications to MRI; however, it may miss small lesions.

TREATMENT

- Discontinuation of potential offending agents.
- Avoidance of excessive breast stimulation.
- Galactorrhea resulting from prolactinoma can be managed medically or with careful surveillance depending on size and growth of tumor, associated symptoms, and prolactin level. Surgical treatment of prolactinomas is usually reserved for medication failures. Please refer to the topic "Prolactinoma" in Section I for additional information.
- No treatment is necessary for normoprolactinemic patients with idiopathic nonbothersome galactorrhea.
- Normoprolactinemic patients with bothersome galactorrhea may respond to low dose dopamine agonist (e.g., cabergoline 0.25 mg twice weekly).
- If patient is experiencing anovulatory dysfunction, consider treatment with bromocriptine (discontinue with confirmation of pregnancy).

REFERRAL

Endocrine and surgical consultation if prolactinoma is detected

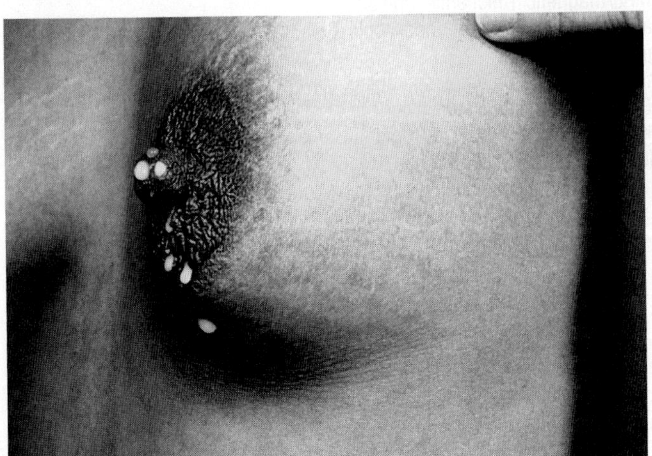

FIG. 1 Galactorrhea. Milk production in a nonpregnant woman resulting from a prolactinoma. (From Haines DE: *Fundamental neuroscience for basic and clinical applications,* ed 3, Philadelphia, 2006, Churchill Livingstone.)

SUGGESTED READING

Available at ExpertConsult.com

RELATED CONTENT

Galactorrhea (Patient Information)
Pituitary Adenoma (Related Key Topic)
Prolactinoma (Related Key Topic)

AUTHOR: **SIRI M. HOLTON, M.D.**

DEFINITION

Gallbladder cancer (GBC) originates from the epithelial lining of the gallbladder. Nearly all of these cancers are adenocarcinomas. Rare pathological types include adenosquamous carcinoma, squamous cell carcinoma, small-cell carcinoma, and carcinosarcoma.

ICD 10-CM CODES
C23 Malignant neoplasm of gallbladder

EPIDEMIOLOGY & DEMOGRAPHICS

INCIDENCE:

- The fifth most common gastrointestinal cancer in the U.S. An estimated 12,190 new cases of gallbladder cancer and cancers of large bile ducts will be diagnosed in 2018, with fewer than 4 in 10 will be gallbladder cancers.
- 1 to 2 cases per 100,000 population in the United States.
- Most prevalent in South American countries and some Asian counties, such as Japan and Korea, due to high incidence of cholelithiasis.

PREDOMINANT SEX AND AGE:

- Female:male ratio 2.5:1 to 3.1:1. Incidence increases with age.

GENETICS: Increased incidence occurs in hereditary syndromes such as Gardner syndrome, neurofibromatosis type I, and hereditary nonpolyposis colon cancer (HNPCC).

RISK FACTORS (BOX 1):

- Gallstone disease
- Porcelain gallbladder
- Female gender
- Older age
- Gallbladder polyps
- Primary sclerosing cholangitis
- Chronic infection from salmonella or helicobacter
- Obesity

BOX 1 Risk Factors for Gallbladder Carcinoma

Anomalous union of the pancreaticobiliary ductal system
Carcinogens*
Cholangiocarcinoma
Cholelithiasis (stone size >1 cm)
Chronic *Salmonella typhi* or *paratyphi* carrier status
First-degree relative with gallbladder cancer
IBD
Intrahepatic biliary dysplasia
Lynch syndrome
Porcelain gallbladder
PSC
Segmental adenomyomatosis in patients ≥60 years of age

*Methylcholanthrene, O-aminoazotoluene, nitrosamines, and possibly others.
IBD, Inflammatory bowel disease; *PSC,* primary sclerosing cholangitis.
From Feldman M et al: *Sleisenger and Fordtran's gastrointestinal and liver disease*, ed 10, Philadelphia, 2016, Elsevier.

PHYSICAL FINDINGS & CLINICAL PRESENTATION

- Early stage: Most patients are asymptomatic.
- Late stage: Right-upper-quadrant pain, weight loss, malaise, nausea, vomiting, and obstructive jaundice. Patients can also present with symptoms of cholecystitis including fever and pain.
- Physical exam may reveal Courvoisier law (palpable gallbladder and mild painless jaundice).

ETIOLOGY

Chronic inflammation of gallbladder from any cause

Dx DIAGNOSIS

DIFFERENTIAL DIAGNOSIS

- Cholangiocarcinoma
- Acalculous cholecystitis
- Carcinoma of the ampulla of Vater
- Gallbladder mucocele
- Gallstones
- Gallbladder volvulus

WORK-UP

- Initial work consists of laboratory evaluation and sonogram of abdomen.
- Liver function tests might reveal bile duct obstruction with an elevated serum bilirubin or alkaline phosphatase.
- Cancer antigen 19-9 (CA 19-9) or carcinoembryonic antigen (CEA) is frequently elevated, but they both have low sensitivity and specificity for diagnostic purposes.
- Suspicious ultrasonographic findings, including calcification, thickened gallbladder wall, gallbladder polyps ≥10 mm, and protruding mass, are warranted for additional imaging studies with computed tomography (CT) of abdomen (Fig. E1), magnetic resonance imaging (MRI)/magnetic resonance cholangiopancreatography (MRCP), or endoscopic ultrasonography (EUS).
- Chest CT should be done to complete staging work-up. PET/CT has limited sensitivity but high specificity in the detection of regional lymph node metastases. PET/CT may be considered when there is an equivocal finding on CT/MRI.
- Staging laparoscopy is very useful to determine resectability state.
- Staging (Table 1).

Rx TREATMENT

- Surgery (Table 2) is the mainstay of treatment for curative intent. Incidental GBC is often operated by laparoscopic cholecystectomy and detected by pathology review postoperatively. In these cases, a radical re-resection is indicated depending on tumor stage.
- Extended cholecystectomy is the preferred approach when GBC is suspected pre-operatively.
- Adjuvant therapy:
  1. T_{1a} with negative margins: no adjuvant chemotherapy.
  2. T_{1b} or higher: adjuvant chemotherapy with fluoropyrimidine-based or gemcitabine-based chemotherapy alone or fluoropyrimidine chemoradiotherapy.
- Unresectable or metastatic disease: Gemcitabine/cisplatin is considered first-line standard of care. Taxanes and fluoropyrimidine-containing regimens can be used upon disease progression. The role of immunotherapy is investigational. Pembrolizumab (PD-1 inhibitor) is appropriate for microsatellite instability high (MSI-H) tumors.

SURVEILLANCE

- Consider imaging every 6 months for 2 yr if clinically indicated, and then annually up to 5 yr.
- Consider CEA and CA 19-9 as clinically indicated.

SUGGESTED READINGS
Available at ExpertConsult.com

AUTHOR: **PATAN GULTAWATVICHAI, M.D.**

TABLE 1 TNM and American Joint Committee on Cancer (AJCC)/International Union Against Cancer (UICC) Staging Systems for Gallbladder Carcinoma

TNM Stage	Criteria		
T_x	Primary tumor cannot be assessed		
T_0	No evidence of primary tumor		
T_{is}	Carcinoma in situ		
T_{1a}	Tumor invades lamina propria		
T_{1b}	Tumor invades muscularis propria		
T_2	Tumor invades perimuscular connective tissue without extension beyond serosa or into liver		
T_3	Tumor perforates the serosa *AND/OR* Tumor directly invades the liver *AND/OR* Tumor invades one other adjacent organ (i.e., stomach, duodenum, colon, pancreas, omentum, extrahepatic bile ducts)		
T_4	Tumor invades the portal vein or hepatic artery *OR* Tumor invades ≥2 extrahepatic organs or structures		
N_x	Regional lymph nodes cannot be assessed		
N_0	No regional lymph node metastases		
N_1	Lymph node metastases along the cystic duct, bile duct, hepatic artery, *AND/OR* portal vein		
N_2	Metastases to periaortic, pericaval, superior mesenteric artery, *AND/OR* celiac artery lymph nodes		
M_0	No distant metastases		
M_1	Distant metastases		
AJCC/UICC Stage	**Tumor**	**Node**	**Metastasis**
0	T_{is}	N_0	M_0
I	T_1	N_0	M_0
II	T_2	N_0	M_0
III_A	T_3	N_0	M_0
III_B	T_{1-3}	N_1	M_0
IV_A	T_4	N_{0-1}	M_0
IV_B	Any T	N_2	M_0
	Any T	Any N	M_1

TNM, tumor, node, metastasis.
From Feldman M et al: *Sleisenger and Fordtran's gastrointestinal and liver disease*, ed 10, Philadelphia, 2016, Elsevier.

TABLE 2 Recommended Management by Stage

Stage	Surgical Management	Postoperative Management
T_{1a}	Simple cholecystectomy	Review pathology report to confirm negative cystic duct margins No routine follow-up advised
T_{1b}	Radical cholecystectomy (i.e., segment IVb/V resection [preferred], hepatic wedge resection, right hepatic lobectomy, or trisectionectomy with R0 resection) and portal lymphadenectomy	Staging workup with CT chest/abdomen/pelvis (or CT chest and MRI abdomen/pelvis) Adjuvant fluoropyrimidine chemoradiation versus gemcitabine-based or fluoropyrimidine-based chemotherapy Surveillance imaging
II	See above for T_{1b} tumors	See above for T_{1b} tumors
III	Consider diagnostic staging laparoscopy followed by operation for T_{1b} tumors if no metastatic disease is identified	See above for T_{1b} tumors
IV_A	Stage IV_A (T_4 $N_{0\text{-}1}$ M_0) disease may be amenable to resection (see stage III)	Adjuvant fluoropyrimidine chemoradiation versus gemcitabine-based or fluoropyrimidine-based chemotherapy
IV_B	N_2 and M_1 disease is a contraindication to attempts at curative resection. Patients may require palliative operation for relief of biliary obstruction but attempts at endoscopic/ percutaneous drainage should be considered first-line treatment	Unresectable disease: combined gemcitabine/cisplatin therapy, fluoropyrimidine-based or gemcitabine-based chemotherapy regimens current

CT, Computed tomography; *MRI,* magnetic resonance imaging.
From Cameron JL, Cameron AM: *Current surgical therapy*, ed 12, Philadelphia, 2017, Elsevier.

BASIC INFORMATION

DEFINITION

Gastric cancer is an adenocarcinoma arising from the stomach. Cancers in the cardia arising within 5 cm of the gastroesophageal junction (GEJ) are typically classified as GEJ cancers. It is subdivided into intestinal and diffuse histology. The diffuse form of gastric cancer is more common in women and young patients, whereas the intestinal type is predominantly related to environmental factors (smoking, diet high in smoked, salted, and pickled food, nitrates and nitrites) and ethnicity (Asian and Pacific descent). The classification of gastric adenocarcinoma by depth of invasion is illustrated in Fig. 1.

SYNONYMS

Gastric adenocarcinoma
Stomach cancer
Linitis plastica

ICD-10CM CODES

C16	Malignant neoplasm of stomach
C16.0	Malignant neoplasm of cardia of stomach
C16.1	Malignant neoplasm of stomach
C16.2	Malignant neoplasm of body of stomach
C16.3	Malignant neoplasm of pyloric antrum
C16.5	Malignant neoplasm of lesser curvature of stomach, unspecified
C16.6	Malignant neoplasm of greater curvature of stomach, unspecified
C16.8	Malignant neoplasm of overlapping sites of stomach

EPIDEMIOLOGY & DEMOGRAPHICS

- Gastric cancer is the fourth commonest cancer in the world, with an annual incidence of approximately 950,000 cases annually; of these, 70% occur in developing countries. The highest incidence is in Asia and the lowest in North America. Annual estimated deaths due to gastric cancer are 723,000 worldwide.
- In the U.S., an estimated 26,240 new cases and 10,800 deaths are expected in 2018.
- Incidence rate of stomach adenocarcinoma is 6.7 in 100,000 persons in the U.S. Mortality rate is 3.4 per 100,000 persons. The incidence of distal stomach tumors has greatly declined, whereas that of proximal tumors of the cardia and fundus is on the rise.
- Gastric cancer is more common in male patients >65 yr (70% of patients are >50 yr).
- Incidence of gastric cancer has been declining over the past 30 yr.
- Male/female ratio is 3:2.
- Hereditary diffuse gastric cancer (HDGC) has an autosomal-dominant inheritance, and cancer develops at a young age (average age 37 yr). Germ-line truncating mutations in the tumor-suppressor E-cadherin gene *(CDH1)* are found in up to 50% of these families. It is associated with an 80% lifetime risk of gastric cancer.
- Increased risk of gastric cancer is also seen with Lynch syndrome, FAP, Peutz-Jeghers, juvenile polyposis syndrome, and hyperplastic gastric polyps.

PHYSICAL FINDINGS & CLINICAL PRESENTATION

- Medical history may reveal complaints of postprandial fullness with significant weight loss (70% to 80%), nausea/emesis (20% to 40%), dysphagia (20%), and dyspepsia, usually unrelieved by antacids; epigastric discomfort, usually lessened by fasting and exacerbated by food intake, is also common.
- Epigastric or abdominal mass (30% to 50%), epigastric pain.
- Anemia from tumor bleeding and hemoccult-positive stools.
- Hard, nodular liver: May indicate metastatic disease to the liver.
- Ascites, lymphadenopathy, or pleural effusions: May indicate metastases.

ETIOLOGY

RISK FACTORS:

- Chronic *Helicobacter pylori* gastritis. Gastric cancer develops in persons infected with *H. pylori* but not in uninfected persons. Those with histologic findings of severe gastric atrophy, corpus-predominant gastritis, or intestinal metaplasia are at increased risk. Persons with *H. pylori* infection and duodenal ulcer are not at risk, whereas those with gastric ulcers, nonulcer dyspepsia, and gastric hyperplastic polyps are. Eradication of *H. pylori* reduces gastric cancer risk.
- Tobacco abuse, heavy alcohol consumption.
- Food additives (nitrosamines), smoked foods, occupational exposure to heavy metals, rubber, asbestos.
- Chronic atrophic gastritis with intestinal metaplasia, hypertrophic gastritis, and pernicious anemia.
- Box 1 summarizes risk factors for gastric adenocarcinoma.

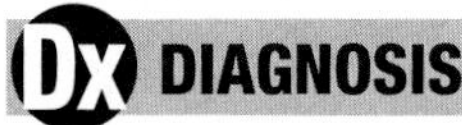

DIAGNOSIS

DIFFERENTIAL DIAGNOSIS

- Gastric lymphoma (5% of gastric malignancies)
- Hypertrophic gastritis
- Peptic ulcer
- Reflux esophagitis

WORKUP

Upper endoscopy (Fig. E2) with biopsy will confirm diagnosis. Endoscopic ultrasonography in combination with PET/CT scanning and operative lymph node dissection can be used in staging of the tumor. Table 1 and Fig. 1 describe staging systems for gastric carcinoma.

LABORATORY TESTS

- Microcytic anemia
- Hemoccult-positive stools
- Hypoalbuminemia

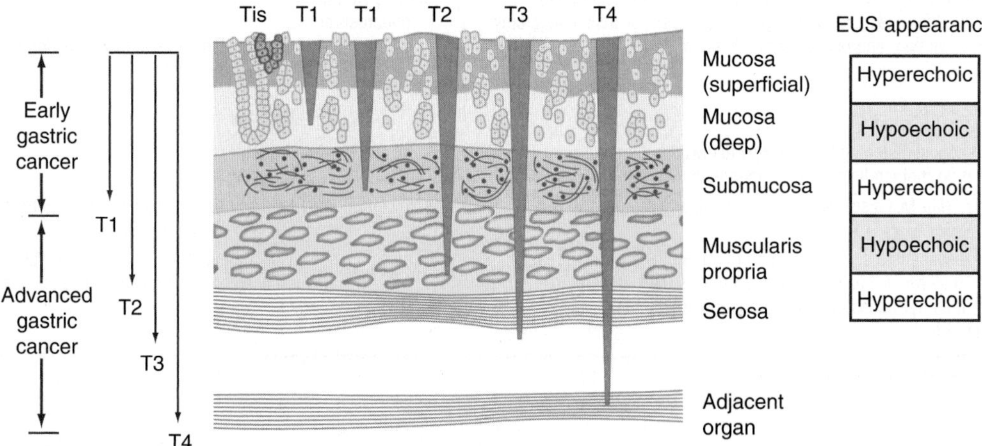

FIG. 1 Classification of gastric adenocarcinoma by depth of invasion (T classification). In the TNM classification, T denotes depth of invasion: T_{is} designates carcinoma in situ; T_1 tumors are confined to the mucosa (T_{1a}) and submucosa (T_{1b}); T_2 tumors invade the muscularis propria but not the serosa; T_3 tumors penetrate the subserosal connective tissue without involving the visceral peritoneum or contiguous structures; and T_4 tumors invade the serosa (visceral peritoneum) and may involve adjacent organs and tissues. In early gastric cancer, the disease is confined to the mucosa and submucosa (T_1), regardless of nodal involvement. *EUS*, Endoscopic ultrasound. (From Feldman M et al [eds]: *Sleisenger and Fordtran's gastrointestinal and liver disease*, ed 10, Philadelphia, 2016, Saunders.)

BOX 1 Risk Factors for Gastric Adenocarcinoma

Definite
H. pylori infection
Chronic atrophic gastritis
Intestinal metaplasia
Dysplasia*
Adenomatous gastric polyps
Cigarette smoking
History of gastric surgery (esp. Billroth II)
Genetic factors:
- Family history of gastric cancer (first-degree relative)
- Familial adenomatous polyposis (with fundic gland polyps)
- Hereditary nonpolyposis colorectal cancer
- Peutz-Jeghers syndrome
- Juvenile polyposis

Probable
High salt intake
Obesity (adenocarcinoma of the cardia only)
Snuff tobacco use
History of gastric ulcer
Pernicious anemia
Regular aspirin or other NSAID use (protective)

Possible
Statin use (protective)
Heavy alcohol use
Low socioeconomic status
Ménétrier disease
High intake of fresh fruits and vegetables (protective)
High ascorbate intake (protective)

Questionable
Hyperplastic and fundic gland polyps
Diet high in nitrates
High green tea consumption (protective)

*Surveillance for cancer is recommended in patients with this risk factor.
NSAID, Nonsteroidal antiinflammatory drug. From Feldman M et al (eds): *Sleisenger and Fordtran's gastrointestinal and liver disease*, ed 10, Philadelphia, 2016, Saunders.

- Abnormal liver enzymes in patients with metastasis to the liver
- Up to 25% of gastric cancers overexpress the HER2 growth factor receptor, and it is now standard practice to evaluate gastroesophageal tumors for HER2 overexpression.
- Mutation-specific predictive genetic testing by polymerase chain reaction amplification followed by restriction: Enzyme digestion and DNA sequencing for truncating mutations in *CDH1* is recommended in families of patients with familial diffuse cancer because gastric cancer develops in three of every four carriers of a mutant *CDH1* gene. Genetic abnormalities in gastric adenocarcinoma are summarized in Table E2.

IMAGING STUDIES

Chest and abdomen PET/CT scan (Fig. E3) to evaluate for metastases

TABLE 1 TNM Staging Criteria and Stages for Gastric Carcinoma based on AJCC 8th Edition

T category	T criteria
T_X	Primary tumor cannot be assessed
T_0	No evidence of primary tumor
T_{is}	Carcinoma *in situ*: Intraepithelial tumor without invasion of the lamina propria, high-grade dysplasia
T_1	Tumor invades the lamina propria, muscularis mucosae, or submucosa
T_{1a}	Tumor invades the lamina propria or muscularis mucosae
T_{1b}	Tumor invades the submucosa
T_2	Tumor invades the muscularis propria
T_3	Tumor penetrates the subserosal connective tissue without invasion of the visceral peritoneum or adjacent structures
T_4	Tumor invades the serosa (visceral peritoneum) or adjacent structures
T_{4a}	Tumor invades the serosa (visceral peritoneum)
N Category	**N Criteria**
N_X	Regional lymph node(s) cannot be assessed
N_0	No regional lymph node metastasis
N_1	Metastasis in one or two regional lymph nodes
N_2	Metastasis in three to six regional lymph nodes
N_3	Metastasis in seven or more regional lymph nodes
N_{3a}	Metastasis in 7 to 15 regional lymph nodes
M Category	**M Criteria**
M_0	No distant metastasis
M_1	Distant metastasis

Stage	pT	pN	M
Stage 0	T_{is}	N_0	M_0
Stage I_A	T_1	N_0	M_0
Stage I_B	T_1	N_1	M_0
	T_2	N_0	M_0
Stage II_A	T_1	N_2	M_0
	T_2	N_1	M_0
	T_3	N_0	M_0
Stage II_B	T_1	N_{3a}	M_0
	T_2	N_2	M_0
	T_3	N1	M_0
	T_{4a}	N_0	M_0
Stage III_A	T_2	N_{3a}	M_0
	T_3	N_2	M_0
	T_{4a}	N_1 or N_2	M_0
	T_{4b}	N_0	M_0
Stage III_B	T_1	N_{3b}	M_0
	T_2	N_{3b}	M_0
	T_3	N_{3a}	M_0
	T_{4a}	N_{3a}	M_0
	T_{4b}	N_1 or N_2	M_0
Stage III_C	T_3	N_{3b}	M_0
	T_{4a}	N_{3b}	M_0
	T_{4b}	N_{3a} or N_{3b}	M_0
Stage IV	Any T	Any N	M_1

AJCC, American Joint Committee on Cancer; *M,* metastases; *pN,* pathologic nodal; *pT,* pathologic tumor; *TNM, tumor, node, metastases.*

Rx TREATMENT

ACUTE GENERAL Rx

- Gastrectomy with regional lymphadenectomy is performed in patients who have early cancers with curative potential (<30% of patients at time of diagnosis). Routine or prophylactic splenectomy is not recommended.
- In advanced cases, palliative gastrectomy (bleeding, obstruction) can be performed. Outlet obstruction can be addressed by performing a gastrojejunostomy.
- In patients with operable gastric cancer, the perioperative regimen chemotherapy can decrease tumor size and stage while improving progression-free and overall survival. The older ECF regimen (epirubicin, cisplatin,

5-fluorouracil) has been now superseded by the FLOT (5-fluorouracil, leucovorin, oxaliplatin, docetaxel) regimen.

- Postoperative adjuvant chemoradiotherapy using 5-fluorouracil (5-FU) and leucovorin improves overall survival and is now the standard of care for stage II–III patients able to tolerate such treatment. Alternatively, combination chemotherapy with FOLFOX (5-fluorouracil, leucovorin, oxaliplatin) or CAPOX (capecitabine, oxaliplatin) regimens can be used in this setting.
- In metastatic gastric cancer, the use of chemotherapy with triplet or doublet regimens results in improved overall survival.
- In the subset of patients with gastric cancer expressing HER2-2/neu oncogene (20%-25% of patients), the addition of trastuzumab to cisplatin plus 5-FU or capecitabine prolongs overall survival. Patients progressing after first-line chemotherapy can derive a survival benefit with the use of chemotherapy in combination with antivascular endothelial growth factor receptor-2 antibody ramucirumab. Immunotherapy with program death receptor-1 antibodies (nivolumab, pembrolizumab) has been shown to improve survival in previously treated patients with high-MSI tumors.

DISPOSITION

- Median survival rate of metastatic or recurrent gastric carcinoma is 10 to 15 months overall.
- The 5-yr survival for early gastric cancers is >35%.

PEARLS & CONSIDERATIONS

COMMENTS

- Gastrectomy patients will need vitamin B_{12} replacement. They are also at risk for dumping syndrome and should be advised to ingest frequent, small meals.
- Prophylactic gastrectomy should be considered in young, asymptomatic carriers of germ-line truncating *CDH1* mutations who belong to families with highly penetrant heredity diffuse gastric cancer.
- Gastric cancer screening for average-risk patients is not recommended in the U.S.

SUGGESTED READINGS

Available at ExpertConsult.com

RELATED CONTENT

Stomach Cancer (Patient Information)

AUTHOR: **RITESH RATHORE, M.D.**

BASIC INFORMATION

DEFINITION

Histologically, *gastritis* refers to inflammation in the stomach. Endoscopically, gastritis refers to a number of abnormal features such as erythema, erosions, and subepithelial hemorrhages. Gastritis can also be subdivided into erosive, nonerosive, and specific types of gastritis with distinctive features both endoscopically and histologically.

SYNONYMS

Erosive gastritis
Hemorrhagic gastritis
Helicobacter pylori gastritis

ICD-10CM CODES

K29.00	Acute gastritis without bleeding
K29.01	Acute gastritis with bleeding
K29.20	Alcoholic gastritis without bleeding
K29.21	Alcoholic gastritis with bleeding
K29.30	Chronic superficial gastritis without bleeding
K29.31	Chronic superficial gastritis with bleeding
K29.40	Chronic atrophic gastritis without bleeding
K29.41	Chronic atrophic gastritis with bleeding
K29.50	Unspecified chronic gastritis without bleeding
K29.51	Unspecified chronic gastritis with bleeding
K29.60	Other gastritis without bleeding
K29.61	Other gastritis with bleeding
K29.70	Gastritis, unspecified, without bleeding
K29.71	Gastritis, unspecified, with bleeding
K52.81	Eosinophilic gastritis or gastroenteritis

EPIDEMIOLOGY & DEMOGRAPHICS

- Erosive and hemorrhagic gastritis is most commonly seen in patients taking nonsteroidal antiinflammatory drugs (NSAIDs), alcoholics, and critically ill patients (usually on ventilator support).
- *H. pylori* infection with gastritis is believed to be present in 30% to 50% of the population; however, the majority are asymptomatic.
- The prevalence of *H. pylori* infection increases with age from <10% in whites <40 yr to >50% in patients >50 yr.

PHYSICAL FINDINGS & CLINICAL PRESENTATION

- Patients with gastritis generally present with nonspecific clinical signs and symptoms (e.g., epigastric pain, abdominal tenderness, bloating, anorexia, nausea [with or without vomiting]). Symptoms may be aggravated by eating.
- Epigastric tenderness in acute alcoholic gastritis (may be absent in chronic gastritis).
- Foul-smelling breath.
- Hematemesis ("coffee grounds" emesis).

ETIOLOGY

- Alcohol, NSAIDs, stress (critically ill patients usually on mechanical respiration), hepatic or renal failure, multiorgan failure
- *H. pylori* infection
- Bile reflux, pancreatic enzyme reflux
- Gastric mucosal atrophy, portal hypertension gastropathy
- Irradiation

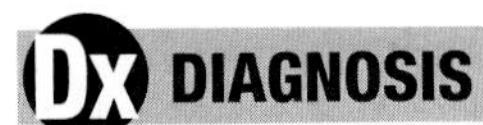

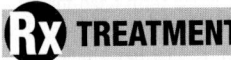

DIAGNOSIS

DIFFERENTIAL DIAGNOSIS

- Peptic ulcer disease
- Gastroesophageal reflux disease
- Nonulcer dyspepsia
- Gastric lymphoma or carcinoma
- Pancreatitis
- Gastroparesis

WORKUP

Diagnostic workup includes a comprehensive history and endoscopy with biopsy.

LABORATORY TESTS

- *H. pylori* testing by urea breath test, stool antigen test (*H. pylori* stool antigen), endoscopic biopsy, or specific antibody test is recommended.
  1. The urea breath test documents active infection (sensitivity and specificity >90%). It uses a flat breath card read by a small analyzer.
  2. The stool antigen test is an enzymatic immunoassay (ELISA) that identifies *H. pylori* antigen in a stool specimen with a polyclonal anti–*H. pylori* antibody. It is as accurate as the urea breath test for diagnosis of active infection and follow-up evaluation of patients treated for *H. pylori.* A negative result on the stool antigen test 8 wk after completion of therapy identifies patients in whom eradication of *H. pylori* was successful.
  3. Histologic evaluation of endoscopic biopsy samples is considered by many the gold standard for accurate diagnosis of *H. pylori* infection. However, detection of *H. pylori* depends on the site and number of biopsy samples, the method of staining, and experience of the pathologist.
  4. Serologic testing for antibodies to *H. pylori* is easy and inexpensive; however, the presence of antibodies demonstrates previous but not necessarily current infection. Antibodies to *H. pylori* can remain elevated for months to yrs after infection has cleared; therefore antibody levels must be interpreted in light of patient's symptoms and other test results (e.g., peptic ulcer disease [PUD] seen on upper gastrointestinal series).
- Vitamin B_{12} level in patients with atrophic gastritis.
- Hematocrit (low if significant bleeding has occurred).

TREATMENT

NONPHARMACOLOGIC THERAPY

- Avoidance of mucosal irritants such as alcohol and NSAIDs
- Lifestyle modifications with avoidance of tobacco and foods that trigger symptoms

ACUTE GENERAL Rx

- Eradication of *H. pylori,* when present, can be accomplished with various regimens:
  1. Quadruple therapy: Proton pump inhibitor (PPI) (omeprazole 20 mg, lansoprazole 30 mg, pantoprazole 40 mg, rabeprazole 20 mg) bid *plus* clarithromycin 500 mg BID plus amoxicillin 1000 mg bid *plus* metronidazole 500 mg BID for 14 days.
  2. Triple therapy: PPI bid *plus* clarithromycin 500 mg bid *and* metronidazole 500 mg bid for 14 days. This regimen is useful in those with penicillin allergy.
  3. Triple therapy: Clarithromycin 500 mg BID plus amoxicillin 1 g BID plus PPI BID for 14 days. Useful only in areas with clarithromycin resistance <15%.
  4. Bismuth quadruple therapy: Bismuth subsalicylate (e.g., Pepto-Bismol) 525 mg QID plus metronidazole 500 mg QID plus tetracycline 500 mg QID plus PPI BID for 14 days.
- Prophylaxis and treatment of stress gastritis with sucralfate suspension 1 g orally q4-6h, H_2-receptor antagonists, or PPIs in patients on ventilator support.

CHRONIC Rx

- Omeprazole, H2RB, or sucralfate in patients receiving long-term NSAIDs.
- Avoidance of alcohol, tobacco, and prolonged NSAID or corticosteroid use.

DISPOSITION

- Patients should be tested for eradication ≥4 weeks after completion of therapy. Undetectable stool antigen tested at least 4 wk after therapy accurately confirms cure of *H. pylori* infection in initially seropositive healthy subjects with reasonable sensitivity. PPI therapy should be stopped at least 2 weeks prior to testing.
- Surveillance gastroscopy in patients with atrophic gastritis (increased risk of gastric cancer).

RELATED CONTENT

Gastritis (Patient Information)
Helicobacter pylori Infection (Related Key Topic)
Peptic Ulcer Disease (Related Key Topic)

AUTHOR: **FRED F. FERRI, M.D.**

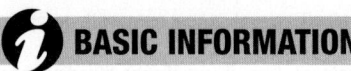

BASIC INFORMATION

DEFINITION

- Gastroenteritis is a broad term used for various gastrointestinal pathologic states. The main manifestation is diarrhea, defined as daily stool of at least 200 g, often accompanied by nausea, vomiting, malaise, anorexia, fever, abdominal pain, and dehydration. Gastroenteritis is usually self-limited, but if it is not managed properly, it can lead to a prolonged course. It usually lasts less than 7 days and not longer than 2 weeks. Diarrhea lasting more than 14 days is chronic or persistent.
- May be caused by viruses, bacteria, or parasites. Viruses are responsible for acute gastroenteritis in most patients.
- Gastroenteritis is a common cause of morbidity/mortality around the world. In the developing world, it is a leading cause of death.

ICD-10CM CODES

K52.9	Non-infective gastroenteritis and colitis
558.3	Allergic gastroenteritis and colitis
K52.1	Infectious gastroenteritis and colitis
K52.0	Gastroenteritis and colitis due to radiation

EPIDEMIOLOGY & DEMOGRAPHICS

- Frequency is difficult to determine. Gastroenteritis is underreported in adults.
- Statistics on sporadic cases of adult viral gastroenteritis are not known. Norovirus is the leading cause of medically attended acute gastroenteritis in U.S. children and is associated with nearly 1 million health care visits annually.
- It is estimated that there are 1.5 billion cases a yr worldwide.
- It is the leading cause of death in many developing countries. Children under the age of 5 yr are most vulnerable.
- Viral gastroenteritis may be transmitted by the fecal-oral route, by asymptomatic carriers, or by symptomatic patients before the symptoms start.
- Traveler's diarrhea affects 20% to 50% of residents of industrialized countries who travel to developing countries.

SEX: Higher mortality seen in women. Females have a higher incidence of *Campylobacter* infections.

AGE:

- May occur at any age
- High morbidity and mortality in the very young (younger than 5 yr), the elderly (people aged 65 or older), and the immunosuppressed

PHYSICAL FINDINGS & CLINICAL PRESENTATION

- Diagnosis is made clinically. Laboratory studies are not routinely necessary.
- A well-taken history is important. The onset, duration, and frequency of diarrhea should be noted. The aim of the physical examination is to assess the patient's degree of hydration. This also helps to identify the cause of diarrhea and identify patients at risk of complications.
- Viral gastroenteritis has a short prodome with vomiting, mild fever, nonbloody and watery diarrhea, usually for 1 to 4 days.
- Bacterial gastroenteritis presents with high fever, bloody diarrhea, severe abdominal pain, and at least 6 stools in a 24-hour period.
- Patients usually present with:
  1. Diarrhea: Usually more than 6 stools a day indicates bacterial cause of gastroenteritis.
  2. Vomiting.
  3. Abdominal pain.
  4. Mucus and/or blood in stool: Indicating bacterial or parasitic infection.
  5. Fever.
  6. Dehydration: This is the main cause of morbidity and mortality. Check for lethargy, dry mucous membrane, poor skin turgor, sunken eyes as signs of dehydration.
  7. Malnutrition: This occurs when diarrhea is chronic. There is reduced muscle and fat mass.
  8. Abdominal pain: This is a very common symptom in gastroenteritis.
  9. Borborygmi: There is significantly increased peristaltic activity, which may cause audible or palpable bowel activity.
  10. Perianal erythema: Secondary to constantly wet area. Wet buttock and perianal area may result in redness and skin breakdown.

ETIOLOGY

- Viral gastroenteritis (in adults)
  1. The caliciviruses, such as *Norovirus* genogroup I (e.g., Norwalk), *Norovirus* genogroup II (e.g., South Hampton), *Sapovirus* (e.g., Sapporo)
  2. Nongroup A *Rotavirus*
  3. *Astrovirus*
  4. Adenovirus
- Bacterial gastroenteritis: The top three leading causes of bacterial diarrhea worldwide are *Salmonella, Shigella,* and *Campylobacter* spp.
  1. *Salmonella* (eggs, dairy)
  2. *Shigella*
  3. *Campylobacter* (dairy, poultry)
  4. *Aeromonas species* (seafood, oysters)
  5. *Yersinia* (pork)
  6. Enterohemorrhagic *Escherichia coli* (ground beef)
  7. *E. coli*
  8. *Clostridium perfringens* (pork, vegetables)
- Parasitic gastroenteritis
  1. Gardia
  2. Cryptosporidium
  3. Microsporidia
  4. Cyclospora
- Traveler's diarrhea

  Usually caused by Enterotoxigenic *E. coli,* but other organisms implicated include *Salmonella, Shigella,* and *Campylobacter.*

  Risk is highest in travelers to Africa, but it is also common in travelers to Portugal, Spain, and some Eastern European countries.

Dx DIAGNOSIS

DIFFERENTIAL DIAGNOSIS

- Amebiasis
- Appendicitis
- Celiac disease
- Inflammatory bowel disease
- Colon cancer
- Bowel obstruction
- Botulism
- Hemolytic uremic syndrome
- Food poisoning
- Intraabdominal abscess
- Crohn disease

WORKUP

- In most cases laboratory tests are not indicated.
- Further workup is indicated in patients who:
  1. Have persistent diarrhea
  2. Are extremely dehydrated
  3. Appear seriously ill
  4. Have high fever
  5. Present with severe abdominal pain
  6. Have bloody diarrhea
  7. Have persistent nausea

LABORATORY TESTS

- Routine laboratory tests:
  1. Tests such as CBC and BMP may not be indicated in making a diagnosis. However, electrolytes and BUN are indicated in patients with severe diarrhea or dehydration.
  2. CBC is indicated with severe diarrhea or toxicity. WBC is increased in *Salmonella* infection; eosinophilia is present in parasitic infections.
- Stool studies:
  1. Presence of blood/leukocytes in stool may indicate inflammatory diarrhea.
  2. In *Salmonella* or *Shigella* infections there is an increased fecal leukocyte.
  3. Stool leukocytes are absent in viral diarrhea.
- Stool culture:
  1. Are only useful when positive.
  2. Usually not necessary in most cases of diarrhea.
  3. Indications for stool cultures include: Bloody stools; prolonged, untreated diarrhea; fever; leukocytes in stool; immunosuppressed patients; immunocompromised patients; and patients who have traveled to remote, exotic, or developing nations. It should also be considered in patients with concurrent or very recent use of antibiotics to rule out *Clostridium difficile* infection as a cause of the diarrhea.
- Examination for ova and parasites (O&P) is indicated in immunosuppressed patients, immunocompromised patients, and patients who have traveled to remote, exotic, or developing nations.

IMAGING STUDIES

- In patients with suspected bowel obstruction, perforation, or toxic megacolon, abdominal series is warranted.

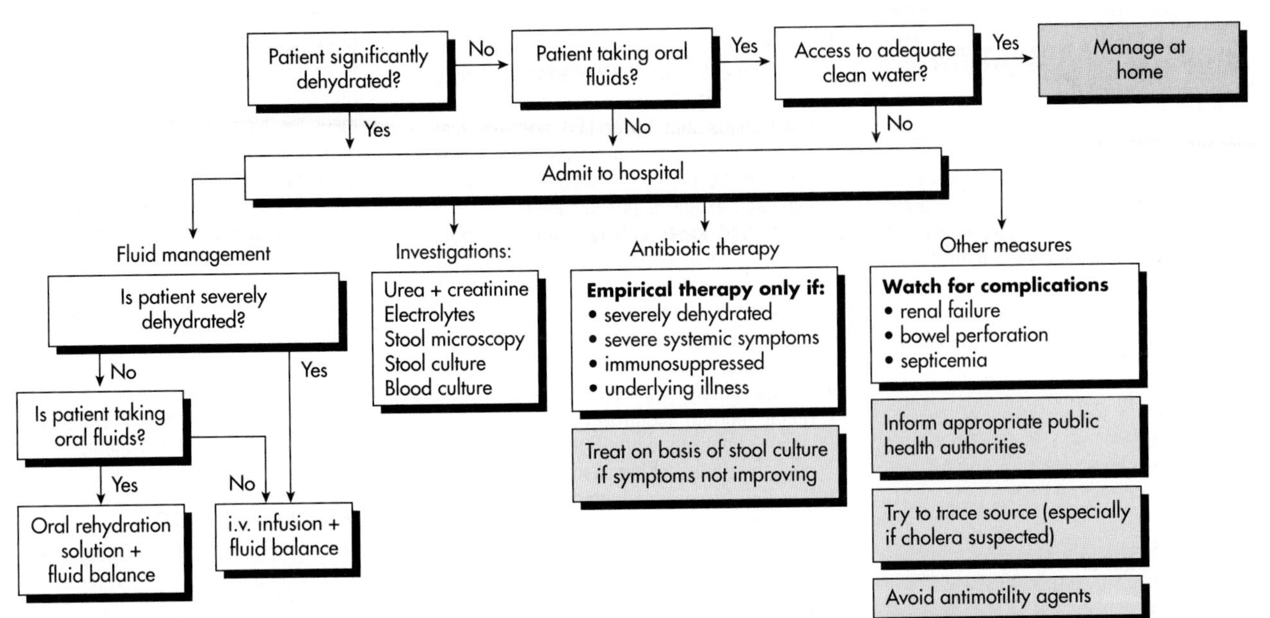

FIG. 1 Management of gastroenteritis. (From Currie G, Douglas G: *Flesh and bones of medicine*, St. Louis, 2011, Mosby, pp 8-9.)

- Consider CT scan of the abdomen in older patients with severe abdominal pain.

Rx TREATMENT

GENERAL CONSIDERATIONS

- Most infectious diarrhea is self-limited. Medical care is mainly supportive. Fig. 1 describes an approach to the management of gastroenteritis.
- It is important to assess the degree of dehydration by checking BP, pulse, HR, skin turgor, mucous membrane, thirst, urine output, and mental status change.
- Oral rehydration therapy is very important in diarrhea treatment.
- Consider intravenous rehydration when oral rehydration fails. Watch out for potassium depletion.
- Early re-feeding decreases recovery time.

Principles of treatment include:

- Rehydration: Orally or intravenously, PRN
- Treatment of symptoms such as fever, abdominal pain, nausea, vomiting as needed
- Identify and treat complications

REHYDRATION:

- Oral hydration products include Naturalyte, Rehydralyte.
- Intravenous solutions used include dextrose 5% in 0.5 isotonic NaCl with 50 mEq $NaHCO_3$ and 10-20 mEq KCl.
  1. Indications for IV hydration include intractable vomiting, severe dehydration, change in mental status or consciousness, and ileus.
  2. Oral hydration is not appropriate due to environmental conditions.

TREATMENT OF SYMPTOMS:

- Infectious diarrhea sometimes requires empiric treatment with antibiotics. Food-borne toxigenic diarrhea usually does not.
- Traveler's diarrhea: Patients without fever or dysentery may be treated with rifaximin 200 mg thrice daily for 3 days, or ciprofloxacin 500 mg twice daily or 750 mg daily for 1 to 3 days; patients with fever or dysentery can be treated with azithromycin 1000 mg in a single dose.
- *C. difficile* diarrhea and parasitic infestations with *Giardia* or *Entamoeba* are treated with metronidazole or vancomycin. For *C. difficile*, it is important to discontinue the causative antibiotic.
- Treat severe nausea and vomiting with antiemetics.
- Antidiarrheal agents may be useful for systemic relief in mild to moderate diarrhea.
- Loperamide (Imodium) or bismuth subsalicylate (Pepto-Bismol) may provide limited relief in traveler's or nonbloody diarrhea.

Dietary measures may include:

- Start with banana, rice, applesauce, toast diet (BRAT diet)
- As early as possible introduce lean meats and clear liquid

In recent yrs the use of probiotics (nonpathogenic live microorganism) has increased; however, recent multicenter trials of combination probiotic (combined *L. rhamnosus-L. helveticus* given twice/day) for children with gastroenteritis did not show any significant benefit and should not be recommended in young children with acute gastroenteritis.[1]

REFERRAL

Referral to infectious disease or gastroenterologist specialist may be indicated in patients:

- With diarrhea lasting more than 7 days
- Hypernatremia
- Severe dehydration associated with cardiovascular symptoms
- In whom a parasitic etiology is suspected
- With *C. difficile* resistant to treatment with metronidazole and vancomycin
- With HIV/AIDS, immunocompromised
- With clinical features indicating extraintestinal involvement (e.g., meningitis, sepsis, pneumonia) or another etiology (e.g., HUS)
- Who relapse

[1] Freedman SB, et al.: Multicenter trial of a combination probiotic for children with gastroenteritis, *N Engl J Med* 379:2015-26, 2018.

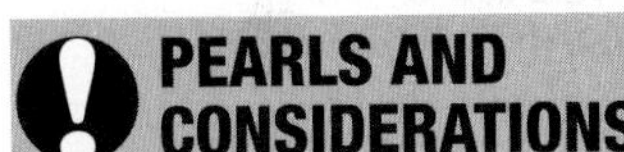

PEARLS AND CONSIDERATIONS

PREVENTION

- Perform proper hand washing before and after eating and after each bowel movement to prevent spread to family members.
- Avoid (raw) shellfish served in certain unregulated places.
- Avoid raw or undercooked eggs and/or poultry.
- Wash all produce before consumption.
- For travelers to high-risk areas:
  1. Eat only cooked foods.
  2. Drink hot or carbonated beverages.
  3. Avoid water, raw peeled fruits/vegetables, green leafy vegetables, and street food sold by street vendors.
  4. Vaccines are available for *Salmonella typhi* and *Vibrio cholerae* (the latter provides about 50% protection for 3-6 months).

PATIENT EDUCATION

- Stress the importance of oral rehydration.
- Stress the need for early appropriate feeding.
- Relapse occurs due to dietary noncompliance.
- Travelers to developing areas should be educated on proper avoidance measures and treatment.
- Also stress the importance of good hygiene, hand washing, safe food preparation, and access to clean water as key in preventing gastroenteritis.

SUGGESTED READINGS

Available at ExpertConsult.com

RELATED CONTENT

Clostridium Difficile Infection
Gastroenteritis (Patient Information)
Giardiasis
Traveler's Diarrhea

AUTHOR: **DANIEL K. ASIEDU, M.D., PH.D., F.A.C.P.**

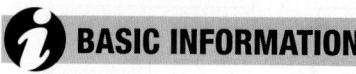

BASIC INFORMATION

DEFINITION

Gastroesophageal reflux disease (GERD) is a motility disorder characterized primarily by heartburn and caused by the reflux of gastric contents into the esophagus. A current definition is a condition that develops when the reflux of stomach contents causes at least two heartburn episodes per week and/or complications. Table 1 describes a classification system for esophagitis.

SYNONYMS

Peptic esophagitis
Reflux esophagitis
GERD

ICD-10CM CODES

K21.9	Gastroesophageal reflux disease without esophagitis
R12	Heartburn

EPIDEMIOLOGY & DEMOGRAPHICS

- GERD is one of the most prevalent gastrointestinal disorders. It is the most common GI diagnosis recorded during visits to outpatient clinics. From 14% to 20% of adults are affected.
- Nearly 7% of persons in the United States have heartburn daily, 20% have it monthly, and 60% have it intermittently. Incidence in pregnant women exceeds 80%.
- Nearly 20% of adults use antacids or over-the-counter H_2 blockers at least once a week for relief of heartburn.

PHYSICAL FINDINGS & CLINICAL PRESENTATION

- Physical examination: Generally unremarkable
- Clinical signs and symptoms: Heartburn, dysphagia, sour taste, regurgitation of gastric contents into the mouth
- Chronic cough and bronchospasm
- Chest pain, laryngitis, early satiety, abdominal fullness, and bloating with belching
- Dental erosions in children

TABLE 1 Los Angeles Endoscopic Classification System for Esophagitis

Grade A	One or more mucosal breaks confined to folds, ≤5 mm
Grade B	One or more mucosal breaks >5 mm confined to folds but not continuous between the tops of mucosal folds
Grade C	Mucosal breaks continuous between tops of two or more mucosal folds but not the circumferential
Grade D	Circumferential mucosal break

From Feldman M, Friedman LS, Brandt LJ: *Sleisenger and Fordtran's gastrointestinal and liver disease*, ed 10, Philadelphia, 2016, Elsevier.

ETIOLOGY

- Incompetent lower esophageal sphincter (LES) (see Fig. 1).
- Medications that lower LES pressure (calcium channel blockers, alpha-adrenergic antagonists, nitrates, theophylline, anticholinergics, sedatives, prostaglandins).
- Foods that lower LES pressure (chocolate, yellow onions, peppermint). Table 2 summarizes modulators of lower esophageal sphincter (LES) pressure.
- Tobacco abuse, alcohol, coffee.
- Pregnancy.
- Gastric acid hypersecretion.
- Hiatal hernia (controversial) present in >70% of patients with GERD; however, most patients with hiatal hernia are asymptomatic.
- Obesity is associated with a statistically significant increase in the risk for GERD symptoms, erosive esophagitis, and esophageal carcinoma.

Dx DIAGNOSIS

DIFFERENTIAL DIAGNOSIS

- Peptic ulcer disease
- Unstable angina
- Esophagitis (from infections such as herpes, *Candida*), medication induced (doxycycline, potassium chloride), eosinophilic esophagitis
- Esophageal spasm (nutcracker esophagus)
- Cancer of esophagus

WORKUP

- Aimed at eliminating the conditions noted in the differential diagnosis and documenting the type and extent of tissue damage. Generally, when symptoms of GERD are typical and the patient responds to therapy, there is no need for further diagnostic tests to verify the diagnosis.
- Upper GI endoscopy (Fig. E2) is useful to document the type and extent of tissue damage in persistent GERD and to exclude potentially malignant conditions such as Barrett esophagus. The American College of Physicians recommends endoscopy in the setting of GERD in people with heartburn and alarm symptoms (dysphagia, bleeding, anemia, weight loss, and recurrent vomiting). It is also indicated in people with GERD symptoms that persist despite a therapeutic trial of 4 to 8 weeks of bid proton pump inhibitor (PPI) therapy in patients with severe erosive esophagus after a 2-month course of PPI therapy to assess healing and rule out Barrett esophagus.

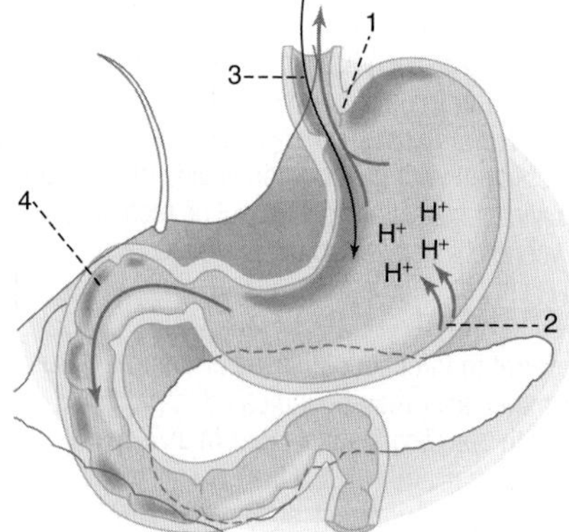

FIG. 1 Pathogenesis of gastroesophageal reflux disease: *(1)* impaired lower esophageal sphincter—low pressures or frequent transient lower esophageal sphincter relaxation; *(2)* hypersecretion of acid; *(3)* decreased acid clearance resulting from impaired peristalsis or abnormal saliva production; *(4)* delayed gastric emptying or duodenogastric reflux of bile salts and pancreatic enzymes. (From Andreoli TE et al: *Andreoli and Carpenter's Cecil essentials of medicine,* ed 8, Philadelphia, 2010, Saunders.)

LABORATORY TESTS

- 24-hr esophageal pH monitoring with transnasal catheter or a 48-hr wireless capsule are sensitive diagnostic tests to assess the degree of acid exposure in the esophagus in patients not responding to acid-reducing therapy; however, they are not practical and generally not done. They are useful in patients with atypical manifestations of GERD, such as chest pain or chronic cough.
- High-resolution esophageal manometry (HRM) is indicated in patients with refractory reflux in whom surgical therapy is planned.
- *Helicobacter pylori* testing is not indicated in GERD.

IMAGING STUDIES

An upper GI series is useful in patients unwilling to have endoscopy or with medical contraindications to the procedure. It can identify ulcerations and strictures; however, it may miss mucosal abnormalities. Only one third of patients with GERD have radiographic signs of esophagitis on an upper GI series.

Rx TREATMENT

NONPHARMACOLOGIC THERAPY

- Lifestyle modifications with avoidance of foods (e.g., citrus- and tomato-based products, onions, spicy foods, carbonated beverages, mint, chocolate, fried foods) and drugs that exacerbate reflux (e.g., caffeine, β-blockers, calcium channel blockers, α-adrenergic agonists, theophylline)
- Avoidance of tobacco and alcohol use
- Elevation of head of bed (4 to 8 in) with blocks
- Avoidance of lying down directly after late or large evening meals, consumption of smaller and more frequent meals
- Weight reduction to BMI <25, decreased fat intake
- Avoidance of clothing that is tight around the waist

GENERAL Rx

- PPIs (esomeprazole 40 mg qd, omeprazole 20 mg qd, lansoprazole 30 mg qd, rabeprazole 20 mg qd, or pantoprazole 40 mg

TABLE 2 Modulators of Lower Esophageal Sphincter (LES) Pressure

	Increase LES Pressure	Decrease LES Pressure
Hormones/peptides	Gastrin	CCK
	Motilin	Secretin
	Substance P	Somatostatin
		Vasoactive intestinal peptide
Neural agents	α-Adrenergic agonists	α-Adrenergic antagonists
	β-Adrenergic antagonists	β-Adrenergic agonists
	Cholinergic agonists	Cholinergic antagonists
Foods and nutrients	Protein	Chocolate
		Fat
		Peppermint
Other factors	Antacids	Barbiturates
	Baclofen	Calcium channel blockers
	Cisapride	Diazepam
	Domperidone	Dopamine
	Histamine	Meperidine
	Metoclopramide	Morphine
	Prostaglandin $F_2\alpha$	Prostaglandins E_2 and I_2
		Serotonin
		Theophylline

CCK, Cholecystokinin.
From Feldman M, Friedman LS, Brandt LJ: *Sleisenger and Fordtran's gastrointestinal and liver disease*, ed 10, Philadelphia, 2016, Elsevier.

TABLE 3 Drug Therapy for Esophageal Disorders

Agent	Dose
Antacids: Liquid (to Buffer Acid and Increase LESP)	
For example, Mylanta II/Maalox TC (acid-neutralizing capacity, 25 mEq/5 ml)*	15 ml qid 1 hr after meals and at bedtime or as needed
Gaviscon (to Decrease Reflux via a Viscous Mechanical Barrier and Buffer Acid)	
$Al(OH)_3$, $NaHCO_3$, Mg trisilicate, alginic acid	2-4 tablets qid at bedtime or as needed
H_2-Receptor Antagonists (to Decrease Acid Secretion)	
Cimetidine	800 mg bid, 400 mg qid, ≈13 ml bid
Ranitidine	150 mg qid or 10 ml qid; maintenance dose, 150 mg bid, 10 ml bid
Famotidine	20-40 mg bid or 2.5-5 ml bid
Nizatidine	150 mg bid
Proton Pump Inhibitors (to Decrease Acid Secretion and Gastric Volume)†	
Omeprazole	20 mg/day; maintenance dose, 20 mg/day
Lansoprazole	30 mg/day; maintenance dose, 15 mg/day
Pantoprazole	40 mg/day; maintenance dose, 40 mg/day
Rabeprazole	20 mg/day; maintenance dose, 20 mg/day
Esomeprazole	20-40 mg/day; maintenance dose, 20 mg/day
Dexlansoprazole	30-60 mg/day; maintenance dose, 30 mg/day

bid, Twice a day; *LESP,* lower esophageal sphincter pressure; *mEq,* milliequivalent; *qid,* four times a day.
*Patients with reflux are not generally hypersecretors of gastric acid, so the therapeutic doses of antacids are based on their capacity to buffer (normal) basal acid secretion rates of approximately 1 to 7 mEq/hr (mean, 2 mEq/hr) and peak meal-stimulated acid secretion rates of about 10 to 60 mEq/hr (mean, 30 mEq/hr).
†High-dose therapy is a twice-daily administration of the usual daily dose.
From Goldman L, Schafer AI: *Goldman's Cecil medicine*, ed 24, Philadelphia, 2012, Saunders.

qd, or dexlansoprazole 30 mg) are generally safe, tolerated, and highly effective in most patients when used on a short-term basis (Table 3). Omeprazole and esomeprazole are inhibitors of CYP2C19 and can increase serum concentrations of phenytoin and diazepam. Concomitant use of clopidogrel should also be avoided with omeprazole and esomeprazole. Increased risk of pneumonia has been documented in hospitalized patients. Long-term use of PPIs has been associated with increased risk of osteoporosis and patients should be warned about an increased risk of fractures with long-term use. Use of PPIs in patients with cirrhosis increases risk of spontaneous bacterial peritonitis and hepatic encephalopathy. Rare side effects of PPIs include acute interstitial nephritis, hypomagnesemia, and QT prolongation.

- H_2 blockers (nizatidine 300 mg qhs, famotidine 40 mg qhs, ranitidine 300 mg qhs, or cimetidine 800 mg qhs) can be used but are generally much less effective than PPIs.
- Antacids (may be useful for relief of mild symptoms; however, they are generally ineffective in severe cases of reflux).
- Prokinetic agents (metoclopramide) are indicated only when PPIs are not fully effective. They can be used in combination therapy; however, side effects limit their use.
- For refractory cases: Surgery with Nissen fundoplication (Fig. 3). Potential surgical candidates should have reflux esophagitis documented by esophagogastroduodenoscopy and normal esophageal motility as evaluated by manometry. Surgery generally consists of reduction of hiatal hernia when present and placement of a gastric wrap around the gastroesophageal (GE) junction (fundoplication). Although laparoscopic fundoplication is now widely used, long-term medical therapy is a better choice for most patients who are willing to remain on daily acid-reduction medication. In patients preferring surgical intervention, surgery should not be advised with the expectation that patients with GERD will no longer need to take antisecretory medications or that the procedure will prevent esophageal cancer among those with GERD and Barrett esophagus. Approximately 17.7% of patients who undergo primary laparoscopic antireflux surgery will experience recurrent gastroesophageal reflux requiring long-term medication use or secondary antireflux surgery. Risk factors for recurrence are older age, female sex, and comorbidity.
- Endoscopic radiofrequency heating of the GE junction (Stretta procedure) is a treatment modality for GERD patients unresponsive to traditional therapy. Its mechanism of action remains unclear. Endoscopic gastroplasty (EndoCinch procedure) is also aimed at treating GERD. Initial results appear encouraging; however, long-term studies are needed before recommending these procedures. A newer surgical approach to GERD is the LINX antireflux device (Figs. E4 and E5).
- Lifestyle modification must be followed for life because GERD is generally an irreversible condition in most patients.

DISPOSITION

- Recurrence of reflux is common if treatment is discontinued. Preliminary trials have shown that in patients with severe reflux esophagitis successfully treated with PPI therapy, stopping PPI medication was associated with T lymphocyte–predominant esophageal inflammation and basal cell and papillary hyperplasia without loss of surface cells. If replicated, these findings suggest that the pathogenesis of reflux esophagitis may be cytokine mediated rather than the result of chemical injury.[1]

[1] Dunbar KB et al: Association of acute gastroesophageal reflux disease with esophageal histologic changes, *JAMA* 315(19):2104–2112, 2016.

 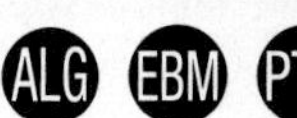

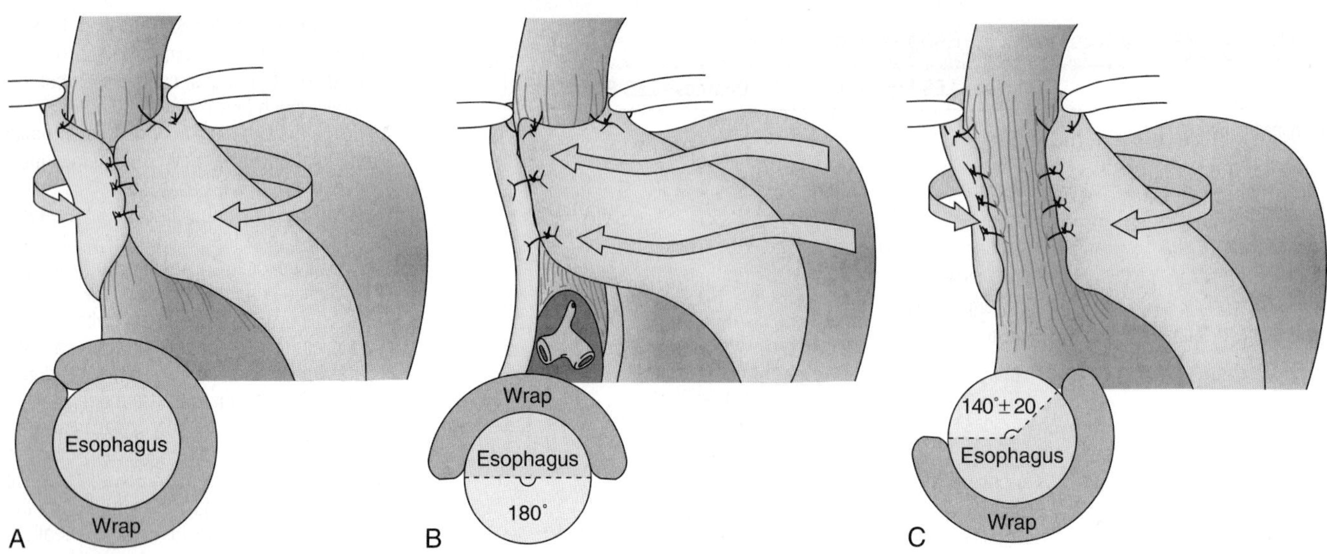

FIG. 3 Three types of fundoplication. A, A 360-degree fundoplication. **B,** Partial anterior fundoplication. **C,** Partial posterior fundoplication. (From Yates RB et al: Gastroesophageal reflux disease and hiatal hernia. In Townsend CM et al [eds]: *Sabiston textbook of surgery,* ed 20, Philadelphia, 2017, Elsevier.)

- The majority of patients respond well to therapy. In patients with chronic GERD, long-term outcomes are similar between medical therapy with PPIs and anti-reflux surgery. Prolonged use of PPIs is associated with increased risk of fractures of hip, wrist, and spine; increased risk of diarrhea from *Clostridium difficile;* pneumonia; and possible iron deficiency from impaired iron absorption. PPIs also block the effects of clopidogrel by inhibiting cytochrome P450 2C19 isozyme. Therefore all PPIs (other than pantoprazole) should be avoided in patients using clopidogrel. H_2 blockers (e.g., ranitidine) can be used for patients with GERD taking clopidogrel.
- Postsurgical complications occur in nearly 20% of patients (dysphagia, gas, bloating, diarrhea, nausea). Long-term follow-up studies also reveal that within 3 to 5 yr, 52% of patients who had undergone antireflux surgery are taking antireflux medications again.

REFERRAL

- There is a strong and probably causal relation between symptomatic prolonged and untreated GERD, Barrett esophagus, and esophageal adenocarcinoma. GI referral for upper endoscopy is needed when there are concerns about associated peptic ulcer disease, Barrett esophagus, or esophageal cancer.
- Patients with Barrett esophagus should undergo surveillance endoscopy with mucosal biopsy every 2 yr or less because the risk of developing adenocarcinoma of esophagus is at least 30 times greater than that of the general population.
- Testing and treating for *Helicobacter pylori* in patients with GERD has not been shown to improve symptoms.
- All children with dental erosions should be evaluated for GERD.

SUGGESTED READINGS

Available at ExpertConsult.com

RELATED CONTENT

Gastroesophageal Reflux Disease (GERD) (Patient Information)
Achalasia (Related Key Topic)
Dysphagia (Related Key Topic)

AUTHOR: **FRED F. FERRI, M.D.**

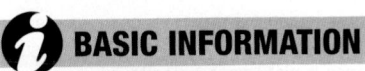

BASIC INFORMATION

DEFINITION

Genito-pelvic pain/penetration disorder, previously referred to as the separate conditions of "vaginismus" or "dyspareunia," is described in DSM-5 as encompassing "persistent or recurrent" difficulty in having intercourse, genital or pelvic pain associated with attempts at intercourse, fear or anxiety associated with the pain of intercourse, or tensing or tightening the pelvic floor muscles while attempting vaginal intercourse.

SYNONYM

Vaginismus

ICD-10CM CODES

N94.1	Unspecified dyspareunia
N94.2	Vaginismus
F52.5	Vaginismus not due to a substance or known physiological condition
F52.6	Dyspareunia not due to a substance or known physiological condition

EPIDEMIOLOGY & DEMOGRAPHICS

INCIDENCE: Estimated at 11.7% to 42% of women presenting to sexual dysfunction clinics.
PREVALENCE: Affects 14% to 34% of younger women and 6.5% to 45% of older women
PREDOMINANT SEX: Affects people with vulvas
RISK FACTORS: Any previous sexual trauma, including incest or rape.

PHYSICAL FINDINGS & CLINICAL PRESENTATION

- Fear of pain with coitus
- Dyspareunia
- Orgasmic dysfunction

ETIOLOGY

- Learned conditioned response (Fig. 1) to real or imagined painful vaginal experience (e.g., traumatic speculum examination, incest, rape)
- Vaginitis
- Pelvic inflammatory disease
- Endometriosis
- Anatomic anomalies
- Atrophic vaginitis
- Mucosal tears
- Inadequate lubrication
- Focal vulvitis
- Painful hymenal tags
- Scarring secondary to episiotomy
- Skin disorders
- Topical allergies
- Postherpetic neuralgia

Dx DIAGNOSIS

WORKUP

- Thorough history (including sexual history)
- Careful pelvic examination
- Behavioral therapy

Rx TREATMENT

NONPHARMACOLOGIC THERAPY

- Deconditioning the response by systematic self-administered progressive dilation techniques using fingers or dilators
- Behavioral and/or psychosexual therapy

ACUTE GENERAL Rx

- Botulinum toxin therapy given locally has been shown to relieve the perineal muscle spasms associated with vaginismus, allowing resumption of intercourse.
  1. Acts by preventing neuromuscular transmission, causing muscle weakness.
  2. Considered experimental treatment for vaginismus at this time.
- Cause should be determined by history and explained to the patient so that she understands the possible mechanics of this disorder.
- Patient must be motivated to desire painless vaginal insertion for such reasons as pleasurable coitus, tampon insertion, or gynecologic examination.
- Patient (and her partner) must be willing to patiently undergo the process of systematic desensitization and counseling.

DISPOSITION

A high percentage of successfully treated patients

REFERRAL

To a gynecologist or sex therapist

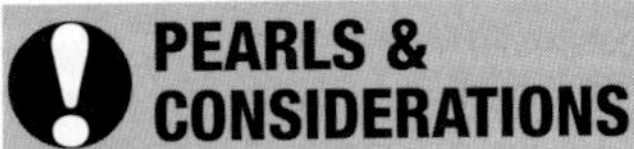

PEARLS & CONSIDERATIONS

COMMENTS

- May uncover early sexual abuse or an aversion to sexuality in general
- American Association of Sex Educators, Counselors and Therapists, 11 Dupont Circle, NW, Washington, DC, 20036
- Sex Information and Education Council of the United States (SIECUS), 90 John St., New York, NY 10038

RELATED CONTENT

Dyspareunia (Related Key Topic)

AUTHOR: **CAITLIN INGRAHAM, M.D.**

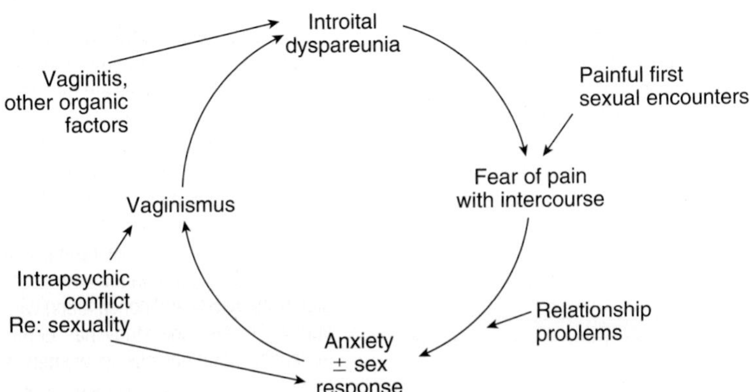

FIG. 1 Dyspareunia and vaginismus cycle. (From Lentz GM: *Emotional aspects of gynecology sexual dysfunction, eating disorders, substance abuse, depression, grief, loss; comprehensive gynecology*, St Louis, 2007, Mosby. Reference: Bergeron S et al: Female sexual pain disorders: a review of the literature on etiology and treatment, *Curr Sex Health Rep* 7:3, 2015.)

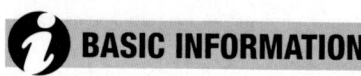

BASIC INFORMATION

DEFINITION

Gestational diabetes mellitus is hyperglycemia occurring during the second or third trimester in absence of a prepregnancy diagnosis of type 1 or type 2 diabetes.

Screening for gestational diabetes mellitus in asymptomatic pregnant women after 24 weeks' gestation is a grade B recommendation by the U.S. Preventive Services Task Force (USPSTF). In the U.S., a two-step approach to screening is commonly used and is currently endorsed by the American College of Obstetricians and Gynecologists (ACOG) and the National Institutes of Health (NIH). The International Association of Diabetes in Pregnancy Study Group has recommended a simplified one-step approach for screening and diagnosing GDM, which has been endorsed by the American Diabetes Association since 2011, with the acknowledgment that the one-step approach increases the prevalence of GDM without clear evidence of benefit. Pregnant women with diabetes mellitus (DM) (gestational or preexisting) are classified according to White's classification (Table 1).

SYNONYMS

Gestational diabetes
Diet-controlled gestational diabetes (A1)
Medication-treated gestational diabetes (A2)

ICD-10CM CODES

024.410 Gestational diabetes mellitus in pregnancy, diet controlled
024.414 Gestational diabetes mellitus in pregnancy, insulin controlled
024.419 Gestational diabetes mellitus in pregnancy, unspecified control
099.810 Abnormal glucose complicating pregnancy

EPIDEMIOLOGY & DEMOGRAPHICS

INCIDENCE: Approximately 5% of pregnant women in the U.S. will be diagnosed with GDM using the two-step approach and 18% using the one-step approach.

PREDOMINANT SEX AND AGE: Women of childbearing age; increased risk is observed in women over the age of 35 yr.

GENETICS: Higher rate in women with a family history of GDM or type 2 diabetes in a first-degree relative; specific HLA alleles (DR3 or DR4) predispose to the development of DM type 2 after pregnancy.

RISK FACTORS

- Overweight or obesity
- Family history of GDM or type 2 diabetes, particularly in first-degree relatives
- Polycystic ovarian syndrome
- Multiple gestation
- Hypertensive disorder of pregnancy or chronic hypertension
- Chronic systemic steroid use
- History of macrosomia in prior pregnancy
- Personal history of abnormal glucose tolerance or GDM in previous pregnancy
- Hispanic, Native American, African American, Asian, or Pacific Islander ethnicity
- Advanced maternal age (over age 25)
- Unexplained perinatal loss or malformation in previous or current pregnancy may be suggestive of preexisting diabetes

PHYSICAL FINDINGS & CLINICAL PRESENTATION

Suspect GDM if:

- Fetal size greater than dates on Leopold's or increased fundal height measurement
- Ultrasound findings of fetal macrosomia (especially enlarged abdominal circumference) or polyhydramnios
- Marked maternal obesity or weight gain above expected range
- Acanthosis nigricans (as underlying insulin resistance increases risk)
- Symptoms of diabetes
- Glucosuria
- Hemoglobin A1C greater than or equal to 5.7 in the first trimester

ETIOLOGY

During normal pregnancy several mechanisms contribute to increased insulin resistance. Placental secretion of human placental lactogen (hPL) decreases maternal insulin sensitivity, decreases maternal glucose utilization, and increases lipolysis, all to ensure adequate glucose availability to the growing fetus. Maternal pancreatic beta cells are increased in order to secrete additional insulin to compensate for the increased circulating blood glucose. Insulin resistance is also exacerbated by an increase in maternal adipose deposition, decreased exercise, and increased caloric intake. GDM occurs when maternal insulin secretion cannot meet the increased glucose burden, resulting in carbohydrate intolerance and hyperglycemia.

TABLE 1 White's Classification for Pregnant Women with Diabetes (Gestational or Preexisting)

Class	Description
A1	DM diagnosed during pregnancy and controlled by diet
A2	DM diagnosed during pregnancy and requiring medication
B	Insulin-requiring DM diagnosed before pregnancy, age >20 yr, lasting <10 yr
C	Insulin-requiring DM, onset at age 10 to 19 yr, with a duration 10 to 19 yr
D	Onset >10 yr or duration >20 yr, or associated with hypertension or background retinopathy
F	DM with renal disease
H	DM with coronary artery disease
R	DM with proliferative retinopathy
T	DM with renal transplant

DM, Diabetes mellitus.

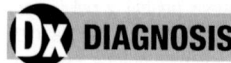

DIAGNOSIS

DIFFERENTIAL DIAGNOSIS

Preexisting type 1 or 2 DM not previously diagnosed

WORKUP

- History with focus on personal medical history, prior pregnancy history, and family history
- Routine prenatal examination
- Laboratory evaluation (see the following)

LABORATORY TESTS

- Exclude preexisting diabetes.
- For women with risk factors (see above), order a 1-hr glucose tolerance test at the first prenatal visit, then repeat at 24 to 28 weeks if initial screen was normal. If abnormal at intake, consider the probability of undiagnosed preexisting DM or underlying insulin resistance and check hemoglobin A1c. A diagnosis of diabetes is made if a woman meets any of the following criteria: fasting plasma glucose >126 mg/dl, A1c >6.5%, random plasma glucose >200 mg/dl. The authors consider a first-trimester A1c of ≥5.7 suggestive of preexisting insulin resistance, and would be inclined to monitor closely for hyperglycemia.
- Two-step approach:
    1. For screening without risk factors, a 1-hr, nonfasting 50-g oral glucose tolerance test (OGTT) is appropriate. If the result is abnormal (≥130 mg/dl, as defined by Carpenter and Coustan), a 3-hr, 100-g oral glucose tolerance test is performed. The diagnosis of GDM is made if two or more of the following glucose values are met or exceeded:
        a. Fasting: 95 mg/dl
        b. 1-hr plasma glucose: 180 mg/dl
        c. 2-hr plasma glucose: 155 mg/dl
        d. 3-hr plasma glucose: 140 mg/dl
- If one of four values on 3-hr glucose tolerance test is abnormal, consider repeat testing in 1 month and recommend a low-carbohydrate diet immediately and consultation with a nutritionist. At least one study has demonstrated increased perinatal risk in women with only one of four abnormal values on 3-hr OGTT.
- One-step approach:
    1. Like the two-step, a one-step screening is performed at 24 to 28 weeks on all pregnant patients who have not already been diagnosed with diabetes. This is a 2-hr, 75-g oral glucose tolerance test performed after an overnight, 8-hr fast. A diagnosis of GDM is made if one or more of the following values are met or exceeded:
        a. Fasting: ≥92 mg/dl

b. 1-hr plasma glucose ≥180 mg/dl
c. 2-hr plasma glucose ≥153 mg/dl

After pregnancy, women with GDM have an increased risk of developing diabetes during their lifetime. Women with GDM should be screened at or after 6 weeks postpartum with a 75-g 2-hour GTT to diagnose type 2 diabetes using the same criteria as nonpregnant patients. Alternatively, an HgbA1c can be performed at or after 12 weeks postpartum.

IMAGING STUDIES

Ultrasound for fetal size is performed in women with GDM. It may be initiated at the time of diagnosis and repeated every 3 to 4 weeks if macrosomia is suspected. Clinicians should consider local standards of care.

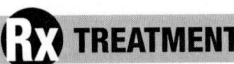

TREATMENT

NONPHARMACOLOGIC THERAPY

- Glucose monitoring:
  1. Four times daily: Fasting and 2-hr postprandial (defined as 2 hr after the start of each meal).
  2. Goals: Fasting <95 mg/dl; 2-hr postprandial <120 mg/dl.
  3. Can also use 1-hr postprandial goal of <140 mg/dl.
- Dietary modifications for glycemic control:
  1. Follow a low-carbohydrate diet; avoid sugar and concentrated sweets; and eat small, frequent meals (three meals with two snacks is often recommended).
  2. Complex carbohydrates should be consumed over simple carbohydrates to prevent glucose fluctuations.
  3. Diet should adequately meet the needs of pregnancy (below) while restricting carbohydrates to 33% to 40% of daily calories. Caloric needs in pregnancy:
     a. BMI <30: 30 kcal/kg/day
     b. BMI >30: 25 kcal/kg/day
     c. BMI >40: 12 to 14 kcal/kg/day
  4. Regular moderate exercise, defined as 30 minutes five times per week.
  5. Ongoing nutrition counseling throughout pregnancy.

PHARMACOLOGIC Rx

Initiate if >20% of glucose values are elevated after trial of diet control:

- Insulin: Considered the gold standard in GDM management.
  1. There are no randomized controlled trials on insulin regimens, and therapy is largely guided by expert opinion.
  2. Insulin is the only FDA-approved medication for GDM (Pregnancy Class B) and does not cross placenta.
  3. Insulin may be started first line or added when oral medications have failed to achieve glycemic control. The authors consider factors such as the degree of hyperglycemia, obstacles to medication adherence, and gestational age at time of diagnosis (with early-onset diagnosis more likely to progress and require insulin) when initiating therapy. The ADA recommends insulin as first-line pharmacotherapy for GDM, and ACOG (2017) mirrors this recommendation (Level A).
  4. Regardless of insulin regimen initiated, blood glucose values should be reviewed frequently, and the regimen adjusted and customized to optimize each woman's blood glucose levels; using a single agent or combination of long, intermediate and/or short-acting insulins.
  5. One commonly used regimen:
     - Insulin 0.7 to 1.0 U/kg/day SQ (based on current pregnant weight), with two thirds of the total daily dose given in the morning and one third of the total daily dose given in the evening
     - One third of each dose is given as short-acting insulin and the remaining two thirds as long-acting insulin
- Oral hypoglycemics:
  1. Oral antidiabetic agents continue to be used in the management of GDM, despite a lack of FDA approval for this indication.
  2. Several recent studies have examined the potential benefits and harms of metformin and glyburide, comparing them with the gold-standard insulin and with each other. Metformin (compared with insulin) has been demonstrated to decrease maternal glucose levels, maternal weight gain, and the risk of gestational hypertension. Evidence grows that it may decrease the risk of preeclampsia as well. Although known to cross the placenta, concerns about the long-term risk in exposed offspring have been mitigated by at least one recent study showing no neurodevelopmental differences with intrauterine exposure to metformin versus insulin. Meanwhile, recent meta-analyses have demonstrated worse neonatal outcomes with the use of glyburide compared with insulin. With both metformin and glyburide, many women go on to require insulin therapy.
  3. As of 2017, ACOG recommends "in women who decline insulin therapy or for those women whom the obstetrician or obstetric care provider believes the patient will be unable to safely administer insulin, metformin is a reasonable second-line choice" (Level B); while suggesting that glyburide should not be recommended as a first-line agent due to a failure to achieve equivalent outcomes to insulin in most studies (also Level B).
  4. Metformin: Begin at 500 mg PO nightly or bid, and titrate up to a maximum of 2500 mg daily in divided doses.
  5. Glyburide: Begin at 2.5 mg qd, and titrate up to a maximum of 20 mg qd (10 mg bid). Increase dose as needed by 2.5 to 5 mg/wk.

ANTENATAL TESTING

Antepartum testing is recommended for women with pregestational diabetes and gestational diabetes. There is no consensus regarding initiation, frequency or modality of antepartum testing in gestational diabetes, and this should be guided by local standards.

ONE COMMONLY USED REGIMEN

- Weekly NST/AFI beginning at 32 weeks or when medications are initiated in women with GDMA2. Less frequent testing or delayed initiation of testing may be considered in women who maintain glycemic control with diet alone (GDMA1), as increased rates of stillbirth have not been observed in these women before 40 weeks' gestation.
- Preexisting or poorly controlled diabetes, vascular complications, or concomitant hypertension: Twice weekly NST/AFI beginning at 28 weeks. Consider hospital admission to obtain glycemic control.

TIMING AND ROUTE OF DELIVERY

- Women with preexisting diabetes should be induced at 39 weeks.
- Women with GDMA2 may also be induced at 39 weeks unless otherwise indicated, with decisions regarding induction guided by local standards of care.
- In women with GDMA1, ACOG supports expectant management of up to 40 and 6/7 weeks with appropriate antepartum testing.
- Counsel regarding elective cesarean section at or after 39 weeks if estimated fetal weight is over 4500 g.
- Consider delivery earlier than 39 weeks if poor glycemic control or other medical indications such as growth restriction or preeclampsia.

INTRAPARTUM MANAGEMENT

- Goal is normoglycemia (80 to 120 mg/dl) using insulin and D5 lactated Ringer IV fluid if needed.
- Monitor glucose every 1 to 2 hours in active labor.
- Preparation for shoulder dystocia.
- If on glyburide, discontinue in labor or 12 hr before a scheduled induction.
- If on insulin consider decreased long-acting insulin by one third to one half before scheduled induction. Most experts recommend holding insulin entirely the morning of a scheduled cesarean delivery.

POSTPARTUM MANAGEMENT

- Class A2: Check fasting blood glucose level before discharge; if abnormal, continue checking at home and schedule early follow-up with primary care physician to confirm diagnosis of DM.
- 6-wk postpartum visit: Screen for impaired glucose tolerance and diabetes with a 75 g, 2-hr glucose tolerance test. Alternatively, an HgbA1c may be performed at or after 12 weeks postpartum.

- If no evidence of DM, screen annually for DM and counsel on risk factor modification.

REFERRALS

- Nutritionist
- Maternal-fetal medicine
- Diabetes educator
- Nurse care manager, when available

COMPLICATIONS

- Maternal: Preeclampsia, future type 2 DM or GDM, operative delivery
- Fetal: Polyhydramnios, macrosomia, congenital malformations, shoulder dystocia, birth trauma, IUFD
- Neonatal: Hypoglycemia, hypocalcemia, hyperbilirubinemia, polycythemia, perinatal death, respiratory distress, future obesity, and DM

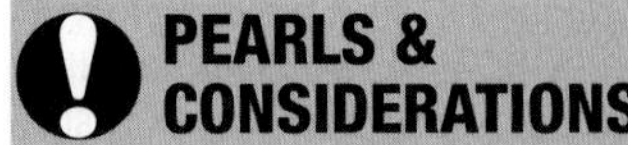

PEARLS & CONSIDERATIONS

- Trials have shown that although treatment of mild gestational DM did not significantly reduce the frequency of a composite outcome that included stillbirth or perinatal death and several neonatal complications, it did reduce the risks of fetal overgrowth, shoulder dystocia, cesarean delivery, and hypertensive disorders.
- Lactation improves maternal glucose metabolism and may prevent or delay the development of type 2 DM following GDM. Higher lactation intensity and longer duration are independently associated with lower 2-yr incidences of DM after a GDM-affected pregnancy.

PREVENTION

Regular exercise, maintenance of ideal body weight, and high-fiber low-glycemic diet

SUGGESTED READINGS

Available at ExpertConsult.com

RELATED CONTENT

Gestational Diabetes (Patient Information)
Diabetes Mellitus (Related Key Topic)

AUTHORS: **ASHLEY LAKIN, D.O., M.A.,** and **SUSANNA R. MAGEE, M.D., M.P.H.**

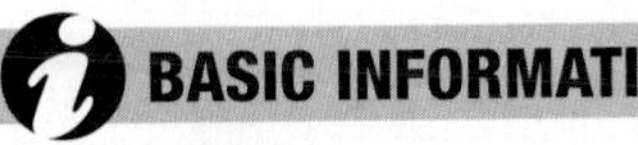

BASIC INFORMATION

DEFINITION

Giant cell arteritis (GCA) is a segmental systemic granulomatous arteritis affecting medium and large arteries in individuals >50 yr. Inflammation primarily targets branches of the extracranial head and neck blood vessels (external carotids, temporal arteries, ciliary and ophthalmic arteries). The aorta and subclavian and brachial arteries can also be affected. Intracranial arteritis is rare.

SYNONYMS

Temporal arteritis
Cranial arteritis
GCA
Horton disease

ICD-10CM CODES

M31.5 Giant cell arteritis with polymyalgia rheumatica
M31.6 Other giant cell arteritis

EPIDEMIOLOGY & DEMOGRAPHICS

INCIDENCE: Approximately 20 new cases per 100,000 persons >50 yr; peak incidence is in patients ages 60 to 80 yr.

PREVALENCE: 200 cases per 100,000 persons; it is the most common primary vasculitis; female/male predominance of twofold to fourfold; more common in Caucasians.

PHYSICAL FINDINGS & CLINICAL PRESENTATION

GCA can present with the following clinical manifestations:

- Headache, often associated with marked scalp tenderness—noticed while brushing hair (hair comb allodynia).
- Constitutional symptoms (fever, weight loss, anorexia, fatigue).
- Polymyalgia rheumatica (aching and stiffness of the trunk and proximal muscle groups).
- Visual disturbances (transient or permanent monocular or binocular visual loss).
- Intermittent claudication of jaw and tongue on mastication that is especially prominent when solid food such as steak is chewed.
- Table 1 describes atypical manifestations of GCA.

Important physical findings in GCA:

- Vascular examination: The temporal artery demonstrates tenderness, decreased pulsation, and nodularity (ropy) (Fig. 1); diminished or absent pulses in upper extremities may be seen.

ETIOLOGY

Vasculitis of unknown etiology. An association with HLA-DRB*04 has been identified. Recent demonstration of varicella zoster virus virion, antigen, and DNA within the vessel walls of the temporal arteries on histopathologic specimens of giant cell arteritis suggest an association.

TABLE 1 Atypical Manifestations of Giant Cell Arteritis

Fever of unknown origin
Respiratory symptoms (especially cough)
Otolaryngeal manifestations
Glossitis
Lingual infarction
Throat pain
Hearing loss
Large-artery disease
Aortic aneurysm
Aortic dissection
Limb claudication
Raynaud's phenomenon
Neurologic manifestations
Peripheral neuropathy
Transient ischemic attack (TIA) or stroke
Dementia
Delirium
Myocardial infarction
Tumorlike lesions
Breast mass
Ovarian and uterine mass
Syndrome of inappropriate antidiuretic hormone secretion (SIADH)
Microangiopathic hemolytic anemia

From Harris ED, et al.: *Kelly's textbook of rheumatology,* ed 7, Philadelphia, 2005, Saunders.

Dx DIAGNOSIS

Clinical history and vascular examination remain cornerstones of diagnosis. An algorithm for diagnosing GCA is described in Fig. 2. The American College of Rheumatology has proposed classification criteria to aid in the diagnosis of GCA. Presence of three or more of these criteria in a patient with suspected vasculitis is considered to be suggestive of GCA.

- Age of onset of symptoms >50 yr.
- New-onset of or new type of localized headache.
- Temporal artery abnormalities including tenderness or decreased pulsation.
- Westergren erythrocyte sedimentation rate (ESR) elevated (typically >50 mm/hr).
- Temporal artery biopsy with vasculitis and mononuclear cell infiltrate or granulomatous changes.

DIFFERENTIAL DIAGNOSIS

- Other vasculitic syndromes
- Nonarteritic anterior ischemic optic neuropathy (NAION)
- Pituitary apoplexy
- Primary amyloidosis
- Transient ischemic attack, stroke
- Infections
- Occult neoplasm, multiple myeloma

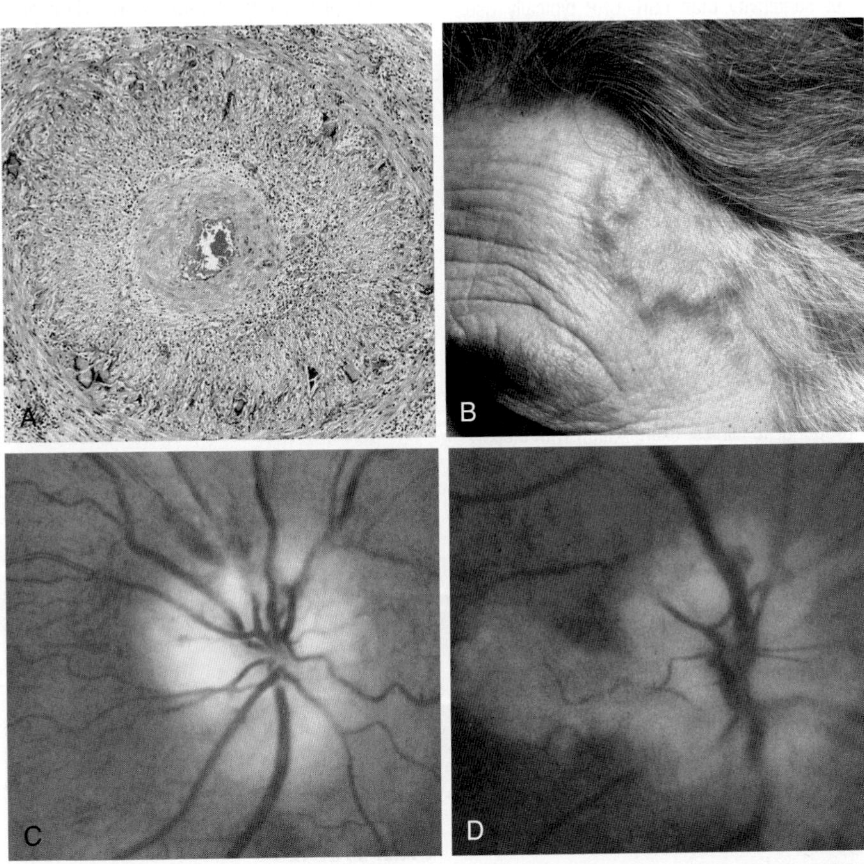

FIG. 1 Giant cell arteritis. A, Histology shows transmural granulomatous inflammation, disruption of the internal elastic lamina, proliferation of the intima, and gross narrowing of the lumen. **B,** The superficial temporal artery is pulseless, nodular, and thickened. **C,** Ischemic optic neuropathy. **D,** Ischemic optic neuropathy and cilioretinal artery occlusion. (From Kanski JJ, Bowling B: *Clinical ophthalmology, a systematic approach,* ed 7, Philadelphia, 2010, Saunders.)

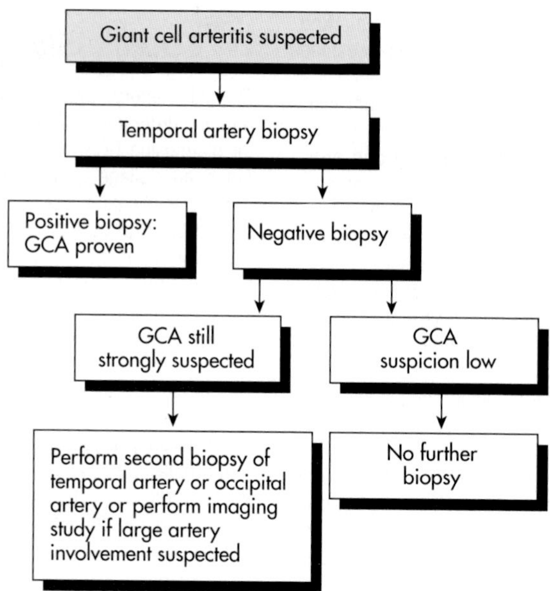

FIG. 2 Algorithm for diagnosing giant cell arteritis *(GCA)*. (From Firestein GS, et al.: *Kelly's textbook of rheumatology,* ed 9, Philadelphia, 2013, Saunders.)

LABORATORY TESTS

- ESR elevated although up to 22% of patients with GCA have normal ESR before treatment.
- C-reactive protein (CRP) is typically included in laboratory investigation; it may have greater sensitivity than ESR. CRP typically rises before the ESR.
- Mild to moderate normochromic normocytic anemia, elevated platelet count.

IMAGING STUDIES

Imaging studies do not play a major role in diagnosing GCA and are rarely indicated:

- Color duplex ultrasonography (CDUS) of temporal artery produces three characteristic features—periluminal "halo" over the temporal artery involved, segmental arterial stenosis, and arterial luminal occlusion in severe cases. CDUS of the temporal artery has 40% to 75% sensitivity and 79% to 83% specificity for diagnosis of GCA. Clinical utility is not superior to clinical examination with biopsy.
- Contrasted MRI of temporal artery may be performed in patients with contraindications to surgical biopsy of the superficial temporal artery if treatment with steroids has not been initiated. MRI has a 78.4% sensitivity and 90.4% specificity in detecting temporal artery involvement in patients with a clinical diagnosis of GCA.
- Angiography of the arms is indicated in patients with peripheral vascular insufficiency.
- FDG-PET imaging may be used to detect large-vessel inflammation in GCA.

Rx TREATMENT

ACUTE GENERAL Rx

- If there is clinical suspicion of GCA, treatment should be initiated without waiting for results of laboratory or imaging studies.
- IV methylprednisolone (250-1000 mg for 1-3 days) is considered standard of care in patients with severe clinical manifestations such as visual loss from ischemic optic neuropathy.
- Oral prednisone (1 mg/kg/day): High-dose oral regimen should be continued at least until symptoms resolve and ESR returns to normal; usually 3 to 4 wk after treatment initiation. Steroid taper is very slow (10% to 20% per mo) with monitoring of clinical features as well as ESR and CRP. When dose <10 mg/day, taper by 1 mg/mo. Treatment may last up to 2 yr or more.

Although corticosteroids have traditionally been the treatment of choice, tocilizumab, an IL-6 receptor blocker, was recently approved by the FDA for the treatment of GCA. Patients treated with tocilizumab and prednisone achieved remission faster, had a greater reduction in steroid dosage, and had prolonged maintenance of remission when compared with those treated with prednisone alone.

There is no evidence for the role of other steroid-sparing agents.

DISPOSITION

With steroid therapy there is a dramatic improvement of systemic symptoms, but not vision in patients with ischemic optic neuropathy. In one study only 4% of eyes improved in both visual acuity and central visual field.

Management of flares: Repeat prednisone induction if patient experiences severe flare. If mild flare, increase prednisone by 10% to 20% and slow down prednisone taper.

REFERRAL

- Surgical or ophthalmologic referral for biopsy of temporal artery.
- Rheumatology referral for long-term immunosuppressive treatment management.

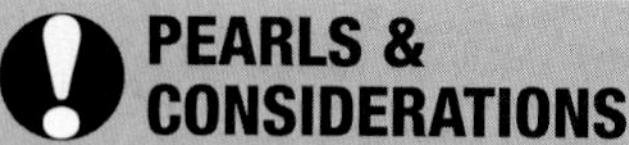

PEARLS & CONSIDERATIONS

- Treatment of GCA should be started if there is clinical suspicion of the disease. This usually includes patients above the age of 50 presenting with a severe headache and systemic features that suggest GCA as well. Physicians should not wait for laboratory or pathologic confirmation before starting treatment as the risk of visual loss increases. Blindness from untreated GCA is permanent.
- Temporal artery biopsy should be performed as soon as possible, but within 2 wk of initiating treatment with steroids. The biopsy may remain positive for 2 to 6 wk after initiation of corticosteroids.
- Treatment should not be withheld pending temporal artery biopsy.
- Temporal artery biopsy may not be required in patients with typical disease features accompanied by characteristic ultrasound or MRI findings.

COMMENTS

- The relation between polymyalgia rheumatica and GCA is unclear, but the two frequently coexist. They are considered to be different points along the gradient or spectrum of the same disease.
- Clinical picture rather than ESR should be the prime yardstick for continuing prednisone therapy. A rising ESR in a clinically asymptomatic patient with normal hematocrit should raise suspicion for alternate explanations (e.g., infections, neoplasms).
- GCA is associated with a markedly increased risk for the development of aortic aneurysm, which is often a late complication and may cause death. Annual chest radiograph in chronic CGA patients has been suggested, as well as emergent chest CT or MRI for clinical suspicion.
- GCA is also associated with increased risk of myocardial infarction, stroke, and peripheral vascular disease.
- Coadministration of low dose aspirin (81 mg/day) has been reported by some as effective for further reduction of risk of blindness. Additional trials may be needed before it can be recommended as standard therapy.

SUGGESTED READINGS

Available at ExpertConsult.com

RELATED CONTENT

Giant Cell Arteritis (Patient Information)
Temporal Arteritis (Patient Information)

AUTHORS: **JOSEPH S. KASS, M.D., J.D., ARUN SWAMINATHAN, M.B.B.S.,** and **SACHIN KEDAR, M.B.B.S., M.D.**

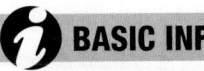

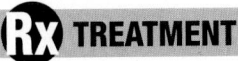

BASIC INFORMATION

DEFINITION

Giardiasis is an intestinal and/or biliary tract infection caused by the non-invasive protozoal parasite *Giardia intestinalis* (also known as *G. lamblia* or *G. duodenalis*). The organism is a widespread zoonotic parasite and frequently contaminates fresh water sources worldwide.

SYNONYMS

Giardiasis
Giardia duodenalis (accepted species name by the CDC)
Giardia intestinalis

ICD-10CM CODE
A07.1 Giardiasis [lambliasis]

EPIDEMIOLOGY & DEMOGRAPHICS

INCIDENCE (IN U.S.):
- Exact incidence unknown. CDC estimates 20,000 cases a year in the U.S.
- Frequently occurs as waterborne outbreaks in international adoptees, travelers, immunocompromised patients, and those with cystic fibrosis.
- *G. lamblia* has been demonstrated in 4% to 7% of submitted stool specimens, making it the most commonly identified intestinal parasite.

PREVALENCE (IN U.S.): 4%
PREDOMINANT SEX: Male = female
PREDOMINANT AGE:
- Preschool children, especially if in day care
- 20 to 40 yr of age, especially among sexually active homosexual men (oral-anal contact)

PEAK INCIDENCE:
- Varies with risk factors, outbreaks, but peak onset from early summer through early fall
- All age groups affected

GENETICS: Familial disposition: Patients with common variable immunodeficiency or X-linked agammaglobulinemia are at increased risk of infection.

PHYSICAL FINDINGS & CLINICAL PRESENTATION

- More than 70% with one or more intestinal symptoms (diarrhea, flatulence, cramps, bloating, nausea). Table 1 summarizes clinical signs and symptoms of giardiasis
- Incubation period averages 7 to 21 days
- Fever in <30%
- Chronic diarrhea, malabsorption, and weight loss, which can be up to 10% of body weight, are common
- GI bleeding is unusual
- Continuous or intermittent symptoms, lasting for 2 to 4 weeks
- Of infected patients, 20% to 25% are asymptomatic and can shed cysts for months

TABLE 1 Symptoms of Giardiasis

Symptom	Frequency (%)
Flatulence	56–74
Anorexia	40–64
Abdominal cramps	55–80
Foul-smelling stool	57–72
Abdominal distention	31
Bloating	55–69
Nausea	58–68
Malaise	84
Diarrhea	89
Belching	30
Weight loss	48–64
Fever	17–28

From Cherry JD, et al.: *Feigin and Cherry's pediatric infectious diseases*, ed 8, Philadelphia, 2019, Elsevier.

ETIOLOGY

Infection is acquired by ingestion of viable cysts of the organism (Fig. 1), typically in contaminated water or food or by fecal-oral contact. *Giardia* cysts are resistant to chlorination and survive well in cold mountain streams.

DIAGNOSIS

DIFFERENTIAL DIAGNOSIS

- Other agents of infective diarrhea (amebae, *Salmonella* sp., *Shigella* sp., *Staphylococcus aureus, Cryptosporidium*, etc.)
- Noninfectious causes of malabsorption

WORKUP

- Stool specimen (three specimens yield 90% sensitivity) as a saline suspension or duodenal aspirate for microscopic examination to establish diagnosis and exclude other pathogens
- Immunoassays for *Giardia* sp. Antigens in stool samples such as the DFA or ELISA are now routinely used in most clinical laboratories. These assays are 85% to 98% sensitive and 90% to 100% specific. They are more sensitive than stool microscopy for confirming the diagnosis. They also have a faster turnaround time.

LABORATORY TESTS

Serum albumin, vitamin B_{12} levels, and stool fat test to exclude malabsorption

IMAGING STUDIES

- Not necessary unless biliary obstruction is suspected
- In detection of organism, possible interference by barium in stool from radiographic studies

TREATMENT

NONPHARMACOLOGIC THERAPY

Avoidance of milk products to reduce symptoms of transient lactase deficiency that occur in many patients and can last for weeks to months

GENERAL Rx

Adult and pediatric (Table E2):
- Metronidazole 250 mg PO three times daily for 5 to 10 days. Pediatric dose: 5 mg/kg tid × 7 days (metronidazole should be avoided in pregnancy)
- Alternative regimen: Tinidazole: 2 g single dose (50 mg/kg in children over 3 years of age)
- Nitazoxanide: aged 12 to 47 mo: 100 mg bid × 3 days. Aged 4 to 11 yr: 200 mg bid × 3 days
- Quinacrine: 100 mg po TID × 5 to 7 days
- Albendazole 400 mg PO qd × 5 days
- Paromomycin 25 to 35 mg/kg/day in three doses for 5 to 10 days. Safe for pregnancy.

DISPOSITION

Reinfection is possible. Post-infection lactose intolerance is common and is frequently mistaken for recurrent infection.

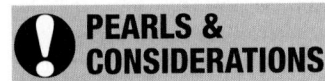

PEARLS & CONSIDERATIONS

COMMENTS

Travelers to endemic areas (developing world, wilderness areas) should be cautioned to boil drinking water or use water purification tablets (for iodine-containing products, chlorination is not effective). Chronic giardiasis as seen in developing nations can cause delays in growth and development in children due to malabsorption and diarrhea.

SUGGESTED READINGS
Available at ExpertConsult.com

RELATED CONTENT

Giardiasis (Patient Information)

AUTHOR: **GLENN G. FORT, M.D., M.P.H.**

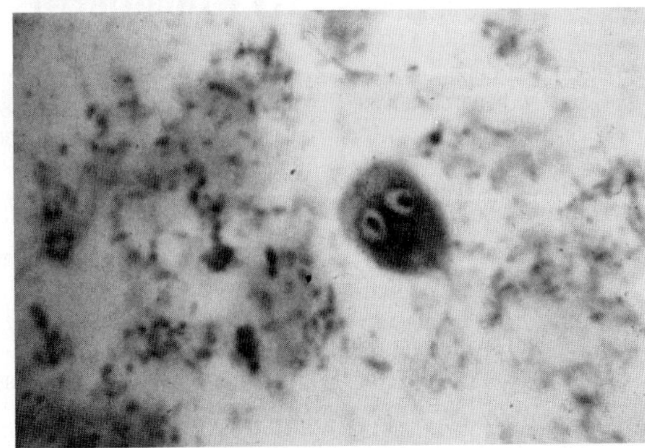

FIG. 1 ***Giardia lamblia*** **trophozoite is demonstrated in a trichrome stain of fecal material.** Note the prominent nuclei in the trophozoite. (From Bennett JE, Dolin R, Blaser MJ: *Mandell, Douglas, and Bennett's principles and practice of infectious diseases*, ed 8, Philadelphia, 2015, Saunders.)

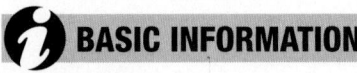

BASIC INFORMATION

DEFINITION

Gilbert syndrome is an autosomal-dominant disorder characterized by indirect hyperbilirubinemia caused by impaired glucuronyl transferase activity.

SYNONYM

Gilbert disease

ICD-10CM CODE
E80.4 Gilbert syndrome

EPIDEMIOLOGY & DEMOGRAPHICS

INCIDENCE (IN U.S.): Probable autosomal-dominant disease affecting >5% of the U.S. population

PREDOMINANT SEX: Male:female ratio of 3:1

GENETICS: Most common hereditary hyperbilirubinemia (genotypic prevalence 12%)

PHYSICAL FINDINGS & CLINICAL PRESENTATION

- No abnormalities on physical examination other than mild jaundice when bilirubin exceeds 3 mg/dl.
- A family history of unconjugated hyperbilirubinemia may be present.

ETIOLOGY

- Decreased elimination of bilirubin in bile is caused by inadequate conjugation of bilirubin.
- Alcohol consumption and starvation diet can increase bilirubin level.
- The pathogenesis of Gilbert syndrome has been linked to a reduction in the bilirubin UGT-1 gene *(HUG-Brl)* transcription, resulting from a mutation in the promoter region.

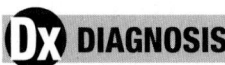

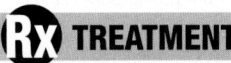

DIAGNOSIS

DIFFERENTIAL DIAGNOSIS

- Hemolytic anemia
- Liver disease (chronic hepatitis, cirrhosis)
- Crigler-Najjar syndrome

WORKUP

- Most patients are diagnosed during or after adolescence, when isolated hyperbilirubinemia is detected as an incidental finding on routine biochemical testing.
- Laboratory evaluation to exclude hemolysis and liver diseases as a cause of the elevated bilirubin level (Table 1 and Fig. 1).

LABORATORY TESTS

Elevated indirect (unconjugated) bilirubin (rarely exceeds 5 mg/dl)

TABLE 1 Characteristic Patterns of Liver Function Tests

Disorder	Bilirubin	Alkaline Phosphatase	AST	ALT	Prothrombin Time	Albumin
Gilbert syndrome (abnormal bilirubin metabolism)	↑	NL	NL	NL	NL	NL
Bile duct obstruction (pancreatic cancer)	↑↑↑	↑↑↑	↑	↑	↑-↑↑	NL
Acute hepatocellular damage (toxic, viral hepatitis)	↑-↑↑↑	↑-↑↑	↑↑↑	↑↑↑	NL-↑↑↑	NL-↓↓
Cirrhosis	NL-↑	NL-↑	NL-↑	NL-↑	NL-↑↑	NL-↓↓

ALT, Alanine aminotransferase; *AST,* aspartate aminotransferase; *NL,* normal; ↑, increase; ↓, decrease (arrows indicate extent of change: ↑-↑↑↑, slight to large).
From Andreoli TE (ed): *Cecil essentials of medicine,* ed 6, Philadelphia, 2005, Saunders.

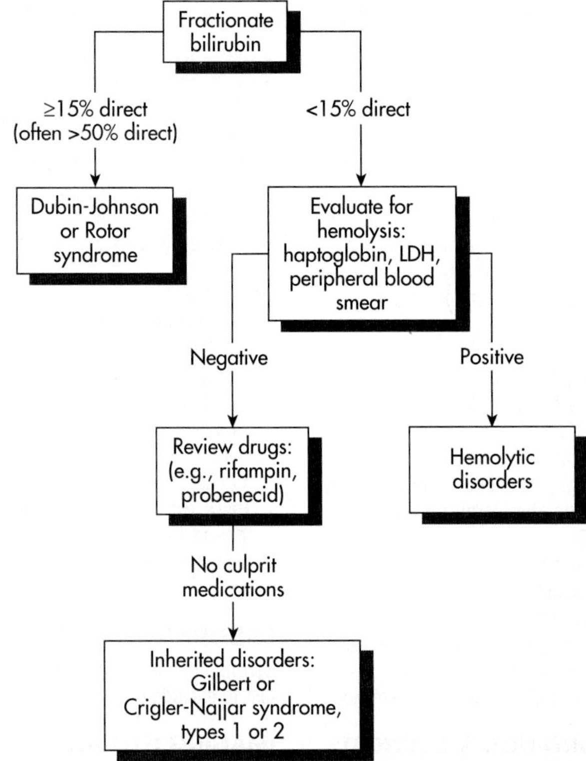

FIG. 1 Evaluation of an isolated elevation of the serum bilirubin level. *LDH,* Lactic dehydrogenase. (From Feldman M et al [eds]: *Sleisenger and Fordtran's gastrointestinal and liver disease,* ed 10, Philadelphia, 2016, Saunders.)

TREATMENT

ACUTE GENERAL Rx

Treatment is generally unnecessary. Phenobarbital (if clinical jaundice is present) can rapidly decrease serum indirect bilirubin level.

DISPOSITION

Prognosis is excellent. Treatment is generally unnecessary.

REFERRAL

Referral is generally not necessary.

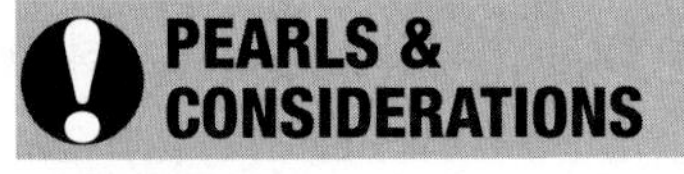

PEARLS & CONSIDERATIONS

COMMENTS

- Patients should be reassured about the benign nature of the condition.
- Fasting for 2 days or significant dehydration may raise the bilirubin level and result in the clinical recognition of jaundice.

AUTHOR: **FRED F. FERRI, M.D.**

BASIC INFORMATION

DEFINITION

Glaucoma is a chronic degenerative optic neuropathy (or the high potential for such degeneration due to risk factors) in which the neuro-retinal rim of the optic nerve becomes progressively thinner, thereby enlarging the optic-nerve cup. The classification of glaucoma is based on the appearance of the iridocorneal angle (open angle vs. narrow or closed angle) and is further subdivided into primary and secondary types. Fig. 1 and Table 1 illustrate the difference between open-angle and narrow-angle glaucoma. Primary open-angle glaucoma can occur with or without elevated intraocular pressure (IOP). Normal tension glaucoma refers to primary open-angle glaucoma without elevated intraocular pressure.

SYNONYMS

Primary open-angle glaucoma (POAG)
Open-angle glaucoma or chronic open-angle glaucoma (OAG, COAG)
Secondary open-angle glaucoma (e.g., pseudoexfoliation, pigment dispersion, trauma, inflammatory)
Ocular hypertension (elevated intraocular pressure with no evidence of optic nerve damage)
Optic nerve cupping, glaucoma suspect

ICD-10CM CODES

H40.10X0	Unspecified open-angle glaucoma, stage unspecified
H40.10X1	Unspecified open-angle glaucoma, mild stage
H40.10X2	Unspecified open-angle glaucoma, moderate stage
H40.10X3	Unspecified open-angle glaucoma, severe stage
H40.10X4	Unspecified open-angle glaucoma, indeterminate stage
H40.11X0	Primary open-angle glaucoma, stage unspecified
H40.11X1	Primary open-angle glaucoma, mild stage
H40.11X2	Primary open-angle glaucoma, moderate stage
H40.11X3	Primary open-angle glaucoma, severe stage
H40.11X4	Primary open-angle glaucoma, indeterminate stage

EPIDEMIOLOGY & DEMOGRAPHICS

INCIDENCE (IN U.S.): Third most common cause of vision loss (75% to 95% of all forms of glaucoma are open angle)

PEAK INCIDENCE:
- Increases after age 40 yr
- Three million cases expected by 2020 because of the rapid increase in aging population

PREVALENCE (IN U.S.):
- Overall prevalence in U.S. population aged >40 yr is estimated to be 1.86%, with 1.57 million white and 398,000 black patients affected. By 2020, we may expect more than 3 million cases in the U.S.
- 150,000 patients have bilateral blindness.
- Prevalence is higher in diabetics, those with high myopia, and older persons.
- More common in African-American population (three times the age-adjusted prevalence than whites). There is a genetic tendency to OAG; multiple genes have been isolated that are associated with development of high IOP and optic nerve damage.

PREDOMINANT AGE:
- Persons >50 yr
- Can occur in 30s and 40s, and juvenile forms are rare

PHYSICAL FINDINGS & CLINICAL PRESENTATION

- High intraocular pressures and/or large optic nerve cup (Fig. E2). Ocular Hypertension Treatment Study results help to delineate important risk factors.
- Abnormal visual fields (with advanced glaucoma damage to the optic nerve).
- Open anterior chamber angle—evaluated with gonioscopy at slit lamp
- Figs. E3 and E4 illustrate stages of open-angle glaucoma.
- Since early treatable stages of OAG normally have no symptoms, it's important to have routine eye exams, especially patients with family history and patients over 60 yr.
- Secondary forms of OAG may exhibit ocular findings such as pseudo-exfoliation, pigment dispersion, blood in anterior chamber, inflammation.

ETIOLOGY

- Uncertain hereditary tendency (multifactorial genetics)
- Topical steroids can induce high IOP and cause glaucoma
- Trauma
- Inflammatory (e.g., history of uveitis)
- High-dose oral corticosteroids taken for prolonged periods

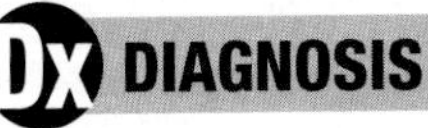

DIAGNOSIS

DIFFERENTIAL DIAGNOSIS

- Other optic neuropathies (previous retinal vascular disorders, optic nerve pits, or coloboma).
- Physiologic cupping of the optic nerve: The optic nerve may appear similar to glaucoma damage but does not progress. This is followed for any signs of progression.
- Ocular hypertension: IOP is chronically elevated, but not causing optic nerve damage, must monitor closely.
- Secondary glaucoma from inflammation and steroid therapy.
- Trauma

WORKUP

- Comprehensive eye examination
- Intraocular pressure
- Slit lamp examination
- Visual fields
- Gonioscopy: To determine the type of glaucoma (narrow, open, or closed angles)
- Nerve fiber analysis (e.g., GDx, OCT, and HRT)
- Corneal thickness (thick central cornea will result in possible overestimation of the true physiologic IOP, and vice versa, so this is

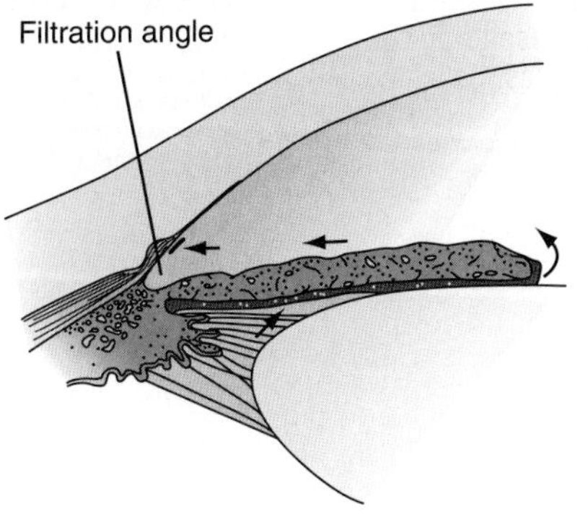

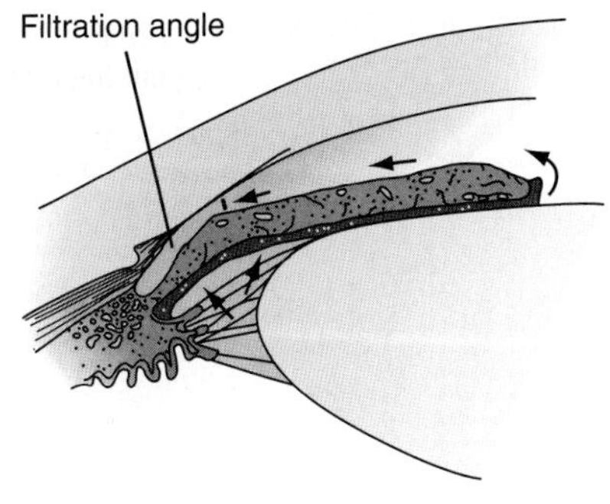

FIG. 1 A, Open-angle glaucoma: Drainage of the aqueous humor becomes obstructed, and impaired flow from the eye leads to gradually increased intraocular pressure. **B,** Narrow-angle glaucoma: When the iris moves forward, as may occur during pupil dilation, the angle is narrowed or even closed. Obstruction of aqueous humor flow leads to angle-closure glaucoma. (From Kaufman DM, Geyer HL, Milstein MJ: *Kaufman's clinical neurology for psychiatrists*, ed 8, Philadelphia, 2017, Elsevier.)

TABLE 1 Characteristics of Glaucoma

Feature	Primary Open-Angle Glaucoma	Narrow-Angle Glaucoma
Occurrence	85% of all glaucoma cases	15% of all glaucoma cases
Cause	Unclear*	Closed angle prevents aqueous drainage
Age at onset	Variable	50 to 85 years
Anterior chamber	Usually normal	Shallow
Chamber angle	Normal	Narrow
Symptoms	Usually none Decreased vision, late	Headache Seeing halos around lights Sudden onset of severe eye pain Vomiting during attack
Cupping of disc	Progressive if not treated	After one or more untreated attacks
Visual fields	Peripheral fields are involved early Central involvement is a very late sign	Involvement is a late sign
Ocular pressure	Progressively higher if not medically controlled Late: High	Early: Detected with provocative tests only
Other signs		Fixed, partially dilated pupil Conjunctival injection "Steamy" cornea†
Treatment	Medical Laser surgery	Surgical
Prognosis	Good if recognized early Very dependent on patient compliance	Good

*Thought to be a defect in the trabecular network ultrastructure.
†Like looking through a steamy window.
From Swartz MH: *Textbook of physical diagnosis, history and examination*, ed 7, Philadelphia, 2014, Elsevier.

important information in diagnosis and treatment of OAG)

LABORATORY TESTS

Blood sugar

IMAGING STUDIES

- Optic nerve photography—stereo photographs
- Visual field testing
- Laser scan of nerve fiber layer, OCT, HRT. Rarely, MRI of orbits if the glaucoma findings are atypical or suspicious of other causes of optic nerve atrophy.

ACUTE GENERAL Rx

- β-Blockers (e.g., timolol) qd to bid depending on individual response to drug.
- Carbonic anhydrase inhibitors (e.g., Diamox 250 mg qid or 500 mg bid).
- Prostaglandin analogues (latanoprost, bimatoprost, travoprost, tafluprost) are commonly used as first-line treatment. They lower intraocular pressure by 25% to 30% by increasing uveoscleral outflow and reducing aqueous production.
- Alpha-2 agonists and cholinergic agonists.
- Hyperosmotic agents (mannitol) in acute treatment (IV).
- Selective laser trabeculoplasty (SLT) may delay or forestall need for second eye drop. The effect may be temporary but the laser can be repeated.

CHRONIC Rx

- At least biannual checks of intraocular pressure and adjustment of medication.
- Surgical trabeculectomy and filter valve surgeries can be considered for glaucoma that progresses (optic nerve changes or visual field progression) despite maximal tolerated medical therapies. Recently, minimally invasive glaucoma surgeries (MIGS) have been advocated for IOP control. Some are performed at the time of cataract procedures and some are independent procedures. The effort is to reduce the risks associated with traditional trabeculectomy.

DISPOSITION

Must be followed by ophthalmologist

REFERRAL

Immediately to ophthalmologist

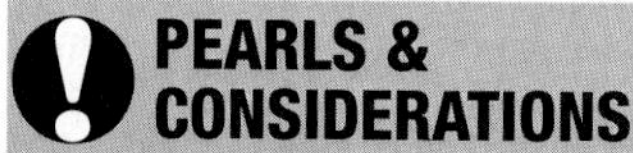

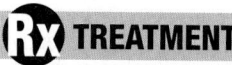

COMMENTS

- Glaucoma is a serious blinding disease that must be monitored professionally by an ophthalmologist. It is mostly asymptomatic until late in the disease when visual problems arise. Even in developed countries half of glaucoma cases are undiagnosed.
- Risk factors that should prompt referral to an ophthalmologist for evaluation of glaucoma are high intraocular pressure, family history of glaucoma, use of systemic or topical corticosteroids, older age, and black race.
- Vision loss from glaucoma cannot be recovered. Early diagnosis and treatment may minimize visual loss.
- Glaucoma is not solely caused by increased intraocular pressure because approximately 20% of patients with glaucoma have normal intraocular pressure. However, high pressure is definitely a risk factor to be considered.

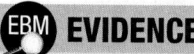

Available at ExpertConsult.com

SUGGESTED READINGS

Available at ExpertConsult.com

RELATED CONTENT

Glaucoma (Patient Information)

AUTHOR: **R. SCOTT HOFFMAN, M.D.**

BASIC INFORMATION

DEFINITION

Primary angle-closure glaucoma occurs when elevated intraocular pressure is associated with closure of the filtration angle or obstruction in the circulating pathway of the aqueous humor.

SYNONYMS

Acute glaucoma, angle-closure glaucoma (ACG)
Pupillary block glaucoma
Narrow-angle glaucoma
Angle-closure glaucoma

ICD-10CM CODES

H40.061	Primary angle closure without glaucoma damage, right eye
H40.062	Primary angle closure without glaucoma damage, left eye
H40.063	Primary angle closure without glaucoma damage, bilateral
H40.069	Primary angle closure without glaucoma damage, unspecified eye

EPIDEMIOLOGY & DEMOGRAPHICS

INCIDENCE (IN U.S.):
- 2% to 8% of all patients with glaucoma.
- Higher incidence among those with hyperopia, small eyes, dense cataracts, shallow anterior chambers.

PEAK INCIDENCE: Greater >50 yr; high association with hyperopia, cataracts, and eye trauma
PREDOMINANT SEX: Females are affected more often than males.
PREDOMINANT AGE: 50 to 60 yr
GENETICS: Family history is not particularly helpful; far-sighted (hyperopes) individuals with thickening lenses (i.e., cataracts) are often those with angle-closure attacks.

PHYSICAL FINDINGS & CLINICAL PRESENTATION

- Although angle-closure glaucoma can present with an acute painful crisis associated with blurred vision, more than 75% of patients present with an asymptomatic course with progressive loss of the visual field (similar to that in patients with primary open-angle glaucoma; referred to as intermittent, subacute, or chronic angle closure)
- Hazy cornea
- Narrow angle
- Pain may be present (supraorbital headache is typical)
- Injection of conjunctiva, red eye (often severe limbal conjunctival injection with very high intraocular pressure [IOP])
- Shallow anterior chamber (one can shine a light from the side to perceive the forward position of the iris with narrow AC angles)
- Thick cataract
- Pupil may be mid-dilated and nonreactive to light
- Figs. E1 and E2 illustrate gonioscopy in primary angle-closure glaucoma

ETIOLOGY

- Narrow angles with acute closure: Blockage of circulatory path of the aqueous humor (Fig. E3) causing increase in IOP. ACG (primary angle closure glaucoma) occurs more commonly in eyes with shorter axial length (farsightedness), shallower anterior chamber, and a relatively larger lens (enlarging cataract).
- Secondary angle-closure glaucoma (more rare) resulting from neovascularization of iris, iris tumors, lens induced, iris scarring, trauma, chronic inflammation with scarring, malignant glaucoma with aqueous misdirection.

DIAGNOSIS

DIFFERENTIAL DIAGNOSIS

- Open-angle glaucoma: Angle-closure glaucoma is distinguished from open-angle glaucoma by the closure of the angle between the iris and cornea, obstructing outflow of aqueous humor
- High intraocular pressure (normal IOP is usually 8 to 21 mm Hg)
- Optic nerve cupping
- Shallow chamber
- Open-angle glaucoma
- Conjunctivitis
- Corneal disease, keratitis
- Uveitis
- Scleritis
- Allergies
- Contact lens wearing with irritation

WORKUP

Comprehensive eye examination: If one suspects narrow angle or angle closure, avoid pupil dilation, as this may exacerbate the attack.
- Intraocular pressure (with ACG, IOP can be extremely high, >60 mm Hg)
- Gonioscopy for direct visualization of the chamber angle
- Slit lamp examination
- Visual field examination
- GDx examination (laser scan of nerve fiber layer), optical coherence tomography (OCT)
- Optic nerve evaluation
- Anterior chamber depth

LABORATORY TESTS

- Blood sugar and complete blood count (if diabetes or inflammatory disease is suspected)
- Visual field
- GDx nerve fiber analysis, OCT, Heidelberg retinal tomography

IMAGING STUDIES

- Fundus photography (optic nerve photos)
- Fluorescein angiography for neovascular disease such as diabetic retinopathy, retinal vein occlusions
- Ultrasound biomicroscopy and anterior OCT can show relationships of anterior eye structures

TREATMENT

The goal of treatment is to acutely lower pressure on the eye and keep it down.

NONPHARMACOLOGIC THERAPY

Laser iridotomy early in disease process

ACUTE GENERAL Rx

- IV mannitol
- Pilocarpine
- β-Blockers
- Diamox
- Laser iridotomy
- Anterior chamber paracentesis (as emergency treatment)

CHRONIC Rx

- Iridotomy: When there is an adequate peripheral hole in the iris, the chance for future angle closure is usually eliminated.
- Lens removal (cataract extraction) can also eliminate the possibility of ACG.
- Trabeculectomy and filter valve procedures for non-responsive cases.
- Other laser procedures, such as gonioplasty for atypical angle closures.

DISPOSITION

Refer to ophthalmologist immediately.

REFERRAL

If acute angle-closure episode is suspected, should refer emergently to ophthalmologist.

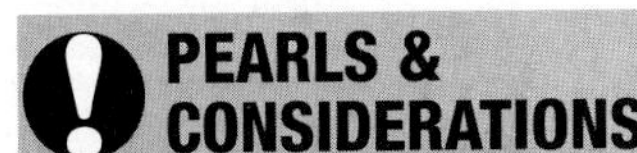

PEARLS & CONSIDERATIONS

COMMENTS

- Do not use antihistamines or vasodilators with narrow-angle glaucoma.
- After iridotomy, the majority of patients will be totally cured and will need no further medication and have no visual loss.
- Lower socioeconomic status and higher levels of social deprivation are risk factors for delayed detection and probable worse outcomes in glaucoma.
- Risk factors that should prompt referral to an ophthalmologist for evaluation of glaucoma are high intraocular pressure, family history of glaucoma, use of systemic or topical corticosteroids, older age, and black race.
- Glaucoma is undiagnosed in 9 out of 10 affected people worldwide and is undiagnosed in 50% of those in developed countries.
- Angle closure has become rarer because most people have cataract extractions at an earlier stage than in the past.

SUGGESTED READINGS

Available at ExpertConsult.com

RELATED CONTENT

Glaucoma (Patient Information).
Glaucoma, Open Angle (Related Key Topic)

AUTHOR: **R. SCOTT HOFFMAN, M.D.**

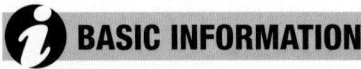

BASIC INFORMATION

DEFINITION

Gonorrhea is a sexually transmitted bacterial infection with a predilection for columnar and transitional epithelial cells. It commonly manifests as urethritis, cervicitis, or salpingitis. Infection may be asymptomatic. It differs between males and females in course, severity, and ease of recognition.

SYNONYMS

Gonococcal urethritis
Gonococcal vulvovaginitis
Gonococcal cervicitis
Gonococcal bartholinitis
GC

ICD-10CM CODES

A54.9	Gonococcal infection, unspecified
O98.211	Gonorrhea complicating pregnancy, first trimester
O98.212	Gonorrhea complicating pregnancy, second trimester
O98.213	Gonorrhea complicating pregnancy, third trimester
O98.219	Gonorrhea complicating pregnancy, unspecified trimester
O98.22	Gonorrhea complicating childbirth
O98.23	Gonorrhea complicating the puerperium
A54.03	Gonococcal cervicitis, unspecified
A54.00	Gonococcal infection of lower genitourinary tract, unspecified

EPIDEMIOLOGY & DEMOGRAPHICS

- The disease is common worldwide, affects both sexes and all ages, especially younger adults; highest incidence is in inner-city areas. Per CDC reports, approximately 470,000 new cases were found in the United States in 2016 with over 60% found in metropolitan statistical centers. Gonorrhea is the second most commonly reported communicable disease.
- Asymptomatic anterior urethral carriage may occur in 12% to 50% of cases in men.
- Asymptomatic in 50% to 80% of cases in women. Most common dissemination by mucosal passage to fallopian tubes, resulting in pelvic inflammatory disease (PID) in 10% to 15% of infected women. Hematogenous spread may result in septic arthritis and skin lesions. Conjunctivitis rarely occurs, but may result in blindness if not rapidly treated. Infection can occur in both men and women in oropharynx and anorectally.
- The World Health Organization (WHO) reports that there were 78 million new cases of gonorrhea worldwide among adults in 2012.

PHYSICAL FINDINGS & CLINICAL PRESENTATION

- Males: Purulent discharge from anterior urethra (Fig. E1, with dysuria appearing 2 to 7 days after infecting exposure. May have rectal infection causing pruritus, tenesmus, and discharge or may be asymptomatic.
- Females: Initial urethritis or cervicitis may occur a few days after exposure, frequently mild. Infections may be asymptomatic or may not produce recognizable symptoms until complications have occurred. In approximately 20% of cases uterine invasion occurs after menstrual period with signs and symptoms of endometritis, salpingitis, or pelvic peritonitis. The patient may have purulent discharge or inflamed Skene or Bartholin glands.
- Classic presentation of acute gonococcal PID is fever, abdominal and adnexal tenderness, and often absence of purulent discharge. Physical examination may be normal if asymptomatic. Disseminated gonococcal infection (DGI) may manifest with petechial or pustular acral skin lesions (Fig. E2), asymmetric polyarthralgia, tenosynovitis, or oligoarticular septic arthritis. The infection is complicated occasionally by perihepatitis and rarely endocarditis or meningitis.

ETIOLOGY

- *Neisseria gonorrhoeae* is the gonococcus. Plasmids coding for β-lactamase render some strains resistant to penicillin or tetracycline. There is an increasing frequency of chromosomally mediated resistance to penicillin, tetracycline, fluoroquinolones, and cefoxitin. In the Far East, high-level resistance to spectinomycin is endemic.
- There are a rising number of cases of quinolone-resistant *N. gonorrhoeae* worldwide, with the expected number to rise in the U.S. from importation.
- Men who have sex with men are vulnerable to the emerging threat of antimicrobial-resistant *N. gonorrhoeae.*

DIAGNOSIS

DIFFERENTIAL DIAGNOSIS

- Nongonococcal urethritis (NGU)
- Nongonococcal mucopurulent cervicitis
- *Chlamydia trachomatis*

WORKUP

Diagnosis depends on bacteriologic investigation. Culture and nucleic acid amplification tests (NAAT) are available for the detection of genitourinary infection with *N. gonorrhoeae.*

- NAATs are preferred testing modalities for the detection of genitourinary infection with *N. gonorrhoeae*. The performance of NAATs with respect to overall sensitivity, specificity, and ease of specimen transport is better than that of any of the other tests available for the diagnosis of gonococcal infections. NAATs should be used to detect gonorrhea except in cases of child sexual assault involving boys and rectal and oropharyngeal infections in prepubescent girls and when evaluating a potential gonorrhea treatment failure, in which case culture and susceptibility testing might be required. NAATs allow testing of the widest variety of specimen types, including endocervical swabs, vaginal swabs, urethral swabs (men), and urine (from both men and women).
- Culture: Gonorrhea culture on Thayer-Martin medium (organism is fastidious; requires aerobic conditions with increased carbon dioxide atmosphere; incubate ASAP). Culture has a sensitivity of 95% or more for urethral specimens from men with symptomatic urethritis and 80% to 90% for endocervical infection in women. Gram-negative intracellular diplococci are diagnostic in male urethral smears (Fig. E3). There is a false-negative rate of 60% to 70% in female cervical or urethral smears.
  1. Concomitant serologic testing for syphilis for all patients
  2. Concomitant *Chlamydia* testing for all patients
  3. Offer of HIV testing and counseling to all patients

LABORATORY TESTS

- First-catch urine (or genital swab) sample NAAT is the preferred screening and diagnostic test for gonorrhea. These tests have largely replaced culture in many settings where persons are screened for asymptomatic genital infection. They are not more sensitive than culture for detecting *N. gonorrhoeae* in cervical or urethral specimen; however, they have specificities >99% and retain sensitivity when used to test voided urine or self-collected vaginal swabs.
- Gonorrhea culture on Thayer-Martin medium (organism is fastidious; requires aerobic conditions with increased carbon dioxide atmosphere; incubate ASAP). Culture has a sensitivity of 95% or more for urethral specimens from men with symptomatic urethritis and 80% to 90% for endocervical infection in women.
- Nonamplified DNA probe tests are less sensitive than culture or NAATs and are not useful in the diagnosis of rectal or pharyngeal infection or for testing urine; however, they are inexpensive, readily available and offered in many laboratories in combination assays for *C. trachomatis.*
- Concomitant serologic testing for syphilis on all patients.
- Concomitant *Chlamydia* testing on all patients.
- Offer of HIV testing and counseling to all patients.

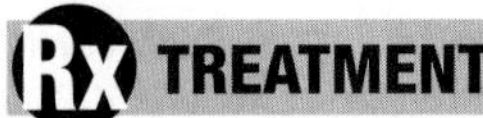

TREATMENT

ACUTE GENERAL Rx

Uncomplicated infections of the cervix, urethra, and rectum. Critical for the practitioner to know local resistance characteristics to best treat the patient:

- Ceftriaxone 250 mg IM × 1 dose *plus* azithromycin 1 g PO single dose. Doxycycline 100 mg PO bid for 7 days can be substituted for azithromycin in patients with azithromycin allergy.

Alternative regimens if ceftriaxone is not available:

- Ceftizoxime, cefoxitin with probenecid, and cefotaxime. None of these injectable cephalosporins offer any advantage over ceftriaxone.
- Cefixime 400 mg PO × 1 dose *plus* azithromycin 1 g orally single dose. Doxycycline 100 mg PO bid for 7 days can be substituted for azithromycin in patients with azithromycin allergy.
- If the patient has severe cephalosporin allergy, then azithromycin 2 g PO single dose *plus* single-dose gemifloxacin 320 mg PO or gentamicin 240 mg IM.
- A test-of-cure is not needed for persons who receive a diagnosis of uncomplicated urogenital or rectal gonorrhea who are treated with any of the recommended or alternative regimens.

Uncomplicated gonococcal infections of the pharynx:

- Ceftriaxone 250 mg IM × 1 dose *plus* azithromycin 1 g PO single dose. Doxycycline 100 mg PO bid for 7 days can be substituted for azithromycin in patients with azithromycin allergy.
- Treatment of the cephalosporin-allergic patient: Oral azithromycin 2 g *plus* single dose gemifloxacin 320 mg PO *or* 240 mg IM of gentamicin is effective.
- Any person with pharyngeal gonorrhea who is treated with an alternative regimen should return 14 days after treatment for a test-of-cure using either culture or NAAT.

Treatment of arthritis and arthritis-dermatitis syndrome:

- Recommended regimen: Ceftriaxone 1 g IM or IV every 24 hours plus azithromycin 1 g orally as a single dose.
- Alternative regimens: Cefotaxime 1 g IV every 8 hours or ceftizoxime 1 g IV every 8 hours *plus* azithromycin 1 g orally in a single dose.

DISPOSITION

- Pregnant women infected with *N. gonorrhoeae* should be treated with dual therapy consisting of ceftriaxone 250 mg in a single IM dose or azithromycin 1 g PO as a single dose. When cephalosporin allergy or other considerations preclude treatment and spectinomycin is not available, consultation with an ID specialist is recommended.
- To reduce development of drug resistance, reculture should be done for patients who show continued symptoms despite treatment. These patients should be tested with a culture-based gonorrhea test that can detect antibiotic resistance.
- All sexual partners should be identified, examined, tested, and receive presumptive treatment.
- Patients should be counseled to avoid unprotected intercourse with partners for 1 week after all partners have completed treatment.

REFERRAL

PID requiring hospitalization, disseminated gonococcal infection

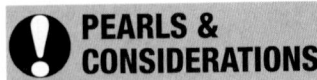

PEARLS & CONSIDERATIONS

COMMENTS

- This is a reportable disease.
- The proportion of gonorrhea cases in heterosexual men who are fluoroquinolone resistant (QRNG) has reached 6.7%, an elevenfold increase from 0.6% in 2001. Fluoroquinolone antibiotics are no longer recommended to treat gonorrhea in the U.S.
- The use of azithromycin as the second antimicrobial is preferred over doxycycline due to the high prevalence of tetracycline resistance.
- The U.S. Preventive Services Task Force (USPSTF) recommends screening for gonorrhea in sexually active females younger than 25 yr and in older women who are at increased risk for infection (multiple partners, new partner, partner who has concurrent partners). The USPSTF also concludes that the current evidence is insufficient to assess the balance of benefits and harms of screening for gonorrhea in men.
- High-intensity counseling on sexual risk reduction has been shown to reduce sexually transmitted infections (STIs) in primary care and related settings.

SUGGESTED READINGS

Available at www.expertconsult.com

RELATED CONTENT

Gonorrhea (Patient Information)
Cervicitis (Related Key Topic)
Chlamydia Genital Infections (Related Key Topic)
Pelvic Inflammatory Disease (Related Key Topic)

AUTHOR: **BETH LEOPOLD, M.D.**

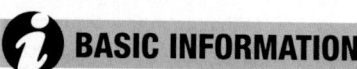

BASIC INFORMATION

DEFINITION

Gout is a term used to refer to a group of disease states caused by tissue deposition of monosodium urate due to prolonged hyperuricemia. Clinical manifestations of gout include acute and chronic arthritis, soft tissue inflammation, tophus formation, gouty nephropathy, and nephrolithiasis. Untreated hyperuricemia in patients with gout may lead to chronic destructive deforming arthritis.

ICD-10CM CODES

M10	Gout
M10.0	Idiopathic gout
M10.2	Drug-induced gout
M10.3	Gout due to impairment of renal function
M10.4	Other secondary gout
M10.9	Gout, unspecified
M10.1	Lead-induced gout

EPIDEMIOLOGY & DEMOGRAPHICS

PREVALENCE: 5 cases per 1000 persons in the U.S. Globally 8 cases per 10,000. Incidence is rising.
PREDOMINANT SEX: Male:female ratio ~4:1
PREDOMINANT AGE: 30 to 50 yr in men. Older than 60 yr in women

ETIOLOGY

- Gout is induced by inflammation from monosodium urate (MSU) crystal deposition. The primary risk factor for MSU deposition is hyperuricemia, though local factors such as temperature, pH, and mechanical stress may play a role.
- Hyperuricemia and gout develop from excessive uric acid production, a decrease in the renal excretion of uric acid, or both.
- Primary hyperuricemia results from an inborn error of metabolism and may be attributed to several biochemical defects.
- Secondary hyperuricemia may develop as a complication of acquired disorders (e.g., leukemia) or as a result of the use of certain drugs (e.g., diuretics). Consumption of alcohol, especially beer, increases the risk of gout, and fructose-rich beverage intake is associated with hyperuricemia.

PHYSICAL FINDINGS & CLINICAL PRESENTATION

ACUTE GOUT:

- Rapid onset of pain and swelling and erythema of a distal joint and/or periarticular soft tissue. Table 1 summarizes key components of gout flares.
- May present as monoarthritis of any joint. Acute gout of the first metatarsophalangeal (MTP) joint (Fig. E1) is known as *podagra*.
- 10% to 15% of attacks are polyarticular.
- Spontaneous resolution occurs over days to weeks.

CHRONIC TOPHACEOUS GOUT (FIG. E2):

- Insidious onset of painless arthritis and soft tissue swelling
- Distal small joints characteristic
- May be confused with nodal osteoarthritis

TABLE 1 Key Components of Gout Flares

- Marked tenderness and swelling of affected joint
- Acute onset with maximum pain in 4-12 hr
- Recurrent pattern of similar attacks
- Marked impairment of physical function
- Resolution of symptoms within 3-14 days

From Hochberg MC, et al.: *Rheumatology*, ed 5, St Louis, 2011, Mosby.

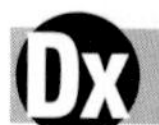

DIAGNOSIS

DIFFERENTIAL DIAGNOSIS OF ACUTE GOUT

- Infectious arthritis cellulitis
- Pseudogout
- Trauma

DIFFERENTIAL DIAGNOSIS OF CHRONIC GOUT

- Osteoarthritis (especially nodal OA in women)
- Rheumatoid arthritis
- Psoriatic arthritis

  Section II describes the differential diagnosis of acute monoarticular and oligoarticular arthritis.

WORKUP

Arthrocentesis and examination of synovial fluid

LABORATORY TESTS

- Uric acid: All patients with gout are hyperuricemic at some time, but during an acute attack the serum uric acid may be normal or low.
- Synovial aspirate: Usually cloudy and markedly inflammatory in nature. Urate crystals in fluid are needle-shaped and strongly negatively birefringent under polarized microscopy (Fig. E3).
- CBC: Mild leukocytosis often present.
- Inflammatory markers: ESR and CRP often elevated.

IMAGING STUDIES

- Plain radiography for diagnosis and evaluation. No typical findings in early gouty arthritis, but late disease is associated with characteristic punched-out marginal erosions and overhanging edges.
- Musculoskeletal ultrasound has been shown to be an effective means of detecting monosodium urate crystal deposition. Ultrasound can differentiate urate crystals that are found on the surface of articular cartilage from CPPD crystals that are seen within the substance of the cartilage (Fig. E4).

TREATMENT OPTIONS FOR ACUTE GOUT

- Nonsteroidal antiinflammatory medication (see Table 2).
  1. Indomethacin 75 mg bid
  2. Ibuprofen 800 mg tid
  3. Naproxen 500 mg bid
  4. Celecoxib 800 mg, then 400 mg/day
- Low-dose colchicine (less toxic and as effective as traditional high-dose colchicine): 1.2 mg colchicine PO, followed by 0.6 mg PO 1 hr later.
- Intraarticular corticosteroid injection (treatment of choice for monoarticular large joint attack): Triamcinolone acetonide 40 mg or equivalent for knee.
- Systemic corticosteroid therapy: Prednisone 40 mg PO for 3 days, then taper over 10 days (effective and safe, but evidence is lacking).

TREATMENT OF HYPERURICEMIA IN PATIENTS WITH GOUT

The American College of Rheumatology and most international rheumatology guidelines recommend that every patient with gout who has tophi, more than two attacks of gout per year, chronic kidney disease, or nephrolithiasis be treated with pharmacologic urate-lowering therapy. Serum uric acid should be monitored on a regular basis and urate-lowering therapy intensified until a target of less than 6 mg/dl is reached. In most cases, urate-lowering therapy should be continued for life.

The American College of Physicians Guidelines recommends a more conservative approach based on recurrence of symptoms. These guidelines have been criticized as ignoring the progressive nature of gout and perpetuating the well-documented underutilization and underdosing of urate-lowering therapy.

NONPHARMACOLOGIC THERAPY

Lifestyle and dietary modification should always be a component of therapy for patients with gout, but this is rarely effective without concomitant pharmacologic urate-lowering therapy, as dietary modification can only lower uric acid by about 1 mg/dl. Recommendations include reducing ingestion of red meat, kidney, liver, yeast extract, shellfish, and overall protein along with restricting alcohol intake. Discontinuation of diuretic therapy may help lower serum uric acid.

PHARMACOLOGIC TREATMENT OF SYMPTOMATIC HYPERURICEMIA

ALLOPURINOL: Allopurinol is very effective and safe when used properly. Correct dosing and patient compliance are essential elements in the prevention of erosive and tophaceous gout. Patients with renal insufficiency are at increased risk for allopurinol hypersensitivity, which manifests as fever, rash, and hepatitis occurring most commonly in the first 3 months of therapy. The rash may progress to life-threatening toxic epidermal necrolysis if not recognized early.

Traditionally, therapy with allopurinol is initiated several weeks after the acute attack has resolved. However, initiation of allopurinol at presentation may improve long-term compliance without reducing the efficacy of acute treatment. The initial dose should be low (≤100 mg/day depending on creatinine clearance) in patients with renal insufficiency and those with very high uric acid levels. High initial doses are associated with increased incidence of allopurinol hypersensitivity. The serum uric acid should

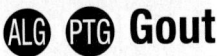

TABLE 2 Treatment of Gout

Acute Gout	Interval Gout	Treatment of Hyperuricemia
NSAIDs (preferred): Indomethacin 50 mg qid or ibuprofen 800 mg tid (or other NSAID in full doses). Contraindicated in patients with renal insufficiency and gastrointestinal disorders. *Or* **Colchicine, oral:** 1.2 mg followed by a second dose of 0.6 mg 1 hr later. Contraindicated in patients with renal insufficiency and gastrointestinal disorders *Or* **Intraarticular steroids** (Treatment of choice for large joint monoarthritis): Triamcinolone 40 mg or equivalent for knee *Or* Systemic steroid therapy (for patients in whom NSAIDs and colchicine are contraindicated) Prednisone 30-50 mg PO daily or in divided doses. May use lower dose in diabetic or postsurgical patients.	**Colchicine, oral:** 0.6-1.2 mg/day as prophylaxis against recurrent attacks. **NSAIDs may also be used for prophylaxis.** **Hypouricemic agent:** Indicated for patients with recurrent attacks despite prophylaxis, severe hyperuricemia, presence of tophi, urolithiasis, or gouty arthritis **Other:** Weight loss, reduce alcohol (especially beer), diet low in seafood, red meat, organ meat, and fructose	**Colchicine, oral:** 0.6-1.2 mg/day for 4-6 wk before initiating hypouricemic therapy and for several months afterward to prevent recurrent attacks during initiation of hypouricemic therapy. *And* **Allopurinol:** Initial dose 100 mg/day in patients with renal insufficiency or very high uric acid levels. Increase dose as needed to attain uric acid less than 6 mg/dl. *Or* **Uricosuric agent** (Use only in patients with good renal function and <600 mg uric acid in a 24-hr collection): probenecid, 0.5-1 g bid, or sulfinpyrazone 100 mg tid or qid **Other:** Consider febuxostat for patients allergic to allopurinol and the addition of lesinurad in patients resistant to xanthine oxidase inhibitors. Pegloticase may be useful for selected patients with severe tophaceous gout.

NSAIDs, Nonsteroidal antiinflammatory drugs.

be reevaluated after 4 to 6 weeks of therapy, and the allopurinol dose adjusted to reduce the serum uric acid to less than 6 mg/dl. The most common therapeutic dosage of allopurinol is 300 mg/day, but dose may be increased by 50 to 100 mg every 2 to 3 weeks until the target serum uric acid level is achieved. There is evidence that increasing allopurinol doses in patients with renal insufficiency does not result in significant toxicity, but concurrent use with statins and colchicine is associated with a higher incidence of adverse effects. Some authors have reported using doses as high as 800 mg daily without excess toxicity. It is recommended that patients of Han Chinese, Thai, and Korean ancestry be tested for HLA-B*5801 before initiating allopurinol as these individuals are at high risk of allopurinol hypersensitivity if this antigen is present.

FEBUXOSTAT: Febuxostat is a xanthine oxidase inhibitor that has been shown to be more potent than allopurinol 300 mg daily for reducing serum uric acid. The chemical structure of febuxostat is different from allopurinol, making cross-reactive allergy unlikely. The metabolism of febuxostat is primarily hepatic, which obviates the need for dose adjustments due to renal insufficiency. Some cases of hepatic toxicity have been reported, and it is recommended that liver function tests be monitored periodically. Febuxostat may help preserve renal function in patients with chronic kidney disease (CKD) but has not been tested in patients with severe renal failure.

The primary indication for febuxostat is demonstrated allergy to allopurinol. The cost of febuxostat may be as much as 40 times that of allopurinol, and there is some evidence suggesting that febuxostat may be associated with higher cardiovascular and all-cause mortality than allopurinol in patients with cardiovascular risk factors. It should be only used when allopurinol is not tolerated.

PROBENECID: Uricosuric agents may be used in patients with good renal function and urinary uric acid less than 600 mg in a 24-hr collection. Probenecid can be used in patients with intolerance to xanthene-oxidase inhibitors. Compliance is poor due to the necessity of taking the drug more often than once daily. In December 2015, the U.S. Food and Drug Administration (FDA) approved lesinurad, which is an inhibitor of the URAT1 transport enzyme, for treatment of hyperuricemia in patients with gout who have not achieved target serum acid levels with xanthine oxidase inhibitors alone. The approved dose is 200 mg PO qd, and lesinurad must be taken in combination with a xanthene oxidase inhibitor.

LESINURAD: A URAT1 and OAT4 inhibitor is FDA approved for gout-associated hyperuricemia unresponsive to xanthine oxidase inhibitor monotherapy. It prevents reuptake of uric acid at the proximal renal tubule. Dosage is 200 mg once daily taken with allopurinol or febuxostat. Increased fluid intake (at least 2 L of liquid per day) and frequent monitoring of renal function is necessary. This drug should not be used in patients with CrCl <45 ml/min.

PEGLOTICASE: Intravenous PEGylated uricase is FDA approved for treatment of severe refractory tophaceous gout. It is a PEGylated recombinant mammalian uricase that rapidly degrades urate when given intravenously. Use is limited by very high cost and significant toxicities, including frequent gout flares and anaphylaxis.

PATIENT/FAMILY EDUCATION

It is essential that patients, families, physicians, and other members of the health care team appreciate the importance of compliance with a daily allopurinol regimen if recurrent flares and progression to chronic arthritis and tophi are to be avoided. Allopurinol should be discontinued only for symptoms suggesting the hypersensitivity syndrome. It should be continued during flares, medical illnesses, and surgical procedures.

REFERRAL

- Rheumatologist if diagnosis is not clear or therapy is complicated
- Podiatrist for management of pedal complications

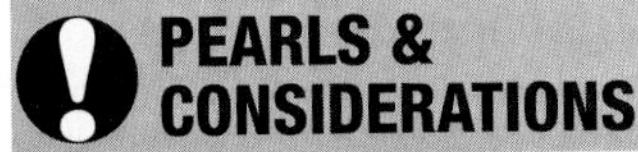

PEARLS & CONSIDERATIONS

Do not stop allopurinol during hospitalizations, surgery, or acute attacks unless there is evidence of drug allergy. The dosage of allopurinol should be adjusted in patients with acute kidney injury.

SUGGESTED READINGS

Available at ExpertConsult.com

RELATED CONTENT

Gout (Patient Information)
Hyperuricemia (Related Key Topic)

AUTHOR: **BERNARD ZIMMERMANN, M.D.**

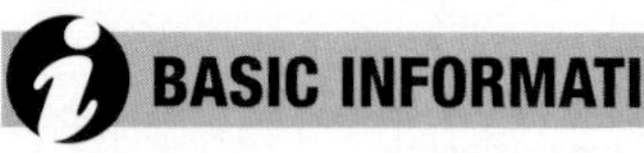

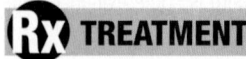

BASIC INFORMATION

DEFINITION

Graft-versus-host disease (GVHD) is a complication of allogeneic hematopoietic stem cell transplant where the patient's bone marrow is replaced by the donor's and the latter recognizes the patient's organ as foreign and launches an immunological attack. GVHD is reported rarely after autologous bone marrow transplant and blood transfusion. GVHD occurring between the time of engraftment through 100 days after transplant is termed *acute GVHD* and that occurs beyond 100 days is termed *chronic GVHD*.

SYNONYM

GVHD

ICD 10-CM CODE

D89.813 Graft-versus-host disease, unspecified

EPIDEMIOLOGY & DEMOGRAPHICS

INCIDENCE The incidence of acute GVHD is 25% to 35% in recipients of fully matched sibling donor grafts and 40% to 50% in recipients of matched unrelated donor grafts. The incidence of chronic GVHD is 30% in recipients of fully histocompatible transplants and 60% to 70% in mismatched or unrelated donor recipients.

PREDOMINANT SEX AND AGE Older age and female donor–to–male recipient transplant are risk factors for GVHD.

GENETICS Degree of HLA mismatch is a risk factor for GVHD.

RISK FACTORS

- Degree of HLA mismatches is the strongest risk factor: HLA-A, -B, -C, -DRB1, HLA-DQ, and -DP
- Source of graft (peripheral blood or bone marrow greater than umbilical cord blood)
- Female donor to male recipient
- Multiparous donors
- Intensity of the transplant conditioning regimen
- Acute GVHD prophylactic regimen
- Transplants that achieve full donor chimerism
- CMV mismatches
- Older patients, those with poor functional status

PHYSICAL FINDINGS & CLINICAL PRESENTATION

- Acute GVHD: Median onset is 21 to 25 days after transplantation.
- Skin is affected in about 80% of patients, gastrointestinal (GI) tract in 50%, and liver in 50%.
- Chronic GVHD is mostly seen within the first yr after HCT, but 5% to 10% of patients develop this after 1 yr. About 30% of chronic GVHD is de novo without history of acute GVHD. The median time of diagnosis of chronic GVHD is 4.5 months. Common clinical manifestations of chronic GVHD are summarized in Table 1.
- Skin lesions include maculopapular rash commonly around the neck, shoulders, palms, and soles.
- More severe lesions include blisters, ulcers, and bullae.
- GI manifestations include anorexia, nausea, vomiting, abdominal pain, ileus, voluminous secretory diarrhea, and hematochezia. Volume of the diarrhea determines the severity of the disease.
- Liver involvement occurs as a result of damage to biliary canaliculi, causing cholestasis with hyperbilirubinemia and elevated alkaline phosphatase. Severity of liver disease is assessed based on serum bilirubin levels.

ETIOLOGY

GVHD occurs when immune cells transplanted from a donor (the graft) recognize the transplant recipient (the host) as foreign, and initiate an immune attack against the recipient organs. The pathophysiology of GVHD is illustrated in Fig. 1.

TABLE 1 Common Clinical Manifestations of Chronic Graft-Versus-Host Disease

Organ System	Clinical Manifestations
Cutaneous	Poikiloderma, lichen planus, dermal sclerosis, morphea-like features, hypopigmentation or hyperpigmentation, ichthyosis, nail dystrophy, onycholysis
Ocular	Keratoconjunctivitis sicca, conjunctivitis, corneal ulcerations
Oral	Lichen planus, hyperkeratotic plaques, xerostomia, mucosal atrophy, ulcers, restriction of mouth opening from sclerosis
Pulmonary	Bronchiolitis obliterans, bronchiolitis obliterans-organizing pneumonia
Gastrointestinal	Esophageal web and strictures, malabsorption syndrome, exocrine pancreatic insufficiency
Hepatic	Cholestasis
Genitourinary	Vaginal stenosis or scarring, lichen planus
Musculoskeletal	Fasciitis, joint contractures from sclerosis, myositis or polymyositis, arthritis
Hematopoietic	Thrombocytopenia, eosinophilia, lymphopenia, hemolytic anemia, hypogammaglobulinemia

From Hoffman R et al: *Hematology: basic principles and practice*, ed 7, Philadelphia, 2018, Elsevier.

Dx DIAGNOSIS

The National Institutes of Health (NIH) consensus criteria used to diagnose GVHD classify manifestations of GVHD as "diagnostic" or "distinctive" of chronic GVHD, or as common to both acute and chronic GVHD.

Common diagnostic criteria sufficient to establish a diagnosis of chronic GVHD:

- Poikiloderma
- Lichen planus-like features
- Esophageal web
- Strictures or stenosis in the upper to midthird of the esophagus
- Bronchiolitis obliterans diagnosed with lung biopsy

Common distinctive criteria that are encountered in chronic GVHD but are insufficient by themselves to establish a diagnosis include the following:

- Depigmentation
- Cicatricial conjunctivitis
- Keratoconjunctivitis sicca
- Bronchiolitis obliterans diagnosed with pulmonary function tests (PFTs) and radiology
- Myositis or polymyositis

To make a diagnosis of chronic GVHD, at least one diagnostic clinical sign of chronic GVHD must be present or at least one distinctive manifestation must be confirmed by pertinent biopsy or other relevant tests in the same or another organ. The clinical features, staging, and grading of acute GVHD are summarized in Tables 2 and 3.

DIFFERENTIAL DIAGNOSIS

- Engraftment syndrome
- Erythema multiforme
- Malignancy
- Hepatic sinusoidal obstructive syndrome
- Drug eruptions and toxicities
- Dermatomyositis
- Systemic sclerosis

WORKUP

Although diagnosis of GVHD is mostly made based on clinical signs and symptoms, biomarkers and organ-specific histology may help establish diagnosis.

LABORATORY TEST(S)

A panel of plasma biomarkers, including IL-2-receptor-α, TNF receptor-1, IL-8, and hepatocyte growth factor, has been suggested as a confirmatory tool for the diagnosis of GVHD at the onset of clinical manifestations, but this is still an active area of investigation.

IMAGING STUDIES

Positron emission tomography (PET) scanning may be used to distinguish intestinal GVHD from other diagnoses in patients with intestinal GVHD.

TREATMENT

Treatment of GVHD:

- Treatment depends on the organs involved and the severity of GVHD. Commonly administered drugs for GVHD are summarized in Table 4.

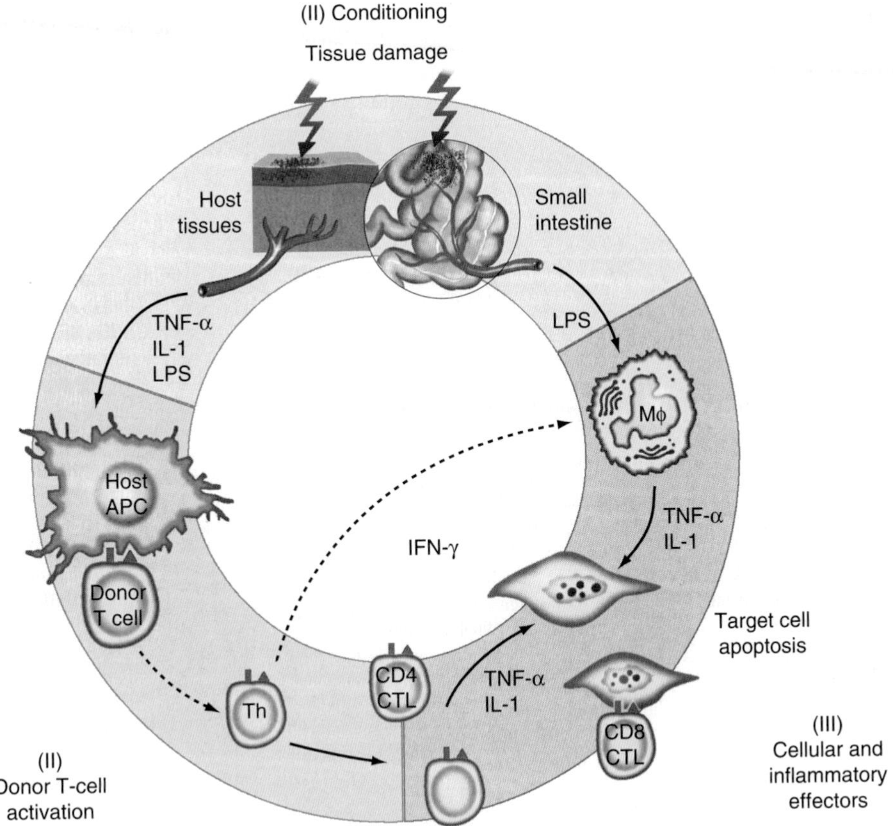

FIG. 1 Pathophysiology of GVHD. During step 1, both irradiation and chemotherapy damage and activate host tissues, including intestinal mucosa, liver, and the skin. Activated cell hosts then secrete inflammatory cytokines (e.g., TNF-α and IL-1), which can be measured in the systemic circulation. The cytokine release has important effects on APCs of the host, including increased expression of adhesion molecules (e.g., ICAM-1, VCAM-1) and of MHC class II antigens. These changes in the APCs enhance the recognition of host MHC and/or minor H antigens by mature donor T cells. During step 2, donor T-cell activation is characterized by proliferation of GVHD T cells and secretion of the Th1 cytokines IL-2 and IFN-γ. Both of these cytokines play central roles in clonal T-cell expansion, induction of CTL and NK cell responses, and the priming of mononuclear phagocytes. In step 3, mononuclear phagocytes primed by IFN-γ are triggered by a second signal such as endotoxin LPS to secrete cytopathic amounts of IL-I and TNF-α. LPS can leak through the intestinal mucosa damaged by the conditioning regimen to stimulate gut-associated lymphoid tissue or Kupffer cells in the liver; LPS that penetrates the epidermis may stimulate keratinocytes, dermal fibroblasts, and macrophages to produce similar cytokines in the skin. This mechanism results in the amplification of local tissue injury and further production of inflammatory effectors such as nitric oxide, which, together with CTL and NK effectors, leads to the observed target tissue destruction in the stem cell transplant host. CTL effectors use Fas/FasL, perforin/granzyme B, and membrane-bound cytokines to lyse target cells. *APC,* Antigen-presenting cell; *CTL,* cytotoxic T lymphocyte; *GVHD,* graft-versus-host disease; *ICAM,* intercellular adhesion molecule; *IFN,* interferon; *IL,* interleukin; *LPS,* lipopolysaccharide; *MHC,* major histocompatibility complex; *NK,* natural killer; *TNF,* tumor necrosis factor; *VCAM,* vascular cell adhesion molecule. (From Hoffman R et al: *Hematology, basic principles and practice*, ed 7, Philadelphia, 2018, Elsevier.)

TABLE 2 Clinical Manifestations and Staging of Acute Graft-Versus-Host Disease

Organ	Clinical Manifestations	Staging
Skin	Erythematous, maculopapular rash involving palms and soles; may become confluent Severe disease: Bullae	Stage 1: <25% rash Stage 2: 25%-50% rash Stage 3: Generalized erythroderma Stage 4: Bullae
Liver	Painless jaundice with conjugated hyperbilirubinemia and increased alkaline phosphatase	Stage 1: Bili 2-3 mg/dl Stage 2: Bili 3.1-6 mg/dl Stage 3: Bili 6.1-15 mg/dl Stage 4: Bili >15 mg/dl
Gastrointestinal tract	Upper: Nausea, vomiting, anorexia Lower: Diarrhea, abdominal cramps, distension, ileus, bleeding	Stage 1: Diarrhea >500 ml/day Stage 2: Diarrhea >1000 ml/day Stage 3: Diarrhea >1500 ml/day Stage 4: Ileus, bleeding

From Hoffman R et al: *Hematology, basic principles and practice*, ed 7, Philadelphia, 2018, Elsevier.

- In mild cutaneous GVHD, topical steroids may be used along with and the optimization of prophylactic regimen.
- Systemic methyl prednisone 2 mg/kg per day in divided doses should be used for grade II or higher GVHD, in addition to the optimization of prophylactic measures. Corticosteroid can be tapered over several months.
- In GVHD with gastrointestinal involvement, systemic glucocorticoids plus oral nonabsorbable steroids should be used. In addition, octreotide may help with diarrhea.
- Patients who demonstrate progression of disease by day 5 of therapy or no response by day 7 are considered to have glucocorticoid resistance. There is no standard therapy

TABLE 3 Glucksberg Criteria for Staging of Acute Graft-Versus-Host Disease[a]

Overall Grade	Skin	Liver		Gut
I	1-2	0		0
II	1-3	1	*and/or*	1
III	2-3	2-4	*and/or*	2-3
IV	2-4	2-4	*and/or*	2-4

[a]See Table 2 for individual organ staging. Traditionally, individual organs are staged without regard to attribution. The overall grade of graft-versus-host disease, however, reflects the actual extent of graft-versus-host disease. To achieve each overall grade, skin disease, liver, and/or gut involvement are required.

From Hoffman R et al: *Hematology, basic principles and practice*, ed 7, Philadelphia, 2018, Elsevier.

TABLE 4 Commonly Administered Drugs for Graft-Versus-Host Disease Prophylaxis and Treatment

Drug	Mechanism	Adverse Effects
Corticosteroids	Direct lymphocyte toxicity; suppress proinflammatory cytokines such as TNF-α	Hyperglycemia, acute psychosis, severe myopathy, neuropathy, osteoporosis, cataract development
Methotrexate (MTX)	Antimetabolite: Inhibit T-cell proliferation	Significant renal, hepatic, and gastrointestinal toxicities
Cyclosporine A (CSA)	IL-2 suppressor; blocks Ca^{2+}-dependent signal transduction distal to TCR engagement	Renal and hepatic insufficiency, hypertension, hyperglycemia, headache, nausea and vomiting, hirsutism, gum hypertrophy, seizure with severe toxicity
Tacrolimus (FK506)	IL-2 receptor; blocks Ca^{2+}-dependent signal transduction distal to TCR engagement	Similar to CSA
Mycophenolate mofetil (MMF)	Inhibits de novo purine synthesis	Body aches, abdominal pain, nausea and vomiting, diarrhea, neutropenia
Sirolimus	mTOR inhibitor	Thrombocytopenia, hyperlipidemia, TTP
Antithymocyte globulin (ATG)	Polyclonal immunoglobulin	Anaphylaxis, serum sickness

Ca^{2+}, Calcium ion; IL-2, interleukin-2; *mTOR,* mammalian target of rapamycin; *TCR,* T-cell receptor; *TNF-α,* tumor necrosis factor-α; *TTP,* thrombotic thrombocytopenic purpura.

From Hoffman R et al: *Hematology, basic principles and practice*, ed 7, Philadelphia, 2018, Elsevier.

for steroid refractory GVHD. Second-line agents in treatment of GVHD include mycophenolate mofetil, etanercept, pentostatin, alpha-1 antitrypsin, sirolimus, ruxolitinib antithymocyte globulin, and extracorporeal photopheresis.

ACUTE GENERAL Rx

Acute treatment involves topical or systemic corticosteroids. Second-line agents can be used in steroid-resistant cases.

CHRONIC Rx

Corticosteroids tapered over several months can be used in chronic treatment of GVHD.

DISPOSITION

Patients should be directed to individuals who originally initiated organ or bone marrow transplantation surgery.

REFERRAL

Physicians with expertise in immunosuppression

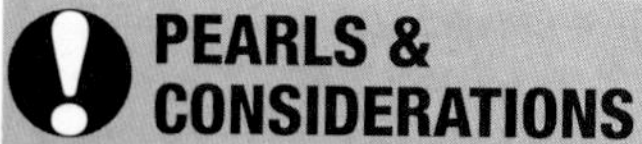

PEARLS & CONSIDERATIONS

COMMENTS

GVHD is a potentially fatal disorder that occurs after an allogeneic transplant of bone marrow, peripheral blood stem cells, or solid organs. The donor bone marrow or peripheral blood stem cells attack the recipient's organs. Immunosuppression is required to prevent and treat this disorder.

GRADING OF GVHD: Severity is defined by the International Blood and Marrow Transplant Research (IBMTR) grading system:

- Grade A—Stage 1 skin involvement alone (maculopapular rash over <25% of the body) with no liver or gastrointestinal involvement
- Grade B—Stage 2 skin involvement; stage 1 to 2 gut or liver involvement
- Grade C—Stage 3 involvement of any organ system (generalized erythroderma; bilirubin 6.1 to 15.0 mg/dl; diarrhea 1500 to 2000 ml/day)
- Grade D—Stage 4 involvement of any organ system (generalized erythroderma with bullous formation; bilirubin >15 mg/dl; diarrhea >2000 ml/day or pain or ileus)

PREVENTION

- Prophylactic regimen should be decided based on underlying disease, the degree of HLA disparity, the conditioning regimen, and patient characteristics.
- Mycophenolate and calcineurin inhibitors should be used in patients undergoing reduced intensity allogeneic hematopoietic cell transplantation.
- For patients who receive myeloablative or reduced intensity conditioning, antithymocyte globulin can be added to the prophylactic regimen.

SUGGESTED READINGS

Available at ExpertConsult.com

AUTHORS: **VANJI KARTHIKEYAN, M.D., and ROHINI PRASHAR, M.D.**

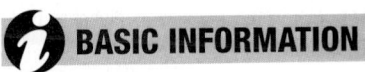

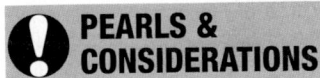

BASIC INFORMATION

DEFINITION

Granuloma annulare (GA) is a chronic, usually self-limited, inflammatory disorder of the dermis that classically presents as arciform to annular plaques located on the extremities.

SYNONYMS

Pseudorheumatoid nodule—subcutaneous granuloma annulare
GA

ICD-10CM CODE
L92.0 Granuloma annulare

EPIDEMIOLOGY & DEMOGRAPHICS

- Most common in children and young adults; most cases of localized GA are diagnosed in patients <30 yr.
- Female predominance (2:1).
- Disseminated form associated with diabetes mellitus.
- Recurrent in 40% of affected individuals.
- A generalized form of GA can occur in up to 15% of patients.

PHYSICAL FINDINGS & CLINICAL PRESENTATION

- The main clinical variants of GA are localized (75%), disseminated (>10 lesions), subcutaneous (occurring primarily in children aged 2-5 yr), patch-type or macular GA, and perforating (rare form manifesting with 1- to 4-mm papules with a central crust usually appearing on the dorsal hands).
- Localized GA starts as a small ring of colored skin or pale erythematous papules. More common in children and young to middle-age adults. Usually, only one or a few lesions occur at any one time.
- Lesions coalesce and evolve into annular plaques over several weeks.
- Plaques undergo central involution and increase in diameter over several months (0.5-5 cm).
- Most frequently found on the lateral and dorsal surfaces of the hands and feet (Fig. 1 and Fig. E2).
- Most lesions resolve spontaneously after several months.
- The generalized form of GA is characterized by hundreds of small (lesions rarely exceed 5 cm in diameter), flesh-colored papules in a symmetric distribution on the trunk and extremities. It most commonly affects women in the fifth or sixth decades but can also be seen in adolescents and children. Some patients are completely asymptomatic, whereas others complain of severe pruritus.
- Macular GA is more common in women between ages 30 to 70 and manifests with flat or slightly palpable erythematous or red-brown lesions on upper medial thighs and in bathing-trunk distribution.
- Deep dermal GA (subcutaneous GA) presents as large, painless, skin-colored nodules that are frequently mistaken for rheumatoid nodules.

ETIOLOGY

Unknown, but may be related to vasculitis, trauma, monocyte activation, or delayed hypersensitivity.

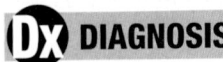

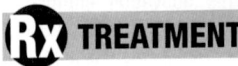

DIAGNOSIS

DIFFERENTIAL DIAGNOSIS

- Tinea corporis
- Lichen planus
- Necrobiosis lipoidica diabeticorum
- Sarcoidosis
- Rheumatoid nodules
- Late secondary or tertiary syphilis
- Arcuate and annular plaques of mycosis fungoides
- Papular GA can simulate insect bites, secondary syphilis, xanthoma
- Annular elastolytic giant cell granuloma

WORKUP

- Diagnosis based on clinical appearance and presentation
- Biopsy when diagnosis is unclear

LABORATORY TESTS

- No laboratory tests will help confirm the diagnosis.
- Biopsy shows focal degeneration of collagen and elastic fibers, mucin deposition, and perivascular and interstitial lymphohistiocytic infiltrate in the upper and middle dermis.

TREATMENT

NONPHARMACOLOGIC THERAPY

Reassurance, given the self-limited and benign nature of GA

CHRONIC Rx

High-potency topical corticosteroids with or without occlusion and intralesional steroid injection into elevated border with triamcinolone 2.5 to 10 mg/ml are useful first-line local therapies.

- Cryosurgery, psoralen ultraviolet-A (UVA) range or UVA-1 therapy, and carbon dioxide laser treatment can also be used.
- Systemic agents (e.g., niacinamide, hydroxychloroquine, chloroquine, cyclosporine, dapsone) are generally reserved for severe cases. Recent case reports indicate positive outcomes with tacrolimus and pimecrolimus and the tumor necrosis factor infliximab.

DISPOSITION

Most lesions resolve spontaneously within 2 yr.

REFERRAL

Dermatology referral recommended for symptomatic, disseminated disease

PEARLS & CONSIDERATIONS

COMMENTS

GA has been described as a paraneoplastic granulomatous reaction to Hodgkin's disease, non-Hodgkin's lymphoma, solid organ tumors, and mycosis fungoides.

RELATED CONTENT

Granuloma Annulare (Patient Information)

AUTHOR: **FRED F. FERRI, M.D.**

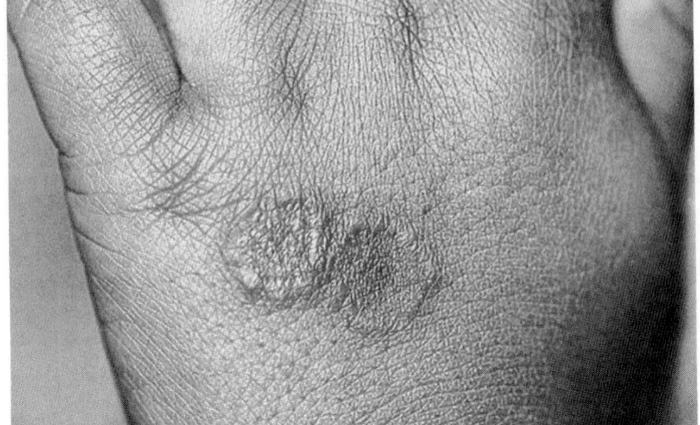

FIG. 1 Granuloma annulare. Annular, flesh-colored, nonscaly plaques. (From Paller AS, Mancini AJ: *Hurwitz clinical pediatric dermatology, a textbook of skin disorders of childhood and adolescence*, ed 5, Edinburgh, 2016, Elsevier.)

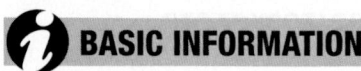

BASIC INFORMATION

DEFINITION

Graves disease is a hypermetabolic state caused by circulating IgG antibodies that bind to and activate the G-protein–coupled thyrotropin receptor. This activation stimulates follicular hypertrophy and hyperplasia, causing thyroid enlargement as well as increases in thyroid hormone production. It affects the thyroid, ocular muscles and shin. It is characterized by thyrotoxicosis, diffuse goiter, and infiltrative ophthalmopathy (edema and inflammation of the extraocular muscles and an increase in orbital connective tissue and fat); infiltrative dermopathy characterized by lymphocytic infiltration of the dermis; accumulation of glycosaminoglycans; and occasionally edema.

SYNONYM

Thyrotoxicosis

ICD-10CM CODES

E05.00	Thyrotoxicosis with diffuse goiter without thyrotoxic crisis or storm
E05.01	Thyrotoxicosis with diffuse goiter with thyrotoxic crisis or storm

EPIDEMIOLOGY & DEMOGRAPHICS

INCIDENCE/PREVALENCE: Graves disease is the most common cause of hyperthyroidism. It affects 3% of women and 0.5% of men during their lifetime. There is a slight increased incidence among young African Americans. The annual incidence of Graves disease-associated ophthalmopathy is 16 cases per 100,000 women and 3 cases per 100,000 men. It is more common in whites than Asians. Cigarette smoking is a risk factor.

PREDOMINANT AGE: Peak incidence is between 30 and 60 yr.

GENETICS: Patients often report a family history of Hashimoto thyroiditis, Graves disease, or other autoimmune conditions. Increased prevalence of HLA-B8 and HLA-DR3 in whites with Graves disease. Concordance rate is 20% among monozygotic twins.

PHYSICAL FINDINGS & CLINICAL PRESENTATION

- Diffusely enlarged thyroid. Thyroid bruit may be present. Cervical lymphadenopathy may also be present.
- Elevated systolic blood pressure with a widened pulse pressure.
- Tachycardia, palpitations, tremor, hyperreflexia.
- Exophthalmos (50% of patients) (Fig. 1), lid retraction (lid lag), in which contraction of the levator palpebrae muscles of the eyelids shows immobility of the upper eyelid with downward rotation of the eye.
- Nervousness, weight loss (weight gain in 10% of patients), heat intolerance, pruritus, muscle weakness, atrial fibrillation.
- Increased sweating, brittle nails, clubbing of fingers.
- Localized infiltrative dermopathy (1% to 2% of patients) is most frequent over the anterolateral aspects of the legs, commonly over the pretibial area (pretibial myxedema) but can be found at other sites (especially after trauma). It is nonpitting and indurated. It is typically patchy with a peau d'orange appearance to the skin.
- Men may have gynecomastia, reduced libido, and erectile dysfunction. Women often have irregular menses.

ETIOLOGY

Autoimmune etiology: Thyrotropin receptor antibodies (TRAb) mediated activation of TSH receptor (TSHR). The activity of the thyroid gland is stimulated by the action of T cells, which induce specific B cells to synthesize antibodies against thyroid-stimulating hormone (TSH) receptors in the follicular cell membrane.

Dx DIAGNOSIS

DIFFERENTIAL DIAGNOSIS

- Anxiety disorder
- Premenopausal state
- Thyroiditis
- Other causes of hyperthyroidism (e.g., toxic multinodular goiter, toxic adenoma)
- Other: Metastatic neoplasm, diabetes mellitus, pheochromocytoma

WORKUP

- The diagnosis is made clinically on most instances.
- The diagnostic workup includes a detailed medical history followed by laboratory and imaging studies and ECG. Patients often present with anxiety, heat intolerance, menstrual dysfunction, increased appetite, and weight loss. Elderly patients can have an atypical presentation (apathetic hyperparathyroidism). For additional information, refer to the topic "Hyperthyroidism."
- Table 1 describes the clinical assessment of the patient with Graves ophthalmopathy.

LABORATORY TESTS

- Increased free thyroxine (T_4) and free triiodothyronine (T_3).
- Decreased TSH.
- Measurement of thyroid-stimulating antibodies (TSI) and TRAb.

IMAGING STUDIES

- 24-hr radioactive iodine uptake (RAIU): Increased homogeneous uptake.
- CT or MRI of the orbits (Fig. E2) is useful if there is uncertainty about the cause of ophthalmopathy.

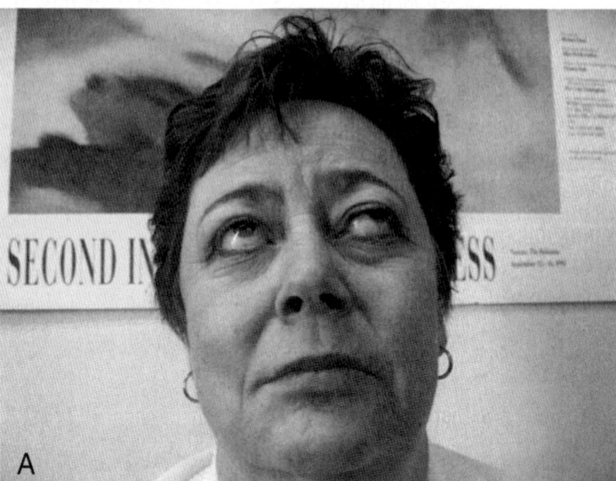

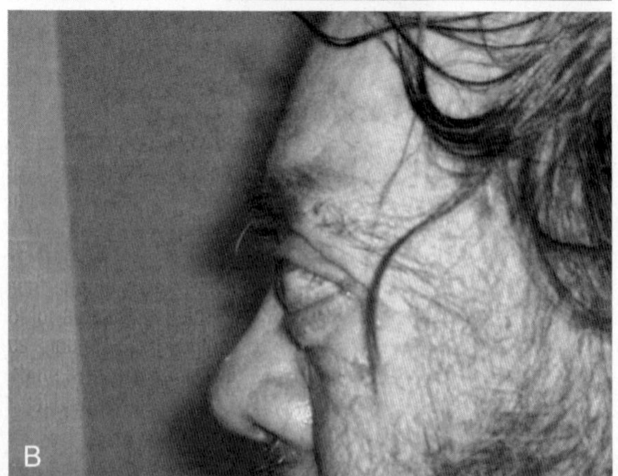

FIG. 1 Proptosis seen in the setting of Graves disease. **A,** Eye signs in Graves disease. **B,** Severe proptosis in Graves disease. (**A** and **B,** Courtesy Dr. Meir H. Kryger.) (From Kryger M, Roth T, Dement WC: *Principles and practice of sleep medicine*, ed 6, Philadelphia, 2017, Elsevier.)

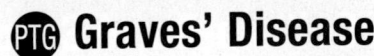

Rx TREATMENT

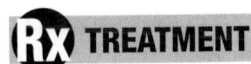

NONPHARMACOLOGIC THERAPY

- Patient education and discussion of therapeutic options.
- Smoking cessation: Smoking is associated with an increased risk of progression of Graves ophthalmopathy.

ACUTE GENERAL Rx

- Antithyroid drugs (thionamides, ATDs) to inhibit thyroid hormone synthesis or peripheral conversion of T_4 to T_3:
  1. Methimazole or propylthiouracil (PTU) are available. Methimazole is generally preferred because it has a longer half-life, allowing for once-daily dosing. PTU is preferred during pregnancy.
  2. Side effects: Skin rash (3% to 5%), arthralgias, myalgias, granulocytopenia (0.5%); rare side effects: Aplastic anemia, hepatic necrosis (PTU), cholestatic jaundice.
  3. Thionamide antithyroid drug therapy results in a remission in 40% to 50% of patients treated for 12 to 18 months.
- Radioactive iodine (RAI):
  1. Treatment of choice for patients >21 yr and younger patients who have not achieved remission after 1 yr of ATD therapy
  2. Contraindicated during pregnancy and lactation
  3. Following radioactive therapy there may be an acute elevation of thyroid antibody titers and exacerbation of ocular symptoms in 15% to 20% of patients.
- Surgery: Near-total thyroidectomy. Indications: Obstructing goiters despite RAI and ATD therapy, patients who refuse RAI and cannot be adequately managed with ATDs, and pregnant women inadequately managed with ATDs. Complications of surgery include hypoparathyroidism (4%) and vocal cord paralysis (1%).
- Adjunctive therapy: Beta-adrenergic receptor blockers (e.g., atenolol 50-100 mg/day) to alleviate the beta-adrenergic symptoms of hyperthyroidism (tachycardia, tremor); contraindicated in patients with bronchospasm.
- Graves ophthalmopathy: Methylcellulose eye drops to protect against excessive dryness, sunglasses to decrease photophobia, intraocular and systemic high-dose corticosteroids for severe exophthalmos. Worsening of ophthalmopathy after RAI therapy is often transient and can be prevented by the administration of prednisone. Other treatment options include antiinflammatory and immunosuppressive agents, radiation, and corrective surgical procedures. The administration of the antioxidant selenium (100 μg PO bid) has been recently reported as effective in improving quality of life, reducing ocular involvement, and slowing progression of the disease in patients with mild Graves orbitopathy. Its mechanism of action is believed to be an effect on the oxygen free radicals and cytokines that play a pathogenic role in Graves orbitopathy. Inhibition of the insulin-like growth factor I receptor (IGF-IR) is a new therapeutic strategy to combat the underlying autoimmune etiology of ophthalmopathy. Trials with teprotumumab, a human monoclonal antibody inhibitor of IGF-IR, in patients with active, moderate-to-severe ophthalmopathy have shown effectiveness in reducing proptosis.[1]
- Dermopathy and acropachy: Topical corticosteroids are often used but are generally ineffective. Trials using rituximab infusion for dermopathy have shown striking improvement.

CHRONIC Rx

Patients undergoing treatment with ATDs should be seen every 1 to 3 mo until euthyroidism is achieved and every 3 to 4 mo while they are receiving ATDs.

DISPOSITION

- ATDs induce sustained remission in <60% of cases.
- The incidence of hypothyroidism after RAI is >50% within the first yr and 2% per yr thereafter.
- Complications of surgery include hypothyroidism (28% to 43% after 10 yr), hypoparathyroidism (4%), and vocal cord paralysis (1%).
- Successful treatment of hyperthyroidism requires lifelong monitoring for the onset of hypothyroidism or the recurrence of thyrotoxicosis.
- RAI therapy is followed by the appearance or worsening of ophthalmopathy more often than is therapy with methimazole, particularly in patients who are cigarette smokers. It can be prevented with the administration of prednisone 0.5 mg/kg body weight per day starting 2 to 3 days after RAI, continued for 1 mo, then tapered off over 2 mo.
- Mild to moderate ophthalmopathy often improves spontaneously. Severe cases can be treated with high-dose glucocorticoids, orbital irradiation, or both. Orbital decompression may be used in patients with optic neuropathy and exophthalmos (see "Hyperthyroidism").

TABLE 1 Clinical Assessment of the Patient with Graves Ophthalmopathy

Activity Measures*
Spontaneous retrobulbar pain
Pain on attempted up or down gaze
Redness of the eyelids
Redness of the conjunctiva
Swelling of the eyelids
Inflammation of the caruncle and/or plica
Conjunctival edema
Severity Measures
Lid aperture: Distance between lid margins in millimeters with the patient looking in the primary position, sitting relaxed, and with distant fixation
Swelling of the eyelids (absent/equivocal, moderate, severe)
Redness of the eyelids (absent/present)
Redness of the conjunctivae (absent/present)
Conjunctival edema (absent, present)
Inflammation of the caruncle or plica (absent, present)
Exophthalmos: Measured in millimeters using the same Hertel exophthalmometer and the same intercanthal distance for an individual patient
Subjective diplopia score†
Eye muscle involvement (ductions in degrees)
Corneal involvement (absent/punctate keratopathy/ulcer)
Optic nerve involvement: Best-corrected visual acuity, color vision, optic disk, relative afferent pupillary defect (absent/present), plus visual fields if optic nerve compression is suspected

*Based on the seven classic features of inflammation in Graves' ophthalmopathy. The clinical activity score (CAS) is the total number of items present; a CAS ≥3 indicates active ophthalmopathy.
†Subjective diplopia score: 0 = no diplopia; 1 = intermittent (i.e., diplopia in primary position of gaze, when tired, or when first awakening); 2 = inconstant (i.e., diplopia at extremes of gaze); 3 = constant (i.e., continuous diplopia in primary or reading position).
From Melmed S, Polonsky KS, Larsen PR, Kronenberg HM: *Williams textbook of endocrinology,* ed 12, Philadelphia, 2011, Saunders.

SUGGESTED READINGS

Available at ExpertConsult.com

RELATED CONTENT

Graves' Disease (Patient Information)
Hyperthyroidism (Related Key Topic)

AUTHOR: **FRED F. FERRI, M.D.**

[1] Smith TJ et al: Teprotumumab for thyroid-associated ophthalmopathy, *N Engl J Med* 376:1748-1761, 2017.

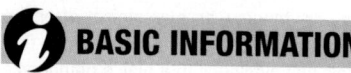

BASIC INFORMATION

DEFINITION

Guillain-Barré syndrome (GBS) is an acute immune-mediated polyradiculoneuropathy (affects nerve roots and peripheral nerves), with predominant motor involvement. It is the most common cause of acute flaccid paralysis in the Western hemisphere and probably worldwide. By definition, maximal clinical weakness, the clinical nadir, occurs within 4 weeks of disease onset.

SYNONYMS

AIDP (acute inflammatory demyelinating polyradiculoneuropathy)
Acute polyneuropathy
Ascending paralysis
GBS
Postinfectious polyneuritis

ICD-10CM CODE
G61.0 Guillain-Barré syndrome

EPIDEMIOLOGY & DEMOGRAPHICS

INCIDENCE: 0.6 to 1.9 cases/100,000 persons annually without geographic variation. Incidence increases with age. A slight peak in incidence occurs between late adolescence and early adulthood. A slight male preponderance (1.25:1) also exists.

PREDISPOSING FACTORS: Viral (HIV, CMV, EBV, influenza) and bacterial *(Campylobacter jejuni, Mycoplasma pneumoniae)* infections; systemic illness (Hodgkin's lymphoma, immunizations). Major antecedents of GBS are described in Box 1.

ETIOLOGY

- Unknown, but believed to be caused by infection-induced aberrant immune response.
- Preceding infectious illness 1 to 4 weeks before disease onset has been noted. The most frequent antecedent infection is *C. jejuni* infection (associated with 30% of cases of GBS and 20% of cases of Miller-Fisher syndrome).
- Humoral and cell-mediated immune attack of peripheral nerve myelin, Schwann cells; sometimes with primary axonal involvement.

PHYSICAL FINDINGS & CLINICAL PRESENTATION

- Symmetric weakness, most commonly involving proximal muscles initially, subsequently involving both proximal and distal muscles; difficulty in ambulating, getting up from a chair, or climbing stairs (Box 2)
- Depressed or absent reflexes bilaterally
- Minimal to moderate glove and stocking paresthesias/dysesthesia/anesthesia or back pain
- Pain (caused by involvement of posterior nerve roots) may be prominent
- Autonomic abnormalities (bradyarrhythmias or tachyarrhythmias, hypotension or hypertension)
- Respiratory insufficiency (caused by weakness of bulbar/intercostal muscles)

BOX 1 Major Antecedents of Guillain-Barré Syndrome

Frequent
Upper respiratory tract infections
Campylobacter jejuni enteritis
Cytomegalovirus infection
Epstein-Barr virus infection
Hepatitis A infection
Hepatitis B infection
Hepatitis C infection
HIV infection

Infrequent
Mycoplasma pneumoniae infection
Haemophilus influenzae infection
Leptospira icterohaemorrhagiae infection
Salmonellosis
Rabies vaccine
Tetanus toxoid
Bacille Calmette-Guérin immunization
Sarcoidosis
Systemic lupus erythematosus
Lymphoma
Trauma
Surgery

Questionable
Hepatitis B vaccine
Influenza vaccine
Hyperthermia
Epidural anesthesia

From Vincent JL et al: *Textbook of critical care*, ed 6, Philadelphia, 2011, Saunders.

BOX 2 Findings Suggesting Guillain-Barré Syndrome

Relative symmetry of symptoms
Mild sensory signs and symptoms
Cranial nerve involvement
Autonomic dysfunction
Absence of fever at onset
Cytoalbuminologic dissociation of cerebrospinal fluid
Typical electrodiagnostic findings
Progression over days to weeks
Recovery beginning 2 to 4 weeks after cessation of progression

From Adams JG: *Emergency medicine: clinical essentials*, Philadelphia, 2013, Saunders.

- Facial paresis, ophthalmoparesis, dysphagia (secondary to cranial nerve involvement)
- GBS consists of several clinical variants based on the pattern of clinical involvement and electrophysiologic findings. These include:
  1. AIDP (most common form in Europe and North America)
  2. Acute motor axonal neuropathy (AMAN; most prevalent form in China and Japan)
  3. Acute motor and sensory axonal neuropathy (AMSAN; has more severe sensory involvement and is associated with more severe clinical course and poorer prognosis)
  4. **Miller Fisher syndrome** (MFS; triad of ophthalmoplegia, ataxia, and areflexia)
  5. Acute pandysautonomia (rapid onset of parasympathetic and sympathetic failure without motor or sensory involvement)
  6. Regional variants (e.g., pharyngeal-cervical-brachial GBS, pure ataxic GBS)

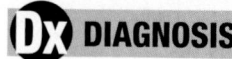

DIAGNOSIS

DIFFERENTIAL DIAGNOSIS

- Toxic peripheral neuropathies: Heavy metal poisoning (lead [microcytic anemia], thallium [alopecia], arsenic [typically accompanied by acute GI illness]), medications (vincristine, disulfiram), organophosphate poisoning, hexacarbon (glue sniffer's neuropathy)
- Nontoxic peripheral neuropathies: Acute intermittent porphyria, fulminant vasculitic polyneuropathy, infectious (poliomyelitis, diphtheria, Lyme disease, West Nile virus), tick paralysis
- Neuromuscular junction disorders: Myasthenia gravis, botulism, snake envenomation
- Myopathies such as polymyositis and acute necrotizing myopathies caused by drugs
- Metabolic derangements such as hypermagnesemia, hypokalemia, hypophosphatemia
- Acute CNS disorders such as basilar artery thrombosis with brainstem infarction, brainstem encephalomyelitis, transverse myelitis, or spinal cord compression
- Conversion disorder
- Malingering

WORKUP

- Exclude other causes based on clinical history, examination, and laboratory tests.
- Lumbar puncture (may be normal in the first 1 to 2 weeks of the illness). Typical findings include elevated CSF protein with few mononuclear leukocytes (albuminocytologic dissociation) in 80% to 90% of patients. Elevated CSF cell counts is an expected feature in cases associated with HIV seroconversion.
- EMG/nerve conduction study (NCS) may be normal in the first 10 to 14 days of the disease. The earliest electrodiagnostic abnormality is prolongation or absence of H-reflexes. NCS evidence of demyelination (prolonged distal latency, conduction velocity slowing, conduction block, temporal dispersion, and prolonged F-waves) in two or more motor nerves confirms diagnosis of AIDP in the appropriate clinical context.

LABORATORY TESTS

- CBC may reveal early leukocytosis with left shift. Electrolytes are tested to exclude metabolic causes of weakness.
- Heavy metal testing; urine porphyria screen; creatine kinase; HIV testing, including tests for HIV seroconversion, especially if CSF demonstrates lymphocytic pleocytosis. MRI brain and spinal cord with and without contrast may be indicated if diagnosis is uncertain. In GBS, a gadolinium-enhanced MRI of the lumbosacral spine may reveal nerve root enhancement.
- Antibodies against ganglioside GQ1b may be present in up to 90% of patients with MFS. IgG antibodies against ganglioside GM1 may be associated with AMAN. There are no antiganglioside antibodies commonly associated with AIDP.

- In equivocal cases, especially if peripheral nerve vasculitis is a concern, nerve biopsy may aid in confirming a diagnosis of GBS. Sensory nerve biopsy demonstrates segmental demyelination with infiltration of monocytes and T cells into the endoneurium. Axonal loss is commonly seen in sensory nerve biopsy specimens in GBS.

Rx TREATMENT

NONPHARMACOLOGIC THERAPY

- Close monitoring of respiratory function (frequent measurements of vital capacity, negative inspiratory force, and tidal volume) and pulmonary toilet should be done because respiratory failure is the major complication in GBS (Fig. E1).
- Frequent repositioning of patient to minimize formation of pressure sores.
- Prevention of venous thromboembolism with antithrombotic stockings as a supplement to pharmacologic venous thromboembolism prevention.
- Emotional support and social counseling for patient and family.
- Pain control.
- Cardiac monitoring to detect arrhythmias.
- Physical and occupational therapy once patient is medically stable and able to participate.
- Avoidance of drugs that may worsen myasthenia gravis or interfere with neuromuscular transmission (Box 3).

BOX 3 Drugs That May Worsen Myasthenia Gravis or Interfere with Neuromuscular Transmission

Antibiotic Agents
- Aminoglycosides
- Erythromycin
- Tetracycline
- Penicillins
- Sulfonamides
- Fluoroquinolones
- Clindamycin
- Lincomycin
- Telithromycin

Anesthetic Agents
- Neuromuscular blocking agents
- Lidocaine
- Procaine

Anticonvulsant Agents
- Phenytoin
- Mephenytoin
- Trimethadione

Cardiovascular Drugs
- Beta blockers
- Procainamide
- Quinidine

Rheumatologic Drugs
- Chloroquine
- D-penicillamine

Miscellaneous
- Iodinated contrast
- Chlorpromazine
- Corticosteroids
- Lithium

Swaiman KF et al: *Swaiman's pediatric neurology, principles and practice,* ed 6, Philadelphia, 2017, Elsevier.

ACUTE GENERAL Rx

- Option 1: Infusion of IV immunoglobulins (IVIG; 0.4 g/kg/day for 5 days). Always check serum IgA levels before infusion to prevent anaphylaxis in IgA-deficient patients.
- Option 2: Early therapeutic plasma exchange (TPE or plasmapheresis: 200–250 ml/kg over five sessions every other day), started within 7 days of onset of symptoms, is beneficial in reducing the need for mechanical ventilation in patients with rapidly progressive disease and results in improved rate of recovery. It is contraindicated in patients with cardiovascular disease (recent MI, unstable angina), active sepsis, and autonomic dysfunction.
- Both therapies are equally effective and may shorten recovery time by 50%. There is no proven benefit from combining IVIG and plasma exchange. Glucocorticoids are contraindicated.
- Mechanical ventilation may be needed if FVC is <12 to 15 ml/kg, vital capacity is rapidly decreasing or is <1000 ml, negative inspiratory force is <20 cm H_2O, PaO_2 is <70, or the patient is having significant difficulty clearing secretions or is aspirating.

CHRONIC Rx

- Ventilatory support may be necessary in 10% to 20% of patients. Adequate fluid/electrolyte support and nutrition are necessary, especially in patients with dysautonomia or bulbar dysfunction.
- Aggressive nursing care to prevent decubitus, infections, fecal impactions, and pressure nerve palsies.
- Monitoring and treatment of autonomic dysfunction (bradyarrhythmias or tachyarrhythmias, orthostatic hypotension, systemic hypertension).
- Treatment of back pain and dysesthesia with low-dose tricyclics, gabapentin, and so on. Opiate narcotics can be used cautiously in the short term but may compound dysautonomia.
- Pharmacologic venous thromboembolism prevention with agents such as heparin (5000 U SC q12h) or enoxaparin (40 mg SC daily) in poorly ambulating and nonambulatory patients.
- Stress ulcer prevention in patients receiving ventilator support.
- Physical and occupational therapy rehabilitation, including supportive devices.

DISPOSITION

- Mortality rate is approximately 5% to 10% worldwide. Causes of death include cardiac arrest, pulmonary embolism, and fulminant infections. A recent study showed 62% complete motor recovery, 14% mild weakness, 9% moderate weakness, 4% bed-bound or ventilated, and 8% dead at 1 yr. Another study suggested that about 33% of patients were free from sensory symptoms at 1 yr, with residual sensory loss present in the lower extremities in 67% and 36% in the upper extremities. About 32% had to change their work, 30% were unable to function at home as well as they could before the disease, and 52% had to alter their leisure activities 1 yr after GBS onset. Excessive fatigue is a common complaint in patients during the recovery phase of GBS. This may be treated with exercise therapy (e.g., bicycle exercise training).
- Predictors for poor recovery (inability to walk independently at 1 yr): Age >60 yr, preceding diarrheal illness, recent CMV infection, fulminant or rapidly progressing course, ventilatory dependence, reduced motor amplitudes (<20% normal), or unexcitable nerves on NCS. Outcomes may also be influenced by complications of medical therapy.
- GBS is typically a monophasic illness. Recurrence may occur in <5% of patients following full recovery.

REFERRAL

- Neurology to aid in diagnosis and direct treatment
- Pulmonary/critical care for ICU management
- Otolaryngology or general surgery for tracheostomy in patients requiring prolonged ventilatory support
- Gastroenterology for percutaneous endoscopic gastrostomy for patients with prolonged inability to obtain nutrition orally

PEARLS & CONSIDERATIONS

- GBS is the most common cause of acute flaccid paralysis.
- Close monitoring of ventilatory function with respiratory mechanics (FVC and NIF) is of paramount importance in all patients with suspected GBS.
- Glucocorticoids are not indicated in GBS and may even slow recovery.

PATIENT/FAMILY EDUCATION

Patient education information may be obtained from the Guillain-Barré Foundation International, The Holly Building, 104 1/2 Forrest Avenue, Narberth, PA 19072; phone: (610) 667-0131; fax: (610) 667-7036; toll-free: (866) 224-3301; E-mail: info@gbs-cidp.org

SUGGESTED READINGS

Available at ExpertConsult.com

RELATED CONTENT

Guillain-Barre Syndrome (Patient Information)

AUTHOR: **DIVYA SINGHAL, M.D.**

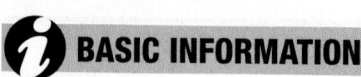

BASIC INFORMATION

DEFINITION

Hallucinations are false perceptions that have no basis in the external environment. Overdoses of hallucinogenic drugs cause symptoms including anxiety, dysphoria, tachycardia, fever, hypertension, seizure, and rhabdomyolysis. Commonly used drugs that cause hallucinations include lysergic acid diethyl amide (LSD), psilocybin (hallucinogenic mushrooms, "magic mushrooms"), mescaline, peyote, methylenedioxymethamphetamine (ecstasy), phencyclidine (PCP, angel dust), cathinone derivatives ("bath salts"), salvia, Datura species (Jimson weed, angel's trumpet), dextromethorphan, and ketamine ("special K," "vitamin K").

SYNONYMS

Overdose, "OD"
Psychedelics
Entheigeon (substance that generates the god/spirit within)
Enactogens (awareness of "the touch within")

ICD-10CM CODES

F16.20	Hallucinogen dependence, uncomplicated
F16.90	LSD reaction (acute) (without dependence)
T40.901	A poisoning by unspecified psychodysleptics [hallucinogens], accidental (unintentional), initial encounter

EPIDEMIOLOGY & DEMOGRAPHICS

INCIDENCE: Used by people of all ages. The drugs commonly are used in group settings such as raves, parties, and college events.
PEAK INCIDENCE: Most commonly between the ages of 17 and 25 yr old
PREVALENCE:
- LSD lifetime prevalence of use >12 yr old: 9.5%
- Hallucinogens prevalence of use >12 yr old: 15.3%
- Overdose or seeking medical treatment is rare

PHYSICAL FINDINGS & CLINICAL PRESENTATION

- Clinical presentation varies by amount and type of drug used.
- Overall presentation includes distortions in body image and sensory perception, as well as rapid, intense alterations in mood; emotions; and suggestibility.
- Overdose symptoms may range from acute anxiety, agitation, tachycardia, hypertension, hyponatremia, hyperthermia, severe agitation, rhabdomyolysis, seizure, cardiac dysrhythmia, respiratory failure, and death.
- Classic pure hallucinogens: Lysergic acid diethyl amide (LSD), psilocybin (hallucinogenic mushrooms, "magic mushrooms"). Individuals rarely present for medical treatment. The patient usually is conscious, alert, and can provide history of drug ingestion. Serious medical problems have been reported to include seizures, hyperthermia, rhabdomyolysis, and acute renal failure. New trends in self-administered "microdosing" of psilocybin or LSD for treatment of depression or other psychological disorders may present as inadvertent overdosing.
- Mescaline: Found in many cacti. Similar structure to LSD; however, there have not been reports of medically significant adverse effects directly from the drug.
- Peyote: Legal for use by the Native American Church. Adverse effects occur first, prior to hallucinations, and within 1 hour of ingestion include severe nausea, vomiting, abdominal pain, dizziness, ataxia, nystagmus, and headache. Mild adrenergic effects of increased temperature, pulse, and blood pressure occurs after the initial symptoms. Hallucinations begin several hours later.
- Methylenedioxymethamphetamine (ecstasy): Not a true hallucinogenic but with similar effects of increased stimulation. Mild increase in temperature, pulse, hypertension, nausea, bruxism, jaw-clenching, dry mouth, muscle aches, ataxia. Severe effects include significant increases in blood pressure leading to intracranial hemorrhage, brain or heart ischemia, arrhythmia, sudden cardiac death, hyponatremia, malignant hyperthermia, DIC, seizures, and rhabdomyolysis. Symptoms are similar to serotonin syndrome.
- Phencyclidine (PCP, angel dust): Similar to ketamine with multiple effects that include features of hallucinations. Patients may have CNS stimulation or depression. The most common signs are mild hypertension and vertical nystagmus in 60% of patients. Other important warning signs for the safety of staff and physicians include severe agitation, physical violence, unpredictable behavior, and decreased response to pain. Disassociation, seizures (up to 3%), rhabdomyolysis with resulting acute renal failure, dystonic reactions, hyperthermia causing hepatic necrosis, and multiorgan failure are also possible.
- Cathinone derivatives (bath salts): Similar to PCP, with sympathomimetic effects of elevated temperature, blood pressure, pulse, sweating. Patients also may be severely agitated, aggressive, and violent toward staff. Severe medical effects include severe hyperthermia, hyponatremia, seizures, and rhabdomyolysis.
- Salvia: Adverse effects are mild and may include slurred speech, dysphoria, headache, nausea, vomiting, dizziness.
- *Datura* species (Jimson weed, angel's trumpet): Anticholinergic alkaloids with symptoms consistent with anticholinergic poisoning: Hyperthermia, delirium, hallucinations, mydriasis, blurry vision, dry mouth, tachycardia, urinary retention.
- Dextromethorphan: Most commonly used by adolescents due to availability in over-the-counter cold and flu products; likely to be associated with salicylate, antihistamine, and acetaminophen overdose due to combination of cold and flu product ingredients.

ETIOLOGY

Usually caused by stimulation of various receptors in the brain, including serotonin type 2, dopamine, norepinephrine, acetylcholine, beta2-adrenergic, NMDA, opioids, and voltage-gated electrolyte channels.

Dx DIAGNOSIS

DIFFERENTIAL DIAGNOSIS

- Alcohol use or withdrawal
- Benzodiazepine withdrawal
- Anticholinergic poisoning
- Serotonin syndrome
- Thyrotoxicosis
- Central nervous system infections
- Structural brain lesions
- Acute psychosis
- Hypoglycemia
- Hypoxia
- Sepsis
- Acute ischemic or hemorrhagic stroke
- Polysubstance use
- Acute psychosis
- Incidental trauma

WORKUP

- Must rule out nontoxic causes of altered mental status. Vital signs should be examined immediately. History of drug use, dementia, delirium, and risk factors for CNS infection should be considered. Patients should also be examined for occult and incidental trauma that occurred while under the influence of the drugs.

LABORATORY TESTS

- Consider:
  1. Complete blood count
  2. Glucose level
  3. Comprehensive metabolic panel
  4. Thyroid-stimulating hormone
  5. Creatine phosphokinase
  6. Arterial blood gas
  7. Toxicologic screening for other illegal drugs, acetaminophen, salicylate

IMAGING STUDIES

- Consider:
  1. ECG
  2. CT of head
  3. MRI of brain

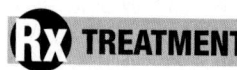

TREATMENT

Because most symptoms are not life or limb threatening, most treatment revolves around supportive treatment.

NONPHARMACOLOGIC THERAPY

- Place patient in a calm and quiet area with limited auditory and visual stimulation.
- Patients may benefit from a sitter to reorient patient and provide and calming presence.
- Physical restraints should be used only if absolutely necessary due to the increased risk of agitation, hyperthermia, and rhabdomyolysis. Severely violent patients may require chemical restraint in addition to physical restraint.

- Severe hypothermia may require active cooling measures.
- Supplemental oxygen should be considered.
- Bowel irrigation not usually recommended after 60 minutes of ingestion; unlikely to be beneficial for most compounds.

ACUTE GENERAL Rx

- Benzodiazepines are the mainstay of medical treatment
- Aggressive intravenous hydration with isotonic crystalloids
- Naloxone
- Dextrose
- Dantrolene if refractive hyperthermia
- Hypertonic saline if hyponatremic
- Cyproheptadine for serotonin syndrome
- IV nitroprusside or nicardipine for blood pressure control
- Propofol, barbiturate for refractive seizure
- Paralytics for hyperthermia secondary to dystonic reactions
- Physostigmine for severe anticholinergic poisoning

DISPOSITION

- Patients should be monitored for several hours for resolution of symptoms. If symptoms improve, patients who are mentally lucid and steady on their feet may be discharged under the close supervision of family or friends.
- Patients not improving mentally may require further workup.
- If no organic cause is found, patients may require psychiatric evaluation.
- Patients may need to be admitted until resolution of organ injury.

REFERRAL

- Psychiatric referral may be required
- Substance abuse or rehab

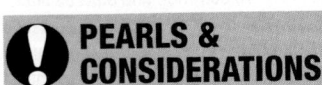

PEARLS & CONSIDERATIONS

COMMENTS:

- Actual substance used may be unclear.
- Most treatment is supportive care.
- Treat symptoms of hyperthermia, severe hypertension, and possible rhabdomyolysis.
- Chemical restraint with benzodiazepines is safe and effective.

SUGGESTED READINGS

Available at ExpertConsult.com

RELATED CONTENT

Alcohol Abuse (Related Key Topic)
Delirium (Related Key Topic)
Delirium Tremens (Related Key Topic)
Opioid Overdose (Related Key Topic)
Serotonin Syndrome (Related Key Topic)

AUTHORS: **DANNY H. VANVALKINBURGH, M.D.**, and **BENJAMIN BAKER, M.D.**

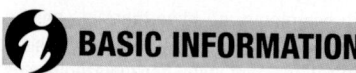

BASIC INFORMATION

DEFINITION

Hand-foot-mouth disease (HFMD) is a viral illness characterized by superficial lesions of the oral mucosa and skin of the extremities. HFMD is primarily caused by coxsackie or enterovirus infection and can be transmitted by either respiratory droplet contact or fecal-oral contact. Although young children are predominantly affected, adults are also at risk. This disease is usually self-limited and benign, although outbreaks in the Asia Pacific region have been increasingly complicated by neurologic and cardiopulmonary sequelae.

SYNONYMS

HFMD
Vesicular stomatitis with exanthema
Coxsackie virus infection
Enterovirus infection

ICD-10CM CODE
B08.4 Enteroviral vesicular stomatitis with exanthem

EPIDEMIOLOGY & DEMOGRAPHICS

- HFMD most often affects children <10 yr.
  1. Children <5 yr are at the highest risk of infection and have the most severe cases.
- HFMD is contagious. Close contacts of affected children, including family members and health care workers, are the most commonly infected adults. Outbreaks can also occur in clustered populations of young adults (a recent outbreak at a military base affected 4.7% of the exposed population).
- Infection is spread from person to person by direct contact with saliva, respiratory secretions, fluid in vesicles, or stool.
- Outbreaks in daycares, schools, summer camps, hospital cohorts, and other groups with close contact are common.
- A person is most contagious during the first week of illness.
- Outbreaks tend to occur during the summer.
- Infection leads to immunity, but a subsequent episode may occur after infection with a different etiologic virus or type.

PHYSICAL FINDINGS & CLINICAL PRESENTATION

Symptoms:

- After a 3- to 5-day incubation period (range 2 to 7 days), patients may report odynophagia, sore throat, malaise, and fever (38.3° to 40° C).
- 1 to 2 days later, the characteristic oral lesions appear (small red spots that blister and may ulcerate). The fluid from these lesions is infectious, and disease can be transmitted through contact with the fluid.
- In 75% of cases, skin lesions on the extremities accompany these oral manifestations (small flat or raised red bumps, sometimes with blisters—they can be macular, maculopapular, or vesicular), but the lesions may be absent. The skin lesions are usually not painful or pruritic, but can be painful.
- Only 11% of adults have cutaneous findings.
- Lesions appear over the course of 1 or 2 days and resolve over 3 to 4 days.

Physical findings:

- Oral lesions are common and are usually found on the tongue, buccal mucosa, gingivae, and hard palate.
- Oral lesions initially start as 1- to 3-mm erythematous macules and evolve into gray vesicles on an erythematous base.
- Vesicles are frequently broken by the time of presentation and appear as superficial, gray ulcers with surrounding erythema.
- Skin lesions of the palms of the hands and soles of the feet are common and start as linear erythematous papules (3 to 10 mm in diameter) that evolve into gray vesicles that may be mildly painful (Fig. 1). These vesicles are usually intact at presentation and remain so until they desquamate within 2 wk. They are nonpruritic.
- Involvement of the buttocks and genital area is also common (present in 31% of cases).
- Although rare, atypical findings such as fingernail or toenail loss (nail separation from the nail matrix, otherwise known as onychomadesis) after HFMD (notably with the A6 strain of coxsackie virus) has been reported in children. The nail loss is temporary, and nails grow back without intervention.
- Another atypical skin manifestation is that of "eczema coxsackium," which is described as the typical skin lesions of coxsackie virus but with a more extensive distribution involving the trunk and extremities, localized to areas of active or past atopic dermatitis.
- In rare cases, encephalitis, meningitis, myocarditis, poliomyelitis-like paralysis, and pulmonary edema may develop. Sporadic acute paralysis and long-term neurologic sequelae have been reported with enterovirus 71.
- Although information is limited, there is no clear evidence that pregnancy outcomes are affected in the setting of maternal infection.

ETIOLOGY

- Coxsackie virus group A, type 16, was the first and is the most common cause of HFMD.
- Enterovirus 71 is the second leading cause of HFMD. Enterovirus 71 is neurotropic and has a predilection for the brainstem, leading to more severe cases of the disease and more complications than with other strains or viruses. Clusters of severe disease have been reported in the Asia Pacific region.
- Coxsackie virus strains A5, A6, A7, A9, A10, B1, B2, B3, and B5 have also been implicated.
- Coxsackie A6 has been known to cause a severe skin rash and self-limited nail abnormalities (onychomadesis). Patients with this strain may lack oral lesions.
- Epidemic outbreaks have been reported with coxsackie A16 and enterovirus 71.

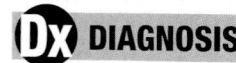

DIAGNOSIS

DIFFERENTIAL DIAGNOSIS

- Aphthous stomatitis
- Herpes simplex infection
- Herpangina
- Behçet's syndrome
- Erythema multiforme
- Pemphigus
- Gonorrhea
- Acute leukemia
- Lymphoma
- Allergic contact dermatitis

WORKUP

The diagnosis is made on the basis of typical history and characteristic physical examination.

LABORATORY TESTS

- Not indicated unless the diagnosis is in doubt such as for a suspected case with an atypical presentation.
  1. Oropharyngeal specimen, stool specimen, or vesicular fluid may be obtained to identify the presence of enterovirus or

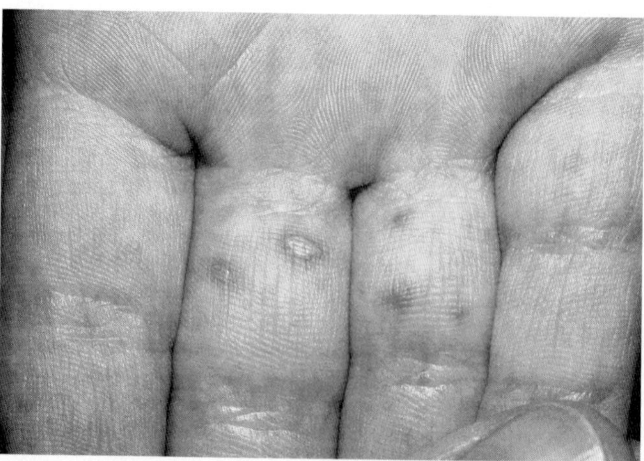

FIG. 1 Hand-foot-mouth disease. Deep-seated vesicles with erythema involving the palmar surface of the fingers. (From Paller AS, Mancini AJ: *Hurwitz clinical pediatric dermatology: a textbook of skin disorders of childhood and adolescence*, ed 5, Edinburgh, 2016, Elsevier.)

coxsackievirus by polymerase chain reaction (PCR), but may take from 2 to 4 weeks for results. Due to prolonged shedding of the virus (weeks to months), detection of virus in secretions may not be responsible for current symptoms.
- Identification of a certain strain is only available in public health laboratories.

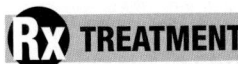

TREATMENT

ACUTE GENERAL Rx

- Symptomatic therapy is given for this usually self-limited disease.
- There are currently no available approved therapies for more severe cases. Antivirals and IV immunoglobulin have been evaluated for enterovirus 71 infections, but these treatments have not been evaluated in randomized, placebo-controlled studies.
- Systemic steroids should be avoided because they have been associated with more severe disease and higher viral loads.

DISPOSITION

Prognosis is excellent except in rare cases of central nervous system or cardiac involvement. Most are managed as outpatients. Hospitalization should be considered if the patient is unable to maintain adequate hydration due to painful oral lesions and in cases of neurologic manifestations such as meningitis, encephalitis, or flaccid paralysis, or cardiac complications such as myocarditis.

REFERRAL

Not usually needed, although dermatology or infectious disease consultation can be considered for diagnostic or therapeutic input for an atypical or severe case

PEARLS & CONSIDERATIONS

- Frequent handwashing, disinfection of contaminated surfaces, and washing of soiled articles of clothing can help reduce transmission.
- HFMD has no relation to hoof and mouth disease in cattle.

SUGGESTED READINGS

Available at ExpertConsult.com

RELATED CONTENT

Hand, Foot, and Mouth Disease (Patient Information)

AUTHOR: **ERICA HARDY, M.D., M.M.S.**

BASIC INFORMATION

DEFINITION

Head and neck squamous cell carcinoma is a malignant disease entity that arises from the epithelium of the mucosal surfaces of the upper aerodigestive tract and accounts for about 90% of head and neck cancers. This disease results from exposure to carcinogens and from the accumulation of genetic alterations. The workup and management of these patients depends upon the specific subsite of the aerodigestive tract in the head and neck from which the primary tumor arises. These subsites are the oral cavity, oropharynx, nasopharynx, hypopharynx, and larynx. Cutaneous malignancies, thyroid neoplasms, and salivary gland neoplasms also occur in the head and neck but are beyond the scope of this chapter.

SYNONYMS

HNC
Head and neck cancer
HNSCC
Head and neck squamous cell carcinoma

ICD-10CM CODES	
C77.0	Secondary and unspecified malignant neoplasm of lymph nodes of head, face, and neck
C00-C14	Malignant neoplasms of lip, oral cavity, and pharynx
C30	Malignant neoplasm of nasal cavities, middle ear, and accessory sinuses
C32	Malignant neoplasm of larynx

EPIDEMIOLOGY & DEMOGRAPHICS

INCIDENCE:

- U.S. annual incidence of head and neck cancer (90% of which is squamous cell carcinoma) is approximately 62,000 persons per yr.
- Annual mortality is approximately 13,000 persons per yr.
- Accounts for approximately 3% of all cancers in the U.S.
- Human papilloma virus (HPV)-associated squamous cell carcinoma of the head and neck accounts for 5% to 20% of all HNSCCs, and 40% to 90% of those arise in oropharynx.
- Incidence of all forms of HNSCC is on the decline, except oropharyngeal squamous cell carcinoma, which is increasing in incidence, likely related to the rise in human papilloma virus (HPV) associated HNSCC.

PEAK INCIDENCE: Sixth decade of life

PREDOMINANT SEX AND AGE: Male:female ratio is about 3:1. Risk increases significantly over the age of 40.

GENETICS: Research is ongoing in genetic factors that lead to the development and progression of HNSCC. Tumor suppressor genes including *p53*, *NOTCH1*, and *CDKN2A*, among others, have been shown to harbor mutations in patients with HNSCC.

RISK FACTORS: The two most strongly implicated risk factors associated with HNSCC are tobacco and alcohol use. These carcinogens place the entire epithelium of the upper respiratory tract at risk for multiple primary tumors via a process known as field cancerization. More recently, a new subset of HNSCC caused by the HPV has been increasing in prevalence. HPV 16 is the most common genotype detected. Patients are more likely to be white middle-aged men, nonsmokers, with minimal alcohol use and higher socioeconomic status.

PHYSICAL FINDINGS & CLINICAL PRESENTATION

- Presenting signs and symptoms are related to local effects of the primary tumor, regional spread, metastatic disease, or paraneoplastic phenomena.
  1. Oral cavity, oropharynx, hypopharynx: Painful mass or ulceration (Fig. 1), dysphagia, odynophagia, weight loss.
  2. Larynx: Hoarseness, voice change, shortness of breath, stridor.
  3. Nasal cavity, paranasal sinus, nasopharynx—referred otalgia, conductive hearing loss from middle ear effusion, epistaxis, cranial nerve palsies.
  4. All sites: Cranial nerve palsies, painless neck mass from regional metastases to cervical lymph nodes. Most common site of distant metastases is the lung, with bone and liver being much less common.
- Physical exam: A thorough examination of the head and neck, including cranial nerve exam, otoscopy, inspection and palpation of oral cavity, oropharynx, and neck, and general physical exam.
  1. Concerning exam findings: Unilateral middle ear effusion, ulcerated mass of the oral cavity (Fig. E2) or oropharynx, trismus, painless neck mass.

ETIOLOGY

Exposure to carcinogens including tobacco and alcohol causes genetic alterations in the epithelium of mucosal surfaces lining the upper aerodigestive tract, leading to malignant transformation of epithelial cells. HPV-associated HNSCC is a direct result of the carcinogenic effects of the virus and is not related to alcohol and tobacco use. Primary nasopharyngeal carcinoma has a weak association with tobacco and alcohol and is endemic to southern China, Southeast Asia, and northern Africa. There is a strong association between Epstein-Barr virus infection and primary nasopharyngeal carcinoma.

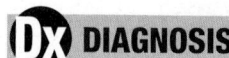

DIAGNOSIS

DIFFERENTIAL DIAGNOSIS

Lymphoma, primary salivary gland malignancy, thyroid malignancy, benign tumors of the upper aerodigestive tract, metastases.

WORKUP

- Initial workup includes incudes a full physical examination, indirect and/or direct laryngoscopy, imaging studies of the head and neck as well as the chest and/or body to assess for metastases, laboratory tests as indicated, and referral to a head and neck cancer specialist.
- Additional workup by head and neck cancer specialist:
  1. Flexible fiber-optic laryngoscopy or mirror laryngoscopy
  2. Biopsy of the tumor in office or under anesthesia
  3. Fine-needle aspiration (FNA) and biopsy for patient who presents with a suspicious neck mass
  4. Panendoscopy with biopsy under anesthesia, which may include direct laryngoscopy, esophagoscopy, and/or bronchoscopy

LABORATORY TESTS

Complete blood count (CBC), coagulation studies, electrolytes, ECG, liver function tests (albumin, transaminases, alkaline phosphatase), TSH

IMAGING STUDIES

- CT scan of the neck with contrast: Necessary to evaluate extent of primary tumor and nodal metastases in neck (Fig. 3).

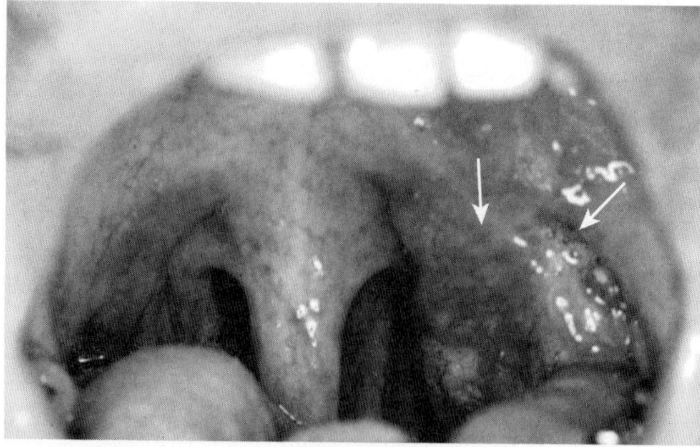

FIG. 1 Squamous cell carcinoma of the left tonsil (*arrows*). (From Richardson MA, et al.: *Cummings otolaryngology–head and neck surgery*, ed 5, Philadelphia, 2010, Mosby, pp. 1358-1374, Figure 100-8.)

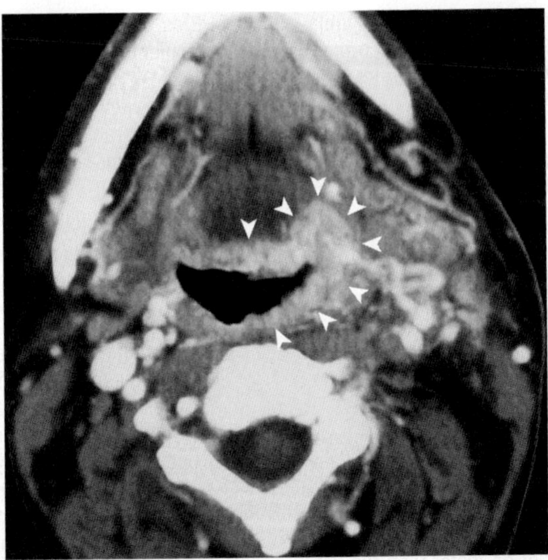

FIG. 3 CT scan with contrast showing tumor of the base of the left oropharynx *(arrowheads).* (From Richardson MA, et al.: *Cummings otolaryngology–head and neck surgery*, ed 5, Philadelphia, 2010, Mosby, pp. 1393-1420, Figure 102-47.)

- MRI of head and neck (optional): Useful for nasopharyngeal, infratemporal fossa, temporal bone, parotid, parapharyngeal, skull base, or intracranial involvement.
- Chest x-ray or CT chest with contrast: To evaluate for lung metastases.
- PET/CT: Highlights areas in the body with increased metabolic uptake. Useful initially to assess extent of primary tumor, location of unknown primary tumor, cervical metastases, distant metastases, and second primary tumors. Can be used to monitor for recurrence in the posttreatment setting.

STAGING

Staging is based on the tumor, node, metastasis (TNM) staging system provided by the AJCC. Staging varies depending on the head and neck subsite that is involved. Any nodal metastasis in the neck automatically classifies as advanced disease (Stage III or IV). Distant metastases place patients at Stage IVC. The exception to this is HPV-positive cancer of the oropharynx, in which the most recent staging system allows for a patient to be classified as low as Stage II even with cervical nodal metastases given the excellent response to treatment and prognosis for these tumors.

Rx TREATMENT

- Treatment consists of surgery, radiation, chemotherapy, or a combination of any or all of the three modalities. The goal is to use as few modalities as possible to minimize side effects of treatment without compromising oncologic success.
  1. Surgery: Complete surgical resection of the primary tumor along with unilateral or bilateral neck dissections to remove involved or potentially involved lymph nodes as clinically indicated.
  2. Radiation: Allows for easier access to poorly exposed tumors such as those of the larynx, oropharynx, nasopharynx, or hypopharynx. Disadvantages include lengthy, time-intensive treatment course, xerostomia, pain, and higher surgical morbidity if salvage surgery is needed.
  3. Chemotherapy: Useful only as an adjuvant to radiation therapy or for palliation. Single-agent cisplatin therapy is widely accepted in the U.S. as a standard for chemoradiation regimens for head and neck cancers of any site. Major toxicities include nausea, vomiting, renal toxicity, ototoxicity, and myelosuppression.
  4. Reconstruction: Performed with the goal of optimizing functional and cosmetic outcomes. Options include primary closure, local flaps, regional flaps, skin grafts, and microvascular free flaps from other parts of the body (e.g., radial forearm, fibula, anterolateral thigh, latissimus, etc.).

ACUTE GENERAL Rx

- Early-stage disease (Stage I or II):
  1. Single-modality treatment with surgery or radiation alone may be appropriate for early-stage head and neck cancer. The choice between one or the other depends on the specific subsite of the head and neck that is involved and the side effects profile for each modality.
  2. Treatment of the potentially involved lymph nodes in the neck with either neck dissection or radiation is controversial and depends on the clinical scenario and the judgment of the treatment team.
- Locoregionally advanced disease (Stage III or IV):
  1. In general, these patients have large tumors >4 cm and/or cervical nodal metastases. Treatment typically involves multimodality therapy with either surgery followed by radiation therapy or upfront chemoradiation alone. Depending on the presence of certain adverse pathologic features of the surgical specimen, adjuvant chemoradiation may be necessary. If chemoradiation is the initial treatment modality, surgery may be needed in the adjuvant setting for residual or recurrent disease.
  2. Laryngeal cancers are the exception where select advanced disease with T3 or N1 tumors can be managed with single-modality therapy with surgery or radiation alone.
  3. Nasopharyngeal cancer is also an exception. This is not a surgical disease. Managed primarily by radiation to primary site and neck for early-stage disease. Chemoradiation is primary treatment for advanced disease. Surgery is reserved for recurrent or residual disease of primary site or neck following radiation therapy.
- Metastatic disease (Stage IVC):
  1. Palliation of symptoms is the primary goal of treatment.
- All patients should be counseled on smoking cessation and avoidance of alcohol.

DISPOSITION

- Prognosis depends on the specific subsite of the head and neck that is involved. Overall 5-yr survival rate for head and neck squamous cell carcinoma is about 55%. This varies with 5-yr survival rates for carcinoma of the lip as high as 89.7% and carcinomas of the hypopharynx as low as approximately 30%.
- Patients are followed on a regular basis multiple times a yr by a head and neck cancer specialist. After a 5-yr disease-free survival, patients are followed on a yearly basis.

REFERRAL

Referral should be made to an otolaryngologist or oral surgeon who specializes in head and neck cancer.

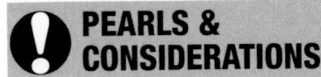

PEARLS & CONSIDERATIONS

PREVENTION

- Encourage all patients to cease using tobacco and to limit alcohol consumption.
- Examine the oral cavity and palpate the neck during the annual physical examination. Work up any suspicious masses or lesions.

PATIENT/FAMILY EDUCATION

http://www.entnet.org/content/head-and-neck-cancer

http://www.cancer.gov/types/head-and-neck

SUGGESTED READINGS

Available at ExpertConsult.com

RELATED CONTENT

Laryngeal Carcinoma (Related Key Topic)
Oral Cancer (Related Key Topic)

AUTHOR: **LOUIS INSALACO, M.D.**

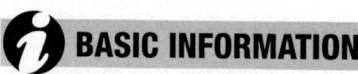

BASIC INFORMATION

DEFINITION

Complete heart block (CHB) is the absence of electrical impulse transmission from the atria to the ventricles when atrioventricular (AV) junction is not physiologically refractory, due to a functional or anatomical impairment of the conduction system, resulting in a bradycardia characterized by AV dissociation. It may be acquired or congenital. CHB can be permanent or reversible.

SYNONYMS

Third-degree AV block
CHB
Complete AV block

ICD-10CM CODE

I44.2 Atrioventricular block, complete

EPIDEMIOLOGY & DEMOGRAPHICS

- The prevalence of CHB is 0.04%.
- The prevalence of CHB increases with age.

PHYSICAL FINDINGS & CLINICAL PRESENTATION

Physical examination may be normal. Cannon A waves may appear in the jugular vein periodically due to the right atrium contracting during ventricular systole. Patients may present with the following clinical manifestations:

- Dizziness, palpitations
- Syncope or presyncope (due to reduced cardiac output)
- Fatigue, impaired exercise tolerance
- Mental status changes
- Congestive heart failure
- Angina pectoris
- Some patients may be asymptomatic (e.g., congenital CHB)

ETIOLOGY

- Fibrosis or sclerosis of the conduction system, Lenegre and Lev disease
- Acute myocardial infarction—inferior (14%) or anterior (2%) wall of patients, usually within 24 hours
- Drug effect (digitalis, calcium channel blockers, beta-blockers, amiodarone)
- Cardiomyopathy and myocarditis
- Infiltrative processes of the myocardium (amyloidosis, sarcoidosis, scleroderma, tumor)
- Metabolic abnormalities (hyperkalemia, hypoxia, hypothyroidism)
- Lyme carditis, rheumatoid nodules, polymyositis, Chagas' disease
- Neuromuscular disorders (Becker muscular dystrophy, myotonic muscular dystrophy)
- Congenital (birth from mothers with systemic lupus)
- Hyperkalemia
- Familial: SCN5 sodium channel mutations have been associated with CHB
- Iatrogenic (cardiac surgery, catheter ablation of arrhythmias, percutaneous coronary intervention). Transcatheter aortic valve implantation (TAVI) is shown to be frequently associated with new conduction abnormalities; patients with preexisting right bundle branch block are at increased risk of CHB (resolves over time in most patients).
- Paroxysmal due to phase 4 block of the His-Purkinje system

Dx DIAGNOSIS

DIFFERENTIAL DIAGNOSIS

- The differential diagnosis includes lesser degree of AV block, automatic accelerated junctional rhythms, and nonconducted premature atrial contractions.
- The atrial rate must be faster than the ventricular rate (more As than Vs), and the junctional or ventricular rate is regular. Episodes of AV dissociation with an accelerated ventricular or junctional pacemaker overtaking the sinus node can often look like heart block on a single electrocardiogram.

WORKUP

- Workup such as routine labs, cardiac biomarkers, and cardiac imaging should be dictated by the clinical circumstances.
- ECG: Diagnostic of the disease (Figs. 1 and 2):
  1. P waves are present with a regular atrial rate that is faster than the ventricular rate.
  2. P waves are not related to the QRS complexes. The PR intervals are variable.
  3. RR intervals are regular.
  4. QRS complexes may be narrow with a rate of 40 to 60 beats/min (block proximal to His bundle) or wide with a rate of <40 beats/min (block distal to His bundle), depending on the location of the block in the conduction system.
  5. Complete AV block can result from block at the level of AV node, within the His bundle, or distal to it, in the Purkinje system.

Rx TREATMENT

ACUTE GENERAL Rx

- Initial treatment should focus on the hemodynamic stability and symptoms of the patient.
- Fig. 3 illustrates the evaluation and management of third degree AV block.
- Consider temporary pacemaker insertion if ventricular escape rate is slow (<40 beats/min) and associated with symptoms or hemodynamic compromise as well as wide QRS escape rhythms, which can be unstable, and QT prolongation above 500 ms, increasing the risk of torsade de pointes ventricular tachycardias.
- CHB as a complication of inferior MI usually only requires temporary pacing; however, a CHB as a result of anterior MI often requires permanent pacing (Table 1).
- Acquired CHB usually requires pacing, but patients with congenital CHB often have sufficiently rapid escape rhythm to prevent symptoms and avoid permanent pacemaker implantation.
- Withdraw AV-nodal blocking agents if any.
- Short-term therapy (until adequate pacing therapy is established):
  1. Vagolytic agents such as atropine may be used to increase the rate of the escape rhythm (for AV nodal level blocks).
  2. Catecholamines such as isoproterenol transiently used for a CHB at any site (use with extreme caution or not at all in patients with coronary artery disease or in patients with digitalis toxicity).
  3. Percutaneous external cardiac pacing (uncomfortable for patients and not always reliably capturing the ventricle).
- Drugs cannot be relied on to increase HR for more than several hours or days without side effects; therefore, temporary or permanent pacemaker insertion is indicated.
- Symptomatic CHB in the absence of a condition that is likely to resolve is an ACC/AHA/HRS Class I indication for permanent pacemaker (PPM) placement.
- Class I indications for PPM placement in asymptomatic patients according to the ACC/AHA guidelines include:
  1. Patients in sinus rhythm, with documented asystolic pauses greater than or equal to 3.0 sec or an escape rate <40 beats/min, or with an escape rhythm that is below the AV node
  2. Patients with atrial fibrillation and bradycardia with one or more pauses of at least 5 sec or longer
  3. After catheter ablation of the AV junction
  4. If cardiomegaly or LV dysfunction is present with ventricular rates of 40 beats/min or faster
  5. Postoperative CHB that is not expected to resolve
  6. When it is associated with neuromuscular diseases, such as Erb dystrophy (limb-girdle muscular dystrophy), Kearns-Sayre syndrome, myotonic muscular dystrophy, and peroneal muscular atrophy
  7. CHB present during exercise in the absence of myocardial ischemia
- Therapy is directed toward the underlying etiology if there is a reversible source (i.e., IV antibiotics for Lyme disease).
- Table 2 summarizes the management of complete heart block.

CHRONIC Rx

Dual-chamber pacemaker implantation. Patients with a pacemaker need regular follow-up and pacemaker monitoring to ensure proper device functioning. Interest has developed recently in placing the ventricular pacing lead in the His bundle region, which can result in a narrow-paced QRS and may prevent ventricular dyssynchrony associated with traditional RV pacing.

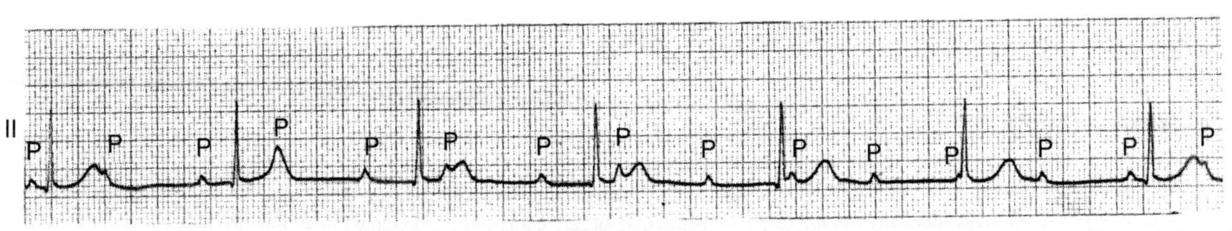

FIG. 1 Third-degree (complete) atrioventricular heart block is characterized by independent atrial (P) and ventricular (QRS) activity. The atrial rate is always faster than the ventricular rate. The PR intervals are completely variable. Some P waves fall on the T wave, distorting its shape. Others may fall in the QRS complex and be "lost." Notice that the QRS complexes are of normal width, indicating that the ventricles are being paced from the atrioventricular junction. (From Goldberger AL, editor: *Clinical electrocardiography*, ed 5, St Louis, 1994, Mosby.)

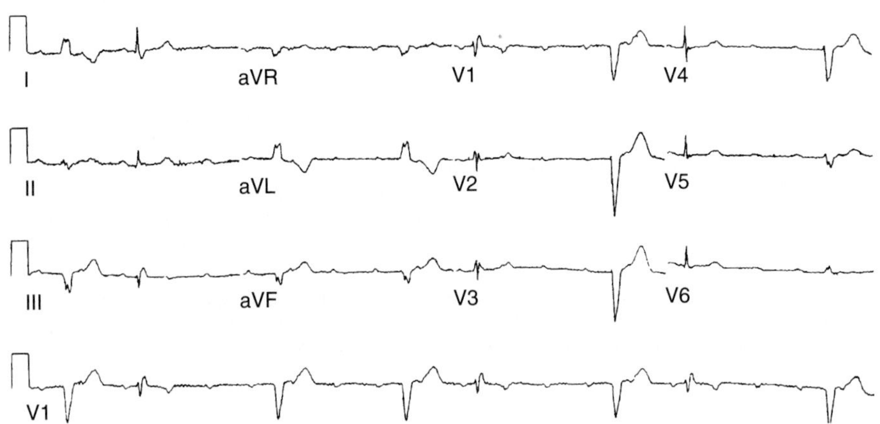

FIG. 2 High-grade atrioventricular block. Note that only three P waves conducted to the ventricle in the whole tracing. Conducted P waves were associated with normal PR intervals and right bundle branch block, a finding suggesting infranodal block. All other P waves were blocked, and ventricular escape rhythm with a left bundle branch block pattern is observed. Note that the block is not caused by retrograde concealment in the atrioventricular node or His-Purkinje system from the ventricular escape complexes because the conducted P waves occurred at a short cycle following the escape complexes. (From Issa Z et al: *Clinical arrhythmology and electrophysiology*, ed 2, Philadelphia, 2012, Saunders.)

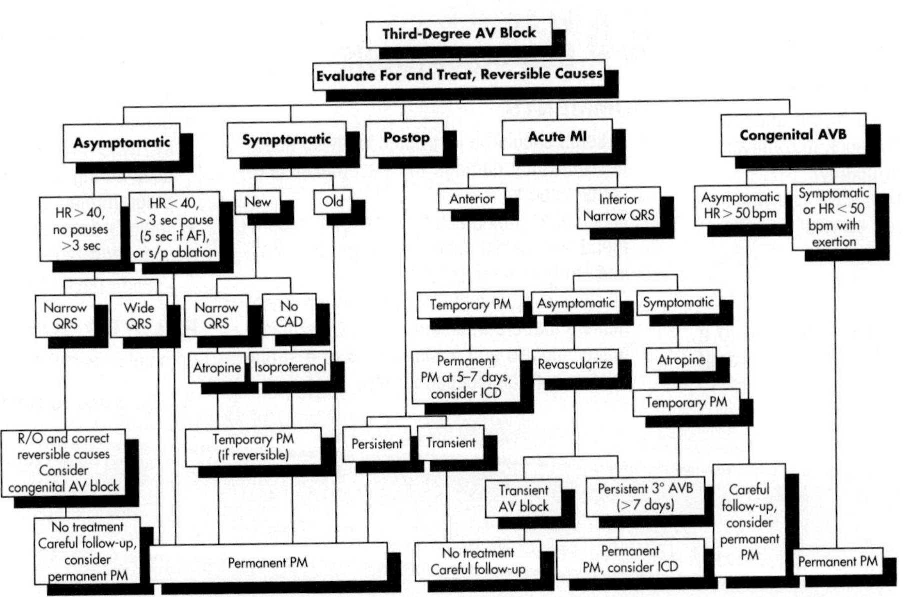

FIG. 3 Evaluation and management of third degree AV block. *AF,* Atrial flutter; *AVB*, atrioventricular block; *bpm,* beats per minute; *CAD*, coronary artery disease; *HR,* heart rate; *ICD*, implantable cardioverter defibrillator; *MI*, myocardial infarction; *PM*, pacemaker *R/O,* rule out. (From Olshansky B, Chung MK, Pogwizd SM et al: *Arrhythmia essentials*, ed 2, Philadelphia, 2017, Elsevier.)

TABLE 1 Indications for Pacing in AV Block

Class I

1. Third-degree or advanced second-degree AV block at any anatomic level associated with any one of the following conditions:
   a. Symptoms (including heart failure) attributable to AV block (Level of Evidence: C)
   b. Arrhythmias and other medical conditions that require drugs that result in symptomatic bradycardia (Level of Evidence: C)
   c. Documented periods of asystole >3.0 seconds, any escape rate <40 beats/min, or any escape rhythm below the AV junction (e.g., a wide QRS morphology) in awake, asymptomatic patients in sinus rhythm (Level of Evidence: C)
   d. A documented period of asystole >5 seconds in awake, asymptomatic patients in atrial fibrillation (Level of Evidence: C)
   e. After catheter ablation of the AV junction (Level of Evidence: C)
   f. Postoperative AV block that is not expected to resolve after cardiac surgery (Level of Evidence: C)
   g. Neuromuscular diseases, such as myotonic muscular dystrophy, Kearns–Sayre syndrome, Erb (limb-girdle) dystrophy, and peroneal muscular atrophy, with or without symptoms of bradycardia (Level of Evidence: B)
2. Asymptomatic third-degree AV block at any anatomic site with an average awake ventricular rate >40 beats/min in patients with cardiomegaly or left ventricular dysfunction
3. Second-degree or third-degree AV block during exercise in the absence of myocardial ischemia (*Level of Evidence: C*)
4. Symptomatic second-degree AV block regardless of type or site of block (*Level of Evidence: B*)

Class IIa

1. Advanced second-degree or third-degree AV block at any anatomic site with an average ventricular rate >40 beats/min in the absence of cardiomegaly (*Level of Evidence: C*)
2. Asymptomatic second-degree AV block at intra- or infra-His levels found at electrophysiologic study (*Level of Evidence: B*)
3. First-degree or second-degree AV block with symptoms similar to those of pacemaker syndrome (*Level of Evidence: B*)
4. Asymptomatic type II second-degree AV block with a narrow QRS. When type II second-degree AV block occurs with a wide QRS, including isolated right bundle branch block, pacing becomes a Class I recommendation. (*Level of Evidence: B*)

Class IIb

1. AV block due to drug use or toxicity when the block is expected to recur even after withdrawal of the drug (*Level of Evidence: B*)
2. Neuromuscular diseases, such as myotonic muscular dystrophy, Kearns–Sayre syndrome, Erb (limb-girdle) dystrophy, and peroneal muscular atrophy with any degree of AV block (including first-degree AV block), with or without symptoms of bradycardia (*Level of Evidence: B*)

Class III

1. Asymptomatic first-degree AV block (*Level of Evidence: B*)
2. Asymptomatic type I second-degree AV block at a site above the His (i.e., the AV node) level or not known to be intra- or infra-Hisian by electrophysiologic study (*Level of Evidence: B*)
3. AV block expected to resolve and unlikely to recur (e.g., drug toxicity, Lyme disease, nocturnally in sleep apnea, early postoperative status, transient increases in vagal tone) (*Level of Evidence: B*)

AV, Atrioventricular.
From Bonow RO et al: *Braunwald's heart disease: a textbook of cardiovascular medicine,* ed 9, Philadelphia, 2012, Saunders.

DISPOSITION

- Mortality is highest in the neonatal period in congenital CHB.
- Prognosis is favorable after insertion of a pacemaker and is related to the underlying etiology of complete AV block (e.g., myocardial infarction, cardiomyopathy).
- Nonrandomized studies have shown that PPM insertion improves survival in patients with CHB.

REFERRAL

All patients with CHB should be referred to a cardiologist for consideration of temporary and/or PPM implantation.

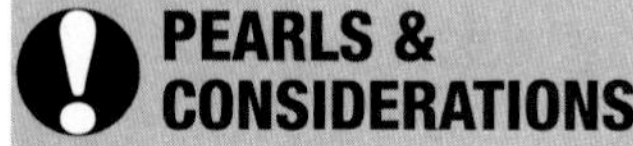

PEARLS & CONSIDERATIONS

COMMENTS

- Patients should be instructed to avoid activities that may damage the pacemaker (e.g., contact sports).
- Pacemaker manufacturers do not recommend any special restrictions regarding proximity to typical household items.
- All pacemaker manufacturers offer pacemakers that are MRI compatible. Older pacemaker models and leads may have a strong relative contraindication for MRI.
- Leadless pacemakers that are implanted directly into the right ventricle using a special delivery system are available for special indications.
- Some medical procedures, such as lithotripsy, hyperbaric chamber, and electrocautery used during surgery, may require pacemaker programming and testing perioperatively.
- Table 3 describes the five-letter pacemaker code, and Table 4 summarizes common permanent pacemakers.

RELATED CONTENT

Complete Heart Block (Patient Information)

AUTHOR: **HEIKO SCHMITT, M.D., PH.D.**

TABLE 2 Complete Heart Block Management

Setting	Therapy
Asymptomatic–Acquired	• Rule out reversible causes, including: Hyperkalemia Acute inferior MI Digoxin toxicity Excess calcium channel blocker therapy Lyme disease • If HR <40 bpm, first-line therapy is a permanent DDD pacemaker. • Temporary pacing is indicated if heart rate <40 bpm. The patient has impaired hemodynamics, and if permanent, pacing cannot be accomplished expeditiously. The CHB has an identifiable and reversible cause, while awaiting recovery. Temporary transvenous pacing must be used with caution in patients with any escape rhythm, particularly if wide QRS complex and slow. Overdrive suppression can occur rapidly. • If the rate of escape rhythm >40 bpm, permanent pacemaker insertion is controversial. • Temporary pacing is to be avoided in asymptomatic patients whose ventricular rates are >40 bpm, especially if the QRS complex is narrow. • CHB due to radio frequency ablation of the AV junction to control ventricular response rate in atrial fibrillation requires permanent pacing. May occur even if the patient is asymptomatic from a slow ventricular rate (40 bpm) that may be quite stable over time. Acquired CHB is associated with a poor short-term prognosis (>50% mortality in the first 6-12 mo after diagnosis). If irreversible, pacing is indicated.
Symptomatic	• A permanent pacemaker is indicated. • Temporary pacing is indicated if permanent pacing cannot be done expeditiously or if CHB has an identifiable and reversible cause (e.g., drug overdose).
Congenital	• Usually associated with a narrow QRS complex with an escape rhythm arising in the AVN. • Patients are usually asymptomatic. • In patients who are asymptomatic, the indications for a pacemaker are controversial. • Patients will need close follow-up, at least annually, for evaluation of symptoms suggesting chronotropic incompetence. • If symptomatic bradycardia, a permanent pacemaker is indicated. • If rate is consistently <50 bpm and does not increase with exercise (chronotropic incompetence), a permanent pacemaker is indicated.
MI	• If symptomatic bradycardia, a temporary pacemaker is indicated. • If CHB block occurs in the setting of an anterior infarction, permanent pacing is indicated if AVB persists. • CHB in inferior MI is generally in the AVN. There is usually no need for a permanent pacemaker, as it usually resolves. If it does not resolve, a permanent pacemaker may be indicated in some cases.
Preoperative	• Permanent pacemaker first, unless the surgery is emergent. • If surgery is emergent, insert a temporary pacemaker pre-op with the plan for a permanent pacemaker after surgery.
Postoperative	• Transcutaneous or temporary transvenous pacing. • A permanent pacemaker is indicated if there is permanent damage to the AV conduction system (e.g., after aortic valve surgery or VSD repair).

AV, Atrioventricular; *AVB,* atrioventricular block; *AVN,* atrioventricular node; *bpm,* beats per minute; *CHB,* complete atrioventricular block; *HR,* heart rate; *MI,* myocardial infarction; *VSD,* ventricular septal defect.
From Olshansky B, Chung MK, Pogwizd SM et al: *Arrhythmia essentials,* ed 2, Philadelphia, 2017, Elsevier.

TABLE 3 Five-Letter Pacemaker Code

Letter 1 Chamber Paced	Letter 2 Chamber Sensed	Letter 3 Sensing Response	Letter 4 Programmability	Letter 5 Antitachycardia Functions
A = atrium	A = atrium	T = triggered*	P = simple	P = pacing
V = ventricle	V = ventricle	I = inhibited	M = multiprogrammable	S = shock
D = dual	D = dual	D = dual (A and V inhibited)	R = rate adaptive	D = dual (shock pace)
0 = none	0 = none	0 = none	C = communicating	
			0 = none	

*In the triggered response mode, the pacemaker discharges or fires when it recognizes an intrinsic depolarization. As a result, pacemaker spikes occur during inscription of the QRS complex. Because this mode results in high energy consumption and a shortened battery life and because the sensing response can be misinterpreted as pacemaker malfunction, this sensing mode is not used with modern pacemakers.
From Marx JA et al: *Rosen's emergency medicine,* ed 8, Philadelphia, 2014, Saunders.

TABLE 4 Common Permanent Pacemakers

Code	Indication	Advantages	Disadvantages
VVI	Intermittent backup pacing; inactive patient	Simplicity; low cost	Fixed rate; risk of pacemaker syndrome
VVIR	Atrial fibrillation	Rate responsive	Requires advanced programming
DDD	Complete heart block	Atrial tracking restores normal physiology	No rate responsiveness; requires two leads and advanced programming
DDDR	Sinus node dysfunction; for rate responsiveness atrioventricular block and need	Universal pacer; all options available by programming	Complexity, cost, programming, and follow-up evaluation

From Marx JA et al: *Rosen's emergency medicine,* ed 8, Philadelphia, 2014, Saunders.

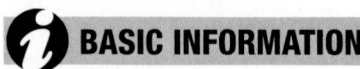

BASIC INFORMATION

DEFINITION

Second-degree heart block or second-degree atrioventricular (AV) heart block is characterized by a failure of one or more, but not all, atrial impulses to conduct to the ventricles. The block may be at any level of the AV conduction system. In both types of second-degree heart block, the sinus rate will continue at regular intervals, resulting in a constant sinus rate. When more than one atrial impulse is present for each ventricular complex, the rhythm may be described as a ratio of the number of atrial impulses to the number of ventricular complexes. Electrocardiographically there are three types of second-degree block:

- Mobitz type I (Wenckebach):
    1. Characterized by a progressive prolongation of the PR interval prior to a blocked nonconducted beat and a shorter PR interval after that blocked beat; the conducted impulse will generally be narrow. The cycle may repeat periodically, leading to "grouped beating."
    2. Site of block is usually AV node (proximal to the His bundle).
- Mobitz type II:
    1. Characterized by fixed PR intervals before and after blocked beats and may be associated with a wide QRS morphology (right bundle branch block [RBBB] or left bundle branch block [LBBB] patterns).
    2. Site of block is usually infranodal, especially when QRS is wide.
    3. It has a greater propensity for progressing to third-degree AV block.
- Pure 2:1 conduction patterns cannot be reliably classified as Mobitz type I or type II because there are not enough P waves to characterize prolongation of the PR interval.

SYNONYMS

Wenckebach block (Mobitz type I block)
Mobitz type II block
AV block

ICD-10CM CODES

I44.1	Atrioventricular block, second degree
I45.5	Other specified heart block
Q24.6	Congenital heart block

EPIDEMIOLOGY & DEMOGRAPHICS

Mobitz type I block is more common and may occur in individuals with heightened vagal tone or as a side effect of medications, such as β-blockers or calcium channel blockers.

PHYSICAL FINDINGS & CLINICAL PRESENTATION

- Patients with Mobitz type I are usually asymptomatic. Patients with either type may feel palpitations or the feeling of "missing a beat." Sudden loss of consciousness without warning (Adams-Stokes attack) can occur in patients with Mobitz type II; however, it is much more common in patients with complete heart block.
- Type I block: There is gradual decrease in the intensity of the first heart sound with widening of the a-c interval in the central venous waveform, ending in a pause, and an a wave not followed by a v wave in the neck along with an irregular pulse.
- Type II block: The first heart sound retains a constant intensity, with intermittent ventricular pauses and a waves not followed by v waves in the neck. There is an irregular pulse for most times with intermittent pauses.

ETIOLOGY

- High vagal tone (young patients, athletes at rest)
- Degenerative changes in the AV conduction system
- Ischemia at the AV nodes (type I with inferior wall myocardial infarction [MI] and type II with anterior wall MI)
- Drugs (digitalis, quinidine, procainamide, adenosine, calcium channel blockers [nondihydropyridines], β-blockers)
- Cardiomyopathies, collagen vascular diseases, infiltrative diseases (amyloidosis, sarcoidosis, hematochromatosis)
- Myocarditis/endocarditis (infectious, e.g., Lyme disease, Chagas' disease; and noninfectious, e.g., systemic lupus erythematosus)
- Hyperkalemia, hypermagnesemia
- Hypothyroidism
- Prior cardiac valve surgery
- Catheter trauma, catheter ablation for arrhythmias

Dx DIAGNOSIS

DIFFERENTIAL DIAGNOSIS

The ECG easily and reliably distinguishes Mobitz type I from Mobitz type II block and from other conduction abnormalities. It should be distinguished from the less common phenomenon of second-degree sinoatrial node exit block.

Mobitz type I block with a normal QRS complex tends to be benign and usually does not progress to more advanced forms of AV conduction within a short period of time because the disease is mostly confined to within the AV node. Mobitz type II block often precedes the development of Adams-Stokes syncope, symptoms are frequent, prognosis is compromised, and progression to third-degree AV block is common and sudden. Thus, type II second-degree AV block with a wide QRS typically indicates diffuse conduction system disease involving even the infranodal His-Purkinje system.

WORKUP

ECG, ambulatory monitoring (Holter or external loop recorders) in selected patients

- Mobitz type I (Fig. 1) ECG shows:
    1. Sequential and gradual prolongation of PR interval leading to a nonconducted P wave
    2. Shortened PR interval following the pause as compared to the pre-pause PR interval
    3. Progressive shortening of the R-R interval prior to nonconducted atrial impulse
    4. Usually see "grouped beating" pattern
- Mobitz type II ECG shows (Fig. 2):
    1. Fixed duration of PR interval with constant P-P and R-R intervals
    2. Sudden nonconducted P wave
    3. Abnormal QRS duration or fascicular blocks are common
- In 2:1 AV block (Fig. 3), it cannot be determined based on the 12-lead ECG whether there is Mobitz type I or type II AV block, although a wide QRS complex is suggestive of Mobitz type II.
    1. Administering atropine can improve AV conduction if the AV block is type I or within the AV node; however, if it is infranodal (i.e., type II), the increased sinus rate caused by atropine may worsen the ratio of AV conduction, resulting in worsening bradycardia.
    2. Exercise stress testing may function in the same way as atropine above. If the disease is confined to the AV node, it may improve with exercise, but in cases of Mobitz type II AV block, the degree of AV block will worsen.
    3. Carotid sinus stimulation and other vagal maneuvers may worsen the AV block if it is at the level of the AV node (i.e., Mobitz type I) but will paradoxically improve the ratio of AV conduction by slowing down the sinus rate if it is a Mobitz type II or infranodal AV block.
    4. An algorithm for evaluation of patients with 2:1 AV block is illustrated in Fig. 4.

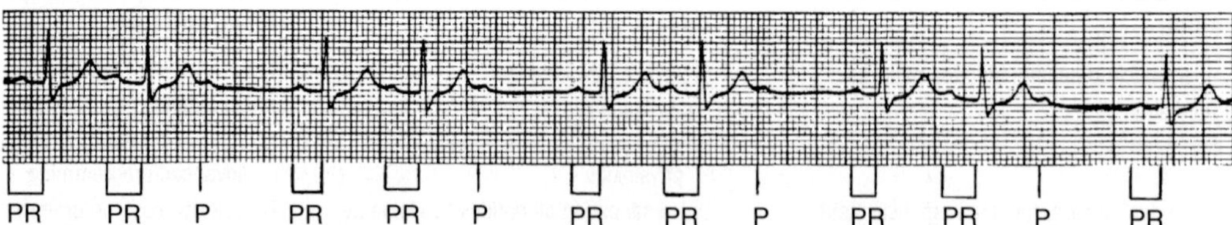

FIG. 1 Wenckebach (Mobitz type I) second-degree atrioventricular block. Notice the progressive increase in PR intervals, with the third P wave in each sequence not followed by a QRS. Wenckebach block produces a characteristically syncopated rhythm with grouping of the QRS complexes (group beating).

Rx TREATMENT

NONPHARMACOLOGIC THERAPY

Elimination of drugs that may induce AV block such as digoxin, beta-blockers, and calcium channel blockers

ACUTE GENERAL Rx

- Treatment is usually not necessary unless the resting heart rate is <40 beats per min (bpm) while awake.
- If symptomatic (e.g., dizziness), atropine 1 mg (may repeat once after 5 min) may be tried to increase AV conduction; if no response, trial of dobutamine or isoproterenol may be helpful prior to insertion of a pacemaker.
- Atropine:
  1. Reduces heart block due to hypervagotonia but not due to AV node ischemia
  2. Does not increase infranodal conduction (third-degree and second-degree AV block that is below the AV node)
  3. Should be used with caution in Mobitz type II AV block due to possible paradoxical decrease in heart rate (as atrial rate increases, AV conduction decreases)
  4. Is ineffective in heart transplantation patients
- If associated with anterior wall MI and wide QRS complex, consider insertion of a temporary pacemaker.
- Indications for permanent pacemaker (PPM) implantation by ACC/AHA/HRS 2008 guidelines:
  1. Second-degree AV block with associated symptomatic bradycardia regardless of the type or site of the block (class I; level of evidence: B).
  2. Second-degree AV block provoked by exercise in the absence of myocardial ischemia (class I; level of evidence: C).
  3. Asymptomatic second-degree AV block at intra- or infra-His levels found at electrophysiologic study (class IIa; level of evidence: B).
  4. First- or second-degree AV block with symptoms similar to those of pacemaker syndrome or hemodynamic compromise (class IIa; level of evidence: B).
  5. Asymptomatic type II second-degree AV block with a wide QRS, including isolated right bundle branch block (class I; level of evidence: B).

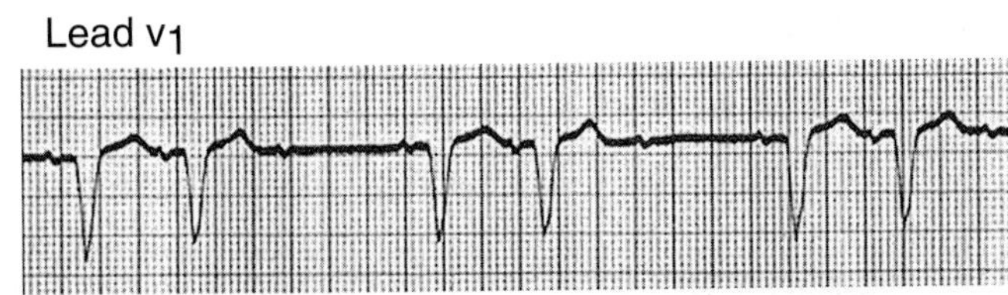

FIG. 2 Mobitz type II atrioventricular (AV) block with left bundle branch block (LBBB). Note the fixed P-P intervals with no change in PR intervals followed by a sudden nonconducted P wave. The LBBB indicates infranodal disease in the His-Purkinje system that is suggestive of Mobitz type II block.

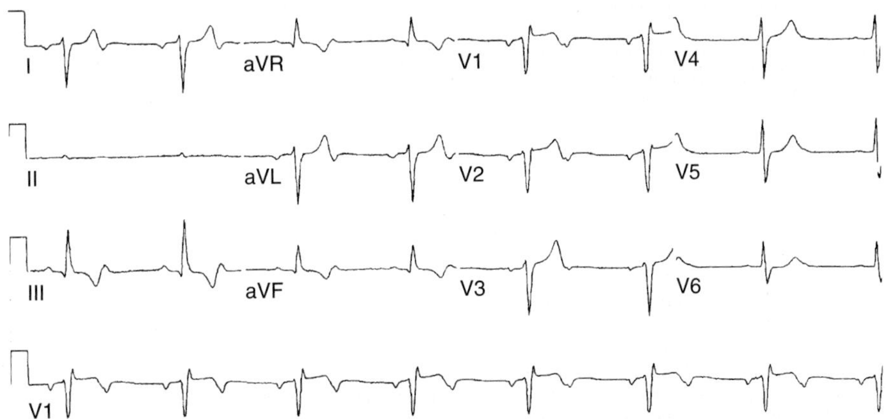

FIG. 3 Second-degree 2:1 atrioventricular block. Notice the short PR interval during conducted complexes and the wide QRS complexes, suggesting block in the His-Purkinje system. (From Issa Z et al: *Clinical arrhythmology and electrophysiology,* ed 2, Philadelphia, 2012, Saunders.)

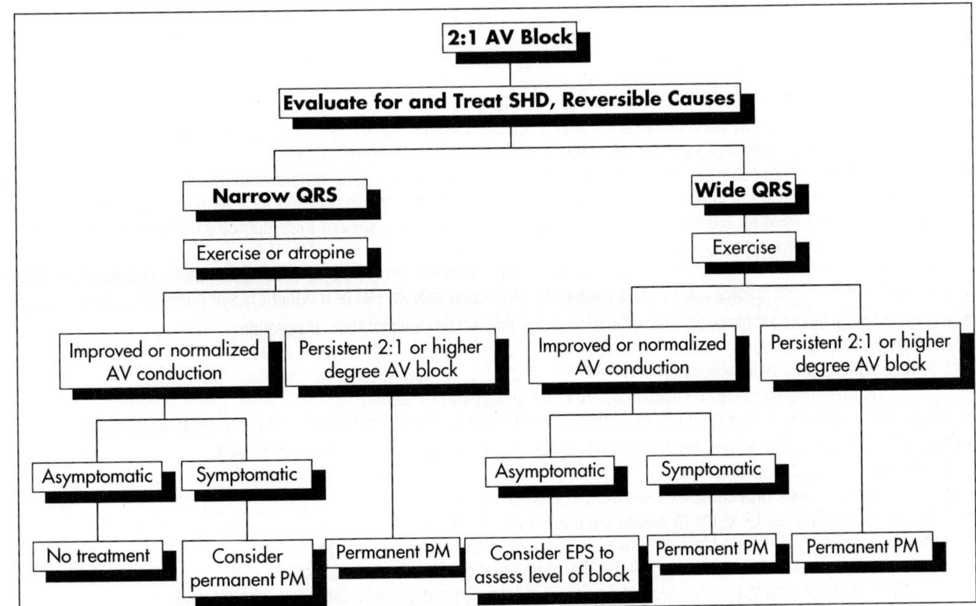

FIG. 4 Evaluation and management of 2:1 AV block. *AV,* Atrioventricular; *EPS,* electrophysiology study; *PM,* pacemaker; *SHD,* structural heart disease (no overt evidence of myocardial, valvular, congenital, or coronary heart disease.) (From Olshansky B et al: *Arrhythmia essentials,* ed 2, Philadelphia, 2017, Elsevier.)

6. PPM is not indicated for asymptomatic type I second-degree AV block at supra-His (AV node) level or that which is not known to be intra- or infra-Hisian (class III; level of evidence: C)

- Table 1 summarizes the management of Mobitz type I second-degree AV block.
- Table 2 summarizes the management of Mobitz type II second-degree AV block.

DISPOSITION

Prognosis is good with insertion of a pacemaker.

REFERRAL

Referral for pacemaker insertion (see "Acute General Rx")

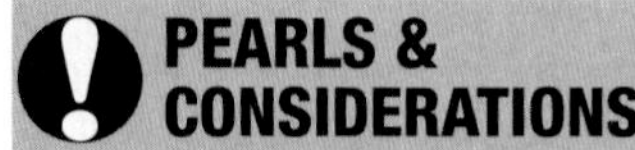

PEARLS & CONSIDERATIONS

COMMENTS

Patients with symptomatic Mobitz type II should be referred for a pacemaker. Asymptomatic patients should be referred if the AV block worsens with exercise and should be followed up routinely for potential development of high-grade AV block.

RELATED CONTENT

Second-Degree Heart Block (Patient Information)

AUTHOR: **ALEEM I. MUGHAL, M.D.**

TABLE 1 Mobitz Type I Second-Degree Atrioventricular Block Management

Setting	Therapy
Outpatient—Asymptomatic	• Treadmill testing will help assess chronotropic competence (if this rhythm is not related to myocardial ischemia), as well as enhance AVN conduction, thereby reducing the degree of Wenckebach block (e.g., from 5:4 to 8:7 or producing first-degree AVB only). • Holter monitoring can assess the degree and level of AVB and the persistence of the problem during activities of daily living and any diurnal variation. • If the QRS duration is wide and Holter monitoring or stress testing suggests infranodal block, an electrophysiology study may help to confirm the level of AVB. • If block is demonstrated to be intra- or infra-Hisian, permanent pacemaker implantation is reasonable, even in an asymptomatic patient. On occasion, intra-Hisian block can be demonstrated in a patient with a narrow, normal-appearing QRS complex by the production of higher degrees of AV block during treadmill testing with the increase in sinus rate. • No therapy. ○ If not due to reversible cause (e.g., drugs or transient damage to the AV node from Lyme disease) and the QRS duration is normal, as more advanced or complete heart block rarely develops. ○ There may be increased risk of syncope and symptoms in the future.
Outpatient—Symptomatic	• Some AV nodal blocking drugs (digoxin, β-adrenergic blockers, calcium blockers) may be the cause and should be reduced or stopped, if possible, and then only if severe symptomatic bradycardia occurs. • If older or at high risk for structural heart disease, consider an echocardiogram to assess LV function (even if no physical findings are present). • If due to a correctable cause such as AV nodal blocking drugs, stop the drug, if possible. • If there is a wide QRS or bundle branch block, it is possible that Wenckebach can be due to a block below the AV node (in the His-Purkinje system). ○ In this case, permanent pacemaker implantation is indicated. ○ Acutely, intravenous atropine or oral theophylline usually increases conduction through the AV node. ○ These may paradoxically decrease ventricular rate and increase the degree of block if the block is below the bundle of His. • Permanent pacemaker implantation is indicated if symptomatic second-degree AVB is not otherwise correctable.
MI	• Is often reversed during thrombolysis or angioplasty • May also appear for the first time concomitantly with these procedures. • Transient in nature • Temporary DDD pacing for the following: ○ Persistent low heart rate (<40 bpm) ○ Low cardiac output ○ Ischemia ○ Refractory hypotension ○ Symptoms of lightheadedness and dizziness • Atropine or theophylline may reverse the block but can cause unwanted tachycardia during drug administration. These drugs are only rarely indicated except at the time of presentation of the patient. • Atypical AV block is more common in inferior-posterior MIs due to the Bezold-Jarisch reflex and the effect of increased vagal tone on the AV node. ○ This is usually transient, and unless there is hemodynamic collapse, there is no need for a temporary pacemaker. ○ Rarely is there a need for a permanent pacemaker. This is true even if transient third-degree (complete) AV block occurs, as high degrees of block tend to resolve over 5-7 days. ○ If the AV block does not resolve but the ventricular rate is >40 bpm, no therapy is required if patient is asymptomatic. ○ If the block does not resolve after 7 days and/or the ventricular rate is <40 or if patient is symptomatic, a permanent pacemaker is indicated.
Preoperative	• Assess drugs given and their need; stop offending drugs that enhance vagal tone, if possible. • If no symptoms, no therapy. • If symptomatic and no reversible causes, provide temporary pacing before surgery. • Need for permanent pacing can be accomplished in the postoperative setting. • Atropine or isoproterenol may be given to increase AV node conduction if symptomatic or hemodynamically significant.
Postoperative	• Rare after CABG but, if it occurs, consider an offending drug or transient ischemia to the AV node. • No therapy is generally needed. • If associated with wide QRS complex, consider block below the His. • If it persists, consider an EP study to assess the level of the block. • If patient is asymptomatic and block is above His, no need for permanent pacemaker. • If patient is symptomatic or block is below the His, permanent pacemaker is indicated. • If the block is associated with valve (especially aortic) surgery, consider direct damage to the AV node. • If persistent, a pacemaker is indicated for symptoms or persistent slow rate (<40 bpm or no increase in rate with exercise).

AV, Atrioventricular; *AVB*, atrioventricular block; *AVN*, atrioventricular node; *CABG*, coronary artery bypass graft; *DDD*, dual-chamber; *EP*, electrophysiology; *LV*, left ventricular; *MI*, myocardial infarction.
From Olshansky B et al: *Arrhythmia essentials*, ed 2, Philadelphia, 2017, Elsevier.

TABLE 2 Mobitz Type II Second-Degree Atrioventricular Block Management

Setting	Therapy
Outpatient—Asymptomatic	• Risk for complete heart block and death is significant (approximately 50%). • A dual-chamber permanent pacemaker is recommended as the pacing system of choice. ○ Admit the patient for a permanent pacemaker and place on a cardiac monitor. ○ In the absence of symptoms or progressive (higher-degree AVB), there is no need for a temporary pacemaker before permanent pacemaker implantation. ○ Avoid atropine. ○ Evaluate for the presence of underlying cardiac disease, such as infiltrative processes (e.g., amyloid) or MI.
Outpatient—Symptomatic	• Dual-chamber permanent pacemaker implantation is indicated. • Admit the patient and place on a cardiac monitor. ○ If symptomatic or hemodynamically detrimental ventricular bradycardia is present, a temporary pacemaker is indicated if a permanent system cannot be placed expeditiously. ○ Do not give atropine because this may worsen the AVB and produce a slower ventricular rate. ○ Exercise, sinus tachycardia, and catecholamines also can worsen the degree of block by enhancing AV nodal conduction and impinging on the refractory period of the His-Purkinje system.
MI	• Place temporary pacemaker. ○ Mobitz type II second-degree AVB is associated with a high rate of heart failure in this setting. ○ A permanent pacemaker is indicated if the AVB is persistent because the risk of complete heart block is >50%. ○ Long-term prognosis may not be improved. ○ Avoid the use of antiarrhythmic drugs (including lidocaine) in the absence of a pacemaker, unless there is sustained ventricular tachyarrhythmia, as these drugs may worsen the degree of AVB. ○ Do not give atropine. ○ Mobitz type II second-degree AVB has a lower (albeit not known with certainty) incidence in the current early revascularization era, but if present or of new onset may improve with time, but this is rare. After being present and persistent, a pacemaker will likely be needed.
Preoperative	• Place permanent pacemaker. ○ If urgent or emergent surgery, place a temporary pacemaker with the plan for a permanent pacemaker after surgery. ○ If CABG, epicardial atrial and ventricular wires can be placed, with temporary pacing as standby, until a permanent transvenous pacemaker can be placed. ○ It is best to place the permanent pacemaker after CABG or other cardiac surgery as leads otherwise tend to dislodge. ○ If endocarditis, temporary pacemaker until infection resolves and after cardiac surgery. ○ Avoid antiarrhythmic drugs and atropine.
Postoperative	• If bradycardia, temporary pacing (via epicardial wires, if present, after cardiac surgery). ○ Temporary Mobitz type II AV block may resolve after cardiac surgery. ○ It may be due to trauma near the His-Purkinje system (e.g., with aortic valve surgery, where left bundle branch block is a not-infrequent accompaniment). ○ Persistent (e.g., more than 3-5 days) Mobitz type II block will require permanent pacing. ○ No antiarrhythmic drugs should be given unless an adequate backup ventricular pacing is available. ○ Endocarditis with abscess near the septum can destroy the His-Purkinje system. ○ Despite surgical repair, permanent pacing will likely be required. ○ For patients having tricuspid valve replacement, an endocardial lead can occasionally be placed across a porcine bioprosthesis without producing tricuspid regurgitation but should be avoided if there is a mechanical valve. ○ Tricuspid valve repair (e.g., annuloplasty) should not pose a problem in positioning a right ventricular lead.

AV, Atrioventricular; *AVB*, atrioventricular block; *CABG*, coronary artery bypass graft; *MI*, myocardial infarction.
From Olshansky B et al: *Arrhythmia essentials*, ed 2, Philadelphia, 2017, Elsevier.

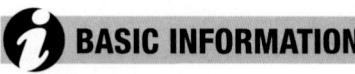

BASIC INFORMATION

DEFINITION

Heart failure (HF) is a complex clinical syndrome that can result from any structural or functional cardiac disorder that impairs the ability of the ventricle to fill with or eject blood. The cardinal manifestations of heart failure are dyspnea and fatigue that can limit exercise tolerance. The pathophysiology of HF (Fig. E1) is related to progressive activation of the neuroendocrine system to compensate for decreased effective circulating volume (Table 1), leading to total body volume overload and circulatory insufficiency. These events culminate in the development of pulmonary congestion as well as peripheral edema. Specifically, the renin-angiotensin-aldosterone system (RAAS) is implicated as being activated in HF, leading to volume expansion (sodium retention) and cardiac fibrosis (mediated through angiotensin II). Disordered adrenergic stimulation has also been recognized as a key component of progression of disease. The term *congestive heart failure* (CHF) usually denotes a volume-overloaded status as a result of HF. Given that not all patients have volume overload at the time of the evaluation, *congestive heart failure* should be distinguished from the broader term *heart failure*.

CLASSIFICATION: The American College of Cardiology/American Heart Association (ACC/AHA) describes the following four stages of HF. This staging model was designed to emphasize the evolution and progression of HF over a continuum and the preventability of HF in at-risk patients.

Stage A: Patients at high risk (e.g., with hypertension, atherosclerotic disease, diabetes mellitus, metabolic syndrome, cytotoxin, family history) for HF but without structural heart disease or symptoms of HF

Stage B: Patients with structural heart disease (e.g., left ventricular [LV] dysfunction) but without symptoms of HF

Stage C: Patients with structural heart disease with prior or current symptoms of HF

Stage D: Patients with refractory HF requiring specialized interventions

In addition to the ACC/AHA stages described above, the New York Heart Association (NYHA) defines four functional classes of HF designed to describe the symptoms of stage C and D HF. The functional classes are intended to assess the symptoms of HF and may fluctuate with therapy. It should be noted that current guidelines employ the functional classes to aid in determination of appropriate treatment.

I. Asymptomatic or symptomatic only at activity levels that would limit normal individuals
II. Symptomatic with ordinary exertion (e.g., 2 city blocks or 1 flight of stairs in a faster than usual pace)
III. Symptomatic with less than ordinary exertion (e.g., less than 2 city blocks or 1 flight of stairs)
IV. Symptomatic at rest

Table 2 compares the ACC/AHA and the NYHA classification. Table 3 describes a simplified classification and common clinical characteristics of patients with acute heart failure.

TERMINOLOGY: HF has been traditionally dichotomized as systolic vs. diastolic, which has now been replaced with the terms *HF with reduced ejection fraction* (HFrEF) and HF with *preserved ejection fraction* (HFpEF), respectively. Other common classifications include right-sided vs. left-sided and high-output vs. low-output. Systolic HF or HFrEF is defined by the presence of impaired contractility of the LV, as measured by ejection fraction (EF) ≤40% with clinical signs or symptoms of HF. In contrast, HFpEF has been described as evidence (clinical) of HF with an EF ≥50% with or without evidence of diastolic dysfunction. The term *HF with preserved EF* is preferred over the term *diastolic HF*, given that many of the physiologic derangements in this subset of HF are not solely restricted to diastolic function of the heart. Patients with an EF in the range of 40% to 50% represent an intermediate group. Right-sided HF denotes peripheral signs and symptoms of HF without evidence of pulmonary congestion, as opposed to left-sided HF, which typically manifests with pulmonary congestion and subsequent signs and symptoms of right-sided HF. The most common cause of right-sided HF is left-sided HF. High-output HF involves signs and symptoms of HF but features an elevated cardiac output unable to meet the abnormally high metabolic demands of peripheral tissues and is the result of myriad systemic disorders (e.g., systemic arteriovenous fistulas, hyperthyroidism, anemia). The term *acute decompensated HF* (ADHF) refers to worsening of signs or symptoms of HF due to a wide range of causes. Of note, HF is not equivalent to cardiomyopathy or LV dysfunction. These latter terms describe the possible structural or functional reasons for the development of HF, whereas HF is a clinical syndrome characterized by specific symptoms and signs.

SYNONYMS

HF
Congestive heart failure
CHF
Cardiac failure
Cardiogenic shock
Cardiogenic pulmonary edema

ICD-10CM CODES

I50.20	Unspecified systolic (congestive) heart failure
I50.21	Acute systolic (congestive) heart failure
I50.22	Chronic systolic (congestive) heart failure
I50.23	Acute on chronic systolic (congestive) heart failure
I50.30	Unspecified diastolic (congestive) heart failure
I50.31	Acute diastolic (congestive) heart failure
I50.32	Chronic diastolic (congestive) heart failure
I50.33	Acute on chronic diastolic (congestive) heart failure
I50.40	Unspecified combined systolic (congestive) and diastolic (congestive) heart failure
I50.41	Acute combined systolic (congestive) and diastolic (congestive) heart failure
I50.42	Chronic combined systolic (congestive) and diastolic (congestive) heart failure
I50.43	Acute on chronic combined systolic (congestive) and diastolic (congestive) heart failure
I50.9	Heart failure, unspecified

EPIDEMIOLOGY & DEMOGRAPHICS

- There is variability in the reported demographics of HF due to heterogeneous definitions and classifications of HF. African Americans have the highest risk for HF of the demographic groups. Incidence rate is lowest among white women and highest among black men, with blacks having a higher 5-yr mortality rate than whites.
- The lifetime risk of developing HF is 20% for Americans ≥40 yr of age.
  1. In the United States, HF incidence has largely remained stable over the past several decades, with >650,000 new HF cases diagnosed annually.
  2. There has been an increase in the prevalence of HF in the population over time. This is primarily due to improved treatment of hypertension and valvular and coronary disease, allowing patients to survive an early death only to later develop HF.
- HF is primarily a condition of the elderly. Approximately 80% of patients hospitalized with HF are older than 65 yr. HF is the most common inpatient diagnosis in the U.S. for patients aged >65 yr.
- HF incidence increases with age, rising from approximately 20 per 1,000 individuals 65 to 69 yr to >80 per 1,000 individuals among those >85 yr. Before age 75, the incidence of HF is higher in males, but both sexes are equally affected after this age cutoff.
- In the U.S., 1.1 million hospital discharges and 3.2 million hospitalizations/ambulatory care visits were associated with HF in 2007.
- Prevalence: 5.1 million persons in the U.S. and an estimated 23 million persons worldwide. The prevalence of HF is rising, especially in the elderly, particularly due to aging of the population and improved survival from other conditions.
- The estimated (direct and indirect) cost of HF in the U.S. was >$40 billion in 2012, with over half of these costs spent on hospitalizations. The mean cost of HF-related hospitalizations is $23,077 per patient and is higher when HF was a secondary rather than the primary diagnosis.
- HFrEF and HFpEF each make up about half of the overall HF burden.
- Among patients with HF in one large population study, hospitalizations were common after

TABLE 1 Compensatory Mechanisms in Heart Failure

Compensatory Response	Stimuli	Beneficial Effects	Adverse Effects	Potential Pharmacologic Interventions
Renin-angiotensin system activation	↓CO/BP ↓Renal blood flow ↑β-adrenergic activity	Maintain vital organ perfusion through vasoconstriction and sodium retention	↑Afterload → worsened LV function Adverse LV remodeling (apoptosis, myocyte hypertrophy)	ACE inhibitors ARBs
Adrenergic activation	↓CO/BP	↑CO through ↑ in heart rate and contractility ↑BP	↑Ischemia ↑Afterload → worsened LV function ↑LVEDP → pulmonary congestion Adverse LV remodeling (apoptosis, myocyte hypertrophy)	β-adrenergic blocking agents
Renal salt and water retention	↑Antidiuretic hormone ↑Norepinephrine ↑Angiotensin II ↑Aldosterone ↓Renal blood flow	↑Preload → ↑stroke volume and CO	Pulmonary and systemic congestion Adverse LV remodeling	Diuretics Aldosterone inhibitors ACE inhibitors, ARBs β-adrenergic blocking agents
↑Natriuretic peptide secretion	Volume expansion (atrial stretch)	Diuresis Natriuresis Partial inhibition of renin-angiotensin system and norepinephrine	None known	Natriuretic peptides

ACE, Angiotensin-converting enzyme; *ARB*, angiotensin receptor blocker; *BP*, blood pressure; *CO*, cardiac output; *LV*, left ventricular; *LVEDP*, left ventricular end-diastolic pressure.
(From Sellke FW et al: *Sabiston & Spencer surgery of the chest*, ed 9, 2016, Elsevier.)

TABLE 2 American College of Cardiology/American Heart Association (ACC/AHA) Stages of Heart Failure (HF) Compared with the New York Heart Association (NYHA) Functional Classification

ACC/AHA Stages		NYHA Functional Classification	
A	At high risk for HF but without structural heart disease or HF symptoms	None	
B	Structural heart disease but without signs or symptoms of HF	I	No limitation of physical activity Ordinary physical activity does not cause symptoms of HF
C	Structural heart disease with previous or current symptoms of HF	I	No limitation of physical activity Ordinary physical activity does not cause symptoms of HF
		II	Slight limitation of physical activity Comfortable at rest, but ordinary physical activity results in symptoms of HF
		III	Marked limitation of physical activity Comfortable at rest, but less than ordinary activity causes symptoms of HF
D	Refractory HF requiring specialized interventions	IV	Unable to carry on any physical activity without symptoms of HF, or symptoms of HF at rest

(From Mann DL, Zipes DP, Libby P, Bonow RO: *Braunwald's heart disease*, ed 10, Philadelphia, 2015, Elsevier.)

HF diagnosis, with 83% of patients hospitalized at least once and 43% hospitalized at least 4 times. More than half of the hospitalizations were related to non-cardiovascular causes.

PHYSICAL FINDINGS & CLINICAL PRESENTATION

The clinical and physical exam findings (Tables 4 and 5) should be given the highest priority when determining the diagnosis of HF. These signs and symptoms are dependent on the severity of disease, precipitant factors, comorbid conditions, and whether the HF symptoms are predominantly right-sided or left-sided.

- Common clinical manifestations are:
  1. Dyspnea on exertion, that can progress to dyspnea at rest, caused by increasing pulmonary vascular congestion
  2. Orthopnea, caused by increased venous return in the recumbent position and further elevated pulmonary venous pressure
  3. Paroxysmal nocturnal dyspnea (PND) resulting from multiple factors including increased venous return in the recumbent position, decreased PaO_2, and decreased adrenergic stimulation of myocardial function during sleep
  4. Nocturnal angina resulting from increased myocardial oxygen demand (secondary to increased venous return in the recumbent position causing increased preload) in patients with concomitant coronary artery disease (CAD)
  5. ***Cheyne-Stokes respiration*** (alternating phases of apnea and hyperventilation) caused by prolonged circulation time from lungs to brain as a result of impaired cardiac output
  6. Fatigue, lethargy, and decreased functional capacity resulting from low cardiac output and hypoperfusion of peripheral tissues
  7. Table 6 summarizes common presenting symptoms and signs of decompensated heart failure.
- Physical examination:
  1. Fine pulmonary crackles, wheezes, tachypnea, hypoxia (due to elevated pulmonary pressures). Crackles may be absent in chronic and longstanding high pulmonary venous pressure because it allows for lymphatic drainage in the lungs to increase.
  2. Tachycardia and narrowed pulse pressure (due to increased sympathetic tone)
  3. S_3 gallop, paradoxical splitting of S_2, jugular venous distention, peripheral edema in dependent tissues, congestive hepatomegaly, ascites, and hepatojugular reflux (due to volume overload)
  4. Perioral and peripheral cyanosis, decreased capillary refill, pulsus alternans, and cool extremities (due to decreased cardiac output)
- Six common clinical presentations identified by European Society of Cardiology of Acute Heart Failure Syndromes:
  1. ADHF presenting with hypertension (SBP >160): The hypertension leads to increased afterload causing pulmonary vascular congestion.
  2. Worsening or decompensation of chronic HF
  3. Flash pulmonary edema

TABLE 3 Simplified Classification and Common Clinical Characteristics of Patients with Acute Heart Failure

Clinical Classification	Symptom Onset	Triggers	Signs and Symptoms	Clinical Assessment	Course
Decompensated heart failure	Usually gradual	Noncompliance, ischemia, infections	Peripheral edema, orthopnea, dyspnea on exertion	SBP: Variable CXR: Often clear despite elevated filling pressures	Variable; high rehospitalization rate
Acute hypertensive heart failure	Usually sudden	Hypertension, atrial arrhythmias, ACS	Dyspnea (often severe), tachypnea, tachycardia, rales common	SBP: High (>180/100 mm Hg) CXR: Evidence of pulmonary edema Hypoxemia common	High acuity but often responds quickly to therapy with vasodilators, noninvasive ventilation; low postdischarge mortality
Cardiogenic shock	Variable	Progression of advanced HF or major myocardial insult (e.g., large-infarct AMI, acute myocarditis)	End-organ hypoperfusion; oliguria, confusion, cool extremities	SBP: Low or low-normal LV function usually severely depressed RV dysfunction common Laboratory evidence of end-organ dysfunction (renal, hepatic)	High inpatient mortality; poor prognosis except with readily reversible cause or mechanical support/transplantation

AMI, Acute myocardial infarction; *CXR*, chest x-ray [film/examination]; *HF*, heart failure.
(From Mann DL, Zipes DP, Libby P, Bonow RO: *Braunwald's heart disease*, ed 10, Philadelphia, 2015, Elsevier.)

4. Cardiogenic shock
5. Acute coronary syndrome (ACS) and ADHF
6. Isolated RV failure

- Each of these scenarios may require different therapies to effectively stabilize and treat the patient.

Acute precipitants of HF decompensation include noncompliance with salt restriction or medications (most common cause), infection, arrhythmias (e.g., atrial fibrillation), ischemia or infarction, uncontrolled hypertension, new medications (e.g., negative inotropic agents such as calcium channel blockers/antiarrhythmic agents), nonsteroidal antiinflammatory drugs (NSAIDs), renal dysfunction, toxins (e.g., ethanol and anthracyclines), cardiac surgery, or valvular catastrophe.

ETIOLOGY

LEFT VENTRICULAR FAILURE: The dichotomy of whether HF occurs in the setting of preserved or reduced LV systolic function plays an important role in treatment strategies. Patients with HFpEF may have significant abnormalities in active relaxation and passive stiffness of the LV as well as valvular disease. HFrEF denotes poor pump function.

- Abnormal LV systolic function:
  1. CAD (acute or chronic ischemia, myocardial infarction [MI], LV aneurysm), the most common cause of cardiomyopathy in the U.S., comprising 50% to 75% of HF patients.
  2. Increased afterload or pressure overload (severe hypertension, aortic stenosis)
  3. Increased preload or volume overload (mitral regurgitation, aortic regurgitation)
  4. Cardiomyopathy: Idiopathic, infiltrative (non-ischemic)
  5. Infectious (Chagas, myocarditis)
  6. Infiltrative (amyloidosis, sarcoidosis, hemochromatosis)
  7. Toxins (ethanol, cocaine, anthracyclines)
  8. Tachycardia induced (e.g., with atrial fibrillation)
- Preserved LV systolic function (Table 7):
  1. Impaired relaxation (myocardial ischemia, diabetes mellitus, metabolic syndrome)
  2. Tachyarrhythmia (featuring reduced diastolic filling time)
  3. Restrictive cardiomyopathy (myocardial stiffness, such as hypereosinophilic syndrome, amyloidosis, hemochromatosis)
  4. High cardiac output (thiamine deficiency, anemia, thyrotoxicosis, arteriovenous malformations)
  5. Increased afterload (uncontrolled hypertension, aortic stenosis, hypertrophic obstructive cardiomyopathy)
  6. Hypervolemia (oliguric renal failure, iatrogenic)

RIGHT VENTRICULAR FAILURE:

- Left-sided HF
- Chronic hypoxemic pulmonary disease

TABLE 4 Using the Medical History to Assess the Patient with Heart Failure (HF)

Symptoms and Signs Associated with HF

Fatigue
Shortness of breath at rest or during exercise
Dyspnea
Tachypnea
Cough
Diminished exercise capacity
Orthopnea
Paroxysmal nocturnal dyspnea
Nocturia
Weight gain/weight loss
Edema (of the extremities or scrotum or elsewhere)
Increasing abdominal girth or bloating
Abdominal pain (particularly if confined to the right upper quadrant)
Loss of appetite or early satiety
Cheyne-Stokes respirations (often reported by a family member rather than the patient)
Somnolence or diminished mental acuity

Historical Information Helpful in Determining Whether Symptoms Are Due to HF

A past history of HF
Cardiac disease (e.g., coronary artery, valvular or congenital disease, previous myocardial infarction)
Risk factors for HF (e.g., diabetes, hypertension, obesity)
Systemic illnesses that can involve the heart (e.g., amyloidosis, sarcoidosis, inherited neuromuscular diseases)
Recent viral illness or history of HIV infection or Chagas disease
Family history of HF or sudden cardiac death
Environmental and/or medical exposure to cardiotoxic substances
Substance abuse
Noncardiac illnesses that could affect the heart indirectly (including high-output states such as anemia, hyperthyroidism, and arteriovenous fistulas)

(From Mann DL, Zipes DP, Libby P, Bonow RO: *Braunwald's heart disease*, ed 10, Philadelphia, 2015, Elsevier.)

TABLE 5 Physical Findings in Heart Failure

Tachycardia
Extra beats or irregular rhythm
Narrow pulse pressure or thready pulse*
Pulsus alternans*
Tachypnea
Cool and/or mottled extremities*
Elevated jugular venous pressure
Dullness and diminished breath sounds at one or both lung bases
Rales, rhonchi, and/or wheezes
Apical impulse displaced leftward and/or inferiorly
Sustained apical impulse
Parasternal lift
S3 and/or S4 heart sounds (either palpable and/or audible)
Tricuspid or mitral regurgitant murmur
Hepatomegaly (often accompanied by right upper quadrant discomfort)
Ascites
Presacral edema
Anasarca*
Pedal edema
Chronic venous stasis changes

*Indicative of more severe disease.
(From Mann DL, Zipes DP, Libby P, Bonow RO: *Braunwald's heart disease*, ed 10, Philadelphia, 2015, Elsevier.)

TABLE 6 Common Presenting Symptoms and Signs of Decompensated Heart Failure

Symptoms	Signs
Predominantly Related to Volume Overload	
Dyspnea (exertional, paroxysmal nocturnal dyspnea, orthopnea, or at rest); cough; wheezing	Rales, pleural effusion
Foot and leg discomfort	Peripheral edema (legs, sacral)
Abdominal discomfort/bloating; early satiety or anorexia	Ascites/increased abdominal girth, right upper quadrant pain or discomfort, hepatomegaly/splenomegaly, scleral icterus Increased weight Elevated jugular venous pressure, abdominojugular reflux Increasing S_3, accentuated P_2 heart sounds
Predominantly Related to Hypoperfusion	
Fatigue	Cool extremities
Altered mental status, daytime drowsiness, confusion, or difficulty concentrating	Pallor, dusky skin discoloration, hypotension
Dizziness, presyncope, or syncope	Pulse pressure (narrow)/proportional pulse pressure (low) Pulsus alternans
Other Signs and Symptoms of Acute Heart Failure	
Depression	Orthostatic hypotension (hypovolemia)
Sleep disturbances	S_4
Palpitations	Systolic and diastolic cardiac murmurs

(From Mann DL, Zipes DP, Libby P, Bonow RO: *Braunwald's heart disease*, ed 10, Philadelphia, 2015, Elsevier.)

- Valvular heart disease (mitral stenosis or regurgitation)
- Pulmonary embolism
- Primary pulmonary hypertension
- Right-to-left shunts that cause systemic hypoxemia (e.g., large patent foramen ovale and tetralogy of Fallot)
- Left-to-right shunts that cause volume overload (e.g., atrial and ventricular septal defects)
- Bacterial endocarditis (right-sided)
- Right ventricular infarction

Dx DIAGNOSIS

DIFFERENTIAL DIAGNOSIS

- COPD, asthma
- Cirrhosis
- Nephrotic syndrome
- Venous insufficiency
- Pulmonary embolism
- ARDS (adult respiratory distress syndrome)
- Pneumonia
- Heroin overdose

WORKUP

- ACC/AHAA guidelines for initial and serial evaluation of heart failure are summarized in Table 8. A flowchart for the evaluation of patients with HF is described in Fig. 2.
- Blood work (to diagnose potentially reversible causes, identify comorbidities, and assess disease severity):
  1. CBC (to evaluate for anemia, infections), urinalysis, blood urea nitrogen (BUN), creatinine, electrolytes (worsening hyponatremia is a marker of disease severity and is associated with higher mortality rates), liver enzymes (hepatic congestion), thyroid function (especially in the elderly or patients with comorbid atrial fibrillation or known thyroid disease)
  2. B-type natriuretic peptide (BNP) is a cardiac neurohormone secreted from the ventricles in response to elevated LV end-diastolic pressure. The sensitivity is low in asymptomatic patients (but low BNP levels have been shown to have a negative predictive value up to 90% in symptomatic patients), and BNP elevation generally correlates with severity of disease and parallels closely morbidity and mortality outcome measures. The cleavage remnant N-terminal-pro-BNP (NT-pro-BNP) has a longer half-life and is cleared through the kidneys, making it susceptible to alterations in renal function. A level of <300 pg/ml has an age-independent 98% negative predictive value. There are new data to suggest that BNP screening and early intervention with risk factor modification in patients at risk of developing heart failure may prevent development of left ventricular dysfunction (class IIa recommendation). Natriuretic peptide biomarkers are also useful (class IA recommendation) both for diagnosis in patients presenting with dyspnea and for prognosis in patients with acute decompensated heart failure and chronic heart failure. Measurement of baseline levels of natriuretic peptide biomarkers on admission to the hospital is useful to establish a prognosis in acutely decompensated HF, and predischarge natriuretic peptide level can be useful to establish a postdischarge prognosis. There are insufficient data to recommend natriuretic peptide biomarker–guided therapy or serial measurements for the purpose of reducing hospitalization or deaths.
  3. Cardiac biomarkers may be elevated if ischemia is the precipitant factor. However, slight elevations are very common and may not always be due to obstructive coronary artery disease. These elevations could be due to subendocardial ischemia (due to increased end-diastolic pressure resulting in decreased perfusion) and necrosis, or cardiomyocyte damage from the inflammatory cytokines or oxidative stress. Impaired renal function is very common, and decreased clearance of the biomarkers can contribute to their elevation. Therefore these elevations should be interpreted in the context of the clinical setting. Despite that, in patients with acute decompensated heart failure (ADHF), a positive cardiac troponin test (from whatever mechanism) is associated with worse prognosis.
  4. Screening for dyslipidemia and glucose intolerance, which are risk factors for CAD.
  5. If hemochromatosis is suspected (specifically in Northern European patients), consider checking a transferrin saturation and ferritin level.
  6. Consider HIV testing in high-risk patients.
- Electrocardiogram (ECG):
  1. Look for signs of prior MI, chamber enlargement, hypertrophy, heart block, arrhythmia, and evidence of pericardial effusion.
  2. More than 25% of patients with HF have some form of intraventricular conduction abnormality that manifests as an increased QRS duration. The most

TABLE 7 Mechanisms/Factors Contributing to the Pathophysiology of Heart Failure with Preserved Ejection Fraction

Cardiovascular

LV Structure

Concentric remodeling, LV hypertrophy

LV Function

Diastolic dysfunction: Abnormal relaxation, decreased recoil, abnormal filling, decreased distensibility, increased diastolic pressure
Systolic dysfunction: Abnormal midwall and long-axis shortening, decreased twist
Hemodynamic load
  Increased afterload and filling load
Heterogeneity
  Dyssynergy, dyssynchrony
Left atrial structure and function
  Increased LA volume and stiffness, decreased LA reservoir function, passive conduit function and active booster pump function
Ischemia
  Subendocardial and microvascular disease, impaired coronary, pulmonary, and peripheral flow reserve
Rate and rhythm abnormalities
  Chronotropic incompetence, atrial fibrillation, supraventricular tachycardia
Vascular dysfunction
  Arterial stiffening, endothelial dysfunction

Cardiomyocyte

Abnormal calcium homeostasis (↑ diastolic calcium or ↓ rate of calcium reuptake → incomplete or impaired relaxation)
  Sarcolemmal calcium channels (Na^+/Ca^{2+} exchanger and calcium pump)
  Sarcoplasmic reticulum Ca^{2+}ATPase (SERCA) abundance and function
  Proteins modifying SERCA activity: Phospholamban, calmodulin, calsequestrin abundance, and phosphorylation state
  Sarcoplasmic reticulum calcium release channels
Energetics (↓ ATP or ↑ ADP slows actin-myosin cross-bridge release)
  ADP/ATP ratio, ADP and P_i concentration, phosphocreatine shuttle function
Proteins regulating cross-bridge formation and calcium sensitivity
  Troponin C: Calcium binding
  Troponin I: Phosphorylation state
Cytoskeletal proteins
  Microtubules (increased density) → ↑ diastolic stiffness
  Titin isoforms (↑ noncompliant isoform and phosphorylation state) → ↑ diastolic stiffness

Extracellular Matrix

Collagen structure, geometry, content, collagen I/III ratio
Collagen homeostasis, synthesis, postsynthetic processing, posttranslational crosslinking, degradation
Basement membrane proteins
Bioactive proteins and peptides: MMP/TIMP, SPARC, TGF-β
Fibroblast structure, function, phenotype
Myofibroblast transdifferentiation

Extra Cardiac

Extrinsic forces (RV-LV interaction and pericardial constraint)
Peripheral muscle and ergoreflex dysfunction
Pulmonary hypertension (secondary to chronic pulmonary venous hypertension)
Neurohormonal activation
Comorbid conditions (renal dysfunction, anemia, chronic lung disease)

ADP, Adenosine diphosphate; *ATP,* adenosine triphosphate; *LA,* left atrium; *LV,* left ventricle; *RV,* right ventricle; *SPARC,* secreted protein, acidic and rich in cysteine [osteonectin]; *TGF,* transforming growth vector.
(From Mann DL, Zipes DP, Libby P, Bonow RO: Braunwald's heart disease, ed 10, Philadelphia, 2015, Elsevier.)

common pattern seen is left bundle-branch block.
- Chest x-ray (Fig. 3):
  1. Evaluate for pulmonary venous congestion, pulmonary edema, pleural effusion, cardiomegaly, chamber dilation, and Kerley B lines.
- Echocardiography:
  1. Plays a critical diagnostic role in patients with HF and is useful in assessment of systolic, diastolic function in addition to assessment of valvular structure and function
- Exercise stress testing:
  1. May be useful in evaluating concomitant ischemic etiologies and assessment of degree of disability in stable compensated patients.
- Cardiac catheterization:
  1. Left heart catheterization can help to identify coronary artery disease as a cause of HF. Right heart catheterization can help to evaluate intracardiac filling pressures, estimates of valvular areas, presence of intracardiac shunts, and calculation of hemodynamic properties such as cardiac output, systemic vascular resistance, and pulmonary artery wedge pressure to further guide management.
- Cardiac MRI:
  1. Useful modality in accurately estimating EF (with less variability than conventional 2D echocardiography). MRI is also useful in excluding pericardial disease, identifying infiltrative disease, and assessing viability in cases of HF caused by underlying ischemic heart disease.

Rx TREATMENT

NONPHARMACOLOGIC GENERAL MEASURES

- Assess the etiology and severity of disease. Educate the patient and family about the nature of the disorder. Assess the home setting and if patient has social support to ensure compliance, especially for patients with dementia.
- Identify and correct precipitating factors (e.g., increased sodium load, medication noncompliance, ischemia, infections, anemia, thyrotoxicosis) and address lifestyle modification (e.g., smoking and alcohol cessation, weight reduction, avoiding use of nonsteroidal antiinflammatory drugs [NSAIDs]). Anemia is common in patients with HF. In patient with NYHA class II and III symptoms and iron deficiency, IV iron replacement may be reasonable to improve functional status and quality of life (class IIb recommendation). Treatments with erythropoiesis-stimulating agents (ESAs) have not shown improved clinical outcomes in patients with systolic HF and mild-to-moderate anemia and are thus not recommended. Table 9 describes ACC/AHA guidelines for treating patients at high risk for development of heart failure.
- Review list of medications and discontinue the ones that can contribute to HF (e.g., NSAIDs, antiarrhythmic drugs, calcium channel blockers, thiazolidinediones)
- Dietary sodium restriction of <2 g/day is commonly recommended to patients with HF and is endorsed by many guidelines.
- Restrict fluid intake to <2 L/day in patients with hyponatremia.
- Caloric supplementation should be provided to patients with advanced HF with weight loss and muscle wasting due to cardiac cachexia. Weight loss may reflect cachexia caused by the higher total energy expenditure associated with HF compared with that of healthy sedentary subjects. The diagnosis of cardiac cachexia independently predicts a worse prognosis.
- For patients with coexisting obstructive sleep apnea, continuous positive airway pressure (CPAP) may be reasonable after polysomnography (class IIb recommendation).
- Exercise training (or regular physical activity) is recommended as safe and effective for patients with class I to III HF who are able to participate to improve functional status (class I recommendation). Cardiac

TABLE 8 ACC/AHA Guidelines for Initial and Serial Evaluation of Heart Failure

Class	Indication	Level of Evidence
	History, Physical Examination, and Risk Scoring	
I	A thorough history and physical examination should be obtained/performed in patients presenting with HF to identify cardiac and noncardiac disorders or behaviors that might cause or accelerate the development or progression of HF.	C
	In patients with idiopathic DCM, a three-generational family history should be obtained to aid in establishing the diagnosis of familial DCM.	C
	Volume status and vital signs should be assessed at each patient encounter. This includes serial assessment of weight, as well as estimates of jugular venous pressure and the presence of peripheral edema or orthopnea.	B
IIa	Validated multivariable risk scores can be useful to estimate subsequent risk of mortality in ambulatory or hospitalized patients with HF.	C
	Diagnostic Tests and Biomarkers	
I	Initial laboratory evaluation of patients presenting with HF should include complete blood count, urinalysis, serum electrolytes (including calcium and magnesium), blood urea nitrogen, serum creatinine, glucose, fasting lipid profile, liver function tests, and thyroid-stimulating hormone.	C
	Serial monitoring, when indicated, should include serum electrolytes and renal function.	C
	A 12-lead ECG should be performed initially on all patients presenting with HF.	C
	In ambulatory patients with dyspnea, measurement of BNP or N-terminal pro-B-type natriuretic (NT-proBNP) is useful to support clinical decision making regarding the diagnosis of HF, especially in the setting of clinical uncertainty, and measurement of BNP or NT-proBNP is useful for establishing prognosis or disease severity in chronic HF.	A
IIa	Screening for hemochromatosis or HIV is reasonable in selected patients who present with HF.	C
	Diagnostic tests for rheumatologic diseases, amyloidosis, or pheochromocytoma are reasonable in patients presenting with HF in whom there is a clinical suspicion of these diseases.	C
	BNP- or NT-proBNP–guided HF therapy can be useful to achieve optimal dosing of GDMT in select clinically euvolemic patients followed in a well-structured HF disease management program.	B
IIb	The usefulness of serial measurement of BNP or NT-proBNP to reduce hospitalization or mortality in patients with HF is not well established. The measurement of other clinically available tests such as biomarkers of myocardial injury or fibrosis may be considered for additive risk stratification in patients with chronic HF.	B
	Noninvasive Cardiac Imaging	
I	Patients with suspected or new-onset HF, or those presenting with acute decompensated HF, should undergo a chest x-ray to assess heart size and pulmonary congestion and to detect alternative cardiac, pulmonary, and other diseases that may cause or contribute to the patient's symptoms.	C
	A 2-dimensional echocardiogram with Doppler should be performed during initial evaluation of patients presenting with HF to assess ventricular function, size, wall thickness, wall motion, and valve function.	C
	Repeat measurement of EF and measurement of the severity of structural remodeling are useful to provide information in patients with HF who have had a significant change in clinical status; who have experienced or recovered from a clinical event; who have received treatment, including GDMT, that might have had a significant effect on cardiac function; or who may be candidates for device therapy.	C
IIa	Noninvasive imaging to detect myocardial ischemia and viability is reasonable in patients presenting with de novo HF who have known CAD and no angina unless the patient is not eligible for revascularization of any kind.	C
	Viability assessment is reasonable in select situations when planning revascularization in patients with HF and CAD.	B
	Radionuclide ventriculography or magnetic resonance imaging can be useful to assess LVEF and volume when echocardiography is inadequate.	C
	Magnetic resonance imaging is reasonable when assessing myocardial infiltrative processes or scar burden.	B
III: No benefit	Routine repeat measurement of LV function assessment in the absence of clinical status change or treatment interventions should not be performed.	B
	Invasive Evaluation	
I	Invasive hemodynamic monitoring with a pulmonary artery catheter should be performed to guide therapy in patients who have respiratory distress or clinical evidence of impaired perfusion in whom the adequacy or excess of intracardiac filling pressures cannot be determined from clinical assessment.	C
IIa	Invasive hemodynamic monitoring can be useful for carefully selected patients with acute HF who have persistent symptoms despite empirical adjustment of standard therapies and (1) whose fluid status, perfusion, or systemic or pulmonary vascular resistance is uncertain; (2) whose systolic pressure remains low, or is associated with symptoms, despite initial therapy; (3) whose renal function is worsening with therapy; (4) who require parenteral vasoactive agents; or (5) who may need consideration for mechanical circulatory support or transplantation.	C
	When ischemia may be contributing to HF, coronary arteriography is a reasonable test for patients eligible for revascularization.	C
	Endomyocardial biopsy can be useful in patients presenting with HF when a specific diagnosis is suspected that would influence therapy.	C
III (no benefit)	Routine use of invasive hemodynamic monitoring is not recommended in normotensive patients with acute decompensated HF and congestion with symptomatic response to diuretics and vasodilators.	B
III (harm)	Endomyocardial biopsy should not be performed in the routine evaluation of patients with HF.	C

ACC, American College of Cardiology; *AHA,* American Heart Association; *BNP,* B-type natriuretic peptide; *CAD,* coronary artery disease; *DCM,* dilated cardiomyopathy; *ECG,* electrocardiogram; *EF,* ejection fraction; *GDMT,* guideline-directed medical therapy; *HF,* heart failure; *LVEF,* left ventricular EF; *LV* left ventricle.

(From Mann DL, Zipes DP, Libby P, Bonow RO: *Braunwald's heart disease*, ed 10, Philadelphia, 2015, Elsevier.)

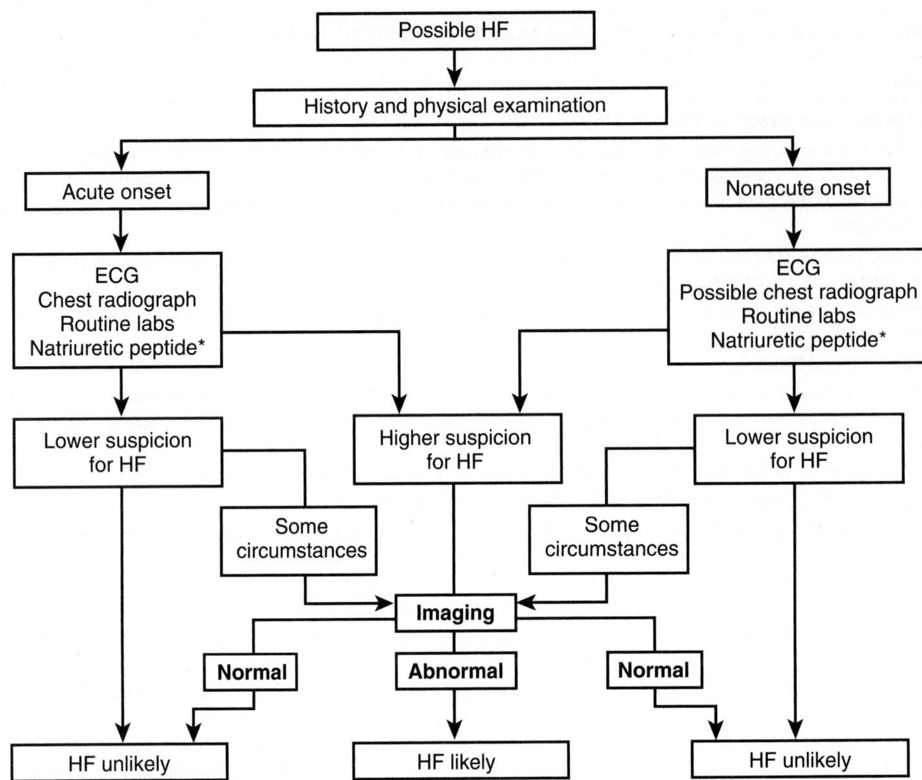

FIG. 2 Flowchart for the evaluation of patients with heart failure *(HF)*. Appropriate criteria for natriuretic peptide testing (*) to identify or exclude HF are summarized in Mann et al. (Table 23-6). The diagnosis of HF is made using a combination of clinical judgment and initial and subsequent testing. After a thorough history and physical examination, along with initial diagnostic testing, imaging (such as with echocardiography) may still be necessary in ambiguous cases to definitively identify or exclude HF. Cut-off values for BNP and NT-proBNP are displayed in Mann et al. (Table 23-6). *ECG*, Electrocardiogram. (From Mann DL, Zipes DP, Libby P, Bonow RO: *Braunwald's heart disease*, ed 10, Philadelphia, 2015, Elsevier.)

rehabilitation is unfortunately an underused preventive measure, although it has been shown to reduce morbidity and mortality. Cardiac rehabilitation can be useful in clinically stable patients with HF to improve functional capacity, exercise duration, health-related quality of life, and mortality (class IIa recommendation).

- Pneumococcal vaccination and annual influenza vaccination.
- ACC/AHA guidelines for treatment of asymptomatic left ventricular systolic dysfunction are summarized in Table 10.

TREATMENT OF ADHF

- Four phases in treatment of ADHF:
  1st phase: Initial stabilization and management (Table 11)
  2nd phase: Inpatient hospital care (Table 12)
  3rd phase: Early discharge planning and care
  4th phase: Early post-discharge care
- 1st phase: Initial stabilization and management

Short-term goals: Hemodynamic stabilization, stabilization of respiratory status, symptom relief, optimization of tissue perfusion, and recognition of more immediately life-threatening conditions (e.g., arrhythmias, valvular catastrophe, MI, cardiac tamponade). Initial therapy of ADHF is contingent on appropriate determination of clinical scenario.

Management as per clinical scenario:

1. ADHF-associated hypertension: Goal is afterload reduction and decrease of systemic hypervolemia. Mode of treatment: Diuresis (IV loop diuretics) and vasodilators (acutely nitrates and morphine followed by treatment with ACE inhibitors or angiotensin receptor blockers [ARBs])
2. Worsening or decompensation of chronic HF (HFrEF or HFpEF): Goal is control of volume status. Treatment is accomplished with vasodilators and diuretics.
3. Flash pulmonary edema: Goal is afterload reduction (vasodilators such as nitrates acutely), respiratory status stabilization, and diuresis (IV loop diuretics). Rate control can be initiated in patients with atrial fibrillation or tachyarrhythmias as it may improve cardiac filling and function.
4. Cardiogenic shock: Goal is hemodynamic stabilization. Treatment consists of inotropes + vasopressors ± mechanical circulatory support ± emergent revascularization if indicated.
5. ACS and ADHF: Goal is hemodynamic stabilization + emergent restoration of coronary perfusion. See "Acute Coronary Syndromes."
6. Isolated RV failure: Goals are identification of etiology: (1) valvular, (2) pulmonary hypertension, and (3) primary RV failure secondary to ischemia. Treatment: Depends on etiology, either corrective surgery vs. treatment of pulmonary hypertension (endothelin antagonists, calcium channel blockers, phosphodiesterase inhibitors) vs. coronary reperfusion therapies.

ACUTE PHARMACOLOGIC TREATMENTS:

- Vasodilators (Table 13) are appropriate in most patients with ADHF (contraindicated in cardiogenic shock and severe aortic stenosis)
  1. Nitroglycerin (0.4 to 0.8 mg sublingually every 3 to 5 min, or by intravenous infusion starting at 0.2 to 0.4 mcg/kg/min with subsequent up titration) may be administered in the emergency setting until relative hypotension ensues. Nitrates are contraindicated after use of phosphodiesterase inhibitors such as sildenafil due to risk of hypotension.
  2. Sodium nitroprusside (0.1 to 0.2 mcg/kg/min as an intravenous infusion) is a potent vasodilator with balanced venous and arteriolar effects that usually requires hemodynamic monitoring with an arterial line and may precipitate coronary steal and thiocyanate toxicity (elevated risk in renal failure).
  3. When given intravenously, loop diuretics have an immediate vasodilator effect that provides clinical relief of symptoms before diuresis begins. Due to gut edema and unpredictable patterns of absorption, oral formulation may become less

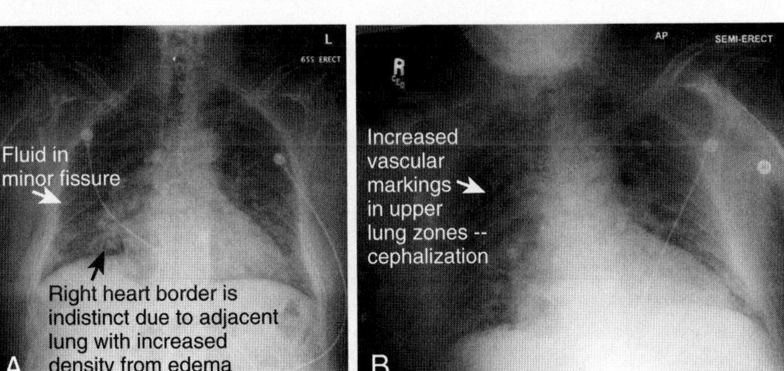

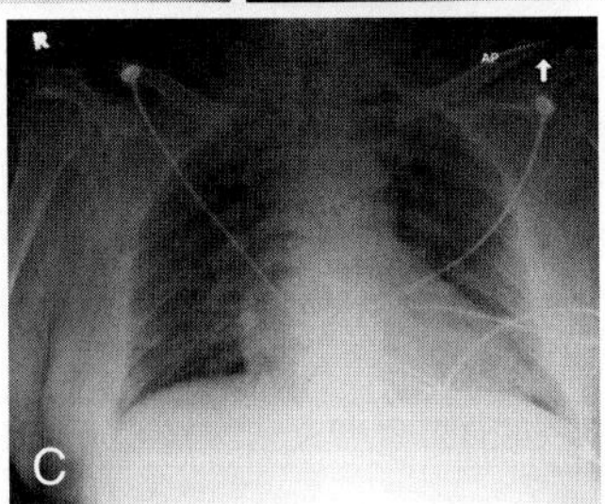

FIG. 3 Congestive heart failure. Mild left ventricular hypertrophy with restricted filling, ejection fraction >55%, and no pericardial effusion. This 63-year-old man with coronary artery disease, chronic renal insufficiency, and diastolic heart failure (ejection fraction >55%) presented multiple times for dyspnea (**A, B,** and **C,** first through third clinical presentations). Each of these three radiographs shows signs of moderate pulmonary edema. The diaphragms and costophrenic angles are clear, suggesting no pleural effusion. The right heart border in all three images is indistinct because of interstitial edema in these locations. Portions of the left heart border are also indistinct. The upper lung fields have a hazy appearance indicating mild edema. Fluid is visible in the minor fissure on all three images. Does the similarity of these radiographs mean that edema is not the cause of the patient's dyspnea? No, he simply presented with pulmonary edema on all three occasions. (From Broder JS: *Diagnostic imaging for the emergency physician,* Philadelphia, 2011, Saunders.)

effective. Therefore intravenous formulation should be used in the acute setting. Studies showed no difference in outcome when using bolus dosing vs. continuous IV infusion. Administration of smaller doses of short-acting loop diuretics multiple times daily is preferable to a single large dose because the kidneys can avidly reabsorb sodium after the initial diuresis. However, if a certain dose is not adequate to force diuresis, the dose, rather than the frequency, should be increased until a single effective dose is reached; more frequent doses can be added as needed. Therefore monitoring of urine output, renal function, and electrolytes is key. The addition of a distal tubule inhibitor such as metolazone 30 min prior to loop diuretic dosing has a synergistic effect and often enhances diuresis because it inhibits sodium reabsorption in the distal segment in the face of increased sodium delivery from the loop. Diuretics should be used with caution in patients with aortic stenosis and are contraindicated in patients with severe hypotension or cardiogenic shock.

- Inotropic agents are used for temporary hemodynamic support in cardiogenic shock, but have not been shown to improve survival. Many of these agents have serious associated adverse events including myocardial necrosis and malignant arrhythmias.

TABLE 9 ACC/AHA Guidelines for Treating Patients at High Risk for Development of Heart Failure (Stage A)

Class	Indication	Level of Evidence
I	Hypertension and lipid disorders should be controlled in accordance with contemporary guidelines to lower the risk of HF.	A
	Other conditions that may lead to or contribute to HF, such as obesity, diabetes mellitus, tobacco use, and known cardiotoxic agents, should be controlled or avoided.	C

ACC, American College of Cardiology; *AHA,* American Heart Association; *HF,* heart failure. (From Mann DL, Zipes DP, Libby P, Bonow RO: *Braunwald's heart disease,* ed 10, Philadelphia, 2015, Elsevier.)

TABLE 10 ACC/AHA Guidelines for Treatment of Asymptomatic Left Ventricular Systolic Dysfunction (Stage B)

Class	Indication	Level of Evidence
I	In all patients with a recent or remote history of MI or ACS and reduced EF, ACE inhibitors should be used to prevent symptomatic HF and reduce mortality. In patients intolerant of ACE inhibitors, ARBs are appropriate unless contraindicated.	A
	In all patients with a recent or remote history of MI or ACS and reduced EF, evidence-based beta-blockers should be used to reduce mortality.	B
	Beta blockade and ACE inhibition should be used in all patients with a recent or remote history of MI regardless of ejection fraction or presence of HF.	
	In all patients with a recent or remote history of MI or ACS, statins should be used to prevent symptomatic HF and cardiovascular events.	A
	Blood pressure should be controlled in accordance with clinical practice guidelines for hypertension to prevent symptomatic HF.	A
	ACE inhibitors should be used in all patients with a reduced EF to prevent symptomatic HF.	A
	Beta-blockers should be used in all patients with a reduced EF to prevent symptomatic HF.	C
IIa	To prevent sudden death, placement of an ICD is reasonable in patients with asymptomatic ischemic cardiomyopathy who are at least 40 days post-MI, have an LVEF of ≤30%, are on appropriate medical therapy, and have reasonable expectation of survival with a good functional status for more than 1 yr.	B
III: Harm	Nondihydropyridine calcium channel blockers with negative inotropic effects may be harmful in asymptomatic patients with low LVEF and no symptoms of HF after MI.	B

ACC, American College of Cardiology; *ACE,* angiotensin-converting-enzyme; *ACS,* acute coronary syndrome; *AHA,* American Heart Association; *EF,* ejection fraction; *HF,* heart failure; *ICD,* implantable cardioverter-defibrillator; *MI,* myocardial infarction; *LVEF,* left ventricular EF. (From Mann DL, Zipes DP, Libby P, Bonow RO: *Braunwald's heart disease,* ed 10, Philadelphia, 2015, Elsevier.)

TABLE 11 ACC/AHA Guidelines for Treatment of Symptomatic Left Ventricular Systolic Dysfunction (Stage C)

Class	Indication	Level of Evidence
	Nonpharmacologic Interventions	
I	Patients with HF should receive specific education to facilitate HF self-care.	B
	Exercise training (or regular physical activity) is recommended as safe and effective for patients with HF who are able to participate to improve functional status.	A
IIa	Cardiac rehabilitation can be useful in clinically stable patients with HF to improve functional capacity, exercise duration, HRQOL, and mortality.	B
	Sodium restriction is reasonable for patients with symptomatic HF to reduce congestive symptoms.	C
	Continuous positive airway pressure (CPAP) can be beneficial to increase LVEF and improve functional status in patients with HF and sleep apnea.	B
	Pharmacologic Interventions	
I	Measures listed as class I recommendations for patients in stages A and B are recommended where appropriate.	A, B, C
	GDMT should be the mainstay of pharmacologic therapy for HFrEF.	A
	Diuretics	
I	Diuretics are recommended in patients with HFrEF who have evidence of fluid retention, unless contraindicated, to ameliorate symptoms.	C
	Angiotensin-Converting Enzyme Inhibitors/Adrenergic Receptor Blockers	
I	ACE inhibitors are recommended in patients with HFrEF and current or previous symptoms, unless contraindicated, to reduce morbidity and mortality.	A
	ARBs are recommended in patients with HFrEF with current or previous symptoms who are ACE inhibitor–intolerant, unless contraindicated, to reduce morbidity and mortality.	A
IIa	ARBs are a reasonable choice to reduce morbidity and mortality as alternatives to ACE inhibitors for first-line therapy in patients with HFrEF, especially in those already taking ARBs for other indications, unless contraindicated.	A
IIb	Addition of an ARB may be considered in persistently symptomatic patients with HFrEF who are already being treated with an ACE inhibitor and a beta-blocker in whom an aldosterone antagonist is not indicated or tolerated.	A
III: Harm	Routinely combining an ACE inhibitor, an ARB, and an aldosterone antagonist.	C
	Beta-Blockers	
I	Use of one of the three beta-blockers proven to reduce mortality (i.e., bisoprolol, carvedilol, and sustained-release metoprolol succinate) is recommended for all patients with current or previous symptoms of HFrEF, unless contraindicated, to reduce morbidity and mortality.	A
	Aldosterone Receptor Antagonists	
I	Aldosterone receptor antagonists (or mineralocorticoid receptor antagonists) are recommended in patients with NYHA class II-IV and LVEF of ≤35%, unless contraindicated, to reduce morbidity and mortality.	A
I	Aldosterone receptor antagonists are recommended to reduce morbidity and mortality after an acute MI in patients with LVEF of ≤40% who develop symptoms of HF or who have a history of diabetes mellitus, unless contraindicated.	B
III: Harm	Inappropriate use of aldosterone receptor antagonists is potentially harmful because of life-threatening hyperkalemia or renal insufficiency when serum creatinine is >2.5 mg/dl in men or >2.0 mg/dl in women (or estimated glomerular filtration rate <30 ml/min/1.73 m^2), and/or potassium >5.0 mEq/liter.	B
	Hydralazine and Isosorbide Dinitrate	
I	The combination of hydralazine and isosorbide dinitrate is recommended to reduce morbidity and mortality for patients self-described as African Americans with NYHA class III-IV HFrEF receiving optimal therapy with ACE inhibitors and beta-blockers, unless contraindicated.	A
IIa	A combination of hydralazine and isosorbide dinitrate can be useful to reduce morbidity or mortality in patients with current or previous symptomatic HFrEF who cannot be given an ACE inhibitor or ARB because of drug intolerance, hypotension, or renal insufficiency, unless contraindicated.	B
	Digoxin	
IIa	Digoxin can be beneficial in patients with HFrEF, unless contraindicated, to decrease hospitalizations for HF.	B
	Anticoagulation	
I	Patients with chronic HF with permanent/persistent/paroxysmal atrial fibrillation and an additional risk factor for cardioembolic stroke (history of hypertension, diabetes mellitus, previous stroke or transient ischemic attack, or ≥75 years of age) should receive chronic anticoagulant therapy.	A
I	The selection of an anticoagulant agent (warfarin, dabigatran, apixaban, or rivaroxaban) for permanent/persistent/paroxysmal atrial fibrillation should be individualized on the basis of risk factors, cost, tolerability, patient preference, potential for drug interactions, and other clinical characteristics, including time in the international normalized ratio therapeutic range if the patient has been taking warfarin.	C
IIa	Chronic anticoagulation is reasonable for patients with chronic HF who have permanent/persistent/paroxysmal atrial fibrillation but no additional risk factor for cardioembolic stroke.	B
III: No benefit	Anticoagulation is not recommended in patients with chronic HFrEF without atrial fibrillation, a previous thromboembolic event, or a cardioembolic source.	B
	Statins	
III: No benefit	Statins are not beneficial as adjunctive therapy when prescribed solely for HF.	A
	Omega-3 Fatty Acids	
IIa	Omega-3 PUFA supplementation is reasonable to use as adjunctive therapy in patients with NYHA class II-IV symptoms and HFrEF or HFpEF, unless contraindicated, to reduce mortality and cardiovascular hospitalizations.	B

Continued

TABLE 11 ACC/AHA Guidelines for Treatment of Symptomatic Left Ventricular Systolic Dysfunction (Stage C)—cont'd

Class	Indication	Level of Evidence
	Drugs of Unproven Value or That May Cause Harm	
III: No benefit	Nutritional supplements as treatment for HF are not recommended in patients with current or previous symptoms of HFrEF.	B
	Hormonal therapies other than to correct deficiencies are not recommended for patients with current or previous symptoms of HFrEF.	C
III: Harm	Drugs known to adversely affect the clinical status of patients with current or previous symptoms of HFrEF are potentially harmful and should be avoided or withdrawn whenever possible (e.g., most antiarrhythmic drugs, most calcium channel blocking drugs [except amlodipine], NSAIDs, or thiazolidinediones).	B
	Long-term use of infused positive inotropic drugs is potentially harmful for patients with HFrEF, except as palliation for patients with end-stage disease who cannot be stabilized with standard medical treatment (see recommendations for stage D).	C
	Calcium Channel Blockers	
III: No benefit	Calcium channel blocking drugs are not recommended for routine therapy in patients with HFrEF.	A

ACC, American College of Cardiology; *ACE,* angiotensin-converting-enzyme; *AHA,* American Heart Association; *ARB,* agiotensin-receptor blocker; *HF,* heart failure; *HFrEF,* heart failure with reduced ejection fraction; *HRQOL,* health-related quality of life; *LVEF,* left ventricular ejection fraction; *NYHA,* New York Heart Association; *NSAID,* nonsteroidal antiinflammatory drug; *PUFA,* polyunsaturated fatty acid.
(From Mann DL, Zipes DP, Libby P, Bonow RO: *Braunwald's heart disease,* ed 10, Philadelphia, 2015, Elsevier.)

TABLE 12 ACC/AHA Recommendations for the Patient Hospitalized with Acute Heart Failure

Class	Indication	Level of Evidence
	Biomarkers	
I	Measurement of BNP or NT-proBNP is useful to support clinical judgment for the diagnosis of acutely decompensated HF, especially in patients in whom the diagnosis is uncertain.	A
I	Measurement of BNP or NT-proBNP and/or cardiac troponin is useful for establishing prognosis or disease severity in acutely decompensated HF.	A
IIB	The usefulness of BNP- or NT-proBNP-guided therapy for acutely decompensated HF is not well established.	C
IIB	Measurement of other clinically available tests such as biomarkers of myocardial injury or fibrosis may be considered for additive risk stratification in patients with acutely decompensated HF.	A
	Precipitating Causes of Acute Heart Failure	
I	ACS precipitating acute HF decompensation should be promptly identified by ECG and serum biomarkers, including cardiac troponin testing, and treated optimally as appropriate to the overall condition and prognosis of the patient.	C
I	Common precipitating factors for acute HF should be considered during initial evaluation, as recognition of these conditions is critical to guide appropriate therapy.	C
	Invasive Evaluation	
I	Invasive hemodynamic monitoring with a pulmonary artery catheter should be performed to guide therapy in patients who have respiratory distress or clinical evidence of impaired perfusion in whom the adequacy or excess of intracardiac filling pressures cannot be determined from clinical assessment.	C
IIA	Invasive hemodynamic monitoring can be useful for carefully selected patients with acute HF who have persistent symptoms despite empirical adjustment of standard therapies and: a. Whose fluid status, perfusion, or systemic or pulmonary vascular resistance is uncertain; b. Whose systolic pressure remains low, or is associated with symptoms, despite initial therapy; c. Whose renal function is worsening with therapy; d. Who require parenteral vasoactive agents; or e. Who may need consideration for MCS or transplantation.	C
III	Routine use of invasive hemodynamic monitoring is not recommended in normotensive patients with acute decompensated HF and congestion with symptomatic response to diuretics and vasodilators.	B
	Maintenance of Guideline-Directed Medical Therapy (GDMT) During Hospitalization	
I	In patients with HFrEF experiencing a symptomatic exacerbation of HF requiring hospitalization during chronic maintenance treatment with GDMT, it is recommended that GDMT be continued in the absence of hemodynamic instability or contraindications.	B
I	Initiation of beta-blocker therapy is recommended after optimization of volume status and successful discontinuation of intravenous diuretics, vasodilators, and inotropic agents. Beta-blocker therapy should be initiated at a low dose and only in stable patients. Caution should be used in initiating beta-blockers in patients who have required inotropes during their hospital course.	B
	Diuretics	
I	Patients with HF admitted with evidence of significant fluid overload should be promptly treated with intravenous loop diuretics to reduce morbidity.	B
I	If patients are already receiving loop diuretic therapy, the initial intravenous dose should equal or exceed their chronic oral daily dose and should be given as either intermittent boluses or continuous infusion. Urine output and signs and symptoms of congestion should be serially assessed, and the diuretic dose should be adjusted accordingly to relieve symptoms, reduce volume excess, and avoid hypotension.	B
I	The effect of HF treatment should be monitored with careful measurement of fluid intake and output, vital signs, body weight that is determined at the same time each day, and clinical signs and symptoms of systemic perfusion and congestion. Daily serum electrolytes, urea nitrogen, and creatinine concentrations should be measured during the use of intravenous diuretics or active titration of HF medications.	C
IIA	When diuresis is inadequate to relieve symptoms, it is reasonable to intensify the diuretic regimen using: a. Higher doses of intravenous loop diuretics or b. Addition of a second (e.g., thiazide) diuretic.	B

TABLE 12 ACC/AHA Recommendations for the Patient Hospitalized with Acute Heart Failure—cont'd

Class	Indication	Level of Evidence
IIB	Low-dose dopamine infusion may be considered in addition to loop diuretic therapy to improve diuresis and better preserve renal function and renal blood flow.	B
	Venous Thromboembolism Prophylaxis	
I	A patient admitted to the hospital with decompensated HF should receive venous thromboembolism prophylaxis with an anticoagulant medication if the risk-benefit ratio is favorable.	B
	Ultrafiltration	
IIB	Ultrafiltration may be considered for patients with obvious volume overload to alleviate congestive symptoms and fluid weight.	B
IIB	Ultrafiltration may be considered for patients with refractory congestion not responding to medical therapy.	C
	Parenteral Therapy	
IIB	If symptomatic hypotension is absent, intravenous nitroglycerin, nitroprusside, or nesiritide may be considered an adjuvant to diuretic therapy for relief of dyspnea in patients admitted with acutely decompensated HF.	A
	Inotropic Support and Mechanical Circulatory Support (MCS)	
I	Until definitive therapy (e.g., coronary revascularization, MCS, heart transplantation) or resolution of the acute precipitating problem, patients with cardiogenic shock should receive temporary intravenous inotropic support to maintain systemic perfusion and preserve end-organ performance.	C
IIA	Nondurable MCS is reasonable as a "bridge to recovery" or "bridge to decision" for carefully selected patients with HF and acute profound disease.	B
IIB	Short-term, continuous intravenous inotropic support may be reasonable in those hospitalized patients with documented severe systolic dysfunction who present with low blood pressure and significantly depressed cardiac output, to maintain systemic perfusion and preserve end-organ performance.	B
III	Use of parenteral inotropic agents in hospitalized patients without documented severe systolic dysfunction, low blood pressure, or impaired perfusion who present with evidence of significantly depressed cardiac output, with or without congestion, is potentially harmful.	B
	Arginine Vasopressin Antagonists	
IIB	In patients hospitalized with volume overload, including HF, who have persistent severe hyponatremia and have or are at risk for having active cognitive symptoms despite water restriction and maximization of GDMT, vasopressin antagonists may be considered in the short term to improve serum sodium concentration in hypervolemic, hyponatremic states with either a V2 receptor–selective or a nonselective vasopressin antagonist.	B
	Transitions of Care	
I	The use of performance improvement systems and/or evidence-based systems of care is recommended in the hospital and early postdischarge outpatient setting to identify appropriate HF patients for GDMT, provide clinicians with useful reminders to advance GDMT, and assess the clinical response.	B
I	Throughout the hospitalization as appropriate, before hospital discharge, at the first postdischarge visit, and in subsequent follow-up visits, the following should be addressed: a. Initiation of GDMT if not done or contraindicated b. Causes of HF, barriers to care, and limitations in support c. Assessment of volume status and blood pressure with adjustment of HF therapy d. Optimization of chronic oral HF therapy e. Renal function and electrolytes f. Management of comorbid conditions g. HF education, self-care, emergency plans, and adherence h. Palliative or hospice care	B
I	Multidisciplinary HF disease management programs are recommended for patients at high risk for hospital readmission, to facilitate the implementation of GDMT, to address different barriers to behavioral change, and to reduce the risk of subsequent rehospitalization for HF.	B
IIA	Scheduling an early follow-up visit (within 7 to 14 days) and early telephone follow-up (within 3 days) of hospital discharge is reasonable.	B
IIA	Use of clinical risk prediction tools and/or biomarkers to identify patients at higher risk for postdischarge clinical events is reasonable.	B

ACC, American College of Cardiology; *AHA*, American Heart Association; *BMP*, basic metabolic panel; *ECG*, electrocardiogram; *HF*, heart failure; *HFrEF*, heart failure with reduced ejection fraction; *GDMT*, guideline-directed medical therapy.
(From Mann DL, Zipes DP, Libby P, Bonow RO: *Braunwald's heart disease*, ed 10, Philadelphia, 2015, Elsevier.)

1. Dobutamine (starting at 2.5 to 5 mcg/kg/min) can be used for inotropic support but is associated with increased myocardial oxygen demand and cardiac arrhythmias and may result in hypotension from decreased systemic vascular resistance.
2. Milrinone (37.5 to 75 mcg/kg loading dose, followed by 0.375 to 0.75 mcg/kg/min) can be used as a vasodilator and inotropic agent, but is associated with increased oxygen demand and cardiac arrhythmias, and may result in hypotension from decreased systemic vascular resistance.

- Renal replacement therapy or ultrafiltration (can be used as an alternative to pharmacologic diuresis in ADHF when renal function is significantly compromised).
- ACE inhibitors or ARBs, if part of a patient's chronic medication regimen, should be continued in the absence of hypotension, acute renal failure, or hyperkalemia.
- Beta-blockers, if part of a patient's chronic medication regimen, may be continued or reduced in dosage in mild exacerbations of HF but should be discontinued in patients with hypotension or those requiring inotropic support. Beta-blockers should not be initiated in patients who are not on chronic beta-blocker therapy until euvolemia is achieved unless used for rate control.
- Morphine sulfate can cause venodilation and thus reduce cardiac preload. It may be used to reduce patient work of breathing and anxiety, but recent retrospective studies have suggested increased incidence of mechanical ventilation and in-hospital mortality in patients who received morphine.
- If ADHF with preserved EF is suspected, therapy is usually aimed at relief of symptoms

TABLE 13 Intravenous Vasoactive Agents for the Treatment of Acute Heart Failure

Intravenous Medication	Initial Dose	Effective Dose Range	Comments
Vasodilators			
Nitroglycerin; glyceryl trinitrate	20 μg/min	40-200 μg/min	Hypotension, headache; tolerance with continuous use after 24 hr
Isosorbide dinitrate	1 mg/h	2-10 mg/h	Hypotension, headache; tolerance with continuous use within 24 hr
Nitroprusside	0.3 μg/kg/min	0.3-5 μg/kg/min (usually <4 μg/kg/min)	Caution in patients with active myocardial ischemia; hypotension; cyanide side effects (nausea, dysphoria); thiocyanate toxicity; light sensitivity
Nesiritide	2 μg/kg bolus with 0.010-0.030 μg/kg/min infusion	0.010-0.030 μg/kg/min	Uptitration: 1 μg/kg bolus, then increase infusion rate by 0.005 μg/kg/min no more frequently than every 3 hr, up to a maximum of 0.03 μg/kg/min Hypotension, headache (less than with organic nitrates)
Inotropes			
Dobutamine	1-2 μg/kg/min	2-20 μg/kg/min	For inotropy and vasodilation; hypotension, tachycardia, arrhythmias; ?mortality
Dopamine	1-2 μg/kg/min	2-4 μg/kg/min	For inotropy and vasodilation; hypotension, tachycardia, arrhythmias; ?mortality
	4-5 μg/kg/min	5-20 μg/kg/min	For inotropy and vasoconstriction; tachycardia, arrhythmias; ?mortality
Milrinone	25-75 μg/kg bolus* over 10-20 min followed by infusion	0.10-0.75 μg/kg/min	For vasodilation and inotropy; hypotension, tachycardia, arrhythmias; renal excretion; ?mortality
Enoximone†	0.5-1 mg/kg	5-20 μg/kg/min	For vasodilation and inotropy; hypotension, tachycardia, arrhythmias; ?mortality
Levosimendan†	12 μg/kg bolus over 10 min followed by infusion	0.1-0.2 μg/kg/min	For vasodilation and inotropy; active metabolite present for ~84 hr; hypotension, tachycardia, arrhythmias; ?mortality
Epinephrine		0.05-0.5 μg/kg/min	For vasoconstriction and inotropy; tachycardia, arrhythmias, end-organ hypoperfusion; ?mortality
Norepinephrine		0.2-1.0 μg/kg/min	For vasoconstriction and inotropy; tachycardia, arrhythmias, end-organ hypoperfusion; ?mortality

*Some clinicians do not administer a bolus dose, so as to decrease the risk of hypotension. Bolus not recommended in patients with hypotension.
†Not approved for use in all countries.
(From Mann DL, Zipes DP, Libby P, Bonow RO: *Braunwald's heart disease*, ed 10, Philadelphia, 2015, Elsevier.)

and correction of any potential precipitating etiologies (e.g., tachycardia, hypertension, ischemia). Treatment generally involves diuretics to reduce pulmonary congestion with caution to not overdiurese given the need for elevated filling pressures in these patients to ensure adequate stroke volume and cardiac output. Nitrates may be useful in providing symptomatic relief but may precipitate hypotension. Ventricular rate should be controlled in the presence of atrial fibrillation, which, at rapid rates, is poorly tolerated in patients with impaired diastolic filling. Negative inotropic agents such as beta-blockers and calcium channel blockers can be used with caution.

- Nesiritide (recombinant brain natriuretic protein) does not reduce morbidity or mortality (ASCEND-HF trial).
- 2nd phase: Inpatient hospital care.
  1. This phase of treatment includes further diuresis and stabilization of volume status (Table 14). The patient should be carefully brought to euvolemia with daily volume status and electrolyte monitoring. The patient should also be transitioned to oral diuretics when stabilized. Whilst inpatient, the patient should have his/her medical and device management optimized with the therapies discussed later.
- 3rd phase: Early discharge planning and care.
  1. The patient should be transitioned to oral diuretics and be placed on optimum outpatient maintenance therapy. If the patient was on IV inotropic therapy, oral regimens should be adjusted while these infusions are tapered off. Prolonged physiologic effects of these IV inotropic agents after their discontinuation before discharge may mask the inadequate diuretic regimen and intolerance to the vasodilator doses. This can result in readmission, especially with milrinone due to its long half-life that can be further prolonged by the common coexisting impaired renal function. Therefore it may be recommended that patients who received inotropic infusions remain hospitalized for at least 48 hours after inotropic agents are discontinued and optimize the oral regimen.
- 4th phase: Early post-discharge care
  1. The patient will require reevaluation and constant monitoring in order to avoid another episode of ADHF. Emphasis should be placed on importance of compliance with instructions regarding dietary restrictions and daily body weight monitoring. Early follow-up should be scheduled as well as outpatient electrolyte monitoring if required after medication adjustments.

CHRONIC TREATMENT OF HFrEF: The goals of HF therapy are clinical improvement followed by stabilizing, slowing, or even reversing deterioration in myocardial function, and ultimately a reduction in risk of morbidity (including hospitalization rates) and mortality.

- ACE inhibitors:
  1. Reduce morbidity and mortality.
  2. Produce both venous and arterial vasodilation acutely, thereby reducing both preload and afterload.
  3. Potential mechanism of long-term benefit is attenuation of RAAS activation and decreased myocardial remodeling and fibrosis.
  4. Used as first-line therapy for asymptomatic LV dysfunction (LVEF <40%) and symptomatic systolic HF (ACC/AHA grades A-D).
  5. Therapy should be initiated at low doses to prevent hypotension and rapidly titrated to higher doses as tolerated.
  6. Contraindications to the use of ACE inhibitors are renal insufficiency (creatinine clearance <30 ml/min), bilateral renal artery stenosis, hyperkalemia, hypotension, or adverse reactions (e.g., angioedema).
- ARBs:
  1. Receptor antagonists to the angiotensin II receptor.

TABLE 14 Therapeutic Approaches for Volume Management in Acute Heart Failure

Severity of Volume Overload	Diuretic/Device	DOSE (mg)	Comments
Moderate	Furosemide or	20-40 or up to 2.5 times oral dose	Intravenous administration preferable in symptomatic patients
	Bumetanide or	0.5-1.0	Titrate dose according to clinical response
	Torsemide	10-20	Monitor Na^+, K^+, creatinine, blood pressure
Severe	Furosemide or	40-160 or 2.5 times oral dose 5-40 mg/hr infusion	Intravenously
	Bumetanide or	1-4/0.5-2 mg/hr infusion (max 2-4 mg/hr, limit 2-4 hr)	Bumetanide and torsemide have higher oral bioavailability than furosemide, but intravenous administration preferable in AHF
	Torsemide	20-100/5-20 mg/hr	
	Ultrafiltration	200-500 ml/hr	Adjust ultrafiltration rate to clinical response, monitor for hypotension; consider hematocrit sensor
Refractory to loop diuretics	Add HCTZ or	25-50 twice daily	Combination with loop diuretic may be better than very high dose of loop diuretics alone
	Metolazone or	2.5-10 once daily	Metolazone more potent if creatinine clearance <30 ml/min
	Chlorothiazide	250-500 IV 500-1000 PO	

AHF, Acute heart failure; *HCTZ*, hydrochlorothiazide.
(From Mann DL, Zipes DP, Libby P, Bonow RO: *Braunwald's heart disease*, ed 10, Philadelphia, 2015, Elsevier.)

2. Clinical trials have not shown any superiority compared to ACE inhibitors in patients with systolic HF (LVEF <40%).
3. Reserved for patients who are ACE inhibitor intolerant.
4. Combination therapy with ARBs and ACE inhibitors is generally not recommended.
5. Have a similar contraindication profile to ACE inhibitors. Routine combined use of an ACE inhibitor, ARB, and aldosterone antagonist is potentially harmful for patients with HFrEF.

- Angiotensin receptor–neprilysin inhibitor (ARNI) (valsartan/sacubitril or Entresto):
  1. Neprilysin is an enzyme that degrades natriuretic peptides, bradykinin, adrenomedullin, and other vasoactive peptides.
  2. Reduces morbidity and mortality. In a randomized controlled trial (PARADIGM-HF) that compared valsartan/sacubitril with enalapril in symptomatic patients with HFrEF tolerating an adequate dose of either ACE inhibitor or ARB, the ARNI reduced the composite end point of cardiovascular death or HF hospitalization significantly, by 20%.
  3. In patients with chronic symptomatic HFrEF NYHA class II or III who tolerate an ACE inhibitor or ARB, replacement by an ARNI is recommended to further reduce morbidity and mortality (class I).
  4. ARNI should not be administered concomitantly with ACE inhibitors or within 36 hours of the last dose of an ACE inhibitor (class III: Harm).
  5. ARNI should not be administered to patients with a history of angioedema (class III: Harm).
- Beta-adrenergic blockers (beta-blockers):
  1. Reduce morbidity and mortality. Such benefits observed with bisoprolol (CIBIS II trial), metoprolol succinate (MERIT-HF trial), and carvedilol (COPERNICUS trial).
  2. Benefit is believed to be conferred by blockade of sympathetic effects of neurohormonal stimulation due to HF.
  3. Are considered first-line therapy for symptomatic patients with systolic HF (NYHA class ≥II and LVEF <35%).
  4. Only carvedilol, bisoprolol, and metoprolol succinate (long acting) have been approved for the medical treatment of chronic HF; these agents are generally started in patients judged to be euvolemic and dosage is to be slowly uptitrated as tolerated.
  5. Adverse effects include worsening HF (due to negative inotropic effects), fatigue, dizziness, bradycardia, hypotension, and bronchospasm.
- Aldosterone receptor antagonists:
  1. Reduce morbidity and mortality
  2. Indicated in patients with NYHA class II-IV HF, with LVEF ≤35%, already treated with ACE inhibitors and beta-blockers without significant renal insufficiency or hyperkalemia. Patients with NYHA class II should have a history of prior cardiovascular hospitalization or elevated plasma natriuretic peptide levels to be considered for aldosterone receptor antagonists. Creatinine should be ≤2.5 mg/dl in men or ≤2.0 mg/dl in women (or estimated glomerular filtration rate >30 ml/min/1.73 m^2), and potassium should be <5.0 mEq/L. They are also indicated for post-MI patients with EF ≤40% who have either symptomatic HF or diabetes mellitus.
  3. Spironolactone may cause gynecomastia, galactorrhea, and hyperkalemia (especially in patients with baseline renal insufficiency or type 4 renal tubular acidosis). It has been best studied in chronic HF with NYHA class III to IV symptoms (RALES study).
  4. Eplerenone is associated with fewer endocrine side effects and has especially been studied in postmyocardial infarction left ventricular dysfunction (EPHESUS trial) and in chronic systolic HF with only class II symptoms (EMPHASIS-HF trial).
  5. Inappropriate use of aldosterone receptor antagonists is potentially harmful because of life-threatening hyperkalemia or renal insufficiency when serum creatinine is >2.5 mg/dl in men or >2.0 mg/dl in women (or estimated glomerular filtration rate <30 ml/min/1.73 m^2), and/or potassium >5.0 mEq/L.
- Diuretics:
  1. Are used to maintain euvolemia and to improve symptoms as discussed previously.
  2. Although data on diuretic efficacy are limited, a meta-analysis of a few small trials found that they were associated with reduction in mortality as well as reduced hospitalization for HF.
  3. Of note, loop diuretics with better bioavailability, such as torsemide and bumetanide, may be used in diuretic-resistant patients but are generally more expensive.
- Combination of isosorbide dinitrate and hydralazine:
  1. Cause venous (nitrates) and arteriolar (hydralazine) vasodilation resulting in decreased preload and afterload.
  2. The combination of hydralazine and isosorbide dinitrate is recommended to reduce morbidity and mortality for patients self-described as African Americans with

NYHA class III–IV HFrEF receiving optimal therapy with ACE inhibitors and beta-blockers, unless contraindicated.

3. A combination of hydralazine and isosorbide dinitrate can be useful to reduce morbidity or mortality in patients with current or prior symptomatic HFrEF who cannot be given an ACE inhibitor or ARB because of drug intolerance, hypotension, or renal insufficiency, unless contraindicated.
4. Adverse effects of nitrates include hypotension, headaches, and tolerance as well as reflex tachycardia and lupus-like syndrome with hydralazine.

- Digoxin:
  1. Positive inotropic and negative chronotropic drug that works by inhibition of the sodium-potassium transmembrane exchange pump and through its vagomimetic action
  2. Commonly used in patients with concomitant atrial fibrillation
  3. Has been shown to reduce HF-related hospitalizations but does NOT confer any mortality benefit (DIG trial). However, there is evidence suggesting that digoxin may actually have an effect on survival that varies with the serum digoxin level; survival was improved when the level was between 0.5 and 0.8 ng/ml (most often in men) and significantly worsened when it was ≥1.2 ng/ml and >0.9 mg/ml in women.
  4. Caution must be used in patients with abnormal renal function to avoid digoxin toxicity and life-threatening arrhythmia. Avoid hypokalemia because potassium competes with digoxin on the same site of the Na^+-K^+-ATPase pump.
- I_f channel inhibitor (ivabradine):
  1. Ivabradine is a new therapeutic agent that selectively inhibits the I_f current in the sinoatrial node, providing heart rate reduction.
  2. Ivabradine can be beneficial to reduce HF hospitalization for patients with symptomatic (NYHA class II-III) stable chronic HFrEF (LVEF ≤35%) who are receiving guideline-directed therapy, including a beta-blocker at maximum tolerated dose, and who are in sinus rhythm with a heart rate of 70 bpm or greater at rest (class IIa).
- Cardiac resynchronization therapy (CRT):
  1. Improves morbidity and mortality rates in selected patients.
  2. The presence of a bundle-branch block or other intraventricular conduction delay (IVCD) can cause ventricular dyssynchrony, which induces regional loading disparities and reduces the efficiency of ventricular contraction, thereby further impairing the systolic function of a failing ventricle.
  3. CRT is indicated for patients who have LVEF ≤35%, sinus rhythm, left bundle-branch block with a QRS duration of 150 ms or greater, and NYHA class II, III, or ambulatory IV symptoms on guideline-directed medical therapy. CRT is NOT indicated in patients whose functional status and life expectancy are limited predominantly by chronic noncardiac conditions. Life expectancy should be >1 yr.
  4. In the appropriate subset of patients, CRT in addition to optimal medical therapy has been shown in numerous clinical trials to improve symptoms by at least one NYHA class, improve 6-min walk distance and quality of life, reduce rate of HF-related hospitalization, and reduce rate of all-cause and cardiovascular mortality.
  5. Detailed guidelines for CRT are beyond the scope of this chapter. Consultation with cardiology service may be indicated.
- Implantable cardioverter-defibrillators (ICDs):
  1. Sudden cardiac death (SCD) is a common cause of death in patients with HF in both ischemic and nonischemic cardiomyopathies. Ventricular tachycardia (VT) degenerating into ventricular fibrillation (VF) is the culprit in the majority of patients with SCD, although bradyarrhythmias do also occur with less frequency.
  2. ICD therapy is recommended for primary prevention of SCD to reduce total mortality in selected patients with nonischemic dilated cardiomyopathy or ischemic heart disease at least 40 days post-MI with LVEF ≤35% and NYHA class II or III symptoms on chronic guideline-directed medical therapy, who have reasonable expectation of meaningful survival for >1 year.
  3. Patients with HF who survive an episode of sudden cardiac arrest or experience sustained VT in the presence of LVEF <35% are at high risk for future arrhythmic events and SCD and obtain a mortality benefit from ICD placement for secondary prevention, with or without adjunctive therapies such as antiarrhythmic drugs, radiofrequency ablation, surgery, or transplant.
- In the absence of an indication (e.g., atrial fibrillation), routine use of anticoagulation is currently not recommended in patients with HF. Even with the increased risk for LV thrombus formation in dilated cardiomyopathy and subsequent thromboembolization, data are conflicting about benefits of antithrombotic (antiplatelet or anticoagulant) therapy for primary prevention to reduce thromboembolic events or mortality in patients with systolic HF who are in sinus rhythm (SOLVD, V-HeFT, SAVE, HELAS, and WASH trials). It may be reasonable to consider anticoagulation for secondary prevention in patients with HF who had a prior thromboembolic event; however, risks and benefits should be carefully assessed.
- Antiplatelet agents are recommended for patients with concomitant CAD.
- Statins are not beneficial as adjunctive therapy when prescribed solely for the diagnosis of HF in the absence of other indications for their use.
- Calcium channel blocking drugs are not recommended as routine treatment for patients with HFrEF.
- Omega-3 polyunsaturated fatty acid supplementation is reasonable to use as adjunctive therapy in patients with NYHA class II-IV symptoms and HFrEF or HFpEF, unless contraindicated, to reduce mortality and cardiovascular hospitalizations.
- Percutaneous coronary intervention (PCI) or surgical revascularization should be considered in patients with HF and significant CAD who are revascularization candidates.
- In general, the following sequence of drugs is recommended:
  1. Loop diuretics to provide symptom relief and achieve a euvolemic state.
  2. ACE inhibitor or ARB started at low doses, then increased to a moderate dose in 1-2 wk. Replace with ARNI in those tolerating ACE inhibitor or ARB.
  3. Beta-blockers after the patient is stable on ACE/ARB treatment. Start a low dose, then uptitrate to goal based on trial data or maximal dose tolerated. Once achieved, uptitration of ACE or ARB to goal doses can be completed.
- The following drugs can be added in selected patients in the absence of contraindications:
  1. Aldosterone antagonists improve survival in NYHA class II with LVEF <30% or NYHA class III-IV with EF <35%. Kidney function should be stable with eGFR ≥30 ml/min and potassium <5 mEq/L.
  2. Combination of hydralazine with a nitrate in patients (particularly African Americans) with a reduced EF.
  3. Digoxin reduces hospitalizations for HF and controls HR in atrial fibrillation. It can also help control symptoms.

CHRONIC TREATMENT OF HFpEF:

- To date, there is a relative dearth of clinical trials examining effective chronic treatment strategies in this subset of patients with HFpEF. Current therapies are mainly for symptomatic relief. ACC/AHA guidelines for treatment of patients with end-stage heart failure are summarized in Table 15.
- Therapy centers on relief of volume overload with judicious diuretic use, treatment of ischemia via coronary revascularization (Table 16), management of atrial fibrillation, controlling heart rate and blood pressure to prevent acute decompensation, and restriction of sodium and fluid to prevent volume overload.
- Diuretics should be used for relief of symptoms due to volume overload in patients with HFpEF.
- The use of beta-blocking agents, ACE inhibitors, and ARBs in patients with hypertension is reasonable to control blood pressure in patients with HFpEF.
- The use of ARBs might be considered to decrease hospitalizations for patients with HFpEF.
- Aldosterone antagonists may be used in appropriate patients with HFpEF (EF >45%, elevated BNP or HF admission in the past year, potassium <5.0 mEq/L, estimated

TABLE 15 ACC/AHA Guidelines for Treatment of Patients with End-Stage Heart Failure (Stage D)

Class	Indication	Level of Evidence
	Nonpharmacologic Interventions	
IIa	Fluid restriction (1.5-2 L/day) is reasonable in stage D, especially in patients with hyponatremia.	B
	Inotropic Support	
I	Until definitive therapy (e.g., coronary revascularization, MCS, heart transplantation) or resolution of the acute precipitating problem, patients with cardiogenic shock should receive temporary intravenous inotropic support to maintain systemic perfusion and preserve end-organ performance.	C
IIa	Continuous intravenous inotropic support is reasonable as "bridge therapy" in patients with stage D refractory to GDMT and device therapy who are eligible for and awaiting MCS or cardiac transplantation.	B
IIb	Short-term, continuous intravenous inotropic support may be reasonable in those hospitalized patients presenting with documented severe systolic dysfunction who present with low blood pressure and significantly depressed cardiac output to maintain systemic perfusion and preserve end-organ performance.	B
	Long-term, continuous intravenous inotropic support may be considered as palliative therapy for symptom control in select patients with stage D disease despite optimal GDMT and device therapy who are not eligible for either MCS or cardiac transplantation.	B
III: Harm	Long-term use of either continuous or intermittent, intravenous parenteral positive inotropic agents, in the absence of specific indications or for reasons other than palliative care, is potentially harmful in the patient with HF.	B
	Use of parenteral inotropic agents in hospitalized patients without documented severe systolic dysfunction, low blood pressure, or impaired perfusion, and evidence of significantly depressed cardiac output, with or without congestion, is potentially harmful.	B
	Mechanical Circulatory Support (MCS)	
IIa	MCS is beneficial in carefully selected patients with stage D HFrEF in whom definitive management (e.g., cardiac transplantation) or cardiac recovery is anticipated or planned).	B
	Nondurable MCS, including the use of percutaneous and extracorporeal ventricular assist devices (VADs), is reasonable as a "bridge to recovery" or "bridge to decision" for carefully selected patients with HFrEF with acute, profound hemodynamic compromise.	B
	Durable MCS is reasonable to prolong survival for carefully selected patients with stage D HFrEF.	B
	Cardiac Transplantation	
I	Evaluation for cardiac transplantation is indicated for carefully selected patients with stage D HF despite GDMT, device, and surgical management.	C

ACC, American College of Cardiology; *AHA,* American Heart Association; *GDMT,* guideline-directed medical therapy; *HF,* heart failure; *HFrEF,* HF with reduced ejection fraction. (From Mann DL, Zipes DP, Libby P, Bonow RO: *Braunwald's heart disease*, ed 10, Philadelphia, 2015, Elsevier.)

TABLE 16 ACC/AHA Guidelines for Surgical/Percutaneous/Transcatheter Interventional Treatments of Heart Failure

Class	Indication	Level of Evidence
I	Coronary artery revascularization via CABG or percutaneous intervention is indicated for patients (HFpEF and HFrEF) on GDMT with angina and suitable coronary artery anatomy, especially for a left main artery stenosis (>50%) or left main–equivalent disease.	C
IIa	CABG to improve survival is reasonable in patients with mild to moderate LV systolic dysfunction (EF 35%-50%) and significant (≥70% diameter stenosis) multivessel CAD or proximal left anterior descending coronary artery stenosis when viable myocardium is present in the region of intended revascularization.	B
	CABG or medical therapy is reasonable to improve morbidity and cardiovascular mortality for patients with severe LV dysfunction (EF <35%), HF, and significant CAD.	B
	Surgical aortic valve replacement is reasonable for patients with critical aortic stenosis and a predicted surgical mortality of no greater than 10%.	B
	Transcatheter aortic valve replacement after careful candidate consideration is reasonable for patients with critical aortic stenosis who are deemed inoperable.	B
IIb	CABG may be considered with the intent of improving survival in patients with ischemic heart disease with severe LV systolic dysfunction (EF <35%) and operable coronary anatomy whether or not viable myocardium is present.	B
	Transcatheter mitral valve repair or mitral valve surgery for functional mitral insufficiency is of uncertain benefit and should only be considered after careful candidate selection and with a background of GDMT.	B
	Surgical reverse remodeling or LV aneurysmectomy may be considered in carefully selected patients with HFrEF for specific indications, including intractable HF and ventricular arrhythmias.	B

ACC, American College of Cardiology; *AHA,* American Heart Association; *CABG,* coronary artery bypass grafting, *CAD,* coronary artery disease; *EF,* ejection fraction; *GDMT,* guideline-directed medical therapy; *HF,* heart failure; *HFrEF,* HF with reduced ejection fraction; *LV,* left ventricle. (From Mann DL, Zipes DP, Libby P, Bonow RO: *Braunwald's heart disease*, ed 10, Philadelphia, 2015, Elsevier.)

glomerular filtration rate >30 and creatinine <2.5 mg/dl) to decrease hospitalizations (class IIb recommendation).

- Routine use of nitrates or phosphodiesterase-5 inhibitors to increase activity or quality of life in patients with HFpEF is not recommended as there is no benefit.
- There is no evidence to support routine use of nutritional supplements and they are not recommended for patients with HFpEF.
- Surgical options for contributing critical aortic stenosis, constrictive pericarditis, and hypertrophic cardiomyopathy (HCM) should be entertained in appropriate patients.
- In patients with comorbidities including anemia, hypertension, and sleep apnea, the following recommendations are made:
  1. Intravenous iron replacement in patients with NYHA class II and III HF and iron deficiency (ferritin <100 ng/ml or 100-300 ng/ml with transferrin saturation <20%) to improve functional status and quality of life (class IIb recommendation).
  2. Titration of medical therapy to attain systolic blood pressure <130 mm Hg is recommended in patients with HFrEF and hypertension, as well as in patients with HFpEF and persistent hypertension after treatment of volume overload (class I recommendation).

TABLE 17 Coordinating Care for Patients with Chronic Heart Failure

Class	Indication	Level of Evidence
I	Effective systems of care coordination with special attention to care transitions should be deployed for every patient with chronic HF that facilitate and ensure effective care that is designed to achieve GDMT and prevent hospitalization.	B
	Every patient with HF should have a clear, detailed, and evidence-based plan of care that ensures the achievement of GDMT goals, effective management of comorbid conditions, timely follow-up with the health care team, appropriate dietary and physical activities, and compliance with secondary prevention guidelines for cardiovascular disease. This plan of care should be updated regularly and made readily available to all members of the patient's health care team.	C
	Palliative and supportive care is effective for patients with symptomatic advanced HF to improve quality of life.	B

GDMT, Guideline directed medical therapy; *HF,* heart failure. (From Mann DL, Zipes DP, Libby P, Bonow RO: *Braunwald's heart disease*, ed 10, Philadelphia, 2015, Elsevier.)

3. A formal sleep assessment should be obtained in patients with NYHA class II-IV HF with suspicion of sleep-disordered breathing. Continuous positive airway pressure should be used in patients with HF and obstructive sleep apnea to improve sleep quality and daytime sleepiness (class IIb recommendation).

DISPOSITION

- Coordination of care (Table 17) is essential in patients with chronic heart failure.
- Annual mortality of systolic HF ranges from 10% in stable patients with mild symptoms to 50% in patients with NYHA class IV disease (a mortality rate rivaling some malignancies). The Seattle Heart Failure Model provides an accurate estimate of 1-, 2-, and 3-yr survival before and after different therapies. This model can be useful to assess the need for LV assist device implantation or urgent transplantation. The calculator is available online at http://depts.washington.edu/shfm/.
- Cardiac transplantation has a 5-yr survival rate of ~70% and represents a viable option in selected patients. Fig. 4 describes an algorithm for evaluation of potential heart transplant recipient.
- The use of an LV assist device (LVAD) in patients with advanced HF can result in a clinically meaningful survival benefit and improve quality of life in patients who are not candidates for cardiac transplantation. There are two approved uses of LVADs specifically as a bridge to transplant and as destination therapy. There are two major categories of LVAD pulsatile flow devices vs. continuous flow devices. Continuous flow devices are associated with increased survival as destination therapy as compared to medically managed controls (REMATCH trial).

SUGGESTED READINGS

Available at ExpertConsult.com

RELATED CONTENT

Heart Failure (Patient Information)

AUTHORS: **HANNAH CHAUDRY, M.D.,** and **ARAVIND RAO KOKKIRALA, M.D. FACC**

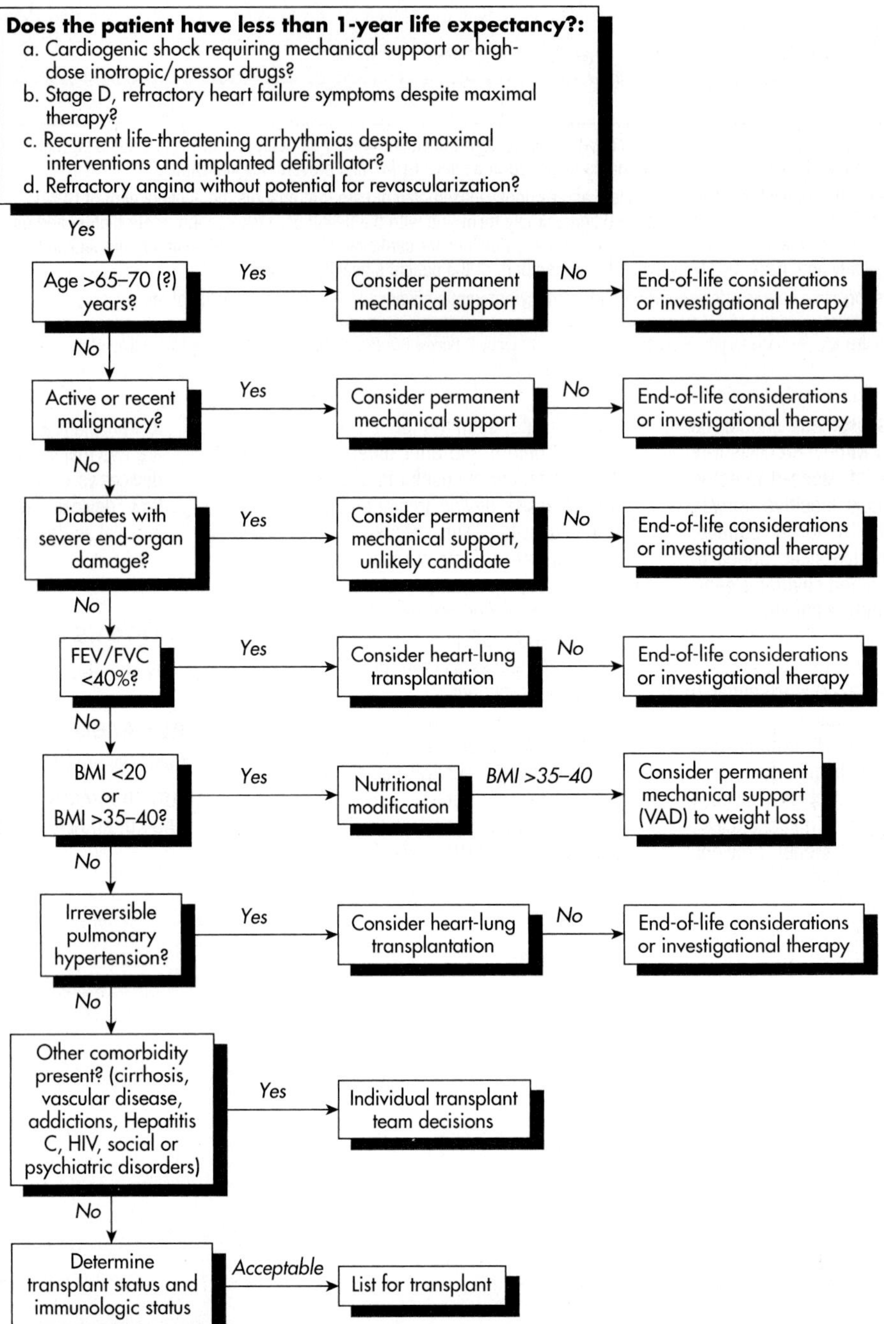

FIG. 4 Evaluation of the potential heart transplant recipient. *FVC*, Forced vital capacity; *FEV*, forced expiratory volume. (From Mann DL, Zipes DP, Libby P, Bonow RO: *Braunwald's heart disease*, ed 10, Philadelphia, 2015, Elsevier.)

BASIC INFORMATION

DEFINITION

Heat exhaustion and heat stroke are part of a continuum of heat-related illness, and unless factors leading to heat exhaustion are corrected swiftly, affected patients can progress to heat stroke.

- ***Heat exhaustion:*** An illness resulting from prolonged, heavy activity in a hot environment with subsequent dehydration, electrolyte depletion, and rectal temperature >37.8° C but ≤40° C.
- ***Heat stroke:*** A life-threatening heat illness characterized by extreme hyperthermia (core temperature >40° C [104.0° F]), dehydration, and neurologic manifestations. Heat stroke can be further subdivided into "exertional heat stroke" occurring in generally healthy individuals undergoing strenuous physical activity in warm conditions and "non-exertional heat stroke" often seen in elderly and/or debilitated patients with impaired thermal regulations due to illness or medications (see Etiology).

SYNONYMS

Heat illness
Hyperthermia

ICD-10CM CODES

T67.5	Heat exhaustion, unspecified
T67.0	Heatstroke and sunstroke
T67.1	Heat syncope
T67.2	Heat cramp
T67.3	Heat exhaustion, anhydrotic
T67.6	Heat fatigue, transient

EPIDEMIOLOGY & DEMOGRAPHICS

INCIDENCE (IN U.S.): Incidence of heat stroke is approximately 20 cases/100,000 population.

PREDOMINANT AGE: Heat exhaustion and stroke occur more frequently in elderly patients, especially those taking diuretics or medications that impair heat dissipation (e.g., phenothiazines, anticholinergics, antihistamines, beta-blockers). Table 1 describes factors predisposing to serious heat illness.

PHYSICAL FINDINGS & CLINICAL PRESENTATION

Heat exhaustion:

- Generalized malaise, weakness, headache, muscle and abdominal cramps, nausea, vomiting, hypotension, tachycardia.
- Rectal temperature is usually normal.
- Sweating is usually present.

Heat stroke:

- Neurologic manifestations (seizures, tremor, hemiplegia, coma, psychosis, other bizarre behavior).
- Evidence of dehydration (poor skin turgor, sunken eyeballs).
- Tachycardia, hyperventilation.
- Skin is hot, red, and flushed.
- Sweating is often (not always) absent, particularly in elderly patients.
- Classic heat stroke generally develops slowly over days and occurs predominantly in older persons and in those with chronic illness. Exertional heat stroke is more common in young, healthy persons, has a more rapid onset, and is associated with higher core temperatures. Table 2 compares classic and exertional heat stroke. Box 1 summarizes organ dysfunction seen in patients with heat stroke.

ETIOLOGY

- Exogenous heat gain (increased ambient temperature)
- Increased heat production (exercise, infection, hyperthyroidism, drugs)
- Impaired heat dissipation (high humidity, heavy clothing, neonatal or elderly patients, drugs [phenothiazines, anticholinergics, antihistamines, butyrophenones, amphetamines, cocaine, alcohol, β-blockers])
- Diuretics, laxatives
- Fig. E1 describes an algorithm of the pathophysiology of heat stroke

TABLE 1 Factors Predisposing to Serious Heat Illness

Individual Factors
Lack of acclimatization
Low physical fitness
Excessive body weight
Dehydration
Advanced age
Young age
Health Conditions
Inflammation and fever
Viral infection
Cardiovascular disease
Diabetes mellitus
Gastroenteritis
Rash, sunburn, and previous burns to large areas of skin
Seizures
Thyroid storm
Neuroleptic malignant syndrome
Malignant hyperthermia
Sickle cell trait
Cystic fibrosis
Spinal cord injury
Drugs
Anticholinergic properties (atropine)
Antiepileptic (topiramate)
Antihistamines
Glutethimide (Doriden)
Phenothiazines
Tricyclic antidepressants
Amphetamines, cocaine, "Ecstasy"
Ergogenic stimulants (e.g., ephedrine, ephedra)
Lithium
Diuretics
β-Blockers
Ethanol
Environmental Factors
High temperature
High humidity
Little air motion
Lack of shade
Heat wave
Physical exercise
Heavy clothing
Air pollution (nitrogen dioxide)

From Goldman L, Schafer AI: *Goldman's Cecil medicine*, ed 24, Philadelphia, 2012, Saunders.

DIAGNOSIS

DIFFERENTIAL DIAGNOSIS

- Infections (meningitis, encephalitis, sepsis)
- Head trauma
- Epilepsy
- Thyroid storm
- Acute cocaine intoxication
- Malignant hyperthermia
- Heat exhaustion can be differentiated from heat stroke by the following:
  1. Essentially intact mental function and lack of significant fever in heat exhaustion
  2. Mild or absent increases in creatine phosphokinase (CPK), aspartate aminotransferase (AST), lactate dehydrogenase (LDH), and alanine aminotransferase (ALT) in heat exhaustion

WORKUP

- Heat stroke: Comprehensive history, physical examination, and laboratory evaluation.
- Heat exhaustion: In most cases, laboratory tests are not necessary for diagnosis.

LABORATORY TESTS

Laboratory abnormalities may include the following:

- Elevated blood urea nitrogen (BUN), creatinine, hematocrit
- Hyponatremia or hypernatremia, hyperkalemia or hypokalemia
- Elevated LDH, AST, ALT, CPK, bilirubin
- Lactic acidosis, respiratory alkalosis (from hyperventilation)
- Myoglobinuria, hypofibrinogenemia, fibrinolysis, hypocalcemia

TREATMENT

- Treatment of heat exhaustion consists primarily of placing the patient in a cool, shaded area and providing rapid hydration and salt replacement.
  1. Fluid intake should be at least 2 L q4h in patients without history of CHF.
  2. Salt replacement can be accomplished by using one-quarter teaspoon of salt or two 10-grain salt tablets dissolved in 1 L of water.
  3. If IV fluid replacement is necessary, young athletes can be given normal saline IV (3 to 4 L over 6 to 8 hr); in elderly patients, consider using D5½NS IV with the rate titrated to cardiovascular status.
- Patients with heat stroke should undergo rapid cooling.
  1. Remove the patient's clothes and place the patient in a cool and well-ventilated room.
  2. If patient is unconscious, position on his or her side and clear the airway. Protect airway and augment oxygenation (e.g., nasal O_2 at 4 L/min to keep oxygen saturation >90%).

TABLE 2 Comparison of Classic and Exertional Heat Stroke

Patient Characteristics	Classic	Exertional
Age	Young children or elderly	15-55 yr
Health	Chronic illness	Usually healthy
Fever	Unusual	Common
Prevailing weather	Frequent in heat waves	Variable
Activity	Sedentary	Strenuous exercise
Drug use	Diuretics, antidepressants, anticholinergics, phenothiazines	Ergogenic stimulants or cocaine
Sweating	Often absent	Common
Acid-base disturbances	Respiratory alkalosis	Lactic acidosis
Acute renal failure	Uncommon	Common (≈15%)
Rhabdomyolysis	Uncommon	Common (≈25%)
CK	Mildly elevated	Markedly elevated (500-1000 U/L)
ALT, AST	Mildly elevated	Markedly elevated
Hyperkalemia	Uncommon	Common
Hypocalcemia	Uncommon	Common
DIC	Mild	Marked
Hypoglycemia	Uncommon	Common

ALT, Alanine aminotransferase; *AST,* aspartate aminotransferase; *CK,* creatine kinase; *DIC,* disseminated intravascular coagulation.
From Goldman L, Schafer AI: *Goldman's Cecil medicine,* ed 24, Philadelphia, 2012, Saunders.

BOX 1 Organ Dysfunction Seen in Patients With Heat Stroke

Encephalopathy
Rhabdomyolysis
Acute renal failure
Acute respiratory distress syndrome
Myocardial injury
Hepatocellular injury
Intestinal ischemia and infarction
Pancreatic injury
Hemorrhagic complication (e.g., disseminated intravascular coagulation)

From Adams JG et al: *Emergency medicine, clinical essentials,* ed 2, Philadelphia, 2013, Elsevier.

3. Monitor body temperature every 5 min. Measurement of the patient's core temperature with a rectal probe is recommended. The goal is to reduce the body temperature to 39° C (102.2° F) in 30 to 60 min. Advantages, disadvantages, and efficacy of various cooling methods are described in Table E3.
4. Spray the patient with a cool mist and use fans to enhance airflow over the body (rapid evaporation method).
5. Immersion of the patient in ice water, stomach lavage with iced saline solution, intravenous administration of cooled fluids, and inhalation of cold air are advisable only when the means for rapid evaporation are not available. Immersion in tepid water (15° C, 59° F) is preferred over ice water immersion to minimize risk of shivering.
6. Use of ice packs on axillae, neck, and groin is controversial because they increase peripheral vasoconstriction and may induce shivering.
7. Antipyretics are ineffective because the hypothalamic set point during heat stroke is normal despite the increased body temperature.
8. Intubate a comatose patient, insert a Foley catheter, and start nasal O_2. Continuous ECG monitoring is recommended.
9. Insert at least two large-bore IV lines and begin IV hydration with normal saline (NS) or Ringer lactate.
10. Draw initial laboratory studies: Electrolytes, complete blood count, blood urea nitrogen, creatinine, AST, ALT, CPK, LDH, glucose, PT (INR), PTT, platelet count, Ca^{2+}, lactic acid, and arterial blood gases.
11. Treat complications as follows:
    a. Hypotension: Vigorous hydration with normal saline or Ringer lactate.
    b. Convulsions: Diazepam 5 to 10 mg IV (slowly).
    c. Shivering: Chlorpromazine 10 to 50 mg IV.
    d. Acidosis: Use bicarbonate judiciously (only in severe acidosis).

- Observe for evidence of rhabdomyolysis and hepatic, renal, or cardiac failure and treat accordingly.

DISPOSITION

Most patients recover completely within 48 hr. Central nervous system injury is permanent in 20% of cases. Mortality rate can exceed 30% in patients with prolonged and severe hyperthermia. Delayed access to cooling is the leading cause of morbidity and mortality in persons with heat stroke.

SUGGESTED READINGS

Available at ExpertConsult.com

RELATED CONTENT

Acute Kidney Injury (Related Key Topic)
Heat Exhaustion and Heat Stroke (Patient Information)
Rhabdomyolysis (Related Key Topic)

AUTHOR: **FRED F. FERRI, M.D.**

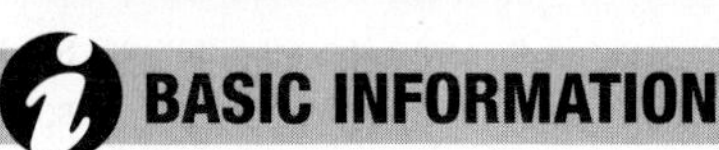

BASIC INFORMATION

DEFINITION

Abnormal uterine bleeding (AUB) is a broad term for variations in normal menses. Normal duration of menstrual flow is 5 days; normal menstrual cycle is 21 to 35 days. Heavy menstrual bleeding, or menorrhagia, is a large volume of menstrual blood loss (i.e., >80 ml per cycle). Bleeding may also be prolonged, intermenstrual, frequent, and irregular. This language replaces prior terms such as *metrorrhagia, polymenorrhea,* or *oligomenorrhea.*

PALM-COEIN classification of abnormal uterine bleeding was adopted in 2011 to standardize terminology and reflect etiology: polyp, adenomyosis, leiomyoma, malignancy and hyperplasia, coagulopathy, ovulatory dysfunction, endometrial, Iatrogenic, and not yet classified. AUB-P would refer to abnormal uterine bleeding due to polyps.

SYNONYMS

Abnormal uterine bleeding
Heavy menstrual bleeding/menorrhagia
Menometrorrhagia
Dysfunctional uterine bleeding
Irregular menstrual cycle

ICD-10CM CODES

N92.0 Excessive and frequent menstruation with regular cycle
N92.1 Excessive and frequent menstruation with irregular cycle
N92.2 Excessive menstruation at puberty
N92.4 Excessive bleeding in the premenopausal period
N92.6 Irregular menstruation, unspecified

EPIDEMIOLOGY & DEMOGRAPHICS

INCIDENCE: 10% to 15% of reproductive-aged women; 30% of outpatient office visits; 70% of all gynecologic consults
PEAK INCIDENCE: Reproductive-aged women, ages 13 to 50
PREVALENCE: 9% to 14% of all women
PREDOMINANT SEX AND AGE: Female; peak in adolescence and perimenopausal periods
GENETICS: Hereditary coagulopathy (most commonly Von Willebrand's disease, platelet dysfunction disorders) in 20% of women with heavy menstrual bleeding
RISK FACTORS: Genetic predisposition, anticoagulation treatment, obesity, endocrinopathies, autoimmune disease, liver disease, renal disease

PHYSICAL FINDINGS & CLINICAL PRESENTATION

- History: Age, age at menarche or menopause, menstrual bleeding patterns, severity of bleeding, pain, underlying medical conditions, surgical history, medications, family history, hirsutism, acne, symptoms of thyroid dysfunction or other endocrinopathy
  1. If heavy bleeding since menarche, screen for signs and symptoms of hemostatic disorder, including postpartum hemorrhage, surgery-related bleeding, bleeding from dental work, easy bruising, epistaxis, and frequent gum bleeding
- Physical exam: Weight, hirsutism, acne, thyroid nodules, signs of insulin resistance (acanthosis nigricans), signs of bleeding disorder (petechiae, ecchymoses, pallor, swollen joints), pelvic examination including external, speculum, and bimanual exam of uterus

ETIOLOGY

- Pregnancy/miscarriage
- Endometrial polyps
- Adenomyosis
- Uterine leiomyoma
- Endometrial hyperplasia or carcinoma
- Coagulopathy, inherited or acquired
- Ovulatory dysfunction, most likely PCOS
- Endometrial
- Iatrogenic

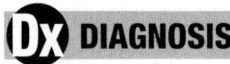

DIAGNOSIS

DIFFERENTIAL DIAGNOSIS

Pregnancy, sexually transmitted infection, polycystic ovary syndrome (PCOS), thyroid dysfunction, anovulation due to immature hypothalamic-pituitary-ovarian axis or perimenopausal transition, uterine pathology including endometrial hyperplasia or carcinoma, leiomyoma, adenomyosis, or endometrial polyp, coagulopathy, iatrogenic due to medications including oral contraceptives or anticoagulants (warfarin), nonuterine bleeding (urinary, gastrointestinal, vaginal, or cervical source)

WORKUP

- History
- Physical exam
- Laboratory, pathology, and imaging studies to determine etiology

LABORATORY TESTS

- Pregnancy test
- Complete blood count (CBC)
- Thyroid-stimulating hormone (TSH)
- *Chlamydia trachomatis* testing if high risk
- Pap smear if indicated
- Targeted screening for bleeding disorders
- Endometrial sampling by endometrial biopsy or hysteroscopic sampling for women >45 yr or <45 yr with history of unopposed estrogen (PCOS, obesity), failed medical management, or persistent abnormal bleeding
- Iron studies if anemia is suspected

IMAGING STUDIES

- Pelvic ultrasound, transabdominal and transvaginal
- Sonohysterography or hysteroscopy if ultrasound is not adequate or further evaluation of the cavity is required
- MRI if needed for surgical planning or further evaluation of structural abnormality

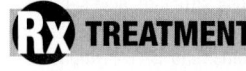

TREATMENT

SURGICAL MANAGEMENT

- Dilation and curettage
- Hysteroscopic resection of uterine pathology including endometrial polyps and submucosal leiomyoma
- Myomectomy
- Endometrial ablation
- Uterine artery embolization
- Hysterectomy

ACUTE GENERAL Rx

Acute severe bleeding may be managed medically with oral progestins, combined oral contraceptive pills, IV estrogen, tranexamic acid, and/or blood transfusion as indicated. Surgical management includes dilation and curettage, uterine artery embolization, or hysterectomy.

CHRONIC Rx

- Combined hormonal contraceptives (pill, transdermal patch, vaginal ring) in a cyclic or continuous regimen
- Progesterone intrauterine device
- Oral or injected progesterone
- Gonadotropin-releasing hormone agonist
- Nonsteroidal antiinflammatory drugs
- Tranexamic acid, aminocaproic acid
- Danazol (significant side-effect profile requires justification for use; this is rare)
- Selective progesterone receptor modulators (investigational for bleeding related to leiomyomas)
- Surgery for anatomic causes, including polypectomy or myomectomy
- Uterine artery embolization for leiomyomatous uterus
- Endometrial ablation or hysterectomy if completed childbearing
- Replacement of or treatment for any abnormal bleeding factors (i.e., DDAVP)

REFERRAL

- If unresponsive to initial hormonal management, referral to gynecologist is warranted.
- If concern for a structural etiology or malignancy, referral to a gynecologist for surgical management is indicated.
- If endometrial sampling reveals endometrial hyperplasia or malignancy, referral to a gynecologist or gynecologic oncologist is indicated. Resampling is necessary with progestin therapy for hyperplasia. If endometrial hyperplasia associated with complex glands or atypia, consultation with gynecologic oncologist is warranted due to high degree of progression to malignancy.

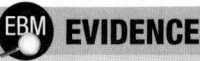

EVIDENCE

Available at ExpertConsult.com

SUGGESTED READINGS

Available at ExpertConsult.com

RELATED CONTENT

Menorrhagia (Patient Information)
Dysfunctional Uterine Bleeding (Related Key Topic)

AUTHORS: **CHRISTINA M. JOHNSON, M.D.,** and **NIMA R. PATEL, M.D., M.S.**

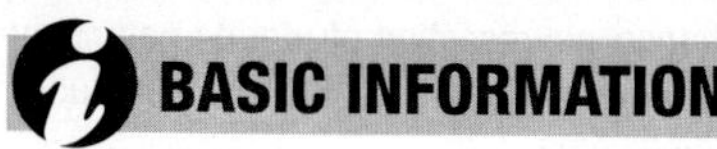

DEFINITION

Infection of the human gastric mucosa with the organism *Helicobacter pylori,* a spiral-shaped gram-negative organism with unique features that allow it to survive in the hostile gastric environment.

SYNONYM

Previously known as *Campylobacter pylori*

ICD-10CM CODE
B96.81 *Helicobacter pylori* [*H. pylori*] as the cause of diseases classified elsewhere

EPIDEMIOLOGY & DEMOGRAPHICS

H. pylori is the most common chronic bacterial infection in human beings, probably affecting 50% of the earth's population in all age groups as well as 30% to 40% of the U.S. population. In developing nations, infection is acquired at an earlier age and occurs more frequently.

CLINICAL PRESENTATION

- *H. pylori* causes histologic gastritis in all affected individuals. The majority of cases are asymptomatic and unlikely to proceed to serious consequences.
- *H. pylori* is a causative agent in peptic ulcer disease (PUD), gastric adenocarcinoma, and gastric mucosa-associated lymphoid tissue lymphoma, as well as a risk factor for iron-deficiency anemia and likely chronic idiopathic thrombocytopenic purpura. It may present with the signs and symptoms of these disorders, including abdominal pain, bloating, anorexia, and early satiety. Fig. 1 describes association of *H. pylori* infection and disease states.
- "Alarm symptoms" that should prompt more immediate and aggressive workup include weight loss, dysphagia, protracted nausea or vomiting, anemia, melena, and palpable abdominal mass, particularly in older individuals.

ETIOLOGY

- Route of acquisition is unknown but is presumed to be person to person by fecal-oral or possibly oral-oral transmission.
- The majority of cases are acquired in childhood. Socioeconomic status and living conditions in childhood affect risk of acquisition of infection. These factors include housing density, number of siblings, overcrowding, sharing a bed, and lack of running water.
- Iatrogenic transmission has been documented.
- *H. pylori* does not invade gastroduodenal tissue, but disrupts the mucous layer, causing the underlying mucosa to be more vulnerable to acid peptic damage.
- It is unclear what differentiates the subset of patients with *H. pylori* who go on to develop ulcers or cancer.

Dx DIAGNOSIS

DIFFERENTIAL DIAGNOSIS

- Infection with *H. pylori* should be considered in the face of PUD, gastric cancer, gastritis, and gastric mucosa-associated lymphoid tissue (MALT) lymphoma.
- *H. pylori* should be considered in the differential diagnosis of upper gastrointestinal (GI) tract disease, along with non-ulcer dyspepsia, reflux esophagitis, biliary tract disease, gastroparesis, pancreatitis, ischemic bowel, and unexplained iron deficiency anemia.

WORKUP

- Workup is indicated in patients with active PUD, a past history of documented peptic ulcer, or gastric MALT lymphoma, as well as those with immune thrombocytopenic purpura (ITP), and otherwise unexplained iron deficiency. The role of routine screening in high-risk populations is not clear. However, numerous studies suggest that *H. pylori* eradication is protective against progression of premalignant gastric lesions. Consider testing those starting long-term NSAID, low-dose aspirin, or proton pump inhibitor (PPI) therapy. Consider a test-and-treat approach in asymptomatic first-degree relatives of gastric cancer patients.
- Routine identification and treatment of *H. pylori* in cases of nonulcer dyspepsia, gastroesophageal reflux disease (GERD), and in asymptomatic individuals in populations at high risk for gastric cancer is considered controversial, although it may be indicated in specific cases. A test-and-treat strategy may be used in patients younger than 55 with uncomplicated dyspepsia who have no alarm symptoms.
- Results of testing must be interpreted in relation to the individual patient's likelihood of *H. pylori* infection based on demographic risk factors. In the U.S. population, increased probability of infection exists in African Americans, Hispanics/Latinos, immigrants from developing nations, patients with poor socioeconomic status, Native Americans from Alaska, and persons >50 yr.
- Routine screening for *H. pylori* is not indicated in asymptomatic patients who are at low risk of infection.
- Infected patients with functional dyspepsia often benefit from treatment and should be evaluated for *H. pylori.*

LABORATORY TESTS

- Testing may be invasive or noninvasive depending on the need for endoscopy for other indications. There is no indication for endoscopy solely to diagnose *H. pylori.*
- Tests for *H. pylori* are differentiated as active or passive. Active tests provide direct evidence that *H. pylori* infection is currently present and include urea breath testing and stool antigen testing. Passive testing, which includes all serologic testing for *H. pylori,* gives indirect evidence of its presence by detecting the presence of antibodies to the organism. Serologic testing is limited by its inability to distinguish between active current infection and prior infection that has resolved.
- Tests that use urease as a marker (urea breath and stool antigen tests and biopsy for urease activity) may result in false-negative results in patients taking antibiotics, bismuth, or antisecretory therapy, as well as those with active ulcer bleeding. Patients should be off antibiotics for 4 wk and off protein pump inhibitors for 2 wk before urea breath or stool antigen testing.

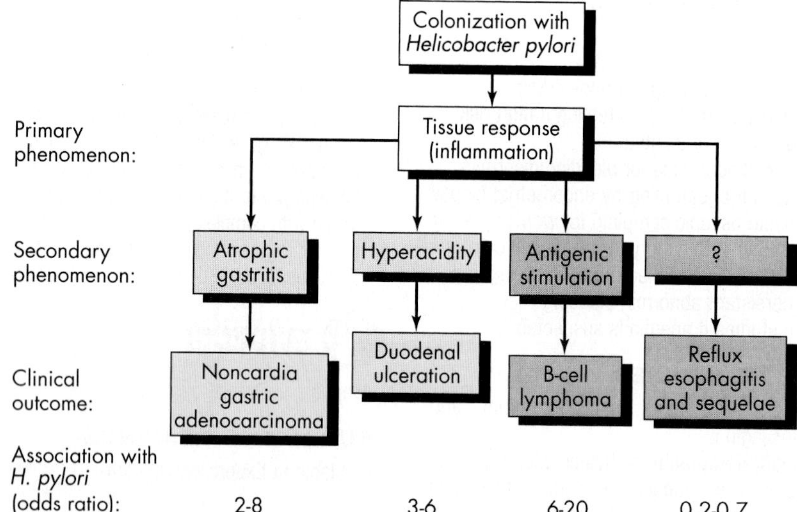

FIG. 1 Association of *Helicobacter pylori* colonization and disease states. After *H. pylori* acquisition, virtually all persons develop persistent colonization that lasts for life. Colonization induces tissue responses termed *chronic gastritis.* This process affects gastric physiology, including glandular structure, acid secretion, and antigen processing, which in turn affect disease risk. Colonization with *H. pylori* increases the risk for certain diseases (duodenal ulcer, gastric ulcer, noncardiac gastric adenocarcinoma, and B-cell lymphomas) but appears to decrease the risk for gastroesophageal reflux disease and its complications, including Barrett esophagus, and adenocarcinoma of the esophagus or gastric cardia. (From Mandell GL, et al.: *Principles and practice of infectious diseases,* ed 7, Philadelphia, 2010, Churchill Livingstone.)

- When diagnostic endoscopy is indicated (for suspicion or follow-up of PUD or gastric MALT), antral biopsy should be tested for urease activity. If urease testing is likely to show a false-negative result because of recent proton pump inhibitor (PPI), bismuth, or antibiotic use or active ulcer bleeding, the sample should undergo histologic examination.
- In cases in which biopsy is not indicated, urea breath testing or stool antigen testing is indicated to evaluate for active infection. The sensitivities and specificities of these two tests are similar (>90%). Urea breath testing is slightly more expensive than stool antigen testing, but both costs are in the modest range. Choice can be made based on patient preference and availability.
- Serologic testing should be avoided. However, it may be useful in low-risk patients in areas with low prevalence to confirm lack of infection. In this situation, positive results should be confirmed with an active testing method.

Rx TREATMENT

ACUTE GENERAL Rx

- Test only patients whom you intend to treat if positive (see "Workup"). At this time, the value of eradicating *H. pylori* infection has been clearly demonstrated in patients with PUD or gastric MALT lymphoma.
- The optimal antibiotic regimen remains undefined. In addition to efficacy, side effects, cost, and ease of administration must be considered.
- Due to increasing resistance to clarithromycin, decisions regarding appropriate regimens should take into account local rates of clarithromycin resistance, as well as any prior macrolide exposure for the patient. Clarithromycin resistance can be assumed to be >15% in the U.S., unless local resistance information is available.
- The following regimens may be considered for first-line therapy:
  1. Quadruple therapy: PPI (esomeprazole 20 mg, lansoprazole 30 mg, pantoprazole 40 mg, omeprazole 40 mg, or rabeprazole 20 mg, all given bid), with twice-daily clarithromycin (500 mg) amoxicillin (1 g bid), and metronidazole 500 mg bid for 10 to 14 days.
  2. Bismuth quadruple therapy: PPI twice daily (see above) combined with bismuth subsalicylate (Pepto-Bismol and others) 262 or 525 mg four times daily, as well as tetracycline (500 mg qid) and metronidazole (250 mg qid or 500 mg tid-qid) for 10 to 14 days This is now recommended as first-line therapy in areas of high clarithromycin resistance and in patients with penicillin allergy.
- Duration of treatment remains controversial. Extending therapy to 10 to 14 days may improve eradication rates. Use of combination capsules may improve compliance but is likely to be more expensive.
- Recent guidelines suggest multiple other regimens that can be considered based on local resistance patterns and patient's allergy profile.
- Prior exposure to a macrolide or metronidazole, for any reason, is associated with increased resistance. A preferable regimen would include medications to which the patient has not been previously exposed.
- Diarrhea and abdominal cramping are commonly observed with many of the regimens. (Probiotics may diminish this effect.) Other side effects may include a metallic taste with metronidazole or clarithromycin, neuropathy, seizures, and disulfiram-like reaction with metronidazole, diarrhea with amoxicillin, photosensitivity with tetracycline, and *Clostridium difficile* infection with any antibiotic exposure. Bismuth may cause black stool and constipation. Tetracycline is contraindicated in pregnant patients.
- 20% of patients may not respond to initial therapy. Optimal retreatment regimens are under investigation. It is important to reinforce compliance. Second-line therapy should avoid antibiotics used in initial treatment and should include either bismuth-containing quadruple therapy or levofloxacin-containing triple therapy (regardless of local clarithromycin resistance patterns). When possible, management of those who do not respond to two courses of therapy should be guided by antimicrobial sensitivity testing (although this is not indicated before initial treatment).

CHRONIC Rx

- It is essential to document clearance of infection after the completion of treatment. Repeat testing is generally performed 1 mo after completion of antibiotics and at least 2 wk after cessation of PPI therapy.
- Serology does not reliably revert to undetectable levels after treatment and should not be used to determine eradication.
- Active tests (urea breath test and stool antigen testing) are preferable. They are equally accurate in confirming eradication, and either may be used depending on availability and patient preference.

DISPOSITION

Consider further evaluation in patients with recurrent symptoms after appropriate treatment.

REFERRAL

- Patients with gastric MALT lymphoma should be followed by a gastroenterologist and oncologist with expertise in the care of lymphoid neoplasms.
- Patients with dyspepsia who have tested positive for *H. pylori* and been treated without resolution should be referred for endoscopy.
- Consider referral for biopsy for culture and sensitivity in patients who have not responded to two attempts at treatment.

PEARLS & CONSIDERATIONS

- It remains unclear whether *H. pylori* eradication reduces the risk of progression to gastric cancer.
- Outcomes in PUD and gastric MALT lymphoma are improved with treatment of associated *H. pylori* infection.
- Tests that provide direct evidence of active *H. pylori* infection (urea breath and stool antigen testing) are preferred. These may result in false-negative results in patients taking antibiotics, bismuth, or antisecretory agents, which should be stopped at an appropriate time interval before testing.
- Serologic testing does not differentiate active from prior infection. If performed, positive results should be confirmed with active testing.
- Be aware of high-risk populations in low-prevalence settings, including immigrants from Mexico, South America, Southeast Asia, and Eastern Europe.

SUGGESTED READINGS

Available at ExpertConsult.com

RELATED CONTENT

Helicobacter pylori Infection (Patient Information)
Gastritis (Related Key Topic)
Peptic Ulcer (Related Key Topic)

AUTHOR: **MARGARET TRYFOROS, M.D.**

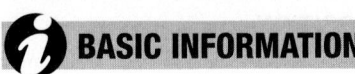

BASIC INFORMATION

DEFINITION

Hemochromatosis is an autosomal-recessive disorder that disrupts the body's regulation of iron and is characterized by increased accumulation of iron in various organs (adrenals, liver, pancreas, heart, testes, kidneys, pituitary) and eventual dysfunction of these organs if not treated appropriately.

SYNONYM

Bronze diabetes

ICD-10CM CODES

E83.110	Hereditary hemochromatosis
E83.111	Hemochromatosis due to repeated red blood cell transfusions
E83.118	Other hemochromatosis
E83.119	Hemochromatosis, unspecified

EPIDEMIOLOGY & DEMOGRAPHICS

INCIDENCE: In whites, approximately 1 in 385 persons.

PREDOMINANT SEX AND AGE: Generally diagnosed in males in their fifth decade. Diagnosis in females is generally not made until 10 to 20 yr after menopause.

GENETICS: Most common genetic disorder in North European ancestry. Homozygosity for the *C282Y* mutation is now found in approximately 5 of every 1000 persons of European descent.

PHYSICAL FINDINGS & CLINICAL PRESENTATION

- In earlier stages patients completely asymptomatic and diagnosed due to abnormal laboratory tests
- Hepatic dysfunction leading to hepatomegaly, fibrosis, and eventually cirrhosis
- Arthritis
- Gonadal insufficiency leading to loss of libido and testicular atrophy
- Diabetes mellitus: Risk greater in patients with family history
- Iron-induced cardiac disease resulting in cardiomyopathy, heart failure, and arrhythmias
- Skin pigmentation

ETIOLOGY

- The majority of the patients diagnosed with hemochromatosis have mutation in the *HFE* gene and are either homozygous for the *C282Y* mutation *(C282Y/C282Y)* or compound heterozygote for the *C282Y* mutation and either the mutation *H63D (C282Y/H63D)* or less commonly the *S65C (C282Y/S65C)*.
- The remainder of the patients are classified as non–*HFE*-associated hemochromatosis.

Dx DIAGNOSIS

DIFFERENTIAL DIAGNOSIS

- Hereditary anemias with defect of erythropoiesis
- Cirrhosis, chronic liver disease, porphyria cutanea tarda
- Repeated blood transfusions
- Table 1 summarizes hereditary causes of iron overload

WORKUP

Medical history, physical examination, and laboratory evaluation should be focused on affected organ systems (see "Physical Findings & Clinical Presentation"). Fig. E1 outlines evaluation for possible hereditary hemochromatosis in an individual with negative family history. Liver biopsy is the gold standard for diagnosis; it reveals iron deposition in hepatocytes, bile ducts, and supporting tissues.

LABORATORY TESTS

- Transferrin saturation is the best screening test. Values >45% are an indication for further testing.
- Elevated serum ferritin is good evidence of iron overload, but other causes like chronic inflammatory conditions, malignancy, and so forth need to be ruled out as ferritin is also an acute phase reactant.
- Genotypical screening for *C282Y* and *H63D* mutation in *HFE* gene should be done in patients with high transferrin saturation, elevated ferritin, or both.
- Liver biopsy (Fig. E2) is the gold standard but is not needed in somebody who has a persistently elevated transferrin saturation, elevated ferritin, or both.
- Hepatic iron index can help differentiate between various causes of iron overload.
- Elevated aspartate aminotransferase, alanine aminotransferase, and alkaline phosphatase are seen.
- Hyperglycemia is found.
- Endocrine abnormalities (decreased testosterone, luteinizing hormone, follicle-stimulating hormone) are noted.
- Table 2 describes laboratory findings in patients with hereditary hemochromatosis.

IMAGING STUDIES

Routine radiologic imaging is not needed. MRI (Fig. E3) may show low signal intensity in the liver.

Rx TREATMENT

The goal of therapy is the removal of excess iron and maintaining it at a normal or near-normal level. Box E1 summarizes the treatment of *HFE*-related hereditary hemochromatosis.

NONPHARMACOLOGIC THERAPY

Phlebotomy is the treatment of choice.

ACUTE GENERAL Rx

- The timing and frequency of phlebotomy needs to be individualized for each patient.
- For patients with heavy iron overload, twice-weekly phlebotomies should be started. In most patients, weekly phlebotomy is adequate.
- The effectiveness of treatment is monitored by periodic ferritin measurement. The goal is to bring ferritin level below 50 ng/ml.
- Patients with iron overload due to transfusion-dependent anemias may not tolerate phlebotomy. For these patients iron chelation may be needed.
- The chelating agent deferoxamine has to be given daily as a 9- to 12-hr IV or SC infusion, and compliance is difficult.
- The oral chelating agent deferasirox (Exjade) is effective, but should not be used in patients with high-risk myelodysplastic syndrome because it can cause renal impairment, hepatic impairment, or gastrointestinal hemorrhage, which can be fatal.

CHRONIC Rx

After the ferritin has been brought to less than 50 ng/ml, phlebotomy is needed on an as-needed basis to keep the ferritin at that level.

DISPOSITION

- Serum ferritin measurement is the most useful prognostic indicator of disease severity.
- Prognosis is good if phlebotomy is started early (before onset of cirrhosis or diabetes mellitus); women can have the full phenotypic expression of the disease, including cirrhosis, and should also be aggressively treated.

REFERRAL

For liver biopsy if diagnosis is uncertain.

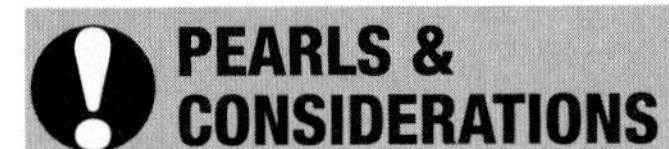

PEARLS & CONSIDERATIONS

COMMENTS

- Persons who are homozygous for the *HFE* gene mutation *C282Y* comprise 85% to 90% of phenotypically affected individuals.
- Patients with hemochromatosis and serum ferritin levels <1000 ng/ml are unlikely to have cirrhosis. Liver biopsy to screen for cirrhosis may be unnecessary in such patients.
- Cirrhotic patients must be periodically monitored (ultrasound or CT scan) because of their increased risk of hepatocellular carcinoma.
- *HFE* gene testing for *C282Y* mutation is a cost-effective method of screening relatives of patients with hereditary hemochromatosis. The American College of Gastroenterology recommends genotyping persons who have abnormal iron screening tests and first-degree relatives of those identified with *C282Y* homozygosity.
- Established cirrhosis, hypogonadism, destructive arthritis, and insulin-dependent diabetes mellitus secondary to hemochromatosis cannot be reversed with repeated phlebotomy, but their progress can be slowed.
- In patients who are heterozygous for *C282Y* or *H63D* mutation, clinically meaningful iron overload does not develop.
- Screening for hepatocellular carcinoma is reserved for those with hereditary hemochromatosis and cirrhosis.

TABLE 1 Hereditary Iron Overload Disorders

Disorder	Gene, Chromosome Location	Inheritance	Plasma Transferrin Saturation	Plasma Ferritin	Iron Deposition Sites	Clinical Manifestations
Hereditary hemochromatosis, *HFE*-associated (type 1; OMIM235200)	*HFE,* 6p21	Autosomal recessive	Early increase; >45%	Later increase after third decade of life	Parenchymal iron overload affecting hepatocytes, heart, pancreas, other organs	Liver and heart disease, diabetes, gonadal failure, arthritis, skin pigmentation
Hereditary hemochromatosis, TfR2-associated (type 3; OMIM604250)	*TFR2,* 7q22	Autosomal recessive	Early increase; >45%	Later increase after third decade of life	Parenchymal iron overload affecting hepatocytes, heart, pancreas, other organs	Liver and heart disease, diabetes, gonadal failure, arthritis, skin pigmentation
Juvenile hemochromatosis, hemojuvelin-associated (type 2A; OMIM 602390)	*HJV,* 1q21	Autosomal recessive	Early increase; >45%	Increased by second decade of life	Parenchymal iron overload affecting hepatocytes, heart, pancreas, other organs	As for hereditary hemochromatosis, but liver involvement less prominent
Juvenile hemochromatosis, hepcidin-associated (type 2B; OMIM613313)	*HAMP,* 19q13	Autosomal recessive	Early increase; >45%	Increased by second decade of life	Parenchymal iron overload affecting hepatocytes, heart, pancreas, other organs	As for hereditary hemochromatosis, but liver involvement less prominent
Hemochromatosis, DMT1-associated (OMIM 206100)	*SCL11A2,* 12q13	Autosomal recessive	Early increase; >45%	Normal to moderately elevated	Hepatic iron overload, predominantly in hepatocytes	Severe microcytic anemia, liver dysfunction
Atransferrinemia (OMIM 209300)	*TF,* 3q22	Autosomal recessive	No plasma transferrin	Increased	Parenchymal iron overload affecting hepatocytes, heart, pancreas; no iron stores in bone marrow or spleen	Transfusion-dependent iron-deficiency anemia, growth retardation, poor survival
Aceruloplasminemia (OMIM 604290)	*CP,* 3q24-q25	Autosomal recessive	Decreased	Increased	Marked iron accumulation in basal ganglia, liver, pancreas	Diabetes, progressive neurologic disease, retinal degeneration
Hemochromatosis, ferroportin-associated, with impaired iron export (type 4A; OMIM606069)	*SLC40A1,* 2q32	Autosomal dominant	Remains normal or low	Early increase	Predominantly macrophage iron deposition	None
Hemochromatosis, ferroportin-associated, with hepcidin resistance (type 4B; OMIM606069)	*SLC40A1,* 2q32	Autosomal dominant	Early increase; >45%	Early increase	Parenchymal iron overload affecting hepatocytes, heart, pancreas, other organs	Similar to *HFE*-associated hemochromatos

From Hoffman R et al: *Hematology: basic principles and practice,* ed 7, Philadelphia, 2018, Elsevier.

TABLE 2 Laboratory Findings in Patients With Hereditary Hemochromatosis

Measurements	Normal Subjects	Patients With Hereditary Hemochromatosis: Asymptomatic	Patients With Hereditary Hemochromatosis: Symptomatic
Blood (Fasting)			
Serum iron level (μg/dl)	60-180	150-280	180-300
Serum transferrin level (mg/dl)	220-410	200-280	200-300
Transferrin saturation (%)	20-45	45-100	80-100
Serum ferritin level (ng/ml)			
Men	20-200	150-1000	500-6000
Women	15-150	120-1000	500-6000
Genetic (*HFE* Mutation Analysis)			
C282Y/C282Y	wt/wt‡	*C282Y/C282Y*	*C282Y/C282Y*
*C282Y/H63D**	wt/wt	*C282Y/H63D*	*C282Y/H63D*
Liver			
Hepatic iron concentration			
μg/g dry weight	300-1500	2000-10,000	8000-30,000
μmol/g dry weight	5-27	36-179	140-550
Hepatic iron index†	<1	1 to >1.9	>1.9
Liver histology			
Perls Prussian blue stain	0, 1+	2+ to 4+	3+, 4+

*Compound heterozygote.
†Calculated by dividing the hepatic iron concentration (in μmol/g dry weight) by the age of the patient (in yr). With the increased use of genetic testing in patients with iron overload, the specificity of the hepatic iron index has diminished.
‡wt/wt: wild type (normal).
From Goldman L, Schafer AI: *Goldman's Cecil medicine,* ed 24, Philadelphia, 2012, Saunders.

SUGGESTED READINGS

Available at ExpertConsult.com

RELATED CONTENT

Hemochromatosis (Patient Information)

AUTHOR: **FRED F. FERRI, M.D.**

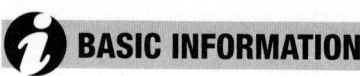

BASIC INFORMATION

DEFINITION

Hemophilia is a hereditary bleeding disorder caused by low levels of factor VIII (hemophilia A) or factor IX coagulant activity (hemophilia B).

SYNONYMS

Hemophilia A: Classic hemophilia, factor VIII deficiency hemophilia

Hemophilia B: Christmas disease, factor IX hemophilia

ICD-10CM CODES	
D66	Hereditary factor VIII deficiency
D67	Hereditary factor IX deficiency
D68.311	Acquired hemophilia
Z14.01	Asymptomatic hemophilia A carrier
Z14.02	Symptomatic hemophilia A carrier

EPIDEMIOLOGY & DEMOGRAPHICS

INCIDENCE/PREVALENCE (IN U.S.): Hemophilia A: 100 cases per 1 million males; it is the most common severe inherited bleeding disorder in humans. Hemophilia B: 20 cases per 1 million males. There are approximately 400,000 patients with severe hemophilia worldwide.

GENETIC: Both hemophilias have an X-linked recessive pattern of inheritance with only males affected.

PHYSICAL FINDINGS & CLINICAL PRESENTATION

- The clinical features of hemophilia A and B are generally indistinguishable from each other. The clinical symptoms are determined by the baseline factor activity in each patient. Spontaneous bleeding can occur with those with *severe* hemophilia (<1% factor VIII or IX activity). Trauma-induced bleeding can occur in those with *moderate* hemophilia (factor levels 1% to 5%) and *mild* hemophilia (factor levels >5%).
- Bleeding is most commonly seen in joints (knees, ankles, elbows), resulting in hot, swollen, painful joints (Fig. 1) and subsequent crippling joint deformity (Fig. 2).
- Bleeding can also occur into the muscles and the gastrointestinal tract.
- Compartment syndrome can occur from large hematomas.
- Hematuria may be present.

ETIOLOGY

- Both disorders are congenital X-linked recessive disorders of hemostasis.
- Hemophilia A: Low factor VIII coagulant (VIII:C) activity; can be classified as mild if factor VIII:C levels are >5%, moderate if levels are 1% to 5%, and severe if levels are <1%.
- Hemophilia B: Low levels of factor IX coagulant activity.
- Spontaneous acquisition of factor VIII inhibitors (acquired hemophilia) is rare.

DIAGNOSIS

DIFFERENTIAL DIAGNOSIS

- Other clotting factor deficiencies
- Platelet function disorders
- Vitamin K deficiency

WORKUP

Patients with mild hemophilia bleed only in response to major trauma or surgery and may not be diagnosed until young adulthood. Diagnostic workup includes laboratory evaluation, as below:

- Partial thromboplastin time (aPTT) is prolonged. Prothrombin time (PT) is normal, and the aPTT mixing study will fully correct.
- Factor VIII (Table 1) Reduced factor VIII:C level distinguishes hemophilia A from other causes of prolonged PTT.
- Factor VIII antigen, fibrinogen level, and bleeding time are normal.
- Factor IX coagulant activity levels are reduced in patients with hemophilia B.
- Coagulation factor activity measurement is useful to correlate with disease severity. Normal range is 50 to 150 U/dl; 5 to 20 U/dl indicates mild disease, 2 to 5 U/dl indicates moderate disease, and <2 U/dl indicates severe disease with spontaneous bleeding episodes.

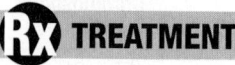

TREATMENT

NONPHARMACOLOGIC THERAPY

- Avoidance of contact sports
- Patient education regarding the disease; promotion of exercises such as swimming
- Avoidance of aspirin or other NSAIDs
- Orthopedic evaluation and physical therapy evaluation in patients with joint involvement
- Hepatitis vaccination

ACUTE GENERAL Rx

(See Box 1 and Box 2)

HEMOPHILIA A:

- Reversal and prevention of acute bleeding in hemophilia A and B are based on adequate replacement of deficient or missing factor protein. Table 2 summarizes recommendations for clotting factor replacement.

TABLE 1 Differential Diagnosis of a Low Factor VIII Level

- FVIII <10%
  1. Severe or moderately severe hemophilia A
  2. Severe type 1 VWD
  3. Type 3 VWD
  4. Type 2N VWD
  5. Acquired hemophilia A
  6. Acquired VWD
- FVIII: 10% to 50%
  1. Mild hemophilia A
  2. Type 1 VWD
  3. Type 2N VWD
  4. Combined FVIII and FV deficiency

FV, Factor V; *FVIII*, factor VIII; *VWD*, von Willebrand disease.

From Hoffman R et al: *Hematology, basic principles and practice*, ed 7, Philadelphia, 2018, Elsevier.

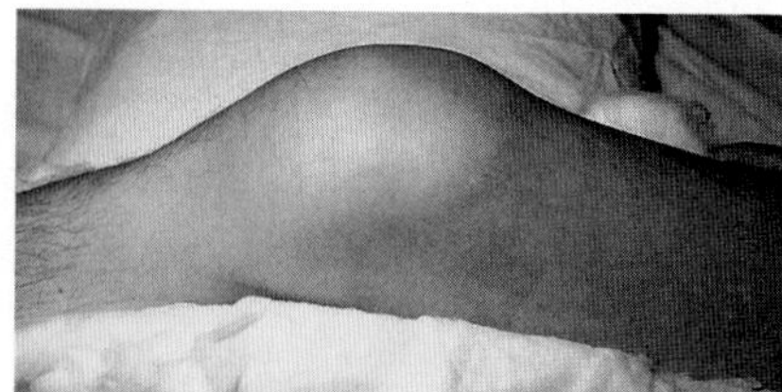

FIG. 1 Acute hemarthrosis of the knee is a common complication of hemophilia. It may be confused with acute infection unless the patient's coagulation disorder is known because the knee is hot, red, swollen, and painful. (From Forbes CD, Jackson WF: *Color atlas and text of clinical medicine*, ed 3, London, 2003, Mosby.)

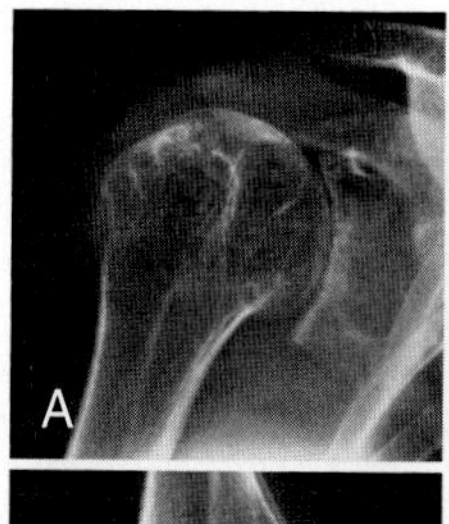

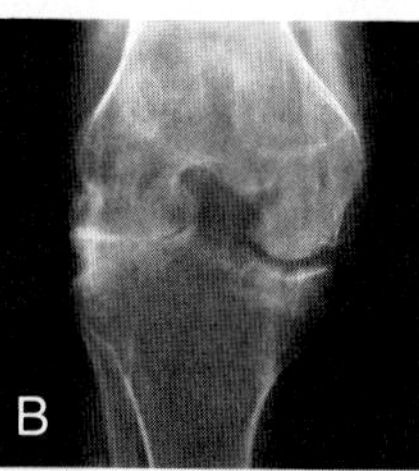

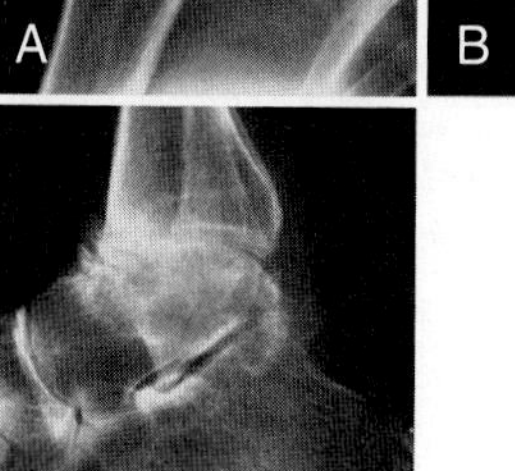

FIG. 2 Radiographic changes associated with hemophilic arthropathy. A, Radiograph of the shoulder showing multiple subchondral cysts in the head of the humerus, an early finding in hemophilic arthropathy. The glenohumeral joint space is fairly well preserved, and range of motion is normal. **B,** Widening of the intercondylar notch and near fusion of the femur and medial tibial condyle in the knee joint affected by hemophilic arthropathy. **C,** Narrowing and fusion of the tibiotalar joint in the ankle. (From Hoffman R et al: *Hematology, basic principles and practice*, ed 5, Philadelphia, 2009, Churchill Livingstone.)

- The choice of the product for replacement therapy is guided by availability, capacity, concerns, and cost. Recombinant factors cost two to three times as much as plasma-derived factors, and the limited capacity to produce recombinant factors often results in periods of shortage. In the United States, the majority of patients with severe hemophilia use recombinant products.
- Factor VIII concentrates are effective in controlling spontaneous and traumatic hemorrhage in severe hemophilia. The new recombinant factor VIII is stable without added human serum albumin (decreased risk of transmission of infectious agents).
- Emicizumab is a bispecific monoclonal antibody that bridges activated factor IX and factor X to replace the function of missing activated factor VIII, thereby restoring hemostasis. In a recent clinical trial,[1] emicizumab prophylaxis administered subcutaneously once weekly or every 2 weeks led to a significantly lower bleeding rate than no prophylaxis among persons with hemophilia A without inhibitors; more than half the participants who received prophylaxis had no treated bleeding events.
- Alloantibodies (inhibitors) that neutralize factor VIII clotting function occur in nearly 30% of patients with severe hemophilia A after exposure to factor VIII. In these patients, bypassing agents (anti-inhibitor coagulant complex [AICC] and recombinant activated factor VII [rFVIIa]) can be used to treat bleeding. AICC can also be used prophylactically to decrease the frequency of joint and other bleeding events in patients with severe hemophilia A and factor VIII inhibitors. Trials with emicizumab have shown that prophylaxis with it significantly lowers the rate of bleeding events among patients with hemophilia A who have developed inhibitors.
- Recombinant activated factor VII is useful to stop spontaneous hemorrhages and prevent excessive bleeding during surgery in 75% of patients with inhibitors. Recommended dose is 90 µg/mg of body weight every 2 to 3 hr for treatment of life-threatening hemorrhage.
- Desmopressin acetate 0.3 µg/kg q24h (causes release of factor VIII:C) may be used in preparation for minor surgical procedures in mild hemophiliacs.
- Aminocaproic acid (EACA, Amicar) 4 g PO q4h can be given for persistent bleeding that is unresponsive to factor VIII concentrate or desmopressin.

HEMOPHILIA B:

- Infuse factor IX concentrates. It is important to remember that factor IX concentrates contain other proteins that may increase the risk of thrombosis with recurrent use; thus factor IX concentrates must be used only when clearly indicated.
- Daily administration of oral cyclophosphamide and prednisone without empirical factor VIII therapy is an effective and well-tolerated treatment for acquired hemophilia.

[1] Mahlangu J et al: Emicizumab prophylaxis in patients who have hemophilia A without inhibitors, *N Engl J Med* 379(9):811–822, 2018

BOX 1 Treatment Options for Bleeding in a Patient with Factor VIII Deficiency and an Inhibitor

- Low Titer, Low Responder
- Mild Bleeding
  1. Local and conservative measures, such as rest, ice, compression, and elevation
  2. If the patient is known to respond to DDAVP (i.e., mild hemophilia A), 0.3 µg/kg IV or 300 µg intranasal (150 µg per nostril; 150 µg for patients <50 kg) for minor bleeding or treatment before minor surgery
  3. Oral antifibrinolytic therapy (ε-aminocaproic acid or tranexamic acid) for mucosal bleeding
  4. FVIII dosing to raise the level to 50%
  5. Recombinant FVIIa (90 to 120 µg/kg, followed by 90 µg/kg every 2 to 3 hours)
  6. Activated prothrombin complex concentrates (50 to 100 units/kg, with maximum daily dose of 200 units/kg)
  7. Concurrent treatment with antifibrinolytics should be administered with caution
- Life- or Limb-Threatening Bleeding
  1. FVIII dosing to maintain FVIII activity levels at 100%
  2. Recombinant FVIIa (270 µg/kg for one dose may be considered with caution versus 90 µg/kg every 2 to 3 hours)
  3. Activated prothrombin complex concentrates (100 units/kg, with maximum daily dose of 200 units/kg)
  4. Concurrent treatment with antifibrinolytics should be administered with caution
- Low Titer, High Responder
- Mild Bleeding
  1. Local and conservative measures, such as rest, ice, compression, and elevation
  2. If the patient is known to respond to DDAVP (i.e., mild hemophilia A), 0.3 µg/kg IV or 300 µg intranasal (150 µg for patients <50 kg) for minor bleeding or treatment before minor surgery
  3. Oral antifibrinolytic therapy (ε-aminocaproic acid or tranexamic acid) for mucosal bleeding
  4. Recombinant factor VIIa (270 µg/kg, bolus may be considered with caution versus 90 µg/kg every 2 to 3 hours)
  5. Activated prothrombin complex concentrates (100 units/kg, with a maximum daily dose of 200 units/kg, may induce anamnesis)
- Life- or Limb-Threatening Bleeding
  1. FVIII in high doses to maintain levels of 100%
  2. Frequent monitoring for an anamnestic response, usually within 5 to 7 days
  3. After the anamnestic response develops:
     a. Recombinant FVIIa (270 µg/kg, may be considered with caution versus 90 µg/kg every 2 to 3 hours)
     b. Activated prothrombin complex concentrates (50 to 100 units/kg, with a maximum daily dose of 200 units/kg)
- High Titer, High Responder
- Mild Bleeding
  1. Local and conservative measures, such as rest, ice, compression, and elevation
  2. Oral antifibrinolytic therapy (ε-aminocaproic acid or tranexamic acid) for mucosal bleeding
  3. Recombinant FVIIa (270 µg/kg, should be considered with caution versus 90 µg/kg every 2 to 3 hours)
  4. Activated prothrombin complex concentrates (100 units/kg, with a maximum daily dose of 200 units/kg)
  5. Concurrent treatment with antifibrinolytics should be administered with caution
- Life- or Limb-Threatening Bleeding
  1. Recombinant FVIIa (270 µg/kg, should be considered with caution versus 90 µg/kg IV every 2 to 3 hours)
  2. Activated prothrombin complex concentrates (100 units/kg, with a maximum daily dose of 200 units/kg)
  3. If available, immunoadsorption can be attempted to rapidly lower the inhibitor titer so as to allow use of FVIII
- Main Features of the Agents Effective for Inhibitor Treatment/Prophylaxis
  1. **Content** APCC: Activated vitamin k–dependent clotting factors; rFVIIa: Recombinant FVIIa alone
  2. **Mechanism of action** APCC: Activate plasma FX and FII; rFVIIa: activates FX on platelets
  3. **Half-Life** APCC: Putatively 8 to 12 hours; rFVIIa: 2 to 3 hours
  4. **Efficacy** APCC: About 80%; rFVIIa: About 80%

APCC, activated prothrombin complex concentrate; *DDAVP,* desmopressin acetate; *FII,* factor II; *FIII,* factor III; *FVIIa,* activated factor VIIa; *FX,* factor X; *IV,* intravenous; *rFVIIa,* recombinant activated clotting factor VII.

Hoffman R et al: *Hematology, basic principles and practice,* ed 7, Philadelphia, 2018, Elsevier.

BOX 2 Treatment of Life-Threatening Bleeding Episodes in Patients with Inhibitors Against Factor VIII or Factor IX

Concentrates

- Factor VIII containing concentrates in high doses (as high as 150-200 IU/kg) if inhibitor titer is low (<5-10 BU). High-dose continuous infusion of factor VIII (≈10 IU/kg per hour) after a high-dose bolus may be useful.
- Recombinant factor VIIa. Dose is 90 μg/kg (or a dose up to 320 μg/kg) administered every 2 hours. Risk of thrombosis exists with this product.
- Activated PCCs at a dose of 50-75 IU/kg every 8-12 hours. Risk of thrombosis exists with this product.

Immunomodulation

- Antibody depletion
  1. Plasmapheresis
  2. Extracorporeal immunoadsorption of plasma (staphylococcal protein A column therapy and other methods)
- Suppression of antibody production
  1. High-dose steroids (equivalent of prednisone 80 mg/day)
  2. Cyclophosphamide (10-15 mg/kg load and 2-3 mg/kg per day)
  3. Intravenous immunoglobulin (1 g/kg daily for 2 days)
  4. More aggressive regimens that may include vincristine, azathioprine, cyclosporine, or interferon-γ

Conservative Measures

- Immobilization
- Compression
- Local application of hemostatic agents
- Antifibrinolytics
- Avoid venipunctures, intramuscular injections, arterial puncture, and lumbar punctures
- Avoid use of medications that inhibit platelet function (ASA, NSAIDs)
- DDAVP may be effective in some patients with low-titer inhibitors

ASA, Aspirin; *BU*, Bethesda unit; *DDAVP*, desmopressin acetate; *NSAIDs*, nonsteroidal antiinflammatory drugs; *PCC*, prothrombin complex concentrate. Hoffman R et al: *Hematology, basic principles and practice*, ed 7, Philadelphia, 2018, Elsevier.

TABLE 2 Recommendations for Clotting Factor Replacement

Site of Bleed	Level Desired (%)	Hemophilia A (rFVIII) (U/kg)	Hemophilia B (rFIX) (U/kg)
Oral mucosa	>30	20	40
Epistaxis	>30	20	40
Joint or muscle	>50	30	50
GI	>50	30	50
GU	>50	50	75
CNS	>100	75	125
Trauma or surgery	>100	75	125

CNS, Central nervous system; *GI*, gastrointestinal; *GU*, genitourinary; *rFIX*, recombinant factor IX; *rFVIII*, recombinant factor VIII. Hoffman R et al: *Hematology, basic principles and practice*, ed 7, Philadelphia, 2018, Elsevier.

TABLE 3 Alternative, Nonclotting Factor Concentrate Therapies for Treating Hemophilia

- Rebalancing hemostasis strategies:
  1. TFPI Inhibition approaches: Anti-TFPI aptamer, antibody and peptide.
  2. Antithrombin siRNA biosynthesis inhibition.
- Both approaches can be delivered by infrequent (weekly or less often) subcutaneous injections.
  1. Factor VIII mimetic molecule: Bispecific antibody to FIXa and FX.
- Can be administered by subcutaneous injection and has shown activity in FVIII inhibitor patients.

FX, Factor X; *FIXa*, Factor IXa; *FVIII*, factor VIII; *siRNA*, small interfering ribonucleic acid; *TFPI*, tissue factor pathway inhibitor. Hoffman R et al: *Hematology, basic principles and practice*, ed 7, Philadelphia, 2018, Elsevier.

CHRONIC Rx

- The aim of chronic treatment is to prevent spontaneous bleeding and excessive bleeding during any surgical intervention. Monitoring and treatment of patients with hemophilia at comprehensive hemophilia treatment centers is cost-effective and decreases morbidity and mortality.
- Prophylaxis with recombinant factor VIII can prevent joint damage and decrease the frequency of joint and other hemorrhages in young boys with severe hemophilia A. The estimated annual cost for treatment of one patient with recombinant factor VIII is $300,000.
- Implantation of genetically altered fibroblasts that produce factor VIII is safe and well tolerated. This form of therapy is feasible in patients with severe hemophilia. Hemophilia will likely be the first common, severe genetic disease to be cured by gene therapy.
- Table 3 summarizes alternative, nonclotting factor concentrate therapies for treating hemophilia.

DISPOSITION

- In the 1980s, approximately 90% of patients with hemophilia were infected with the hepatitis C virus (HCV), and more than 55% of this cohort was coinfected with HIV. The development of genetically engineered recombinant factor therapy in the 1990s virtually eliminated the risk of acquiring HCV and HIV from factor replacement therapy.
- Despite the advent of virally safe blood products and blood treatment programs, many hemophiliacs are HCV and HIV seropositive.
- Intracranial bleeds are a common cause of death in hemophiliacs. They are fatal in 30% of patients, occur in 10% of patients, and are generally the result of trauma.

REFERRAL

To a specialized center with multidisciplinary teams that can treat the disease and comorbidities

SUGGESTED READINGS

Available at ExpertConsult.com

RELATED CONTENT

Hemophilia (Patient Information)

AUTHOR: **BHARTI RATHORE, M.D.**

H

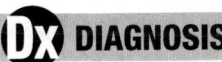

BASIC INFORMATION

DEFINITION

Hemoptysis is coughing up of blood originating from the lower respiratory tract, ranging from blood-streaked sputum to gross blood. If greater than 400 to 600 ml in 24 hours or if the bleeding rate is >100 ml/hr, it is considered massive hemoptysis.

ICD-10CM CODE

R04.2 Hemoptysis

EPIDEMIOLOGY & DEMOGRAPHICS

INCIDENCE: Unknown, varies based on underlying pathology

RISK FACTORS: Tobacco smoking predisposes to lung cancer, a common cause of hemoptysis. Systemic processes (rheumatologic, renal, hematologic) may contribute to alveolar hemorrhage or vasculitis. Anticoagulation can worsen bleeding.

PHYSICAL FINDINGS & CLINICAL PRESENTATION

- Presentation of hemoptysis is variable and can range from minimal blood-tinged sputum to more than 500 ml of gross blood in 24 hr. Other symptoms depend on the underlying etiology and can include cough, sputum production, fever, shortness of breath, weight loss, night sweats, wheezing, and chest pain.
- There are no specific exam findings, but clues to the etiology may be present, for example, focal wheezing, rhonchi or rales on pulmonary exam, murmur of mitral stenosis on cardiac exam.

ETIOLOGY

- There are many potential causes of hemoptysis including airway disease (bronchitis, bronchiectasis, lung neoplasm), infection (necrotizing pneumonia, lung abscess, tuberculosis, fungal infection), inflammatory diseases (granulomatosis with polyangiitis, Goodpasture syndrome, lupus), cardiac disease (mitral stenosis after rheumatic heart disease, congenital heart diseases), and others (pulmonary embolism, cocaine use, foreign body, airway trauma, iatrogenic and cryptogenic).
- Acute respiratory tract infections, asthma, COPD, malignancy, and bronchiectasis are the most common diagnoses in outpatient primary care.
- Worldwide, tuberculosis accounts for 7% to 85% of cases of massive hemoptysis. Highest incidence is in South Africa; lowest incidence is in the U.S.

DIAGNOSIS

DIFFERENTIAL DIAGNOSIS

- Various potential causes of lower respiratory tract bleeding
  1. Airway disease (bronchitis, bronchiectasis, lung neoplasm)
  2. Infection (necrotizing pneumonia, lung abscess, tuberculosis, fungal infection)
  3. Inflammatory diseases (granulomatosis with polyangiitis, Goodpasture syndrome, lupus)
  4. Cardiac disease (mitral stenosis after rheumatic heart disease, congenital heart diseases)
  5. Pulmonary embolism
  6. Cocaine use
  7. Foreign body
- Bleeding from upper respiratory tract
- Hematemesis or epistaxis
- Coagulopathy

WORKUP

- The initial history should focus on determining the anatomic origin of the bleeding and on quantifying the volume of the hemoptysis in order to triage appropriately.
- Complete history and physical exam may suggest a particular etiology; important to ask about duration and quantity of hemoptysis and smoking history.

LABORATORY TESTS

- Complete blood count
- Coagulation profile
- Serum chemistries, including creatinine, urinalysis
- If indicated, consider vasculitis serologies (i.e., ANA, ANCA, anti-GBM)
- Arterial blood gas to assess oxygenation
- Sputum for cultures and cytologic studies
- PPD

IMAGING STUDIES

- Chest x-ray: All patients with hemoptysis should have a chest x-ray but will likely need additional studies to localize site of bleeding.
- Chest CT: Chest CT scan combined with flexible bronchoscopy has the highest yield for localizing the site of bleeding.

TREATMENT

Varies based on underlying etiology and nonmassive versus massive hemoptysis

NONPHARMACOLOGIC THERAPY

Massive hemoptysis:

- Arteriographic embolization of bronchial arteries and/or collateral systemic vessels
- Surgical resection of affected lung

ACUTE GENERAL Rx

Massive hemoptysis (Fig. 1):

- Stabilize hemodynamic status and oxygenation.
- Reverse any coagulopathy.
- Bronchoscopy can be used to identify cause of hemoptysis (e.g., neoplasm), as well as to help isolate a site/segment of bleeding.
- If site of bleeding is known, place patient with bleeding lung in dependent position to prevent blood from spilling into non-affected lung, and consider selective intubation with large-bore, single-lumen endotracheal tube or double-lumen endotracheal tube.
- Bronchoscopic lavage with iced saline or topical application of epinephrine can be tried as a temporizing measure.
- Bronchoscopic balloon tamponade of bleeding site can be used as temporizing measure.
- Early consultation with interventional radiology, interventional pulmonology, and/or thoracic surgery for definitive intervention is recommended.

Submassive hemoptysis:

For submassive hemoptysis, identify and treat underlying condition. Refer to pulmonologist or hematologist if indicated.

CHRONIC Rx

For patients requiring anticoagulation or antiplatelet therapy for another disorder, consider risks/benefits of continued anticoagulation or antiplatelet therapy.

DISPOSITION

Generally, patients have a good prognosis after an episode of hemoptysis, but those with massive bleeding and/or malignancy tend to have a poorer prognosis.

SUGGESTED READING

Available at ExpertConsult.com

RELATED CONTENT

Evaluation of hemoptysis (Algorithm, Section III)

AUTHOR: **GAETANE MICHAUD, M.D.**

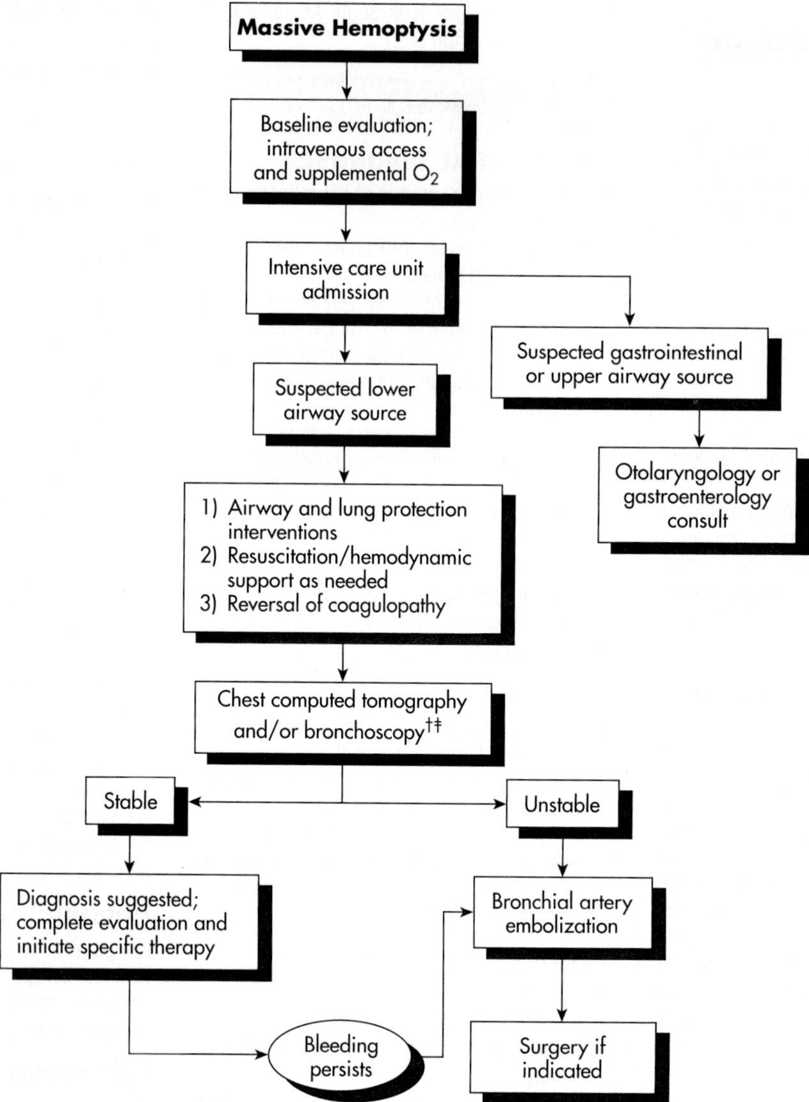
Massive Hemoptysis
Baseline evaluation; intravenous access and supplemental O_2
Intensive care unit admission
Suspected gastrointestinal or upper airway source
Otolaryngology or gastroenterology consult
Suspected lower airway source
1) Airway and lung protection interventions
2) Resuscitation/hemodynamic support as needed
3) Reversal of coagulopathy
Chest computed tomography and/or bronchoscopy†‡
Stable
Unstable
Diagnosis suggested; complete evaluation and initiate specific therapy
Bronchial artery embolization
Bleeding persists
Surgery if indicated

FIG. 1 Massive hemoptysis. *History and physical examination, complete blood count, coagulation studies, type and cross-match, chest radiograph, and arterial blood gas. †Local availability and patient stability should guide choice; computed tomography is preferred for the initial evaluation of a stable patient. ‡Local measures, including topical vasoconstrictors, bronchial blockers, laser photocoagulation, electrocautery, and hemostatic agents, can be used endobronchially. (From Parrillo JE, Dellinger RP: *Critical care medicine: principles of diagnosis and management in the adult*, ed 4, Philadelphia, 2014, Saunders.)

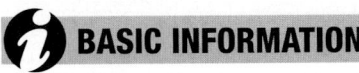

BASIC INFORMATION

DEFINITION

There are two forms of heparin-induced thrombocytopenia (HIT). Type I HIT is a mild, transient decrease in platelet count that occurs during the first 2 days of heparin exposure due to non–immune-mediated platelet aggregation. This is a benign reaction, and the platelet count will return to normal while heparin is continued. This chapter will address Type II HIT, an antibody-mediated thrombocytopenia with risk of thrombosis.

SYNONYMS

Type II heparin-induced thrombocytopenia
Heparin-induced thrombocytopenia and thrombosis (HITT)
Heparin-associated immune thrombocytopenia

ICD-10CM CODE
D75.82 Heparin-induced thrombocytopenia (HIT)

EPIDEMIOLOGY & DEMOGRAPHICS

INCIDENCE: Occurs in 0.2% to 5% of patients exposed to heparin in various clinical settings. Initially, there was an overwhelming underdiagnosis of HIT; however, since the introduction of HIT antibody ELISA test, there is a propensity to overdiagnose HIT irrespective of the clinical scenario.

PREDOMINANT SEX AND AGE: Females are at slightly higher risk than males. More common in adults, but may also occur in children.

RISK FACTORS: Heparin type (unfractionated heparin has up to 10 times greater risk than low–molecular-weight heparin), dose (therapeutic dose may have a greater risk than prophylactic dose, though no dose is considered too low to cause HIT), and duration (longer duration of exposure confers greater risk); type of patient (surgical patients, especially cardiac and orthopedic, are at higher risk than medical patients). Risk factors for HIT are summarized in Table 1

PHYSICAL FINDINGS & CLINICAL PRESENTATION

Suspect in a patient with:

- Exposure to heparin in the last 5 to 10 days OR exposed to heparin in the prior 3 mo
- Unexplained platelet count decrease to 50% below pretreatment baseline
- Onset of thrombocytopenia 5 to 10 days after heparin initiation
- Venous or arterial thrombosis (e.g., DVT or phlegmasia cerulea dolens, pulmonary embolism, skin necrosis at heparin injection sites, limb gangrene, adrenal hemorrhage, stroke or cavernous sinus thrombosis, myocardial infarction)
- Acute anaphylaxis during administration of heparin bolus

ETIOLOGY

Occurs when IgG antibodies bind to complexes of heparin and platelet factor 4 (PF4), a prothrombotic cytokine released from platelets during their activation. The resulting immune complexes activate adjacent platelets, leading to further PF4 release, additional antibody production, and eventual platelet aggregation with premature removal from circulation (causing thrombocytopenia). This process also leads to increased thrombin generation, though the full mechanism of thrombosis in HIT is not completely understood.

DIAGNOSIS

DIFFERENTIAL DIAGNOSIS

Thrombocytopenia due to other causes including:

- Sepsis or infection
- Disseminated intravascular coagulation
- Immune thrombocytopenia
- Thrombocytopenic thrombotic purpura
- Hemolytic uremic syndrome
- Drug-induced thrombocytopenia (other than heparin)
- Antiphospholipid antibody syndrome
- Liver failure
- Splenic sequestration
- Intravascular devices

WORKUP

HIT is, first and foremost, a clinical diagnosis that is confirmed with laboratory testing. See Table 2 for workup based on pretest probability. If the patient has a low pretest probability score, heparin can be safely continued, and there is no need to send further testing for HIT. A patient with moderate-to-high pretest probability requires HIT testing (Table 3), imaging studies for lower-extremity deep venous thrombosis (also consider imaging of upper extremities if swelling is present or venous catheters are in place), cessation of heparin products, and initiation of alternative anticoagulation. Patients with moderate-to-high pretest probability without HIT antibodies or intermediate pretest probability with only weakly positive HIT antibodies (based on optical density, discussed below) can resume heparin, as HIT is unlikely in these scenarios. Patients with high pretest probability with weakly positive antibodies or moderate-to-high pretest probability with moderate to strongly positive antibodies likely have HIT and should be treated as such.

LABORATORY TESTS

These can be broadly divided into two categories: immunoassays (high sensitivity) and functional assays (high specificity).

In the appropriate clinical setting, testing for HIT antibodies with an ELISA can be useful. This test is very sensitive, but not specific. The majority of patients with positive testing for HIT antibodies will not develop clinical HIT. Thus, HIT antibody testing is more effective for ruling out rather than confirming the diagnosis of HIT.

HIT antibody optical density (OD) can be used as a correlate for HIT antibody concentration. OD range is defined as weakly positive (0.4 to 1.0), moderately positive (1.0 to 2.0), or strongly positive (>2.0). A weakly positive OD (0.4 to 1.0) is only rarely associated with functional assay positivity (1% to 5%), whereas an OD >2.0 almost always shows functional assay positivity (89% to 100%). A higher OD is also associated with a higher pretest probability score and increased risk of thrombosis. Of note, the HIT antibody IgG subtype is the pathologic antibody for HIT, and thus the use of IgG-specific ELISA kits increases the test specificity over the polyspecific (IgA/M/G) antibody. In general, patients with low pretest probability via the 4T clinical prediction score should not have HIT antibody testing performed because it has a more than 99% negative predictive value, while all patients with intermediate and high pretest probability of HIT benefit from HIT antibody testing.

The gold standard test for HIT is to measure heparin-dependent platelet activation via the functional serotonin release assay (14C-SRA). This is both a highly sensitive and specific test. Donor platelets are radiolabeled with serotonin and then incubated with patient serum and heparin. If antibodies to the platelet factor 4-heparin complex are present in the patient's serum, the platelets react and release the radiolabeled serotonin, which is then measured. Availability and turnaround time of this test is dependent on the institution, which can influence the test's clinical utility. Cases where there is intermediate pretest probability with only a weakly positive HIT antibody OD most benefit from confirmatory SRA testing.

Overall, the diagnosis of HIT can be considered confirmed by (1) a positive ELISA with OD >2.00 or (2) a positive functional assay.

IMAGING STUDIES

Doppler ultrasonography of the extremities in the correct clinical setting.

TREATMENT

- For patients with a moderate or high pretest probability, discontinue all heparin exposure. Even if the patient does not have a clinically evident thrombosis, there is a significant risk of developing an incident clot within the

TABLE 1 Risk Factors for Heparin-Induced Thrombocytopenia

Heparin type	Unfractionated > low-molecular-weight heparin > fondaparinux
Patient type	Postoperative (major > minor surgery) > medical > obstetric/pediatric
Dose[a]	Prophylactic dose > therapeutic dose > flushes
Duration	11-14 days[b] > 5-10 days > 4 days or fewer
Sex	Female > male

From Hoffman R, et al.: *Hematology, basic principles and practice,* ed 7, Philadelphia, 2018, Elsevier.

TABLE 2 The 4Ts Score for Estimating the Pretest Probability of Heparin-Induced Thrombocytopenia[1]

	POINTS (0, 1, or 2 for each of the four parameters; maximum points = 8)		
	2	**1**	**0**
Thrombocytopenia (acute)	>50% platelet count fall to nadir ≥20 × 10^9/L	30%-50% platelet count fall; or nadir 10-19 × 10^9/L	<30% platelet count fall; or nadir ≤10 × 10^9/L
Timing of fall in platelet count or other sequelae	Onset day 5-10 or <1 day (if heparin exposure within 30 days)	>Day 10, timing unclear, or <day 1 with recent heparin 31-100 days	Platelet count fall <day 4 (without recent heparin exposure)
Thrombosis or other sequelae	New thrombosis; skin necrosis; post-heparin bolus acute systemic reaction	Progressive or recurrent thrombosis; erythematous skin lesions; suspected thrombosis—not confirmed	None
Other cause for thrombocytopenia	No other cause for platelet count fall is evident	Possible other cause is evident	Definite other cause is present
Pretest probability score: 6-8 = High; 4-5 = Intermediate; 0-3 = Low			

From Vincent JL, et al.: *Textbook of critical care*, ed 7, Philadelphia, 2017, Elsevier.

TABLE 3 Laboratory Assays for Heparin-Induced Thrombocytopenia

Assay	Sensitivity (%)	Specificity (%)	Positive Predictive Value (%)	Negative Predictive Value (%)
Functional assay (e.g., serotonin release assay)	88	~100	~100	81
PF4/heparin enzyme immunoassay (ELISA)	95-98	86	93	95

ELISA, Enzyme-linked immunosorbent assay; *PF4,* platelet factor 4.
From Goldman L, Schafer AI: *Goldman's Cecil medicine,* ed 24, Philadelphia, 2012, Saunders.

TABLE 4 Treatment Schedules for Lepirudin, Desirudin, Bivalirudin, and Argatroban

Anticoagulant	Dosing Protocol for HIT-Associated Thrombosis	Anticoagulant Monitoring[a]	Clearance	Half-Life (min)	Comment
Lepirudin	No bolus; initial infusion rate: 0.05-0.10 mg/kg per hour[b,c]	1.5-2.5 × baseline aPTT	Renal[c]	80	Approved dosing regimen (not shown) is too high; no longer available (withdrawn by manufacturer)
Desirudin	Not established	aPTT	Renal	120	Half-life shown is for subcutaneous administration; minimal experience for treating HIT
Bivalirudin	No bolus; initial infusion rate: 0.15-0.20 mg/kg per hour	1.5-2.5 × baseline aPTT	Enzymic (80%); renal (20%)	25	Off-label treatment for HIT (although approved for PCI in patient with HIT); minor prolongation of INR (compared with argatroban)
Argatroban	No bolus; initial infusion rate: 2 μg/kg per minute	1.5-3.0 × baseline aPTT	Hepatobiliary	40-50	Initial dose 0.5 μg/kg per minute in hepatic insufficiency[d]; moderate or marked prolongation of INR, which complicates overlap with warfarin anticoagulation

Dosing protocols shown are appropriate for most patients with strongly suspected or confirmed HIT whether or not complicated by thrombosis. (Dosing for bivalirudin and argatroban is substantially different when given for PCI.)
aPTT, Activated partial thromboplastin time; *HIT,* heparin-induced thrombocytopenia; *INR,* international normalized ratio; *PCI,* percutaneous coronary intervention.
[a]In general, the patient's baseline aPTT should be used for calculating target range when appropriate; otherwise the mean laboratory normal range can be used.
[b]This dosing protocol differs from the package insert (which advises initial bolus of 0.4 mg/kg and initial infusion rate [assuming normal renal function] of 0.15 mg/kg per hour); however, this dosing regimen is now considered too high.[26]
[c]Major dose reduction in renal insufficiency is required.[26]
[d]Reduced initial dosing (e.g., 0.5–1.2 μg/kg per minute) is also appropriate in patients in intensive care units, with cardiac failure, or postcardiac surgery).
From Hoffman R, et al.: *Hematology, basic principles and practice,* ed 7, Philadelphia, 2018, Elsevier.

subsequent 30 days. Thus, the patient must be started on an alternative anticoagulant.

- Two agents, both direct thrombin inhibitors, are approved for this indication (Table 4):
  1. Argatroban (preferred agent in renal failure and in hemodialysis patients; avoid in liver dysfunction).
  2. Bivalirudin (approved only for patients with HIT or at risk of HIT who are undergoing PCI; dose adjustment is required in renal failure).
- NOTE: Lepirudin is no longer available. Outside of the U.S., the factor Xa inhibitor danaparoid may be used.
- Platelet transfusion in the absence of life-threatening hemorrhage or extreme thrombocytopenia should be avoided. Risk of bleeding is low, and platelet transfusions in HIT can increase risk of arterial thrombosis.
- A direct thrombin inhibitor should be continued as a single agent until the platelet count returns to baseline (generally 150 × 109/L, but consider the individual patient's baseline).
- Warfarin can be added after platelet recovery (maximum dose of 5 mg/day to reduce risk of warfarin-induced skin necrosis and venous limb gangrene). This overlap therapy should continue until the platelet count has reached a stable plateau, the INR has reached goal (typically 2 to 3, though guidelines may vary with argatroban as it artificially elevates the INR), and after a minimum overlap of 5 days

TABLE 5 Treatment Schedules for Danaparoid and Fondaparinux

Anticoagulant	Therapeutic Dosing Protocol for HIT-Associated Thrombosis[a]	Anticoagulant Monitoring	Clearance	Half-Life (h)	Comment
Danaparoid	Initial bolus, 2250 units[b] IV; accelerated infusion (400 units/h × 4 h, 300 units/h × 4 h; then 200 units/h IV, subsequently adjusted by antifactor Xa levels)	Antifactor Xa levels (target, 0.5–0.8 units/ml)	Renal (minor)	25	Widely approved for HIT treatment (although not in the United States); not available in the United States; low risk for in vivo cross-reactivity; prophylactic-dose therapy[c] may be appropriate when clinical suspicion for HIT is low
Fondaparinux	7.5 mg[d] subcutaneous once daily	Anti–Xa factor levels (target levels not well established)	Renal (major)	17	Not approved for HIT treatment (although increasingly used as off-label therapy). Prophylactic-dose therapy[e] may be appropriate when clinical suspicion for HIT is low, or if there is renal insufficiency

HIT, Heparin-induced thrombocytopenia; *IV*, intravenous.
[a]Therapeutic dosing is usually appropriate for strongly suspected or confirmed HIT (including "isolated" HIT, i.e., HIT without apparent thrombosis), or when thrombosis is documented.
[b]Adjust IV danaparoid bolus for body weight: <60 kg, 1500 units; 60-75 kg, 2250 units; 75-90 kg, 3000 units; >90 kg, 3750 units.
[c]Prophylactic-dose regimen, 750 units subcutaneous every 8 h (for renal failure, reduce to 750 units every 12 h).
[d]Five milligrams for body weight <50 kg and 10 mg for body weight >100 kg; the author sometimes gives 10 mg as the first and/or second dose (rather than 7.5 mg) for severe HIT. Because HIT treatment is usually started in the afternoon, the author usually gives the second dose (and subsequent doses) at 8 am (i.e., the interval between first and second doses is often only 14-20 h rather than 24 h), which helps to achieve steady-state therapy more quickly. Dose reduction and antifactor Xa monitoring (if available) is appropriate if being used in a patient with renal insufficiency.
[e]Prophylactic-dose regimen, 2.5 mg subcutaneous every day (assumes normal renal function).
From Hoffman R, et al.: *Hematology, basic principles and practice,* ed 7, Philadelphia, 2018, Elsevier.

with both the direct thrombin inhibitor and warfarin.
- The length of treatment is controversial, but most clinicians agree that at least 1 mo of alternative anticoagulation is required in the absence of thrombosis, while at least 3 to 6 mo of treatment are required in the presence of thrombosis.
- Fondaparinux, a synthetic pentasaccharide that inhibits factor X but not thrombin, is being increasingly used for treatment of HIT despite not yet being FDA approved (Table 5). Emerging data suggest it has similar efficacy as direct thrombin inhibitors, with the additional advantages of lower bleeding risk, easier administration (subcutaneous), and lower cost. Rare cases of fondaparinux-induced HIT have been reported, however.
- The use of direct oral anticoagulants (e.g., rivaroxaban, dabigatran, apixaban) is being studied. Retrospective reviews have shown DOACs to be safe and effective for the treatment of HIT.

REFERRAL

Request a hematology consultation.

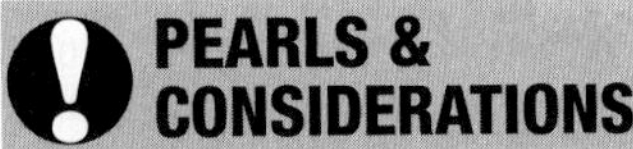

PEARLS & CONSIDERATIONS

COMMENTS

- HIT paradoxically causes thrombocytopenia and *clotting*, not bleeding.
- It is unclear whether patients with HIT should be considered heparin allergic lifelong. Risk of recurrent HIT with heparin rechallenge years later is relatively low, about 5% in one small study (though recurrence risk is higher perioperatively). If such a patient requires surgery with heparin (e.g., on-pump cardiac bypass), consider perioperative argatroban.
- Consult the coagulation laboratory and/or hematology when bridging patients on argatroban to warfarin, as argatroban concomitantly raises the INR in most assays. Some clinicians will use a higher target than 2 to 3 during the bridging period for this reason.
- Be alert to heparin exposure in the absence of anticoagulation or DVT prophylaxis: Hospitalized patients are often exposed to heparin lock flushes, heparin-coated catheters, or heparin-coated guidewires—any of which could precipitate HIT.

PREVENTION

Strongly consider the use of low-molecular-weight heparin in place of unfractionated heparin in hospitalized patients with a stable creatinine clearance of 30 ml/min or greater. Such a preventive strategy can reduce the risk of HIT by over 90% and yield cost savings in testing and treatment.

SUGGESTED READINGS

Available at ExpertConsult.com

AUTHOR: **JOHN L. REAGAN, M.D.**

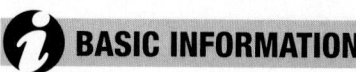

BASIC INFORMATION

DEFINITION

Hepatic encephalopathy is a neuropsychiatric syndrome occurring in patients with severe impairment of liver function and consequent accumulation of toxic products not metabolized by the liver. It is characterized by gradual impairment of the ability to perform mental tasks and to react to external stimuli. Fig. 1 illustrates the hepatic encephalopathy grades in acute liver failure. ***Minimal hepatic encephalopathy*** refers to patients with hepatic cirrhosis and mild cognitive impairment, but no history of overt encephalopathy.

SYNONYMS

Hepatic coma
Portal systemic encephalopathy
HE

ICD-10CM CODES

K72.0	Acute and subacute hepatic failure
K72.1	Chronic hepatic failure
K72.9	Hepatic failure, unspecified
G92	Toxic encephalopathy
G93.40	Encephalopathy, unspecified
G93.41	Metabolic encephalopathy
K70.40	Alcoholic hepatic failure without coma
K70.41	Alcoholic hepatic failure with coma
K72.00	Acute and subacute hepatic failure without coma
K72.01	Acute and subacute hepatic failure with coma
K72.10	Chronic hepatic failure without coma
K72.11	Chronic hepatic failure with coma
K72.90	Hepatic failure, unspecified without coma
K72.91	Hepatic failure, unspecified with coma
K91.82	Postprocedural hepatic failure

EPIDEMIOLOGY & DEMOGRAPHICS

INCIDENCE/PREVALENCE: Hepatic encephalopathy occurs in >40% of all cases of cirrhosis.

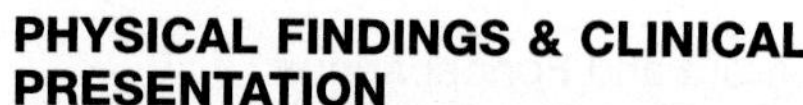

PHYSICAL FINDINGS & CLINICAL PRESENTATION

Hepatic encephalopathy can be classified by clinical stages described in Table 1. Other widely used scales are the four score criteria and the West Haven criteria. The West Haven criteria for grading hepatic encephalopathy is as follows:

- Grade (0): No abnormalities noted
- Grade (1): Unawareness (mild), euphoria or anxiety, shortened attention span, impairment of calculation ability, lethargy, or apathy
- Grade (2): Disorientation to time, obvious personal change, inappropriate behavior
- Grade (3): Somnolence to stupor, responsiveness to stimuli, gross disorientation, bizarre behavior
- Grade (4): Coma

The physical examination in hepatic encephalopathy varies with the stage and may reveal the following abnormalities:

- Skin: Jaundice, palmar erythema, spider angiomata, ecchymosis, dilated superficial periumbilical veins (caput medusae) in patients with cirrhosis
- Eyes: Scleral icterus, Kayser-Fleischer rings (Wilson disease)
- Breath: Fetor hepaticus
- Chest: Gynecomastia in men with chronic liver disease
- Abdomen: Ascites, small nodular liver (cirrhosis), tender hepatomegaly (congestive hepatomegaly)
- Rectal examination: Hemorrhoids (portal hypertension), guaiac-positive stool (alcoholic gastritis, bleeding esophageal varices, peptic ulcer disease, bleeding hemorrhoids)
- Genitalia: Testicular atrophy in males with chronic liver disease
- Extremities: Pedal edema from hypoalbuminemia
- Neurologic: Flapping tremor (asterixis), obtundation, coma with or without decerebrate posturing

ETIOLOGY

- Hepatic encephalopathy is thought to be caused mainly by accumulation of unmetabolized ammonia. The shunting of ammonia into the systemic circulation results in neuronal dysfunction leading to hepatic encephalopathy
- Precipitating factors in patients with underlying cirrhosis (upper gastrointestinal bleeding, hypokalemia, hypomagnesemia, analgesic and sedative drugs, sepsis, alkalosis, increased dietary protein)
- Acute fulminant viral hepatitis
- Drugs and toxins (e.g., isoniazid, acetaminophen, diclofenac and other NSAIDs, statins, methyldopa, loratadine, propylthiouracil, lisinopril, labetalol, halothane, carbon tetrachloride, erythromycin, nitrofurantoin, troglitazone, herbal products, flavocoxid)
- Reye syndrome
- Shock and/or sepsis
- Fatty liver of pregnancy
- Metastatic carcinoma, hepatocellular carcinoma
- Other: Autoimmune hepatitis, ischemic veno-occlusive disease, sclerosing cholangitis, heat stroke, amebic abscesses

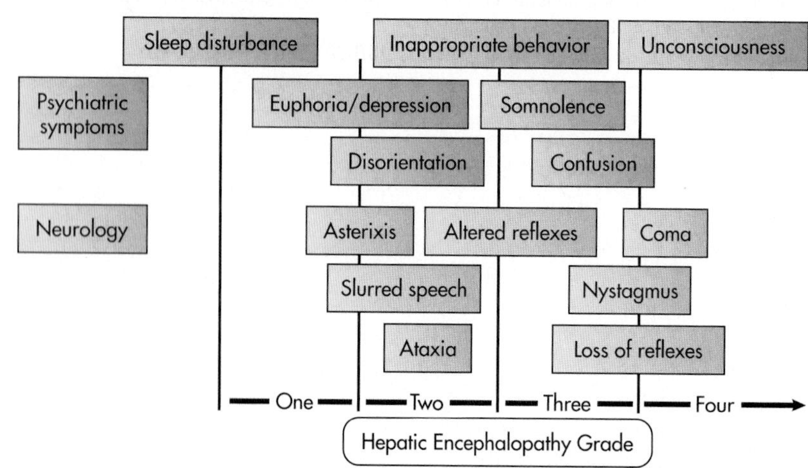

FIG. 1 Hepatic encephalopathy grade in acute liver failure. (From Parrillo JE, Dellinger RP: *Critical care medicine, principles of diagnosis and management in the adult,* ed 4, Philadelphia, 2014, Elsevier.)

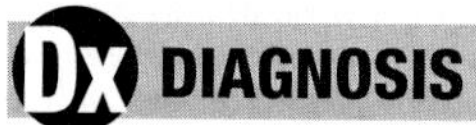

DIAGNOSIS

DIFFERENTIAL DIAGNOSIS

- Delirium caused by medications or illicit drugs
- Cerebrovascular accident, subdural hematoma
- Meningitis, encephalitis
- Hypoglycemia
- Uremia
- Cerebral anoxia
- Hypercalcemia
- Metastatic neoplasm to brain
- Alcohol withdrawal syndrome/Wernicke-Korsakoff syndrome
- Hyponatremia
- Postictal state

WORKUP

Hepatic encephalopathy should be considered in any patient with cirrhosis who presents with neuropsychiatric manifestations. Exclude other etiologies with comprehensive history (obtained from patient, relatives, and others), physical examination, and laboratory and imaging studies. A pertinent history should include exposure to hepatitis, ethanol intake, drug history, exposure to toxins, IV drug abuse, measles or influenza with aspirin use (Reye syndrome), and history of carcinoma (primary or metastatic). Minimal hepatic encephalopathy may not be obvious on clinical examination, but can be detected with neurophysiologic and neuropsychiatric testing.

LABORATORY TESTS

- Alanine aminotransferase, aspartate aminotransferase, bilirubin, alkaline phosphatase, glucose, calcium, electrolytes, blood urea nitrogen, creatinine, albumin
- Complete blood count, platelet count, prothrombin time, partial thromboplastin time
- Serum and urine toxicology screen in suspected medication or illegal drug use
- Blood and urine cultures, urinalysis

TABLE 1 Clinical Stages of Hepatic Encephalopathy

Stage	Asterixis	EEG Changes	Clinical Manifestations
I (prodrome)	Slight	Minimal	Mild intellectual impairment, disturbed sleep-wake cycle
II (impending)	Easily elicited	Usually generalized	Drowsiness, confusion, coma/inappropriate behavior, disorientation, mood swings
III (stupor)	Present if patient cooperative	Grossly abnormal slowing of rhythm	Drowsy, unresponsive to verbal commands, markedly confused, delirious, hyperreflexia, positive Babinski sign
IV (coma)	Usually absent	Appearance of delta waves, decreased amplitudes	Unconscious, decerebrate or decorticate response to pain present (stage IVA) or absent (stage IVB)

EEG, Electroencephalogram.
From Fuhrman BP, et al.: *Pediatric critical care,* ed 4, Philadelphia, 2011, Saunders.

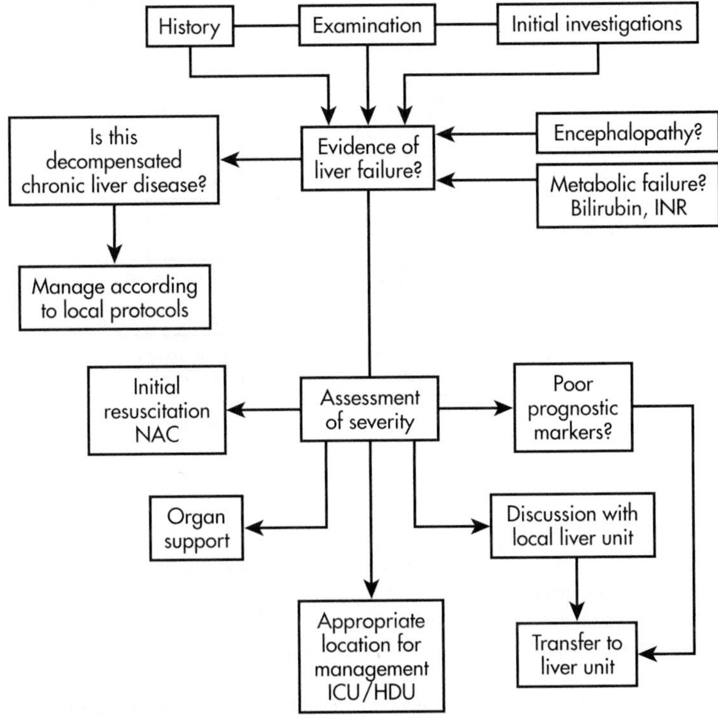

FIG. 2 Initial management of a patient presenting with liver failure. *HDU,* high dependency unit; *ICU,* intensive care unit; *INR,* international normalized ratio; *NAC, N*-acetylcysteine. (From Parrillo JE, Dellinger RP: *Critical care medicine, principles of diagnosis and management in the adult,* ed 4, Philadelphia, 2014, Elsevier.)

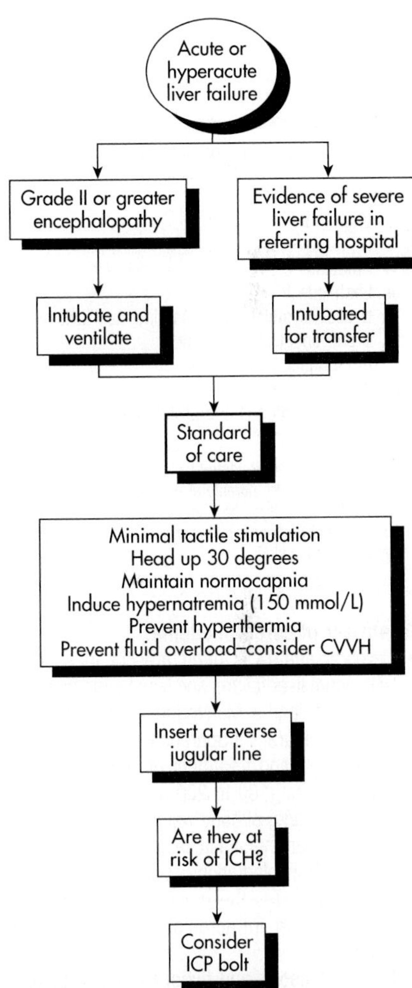

FIG. 3 Initial management of patient with high-grade encephalopathy. *CVVH,* continuous venovenous hemofiltration; *ICH,* intracranial hypertension; *ICP,* intracranial pressure. (From Parrillo JE, Dellinger RP: *Critical care medicine: principles of diagnosis and management in the adult,* ed 4, Philadelphia, 2014, Saunders.)

- Venous ammonia level. Measurement of serum ammonia level is useful in the evaluation of acute liver failure because levels correlate with the severity of encephalopathy and elevated levels are predictive of severe encephalopathy and cerebral edema. It is not useful for the evaluation or screening of hepatic encephalopathy in patients with chronic liver disease because it can neither rule in nor rule out hepatic encephalopathy, and levels do not correlate with the degree of encephalopathy
- Arterial blood gases

IMAGING STUDIES

CT scan or MRI of the brain may be useful in selected patients to exclude other etiologies when diagnosis is unclear.

Rx TREATMENT

NONPHARMACOLOGIC THERAPY

- Identification and treatment of precipitating factors.
- Restriction of protein intake is ill-advised and not necessary, since normal protein intake does not appear to exacerbate hepatic encephalopathy.

ACUTE GENERAL Rx

Fig. 2 illustrates the initial management of a patient presenting with liver failure. The approach to patients with high grade hepatic encephalopathy is shown in Fig. 3. Table 2 summarizes the management of fulminant hepatic failure.

Reduction of colonic ammonia production:

- Lactulose 25 ml twice daily initially; dose is subsequently adjusted depending on clinical response to achieve production of 3 bowel movements daily. IV ornithine aspartate should be considered for those not responding to lactulose.
- The oral antibiotic rifaximin (550 mg PO bid) is effective in reducing the risk of recurrent hepatic encephalopathy in patients with cirrhosis. It can be taken with lactulose, and the combination of lactulose and rifaximin is superior to lactulose alone in reversing hepatic encephalopathy. Rifaximin has also been shown to be effective in improving psychometric performance and health-related quality of life in patients with minimal hepatic encephalopathy. It is well tolerated but expensive.
- Probiotics (e.g., 1 capsule containing 112.5 billion viable lyophilized bacteria tid) might also be beneficial in altering gut flora to reduce ammonia production.

TABLE 2 Management of Fulminant Hepatic Failure

No sedation except for procedures
Minimal handling
Enteric precautions until infection ruled out
Monitor:
1. Heart and respiratory rate
2. Arterial BP, CVP
3. Core/toe temperature
4. Neurologic observations
5. Gastric pH (>5.0)
6. Blood glucose (>4 mmol/L)
7. Acid-base
8. Electrolytes
9. PT, PTT

Fluid balance
1. 75% maintenance
2. Dextrose 10%-50% (provide 6-10 mg/kg/min)
3. Sodium (0.5-1 mmol/L)
4. Potassium (2-4 mmol/L)

Maintain circulating volume with colloid/FFP
Coagulation support only if required
Drugs
1. Vitamin K
2. H2 antagonist
3. Antacids
4. Lactulose
5. N-acetylcysteine for acetaminophen toxicity
6. Broad-spectrum antibiotics
7. Antifungals

Nutrition
1. Enteral feeding (1-2 g protein/kg/day)
2. PN if ventilated

BP, Blood pressure; *CVP,* central venous pressure; *FFP,* fresh frozen plasma; *PN,* parenteral nutrition; *PT,* prothrombin time; *PTT,* partial thromboplastin time.
From Fuhrman BP, et al.: *Pediatric critical care,* ed 4, Philadelphia, 2011, Saunders.

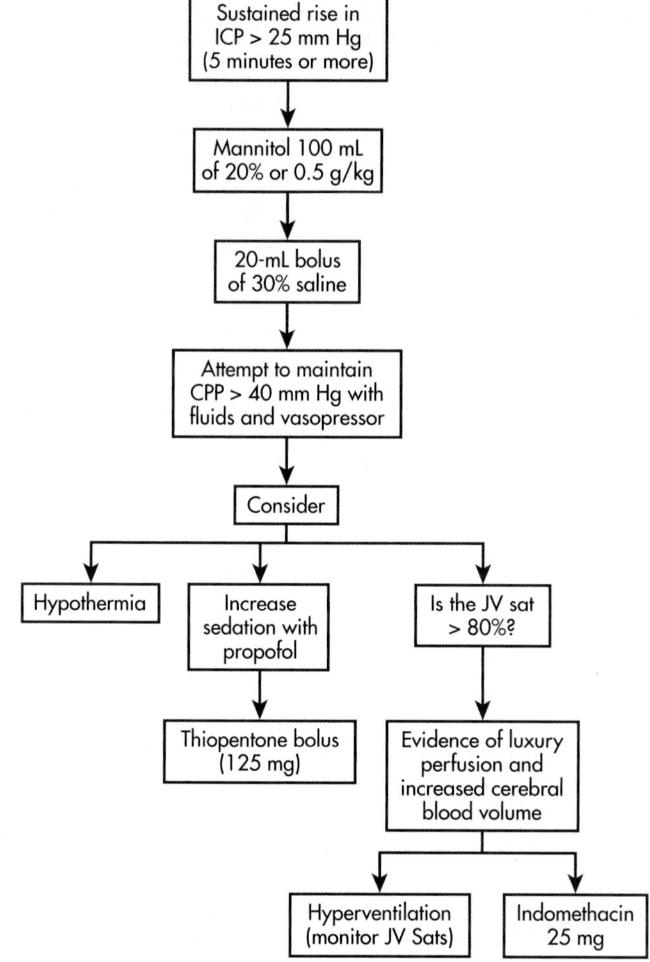

FIG. 4 Management of a sustained rise in intracranial pressure. *CPP,* cerebral perfusion pressure; *ICP,* intracranial pressure; *JV,* jugular venous; *Sats,* saturation. (From Parrillo JE, Dellinger RP: *Critical care medicine, principles of diagnosis and management in the adult,* ed 4, Philadelphia, 2014, Elsevier.)

Treatment of cerebral edema:

- Cerebral edema is often present in patients with acute liver failure, and it accounts for nearly 50% of deaths. Monitoring intracranial pressure by epidural, intraparenchymal, or subdural transducers and treatment of cerebral edema with mannitol (100 to 200 ml of 20% solution [0.3 to 0.4 g/kg of body weight]) given by rapid IV infusion are helpful in selected patients (e.g., potential transplantation patients).
- Fig. 4 illustrates the management of a sustained rise in intracranial pressure in liver failure.
- Dexamethasone and hyperventilation (useful in head injury) are of little value in treating cerebral edema from liver failure.

CHRONIC Rx

- Avoidance of any precipitating factors (e.g., high-protein diet, medications).
- Consideration of liver transplantation in selected patients with progressive or recurrent encephalopathy (Box E1). Liver transplantation remains the only curative therapeutic option.

DISPOSITION

Prognosis varies with the underlying etiology of the liver failure and the grade of encephalopathy (generally good for grades 1 or 2; poor for grades 3 or 4). Without proper therapy, the survival rate at 1 yr is 42% and decreases to 23% at 3 yr.

REFERRAL

The early stages of hepatic encephalopathy can be managed in the outpatient setting, whereas stages III or IV require hospital admission.

PEARLS & CONSIDERATIONS

COMMENTS

- Trials have shown that adding IV albumin to lactulose may improve outcomes in severe hepatic encephalopathy by reducing oxidative stress through reduction of levels of circulating cytokines and endotoxins.
- Long-acting benzodiazepines should not be used to treat anxiety and sleep disorders in patients with cirrhosis, as they may precipitate encephalopathy.
- Patients not responding to supportive therapy should be evaluated for liver transplantation.
- Not all patients with cirrhosis develop hepatic encephalopathy. It has been shown that 40% of persons with cirrhosis and minimal hepatic encephalopathy do not develop overt hepatic encephalopathy in long-term follow-up. There are genetic factors associated with development of hepatic encephalopathy in patients with cirrhosis. Genetic analyses have shown that glutaminase TACC and CACC haplotypes are linked to the risk for overt hepatic encephalopathy.

SUGGESTED READINGS

Available at ExpertConsult.com

RELATED CONTENT

Encephalopathy (Patient Information)
Cirrhosis (Related Key Topic)
Hepatic Encephalopathy (Related Key Topic)

AUTHOR: **FRED F. FERRI, M.D.**

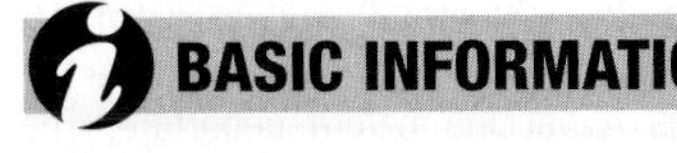

BASIC INFORMATION

DEFINITION

Hepatitis A is generally an acute self-limiting infection of the liver by an enterically transmitted picornavirus, hepatitis A virus (HAV). Infection may range from asymptomatic to fulminant hepatitis.

SYNONYMS

Infectious hepatitis
Short incubation hepatitis
Type A hepatitis
HAV (hepatitis A virus)

ICD-10CM CODES
B15.9 Hepatitis A without hepatic coma
B15.0 Hepatitis A with hepatic coma

EPIDEMIOLOGY & DEMOGRAPHICS

INCIDENCE:
- Hepatitis A occurs worldwide, affecting 1.4 million people annually and accounting for 20% to 40% of cases of viral hepatitis in the United States.
- The seroprevalence increases with age, ranging from 10% in individuals aged <5 yr to 74% in those aged >50 yr.
- In the United States, average disease rate was ~15 cases/100,000 persons/yr before routine vaccination of all children in certain states. The incidence after 2005 is about 1 case/100,000.
- The incidence is relatively higher in some regions in the United States, including Arizona, Alaska, California, Idaho, Nevada, New Mexico, Oklahoma, Oregon, South Dakota, and Washington.
- At-risk groups include:
  1. Residents and staff of group homes.
  2. Children and employees of day care centers.
  3. People who engage in oral-anal contact, regardless of sexual orientation.
  4. IV drug abusers.
  5. Travel to endemic areas.
  6. Areas of overcrowding, poor sanitation, inadequate sewage treatment.

PREVALENCE:
- Approximately threefourths of the U.S. population has serologic evidence of prior infection.
- Anti-HAV prevalence has an inverse relation to income and household size.

PREDOMINANT SEX: None, except higher infection rates seen in homosexual males who engage in oral–anal contact.

PREDOMINANT AGE/PEAK INCIDENCE:
- In areas of high rates of hepatitis A, virtually all children are infected while younger than 10 yr, but disease is rare.
- In areas of moderate rates of hepatitis A, disease occurs in late childhood and young adults.
- In areas of low rates of hepatitis A, most cases occur in young adults.

INCUBATION PERIOD: Averages 30 days (15 to 50)

PHYSICAL FINDINGS & CLINICAL PRESENTATION

- Infection with HAV may have acute or subacute presentation, icteric or anicteric. Severity of illness seems to increase with age (90% of infection in children aged <5 yr may be subclinical).
- The incubation period of HAV is 2 to 6 wk.
- A preicteric, prodromal phase of approximately 1 to 14 days; 15% no apparent prodrome. Symptoms are usually abrupt in onset and may include anorexia, fatigue, malaise, nausea, vomiting, fever, headache, and mild abdominal pain.
- Less common symptoms are chills, myalgias, arthralgias, upper respiratory symptoms, constipation, diarrhea, pruritus, urticaria.
- Jaundice occurs in >70% of patients. Patients older than 30 yr are more likely than younger individuals to have jaundice.
- The icteric phase is preceded by dark urine.
- Bilirubinuria is typically followed a few days later by clay-colored stools and icterus.

PHYSICAL EXAMINATION

- Jaundice: Peaks in severity 2 wk after onset
- Hepatomegaly
- Splenomegaly
- Cervical lymphadenopathy
- Evanescent rash
- Petechiae
- Cardiac arrhythmias

COMPLICATIONS

- Cholestasis
- Fulminant hepatitis
- Arthritis
- Myocarditis
- Optic neuritis
- Transverse myelitis
- Thrombocytopenic purpura
- Aplastic anemia
- Red cell aplasia
- Henoch-Schönlein purpura
- IgA dominant glomerulonephritis

ETIOLOGY

- Caused by HAV, a 27-nm, nonenveloped, icosahedral, positive-stranded RNA virus.
- Transmission is fecal-oral route, from person to person. Transmission occurs with close contact or with food- or water-borne outbreaks with inadequately purified water or cooked foods. Recent outbreaks have involved green onions and tomatoes.
- Parenteral transmission is considered rare.
- Vertical transmission has also been reported.

Dx DIAGNOSIS

DIFFERENTIAL DIAGNOSIS

- Other hepatitis virus (B, C, D, E)
- Infectious mononucleosis
- Cytomegalovirus infection
- Herpes simplex virus infection
- Leptospirosis
- Brucellosis
- Drug-induced liver disease
- Ischemic hepatitis
- Autoimmune hepatitis

WORKUP

- IgM antibody specific for HAV.
- Liver function tests; ALT and AST elevations are sensitive for liver damage but not specific for HAV.
- Elevated ESR.
- CBC; may find mild lymphocytosis.

LABORATORY TESTS

- Diagnosis confirmed by IgM anti-HAV; it is detectable in almost all infected patients at presentation and remains positive for 3 to 6 mo.
- A fourfold rise in titer of total antibody (IgM and IgG) to HAV confirms acute infection.
- HAV detection in stool and body fluids by electron microscopy.
- HAV RNA detection in stool, body fluids, serum, and liver tissue.
- ALT and AST usually more than 8 times normal in acute infection.
- Bilirubin usually 5 to 15 times normal.
- Alkaline phosphatase minimally elevated, but higher level in cholestasis.
- Albumin and prothrombin time are generally normal; if elevated, they may herald hepatic necrosis.
- Fig. 1 illustrates the typical course of hepatis A.

IMAGING STUDIES

- Rarely useful
- Sonogram (fulminant hepatitis)

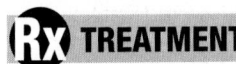

TREATMENT

- Usually self-limited.
- Supportive care.
- Those with fulminant hepatitis may require hospitalization and treatment of associated complications.
- Activity as tolerated.
- Advise to avoid alcohol and hepatotoxic drugs.
- Patients with fulminant hepatitis should be assessed for liver transplantation.

CHRONIC Rx

No chronic HAV and no chronic carrier state. The majority of patients have resolution of symptoms and liver abnormalities within 3 months.

DISPOSITION

- Follow-up as outpatient.
- Most patients recover within 3 mo of infection, although 5% to 10% of patients will experience a relapse in the first 6 mo.
- HAV is a self-limited infection and does not cause chronic hepatitis.

REFERRAL

- To a hepatologist if severe, fulminant hepatitis develops
- To a transplant surgeon if liver transplant becomes a consideration for fulminant hepatitis and liver failure

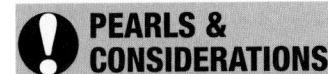

PEARLS & CONSIDERATIONS

- All cases of hepatitis A should be reported to the public health authorities because food-borne or water-borne outbreaks may occur,

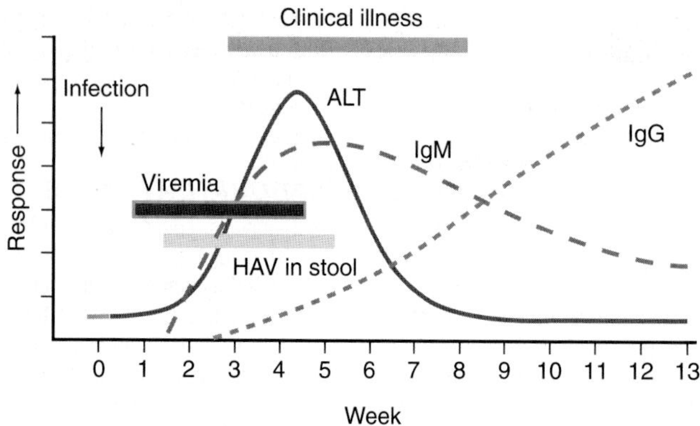

FIG. 1 Immunologic, virologic, and biochemical events during the course of a typical hepatitis A virus *(HAV)* infection. *ALT,* Alanine transaminase; *IgG,* immunoglobulin G; *IgM,* immunoglobulin M. (From Cherry JD et al: *Feigin and Cherry's pediatric infectious diseases,* ed 8, Philadelphia, 2019, Elsevier.)

TABLE 1 Recommendations for Routine Preexposure Use of Hepatitis A Virus Vaccine

Group	Comments
Children	Vaccine should be given to all children at age 1 yr (12-23 mo). * Vaccination of children 2-18 yr may also be warranted.†
International travelers‡	IG may be given in addition to or instead of vaccine; children <12 mo should receive IG.
Close contacts of newly arriving international adoptees	All persons who anticipate close personal contact (e.g., household contact or regular babysitter) during the first 60 days after arrival
Men who have sex with men	Includes adolescents
Illicit drug users	Includes adolescents
Persons with chronic liver disease, such as those with hepatitis B or C	Increased risk of fulminant hepatitis A with HAV infection
Persons receiving clotting factor concentrates	
Persons who work with HAV in research laboratory settings	

HAV, hepatitis A virus; *IG,* immunoglobulin.
*Hepatitis A vaccine is not licensed for children <12 months.
†States and communities with existing vaccination programs for children ages 2 to 18 years are encouraged to maintain these programs. Catch-up vaccination for this age group may be warranted elsewhere in the context of ongoing outbreaks among children.
‡Persons traveling to Canada, Western Europe, Japan, Australia, or New Zealand are at no greater risk than in the U.S.
From Bennett JE et al: *Mandell, Douglas, and Bennett's principles and practice of infectious diseases,* ed 8, Philadelphia, 2015, Saunders.

and public health efforts (mass vaccination or immunoglobulin therapy) may prevent secondary cases.

- Hepatitis A is a common illness in internationally traveled and developing countries. Pretravel vaccination is strongly recommended for travelers who are HAV susceptible. Table 1 summarizes recommendations for preexposure use of hepatitis A virus vaccine.
- Handwashing is important, as the hepatitis A virus may survive for up to 4 hours on the fingertips.

PREVENTION

- Improvement in hygiene and sanitation
- Heating food
- Avoidance of water and foods from endemic area.

PASSIVE IMMUNIZATION

- Immunoglobulin provides protection against HAV through passive transfer of antibody.
- Preexposure prophylaxis indicated for people traveling to endemic areas with immune globulin (Ig 0.02 or 0.06 ml/kg given IM) who have not received or cannot receive the hepatitis A vaccine before departure. The lower dose is effective for up to 3 mo, and the higher dose is effective for up to 5 mo.
- Postexposure prophylaxis (PEP): For individuals with a recent exposure to hepatitis A who have not received the vaccine, post-exposure prophylaxis is warranted with either immune globulin (Ig 0.02 ml/kg given IM) or a single dose of the hepatitis A vaccine within 2 wk of the exposure. For healthy persons ages 12 mo to 40 yr of age, a single dose of the hepatitis A vaccine should be given. Children <12 mo, adults >40 yr of age, and persons who have chronic liver disease and who are immunocompromised should receive immunoglobulin.

ACTIVE IMMUNIZATION

- There are several inactivated and attenuated hepatitis vaccines; only the inactivated vaccines are currently available for use and they have been found to be safe and highly immunogenic: HAVRIX or VAQTA. These can be used in adults and children older than 12 mo. They are given as a two-dose regimen 6 mo to 1 yr apart. A combined hepatitis A and hepatitis B vaccine called TWINRX is also available.
- Protective antibody levels were reached in 94% to 100% of adults 1 mo after the first dose; similar results have been found for children and adolescents.
- Theoretic analyses of antibody levels estimate duration of immunity to be 10 to 20 yr.
- Vaccine should be considered for persons who are at risk. Those traveling to or working in endemic areas, homosexual men, illegal drug users, persons with chronic liver disease, and children in areas with high rates of hepatitis A infection.
- The Advisory Committee on Immunization Practices recommends routine hepatitis A vaccination for all children beginning at 12 to 23 mo of age. Simultaneous administration of MMR and HCPA vaccines is recommended for infants aged 6 to 11 mo traveling internationally. The travel-related dose for infants aged 6 to 11 mo should not be counted towards the routine 2-dose series.

SUGGESTED READINGS

Available at ExpertConsult.com

RELATED CONTENT

Hepatitis A (Patient Information)

AUTHOR: **GLENN G. FORT, M.D., M.P.H.**

BASIC INFORMATION

DEFINITION

Hepatitis B is an acute infection of the liver parenchymal cells caused by the hepatitis B virus (HBV).

SYNONYMS

Serum hepatitis
Long incubation (30 to 180 days) hepatitis HBV
HBV

EPIDEMIOLOGY & DEMOGRAPHICS

INCIDENCE:

- ~200,000 to 300,000 infections annually in the U.S.
- Much higher incidence in Europe (~1 million new cases annually) and in areas of high endemicity.
- In the U.S., transmission is mainly horizontal (percutaneous and mucous membrane exposure to infectious blood and other body fluids [e.g., sexual transmission, either homosexual or heterosexual]); also from needle sharing among drug abusers; occupational exposure to contaminated blood and blood products; persons receiving transfusions of blood and blood products; and hemodialysis patients.

NOTE: Improved screening of blood and blood products has greatly reduced, although not eliminated, the risk of posttransfusion HBV infection.

- In areas of high endemicity, transmission is largely vertical (perinatal): HBV exists in the blood and body fluids. Perinatal transmission from HBsAg-positive mothers is as high as 90% unless immunoprophylaxis is given.

PREVALENCE:

- The WHO estimates that 400 million people worldwide (6% of the population) are chronic HBV carriers. North America, Western Europe, and Australia are areas of low prevalence, <2%. In the United States an estimated 800,000 to 1.4 million people have chronic HBV infection. About two thirds of them are unaware that they are infected.
- Africa, Asia, and the Western Pacific region are areas of high prevalence, ≥8%.
- Southern and Eastern Europe have intermediate rates, 2% to 7%.
- Chronically infected persons, those with positive HBsAg for >6 mo, represent the major source of infection.
- As many as 95% of infants and children aged <5, who typically have subclinical acute infection, will become chronic HBV carriers.
- Adults are more likely to have clinically evident acute infection, but only 1% to 5% will develop chronic infection.
- ~0.1% of patients with acute infection will develop fulminant acute hepatitis resulting in death.

PREDOMINANT SEX:

- Predominant in males because of increased IV drug abuse, homosexuality.
- Females more commonly terminate in chronic carrier state.

PREDOMINANT AGE: 20 to 45 yr.
PEAK INCIDENCE: 30 to 45 yr of age, at rates of 5% to 20%.
GENETICS: Neonatal infection:

- Rare in the United States.
- High (up to 90%) in areas of high endemicity (only 5% to 10% of perinatal infections occur in utero).

PHYSICAL FINDINGS & CLINICAL PRESENTATION (FIG. 1)

- The incubation period of HBV infection is 4 to 24 weeks. HBV infection presents as acute hepatitis in a minority of patients.
- Patients often present with nonspecific symptoms.
- Profound malaise.
- Many asymptomatic cases.
- Prodrome:
  1. 15% to 20% serum sickness (urticaria, rash, arthralgia) during early HBsAg.
  2. HBsAg-Ab complex disease (polyarteritis nodosa–arthritis, arteritis, glomerulonephritis).
- Hepatomegaly (87%) with right upper quadrant (RUQ) tenderness:
  1. Hepatic punch tenderness.
  2. Splenomegaly: Rare (10% to 15%).
- Jaundice (30% of patients), dark urine, with occasional pruritus.
- Variable fever (when present, generally precedes jaundice and rapidly declines following onset of icteric phase).
- Spider angiomata: Rare; resolves during recovery.
- Rare polyarteritis nodosa, cryoglobulinemia.

ETIOLOGY

- Caused by HBV (42-nm hepadnavirus with an outer surface coat [HBsAg], inner nucleocapsid core [HBcAg; HBeAg]; DNA polymerase; and partially double-stranded DNA genome). There are eight genotypes (A to H) based on nucleotide sequence. The prevalence of each genotype varies widely.
- Transmission by parenteral route (needle use, tattooing, ear piercing, acupuncture, transfusion of blood and blood products, hemodialysis, sexual contact), perinatal transmission.
- Infection may result from contact of infectious material with mucous membranes and open skin breaks (e.g., HBV is stable and can be transmitted from toothbrushes, utensils, razors, baby toys, assorted medical equipment [respirators, endoscopes]).
- Oral intake of infectious material may result in infection through breaks in the oral mucosa.
- Food or water are virtually never found to be sources of HBV infection.
- Infection occurs primarily in liver, where necrosis probably results from cytotoxic T-cell response, direct cytopathic effect of HBcAg (core antigen), high-level HBsAg (surface antigen) expression, or coinfection with delta (D) hepatitis virus (RNA delta core within HBsAg envelope).
- Recovery (>90%):
  1. Fulminant hepatitis occurring in <1% (especially if coinfected with hepatitis D); 80% fatal.
  2. Unusual (5%) prolonged acute disease for 4 to 12 mo, with recovery.
  3. Overall fatality increases with age and viral inoculation (e.g., transfusions).
- Chronic hepatitis B (CHB) infection (1% to 2%), four phases:
  1. Immune-tolerant phase: A highly replicative/low-inflammatory phase where HBV DNA levels are high (typically >1 million IU/ml), ALT levels are normal, and biopsies have minimal signs of significant inflammation or fibrosis.
     a. This phase can persist for yrs, especially in those infected prenatally.
     b. With age there is a likely transformation to an HBeAg-positive immune-active phase.
  2. HBeAg-positive immune-active phase: Elevated ALT and HBV DNA levels in conjunction with liver injury (≥ 20,000 IU/ml).

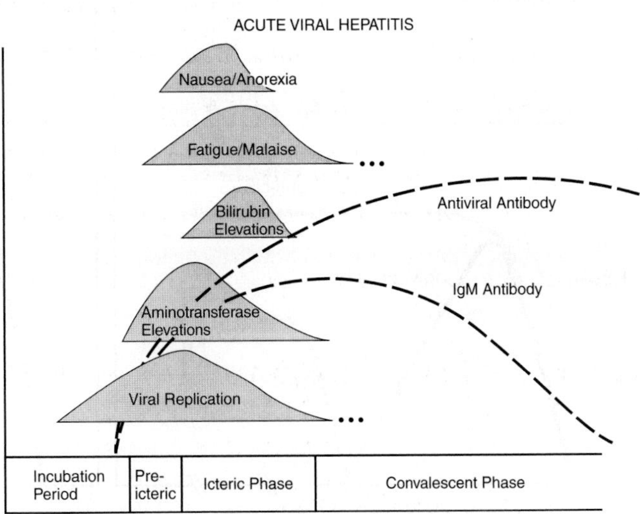

FIG. 1 The typical course of acute viral hepatitis. *IgM,* Immunoglobulin M. (From Goldman L, Ausiello D [eds]: *Cecil textbook of medicine,* ed 22, Philadelphia, 2004, Saunders.)

Median age of onset is 30 yr in those infected at a young age. Biopsy will show moderate to severe inflammation or fibrosis.
3. Inactive CHB phase: HBV DNA levels are low or undetectable (<2000 IU/ml), ALT levels are normal, and anti-HBe is present. Biopsy shows minimal necroinflammation but variable fibrosis.
4. HBeAg-negative immune reactivation phase: Elevated ALT and elevated HBV DNA (≥2000 IU/ml). Biopsy will show moderate to severe necroinflammation and fibrosis.

- Table 1 summarizes causes of hepatitis flares in patients with CHB.
- The most feared complications of CHB are cirrhosis and hepatocellular carcinoma (HCC), which kill more than 300,000 people/yr globally. One quarter to one third of patients will go on to develop these complications. The risk of developing HCC appears to be greatest among individuals with the highest serum levels of HBV DNA.

Dx DIAGNOSIS

DIFFERENTIAL DIAGNOSIS

- Acute disease confused with other viral hepatitis infections (A, C, D, E).
- Any viral illness producing systemic disease and hepatitis (e.g., yellow fever, EBV, CMV, HIV, rubella, rubeola, coxsackie B, adenovirus, herpes simplex or zoster).
- Nonviral causes of hepatitis (e.g., leptospirosis, toxoplasmosis, alcoholic hepatitis, drug-induced [e.g., acetaminophen, INH], toxic hepatitis [carbon tetrachloride, benzene]).

WORKUP

- Acute serum specimen for hepatitis B serology (HBsAg, HBsAb, HBcAb, HBeAg, HBeAb), HBDNA by PCR
- LFTs
- CBC
- Liver biopsy: Rarely indicated for diagnosis of fulminant viral hepatitis, chronic hepatitis, cirrhosis, carcinoma

LABORATORY TESTS

- Diagnosis of acute HBV infection is best confirmed by IgM HBcAb in acute or early convalescent serum or by HBDNA by PCR.
  1. Generally, IgM present during onset of jaundice.
  2. Coexisting HBsAg.
- HBsAg and IgG-HBcAb during acute jaundice are strongly suggestive of remote HBV infection and another cause for current illness (Fig. 2).
- HBsAb alone is suggestive of immunization response.
- With recovery, HBeAg is rapidly replaced by HBeAb in 2 to 3 mo, and HBsAg is replaced by HBsAb in 5 to 6 mo.
- In chronic HBV hepatitis, HBsAg and HBeAg are persistent without corresponding Ab.

TABLE 1 Causes of Hepatitis Flares in Patients with Chronic Hepatitis B

Cause of Flare	Comment
Spontaneous	Factors that precipitate viral replication are unclear
Immunosuppressive therapy	Flares are often observed during withdrawal of the agent; preemptive antiviral therapy is required
Antiviral therapy for HBV	
Interferon	Flares are often observed during the second to third month of therapy in 30% of patients; may herald virologic response
Nucleoside analog	
During treatment	Flares are no more common than with placebo
Drug-resistant HBV	Severe consequences can occur in patients with advanced liver disease
On withdrawal	Flares are caused by the rapid reemergence of wild-type HBV; severe consequences can occur in patients with advanced liver disease
HIV treatment	Flares can occur as a result of the direct toxicity of HAART or with immune reconstitution; HBV increases the risk of antiretroviral drug hepatotoxicity
Genotypic variation	
Precore and core promoter mutants	Fluctuations in serum ALT levels are common with precore mutants
Superinfection with other hepatitis viruses	May be associated with suppression of HBV replication

ALT, Alanine aminotransferase; *HAART,* highly active antiretroviral therapy; *HBV,* hepatitis B virus; *HIV,* human immunodeficiency virus.
From Feldman M, et al. [eds]: *Sleisenger and Fordtran's gastrointestinal and liver disease,* ed 10, Philadelphia, 2016, Saunders.

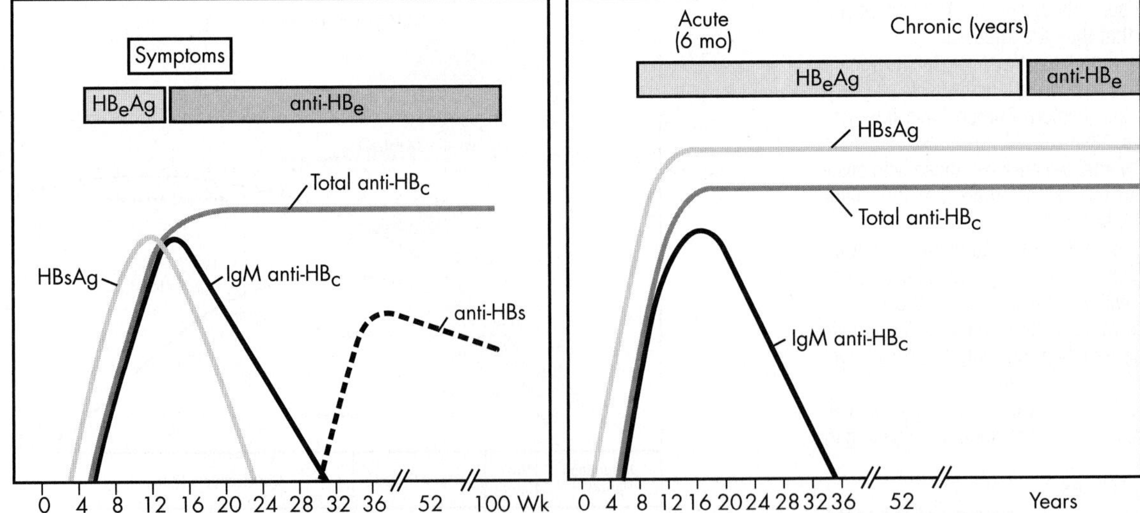

FIG. 2 Typical course of hepatitis B. *Left,* Typical course of acute hepatitis B. *Right,* Chronic hepatitis B. *HBc,* Hepatitis B core; *HBe,* hepatitis B early; *HBeAg,* hepatitis B early antigen; *HBs,* hepatitis B surface; *HBsAg,* hepatitis B surface antigen; *IgM,* immunoglobulin M. (From Mandell GL, et al.: *Principles and practice of infectious diseases,* ed 7, Philadelphia, 2010, Saunders.)

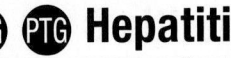

- In chronic carrier state, HBsAg is persistent, but HBeAg is replaced by HBeAb.
- HBcAb develops in all outcomes.
- HBeAg correlation with highest infectivity; appearance of HBeAb heralds recovery.
- LFTs:
  1. ALT and AST: Usually more than eight times normal (often 1000 U/L) at onset of jaundice (minimal acute ALT/AST rises often followed by chronic hepatitis or hepatocellular carcinoma).
  2. Bilirubin: Variably elevated in icteric viral hepatitis.
  3. Alkaline phosphatase: Minimally elevated (one to three times normal) acutely.
- Albumin and prothrombin time:
  1. Generally normal.
  2. If abnormal, possible harbinger of impending hepatic necrosis (fulminant hepatitis).
- WBC and ESR: Generally normal.

IMAGING STUDIES

- Sonogram to document rapid reduction in liver size during fulminant hepatitis or mass in hepatocellular carcinoma
- Fibroscan (transient elastography): A noninvasive specialized ultrasound test to quantify liver fibrosis without liver biopsy

Rx TREATMENT

NONPHARMACOLOGIC THERAPY

- Symptomatic treatment as necessary
- Activity as tolerated
- High-calorie diet preferred; often best tolerated in morning

ACUTE GENERAL Rx

- In most cases of acute HBV infection no treatment necessary; >90% of adults will spontaneously clear infection.
- Hospitalization advisable for any patient in danger from dehydration caused by poor oral intake, whose PT is prolonged, who has rising bilirubin level >15 to 20 μg/dl, or who has any clinical evidence of hepatic failure. Table 2 summarizes indications for prompt or urgent treatment of hepatitis B.
- IV therapy needed (rarely) for hydration during severe vomiting.
- Avoid hepatically metabolized drugs.
- No therapeutic measures are beneficial.
- Steroids not shown helpful.

CHRONIC Rx

- Treatment of chronic HBV infection is dependent on which phase the patient is found to be in:
  1. Therapy is warranted for patients in immune-active CHB stage (HBeAg negative or HBeAg positive) to decrease the risk of liver-related complications. Treatment options include:
     a. Pegylated interferon 2a: 180 micrograms subcutaneously weekly for 48 weeks. This will lead to seroconversion rates of 20% to 30% (HBeAg to anti-HBe), and 65% of patients will have HBV DNA <2000 IU/ml off therapy but cure rates remain low at 3–7% and has significant side effects: bone marrow suppression and exacerbation of existing neuropsychiatric symptoms, including depression. Candidates for interferon therapy should not have significant psychiatric disease, cardiac disease, cytopenia, seizure disorder, autoimmune disease, or pregnancy.
     b. Entecavir: A nucleotide analogue. Dose 0.5 to 1 mg daily, suppresses HBV DNA replication and improves liver inflammation and fibrosis
     c. Tenofovir disoproxil: 300 mg daily, is another nucleotide analogue. A newer formulation, tenofovir alafenamide (Vemlidy) 25 mg a day, has less renal and bone toxicity in long-term use.
     d. Other nucleotide agents: Lamivudine, telbivudine, and adefovir are less frequently used due to issues of resistance.
     e. Cure rates with nucleotide agents are between 1% and 12%, and thus most patients will require treatment indefinitely but are considered first line of therapy.
  2. Therapy is not warranted in adults with immune-tolerant CHB. LFTs should be checked every 6 months to look for conversion to immune-active or inactive status.
     a. Therapy may be warranted for select adults >40 with normal ALT and elevated HBV DNA (≥1 million IU/ml) with liver biopsy showing significant necroinflammation or fibrosis.
  3. HBeAg-positive adults without cirrhosis who seroconvert to anti-HBe on therapy with entecavir or tenofovir disoproxil can discontinue treatment after a period of treatment consolidation.
  4. It is recommended that patients receive indefinite therapy with entecavir or tenofovir disoproxil if HBeAg-negative immune-active CHB is present, unless there is a competing rationale for treatment discontinuation.
  5. Adults with compensated cirrhosis and low levels of viremia (<2000 IU/ml) should be treated with entecavir or tenofovir disoproxil to reduce the risk of decompensation, regardless of ALT level.

DISPOSITION

- Follow-up as outpatient
- Acute disease: Infection will resolve (defined as clearance of hepatitis B surface antigen within 6 months) in 90% of adult patients.
- Rare fatalities (fulminant hepatitis)
- Possible chronic carrier state, cirrhosis, hepatocellular carcinoma
- Cure of HBV is an unrealistic goal for most patients with chronic infection since only a few patients will become HBsAb with current treatment modalities

REFERRAL

To infectious disease specialist and gastroenterologist for consultation regarding fulminant hepatitis or prolonged cholestasis, for cases of uncertain etiology, or for treatment of CAH

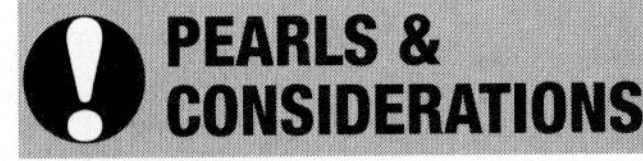

PEARLS & CONSIDERATIONS

COMMENTS

- Virus and HBsAg in high titers in blood for 1 to 7 wk before jaundice and for a variable time thereafter.

TABLE 2 Indications for Prompt or Urgent Treatment of Hepatitis B

	Indications	Preferred Agent	Principal Supportive Data
Cirrhosis*			
Decompensated	Clinical stabilization; minimizing risk for recurrence after transplant	Entecavir (0.5 mg) or tenofovir (300 mg)†	Open label; multiple large case series
Borderline compensated	Forestalling disease progression; avoidance of transplantation	As above	Undefined
Well compensated	As above	As above	Randomized controlled trials
Acute Liver Failure			
HBV reactivation	Minimizing further liver injury; reducing risk of recurrence after liver transplantation, if needed	Entecavir (0.5 mg) or tenofovir (300 mg)†	Open label with comparison with historical controls
Severe acute hepatitis	Minimizing further liver injury and enhancing full recovery	Consider lamivudine or telbivudine‡	Small case series

*It has been the author's (RP) practice to use maintenance antiviral therapy for all hepatitis B surface antigen (HBsAg)-positive patients with cirrhosis to prevent reactivation of hepatitis B.

†Daily dose should be adjusted according to the patient's renal function, as indicated in the manufacturer's recommendations.

‡Either agent can be used if the anticipated duration of therapy is 6 mo or less.

HBV, Hepatitis B virus. From Feldman M, Friedman LS, Brandt LJ: *Sleisenger and Fordtran's gastrointestinal and liver disease*, ed 10, Philadelphia, 2016, Elsevier.

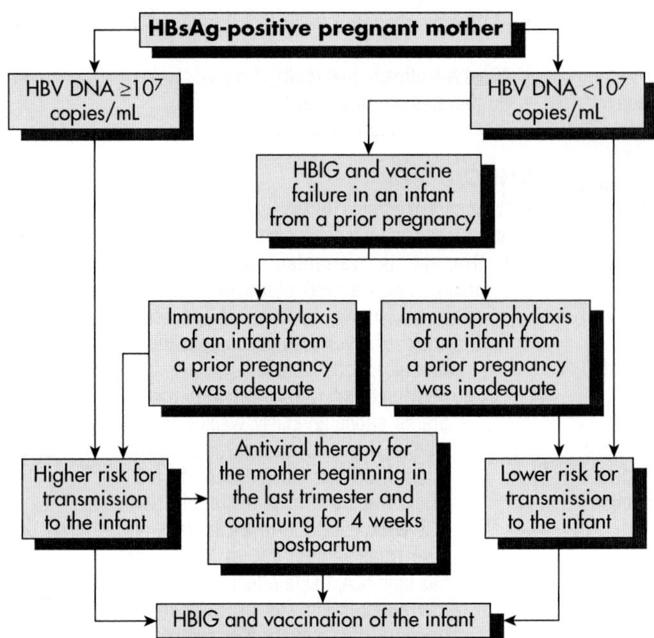

FIG. 3 Algorithm for the treatment of hepatitis B surface antigen (HBsAg)–positive mothers during pregnancy. The goal of treatment in highly viremic mothers is to lower the serum HBV DNA level by several $\log_{10}$ IU/ml by the time of delivery to minimize the chance of newborn infection. The choice of antiviral agent is less important if treatment of the mother is not needed long term. In the event that the treatment needs to be continued after delivery, the patient should be started on a high-genetic-barrier drug initially or switched to one immediately after delivery. See text for further details about drug selection. *DNA,* Deoxyribonucleic acid; *HBIG,* hepatitis B immune globulin; *HBV,* hepatitis B virus. (From Feldman M, et al. [eds]: *Sleisenger and Fordtran's gastrointestinal and liver disease,* ed 10, Philadelphia, 2016, Saunders.)

TABLE 3 Interpretation of Serologic Markers and Serum DNA in Hepatitis B

	HBsAg	HBeAg	Anti-HBc IgM	Anti-HBc IgG	Anti-HBs	Anti-HBe	HBV DNA*
Acute hepatitis	+	+/−	+				+
Acute hepatitis, window period			+				
Recovery from acute hepatitis			+	+	+	+/−	
Chronic hepatitis	+	+					+
Chronic hepatitis (precore mutant)	+					+	+
Inactive carrier	+					+/−	
Vaccinated					+		

anti-HBc IgG, Hepatitis B core antibody (IgG type); *anti-HBc IgM,* hepatitis B core antibody (IgM type); anti-HBe, hepatitis B early antibody; *anti-HBs,* hepatitis B surface antibody; *DNA,* deoxyribonucleic acid; *HBeAg,* hepatitis Be antigen; *HBsAg,* hepatitis B surface antigen; *HBV DNA,* hepatitis B viral DNA.
*HBV DNA >10^5 copies/ml.
From Andreoli TE, et al.: *Andreoli and Carpenter's Cecil essentials of medicine,* ed 8, Philadelphia, 2010, Saunders.

- Screening (HBV surface antigen [HBsAg], HBV core antigen antibody, antibody to HBsAg) should be offered to high risk groups.
- Transmission is possible during entire period of HBsAg (and especially during HBeAg) in serum.
- Universal precautions should be followed for all contacts with blood or secretions/excretions contaminated with blood.
- Antiviral therapy is recommended in pregnancy to reduce perinatal transmission if HBsAg positive and HBV DNA >200,000 IU/ml. Can use tenofovir disoproxil, lamivudine, or telbivudine. Fig. 3 describes an algorithm for the treatment of hepatitis B surface antigen (HBsAg)–positive mothers during pregnancy.
- Preventing before exposure:
  1. Lifestyle changes.
  2. Meticulous testing of blood supply (although some chronically infected, infectious donors are HBsAg negative).
  3. Sterilization via steam or hypochlorite.
  4. Hepatitis B vaccine for high-risk groups given IM in deltoid to induce HBsAb (response should be confirmed) is protective (>90% effective). The FDA has recently approved a two-dose hepatitis B virus vaccine (HEPLISAV-B) for use in adults ≥ 18 yr old, administered at 0 and 1 month.
  5. Recommendation for universal childhood immunization with doses at birth, 1 mo, and 6 mo.
- Prevention after exposure:
  1. HBV hyperimmune globulin (HBIG) (0.06 ml/kg IM) given immediately after needlestick, within 14 days of sexual exposure, or at birth, followed by HBV vaccination. A second dose of HBIG is given in 28 days for those refusing vaccine or vaccine nonresponders.
  2. Standard immune globulin: Nearly as effective as HBIG.
- Preventive therapy with entecavir or tenofovir disoproxil for patients who test positive for HBsAg and are undergoing chemotherapy may reduce the risk for HBV reactivation and HBV-associated morbidity and mortality.
- Hepatitis B prophylaxis is described in Section V.
- Table 3 summarizes interpretation of serologic markers and serum DNA in hepatitis B.

SUGGESTED READINGS

Available at ExpertConsult.com

RELATED CONTENT

Hepatitis B (Patient Information)

AUTHOR: **GLENN G. FORT, M.D., M.P.H.**

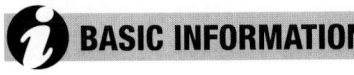

BASIC INFORMATION

DEFINITION

Hepatitis C is an acute liver parenchymal infection caused by hepatitis C virus (HCV).

SYNONYM

Transfusion-related non-A, non-B hepatitis (incubation period averages 6 wk, intermediate between hepatitis A and B)

ICD-10CM CODES

B17.1	Acute hepatitis C
B18.2	Chronic viral hepatitis C
B17.10	Acute hepatitis C without hepatic coma
B17.11	Acute hepatitis C with hepatic coma
B19.20	Unspecified viral hepatitis C without hepatic coma
B19.21	Unspecified viral hepatitis C with hepatic coma

EPIDEMIOLOGY & DEMOGRAPHICS

Hepatitis C infection is the most common chronic blood-borne infection in the United States. About 3% of baby boomers test positive for the virus. The CDC now recommends testing for hepatitis C for anyone born from 1945 to 1965.

INCIDENCE: HCV infects more than 185 million individuals worldwide. Approximately 20% of patients chronically infected with HCV progress to cirrhosis.

- 150,000 new cases/yr (37,500 symptomatic; 93,000 later chronic liver disease; 30,700 cirrhosis). The incidence of acute HCV has declined substantially over the past 30 yr (from 7.4/100,000 to 0.7/100,000).
- ~9000 of these ultimately die of HCV infection; most common (40%) cause of nonalcoholic liver disease in the United States

PREVALENCE (IN U.S.):

- Overall prevalence of anti-HCV antibody is 1% to 1.2% (an estimated 2.7 million persons nationwide).
- Highest prevalence in hemophiliacs transfused before 1987 and users of injection drugs, 72% to 90%. Over past 30 yr, blood transfusion as a risk factor declined from 15% of cases to 1.9%.
- Among low-risk groups, prevalence 0.6%.

PREDOMINANT SEX: Slight male predominance.

PREDOMINANT AGE: Highest prevalence in 30- to 49-yr age group (65%).

PEAK INCIDENCE:

- 20 to 39 yr of age.
- African Americans and whites have similar incidence of acute disease; Hispanics have higher rates.
- Prevalence is substantially higher among non-Hispanic blacks than among non-Hispanic whites.

GENETICS: Neonatal infection is rare; increased risk with maternal HIV-1 coinfection.

PHYSICAL FINDINGS & CLINICAL PRESENTATION

- Symptoms usually develop 7 to 8 wk after infection (range of 2 to 26 wk), but 70% to 80% of cases are subclinical.
- 10% to 20% report acute illness with jaundice and nonspecific symptoms (abdominal pain, anorexia, malaise).
- Fulminant hepatitis may rarely occur during this period.
- After acute infection, 15% to 25% have complete resolution (absence of HCV RNA in serum, normal ALT).
- Progression to chronic infection is common, 50% to 84%. 74% to 86% have persistent viremia; spontaneous clearance of viremia in chronic infection is rare. 60% to 70% of patients will have persistent or fluctuating ALT levels; 30% to 40% with chronic infection have normal ALT levels.
- 15% to 20% of those with chronic HCV will develop cirrhosis over a period of 20 to 30 yr; in most others, chronic infection leads to hepatitis and varying degrees of fibrosis. Table 1 summarizes factors associated with progression of hepatic fibrosis in patients with chronic HCV infection. Table 2 describes factors associated with cirrhosis in persons with hepatitis C infection.
- 0.4% to 2.5% of patients with chronic infection develop hepatocellular carcinoma (HCC).
- 25% of patients with chronic infection continue to have an asymptomatic course with normal LFTs and benign histology.
- In chronic HCV infection, extrahepatic sequelae include a variety of immunologic and lymphoproliferative disorders (e.g., cryoglobulinemia, membranoproliferative glomerulonephritis, and possibly Sjögren's syndrome, autoimmune thyroiditis, polyarteritis nodosa, aplastic anemia, lichen planus, porphyria cutanea tarda, B-cell lymphoma, others).
- Fig. 1 illustrates the natural history of HCV infection.

ETIOLOGY

- Caused by HCV (single-stranded RNA flavivirus). HCV genotype 1 accounts for about 75% of HCV in the US. Genotypes 2 and 3 account for about 20-25% of infections, genotype 4 for 6%, and genotypes 5 and 6 for about 1%.
- Most HCV transmission is parenteral.
- In the United States, advances in screening of blood and blood products have made transfusion-related HCV infection rare (the risk is estimated to be 0.001% per unit transfused).
- Injecting-drug use accounts for most HCV transmission in the United States (60% of newly acquired cases, 20% to 50% of chronically infected persons).
- Occupational needlestick exposure from an HCV-positive source has a seroconversion rate of 1.8% (range 0% to 7%).
- Nosocomial transmission rates (from surgery and procedures such as colonoscopy and hemodialysis) are extremely low.
- Sexual transmission and maternal-fetal transmission are infrequent (estimated at 5%).
- No identifiable risk in 40% to 50% of community-acquired hepatitis C, but snorting of cocaine by shared use of straw or rolled-up paper has been identified as a risk factor because it causes microscopic bleeding of nasal mucosa.
- HCV infection may stimulate production of cytotoxic T lymphocytes and cytokines (INF-γ), which probably mediate hepatic necrosis.

Dx DIAGNOSIS

DIFFERENTIAL DIAGNOSIS

- Other hepatitis viruses (A, B, D, E).
- Other viral illnesses producing systemic disease (e.g., yellow fever, EBV, CMV, HIV, rubella, rubeola, coxsackie B, adenovirus, HSV, HZV).
- Nonviral hepatitis (e.g., leptospirosis, toxoplasmosis, alcoholic hepatitis, drug-induced hepatitis [acetaminophen, INH], toxic hepatitis).

WORKUP

- Acute hepatitis C antibody, viral genotyping, viral titers.
- LFTs; CBC.

NOTE: ALT is an easy and inexpensive test to monitor infection and efficacy of therapy. However, ALT levels may fluctuate or even be normal in active or chronic infection and even with cirrhosis, and ALT may remain elevated even after clearance of viremia.

TABLE 1 Factors Associated With Progression of Hepatic Fibrosis in Patients With Chronic Hepatitis C Virus Infection

Established	Possible	Not Associated
Age >40 years	Increased hepatic iron concentration	Viral genotype
Alcohol consumption	Male gender	Viral load
Hepatitis B virus coinfection	Serum ALT level	
HIV coinfection		
Immunosuppressed state		
Insulin resistance		
Marijuana use		
Obesity		
Schistosomiasis		
Severe hepatic necroinflammation		
Smoking		
White race		

From Feldman M et al [eds]: *Sleisenger and Fordtran's gastrointestinal and liver disease*, ed 10, Philadelphia, 2016, Saunders.

TABLE 2 Factors Associated With Cirrhosis in Persons With Hepatitis C Infection

Factor	Impact	Comment
Environmental		
Alcohol use	+4	The importance of minimal alcohol ingestion (<20 g/day) has not been established
Host		
HIV infection	+4	Increasingly important as HIV-related survival improves; may be masked by competing mortality
HBV infection	+3	Strong effect when HBsAg positive; relatively uncommon
Age	+4	Strong effect; increases as low as 40 yr. Hard to distinguish from infection duration
Body mass index	+2	Associated with metabolic syndrome
Duration of HCV infection	+3	Cirrhosis is rare before 10 yr
HLA type	+1?	HLA B54 is correlated with increased risk of cirrhosis; DRB1*0301 with lack of cirrhosis
Viral		
Quasispecies complexity	+1	Cross-sectional studies cannot assess causality, and complexity may be confounded by duration of infection
HCV genotype 1	+1?	Genotype 1b in some, but not other studies, could be confounded by longer duration of 1b infections
Quantitative measures of viremia (serum or plasma HCV RNA level)	+2	Not always detected or lost in multivariate analysis of age or HIV

HCV, Hepatitis C virus; *HIV,* human immunodeficiency virus; *HLA,* human leukocyte antigen; *RNA,* ribonucleic acid.
From Bennett JE et al: *Mandell, Douglas, and Bennett's principles and practice of infectious diseases*, ed 8, Philadelphia, 2015, Saunders.

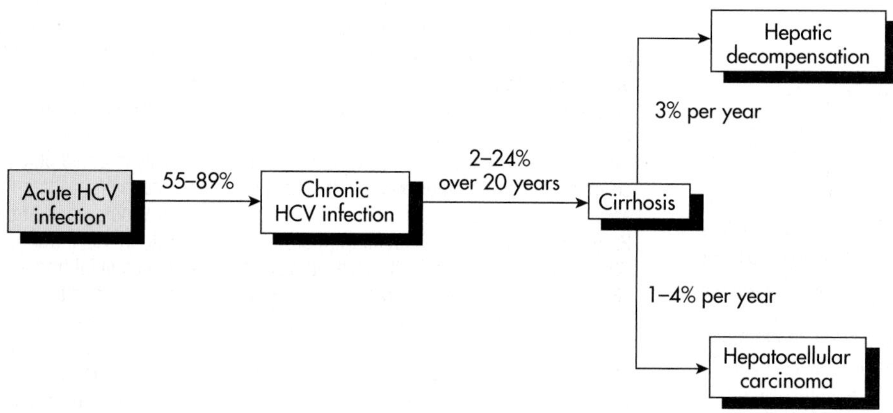

FIG. 1 Natural history of HCV infection. Hepatic decompensation includes ascites, hepatic encephalopathy, variceal hemorrhage, hepatorenal syndrome, or hepatic synthetic dysfunction. (From Feldman M et al [eds]: *Sleisenger and Fordtran's gastrointestinal and liver disease*, ed 10, Philadelphia, 2016, Saunders.)

- Liver biopsy with histologic staging is the gold standard for assessing the degree of disease activity and the likelihood of disease progression, and also to help rule out other causes of liver disease.
- Transient elastography (Fibroscan) is a noninvasive specialized ultrasound assessment that quantifies liver fibrosis and corresponds it to the equivalent in the METAVIR scoring system traditionally used in liver biopsies. It is being increasingly used in place of liver biopsy in many institutions.

LABORATORY TESTS

- Diagnosis is often by exclusion, because it takes 6 wk to 12 mo to develop anti-HCV antibody (70% positive by 6 wk, 90% positive by 6 mo).
- Diagnostic tests include serologic assays for antibodies and molecular tests for viral particles.
  1. Enzyme immunoassay is the test for anti-HCV antibody:
     The current version can detect antibody within 4 to 10 wk after infection.
     False-negative rate in low-risk populations is 0.5% to 1%.
     False negatives also occur in immunecompromised persons, HIV-1, renal failure, HCV-associated essential mixed cryoglobulinemia.
     False positives in autoimmune hepatitis, paraproteinemia, and persons with no risk factors.
- The recombinant immunoblot assay that was previously recommended as a follow-up to positive antibody test is no longer available. The CDC now recommends that anyone who tests positive for HCV antibodies receive a follow-up HCV RNA test.
- Qualitative and quantitative HCV RNA tests using PCR: Lower limit of detection is <43 IU/ml.
- Used to confirm viremia and to assess response to treatment.
- Qualitative polymerase chain reaction (PCR) useful in patients with negative enzyme immunoassay in whom infection is suspected.
- Quantitative tests use either branched-chain DNA or reverse transcription PCR; the latter is more sensitive.
- Viral genotyping can distinguish among genotypes 1, 2, 3, 4, 5, and 6, which is helpful in choosing therapy; most of these tests use PCR. Genotypes 1, 2, 3, and 4 predominate in the United States and Europe (genotype 1 is especially common in North America [60% to 75% of Hep C infections in the United States]).
- FibroSure score uses a combination of six serum markers of liver function plus age and gender in a patented algorithm to generate a measure of fibrosis and necroinflammatory activity in the liver as a quantitative surrogate marker for the corresponding METAVIR scoring system.
- LFTs: ALT and AST may be elevated to more than eight times normal in acute infection; in chronic infection ALT may be normal or fluctuate.
- Bilirubin may be five to 10 times normal.
- Albumin and prothrombin time generally normal; if abnormal, may be harbinger of impending hepatic necrosis.
- WBC and erythrocyte sedimentation rate (ESR) are generally normal.
- HIV testing. Infection with HCV is seen in 15% to 30% of individuals with HIV infection due to shared risk factors.
- All patients infected with HCV should be tested for Hepatitis B. HBV vaccination is recommended for susceptible individuals,

because HBV reactivation may occur during treatment of HCV with direct-acting antiviral therapy.

IMAGING STUDIES

- Transient elastography (Fibroscan) to quantify liver fibrosis as an absolute score. Some insurance companies use this score as a basis to determine eligibility for treatment.
- Sonogram: Rapid liver size reduction during fulminant hepatitis or mass in HCC.

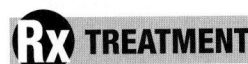

TREATMENT

NONPHARMACOLOGIC THERAPY

Activity and diet as tolerated; avoid saw palmetto and green tea leaf herbs.

ACUTE GENERAL Rx

- Supportive care.
- Avoid hepatically metabolized drugs.

CHRONIC Rx

Response to therapy is influenced by HCV genotype. Recommendations for the treatment of hepatitis C in adults are changing constantly as new therapies come to the market. The advent of direct-acting antiviral agents (DAAs) has drastically changed treatment options and improved cure rates to greater than 95%. The most up-to-date guidance is available at the website www.hcvguidelines.org. The following is a brief summary of the guidelines based on genotype. Newer agents containing fixed-dose combinations of direct-acting antiviral (DAA) drugs have been approved for HCV infections caused by any of the six major HCV genotypes in patients without cirrhosis or with compensated cirrhosis. These agents are Mavyret (combination of glecaprevir, an HCV NS3/4A protease inhibitor, and pibrentasvir, an NS5A inhibitor) and Vosevi (combination of the NS5B nucleotide polymerase inhibitor sofosbuvir, the NS5A inhibitor velpatasvir, and the NS3/4A protease inhibitor voxilaprevir). Both agents are approved for use in treatment-experienced patients and Mavyret is also approved for treatment-naïve patients. Currently, these treatment regimens are extremely expensive.

Genotype 1a: Options for treatment-naïve patients without cirrhosis, listed by level of evidence:

- Daily fixed-dose combination of elbasvir (50 mg)/grazoprevir (100 mg) [Zepatier] for 12 wk and in those who do not have baseline NS5A RAVs (amino acid substitutions at 28, 30, 31, or 93 that confer resistance to elbasvir). Rating: Class I, Level A.
- Daily fixed-dose combination of glecaprevir (300 mg)/pibrentasvir (120 mg) [Mavyret] for 8 weeks. Rating: Class I, Level A
- Daily fixed-dose combination of ledipasvir (90 mg)/sofosbuvir (400 mg) [Harvoni] for 12 wk. Rating: Class I, Level A. (Can also use this regimen for only 8 wk for patients who are non-black, HIV-uninfected, and whose HCV RNA level is <6 million IU/ml. Rating: Class I, Level B.)
- Daily fixed-dose combination of sofosbuvir (400 mg)/velpatasvir (100 mg) [Epclusa] for 12 weeks. Rating: Class I, Level A
- Alternative regimens:
  1. Daily fixed-dose combination of paritaprevir (150 mg)/ritonavir (100 mg)/ombitasvir (25 mg) with dasabuvir (600 mg) as part of an extended-release regimen or plus twice-daily dosed dasabuvir (250 mg) with weight-based ribavirin for 12 weeks. Rating: Class I, Level A.
  2. Daily simeprevir (150 mg) plus sofosbuvir (400 mg) for 12 weeks. Rating: Class I, Level A
  3. Daily daclatasvir (60 mg) plus sofosbuvir (400 mg) daily for 12 weeks. Rating: Class I, Level B
  4. Daily fixed-dose combination of elbasvir (50 mg)/grazoprevir (100 mg) [Zepatier] with weight-based ribavirin for patients with baseline NS5A RADs for elbasvir for 16 weeks. Rating; Class IIa, Level B

Genotype 1a: Options for treatment-naïve patients with compensated cirrhosis:

- Daily fixed-dose combination of elbasvir (50 mg)/grazoprevir (100 mg) [Zepatier] and in those in whom no baseline NS5A RAVs for elbasvir are detected for 12 wk. Rating: Class I, Level A.
- Daily fixed-dose combination of glecaprevir (300 mg)/pibrentasvir (120 mg) [Mavyret] for 12 weeks. Rating: Class I, Level A
- Daily fixed-dose combination of ledipasvir (90 mg)/sofosbuvir (400 mg) [Harvoni] for 12 wk. Rating: Class I, Level A.
- Daily fixed-dose combination of sofosbuvir (400 mg)/velpatasvir (100 mg) [Epclusa] for 12 wk. Rating: Class I, Level A.
- Alternative regimen:
  1. Daily fixed-dose combination of elbasvir (50 mg)/grazoprevir (100 mg) [Zepatier] with weight-based ribavirin for 16 wk for patients who have baseline NS5A RASs. Rating: Class IIa, Level B.

Genotype 1b: Treatment-naïve patients without cirrhosis:

- Daily fixed-dose combination of elbasvir (50 mg)/grazoprevir (100 mg) [Zepatier] for 12 wk. Rating: Class I, Level A.
- Daily fixed-dose combination of glecaprevir (300 mg)/pibrentasvir (120 mg) [Mavyret] for 8 weeks. Rating: Class I, A
- Daily fixed-dose combination of ledipasvir (90 mg)/sofosbuvir (400 mg) [Harvoni] for 12 wk. Rating: Class I, Level A. (Can treat for 8 wk in patients who are non-black, HIV-uninfected, and whose HCV RNA level is <6 million IU/ml. Class I, Level B.)
- Daily fixed-dose combination of sofosbuvir (400 mg)/velpatasvir (100 mg) [Epclusa] for 12 weeks. Rating: Class I, Level A
- Alternative regimens:
  1. Daily fixed-dose combination of paritaprevir (150 mg)/ritonavir (100 mg)/ombitasvir (25 mg) with dasabuvir (600 mg) as part of an extended-release regimen or plus twice-daily dosed dasabuvir (250 mg) for 12 weeks. Rating: Class I, Level A
  2. Daily simeprevir (150 mg) plus sofosbuvir (400 mg) daily for 12 weeks. Rating: Class I, Level A
  3. Daily daclatasvir (60 mg) plus sofosbuvir (400 mg) for 12 weeks. Rating: Class I, Level B

Genotype 1b: Treatment-naïve patients with compensated cirrhosis:

- Daily fixed-dose combination of elbasvir (50 mg)/grazoprevir (100 mg) [Zepatier] for 12 wk. Rating: Class I, Level A.
- Daily fixed-dose combination of glecaprevir (300 mg)/pibrentasvir (120 mg) [Mavyret] for 12 weeks. Rating: Class I, Level A
- Daily fixed-dose combination of ledipasvir (90 mg)/sofosbuvir [Harvoni] for 12 wk. Rating: Class I, Level A.
- Daily fixed-dose combination of sofosbuvir (400 mg)/velpatasvir (100 mg) [Epclusa] for 12 wk. Rating: Class I, Level A.
- Alternative regimens:
  1. Daily fixed-dose combination of paritaprevir (150 mg)/ritonavir (100 mg)/ombitasvir (25 mg) with dasabuvir (600 mg) as part of an extended-release regimen or plus twice-daily dosed dasabuvir (250 mg) for 12 weeks Rating: Class I, Level A.

Genotype 2: Treatment-naïve regimens without cirrhosis:

- Daily fixed-dose combination of glecaprevir (300 mg)/pibrentasvir (120 mg) [Mavyret] for 8 weeks. Rating: Class I, Level A
- Daily fixed-dose combination of sofosbuvir (400 mg)/velpatasvir (100 mg) [Epclusa] for 12 wk. Rating: Class I, Level A.
- Alternative regimen: Daily daclatasvir (60 mg) plus sofosbuvir (400 mg) for 12 wk. Rating: Class IIa, Level B.

Genotype 2: Treatment-naïve patients with compensated cirrhosis:

- Daily fixed-dose combination of sofosbuvir (400 mg)/velpatasvir (100 mg) [Epclusa] for 12 wk. Rating: Class I, Level A.
- Daily fixed-dose combination of glecaprevir (300 mg)/pibrentsavir (120 mg) for 12 weeks. Rating: Class I, Level B
- Alternative regimen: Daily daclatasvir (60 mg) plus sofosbuvir (400 mg) for 16 to 24 wk. Rating: Class IIa, Level B.

Genotype 3: Treatment-naïve patients without cirrhosis:

- Daily fixed-dose of glecaprevir (300 mg)/pibrentasvir (120 mg) for 8 weeks. Rating: Class I, Level A
- Daily fixed-dose combination of sofosbuvir (400 mg)/velpatasvir (100 mg) [Epclusa] for 12 weeks. Rating: Class I, Level A.
- Alternative regimen: Daily daclatasvir (60 mg) plus sofosbuvir (400 mg) for 12 weeks. Rating: Class I, Level A

Genotype 3: Treatment-naïve patients with compensated cirrhosis:

- Daily fixed-dose combination of glecaprevir (300 mg)/pibrentasvir (120 mg) [Mavyret] for 12 weeks. Rating: Class I, Level A
- Daily fixed-dose combination of sofosbuvir (400 mg)/velpatasvir (100 mg) [Epclusa] for 12 wk. Rating: Class I, Level A.

- Alternative regimens:
  1. Daily fixed-dose combination of sofosbuvir (400 mg)/velpatasvir (100 mg)/voxilaprevir (100 mg) [Vosevi] when Y93H amino acid substitution is present for 12 weeks. Rating: IIa, Level B.
  2. Daily daclatasvir (60 mg) plus sofosbuvir (400 mg) with or without weight-based ribavirin for 24 weeks. Rating: Class IIa, Level B

Genotype 4: Treatment-naïve patients without cirrhosis:

- Daily fixed-dose combination of glecaprevir (300 mg)/pibrentasvir (120 mg) {Mavyret] for 8 weeks. Rating: Class I Level A.
- Daily fixed-dose combination of sofosbuvir (400 mg)/velpatasvir (100 mg) [Epclusa] for 12 weeks. Rating: Class I, Level A.
- Daily fixed-dose combination of elbasvir (50 mg)/grazoprevir (100 mg) [Zepatier] for 12 weeks. Rating: Class IIa, Level B.
- Daily fixed-dose combination of ledipasvir (90 mg)/sofosbuvir (400 mg) [Harvoni] for 12 weeks. Rating: Class IIa, Level B.
- Alternative regimen: Daily fixed-dose combination of paritaprevir (150 mg)/ritonavir (100 mg)/ombitasvir (25 mg) and weight-based ribavirin for 12 weeks. Rating: Class I, Level A

Genotype 4: Treatment-naïve patients with compensated cirrhosis:

- Daily fixed-dose combination of sofosbuvir (400 mg)/velpatasvir (100 mg) [Epclusa] for 12 weeks. Rating: Class I, Level A.
- Daily fixed-dose combination of glecaprevir (300 mg)/pibrentasvir (120 mg) [Mavyret] for 12 weeks. Rating: Class I, Level B.
- Daily fixed-dose combination of elbasvir (50 mg)/grazoprevir (100 mg) [Zepatier] for 12 wk. Rating: Class IIa, Level B.
- Daily fixed-dose combination of ledipasvir (90 mg)/sofosbuvir (400 mg) [Harvoni] for 12 wk. Rating: Class IIa, Level B.
- Alternative regimen: Daily fixed-dose combination of paritaprevir (150 mg)/ritonavir (100 mg)/ombitasvir (25 mg) and weight-based ribavirin for 12 weeks. Rating: Class I, Level A

Genotypes 5 and 6: Treatment-naïve patients with and without cirrhosis:

- Daily fixed-dose combination of glecaprevir (300 mg)/pibrentasvir (120 mg) for 8 weeks with no cirrhosis. Rating: Class I, Level A and 12 weeks with compensated cirrhosis. Rating: Class I, Level A
- Daily fixed-dose combination of sofosbuvir (400 mg)/velpatasvir (100 mg) [Epclusa] for 12 wk. Rating: Class I, Level B.
- Daily fixed-dose combination of ledipasvir (90 mg)/sofosbuvir (400 mg) [Harvoni] for 12 wk. Rating: Class IIa, Level B.

Drug interactions can be significant with these regimens (http://www.hepdruginteractions.org). With DAA regimens, viral loads are measured at 4 wk into the therapy to monitor success and at the end of therapy. A final viral load is measured 12 wk after completing the treatment, and if undetectable, the patient is considered to have a sustained virologic response (SVR), which equates to a cure.

For *treatment-experienced* patients there are guidelines per genotype as well (www.hcvguidelines.org). Treatment is based on genotype and whether the patient is without cirrhosis or with compensated cirrhosis. Regimen will depend on whether the patient had been exposed in the past to interferon/ribavirin-based regimens, NS3 protease inhibitors regimens (telaprevir, boceprevir, simeprevir), or DAA agents.

In 2017, a new salvage regimen was approved: Once-daily Vosevi (fixed-dose combination of 100 mg voxilaprevir (HCV NS3/4A protease inhibitor) plus 400 mg sofosbuvir and 100 mg velpatasvir. Eligible patients include:

- Genotypes 1, 2, 3, 4, 5, or 6 in patients previously treated with a regimen containing an NS5A inhibitor for 12 wk (Note: In clinical trials, prior experience with NS5A inhibitors included daclatasvir, elbasavir, ledipasvir, ombitasvir, or velpatasvir)
- Genotype 1a or 3 in patients previously treated with sofosbuvir without an NS5A inhibitor for 12 wk. (Note: In clinical trials, prior treatment experience included sofosbuvir with or without any of the following: peginterferon alfa/ribivirin, ribivirin, HCV NS3/4A protease inhibitors: boceprevir, simeprevir, or telaprevir.)
- Liver transplantation:
  1. Hepatitis C is the main indication for liver transplantation in the United States.
  2. It is the only option for patients with deteriorating HCV-related cirrhosis and for some patients with HCC.
  3. Recurrent infection occurs in almost all patients with progressive fibrosis and cirrhosis; as many as 20% progress to cirrhosis within 5 yr posttransplant.

DISPOSITION

- The absence of HCV RNA in blood 12 wk after completion of treatment is considered a cure. There is no need to check HCV antibodies since they will remain positive indefinitely.
- SVR after treatment among HCV-infected persons at any stage of fibrosis is associated with reduced HCC.
- Periodic abdominal ultrasonography for HCC screening.
- Recent guidelines recommend against measurement of alpha-fetoprotein (AFP) to screen for HCC in patients with chronic hepatitis C due to lack of sensitivity, specificity, and predictive values.

REFERRAL

- To a hepatologist or infectious disease specialist for treatment for hepatitis C in patients who have been previously treated or for treatment failures with DAA agents.
- To a transplant surgeon for consideration of liver transplant if indicated.

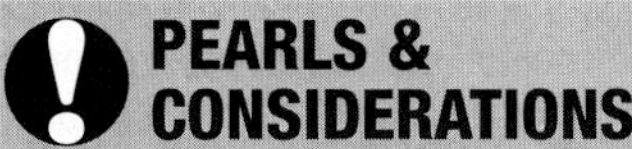

PEARLS & CONSIDERATIONS

- More rapid progression of disease in persons who drink alcohol regularly, persons of advanced age at time of infection, and those coinfected with other viruses (HIV, hepatitis B). All persons with identified HCV infection should receive a brief alcohol screening and intervention as clinically indicated.
- Regression of cirrhosis has been demonstrated after antiviral therapy in some patients with chronic hepatitis C. Regression is associated with decreased disease-related morbidity and improved survival.
- The presence of interleukin (IL)-28B and HLA class II is independently associated with spontaneous resolution of HCV infection, and single nucleotide polymorphism IL-28B and DQB1*03:01 may explain approximately 15% of spontaneous resolution of HCV infection.

SUGGESTED READINGS

Available at ExpertConsult.com

RELATED CONTENT

Hepatitis C (Patient Information)

AUTHOR: **GLENN G. FORT, M.D., M.P.H.**

H

Diseases and Disorders

BASIC INFORMATION

DEFINITION

Hepatocellular carcinoma (HCC) is a malignant neoplasm of the hepatocytes.

SYNONYMS

Hepatoma
HCC

EPIDEMIOLOGY & DEMOGRAPHICS

HCC is the fifth most common cancer worldwide (~600,000 new cases/yr) and the second most common cause of cancer deaths. Incidence varies worldwide:

- 85% of patients with hepatocellular carcinoma have cirrhosis.
- Areas with high rates of hepatitis B and C (East Asia, sub-Saharan Africa) have highest incidence.
- Males more affected than females, with ratios between 2:1 and 4:1.
- Peak incidence: Fifth and sixth decades in Western countries, earlier in areas with perinatal transmission of hepatitis B.
- Incidence has grown in the U.S. due to chronic hepatitis C, increasing obesity, and diabetes mellitus.
  1. During the past two decades, the incidence in the U.S. doubled. In 2013, an estimated 25,600 cases were recorded. The greatest proportional increase has been among Hispanics and whites between 45 and 60 yr of age.
  2. Mean age of diagnosis approximately 65 yr.
  3. HCC is the fastest-rising cause of cancer-related deaths in the U.S.
  4. The incidence in the U.S. is expected to increase to 38,350 cases by 2020 and 56,200 cases by 2030.
- Risk factors:
  1. Chronic hepatitis B infection accounts for 50% of all cases and most childhood cases.
  2. Chronic hepatitis C infection markers are found in 80% to 90% of patients with HCC in Japan and 30% to 50% in the U.S.
  3. Cirrhosis from other causes: Alcoholic liver disease, nonalcoholic steatohepatitis, primary biliary cirrhosis, hemochromatosis, α1-antitrypsin deficiency, and autoimmune hepatitis.
  4. Hepatotoxins: Aflatoxin B1.
  5. Systemic diseases affecting the liver: Tyrosinemia.
  6. Obesity and diabetes mellitus.

PHYSICAL FINDINGS & CLINICAL PRESENTATION

- One third of patients are asymptomatic.
- Abdominal pain may be the initial presentation.
- Signs of underlying cirrhosis and portal hypertension are often present.
- Previously compensated cirrhosis with new ascites, encephalopathy, jaundice, or bleeding.
- Paraneoplastic syndromes (hypoglycemia, erythrocytosis, hypercalcemia, severe diarrhea, dermatomyositis) may be present. Box 1 summarizes paraneoplastic syndromes associated with hepatocellular carcinoma.
- Table 1 summarizes symptoms and signs of hepatocellular carcinoma.

DIAGNOSIS

DIFFERENTIAL DIAGNOSIS

- Metastatic cancers to liver
- Intrahepatic cholangiocarcinoma
- Benign liver neoplasms (adenomas, focal nodular hyperplasia, and hemangiomas)
- Focal fatty infiltration

WORKUP

- History regarding risk factors
- Physical examination with attention to signs of chronic liver disease
- Laboratory evaluation and imaging studies
- Imaging studies: Ultrasound for initial testing; 3-phase CT scan or dynamic contrast-enhanced MRI

BOX 1 Paraneoplastic Syndromes Associated with Hepatocellular Carcinoma

Carcinoid syndrome
Hypercalcemia
Hypertension
Hypertrophic osteoarthropathy
Hypoglycemia
Neuropathy
Osteoporosis
Polycythemia (erythrocytosis)
Polymyositis
Porphyria
Sexual changes—isosexual precocity, gynecomastia, feminization
Thyrotoxicosis
Thrombophlebitis migrans
Watery diarrhea syndrome

From Feldman M, Friedman LS, Brandt LJ: *Sleisenger and Fordtran's gastrointestinal and liver disease*, ed 10, Philadelphia, 2016, Elsevier.

TABLE 1 Symptoms and Signs of Hepatocellular Carcinoma

Symptom	Frequency (%)
Abdominal pain	59-95
Weight loss	34-71
Weakness	22-53
Abdominal swelling	28-43
Nonspecific GI symptoms	25-28
Jaundice	5-26
Sign	
Hepatomegaly	54-98
Ascites	35-61
Fever	11-54
Splenomegaly	27-42
Wasting	25-41
Jaundice	4-35
Hepatic bruit	6-25

GI, Gastrointestinal. From Feldman M, Friedman LS, Brandt LJ: *Sleisenger and Fordtran's gastrointestinal and liver disease*, ed 10, Philadelphia, 2016, Elsevier.

LABORATORY TESTS

- Liver function tests.
- α-Fetoprotein (AFP) levels can be elevated in 70% of patients. An AFP level >400 ng/ml is highly suggestive of HCC; however, elevations may not be seen in up to 40% of patients with small lesions (1-2 cm).
- Paraneoplastic syndromes associated with HCC may cause hypercalcemia, hypoglycemia, and polycythemia.
- Elevated serum HBV DNA level (≥10,000 copies/ml) is a strong risk predictor of HCC independent of HBeAg, serum aminotransferase level, and liver cirrhosis.

IMAGING STUDIES

Ultrasound (US), CT scan (Fig. 1), or MRI. Ultrasound is most commonly used as a screening test for HCC in high-risk patients every 6 months. Fig. E2 shows a laparoscopic view of a cirrhotic liver with a nodular hepatoma.

The following imaging modalities are recommended based on US findings:

- Hepatic lesion <1 cm needs to be followed with a repeat US every 3 months to ensure the lesion does not change in size. If stable for 24 months, the interval for US can be increased back to every 6 months.
- Hepatic lesion >1 cm needs further confirmatory imaging with either a CT scan or an MRI scan. If the chosen imaging modality shows characteristics typical of HCC (hypervascular in the arterial phase with washout in the portal venous or delayed phase) the diagnosis of HCC is confirmed with no need for additional diagnostic testing or biopsy. If the imaging modality is inconclusive or atypical for HCC then the alternate imaging test must be performed. If the second imaging modality is also inconclusive, an image-guided biopsy is recommended.

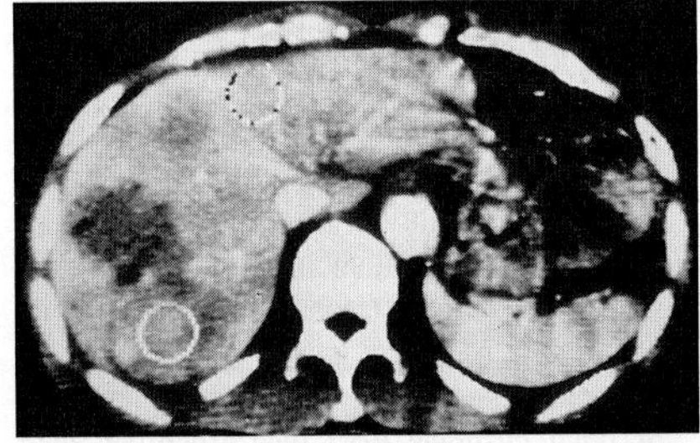

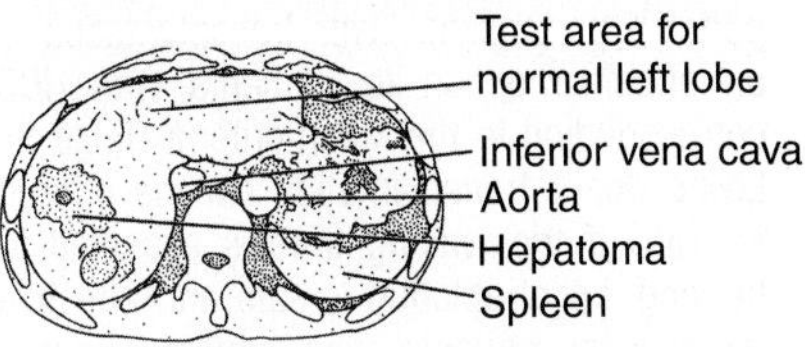

FIG. 1 Hepatoma. CT scan shows a diffuse lesion in the right lobe of an otherwise normal liver. (From Skarin AT: *Atlas of diagnostic oncology*, ed 3, St Louis, 2003, Mosby.)

BIOPSY: Percutaneous biopsy under ultrasound or CT scan is obtained in the event that imaging studies are nondiagnostic or atypical for HCC, or if no cirrhosis is present. Negative biopsy results should be followed and the hepatic nodule reassessed every 3 to 6 months until it is no longer seen, enlarges, or shows diagnostic characteristics.

SCREENING: Screening high-risk patients with US every 6 months is currently recommended to identify early-stage HCC. The use of AFP in addition to US is debatable; though it does increase detection rate it also increases false-positive results. The use of AFP alone should be discouraged due to limited sensitivity and specificity. Patients on transplant waiting lists should be regularly screened for HCC because in the U.S. the development of HCC gives increased priority for liver transplantation. Screening for HCC is recommended in the following groups:

- Hepatitis B carriers (HBsAg positive): Asian males >40 yr, Asian females >50 yr, all cirrhotic hepatitis B carriers, family history of HCC and North American blacks/Africans older than age 20 yr
- Cirrhosis (nonhepatitis B): Hepatitis C, alcoholic cirrhosis, hemochromatosis, primary biliary cirrhosis, and possibly α1-antitrypsin deficiency, autoimmune hepatitis, and nonalcoholic steatohepatitis

STAGING: The commonly used Barcelona Clinic Liver Cancer (BCLC) staging system includes patient performance status, cancer symptoms, number and size of nodules, and liver function. Treatment is determined according to stage:

- Early stage (A): Asymptomatic single tumor 5 cm or 3 nodules, each ≤3 cm
- Intermediate stage (B): Patients with tumors that exceed early criteria but do not yet show cancer-related symptoms, vascular invasion, or metastases
- Advanced stage (C): Patients with mild cancer-related symptoms and/or vascular invasion or extrahepatic spread
- End-stage (D): Patients with advanced, symptomatic disease

TABLE 2 Treatment Options for Hepatocellular Carcinoma

Treatment Modality	Comments
Surgical resection	Curative but limited to noncirrhotic patients and cirrhotic patients without portal hypertension
Liver transplantation	Successful in selected patients with limited disease; requires lifelong immunosuppression
Radiofrequency ablation or ethanol injection	Potentially curative for small tumors, including multiple tumors
Transarterial chemoembolization (TACE)	Prolongs survival in unresectable tumors if hepatic function is preserved; not curative
Immunotherapy	Checkpoint inhibitors improve survival in previously treated patients
Targeted molecular therapies	Sorafenib and lenvatinib improve patient survival in previously untreated patients Regorafenib and cabozantinib improve patient survival in previously treated patients

Rx TREATMENT

- Treatment options for hepatocellular carcinoma are summarized in Table 2. Fig. 3 describes a treatment algorithm for HCC.
- Early stage: Curative treatment (surgical resection or liver transplantation). Patients who have a single lesion can be offered surgical resection if they are noncirrhotic or have cirrhosis with well-preserved liver function, normal bilirubin, and no significant portal hypertension. Liver transplantation is an effective option for patients with HCC corresponding to the Milan criteria (Table 3). Living donor transplantation can be offered for HCC if the waiting time is expected to be long. Local ablation is safe and effective therapy for patients who cannot undergo resection or as a bridge to transplantation. With these options, survival at 5 yr ranges from 50% to 70%. Radiofrequency ablation (RFA) is used in patients with early HCC who are not surgical candidates, and very high local control rates at 2 yr are obtained (>90%), but eventual recurrence rates can approach 70% at 5 yr.
- Intermediate stage: Transarterial chemoembolization (TACE) is recommended as first-line, noncurative therapy for nonsurgical patients with large/multifocal HCC who do not have vascular invasion or extrahepatic spread. More recently, transarterial use of selective internal radiation therapy (SIRT) with yttrium-90 radiolabeled glass microspheres is an alternative to traditional TACE approaches in this setting. Median survivals exceed 2 yr.
- Advanced stage: Palliative targeted therapy, immunotherapy, or clinical trials are used in this stage. Sorafenib, an oral multikinase inhibitor, is the standard of care and improves overall survival. The effectiveness has been demonstrated in patients with Child-Pugh A cirrhosis, and the greatest benefit is seen in patients with hepatitis C related HCC. The oral targeted inhibitor, lenvatinib, has recently been approved based on improvement in response rates and progression-free survival.
- In patients who have previously received first-line targeted therapy, the oral tyrosine kinase inhibitors regorafenib and cabozantinib have shown improved survival. In addition, the immune checkpoint inhibitors nivolumab and pembrolizumab have demonstrated improved survival when used in the second-line setting.

DISPOSITION

- For resectable HCC, the 5-yr survival after liver transplantation is 50% to 70% and 30% to 50% with surgical resection. For unresectable HCC, the overall prognosis is poor.
- Tumor size is an independent prognostic factor for resected small HCC (≤50 mm in diameter). Patients with tumors of 0-35 mm diameter have a better 60-month HCC specific survival rate than do those with larger tumors (36-50 mm).[1]
- In the U.S. the 5-yr overall survival rate for HCC is approximately 10%.

REFERRAL

Multidisciplinary gastrointestinal cancer team for treatment planning

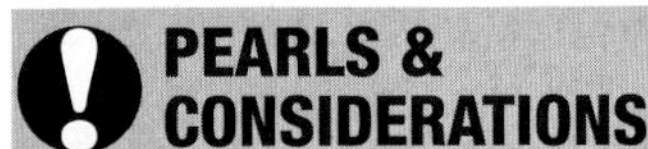

PEARLS & CONSIDERATIONS

PREVENTION

- Universal hepatitis B vaccination in children in endemic areas has been shown to decrease the incidence of HCC.
- Treatment of patients with chronic hepatitis B–associated cirrhosis with lamivudine reduces the incidence of HCC. Treatment with entecavir in chronic hepatitis B-HCC can improve hepatic function and MELD score.
- Treatment with interferon-based therapy in patients with noncirrhotic hepatitis C reduces risk of HCC in patients demonstrating a sustained viral response.
- HCC screening is recommended in high-risk patients because curative therapies are available only for small and early HCC.
- Patients diagnosed with HCC with an AFP >1000 are at increased risk for recurrence after transplantation regardless of tumor size.
- There are numerous ongoing trials with tyrosine kinase inhibitors and monoclonal antibodies for advanced HCC in patients who are intolerant or resistant to sorafenib. The future of therapy for advanced HCC will likely lead to the personalized combination of multiple agents targeting different oncogenic pathways to optimize treatment success.

[1] Zhang W, et al.: Effect of tumor size on cancer-specific survival in small hepatocellular carcinoma, *Mayo Clin Proc* 90(9):1187–1195, 2015.

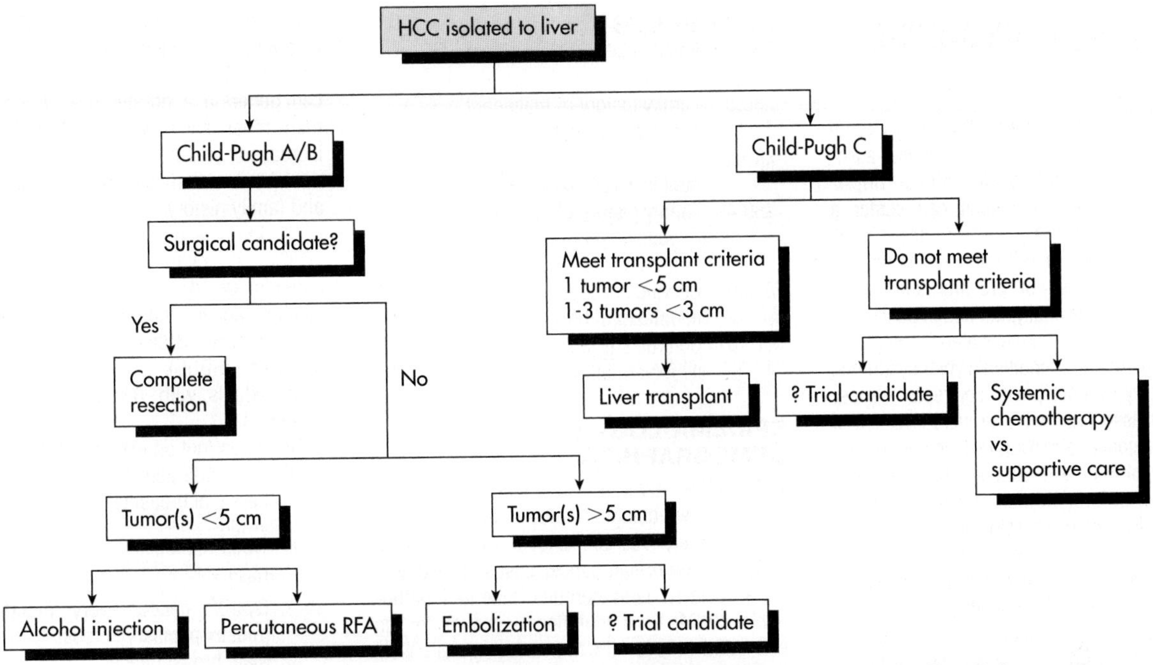

FIG. 3 Treatment algorithm for hepatocellular carcinoma (HCC). *RFA,* Radiofrequency ablation. (From Bruix J, Sherman M; AASLD: Management of hepatocellular carcinoma: an update, *Hepatology* 53(3):1020-1022, 2011.)

TABLE 3 Milan Criteria of Eligibility for Liver Transplantation

Presence of a tumor ≤5 cm in diameter in patients with single hepatocellular carcinomas
Or
≤3 tumor nodules, each 3 cm or less in diameter, in patients with multiple tumors

From Cameron JL, Cameron AM: *Current surgical therapy,* ed 10, Philadelphia, 2011, Saunders.

SUGGESTED READINGS

Available at ExpertConsult.com

RELATED CONTENT

Liver Cancer (Patient Information)

AUTHOR: **BHARTI RATHORE, M.D.**

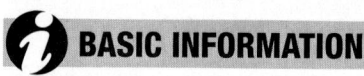

BASIC INFORMATION

DEFINITION

Hereditary breast and ovarian cancer syndrome (HBOC) patients carry a significant cancer-associated alteration in the *BRCA1* and/or *BRCA2* gene. These genetic mutations can confer a heightened risk of malignancy in the breast, ovary, fallopian tube, and peritoneum in women and an elevated risk of prostate and breast cancer in men. Additionally, the risk of pancreatic cancer and skin cancer are elevated for both men and women. Another condition, Lynch syndrome, or hereditary nonpolyposis colorectal cancer (HNPCC) is associated with an increased risk of endometrial cancer and ovarian cancer in women and cancer of the colon, stomach, pancreas, and small bowel in both women and men. Patients with Lynch syndrome carry significant pathogenic alterations in five genes, as noted below.

The risk for a particular verified genetically associated cancer is significantly greater than the cancer risk associated with the general population or with one's personal and/or family cancer history alone, without a positive genetic test. Frequently, a cancer that is associated with a heritable genetic mutation presents at a younger age than that seen in the general population is a relatively rare type of cancer and/or affects multiple same-side family members. Identifying carriers can significantly reduce the morbidity and mortality of the patient and her/his close family members.

SYNONYMS

Hereditary breast and ovarian cancer syndrome (HBOC)
Lynch syndrome/hereditary nonpolyposis colorectal cancer (HNPCC)
Hereditary cancer syndrome

ICD-10CM CODES

Z84.81 Family history of carrier of genetic disease
Z80.3 Family history of malignant neoplasm of breast
Z80.41 Family history of malignant neoplasm of ovary
Z80.49 Family history of malignant neoplasm of other genital organs (uterus, vagina, for example)
Z15.01 Genetic susceptibility to malignant neoplasm of breast
Z15.02 Genetic susceptibility to malignant neoplasm of ovary

EPIDEMIOLOGY & DEMOGRAPHICS

INCIDENCE: Overall, an estimated 6% to 10% of gynecologic cancers are heritable. Approximately 7% to 10% of the estimated 235,000 new breast cancer cases are likely to be associated with heredity. Inherited pathogenic *BRCA 1, 2* mutations account for an estimated 11% to 15% of ovarian cancer cases. Less than 1% of the general population has a pathogenic mutation in the *BRCA 1* or *2* gene. As noted above, Lynch syndrome–associated mutations increase ovarian and uterine cancer as well as colorectal (up to 5% of colorectal cancers are considered heritable), pancreatic, and gastric cancers. This article will, however, focus on gynecologic disease. Table 1 provides examples of hereditary cancer syndromes and their associated genes.

PREDOMINANT SEX AND AGE: Although females are predominantly affected, males who carry deleterious mutations in *BRCA 1, 2* are at a significantly higher risk for cancer. Both sexes can transmit the altered gene to their offspring.

GENETICS: The transmission pattern is autosomal dominant. A child whose father or mother has a *BRCA* mutation has a 50% chance of inheriting that genetic mutation.

RISK FACTORS: *BRCA1* and *BRCA2* mutations can generate a greater risk of breast cancer than other such well-established factors as increased breast density, history of atypical ductal or lobular hyperplasia, nulliparity, obesity, and family history.

Up to 37% of breast cancer patients and 100% of ovarian/tubal/peritoneal cancer patients are at risk for hereditary breast and ovarian cancer syndrome.

Hereditary Breast and Ovarian Cancer Syndrome (HBOC):

- Individuals with *BRCA1, BRCA2* mutations (Fig. 1)
- Red flags (not an exhaustive list) for possible HBOC include personal or family history of:
  1. Personal breast cancer diagnosed at $\leq$45 yr old
  2. Triple-negative breast cancer (ER-, PR-, Her2-)
  3. Ovarian cancer—very important factor (mostly papillary serous)
  4. Male breast cancer
  5. Two primary breast cancers
  6. Ashkenazi Jewish ancestry
  7. Breast cancer with $\geq$2 relatives with an HBOC-associated cancer (breast, ovary, prostate, pancreatic cancers)
  8. A previously identified HBOC mutation
  9. Two or more close relatives with breast cancer, one of whom was diagnosed at age 50 yr or younger
  10. Three or more HBOC-associated cancers at any age

NOTE:

- One half of *BRCA* carriers inherit the mutation from their father.
- Early onset of cancer may be a more important red flag than the number of affected

TABLE 1 Examples of Hereditary Cancer Syndromes and Their Associated Genes

	Breast Cancer	Ovarian Cancer	Colorectal Cancer	Uterine Cancer	Melanoma	Pancreatic Cancer	Stomach Cancer	Prostate Cancer	Leukemia
Hereditary Breast Ovarian Cancer Syndrome									
BRCA1	*	*				*		*	
BRCA2	*	*			*	*		*	
Lynch Syndrome									
MLH1		*	*	*		*	*		
MSH2		*	*	*		*	*		
MSH6		*	*	*		*	*		
PMS2		*	*	*		*	*		
Familial Adenomatous Polyposis Syndrome									
APC			*			*	*		
Li-Fraumeni Syndrome									
TP53	*	*	*	*	*	*	*	*	*
Cowden's Syndrome									
PTEN	*		*	*	*				
Peutz-Jeghers Syndrome									
STK11	*	*	*	*		*	*		
Hereditary Diffuse Gastric Cancer Syndrome									
CDH 1	*		*				*		

From Cameron JL, Cameron AM: *Current surgical therapy*, ed 12, Philadelphia, 2017, Elsevier.

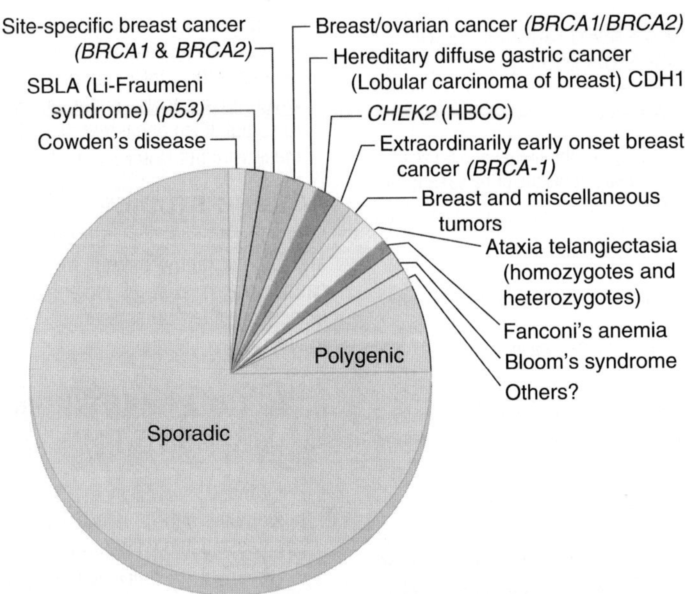

FIG. 1 Schematic depicting heterogeneity in breast cancer. *HBCC,* hereditary breast and colorectal cancer; *SBLA,* sarcoma, breast and brain tumors, leukemia, laryngeal and lung cancer, and adrenal cortical carcinoma. (From Goldman L, Schafer AI: *Goldman's Cecil medicine*, ed 24, Philadelphia, 2012, Saunders.)

TABLE 2 Testing Criteria for Breast Ovarian Cancer Syndrome*
Individual from a family with a known deleterious *BRCA1* or *BRCA2* gene mutation
Personal history of breast cancer plus one or more of the following:
Diagnosed at ≤45 years of age
Diagnosed at ≤50 years of age with
An additional breast cancer primary
At least one close blood relative with breast cancer at any age
At least one close relative with pancreatic cancer
At least one close relative with prostate cancer
An unknown or limited family history
Diagnosed at of age 60 with
Triple-negative breast cancer
Diagnosed at any age with
At least one close blood relative with breast cancer before 50 years of age
At least two close blood relatives with breast cancer at any age
At least one close blood relative with ovarian cancer
At least one close blood relative with pancreatic cancer
At least two close blood relatives with prostate cancer
A close female blood relative with ovarian cancer
An individual of ethnicity associated with a higher mutation frequency
Personal history of ovarian cancer
Personal history of male breast cancer
Personal history of prostate cancer at any age with a close relative with breast, ovarian, or pancreatic cancer at any age
Personal history of pancreatic cancer and Ashkenazi Jewish ancestry
Family history meeting any of the above criteria
See NCCN guidelines for the most up-to-date and detailed description for counseling and testing.

*For more detailed information, see the National Comprehensive Cancer Network (NCCN) guidelines.
From Disaia PJ et al: *Clinical gynecologic oncology*, ed 9, Philadelphia, 2017, Elsevier.

family members, especially if the number of family members is small to begin with.

- Testing criteria (Tables 2 and 3), as per National Comprehensive Cancer Network (NCCN) guidelines, may differ from the red flags noted previously.
- Family history extends to first-, second-, and third-degree relatives.
- Consider Lynch syndrome–associated cancers (e.g., colorectal, gastric, brain, pancreas, small bowel, skin, ureter, renal pelvis, GI polyps), as Lynch syndrome is associated also with ovarian and uterine (endometrial) cancer.
- *BRCA* stands for BReast CAncer.
  1. The majority (84%) of the approximately 7% of breast cancers and 14% of ovarian cancers that result from a heritable mutation are due to a *BRCA1* (52%) and *BRCA2* (32%) gene mutation.
  2. By age 70, in comparison to the 7.3% risk of breast cancer in the general population, or approximately double that risk if one has an affected first-degree relative, *BRCA1* and *BRCA2* mutation carriers have up to an 87% reported risk of developing breast cancer. As opposed to a general-population risk of 2% for developing a second breast primary within 5 yr of a first diagnosis, women with HBOC mutations have a 12% to 27% risk. This risk climbs to a reported 50% (*BRCA2*) and up to 64% (*BRCA1*) by age 70.
  3. By age 70, in contrast to the 0.7% risk of ovarian cancer in the general population, there is a reported risk of up to 27% to 63% for *BRCA2* and *BRCA1* mutation carriers, respectively. The risk for ovarian cancer within 10 yr of a breast cancer diagnosis is 6.8% (*BRCA2*) to 12.7% (*BRCA1*) as opposed to a general-population risk of less than 1.0%.
  4. Men with HBOC have an up to tenfold increased risk for breast cancer and a more than twofold increase in prostate cancer in comparison to the general-population risk. In men, the *BRCA2* mutation increases the cancer risk more than the *BRCA1* mutation. In fact, the breast cancer risk for a male with a *BRCA2* mutation is up to 80 times the risk seen in the general population.
  5. Both men and women have an elevated risk (up to sevenfold) for pancreatic cancer (*BRCA2* >1) and for melanoma (2.5-fold increase with *BRCA2*).
  6. Ashkenazi Jewish ancestry is associated with founder mutations 187delAG (*BRCA1*), 5382insC (*BRCA1*), and 6174delT (*BRCA2*), which confer a significantly elevated risk for breast and ovarian cancer. As opposed to the 1 in 400 risk in the general population, 1 in 40 individuals of Ashkenazi Jewish descent have a *BRCA 1* or *2* mutation.

Lynch Syndrome (Hereditary Nonpolyposis Colorectal Cancer):

- Individuals with *MLH1, MSH2, MSH6, PMS2, EPCAM* mutations.
- By age 70, Lynch syndrome carriers have—in addition to an increased risk for colorectal, gastric, hepatobiliary, urinary tract, small bowel, brain, skin, and pancreatic cancers— up to an approximately twentyfold increase in ovarian cancer (4%-12% risk vs. the general-population risk of 0.7%) and up to an approximately fortyfold increase in uterine cancer (25%-60+% risk vs. the general-population risk of 1.6%).
- The previously listed genes and others (e.g., *PTEN, TP53, CDH1, STK11*) that are found less frequently are considered high-penetrance genes, as they can increase the relative risk of their respective syndromes by greater than four- to fivefold.
- Other, more moderate-penetrant genes (e.g., *CHEK2, ATM, PALB2, BRIP1, RAD51C, RAD51D*), that is, those that are associated with a two- to fourfold increase in the relative risk of cancer, should be considered when assessing risk and ordering genetic tests.
- More than 12 known gene mutations are associated with an elevated risk for breast cancer, and a similar number are associated with an elevated risk for ovarian cancer. As such, screening for *BRCA 1, BRCA2* alone will miss these mutations.

TABLE 3 National Comprehensive Cancer Network (NCCN) Guidelines for Recommending Genetic Testing for *BRCA1* or *BRCA2* Mutations*

Personal history of breast cancer and one or more of the following:

- Diagnosed at age ≤45 years
- Diagnosed with at least two breast cancer primaries (bilateral, separate ipsilateral), the first at age 50 years
- Diagnosed at age ≤50 years with one or more close relatives† with breast cancer (prostate or pancreatic) at any age
- Diagnosed with triple-negative breast cancer at age ≤60 years
- Diagnosed at any age with one or more close relatives with breast cancer at age ≤50 years
- Diagnosed at any age with two or more close relatives at any age
- Diagnosed at any age with one or more close relatives with invasive ovarian cancer (including fallopian tube and primary peritoneal) at any age
- Diagnosed at any age with two or more close relatives with pancreatic and/or prostate cancer
- Having a close male relative with breast cancer at any age

*Individuals with a limited or unknown family history may have an underestimated probability of a familial gene mutation detection.
†Close relative pertains to first-, second- or third-degree blood relatives on the same side (either maternal or paternal) of the family.
From Disaia PJ et al: *Clinical gynecologic oncology*, ed 9, Philadelphia, 2017, Elsevier.

- In addition to established deleterious mismatch repair gene mutations, gene alterations that are categorized in the literature as emerging risk mutations are also associated with hereditary gynecologic and other cancers.

PHYSICAL FINDINGS & CLINICAL PRESENTATION

- Present at a younger age
- Bilaterality more likely
- Multiple primaries in one individual

ETIOLOGY

Hereditary cancers are typically due to a genetic mutation in a tumor suppression gene that interferes with DNA repair and allows an otherwise potentially avoidable cancer to develop. This is distinct from familial cancers in which there is no isolated gene mutation but, nonetheless, cancers appear in the family to a degree more than that which would be statistically seen in the general population. Nongenetic factors such as lifestyle habits and environmental influences contribute to cancer risk as well.

Dx DIAGNOSIS

DIFFERENTIAL DIAGNOSIS

- General (sporadic) population or familial basis for the cancer in question.
- Hereditary cancer is more likely to present at a younger age, to span a number of generations, to affect more family members than would be expected (if a large enough family), especially in a suspicious pattern, and to include some rare (ovary, male breast cancer, for example) presentations.
- In addition to the more common syndromes listed previously, consider Cowden (*PTEN*), Peutz-Jeghers (*STK11*), Li-Fraumeni (*TP53*), and others.

WORKUP

Family history questionnaire, patient and family interviews, genetic counseling/risk assessment (including tools such as Tyrer-Cuzick/Gail/Claus models), and tailored genetic testing.

LABORATORY TESTS

- A simple blood or saliva sample drawn in the office or a lab, after informed consent, is needed. This specimen should be sent to a reliable laboratory recognized nationally for its genetic cancer testing accuracy (technologic and interpretative), reporting format, and the support staff ability and availability for consultation, office counseling, and testing integration. Look for a laboratory that has published peer-reviewed data and has an accurate classification methodology that relies on an extensive database. Realize that these labs are not FDA approved and that CLIA certification, while needed, relies on just in-house data. Remember also that most patients get tested only once in their lifetime, and so accuracy is imperative.
- Options include:
  1. Syndrome specific: For example, HBOC-*BRCA* testing (including large rearrangement detection); Lynch syndrome; founder mutation testing (187delAG, 5382insC, 6174delT)—Ashkenazi Jewish population (often recommended as the first test for this population); single-site testing (if a previously identified gene mutation is known in the family); cancer specific, for example, breast cancer panel–*BRCA 1, 2* with/without reflex to broader panel (i.e., sequential testing).
  2. Comprehensive panel testing (can include HBOC syndrome *BRCA1*, *BRCA2*), Lynch syndrome (*MLH1, MSH2, MSH6, PMS2, EPCAM*), Li-Fraumeni (*TP53*), Cowden (*PTEN*), Peutz-Jeghers (*STK11*), *PALB2, CHEK2, ATM, BRIP1, RAD51C*, and others [upward of 28+ genes]).
- Choice of the test is generally based on personal/family history, although thoroughness of the risk assessment may be limited by attempting to choose a gene test based on history/phenotype alone.
- Comprehensive panel testing has been shown to increase mutation detection and to aid in test selection when patients qualify for more than one syndrome/cancer-specific test, or it can be used to capture a potentially broader view of risk. There is a concern, however, for detecting mutations that are not clinically actionable, at this time.
- Categories of results include (1) positive or negative for a deleterious mutation or (2) a genetic variant of uncertain significance, in which a cancer risk is not yet established or ruled out. It is critical that the classification of these variants is accurate.

IMAGING STUDIES

Screening transvaginal ultrasonography, annual mammography, annual MRI (when breast cancer risk is 20% or more based on Tyrer-Cuzick or other breast cancer risk screening models)

Rx TREATMENT/RISK REDUCTION

- Heightened surveillance, judicious chemoprevention, and prophylactic surgery have been associated with improved outcomes.
- Surveillance includes patient breast awareness, clinical breast exam, mammography, MRI, transvaginal ultrasonography, and CA-125 blood testing, for example.
- Chemopreventive approaches have been shown to reduce the risk of ovarian cancer by up to 60% (with an oral contraceptive) and risk of contralateral breast cancer by as much as 53% (with tamoxifen).
- In HBOC patients, prophylactic total mastectomy can reduce the risk for breast cancer by 90%, and a bilateral salpingo-oophorectomy, after childbearing or by age 40, can reduce the risk of ovarian cancer by up to 96% and the risk of breast cancer by up to 68%.
- Consider preimplantation genetic diagnosis in conjunction with in vitro fertilization.

REFERRAL

If services are needed beyond one's practice or comfort level, consider consulting with knowledgeable genetic counselors, gynecologists, gynecologic oncologists, breast surgeons, and gastroenterology specialists, among others.

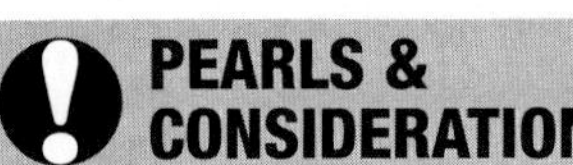

PEARLS & CONSIDERATIONS

- Be vigilant. Be motivated by the risks: Women with these mutations are approximately 10 times more likely to develop breast cancer and 20 to 30 times more likely to develop ovarian cancer. Look for red flags during every encounter, regardless of the patient's chief complaint or scheduled visit type, and inquire and regularly update information about the patient's personal and family history of cancer. Consider that approximately 10% of general practice patients have a significant family history. Supply a printed family history questionnaire. Always consider your patient's cancer risk, especially when charting a new treatment course or planning a surgical procedure. Oftentimes, a more comprehensive approach may be taken if a patient proves to be a mutation carrier.

- Adjust the age at which screening/treatment is initiated and the frequency of the visits depending on the age of the youngest affected family member, the at-risk cancer site, and the carrier status of the patient.
- Encourage input from the patient during the screening, workup, follow-up, and treatment.
- Recommend that the patient verify any questionable family history, collect appropriate family documentation/testing, and involve her family in the process; this involvement can include advising, counseling, and testing for close relatives.
- Try to counsel and test (if appropriate) those family member(s) who, if tested, would render testing of progeny/other family members less necessary. Testing an affected family member is oftentimes the most appropriate, efficient, cost-effective, and informative approach.
- Genetic testing can more accurately predict risk and enable a more tailored management approach than relying on one's family history alone. Be mindful that there may be other, although as yet unidentified, mutations at the root of one's patient's personal or family cancer history.
- Refer to your professional societies and the NCCN for screening and surveillance/imaging/treatment guidelines. Don't hesitate to engage the assistance of a genetic counselor, gynecologist, oncologist, breast surgeon, and/or a gastroenterologist during this initial phase.
- Involve other appropriate specialists in the patient's short- and long-term care, depending on the at-risk anatomic systems.
- Remember that *BRCA1*- and *BRCA2*-positive men are at a significantly higher risk for breast and prostate cancer.
- Consider prophylactic bilateral mastectomy or bilateral salpingo-oophorectomy.
- Encourage high-risk patients to complete childbearing at a younger age and consider, as appropriate, subsequent prophylactic bilateral salpingo-oophorectomy and menopause hormone therapy options.
- Recommend prophylactic bilateral salpingectomy for at-risk patients during any other surgical procedure—once childbearing is complete. Consider such assistive reproductive options as preimplantation genetic diagnosis.
- Genetic information cannot be used as the basis for a "preexisting condition" with regard to health insurance or employment, according to federal and state laws. It may play a role in life insurance, disability insurance, and long-term care insurance.
- While insurance coverage generally is available, panel testing reimbursement may occasionally be challenged. Vocalize and document your support of the appropriate testing and management, with both your patient and her/his insurance company. Enlist the assistance of your local professional society, as needed.
- There may be a medical-legal risk if a failure to identify and/or genetically counsel or test a high-risk patient and/or her family results in a delay in the diagnosis of breast or ovarian cancer. The provider, laboratory, insurance company, and the employer may have legal exposure for failing to order testing, for providing inaccurate results, or for denial of coverage, respectively.
- Being aware of a patient's cancer risk facilitates initiation of those preventive screenings and management strategies that have been shown to reduce the likelihood of cancer and improve early cancer detection rates. This can be of tremendous benefit for the patient's family members as well as the patient.

PREVENTION

Consider appropriate screening and surveillance (awareness/physical exam by patient and health care provider, imaging studies, diagnostic procedures, counseling, and genetic testing) as well as prophylactic surgery and chemopreventive measures.

PATIENT/FAMILY EDUCATION

Always encourage patients to revisit their personal and family history and to update this information with all of their health care providers and their family members. Recommend that patients initiate discussions with their family members and other health care providers in an ongoing effort to reduce their and their loved ones' risk of heritable cancer.

Refer to NCCN guidelines (www.nccn.org) and national specialty society recommendations.

SUGGESTED READINGS

Available at ExpertConsult.com

RELATED CONTENT

Breast Cancer (Related Key Topic)
Lynch Syndrome (Related Key Topic)
Ovarian Cancer (Related Key Topic)

AUTHOR: **DAVID I. KURSS, M.D., F.A.C.O.G., N.C.M.P.**

BASIC INFORMATION

DEFINITION

Herpes simplex is a viral infection caused by the herpes simplex virus (HSV). HSV-1 is associated primarily with oral infections, and HSV-2 causes mainly genital infections. However, either type can infect any site. After the primary infection, the virus enters the nerve endings in the skin directly below the lesions and ascends to the dorsal root ganglia, where it remains in a latent stage until it is reactivated.

SYNONYMS

Genital herpes
Herpes labialis
Herpes gladiatorum
Herpes digitalis
Oral herpes

EPIDEMIOLOGY & DEMOGRAPHICS

- More than 85% of adults have serologic evidence of HSV-1 infection. The seroprevalence of adults with HSV-2 in the United States is 25%; however, only approximately 20% of these persons recall having symptoms of HSV infection.
- Most cases of eye or digital herpetic infections are caused by HSV-1.
- Worldwide, more than 400 million persons have genital herpes caused by HSV-2. In the U.S., 1 in 5 adults is infected with HSV-2, and 1 million new infections occur yearly.
- Frequency of recurrence of HSV-2 genital herpes is higher than HSV-1 oral labial infection.
- The frequency of recurrence is lowest for oral labial HSV-2 infections.
- The incidence of complications from herpes simplex (e.g., herpes encephalitis) is highest in immunocompromised hosts.
- Male circumcision significantly reduces the incidence of HSV-2.

PHYSICAL FINDINGS & CLINICAL PRESENTATION

PRIMARY INFECTION:

- Symptoms occur from 3 to 7 days after contact (respiratory droplets, direct contact).
- Constitutional symptoms include low-grade fever, headache and myalgias, regional lymphadenopathy, and localized pain.
- Pain, burning, itching, and tingling last several hours.
- Grouped vesicles, usually with surrounding erythema, appear and generally ulcerate or crust within 48 hr (Fig. 1).
- The vesicles are uniform in size (differentiating it from herpes zoster vesicles, which vary in size). Scattered erosions covered with exudate may be noted on genitals (Fig. E2).
- During the acute eruption the patient is uncomfortable; involvement of lips and inside of mouth (Fig. 3) may make it unpleasant for the patient to eat; urinary retention may complicate involvement of the genital area.
- Lesions generally last from 2 to 6 wk and heal without scarring.

RECURRENT INFECTION:

- Generally caused by alteration in the immune system; fatigue, stress, menses, local skin trauma, and exposure to sunlight are contributing factors.
- The prodromal symptoms (fatigue, burning and tingling of the affected area) last 12 to 24 hr.
- A cluster of lesions generally evolves within 24 hr from a macule to a papule and then vesicles surrounded by erythema; the vesicles coalesce and subsequently rupture within 4 days, revealing erosions covered by crusts.
- The crusts are generally shed within 7 to 10 days, revealing a pink surface.
- The most frequent location of the lesions is on the vermilion border of the lips (HSV-1), the penile shaft or glans penis and the labia (HSV-2), buttocks (seen more frequently in women), fingertips (herpetic whitlow), and trunk (may be confused with herpes zoster).
- Rapid onset of diffuse cutaneous herpes simplex (eczema herpeticum) may occur in certain atopic infants and adults. It is a medical emergency, especially in young infants, and should be promptly treated with acyclovir.
- Herpes encephalitis, meningitis, and ocular herpes can occur in patients with immunocompromised status and occasionally in normal hosts.

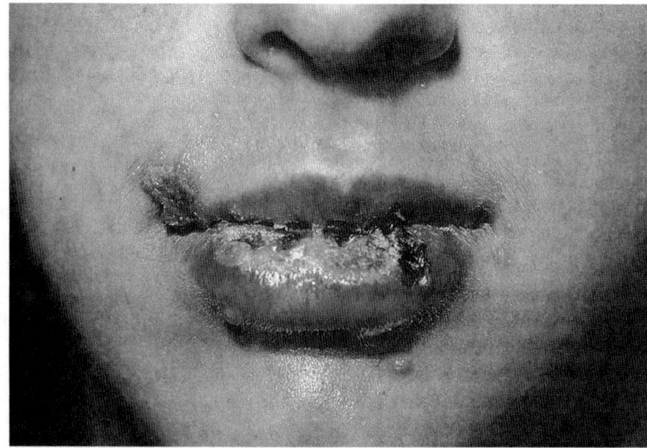

FIG. 1 Herpetic gingivostomatitis. Multiple erosions with crusting. Note the associated lesions involving the chin. (From Paller AS, Mancini, AJ: *Hurwitz clinical pediatric dermatology: a textbook of skin disorders of childhood and adolescence*, ed 5, 2016, Elsevier.)

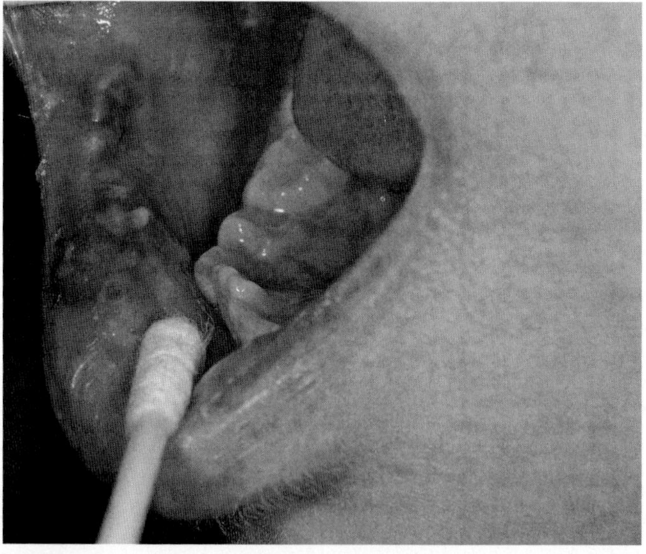

FIG. 3 Herpes labialis. Erythematous erosions clustered on the right lower lip in a patient with labial herpes. This young girl also had herpes-associated erythema multiforme. (From Paller AS, Mancini, AJ: *Hurwitz clinical pediatric dermatology: a textbook of skin disorders of childhood and adolescence*, ed 5, 2016, Elsevier.)

ETIOLOGY

HSV-1 and HSV-2 are both DNA viruses.

Dx DIAGNOSIS

DIFFERENTIAL DIAGNOSIS

- Impetigo
- Behçet syndrome
- Coxsackie virus infection
- Syphilis
- Stevens-Johnson syndrome
- Herpangina
- Aphthous stomatitis
- Varicella
- Herpes zoster

WORKUP

Diagnosis is based on clinical presentation. Laboratory evaluation confirms diagnosis.

LABORATORY TESTS

- Direct immunofluorescent antibody slide tests provide a rapid diagnosis.
- Viral culture is the most definitive method for diagnosis; results are generally available in 1 or 2 days. The lesions should be sampled during the vesicular or early ulcerative stage; cervical samples should be taken from the endocervix with a swab.
- Pap smear will detect HSV-infected cells in cervical tissue from women without symptoms.
- Serologic tests for HSV: Immunoglobulin (Ig) G and IgM serum antibodies. Antibodies to HSV occur in 50% to 90% of adults. The presence of IgM or a fourfold or greater rise in IgG titers indicates a recent infection (convalescent sample should be drawn 2 to 3 wk after the acute specimen is drawn).
- Tzanck smear is a readily available test that will demonstrate multinucleated giant cells. However, it is not a highly sensitive test.

Rx TREATMENT

- Table 1 summarizes antiviral chemotherapy for HSV infection.
- Topical acyclovir, penciclovir, and docosanol are optional treatments for recurrent herpes labialis, but they are less effective than oral treatments.

DISPOSITION

Most patients recover from the initial episode or recurrences without complications; immunocompromised hosts are at risk for complications (e.g., disseminated herpes simplex infection, herpes encephalitis).

REFERRAL

- Hospital admission in patients with herpes encephalitis or herpes meningitis and in immunocompromised hosts with diffuse herpes simplex infection
- Ophthalmology referral in patients with suspected ocular herpes

TABLE 1 Topical and Oral Antiviral Medications Used for Herpes Simplex Virus Infections*

Drug	Formulation	Regimen	Indication/Comment
Topical			
Acyclovir	5% cream (2 g, 5 g)	Apply 5 times/day	Recurrent HL; A: ≥12 years; 4 days; Rx
	5% ointment (15 g, 30 g)	Apply 6 times/day	Initial GH, localized HSV; A: adults; 7 days; Rx
Penciclovir	1% cream (1.5 g, 5 g)	Apply q. 2 h (awake)	Recurrent HL; A: ≥12 years; 4 days; Rx
Docosanol	10% cream (2 g)	Apply 5 times/day	HL; A: ≥12 years; treat until healed; OTC
Oral (all Rx)			
Acyclovir	200 mg capsule 400 mg, 800 mg tablet 200 mg/5 ml susp		A: ≥2 years
		200 mg 5 times/day	Initial GH; 10 days
		200 mg 5 times/day	Recurrent GH; 5 days
		400 mg 2 times/day	Suppression, recurrent GH; up to 12 mo, then reevaluate
Famciclovir	125, 250, 500 mg tablet		A: ≥18 yr
		1500 mg single dose	Recurrent HL
		1000 mg 2 times/day	Recurrent GH; 1 day
		250 mg 2 times/day	Suppression, recurrent GH; up to 12 mo
Valacyclovir	500 mg, 1 g caplet		A: adults and ≥12 years for HL
		1 g 2 times/day	Initial GH; 10 days
		500 mg 2 times/day	Recurrent GH; 3 days
		500 mg–1 g once daily	Suppressive GH
		2 g 2 times/day	HL; 1 day; both adults and children ≥12 yr

A, Approved; *GH*, genital herpes; *HL*, herpes labialis; *HSV*, herpes simplex virus; *Rx*, by prescription; *OTC*, over-the-counter.
*Approved indications and regimens listed; often used off-label.
From Paller AS, Mancini AJ: *Hurwitz clinical pediatric dermatology: a textbook of skin disorders of childhood and adolescence*, ed 5, 2016, Elsevier.

PEARLS & CONSIDERATIONS

COMMENTS

- Provide patient education regarding transmission of HSV.
- Condom use offers significant protection against HSV-1 infection in susceptible women.
- Patients should be instructed on the use of condoms for sexual intercourse and on avoiding kissing or sexual intercourse until lesions are crusted. Pericoital application of tenofovir gel, an antiretroviral vaginal gel, has also been shown to reduce the risk of HSV-2 in women. This may be useful in regions of the world where use of condoms is shunned.
- Patients should also avoid contact with immunocompromised hosts or neonates while lesions are present.
- Proper handwashing techniques should be explained.
- Patients with herpes gladiatorum (cutaneous herpes in athletes involved in contact sports) should be excluded from participation in active sports until lesions have resolved.
- Many new HSV-2 infections are asymptomatic. Since HSV-2 antibody tests have become commercially available, an increasing number of persons have learned that they have genital herpes through serologic testing. Persons with asymptomatic HSV-2 infection shed virus in the genital tract less frequently than persons with symptomatic infection, but much of the difference is attributable to less frequent genital lesions because genital lesions are accompanied by frequent viral shedding. The U.S. Preventive Services Task Force (USPSTF) recommends against routine serologic screening for genital HSV infection in asymptomatic adolescents and adults, including those that are pregnant.
- Suppressive treatment of HSV-2 infection lowers the incidence of genital lesions by 70% to 80%, but cuts the rate of HSV-2 transmission to uninfected partners by only 50%.

- Pregnancy: Antiviral prophylaxis with acyclovir is recommended from 36 weeks of gestation until delivery in women with a history of genital herpes. Elective cesarean delivery should be performed in laboring patients with active lesions to decrease the risk of neonatal herpes.
- Trials involving investigational herpes simplex vaccine have found it to be effective in preventing HSV-1 genital disease and infection, but not in preventing HSV-2 disease or infection.

RELATED CONTENT

Genital Herpes (Patient Information)
Oral Herpes (Patient Information)

AUTHOR: **FRED F. FERRI, M.D.**

BASIC INFORMATION

DEFINITION

Herpes zoster is a disease caused by reactivation of the varicella-zoster virus, with spread of the virus alone from the sensory nerve to the dermatome. After the primary infection (chickenpox), the virus becomes latent in the dorsal root ganglia and reemerges when there is a weakening of the immune system (as a result of disease or advanced age). Over 90% of the adult U.S. population is latently infected with varicella zoster virus.

SYNONYMS

Shingles
HZ

ICD-10CM CODES

B02	Herpes zoster
B02.7	Disseminated zoster
B02.8	Zoster with other complications
B02.9	Zoster without complications
B02.39	Other herpes zoster eye disease
B02.0	Zoster encephalitis
B02.1	Zoster meningitis
B02.30	Zoster ocular disease, unspecified
B02.31	Zoster conjunctivitis
B02.32	Zoster iridocyclitis
B02.33	Zoster keratitis
B02.34	Zoster scleritis
B02.39	Other herpes zoster eye disease

EPIDEMIOLOGY & DEMOGRAPHICS

- Herpes zoster occurs during the lifetime of 10% to 20% of the population. There are approximately 1 million cases annually in the U.S. The incidence of herpes zoster has increased four fold over the past 6 decades,
- There is an increased incidence in immunocompromised patients (chemotherapy, radiotherapy, immunosuppression due to corticosteroids, AIDS, DM, malignancy), the elderly (most common after age 60) (Fig. 1), and children who acquired chickenpox when younger than 2 mo.

PHYSICAL FINDINGS & CLINICAL PRESENTATION

- Pain generally precedes skin manifestation by 3 to 5 days and is generally localized to the dermatome that will be affected by the skin lesions.
- Constitutional symptoms are often present (malaise, fever, headache).
- The initial rash consists of erythematous maculopapules generally affecting one dermatome (thoracic region in majority of cases [Fig. 2]). Typically the rash does not cross the midline. Some patients (<30%) may have scattered vesicles outside the affected dermatome. In rare cases the rash can be generalized (Fig. 3).
- The initial maculopapules evolve into vesicles and pustules by the third or the fourth day.
- The vesicles have an erythematous base (Fig. 4), are cloudy, of various sizes (a distinguishing characteristic from herpes simplex, in which the vesicles are of uniform size), and may have a classic appearance of grouped vesicles (Fig. 5).
- The vesicles subsequently become umbilicated and then form crusts that generally fall off within 3 wk; scarring may occur.
- Pain during and after the rash is generally significant. Postherpetic neuralgia occurs after herpes zoster in approximately one third of patients aged 60 yr and older and can persist for months or years.
- Secondary bacterial infection with *Staphylococcus aureus* or *Streptococcus pyogenes* may occur.
- Regional lymphadenopathy may occur.
- Herpes zoster may involve the trigeminal nerve (most frequent cranial nerve involved); involvement of the first division of the trigeminal nerve is known as "herpes zoster ophthalmicus" and can result in blindness. The appearance of blisters on the tip of the nose (Huchinson sign) is a common manifestation of herpes zoster ophthalmicus. Involvement of the geniculate ganglion can cause facial palsy and a painful ear, with the presence of vesicles on the pinna and external auditory canal (Ramsay Hunt syndrome).
- Pain typical of herpes zoster in the absence of cutaneous lesions is known as "Zoster sine herpete" is rare.

ETIOLOGY

Reactivation of varicella virus (human herpes virus III)

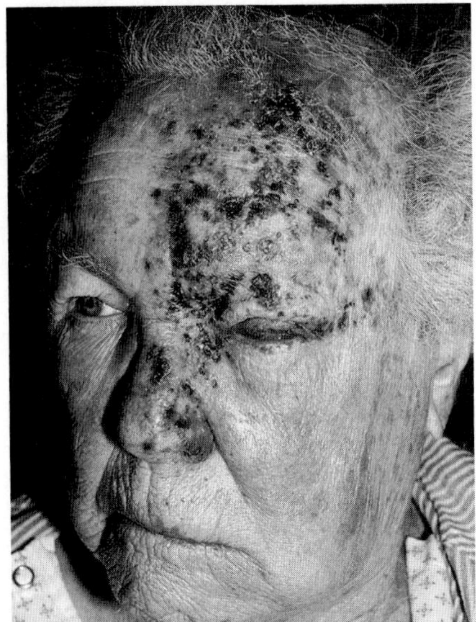

FIG. 1 Herpes zoster, involvement of the V1 dermatome. (From James WD, et al.: *Andrews' diseases of the skin: clinical dermatology*, ed 12, Philadelphia, 2016, Elsevier.)

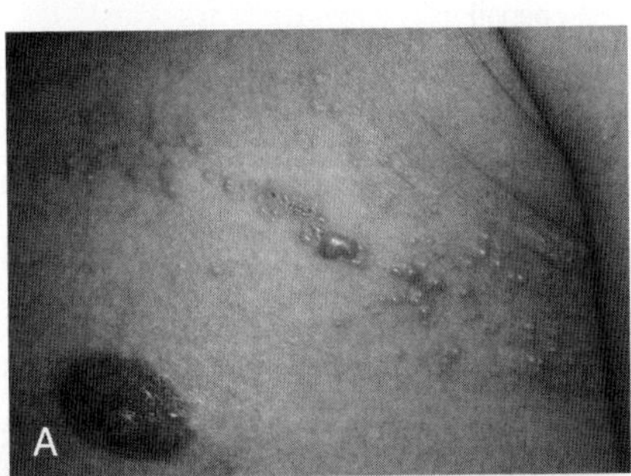

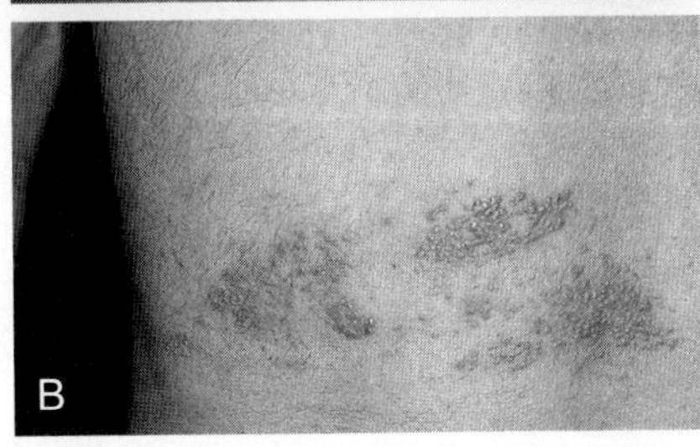

FIG. 2 A and B, Herpes zoster lesions in T3 distribution. (From Swartz, MH: *Textbook of physical diagnosis*, ed 7, Philadelphia, 2014, Saunders.)

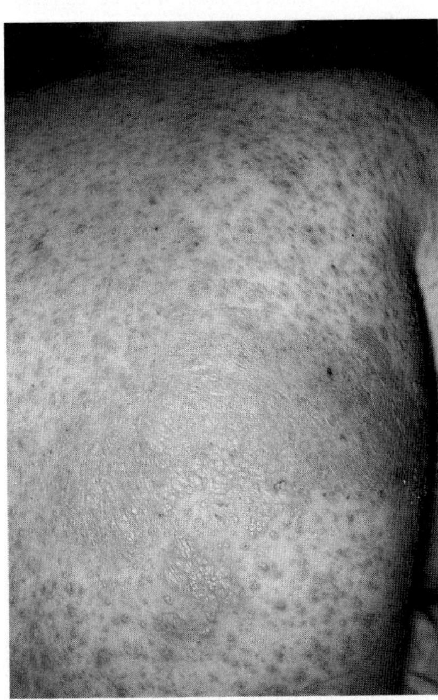

FIG. 3 Herpes zoster, generalized. (From Swartz, MH: *Textbook of physical diagnosis*, ed 7, Philadelphia, 2014, Saunders.)

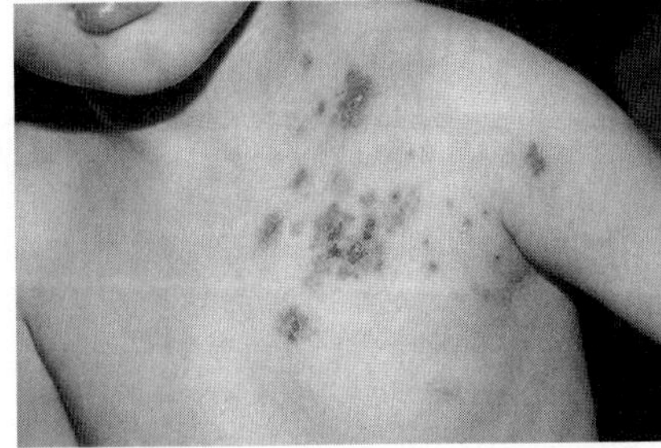

FIG. 4 Herpes zoster occurred in this 3-year-old. She had chickenpox at age 18 months. The varicella-zoster virus causes both conditions. Spontaneous resolution can be expected. (From White GM, Cox NH [eds]: *Diseases of the skin, a color atlas and text*, ed 2, St Louis, 2006, Mosby.)

 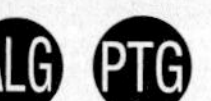

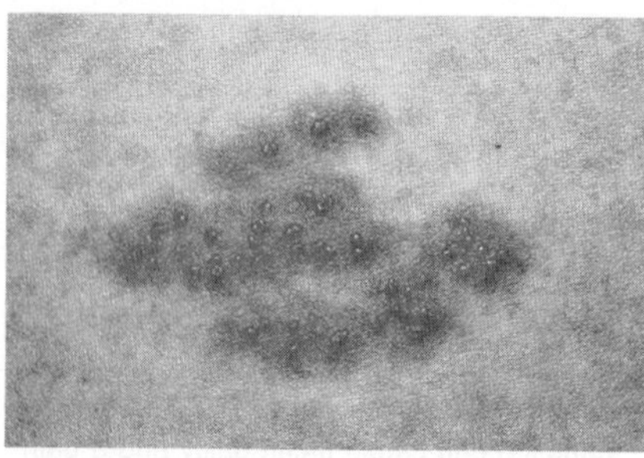

FIG. 5 Herpes zoster. Classic appearance of grouped vesicles. (From White GM, Cox NH [eds]: *Diseases of the skin, a color atlas and text,* ed 2, St Louis, 2006, Mosby.)

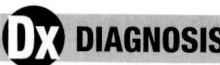

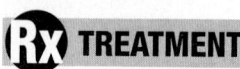

DIAGNOSIS

DIFFERENTIAL DIAGNOSIS

- Rash: Herpes simplex and other viral infections, contact dermatitis
- Pain from herpes zoster: May be confused with acute myocardial infarction, pulmonary embolism, pleuritis, pericarditis, renal colic

WORKUP

The diagnosis of herpes zoster is usually made by the characteristic dermatomal presentation.

LABORATORY TESTS

Laboratory tests are generally not necessary. In cases where the clinical diagnosis is not obvious, PCR testing for varicella zoster virus is has high sensitivity and specificity. It is readily available and results can usually be obtained in less than 24 hours. Other laboratory studies for diagnosis of herpes zoster include viral culture, DFA, and serologic testing.

TREATMENT

NONPHARMACOLOGIC THERAPY

- Wet compresses (using Burow solution or cool tap water) applied for 15 to 30 min five to ten times a day may be useful to break vesicles and remove serum and crust. Then carefully pat dry.
- Care must be taken to prevent any secondary bacterial infection by keeping cutaneous lesions clean and dry

ACUTE GENERAL Rx

- Oral antiviral agents can shorten the disease course and help prevent post-herpetic neuralgia. They can decrease acute pain, inflammation, and vesicle formation when treatment is begun within 72 hr of onset of rash. Treatment options are:
  1. Valacyclovir 1000 mg tid for 7 days
  2. Famciclovir 500 mg tid for 7 days
  3. Acyclovir 800 mg 5 times daily for 7 to 10 days
- The role of corticosteroids in herpes zoster is controversial. Many physicians prescribe them to improve rash healing and reduce pain severity; however, a Cochrane review failed to show sufficient evidence to support the use of corticosteroids for the prevention of postherpetic neuralgia. Corticosteroids can be considered in older patients within 72 hr of clinical presentation or if new lesions are still appearing if there are no contraindications to their use. Initial dose is prednisone 60 mg/day decreased by 5 mg/day until finished.
- Immunocompromised patients and patients with herpes zoster complicated by CNS involvement should be treated with IV acyclovir 10–15 mg/kg q8h in 1-hr infusions for 7 days, with close monitoring of renal function and adequate hydration; vidarabine (continuous 12-hr infusion of 10 mg/kg/day for 7 days) is also effective for treatment of disseminated herpes zoster in immunocompromised hosts.
- Patients with AIDS and transplant recipients may develop acyclovir-resistant varicella-zoster; these patients can be treated with foscarnet (40 mg/kg IV q8h) continued for at least 10 days or until lesions are completely healed.
- Postherpetic neuralgia:
  1. Gabapentin 100 to 600 mg tid is effective in the treatment of pain and sleep interference associated with postherpetic neuralgia. Other effective agents are pregabalin, duloxetine, and tricyclic antidepressants.
  2. Lidocaine patch 5% is also effective in relieving postherpetic neuralgia. Patches are applied to intact skin after resolution of blisters and crusts to cover the most painful area for up to 12 hr within a 24-hr period.
  3. Capsaicin cream can be useful for treatment of postherpetic neuralgia. It is generally applied 3 to 5 times daily for several weeks after the crusts have fallen off. A topical 8% patch formulation of capsaicin is now available by prescription for postherpetic neuralgia.
  4. Sympathetic blocks (stellate ganglion or epidural) with 0.25% bupivacaine and rhizotomy are reserved for severe cases unresponsive to conservative treatment.

DISPOSITION

- The incidence of postherpetic neuralgia (defined as pain that persists more than 90 days after onset of rash) increases with age (<30% by age 40 yr, >70% by age 70 yr); antivirals reduce the risk of postherpetic neuralgia.
- Incidence of disseminated herpes zoster is increased in immunocompromised hosts (e.g., 15% to 50% of patients with active Hodgkin's disease).
- Immunocompromised hosts are also more prone to neurologic complications (encephalitis, myelitis, cranial and peripheral nerve palsies, acute retinal necrosis). The mortality rate is 10% to 20% in immunocompromised hosts with disseminated zoster.
- Motor neuropathies occur in 5% of all cases of zoster; complete recovery occurs in >70% of patients.
- Rates of HZ recurrence are more frequent than previously reported and are comparable to rates of first HZ occurrence in immunocompetent individuals.

REFERRAL

- Hospitalization for IV acyclovir in patients with disseminated herpes zoster.
- Patients with herpes zoster ophthalmicus should be referred to an ophthalmologist.
- Consultation with an otolaryngologist is advisable in patients with Ramsey-Hunt syndrome.
- Vaccination: In the absence of the herpes zoster vaccine, persons who live to 85 yr of age have a 50% risk of herpes zoster. Immunocompetent adults ≥50 yr (including those who have already received Zostavax) are appropriate candidates for recombinant varicella zoster virus vaccine (Shingrix). It consists of 2 doses 2-6 months apart and is preferred over zostavax for herpes zoster prevention. Adults who are VZV seronegative (never had varicella) should be immunized against varicella with two doses of varicella vaccine (Varivax). Despite its efficacy and safety, use of this vaccine remains low (<8% of potential recipients).

SUGGESTED READINGS

Available at ExpertConsult.com

RELATED CONTENT

Shingles (Patient Information)
Post-Herpetic Neuralgia (Related Key Topic)
Ramsey-Hunt Syndrome (Related Key Topic)

AUTHOR: **FRED F. FERRI, M.D.**

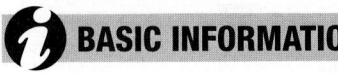

BASIC INFORMATION

DEFINITION

Hidradenitis suppurativa (HS) is a chronic, relapsing suppurative cutaneous disease affecting skin that bears apocrine glands and is manifested by abscesses, fistulating sinus tracts, and chronic infection leading to scarring.

SYNONYMS

Acne inversa
Apocrinitis
Verneuil disease
HS

ICD-10CM CODE

L73.2 Hidradenitis suppurativa

EPIDEMIOLOGY & DEMOGRAPHICS

Onset is postpubertal, with an average age of onset of 23 yr; rates decline after age 55 yr.

PREVALENCE: Overall prevalence in the United States is ~1% to 2%.

PREDOMINANT SEX: Female: male ratio is 3:1.

PREDOMINANT AGE: HS most often manifests after puberty, usually in the second or third decade of life. It is rare in the elderly.

RISK FACTORS:

- Obesity and metabolic syndrome
- Family history (approximately 30%)
- Hyperandrogenism in women
- Cigarette smoking

PHYSICAL FINDINGS & CLINICAL PRESENTATION

The diagnosis is primarily clinical, based on the development of typical lesions in a characteristic distribution, with a relapsing nature. The course of HS is prolonged and marked by intermittent periods of activity and remission.

- Early symptoms include pain, itching, burning, erythema, and hyperhidrosis.
- Typical lesions include:
  1. Painful erythematous papules and nodules leading to painful abscesses with foul-smelling discharge.
  2. Dermal contractures and ropelike elevation of the skin.
  3. Comedones in the apocrine, gland-bearing skin.
- Classified into Hurley Stages (Table 1):
  1. Stage I: Abscesses without sinus tracts or scarring.
  2. Stage II: Multiple abscesses plus sinus tracts and scarring.
  3. Stage III: Diffuse involvement of entire area with abscesses, sinus tracts, and scarring.
- The axilla is the most common site (Fig. 1).
- Less common sites include the inguinal region, the breasts (more often in women), and the perineal or perianal skin (more often in men).
- There is a strong tendency toward relapse and recurrence.
- There is often a poor response to conventional antibiotics and no pathogens isolated from cultures of lesions.
- The disease is often mistaken for a simple infection and a long delay in diagnosis is common.
- Three clinical subtypes of HS have been recently proposed[1]:
  1. A classic axillary-mammary HS subtype, representing 48% of cases and characterized by breast and axillary involvement and hypertrophic scarring.
  2. A follicular HS subtype, representing 26% of cases manifesting primarily in male smokers with a family history of HS and characterized by follicular lesions, including epidermal cysts, pilonidal sinus, comedones, and severe acne.
  3. A gluteal HS subtype, representing 26% of cases, most often seen in smokers with lower body mass index (BMI) and with a morphology characterized by follicular papules, folliculitis, and gluteal involvement.

[1] Woodruff CM, Charlie AM, Leslie KS: Hidradenitis suppurative: a guide for the practicing physician, *Mayo Clin Proc* 90(12):1679-1693, 2015.

ETIOLOGY

- Keratinous materials plug apocrine glands in hair follicles leading to stasis, dilation, rupture, and re-epithelialization. Fig. 2 illustrates the pathogenesis of hidradenitis suppurativa.
- Bacteria are trapped and multiply, leading to gland rupture with surrounding inflammation and local bacterial infection.
- Over time, repeated nodules and infections cause scarring, which can lead to deep tissue damage and sinus tracts.
- Infectious agents such as *Streptococcus, Staphylococcus,* and *Escherichia coli,* and enteric flora have been identified in cultures but are likely a secondary component of the disease.
- There is likely a significant genetic component to the disease. 35% to 40% of patients report a family history of HS. An HS spectrum of different phenotypes has been

TABLE 1 Hidradenitis Suppurativa—Grading Systems and Therapeutic Ladder

Hurley staging system

- Stage I—one or more abscesses with no sinus tract or scar formation
- Stage II—one or more widely separated recurrent abscesses, with sinus tract and scar formation
- Stage III—multiple interconnected sinus tracts and abscesses throughout an affected region; more extensive scarring

Sartorius grading system

- Anatomical regions involved: Axilla (left and/or right), groin (left and/or right), gluteal (left and/or right), or other region (e.g., inframammary): 3 points per region involved
- Number and scores of lesions for each region: Nodules = 1; fistulae = 6
- The longest distance between two relevant lesions* (i.e., nodules and fistulae) in each region: <5 cm = 1; 5–10 cm = 3; >10 cm = 9
- Are all lesions clearly separated by normal skin? In each region—yes 0/no (Hurley III) 9

Therapeutic ladder

Indication	Therapeutic interventions
General measures	• If obese or overweight, weight reduction • Reduce friction and moisture via loose undergarments, absorbent powders, and topical aluminum chloride • Antiseptic soaps • Smoking cessation
Hurley Stage I	• Intralesional triamcinolone (5 mg/ml) injections into early inflammatory lesions • Topical clindamycin • Eradication of *S. aureus* carriage with topical mupirocin in nose, axillae, umbilicus, and perianal regions • Oral antibiotics tailored to results of bacterial cultures from pustular discharge or abscess contents • Oral antibiotic therapy (alone or in combination) for its anti-inflammatory effect (rifampin + clindamycin, tetracycline, doxycycline, minocycline, dapsone, trimethoprim–sulfamethoxazole) • Oral anti-androgen therapy (e.g., finasteride)
Hurley Stage II	• Oral antibiotic therapy (see Stage I) • Acitretin • Systemic immunosuppressive agents including adalimumab,† infliximab, and cyclosporine Surgical treatments‡ • Limited local excisions with second intention healing • CO_2 laser ablation with second intention healing • Nd:YAG laser treatments, at least 3–4 monthly sessions
Hurley Stage III	Medical treatments outlined for Stages I and II Surgical treatments‡ • Early wide surgical excision of involved areas • CO_2 laser ablation with second intention healing

*Or size if only one lesion.
†FDA-approved dosing regimen: 160 mg (four 40 mg injections) on day 1, *or* 80 mg daily on days 1 and 2 followed by 80 mg on day 15 and then 40 mg on day 29 and weekly thereafter.
‡Incision and drainage are discouraged given high rate of recurrence.
From Bolognia J: *Dermatology,* ed 4, 2018, Elsevier

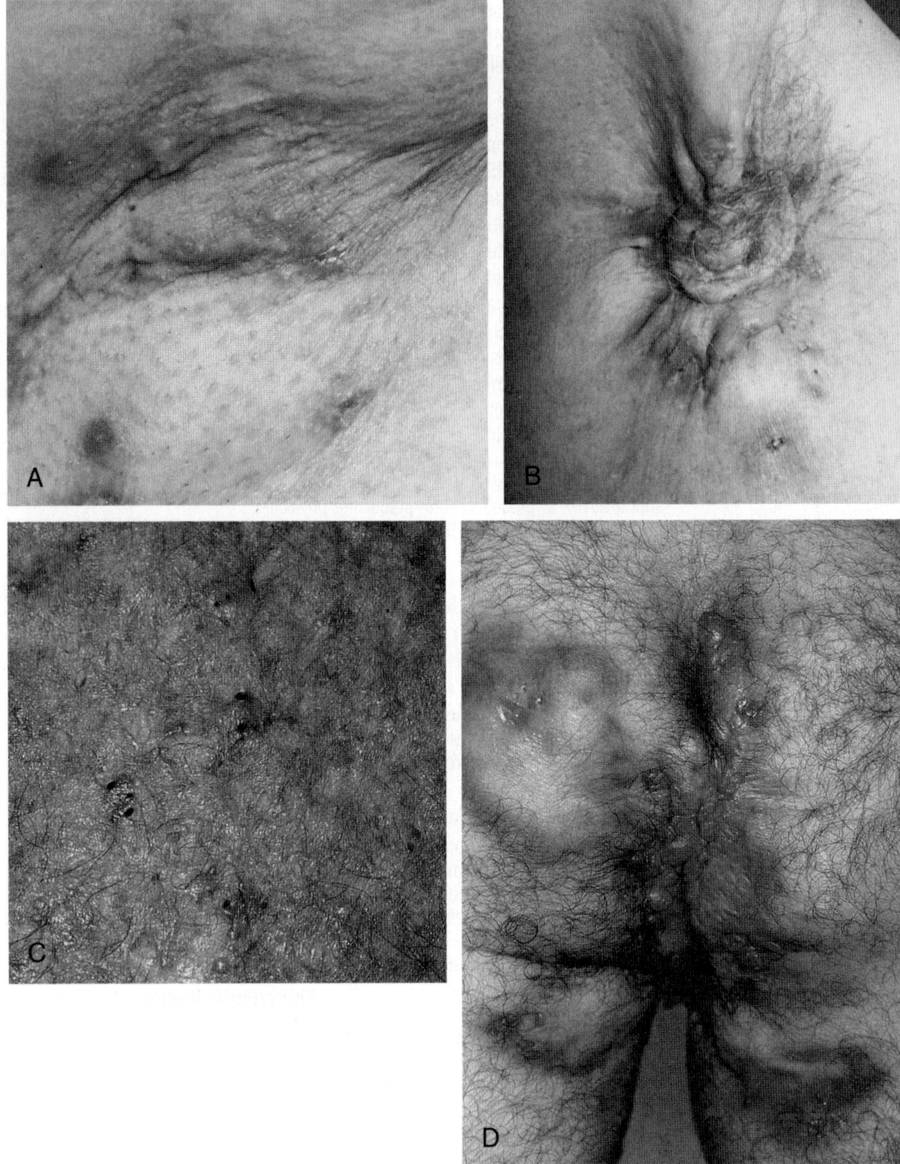

FIG. 1 Hidradenitis suppurativa. A and **B,** Papulopustules, nodules, sinus tracts, and scarring in the axilla (Hurley stage II [A] and III [B]). **C,** Superficial sinus tracts that serve as a clue to the diagnosis, even in the absence of active disease. **D,** Severe disease with inflammatory nodules, hypertrophic scarring, draining fistulae, and sinus tract formation of the perianal region, buttocks, and upper thighs. This is the type of patient who is at risk for the development of squamous cell carcinoma and secondary amyloidosis. (**A,** Courtesy, Kalman Watsky, MD; **B,** Courtesy, Marco Romanelli, MD. In Bolognia J: *Dermatology,* ed 4, 2018, Elsevier.)

characterized involving genetic factors that are not yet well described but may be important for future therapy.

- HS has been associated with other endocrine and autoimmune disorders such as diabetes, Cushing's syndrome, acromegaly, Crohn disease, and inflammatory arthritis.
- Metabolic syndrome affects as many as 50% of patients with HS and may exacerbate the associated inflammation.

Dx DIAGNOSIS

DIFFERENTIAL DIAGNOSIS

- Follicular pyodermias such as folliculitis, furuncles, carbuncles, and pilonidal cysts
- Noduloulcerative syphilis
- Cat scratch disease
- Granuloma inguinale
- Perianal and vulvar manifestations of Crohn disease
- Actinomycosis
- Lymphogranuloma venereum
- Dermoid, epidermoid, or Bartholin cysts
- Tuberculous inflammation of the skin
- Lymphadenitis
- Erysipelas

WORKUP

Primarily a clinical diagnosis based on typical lesions (see "Physical Findings & Clinical Presentation").

LABORATORY TESTS

- Patients with acute lesions may have an elevated erythrocyte sedimentation rate or WBC.
- Febrile and toxic-appearing patients should have complete blood count, chemistries, and blood cultures.
- Any pus should be sampled for bacterial culture and sensitivity.

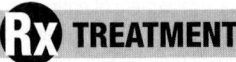

Rx TREATMENT

There is no definitive cure for hidradenitis.

NONPHARMACOLOGIC THERAPY

- Weight loss and control of metabolic syndrome.
- Smoking cessation.
- Avoidance of shaving, depilatory creams, deodorants.
- Avoidance of tight-fitting clothing.
- Warm compresses.

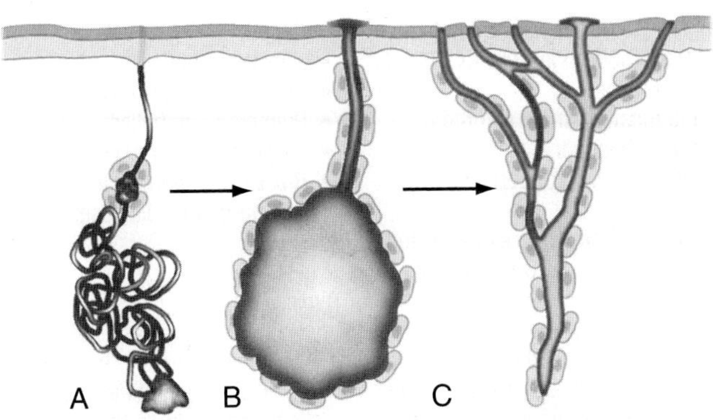

FIG. 2 Pathogenesis of hidradenitis suppurativa, an inflammatory disease of the apocrine sweat glands and adjacent connective tissue. ***A***, The initiating event is occlusion of the apocrine duct by a keratinous plug. ***B***, Bacteria are trapped beneath the keratinous plug and multiply to form an abscess, which can rupture into adjacent tissue. ***C***, The end result is recurrent abscesses, chronic draining sinuses, and indurated scarred skin and subcutaneous tissues. Often, multiple tracts are interconnected and lead to the skin. (From James WD et al: *Andrews' diseases of the skin*, ed 12, Philadelphia, 2016, Elsevier.)

- Incision and drainage of nonpurulent lesions is *not* recommended due to recurrence and scarring.
- Laser therapy, radiotherapy, and cryotherapy currently under study.
- Wide local excision for stage III disease with or without vacuum-assisted closure device.

ACUTE AND CHRONIC Rx

- NSAIDs for inflammation and pain, consider gabapentin, pregabalin, SSRIs for chronic pain management.
- Antibiotics never proven to be effective; however, they are a mainstay of treatment. Can base treatment on the basis of aspirate culture and sensitivities or empirically.
  1. Clindamycin is the only topical antibiotic proven to be effective in randomized controlled trial and is appropriate for stage I disease.
  2. For oral therapy in stage II: Consider clindamycin and rifampin in combination. Cephalosporins, dicloxacillin, erythromycin, minocycline, and tetracycline have also been used.
  3. Severe, recurrent disease can require up to 3 to 6 mo of antibiotics.
- Oral contraceptives with low androgenic progesterone (norgestimate, desogestrel, or gestodene) for women show mixed effectiveness. They are especially advantageous for female patients of childbearing age who also require some form of birth control.
- Isotretinoin has been used with mixed effectiveness. It should be avoided in women of childbearing age.
- Metformin has mixed effectiveness, possibly due to related metabolic syndrome and hyperandrogenism.
- Trials using zinc gluconate 75 to 118 mg/day in patients with mild (grade 1) disease have shown mixed effectiveness.
- Corticosteroids and other immune suppressants such as cyclosporin, infliximab, and etanercept have been used for stage II disease, with mixed results.
- Adalimumab, an antitumor necrosis factor-α antibody given once per week (dose 40 mg/wk) has shown significantly higher clinical response as compared to placebo in phase 3 trials. Infliximab has also been used in trials with variable success rates, with most patients exhibiting clinical improvement within 8 wk.

COMPLICATIONS

- Squamous cell carcinoma
- Scarring leading to restricted limb mobility or lymphedema
- Rectal or urethral fistulas
- Psychological effects related to disfiguring nature of disease

REFERRAL

- Referral to dermatology during stage I to II disease.
- Referral to a surgeon is indicated for stage III disease.
- Surgical approaches include laser surgery and excisional surgery.

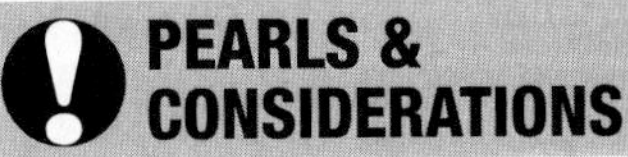

PEARLS & CONSIDERATIONS

COMMENTS

- Patients with hidradenitis are at risk for severe depression, social isolation, and negatively impacted sexuality as a result of their disease.
- There is an average delay in diagnosis of 12 yr and most patients are diagnosed in stage II of the disease.
- It is important to maximize nonmedical treatment, start medical treatment, and refer to a surgeon early in the disease course to ensure the best quality of life for patients.
- The only definitive treatment for hidradenitis is wide excision of the involved skin.

SUGGESTED READINGS

Available at ExpertConsult.com

AUTHOR: **FRED F. FERRI, M.D.**

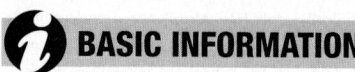

DEFINITION

High-altitude illness refers to a spectrum of cerebral and pulmonary syndromes related to hypoxemia occurring during rapid ascent to high altitudes in unacclimatized individuals. Common acute syndromes include high-altitude pulmonary edema (HAPE), acute mountain sickness (AMS), and high-altitude cerebral edema (HACE). The latter two are thought to represent different points of severity along the same pathophysiologic process in the brain.

SYNONYMS

Altitude sickness
High-altitude headache
Acute mountain sickness
AMS
High-altitude pulmonary edema
High-altitude cerebral edema

ICD-10CM CODES

W94	Exposure to high and low air pressure and changes in air pressure
T70.29	Other and unspecified effects of high altitude

EPIDEMIOLOGY & DEMOGRAPHICS

- Millions of people worldwide are at risk of developing altitude sickness annually.
- 80% of people who ascend to high altitudes have high-altitude headache (HAH_2).
- AMS is the most common of the altitude diseases. It affects approximately 40% to 50% of people ascending to 14,000 ft (4200 m) from lowland and 25% of visitors to an altitude of 2000 meters (6560 feet).
- The incidence of HACE is reported to be 0.1% to 2% at elevations in excess of 12,000 ft (3000 m). HACE is often complicated by concomitant HAPE.
- Men are five times more likely to develop HAPE than are women.
- AMS and HACE affect men and women equally.
- Some studies have suggested that climbers with a prior history of HAPE have a roughly 60% chance of recurrence if they ascend to the same elevation at the same rate.

PHYSICAL FINDINGS & CLINICAL PRESENTATION (TABLE E1)

HAH_1

- Headache that develops within 24 hr of ascent.
- Bilateral, frontal or frontotemporal, dull or pressing quality.
- Mild to moderate intensity and aggravated by exertion, movement, straining, coughing, or bending.
- Headache resolves within 8 hr of descent.
- HAH should resolve with analgesics and/or 10 to 15 min of supplementary oxygen.
- Difficult to distinguish from headaches secondary to dehydration.

AMS

- AMS is thought to be a progression of HAH_2.
- Occurs within 6 to 12 hours after rapid ascent to 8000 ft (2500 m) in 10% to 25% of unacclimatized persons.
- Headache is the most common symptom.
- Dizziness and light-headedness.
- Nausea, vomiting, and loss of appetite.
- Fatigue.
- Sleep disturbance from an exaggerated hyperventilatory phase of Cheyne-Stokes respiration in response to hypoxemia and alkalosis.
- AMS can evolve into HAPE and HACE.
- Retinal hemorrhages can be present from increased blood flow or breakdown in the blood-retinal barrier.
- Supplemental oxygen may be used to support the clinical diagnosis.

HACE

- Usually presents several days after AMS.
- Headache, nausea, vomiting, mild fever, confusion, irritability, drowsiness, stupor, hallucinations, seizures, and paralysis.
- Truncal ataxia and encephalopathy.
- Coma and death from brain herniation may develop within hours of the first symptoms.

HAPE (Fig. E1)

- Typically occurs 2 to 4 days after ascent to more than 8000 ft (2500 m).
- It can occur at a lower elevation in patients with pulmonary hypertension.
- Dyspnea out of proportion to the level of exertion, loss of stamina.
- Dry cough or cough with frothy rust- or pink-tinged sputum.
- Chest tightness.
- Tachycardia, tachypnea, rales, cyanosis.

ETIOLOGY

- During ascent to altitudes above sea level, the atmospheric pressure decreases. Although the percentage of oxygen in the air remains the same, the partial pressure of oxygen decreases with increased altitude, and can cause hypoxemia. Fig. E2 illustrates the effect of altitude on alveolar Pao_2 and oxygen saturation.
- Increased cerebral blood flow and the loss of autoregulation of intracranial pressure may contribute to increased cerebral vascular permeability and subsequent brain edema (HACE).
- Hypobaric hypoxia can trigger elevated pulmonary pressures, resulting in protein-rich, hemorrhagic exudates into the lung alveoli due to a breakdown in the pulmonary blood-gas barrier (HAPE).
- The body responds to low oxygen partial pressures through a process of acclimatization (see "Comments").

Dx DIAGNOSIS

Made by clinical presentation and physical findings

DIFFERENTIAL DIAGNOSIS

- Dehydration
- Carbon monoxide poisoning
- Hypothermia
- Infection
- Substance abuse
- Congestive heart failure
- Pulmonary embolism
- Cerebrovascular accident
- Box E1 summarizes the differential diagnosis of high-altitude illnesses

WORKUP

Typically the diagnosis is self-evident after history and physical examination. Laboratory tests and imaging studies help monitor cardiopulmonary and central nervous system status in patients admitted to the intensive care unit for pulmonary and/or cerebral edema. In patients with HAPE occurring at lower altitudes (<8000 ft), an evaluation of preexisting pulmonary hypertension or a left-to-right shunt should be considered.

LABORATORY TESTS

Not useful, unless to rule out an alternative diagnosis

IMAGING STUDIES

- Chest x-ray showing Kerley B-lines and patchy edema (see Fig. E1)
- CT scan of the head showing diffuse or patchy edema
- MRI of the head showing characteristic intense T2 signal in the white matter

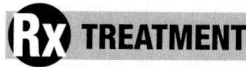

NON-PHARMACOLOGIC THERAPY

- Stop the ascent to allow acclimatization or start to descend until symptoms have resolved.
- Patient with AMS can stay at the same height and may ascend once symptoms resolve but should strongly consider using acetazolamide for the remainder of the trip.
- If the symptoms recur or fail to resolve after 2 to 3 days, descent is indicated.
- Descent is the definitive treatment and should begin immediately at the first suspicion of HACE.
- Oxygen 4 to 6 L/min is used for severe AMS, HAPE, and HACE.
- Portable hyperbaric bags are useful if available at the site.
- Altitude can cause diuresis that may be mediated by enhanced release of atrial natriuretic peptide. When coupled with the increased fluid loss through increased ventilation, there is a higher risk for dehydration, and adequate hydration should be maintained.

ACUTE PHARMACOLOGIC Rx

- Nonsteroidal anti-inflammatory drugs (e.g., ibuprofen 600 mg every 6 hours, beginning 6 hours before ascending) are often used for prophylaxis of traditional altitude sickness and in treating headaches in AMS. However trials have shown that ibuprofen is slightly inferior to acetazolamide for acute mountain sickness prevention, and should not be recommended over acetazolamide for rapid ascent.[1]

[1] Burns P et al: Altitude sickness prevention with ibuprofen relative to acetazolamide, Am J Med 132(2):247-251, 2019.

- Acetazolamide 125 to 250 mg PO bid is the preferred agent and has been effective for both prevention and acute therapy in patients with AMS and HACE. Dexamethasone is equally effective to reduce symptoms of AMS and can be used as an alternative to acetazolamide. It should also be added to acetazolamide in patients with HACE.
- Nifedipine 10 mg sublingual followed by long-acting nifedipine 30 mg bid is used for patients with HAPE who cannot descend immediately. Salvage therapy in absence of supplemental oxygen and descent also includes phosphodiesterase-5 inhibitors (sildenafil or tadalafil).
- Dexamethasone 4 mg PO every 6 hr is used in patients with severe AMS, HAPE, or HACE.

CHRONIC Rx

Prevention is the most prudent therapy.

- Slow, staged ascent to avoid altitude sickness.
- Start the ascent below 8000 feet.
- Ascend 1000 feet/day (300 m/day).
- Spend two nights at the same altitude every 3 days.
- Sleep at lower heights than the altitude climbed ("climb high, sleep low").
- Prophylactic therapy with NSAIDs (ibuprofen 600 mg every 6 hours, beginning 6 hours before ascending) or acetazolamide up to 750 mg daily and/or dexamethasone 8 to 16 mg daily decreases the risk of developing AMS (combination may have additive benefit). The drugs should be used until acclimatization occurs.
- Prophylactic inhalation of a β-adrenergic agonist, salmeterol 125 mcg q12h, or the use of slow-release nifedipine 20 mg bid have both been shown to reduce the risk of HAPE in susceptible individuals.
- Tadalafil, a long-acting phosphodiesterase inhibitor, has recently been shown to decrease the incidence of HAPE in susceptible individuals.
- Box 2 summarizes field treatment of high-altitude illness.

DISPOSITION

- AMS improves over a period of 2 to 3 days.
- HAPE is the most common cause of death among patients with altitude illnesses.
- More than 60% of patients with HAPE will have recurrence of symptoms on subsequent climbs.
- In HACE, neurologic deficits may persist for weeks but eventually resolve. If coma occurs, prognosis is poor.

REFERRAL

Cardiology and neurology referrals are made in patients with pulmonary edema and central nervous system findings, respectively.

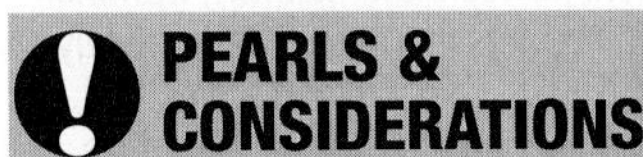

PEARLS & CONSIDERATIONS

COMMENTS

- Acclimatization is the process in which an individual who normally resides at low altitudes adapts to hypobaric hypoxia to improve tolerance and performance at higher altitudes. These mechanisms include:
  1. An increase in respiratory rate and tidal volume. This hyperventilation allows lowering of arterial carbon dioxide to preserve oxygen delivery, even at extreme altitudes.
  2. An early increase in heart rate and stroke volume to improve oxygen delivery. After 1 week, both parameters decrease because of diuresis and lower catecholamine levels.
  3. Pulmonary hypertension develops in response to hypoxemia, resulting in improvement of the ventilation-perfusion mismatch but may be maladaptive and lead to the development of HAPE.
  4. Cerebral vasodilation to increase blood flow to the brain.
  5. Rise in hemoglobin and hematocrit. This is a long-term process that takes up to 1 week to occur in response to the need for improved oxygen delivery.
- Adaptation to altitude is different from acclimatization and refers to physiologic differences in permanent residents at high altitude (e.g., an increased oxygen diffusion capacity).
- High-altitude illness can generally be prevented by ascending to 300 to 500 meters per day at altitudes above 3000 meters and including a rest day every 3 to 4 days.
- Risk factors for the development of altitude sicknesses are:
  1. Rapid ascent.
  2. Previous history of altitude sickness.
  3. Strenuous exertion on arrival.
  4. Obesity.
  5. Male gender.
- Physical fitness is not protective against high-altitude illness.
- Both dexamethasone and tadalafil decrease systolic pulmonary artery pressure and may reduce the incidence of HAPE in adults with a history of HAPE. Dexamethasone prophylaxis may also reduce the incidence of AMS in these adults.
- Descent is mandatory for all persons with HACE or HAPE.
- The American College of Chest Physicians has released a primer on caring for passengers with a variety of health conditions who are traveling to high-altitude places or areas (http://www.accpstorage.org/newOrganization/patients/TravelingwithOxygen.pdf). Specific indications for supplemental oxygen are provided in the document.

BOX 2 Field Treatment of High-Altitude Illness

High-Altitude Headache and Mild Acute Mountain Sickness
- Stop ascent, rest, acclimatize at same altitude.
- Symptomatic treatment as necessary with analgesics and anti-emetics.
- Consider acetazolamide, 125 to 250 mg bid, to speed acclimatization.
- OR descend 500 m (1640 feet) or more.

Moderate to Severe Acute Mountain Sickness
- Low-flow oxygen, if available.
- Acetazolamide, 125 to 250 mg bid, with or without dexamethasone, 4 mg PO, IM, or IV q6h.
- Hyperbaric therapy.
- OR immediate descent.

High-Altitude Cerebral Edema
- Immediate descent or evacuation.
- Oxygen, 2 to 4 L/min.
- Dexamethasone, 8 mg PO, IM, or IV, then 4 mg q6h.
- Hyperbaric therapy.

High-Altitude Pulmonary Edema
- Minimize exertion and keep warm.
- Immediate descent or hyperbaric therapy.
- Oxygen, 4 to 6 L/min until improving, then 2 to 4 L/min.

If above unavailable, one of the following:
- Nifedipine, 30 mg extended release q12h.
- Sildenafil 50 mg q8h.
- Tadalafil 10 mg q12h.
- β-agonists may be helpful.

Periodic Breathing
- Acetazolamide, 62.5 to 125 mg at bedtime as needed.

bid, Twice a day; *IM,* intramuscularly; *IV,* intravenously; *PO,* orally.
From Auerbach P: *Wilderness medicine, expert consult* Premium Edition—Enhanced Online Features and Print, Philadelphia, 2012, Saunders.

SUGGESTED READINGS

Available at ExpertConsult.com

RELATED CONTENT

Altitude Sickness (Patient Information)

AUTHORS: **JAVERYAH SAFI, M.D.,** and **SAMAAN RAFEQ, M.D.**

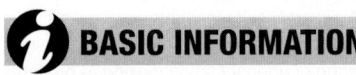

BASIC INFORMATION

DEFINITION

Hirsutism is the development of stiff, pigmented (terminal) facial and body hair (male distribution) in women as a result of excess androgen production.

SYNONYM

Excessive hair growth

ICD-10CM CODE

L68.0 Hirsutism

EPIDEMIOLOGY & DEMOGRAPHICS

- Overall prevalence unknown, estimated 5% to 10% in reproductive age women.
- Race and genetics should be considered. Some distinct ethnic populations have minimal body hair and others (Mediterranean, Middle Eastern, South Asian) have moderate to large amounts of body hair while serum androgen levels are similar.
- Social norms and culture also determine how much body hair is cosmetically acceptable.
- Half of all cases of mild hirsutism do not have hyperandrogenemia. "Patient-important hirsutism" refers to hirsutism causing woman sufficient distress to seek care.
- Incidence and presentation of hirsutism is dependent on underlying cause of androgen excess (see "Differential Diagnosis").
- Most women with hirsutism have polycystic ovary syndrome (PCOS). PCOS accounts for 95% of cases of hirsutism.

PHYSICAL FINDINGS & CLINICAL PRESENTATION

- Timing of symptoms: Abrupt onset, short duration, rapid progression, progressive worsening, more severe signs of virilization (Fig. 1), or later age of onset suggest androgen-producing tumor, late-onset congenital adrenal hyperplasia, or Cushing's syndrome. Weight increases may produce increased androgen production.
- Menstrual history: Menarche, cycle regularity and symptoms of ovulation, fertility, and contraception use. Anovulatory cycles are the most common underlying cause of androgen excess.
- Medication use history: Some drugs cause hirsutism or produce androgenic effects (danazol, phenytoin, valproic acid, androgenic progestins [e.g., norgestrel], cyclosporin, minoxidil, metoclopramide, phenothiazines, methyldopa, diazoxide, and penicillamine).
- Family history: Known or suspected family history of hirsutism, congenital adrenal hyperplasia, insulin resistance, polycystic ovary syndrome (PCOS), infertility, obesity, menstrual irregularity may be found.
- Physical exam reveals deepening voice, body habitus, increased muscle mass, galactorrhea; abdominal and pelvic exam.
- Associated cutaneous manifestations (Fig. 2) are acne, acanthosis nigricans, striae, hair distribution, location and quantity, frontotemporal balding, muscle mass, clitoromegaly.
- Ferriman-Gallwey scale, a simple, pictorial system of scoring nine body areas, is the most common tool used to quantify hirsutism. It may be unreliable in non-Caucasian women of other ethnicities.

ETIOLOGY

- Presence of hirsutism indicates androgen excess. Total testosterone may be normal, but free testosterone is elevated.
- Androgens induce vellus hair follicles (soft, unpigmented hair) in sex-specific areas (upper lip, chin, midsternum, upper abdomen, back, buttocks) to develop into thicker, more heavily pigmented terminal hairs.
- Anovulatory ovaries are usual source of excess androgens through thecal cell steroidogenesis and conversion of androstenedione to testosterone. The most common cause of hirsutism is polycystic ovary syndrome, which accounts for three out of every four cases.
- Conditions that decrease hepatic production of sex hormone binding globulin (SHBG) decrease protein-bound testosterone and increase free testosterone fraction (e.g., low estrogen, high androgen, and hyperinsulinemic states).
- Late-onset, congenital adrenal hyperplasia enzyme deficiency (most commonly 21-hydroxylase deficiency) produces excess 17 hydroxyprogesterone (17-OHP) and overproduction of androstenedione.
- Rare ovarian tumors primarily derived from Sertoli-Leydig cells, granulosa theca cells, or hilus cells produce excess androgens.
- Rare adrenal tumors produce excess androgens.
- Rare pituitary or hypothalamic tumors produce excess prolactin and can lead to anovulation.
- Box 1 summarizes causes of androgen excess in women of reproductive age.

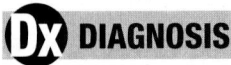

DIAGNOSIS

DIFFERENTIAL DIAGNOSIS

- Androgen-independent vellus hair: Soft, unpigmented hair that covers entire body
- Hypertrichosis: Diffusely increased total body hair (vellus or lanugo-type) not restricted to androgen-dependent areas often an adverse response to a medication or systemic illness (e.g., anorexia nervosa, porphyria, malnutrition, hypothyroidism)
- PCOS 75%
- Idiopathic 5% to 15%
- Congenital adrenal hyperplasia 1% to 8%
- Insulin resistance syndrome 3% to 4%
- Cushing's syndrome <1%
- Drug induced <1%
- Ovarian tumor <1%
- Adrenal tumor <1%
- Hyperthecosis <1%
- Hyperprolactinemia <1%

WORKUP

- Hirsutism is a clinical diagnosis.
- Management of hirsutism is largely independent of the etiology.
- Workup in selected hirsute women is directed to determine underlying cause of androgen excess.
- See specific conditions for more detailed workup of individual diagnoses.

LABORATORY TESTS

Establishing laboratory evidence of excess androgens in women with moderate or severe hirsutism, sudden onset, rapid progression, or associated menstrual dysfunction, central obesity, clitoromegaly, or acanthosis nigricans is an approach consistent with guidelines from the Endocrine Society, the American College of Obstetricians and Gynecologists, the Androgen Excess and Polycystic Ovary Syndrome Society, and the American Association of Clinical Endocrinologists.

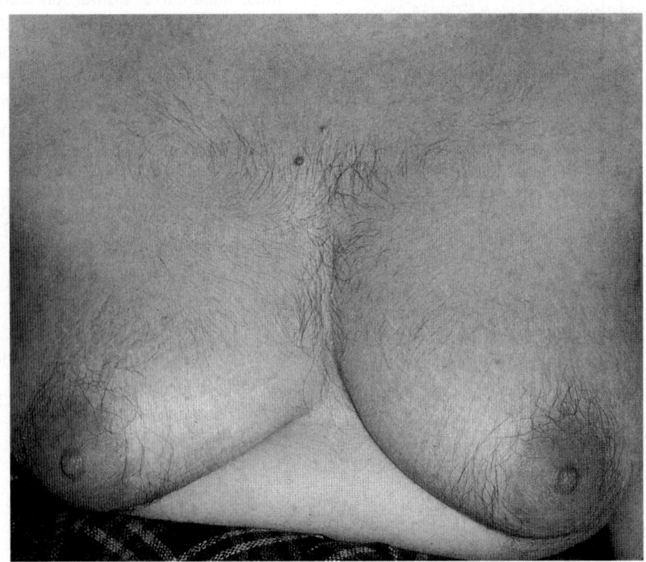

FIG. 1 Hirsutism. (From James WD et al: *Andrews' diseases of the skin*, ed 12, Philadelphia, 2016, Saunders.)

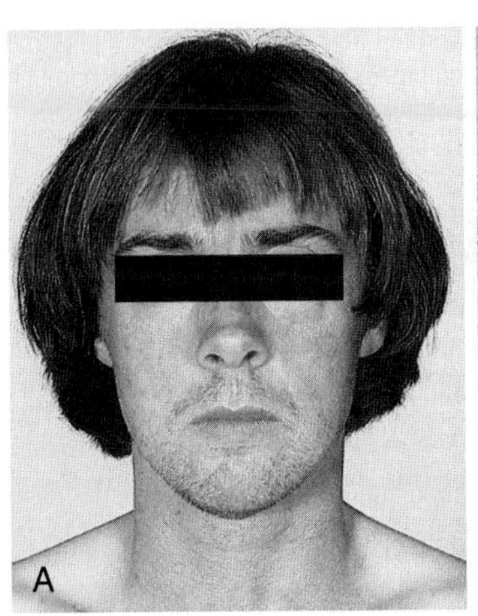

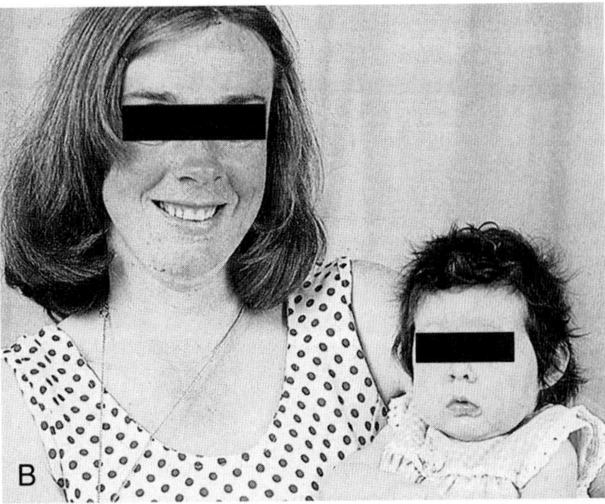

FIG. 2 A patient with an arrhenoblastoma with associated polycystic ovaries before and after treatment. A, Before treatment, the patient had marked facial hirsutism. **B,** The patient is shown successfully treated. The tumor was resected and ovulation ensued with clomiphene and human chorionic gonadotropin therapy. (From Besser CM, Thorner MO: *Comprehensive clinical endocrinology,* ed 3, St Louis, 2002, Mosby.)

BOX 1 Causes of Androgen Excess in Women of Reproductive Age

Ovarian
Polycystic ovary syndrome (PCOS)
Hyperthecosis (a severe PCOS variant)
Ovarian tumor (e.g., Sertoli-Leydig cell tumor)

Adrenal
Nonclassic adrenal hyperplasia
Cushing's syndrome
Glucocorticoid resistance
Adrenal tumor (e.g., adenoma, carcinoma)

Specific Conditions of Pregnancy
Luteoma of pregnancy
Hyperreaction luteinalis
Aromatase deficiency in fetus

Other
Hyperprolactinemia, hypothyroidism
Medications (danazol, testosterone, anabolizing agents)
Idiopathic hirsutism (normal serum testosterone in an ovulatory woman)
Idiopathic hyperandrogenism (patients who do not fall into any of the other categories listed)

From Melmed S et al: *Williams textbook of endocrinology,* ed 12, Philadelphia, 2011, Saunders.

- Total plasma testosterone (normal range 20-60 ng/dl [0.69-2.1 nmol/L]) or free testosterone: Early morning on day 4 to 10 of menstrual cycle to screen for testosterone-secreting tumors. If moderately or markedly elevated (total testosterone >150 ng/dl [5.2 nmol/L], free testosterone >2 ng/dl [0.07 nmol/L]) may image adrenals and ovaries for androgen-secreting tumors.

Other laboratory test considerations if appropriate:
- Prolactin: Moderately elevated values should prompt imaging of pituitary-hypothalamic region.
- 17-OHP (17 α-hydroxyprogesterone): Screen for adrenal enzyme deficiencies. Morning value >200 ng/dl in early follicular phase suggests nonclassic (late onset) congenital adrenal hyperplasia due to 21-hydroxylase deficiency and may be confirmed with high-dose (250 mcg) ACTH stimulation test.
- Thyroid-stimulating hormone (TSH): Rule out hypothyroidism.
- Dehydroepiandrosterone sulfate (DHEA-S): Screen for adrenal androgen production as almost entirely produced by adrenals. Levels >700 mcg/dl (13.6 nmol/L) raise suspicion for adrenal androgen-secreting tumor.

Additional laboratory test considerations if appropriate:
- Follicle-stimulating hormone (FSH): Rule out hypoestrogenic state (perimenopausal).
- Luteinizing hormone (LH): Typically elevated in PCOS with low or normal FSH.
- 24-hour urinary free cortisol: Rule out Cushing's syndrome and overproduction of cortisol.
- Overnight single-dose dexamethasone suppression test: Rule out Cushing's syndrome and adrenal hyperfunction.
- Fasting blood sugar (FBS), 2-hr 75-g oral glucose tolerance test, fasting insulin levels: Rule out insulin resistance syndrome.
- Table 1 summarizes laboratory tests for the differential diagnosis of androgen excess.

IMAGING STUDIES

Imaging study considerations if appropriate:
- Pelvic ultrasound (high resolution, transvaginal): Rule out ovarian tumor if total testosterone is elevated.
- Abdominal CT/MRI: Rule out adrenal tumor if elevated DHEAS.
- Pituitary-hypothalamic region CT/MRI: Rule out pituitary tumor if prolactin elevated.
- Laparoscopy/laparotomy: Rule out small ovarian tumor in cases of elevated testosterone levels without radiologic evidence of adrenal or ovarian pathology.

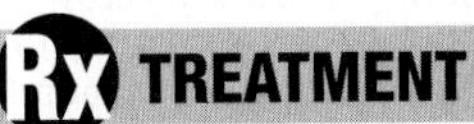

Rx TREATMENT

NONPHARMACOLOGIC THERAPY

- Weight reduction: Can reduce androgen production indirectly by reducing insulin-stimulated theca cell androgen production and improve menstrual function, and slow hair growth in obese women.
- Cosmetic: Temporary.
  1. Shaving: Does not stimulate hair growth; lasts days, leaves stubble.
  2. Epilation: Electronic plucking.
  3. Bleaching: Removes hair pigment. May cause skin irritation.
  4. Mechanical waxing/plucking.
  5. Depilatories: Gels, lotions, or creams that chemically disrupt sulfide bonds of hair causing dissolution of hair shaft. No stubble.
  6. Photoepilation (laser and intense pulsed light [IPL]): Hair follicles destroyed by wavelengths of light absorbed by melanin. Good for pigmented hair; laser treatment is more effective than shaving, waxing, and electrolysis. It lasts 3 to 6 months as vellus follicles remain and can be converted to terminal pigmented hair under excess androgens.
- Cosmetic: Permanent. Electrolysis: Destroys individual hair follicles. May be expensive and time consuming.

ACUTE GENERAL Rx

See "Pharmacologic Therapy."

CHRONIC Rx

See "Pharmacologic Therapy."

PHARMACOLOGIC THERAPY

- Usually second-line treatment following nonpharmacologic, physical methods of hair control, and in consideration of patient's comorbidities and risk factors, patient preferences, area of excess hair amenable to treatment, and access and affordability of treatments.
- Pharmacologic treatments categorized as topical, oral contraceptive pills (OCPs), antiandrogens (potential adverse effects on a developing male fetus, so use with reliable contraception), other treatments directed at specific underlying etiology.
- Topical: Eflornithine topical cream 13.9%: Unclear mechanism of action; may

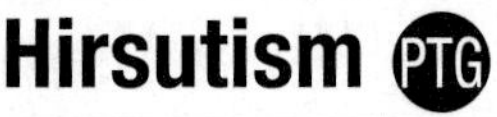

TABLE 1 Laboratory Tests for the Differential Diagnosis of Androgen Excess

Initial Testing

Total testosterone
Prolactin
Thyroid-stimulating hormone

Further Testing Based on Clinical Presentation

17-Hydroxyprogesterone (8:00 a.m.)
17-Hydroxyprogesterone 60 min after IV ACTH
Cortisol (8:00 a.m.) after 1 mg dexamethasone at midnight
DHEAS
Androstenedione
Imaging of ovaries (transvaginal ultrasonography)
Imaging of adrenals (abdominal ultrasonography, CT, MRI)
Nuclear imaging after IV administration of radiolabeled cholesterol

ACTH, Adrenocorticotropic hormone; *CT,* computed tomography; *DHEAS,* dehydroepiandrosterone sulfate *IV,* intravenous; *MRI,* magnetic resonance imaging.
From Melmed S et al: *Williams textbook of endocrinology,* ed 12, Philadelphia, 2011, Saunders.

inhibit ornithine decarboxylase, retarding hair growth. Temporary cosmetic treatment for facial hair. Applied directly to unwanted facial hair bid with at least 8-hr spaced applications. Does not remove hair, rather slows growth. Slow response over 4 to 8 wk. Hair growth returns upon discontinuation of treatment.

- OCPs: Suppress ovarian steroidogenesis and LH through low-dose estrogen and low androgenic progestational agents. Slow response to treatment. Suppresses new hair growth. Established hair unaffected. Low-dose OCPs with low androgenic progestational agents, for example, desogestrel, drospirenone, norgestimate. Avoid norgestrel and levonorgestrel (higher androgenic progestational agents).
- Antiandrogens: Spironolactone: When OCPs unacceptable or may be added for disappointing results after 6 mo of OCP treatment.
  1. Aldosterone-antagonist diuretic inhibits adrenal and ovarian biosynthesis of androgens. May result in ovulation, so consider contraception needs.
  2. Slow response usually 6 mo or more.
  3. 200 mg PO qd, then decrease to 25 to 50 mg qd maintenance.
  4. May cause hyperkalemia.
  5. Anovulatory, unopposed estrogen states require progestin management.

REFERRAL

- To endocrinologist if difficulty in determining diagnosis, achieving therapeutic goals, or resistant to first-line therapies. Prepubertal and postmenopausal hirsutism is suspicious for neoplastic or secondary endocrine causes and should be referred for further evaluation.
- Consider referral or consultation for following therapies:
  1. Finasteride: Antiandrogen, in hair follicle blocks 5α-reductase conversion of testosterone to intranuclearly active 5α-dihydrotestosterone (DHT).
     a. Use only with reliable contraception because DHT necessary for normal male fetus urogenital development.
     b. Not FDA approved for treatment of hirsutism.
     c. 1 to 5 mg PO qd.
  2. Flutamide: Inhibits androgen uptake and receptor binding
     a. Not recommended by Endocrine Society Clinical Practice Guidelines and not FDA approved for treatment of hirsutism, but used by some European endocrinologists.
     b. Use only with reliable contraception.
     c. Reserved for women with severe, resistant hirsutism because of risk of hepatic dysfunction.
  3. Cyproterone acetate: Antiandrogen that competes with DHT for binding androgen receptors. Used as progestin component of OCPs outside the United States.
- Other treatments directed at specific underlying etiology:
  1. Metformin/thiazolidinediones: Therapy reserved for documented insulin-resistant states.
  2. GnRH agonists: Recommended only in women with severe hyperandrogenemia (e.g., ovarian hyperthecosis) with suboptimal response to combination low-dose estrogen/progestin pills and antiandrogen treatment. Inhibits gonadotropin and consequently ovarian androgen and estrogen secretion.
  3. Dexamethasone: Adrenal glucocorticoid suppression is reserved for diagnosis of adrenal enzyme deficiency.
  4. Total abdominal hysterectomy/bilateral salpingo-oophorectomy reserved for recalcitrant hirsutism in older female with hyperthecosis and undesired fertility.

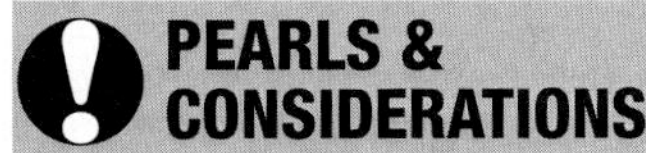

PEARLS & CONSIDERATIONS

COMMENTS

- Hirsutism is both an endocrine and cosmetic problem for patients.
- Ovulation induction therapy is indicated in women desiring pregnancy.
- Delay checking serum androgens until oral contraceptives have been discontinued for 2 to 3 mo.
- Evaluation of incidental adrenal mass is always warranted.

SUGGESTED READINGS

Available at ExpertConsult.com

RELATED CONTENT

Hirsutism (Patient Information)
Polycystic Ovary Syndrome (Related Key Topic)

AUTHOR: **FRED F. FERRI, M.D.**

BASIC INFORMATION

DEFINITION

Hodgkin lymphoma is a malignant disorder arising from germinal center B cells and characterized histologically by the presence of multinucleated giant cells (Reed-Sternberg cells) in a mixed inflammatory background.

ICD-10CM CODES

C81.90	Hodgkin lymphoma, unspecified, unspecified site
C81.00	Nodular lymphocyte predominant Hodgkin lymphoma, unspecified site
C81.10	Nodular sclerosis classical Hodgkin lymphoma, unspecified site
C81.20	Mixed cellularity classical Hodgkin lymphoma, unspecified site
C81.30	Lymphocyte depleted classical Hodgkin lymphoma, unspecified site
C81.79	Other classical Hodgkin lymphoma, extranodal and solid organ sites
C81.90	Hodgkin lymphoma, unspecified, unspecified site
C81.91	Hodgkin lymphoma, unspecified, lymph nodes of head, face, and neck
C81.92	Hodgkin lymphoma, unspecified, intrathoracic lymph nodes
C81.93	Hodgkin lymphoma, unspecified, intra-abdominal lymph nodes
C81.94	Hodgkin lymphoma, unspecified, lymph nodes of axilla and upper limb
C81.95	Hodgkin lymphoma, unspecified, lymph nodes of inguinal region and lower limb
C81.96	Hodgkin lymphoma, unspecified, intrapelvic lymph nodes
C81.97	Hodgkin lymphoma, unspecified, spleen
C81.98	Hodgkin lymphoma, unspecified, lymph nodes of multiple sites
C81.99	Hodgkin lymphoma, unspecified, extranodal and solid organ sites

EPIDEMIOLOGY & DEMOGRAPHICS

- There is a bimodal age distribution (15-34 yr and >50 yr).
- Incidence is 4 in 100,000 cases; >8000 new cases of Hodgkin lymphoma diagnosed annually in the U.S.
- Concordance for Hodgkin lymphoma in identical twins suggests that a genetic susceptibility underlies Hodgkin lymphoma in young adulthood.
- There is association between certain HLA haplotypes, especially HLA-A1.
- The disease is more common in males (in childhood Hodgkin lymphoma, >80% occur in males), whites, and higher socioeconomic groups.
- There is an increased risk in smokers and HIV-infected individuals.

PHYSICAL FINDINGS & CLINICAL PRESENTATION

- Painless palpable lymphadenopathy is the most common presenting symptom.
- The most common site of involvement is the neck region.
- Fever and night sweats: Fever in a cyclical pattern (days or weeks of fever alternating with afebrile periods) is known as Pel-Ebstein fever.
- Unexplained weight loss, generalized malaise.
- Persistent, nonproductive cough.
- Lymph node pain associated with alcohol ingestion often because of heavy eosinophil infiltration of the tumor sites is relatively uncommon.
- Generalized pruritus.
- Hepatosplenomegaly.
- Other: Superior vena cava syndrome, spinal cord compression (rare), erythema nodosum (very rare), ichthyosis (very rare).

ETIOLOGY

- Evidence implicating Epstein-Barr virus remains controversial.
- Cigarette smoking has also been implicated.

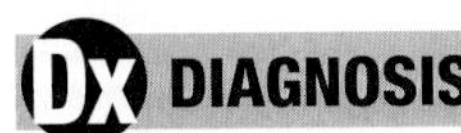

DIAGNOSIS

DIFFERENTIAL DIAGNOSIS

- Non-Hodgkin's lymphoma
- Sarcoidosis
- Infections (e.g., cytomegalovirus, Epstein-Barr virus, toxoplasmosis, HIV, tuberculosis)
- Drug reaction

WORKUP

Diagnosis is confirmed by lymph node biopsy. The World Health Organization classifies Hodgkin lymphoma into two groups: classical Hodgkin lymphoma (92% to 97%) and nodular lymphocyte-predominant Hodgkin lymphoma (3% to 8%). Classical Hodgkin lymphoma has four main histologic subtypes based on the number of lymphocytes, Reed-Sternberg cells, and the presence of fibrous tissue (Table 1):

- Nodular sclerosis (Fig. E1)
- Mixed cellularity (Fig. E2)
- Lymphocyte rich
- Lymphocyte depleted

Nodular sclerosis occurs mainly in young adulthood, whereas the mixed cellularity type is more prevalent after age 50 yr. Table 2 summarizes key features of Hodgkin lymphomas.

Staging: Table 3 describes the Cotswolds staging classification.

Proper staging requires the following:

- Detailed history (with documentation of "B symptoms" and physical examination).
- Excisional biopsy with histologic, immunophenotypic and immunohistochemical analysis.
- Laboratory evaluation (complete blood count, erythrocyte sedimentation rate [ESR], blood urea nitrogen, creatinine, liver function tests, albumin, lactate dehydrogenase, HIV test), immunophenotypic markers (see Table 4).
- Positron emission tomography (PET)/computed tomography (CT) scan of the chest, abdomen, and pelvis.
- Unilateral bone marrow biopsy in selected patients.

Box 1 summarizes recommended staging procedures for Hodgkin lymphoma.

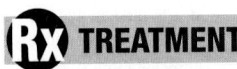

TREATMENT

ACUTE GENERAL Rx

The main therapeutic modality includes chemotherapy with or without radiotherapy depending on stage and other risk factors (Table 5). In general, chemotherapy plus involved-site radiotherapy is standard treatment for Hodgkin lymphoma in the early stages; however, recent data suggest that chemotherapy alone is appropriate for a significant proportion of patients. Chemotherapy (Table 6) is used for advanced stage disease with radiotherapy in selected patients, such as those with bulky disease.

Most oncologists prefer the combination of adriamycin (doxorubicin), bleomycin, vinblastine, and dacarbazine (ABVD). ABVD does not cause infertility or stem cell damage and has also shown to be effective in patients with HIV infection and Hodgkin lymphoma. Table 7 describes characteristics of the ABVD regimen.

Recent trials have shown that in patients with early-stage Hodgkin lymphoma and favorable prognosis, defined by fewer than three nodal sites without bulky or extranodal disease in the absence of ESR >50 without symptoms or 30 with symptoms, treatment with two cycles of ABVD followed by 20 Gy of involved-field radiation therapy may be as effective as, and less toxic than, four cycles of ABVD followed by 30 Gy of involved-field radiation therapy. For patients with early stage disease who do not meet these criteria, options include three or four cycles of ABVD plus involved site radiotherapy to 30 Gy. In addition, chemotherapy alone, in the absence of bulky disease, is an alternative approach, especially in women younger than 30 yr given the increased risk of including breast cancer, as well as cardiac and thyroid disease. Although the risk of disease recurrence is slightly higher in patients who receive chemotherapy alone, there is no difference in overall survival.

TABLE 1 Frequency of Histologic Subtypes of Hodgkin Lymphoma According to the 2008 WHO Classification

Classic Hodgkin Lymphoma (cHL)	95%
• Nodular sclerosis classic Hodgkin lymphoma (NSCHL)	70%
• Mixed cellularity classic Hodgkin lymphoma (MCCHL)	20%–25%
• Lymphocyte-rich classic Hodgkin lymphoma (LRCHL)	5%
• Lymphocyte-depleted classic Hodgkin lymphoma (LDCHL)	<1%
Nodular Lymphocyte Predominant Hodgkin Lymphoma (NLPHL)	5%

From Hoffman R et al: *Hematology, basic principles and practice*, ed 7, Philadelphia, 2018, Elsevier.

TABLE 2 Key Features of Hodgkin Lymphomas

Lymphoma	Demographics, Clinical Presentation	Morphology	Cell Surface Markers	Prognosis
Nodular, lymphocyte predominant (NLPHL)	M > F, 30-50 years, with peripheral lymphadenopathy	Mononuclear cells with convoluted nuclei (popcorn or L&H cells) loosely aggregated in nodules of small B cells	CD45, CD20, bcl-6, J-chain, Oct-2, BOB.1, EBV absent in LP cells	Excellent for stages I, II
Nodular sclerosis	M = F, <30 years with mediastinal mass, occasional spleen or lung involvement; 40% have B symptoms; most patients present with stage II disease	Broad bands of collagen, nodules of lymphoid tissue with aggregates of HRS cells and lacunar cells, multinucleated variants	CD15, CD30, CD45-EBV in 1%-40%	Good with systemic therapy
Mixed cellularity	M > F; median age, 38 years; peripheral lymphadenopathy common, spleen, BM; B symptoms common; patients often stage III or IV	Classic HRS cells in mixture of lymphocytes, plasma cells, eosinophils, histiocytes	CD15, CD30, CD45-EBV in 75%	Good with systemic therapy
Lymphocyte depletion	M > F; median age, 30-37 years; B symptoms, advanced stage common; associated with HIV	Classic HRS cells common with paucity of background lymphocytes; pleomorphic HRS cells mimic sarcoma	CD15, CD30, CD45-EBV positive in HIV-affected patients	Associated with advanced stage
Lymphocyte-rich classical	M > F, older age; peripheral lymphadenopathy; B symptoms rare; most patients with stage I or II disease	Scattered classic HRS cells among numerous small lymphocytes; nodular growth pattern	CD15, CD30; Oct2 and BOB.1 vary; J-chain absent; EBV in 40%-75%	Good, similar to NLPHL

BM, Bone marrow; *CHL,* classical Hodgkin lymphoma; *EBV,* Epstein-Barr virus; *F,* female; *HIV,* human immunodeficiency virus; *HRS,* Hodgkin Reed-Sternberg; *L&H,* lymphocytic and histiocytic; *LP,* lymphoplasmacytic; *M,* male.
From McPherson RA, Pincus MR: *Henry's clinical diagnosis and management by laboratory methods,* ed 23, St Louis, 2017, Elsevier.

TABLE 3 Cotswold-Modified Ann Arbor Staging System for Hodgkin Lymphoma

Stage	Criteria
I	Disease affecting a single lymph node region or lymphoid structure (e.g., spleen, thymus, Waldeyer ring)
II	Disease affecting two or more discrete lymph node regions confined to the same side of the diaphragm
III	Disease affecting two or more discrete lymph node regions or lymphoid structures on both sides of the diaphragm
IV	Disease that has spread to one or more extranodal sites (that do not meet the criteria for E) or extralymphatic structure including involvement of the bone marrow, liver, or lungs
Designation	**Criteria**
A	Absence of B symptoms[a]
B	Presence of B symptoms[a]
S	Involvement of the spleen
E	Single extranodal site or involvement of an extranodal site that is contiguous to an involved nodal region
X	Bulky disease as defined as >1/3 mediastinum at its widest part or a nodal mass >10 cm at its greatest diameter

[a]B symptoms: Constitutional symptoms including night sweats, fevers, or weight loss (>10% over 6 months).
From Hoffman R et al: *Hematology, basic principles and practice,* ed 7, Philadelphia, 2018, Elsevier.

TABLE 4 Selected Immunophenotypic Markers and Histologic Characteristics of Use in the Differential Diagnosis of Hodgkin Lymphoma and Other Lymphoid Neoplasms

Marker	Classical HL	Nodular Lymphocyte Predominant HL	TCRBCL	ALCL
CD30	+	–	–	+
CD15	+	–	–	–
CD20	–/+*	+	+	–
CD45	–	+	+	+/–
CD79a	–	+	+	–
ALK	–	–	–	+/–
EMA	–	+	+	+
Nodular growth protein	+/–†	+	–	–

+, >90% of cases positive; +/–, majority of cases positive; –/+, minority of cases positive; –, <10% of cases positive; *ALCL,* anaplastic large cell lymphoma; *HL,* Hodgkin lymphoma; *TCRBCL,* T-cell rich B-cell lymphoma.
*CD20 positivity in classical Hodgkin lymphoma is quite heterogeneous, with a wide range in brightness of staining.
†In classical Hodgkin lymphoma, a nodular growth pattern is confined to the nodular sclerosing subtype.
From Abeloff MD: *Clinical oncology,* ed 3, Philadelphia, 2004, Saunders.

BEACOPP, an intensified regimen consisting of bleomycin, etoposide, doxorubicin, cyclophosphamide, vincristine, procarbazine, and prednisone, has been advocated by some as the new standard for treatment of advanced Hodgkin lymphoma in place of ABVD. Recent trials have shown that treatment with BEACOPP, as compared with ABVD, results in better initial tumor control, but the long-term clinical outcome does not differ significantly between the two regimens. In addition, with the use of the escalated BEACOPP regimen, the rate of complications is higher (3% treatment-related death, 20% rate of hospitalization, and 3% rate of secondary leukemia, and near-universal infertility). Thus, if the goal is cure with the least overall toxic effects, it is best to favor ABVD therapy, reserving rescue therapy with high-dose chemotherapy and autologous hematopoietic stem-cell transplantation for the small number of patients in whom the primary treatment fails.

In March 2018, the FDA approved the combination of brentuximab vedotin and doxorubicin, vinblastine and dacarbazine (AVD) for previously untreated, stage III or IV Hodgkin lymphoma patients. The combination of brentuximab vedotin and AVD was associated with a longer median modified progression-free survival than ABVD, but also was associated with higher rates of neutropenia and neuropathy.

- Definitions of treatment groups are described in Table 8.
- Recommendations for the primary treatment of Hodgkin lymphoma outside of clinical trials are described in Table 9.
- In 2011, the FDA approved the use of the anti-CD30 antibody drug conjugate brentuximab vedotin for the treatment of patients with Hodgkin lymphoma who have relapsed after autologous stem cell transplant and for patients who have relapsed but are not candidates for transplant. Brentuximab vedotin is associated with an overall response rate of 75%.

BOX 1 Recommended Staging Procedures for Hodgkin Lymphoma

The following staging procedures are recommended for the initial workup of Hodgkin lymphoma:

1. Adequate surgical biopsy reviewed by an experienced hematopathologist
2. Cytologic examination of any effusion in selected cases
3. Detailed history, with attention to the presence or absence of systemic symptoms, and a careful physical examination, emphasizing node chains, size of the liver and spleen, and inspection of Waldeyer ring
4. Routine laboratory tests: Complete blood cell count, erythrocyte sedimentation rate, and liver function tests
5. Neck, chest, and abdominal CT imaging fused with 18-FDG PET scan (Fig. E3)

From Hoffman R et al: *Hematology: basic principles and practice,* ed 5, Philadelphia, 2009, Churchill Livingstone.

TABLE 5 Standard Treatment Approach According to Prognostic Group

Early-favorable HL	Combined modality therapy • 2–4 cycles of chemotherapy followed by involved-field radiotherapy
Early-unfavorable HL (intermediate-stage)	Combined modality therapy • 4–6 cycles of chemotherapy followed by involved-field radiotherapy
Advanced HL	Extensive chemotherapy • 6–8 cycles of chemotherapy ± consolidation with localized radiotherapy

From Hoffman R et al: *Hematology, basic principles and practice*, ed 7, Philadelphia, 2018, Elsevier.

TABLE 6 Standard Chemotherapy Regimens for the Treatment of Advanced Hodgkin Lymphoma

Regimen	Drugs	Route	Schedule
ABVD	Adriamycin 25 mg/m^2	IV	Day 1 and 15
	Bleomycin 10 mg/m^2	IV	Day 1 and 15
	Vinblastine 6 mg/m^2	IV	Day 1 and 15
	Dacarbazine 375 mg/m^2	IV	Day 1 and 15
			Every 28 days
BEACOPP (escalated)	Bleomycin 10 mg/m^2	IV	Day 8
	Etoposide 200 mg/m^2	IV	Day 1–3
	Adriamycin 35 mg/m^2	IV	Day 1
	Cyclophosphamide 1250 mg/m^2	IV	Day 1
	Vincristine 1.4 mg/m^2	IV	Day 8
	Procabazine 100 mg/m^2	PO	Days 1–7
	Prednisolone 40 mg/m^2	PO	Days 1–14
	G-CSF	SC	From day 8
			Every 21 days

G-CSF, Granulocyte colony-stimulating factor.
From Hoffman R et al: *Hematology, basic principles and practice*, ed 7, Philadelphia, 2018, Elsevier.

TABLE 7 Characteristics of the ABVD Regimen

Agents: Doxorubicin, bleomycin, vinblastine, dacarbazine
All intravenous, total compliance
80% complete response rate
10% primary refractory disease
60%-65% overall disease-free survival
Most relapses occur within the first 4 yr; however, about 10% of all relapses occur beyond 5 yr
Major side effects are nausea, phlebitis, myelosuppression, less cumulative myelotoxicity than MOPP
No infertility
No leukemia

ABVD, Adriamycin (doxorubicin), bleomycin, vinblastine, dacarbazine; *MOPP,* mechlorethamine, Oncovin (vincristine), procarbazine, prednisone.
From Abeloff MD: *Clinical oncology*, ed 3, Philadelphia, 2004, Saunders.

- In August 2015, brentuximab vedotin was approved as consolidation therapy after autologous transplant in patients at high risk for relapse. The median progression-free survival with brentuximab vedotin was 43 mo vs. 24 mo in patients who received placebo.
- In May 2016, the FDA approved the anti-PD-1 monoclonal antibody nivolumab for patients with Hodgkin lymphoma who relapsed after autologous stem cell transplant and post-transplant brentuximab vedotin. The overall response rate to nivolumab was 65%, and the complete response rate was 7%.
- In March 2017, the FDA approved the anti-PD-1 monoclonal antibody pembrolizumab in patients with refractory disease or those who have relapsed after three or more lines of therapy. The overall response rate was 69%, and the complete response rate was 22%.

DISPOSITION

- Cure rates as high as 85% to 90% in early stage patients and 75% in stage III/V disease are now possible with appropriate initial therapy.
- Poor prognostic features (Table 10, Table 11) include presence of B symptoms, advanced age, advanced stage at initial presentation, male sex, low albumin, high ESR, lymphocyte depletion histology, and increased number of tumor-associated macrophages.
- Unlike escalated BEACOPP, ABVD is not associated with a risk of leukemia.
- Mediastinal irradiation increases the risk of subsequent cardiac disease, including valvular and pericardial disease, accelerated coronary artery disease, and conduction abnormalities.
- Radiation therapy increases the risk of developing secondary solid tumors, especially breast cancer in women younger than age 30 yr (Table 12).
- Table 13 describes potential late complications of Hodgkin lymphoma treatment and appropriate clinical responses and preventive strategies.

REFERRAL

- To surgery for lymph node biopsy
- Fertility clinic for sperm banking
- Hematology/oncology
- Radiation oncology, in selected cases

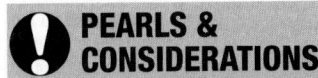

PEARLS & CONSIDERATIONS

COMMENTS

- Young male patients should consider sperm banking before the initiation of therapy even though the risk of infertility with ABVD is low. Symptomatic males, particularly with advanced stage Hodgkin lymphoma, may have disease-related oligospermia at diagnosis.
- Chemotherapy with or without involved-field radiotherapy should be the standard treatment for Hodgkin lymphoma with early stage disease. Chemotherapy with radiation in selected cases should be the standard of care for advanced stage.
- After failure of ABVD therapy, more than 60% of patients who have had a relapse and about

TABLE 8 Definition of Treatment Groups According to the EORTC/GELA and GHSG

Treatment Group	EORTC/GELA	GHSG	NCIC/ECOG
Early-stage favorable	CS I-II without risk factors (supra-diaphragmatic)	CS I-II without risk factors	Standard risk group: Favorable CSD I-II (without risk factors)
Early-stage unfavorable (intermediate)	CS I-II with ≥1 risk factors (supra-diaphragmatic)	CS I, CSIIA ≥1 risk factors; CS IIB with C/D but without A/B	Standard risk group: Unfavorable CS I-II (at least one risk factor)
Advanced stage	CS III-IV	CS IIB with A/B;CS III-IV	High-risk group: CS I or II with bulky disease; intraabdominal disease; CS III, IV
Risk factors (RF)	A large mediastinal mass B age ≥50 yr C elevated ESR* D ≥4 involved regions	A large mediastinal mass B extranodal disease C elevated ESR* D ≥3 involved areas	A ≥40 years B not NLPHL or NS histology C ESR ≥50 mm/h D ≥4 involved nodal regions

CS, Clinical stage; *ECOG,* Eastern Cooperative Oncology Group; *EORTC,* European Organization for Research and Treatment of Cancer; *GELA,* Groupe d'Etude des Lymphomes de l'Adulte; *GHSG,* German Hodgkin Study Group; *NCIC,* National Cancer Institute of Canada.
*Erythrocyte sedimentation rate (ESR) (≥50 mm/h without or ≥30 mm/h with B-symptoms).
From Hoffman R et al: *Hematology, basic principles and practice*, ed 5, New York, 2009, Churchill Livingstone.

TABLE 9 Recommendations for the Primary Treatment of Hodgkin Lymphoma Outside of Clinical Trials

Group	Stage	Recommendation
Early stages (favorable)	CS I-II A/B, no RFs	2 cycles ABVD + ISRT (20 Gy)
	Early stages (unfavorable, intermediate)	4-6 cycles ABVD ±30 Gy for nonbulky disease
	CS I-II A/B + RFs	4-6 cycles ABVD + 30 Gy for bulky disease
Advanced stages	CS IIB + RFs, CS III A/B, CS IV A/B	6 cycles ABVD; BEACOPP-escalated *or* BEACOPP-14 ± RT, 20-30 Gy for residual tumor (PET positive) and/or bulky disease

ABVD regimen, Adriamycin (doxorubicin), vinblastine, bleomycin, and dacarbazine; *BEACOPP-baseline* regimen, bleomycin, etoposide, Adriamycin (doxorubicin), cyclophosphamide, Oncovin (vincristine), procarbazine, and prednisone; *BEACOPP-escalated* regimen, bleomycin, etoposide, Adriamycin (doxorubicin), cyclophosphamide, Oncovin (vincristine), procarbazine, prednisone, and G-CSF; *BEACOPP-14* regimen, bleomycin, etoposide, Adriamycin (doxorubicin), cyclophosphamide, Oncovin (vincristine), procarbazine, prednisone, and G-CSF; *CS,* clinical stage; *IF,* involved field; *MOPP* regimen, mechlorethamine, Oncovin (vincristine), procarbazine, and prednisone; *PET,* positron emission tomography; *RF,* risk factors; *RT,* radiation therapy; *Stanford V* regimen, nitrogen mustard, doxorubicin, vinblastine, bleomycin, vincristine, etoposide, and prednisone.
From Hoffman R et al: *Hematology, basic principles and practice*, ed 5, New York, 2009, Churchill Livingstone.

TABLE 10 Prognostic Factors in Early and Advanced-Stage Hodgkin Lymphoma

Prognostic Group	EORTC	GHSG	NCCN
Early-favorable	CS I-II without risk factors (supra-diaphragmatic)	CS I-II without risk factors	CS IA-IIA without risk factors
Early-unfavorable (Intermediate)	CS I-II with ≥1 risk factor (supra-diaphragmatic)	CS I-IIA with ≥1 risk factor C/D but not A/B	CS I-II with ≥1 risk factor
Advanced	CS III-IV	CS IIB with risk factors A/B CS III/IV	CS III-IV
Prognostic factors	(A) Bulky mediastinal mass[a] (B) Age ≥50 years (C) Elevated ESR (>50 mm/h without B symptoms; >30 mm/h with B symptoms)[b] (D) ≥4 nodal areas (out of 5 supra-diaphragmatic EORTC areas)	(A) Bulky mediastinal mass[a] (B) Extranodal disease (>1 lesion) (C) Elevated ESR (>50 mm/h without B symptoms; >30 mm/h with B symptoms)[b] (D) (D) ≥3 nodal areas (out of 11 GHSG areas)	(A) Bulky mediastinal mass[a] (B) Bulk >10 cm (C) Elevated ESR (>50 mm/h without B symptoms) (D) B symptoms (E) ≥4 nodal areas (out of 17 Ann Arbor regions)

CS, Clinical stage; *EORTC,* European Organization for Research and Treatment of Cancer; *ESR,* estimated sedimentation rate; *GHSG,* German Hodgkin Study Group; *NCCN,* National Comprehensive Cancer Network.
[a]Bulky mediastinal mass: Ratio ≥0.035 of the maximum horizontal chest diameter (*EORTC*); ratio ≥1/3 of the maximum horizontal chest diameter (*GHSG*); ratio >1/3 of the maximum horizontal chest diameter (*NCCN*).
[b]B symptoms: Night-sweats, fever, weight loss (unexplained, >10% over 6 months).
From Hoffman R et al: *Hematology, basic principles and practice*, ed 7, Philadelphia, 2018, Elsevier.

TABLE 11 International Prognostic Score (IPS) for Advanced Hodgkin Lymphoma

No. of Prognostic Factors	% of patients	5-year FFP (%)	5-year OS (%)
0–1 (low-risk)	29	79	90
2–3 (intermediate-risk)	52	64	80
4–7 (high-risk)	19	47	59

FFP, Freedom from progression; *OS,* overall survival.
From Hoffman R et al: *Hematology, basic principles and practice*, ed 7, Philadelphia, 2018, Elsevier.

TABLE 12 Second Neoplasms Seen With Increased Frequency After Successful Hodgkin Lymphoma Treatment

Acute myelogenous leukemia/myelodysplasia (BEACOPP)
Non-Hodgkin's lymphoma
Melanoma
Soft tissue sarcoma
Adenocarcinoma
Breast
Thyroid
Lung
Stomach and esophagus
Squamous cell carcinoma
Skin
Uterine cervix
Head and neck

From Abeloff MD: *Clinical oncology*, ed 3, Philadelphia, 2004, Saunders.

30% of patients with initially refractory lymphoma can be reliably cured with high-dose chemotherapy and autologous hematopoietic stem-cell transplantation.

SUGGESTED READINGS

Available at ExpertConsult.com

RELATED CONTENT

Hodgkin Lymphoma (Patient Information)

AUTHORS: **JORGE J. CASTILLO, M.D.,** and **ANN S. LACASCE, M.D., M.M.SC.**

TABLE 13 Potential Late Complications of Hodgkin Lymphoma Treatment and Appropriate Clinical Responses and Preventive Strategies

Risk/Problem	Incidence/Response
Dental caries	Neck or oropharyngeal irradiation can cause decreased salivation. Patients should have careful dental care follow-up and should make their dentist aware of the previous irradiation.
Hypothyroidism	After external beam irradiation that encompasses the thyroid with doses sufficient to cure Hodgkin lymphoma, at least 50% of patients will eventually become hypothyroid. All patients whose TSH level becomes elevated should be treated with lifelong thyroxine replacement in doses sufficient to suppress TSH levels to low normal. This is also necessary to ensure that the radiation-damaged thyroid is not subjected to long-term stimulation by thyroid-stimulating hormone, which can increase the risk of thyroid neoplasm.
Infertility	ABVD is not known to cause any permanent gonadal toxicity, although oligospermia for 1-2 yr after treatment is common. Direct or scatter radiation to gonadal tissue can cause infertility, amenorrhea, or premature menopause, but this seldom occurs with the current fields used for the treatment of Hodgkin lymphoma. Thus, with the current chemotherapy regimens and radiation fields used, most patients will not develop these problems. In general, after treatment, women who continue menstruating are fertile, but men require semen analysis to provide a specific answer. High-dose chemoradiotherapy and hematopoietic stem cell transplantation almost always cause permanent infertility in both genders, although some young women occasionally recover fertility.
Impaired immunity to infections	Hodgkin lymphoma and its treatment can lead to lifelong impairment of full immunity to infection. All patients should be given annual influenza immunization and pneumococcal immunization every 5 years. Patients whose spleen has been irradiated or removed should also be immunized against meningococcal types A and C and *Haemophilus influenza* type B. As for all adults, diphtheria and tetanus immunizations should be kept up-to-date.
Secondary neoplasms	Although uncommon, certain secondary neoplasms occur with increased frequency in patients who have been treated for Hodgkin lymphoma. These include acute myelogenous leukemia, thyroid, breast, lung, and upper gastrointestinal carcinoma and melanoma, and cervical carcinoma in situ. It is appropriate to screen for these neoplasms for the rest of the patient's life because they might have lengthy induction periods.

ABVD, Adriamycin, bleomycin, vinblastine, dacarbazine; *TSH,* thyroid-stimulating hormone.
From Abeloff MD: *Clinical oncology*, ed 3, Philadelphia, 2004, Saunders.

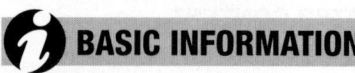

BASIC INFORMATION

DEFINITION

Hookworm is a parasitic infection of the intestine caused by the soil helminths *Necator americanus* (North and South America, Central Africa and parts of Asia) and *Ancylostoma duodenale* (Mediterranean nations, India, Iran, Far East). The hookworm of dogs and cats, *Ancylostoma ceylanicum*, (India, Southeast Asia) also can affect humans

SYNONYMS

Ground itch
Ancylostoma duodenale infection
Necator americanus infection

EPIDEMIOLOGY & DEMOGRAPHICS

INCIDENCE (IN U.S.):

- Varies greatly in different areas of the United States.
- Most common in rural areas of southeastern United States.
- Poor sanitation and increased rainfall increase incidence.

PREVALENCE (IN U.S.): Varies from 10% to 90% in regions where it is found.

PREDOMINANT AGE: Schoolchildren

PHYSICAL FINDINGS & CLINICAL PRESENTATION

- Nonspecific abdominal complaints
- Symptoms related to iron deficiency anemia depending on the amount of iron in the diet and worm burden (these organisms consume host's RBCs)
- Fatigue, tachycardia, dyspnea, and high-output failure
- Hypoproteinemia and edema from loss of proteins into the intestinal tract
- Unusual for pulmonary manifestations to occur when the larvae migrate through the lungs
- Skin rash at sites of larval penetration in some individuals without prior exposure: Ground itch

ETIOLOGY

Two main species can cause this disease: *N. americanus* and *A. duodenale. N. americanus* is the predominant cause of hookworm in the United States. They are soil nematodes (geohelminthic infections) that are acquired by skin contact (i.e., bare feet) with contaminated soils in moist, warm climate. Worldwide, over 700 million people are infected.

- Infection occurs via penetration of the skin by the larval form, with subsequent migration via the bloodstream to the alveoli, up the respiratory tract, then into the GI tract (Fig. 1).
- *Ancylostoma* spp. infection can also occur via the oral route through ingestion of contaminated water supplies.
- Sharp mouth parts allow for attachment to intestinal mucosa.
- *Ancylostoma* spp. are more likely to cause iron deficiency anemia because they are larger and remove more blood daily from the bowel wall than the other hookworm species, *N. americanus.*

DIAGNOSIS

DIFFERENTIAL DIAGNOSIS

- Strongyloidiasis
- Ascariasis
- Other causes of iron deficiency anemia and malabsorption

WORKUP

Examine stool for hookworm eggs. Shedding of eggs starts around 8 weeks after skin penetration in *N. americanum* infections and longer with *A. duodenale,* but eggs are indistinguishable between the two species. PCR stool assays are available in reference labs.

LABORATORY TESTS

CBC to show hypochromic, microcytic anemia; possible mild eosinophilia and hypoalbuminemia

IMAGING STUDIES

Chest x-ray: Generally not helpful, occasionally shows opacities.

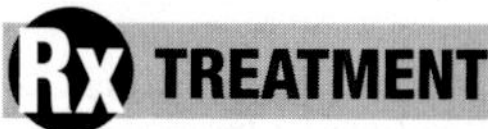

TREATMENT

NONPHARMACOLOGIC THERAPY

- Prevention of disease by not walking barefoot and by improving sanitary conditions.
- Vaccines are in development.

ACUTE GENERAL Rx

- Albendazole 400 mg PO as a single dose or daily for 3 days is the preferred treatment.
- Mebendazole 100 mg PO bid for 3 days is more effective than as a 500-mg single dose.
- Pyrantel pamoate 11 mg/kg (to max dose of 1 g) PO qd × 3 days.
- Iron supplementation may be helpful in patients with iron deficiency.

DISPOSITION

Easily treated

REFERRAL

To gastroenterologist and infectious disease specialist if diagnosis uncertain

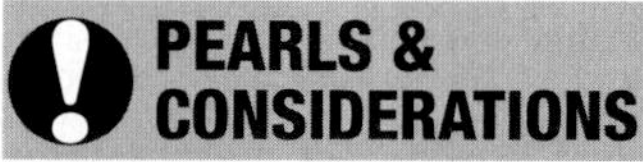

PEARLS & CONSIDERATIONS

COMMENTS

- Appropriate disposal of human waste is important in controlling the disease in areas with a high prevalence of hookworm infestation.
- Wearing shoes will avoid contact with contaminated soil, and the provision of safe water and sanitation for disposing human excreta is important in control of hookworm.

SUGGESTED READING

Available at ExpertConsult.com

RELATED CONTENT

Hookworm Infection (Patient Information)

AUTHOR: **GLENN G. FORT, M.D., M.P.H.**

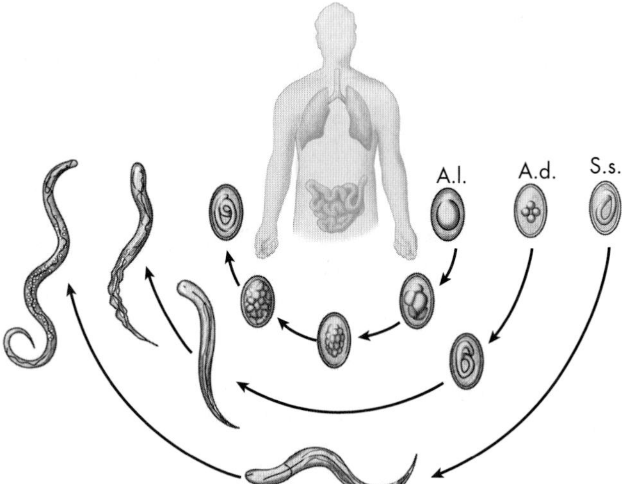

FIG. 1 Life cycle of intestinal nematodes with a migratory phase through the lungs. Eggs are passed with stools in *Ascaris lumbricoides (A.l.), Necator americanus,* or *Ancylostoma duodenale (A.d.),* or they hatch on their way out in *Strongyloides stercoralis (S.s.).* Ascaris eggs mature in soil, and humans are infected upon ingestion of these eggs. With hookworm and strongyloidiasis, humans are infected via skin penetration by filariform larvae. In all three infections, larvae pass through a migratory phase via the lungs before reaching maturity at their final habitat in the small intestine. (From Mandell GL et al: *Principles and practice of infectious diseases,* ed 7, Philadelphia, 2010, Churchill Livingstone.)

BASIC INFORMATION

DEFINITION

Hot flashes are sudden onset of intense warmth that begins in the neck or face, or in the chest and progresses to the neck and face; often associated with profuse sweating, flushing, clamminess, anxiety, and palpitations.

SYNONYMS

HFs
Vasomotor symptoms (VMSs)
Hot flushes
Night sweats

ICD-10CM CODES

N95.1	Menopausal and female climacteric states
R23.2	Flushing

EPIDEMIOLOGY & DEMOGRAPHICS

- Hot flashes affect up to 75% of women who are in the menopausal transition.
- Hot flashes typically start during late perimenopause, increase in frequency and severity throughout the menopausal transition, and finally decline over time after the final menstrual period.
- Median total duration of hot flashes around 7 yr with symptoms lasting for a median of 4.5 yr after the last menstrual period. Women who have hot flashes early in the menopause transition can experience symptoms for more than 12 yr.
- Prevalence of hot flashes differs among racial and ethnic groups in the U.S. with highest frequency among African American women and lowest frequency among Chinese and Japanese women.

PHYSICAL FINDINGS & CLINICAL PRESENTATION

- Profuse sweating and red blotching of skin may be noted during the vasomotor event.
- Palpitations and hyperreflexia may be present during the hot flash.
- Hot flashes typically last 1 to 5 min.
- Each hot flash is associated with increase in temperature, increased pulse rate, and increased blood flow into the hands and face.
- Hot flashes during sleep are common and are referred to as *night sweats.*
- There is considerable variation in the frequency of hot flashes. One third of women report more than 10 flashes per day.

ETIOLOGY

- Dysfunction of central thermoregulatory centers caused by reduction of estrogen levels at the time of menopause
- Tamoxifen use
- Chemotherapy-induced ovarian failure
- Androgen ablation therapy for prostate carcinoma

DIAGNOSIS

DIFFERENTIAL DIAGNOSIS

- Carcinoid syndrome
- Anxiety disorder
- Idiopathic flushing
- Malignancy (lymphoma, solid tumors)
- Hyperthyroidism
- Hyperhidrosis
- Infection

WORKUP

Evaluation of hot flashes is aimed at excluding the conditions listed in the differential diagnosis.

LABORATORY TESTS

- Follicle-stimulating hormone (FSH), luteinizing hormone, estradiol level. The serum FSH levels rather than estradiol levels are associated with greater severity of hot flashes in older postmenopausal women, suggesting that nonestrogen feedback systems may be important in modulating the severity of hot flashes. It is not necessary to obtain an FSH to make the diagnosis of menopausal status, however. An amenorrheic woman over age 50 with vasomotor symptoms is assumed to have made the menopausal transition, and serum markers of menopause are not required to complete the diagnosis.
- Thyroid-stimulating hormone (TSH).

TREATMENT

NONPHARMACOLOGIC THERAPY

- Behavioral interventions such as relaxation training and paced respiration have been reported effective in reducing symptoms in some women.
- Lifestyle changes such as maintaining a healthy body weight, exercising regularly, and avoiding caffeine, alcohol, tobacco, and spicy foods may be beneficial.

GENERAL Rx

- Systemic hormone therapy with estrogen alone or in combination with progestin is the most effective way to manage menopausal hot flashes with up to a 75% reduction in weekly episodes. Women receiving hormone therapy are at increased risk of thromboembolic disease and breast cancer; therefore, use should be limited to the shortest duration and smallest possible dose to control symptoms, and only after considering potential risks and benefits for each individual patient.
- While there is some evidence that progestin-only medications may improve hot flashes, it is not considered first-line treatment for vasomotor symptom management.
- The only nonhormonal method that is FDA-approved for management of hot flashes is the SSRI Paroxitine (7.5 mg daily). Other antidepressants shown to be effective for treatment of hot flashes include escitalopram (10 mg to 20 mg per day), venlafaxine (37.5 mg to 75 mg per day), and desvenlafaxine (100 mg to 150 mg per day). Caution should be taken in prescribing SSRIs and SSNRIs in women taking tamoxifen, as these antidepressants interfere with the cytochrome P-450 metabolism of tamoxifen, reducing its efficacy.
- Duavee is a new FDA-approved treatment of moderate to severe vasomotor menopausal symptoms. It consists of a combination of conjugated estrogens and bazedoxifene, a new selective estrogen receptor modulator (SERM).
- The anticonvulsant gabapentin (300-1200 mg/day) represents another nonhormonal alternative in the treatment of hot flashes. It can be used alone or in combination with an antidepressant; however, combining the two medications does not appear to be more effective than just gabapentin alone.
- The antihypertensive clonidine is also somewhat effective in reducing the frequency of hot flashes in mild cases. Adverse effects include dry mouth, sedation, and dizziness.
- Recent trials with the anti-cholinergic drug oxybutynin have shown effectiveness in reducing the frequency and severity of hot flashes in women with a history of breast cancer.
- Vitamin E (800 IU/day) may be effective in patients with mild symptoms that do not interfere with sleep or daily function.
- Soy protein (use of soy extracts that contain plant-derived estrogens [phytoestrogens]) is often used; however, clinical trials have not shown clear efficacy.
- Several classes of herbal remedies are available to patients and are commonly used, generally without significant benefit. Frequently used agents are *Cimicifuga racemosa* (black cohosh, snakeroot, bugbane), *Angelica sinensis,* and evening primrose (evening star). Recent trials using the isopropanolic extract of black cohosh rootstock (Remifemin) did show some improvement in controlling menopausal symptoms. Such alternative medications may be used to treat mild to moderate symptoms, but it is possible that symptomatic improvements may derive in part from a placebo effect. Acupuncturists are the second most consulted therapists by menopausal women. Evidence of acupuncture efficacy as an HF treatment is conflicting. A recent randomized trial[1] revealed that Chinese medicine acupuncture was not superior to noninsertive sham acupuncture for women with moderately severe menopausal HFs.

SUGGESTED READING

Available at ExpertConsult.com

RELATED CONTENT

Hot Flashes (Patient Information)
Menopause (Related Key Topic)

AUTHOR: **HELEN VALERIE TOMA, MD, MSPH**

[1] Ee C et al: Acupuncture for menopausal hot flashes: a randomized trial, *Ann Intern Med* 164:146-154, 2016.

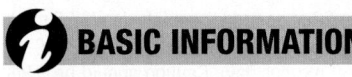

BASIC INFORMATION

DEFINITION

The human immunodeficiency virus (HIV) is a retrovirus that is responsible for causing acquired immunodeficiency syndrome (AIDS). HIV infection does not necessarily mean a person has AIDS. Table 1 summarizes surveillance case definition for HIV.

SYNONYMS

HIV

AIDS: The result of progressive HIV infection in which a person has a weakened immune system and meets specific diagnostic criteria (See "Acquired Immunodeficiency Syndrome" in Section I and Table 2.)

EPIDEMIOLOGY & DEMOGRAPHICS (IN U.S.)

- There are an estimated 1.1 million people infected with HIV in the United States, with approximately 1 out of 7 (15%) who do not know they are infected.
- In 2015, there were an estimated 38,500 new HIV infections, according to the CDC.
- Incidence is highest among gay, bisexual, and other men who have sex with men (MSM) and in minority racial and ethnic populations.

PREDOMINANT RISK GROUPS:

- Gay, bisexual, and other MSM is the group most affected by HIV.
- In 2015, MSM accounted for approximately 68% of all new infections, according to the CDC.
- HIV disproportionately affects MSM of younger age and black/African American and Hispanic/Latino background.
- Heterosexual transmission and injection drug use accounted for 23% and 9%, respectively, of new HIV infections in 2015.
- Table 3 summarizes risk factors associated with sexual transmission of HIV.

RACIAL DATA:

- In 2016, black/African Americans accounted for 44% of new HIV infections despite being 12% of the U.S. population.
- In 2016, Hispanics/Latinos accounted for 25% of new HIV infections despite being 18% of the U.S. population.

GENETICS

Familial Disposition:

Individuals with deletions in the *CCR5* gene are immune from infection with macrophage tropic virus (the predominant virus in sexual transmission). Other genetic variants may contribute to rapid progression or long-term control of the virus once infected. One in 300 individuals infected with HIV is an "elite controller," which means they are able to maintain a normal CD4 count and undetectable viral load through immune control.

Congenital Infection:

- In 2016, 99 children under the age of 13 received a diagnosis of perinatally acquired HIV according to the CDC, which may occur in utero, during delivery, or after delivery via breastfeeding.
- No specific congenital abnormalities are associated with HIV infection, although there is a higher risk of spontaneous abortion and low birth weight.

Neonatal Infection:

- May occur during delivery or via breastfeeding.
- Typically asymptomatic.
- All pregnant women should be tested for HIV and, if positive, take antiretrovirals (ARVs).

PHYSICAL FINDINGS & CLINICAL PRESENTATION

- Signs and symptoms are variable with stage of disease.
- Acute HIV infection (0 to 3 months, usually within several weeks):
  1. Causes a self-limited mononucleosis-like illness in 50% to 80% of individuals, characterized by fever, sore throat, lymphadenopathy, headache, and a rash resembling roseola. Individuals may also be asymptomatic.
  2. In a minority of acute cases, aseptic meningitis, Bell palsy, or peripheral neuropathy may occur.
  3. Opportunistic infections such as thrush or *Pneumocystis jiroveci* pneumonia (PJP) may occur.
- Chronic HIV infection is usually characterized by a prolonged asymptomatic "latent" phase followed by nonspecific symptoms of lymphadenopathy, fatigue, weight loss, diarrhea,

TABLE 1 Surveillance Case Definition for HIV Infection in Adults and Adolescents (Age >13 Years)

Stage	Laboratory Evidence	Clinical Evidence
Stage1	Laboratory confirmation of HIV infection and CD4+T lymphocyte count of ≥500 cells/μL or CD4+T-lymphocyte percentage of ≥29%[a]	No AIDS-defining condition (see Table 2)
Stage 2	Laboratory confirmation of HIV infection and CD4+T lymphocyte count of 200–499 cells/μL or CD4+T-lymphocyte percentage of 14%–28%[a]	No AIDS-defining condition (see Table 2)
Stage 3	Laboratory confirmation of HIV infection and CD4+T lymphocyte count of <200 cells/μL or CD4+T-lymphocyte percentage of <14%[a]	Documentation of an AIDS-defining condition with laboratory confirmation of HIV infection (see Table 2)
Stage unknown	Laboratory confirmation of HIV infection and no information on CD4+T-lymphocyte count or percentage	No information on presence of an AIDS-defining condition

[a]The CD4+T-lymphocyte percentage is percentage of the total lymphocyte count.
From Hoffman R, et al.: *Hematology, basic principles and practice,* ed 7, Philadelphia, 2018, Elsevier.

TABLE 2 Surveillance Definitions of AIDS-Defining Conditions

Opportunistic Infections:

- *Pneumocystis jirovecii (carinii)*
- *Mycobacterium avium* complex
- *Mycobacterium tuberculosis*
- Toxoplasmosis
- Candidiasis: Esophageal and systemic
- Histoplasmosis
- Cryptococcosis
- Cryptosporidiosis and isosporiasis
- Leishmaniasis
- Cytomegalovirus disease
- Recurrent bacterial infections (≥2 episodes/yr)

Lymphomas

Kaposi Sarcoma

Cervical Cancer

AIDS Dementia Syndrome

Wasting Syndrome

From Hoffman R, et al.: *Hematology, basic principles and practice,* ed 7, Philadelphia, 2018, Elsevier.

TABLE 3 Risk Factors Associated with Sexual Transmission of HIV

Sexually transmitted infections
- Ulcerative or nonulcerative diseases

Genital tract inflammation

HIV disease
- Higher viral loads
- Lower CD4+ levels
- Acute HIV infection
- Lack of effective antiretroviral therapy
- Lack of heterozygosity or homozygosity for the inactivating 32-base pair deletion in the chemokine receptor gene *(CCR5)*

Anatomic factors
- Lack of circumcision
- Cervical ectopy
- Leukocytospermia
- Hormonal contraception

Sexual practices
- Receptive anal intercourse
- Sexual activity during menses
- Bleeding during intercourse (disruption of vaginal mucosa through trauma)
- Lack of barrier protection

HIV viral features
- Syncytium formation
- Certain viral clades

HIV, Human immunodeficiency virus.
From Bennett JE, Dolin R, Blaser MJ: *Mandell, Douglas, and Bennett's principles and practice of infectious diseases,* ed 8, Philadelphia, 2015, Saunders.

H

Diseases and Disorders

TABLE 4 Etiology of Anemia in Human Immunodeficiency Virus

HIV Related

HIV Infection

- Anemia of chronic disease
- Blunted production/response to erythropoietin
- Suppression of CFU-GEMM (HIV/inflammatory cytokines)

Neoplasms Infiltrating BM

Non-Hodgkin lymphoma, KS, Hodgkin lymphoma

Infections of the BM

- Parvovirus B19
- Atypical mycobact (MAI/MAC)
- M. TB
- Histoplasma
- CMV

Medications Causing Decreased Production	Medications Causing Hemolysis
• RT inhibitors • Ganciclovir • Bactrim • Amphotericin B	• Indinavir • Bactrim and Dapsone in G6PD deficiency

HIV Unrelated

- B_{12} and/or folic acid deficiencies
- Iron deficiency caused by chronic blood loss

BM, Bone marrow; *CFU-GEMM,* colony-forming unit–granulocyte, erythrocyte, macrophage, megakaryocyte; *CMV,* cytomegalovirus; *G6PD,* glucose-6-phosphate dehydrogenase; *HIV,* human immunodeficiency virus; *KS,* Kaposi sarcoma; *MAC,* mycobacterium avium complex; *MAI,* mycobacterium avium-intracellulare; *M. TB,* Mycobacterium tuberculosis, *RT,* reverse transcriptase.

From Hoffman R, et al.: *Hematology, basic principles and practice,* ed 7, Philadelphia, 2018, Elsevier.

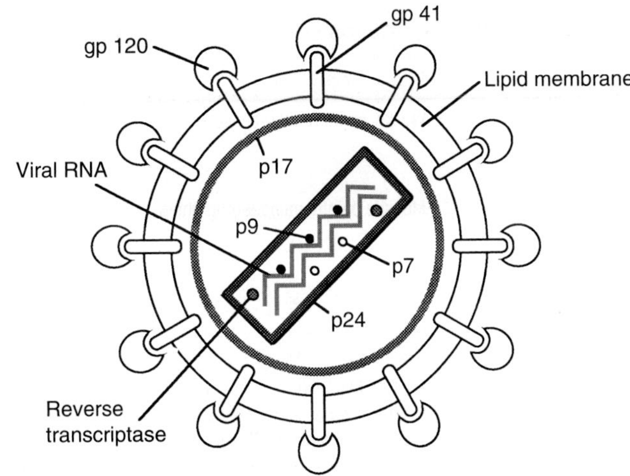

FIG. 1 Structure of the HIV Virion. Two coding strands of genomic ribonucleic acid (RNA) are packaged in the nucleoid core with p7, p9, and p24 proteins and reverse transcriptase. The core is surrounded by the p17 matrix protein lining the inner surface of the envelope. The envelope consists of a lipid bilayer derived from the infected cell and glycoprotein spikes that consist of the outer glycoprotein (GP) 120 molecule, which contains the binding site for CD4, and GP41, which anchors the glycoprotein complex to the envelope and mediates fusion of the viral membrane with the cell membrane during viral penetration. (From Hoffman R, et al.: *Hematology, basic principles and practice,* ed 7, Philadelphia, 2018, Elsevier.)

and skin changes including seborrheic dermatitis, localized herpes zoster, and/or fungal infection.

- Advanced disease is characterized by AIDS-associated diseases, including infections and malignancies (see specific disorders). Anemia may be multifactorial (Table 4).
- HIV infection in women may be associated with lower levels of viral load at comparable degrees of immunosuppression when compared with men. Furthermore, women may, on average, have higher CD4 counts at the time of HIV diagnosis.
- Another special consideration in women infected with HIV is the high incidence of human papillomavirus (HPV) co-infection and risk for cervical cancer. HIV-positive women should be screened for cervical cancer at time of initial HIV diagnosis and annually thereafter if pap testing is normal. If the results of three consecutive Pap tests are normal, then follow-up testing can occur every 3 years. HPV vaccination is also recommended in men and women 9- to 26-years-old who are HIV positive.
- Co-infection with HIV and hepatitis C virus is common because of similar transmission risk. Hepatitis C is most commonly transmitted by contaminated needles or blood exposure. Hepatitis C can be transmitted sexually, but the risk is low. Patients with HIV and hepatitis C progress faster to cirrhosis. Patients may already have signs of advanced liver disease at the time of diagnosis.

ETIOLOGY

- HIV is a single-stranded RNA retrovirus (Fig. 1) that is categorized as type 1 or 2.
- HIV-1 was derived from transmission of a simian immunodeficiency virus (SIV) from chimpanzees in Central Africa; HIV-2 was derived from an SIV found in sooty mangabey monkeys from West Africa.
- HIV-1 is the predominant pathogenic retrovirus in human populations; HIV-2 has limited distribution (primarily West Africa) and tends to progress less rapidly than HIV-1. HIV-2 should be considered in individuals from West Africa or whose sexual partners are from West Africa.
- HIV is transmitted by sexual contact, shared needles, blood transfusion, or from mother to child during pregnancy, delivery, or breastfeeding.
- Primary target of infection: CD4 lymphocytes.

Dx DIAGNOSIS

DIFFERENTIAL DIAGNOSIS

- Acute HIV infection: Often diagnosed or confused with mononucleosis or other respiratory viral infections.
- Late symptoms: Similar to those produced by other wasting/chronic illnesses such as neoplasms, tuberculosis (TB), disseminated fungal infection (such as *Candida*), malabsorption, or depression.
- HIV-related encephalopathy: Confused with Alzheimer's disease or other causes of chronic dementia (cognitive impairment in HIV infection is described in another chapter in Section I); myelopathy and neuropathy possibly resembling other demyelinating diseases such as multiple sclerosis.
- Direct central nervous system (CNS) involvement: Manifests as encephalopathy, myelopathy, or neuropathy in advanced cases. Table 5 summarizes neuromuscular syndromes in HIV infection.
- Renal failure, rheumatologic disorders, thrombocytopenia, or cardiac abnormalities (Table 6) may be seen in association with HIV-1.

WORKUP

Diagnosis is established by testing for HIV antibodies in the blood. The CDC recommends routine testing for patients in all health care settings unless the patient declines (opt-out screening). This includes routine testing of pregnant women. It is also recommended that separate written consent should no longer be required, although by law this is being addressed on a state-by-state basis. Generally, all persons aged 13 to 64 yr should undergo HIV testing at least once, and more frequently (at least once a yr) if sexually active. For individuals who may be at higher risk (e.g., men who are having sex with multiple other men), 3 to 6 months may be recommended.

An FDA-approved at-home rapid HIV screening test is available. It uses swabs of oral fluids from upper and lower gums. A positive test requires confirmatory testing.

LABORATORY TESTS

HIV antibodies are detected by a two-step technique:

- ELISA (enzyme-linked immunosorbent assay), which is a sensitive screening test.

TABLE 5 Neuromuscular Syndromes in Human Immunodeficiency Virus Type–1 Infection

Diagnosis	Disease Stage	Clinical Features	Diagnostic Studies	Treatment
AIDP CIDP	Early > late	Weakness more than sensory loss	CSF: ↑ WBCs ↑↑ Protein NCSs: Demyelination	Early: IVIG, steroids, plasmapheresis Late: Consider ganciclovir/foscarnet
MM	Early or late	Multiple painful mononeuropathies	NCSs: Multifocal axonal neuropathy Biopsy: Inflammation/vasculitis CMV	Early: None Late: Steroids/cyclophosphamide Ganciclovir/foscarnet
Nucleoside Neuropathy	Any stage	Distal sensory loss Neuropathic pain	NCSs: Distal axonopathy Increased serum lactate	Nucleoside withdrawal
DSPN	Late	Distal sensory loss Neuropathic pain	NCSs: Distal axonopathy	NSAIDs, capsaicin AED, tricyclics
PP	Late	Progressive flaccid paraparesis, urinary dysfunction, LS pain	CSF: IncreasedWBCs (PMNs), CMV PCR+	Ganciclovir/foscarnet Cidofovir
DILS	Late	Sjögren's syndrome, distal motor and sensory loss, pain	NCSs: Axonal neuropathy Biopsy: CD8+ T cells, HIV-1	Zidovudine/ART Steroids
Zidovudine Myopathy	Any stage	Proximal weakness Myalgias	EMG: ± irritative Biopsy: Ragged red fibers	Zidovudine withdrawal
Polymyositis	Any stage	Proximal weakness Myalgias	EMG: ± irritative Biopsy: Inflammatory infiltrates	Steroids, IVIG Immunosuppressants
ALS-like	Late	Weakness, dysphagia	EMG: Neurogenic	ART

AED, Antiepileptic drug; *AIDP*, acute inflammatory demyelinating polyneuropathy; *ALS*, amyotrophic lateral sclerosis; *ART*, antiretroviral therapy; *CIDP*, chronic inflammatory demyelinating polyneuropathy; *CMV*, cytomegalovirus; *CSF*, cerebrospinal fluid; *DILS*, diffuse infiltrative lymphocytosis syndrome; *DSPN*, distal sensory polyneuropathy; *EMG*, electromyography; *HIV*, human immunodeficiency virus; *IVIG*, intravenous immunoglobulin; *LS*, lumbosacral; *MM*, mononeuritis multiplex; *NCS*, nerve conduction studies; *NSAID*, nonsteroidal anti-inflammatory drug; *PCR*, polymerase chain reaction; *PMNs*, polymorphonuclear leukocytes; *PP*, progressive polyradiculopathy; *WBCs*, white blood cells.

From Bennett JE, Dolin R, Blaser MJ: *Mandell, Douglas, and Bennett's principles and practice of infectious diseases*, ed 8, Philadelphia, 2015, Saunders.

TABLE 6 Summary of HIV-Associated Cardiovascular Diseases

Disease	Possible Causes	Incidence/Prevalence	Diagnosis	Treatment
Accelerated atherosclerosis	Protease inhibitors, atherogenesis with virus-infected macrophages, chronic inflammation, glucose intolerance, dyslipidemia, endothelial dysfunction	Up to 8%	ECG, stress testing, echocardiography, lipid profile, CT angiography, calcium scoring	Smoking cessation, low-fat diet, aerobic exercise, blood pressure control, guideline-based statin use, percutaneous coronary intervention, coronary artery bypass surgery
Dilated cardiomyopathy	Coronary artery disease	Up to 8% of asymptomatic patients	Chest radiographic findings	Diuretics, digoxin, ACE inhibitors, beta blockers
LV systolic dysfunction	Drug related: Cocaine, AZT, IL-2, doxorubicin, interferon Infectious: HIV, *Toxoplasma*, coxsackievirus group B, EBV, CMV, adenovirus Metabolic or endocrine: selenium or carnitine deficiency, anemia, hypocalcemia, hypophosphatemia, hyponatremia, hypokalemia, hypoalbuminemia, hypothyroidism, growth hormone deficiency, adrenal insufficiency, hyperinsulinemia Cytokines: TNF-β, nitric oxide, TGF-β, endothelin-1, interleukins Immunodeficiency: CD4 count <100 Autoimmune	Up to 25% of autopsy cases	ECG: Nonspecific conduction abnormalities, PVCs, PACs Echocardiographic findings: Low to normal LV wall thickness, increased LV mass, LV dilation, systolic LV dysfunction Possible laboratory studies: Troponin T, brain natriuretic peptide concentration, CD4 count, viral load, viral PCR, *Toxoplasma* serology, thyroid-stimulating hormone, cortisol, carnitine, selenium, serum ACE, stress testing, myocardial biopsy, cardiac catheterization	Adjunctive treatment in HIV patients Treatment of infection Nutritional replacement IVIG Intensify antiretroviral therapy Follow-up serial echocardiograms
LV diastolic dysfunction	TNF, IL-6 Hypertension Chronic viral infection	Up to 37% asymptomatic	Echocardiography Tissue Doppler imaging	Treat hypertension Intensify antiretroviral therapy
Primary pulmonary hypertension	Plexogenic pulmonary arteriopathy	0.5%	ECG, echocardiography, right-heart catheterization	Anticoagulation, vasodilators, prostacyclin analogues Endothelin antagonists PDE-5 inhibitors

Continued

TABLE 6 Summary of HIV-Associated Cardiovascular Diseases—cont'd

Disease	Possible Causes	Incidence/Prevalence	Diagnosis	Treatment
Pericardial	Bacteria: *Staphylococcus, Streptococcus, Proteus, Klebsiella, Enterococcus, Listeria, Nocardia, Mycobacterium* Viral pathogens: HIV, HSV, CMV, adenovirus, echovirus Other pathogens: *Cryptococcus, Toxoplasma, Histoplasma* Malignancy: Kaposi sarcoma, lymphoma, capillary leak/wasting/malnutrition Hypothyroidism Immunodeficiency Uremia Autoimmune	11%/yr, markedly reduced in post-HAART studies Spontaneous resolution in 42% of affected patients Approximately 30% increase in 6-mo mortality	Pericardial rub on examination Echocardiography Fluid analysis for Gram stain, culture, and cytology ECG—low voltage/PR depression Associated pleural and peritoneal fluid analysis Pericardial biopsy	Treat the cause Follow-up: Serial echocardiograms Intensify antiretroviral therapy Pericardiocentesis or window
Infective endocarditis	Bacteria: *Staphylococcus aureus* or *Staphylococcus epidermidis, Salmonella, Streptococcus, Haemophilus parainfluenzae, Pseudallescheria boydii*, HASEK organisms Fungal: *Aspergillus fumigatus, Candida, Cryptococcus neoformans*	6% increased incidence in IVDAs, regardless of HIV status	Blood cultures; echocardiography	Intravenous antibiotics, valve replacements
Nonbacterial thrombotic endocarditis	Valvular damage, vitamin C deficiency, malnutrition, wasting, DIC, hypercoagulable state, prolonged acquired immunodeficiency	Rare condition, but clinically relevant emboli in 42% of cases	Echocardiography	Anticoagulation Treat vasculitis or underlying illness
Malignancy	Kaposi sarcoma, non-Hodgkin lymphoma, leiomyosarcoma, low CD4 count, prolonged immunodeficiency HHV-8, EBV	Approximately 1% Usually metastatic in HIV-positive patients	Echocardiography, biopsy	Chemotherapy possible
Right ventricular disease	Recurrent pulmonary infections, pulmonary arteritis, microvascular pulmonary emboli, COPD		ECG, echocardiography, right-heart catheterization	Diuretics, treat underlying lung infection or disease, anticoagulation as clinically indicated
Vasculitis	Drug therapy with antibiotics and antivirals	Increasing incidence	Clinical diagnosis	Systemic corticosteroids, withdrawal of drug
Autonomic dysfunction	CNS disease, drug therapy, prolonged immunodeficiency, malnutrition, sedentary lifestyle	Increased in patients with CNS disease	Tilt-table test, Holter or event monitoring	Procedural precautions
Arrhythmias	Drug therapy, pentamidine, autonomic dysfunction, acidosis electrolyte abnormalities		ECG—long QT, Holter monitoring, exercise stress testing	Discontinue drug, procedural precautions, electrolyte replacement
Lipodystrophy	Drug therapy: Protease inhibitors		Echocardiography, lipid profile, cardiac catheterization, coronary calcium score	Lipid therapy (beware of drug interactions), aerobic exercise, altered antiretroviral therapy, cosmetic surgery/fat implantation

ACE, Angiotensin-converting enzyme; *AZT*, zidovudine (azidothymidine); *CMV*, cytomegalovirus; *CNS*, central nervous system; *COPD*, chronic obstructive pulmonary disease; *CT*, computed tomography; *DIC*, disseminated intravascular coagulation; *EBV*, Epstein-Barr virus; *ECG*, electrocardiogram; *HASEK*, *Haemophilus* species (*Haemophilus parainfluenzae, Haemophilus aphrophilus, Haemophilus paraphrophilus*), *Actinobacillus actinomycetemcomitans, Cardiobacterium hominis, Eikenella corrodens*, and *Kingella* species; *HHV*, human herpesvirus; *HSV*, herpes simplex virus; *IVDA*, intravenous drug abuser; *IVIG*, intravenous immunoglobulin; *PAC*, premature atrial complex; *PCR*, polymerase chain reaction; *PDE*, phosphodiesterase; *PVC*, premature ventricular complex; *TGF*, transforming growth factor.

From Mann DL, et al.: *Braunwald's heart disease*, ed 10, Philadelphia, 2015, Elsevier.

- Confirmation of positive ELISA tests with more specific assays. The classic confirmatory test is the Western blot, but other modalities may be used. Fig. E2 summarizes the laboratory diagnosis of HIV infection.
- Screening ELISA antibody tests will measure HIV-1 and HIV-2 antibodies. Confirmatory tests will generally differentiate between HIV-1 and HIV-2 as well. However, the viral load assays (HIV RNA PCR) are specific only for HIV-1.
- Fourth-generation antibody/antigen tests can detect the "p24" antigen, which is present early in HIV infection and can be used to diagnose HIV earlier than previous generations. An HIV RNA PCR should still be sent if acute HIV is suspected.
- Baseline viral resistance testing (e.g., genotype) is recommended for all newly diagnosed patients with HIV to guide choice of ART.
- The CD4 count and HIV viral load (e.g., HIV RNA PCR) should be measured in all patients.
- The CD4 count is a marker of current immune status. Table 7 describes the World Health Organization (WHO) immunologic classification for established HIV infection.
- The HIV RNA PCR (viral load) is predictive of disease progression.
- Rapid serologic tests have been increasingly used and are useful in specific settings: occupational exposures, pregnant women in labor without previous testing, and patients in high seroprevalence areas (for immediate results). Specimens are either blood or saliva and results are given within 1 to 20 min. Although sensitivity is high (99%), false-positive tests are more common in low seroprevalence populations. Thus, all positive results must be confirmed with standard serology.
- Early during infection (i.e., acute HIV infection), standard antibody tests may be negative ("window period"). The standard for diagnosing HIV during acute HIV infection is by testing for HIV RNA (viral load).
- In 2014, the CDC released a revised surveillance case definition for HIV infection. This information has been added in the EBM section of this topic. Table 8 describes the WHO clinical staging of HIV/AIDS for adults and adolescents with confirmed HIV infection. Table 9 compares the WHO and CDC staging systems.

TABLE 7 World Health Organization Immunologic Classification for Established HIV Infection

HIV-Associated Immunodeficiency	Age-Related CD4 Values			
	<11 mo (% CD4+)	12-35 mo (% CD4+)	36-59 mo (% CD4+)	>5 yr (Absolute No./mm³ or % CD4+)
None or not significant	>35	>30	>25	>500
Mild	30-35	25-30	20-25	350-500
Advanced	25-29	20-24	15-19	200-349
Severe	<25	<20	<15	<200 or <15%

From Bennett JE, Dolin R, Blaser MJ: *Mandell, Douglas, and Bennett's principles and practice of infectious diseases,* ed 8, Philadelphia, 2015, Saunders.

TABLE 8 World Health Organization Clinical Staging of HIV/AIDS for Adults and Adolescents With Confirmed HIV Infection

Clinical Stage 1
Asymptomatic
Persistent generalized lymphadenopathy
Clinical Stage 2
Moderate unexplained weight loss (<10% of presumed or measured body weight)*
Recurrent respiratory tract infections (e.g., sinusitis, tonsillitis, otitis media, pharyngitis)
Herpes zoster
Angular cheilitis
Recurrent oral ulceration
Papular pruritic eruptions
Seborrheic dermatitis
Fungal nail infections
Clinical Stage 3
Unexplained* severe weight loss (>10% of presumed or measured body weight)
Unexplained chronic diarrhea for longer than 1 month
Unexplained persistent fever (>37.6° C [99.7° F]), intermittent or constant, for longer than 1 month
Persistent oral candidiasis
Oral hairy leukoplakia
Pulmonary tuberculosis (current)
Severe bacterial infections (e.g., pneumonia, empyema, pyomyositis, bone or joint infection, meningitis, or bacteremia)
Acute necrotizing ulcerative stomatitis, gingivitis, or periodontitis
Unexplained anemia (<8 g/dl), neutropenia (<0.5 × 10^9/L), or chronic thrombocytopenia (<50 × 10^9/L)
Clinical Stage 4†
HIV wasting syndrome
Pneumocystis jirovecii
Recurrent severe bacterial pneumonia
Chronic herpes simplex infection (orolabial, genital or anorectal, longer than 1 month's duration, or visceral at any site)
Esophageal candidiasis (or candidiasis of trachea, bronchi, or lungs)
Extrapulmonary tuberculosis
Kaposi sarcoma
Cytomegalovirus infection (retinitis or infection of other organs)
Central nervous system toxoplasmosis
HIV encephalopathy
Extrapulmonary cryptococcosis, including meningitis
Disseminated nontuberculous mycobacterial infection
Progressive multifocal leukoencephalopathy
Chronic cryptosporidiosis (with diarrhea)
Chronic isosporiasis
Disseminated mycosis (coccidioidomycosis or histoplasmosis)
Recurrent nontyphoidal *Salmonella* bacteremia
Lymphoma (cerebral or B-cell non-Hodgkin's) or other solid HIV-associated tumors
Invasive cervical carcinoma
Atypical disseminated leishmaniasis
Symptomatic HIV-associated nephropathy or symptomatic HIV-associated cardiomyopathy

*Unexplained refers to when the condition is not explained by other causes.
†Some additional specific conditions can also be included in regional classifications (e.g., reactivation of American trypanosomiasis [meningoencephalitis or myocarditis]) in the World Health Organization region of the Americas and disseminated penicilliosis in Asia.
From Bennett JE, Dolin R, Blaser MJ: *Mandell, Douglas, and Bennett's principles and practice of infectious diseases,* ed 8, Philadelphia, 2015, Saunders.

TABLE 9 Comparison of WHO and CDC Staging Systems*

WHO Stage†	WHO T-Lymphocyte Count and Percentage‡	CDC Stage§	CDC T-Lymphocyte Count and Percentage
Stage 1 (HIV infection)	$CD4^+$ T-lymphocyte count of ≥500 cells/mm^3	Stage 1 (HIV infection)	$CD4^+$ T-lymphocyte count of ≥500 cells/mm^3 or $CD4^+$ T-lymphocyte percentage of ≥29
Stage 2 (HIV infection)	$CD4^+$ T-lymphocyte count of 350-499 cells/mm^3	Stage 2 (HIV infection)	$CD4^+$ T-lymphocyte count of 200-499 cells/mm^3 or $CD4^+$ T-lymphocyte percentage of 14-28
Stage 3 (advanced HIV disease [AHD])	$CD4^+$ T-lymphocyte count of 200-349 cells/mm^3	Stage 2 (HIV infection)	$CD4^+$ T-lymphocyte count of 200-499 cells/mm^3 or $CD4^+$ T-lymphocyte percentage of 14-28
Stage 4 (acquired immunodeficiency syndrome [AIDS])	$CD4^+$ T-lymphocyte count of <200 cells/mm^3 or $CD4^+$ T-lymphocyte percentage of <15	Stage 3 (AIDS)	$CD4^+$ T-lymphocyte count of <200 cells/mm^3 or $CD4^+$ T-lymphocyte percentage of <14

CDC, Centers for Disease Control and Prevention; *WHO,* World Health Organization.
*For reporting purposes only.
†Among adults and children aged ≥5 years.
‡Percentage applicable for stage 4 only.
§Among adults and adolescents (ages ≥13 years). CDC also includes a fourth stage, stage unknown; laboratory confirmation of HIV infection but no information on $CD4^+$ T-lymphocyte count or percentage and no information on AIDS-defining conditions.
From Bennett JE, Dolin R, Blaser MJ: *Mandell, Douglas, and Bennett's principles and practice of infectious diseases,* ed 8, Philadelphia, 2015, Saunders.

Rx TREATMENT

NONPHARMACOLOGIC THERAPY

Maintenance of adequate nutrition

ACUTE GENERAL Rx

Acute management of opportunistic infections and malignancies (see AIDS-associated disorders, "*Pneumocystis jiroveci* Pneumonia," "Cryptococcosis," "Tuberculosis," "Cryptosporidiosis," "Toxoplasmosis," etc., elsewhere in this text).

CHRONIC Rx

All HIV-infected patients should be considered for ART regardless of CD4 cell count. The benefit of ART is well established in preventing progression to AIDS and associated comorbidities. Furthermore, individuals who are on ART and undetectable are highly unlikely to transmit HIV to others. Identifying individuals with HIV as soon as possible and administering ART is the basis of effective public health approaches to addressing HIV (i.e. "Treatment as Prevention").

- Therapy is strongly recommended for all patients with symptomatic established HIV disease regardless of the CD4 count. Symptomatic HIV disease is defined as the presence of any of the following: thrush, vaginal candidiasis, herpes zoster, peripheral neuropathy, bacillary angiomatosis, cervical dysplasia in situ, constitutional symptoms such as fever or diarrhea for more than 1 month, ITP, PID, or listeriosis.
- In asymptomatic individuals, ART is recommended regardless of CD4 cell counts. The recommendations are due to the safety and benefit of newer antivirals in preventing AIDS and decreasing both morbidity and mortality. Earlier treatment may also help reduce transmission of the virus to others due to reductions in viral loads.
- ART generally consists of using a 3-drug regimen to treat HIV infection. Classes of antiretrovirals include:
  1. Nucleoside/nucleotide reverse transcriptase inhibitor (NRTI): Zidovudine (AZT), lamivudine (3TC), emtricitabine (FTC), tenofovir disoproxil fumarate (TDF), tenofovir alafenamide (TAF), abacavir (ABC), stavudine (D4T), or didanosine (DDI).
  2. Protease inhibitors (PI): Lopinavir/ritonavir, atazanavir, fosamprenavir, darunavir, saquinavir, amprenavir, tipranavir, nelfinavir, and indinavir. These PIs may be "boosted" by ritonavir or cobicistat to increase levels.
  3. Non-nucleoside reverse transcriptase inhibitors (NNRTI): Nevirapine, efavirenz, etravirine, delavirdine, or rilpivirine.
  4. Integrase inhibitors (II): Raltegravir, elvitegravir, bictegravir and dolutegravir.
  5. Fusion inhibitors: Enfuvirtide (T-20). This drug is administered through subcutaneous injections and is only used as part of a salvage regimen for individuals who have failed multiple other regimens.
  6. CCR5 inhibitors: Maraviroc. Before using this drug, a viral trophism assay should be checked to determine if the virus uses the CCR5 co-receptor to infect cells. If the virus uses the CXCR4 co-receptor, this drug will not be effective.
  7. Post-attachment inhibitors: Ibalizumab. Blocks CD4 receptors that HIV needs to enter cells with.
- Adding a fourth drug to the three-drug regimen does not improve viral suppression or outcomes and is not recommended. Treatment interruptions based upon CD4 responses appear harmful in recent comparative studies versus standard continuous treatment protocols and should be avoided. Antiretroviral regimens for initial therapy are summarized in Table 10.
- Typical dosing regimen consists of two NRTIs and either a NNRTI, PI, or II. IIs are now the preferred third drug because of tolerability. Data support inclusion of lamivudine or emtricitabine as one of the two NRTIs.
- Individuals with drug resistant HIV may be on more complex and atypical regimens. Consultation with an HIV specialist is recommended.

Standard NRTIs include:

- Tenofovir disoproxil fumarate/emtricitabine 1 tablet once daily. Individuals with underlying renal dysfunction or requiring other nephrotoxic agents may be at increased risk of renal toxicity while taking tenofovir. TDF may also be associated with reductions in bone mineral density.
- Tenofovir alafenamide/emtricitabine 1 tablet once daily. TAF is a newer formulation of TDF with less nephrotoxicity and bone mineral density effects. Both TDF/FTC, and TAF/FTC are recommended components of the initial regimen (with a "backbone" medication). TDF should be avoided in patients with a creatinine clearance (CrCl) <60 ml/min. TAF should be avoided in patients with a CrCl <30 ml/min.
- Abacavir/lamivudine 1 tablet once daily. Abacavir may be associated with increased risk of myocardial infarction. Before using this drug, individuals should be checked for HLA-B*5701. Individuals with this allele are at higher risk of serious hypersensitivity reactions, and this drug should be avoided.
- Zidovudine/lamivudine)1 tablet twice daily. Once widely prescribed; now rarely used due to lower efficacy compared with tenofovir-emtricitabine; zidovudine is associated with lipoatrophy and anemia, as well as GI and CNS side effects.

Standard backbone regimens include:

- IIs (These are now considered first line.):
  1. Dolutegravir (50 mg once daily): The FDA has approved a fixed-dose combination of the integrase strand inhibitor dolutegravir and the NRTIs abacavir and lamivudine for once-daily treatment of HIV-1 infection. HLA-B*5701 should be checked first.
  2. Elvitegravir: Given with cobicistat (booster) and tenofovir/emtricitabine in a fixed-dose combination.
  3. Raltegravir (400 mg twice a day).
- NNRTIs
  1. Efavirenz 600 mg daily: Should be used in caution in women in the first trimester or those who are contemplating pregnancy.

TABLE 10 What Antiretroviral Regimen to Choose for Initial Therapy

Preferred Regimens	Comments
Integrase inhibitor-based regimen Raltegravir + TDF/FTC or TAF/FTC Dolutegravir + TDF/FTC or TAF/FTC Dolutegravir/ABC/3TC Elvitegravir/cobicistat/TDF/FTC Elvitegravir/cobicistat/TAF/FTC	Use abacavir only in individuals who are HLA-B*5701 negative.
PI-based regimen Darunavir/r (once daily) + TDF/FTC or TAF/FTC	Use if there is a concern for drug resistance.
Preferred regimen for pregnant women ABC/3TC or TDF/FTCPlus Raltegravir or Darunavir/r or Atazanavir/r	TDF should be avoided in renal impairment.
Alternative Regimens	**Comments**
NNRTI-based regimens (in alphabetical order) EFV/TDF/FTC or EFV + TAF/FTC EFV + ABC/3TC RPV/TDF/FTC or RPV/TAF/FTC RPV + ABC/3TC PI-based regimens (in alphabetical order) ATV/r + ABC/3TC ATV/r + TDF/FTC or TAF/FTC DRV/c or DRV/r + ABC/3TC DRV/c + TDF/FTC or TAF/FTC	EFV should not be used with caution in the first trimester of pregnancy or in women trying to conceive. NVP should not be used in patients with moderate to severe hepatic impairment (Child-Pugh B or C) Should not be used in women with pre-treatment CD4 >250 cells/mm^3 or men with CD4 >400 cells/mm^3 ABC should not be used in patients who test positive for HLA-B*5701 Use with caution in patients with high risk of cardiovascular disease or with pretreatment HIV RNA >100,000 copies/ml Once-daily LPV/r is not recommended in pregnant women.

3TC, Lamivudine; *ABC,* abacavir; *ATV,* atazanavir; *ddI,* didanosine; *DRV,* darunavir; *EFV,* efavirenz; *FPV,* fosamprenavir; *FTC,* emtricitabine; *INSTI,* integrase strand transfer inhibitor; *MRV,* maraviroc; *NNRTI,* nonnucleoside reverse transcriptase inhibitor; *NRTI,* nucleos(t)ide reverse transcriptase inhibitor; *NVP,* nevirapine; *PI,* protease inhibitor; *r,* low dose ritonavir; *RAL,* raltegravir; *RVP,* rilpivirine; *SQV,* saquinavir; *TDF,* tenofovir disoproxil fumarate; *TAF,* tenofovir alafenamide; *ZDV,* zidovudine. The following combinations in the recommended list are available as fixed-dose combination formulations: ABC/3TC, EFV/TDF/FTC, LPV/r, TDF/FTC, RPV/TDF/FTC, and ZDV/3TC.

Modified from Panel on Antiretroviral Guidelines for Adults and Adolescents. Guidelines for the use of antiretroviral agents in HIV-1–infected adults and adolescents. Department of Health and Human Services 1-161, 2018. http://www.aidsinfo.nih.gov/ContentFiles/AdultandAdolescentGL.pdf.

2. Rilpivirine: Given with tenofovir and emtricitabine as part of a fixed-dose combination.
3. Nevirapine 200 mg two times a day: Avoid with CD4 count >250 in men and >350 cells per cubic millimeter in women because of the risk of hepatitis. The newer agent rilpivirine had higher virologic failures and should be considered an alternative agent.
4. Etravirine 200 mg two times a day: This drug is generally used in patients for whom other regimens have failed. Etravirine retains activity in many patients who have developed resistance against efavirenz and nevirapine.

- PIs (ritonavir boosted)
  1. Lopinavir and ritonavir (200 mg/50 mg) 2 tablets twice a day (or 4 tablets once a day): Most likely to cause diarrhea and has the greatest negative effect on triglyceride levels.
  2. Atazanavir and ritonavir (300 mg and 100 mg) 2 tablets a day: Lower pill burden but use with caution with acid-reducing agents—can alter absorption.
  3. Fosamprenavir and ritonavir (700 mg and 100 mg) 2 tablets twice a day (or 4 tablets once a day): Cannot take fosamprenavir with sulfa allergy.
  4. Darunavir and ritonavir (800 mg and 100 mg a day): This is considered a preferred PI regimen within the DHHS guidelines with either tenofovir disoproxil fumarate or TAF and emtricitabine.
  5. Saquinavir and ritonavir: Saquinavir is no longer recommended for initial treatment of any patient and should be prescribed only in consultation with a specialist.
- All these drugs have their own unique, as well as class-specific, side effects and require careful follow-up to achieve optimal antiviral effects. Compliance with the drug regimen and tolerance of common side effects are critically important to maintain drug efficacy. Antiviral response should be monitored by baseline HIV viral load and CD4 count and repeat measurement at 2 and 4 weeks into treatment and then periodically (every 3-6 months) to ensure viral suppression.
- All patients should have genotypic resistance testing upon entry into medical care and before initiation of ART.
- In experienced patients, an antiretroviral regimen should be constructed based on past antiretroviral use and the results of genotypic or phenotypic testing.
- Patients with a CD4 count <200/mm^3 should be given preventive therapy for PJP (Table 11).
- Evaluation of chronic diarrhea in patients with HIV is described in the AIDS topic in Section I.
- Criteria for discontinuing and restarting opportunistic infection prophylaxis for adults and adolescents with HIV infection is described in Table 12.
- HIV infection in a pregnant woman poses special challenges and considerations. Appropriate and timely ART given to mother and newborn has been shown to dramatically reduce the risk of perinatal transmission of HIV. The goal of therapy is to achieve an undetectable viral load. For HIV-infected pregnant women who are already receiving ART: (1) continue therapy if suppressing viral replication, but avoid use of efavirenz in the first trimester (substitution is recommended in the first trimester); (2) if viremia on therapy, genotypic testing is recommended; (3) nevirapine should be continued, regardless of CD4 count, if there is viral suppression. For HIV-infected pregnant women who have never received ART: (1) women who require ART for their own health should start on ART in the first trimester. Most antiretrovirals are safe in pregnancy, however, efavirenz should be avoided because of possible teratogenicity (Class D), DDI and D4T should be avoided (potential of lactic acidosis), and some protease inhibitors may be dose-altered in pregnancy. Nevirapine should not be initiated in an antiretroviral-naive pregnant patient with CD4 counts >250 cells/mm^3 because of the risk of hepatotoxicity. (2) Women who do not need ART for their own health should also initiate three-drug therapy, but may do so at the end of the first trimester.
- Dolutegravir should also be used with caution in women who are pregnant or of childbearing age.
- ART should continue through the baby's birth. Zidovudine should also be given intravenously to the woman at the time of labor if the woman has an HIV RNA >1000 copies/ml or there is a concern for poor adherence, regardless of whether it is an existing component of her three-drug regimen. In women with viral loads persistently >1000 copies/ml despite appropriate ART, cesarean section may further lower risk of transmission. For women with HIV RNA <1000 copies/ml zidovudine (AZT) should also be given to the newborn for the first six weeks of life. If HIV RNA levels are >1000 copies/ml, infants should receive combination ART which may include zidovudine, lamivudine and nevirapine for six weeks. Mothers should completely avoid nursing.

DISPOSITION

- Ongoing care consisting of frequent medical evaluations and monitoring of CD4 counts and HIV viral loads.
- Long-term care focused on providing up-to-date ART and prophylaxis of PJP and other opportunistic infections, as well as early detection of complications.
- Ongoing assessment for cardiovascular risk and other primary prevention interventions.

H

TABLE 11 Criteria for Discontinuing and Restarting Opportunistic Infection Prophylaxis for Adults and Adolescents with Human Immunodeficiency Virus Infection

Opportunistic Infection	Criteria for Discontinuing Primary Prophylaxis	Criteria for Restarting Primary Prophylaxis	Criteria for Discontinuing Secondary Prophylaxis/Chronic Maintenance Therapy	Criteria for Restarting Secondary Prophylaxis/Chronic Maintenance Therapy
Pneumocystis pneumonia (PJP)	CD4+ count >200 cells/mm³ for >3 mo in response to ART	CD4+ count <200 cells/mm³	CD4+ count increased from <200 cells/mm³ to >200 cells/mm³ for ≥3 mo in response to ART If PJP is diagnosed when CD4+ count >200 cells/mm³, prophylaxis should probably be continued for life regardless of CD4+ count rise in response to ART.	CD4+ count <200 cells/mm³, or if PCP recurred at a CD4+ count >200 cells/mm³
Toxoplasma gondii encephalitis (TE)	CD4+ count >200 cells/mm³ for >3 mo in response to ART	CD4+ count <100-200 cells/mm³	Successfully completed initial therapy, remain asymptomatic of signs and symptoms of TE, and CD4+ count >200 cells/mm³ for >6 mo in response to ART	CD4+ count <100 cells/mm³
Microsporidiosis	Not applicable	Not applicable	No signs and symptoms of non-ocular microsporidiosis and CD4+ count >200 cells/mm³ for >6 mo in response to ART Patients with ocular microsporidiosis should be on therapy indefinitely regardless of CD4+ count.	No recommendation
Disseminated *Mycobacterium avium* complex (MAC) disease	CD4+ count >100 cells/mm³ for ≥3 mo in response to ART	CD4+ count <50 cells/mm³	If fulfill the following criteria Completed ≥12 mo therapy, and No signs and symptoms of MAC, and Have sustained (≥6 mo) CD4+ count >100 cells/mm³ in response to ART	CD4+ count <50 cells/mm³
Bartonellosis	Not applicable	Not applicable	If fulfill the following criteria Received 3-4 mo of treatment CD4+ count >200 cells/mm³ for ≥6 mo Certain specialists would discontinue therapy only if *Bartonella* titers have also decreased by fourfold.	No recommendation
Mucosal candidiasis	Not applicable	Not applicable	If used, reasonable to discontinue when CD4+ count >200 cells/mm³	No recommendation
Cryptococcal meningitis	Not applicable	Not applicable	If fulfill the following criteria Completed course of initial therapy Remain asymptomatic of cryptococcosis CD4+ count ≥200 cells/mm³ for >6 mo in response to ART Certain specialists would perform a lumbar puncture to determine if cerebrospinal fluid is culture and antigen negative before stopping therapy.	CD4+ count <100 cells/mm³
Histoplasma capsulatum infection	If used, CD4+ count >150 cells/mm³ for 6 mo on ART	For patients at high risk for acquiring histoplasmosis, restart at CD4+ count ≤150 cells/mm³.	If fulfill the following criteria received itraconazole for ≥1 yr Negative blood cultures CD4+ count >150 cells/mm³ for ≥6 mo in response to ART Serum *Histoplasma* antigen <2 units	CD4+ count ≤150 cells/mm³
Coccidioidomycosis	If used, CD4+ count ≥250 cells/mm³ for ≥6 mo	If used, restart at CD4+ count <250 cells/mm³	**Only for patients with focal coccidioidal pneumonia:** Clinically responded to ≥12 mo of antifungal therapy CD4+ count >250 cells/mm³ Receiving ART Suppressive therapy should be continued indefinitely, even with increase in CD4+ count on ART for patients with diffuse pulmonary, disseminated, or meningeal diseases.	No recommendation
Cytomegalovirus retinitis	Not applicable	Not applicable	CD4+ count >100 cells/mm³ for >3-6 mo in response to ART. Therapy should be discontinued only after consultation with an ophthalmologist, taking into account magnitude and duration of CD4+ count increase, anatomic location of the lesions, vision in the contralateral eye, and the feasibility of regular ophthalmologic monitoring.Routine (every 3 mo) ophthalmologic follow-up is recommended for early detection of relapse or immune restoration uveitis.	No recommendation
Isospora belli infection	Not applicable	Not applicable	Sustained increase in CD4+ count to >200 cells/mm³ for >6 mo in response to ART and without evidence of *I. belli* infection	No recommendation

Modified from Centers for Disease Control and Prevention. Guidelines for prevention and treatment of opportunistic infections in HIV-infected adults and adolescents. Recommendations from CDC, the National Institutes of Health, and the HIV Medicine Association of the Infectious Disease Society of America. *MMWR Morb Mortal Wkly Rep* 58(RR-4), 2009.

TABLE 12 Prophylaxis to Prevent First Episode of HIV-related Opportunistic Disease

Pathogen	Indication	First Choice	Alternative
Pneumocystis jiroveci pneumonia (PJP, previously referred to as *Pneumocystis carinii,* PCP)	CD4+ count <200 cells/mm^3 or oropharyngeal candidiasisCD4+ <14% or history of AIDS-defining illness CD4+ count >200 but <250 cells/mm^3 if monitoring CD4+ count every 1-3 mo is not possible	Trimethoprim-sulfamethoxazole (TMP-SMX) double-strength PO daily; *or* single-strength daily	TMP-SMX 1 double-strength PO 3 times weekly; *or* Dapsone 100 mg PO daily or 50 mg PO bid; *or* Aerosolized pentamidine 300 mg via Respirgard II nebulizer every month; *or* Atovaquone 1500 mg PO daily
Toxoplasma gondii encephalitis	*Toxoplasma* IgG–positive patients with CD4+ count <100 cells/mm^{3}Seronegative patients receiving PCP prophylaxis not active against toxoplasmosis should have *Toxoplasma* serology retested if CD4+ count declines to <100 cells/mm^3. Prophylaxis should be initiated if seroconversion occurred.	TMP-SMX, 1 double-strength PO daily	TMP-SMX 1 double-strength PO 3 times weekly; *or* TMP-SMX 1 single-strength PO daily; *or* Dapsone 50 mg PO daily + pyrimethamine 50 mg PO weekly + leucovorin 25 mg PO weekly; *or* Dapsone 200 mg PO weekly + pyrimethamine 75 mg PO weekly + leucovorin 25 mg PO weekly
Mycobacterium tuberculosis infection (TB) (treatment of latent TB infection or LTBI)	(1) Diagnostic test for LTBI, no evidence of active TB, and no prior history of treatment for active or latent TB (2) Diagnostic test for LTBI, but close contact with a person with infectious pulmonary TB and no evidence of active TB (3) A history of untreated or inadequately treated healed TB (i.e., old fibrotic lesions) regardless of diagnostic tests for LTBI and no evidence of active TB	Isoniazid (INH) 300 mg PO daily or 900 mg PO twice weekly for 9 mo—both plus pyridoxine 25 mg PO daily; *or* For persons exposed to drug-resistant TB, selection of drugs after consultation with public health authorities	Rifampin (RIF) 600 mg PO daily × 4 mo; or Rifabutin (dosage depends on ART regimen) . Be careful of drug interactions with these medications (PIs and NNRTIs).
Disseminated *Mycobacterium avium* complex (MAC) disease	CD4+ count <50 cells/mm^3—after ruling out active MAC infection	Azithromycin 1200 mg PO once weekly; *or* Clarithromycin 500 mg PO bid; *or* Azithromycin 600 mg PO twice weekly	RFB 300 mg PO daily (dosage adjustment based on drug-drug interactions with antiretroviral therapy); rule out active TB before starting RFB
Streptococcus pneumoniae infection	CD4+ count >200 cells/mm^3 and no receipt of pneumococcal vaccine in the past 5 yrCD4+ count <200 cells/mm^3—vaccination can be offered In patients who received polysaccharide pneumococcal vaccination (PPV) when CD4+ count <200 cells/mm^3 but has increased to >200 cells/mm^3 in response to antiretroviral therapy	A single dose of PCV13 followed by a single dose of PPSV23 at least 8 wk later. A second dose of PPSV23 should be given 5 yr after the initial PPSV23 dose.	
Influenza A and B virus infection	All HIV-infected patients	Inactivated influenza vaccine 0.5 ml IM annually	
Histoplasma capsulatum infection	CD4+ count ≤150 cells/mm^3 and at high risk because of occupational exposure or live in a community with a hyperendemic rate of histoplasmosis (>10 cases/100 patient-yr)	Itraconazole 200 mg PO daily	
Coccidioidomycosis	Positive IgM or IgG serologic test result in a patient from a disease-endemic area; and CD4+ count <250 cells/mm^3	Fluconazole 400 mg PO dailyItraconazole 200 mg PO bid	
Varicella-zoster virus (VZV) infection	*Pre-exposure prevention:* Patients with CD4+ count ≥200 cells/mm^3 who have not been vaccinated, have no history of varicella or herpes zoster, or who are seronegative for VZV NOTE: Routine VZV serologic testing in HIV-infected adults is not recommended. *Postexposure—close contact with a person who has active varicella or herpes zoster* For susceptible patients (those who have no history of vaccination or of either condition, or are known to be VZV seronegative)	*Pre-exposure prevention:* Primary varicella vaccination (Varivax), 2 doses (0.5 ml SC) administered 3 mo apart. If vaccination results in disease because of vaccine virus, treatment with acyclovir is recommended. *Postexposure therapy:* Varicella-zoster immune globulin (VariZIG) 125 IU per 10 kg (maximum of 625 IU) IM, administered within 96 hr after exposure to a person with active varicella or herpes zoster NOTE: As of June 2007, VariZIG can be obtained only under a treatment IND (1-800-843-7477, FFF Enterprises).	VZV-susceptible household contacts of susceptible HIV-infected persons should be vaccinated to prevent potential transmission of VZV to their HIV-infected contacts.Alternative postexposure therapy: Postexposure varicella vaccine (Varivax) 0.5 ml SC × 2 doses, 3 mo apart if CD4+ count >200 cells/mm^3; *or* Preemptive acyclovir 800 mg PO 3×/day for 5 days These two alternatives have not been studied in the HIV population.
Human papillomavirus (HPV) infection	Women aged 11-26 yr. Men aged 11-26 yr	HPV quadrivalent vaccine 0.5 ml IM mo 0, 2, and 6	
Hepatitis A virus (HAV) infection	HAV-susceptible patients with chronic liver disease or who are injection-drug users, or men who have sex with men. Certain specialists might delay vaccination until CD4+ count >200 cells/mm^3.	Hepatitis A vaccine 1 ml IM × 2 doses—at 0 and 6-12 mo IgG antibody response should be assessed 1 mo after vaccination; nonresponders should be revaccinated	

Continued

TABLE 12 Prophylaxis to Prevent First Episode of HIV-related Opportunistic Disease—cont'd

Pathogen	Indication	First Choice	Alternative
Hepatitis B virus (HBV) infection	All HIV patients without evidence of prior exposure to HBV should be vaccinated with HBV vaccine, including patients with CD4+ count <200 cells/mm³. *Patients with isolated anti-HBc:* Consider screening for HBV DNA before vaccination to rule out occult chronic HBV infection	Hepatitis B vaccine IM (Engerix-B 20 μg/ml or Recombivax HB 10 μg/ml) at 0, 1, and 6 mo Anti-HBs should be obtained 1 mo after completion of the vaccine series.	Some experts recommend vaccinating with 40-μg doses of either vaccine.
	Vaccine nonresponders: Defined as anti-HBs <10 IU/ml 1 mo after a vaccination series For patients with low CD4+ count at the time of first vaccination series, certain specialists might delay revaccination until after a sustained increase in CD4+ count with antiretroviral therapy.	Revaccinate with a second vaccine series.	Some experts recommend revaccinating with 40-μg doses of either vaccine.

Modified from Centers for Disease Control and Prevention. Guidelines for prevention and treatment of opportunistic infections in HIV-infected adults and adolescents: Recommendations from CDC, the National Institutes of Health, and the HIV Medicine Association of the Infectious Disease Society of America, *MMWR Morb Mortal Wkly Rep* 58(RR-4), 2009.

- Screening for hepatitis A, B, and C. Treatment when indicated. Drugs such as TDF and lamivudine have activity against both HIV and hepatitis B and may be used in patients with co-infection.
- Vaccinations including hepatitis A and B (when susceptible), pneumococcus (PCV13 and PPSV23), tetanus/diphtheria/pertussis, meningococcal, and influenza. Box 1 summarizes vaccinations in HIV-positive adults.
- Yearly screening for other sexually transmitted infections (chlamydia, gonorrhea, syphilis).
- Consideration of AIDS (lymphomas, HPV) and non-AIDS related (screening for general population, age-specific cancers).

BOX 1 Vaccination in HIV-Positive Adults

Generally Avoid
- VZV
- BCG
- Oral polio
- Oral typhoid

Avoid if CD4+ Cells <200
- Yellow fever
- Measles

Give Routinely
- Tetanus/diphtheria (or Tdap)
- Hepatitis A/B
- *Streptococcus pneumoniae*
- Hib
- Meningococcal
- Influenza, yearly

Give if Indicated for Travel
- Typhoid Vi
- Meningococcal
- Polio, IPV
- Rabies
- Japanese encephalitis
- Tick-borne encephalitis

From Auerbach P: *Wilderness medicine, expert consult* Premium Edition—Enhanced Online Features and Print, Philadelphia, 2012, Saunders.

REFERRAL

To a physician knowledgeable and experienced in the management of HIV infection and its complications.

PREVENTION:
- TDF/FTC may be used as pre-exposure prophylaxis (PrEP). Individuals who are HIV negative may take TDF/FTC once a day to prevent HIV infection. PrEP has been demonstrated to be effective in MSM, heterosexuals, and injection drug users. Individuals on PrEP should be monitored every three months for renal dysfunction, HIV status, and adherence.
- Post-exposure prophylaxis (PEP) is an effective prevention intervention for individuals exposed to HIV infection, either occupationally or through a sexual exposure. PEP should be taken within 72 hours of an exposure and continued for 28 days. Baseline HIV status, renal function, hepatitis B/C, and liver function should be assessed. The recommended first-line regimen is tenofovir-emtricitabine 300/200 mg once daily plus raltegravir 400 mg orally twice daily or Dolutegravir 50mg once daily. Dolutegravir should be avoided in women of childbearing potential or who are pregnant.

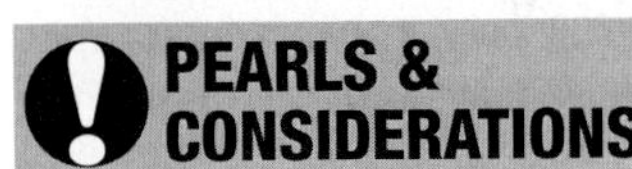

PEARLS & CONSIDERATIONS

COMMENTS

- ART should be initiated in all HIV-infected individuals regardless of CD4 cell counts.
- ART in combination with avoidance of breast-feeding and elective cesarean section in women with viremia reduces risk for mother-to-child transmission.

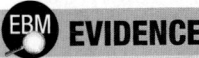

EVIDENCE

Available at ExpertConsult.com

SUGGESTED READINGS

Available at ExpertConsult.com

RELATED CONTENT

Human Immunodeficiency Virus (HIV) Infection (Patient Information)
Acquired Immunodeficiency Syndrome (Related Key Topic)

AUTHOR: **PHILIP A. CHAN, M.D., M.S.**

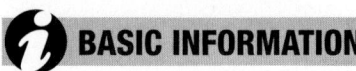

BASIC INFORMATION

DEFINITION

Normal pressure hydrocephalus (NPH) is a syndrome of symptomatic hydrocephalus in the setting of normal cerebrospinal fluid (CSF) pressure. The classic clinical triad of NPH includes gait disturbance, cognitive decline, and incontinence.

SYNONYMS

Normal pressure hydrocephalus
NPH
Occult hydrocephalus
Extraventricular obstructive hydrocephalus
Chronic hydrocephalus

ICD-10CM CODES
G91.2 Normal pressure hydrocephalus
G91.8 Other hydrocephalus

EPIDEMIOLOGY & DEMOGRAPHICS

INCIDENCE: The exact incidence is not known. In one study the incidence was found to be 5.5 per 100,000, but it may account for up to 5% of dementia in the U.S. Hospital discharge data suggest approximately 11,500 new cases diagnosed annually (may be overestimated). The prevalence of NPH may be as high as 14% among extended care facility patients.
PREDOMINANT SEX: Males = females
PREDOMINANT AGE: NPH is more common with increasing age. In one study of 1238 patients who had undergone a head CT and neuropsychiatric evaluation, 0.2% of patients between 70 and 79 had probable NPH, and 5.9% of those 80 yr old and older had probable NPH.

PHYSICAL FINDINGS & CLINICAL PRESENTATION

- Gait difficulty: A "magnetic" gait in which patients have difficulty initiating ambulation, and the gait may be broad-based and shuffling, with the appearance that the feet are stuck to the floor.
- Cognitive decline: Mental slowing, forgetfulness, and inattention, typically without agnosia, aphasia, or other cortical disturbances.
- Incontinence: Initially may have urinary urgency; incontinence later develops. Fecal incontinence also occasionally occurs. In one prospective study of 55 consecutive patients with idiopathic NPH, nocturia was the most common symptom, urge incontinence was the most bothersome, and 100% had detrusor overactivity on urodynamic studies.
- *Gegenhalten* (paratonia or involuntary resistance with passive movement) or other frontal lobe signs may be seen.

ETIOLOGY

- Approximately 50% of cases are idiopathic; the remaining cases have a variety of causes, including prior subarachnoid hemorrhage, meningitis, head trauma, or intracranial surgery.
- Symptoms are presumed to result from stretching of sacral motor and limbic fibers that lie near the ventricles as dilation occurs.

Dx DIAGNOSIS

DIFFERENTIAL DIAGNOSIS

- Alzheimer's disease with extrapyramidal features
- Cognitive impairment in the setting of Parkinson's disease or parkinsonism-plus syndromes
- Dementia with Lewy bodies
- Frontotemporal dementia
- Cervical spondylosis with cord compromise in the setting of degenerative dementia
- Multi-infarct dementia
- HIV-associated dementia

WORKUP

- Large-volume lumbar puncture:
  1. Time to walk a prespecified distance (usually 25 feet) is measured, followed by removal of 40 to 50 ml of CSF.
  2. Retest of timed walking is done later (sometimes at 1 and 4 hr). Patients who have significant improvement in gait are more likely to be shunt-responsive; those with mild or negative response can have variable outcomes.
  3. Opening and closing pressure are measured; if pressure is elevated, alternative causes must be considered. Higher *normal* pressure may predict a good outcome from CSF shunting (normal CSF pressure: 8-15 mm Hg or 10-18 cm H_2O).
- Measurement of CSF outflow resistance by an infusion test or CSF pressure monitoring is sometimes used to help predict surgical outcome. External lumbar drainage (ELD) is being used more commonly.

LABORATORY TESTS

- CSF should be sent for routine fluid analysis to exclude other pathologies.
- CSF biomarkers may be useful in excluding Alzheimer's disease (e.g., Tau/A beta 42).

IMAGING STUDIES

- CT scan or MRI (Fig. 1) can be used to document ventriculomegaly. The distinguishing feature of NPH is ventricular enlargement out of proportion to sulcal atrophy (Fig. E2), and typically the frontal horn ratio (Evans ratio) exceeds 0.40. An algorithm for evaluation of patients with enlarged ventricles is described in Fig. 3.
- MRI has advantages over CT, including better ability to visualize structures in the posterior fossa, visualize transependymal CSF flow (seen as periventricular T2 FLAIR hyperintensity), and document extent of white matter lesions. On MRI a flow void in the aqueduct and third ventricle ("jet sign"), thinning and elevation of the corpus callosum on sagittal images, rounding of the frontal horns, and a narrow CSF space at the high convexity/midline areas relative to Sylvian fissure size may be seen. MRI time-resolved 2D phase contrast imaging with velocity encoding can also be used to visualize CSF flow.
- Isotope cisternography and dynamic MRI studies have not been shown to be superior in predicting shunt outcome.

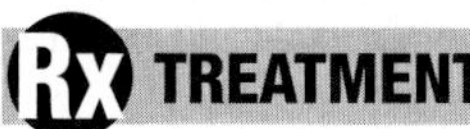

TREATMENT

There is no evidence that NPH can be effectively treated with medications. CSF diversion via a ventriculoperitoneal shunt is a definitive treatment.

NONPHARMACOLOGIC THERAPY

Response to ventriculoperitoneal shunting is variable. Some patients (variable depending on series reported) show significant improvement

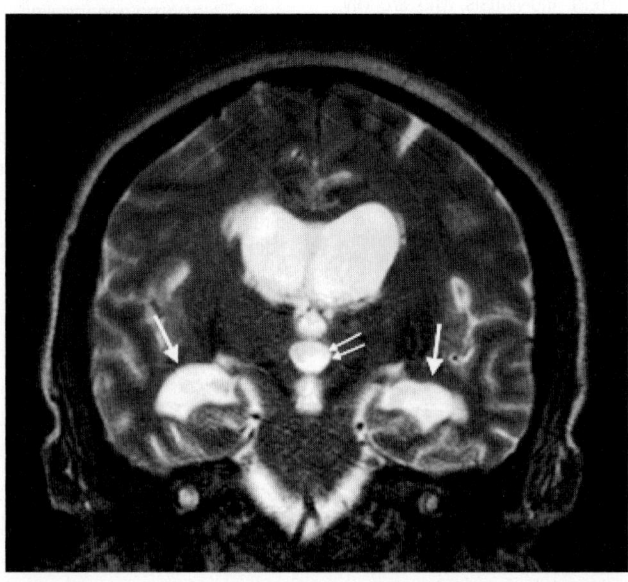

FIG. 1 This MRI study shows a coronal view of the brain of a patient with NPH. It demonstrates the classic findings: dilation of the lateral ventricles, their temporal horns (*large arrows*), and the third ventricle (*pair of arrows*), and absence of cerebral atrophy. (From Kaufman DM, Geyer HL, Milstein MJ: *Kaufman's clinical neurology for psychiatrists*, ed 8, Philadelphia, 2017, Elsevier)

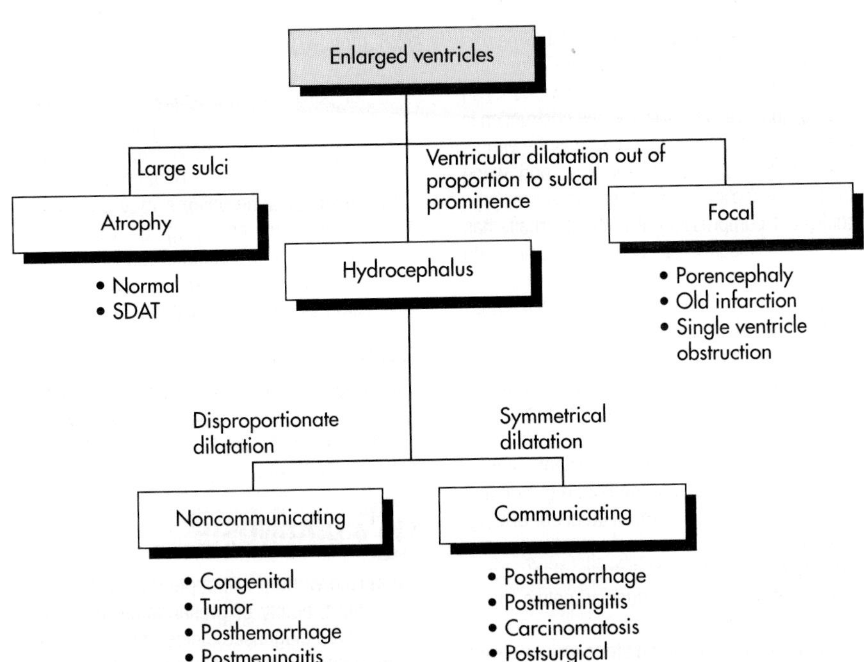

FIG. 3 Radiographic differential diagnosis of enlarged ventricles. *SDAT,* Senile dementia of the Alzheimer's type. (From Weissleder R, et al.: *Primer of diagnostic imaging,* ed 5, St Louis, 2011, Mosby.)

from shunting; however, effectiveness of shunting has never been demonstrated in a randomized controlled trial. Gait is most likely to improve.

Factors that may predict positive outcome with surgery:

- NPH caused by prior trauma, subarachnoid hemorrhage, or meningitis
- History of mild impairment in cognition <2 yr duration
- Onset of gait abnormality before cognitive decline
- Imaging demonstrates hydrocephalus without sulcal enlargement, including normal-sized sylvian fissures and cortical sulci, and absent or mild white matter lesions
- Transependymal CSF flow visualized on MRI
- Large-volume tap or ELD produces dramatic but temporary relief of symptoms
- High *normal* opening pressure

Factors that may predict negative outcome with surgery:

- Extensive white matter lesions or diffuse cerebral atrophy on MRI
- Moderate to severe cognitive impairment
- Onset of cognitive impairment before gait disorder
- History of alcohol abuse

ACUTE GENERAL Rx

Shunting in selected patients

DISPOSITION

Symptoms of NPH may progress over time. Prompt diagnosis may improve chances for treatment success.

REFERRAL

To neurologist for initial evaluation, including lumbar puncture, followed by neurosurgeon for shunting in appropriate patients

PEARLS & CONSIDERATIONS

Each of the cardinal symptoms of NPH is commonly seen in the elderly and occurs in multiple disease processes; therefore, differential diagnoses should always be considered carefully.

CAUTION

Shunt complications, including subdural or intracerebral hematoma, may occur in 30% to 40% of patients. In one retrospective study spanning 10 yr, which included patients with idiopathic as well as other forms of adult hydrocephalus, the shunt failure rate was 32%.

SUGGESTED READINGS

Available at ExpertConsult.com

RELATED CONTENT

Normal Pressure Hydrocephalus (Patient Information)

AUTHORS: **TAMARA G. FONG, M.D., PH.D.,** and **IRINA A. SKYLAR-SCOTT, M.D.**

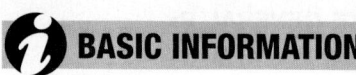

DEFINITION

Hydronephrosis means "water inside the kidney" in Greek and is an anatomic dilation of the collecting system of the kidneys (renal pelvis and/or calyces). When combined with dilation of the ureters, this is known as hydroureteronephrosis. Hydronephrosis is not a specific diagnosis and is *not* synonymous with obstruction. Hydronephrosis can occur with complete, partial, or no obstruction of urine flow.

SYNONYMS

Pelviectasis
Caliectasis
Pelvocaliectasis
Pyelocaliectasis

ICD-10-CM CODES

N13.0	Hydronephrosis with ureteropelvic junction obstruction
N13.1	Hydronephrosis with ureteral stricture, not elsewhere classified
N13.2	Hydronephrosis with renal and ureteral calculous obstruction
N13.30	Unspecified hydronephrosis
N13.39	Other hydronephrosis
Q62.0	Congenital hydronephrosis

EPIDEMIOLOGY & DEMOGRAPHICS

Prevalence from multiple autopsy series ranges from 2% to 4%, with subjects ranging in age from neonates to geriatric patients. Antenatal hydronephrosis is one of the most common findings in prenatal ultrasound scans, affecting up to 5% of pregnancies, with 30% to 40% persisting postnatally. Of these, 40% resolving spontaneously. Hydronephrosis in children is often caused by congenital and structural abnormalities of the kidneys and ureters as with ureteropelvic junction obstruction (UPJO) and vesicoureteral reflux (VUR). Hydronephrosis in adults is often a result of obstruction of one or both kidneys, usually caused by stones, tumors, infections, and trauma. Stones remain the commonest cause overall of upper urinary tract obstruction. In adults 20 to 60 yr in age, hydronephrosis is more common in women, secondary to pregnancy/gynecological causes. During pregnancy, physiologic hydronephrosis (more commonly on the right) can occur in up to 90% of cases, and is often asymptomatic. In older patients (age >60 yr), obstructions from prostate enlargement or malignancy are the most common causes.

CLINICAL PRESENTATION

Hydronephrosis may present as an asymptomatic, incidental finding during imaging performed for another purpose. Symptoms often indicate an element of obstruction, and the presentation will depend on the *degree* of obstruction (complete or partial), *chronicity* of obstruction (acute or chronic), and *anatomic* factors (unilateral, bilateral and intrinsic or extrinsic in the ureter).

HISTORY:

- Pain is usually present along the flank with radiation toward the ipsilateral groin or lower abdominal quadrant. If sudden and severe in onset, consider a ureteral stone. If the pain is induced by diuresis (e.g., following consumption of alcohol), consider ureteropelvic junction obstruction ("Dietl's crisis"). When obstruction is subacute to chronic, symptoms may be vague, less intense, or absent, and wax and wane in severity (colic). Extrinsic compression (e.g., malignant compression of ureters) usually has a more insidious onset compared to intrinsic obstruction (e.g., ureteral stone or blood clot).
- Nausea and vomiting are typically associated with acute obstruction, most often from an intrinsic obstructing process.
- Oliguria/anuria may occur with complete, bilateral obstruction, or with an obstructed solitary kidney.
- Urinary symptoms are often absent, unless there is an associated condition, e.g., urinary tract infection, distal ureteral stone, or urinary retention. Irritating urinary symptoms may predominate, including dysuria, flank pain, urinary urgency and frequency, pelvic pressure and discomfort.
- Hematuria: May indicate a stone, urinary tract infection or malignancy.
- Site of obstruction can relate to the presentation: Upper tract obstruction will frequently present with flank pain, whereas lower tract obstruction is often associated with obstructive voiding symptoms.

PHYSICAL EXAMINATION: A complete physical examination is warranted, but may not be helpful in the assessment of hydronephrosis. Areas to pay special attention to include:

- Blood pressure measurement
- Palpable abdominal masses are rare, except in children or very thin patients with massive hydronephrosis. Costovertebral angle tenderness is not a particularly helpful finding. Palpate and percuss for an enlarged bladder.
- Complete genitourinary and pelvic exams
  1. Pelvic exam will assess for pelvic masses or pelvic organ prolapse, which could be related to ureteral prolapse.
  2. Digital rectal exam will assess for prostatic abnormality or rectal mass.
  3. Residual urine volume may demonstrate incomplete emptying of the bladder. Residual urine volume can be evaluated indirectly by bedside ultrasonography or directly by catheterization.

ETIOLOGY

Hydronephrosis can be caused by extrinsic or intrinsic factors relative to the urinary tract (Table 1). Causes can also be grouped as congenital or acquired.

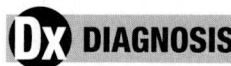

Diagnostic workup will depend upon the age of the patient, acuity of presentation, if hydronephrosis was diagnosed incidentally, and whether associated symptoms are present.

DIFFERENTIAL DIAGNOSIS

- Extrarenal pelvis where no true obstruction exists, but is confused with obstruction
- Urinary stones
- Neoplastic disease: Kidney, ureter, bladder, urethra
- Prostatic hyperplasia
- Urethral stricture
- Neurologic disease producing voiding dysfunction
- Urinary reflux
- Urinary tract infection
- Medication effects
- Trauma
- Congenital abnormality of urinary tract

TABLE 1 Causes of Hydronephrosis

Obstructive	
Intrinsic to the Urinary Tract	Ureter: Ureteropelvic junction obstruction, ureterovesical junction obstruction, stricture, tumor, ureterocele, stone, blood clot, sloughed papilla, infection, hyperplastic polyp
	Bladder: Malignancy, stone, bladder neck obstruction, urine retention
	Prostate: Benign prostatic enlargement, prostatitis, calculus, abscess, malignancy
	Urethra: Stricture, stone, diverticulum, malignancy, posterior urethral valves, phimosis
Extrinsic to the Urinary Tract	Reproductive System:
	Uterus: Pregnancy, prolapse, fibroids, malignancy
	Ovary: Malignancy, cyst, abscess
	Vascular System:
	Aneurysm: Abdominal aorta, iliac vessel
	Aberrant vessels: Ureteropelvic junction
	Venous: Retrocaval ureter, ovarian vein syndrome
	Gastrointestinal System:
	Inflammatory bowel disease, GI malignancy, abscesses, cysts
	Diseases of the Retroperitoneum
	Retroperitoneal fibrosis
	Retroperitoneal malignancy (primary or metastatic deposits)
	Hematoma
	Lymphocele
	Iatrogenic injury
Nonobstructive	
	Vesicoureteral reflux
	Extrarenal pelvis
	Megaureter/megacalycosis
	Pyelonephritis

- Urinary retention
- Retroperitoneal fibrosis
- Urinary Trauma
- Iatrogenic injuries

LABORATORY TESTS

- **Evaluation of kidney function** by blood urea nitrogen and creatinine. If azotemia is present, bilateral obstruction or unilateral obstruction of a solitary kidney has occurred.
- **Evaluation of electrolyte abnormalities** including hypo- or hypernatremia, hyperkalemia, and low bicarbonate concentration.
- **Urinalysis and sediment examination** may reveal white blood cells, red blood cells, or bacteria in the appropriate setting (e.g., infection, stones). Urine microscopy facilitates crystal identification, which may suggest urinary stone disease. The sediment may be normal in obstructive renal disease.
- **Urine culture** should be sent if urinalysis or presentation suggests urinary tract infection.
- **Urine cytology** if urothelial cancer is suspected.

IMAGING STUDIES

- Ultrasound is an excellent initial test, especially for children and pregnant women. It is a screening test that permits evaluation of the kidneys, portions of the ureters, bladder wall, and bladder volume, as well as the contour of the collecting system and ureters. Point-of-care ultrasound provides early, rapid imaging and aids patient triage and justification for additional imaging. Ultrasound is >90% sensitive and specific for hydronephrosis. The absence of ureteral jets on ultrasound may be an indirect sign of obstruction, but is not definitive (Fig. E1).
- Abdominal, plain film, or kidney, ureter and bladder (KUB) radiographs are of limited value in isolation. These tests complement ultrasound and may be helpful in diagnosing radiopaque kidney or ureteral stones
- Abdominal CT scan without intravenous contrast medium provides excellent localization of sites of obstruction (Figs. E2 and E3), especially if a ureteral calculus is the cause of obstruction. A normal ureter on an unenhanced CT is considered 2 to 3 mm wide in adults. If kidney function is normal, CT urography (without and then with contrast, and with delayed images of the ureters), provides excellent anatomic information, and is modality of choice for assessment of possible upper tract tumors or evaluation of incidental hydronephrosis.
- MRI is an alternative to CT. MRI provides detail, but cannot directly detect a stone, expensive. Impaired renal function may preclude gadolinium administration. MRI is considered after other tests are inconclusive or contraindicated, such as in pregnant patients, those with renal insufficiency, and those with contrast allergy.
- Antegrade or retrograde ureterograms/pyelograms are invasive procedures, but can be used if there are contraindications to CT or MRI scans with contrast (e.g., contrast allergy, renal impairment).
- Voiding cystourethrography can diagnose vesicoureteral reflux and bladder neck or urethral obstruction.
- Diuretic renography (MAG3 renogram) is a functional radioisotopic test that provides differential function of each kidney, and determines if functional obstruction is present.

Rx TREATMENT

ACUTE GENERAL Rx

- Analgesics, antiemetics, and fluids for treatment of pain, nausea, and vomiting
- Antibiotics for urinary tract infection/pyelonephritis

Definitive management:

- Management depends on presence of obstruction, etiology, and location of hydronephrosis. Prompt treatment of infection and relief of obstruction prevent long-term loss of kidney function. Chronic, bilateral obstruction, such as from any cause may produce permanent functional deterioration.
- General principles include:
  1. Observation and outpatient workup for asymptomatic or minimally symptomatic patients with no infection, electrolyte derangements, or acute kidney injury.
  2. Surgical treatment is aimed at relieving obstruction, and indicated if there is acute obstruction with urinary tract infection, acute kidney injury, uncontrollable pain, or nausea and vomiting.
  3. Urethral urinary catheter or suprapubic catheter placement is indicated for bladder outlet obstruction.
  4. Ureteral stenting is carried out for decompression of one or both kidneys.
  5. Percutaneous nephrostomy tubes may be required in the setting of extrinsic ureteral compression or when ureteral stenting is not possible or fails.

REFERRAL

Prompt, emergent referral is paramount in the setting of severe symptoms, infection, or impaired renal function.

- Urology for diagnostic and/or therapeutic procedures (pediatric urologist for antenatal or postnatal hydronephrosis)
- Oncology if neoplasm diagnosed
- Gynecology if pregnancy or female pelvic anatomy is involved
- Nephrology for electrolyte/acid-base disturbances

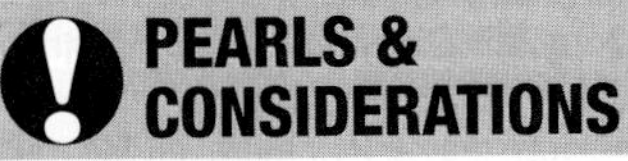

PEARLS & CONSIDERATIONS

COMMENTS

- Hydronephrosis is not a primary disorder; an underlying etiology must be sought.
- Children often have congenital causes; adults generally have acquired intrinsic or extrinsic causes.
- There are obstructive and nonobstructive causes of hydronephrosis. Further evaluation can be performed without specialty consultation with a computed tomography urogram, magnetic resonance urogram, or diuretic renogram.
- Prompt renal decompression is critical when hydronephrosis is associated with infection, severe kidney injury, and/or electrolyte abnormalities.

PREVENTION

Timely and appropriate management of acute kidney obstruction prevents long-term kidney damage. Hydronephrosis may persist after relief of the obstructing cause.

SUGGESTED READINGS

Available at ExpertConsult.com

AUTHORS: **LEE BAUMGARTEN, M.D.**, and **DAVID A. LEAVITT, M.D.**

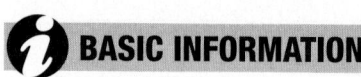

BASIC INFORMATION

DEFINITION

Hypercholesterolemia refers to a blood cholesterol measurement ≥200 mg/dl.

SYNONYMS

Hyperlipidemia
Hypercholesteremia
Dyslipidemia
Type II familial hyperlipoproteinemia

ICD-10CM CODES
E78.0 Pure hypercholesterolemia

EPIDEMIOLOGY & DEMOGRAPHICS

- Over 105 million (37%) adults in the U.S. have total blood cholesterol levels higher than 200 mg/dl. Of this group, more than 36 million adults have extremely high-risk cholesterol levels over 240 mg/dl (13%).
- For men over the age of 20 yr, approximately 48% of white men, 45% of black men, and 50% of Hispanic men have high blood cholesterol.
- For women over the age of 20, approximately 50% of white women, 42% of black women, and 50% of Hispanic women have hypercholesterolemia.
- Prevalence of hypercholesterolemia increases with increasing age.
- According to NHANES data for 2009-2010, about 47% of adults had at least one of three risk factors for cardiovascular disease—uncontrolled high blood pressure, uncontrolled high levels of low-density lipoproteins (LDL) cholesterol, or current smoking.

PHYSICAL FINDINGS & CLINICAL PRESENTATION

- A detailed medication history should be performed because some medications may affect lipid levels (e.g., thiazides, corticosteroids, beta-blockers, and estrogens).
- The physical examination should include measurements of BMI and BP, thyroid and liver assessments, and examining peripheral pulses including carotids for bruits.
- Physical findings, particularly in the familial forms may include:
  1. Tendon xanthomas
  2. Xanthelasma
  3. Arcus corneae
  4. Arterial bruits (young adulthood)

ETIOLOGY

Primary:
- Genetics
- Obesity
- Dietary intake

Secondary:
- Hypothyroidism
- Diabetes mellitus
- Nephrotic syndrome
- Obstructive liver disease: Hepatoma, extrahepatic biliary obstruction, primary biliary cirrhosis
- Alcohol or tobacco use
- Dysgammaglobulinemia (multiple myeloma, SLE)
- Drugs: Oral contraceptives, progesterone, corticosteroids, thiazide diuretics, β-blockers, androgenic steroids, retinoic acid derivatives, protease inhibitors

Dx DIAGNOSIS

DIFFERENTIAL DIAGNOSIS

- Always consider underlying secondary causes for the elevated cholesterol.
- Patients with very high LDL cholesterol usually have genetic forms of hypercholesterolemia (see "Hyperlipoproteinemia, Primary"). Early detection of these cases and family testing to identify similarly affected relatives is important.
- Metabolic syndrome:
  1. A constellation of lipid and nonlipid risk factors of a metabolic origin
  2. Diagnosed when three or more of the following are present: abdominal obesity (waist circumference >40 in in men and >35 in in women); fasting triglycerides >150 mg/dl; HDL <40 mg/dl in males and <50 mg/dl in females; systolic BP >130 mmHg and diastolic BP >85 mmHg; fasting glucose >110 mg/dl

WHO SHOULD BE SCREENED:
- AACE recommends screening of patients >20 yr of age for elevated cholesterol every 5 yr, males >45 yr and females >55 yr of age every 1-2 yr, and >65 yr of age every yr up to 75 yr of age regardless of CAD risk status. Patients above 75 yr of age with multiple CAD risk factors should still continue to get screened annually.
- The USPSTF supports routine screening for men aged >35 yr and women aged >45 yr by measurement of nonfasting total and HDL cholesterol alone.
- In 2010, the USPSTF recommended routine screening for overweight and obesity in persons aged <20 yr.
- In 2011, ACC/AHA recommended screening for hypertriglyceridemia by a nonfasting measurement. A nonfasting level of <200 mg/dl is commensurate with an optimal level of <100 mg/dl and no further testing is required. However, a nonfasting level of >200 mg/dl warrants further testing with a fasting lipid profile.

LABORATORY TESTS

- Obtain a lipid profile. A fasting lipid panel has been traditionally preferred over a nonfasting lipid profile; however, this recommendation has come into question, and expert consensus statements from Canada and Europe recommend nonfasting lipid testing as the new standard for lipid measurement. In nonfasting patients, triglyceride levels ≥175 mg/dl should be considered elevated as compared with 15- mg/dl for fasting panels. Fasting lipid panels are preferred for patients with triglycerides over 400 mg/dl.
- Perform a workup for secondary causes if clinically indicated, such as TSH, metabolic profile, LFTs, and fasting glucose.

Rx TREATMENT

NONPHARMACOLOGIC THERAPY

- First line of treatment: Dietary therapy can result in 5% to 15% reduction in LDL cholesterol level.
- Composition of the **TLC diet:**
  1. Total fat 25% to 30% of total calories
  2. Polyunsaturated fat up to 10% of total calories
  3. Monounsaturated fat up to 20% of total calories
  4. Saturated fats <7% of total calories
  5. Carbohydrate 50% to 60% of total calories
  6. Protein 15% of total calories
  7. No more than 200 mg/day of cholesterol
  8. Fiber 20 to 30 g/day
- Increased physical activity: Encourage 30 min of moderately intense physical activity, four to six times a week (e.g., brisk walking, riding stationary bike, water aerobics)
- Maintenance of a healthy weight
- Avoidance of tobacco products
- Counseling on CAD risk factors (Table 1)
- Plant-based diets (including stanol-containing margarines, oat bran, and nuts) have shown effectiveness in controlling lipids.

ACUTE GENERAL Rx

No acute treatment needed

CHRONIC Rx

- Box 1 summarizes the key recommendations for the treatment of blood cholesterol to reduce ASCVD (atherosclerotic cardiovascular disease) risk in adults.
- The guidelines identify four high-risk groups that benefit from statin therapy:
  1. Patients with clinical ASCVD (Table 2, Fig. 1)
  2. LDL ≥190 mg/dl
  3. DM aged 40-75 yr and LDL 70-189 mg/dl
  4. Ten-yr risk for ASCVD ≥7.5% and LDL 70-189 mg/dl
- The 10-yr risk of ASCVD is calculated with the risk calculator available at http://my.americanheart.org/cvriskcalculator
- ASCVD events are reduced by using the maximum tolerated statin intensity in the above groups shown to benefit the most (Tables 3 and 4).

TABLE 1 Risk Factors for Heart Disease

1. Cigarette smoking
2. Hypertension (BP ≤140/90 mm Hg or on medications)
3. Low HDL cholesterol (<40 mg/dl)*
4. Family history of premature CHD (<55 yr in first-degree male relative or <65 yr in first-degree female relative)
5. Age (men ≥45 yr, women ≥55 yr)

BP, Blood pressure; *CHD*, congenital heart disease; *HDL*, high-density lipoprotein cholesterol.
*HDL cholesterol >60 mg/dl counts as a negative risk factor; its presence removes one risk factor from the total count.

BOX 1 2013 ACC/AHA Summary of Key Recommendations for the Treatment of Blood Cholesterol to Reduce ASCVD Risk in Adults

A. Heart-healthy lifestyle habits should be encouraged for all individuals.
B. The appropriate intensity of statin therapy should be initiated or continued:
 1. Clinical ASCVD*
  a. Age 75 years or less and no safety concerns: High-intensity statin (class I, level A)
  b. Age 75 years or safety concerns: Moderate-intensity statin (class I, level A)
 2. Primary prevention: Primary LDL-C 190 mg/dl or greater
  a. Rule out secondary causes of hyperlipidemia (class I, level B)
  b. Age 21 years or older: High-intensity statin (class I, level B)
  c. Achieve at least a 50% reduction in LDL-C (class IIa, level B)
  d. LDL-C lowering nonstatin therapy may be considered to further reduce LDL-C (class IIb, level C)
 3. Primary prevention: Diabetes, 40 to 75 years of age, and LDL-C 70 to 189 mg/dl
  a. Moderate-intensity statin (class I, level A)
  b. Consider high-intensity statin when 7.5% or greater 10-year ASCVD risk using the Pooled Cohort Equations‡† (class IIa, level B)
 4. Primary prevention: No diabetes, 40 to 75 years of age, and LDL-C 70 to 189 mg/dl
  a. Estimate 10-year ASCVD risk using the Risk Calculator based on the Pooled Cohort Equations in those *not* receiving a statin; estimate risk every 4 to 6 years (class I, level B)
  b. To determine whether to initiate a statin, engage in a clinician-patient discussion of the potential for ASCVD risk reduction, adverse effects, drug-drug interactions, and patient preferences
  c. Reemphasize heart-healthy lifestyle habits and address other risk factors (class IIa, level C)
   i. 7.5% or greater 10-year ASCVD risk: Moderate- or high-intensity statin (class I, level A)
   ii. 5% to 7.5% 10-year ASCVD risk: Consider moderate-intensity statin (class IIa, level B)
   iii. Other factors may be considered: LDL-C 160 mg/dl or greater, family history of premature ASCVD, hs-CRP 2.0 mg/L or greater, CAC score 300 Agatston units or greater, ABI less than 0.9, or lifetime ASCVD risk (class IIb, level C)
 5. Primary prevention when LDL-C is less than 190 mg/dl and age is less than 40 or more than 75 years, or less than 5% 10-year ASCVD risk
  a. Statin therapy may be considered in selected individuals (class IIb, level C)
 6. Statin therapy is not routinely recommended for individuals with NYHA class II-IV heart failure or who are receiving maintenance hemodialysis
C. Regularly monitor adherence to lifestyle and drug therapy with lipid and safety assessments
 1. Assess adherence, response to therapy, and adverse effects within 4 to 12 weeks following statin initiation or change in therapy (class I, level A)
  a. Measure a fasting lipid panel (class I, level A)
  b. Do not routinely monitor ALT or CK unless symptomatic (class IIa, level C)
  c. Screen and treat type 2 diabetes according to current practice guidelines. Heart-healthy lifestyle habits should be encouraged to prevent progression to diabetes (class I, level B)
  d. Anticipated therapeutic response: Approximately 50% or greater reduction in LDL-C from baseline for high-intensity statin and 30% to 50% for moderate-intensity statin (class IIa, level B)
   i. Insufficient evidence for LDL-C or non–HDL-C treatment targets from RCTs
   ii. For those with unknown baseline LDL-C, an LDL-C less than 100 mg/dl was observed in RCTs of high-intensity statin therapy
  e. Less than anticipated therapeutic response:
   i. Reinforce improved adherence to lifestyle and drug therapy (class I, level A)
   ii. Evaluate for secondary causes of hyperlipidemia if indicated (class I, level A)
   iii. Increase statin intensity, or if on maximally tolerated statin intensity, consider addition of nonstatin therapy in selected high-risk individuals§ (class IIb, level C)
  f. Regularly monitor adherence to lifestyle and drug therapy every 3 to 12 months once adherence has been established. Continue assessment of adherence for optimal ASCVD risk reduction and safety (class I, level A)
D. In individuals intolerant of the recommended intensity of statin therapy, use the maximally tolerated intensity of statin (class I, level B). If there are muscle or other symptoms, establish that they are related to the statin (class IIa, level B)

ABI, Ankle-brachial index; *ACC*, American College of Cardiology; *AHA*, American Heart Association; *ALT*, alanine aminotransferase, a test of hepatic function; *ASCVD*, atherosclerotic cardiovascular disease; *CAC*, coronary artery calcium; *CHD*, coronary heart disease; *CK*, creatine kinase, a test of muscle injury; *HDL-C*, high-density lipoprotein cholesterol; *hs-CRP*, high-sensitivity C-reactive protein; *LDL-C*, low-density lipoprotein cholesterol; *MI*, myocardial infarction; *NYHA*, New York Heart Association; *RCTs*, randomized controlled trials; and *TIA*, transient ischemic attack.

*Clinical ASCVD includes acute coronary syndromes, history of MI, stable or unstable angina, coronary or other arterial revascularization, stroke, TIA, or peripheral arterial disease presumed to be of atherosclerotic origin.

†Estimated 10-year or "hard" ASCVD risk includes first occurrence of nonfatal MI, CHD death, and nonfatal and fatal stroke as used by the Risk Assessment Work Group in developing the Pooled Cohort Equations on the basis of age, sex, smoking status, total cholesterol level, HDL-C level, systolic blood pressure, and the use of antihypertensive therapy.

‡These factors may include primary LDL-C of 160 mg/dl or greater or other evidence of genetic hyperlipidemias; family history of premature ASCVD with onset at less than 55 years of age in a first-degree male relative or at less than 65 years of age in a first-degree female relative; hs-CRP 2 mg/L or greater; CAC score 300 Agatston units or greater or 75th percentile or greater for age, sex, and ethnicity; ABI less than 0.9; or lifetime risk of ASCVD. Additional factors that might aid in individual risk assessment could be identified in the future.

§High-risk individuals include those with clinical ASCVD, an untreated LDL-C 190 mg/dl or greater, suggesting genetic hypercholesterolemia, or individuals with diabetes 40 to 75 years of age and LDL-C 70 to 189 mg/dl.

From 2013 ACC/AHA guideline on the treatment of blood cholesterol to reduce atherosclerotic cardiovascular risk in adults: a report of the American College of Cardiology/American Heart Association Task Force on Practice Guidelines, *J Am Coll Cardiol* 63(25 Pt B):2889-2934, 2014.

TABLE 2 Atherosclerotic Cardiovascular Disease

1. Coronary heart disease: Acute coronary syndromes, history of myocardial infarction, stable or unstable angina, coronary or other arterial revascularization
2. Stroke or transient ischemic attack
3. Peripheral arterial disease

- Additional factors such as CRP >2 mg/L, primary LDL >160, genetic hyperlipidemias, family history of premature CHD, ABI <0.9, and CAD score >300 Agatston units may be used in patients who are not in one of four statin benefit groups and for whom a decision to initiate statin therapy is otherwise unclear.
- Percent reduction in LDL cholesterol is used as a guide to compliance and adherence to therapy but is not considered a treatment goal. Studies have shown that compared with less-intensive LDL-C lowering, more intensive lowering reduces all-cause mortality and cardiovascular mortality; patients with higher baseline LDL-C have greater benefit.

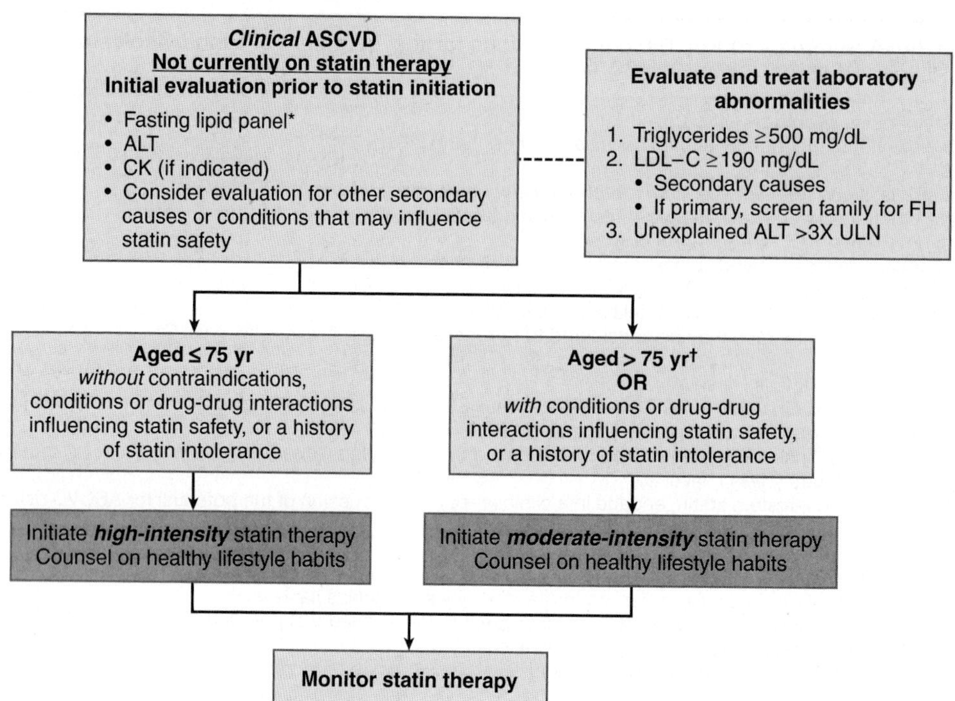

Clinical ASCVD
Not currently on statin therapy
Initial evaluation prior to statin initiation
• Fasting lipid panel*
• ALT
• CK (if indicated)
• Consider evaluation for other secondary causes or conditions that may influence statin safety
Evaluate and treat laboratory abnormalities
1. Triglycerides ≥500 mg/dL
2. LDL–C ≥190 mg/dL
• Secondary causes
• If primary, screen family for FH
3. Unexplained ALT >3X ULN
Aged ≤ 75 yr
without contraindications, conditions or drug-drug interactions influencing statin safety, or a history of statin intolerance
Aged > 75 yr†
OR
with conditions or drug-drug interactions influencing statin safety, or a history of statin intolerance
Initiate ***high-intensity*** statin therapy
Counsel on healthy lifestyle habits
Initiate ***moderate-intensity*** statin therapy
Counsel on healthy lifestyle habits
Monitor statin therapy

FIG. 1 Initiating statin therapy in individuals with clinical ASCVD. Colors correspond to the class of recommendations in the ACC/AHA Table 1. *Fasting lipid panel is preferred. In a nonfasting individual, a nonfasting non-HDL-C >220 mg/dl may indicate genetic hypercholesterolemia that requires further evaluation or a secondary etiology. If nonfasting triglycerides are >500 mg/dl, a fasting lipid panel is required. †It is reasonable to evaluate the potential for ASCVD benefits and for adverse effects and to consider patient preferences in initiating or continuing a moderate- or high-intensity statin in individuals with ASCVD >75 years of age. *ACC*, American College of Cardiology; *AHA*, American Heart Association; *ALT*, alanine transaminase; *ASCVD*, atherosclerotic cardiovascular disease; *CK*, creatine kinase; *FH*, familial hypercholesterolemia; *HDL–C*, high-density lipoprotein cholesterol; *LDL–C*, low-density lipoprotein cholesterol; *ULN*, upper limit of normal. (Modified from Stone NJ, Robinson J, Lichtenstein AH, et al.: 2013 ACC/AHA guideline on the treatment of blood cholesterol to reduce atherosclerotic cardiovascular risk in adults: a report of the American College of Cardiology/American Heart Association Task Force on Practice Guidelines, *J Am Coll Cardiol*, 2013.)
(From Mann DL, et al.: *Braunwald's heart disease*, ed 10, Philadelphia, 2015. Elsevier.)

TABLE 3 Statin Intensity Therapies

High Intensity (Decrease LDL-C ≥50%)	Moderate Intensity (Decrease LDL-C 30%-49%)
Atorvastatin 40-80 mg	Atorvastatin 10-20 mg
Rosuvastatin 20-40 mg	Rosuvastatin 5-10 mg
—	Simvastatin 20-40 mg
—	Pravastatin 40-80 mg
—	Lovastatin 40 mg
—	Fluvastatin XL 80 mg
—	Fluvastatin 40 mg bid
—	Pitavastatin 2-4 mg

LDL-C, Low-density lipoprotein cholesterol.
From Stone N, et al.: 2013 ACC/AHA guideline on the treatment of blood cholesterol to reduce atherosclerotic cardiovascular risk in adults: a report of the American College of Cardiology/American Heart Association Task Force on Practice Guidelines, *J Am Coll Cardiol* 63(25 Pt. B):2889, 2014.

TABLE 4 Statin Benefit Groups and Recommended Therapy

Statin Benefit Group	High Intensity	Moderate Intensity	Additional Testing
Clinical ASCVD	Yes	Consider†	None
Primary LDL-C >190 mg/dl	Yes	Consider†	None
Diabetes without ASCVD and 10-year risk ≥7.5%*	Yes	Consider†	None
Diabetes without ASCVD and 10-year risk <7.5%*	Consider‡	Yes	Case-by-case
Primary prevention and 10-year risk ≥7.5%*	Consider‡	Yes	Case-by-case
Primary prevention and 10-year risk <7.5%*	Consider‡	Consider‡	Case-by-case

ASCVD, Atherosclerotic cardiovascular disease; *LDL-C*, low-density lipoprotein cholesterol.
*Based on Pooled Cohort Risk Equations.
†If age >75 years or not candidate for high intensity.
‡If abnormal high-sensitivity C-reactive protein, coronary artery calcium, ankle-brachial index, lifetime risk.
From Boyden TF, et al.: Implementing new guidelines in the management of blood cholesterol, *Am J Med* 127:705, 2014.

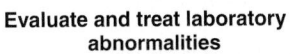

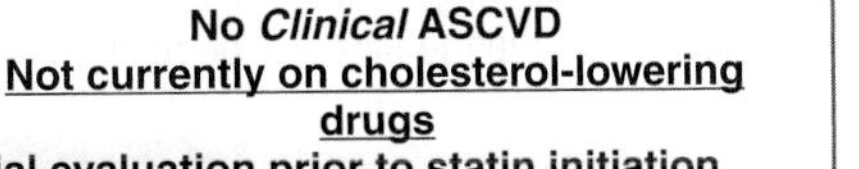

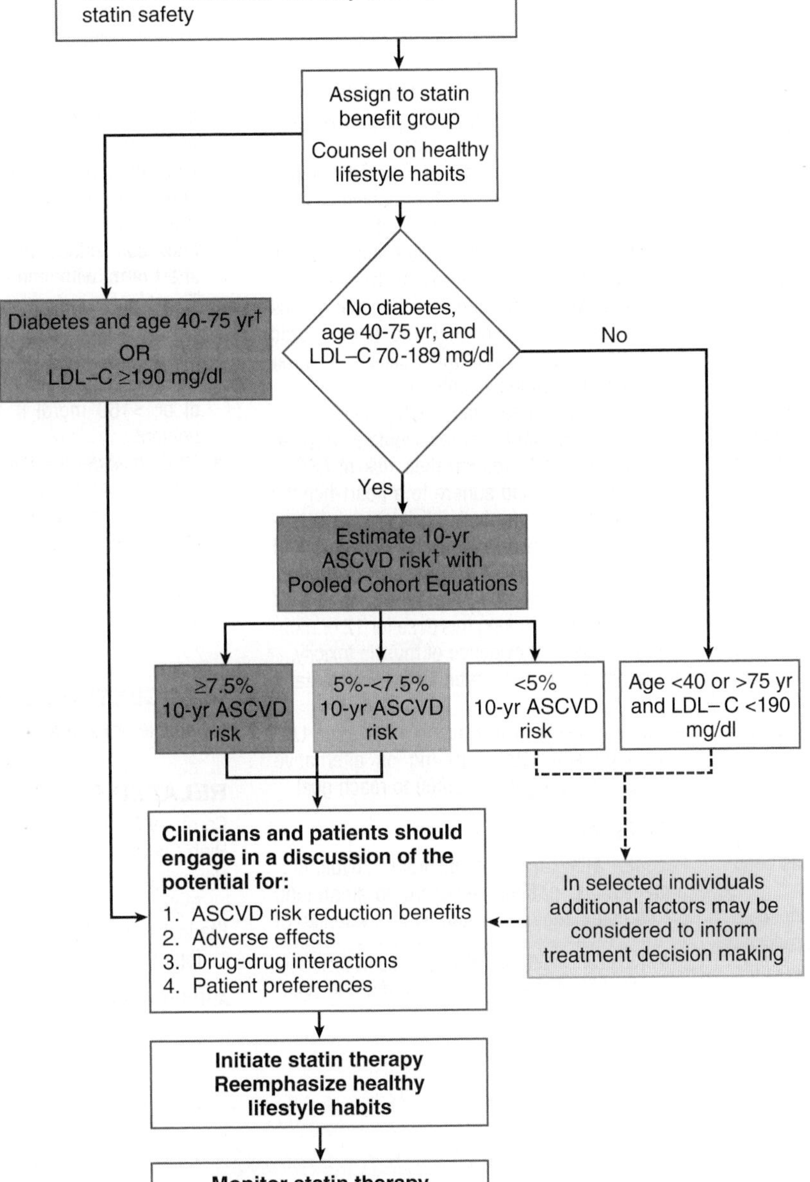

No *Clinical* ASCVD
Not currently on cholesterol-lowering drugs
Initial evaluation prior to statin initiation
• Fasting lipid panel*
• ALT
• Hemoglobin A1c (if diabetes status unknown)
• CK (if indicated)
• Consider evaluation for other secondary causes or conditions that may influence statin safety
Evaluate and treat laboratory abnormalities
1. Triglycerides ≥500 mg/dl
2. LDL–C ≥190 mg/dl
• Secondary causes
• If primary, screen family for FH
3. Unexplained ALT >3X ULN
Assign to statin benefit group
Counsel on healthy lifestyle habits
Diabetes and age 40-75 yr†
OR
LDL–C ≥190 mg/dl
No diabetes, age 40-75 yr, and LDL–C 70-189 mg/dl
No
Yes
Estimate 10-yr ASCVD risk† with Pooled Cohort Equations
≥7.5% 10-yr ASCVD risk
5%-<7.5% 10-yr ASCVD risk
<5% 10-yr ASCVD risk
Age <40 or >75 yr and LDL–C <190 mg/dl
Clinicians and patients should engage in a discussion of the potential for:
1. ASCVD risk reduction benefits
2. Adverse effects
3. Drug-drug interactions
4. Patient preferences
In selected individuals additional factors may be considered to inform treatment decision making
Initiate statin therapy
Reemphasize healthy lifestyle habits
Monitor statin therapy

FIG. 2 Initiating statin therapy in individuals without clinical ASCVD. *Fasting lipid panel is preferred. In a nonfasting individual, a nonfasting non-HDL–C>220 mg/dl may indicate genetic hypercholesterolemia that requires further evaluation or a secondary etiology. If nonfasting triglycerides are >500 mg/dl, a fasting lipid panel is required. †The Pooled Cohort Equations can be used to estimate 10-year ASCVD risk in individuals with and without diabetes. *ALT*, Alanine transaminase; *ASCVD*, atherosclerotic cardiovascular disease; *CK*, creatine kinase; *FH*, familial hypercholesterolemia; *LDL–C*, low-density lipoprotein cholesterol; *ULN*, upper limit of normal. (Modified from Stone NJ, Robinson J, Lichtenstein AH et al: 2013 ACC/AHA guideline on the treatment of blood cholesterol to reduce atherosclerotic cardiovascular risk in adults: a report of the American College of Cardiology/American Heart Association Task Force on Practice Guidelines, *J Am Coll Cardiol*, 2013.)
(From Mann DL, et al.: *Braunwald's heart disease*, ed 10, Philadelphia, 2015. Elsevier.)

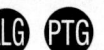

- Moderate-intensity statin therapy should be continued for individuals >75 yr of age for secondary prevention. However, factors such as comorbidities, safety, and priorities of care should be considered before initiating statins for primary prevention of ASCVD.
- Fig. 2 illustrates initiating statin therapy in individuals without clinical ASCVD.
- Adherence to lifestyle and to statin therapy should be reiterated with patients before the addition of a nonstatin drug.
- High-risk patients with a suboptimal response to statins who are unable to tolerate a recommended intensity or who are completely statin intolerant may benefit from the addition of a nonstatin cholesterol-lowering agent such as ezetimibe.
- Table E5 summarizes oral drugs affecting lipoprotein metabolism.
- PCSK9 (proprotein convertase subtilisin/kexin type 9) inhibitors (alirocumab [Praluent], evolocumab [Repatha]) are indicated as adjunct to diet and maximally tolerated statin therapy for the treatment of adults with heterozygous familial hypercholesterolemia or clinical atherosclerotic cardiovascular disease, who require additional lowering of LDL cholesterol. PCSK9 inhibitors lower risk for ischemic cardiovascular events in persons with stable CAD and elevated atherogenic lipoproteins despite statin therapy. These medications are administered by subcutaneous injection and are expensive.
- The management of metabolic syndrome includes weight reduction, increased physical activity, and treatment of hypertension, elevated triglycerides, and low HDL cholesterol.
- According to recent studies, each 40 mg/dl reduction in LDL cholesterol by statin therapy confers a 20% reduction in ASCVD. In other words, a relative risk reduction of 30% in ASCVD by moderate-intensity therapy and 45% by high-intensity therapy has been approximated.
- Recent trials have shown that bempedoic acid, an inhibitor of ATP citrate lyase, reduces LDL cholesterol. The addition of bempedoic acid to maximally tolerated statin therapy did not lead to a higher incidence of overall adverse events than placebo and led to significant lowering of LDL cholesterol.[1]

DISPOSITION AND FOLLOW-UP

- Baseline LFT testing should be done before initiation of statin therapy and as clinically indicated thereafter.
- CK level monitoring is not recommended unless a patient reports muscle weakness or myalgias.
- Statin therapy should be monitored by repeating a lipid profile within 4 to 12 weeks after initiation of therapy.
- Counseling about behavioral lifestyle changes and risk factors for CHD should be provided at every follow-up visit.
- Adverse effects of statin-associated diabetes varies by statin intensity: 1 excess case of diabetes per 1000 treated individuals with moderate-intensity statin and 3 excess cases of diabetes per 1000 treated individuals with high-intensity statin per yr has been reported. Myopathy and hemorrhagic stroke incidence is around 1 excess case per 10,000 treated individuals.
- Per new guidelines, those who develop diabetes during statin therapy should be advised to continue it to reduce their risk of ASCVD events and should adhere to a heart-healthy diet, engage in physical activity, cease tobacco use, and maintain a healthy body weight (Table E5).
- Maintain patients on simvastatin 80 mg only if they have been taking this dose for 12 or more months without evidence of muscle toxicity.
- Do not start new patients on simvastatin 80 mg.
- Place patients who do not meet their LDL goal on simvastatin 40 mg on alternative LDL-C-lowering treatment(s) to reach goal.

REFERRAL

Patients with rare lipid disorders, hyperlipoproteinemias, patients resistant to treatment, on complex regimens, and with evidence of disease progression despite treatment should be referred to a lipid specialist.

[1] Ray KK, et al.: Safety and efficacy of bempedoic acid to reduce LDL cholesterol, *N Engl J Med* 380:1022-1032, 2019.

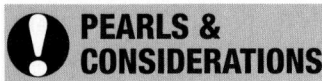

PEARLS & CONSIDERATIONS

COMMENTS

- Coronary artery calcium (CAC) measurement may be useful in selected patients when decision on statin initiation is uncertain. In patients with CAC scores ≥ 100, initiation of statins is reasonable.
- Familial hypercholesterolemia (FH) is characterized by elevated cholesterol concentrations early in life. Untreated FH is associated with premature cardiovascular disease in adulthood. Screening can detect FH in children, and lipid-lowering treatment in childhood can reduce lipid concentrations in the short term, with little evidence of harm.
- The American Academy of Pediatrics (AAP) guideline (*Pediatrics* 122:198, 2008) recommends consideration toward pharmacologic treatment for children with LDL >190 mg/dl or >160 mg/dl if other risk factors are present.
- *HDL cholesterol efflux capacity* refers to the ability of HDL to accept cholesterol from macrophages, which is a key step in reverse cholesterol transport. It is inversely associated with the incidence of cardiovascular events and may be a useful biomarker when added to traditional risk factors.

SUGGESTED READINGS

Available at ExpertConsult.com

RELATED CONTENT

Coronary Artery Disease (Related Key Topic)
High Cholesterol (Patient Information)
Hyperlipoproteinemia, Primary (Related Key Topic)
Statin Induced Muscle Syndrome (Related Key Topic)

AUTHOR: **FRED F. FERRI, M.D.**

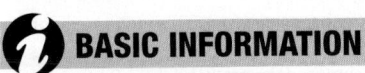

DEFINITION

Hypercoagulable state is an inherited or acquired condition associated with an increased risk of thrombosis. A classification of hypercoagulable states is described in Table 1.

SYNONYM

Thrombophilia

ICD-10CM CODES
D68.5 Primary thrombophilia
D68.6 Other thrombophilia
D68.8 Other specified coagulation defects
D68.9 Coagulation defect, unspecified

EPIDEMIOLOGY & DEMOGRAPHICS

INCIDENCE, PREVALENCE, PREDOMINANT SEX, AND AGE: See Table 2. Significant variations in the prevalence rates and thrombotic risks for hypercoagulable states are reported. This may reflect geographic variation in the prevalence of genetic defects, different populations, or the presence of other unidentified thrombophilic risk factors. When thrombosis occurs, it is often associated with an acquired risk factor (e.g., surgery, pregnancy, oral contraceptive [OC] use).

GENETICS:
- Most people with a genetic defect will not have thrombotic disease.
- Approximately half of patients with unprovoked thrombosis have an identifiable inherited thrombophilia. There is a low risk of recurrent thrombosis in patients with a single genetic defect. Multiple genetic defects are not uncommon (1% to 2% prevalence in patients with idiopathic venous thromboembolism [VTE]); a strong synergistic effect occurs when multiple defects are present.

RISK FACTORS: Family history of thrombosis, increasing age, tobacco use, immobility, surgery, prior history of DVT, pregnancy, hormone replacement therapy, trauma, connective tissue disease, underlying malignancy, medications (megestrol acetate, tamoxifen, oral contraceptives). Potential prothrombotic states are summarized in Table 3.

PHYSICAL FINDINGS & CLINICAL PRESENTATION

- Inherited thrombophilia is usually associated with VTE, most commonly deep vein thrombosis (DVT)
- Some acquired thrombophilias are associated with arterial thrombosis. Table 2 describes sites of thrombosis according to coagulation defect
- Pregnancy complications
- Medical conditions associated with increased risk of thrombosis

ETIOLOGY

- Thrombosis is often a multifactorial process with genetic, environmental, and acquired factors. Table E4, Table E5, Table E6, and Table E7 describe causes of acquired and inherited deficiencies in antithrombin, protein C, and protein S.
- Thrombotic risk increases with use of OCs or hormone replacement therapy (HRT) and during the pregnancy/postpartum period.
- Adverse pregnancy outcomes may be caused by thrombosis of the uteroplacental circulation.

TABLE 1 Classification of Hypercoagulable States

Hereditary	Mixed	Acquired
Loss of Function		
Antithrombin deficiency	Hyperhomocysteinemia	Previous venous thromboembolism
Protein C deficiency	Obesity	Pregnancy, puerperium
Protein S deficiency	Cancer	
		Drug-induced:
		Heparin-induced thrombocytopenia
		Prothrombin complex concentrates
		l-asparaginase
		Hormonal therapy
Gain of Function		
Factor V Leiden	Postoperative	
Prothrombin FII G20210A	Myeloproliferative disorders	
Elevated factor VIII, IX, or XI		

Hoffman R et al: *Hematology, basic principles and practice*, ed 7, Philadelphia, 2018, Elsevier.

TABLE 3 Potential Prothrombotic States

Congenital
Deficiency of anticoagulants
AT-III, protein C or protein S, plasminogen
Resistance to cofactor proteolysis
Factor V Leiden
High levels of procoagulants
Prothrombin 20210 mutation
Damage to endothelium
Acquired
Obstruction to flow indwelling lines
Pregnancy
Polycythemia/dehydration
Immobilization
Injury
Trauma, surgery, exercise
Inflammation
IBD, vasculitis, infection, Behçet's syndrome
Hypercoagulability
Pregnancy
Malignancy
Antiphospholipid syndrome
Nephrotic syndrome
Oral contraceptives L-Asparaginase
Rare Other Entities
Congenital dysfibrinogenemia
Acquired
Paroxysmal nocturnal hemoglobinuria
Thrombocythemia
Vascular grafts

AT-III, Antithrombin III; *IBD*, inflammatory bowel disease.
From Kliegman RM et al: *Nelson textbook of pediatrics*, ed 19, Philadelphia, 2011, Saunders.

TABLE 2 Hypercoagulable Conditions

	Prevalence in General Population (%)	Prevalence in Population With Thrombosis (%)	A/V Events	Relative Risk of Thrombosis
FVL mutation	5% of whites; rare in nonwhites	12%-40%	V	Heterozygous: 3-7; homozygous: 80
Prothrombin G20210A mutation	3% of whites; rare in nonwhites	6%-18%	V	3
AT deficiency	0.02%	1%-3%	V	20-50
PC deficiency	0.2%-0.4%	3%-5%	V	7-15
PS deficiency	0.03%-0.1%	1%-5%	V	5-11
Antiphospholipid antibody syndrome	1%-2%	5%-21%	V + A	2-11

A, Arterial; *AT*, antithrombin; *FVL*, factor V Leiden; *PC*, protein C; *PS*, protein S; *V*, venous.

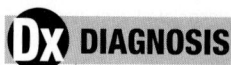

DIAGNOSIS

DIFFERENTIAL DIAGNOSIS

INHERITED: Factor V Leiden (FVL) mutation:
- Autosomal-dominant mutation with low penetrance.
- Causes activated protein C resistance (APCR); 90% of APCR is caused by FVL mutation.
- Most common inherited thrombophilia; accounts for 40% to 50% of cases.
- OC use in heterozygous carriers is associated with an eightfold increased risk of VTE compared with noncarriers and a thirty-fivefold increased risk of VTE compared with noncarriers not using OCs.
- May be associated with cardiovascular disease in select high-risk subgroups.

Prothrombin G20210A mutation:
- Autosomal-dominant mutation with low penetrance.
- OC use in heterozygous carriers is associated with a sixteenfold increased risk of VTE compared with noncarriers not using OCs.
- May be associated with cardiovascular disease in select high-risk subgroups and young patients with ischemic stroke.
- Causes increased mRNA accumulation and protein synthesis, leading to elevated prothrombin plasma concentrations.

Protein C, protein S, antithrombin (AT) deficiency:
- Autosomal-dominant inheritance; many mutations identified for each of these conditions.
- Decreased level (type I deficiency) or abnormal function (type II deficiency).
- First episode of thrombosis is usually in young adults.

Protein C and protein S:
- Homozygous condition is very rare; usually associated with lethal thrombosis in infancy.
- Associated with warfarin-induced skin necrosis, which occurs secondary to depletion of vitamin K–dependent anticoagulant factors sooner than procoagulant factors in the first few days of therapy.

AT deficiency:
- Most thrombogenic of the inherited thrombophilias; 50% lifetime risk of thrombosis.
- Homozygous condition is very rare, probably not compatible with normal fetal development.
- Arterial thrombosis can occur rarely.
- Can cause heparin resistance.

Other possible causes: Non-O blood group, dysfibrinogenemia, elevated thrombin-activatable fibrinolysis inhibitor, elevated factor IX and factor XI levels

ACQUIRED: Antiphospholipid antibody syndrome (APS):
- Most common cause of acquired thrombophilia.
- Can present as arterial or venous thrombosis, recurrent pregnancy loss, and adverse pregnancy outcomes.
- Thromboembolic events occur in up to 30% of population; high risk of recurrent thrombosis (up to 70% reported).
- See "Antiphospholipid Antibody Syndrome" for more information.

Conditions associated with increased risk of thrombosis:
- Prior thrombosis
- Trauma
- Medical illness: Heart failure, respiratory failure, infection, diabetes mellitus, obesity, nephrotic syndrome, inflammatory bowel disease
- Chronic hemolysis–paroxysmal nocturnal hemoglobinuria, atypical hemolytic uremic syndrome, sickle cell anemia
- Pregnancy (sixfold increased risk of VTE), postpartum, OC use (fourfold increased risk, higher risk with third-generation OCs), transdermal contraceptive patch, HRT (twofold increased risk), tamoxifen, raloxifene
- Immobilization, travel
- Surgery (especially orthopedic), central venous catheters
- Hyperviscosity syndromes
- Myeloproliferative disorders
- Malignancy: Disease or treatment related
- Heparin-induced thrombocytopenia and thrombosis
- Smoking

WORKUP

- History (presence of conditions or use of medications predisposing to thrombosis, family history of thrombosis), physical examination, laboratory tests, imaging studies. Routine investigations to evaluate a patient with thrombosis are summarized in Box 1.
- Age-appropriate cancer screening.
- No consensus exists regarding screening for thrombophilia; few cost-effectiveness or outcomes data are available. Thrombophilia screening is probably overused, as results usually do not change management.
- Thrombophilia screening is not recommended for primary prevention of VTE; some advocate testing prior to OC use or pregnancy in women with a strong family history of thrombosis or thrombophilia. Box 2 summarizes recommendations regarding when to perform a thrombophilia screen. Essential tests for thrombophilia screening are described in Box 3.
- Screening not recommended if VTE was associated with an identified risk factor. A possible exception is thrombosis associated with pregnancy, the postpartum period, or with OC use.
- Provoked by weak triggers in a patient with a strong family history and female family members of childbearing age; consider testing for FVL, prothrombin G20210A mutation, protein C, protein S, and AT deficiency. Consider testing for APS if extensive DVT or PE.
- Unprovoked VTE:
  1. Screen individuals for APCR, prothrombin G20210A mutation, protein C, protein S, AT deficiency, and APS if any of the following are present: <50 yr of age at first episode of thrombosis + strong family history of thrombosis or female family member of childbearing age, thrombosis in unusual anatomic location (cerebral veins or splanchnic veins; if splanchnic veins, consider testing as well for MPN and PNH).
  2. Screen all others for APS.
- Arterial thrombosis: Screen for APS.
- Note: Routine screening for factor VIII level or hyperhomocysteinemia is not recommended.

BOX 1 Routine Investigations to Evaluate a Patient with Thrombosis

Test	Abnormality	Diagnostic Information
Complete blood count	Elevated hematocrit Increased white count Increased platelet count Leukopenia Thrombocytopenia	Myeloproliferative disorder (e.g., essential thrombocythemia, polycythemia vera); may be found in paroxysmal nocturnal hemoglobinuria; if associated with heparin administration, consider heparin-induced thrombocytopenia
Blood film	Leukoerythroblastic changes	Underlying neoplasm invading bone marrow
Liver function tests	Abnormal tests	May point to malignancy
Renal function	Impaired renal function	Assess prior to anticoagulation with heparin, low-molecular-weight heparin or new oral anticoagulants
Urinalysis	Proteinuria	Nephrotic syndrome; may be associated with venous thromboembolism or renal vein thrombosis
PT and aPTT	Prolonged PT and aPTT	To enable safe anticoagulation to proceed if required Need to exclude lupus anticoagulant

aPTT, Activated partial thromboplastin time; PT, prothrombin time.

Hoffman R et al: *Hematology, basic principles and practice*, ed 7, Philadelphia, 2018, Elsevier.

BOX 2 When to Perform a Thrombophilia Screen

Clinical Scenario
- First episode of unprovoked venous thromboembolism in individuals younger than 40 years of age
- Thrombosis in an unusual site (e.g., cerebral or mesenteric thrombosis)
- Two or more first-degree relatives with unprovoked thrombosis
- Three or more early pregnancy losses, or one or more fetal deaths after 10 weeks gestation

Hoffman R et al: *Hematology, basic principles and practice*, ed 7, Philadelphia, 2018, Elsevier.

BOX 3 Essential Tests for Thrombophilia Screening

- Basic coagulation screen
  - International normalized ratio (INR): To exclude warfarin effect—warfarin will lower protein C and S levels
  - Activated partial thromboplastin time (aPTT): To exclude heparin effect—heparin will lower antithrombin levels
- Functional assay for antithrombin (with heparin to detect type II defects)
- Functional assay for protein C
- Functional assay for protein S (immune assays for total and free protein S)
- APC resistance assay: With genetic test for factor V_{Leiden} for confirmation of abnormal results
- Genetic test for FIIG 20210A gene mutation
- Anticardiolipin and β_2-glycoprotein-1 antibodies (IgG and IgM) and lupus anticoagulant assay

Hoffman R et al: *Hematology, basic principles and practice*, ed 7, Philadelphia, 2018, Elsevier.

TIMING OF WORKUP:
- Ideally >3 wk after discontinuation of VKA and >2 days after discontinuation of DOAC (except for APS, which requires prolonged anticoagulation).
- Note: Acute thrombosis, anticoagulation, pregnancy, and many medical conditions can affect the results and must be considered in the timing and interpretation of the workup.

LABORATORY TESTS

- CBC with peripheral smear, electrolytes, calcium, creatinine, BUN and liver function tests, prothrombin time/partial thromboplastin time, prostate-specific antigen (in men aged >50 yr), urinalysis.
- Note: Genetic counseling and written informed consent should be obtained before genetic testing. Abnormal nongenetic tests should be repeated after 6 wk to decrease false-positive results.
- APCR: APC-resistance assay (using factor V–deficient plasma). Presence of lupus anticoagulant causes false positives. Follow-up positive APCR assay with genetic test for FVL.
- Prothrombin G20210A mutation testing.
- AT, protein C, and protein S deficiency: Functional assays; if decreased perform antigenic assay to determine type of deficiency. Antigenic assays for protein S should measure free and total levels. In protein C and protein S deficiency, the functional assay may be falsely low in the presence of APCR or elevated factor VIII level and falsely high if lupus anticoagulant is present.
- APS: Any one of the following found on two occasions at least 12 weeks apart: Lupus anticoagulant, anticardiolipin antibodies, or anti–B_2-glycoprotein-I antibodies.

IMAGING STUDIES

Chest radiograph and other tests as appropriate to diagnose thrombosis and rule out associated conditions

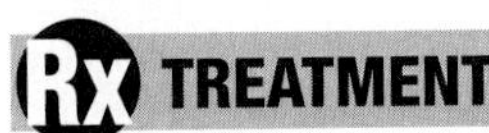

TREATMENT

NONPHARMACOLOGIC THERAPY

OC/HRT use and smoking should be avoided.

PROPHYLAXIS

- Prophylactic anticoagulation in high-risk situations.
- Patients with AT deficiency may benefit from antithrombin concentrates in high-risk situations.
- Pregnancy prophylaxis: Timing and intensity of therapy is based on the patient's risk (genetic or acquired defect and clinical history). Women with thrombophilia and recurrent adverse pregnancy outcomes may benefit from prophylaxis with heparin (low-molecular-weight heparin most commonly used) and low-dose aspirin.

ACUTE GENERAL Rx

Initial therapy is the same as for individuals with and without thrombophilia, with exceptions for protein C and AT deficiency as detailed in the following.

Venous thrombosis:
- Direct oral anticoagulants (DOACs) such as Xa inhibitors (rivaroxaban and apixaban) have been FDA-approved for treatment in acute DVT and are currently recommended as first-line therapy. They have been found to be noninferior to warfarin, appear easier to use with fewer drug interactions, and have a trend toward less major bleeding.
- In patients unable to take DOACs, begin low-molecular-weight heparin (LMWH) and warfarin simultaneously. Continue heparin for at least 5 days and until international normalized ratio (INR) is therapeutic for 2 consecutive days; continue warfarin for at least 3 months. Aim for INR of 2 to 3. Unfractionated heparin (UH) or fondaparinux (factor Xa inhibitor) may be used as alternatives to LMWH. LMWH is preferred over UH (except in patients with massive pulmonary embolism, increased risk of bleeding, or renal failure) because of equivalent or superior effectiveness and a better safety profile.
- Thrombophilia is not associated with a higher risk of recurrent VTE during warfarin therapy, with the exception of cancer patients in whom LMWH for 3 to 6 mo is associated with lower rates of recurrence than warfarin therapy.
- In pregnancy, anticoagulate with heparin throughout pregnancy and for at least 6 wk postpartum. Minimum duration of anticoagulation should be 6 mo. LMWH is preferred over UH. Warfarin may be used postpartum.
- Consider thrombolysis or thrombectomy in patients with massive pulmonary embolism or large proximal lower extremity DVT.

Protein C deficiency:
- Warfarin-induced skin necrosis: Discontinue warfarin, give vitamin K, and start heparin anticoagulation. Consider protein C replacement with protein C concentrate or fresh frozen plasma. Warfarin may be restarted at a low dose (2 mg daily for 3 days and increase by 2 to 3 mg daily until target INR is reached). Continue heparin for at least 5 days and until warfarin-induced anticoagulation is achieved.

AT deficiency:
- AT concentrates may be used if difficulty achieving anticoagulation (heparin resistance), severe thrombosis, or recurrent thrombosis despite adequate anticoagulation.

Arterial thrombosis:
- Anticoagulation and evaluation for thrombolysis or surgery.

CHRONIC Rx

- Optimal duration of anticoagulation remains unknown. Length of therapy may be individualized by assessing the risk of recurrence. Residual thrombosis (on ultrasonography) or elevated D-dimer levels after completion of anticoagulation are associated with an increased risk of recurrence. With these findings, consider prolonging anticoagulation.
- Must consider risk and benefit; risk of major bleeding 2% to 3% annually in general population on anticoagulation but higher in the elderly (7% to 9% per yr). Long-term anticoagulation is usually not indicated given the low risk of recurrent thrombosis for most conditions and the bleeding risk associated with anticoagulation.
- Indefinite anticoagulation considered if any of the following:
  1. Life-threatening thrombosis or thrombosis at an unusual site
  2. More than a single genetic defect
  3. Presence of AT deficiency or APS

TABLE 8 Management of Women with a History of Venous Thrombosis During Pregnancy and the Puerperium

Clinical History	Thrombophilia	Antepartum	Postpartum[a]
Prior VTE due to a transient risk factor	No	Surveillance	Yes
Prior VTE due to pregnancy or estrogens	Yes or no	Prophylactic LMWH	Yes
Prior idiopathic VTE	Yes or no	Prophylactic LMWH	Yes
Recurrent VTE	Yes or no	Treatment dose LMWH	Resume long-term anticoagulation
No prior VTE	Antithrombin deficiency; homozygous FII G20210A; or Factor V_{Leiden}; or dual heterozygosity for both mutations	Prophylactic or intermediate dose LMWH	Yes
Positive family history			

LMWH, low-molecular-weight heparin; *VTE*, venous thromboembolism.
[a]Postpartum prophylaxis involves a 6-week course of prophylactic doses of LMWH or dose-adjusted warfarin (target INR: 2.0 to 3.0).
Hoffman R et al: *Hematology, basic principles and practice*, ed 7, Philadelphia, 2018, Elsevier.

4. Unprovoked DVT or PE with low bleeding risk
5. >1 Provoked DVT or PE with low bleeding risk

- Patients with active cancer may benefit from indefinite anticoagulation.

DISPOSITION

Depends on underlying condition

REFERRAL

Hematology, maternal-fetal medicine, obstetric medicine

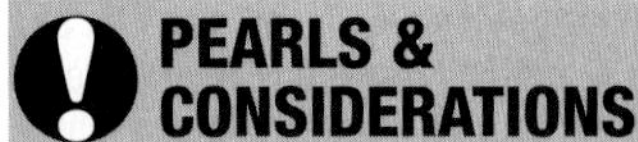

PEARLS & CONSIDERATIONS

COMMENTS

- Women with thrombophilic defects but no prior history of venous thromboembolism, or family history of the same, likely do not require antepartum prophylaxis or postpartum treatment, but definitive data are lacking. A summary of these recommendations is provided in Table 8.
- DOACs and warfarin therapy effectively reduce the risk of recurrent VTE; when therapy is discontinued VTE risk increases.
- Previous episode of VTE is a major risk factor for recurrence regardless of the presence of thrombophilia. Risk is greatest in the first 2 yr after thrombosis. 20% of all patients with unprovoked VTE have recurrence within 5 yr.
- Genetic risk factors for thrombosis in nonwhites remain largely unknown.
- Interpreting workup: Many medical conditions cause acquired abnormalities.
  1. Acute thrombosis may be associated with lupus anticoagulant, increased anticardiolipin antibodies, and elevated factor VIII levels
  2. Heparin therapy: Antithrombin levels decrease by up to 30%; can affect lupus anticoagulant testing
  3. Warfarin therapy: Cannot measure protein C and protein S (levels and function decrease); antithrombin levels may increase; can affect lupus anticoagulant testing
  4. Protein C, protein S, and antithrombin levels decrease with acute thrombosis (<2 wk), surgery, liver disease, disseminated intravascular coagulation, and chemotherapy. Protein C level also decreases with severe infection but levels increase with age and hyperlipidemia. Protein S and antithrombin levels also decrease with nephrotic syndrome, pregnancy, and estrogen therapy (HRT, OC)
  5. APCR is increased with pregnancy, estrogen therapy (HRT, OCs), and certain cancers; elevated factor VIII level and antiphospholipid antibodies can cause APCR

PREVENTION

Risk of post-thrombotic syndrome decreases if compression stockings are worn for at least 1 yr, starting in the first month after the DVT.

PATIENT & FAMILY EDUCATION

National Blood Clot Alliance
120 White Plains Road, Suite 100
Tarrytown, NY 10591
http://www.stoptheclot.org/contact.htm
National Collaborative Outreach Project of the Blood Clot Outreach Program at the Hemophilia and Thrombosis Center University of North Carolina at Chapel Hill
http://www.clotconnect.org/about-clot-connect/about
Factor V Leiden Resources
http://www.fvleiden.org/resources/index.html
APS Foundation of America, Inc.
P. O. Box 801
LaCrosse, WI 54602-0801
http://www.apsfa.org/

SUGGESTED READINGS

Available at ExpertConsult.com

RELATED CONTENT

Thrombophilia (Patient Information)
Antiphospholipid Syndrome (Related Key Topic)
Deep Vein Thrombosis (Related Key Topic)
Pulmonary Embolism (Related Key Topic)

AUTHOR: **JOHN L. REAGAN, M.D.**

BASIC INFORMATION

DEFINITION

Hyperemesis gravidarum refers to a severe and persistent form of nausea and vomiting in pregnancy. While no precise criteria exist to define the severity, it may be characterized by at least a 5% weight loss from prepregnancy weight, dehydration, ketonuria, and electrolyte imbalance. Typical onset occurs at week 4 to 8 of pregnancy, continuing through week 14 to 16 of pregnancy.

ICD-10CM CODES

O21.0	Mild hyperemesis gravidarum
O21.1	Hyperemesis gravidarum with metabolic disturbance

EPIDEMIOLOGY & DEMOGRAPHICS

INCIDENCE: 0.5% to 2% of pregnancies

GENETICS: A genetic predisposition may exist; hyperemesis gravidarum is more common among first-degree relatives of those diagnosed with the condition.

RISK FACTORS: Women with increased placental mass, including molar pregnancy or multiple gestation, family history or personal history of hyperemesis gravidarum, prior miscarriage, nulliparity, young age, hyperthyroidism, gastrointestinal disorders, vestibular disease, motion sickness, long interpregnancy interval, and supertaster status. Alcohol use, smoking, and anosmia may be protective. A female fetus increases the risk by 1.27-fold.

PHYSICAL FINDINGS & CLINICAL PRESENTATION

- Weight loss of more than 5% from pregravid weight
- Symptoms—nausea, vomiting, spitting, enhanced olfactory senses, food and/or fluid intolerance, lethargy
- Signs—poor skin turgor, dry mucous membranes, hypotension, tachycardia
- Complications include inadequate caloric and nutritional intake, dehydration, and electrolyte abnormalities, including hyponatremia, hypocalcemia, hypokalemia, and, in severe cases, hypochloremic metabolic acidosis or Wernicke encephalopathy from thiamine deficiency. Severe hyperemesis gravidarum also has been shown to correlate with higher rates of anxiety and depression.

ETIOLOGY

Unknown, but likely multifactorial. Theories include interactions between hCG and the thyroid, gestational hyperestrogenemia, and gastric dysrhythmias.

DIAGNOSIS

DIFFERENTIAL DIAGNOSIS

- Gastrointestinal conditions—gastroenteritis, gastroparesis, biliary tract disease, hepatitis, intestinal obstruction, peptic ulcer disease, appendicitis, inflammatory bowel disease
- Genitourinary tract conditions—pyelonephritis, nephrolithiasis
- Metabolic disease—hyperthyroidism, hyperparathyroidism, diabetic ketoacidosis, cannabinoid hyperemesis syndrome, porphyria, adrenal insufficiency
- Neurologic conditions—pseudotumor cerebri, vestibular lesions, migraines, tumors of the central nervous system, cyclic vomiting syndrome
- Miscellaneous—drug toxicity or intolerance, psychogenic
- Pregnancy-related conditions—acute fatty liver of pregnancy, preeclampsia

WORKUP

Diagnosis is one of exclusion. History and physical examination along with laboratory tests to rule out other causes of vomiting should be performed.

LABORATORY TESTS

- BMP may reveal hyponatremia, hypokalemia, low serum urea
- Urinalysis may show elevated specific gravity, ketonuria, or proteinuria
- Liver enzymes (ALT typically more elevated than AST, both usually only reaching 2-3 times the upper limit of normal)
- Serum bilirubin (<4 mg/dl)
- Serum amylase or lipase (up to 5× greater than normal)
- CBC may show an increase in hematocrit from volume depletion
- Magnesium and calcium may be low
- TSH and free T4 (transient hyperthyroidism occurs in 2/3 of women with hyperemesis gravidarum; this is biochemical hyperthyroidism that usually resolves by 18 weeks of gestation; testing and treatment should not be undertaken without additional clinical evidence of intrinsic thyroid disease)

IMAGING STUDIES

- Ultrasound to evaluate for multiple gestation or molar pregnancy
- If the patient is having associated pain, a right upper quadrant ultrasound may be indicated to evaluate biliary tract disease

TREATMENT

NONPHARMACOLOGIC THERAPY

- Avoidance of foods and smells that trigger nausea
- Ginger (200 to 500 mg q8h)
- Protein-heavy meals
- Reassurance and support, in some cases intensive cognitive-behavioral therapy

ACUTE GENERAL Rx

- Pyridoxine (vitamin B_6) 10-25 mg PO q8h
- Doxylamine 12.5-25 mg qhs
- Pyridoxine (10 mg)/doxylamine (10mg) combination, starting with 2 tablets qhs and adding an additional 1 tablet q am and 1 tablet q pm if needed
- Antiemetics including promethazine, prochlorperazine, metoclopramide, and ondansetron have been shown to be generally safe and effective in improving pregnancy outcome
- Corticosteroids (methylprednisolone, prednisone) may be considered after 10 weeks of gestation
- IV fluid and electrolyte administration if evidence of deficiency is found
- Thiamine prior to dextrose administration to avoid Wernicke encephalopathy
- Restart oral intake gradually no less than 48 hr after vomiting has stopped

CHRONIC Rx

- If unable to tolerate oral intake, consider replacing with enteral or parenteral feeding
- Repeated IV fluid and electrolyte replacement can be conducted through outpatient visits

COMPLEMENTARY & ALTERNATIVE MEDICINE

- Supportive psychotherapy
- Acupuncture
- Acupressure with use of a wrist band

DISPOSITION

- Infants born from pregnancies complicated by hyperemesis may have a higher risk of being small for gestational age or low-birth-weight than those not; however, this may be limited to infants of women who have experienced significant weight loss in the setting of hyperemesis.
- Women with hyperemesis gravidarum should be counseled that they have a higher risk than other women of developing similar symptoms in future pregnancies.

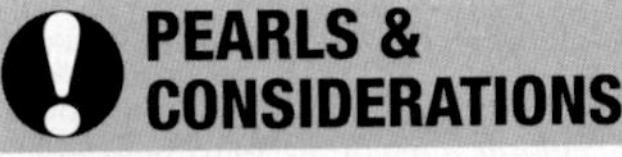

PEARLS & CONSIDERATIONS

COMMENTS

Nausea and vomiting in early pregnancy are associated with psychosocial morbidity.

RELATED CONTENT

Hyperemesis Gravidarum (Patient Information)

AUTHOR: **T. CAROLINE BANK, M.D.**

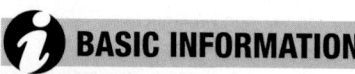

BASIC INFORMATION

DEFINITION

Hyperglycemic hyperosmolar syndrome (HHS) is a life-threatening complication of diabetes mellitus characterized by marked hyperglycemia, dehydration, and hyperosmolality with or without mental obtundation, in the absence of significant ketoacidosis.

SYNONYMS

HHS
Hyperosmolar hyperglycemic syndrome
Diabetic hyperosmolar syndrome
Hyperglycemic hyperosmolar nonketotic syndrome
Hyperglycemic hyperosmolar nonketotic coma
Hyperosmolar hyperglycemic state
Nonketotic hyperosmolar syndrome

ICD-10CM CODES

E08.00	Diabetes mellitus due to underlying condition with hyperosmolarity without nonketotic hyperglycemic-hyperosmolar coma (NKHHC)
E08.01	Diabetes mellitus due to underlying condition with hyperosmolarity with coma
E09.00	Drug or chemical induced diabetes mellitus with hyperosmolarity without nonketotic hyperglycemic-hyperosmolar coma (NKHHC)
E09.01	Drug or chemical induced diabetes mellitus with hyperosmolarity with coma
E11.00	Type 2 diabetes mellitus with hyperosmolarity without nonketotic hyperglycemic-hyperosmolar coma (NKHHC)
E11.01	Type 2 diabetes mellitus with hyperosmolarity with coma
E13.00	Other specified diabetes mellitus with hyperosmolarity without nonketotic hyperglycemic-hyperosmolar coma (NKHHC)
E13.01	Other specified diabetes mellitus with hyperosmolarity with coma

EPIDEMIOLOGY & DEMOGRAPHICS

HHS is a rare condition that most commonly affects patients with type 2 diabetes mellitus. Approximately 20% of patients have no history of diabetes. Elderly individuals with new-onset diabetes or those with poorly controlled type 2 diabetes predisposed to dehydration are at increased risk. Mortality from HHS is estimated at 5% to 20%, higher than mortality from diabetic ketoacidosis.

PHYSICAL FINDINGS & CLINICAL PRESENTATION

- Polyuria, polydipsia, weight loss, weakness
- Mental obtundation (can range from full alertness to coma)
- Focal neurologic signs (e.g., hemiplegia, hemianopsia) or seizures (focal or generalized), aphasia, visual hallucinations
- Symptoms of coexisting illnesses or comorbidities that may have precipitated the event
- Signs of dehydration such as dry mucous membranes, poor skin turgor, sunken eyes, hypotension, tachycardia
- Normo- or hypothermia even in the presence of infection, due to peripheral vasodilation

ETIOLOGY

HHS can be precipitated by various conditions:

- Infection (most common precipitant)
- Insulin deficiency (undiagnosed diabetes, inadequate insulin, or medication nonadherence)
- Inflammatory conditions (e.g., acute pancreatitis, acute cholecystitis)
- Ischemia/infarction (e.g., myocardial infarction, stroke, bowel ischemia)
- Renal failure
- Severe dehydration (e.g., burns, heatstroke)
- Drugs (e.g., steroids, thiazides, atypical antipsychotics, sympathomimetics including cocaine, alcohol, pentamidine)

A relative insulin deficiency provides enough insulin to inhibit ketogenesis but not enough to inhibit hepatic gluconeogenesis, glycogenolysis, or peripheral glucose uptake, thereby resulting in hyperglycemia. With underlying illness, counterregulatory hormone excess leads to further blood glucose rise. The resultant extreme hyperglycemia leads to osmotic diuresis. If adequate hydration is not maintained, dehydration and worsening renal function ensue. Diminished renal filtration further impairs glucose excretion, thus exacerbating the hyperglycemia, dehydration, and hyperosmolality.

Dx DIAGNOSIS

DIFFERENTIAL DIAGNOSIS

- Diabetic ketoacidosis
- Stroke (especially in the elderly with neurologic abnormalities)
- Hypovolemic or septic shock
- Encephalopathy

WORKUP

After the initial history is obtained, perform a physical exam that includes immediate evaluation of airway, breathing, circulation, mental status, volume status, and signs suggestive of precipitating event including infection, myocardial infarction, or stroke.

LABORATORY TESTS

- Hyperglycemia: Blood glucose >600 mg/dl (Box 1).
- Serum osmolality: Typically >320 mOsm/kg.
- Complete metabolic panel including serum creatinine, blood urea nitrogen (BUN), electrolytes, glucose.
- Serum sodium: May be low, normal, or high. Hyperglycemia increases plasma osmolality, which attracts intracellular water to the extracellular compartment, decreasing serum sodium. Serum sodium can be corrected by adding 1.6 mEq/L to the measured serum sodium for every 100 mg/dl rise in serum glucose above 100 mg/dl. Marked osmotic diuresis induced by hyperglycemia may cause the serum sodium to be normal or high.
- Serum potassium and phosphate: Total body potassium and phosphate deficit typically occur due to urinary losses from osmotic diuresis. However, the levels may be acutely normal or high due to extracellular shift secondary to insulin deficiency and hyperosmolality.
- Anion gap and serum lactate: Anion gap may be normal or elevated in the setting of lactic acidosis.
- Arterial blood gas: pH >7.3.
- Serum and urine ketones: Negative or small.
- Serum bicarbonate: >15 mEq/L.
- Hemoglobin A1c (if not performed in past 3 months).
- Complete blood count with differential (may indicate presence of underlying infection [leukocytosis >25,000 mm^3], inflammatory condition, hemoconcentration. A leukocytosis of 10,000 to 15,000 mm^3 is expected from the stress of illness alone.)
- Urinalysis, urine/sputum/blood cultures as indicated based on the physical exam findings to evaluate the precipitating illness and other comorbidities.

IMAGING STUDIES

ECG, chest radiograph, and other imaging studies as indicated to evaluate the precipitating causes

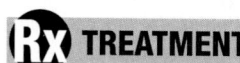

TREATMENT

ACUTE GENERAL Rx

- Aggressive fluid resuscitation, IV insulin, and electrolyte correction are the mainstays of treatment. Patients with HHS are very ill, and many are elderly; therefore, slower correction of osmolality may be required to limit cerebral edema.

BOX 1 Diagnostic Testing Criteria for Patients with Hyperglycemic Hyperosmolar State

Glucose higher than 600 mg/dl
Normal pH (classically, however, patients are often mildly acidotic)
No significant ketosis*
Serum osmolarity

- >320 mOsm/L with any mental status changes, *or*
- >350 mOsm/L

From Adams JG, et al. (eds): *Emergency medicine: clinical essentials*, ed 2, Philadelphia, 2013, Saunders.
*Serum acetoacetate is often present, typically an absent or low β-hydroxybutyrate level.

Aggressive IV fluid replacement

- Due to trivial ketonemia and the insulin sensitivity of most HHS patients, initial treatment is IV fluid alone without insulin. Insulin used prior to IV hydration or early in resuscitation risks a precipitous drop in serum osmolality. In the absence of cardiac compromise or end-stage renal disease, infuse 0.9% normal saline (NS) at an initial rate of 1 L/hour. A lower rate of 250 to 500 ml/hr may be adequate in the absence of severe dehydration. If the corrected serum sodium is high, 0.45% NS may be infused instead. Reassess corrected sodium needs by frequent checks and calculation. Recommended sodium decline is 0.5 mEq/L/hr and should not surpass 10 to 12 mEq/L per day. Use measured or calculated osmolality to guide rate of fluid resuscitation for gradual normalization of osmolality. Once serum glucose decreases to 300 mg/dl, change the IV fluid to 5% dextrose with 0.45% NS at 150 to 250 ml/hr.

Insulin

- Once glucose is no longer significantly improving with fluids alone, reassess patient's fluid status and initiate IV insulin. Administer initial bolus of IV regular insulin 0.1 units/kg followed by 0.1 units/kg/hr infusion or a continuous infusion of 0.14 units/kg/hr without initial bolus. If serum glucose declines by less than 50 to 75 mg/dl in the first hour, increase the insulin infusion rate. Once the serum glucose reaches 300 mg/dl, decrease the insulin infusion rate to 0.02 to 0.05 units/kg/hr to maintain serum glucose between 200 to 300 mg/dl until resolution of HHS.

Potassium replacement

- Insulin therapy shifts potassium intracellularly, frequently causing hypokalemia. If serum potassium at presentation is between 3.3 to 5.2 mEq/L, infuse 20 to 30 mEq of potassium chloride (KCl) with each liter of IV fluid to maintain serum potassium between 4 to 5 mEq/L. If serum potassium at presentation is <3.3 mEq/L, replace potassium by administering KCl infusion at 20 to 30 mEq/hr and hold insulin until serum potassium is >3.3 mEq/L. If serum potassium at presentation is >5.2 mEq/L, monitor serum potassium level every 2 hr without replacement.

Phosphate and magnesium replacement

- Phosphate and magnesium replacement are not routinely recommended. There are no studies on phosphate use in the treatment of HHS. Very low phosphorus levels may limit adenosine triphosphate (ATP) generation, thus limiting adequate diaphragm function. In patients with cardiac dysfunction, respiratory depression, or anemia and serum phosphate <1 mg/dl, add 20 to 30 mEq/L of potassium phosphate to the IV fluids.
- Monitor serum glucose hourly and serum electrolytes, blood urea nitrogen (BUN), and creatinine every 2 to 4 hr until resolution of HHS.

Transition to subcutaneous insulin

- Normalization of serum osmolality and mental status indicate resolution of HHS. At this point, transition to subcutaneous insulin. Overlap initiation of subcutaneous long- or intermediate-acting insulin and discontinuation of IV insulin by 2 to 4 hours to ensure adequate insulin levels and prevent rebound hyperglycemia. In patients with a known history of diabetes, their home insulin regimen may be initiated if it was adequate prior to presentation. In patients with poorly controlled diabetes, the subcutaneous insulin dose can be determined based on their stable insulin drip requirement. Insulin-naïve patients may be started on basal-bolus insulin therapy, starting with a total daily dose of 0.5 to 0.8 units/kg (split as half-basal and half-bolus: administer one third total bolus for each meal). Their stable insulin drip requirement will also help guide initial doses of subcutaneous insulin. Further subcutaneous insulin dose titration will be based on resultant blood glucoses. Resolution of glucotoxicity and the inciting condition(s) will decrease insulin requirements. The underlying infection/inflammatory condition or precipitating event must be adequately treated.

Chronic therapy

- Most patients will need insulin at discharge, at least short-term. Patients whose diabetes was previously well controlled on oral agents may resume oral therapy after stabilization of blood glucose with the use of insulin.

Disposition

- Most patients will need to be managed in an emergency care setting such as the intensive care unit or in a step-up facility where close supervision and monitoring are feasible.

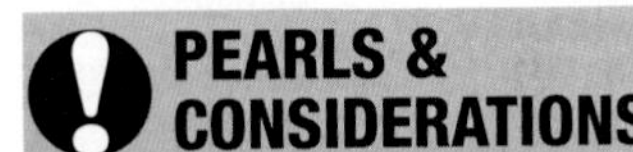

PEARLS & CONSIDERATIONS

COMMENTS

Educating the patient, family, and caregivers at chronic care facilities regarding optimal glycemic control, limiting modifiable risk factors for HHS, and prevention of dehydration are paramount.

SUGGESTED READINGS

Available at ExpertConsult.com

AUTHOR: **JESSICA E. SHILL, M.D.**

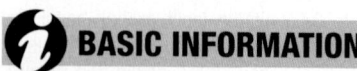

BASIC INFORMATION

DEFINITION

Abnormal elevation of potassium (K^+) in the blood associated with either normal or altered total body stores of potassium. Normal K^+ level in the blood is 3.5-5.0 milliequivalents per liter (mEq/L). Hyperkalemia can be defined as mild (levels 5.1-6.0 mEq/L), moderate (levels 6.0-7.0 mEq/L) and severe (levels >7.0 mEq/L). Levels higher than 7 mEq/L can lead to significant hemodynamic and neurologic consequences, whereas levels exceeding 8.5 mEq/L can cause respiratory paralysis or cardiac arrest and quickly be fatal.

SYNONYM

High potassium

ICD-10CM CODE
E87.5 Hyperpotassemia

EPIDEMIOLOGY & DEMOGRAPHICS

INCIDENCE & PREVALENCE:

- Overall incidence and prevalence of hyperkalemia is unknown. The rate is low in uncomplicated hypertensives on the inhibitors of renin-angiotensin-aldosterone system (RAASi), but it rises in the setting of other comorbidities listed below.
- Rarely detected in the general population, it is seen in only 2.6% of emergency room visits and 3.5% of hospital admissions in a Canadian study, with similar results in two U.S. studies.
- Chronic kidney disease (CKD) patients are most prevalent at 10%. Increased risk depends on the underlying conditions present. Is also seen with end-stage kidney disease (ESKD), acute kidney injury (AKI), cardiovascular disease (CVD), diabetes mellitus (DM), or metabolic acidosis (especially associated with non-gap inorganic acidosis), and on medications such as RAASi and mineralocorticoid receptor inhibitors (MRA) and other potassium-sparing diuretics.
- The prevalence of ICD10 diagnosis for hyperkalemia was found to be very low (14.6%).

PREDOMINANT SEX & AGE:

- More common with increasing age due to increased prevalence of etiological factors such as CKD, DM, CVD, and concomitant use of medications that predispose to hyperkalemia.
- Lower socioeconomic groups also have an increased prevalence, where monitoring of drug therapy and control of DM and hypertension are often inadequate.

GENETICS: Other syndromes that may be associated with hyperkalemia include:

- Pseudohyperparathyroidism type II (Familial hyperkalemic hypertension also known as Gordon syndrome)
  1. Characterized by hypertension and hyperkalemia
  2. Mutations of several genes can be seen affecting sodium, potassium, and chloride transport in the tubule of the kidney
  3. All forms respond to treatment with thiazide-like diuretics
- Hyperkalemic periodic paralysis
  1. Autosomal dominant mutation resulting in flaccid generalized weakness and hyperkalemia
- Glomerulopathy with fibronectin deposits (GFND)
  1. Autosomal dominant disorder manifested by proteinuria, hypertension, and Type IV RTA
- Disorders of steroid metabolism and mineralocorticoid receptors
  1. 21-hydroxylase deficiency and aldosterone synthase deficiency both associated with low aldosterone levels
- Congenital hypoaldosteronism
  1. Autosomal recessive mutation associated with low aldosterone and salt wasting
  2. Increased serum ratio of 18-hydroxycorticosterone-to-aldosterone
- Nephronophthisis
  1. Manifested by enlargement of kidneys, inflammatory portal fibrosis, and development of ESKD. Results in progressive interstitial fibrosis and tubulopathy.
- Disorders of chloride homeostasis
  1. Autosomal recessive mutation causing isolated hyperchlorihidrosis with excessive salt wasting in sweat resulting in severe hyponatremic dehydration and hyperkalemia

RISK FACTORS: Primary risk factor is CKD, especially if eGFR is <45 ml/min/1.73 m^2 more commonly associated with diabetes mellitus type 1 or 2, or urinary tract obstruction with obstructive nephropathy (especially if associated with chronic interstitial nephritis).

Medications associated with hyperkalemia

- Potassium-sparing diuretics (e.g., spironolactone, triamterene, amiloride, eplerenone)
- Nonsteroidal anti-inflammatory drugs (NSAIDs)
- Angiotensin-converting enzyme inhibitors (ACEIs)
- Angiotensin receptor blockers (ARBs)
- Direct renin inhibitors
- Calcineurin inhibitors (cyclosporine and tacrolimus)
- Pentamidine
- Trimethaphan-sulfamethoxazole
- Heparin
- Ketoconazole
- Metyrapone
- Herbs

Clinical risk factors

- Male sex
- Non-black
- DM
- CVD
- CHF
- AKI
- CKD
- Acidosis (nonorganic)
- Urinary obstruction

PHYSICAL FINDINGS & CLINICAL PRESENTATION

Most patients presenting with hyperkalemia are asymptomatic, with the abnormal laboratory study discovered inadvertently. The symptoms when present are nonspecific and mostly related to muscular or cardiac dysfunction.

- Muscle paralysis
- Dyspnea
- Palpitations
- Chest pain
- Nausea or vomiting
- Paresthesias

The physical exam typically does not alert the physician to a diagnosis of hyperkalemia, other than bradycardia, if present, or muscle tenderness accompanied by muscle weakness, suggesting rhabdomyolysis. Flaccid paralysis and/or depressed or absent deep tendon reflexes may be present.

ETIOLOGY

- Potassium is maintained in a narrow range of normal (3.8–5.0 mEq/L) by redundant and highly efficient homeostatic mechanisms that simultaneously control internal K^+ redistribution while regulating net K^+ excretion especially in the face of increased K^+. When a defect occurs in one or both of these two processes, a net rise in extracellular K^+ concentration occurs, resulting in hyperkalemia. We often see a blunting of the redistribution process with insulin deficiency, decrease in aldosterone production or action, decreased adrenergic activity, and osmolar disturbances associated with an increase in extracellular osmolality such as with hyperglycemia.
- The kidney is responsible for most of the regulation of potassium absorption and excretion (95%), which is dependent on the functional renal mass, thus the prominent association with CKD and reduced renal mass. Kidney failure or failure of the renal tubule to augment K^+ secretion plays a role in the maintenance of hyperkalemia. The importance of cell shifts is illustrated by the observation that if only 2% of potassium is shifted out of the cells to the extracellular fluid, it would raise the level from 4 mEq/L to 8 mEq/L, which would be critical.
- CKD is the single most important condition predisposing to hyperkalemia due to progressively decreasing GFR (falling clearance) and development of tubulointerstitial dysfunction (lower tubular secretion). Patients with progressive CKD are commonly associated with CVD, DM, HBP, and proteinuria, and they therefore are instructed to consume a diet very low in sodium, typically associated with a higher potassium intake. Low-sodium diets may be compensated for by an increase in salt-substitute intake, in many cases without the patients realizing that potassium chloride may further increase potassium intake. Another condition not uncommonly associated with CKD acutely increasing the risk of hyperkalemia is AKI, which, in addition to acutely reducing the capacity of the kidney to excrete a potassium load, can be associated with an acute potassium load, especially if in the presence of tissue breakdown (e.g., rhabdomyolysis), gastrointestinal bleeding, or transfusions with outdated blood. Metabolic acidosis commonly acutely worsens in AKI, facilitating shift of potassium out of cells.

These processes can often result in the development of severe and life-threatening hyperkalemia.

- DM (characterized by insulin deficiency and hypertonicity when uncontrolled, both of which shift potassium out of cells) and CVD (especially myocardial infarctions, left ventricular hypertrophy, and congestive heart failure, often associated with various pharmacologic interventions that may induce or worsen hyperkalemia). CVD often clusters with CKD and hence their concomitant presence may contribute to a higher prevalence of hyperkalemia. Among the relevant CVD medications, recall that β_2-2 receptor blockers inhibit renin production (decreasing ability of potassium to shift into cells); heparin inhibits aldosterone production (decreasing ability to excrete a potassium load); and digitalis impairs potassium excretion (by blocking Na-K-ATPase, which is important in potassium secretion by the tubule). The magnitude of impact on potassium by these medications, however, is limited, typically in the range of ~0.2–0.5 mEq/L. A much more relevant class is RAASi and potassium-sparing diuretics (Amiloride), with hyperkalemia seen in <2 % of patients without CKD, increasing to 5% with dual RAASi therapy, and up to 10% in the presence of CKD (especially stages >3b). In those patients at risk for hyperkalemia, it is recommended not to use dual RAASi therapy and to be very cautious with the use of RAASi and MRA.

Dx DIAGNOSIS

DIFFERENTIAL DIAGNOSIS

Hyperkalemia develops due to three mechanisms: redistribution, decreased secretion, and increased intake. (In the presence of normal renal and adrenal function, it is very difficult to ingest enough potassium to become hyperkalemic, so hyperkalemia is rarely seen in people without advanced CKD.) The differential diagnosis is listed in Table 1.

TABLE 1 Differential Diagnosis of Hyperkalemia

- Pseudohyperkalemia
- Cellular redistribution from intra- to extracellular space
    1. Mineral acid acidosis (not endogenous organic acidosis)
        a. Hyperkalemia inhibits ammoniagenesis, reducing net acid secretion and compounding metabolic acidosis
    2. Hypertonicity (hyperglycemia, sucrose, mannitol)
    3. DM: Insulin deficiency
    4. Hyperkalemic periodic paralysis
    5. β2-adrenergic antagonists
    6. α-adrenergic agonists
    7. Drugs
        a. Glucagon
        b. Digoxin overdose
        c. Aminocaproic acid-A
        d. Tetrodotoxin
        e. Succinyl choline
    8. Rebound after labile and or per
    9. Extreme exercise
    10. Crush and tissue injury
        a. Rhabdomyolysis
        b. Hemolysis
        c. Tumor lysis syndrome
- Decreased renal excretion
    1. CKD
        a. Use of nonsteroidal antiinflammatory drugs (NSAIDs)
    2. ESKD
    3. Type 4 Renal Tubular Acidosis
        a. Diabetes mellitus
        b. Obstructive nephropathy
        c. Amiloride
        d. Trimethoprim
        e. Pentamidine
        f. Suxamethonium
        g. Volume depletion
        h. HIV infections
- Excess intake (rare except in advanced CKD or ESKD)
    1. Salt substitute (typically KCl)
    2. Potassium-enriched foods (melons, citrus juice, raw coconut juice has 44.3 mEq/L [44.3 mmol/L], noni juice has 56 mEq/L [56 mmol/L] K)
    3. River bed clay (red clay) very enriched, with 100 mEq K/100 g clay)
- Mineralocorticoid deficiency (Addison disease)
    1. Hypoaldosteronism: Primary or secondary
    2. HIV infection
- Defect of tubular function or voltage defect resulting in hyperkalemia and hypertension
    1. Genetic
        a. Pseudohyperaldosteronism type 2
- Also known as familial hyperkalemic hypertension or Gordon syndrome
    1. Acquired
        a. Calcineurin inhibitors (tacrolimus and cyclosporine)

CKD, Chronic kidney disease; *DM*, diabetes mellitus; *ESKD*, end-stage kidney disease; *KCl*, potassium chloride.

WORKUP

Fig. 1 illustrates a clinical approach to hyperkalemia. The following steps should be followed in the workup of hyperkalemia:

- R/O pseudohyperkalemia

An in vitro phenomenon caused by mechanical release of potassium from cells during phlebotomy or specimen processing. This may be seen with severe leukocytosis (>70,000/cm^3 or thrombocytosis (platelet count >500,000 cm^3), severe fist clenching during phlebotomy, prolonged application of a tight tourniquet, and use of a small-bore needle. The diagnosis is made when serum potassium concentration exceeds the plasma potassium concentration by >0.5 mEq/L (>0.5 mmol/L). Contamination with potassium EDTA in certain tubes can spuriously increase plasma potassium concentration accompanied by a very low plasma calcium concentration.

- If no predisposition to hyperkalemia, repeat the blood test before taking action, unless ECG changes are present.
- Perform an ECG to look for the hallmark changes seen with hyperkalemia, which commonly have a sequential progression that historically seemed to correlate with the potassium level, if present. Some studies seem to indicate inconsistent findings of the ECG in hyperkalemia, especially with K^+ levels <6.5 mEq/L and more predictive at levels >7.2 to 9.4 mEq/L.
    1. Early ECG changes seen with serum potassium level of 5.5–6.5 mEq/L: Peaked T waves (Fig. E2), especially in the precordial leads; shortened QT interval; and occasionally ST segment depression.
    2. K >6.5 mEq/L: Widening of the QRS complex (nonspecific intraventricular conduction delay [IVCD]) of >120 milliseconds that does not meet the criteria for right or left bundle branch block. If you see an IVCD, think hyperkalemia. May also see amplified R waves.
    3. K >7 mEq/L: Associated with decreased amplitude of P waves with increase in PR interval and development of bradycardia, which is associated with atrioventricular blocks.
    4. K >8.0 mEq/L: Develops absence of P waves and the progressively widened QRS eventually merges with the T waves, forming a sine wave pattern followed by ventricular fibrillation or asystole.

In hemodialysis patients with hyperkalemia, T wave "tenting" was nonpredictive of serum K^+ level, especially in the elderly and diabetics. There have even been case reports of severe hyperkalemia with no ECG changes.

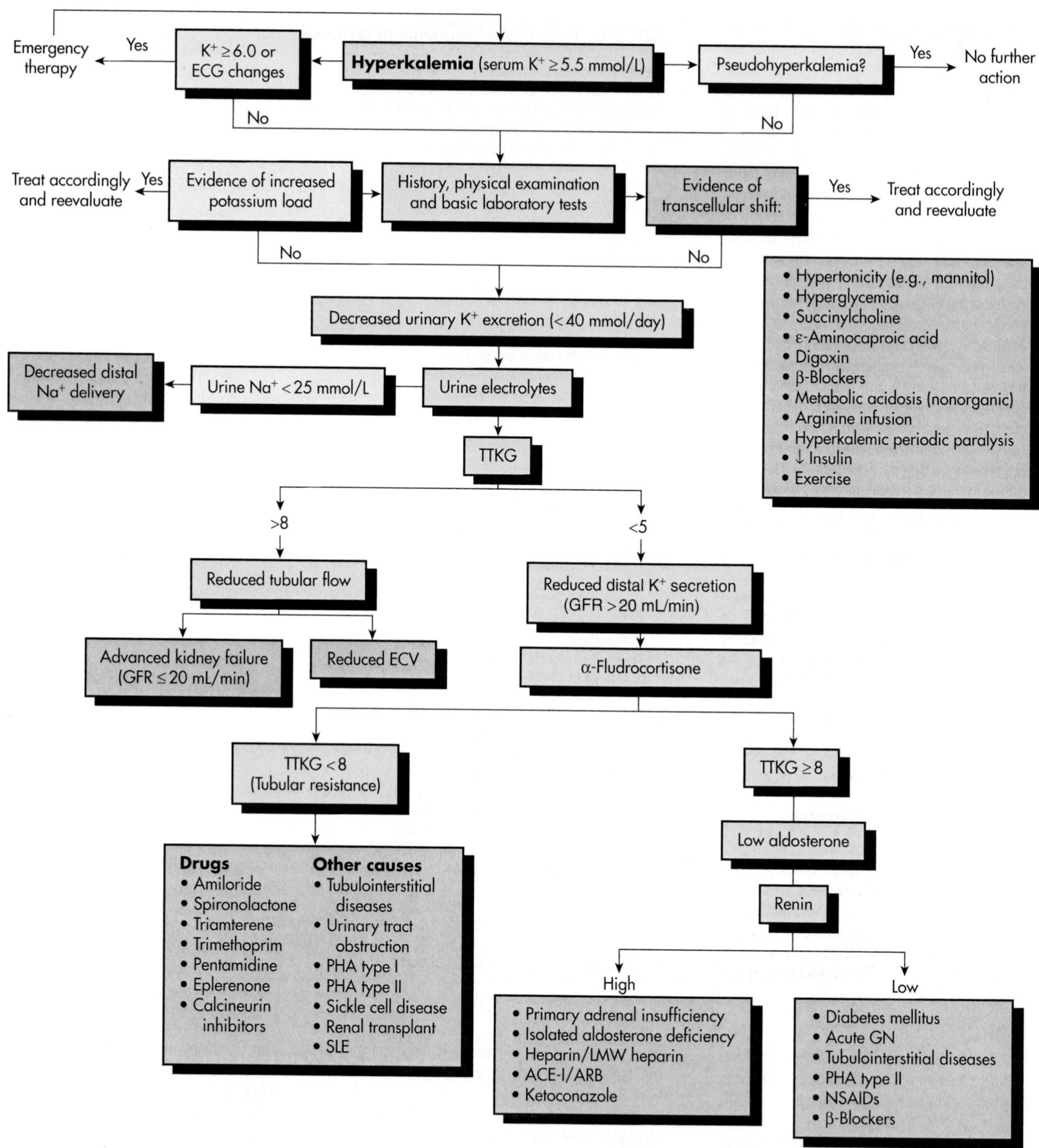

FIG. 1 Clinical approach to hyperkalemia. *ACE-I*, Angiotensin-converting enzyme inhibitor; *EC*, electrocardiogram; *GN*, glomerulonephritis; *ARB*, angiotensin II receptor blocker; *CCD*, cortical collecting duct; *ECV*, effective circulatory volume; *GFR*, glomerular filtration rate; *HIV*, human immunodeficiency virus; *LMW heparin*, low-molecular-weight heparin; *NSAIDs*, nonsteroidal anti-inflammatory drugs; *PHA*, pseudohypoaldosteronism; *SLE*, systemic lupus erythematosus; *TTKG*, transtubular potassium gradient. (From Skorecki K et al: *Brenner & Rector's the kidney*, ed 10, Philadelphia, 2016, Elsevier.)

- Look for the symptoms or physical findings noted above and then do the basic studies:
  1. ECG
  2. Urine potassium, sodium, and osmolality
  3. Complete blood count and platelet count
  4. Basic metabolic profile with a calculated estimated GFR (eGFR) (CKD alone should not develop hyperkalemia until eGFR is <20–25 ml/min.)

  Depending on the history and results of the initial blood tests, the following may be indicated:
  a. Glucose to r/o hypertonicity in uncontrolled diabetics
  b. Digoxin level if patient is on digoxin
  c. Arterial or venous blood gas if acidosis is suspected
  d. Urinalysis if renal insufficiency is present to r/o AKI or acute glomerulonephritis

TABLE 2 Defining Renal Origin of Hyperkalemia

Application of TTKG, FE_K, and Urine K:Cr Ratio
Expected values for TTKG* or FE_K
Nonrenal forms of hyperkalemia
TTKG >5-7, FE_K >10%
Urine K:Cr ratio >30 mEq/L
Spot urine [K^+] >25 mEq/L
Renal hyperkalemia
TTKG <5 or FE_K <10% (inappropriately low)
Urine K:Cr ratio <30 mEq/g Cr
Urine [K^+] <25 mEq/24 h

Cr, creatinine; *FE_K*, fractional excretion of K^+; *TTKG*, transtubular potassium gradient.
*Prerequisites for use: U_{Na} >25 mEq/L and urine not dilute.
Formulae:
TTKG = (Urine K ÷ [Urine osmolality/Plasma osmolality]) ÷ Plasma K
FE_K = ([urine K^+]/[serum K^+])/(urine creatinine/serum creatinine)
Multiply by 100 for percentage

e. Serum cortisol and aldosterone levels to check for deficiency when other causes are eliminated
f. Serum uric acid and phosphorus to r/o tumor lysis syndrome
g. Serum creatinine phosphokinase (CPK) and calcium measurements for rhabdomyolysis
h. Urine myoglobin test (if you see a very + dipstick of urine for blood and no RBCs, be suspicious of this) for crush injury and rhabdomyolysis

- Accurately assess kidney function with a serum creatinine and calculated GFR to define the risk of hyperkalemia as well as the acid base status, especially identifying the presence of a non-anion gap mineral metabolic acidosis.
- Look for the presence of a non-anion gap mineral metabolic acidosis associated with the hyperkalemia typically diagnosing a Type 4 RTA. This is typically seen with a hyporeninemic hypoaldosterone state (seen in diabetic nephropathy of chronic interstitial nephropathy) or obstructive nephropathy.
- Determine the presence of a renal origin for hyperkalemia using the urine potassium concentration.

This will determine the presence of a renal tubule dysfunction in a hyperkalemic patient. There are four types of urine chemistry analysis available to determine this: (1) Urine potassium (K) concentration, (2) the fractional excretion of potassium, (3) the urine potassium/creatinine ratio, and (4) the "transtubular potassium gradient" (TTKG). See Table 2 for the expected values of each in both renal and nonrenal causes of hyperkalemia.

LABORATORY TESTS

- Serum electrolytes, BUN, and creatinine
- Urinalysis and urine protein–creatinine ratio
- Serum and plasma potassium
- Plasma and urine osmolality
- Serum and urine creatinine
- Cortisol level
- Aldosterone level
- 18-hydroxycorticosterone

IMAGING STUDIES

- Ultrasound of the kidneys and bladder
- CT scan of the abdomen

Rx TREATMENT

- Supportive measurements such as fluids, pacing, and pressers do not work in the setting of hyperkalemia. In acute, severe, life-threatening hyperkalemia, the approach is divided into two components. First stabilize the myocardium to prevent a fatal arrhythmia. Giving IV calcium is cardioprotective in the setting of hyperkalemia, commonly reversing all hyperkalemic ECG changes within seconds of administration. However, it does not decrease the potassium levels; therefore, other therapies are needed to reduce the potassium level.
- Before giving calcium, make sure digoxin toxicity is not present, as calcium administration can be fatal in the face of digoxin-induced hyperkalemia.
- The aggressiveness of the treatment should be directly related to the rapidity with which the hyperkalemia developed, the absolute level of the potassium, and the evidence of toxicity by symptoms and/or examination and ECG changes. The more rapid the rise in potassium, the higher the level; and the more severe the cardiotoxicity depicted by the ECG changes, the more aggressive the therapy should be.

NONPHARMACOLOGIC THERAPY

- The mainstay of therapy should be educating the patient and the family regarding a low-potassium diet (<3 g/day), as well as providing a list of high-potassium foods to avoid.
- Maintaining adequate hydration and preventing volume depletion, which limits potassium excretion by the kidney.

ACUTE GENERAL Rx

In patients with severe hyperkalemia, treatment is as follows:

- IV calcium (Fig. 3) to ameliorate cardiac toxicity (if not digoxin toxic).
- Identify and remove sources of potassium intake.
- IV glucose and insulin infusion to enhance cellular uptake of potassium.
  1. Make sure to monitor closely for several hours for hypoglycemia, especially in advanced CKD patients.
- Correct severe acidosis with IV sodium bicarbonate.
- Consider beta-adrenergic agonist therapy (e.g., nebulized albuterol, 10 mg via venti mask), which is preferred over alkali therapy in patients with renal failure.
- Increase potassium excretion with administration of loop diuretic IV or cation-exchange medications mentioned previously.
  1. Medications that increase potassium excretion in addition to IV saline and loop diuretics include use of an aldosterone analogue (e.g., 9-alpha fludrocortisone acetate [Florinef]) in patients with hyporeninemia or hypoaldosteronism or patients with solid organ transplant on CNI and hyperkalemia.
- Emergency dialysis in potentially lethal hyperkalemia unresponsive to conservative measures or with acute kidney failure.

CHRONIC Rx

In the presence of a moderate elevation of potassium and no ECG abnormalities:

- Correct the source of increase potassium (e.g., inhibited excretion or increased intake)
  1. Historical therapy is sodium polystyrene sulfate with or without sorbitol. This may fall to the wayside in the face of the newer therapies with more consistent results and less potential toxicity (dose is 15 g to 30 g orally and may be repeated in 3–4 hours). Do not give as an enema (especially with sorbitol).
  2. Patiromer is a non-reabsorbed oral calcium-containing potassium-binding polymer suspension (dose 4.2 grams BID).
     a. Shown to lower serum potassium in hyperkalemia associated with diabetic nephropathy and CHF on RAASi
  3. Sodium zirconium cyclosilicate, now available in the U.S., is a nonabsorbed inorganic polymer selectively exchanging potassium for sodium and hydrogen ions (dose 10 grams tid for up to 48 hours followed by 5 g to 10 g daily for chronic use).
- Increase potassium excretion using cation exchange resin or diuretics.

Management of nonurgent hyperkalemia:

- Discontinue or reduce medications that interfere with potassium excretion.
  1. Stop RAASi (special care if in combination)
  2. Stop spironolactone, eplerenone, amiloride, triamterene
  3. Stop all NSAIDs (including OTC) and Cox 2 inhibitors
  4. Herbal medicine: stop Chan su and Noni juice
  5. If possible, address whether patient is on a calcineurin inhibitor (CNI)
- Prescribe a low-potassium diet (70 mEq/day).
- Give a loop diuretic (or thiazide of CNI-induced hyperkalemia).
- If bicarbonate <22, give $NaHCO_3$ tablets (650 mg tablet [7.6 mEq] or Shohl solution (sodium citrate) (3–60 ml tid).
- Patiromer or sodium zirconium cyclosilicate avoids use of SPS for chronic hyperkalemia.
  1. Patiromer not effective for urgent hyperkalemia: SPS empirically used, some ongoing studies looking at sodium zirconium cyclosilicate
- ZS-9 has application in chronic hyperkalemia and may have application in acute/urgent hyperkalemia (studies pending).
- May be able to continue RAASi with either patiromer or sodium zirconium cyclosilicate.

DISPOSITION

Patients with acute symptomatic hyperkalemia with ECG changes should be admitted to a hospital in a monitored bed/intensive care unit.

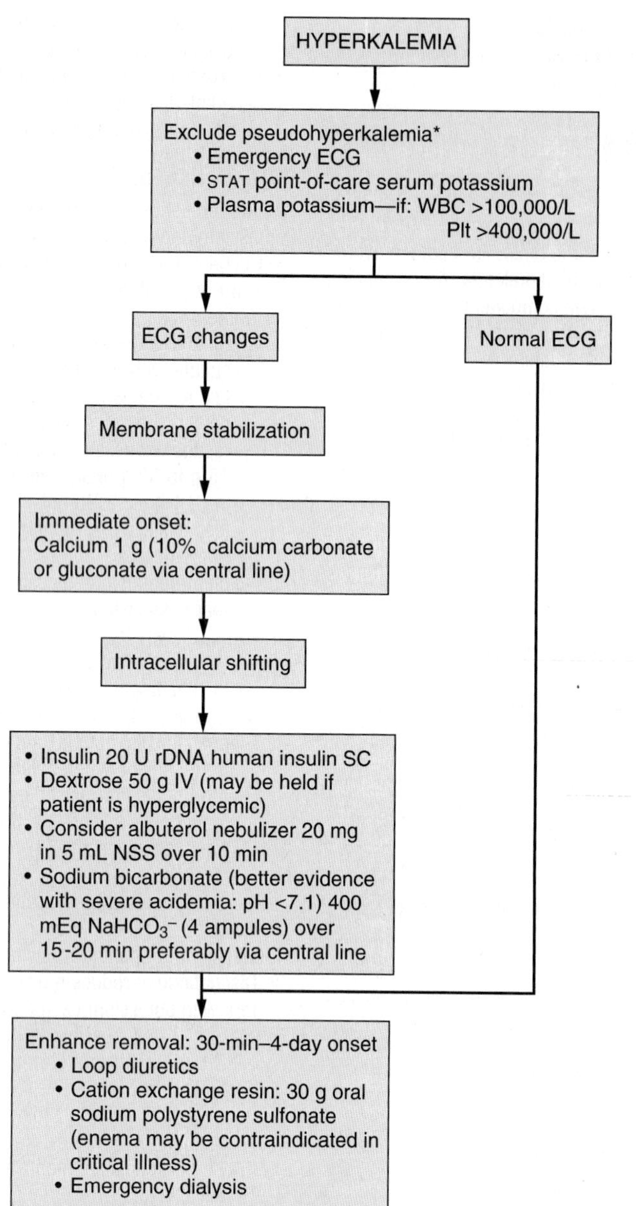

FIG. 3 Algorithm for treatment of hyperkalemia. *ECG,* Electrocardiogram; *IV,* intravenously; *NSS,* normal saline solution; *Plt,* platelet count; *SC,* subcutaneously; *WBC,* white blood cell count. (From Ronco C et al: *Critical Care Nephrology*, ed 3, Philadelphia, 2019, Elsevier.)

Asymptomatic patients with no ECG changes can be treated as outpatients and educated extensively regarding a low-potassium diet with close follow-up including a repeat potassium in 24–48 hr, depending on the severity, and a week later.

REFERRAL

Patients with associated hypertension, proteinuria, CKD, or persistent hyperkalemia should be referred to a nephrologist for more intensive evaluation and to assess for a genetic etiology.

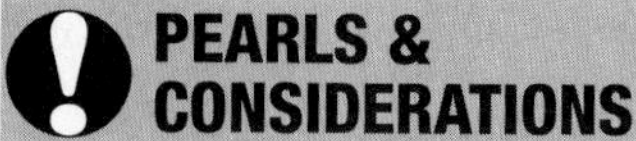

PEARLS & CONSIDERATIONS

COMMENTS

- Ensure that specimen is not hemolyzed.
- When in doubt, repeat the test.
- Rule out pseudohyperkalemia.
- Risk associated with comparable levels of hyperkalemia is higher in individuals with normal kidney function compared to those with increasingly severe CKD.
- Do not give IV calcium or insulin/dextrose if no ECG changes for hyperkalemia.
- Don't forget to educate and encourage dietary restriction of potassium. (Avoid salt substitutes.)
- Evaluate for urinary obstruction, especially in diabetics (neurogenic bladder) and in elderly males (prostatic hypertrophy).

PREVENTION

- Avoid dual therapy with ARB and ACEI or direct renin inhibitor.
- In patients with type 4 RTA, educate to reduce high-potassium food intake during their seasons (e.g., tomatoes, citrus fruits), avoid travel to areas where these foods are endemic and avoid volume depletion.
- In CKD patients or in patients with type 4 RTA, avoid using a salt substitute (which is potassium chloride).

PATIENT/FAMILY EDUCATION

Education regarding potassium content of foods is of high, practical importance. A renal nutritionist should review the patient's medical records for potential dietary interventions.

SUGGESTED READINGS

Available at ExpertConsult.com

RELATED CONTENT

Chronic Kidney Disease (Related Key Topic)

AUTHORS: **NELSON KOPYT, D.O.,** and **JERRY YEE, M.D.**

BASIC INFORMATION

DEFINITION

- Primary hyperlipoproteinemia is a group of genetic disorders of the lipid transport proteins in the blood that manifests as abnormally elevated levels of cholesterol, triglycerides, or both in the serum of affected patients.
- Usually defined as total cholesterol, LDL, triglycerides, or lipoprotein A levels above 90th percentile or HDL or apo A-1 levels below the 10th percentile for the general population. Fig. E1 illustrates the structure of lipoproteins. Plasma lipoprotein composition is described in Table E1.

SYNONYM

Hyperlipidemia

ICD-10CM CODES

E78.0 Pure hypercholesterolemia
E78.2 Mixed hyperlipidemia
E78.1 Pure hyperglyceridemia
E78.4 Other hyperlipidemia
E78.3 Hyperchylomicronemia

EPIDEMIOLOGY & DEMOGRAPHICS

INCIDENCE: The most common types are lipoprotein A excess, hypertriglyceridemia, and combined hyperlipidemia.

- Incidence of heterozygous familial hypercholesterolemia: 1:500.
- Incidence of homozygous familial hypercholesterolemia: 1:1 million.
- Familial hypercholesterolemia: Autosomal-dominant disorder.
- Familial combined hyperlipidemia: Possibly an autosomal-dominant disorder.
- Multifactorial predilection: Apparent in majority of affected individuals.

GENETICS:

- Familial lipoprotein lipase deficiency: Autosomal recessive, resulting in an elevation in the plasma chylomicrons and triglycerides
- Familial apoprotein CII deficiency: Autosomal recessive, resulting in increased serum chylomicrons, very-low-density lipoprotein (VLDL), and hypertriglyceridemia
- Familial type 3 hyperlipoproteinemia: Single-gene defect requiring contributory factors to manifest
- Familial hypercholesterolemia: Autosomal-dominant defect of the LDL receptor, resulting in an elevated serum cholesterol level and normal triglycerides
- Familial hypertriglyceridemia: Common, autosomal-dominant defect resulting in elevated VLDL and triglycerides
- Multiple lipoprotein–type hyperlipidemia: Autosomal dominant, manifesting as isolated hypercholesterolemia, isolated hypertriglyceridemia, or hyperlipidemia
- Polygenic hypercholesterolemia: Multifactorial
- Polygenic hyperalphalipoproteinemia: Autosomal dominant or polygenic, causing an elevated high-density lipoprotein
- A classification of lipoprotein disorders and their clinical findings and management are summarized in Table 2.

PHYSICAL FINDINGS & CLINICAL PRESENTATION

- Familial lipoprotein lipase deficiency: Recurrent bouts of abdominal pain in infancy, eruptive xanthomas, hepatomegaly, splenomegaly, lipemia retinalis
- Familial apoprotein CII deficiency: Occasional eruptive xanthomas
- Familial type 3 hyperlipoproteinemia: Xanthoma striata palmaris or tuberoeruptive xanthomas, xanthelasmas, arterial bruits at a young age, gangrene of the lower extremities at a young age
- Familial hypercholesterolemia: Tendon xanthomas, arcus corneae, xanthelasma
- Familial hypertriglyceridemia: Associated obesity; eruptive xanthomas can develop with exacerbations

ETIOLOGY

- Genetic defects causing lipid abnormalities
- Environmental influences, including diet, drugs, and alcohol intake

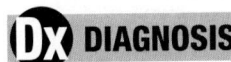

DIAGNOSIS

DIFFERENTIAL DIAGNOSIS

Secondary causes of hyperlipoproteinemias:

- Hypothyroidism
- Diabetes mellitus
- Pancreatitis
- Autoimmune hyperlipoproteinemia
- Nephrotic syndrome
- Biliary obstruction. Table E3 describes the differential diagnosis of hyperlipidemia and dyslipidemia.

WORKUP

- Family history for premature cardiac disease
- Personal history of recurrent pancreatitis
- Detailed physical examination

LABORATORY TESTS

- Standard lipid profile. Table 4 summarizes laboratory findings in lipid disorders.
- If normal, further testing with measurement of lipoprotein A, apo B, and apo A-1
- Lipoprotein electrophoresis and ultracentrifugation (for phenotypic classification)
- Workup for secondary causes: TSH, fasting glucose, liver function, renal function, urinary protein

TREATMENT

NONPHARMACOLOGIC THERAPY

- Cornerstone of treatment: Dietary therapy
  1. TLC diet (**t**herapeutic **l**ifestyle **c**hanges): See "Hypercholesterolemia" topic
- Risk factor reduction includes smoking cessation, treatment of hypertension, exercise
- Familial lipoprotein lipase deficiency and familial apoprotein CII deficiency: Fat-free diet
- Remainder of cases, except those with polygenic hyperalphalipoproteinemia: Fat- and cholesterol-restricted diets

ACUTE GENERAL Rx

No acute treatment needed.

CHRONIC Rx

- Familial lipoprotein lipase deficiency, polygenic hyperalphalipoproteinemia, or familial apoprotein CII deficiency: No chronic drug therapy
- Familial type 3 hyperlipoproteinemia: Usually responds well to secondary causes being treated and diet therapy; if not, fibric acids may be tried
- Familial hypercholesterolemia: Statins, bile acid sequestrants, or niacin. Ezetimibe can be added to statins to achieve LDL goals. Alirocumab and evolocumab are subcutaneously injected PCSK9 (protein convertase subtilisin kexin type 9) inhibitors available as an adjunct diet and maximally tolerated statin therapy for adults with heterozygous familial hypercholesterolemia (HeFH). They can be added to statins and ezetimibe
- Familial hypertriglyceridemia: Fibric acids (fenofibrate), niacin, omega-3 PUFA-containing fish oil capsules. Icosapent ethyl, a highly purified eicosapentaenoic acid esther, has been shown to lower triglyceride levels and cardiovascular risk in patients with hypertriglyceridemia
- Multiple lipoprotein–type hyperlipidemia: Drug therapy aimed at the predominant lipid abnormality noted
- Recent data suggest in patients with lipoprotein abnormalities that treatment goals should be based on non-HDL cholesterol rather than LDL cholesterol
- The FDA has approved mipomersen and lomitapide in patients with homozygous familial hypercholesterolemia already taking maximum doses of other lipid-lowering drugs. Both medicines are hepatotoxic and very expensive
- Recent trials with bempedoic acid, an inhibitor of ATP citrate lyase that lowers LDL cholesterol, have shown to significantly lower LDL when bempedoic acid was added to maximally tolerated statin therapy

DISPOSITION

- Those with polygenic hyperalphalipoproteinemia: Excellent prognosis for longevity
- Those with familial hypercholesterolemia, familial type 3 hypercholesterolemia, or multiple lipoprotein–type hyperlipidemia: Even with aggressive treatment, at high risk for accelerated atherosclerosis and coronary artery disease

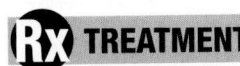

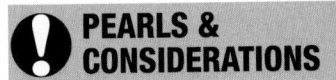

PEARLS & CONSIDERATIONS

COMMENTS

- Patient information is available through the American Heart Association.
- Lipid-lowering drug therapy is recommended for children ≥10 yr whose LDL-C levels remain extremely elevated after 6 mo to 1 yr of dietary modification. Drug therapy also can be considered for children with LDL-C levels of ≥190 mg/dl.

SUGGESTED READINGS

Available at ExpertConsult.com

RELATED CONTENT

Hypercholesterolemia (Related Key Topic)

AUTHOR: **FRED F. FERRI, M.D.**

TABLE 2 Disorders of Lipids: Clinical Findings and Management

Disorder	Xanthomas	Cardiovascular	Gastrointestinal	Neurologic	Ophthalmologic	Other Findings	Management
Type I	Eruptive, tendinous, xanthelasmas	None	Acute abdomen, hepatosplenomegaly, pancreatitis	None	Lipemia retinalis, retinal vein occlusion	Diabetes, lipemic plasma	Diet, plasmapheresis
Type II	Planar, especially intertriginous, tendinous, tuberous	Generalized atherosclerosis	None	None	Arcus cornea	None	Type IIa: bile acid sequestrants, statins, niacin, fish oil Type IIb: statins, niacin, fibrate
Type III	Planar, especially palmar, tuberous	Atherosclerosis	None	None	None	Abnormal glucose tolerance, hyperuricemia	Statins, fibrate
Type IV	Eruptive, tuberous	Atherosclerosis	Acute abdomen, hepatosplenomegaly, pancreatitis	None	Lipemia retinalis	Obesity	Statins, fibrate, niacin
Type V	Eruptive, tuberous	Atherosclerosis	Acute abdomen, hepatosplenomegaly, pancreatitis	None	Lipemia retinalis	Obesity, hyperinsulinemia	Niacin, fibrate
Tangier	Macular rash, foam cells in biopsies	Atherosclerosis	Acute abdomen, hepatosplenomegaly	Peripheral neuropathy	Corneal infiltration	Enlarged orange tonsils, lymphadenopathy	
Apolipoprotein A-I and C-III deficiency	Planar and tendon xanthomas, foam cells in biopsies	Atherosclerosis	Normal	Normal	Corneal clouding	None	
HDL deficiency with planar xanthomas	Planar xanthomas, foam cells in biopsies	Atherosclerosis	Hepatomegaly	Normal	Corneal opacity	None	

HDL, High-density lipoprotein.
From Paller AS, Mancini, AJ: *Hurwitz clinical pediatric dermatology: a textbook of skin disorders of childhood and adolescence,* ed 5, 2016, Elsevier.

TABLE 4 Laboratory Findings in Lipid Disorders

Disorder	Inheritance	OMIM No.	Prevalence	Cholesterol	Triglycerides	VLDL	Chylomicrons	LDL	HDL	Serum	Cause
Type I	AR		1/million	↑	↑↑↑	↑	↑	↓	↓↓↓	Creamy top	
a: Familial hyperchylomicronemia		239600, 246650, 615947									a: Deficiency from mutations in lipoprotein lipase; *LMF1*; *GPIHBP1*
b: Familial apoprotein C2 or A-V deficiency		207750, 133650									b. Deficient ApoC2 or ApoA5 (see Type 5)
c: —		118830									c. LP lipase inhibitor in blood
Type II			1 in 500 for heterozygotes	↑	Nl or ↑	↑	Nl	↓	↓	Clear	
a: Familial hypercholesterolemia	AD	143890, 144010, 603776									LDL receptor defect in 60%-80%; *APOB, PCSK9,* each <5%
	AR	603813									*LDLRAP1*
b: Familial combined hyperlipidemia	AD, AR	144250	1 in 100							Clear	Polygenic Decreased LDL receptor and ApoB100 dysfunction
Type III Familial dysbetalipoproteinemia	AR	107741	1 in 10,000	↑	↑	↑	↑	↓	Nl	Turbid	ApoE2 synthesis
Type IV Familial hypertriglyceridemia	AD	144600	1 in 100	↑	Nl ↑	↑	Nl	↓	↓↓	Turbid	Renal disease, diabetes
Type V	AR	144650	Very rare	↑	↑↑↑	↑	↑	↓	↓↓↓	Creamy top, turbid bottom	Apo A-V (ApoA5) deficiency

AD, Autosomal dominant; *Apo,* apolipoprotein; *AR,* autosomal recessive; *HDL,* high-density lipoprotein; *LDL,* low-density lipoprotein; *LP,* lipoprotein; *Nl,* normal; *OMIM,* Online Mendelian Inheritance in Man; *VLDL,* very low-density lipoprotein; *↑,* increased; *↓,* decreased.

From Paller AS, Mancini, AJ: *Hurwitz clinical pediatric dermatology: a textbook of skin disorders of childhood and adolescence,* ed 5, 2016, Elsevier.

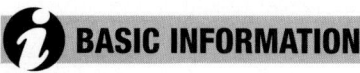

BASIC INFORMATION

DEFINITION

Hypernatremia is a clinical disorder that results from a net water deficit (i.e., dehydration). It is identified clinically when serum sodium concentration (S_{Na}) exceeds the upper limit of normal (145 mEq/L). Hypernatremia does not reflect the net total body sodium content or volume status. Consequently, patients may be hypovolemic, hypervolemic, or euvolemic.

SYNONYMS

Hyperosmolality
Hypertonicity
High serum sodium concentration

ICD-10CM CODES

E87.0 Hyperosmolality and/or hypernatremia
E86.0 Dehydration

EPIDEMIOLOGY & DEMOGRAPHICS

The prevalence of hypernatremia varies based on the defined population and clinical setting. In the outpatient setting, it is reported at the extremes of age. Sixty percent of hypernatremia cases develop in hospitalized patients, and about 80% of these cases occur in intensive care units.

Among noncritical hospitalized patients, prevalence ranges from 0.2% to 2.5%. The incidence of hypernatremia is higher in critically ill and elderly patients. Prevalence ranges from 10% to 26% in this population. Hypernatremia is independently associated with mortality.

RISK FACTORS:

- Age >60 yr
- Acute kidney injury on admission
- Altered mental status
- Mechanical ventilation
- Enteral tube feeding
- Negative fluid balance
- Hyperglycemia/uncontrolled diabetes mellitus
- Hypertonic bicarbonate or mannitol administration
- Hypokalemia
- Hypercalcemia
- Underlying polyuric disorders

PHYSICAL FINDINGS & CLINICAL PRESENTATION

- Symptoms generally correlate with the severity of hypernatremia, rapidity of development, and underlying cause. In the elderly, symptoms do not generally develop until S_{Na} >160 mEq/L.
- In mild hypernatremia, symptoms can include generalized muscle weakness, restlessness, anorexia, nausea, and vomiting.
- With severe hypernatremia, symptoms can begin with lethargy and irritability with progression to confusion, seizures, and, rarely, coma.
- In extreme scenarios, particularly in infants, hypernatremia-induced brain cell shrinkage can lead to intracranial bleeding from vascular stretching and subsequent vessel rupture.
- Polydipsia and polyuria may be present in certain types of hypernatremia such as diabetes insipidus.
- Key elements in history should focus on net fluid and water intake and losses, urine output, thirst response, and patient access to water.
- Clinicians should evaluate the volume status of a patient. Classifying volume status will assist in determining the etiology and management of hypernatremia. (Fig. 1)

ETIOLOGY

The etiology of hypernatremia is understood through the Edelman equation (refer to "Hyponatremia"). As a result, hypernatremia can be a clinical end result of either a net water deficit or excessive sodium intake. Renal water regulation and thirst stimuli are key physiologic components that prevent hypernatremia.

- To prevent hypernatremia, water is retained and urine concentrated by the kidneys under the influence of antidiuretic hormone (ADH) or vasopressin. Impairment of ADH secretion,

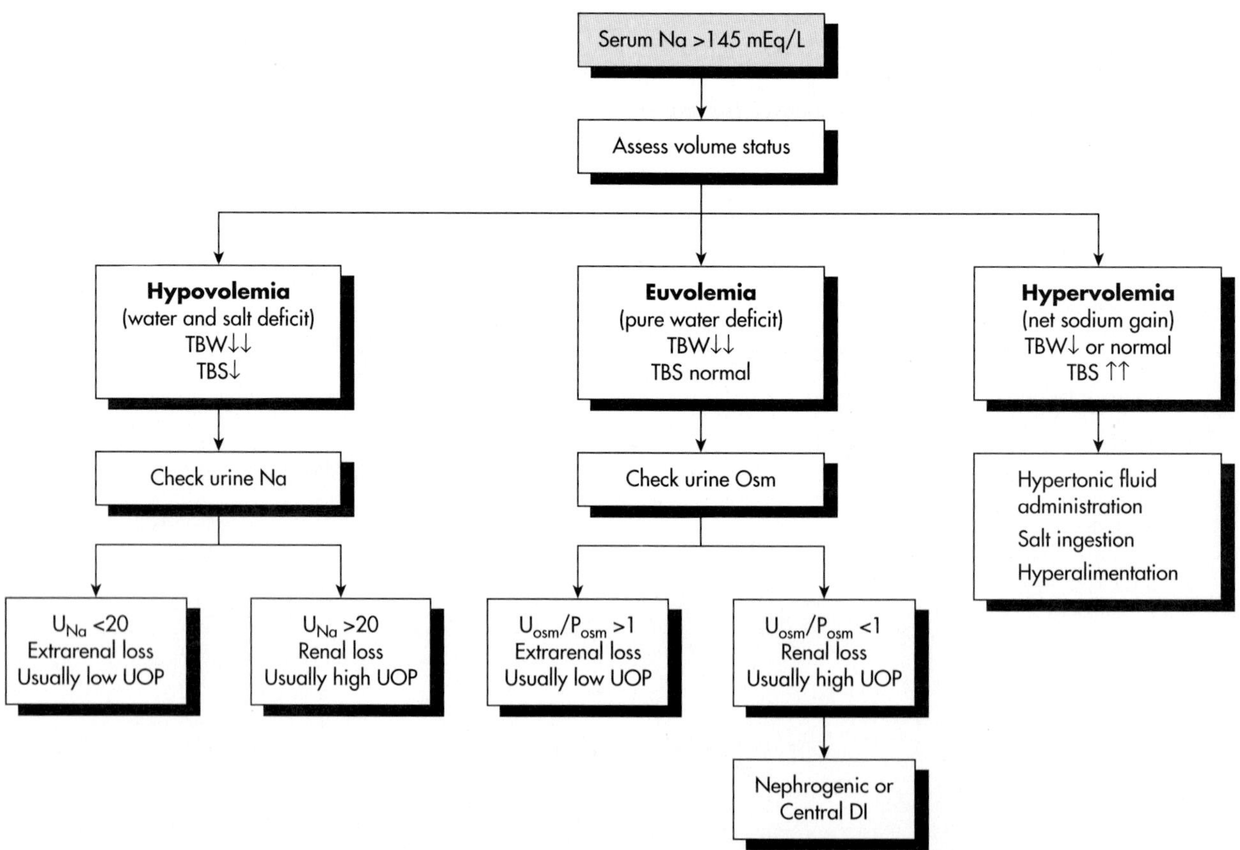

FIG. 1 Diagnostic approach to hypernatremia. *DI*, Diabetes insipidus; *Na*, Sodium; *Osm*, osmolality; *TBW*, total body water; *TBS*, total body salt; *UOP*, urine output. (Adapted from Gilbert SJ, Weiner DE: *National Kidney Foundation primer on kidney disease*, ed 6, Philadelphia, 2017, Elsevier Saunders.)

reduction of the medullary concentration gradient, or inability of ADH to stimulate insertion of aquaporin channels into the luminal membranes of collecting duct cells leads to excessive renal water losses and hypernatremia.

- Elevated plasma osmolality, i.e., hypernatremia, triggers a thirst response by the hypothalamus. If water intake exceeds water loss or net solute gain, hypernatremia is avoided. Hypernatremia develops when the thirst response is impaired or when there is a lack of access to water, a common circumstance for mechanically ventilated patients and the elderly with cognitive impairments and physical limitations.

Hypernatremia can be classified in the following manner:

1. Excessive water loss
   a. Gastrointestinal losses
      i. Vomiting or nasogastric losses
      ii. Ileostomy
      iii. Pancreaticobiliary fistula
      iv. Diarrhea
      v. Laxatives
   b. Renal losses
      i. Osmotic diuresis
         A. Osmotic diuretics (mannitol)
         B. Glycosuria (hyperglycemia or use of SGLT2 inhibitors)
         C. Urea diuresis (e.g., steroid use, high-protein diet)
         D. Postobstructive and post-acute tubular necrosis (post-ATN) diuresis
      ii. Water diuresis
         A. Central diabetes insipidus (DI)
            a. Genetic
               i. Autosomal dominant
               ii. Autosomal recessive
            b. Acquired (e.g., post trauma, iatrogenic, craniopharyngioma, metastatic cancers, encephalitis)
            c. Sarcoidosis
            d. Multifocal Langerhans cell histiocytosis
            e. Eosinophilic granulomatosis
         B. Nephrogenic diabetes insipidus
            a. Genetic
               i. Arginine vasopressin receptor 2 (AVPR2) or aquaporin 2 (AQP2) mutations
               ii. Autosomal dominant polycystic kidney disease
            b. Acquired
               i. Chronic kidney disease
               ii. Post-ATN diuresis
               iii. Hypokalemia
               iv. Hypercalcemia (diverse causes)
               v. Drugs (e.g., lithium, amphotericin, ifosfamide, demeclocycline)
               vi. Gestation (increased placental vasopressinase)
2. Impaired water intake
   a. Adipsia or hypodipsia
      i. Septooptic dysplasia
      ii. Craniopharyngioma
   b. Impaired access to water
      i. Mechanical ventilation
      ii. Dementia
      iii. Cognitive impairment

TABLE 1 Causes of Hypernatremia

Hypovolemic Hypernatremia

Renal Loss
- Loop diuretics
- Post-AKI diuresis
- Postobstructive diuresis
- Osmotic diuresis (hyperglycemia, mannitol, urea)

Extrarenal Loss
- Gastrointestinal (diarrhea, nasogastric suctioning, vomiting)
- Skin (sweating, burns)

Euvolemic Hypernatremia

Renal Loss
- Diabetes Insipidus (ADH-dependent mechanism)
  - Central DI (complete or partial)
  - Nephrogenic DI (X-linked recessive with defect in V2 receptor or aquaporin, unresponsive to ADH)
  - Gestational DI
- Acquired Nephrogenic DI
  - Electrolyte disturbances (hypercalcemia, hypokalemia)
  - Drug-induced (amphotericin B, lithium, foscarnet)
  - Chronic kidney disease (medullary cystic disease, sickle cell anemia, amyloidosis, Sjögren syndrome)
  - Malnutritiono

Extrarenal loss
- Increased insensible loss (fevers, sweating, tachypnea)
- Decreased intake
  - Primary hypodipsia
  - Reset osmostat
  - Decreased access to water (altered mental status, iatrogenic)
- Water loss into cells (seizures, exercise)

Hypervolemic Hypernatremia
- Excessive sodium administration (saline or bicarbonate)
- Hyperalimentation
- Salt ingestion
- Mineralocorticoid excess
- Hypertonic dialysis

ADH, Antidiuretic hormone; *AKI*, acute kidney injury; *DI*, diabetes insipidus.

Adapted from Gilbert SJ, Weiner DE: *National Kidney Foundation primer on kidney disease*, ed 6, Philadelphia, 2017, Elsevier Saunders.

3. Excessive sodium intake
   a. Hypertonic saline or sodium bicarbonate administration
   b. Salt tablet ingestion
   c. Salt-water drowning

An alternative classification based on the volume status of the patient is provided in Table 1.

Dx DIAGNOSIS

DIFFERENTIAL DIAGNOSIS

Dehydration refers to net water deficits, and its clinical result is hypernatremia. Conversely, volume depletion occurs as a result of net loss of total body sodium and water, which results in decreased intravascular volume. Recognizing dehydration and volume depletion as distinct entities that may coexist has management implications. For example, euvolemic hypernatremia is due to pure water loss, and replacing water deficit is adequate therapy. This strategy is not appropriate in hypovolemic hypernatremia because volume (sodium and potassium) and water losses require replacement.

WORKUP

- Workup of hypernatremia begins with a detailed history and physical examination. Historical features that reveal volume depletion and/or dehydration are crucial and include a family history of diabetes insipidus and medication or drug use.
- In hospitalized patients, careful assessments of cumulative fluid balances and fluid losses must be made.
- In adults, hypernatremia usually develops from net water loss and inability to access water (e.g., altered mentation, mechanical ventilation). If access to water is not restricted, etiologies that impair the thirst center should be entertained.
- In the presence of polyuria, the underlying etiology should be sought.

LABORATORY TESTS

- Serum chemistry: S_{Na} with serial repetition based on clinical scenario (e.g., 2–12 hours). Frequent monitoring facilitates an appropriate correction rate of S_{Na} and evaluation of the response to therapy. Derangements of other electrolyte and renal parameters frequently accompany hypernatremia.
- Urine osmolality (U_{osm}): In the presence of a functioning ADH axis, a rise in plasma osmolality leads to ADH-mediated urinary concentration (U_{osm} exceeds P_{osm}, typically, >600–700 mOsm/kg). Thus, U_{osm} may signal the presence of DI.
  1. Low U_{osm} (<300 mOsm/kg) suggests hypernatremia from CDI or NDI. After an initial diagnostic workup is conducted, will need to differentiate CDI from NDI, as outlined in DI section.
  2. High U_{osm} is likely due to extrarenal water losses.
- Urine sodium (U_{Na}) and urine potassium (U_K): U_{NA} assists in assessing intravascular volume (Fig. 1), whereas U_{NA} and U_K help quantify urine electrolyte-free water clearance to guide therapy as explained below. Urinary parameters should be monitored every 12 to 24 hours until S_{Na} is adequately corrected.

Rx TREATMENT

- Treatment of hypernatremia requires the replacement of the existing water deficit and concurrent daily water losses.
- Volume replacement may be required, and may take precedence when volume depletion is present.
- A stepwise approach to the therapy of hypernatremia is depicted in Fig 2.
  1. Step 1: Identify the rate of correction, rate of rise of S_{Na}.

- Step 1: Identify rate of correction
- Step 2: Calculate free water deficit

$$\text{Water deficit} = \text{TBW}\left[\frac{\text{Current } S_{Na} - \text{Desired } S_{Na}}{\text{Desired } S_{Na}}\right]$$

- Step 3: Choose fluid replacement regimen

$$\text{Change in } S_{Na} = \frac{\text{Infusate Na} - \text{Current } S_{Na}}{\text{TBW} + 1}$$

- Step 4: Assess ongoing water losses.
  - Urinary water losses estimated by free water clearance

$$C_{electrolyte\text{-}free} = V\left[1 - \frac{U_{Na} + U_K}{S_{Na}}\right]$$

  - Insensible water losses approximately 15-20 mL/kg/day
- Step 5: Determine underlying cause

FIG. 2 Approach to treatment of hypernatremia. $C_{electrolyte\text{-}free}$, Electrolyte-free water clearance; *Na*, sodium; S_{Na}, serum sodium; *TBW*, total body water; U_{Na}, urine sodium; U_K, urine potassium; *V*, urine volume. (Adapted from Gilbert SJ, Weiner DE: *National Kidney Foundation primer on kidney disease*, ed 6, Philadelphia, 2017, Elsevier Saunders.)

a. Although the exact risk is unknown, rapid correction of chronic hyponatremia (>48 hr) can have deleterious neurologic consequences, namely cerebral edema.
b. Based on clinical data from infants, chronic hypernatremia should not be corrected faster than 10–128 mEq/L per day or 0.5 mEq/L per hour. This rate would apply to most nonhospitalized elderly patients, as hypernatremia develops over several days.
c. In the rare patient with acute hypernatremia (e.g., intentional or accidental massive sodium ingestions), S_{Na} should be corrected rapidly (within 24 hour) to normal levels to prevent osmotic demyelination.

2. Step 2: Calculate free water deficit.
   a. Free water deficit is the volume of free water required to correct S_{Na} to the desired value. This is estimated with the following formula:
      (1) Water Deficit = TBW × [Current S_{Na} – (Desired S_{Na}/Desired S_{Na})]
   b. In the preceding formula, TBW is the estimated total body water. Desired SNa is the target SNa one wishes to achieve in a 24-hr period as determined in Step 1.
   c. As a general estimate, TBW estimates are 50% to 60% of lean body weight in men and women.
3. Step 3: Choose fluid replacement regimen.
   a. In patients with a pure water deficit, the calculated water deficit in Step 2 should be replaced as either enteral water or intravenous D_5W. Never infuse pure water by intravenous route.
   b. When feasible, the enteral route is preferred because rapid glucose infusion-induced hyperglycemia may cause further osmotic diuresis. This pathophysiology occurs when D5W infusion rates exceed approximately 300 ml/hr.
   c. The rate of replacement (ml/hr) of the water deficit is obtained by dividing the calculated water deficit volume by 24 hours. However, the ongoing rate of water losses must be addressed simultaneously.
   d. Because hypovolemia is present in more than 50% of cases of hypernatremia, concurrent volume replacement with isotonic fluid should be administered (0.9% sodium chloride [NaCl]) when appropriate. An alternative strategy is to use a single infusion of 0.45% saline solution that replaces salt and water. For example, 1 L of 0.45% NaCl adds 500 ml of water and 500 ml of 0.9% NaCl to the total body water.
   e. The change in S_{Na} with 1 L of a particular replacement fluid can be predicted by the following formula:
      (1) Change in S_{Na} = (Infusate Sodium – Current S_{Na}) / (TBW + 1)
4. Step 4: Assess ongoing water losses.
   a. Patients have ongoing daily water losses that must be added to the above water-deficit volume. Water losses occur via urinary water excretion and insensible losses from skin, stool, and respiratory tract. Failure to account for these losses will result in undercorrection of hypernatremia.
   b. Urinary losses can be estimated by the electrolyte-free water clearance equation in Fig. 2.
   c. Insensible water losses can be estimated as 15–20 ml/kg/day.

- If hypernatremia is due to hypervolemia, consider the addition of loop diuretics to remove excess sodium.
- Evaluate for any underlying cause of hypernatremia and treat accordingly.
- Replace other electrolyte deficits such as potassium.
- Repeat Steps 1 through 4 until S_{Na} is corrected to 140 to 145 mEq/L.
- The preceding formulas only represent guidance. Largely due to estimation errors in assessing TBW and fluid losses, under- or overestimation is common. As a result, serial measurements of S_{Na} must be made and supplemented by clinical judgement, sometimes as frequently as every 2 hours during initial hours of management.

DISPOSITION

Management of hypernatremia generally warrants inpatient admission because patients have underlying conditions that impair the thirst response.

REFERRAL

Nephrology consultation for management of hypernatremia and evaluation of underlying causes can be considered. Endocrinology consultation may be warranted if central DI is suspected.

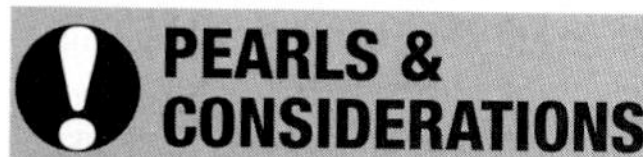

COMMENTS

- Hypernatremia is a water-deficit problem that often is associated with an impaired thirst mechanism.
- Volume deficit may be present simultaneously.
- A judicious rate of correction and water deficit should be applied.

SUGGESTED READINGS

Available at ExpertConsult.com

RELATED CONTENT

Diabetes Insipidus (Related Key Topic)

AUTHOR: **LALATHAKSHA KUMBAR, M.D.**

BASIC INFORMATION

DEFINITION

Hyperparathyroidism is an endocrine disorder caused by excessive secretion of parathyroid hormone (PTH) from the parathyroid glands. Autonomous production of PTH resulting in hypercalcemia defines primary hyperparathyroidism. Secondary hyperparathyroidism occurs when the parathyroid glands appropriately increase PTH production in response to low calcium or vitamin D states. Primary hyperparathyroidism is the focus of this section.

ICD-10CM CODES

E21.0	Primary hyperparathyroidism
E21.1	Secondary hyperparathyroidism, not elsewhere classified
E21.2	Other hyperparathyroidism
E21.3	Hyperparathyroidism, unspecified
N25.81	Secondary hyperparathyroidism of renal origin

EPIDEMIOLOGY & DEMOGRAPHICS

INCIDENCE: Four cases per 100,000 persons per yr. Although malignancy is the most common cause of hypercalcemia in hospitalized patients, primary hyperparathyroidism is the most common cause of hypercalcemia in the outpatient setting.

PREVALENCE: Varies by country and race with approximately nine cases/1000 persons in the United States.

PREDOMINANT SEX AND AGE: Higher prevalence in women (female:male ratio 3 to 4:1) and older age (peaks in the seventh decade of life).

PHYSICAL FINDINGS & CLINICAL PRESENTATION

The majority of patients with primary hyperparathyroidism are asymptomatic. Diagnosis is usually considered in patients after an incidental discovery of hypercalcemia or during the evaluation for decreased bone mass. The development of symptoms varies with severity and rapidity of disease progression and reflects both the hypercalcemic and hyperparathyroid components of the disease process.

- Cardiovascular: Hypertension, shortened QT interval, bradycardia, arrhythmia, valvular calcification, left ventricular hypertrophy, increased mean carotid intima-media thickness
- GI: Anorexia, nausea, vomiting, constipation, abdominal pain, peptic ulcer disease, pancreatitis
- Genitourinary (GU): Nephrolithiasis, nephrocalcinosis, renal insufficiency, polydipsia, polyuria, nocturia, nephrogenic diabetes insipidus, renal tubular acidosis
- Musculoskeletal: Weakness, myopathy, bone pain, osteopenia, osteoporosis, gout, pseudogout, chondrocalcinosis, osteitis fibrosa cystica, subperiosteal bone resorption (Fig. E1)
- CNS: Confusion, anxiety, fatigue, lethargy, obtundation, depression, coma
- Other: Pruritus, metastatic calcifications, band keratopathy

ETIOLOGY

- Most cases of primary hyperparathyroidism are sporadic, but hyperparathyroidism can be associated with rare familial conditions such as multiple endocrine neoplasia (MEN-1 and MEN-2). Mutations in certain genes have been linked to tumor development in both sporadic and familial cases such as hyperparathyroidism-jaw tumor syndrome. Higher prevalence of hyperparathyroidism is noted with head and neck irradiation, chronic low calcium or vitamin D status, and lithium therapy.
- Pathologic characteristics include adenoma (80%), hyperplasia (15% to 20%), or carcinomas (<1%).

DIAGNOSIS

DIFFERENTIAL DIAGNOSIS

- Primary hyperparathyroidism:
  1. Adenoma (80%)
  2. Hyperplasia (15% to 20%)
  3. Carcinomas (<1%)
- Secondary hyperparathyroidism precipitated by conditions that result in hypocalcemia:
  1. Renal calcium loss (i.e., medication: loop diuretics and hypercalciuria)
  2. Calcium deficiency
  3. Vitamin D deficiency
  4. Malabsorption
  5. Chronic kidney disease (most common)
  6. Pseudohypoparathyroidism (PTH resistance)
  7. Inhibition of bone resorption (i.e., bisphosphonates)
- Other causes of hypercalcemia include:
  1. Medications: Thiazide diuretics, lithium therapy
  2. Vitamin D intoxication, milk-alkali syndrome
  3. Familial hypocalciuric hypercalcemia (FHH)
  4. Renal failure (tertiary hyperparathyroidism)
  5. Thyrotoxicosis
  6. Granulomatous disorders (e.g., sarcoidosis)
  7. Malignancy (e.g., lung cancer, lymphoma, multiple myeloma, bone metastasis)
  8. Prolonged immobilization

WORKUP

- Typically, primary hyperparathyroidism is confirmed with an elevated serum calcium and PTH level.
  1. Two measurements of serum calcium are required for the confirmation of hypercalcemia. Total calcium should be corrected for low albumin utilizing the formula: Corrected Calcium = Serum Calcium + $0.8 \times 4 -$ serum albumin. If a reliable laboratory is available, ionized calcium should be considered, especially in conditions associated with acid-base disturbances or low albumin states. Patients with primary hyperparathyroidism can also present with normal calcium levels. The most common reason for this finding is concomitant vitamin D deficiency and primary hyperparathyroidism.
  2. The serum intact PTH (iPTH) level is the single best test to evaluate the etiology of hypercalcemia. PTH is elevated or in the high normal range (i.e., inappropriately normal for an elevated calcium state) in primary hyperparathyroidism. PTH is decreased in most other conditions associated with elevated calcium.
- Other causes of hypercalcemia should be ruled out. These are typically associated with low PTH levels. Exceptions include lithium use and FHH.
  1. Review medication history to determine lithium, thiazide, vitamin D, or calcium intake.
  2. Check 24-hour urine calcium:creatinine to rule out FHH. Urine calcium is usually low in FHH. PTH can be normal or high in FHH.
  3. Consider PTH-related peptide (PTHrP) to evaluate hypercalcemia related to malignancies and vitamin D 1,25 to assess hypercalcemia secondary to granulomatous diseases or lymphomas.
  4. Multiple myeloma and bone metastasis can also result in a high calcium state and therefore must be appropriately evaluated.
- Rule out other causes of elevated PTH (i.e., secondary hyperparathyroidism). Serum calcium is typically low or low-normal in secondary hyperparathyroidism.
  1. Check calcium and 25 OH-vitamin D to rule out deficiency states.
  2. Check serum creatinine to assess renal function and 24-hour urine calcium and creatinine to evaluate renal loss.

LABORATORY TESTS

- Serum calcium (ionized or corrected calcium): Normal or elevated in primary hyperparathyroidism
- Serum phosphorus: Low or low-normal in primary hyperparathyroidism
- PTH: Elevated or high normal in primary hyperparathyroidism
- Serum creatinine and estimated glomerular filtration rate (eGFR)
- 24-hour urine calcium and creatinine: Hypercalcemia is present in up to 30% of patients with primary hyperparathroidism
- PTHrP and 1,25 OH-vitamin D levels 25 OH-vitamin D level
- ECG may reveal shortening of the QT interval secondary to severe hypercalcemia (>12 mg/dl)

IMAGING STUDIES

- Parathyroid localization with technetium-99m sestamibi can identify potential adenomas to help with surgical planning.
- Parathyroid ultrasound is also used to localize the parathyroid adenoma.
- Bone mineral density (BMD) of the spine, hip, and forearm (distal third) is recommended for all patients with hyperparathyroidism in order to assess the risk for osteoporosis and fragility fractures. Cortical bone loss (i.e., forearm or hip) is greater than trabecular bone loss (i.e., spine) in hyperparathyroidism.
- Renal ultrasound can be considered to assess asymptomatic renal stones.

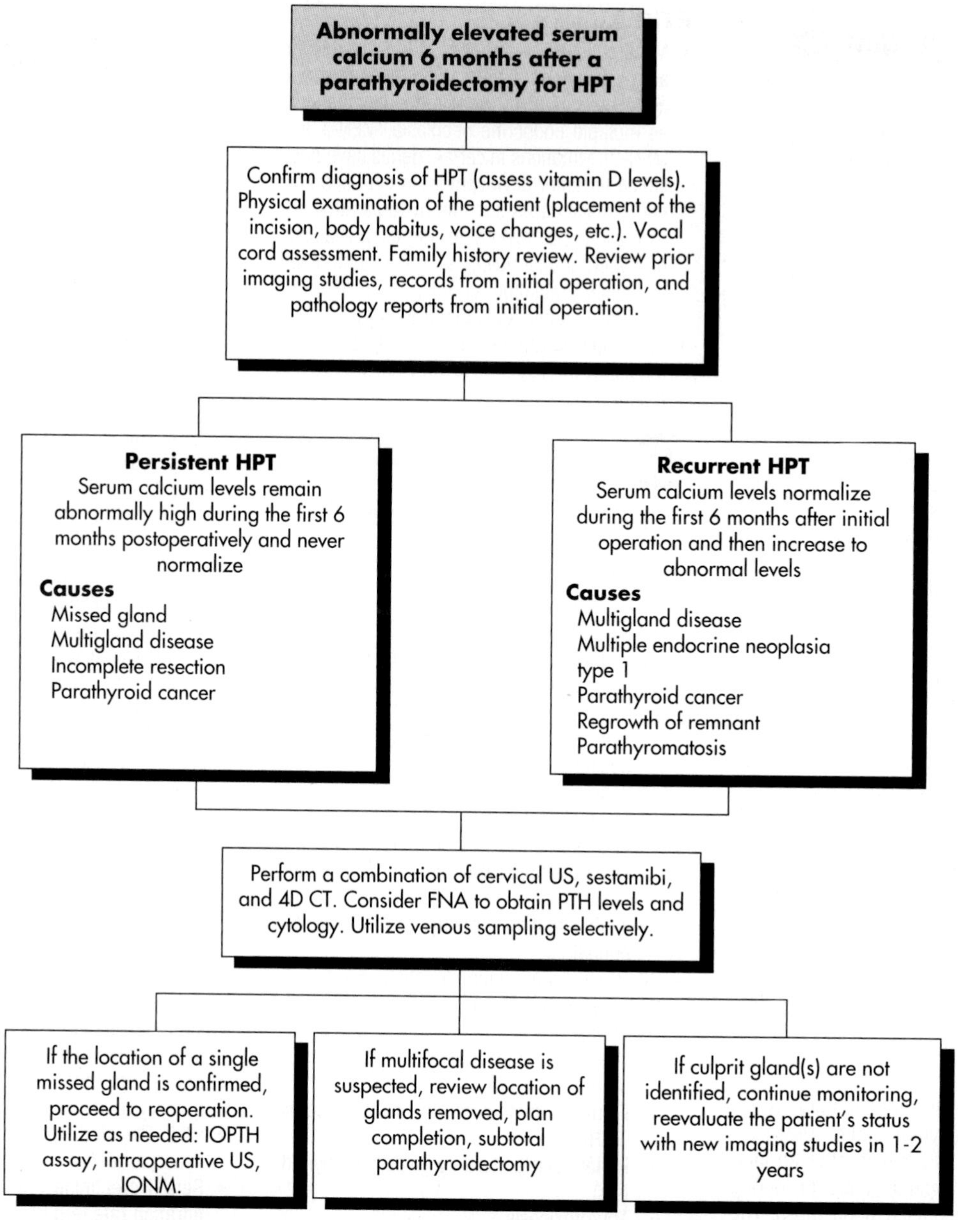

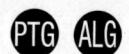

Abnormally elevated serum calcium 6 months after a parathyroidectomy for HPT

Confirm diagnosis of HPT (assess vitamin D levels). Physical examination of the patient (placement of the incision, body habitus, voice changes, etc.). Vocal cord assessment. Family history review. Review prior imaging studies, records from initial operation, and pathology reports from initial operation.

Persistent HPT
Serum calcium levels remain abnormally high during the first 6 months postoperatively and never normalize
Causes
Missed gland
Multigland disease
Incomplete resection
Parathyroid cancer

Recurrent HPT
Serum calcium levels normalize during the first 6 months after initial operation and then increase to abnormal levels
Causes
Multigland disease
Multiple endocrine neoplasia type 1
Parathyroid cancer
Regrowth of remnant
Parathyromatosis

Perform a combination of cervical US, sestamibi, and 4D CT. Consider FNA to obtain PTH levels and cytology. Utilize venous sampling selectively.

If the location of a single missed gland is confirmed, proceed to reoperation. Utilize as needed: IOPTH assay, intraoperative US, IONM.

If multifocal disease is suspected, review location of glands removed, plan completion, subtotal parathyroidectomy

If culprit gland(s) are not identified, continue monitoring, reevaluate the patient's status with new imaging studies in 1-2 years

FIG. 2 Algorithm for managing persistent or recurrent hyperparathyroidism (HPT). *4D CT*, Four-dimensional computed tomography; *FNA*, fine-needle aspiration; *IONM*, intraoperative neurophysiologic monitoring; *IOPTH*, intraoperative parathyroid hormone; *PTH*, parathyroid hormone; *sestamibi*, technetium (^{99m}Tc) sestamibi imaging; *US*, ultrasonography. (From Cameron JL, Cameron AM: *Current surgical therapy*, ed 12, Philadelphia, 2017, Elsevier.)

Rx TREATMENT

Modality of treatment depends on disease progression and which patients are more likely to suffer end-organ effects of hyperparathyroidism or benefit the most from surgery. Fig. 2 illustrates an algorithm for managing persistent or recurrent hyperparathyroidism.

- Surgery is the only definitive treatment for symptomatic primary hyperparathyroidism. Surgery can normalize calcium levels, decrease the risk for kidney stones, improve bone mineral density and fracture risk, and enhance quality of life measures.
  1. Indications for parathyroidectomy (Box 1):
     a. All patients younger than 50 yr
     b. Hypercalcemia (Ca >1 mg/dl above upper limit normal)
     c. Creatinine clearance <60 ml/min
     d. 24-h urine for calcium >400 mg/dl (>10 mmol/dl)
     e. Presence of nephrolithiasis or nephrocalcinosis by x-ray, ultrasound, or CT
     f. Osteoporosis
        a. Bone mineral density (BMD) by dual-energy x-ray absorptiometry (DXA): T-score ≤2.5 at lumbar spine, total hip, femoral neck, or distal one third radius
        b. Vertebral fracture by x-ray, CT, MRI, or vertebral fracture assessment (VFA) by DXA
  2. Surgical approaches include:
     a. Minimally invasive parathyroidectomy has increased in popularity. The surgeon will identify and remove the abnormal gland that was identified on preoperative imaging. This technique has limited dissection and has improved recovery time. Intraoperative monitoring of PTH level is done to ensure the removal of the abnormal gland. Fall of PTH level by 50%, into the normal range, is expected within 10 to 15 min after removal of the abnormal gland.
     b. Bilateral neck exploration under general anesthesia is the traditional surgical approach. All parathyroid glands are identified and compared. An experienced endocrine surgeon cures >95% of patients undergoing bilateral neck exploration. Potential complications include transient and permanent hypocalcemia secondary to hypoparathyroidism and recurrent laryngeal nerve injury.

BOX 1 Indications for Parathyroidectomy in Patients With Secondary and Tertiary Hyperparathyroidism

Indications for Parathyroidectomy in Patients With Secondary Hyperparathyroidism (SHPT)

SHPT refractory to medical therapy:

- Parathyroid hormone >1000 pg/ml
- Calcium × Phosphorus product >55

Renal osteodystrophy

Calciphylaxis

Other retractable symptoms, including uremic pruritus, persistent anemia, bone pain, muscle pain, abdominal pain, fatigue, and weakness

Indications for Parathyroidectomy in Patients With Tertiary Hyperparathyroidism

Severe hypercalcemia (calcium >12.5 mg/dl)

Persistent hypercalcemia ≥2 years after renal transplantation, associated with:

- Decline in renal function, without graft rejection
- Nephrolithiasis
- Progressive bone disease
- Pancreatitis

From Cameron JL, Cameron AM: *Current surgical therapy*, ed 12, Philadelphia, 2017, Elsevier.

- Ablation therapy (e.g., ethanol, angiographic, radiofrequency) can be considered in patients who are not surgical candidates. Limited data are available on efficacy and side effects. Repeat ablations may be required if hypercalcemia persists.
- Medical management:
  1. Avoid medications that precipitate hypercalcemia (e.g., thiazide or lithium)
  2. Because inadequate calcium and vitamin D status stimulates PTH, it is not necessary to significantly restrict calcium and vitamin D intake. Vitamin D replacement safely improves vitamin D level and decreases PTH level without significantly increasing serum calcium level and urinary calcium excretion. Repletion of vitamin D is recommended in patients whose levels are <30 mg/dl (75 mmol/L). Dietary calcium intake should be approximately 1000 mg/day.
  3. Encourage physical activity since immobilization increases bone resorption.
  4. Recommend adequate hydration (at least 2 L) to minimize the risk of nephrolithiasis.
     a. For patients who are not surgical candidates or who refuse surgery, pharmacologic options are available. The choice of pharmacologic agents is dependent on the desired goal. Cinacalcet (Sensipar) is an oral calcimimetic agent that activates the calcium sensing receptor in the parathyroid gland. It decreases PTH production and subsequently normalizes or decreases serum calcium levels, without significant BMD changes. It is indicated for the treatment of severe hypercalcemia in patients with primary hyperparathyroidism who are unable to undergo surgery. It is also indicated for the treatment of secondary hyperparathyroidism associated with chronic kidney disease and for hypercalcemia associated with parathyroid carcinoma.
     b. Agents such as bisphosphonates (e.g., alendronate, zoledronate) that inhibit bone resorption and increase BMD should be considered when improvement in BMD is the primary goal in patients with hyperparathyroidism.
- Medical monitoring is recommended for asymptomatic primary hyperparathyroidism. The majority of patients do not manifest disease progression during observation. However, approximately 25% of asymptomatic patients require surgery over a 10-yr follow-up period.
  1. Indications for medical monitoring:
     a. Clinically asymptomatic and >50 yr old
     b. Serum calcium level only mildly elevated (<1 mg/dl above upper limit normal)
     c. GFR >60 ml/min and no nephrolithiasis or nephrocalcinosis
     d. No evidence of osteoporosis
     e. Medically unfit for surgery or refusing surgery
- Symptoms should be assessed regularly. Serum calcium, PTH, creatinine, and eGFR should be checked semiannually. DXA performed at three sites every 1 to 2 yr or vertebral fracture assessment of the spine is clinically indicated (e.g., height loss, back pain).

ACUTE GENERAL Rx

Severe and/or symptomatic hypercalcemia may require hospitalization, especially if serum calcium >12 mg/dl. Acute management of hypercalcemia includes:

- Vigorous hydration with IV normal saline (2 to 4 L/day). Fluid status must be monitored in patients with cardiac dysfunction or renal insufficiency in order to avoid fluid overload.
- Bisphosphonates can effectively decrease calcium levels. Zoledronate (4 mg IV over 15 min) or pamidronate (60 to 90 mg IV over 4 hours) are both effective. Onset of action is 24 to 48 hours.
- Calcitonin (4 units/kg IM/SC every 12 hours) may be used with bisphosphonates to achieve a more rapid reduction of calcium levels. Onset of action is within hours.

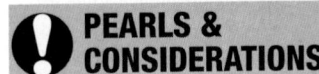

COMMENTS

- Parathyroidectomy should be considered for all patients with symptomatic hyperparathyroidism. If surgery is contraindicated or not desired, cinacalcet and bisphosphonates can be used.
- Asymptomatic patients can be monitored with serial calcium, creatinine, eGFR, and bone mineral density measurements. Disease progression may result in surgery.
- Most patients can be managed medically by limiting factors that result in hypercalcemia (e.g., dehydration, immobilization, thiazide diuretics) and maintaining normal calcium and vitamin D intake.
- Patients with osteopenia and high fracture risk may require antiresorptive therapy such as bisphosphonates.

SUGGESTED READINGS

Available at ExpertConsult.com

RELATED CONTENT

Hyperparathyroidism (Patient Information)

AUTHOR: **THARANI RAJESWARAN, M.D.**

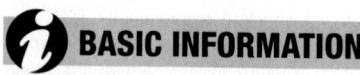

DEFINITION

Hypersensitivity pneumonitis (HP) is a group of immunologically mediated pulmonary diseases, with or without systemic manifestations (e.g., fever, weight loss), caused by the inhalation of an antigen to which the patient is sensitized and hyperresponsive. Sensitization and exposure alone in the absence of symptoms do not define the disease.

SYNONYMS

HP - Extrinsic allergic alveolitis (EAA)
Bird fancier's lung
Farmer's lung
Malt worker's lung
"Ventilation" pneumonitis
Maple bark-stripper's lung
Sauna taker's lung
Hot tub lung

ICD-10CM CODES

J67.x Hypersensitivity pneumonitis due to specific organic dusts
J67.9 Hypersensitivity pneumonitis due to unspecified organic dust

EPIDEMIOLOGY & DEMOGRAPHICS

- Estimates of the prevalence and incidence of HP vary considerably and depend on the definition and methods used to establish the diagnosis.
- Clinical presentation depends on the intensity of exposure, environmental conditions, and genetic risk factors that remain poorly understood.
- More than 300 causative agents have been identified, and the number continues to grow.
- Causative agents in residential and occupational exposures include birds, mold, humidifiers, fountains, steam irons, dry sausage molds, moldy cheese, contaminated wood, biofilm contained within wind instruments (e.g., trombone, saxophone), and organic and inorganic chemicals, including metalworking fluids.
- It is likely that genetic factors are also involved that result in an exaggerated lung response to an offending agent. The major histocompatibility complex is the most studied thus far.

PHYSICAL FINDINGS & CLINICAL PRESENTATION

Vary depending on frequency and intensity of antigen exposure.

- Acute: Fever, cough, malaise, and dyspnea 4 to 6 hours after an intense exposure. Symptoms resolve with removal of the inciting agent, typically within 12 to 24 hours.
- Often misdiagnosed initially as a viral illness or asthma.
- Subacute: Insidious onset of productive cough, dyspnea on exertion, anorexia, and weight loss, usually from a heavy, sustained exposure
- Chronic: Gradually progressive cough, dyspnea, malaise, and weight loss, usually from low-grade or recurrent exposure
- Physical examination: Hypoxemia, cyanosis, rales, possible fever

ETIOLOGY

- Numerous environmental agents, often encountered in occupational settings.
- Common sources of antigens: "Moldy" hay, silage, grain, or vegetables; bird droppings or feathers (including those found commonly in down pillows, blankets, and upholstered furniture); low-molecular-weight chemicals (e.g., isocyanates); pharmaceutical products.
- Fig. E1 illustrates the pathogenesis of hypersensitivity pneumonitis.

Dx DIAGNOSIS

- Accurate diagnosis is important for differentiating HP from other interstitial lung diseases because the prognosis and treatment may differ.
- The clinical syndrome of acute HP is indistinguishable from an acute respiratory infection with a history of illness occurring within hours of exposure to an antigen.
- Need high index of suspicion.
- Detailed occupational and home exposure history is required.
- Lung biopsy is often necessary for diagnosis.

DIFFERENTIAL DIAGNOSIS

Acute Stages	Chronic Stages
Allergic bronchopulmonary aspergillosis	Idiopathic pulmonary fibrosis (IPF)
Pulmonary embolism	Bronchiectasis
Asthma	Chronic bronchitis
Aspiration pneumonia	Nonspecific interstitial pneumonia (NSIP)
Bacterial pneumonia	
Fungal or mycobacterial pneumonia	
Bronchiolitis obliterans–organizing pneumonia	Connective tissue–related lung disease
Eosinophilic pneumonia	Sarcoidosis
Churg-Strauss syndrome	
Wegener granulomatosis	

WORKUP

No single radiologic, physiologic, or immunologic test is specific for the diagnosis of HP. HP must be suspected in any patient presenting with cough, dyspnea, fever, and malaise. A thorough history focusing on potential exposures is essential. Table 1 describes examples of occupational causes of HP.

Environmental and occupational history questions should ask about grain dusts, animal handling, food processing, cooling towers, fountains, metal-working fluids, symptom improvement away from exposure, pets (particularly birds), hobbies involving chemicals, feathers, or fur, organic dusts, presence of humidifiers, dehumidifiers, or hot tubs/saunas, leaking or flooding indoors, visible fungal growth in living or working environment, feather pillows, bedding, or upholstered furniture.

TABLE 1 Examples of Occupational Causes of Hypersensitivity Pneumonitis

Occupation	Cause
Farmer	Thermophilic actinomycetes in moldy hay
Metal worker	Contamination of metal-working fluids with microorganisms such as Mycobacteria immunogens or fungi
Worker exposed to humidifiers	Contamination with microorganisms such as protozoa or fungi
Sugarcane worker	Moldy sugarcane (bagassosis)
Maple bark stripper	Fungi
Chicken or turkey worker	Avian proteins
Pharmaceutical worker	Penicillin
Food handler	Soybeans
Office worker	Microorganisms contaminating air conditioners or humidifiers
Swimming pool attendant	Fungal contamination in sprays around pool area
Animal worker	Rat proteins
Mushroom worker	Fungi
Wheat farmer or handler	Weevil-infested flour
Greenhouse worker	Fungi
Workers spraying urethane paint or adhesives/sealants (or less often, other workers using diisocyanate)	Methylene diphenyl diisocyanate, hexamethylene diisocyanate, toluene diisocyanates
Chemical worker using plastics, resins, paints	Trimellitic anhydride

From Goldman L, Schafer AI: *Goldman's Cecil medicine*, ed 24, Philadelphia, 2012, Saunders.

Major diagnostic criteria:
- History of compatible clinical symptoms, physical exam, changes on chest radiograph or high resolution CT (HRCT) of the chest, and pulmonary function tests. Particularly suspicious if symptoms appear to worsen within hours after antigen exposure
- Confirmation of exposure to the offending agent by history, investigation of the environment, serum precipitin tests to potential agents (often referred to as a "hypersensitivity panel" by many labs)
- BAL fluid lymphocytosis (if performed)
- Compatible histologic changes by lung biopsy (if performed): Poorly formed granulomas or mononuclear cell infiltrate
- Positive natural challenge (reproduction of symptoms and laboratory abnormalities after exposure to the suspected environment) or controlled inhalation challenge

LABORATORY TESTS

- Routine laboratory tests do not make the diagnosis, but typically the erythrocyte sedimentation rate, C-reactive protein, lactate dehydrogenase, and leukocyte count are increased; elevated immunoglobulins IgG and IgM are nonspecific; rheumatoid factor (RF) and immune complexes are often positive; peripheral eosinophil count and serum IgE are generally normal.
- Lactate dehydrogenase (LDH) is increased and tends to decrease with improvement.
- Pulmonary function tests: Restrictive ventilatory pattern is typically seen. Decreased FEV_1, decreased forced vital capacity, decreased total lung capacity, decreased diffusion capacity, and decreased static compliance.
- Arterial blood gases show mild hypoxemia (worsens with exercise).
- A-a gradient shows slight increase.
- Serum precipitin test for IgG antibodies against offending antigen may be positive in serum. Precipitins are sensitive but not specific for HP (asymptomatic patients may have IgG antibodies in serum). HP may also be present without a positive precipitin test.
- Skin testing is generally not helpful in establishing a diagnosis.

IMAGING STUDIES

Chest x-ray: Nonspecific; may be normal in early stage.
- Acute/subacute: Bilateral interstitial and alveolar nodular infiltrates in a patchy or homogeneous distribution.
- Chronic: Diffuse reticulonodular infiltrates and fibrosis.

High-resolution chest CT scan (Fig. 2): No pathognomonic features but demonstrates airspace and interstitial patterns in the acute and subacute stage. The chronic stage reveals honeycombing, air trapping, and bronchiectasis.

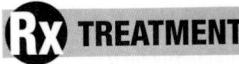

TREATMENT

NONPHARMACOLOGIC THERAPY

Early recognition and avoidance of the causative antigen

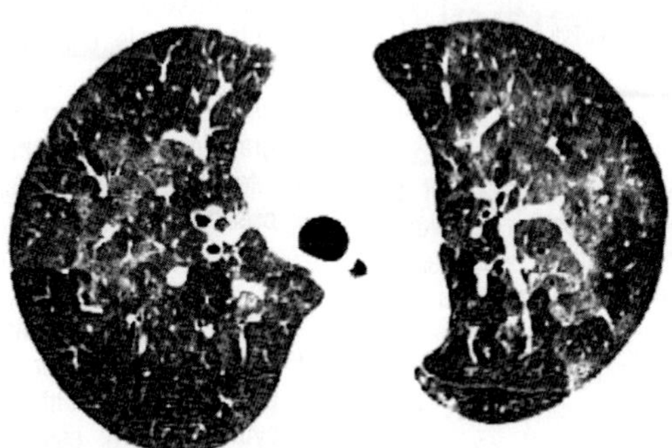

FIG. 2 In this patient with hypersensitivity pneumonitis, patchy ground-glass opacity is visible bilaterally. (From Mason RJ: *Murray & Nadel's textbook of respiratory medicine*, ed 5, Philadelphia, 2010, Saunders.)

ACUTE GENERAL Rx

- Glucocorticoids accelerate initial lung recovery but may have no effect long term (from a controlled study in farmer's lung). No prospective, randomized, placebo-controlled trials for other types of HP or subacute and chronic stages.
- Prednisone 0.5 to 1 mg/kg usually over 1 to 2 wk then tapered over 4 wk. Some patients, particularly those with subacute or chronic presentation, may require a longer course of therapy.

DISPOSITION/PROGNOSIS

Prognosis is generally better in patients with acute or subacute HP. Prognosis is worse in those with older age, desaturation during exercise, and findings of severe fibrosis by lung biopsy.
- Acute: 4 to 48 hours
- Clinical: Fever, chills, cough, hypoxia, malaise
- HRCT: Ground-glass infiltrates
- Immunopathology: Poorly formed, noncaseating granulomas or mononuclear cell infiltration in a peribronchial distribution, frequently with giant cells
- Prognosis: Good

Subacute: Weeks to 4 mo
- Clinical: Dyspnea, cough, episodic flares
- HRCT: Micronodules, air trapping
- Immunopathology: More well-formed, noncaseating granulomas, bronchiolitis, organizing pneumonia, and interstitial fibrosis
- Prognosis: Good

Chronic: 4 mo to yrs
- Clinical: Dyspnea, cough, fatigue, weight loss
- HRCT: Fibrosis (possible), honeycombing, emphysema
- Immunopathology: Granulomatous inflammation may be seen in addition to bronchiolitis obliterans (with or without organizing pneumonia) and honeycombing and fibrosis, lymphocytic infiltration, centrilobular and bridging fibrosis, neutrophil-mediated air space destruction, giant cells
- Prognosis: Generally poor

REFERRAL

- Bronchoscopy: BAL provides useful supportive data in the diagnosis of HP. Usually reveals intense lymphocytosis (typically T cells >50%) of predominantly CD8+ suppressor cells. In the acute stage neutrophils predominate, but as the disease progresses to chronic form the ratio of CD4+ to CD8+ cells increases. When fibrosis is present the number of neutrophils increases.
- Lung biopsy: The histopathologic features of HP are distinctive but not pathognomonic. Bronchiolitis and interstitial pneumonitis with granuloma formation typically is seen. Variable degrees of interstitial fibrosis are seen in the chronic form. Chronic HP may be difficult to distinguish from IPF or NSIP pathologically.
- Laboratory inhalation challenge: Testing to prove a direct relation between a suspected antigen and disease; extract of antigen is inhaled by nebulizer.

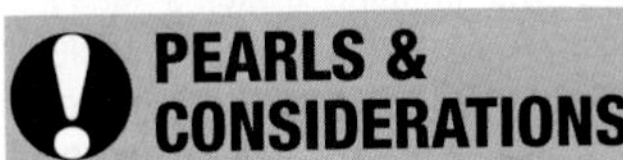

PEARLS & CONSIDERATIONS

A clinical prediction rule using six features has high specificity and sensitivity for the diagnosis of acute and subacute HP:
- Exposure to a known offending agent
- Positive specific precipitating antibody
- Recurrent episodes of symptoms
- Inspiratory crackles
- Symptoms occurring 4 to 8 hr after exposure
- Weight loss

HP occurs more frequently in smokers than nonsmokers (likely from an immunosuppressive effect).

SUGGESTED READINGS

Available at ExpertConsult.com

RELATED CONTENT

Hypersensitivity Pneumonitis (Patient Information)

AUTHOR: **MELISSA H. TUKEY, M.D., M.S.**

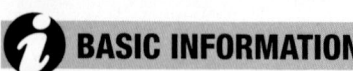

BASIC INFORMATION

DEFINITION

Hypersplenism is a syndrome characterized by splenomegaly, cytopenias (one or more of the following: anemia, thrombocytopenia, or leukopenia), and compensatory hyperplastic bone marrow. These cytopenias are correctable with splenectomy.

ICD-10CM CODE
D73.1 Hypersplenism

EPIDEMIOLOGY & DEMOGRAPHICS

Most often seen in patients with liver disease, hematologic malignancy, and infection

PHYSICAL FINDINGS & CLINICAL PRESENTATION

- Symptoms depend on the size of the spleen, rate of growth, and underlying disease.
- History: Early satiety, abdominal discomfort or fullness, acute left upper quadrant (LUQ) pain (infarction, sequestration crisis), referred pain to left shoulder
- Physical examination: Splenomegaly (normal spleen usually not palpable), LUQ tenderness, presence of a rub in LUQ (suggestive of splenic infarct), stigmata of cytopenias

ETIOLOGY

- The spleen is an important component of the hematologic and immune systems (antigen processing and antibody synthesis). The spleen is responsible for the modification (removal of particles and parasites) and clearance of senescent or poorly deformable red blood cells (RBCs). It also filters blood, removing foreign particles (microorganisms) and other particulates (e.g., complement- or antibody-coated cells) from the circulation. The spleen is a platelet reservoir, storing 30% of platelet mass. It can become the site of hematopoiesis in certain disease states. The spleen's normal activities are augmented when enlarged.
- Splenomegaly increases the proportion of blood channeled through the red pulp, causing inappropriate splenic pooling of both normal and abnormal blood cells. The size of the spleen determines the amount of cell sequestration. Up to 90% of platelets may be pooled in an enlarged spleen. Prolonged sequestration leads to increased destruction of RBCs. Platelets and white blood cells (WBCs) have about normal survival time even when sequestered and may be available if needed.
- Splenomegaly exacerbates cytopenias by dilution, possibly due to plasma volume expansion.

Dx DIAGNOSIS

DIFFERENTIAL DIAGNOSIS

Hypersplenism can be caused by splenomegaly of almost any cause.

- Splenic congestion: Cirrhosis (portal hypertension); congestive heart failure; portal, splenic, or hepatic vein thrombosis
- Hematologic causes: Hemolytic anemia, spherocytosis, elliptocytosis, sickle cell anemia, thalassemia, extramedullary hematopoiesis, chronic transfusions, following use of granulocyte colony-stimulating factor
- Infections: Viral (hepatitis, infectious mononucleosis, cytomegalovirus, HIV/AIDS), bacterial (endocarditis, sepsis, tuberculosis, salmonella, brucella), parasitic (babesiosis, malaria, leishmaniasis, schistosomiasis, toxoplasmosis), fungal
- Malignancy: Acute or chronic leukemia, lymphoma, myeloproliferative diseases (polycythemia vera, essential thrombocythemia, myelofibrosis), splenic or metastatic tumors
- Inflammatory diseases: Rheumatic fever, rheumatoid arthritis (Felty syndrome), systemic lupus erythematosus, sarcoid, serum sickness
- Infiltrative diseases: Amyloidosis, Gaucher disease, Niemann-Pick disease, glycogen storage disease

WORKUP

History (including travel), physical examination, laboratory tests, imaging studies

LABORATORY TESTS

- CBC with differential: Cytopenias, neutrophilia (infection)
- Peripheral smear: RBC and WBC morphology (abnormal cells may suggest infection, malignancy, bone marrow disease, rheumatologic disease), organisms (bacteria, malaria, babesiosis)
- Bone marrow aspiration/biopsy: Hyperplasia of cytopenic cell lines; hematologic, infiltrative, or infectious disorders
- Tests to diagnose suspected cause of splenomegaly: Liver function, hepatitis serology, HIV, rheumatoid factor, antinuclear antibody, tissue biopsy
- Note: Red cell mass (^{51}Cr assay) may be used to assess severity of anemia. RBC mass measurement will differentiate true anemia (decrease in RBCs) from dilutional anemia (plasma volume expansion)

IMAGING STUDIES

Choice of imaging study depends on suspected underlying pathology.

- Ultrasound: Splenic size, presence of cyst or abscess
- CT: Estimate volume, obtain structural information: Cyst, abscess, malignancy
- MRI: Most useful for assessing vascular lesions and infections
- Nuclear medicine: Liver-spleen scan: Assess anatomy and function; may suggest presence of portal hypertension
- Consider additional tests as suggested by history and exam: Chest radiograph, echocardiogram, PET scan

Rx TREATMENT

ACUTE GENERAL Rx

- Treat underlying disease
- Splenectomy is considered if:
  1. Indicated for the management of the underlying cause
  2. Persistent symptomatic disease (severe cytopenia) not responding to therapy
  3. Necessary for diagnosis

Risks:

- Infections (especially encapsulated organisms): Risk greatest in the first 2 yr after splenectomy. Mortality rate from sepsis is fiftyfold greater in asplenic patients. Attempts to decrease risk include:
  1. Immunization with pneumococcal (PCV13 and PPSV23), meningococcal (MenACWY and MenB), and *Haemophilus influenza* type b (Hib) vaccines (if not previously vaccinated) at least 2 wk before splenectomy. Preferred: PCV13 vaccination followed by PPSV23 vaccination at least 8 wk later. If already immunized with PPSV23, PCV13 vaccine should be given at least 1 yr later. Revaccination with PPSV23 in 5 yr and again after age 65 yr (and 5 yr after most recent dose). Revaccination for meningococcal (MenACWY) every 5 yr. Annual inactivated or recombinant influenza vaccination. Note: If unable to vaccinate 2 wk before splenectomy, vaccinate 2 wk after surgery.
  2. Prophylactic antibiotics after splenectomy in highest-risk patients.
  3. Patient education regarding the importance of rapid initiation of antibiotics at the first sign of infection.
- Thromboembolic complications, especially high risk of portal vein thrombosis.
- Possible increased risk of atherosclerotic heart disease and cancer.
- Splenectomy should not be performed if the spleen is the main site of hematopoiesis as a result of bone marrow failure (e.g., myelofibrosis).
- Other options include partial splenectomy, partial splenic embolization, radiofrequency ablation, portosystemic shunting (for congestive splenomegaly).

DISPOSITION

- Cytopenias are usually correctable with splenectomy; normal cell counts return within a few weeks.
- Splenectomy may alleviate portal hypertension.
- Prognosis depends on the underlying disease.

REFERRAL

Hematology

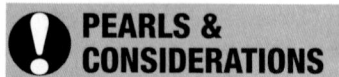

PEARLS & CONSIDERATIONS

Thrombocytopenia in hypersplenism is usually moderately severe ($>50 \times 10^9$/L) and asymptomatic; severe thrombocytopenia ($<20 \times 10^9$/L) suggests another diagnosis.

SUGGESTED READINGS

Available at ExpertConsult.com

RELATED CONTENT

Hypersplenism (Patient Information)
Felty Syndrome (Related Key Topic)

AUTHOR: **SUDEEP K. AULAKH, M.D.**

BASIC INFORMATION

DEFINITION

Normal blood pressure (BP) in adults can be defined as systolic BP <120 mm Hg and diastolic BP <80 mm Hg. Elevated blood pressure is defined as systolic BP between 120 and 129 mm Hg or diastolic BP <80 mm Hg. Hypertension can be divided into stage 1: systolic BP from 130 to 139 mm Hg or diastolic BP from 80 to 89 mm Hg and stage 2: systolic BP ≥140 mm Hg or diastolic BP ≥90 mm Hg. This definition is based on accurate measurements and average of ≥2 readings on ≥2 occasions.

SYNONYMS

Essential hypertension
Idiopathic hypertension
High BP

ICD-10CM CODES	
I10	Essential (primary) hypertension
I15.0	Renovascular hypertension
I15.1	Hypertension secondary to other renal disorders
I15.2	Hypertension secondary to endocrine disorders
I15.8	Other secondary hypertension
I15.9	Secondary hypertension, unspecified
O10.919	Unspecified pre-existing hypertension complicating pregnancy, unspecified trimester
I67.4	Hypertensive encephalopathy

EPIDEMIOLOGY & DEMOGRAPHICS

- In the U.S., 50% of people age 60 to 69 yr and approximately 75% of people >70 yr of age are affected, Worldwide, it is estimated that 41% of people ages 35 to 70 yr have hypertension, and only 46.5% of them are aware of it.
- Peak prevalence increases with age and was highest among non-Hispanic black adults in the U.S.
- Hypertension is linked with a higher risk of heart attack, stroke, heart failure, and kidney disease.

PHYSICAL FINDINGS & CLINICAL PRESENTATION

Physical examination may be entirely within normal limits except for the presence of elevated BP. A proper initial physical examination on a hypertensive patient should include the following:

- The BP should be measured with an appropriately sized cuff (bladder of the cuff should cover at least two thirds of the circumference of the arm) and in both arms (the higher of the readings being used). Table 1 describes blood pressure cuff size and error in measurement.
- The BP should be measured twice on each visit, and separated by at least 1 to 2 min to allow the return of trapped blood.
- The patient should be seated in a calm environment for at least 5 min with the arm in which BP is measured rested on support level with the heart.
- Postural BP change should always be recorded in the elderly to diagnose postural hypotension. This is assessed by taking BP in supine (after 5-min rest) and standing (after 2 min) positions. A drop of ≥20 mm Hg in systolic, a drop of ≥10 mm Hg diastolic BP, or symptoms of cerebral hypoperfusion is suggestive of postural (orthostatic) hypotension.
- A diagnosis of HTN may be established if the BP is markedly elevated (>180/110 mm Hg) or has evidence of end organ damage; otherwise such a diagnosis should wait until BP is found elevated on >2 readings on >2 different occasions.
- Nonoffice (home, workplace, 24-hr ambulatory) BP determination to establish the pattern of HTN (sustained, "white coat," or "masked" HTN) in selected patients.
- Measure heart rate, height, weight, body mass index, and waist circumference.
- Some general clinical clues for when to screen for secondary HTN include:
  1. Severe or resistant HTN.
  2. An acute rise in BP developing in a patient with previous stable BP.
  3. Age less than 30 yr, non-obese, non-black with no family history of HTN.
  4. Sudden onset or accelerated hypertension.
  5. Age of onset before puberty. If above is suspected, additional tests for secondary HTN should be done including renin, aldosterone, cortisol levels, 24-hr urine metanephrines, and serum catecholamines.
- Physical examination should include searching for secondary causes, and sequelae of hypertension.
- Examine skin for the presence of café-au-lait spots (neurofibromatosis), uremic appearance (renal failure), and violaceous striae (Cushing's syndrome).
- Perform careful funduscopic examination; check for papilledema, retinal exudates, hemorrhages, arterial narrowing, arteriovenous compression.
- Examine neck for carotid bruits, distended neck veins, and enlarged thyroid gland.
- Perform extensive cardiopulmonary examination: Check for a laterally displaced point of maximal intensity, an S3 or S4, and valvular murmurs.
- Palpate abdomen for renal masses (pheochromocytoma, polycystic kidneys), and auscultate for bruit over the aorta and renal arteries.
- Examine arterial pulses (dilated or absent femoral pulses and BP greater in upper extremities than lower extremities suggest aortic coarctation).
- Look for truncal obesity (Cushing's syndrome) and pedal edema (congestive heart failure [CHF]).
- Table 2 provides a guide to evaluation of identifiable causes of HTN.
- Table 3 summarizes clinical clues to guide the investigation in young patients with hypertension that has a potentially hereditary cause.

ETIOLOGY

- Essential (primary) HTN (85%)
- Drug induced or drug related (5%)
  1. NSAIDs
  2. Oral contraceptives
  3. Corticosteroids
- Renal HTN (5%)
  1. Renal parenchymal disease (3%)
  2. Renovascular HTN (RVH) (<2%)
- Endocrine (<2%)
  1. Primary aldosteronism (at least 5%)
  2. Pheochromocytoma (0.2%)
  3. Cushing's syndrome and long-term steroid therapy (0.2%)
  4. Hyperparathyroidism or thyroid disease (0.2%)
- Coarctation of the aorta (0.2%)

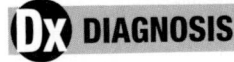

DIAGNOSIS

WORKUP

- The objective for the initial evaluation of HTN is to establish the diagnosis and stage of HTN. Table 4 summarizes initial laboratory evaluation of the hypertensive patient.
- Gather office and nonoffice BP readings, assess presence of target organ damage (TOD), assess the level of global cardiovascular

TABLE 1 Blood Pressure Cuff Size and Error in Measurement*

	Arm Circumference		
Cuff Bladder Size	28 cm or less	29-42 cm	43 cm or more
Regular (12 × 23 cm)	Accurate	Overestimates SBP by 4-8 mm Hg DBP by 3-6 mm Hg	Overestimates SBP by 16-17 mm Hg DBP by 10-11 mm Hg
Large (15 × 33 cm)	Underestimates SBP by 2-3 mm Hg DBP by 1-2 mm Hg	Accurate	Overestimates SBP by 5-7 mm Hg DBP by 2-4 mm Hg
Thigh (18 × 36 cm)	Underestimates SBP by 5-7 mm Hg DBP by 1-3 mm Hg	Underestimates SBP by 5-7 mm Hg DBP by 2-4 mm Hg	Accurate

DBP, Diastolic blood pressure reading; *SBP*, systolic blood pressure reading.
**Overestimation* means that hypertension may be diagnosed in someone with normal blood pressure; *underestimation* means that the blood pressure reading may be normal in someone who actually has high blood pressure. See text for further discussion.
From McGee, S: *Evidence-based physical diagnosis*, ed 4, Philadelphia, 2018, Elsevier.

TABLE 2 Guide to Evaluation of Identifiable Causes of Hypertension

Suspected Diagnosis	Clinical Clues	Diagnostic Testing
Chronic kidney disease	Estimated GFR <60 ml/min/1.73 m^2 Urine albumin-to-creatinine ratio ≥30 mg/g	Renal sonography
Renovascular disease	New elevation in serum creatinine, marked elevation in serum creatinine with ACEI or ARB, drug-resistant hypertension, flash pulmonary edema, abdominal, or flank bruit	Renal sonography (atrophic kidney), CT or MR angiography, invasive angiography
Coarctation of the aorta	Arm pulses > leg pulses, arm BP > leg BP, chest bruits, rib notching on chest radiography	MR angiography, TEE, invasive angiography
Primary aldosteronism	Hypokalemia, drug-resistant hypertension	Plasma renin and aldosterone, 24-hr urine aldosterone and potassium after oral salt loading, adrenal vein sampling
Cushing's syndrome	Truncal obesity, wide and blanching purple striae, muscle weakness	1 mg dexamethasone-suppression test, urinary cortisol after dexamethasone, adrenal CT
Pheochromocytoma	Paroxysms of hypertension, palpitations, perspiration, and pallor; diabetes	Plasma metanephrines, 24-hr urinary metanephrines and catecholamines, abdominal CT or MR imaging
Obstructive sleep apnea	Loud snoring, large neck, obesity, somnolence	Polysomnography

ACEI, Angiotensin-converting enzyme inhibitor; *ARB,* angiotensin receptor blocker; *BP,* blood pressure; *CT,* computed tomography; *GFR,* glomerular filtration rate; *MR,* magnetic resonance; *TEE,* transesophageal echocardiography.
From Goldman L, Schafer AI: *Goldman's Cecil medicine,* ed 24, Philadelphia, 2012, Saunders.

TABLE 3 Clinical Clues to Guide the Investigation in Young Patients with Hypertension That Has a Potentially Hereditary Cause

Specific Conditions	Possible Causes of Familial Hypertension	Clinical Clues
Catecholamine-Producing Tumors		
Pheochromocytoma/paraganglioma	Familial cases are responsible for <30% of cases, including MEN2A and MEN2B, von Hippel-Lindau disease, neurofibromatosis, and familial paraganglioma syndromes (SDH complex mutations)	Paroxysmal palpitations, headaches, diaphoresis, pale flushing; syndromic features of any of the associated disorders
Neuroblastomas (adrenal) Aortic or renovascular lesions	1%-2% of neuroblastomas are familial	
Coarctation of the aorta	Overrepresented in families but no familial distribution	Asymmetry between upper- and lower-extremity BP, radial-formal pulse delay; associated with Turner syndrome, Williams syndrome, and bicuspid aortic valve
Renal artery stenosis caused by fibromuscular dysplasia or inherited arterial wall lesions	<10% familial with AD pattern	Abnormal renal vascular imaging results; vascular disease in the carotid territory at an early age; common in neurofibromatosis and Williams syndrome; also present in tuberous sclerosis, Ehlers-Danlos syndrome, and Marfan syndrome
Parenchymal kidney disease GN	Alport disease (X-linked, AR, or AD), familial IgA nephropathy (AD with incomplete penetrance)	Proteinuria, hematuria, low eGFR
PKD	ADPKD type 1 or 2, ARPKD	Multiple renal cysts (as few as 3 in patients under 30 yr)
Adrenocortical disease Glucocorticoid-remediable aldosteronism (familial hyperaldosteronism type I)	AD chimeric fusion of the 11β-hydroxylase and aldosterone synthase genes	Cerebral hemorrhages at young age, cerebral aneurysms; mild hypokalemia; high plasma aldosterone, low renin
Familial hyperaldosteronism	AD; unknown defect	Severe type 2 hypertension in early adulthood; high plasma aldosterone, low renin; no response to glucocorticoid treatment
Familial hyperaldosteronism type III	AD; unknown defect	Severe hypertension in childhood with extensive target-organ damage; high plasma aldosterone, low renin; marked bilateral adrenal enlargement
Congenital adrenal hyperplasia	AR mutations in 11β-hydroxylase or 21-hydroxylase	Hirsutism, virilization; hypokalemia and metabolic alkalosis; low plasma aldosterone and renin
Monogenic Primary Renal Tubular Defects		
Gordon syndrome	AD mutations of *KLHL3, CUL3, WNK1,* and *WNK4;* AR mutations of *KLHL3*	Hyperkalemia and metabolic acidosis with normal renal function
Liddle syndrome	AD mutations of the epithelial sodium channel	Hypokalemia and metabolic alkalosis; low plasma aldosterone and renin
Apparent mineralocorticoid excess	AD mutation in 11β-hydroxysteroid dehydrogenase type 2	Hypokalemia and metabolic alkalosis; low plasma aldosterone and renin
Geller syndrome Hypertension-brachydactyly syndrome	AD mutation in the mineralocorticoid receptor AD mutations in the phosphodiesterase E3A enzyme	Hypokalemia and metabolic alkalosis; low plasma aldosterone and renin; increased BP during pregnancy or exposure to spironolactone
Unknown Mechanisms		
Hypertension-brachydactyly syndrome	AD	Short fingers (small phalanges) and short stature; brainstem compression from vascular tortuosity in the posterior fossa
Essential Hypertension		
	Polygenic	When obesity or metabolic syndrome is present, the likelihood of essential hypertension is higher

AD, Autosomal dominant; *ADPKD,* autosomal dominant polycystic kidney disease; *AR,* autosomal recessive; *ARPKD,* autosomal recessive polycystic kidney disease; *BP,* blood pressure; *eGFR,* estimated glomerular filtration rate; *GN,* glomerulonephritis; *IgA,* immunoglobulin A; *MEN,* multiple endocrine neoplasia; *PKD,* polycystic kidney disease; *SDH,* succinate dehydrogenase.
From Skorecki K et al: *Brenner and Rector's the kidney,* ed 10, Philadelphia, 2016, Elsevier.

TABLE 4 Initial Laboratory Evaluation of the Hypertensive Patient to Investigate the Presence of Comorbid Conditions, Secondary Causes, or Established Target-Organ Damage

Test	Clinical Usefulness
Serum creatinine (and estimated glomerular filtration rate)	Assessment of renal function. Identifies parenchymal kidney disease as a possible secondary cause as well as established TOD.
Serum potassium	Low potassium (of renal origin) suggests mineralocorticoid excess (primary or secondary), glucocorticoid excess, Liddle syndrome. High potassium with normal renal function suggests Gordon syndrome. Low levels raise caution about the use of thiazides and loop diuretics. High levels preclude the use of ACEIs, ARBs, renin inhibitors, and potassium-sparing diuretics.
Serum sodium	If high, suggests primary aldosteronism. If low, alerts to the need to avoid thiazide diuretics.
Serum bicarbonate	If high, suggests aldosterone excess (primary or secondary). If low with normal renal function, suggests Gordon syndrome (with high potassium) or primary hyperparathyroidism (with high calcium).
Serum calcium	If high, suggests primary hyperparathyroidism.
Serum glucose	Identifies prediabetes or diabetes. In the appropriate setting, suggests glucocorticoid excess, pheochromocytoma, or acromegaly.
Lipid profile	Identifies hyperlipidemia.
Hemoglobin/hematocrit	If high, in the absence of other hematologic abnormalities or underlying lung disease, suggests sleep apnea.
Urinalysis*	Proteinuria and hematuria identify a possible secondary cause (glomerulonephritis). Proteinuria can also be a marker of TOD.
Electrocardiogram	Identifies left ventricular hypertrophy, old myocardial infarction, or other ischemic changes. Identifies conduction abnormalities that may preclude the use of β-blockers or nondihydropyridine CCBs.

The most recent guidelines do not recommend BUN measurement alone.
ACEI, Angiotensin-converting enzyme inhibitor; *ARB,* angiotensin receptor blocker; *CCB,* calcium channel blocker; *TOD,* target-organ damage.
*Some organizations recommend screening microalbuminuria as a more sensitive tool to identify early renal injury.
From Skorecki K et al: *Brenner and Rector's the kidney*, ed 10, Philadelphia, 2016, Elsevier.

disease risk and produce a plan for individualized monitoring and therapy.

- Patient counseling and education should be prominent features of the initial evaluation.
- Pertinent history:
  1. Age of onset of HTN, previous antihypertensive therapy
  2. Family history of HTN, stroke, cardiovascular disease
- Diet, salt intake, caffeine, alcohol, drugs (e.g., oral contraceptives, NSAIDs, decongestants, steroids)
- Occupation, lifestyle, pain, socioeconomic status, psychologic factors
- Other cardiovascular risk factors: Hyperlipidemia, obesity, diabetes mellitus
- Symptoms of secondary HTN:
  1. Headache, palpitations, excessive perspiration (possible pheochromocytoma)
  2. Weakness, polyuria (consider hyperaldosteronism)
  3. Claudication of lower extremities (seen with coarctation of aorta)
  4. Loud snoring, day-time somnolence, morning confusion (may warrant evaluation for sleep apnea)

LABORATORY TESTS

- Routine laboratory tests recommended before initiating therapy include:
  1. Urinalysis with microscopic evaluation; for signs of glomerulopathy.
  2. Basic metabolic panel and calcium; for signs of kidney damage, hypokalemia (primary aldosteronism and Cushing's syndrome), hypercalcemia (hyperparathyroid).
  3. Complete blood count.
  4. Screening for coexisting diseases that may adversely affect prognosis; hemoglobin a1c or fasting glucose level, serum lipid panel.
  5. Optional tests include measurement of urinary albumin or albumin/creatinine ratio.

IMAGING STUDIES

- ECG: Check for presence of left ventricular hypertrophy (LVH) with strain pattern.
- Renal duplex ultrasonography, CT angiography or magnetic resonance angiography of the renal arteries in suspected renovascular hypertension (renal artery stenosis) may be considered.

Rx TREATMENT

NONPHARMACOLOGIC THERAPY

Lifestyle modifications (the initial treatment of hypertension should focus on lifestyle modifications):

- Weight loss if overweight (target BMI <25).
- Limit alcohol intake to 1 oz of ethanol per day (<2 drinks/day) in men or 0.5 oz (<1 drink/day) in women.
- Regular aerobic exercise (at least 30 min/day on most days).
- Reduce sodium intake to <100 mmol/day (<1.5 g of sodium/day).
- Maintain adequate dietary potassium (>3500 mg/day) intake in patients with normal kidney function.
- Smoking cessation.
- The BP reduction seen ranges from 2 to 20 mm Hg, most significant with substantial weight loss and the implementation of the Dietary Approaches to Stop Hypertension (DASH) eating plan, which relies on a diet high in fruits and vegetables, moderate in low-fat dairy products, and low in animal protein but with substantial amount of plant protein from legumes and nuts.

ACUTE GENERAL Rx

- Multiple recent consensus documents regarding blood pressure goals and when to initiate treatment have been published.
- According to the 2017 *ACC/AHA/AAPA/ABC/ACPM/AGS/APhA/ASH/ASPC/NMA/PCNA Guideline for the Prevention, Detection, Evaluation, and Management of High Blood Pressure in Adults*, goals of treatment are as follows[1]:
  1. For adults with confirmed hypertension and known cardiovascular disease (CVD) or 10-yr ASCVD event risk of 10% or higher, a BP target of less than 130/80 mmHG is recommended.
  2. For adults with confirmed hypertension without additional markers of increased CVD risk, a BP target of less than 130/80 mmHG may be reasonable.
- In addition, initiation of therapy recommendations is as follows:
  1. Use of BP-lowering medication is recommended for primary prevention of CVD in adults with no history of CVD and with an estimated 10-yr ASCVD risk <10% and Stage 2 Hypertension.
  2. Use of BP-lowering medications is recommended for secondary prevention of recurrent CVD events in patients with clinical CVD and for primary prevention in adults with an estimated 10-yr atherosclerotic cardiovascular disease (ASCVD) risk of 10% or higher and Stage 1 Hypertension.
  3. Initiate antihypertensive drug therapy with 2 first-line agents of different classes for adults with Stage 2 Hypertension and BP more than 20/10 mmHg higher than their target.
  4. It is reasonable to initiate therapy with a single agent for adults with Stage 1 hypertension and a goal less than 130/80 mmHg.

[1]Whelton P et al: 2017 *ACC/AHA/AAPA/ABC/ACPM/AGS/APhA/ASH/ASPC/NMA/PCNA Guideline for the Prevention, Detection, Evaluation, and Management of High Blood Pressure in Adults* executive summary: a report of the American College of Cardiology/American Heart Association task force on clinical guidelines, *J Am Coll Cardiol* 2017.

5. Patients with diabetes mellitus and chronic kidney disease are considered high risk.

- Additionl guidance may be taken from the writers of the JNC 8 guidelines, published in 2014[2]:
  1. In the general non-black population, preferred initial agents are thiazide-type diuretics, angiotensin-converting enzyme inhibitors (ACEi), calcium channel blockers (CCBs), or angiotensin receptor blockers (ARBs). ACEi or ARBs are preferred initial agents in diabetics and those with CKD in this population.
  2. Preferred initial agents in the black population (including diabetics) are thiazide-type diuretics or CCBs.
  3. When selecting drugs, try to give once per day dosages to improve compliance. Also consider the cost of the medication, metabolic and subjective side effects, and drug-drug interactions.
- The major advantages and limitations of each class of drugs are described as follows:
  1. Thiazide diuretics:
     a. Advantages: Inexpensive, once-daily dosing. Useful in edematous states, CHF, chronic renal disease, elderly patients (decreased incidence of hip fractures in elderly patients)
     b. Disadvantages: Significant adverse metabolic effects (hypokalemia), increased risk of cardiac arrhythmias, sexual dysfunction, gout flares, possible adverse effects on lipids and glucose levels
  2. Beta-blockers:
     a. Advantages: Ideal in hypertensive patients with ischemic heart disease or status post MI. Favored in hyperkinetic, young patients (resting tachycardia, wide pulse pressure, hyperdynamic heart) and stable CHF patients.
     b. Disadvantages: Adverse effect on quality of life (increased incidence of fatigue, depression, impotence), bronchospasm, hypoglycemia, peripheral vascular disease, adverse effects on lipids, masking of signs and symptoms of hypoglycemia in diabetics.
  3. Calcium antagonists:
     a. Advantages: Helpful in hypertensive patients with ischemic heart disease. Generally favorable effect on quality of life; can be used in patients with bronchospastic disorders, renal disease, peripheral vascular disease, metabolic disorders, and salt sensitivity. CCBs BP-lowering effect is independent of Na^+ intake.
     b. Disadvantages: Diltiazem and verapamil should be avoided in patients with CHF due to systolic dysfunction because of their negative inotropic effects; pedal edema may occur with nifedipine and amlodipine; constipation can be severe in elderly patients receiving verapamil. CCB-related edema is positional in nature, it improves with lying position; additional strategies include switching CCB classes, reducing dosage, giving the medication later in the day, and adding a venodilator (nitrates, an ACE, or an ARB); diuretics may improve edema, but at the expense of a reduction in plasma volume.
  4. ACE inhibitors:
     a. Advantages: First-line therapy for patients with left ventricular dysfunction, helpful in prevention of diabetic renal disease; effective in decreasing LVH, and remodeling.
     b. Disadvantages: Dry cough is a frequent side effect (5%-20% of patients); hyperkalemia may occur in patients with diabetes or severe renal insufficiency; hypotension may occur in volume-depleted patients; increased risk of renal failure in patients with renal artery stenosis; contraindicated in pregnancy.
  5. ARBs:
     a. Advantages: Well tolerated, favorable impact on quality of life; useful in patients unable to tolerate ACE inhibitors because of persistent cough and in CHF and diabetic patients; single daily dose. An episode of renal insufficiency with ACE inhibitors does not rule out future therapy with an ARB unless high-grade bilateral renal artery stenosis exists.
     b. Disadvantages: Hypotension may occur in volume-depleted patients; hyperkalemia; risk of renal failure in renal artery stenosis; contraindicated in pregnancy.
  6. Alpha-adrenergic blockers:
     a. Advantages: No adverse effect on blood lipids or insulin sensitivity; helpful in benign prostatic hypertrophy.
     b. Disadvantages: Postural hypotension, sedation; syncope can be avoided by giving an initial low dose at bedtime. Generally considered third- or fourth-line agent.
  7. Central alpha-antagonists:
     a. Oral clonidine mainstay of therapy for hypertensive urgencies because of the ease of administration and relative safety.
     b. Transdermal clonidine; useful in management of labile HTN, the hospitalized patient who cannot take medications by mouth, and patients subject to early-morning BP surges. At equivalent doses, transdermal clonidine is more apt to precipitate salt and water retention than is the case with oral clonidine.
     c. Dose beyond 0.4 mg causes fatigue, sedation, dry mouth, salt and water retention, and rebound HTN upon abrupt termination of the medication.
  8. Combined alpha- and beta-adrenergic receptor blockers:
     a. Labetalol, nebivolol, and carvedilol: Use is reserved to treat complicated hypertensive patient when an antihypertensive effect beyond beta-blockade is sought. IV labetalol is used for hypertensive emergencies. Carvedilol is shown to have less adverse effect on glycemic control than metoprolol and to reduce urinary protein excretion in hypertensive diabetic patients.
  9. Direct-acting smooth muscle relaxant: Hydralazine
     a. Advantages: Beneficial in black patients when used with isosorbide dinitrate.
     b. Disadvantages: May lead to reflex tachycardia, worsening ischemia (best used with nitrates), at higher doses or with renal failure can lead to a reversible drug-induced lupus.
  10. Renin inhibitors: Newest class of antihypertensives (Aliskiren):
      a. Advantages: Generally well tolerated; once-daily dosing; can be used alone or in combination with other antihypertensive agents (avoid combining with ACEI or ARBs given increase of hyperkalemia).
      b. Disadvantages: Contraindicated in pregnancy; should not be used in patients with impaired renal function; excessive cost; paucity of cardiovascular outcomes data showing benefit.

TREATMENT OF RENOVASCULAR HYPERTENSION: The therapeutic approach varies with the cause of the renovascular hypertension (RVH) (refer to "Renal Artery Stenosis" for additional information).

- Young patients with fibromuscular dysplasia refractory to medical therapy can be treated with percutaneous transluminal renal angioplasty (PTRA).
- Medical therapy is advisable in elderly patients with atheromatous RVH; useful agents are:
  1. Beta-blockers: Highly effective in patients with elevated plasma renin
  2. ACE inhibitors: Highly effective; however, should be avoided in patients with bilateral renal artery stenosis or with a solitary kidney and renal artery stenosis
  3. Diuretics: Often used in combination with ACE inhibitors
- Surgical revascularization: A recent trial revealed that renal-artery stenting does not confer a significant benefit with respect to the prevention of clinical events when added to comprehensive, multifactorial medical therapy in people with atherosclerotic renal-artery stenosis and hypertension or CKD.[3]

[2] James PA et al: 2014 Evidence-based guidelines for the management of high blood pressure in adults. Report from the panel members appointed to the eighth Joint National Committee (JNC8), *JAMA* 311(5):507-520, 2014.

[3] Cooper CJ et al: Stenting and medical therapy for atherosclerotic renal-artery stenosis, *N Engl J Med* 370:13-22, 2014..

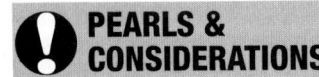

TABLE 5 Drugs Used to Treat Hypertension in Pregnancy

Drug	Starting Dose	Maximum Dose	Comments
Acute Treatment of Severe Hypertension			
Hydralazine	5-10 mg IV every 20 min	20 mg*	Avoid in cases of tachycardia and persistent headaches
Labetalol	20-40 mg IV every 10-15 min	220 mg*	Avoid in women with asthma or congestive heart failure
Nifedipine	10-20 mg oral every 30 min	50 mg*	Avoid in case of tachycardia and palpitations
Long-Term Treatment of Hypertension			
Methyldopa	250 mg bid	4 g/day	
Labetalol	100 mg bid	2400 mg/day	
Nifedipine	10 mg bid	120 mg/day	
Thiazide diuretic	12.5 mg bid	50 mg/day	

*If desired blood pressure levels are not achieved, switch to another drug.
From Gabbe SG: *Obstetrics*, ed 6, Philadelphia, 2012, Saunders.

HTN DURING PREGNANCY:

- HTN complicates 5% to 12% of all pregnancies.
- The American Obstetrical Committee defines BP of 130/80 mm Hg as the upper limit of normal at any time during pregnancy.
- A rise of 30 mm Hg systolic or 15 mm Hg diastolic is also considered abnormal regardless of the absolute values obtained.
- Hypertension during pregnancy can be from chronic HTN, gestational HTN, preeclampsia or preeclampsia superimposed on chronic HTN. It is important to distinguish the etiology because the risk to mother and fetus is much greater in preeclampsia.
- Treatment of chronic HTN during pregnancy is as follows:
  1. Initial treatment with conservative measures (proper nutrition, limited physical activity).
  2. When drug therapy is necessary, initiation of methyldopa, hydralazine, labetalol or nifedipine is preferred. Table 5 summarizes drugs used to treat hypertension in pregnancy.
  3. ACE inhibitors can cause fetal and neonatal complications; their use should be avoided in pregnancy.
  4. The safety of CCBs remains unclear.
  5. Diuretics should be used only if there is a specific reason for initiating and maintaining their use (e.g., HTN associated with severe fluid overload or left ventricular dysfunction).

MALIGNANT HTN, HYPERTENSIVE EMERGENCIES, AND HYPERTENSIVE URGENCIES:

Definitions:

- Malignant HTN occurs with HTN when there are grades III and IV retinopathy (exudates, hemorrhages and papilledema).
  1. The rate of BP rise is a critical factor in the development of malignant HTN.
  2. Complications and mortality rates are much higher in malignant HTN compared to essential HTN.
  3. Requires immediate BP reduction (not necessarily into normal ranges) to prevent or limit target organ disease.
- Hypertensive emergencies occur when the BP elevation is >180 mmHg systolic and/or >120 mmHg diastolic without evidence of new or progressive organ dysfunction. It requires rapid lowering of BP to prevent end-organ damage.
- Hypertensive urgencies are BP elevations >180 mmHg systolic and/or >120 mmHg diastolic with end-organ damage that should be corrected within 24 hrs of presentation.
  1. Most clinicians suggest lowering the BP to <160 mm Hg/<100 mm Hg or to a level no more than 30% lower than the patient's baseline BP.

Therapy: The choice of therapeutic agents varies with the cause. IV medications are preferred in hypertensive emergencies.

- Nitroprusside is the drug of choice in hypertensive encephalopathy, HTN and intracranial bleeding, malignant HTN, HTN and heart failure, dissecting aortic aneurysm (used in combination with propranolol); its onset of action is immediate. Because it is metabolized to cyanide, patients should be carefully monitored for toxicity (mental status changes, acidemia).
- Fenoldopam is a vasodilator agent useful for the short-term (up to 48 hr) management of severe HTN when rapid but quickly reversible reduction of BP is required. It should be avoided in patients with glaucoma.
- Other commonly used agents are the IV CCBs nicardipine and clevidipine (useful for urgent treatment of HTN in the intensive care unit or operating room), the beta-blocker esmolol (useful in aortic dissection or postoperative HTN), labetalol (combined β-adrenergic and α-blocker useful in patients with coronary disease), phentolamine (useful for catecholamine-related emergencies), IV nitroglycerin (used in patients with cardiac ischemia and hypertensive crisis), and hydralazine (used for hypertensive emergencies in pregnancy.
- Table 6 summarizes IV medications useful in hypertensive crisis.

The following are important points to remember when treating hypertensive emergencies:

- Introduce a plan for long-term therapy at the time of the initial emergency treatment.
- Agents that reduce arterial pressure can cause the kidney to retain sodium and water; therefore the judicious administration of diuretics should accompany their use.
- The initial goal of antihypertensive therapy is not to achieve a normal BP, but rather to gradually reduce the BP; cerebral hypoperfusion may occur if the mean BP is hypertension in patients with CKD.

PEARLS & CONSIDERATIONS

COMMENTS

- For patients with hypertension, every 20/10 mm Hg increase in BP doubles the risk of cardiovascular events.
- Most patients will require at least two medications for BP control.
- If BP is greater than 20/10 mm Hg above goal, therapy should be initiated with two drugs.
- Resistant HTN: HTN is considered resistant if the BP cannot be reduced below target levels in patients who are compliant with an optimal triple-drug regimen that includes a diuretic. Terms *refractory* and *resistant* are used interchangeably. Causes include pseudohypertension, measurement artifact, medication nonadherence, volume overload, and secondary HTN.
  1. Pseudohypertension in elderly: Hardened and sclerotic artery is not compressible hence falsely elevates BP measurement artifact.
  2. Measurement artifact: BP taken incorrectly (small cuff, improper support).
- Renal sympathetic denervation: A recent blinded trial did not show a significant reduction of systolic blood pressure in patients with resistant hypertension 6 mo after renal artery denervation as compared with a sham control.
- Barriers to BP control: System issues, provider issues; patient issues, and behavior issues. The rate at which physicians adopt recommended changes based on evidence-based findings can be quite slow and has been properly described as "clinical inertia."
- Indications for specialist referral for patients with HTN are described in Table 7.
- New U.S. guidelines for the treatment of hypertension recommend the following:
  1. Use of blood pressure-lowering medication for secondary prevention in patients with cardiovascular disease and average systolic blood pressure (SBP) ≥130 mm Hg or diastolic blood pressure (DBP) ≥80 mm Hg, and for primary prevention in adults with an estimated 10-yr ASCVD risk of >10% and an average SBP ≥130 mm Hg or DBP ≥80 mm Hg.
  2. In patients with no history of cardiovascular disease and an estimated 10-yr ASCVD risk <10%, blood pressure lowering medication is recommended for those with an average SBP ≥140 mm Hg or an average DBP ≥90 mm Hg.

TABLE 6 Treatment of Hypertensive Crisis: Intravenous Medications

Drug Name and Mechanism of Action	Indications/Advantages/Dose	Disadvantages/Adverse Effects/Metabolism Cautions
Sodium Nitroprusside		
Nitric oxide compound; vasodilation of arteriolar and venous smooth muscle Increases cardiac output by decreasing afterload	Useful in most hypertensive emergencies Onset of action immediate, duration of action 1-2 min Dose: 0.25 μg/kg/min Maximum dose: 8-10 μg/kg/min	Contraindicated in high-output cardiac failure, congenital optic atrophy. Anemia and liver disease at risk of cyanide toxicity: Acidosis, tachycardia, change in mental status, almond smell on breath. Risk of thiocyanate toxicity with renal disease: Psychosis, hyperreflexia, seizure, tinnitus. Cautious use with increased intracranial pressure. Do not use maximum dose for more than 10 min. Crosses the placenta.
Nitroglycerin		
Directly interacts with nitrate receptors on vascular smooth muscle Primarily dilates venous bed Decreases preload	Use with symptoms of cardiac ischemia, perioperative hypertension in cardiac surgery Initial dose: 5 μg/min Maximum dose: 100 μg/min	Contraindicated in angle-closure glaucoma, increased intracranial pressure. Blood pressure decreased secondary to decreased preload, cardiac output—avoid when cerebral or renal perfusion compromised. Caution with right ventricular infarct.
Labetalol		
β- and α-Adrenergic blockade α:β-Blocking ratio is 1:7	Onset of action 2-5 min, duration 3-6 hr Bolus 20 mg, then 20-80 mg every 10 min for maximum dose 300 mg Infuse at 0.5-2 mg/min	Avoid in bronchospasm, bradycardia, congestive heart failure, greater than first-degree heart block, second/third trimester pregnancy. Use caution with hepatic dysfunction, inhalational anesthetics (myocardial depression). Enters breast milk.
Esmolol		
Cardioselective β1-adrenergic blocking agent	Use with aortic dissection Use during intubation, intraoperative, and postoperative hypertension Onset of action 60 sec, duration 10-20 min 200-500 μg/kg/min for 4 min, then infuse 50-300 μg/kg/min	See labetalol. Not dependent on renal or hepatic function for metabolism (metabolized by hydrolysis in red blood cells).
Fenoldopam		
Postsynaptic dopamine-1 agonist; decreases peripheral vascular resistance; 10 times more potent than dopamine as vasodilator	May be advantageous in kidney disease, increases renal blood flow, increases sodium excretion, no toxic metabolites Initial dose: 0.1 μg/kg/min, with titration every 15 min No bolus	Contraindicated in glaucoma (may increase intraocular pressure) or allergy to sulfites; hypotension, especially with concurrent β-blocker. Check serum potassium every 6 hr. Concurrent acetaminophen may significantly increase blood levels. Dose-related tachycardia.
Hydralazine		
Primarily dilates arteriolar vasculature	Primarily used in pregnancy/eclampsia Dose: 10 mg every 20-130 min; maximum dose 20 mg Decreases blood pressure in 10-20 min Duration of action 2-4 hr	Reflex tachycardia; give β-blocker concurrently. May exacerbate angina. Half-life 3 hr, affects blood pressure for 100 hr. Depends on hepatic acetylation for inactivation.
Phentolamine		
α-Adrenergic blockade	Used primarily to treat hypertension from excessive catecholamine excess (e.g., pheochromocytoma) Dose: 5-15 mg Onset of action 1-2 min, duration 3-10 min	β-blockade is generally added to control tachycardia or arrhythmias. As in all catecholamine excess states, β-blockers should never be given first, as the loss of β-adrenergically mediated vasodilatation will leave α-adrenergically mediated vasoconstriction unopposed and result in increased pressure.
Nicardipine		
Dihydropyridine calcium channel blocker; inhibits transmembrane influx of calcium ions into cardiac and smooth muscle	Onset of action 10-20 min, duration 1-4 hr Initial dose: 5 mg/hr to maximum of 15 mg/hr	Avoid with congestive heart failure, cardiac ischemia. Adverse effects include tachycardia, flushing, headache.
Clevidipine		
Short-acting dihydropyridine calcium channel antagonist[101]	Initial dose: 1 mg/hr; can be increased to 21 mg/hr	Reduces blood pressure without affecting cardiac filling pressures or causing reflex tachycardia.
Enalaprilat		
Angiotensin-converting enzyme inhibitor	Onset of action 15-20 min, duration 12-24 hr Dose: 1.25-5 mg every 6 hr	Response not predictable, with high renin states may see acute hypotension. Hyperkalemia in setting of reduced glomerular filtration rate. Avoid in pregnancy.
Trimethaphan		
Nondepolarizing ganglionic blocking agent; competes with acetylcholine for postsynaptic receptors	Used in aortic dissection Dose: 0.5-5 mg/min	Does not increase cardiac output. No inotropic cardiac effect. Disadvantages include parasympathetic blockade, resulting in paralytic ileus and bladder atony and development of tachyphylaxis after 24-96 hr of use.

From Vincent JL et al: *Textbook of critical care*, ed 7, Philadelphia, 2017, Elsevier.

TABLE 7 Indications for Specialist Referral for Patients with Hypertension

Urgent Treatment Needed
Accelerated hypertension (severe hypertension with grade III-IV retinopathy)
Particularly severe hypertension (>220/120 mm Hg)
Impending complications (e.g., transient ischemic attack, left ventricular failure)
Possible Underlying Cause
Any clue in history or examination of a secondary cause (e.g., hypokalemia with increased or high–normal plasma sodium)
Elevated serum creatinine
Proteinuria or hematuria
Sudden onset or worsening of hypertension
Young age (any hypertension <20 yr; needing treatment <30 yr)
Therapeutic Problems
Multiple drug intolerances
Multiple drug contraindications
Persistent nonadherence or nonconcordance
Special Situations
Unusual blood pressure variability
Possible white coat hypertension
Hypertension in pregnancy

From Floege J et al: *Comprehensive clinical nephrology,* ed 4, Philadelphia, 2010, Saunders

SUGGESTED READINGS

Available at ExpertConsult.com

RELATED CONTENT

High Blood Pressure (Patient Information)
High Blood Pressure–Child (Patient Information)
Eclampsia (Related Key Topic)
Pre-Eclampsia (Related Key Topic)
Renal Artery Stenosis (Related Key Topic)

AUTHOR: **TANIA B. BABAR, M.D.**

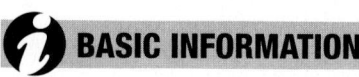

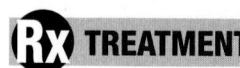

BASIC INFORMATION

DEFINITION

Hyperthyroidism is a hypermetabolic state resulting from excess thyroid hormone.

SYNONYM

Thyrotoxicosis

ICD-10CM CODES	
E05.00	Thyrotoxicosis with diffuse goiter without thyrotoxic crisis or storm
E05.01	Thyrotoxicosis with diffuse goiter with thyrotoxic crisis or storm
E05.10	Thyrotoxicosis with toxic single thyroid nodule without thyrotoxic crisis or storm
E05.11	Thyrotoxicosis with toxic single thyroid nodule with thyrotoxic crisis or storm
E05.20	Thyrotoxicosis with toxic multinodular goiter without thyrotoxic crisis or storm
E05.21	Thyrotoxicosis with toxic multinodular goiter with thyrotoxic crisis or storm
E05.30	Thyrotoxicosis from ectopic thyroid tissue without thyrotoxic crisis or storm
E05.31	Thyrotoxicosis from ectopic thyroid tissue with thyrotoxic crisis or storm
E05.40	Thyrotoxicosis factitia without thyrotoxic crisis or storm
E05.41	Thyrotoxicosis factitia with thyrotoxic crisis or storm
E05.80	Other thyrotoxicosis without thyrotoxic crisis or storm
E05.81	Other thyrotoxicosis with thyrotoxic crisis or storm
E05.90	Thyrotoxicosis, unspecified without thyrotoxic crisis or storm
E05.91	Thyrotoxicosis, unspecified with thyrotoxic crisis or storm
E06.2	Chronic thyroiditis with transient thyrotoxicosis

EPIDEMIOLOGY & DEMOGRAPHICS

INCIDENCE/PREVALENCE:

- Hyperthyroidism affects 2% of women and 0.2% of men in their lifetimes.
- Toxic multinodular goiter usually occurs in women >55 yr and is more common than Graves disease in the elderly.

PHYSICAL FINDINGS & CLINICAL PRESENTATION

- Patients with hyperthyroidism generally present with tachycardia, tremor, hyperreflexia, anxiety, irritability, emotional lability, panic attacks, heat intolerance, sweating, increased appetite, diarrhea, weight loss, menstrual dysfunction (oligomenorrhea, amenorrhea). Presentation may be different in elderly patients (see the following).
- Patients with Graves disease may present with exophthalmos, lid retraction, and lid lag (Graves ophthalmopathy). The following signs and symptoms of ophthalmopathy may be present: blurring of vision, photophobia, increased lacrimation, double vision, and deep orbital pressure. Clubbing of fingers associated with periosteal new bone formation in other skeletal areas (Graves acropachy) and pretibial myxedema may also be noted.
- Clinical signs of hyperthyroidism in the elderly may be masked by manifestations of coexisting disease (e.g., new-onset atrial fibrillation, exacerbation of congestive heart failure).

ETIOLOGY

- Graves disease (diffuse toxic goiter): 80% to 90% of all cases of hyperthyroidism
- Toxic multinodular goiter (Plummer disease)
- Toxic adenoma
- Iatrogenic and factitious
- Transient hyperthyroidism (subacute thyroiditis, Hashimoto thyroiditis)
- Rare causes: Hypersecretion of thyroid-stimulating hormone (TSH) (e.g., pituitary neoplasms), struma ovarii, ingestion of large amount of iodine in a patient with preexisting thyroid hyperplasia or adenoma (Jod-Basedow phenomenon), hydatidiform mole, carcinoma of thyroid, amiodarone therapy

Dx DIAGNOSIS

DIFFERENTIAL DIAGNOSIS

- Anxiety disorder
- Pheochromocytoma
- Metastatic neoplasm
- Diabetes mellitus
- Premenopausal state

WORKUP

Suspected hyperthyroidism requires laboratory confirmation and identification of its etiology because treatment varies with cause. A detailed medical history will often provide clues to the diagnosis and etiology of the hyperthyroidism. Fig. E1 describes a diagnostic approach to suspected hyperthyroidism.

LABORATORY TESTS

- Elevated free thyroxine (T_4)
- Elevated free triiodothyronine (T_3): Generally not necessary for diagnosis
- Low TSH (unless hyperthyroidism is a result of the rare hypersecretion of TSH from a pituitary adenoma)
- Thyroid autoantibodies useful in selected cases to differentiate Graves disease from toxic multinodular goiter (absent thyroid antibodies)

IMAGING STUDIES

- 24-hour radioactive iodine uptake (RAIU) is useful to distinguish hyperthyroidism from iatrogenic thyroid hormone synthesis (thyrotoxicosis factitia) and from thyroiditis.
- An overactive thyroid shows increased uptake, whereas a normal underactive thyroid (iatrogenic thyroid ingestion, painless or subacute thyroiditis) shows normal or decreased uptake.
- The RAIU results also vary with the etiology of the hyperthyroidism:
  1. Graves disease: Increased homogeneous uptake
  2. Multinodular goiter: Increased heterogeneous uptake
  3. Hot nodule: Single focus of increased uptake
- RAIU is also generally performed before the therapeutic administration of radioactive iodine to determine the appropriate dose.

Rx TREATMENT

NONPHARMACOLOGIC THERAPY

Patient education regarding thyroid disease and discussion of the therapeutic options. Patients should be informed that radioiodine, antithyroid drugs, and surgery are all reasonable treatment options for hyperthyroidism. It is crucial for the physician to have a detailed discussion with the patient about the benefits and risks relative to lifestyle, patients' values, and coexisting conditions.

ACUTE GENERAL Rx

ANTITHYROID DRUGS (THIONAMIDES): Propylthiouracil (PTU) and methimazole inhibit thyroid hormone synthesis by blocking production of thyroid peroxidase (PTU and methimazole) or inhibit peripheral conversion of T_4 to T_3 (PTU). Methimazole is favored by most endocrinologists because of the potential for hepatic failure with PTU. PTU is preferred in pregnant women during the first trimester because methimazole has been associated with aplasia cutis and with choanal and esophageal atresia. Complete blood count and differential should be obtained before their use.

- Dosage: Methimazole 15 to 30 mg/day given as a single dose; PTU 50 to 100 mg PO q8h.
- Antithyroid drugs can be used as the primary form of treatment or as adjunctive therapy before radioactive therapy or surgery or afterward if the hyperthyroidism recurs.
- Side effects: Skin rash (3% to 5% of patients), arthralgias, myalgias, granulocytopenia (0.5%). Rare side effects are aplastic anemia, hepatic necrosis from PTU, cholestatic jaundice from methimazole.
- When antithyroid drugs are used as primary therapy, they are usually given for 6 to 18 mo; prolonged therapy may cause hypothyroidism. Monitor thyroid function every 2 mo for 6 mo, then less frequently.
- The use of antithyroid drugs before radioiodine therapy is best reserved for patients in whom exacerbation of hyperthyroidism after radioactive iodine therapy is hazardous (e.g., elderly patients with coronary artery disease or significant coexisting morbidity). In these patients the antithyroid drug can be stopped 2 days before radioactive iodine therapy, resumed 2 days later, and continued for 4 to 6 wk.

RADIOIODINE THERAPY (RADIOACTIVE IODINE [RAI; ^{131}I]):

- RAI is the treatment of choice for patients aged >21 yr and younger patients who have not achieved remission after 1 yr of antithyroid drug therapy. RAI is also used in hyperthyroidism caused by toxic adenoma or toxic multinodular goiter.
- Contraindicated during pregnancy (can cause fetal hypothyroidism) and lactation. Pregnancy should be excluded in women of childbearing age before RAI is administered.
- A single dose of RAI is effective in inducing a euthyroid state in nearly 80% of patients.
- There is a high incidence of post-RAI hypothyroidism (>50% within first yr and 2%/yr thereafter); these patients should be frequently evaluated for the onset of hypothyroidism (see "Chronic Rx").

SURGICAL THERAPY (SUBTOTAL THYROIDECTOMY):

- Indicated in obstructing goiters, in any patient who refuses RAI and cannot be adequately managed with antithyroid medications (e.g., patients with toxic adenoma or toxic multinodular goiter), and in pregnant patients who cannot be adequately managed with antithyroid medication or develop side effects to them. Thyroidectomy can also be considered as primary therapy in refractory cases of amiodarone-induced hyperthyroidism. Thyroidectomy is not indicated for low RAIU hyperthyroidism.
- Patients should be rendered euthyroid with antithyroid drugs before surgery.
- Complications of surgery include hypothyroidism (28% to 43% after 10 yr), hypoparathyroidism, and vocal cord paralysis (1%).
- Most patients should be started on replacement doses of levothyroxine (1.7 mcg/kg/day) before discharge from hospital.
- Hyperthyroidism recurs after surgery in 10% to 15% of patients.

ADJUNCTIVE THERAPY: Propranolol alleviates the beta-adrenergic symptoms of hyperthyroidism; initial dose is 20 to 40 mg PO q6h; dosage is gradually increased until symptoms are controlled. Major contraindications to propranolol are congestive heart failure and bronchospasm. Diagnosis and treatment of thyrotoxic storm are also discussed in Section I.

CHRONIC Rx

- Patients undergoing treatment with antithyroid drugs should be seen every 1 to 3 mo until euthyroidism is achieved and every 3 to 4 mo while they remain on antithyroid therapy. After treatment is stopped, periodic monitoring of thyroid function tests with TSH is recommended every 3 mo for 1 yr, then every 6 mo for 1 yr, then annually.
- Orbital decompression surgery can be used to correct Graves orbitopathy (Fig. E2). The administration of the antioxidant selenium (100 mcg PO bid) has been recently reported as effective in improving quality of life, reducing ocular involvement, and slowing progression of the disease in patients with mild Graves orbitopathy. Its mechanism of action is believed to be an effect on the oxygen free radicals and cytokines that play a pathogenic role in Graves orbitopathy.

DISPOSITION

Successful treatment of hyperthyroidism requires lifelong monitoring for the onset of hypothyroidism or the recurrence of thyrotoxicosis.

REFERRAL

- Endocrinology referral is recommended at the time of initial diagnosis and during treatment.
- Surgical referral in selected patients (see "Surgical Therapy").
- Hospitalization of all patients with thyroid storm.

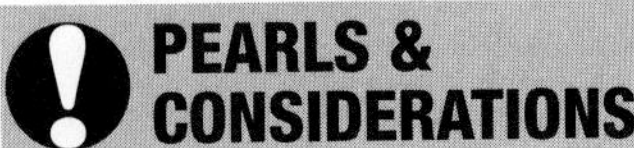

PEARLS & CONSIDERATIONS

COMMENTS

- Elderly hyperthyroid patients may have only subtle signs (weight loss, tachycardia, fine skin, brittle nails). This form is known as ***apathetic hyperthyroidism*** and manifests with lethargy rather than hyperkinetic activity. An enlarged thyroid gland may be absent. Coexisting medical disorders (most commonly cardiac disease) may also mask the symptoms. These patients often have unexplained congestive heart failure, worsening of angina, or new-onset atrial fibrillation resistant to treatment. See the topic "Graves Disease" for additional information on diagnosis and treatment.
- **Subclinical hyperthyroidism** is defined as a normal serum-free thyroxine and free triiodothyronine levels with a TSH level suppressed below the normal range and usually undetectable. Prevalence in the general population is 1% to 2%. These patients usually do not present with signs or symptoms of overt hyperthyroidism. Subclinical hyperthyroidism is associated with an increased risk of atrial fibrillation and heart failure in older adults. Treatment options include observation or a therapeutic trial of low-dose antithyroid agents for 6 mo to attempt to induce remission. The American Thyroid Association and the American Association of Clinical Endocrinologists recommend treatment of patients with TSH levels <0.1 mIU if they are older than 65 or have associated comorbidities (osteoporosis, heart failure).
- ***Thyrotoxic periodic paralysis (TPP)*** is a hyperthyroidism-related hypokalemia and muscle-weakening condition resulting from a sudden shift of potassium into cells. Many patients do not have other symptoms of hyperthyroidism. Typical presentation involves an Asian adult male with acute fatigue and muscle weakness initially presenting in the lower extremities. Physical examination reveals decreased deep tendon reflexes, hypertension, and tachycardia. ECG often reveals U waves, high QRS voltage, and first-degree atrioventricular block. Additional laboratory testing reveals normal acid-base state, hypokalemia with low urinary potassium excretion (spot urinary potassium concentration <20 mEq/L from potassium shift into cells), hypophosphatemia, hypophosphaturia, and hypercalciuria. Electromyography during attacks shows low-amplitude compound muscle action potential of the tested muscle. Therapy consists of cautious potassium supplementation (increased risk of rebound hyperkalemia). Use of nonselective beta-blockers (e.g., propranolol) to counteract hyperadrenergic activity, which may be causing TPP, may also be useful.

SUGGESTED READINGS

Available at ExpertConsult.com

RELATED CONTENT

Hyperthyroidism (Patient Information)
Graves Disease (Related Key Topic)
Thyrotoxic Storm (Related Key Topic)

AUTHOR: **FRED F. FERRI, M.D.**

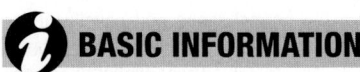

BASIC INFORMATION

DEFINITION

Hypertrophic osteoarthropathy (HOA) is a syndrome of clubbing of the digits, periostitis of long bones, abnormal proliferation of skin, and arthritis. Clubbing may be asymptomatic, but patients with periostitis often have deep aching in long bones which is worse with dependency. HOA may be primary or secondary to other underlying disease processes.

SYNONYMS

Primary hypertrophic osteoarthropathy
Pachydermoperiostosis
Idiopathic clubbing
Touraine-Solente-Golé syndrome
Secondary hypertrophic osteoarthropathy
HOA

ICD-10CM CODES

M89.3	Hypertrophy of bone
M89.40	Other hypertrophic osteoarthropathy, unspecified site
M89.411	Other hypertrophic osteoarthropathy, right shoulder
M89.412	Other hypertrophic osteoarthropathy, left shoulder
M89.419	Other hypertrophic osteoarthropathy, unspecified shoulder
M89.421	Other hypertrophic osteoarthropathy, right upper arm
M89.422	Other hypertrophic osteoarthropathy, left upper arm
M89.429	Other hypertrophic osteoarthropathy, unspecified upper arm
M89.431	Other hypertrophic osteoarthropathy, right forearm
M89.432	Other hypertrophic osteoarthropathy, left forearm
M89.439	Other hypertrophic osteoarthropathy, unspecified forearm
M89.441	Other hypertrophic osteoarthropathy, right hand
M89.442	Other hypertrophic osteoarthropathy, left hand
M89.449	Other hypertrophic osteoarthropathy, unspecified hand
M89.451	Other hypertrophic osteoarthropathy, right thigh
M89.452	Other hypertrophic osteoarthropathy, left thigh
M89.459	Other hypertrophic osteoarthropathy, unspecified thigh
M89.461	Other hypertrophic osteoarthropathy, right lower leg
M89.462	Other hypertrophic osteoarthropathy, left lower leg
M89.469	Other hypertrophic osteoarthropathy, unspecified lower leg
M89.471	Other hypertrophic osteoarthropathy, right ankle and foot
M89.472	Other hypertrophic osteoarthropathy, left ankle and foot
M89.479	Other hypertrophic osteoarthropathy, unspecified ankle and foot
M89.48	Other hypertrophic osteoarthropathy, other site
M89.49	Other hypertrophic osteoarthropathy, multiple sites

EPIDEMIOLOGY & DEMOGRAPHICS

- Fig. 1 provides a classification of HOA.
- Primary HOA is a familial autosomal-dominant disease affecting the age group between 1 and 20 yr and is rare.
- There is a male/female ratio of 9:1 in occurrence.
- Secondary HOA is more common, typically occurs in adults 55 to 75 yr of age. 80% to 90% of secondary HOA is associated with non–small cell lung cancer, most frequently adenocarcinoma; other associated illnesses include:
  1. Pulmonary: Mesothelioma, bronchogenic carcinoma, lung abscesses, empyema, bronchiectasis, cystic fibrosis, pulmonary fibrosis, sarcoidosis, arteriovenous malformations
  2. Gastrointestinal: Carcinoma of esophagus or colon, biliary atresia, peptic ulcer disease, inflammatory bowel disease, hepatocellular carcinoma, liver cirrhosis, amebiasis, laxative abuse, achalasia
  3. Cardiac: Infective endocarditis, right-to-left cardiac shunts, aortic aneurysms, infected aortic bypass graft
  4. Hematologic: Thalassemia, myelofibrosis, Hodgkin lymphoma
  5. Endocrine: Thyroid acropachy, POEMS syndrome (polyneuropathy, organomegaly, endocrinopathy, M component, and skin changes)
  6. Connective tissue diseases
  7. Thymoma
  8. HIV infection
  9. Osteosarcoma
  10. Nasopharyngeal sarcoma

PHYSICAL FINDINGS & CLINICAL PRESENTATION

- Primary HOA typically presents with the insidious onset of clubbing of the hands and feet, described as "spade-like." Finger clubbing is diagnosed by measurement of the digital index (Fig. 2). Other signs and symptoms of HOA include:
  1. Joint pain and swelling
  2. Sensation of warmth or burning in the hands and feet
  3. Coarsening of facial features with grooves or depressions in the scalp, ptosis of the lids
  4. Thickening of the arms and legs
  5. Oily skin, diaphoresis, gynecomastia, and acne
  6. Thin and shiny appearance of the skin around the nail bed
  7. Nail convexity with nail "floating" sensation within the soft tissue is noticed on palpation of the base of the nail bed
  8. Elephant legs: Nonpitting soft tissue swelling with tenderness can be seen
- Secondary HOA patients may present with clinical symptoms before the underlying disorder can be detected. Signs and symptoms are similar to those seen in primary HOA, but there may be findings related to the underlying disease (e.g., bronchogenic carcinoma, infective endocarditis).
- Patients presenting with painful joints prior to developing clubbing can be misdiagnosed as having inflammatory arthritis.

ETIOLOGY

The pathogenesis of HOA is not fully understood; current knowledge suggests that HOA results from the activation of one or more growth factors and inflammatory mediators. Levels of vascular endothelial growth factor (VEGF) have been found to be elevated in both primary and secondary HOA. Platelet-derived growth factor secreted by megakaryocytes that normally are inactivated in the lungs and systemic circulation have been implicated in the etiology of HOA in the setting of pulmonary conditions and right-to-left-shunts. Primary HOA likely has a genetic basis. Mutations in the HPGD gene that encodes for prostaglandin synthesis have been identified in some patients with this condition. The finding of hyperestrogenism in patients with HOA and simple clubbing led to a new hypothesis on the pathogenesis of HOA involving

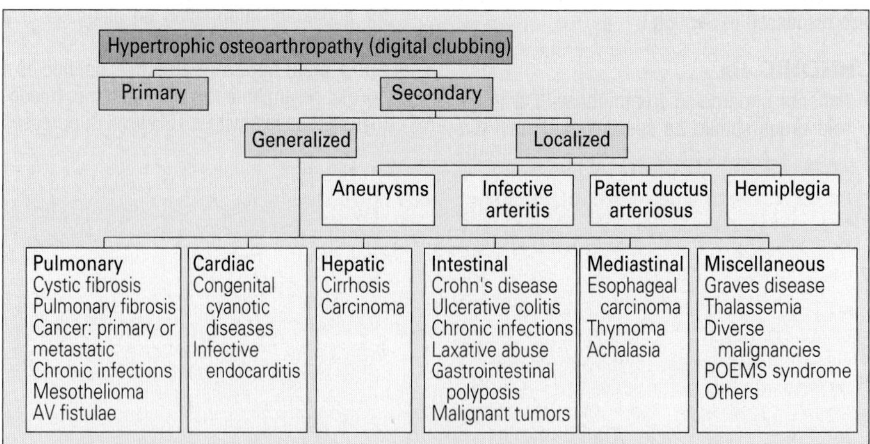

FIG. 1 Classification of hypertrophic osteoarthropathy. *AV,* Arteriovenous; *POEMS,* polyneuropathy, organomegaly, endocrinopathy, monoclonal proteins, and skin changes. (From Hochberg MC, et al.: *Rheumatology,* ed 5, St Louis, 2011, Mosby.)

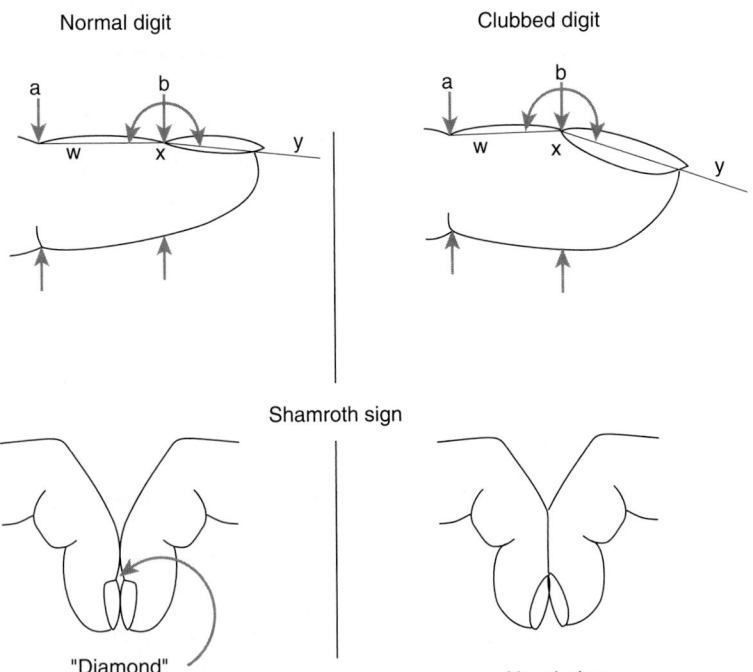

FIG. 2 Clubbing. The normal digit is on the left; the clubbed one, on the right. The distal interphalangeal joint is denoted by **A**; the junction of the nail and skin at the midline is denoted by **B**. The interphalangeal depth ratio is the ratio of the digit's depth measured at **B** divided by that at **A**. The hyponychial angle is the angle *wxy*. In the figure, the depth ratio is 0.9 for the normal digit and 1.2 for the clubbed digit (a ratio >1 indicates clubbing), and the hyponychial angle is 185 degrees for the normal digit and 200 degrees for the clubbed digit (a hyponychial angle >190 degrees indicates clubbing). The Shamroth sign refers to the absence of the diamond-shaped window that normally appears when the terminal phalanges of similar digits are opposed to each other. (From McGee, S: *Evidence-based physical diagnosis,* ed 4, Philadelphia, 2018, Elsevier.)

estrogens, prostaglandin E2, prostaglandin A2, and the inflammatory reflex.

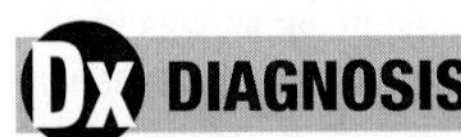

DIAGNOSIS

Diagnosis is primarily clinical; radiographs and bone scans can help confirm the diagnosis.

DIFFERENTIAL DIAGNOSIS

Paget disease, reactive arthritis, psoriatic arthritis, syphilitic periostitis, osteoarthritis, rheumatoid arthritis, osteomyelitis, scleromyxedema, and acromegaly.

WORKUP

HOA warrants an investigation into any associated illnesses.

LABORATORY TESTS

- Routine laboratory studies such as blood count, electrolytes, and urine studies are typically normal in primary and secondary HOA.
- Erythrocyte sedimentation rate is elevated in secondary HOA.
- Liver function tests may be abnormal in patients with secondary HOA from gastrointestinal pathology.
- Alkaline phosphatase may be elevated as a result of periostitis of long bones.
- Analysis of the synovial fluid from joint effusions reveals a low white blood cell count with normal viscosity, color, and complement levels.

IMAGING STUDIES

- A chest radiograph should be obtained to rule out underlying lung cancer.
- Radiographs of the long bones show periosteal new bone formation (Fig. E3).
- Doppler ultrasound may be useful in identifying periostitis.
- Bone scan with technetium-99m reveals cortical uptake
- SPECT/CT can increase specificity by excluding bony metastasis.
- Angiography findings may demonstrate hypervascularization of the finger pads.

Rx TREATMENT

ACUTE GENERAL Rx

- Treatment of primary HOA is symptomatic. Nonsteroidal anti-inflammatory medications, corticosteroids, tamoxifen citrate, or retinoids can be used.
- Colchicine can be helpful for the pain due to subperiosteal new bone formation.
- Reconstructive surgery is indicated for correction of gross disfigurement.
- Case reports of improvement in symptoms of primary HOA with infliximab and arthroscopic synovectomy.
- Treatment of secondary HOA is to eradicate the underlying disease (e.g., antibiotics for infective endocarditis, surgery for bronchogenic carcinoma). Correction of heart malformation or removal of an underlying tumor is rapidly followed by regression of HOA.

CHRONIC Rx

In patients with secondary HOA refractory to NSAIDs and aspirin, octreotide (100 mcg subcutaneously twice daily) and bisphosphonates, including pamidronate (1 mg/kg intravenously to a maximum of 60 mg) and zoledronic acid, which inhibit VEGF expression, have significantly reduced pain.

Vagotomy has been tried with some success. However, the definitive treatment is to treat the underlying disease.

REFERRAL

Referral should be made to rheumatology when the diagnosis of HOA is suspected and the cause remains unclear.

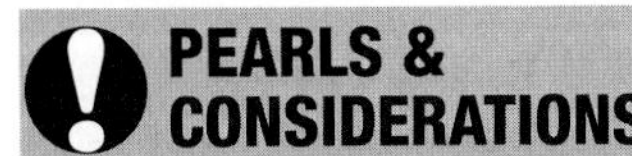

PEARLS & CONSIDERATIONS

- Symptoms of joint pain and swelling in patients with primary HOA often improve with time.
- Prognosis and disease course in patients with secondary HOA will depend on the underlying cause.
- The insidious development of clubbing suggests an infectious process, whereas the rapid progression of clubbing may suggest underlying malignancy.

COMMENTS

- Infections and intrathoracic malignancies are the most common causes of secondary HOA.
- HOA secondary to infection of an arterial graft has been reported.

SUGGESTED READINGS

Available at ExpertConsult.com

AUTHOR: **BERNARD ZIMMERMANN, M.D.**

BASIC INFORMATION

DEFINITION

Hyperuricemia may be defined as serum uric acid >7.0 mg/dl in males or >6.0 mg/dl in females. Some persons who are not hyperuricemic by this definition will have levels of uric acid that exceed the limit of solubility of uric acid in tissue. Data from the Framingham study indicate that hyperuricemia increased from 4.8% of the population in the early 1970s to 9.3% in the mid-1980s. Age is an important risk factor in the increasing incidence of hyperuricemia and gout. Women become hyperuricemic at an older age than men due to the uricosuric effect of estrogen. Most people with hyperuricemia are asymptomatic and will remain so; however, 20% of those with serum uric acid >9 mg/dl will develop gout in 5 yr. Hyperuricemia is strongly associated with gout, obesity, diabetes, hypertension, and cardiovascular disease but has not been proven to cause any of these conditions.

ASYMPTOMATIC HYPERURICEMIA

Definition: Laboratory evidence of elevated serum uric acid without clinical disease known to be caused by hyperuricemia

ICD-10CM CODE
E79.0 Hyperuricemia without signs of inflammatory arthritis and tophaceous disease

ETIOLOGY

Overproduction of uric acid accounts for a minority of cases of hyperuricemia. Most cases are due to decreased renal clearance of uric acid and high dietary purine consumption. Fig. E1 describes factors affecting urate balance. Table 1 describes classification of hyperuricemia and gout.

TABLE 1 Classification of Hyperuricemia and Gout

Impaired Uric Acid Excretion
Primary gout with decreased uric acid clearance
Secondary gout
Clinical conditions
Reduced glomerular filtration rate
Hypertension
Obesity
Systemic acidosis
Familial juvenile hyperuricemic nephropathy
Medullary cystic kidney disease
Lead nephropathy
Drugs
Diuretics
Ethanol
Low-dose salicylates (0.3-3.0 g/day)
Cyclosporine
Tacrolimus
Levodopa
Excessive urate production
Primary metabolic disorders
HPRT deficiency
PRPP synthetase overactivity
Glucose-6-phosphatase deficiency
Fructose-1-phosphate aldolase deficiency
Secondary causes
Clinical conditions
Myelo- and lymphoproliferative disorders
Obesity
Psoriasis
Glycogenoses III, V, VII
Drugs and dietary components
Nicotinic acid
Pancreatic extract
Cytotoxic drugs
Red meat, organ meat, shellfish
Alcoholic beverages (especially beer)
Fructose

HPRT, Hypoxanthine-guanine phosphoribosyltransferase; *PRPP*, phosphoribosyl pyrophosphate.
From Goldman L, Schafer AI: *Goldman's Cecil medicine*, ed 24, Philadelphia, 2012, Saunders.

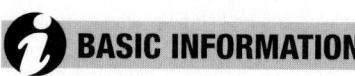

DIAGNOSIS

EVALUATION

The finding of hyperuricemia should prompt a thorough evaluation of potential causes and related diseases. Fig. 2 describes the evaluation of patients with hyperuricemia. If there is no clinical evidence of gout, nephrolithiasis, or acute kidney injury, the patient may be said to have asymptomatic hyperuricemia. Potential causes of elevated uric acid include malignancy, renal insufficiency, toxins, lead toxicity, and dietary indiscretion. If a careful history and physical exam do not reveal an evident cause of persistent hyperuricemia, a 24-hour urine collection for uric acid and creatinine may be considered. Patients with urinary excretion of uric acid >800 mg/24 hours are likely to be overproducers of uric acid and should be investigated more thoroughly for the underlying cause of their hyperuricemia.

LABORATORY TESTS

- CBC with differential
- Blood urea nitrogen (BUN)/creatinine
- Urinalysis
- Lipid profile
- Consider 24-hour urine collection for uric acid

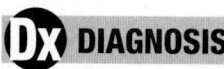

TREATMENT

No specific therapy is indicated for most patients with asymptomatic hyperuricemia. Lifestyle and dietary modification are often advisable.

NONPHARMACOLOGIC THERAPY

- Weight loss
- Reduce alcohol intake, especially beer
- Reduce consumption of foods known to be high in purines such as red meat, organ meat, and high-fructose soft drinks

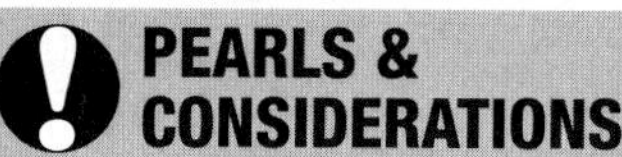

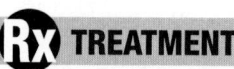

PEARLS & CONSIDERATIONS

- Research suggests there may be a causal relationship between hyperuricemia and early hypertension.
- Very high levels of serum uric acid may warrant treatment even if asymptomatic.
- Patients with hyperuricemia and a family history of gout should be followed closely for the development of gouty arthritis.
- Hyperuricemia in patients with gout should almost always be treated with urate-lowering medication (see "Gout").
- The presence of gouty tophi or arthritis due to gout is an absolute indication for urate-lowering therapy.

There is evidence from several sources suggesting that treatment of hyperuricemia slows the progression of chronic kidney disease (CKD) in patients without gout. However, one large randomized controlled study of febuxostat therapy in stage 3 CKD conducted in Japan was unable to replicate this finding. Current recommendations do not support the use of urate-lowering therapy in CKD unless there is concomitant gout, but the issue needs further study.

Recent studies have suggested that allopurinol use is associated with a reduced risk of myocardial infarction and reduction in all-cause mortality. These preliminary studies have sparked renewed interest in research to evaluate the effects of treatment of asymptomatic hyperuricemia in hopes of improving the many disease states associated with high levels of serum uric acid.

SUGGESTED READINGS
Available at ExpertConsult.com

RELATED CONTENT

Gout (Related Key Topic)

AUTHOR: **BERNARD ZIMMERMANN, M.D.**

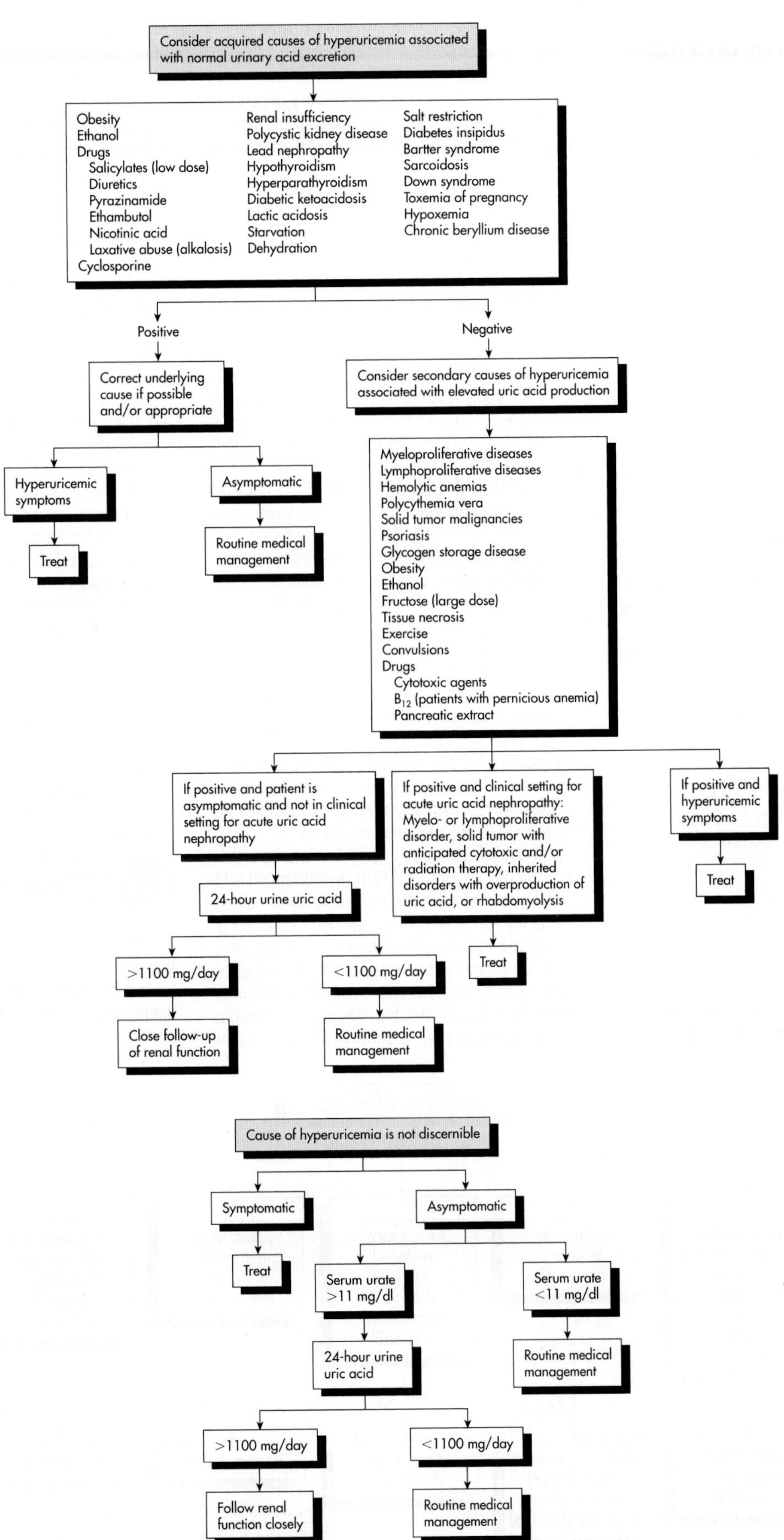

FIG. 2 Evaluation of patients with hyperuricemia. (From Harris ED, et al. [eds]: *Kelley's textbook of rheumatology,* ed 7, Philadelphia, 2005, Saunders.)

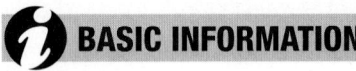

BASIC INFORMATION

DEFINITION

- Persistently or recurrently diminished or absent sexual/erotic thoughts or fantasies and desire for sexual activity.
- The judgment of deficiency is made by the clinician taking into account factors related to age, social context, and general contexts of the individual's life.
- Symptoms must have been present for a minimum of 6 mo, the majority of the time, and be distressing to the individual.
- The lack of desire must not be better explained by a nonsexual mental disorder or by severe relationship distress or other significant stressor.
- Must also not be better attributable to substance/medication or another medical condition.

SYNONYMS

Subsumed in female sexual interest/arousal disorder
Hypoactive sexual desire disorder, situational
Psychosexual desire disorder, situational hypoactive
Psychosexual dysfunction associated with inhibited libido
Psychosexual dysfunction with inhibited libido
Situational hypoactive sexual desire disorder
HSDD

ICD-10CM CODES
F52.0 Hypoactive sexual desire disorder
F52.22 Female sexual arousal disorder
DSM-5 CODES
302.71
302.72

EPIDEMIOLOGY & DEMOGRAPHICS

PEAK INCIDENCE: Prevalence of low sexual desire increases with age. Middle-aged women (45 to 65 yr old) and men over 60 appear at greatest risk of experiencing qualifying distress.

PREVALENCE:

- Among males, rates of HSDD vary depending on country of origin and means of assessment. Generally, 6% of men 18 to 24 and 41% of men 66 to 74 report problems with sexual desire. Persistent lack of sexual interest that lasts longer than 6 mo is seen in approximately 1.8% of men 16 to 44.
- For women, rates of HSDD are more uncertain, especially given the new inclusion of HSDD into female sexual interest/arousal disorder. Prior studies with less stringent criteria suggest approximately 36% of women endorse low sexual desire, but roughly only 8% report experiencing clinical levels of related distress. These rates also vary by country of origin and method of assessment (Fig. 1).

PREDOMINANT SEX AND AGE: HSDD appears to be more prevalent in women; however, men are more likely to be underdiagnosed or misdiagnosed with another sexual dysfunction.

GENETICS: There appears to be a strong influence of genetics in the vulnerability of women to sexual dysfunction. Specifically, women with the ll genotype for the SCL6A4 promoter region (5HTTLPR) appear to be eight times more likely to have selective serotonin reuptake inhibitor (SSRI) associated sexual dysfunction if they are also taking oral contraceptives. Men with the ll genotype have also been found to be at greater risk of sexual dysfunction. Similarly, dopamine (D4) receptor polymorphisms influence all phases of the sexual response cycle.

RISK FACTORS: Temperamental and environmental risk factors for HSDD include mood and anxiety symptoms, negative cognitions about sexuality or relationship, alcohol use, early childhood trauma, interpersonal problems, and lack of adequate sex education. Physiological risk factors include age, medical conditions such as diabetes mellitus, thyroid dysfunction, hyperprolactinemia, coronary disease, renal failure, and androgen deficiency, as well as other neuroendocrine changes.

PHYSICAL FINDINGS & CLINICAL PRESENTATION:

- HSDD can be lifelong or acquired as well as generalized or situational.
- Men appear more likely to present with the acquired, situational subtype.
- For women, lack of pleasure is a common presenting clinical complaint.
- Consideration of initiation of sexual activity and receptivity to sexual activity initiated by the partner should be assessed. Men are often more likely to initiate sexual encounters, and noninitiation may be a signifier of a possible problem, but any shift in pattern of initiation should be investigated further.
- Other sexual activities such as masturbation or partnered sexual activity may still occur even in the context of low sexual desire.
- The interpersonal context of HSDD should be taken into account, as often a desire discrepancy between partners leads to discussions of possible HSDD, but this is not sufficient for diagnosis.
- Symptoms should be present for approximately 6 mo, but clinical judgment can be used if symptoms are of lesser duration.

ETIOLOGY

Best evidence suggests a multifactorial etiology, including factors along the biopsychosocial continuum, including genetic vulnerability, interpersonal distress, cultural factors, mental health, medical conditions, and medical treatments.

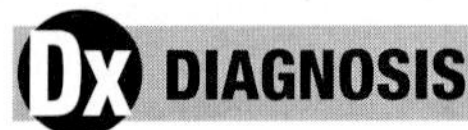

DIAGNOSIS

DIFFERENTIAL DIAGNOSIS

If low sexual desire can be attributed largely to one of these factors, HSDD should not be diagnosed, and the underlying factor should be addressed.

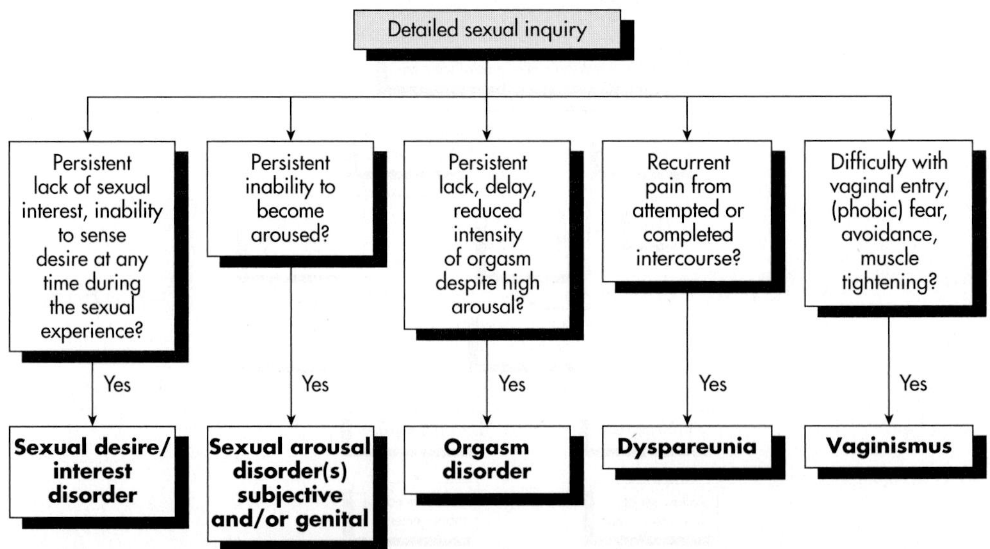

FIG. 1 Currently recommended definitions for women's sexual dysfunction. Comorbidity is usual, especially sexual desire/interest disorder with one of the sexual arousal disorders. (From Melmed S et al: *Williams textbook of endocrinology*, ed 12, Philadelphia, 2011, Saunders.)

- Nonsexual mental disorder: Depression, anxiety, posttraumatic stress disorder, and schizophrenia
- Substance/medication use: Drugs of abuse (e.g., alcohol), anticonvulsants (e.g., carbamazepine), cardiovascular and antihypertensive agents (e.g., clonidine), hormonal medications (e.g., oral contraceptives), and psychotropic medications (e.g., SSRIs).
- Another medical condition: Endocrine disorders (e.g., diabetes mellitus), coronary artery disease, cancer, central nervous system disease, hypertension, and arthritis.
- Interpersonal factors: Relationship discord, partner sexual problems, dissatisfaction with partner or relationship, communication deficits, and intimate partner violence.
- Other sexual dysfunctions: Erectile disorder, female orgasmic disorder, and genitopelvic pain/penetration disorder.

WORKUP

- Clinical interview should include a sexual history, medical history, and psychosocial history. The sexual history should include questions about prior sexual issues, sexual behavior and practices, and patient's treatment goals.
- A physical examination may be warranted for some female patients to identify possible contributing factors to low desire such as vulvovaginal atrophy, genital sensory changes, and pelvic floor prolapse.
- Symptoms of depression and anxiety should be assessed. This can be done with brief screeners such as the PHQ-9 and GAD-7.
- Adequate endocrine functioning can be assessed through a combination of history taking (e.g., menstrual patterns) and laboratory tests when warranted by history.
- Self-rating scales and standardized symptom-specific checklist may be helpful in diagnosis and determining treatment. Example screeners include the Brief Sexual Symptom Checklist (BSSC), the Decreased Sexual Desire Screener (DSDS), and Female Sexual Function Index (FSFI).

LABORATORY TESTS

- Laboratory tests should be undertaken if indicated by history or physical exam.
- Common tests include:
  1. Thyroid function, serum total testosterone, prolactin, follicle-stimulating hormone (FSH), and luteinizing hormone (LH).

Rx TREATMENT

NONPHARMACOLOGIC THERAPY

- Multimodal interventions are often needed to address the complex etiology of HSDD.
- Basic sex education can be a valuable in-office intervention that can alleviate distress that arises from unrealistic norms or misunderstandings related to basic reproductive anatomy and physiology.
- Simple suggestions related to reducing stress, increasing communication with partner, and leading a healthy lifestyle can help to improve sexual function for some.
- Patients should be referred for psychological intervention when medical rule-outs have been completed. Therapist should have experience with treating sexual problems.
- The number of controlled trials studying the efficacy of psychological treatment for HSDD is limited; however, available evidence suggests significant improvements with the use of cognitive behavioral therapy, mindfulness-based approaches, traditional sex therapy, or a combination.
- There is support for both individual- and couple-based treatments.

ACUTE GENERAL Rx

- Currently, only one FDA-approved treatment exists for premenopausal women with HSDD: Flibanserin (Addyi). Addyi is a multifunctional serotonin agonist/antagonist that passes through the blood-brain barrier and selectively affects the prefrontal cortex. Addyi has been shown to increase the number of satisfying sexual events per month.
- Addyi is contraindicated for use with moderate and strong CYP3A4 inhibitors, with alcohol, and in patients with hepatic impairments. Side effects include dizziness, somnolence, fatigue, and nausea.
- The FDA has required a Risk Evaluation and Mitigation Strategy (REMS) for Addyi, which requires prescribers and pharmacies to be certified in the REMS program to prescribe and dispense. More information is available at: https://addyirems.com/AddyiUI/rems/home.action.
- Bupropion hydrochloride is a mild dopamine and norepinephrine reuptake inhibitor and nicotinic acetylcholine receptor antagonist that is used as an antidepressant and smoking cessation aid. There is some empirical evidence for off-label use suggesting that bupropion significantly increases sexual desire in nondepressed women. It has also been shown to be effective in reversing SSRI-induced sexual dysfunction.
- Buspirone is a serotonin 1A partial agonist and is used off-label for treatment of HSDD. It has been shown to reduce low-desire side effects of SSRIs when coadministered.
- Testosterone is widely prescribed off-label for postmenopausal women, with substantial evidence suggesting testosterone therapy improves sexual well-being among postmenopausal women. There is limited evidence for similar effects among premenopausal women.
- Testosterone is a well-established treatment for men with HSDD secondary to low testosterone.

COMPLEMENTARY & ALTERNATIVE MEDICINE

Recent studies have shown good preliminary efficacy of treating both sexual arousal and desire disorders with mindfulness, yoga, and meditation as a complement to psychotherapy.

DISPOSITION

- HSDD is a common sexual dysfunction that affects both men and women across the life span. With appropriate identification and treatment, many patients will experience improvement in sexual desire; however, finding appropriate referrals and support for patients may be challenging.
- Specific types of HSDD can resolve in time untreated if a patient's contextual factors change (e.g., new partner), but for others HSDD will persist or worsen without treatment.
- Patients may be at higher risk for relationship discord and other psychiatric disorders such as depression and anxiety.

REFERRAL

- Most patients presenting with HSDD would benefit from referral to a therapist skilled in treating sexual problems.
- Patients with unresolved physical or sexual trauma should be promptly referred to a specialist.
- Establishing a referral network of specialists in sexual medicine and therapy is important.

PEARLS & CONSIDERATIONS

- Biological and psychological factors often comingle and contribute to the individual picture of HSDD.
- Linguistic and cultural variations can heavily impact the presentation of HSDD and the associated distress as well as treatment.
- New FDA-approved medication Addyi remains controversial among sexual medicine specialists.
- Discussions of potential sexual side effects of medications and of general sexual health with all patients will allow for more open conversations when problems do arise.

SUGGESTED READINGS

Available at ExpertConsult.com

RELATED CONTENT

Ejaculation and Orgasm Disorders (Related Key Topic)

Sexual Dysfunction in Women (Related Key Topic)

AUTHOR: **KARLENE CUNNINGHAM, PH.D.**

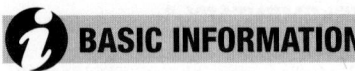

BASIC INFORMATION

DEFINITION

Hypoglycemia refers to abnormally low blood glucose levels in circulating plasma. It is defined as a glucose value less than 70 mg/dl (3.9 mmol/L). "Serious hypoglycemia" refers to values <54 mg/dl (3.0 mmol/L). "Severe hypoglycemia" is any glucose value necessitating external assistance to correct it. "Reactive hypoglycemia" refers to symptoms of hypoglycemia with plasma glucose value greater than 70 mg/dl. A multitude of scenarios can lead to this potentially fatal condition.

SYNONYMS

Glycopenia
Low blood glucose
Low blood sugar
HG

ICD-10CM CODES

E16.1	Other hypoglycemia
E16.2	Hypoglycemia, unspecified
E10.641	Type 1 diabetes mellitus with hypoglycemia with coma
E10.649	Type 1 diabetes mellitus with hypoglycemia without coma
E11.641	Type 2 diabetes mellitus with hypoglycemia with coma
E11.649	Type 2 diabetes mellitus with hypoglycemia without coma
E13.641	Other specified diabetes mellitus with hypoglycemia with coma
E13.649	Other specified diabetes mellitus with hypoglycemia without coma

EPIDEMIOLOGY & DEMOGRAPHICS

- More frequent in type 1 diabetes mellitus (DM). Estimated that glucose levels may be as low as 50 to 60 mg/dl ~10% of the time in T1DM.
- HG occurrence 62 to 320 episodes per 100 patient yr in type 1 diabetes vs. 35 episodes per 100 patient yr in type 2 diabetes.

PHYSICAL EXAMINATION & CLINICAL PRESENTATION

- Symptoms are often nonspecific.
- Early symptoms include sweating, pallor, anxiety, palpitations, hunger, and tremor.
- Late symptoms with lower plasma glucose levels include seizures, altered mental status, and coma.
- Profound or prolonged hypoglycemic episodes can cause irreversible brain injury, cardiopulmonary arrest, and death.

ETIOLOGY

- Medications are the most common cause of hypoglycemia.
  1. Most common causes include exogenous insulin, insulin secretagogues (sulfonylureas [SU] and meglitinides [MG]), and alcohol
- Critical illness
  1. Organ failure (hepatic, cardiac, or renal)
  2. Sepsis
- Hormone deficiency (cortisol, glucagon, and epinephrine)
- Endogenous hyperinsulinism (insulinoma, functional beta-cell disorders, insulin autoimmune hypoglycemia)
- Rare fatal episodes thought to be secondary to ventricular arrhythmias

Dx DIAGNOSIS

Characterized by Whipple triad:

- Symptoms potentially explained by hypoglycemia
- Low blood glucose levels during the symptoms
- Relief of symptoms with administration of glucose or glucagon

DIFFERENTIAL DIAGNOSIS

- Hypoglycemic symptoms in the presence of normal plasma glucose levels (>70 mg/dl) point to other etiologies
  1. Postprandial syndrome, cardiac disease, psychiatric disease, metabolic disorders (hyperthyroidism, pheochromocytoma)

WORKUP

- If Whipple triad is positive, the next step is to consider a patient's medical status.
- Iatrogenic causes are the most common causes of hypoglycemia in hospitalized patients (review the timing of glucose-lowering medications and interactions between medications).
- Detailed history, including past medical history, a thorough medication history, and timing of hypoglycemia (in regard to meals and medications).

LABORATORY TESTS

- An algorithm for recognition and evaluation of hypoglycemia is described in Fig. 1.
- If the cause is not apparent after a thorough history, the following labs are appropriate:

FASTING: If symptoms witnessed when fasting, with verified low blood glucose levels, draw the following labs: plasma glucose, ß-hydroxybutyrate (BHOB), insulin, C-peptide, proinsulin, screen for SU and MG metabolites.

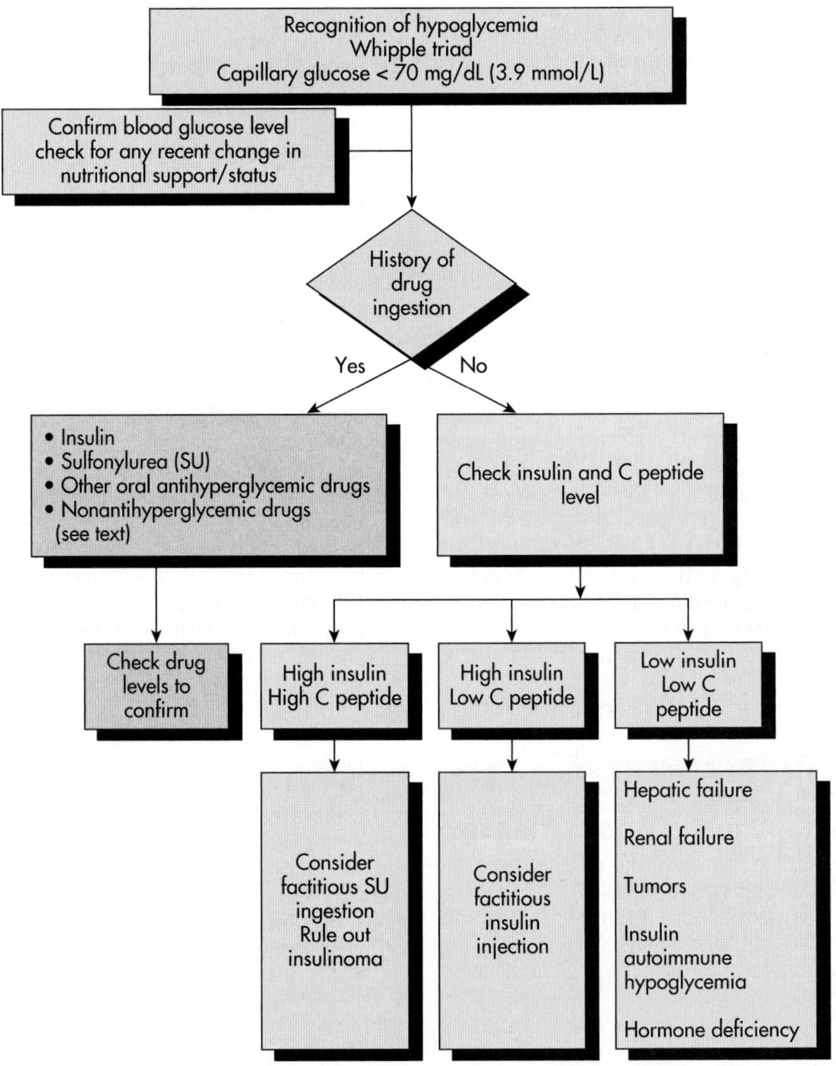

FIG. 1 Recognition and evaluation of hypoglycemia. (From Vincent JL, Abraham E, Moore FA et al: *Textbook of critical care*, ed 7, Philadelphia, 2017, Elsevier.)

POSTPRANDIAL:

- Plasma glucose, insulin, C-peptide, and proinsulin prior to ingestion of the meal and every 30 min thereafter for 5 hr.
- Only evaluate the samples drawn when glucose levels are <60 mg/dl.
- If a patient has a presentation consistent with Whipple triad, then measure SU, MG, and antibodies to insulin.

72-HR FAST:

- Collect blood specimens for measurement of plasma glucose, insulin, C-peptide, proinsulin, and BHOB every 6 hr until the glucose concentration is <60 mg/dl.
- Increase frequency of sampling to every 1 to 2 hr.
- Insulin, C-peptide, and proinsulin are only relevant in those specimens in which the plasma glucose concentration is <60 mg/dl.
- The fast should be ended when any of the following occurs:
  1. The plasma glucose concentration is <45 mg/dl.
  2. The patient has symptoms or signs of hypoglycemia.
  3. 72 hr have elapsed.
  4. The plasma glucose concentration is <55 and Whipple triad has been documented on a prior occasion.
- Insulin antibodies are also measured but do not need to be measured during the hypoglycemic state.

IMAGING

If hypoglycemia is suspected secondary to an insulinoma or malignancy, transabdominal ultrasound (US), CT scan, or endoscopic US can be used to help with diagnosis as well as for staging purposes.

Rx TREATMENT

NONPHARMACOLOGIC THERAPY

- Recognition of signs and symptoms, and self-monitoring of blood glucose are especially important in insulin-deficient patient.
- Avoiding drugs that can exacerbate condition (e.g., alcohol) if it occurs on repeated occasions.
- Bedtime snacks if hypoglycemia occurs at night
- In situations caused by tumor etiologies (e.g., islet cell, insulinoma, and nonislet cell), definitive treatment may require surgical removal.

PHARMACOLOGIC THERAPY

- Treating the underlying etiology that exacerbates hypoglycemia (e.g., infection, proper diabetic regimen)
- Fast-acting carbohydrates (e.g., glucose tablets, hard candy, IV dextrose infusion)
- Pure glucose (dextrose) if caused by insulin secretagogue in addition with alpha-glucosidase inhibitor
- In severe hypoglycemia with seizure activity, 25 g of 50% dextrose IV or 0.5 to 1.0 mg IM/subcutaneous glucagon
- Fig. 2 describes a management algorithm for hypoglycemia

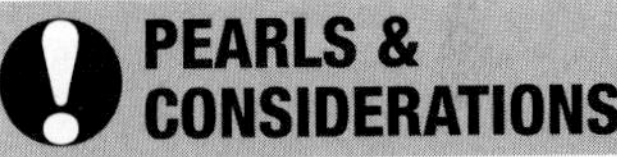

PEARLS & CONSIDERATIONS

- Hypoglycemia can cause severe morbidity and death if not dealt with promptly and effectively.
- Hypoglycemia is very common in patients with diabetes mellitus, especially type 1 DM, and most commonly it is a side effect of medications.
- In patients who are hospitalized, the etiology is often multifactorial.
- Clinically important hypoglycemia is uncommon in nondiabetic patients, and evaluation for a hypoglycemic disorder in these patients should only occur if the Whipple triad is met.

REFERRAL

- Most scenarios of hypoglycemia can be managed by primary care physicians by adjusting medications.
- If the cause is not clear, then endocrinology referral is recommended.

RELATED CONTENT

Insulinoma (Related Key Topic)
Postprandial (Reactive) Hypoglycemia (Related Key Topic)
Diabetes Mellitus (Related Key Topic)

AUTHOR: **JAFET OJEDA RODRIGUEZ, M.D.**

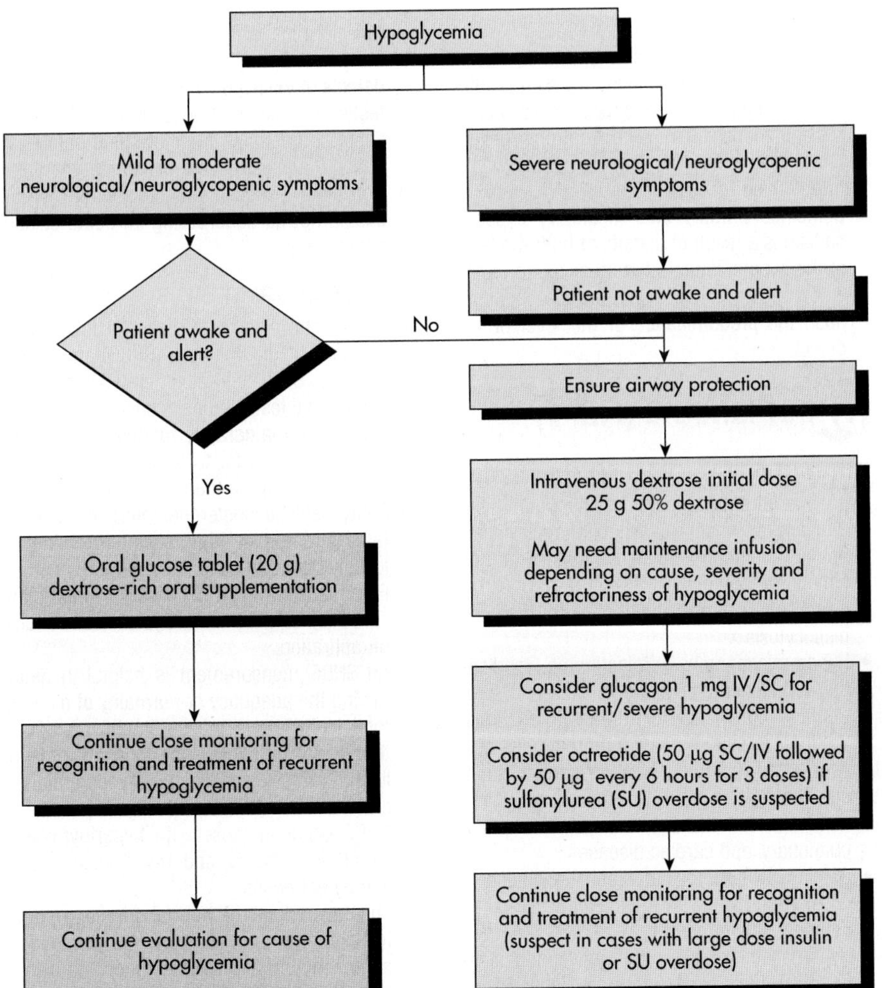

FIG. 2 Management of hypoglycemia. (From Vincent JL, Abraham E, Moore FA et al: *Textbook of critical care*, ed 7, Philadelphia, 2017, Elsevier.)

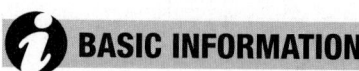

BASIC INFORMATION

DEFINITION

Male hypogonadism is a clinical syndrome involving subnormal testosterone levels and/or impaired sperm production due to dysfunction at one or both levels of the hypothalamic-pituitary-testicular axis.

SYNONYM

Testicular dysfunction

ICD-10CM CODES

E29	Testicular dysfunction
E29.1	Testicular hypofunction
E29.8	Other testicular dysfunction
E29.9	Testicular dysfunction, unspecified
E23.0	Hypopituitarism
E23.1	Drug-induced hypopituitarism
E89.3	Postprocedural hypopituitarism

EPIDEMIOLOGY & DEMOGRAPHICS

INCIDENCE: Hypogonadism is the most common clinical disorder of the testis. Incidence is unclear due to the many possible underlying factors, nonspecificity of symptoms, and questions relating to the adequacy of a diagnostic serum total testosterone threshold.

PREVALENCE: Prevalence of hypogonadism increases with aging, obesity, diabetes mellitus, and other comorbidities. The average decrease in serum total testosterone levels in aging men is 1% to 2% per year. Prevalence rises to 23% among men in their 70s. However, in population-based surveys of community-dwelling middle-aged and older males, prevalence of hypogonadism is approximately 6%.

GENETICS: Genetic abnormalities, underlie a number of hypogonadal disorders including Klinefelter syndrome, Noonan syndrome, hemochromatosis, Kallmann syndrome, and Prader-Willi syndrome.

RISK FACTORS: These are many and include genetic abnormalities; the aging process; pituitary and testicular lesions and disorders; medications; drug abuse; HIV disease; acute illnesses; chronic cardiac, hepatic, renal, and pulmonary diseases; cancer; ionizing radiation; chemotherapy; obesity; and malnutrition.

PHYSICAL FINDINGS & CLINICAL PRESENTATION

Sexual (specific)

- Decrease in frequency of erections
- Erectile dysfunction
- Decrease in libido
- Decreased fertility
- Small or shrinking testes
- Gynecomastia
- Diminished sexual hair
- Hot flushes and sweats

Neuropsychologic (less specific)

- Depression
- Inability to concentrate
- Diminished motivation and vitality
- Decrease in self-confidence
- Diminished energy and stamina
- Sleep disturbances

Physical features and findings

- Diminished capacity for physical activity
- Decrease in physical endurance and performance
- Diminished muscle mass and strength
- Increase in body fat
- Decrease or loss of axillary and pubic hair and decrease in shaving frequency
- Fine wrinkling over the lateral aspects of the face
- Breast enlargement with or without tenderness
- Change in consistency and decrease in size of testes
- Fragility fractures
- Anemia

ETIOLOGY

- The importance of a careful history and examination cannot be overstated to determine the etiology of possible hypogonadism. Primary hypogonadism is a result of a decrease in testicular testosterone secretion and/or a decrease in spermatogenesis with an associated increase in gonadotropin levels as in Klinefelter syndrome, cryptorchidism, and following orchitis, testicular trauma, chemotherapy, and irradiation.
- Secondary hypogonadism is due to hypothalamic-pituitary dysfunction, which results in a decrease in testosterone levels and/or spermatogenesis with gonadotropin levels that are subnormal or inappropriately within the normal range.
- Combined primary and secondary hypogonadism is a result of deficits at both the level of the hypothalamic-pituitary axis and testes with variable gonadotropin levels depending upon the predominance of the level of the defect.

Dx DIAGNOSIS (FIG. 1)

DIFFERENTIAL DIAGNOSIS

Hypogonadotropic or secondary hypogonadism

- Pituitary dysfunction—hypopituitarism, functioning or nonfunctioning pituitary tumor, lymphocytic hypophysitis, infiltrative disease as with sarcoidosis, hemochromatosis, and histiocytosis X
- Hyperprolactinemia—prolactinoma, medication-related, chronic kidney disease
- Genetic—Kallmann syndrome with anosmia, Prader-Willi syndrome with morbid obesity
- Acute and chronic illnesses, malnutrition, emotional disorders, HIV, sleep apnea, aging, malignancies, obesity, and renal, hepatic, pulmonary, and cardiac diseases
- Opioids, CNS—active medications, glucocorticoid excess, and GnRH analogues (androgen deprivation therapy)

Hypergonadotropic or primary hypogonadism

- Genetic—Klinefelter syndrome, Noonan syndrome, myotonic dystrophy
- Gonadal damage due to drugs, alcohol, radiation, chemotherapy, trauma
- Congenital anorchia (vanishing testis syndrome)
- Cryptorchidism
- Mumps orchitis, HIV orchitis
- Diabetes mellitus
- Hodgkin's disease
- Aging

Combined primary and secondary hypogonadism

- Hemochromatosis, sickle cell disease, thalassemia
- Alcoholism, glucocorticoid therapy, aging
- Chronic cardiac, hepatic, renal, pulmonary diseases, and HIV disease

WORKUP

- Determine the presence or absence of male hypogonadism on the basis of history, clinical manifestations and findings, and documentation of consistently low serum total testosterone levels and/or abnormal seminal fluid analysis.
- Morning serum total testosterone levels should be measured on at least 2 or 3 occasions for confirmation of diagnosis and when necessary followed by measurement of serum free or bioavailable testosterone.
- Serum follicle-stimulating hormone (FSH) and luteinizing hormone (LH) levels are measured to determine whether hypogonadism is primary, secondary, or a result of combined defects of the hypothalamic-pituitary axis and testis. The case of testosterone deficiency should be definitively determined before initiation of testosterone replacement therapy.
- Hormonal assessment of gonadal status should not be done during an acute or subacute illness.

LABORATORY TESTS

- Serum total testosterone is tightly bound to sex hormone binding globulin (SHBG) and weakly bound to circulating albumin. 0.5% to 3% of serum total testosterone is unbound or free.
- Liquid chromatography tandem mass spectrometry assays for total serum testosterone are more accurate than immunoassays.
- Bioavailable testosterone refers to unbound testosterone plus the testosterone that is loosely bound to albumin.
- Free testosterone, if necessary, is best measured by equilibrium dialysis or centrifugal ultrafiltration.
- An SHBG measurement is helpful in determining the adequacy or normality of a serum total testosterone measurement. Conditions that lower SHBG include obesity, protein-losing states, androgens, hypothyroidism, and familial SHBG deficiency. Increases in SHBG occur in those with hyperthyroidism, hepatitis, cirrhosis, and HIV disease, aging, and by estrogens.
- The lower limit of normal for serum total testosterone in a healthy young male is approximately 240 to 280 ng/dl and a low-normal serum free testosterone in a young normal male is 9 pg/ml.
- Serum total testosterone levels can vary from day-to-day and there is a diurnal

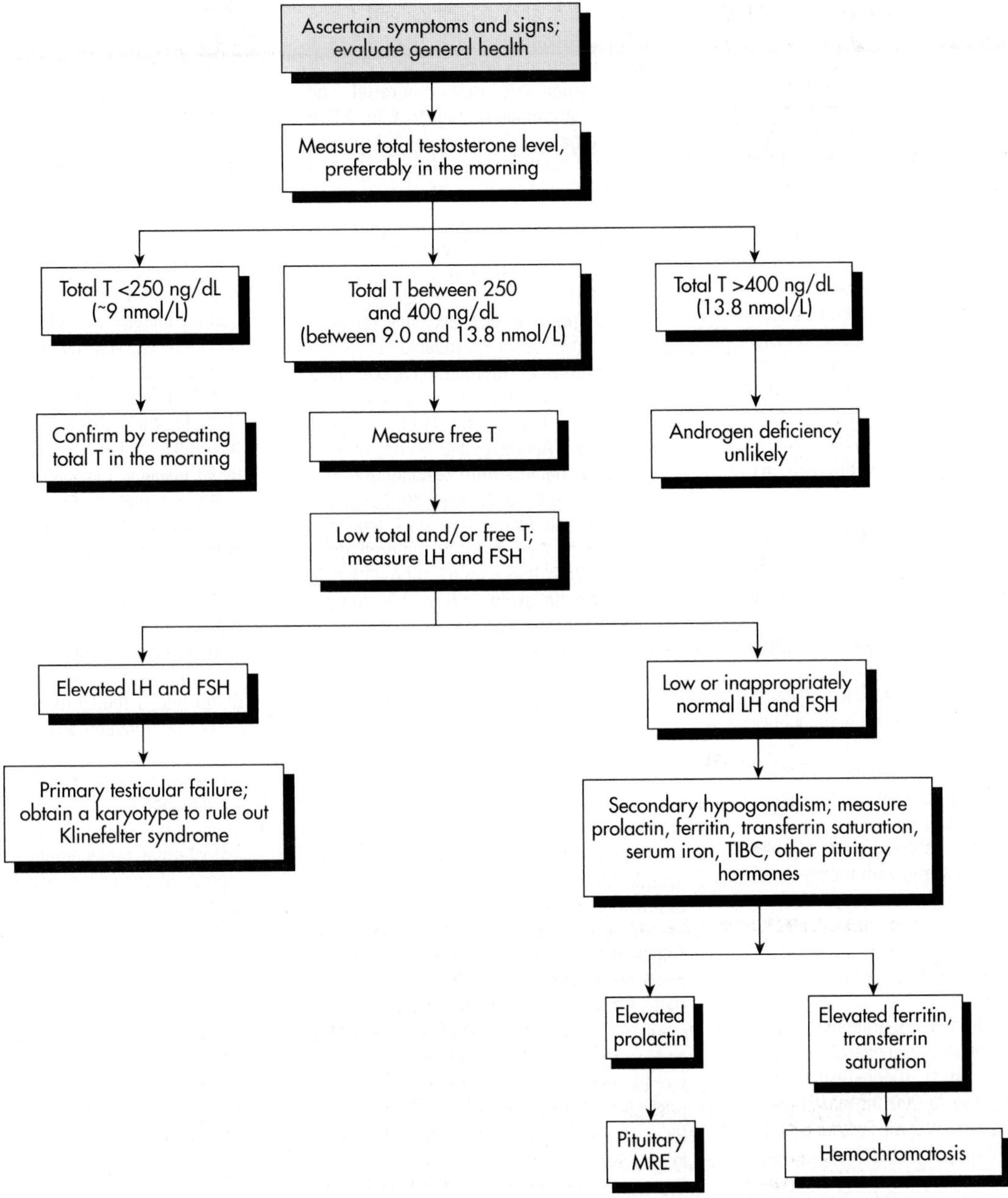

FIG. 1 Algorithm showing an approach for the diagnostic evaluation of adult men suspected of having androgen deficiency. *FSH,* Follicle-stimulating hormone; *LH,* luteinizing hormone; *MRE,* magnetic resonance elastography; *MRI,* magnetic resonance imaging; *TIBC,* total iron-binding capacity. (Modified from Shalender B, Shehzad B: Diagnosis and treatment of hypogonadism in men, *Best Pract Res Clin Endocrin* 25(2):251-270, 2011.)

rhythm in young normal males with morning levels that are higher by approximately 20% to 25% as compared with levels in the afternoon.

- In elderly males, the diurnal rhythm is diminished with levels approximately 10% lower in the afternoon as compared with morning levels.
- Serum FSH and LH measurements are important in delineating primary, secondary, and combined hypogonadism.
- Hypogonadal symptoms are more likely to be seen in those with total serum testosterone level below the lower limit of values for young normal males. Serum total testosterone levels of <150 ng/dl are unequivocally low.
- Transient suppression of total serum testosterone may occur during acute illness, in males that are being treated with glucocorticoid, in those taking opiates or CNS-active medications, in those with malnutrition or poor eating habits, and during excessive physical exercise.
- Quantity and quality of sperm counts and activity can vary in a significant way for a variety of reasons. Therefore, in assessing fertility, seminal fluid analysis should be done on two or more occasions, each separated by two or more weeks, and on semen collected within an hour of ejaculation after more than two days of abstinence.
- Depending on the clinical picture and examination, other studies may be necessary, including a karyotype analysis, for example, for Klinefelter syndrome, or serum prolactin measurement for patients with possible hyperprolactinemia, which may be drug-induced, related to a prolactinoma, or to chronic renal disease.

IMAGING STUDIES

In males with severe androgen deficiency with low serum gonadotropin levels, increased serum prolactin levels, hypopituitarism, severe headaches, and visual defects, an MRI of the pituitary would be appropriate. In males with hypogonadism and a history of fractures, dual energy x-ray absorptiometry (DXA) measurements of spine and hip should be obtained to further delineate the status of the skeletal system.

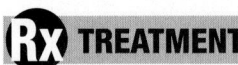

TREATMENT

Testosterone replacement therapy is indicated when patients have symptoms and signs of hypogonadism and serum testosterone levels that are consistently subnormal with levels of <250 ng/dl. The goal of replacement therapy is to restore serum testosterone levels to within the normal range of values and to have a positive effect on the constellation of hypogonadal symptoms and signs. Subnormal spermatogenesis, if present in such patients, is not affected by testosterone therapy. In patients with hypogonadotropic or secondary hypogonadism, chorionic gonadotropin and/or GnRH therapy can optimize spermatogenesis, whereas, generally in patients with primary hypogonadism, subnormal spermatogenesis and infertility are irreversible.

NONPHARMACOLOGIC THERAPY

- Weight reduction, especially when it appears to be a major factor underlying male hypogonadism
- Discontinuation of anabolic steroids, CNS-active medications, and narcotic abuse
- Surgery or radiation therapy for patients with a pituitary functioning or nonfunctioning tumor with visual field abnormality and headaches who are not candidates for further medical therapy or have been unsuccessfully treated with medication
- Surgery indicated for chronic gynecomastia and, occasionally, in cases with recent-onset gynecomastia that has not responded to testosterone replacement therapy

CHRONIC THERAPY

Testosterone formulations:

- Parenteral testosterone preparations:
  1. Testosterone enanthate (generic) and testosterone cypionate (Depo-Testosterone and generic) 150 to 200 mg are injected intramuscularly every 2 wk. Following injections, there are appreciable fluctuations in serum testosterone, with levels rising within the first several days and a subsequent decrease to normal and in some cases to below normal at the end of the 2 wk. As a result of the varying levels of testosterone, patients may have related symptoms. Adjustments in dose and dosing interval may help to alleviate the serum fluctuations and clinical symptoms. Testosterone undecanoate (AUEFD-ENDO) is an injectable depot formulation FDA-approved for male hypogonadism. The recommended dosage is 750 mg injected IM at 0 and 4 wk, and then every 10 wk thereafter.
- Topical testosterone preparations:
  1. Testosterone adhesive patch (Androderm) delivers 2.5 or 5 mg of testosterone when applied nightly to the back, abdomen, upper arms, or thighs. Serum testosterone levels rise to within normal range in a few hours after application and, thereafter, are relatively stable. Daily doses of up to 10 mg may be necessary.
  2. Testosterone 1% gels (AndroGel and Testim). Androgel is available in 2.5 g and 5 g gel units that deliver 2.5 mg and 5 mg of testosterone, respectively. The gel is applied daily in the morning by hand over the shoulder, upper arms, or abdomen. Adjustments in dose to 7.5 g or 10 g of gel may be necessary to optimize serum testosterone levels. AndroGel (1.62%) pump is also available for daily application. Testim is available in 5-g and 10-g tubes and with morning applications over the shoulders or arms delivers 5 mg and 10 mg of testosterone, respectively. Both AndroGel and Testim provide relatively stable serum testosterone levels. Two new transdermal formulations, Fortesta and Axiron, are now available and are applied daily by metered dose pumps. With these preparations, care is necessary to avoid skin-to-skin contact exposure with others.
- Testosterone pellets:
  1. 3 to 6 pellets of testosterone each containing 75 mg of testosterone are surgically inserted subcutaneously every 3 to 6 months and provide relatively stable serum testosterone levels.

RISKS & ADVERSE EFFECTS

- Contraindications to testosterone therapy include prostate cancer and breast cancer. Relative contraindications include severe benign prostatic hyperplasia, hematocrit ≥50% at baseline, sleep apnea, and severe congestive heart failure.
- Patients on chronic testosterone therapy need to be followed carefully with prostate and prostate-specific antigen (PSA) assessments and hematocrit measurements for possible excessive induction of erythrocytosis, initially at 3 to 6 mo and at regular intervals thereafter.
- Current testosterone use for 6 mo or shorter is associated with 63% higher risk for venous thromboembolism (VTE). VTE risk peaks during the first 6 mo and declines to 25% thereafter.[1]

REFERRAL

Endocrinology for full endocrine and metabolic assessment and therapy. Urology for further assessment and follow-up of the prostate and for evaluation and therapy of erectile dysfunction. Neurosurgery for evaluation and possible surgery for a pituitary lesion. Plastic surgery for chronic gynecomastia. Reproductive endocrinology for those with an infertility problem.

[1] Martinez C et al: Testosterone treatment and risk of venous thromboembolism: population based case-control study, *BMJ* 355:596–598, 2016.

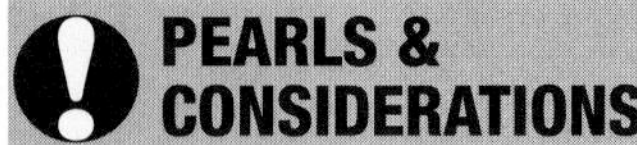

PEARLS & CONSIDERATIONS

COMMENTS

- Do not screen men "routinely" for hypogonadism. Screening men with nonspecific symptoms of hypogonadism (e.g., decreased energy) is also not recommended. Screening should be limited to men with specific signs and symptoms of hypogonadism.
- Male hypogonadism is an important and frequently encountered problem that requires a complete medical history, examination, and hormonal assessment to determine whether a patient has hypogonadism and requires testosterone replacement therapy. Treated patients need to be seen on a regular basis to avoid possible testosterone adverse effects. Patients requiring testosterone replacement should have testosterone, prostate specific antigen, and hematocrit levels monitored.
- A recent trial to evaluate the effects of testosterone treatment in older men revealed that in symptomatic men 65 years of age or older, raising testosterone concentrations for 1 yr from moderately low to the mid-normal range had a moderate benefit with respect to sexual function and some benefit with respect to mood and depressive symptoms but no benefit with respect to vitality or walking distance.[1]
- Controversy exists regarding the safety of testosterone replacement therapy following reports of increased risk of cardiovascular events. However, a recent trial among men with androgen deficiency dispensed testosterone prescriptions revealed lower risk of cardiovascular outcomes over a median follow-up of 3.4 yr.[2]
- Clinical trials have also demonstrated that testosterone replacement in men with low testosterone increases volumetric bone mineral density (vBMD) and estimated bone strength more in trabecular than peripheral bone and more in the spine than the hip.[3]

SUGGESTED READINGS

Available at ExpertConsult.com

AUTHOR: **JOSEPH R. TUCCI, M.D., F.A.C.P., F.A.C.E.**

[1] Snyder PJ et al: Effects of testosterone treatment in older men, *N Engl J Med* 374:611–624, 2016.

[2] Cheetham TC et al: Association of testosterone replacement with cardiovascular outcomes among men with androgen deficiency, *JAMA Int Med* 177(4):491–499, 2017.

[3] Synder PJ et al: Effect of testosterone treatment on volumetric bone density and strength in older men with low testosterone, *JAMA Int Med* 177(4):471–479, 2017.

BASIC INFORMATION

DEFINITION

Magnesium (Mg), after potassium, is the second most abundant cation of the intracellular fluid in living organisms. This ion plays a vital role in nearly every major metabolic and biochemical process within cells. Magnesium is a critical cofactor of the ubiquitous cellular Na^+-K^+-ATPase. Serum magnesium concentration is tightly regulated by a dynamic balance among three organ systems: gut, kidney, and bone. Magnesium has been implicated in and used as treatment for several diseases. Although its importance is widely acknowledged, routine serum magnesium levels generally are not evaluated in clinical medicine.

Magnesium deficiency is defined as a decrease in total body magnesium content. The recommended daily allowance of magnesium is 420 mg for males and 320 mg for females. Fig. 1 illustrates magnesium homeostasis in healthy adults. Poor dietary intake of magnesium usually does not lead to severe magnesium deficiency because the normal kidney prevents it through magnesium conservation. Fig. 2 depicts the renal handling of magnesium by the kidney. Hypomagnesemia is typically defined as a total serum magnesium concentration below 1.8 mg/dl and is categorized as mild (1.5–1.8 mg/dl), moderate (1–1.4 mg/dl), or severe (<1 mg/dl).

SYNONYMS

Magnesium deficiency
Low magnesium

ICD-10CM CODES

E83.40 Disorders of magnesium metabolism, unspecified
E83.42 Hypomagnesemia

EPIDEMIOLOGY & DEMOGRAPHICS

Hypomagnesemia has been estimated to occur in more than 10% of hospitalized patients and is especially common among the critically ill, with an incidence as high as 65%. It may be encountered in 25% to 35% of patients with acute pancreatitis. Low magnesium levels frequently are encountered in chronic alcoholics and poorly controlled diabetics. The incidence and prevalence of hypomagnesemia are similar across sexes, races, and ethnicities, but may be greater in the elderly. This observation may be explained by poorer nutritional intake, greater use of certain medications (e.g., diuretics, laxatives), or comorbidities.

RISK FACTORS

- Alcoholism
- Volume expansion (including pregnancy)
- Poorly controlled diabetes mellitus
- Chronic diuretic use
- Chronic laxative use
- Chronic use of proton pump inhibitors
- Subarachnoid hemorrhage
- Severe sepsis
- Acute phase after liver transplantation
- Large transfusions with citrate-rich blood products
- Postsurgical patients
- Leptospirosis

PHYSICAL FINDINGS & CLINICAL PRESENTATION

- Mild hypomagnesemia is most frequently asymptomatic. Clinical manifestations appear with more severe deficiency.
- Signs and symptoms are not unique and frequently difficult to determine if caused by hypomagnesemia or its complications of hypokalemia or hypocalcemia.
- Symptoms of hypomagnesemia have been reported at modest degrees of depletion, but generally they are more common when serum magnesium levels fall below 1.2 mg/dl.
- Neuromuscular effects include weakness, cramps, and paresthesias. Manifestations may include Trousseau and Chvostek signs. More severe depletion can cause vertical nystagmus, tetany, and seizures.
- Metabolic effects include hypokalemia from renal potassium wasting that may be refractory to potassium supplementation until magnesium deficiency is repaired. Hypocalcemia is also common in hypomagnesemia, which suppresses release of parathyroid hormone (PTH), and end-organ resistance to PTH with low 1, 25 vitamin D levels may occur.
- Cardiovascular effects: Hypomagnesemia is associated with a variety of atrial and ventricular arrhythmias.
- ECG findings: Flattened T-waves, prolonged QT interval, ST depression, and widened QRS complexes.
- The role of magnesium deficiency in the clinical development of seizures and cardiac arrhythmias requires treatment of these conditions with magnesium.

ETIOLOGY

Causes (Table 1)

DIAGNOSIS

WORKUP

- Comprehensive history including medication and dietary history, alcohol use, prior magnesium measurements, and history of disorders associated with hypomagnesemia (e.g., disorders of gastrointestinal tract, vomiting, diarrhea)
- Physical examination and review of vital signs, intake, and output

LABORATORY TESTS

The total serum concentration of magnesium should be measured in hospitalized patients with acute illness to screen for hypomagnesemia. This is indicated for critically ill patients and those deemed at risk of cardiac arrhythmias or seizures. Although the ionized fraction of serum magnesium (typically two-thirds of the total concentration) is the physiologically active form of the cation, measurement of serum ionized magnesium is not recommended because this measurement does not influence clinical management. The etiology of magnesium deficiency is often obvious from the history. When the cause is unknown, the fractional excretion of magnesium (FE_{Mg}) may facilitate diagnosis. With extrarenal magnesium loss from

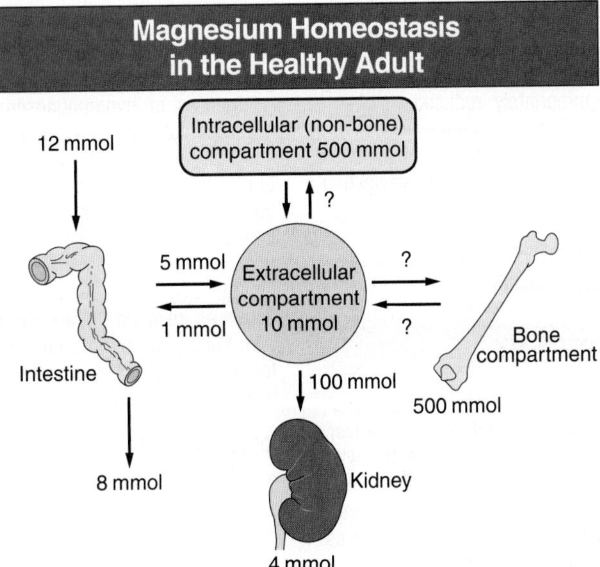

FIG. 1 Magnesium homeostasis in healthy young adults. Net zero balance results from net intestinal uptake (absorption minus secretion) equaling urinary loss. After its passage into the extracellular fluid, Mg^{2+} enters the intracellular space and is deposited in bone or soft tissue or eliminated via the kidneys. Entry and exit fluxes between the extracellular and intracellular spaces (skeletal and nonskeletal compartments) are also of identical magnitude; however, precise values of exchange are still debated. (From Johnson RJ: *Comprehensive clinical nephrology*, ed 6, Philadelphia, 2019, Elsevier.)

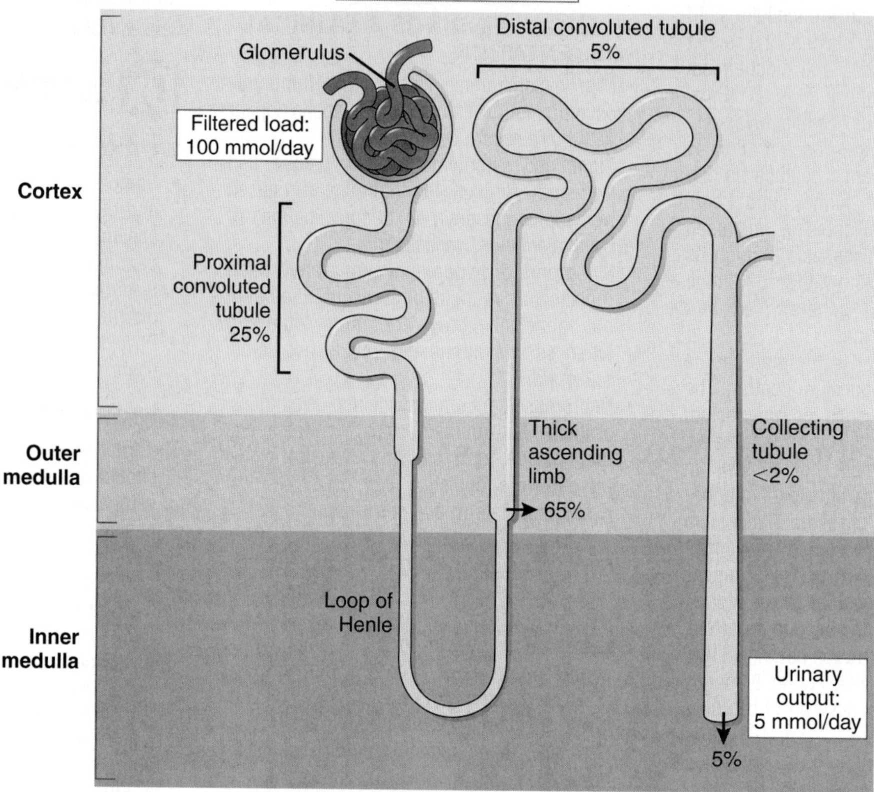

FIG. 2 Sites of magnesium reabsorption in various segments. Percentage absorbed in various segments of the renal tubule from the glomerular ultrafiltrate. (Redrawn from Quamme GA: Control of magnesium transport in the thick ascending limb, *Am J Physiol* 256:F197–F210, 1989. In Johnson RJ: *Comprehensive clinical nephrology*, ed 6, Philadelphia, 2019, Elsevier.)

malabsorption or laxative abuse, the FE_{Mg} should be appropriately reduced (<4%). If FE_{Mg} exceeds 4%, renal magnesium wasting is present, often secondary to surreptitious diuretic use or familial magnesium-wasting disorders.

IMAGING STUDIES

Not routinely recommended

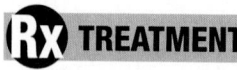

TREATMENT

It is unclear whether mild, asymptomatic hypomagnesemia requires treatment. However, symptomatic hypomagnesemia is treated with intravenous magnesium, typically magnesium sulfate. For treatment of *torsades de pointes*, 1-2 grams of intravenous magnesium sulfate as a bolus over 5 minutes is recommended.

Magnesium repletion in patients with acute or chronic renal insufficiency must be carried out cautiously. Evaluation for depressed deep tendon reflexes, periodic monitoring of serum magnesium levels, and dose reductions from 50% to 75% are recommended.

Oral magnesium supplementation may treat mild cases of hypomagnesemia successfully. In the outpatient setting, oral magnesium salts such as magnesium oxide (250-500 mg 4 times daily) can be used for repletion. However, these agents frequently cause diarrhea, particularly at high doses. Patients with gastrointestinal magnesium-wasting who do not achieve normal levels of repletion with one formulation may respond to an alternative formulation. Potassium-sparing diuretics may be used for renal magnesium-wasting states, provided hyperkalemia does not occur.

DISPOSITION

- Potential contributing factors should be evaluated and treated appropriately.
- Patients with symptomatic or severe hypomagnesemia require monitoring in an intensive care setting until the serum magnesium concentration and associated electrolyte abnormalities are corrected and stabilized at safe levels.
- The risk of recurrence depends primarily on the nature of the underlying disorder. Hypomagnesemia has less chance of recurrence if the offending medication is discontinued and/or when gastrointestinal and renal losses are not chronic. Inherited disorders may necessitate prolonged supplementation.
- In patients with self-limited reasons for magnesium deficiency, repletion therapy can be accomplished easily. However, in patients with persistent magnesium wasting, treatment by oral magnesium therapy may not correct the serum level to normal. Nevertheless, these individuals adapt to their chronic hypomagnesemia and tolerate it fairly well.

REFERRAL

- Outpatient referral to nephrology or endocrinology may be indicated to help manage patients with chronic hypomagnesemia that does not warrant hospital admission.
- Inpatient referral to specialists in nephrology, endocrinology, and /or critical care medicine is recommended in cases of severe or symptomatic hypomagnesemia.
- Consultation with a dietitian can help increase dietary magnesium intake and protein supplementation in malnourished patients.

TABLE 1 Causes of Magnesium Deficiency

Poor intake	Dietary deprivation or malnutrition Insufficient magnesium in tube-feeding formulas Parenteral nutrition preparations with insufficient magnesium
Redistribution of magnesium from extracellular to intracellular space or bone	Treatment of diabetic ketoacidosis Refeeding syndrome Hungry bone syndrome following parathyroidectomy Correction of metabolic acidosis Acute and chronic pancreatitis (soft tissue sequestration and gastrointestinal loss) Severe burns (sequestration in necrotic tissue) Hyperthyroidism
Poor intestinal absorption/increased intestinal loss	Diarrhea Inflammatory bowel disease (*e.g.*, Crohn disease, ulcerative colitis) Intestinal fistula Laxative use Nasogastric suction Proton pump inhibitor administration Severe malabsorption Short bowel syndrome Steatorrhea
Excessive renal loss	Diuretics: Loop diuretics (loss of magnesium and calcium) Thiazide-like diuretics (loss of magnesium with calcium retention) Hypercalciuria Metabolic acidosis Osmotic diuretics (hypertonic solutions) Poorly controlled diabetes and diabetic ketoacidosis (especially during recovery phase after phosphorus replacement) Primary hyperaldosteronism Renal tubular acidosis Syndrome of inappropriate antidiuretic hormone secretion (SIADH) Other drugs: Aminoglycosides Amphotericin B Cisplatin, carboplatin Cyclosporine Foscarnet Monoclonal antibodies that target the epidermal growth factor receptor (*e.g.*, cetuximab, panitumumab) Pentamidine Tacrolimus
Inherited causes	Autosomal-dominant hypocalcemia with hypercalciuria (ADHH) Bartter syndrome Familial hypomagnesemia with hypercalciuria and nephrocalcinosis Gitelman syndrome Hypomagnesemia with secondary hypocalcemia (HSH) Isolated dominant hypomagnesemia Isolated recessive hypomagnesemia

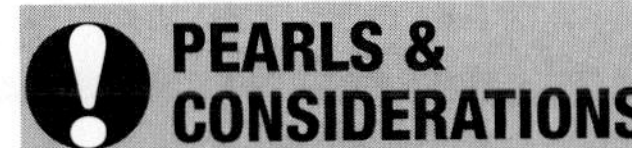

PEARLS & CONSIDERATIONS

COMMENTS

Serum magnesium measurement is the most available and most commonly employed test to evaluate magnesium status.

Routine correction of underlying etiologies and electrolyte and metabolic derangements is recommended for hypomagnesemia while increasing dietary magnesium intake and/or supplementing magnesium. Chronic hypomagnesemia may be associated with various micro- and macrovascular complications.

SUGGESTED READINGS

Available at ExpertConsult.com

RELATED TOPICS

Hypokalemia (Related Key Topic)
Hypoparathyroidism (Related Key Topic)

AUTHOR: **SNIGDHA T. REDDY, M.D.**

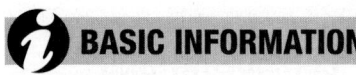

BASIC INFORMATION

DEFINITION

In its broadest sense, hyponatremia is defined as a measured serum sodium concentration (S_{Na}) less than the lower limit of normal (i.e., <135 mEq/L in most clinical labs). Since the clinical manifestations of hyponatremia are due to hypotonicity, appropriate clinical management depends on correctly distinguishing between the majority of patients with hypotonic hyponatremia from patients who are hypertonic or isotonic or have pseudohyponatremia (low measured S_{Na} due solely to laboratory artifact). For this chapter, hyponatremia will be used synonymously with hypotonic hyponatremia. Pseudohyponatremia and hypertonic/isotonic hyponatremia will be identified specifically by those names.

SYNONYMS

Low serum sodium concentration
Hypo-osmolality

ICD-10CM CODE
E87.1 Hypo-osmolality and hyponatremia

EPIDEMIOLOGY & DEMOGRAPHICS

PREVALENCE: The prevalence of hyponatremia varies widely according to setting and population age. In the general U.S. population dataset captured by the National Health and Nutrition Examination Survey (NHANES), the overall prevalence was 1.72%. One study of emergency department patients reported a prevalence of 2.3% in patients 16 to 21 yr and 16.9% in patients >80 yr of age. Following surgery for traumatic hip fracture, the incidence of moderate (<135 mmol/L) and severe (<130 mmol/L) postoperative hyponatremia was 27% (95% CI: 21.7% to 32.5%) and 9% (95% CI: 5.7% to 12.8%), respectively. The prevalence in stable, older outpatients has been reported to be around 8% and as much as 18% to 20% in sicker or frailer populations. The overall incidence (at or after hospital admission) is similar, with even higher rates in patients admitted for congestive heart failure (CHF) or cirrhosis or in elderly patients admitted for fragility fracture.

PREDOMINANT SEX AND AGE: Prevalence of hyponatremia was significantly higher in women in the NHANES dataset (2.09%; P = 0.004) and increased with age.

GENETICS: While rare, a familial gain-of-function mutation of the AVP V2 receptor in the renal collecting duct resulting in hyponatremia has been reported.

RISK FACTORS: In NHANES, hyponatremia was more common in subjects with hypertension, diabetes, coronary artery disease, stroke, chronic obstructive pulmonary disease, cancer, and psychiatric disorders, and less common in those with no comorbidities (1.04%, *P*<0.001). A significant risk of death was associated with hyponatremia in unadjusted (hazard ratio [HR], 3.61; *P*<0.001) and adjusted (HR, 2.43; *P*<.001) Cox models controlling for demographics, smoking, comorbidities, and insurance status. The incidence in outpatients using thiazide diuretics was 15.1%, with a HR of 4.95 (95% CI, 4.12–5.96). Reported incidences in outpatients using selective serotonin reuptake inhibitors (SSRIs) or selective norepinephrine reuptake inhibitors (SNRIs) has varied widely between 0.5% and 32%.

PHYSICAL FINDINGS & CLINICAL PRESENTATION

- Critical historical information that the health care provider needs to obtain includes detailed documentation of fluid consumption and diet, gastrointestinal and insensible losses of fluid and electrolytes, urine outputs, changes in weight, medication use, changes in behavior or cognition, and presence of comorbid conditions that increase the risk of hyponatremia including malignancies, CNS or pulmonary diseases, adrenal or thyroid diseases, CHF, liver disease, or nephrotic syndrome. In the appropriate setting, participation in marathons or other strenuous endurance exercise or attendance at "rave" parties where the use of 3,4-methylenedioxy-methamphetamine (MDMA, "ecstasy") is common should be noted.
- The clinical presentation and physical findings are determined primarily by the acuity and severity of the hyponatremia as well as the underlying etiology. The etiology of hyponatremia may affect the clinical presentation both directly and/or by its effect on the extracellular fluid volume (ECFV). Hypovolemia and hypervolemia (decreased or increased ECFV, respectively) are identified by the usual clinical criteria, although if available vector bioimpedance analysis has been shown to further increase accuracy. Specific manifestations of the precipitating cause or underlying diseases may be evident (e.g., fever and delirium following the use of MDMA, stigmata of alcoholism or malnutrition, fever and/or localizing symptoms related to pneumonia or other pulmonary disease, or headaches and visual field defects from an intracranial mass).
- Neurologic symptoms predominate as the direct clinical manifestations of hyponatremia due to cerebrocyte swelling. Compensatory processes that reduce cerebral edema by extrusion of electrolytes, amino acids, and carbohydrates from brain cells take 24 hours to fully engage and up to 7 days to reach completion. Therefore, patients who develop hyponatremia over less than 24 to 48 hours have the highest degree of brain swelling, the most severe neurologic symptoms, and the highest risk of permanent or fatal brain injury. Postpubertal, premenopausal women appear to undergo cerebral compensation more slowly, placing them at greater risk from acute hyponatremia.
- Acute hyponatremia may result in nausea and malaise as S_{Na} becomes <130 mEq/, and headache, lethargy, obtundation, neurogenic pulmonary edema, and/or seizures occur in cases of S_{Na} <120 mEq/L. In the most severe cases death from brain stem herniation can occur.
- Chronic hyponatremia almost never presents with life-threatening clinical manifestations. However, subtler neurologic disturbances such as ataxia, short-term memory deficits, fatigue, lethargy, and nausea have been commonly reported. Muscular weakness and elevated creatine kinase and even rhabdomyolysis have been reported. Chronic hyponatremia has also been associated with increased risk of falls, fractures, and osteoporosis in elderly patients. Hyponatremia has been associated with increased risk of cardiovascular complications and mortality in elderly outpatients, general hospital admissions, and patients admitted for stroke, subarachnoid hemorrhage, CHF, cirrhosis, pneumonia, hip fracture, and liver transplantation.

ETIOLOGY

- In patients with hypotonic hyponatremia, S_{Na} is closely approximated by the ratio ($TBNa_e$ + TBK_e)/TBW, where $TBNa_e$ and TBK_e represent exchangeable total body sodium and potassium, respectively, and TBW represents total body water. Hypotonic hyponatremia results from decreases in this numerator, increases in this denominator, or both. TBNa is the main determinant of ECFV.
- ECFV depletion (with proportionately greater decrease in $TBNa_e$ and possibly TBK_e than in TBW).
  1. GI losses with intake of hypotonic fluids
  2. Renal losses (diuresis, tubulopathies) with intake of hypotonic fluid
  3. Cerebral salt wasting
- Euvolemic (normal ECFV)
  1. Syndrome of inappropriate antidiuresis (SIAD, see "Syndrome of Inappropriate Antidiuresis")
  2. Medications (thiazide diuretics, SSRIs and SNRIs, narcotics, MDMA/"ecstasy," carbamazepine, cyclophosphamide, nicotine, DDAVP, phenothiazines, terlipressin)
  3. Pain, nausea, stress
  4. Marathon running or other endurance exercise
  5. Primary polydipsia
  6. Solute-limited water excretion (tea-and-toast diet, beer potomania)
  7. Severe potassium deficiency with normal total body sodium
  8. Adrenal insufficiency or hypothyroidism
  9. Reset osmostat
- Increased ECFV (with decreased effective arterial blood volume [EABV]). Hyponatremia results from proportionately greater increase in TBW than in TBNa and TBK.
  1. CHF
  2. Nephrotic syndrome
  3. Cirrhosis

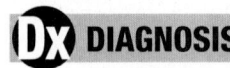

DIAGNOSIS

DIFFERENTIAL DIAGNOSIS

- *Pseudohyponatremia.* Clinical laboratories measure the concentration of sodium (mEq) per liter of plasma, not plasma water. Consequently, conditions (severe hypertriglyceridemia and hyperproteinemia) that significantly reduce the aqueous fraction of plasma (normally 0.93) may lead to a decrease in the reported S_{Na} despite the presence of serum normal osmolality (S_{osm}). However, since the condition can coexist with preexisting hypernatremia or hypotonic hyponatremia (which affects S_{osm}), a more reliable method for identifying the disorder is the presence of an increased osmolal gap (i.e., difference between measured and calculated serum osmolality >10 mOsm/L) and a low S_{Na}. Calculated $S_{osm\ (mOsm/L)} = 2 \times (S_{Na}) + S_{Glu}$ (mg/dl)/18 + BUN (mg/dl)/2.8.

- *Hypertonic hyponatremia.* Small solutes such as glucose (in the absence of insulin), mannitol, sorbitol, and glycine that accumulate in higher concentrations in ECF than ICF induce a shift of water from ICF to ECF compartments. Since ICF is virtually sodium free, this dilutes the ECF sodium concentration and results in hyponatremia. In the case of glucose, a decrease in S_{Na} of 1.6 mEq/L occurs for each increment of serum glucose of 100 mg/dl. The tendency of a solute *in vivo* to shift fluid from ICF to ECF is known as tonicity, which is of clinical importance because increases and decreases in tonicity also result in brain cell shrinkage and edema, respectively. In contrast, solutes such as urea or ethanol that equilibrate across cell membranes affect in vitro osmolality (measured by freezing point depression) but not tonicity or S_{Na+}.

WORKUP

- Comprehensive history, including medication and drug abuse history, psychiatric history, exercise history, prior serum sodium measurements, dietary history, history of external fluid losses, volume and composition of oral and IV fluid intake, and history suggestive of disorders associated with hyponatremia (e.g., disorders of the lungs, CNS, heart, kidney, liver, adrenal gland, or thyroid; malignancies; diabetes mellitus; nausea; vomiting; pain; or stress)
- Comprehensive physical examination including careful review of vital signs, weights, intake and outputs; evidence of increased ECFV (e.g., edema, ascites, or pleural effusions) or ECFV depletion and evidence of comorbid diseases listed previously (e.g., abnormal pulmonary, neurological or cardiovascular exam, hepatomegaly, thyromegaly or nodular thyroid)

LABORATORY TESTS

- Serum osmolality to detect pseudohyponatremia or hypertonic hypernatremia due to solutes other than glucose, in the appropriate clinical circumstances
- Serum triglycerides and total protein, if pseudohyponatremia is suspected
- Serum glucose to adjust for influence on serum sodium (serum sodium decreases approximately 1.6 mEq/L for every additional 100 mg/dl increase in serum glucose)
- Serum potassium: Since $S_{Na} = (TBNa_e + TBK_e)/TBW$, decreases in TBK lower both S_K and S_{Na}
- Random urine osmolality and 24-hour urine volume. U_{osm} <100 mOsm/kg H_2O usually indicates appropriate suppression of ADH, suggesting the diagnoses of solute-limited water excretion, primary polydipsia, or a reset osmostat (if S_{Na} is below the patient's altered setpoint). $U_{osm} \geq 100$ mOsm/kg H_2O usually implies effective ADH bioactivity. However, large quantities of isosmotic urine (U_{osm} ~290 mOsm/kg H_2O with total urine osmolar excretion >900 mOsm/day) are indicative of osmotic diuresis (with accompanying intake of hypotonic fluids)
- Random urine sodium (U_{Na}), and urine potassium (U_K). U_{Na} <20 to 40 mEq/L suggests either decreased ECFV or decreased EABV. U_K must be considered when prescribing and monitoring therapy (see the following)
- Specific testing for comorbid diseases listed previously as clinically indicated (e.g., AM or cosyntropin-stimulated serum cortisol level, BNP, TSH)
- Fig. 1 illustrates an algorithm for diagnosis of hyponatremia

IMAGING STUDIES

Not routinely required but may be indicated to diagnose associated etiologies or to evaluate associated delirium that may be present in acute hyponatremia

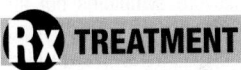

TREATMENT

NONPHARMACOLOGIC THERAPY

Hyponatremic patients excrete less free water than they take in. In most cases, their capacity to excrete free water is insufficient to match even conventional quantities of (hypotonic) fluid intake. Moderate fluid restriction (10-15 ml/kg) is indicated while patients are hyponatremic, especially if free water excretion capacity remains impaired. Diets high in protein, sodium, and potassium (including the use of NaCl tablets) increase osmolar generation and can increase free water excretion modestly. Pharmaceutical-grade urea powder, which has been used widely in Europe as a means of increasing urinary osmolar excretion, recently has been sold as a "food supplement" in the United States in flavored individual

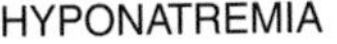

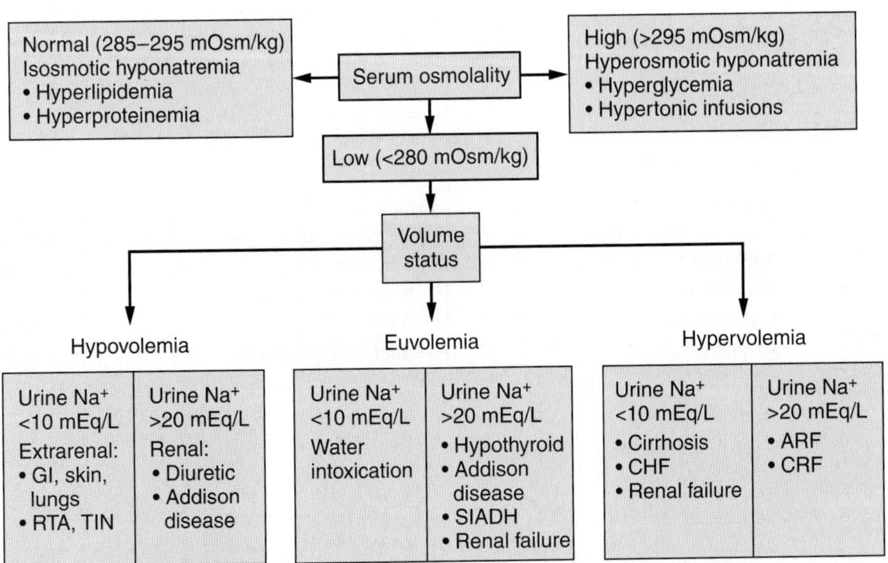

FIG. 1 Algorithm for diagnosis of hyponatremia. *ARF,* Acute renal failure; *CHF,* congestive heart failure; *CRF,* chronic renal failure; *GI,* gastrointestinal; *RTA,* renal tubular acidosis; *SIADH,* syndrome of inappropriate antidiuretic hormone (secretion); *TIN,* tubulointerstitial necrosis. (From Ronco C, et al.: *Critical care nephrology,* ed 3, Philadelphia, 2019, Elsevier.)

packets. 15 g urea provides 250 mOsm, equal to 14.7 500mg NaCl tablets or 7.35 1 g NaCl tablets. A typical dose for a 70 kg patient would be 15 to 30 g daily.

ACUTE GENERAL Rx

- Acute (hypotonic) hyponatremia is defined as developing over <24 hours. Acute hyponatremia results in larger increases in brain water than equivalent changes in S_{Na} developing over longer durations. Consequently, correction of acute hyponatremia is a medical emergency mandating an increase in S_{Na} of 4 to 6 mEq/L in the first 1 to 3 hours depending on the severity of symptoms and the acuity of the increase. Iatrogenic cases (classically children or premenopausal women receiving perioperative hypotonic fluids), fortunately rare now, can present with headache or nausea prior to severe symptoms but still require emergent correction. Acute hyponatremia is rare in patients with high ECFV because the increased TBNa partially offsets the decreased ($TBNa_e$ + TBK_e)/TBW ratio driven by high TBW.
- Controlled increases in S_{Na} at this rapid rate almost always require the use of hypertonic (3%) saline. A useful rule-of-thumb is that 2 ml/kg of 3% saline can be expected to increase S_{Na} by 1.6 to 2 mEq/L. The recommended rate of correction in severe acute hyponatremia is an increase in S_{Na} of 4 to 6 mEq/L in the first hour. In euvolemic patients (i.e., normal TB_{Na}), furosemide at 20 to 40 mg IV has been used with hypertonic saline to lessen ECFV expansion while maintaining a rapid increase in S_{Na} by increasing free water excretion.
- Regardless of the therapy used, patients with acute hyponatremia require monitoring in an intensive care setting with frequent measurements of S_{Na}, urine volume, and U_{osm} until they are neurologically stable and the S_{Na} is near normal.
- Fig.2 summarizes a treatment algorithm for hyponatremia.

CHRONIC Rx

- Chronic hyponatremia develops over 24 to 48 hours. Brain cells adapt by extruding electrolytes and organic osmolytes such as amino acids. Thus, brain edema is minimized while the risks of rapid correction increase. Precipitous increases of S_{Na} in this setting have been associated with serious demyelinating brain injuries. The appropriate target for correction of hyponatremia in this setting is 6 to 8 mEq/L per day.
- In hypovolemic patients with chronic hyponatremia the usual clinical practice is to administer 0.9% saline until patients are euvolemic. The 0.9% saline results in very little direct change in S_{Na} because it proportionately increases Cat_{TB} and TBW, but indirectly can trigger a rapid increase in S_{Na} when hypovolemia-induced (non-osmotic) stimulation of ADH is suppressed. The simultaneous use of DDAVP (1–2 mcg IV every 6–12 hours) is a recommended adjuvant to therapy in these patients to prevent unanticipated and unwanted increases in free water loss than can result in unpredictably high rates of increase in S_{Na}. Once the patient is euvolemic IV fluids can be stopped and the patient monitored. If the rate or magnitude of S_{Na} correction starts to exceed prudent targets, DDAVP may be re-dosed as needed. Since decreased ECFV may not always be recognized, DDAVP administration may also be judiciously administered in some apparently euvolemic patients with chronic hyponatremia treated with 0.9% or 3% saline.
- The treatment of euvolemic patients is covered in detail in "Syndrome of Inappropriate Antidiuresis" and thus is only briefly reviewed here. The goals of therapy in these patients are to restore TBW to normal while keeping TBNa and TBK normal, correcting S_{Na} at a safe rate. Some patients with chronic euvolemic hyponatremia (especially those with drug-induced etiologies or primary polydipsia) have self-limited abnormalities and primarily require monitoring to prevent excessively rapid correction, although active therapy as described below can be started to avoid delays. If required, DDAVP can be administered intermittently to temporarily block further losses of free water to slow the overall rate of correction. If overcorrection has occurred, oral and/or IV hypotonic fluids can be quantitatively given to lower the serum sodium actively. Other disorders may only slowly resolve, if at all, and require more active therapy as outlined in "Syndrome of Inappropriate Antidiuresis," consisting of either a direct V2 receptor antagonist or a loop diuretic with replacement of electrolytes lost in urine.

DISPOSITION

- Patients with symptomatic or severe hyponatremia require monitoring in an ICU setting until the S_{Na} has stabilized at a safe level. Frequent monitoring of serum sodium, urine

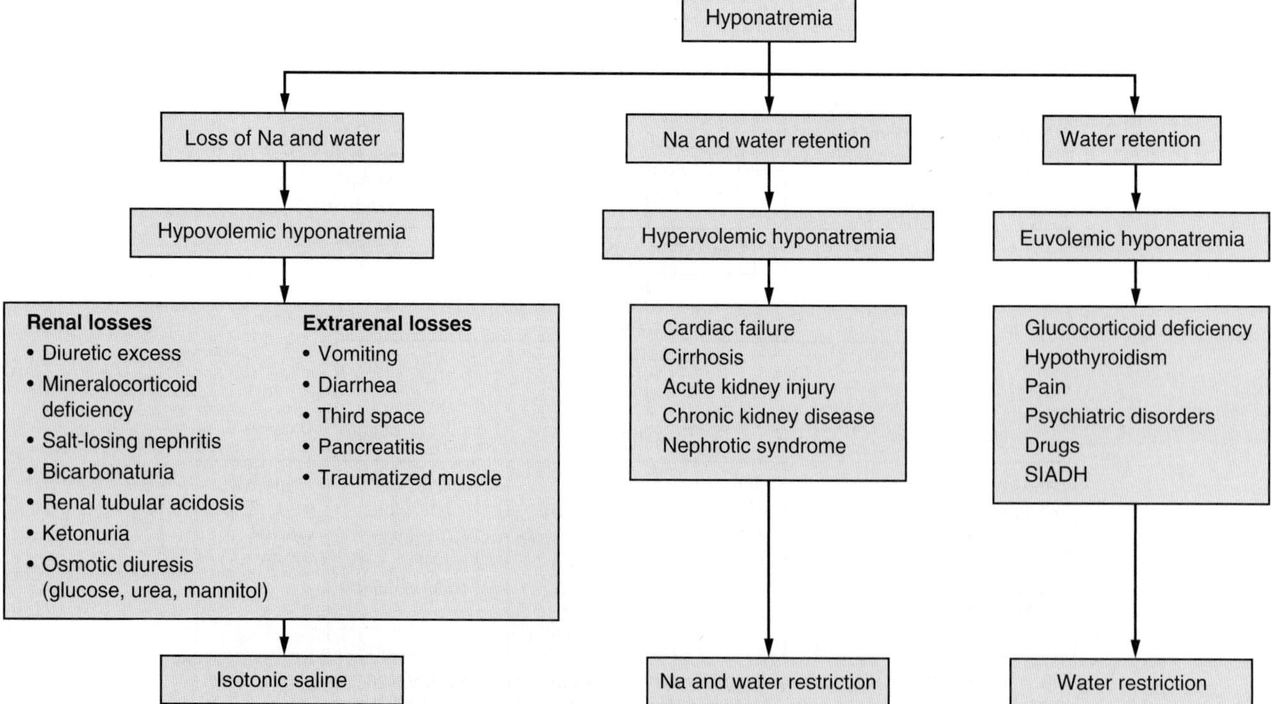

FIG. 2 Algorithm of diagnosis and treatment of hyponatremia. (From Ronco C, et al.: *Critical care nephrology*, ed 3, Philadelphia, 2019, Elsevier.)

volume, and urine osmolality and electrolytes is required, with adjustments in therapy as outlined previously as needed.

- All potential contributing causes should be evaluated and treated appropriately. In addition to obvious disorders, less apparent conditions such as adrenal insufficiency and hypothyroidism should be ruled out.
- The risk of recurrence depends primarily on the nature of the underlying disorders present. Hypovolemic hyponatremia (e.g., diarrheal or diuretic-induced electrolyte and water losses) or drug-induced SIAD may have little chance of recurrence if the offending medication is discontinued or the gastrointestinal losses are not chronic. Elderly patients with solute limited diuresis from low electrolyte and protein intake may be resistant to major changes in diet, but may agree to NaCl tablets and/or protein supplements. In addition to disease-specific management, incurable conditions (e.g., chronic CNS or pulmonary disease, CHF, or cirrhosis) may require lifelong fluid restriction (10–15 ml/kg per day), high protein and electrolyte diets as tolerated, and periodic monitoring of the S_{Na} to reduce the risk of recurrence.

REFERRAL

- Referral to specialists in nephrology, endocrinology, and/or critical care medicine is recommended in cases of severe or symptomatic hyponatremia to aid in setting appropriate rates of correction and to recommend, monitor, and adjust therapeutic regimens to achieve those target rates.
- Outpatient referral to nephrology or endocrinology may be indicated to help manage patients with recurrent hyponatremia or mild hyponatremia that does not warrant hospitalization.

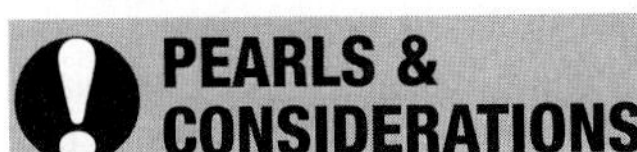

PEARLS & CONSIDERATIONS

COMMENTS

PREVENTION: Well-meaning family members, friends, news media, and even health care providers often direct patients who have chronic kidney disease or who take diuretics to drink large amounts of water. When these patients consume more free water than they can excrete, hyponatremia may develop. Similarly, participants in marathons or other high-intensity endurance activities may ingest so much water that in place of TBW depletion they develop high TBW and hyponatremia. Patients at risk for hyponatremia should receive a specific fluid prescription that avoids both extremes. Conversely, patients with diarrheal losses or who develop decreased ECFV from loop or combination diuretics need to be counseled that intake of water or other hypotonic fluids alone will lead to hyponatremia but not effectively restore ECFV. Safe outpatient correction of ECFV requires the consumption of electrolyte-containing solutions such as those marketed for infants. A more recent alternative is the use of commercial electrolyte tablets or packets used according to manufacturer instructions. Standard sports drinks have high sugar content but relatively low quantities of electrolytes.

SUGGESTED READINGS

Available at ExpertConsult.com

RELATED CONTENT

Syndrome of Inappropriate Antidiuresis (Related Key Topic)

AUTHORS: **MARK D. FABER, M.D.,** and **JERRY YEE, M.D.**

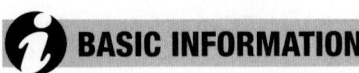

BASIC INFORMATION

DEFINITION

A decrease in parathyroid hormone (PTH) secretion or function results in hypoparathyroidism. In primary hypoparathyroidism, absence or dysfunction of the parathyroid gland results in inadequate PTH secretion and subsequent hypocalcemia and hyperphosphatemia. Surgical hypoparathyroidism is the most common etiology, followed by autoimmune disorders. Individuals with autoimmune polyglandular syndrome 1 typically present in childhood/adolescence with candidiasis, hypoparathyroidism, and adrenal insufficiency. Impaired function of PTH (i.e., PTH resistance) can also cause hypocalcemia and hyperphosphatemia, but the measured PTH level is elevated in this circumstance. A maternally transmitted mutation in the *GNAS1* gene results in PTH resistance (i.e., pseudohypoparathyroidism). It is associated with characteristic features that include developmental delay, short stature, round facies, and short 4th metacarpal known as Albright's hereditary osteodystrophy (AHO). Paternal transmission manifests with AHO without PTH resistance (i.e., pseudopseudohypoparathyroidism; Table 1). Secondary hypoparathyroidism, a condition in which PTH levels are low in response to hypercalcemic states, is discussed in Section IV (see hypercalcemia discussion in the "Calcium" topic).

ICD-10CM CODES

E20.0 Idiopathic hypoparathyroidism
E20.1 Pseudohypoparathyroidism
E20.8 Other hypoparathyroidism
E20.9 Hypoparathyroidism, unspecified
E89.2 Postprocedural hypoparathyroidism
P71.4 Transitory neonatal hypoparathyroidism

EPIDEMIOLOGY & DEMOGRAPHICS

The incidence and prevalence of primary hypoparathyroidism depends on the etiology of the condition. Estimated prevalence in the United States is between 60,000 and 115,000 cases. Postoperative hypoparathyroidism is the most common etiology (75%). This occurs in the setting of thyroid or parathyroid surgery as a result of removal of, or vascular compromise of, the parathyroid glands during surgery. Transient hypoparathyroidism (<6 mon) can be as high as 20% postoperatively, but permanent dysfunction (>6 mon) is less common (3%). Autoimmune disorders are the second most common cause of hypoparathyroidism in adults (female/male ratio of 1.4:1.0). Autoimmune polyglandular syndrome type I is reported to have an incidence worldwide of 1:1,000,000. Other etiologies of hypoparathyroidism are very rare.

PHYSICAL FINDINGS & CLINICAL PRESENTATION

The symptoms of hypoparathyroidism are primarily related to hypocalcemia. The presentation of symptoms varies with the severity and duration of illness.

- Cardiovascular: Prolonged QT intervals, QRS and ST segment changes, ventricular arrhythmias
- Musculoskeletal: Muscle cramps, laryngospasm, osteomalacia (adults), rickets (children), weakened tooth enamel, osteosclerosis
- CNS: Tetany (Chvostek sign and Trousseau sign), seizures, paresthesias, visual impairment from cataract formation, altered mental status, papilledema, and basal ganglia calcifications with longstanding disease
- GI: Abdominal pain
- Renal: Hypercalciuria and nephrolithiasis
- Other: Dry scaly skin, brittle nails, dry hair

In addition to the hypocalcemia-related symptoms, syndromes associated with hypoparathyroidism can have distinct clinical findings. Conditions associated with hypoparathyroidism include:

- Autoimmune polyglandular syndrome type 1: Mucocutaneous candidiasis and adrenal insufficiency
- DiGeorge syndrome: Dysmorphic facies, cleft palate
- Pseudohypoparathyroidism: Developmental delay, short stature, round face, short 4th metacarpal (Albright hereditary osteodystrophy)
- Hypoparathyroidism-retardation-dysmorphism syndrome: Short stature, microcephaly, microphthalmia, small hands and feet, abnormal teeth
- Hypoparathyroidism-deafness-renal dysplasia syndrome: Sensorineural deafness

ETIOLOGY

There are several etiologies of hypoparathyroidism:

- Postoperative hypoparathyroidism; most common cause
- Destruction of the parathyroids:
  1. Autoimmune polyglandular syndrome type 1
  2. Radiation to the neck
  3. Infiltrative disease (e.g., metastatic carcinoma, Wilson disease, hemochromatosis, thalassemia, granulomatous disease)
- Developmental defects of the parathyroids:
  1. Isolated hypoparathyroidism
  2. Branchial dysembryogenesis (DiGeorge syndrome)
  3. Hypoparathyroidism-retardation-dysmorphism syndrome
  4. Hypoparathyroidism-deafness-renal dysplasia syndrome
  5. Mitochondrial dysfunction associated with hypoparathyroidism
- Functional and secretory defects of the parathyroid glands:
  1. Activating mutation of the calcium-sensing receptor alters the set point of the receptor and decreases PTH secretion
  2. Activating antibodies to calcium-sensing receptor alters the set point of the receptor and decreases PTH secretion
  3. PTH resistance (i.e., target organs unresponsive to PTH action)
     a. Pseudohypoparathyroidism (PHP): Heterogeneous disorder presenting in childhood characterized by hypocalcemia, hyperphosphatemia, and elevated PTH levels. Table 2 summarizes the various types of PHP
     b. Hypermagnesemia and hypomagnesemia

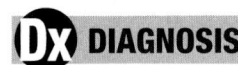

DIAGNOSIS

DIFFERENTIAL DIAGNOSIS

- Secondary hypoparathyroidism as a result of hypercalcemia (discussed in "Hypercalcemia").
- Other conditions associated with hypocalcemia. These conditions are usually associated with an elevated PTH hormone level.

WORKUP

- Hypoparathyroidism is characterized by hypocalcemia and hyperphosphatemia as a result of inadequate PTH secretion.
  1. Two measurements of serum calcium are required for the confirmation of hypocalcemia. Total calcium should be corrected for low albumin utilizing the formula: Corrected calcium = measured calcium + [(4 − albumin) × 0.8]. If a reliable laboratory is available, ionized calcium should be considered especially in conditions associated with acid-base disturbances or low albumin states.
  2. Serum phosphorus is usually high-normal or elevated in primary hypoparathyroidism.
  3. Serum intact PTH (iPTH) level is the single best test to evaluate the etiology of hypocalcemia. Typically, PTH is decreased in primary hypoparathyroidism and elevated in most other conditions associated with

TABLE 1 Types of Hypoparathyroidism

Type	Calcium	PO_4	PTH	Comments
Hypoparathyroidism	↓	↑	↓	Surgical removal (most common cause)
Pseudohypoparathyroidism	↓	↑	Ø↑	End-organ resistance to parathyroid hormone and Albright hereditary osteodystrophy
Pseudo-pseudohypoparathyroidism	Normal	Normal	Normal	Only Albright hereditary osteodystrophy

PO_4, Phosphate; *PTH,* parathyroid hormone. Adapted from Weissleder R, et al.: *Primer of diagnostic imaging,* ed 5, St Louis, 2011, Mosby.

TABLE 2 Types of Pseudohypoparathyroidism (PHP)

Disorder	Urinary cAMP Response to PTH	Urinary PO_4 Response to PTH	Other Hormonal Resistance	AHO	Pathophysiology
PHP type 1A	Decreased	Decreased	Yes	Yes	$G_s\alpha$ mutation
Pseudo-PHP	Normal	Normal	No	Yes	$G_s\alpha$ mutation
PHP type 1B	Decreased	Decreased	No	No	*GNAS1* imprinting mutations
PHP type 1C	Decreased	Decreased	Yes	Yes	$G_s\alpha$ activity normal
PHP type 2	Normal	Decreased	No	No	Vitamin D deficiency or myotonic dystrophy in some cases

AHO, Albright's hereditary osteodystrophy; *cAMP*, cyclic adenosine monophosphate; *GNAS1*, portion of the *GNAS* complex locus encoding $G_s\alpha$; *$G_s\alpha$*, α-subunit of the stimulatory G protein; *PO_4*, phosphate; *PTH*, parathyroid hormone.
From Melmed S, et al.: *Williams textbook of endocrinology*, ed 12, Philadelphia, 2011, Saunders.

low calcium levels. However, PTH is also elevated in disorders associated with impaired PTH function (i.e., pseudohypoparathyroidism). Genetic studies as indicated if medical or family history is suggestive.

The diagnosis is established by concurrent measurements of ionized calcium or corrected calcium that is within the lower limit of normal range and low or undetectable levels of PTH on two separate occasions at least 2 wk apart.

LABORATORY TESTS

- Total and ionized calcium: Low in hypoparathyroidism
- PTH: Low in hypoparathyroidism and high in PTH resistance states like pseudohypoparathyroidism
- Phosphorus: High-normal or high in hypoparathyroidism
- Magnesium: Both hypomagnesemia and hypermagnesemia can cause hypoparathyroidism
- 24-hr urine for calcium and creatinine to evaluate the risk for renal stones
- ECG should be considered. Hypocalcemia is associated with prolonged QT interval, rarely ST-segment elevations

Rx TREATMENT

NONPHARMACOLOGIC THERAPY

Parathyroid autotransplantation:

- Hypoparathyroidism and subsequent hypocalcemia are common problems after neck exploration for total or near-total thyroidectomy or parathyroidectomy. In cases where there is concern for postoperative hypoparathyroidism, parathyroid autotransplantation of one or two parathyroid glands into the forearm or sternocleidomastoid muscle should be performed to prevent postoperative hypoparathyroidism.

PHARMACOLOGIC THERAPY

The mainstay of treatment for primary hypoparathyroidism is pharmacologic therapy with calcium and vitamin D supplementation. The goals of therapy are to control symptoms and minimize complications of therapy. The aim should be to achieve low-normal serum calcium level (8.0-8.5 mg/dl), high-normal serum phosphorus level, 24-hr urinary calcium <300 mg/day, and a calcium-phosphorus product <55 mg^2/dl^2.

- Vitamin D:
  1. There are several vitamin D preparations available on the market, but the treatment of choice for patients with primary hypoparathyroidism is calcitriol. It is an active metabolite that does not require hydroxylation in the liver or kidney and therefore bypasses the PTH-mediated 1-α hydroxylation defect that occurs with hypoparathyroidism.
  2. Dose of 0.25 to 1 μg once or twice daily is usually required to correct hypocalcemia and improve symptoms. Its maximal effect is seen after 10 hr and it lasts for 2 to 3 days.
  3. Vitamin D_2 (ergocalciferol) or vitamin D_3 (cholecalciferol) may also be supplemented if levels are found to be low.
- Calcium:
  1. Calcium carbonate or calcium citrates are common oral agents used for treatment of hypocalcemia associated with hypoparathyroidism. Calcium carbonate contains 40% elemental calcium, and calcium citrate contains 21% elemental calcium. Calcium carbonate requires an acidic environment for effective absorption, and as a result, it must be taken with food. Its effectiveness is decreased with concomitant use of H_2 blockers or proton pump inhibitors. Calcium citrate does not require an acidic environment for effective absorption.
  2. Start with a dose of 500 to 1000 mg of elemental calcium two to three times daily and adjust the dose for a desired calcium in the low-normal range.
- Magnesium:
  1. Hypocalcemia is difficult to correct without normalizing magnesium levels.
  2. Magnesium sulfate IV 2 g over 20 min followed by 1 g/hr infusion can be considered in severe deficiency states. Milder deficiencies can be managed with oral magnesium 100 mg tid.
- Thiazide diuretics:
  1. Thiazide diuretics (25-100 mg daily) decrease urine calcium excretion and decrease kidney stones. They should be considered in individuals with urine calcium >250 mg/day.
- PTH replacement:
  1. Injectable synthetic human PTH (1-84) decreases urinary calcium excretion and maintains serum calcium in the normal range with reduced requirements for calcium and vitamin D supplementation.
  2. PTH (1-84, Natpara, an 84-amino acid single-chain polypeptide identical to native parathyroid hormone) is the first FDA approved for use in the treatment of hypoparathyroidism. PTH (1-84) is recommended for patients who cannot be well controlled on conventional therapy alone. The cost for a 4-wk supply of Natpara exceeds $7000.
  3. PTH (1-84) is recommended for patients who cannot be well controlled on conventional therapy alone.

ACUTE GENERAL Rx

Severe and/or symptomatic hypocalcemia requires hospitalization. Acute management of hypocalcemia includes:

- Telemetry monitoring for arrhythmias associated with severe hypocalcemia
- IV infusion of calcium gluconate 10 ml of 10% solution to receive a bolus of 90 mg of elemental calcium followed by an infusion of 0.5 to 2 mg/kg/hr until calcium levels are in the low-normal range

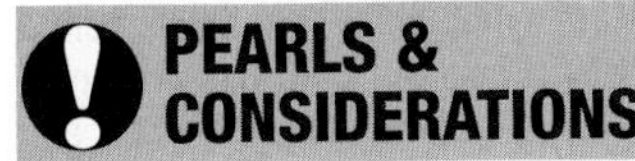

COMMENTS

- The mainstay of treatment for primary hypoparathyroidism is calcitriol and calcium supplementation to maintain a goal serum calcium level in the low-normal range. IV calcium should be considered if calcium <7.0 mg/dl.
- Hypomagnesemia causes functional, reversible parathyroid hypofunction. Magnesium levels should be assessed and appropriately replaced in all patients with hypocalcemia before a low PTH level is attributed to hypoparathyroidism.
- In patients undergoing neck exploration, consideration should be given to the parathyroid glands. Autotransplantation of one or more parathyroid glands should be considered when appropriate to prevent postoperative hypoparathyroidism.

SUGGESTED READINGS

Available at ExpertConsult.com

AUTHORS: **THARANI RAJESWARAN, M.D.**, and **VICKY CHENG, M.D.**

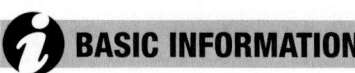

BASIC INFORMATION

DEFINITION

Hypopituitarism (from the Latin *pituita,* meaning "phlegm") is the deficiency of one or more of the hormones of the anterior or posterior pituitary gland resulting from diseases of the hypothalamus or pituitary gland. Panhypopituitarism indicates the loss of all the pituitary hormones but is often used in clinical practice to describe patients deficient in growth hormone (GH), gonadotropins, corticotropin, or thyrotropin in whom posterior pituitary function remains intact.

SYNONYMS

Panhypopituitarism
Pituitary insufficiency

ICD-10CM CODES
E23.0 Hypopituitarism
E23.1 Drug-induced hypopituitarism
E89.3 Postprocedural hypopituitarism

EPIDEMIOLOGY & DEMOGRAPHICS

Incidence of 4.2 cases per 100,000 persons

PHYSICAL FINDINGS & CLINICAL PRESENTATION

Symptoms depend on type of onset, number and severity of hormone deficiencies, their target organs, and age of onset.

- Mass effect of a pituitary tumor can cause headaches and visual disturbances (typically as bitemporal hemianopsia).
- Rhinorrhea.
- Corticotropin deficiency:
  1. Fatigue and weakness, no appetite, abdominal pain, nausea, vomiting, failure to thrive in children, and hyponatremia. If the onset is abrupt, hypotension and shock.
- Thyrotropin deficiency:
  1. Fatigue and weakness, weight gain, cold intolerance, anemia, constipation
  2. Bradycardia, hung-up reflexes, pretibial edema, change in voice, and hair loss
- Gonadotropin deficiency:
  1. Loss of libido, erectile dysfunction, amenorrhea, hot flashes, dyspareunia, infertility, gynecomastia, decreased muscle mass, and anemia
- GH deficiency:
  1. Growth retardation in children
  2. Easy fatigue, hypoglycemia
  3. Lean mass is reduced and fat mass is increased, leading to obesity
  4. Decreased bone mineral density, increased low-density lipoprotein cholesterol, obesity, increased inflammatory cardiovascular markers (interleukin-6 and C-reactive protein)
- Hyperprolactinemia:
  1. Galactorrhea, hypogonadism, inability to lactate after delivery
  2. Posterior pituitary (vasopressin; antidiuretic hormone [ADH] deficiency): Diabetes insipidus with polyuria, polydipsia, nocturia, hypotension, and dehydration

ETIOLOGY

It can be congenital or acquired:

- Congenital: Mutations in transcription factors produce multiple hormonal deficiencies. Mutations in genes produce single hormonal deficiency.
- Acquired: The result of destruction of pituitary cells caused by:
  1. Pituitary apoplexy: Hemorrhage or infarction of the pituitary gland. Predisposing factors include diabetes mellitus, anticoagulation therapy, head trauma, and radiation therapy. Sheehan syndrome: Postpartum necrosis, a rare complication after pregnancy.
  2. Infiltrative disease, including sarcoidosis, hemachromatosis, histiocytosis X, Wegener granulomatosis, lymphocytic hypophysitis, and infection of the pituitary (tuberculosis, mycosis, syphilis).
  3. Primary empty sella syndrome: Flattening of the pituitary gland caused by extension of the subarachnoid space and filling of cerebrospinal fluid into the sella turcica.
  4. Pituitary tumors: Classified by size (microadenomas, <10 mm; macroadenomas, >10 mm) and function. Prolactin-secreting tumors and nonfunctioning tumors account for the majority of pituitary adenomas.
  5. Suprasellar tumors: Craniopharyngiomas are the most common.

Dx DIAGNOSIS

The diagnosis of hypopituitarism is suspected by clinical history and physical findings and is established by blood tests to confirm the presence of hormone deficiency.

DIFFERENTIAL DIAGNOSIS

The differential diagnosis is as outlined under "Etiology."

WORKUP

Includes baseline determination of each anterior pituitary hormone followed by dynamic provocative stimulation tests, radiograph imaging, and formal visual field testing. Table 1 summarizes testing for assessment of anterior pituitary function.

LABORATORY TESTS

- Corticotropin deficiency:
  1. The presence of a 9:00 am cortisol level >20 mcg/dl or <4 mcg/dl usually confirms sufficiency or deficiency, respectively.
  2. Corticotropin stimulation test using 250 mcg of corticotropin given IV and measuring serum cortisol before and 30 and 60 min after administration. A normal response is an increase in serum cortisol level >20 mcg/dl.
  3. With pituitary disease these test results may be indeterminate, and more dynamic testing such as an insulin-tolerance or metyrapone test may be necessary.
- Thyrotropin deficiency:
  1. Thyroid-stimulating hormone (TSH) and free T_4 measurements
  2. Primary hypothyroidism shows elevated TSH with low free T_4. Secondary hypothyroidism shows normal or low TSH with low free T_4 and low T_3 resin uptake.
- Gonadotropin deficiency:
  1. Follicle-stimulating hormone (FSH), luteinizing hormone (LH), estrogen, and testosterone measurements.
  2. In men, hypogonadotropic hypogonadism is seen with low testosterone levels and normal or low FSH and LH levels (ideally measured at 9:00 AM because of diurnal rhythm). Check free testosterone if patient is obese.
  3. In premenopausal women with amenorrhea, low estrogen with normal or low FSH and LH levels is typically seen.
- GH deficiency:
  1. Insulin-induced hypoglycemia stimulation test using 0.1 to 0.15 unit/kg regular insulin given IV and measuring GH 30, 60, and 120 min after administration. A normal response is a GH level >3 mcg/dl. This test is contraindicated in seizure disorder or ischemic heart disease.
  2. Combination of GH-releasing hormone plus arginine is an alternative test, with a diagnostic threshold of 9 mcg/L.
  3. Because the relation between serum insulin-like growth factor (IGF)-1 and GH levels blurs with age, a normal serum IGF-1 does not exclude the diagnosis in older adults.
- Hyperprolactinemia: Prolactin levels may be elevated in prolactin-secreting pituitary adenomas.
- Vasopressin deficiency:
  1. Urinalysis shows low specific gravity.
  2. Urine osmolality is low.
  3. Serum osmolality is high.
  4. Fluid deprivation test over 18 hr with inability to concentrate the urine.
  5. Serum vasopressin level is low.
  6. Electrolytes may show hyponatremia and exclude hyperglycemia.

IMAGING STUDIES

- Imaging is the first step in identifying an underlying cause.
- MRI (Fig. 1) is more sensitive than CT in visualizing the pituitary fossa, sella turcica, optic chiasm, pituitary stalk, and cavernous sinuses. It is also more sensitive in detecting pituitary microadenomas. CT with contrast can be used if MRI is not available.
- Surveillance scan at baseline and 12 mo thereafter depending on protocol and clinical symptoms.

TABLE 1 Assessment of Anterior Pituitary Function

Test	Dose	Normal Response	Side Effects
ACTH			
Insulin tolerance	0.1-0.15 U/kg IV	Peak cortisol response >18 μg/dl, or ≥5 μg/dl	Sweating, palpitation, tremor
Metyrapone	30 mg/kg PO at 11 PM	Peak 11-DOC ≥=7 μg/dl Peak cortisol ≤7 μg/dl Peak ACTH >75 pg/ml	Nausea, insomnia, adrenal crisis
CRH stimulation	100 μg IV	Peak ACTH ≥2-4-fold Peak cortisol ≥20 μg/dl or ↑ ≥=7 μg/dl	Flushing
ACTH stimulation	250 μg IV or IM, or 1 μg IV	Peak cortisol ≥20 μg/dl	Rare
TSH			
Serum T_4 (free T_4) Total T_3 TSH—third-generation TRH stimulation	200-500 μg IV	Peak TSH ≥2.5-fold, or ↑ ≥5-6 mU/L (females) or ≥2-3 mU/L (males)	Flushing, nausea, urge to micturate
PRL			
Serum PRL TRH stimulation	200-500 μg IV	PRL ↑ ≥2.5-fold	Flushing, nausea, urge to micturate
LH/FSH			
Serum LH and FSH Serum testosterone GnRH stimulation	100 μg IV	Elevated in menopause and in men with primary testicular failure (otherwise normal) 300-900 ng/ml LH ≥2-3-fold, or ↑ by 10 IU/L FSH ≥1.5-2-fold, or ↑ ≥2 IU/L	Rare
GH			
Insulin tolerance	0.1-0.15 U/kg	GH peak >5 μg/L	Sweating, palpitation, tremor
L-Arginine	Arginine 0.5 g/kg (maximum, 30 g) IV over 30-120 min	GH peak >0.4 μg/L	Nausea
Plus			
GHRH	GHRH 1-5 μg/kg	GH peak >4 μg/L	Flushing

ACTH, Adrenocorticotropic hormone; *CRH,* corticotropin-releasing hormone; *11-DOC,* 11-deoxycorticosterone; *FSH,* follicle-stimulating hormone; *GH,* growth hormone; *GHRH,* growth hormone–releasing hormone; *GnRH,* gonadotropin-releasing hormone; *LH,* luteinizing hormone; *PRL,* prolactin; *T_3,* triiodothyronine; *T_4,* thyroxine; *TSH,* thyroid-stimulating hormone; *TRH,* thyrotropin-releasing hormone.
From Melmed S, Polonsky KS, Larsen PR, Kronenberg HM: *Williams textbook of endocrinology,* ed 12, Philadelphia, 2011, Saunders, Elsevier Inc.

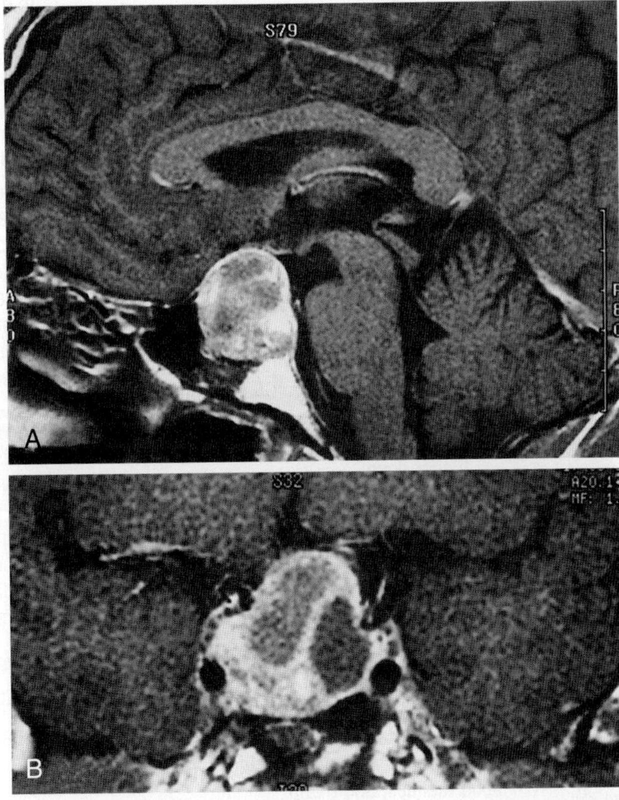

FIG. 1 T1-weighted gadolinium-enhanced MR of a pituitary adenoma. (A) Sagittal and **(B)** coronal images. (Courtesy of D. Thomas. From Bowling B: *Kanski's clinical ophthalmology,* ed 8, Philadelphia, 2016, Elsevier.)

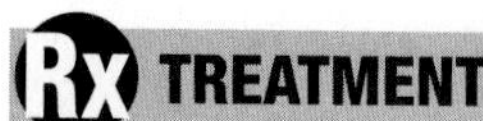

TREATMENT

Threefold: Removing underlying cause (surgery or radiation), treating hormonal deficiencies, and addressing any other repercussions from deficiency. Table 2 summarizes replacement therapy for adult hypopituitarism.

NONPHARMACOLOGIC THERAPY

- IV fluid resuscitation, correction of electrolyte and metabolic abnormalities with potassium bicarbonate, and oxygen therapy.
- Transsphenoidal surgery for tumors causing specific symptoms.
- Radiation or stereotactic radiosurgery ("gamma knife") for medically unresponsive, surgically unresectable tumors and tumors for which other modalities are contraindicated. It is both safe and effective for recurrent or residual pituitary adenomas.

TABLE 2 Replacement Therapy for Adult Hypopituitarism*

Deficient Hormone
Treatment
ACTH
Hydrocortisone: 10-20 mg/day in divided doses
Cortisone acetate: 15-25 mg/day in divided doses
TSH
L-Thyroxine: 0.05-0.2 mg/day according to T_4 levels
FSH/LH (in males)
Testosterone enanthate: 200 mg IM q2-3 wk
Testosterone skin patch: 2.5-5.0 mg/day (or up to 7.5 mg/day)
Testosterone gel: 3-6 g/day
For fertility: hCG three times weekly, or hCG + either FSH or menopausal gonadotropin or GnRH
FSH/LH (in females)
Conjugated estrogen: 0.3-0.625 mg/day
Micronized estradiol: 1 mg/day
Estradiol valerate: 2 mg
Piperazine estrone sulfate: 1.25 mg
Estradiol skin patch: 4-8 mg twice weekly
All of the estrogens are administered with progesterone or progestin sequentially or in combination if uterus is present
For fertility: Menopausal gonadotropin, and hCG, or GnRH
Growth hormone
Somatotropin (in adults): 0.2-1.0 mg/day SC
Somatotropin (in children): 0.02-0.05 mg/kg per day
Vasopressin
Intranasal desmopressin: 10-20 μg bid
Oral DDAVP: 300-600 μg/day, usually in divided doses

ACTH, Adrenocorticotropic hormone; *DDAVP,* desmopressin acetate; *FSH,* follicle-stimulating hormone; *GnRH,* gonadotropin-releasing hormone; *hCG,* human chorionic gonadotropin; *LH,* luteinizing hormone; T_4, thyroxine; *TSH,* thyroid-stimulating hormone.

From Melmed S, Polonsky KS, Larsen PR, Kronenberg HM: *Williams textbook of endocrinology,* ed 12, Philadelphia, 2011, Saunders, Elsevier Inc.

ACUTE GENERAL Rx

Acute situations such as adrenal crisis or myxedema coma can occur in untreated hypopituitarism and should be treated accordingly with IV corticosteroids (e.g., hydrocortisone 100 to 250 mg bolus followed by hydrocortisone 100 mg IV q6h for 24 hr) and levothyroxine (e.g., 5 to 8 mcg/kg IV over 15 min, then 100 mcg IV q24h).

CHRONIC Rx

Treatment is lifelong:

- Adrenocorticotropic hormone (ACTH) deficiency: Hydrocortisone 10 mg PO every morning and 5 mg PO every evening or prednisone 5 mg PO every morning and 2.5 mg PO every evening. Dexamethasone or prednisone is often preferred because of longer duration of action.
- LH and FSH deficiency:
  1. In men, testosterone enanthate or propionate 200 to 300 mg IM every 2 to 3 wk, or transdermal testosterone scrotal patches can be tried.
  2. In women who are not interested in fertility, conjugated estrogen 0.3 to 1.25 mg/day and held the last 5 to 7 days of each month with the addition of medroxyprogesterone 10 mg/day given during days 15 to 25 of the normal menstrual cycle. In those who have secondary hypogonadism and wish to become pregnant, pulsatile gonadotropic-releasing hormone may be of benefit.
- TSH deficiency: Levothyroxine 0.05 to 0.2 mg/day. Only free thyroxine should be used to monitor appropriate dosing to maintain thyroxine level in the mid to upper half of normal range.
- GH deficiency:
  1. GH replacement in children is universally accepted.
  2. GH replacement in adults is not generally recommended and requires careful consideration of each individual case. It may have effects on quality of life, body composition, bone density, and cardiovascular risk factors.
  3. Side effects of replacement include peripheral edema, arthralgia, and headaches.
  4. Usual GH dose is between 0.2 and 0.4 mg, determined by the age and gender of a patient and increments of 0.1 mg every 2 to 4 wk until serum IGF-1 is in the upper part of the normal range. Young adults and women taking estrogen require a higher dose.
- ADH deficiency:
  1. Desmopressin (DDAVP) 10 to 20 mcg by intranasal spray or 0.05 to 0.1 mg PO bid is used in patients with diabetes insipidus.
  2. Vasopressin: 5 to 10 U given IM or SC q6h.

DISPOSITION

- Hormone replacement therapy is adjusted according to serum hormone monitoring.
- If untreated can lead to adrenal crisis, severe hyponatremia and hypothyroidism, metabolic abnormalities, and death.
- Complications: Visual deficit, adrenal crisis, susceptibility to infection and other stressors.
- Prognosis: Stable patients have a favorable prognosis with replacement hormone therapy. Patients with acute decompensation are in critical condition with a high mortality rate.

REFERRAL

Consultation with an endocrinologist and neurosurgeon for surgical treatment

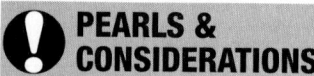

PEARLS & CONSIDERATIONS

- All patients sustaining moderate to severe head injury should undergo assessment of anterior pituitary function during the acute phase and at 6 mo.
- IGF-1 can be used as a marker of GH deficiency.
- All tests of GH secretion are more likely to give false-positive results in obese patients.
- The GH axis is the most vulnerable to the effects of radiotherapy; doses as low as 18 Gy in children have caused GH deficiency.
- Sequence of hormonal disruption: GH secretion then gonadotropin secretion. TSH and adrenocorticotropic hormone secretion are somewhat resistant.
- Thyroxine supplementation increases the rate of cortisol metabolism and can lead to adrenal crisis, so corticosteroids should be replaced first.
- All patients receiving glucocorticoid replacement therapy should wear proper identification stating the need for this therapy.
- Stress doses of corticosteroids are indicated before surgery or for any medical emergency (e.g., sepsis, acute myocardial infarction).
- Antidiuretic hormone deficiency may be masked if there is ACTH deficiency with symptoms only appearing when cortisol has been replaced.

COMMENTS

- Mineralocorticoid replacement is not necessary in secondary adrenal insufficiency because the renin-angiotensin-aldosterone system is unaffected by pituitary failure.
- Patients with adult-acquired GH deficiency must meet at least two criteria before replacement therapy: a poor GH response to at least two standard stimuli and hypopituitarism from pituitary or hypothalamic damage. The criteria are different in children in whom GH is required for normal growth.
- Prevention of acute decompensation can be accomplished by reminding patients to increase the dose of hydrocortisone in response to stress.
- Medical therapy should precede surgical therapy.

RELATED CONTENT

Hypopituitarism (Patient Information)

AUTHOR: **FRED F. FERRI, M.D.**

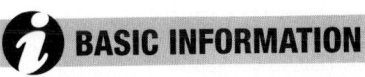

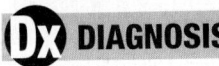

BASIC INFORMATION

DEFINITION

Hypothermia is a rectal temperature <35° C (95.8° F). "Accidental hypothermia" is an unintentionally induced decrease in core temperature in the absence of preoptic anterior hypothalamic conditions.

ICD-10CM CODES

T68 Hypothermia

R68.0 Hypothermia, not associated with low environmental temperature

EPIDEMIOLOGY & DEMOGRAPHICS

- Hypothermia occurs most frequently in the following groups: alcoholics; homeless; learning-impaired; patients with cardiovascular, cerebrovascular, or pituitary disorders; those using sedatives or tranquilizers; and elderly patients.
- >700 persons in the United States die from hypothermia annually.

PHYSICAL FINDINGS & CLINICAL PRESENTATION

The clinical presentation varies with the severity of hypothermia. Shivering may be absent if body temperature is <33.3° C (92° F) or in patients taking phenothiazines.

Hypothermia may masquerade as cerebrovascular accident, ataxia, or slurred speech, or the patient may appear comatose or clinically dead. Signs of hypothermia are summarized in Box E1. Physiologic stages of hypothermia:

- Stage HT I: Mild hypothermia (typical core temperature 32.2° to 35° C [90° to 95° F]): arrhythmias, ataxia
- Stage HT II: Moderate hypothermia (core temperature 28° to 32.2° C [82.4° to 90° F]):
  1. Progressive decrease of level of consciousness, pulse, cardiac output, and respiration
  2. Fibrillation, dysrhythmias (increased susceptibility to ventricular tachycardia)
  3. Elimination of shivering mechanism for thermogenesis
- Stage HT III: Severe hypothermia (core temperature ≤28° C to 24° C [82.4° F to 75° F]):
  1. Absence of reflexes or response to pain
  2. Decreased cerebral blood flow, decreased CO_2
  3. Increased risk of ventricular fibrillation or asystole
  4. Vital signs present
- Stage IV: No vital signs (core temperature <24° C [75° F])

ETIOLOGY

Exposure to cold temperatures for a prolonged period. Contributing factors include:

- Drugs: Ethanol, phenothiazines, sedative-hypnotics
- Skin disorders: Extensive burns, severe psoriasis, exfoliative dermatitis
- Metabolic disorders: Hypopituitarism, hypothyroidism, hypoadrenalism
- Neurologic abnormalities: Stroke, head trauma, acute spinal cord transection, impaired shivering
- Other: Lack of acclimatization, aggressive fluid resuscitation, sepsis, heat stroke treatment
- Box E2 summarizes factors predisposing to hypothermia

Dx DIAGNOSIS

DIFFERENTIAL DIAGNOSIS

- It is crucial to determine an accurate core temperature measurement. Advantages and considerations of various methods to determine core temperature are summarized in Table 1. Core temperature is best monitored with an esophageal probe. Rectal and bladder temperature generally lag behind core temperatures during the rewarming process.
- Cerebrovascular accident
- Myxedema coma
- Drug intoxication
- Hypoglycemia

LABORATORY TESTS

- Metabolic and respiratory acidosis are usually present.
  1. When blood cools, the arterial pH increases, oxygen tension (Po_2) increases, and the Pco_2 falls:
     a. pH increases 0.008 U/° F (or 0.015 U/° C), causing a decrease in temperature.
     b. Pao_2 increases 3.3%/° F, causing a decrease in temperature. Oxygenation considerations during hypothermia are described in Box 3.
     c. $Paco_2$ decreases 2.4%/° F, causing a decrease in temperature.
  2. Blood gas analyzers warm the blood to 37° C (98.6° F), increasing the partial pressure of dissolved gases, resulting in higher oxygen and carbon dioxide levels and a lower pH than the patient's actual values. Correction of arterial blood gases for temperature is unnecessary as a guide to therapy. The use of uncorrected values also permits reference to the standard acid–base nomograms.
- A decrease in K^+ initially, then an increase in K^+ with increasing hypothermia; extreme hyperkalemia indicates a poor prognosis.
- Hematocrit increases (caused by hemoconcentration), decreasing leukocytes and platelets (caused by splenic sequestration).
- Blood viscosity, increased clotting time.

TABLE 1 Core Temperature Measurements

Type	Advantages	Considerations
Rectal	Convenient Continuous monitoring	Insert 15 cm (6 inches) Lags during transition from cooling to rewarming Falsely elevated with peritoneal lavage Falsely low if probe is in cold feces or when lower extremities are frozen
Esophageal	Convenient Continuous monitoring	Insert 24 cm (9.5 inches) below larynx Tracheal misplacement Aspiration Falsely elevated with heated inhalation
Tympanic	Approximates hypothalamic temperature via internal carotid artery	Probe: Tympanic membrane perforation; canal hemorrhage Infrared: Unreliable; cerumen effect
Bladder	Convenient Continuous monitoring	Unreliable Falsely elevated with peritoneal lavage Falsely low with cold diuresis

From Auerbach P: *Wilderness medicine, expert consult premium edition—enhanced online features and print*, Philadelphia, 2012, Saunders.

BOX 3 Oxygenation Considerations During Hypothermia

Detrimental Factors

Oxygen consumption increases with rise in temperature; caution if rapid rewarming; shivering also increases demand
Decreased temperature shifts oxyhemoglobin dissociation curve to the left
Ventilation-perfusion mismatch; atelectasis; decreased respiratory minute volume; bronchorrhea; decreased protective airway reflexes
Decreased tissue perfusion from vasoconstriction; increased viscosity
"Functional hemoglobin" concept: Capability of hemoglobin to unload oxygen is lowered
Decreased thoracic elasticity and pulmonary compliance

Protective Factors

Reduction of oxygen consumption: 50% at 28° C (82.4° F); 75% at 22° C (71.6° F); 92% at 10° C (50° F)
Increased oxygen solubility in plasma
Decreased pH and increased $Paco_2$ shift oxyhemoglobin dissociation curve to right

From Auerbach P: *Wilderness medicine*, ed 4, St Louis, 2001, Mosby.

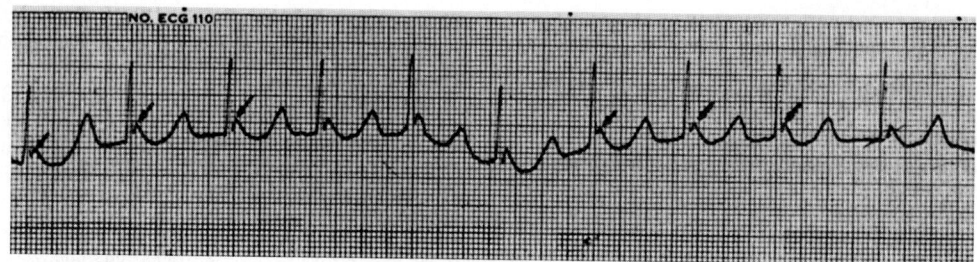

FIG. 1 Hypothermic J waves (Osborne waves) *(arrows)* in an 80-year-old man with core temperature of 86° F (30° C). These waves disappeared with rewarming. (From Morse CD, Rial WY: Emergency medicine.)

BOX 4 Preparing Hypothermic Patients for Transport

1. The patient must be dry. Gently remove or cut off wet clothing, and replace it with dry clothing or a dry insulation system. Keep the patient horizontal, and do not allow exertion or massage of the extremities.
2. Stabilize injuries (i.e., the spine; place fractures in the correct anatomic position). Open wounds should be covered before packaging.
3. Initiate heated intravenous infusions (IVs) if feasible; bags can be placed under the patient's buttocks or in a compressor system. Administer a fluid challenge.
4. Active rewarming should be limited to heated inhalation and truncal heat. Insulate hot water bottles in stockings or mittens, and then place them in the patient's axillae and groin.
5. The patient should be wrapped. Begin building the wrap by placing a large plastic sheet on the available surface (floor, ground), and on it place an insulated sleeping pad. A layer of blankets, a sleeping bag, or bubble wrap insulating material is laid over the sleeping pad. The patient is then placed on the insulation. Heating bottles are put in place along with IVs, and the entire package is wrapped layer over layer, with the plastic as the final closure. The patient's face should be partially covered, but a tunnel should be created to allow access for breathing and monitoring.

From Auerbach P: *Wilderness medicine, expert consult premium edition—enhanced online features and print*, Philadelphia, 2012, Elsevier.

IMAGING STUDIES

- Chest x-ray: Generally not helpful; may reveal evidence of aspiration (e.g., intoxicated patient with aspiration pneumonia).
- ECG: Prolonged PR, QT, and QRS segments, depressed ST segments, inverted T waves, atrioventricular block, and hypothermic J waves (Osborne waves) may appear at temperatures less than 33.0° C (91.4° F); characterized by notching of the junction of the QRS complex and ST segments (Fig. 1).

Rx TREATMENT

NONPHARMACOLOGIC THERAPY

- The first critical step in management of accidental hypothermia is initiating passive external rewarming by removing wet clothing and covering the patient with insulating material.
- Specific treatment of hypothermia varies with the following:
  1. Degree of hypothermia
  2. Existence of concomitant diseases (e.g., cardiovascular insufficiency)
  3. Patient's age and medical condition (e.g., elderly, debilitated patients vs. young, healthy patients)
- General measures:
  1. Secure an airway before warming all unconscious patients; precede endotracheal intubation with oxygenation (if possible) to minimize the risk of arrhythmias during the procedure.
  2. Peripheral vasoconstriction may impede placement of a peripheral intravenous catheter; consider femoral venous access as an alternative to the jugular or subclavian sites to avoid ventricular stimulation.
  3. A Foley catheter should be inserted, and urinary output should be monitored and maintained >0.5 to 1 ml/kg/hr with intravascular volume replacement.
  4. Box 4 summarizes measures for preparing hypothermic patients for transport.

ACUTE GENERAL Rx

- Continuous ECG monitoring of patients is recommended. Ventricular arrhythmias can be treated with bretylium; lidocaine is generally ineffective, and procainamide is associated with an increased incidence of ventricular fibrillation in hypothermic patients.
- Correct severe acidosis and electrolyte abnormalities.
- Hypothyroidism, if present, should be promptly treated (see "Myxedema Coma").
- If clinical evidence suggests adrenal insufficiency, administer IV methylprednisolone.

In patients unresponsive to verbal or noxious stimuli or with altered mental status, 100 mg of thiamine, 0.4 mg of naloxone, and 1 ampule of 50% dextrose may be given.

Warm (104° to 113° F [40° to 45° C]), humidified oxygen should also be given if available.

- Specific treatment:
  1. Mild hypothermia (rectal temperature <32.3° C [90° F]): Passive external rewarming is indicated. Place the patient in a warm room (temperature >21° C [69.8° F]), and cover with insulating material after gently removing wet clothing; recommended rewarming rates vary between 0.5° and 20° C/hr but should not exceed 0.55° C/hr in elderly persons.
  2. Moderate to severe hypothermia:
     a. Active core rewarming
        (1) Delivery of heat by way of fluids: Warm gastrointestinal irrigation (with saline enemas and by nasogastric tube); IV fluids (usually D_5NS without potassium) warmed to 104° to 107.6° F (40° to 42° C), peritoneal dialysis with dialysate heated to 40.5° to 42.5° C.
        (2) Inhalation of heated, humidified oxygen (warmed to 40° C [104° F]) increases core temperature by 1° C (1.8° F) per hr and decreases evaporative heat loss from respiration.
  3. Active external rewarming: Immersion in a bath of warm water (40° to 41° C); active external rewarming may produce shock because of excessive peripheral vasodilation. Ideal candidates are previously healthy, young patients with acute immersion hypothermia.
  4. Extracorporeal blood warming with cardiopulmonary bypass appears to be an efficacious rewarming technique in young, otherwise healthy persons.
  5. Patients with cardiac instability and those in cardiac arrest should be transported to a center capable of providing extracorporeal membrane oxygenation (ECMO) unless other conditions (e.g., trauma) require transport to a closer facility.

SUGGESTED READING

Available at ExpertConsult.com

RELATED CONTENT

Hypothermia (Patient Information)

AUTHOR: **FRED F. FERRI, M.D.**

BASIC INFORMATION

DEFINITION

Hypothyroidism is a disorder caused by the inadequate secretion of thyroid hormone.

SYNONYM

Myxedema

ICD-10CM CODES

E03.9	Hypothyroidism, unspecified
E00.9	Congenital iodine-deficiency syndrome, unspecified
E89.0	Postprocedural hypothyroidism
E03.2	Hypothyroidism due to medicaments and other exogenous substances
E02	Subclinical iodine-deficiency hypothyroidism
E03.0	Congenital hypothyroidism with diffuse goiter
E03.1	Congenital hypothyroidism without goiter
E03.3	Postinfectious hypothyroidism
E03.8	Other specified hypothyroidism

EPIDEMIOLOGY & DEMOGRAPHICS

INCIDENCE/PREVALENCE: 1.5% to 2% of women and 0.2% of men. Overall, about 1 in 300 persons in the U.S. has hypothyroidism.

PREDOMINANT AGE: Incidence of hypothyroidism increases with age; among persons older than 60 yr, 6% of women and 2.5% of men have laboratory evidence of hypothyroidism (thyroid-stimulating hormone [TSH] more than twice normal level).

PHYSICAL FINDINGS & CLINICAL PRESENTATION

- Hypothyroid patients generally present with the following signs and symptoms: fatigue, lethargy, weakness, constipation, weight gain, cold intolerance, muscle weakness, slow speech, slow cerebration with poor memory
- Skin: Dry, coarse, thick, cool, sallow (yellow color caused by carotenemia); nonpitting edema in skin of eyelids and hands (myxedema) secondary to infiltration of subcutaneous tissues by a hydrophilic mucopolysaccharide substance (Fig. E1, *A* and *B*)
- Hair: Brittle and coarse; loss of outer third of eyebrows
- Faces: Dulled expression, thickened tongue, thick and slow-moving lips
- Thyroid gland: May or may not be palpable (depending on the cause of the hypothyroidism)
- Heart sounds: Distant, possible pericardial effusion
- Pulse: Bradycardia
- Neurologic: Delayed relaxation phase of the deep tendon reflexes, cerebellar ataxia, hearing impairment, poor memory, peripheral neuropathies with paresthesia
- Musculoskeletal: Carpal tunnel syndrome, muscular stiffness, weakness

ETIOLOGY

- Primary hypothyroidism (thyroid gland dysfunction): The cause of >90% of the cases of hypothyroidism
  1. Hashimoto thyroiditis is the most common cause of hypothyroidism after age 8 yr
  2. Idiopathic myxedema (nongoitrous form of Hashimoto thyroiditis)
  3. Previous treatment of hyperthyroidism (radioiodine therapy, subtotal thyroidectomy)
  4. Subacute thyroiditis
  5. Radiation therapy to the neck (usually for malignant disease)
  6. Iodine deficiency or excess
  7. Drugs (lithium, para-aminosalicylate, sulfonamides, phenylbutazone, amiodarone, thiourea)
  8. Congenital (approximately one case per 2000 to 4000 live births)
  9. Prolonged treatment with iodides
- Secondary hypothyroidism: Pituitary dysfunction, postpartum necrosis, neoplasm, infiltrative disease causing deficiency of TSH
- Tertiary hypothyroidism: Hypothalamic disease (granuloma, neoplasm, or irradiation causing deficiency of thyrotropin-releasing hormone)
- Tissue resistance to thyroid hormone: Rare

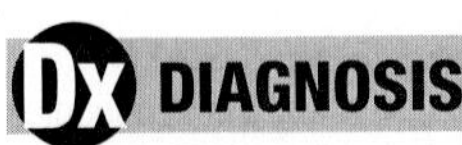

DIAGNOSIS

DIFFERENTIAL DIAGNOSIS

- Depression
- Dementia from other causes
- Systemic disorders (e.g., nephrotic syndrome, congestive heart failure, amyloidosis)

LABORATORY TESTS

- TSH, free T_4, thyroid peroxidase antibodies (TPO_{AB}).
- Increased TSH: TSH may be normal if patient has secondary or tertiary hypothyroidism, is receiving dopamine or corticosteroids, or the level is obtained after severe illness.
- Decreased free T_4 in hypothroidism, normal free T_4 in subclinical hypothyroidism.
- Other common laboratory abnormalities: Hyperlipidemia, hyponatremia, and anemia.
- Increased antimicrosomal and antithyroglobulin antibody titers: Useful when autoimmune thyroiditis is suspected as the cause of the hypothyroidism. The American Thyroid Association recommends treatment of pregnant patients with subclinical hypothyroidism and anti-thyroid peroxidase (anti-TPO) antibody positivity.
- Fig. 2 describes a strategy for the laboratory evaluation of patients with suspected hypothyroidism.

TREATMENT

NONPHARMACOLOGIC THERAPY

Patients should be educated regarding hypothyroidism and its possible complications. Patients should also be instructed about the need for lifelong treatment and monitoring of their thyroid abnormality.

ACUTE GENERAL Rx

Start replacement therapy with levothyroxine (L-thyroxine) 25 to 100 μg/day, depending on the patient's age and the severity of the disease. Physiologic combinations of L-thyroxine plus liothyronine do not offer any objective advantage over L-thyroxine alone. The levothyroxine dose may be increased every 6 to 8 wk, depending on the clinical response and serum TSH level. Elderly patients and patients with coronary artery disease should be started with 12.5 to 25 μg/day (higher doses may precipitate angina). The average maintenance dose of levothyroxine is 1.7 μg/kg/day (100 to 150 μg/day in adults). The elderly may require <1 μg/kg/day, whereas children generally require higher doses (up to 3 to 4 μg/kg/day). Pregnant patients also have increased requirements. Estrogen therapy may also increase the need for thyroxine. Women with hypothyroidism should increase their levothyroxine dose by approximately 30% as soon as pregnancy is confirmed. Close monitoring of serum thyrotropin levels and adjustment of levothyroxine dose to maintain a TSH level of 4.0 mU per liter as upper limit is recommended throughout pregnancy. Table 1 summarizes conditions that alter levothyroxine requirements.

CHRONIC Rx

- Periodic monitoring of TSH level is an essential part of treatment. Patients should be evaluated initially with office visit and TSH levels every 6 to 8 wk until the patient is clinically euthyroid and the TSH level is normalized. The frequency of subsequent visits and TSH measurement can then be decreased to every 6 to 12 mo. Pregnant patients should be checked every trimester.
- For monitoring therapy in patients with central hypothyroidism, measurement of serum free thyroxine (free T_4 level) is appropriate and should be maintained in the upper half of the normal range.

REFERRAL

Admission to the hospital intensive care unit is recommended in all patients with myxedema coma. Additional information on the diagnosis and treatment of this life-threatening complication of hypothyroidism is available under "Myxedema Coma" in Section I.

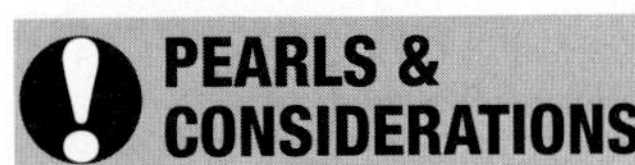

PEARLS & CONSIDERATIONS

COMMENTS

Subclinical hypothyroidism occurs in as many as 20% of elderly patients and is characterized by an elevated serum TSH and a normal free T_4 level. Subclinical hypothyroidism can progress to overt

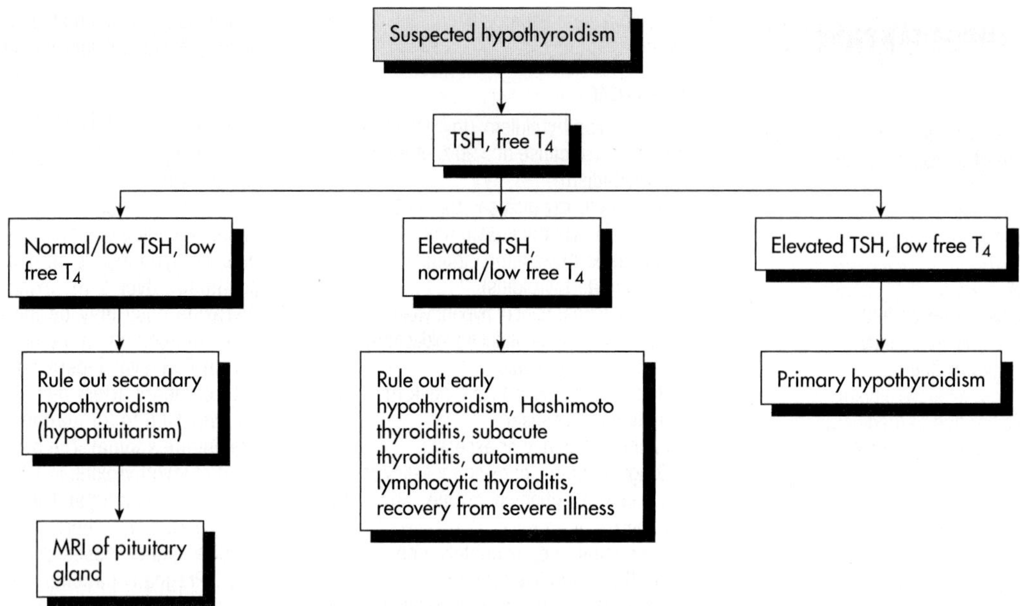

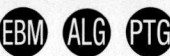

FIG. 2 Strategy for the laboratory evaluation of patients with suspected hypothyroidism. The principal differential diagnosis is between primary and central hypothyroidism. The serum thyrotropin (TSH) concentration is the critical laboratory determination that, in general, allows recognition of the cause of the disease. An exception is the individual with a recent history of thyrotoxicosis (and suppressed TSH), in whom a low free thyroxine (T_4) level may be associated with a reduced TSH level for several months after relief of the thyrotoxicosis. In patients with primary hypothyroidism, the absence of thyroid peroxidase (TPO) antibodies raises a possible diagnosis of transient hypothyroidism after an undiagnosed episode of subacute or postviral thyroiditis. In such patients, a trial of levothyroxine in reduced dosage after 4 months may reveal recovery of thyroid function, thus avoiding permanent levothyroxine replacement. *MRI,* Magnetic resonance imaging. (From Melmed S, et al.: *Williams textbook of endocrinology,* ed 12, Philadelphia, 2011, Saunders.)

TABLE 1 Conditions That Alter Levothyroxine Requirements

Increased Levothyroxine Requirements
Pregnancy
Gastrointestinal Disorders
Mucosal diseases of the small bowel (e.g., sprue)
After jejunoileal bypass and small-bowel resection
Impaired gastric acid secretion (e.g., atrophic gastritis)
Diabetic diarrhea
Drugs That Interfere with Levothyroxine Absorption
Cholestyramine
Sucralfate
Aluminum hydroxide
Calcium carbonate
Ferrous sulfate
Drugs That Increase the Cytochrome P450 Enzyme (CYP3A4) Activity
Rifampin
Carbamazepine
Estrogen
Phenytoin
Sertraline
Drugs That Block T_4-to-T_3 Conversion
Amiodarone
Conditions That May Block Deiodinase Synthesis
Selenium deficiency
Cirrhosis
Decreased Levothyroxine Requirements
Aging (≥65 yr)
Androgen therapy in women

T_3, Triiodothyronine; *T_4,* thyroxine.
From Melmed S, et al.: *Williams textbook of endocrinology,* ed 12, Philadelphia, 2011, Saunders

hypothyroidism, especially if antithyroid antibodies are present. It is associated with an increased risk of coronary heart disease events and mortality, particularly in those with a TSH concentration of 10 mU/L or greater. Treatment is individualized and controversial. Some trials[1] have shown that levothyroxine provides no apparent benefit in older persons with subclinical hypothyroidism. The management of subclinical hypothyroidism should be individualized on the basis of TSH level, comorbid conditions, risk factors, and patient preference. In general, replacement therapy is recommended by most physicians for patients with serum TSH >10 mU/L and with presence of goiter or thyroid autoantibodies or patient has risk factors.

Congenital hypothyroidism is a pediatric disorder with an observed prevalence of one in 2000 to 4000 live births in the U.S. Screening is conducted in all newborns in all states and accomplished by measuring TSH from dried whole blood spots collected on a newborn by heel stick within the first 24 to 48 hours of life. Currently 14 states perform a routine second screen at approximately 2 weeks of age. A two-screen approach is preferred because retrospective analysis found that 20% of congenital hypothyroidism cases were in infants who had normal TSH on the first screen but elevated TSH concentrations on the second screen.

[1] Stott DJ, et al.: Thyroid hormone therapy for older adults with subclinical hypothyroidism, *N Engl J Med* 376:2534-2544, 2017.

SUGGESTED READINGS

Available at ExpertConsult.com

RELATED CONTENT

Hypothyroidism (Patient Information)
Myxedema Coma (Related Key Topic)

AUTHOR: **FRED F. FERRI, M.D.**

BASIC INFORMATION

DEFINITION

Idiopathic pulmonary fibrosis (IPF) is a specific form of chronic fibrosing interstitial pneumonia with histopathologic characteristics of usual interstitial pneumonia (UIP) occurring in the absence of an identifiable cause of lung injury. Clinically, it is characterized by progressive parenchymal scarring and loss of pulmonary function.

SYNONYMS

Cryptogenic fibrosing alveolitis
IPF
Pulmonary fibrosis
Usual interstitial pneumonia

ICD-10CM CODE

J84.112 Idiopathic pulmonary fibrosis

EPIDEMIOLOGY & DEMOGRAPHICS

- Incidence: 7 to 16 cases/100,000 persons worldwide. Clinically IPF affects >50,000 people in the U.S. and accounts for 20% to 30% of interstitial lung diseases. It is the most common idiopathic interstitial pneumonia.
- Most commonly presents in sixth and seventh decades
- More common in men than women
- More common in current and past smokers
- Familial forms account for 3% to 25% of cases. Genetic variants: Include mutations in surfactant protein C and telomerase as well as polymorphisms of the *MUC5B* gene.
- No distinct geographic distribution; no clear racial predilection

PHYSICAL FINDINGS & CLINICAL PRESENTATION

- Most present with gradual onset (>6 mo) of exertional dyspnea and nonproductive cough. Progressive dyspnea is usually the most prominent symptom. Cough affects up to 80% of patients with IPF, is frequently disabling, and lacks effective therapy.
- Fine bibasilar inspiratory crackles, "velcro inspiratory crackles" in >80% of patients, with progression upward as the disease advances.
- Clubbing is found in 25% to 50% of patients.
- Cyanosis and right heart failure (cor pulmonale) may occur late in the disease course.
- There are no extrapulmonary manifestations beyond clubbing and complications of right heart failure. Fever and wheezing are rare and suggest alternative diagnosis.
- Fig. 1 is a chest radiograph showing diffuse bilateral lower lung predominant reticular opacities in a patient with IPF.

ETIOLOGY

- Unknown
- Cigarette smoking, environmental exposures, gastroesophageal reflux and microaspiration have been associated with IPF.
- Aberrant tissue repair and fibrosis are believed to play a greater role in the pathogenesis than generalized inflammation. Immune system activation and increased vascular permeability contribute to the underlying pathology.

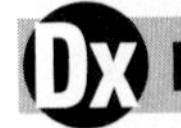

DIAGNOSIS

DIFFERENTIAL DIAGNOSIS

- Sarcoidosis
- Drug-induced interstitial lung disease
- Pulmonary manifestations of collagen vascular diseases (e.g., rheumatoid arthritis [RA], systemic sclerosis); ILD may be an initial sign of disease
- Hypersensitivity pneumonitis (HP)
- Occupational exposures (e.g., asbestos, silica) may cause pneumoconiosis that mimics IPF
- Other idiopathic interstitial pneumonias:
    1. Desquamative interstitial pneumonia (DIP)
    2. Respiratory bronchitis–interstitial lung disease (RB-ILD)
    3. Acute interstitial pneumonia (AIP)
    4. Nonspecific interstitial pneumonia (NSIP)
    5. Cryptogenic organizing pneumonia (COP)
- IPF is considered a diagnosis of exclusion.

WORKUP

- Almost all patients have abnormal chest radiograph at presentation, with bilateral reticular opacities most prominent in the periphery and lower lobes. Peripheral honeycombing may be seen.
- High-resolution CT scan (Fig. 2) is the best diagnostic test. It shows patchy peripheral reticular abnormalities with intralobular linear opacities, irregular septal thickening, subpleural honeycombing, and minimal, if any, ground-glass opacities.
- Pulmonary function testing shows restrictive pattern and reduced carbon monoxide diffusion into the lung.
- Six-minute walk test may show reduced exercise tolerance and/or exertional hypoxia.
- Laboratory abnormalities (nondiagnostic): Mild anemia; increases in erythrocyte sedimentation rate, lactate dehydrogenase, C-reactive protein; low titer antinuclear antibody seen in up to 30% of patients.
- The need for autoimmune serologies is not well defined. Any signs or symptoms that might suggest underlying autoimmunity should be evaluated fully.
- There is a limited role for bronchoalveolar lavage either in diagnosis or monitoring IPF.
- Gold standard for diagnosis is lung biopsy (open thoracotomy or video-assisted thoracoscopy). Hallmark features: Heterogeneous distribution of parenchymal fibrosis against background of mild inflammation (UIP). In patients with characteristic chest CTs, lung biopsies can be avoided.
- When there is uncertainty, lung biopsy is critical to distinguish IPF from diseases with better prognosis and different treatment options.
- Table 1 summarizes histologic findings for immunologic diseases.
- A multidisciplinary approach involving the collaboration of pulmonology, radiology and pathology to secure a diagnosis is considered standard of care.

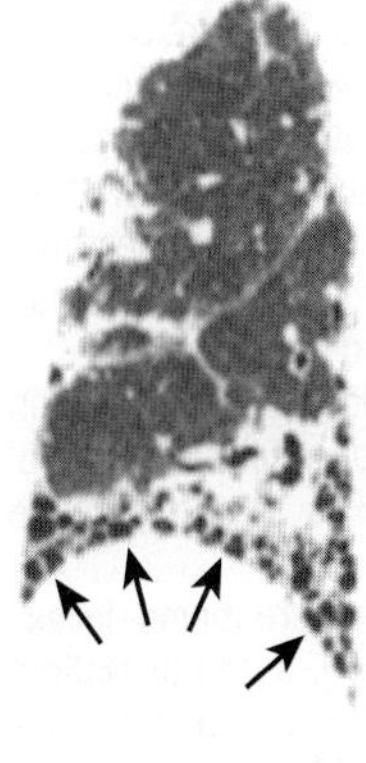
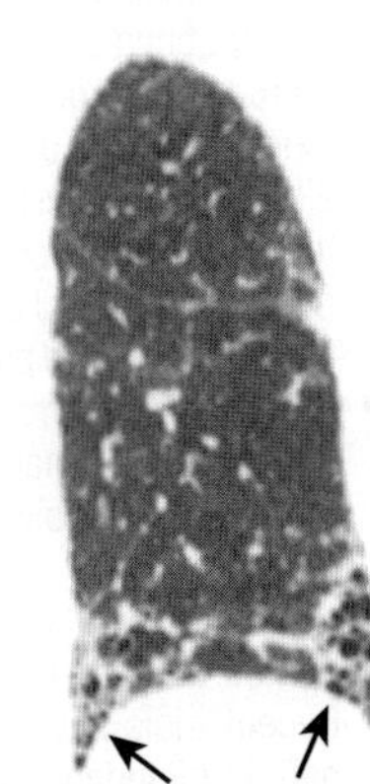

FIG. 2 Pulmonary fibrosis, honeycombing, and a usual interstitial pneumonia (UIP) pattern in idiopathic pulmonary fibrosis (IPF). Coronal high-resolution computed tomography reconstruction shows honeycombing (*arrows*) with a basal and subpleural predominance. This is typical of a UIP pattern. (Webb WR, Brant WE, Major NM: *Fundamentals of body CT*, ed 4, Philadelphia, 2015, Saunders.)

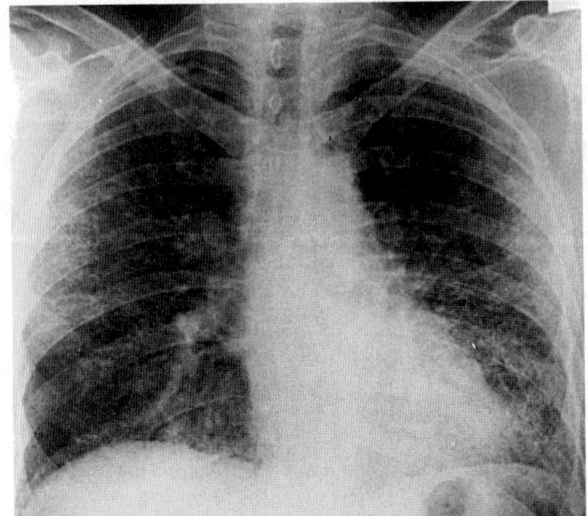

FIG. 1 Chest radiograph shows diffuse bilateral lower lung predominant reticular opacities in a patient with idiopathic pulmonary fibrosis (IPF). (From Mason RJ: *Murray & Nadel's textbook of respiratory medicine*, ed 5, Philadelphia, 2010, Saunders.)

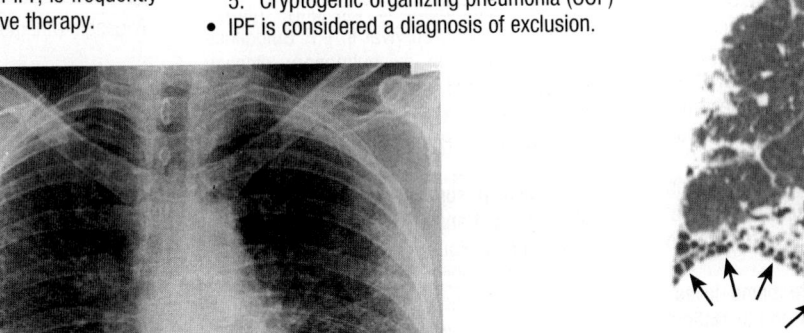

TABLE 1 Summary of Histologic Findings for Immunologic Lung Diseases

Disease	Histology
Granulomatous	
Foreign body, inorganic dust	Simple granuloma
Hypersensitivity pneumonitis	Granulomas with CD4+/CD8+ T cells; interstitial edema; fibrosis in later stages
Infections	
Tuberculosis	Caseating granulomas
Sarcoidosis	Noncaseating granulomas
Granulomatous Vasculitides	
Wegener granulomatosis	Necrotizing granulomas involving vasculature
Churg-Strauss syndrome	Necrotizing granulomas involving vasculature
Eosinophilic pneumonias	Granulomas with eosinophilic predominance; interstitial edema
Histiocytosis X	Granulomas with Langerhans cells
Alveolitic	
Drug-associated injury	Interstitial edema with inflammatory cells
Goodpasture syndrome	Linear staining of basement membrane with anti-IgG antibodies typically seen on renal biopsy; interstitial edema with inflammatory cells
Idiopathic Interstitial Pneumonias	
Idiopathic pulmonary fibrosis	Interstitial edema and/or fibrosis with inflammatory cells; patchy fibrotic change
Desquamative interstitial pneumonia	Interstitial edema with sparse inflammatory cells; mild diffuse fibrotic change
Idiopathic nonspecific interstitial pneumonia	Thickened interstitium with inflammatory cells; some patchy fibrosis
Acute interstitial pneumonia	Diffuse alveolar damage with thickened fibrotic interstitium; proliferating fibroblasts
Respiratory bronchiolitis–associated interstitial lung disease	Macrophages infiltrating distal bronchioles
Cryptogenic organizing pneumonia	Chronically inflamed alveoli with granulation tissue in bronchioles and macrophages in alveoli
Lymphocytic interstitial pneumonia	Diffuse lymphocytic and plasma cell infiltration; minimal alveolar injury
Idiopathic pleuroparenchymal fibroelastosis	Diffuse alveolar damage with fibrosis

From Sellke FW et al: *Sabiston & Spencer Surgery of the Chest*, ed 9, 2016, Elsevier.

TREATMENT

- Two FDA-approved oral therapies have proven efficacy in slowing disease progression. Combination therapy with both medications has not been investigated. They are suspected to have roughly similar clinical efficacies.
- Pirfenidone is an antifibrotic medication without a known mechanism of action. It is taken three times a day with food. Its major side effects are nausea, abdominal discomfort, and photosensitivity. LFTs require periodic surveillance.
- Nintedanib is a tyrosine kinase inhibitor taken twice daily. Its major side effect is diarrhea, which often resolves. LFTs also need to be followed.
- Additional new therapies are being investigated and are in phase I, II and III testing. Recent trials have shown that adding sildenafil to nintedanib did not improve quality of life or lessen 24-week mortality.[2]
- In patients with advanced disease, treatment options include supportive care (pulmonary rehabilitation, supplemental oxygen, influenza and pneumococcal vaccination) and potential lung transplantation.
- Treatment of asymptomatic gastroesophageal reflux may be reasonable given association between pulmonary fibrosis and reflux or microaspiration.
- Lung transplantation is the only therapy shown to prolong survival in IPF. Guidelines for transplantation by pulmonary disease are summarized in Box 1. Box 2 summarizes absolute contraindications to lung transplantation. Posttransplant 5-yr survival for IPF patients is approximately 50% to 60%. Median survival time is longer after bilateral lung transplantation than single lung transplantation but is associated with more complications during the first yr.
- Acute exacerbation of IPF, defined as worsening dyspnea (<1 mo), the presence of new opacities on radiograph, and the lack of evidence of infection, has a yearly incidence of 10% to 20%. Progressive respiratory failure may require mechanical ventilation; however, a palliative care approach is often chosen instead. Treatment for exacerbations typically includes high-dose corticosteroids and broad-spectrum antibiotics, although the efficacy of this approach is unproven and questionable.

DISPOSITION

- Spontaneous remissions do not occur, although long periods of stability can occur.
- Natural history includes progressive loss of pulmonary function. Predictors of poor outcome include older age, male gender, moderately to severely abnormal PFTs and presence of pulmonary hypertension.
- There is an increased risk of lung cancer.
- Mean survival after the diagnosis of biopsy-confirmed IPF is 3 to 5 yr, although with new therapies available, survival is less defined.
- Respiratory failure is the most common cause of death.

REFERRAL

- To pulmonologist for review of abnormal chest imaging and establishing diagnosis.
- Encouraging participation in clinical trials is a priority.
- Early referral for lung transplant.
- Later stage management should include palliative care or hospice services.

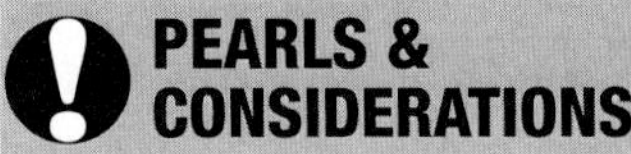

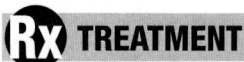

PEARLS & CONSIDERATIONS

- The course is progressive, with a high mortality rate. The most common cause of death in IPF is respiratory failure.
- Critical to differentiate IPF from other interstitial lung diseases because prognosis and treatment approaches differ.
- Two oral therapies shown to slow disease progression are available. Combination therapy has not been investigated. Additional novel treatments are being investigated.[1]

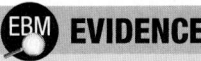

EVIDENCE

Available at ExpertConsult.com

SUGGESTED READINGS

Available at ExpertConsult.com

RELATED CONTENT

Idiopathic Pulmonary Fibrosis (Patient Information)

AUTHOR: **PETER LACAMERA, M.D.**

[1] Peljto AL et al: Association between the MUC5B promoter polymorphism and survival in patients with idiopathic pulmonary fibrosis, *JAMA* 309(21):2232-2239, 2013.

[2] Kolb M et al: Nintedanib plus sildenafil in patients with idiopathic pulmonary fibrosis, *N Engl J Med* 379:1722-31, 2018.

BOX 1 Guidelines for Transplantation by Pulmonary Disease

Chronic Obstructive Pulmonary Disease
Patients with a BODE index* of 7 to 10 or at least one of the following:
- History of hospitalization for exacerbation associated with acute hypercapnia (Pco_2 >50 mm Hg)
- Pulmonary hypertension or cor pulmonale, or both, despite oxygen therapy
- FEV_1 <20% predicted and either DLCO <20% predicted or homogeneous distribution of emphysema

Cystic Fibrosis and Other Causes of Bronchiectasis
Oxygen-dependent respiratory failure
Hypercapnia
Pulmonary hypertension

Idiopathic Pulmonary Fibrosis and NSIP
Histologic or radiographic evidence of usual interstitial pneumonia and any of the following:
- DLCO <39% predicted
- 10% or greater decrement in FVC during 6 months of follow-up
- A decrease in pulse oximetry below 88% during a 6-MWT
- Honeycombing on high-resolution computed tomography (fibrosis score >2)

Histologic evidence of NSIP and any of the following:
- DLCO <35% predicted
- 10% or greater decrement in FVC or 15% decrease in DLCO during 6 months of follow-up

Pulmonary Arterial Hypertension
Persistent New York Heart Association class III or IV on maximal medical therapy
Low (<350 m) or declining 6-MWT
Failing therapy with intravenous epoprostenol or equivalent
Cardiac index <2 L/min/m^2
Right atrial pressure >15 mm Hg

6-MWT, 6-minute walk test; *DLCO,* diffusing capacity of the lungs for carbon monoxide; *FVC,* forced vital capacity; *NSIP,* nonspecific interstitial pneumonia.
*BODE index includes body mass index, degree of airflow obstruction (assessed by percent predicted FEV_1), degree of dyspnea (assessed by the modified Medical Research Council [MMRC] dyspnea scale), and exercise capacity (assessed by the 6-minute walk distance). The index increases as body mass index, FEV_1, and distance walked decrease and as the MMRC scale increases.
From Sellke FW, del Nido PJ, Swanson SJ: *Sabiston & Spencer surgery of the chest*, ed 9, Philadelphia, 2016, Elsevier.

BOX 2 Absolute Contraindications to Lung Transplantation

- Malignancy within the last 2 yr, with the exception of cutaneous squamous and basal cell carcinomas; the role of lung transplantation in patients with focal pulmonary adenocarcinoma in situ (formerly known as *bronchoalveolar carcinoma*)
- Untreatable advanced dysfunction of another organ system (heart, liver, kidney); coronary artery disease not amenable to percutaneous intervention or bypass grafting, or associated with significant impairment of left ventricular function, is an absolute contraindication to lung transplantation, but heart-lung transplantation could be considered in some cases
- Incurable chronic extrapulmonary infection, including chronic active viral hepatitis B, hepatitis C, and human immunodeficiency virus
- Significant chest-wall or spinal deformity
- Nonadherence or inability to follow through with medical therapy or office follow-up
- Untreatable psychiatric or psychological condition associated with the inability to cooperate or comply with medical therapy
- Absence of a consistent or reliable social support system
- Substance addiction (alcohol, tobacco, or narcotics) that is either active or has been within the last 6 mo

From Sellke FW, del Nido PJ, Swanson SJ: *Sabiston & Spencer surgery of the chest*, ed 9, Philadelphia, 2016, Elsevier.

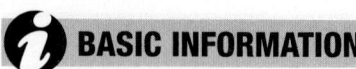

DEFINITION

Immune thrombocytopenic purpura (ITP) is an autoimmune disorder in which antibody-coated or immune complex-coated platelets are destroyed prematurely, producing defects in cellular immunity that result in peripheral thrombocytopenia. In primary ITP, the thrombocytopenia is isolated, whereas in secondary ITP, the condition is associated with other disorders (e.g., SLE, HIV, CLL, lymphomas).

ICD-10CM CODE
D69.3 Immune thrombocytopenic purpura

EPIDEMIOLOGY & DEMOGRAPHICS

INCIDENCE: Primary ITP occurs in 10 in 100,000 adults, 5 in 100,000 children.

PREVALENCE: Five to 10 cases per 100,000 persons.

PREDOMINANT SEX: 72% of patients >10 yr are female; among children, males are more commonly affected.

PREDOMINANT AGE: Children ages 1 to 6 yr and young women (70% are <40 yr). New onset of ITP after age 60 yr is uncommon; comprehensive workup may be required.

PHYSICAL FINDINGS & CLINICAL PRESENTATION

The presentation of ITP is different in children and adults:

- Children generally present with sudden onset of bruising and petechiae from severe thrombocytopenia.
- In adults, the presentation is insidious; a history of prolonged purpura may be present; many patients are diagnosed incidentally on the basis of automated laboratory tests that now routinely include platelet counts.
- The physical examination may be entirely normal.
- Patients with severe thrombocytopenia may have petechiae, purpura, epistaxis, or heme-positive stool from gastrointestinal bleeding. Life-threatening bleeding is uncommon and generally confined to patients with platelets <10,000/mm^3.
- Splenomegaly is unusual; its presence should alert to the possibility of other etiologies of thrombocytopenia.
- The presence of dysmorphic features (skeletal anomalies, auditory abnormalities) may indicate a congenital disorder as the cause of the thrombocytopenia.

ETIOLOGY

Increased platelet destruction is caused by autoantibody targets to platelet-membrane antigens, in particular, antibodies against platelet GPIIb/IIIa or GPIb/IX. The spleen has a major role in ITP by producing autoantibodies in the white pulp and removing autoantibody-coated platelets in the red pulp. Production of antibodies could be triggered either by immunogenicity of membrane glycoproteins (GPs) on the platelet surface or by external factors such as infections or medications.

Dx DIAGNOSIS

DIFFERENTIAL DIAGNOSIS

- Falsely low platelet count due to aggregation (resulting from EDTA-dependent or cold-dependent agglutinins). Platelet count is corrected by using heparin or citrate anticoagulated tube.
- Viral infections (e.g., HIV, hepatitis C, mononucleosis, rubella).
- Drugs commonly implicated are quinidine, heparin, antibiotics (linezolid, vancomycin, sulfonamides, rifampin), platelet inhibitors (tirofiban, abciximab, eptifibatide), cimetidine, NSAIDs, thiazide diuretics, antirheumatic agents (gold salts, penicillamine), and many chemotherapeutic agents (cyclosporine, fludarabine, carboplatin, oxaliplatin).
- Hypersplenism resulting from liver disease.
- Myelodysplastic and lymphoproliferative disorders.
- Pregnancy, hypothyroidism.
- SLE, TTP, hemolytic-uremic syndrome.
- Congenital thrombocytopenia (e.g., Fanconi syndrome, May-Hegglin anomaly, Bernard-Soulier syndrome).

LABORATORY TESTS

- Complete blood count, platelet count, and peripheral smear: Platelets are decreased. The peripheral smear should show large platelets and no schistocytes (Fig. E1). Red blood cells and white blood cells have a normal morphology. Unless the patient has been bleeding, the hemoglobin level and leukocyte count should be normal.
- Additional tests may be ordered to exclude other causes of the thrombocytopenia when clinically indicated (e.g., HIV, ANA, TSH [hypothyroidism and hyperthyroidism can cause thrombocytopenia], liver enzymes, Hep C ab).
- Direct assay of platelet-bound antibodies has an estimated positive predictive value of only 80% to 83%. A negative test cannot be used to rule out the diagnosis.
- Bone marrow aspiration and biopsy are recommended in adults older than 60 yr; evidence of immature cells on peripheral smear, or persistent neutropenia.

IMAGING STUDIES

CT scan of abdomen/pelvis in patients with splenomegaly to exclude other disorders causing thrombocytopenia

Rx TREATMENT

NONPHARMACOLOGIC THERAPY

- Minimize activity to prevent injury or bruising (e.g., contact sports should be avoided).
- Stop any potentially offending drugs (see "Etiology"). Avoid medications that increase the risk of bleeding (e.g., aspirin and other NSAIDs).

ACUTE GENERAL Rx

- Treatment varies with the platelet count, patient's age, and bleeding status (Fig. 2).
- Observation and frequent monitoring of platelet count are needed in asymptomatic patients with platelet counts >30,000/mm^3.
- Oral prednisone 1 mg/kg/day in a tapering dose generally for 4 to 6 wk is the most common initial regimen. Methylprednisolone 30 mg/kg/day IV infused over a period of 20 to 30 min (maximum dose of 1 g/day for 2 or 3 days) plus IV immunoglobulin (1 g/kg/day for 2 or 3 days) and infusion of platelets should be given to patients with neurologic symptoms, internal bleeding, or those undergoing emergency surgery.
- Prednisone is continued until the platelet count is >100, 000/mm^3 and then slowly tapered off. Response rates range from 50% to 75%, and most responses occur within the first 3 wk.
- Pulsed oral dexamethasone given at a dosage of 40 mg/day for 4 consecutive days when given for three to four cycles every 4 wk results in a high response rate (80%-85%) and has been shown to have fewer side effects when compared to longer courses of prednisone. A meta-analysis of nine randomized trials reveled no major increase in efficacy but confirmed less toxicity and faster increases in platelet counts using high-dose dexamethasone. Continuation of corticosteroids is limited by long-term complications associated with its use (osteoporosis, weight gain, opportunistic infections, emotional lability).
- IV immunoglobulin (typically 1-2 g/kg in divided doses) is used in patients who have not responded to corticosteroids and often in pregnant patients. It rapidly increases platelet count in nearly 80% of patients, but its effect is transient.
- Anti-D immunoglobulin, a pooled IgG product derived from the plasma of Rh(D)-negative donors, is also effective. It can be given only to patients who are Rh(D) positive with hemoglobin >8 mg/dl with a usual dose of 50 to 75 mcg/kg.
- Rituximab, a monoclonal antibody directed against the CD20 antigen, is used as a second-line agent. Usual dose is 375 mg/m^2 weekly × 4 wk.
- Splenectomy is considered a subsequent option in case of rituximab failure. Previously, it was considered in adults with platelet count <20,000/mm^3 after 6 wk of medical treatment or after 6 mo if more than 10 to 20 mg of prednisone per day is required to maintain a platelet count >30,000/mm^3. In children, splenectomy is generally reserved for persistent thrombocytopenia (>1 yr) and clinically significant bleeding. Appropriate immunizations (pneumococcal vaccine in adults and children, *Haemophilus influenzae* vaccine, meningococcal vaccine in children) should be administered earlier than 2 wk before planned splenectomy. Postsplenectomy vaccinations should be performed in all cases.
- Additional second-line agents are thrombopoietin receptor agonists (TPO-RA), azathioprine, cyclosporin A, cyclophosphamide, danazol, dapsone, mycophenolate mofetil, and *Vinca* alkaloids. Romiplostim, a recombinant fusion protein, and the oral TPO-RA eltrombopag are effective in increasing platelet count in adult patients with chronic ITP refractory to corticosteroids and/or splenectomy. American Society of Hematology guidelines, revised in

2011, recommend the use of TPO-RA for adult patients with ITP at risk for bleeding who have a contraindication to splenectomy, or who do not have a response to at least one other therapy.

- Fostamatinib is an inhibitor of the enzyme spleen tyrosine kinase (Syk). Syk plays an important role in phagocytosis of FcγR-mediated signal transduction and inflammatory propagation. It received FDA approval of chronic ITP in adults who had an insufficient response to previous treatment including corticosteroids, IVIG, splenectomy and/or a TPO-RA. The recommended dose initially is 100 mg orally twice daily. It can be increased to 150 mg twice a day if the platelet count has not responded to at least $50x10^9/mm^3$ at one month.
- Platelet transfusion is needed only in case of life-threatening hemorrhage.

PREGNANCY Rx

- No treatment is required when platelet count is $>30,000/mm^3$ or higher until 36 weeks' gestation, except anticipating premature labor.
- Oral corticosteroids and intravenous immunoglobulin (IVIG) are first-line treatments.
- Refractory ITP may require splenectomy in the second trimester.

DISPOSITION

- More than 80% of children have a complete remission within 8 wk.
- In adults, the course of the disease is chronic; only 5% of adults have spontaneous remission.
- The principal cause of death from ITP is intracranial hemorrhage (1% of children, 5% of adults).

SUGGESTED READINGS

Available at ExpertConsult.com

RELATED CONTENT

Immune Thrombocytopenic Purpura (Patient Information).

AUTHOR: **PATAN GULTAWATVICHAI, M.D.**

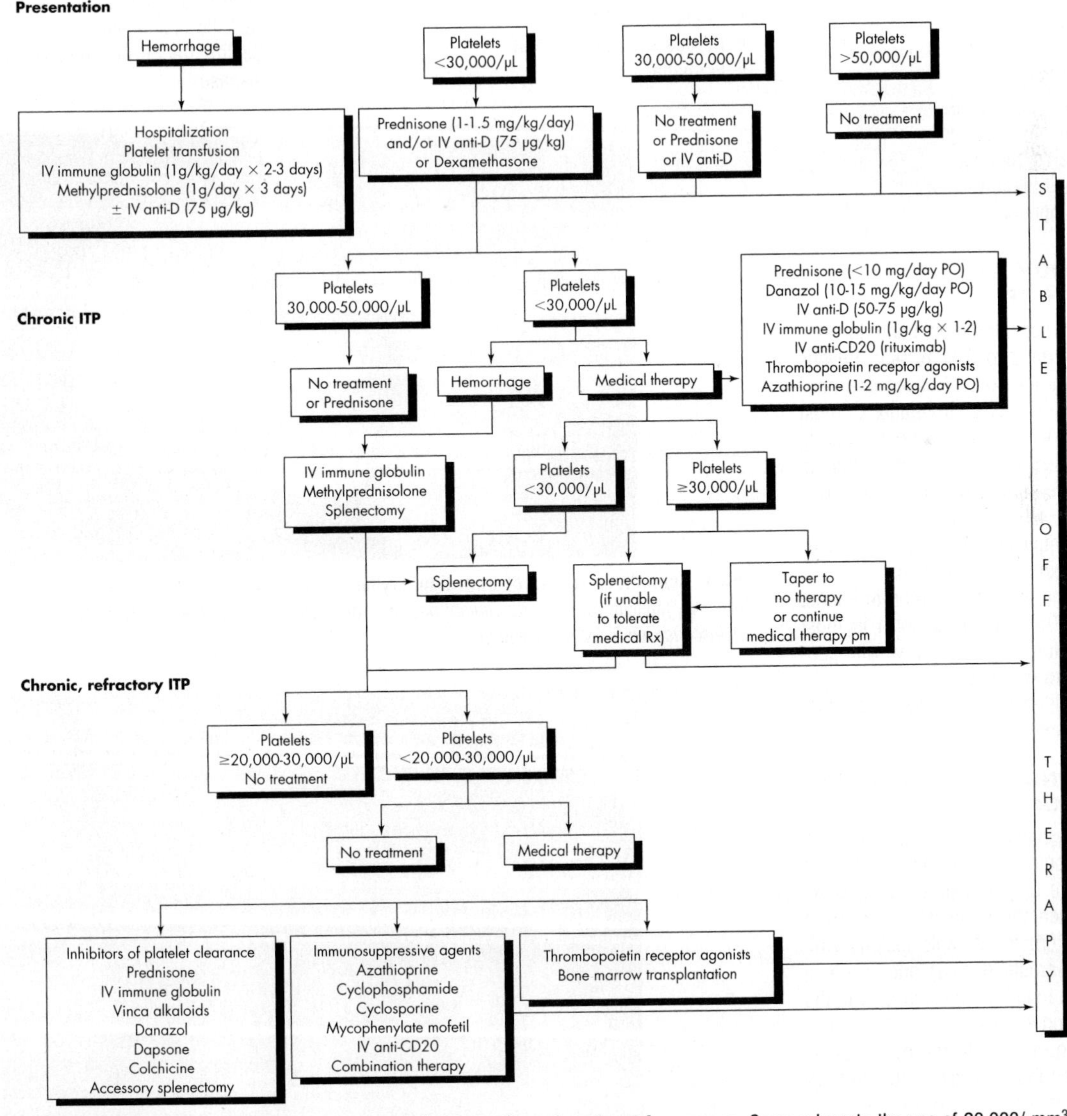

FIG. 2 Treatment algorithm for management of adult-onset immune thrombocytopenic purpura. Some advocate the use of 20,000/ mm^3 as a guideline for therapy. The decision to treat patients with platelet counts lower than 50,000/ mm^3 is based in part on evidence of bleeding, a history of bleeding, comorbid risk factors, lifestyle, and tolerance of therapy. There is no consensus as to duration of steroid therapy. The use of anti-D as initial therapy is appropriate only for Rh(D)-positive individuals who are not markedly anemic or hemolyzing. The goal of medical therapy is to attain a hemostatic platelet count, generally >20,000 to 30,000/ mm^3. The threshold for treatment depends on comorbid risk factors for bleeding and risk of trauma. Higher platelet counts may be appropriate for surgery or after trauma. Medications can be used individually, but combinations of azathioprine and danazol (or corticosteroids) may provide added benefit and allow lower doses to be used. IVIG and anti-D are generally reserved for severe thrombocytopenia unresponsive to oral agents. The decision to proceed to splenectomy depends on intensity of therapy required, tolerance to side effects, risk of surgery, and patient preference. IVIG and/or methylprednisolone may help to increase the platelet count immediately before splenectomy. Laparoscopic and open splenectomy have comparable outcomes. The decision to treat patients who have platelet counts lower than 20,000 to 30,000/ mm^3 after splenectomy involves an assessment of the risk of hemorrhage versus the side effects of each form of therapy. *IV,* Intravenous; *PO,* by mouth; *Rx,* prescription. (Modified from Hoffman R, et al.: *Hematology, basic principles and practice,* ed 7, Philadelphia, 2018, Churchill Livingstone.)

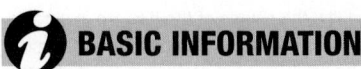

BASIC INFORMATION

DEFINITION

Impetigo is a superficial skin infection generally caused by *Staphylococcus aureus* and/or *Streptococcus* spp.

Common presentations are bullous impetigo (generally caused by staphylococcal disease) and nonbullous impetigo (from streptococcal infection and possible staphylococcal infection); the bullous form is caused by an epidermolytic toxin produced at the site of infection.

SYNONYMS

Impetigo vulgaris
Pyoderma
Impetigo contagiosa
Bullous impetigo

ICD-10CM CODES

L01.00	Impetigo, unspecified
L01.01	Non-bullous impetigo
L01.02	Bockhart's impetigo
L01.03	Bullous impetigo
L01.09	Other impetigo

EPIDEMIOLOGY & DEMOGRAPHICS

Impetigo is the most common bacterial skin infection in children 2 to 5 yr of age. Bullous impetigo accounts for 30% of cases and nonbullous for 70% of cases. Impetigo is most common in temperate zones, mostly during the summer in hot, humid weather. Common sources for children are dirty fingers, pets, and other children in school or day care centers. Impetigo often complicates insect bites, pediculosis, scabies, eczema, and poison ivy.

- Bullous impetigo is most common in infants and children. The nonbullous form is most common in children ages 2 to 5 yr with poor hygiene in warm climates.
- The overall incidence of acute nephritis with impetigo varies between 2% and 5%.

PHYSICAL FINDINGS & CLINICAL PRESENTATION

- Nonbullous impetigo begins as a single red macule or papule that quickly becomes a vesicle. Rupture of the vesicle produces an erosion of which the contents dry to form honey-colored crusts. Multiple lesions with golden yellow crusts (Fig. 1) and weeping areas are often found on the skin around the nose, mouth, and limbs.
- Bullous impetigo is manifested by the presence of vesicles that enlarge rapidly to form bullae with contents that vary from clear to cloudy. There is subsequent collapse of the center of the bullae (Fig. 2); the peripheral areas may retain fluid, and a honey-colored crust may appear in the center (Fig. 3). As the lesions enlarge and become contiguous with the others, a scaling border replaces the fluid-filled rim; there is minimal erythema surrounding the lesions.
- Regional lymphadenopathy is most common with nonbullous impetigo.
- Constitutional symptoms are generally absent.

ETIOLOGY

- *S. aureus* coagulase positive is the dominant microorganism (50% to 70% of cases).
- *S. pyogenes* (group A β-hemolytic streptococci): M-T serotypes of this organism associated with acute nephritis are 2, 49, 55, 57, and 60. Group B streptococci are associated with newborn impetigo.

Dx DIAGNOSIS

DIFFERENTIAL DIAGNOSIS

- Atopic dermatitis
- Herpes simplex infection
- Ecthyma
- Folliculitis
- Dermatitis herpetiformis
- Insect bites
- Scabies, pediculosis
- Tinea corporis, cutaneous candidiasis
- Pemphigus vulgaris and bullous pemphigoid
- Chickenpox
- Thermal burns
- Contact dermatitis
- Stevens-Johnson syndrome, Sweet syndrome

WORKUP

Diagnosis is clinical.

LABORATORY TESTS

- Generally not necessary.
- Gram stain and culture and sensitivity to confirm the diagnosis when the clinical presentation is unclear.
- Sedimentation rate parallel to activity of the disease.

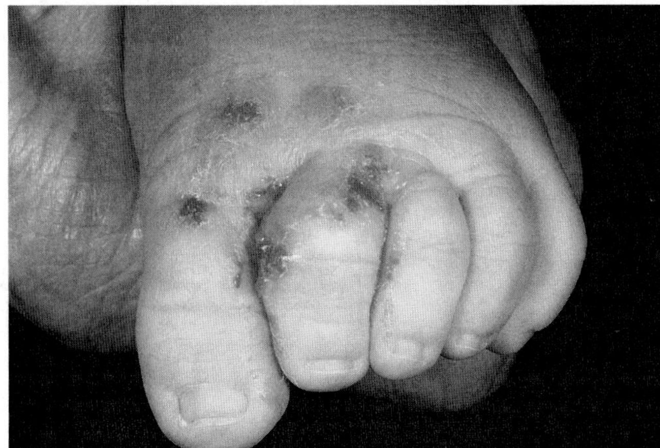

FIG. 1 Nonbullous (crusted) impetigo. Erythematous papules with honey yellow–colored crusting. (From Paller AS, Mancini AJ: *Hurwitz clinical pediatric dermatology, a textbook of skin disorders of childhood and adolescence*, ed 5, 2016, Elsevier.)

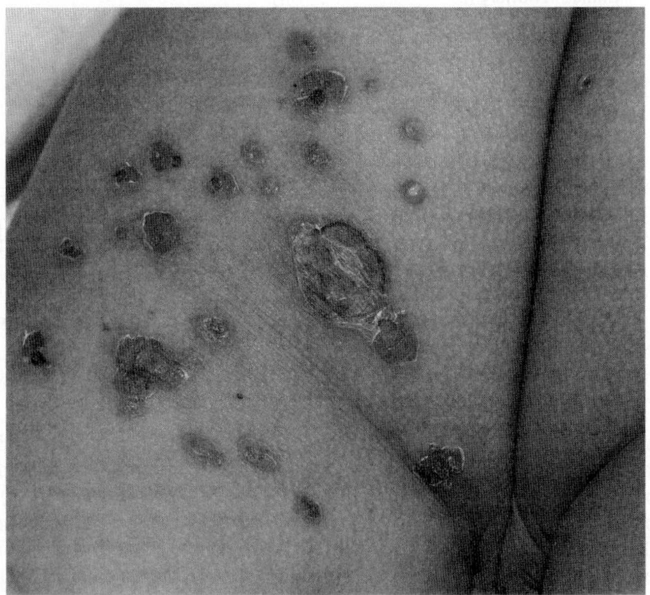

FIG. 2 Bullous impetigo. Thin-walled vesicles and shallow erosions with peripheral collarettes and mild crusting on the buttock and posterior thigh. (From Paller AS, Mancini AJ: *Hurwitz clinical pediatric dermatology, a textbook of skin disorders of childhood and adolescence*, ed 5, 2016, Elsevier.)

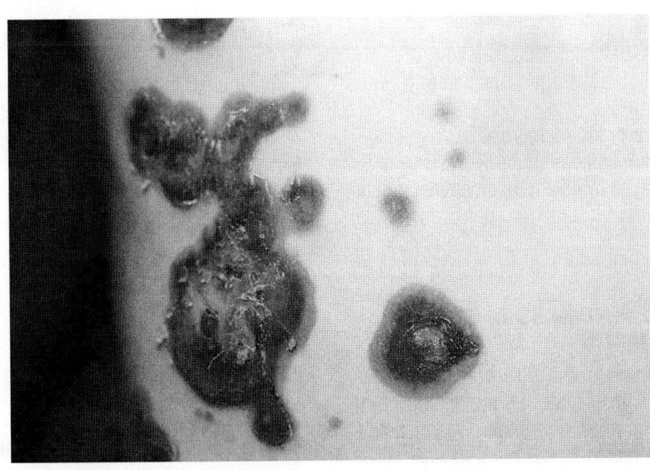

FIG. 3 Bullous impetigo. Multiple tender, erythematous patches with a peripheral collarette, representing remnants of the blister roof. (From Paller AS, Mancini AJ: *Hurwitz clinical pediatric dermatology, a textbook of skin disorders of childhood and adolescence*, ed 5, 2016, Elsevier.)

- Increased anti-DNAse B and antihyaluronidase.
- Urinalysis revealing hematuria with erythrocyte casts and proteinuria in patients with acute nephritis (most frequently occurring in children between ages 2 and 4 yr in the southern part of the U.S.).
- If recurrent staphylococcal impetigo develops, a culture of the anterior nares should be done to rule out a carrier state.

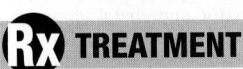

TREATMENT

NONPHARMACOLOGIC THERAPY

Remove crusts by soaking with wet cloth compresses (crusts block the penetration of antibacterial creams).

GENERAL Rx

- Application of 2% mupirocin ointment tid for 10 days or retapamulin 1% applied bid for 5 days to the affected area or until all lesions have cleared.
- Oral antibiotics are used in severe cases: Commonly used agents are dicloxacillin 250 mg qid for 7 to 10 days, cephalexin 250 mg qid for 7 to 10 days, azithromycin 500 mg on day 1, 250 mg on days 2 through 5, amoxicillin/clavulanate 500 mg q8h.
- Impetigo can be prevented by prompt application of mupirocin or triple-antibiotic ointment (bacitracin, Polysporin, and neomycin) to sites of skin trauma.
- Patients who are carriers of *S. aureus* in their nares should be treated with mupirocin ointment applied to their nares bid for 5 days or a 10-day course of rifampin, 600 mg/day, combined with dicloxacillin (for MSSA) or TMP-SMX (for MRSA).
- Fingernails should be kept short, and patients should be advised not to scratch any lesions to avoid spread of infection.

DISPOSITION

Most cases of impetigo resolve promptly with appropriate treatment. Both bullous and nonbullous forms of impetigo heal without scarring.

REFERRAL

Nephrology referral in patients with acute nephritis

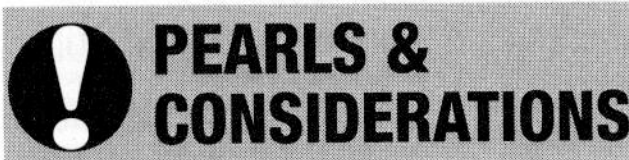

PEARLS & CONSIDERATIONS

COMMENTS

- Patients should be instructed on use of antibacterial soaps and avoidance of sharing of towels and washcloths because impetigo is extremely contagious.
- Children attending day care should be removed until 48 to 72 hr after initiation of antibiotic treatment.
- Bullous impetigo may be an early manifestation of HIV infection.

SUGGESTED READINGS

Available online at ExpertConsult.com

RELATED CONTENT

Impetigo (Patient Information)

AUTHOR: **FRED F. FERRI, M.D.**

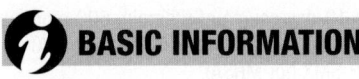

DEFINITION

Fecal incontinence is defined as the involuntary loss of gas or liquid stool (minor incontinence) or the involuntary loss of solid stool (major incontinence).

SYNONYMS

Anal or bowel incontinence
Accidental bowel leakage
Fecal incontinence

ICD-10CM CODES
R15.9 Full incontinence of feces
F98.1 Encopresis not due to a substance or known physiological condition

EPIDEMIOLOGY & DEMOGRAPHICS

INCIDENCE: Affects 0.5% to 1.5% of the population younger than age 65, but >10% older than 65. More common in institutionalized patients.
PREVALENCE: Varies widely depending on definition used and population studied; often underreported. In community-based studies, ranges from 1% to 24%. Increases with age and BMI in women.
PREDOMINANT SEX AND AGE: Slightly more common in females than males and those of advanced age (older than 65 yr).

RISK FACTORS
- Cognitive or behavioral dysfunction
- Structural anorectal abnormalities (e.g., rectal prolapse)
- Neurologic disorders, comorbidities (e.g., diabetes mellitus), inflammatory bowel disease (IBD)
- Poor mobility in female gender, advanced age
- Anal sphincter trauma (surgery, obstetrical injury)
- Fecal impaction from constipation or diarrhea

PHYSICAL FINDINGS & CLINICAL PRESENTATION

- Inspect perianal area to evaluate for the presence of fecal material, prolapsing hemorrhoids, chemical dermatitis, scars, fistula or rectal prolapse.
- Assess for anocutaneous reflex. This may be elicited by stroking skin in each perianal quadrant (normal response is a brisk anal wink). Absent reflex is suggestive of nerve damage.
- Digital rectal examination to assess for impaction, mass, and resting to squeezing anal tone by asking the patient to bear down. Ask patient to bear down to assess for rectal prolapse or excessive perianal descent.

ETIOLOGY

- Usually multifactorial. Table 1 summarizes the mechanisms, causes, and pathophysiology of fecal incontinence. Common types of anorectal dysfunction causing rectal outlet delay in the elderly are summarized in Table 2.
- Overflow due to fecal impaction
- Anal sphincter weakness
  1. Trauma (e.g., anorectal surgery, childbirth).
  2. Nontraumatic (e.g., neurologic, spinal cord lesions, diabetes, scleroderma).
- Anorectal inflammation
  1. Radiation, IBD
- CNS disorders (e.g., dementia, multiple sclerosis, stroke)
- Anatomic disturbance of pelvic floor
  1. Fistula, prolapse
- Idiopathic

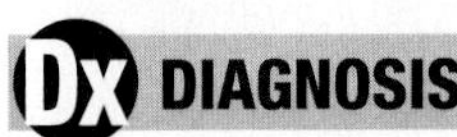

DIFFERENTIAL DIAGNOSIS

- Fecal encopresis
- Irritable bowel syndrome or IBD

WORKUP

- Requires detailed history taking that includes the onset and precipitating events, duration and severity, stool consistency and urgency. Important to evaluate for history of urinary incontinence, anorectal surgery or radiation, neurologic disorders, or prior vaginal deliveries and complete a thorough physical exam. An algorithm for the evaluation and management of patients with fecal incontinence is illustrated in Fig. 1.
- Diagnostic workup may include endoscopy, anorectal manometry, endorectal ultrasound

TABLE 1 Mechanisms, Causes, and Pathophysiology of Fecal Incontinence

Mechanism	Causes	Pathophysiology
Abnormal Anorectal or Pelvic Floor Structures		
Anal sphincter muscles	Hemorrhoidectomy, neuropathy, obstetric injury	Sphincter weakness, loss of sampling reflex
Puborectalis muscle	Aging, excessive perineal descent, trauma	Obtuse anorectal angle, sphincter weakness
Pudendal nerve	Excessive straining, obstetric or surgical injury, perineal descent	Sphincter weakness, sensory loss, impaired reflexes
Nervous system, spinal cord, autonomic nervous system	Avulsion injury, spine surgery, diabetes mellitus, head injury, multiple sclerosis, spinal cord injury, stroke	Loss of sensation, impaired reflexes, secondary myopathy, loss of accommodation
Rectum	Aging, IBD, IBS, prolapse, radiation	Loss of accommodation, loss of sensation, hypersensitivity
Abnormal Anorectal or Pelvic Floor Function		
Impaired anorectal sensation	Autonomic nervous system disorders, central nervous system disorders, obstetric injury	Loss of stool awareness, rectoanal agnosia
Fecal impaction	Dyssynergic defecation	Fecal retention with overflow, impaired sensation
Altered Stool Characteristics		
Increased volume and loose consistency	Drugs, bile salt malabsorption, infection, IBD, IBS, laxatives, metabolic disorders	Diarrhea and urgency, rapid stool transport, impaired accommodation
Hard stools, retention	Drugs, dyssynergia	Fecal retention with overflow
Miscellaneous		
Physical mobility, cognitive function	Aging, dementia, disability	Multifactorial changes
Psychosis	Willful soiling	Multifactorial changes
Drugs*	Anticholinergics	Constipation
	Antidepressants	Altered sensation, constipation
	Caffeine	Relaxation of sphincter tone
	Laxatives	Diarrhea
	Muscle relaxants	Relaxation of sphincter tone
Food intolerance	Fructose, lactose, or sorbitol malabsorption	Diarrhea, flatus

*Pathophysiology is noted for each class of drugs.
Feldman M, Friedman LS, Brandt LJ: *Sleisenger and Fordtran's gastrointestinal and liver disease*, ed 10, Philadelphia, 2016, Elsevier.

TABLE 2 Types of Anorectal Dysfunction Causing Rectal Outlet Delay in Older People

Pathophysiology	Clinical Picture	
Rectal dysmotility	Reduced rectal motility and contractions Increased rectal compliance Variable degree of rectal dilation Impaired rectal sensation with blunting of urge to pass stool Over time, increasing rectal distention required to reflexively trigger the defecation mechanism	Rectal hard or soft stool retention on digital examination of which patient may be unaware Chronic rectal distention leads to relaxation of the internal sphincter and fecal soiling One postulated cause is diminished parasympathetic outflow as a result of impaired sacral cord function (e.g., from ischemia or spinal stenosis). May also develop through persistent disregard or suppression of the urge to defecate as a result of dementia, depression, immobility, or painful anorectal conditions
Pelvic floor dyssynergia	Paradoxical contraction or failure to relax the pelvic floor and external anal sphincter muscles during defecation Manometric studies show paradoxical increases in anal canal pressure on straining	Severe and long-standing symptoms of rectal outlet delay Parkinson disease More common in younger women
Irritable bowel syndrome	Increased rectal tone and reduced compliance Lower pain threshold on distending the rectum during anorectal function tests	Usually constipation-predominant in older people Rome criteria symptoms: Abdominal distention or pain relieved by defecation, passage of mucus, and feeling of incomplete emptying

From Fillit HM: *Brocklehurst's textbook of geriatric medicine and gerontology*, ed 8, 2017, Elsevier.

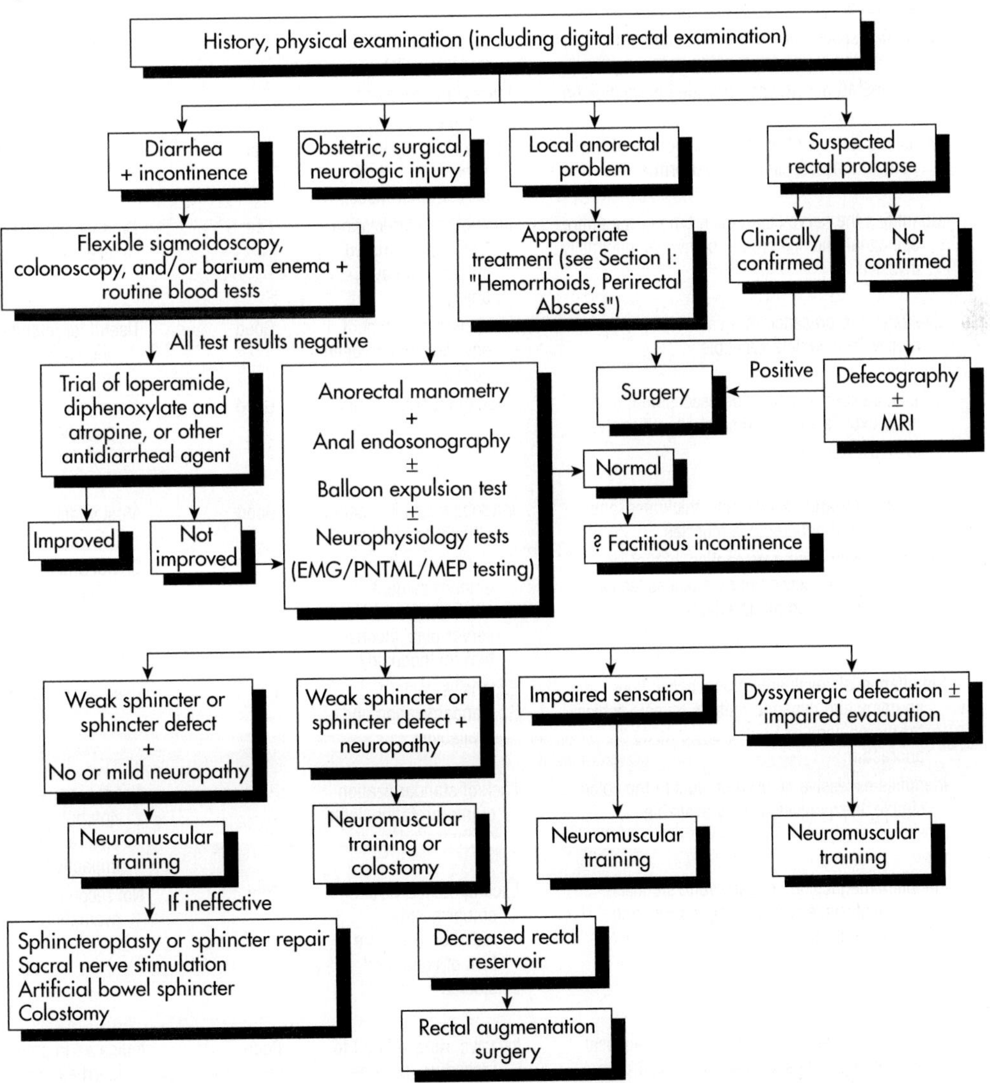

FIG. 1 Algorithm for the evaluation and management of patients with fecal incontinence. *EMG*, Electromyography; *MEP*, motor evoked potential; *PNTML*, pudendal nerve terminal motor latency. (From Feldman M, Friedman LS, Brandt LJ: *Sleisenger and Fordtran's gastrointestinal and liver disease*, ed 10, Philadelphia, 2016, Elsevier.)

(simple and economical), MRI, defecography, pudendal nerve terminal latency, balloon expulsion test, and anal electromyography (EMG), depending on signs and symptoms. Diagnostic tests for fecal incontinence are summarized in Table 3.

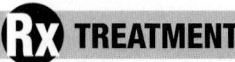

TREATMENT

- Therapy is focused on patient education (Table E4), supportive care, medications, biofeedback, and surgery. Table 5 summarizes bowel preparation in the elderly prior to colonoscopy.
- Medications focus on decreasing stool frequency and improving consistency.
  1. Fiber supplements (e.g., methylcellulose)
  2. Antidiarrheals: Loperamide, diphenoxylate/atropine sulfate, cholestyramine
  3. Topical phenylephrine, oral valproate sodium to increase smooth muscle tone
  4. Injectable anal bulking agent: Dextranomer-hyaluronic acid gel is FDA approved for the treatment of fecal incontinence in adults who fail conservative therapy. Given as four 1-ml injections into the deep submucosal layer of the anal canal. If inadequate response after at least 4 wk, a second course can be attempted.

NONPHARMACOLOGIC THERAPY

- Supportive therapy:
  1. Education, behavioral training, pelvic floor exercises
  2. Dietary modifications (e.g., increased fiber/fluid intake, less caffeine), food diary
  3. Incontinence pads, barrier cream (e.g., zinc oxide)

TABLE 3 Diagnostic Tests for Fecal Incontinence

Test	Clinical Use: Advantages	Clinical Use: Disadvantages	Quality of Evidence	Comments
Physiologic				
Anorectal manometry	Quantifies EAS and IAS pressures; identifies rectal hyposensitivity, rectal hypersensitivity, impaired rectal compliance, dyssynergic defecation	Lack of standardization	Good	Useful for detecting anal sphincter weakness, altered rectal sensation and accommodation, and dyssynergia
Needle EMG	Quantifies spike potentials and re-innervation pattern indicating neuropathy or myopathy	Invasive, painful; not widely available	Fair	Useful but used largely in research laboratories
Surface EMG	Displays EMG activity; can provide information on normal or weak muscle tone	Inaccurate, frequent artifacts	Fair	Used largely for neuromuscular training
Pudendal nerve terminal motor latency (PNTML)	Measures latency of the terminal portion of the pudendal nerve, simple to perform	Minimally invasive, low sensitivity, interobserver differences	Fair	Conflicting data; correlation with other tests and surgical outcome unclear
Translumbar and transsacral motor evoked potentials	Quantifies the nerve conduction time of the entire spinoanal and spinorectal pathways; minimally invasive	Lack of standardization, training, controlled studies, and availability	Fair	Promising noninvasive test; more objective and higher yield than PNTML
Colonic transit study with radiopaque markers	Evaluates the presence of fecal retention; inexpensive and widely available	Inconsistent methodology, validity has been questioned	Good	Useful for identifying patients with fecal seepage and older persons with impaction
Balloon expulsion test (BET)	Simple, inexpensive, bedside assessment of ability to expel a simulated stool; identifies dyssynergic defecation	Lack of standardization	Good	Normal BET does not exclude dyssynergia; should be interpreted in the context of other anorectal test results
Imaging				
Anorectal US	Visualizes IAS and EAS defects, thickness, and atrophy and puborectalis muscles	Interobserver bias; scars difficult to identify	Good	Most widely available
Defecography	Detects prolapse, intussusception, obtuse anorectal angle, and pelvic floor weakness, as well as rectoceles and megarectum	Radiation exposure, embarrassment, availability, interobserver bias, inconsistent methodology	Fair	Useful and complementary with other tests
MRI	Simultaneously evaluates global pelvic floor anatomy and dynamic motion; reveals sphincter morphology and pathology outside the anorectum	Expensive, lack of standardization and availability	Fair	Used as an adjunct to other tests
Plain abdominal film	Identifies excessive amount of stool in the colon; simple, inexpensive, widely available	Lack of standardization of interpretation, lack of controlled studies	Poor	Not recommended for routine evaluation but useful in older adults and children with incontinence and fecal impaction
Barium enema	Identifies megacolon, megarectum, stenosis, diverticulosis, extrinsic compression, and intraluminal masses	Lack of standardization, embarrassment, radiation exposure, lack of controlled studies	Poor	Not recommended as part of routine evaluation
Endoscopy				
Flexible sigmoidoscopy and colonoscopy	Directly visualizes the colon to exclude mucosal lesions (e.g., solitary rectal ulcer syndrome, inflammation, malignancy)	Invasive, risks related to procedure (perforation, bleeding) and sedation	Poor	Indicated in patients with unexplained diarrhea and seepage and patients >age 50

EAS, External anal sphincter; *EMG*, electromyography; *IAS*, internal anal sphincter.
Feldman M, Friedman LS, Brandt LJ: *Sleisenger and Fordtran's gastrointestinal and liver disease*, ed 10, Philadelphia, 2016, Elsevier.

TABLE 5 Bowel Preparation in Older People

- Older age, constipation, reported laxative use, tricyclic antidepressants, stroke, diabetes, and dementia are associated with inadequate preparation and taking longer to perform full colonoscopy.
- Even when patients take 75% to 100% of their prescribed treatments, bowel preparation is satisfactory only 50% of the time.

Guidance

- Give regular laxatives (e.g., Movicol 2 sachets daily) and enemas or suppositories for at least 1 week before the procedure, with a longer run-up period in patients known to have constipation and those with comorbidities such as diabetes.
- Individualize the cathartic regimen (e.g., 1 to 2 L of GoLYTELY daily over 2 to 3 days in those unable to drink 4 L, or use of alternative preparations such as sodium picosulfate).
- Identify potential nonadherence. ("Can the patient drink 4 L of GoLYTELY in 24 hours?")
- Preempt unpleasant side effects. ("Will the patient be able to reach the toilet in time to avoid fecal leakage?")
- Use oral phospho soda with caution as administration in older people increases serum phosphate, even in patients with normal creatinine clearance.
- Consider preprocedure plain abdominal x-ray for evaluation of persistent fecal loading.
- Where possible, give a clear fluid diet before administration of bowel preparation.

From Fillit HM: *Brocklehurst's textbook of geriatric medicine and gerontology,* ed 8, 2017, Elsevier.

- Biofeedback therapy
- Electrical stimulation:
  1. Anal electrodes
  2. Sacral nerve stimulation
  3. Posterior tibial nerve stimulation
- Surgery:
  1. Anal sphincteroplasty
  2. Implanted devices (e.g., artificial anal sphincter).
  3. Colostomy (if intractable symptoms and/or failed all other therapies)
  4. Miscellaneous: Radiofrequency ablation, anal sling

REFERRAL

Colorectal surgery

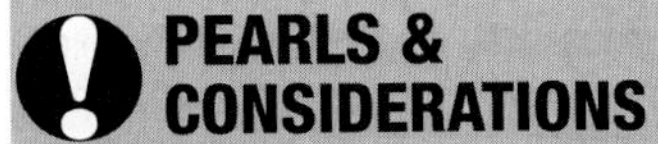

PEARLS & CONSIDERATIONS

COMMENTS

The shame, embarrassment, and stigma associated with fecal and urinary incontinence pose significant barriers to seeking professional treatment, resulting in many people suffering from these conditions without help. Therefore, during routine office visits, asking all patients older than 70 about incontinence may be helpful.

PREVENTION

- Reduce constipation and avoid straining during bowel movements.
- Routine episiotomy is the most easily preventable risk factor for fecal incontinence in females.

PATIENT/FAMILY EDUCATION

http://digestive.niddk.nih.gov/ddiseases/pubs/fecalincontinence/index.aspx

SUGGESTED READINGS

Available at ExpertConsult.com

AUTHOR: **FRED F. FERRI, M.D.**

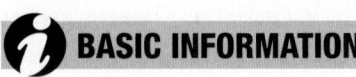

BASIC INFORMATION

DEFINITION

Urinary incontinence is the involuntary loss of urine.

ICD-10CM CODES

R32	Unspecified urinary incontinence
N39.3	Stress incontinence (female) (male)
N39.41	Urgency urinary incontinence
N39.46	Mixed incontinence
N39.49	Disorder of urinary system, unspecified
R39.81	Functional urinary incontinence

EPIDEMIOLOGY & DEMOGRAPHICS

INCIDENCE/PREVALENCE: In the general population between the ages of 15 and 64 yr, 1.5% to 5% of men and 25% to 57% of women have urinary incontinence. In the nursing home population, 75% of the population has some degree of incontinence. Nearly 20% of children through the mid-teenage yrs have episodes of urinary incontinence.

CLINICAL, PSYCHOLOGICAL, & SOCIAL IMPACT

Fewer than 50% of women living with incontinence in the U.S. consult health care professionals for care, resulting in significant physical and psychological limitations. Many women choose to turn to home remedies, commercially available absorbent materials, and supportive aids. As the incontinence worsens, many women become depressed, limit social interaction, refrain from sexual intimacy, and become homebound. It is estimated that $19.5 billion in direct costs is spent annually on incontinence in the U.S. Urinary incontinence contributes to approximately 6% of nursing home admissions in the older population, leading to a cost of $3 billion per yr. With aging populations around the world, this cost is dramatically increasing every yr.

MAJOR TYPES OF INCONTINENCE (FIG. 1)

- **Stress urinary incontinence (SUI)** (Table E1) is the complaint of involuntary loss of urine on effort or physical exertion (sporting activities), or on sneezing or coughing (any activity that increases intraabdominal pressure). SUI may be demonstrated in the office with a simple cough stress test during examination and further characterized with degree of urethral mobility (cotton swab test).
- **Urgency urinary incontinence (UUI)** is the complaint of involuntary loss of urine associated with urgency, a sudden compelling desire to pass urine that is difficult to defer. The diagnosis is often made clinically based on patient's report of symptoms but may also be associated with involuntary detrusor contractions on urodynamic investigation. May be idiopathic or neurogenic.
- **Overactive bladder (OAB)** is described as a constellation of symptoms (Figs. E2 and E3) including urgency, with or without urgency urinary incontinence, usually with urinary frequency and nocturia. It should be distinguished from excessive fluid intake and must exclude urinary tract infection. Can occur in up to 27% of men and up to 43% of women.
- **Mixed urinary incontinence** is the complaint of involuntary leakage of urine associated with urgency and also with exertion, effort, sneezing or coughing (see Fig. E4).
- **Overflow incontinence** is the leakage of urine resulting from urinary retention with resultant overflow or spilling of the urine. Causes include hypotonic bladder resulting from age, neurologic conditions such as diabetes or spinal cord injury, prior surgery, drug effects, or fecal impaction. It may also be caused by obstruction at the bladder neck and urethra, such as from prior anti-incontinence surgery, pelvic organ prolapse, urethral stenosis, or detrusor-sphincter dyssynergia.
- **Functional urinary incontinence** is the complaint of involuntary leakage of urine resulting from chronic impairments of physical and/or cognitive functioning. This is a diagnosis of exclusion and may be cured by improving the patient's functional status, treating comorbidities, changing medications, and reducing environmental barriers.
- **Extraurethral urinary incontinence** is leakage that bypasses the urethral meatus (i.e., vesicovaginal fistula or ectopic ureter).

Dx DIAGNOSIS

HISTORY

- Since many women are hesitant to bring up symptoms of incontinence, these symptoms should be elicited through simple screening.
- History of present illness, psychosocial factors, congenital disorders, access issues for the physically challenged, neurologic disorders, and medication use are coexistent disorders that may affect the urinary tract.
- Urinary incontinence may be characterized by frequency of incontinence episodes, severity, and extent of bother.
- Voiding diary to assess total voided volume, frequency of micturition, mean volume voided, largest single volume, diurnal distribution, nature and severity of incontinence.
- Assessments of the severity of symptoms and goals for treatment are important parts of the history.

WORKUP

- General physical examination:
  1. Confounding conditions including mobility issues. Comorbid conditions that can cause or contribute to urinary incontinence in elderly patients are summarized in Table 2. Table 3 describes medications that can cause or contribute to urinary incontinence.
  2. Neuromuscular deficits (gait of the patient)
- Pelvic exam:
  1. Concurrent pelvic organ prolapse
  2. Vaginal discharge
  3. Estrogen status
  4. Pelvic floor strength assessment
  5. Neurologic examination to assess sacral nerves with anal wink and bulbocavernosus reflex
- Rectal examination to assess sphincter tone and stool impaction
- Simple cough stress test
- Urethral hypermobility
- Postvoid residual check with bladder scan or catheter to exclude retention
- 3-day bladder diary to assess frequency, timing, and volume of voids

LABORATORY TESTS

It is important to rule out urinary tract infection and microscopic hematuria with urinalysis and/or culture prior to more invasive testing for other causes for incontinence.

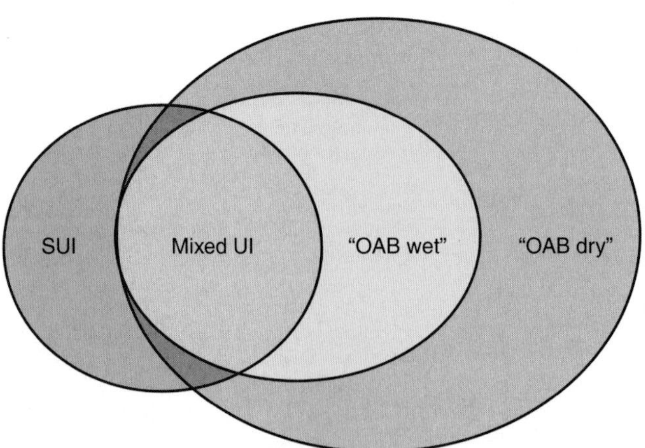

FIG. 1 Incontinence may be stress urinary incontinence *(SUI)*, mixed urinary incontinence *(UI)*, or urgency urinary incontinence ("overactive bladder *[OAB]* wet"), especially in women. SUI can coexist with "OAB dry," giving rise to mixed symptoms of stress incontinence and urgency. (From Wein AJ et al: *Campbell-Walsh urology*, ed 11, Philadelphia, 2016, Elsevier.)

TABLE 2 Comorbid Conditions That Can Cause or Contribute to Urinary Incontinence in Frail Older Adults

Conditions	Comments	Implications for Management
Comorbid Medical Illnesses		
Diabetes mellitus	Poor control can cause polyuria and precipitate or exacerbate incontinence; also associated with increased likelihood of urgency incontinence and diabetic neuropathic bladder	Better control of diabetes can reduce osmotic diuresis and associated polyuria, improve incontinence
Degenerative joint disease	Can impair mobility and precipitate urgency UI	Optimal pharmacologic and nonpharmacologic pain management can improve mobility, toileting ability
Chronic pulmonary disease	Associated cough can worsen stress UI	Cough suppression can reduce stress incontinence and cough-induced urgency UI
Congestive heart failure Lower extremity venous insufficiency	Increased nighttime urine production can contribute to nocturia and UI	Optimizing pharmacologic management of congestive heart failure, sodium restriction, support stockings, leg elevation, and late afternoon dose of rapid-acting diuretic may reduce nocturnal polyuria, associated nocturia, nighttime UI
Sleep apnea	May increase nighttime urine production by increasing production of atrial natriuretic peptide	Diagnosis and treatment of sleep apnea, usually with continuous positive airway pressure devices, may relieve UI, reduce nocturnal polyuria and associated nocturia
Severe constipation and fecal impaction	Associated with "double" incontinence (urine and fecal)	Appropriate use of stool softeners Adequate fluid intake and exercise Disimpaction if necessary
Neurologic and Psychiatric Conditions		
Stroke	Can precipitate urgency UI and, less often, urinary retention; also impairs mobility	UI after acute stroke often resolves with rehabilitation; persistent UI should be further evaluated. Regular toileting assistance essential for those with persistent mobility impairment
Parkinson's disease	Associated with urgency UI; also causes impaired mobility and cognition in late stages	Optimizing management may improve mobility, improve UI Regular toileting assistance essential for those with mobility and cognitive impairment in late stages
Normal-pressure hydrocephalus	Presents with UI, along with gait and cognitive impairments	Patients presenting with all three symptoms should be considered for brain imaging to rule out this condition; may improve with a ventricular-peritoneal shunt
Dementia (Alzheimer's, multi-infarct, others)	Associated with urgency UI; impaired cognition and apraxia interfere with toileting and hygiene	Regular toileting assistance essential for those with mobility and cognitive impairment in late stages
Depression	May impair motivation to be continent; may also be a consequence of incontinence	Optimizing pharmacologic and non-pharmacologic management of depression may improve UI
		Discontinuation or modification of drug regimen
Medications		
Functional Impairments		
Impaired mobility, impaired cognition	Impaired cognition and/or mobility due to a variety of conditions (listed above) and others can interfere with ability to toilet independently and can precipitate UI	Regular toileting assistance essential for those with severe mobility and/or cognitive impairment
Environmental Factors		
Inaccessible toilets Unsafe toilet facilities No contrasting color between toilet and seat Caregivers unavailable for toileting assistance	Frail, functionally impaired persons require accessible and safe toilet facilities and, in many cases, human assistance to be continent	Environmental alterations may be helpful; supportive measures such as pads may be necessary if caregiver assistance not regularly available

UI, Urinary incontinence.
From Fillit HM: *Brocklehurst's textbook of geriatric medicine and gerontology*, ed 8, Philadelphia, 2017, Elsevier.

SPECIALIZED STUDIES

- **Urodynamic testing**: Measures different facets of urine storage and evacuation; usually necessary only if basic office evaluation does not elicit the cause of incontinence, if incontinence is persistent despite treatments, or if there are confounding contributors to incontinence including prior surgery.
  1. Simple cystometrogram: Graph of bladder and abdominal pressures related to fluid volume during filling/storage/voiding to assess sensation and capacity; also assesses presence of detrusor contractions, whether voluntary or involuntary.
  2. Uroflowmetry and pressure-flow studies: Measure the mechanism of bladder emptying and rate of urine flow.
  3. Urethral mechanism and pressure studies.
  4. Electromyography: Studies the neuromuscular activity of pelvic muscles and striated urethral sphincter during filling and micturition.
- **Cystourethroscopy**: Procedure that can be done in the office or the operating room in which an endoscope is inserted into the urethra to view the inside of the bladder and urethra. This procedure is not routinely used to evaluate incontinence unless hematuria is present or prior pelvic surgery is noted on history.

IMAGING STUDIES

- These are usually ordered only if history and/or physical findings suggest other, less common causes of incontinence (i.e., genitourinary fistula) or if microscopic hematuria is present.

TABLE 3 Medications That Can Cause or Contribute to Urinary Incontinence in Frail Older Adults

Medications	Effects on Continence
α-Adrenergic agonists	Increased smooth muscle tone in urethra and prostatic capsule may precipitate obstruction, urinary retention, related symptoms
α-Adrenergic antagonists	Decreased smooth muscle tone in urethra may precipitate stress urinary incontinence in women
Angiotensin-converting enzyme inhibitors	Cause cough that can exacerbate UI
Anticholinergics	May cause impaired emptying, urinary retention, and constipation, which can contribute to UI; may cause cognitive impairment, reduce effective toileting ability
Calcium channel blockers	May cause impaired emptying, urinary retention, and constipation, which can contribute to UI; may cause dependent edema, which can contribute to nocturnal polyuria
Cholinesterase inhibitors	Increase bladder contractility, may precipitate urgency UI
Diuretics	Cause diuresis and precipitate UI
Lithium	Polyuria due to diabetes insipidus
Opioid analgesics	May cause urinary retention, constipation, confusion, immobility, all of which can contribute to UI
Psychotropic drugs Sedatives Hypnotics Antipsychotics Histamine1 receptor antagonists	May cause confusion and impaired mobility and precipitate UI; anticholinergic effects; confusion
Selective serotonin reuptake inhibitors	Increase cholinergic transmission, may lead to urinary UI
Others—gabapentin, glitazones, nonsteroidal antiinflammatory drugs	Can cause edema, which can lead to nocturnal polyuria and cause nocturia and nighttime UI

UI, Urinary incontinence.
From Fillit HM: *Brocklehurst's textbook of geriatric medicine and gerontology*, ed 8, Philadelphia, 2017, Elsevier.

- Renal ultrasound may be used to assess for hydronephrosis.
- CT urogram may be used to assess upper tract abnormalities, congenital anomalies, genitourinary fistula, and microscopic hematuria etiologies.

Rx TREATMENT

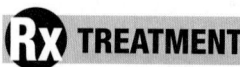

- The recommended approach to urinary incontinence is a stepped care plan first offering noninvasive behavioral modifications such as bladder training, weight loss, and fluid management. Fig. E5 summarizes the diagnosis and treatment of overactive bladder.
- **Pelvic floor muscle training,** including Kegel exercises and often augmented with biofeedback or electrical stimulation, is an important component of first-line therapy for stress, urge, and mixed incontinence.
- **Pharmacotherapy** is usually reserved for urgency urinary incontinence.
  1. Antimuscarinic (anticholinergic) medications: Block parasympathetic muscarinic receptors (detrusor M2/M3 receptors) to inhibit involuntary detrusor contractions.
     a. Agents available: Darifenacin, fesoterodine, oxybutynin (available orally and as a transdermal patch), solifenacin, tolterodine, and trospium.
     b. Efficacy: Shown to improve symptoms and continence but only modestly compared with placebo.
     c. Side effects: High rates of discontinuation due to side effects, most often dry mouth and constipation. May also exacerbate urinary retention, blurred vision, dyspepsia, and impaired cognitive function; contraindicated in narrow-angle glaucoma.
  1. Beta-agonists: Stimulate β3-adrenergic receptor in the detrusor muscle to cause relaxation and increase bladder capacity.
     a. Agent available: Mirabegron
     b. Efficacy: Significant reductions in urgency incontinence in randomized trials
     c. Side effects: Tachycardia, headache, and diarrhea (similar to placebo); not recommended in uncontrolled hypertension
  1. OnabotulinumtoxinA (Botox A): Inhibits the presynaptic release of acetylcholine from motor neurons at the neuromuscular junction to paralyze the muscle; given by cystoscopic injection.
     a. Efficacy: Similar rates of improvement seen when compared with antimuscarinic medications, but more women reporting complete resolution of urgency urinary incontinence with Botox A; third-line treatment due to adverse effects
     b. Adverse effects: Urinary retention or incomplete bladder emptying (5% requiring catheterization) and urinary tract infections (33%)
- **Peripheral tibial nerve stimulation**: 30-minute session of tibial nerve stimulation once per week for 12 weeks followed by a customized maintenance plan to treat OAB. Compared with placebo, pooled success rate was 60% in a guideline published by American Urological Association; fewer adverse events noted when compared with anti-muscarinic medication.
- **Sacral neuromodulation**: Stimulation of bladder and pelvic floor nerves to treat OAB, UUI, and idiopathic urinary retention. The mechanism is unknown. The procedure occurs in a two-stage process: First the electrode is placed near S3 to determine if symptoms are improved; if so, then next the pulse generator is implanted. Evidence suggests 70% of women experience significant improvement in their symptoms with sacral neuromodulation.
- **Devices**:
  1. Continence pessaries: For women with SUI who wish to defer or avoid surgery; help increase urethral resistance during increased intraabdominal pressure. A large randomized controlled trial demonstrated similar outcomes among women who underwent pessary, behavioral therapy, or a combination of both for incontinence; at 12 months, approximately 50% of women still using the assigned treatment reported improvement in symptoms.
  2. Over-the-counter vaginal or urethral inserts: Disposable devices used to support the urethra, especially in women with situational stress incontinence (i.e., only when exercising); however, urethral inserts have been associated with a high rate of urinary tract infection.
- **Surgery**: Indicated for women with SUI without symptom control after conservative management or as first-line treatment in appropriately counseled women who decline more conservative treatment.
  1. Synthetic slings are the most common primary surgical treatment for SUI. Cure rates of 62% to 98% have been reported in a recent systematic review.
     a. Transvaginal/retropubic: Trocars are passed through the retropubic space from the midurethra to the abdomen (or vice versa). Cure rates range from 81% to 84% at all time points with de novo urgency in approximately 6% of patients.
     b. Transobturator: Trocars are passed from the vagina behind the ischium (or vice versa).
     c. Single-incision slings: Only one vaginal incision is needed beneath the urethra; ends of the sling are secured in the internal obturator muscle.

TABLE 4 Transient Causes of Urinary Incontinence (DIAPPERS)

D	Delirium/confusional state
I	Infection—urinary (symptomatic)
A	Atrophic urethritis/vaginitis
P	Pharmaceuticals (diuretics, and so on)
P	Psychological, especially depression
E	Endocrine (hypercalcemia, hypokalemia, glycosuria)
R	Restricted mobility
S	Stool impaction

From Floege J et al: *Comprehensive clinical nephrology*, ed 4, Philadelphia, 2010, Saunders.

2. Autologous fascial slings: Usually considered second line after the failure of synthetic slings due to length and morbidity of the operation. Cure rates estimated to be 90% at 12 to 23 months and 82% at 48 months or greater.
3. Cadaveric slings: Usually second line; use has declined more recently due to concerns with early failure and declining success rate over time. Cure rates of 74% at 12 to 23 months and 80% at 48 months or greater.
4. Retropubic urethropexy, i.e., Burch procedure (open abdominal or laparoscopic): A large meta-analysis estimated cure rates to be 82% at 12 to 23 months and 73% at 48 months or longer for open procedures.

- **Bulking Agents**: For treatment of stress incontinence without hypermobility or in poor surgical candidates.
  1. Available agents: Pyrolytic carbon-coated beads, calcium hydroxylapatite
  2. Effectiveness: Relatively noninvasive but less effective than surgical intervention; cure rate at 63% to 80% at 1 yr
- Treatment for urinary retention and overflow incontinence focuses on reversal of modifiable factors and drainage of urine from the bladder.
  1. Clean intermittent self-catheterization
  2. Sacral neuromodulation

PEARLS & CONSIDERATIONS

COMMENTS

- Weight loss and exercise are helpful for urinary incontinence in obese women. Overweight and obese women with urinary incontinence also have a high prevalence of monthly fecal incontinence (16% found to be associated with low dietary fiber intake after adjustment for other known risk factors for fecal incontinence).
- Transient causes of urinary incontinence in the elderly are described in Table 4.
- Other forms of incontinence:
  1. Nocturnal enuresis: Loss of urine occurring during sleep; can occur as idiopathic or neurogenic.
  2. Postvoid dribble: A postsphincteric collection of urine seen with urethral diverticulum; can be idiopathic.
  3. Extraurethral incontinence: Enterovesical, urethral; also known as *fistula.*
- Conditions that predispose to surgical failure: Advanced age, prior failed incontinence surgery, concurrent detrusor instability, abnormal perineal electromyography, pelvic radiation
- The Women's Preventive Services Initiative (WPSI) recommends screening women for urinary incontinence annually

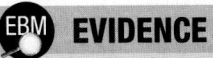

EVIDENCE

Available at ExpertConsult.com

SUGGESTED READINGS

Available at ExpertConsult.com

RELATED CONTENT

Urinary Incontinence (Patient Information)
Pelvic Organ Prolapse (Related Key Topic)

AUTHORS: **MEAGAN CRAMER, M.D.,** and **EMILY K. SAKS, M.D., M.S.C.E.**

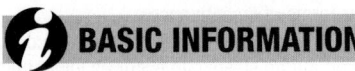

DEFINITION

Infertility in a reproductive-age couple is the inability to conceive after unprotected intercourse for ≥1 yr. When a female is greater than 35 yr of age, an evaluation is justified after 6 months without successful pregnancy. Earlier evaluation at any age is warranted with preexisting symptoms or medical conditions.

SYNONYM

Sterility

ICD-10CM CODES	
N46	Male infertility
N46.8	Other male infertility
N46.9	Male infertility, unspecified
N97.0	Female infertility associated with anovulation
N97.1	Female infertility of tubal origin
N97.2	Female infertility of uterine origin
N97.8	Female infertility of other origin
N97.9	Female infertility, unspecified
009.00	Supervision of pregnancy with history of infertility, unspecified trimester
009.01	Supervision of pregnancy with history of infertility, first trimester
009.02	Supervision of pregnancy with history of infertility, second trimester
009.03	Supervision of pregnancy with history of infertility, third trimester
Z31.81	Encounter for male factor infertility in female patient

EPIDEMIOLOGY & DEMOGRAPHICS

PEAK INCIDENCE: The incidence of infertility increases with age. Subtle decreases in female fertility start as early as age 30. The rate of infertility increases dramatically after age 37, and unassisted pregnancies become extremely uncommon as women reach the mid-40s. There is also a subtle, but still detectable, decrease in male fertility that may start as early as age 30.

PREVALENCE: One in eight reproductive age couples experience infertility. This prevalence is consistent in all developed countries and there is evidence that it is historically stable.

PREDOMINANT SEX AND AGE: By definition this is a diagnosis of reproductive age couples. Infertility increases with aging in both males and females, but more dramatically in women. Male factor is responsible in ~40% of couples and the female factor is responsible in ~40% of couples. The remainder of the cases are either combined male and female, or unexplained infertility, meaning a clear cause is not identified.

RISK FACTORS: Aging is among the most common risk factors, predominantly among females, although there is evidence that aging affects male fertility as well. Women are increasingly deferring pregnancy due to the lack of a partner or career, which is likely associated with increasing prevalence in certain sectors of the population. Tubal factor infertility can be a result of endometriosis, prior tubal surgery, prior ruptured appendix, or sexually transmitted diseases such as chlamydia and gonorrhea. Extremes of weight, particularly obesity, are associated with ovulatory dysfunction. Other causes include polycystic ovarian syndrome (PCOS), hypothalamic dysfunction, thyroid disorders and hyperprolactinemia. Male factor infertility may be idiopathic or due to trauma, infection, varicocele, obstruction, hypothalamic dysfunction, or exposure to environmental toxins. Smoking is the most common lifestyle choice that impairs fertility.

PHYSICAL FINDINGS & CLINICAL PRESENTATION

- Age
- Previous fertility, particularly if no pregnancy has occurred in another relationship despite absence of contraception
- Absence of secondary sexual characteristics
- Abnormal uterine bleeding or absent menstruation
- Clinical signs of androgen excess: Hirsutism, acne, alopecia
- Abnormal pelvic exam: Enlarged uterus, adnexal masses, pelvic/abdominal tenderness
- History of urological surgery in male or trauma to testes

ETIOLOGY

- Female factor:
  1. Advanced age
  2. Tubal factor: Pelvic inflammatory disease, endometriosis, prior pelvic surgery, history of ruptured appendicitis, prior elective sterilization
  3. Anatomic: Uterine fibroids, polyps, intrauterine adhesions, uterine anomalies
  4. Oligo-/anovulation: Most frequently due to polycystic ovarian syndrome (PCOS), but also due to thyroid abnormalities, hyperprolactinemia, nonclassic congenital adrenal hyperplasia, hypothalamic dysfunction
- Male factor:
  1. Abnormal semen analysis
  2. Elective sterilization
- Idiopathic: Both male and female

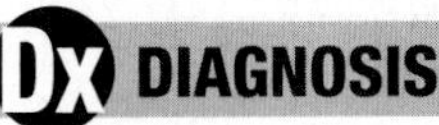

WORKUP

- Confirmation of ovulation: History of regular menstrual cycles, mid-luteal serum progesterone, basal body temperature testing, urinary luteinizing hormone predictor kits
- Complete transvaginal pelvic ultrasound
- Ovarian reserve testing: Anti-müllerian hormone, FSH, and estradiol obtained on cycle day 2-4 and antral follicle count
- Fallopian tube evaluation: Hysterosalpingogram (HSG) (Fig. 1)
- Uterine cavity evaluation: HSG, saline infusion sonohysterography, hysteroscopy, or 3D ultrasound of uterus
- Male factor: Semen analysis

LABORATORY TESTS

- Semen analysis, using Kruger strict morphology. Abstain 2 to 5 days prior to test.
- FSH and estradiol collected cycle day 2, 3, or 4 and anti-müllerian hormone as a measure of ovarian reserve.
- Mid-luteal progesterone (ideally 7 days prior to expected menses). Given variability of serum progesterone measurements throughout the day and absence of a reliable threshold, most practitioners use clinical criteria to diagnose ovulatory dysfunction.
- Urinary luteinizing hormone measurement
- TSH
- In patients with oligo- or anovulation: Prolactin, testosterone, 17-hydroxyprogesterone

IMAGING STUDIES

- Day 2 or 3 transvaginal pelvic ultrasound to assess uterine or adnexal abnormalities and to count the number of small antral follicles (2-9 mm) as a measure of ovarian

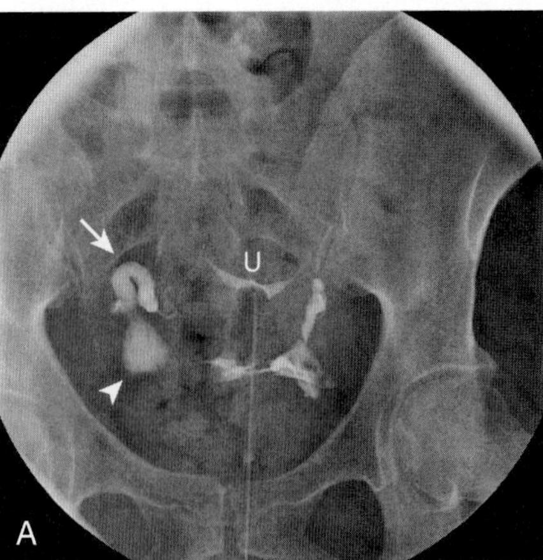

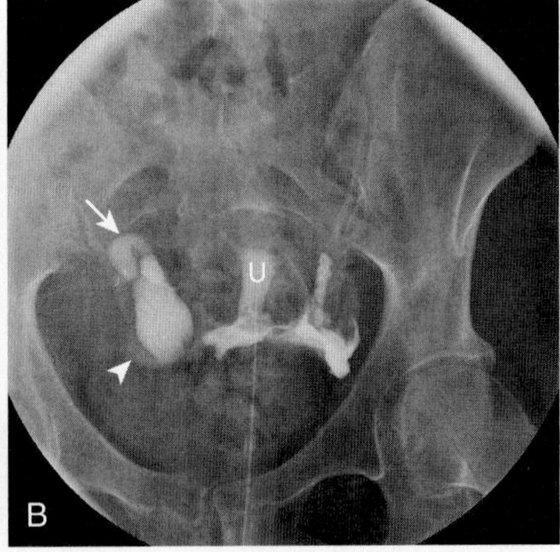

FIG. 1 Hysterosalpingogram spot radiographs early **(A)** and late **(B)** demonstrate a rounded collection of contrast material *(arrowhead)* adjacent to the dilated ampullary portion of the right fallopian tube *(arrow),* caused by peritubal pelvic adhesions related to previous pelvic inflammatory disease. Normal patient left fallopian tube. *U,* Uterus. (From Fielding JR et al: *Gynecologic imaging,* Philadelphia, 2011, Saunders.)

reserve. If oligo- or anovulatory, to assess for polycystic-appearing ovary.
- Hysterosalpingogram (early follicular phase after menses complete but before ovulation, typically between days 5 and 12 of the menstrual cycle).
- Also used for imaging of uterine cavity: Saline infusion sonohysterography, 3D ultrasound of uterus, hysteroscopy.

Rx TREATMENT

Once the patient presents for evaluation, testing should be completed as quickly as possible, ideally within one menstrual cycle. The couple should follow up with the evaluating provider once all testing is completed and treatment initiated as abnormalities are found.

ACUTE GENERAL Rx

- Oligo- or anovulation should be treated with ovulation induction agents, such as clomiphene citrate or aromatase inhibitors. A recent multicenter trial found that aromatase inhibitors achieved higher live birth rates than clomiphene citrate.[1] Historically, clomiphene citrate has been used, but a very well done randomized controlled trial convincingly demonstrated that letrozole is superior. Far less commonly, ovulatory dysfunction is the result of hypothalamic dysfunction. In these patients, once hypothalamic or pituitary abnormalities are excluded with MRI, ovulation can be achieved using injectable gonadotropins.
- Tubal factor infertility may be treated surgically if mild, and if the female patient is young and can afford the time to attempt pregnancy over multiple menstrual cycles. If the patient is older or if the tubal pathology is moderate to severe, in vitro fertilization (IVF) is recommended.
- Uterine anatomic abnormalities such as submucosal fibroids, polyps, intrauterine adhesions, or septate uterus should be corrected if they are identified. Fibroids that do not impact the uterine cavity probably do not interfere with fertility. Removal of intramural or subserosal fibroids is reserved for situations in which these cause excessive vaginal bleeding, pain, or pressure.
- Male infertility: Referral to urologist for complete evaluation. If semen analysis is severely abnormal, the following laboratory testing is recommended: Testosterone, FSH, estradiol, luteinizing hormone, TSH and prolactin, karyotype and Y-chromosome microdeletion.
  1. Mild male factor infertility may be treated with intrauterine insemination (IUI), but severe male factor will usually require assisted reproductive technologies (ART) with intracytoplasmic sperm injection (ICSI) in the laboratory, where sperm is injected directly into the oocyte. ICSI use has increased from 36.4% in 1996 to 76.2% in 2012 with the largest increase among cycles without male factor infertility. Donor sperm may be necessary in cases of azoospermia due to testicular failure, if male partner has a genetic disorder, or if couple is unable to proceed with IVF/ICSI.
- Unexplained infertility can be treated empirically using superovulation with clomiphene citrate, aromatase inhibitors, or gonadotropins combined with intrauterine insemination with partner's or donor sperm. Most providers recommend using an oral ovulation induction agent with insemination as a first-line superovulatory agent because it is inexpensive. After 3 to 4 such cycles, few pregnancies occur and the couple should be advised to become more aggressive. Controversy exists as to whether gonadotropins with insemination or IVF should be used after clomiphene citrate superovulation induction. There is evidence suggesting that moving to IVF after 3 months of clomiphene citrate and insemination shortens the time interval to achieving pregnancy.[2] A randomized trial in women with unexplained infertility revealed ovarian stimulation with letrozole resulted in a significantly lower frequency of multiple gestation but also a lower frequency of live birth, as compared with gonadotropin but not as compared with clomiphene.
- Donor egg or embryo may be required in cases of premature ovarian insufficiency or due to age factor. Some couples may elect to pursue adoption.
- For LGBT couples, many family building options are available, including IUI or IVF utilizing donor sperm, donor oocytes, and/or gestational carrier, depending on the needs of the couple.

COMPLEMENTARY & ALTERNATIVE MEDICINE

Acupuncture is widely used by women being treated for infertility. Limited data suggest some benefit, with possible mechanisms of action including increasing blood flow to the uterus and/or ovaries. Despite these studies, it is unproven whether acupuncture definitely improves IVF outcomes. Patients may additionally benefit from the stress relief that acupuncture provides.

DISPOSITION

- Most couples will achieve a pregnancy, provided that they are willing to proceed with treatment including ovulation induction, superovulation, IUI, IVF, or gamete donation.
- Adoption is also a worthwhile and viable possibility for couples unable to conceive.

REFERRAL

Couples should be referred to a reproductive endocrinologist once the complexity of treatment exceeds the comfort level of the provider, whether a family physician, internist, or general gynecologist. Complex ovulation and superovulation induction and ART are best managed by a board-certified reproductive endocrinologist.

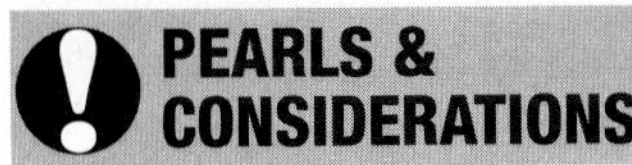

PEARLS & CONSIDERATIONS

COMMENTS

- The incidence of heterotopic pregnancy in patients who have undergone ART is relatively common; identification of a patient with ultrasound-proved intrauterine pregnancy who used ART to conceive should NOT necessarily exclude the possibility of an ectopic gestation.
- Single-embryo transfer is becoming more common in IVF cycles to reduce the rate of multiple gestation.
- Preimplantation genetic diagnosis is used in selected IVF cycles when one or both parents has one or more known genetic abnormalities to test embryos for these specific genetic abnormalities prior to implantation.
- Preimplantation genetic screening is used in IVF cycles to screen embryos for aneuploidy prior to implantation.

PREVENTION

- Techniques that reduce the incidence of pelvic inflammatory disease, such as condom use, can reduce pelvic adhesions that are associated with tubal factor infertility.
- Women should be made aware of the fact that delaying pregnancy into the later reproductive years reduces the likelihood for successful pregnancy. Many women are electing to cryopreserve oocytes or embryos for future use.
- Oocyte, embryo, or sperm cryopreservation is recommended for patients undergoing gonadotoxic chemotherapy or radiation treatment as a means of fertility preservation. Ovarian or testicular tissue cryopreservation may also be performed under a research protocol. All patients should be referred to a reproductive endocrinologist before planned treatment to discuss fertility preservation options.

PATIENT & FAMILY EDUCATION

Patient support groups such as *Resolve* (www.resolve.org) are available to help couples during evaluation and treatment of infertility, which can be extraordinarily stressful.

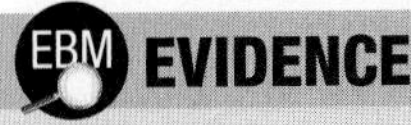

EVIDENCE

Available at ExpertConsult.com

SUGGESTED READINGS

Available at ExpertConsult.com

RELATED CONTENT

Infertility (Patient Information)
Amenorrhea (Related Key Topic)
Pelvic Inflammatory Disease (Related Key Topic)
Polycystic Ovary Syndrome (Related Key Topic)

AUTHOR: **EMELIA ARGYROPOULOS BACHMAN, M.D.**

[1] Legro RS et al: Letrozole versus clomiphene for infertility in the polycystic ovary syndrome, *N Engl J Med* 371:119-129, 2014.

[2] Reindollar RH et al: A randomized clinical trial to evaluate optimal treatment for unexplained infertility: the fast track and standard treatment (FASTT) trial, *Fertil Steril* 94:888-899, 2010.

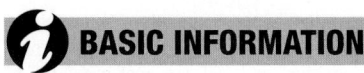

BASIC INFORMATION

DEFINITION

Inflammatory myopathies are idiopathic diseases of muscle characterized clinically by muscle weakness and pathologically by inflammation and muscle fiber breakdown. The four most common are dermatomyositis (DM), necrotizing autoimmune myositis, polymyositis (PM), and inclusion body myositis (IBM). See separate topics on "Inclusion Body Myositis" and "Necrotizing Autoimmune Myopathy" for details regarding these topics.

SYNONYMS

Immune-mediated myopathies
Idiopathic inflammatory myopathies
Myositis syndromes
Polymyositis
Dermatomyositis
IMM

ICD-10CM CODES

M33.90	Dermatopolymyositis, unspecified, organ involvement unspecified
M33.20	Polymyositis, organ involvement unspecified
M33.02	Juvenile dermatopolymyositis with myopathy
M33.12	Other dermatopolymyositis with myopathy
M33.22	Polymyositis with myopathy
M33.92	Dermatopolymyositis, unspecified with myopathy

EPIDEMIOLOGY & DEMOGRAPHICS

Inflammatory myopathies are the largest group of potentially treatable myopathies in children and adults.

DM:
- Occurs in children and in adults (bimodal age peak)
- Average age at diagnosis is 40 yr in adults. Age range in children: 5 to 14 yr
- More common in females than in males (2:1)
- Incidence 1:100,000
- Prevalence 1 to 10 cases/million in adults and 1 to 3.2 cases/million in children
- Up to one third of patients older than 50 with DM have an associated malignancy

PM:
- Occurs mostly in adults, very rare in children
- Average age at diagnosis >20 yr
- More common in females
- Least common inflammatory myopathy
- Exact incidence unknown

PHYSICAL FINDINGS & CLINICAL PRESENTATION

DM and PM:
- Most patients have a subacute onset over weeks to months.
- Pattern is typically symmetric proximal muscle weakness involving the proximal limbs (shoulder and pelvic girdles).
- Weakness of neck flexion and extension is common.
- Difficulty getting up from a chair, climbing stairs, reaching for objects above head, or combing hair.
- Distal muscle and ocular involvement is uncommon.
- Sensation is preserved.
- Reflexes may be preserved or diminished.
- Dysphagia and dysphonia result from involvement of striated muscle of the pharynx and proximal esophagus.
- Esophageal dysmotility is common in DM.
- Respiratory failure from associated pulmonary fibrosis.
- Cardiac conduction abnormalities can be seen with DM.
- Systemic autoimmune disease occurs frequently in PM, and rarely in DM.
- Skin findings in DM:
  1. Heliotrope rash on the upper eyelids (Fig. E1)
  2. Erythematous rash on the face
  3. May also involve the back and shoulders (shawl sign), neck and chest (V-shape), knees (Fig. E2), and elbows
  4. Photosensitivity
  5. Gottron's papules (violaceous papules overlying dorsal interphalangeal or metacarpophalangeal areas, elbow or knee joints (Fig. E3))
  6. Nail cracking, thickening, and irregularity (Fig. E4) with periungual telangiectasia
  7. Mechanic's hand: Fissured, hyperpigmented, scaly, and hyperkeratotic; also associated with increased risk of interstitial lung disease

ETIOLOGY

DM: Complex, immune-mediated microangiopathy. Adaptive immune response via humorally mediated complement attack

PM: Unknown:
- Cell-mediated immune major histocompatibility-I (MHC-1) process directed against muscle fibers is likely, given biopsy features.
- A viral etiology has been proposed secondary to the presence of autoantibodies to histidyl transferase, anti-Jo-1, and signal recognition particle.

Dx DIAGNOSIS

- The diagnosis of each subtype of inflammatory myopathy is based on clinical history, pattern of muscle involvement, electromyographic findings, muscle biopsy, and presence of certain antibodies.
- Myopathic pattern of muscle weakness
- Characteristic rash in DM
- EMG shows myopathic (small-amplitude, short-duration, polyphasic) motor potentials with early recruitment
- Majority of patients have "irritable" features (fibrillations and positive sharp waves) on EMG
- See "Laboratory Tests."
- Biopsy is required for diagnosis and should confirm inflammation before treatment is started. Table 1 describes histologic features of idiopathic inflammatory myopathies. In idiopathic inflammatory myopathies, myopathic features (variation in fiber size, fiber splitting, fatty replacement of muscle tissue, and increased endomysial connective tissue) should be seen in addition to the following:
  1. DM: Perifascicular atrophy, MAC deposition along capillaries
  2. PM: Endomysial infiltrates composed of CD8+ T cells and macrophages invading nonnecrotic muscle fibers that express MHC-I antigen

DIFFERENTIAL DIAGNOSIS

- IBM
- Muscular dystrophies
- Amyloid myoneuropathy
- Amyotrophic lateral sclerosis
- Myasthenia gravis
- Eaton-Lambert syndrome
- Drug-induced myopathies (e.g., quinidine, NSAIDs, penicillamine, HMG CoA-reductase inhibitors)
- Diabetic amyotrophy
- Guillain-Barré syndrome
- Hyperthyroidism or hypothyroidism
- Lichen planus
- Amyopathic DM (rash without weakness)
- DM sine rash (weakness with characteristic biopsy, but no rash)
- Systemic lupus erythematosus (SLE)
- Contact atopic or seborrheic dermatitis
- Psoriasis

LABORATORY TESTS

- Creatine kinase (CK) is the most sensitive muscle enzyme test for muscle breakdown. It should be checked at onset, and serially monitored several times during treatment.
- CK is typically elevated (5-50× normal) in active PM.
- CK may be normal or only slightly elevated in DM.
- Aldolase, AST, ALT, alkaline phosphatase, and LDH may be elevated.
- Anti-Jo-1 antibodies are seen in myositis with associated interstitial lung disease but are not specific for either DM or PM.
- DM: Anti-MDA-5, anti-Mi-2, anti-TIF-1, and anti-NXP2 (implicated in cancer-associated dermatomyositis).
- PM: Antisynthetase antibodies (often seen in overlap myositis) associated with interstitial lung disease, arthritis, fever, and "mechanic's hands."
- Electrolytes, thyroid-stimulating hormone (TSH), Ca, and Mg should be evaluated to exclude other causes of weakness.
- Check ECG for cardiac involvement.

IMAGING STUDIES

- Chest x-ray is used to rule out pulmonary involvement. If suspicious for pulmonary interstitial disease, a high-resolution CT scan of the chest may be helpful.
- Radiography is an efficient means of identifying and characterizing soft-tissue calcinosis (Fig. E5).

TABLE 1 Histologic Features of Idiopathic Inflammatory Myopathies

Feature	Dermatomyositis	Polymyositis	Inclusion Body Myositis
Necrosis of muscle fibers	+	+	+
Variation in fiber diameter	+	+	+
Regeneration of muscle fibers	+	+	+
Proliferation of connective tissue	+	+	+
Infiltration of mononuclear cells*	+	+	+
Perivascular and perimysial inflammation	+	–/+	–/+
Endomysial inflammation	–/+	+	+
Perifascicular atrophy	+	–	–
Abnormally dilated capillaries	+	–/+	–
Reduced capillary density	+	–/+	–
Deposition of complement on vessel walls	+	–/+	–
Microinfarcts	+	–	–
Invasion of non-necrotic fibers by cytotoxic T lymphocytes and macrophages	–	+	+
Expression of major histocompatibility complex class I on muscle fibers	–/+	+	+
Rimmed vacuoles with amyloid deposits and tubulofilaments†	–	–	+
Angulated or atrophic and hypertrophic fibers	–	–	+
Ragged red or cytochrome oxidase–negative fibers	–	–	+

*Inflammation is absent in a small proportion of polymyositis and dermatomyositis biopsies.
†Also seen in chronic neurogenic conditions and distal myopathies.
From Firestein GS, et al.: *Kelley's textbook of rheumatology,* ed 9, Philadelphia, 2013, Saunders, Elsevier.

- Although MRI arguably has greater diagnostic value than electromyography or serum enzyme measurements in cases of suspected idiopathic inflammatory myopathy, MRI findings have not been formalized as a diagnostic criterion for idiopathic inflammatory myopathy. The acceptance of MRI as a diagnostic tool in myositis may be inhibited by the high cost and the need for more reliable and validated methods of summarizing the findings of MRI. MRI evaluation before biopsy, however, has become routine at many tertiary care centers. Fascial disease is manifested on MRI by fascial or perifascial hyperintensity on fluid-sensitive sequences. The edema-like signal in the deep subcutis may accompany fasciitis and can indicate associated panniculitis (Fig. E6).
- Video fluoroscopy or barium swallow study to look for upper esophageal dysfunction in patients with dysphagia and DM.

Rx TREATMENT

Goal: Maintain function, minimize disease/iatrogenic sequelae

NONPHARMACOLOGIC THERAPY

- Sun-blocking agents with SPF 15 or greater for skin protection in patients with DM
- Physical therapy beneficial for gait training and increasing muscle tone and strength
- Occupational therapy assists with activities of daily living
- Speech therapy to monitor patients with swallowing dysfunction

ACUTE GENERAL Rx

- Corticosteroids are the mainstay of therapy. Start prednisone 1 to 2 mg/kg per day, up to a maximum dose of 100 mg/day. Continue until muscle strength improves or muscle enzymes have normalized for at least 4 wk. Begin tapering by 10 mg/month until 60 mg/day, then slowly taper by 5 mg/month. Consider every-other-day prednisone treatment at same dose (may decrease side effects).
- Consider IV immunoglobulin (IVIG) if patient fails to improve on prednisone, or muscle enzymes begin rising when tapering off prednisone. See "Chronic Rx" for specific dosage.
- Hydroxychloroquine can be used to treat the cutaneous lesions of DM.
- A treatment algorithm for adult patients with PM and DM is described in Fig. 7.

CHRONIC Rx

- Chronic prednisone therapy may be needed for years, but other immunosuppressive ("steroid-sparing") agents may be added early to decrease long-term steroid side effects.
- Azathioprine 2 to 3 mg/kg per day tapered to 1 mg/kg per day once steroid is tapered to 15 mg/day. Reduce dosage monthly by 25-mg intervals. Maintenance dosage is 50 mg/day.
- Methotrexate 7.5 to 10 mg PO/wk, increased by 2.5 mg/wk to total of 25 mg/wk; consider IM dosing if PO is ineffective.
- IV immunoglobulin 2 g/kg total dose over 2 to 5 days.
- IV cyclophosphamide 1 g/M^2 monthly for 6 mo is preferred to oral dosing for refractory cases. However, oral dosing of cyclophosphamide is 1 to 3 mg/kg per day PO or 2 to 4 mg/kg per day in conjunction with prednisone.
- Cyclosporine A: Initial dose 2.0 to 2.5 mg/kg bid; long-term maintenance is lowest effective dose.
- Mycophenolate mofetil 500 mg PO bid, titrate to 1500 mg PO bid over 1 to 2 months.
- Hydroxychloroquine 200 mg PO daily; monitor for visual changes.

DISPOSITION

- 30% to 40% of patients achieve clinical remission with treatment.
- In patients with residual weakness, deficits typically remain stable over long-term follow-up.
- 10% experience recurrent disease.
- Serum CK often returns to normal before symptoms improve.
- During exacerbations, enzymes may rise before clinical symptoms appear.
- Poor prognostic indicators include delay in diagnosis, older age, recalcitrant disease, malignancy, interstitial pulmonary fibrosis, dysphagia, leukocytosis, fever, and anorexia.
- Infection, malignancy, and cardiac and pulmonary dysfunction are the most common causes of death.
- With early treatment, 5- and 8-yr survival rates of 80% and 73%, respectively, have been reported.

REFERRAL

Neurology or rheumatology referral should be made to help establish the diagnosis and implement treatment.

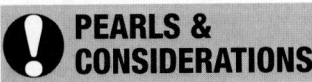

PEARLS & CONSIDERATIONS

- Do not implement treatment before muscle biopsy.
- When assessing response to treatment, clinical muscle strength is more important than muscle enzyme tests.
- The concern for malignancies (ovary, lung, breast, GI) associated with DM is legitimate and merits screening in patients older than age 40 at time of diagnosis and every 2 to 3 yr thereafter.
- No association exists between juvenile DM and malignancy.

- Overlap syndrome refers to patients with DM who also meet criteria for a connective tissue disorder (e.g., rheumatoid arthritis, scleroderma, SLE).
- In any patient taking steroids, closely monitor for:
  1. Diabetes or glucose intolerance (2-hr oral glucose tolerance test)
  2. Osteopenia/osteoporosis (DEXA scan q6mo)
  3. Cataracts (yearly ophthalmologic appointment)
  4. Hypertension
  5. Psychiatric side effects including depression or psychosis
  6. Poor sleep
  7. Peptic ulcer disease (prescribe H_2 antagonist or proton pump inhibitor)
- Clinical and immune response features can be used for categorizing heterogeneous myositis syndromes and mutually exclusive and stable phenotypes and are useful for predicting clinical signs and symptoms, associated environmental and genetic risk factors, and responses to therapy and prognosis.

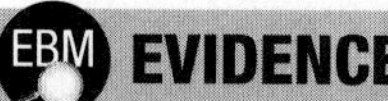

EVIDENCE

Available at ExpertConsult.com

SUGGESTED READINGS

Available at ExpertConsult.com

RELATED CONTENT

Dermatomyositis and Polymyositis (Patient Information)
Inclusion Body Myositis (Related Key Topic)
Necrotizing Autoimmune Myopathy (Related Key Topic)

AUTHORS: **JOSEPH S. KASS, M.D., J.D.** and **GAVIN BROWN, M.D.**

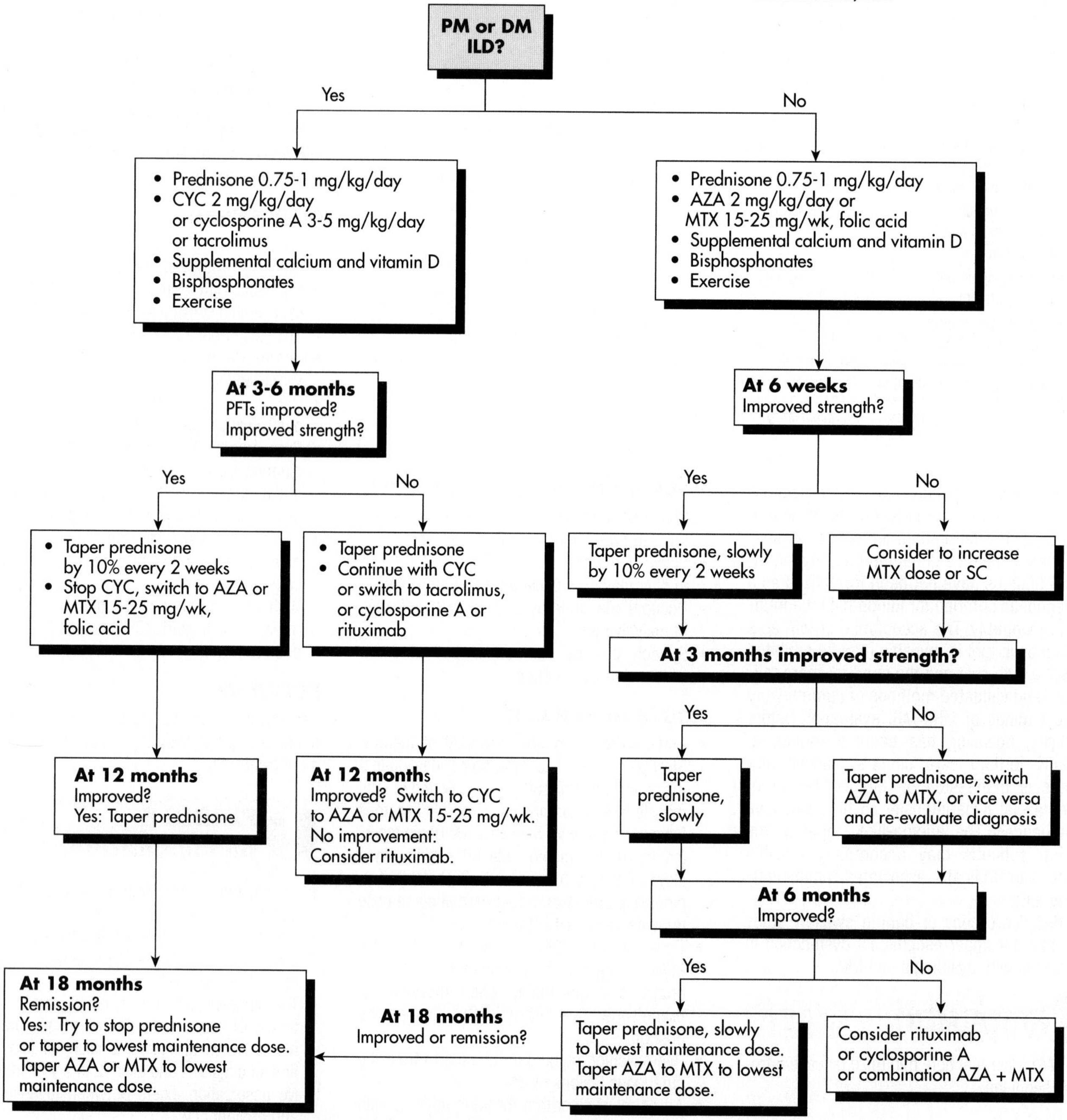

PM or DM ILD?

Yes →
- Prednisone 0.75-1 mg/kg/day
- CYC 2 mg/kg/day or cyclosporine A 3-5 mg/kg/day or tacrolimus
- Supplemental calcium and vitamin D
- Bisphosphonates
- Exercise

At 3-6 months PFTs improved? Improved strength?

- Yes:
  - Taper prednisone by 10% every 2 weeks
  - Stop CYC, switch to AZA or MTX 15-25 mg/wk, folic acid

  At 12 months Improved? Yes: Taper prednisone

  At 18 months Remission? Yes: Try to stop prednisone or taper to lowest maintenance dose. Taper AZA or MTX to lowest maintenance dose.
- No:
  - Taper prednisone
  - Continue with CYC or switch to tacrolimus, or cyclosporine A or rituximab

  At 12 months Improved? Switch to CYC to AZA or MTX 15-25 mg/wk. No improvement: Consider rituximab.

No →
- Prednisone 0.75-1 mg/kg/day
- AZA 2 mg/kg/day or MTX 15-25 mg/wk, folic acid
- Supplemental calcium and vitamin D
- Bisphosphonates
- Exercise

At 6 weeks Improved strength?

- Yes: Taper prednisone, slowly by 10% every 2 weeks
- No: Consider to increase MTX dose or SC

At 3 months improved strength?

- Yes: Taper prednisone, slowly
- No: Taper prednisone, switch AZA to MTX, or vice versa and re-evaluate diagnosis

At 6 months Improved?

- Yes: Taper prednisone, slowly to lowest maintenance dose. Taper AZA to MTX to lowest maintenance dose. → **At 18 months** Improved or remission? → (At 18 months Remission? box)
- No: Consider rituximab or cyclosporine A or combination AZA + MTX

FIG. 7 Treatment algorithm for adult patients with polymyositis *(PM)* or dermatomyositis *(DM)*. *AZA,* Azathioprine; *CYC,* cyclophosphamide; *ILD,* interstitial lung disease; *MTX,* methotrexate; *PFT,* pulmonary function test; *SC,* subcutaneous. (From Firestein GS, et al.: *Kelley's textbook of rheumatology,* ed 9, Philadelphia, 2013, Saunders, Elsevier.)

BASIC INFORMATION

DEFINITION

Influenza is an acute febrile illness caused by infection with influenza type A or B virus. Seasonal influenza can include the H1N1 virus. A similar respiratory illness is severe acute respiratory syndrome (SARS) caused by a coronavirus called SARS-associated coronavirus (SARS-CoV). A new novel coronavirus was recognized in two patients in September 2012. This is a very different virus from the SARS agent; the two patients exhibited acute respiratory distress syndrome, renal failure, consumptive coagulopathy, and/or pericarditis. Now called the Middle East respiratory syndrome (MERS-CoV) virus, it has affected more than 2,200 persons in 27 countries since 2012. Patients have fever and pneumonia requiring hospitalization. Transmission spread in 2015 from the Middle East to Korea and China, resulting in more than 185 cases. There were 558 cases in Saudi Arabia from January 2015 through early June 2016, and 75 in 2018. Persons who are immunocompromised or have diabetes, renal failure, or chronic lung disease are thought to be at greater risk of severe illness. Dromedary camels and their milk are documented to harbor MERS-CoV.

Refer to the "Influenza, Avian" topic for more information.

SYNONYMS

Flu
Influenza-like illness (ILI)

ICD-10CM CODES

J10.00	Influenza due to other identified influenza virus with unspecified type of pneumonia
J10.1	Influenza due to other identified influenza virus with other respiratory manifestations
J11.1	Influenza due to unidentified influenza virus with other respiratory manifestations
J12.9	Viral pneumonia, unspecified

EPIDEMIOLOGY & DEMOGRAPHICS

PEAK INCIDENCE: Winter outbreaks lasting 5 to 6 wk.

PREDOMINANT SEX: Male = female.

PREDOMINANT AGE: Attack rates are usually higher among children than adults, although children are less prone to pulmonary complications. The severity of the 2017-2018 flu season was described by the Centers for Disease Control and Prevention (CDC) as high for all age groups: children, adults and older adults. Of the 171 reported pediatric deaths in the 2017-2018 season, 22% of the vaccine-eligible children had received vaccine.

INCIDENCE (IN U.S.): Annual incidence of influenza-related deaths is between 12,000 and 56,000 deaths/yr.

PHYSICAL FINDINGS & CLINICAL PRESENTATION

- "Classic flu" is characterized by abrupt onset of fever, headache, myalgias, anorexia, and malaise after a 1- to 2-day incubation period.
- Clinical syndromes are similar to those produced by other respiratory viruses, including pharyngitis, common colds, tracheobronchitis, bronchiolitis, and croup.
- Respiratory symptoms such as cough, sore throat, and nasal discharge are usually present at the onset of illness, but systemic symptoms predominate.
- Elderly patients may experience fever, weakness, and confusion without any respiratory complaints.
- Acute deterioration to status asthmaticus may occur in patients with asthma.
- Influenza pneumonia: Rapidly progressive cough, dyspnea, and cyanosis may occur after typical flu onset. This may be caused by primary influenza pneumonia or secondary bacterial pneumonia (often pneumococcal or staphylococcal co-infection).
- For influenza A (H3N2v), children younger than 10 yr lack immunity. People ≥65 yr and those with morbid obesity are at high risk.

ETIOLOGY

- Variation in the surface antigens of the influenza virus, hemagglutinin (HA) and neuraminidase (NA), leading to infection with variants to which immunity is inadequate in the population at risk.
- Droplet transmission by small-particle aerosols and deposited on the respiratory tract epithelium.

Dx DIAGNOSIS

DIFFERENTIAL DIAGNOSIS

- Respiratory syncytial virus, adenovirus, parainfluenza virus infection.
- Secondary bacterial pneumonia or mixed bacterial-viral pneumonia.

WORKUP

- The accuracy of clinical diagnosis of influenza on the basis of symptoms alone is limited because symptoms from illness caused by other pathogens can overlap considerably with influenza. Diagnostic tests available for influenza include viral cultures, serology, rapid influenza diagnostic tests (RIDTs), reverse transcription-polymerase chain reaction (RT-PCR), and immunofluorescence assays.
- Virus isolation from nasal or throat swab or sputum specimens is the most rapid diagnostic method in the setting of acute illness.
- Specimens are placed into virus transport medium and processed by a reference laboratory.
- For serologic diagnosis:
  1. Paired serum specimens, acute and convalescent, the latter obtained 10 to 20 days later
  2. Fourfold rises or falls in the titer of antibodies (various techniques) considered diagnostic of recent infection
  3. Commercial rapid influenza diagnostic tests (RIDTs) are available. They can detect influenza virus antigens within 15 minutes of testing. Rapid flu test should be collected as early as possible, ideally within 4 days of onset. False-negative results are common during the flu season. A negative test result does NOT exclude diagnosis of influenza.
  4. Commercial RIDTs cannot determine if an H3N2 is a variant virus; when suspect H3N2v virus infection, send nasopharyngeal swab or aspirate in viral transport medium to state public health laboratory for rRT-PCR testing using Centers for Disease Control and Prevention (CDC) FLU rRT-PCR diagnostic panel assay. Novel digital immunoassay (DIAs) and rapid nucleic amplification tests (NAATs) have a markedly higher sensitivity for influenza A and B than traditional RIDTs.

LABORATORY TESTS

Septic syndrome presentation: CBC, ABG analysis, blood cultures

IMAGING STUDIES

- Chest x-ray examination when suspecting viral pneumonia: Peribronchial and patchy interstitial infiltrates in multiple lobes with atelectasis. Table 1 describes x-ray pulmonary findings based on virus type.
- Possible progression to diffuse interstitial pneumonitis.

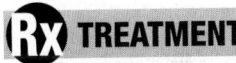

TREATMENT

NONPHARMACOLOGIC THERAPY

- Bed rest.
- Hydration.

ACUTE GENERAL Rx

- Supportive care: Antipyretics; avoid use of aspirin in children because of the association with Reye's syndrome.
- Antibiotics if bacterial pneumonia is proved or suspected.
- Amantadine is NOT recommended due to resistant isolates.
- Neuraminidase inhibitors block release of virions from infected cells, resulting in shortened duration of symptoms and decrease in complications; effective against both influenza A and B, including A (H3N2v) for all hospitalized patients, those with severe and progressive illness, and high-risk patients with suspected or confirmed H3N2v.
  1. Oseltamivir, administered orally:
     a. For treatment, 75 mg PO twice daily for 5 days.
     b. For prevention, 75 mg PO once daily for a minimum of 2 wk in an outbreak setting or 7 days after exposure for an adult.
  2. Zanamivir, administered via inhaler:
     a. For treatment, 10 mg (2 inhalations of 5 mg each) twice daily for 5 days.

TABLE 1 Pulmonary Radiographic Findings Based on Virus Type

Virus	Centrilobular Nodules	Lobar Ground-Glass	Diffuse Ground-Glass	Thickened Interlobular Septa	Consolidation
Influenza	+++	+++	+		+
Epstein-Barr	+	+	+		+
Cytomegalovirus	++	++	++	+	+
Varicella-zoster	+++	+	+		
Herpes simplex	+	+++	+		+++
Measles	++	+	+		+
Hantavirus			+++	+	++
Adenovirus	++	+			+++

From Weissleder R et al: *Primer of diagnostic imaging,* ed 5, St Louis, 2011, Mosby.

b. For prevention in households, 10 mg (2 inhalations of 5 mg each) once daily for 7 days. Not recommended in persons with underlying airways disease such as asthma or chronic obstructive pulmonary disease.
c. Adjust dosing in patients with renal impairment or end-stage renal disease.

3. Baloxavir (Xofluza) was approved by the FDA in 2018 for acute uncomplicated influenza infection in patients ≥ 12 years of age. Its mechanism of action is through inhibition of an endonuclease involved in viral RNA replication. It is a single dose drug.

- Placebo-controlled studies have suggested that antiviral therapy with any of the previously mentioned agents must ideally be initiated within 1 to 2 days of the onset of symptoms and reduces the duration of illness by ~1 day.
- Oseltamivir resistance developed on therapy in individuals with avian flu (H5N1) in Asia, and this is associated with poor outcome.
- Amantadine and rimantadine resistance are documented for novel (H1N1) influenza and H3N2 influenza virus.
- Systemic corticosteroids should not be routinely administered to patients with suspected or confirmed influenza, including H3N2v virus infection, except for patients on chronic corticosteroid therapy for COPD, asthma.
- Recent trials[1] have shown that in patients hospitalized with severe influenza infection, triple therapy with clarithromycin 500 mg, naproxen 200 mg, and oseltamivir 75 mg BID for 30 days reduced mortality and did not increase complications compared with oseltamivir (75 mg BID for 5 days) alone.

DISPOSITION

Patients are hospitalized if signs of pneumonia are present.

REFERRAL

Infectious disease and/or pulmonary consultation when influenza pneumonia is suspected.

[1]Hung IFN et al: Efficacy of clarithromycin-naproxen-oseltamivir combination in the treatment of patients hospitalized for influenza (H3N2) infection: an open-lab, randomized, controlled, phase IIb/III trial, *Chest* 151:1069–1080, 2017.

PEARLS & CONSIDERATIONS

COMMENTS

- Prevention of influenza in patients at high risk is an important goal of primary care.
- Vaccines reduce the risk of infection and the severity of illness.
  1. Antigenic composition of the vaccine is updated annually. The northern hemisphere's 2018-2019 season trivalent vaccine includes an A/Michigan/45/2015 (H1N1) pdm09-like virus, an A/Singapore/INFIMH-16-0019 A(H3N2)-like virus, and a B/Colorado/06/2017-like (B/Victoria lineage) virus.
  2. Quadrivalent vaccines contain these three vaccine viruses, plus a second influenza B vaccine virus strain called B/Phuket/3073/2013-like (B/Yamagata lineage) virus.
  3. Revaccination is recommended annually before onset of influenza activity in the community, even for those who received the vaccine in the previous season.
  4. Delaying vaccination to ensure persistence of vaccine-induced protection during flu season could result in missed opportunities to vaccinate.
  5. Seasonal influenza vaccine does not provide protection against the influenza A (H3N2v) virus that is associated with agricultural fairs.
  6. Vaccination should be given at the start of the flu season (September-October) for all persons aged ≥6 mo. Vaccination is particularly important for persons who are at increased risk for severe complications from influenza. When vaccine supply is limited, vaccination efforts should focus on the following groups:
     a. All children aged 6 mo to 4 yr (59 mo).
     b. People 50 yr and older.
     c. Adults and children with chronic cardiac (except hypertension) or pulmonary (including asthma), renal, hepatic, neurologic, hematologic or metabolic disease (including diabetes mellitus).
     d. Immunocompromised patients (including HIV-infected persons or patients immunosuppressed due to medications).
     e. Women who are or will be pregnant during the influenza season.
     f. Children aged 6 mo to 18 yr who are receiving long-term aspirin therapy.
     g. Residents of nursing homes and other long-term care facilities.
     h. American Indians/Alaska Natives.
     i. Persons who are morbidly obese (BMI ≥40).
     j. Health care workers (HCWs).
     k. Household contacts and caregivers of persons in the previous groups.
  7. Vaccination should be delayed for persons with moderate to severe acute febrile illness. Precautions include:
     a. Guillain-Barré syndrome within 6 wk following a previous dose of influenza vaccine.
     b. Moderate or severe acute illness with or without fever (for trivalent inactivated influenza vaccine).
  8. Contraindication to receiving vaccine is a previous severe allergic reaction to influenza vaccine.
  9. Special efforts should be made to vaccinate high-risk patients <65 yr, only 10% to 15% of whom are vaccinated each yr.
  10. HCW vaccination minimizes transmission to patients and coworkers. Some states mandate vaccination of HCWs; some healthcare facilities and other states require the wearing of face masks by unvaccinated HCWs during the influenza season, particularly when there is widespread flu.
  11. Vaccine efficacy varies by age and by type of circulating virus. Efficacy varies each yr and has ranged from 23% to 60% overall; 2017-2018 efficacy was low. Even with low efficacy, hospitalizations are reduced.
  12. Alternate vaccine formulations:
      a. Intradermal vaccine is available for injection into skin instead of muscle. This uses a smaller needle than the regular flu vaccine and might be preferred by adults aged 18 to 64 yr who do not like shots.
      b. The CDC's Advisory Committee on Immunization Practices (ACIP) found no measurable protective benefit from using nasal spray, live-attenuated influenza vaccine (LAIV) during the

TABLE 2 Antiviral Agents for Influenza

	Amantadine	Rimantadine	Zanamivir	Oseltamivir
Protein target	M2	M2	Neuraminidase	Neuraminidase
Activity	A only (H1N1 and H3N2 are resistant)	A only (H1N1 and H3N2 are resistant)	A and B	A and B
Side effects	CNS (13%) GI (3%)	GI (6%)	? Bronchospasm	GI (9%)
Metabolism	None	Multiple (hepatic)	None	Hepatic
Excretion	Renal	Renal,+ others	Renal	Renal (tubular secretion)
Drug interactions	Antihistamines, anticholinergics	None	None	Probenecid (increased levels of oseltamivir)
Dose adjustments needed	≥65 yr old CrCl <50 ml/min	≥65 yr old CrCl <10 ml/min	None	CrCl <30 ml/min Severe liver dysfunction
Contraindications	Acute-angle glaucoma	Severe liver dysfunction	Underlying airway disease, asthma	
FDA-Approved Indications				
Therapy	Adults and children ≥1 yr old	Adults only	Adults and children ≥7 yr old	Adults and children ≥1 yr old*
Prophylaxis	Yes	Yes	Adults and children ≥5 yr old	Adults and children ≥13 yr old†

CNS, Central nervous system; *CrCl,* creatinine clearance; *FDA,* U.S. Food and Drug Administration; *GI,* gastrointestinal.
*FDA has authorized treatment of S-OIV (novel H1N1) virus with oseltamivir in children ≥3 mo of age.
†FDA has authorized prophylaxis for S-OIV (novel H1N1) virus with oseltamivir in children ≥1 yr.
From Mandell GL et al: *Principles and practice of infectious diseases,* ed 7, Philadelphia, 2010, Churchill Livingstone.

2015-2016 flu season. ACIP recently reviewed more data and found LAIV4 effective against influenza B and influenza A (H3N2). Effectiveness of the updated LAIV4 against currently circulating influenza A (H1N1) pdm09-like viruses is unknown. ACIP recommends any licensed, age-appropriate influenza vaccine, including LAIV4, for the 2018-2019 season.

c. Give TIV if recipient has egg allergy or asthma or cares for immunosuppressed persons who require a protective environment.
d. Thimerosal-free vaccine is available.
e. IIV can be trivalent or quadrivalent, and egg-based or non-egg-based (cell culture or recombinant hemagglutinin).
f. There is no preference for standard dose IIV, high dose IIV (age 65 or over) or intradermal IIV (ages 18-64).
g. ACIP guidance for egg allergies:
   (1) If a person with egg allergy experiences only hives, then administer trivalent recombinant hemagglutinin influenza vaccine (RIV3) if ages 18 to 49, or IIV and observe for at least 30 minutes for reaction following vaccine.
   (2) If a person with egg allergy experiences other symptoms such as cardiovascular (e.g., hypotension), respiratory distress (e.g., wheezing), gastrointestinal (e.g., nausea/vomiting), reaction requiring epinephrine or emergency medical attention, administer RIV3 if age 18 to 49, or refer to a physician with expertise in management of allergic conditions.
   (3) If there is no known history of exposure to egg, but the person is suspected of having egg allergy, consult with a physician who has expertise in the management of allergies before vaccinating, or give RIV3 (if ages 18 to 49).

- Chemoprophylaxis:
  1. Table 2 describes antiviral agents for influenza. Oseltamivir and zanamivir are recommended in the U.S. during the influenza season. Baloxavir marboxil was recently (2018) FDA approved and may eventually replace the other agents as a preferred drug (single dose, low side effects profile).
  2. Consider (after the current circulating strain of influenza has been shown to be sensitive):
     a. For high-risk patients in whom vaccination is contraindicated.
     b. When the available vaccine is known not to include the circulating strain.
     c. To provide added protection to immunosuppressed patients likely to have a diminished response to vaccination.
     d. In the setting of an outbreak, when immediate protection of unvaccinated or recently vaccinated patients at high risk of complications is desired.
  3. Chemoprophylaxis with antiviral drugs is not recommended for healthy persons exposed to seasonal influenza.
  4. Give for 2 wk in the case of late vaccination and for the duration of the flu season in all other patients.
  5. Treatment should not wait for laboratory confirmation of influenza.
  6. Do not give aspirin or aspirin-containing products to children with influenza-like illness due to the risk of Reye's syndrome.
- Other prevention strategies:
  1. Hand hygiene, cough etiquette (cover your cough), respiratory hygiene (use of tissues, facemasks for the ill and proper disposal).
  2. Seasonal flu personal protective equipment (PPE)—wear gloves and gowns as per universal/standard precautions. Per the CDC, wear a facemask, adhering to Droplet Precautions for 7 days after illness onset or until 24 hr after fever and respiratory symptoms are resolved, whichever is longer. Patient placement in a negative pressure room and N95 respirator for health care workers are recommended when conducting aerosol-generating procedures.
  3. Highly pathogenic Asian avian influenza (HPAI) includes H5N1, H7N9, H5N2, and H5N8. CDC recommends wearing eye protection, N95 respirator, gown, and gloves as for airborne and contact precautions.
  4. Management of ill health care workers—exclude from work until at least 24 hr after they no longer have a fever (without the use of fever-reducing medication). Extended exclusion time period when caring for severely immunocompromised patients.
  5. Standard cleaning and disinfection procedures.
- The Centers for Medicare and Medicaid Services links health care worker vaccine acceptance with payment for performance.

SUGGESTED READINGS

Available at ExpertConsult.com

RELATED CONTENT

Influenza (Flu) (Patient Information)

AUTHOR: **MARLENE FISHMAN WOLPERT, M.P.H., C.I.C., F.A.P.I.C.**

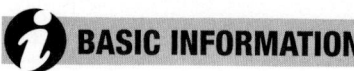

BASIC INFORMATION

DEFINITION

Inguinal hernias are characterized by their location and reducibility. An ***indirect*** inguinal hernia courses from the internal inguinal ring, toward the external inguinal ring, and into the scrotum. A ***direct*** inguinal hernia bulges directly outward and is medial to the internal inguinal ring. An irreducible (i.e., not able to be pushed back into the abdominal cavity) inguinal hernia is ***incarcerated*** and may be associated with moderate to severe pain, tenderness to palpation and/or overlying erythema. A ***strangulated*** inguinal hernia is an incarcerated hernia with a compromised blood supply and ischemia resulting in moderate to severe pain, tenderness to palpation, overlying erythema, +/- fever, and/or nausea and vomiting.

SYNONYMS

Groin hernia
Indirect hernia
Direct hernia

ICD-10CM CODES

K40	Inguinal hernia
K40.9	Inguinal hernia without obstruction or gangrene

EPIDEMIOLOGY & DEMOGRAPHICS

INCIDENCE: Incidence is unknown.
PEAK INCIDENCE: Increases with age
PREVALENCE: Approximately 5% of the population experiences an abdominal hernia, and 75% of these are inguinal hernias. Two thirds of inguinal hernias are indirect, and the rest are direct.
PREDOMINANT SEX AND AGE: Male gender and increasing age are associated with increased incidence of inguinal hernias.
RISK FACTORS: History of hernia repair, older age, male sex, Caucasian race, family history, smoking

PHYSICAL FINDINGS & CLINICAL PRESENTATION

- Patients with asymptomatic or mildly symptomatic inguinal hernias often present with a complaint of groin bulging, discomfort or both.
- Patients with incarcerated or strangulated inguinal hernias present with moderate to severe groin pain and tenderness to palpation and may have overlying erythema, fever, nausea or vomiting.
- The most common physical exam findings are palpable groin bulging within the scrotum (indirect hernia) (Fig. 1) or inguinal region (direct hernia); this may be best appreciated in the standing position. In males, an asymptomatic indirect hernia may be detected by invaginating the scrotal tissue, following the spermatic cord into the external femoral ring and instructing the patient to perform the Valsalva maneuver.

ETIOLOGY

Inguinal hernias are caused by a defect in the abdominal wall that is present at birth or develops with age.

Dx DIAGNOSIS

DIFFERENTIAL DIAGNOSIS

- Other hernias: Femoral, abdominal (Fig. 2)
- Testicular: Testicular torsion, epididymitis
- Pregnant patient: Round ligament varicosity
- Vascular: Femoral aneurysm or pseudoaneurysm
- Lymphatic: Inguinal lymphadenitis, lymphogranuloma venereum

WORKUP

- Uncomplicated inguinal hernias may be diagnosed based on history or physical examination.
- If the diagnosis is unclear and the patient is asymptomatic or mildly symptomatic (mild discomfort), proceed to imaging.
- If the patient is moderately or severely symptomatic, or incarcerated or strangulated hernia is suspected, refer the patient to an emergency department.

LABORATORY TESTS

- Asymptomatic and mildly symptomatic patients require no laboratory testing.
- All other patients should be referred to an emergent setting for a complete blood count, basic metabolic panel, lactate, PT/INR and type and screen.

IMAGING STUDIES

- If there is low concern for incarcerated or strangulated hernia (e.g., groin bulging with mild discomfort), yet the diagnosis remains unclear, obtain a groin ultrasound.
- If there is clinical concern for incarcerated or strangulated hernia (e.g., moderate to severe pain, overlying redness, nausea, vomiting, fever, increased bowel sounds), refer to the emergency department for CT abdomen/pelvis with IV contrast.

Rx TREATMENT

Asymptomatic and mildly symptomatic inguinal hernias can be referred on an outpatient basis to a general surgeon for expectant management.
Suspected incarcerated or strangulated hernias should be referred to an emergency department for reduction and/or emergent surgical consultation.

NONPHARMACOLOGIC THERAPY

Although spring trusses are more commonly used in Europe, a surgeon may fit the patient with one during a period of watchful waiting.

ACUTE GENERAL Rx

- Patients with suspected incarcerated hernias need emergent reduction. This is best accomplished in an emergency department setting given the frequent need for intravenous medications.
- Incarcerated hernias sometimes can be reduced with firm direct pressure when the patient is in the Trendelenburg position; most require intravenous analgesia.

CHRONIC Rx

Patients with easily reducible, mildly symptomatic hernias can be referred to a general surgeon for expectant management.

DISPOSITION

- Patients without suspected incarcerated or strangulated hernia can be dispositioned home.
- Patients with moderate or severely symptomatic hernias or suspected incarcerated or strangulated hernias should be dispositioned to an emergent setting.

REFERRAL

- Mildly symptomatic patients should be referred to a general surgeon on an outpatient basis for watchful waiting.
- Moderately symptomatic patients (with no signs or symptoms of incarceration) should be referred urgently to a general surgeon for consideration of elective repair.
- Patients who present with potential incarceration or strangulation should be referred to an emergency department for reduction and emergent surgical consultation.

FIG. 1 Left indirect inguinal hernia. (From Swartz MH: *Textbook of physical diagnosis, history and examination*, ed 7, 2014, Elsevier.)

SUGGESTED READINGS

Available at ExpertConsult.com

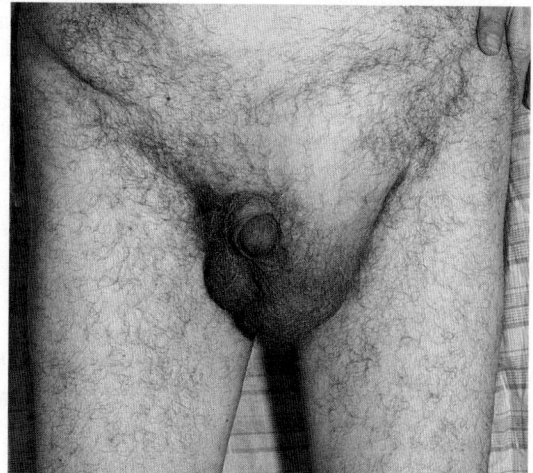

AUTHORS: **RORY MERRITT, M.D.,** and **BRIAN CLYNE, M.D.**

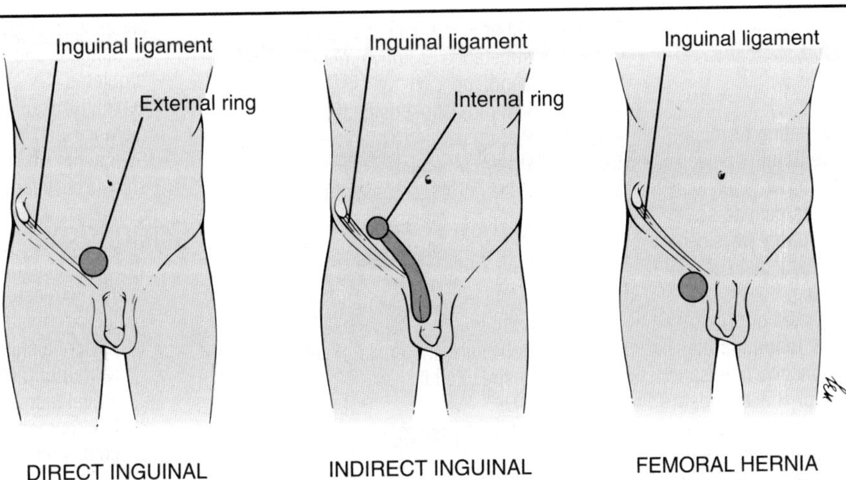

Feature	Direct Inguinal*	Indirect Inguinal†	Femoral
Occurrence	Middle-aged and elderly men	All ages	Least common: more frequently found in women
Bilaterality	55%	30%	Rarely
Origin of swelling	Above inguinal ligament; directly behind and through external ring	Above inguinal ligament; hernial sac enters inguinal canal at internal ring and exits at external ring	Below inguinal ligament
Scrotal involvement	Rare	Common	None
Impulse location	At side of examining finger in ingunal canal	At tip of examining finger in inguinal canal	Not felt by examining finger in inguinal canal; mass below canal

*See Figure 15-43.
†See Figure 15-42.

FIG. 2 Differential diagnosis of hernias. (From Swartz MH: *Textbook of physical diagnosis, history and examination*, ed 7, 2014, Elsevier.)

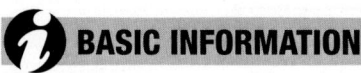

BASIC INFORMATION

DEFINITION

Insomnia is a disturbance of initiating or maintaining sleep. Restless, nonrestorative sleep may also be described as another specified insomnia. The disturbance occurs despite adequate circumstances and opportunity for sleep and is accompanied by significant distress or impairment in daytime functioning.

In the new DSM-5, the diagnosis of primary insomnia has been replaced with **insomnia disorder** in order to avoid the distinction between primary and secondary forms of the disorder. This paradigm shift relates to widely accepted research in the field suggesting that there is a bidirectional and interactive relationship between insomnia and any coexisting medical and/or mental disorders.

SYNONYMS

Sleeplessness

Sleep disorder, sleep disturbance, dyssomnia (NOTE: The terms *sleep disorder, sleep disturbance,* and *dyssomnia* are generic and can refer to disorders of wakefulness [hypersomnia] or sleep-related behavior disorders [parasomnias])

Insomnia disorder

ICD-10CM CODES

F51.01	Primary insomnia
F51.02	Adjustment insomnia
F51.03	Paradoxical insomnia
F51.04	Psychophysiologic insomnia
F51.05	Insomnia due to other mental disorder
F51.09	Other insomnia not due to a substance or known physiological condition
G47.00	Insomnia, unspecified
G47.01	Insomnia due to medical condition
G47.09	Other insomnia
Z73.810	Behavioral insomnia of childhood, sleep-onset association type
Z73.811	Behavioral insomnia of childhood, limit setting type
Z73.812	Behavioral insomnia of childhood, combined type
Z73.819	Behavioral insomnia of childhood, unspecified type

DSM-5 CODES

Depends on specific diagnosis.

EPIDEMIOLOGY & DEMOGRAPHICS

INCIDENCE (IN U.S.): 30% to 45% of adults experience occasional bouts of acute insomnia.

PREVALENCE (IN U.S.): 1% to 15% of all adults and 25% of older adults develop persistent insomnia.

PREDOMINANT SEX: More common in women

PREDOMINANT AGE: Transient insomnia can occur at any age; persistent insomnia can also occur at any age but is more common after age 60 yr.

GENETICS: Can run in families and may be genetically influenced. Circadian rhythm disorders and narcolepsy have been traced to specific genes.

PHYSICAL FINDINGS & CLINICAL PRESENTATION

- Difficulty initiating sleep, inability to maintain sleep, and/or early morning awakening.
- Significant distress or impairment in daytime functioning such as fatigue or low energy, sleepiness, cognitive impairments, mood disturbances, and/or physiologic or behavioral problems.
- Difficulty occurs despite adequate opportunity for sleep.
- Symptoms may be acute and self-limited, chronic but intermittent, or chronic and frequent.

ETIOLOGY

- Transient insomnia:
  1. Any stressful biopsychosocial change in life circumstance (e.g., marriage, divorce, birth of a child, loss of a loved one, illness, retirement, etc.)
  2. Travel (across time zones)
  3. Environmental disruptions (noise, heat, cold, poor bedding, bed partners, unfamiliar surroundings, etc.)
- Persistent insomnia (Fig. 1):
  1. Mood and anxiety disorders (depression, hypomania/mania, PTSD)
  2. Psychophysiologic insomnia (conditioned arousal, extended sleep opportunity, sleep effort, poor sleep hygiene)
  3. Sleep-related breathing disorders (e.g., obstructive apnea and hypopnea, increased upper airway resistance)
  4. Chronobiologic (also known as circadian rhythm) disorder (delayed sleep phase, advanced sleep phase, shift work, non-24-hr sleep-wake disorder secondary to blindness)
  5. Drug and alcohol abuse
  6. Restless legs syndrome and periodic leg movements
  7. Neurodegenerative (Alzheimer's disease, Parkinson's disease, etc.)
  8. Medical (pain, GERD, nocturia, orthopnea, menopause, medications, etc.)

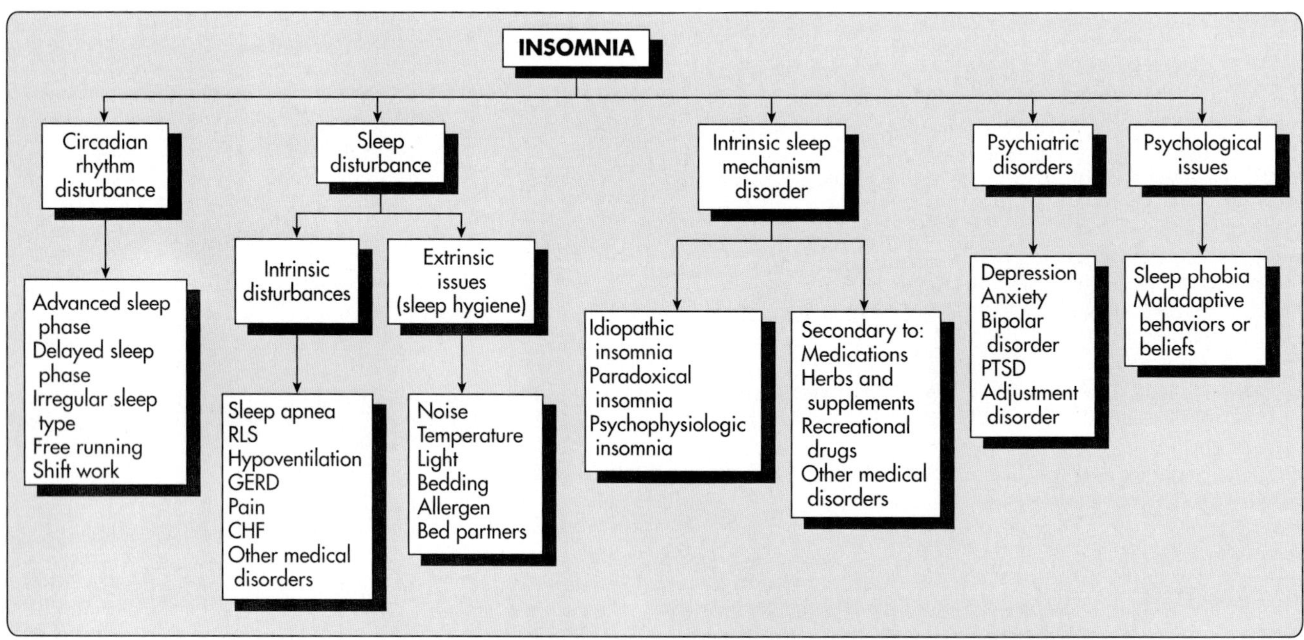

FIG. 1 Diagnostic flowchart to approach insomnia. *CHF,* Congestive heart failure; *GERD,* gastroesophageal reflux disease; *PTSD,* posttraumatic stress disorder; *RLS,* restless legs syndrome. (From Kryger MH et al: *Principles and practice of sleep medicine*, ed 6, Philadelphia, 2017, Elsevier.)

I

Diseases and Disorders

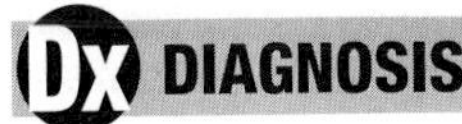

DIAGNOSIS

Diagnostic and Statistical Manual of Mental Disorders (DSM-5) criteria for the diagnosis of insomnia disorder is as follows:[1]

- Dissatisfaction with sleep quantity or quality, with one or more of the following symptoms:
- Difficulty initiating sleep
- Difficulty maintaining sleep, characterized by frequent awakenings or trouble returning to sleep after awakenings
- Early-morning awakening with inability to return to sleep
- The sleep disturbance causes clinically significant distress or impairment in daytime functioning, as evidenced by at least one of the following:
  1. Fatigue or low energy
  2. Daytime sleepiness
  3. Impaired attention, concentration, or memory
  4. Mood disturbance
  5. Behavioral difficulties
  6. Impaired occupational or academic function
  7. Impaired interpersonal or social function
  8. Negative effect on caregiver or family functioning
- The sleep difficulty occurs at least 3 nights per week, is present for at least 3 months, and occurs despite adequate opportunity for sleep

DIFFERENTIAL DIAGNOSIS

Insomnia disorder is only ruled out when the disorder is seen exclusively during other etiologies (see "Etiology"). It can be precipitated by a "primary" medical, mental health, or other sleep-wake disorder, but often continues as a comorbid condition even after the "primary disorder" has been treated. For example, insomnia remains the most resistant symptom following the treatment of depression. Its continued expression complicates the treatment of depression, reduces remission rates, and increases the likelihood of relapse of depression. Once evidence has been established of ongoing perpetuating factors such as conditioned arousal, sleep extension, worry and rumination about sleep, and sleep effort, this predicts that the insomnia will not likely remit even with the remission of the original precipitating stressor or disorder.

Circadian rhythm disturbances such as those seen in shift workers, blind individuals who lack a light-dark cycle to synchronize the body clock, adolescents and young adults with delayed sleep phase syndrome, and people with jet lag can mimic signs and symptoms of insomnia, especially initial and late insomnia. These disorders can be treated with chronobiologic therapies such as chronotherapy, bright light exposure, melatonin, or melatonin agonists. However, the timing of these interventions can be critical to outcome and constitutes therapies that are very different from standard medical and/or behavioral treatment for insomnia.

[1]American Psychiatric Association: *Diagnostic and statistical manual of mental disorders,* 5th ed, American Psychiatric Publishing, Arlington, VA, 2013.

BOX 1 Sleep Habits (Sleep Hygiene Measures) That May Improve Sleep

1. Reduce caffeine, alcohol, or tobacco late in the day or especially evening.
2. Avoid heavy meals at night, but consider a light snack before bed such as toast or a handful of nuts.
3. Increase daytime activity, but avoid exercise within 3-5 hours of bedtime.
4. Increase daytime exposure to natural light.
5. Reduce liquids in the last 4 hours before bedtime.
6. Consider white noise as background sound for the sleep environment.
7. Maintain regular bed and wake times.
8. Go to bed with calm mind; resolve arguments or set a time earlier in the day to review problems and perhaps write down plans, solutions, or things to do.
9. Keep light exposure in the middle of the night to a minimum when awake and attenuate morning light in the bedroom.
10. Avoid pets in the bed.

WORKUP

- History (with bed partner interview, if possible).
- Sleep diary for 2 wk (Consider the Consensus Sleep Diary [Carney CE et al in Suggested Readings]).
- Wrist actigraphy (detects gross limb movements and can distinguish wake from sleep states) as an adjunct to a sleep diary provides some objective verification of the diary data and provides prospective measurement of sleep and wake across the 24-hr day. Actigraphy should not be considered an alternative to prospective sleep diary data.
- Validated sleep-quality rating scale (optional).
  1. Insomnia Severity Index.
  2. Pittsburgh Sleep Quality Index.
  3. Epworth Sleepiness Scale (see Daytime Sleepiness Test at http://www.sleepfoundation.org).

LABORATORY TESTS

- Evaluate for anemia (especially low ferritin level), uremia (for restless legs), thyroid function (if other signs present).
- Polysomnography (in home or in sleep laboratory) is not standard for insomnia but should be reserved for patients whose history suggests specific sleep-related breathing or movement disorders. It is indicated for symptoms suggestive of daytime sleepiness (obstructive sleep apnea, narcolepsy), nonrestorative sleep (periodic leg movements, chronic pain conditions), or sleep behavior suggesting parasomnia (somnambulism, REM sleep behavior).

IMAGING STUDIES

- Not generally helpful
- Brain CT or MRI for severe daytime sleepiness or acute onset

Rx TREATMENT

NONPHARMACOLOGIC THERAPY

- Sleep hygiene measures (Box 1) as a monotherapy are not very effective in cases of persistent insomnia. More useful if combined with procedures described next.
- Cognitive-behavioral therapy (CBT-I) has been shown to reduce time to fall asleep and time awake during the night, can reduce reliance on sleep medications, and has shown lasting effects after treatment has been discontinued. It should be the initial treatment option in persons with chronic insomnia.
- The standard components that comprise CBT-I are as follows:
  1. Stimulus control, which addresses the conditioned cues that create arousal when attempting to sleep by restricting activity in bed to sleep and sex and not permitting sleep effort, worrying, watching TV, reading, etc., in bed (reconditioning of this type can take several days or weeks—patients should not come to expect positive changes on the first night).
  2. Sleep restriction therapy reduces sleep opportunity to the average amount of total sleep time the patient is getting as determined by baseline sleep diary data. Sleep time is increased incrementally, based on improving sleep efficiency. Note that restricted time in bed should never be <5 hr. For the elderly and infirm, average total sleep time plus 30 min is sometimes considered. For patients whose estimated average total sleep time is <4hr, a diagnosis of paradoxical insomnia should be considered and CBT-I would be contraindicated. Caution should also be exercised when using sleep restriction therapy in bipolar disorder and seizure disorders, as sleep deprivation early in treatment can precipitate a manic episode and lower seizure threshold, respectively.
  3. Cognitive therapy targets unhelpful beliefs and worries about sleep, negative and unwanted thoughts, sleep effort, selective attention bias and monitoring, misperception of sleep and daytime deficits, and counterproductive safety behaviors that are thought to maintain insomnia.
  4. Sleep hygiene is aimed at improving sleep habits (e.g., initiating or maintaining exercise, avoiding heavy meals at night, and altering the timing of or eliminating caffeine, nicotine, and alcohol intake). Environmental factors should also be addressed (e.g., using white noise and/or light attenuating bedroom). Caffeine sometimes can prove useful when used judiciously in the morning and early afternoon to combat the increased fatigue and somnolence that are produced early in therapy with sleep restriction and stimulus control. In addition, exercise contin-

gently applied to daytime fatigue can also help to improve alertness during the day and increase sleep pressure at bedtime.

5. Relaxation exercises (e.g., progressive muscle relaxation, diaphragmatic breathing) may be good adjunctive therapy, especially in highly anxious patients, but are not thought to be essential in CBT-I. Increasingly, mindfulness-based practices are being effectively utilized alone and in combination with other elements of CBT-I. Mindfulness may help patients to adopt a more flexible and accepting stance toward insomnia.

ACUTE GENERAL Rx

- Benzodiazepine receptor agonists zolpidem 5 mg and zaleplon 5 mg for sleep-onset insomnia, and zolpidem continuous-release formulation 6.25 to 12.5 mg and eszopiclone 1 to 3 mg for maintenance insomnia.
- Suvorexant is an orexin receptor antagonist FDA approved for insomnia. Signaling of orexin neuropeptides sustains wakefulness. Suvorexant promotes sleep by blocking orexin neuropeptides from binding to their receptors. The initial dose is 10 mg once daily within 30 minutes of bedtime. Most common side effect (10%) is next-day somnolence.
- Benzodiazepine sedative-hypnotics (e.g., temazepam 7.5-30 mg, triazolam 0.125-0.25 mg).
- A low-dose formulation (6 mg) of the tricyclic antidepressant doxepin, brand name Silenor, is also FDA approved for treatment of insomnia associated with sleep maintenance. This dose retains the hypnotic effect of doxepin without the typical tricyclic effects. A generic 10 mg/ml liquid formulation of doxepin is also available.
- In critical care: Lorazepam 0.25 to 0.5 mg PO, SL, or IV as needed for sleep. In patients with acute delirium, haloperidol 0.25 to 0.5 mg IV as needed up to 2 mg/day may be less likely to worsen confusion.
- Melatonin agonist ramelteon 8 mg for sleep-onset insomnia when a mild agent without benzodiazepine side effects is desired.
- Avoid antihistamines except for occasional use.
- Optimize treatment of medical symptoms, especially pain.
- Most prescription and over-the-counter medications carry significant risk of adverse events and drug interactions, especially in the geriatric patient. Preferred pharmacotherapeutic agents in the elderly are zolpidem, zaleplon, eszopiclone, and ramelteon.

CHRONIC Rx

- Considerable research supports the efficacy of CBT-I, with acute treatment outcomes equivalent to pharmacotherapy, and better long-term outcomes and maintenance of treatment gains. Although there is limited availability of CBT-I specialists, especially in certain geographic areas, there are now online interactive evidence-based self-help programs that can serve as an effective base for a stepped model of care. Patients who fail these attempts should still be encouraged to seek more tailored treatment with a specialist, especially when the insomnia is comorbid with other conditions.
- When CBT-I is applied to patients with related comorbidities (e.g., depression, chronic pain), evidence suggests that targeted treatment for insomnia not only results in significant improvement of the insomnia but, in many cases, influences the course of the related comorbidities. For example, when CBT-I is applied concurrently with antidepressants, it has the effect of doubling remission rates in depression and reduces suicidal ideation by up to 65%. In a recent study of patients with comorbid depression and insomnia, head-to-head comparison of Internet-based treatments for depression (dCBT-D) and insomnia (dCBT-I) demonstrated that dCBT-I outperformed dCBT-D for insomnia and matched its efficacy in depression.
- Note that the American College of Physicians recently published clinical guidelines for the management of chronic insomnia disorder, suggesting that CBT-I be the first-line treatment for insomnia and recommending that it be attempted before pharmacologic approaches when possible.
- Three sedative-hypnotics—zolpidem continuous release, eszopiclone, and ramelteon—FDA approved for long-term use.
- Some evidence shows that benzodiazepines and benzodiazepine receptor agonists can be used for chronic insomnia on either intermittent or nightly use with moderate risk of tolerance and dependence but low risk of addiction.
- Sedating antidepressants (e.g., trazodone 25-150 mg, mirtazapine 7.5-30 mg, amitriptyline 25-50 mg, doxepin 10 mg) are in widespread use, with limited data on safety and efficacy. Amitriptyline should be avoided in older adults.
- Sedating antipsychotics (e.g., quetiapine 25-200 mg, olanzapine 2.5-10 mg at night) considered for severe mood or psychotic disorders associated with insomnia.

COMPLEMENTARY & ALTERNATIVE MEDICINE

Melatonin may shorten sleep-onset latency in some individuals. It may have more clinical utility in the management of circadian rhythm disorders. Timing of administration in these types of cases requires careful consideration and would not be often administered at bedtime.

DISPOSITION

- Transient (acute) insomnia: Usually self-limited. May require follow-up if stress-related or illness-related because of risk of depression or persistence. Prophylactic education regarding maladaptive sleep practices such as extending time in bed, and/or remaining in bed when unable to sleep, might be helpful in avoiding a more protracted course of insomnia.
- Persistent insomnia: Patients who respond well to CBT-I often continue to maintain gains at 1-and 2-yr follow-ups. Patients may need periodic follow-up to reinforce good sleep hygiene and stimulus control and for reevaluation of pharmacologic therapies. There is now a compelling amount of evidence that insomnia, if left untreated, is associated with significant negative mental and health effects over time.

REFERRAL

- A referral to a behavioral medicine specialist may be required for CBT-I or for circadian rhythm disturbances (find a directory at http://www.behavioralsleep.org/findspecialist.aspx)
- Excessive daytime sleepiness not obviously caused by insomnia (e.g., narcolepsy, sleep-related breathing disorder)
- Nighttime behavior suggestive of a parasomnia (e.g., somnambulism, REM behavior disorder)
- Severe insomnia not responsive to basic interventions

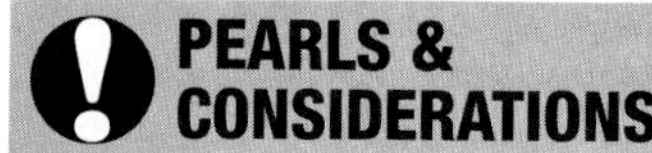

PEARLS & CONSIDERATIONS

COMMENTS

CBT-I often results in worse sleep and more fatigue in the short run. Patients often respond to initial worsening of symptoms as a sign of failure; however, they should be encouraged to see this as an important piece of the therapy and to stay the course as new conditioned patterns begin to emerge, sleep efficiency improves, and total sleep time gradually increases.

Patients should avoid compensating for lost sleep by extending sleep opportunity in the form of going to bed early, sleeping in, or napping. Therefore, early treatment should focus on helping patients to manage daytime fatigue and sleepiness by engaging in activities that help patients stay awake and maintain set bed and wake times.

PREVENTION

It is estimated that 50% to 70% of individuals demonstrating the syndrome of insomnia (e.g., insomnia symptoms more than 3 days per week for a month along with deleterious daytime sequelae) are still syndromic 1 to 5 yr later. Therefore, early intervention with medication or education to prevent the development of maladaptive compensatory behaviors (e.g., napping, sleeping late, tossing and turning in bed, avoiding or decreasing daytime activity) may help to reduce the risk of developing persistent insomnia.

PATIENT & FAMILY EDUCATION

The National Sleep Foundation (http://www.sleepfoundation.org) is a comprehensive resource for health care providers and patients.

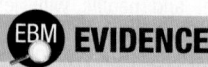

EVIDENCE

Available at ExpertConsult.com

SUGGESTED READINGS

Available at ExpertConsult.com

RELATED CONTENT

Sleep disorders (Algorithm in Section III)
Insomnia (Patient Information)

AUTHOR: **DONN POSNER, PH.D.**

BASIC INFORMATION

DEFINITION

The interstitial lung diseases (ILDs) include more than 150 nonmalignant disorders, characterized by varying degrees of damage to the lung parenchyma or interstitium via inflammation and fibrosis. The term "ILD" can be confusing as processes affecting the alveolar space (e.g., pulmonary alveolar proteinosis) are also lumped under the title. A clinical classification of the interstitial lung diseases is summarized in Table 1. The diseases can generally divided into three subgroups—those that are caused by an identifiable or suspected trigger, those that are associated with an underlying, more systemic disorder, and those that are idiopathic.

SYNONYMS

Interstitial pulmonary disease
ILD
Diffuse parenchymal lung disease (DPLD)
Interstitial pneumonia

ICD-10CM CODES

J84.17	Other interstitial pulmonary diseases with fibrosis in diseases classified elsewhere
J84.89	Other specified interstitial pulmonary diseases
J84.9	Interstitial pulmonary disease, unspecified
J84.115	Respiratory bronchiolitis interstitial lung disease
J84.848	Other interstitial lung diseases of childhood

EPIDEMIOLOGY & DEMOGRAPHICS

INCIDENCE AND PREVALENCE: Varies widely with type of ILD. The most common ILDs are sarcoidosis, cryptogenic organizing pneumonia, and idiopathic pulmonary fibrosis. The prevalence of these syndromes varies widely across different populations as defined by age, gender, and race.

PREDOMINANT SEX & AGE: Some ILDs are more common in women, such as those resulting from connective tissue disorders. Lymphangiomyomatosis occurs exclusively in premenopausal women. ILD caused by occupational exposures are more common in men. Most ILDs occur in people >50 yr; however, sarcoidosis most often presents in younger populations.

RISK FACTORS: Although many ILDs are categorized as idiopathic, the most common identifiable risk factors include environmental exposures such as silicone, asbestos, or bird droppings; reactions to drugs such as chemotherapeutic agents; radiation therapy; cardiac medications; and finally some history of connective tissue disease such as rheumatoid arthritis or scleroderma. Both tobacco and drug use can result in an ILD.

PHYSICAL FINDINGS & CLINICAL PRESENTATION

- Shortness of breath (especially with exertion)
- Cough (dry)
- Tachypnea
- Bibasilar end-inspiratory dry crackles
- Pulmonary hypertension
- Cyanosis, clubbing

Hallmarks of ILD include a restrictive pattern and decreased diffusing capacity for carbon monoxide (DLCO) as demonstrated by pulmonary function testing. The restrictive process can be the result of a number of factors depending on the type of ILD. Different types of ILD are characterized by varying degrees of acute inflammatory changes, which are potentially reversible, and fibrosis, which is largely irreversible.

- Specific changes may be seen:
  1. Granulomatous: Accumulation of T lymphocytes, macrophages, and epithelioid cells into granulomas in lung parenchyma
  2. Inflammation and fibrosis: Injury to epithelium causes inflammation; if chronic, inflammation spreads to interstitium and vascular areas

TABLE 1 Clinical Classification of the Interstitial Lung Diseases

Connective Tissue Diseases
Scleroderma
Polymyositis-dermatomyositis
Systemic lupus erythematosus
Rheumatoid arthritis
Mixed connective tissue disease
Ankylosing spondylitis
Treatment-Related or Drug-Induced Diseases
Antibiotics (nitrofurantoin, sulfasalazine)
Antiarrhythmics (amiodarone, tocainide, propranolol)
Antiinflammatories (gold, penicillamine)
Anticonvulsants (Dilantin)
Chemotherapeutic agents (mitomycin C, bleomycin, busulfan, cyclophosphamide, chlorambucil, methotrexate, azathioprine, BCNU [carmustine], procarbazine)
Therapeutic radiation
Oxygen toxicity
Narcotics
Primary and Idiopathic Diseases
Sarcoidosis
Primary pulmonary Langerhans cell histiocytosis (eosinophilic granuloma)
Amyloidosis
Pulmonary vasculitis
Gaucher disease
Niemann-Pick disease
Hermansky-Pudlak syndrome
Neurofibromatosis
Lymphangioleiomyomatosis
Tuberous sclerosis
Idiopathic pulmonary fibrosis
Nonspecific interstitial pneumonia
Cryptogenic organizing pneumonia
Respiratory bronchiolitis ILD or desquamative interstitial pneumonia
Acute interstitial pneumonia
Lymphocytic interstitial pneumonia
Pleuroparenchymal fibroelastosis
Bone marrow transplantation
Eosinophilic pneumonia
Alveolar proteinosis
Alveolar microlithiasis
Metastatic calcification
Occupational and Environmental Diseases
Inorganic
Silicosis
Asbestosis
Hard-metal pneumoconiosis
Coal worker's pneumoconiosis
Berylliosis
Talc pneumoconiosis
Siderosis (arc welder)
Stannosis (tin)
Organic (hypersensitivity pneumonitis)
Bird breeder's lung
Farmer's lung

AIDS, Acquired immunodeficiency syndrome; *ILD*, interstitial lung disease.
Modified from Mason RJ: *Murray & Nadel's textbook of respiratory medicine*, 5th ed, Philadelphia, 2010, Saunders.

ETIOLOGY

There is a wide range of environmental and workplace exposures that can directly result in an ILD. The mechanism by which underlying autoimmunity can lead to an associated ILD is not clear.

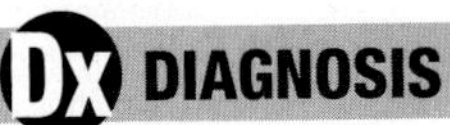

DIAGNOSIS

DIFFERENTIAL DIAGNOSIS

- Congestive heart failure
- Pneumonia: Viral, bacterial, mycobacterial, fungal
- Pulmonary embolism
- COPD
- Pulmonary hypertension
- Vasculitis
- Metastatic malignancy manifesting as lymphangitic carcinomatosis

WORKUP

- Well-defined patterns in pulmonary function tests are usually consistent with restrictive defect (decreased FVC, FRC, RV, and TLC) owing to decreased lung compliance caused by alveolar wall thickening as a result of inflammation and fibrosis. Diffusion capacity is usually reduced also because of inflammation and thickening of alveolar walls, though nonspecific. FEV_1/FVC is usually normal or increased because lung stiffness keeps small airways open, although some conditions (e.g., sarcoidosis, hypersensitivity pneumonitis) may result in air trapping.
- Bronchoscopy and bronchoalveolar lavage (BAL) may help identify type of ILD. However, their role in defining stage of disease and response to therapy is controversial. Histologic patterns in the interstitial lung diseases and their disease associations are summarized in Table 2.
- If laboratory studies and imaging including HRCT fail in yielding a diagnosis, a surgical biopsy may be required. A common objective of performing a biopsy is to evaluate the possibility of idiopathic pulmonary fibrosis, which has a unique approach to treatment.
- Fig. 1 illustrates an algorithm for the approach to a patient with interstitial lung disease.

LABORATORY TESTS

- ABGs may be normal or show respiratory alkalosis and widened Aa gradient.
- Blood tests for connective tissue diseases, such as antinuclear antibodies,

TABLE 2 Histologic Patterns in the Interstitial Lung Diseases and Their Disease Associations

Histologic Patterns	Clinical Associations
Usual interstitial pneumonia	Idiopathic pulmonary fibrosis; connective tissue diseases (uncommon); asbestosis; chronic hypersensitivity pneumonitis; chronic aspiration pneumonia; chronic radiation pneumonitis; Hermansky-Pudlak syndrome
Nonspecific interstitial pneumonia	Idiopathic; connective tissue diseases; drugs; AIDS
Diffuse alveolar damage	Acute interstitial pneumonia (Hamman-Rich syndrome); acute respiratory distress syndrome (ARDS); drugs (cytotoxic agents, heroin, paraquat, ethchlorvynol, aspirin); toxic gas inhalation; radiation therapy; oxygen toxicity; connective tissue disease; infections
Organizing pneumonia	Cryptogenic organizing pneumonia; organizing stage of diffuse alveolar damage; drugs (amiodarone, cocaine); infections; connective tissue diseases
Desquamative interstitial pneumonia/respiratory bronchiolitis	Cigarette smoking; idiopathic DIP of childhood
Lymphocytic interstitial pneumonia	Idiopathic; hypogammaglobulinemia; autoimmune diseases, including Hashimoto thyroiditis, lupus erythematosus, primary biliary cirrhosis, Sjögren's syndrome, myasthenia gravis, chronic active hepatitis; AIDS; allogeneic bone marrow transplantation
Eosinophilic pneumonia	Idiopathic acute and chronic; tropical filarial eosinophilia; parasitic infections; allergic bronchopulmonary aspergillosis; allergic granulomatosis of Churg and Strauss; hypereosinophilic syndrome; AIDS
Alveolar proteinosis	Pulmonary alveolar proteinosis; acute silicosis; aluminum dust; AIDS; myeloproliferative disorder
Diffuse alveolar hemorrhage	
with capillaritis	Wegener granulomatosis; microscopic polyangiitis; systemic lupus erythematosus; polymyositis; scleroderma; rheumatoid arthritis; mixed connective tissue disease; lung transplantation; drugs (retinoic acid, propylthiouracil, Dilantin); Behçet's disease; cryoglobulinemia; Henoch-Schönlein purpura; pauci-immune glomerulonephritis; immune complex glomerulonephritis
Without capillaritis	Idiopathic pulmonary hemosiderosis; systemic lupus erythematosus; Goodpasture syndrome; diffuse alveolar damage; pulmonary venoocclusive disease; mitral stenosis; lymphangioleiomyomatosis
Amyloid deposition	Primary amyloidosis; multiple myeloma; lymphocytic interstitial pneumonia
Granuloma	Sarcoidosis; hypersensitivity pneumonitis; pulmonary Langerhans cell histiocytosis; silicosis; intravenous talcosis; berylliosis; lymphocytic interstitial pneumonia; infections

AIDS, Acquired immunodeficiency syndrome; *DIP,* desquamative interstitial pneumonia.
Modified from Mason RJ: *Murray & Nadel's textbook of respiratory medicine,* 5th ed, Philadelphia, 2010, Saunders.

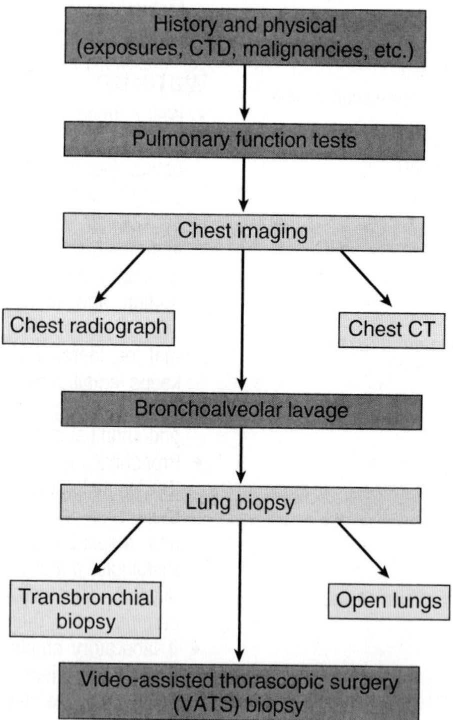

FIG. 1 Algorithm for the approach to a patient with interstitial lung disease. *CT,* computed tomography; *CTD,* connective tissue disease. (From Sellke FW, del Nido PJ, Swanson SJ: *Sabiston & Spencer surgery of the chest,* ed 9, Philadelphia, 2016, Elsevier.)

anti-immunoglobulin antibodies (rheumatoid factors), LDH. Laboratory findings in the interstitial lung diseases are summarized in Table 3.

- Serum precipitins confirm exposure if hypersensitivity pneumonitis is suspected.
- Antineutrophil cytoplasmic antibodies or anti-basement membrane antibodies if vasculitis is suspected.
- Angiotensin-converting enzyme testing (ACE levels) in sarcoidosis is of unclear value.

IMAGING STUDIES

- Chest x-ray may be normal but commonly shows a bibasilar reticular pattern. Table 4 summarizes radiographic features of the interstitial lung diseases.
- High-resolution CT (HRCT) (Fig. 2) is the gold standard for evaluating parenchymal opacities seen on chest x-ray; it is also useful for determining potential biopsy sites.
- Echocardiography may be useful to evaluate cardiac function/dilation or to evaluate for pulmonary hypertension, which can complicate advanced ILDs.

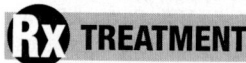

TREATMENT

NONPHARMACOLOGIC THERAPY

Avoidance of tobacco and occupational exposures

ACUTE GENERAL Rx

- Supplemental oxygen in patients with hypoxemia is helpful short and long term.
- Glucocorticoids are the mainstay of therapy for many of the ILDs. Patients should be continuously reevaluated after the initiation of treatment to gauge response. If they are improved or stable, steroids may be tapered. If not, the same course may be maintained 4 additional wk. If patient's condition is unresponsive to steroids or declines as the steroids are tapered, may consider adding second agent (cyclophosphamide, azathioprine, mycophenolate, among other options).

TABLE 3 Radiographic Features of the Interstitial Lung Diseases

Feature	Diseases
Upper zone–predominant disease	Radiation pneumonitis; neurofibromatosis; chronic sarcoidosis; pulmonary Langerhans cell histiocytosis; silicosis; chronic hypersensitivity pneumonitis; chronic eosinophilic pneumonia; ankylosing spondylitis; nodular rheumatoid arthritis; berylliosis; drug-induced (amiodarone, gold, BCNU [carmustine]); radiation
Increased lung volumes	Lymphangioleiomyomatosis; chronic sarcoidosis; chronic pulmonary Langerhans cell histiocytosis; tuberous sclerosis; neurofibromatosis
Radiographic honey-comb lung	Idiopathic pulmonary fibrosis; connective tissue disease; asbestosis; drug-induced; lymphocytic interstitial pneumonia; chronic aspiration pneumonia; hemosiderosis; Hermansky-Pudlak syndrome; alveolar proteinosis
Pneumothorax	Pulmonary Langerhans cell histiocytosis; lymphangioleiomyomatosis; tuberous sclerosis; neurofibromatosis, IPF
Kerley B lines	Lymphangitic carcinomatosis; lymphangioleiomyomatosis; left atrial hypertension (mitral valve disease, venoocclusive disease); lymphoma; amyloidosis
Lymphadenopathy	Sarcoidosis; lymphoma; lymphangitic carcinomatosis; lymphoid interstitial pneumonia; berylliosis; amyloidosis; Gaucher disease
Pleural disease	Lymphangitic carcinomatosis; connective tissue disease; asbestosis (pleural calcification); lymphangioleiomyomatosis (chylous effusion); drug-induced (nitrofurantoin, radiation); sarcoidosis
Eggshell calcification of lymph nodes	Silicosis; sarcoidosis; radiation

IPF, Idiopathic pulmonary fibrosis.
From Mason RJ: *Murray & Nadel's textbook of respiratory medicine*, 5th ed, Philadelphia, 2010, Saunders.

TABLE 4 Laboratory Findings in the Interstitial Lung Diseases

Finding	Diseases
Leukopenia	Sarcoidosis; connective tissue disease; lymphoma; drug-induced
Leukocytosis	Systemic vasculitis; hypersensitivity pneumonitis; lymphoma
Eosinophilia	Eosinophilic pneumonia; sarcoidosis; systemic vasculitis; drug-induced (sulfa, methotrexate)
Thrombocytopenia	Sarcoidosis; connective tissue disease; drug-induced; Gaucher disease; idiopathic pulmonary fibrosis
Hemolytic anemia	Connective tissue disease; sarcoidosis; lymphoma; drug-induced; idiopathic pulmonary fibrosis
Normocytic anemia	Diffuse alveolar hemorrhage syndromes; connective tissue disease; lymphangitic carcinomatosis
Urinary sediment abnormalities	Connective tissue disease; systemic vasculitis; drug-induced
Hypogammaglobulinemia	Lymphocytic interstitial pneumonia
Hypergammaglobulinemia	Connective tissue disease; sarcoidosis; systemic vasculitis; idiopathic pulmonary fibrosis; asbestosis; silicosis; lymphocytic interstitial pneumonia; lymphoma
Serum autoantibodies	Connective tissue disease; systemic vasculitis; sarcoidosis; idiopathic pulmonary fibrosis; silicosis; asbestosis; lymphocytic interstitial pneumonia
Serum immune complexes	Idiopathic pulmonary fibrosis; lymphocytic interstitial pneumonia; systemic vasculitis; connective tissue disease; pulmonary Langerhans cell histiocytosis
Serum angiotensin-converting enzyme	Sarcoidosis; hypersensitivity pneumonitis; silicosis; acute respiratory distress syndrome; Gaucher disease
Antibasement membrane antibody	Goodpasture syndrome
Antineutrophil cytoplasmic antibody	Systemic vasculitis

From Mason, RJ: *Murray & Nadel's textbook of respiratory medicine*, 5th ed, Philadelphia, 2010, Saunders.

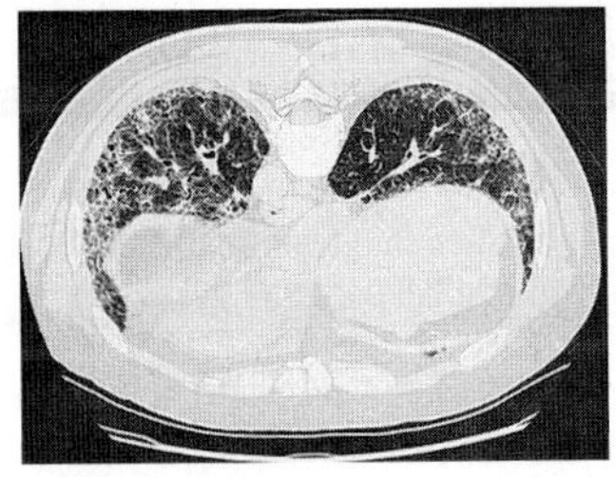

FIG. 2 High-resolution computed tomography scan of the chest shows fibrotic changes in a subpleural distribution with honeycombing consistent with usual interstitial pneumonia. (From Hochberg MC et al: *Rheumatology,* ed 5, St Louis, 2011, Mosby.)

CHRONIC GENERAL Rx

- Outpatient pulmonary rehabilitation may be of value.
- Lung transplantation may be considered in appropriate patients in severe stages of the disease.

DISPOSITION

The prognosis is highly variable and depends on the cause, severity of illness, and initial response to treatment.

REFERRAL

- Pulmonary referral for workup and management
- Surgical referral for biopsy

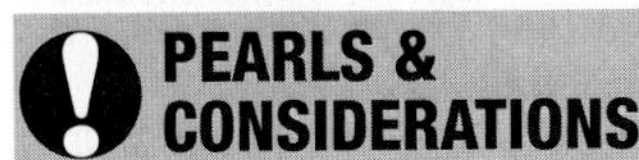

PEARLS & CONSIDERATIONS

COMMENTS

It is very important when working up an ILD to take a thorough history of tobacco and drug use, prior medications, workplace and environmental exposures and pets, as well as a review of systems, including signs and symptoms that might suggest an underlying connective tissue disease.

PREVENTION

Proper industrial hygiene from a respiratory perspective is important as well as close surveillance when patients are given medications with known pulmonary toxicity. Symptoms of an ILD in the setting of an autoimmune condition need to be evaluated thoroughly.

SUGGESTED READINGS

Available at ExpertConsult.com

RELATED CONTENT

Interstitial Pulmonary Disease (Patient Information)

AUTHOR: **PETER LACAMERA, M.D.**

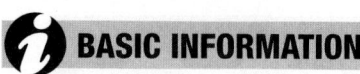

BASIC INFORMATION

DEFINITION

Can be classified into two broad categories:

1. Acute interstitial nephritis (AIN):
   a. Decrease in renal function resulting from delayed hypersensitivity immune-mediated injury, most often drug-induced
   b. Characterized on renal biopsy by edema and leukocyte infiltration of the renal interstitium and tubules (referred to as *tubulitis*), classically sparing glomeruli and blood vessels
2. Chronic interstitial nephritis:
   a. Final common pathway of many chronic kidney diseases including diabetic kidney disease, hypertensive kidney disease, unresolved AIN, chronic obstruction, high-grade vesicoureteral reflux, and chronic bacterial infections
   b. Characterized on renal biopsy by interstitial fibrosis with mononuclear leukocyte infiltration and tubular atrophy

SYNONYMS

Acute tubulo-interstitial nephritis
Contracted kidney
Cirrhosis of the kidney
Granular kidney
Gouty kidney
Renal sclerosis
Chronic productive nephritis without exudation

ICD-10CM CODES

N05.9 Unspecified nephritic syndrome with unspecified morphologic changes
N17.2 Acute kidney failure with medullary necrosis
N05.8 Unspecified nephritic syndrome with other morphologic changes
N10 Acute tubulo-interstitial nephritis
N11.8 Other chronic tubulo-interstitial nephritis
N11.9 Chronic tubulo-interstitial nephritis, unspecified
N12 Tubulo-interstitial nephritis, not specified as acute or chronic

EPIDEMIOLOGY & DEMOGRAPHICS

PREVALENCE:

- Prevalence is significantly underestimated.
- AIN is found in more than 11% of patients biopsied with AKI and may comprise 10% to 27% of all AKI cases.

DEMOGRAPHICS:

- Increasing incidence in the elderly, thought to be due to reduced GFR, immune-mediated dysfunction, increasing medication use, and comorbidities
- Median age at presentation is 65 yr

RISK FACTORS:

- Advanced age (>65 yr)
- Volume depletion
- Underlying kidney disease
- Congestive heart failure
- Diabetes
- HIV infection

PHYSICAL FINDINGS & CLINICAL PRESENTATION

SIGNS AND SYMPTOMS:

- For acute interstitial nephritis, most common presentation is a rise in serum creatinine and BUN that is asymptomatic or associated with nonspecific symptoms of acute renal failure due to any cause, including:
  1. Malaise
  2. Anorexia
  3. Nausea and vomiting
  4. Oliguria or polyuria
  5. Hematuria
  6. Flank pain
- Classic triad (fever, maculopapular rash, and arthralgias) is present in only 5% of cases:
  1. When present, the rash is usually a truncal maculopapular morbilliform eruption.
  2. Triad was characteristic of methicillin-related AIN. This drug has not been used in the U.S. for decades.
- A small minority present with tubulo-interstitial nephritis and uveitis (TINU) syndrome. The uveitis may be symptomatic or subclinical and may develop before, during, or after the renal injury. Adolescent females are most often affected by TINU.
- For chronic interstitial nephritis, there may be a subacute to protracted subtle rise in creatinine without any obvious symptoms as seen with AIN.

ETIOLOGY

ACUTE INTERSTITIAL NEPHRITIS:

- **Drug-induced** (70%). More than 150 agents have been implicated. AKI usually develops 10 to14 days after exposure to the drug, but may develop sooner if there was a previous exposure.
  1. Antibiotics (beta-lactams, sulfonamides, rifampin, fluoroquinolones)
  2. NSAIDs (including selective COX-2 inhibitors)
  3. Proton pump inhibitors and H2 antagonists
  4. Anti-neoplastic agents
  5. Anticonvulsants
  6. Allopurinol (particularly common cause of DRESS with AIN)
  7. Immunotherapy: Checkpoint pathway inhibitors
- **Infection** (10% to 15%). May be systemic or localized to genitourinary system.
  1. Bacterial: Staphylococci, streptococci, *Corynebacterium diphtheria, Legionellae, Yersiniae, Mycobacteria, Mycoplasmas, Rickettsiae*
  2. Viral: Cytomegalovirus, Epstein-Barr virus, hantaviruses, hepatitis C virus, herpes simplex virus, HIV, mumps, polyomavirus, influenza A virus
  3. Other: *Treponema pallidum, Toxoplasma gondii*, Babesia species
- **Other Causes** (15% to 20%)
  1. Idiopathic (10%)
  2. Immune disorders: Systemic lupus erythematosus, Sjögren syndrome, small-vessel vasculitides, autoimmune pancreatitis
  3. Neoplastic disorders (multiple myeloma)
  4. DRESS syndrome
  5. IgG4-related tubulointerstitial nephritis
  6. Hypocomplementemic tubulointerstitial nephritis

CHRONIC INTERSTITIAL NEPHRITIS:

- Metabolic diseases (urate nephropathy, hypercalcemic nephropathy, hypokalemic nephropathy, oxalate nephropathy)
- Sarcoidosis
- Heavy metals
- Chronic urinary tract obstruction
- Aristolochic acid
- Diabetic kidney disease
- Hypertensive kidney disease

OVERLAP OF ACUTE AND CHRONIC INTERSTITIAL NEPHRITIS: Some metabolic processes and autoimmune disorders can present either as acute or chronic interstitial nephritis. For example, oxalate nephropathy can present with acute interstitial nephropathy in the setting of ethylene glycol ingestion, or with chronic interstitial nephritis in patients with prior bariatric surgery and a high oxalate-containing diet.

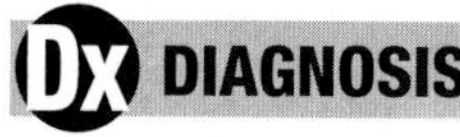

DIAGNOSIS

DIFFERENTIAL DIAGNOSIS

Other causes of AKI or CKD, including ATN, glomerulonephritis, hypertensive nephrosclerosis, prerenal azotemia, obstructive nephropathy, renal vascular disease

WORKUP

- Diagnosis is most often made by defining the temporal relationship between onset and resolution of an AKI episode with use and discontinuation of a known culprit drug.
- Gold standard for diagnosis is the kidney biopsy. This is reserved for clinical situations with unclear diagnoses, when removal of the offending agent does not result in improvement or may impact medical care, or when steroid initiation is being considered.

LABORATORY TESTS

- No single laboratory test has sufficient positive or negative predictive value to be useful in diagnosing interstitial nephritis.
- Diagnosis may be made based on clinical history, constellation of urine and serum abnormalities, and clinical course.

URINE TESTS

- Urine eosinophilia historically was considered a marker of AIN, but this urinary finding is neither sensitive nor specific for AIN and has a low positive and negative predictive value—that is, they do not help diagnose or rule out AIN and should not be used in diagnosis.
- Urinalysis findings may include sterile pyuria, microhematuria, glucosuria, and proteinuria.
- Urine sediment analysis may include leukocytes, leukocyte casts, possible red cells, and possible tubular epithelial cells (Fig. 1). However, a bland urine sediment can also be seen in interstitial nephritis, especially chronic.

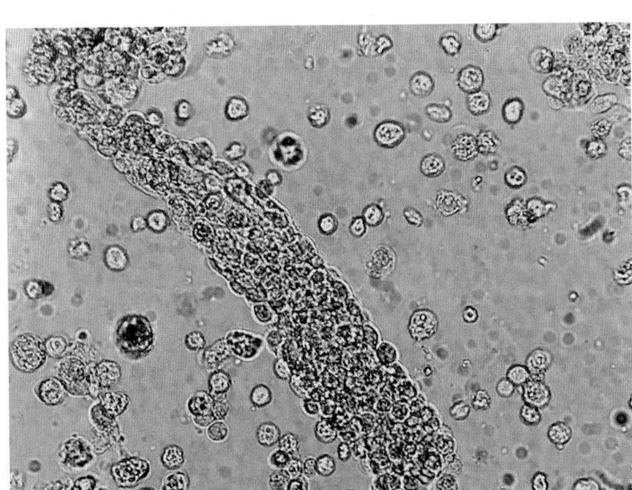

FIG. 1 Urinary sediment showing white blood cells and white blood cell cast. (Courtesy Randy L. Luciano, M.D.)

BLOOD TESTS

- Serum chemistry profile: Elevated BUN, elevated creatinine, low serum phosphorus, low serum urate
- Complete blood count with differential may show:
  1. Eosinophilia (not sensitive, but if present greatly increases clinical suspicion for a systemic drug reaction; may also occur in other causes of AKI including cholesterol emboli, vasculitis, and hematologic or solid organ malignancy).
  2. Anemia (may be out of proportion to degree of AKI because erythropoietin-producing cells reside within the interstitium and may be impacted by the inflammatory cellular congestion).
- If drug-related AIN is not suspected, laboratory workup for infection, vasculitis, and autoimmune disorders may be warranted depending on the clinical context.

IMAGING STUDIES

Gallium scintigraphy and PET/CT have both been used to evaluate AIN in patients. These tests may distinguish between AIN and other forms of AKI in patients too unstable for a renal biopsy.

KIDNEY BIOPSY

Critical in diagnosis of interstitial nephritis in patients in whom the differential of AKI is broad. Biopsy findings include (Fig. E2):

- Predominant lymphocytic and monocytic infiltrate (Fig. E2B).
- Presence of eosinophils is suggestive of drug-induced AIN (Fig. E2C).
- Tubulitis (renal tubular invasion by inflammatory cells) is suggestive of AIN.
- Early on, inflammation is associated with edema, but may transition to fibrosis with underlying tubular atrophy as the process becomes more chronic (Fig. E2D).

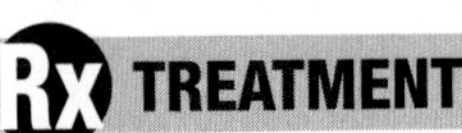

TREATMENT

NONPHARMACOLOGIC THERAPY

Largely supportive; removal of offending agent, if known, will resolve 60% of all cases.

ACUTE GENERAL Rx

- Maintain adequate hydration and urine output but avoid volume overload.
- Identify and treat infection if present.
- Avoid nephrotoxins and medications that impair renal blood flow.
- Uveitis in TINU may be asymptomatic; therefore, ophthalmologic exam is required in idiopathic AIN.
- Initiation of steroids is controversial. Retrospective studies and anecdotal literature have shown that steroid treatment, started within 7 days of diagnosis, may reduce need for chronic dialysis in patients with drug-induced AIN who have not responded to drug withdrawal alone. Steroids are the basis of treatment in idiopathic AIN, AIN associated with systemic disease, and TINU. Dosing is typically pulsed steroids with IV methylprednisolone (250–500 mg daily ×3 days) followed by 0.5 to 1 mg/kg per day, tapering over 4 to 6 weeks.
- Cyclophosphamide, cyclosporine, and mycophenolate mofetil have all been used anecdotally in steroid-resistant disease. Additionally, mycophenolate mofetil has been used as a steroid-sparing agent if AKI recurs when steroids are tapered or discontinued.

CHRONIC Rx

- Limit exposure to known nephrotoxic agents.
- Adjust dosages of all medications as indicated by glomerular filtration rate.
- Tight control of blood pressure, diabetes, and cholesterol.
- Relieve any sources of chronic obstruction (treat BPH).

DISPOSITION

With acute interstitial nephritis (AIN):

- Complete recovery with return to baseline creatinine occurs in 60% to 65% of cases
- Partial recovery is seen in 10% to 20%
- Irreversible damage in 5% to 10%
- Relapse is common with repeated exposure to offending agents

REFERRAL

Renal consultation is often necessary, especially if the diagnosis is unclear, biopsy is required, or there is treatment-resistant disease.

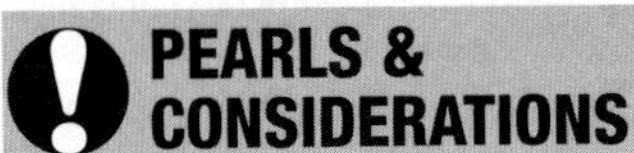

PEARLS & CONSIDERATIONS

COMMENTS

Acute interstitial nephritis is most often due to drugs started in the preceding 30 days. The most common drug classes are beta-lactam antibiotics, NSAIDs, and PPIs. In contrast to ATN, which is often associated with oliguria, early AIN may be associated with polyuria; therefore, a high index of suspicion in this clinical setting is essential for early diagnosis.

PREVENTION

Use known offending agents with care, especially in the elderly and those with known underlying kidney disease.

PATIENT/FAMILY EDUCATION

http://www.nlm.nih.gov/medlineplus/ency/article/000464.htm

SUGGESTED READINGS

Available at ExpertConsult.com

RELATED CONTENT

Interstitial Nephritis (Patient Information)

AUTHOR: **RANDY L. LUCIANO, M.D., PH.D.**

BASIC INFORMATION

DEFINITION

Irritable bowel syndrome (IBS) is a chronic functional disorder manifested by alteration in bowel habits and recurrent abdominal pain and bloating. IBS is a symptom complex influenced by a variety of physiologic determinants from gut to brain and back. The ROME IV criteria for diagnosis of IBS are:

- Patient has recurrent abdominal pain ≥1 day per week, on average, in the previous 3 mo, with an onset ≥6 mo before diagnosis
- Abdominal pain is associated with at least two of the following three symptoms:
  1. Pain related to defecation
  2. Change in frequency of stool
  3. Change in form (appearance) of stool
- Patient has none of the following warning signs:
  1. Age ≥50 yr, no previous colon cancer screening, and presence of symptoms
  2. Recent change in bowel habit
  3. Evidence of overt GI bleeding (e.g., melena or hematochezia)
  4. Nocturnal pain or passage of stool
  5. Unintentional weight loss
  6. Family history of colorectal cancer or inflammatory bowel disease
  7. Palpable abdominal mass or lymphadenopathy
  8. Evidence of iron-deficiency anemia on blood testing
  9. Positive test for fecal occult blood
- The criteria must be fulfilled for at least the past 3 mo with symptom onset at least 6 mo before the diagnosis.
- Table 1 subtypes IBS by predominant stool pattern.

SYNONYMS

Irritable colon
Spastic colon
IBS

ICD-10CM CODES

K58 Irritable bowel syndrome
K58.9 Irritable bowel syndrome without diarrhea
K58.0 Irritable bowel syndrome with diarrhea

EPIDEMIOLOGY & DEMOGRAPHICS

- IBS is the most common functional bowel disorder. An estimated 15 million people in the United States have IBS.
- IBS occurs in 7% to 21% of the general population of industrialized countries and is responsible for >50% of gastrointestinal (GI) referrals. Worldwide adult prevalence is 12%. Incidence increases during adolescence and peaks in third and fourth decades of life.
- Female:male ratio is 2:1. Peak prevalence is from 20 to 39 yr of age.
- Nearly 50% of patients have psychiatric abnormalities, with anxiety disorders being most common.

PHYSICAL FINDINGS & CLINICAL PRESENTATION

- The clinical presentation of IBS consists of abdominal pain and abnormalities of defecation, which may include loose stools, usually after meals and in the morning, alternating with episodes of constipation.
- Physical examination is generally normal.
- Nonspecific abdominal tenderness and distention may be present.

ETIOLOGY

- Unknown, believed to be multifactorial. Fig. 1 illustrates a biopsychological model of IBS pathophysiology
- Associated pathophysiology includes altered GI motility, alteration in gut flora, and increased gut sensitivity
- Risk factors: Anxiety, depression, personality disorders, history of childhood sexual abuse, and domestic abuse in women

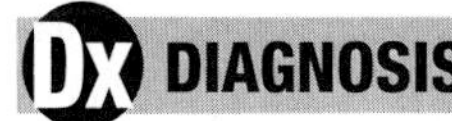

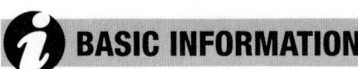

DIAGNOSIS

DIFFERENTIAL DIAGNOSIS

- Inflammatory bowel disease (IBD)
- Diverticulitis
- Colon malignancy
- Endometriosis
- Peptic ulcer disease
- Biliary liver disease
- Chronic pancreatitis
- Constipation caused by medications (opiates, calcium channel blockers, anticholinergics)
- Diarrhea caused by medications (metformin, colchicine, proton pump inhibitors, antacids, antibiotics)
- Small-bowel overgrowth
- Celiac disease
- Parasites
- Lymphoma of GI tract
- Pelvic floor dyssynergia

TABLE 1 Subtyping Irritable Bowel Syndrome by Predominant Stool Pattern

1. IBS with constipation (IBS-C)—hard or lumpy stools* ≥25% and loose (mushy) or watery stools† ≥25% of bowel movements‡
2. IBS with diarrhea (IBS-D)—loose (mushy) or watery stools† ≥25% and hard or lumpy stool* ≥25% of bowel movements‡
3. Mixed IBS—hard or lumpy stools* ≥25% and loose (mushy) or watery stools† ≥25% of bowel movements‡
4. Unsubtyped IBS (IBS unclassified)—insufficient abnormality of stool consistency to meet criteria for IBS with constipation, diarrhea, or mixed‡

IBS, Irritable bowel syndrome.
*Bristol Stool Form Scale 1-2 (separate hard lumps like nuts [difficult to pass] or sausage-shaped but lumpy).
†Bristol Stool Form Scale 6-7 (fluffy pieces with ragged edges, a mushy stool or watery, no solid pieces, entirely liquid).
‡In the absence of use of antidiarrheals or laxatives.
Adapted from Sayuk GS, Gyawali CP: Irritable bowel syndrome: modern concepts and management options. *Am J Med* 128(8):817-827, 2015.

WORKUP

Diagnostic workup (Table 2) is aimed primarily at excluding the conditions listed in the differential diagnoses. A step-wise approach is critical. It is important to identify red flags of other diseases, such as weight loss, rectal bleeding, onset in patients >50 yr, fever, nocturnal pain, and family history of malignancy or IBD. Additional red flags include abnormal examination (e.g., mass, enlarged lymph nodes, stool positive for occult blood, muscle wasting) and abnormal laboratory values (anemia, leukocytosis, abnormal chemistry).

LABORATORY TESTS

- Blood work is generally normal. CBC is reasonable to evaluate for anemia. The presence of anemia should alert to the possibility of a colonic malignancy or IBD.
- Other reasonable tests include C-reactive protein, tissue transglutaminase antibody (rule out celiac disease) and TSH (rule out thyroid abnormalities).
- Fecal calprotectin level is useful to differentiate IBS from inflammatory bowel disease in patients who have IBS with diarrhea or with both diarrhea and constipation. Fecal calprotectin levels less than 40 mcg/g exclude IBD in patients with IBS.
- Testing of stool for ova and parasites should be considered only in patients with chronic diarrhea. Evaluation of stool for *Clostridium difficile* may be helpful in patients with predominant diarrhea symptoms who have recently taken antibiotics.

IMAGING STUDIES

Imaging studies (e.g., flat and upright abdominal radiograph, small-bowel series, sonogram or CT of abdomen and pelvis) are normal and not necessary for diagnosis.

Lower endoscopy is generally normal except for the presence of some spasms. Colonoscopic imaging should be performed only in persons who have alarm features to rule out organic disease and in persons older than 50 yr to screen for colorectal cancer.

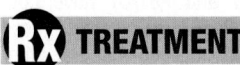

TREATMENT

NONPHARMACOLOGIC THERAPY

- The patient should be encouraged to maintain an adequate fiber intake and to eliminate foods that aggravate symptoms. Avoidance of caffeine, dairy products, fatty foods, and dietary excesses is also helpful. Several clinical trials have shown that a diet low in fermentable oligosaccharides, disaccharides, monosaccharides, and polyols (FODMAPs) improves symptoms in nearly 70% of patients with IBS.
- Cognitive-behavioral therapy is also recommended, particularly in younger patients because psychosocial stressors are important triggers of IBS. Reassurance that the disorder is benign and education about trigger avoidance and stress management are important.
- Importance of regular exercise and adequate fluid intake should be stressed.
- Fig. E2 illustrates the management of irritable bowel syndrome.

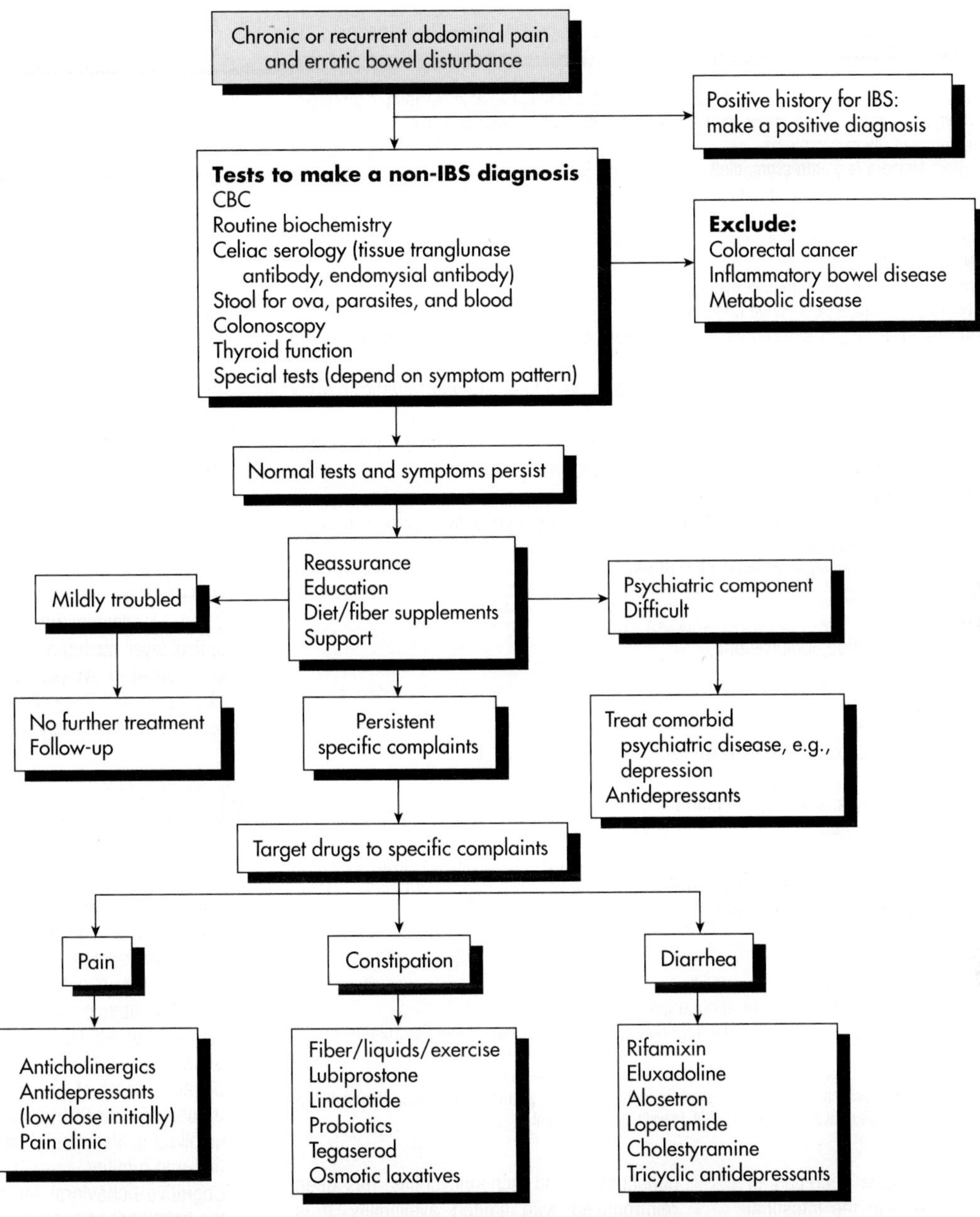

FIG. 1 A biopsychosocial model of irritable bowel syndrome pathophysiology. Irritable bowel syndrome is thought to be a multifactorial disorder, deriving from a potential multitude of etiopathogenic factors, including environmental, psychological, and physiologic factors. This model highlights the complex, often bidirectional interplay of these factors in the experience of irritable bowel syndrome symptoms. *cGMP,* Cyclic guanosine monophosphate; *5-HT3*, serotonin type 3; *5-HT4*, serotonin type 4; *FODMAPS*, fermentable oligosaccharides, disaccharides, monosaccharides, and polyols; *HRQOL*, health-related quality of life; *IBS*, irritable bowel syndrome. (Modified from Sayuk GS, Gyawali CP: Irritable bowel syndrome: modern concepts and management options, *Am J Med* 128(8):817–827, 2015.)

GENERAL Rx

- The mainstay of treatment of IBS is a high-fiber diet. Fiber is helpful for relief of constipation but not for relief of pain. Because symptoms are chronic, the use of laxatives should generally be avoided.
- Soluble fiber (psyllium) is more effective in symptom relief than insoluble fiber (bran). Fiber supplementation with psyllium 1 tbsp bid or calcium polycarbophil (FiberCon) 2 tablets one to four times daily followed by 8 oz of water may be necessary in some patients.
- Patients should be instructed that there might be some increased bloating on initiation of fiber supplementation, which should resolve within 2 to 3 wk. It is important that patients take these fiber products on a regular basis and not only as needed. Fiber is not effective in patients with diarrhea-predominant IBS and may worsen symptoms in these patients.
- Patients who appear anxious can benefit from use of sedatives or selective serotonin reuptake inhibitors (SSRIs). Tricyclic antidepressants in low doses are also effective in some patients with diarrhea-predominant IBS.
- C-2 chloride channel activators: Lubiprostone (Amitiza) is a chloride channel activator that stimulates chloride-rich intestinal fluid secretion and accelerates small intestine and colonic transmit time. It may be effective in chronic constipation-predominant IBS unresponsive to conventional treatment. Usual dose is 8 to 24 mcg bid with food. Side effects include headache and nausea.
- Linaclotide (Linzess) is a guanylate cyclase-C (GC-C) agonist FDA approved for IBS

TABLE 2 Irritable Bowel Syndrome Treatment Strategy: A Way Forward

1. Evaluation
   a. Consider conditions that mimic IBS (e.g., celiac disease, microscopic colitis, bile acid diarrhea, pancreatic insufficiency, carbohydrate intolerances, medication side effects, postsurgical neoanatomy)
   b. Assess for the presence of alarm symptoms
   c. Evaluate for symptom triggers (e.g., stressors, diet)
   d. Explore presence of other functional GI (e.g., functional dyspepsia) and non-GI disorders (e.g., fibromyalgia), psychiatric comorbidity, and drug intolerances
   e. Understand previous IBS treatment experiences
2. Selection of treatment approach
   a. Predicated on symptom severity and dominant symptoms
   b. Symptom severity (intensity, bother, effects on quality of life)
      i. Mild symptoms, intermittent symptoms, low symptom burden: Symptomatic or peripheral therapy
      ii. Moderate symptoms: Centrally acting neuromodulators, especially if symptomatic therapy does not provide adequate benefit
      iii. Severe symptoms and those with comorbidities (non-GI functional disorders, psychiatric): Both centrally acting neuromodulators and peripheral therapy
         a. Concurrent affective disorders need to be managed.
         b. Other central therapies (cognitive and behavioral therapy, hypnosis, stress reduction) may need to be considered.
   b. Dominant symptoms (diarrhea, constipation, pain, other GI symptoms)
      i. Constipation predominant
         a. Laxatives, fiber
         b. Novel agents (linaclotide, lubiprostone)
      ii. Diarrhea predominant
         a. Antidiarrheals
         b. Alosetron
         c. Address dysbiosis (rifaximin, probiotics)
         d. Diet (low FODMAP)
         e. Bile binders (cholestyramine, colesevelam)
         f. Disaccharidases (lactase)
      iii. Pain predominant
         a. Antidepressants (TCAs and SNRIs preferred)
         b. Linaclotide when constipation present
         c. Avoid narcotics
3. Education and therapeutic alliance
   a. Inform patient about etiopathogenesis.
   b. Reaffirm legitimacy of diagnosis; allay concerns about organic disease.
   c. Provide information about support organizations (International Foundation for Functional Gastrointestinal Disorders).

FODMAP, Fermentable oligosaccharides, disaccharides, monosaccharides, and polyols; *GI,* gastrointestinal; *IBS,* irritable bowel syndrome; *SNRI,* serotonin-norepinephrine reuptake inhibitor; *TCA,* tricyclic antidepressant.

with constipation.It stimulates secretion of chloride and bicarbonate into the intestinal lumen, mainly through activation of the CFTR ion channel, resulting in increased intestinal fluid and accelerated transit. Usual dose for IBS is 290 mcg 30 min before eating. The most common adverse effects are diarrhea, abdominal pain, flatulence, and abdominal distension.

- Eluxadoline (Viberzi) is a μ-opioid receptor agonist and Δ-opioid receptor antagonist FDA approved for IBS with diarrhea. It decreases muscle contractility, inhibits water and electrolyte secretion, and increases rectal sphincter tone. Usual dose is 100 mg PO bid taken with food.
- Loperamide is effective for diarrhea. Alosetron, a serotonin type-3 receptor antagonist previously withdrawn because of severe constipation and ischemic colitis, has been reintroduced with limited availability. It is indicated only for women with severe chronic diarrhea-predominant IBS unresponsive to conventional therapy and not caused by anatomic or metabolic abnormality. Starting dose is 1 mg qd.
- Alterations in gut flora have been identified as potentially contributing to IBS (84% of IBS patients have an abnormal lactulose breath test, suggesting small-intestinal bacterial overgrowth). Rifaximin, a gut-selective antibiotic, has been used in recent trials to eradicate bacterial overgrowth (70% eradication rate). A dose of 400 mg tid for 10 days was reported effective in improving IBS symptoms up to 10 wk after discontinuation of therapy. Until additional evidence is available, use of rifaximin or other antibiotics in IBS should be reserved for patients with proven bacterial overgrowth.
- Antispasmodics-anticholinergics (e.g., dicyclomine, hyoscyamine) are often used, but efficacy data from clinical trials are inconclusive.
- Probiotics: Bifidobacteria and some combinations of probiotics have shown some limited efficacy. Lactobacilli do not appear to be effective for the treatment of IBS. Additional data showing efficacy is needed before probiotics can be endorsed for treatment of IBS.
- Antidepressants: SSRIs are more effective than placebo for relief of global IBS symptoms.

DISPOSITION

More than 60% of patients respond successfully to treatment over the initial 12 mo; however, IBS is a chronic, relapsing condition and requires prolonged therapy.

REFERRAL

GI referral is recommended in patients with rectal bleeding, fever, nocturnal diarrhea, anemia, weight loss, or onset of symptoms >40 yr. Consultation is also necessary if specialized diagnostic procedures such as endoscopy are necessary.

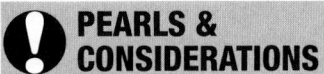

PEARLS & CONSIDERATIONS

COMMENTS

- Patients should be educated regarding maintenance of a high-fiber diet and elimination of stressors, which can precipitate attacks of IBS. They should be reassured that their condition does not lead to cancer.
- Recent drug efforts (alosetron, tegaserod) are aimed at serotonergic receptors in the gut because most of the serotonin in the body is found in the GI tract and is believed to be involved in the mediation of visceral sensation and motility.
- Cognitive-behavioral therapy is effective in the treatment of patients with IBS and should be considered as part of the armamentarium against this disorder.
- Some patients with IBS but without celiac disease show symptom improvement on a wheat-free diet. A 2- to 3-wk trial of wheat avoidance may be reasonable in patients with treatment-resistant IBS.

SUGGESTED READINGS

Available at ExpertConsult.com

RELATED CONTENT

Irritable Bowel Syndrome (Patient Information)

AUTHOR: **FRED F. FERRI, M.D.**

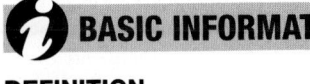

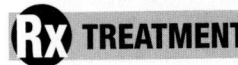

BASIC INFORMATION

DEFINITION

Ischemic colitis (IC) is tissue damage and inflammation of the large intestine due to a reduction in blood flow.

SYNONYMS

Intestinal ischemia
Colonic ischemia
IC

ICD-10CM CODES

K55.0	Acute vascular disorders of intestine
K55.03	Acute (reversible) ischemia of large intestine
K55.9	Vascular disorder of intestine, unspecified
K51.50	Left-sided colitis without complications
K51.51	Left-sided colitis with complications
K51.513	Left-sided colitis with fistula
K51.514	Left-sided colitis with abscess
K51.511	Left-sided colitis with rectal bleeding
K51.512	Left-sided colitis with intestinal obstruction
K51.518	Left-sided colitis with other complication
K51.519	Left-sided colitis with unspecified complications
K52.3	Indeterminate colitis

EPIDEMIOLOGY & DEMOGRAPHICS

INCIDENCE: It is the most common type of intestinal ischemia with an annual incidence of 15.6 to 17.7 per 100,000.

PEAK INCIDENCE: Unknown

PREVALENCE: Unknown

PREDOMINANT SEX AND AGE:

- More common among older patients (60s to 70s)
- Female predominance

RISK FACTORS:

- Older age (60s to 70s)
- Atherosclerotic disease
- Hemodialysis
- Hypertension
- Atrial fibrillation
- Diabetes
- Small vessel disease
- Aortic surgery, endovascular intervention, cardiopulmonary bypass surgery
- Long-distance running, extreme exercise
- Hypercoagulable state
- Myocardial ischemia
- Mechanical obstruction
- Hypoalbuminemia
- Shock

PHYSICAL FINDINGS & CLINICAL PRESENTATION

- Key historical points:
  1. Rapid-onset cramping and abdominal pain (classically thought to involve the left side more often, but newer literature suggests that no one region is affected predominantly)
  2. Urge to defecate may accompany developing abdominal pain
  3. Hematochezia (usually within 24 hrs)
- Physical exam findings suggestive of ischemic colitis:
  1. Abdominal exam may be nonspecific early on
  2. May have peritoneal signs in severe illness or bowel perforation
  3. Hypotension and tachycardia in severe cases
  4. Guaiac positive stool

ETIOLOGY

GENERAL:

- Caused by a reduction in blood flow, usually sudden, to a segment of the large intestine. The resulting blood flow is not enough to provide the oxygen and nutrients necessary for normal cellular metabolism.
- Particularly affected are the watershed regions of the colon (Fig. 1), which have limited collateral circulation (splenic flexure and sigmoid colon).
- Medical and surgical conditions associated with ischemic colitis are summarized in Box 1.

SPECIFIC:

- Non-occlusive disease:
  1. Hypoperfusion: Cardiac failure, septic shock, hemorrhagic shock, hemodialysis
  2. Iatrogenic: Drugs (especially constipation-inducing). Medications associated with ischemic colitis are summarized in Box 2.
  3. Colonic obstruction: Colon cancer, constipation, volvulus
  4. Long-distance running
- Occlusive disease:
  1. Arterial: Thrombus/emboli, cholesterol emboli, small vessel disease (atherosclerosis, diabetes, vasculitis, rheumatoid arthritis, radiation, amyloidosis), trauma
  2. Surgical: Aortic aneurysm repair, cardiac catheterization, cardiopulmonary bypass, colectomy, endoscopy, renal transplant
  3. Venous: Mesenteric venous thrombosis, hypercoagulable state, sickle cell disease, pancreatitis, portal hypertension, lymphocytic phlebitis

Dx DIAGNOSIS

DIFFERENTIAL DIAGNOSIS

- Infectious colitis (e.g., *Clostridium difficile, Salmonella, Shigella*)
- Inflammatory bowel disease
- Diverticulitis
- Bowel obstruction
- Pancreatitis
- Malignancy
- Radiation enteritis

WORKUP

The clinical presentation is often vague and can be variable from patient to patient. A high index of suspicion must be maintained in any patient presenting with abdominal pain and bloody stool. In addition to the physical exam, the following are key to confirming the diagnosis:

- Lab studies
- Computed tomography
- Lower endoscopy

LABORATORY TESTS

- General:
  1. CBC (may see leukocytosis)
  2. Metabolic panel
  3. Liver function panel
- Specific markers: There are no specific laboratory tests for ischemic colitis. However, elevated levels of certain markers suggest inadequate global perfusion:
  1. Lactate
  2. Lactate dehydrogenase
  3. CK
  4. Amylase
- Coagulation studies
- Stool studies: Stool culture, ova and parasite, *C. difficile* toxin assay, tests for *Salmonella, Shigella, Campylobacter,* and *E. coli*

IMAGING STUDIES

- Abdominal CT with contrast: Although findings can be nonspecific, the value of CT is in distinguishing ischemic colitis from nonischemic causes of abdominal pain. It also can assess the degree of ischemia and gauge the need for surgical intervention. It may identify arterial emboli or venous obstruction. Specific findings suggestive of ischemic colitis include, but are not limited to, intestinal wall thickening, thumbprinting, pericolonic stranding, and peritoneal free fluid or free air. Pneumatosis (the presence of gas in the colonic wall), portal venous gas, and the presence of megacolon usually indicate severe disease favoring immediate surgical intervention.
- Abdominal radiograph: X-rays are rarely helpful in diagnosing ischemic colitis. Findings may be subtle or absent unless transmural necrosis and perforation have occurred, causing pneumoperitoneum.
- Lower endoscopy: This is the gold standard for confirming diagnosis of ischemic colitis. In the absence of peritoneal signs, colonoscopy is the test of choice to evaluate the degree of ischemia. If ischemia is suspected, lower endoscopy should be performed within the first 24-48 hrs. In most cases, visual inspection of the colonic wall using this technique will confirm the diagnosis and dictate the need for conservative versus surgical management. However, endoscopy should not be performed in patients with acute peritonitis or evidence of irreversible ischemic damage on CT.

Rx TREATMENT

- Treatment depends on the severity of disease and the specific etiology of colonic ischemia. However, the mainstay of therapy consists of optimizing blood flow to ischemic regions of bowel and removing any potential exacerbating factors. Initial supportive care consists of aggressive IV crystalloid resuscitation, bowel

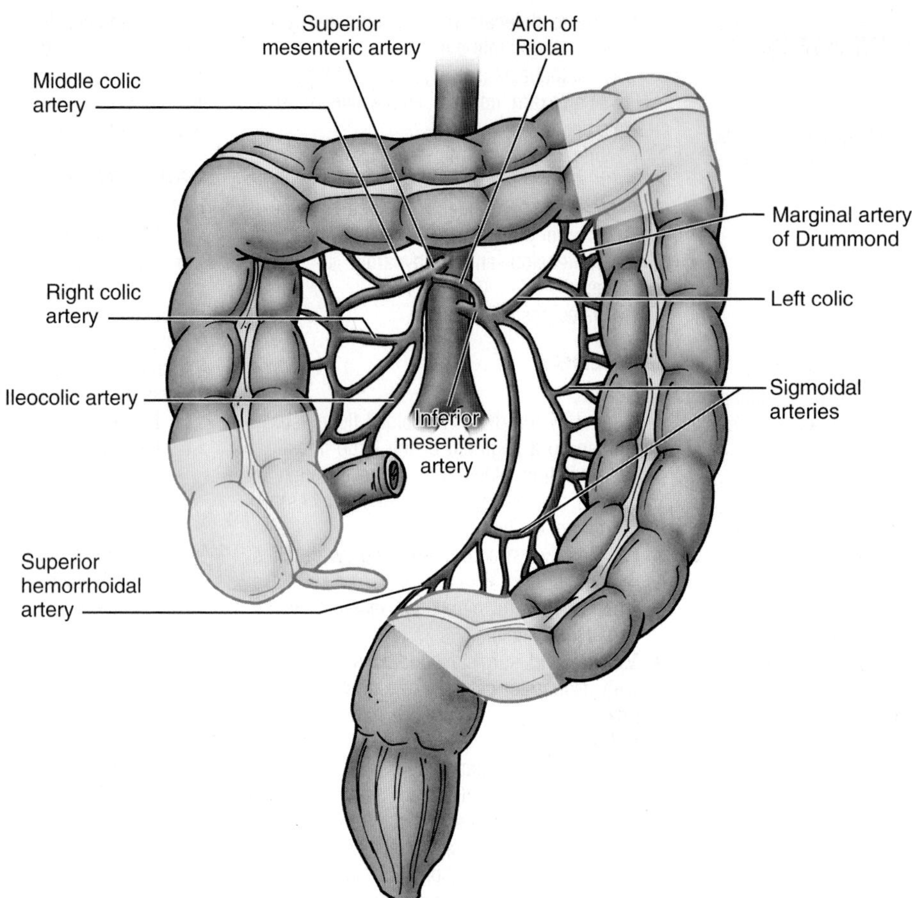

FIG. 1 Arterial supply to the colon. Shaded areas depicting potential watershed regions. (From Cameron JL, Cameron AM: *Current surgical therapy*, ed 12, Philadelphia, 2017, Elsevier.)

BOX 1 Medical and Surgical Conditions Associated with Ischemic Colitis

Cardiovascular/Pulmonary
Atherosclerosis*
Atrial fibrillation
Chronic obstructive pulmonary disease
Hypertension

Gastrointestinal
Constipation
Diarrhea
Irritable bowel syndrome

Low Flow State
Septic shock
Congestive heart failure
Hemorrhagic shock
Hypotension

Surgery
Abdominal surgery
Aortic surgery
Cardiovascular surgery

Invasive Interventions
Postendovascular abdominal manipulations (e.g., chemoembolization)
Postcolonoscopy

Metabolic/Rheumatoid
Diabetes mellitus
Dyslipidemia
Rheumatoid arthritis
Systemic lupus erythematosus

Miscellaneous
Hypercoagulable states†
Sickle cell disease
Long-distance running

*For example, ischemic heart disease, cerebrovascular disease, peripheral vascular disease.
†Antiphospholipid syndrome, factor V Leiden deficiency, protein C and S deficiency.
From Cameron JL, Cameron AM: *Current surgical therapy*, ed 12, Philadelphia, 2017, Elsevier.

BOX 2 Drugs Associated with Ischemic Colitis

Constipation-inducing drugs (opioids and nonopioids)
Immunomodulator drugs (anti-TNFα, type 1 interferon-α, type 1 interferon-β)
Chemotherapeutic drugs (e.g., Taxanes)
Cocaine and methamphetamines
Female hormones
Oral contraceptive medications
Antibiotics
Pseudoephedrine
Serotoninergic (e.g., Alosetron, Sumatriptan)
Diuretics

TNF, Tumor necrosis factor. From Cameron JL, Cameron AM: *Current surgical therapy*, ed 12, Philadelphia, 2017, Elsevier.

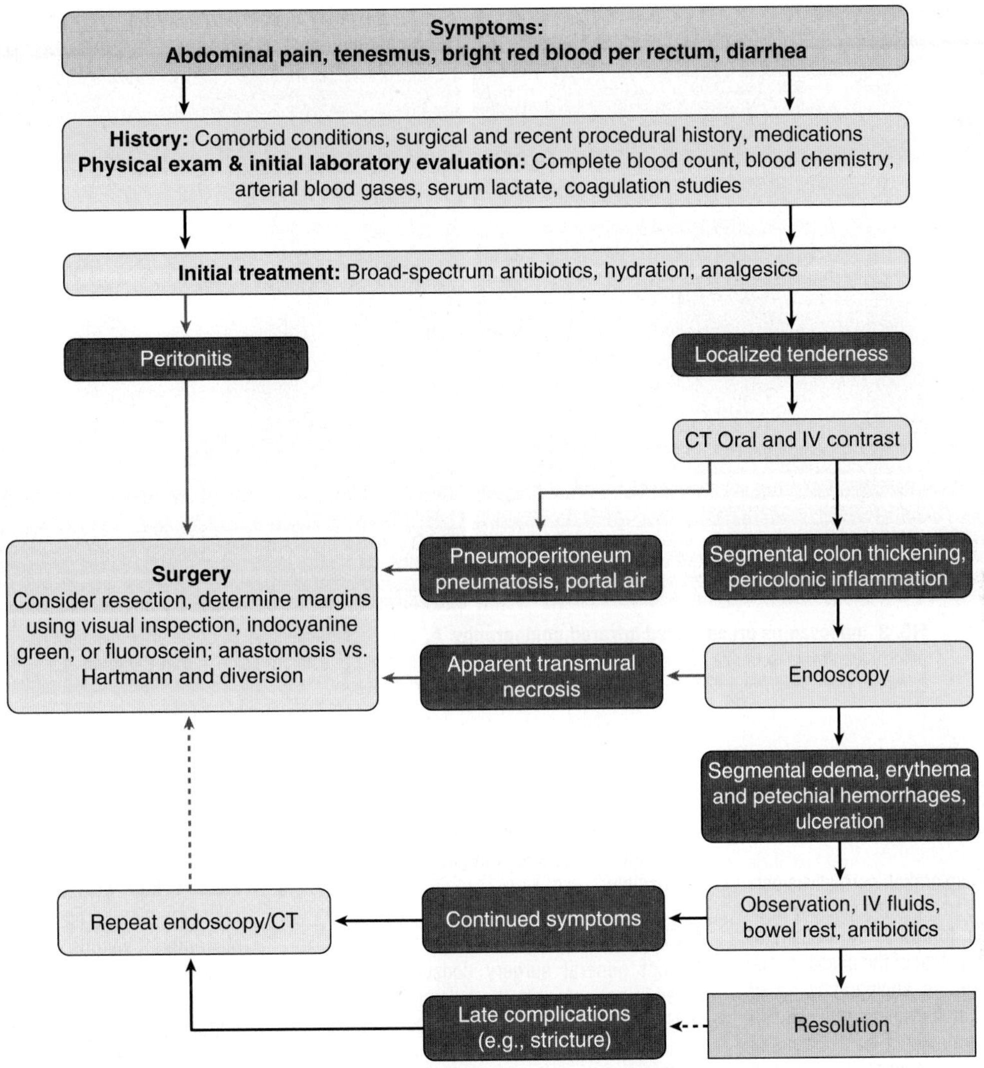

FIG. 2 Treatment algorithm for ischemic colitis. *CT,* Computed tomography; *IV,* intravenous. (From Cameron JL, Cameron AM: *Current surgical therapy*, ed 12, Philadelphia, 2017, Elsevier.)

rest, and broad-spectrum antibiotics with aerobic and anaerobic coverage. A treatment algorithm is illustrated in Fig. 2.

- In mild cases where patients are hemodynamically stable and do not have signs of peritonitis, colonoscopy should be performed. Patients with nonviable bowel seen on endoscopy require immediate operative intervention. However, the remainder of patients should be managed medically with continued IV fluids, bowel rest, and broad-spectrum antibiotics. Consider the use of a nasogastric tube in patients with abdominal distention or signs of ileus or bowel obstruction. Avoid vasoconstrictive medications as these can exacerbate colonic hypoperfusion. Monitor signs of adequate end organ perfusion (e.g., mental status, abdominal pain, urine output).
- In severe cases not responding to supportive therapy, where patients are exhibiting acute peritonitis, sepsis, hypotension, or pain out of proportion to clinical exam, surgical abdominal exploration is warranted. Resection of gangrenous segments of bowel may be necessary. Colonoscopy should be avoided in these patients.

NONPHARMACOLOGIC THERAPY

- Open or laparoscopic abdominal exploration to identify necrotic bowel. Box 3 summarizes indications for surgical intervention in patients with ischemic colitis
- NG tube for bowel decompression if ileus is present

ACUTE GENERAL Rx

- Supportive care:
  1. IV fluids
  2. Bowel rest
  3. Broad-spectrum antibiotics (aerobic and anaerobic coverage)
- Anti-coagulation (not indicated in nonocclusive ischemia but may be considered in proven arterial occlusion or mesenteric vein thrombosis).

BOX 3 Indications for Surgical Intervention in Patients with Ischemic Colitis

Acute
Peritonitis
Bowel perforation
Bowel necrosis
Fulminant colitis
Massive hemorrhage
Sepsis

Chronic
Intractable symptoms (abdominal pain, bloody diarrhea, etc.) lasting >2 weeks
Recurrent sepsis
Chronic colitis
Ischemic stricture
Malnutrition from protein-losing enteropathy

From Cameron JL, Cameron AM: *Current surgical therapy*, ed 12, Philadelphia, 2017, Elsevier.

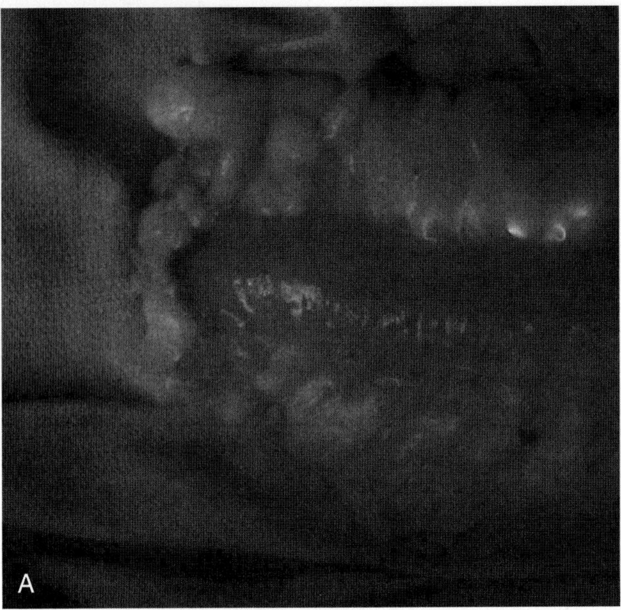

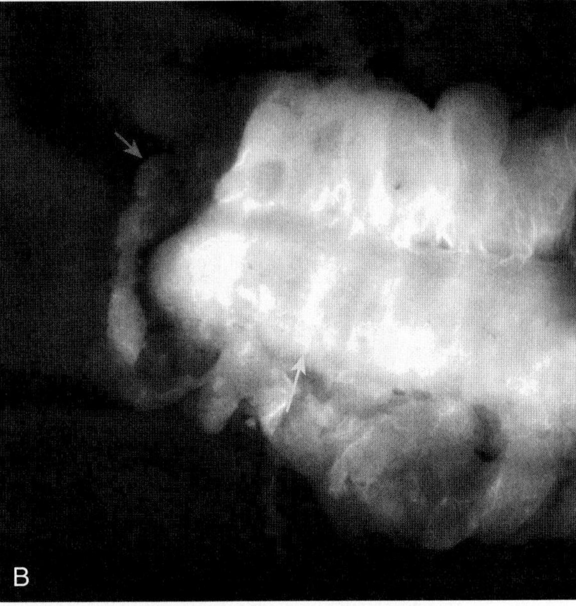

FIG. 3 Indocyanine green-based infrared angiography. A, Colon before injection. **B,** Colon after injection: *(short blue arrow)* ischemia of resection margin; *(yellow arrow)* normal perfusion of colon. (From Cameron JL, Cameron AM: *Current surgical therapy*, ed 12, Philadelphia, 2017, Elsevier.)

- Abdominal exploration:
  1. Bowel prep should be given.
  2. Bowel resection may be indicated in severe colitis.
  3. Repeat surgical exploration normally is performed within 12 to 24 hrs, especially after colonic resection, to assess the viability of colonic tissue and state of the anastomosis. Intraoperative infrared angiography based on IV injection of indo cyanine green (Fig. 3) can be used as an adjunct for decisions of whether to resect in determining margins and the integrity of intestinal anastomoses.
  4. Note that primary anastomosis after colonic resection is contraindicated in certain cases (e.g., presence of aortic or iliac grafts; or when tissue is too friable for stable anastomosis).

CHRONIC Rx

- Avoid overly aggressive hypertension treatment.
- Avoid dehydration.
- Avoid extreme exercise.

DISPOSITION

- Most cases of acute ischemic colitis resolve with medical care in 1 to 2 days. However, the need for surgery in more severe cases portends a worse prognosis and is associated with increased morbidity and mortality. Any risk factors for ischemic colitis should be identified and mitigated as much as possible.

REFERRAL

Prompt general surgery consultation is indicated in patients with the following:

- Hemodynamic instability and peritoneal signs on examination
- CT showing signs of bowel infarction or perforation
- Endoscopy showing nonviable bowel or peritoneal signs

PEARLS & CONSIDERATIONS

COMMENTS

Ischemic colitis typically occurs in older patients who have multiple comorbidities. A high index of suspicion should be maintained for patients with recent endovascular procedures. These patients require close outpatient followup and management by a primary care provider.

PREVENTION

Avoid overly aggressive hypertension treatment, dehydration, and extreme exercise.

RELATED TOPICS

Acute Mesenteric Ischemia (Related Key Topic)
Mesenteric Venous Thrombosis (Related Key Topic)

SUGGESTED READINGS

Available at ExpertConsult.com

AUTHOR: **AMADEO J. DE LUCA-WESTRATE, M.D.**

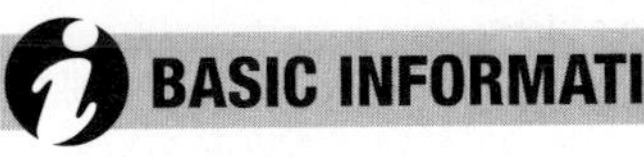

BASIC INFORMATION

DEFINITION

- A common form of vascular liver disease
- Occurs when a severe systemic disturbance leads to decreased perfusion to the liver resulting in tissue hypoxia

SYNONYMS

Hypoxic hepatitis
Shock liver
Ischemic hepatopathy
Hepatic necrosis

ICD-10CM CODES

K76.2	Central hemorrhagic necrosis of liver
K75.89	Other specified inflammatory liver disease

EPIDEMIOLOGY & DEMOGRAPHICS

- Occurs worldwide

INCIDENCE:

- Less than 1% on the inpatient medical wards
- Incidence is higher (2.5%) in intensive care unit

PEAK INCIDENCE: Highest in the cardiac care units

PREVALENCE:

- Recognized as most frequent cause of acute liver injury
- 57% of patients with liver enzymes >1000 IU/L have ischemic hepatitis
- Prevalence up to 10% in the intensive care setting

PREDOMINANT AGE AND SEX:

- Can occur in all ages
- Most common in elderly

GENETICS: No genetic predisposition

RISK FACTORS:

- Most common is cardiovascular disease
- Chronic heart failure
- Cirrhosis

PHYSICAL FINDINGS & CLINICAL PRESENTATION

- Altered mental status may be present due to decreased cerebral perfusion.
- Other symptoms are often masked by the overall disease state.
- Hepatic synthetic function is usually preserved in ischemic hepatitis.

ETIOLOGY

- Cardiac disease in the most common (Fig. E1).
- This includes myocardial infarction, arrhythmias, cardiac tamponade, and cardiogenic shock.
- Majority of patients have markedly increased cardiac filling pressures.
- Respiratory failure and sepsis are the second and third most common.
- Hypovolemic shock from hemorrhage, dehydration, and heat stroke.
- Hypotension (only 1 in 2 patients have documented low blood pressures)
- See Table 1 for a brief summary of the different causes of ischemic hepatitis.

Dx DIAGNOSIS

DIFFERENTIAL DIAGNOSIS (TABLE 2)

- Acute viral hepatitis
- Autoimmune hepatitis
- Drug-induced liver injury
- Other toxins and medications (i.e., acetaminophen toxicity)

WORKUP

- Diagnosed by laboratory parameters and the clinical context of a hospitalized patient.
- Workup is directed at identifying the predisposing cause.
- Liver biopsy is not required.
- Histology shows centrilobular (zone 3) necrosis with preservation of the hepatic architecture.
- Necrosis can extend to the midzonal hepatocytes in the setting of prolonged ischemia.

LABORATORY TESTS

- Extremely elevated aminotransferase levels, often exceeding 200 times the upper limit of normal.
- Aspartate aminotransferase (AST) and alanine aminotransferase (ALT) rapidly rise after the ischemic insult.
- They peak within 1 to 3 days.
- They usually return to normal within 7 to 10 days if the initial ischemic insult is resolved.
- Lactate dehydrogenase (LDH) level is extremely elevated.
- ALT/LDH ratio of less than 1.5 is suggestive.
- Prothrombin time can be slightly prolonged.
- The serum bilirubin can be mildly increased.
- Serum bilirubin peaks after the aminotransferases peak.
- Increased blood urea nitrogen and creatinine levels from acute tubular necrosis and renal dysfunction.

IMAGING STUDIES

Imaging is not required for the diagnosis.

Rx TREATMENT

NONPHARMACOLOGIC THERAPY

Management is directed at treating the underlying illness causing the systemic disturbance.

ACUTE GENERAL TREATMENT

- Hemodynamic resuscitation
- Inotropic agents for cardiogenic shock
- Intravenous fluid resuscitation with or without vasoconstrictors for septic or hypovolemic shock
- Blood transfusions if hypovolemic shock from blood loss
- These measures optimize hepatic perfusion and resolve tissue hypoxia
- There is no role for *N*-acetylcysteine administration

TABLE 1 Causes of Ischemic Hepatitis

Cardiovascular disease (most common): Cardiogenic shock
Respiratory failure
Sepsis/septic shock
Hypovolemic shock: Hemorrhage, volume depletion
Hypotension

TABLE 2 Common Differentials of Ischemic Hepatitis

Acute viral hepatitis (e.g., hepatitis A, hepatitis B)
Autoimmune hepatitis
Toxins (e.g., herbal supplements)
Medications (e.g., acetaminophen)

CHRONIC TREATMENT

- Ensure stability of underlying illness
- No specific liver-directed therapy

DISPOSITION

- Most commonly a self-limited and benign condition if promptly managed.
- Occasionally associated with significant mortality.
- Prognosis is determined by the severity of the underlying illness. In-hospital mortality associated with ischemic hepatitis is roughly 50%.
- Patients with underlying chronic heart failure or cirrhosis have worse outcomes.
- Other poor prognostic factors include persistently elevated aminotransferase and multiorgan failure.

REFERRAL

- Referral to a hepatologist is not required once illness is resolved.
- Referral is appropriate if patient has underlying cirrhosis.

PEARLS AND CONSIDERATIONS

COMMENTS

- Have a high index of suspicion for this diagnosis in a hospitalized patient with severe systemic illness and significantly elevated AST and ALT
- Use ALT/LDH ratio to aid in the diagnosis
- Do not be alarmed if bilirubin continues to rise after AST and ALT peak
- Hypotension is often not documented or not present at all
- Patients with significantly elevated liver enzymes should be evaluated for occult heart failure

PREVENTION

Ensure stability of comorbidities (e.g., cardiac disease)

AUTHOR: **HIRSH D. TRIVEDI, M.D.**

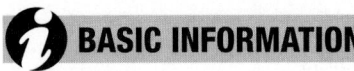

DEFINITION

Jaundice is a yellowish discoloration of the sclera (Fig. E1), skin, and mucous membranes caused by an excessive amount of bilirubin in the bloodstream. Clinically detectable jaundice in adults is a serum bilirubin of 2.5 to 3 mg/dl.

SYNONYM

Icterus

ICD-10CM CODE
R17 Unspecified jaundice

EPIDEMIOLOGY & DEMOGRAPHICS

The prevalent causes of jaundice by age and sex:

- Young adulthood (for either sex): Viral hepatitis, Gilbert disease
- Middle adulthood (for either sex): Drug-induced hepatitis and cirrhosis
- Middle-aged and older men: Alcoholic liver disease, pancreatic cancer, hepatoma, primary hemochromatosis
- Women: Primary biliary cirrhosis, chronic active hepatitis, choledocholithiasis, carcinoma of the gallbladder

PHYSICAL FINDINGS & CLINICAL PRESENTATION

Presentation can vary from an incidental finding to acute and life threatening. History and physical examination give important clues to the underlying condition.

Key history of present illness findings:

- Duration of jaundice
- Associated symptoms: Abdominal pain, fever, nausea, malaise, pruritus, chills, changes in urine and stool color, anorexia and/or weight loss

Key social history/exposure findings:

- Alcohol use, injection of illicit drugs, use of hepatotoxic medication or herbal products, blood transfusions, unprotected sex, ingestion of shellfish, travel, occupational exposure to toxins

Key medical history findings:

- Prior abdominal/biliary surgery, prior episodes of jaundice, prior diagnosis of hepatitis B or C, inflammatory bowel disease

Key physical findings:

- Vital sign abnormalities: Fever, hypotension, tachycardia
- Signs of acute disease: Abdominal tenderness, splenomegaly, abdominal mass, encephalopathy, Murphy's sign
- Signs of chronic liver disease: Palmar erythema, spider angiomas, bruising, gynecomastia, testicular atrophy, ascites, weight loss, Kayser-Fleischer rings (Wilson), caput medusa, internal hemorrhoids, scleral icterus

ETIOLOGY

Disruption in any of the three phases of bilirubin metabolism can lead to jaundice:

- Prehepatic phase: An increase in heme degradation products from red blood cell catabolism, ineffective erythropoiesis, or breakdown of muscle myoglobin and cytochromes; leads to indirect (unconjugated) hyperbilirubinemia
- Intrahepatic phase: Destruction of the hepatocytes or disruption of either of the two separate biochemical processes that conjugate bilirubin in the hepatocyte; may lead to indirect (unconjugated) or direct (conjugated) hyperbilirubinemia
- Posthepatic phase: Blockage of the release of water-soluble bilirubin from the hepatobiliary system, preventing excretion into the stool or urine or recycling within the gut flora; leads to direct (conjugated) hyperbilirubinemia

Dx DIAGNOSIS

DIFFERENTIAL DIAGNOSIS

Prehepatic causes:

- Hemolytic processes (e.g., sickle cell disease, spherocytosis, thalassemia, G6PD, immune hemolysis, HUS), ineffective erythropoiesis (e.g., thalassemia, folate, severe iron deficiency), or large hematoma reabsorption.

Intrahepatic causes:

- If unconjugated hyperbilirubinemia: Enzyme metabolism disorders (Gilbert disease, Crigler-Najjar syndrome), drugs that alter the enzymatic pathways such as rifampin, isoniazid, and probenecid.
- If conjugated hyperbilirubinemia: Intrahepatic cholestasis caused by:
  1. Viruses: hepatitis A, B, and C; Epstein-Barr, hemorrhagic viruses (yellow fever, Ebola)
  2. Other infections: Bacteria (leptospirosis, MAI), parasites (schistosomiasis, malaria, amebiasis), fungal (blastomyces, histoplasma)
  3. Alcohol: Alcoholic hepatitis, alcoholic cirrhosis
  4. Autoimmune: Primary biliary cirrhosis, primary sclerosing cholangitis, autoimmune hepatitis
  5. Hepatotoxic drug-induced: Acetaminophen (most common), penicillins (most commonly Augmentin), chlorpromazine, steroids (estrogenic or anabolic), NSAIDs, valproic acid, some herbals such as kava, ma huang, and off-market weight-loss supplements
  6. Hereditary/metabolic: Sickle cell disease and other RBC dyscrasias, hemochromatosis, Wilson disease, Dubin-Johnson and Rotor syndromes, α-antitrypsin deficiency, glycogen storage disease, NASH (nonalcoholic steatohepatitis), porphyria, benign recurrent intrahepatic cholestasis
  7. Systemic disease: Invading liver: Sarcoidosis, amyloidosis, hemochromatosis, tuberculosis, *Mycobacterium avium intracellulare*
  8. Other: Cirrhosis, sepsis, total parenteral nutrition, intrahepatic cholestasis of pregnancy, graft-versus-host disease, environmental toxins, benign postoperative state

Posthepatic causes:

- Intrinsic or extrinsic obstruction of the biliary system
  1. Blockage within hepatobiliary tree: Strictures, cholangiocarcinoma, gallbladder cancer, carcinoma of ampulla of Vater, infection (e.g., cytomegalovirus, *Cryptosporidium* in patients with AIDS, parasites), choledocholithiasis
  2. Blockage outside of hepatobiliary tree: Pancreatitis, pancreatic carcinoma, pancreatic pseudocyst, lymphoma
- Pseudojaundice: Not related to bilirubin but rather resulting from excessive ingestion of foods containing beta carotene (e.g., carrots, melons, squash)

WORKUP

- History, physical examination, and first-line lab tests can often clarify diagnosis. Fig. 2 describes a clinical approach to jaundice.
- Table 1 summarizes the differential diagnosis of critical and emergent diagnoses in patients with jaundice.

LABORATORY TESTS

- First-line tests:
  1. Serum total and direct bilirubin
  2. Urinalysis
  3. Liver function tests (AST, ALT, GGTP, alkaline phosphatase), CBC, liver synthetic function (albumin, PT, PTT), pancreatic function (amylase, lipase)
- If serum total bilirubin and direct bilirubin are elevated and urine is positive for bilirubin, consider intrahepatic or posthepatic process. If serum total bilirubin is elevated but direct bilirubin is normal (unconjugated hyperbilirubinemia) and urine is negative for bilirubin, consider prehepatic or intrahepatic processes.

Additional tests if diagnosis unclear:

- Screen for hepatitis A, B, and C; if still unclear, then consider following options based on H&P.
- Other viruses: EBV, CMV.
- Autoimmune disorders: Antimitochondrial antibody (elevated in primary biliary cirrhosis); anti-smooth muscle antibody, ANA (elevated in autoimmune hepatitis); antinuclear cytoplasmic antibody (elevated in primary sclerosing cholangitis).
- Ceruloplasmin (elevated in Wilson disease).
- Alpha-1 antitrypsin deficiency (elevated in cirrhosis and emphysema).
- Ferritin, Fe saturation (elevated in hemochromatosis).
- Blood smear (RBC dyscrasias).
- Diagnosis of exclusion: Gilbert syndrome.
- Liver biopsy: Essential in diagnosis of chronic hepatitis. Can be used for diagnosis of liver masses but carries a substantial risk.

IMAGING STUDIES

- Abdominal ultrasound: First-line study (Figs. E3 and E4) may be completed bedside, most sensitive for proximal biliary tract disease; presence of dilated ducts hints at an extrahepatic process.

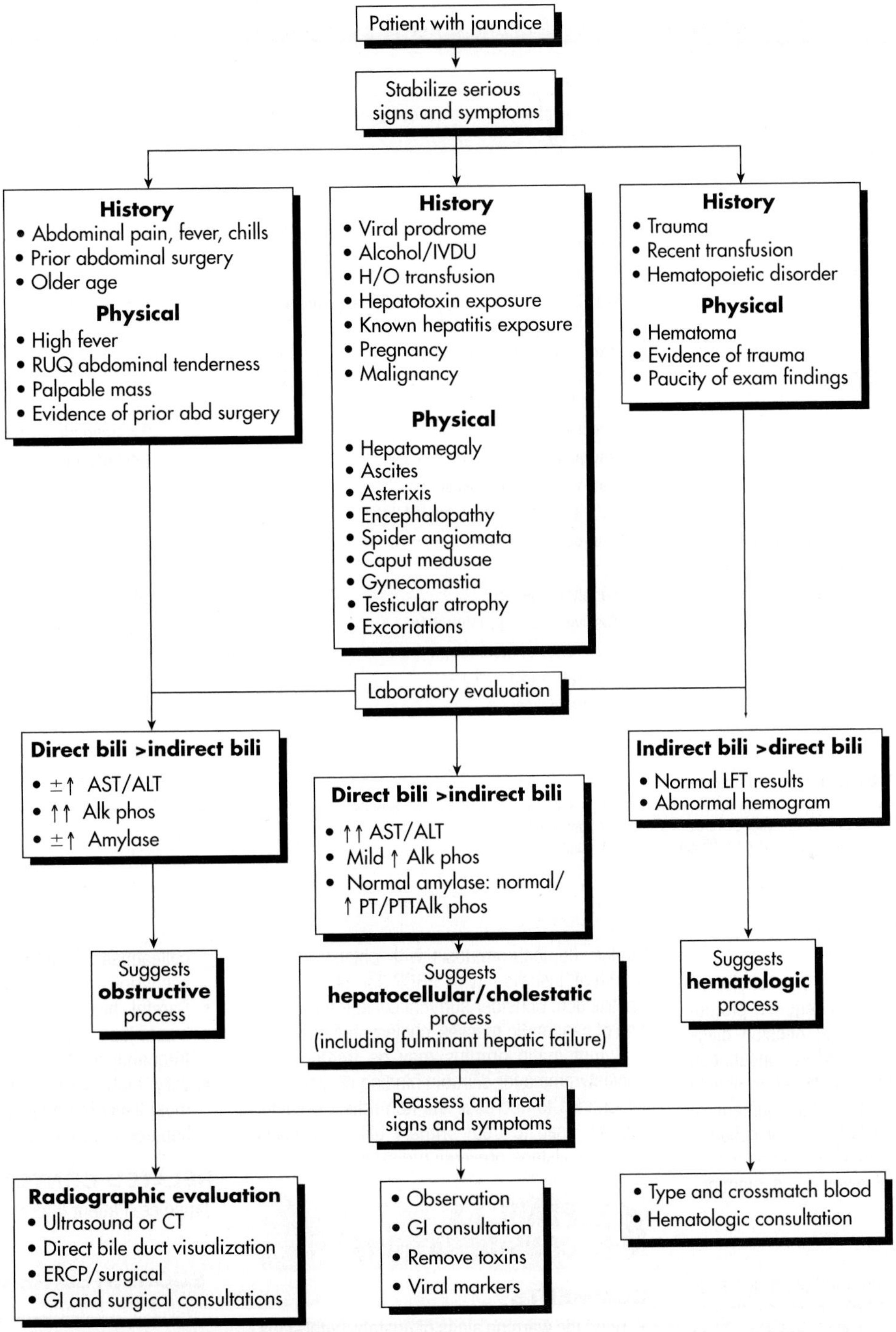

Patient with jaundice

Stabilize serious signs and symptoms

History
- Abdominal pain, fever, chills
- Prior abdominal surgery
- Older age

Physical
- High fever
- RUQ abdominal tenderness
- Palpable mass
- Evidence of prior abd surgery

History
- Viral prodrome
- Alcohol/IVDU
- H/O transfusion
- Hepatotoxin exposure
- Known hepatitis exposure
- Pregnancy
- Malignancy

Physical
- Hepatomegaly
- Ascites
- Asterixis
- Encephalopathy
- Spider angiomata
- Caput medusae
- Gynecomastia
- Testicular atrophy
- Excoriations

History
- Trauma
- Recent transfusion
- Hematopoietic disorder

Physical
- Hematoma
- Evidence of trauma
- Paucity of exam findings

Laboratory evaluation

Direct bili >indirect bili
- ±↑ AST/ALT
- ↑↑ Alk phos
- ±↑ Amylase

Direct bili >indirect bili
- ↑↑ AST/ALT
- Mild ↑ Alk phos
- Normal amylase: normal/↑ PT/PTTAlk phos

Indirect bili >direct bili
- Normal LFT results
- Abnormal hemogram

Suggests **obstructive** process

Suggests **hepatocellular/cholestatic** process (including fulminant hepatic failure)

Suggests **hematologic** process

Reassess and treat signs and symptoms

Radiographic evaluation
- Ultrasound or CT
- Direct bile duct visualization
- ERCP/surgical
- GI and surgical consultations

- Observation
- GI consultation
- Remove toxins
- Viral markers

- Type and crossmatch blood
- Hematologic consultation

FIG. 2 Management of the patient with jaundice. *Alk phos,* Alkaline phosphatase; *ALT,* alanine aminotransferase; *AST,* aspartate aminotransferase; *bili,* bilirubin; *CT,* computed tomography; *ERCP,* endoscopic retrograde cholangiopancreatography; *GI,* gastrointestinal; *H/O,* history of; *IVDU,* intravenous drug use; *LFT,* liver function test; *PT,* prothrombin time; *PTT,* partial thromboplastin time; *RUQ,* right upper quadrant. (From Marx AJ et al: *Rosen's emergency medicine: concepts and clinical practice,* ed 7, Philadelphia, 2010, Elsevier.)

- Abdominal CT: Often necessary to elucidate more information on liver, pancreas, and distal biliary system.
- Endoscopic retrograde cholangiopancreatography: Rarely necessary for diagnostics. Refer to GI consultant.
- Percutaneous transhepatic cholangiography: Rarely necessary for diagnostics. Refer to GI or surgical consultant.
- Magnetic resonance cholangiopancreatography: Noninvasive visualization of bile and pancreatic ducts. Refer to GI consultant.
- Endoscopic ultrasound: Used for characterization and, if needed, biopsy of any focal lesions found within biliary tree and/or pancreas. Refer to GI consultant.

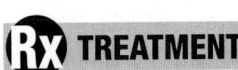

TREATMENT

NONPHARMACOLOGIC THERAPY

Depends on underlying cause of the jaundice and clinical stability of the patient. Generally, obstructive causes require surgical treatment, while nonobstructive causes require medical treatment.

TABLE 1 Jaundice: Differential Diagnosis of Critical and Emergent Diagnoses

System	Critical	Emergent	Nonemergent
Hepatic	Fulminant hepatic failure	Hepatitis of any cause with confusion, bleeding, or coagulopathy	Hepatitis with normal mental status, normal vital signs, and no active bleeding
	Toxin	Wilson disease	
	Virus	Primary biliary cirrhosis	
	Alcohol	Autoimmune hepatitis	
	Ischemic insult	Liver transplant rejection	
	Reye's syndrome	Infiltrative liver disease	
		Drug induced (isoniazid, phenytoin, acetaminophen, ritonavir, halothane, sulfonamides)	
		Toxin ingestion or exposure	
Biliary	Cholangitis	Bile duct obstruction (stone, inflammation, stricture, neoplasm)	
Systemic	Sepsis	Sarcoidosis	Posttraumatic hematoma resorption
	Heatstroke	Amyloidosis	Total parenteral nutrition
		Graft-versus-host disease	
Cardiovascular	Obstructing AAA	Right-sided congestive heart failure	
	Budd-Chiari syndrome	Veno-occlusive disease	
	Severe congestive heart failure		
Hematologic-oncologic	Transfusion reaction	Hemolytic anemia	Gilbert syndrome
		Massive malignant infiltration	Physiologic neonatal jaundice
		Inborn error of metabolism	
		Pancreatic head tumor	
		Metastatic disease	
Reproductive	Preeclampsia or HELLP syndrome	Hyperemesis gravidarum	
	Acute fatty liver of pregnancy		Cholestasis of pregnancy

AAA, Abdominal aortic aneurysm; *HELLP,* hemolysis, elevated liver enzymes, low platelets.
From Marx JA et al: *Rosen's emergency medicine,* ed 8, Philadelphia, 2014, Saunders.

ACUTE GENERAL Rx

Acute, life-threatening illness (e.g., cholecystitis or ascending cholangitis) requires prompt diagnosis with basic labs and bedside diagnostics, with early surgical and GI consultation in conjunction. Suspicious medications should be stopped. Initiate medical management of symptoms with analgesia, IV fluids, correction of coagulopathies, and consideration of antibiotics. *N*-Acetylcysteine can be given for acetaminophen overdose.

CHRONIC Rx

Reversible causes must be ruled out first—suspicious medications and EtOH must be discontinued. Consider GI consult for management of many intrahepatic diseases, such as treatment of hepatitis B or C, Wilson disease with penicillamine, hemochromatosis with phlebotomy, or for stent insertion with ERCP for posthepatic obstruction. Consider surgical consult for resection of pancreatic masses, cholecystectomy, etc.

Symptomatic pruritus may be treated with cholestyramine for bilirubin binding or with antihistamines to decrease the itch reflex. Ursodiol may be used to treat primary biliary cirrhosis and for gallstone prevention/dissolution.

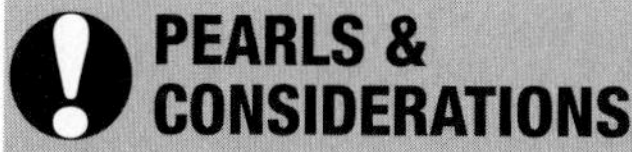

PEARLS & CONSIDERATIONS

COMMENTS

- Heed the warning signs of unstable vital signs to diagnose life-threatening illness; early collaboration with surgical and gastroenterology colleagues is helpful in complex patient care scenarios.
- Careful history and physical examination, basic labs, and prompt bedside imaging frequently lead to accurate diagnosis.
- Very high serum bilirubin (>15 mg/dl) is most likely to be seen in cirrhosis. Watch for hepatorenal syndrome in these patients.

RELATED CONTENT

Jaundice (Patient Information)

SUGGESTED READINGS

Available at ExpertConsult.com

AUTHORS: **ALLA GOLDBURT, M.D.,** and **PAOLO G. PACE, M.A.S.C., M.D.**

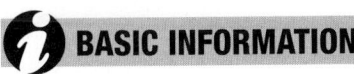

BASIC INFORMATION

DEFINITION

Junctional rhythm is an abnormal cardiac rhythm originating in the His bundle or atrioventricular (AV) node. This diagnosis includes three distinct entities based on rate:

1. A junctional escape rhythm has a rate of 40-60 bpm.
2. Accelerated junctional rhythm has a rate of 60-100 bpm.
3. Junctional ectopic tachycardia (JET) has a rate of >100 bpm.

SYNONYMS

Junctional escape rhythm
Accelerated junctional rhythm
Junctional ectopic tachycardia (JET)
Nodal rhythm disorder
Ectopic rhythm disorder
Junctional premature depolarization

ICD-10CM CODE

I49.2 Junctional premature depolarization

EPIDEMIOLOGY & DEMOGRAPHICS

INCIDENCE: Junctional rhythm occurs more commonly in children due to higher vagal tone (13% of 10- to 13-yr-old boys, 45% of 7- to 10-yr-old children, and 19% of infants have junctional rhythm during sleep).[1] Endurance athletes have a 20% incidence of junctional rhythm, for a similar reason.

PREVALENCE: Junctional tachycardia is a rare cause of supraventricular tachycardia. It is rare in the pediatric population and even less common in adults. On the contrary, junctional rhythm is common although the prevalence is not well defined.

GENETICS: There is no known hereditary component.

RISK FACTORS: Conduction system disease, heart block, digitalis intoxication, heart surgery, endocarditis

PHYSICAL FINDINGS & CLINICAL PRESENTATION

ESSENTIAL HISTORY:

- Previous history of syncope, presyncope, lightheadedness.
- Drugs, especially digoxin. Amount taken, time of ingestion. The digestion time is especially important because the serum digoxin level ideally should be measured at least 6 hours after ingestion to ensure accuracy. Obtain a thorough medication history to determine if any recent additions or dosing changes were made.

SYMPTOMS:

- Lightheadedness
- Syncope
- Palpitations
- Symptoms associated with digitalis intoxication: Gastrointestinal symptoms such as anorexia, nausea, vomiting, and abdominal pain. Neurologic manifestation such as lethargy, fatigue, delirium, confusion, weakness. Visual changes: Alteration in color vision, diplopia, photophobia, decreased visual acuity

PHYSICAL EXAMINATION:

- Vital signs
- Look for evidence of hypoperfusion and end organ dysfunction
- Cannon A-waves on examination of the jugular pulse

ETIOLOGY

Junctional tachycardia can occur as a primary arrhythmia (usually in children-JET), secondary to digitalis intoxication or catecholamine intoxication, or in the setting of injury to the His bundle (e.g., after valve surgery, abscess, sarcoidosis, myocarditis, ischemia, etc.).

DIAGNOSIS

DIFFERENTIAL DIAGNOSIS

- AVNRT (atrioventricular nodal reentrant tachycardia)
- AVRT (atrioventricular reentrant tachycardia)
- Accelerated idioventricular rhythm–in the case of junctional rhythm with aberrant conduction
- Fig. 1 illustrates arrhythmias originating in the atrioventricular node

WORKUP

- Vital signs
- 12 lead ECG. (Figs. 2 and 3). The rhythm is almost perfectly regular and the QRS complex is generally narrow and similar to the complex seen during sinus rhythm. Retrograde P waves with a very short interval from QRS to P wave can be seen
- History of cardiac surgery, fevers, drug ingestion

LABORATORY TESTS

- Serum digoxin concentration
- Serum potassium concentration
- Creatinine and blood urea nitrogen (BUN) to assess renal function
- Troponin

IMAGING STUDIES

Echocardiogram

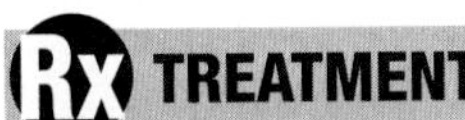

TREATMENT

Junctional tachycardia may be a marker for a serious underlying condition such as digitalis toxicity, postcardiac surgery, endocarditis, hypokalemia, or myocardial ischemia. Underlying conditions should be sought and corrected accordingly.

NONPHARMACOLOGIC THERAPY

- Junctional escape rhythm in the setting of sinus arrest or complete heart block without reversible cause necessitates permanent pacemaker implantation.
- Junctional ectopic tachycardia can be treated with antiarrhythmics or radiofrequency ablation.

ELECTROPHYSIOLOGY STUDY: The origin of this tachycardia is within the His bundle or AV node, and it can be diagnosed definitively by intracardiac recordings. Junctional rhythm most frequently takes the form of escape rhythms in the presence of sinus node dysfunction or AV nodal block, which can be diagnosed on electrophysiology (EP) study. These escape rhythms usually have a QRS morphology identical to that seen during sinus rhythm. In such cases, there is no P wave before the QRS complexes. The P waves can occur simultaneously with the QRS complexes; more commonly, they are retrograde. When the junctional rhythm is faster than 100 beats/min, it is called junctional tachycardia.

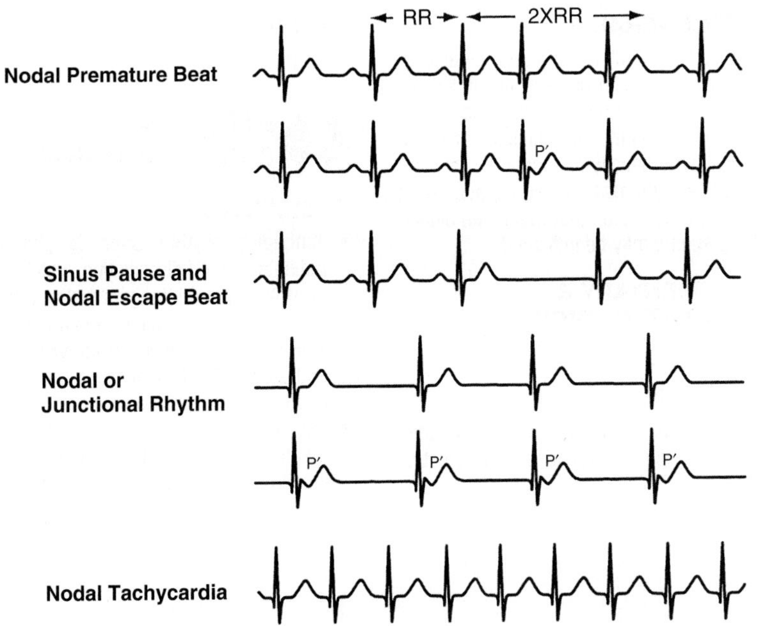

FIG. 1 Arrhythmias originating in the atrioventricular node. (From Park MK: *Park's pediatric cardiology for practitioners*, ed 6, Philadelphia, 2014, Elsevier.)

[1] Drago F et al: Neonatal and pediatric arrhythmias: clinical and electrocardiographic aspects, *Card Electrophysiol Clin* 10(2):397-412, 2018.

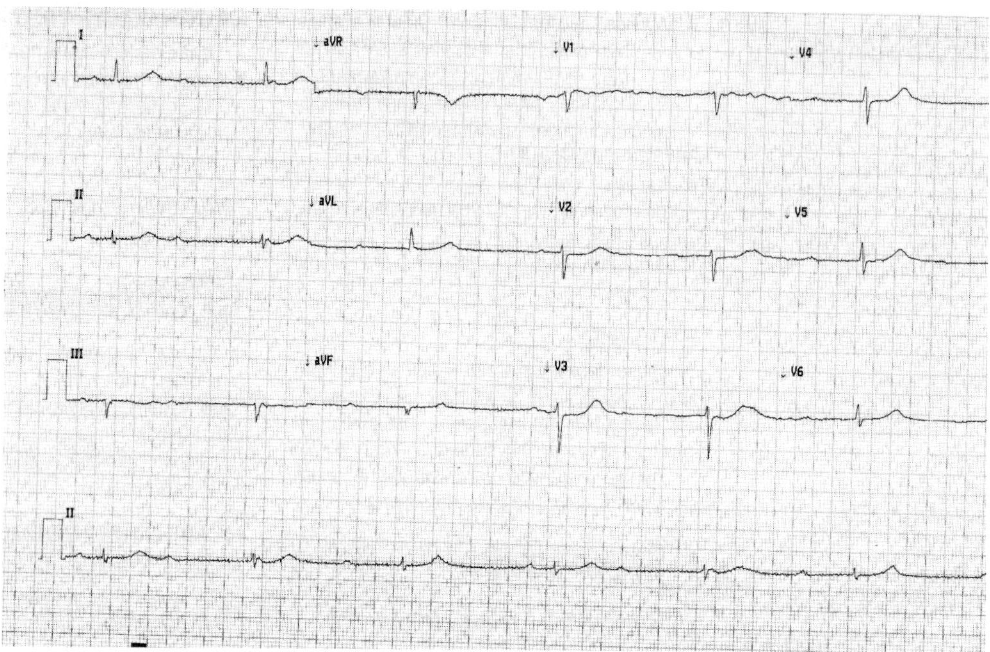

FIG. 2 Electrocardiogram of a patient with junctional rhythm and complete heart block. Note the narrow QRS complex and dissociated P waves. *aVF,* Augmented vector foot; *aVL,* augmented vector left; *aVR,* augmented vector right.

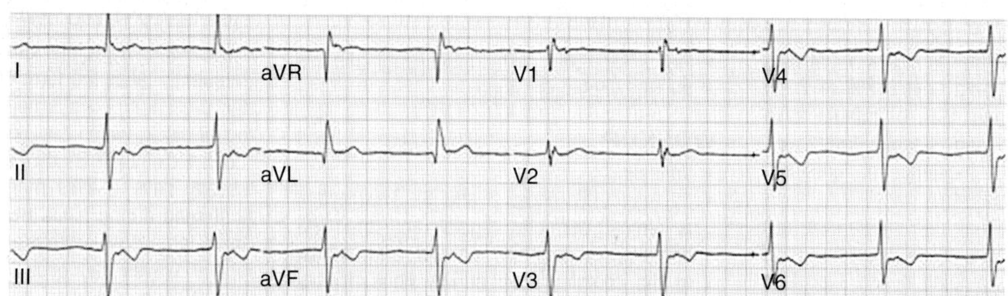

FIG. 3 Junctional rhythm with retrograde P waves that are negative in the inferior leads. *aVF,* Augmented vector foot; *aVL,* augmented vector left; *aVR,* augmented vector right. (From Parrillo JE, Dellinger RP: *Critical care medicine: principles of diagnosis and management in the adult,* ed 4, Philadelphia, 2014, Elsevier.)

ACUTE GENERAL Rx

The mainstay of managing nonparoxysmal junctional tachycardia is to correct the underlying abnormality. Withholding digitalis when junctional tachycardia is the only clinical manifestation of toxicity is usually adequate. If, however, ventricular arrhythmias or high-grade heart block are observed, then treatment with digitalis-binding agents may be indicated.

COMPLEMENTARY & ALTERNATIVE MEDICINE

N/A

DISPOSITION

Admit to cardiac telemetry if symptomatic. Consider specialty referral to cardiac electrophysiology.

REFERRAL

Refer to cardiologist.

PEARLS & CONSIDERATIONS

COMMENTS

- Junctional rhythm often is observed in patients with AV dissociation, which can lead to atrial contraction against closed atrioventricular valves, resulting in cannon A waves. This wave will cause pulsation in the neck and abdomen, headache, cough, jaw pain and possible hypotension.
- The presence of a perfectly regular rhythm in a patient with atrial fibrillation often indicates junctional rhythm with complete heart block.

PREVENTION

N/A

SUGGESTED READING

Available at ExpertConsult.com

RELATED CONTENT

Digitalis Overdose (Related Key Topic)
Sick Sinus Syndrome (Related Key Topic)
Heart Block, Complete (Related Key Topic)
Heart Block, Second Degree (Related Key Topic)

AUTHORS: **AHARON EREZ, M.D.,** and **JOHN WYLIE, M.D.**

BASIC INFORMATION

DEFINITION

Juenile idiopathic arthritis (JIA), previously referred to as juvenile rheumatoid arthritis (JRA), is a diverse spectrum of chronic arthritides, involving ≥1 joints for at least 6 weeks in a patient ≤16 yr of age. Other causes of arthritis must be excluded.

SYNONYMS

JIA
JRA
Juvenile rheumatoid arthritis (JRA)
Still's disease (specifically systemic JIA)

ICD-10CM CODES

M08.00 Unspecified juvenile rheumatoid arthritis of unspecified site
M08.29 Juvenile rheumatoid arthritis with systemic onset, multiple sites
M08.40 Pauciarticular juvenile rheumatoid arthritis, unspecified site
M08.09 Unspecified juvenile rheumatoid arthritis, multiple sites
M08.20 Juvenile rheumatoid arthritis with systemic onset, unspecified site

EPIDEMIOLOGY & DEMOGRAPHICS

PREVALENCE: 1 per 1000 children in the U.S.; more common in children of European ancestry

PHYSICAL FINDINGS & CLINICAL PRESENTATION

- JIA is subdivided into seven categories based on the International League of Associations for Rheumatology (ILAR) classification criteria (summarized in Table 1).
  1. Systemic onset JIA (4% to 17%)
     a. Arthritis in ≥1 joints with or preceded by fever of at least 2-wk duration that is quotidian (once daily) for at least 3 days and associated with at least one of the following: (1) evanescent erythematous rash (Fig. E1); (2) generalized lymphadenopathy; (3) hepatomegaly, splenomegaly, or both; and (4) serositis.
- Oligoarticular JIA (Fig. 2) (27% to 56%)
  1. Arthritis in <4 joints in the first 6 mo of disease. There are two subtypes:
     a. Persistent: ≤4 joints throughout the disease course.
     b. Extended: ≤4 joints during the first 6 mo extending to >4 joints after 6 mo.
- Polyarthritis, rheumatoid factor (RF) negative (11% to 28%)
  1. Arthritis in >5 joints during first 6 mo of the disease with negative RF.
- Polyarthritis, RF positive (2% to 7%)
  1. Arthritis involves ≥5 joints during first 6 mo of the disease with positive RF on at least two tests run 3 mo apart.
  2. Anti–cyclic citrullinated (CCP) antibodies may also be present.
  3. Most similar to adult rheumatoid arthritis; most likely to progress.
- Psoriatic arthritis (2% to 11%)
  1. Psoriasis and arthritis or psoriasis and ≥2 of the following:
     a. Dactylitis, nail pitting, onycholysis, and psoriasis in a first-degree relative.
- Enthesitis-related arthritis (3% to 11%)
  1. Arthritis or enthesitis and ≥2 of the following:
     a. Sacroiliac tenderness, positive HLA-B27, male age >6 yr, acute anterior uveitis, or first-degree relative with HLA-B27-associated disease
- Undifferentiated arthritis (11% to 21%)
  1. Fulfills criteria in ≥2 categories above, or none of them

ETIOLOGY

Genetically susceptible individuals may develop an inappropriate immune response toward a self-antigen after exposure to an environmental trigger. Variants in HLA, PTPN22, and STAT4 loci may be associated with disease.

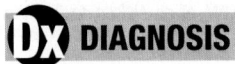

DIAGNOSIS

DIFFERENTIAL DIAGNOSIS

- Infection: Viral (parvovirus, toxic synovitis) or bacterial (Lyme, osteomyelitis, septic joints)
- Inflammation: Lupus, serum sickness, inflammatory bowel disease

TABLE 1 Overview of the Main Features of the Subtypes of Juvenile Idiopathic Arthritis

ILAR Subtype	Peak Age of Onset (yr)	Female: Male; % of All JIA	Arthritis Pattern	Extraarticular Features	Investigations	Notes on Therapy
Systemic arthritis	2-4	1:1; ~10% of JIA cases	Polyarticular, often knees, wrists, and ankles; also fingers, neck, and hips	Daily fever; evanescent rash; pericarditis; pleuritis	Anemia; WBC↑↑; ESR↑↑; CRP↑↑; ferritin;↑ platelets↑↑ (normal or ↑ in MAS)	Less responsive to standard treatment with MTX and anti-TNF agents; consider IL-1Ra in resistant cases
Oligoarthritis	>6	4:1; 50%-60% of JIA (but ethnic variation)	Knees ++; ankles, fingers +	Uveitis in ~30%	ANA positive in 60%; other tests usually normal; may have mildly ↑ ESR/CRP	NSAIDs and intraarticular steroids; occasionally require MTX
Polyarthritis, RF negative	6-7	3:1; 30% of JIA cases	Symmetric or asymmetric; small and large joints; cervical spine; TMJ	Uveitis in ~10%	ANA positive in 40%; RF negative; ESR ↑ or; ↑↑ CRP↑/normal; mild anemia	Standard therapy with MTX and NSAIDs, then if nonresponsive, anti-TNF agents or other biologics
Polyarthritis, RF positive	9-12	9:1; >10% of JIA cases	Aggressive symmetric polyarthritis	Rheumatoid nodules in 10%; low-grade fever	RF positive; ESR ↑↑; CRP ↑/normal; mild anemia	Long-term remission unlikely; early aggressive therapy is warranted
Psoriatic arthritis	7-10	2:1; >10% of JIA cases	Asymmetric arthritis of small or medium sized joints	Uveitis in 10%; psoriasis in 50%	ANA positive in 50%; ESR ↑; CRP ↑/normal; mild anemia	NSAIDs and intraarticular steroids; second-line agents less commonly
Enthesitis-related arthritis	9-12	1:7; 10% of JIA cases	Predominantly lower limb joints affected; sometimes axial skeleton (but less than adult AS)	Acute anterior uveitis; association with reactive arthritis and IBD	80% HLA-B27[1]	NSAIDs and intraarticular steroids; consider sulfasalazine as alternative to MTX

ANA, Antinuclear antibody; *AS,* ankylosing spondylitis; *CRP,* C-reactive protein; *ESR,* erythrocyte sedimentation rate; *IBD,* inflammatory bowel disease; *ILAR,* International League of Associations for Rheumatology; *IL-1Ra,* interleukin-1 receptor antagonist; *JIA,* juvenile idiopathic arthritis; *MAS,* macrophage activation syndrome; *MTX,* methotrexate; *NSAID,* nonsteroidal anti-inflammatory drug; *RF,* rheumatoid factor; *TMJ,* temporomandibular joint; *TNF,* tumor necrosis factor; *WBC,* white blood cell count.
From Firestein G et al: *Kelley's textbook of rheumatology,* ed 9, Philadelphia, 2013, Saunders.

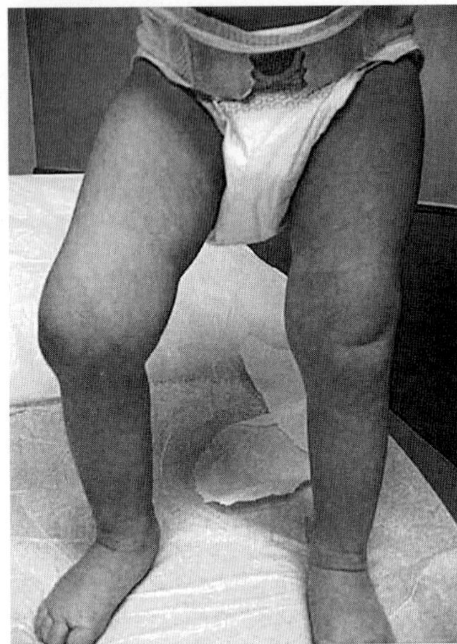

FIG. 2 Oligoarticular juvenile idiopathic arthritis with swelling and flexion contracture of the right knee. (From Kliegman RM et al: *Nelson textbook of pediatrics,* ed 19, Philadelphia, 2011, Saunders.)

- Reactive: Post-streptococcal, rheumatic fever
- Malignancy: Leukemia, bone tumors

LABORATORY TESTS

- No single diagnostic test. Rule out other causes of arthritis
- Elevated sedimentation rate and C-reactive protein
- Mild anemia, leukocytosis
- Rheumatoid factor: Rarely positive in children
- Antinuclear antibodies: Elevation associated with ocular complications
- Pancytopenia, a consumptive coagulopathy, elevated ferritin, and liver enzymes are indicative of macrophage activation syndrome in systemic JIA. Bone marrow biopsy is needed to confirm diagnosis

IMAGING STUDIES

- Radiographs show soft tissue swelling and periarticular osteopenia early in the disease (Fig. 3).
- Joint destruction (Fig. 4) is less frequent, but bony erosion and cyst formation may be present.

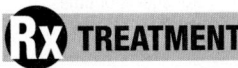

TREATMENT

NONPHARMACOLOGIC THERAPY

Collaboration among the patient's pediatrician, rheumatologist, orthopedist, and physical therapist yields the best outcome. Education regarding diet and weight management (Fig. 5).

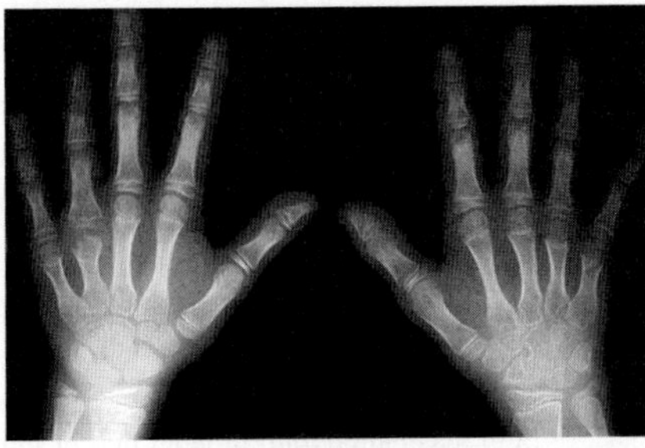

FIG. 3 Juvenile idiopathic arthritis (JIA). Oligoarticular-onset JIA in an 8-yr-old. Epiphyseal destruction and undergrowth of the third metacarpophalangeal joint of the left hand are seen, as well as overgrowth of the carpal bones of the right wrist compared with the left wrist. Also note the widened appearance of the third phalanges caused by periosteal new bone formation. (From Hochberg MC et al: *Rheumatology,* ed 5, St Louis, 2011, Mosby.)

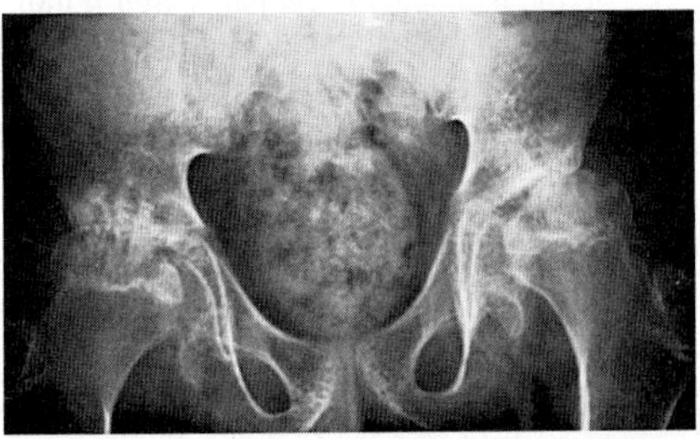

FIG. 4 Severe hip disease in a 13-yr-old boy with active, systemic-onset juvenile idiopathic arthritis. Radiograph shows destruction of the femoral head and acetabula, joint space narrowing, and subluxation of left hip. The patient had received corticosteroids systemically for 9 yr. (From Kliegman RM et al: *Nelson textbook of pediatrics,* ed 19, Philadelphia, 2011, Saunders.)

CHRONIC GENERAL Rx

- NSAIDs: Used as monotherapy or in conjunction with intraarticular steroids
- DMARDs: Methotrexate, leflunomide, sulfasalazine
  1. Required by two thirds of children
  2. Axial involvement is less responsive to methotrexate
- Biologics: Improve morbidity associated with JIA. Individual subtypes show varying responses to therapy
  1. Tumor necrosis factor antagonists such as etanercept and adalimumab
  2. T-cell modulator, abatacept
  3. IL-1 and IL-6 antagonists, anakinra, and tocilizumab for those with systemic JIA

  Meta-analysis of randomized controlled trials did not show statistically significant differences in the efficacy or safety profile of these agents.
- Systemic corticosteroids should be limited when possible.

DISPOSITION

- More than 50% continue to have active disease into adulthood.
- Patients with persistent oligoarticular disease are most likely to achieve remission, while those who are RF positive are least likely to achieve remission.
- Macrophage activation syndrome is a life-threatening complication in systemic JIA.
- Asymmetric joint involvement can lead to growth failure and limb length discrepancies.

REFERRAL

- Early rheumatology consultation.
- Ophthalmology consultation at diagnosis and at least annually.
- Children age <7 yr, with + ANA are at the highest risk for ocular inflammation and require screening every 3 to 4 mo.

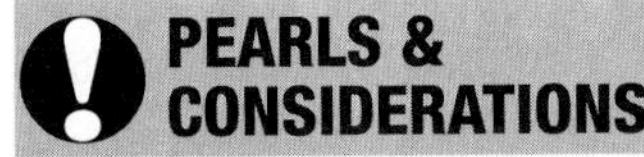
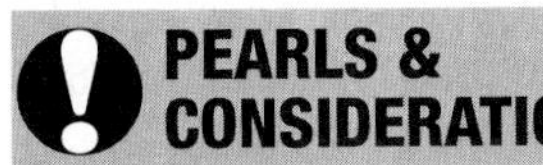

PEARLS & CONSIDERATIONS

COMMENTS

JIA is an autoinflammatory disease with a strong genetic component. Genomics is increasingly used to identify susceptibility loci. Immunomodulators have improved therapy in refractory disease. Normalization of the immune response early in the disease can limit disease progression. Children with JIA have an increased rate of malignancy compared with the general population. It is unclear if treatment with TNFi significantly increases the risk compared with no TNFi use.

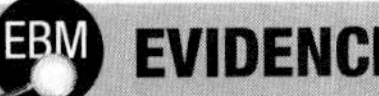

EVIDENCE

Available at ExpertConsult.com

SUGGESTED READINGS

Available at ExpertConsult.com

RELATED CONTENT

Juvenile Rheumatoid Arthritis (Patient Information)

AUTHOR: **MICHELLE C. MACIAG, M.D.**

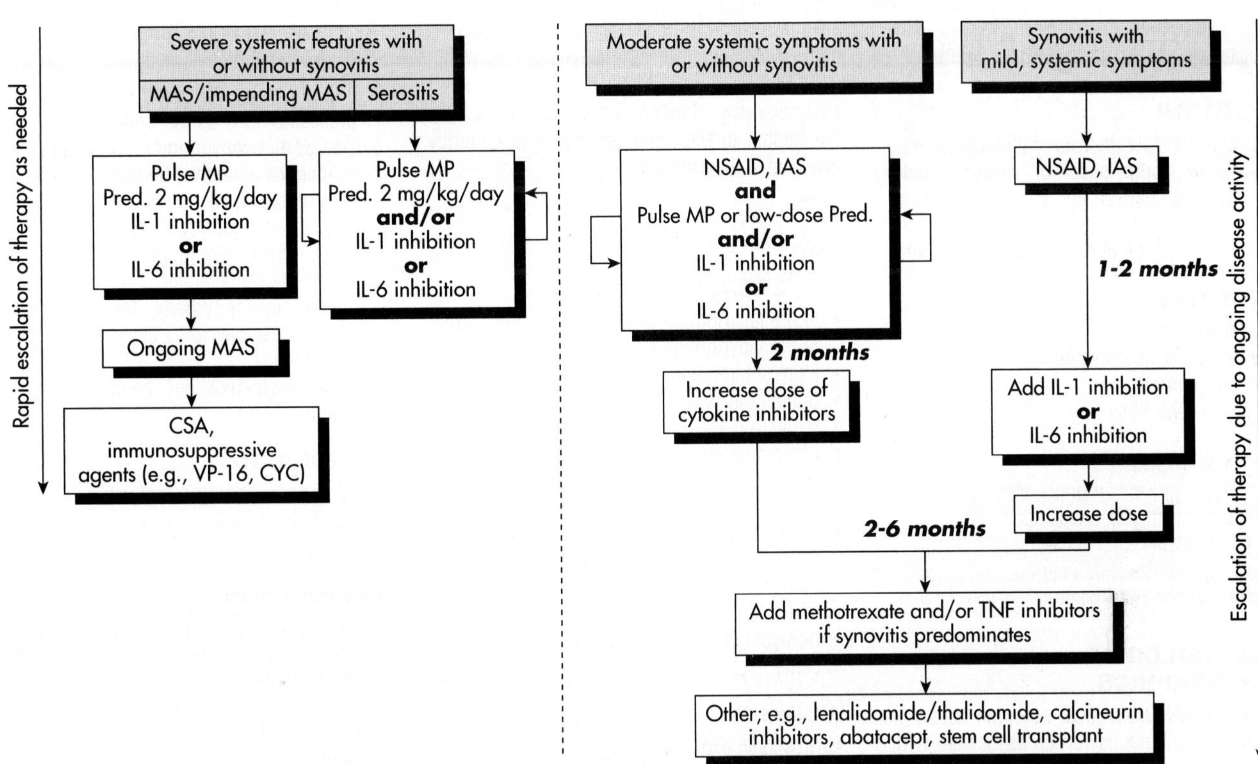

FIG. 5 Systemic juvenile idiopathic arthritis treatment algorithm. The treatment goal is remission of disease activity, both systemic and articular, and is stratified by severity of disease. Algorithm is divided into severe systemic disease manifestations (macrophage activation syndrome [MAS], serositis) or synovitis with milder systemic disease. Currently there is significant variability in practice regarding using corticosteroid as initial systemic therapy or moving directly to inflammatory cytokine inhibitors. At the time of this writing, interleukin (IL)-1 inhibition and IL-6 inhibition are currently in trials, and more information is likely to be available in the future. *CSA*, cyclosporine A; *CYC*, cyclophosphamide; *IAS*, intraarticular steroid; *MP*, methylprednisolone; *NSAID*, nonsteroidal antiinflammatory drug; *Pred.*, prednisone; *TNF*, tumor necrosis factor. (From Firestein GS et al: *Kelley's textbook of rheumatology*, ed 9, Philadelphia, 2013, Saunders.)

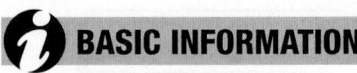

BASIC INFORMATION

DEFINITION

Labyrinthitis is a peripheral vestibulopathy characterized by acute onset of vertigo usually associated with nausea and vomiting. It can be associated with hearing loss and gait abnormalities and may be either serous or purulent.

SYNONYMS

Acute labyrinthitis
Acute vestibular neuronopathy
Vestibular neuronitis
Viral neurolabyrinthitis

ICD-10CM CODES

H81.23 Vestibular neuronitis, bilateral
H83.09 Labyrinthitis, unspecified ear
H83.01 Labyrinthitis, right ear
H83.02 Labyrinthitis, left ear
H83.03 Labyrinthitis, bilateral

EPIDEMIOLOGY & DEMOGRAPHICS

INCIDENCE (IN U.S.): Most common cause of prolonged spontaneous vertigo associated with nausea at any age
PREDOMINANT AGE: Any

CLINICAL PRESENTATION

- Vertigo, nausea, and vomiting with onset over several hours
- Symptoms usually peak within 24 hours, then resolve gradually over several weeks
- During the first day, the patient usually has difficulty focusing the eyes because of spontaneous nystagmus
- Usually has benign course with complete recovery within 1 to 3 mo, though older patients may have intractable dizziness that persists for many months

PHYSICAL FINDINGS

- Nystagmus
- Nausea
- Vomiting
- Vertigo worsening with head movement
- Abnormal caloric ENG tests
- May have hearing loss in the affected ear or ears
- Normal otoscopic exam typically
- Normal neurologic exam; may have signs of vestibular loss, such as a positive head thrust test

ETIOLOGY

Symptoms often preceded for 1 to 2 wk by a viral-like illness. Labyrinthitis may be either bacterial or viral and may be either tympanogenic (i.e., resulting from spread of infection into the inner ear from the middle ear, antrum, or petrous apex), meningogenic, or hematogenic from encephalitis or brain abscess. The round window membrane is considered the most likely pathway of inflammatory mediators from the middle to the inner ear that subsequently give rise to labyrinthitis.

DIAGNOSIS

DIFFERENTIAL DIAGNOSIS

- Acute labyrinthine ischemia (ischemic stroke of the labyrinthine artery)
- Labyrinthine fistula
- Benign paroxysmal positional vertigo
- Ménière disease
- Cholesteatoma
- Drug-induced vestibulocochlear nerve damage
- Vestibulocochlear nerve (cranial nerve VIII) tumor
- Head trauma
- Vertebrobasilar stroke
- Dehiscence of the superior semicircular canal

WORKUP

- Otoscopic examination
- Neurologic examination, with close attention to cranial nerves
- Bedside test of vestibular function, specifically head thrust or head heave test
- Audiogram if symptoms accompanied by hearing loss
- Caloric test if presentation is atypical

LABORATORY TESTS

- Routine laboratory tests are generally not helpful.
- If there is a history of significant emesis, check electrolytes, BUN, and creatinine.

IMAGING STUDIES

- Imaging studies are usually not necessary.
- Gadolinium-enhanced MRI may show enhancement of bony labyrinth. MRI of the brain with and without contrast with fine cuts through the internal auditory canal is indicated if there is an abnormal cranial nerve exam, headache, concern for stroke, or suspicion of cranial nerve VIII nerve tumor.
- Head CT with fine cuts through temporal bones is indicated if there is a history of trauma or suspicion of cholesteatoma.

TREATMENT

NONPHARMACOLOGIC THERAPY

- Reassurance
- Initial bed rest, then encourage increase in activity as tolerated

ACUTE GENERAL Rx

- Treatment is with antiemetics such as promethazine or ondansetron; vestibular suppressants such as the antihistamines meclizine or diphenhydramine; the anticholinergic scopolamine; and the benzodiazepines diazepam or lorazepam. These medications should only be continued for a few days during the acute phase. Some of these medications, especially scopolamine, should be used with caution in the elderly. Methylprednisolone 100 mg per day for 3 days, with slow taper over 3 wk.
- Valacyclovir has not been shown to be helpful.

CHRONIC Rx

- No specific pharmacologic chronic therapy.
- Vestibular rehabilitation is useful for patients with persistent symptoms.

DISPOSITION

Usually does not require hospital admission unless the patient is unable to tolerate oral intake of liquids

REFERRAL

- Refer if symptoms persist or neurologic abnormalities are present.
- Consider vestibular rehabilitation, particularly in the elderly.

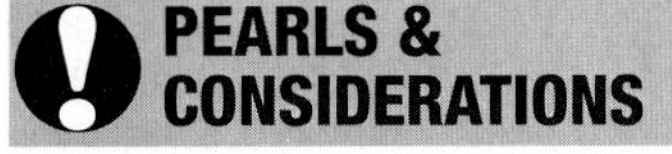

PEARLS & CONSIDERATIONS

COMMENTS

Labyrinthitis is a term that usually implies peripheral vestibulopathy associated with hearing loss. The term *vestibular neuronitis* is typically used when hearing is not affected. Despite this technical distinction, many physicians use these terms interchangeably.

RELATED CONTENT

Labyrinthitis (Patient Information)
Benign Paroxysmal Positional Vertigo (Related Key Topic)
Vestibular Neuronitis (Related Key Topic)

AUTHORS: **MICHAEL POHLEN, M.D., JOSEPH S. KASS, M.D., J.D.,** and **SHARON S. HARTMAN POLENSEK, M.D., PH.D.**

BASIC INFORMATION

DEFINITION

Lactose intolerance is the insufficient concentration of lactase enzyme, leading to fermentation of malabsorbed lactose by intestinal bacteria with subsequent production of intestinal gas and various organic acids, manifesting clinically with diarrhea, abdominal pain, flatulence, or bloating after lactose intake. *Lactose malabsorption* occurs when a substantial amount of lactose is not absorbed in the intestine. *Lactase deficiency* is defined as brush-border lactase activity that is markedly reduced relative to the activity observed in infants.

SYNONYMS

Lactose malabsorption
Lactase deficiency
Milk intolerance
Carbohydrate malabsorption

ICD-10CM CODES
E73.9 Lactose intolerance, unspecified
E73.8 Other lactose intolerance

EPIDEMIOLOGY & DEMOGRAPHICS

- Nearly 50 million people in the United States have partial or complete lactose intolerance. There are racial differences, with <25% of white adults being lactose intolerant but >85% of Asian Americans and >60% of African Americans having some form of lactose intolerance.
- There are geographic variations: Highest in Asians (up to 90%), lowest in northern Europeans (approximately 10%), intermediate in southern Europeans and Middle Eastern populations (up to 40%).

PHYSICAL FINDINGS & CLINICAL PRESENTATION

- Abdominal tenderness and cramping, bloating, flatulence.
- Diarrhea.
- Symptoms are directly related to the osmotic pressure of substrate in the colon and occur approximately 2 hr after ingestion of lactose.
- Physical examination: May be entirely within normal limits.

ETIOLOGY

- Before it can be absorbed, lactose is cleared to glucose and galactose by the enzyme lactase in the brush border of the small intestine. If the amount of lactase is marginal or its expression is left, lactose intolerance will results.
- Congenital lactase deficiency: Common in premature infants; rare in term infants and generally inherited as a chromosomal recessive trait.
- Secondary lactose intolerance: Usually a result of injury of the intestinal mucosa (Crohn disease, viral gastroenteritis, AIDS enteropathy, cryptosporidiosis, Whipple disease, sprue).
- Acquired primary lactase deficiency (adult-type hypolactasia OMIM # 223100) is the most common form of lactase deficiency worldwide. The decline in lactase activity is a multifactorial process that is regulated at the gene transcription level and leads to decreased biosynthesis, retardation of intracellular transport, or maturation of the enzyme lactase-phlorizin hydrolase.

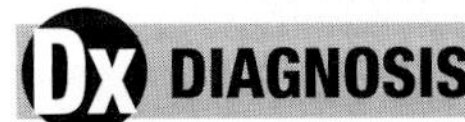

DIAGNOSIS

DIFFERENTIAL DIAGNOSIS

- Inflammatory bowel disease
- Irritable bowel syndrome
- Pancreatic insufficiency
- Nontropical and tropical sprue
- Cystic fibrosis
- Diverticular disease
- Bowel neoplasm
- Laxative abuse
- Celiac disease
- Parasitic disease (e.g., giardiasis)
- Viral or bacterial infections

WORKUP

- A detailed dietary history is essential in the evaluation of patients with suspected carbohydrate malabsorption.
- The diagnosis can usually be made on the basis of the history and improvement with dietary manipulation.
- Diagnostic workup may include confirming the diagnosis with hydrogen breath test and excluding other conditions listed in the differential diagnosis that may also coexist with lactase deficiency.

LABORATORY TESTS

- Laboratory evaluation may not be necessary in patients with significant history.
- Lactose breath hydrogen test: A rise in breath hydrogen >20 ppm within 90 min of ingestion of 50 g of lactose is positive for lactase deficiency. This test is positive in 90% of patients with lactose malabsorption. Common causes of false-negative results are recent use of oral antibiotics or recent high colonic enema. Fig. E1 illustrates the role of symptoms in determining the clinical importance of lactose malabsorption.
- The lactose tolerance test is an older and less accurate testing modality (20% rate of false-positive and false-negative results). The patient is administered an oral dose of 1 to 1.5 g of lactose/kg body weight. Serial measurement of blood glucose level on an hourly basis for 3 hr is then performed. The test is considered positive if the patient develops intestinal symptoms and the blood glucose level rises <20 mg/dl above the fasting baseline level.
- Diarrhea associated with lactase deficiency is osmotic in nature with an osmotic gap and a pH <6.5.

IMAGING STUDIES

Imaging studies are generally not indicated. A small bowel series may be useful in patients with significant malabsorption.

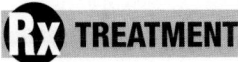

TREATMENT

NONPHARMACOLOGIC THERAPY

Management consists of reducing lactose exposure by avoiding milk and milk-containing products or using milk in which the lactose has been prehydrolyzed with lactase. A lactose-free diet generally results in prompt resolution of symptoms. Lactose is primarily found in dairy products but may be present as an ingredient or component of common foods and beverages. Possible sources of lactose include breads, candies, cold cuts, dessert mixes, cream soups, bologna, commercial sauces and gravies, chocolate, drink mixes, salad dressings, and medications. Labels should be read carefully to identify sources of lactose.

ACUTE GENERAL Rx

- Addition of lactase enzyme supplement (Lactaid tablets, Dairy Ease) before the ingestion of milk products may prevent symptoms in some patients. However, it is not effective for all lactose-intolerant patients.
- Lactose-intolerant patients must ensure adequate calcium intake. Calcium supplementation is recommended to prevent osteoporosis.

CHRONIC Rx

Patient education regarding foods high in lactose, such as milk, cottage cheese, or ice cream, is recommended.

DISPOSITION

Clinical improvement with restriction or elimination of milk products

REFERRAL

GI referral for endoscopic procedures if concomitant GI disorders are suspected.

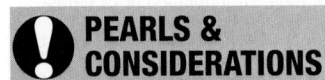

PEARLS & CONSIDERATIONS

COMMENTS

- There is great variability in signs and symptoms in patients with lactose intolerance depending on the degree of lactase deficiency. Most individuals with presumed lactose malabsorption can tolerate 12 to 15 g of lactose or up to 12 oz of milk daily without symptoms.
- Nondairy synthetic drinks (e.g., Coffee-Mate) and use of rice milk are generally well tolerated.

SUGGESTED READING

Available at ExpertConsult.com

RELATED CONTENT

Lactose Intolerance (Patient Information)

AUTHOR: **FRED F. FERRI, M.D.**

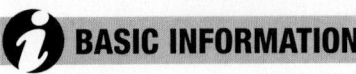

BASIC INFORMATION

DEFINITION

A mechanical or functional interruption of normal intraluminal flow through the colon

SYNONYM

Colorectal obstruction

ICD-10CM CODES
K56.60 Unspecified intestinal obstruction
K56.69 Other intestinal obstruction

EPIDEMIOLOGY & DEMOGRAPHICS

PEAK INCIDENCE: 73 yr of age, higher in the elderly due to increased rates of colorectal cancer

PREVALENCE: 25% of intestinal obstructions

PREDOMINANT SEX AND AGE: Affects males and females equally, more common in the elderly

RISK FACTORS: Colorectal cancer, prior abdominal surgery, prior colorectal resection, chronic constipation, radiation

PHYSICAL FINDINGS & CLINICAL PRESENTATION:

- History:
  1. Patients commonly present with abdominal pain, abdominal distension, and obstipation.
  2. Patients may have nausea and vomiting, but these are very late-presenting symptoms.
  3. Patients may report a history of bloating or constipation prior to the onset of more severe symptoms.
  4. Inquiries should be made concerning recent weight loss or gain, bowel habits, narcotic use, prior surgery, and malignancy.
- Physical exam:
  1. Patient may be tachycardic or febrile from perforation, strangulation or ischemia.
  2. Exam should include palpation of the abdomen, investigation for umbilical, inguinal and femoral hernias, as well as a rectal exam.
  3. Physical exam findings may include:
     a. Distended, tympanitic abdomen.
     b. Nonspecific tenderness to palpation of the lower abdomen.
     c. A palpable hernia.
     d. Rectal mass or frank blood on rectal exam.
  4. If possible, proctoscopy should be performed in the office to evaluate for volvulus or sigmoid mass.

ETIOLOGY

- Colorectal cancer, volvulus, diverticulitis, abscess, adhesions, anastomotic strictures, hernia, fecal impaction, inflammatory bowel disease, ischemic colitis, intussusception, colonic pseudo-obstruction, narcotic associated adynamic ileus, sepsis or *C. difficile* infection.
- Box 1 summarizes causes of adult large bowel obstruction.

DIAGNOSIS

DIFFERENTIAL DIAGNOSIS

- Colorectal cancer
- Volvulus
- Diverticulitis
- Abdominal abscess
- Abdominal adhesions
- Anastomotic stricture
- Hernia
- Fecal impaction
- Crohn's disease
- Ischemic colitis
- Intussusception
- Pseudo-obstruction (Ogilvie syndrome)
- Constipation

WORKUP

- Establish IV access with two large bore IVs.
- Make the patient NPO.
- Flexible sigmoidoscopy or colonoscopy in stable patients.

LABORATORY TESTS

- Complete blood count
- Basic metabolic panel

IMAGING STUDIES

- Acute abdominal series should demonstrate dilation of the colon (Fig. 1):
  1. Sensitivity 84%
  2. Specificity 72%
- CT abdomen and pelvis imaging is useful to pinpoint the obstruction and possibly identify the etiology (Fig. 2):
  1. Sensitivity 83%
  2. Specificity 93%
- Water contrast enema is useful for evaluating volvulus or distal obstruction cancer:
  1. Sensitivity 96%
  2. Specificity 98%
  3. Occasionally therapeutic

BOX 1 Causes of Adult Large Bowel Obstruction

Mechanical
- Neoplasm
- Volvulus (sigmoid, cecal, transverse colon)
- Diverticulitis
- Cecal bascule
- Intussusception
- Inflammatory bowel disease
- Incarcerated hernia
- Infection (abscess, inflammation)
- Fecal impaction
- Adhesion-related obstruction
- Foreign body

Functional
- Acute toxic or chronic megacolon
- Colonic pseudo-obstruction (Ogilvie's syndrome)

From Cameron JL, Cameron AM: *Current surgical therapy*, ed 12, Philadelphia, 2017, Elsevier.

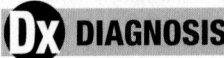

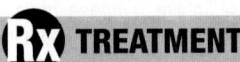

TREATMENT

- IV fluid resuscitation
  1. Consider placing Foley catheter to monitor UOP
- Correction of electrolyte abnormalities
- Nasogastric tube to decompress the GI tract
- Cessation of narcotics and antihistamines

NONPHARMACOLOGIC THERAPY

- Emergent laparotomy for perforation, closed loop obstruction, peritonitis, or ischemia
  1. Placement of loop colostomy
- Rectal cancer: Loop colostomy for cancer, then neoadjuvant chemoradiation
- Colon cancer: Depends on location; Hartmann's for sigmoid colon cancer, partial or total colectomy for other colon cancers
- Colonoscopy for colonic decompression of volvulus
- Endoscopic stenting for palliation or as a bridge to surgery

ACUTE GENERAL Rx

Neostigmine for pseudo-obstruction

CHRONIC Rx

Not indicated

DISPOSITION

Immediate referral to general surgery and hospital admission

REFERRAL

General surgery

SUGGESTED READINGS
Available at ExpertConsult.com

RELATED CONTENT

Acute Colonic Pseudo-Obstruction (Ogilvie Syndrome) (Related Key Topic)
Constipation (Related Key Topic)
Colorectal Cancer (Related Key Topic)

AUTHORS: **DANIEL C. NEUBAUER, M.D.,** and **MARK F. BRADY, M.D., M.P.H., M.M.S.**

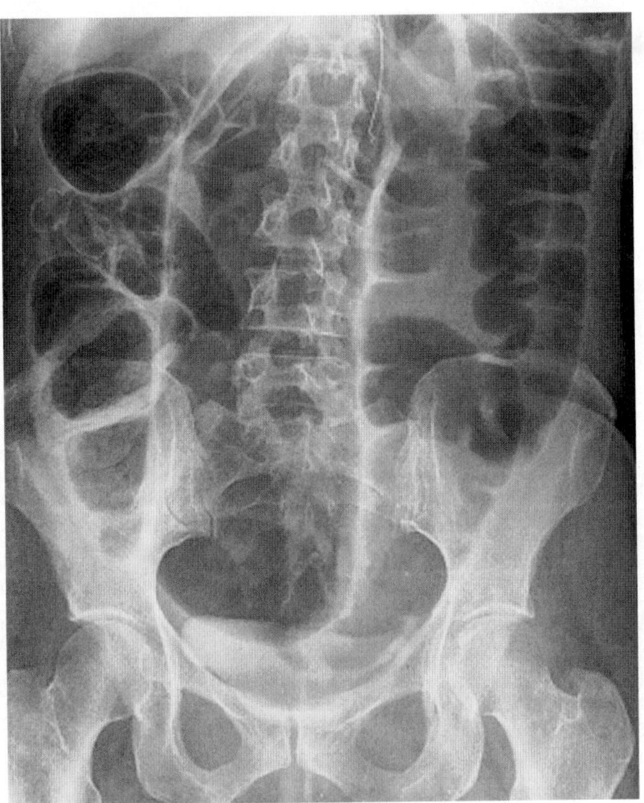

FIG. 1 Sigmoid volvulus. (Courtesy Harisinghani Mukesh, MD, MGH Radiology. In Cameron JL, Cameron AM: *Current surgical therapy*, ed 12, Philadelphia, 2017, Elsevier.)

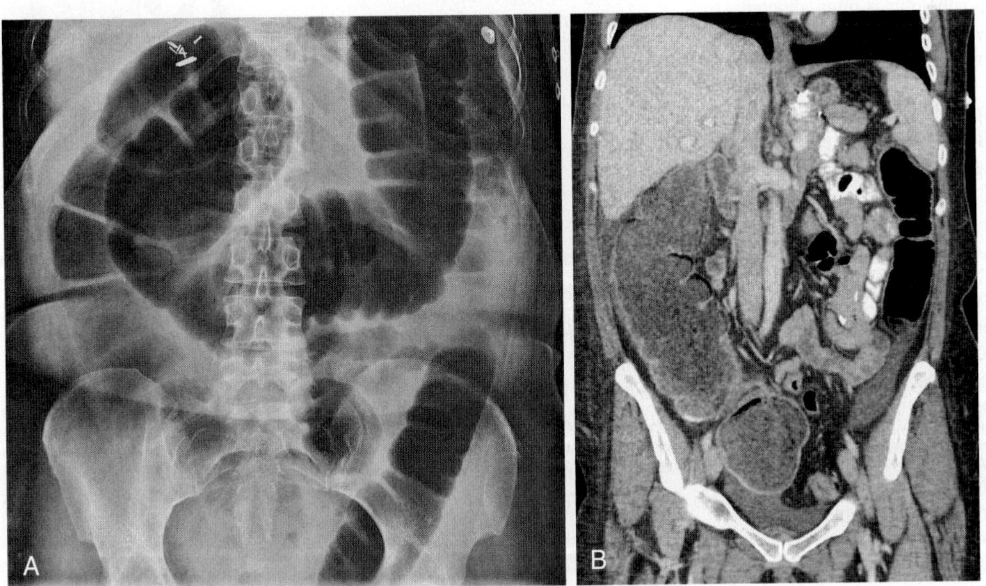

FIG. 2 A and **B,** Obstructing sigmoid colon cancer. (Courtesy Harisinghani Mukesh, MD, MGH Radiology. In Cameron JL, Cameron AM: *Current surgical therapy*, ed 12, Philadelphia, 2017, Elsevier.)

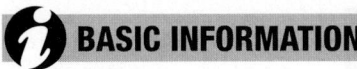

BASIC INFORMATION

DEFINITION

Laryngitis is an acute or chronic inflammation of the laryngeal mucous membranes.

SYNONYM

Lower respiratory tract infection

ICD-10CM CODES
J04.0 Acute laryngitis
J37.0 Chronic laryngitis

EPIDEMIOLOGY & DEMOGRAPHICS

It is a common illness worldwide in both genders and all age groups, but the diagnosis is imprecise and, therefore, statistics are not readily available with respect to incidence and prevalence.

PHYSICAL FINDINGS & CLINICAL PRESENTATION

ACUTE LARYNGITIS:

- Clinical syndrome characterized by the onset of hoarseness, voice breaks, or episodes of aphonia; may also have accompanying sore throat, cough, nasal congestion, and rhinorrhea.
- Usually associated with viral upper respiratory infection.
- Larynx with diffuse erythema, edema, and vascular engorgement of the vocal folds, and occasionally mucosal ulceration.
- In young children subglottis is often affected, resulting in airway narrowing with marked hoarseness, inspiratory stridor, dyspnea, and restlessness.
- Respiratory compromise rare in adults.

CHRONIC LARYNGITIS: Characterized by hoarseness or dysphonia persisting for longer than 2 wk.

ETIOLOGY

ACUTE LARYNGITIS:

- Most often caused by viruses so treatment consists of supportive measures as outlined in "Nonpharmacologic Therapy" section.
- Studies evaluating the use of antibiotics (erythromycin, penicillin) in acute laryngitis failed to show objective clinical benefit over placebo so they are not routinely recommended. Antibiotics and other antimicrobials may be indicated in cases in which specific treatable pathogens are identified.
- Avoid decongestants because of their drying effect.
- Guaifenesin may be a useful adjunct as a mucolytic agent.
- In gastroesophageal reflux disease (GERD)-associated laryngitis use acid-suppressive therapy (H_2 blockers, proton pump inhibitors) and nocturnal antireflux precautions.

CHRONIC LARYNGITIS:

- Results from any of the following: tuberculosis, usually through bronchogenic spread; leprosy, from nasopharyngeal or oropharyngeal spread; syphilis, in secondary and tertiary stages; rhinoscleroma, extending from the nose and nasopharynx; actinomycosis; cryptococcosis; histoplasmosis; blastomycosis; paracoccidioidomycosis; coccidiosis; candidiasis; aspergillosis; sporotrichosis; rhinosporidiosis; parasitic infections including leishmaniasis and *Clinostomum* infection following raw fresh-water fish ingestion.
- Noninfectious causes of both acute and chronic laryngitis include malignancy, voice abuse (singers), GERD, and chemical or environmental irritants such as cigarettes and allergens. Other causes of inflammatory or granulomatous lesions of the larynx include relapsing polychondritis, Wegener granulomatosis, and sarcoidosis.

Dx DIAGNOSIS

DIFFERENTIAL DIAGNOSIS

- Young children with signs of airway obstruction:
  1. Supraglottitis (epiglottitis).
  2. Laryngotracheobronchitis.
  3. Tracheitis.
  4. Foreign body aspiration.
- In adults with persistent hoarseness, consider noninfectious causes of laryngitis as listed previously.
- Table E1 summarizes the classification and definition of infectious illnesses involving the larynx and supraglottic and infraglottic regions.

WORKUP

- History and physical examination: Diagnosis is usually apparent.
- Laryngoscopy for severe or persistent cases.
- Laryngeal cultures should be performed if a cause other than acute viral infection is suspected.
- Imaging not indicated unless there is evidence of airway compromise. Obtain plain radiographs of neck, anteroposterior and lateral views, to differentiate laryngitis from acute laryngotracheobronchitis or supraglottitis.

Rx TREATMENT

NONPHARMACOLOGIC THERAPY

- Rest the voice.
- Use an air humidifier.
- Ensure adequate hydration. Avoid alcohol and caffeine because of diuretic effect.

ACUTE GENERAL Rx

- Antibiotics and other antimicrobials should generally not be used. They are indicated only when a specific pathogen is isolated; commonly employed antibacterial agents are macrolides; clarithromycin 500 mg by mouth bid for 5 to 7 days or azithromycin 500 mg followed by 250 mg once daily for 4 to 5 days if the cause of laryngitis is found to be *Mycoplasma pneumoniae* or *Chlamydophila pneumoniae* (the new name for what was formerly known as *Chlamydia pneumoniae*).
- Avoid decongestants because of their drying effect.
- Guaifenesin may be a useful adjunct as a mucolytic agent.
- In GERD-associated laryngitis use acid-suppressive therapy (H_2 blockers, proton pump inhibitors) and nocturnal antireflux precautions.

DISPOSITION

Uncomplicated laryngitis is usually benign, with gradual resolution of symptoms.

REFERRAL

- If symptoms persist for >2 wk, refer to otolaryngologist for laryngoscopy.
- Consider referral to gastroenterologist if GERD is suspected.

PEARLS & CONSIDERATIONS

- Most cases of uncomplicated acute laryngitis are viral in origin, and antibacterial agents should not be routinely administered.
- A recent Cochrane analysis in 2013 found no evidence for the use of empiric antibiotics in adults with laryngitis.
- The most difficult clinical challenge is often convincing patients with acute laryngitis that they do not need and will not benefit from antibacterial agents.

SUGGESTED READING

Available at Expertconsult.com

RELATED CONTENT

Laryngitis (Patient Information)

AUTHOR: **GLENN G. FORT, M.D., M.P.H.**

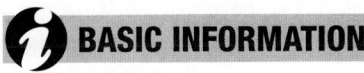

BASIC INFORMATION

DEFINITION

Lead is a potent, pervasive neurotoxicant. Lead poisoning refers to multisystem abnormalities resulting from excessive lead exposure.

SYNONYM

Plumbism

ICD-10CM CODES

T56.0X1A	Toxic effect of lead and its compounds, accidental (unintentional), initial encounter
T56.0X1D	Toxic effect of lead and its compounds, accidental (unintentional), subsequent encounter
T56.0X1S	Toxic effect of lead and its compounds, accidental (unintentional), sequela
T56.0X2A	Toxic effect of lead and its compounds, intentional self-harm, initial encounter
T56.0X2D	Toxic effect of lead and its compounds, intentional self-harm, subsequent encounter
T56.0X2S	Toxic effect of lead and its compounds, intentional self-harm, sequela
T56.0X3A	Toxic effect of lead and its compounds, assault, initial encounter
T56.0X3D	Toxic effect of lead and its compounds, assault, subsequent encounter
T56.0X3S	Toxic effect of lead and its compounds, assault, sequela
T56.0X4A	Toxic effect of lead and its compounds, undetermined, initial encounter
T56.0X4D	Toxic effect of lead and its compounds, undetermined, subsequent encounter
T56.0X4S	Toxic effect of lead and its compounds, undetermined, sequela

EPIDEMIOLOGY & DEMOGRAPHICS

- Lead poisoning is most common in children ages 1 to 5 yr (17,000 cases/100,000 persons). The highest rates are among blacks, those with low income, and urban children.
- In 1991 the Centers for Disease Control and Prevention (CDC) lowered the definition of a safe blood lead level to <10 mcg/dl of whole blood (a blood lead level of 25 mcg/dl was considered acceptable before 1991).
- It is estimated that >15% of preschoolers in the U.S. have a blood lead level >15 mcg/dl.

PHYSICAL FINDINGS & CLINICAL PRESENTATION

- Findings vary with the degree of toxicity (Table 1). Examination may be normal in patients with mild toxicity.
- Myalgias, irritability, headache, and general fatigue may be present initially.
- Abdominal cramping, constipation, weight loss, tremor, paresthesias and peripheral neuritis, seizures, and coma may occur with severe toxicity.
- Motor neuropathy is common in children with lead poisoning; learning disorders are also frequent.

ETIOLOGY

Chronic, repeated exposure to paint containing lead, plumbing, storage of batteries, pottery, or lead soldering. Concentration of lead is generally highest in lead-based paint on exterior surfaces. Among interior surfaces, windows are most likely to have the highest lead content.

DIAGNOSIS

DIFFERENTIAL DIAGNOSIS

- Polyneuropathies from other sources
- Anxiety disorder, attention deficit disorder
- Malabsorption, acute abdomen
- Iron-deficiency anemia

WORKUP

Laboratory screening: All U.S. children should be considered to be at risk for lead poisoning and should be screened routinely starting at age 1 yr for low-risk children and age 6 mo for high-risk children.

LABORATORY TESTS

- Venous blood lead level: Normal level, <5 mcg/dl; levels of 50 to 70 mcg/dl, indicative of moderate toxicity; levels >70 mcg/dl, associated with severe poisoning
- Mild anemia with basophilic stippling on peripheral smear
- Elevated zinc protoporphyrin levels or free erythrocyte protoporphyrin level
- An increased body burden of lead with previous high-level exposure in patients with occupational lead poisoning can be demonstrated by measuring the excretion of lead in urine after premedication with calcium ethylenediamine tetraacetic acid (EDTA) or another chelating agent

IMAGING STUDIES

- Imaging studies are generally not necessary.
- A plain abdominal film can visualize lead particles in the gut.
- "Lead lines" may be noted on x-ray films of long bones.

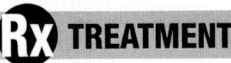

TREATMENT

NONPHARMACOLOGIC THERAPY

- Provide adequate amounts of calcium, iron, zinc, and protein in patient's diet.
- Family education on sources of lead exposure and potential adverse health effects.

ACUTE GENERAL Rx

- The use of chelation in cases of acute lead poisoning is guided by the patient's clinical status and the blood lead level (BLL). For children with blood levels of 10 to 19 mcg/dl, the CDC recommends nonpharmacologic interventions (see "Nonpharmacologic Therapy").
- For children with blood levels between 20 and 44 mcg/dl, the CDC recommendations include case management by a qualified social worker, clinical management, environmental assessment, and lead hazard control. Chelation therapy should be considered in children with refractory blood lead levels.

Chelation therapy (Table 2) is indicated in children with blood lead levels >45 mcg/dl:

- Succimer (DMSA) 10 mg/kg PO q8h for 5 days then q12h for 2 wk can be used in patients with levels between 45 and 70 mcg/dl.

TABLE 1 Serum Lead Levels and Symptoms

	Symptoms	
Level (μg/dl)	Adults	Children
10	None	Decreased IQ Decreased hearing Decreased growth
20	Increased protoporphyrin No symptoms	Decreased nerve conduction velocity Increased protoporphyrin
30	Increased blood pressure Decreased hearing	Decreased vitamin D metabolism
40	Peripheral neuropathies Nephropathy Infertility (men)	Decreased hemoglobin synthesis
50	Decreased hemoglobin synthesis	Lead colic
70	Anemia	Anemia Encephalopathy Nephropathy
100	Encephalopathy	Death

IQ, Intelligence quotient.
From Marx JA et al: *Rosen's emergency medicine*, ed 8, Philadelphia, 2014, Saunders.

TABLE 2 Chelators*

Chelator	Dose	Indications	Contraindications
Deferoxamine	15 mg/kg/hr up to 24 hr (titrate up slowly because of hypotension)	Iron level >500 g/dl or systemic symptoms	
Dimercaprol (British anti-Lewisite [BAL])	Lead encephalopathy: 75 mg/m^2 deep IM injection every 4 hr for 5 days in children or 4 mg/kg every 4 hr for adults Arsenic (severe): No established regimen; consider 3 mg/kg IM every 4 hr for 48 hr; then twice daily for 7-10 days Mercury: 5 mg/kg IM first; then 2.5 mg/kg every 12-24 hr	Lead level >70 g/dl or encephalopathy Arsenic: symptomatic patient with known exposure Mercury: Inorganic	Peanut allergy Organic mercury poisoning
$CaNa_2EDTA$	1500 mg/m^2/day continuous IV infusion 50 mg/kg/day or 1000 mg/m^2/day in 2-4 divided doses for up to 5 days if less severe symptoms	Lead: Given after first dose of BAL for blood lead level above 70 g/dl or encephalopathy	
Succimer (DMSA)	10 mg/kg q8h × 5 days; then q12h for 14 days	Lead level of 45-69 g/dl Arsenic: If tolerated orally for subacute and chronic toxicity Mercury: Acute and chronic	
D-Penicillamine	25 mg/kg q6h × 5 days	Lead level of 45-69 g/dl, succimer not tolerated Arsenic: Only if BAL and DMSA are unavailable Mercury: If BAL and DMSA are unavailable or not tolerated	Penicillin allergy
DMPS (investigational)	5 mg/kg/dose IM q6-8h day 1, q8-12h day 2, q12-24h day 3 and until 24-hr urine is <50 μg/L	Lead (chronic) Arsenic Mercury	

BAL, Dimercaprol; *DMPS*, 2,3-Dimercapto-1-propanesulfonic acid; *DMSA*, dimercaptosuccinic acid; *EDTA*, edetate calcium disodium; *IM*, intramuscular; *IV*, intravenous.
*Indications for chelation and dosing regimens may change. Consult with a toxicologist or poison control center for the most up-to-date recommendations.
From Marx JA et al: *Rosen's emergency medicine*, ed 8, Philadelphia, 2014, Saunders.

- Edetate calcium disodium (EDTA) and dimercaprol (BAL) are effective in patients with severe toxicity.
- Use of both EDTA and DMSA is indicated in children with blood levels >70 mcg/dl.
- d-Penicillamine (Cuprimine) can also be used for lead poisoning, but it is not FDA approved for this condition.

CHRONIC Rx

- Reduce exposure, remove any potential lead sources.
- Correct iron deficiency and any other nutritional deficiencies.
- Recheck blood lead level 7 to 21 days after chelation therapy.

DISPOSITION

Patients with mild to moderate toxicity generally improve without any residual deficits. The presence of encephalopathy at diagnosis is a poor prognostic sign. Residual neurologic deficits may persist in these patients. Chelation therapy seems to slow the progression of renal insufficiency in patients with mildly elevated body lead burden.

REFERRAL

If exposure to lead is work related, it should be reported to the Office of the United States Occupational Safety and Health Administration (OSHA). Follow-up testing is mandatory in all patients after an abnormal screening blood lead level.

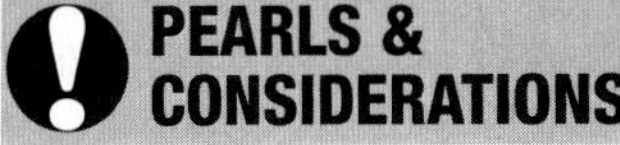

PEARLS & CONSIDERATIONS

COMMENTS

- Even blood lead concentrations as low as 5-10 mcg/dl are inversely associated with children's IQ scores at age 3 and 5 yr. A recent study evaluating long-term ramifications of childhood lead exposure revealed that childhood lead exposure was associated with lower cognitive function and socioeconomic status at age 38 yr, with declines in IQ, and downward social mobility.[1]
- Screening of household members of affected individuals is recommended.
- In children with blood lead levels of >45 mg/dl, treatment with succimer does not improve scores on tests of cognition, behavior, or neuropsychological function.

[1] Reuben A et al: Association of childhood blood lead levels with cognitive function and socioeconomic status at age 38 and with IQ change and socioeconomic mobility between childhood and adulthood, *JAMA* 317(12):1244–1251, 2017.

- Lead toxicity may delay growth and pubertal development in girls.
- Low-level environmental lead exposure may accelerate progressive renal insufficiency in patients without diabetes who have chronic renal disease. Repeated chelation therapy may improve renal function and slow the progression of renal failure.

RELATED CONTENT

Lead Poisoning (Patient Information)

AUTHOR: **FRED F. FERRI, M.D.**

BASIC INFORMATION

DEFINITION

Legg-Calvé-Perthes disease (LCPD) is characterized by vascular compromise to the immature proximal femoral head leading to avascular necrosis of the femoral head. The classification of LCPD is outlined in Fig. 1.

SYNONYMS

Perthes disease
Coxa plana
Capital femoral osteochondrosis
Osteonecrosis of the proximal femoral epiphysis
LCPD

ICD-10CM CODE

M91.10 Juvenile osteochondrosis of head of femur [Legg-Calvé-Perthes], unspecified leg

EPIDEMIOLOGY & DEMOGRAPHICS

PREVALENCE: One case in 1300 children. More common in Caucasians.
INCIDENCE: One in 1200 children younger than 15 yr of age
PREDOMINANT SEX: Male:female ratio of 4:1
PREDOMINANT AGE: 4 to 10 yr old

PHYSICAL FINDINGS & CLINICAL PRESENTATION

- Initial symptom: Usually a mildly painful limp.
- Pain may be referred down the medial aspect of the thigh to the knee.
- Positive roll test: With the patient in the supine position, rolling of the affected extremity into internal and external rotation elicits guarding, with limited range of motion.
- Pain at the extremes of motion and tenderness over the anterior aspect of the hip joint.
- No history of trauma.
- Condition is bilateral in 10% to 20% of patients.

ETIOLOGY

Unknown. Increased association with ADHD, delayed bone age

DIAGNOSIS

DIFFERENTIAL DIAGNOSIS

Unilateral disease:
- Transient synovitis
- Sickle cell disease
- Septic arthritis
- Neoplastic process
- Spondyloepiphyseal dysplasia tarda
- Slipped capital femoral epiphysis

BILATERAL DISEASE

- Multiple epiphyseal dysplasia
- Sickle cell disease
- Juvenile idiopathic arthritis

WORKUP

Diagnosis is usually based on physical examination findings and radiographic evaluation.

IMAGING STUDIES

- MRI is most sensitive for early LCPD.
- Plain x-ray (AP and frog-leg lateral x-rays) (Fig. 2) will show late changes.
- Technetium bone scan may help confirm the diagnosis in early cases.

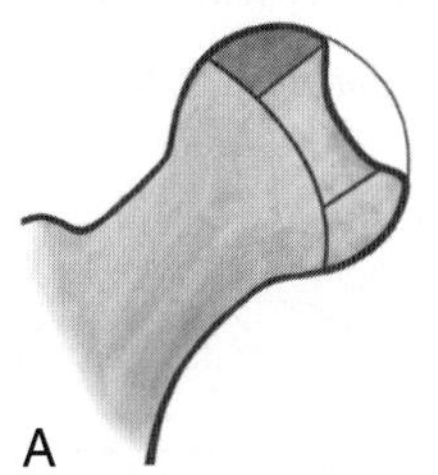

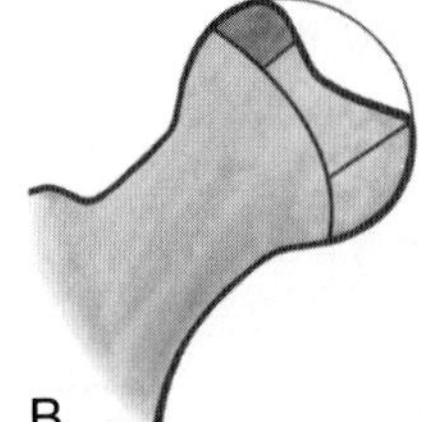

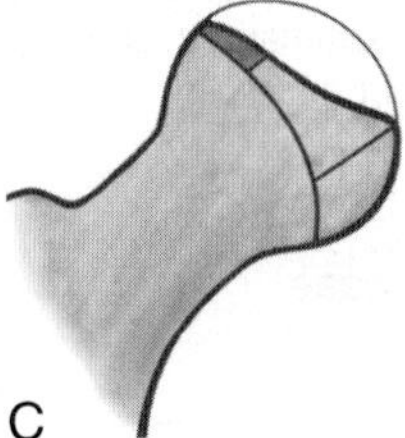

FIG. 1 Lateral pillar classification for Legg-Calvé-Perthes disease. A, There is no involvement of the lateral pillar. **B,** >50% of the lateral pillar height is maintained. **C,** <50% of the lateral pillar height is maintained. (From Kliegman RM et al: *Nelson textbook of pediatrics,* ed 19, Philadelphia, 2011, Saunders.)

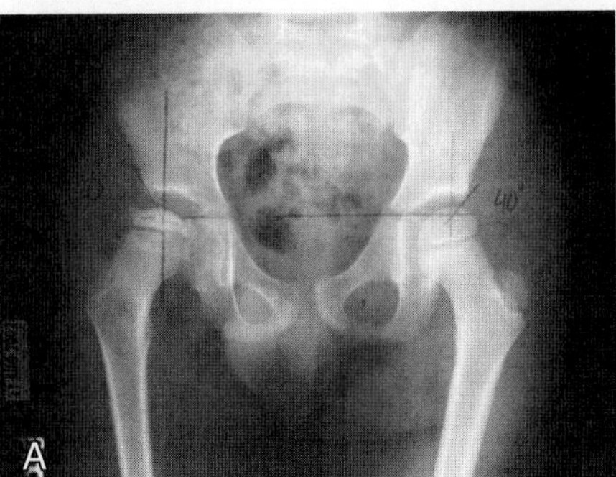

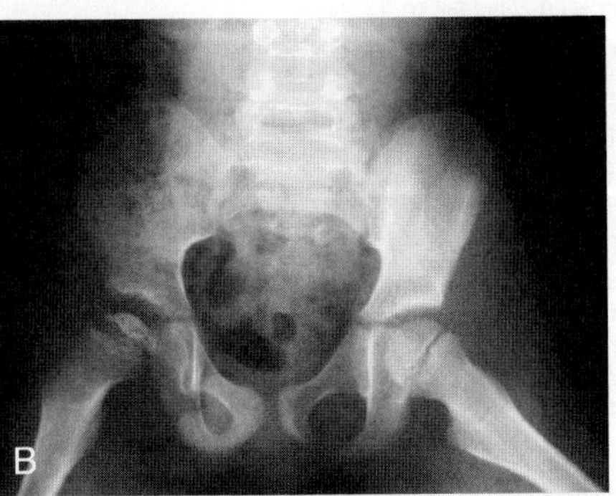

FIG. 2 A, Anteroposterior radiograph of the pelvis shows epiphyseal fragmentation in the right hip, characteristic of the fragmentation phase of Legg-Calvé-Perthes disease. **B,** The frog-leg lateral view demonstrates subchondral fracture, increased density of the femoral head, and some collapse. (From Kliegman RM et al: *Nelson textbook of pediatrics,* ed 19, Philadelphia, 2011, Saunders.)

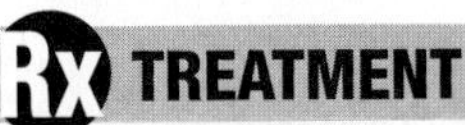

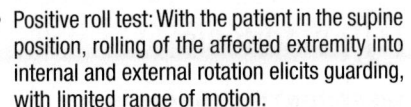

TREATMENT

ACUTE GENERAL Rx

- Non-weight bearing followed by bracing.
- Bracing may be required for 2 to 3 yr in a small subset of patients.
- NSAIDs for pain control.
- Range-of-motion physical therapy exercises.
- Surgery may be required in refractory cases, usually femoral or pelvic osteotomies.

DISPOSITION

- Prognosis depends on the age of patient and the degree of involvement of the femoral head at onset.
- In patients younger than 6 yr, outcome is generally favorable, regardless of treatment.
- Patients over the age of 8 yr at onset often have less favorable outcomes. Females tend to do worse than males in this age group.
- A subset of patients may go on to develop degenerative arthritis.

REFERRAL

Referral to pediatric orthopedist when diagnosis is suspected.

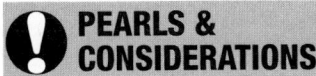

PEARLS & CONSIDERATIONS

Both the etiology and treatment of LCPD remain controversial. Treatment recommendations vary widely and continue to evolve. Children over the age of 8 yr at onset may benefit from early surgical intervention.

SUGGESTED READINGS

Available at ExpertConsult.com

RELATED CONTENT

Legg-Calvé-Perthes Disease (Patient Information)

AUTHOR: **ANDREW P. THOME JR., M.D.**

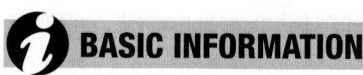

DEFINITION

Pneumonia caused by *Legionella pneumophila*

SYNONYM

Legionella pneumonia

ICD-10CM CODE
A48.1 Legionnaires' disease

EPIDEMIOLOGY & DEMOGRAPHICS

PREVALENCE: Rough estimates of 18–36 cases per 100 000, mostly sporadic cases, occasional community outbreaks due to contaminated fresh water sources. Nosocomial outbreaks have been reported.

PREDOMINANT SEX AND AGE: Male gender with twofold increased risk, age >50

RISK FACTORS: Chronic heart disease, smoking, ESRD, immunosuppression, cancer. No person-to-person transmission

PHYSICAL FINDINGS & CLINICAL PRESENTATION

- Acute respiratory illness similar to other forms of community acquired pneumonia.
- Hypoxia, cough, physical exam with localizing chest findings.
- A febrile prodrome with myalgia, anorexia, and headaches can occur, which may be confused with influenza.
- Gastrointestinal symptoms such as diarrhea and abdominal pain are common.

ETIOLOGY

Legionella pneumophila, atypical agent. Grows in warm water sources and can cause outbreaks

Dx DIAGNOSIS

DIFFERENTIAL DIAGNOSIS

Clinically indistinguishable from other typical and atypical pneumonias

WORKUP

Similar to other pneumonias. CURB 65 or PSI may be used to stratify patients according to severity.

LABORATORY TESTS

- Legionella urinary antigen highly sensitive for Legionella serotype 1 (80% of Legionella strains).
- Additional lab abnormalities such as LFTs, hyponatremia, elevated creatine kinase, coagulopathy are commonly seen.

IMAGING STUDIES

CXR (Fig. E1) with focal or diffuse consolidation, indistinguishable from other pneumonias

Rx TREATMENT

NONPHARMACOLOGIC THERAPY

Supportive therapy: Oxygen, may require intubation for severe hypoxia, fluid management in case of diarrhea

ACUTE GENERAL Rx

- Antibiotic coverage for atypical pneumonia. Azithromycin or levofloxacin are recommended. Treatment duration similar to other forms of community acquired pneumonia, with the exception of severely immunosuppressed patients who are treated for up to 21 days.
- Table 1 summarizes preferred therapy for Legionnaire's disease.

DISPOSITION

- Mild cases managed as outpatient are likely under-diagnosed due to lack of specific testing.
- Recognized as cause of severe pneumonia with high rates of ICU admission.

REFERRAL

- Pulmonologist/infectious disease specialist in severe cases.
- Identified cases should be reported to public health authorities for prompt recognition of outbreaks.

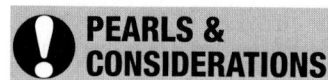

COMMENTS

Pontiac fever is an acute systemic illness caused by Legionella without specific pneumonia features. Local outbreaks have been reported.

PREVENTION

Prompt recognition of clusters to identify water source is pivotal to contain an outbreak.

PATIENT/FAMILY EDUCATION

To be recognized as potential public health problem. No risk for transmission to other family members.

SUGGESTED READINGS
Available at ExpertConsult.com

RELATED TOPICS

Pneumonia, Bacterial (Related Key Topic)

AUTHOR: **SEBASTIAN G. KURZ, M.D.**

TABLE 1 Preferred Therapy for Legionnaires' Disease

Clinical Condition	First Choices	Dosage* †	Second Choices	Dosage* †
Mild pneumonia inpatient or outpatient, not immunocompromised	Azithromycin *or*	500 mg 1×/day for 3-5 days	Doxycycline	200 mg load, then 100 mg 2×/day for 10-14 days
	Levofloxacin *or*	500 mg 1×/day for 7-10 days	Erythromycin	500 mg 4×/day for 10-14 days
	Ciprofloxacin *or*	500 mg 2×/days for 7-10 days		
	Moxifloxacin *or*	400 mg 1×/day for 7-10 days		
	Clarithromycin	500 mg 2×/day for 10-14 days		
Moderate to severe pneumonia or immunocompromised‡	Azithromycin *or*	500 mg 1×/day for 5-7 days	Ciprofloxacin *or*	750 mg 2×/day for 14 days
			Moxifloxacin *or*	400 mg 1×/day for 14 days
	Levofloxacin	500 mg 1×/day for 7-10 days 750 mg 1×/day for 5-7 days	Erythromycin *or*	750-1000 mg IV 4×/day for 3-7 days, then 500 mg 4×/day for a total course of 21 days
			Clarithromycin	500 mg IV 2×/day for 3-7 days, and then 500 mg 2×/day for a total course of 21 days

*Dosage adjustments have to be made for renal insufficiency for some of these drugs. Patients with mild disease may be treated entirely with oral therapy, whereas for severely ill patients parenteral therapy is advised until improvement is seen and oral absorption is sufficient.
†Therapy duration may need to be considerably longer for patients with lung abscesses, empyema, endocarditis, or extrathoracic infection.
‡Severely immunocompromised patients may require courses of therapy at the high end of the duration ranges given, or even longer. Close clinical follow-up is required to detect possible relapse after antibiotics have been discontinued.
IV, Intravenous.
From Bennett JE et al: *Mandell, Douglas, and Bennett's principles and practice of infectious diseases*, ed 8, Philadelphia, 2015, Elsevier.

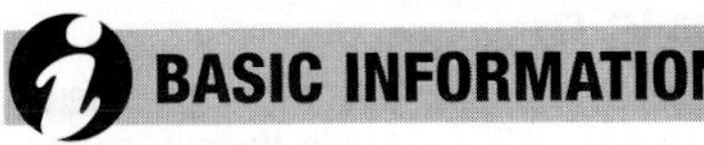

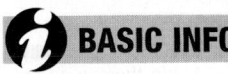

BASIC INFORMATION

DEFINITION

Liver abscess is a necrotic infection of the liver usually classified as pyogenic or amebic.

SYNONYMS

Pyogenic hepatic abscess
Amebic hepatic abscess

ICD-10CM CODE
K75.0 Abscess of liver

EPIDEMIOLOGY & DEMOGRAPHICS

INCIDENCE: Incidence of pyogenic liver abscess is 2.3 cases per 100,000 population.
PREVALENCE (WORLDWIDE): Amebic liver abscess is more common than pyogenic liver abscess.
PREVALENCE (IN U.S.): Pyogenic liver abscess is more common than amebic liver abscess.
PREDOMINANT SEX AND AGE: More common in men than women; male/female ratio of 2:1; most common in fourth to sixth decades of life.

PHYSICAL FINDINGS & CLINICAL PRESENTATION

- Fever, chills, and sweats
- Weakness/malaise
- Anorexia with weight loss
- Nausea, vomiting, and diarrhea
- Cough with pleuritic chest pain
- Right upper quadrant abdominal pain
- Hepatomegaly
- Splenomegaly
- Jaundice
- Pleural effusions, rales, and friction rubs may be present
- Most abscesses occur on the right lobe of the liver

ETIOLOGY

- Pyogenic liver abscess is usually polymicrobial (*Klebsiella pneumoniae* [43%], *Escherichia coli* [33%], *Streptococcus* spp. [37%], *Pseudomonas aeruginosa, Proteus* spp., *Bacteroides* spp. [24%], *Fusobacterium* spp., *Actinomyces* spp., gram-positive anaerobes, and *Staphylococcus aureus*).
- Pyogenic liver abscess occurs from:
    1. Biliary disease with cholangitis (accounts for approximately 40% to 60%).
    2. Gallbladder disease with contiguous spread to the liver.
    3. Diverticulitis or appendicitis with spread via the portal circulation.
    4. Hematogenous spread via the hepatic artery, though uncommon; if a solitary organism is isolated, a distant source of hematogenous seeding should be sought.
    5. Penetrating wounds.
    6. Cryptogenic.
    7. Infection by way of portal system (portal pyemia).
    8. No causes found in approximately half of cases.
    9. Incidence increased in patients with diabetes and metastatic cancer.
    10. Table 1 summarizes underlying etiology and bacteriology of liver abscesses.
- Amebic hepatic abscess is caused by the parasite *Entamoeba histolytica.* Amebiasis is usually due to fecal-oral contamination and invades the intestinal mucosa, gaining entry into the portal system to reach the liver. Amebic abscess occurs in 3% to 7% of patients with amebiasis.
- A comparison of pyogenic and amebic liver abscess is summarized in Table 2.

Box 1 describes pearls for amebic liver abscesses. The abscess is usually solitary (85%) and in the right lobe (72%).

Dx DIAGNOSIS

The diagnosis of liver abscess requires a high index of suspicion after a detailed history and physical examination. Imaging studies and microbiologic, serologic, and percutaneous techniques (e.g., aspiration) confirm the presence of a liver abscess.

TABLE 1 Underlying Etiology and Bacteriology

Etiology	Bacteriology
Biliary, benign	*Escherichia coli* *Klebsiella* spp. *Enterococcus*
Biliary, malignant	*Pseudomonas* spp. Multiply resistant GN aerobes VRE Yeast
Diverticulitis/appendicitis	GN aerobes *Bacteroides fragilis*
Severe cholecystitis	See Biliary, benign *Clostridium perfringens* *Bacteroides* spp.
Subcutaneous abscess	*Staphylococcus* spp. MRSA
Endocarditis	*Enterococcus* spp. *Staphylococcus* spp.
Cryptogenic	Anaerobes

GN, Gram-negative; *MRSA,* methicillin-resistant Staphylococcus aureus; *VRE,* Vancomycin-resistant Enterococcus.
From Cameron, JL, Cameron AM: *Current surgical therapy,* ed 10, Philadelphia, 2011, Saunders.

DIFFERENTIAL DIAGNOSIS

- Cholangitis
- Cholecystitis
- Diverticulitis
- Appendicitis
- Perforated viscus
- Mesentery ischemia
- Pulmonary embolism
- Pancreatitis

WORKUP

- The workup of a liver abscess should focus on differentiating between amebic and pyogenic causes.
- Features suggesting an amebic cause include travel to an endemic area, single abscess rather than multiple abscesses, subacute onset of symptoms, and absence of conditions predisposing to pyogenic liver abscess, as highlighted under "Etiology."
- Laboratory studies are not specific but are useful as adjunctive tests.
- Imaging studies cannot differentiate between the two, and bacteriologic cultures may be sterile in 50% of the cases.

LABORATORY TESTS

- Complete blood count: Leukocytosis
- Liver function tests: Alkaline phosphatase is most commonly elevated (95% to 100%); aspartate transaminase (AST) and alanine transaminase (ALT) elevated in 50% of cases; elevated bilirubin (28% to 30%); decreased albumin
- Prothrombin time (INR): Prolonged (70%)
- Blood cultures: Positive in 50% of cases
- Aspiration (50% sterile)
- Stool samples for *E. histolytica* trophozoites (positive in 10% to 15% of amebic liver abscess cases)
- Serologic testing for *E. histolytica* should be done on all patients, but it is important to remember that it does not differentiate acute from old infections

IMAGING STUDIES

- Ultrasound (80% to 100% sensitivity in detecting abscesses) shows round or oval hypoechogenic mass (Fig. E1, *A*).

TABLE 2 Comparisons of Pyogenic and Amebic Liver Abscess

Parameter	Pyogenic Liver Abscess	Amebic Liver Abscess
Number	Often multiple	Usually single
Location	Either lobe of liver	Usually right hepatic lobe, near the diaphragm
Presentation	Subacute	Acute
Jaundice	Mild	Moderate
Diagnosis	US or CT ± aspiration	US or CT and serology
Treatment	Drainage (if technically feasible) + IV antibiotics (see text)	Metronidazole, 750 mg 3 times daily for 7-10 days orally or IV; or tinidazole, 2 g orally for 3 days, followed by iodoquinol, 650 mg orally 3 times daily for 20 days; diloxanide furoate, 500 mg orally 3 times daily for 10 days; or aminosidine (paromomycin) 25-35 mg/kg/day orally in 3 divided doses for 7-10 days

CT, Computed tomography; *IV,* intravenous; *US,* ultrasonography.
From Feldman M, Friedman LS, Brandt LJ: *Sleisenger and Fordtran's gastrointestinal and liver disease,* ed 10, Philadelphia, 2016, Elsevier.

BOX 1 Pearls for Amebic Liver Abscesses

- Only 10%-20% of patients with amebic liver abscess have a history of diarrhea.
- Treat the intestinal infection to prevent relapse of amebic liver abscess. Failure to use luminal amebicidal agents after metronidazole in cases of amebic abscess results in a 10% relapse rate.
- Failure to show response to antiamebic medication requires evaluation for polymicrobial infection with bacteria.
- Amebic abscess usually responds clinically to antimicrobial therapy in 3 to 7 days, although imaging takes several months to show resolution.
- Percutaneous drainage is rarely required.

From Cameron, JL, Cameron AM: *Current surgical therapy*, ed 10, Philadelphia, 2011, Saunders.

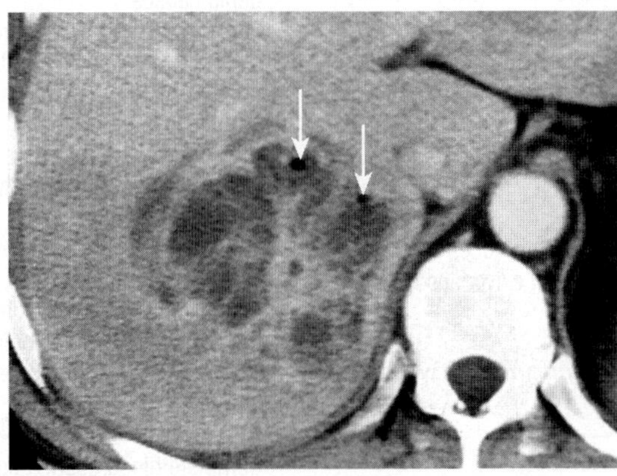

FIG. 2 Pyogenic liver abscess. A liver abscess containing *Escherichia coli* has irregular septations and contains a few bubbles of air (*arrows*). Because of the multiple loculations, this abscess did not respond to a percutaneous catheter for drainage and required surgical debridement. (From Webb WR, Brant WE, Major NM: *Fundamentals of body CT*, ed 4, Philadelphia, 2015, Saunders.)

- CT scan is more sensitive in detecting hepatic abscesses and contiguous organ extension and is the imaging study of choice (Fig. E1, *B*, and Fig. 2).
- Chest x-ray: Abnormal in 50% of the cases, may reveal elevated right hemidiaphragm, subdiaphragmatic air-fluid levels, pleural effusions, and consolidating infiltrates.
- Most liver abscesses are single; however, multiple liver abscesses can occur with systemic bacteremia.

Rx TREATMENT

NONPHARMACOLOGIC THERAPY

- The management of pyogenic liver abscess differs from that of amebic liver abscess.
- Medical management is the cornerstone of therapy in amebic liver abscess, whereas early intervention in the form of surgical therapy or catheter drainage and parenteral antibiotics is the rule in pyogenic liver abscess greater than 3 cm. Smaller abscesses (<3 cm) can generally be treated with broad-spectrum antibiotics.

ACUTE GENERAL Rx

- Percutaneous drainage under CT or ultrasound guidance is essential in the treatment of pyogenic liver abscesses.
- Aspiration of hepatic amebic abscesses is not required unless there is no response to treatment or a pyogenic cause is being considered.
- Empiric broad-spectrum antibiotics are recommended initially until culture results are available. Common choices include:
  1. Metronidazole (500 mg IV q8h) plus ceftriaxone or levofloxacin.
  2. Monotherapy with a beta-lactam/beta-lactamase inhibitor, such as piperacillin/tazobactam (4.5 g q6h), ticarcillin-clavulanate (3.1 g q4h), or ampicillin-sulbactam (3 g q6h).
  3. Monotherapy with a carbapenem, such as imipenem (500 mg IV q6h), meropenem (1 g q8h), or ertapenem (1 g daily).
  4. Duration of antibiotic treatment is usually 4 to 6 wk with IV antibiotics used for the first 1 to 2 wk or until a favorable clinical response, followed thereafter with oral antibiotics (e.g., metronidazole 500 mg PO q8h plus ciprofloxacin 500 mg PO q12h).
  5. Third-generation cephalosporins should not be used as single agents for empiric therapy because of risk of the emergence of beta-lactamase-producing bacteria.
- Antibiotic coverage for amebic liver abscesses includes:
  1. Metronidazole 750 mg PO tid for 10 days or tinidazole.
  2. Eradication of the coexistent intestinal infection with paromomycin for 10 days.

CHRONIC Rx

- If fever persists for 2 wk despite percutaneous drainage and antibiotic therapy as outlined under "Acute General Rx," or if there is failure of aspiration or failure of percutaneous drainage, surgery is indicated.
- In patients not responding to intravenous antibiotics and percutaneous drainage, hepatic artery antibiotic infusion can be considered.
- In patients with evidence of metastatic disease that is causing biliary obstruction, a gastroenterology consultation for endoscopic retrograde cholangiopancreatography and stenting should be considered.

DISPOSITION

- Most patients with pyogenic liver abscesses defervesce within 2 wk of treatment with antibiotics and drainage.
- No randomized controlled studies have evaluated the optimal duration of antibiotic therapy for pyogenic liver abscess. Typical duration of antibiotic therapy is at least 4 to 6 wk.
- Pyogenic liver abscess cure rates using percutaneous drainage and antibiotics have been reported to be between 88% and 100%.
- Mortality rate of untreated pyogenic liver abscess is nearly 100%.
- Most patients with amebic liver abscesses defervesce within 4 to 5 days of treatment.
- Amebic liver abscess mortality rate is <1% unless complications occur (see "Comments").
- Follow-up imaging should be used to monitor response to therapy; continue treatment until CT scan shows complete or near-complete resolution of cavity.

REFERRAL

Infectious disease, gastroenterology, interventional radiology, and general surgical consultations are recommended in any patient with hepatic abscess.

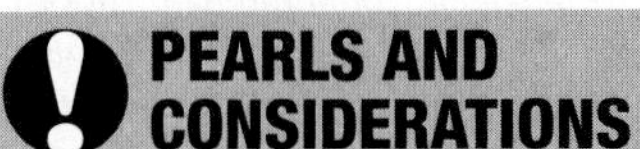

PEARLS AND CONSIDERATIONS

COMMENTS

- Complications of pyogenic and amebic liver abscesses include:
  1. Pleuropulmonary extension, resulting in empyema, abscess, and fistula formation
  2. Peritonitis
  3. Purulent pericarditis
  4. Sepsis
- Amebic liver abscesses complicate amebic colitis in nearly 10% of cases.

RELATED CONTENT

Liver Abscess (Patient Information)
Amebiasis (Related Key Topic)

AUTHOR: **FRED F. FERRI, M.D.**

BASIC INFORMATION

DEFINITION

Long QT syndrome (LQTS) is a disorder of myocardial repolarization characterized by a prolongation of the QT interval on the ECG associated with an increased risk of developing life-threatening ventricular arrhythmias, most commonly torsades de pointes (a specific type of polymorphic ventricular tachycardia), which may lead to ventricular fibrillation and sudden cardiac death (SCD). This syndrome may be either genetic or acquired.

SYNONYMS

LQTS

Congenital forms:

Jervell and Lange-Nielsen syndrome (associated with deafness)

Romano-Ward syndrome (associated with normal hearing)

ICD-10CM CODE

I45.81 Long QT syndrome

EPIDEMIOLOGY & DEMOGRAPHICS

- Congenital LQTS is thought to account for >3000 deaths in childhood per yr in the United States.
- Prevalence is felt to be 1:2000 of apparently healthy white young births. It may be higher because this is based on genetic testing of infants in whom the QTc was in excess of 470 and 460 milliseconds, respectively (Schwartz, 2009).
- Presence of LQTS has been shown in all racial groups. Review of data from the US portion of the international LQTS registry found a lower incidence but higher severity of QT prolongation among African Americans. These findings could be in part attributable to socioeconomic factors (Fugate, 2010).
- Incidence of LQTS is thought to be between 1:2500 and 1:10,000 in the general population, although it has been difficult to estimate due to incomplete penetrance. Congenital form associated with deafness is autosomal recessive (Jervell and Lange Nielsen syndrome) and is less common than the autosomal dominant form as well as more severe.
- Congenital form associated with normal hearing (Romano-Ward syndrome) is autosomal dominant. Although inheritance of LQTS is autosomal dominant, female predominance has often been observed and has been attributed to an increased susceptibility to cardiac arrhythmias in women. LQTS is more likely to express itself before puberty in males and after puberty in females.
- At least 17 different LQTS genes have been identified to date. LQTS is more common in women than in men.
- Mortality rate is estimated to be about 1% per yr.
- Multiple mutations causing congenital LQTS have been described. The most common types of LQTS are described in Table 1.

PHYSICAL FINDINGS & CLINICAL PRESENTATION

- Many episodes are stress mediated.
- Palpitations, presyncope.
- Syncope caused by ventricular tachycardia.
- SCD.
- Seizure.
- Family history of LQTS, but a family history of SCD has not been proved to be a risk factor for SCD in patients with LQTS.
- Abnormal ECG (prolonged QT) in asymptomatic relatives of known case.
- Prolonged QTc interval on ECG (QTc should be >460 ms in women and >440 ms in men). Notably, 20% to 25% genotype positive LQTS may have normal QTc on resting ECG.
- In case of congenital LQTS, the presentation of syncope or SCD is typically triggered by exercise and swimming in LQT1 patients, in LQT2 patients by emotion, pregnancy, or noise, and patients with LQT3 are at highest risk of events when at rest or asleep.

ETIOLOGY

- Cardiac repolarization abnormality
- Congenital cause (hundreds of mutations on more than 10 genes have been identified)
- Most of the gene mutations affect function of ion channels leading to prolonged repolarization (i.e., sodium and potassium channels resulting in either increased Na^+ influx or decreased K^+ efflux). These mutations prolong depolarization and predispose the patient to torsades de pointes
- Acquired causes:
  1. Drugs: Dofetilide, ibutilide, bepridil, quinidine, procainamide, sotalol, amiodarone, ranolazine, disopyramide, phenothiazines and antiemetic agents (droperidol, domperidone), tricyclic antidepressants, antipsychotics (quetiapine, ziprasidone, iloperidone), citalopram, antihistamines, quinolones, azithromycin, astemizole or cisapride given with ketoconazole or erythromycin, clarithromycin, and antimalarials, particularly among patients with asthma or those using potassium-lowering medications; also common in patients receiving methadone
  2. Hypokalemia, hypomagnesemia, hypocalcemia (especially in patients with malabsorption syndrome)
  3. Liquid protein diet
  4. Central nervous system lesions
  5. Ischemia
  6. Hypothyroidism

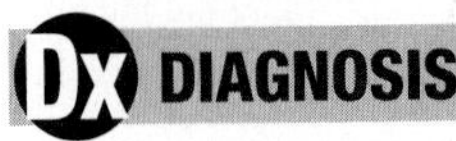

DIAGNOSIS

DIFFERENTIAL DIAGNOSIS

See "Syncope." Brugada syndrome, arrhythmogenic right ventricular dysplasia, and LQTS are major causes of genetic sudden death syndromes (Fig. 1).

TABLE 1 Common Types of Long QT (LQT) Syndrome

	LQT1	LQT2	LQT3
Pathophysiology			
Gene	*KCNQ1 (KvLQT1)*	*KCNH2 (HERG)*	*SCN5A*
Protein	$K_v7.1$	$K_v11.1$	$Na_v1.5$
Ionic current	Decreased I_{Ks}	Decreased I_{Kr}	Increased late I_{Na}
Clinical Presentation			
Incidence of cardiac events	63%	46%	18%
Incidence of SCD	4%	4%	4%
Arrhythmia triggers	Emotional/physical stress (swimming, diving)	Emotional stress, arousal (alarm clock, telephone), rest, postpartum period	Sleep/rest
ECG	Broad-based T wave	Low-amplitude, bifid T wave	Long isoelectric ST segment
QT response to exercise	Attenuated QTc shortening and an exaggerated QTc prolongation during early and peak exercise	Normal QT during exercise but with exaggerated QT hysteresis	Supernormal QT shortening
Management			
Exercise restriction	+++	++	?
Response to beta blockers	+++	+++	?
Potassium supplement	+	++	+
Left cervicothoracic sympathectomy	++	++	++
Response to mexiletine	+	+	++

From Issa Z, et al.: *Clinical arrhythmology and electrophysiology,* ed 2, Philadelphia, 2012, Saunders.

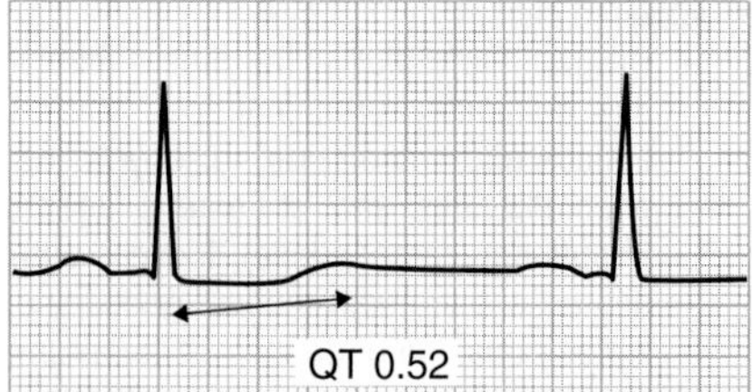

A

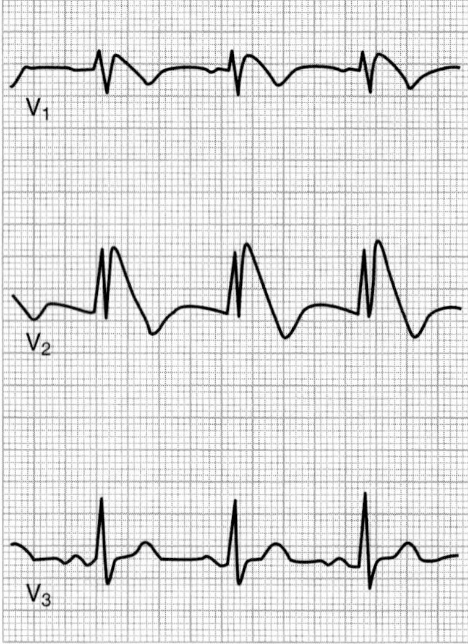

B

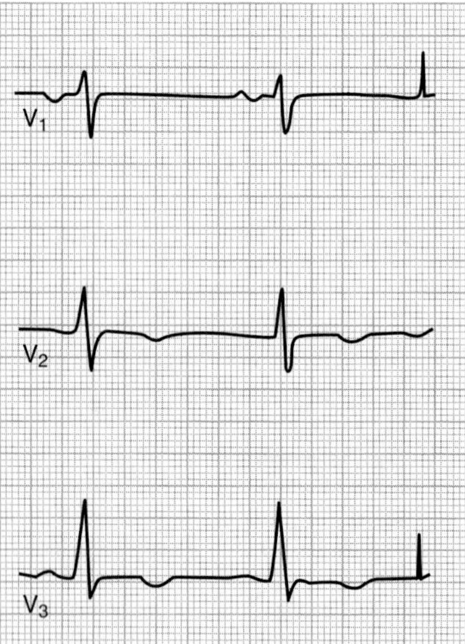

C

FIG. 1 Sinus rhythm electrocardiogram findings in three genetic sudden death syndromes. A, QT prolongation during sinus rhythm in a patient with long QT syndrome. **B,** ST elevation in V_1 and V_2 in a patient with Brugada syndrome. **C,** T wave inversion in V_1-V_3 in a patient with arrhythmogenic right ventricular dysplasia. (From Goldman L, Schafer AI: *Goldman's Cecil medicine,* ed 24, Philadelphia, 2012, Saunders.)

Diagnostic criteria for the congenital LQTS as per 2013 HRS Guidelines:

LQTS is diagnosed:

- In the presence of an LQTS risk score ≥3.5 in the absence of a secondary cause for QT prolongation and/or
- In the presence of an unequivocally pathogenic mutation in one of the LQTS genes or
- In the presence of a QT interval corrected for heart rate using Bazett formula (QTc) ≥500 ms in repeated 12-lead electrocardiogram (ECG) and in the absence of a secondary cause for QT prolongation.
- LQTS can be diagnosed in the presence of a QTc between 480 and 499 ms in repeated 12-lead ECGs in a patient with unexplained syncope in the absence of a secondary cause for QT prolongation and in the absence of a pathogenic mutation.

LQTS Risk Score (Schwartz 2011):

ECG Criteria	
QTc >480 ms	3 points
QTc 460-480 ms	2 points
QTc 450-460 ms (males)	1 point
QTc 4th minute of recovery from exercise stress test >480 ms	1 point
Torsades de pointes	2 points
T-wave alternans	1 point
Notched T wave in three leads	1 point
Bradycardia	0.5 point
History	
Syncope with stress	2 points
Syncope without stress	1 point
Congenital deafness	0.5 point
Definite family history of long QT	1 point
Unexplained cardiac death in first-degree relative <30 yr	0.5 point

Total score: 1 point: Low probability of LQTS. 1.5 to 3 points: Intermediate probability of LQTS. ≥ 3.5 points high probability.

WORKUP

Cardiology referral is recommended for all cases.

Genetic analysis is an essential step for risk stratification of patients with congenital prolonged QT and is important for identification of potential mutation carriers within the proband family. There is evidence for gene-specific triggers of events and therapeutic efficacy. Molecular screening should become part of the routine clinical management of LQTS.

In relatives of known patients with LQTS or in young patients with syncope:

- Stress test may prolong the QT interval or cause T-wave alternans.
- Valsalva maneuver: May prolong the QT interval or cause T-wave alternans.
- Prolonged ECG monitoring with various stimulations aimed at increasing catecholamines and assess for QT prolongation (perform in a setting that can provide resuscitation with α- and β-antagonists readily available).
- Epinephrine-induced prolongation of the QT interval (epinephrine infusion QT stress test)
- Genetic analysis:
  1. *LQT1* locus of *KCNQ1* potassium channel gene.
  2. *LQT2* locus of *KCNH2* potassium channel gene.
  3. *LQT3* locus of *SCN5A* sodium channel gene.
  4. These three variants account for >90% of all genotyped LQTS patients, whereas the remaining genes are responsible for a minority of cases.
- Risk stratification for each genetic variant on the basis of gender and QTc: Groups are defined on the basis of the probability of the first cardiac event (syncope, cardiac arrest, or sudden death) before the age of 40 yr or before therapy. Specific mutations, depending on type, location, and degree, may confer a high risk even if the ECG abnormalities are mild. Clinically, QT interval duration was the strongest predictor of risk for cardiac events; a QTc exceeding 500 ms identifies patients with the highest risk.
  1. High risk (>50% of cardiac event): QTc ≥ 500 ms and LQT1 or LQT2, or male with LQT3.
  2. Moderate risk (30%-50%): QTc <500 ms in male with LQT3 or in female with LQT2 or LQT3, and female with LQT3 with QTc ≥500 ms.
  3. Low risk (<30%): QTc <500 ms and LQT1 or male LQT2 with QTc <500 ms.
  4. Prophylactic treatment should be considered in all patients with moderate or high risk for cardiac events based on the above risk stratification scheme (Table 2).

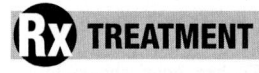

TREATMENT

NONPHARMACOLOGIC

- Focuses on exclusion of triggers of life-threatening arrhythmia—there are gene-specific triggers for symptoms:
  1. *LQT1* patients experience 90% of lethal events under physical and emotional stress. Swimming and diving should be avoided or performed under supervision.
  2. *LQT2* patients are at highest risk during arousal or emotions, also during sleep and at rest but not at all during exercise; avoid sudden or excessive acoustic stimuli, especially during sleep (e.g., avoid telephone and/or alarm clock in the proximity)—as opposed to *LQT3* patients, in whom 80% of the events occur at rest or while asleep.
- Previously, all patients with LQTS have been instructed to avoid competitive sports. More recently, low-risk, genetically confirmed LQTS with borderline QTc prolongation, without prior cardiac symptoms and no familial history of SCD are thought to be safe to participate in competitive sports where AED and BLS personnel is available. ICD implantation solely for the purpose of participating in sports is deemed inappropriate. For athletes with ICD implanted for another indication, returning to a low level of exertion is deemed reasonable, and a higher level of exertion may be considered after extensive discussion of potential risks.

TABLE 2 Cardiac Event Risk Stratification Scheme Based on Genes, Gender, and QTc

	QTc <500 ms		QTc ≥550 ms	
Genetic Subtype	**Male**	**Female**	**Male**	**Female**
LQT1	Low	Low	High	High
LQT2	Low	Intermediate	High	High
LQT3	Intermediate	Intermediate	High	Intermediate

Probability of the first cardiac event (syncope, cardiac arrest, or sudden death) before the age of 40 years or before therapy. High = >50%, Intermediate = 30%-50%, Low = <30%.

TABLE 3 Management of Patients with Long QT Syndrome

Type of Syndrome	Management	Indication
Congenital	Beta-blockers	Asymptomatic patients, symptomatic patients (who do not have bronchospasm)
	Cervicothoracic sympathectomy	Refractory symptoms, especially in pediatric patients
	Cardiac pacing	Refractory symptoms associated with bradycardia, pauses
	Implantable cardioverter-defibrillator	Cardiac arrest, refractory syncope, prophylaxis for moderate- to high-risk patients for cardiac events
Acquired	Elimination of causative drug or condition	All patients
	Magnesium sulfate	Nonsustained ventricular tachycardia, torsades de pointes (even with a normal serum magnesium concentration)
	Administration of potassium (to keep serum K^+ >4.5 mEq/L)	Serum K^+ <4.5 mEq/L
	Maneuvers to increase heart rate (cardiac pacing, isoproterenol)	Bradycardia, arrhythmias refractory to magnesium sulfate

K^+, Potassium.
Adapted from Crawford MH et al (eds): *Cardiology*, ed 2, St Louis, 2004, Mosby.

- Implantation of an implantable cardioverter-defibrillator (ICD) is recommended according to the ACC/AHA guidelines for patients with a good functional status for more than 1 yr and the following conditions (Table 3):
  1. Survivors of cardiac arrest (class 1).
  2. Patients with syncope or ventricular tachycardia while receiving β-blockers (class IIa).
  3. Prophylaxis of SCD with use of β-blocker in patients with characteristics that suggest high risk (such as *LQT2* and *LQT3, QTc >500 ms*) (class IIb).

PHARMACOLOGIC

- With few exceptions (mostly borderline QTc and LQT1 males aged >25 to 30 yr), all mutation carriers should be treated because of the risk of SCD during first cardiac event. All symptomatic patients should be treated as well.
- Beta-blockers, chiefly propranolol and nadolol, are an initial therapy of choice—there are differential responses to β-blocker therapy among different genetic variants; especially effective among LQT1 patients. Studies showed the efficacy of β-blockers with an overall mortality <2% over a mean follow-up exceeding 5 yr.
- In patients with LQT3, mexiletine shortens the QTc and can be given with a β-blocker.
- In the 20% to 30% of patients who continue to have symptoms on a β-blocker, the main options are either left cardiac sympathetic denervation (LCSD) or the prophylactic implantation of an ICD.
- In patients with frequent ICD shocks or in those with high risk for SCD where ICD placement cannot be performed, cardiac pacing and/or LCSD may be indicated.
- In patients with recurrent syncope and/or aborted cardiac arrest despite combined ICD and β-blocker, LCSD as adjunctive therapy can be performed.
- Correctable factors including electrolyte disorder—hypokalemia and hypomagnesemia—and avoidance of precipitating drugs that may further prolong the QT interval is mandatory. A complete list of drugs that can potentially prolong QT may be found at www.crediblemeds.org.
- For patients with acquired form and torsades de pointes, IV magnesium and atrial or ventricular pacing are initial choices.
- Table 3 summarizes management of patients with LQTS.

PROGNOSIS

In carefully treated patients, mortality is around 0.5% to 1% over 20 yr.

The timing and frequency of syncope, QTc prolongation, and gender are predictive of risk for aborted cardiac arrest and SCD during adolescence. Higher risk is present in those with one or two or more episodes of syncope in the last 10 yr compared with those with no syncopal episodes, those with QTc >530 ms, and males aged 10 to 12 yr.

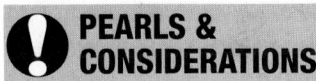

COMMENTS

Family history should be assessed for a history of sudden death and other deaths that may have occurred as manifestations of LQTS (e.g., sudden infant death, drowning, and loss of consciousness while driving).

RELATED CONTENT

Long QT Syndrome (Patient Information)
Torsades des Pointes (Related Key Topic)

SUGGESTED READINGS

Available at ExpertConsult.com

AUTHOR: **SIMON GRINGUT, M.D.**

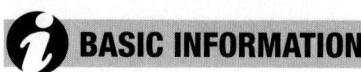

BASIC INFORMATION

DEFINITION

A lung abscess is an infection of the lung parenchyma resulting in a necrotic cavity containing pus.

SYNONYM

Pulmonary abscess

ICD-10CM CODES
J85.1 Abscess of lung with pneumonia
J85.2 Abscess of lung without pneumonia
A06.5 Amebic lung abscess

EPIDEMIOLOGY & DEMOGRAPHICS

INCIDENCE: Has decreased over the last 30 yr as a result of antibiotic therapy.

- Lung abscess in patients age 50 and over is associated with primary lung neoplasia in 30% of the cases.
- Lung abscesses commonly coexist with empyemas (pus in the pleural space).

RISK FACTORS (SEE TABLE 1):

1. Alcohol-related problems
2. Seizure disorders
3. Cerebrovascular disorders with dysphagia
4. Drug abuse
5. Esophageal disorders (e.g., scleroderma, esophageal carcinoma)
6. Poor oral hygiene
7. Obstructive malignant lung disease
8. Bronchiectasis

PHYSICAL FINDINGS & CLINICAL PRESENTATION

- Symptoms are generally insidious and prolonged, occurring for weeks to months
- Fever, chills, and sweats
- Cough
- Sputum production (purulent with foul odor)
- Pleuritic chest pain
- Hemoptysis
- Dyspnea
- Malaise, fatigue, and weakness
- Tachycardia and tachypnea
- Dullness to percussion, whispered pectoriloquy, and bronchophony
- Amphoric breath sounds (low-pitched sound of air moving across a large open cavity)

ETIOLOGY

- The most important factor predisposing to lung abscess is aspiration.
- Following aspiration as a major predisposing factor is periodontal disease.
- Lung abscess is rare in an edentulous person.
- Approximately 90% of lung abscesses are caused by anaerobic microorganisms (peptostreptococci, microaerophilic streptococci such as *Streptococcus milleri, Bacteroides* species, *Fusobacterium nucleatum, Prevotella*). Pulmonary actinomycosis will also generate lung abscess.
- In most cases anaerobic infection is mixed with aerobic or facultative anaerobic organisms *(S. aureus, E. coli, K. pneumoniae, P. aeruginosa).*
- Parasitic organisms including *Paragonimus westermani* and *Entamoeba histolytica.*
- Fungi including *Aspergillus, Cryptococcus, Histoplasma, Blastomyces,* and *Coccidioides* spp.
- Immunocompromised hosts may become infected with *Aspergillus,* mycobacteria, *Nocardia, Legionella micdadei,* and *Rhodococcus equi.*
- Lung necrosis caused by community strains of MRSA (USA 300 strain) in young adults or adolescents after acute influenza was initially reported in 2002 and can be quite fulminant.

Dx DIAGNOSIS

Lung abscess may be primary or secondary.

- *Primary lung abscess* refers to infection from normal host organisms within the lung (e.g., aspiration, pneumonia).
- Secondary lung abscess results from other preexisting conditions (e.g., endocarditis, underlying lung cancer, pulmonary emboli).

Lung abscess may be acute or chronic.

- Acute lung abscess is present if symptoms are of less than 4 to 6 wk.
- Chronic lung abscess is present if symptoms last longer than 6 wk.

DIFFERENTIAL DIAGNOSIS

The differential diagnosis is similar to that for cavitary lung lesions:

- Bacterial (anaerobic, aerobic, infected bulla, empyema, actinomycosis, tuberculosis)
- Fungal (histoplasmosis, coccidioidomycosis, blastomycosis, aspergillosis, cryptococcosis, Zygomycetes)
- Parasitic (amebiasis, echinococcosis)
- Malignancy (primary lung carcinoma, metastatic lung disease, lymphoma, Hodgkin's disease)
- Granulomatosis with polyangiitis, sarcoidosis, endocarditis, and septic pulmonary emboli

WORKUP

- The workup of a patient with lung abscess attempts to elicit a primary or a secondary cause.
- Blood tests are not specific in diagnosing lung abscesses.
- Most diagnoses are made from imaging studies; however, to diagnose a specific cause bacteriologic studies are needed.

LABORATORY TESTS

- CBC with leukocytosis.
- Bacteriologic studies:
  1. Sputum Gram stain and culture (commonly contaminated by oral flora).
  2. Percutaneous transtracheal aspiration.
  3. Percutaneous transthoracic aspiration.
  4. Fiberoptic bronchoscopy using bronchial brushings or bronchoalveolar lavage is the most widely used intervention when trying to obtain diagnostic bacteriologic cultures.
- Blood cultures on some occasions (<30%) may be positive.
- If an empyema is present, obtaining empyema fluid via thoracentesis may isolate the organism.

IMAGING STUDIES

- Chest x-ray makes the diagnosis of lung abscess showing the cavitary lesion with an air-fluid level.
- Lung abscesses are most commonly found in the posterior segment of the right upper lobe.
- Chest CT scan can localize and size the lesion and assist in differentiating lung abscesses from other pathologic processes (e.g., tumor, empyema, infected bulla) (Fig. 1).

Rx TREATMENT

NONPHARMACOLOGIC THERAPY

- Oxygen therapy
- Postural drainage
- Respiratory therapy maneuvers

ACUTE GENERAL Rx

- Piperacillin/tazobactam 3.375 g IV q6h in aspiration pneumonia with lung abscess.
- Ceftriaxone 1 to 2 g IV q24h plus metronidazole: 500 mg IV q8h.
- Clindamycin is more effective for anaerobic lung abscess than penicillin alone. Dose: 900 mg IV q8h until improved, then 300 to 600 mg PO q6h.
- Penicillin 1 to 2 million units IV q4h until improvement (afebrile, decreased phlegm production, followed by penicillin VK 500 mg

TABLE 1 Risk Factors for Aspiration Pneumonia and Lung Abscess

Increased bacterial inoculum	Periodontal disease, gingivitis, tonsillar or dental abscess, drugs that decrease gastric acidity
Impairment of consciousness	Drugs, alcohol, general anesthesia, metabolic encephalopathy, coma, shock, cerebrovascular accident, cardiopulmonary arrest, seizures, surgery, trauma
Impaired cough and gag reflexes	Vocal cord paralysis, intratracheal anesthesia, endotracheal tube, tracheostomy, myopathy, myelopathy, other neurologic disorders
Impairment of esophageal function	Diverticula, achalasia, strictures, disorders of gastrointestinal motility, neoplasm, tracheoesophageal fistula, pseudobulbar palsy
Emesis	Nasogastric tube, gastric dilation, ileus, intestinal obstruction

From Cohen J, Powderly WG: *Infectious diseases,* ed 2, St Louis, 2004, Mosby.

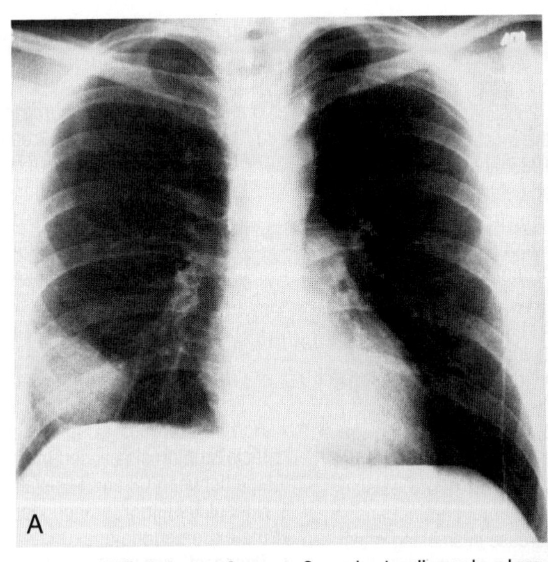

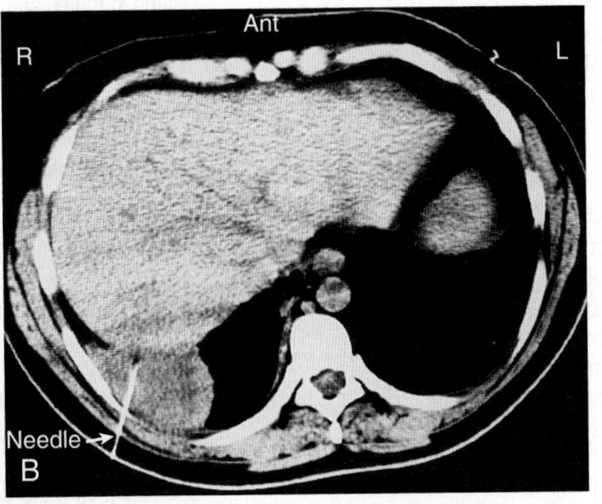

FIG. 1 Lung abscess. On a chest radiograph, a lung abscess may look to be a solid rounded lesion **(A),** or, if it has a connection with the bronchus, there may be an air-fluid level in a thick-walled cavitary lesion. CT scanning **(B)** can be used to localize the lesion and to place a needle for drainage and aspiration of contents for culture. (From Mettler FA [ed]: *Primary care radiology,* Philadelphia, 2000, Saunders.)

PO q6h for 2 to 3 wk but often up to 6 to 8 wk) can be given with metronidazole doses of 7.5 mg/kg IV q6h followed by PO 500 mg bid to qid dosing as an alternative to clindamycin.

- Penicillin should not be used alone because many mouth flora anaerobes now produce penicillinase enzymes. Metronidazole should not be used alone because it is not active against microaerophilic streptococci and some anaerobic cocci.
- Other alternatives are ampicillin/sulbactam and carbapenems such as ertapenem and meropenem.

CHRONIC Rx

- Bronchoscopy to assist with drainage and/or diagnosis is indicated in patients who fail to respond to antibiotics or if there is suspected underlying malignancy.
- Surgery is indicated on rare occasions (<10%) in patients with complications of lung abscess (see "Comments").

DISPOSITION

- More than 95% of patients are cured with the use of antibiotics alone.
- Complications of lung abscesses include:
  1. Empyema
  2. Massive hemoptysis
  3. Pneumothorax
  4. Bronchopleural fistula
  5. Hepatobronchial fistula
  6. Brain abscess
  7. Bronchiectasis
- Mortality is low in community-acquired lung abscess (2.5%).
- Hospital-acquired lung abscess carries a high mortality rate (65%).

REFERRAL

If lung abscess is present, consultation with pulmonary and infectious disease specialist is recommended. An interventional radiologist also may be able to perform drainage and obtain cultures.

PEARLS & CONSIDERATIONS

COMMENTS

- Refractory cases are usually the result of:
  1. Large cavity size (>6 cm)
  2. Recurrent aspiration
  3. Thick-walled cavities
  4. Underlying lung carcinoma
  5. Empyema formation
- Necrotizing pneumonia is similar to a lung abscess but differs in size (<2 cm in diameter) and number (usually multiple suppurative cavitary lesions).

SUGGESTED READING

Available at ExpertConsult.com

RELATED CONTENT

Lung Abscess (Patient Information)
Aspiration Pneumonia (Related Key Topic)

AUTHOR: **GLENN G. FORT, M.D., M.P.H.**

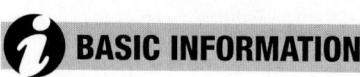

DEFINITION

A primary lung neoplasm is a malignancy arising from lung tissue. The different types are non–small cell lung cancer (NSCLC , 85% of all lung cancers; squamous cell carcinoma, adenocarcinoma, and large cell carcinoma) and small cell lung cancer (SCLC, 15% of all lung cancers).

ADENOCARCINOMA: Represents 35% to 40% of lung carcinomas; frequently located in midlung and periphery; initial metastases are to lymphatics; frequently associated with peripheral scars; adenocarcinoma is described as preinvasive, minimally invasive, or invasive

SQUAMOUS CELL: Represents 20% to 30% of lung cancers; central location; metastasis by local invasion; frequent cavitation and obstructive phenomena

SMALL CELL: Represents 15% of lung carcinomas; central location; metastasis through lymphatics; associated with lesion of the short arm of chromosome 3; high cavitation rate

LARGE CELL: Represents 10% to 15% of lung carcinomas; frequently located in the periphery; metastasis to central nervous system and mediastinum; rapid growth rate with early metastasis

LEPIDIC-PREDOMINANT PATTERN (BRONCHOALVEOLAR): Represents 5% of lung carcinomas; frequently located in the periphery; may be bilateral; initial metastasis through lymphatic, hematogenous, and local invasion; no correlation with cigarette smoking; cavitation rare

SYNONYM

Lung cancer

ICD-10CM CODES

C34.10 Malignant neoplasm of upper lobe, unspecified bronchus or lung
C34.11 Malignant neoplasm of upper lobe, right bronchus or lung
C34.12 Malignant neoplasm of upper lobe, left bronchus or lung
C34.2 Malignant neoplasm of middle lobe, bronchus or lung
C34.30 Malignant neoplasm of lower lobe, unspecified bronchus or lung
C34.31 Malignant neoplasm of lower lobe, right bronchus or lung
C34.32 Malignant neoplasm of lower lobe, left bronchus or lung
C34.80 Malignant neoplasm of overlapping sites of unspecified bronchus and lung
C34.81 Malignant neoplasm of overlapping sites of right bronchus and lung
C34.82 Malignant neoplasm of overlapping sites of left bronchus and lung
C34.90 Malignant neoplasm of unspecified part of unspecified bronchus or lung
C34.91 Malignant neoplasm of unspecified part of right bronchus or lung
C34.92 Malignant neoplasm of unspecified part of left bronchus or lung

EPIDEMIOLOGY & DEMOGRAPHICS

- Lung cancer is responsible for >30% of cancer deaths in males and >25% of cancer deaths in females. It has been the most common cancer in the world since 1985 and is the leading cause of cancer-related death in both sexes.
- Tobacco smoke is implicated in 90% of cases; of these, secondhand smoke is responsible for approximately 20% of cases.
- In the U.S., there will be an estimated 234,030 new cases of lung cancer and 154,050 deaths from lung cancer in 2018. Worldwide 1.6 million tumor-related deaths are attributed annually to lung cancer.
- From 1990 through 2013 the percentage of patients with non-small-cell lung cancer who never smoked rose from 8% to 16%, raising concerns about environmental carcinogens.
- Coincident with the decrease in smoking rates, the incidence of new cases and the rate lung cancer deaths in the U.S. continue to decrease. However, death rates among African Americans continue to be disproportionately higher.

PHYSICAL FINDINGS & CLINICAL PRESENTATION

- Weight loss, fatigue, fever, anorexia, dysphagia
- Cough, hemoptysis, dyspnea, wheezing
- Chest, shoulder, and bone pain
- Paraneoplastic syndromes (see Table 1):
  1. *Lambert-Eaton myasthenic syndrome:* Myopathy involving proximal muscle groups
  2. Endocrine manifestations: Hypercalcemia, ectopic adrenocorticotropic hormone secretion, syndrome of inappropriate excretion of adrenocorticotropic hormone (SIADH)
  3. Neurologic: Subacute cerebellar degeneration, peripheral neuropathy, cortical degeneration
  4. Musculoskeletal: Polymyositis, clubbing, hypertrophic pulmonary osteoarthropathy
  5. Hematologic or vascular: Migratory thrombophlebitis, marantic thrombosis, anemia, thrombocytosis, or thrombocytopenia
  6. Cutaneous: Acanthosis nigricans, dermatomyositis
- Pleural effusion (10% of patients), recurrent pneumonias (from obstruction), localized wheezing
- *Superior vena cava syndrome:*
  1. Obstruction of venous return of the superior vena cava is most commonly caused by bronchogenic carcinoma or metastasis to paratracheal nodes.
  2. The patient usually reports headache, nausea, dizziness, visual changes, syncope, and respiratory distress.
  3. Physical examination reveals distention of thoracic and neck veins, edema of face and upper extremities, facial plethora, and cyanosis.
- *Horner syndrome:* Constricted pupil, ptosis, facial anhidrosis caused by spinal cord damage between C8 and T1 as a result of a superior sulcus tumor (bronchogenic carcinoma of the extreme lung apex)
- *Pancoast tumor:* A superior sulcus tumor (Fig. 1) associated with ipsilateral Horner syndrome and shoulder pain

ETIOLOGY

- Tobacco abuse; the chance of developing lung cancer for a 40-pack-yr persistent smoker is 20 times that of someone who never smoked
- Environmental agents (e.g., radon) and industrial agents (e.g., ionizing radiation, asbestos, nickel, uranium, vinyl chloride, chromium, arsenic, coal dust)
- Lung cancer susceptibility and risk increased in inherited cancer syndromes caused by germ-line mutations in p53, retinoblastoma, and epidermal growth factor receptor *(EGFR)* genes

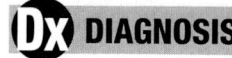

DIFFERENTIAL DIAGNOSIS

- Pneumonia
- Tuberculosis (TB)
- Metastatic carcinoma to the lung
- Lung abscess
- Granulomatous disease

TABLE 1 Paraneoplastic Syndromes Associated with Bronchogenic Carcinoma

Syndrome	Cell Type	Mechanism
Hypertrophic pulmonary osteoarthropathy and clubbing	All types	Unknown
Hyponatremia	SCLC most common; may be any type	SIADH, ectopic antidiuretic hormone production by tumor
Hypercalcemia	Usually squamous cell	Bone metastases, osteoclast-activating factor, parathyroid hormone–like hormone, prostaglandins
Cushing's syndrome	Usually SCLC	Ectopic ACTH production
Lambert-Eaton myasthenic syndrome	Usually SCLC	Voltage-sensitive calcium channel antibodies in >75%; affects presynaptic neuronal calcium channel activity
Other neuromyopathic disorders	SCLC most common; may be any type	Antineuronal nuclear antibodies, also known as anti-Hu; others unknown
Thrombophlebitis	All types	Unknown

ACTH, Adrenocorticotropic hormone; *SCLC,* small cell lung cancer; *SIADH,* syndrome of inappropriate secretion of antidiuretic hormone.
Adapted from Andreoli TE, et al.: *Andreoli and Carpenter's Cecil essentials of medicine,* ed 8, Philadelphia, 2010, Saunders.

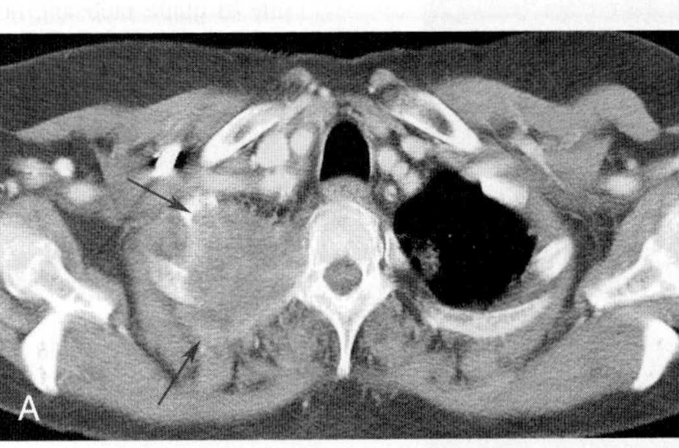

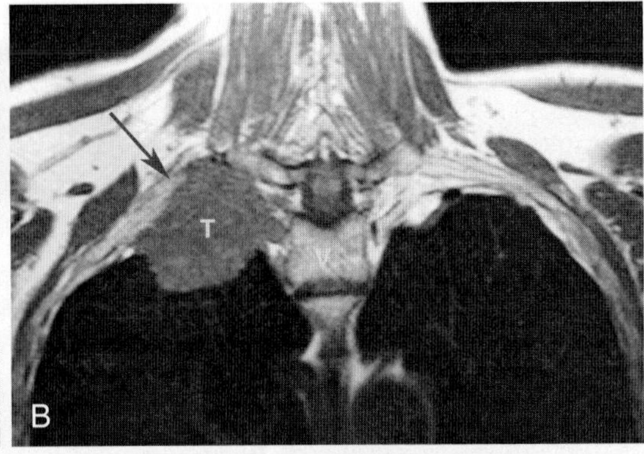

FIG. 1 Pancoast tumor with chest wall invasion. A, On computed tomography, a right apical mass is associated with invasion of the chest wall and rib destruction *(arrows)*. Although the tumor appears to contact the vertebral body, it appears intact. **B,** Coronal magnetic resonance imaging shows the relationship of the tumor (*T*) to the vertebral body (*V*) and the brachial plexus (*arrow*), which appears to be involved. (From Webb WR, et al.: *Fundamentals of body CT*, ed 4, Philadelphia, 2015, Elsevier.)

- Carcinoid tumor
- Sarcoidosis
- Benign lesions that simulate thoracic malignancy:
  1. Lobar atelectasis: Pneumonia, chronic inflammatory disease, allergic bronchopulmonary aspergillosis
  2. Multiple pulmonary nodules: Septic emboli, Wegener's granulomatosis, sarcoidosis, rheumatoid nodules, fungal disease, multiple pulmonary atrioventricular fistulas
  3. Mediastinal adenopathy: Sarcoidosis, lymphoma, primary TB, fungal disease, silicosis, pneumoconiosis, drug-induced (e.g., phenytoin, trimethadione)
  4. Pleural effusion: Congestive heart failure, pneumonia with parapneumonic effusion, TB, viral pneumonitis, ascites, pancreatitis, collagen-vascular disease

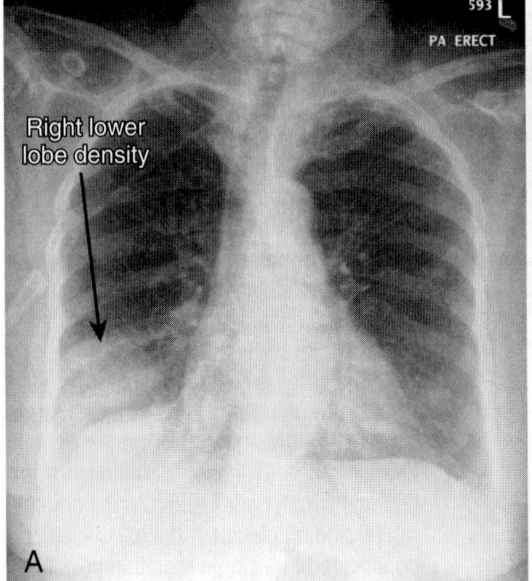

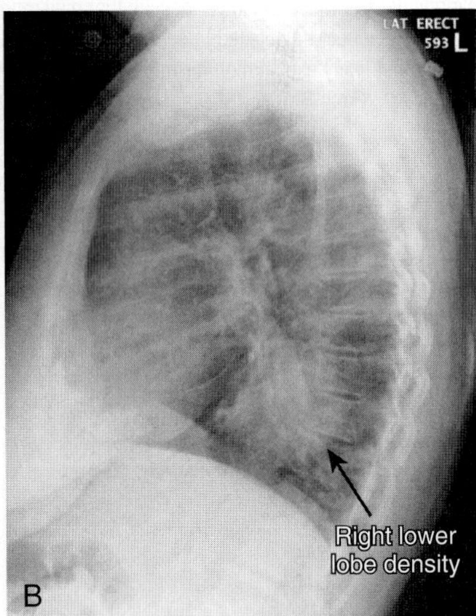

FIG. 2 Lung neoplasm, primary. Lung mass presenting with hemoptysis. **A,** Posterior-anterior (PA) chest x-ray. **B,** Lateral chest x-ray. This 83-year-old female presented with hemoptysis of a quarter-sized clot. Her posterior-anterior chest x-ray shows a rounded right lower lobe density. On the lateral view, this is visible in the retrocardiac space. This density measures 7.6 cm in diameter. Pneumonia, neoplasm, or abscess could have this appearance on chest x-ray. Computed tomography was performed to further delineate the pathology (see Fig. 3). (From Broder JS: *Diagnostic imaging for the emergency physician,* Philadelphia, 2011, Saunders.)

WORKUP

The workup generally includes chest CT, positron-emission tomographic (PET) scan, and tissue biopsy. Molecular testing for treatable oncogenic alterations should be performed to further classify NSCLC. This includes testing for mutations in the gene encoding epidermal growth factor receptor (eGFR) and in BRAF v600e, searching for translocations in the genes encoding anaplastic lymphoma kinase (ALK) and rat osteosarcoma (ROS1), and assessing expression of programmed geath ligand-1 (PD-L1).[1] Additional lab tests include CBC, serum chemistry studies. Diagnosis and staging of lung cancer should be performed simultaneously to minimize invasive testing.

LABORATORY TESTS

Various modalities are available to obtain a tissue diagnosis:

- Biopsy of any suspicious lymph nodes (e.g., supraclavicular or mediastinal node)
- Flexible fiberoptic bronchoscopy: Brush and biopsy specimens are obtained from any visualized endobronchial lesions. The use of a gene-expression classifier has a high sensitivity across different lesion sizes, locations, stages, and cell type of lung cancer. The combination of the classifier plus bronchoscopy has a sensitivity of >85%. In intermediate-risk patients with a nondiagnostic bronchoscopic examination, a negative classifier score provides support for a more conservative diagnostic approach.[2]
- Transbronchial needle aspiration: Done with a special needle passed through the bronchoscope; this technique is useful to sample mediastinal masses or paratracheal lymph nodes
- Transthoracic fine-needle aspiration biopsy with fluoroscopic or CT scan guidance to evaluate peripheral pulmonary nodules
- Endobronchial ultrasound (EBUS) guided biopsy and staging is now routinely used to evaluate suspected mediastinal and hilar nodes
- Mediastinoscopy and anteromedial sternotomy in suspected tumor involvement of the mediastinum
- Pleural biopsy in patients with pleural effusion
- Thoracentesis of pleural effusion and cytologic evaluation of the obtained fluid may confirm diagnosis

IMAGING STUDIES

- Chest x-ray (Fig. 2): The radiographic presentation often varies with the cell type. Presence of pleural effusion, lobar atelectasis, and mediastinal adenopathy can occur in any cell type.
- CT scan of the chest (Fig. 3) can evaluate mediastinal and pleural extension. The chest CT should include liver and adrenal glands (common sites of metastases). CT or MRI of brain should be considered in a patient presenting with neurologic symptoms (e.g., headaches, vision disturbances).
- PET with ^{18}F-fluorodeoxyglucose (^{18}FDG-PET) (Fig. E4) is superior to CT in detecting

[1] Reck M, Rabe KF: Precision diagnosis and treatment for advanced non-small-cell lung cancer, N Engl J Med, 377(9):849-861, 2017.

[2] Silvestri GA, et al.: A bronchial genomic classifier for the diagnostic evaluation of lung cancer, *N Engl J Med* 373:243–251, 2015..

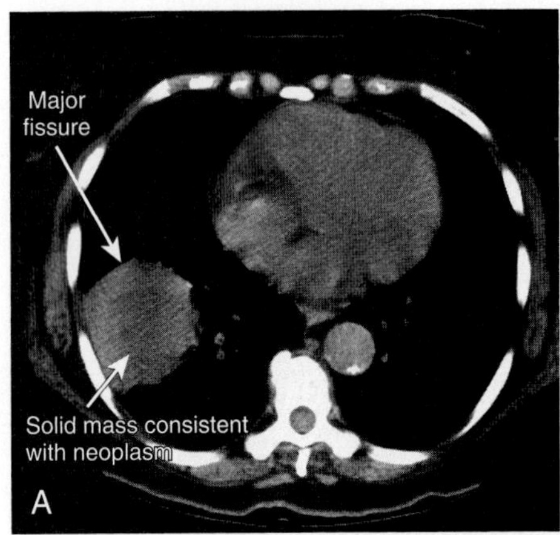

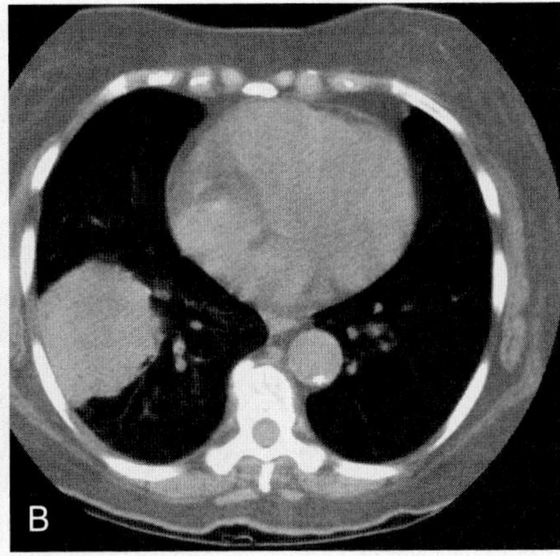

FIG. 3 Lung neoplasm, primary. Lung mass presenting with hemoptysis. Same patient as in Fig. 2. Noncontrast computed tomography was performed (contrast was withheld as a consequence of the patient's renal dysfunction) and shows a 6 by 6 cm round lesion abutting the oblique fissure (also called the major fissure) and lateral chest wall. **A,** Soft tissue windows. **B,** Lung windows. On soft tissue windows, the center appears slightly darker, indicating lower density that may represent central necrosis. If IV contrast had been given, an area of necrosis would have failed to enhance. Infection or infarction is technically possible, but a pulmonary neoplasm is the most likely explanation for this lesion. Biopsy showed this to be a moderately differentiated squamous cell carcinoma. (From Broder JS: *Diagnostic imaging for the emergency physician,* Philadelphia, 2011, Saunders.)

TABLE 2 TNM Stage Groups for Non-Small Cell Lung Cancer

Stage	T	N	M
Stage 0	T_{is}	N_0	M_0
Stage I_{A1}	T_{mi} or T_{1a}	N_0	M_0
Stage I_{A2}	T_{1b}	N_0	M_0
Stage I_{A3}	T_{1c}	N_0	M_0
Stage I_B	T_{2a}	N_0	M_0
Stage II_A	T_{2b}	N_0	M_0
Stage II_B	$T_{1a\text{-}c}$	N_1	M_0
	$T_{2a\text{-}b}$	N_1	M_0
	T_3	N_0	M_0
Stage III_A	$T_{1a\text{-}c}$	N_2	M_0
	$T_{2a\text{-}b}$	N_2	M_0
	T_3	N_1	M_0
	T_4	$N_{0\text{-}1}$	M_0
Stage III_B	$T_{1a\text{-}c}$	N_3	M_0
	$T_{2a\text{-}b}$	N_3	M_0
	$T_{3\text{-}4}$	N_2	M_0
Stage III_C	$T_{3\text{-}4}$	N_3	M_0
Stage IV_A	Any T	Any N	$M_{1a\text{-}1b}$
Stage IV_B	Any T	Any N	M_{1c}

TNM, Tumor, node, matastases.

mediastinal and distant metastases in NSCLC. It is useful for preoperative staging of NSCLC.

- The use of PET-CT for preoperative staging of NSCLC reduces both the total number of thoracotomies and the number of futile thoracotomies.

STAGING

After confirmation of diagnosis, patients should undergo staging:

- In NSCLC, the TNM staging system is used. Table 2 summarizes TNM stage groups. Both stage I (no lymph node involvement) and stage II (ipsilateral bronchopulmonary/ hilar lymph nodes or T_3 tumor) include localized tumors for which surgical resection is the preferred treatment. Stage III is subdivided into III_A (potentially resectable) and II_B/III_C (unresectable). Stage IV indicates metastatic disease with stage IV_A referring to intrathoracic metastases or pleural involvement or single extra-thoracic metastasis. stage IV_B includes tumors with multiple extra-thoracic metastases.
- In SCLC, the staging system developed by the Veterans Administration Lung Cancer Study Group is used. It contains two stages:
  1. Limited-stage disease: Confined to the regional lymph nodes and to one hemithorax (excluding pleural surfaces), which can be included in a single radiation portal
  2. Extensive-stage disease: Spread beyond the confines of limited-stage disease
- Pretreatment staging procedures for lung cancer patients, in addition to complete history and physical examination, generally include the following tests:
  1. Chest radiograph (posteroanterior and lateral), ECG.
  2. Laboratory evaluation: Complete blood count, complete metabolic panel; arterial blood gases and pulse oximetry in selected cases.
  3. Pulmonary function studies.
  4. CT scan of chest and PET scan: Trials have shown a reduction in futile thoracotomies for patients with suspected NSCLC who undergo preoperative assessment with PET in addition to conventional workup.
  5. Mediastinoscopy or anterior mediastinotomy in patients being considered for possible curative lung resection.
  6. Biopsy of any accessible suspect lesions.
  7. CT scan to include liver and brain.
  8. Bone marrow aspiration and biopsy only in selected patients with small cell carcinoma of the lung. In the absence of an increased lactate dehydrogenase or cytopenias, routine bone marrow examination is not recommended.
  9. Newer technologies in preoperative staging include endoscopic bronchial ultrasonography and esophageal ultrasonography to guide biopsies; however, cervical mediastinoscopy is standard criterion in preoperative nodal staging (sensitivity >93%, specificity >95%).

Rx TREATMENT

NONPHARMACOLOGIC THERAPY

- Nutritional support
- Avoidance of tobacco and other substances toxic to the lungs
- Supplemental oxygen

ACUTE GENERAL Rx

NON–SMALL CELL CARCINOMA:

- Surgical resection is standard in patients with operable NSCLC (stage I or II) who are surgical candidates. Lobectomy is the best standard surgical approach. Lesser resections may be necessary in patients with marginal pulmonary reserve. Video-assisted thoracic surgery (VATS) is helpful in decreasing morbidity and shortening hospital stay.
  1. Surgical resection is indicated in patients with limited disease (not involving mediastinal nodes, ribs, pleura, or distant sites). This represents approximately 15% to 30% of diagnosed cases. Stereotactic ablative radiotherapy is a reasonable option for patients with localized NSCLC who are not surgical candidates. Multimodality treatment guidelines are summarized in Table 3.
  2. Preoperative evaluation includes cardiac status and pulmonary function assessment. Pneumonectomy is possible if the patient has a preoperative $FEV_1 = 2$ L or if the maximal voluntary ventilation is >50% of predicted capacity. Individuals with FEV_1 >1.5 L are suitable for lobectomy without further evaluation unless there is evidence of interstitial lung disease or undue dyspnea on exertion. In that case, carbon dioxide diffusion in the lung (DLCO) should be measured. If the DLCO is <80% predicted normal, the individual may not be clearly operable.
  3. Conventional radiotherapy fails to durably control the primary lung tumor in nearly 70% of patients and 2-yr survival is less than 40%. Stereotactic body radiation (SBRT) uses several highly focused radiation beams to deliver high doses in 3 to 5 fractions and appears to be more effective than conventional radiotherapy, with a local control rate equivalent to that with surgery in inoperable early stage lung cancer.
  4. Preoperative chemotherapy should be considered in patients with more advanced disease (stage IIIA) who are being considered for surgery because it increases the median survival time in patients with NSCLC compared with the use of surgery alone.
  5. Postoperative adjuvant chemotherapy significantly increases 5-yr survival (69% vs. 54%) in patients with completely resected stage II-IIIA NSCLC.

TABLE 3 Summary of Multimodality Guidelines

Stage	Surgery	Adjuvant Therapy	Radiation	Chemotherapy	Level of Evidence
I	Yes	No	No	No	1B—Surgical resection 1B—Against postoperative chemotherapy 1A—Against postoperative radiation therapy
II	Yes	Yes	No	Yes	1B—Surgical resection 1A—Postoperative chemotherapy 2A—Against postoperative radiation therapy
IIIA					
(N2-occult)	Yes	Yes	May be considered	Yes	1A—Adjuvant chemo 2C—Adjuvant radiation
(N2-discrete)	Yes	No	Yes	Yes	1A—Definite or induction followed by surgery
			(Definitive or induction recommended)		1C—Against primary resection followed by adjuvant therapy
IIIB	No	No	Yes	Yes	1A—Definitive concurrent
(N2, N3)			(Definitive concurrent)		1A—Against induction followed by surgery

From Sellke FW, et al.: *Sabiston & Spencer surgery of the chest*, ed 9, 2016, Elsevier.

- Treatment of unresectable NSCLC:
  1. Radiotherapy alone is used primarily for treatment of central nervous system and skeletal metastases, superior vena cava syndrome. Thoracic radiotherapy in combination with chemotherapy is standard therapy for unresectable stage 3 disease.
  2. Chemotherapy, targeted therapy, and immune checkpoint therapy are the mainstays of treatment for advanced stage IV or metastatic NSCLC. Initial stratification is done based on pathology (squamous vs. nonsquamous cancers), presence of driver mutations (e.g., *EGFR, ALK, ROS1,* and *BRAF* mutations in adenocarcinomas), and expression of programmed death receptor ligand-1 (PDL-1). Table 4 summarizes selected NSCLC oncogenes and targeted therapy.
  3. A platinum-based chemotherapy doublet regimen is recommended for fit patients, and single agents are offered to elderly patients and those with poor performance status. Various combination regimens are available with platinum plus pemetrexed preferred for nonsquamous cancers while other for squamous cancers other doublets such as paclitaxel plus carboplatin, cisplatin plus vinorelbine, gemcitabine plus cisplatin, and cisplatin plus docetaxel are utilized with none being clearly superior to the others. The addition of bevacizumab to paclitaxel plus carboplatin results in significant survival benefit in nonsquamous cancers.
  4. Upfront therapy with pembrolizumab, a PD-1 immune-checkpoint inhibitor antibody that disrupts PD-1 mediated signaling and restores antitumor immunity, is superior to chemotherapy in patients with >50% PD-L1 expression. When pembrolizumab is combined with chemotherapy in patients with 1-50% PD-L1 expression, there is an improvement in overall survival. In addition, atezolizumab and nivolumab (other checkpoint inhibitors) have been shown to have superior survival benefit versus docetaxel in advanced NSCLC that had previously received chemotherapy.
  5. Tyrosine kinase inhibitors targeting activating mutations are of use in patients whose adenocarcinomas harbor the EGFR mutations. Gefitinib, erlotinib, afatinib, osimertinib, and dacomitinib are oral EGFR inhibitors that have showed impressive responses and improvements in median overall survival to the range of 30 months. (These mutations are more common in adenocarcinomas found in patients who are never or light smokers and in Asian patients). Patients with EGFR mutations can acquire secondary T790M mutations that can be targeted with the oral inhibitor osimertinib.
  6. Oncogenic fusion genes consisting of *EML4* and anaplastic lymphoma kinase (ALK) are present in 4% to 5% of adenocarcinomas and can be treated with inhibitors crizotinib, ceritinib, alectinib, or brigantinib. Approximately 2% of adenocarcinomas have genetic rearrangements involving the ROS1 proto-oncogenic receptor tyrosine kinase (ROS1), and these patients can be treated with the oral inhibitors crizotinib and ceritinib.
  7. The addition of chemotherapy to radiotherapy (CRT) improves survival in patients with locally advanced, unresectable stages III NSCLC. The addition of the checkpoint inhibitor durvalumab has recently shown improvement in overall survival in this population when administered sequentially after CRT.
  8. Early initiation of palliative care focusing on management of symptoms, psychosocial support, and assistance with decision making in patients with metastatic NSCLC leads to improved quality of life, longer survival, and less use of aggressive end-of-life care.

SMALL CELL LUNG CANCER:
- Limited-stage disease: Standard treatments include thoracic radiotherapy and chemotherapy (cisplatin and etoposide).
- Extensive-stage disease: Standard treatments include combination chemotherapy (platinum plus etoposide or platinum plus irinotecan).
- Prophylactic cranial irradiation for patients in complete remission to decrease the risk of central nervous system metastasis.
- Despite high initial response rates, most patients eventually relapse. Topotecan or irinotecan may be an option for these patients.
- The anti-PD-1 antibody, nivolumab, has demonstrated survival benefit in SCLC patients who have failed standard therapies.

DISPOSITION
- The 5-yr survival of patients with NSCLC when the disease is resectable is approximately 30%.
- Median survival time in patients with limited-stage disease SCLC is 15 mo; in patients with extensive-stage SCLC, it is 9 mo.
- Among patients with metastatic NSCLC, early palliative care results in longer survival and significant improvements in both quality of life and mood.

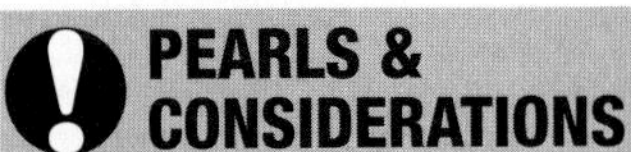

PEARLS & CONSIDERATIONS

CT screening with use of low-dose computed tomography (LDCT) for detection of lung cancer among persons with a heavy history of smoking increases the percentage of lung cancer cases that are diagnosed in stage 1 and reduces mortality from lung cancer. The National Lung Screening Trial (NLST) showed that lung cancer screening with LDCT resulted in a 20% reduction in lung cancer mortality. New guidelines recommend annual LDCT for those who are current or former smokers aged 55 to 74. Screening should be discontinued once a person has not smoked for 15 yr or develops a health problem that substantially limits life expectancy or the ability or willingness to have curative lung surgery.

SUGGESTED READINGS
Available at ExpertConsult.com

RELATED CONTENT
Lung Cancer (Patient Information)
Lung Cancer Screening (Patient Information)
Horner Syndrome (Related Key Topic)
Lambert-Eaton Myasthenic Syndrome (Related Key Topic)
Paraneoplastic Syndromes (Related Key Topic)
Superior Vena Cava Syndrome (Related Key Topic)

AUTHOR: **RITESH RATHORE, M.D.**

TABLE 4 Selected Non-Small Cell Lung Cancer Oncogenes and Targeted Therapy

Oncogene Alteration	Incidence (%)	Clinical Relevance	Treatment
BRAF			
Mutation	1-3	V600E mutation: Most common, equal association with smokers and nonsmokers May be mechanism of acquired EGFR TKI resistance	dabrafenib plus trametinib
EGFR (ErbB1, HER1)			
Mutation	13-50	Exon 19 deletion and Exon 21 point mutation are the most common Predominantly adenocarcinoma and nonsmokers; up to 50% frequency in Asians	TKI: Gefitinib, erlotinib, afatinib, osimertinib
EML4-ALK			
Fusion	3-7	Most frequent in adenocarcinomas, nonsmokers, men, and younger patients	Nonspecific TKI: Crizotinib, certinib, alectinib, brigantinib
Her2/neu (ErbB2)			No approved therapy
Mutation	2-6	Mostly adenocarcinomas and nonsmokers	
Amplification	23	Mechanism of resistance to EGFR TKI	
KRAS			
Mutation	5-30	Mostly adenocarcinomas and smokers May contribute to resistance to ALF, BRAF, and PI3K inhibitors	No approved therapy
MET			No approved therapy
Mutation	<5		
Amplification	21	Mechanism of resistance to EGFR TKI	
PIK3CA			No approved therapy
Mutation	<10	Frequently occurs in association with other mutations; more common in squamous cell	
Amplification	5-43	Mechanism of resistance to EGFR TKI	
PTEN			
Mutation	1.7-10	Associated with PI3K activation, resistance to EGFR TKI, and sensitivity to PI3K inhibitors More frequent in squamous cell	
Loss of function	4-21	Associated with PI3K activation, resistance to EGFR TKI, and sensitivity to PI3K inhibitors More frequent in squamous cell	
RET fusion gene	1-2	Mostly adenocarcinomas and nonsmokers	No approved therapy
ROS1 fusion gene	2	Mostly adenocarcinomas, nonsmokers, and younger patients	TKI: Crizotinib
VEGF			Monoclonal antibodies: Bevacizumab VEGFR TKI

BRAF, v-raf murine sarcoma viral oncogene homolog B1; *EGFR,* epidermal growth factor receptor; *EML4-ALK,* echinoderm microtubule-associated protein-like 4 anaplastic lymphoma kinase; *ERBB,* avian erythroblastosis oncogene B; *Her2,* human epidermal growth factor receptor 2; *KRAS,* Kirsten Rat sarcoma viral oncogene homolog; *MET,* mesenchymal-epithelial transition; *PIK3CA,* phosphoinositide-3-kinase catalytic alpha polypeptide; *PTEN,* phosphatase and tensin homolog; *RET,* rearranged during transfection; *ROS1,* reactive oxygen species 1; *TKI,* tyrosine kinase inhibitor; *VEGF,* vascular endothelial growth factor; *VEGFR,* vascular endothelial growth factor receptor.

From Sellke FW, et al.: *Sabiston & Spencer surgery of the chest,* ed 9, 2016, Elsevier

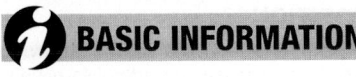

BASIC INFORMATION

DEFINITION

Lyme disease is a multisystem inflammatory disorder caused by the transmission of a spirochete, *Borrelia burgdorferi,* via the bite of infected *Ixodes* ticks, taking 36 to 48 hr for a tick to take a blood meal and transmit the infecting organism to the host.

SYNONYMS

Bannwarth's syndrome (Europe)
Acrodermatitis chronica atrophicans

ICD-10CM CODES

A69.20	Lyme disease, unspecified
A69.21	Meningitis due to Lyme disease
A69.22	Other neurologic disorders in Lyme disease
A69.23	Arthritis due to Lyme disease
A69.29	Other conditions associated with Lyme disease

EPIDEMIOLOGY & DEMOGRAPHICS

INCIDENCE (IN U.S.): In the U.S., 4.4 cases/100,000 persons; it is the most common vector-borne infection in the U.S., with more than 30,000 new cases reported each yr. 90% of cases are found in: Massachusetts, Connecticut, Rhode Island, New York, New Jersey, Pennsylvania, Minnesota, Wisconsin, and California. The area of transmission in the U.S. is expanding farther into the South and upper Northeast (Fig. E1). The disease also occurs in Europe and Asia with a different *Ixodes* tick vector. Table E1 summarizes principal vector ticks and spirochetes associated with Lyme borreliosis.

PEAK INCIDENCE: May to November
PREDOMINANT SEX: Male = female
PREDOMINANT AGE: Median age of 28 yr

PHYSICAL FINDINGS & CLINICAL PRESENTATION

Lyme disease may present in the following stages:

- *Early localized stage (incubation period 3-30 days):* Early Lyme disease, erythema migrans (EM); skin rash, often at site of tick bite (the CDC has defined EM rash as an expanding red macule or papule that must reach at least 5 cm in size, with or without central clearing); target lesions from ECM can be found in 60% to 80% of localized infections; possible fever, myalgias 3 to 32 days after tick bite
- *Early disseminated stage (incubation period 3-6 weeks):* Days to weeks later; multiorgan system involvement, including CNS with aseptic meningitis–type picture or Bell's palsy, joints (arthritis or arthralgias), cardiac including varying degrees of heart block; related to dissemination of spirochete
- *Late stage (incubation period months to yrs):* Mo to yr after tick exposure; affects central and peripheral nervous system, cardiac, joints

Common presenting signs and symptoms include:

- EM (Fig. 2). Most patients with EM (about 80%) have a single lesion but the bacteria can disseminate hematogenously to other sites in the skin and result in often smaller erythema migrans lesions.
- Lymphadenopathy, neck pains, pharyngeal erythema, myalgias, hepatosplenomegaly.
- Patients will complain of malaise, fatigue, lethargy, headache, fever/chills, neck pain, myalgias, back pain.

ETIOLOGY

B. burgdorferi transmitted from bite of an *Ixodes* tick (mostly in the nymph stage, but can also be from adult ticks). Human infection occurs through inoculation of spirochetes in infected

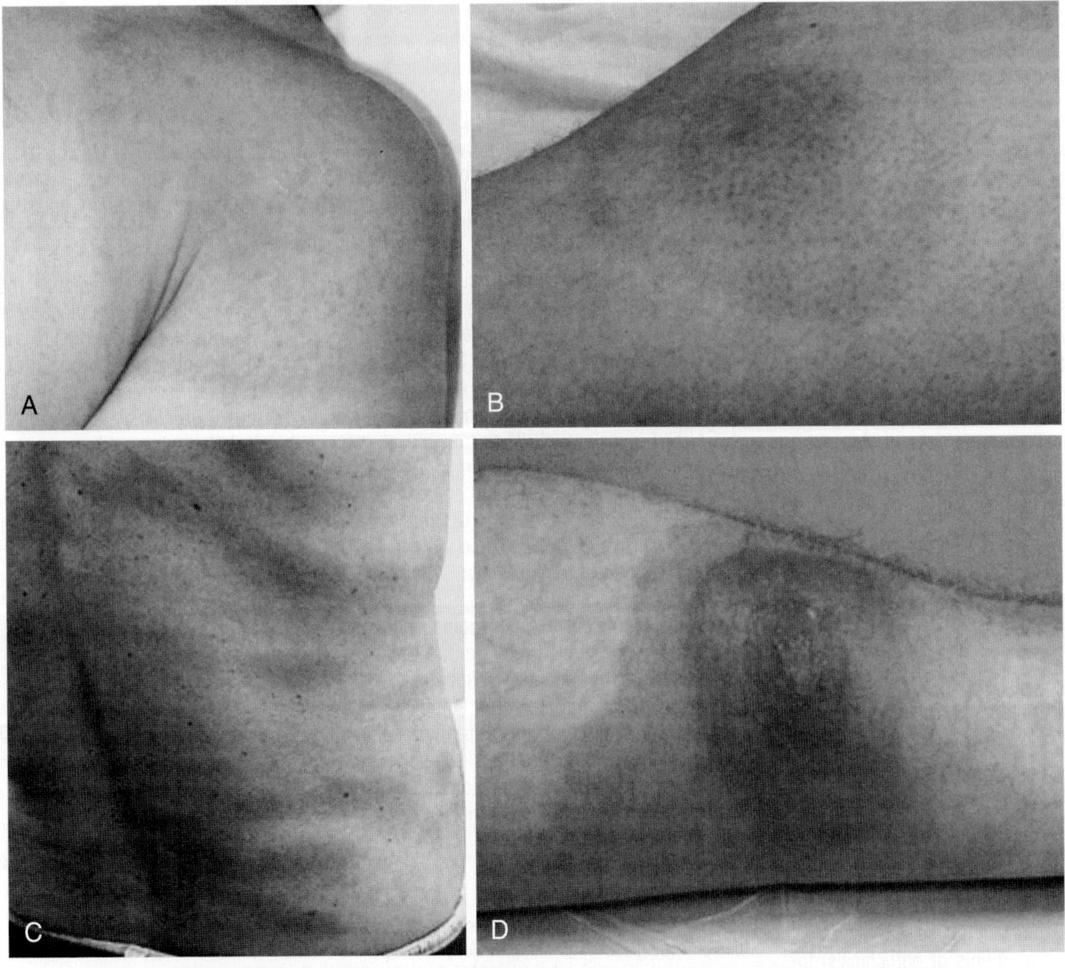

FIG. 2 Erythema migrans rash of Lyme disease. A, Typical macular lesion on left shoulder. **B,** Bull's eye lesion on lateral thigh with central punctum. **C,** Multiple lesions on back. **D,** Lesion with vesicular center on posterior thigh. (Courtesy Juan Salazar, M.D., University of Connecticut Health Center.)

TABLE 2 Criteria for Western Blot Interpretation in the Serologic Confirmation of Lyme Disease

Duration of Disease	Isotype Tested	Criteria for Positive Test
First month of infection	IgM	2 of the following 3 bands are present: 23 kD (OspC), 39 kD (BmpA), and 41 kD (Fla)
After first month of infection	IgG	5 of 10 bands are present: 18 kD, 21 kD, 28 kD, 30 kD, 39 kD, 41 kD, 45 kD, 58 kD (not GroEL), 66 kD, and 93 kD

Ig;Immunoglobulin.
Modified from Centers for Disease Control and Prevention: Recommendations for test performance and interpretation from the Second National Conference on Serologic Diagnosis of Lyme Disease, *MMWR Morb Mortal Wkly Rep* 44:590–591, 1995.

saliva and usually requires tick attachment for more than 36 hours.

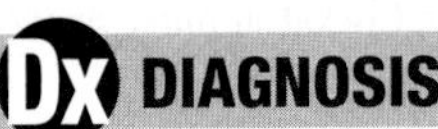

DIAGNOSIS

Clinical presentation, exposure to ticks in endemic area, and diagnostic testing for antibody response to *B. burgdorferi.* Serologic testing at early stages is usually negative; therefore, in early stage, documentation of erythema migrans lesion with a compatible epidemiologic history is sufficient for diagnosis, and laboratory testing is not indicated.

DIFFERENTIAL DIAGNOSIS

- Chronic fatigue/fibromyalgia
- Acute viral illnesses
- Babesiosis
- Human granulocytic anaplasmosis

WORKUP

- ELISA testing and if positive or equivocal then followed by a Western blot IgM and IgG (Table 2). A Western blot IgM assay is positive if 2 of 3 bands present. The Western blot IgG is positive if 5 of 10 bands present.
- An alternative serologic test is the VlsE C6 ELISA (C6 peptide), which detects an IgG response earlier and may be more sensitive than the ELISA, but its specificity is lower than the two-tier testing method.
- Early disease often is difficult to diagnose serologically, secondary to slow immune response.
- Culturing of skin lesions (EM) and polymerase chain reaction (PCR) of synovial fluid or CSF can also give the diagnosis of active infection.

IMAGING STUDIES

- ECG
- Echocardiogram if conduction abnormalities are present with cardiac involvement
- CT scan, MRI of head for CNS involvement

Rx TREATMENT

Early localized Lyme disease:

- Doxycycline 100 mg bid in adults (children: 2 mg/kg twice daily if ≥8 yr) [doxycycline offers the advantage of treating possible coinfection with the bacterial agents of ehrlichiosis] for 10 to 14 days or amoxicillin 500 mg tid for adults (children: 50 mg/kg per day in three divided doses) for 14 to 21 days.
- Alternative treatments for pregnancy and children ≦8 yr: Cefuroxime axetil 500 mg bid for 14 to 21 days (children: 30 mg/kg per day in two divided doses), azithromycin 500 mg PO for 7 to 10 days but should **not** be used as a first-line agent, as it is less effective than doxycycline and amoxicillin.
- A single dose of 200 mg doxycycline given within 72 hr of removing an engorged *Ixodes* tick can significantly reduce the risk of developing of Lyme disease in endemic areas and is reasonable prophylaxis in nonpregnant adults and children ≥8 yr old.

Early disseminated and late persistent infection:

- 28 days of treatment is often prescribed, although recent evidence supports treating patients with a 14-day course of oral doxycycline for early neurologic Lyme disease in ambulatory patients. Doxycycline and ceftriaxone appear equally effective for acute disseminated Lyme disease.[1]
- Arthritis: 28 days of doxycycline or amoxicillin plus probenecid.
- Neurologic involvement requires parenteral antibiotics. Those who fail to respond should be treated with IV ceftriaxone or cefotaxime.
- Ceftriaxone 2 g/day IV for 21 to 28 days; alternative: cefotaxime 2 g q8h IV; alternative: penicillin G 5 million U qid.
- Cardiac involvement: IV ceftriaxone or cefotaxime plus cardiac monitoring.
- Prolonged treatment with IV or PO antibiotic therapy for up to 90 days did not improve symptoms more than placebo.

Post–Lyme disease syndrome:

- Presence of disabling symptoms such as fatigue, malaise, diffuse pains, and poor concentration, which may be due to an exuberant host inflammatory response
- Antibiotics are not indicated. Antibiotic treatment of patients with persistent unexplained symptoms despite previous antibiotic treatment of Lyme disease provides little, if any, benefit and carries significant risk
- Supportive care

[1] Sanchez E, et al.: Diagnosis, treatment, and prevention of Lyme disease, human granulocytic anaplasmosis, and babesiosis: a review, *JAMA* 315(16):1767–1777, 2016..

DISPOSITION

- The patient often needs careful follow-up and supportive care for the arthralgia-neuritis symptoms.
- 10% to 20% of treated patients may have lingering symptoms of fatigue, disrupted sleep, and musculoskeletal complaints. Repeat episodes of EM in appropriately treated patients are due to reinfection and not to relapse.

REFERRAL

- To a neurologist if significant neurologic complications (meningitis, myelitis, ophthalmoplegia, Bell's palsy)
- To a cardiologist if the patient develops evidence of cardiac conduction disturbances or pericarditis

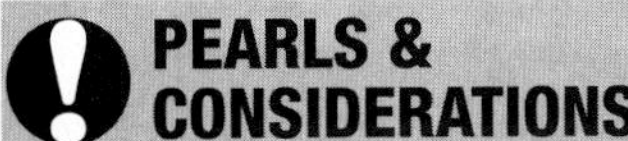

PEARLS & CONSIDERATIONS

- A physician diagnosis of classic EM in an endemic region of Lyme disease is sufficient to make a definitive diagnosis.
- In some patients with Lyme disease, nonspecific complaints such as headache, fatigue, and arthralgia may persist for months after appropriate (and ultimately successful) antibiotic treatment. Long-term antibiotic treatment does not provide additional beneficial effects.
- There is no evidence of current or previous *Borrelia burgdorferi* infection in most patients evaluated at university-based Lyme disease referral centers. Psychiatric comorbidity and other psychological factors are prominent in the presentation and outcome of some patients who inaccurately ascribe longstanding symptoms to "chronic Lyme disease."
- It is important to realize that one tick bite can transmit Lyme disease *and* the bacterial agents of either ehrlichiosis or babesiosis, or even both, and these latter agents require separate serologic testing and possibly therapy. *Ehrlichiosis* is treated with doxycycline, but *Babesia* would require a different therapy.
- Tick bite protection: EPA-registered insect repellents containing DEET, picaridin, IR3535, oil of lemon eucalyptus (OLE), para-menthane-diol (PMD), or 2-undecanone can prevent ticks from attaching when applied, and can last for several hours. OLE and PMD products cannot be used on children under 3 yr of age.

SUGGESTED READINGS

Available at ExpertConsult.com

RELATED CONTENT

Lyme Disease (Patient Information)

AUTHOR: **GLENN G. FORT, M.D., M.P.H.**

BASIC INFORMATION

DEFINITION

Lymphangitis refers to the inflammation of lymphatic vessels due to infectious or noninfectious causes. Infectious causes include bacteria, mycobacteria, viruses, fungi, and parasites.

SYNONYMS

Nodular lymphangitis
Sporotrichoid lymphangitis

ICD-10CM CODE

I89.1 Lymphangitis

EPIDEMIOLOGY & DEMOGRAPHICS

INCIDENCE (IN U.S.): Several hundred cases/yr of sporotrichoid lymphangitis, which is a fungal infection; bacterial lymphangitis more common but not reported.

PHYSICAL FINDINGS & CLINICAL PRESENTATION

ACUTE LYMPHANGITIS:

- Commonly associated with a bacterial cellulitis
- Usually develops after cutaneous inoculation of microorganisms into the lymphatic vessels through disrupted skin or as a result of spread from a distal infection
- May or may not recognize a site of skin trauma (i.e., laceration, puncture, ulcer)
- In hours to days, distal appearance of erythema, edema, and tenderness, with linear erythematous streaks extending proximally to regional lymph nodes
- Possible lymphadenitis and fever
- Predisposition to group A streptococcal infection of the skin in those with uncontrolled diabetes mellitus, chronic lymphedema, and superficial fungal infections (e.g., tinea pedis)

SPOROTRICHOID OR NODULAR LYMPHANGITIS:

- Includes subcutaneous nodules that develop along the path of involved lymphatics
- Usually preceded by an episode of cutaneous inoculation or trauma to the hand
- Lesions apparent from one to several weeks after inoculation
- Initially, nodular or papular lesion; may ulcerate
- Pain is organism-dependent
- May have frank pus or a serosanguineous discharge
- Systemic complaints uncommon, but infection with certain microorganisms associated with fever, chills, myalgias, and headache

ETIOLOGY

- Acute lymphangitis: Usually associated with *Streptococcus pyogenes* (group A streptococcus), and to a lesser extent staphylococcus species, including community-acquired methicillin-resistant *S. aureus* (CA-MRSA)
- Nodular lymphangitis caused by one of several organisms:
  1. *Sporothrix schenckii* ("Rose gardener's disease," corn cultivation)
     a. Most common recognized cause in the U.S., usually in the Midwest.
     b. Fungus found in soil and plant debris
  2. *Nocardia brasiliensis:* Gram-positive rod-shaped bacteria found in soil
  3. *Mycobacterium marinum:* Associated with trauma related to water (e.g., aquariums, swimming pools, fish)
  4. *Leishmania brasiliensis:*
     a. Protozoal parasite transmitted to humans by sand flies, mostly to travelers in endemic areas (Texas, rural Central and South America, Africa, subtropical Asia)
  5. *Francisella tularensis:* Gram-negative bacteria. Also causes lymphadenitis:
     a. Most often in Southern/Midwestern states (Arkansas, Missouri, Oklahoma)
     b. Associated with contact with infected mammals (e.g., rabbits, squirrels, cats), tick bites, and (rarely) water exposure

DIAGNOSIS

DIFFERENTIAL DIAGNOSIS

- Nodular lymphangitis
  1. Blastomyces or Coccidiodes, Histoplasma, *Bacillus anthracis*, Mycetoma
- Insect or snake bites
- Filariasis

WORKUP

- Acute lymphangitis: Blood cultures
- Nodular lymphangitis: Various stains and cultures of drainage or biopsy specimens of inoculation sites

LABORATORY TESTS

- WBCs possibly elevated with cellulitis
- Eosinophilia common with helminthic infections
- Skin biopsy and microbiologic cultures may be necessary to confirm diagnosis in nodular lymphangitis

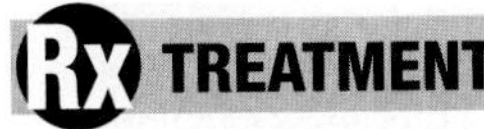

TREATMENT

NONPHARMACOLOGIC THERAPY

Limb elevation

ACUTE GENERAL Rx

- Penicillin possibly sufficient, but 1 wk of dicloxacillin or cephalexin 500 mg PO qid commonly used to ensure antistaphylococcal coverage; if CA-MRSA suspected, then use oral Bactrim DS one PO bid or clindamycin 300 mg PO q6H. Reserve vancomycin 1 g IV every 12 hr for patients requiring IV therapy.
- If allergic to penicillin:
  1. Clindamycin 300 mg PO qid for 7 days *or*
  2. Erythromycin 500 mg PO qid for 7 days
  3. Levofloxacin 500 mg PO daily or moxifloxacin 400 mg PO daily for 7 days
- Nodular lymphangitis: Specific therapy directed at etiologic agent.
- For superficial fungal infections: Treatment may prevent recurrence of acute lymphangitis.

DISPOSITION

- Acute lymphangitis: Usually resolves with therapy
- Recurrent attacks: May lead to chronic lymphedema of limb, rarely resulting in elephantiasis nostras (nonfilarial elephantiasis)
- Nodular lymphangitis: Usually responds to appropriate therapy

REFERRAL

- If acute lymphangitis is more than a mild disease or if it involves the face
- If nodular lymphangitis or filariasis is suspected

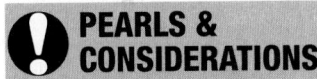

PEARLS & CONSIDERATIONS

COMMENTS

- Outside of the U.S., initial episodes of filariasis caused by Brugia malayi resemble acute lymphangitis.
- Chronic lymphedema or elephantiasis results from recurrent episodes.
- For chronic lymphedema, adherence to limb elevation, compression/support stockings, and adequate glycemic control (for patients with diabetes) all can reduce risk of acute lymphangitis.

SUGGESTED READINGS

Available at www.ExpertConsult.com

RELATED CONTENT

Lymphangitis (Patient Information)

AUTHORS: **ALEISHA M. NABOWER, M.D.,** and **RUSSELL J. MCCULLOH, M.D.**

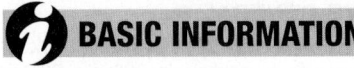

BASIC INFORMATION

DEFINITION

A primary role of the lymphatic system is to transport proteins from the interstitium to the heart. When the transport capacity of the lymphatic system is reduced, proteins accumulate in the interstitium. Accumulated proteins attract water, which creates a high protein swelling in the subcutaneous tissues called lymphedema.

SYNONYM

Elephantiasis

ICD-10CM CODES
I97.2 Postmastectomy lymphedema syndrome
I89.0 Lymphedema, not elsewhere classified
Q82.0 Hereditary lymphedema

EPIDEMIOLOGY & DEMOGRAPHICS

PRIMARY LYMPHEDEMA:
- Found in 1.1/100,000 people aged <20 yr
- Females outnumber males 3.5:1
- Incidence peaks between ages 12 and 16 (puberty)

SECONDARY LYMPHEDEMA: See specific etiology in the following.

PHYSICAL FINDINGS & CLINICAL PRESENTATION

Lymphedema is a slow-onset, progressive disease characterized by an asymmetrical, inflammatory swelling, traveling distal to proximal, that can affect any body part including limbs, trunk, head/neck, and genitals (Fig. 1). Box 1 summarizes lymphedema staging from the International Society of Lymphology.

STAGE 0: LATENCY:
- Decreased lymphatic system transport capacity due to primary or secondary etiology.

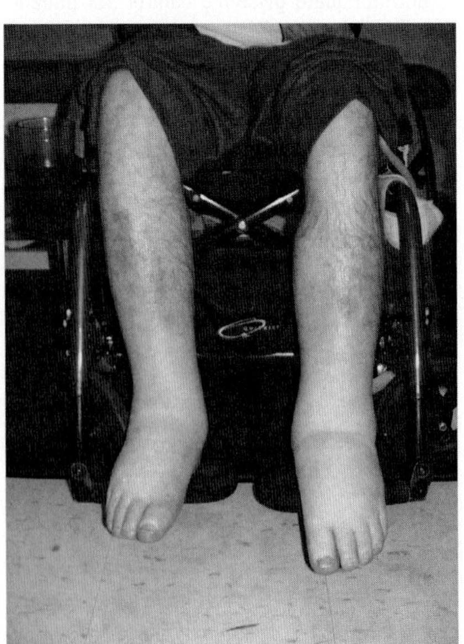

FIG. 1 Lymphedema before treatment.

- Subjective complaints of affected body part feeling heavy or achy.
- No objective findings, no apparent swelling.

STAGE I: REVERSIBLE:
- Edema is observable, soft, pitting and reversible with elevation.
- No secondary skin changes are present.

STAGE II: SPONTANEOUSLY IRREVERSIBLE:
- Skin becomes more firm/fibrotic, therefore less pitting.
- Edema does not reverse to normal with elevation.
- Possibility of infections (cellulitis), wounds, or weeping (lymphorrhea).

STAGE III: ELEPHANTIASIS:
- Skin becomes very firm/fibrotic, therefore nonpitting.
- Evidence of substantial skin changes (e.g., papillomas, lobules, "peau d' orange").

ETIOLOGY: Lymphedema is caused by a reduction in lymphatic system transport and is classified into primary and secondary forms.

Primary Lymphedema:
- Occurs when the lymphatic system does not mature properly during fetal development
  1. Aplasia
  2. Hypoplasia
  3. Hyperplasia
- Can be familial, genetic, or hereditary
- Lymphedema congenital: Symptoms present at birth
- Lymphedema praecox: Symptoms onset before the age of 35 (commonly during puberty)
- Lymphedema tardum: Symptoms onset at the age of 35 or after

Secondary Lymphedema:
- Occurs secondary to a disruption or obstruction of the lymphatic system caused by:
  1. Filariasis (#1 cause worldwide)
  2. Lymph node surgery/radiation due to cancer (#1 cause in the U.S.)
  3. Other: Chronic venous insufficiency (CVI), deep vein thrombosis (DVT), infection, surgery/trauma, lipedema, and obesity

BOX 1 Lymphedema Staging

Stage 0: Latent
- Impaired lymphatic function
- No evident edema; subclinical
- May last months or years before progression

Stage I: Spontaneously Reversible
- Early accumulation of protein-rich fluid
- Pitting edema
- Subsides with elevation

Stage II: Spontaneously Irreversible
- Accumulation of protein-rich fluid
- Pitting edema progresses to fibrosis
- Does not resolve with elevation alone

Stage III: Lymphostatic Elephantiasis
- Nonpitting
- Significant fibrosis
- Trophic skin changes

From International Society of Lymphology: The diagnosis and treatment of peripheral edema: 2009 consensus document of the International Society of Lymphology, *Lymphology* 42(2):51–60, 2009.

DIAGNOSIS

- Lymphedema is primarily a clinical diagnosis made on the basis of past medical history and objective findings that distinguish it from other causes of chronic edema.
- A Stemmer sign is often used to identify lymphedema (inability to pick up or pinch a fold of skin at the base of the second toe or finger).
- When physical examination is inconclusive, other available imaging tests can help make the diagnosis (see "Imaging Studies").

DIFFERENTIAL DIAGNOSIS

Other causes of edema that should be ruled out before treatment for lymphedema include cardiac, renal, hepatic, and thyroid dysfunction.

WORKUP

A detailed history and physical examination should help exclude most of the differential diagnoses.

LABORATORY TESTS

- Blood urea nitrogen, creatinine, liver function tests, albumin, urine analysis, and thyroid function tests are obtained to exclude possible systemic causes of edema.
- Genetic testing may be practical in defining a specific hereditary syndrome with a discrete gene mutation such as lymphedema distichiasis (*FOXC2*), Milroy's disease (*VEGFR-3*), Meige disease, or Klippel-Trenaunay-Weber syndrome.

IMAGING STUDIES

- Lymphoscintigraphy: Diagnostic image of choice for lymphedema (if needed)
- Indocyanine green (ICG) fluorescent lymphography: Can now be used to identify sentinel nodes, to demonstrate superficial lymph channels and functional lymphatics, to indicate treatment pathways, and to confirm the effectiveness of therapeutic techniques
- Magnetic resonance imaging (MRI): Primarily used in tumor diagnosis
- Duplex ultrasound: Determines venous involvement in the edema
- Computed axial tomography (CAT): Distinguishes between fatty tissue and accumulations of protein-rich fluids
- Lymphography: Phased out in favor of less invasive techniques

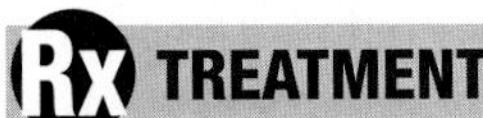

TREATMENT

NONPHARMACOLOGIC THERAPY

- Complete decongestive therapy (CDT) is backed by longstanding research and experience as the primary treatment of choice for lymphedema in both children and adults (Fig. 2). It should be delivered by a certified

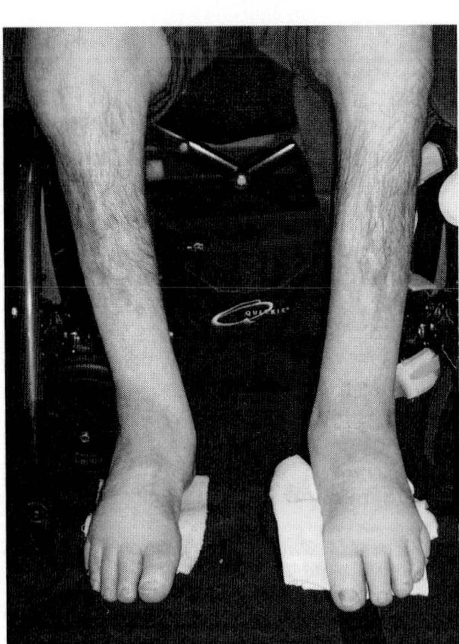

FIG. 2 Lymphedema after treatment.

lymphedema therapist (CLT). CDT involves a two-phase treatment program:

1. Phase 1—Reduce tissue congestion of affected body part with daily treatments:
   a. Manual lymph drainage
   b. Skin care
   c. Compression wrapping of limb
   d. Decongestive exercises
2. Phase 2—Maintain decongestion with Home Maintenance Program:
   a. Daily use of elastic and inelastic compression garments that are properly fitted according to circumference and length to prevent lymphedema from returning.
   b. Compression is graduated; most of the compression is distal with decreasing compression in the stocking proximally.
   c. Different knits and compression classes are available for different stages of lymphedema.
   d. Choices of garments include below-the-knee stockings, thigh-high stockings, pantyhose, sleeves, bras, and truncal garments.

- Massage (or any modality that increases blood flow) can have negative effects on lymphedema by increasing vasodilation. Therefore it is contraindicated on the lymphedematous quadrants.
- Compression pumps have not been found to be effective in removing proteins from lymphedematous quadrants.
- Nutritional therapy (reducing the amount of proteins ingested) is ineffective in the treatment of lymphedema.

PHARMACOLOGIC THERAPY

No drugs have been shown to be beneficial in the treatment of lymphedema. Diuretics, in particular, have not been found to be effective in removing proteins from lymphedematous quadrants and may promote the development of volume depletion.

SURGERY

Surgery for lymphedema has been proven largely unsuccessful and should not be considered before CDT. Surgical procedures are divided into two types:

- Physiologic procedures: Those performed to improve lymph node drainage (e.g., anastomoses of the lymph system with the venous system, lymph node transplant).
- Excisional or debulking procedures: Those performed to excise the subcutaneous tissue (e.g., Charles' procedure, Thompson's procedure, the modified Homans' procedure, and liposuction). Liposuction-circumferential suction-assisted lipectomy represents a newly proposed method to reduce morbidity involved in the traditional excisional techniques.

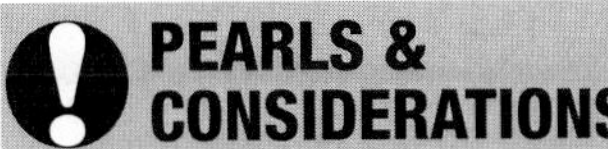

PEARLS & CONSIDERATIONS

- Lymphedema is a chronic, generally incurable but very manageable condition that requires lifelong care and attention along with psychosocial support.
- Children and adolescents (along with parents and adults) should be encouraged to pursue a normal life, participating in school activities and sports (preferably noncontact, such as swimming).
- Infections such as cellulitis should be treated promptly.
- If the etiology is filariasis caused by the parasites *Wuchereria bancrofti* or *Brugia malayi*, treatment is diethylcarbamazine citrate 5 mg/kg in divided doses for 3 wk.
- Patients with lymphedema commonly manifest psychiatric comorbidities as a result of their disease, such as anxiety, depression, adjustment problems, and difficulty in vocational, domestic, or social domains.
- Lymphedema can be complicated in rare cases by development of lymphangiosarcomata or other cutaneous malignancies.
- Gene therapy to develop new lymphangioses in the affected body parts is a potential clinical remedy in the future.

SUGGESTED READINGS

Available at ExpertConsult.com

RELATED CONTENT

Lymphedema (Patient Information)

AUTHORS: **FRANK G. FORT, M.D., M.P.H.,** and **KATHRYN TAYLOR ANILOWSKI, M.S., P.T., C.L.T.-L.A.N.A.**

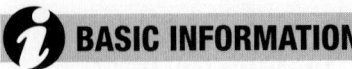

BASIC INFORMATION

DEFINITION

Lymphocytic colitis, also known as microscopic colitis (MC), is an inflammatory condition of the colon that most often presents as chronic watery diarrhea. Although clinically similar, lymphocytic colitis and collagenous colitis represent two histopathologic subtypes of microscopic colitis.

SYNONYMS

Microscopic colitis (MC)
Collagenous colitis

ICD-10CM CODES	
K52.839	Microscopic colitis
K52.838	Other microscopic colitis
K52.832	Lymphocytic colitis
K52.831	Collagenous colitis
K52.9	Colitis, nonspecific

EPIDEMIOLOGY & DEMOGRAPHICS

INCIDENCE: Incidence of microscopic colitis is 24 to 103 in 100,000 person yrs.
PEAK INCIDENCE: Most cases of microscopic colitis are diagnosed in patients 60 to 70 yrs of age.
PREVALENCE: Approximately 7.5% of patients who undergo workup for chronic watery diarrhea are diagnosed with MC.
PREDOMINANT SEX AND AGE: Microscopic colitis, more specifically the collagenous variant, affects females most commonly and occurs later in life (>65 yrs).
GENETICS: It is unclear how important specific genetic polymorphisms are in the pathophysiology of MC.
RISK FACTORS:
- Increased age
- Smoking: One study demonstrated that patients who smoke are diagnosed with MC an average of 10 yrs earlier than their nonsmoker counterparts
- Autoimmune disorders such as rheumatoid arthritis, thyroid disease, type I diabetes
- Celiac disease
- Medications: NSAIDs, proton pump inhibitors (PPIs), selective serotonin reuptake inhibitors (SSRIs), HMG-COA reductase inhibitors (statins)

PHYSICAL FINDINGS & CLINICAL PRESENTATION

- Most often presents with chronic watery diarrhea (>3 BM daily). Classically, patients with microscopic colitis will experience nocturnal bowel movements.
- Other symptoms include abdominal pain, fecal incontinence, urgency, and less commonly, weight loss.
- Melena and hematochezia are not hallmarks of this disease.

ETIOLOGY

- The pathophysiology of MC remains unclear. Some studies suggest that colonic inflammation promotes a breakdown in electrolyte transport, leading to a combined osmotic and secretory diarrhea. Luminal agents including dietary items, bacterial flora, and medications may influence inflammation.
- Serotonin signaling also may play an important role in the development of MC as patients with a specific polymorphism in a serotonin receptor show a higher incidence of the disease.

Dx DIAGNOSIS

DIFFERENTIAL DIAGNOSIS

- Irritable bowel syndrome (IBS)
- Inflammatory bowel disease (IBD)
- Ischemic colitis
- Infectious colitis (*C. difficile, E. coli*, giardia, cryptosporidium, entamoeba histolytica)
- Pancreatic insufficiency
- Celiac sprue
- Intestinal lymphoma
- Carcinoid tumor
- Diverticulitis
- Small intestine bacterial overgrowth

WORKUP

- Given the breadth of causes of watery diarrhea, the diagnostic workup is largely guided by history.
- Infectious causes of symptoms should be ruled out first, particularly if the patient has specific risk factors including recent travel, consumption of untreated water, recent antibiotic use or hospitalization.
- A careful history may elucidate specific dietary triggers such as lactose intolerance.
- Celiac disease is often comorbid with MC and should be ruled out in all patients with chronic watery diarrhea.

LABORATORY TESTS

- CBC
- Hepatic function panel
- Electrolyte panel
- *C. difficile* stool PCR
- If the patient has been exposed to untreated drinking water, testing for giardia, cryptosporidium, and *E. hisolytica* is indicated
- IgA tissue transglutaminase
- Consider fecal elastase if history is concerning for pancreatic insufficiency
- Fecal calprotectin: Unclear diagnostic benefit

IMAGING STUDIES

- MC is both a clinical and histopathologic diagnosis.
- Abdominal imaging is not helpful in diagnosing MC but may be warranted in patients with severe abdominal pain, evidence of obstruction, or a clinical history suggestive of infectious colitis or diverticulitis. Perforation is a rare complication of MC.
- Colonoscopy is a necessary part of MC diagnosis. On gross endoscopic examination, the colonic mucosa most often appears normal. Nonspecific findings such as erythema or mucosal cracking can be observed in a rare subset of patients.
- Obtaining multiple biopsies of each part of the large colon is foundational for endoscopic evaluation and maximizes diagnostic sensitivity. Lymphocytic colitis and collagenous colitis represent two histologic subtypes of MC. Lymphocytic colitis is marked by >20 intraepithelial lymphocytes to 100 surface epithelial cells in the presence of normal colonic mucosa. Collagenous colitis is characterized by increased intraepithelial lymphocytes and a thickened (>1mm) subepithelial collagen band in the setting of normal colonic mucosa.

Rx TREATMENT

There is no evidence to suggest that MC increases one's risk of colorectal cancer, nor is it believed to portend increased mortality. However, treatment is important to limit the significant burden on quality of life and healthcare costs. Both histopathologic subtypes of MC are clinically similar and managed using the same modalities. A treatment algorithm for collagenous and lymphocytic colitis is shown in Fig. 1.

NONPHARMACOLOGIC THERAPY

- The first step in management is to withdraw any medications that can provoke disease activity. NSAIDs are most notably associated with microscopic colitis and should be withheld. Other medications that may be associated with microscopic colitis include SSRIs, PPIs, statins, and bisphosphonates. Many of these medications are both common and effective, and a careful consideration of risk vs. benefit should occur before withdrawal.
- Smoking cessation.

ACUTE GENERAL Rx

- Antidiarrheal agents including loperamide can be used in patients with mild symptoms. Nighttime dosing of these meds may curb nocturnal diarrhea.
- Budesonide
  1. Shown to be most effective as first-line induction therapy and often is given for up to eight weeks.
- Mesalamine
  1. Although several studies demonstrate that it is less effective than budesonide, mesalamine also can be used for induction therapy.
- Bismuth salicylate
  1. For those with contraindications to budesonide and mesalamine, bismuth salicylate is another medication shown to be superior to watchful waiting in patients with mild symptomatic disease.
- Bile acid sequestrants
  1. There is limited data to suggest that bile acid sequestrants such as cholestyramine may be useful as single-agent or adjuvant induction therapy in patients with mild symptoms.
- Immune modulators
  1. Although limited supporting evidence exists for their use, immune modulators such as

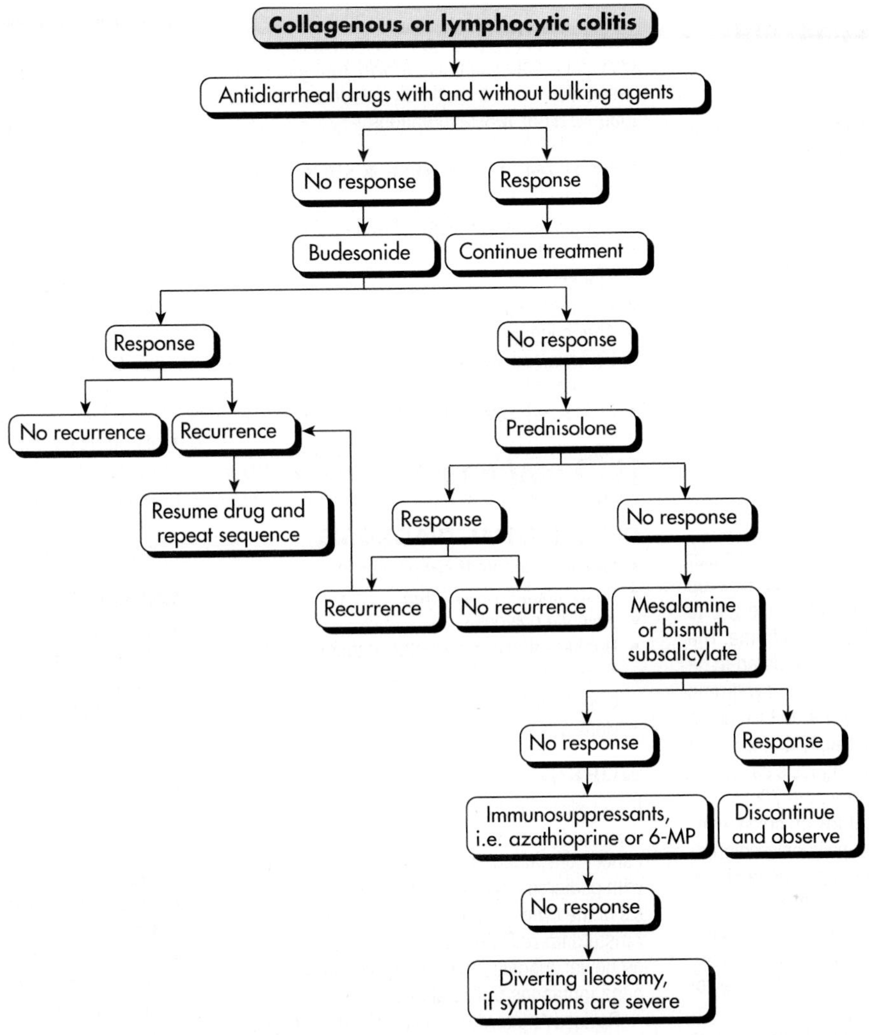

FIG. 1 Algorithm for the treatment of collagenous or lymphocytic colitis. *6-MP,* 6-Mercaptopurine. (From Feldman M, et al.: *Sleisenger and Fordtran's gastrointestinal and liver disease,* ed 10, Philadelphia, 2016, Elsevier.)

azathioprine and anti-TNF-alpha inhibitors also may have a role for induction therapy in budesonide refractory disease.

- There is no role for systemic steroids such as prednisone in the treatment of microscopic colitis.
- Rarely, patients require surgical intervention with colonic diversion.

CHRONIC Rx

Approximately two thirds of patients with microscopic colitis experience relapsed disease and require maintenance therapy. Budesonide is the most studied maintenance agent that can be administered for up to 12 months at doses lower than those used for induction. For less severe disease, patients also can continue using bismuth salicylate or cholestyramine.

COMPLEMENTARY & ALTERNATIVE MEDICINE

It is unclear whether probiotics provide benefit.

DISPOSITION

Symptoms associated with MC are often episodic. While induction therapy is highly effective, 66% of patients in remission will experience a subsequent disease flare.

REFERRAL

- Gastroenterology referral should be offered to patients with long standing chronic diarrhea whose workups have ruled out acute infectious causes.
- Nutrition referrals also may be helpful in patients with severe symptoms such as weight loss.

PEARLS & CONSIDERATIONS

COMMENTS

- MC poses a significant burden on patient quality of life and is often under-recognized.
- Chronic watery diarrhea in the older adult, particularly with nighttime symptoms, should prompt the provider to consider MC. Identification of MC through clinical history and endoscopic evaluation should not be delayed as induction therapy is highly effective at improving disease morbidity.
- Budesonide remains the most effective mainstay medication for both induction and maintenance therapy. Other medications such as bismuth salicylate and cholestyramine are well tolerated and suitable as adjunct or single-agent therapies. Refractory cases may require immunomodulator therapy such as azathioprine or anti-tumor necrosis factor biologic agents such as infliximab.

PREVENTION

As with many other chronic illnesses, smoking cessation is an important part of both management and prevention.

PATIENT/FAMILY EDUCATION

There is no known genetic abnormality, but presentation may trend in families.

SUGGESTED READINGS

Available at ExpertConsult.com

RELATED CONTENT

Irritable Bowel Syndrome (Related Key Topic)
Crohn Disease (Related Key Topic)
Ulcerative Colitis (Related Key Topic)
Traveler Diarrhea (Related Key Topic)

AUTHORS: **BRETON ROUSSEL, M.D.,** and **SARAH HYDER, M.D.**

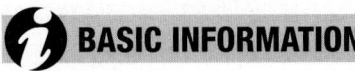

BASIC INFORMATION

DEFINITION

Lynch syndrome is a hereditary predisposition to malignancy of the colon that is explained by a germline mutation in a DNA mismatch repair gene.

SYNONYMS

Hereditary non-polyposis colorectal cancer
HPNCC
Hereditary site-specific colon cancer

ICD-10 CM CODE

C18.9 Malignant neoplasm of colon, unspecified

EPIDEMIOLOGY & DEMOGRAPHICS

The lifetime risk for developing colon cancer in the United States is approximately 6%. Up to 30% of colon cancer is inherited and 2% to 4% may be attributable to Lynch syndrome. The incidence of Lynch syndrome is estimated to be between 1:660 and 1:2000. Lynch syndrome is the most common form of hereditary colon cancer. The average age of diagnosis for Lynch syndrome is 45 yr, although diagnosis can occur as early as the 20s or as late as the 70s.

RISK FACTORS: Family history of colon cancer or other hereditary non-polyposis colorectal cancer (HNPCC)-related cancers such as endometrial (up to 40% of women with Lynch syndrome may develop endometrial cancer), biliary tract, ovarian, stomach, upper urinary tract, or brain. Table 1 summarizes the risk of Lynch syndrome.

GENETICS: Autosomal-dominant inheritance pattern.

ETIOLOGY

Lynch syndrome is thought to be secondary to germline mutations in DNA mismatch repair genes. The predominant genes involved are *MSH2* and *MLH1,* which are tumor suppressor genes, although other genes have documented involvement (*PMS1, PMS2, MSH6,* and *EpCAM*). Mutations in these genes prevent repair of DNA mismatches during DNA replication. This is most prevalent in regions of DNA called microsatellites, causing DNA microsatellite instability and leading to an increased risk for malignancy, especially colon cancer. *MSH6* mutations are associated with a markedly lower cancer risk than *MLH1* or *MSH2* mutations.

PHYSICAL FINDINGS & CLINICAL PRESENTATION

- Changes in bowel habits (prolonged constipation)
- Melena
- Hematochezia
- Abdominal pain
- Unexplained weight loss
- Decreased appetite
- Right sided colon cancer (70% to 85% of cases)

Dx DIAGNOSIS

DIFFERENTIAL DIAGNOSIS

- Familial adenomatosis polyposis
- Peutz-Jeghers syndrome
- Juvenile polyposis
- Nonhereditary colorectal cancer. Table 2 compares Lynch syndrome and sporadic colorectal cancer
- Gardner syndrome

WORKUP

If an individual presents with numerous adenomatous polyps or has multiple relatives with cancer at a young age, a family history complete with pedigree must be obtained. Clinical diagnosis of the Lynch syndrome can be made with the Amsterdam or Bethesda criteria (Box 1) as well as newer models such as prediction model for gene mutations 5 (PREMM$_5$).

- Revised Amsterdam (II) criteria (must meet all criteria):
  1. HNPCC-associated carrier diagnosis in at least three individuals in the family
  2. One of the patients is a first-degree family member of two other patients
  3. Involved patients occur in at least two successive generations with diagnosis of HNPCC
  4. At least one diagnosis in family of HNPCC was made before age 50
  5. The diagnoses are histologically confirmed.
  6. Familial adenomatous polyposis is excluded.
- Bethesda criteria (must meet all criteria):
  1. Colorectal cancer before age 50
  2. Multiple colorectal cancers or other HNPCC-related cancers such as biliary tract, endometrial, stomach, or ovary
  3. Colorectal cancer with microsatellite instability histology <60 yr of age
  4. Colorectal cancer or HNPCC-related cancer in first-degree relative <50 yr of age
  5. Colorectal cancer or HNPCC-related cancer in at least two first- or second-degree relatives, any age
- If criteria for the Lynch syndrome are not met, no further analysis is necessary (although a genetic syndrome cannot be definitively excluded and genetic referral may be warranted).

LABORATORY TESTS

- If a patient meets criteria for Lynch syndrome, immunohistochemistry can be performed for the presence or absence of mismatch repair genes *MLH1, MSH2, MSH6,* and *PMS2.* Rarely, *MLH3* is identified.
- Microsatellite instability analysis should also be performed if criteria for Lynch syndrome are met.

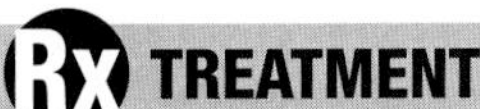

TREATMENT

- If the mutation has been identified in a family member, screening for this mutation can be performed via genetic testing. Informed consent must be obtained after a thorough explanation has been provided to each individual. Criteria for referral to a genetic counselor for suspected Lynch syndrome is summarized in Table 3.
- Surveillance using colonoscopy can be performed in individuals who screen positive, while those who screen negative can be discharged. The mismatch repair gene that is mutated guides screening.

TABLE 1 Risk of Lynch Syndrome

Condition	Risk (%)
Endometrial cancer at any age	1.8
Endometrial cancer diagnosed before 50 years of age	9
Endometrial and colon cancer at any age	18
Endometrial and colon cancer before 50 years of age	43
Endometrial and ovarian cancer	7

From Disaia PJ et al: *Clinical gynecologic oncology,* ed 9, Philadelphia, 2017, Elsevier.

TABLE 2 Comparison of Clinical Features in Lynch Syndrome and Sporadic Colorectal Cancer

Clinical Feature	Lynch Syndrome	Sporadic Colorectal Cancer
Mean age at diagnosis (years)	45	67
Multiple colon cancers	35%	4%-11%
Synchronous colon cancers	18%	3%-6%
Metachronous colon cancers	24%	1%-5%
Proximal location of the initial cancer*	72%	35%
Increased risk of malignant tumors at other sites	Yes	No
Mucinous and poorly differentiated colon cancers	Common	Infrequent
Prognosis	Favorable[†]	Variable

*Proximal to the splenic flexure.
[†]Patients whose tumors demonstrate microsatellite instability have a more favorable prognosis than those with microsatellite-stable tumors.
From Feldman M, Friedman LS, Brandt LJ: *Sleisenger and Fordtran's gastrointestinal and liver disease,* ed 10, Philadelphia, 2016, Elsevier.

BOX 1 Amsterdam II Criteria for Hereditary Nonpolyposis Colorectal Cancer (Lynch Syndrome)

Criteria defined by the International Collaborative Group on Hereditary Nonpolyposis Colorectal Cancer
- At least 3 relatives with CRC (one must be a first-degree relative of the other two) or a Lynch syndrome–associated cancer*
- CRC involving at least 2 successive generations
- One or more cancer cases before age 50 years
- Familial adenomatous polyposis should be excluded
- Tumors should be verified by histologic examination

CRC, Colorectal cancer
*Endometrium, ovary, stomach, ureter/renal pelvis, pancreas, brain, hepatobiliary tract, small intestine, and multiple sebaceous adenomas and carcinomas and keratoacanthomas in the Muir-Torre variant of Lynch syndrome.
From Feldman M, Friedman LS, Brandt LJ: *Sleisenger and Fordtran's gastrointestinal and liver disease*, ed 10, Philadelphia, 2016, Elsevier.

TABLE 3 Criteria for Referral to a Genetic Counselor for Suspected Lynch Syndrome

Bethesda guidelines
Amsterdam Criteria fulfilled
Persons with two relatives with Lynch syndrome
Colorectal cancer and first-degree relative with a Lynch cancer before 45 years or a first-degree relative with an adenoma before 40 years of age
Colorectal cancer or endometrial cancer before 45 years of age
Right-sided, undifferentiated colon cancer before 45 years of age
Signet ring colon cancer before 45 years of age
Adenoma before 40 years of age

From Feldman M, Friedman LS, Brandt LJ: *Sleisenger and Fordtran's gastrointestinal and liver disease*, ed 10, Philadelphia, 2016, Elsevier.

- According to the Netherlands Surveillance Protocol, for example, individuals with mutations in *MLH1, MSH2,* or *MSH6* should have colonoscopies every 1 to 2 yr starting at age 20 to 25 yr; urine cytology every 1 to 2 yr starting at age 30 to 35 yr; esophagogastroduodenoscopy every 1 to 2 yr starting at age 30 to 35 yr; and, in females, ultrasound of endometrium and CA-125 every 1 to 2 yr starting at age 30 to 35 yr.
- *Helicobacter pylori* testing is also indicated in patients with Lynch syndrome or at high risk for it.
- Aspirin may be protective against colorectal cancer in Lynch syndrome patients.

REFERRALS

- To gastroenterology for surveillance colonoscopies
- To genetic counselor if patient satisfies Bethesda criteria
- To psychologist as necessary for psychological support

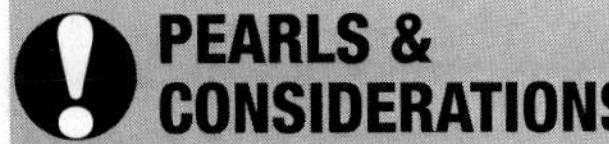

PEARLS & CONSIDERATIONS

- Before genetic testing is instituted, informed consent must be obtained because consequences of this testing include the necessity of lifelong screenings such as colonoscopies.
- The risk of pancreatic cancer is increased in families with Lynch syndrome compared with the U.S. population.
- **Familial Colorectal Cancer Type X** refers to patients who meet the Amsterdam criteria for HPNCC but have no molecular evidence of a MMR deficiency. These patients have a lower risk of colon cancer and no increased risk of extracolonic cancer compared to those with Lynch syndrome.

PATIENT & FAMILY EDUCATION

- For information on local genetic counselors, visit the National Society of Genetic Counselors website at www.nsgc.org.
- For information on Lynch syndrome, visit www.mayoclinic.com/health/lynch-syndrome/DS00669.

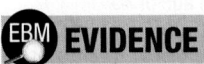

EVIDENCE

Available at ExpertConsult.com

SUGGESTED READINGS

Available at ExpertConsult.com

RELATED CONTENT

Colorectal Cancer (Related Key Topic)
Familial Adenomatous Polyposis and Gardner Syndrome (Related Key Topic)
Peutz-Jeghers Syndrome and Other Polyposis Syndromes (Related Key Topic)

AUTHOR: **FRED F. FERRI, M.D.**

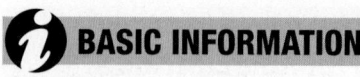

BASIC INFORMATION

DEFINITION

Malabsorption is the diminished intestinal absorption of dietary nutrients. The majority of malabsorption is due to either congenital or acquired defects in the membrane transport system, absorption, and brush border processing in the intestinal epithelium.

SYNONYM

Maldigestion

ICD-10CM CODES

K90.9	Intestinal malabsorption, unspecified
K90.4	Malabsorption due to intolerance, not elsewhere classified
K90.89	Other intestinal malabsorption
K91.2	Postsurgical malabsorption, not elsewhere classified

EPIDEMIOLOGY & DEMOGRAPHICS

PREDOMINANT SEX AND AGE: More common in females, with a mean age of 40

GENETICS:

- HLA-DQ2 present in 95% of celiac disease

RISK FACTORS:

- Excessive alcohol consumption
- History of celiac disease
- History of IBD
- Intestinal surgery

PHYSICAL FINDINGS & CLINICAL PRESENTATION

- Most commonly nonspecific symptoms such as abdominal flatulence and distention are seen.
- Due to the osmotic load from maldigestion/malabsorption, watery diarrhea may be present. In the case of fat digestive disorder, steatorrhea ensues.
- Weight loss is very common but many patients are able to compensate by increased caloric load. Diffuse disease often has much more pronounced weight loss.
- Chronic protein malabsorption can cause hypoalbuminemia, leading to edema and ascites.
- Both microcytic and macrocytic anemia can result from micronutrient deficiency (iron/B_{12}). These patients can be pale and present with fatigue.
- Bleeding disorders from vitamin K deficiency can lead to ecchymosis, melena, and hematuria.
- Vitamin D deficiency can lead to bone disorders. Secondary hyperparathyroidism can be a presenting feature.
- Electrolyte and vitamin deficiency can lead to neurologic disorders such as ataxia, weakness, and neuropathy, and may have positive Chvostek or Trousseau sign.
- Autoimmune disease-specific dermatologic findings such as alopecia, pellagra, erythema nodosum, pyoderma gangrenosum, cheilosis, glossitis, and aphthous ulcers may be present.
- Cardinal clinical features of specific malabsorptive disorders are summarized in Table 1.

ETIOLOGY

- Can be congenital or acquired.
- Disease-specific etiology. Mechanisms of malabsorption, malabsorbed substrates, and representative causes are summarized in Table 2.

DIFFERENTIAL DIAGNOSIS

- Crohn disease
- Celiac disease
- Hartnup disease
- Chronic pancreatitis
- Pancreatic insufficiency
- Cystic fibrosis
- Short bowel syndrome

TABLE 1 Cardinal Clinical Features of Specific Malabsorptive Disorders

Disorder	Cardinal Clinical Features
Adrenal insufficiency	Skin darkening, hyponatremia, hyperkalemia
Amyloidosis	Renal disease, nephrotic syndrome, cardiomyopathy, neuropathy, carpal tunnel syndrome, macroglossia, hepatosplenomegaly
Bile acid deficiency	Ileal resection or disease, liver disease
Carcinoid syndrome	Flushing, cardiac murmur
Celiac disease	Variable symptoms: dermatitis herpetiformis, alopecia, aphthous mouth ulcers, arthropathy, neurologic symptoms, and (life-threatening) malnutrition; elevated liver biochemical test levels, mild iron deficiency
Crohn disease	Arthritis, aphthous mouth ulcers, episcleritis, uveitis, pyoderma gangrenosum, erythema nodosum, abdominal mass, fistulas, perianal fistulae, primary sclerosing cholangitis (PSC), laboratory signs of inflammation
CF	Chronic sinopulmonary disease, meconium ileus, distal intestinal obstruction syndrome (DIOS), elevated sweat chloride
Cystinuria, Hartnup's disease	Kidney stones, dermatosis
Diabetes mellitus	Long history of diabetes and diabetic complications
Disaccharidase deficiency	Bloating and cramping, intermittent diarrhea
GI fistulas	Previous intestinal surgery or trauma, Crohn disease
Glucagonoma	Migratory necrolytic erythema, enlarged gallbladder
Hyperthyroidism, hypothyroidism	Symptoms and signs of thyroid disease
Hypogammaglobulinemia	Recurrent infections
Intestinal ischemia	Other ischemic organ manifestations; abdominal pain with eating (chronic mesenteric ischemia)
Lymphoma	Enlarged mesenteric or retroperitoneal lymph nodes, abdominal mass, abdominal pain, fever
Mastocytosis	Urticaria pigmentosum, peptic ulcer
Mycobacterium avium complex infection	AIDS
Pancreatic insufficiency	History of pancreatitis, abdominal pain, or alcoholism; large-volume fatty, oily stools; passage of orange oil
Parasitic infection	History of travel to endemic areas
PBC	Jaundice, itching
Scleroderma	Dysphagia, inability to open the mouth widely, Raynaud's phenomenon, skin tightening
SIBO	Previous intestinal surgery, motility disorder (scleroderma, pseudo-obstruction), small intestinal diverticula, strictures
Tropical sprue	History of travel to endemic area
Tuberculosis	Specific history of exposure, living in or travel to endemic area, immunosuppression, abdominal mass or intestinal obstruction, ascites
Whipple disease	Lymphadenopathy, fever, arthritis, cerebral symptoms, heart murmur (pulmonary valve), oculomasticatory myorhythmia
ZES	Peptic ulcers, diarrhea

AIDS, Acquired immunodeficiency syndrome; *CF,* cystic fibrosis; *GI,* gastrointestinal; *PBC,* primary biliary cholangitis; *SIBO,* small intestinal bacterial overgrowth; ZES, Zollinger-Ellison syndrome.
From Feldman M et al: *Sleisenger and Fordtran's gastrointestinal and liver disease*, ed 10, Philadelphia, 2016, Elsevier.

TABLE 2 Mechanisms of Malabsorption, Malabsorbed Substrates, and Representative Causes

Pathophysiologic Mechanism	Malabsorbed Substrate(s)	Representative Causes
Maldigestion		
Conjugated bile acid deficiency	Fat Fat-soluble vitamins Calcium Magnesium	Hepatic parenchymal disease Biliary obstruction SIBO with bile acid deconjugation Ileal bile acid malabsorption CCK deficiency
Pancreatic insufficiency	Fat Protein Carbohydrate Fat-soluble vitamins Vitamin B_{12} (cobalamin)	Congenital defects Chronic pancreatitis Pancreatic tumors Inactivation of pancreatic enzymes (e.g., ZES)
Reduced mucosal digestion	Carbohydrate	Congenital defects Acquired lactase deficiency
	Protein	Generalized mucosal disease (e.g., celiac disease, Crohn disease)
Intraluminal consumption of nutrients	Vitamin B_{12} (cobalamin)	SIBO Helminthic infections (e.g., *Diphyllobothrium latum* infection)
Malabsorption		
Reduced mucosal absorption	Fat Protein Carbohydrate Vitamins Minerals	Congenital transport defects Generalized mucosal diseases (e.g., celiac disease, Crohn disease) Previous intestinal resection or bypass Infections Intestinal lymphoma
Decreased transport from the intestine	Fat Protein	Intestinal lymphangiectasia Primary Secondary (e.g., solid tumors, Whipple disease, lymphomas) Venous stasis (e.g., from heart failure)
Other Mechanisms		
Decreased gastric acid and/or intrinsic factor secretion	Vitamin B_{12}	Pernicious anemia Atrophic gastritis Previous gastric resection
Decreased gastric mixing and/or rapid gastric emptying	Fat Calcium Protein	Previous gastric resection Autonomic neuropathy
Rapid intestinal transit	Fat	Autonomic neuropathy Hyperthyroidism

CCK, Cholecystokinin; *SIBO,* small intestinal bacterial overgrowth; *ZES,* Zollinger-Ellison syndrome.
From Feldman M et al: *Sleisenger and Fordtran's gastrointestinal and liver disease,* ed 10, Philadelphia, 2016, Elsevier.

- Neoplasm
- Abetalipoproteinemia
- Lactose intolerance
- Small intestine bacterial overgrowth
- Chronic atrophic gastritis
- Zollinger-Ellison syndrome
- Chronic cholestasis
- Cirrhosis

WORKUP

- A detailed history including alcohol consumption, surgical history as well as autoimmune disease can help diagnose the underlying disease. It is important to screen for anemia and electrolyte abnormalities due to malabsorption.
- Table 3 summarizes malabsorptive diseases or conditions in which noninvasive tests can establish malabsorption or provide a diagnosis.

LABORATORY TESTS

- CBC, serum iron, Vitamin B_{12}, and folate to detect for anemia.
- **Prothrombin time:** Elevated PT can suggest vitamin K deficiency.
- **Fat malabsorption:** The gold standard is the 72-hour stool elastase or fat collection. More than 6/g day in the stool is pathologic. This test can be cumbersome so other options are available. Sudan III stain and acid steatocrit tests are qualitative measures of steatorrhea. Serologic testing for celiac disease should be considered as well.
- **Carbohydrate malabsorption:** Carbohydrate malabsorption leads to fermentation of the undigested carbohydrates by intestinal bacteria.
- The urinary D-xylose test for carbohydrate absorption in the small intestine. After loading with D-xylose, urinary D-xylose levels are measured. Low levels suggest intestinal malabsorption.
- Lactose intolerance can be tested by the lactose tolerance test or the breath test. The lactose tolerance test measures blood glucose after lactose administration. Development of symptoms or inadequate increase in blood sugar is indicative of lactose intolerance. H_2/CO_2 breath tests using specific forms of carbohydrates can detect malabsorption as well.
- **Protein malabsorption:** Protein malabsorption is likely due to small intestinal bacterial overgrowth or protein gastroenteropathies. Alpha-1 antitrypsin clearance or 99mTc-albumin gamma camera scintigraphy may aid in this diagnosis.
- **Pancreatic insufficiency:** Fecal elastase and chymotrypsin levels can distinguish from pancreatic and intestinal causes.
- **Vitamin deficiency:** It is important to assess serum vitamin B_{12} and methylmalonic acid levels. Schilling's test is rarely used but can be useful in some cases.
- **Bile acid malabsorption:** Quantitative stool bile acid measurement is the preferred method of diagnosis. SeHCAT test (selenium homocholic acid taurine test) is another option but less likely used.
- **Bacterial overgrowth:** This can be detected with endoscopic jejunal aspirate culture or a less invasive hydrogen breath test.
- Table 4 summarizes useful laboratory tests for evaluating patients with suspected malabsorption and for establishing possible nutrient deficiencies.

IMAGING STUDIES

- Abdominal US can identify thickened small bowel wall
- Endoscopy for visualization and biopsy
- Small bowel follow through
- Abdominal CT/MRI
- ERCP/MRCP/EUS for identification of pancreatic abnormalities
- Capsule endoscopy

Rx TREATMENT

Involves identification and treatment of the underlying illness, treatment of diarrhea, and nutritional repletion

NONPHARMACOLOGIC THERAPY

- A gluten-free diet in patients with celiac disease. Avoidance of lactose-containing product in lactose intolerance.
- Avoidance of caffeine and high sugar containing compounds has been found to decrease diarrhea in some cases.

ACUTE GENERAL Rx

- Control of the underlying disease should be primary goal.
- It is also essential to control any volume and electrolyte abnormalities that might exist.

CHRONIC Rx

- Control of chronic diarrhea with loperamide should be one of the goals in a chronic malabsorptive state.
- Correction of volume and electrolyte disturbance with oral rehydration therapy should be made a priority.
- Bile acid conjugates can decrease steatorrhea in some cases.

TABLE 3 Malabsorptive Diseases or Conditions in Which Noninvasive Tests Can Establish Malabsorption or Provide a Diagnosis

Disease or Condition	Diagnostic Test(s)	Comment(s)
Lactose malabsorption	Lactose hydrogen breath test Lactose tolerance test	Tests do not differentiate between primary and secondary lactose malabsorption.
Incomplete fructose absorption	Fructose hydrogen breath test	
SIBO	^{14}C-D-xylose breath test Glucose hydrogen breath test Schilling test with and without antibiotics	A predisposing factor should be sought if the result of any of the tests is positive.
Bile acid malabsorption	SeHCAT test, ^{14}C-TCA test	Does not differentiate between primary and secondary causes.
Exocrine pancreatic insufficiency	Quantitative fecal fat determination	Used to establish malabsorption in chronic pancreatitis.
	Fecal elastase or chymotrypsin, tubeless tests	Variable sensitivity and specificity, depending on the type of test and stage of the disease.
Vitamin B_{12} malabsorption	Schilling test	The test is performed without intrinsic factor and, depending on the result with intrinsic factor, with antibiotics or pancreatic enzymes. Further tests are necessary if SIBO, terminal ileal disease, or pancreatic disease is suspected.

SeHCAT, Seleniu-75-homotaurocholic acid test; *SIBO,* small intestinal bacterial overgrowth; *TCA,* taurocholic acid.
From Feldman M et al: *Sleisenger and Fordtran's gastrointestinal and liver disease*, ed 10, Philadelphia, 2016, Elsevier.

TABLE 4 Useful Laboratory Tests for Patients with Suspected Malabsorption and for Establishing Possible Nutrient Deficiencies

Test	Comment(s)
Blood Cell Count	
Hematocrit, hemoglobin	Decreased in iron, vitamin B_{12}, and folate malabsorption or with blood loss
Mean corpuscular hemoglobin or mean corpuscular volume	Decreased in iron malabsorption; increased in folate and vitamin B_{12} malabsorption
White blood cells, differential	Decreased in vitamin B_{12} and folate malabsorption; low lymphocyte count in lymphangiectasia
Biochemical Tests (Serum)	
TGs	Decreased in severe fat malabsorption
Cholesterol	Decreased in bile acid malabsorption or severe fat malabsorption
Albumin	Decreased in severe malnutrition, lymphangiectasia, protein-losing enteropathy
Alkaline phosphatase	Increased in calcium and vitamin D malabsorption (severe steatorrhea); decreased in zinc deficiency
Calcium, phosphorus, magnesium	Decreased in extensive small intestinal mucosal disease, after extensive intestinal resection, or in vitamin D deficiency
Zinc	Decreased in extensive small intestinal mucosal disease or intestinal resection
Iron, ferritin	Decreased in celiac disease, in other extensive small intestinal mucosal diseases, and with chronic blood loss
Other Serum Tests	
Prothrombin time	Prolonged in vitamin K malabsorption
β-Carotene	Decreased in fat malabsorption from hepatobiliary or intestinal diseases
Immunoglobulins	Decreased in lymphangiectasia, diffuse lymphoma
Folic acid	Decreased in extensive small intestinal mucosal diseases, with anticonvulsant use, in pregnancy; may be increased in SIBO
Vitamin B_{12}	Decreased after gastrectomy, in pernicious anemia, terminal ileal disease, SIBO, and infection with *Diphyllobothrium latum*
Methylmalonic acid	Markedly elevated in vitamin B_{12} deficiency
Homocysteine	Markedly elevated in vitamin B_{12} or folate deficiency
Citrulline	May be decreased in destructive small intestinal mucosal disease or intestinal resection
Stool Tests	
Fat	Qualitative or quantitative increase in fat malabsorption
Elastase, chymotrypsin	Decreased concentrations and output in exocrine pancreatic insufficiency
pH	Less than 5.5 in carbohydrate malabsorption

SIBO, Small intestinal bacterial overgrowth; *TGs,* thyroglobulins.
From Feldman M et al: *Sleisenger and Fordtran's gastrointestinal and liver disease*, ed 10, Philadelphia, 2016, Elsevier.

- Pancreatic insufficiency is typically treated with a low-fat diet and exogenous pancreatic enzymes.
- Teduglutide-homolog of GLP-2 has been shown to increase absorptive surface area in short bowel syndrome.
- Periodic DEXA scans are indicated in chronic malabsorption in the setting of vitamin D deficiency.
- Oral supplementation with vitamins and minerals is important, sometimes requiring parenteral therapy.

REFERRAL

- Gastroenterology consultation can help in diagnosis when initial laboratory testing is unclear.
- Nutrition consultation can help patients with diet modification to alleviate symptoms.

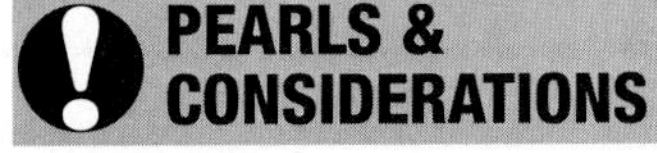

PEARLS & CONSIDERATIONS

COMMENTS

- Malabsorption should be considered a sign of an underlying disease.
- Treatment should focus on treating the underlying disorder.
- Nutrient and volume repletion should be priority in any treatment plan of malabsorption.

RELATED CONTENT

Celiac Disease (Related Key Topic)
Crohn Disease (Related Key Topic)
Cystic Fibrosis (Related Key Topic)
Irritable Bowel Syndrome (Related Key Topic)
Lactose Intolerance (Related Key Topic)
Pancreatitis, Chronic (Related Key Topic)
Short Bowel Syndrome (Related Key Topic)
Small Intestinal Bacterial Overgrowth (Related Key Topic)
Ulcerative Colitis (Related Key Topic)

AUTHORS: **ROSANN CHOLANKERIL, M.D., GEORGE CHOLANKERIL, M.D., DIMITRI GITELMAKER, M.D.,** and **ALAN EPSTEIN, M.D.**

BASIC INFORMATION

DEFINITION

Malaria is a protozoan disease caused by intraerythrocytic protozoa of the genus *Plasmodium* and transmitted by female *Anopheles* spp. mosquitoes. It is endemic throughout most of the tropics and is characterized by hectic fever and often presents with classic malarial paroxysm. Five species of genus *Plasmodium* usually infect humans (Table 1):

- *P. falciparum*
- *P. vivax*
- *P. malariae*
- *P. ovale*
- *P. knowlesi*

SYNONYMS

Periodic fever
Tertian malaria
Quartan malaria
Tropical splenomegaly

ICD-10CM CODES

B54 Unspecified malaria
B50.9 *Plasmodium falciparum* malaria, unspecified
B51.9 *Plasmodium vivax* malaria without complications
B52.9 *Plasmodium malariae* malaria without complications
53.0 *Plasmodium ovale* malaria
B53.8 Other parasitologically confirmed malaria, not elsewhere classified

EPIDEMIOLOGY & DEMOGRAPHICS

Global:

- ~300 million cases/yr in more than 100 countries
- Around 900,000 deaths/yr, with more than 80% of the deaths occurring in children of sub-Saharan Africa
- 3 billion people live in malaria-endemic areas

U.S.:

- ~1500 cases reported to the CDC in the U.S. each yr (Fig. E1). In the majority of reported cases, U.S. civilians who acquired infection abroad had not adhered to a chemoprophylaxis regimen that was appropriate for the country in which they acquired malaria
- More than 50% of the reported cases in the U.S. are *P. falciparum.* On average, there are six deaths per yr in the U.S.
- Most infections limited to:
  1. Immigrant population
  2. Returned travelers or troops from endemic area
- Occasionally, transmission through exposure to infected blood product or shared intravenous needles by users of injection drugs
- Congenital transmission possible
- Local mosquito-borne transmission reported
- Competent mosquito vectors present
  1. *A. albimanus* in Eastern U.S.
  2. *A. freeborni* in Western U.S.

Geographic distribution:

- *P. falciparum:* Sub-Saharan Africa, Papua New Guinea, Solomon Islands, Haiti, Indian subcontinent
- *P. vivax:* Central America, South America, North Africa, Middle East, Indian subcontinent
- *P. ovale:* West Africa
- *P. malariae:* Worldwide

Parasite life cycle (Fig. 2):

- Human infection begins when a female anopheline mosquito bites (only female anopheline mosquito takes blood meal) and inoculates plasmodial sporozoites into bloodstream. The bite usually occurs between dusk and dawn.
- The sporozoites then travel to liver and invade to hepatocytes.
- In the hepatocytes, the sporozoites mature to tissue schizont or become dormant hypnozoites.
- The tissue schizonts amplify the infection by producing a large number of merozoites (10,000-30,000).
- Each merozoite is capable of invading an RBC and can establish the asexual cycle of replication in RBCs.
- Asexual cycles produce and release 24 to 32 merozoites at the end of 48- or 72-hr *(P. malariae)* cycles.
- The hypnozoites are only found in relapsing malaria *P. vivax* or *P. ovale* and may remain dormant for up to 5 yr.
- Eventually some intraerythrocytic parasites develop into gametocytes. Male and female gametocytes are taken up by a female anopheline mosquito with a blood meal where they fertilize in the mosquito gut to produce a diploid zygote that matures to an ookinete; haploid sporozoites are generated that migrate to the salivary gland of the mosquito to infect another human.

PHYSICAL FINDINGS & CLINICAL PRESENTATION

- Fever is the hallmark of malaria, known as malarial paroxysm, initially daily until synchronization of infection after several wk, when fever may occur every other day (tertian) in *P. vivax, P. ovale,* or *P. falciparum* malaria or every third day (quartan) in *P. malariae* malaria. Table 2 describes the WHO criteria for severe malaria.
- Classic malarial paroxysm characterized by:
  1. Cold stage: Abrupt onset of cold feeling associated with rigors, shakes
  2. Hot stage: High fever (~40° C; 104° F) associated with restlessness
  3. Sweating stage: Patient defervesces
- Nonspecific symptoms are:
  1. Headache
  2. Cough
  3. Myalgia
  4. Vomiting
  5. Diarrhea
  6. Jaundice
- *P. falciparum:*
  1. Most pathogenic of the four species.
  2. Rapidly progresses to high-level parasitemia.
  3. Important cause of the fatal malaria.

TABLE 1 Characteristics of the *Plasmodium* Species Responsible for Human Malaria

	SPECIES				
Characteristic	***P. falciparum***	***P. vivax***	***P. ovale***	***P. malariae***	***P. knowlesi***
Incubation period in days (range)	12 (8–25)	14 (8–27)	17 (15 to ≥18)	28 (15 to ≥40)	11 (9 to >12)
Periodicity of febrile attacks (hours)	None	48	48	72	24
Earliest appearance of gametocytes (days)	10	3	?	?	?
Relapse	No	Yes	Yes	No	No
Duration of untreated infection (years)	1–2	1.5–4	1.5–4	3–50	?
RBC preference	Younger cells (but can invade cells of all ages)	Reticulocytes	Reticulocytes	Older cells	?
Characteristic morphology	Ring forms	Schüffner dots	Schüffner dots	Normal-sized cells	Ring forms
	Multiply infected cells	Enlarged RBCs	Enlarged RBCs	Band or rectangular forms of trophozoites	Occasional multiply infected cells
	Banana-shaped gametocytes				Band forms

RBC, Red blood cell.
From Cherry JD et al: *Feigin and Cherry's textbook of pediatric infectious diseases*, ed 8, Philadelphia, 2019, Elsevier.

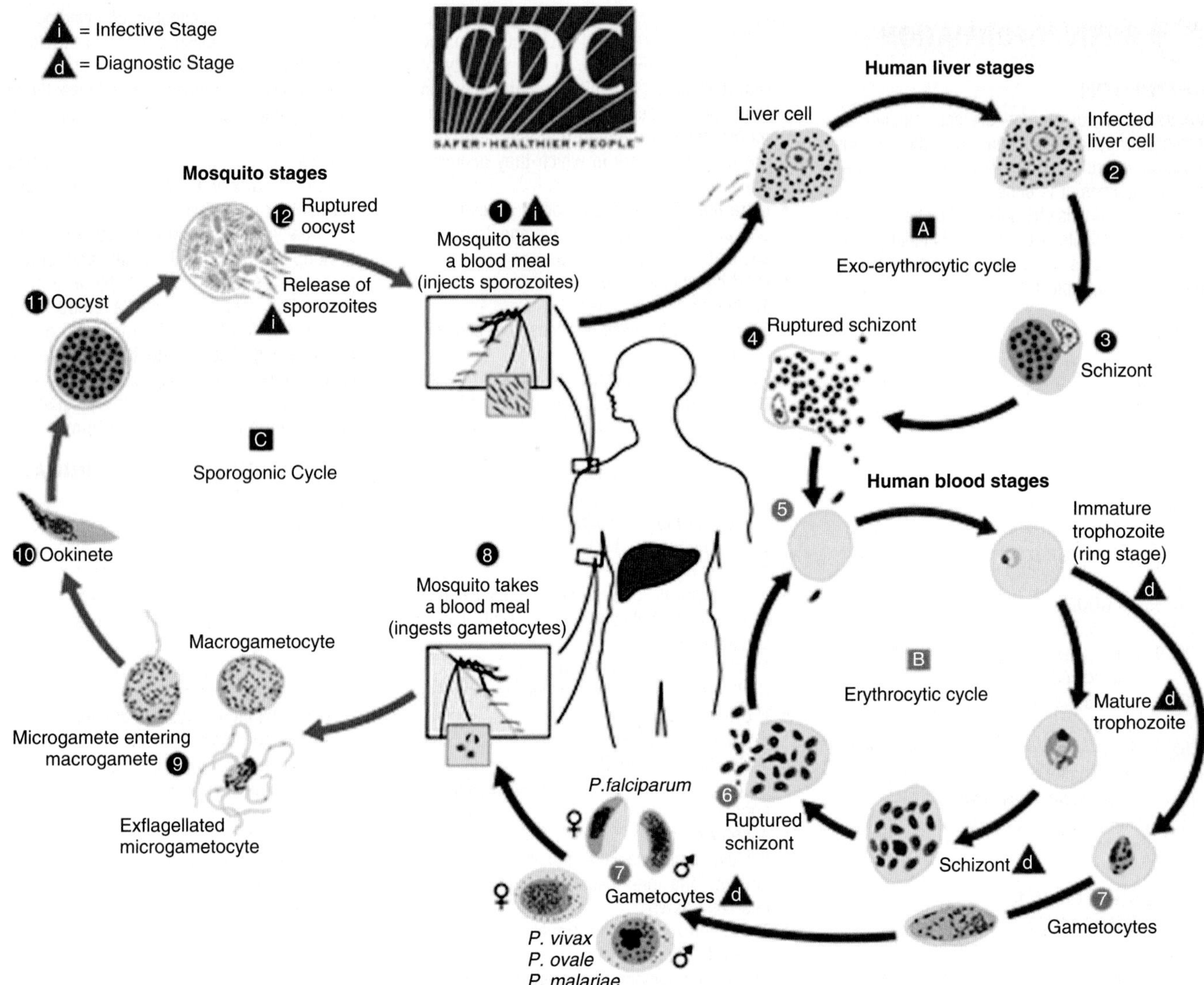

FIG. 2 Life cycle of human malaria parasites. The malaria parasite life cycle involves two hosts. During a blood meal, a malaria-infected female *Anopheles* mosquito inoculates sporozoites into the human host *(1)*. Sporozoites infect liver cells *(2)* and mature into schizonts *(3)*, which rupture and release merozoites *(4)*. (Of note, in *P. vivax* and *P. ovale* a dormant stage [hypnozoites] can persist in the liver and cause relapses by invading the bloodstream weeks, or even years, later.) After this initial replication in the liver (exo-erythrocytic schizogony *[A]*), the parasites undergo asexual multiplication in the erythrocytes (erythrocytic schizogony *[B]*). Merozoites infect red blood cells *(5)*. Ring stage trophozoites mature into schizonts, which rupture, releasing merozoites *(6)*. Some parasites differentiate into sexual erythrocytic stages (gametocytes) *(7)*. Blood stage parasites are responsible for clinical manifestations of the disease. The gametocytes, male (microgametocytes) and female (macrogametocytes), are ingested by an *Anopheles* mosquito during a blood meal *(8)*. The parasites' multiplication in the mosquito is known as the sporogonic cycle *(C)*. While in the mosquito's stomach, the microgametes penetrate the macrogametes, generating zygotes *(9)*. The zygotes in turn become motile and elongated (ookinetes) *(10)* and invade the midgut wall of the mosquito, where they develop into oocysts *(11)*. The oocysts grow, rupture, and release sporozoites *(12)*, which make their way to the mosquito's salivary glands. Inoculation of the sporozoites *(1)* into a new human host perpetuates the malaria life cycle. (From Centers for Disease Control and Prevention. About Malaria: Biology; http://www.cdc.gov/malaria/about/biology/ in Cherry JD et al: *Feigin and Cherry's textbook of pediatric infectious diseases*, ed 8, Philadelphia, 2019, Elsevier.)

4. Classic malarial paroxysm is usually absent.
5. Incubation period after exposure is 12 days (range: 9-60 days).
6. Cytoadherence and resetting of RBCs play central role in pathogenesis.
7. The sequestration of RBCs in vital organs leads to fatal complications.
8. Cerebral malaria is a feared complication.
9. Invades erythrocytes of all ages.
10. Lacks hypnozoites (intrahepatic stage), does not relapse.
11. Blood smear usually shows ring form only.
12. Pigment color is black.
13. Banana-shaped gametocytes; if seen in blood, smear is diagnostic.
14. Chloroquine resistance is widely present.

- *P. vivax:*
  1. Known as tertian malaria: Fever occurs every other day.

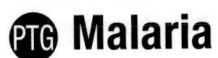

TABLE 2 World Health Organization Criteria for Severe Malaria, 2000

Impaired consciousness
Prostration
Respiratory distress
Multiple seizures
Jaundice
Hemoglobinuria
Abnormal bleeding
Severe anemia
Circulatory collapse
Pulmonary edema

From Kliegman RM et al: *Nelson textbook of pediatrics,* ed 19, Philadelphia, 2011, Saunders.

2. Duffy blood-group antigen FYA- or FYB-related receptor is needed for attachment to RBC.
3. FyFy phenotype (most West African) individuals are resistant to *P. vivax* malaria.
4. Incubation period after exposure is 14 days (range: 8-27 days).
5. Hypnozoites may cause relapse of infection after yrs.
6. Infects mainly reticulocytes.
7. Irregularly shaped large rings and trophozoites, enlarged RBCs, and Schüffner's dots are seen in peripheral blood smear.
8. Pigment color is yellow-brown.
9. *P. vivax* from Papua New Guinea has reduced sensitivity to chloroquine.
10. Primaquine is needed to eradicate the hypnozoites.

- *P. ovale:*
  1. Also known as tertian malaria; fever occurs every other day.
  2. Occurs mainly in tropical Africa.
  3. Incubation period after exposure is 14 days (range: 8-27 days).
  4. Hypnozoites may cause relapse of infection.
  5. Infects mainly reticulocytes.
  6. Infected RBC is seen as enlarged, oval shape containing large ring or trophozoites with Schüffner's dots.
  7. Pigment color is dark brown.
  8. Primaquine needed to eradicate the hypnozoites.
  9. No chloroquine resistance has been encountered.
- *P. malariae:*
  1. Known as quartan malaria; fever occurs every third day.
  2. Common cause of chronic malarial infection.
  3. May persist for 20 to 30 yr after leaving the endemic area.
  4. Worldwide distribution.
  5. Incubation period after exposure is 30 days (range: 16-60 days).
  6. Lacks hypnozoites (intrahepatic stage).
  7. May persist in blood for many yrs if treated inadequately.
  8. Chronic infection may cause soluble immune-complex, resulting in nephritic syndrome.
  9. Infects mainly mature RBCs.
  10. Band or rectangular forms of trophozoites are commonly seen in peripheral blood smear.
  11. Pigment color is brown-black.
- Cerebral malaria:
  1. Feared complication of *P. falciparum* infection.
  2. Mortality is ~20%.
  3. Pathogenesis is poorly understood.
  4. Ischemia as a result of sequestration of parasites or cytokines induced by parasite toxin(s) is the key debate.
  5. Seizure and altered mental status leading to coma are cardinal manifestation.
  6. Hypoglycemia, lactic acidosis, and elevated circulating TNF-α may be present.
  7. CSF studies: No increase of WBC count or protein, raised lactate concentrate, and increased opening pressure, especially in children, may be present.

Dx DIAGNOSIS

DIFFERENTIAL DIAGNOSIS

- Typhoid fever
- Dengue fever
- Yellow fever
- Viral hepatitis
- Influenza
- Brucellosis
- Urinary tract infection
- Leishmaniasis
- Trypanosomiasis
- Rickettsial diseases
- Leptospirosis

WORKUP

- Clinical diagnosis is notoriously inaccurate.
- Demonstration of malarial parasites in blood smear is essential.
- Newer molecular diagnostic techniques (polymerase chain reaction, rapid diagnostic tests) are promising (Table 3).

LABORATORY TESTS

- The thick and thin blood film is required to identify malarial parasites (Fig. E3). A Giemsa-stained film of the patient's peripheral blood should be examined for parasites as soon as possible.
- The thick smears are more sensitive and primarily used to detect the presence of parasites.
- The thin smears are used for species differentiation and parasite density estimation.
- A patient who is suspected of having malaria but who has no parasite seen in blood smears should have blood smears repeated every 12 to 24 hr for 3 consecutive days.

PREPARATION OF BLOOD SMEAR:

- Must be prepared from fresh blood obtained by pricking the finger.
- The thin smear is fixed in methanol before staining.
- The thick smear is stained unfixed.
- The smear should be stained with a 3% Giemsa solution (pH of 7.2) for 30 to 45 min.
- The parasite density should be estimated by counting the percentage of RBCs infected, not the number of parasites, under an oil immersion lens on thin film.

COMMON ERRORS IN READING MALARIAL SMEARS:

- Platelets overlying an RBC
- Misreading artifacts as parasites
- Concern about missing a positive slide

MOLECULAR DIAGNOSIS OF MALARIA:

- Rapid diagnostic tests (RDT):
  1. Employ immunochromatographic lateral flow technology for antigen detection.
  2. Thus far only one RDT has been FDA approved: BinaxNOW Malaria test kit.
  3. This kit is based on antigens HRP-2 and aldolase.
  4. For *P. falciparum:* Sensitivity 95% and specificity 94%.
  5. For *P. vivax:* Sensitivity 69% and specificity 100%.
- Limitations of the BinaxNOW Malaria test:
  1. Not approved for mixed infections.
  2. Should not be used for *P. malariae* and *P. ovale* as data are limited.
  3. Positive test must be confirmed by microscopy.
  4. Negative results require confirmation by thick and thin smears.
  5. This test cannot be used to monitor therapy as antigen persists after the elimination of the parasite, causing false positives.
- Other diagnostic tests available include:
  1. Tagged monoclonal antibodies for malaria antigen detection.
  2. Nucleic acid amplification and detection: PCR can detect parasites down to a level of 1 to 5 parasites per microliter of blood. PCR can detect mixed species infection.
  3. Fluorescence microscopy with acridine orange or other staining.
  4. Dark field microscopy.

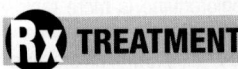

Rx TREATMENT

NONPHARMACOLOGIC THERAPY

ANTIMOSQUITO MEASURES:

- Eradication of mosquito breeding places by chemical spray
- Use of mosquito nets properly in the endemic areas
- Use of protective clothing
- Use of insect spray (permethrin), mosquito coils, or repellents such as diethyltoluamide (DEET). For adults, DEET (30% to 50%) is generally protective for at least 4 hr. For smaller children, use DEET at ≤20% concentration.

TABLE 3 Malaria Rapid Diagnostic Tests Available in the U.S.[a]

RDT Name	Malaria Antigen Target	Malaria Species Detected	Sensitivity	Comment
Binax Now	HRP-2 and aldolase	*P. falciparum, P. vivax, P. malariae,* and *P. ovale*	94% for *P. falciparum* 84% for non- *P. falciparum* 87% for pure *P. vivax* infections 62% for pure *P. ovale* and *P. malariae* infections	Sensitivity increased to 96% for pure *P. falciparum* infection Overall specificity of 99% FDA-approved for use in the U.S.
Parasight F	HRP-2	*P. falciparum*	96.5–100 in Kenya when >60 parasites/μL, lower with less parasitemia 40% in travelers when <50 parasites/μL, >93% when >100 parasites/ μL	Antigen persists for 6–7 days 6 in 11.9%–20% of subjects whose blood smears had cleared Not FDA approved for use in the U.S.
ICT Malaria Pf/Pv	HRP-2 and aldolase	*P. falciparum* and *P. vivax*	97% for *P. falciparum* 44% for *P. vivax*	Specificity of 90% for *P. falciparum* Specificity of 100% for *P. vivax* Not FDA-approved for use in the U.S.
OptiMAL-IT	LDH	*P. falciparum, P. vivax, P. malariae,* and *P. ovale*	85-95%; decreased with lower parasite density	Specificity of 100% *P. falciparum*, 75%–85% for *P. vivax* Not FDA approved for use in the U.S.
Clearview	LDH	*P. falciparum, P. vivax, P. malariae,* and *P. ovale*	93% specificity of 100%, with sensitivities of 99%, 90.0%, 86%, and 60%, respectively, for *P. falciparum, P. vivax, P. malariae,* and *P. ovale*	Specificity of 100% for *P. falciparum*, 99% for *P. vivax*, 90% for *P. malariae*, and 60% for *P. ovale* Not FDA-approved for use in the U.S.

FDA, Food and Drug Administration; *HRP-2*, histidine-rich protein-2; *RDT*, rapid diagnostic test.
[a]Direct microscopy should be performed where available with a negative RDT, given higher false-negative rates with low parasitemia, and when severe malaria is suspected.
From Cherry JD et al: *Feigin and Cherry's textbook of pediatric infectious diseases*, ed 8, Philadelphia, 2019, Elsevier.

ACUTE GENERAL Rx

A definitive diagnosis of malaria is essential for specific antimalarial chemotherapy.

NON-FALCIPARUM MALARIA:

- Chloroquine 600 mg base (1000 mg chloroquine phosphate) PO loading dose, 6 hr later 300 mg base (500 mg salt), then 300 mg base (500 mg salt) daily for 2 days.
- In the case of *P. vivax* and *P. ovale,* treatment with primaquine 15 mg daily for 14 days is needed to eradicate the exoerythrocytic forms, especially the hypnozoites responsible for relapses.
- G6PD should be measured before primaquine is given. Primaquine is not recommended for those who are glucose-6-phosphate dehydrogenase deficient, because primaquine can cause hemolysis and even death in G6PD-deficient persons. Normal G6PD levels must be documented before using primaquine for either chemoprophylaxis or treatment.
- Chloroquine-resistant *P. vivax* has been documented; in that case, quinine is given.

FALCIPARUM MALARIA:

- Chloroquine can be used cautiously for falciparum malaria acquired in chloroquine-sensitive areas (chloroquine is more rapidly effective than quinine).
- For uncomplicated *P falciparum,* an oral artemisin combination therapy (ACT) is recommended by the CDC. The only ACT approved in the U.S. is artemether-lumefantrine (Coartem), which is not widely available. Do not delay therapy in trying to obtain it; use another first-line agent. Dosage for adults: 4 tablets atemether-lumefantrine (20/120 mg) as a single dose, then 4 tablets again after 8 hr, then 4 tablets q12h for 2 days (take with food). Can cause prolongation of Q-T interval. Not recommended in infants <5 kg. Dose dependent on weight in children:
  1. 5 to 15 kg: 1 tablet (20/120 mg) as a single dose, then 1 tablet again after 8 hr, then 1 tablet q12h for 2 days
  2. 16 to 25 kg: 2 tablets (40/240 mg) as a single dose, then 2 tablets again after 8 hr, then 2 tablets q12h for 2 days
  3. 26 to 35 kg: 3 tablets (60/360 mg) as a single dose, then 3 tablets again after 8 hr, then 3 tablets q12h for 2 days
  4. >35 kg: Treat as adult
- Atovaquone-proguanil (Malarone): 250 mg atovaquone/100 mg proguanil): 4 adult tabs PO once a day for 3 days with food. Pediatric dosage: Pediatric tablets (62.5 mg atovaquone/25 mg proguanil) are used based on weight:
  1. 5 to 8 kg: 2 pediatric tabs PO once daily for 3 days
  2. 9 to 10 kg: 3 pediatric tabs PO once daily for 3 days
  3. 11 to 20 kg: 1 adult tab PO once daily for 3 days
  4. 21 to 30 kg: 2 adult tabs PO once daily for 3 days
  5. 31 to 40 kg: 3 adult tabs PO once daily for 3 days
  6. >40 kg: 4 adult tabs PO once daily for 3 days
- Another first-line option for treatment in adults is oral quinine sulfate 10 mg (salt)/kg (usually 650 mg) q8h for 3 to 7 days plus doxycycline 100 mg PO bid, both for 7 days. Pediatric dosage: Quinine sulfate 10 mg/kg PO tid plus clindamycin 20 mg/kg per day divided tid, both for 7 days.
- Table 4 summarizes some treatment guidelines for severe *Plastidium falciparum* malaria.

ALTERNATIVES:

- Quinine sulfate plus clindamycin 900 mg tid for 7 days in adults
- Mefloquine 750 mg PO, then 500 mg PO 6 to 12 hr later in adults
- Atovaquone-proguanil (Malarone) or quinine sulfate plus doxycycline can be used when species is unknown. Artemether-lumefantrine is also recommended by WHO for treatment of unknown species, but in U.S. is only approved for *P.* falciparum

NOTE: Parasitemia may paradoxically rise in the first 24 to 36 hr and is not an indication of treatment failure.

SEVERE FALCIPARUM MALARIA:

- It is a medical emergency; intensive care is preferred.
- Measurement of blood glucose, lactate, ABG is important.
- IV quinidine gluconate 10 mg salt/kg loading dose (maximum 600 mg) in NS; infuse slowly over 1 to 2 hr, followed by continuous infusion of 0.02 mg/kg/min until patient can swallow.
- Need to monitor ECG for observation of QT interval as can prolong. Also need to monitor blood pressure and glucose to avoid hypoglycemia.
- Alternatively, IV artesunate: 2.4 mg/kg IV first dose, then at 12 and 24 hr followed by 2.4 mg/kg once daily. One recent study showed the superiority of parenteral artesunate over parenteral quinine in adults and children who could not take an oral medication.
- Plasmapheresis is an option for parasitemia >30% or in pregnant women and in elderly with severe malaria.

NOTE: WHO recommends IV artesunate as the treatment of choice for severe malaria in adults and children in area of low transmission. Data on children in high-transmission regions are limited, and WHO recommends treatment with artesunate, artemether, or quinine.

MULTIDRUG-RESISTANT MALARIA:

- Mefloquine 1250 mg as a single dose, *or*
- Halofantrine 500 mg every 6 hr for 3 doses, repeat same course after 1 wk
- Combination therapy usually preferred

DISPOSITION

RISK FACTORS FOR FATAL MALARIA:

- Failure to take chemoprophylaxis

TABLE 4 Treatment Guidelines for Severe *Plasmodium falciparum* Malaria

Drug	Dose	Comments
Artemisinin compounds		
ArtesunateArtemether	2.4 mg/kg IV bolus at 0, 12, 24 hours, then daily until patient is able to transition to the following oral regimen: 1. Artemether + lumefantrine: Tablets containing 20 + 120 mg, 40 + 240 mg of artemether and lumefantrine, respectively • Adults ≥35 kg: 80 + 480 mg twice daily for 3 days • Children: • 5 to <15 kg: 20 + 120 mg twice daily for 3 days • 15 to <25 kg: 40 + 240 mg twice daily for 3 days • 25 to <35 kg: 60 + 360 mg twice daily for 3 days 2. Artesunate + amodiaquine: A fixed-dose combination tablet containing 25 + 67.5 mg, 50 + 135 mg, 100 + 270 mg of artesunate and amodiaquine, respectively • Adults ≥36 kg, 200 + 540 mg daily for 3 days • Children: • 4.5 to <9 kg: 25 + 67.5 mg daily for 3 days • 9 to <18 kg: 50 + 135 mg daily for 3 days • 18 to <36 kg: 100 + 270 mg daily for 3 days 3. Dihydroartemisinin (DHA) + piperaquine (PPQ): Tablets containing 20 + 160 mg, 40 + 320 mg of DHA and PPQ, respectively • Adults: • 36 to <75 kg: 120 + 960 mg daily for 3 days • ≥75 kg: 160 + 1280 mg daily for 3 days (no data on dose recommendation >100 kg) • Children • 5 to<7 kg: 10 + 80 mg daily for 3 days • 7 to <13 kg: 20 + 160 mg daily for 3 days • 13 to <24 kg: 40 + 320 mg daily for 3 days • 24 to <36 kg: 80 + 640 mg daily for 3 days 4. Artesunate or quinine PO to complete 7 days plus doxycycline, 100 mg PO BID × 7 days 5. Artesunate or quinine PO to complete 7 days plus clindamycin, 20 mg base/kg/d PO, TID × 7 days Initial dose: 3.2 mg/kg IM (anterior tight); maintenance dose: 1.6 mg/kg IM daily until patient is able to transition to oral regimen as described earlier for artesunate	Artesunate has "investigational new drug" status in the U.S. and is available only on request to the CDC (770-488-7788). Eligibility requirements include inability to take oral medications, high levels of parasitemia, clinical evidence of severe malaria, intolerance of or contraindication to quinidine, failure of quinidine therapy, and lack of rapid access to quinidine. Where available, artesunate rectal suppositories (10 mg/kg) may be used in children <5 years of age if IV or IM administration is not possible. Doxycycline is contraindicated in children <8 years of age and in pregnancy. Atovaquone/proguanil is packaged in the U.S. in fixed-dose combination tablets of 250 mg atovaquone/100 mg proguanil for adults and 62.5 mg atovaquone/25 mg proguanil for children. Safety of atovaquone/proguanil in pregnancy has not been established.
Cinchona Alkaloid Regimens		
Quinine dihydrochloride	20 mg salt/kg IV or IM on admission, then 10 mg/kg q 8 h. Can be given IM if IV administration is not possible. One of the following drugs should also be given concurrently: 1. ACT as listed earlier. 2. Doxycycline as listed earlier. If patient unable to take PO, give 100 mg IV q 12 h and switch to PO when possible. Avoid rapid IV administration. 3. Clindamycin as listed earlier. If patient unable to take PO, give 10 mg base/kg loading dose IV followed by 5 mg base/kg IV q 8 h and switch to PO when possible. Avoid rapid IV administration.	The infusion rate of IV quinine should be rate controlled and not exceed 5 mg salt/kg per hour. The drug is usually diluted in 5% dextrose and infused over 4 hours. IV quinine is not available in the U.S. When administering IM, the dose should be split and diluted to a concentration of 60-100 mg/kg and delivered to each thigh. Reduce the quinine dose by one third (to 10 mg salt/kg q 12 h) after 48 hours in patients with severe renal and/or hepatic dysfunction. Doxycycline is contraindicated in children <8 years old and in pregnancy.
Quinidine gluconate	6.25 mg base/kg (= 10 mg salt/kg) IV on admission over 1-2 hours, then 0.0125 mg base/kg minute (= 0.02 mg salt/kg per minute) continuous infusion. An alternative regimen is 15 mg base/kg (= 24 mg salt/kg) loading dose IV infused over 4 hours, followed by 7.5 mg base/kg (= 12 mg salt/kg) infused over 4 hours q 8 h, starting 8 hours after the loading dose. A second drug should be given concurrently as listed earlier for quinine.	The loading dose should be omitted if the patient received >40 mg/kg quinine in the preceding 48 hours or mefloquine in the previous 12 hours. Reduce the dose by one third after 48 hours in patients with severe renal and/or hepatic dysfunction.

BID, Twice a day; *CDC,* Centers for Disease Control and Prevention; *DHA,* dihydroartemisinin; *IM,* intramuscular; *IV,* intravenous; *PO,* by mouth; *PPQ,* piperaquine; q8h, every 8 hours; *TID,* thrice a day.
From Vincent JL et al: *Textbook of critical care,* ed 7, Philadelphia, 2017, Elsevier.

- Delay in seeking medical care
- Misdiagnosis

COMPLICATIONS OF MALARIA:

- Anemia
- Acidosis
- Hypoglycemia
- Respiratory distress
- Disseminated intravascular coagulation
- Blackwater fever
- Renal failure
- Shock

REFERRAL

- To an infectious disease specialist or travel medicine expert for severe malaria complications
- To an intensive care specialist if severe cerebral malaria or other major organ failure develops
- All malaria cases are mandated to be reported to local and state health departments by health care providers or laboratory staff

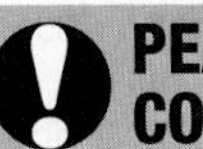

PEARLS & CONSIDERATIONS

HOST RESPONSE

- The specific immune response to malaria confers protection from high-level parasitemia and disease, but not from infection.
- Asymptomatic parasitemia without illness (premunition) is common among adults in endemic areas.

TABLE 5 Drug Regimens Used for Prevention of Malaria

Drug	Adult Dosage	Pediatric Dosage	Comments
Chloroquine-Sensitive Areas			
Chloroquine phosphate (drug of choice)	500 mg salt (300 mg base) orally once/wk	8.3 mg/kg salt (5 mg/kg base) once/wk, up to adult dose of 300 mg base	Begin 1–2 wk before exposure, continue during exposure, and continue for 4 wk after exposure May be used in pregnant women
Hydroxychloroquine sulfate	400 mg salt (310 mg base) orally once/wk	6.5 mg/kg salt (5 mg/kg base) orally once/wk	Begin 1–2 wk before exposure, continue during exposure, and continue for 4 wk after exposure An alternative to chloroquine for use only in areas with chloroquine-sensitive malaria
Chloroquine-Resistant Areas			
Atovaquone-proguanil	250 mg/100 mg (1 tablet) daily	5–8 kg: Pediatric tablet daily 9–10 kg: Pediatric tablet daily 11-20 kg: 1 pediatric tablet daily 21-30 kg: 2 pediatric tablets daily 31-40 kg: 3 pediatric tablets daily >40 kg: 1 adult tablet daily	Begin 1–2 days before exposure, continue during exposure, and continue for 7 days after exposure Pediatric tablets contain 62.5 mg atovaquone and 25 mg proguanil hydrochloride See text for contraindications
Mefloquine	250 mg salt (228 mg base) orally once/wk	≤9 kg: 5 mg/kg salt (4.6 mg/kg base) orally once/wk 10-19 kg: Tablet orally once/wk 20-30 kg: Tablet orally once/wk 31–45 kg: Tablet orally once/wk >45 kg: 1 Tablet orally once/wk	Begin 1–2 wk before exposure, continue during exposure, and continue for 4 wk after exposure
Or			
Doxycycline	100 mg daily	2.2 mg/kg/day up to 100 mg/day	Begin 1–2 days before exposure, continue during exposure, and for 4 wk after exposure; not to be used in children >8 yr or pregnant women
Or			
Alternative			
Primaquine	52.6 mg salt (30 mg base) orally daily	0.8 mg/kg salt (0.5 mg/kg base) up to adult dose orally daily	Begin 1–2 days before exposure, continue during exposure, and continue for 7 days after exposure Contraindicated in people with G6PD deficiency, in pregnancy, and during lactation Prophylaxis to areas principally with *P. vivax*

From Cherry JD et al: *Feigin and Cherry's textbook of pediatric infectious diseases*, ed 8, Philadelphia, 2019, Elsevier.

- Immunity is specific for both the species and the strain of infecting malarial parasites.
- Immunity to all strains is never achieved.
- Normal spleen function is an important host factor because of immunologic as well as filtering functions of the spleen.
- Both humoral and cellular immunity is necessary for protection.
- Polyclonal increase in serum level of IgG, IgM, and IgA occurs in immune individuals.
- Antibody to antigenically variant protein PfEMP1 is important for protection in case of *P. falciparum* malaria.
- Passively transferred IgG from immune individuals has been shown to be protective.
- Maternal antibody confers relative protection of infants from severe disease.
- Genetic disorders (sickle cell disease, thalassemia, and G6PD deficiency) confer protection from death because parasites are unable to grow efficiently in low-oxygen tensions, thus preventing high-level parasitemias.
- Individuals deficient of Duffy factor in RBCs are resistant to infection by *P. vivax.*
- Nonspecific defense mechanisms, such as cytokines (TNF-α, IL-1, -6, -8), also play an important role in protection, causing fever (temperatures of 40° C damage mature parasites) and other pathologic effects.

PREVENTION OF MALARIA: Medications are available for the prophylaxis of malaria and will vary depending on level of chloroquine resistance in a given area (Table 5).

Areas free of chloroquine-resistant Falciparum malaria

Chloroquine 300 mg base (500 mg chloroquine phosphate) PO/wk. Start 1 wk prior to arrival in malaria area, then weekly while there and for 4 wk on leaving malaria area. Pediatric dose: 8.3 mg/kg (5 mg/kg base). Alternatives for adults include atovaquone-proguanil (Malarone): 1 adult tablet per day starting 1 to 2 days prior to arriving in malaria area, then daily while there and then for 7 days daily on leaving malaria area. For children, atovaquone-proguanil pediatric tablets based on weight:

- 11 to 20 kg: 1 pediatric tablet
- 21 to 30 kg: 2 pediatric tablets
- 31 to 40 kg: 3 pediatric tablets
- >40 kg: 1 adult tablet

Areas with chloroquine-resistant Falciparum malaria

- Atovaquone-proguanil (Malarone): Dosing as previously
- Mefloquine 250 mg (228 mg base) PO/wk, starting 1 wk before arriving in malaria area, weekly while there and then weekly for 4 wk on return. In children, mefloquine dose is based on weight:
  1. <15 kg: 5 mg/kg
  2. 16 to 19 kg: ¼ adult dose
  3. 20 to 30 kg: ½ adult dose
  4. 31 to 45 kg: ¾ adult dose
  5. >45 kg: Adult dose
- Doxycycline 100 mg PO/day for adults and children aged >8. Start 1 to 2 days before travel, daily while in malaria area, and then daily for 4 wk on return.

SPECIAL CONSIDERATIONS:

- Long-term visitors or travelers
- Children aged <12 yr
- Immunocompromised host
- Pregnant women: Chloroquine and mefloquine are safe in pregnancy but not atovaquone-proguanil. A recent trial revealed that the burden of malaria in pregnancy was significantly lower among adolescent girls or women who received intermittent preventive treatment with dihydroartemisinin-piperaquine than among those who received sulfadoxine-pyrimethamine, and monthly treatment with dihydroartemisinin-piperaquine was superior to three-dose dihydroartemisinin-piperaquine with regards to several outcomes.[1] Avoid doxycycline and primaquine.
- An increasing number of areas in southeast Asia have mefloquine-resistant malaria, including Cambodia, Thailand, and Vietnam.

[1] Kakuru A et al: Dihydroartemisinin-piperaquine for the prevention of malaria in pregnancy, *N Engl J Med* 374:928-939, 2016.

TABLE 6 Sources for Malaria Prophylaxis, Diagnosis, and Treatment Recommendations

Type of Information	Source	Availability	Telephone Number, Internet Address, or Electronic Mail Address
Prophylaxis	CDC's Traveler's Health Internet site (includes online access to Health Information for International Travel)	24 hours/day	http://www.nc.cdc.gov/travel
	(The Yellow Book)	Order from Oxford University Press, Inc. Order Fulfillment 198 Madison Avenue, New York, NY 10016-4314	800-451-7556 or http://www.oup.com/us/
	CDC's Malaria Branch Internet site with Malaria Information and Prophylaxis, By Country (Red Pages)	24 hours/day	http://www.cdc.gov/malaria/travelers/country_table/a.html
	CDC Malaria Map Application	24 hours/day	http://www.cdc.gov/malaria/map
Diagnosis	CDC's Division of Parasitic Diseases and Malaria diagnostic internet site (DPDx)	24 hours/day	http://www.dpd.cdc.gov/dpdx
	CDC's Division of Parasitic Diseases and Malaria diagnostic CD-ROM (DPDx)	Order by electronic mail from CDC Division of Parasitic Diseases and Malaria	dpdx@cdc.gov
Treatment	CDC Malaria Branch	9:00 A.M.–5:00 P.M. Eastern time, Monday–Friday	770-488-7788 or toll-free 855-856-4713*
	CDC Malaria Branch	5:00 P.M.–9:00 A.M. Eastern time on weekdays and all day weekends and holidays	770-488-7100* (This number is for the CDC's Emergency Operations Center. Ask a staff member to page the person on call for the Malaria Branch.) http://www.cdc.gov/malaria/ diagnosis_treatment/treatment.html

CDC, Centers for Disease Control & Prevention.
*These numbers are intended for health care professionals only.
Cullen KA et al: Malaria surveillance—United States, 2013, *MMWR Surveill Summ* 65:1–22, 2016

Therefore, in specific regions of these countries, mefloquine cannot be used for prophylaxis or treatment.

PREVENTION OF RELAPSE[2]:

- Treatment of *P. vivax* requires the clearing of asexual parasites, but relapse can be prevented only if dormant hypnozoites are cleared from the liver (a treatment termed "radical cure")
- Tafenoquine, slowly eliminated, single dose 8-aminoquinoline is effective in significantly lowering the risk of *P. vivax* recurrence in patients with phenotypically normal GG PD activity

VACCINATION:

- In 2015, Mosquirix (RTS,S), a recombinant protein-based vaccine, was approved in Europe to prevent malaria in babies in Africa. It showed an efficacy of about 30% in babies 6 to 12 weeks old and about 46% in babies 5 to 17 months old.
- New DNA-based vaccines are in development.

MALARIA INFORMATION:

- CDC Travelers' Health Hotline (877) 394-8747; CDC Travelers' Health Fax (888) 232-3299
- CDC Malaria Epidemiology (770) 488-7788; internet: www.cdc.gov
- Table 6 summarizes sources for malaria prophylaxis, diagnosis, and treatment recommendations.

SUGGESTED READINGS

Available at ExpertConsult.com

RELATED CONTENT

Malaria (Patient Information)

AUTHOR: **GLENN G. FORT, M.D., M.P.H.**

[2]Lacerda MVG et al: Single-dose tafenoquine to prevent relapse of *Plasmodium vivax* malaria, *N Engl J Med* 380:215–218, 2019.

BASIC INFORMATION

DEFINITION

Malignant hyperthermia (MH) is a rare life-threatening subclinical myopathy that can manifest clinical symptoms in MH-susceptible (MHS) individuals after exposure to triggering medications. These drugs include halogenated anesthetic gases, such as halothane, isoflurane, sevoflurane, and desflurane, as well as the depolarizing agent succinylcholine. When given to genetically susceptible individuals, these agents may cause excessive skeletal muscle contraction. Initial signs include rising end-tidal carbon dioxide ($ETCO_2$) levels and tachycardia, with subsequent hyperthermia, acidemia, and skeletal muscle rigidity. Symptomology may be variable, especially during surgery and general anesthesia. Mortality has recently been reported to be 1.4% to 5%, down from 70% in the past, likely due to the prevalence of intraoperative temperature and $ETCO_2$ monitoring and the use of dantrolene for treatment. Advanced age, muscularity, comorbidities, and disseminated intravascular coagulation (DIC) increase risk of death.

SYNONYMS

Anesthesia related hyperthermia
Hyperpyrexia, Malignant
Hyperthermia, Malignant
Malignant Hyperpyrexia
MHS
MH

ICD-10CM Codes

T88.3	Malignant hyperthermia due to anesthesia
T88.3XXA	initial encounter
T88.3XXD	subsequent encounter
T88.3XXS	sequelae

EPIDEMIOLOGY & DEMOGRAPHICS

Malignant hyperthermia results from excess calcium accumulation in the skeletal muscle tissue of MHS individuals, following exposure to one or more "triggering" medications, including the halogenated volatile anesthetics and the skeletal muscle relaxant, succinylcholine. This is due to excessive release of sarcoplasmic calcium, which occurs because of a genetic anomaly. The result is a hypermetabolic and prolonged contractile state, with subsequent serious morbidity and possible mortality, especially when untreated.

All ethnic groups are at risk. MH susceptibility is associated with, although distinct from, two other diseases: central core and multiminicore disease.

PEAK INCIDENCE: Among patients undergoing general anesthesia, the incidence is approximately 1:100,000. It is widely believed that unrecognized events occur and that half of afflicted patients have had a prior uneventful exposure to a triggering agent.

GENETICS: Susceptibility to MH is due to at least six known genetic variations of MH, all of which are inherited in an autosomal dominant pattern. The most common is a mutation of the ryanodine receptor RYR1, causing MHS1. A CACNA1S mutation causes another form, MHS5. Other types are much less common, and in some cases (a CACNA2D mutation and RYR1) may interact (MHS3). Of note, patients with genetic susceptibility to MH may have an uneventful anesthesia while receiving known triggering agents; previous exposure does not exclude the possibility of a future MH crisis.

PREVALENCE: In the general population, between 1:2000-1:3000 are thought to carry a defective gene for the ryanodine receptor. However, the prevalence of MHS is estimated to be 1:2000. In family cohorts of patients who are susceptible, the prevalence of susceptibility ranges from 1:200 to 1:5000 due to incomplete penetrance and variable expressivity. The majority of these MHS individuals are never exposed to a triggering agent such that a MH clinical event following exposure occurs with a frequency between 1:15,000-1:75,000.

PREDOMINANT SEX AND AGE: MH male to female ratio is 2:1. Children account for up to half of cases.

RISK FACTORS:

- Preoperatively, the patient and family history is used to evaluate the risk of MH and other myopathies. Patients with other RYR1 abnormalities, such as central core myopathy or multiminicore disease (RYR1 or SELENON), though not true MHS, should not receive succinylcholine or volatile anesthetics.
- Patients with dystrophinopathies such as Duchenne and Becker muscular dystrophy, enzymopathies of skeletal muscle such as McArdle disease, or exercise- and heat-induced rhabdomyolysis, may develop rhabdomyolysis when exposed to these agents, especially succinylcholine. Osteogenesis imperfecta, myotonia, and neuroleptic malignant syndrome are no longer felt to be associated with MHS.

PHYSICAL FINDINGS & CLINICAL PRESENTATION

- Within minutes to hours after a triggering agent is administered, the patient may develop muscle rigidity, with resulting tachypnea and tachycardia. In the operating room, MH is often difficult to recognize and rigidity may be attributed to inadequate sedation or absent due to general anesthesia and muscle paralysis. Vital sign perturbations may be missed due to ongoing surgery.
- Masseter muscle rigidity is rare now that succinylcholine is used rarely for muscle relaxation and is not related to MHS.
- Manifestations of increased skeletal muscle metabolism include increased CO_2 production, leading to elevated mixed venous and arterial pCO_2, and an elevated $ETCO_2$; tachycardia is common.
- Hyperthermia or a rapidly increasing temperature from an anesthesia-induced hypothermic state, also a result of hypermetabolism, is present in more than 50% of MH events. Hyperthermia is not always present early in MH crisis, eliminating increasing core body temperature as a definitive inclusion factor in diagnosing MH at an early stage. Higher core body temperature correlates with increased morbidity.
- Muscle injury with an elevated creatine kinase (CK) may lead to rhabdomyolysis, observed myoglobinuria (if a urinary catheter is present), and subsequent acute renal failure. Disseminated intravascular coagulation (DIC) may develop.
- The skin may be erythematous initially, progressing to a mottled, cyanotic appearance.
- Box 1 summarizes the findings consistent with MH.

ETIOLOGY: Approximately 50% of cases of MH susceptibility (MHS) are inherited (primarily MH1 and MH5); the remainder are presumed to be the result of a new mutations. The majority of the mutations, either inherited or de novo, are on chromosome 19 (19q13.2, with at least 35 variants), but other mutations may be found

BOX 1 Positive Findings Consistent with Malignant Hyperthermia (MH)

History of recent exposure to trigger agent, including volatile anesthetic agents or succinylcholine
Family or personal history of MH susceptibility
Total body rigidity
Inappropriately elevated (38.8° C; 101.8° F) or rapidly increasing temperature (>1.5° C over 5 min)
Inappropriate tachypnea
Profuse sweating
Mottled, cyanotic skin
Dark urine, urine dipstick testing shows a positive result from blood without red cells in the sediment and no hemolysis
Unexplained, excessive bleeding
Unexplained ventricular tachycardia or fibrillation
Inappropriate hypercarbia (venous $Paco_2$ >65 mm Hg, arterial $Paco_2$ >55 mm Hg) if the patient is receiving positive-pressure ventilation or is spontaneously breathing with greater than normal minute ventilation
Arterial base excess more negative than −8 mEq/L
Arterial pH <7.25
Potassium concentration >6 mEq/L
Creatine kinase >10,000 IU/L

From Fuhrman BP, et al.: *Pediatric critical care*, ed 4, Philadelphia, 2011, Saunders.

at 1q32.1 (CACNA1S with at least five variants), 17q11.2-q24, 7q21.2, 3q13.1, or 5p. The result is the abnormality of skeletal muscle calcium homeostasis and susceptibility to MH, with significant clinical variability due to incomplete penetrance and variable expressivity.

Dx DIAGNOSIS

DIFFERENTIAL DIAGNOSIS

- Exertional heatstroke
- MH symptomology following excessive heat exposure to a MHS patient who did not receive a triggering agent
- Neuroleptic malignant syndrome
- Fever
- Thyrotoxicosis
- Pheochromocytoma
- Central nervous system infection or space-occupying lesion
- MDMA (Ecstasy), cocaine, alcohol withdrawal, or amphetamine use
- Serotonin syndrome
- Adverse reaction to MAOIs or anticholinergic drug
- Strychnine poisoning
- Sepsis
- Drug withdrawal
- Rhabdomyolysis
- Transfusion reactions

WORKUP

MH can often be distinguished from other causes of hyperthermia based on a history of exposure to a triggering agent. A rapid rise in $ETCO_2$ with no change in minute ventilation, especially in the setting of tachycardia, should prompt consideration of MH until proven otherwise.

LABORATORY TESTS

Considerations for laboratory testing fall into three scenarios:

- In the acute setting, important studies include electrolytes, arterial blood gas, and urine myoglobin to help confirm the diagnosis.
- Once the diagnosis is presumptive, it is important to monitor serial lab data including blood gases and electrolytes, especially potassium and creatinine. Creatine kinase and urine myoglobin should also be followed. Coagulation studies should be obtained to evaluate for DIC.
- If hyperthermia is less acute or the presentation atypical, thyroid function studies, CBC, toxicology screen, and urine vanillylmandelic acid (VMA) may be useful. Treatment should not be delayed while these labs are pending.

IMAGING STUDIES

A CT scan of the head may be obtained to evaluate for space-occupying lesion if clinically indicated. Imaging should never delay prompt treatment of strongly suspected MH.

SUSCEPTIBILITY TESTING: Testing for MH susceptibility involves genetic evaluation or the *in vitro* muscle contracture test. The latter involves placing a muscle biopsy specimen in a bath of caffeine or halothane. Significant muscle contraction is 97% to 99% sensitive for MH susceptibility, with a specificity of 78% to 94% and a cost of $6 to $10,000. It is performed in only a few sites in the U.S. Genetic testing, while noninvasive, has a sensitivity of <50% and a cost of $1 to $4000. Generally, a positive contracture test leads to genetic testing, unless there is a positive family history, in which case the patient may choose genetic testing directly.

Testing for MHS can be performed preoperatively in patients deemed to be at risk or those with a personal or family history of anesthesia-induced complications suggestive of MH. Depending on the wishes of the patient and/or family following a thorough history and counseling, a decision to proceed with anesthesia and surgery without prior testing may be reasonable, with the avoidance of volatile agents or succinylcholine. In such a case, the patient should be counseled that forgoing testing may place them at risk if an intubation is required in an emergency setting, succinylcholine is used unknowingly, and the patient is truly MHS.

After an acute event, the patient should undergo susceptibility testing to confirm the diagnosis and the need for testing other immediate family members at risk. If positive, the patient should be given a letter and wear a medical alert bracelet.

BOX 2 Management of an Acute Malignant Hyperthermia Episode in the Intensive Care Unit

1. Administer high-flow 100% oxygen via a nonrebreathing mask and consider endotracheal intubation.
2. For ventilated patients, administer an FiO_2 of 1.0 and increase minute ventilation to control $PaCO_2$.
3. Administer dantrolene (2.5 mg/kg intravenously) over 10 min, and repeat until acidosis and muscle rigidity have resolved. Repeat dantrolene (1 mg/kg) every 6 hr.
4. Initiate cooling with ice packs in the axillae and groin; decrease room temperature; use hypothermia blankets, iced intravenous saline solution (10 ml/kg over 10 min, repeated as needed), and lavage body cavities with cold saline solution if temperature is greater than 39° C. Stop cooling when core temperature falls to 38° C.
5. Correct metabolic acidosis with sodium bicarbonate (1-2 mEq/kg initially), and give subsequent doses based on base excess and body weight.
6. Administer calcium chloride (10 mg/kg) or calcium gluconate (100-200 mg/kg) for cardiotoxicity associated with hyperkalemia.
7. Give regular insulin (0.1 U/kg) and glucose (0.3-0.5 g/kg) to correct hyperkalemia.
8. Administer lidocaine (1 mg/kg) to treat ventricular arrhythmias. Consider amiodarone (5 mg/kg IV) for refractory, stable ventricular tachycardia. Do not delay defibrillation or cardiopulmonary resuscitation if indicated by cardiovascular instability.
9. Maintain urine output of 2 ml/kg/hr with aggressive cold fluid administration, furosemide (0.5-1 mg/kg), and additional mannitol (0.25-0.3 g/kg) if needed.
10. Consider quantitative end-tidal CO_2 monitoring.
11. Monitor core temperature (pulmonary artery, esophageal temperature probe, rectal probe).
12. Place arterial catheter for invasive blood pressure monitoring and frequent blood sampling. Consider central venous catheter and/or pulmonary artery catheter if indicated by cardiovascular instability.
13. Repeat venous blood gas and electrolytes until these normalize. Repeat CK at least every 6 hr while the patient is in ICU and then daily until CK returns to normal. Assess glucose, clotting function, and hepatic and renal functions, and treat symptomatically. Repeat lactic acid measurement after each dantrolene administration.
14. Consider hemodialysis if indicated.
15. Consider intensive care monitoring for at least 24 hr after MH episode or after recrudescence of MH.
16. Refer the patient for muscle caffeine-halothane contracture testing and consider genetic testing. Pursue a pathologic diagnosis for other occult myopathies.

CK, Creatine kinase; *ICU,* intensive care unit; *MH,* malignant hyperthermia.
From Fuhrman BP, et al.: *Pediatric critical care,* ed 4, Philadelphia, 2011, Saunders.

Rx TREATMENT

NONPHARMACOLOGIC THERAPY

- The patient should be cooled to 38°C. This can be accomplished with ice packs to the axillae and groin, a cooling blanket, a fan with cool mist, or chilled IV fluids. In extreme situations, partial extracorporeal bypass or iced peritoneal lavage have proven helpful.
- Frequent evaluation of core temperature, hemodynamics, and gas exchange are imperative.

ACUTE GENERAL Rx (SEE BOX 2)

- Notify the surgeon to stop surgery immediately. Discontinue all triggering agents and switch to nontriggering agents if surgery must be continued.
- Get dantrolene and your hospital's MH cart; call for help.
- Hyperventilate with 100% oxygen at flows of 10 L/min to flush volatile anesthetics and decrease ETCO2. Insert charcoal filters in line if available to further absorb agent.
- Administer dantrolene as a rapid IV bolus at a dose of 2.5 mg/kg through a large bore catheter. Repeat every five minutes until an observable decrease is seen in muscle rigidity, tachycardia, or ETCO2; a total dose greater

than 10mg/kg may be required, especially in patients with greater muscle mass.
- Up to 25% of patients will have recrudescence of their symptoms, on average 13 hours after the initiation of MH. Dantrolene, 1mg/kg IV every 4 to 6 hours or by continuous infusion at 0.1 to 0.3 mg/kg/hr IV, is recommended for at least 24 to 48 hours. Additional boluses may be needed for breakthrough signs.
- Aggressive hydration with forced diuresis and alkalization of the urine should be instituted for rhabdomyolysis. Observe closely for the development of compartment syndrome, renal failure, and DIC.
- Beta-blockers and lidocaine may be useful for dysrhythmias. Use of calcium channel blockers should be avoided as the combination with dantrolene may produce profound hyperkalemia and significantly depress cardiac function.

CHRONIC Rx

- This is an acute disease, resolving in 24 to 48 hours with appropriate treatment.
- The MHS patient should be aware that exercise in excessive heat and/or humidity could trigger an episode of MH without exposure to a pharmacologic triggering agent.
- The patient as well as immediate family members should be advised to undergo susceptibility testing.
- The patient should be given a letter by his/her anesthesiologist and wear a medical alert bracelet.

COMPLEMENTARY & ALTERNATIVE MEDICINE

None

DISPOSITION

After MH crisis, patients should be admitted to the intensive care unit for at least 24 hrs where close monitoring and supportive care can be maximized.

BOX 3 Anesthetics Associated with the Development of Malignant Hyperthermia and Neuroleptic Malignant Syndrome

Malignant Hyperthermia

Volatile Anesthetics

Desflurane, isoflurane, sevoflurane

Muscle Relaxants

Succinylcholine

Neuroleptic Malignant Syndrome

Phenothiazines

Fluphenazine, chlorpromazine, levomepromazine, thioridazine, trimeprazine, trifluoperazine, prochlorperazine

Butyrophenones

Haloperidol, bromperidol, droperidol

Dibenzoxepine

Loxapine

Dopamine-Depleting Drugs

Alpha-methyltyrosine, tetrabenazine

Dopaminergic Agent Withdrawal

Levodopa-carbidopa, amantadine

Modified from Parrillo JE, Dellinger RP: *Critical care medicine: principles of diagnosis and management in the adult*, ed 4, Philadelphia, 2014, Saunders.

REFERRAL

Anesthesiology, cardiology, nephrology, and hematology consultation as appropriate. After the acute event, a genetics consult may be warranted to facilitate testing

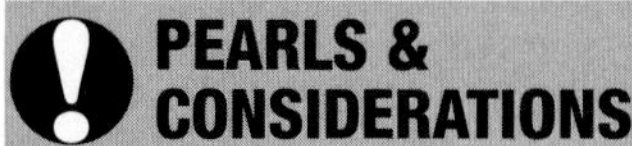

PEARLS & CONSIDERATIONS

COMMENTS

- MH is a life-threatening condition that requires prompt recognition to minimize illness, end-organ damage, and/or death.
- Family or personal history of problems with general anesthesia in the past are clues to susceptibility and should prompt careful preoperative evaluation.
- Prophylactic dantrolene is no longer recommended for known MHS patients undergoing general anesthesia with nontriggering agents.
- Box 3 summarizes anesthetics associated with the development of malignant hyperthermia and neuroleptic malignant syndrome.

PATIENT & FAMILY EDUCATION

The patient and his/her family should be made aware of the diagnosis so that they can provide information to the anesthesiologist and other intraoperative caregivers when undergoing any type of surgery or procedure under sedation. The patient should be given a letter that can be shown to future care givers. A medical alert bracelet should be recommended.

SUGGESTED READINGS

Available at ExpertConsult.com

AUTHOR: **RICHARD GILLERMAN, M.D., PH.D.**

BASIC INFORMATION

DEFINITION

A Mallory-Weiss tear (MWT) is a longitudinal mucosal laceration in the region of the gastroesophageal junction and gastric cardia typically occurring after repeated episodes of severe vomiting or retching.

SYNONYMS

Mallory-Weiss syndrome
MWT

ICD-10CM CODE

K22.6 Mallory-Weiss syndrome

EPIDEMIOLOGY & DEMOGRAPHICS

- Accounts for 5% to 15% of cases of upper gastrointestinal (GI) bleeding
- Reported from early childhood to old age; the majority of patients are age 40 to 60 yr
- More common in males
- Alcohol use is present in 30% to 60%

PHYSICAL FINDINGS & CLINICAL PRESENTATION

- Vomiting, retching, or vigorous coughing will often, but not always, precede hematemesis.
- Patients may be clinically stable or present with tachycardia, hypotension, melena, hematochezia, epigastric pain, or back pain.
- Bleeding may be self-limited or severe. Rebleeding is more common in patients with advanced alcoholic liver disease.
- Tears may be seen in association with other upper GI tract lesions, including hiatal hernia (present in as many as 90% of patients), ulcers, and esophageal varices, particularly in alcoholics.

ETIOLOGY

- An acute increase in intragastric and intraabdominal pressure is transmitted to the gastroesophageal junction and esophagus, resulting in mucosal laceration.
- Vomiting may be associated with alcohol use, cannabinoid use, ketoacidosis, ulcer disease, uremia, pancreatitis, chemotherapy, cholecystitis, pregnancy (in particular associated with hyperemesis gravidarum), myocardial infarction, or the postoperative period.
- Infrequently reported causes include chest wall trauma (including CPR), hiccups, coughing, seizures, lifting/straining, blunt abdominal trauma, acute severe asthma, and labor and delivery.
- Tears may be iatrogenic, related to routine endoscopy (especially in struggling, retching, or older patients, or in association with hiatal hernias or distal gastrectomy), enteroscopy with or without overtubes, esophageal dilation, lower esophageal pneumatic disruption therapy for achalasia, endoscopic submucosal dissection, transesophageal echocardiography, or in association with polyethylene glycol electrolyte colonic lavage preparation.
- Tears are frequently found on the right lateral wall of the esophagus.

DIAGNOSIS

DIFFERENTIAL DIAGNOSIS

- Esophageal or gastric varices
- Esophagitis or esophageal ulcers (peptic or pill-induced)
- Gastric erosions
- Gastric or duodenal ulcer
- Dieulafoy lesion
- Arteriovenous malformations
- Neoplasms (usually gastric)
- Boerhaave syndrome

WORKUP

Endoscopy is the diagnostic method of choice.

LABORATORY TESTS

- Complete blood count, prothrombin time, partial thromboplastin time
- Electrolytes, blood urea nitrogen, creatinine, liver function tests, pregnancy test, tests to evaluate for predisposing conditions

IMAGING STUDIES

- Upper GI series is usually not sensitive.
- Patients with concurrent chest pain, dyspnea, shock, or physical examination findings of crepitus or pleural effusion should have a chest radiograph or CT to exclude Boerhaave syndrome.

TREATMENT

NONPHARMACOLOGIC THERAPY

- Supportive care
- Avoidance of aspirin, nonsteroidal antiinflammatory drugs, and anticoagulants

ACUTE GENERAL Rx

- Patients with active bleeding or hemodynamic instability require large-bore IVs, fluid resuscitation, transfusion of blood products (red blood cells, fresh frozen plasma, platelets), and holding or reversal of anticoagulation as appropriate.
- Nasogastric decompression and antiemetics may be considered.
- Endoscopic therapy for patients with active or ongoing hemorrhage (Fig. E1). Therapeutic modalities include electrocoagulation, argon plasma photocoagulation, heater probe coagulation, injection (e.g., 1:10,000 epinephrine, polidocanol), sclerotherapy (for bleeding associated with esophageal varices), band ligation, endoscopic hemoclips (Fig. E2), over-the-scope clips, and hemostatic sprays (therapies may be used alone or in combination) (Fig. E3). Hemoclips combined with a nylon snare ("tulip-bundle" technique) have been successfully used for refractory bleeding.
- Arterial embolization in patients with active bleeding who are poor surgical candidates.
- Laparotomy, with gastrotomy and oversewing of the tear, is required in a small percentage of patients with uncontrolled bleeding.

CHRONIC Rx

- Healing will usually occur without specific therapy.
- H_2 blockers or proton pump inhibitors may be given to help facilitate healing but should not be used long term unless appropriate indications are present.

DISPOSITION

- Prognosis is good, with spontaneous cessation of bleeding in upward of 90% of patients. Endoscopic features can guide treatment. Blatchford score <6 suggests no need for transfusion or endoscopic intervention.
  1. Blatchford score is calculated by certain indices (sex, blood urea nitrogen, hemoglobin, systolic blood pressure, pulse, and the presence of melena, syncope, hepatic disease, or cardiac failure) and is used to determine which patients need clinical intervention for acute upper gastrointestinal bleeding.
- Delayed rebleeding is described in patients with high-risk stigmata (shock at initial presentation, spurting, or oozing at initial endoscopy).
- Death has been reported in 3% to 12%, often in association with severe bleeding and underlying comorbid conditions such as advanced age, coagulopathy, elevated transaminases, thrombocytopenia, alcohol use, presentation with a very low hemoglobin level or melena, and multi-system organ failure. Over the past decade, associated mortality appears to be significantly declining.

REFERRAL

- Gastrointestinal referral for endoscopy
- Surgical referral for bleeding unresponsive to endoscopic treatment or in the setting of coexistent perforation

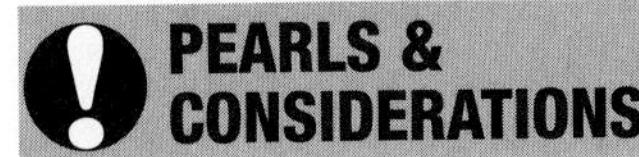

PEARLS & CONSIDERATIONS

Conditions predisposing to retching or vomiting should be identified and treated at presentation.

SUGGESTED READINGS

Available at ExpertConsult.com

RELATED CONTENT

Mallory-Weiss Tear (Patient Information)

AUTHOR: **HARLAN G. RICH, M.D., FACP, AGAF.**

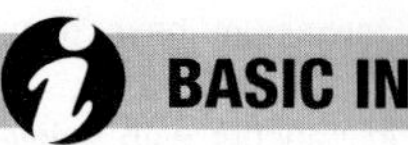

BASIC INFORMATION

DEFINITION

Mastitis is local painful inflammation of the breast that may or may not be accompanied by infection, flulike symptoms, and abscess formation.

ICD-10CM CODES

N61	Inflammatory disorders of breast
091.12	Abscess of breast associated with the puerperium
091.22	Nonpurulent mastitis associated with the puerperium

EPIDEMIOLOGY & DEMOGRAPHICS

- Mastitis is the most common cause of inflammatory breast disease, and most cases are related to lactation.
  1. Nonpuerperal cases of mastitis can affect either the periareolar (periductal) region or peripheral breast tissue.
  2. Periductal mastitis is most common in younger, reproductive-age women. The majority of those affected are active smokers.
- In lactating mothers, mastitis typically occurs in the first 3 mo of the postpartum period (74% to 95% of cases).
- When severe, mastitis can lead to a breast abscess (5% to 11%) or septicemia.
- Delayed diagnosis and treatment of lactational mastitis can lead to discontinuation of breastfeeding, breast tissue damage, or recurrence.
- In younger, nonlactating women, infection often presents as periductal mastitis (PM) and is caused by inflamed milk ducts near the nipple.
- Granulomatous mastitis (GM) is a rarer form of benign inflammation of the breast and also most commonly occurs in reproductive-age women. It generally affects the breast peripherally.
- Mastitis also can occur in infancy when there is breast hypertrophy from maternal hormone.

PREVALENCE: Lactational mastitis occurs in up to 33% of mothers.

PREDOMINANT SEX: Females

RISK FACTORS:

- Previous mastitis
- Milk stasis and missed feedings
- Cracked, fissured, or sore nipples
- Primiparity and infant attachment difficulties
- Cleft lip or palate or short frenulum in infant
- Use of manual breast pump
- Diabetes
- Breast implants
- Nipple piercings
- Rapid weaning
- Smoking (periductal mastitis)

PHYSICAL FINDINGS & CLINICAL PRESENTATION

- Warmth, redness, tenderness in breast
- Unilateral or bilateral
- Malaise, myalgias, fevers, chills
- Decreased milk output
- Breast is hard and swollen in a wedge-shaped area
- In PM, breast mass near nipple with retraction or discharge
- In GM, enlarged axillary lymph nodes or sinus tract formation

ETIOLOGY

- In lactational mastitis, infection occurs a result of milk stasis and irritation of the milk ducts due to local immune response to milk proteins.
  1. Bacterial infection of subcutaneous tissue due to breaks in skin.
- Most commonly, *S. aureus;* less common, *S. epidermidis*, group A beta-hemolytic streptococci, *S. pneumoniae, E. coli, Candida albicans, M. tuberculosis.* GM results from inflammation with epithelioid histiocytes and multinucleated giant cells and can be caused by etiologies like tuberculosis, sarcoidosis, foreign body reaction, parasitic and mycotic infections, or idiopathic.
- Periductal mastitis occurs following inflammation around nondilated subareolar ducts and often can progress to abscess formation. Peripheral abscesses can result from trauma, usually in the setting of comorbid conditions impairing immunity such as diabetes or use of immunosuppressive medications.
- Neonatal mastitis caused by *S. aureus* or gram-negative enteric bacteria.

DIAGNOSIS

DIFFERENTIAL DIAGNOSIS

- Engorgement, plugged duct (see Table 1)
- Breast abscess
- Inflammatory or other breast cancer (3% of women diagnosed with breast cancer are lactating)
- Mastitis as a symptom of hyperprolactinemia or galactorrhea
- GM can be manifestation of systemic disease (sarcoidosis, Wegener granulomatosis, GCA, polyarteritis nodosa, TB, syphilis)

WORKUP

- History and clinical exam with thorough breast exam and assessment of axillary nodes and nipple discharge are sufficient for diagnosis.
- Recurrent mastitis should include workup for underlying breast disease.

LABORATORY TESTS

- Simple lactational mastitis requires no milk culture or laboratory studies.
- Obtain midstream sample of milk for culture and sensitivities in refractory mastitis or in MRSA-suspected cases.
- CBC and blood cultures in toxic patients.
- In abscess formation, culture of drainage or aspirate fluid.
- Gram stain and culture indicated in infant mastitis.

IMAGING STUDIES

- Not necessary unless refractory mastitis or abscess suspected
- Consider US (Fig. 1) to evaluate for abscess or mammogram when appropriate to exclude carcinoma
- In GM, mammogram and US-guided FNA are standard

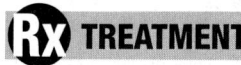

TREATMENT

NONPHARMACOLOGIC THERAPY

- Mainstay of therapy is effective milk removal through continued breastfeeding or pumping.
- Consider referral to a certified lactation consultant to improve breastfeeding technique.
- Warm compresses, increased fluid intake, good nutrition, and rest.
- In abscess formation (10% of women who are treated for bacterial mastitis), surgical drainage or needle aspiration is necessary, followed by antibiotic therapy based on sensitivities of culture.

ACUTE GENERAL Rx

- NSAIDs and analgesics (e.g., acetaminophen, ibuprofen). There is insufficient evidence to support or refute the effectiveness of antibiotic therapy. Common regimens include:
- No history of MRSA:
  1. Dicloxacillin 250 mg 4×/d for 7 d
  2. Cephalexin 500 mg 4×/d for 10-14 d
  3. Inpatient: Nafcillin or oxacillin 2 g IV q4h
  4. Erythromycin may be used in patients allergic to penicillin
- Suspected MRSA or high-risk penicillin allergy:
  1. Trimethoprim/sulfamethoxazole 160 mg/800 mg 2×/d for 10 to 14 d; should not be used when breastfeeding healthy infants <2 mo or compromised infants
  2. Clindamycin 300 mg 4×/d for 10 to 14 d
  3. Inpatient: Vancomycin 1 g IV q12h
- Oxytocin nasal spray if letdown reflex disturbed

TABLE 1 Comparison of Findings of Engorgement, Plugged Duct, and Mastitis

Characteristics	Engorgement	Plugged Duct	Mastitis
Onset	Gradual, immediately	Gradual, after feedings	Sudden, after 10 days postpartum
Site	Bilateral	Unilateral	Usually unilateral
Swelling and heat	Generalized	May shift/little or no heat	Localized red, hot, and swollen
Body temperature	<38.4° C; 101.1° F	<38.4° C; 101.1° F	>38.4° C; 101.1° F
Systemic symptoms	Feels well	Feels well	Flulike symptoms

From Lawrence RA, Lawrence RM: *Breastfeeding: a guide for the medical profession,* ed 5, St Louis, 1999, Mosby.

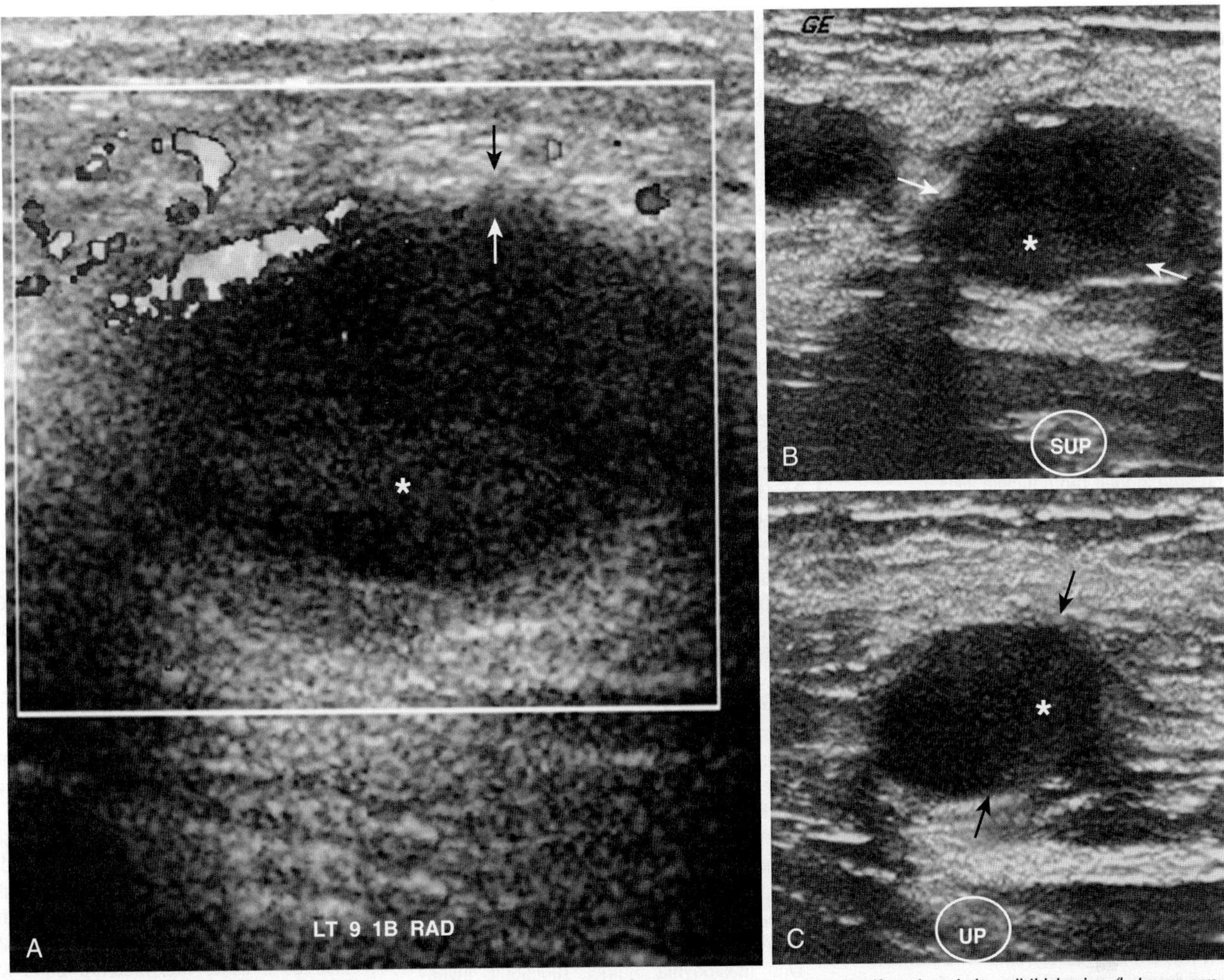

FIG. 1 Inflamed or infected cyst. A, Acutely inflamed or infected cysts demonstrate three findings: (1) abnormal uniform isoechoic wall thickening *(between arrows),* (2) dependent debris *(asterisk),* and (3) hyperemia of the thickened wall. **B,** Supine and **C,** upright images show the debris *(asterisk),* resembling sludge within a gallbladder, shifting to the dependent part of the cyst when the position of the patient is changed from supine to upright or lateral decubitus positions. Note the change in the position of the interface between the nondependent fluid and the dependent debris or pus *(between arrows).* (From Rumack CM, et al.: *Diagnostic ultrasound,* ed 4, Philadelphia, 2011, Mosby.)

- Consider treatment for candidal infection if bilateral symptoms and infant with thrush
  1. Topical clotrimazole for mother and oral nystatin for infant, with careful washing of all pacifiers and nipples
  2. If resistant to topical treatment, can consider oral fluconazole; however, data in breastfeeding are limited
- Infant mastitis typically is treated in an inpatient setting with parenteral antibiotics based on results of gram stain.
- Most PM cases are treated adequately with a combination of antibiotics, needle aspiration/incision, and drainage. In recurrent cases, surgical removal of diseased ducts may be needed.
- If antibiotic and NSAID treatment for GM fails, immunosuppressive drugs (steroids, methotrexate) can be used. Surgical management is not recommended due to associated slow wound healing.

CHRONIC Rx

- No evidence proving benefit of prophylactic antibiotics to prevent lactational mastitis
- In GM, systemic corticosteroids or wide surgical resection

COMPLEMENTARY & ALTERNATIVE MEDICINE

- Complementary therapies not assessed in prospective studies: *Belladonna, Phytolacca, Chamomilla,* sulfur, *Bellis perennis.*
- Several strains of lactobacilli have shown promise as probiotic agents that might be useful in treating mastitis, including *L. fermentum* and *L. salivarius.* These results should be replicated before this approach is adopted widely.

REFERRAL

Refer to surgeon for severe PM or significant lactational abscess that does not resolve with conservative measures

PEARLS & CONSIDERATIONS

COMMENTS

- 25% of breastfeeding mothers with one episode of mastitis stop breastfeeding.
- Increasing incidence of MRSA mastitis.
- Lactational mastitis is a risk factor for vertical transmission of infections (i.e., HIV-1, CMV, measles, hepatitis B and C).
- When reassessing refractory nonlactational mastitis, the most important consideration is the possibility of cancer.
- Nonlactational mastitis can be a manifestation of systemic disease.
- GM mimics breast cancer both clinically and radiologically (>50% of reported cases are initially mistaken for carcinoma). This includes fine needle aspiration, which is sometimes interpreted as malignant.

SUGGESTED READINGS

Available at ExpertConsult.com

RELATED CONTENT

Lactational Mastitis (Patient Information)
Breast Abscess (Related Key Topic)
Fibrocystic Breast Disease (Related Key Topic)
Mastitis (Patient Information)

AUTHOR: **JHENETTE LAUDER, M.D.**

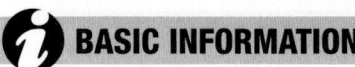

BASIC INFORMATION

DEFINITION

- Pain in the breast
- Usually cyclic but may be noncyclic or extramammary

SYNONYM

Mastalgia

ICD-10CM CODE
N64.4 Mastodynia

EPIDEMIOLOGY & DEMOGRAPHICS

- Mastodynia affects up to 70% of women at some time in their reproductive lives.
- Severe cyclic mastodynia lasting more than 5 days/mo and of sufficient intensity to interfere with sexual, physical, social, and work-related activities is reported among 30% of premenopausal women.
- Underlying fear of breast cancer is the reason most of these women seek medical consultation.
- One tenth of women with mastodynia require pain-relieving therapy.

PHYSICAL FINDINGS & CLINICAL PRESENTATION

- Usually the breasts are normal bilaterally.
- Generalized breast nodularity without discrete lumps.
- Chest wall tenderness: Extramammary breast pain, unilateral, aggravated by activity.
- Distinguishing mammary from extramammary pain can be difficult.
- With the patient lying on her side so that the breast tissue falls away from the chest wall, tenderness can then be reproduced by direct pressure over the offending site.
- Cyclic mastodynia presents in the luteal phase of the menstrual cycle one week prior to onset of menses and resolves with menstruation.
- Women with cyclic mastodynia tend to have abdominal bloating, leg swelling, and other symptoms of premenstrual syndrome.
- Noncyclic mastodynia is unrelated to the menstrual cycle.
- Extramammary breast pain simulates noncyclic mastodynia.

ETIOLOGY

- Hormonal imbalance: Theories include increased estrogen, decreased progesterone, and increased prolactin
- Abnormal lipid metabolism, increased saturated fatty acids
- Premenstrual syndrome (20%)
- Fibrocystic breast disease
- Emotional abuse and anxiety
- Excessive caffeine intake has not been proven
- Breast cancer (10%)
- Tietze syndrome (idiopathic costochondritis)

Dx DIAGNOSIS

DIFFERENTIAL DIAGNOSIS

- See "Etiology."
- The majority of women with mastodynia have no underlying abnormality.
- Breast fullness and tenderness associated with hormonal changes fluctuate with the menstrual cycle.
- Similarly, breast nodularity, which may or may not be the result of fibrocystic breast disease, also fluctuates with the menstrual cycle.
- Discrete breast lumps need full evaluation to rule out malignancy.
- Tietze syndrome is usually unilateral and may be associated with chest wall swelling.

LABORATORY TESTS

Although hormonal imbalance and abnormal lipid metabolism have been implicated in the etiopathogenesis of mastodynia, there is no good evidence to support any consistent pattern of serum hormonal or lipid profile in women with mastodynia. These tests are therefore not recommended.

IMAGING STUDIES

- Mammography should be part of the baseline investigation if the woman is >35 yr.
- Ultrasound is helpful in the assessment of cystic breast lesions.
- In women <35 yr, imaging is not helpful unless a lump has been palpated clinically. Consideration of family history for breast disease is important.
- There are no radiologic features associated with mastodynia: Rather, radiologic investigations are performed to exclude the rare presence of a subclinical carcinoma.

Rx TREATMENT

NONPHARMACOLOGIC THERAPY

- 78% to 85% of women with mastodynia can be reassured after full clinical evaluation. In fact, reassurance can be considered first-line therapy for mastodynia since many women who present are concerned about significant pathology, especially cancer.
- The remaining women require some form of therapy in addition to reassurance.
- A firm, supportive brassiere designed for postpartum use is particularly helpful if mastodynia is associated with breast swelling.
- Follow a low-fat, high-carbohydrate diet.
- Reducing caffeine intake has not been proven effective but may help some women.

ACUTE GENERAL Rx

- There is limited evidence supporting the use of evening primrose oil, which contains gamma-linolenic acid, but this may be offered to patients as it is generally benign.
- Topical NSAID preparations (Diclofenac, salicylate) may confer some benefit and can be prescribed for these women.
- Hormonal therapy is the mainstay of treatment and may include progesterone-only oral contraceptives or cyclic Provera.
- Danazol is the only drug approved by the FDA for the treatment of mastodynia. Danazol has some androgenic and peripheral antiestrogenic effects. Its efficacy is well established, with significant relief of mastodynia in 70% to 93% of cases.
    1. Widespread use of danazol is limited because of its adverse side effects. These include menstrual irregularities, depression, acne, hirsutism, and, in severe cases, voice deepening. Women should be advised to use effective nonhormonal contraception because of the drug's potential adverse effects on the fetus. It is imperative to rule out pregnancy prior to drug initiation.
    2. The side effects of danazol can be significantly reduced by using a low dose (100 mg daily) and confining treatment to 2 wk preceding menstruation. However, alternatives should be explored.
- Tamoxifen, a synthetic antiestrogen, has also been shown to be effective in the treatment of mastodynia. Although effective in relieving symptoms, its use is extremely limited because of side effects, although it has fewer than Danazol. When used, it should be at a low dosage of 10 mg/day and duration should be limited to 6 mo at a time. In the U.S. this agent is not approved for use in women with mastodynia.
- Bromocriptine is a dopamine-receptor agonist whose primary action is inhibition of prolactin release. It has been used extensively in the treatment of severe cyclic mastodynia and is effective. Again, side effects such as headache and lightheadedness have limited its use and it is less effective than Danazol.
- Lisuride maleate was recently found to be effective by one study.
- Other hormonal agents that have been reported to be effective in small studies cannot be recommended. Either they have unacceptable side effect profiles or their efficacy is not established. These agents include gestrinone, gonadotropin-releasing hormone analogues, progesterone, and hormone replacement therapy.
- Investigational treatments: Phytoestrogens, agnus cactus, chamomile.

CHRONIC Rx

- Longstanding cases of mastodynia can be managed with intermittent low-dose danazol therapy to limit side effects. In between these courses of hormone, nonpharmacologic and nonhormonal therapy can be used.
- Severe, unremitting mastodynia that does not respond to medical treatment may require mastectomy; this is rare.

DISPOSITION

- Cyclic mastodynia resolves spontaneously in 20% to 30% of women.
- Noncyclic mastodynia responds poorly to treatment but may resolve spontaneously in up to 50% of women.

RELATED CONTENT

Breast Pain (Patient Information)
Fibrocystic Breast Disease (Related Key Topic)

AUTHOR: **GINA RANIERI, D.O.**

BASIC INFORMATION

DEFINITION

Mastoiditis is inflammation of the mastoid process and air cells, a complication of otitis media.

SYNONYM

Mastoid abscess

ICD-10CM CODES
H70.0 Acute mastoiditis
H40.1 Chronic mastoiditis
H70.8 Other mastoiditis and related conditions
H70.9 Mastoiditis, unspecified

EPIDEMIOLOGY & DEMOGRAPHICS

INCIDENCE (IN U.S.): Since the introduction of antibiotic therapy and use of broad-spectrum antibiotics, there has been a marked decline in the incidence of acute mastoiditis.
PREDOMINANT SEX: More common in males
PREDOMINANT AGE: 2 mo to 18 yr
PEAK INCIDENCE: Early childhood

PHYSICAL FINDINGS & CLINICAL PRESENTATION

- Acute mastoiditis is usually a complication of acute otitis media.
- Most common presenting symptom is pain and tenderness in the postauricular region.
- Other signs or symptoms include:
  1. Fever
  2. Postauricular erythema and edema
  3. Protrusion of the pinna inferiorly and anteriorly
  4. Tympanic membrane usually intact with signs of acute otitis media
- Complications of acute mastoiditis include:
  1. Subperiosteal abscess (most common complication)
  2. Hearing loss
  3. Facial nerve palsy
  4. Labyrinthitis
  5. Intracranial complications such as hydrocephalus, meningitis, encephalitis, intracranial abscess, and lateral sinus thrombosis
- Chronic mastoiditis is characterized by chronic otorrhea and chronic tympanic membrane perforation.

ETIOLOGY

- Continuity exists between the middle air space and the mastoid cavity.
- Initial hyperemia and edema of the mucosal lining of the air cells result in accumulation of purulent exudate.
- Dissolution of calcium from bony septa and osteoclastic activity in the inflamed periosteum lead to bone necrosis and coalescence of air cells.
- Most common bacterial isolates are:
  1. *Streptococcus pneumoniae*
  2. *Streptococcus pyogenes*
  3. *Haemophilus influenzae*
  4. *Moraxella catarrhalis*
  5. *Staphylococcus aureus*
- Often, there are multiple organisms in chronic mastoiditis, with predominance of anaerobes and gram-negative bacteria.
- *Mycobacterium tuberculosis,* nontuberculous mycobacteria, *Aspergillus,* and *Rhodococcus equi* have been reported in cases of mastoiditis in severely immunocompromised individuals.

Dx DIAGNOSIS

DIFFERENTIAL DIAGNOSIS

- Children:
  1. Rhabdomyosarcoma
  2. Histiocytosis X
  3. Leukemia
  4. Kawasaki syndrome
- Adults:
  1. Fulminant otitis externa
  2. Histiocytosis X
  3. Metastatic disease

WORKUP

A thorough history and physical examination are important in establishing diagnosis.

LABORATORY TESTS

- Fluid for gram stain and culture may be obtained by myringotomy.
- If there is a perforation in the tympanic membrane with drainage, cultures of this may be taken after carefully cleaning the external canal.

IMAGING STUDIES

- Plain x-rays of the mastoid region may demonstrate clouding or opacification in areas of pneumatization.
- CT scan can demonstrate early involvement of bone (mastoiditis with bone destruction).
- MRI is more sensitive than CT scan in evaluating soft-tissue involvement and is useful in conjunction with CT scan to investigate other complications of mastoiditis.

Rx TREATMENT

NONPHARMACOLOGIC THERAPY

Myringotomy, if the ear is not already draining

ACUTE GENERAL Rx

- Initiated with IV antibiotics directed against the common organisms *S. pneumoniae* and *H. influenzae.* Useful agents are amoxicillin/clavulanate, ceftriaxone, and cefotaxime. If the disease in the mastoid has had a prolonged course, coverage for *S. aureus* with gram-negative enteric bacilli may be considered for initial therapy until results of cultures become available. Add vancomycin if methicillin-resistant *Staphylococcus aureus* (MRSA) suspected or nafcillin/oxacillin if culture is positive for *S. aureus*, methicillin susceptible.
- Antibiotics continued until all signs of mastoiditis have resolved
- Directed against enteric gram-negative organisms and anaerobes in chronic mastoiditis
- Indications for mastoidectomy:
  1. Failure to improve after 72 hr of therapy
  2. Persistent fever
  3. Imminent or overt signs of intracranial complications
  4. Evidence of a subperiosteal abscess in the mastoid bone

DISPOSITION

Proceed with mastoidectomy when medical therapy fails.

REFERRAL

- To otorhinolaryngologist:
  1. If diagnosis is in doubt
  2. If aural complications present
  3. To evaluate for surgical intervention
- To neurosurgeon if intratemporal or intracranial extension of infection suspected:
  1. Aural complications: Bone destruction, subperiosteal abscess, petrositis, facial paralysis, labyrinthitis
  2. Intracranial complications: Extradural abscess, lateral sinus thrombophlebitis or thrombosis, subdural abscess, meningitis, brain abscess, otitic hydrocephalus

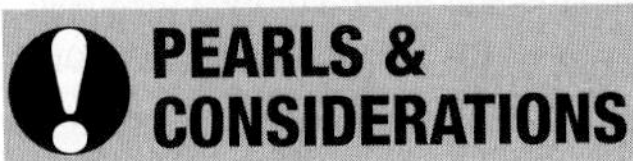

PEARLS & CONSIDERATIONS

Mastoiditis is particularly difficult to eradicate because the mastoid air cells are poorly vascularized and difficult to drain.

SUGGESTED READINGS

Available at ExpertConsult.com

RELATED CONTENT

Mastoiditis (Patient Information)

AUTHOR: **GLENN G. FORT, M.D., M.P.H.**

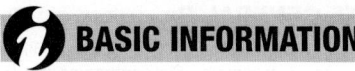

DEFINITION

Mediastinitis is an infection involving the connective mediastinal tissue that fills the interpleural spaces and surrounds the mediastinal organs. It can be acute or chronic.

SYNONYMS

Fibrosing mediastinitis
Sclerosing mediastinitis
Granulomatous mediastinitis

ICD-10CM CODE
J98.5 Mediastinitis

EPIDEMIOLOGY

Acute mediastinitis (Box 1) occurs most frequently as a postoperative infection after a median sternotomy and can be a life-threatening infection. Most infections are bacterial in nature.

Chronic mediastinitis is a chronic form of infection in the mediastinum characterized by an invasive and compressive inflammatory infiltrate. It is mostly caused by fungi and some bacteria.

INCIDENCE: Incidence of postoperative mediastinitis ranges from 0.4 to 5%.

RISK FACTORS: Mediastinal infections have four possible sources:
- Direct contamination as seen in trauma or surgery (e.g., open heart, esophageal)
- Hematogenous or lymphatic spread
- Extension of infection from the neck or retroperitoneum
- Extension from the lung, pleura, or chest wall

PHYSICAL FINDINGS & CLINICAL PRESENTATION

- Patients with acute mediastinitis present with acute onset of fever, tachycardia, chest pain, dysphagia, or respiratory distress. There may be signs of sternal wound infection or cellulitis and/or crepitus and edema of the chest wall.
- Patients with chronic mediastinitis are mostly asymptomatic until symptoms develop related to invasion or obstructions of structures within the mediastinum or adjacent to the mediastinum, such as cough, dyspnea, wheezing, chest pain, dysphagia, or hemoptysis. Complications of chronic or sclerosing mediastinitis include:
  1. Superior vena cava syndrome. Histoplasma is the most common nonmalignant cause of this syndrome, marked by edema of face, neck and torso; neck vein distention; and headache.
  2. Pulmonary venous or arterial obstruction.
  3. Esophageal obstruction, cor pulmonale, constructive pericarditis.
  4. Thoracic duct obstruction.

BOX 1 Classification of Mediastinitis

Acute Mediastinitis
- A. Due to traumatic perforation of the esophagus
  1. Spontaneous or postemetic
  2. Foreign body–associated
  3. Instrumentation or surgery
- B. Due to extension of infection from adjacent structures
  1. Infection of the head and neck
  2. Infections of lungs, pleura, lymph nodes, or pericardium
  3. Subphrenic infection
  4. Vertebral osteomyelitis
  5. Hematogenous dissemination
- C. Postoperative

Chronic Mediastinitis

From Cherry JD et al: *Feigin and Cherry's textbook of pediatric infectious diseases*, ed 8, Philadelphia, 2019, Elsevier.

ETIOLOGY (TABLE 1)

Acute mediastinitis:
- Related to head and neck infections or esophageal perforation
  1. Anaerobic bacteria: *Peptostreptococci, Veillonella, Fusobacterium, Actinomyces, Prevotella, Eubacterium, Bacteroides*
  2. Aerobic bacteria: *Streptococcus, Staphylococcus, Corynebacterium, Moraxella*, enteric gram-negative rods
  3. Fungi: *Candida albicans*
  4. Related to cardiothoracic surgery
  5. Gram-positive bacteria: *Staphylococcus aureus, Staphylococcus epidermidis, Enterococcus, Streptococcus*
  6. Gram-negative bacteria: *Escherichia coli, Enterobacter, Klebsiella, Proteus, Pseudomonas*, other Enterobacteriaceae
  7. Fungi: *Candida albicans*

Chronic mediastinitis:
- *Histoplasma capsulatum,* a dimorphic fungus, is the most common and can cause mediastinal granuloma or fibrosing mediastinitis. A leakage of fungal antigens from lymph nodes into the mediastinal space is believed to cause a hypersensitivity reaction and subsequent exuberant fibrotic response.
- Other: *Mycobacterium tuberculosis, Nocardia,* actinomycosis, aspergillosis.

Dx DIAGNOSIS

DIFFERENTIAL DIAGNOSIS

For chronic mediastinitis:
- Tumors that can also cause superior vena cava syndrome (e.g., Hodgkin's and non-Hodgkin's lymphomas, mesothelioma)
- Sarcoidosis
- Behçet's syndrome
- Mediastinal fibrosis associated with radiation
- Silicosis

LABORATORY TESTS

- CBC with differential, C-reactive protein, and procalcitonin can point to bacterial infection
- Obtain cultures: Aerobic and anaerobic bacteria and fungi, intraoperatively or of any purulent drainage
- Pathologic examination: Distinguish between cancer and infection for chronic mediastinitis and allow for specific fungal stains on tissues

IMAGING STUDIES

- Chest x-ray: Can show diffuse mediastinal widening or evidence of mediastinal abscess, including gas bubbles or fluid level. Pneumomediastinum (Fig. E1) or pneumothorax can be seen with esophageal perforation (Table 2).
- Chest CT (Fig. E2): Can show the same as x-ray but is more sensitive in determining degree of mediastinal involvement and may guide drainage procedures for treatment or diagnosis.
- MRI may be superior to CT for sclerosing mediastinitis.

TABLE 1 Microbiology of Mediastinitis

Organisms Frequently Recovered in Mediastinitis Secondary to Infection of the Head and Neck or Esophageal Perforation

Anaerobic

Gram-positive cocci—*Peptostreptococcus* spp.
Gram-positive bacilli—*Actinomyces, Eubacterium, Lactobacillus*
Gram-negative cocci—*Veillonella*
Gram-negative bacilli—*Bacteroides* spp., *Fusobacterium* spp., *Prevotella* spp., *Porphyromonas* spp.

Aerobic or Facultative

Gram-positive cocci—*Streptococcus* spp., *Staphylococcus* spp.
Gram-positive bacilli—*Corynebacterium*
Gram-negative cocci—*Moraxella*
Gram-negative bacilli—Enterobacteriaceae, *Pseudomonas* spp., *Eikenella corrodens*
Fungi—*Candida albicans*

Representative Organisms Recovered in Mediastinitis Secondary to Cardiothoracic Surgery, with Representative Rate and Range

Gram-Positive Cocci

Staphylococcus aureus, 25% (7.1%-66.7%)
Staphylococcus epidermidis, 30% (6%-45.5%)
Enterococcus spp., 10% (8%-18.8%)
Streptococcus spp., 2% (0%-18.2%)

Gram-Negative Bacilli

Escherichia coli, 5% (0%-12.5%)
Enterobacter spp., 10% (4%-21.4%)
Klebsiella spp., 3% (0%-21.1%)
Proteus spp., 2% (0%-7.1%)
Other Enterobacteriaceae, 2% (0%-20%)
Pseudomonas spp., 2% (0%-54%)

Fungi

C. albicans, <2 (0%-20.5%)
Polymicrobial, 10% (0%-40%)

Others Occasionally Reported

Acinetobacter, Salmonella spp., *Legionella* spp., *Bacteroides fragilis, Corynebacterium* spp., *Burkholderia cepacia, Mycoplasma hominis, Candida tropicalis, Aspergillus* spp., *Nocardia* spp., *Kluyvera, Gordonia sputi, Mycobacterium fortuitum, Mycobacterium chelonae, Rhodococcus bronchialis*

Other Unusual Causes of Mediastinitis

Anthrax, brucellosis, actinomycosis, paragonimiasis, *Streptococcus pneumonia*

From Bennett JE et al: *Mandell, Douglas, and Bennett's principles and practice of infectious diseases*, ed 8, Philadelphia, 2015, Saunders.

TABLE 2 Risk Factors for Surgical Site Infection/Mediastinitis Post–Cardiac Surgery

Preoperative Risk Factors	Operative Risk Factors	Postoperative Risk Factors
Increasing age	Emergent surgery	Need for reexploration
Diabetes	Heart transplant	Prolonged ICU stay
Staphylococcus aureus nasal colonization	Increasing complexity of surgery	Need for mechanical ventilation >48 hr
Previous sternotomy	Use of internal thoracic arteries in CABG	Lack of perioperative glucose control
COPD	Prolonged operative time	Placement of tracheostomy
Peripheral vascular disease	Hair removal by razor, not clippers	Postoperative myocardial infarction
Class 3-4 angina	Inappropriate timing of antibiotics	Receipt of multiple blood products
Renal failure requiring hemodialysis	Prolonged time on cardiopulmonary bypass	Postoperative low cardiac output state
History of endocarditis	High core temperature during bypass (>38°C; 100.4° F)	
Cigarette smoking		
Low cardiac output		
Concurrent infection		
Prolonged preoperative hospitalization		
Preoperative use of a ventricular assist device		

CABG, Coronary artery bypass grafting; *COPD*, chronic obstructive pulmonary disease; *ICU*, intensive care unit.
From Bennett JE et al: *Mandell, Douglas, and Bennett's principles and practice of infectious diseases*, ed 8, Philadelphia, 2015, Saunders.

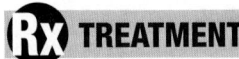

TREATMENT

NONPHARMACOLOGIC THERAPY

Surgery remains the gold standard treatment of mediastinitis for optimal drainage and debridement.

- Open techniques: Debridement of infected tissue and open packing of the wound with delayed closure or use of vacuum-assisted closure for acute mediastinitis
- Closed techniques: Debridement of infected tissues, closure of the sternum, and postoperative irrigation through drainage tubes for acute mediastinitis

ACUTE GENERAL Rx

- Intravenous antibiotics: Also a cornerstone of therapy but without surgery may fail. Broad-spectrum antibiotics should be used until cultures are finalized. Combination of piperacillin-tazobactam or meropenem plus vancomycin offers good initial coverage for acute mediastinitis. Other options include ciprofloxacin or cefepime for gram-negative rods, linezolid for gram-positive bacteria, metronidazole for anaerobic bacteria.
- Therapy is 2 to 3 wk, but some cases may require 4 to 6 wk.

CHRONIC Rx

There is no definitive cure for chronic fibrosing or sclerosing mediastinitis. Antifungal agents and steroids generally do not work. The goal of therapy is to palliate symptoms by relieving airway, vascular, or esophageal obstruction. Surgery in patients with extensive fibrosis has high morbidity and mortality.

DISPOSITION

Patients may need extensive wound care and possible vacuum-assisted closure and prolonged intravenous antibiotics.

REFERRAL

- Thoracic surgeon and/or head and neck surgeon for surgery and debridement
- Infectious diseases consultant for antibiotic selection and long-term management

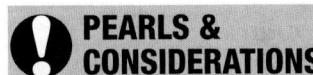

PEARLS & CONSIDERATIONS

COMMENTS

Histoplasma capsulatum is a dimorphic fungus found commonly in bird and bat fecal material and is most prevalent in the Ohio and Mississippi river valleys of the United States.

PREVENTION

Antibiotic prophylaxis should be given within 60 minutes before incision for surgeries requiring sternotomy. Options include cefazolin 1 g IV if <80 kg and 2 g if >80 kg, or cefuroxime 1.5 g IV. If the patient is penicillin allergic or has a history of methicillin-resistant *S. aureus* (MRSA) infection or surgery is to be done in a hospital where MRSA infection is common, use vancomycin 1 g IV.

SUGGESTED READINGS

Available online at ExpertConsult.com

AUTHOR: **GLENN G. FORT, M.D., M.P.H.**

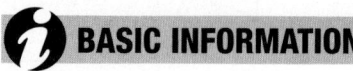

BASIC INFORMATION

DEFINITION

Medical cannabis refers to the use of cannabis or cannabinoids as medical therapy to treat disease or alleviate symptoms.

SYNONYMS

Medical cannabis
Cannabinoids
CBD
THC

ICD-10CM CODES

F12.9	Cannabis use, unspecified
Z02.79	Encounter for issue of other medical certificate
Z79.899	Other long term (current) drug therapy

BACKGROUND

- First medical marijuana law (MML) was enacted in California in 1996, allowing for use of medical cannabis despite lack of Food and Drug Administration (FDA) testing for safety and efficacy.
- In 2014, 0.8% of the U.S. population used medical marijuana exclusively, and 0.5% used medical and recreational marijuana.
- Of 2014 marijuana smokers, 6.2% used medical marijuana only and 3.6% used medical and recreational marijuana.
- In 2015, 1.57% U.S. population used medical marijuana; highest increase in prevalence noted to be in 2015.
- Residents of medical marijuana states were 1.3 times more likely to use medical marijuana in 2015 compared to 2013.
- As of July 2018, state-level referendum and legislation resulted in 31 U.S. states, DC, Guam, and Puerto Rico with policies that legalized marijuana use for medical purposes.

MECHANISM OF ACTION

- Cannabinoids elicit their effects by interacting with cannabinoid receptors in various central nervous system (CNS) locations, eliciting diverse CNS and peripheral nervous system (PNS) effects.
- Primarily bind to CB1 G-protein-coupled receptors in the basal ganglia, hippocampus, cortex, and cerebellum, eliciting antinociception, locomotor, and psychoactive effects.
- Marijuana contains roughly 60 plant-derived cannabinoid compounds, with the major phytocannabinoids being cannabidiol (CBD) and Δ^9-tetrahydrocannabinol (THC).

FORMULATIONS

Research has demonstrated a wide range of THC and CBD concentrations in various formulations, with frequent inaccurate labelling.

- Cigarettes
- Tinctures
- Capsules
- Vaporization cartridges
- Purified cannabinoids butane hash oil
- Supercritical fluid extracts (SFEs or "dabs")
- Buccal sprays
- Edibles
- Lozenges
- Transdermal patches

INDICATIONS

- Variable evidence for treatment of
  1. Chronic pain
  2. Chemotherapy-induced nausea/vomiting
  3. HIV related anorexia
  4. Glaucoma
  5. Anxiety
  6. Multiple sclerosis
  7. Seizures
- Marijuana has not been FDA approved as safe and effective for any indication and remains a Schedule I drug.
- However, there are phytocannabinoids and synthetic phytocannabinoid analogs that are FDA approved.
  1. Dronabinol and Nabilone (synthetic THC analogs) are schedule II FDA approved medications for AIDS associated anorexia and chemotherapy induced nausea, respectively.
  2. Purified cannabidiol (CBD) is FDA approved for seizures associated with Dravet or Lennox-Gastaut syndrome.
- Qualifying diagnoses for certification for prescription medical marijuana vary by state, but typically include
  1. Cancer
  2. Glaucoma
  3. HIV/AIDS
  4. Hepatitis C
  5. Cachexia
  6. Severe, debilitating, chronic pain
  7. Severe nausea
  8. Seizures
  9. Severe muscle spasms
  10. Crohn disease
  11. Alzheimer's disease
  12. PTSD
  13. Sickle cell disease

EFFICACY

- There is evidence in the medical literature demonstrating that marijuana improves non–cancer-related pain, chemotherapy-induced nausea and vomiting, and spasticity in multiple sclerosis.
  1. A 2011 systematic review of randomized controlled trials (RCTs) demonstrated statistically significant improvement in pain scores for non–cancer-related chronic pain in 15 of 18 trials with no serious adverse effects.
  2. A 2015 systematic review and meta-analysis showed improved response in nausea and vomiting compared to placebo (OR 3.82).
  3. A 2018 systematic review of systematic reviews demonstrated a decrease in nausea and vomiting following chemotherapy (RR 3.60 compared to placebo), improved spasticity with MS (RR 1.45 compared to placebo), and a modest benefit with primarily neuropathic pain (RR 1.37 compared to placebo) with frequent adverse effects including psychosis, "feeling high," and somnolence (number needed to harm = 5-8).
     a. No statistically significant improvement was noted in acute pain.
  4. A Cochrane review in 2013 found no statistically significant weight gain with dronabinol in HIV/AIDS patients, and multiple RCTs have identified megestrol acetate as superior to dronabinol for weight gain in cancer patients.

RISKS OF USE

- Marijuana use has been demonstrated to impair short-term memory consolidation, reaction time, and concept formation, and to increase incidence of road traffic accidents, ataxia, euphoria, disorientation, dry mouth, somnolence, and, at high doses, psychosis, panic, and paranoia.
- Meta-analyses demonstrate increased respiratory symptoms of cough, sputum production, and wheeze with smoking marijuana; however, there was no statistical difference in pulmonary function.
- Concomitant use of other medications such as opiates and benzodiazepines should be avoided as it could lead to somnolence and respiratory suppression.
- Medical marijuana should be stored away from children given the risk of toxic ingestion.

PRESCRIBING

- Marijuana remains classified as a schedule I drug under the Controlled Substance Act of 1970.
- However, the Justice Department declared it would not prosecute any physician who recommends medical marijuana for a legitimate medical indication in a state where it has been legalized.
- Medical marijuana card (MMC)
  1. MMC allows a patient to possess a certain amount of marijuana for medical use and not be prosecuted for possession of marijuana.
  2. In order to obtain an MMC, a patient must obtain physician certification confirming a clinical indication for medical marijuana.
  3. With an MMC, the patient can go to a licensed medical marijuana compassion center (dispensary), which will dispense a dose and formulation of medical marijuana appropriate for the patient's medical condition.
  4. Physicians do not prescribe the dose or formulation of medical marijuana.
- To certify a patient for a medical marijuana card, physicians must
  1. Complete a Department of Health certification form.
     a. Forms vary by state, but typically consist of a single-page form indicating a qualifying diagnosis that is to be signed by the physician.
  2. Complete and document a full medical history and physical exam.

3. Explain the risks, benefits, and side effects of medical marijuana.
4. Continue an ongoing role on the patient's health care team.
5. Maintain accurate medical records and documentation of the patient's clinical indication for medical marijuana.

- Some states require additional physician training and registration with the state medical marijuana program prior to being able to certify patients.
- Physicians are under no obligation to issue medical marijuana certifications.

PEARLS & CONSIDERATIONS

- Medical marijuana has been shown to improve non–cancer-related pain, chemotherapy-induced nausea and vomiting, and spasticity in multiple sclerosis.
    1. However, qualifying diagnoses for a medical marijuana card include cancer, glaucoma, HIV/AIDS, hepatitis C, cachexia, debilitating chronic pain, severe nausea, seizures, severe muscle spasms, Crohn disease, Alzheimer's disease, PTSD, and sickle cell disease. Qualifying diagnoses may vary from state to state.
    2. Adverse effects include increased incidence of road traffic accidents and pulmonary and cognitive side effects. At high doses, psychosis, panic, and paranoia can occur.
    3. Hospitals may also have specific restrictions and policies regarding medical marijuana for inpatient stays.
- Medical marijuana laws and regulations permit patients to use medical marijuana if certified by a physician but vary by state.
    1. Physician certification involves documentation that a patient has a qualifying clinical condition.
    2. A medical marijuana card entitles a patient or designated caregiver to possess a given amount of marijuana and therefore will not be prosecuted for possession of marijuana.
    3. Medical marijuana can be obtained at state regulated medical marijuana compassion centers (dispensaries). Compassion centers obtain marijuana from licensed cultivators and offer a variety of formulations that are regulated by the state.
    4. There is no FDA oversight of the compassion centers.
- Physicians do not prescribe the dose or formulation of medical marijuana.
- Physicians are under no obligation to issue medical marijuana certifications.

PATIENT/FAMILY EDUCATION

- Patients must possess a valid state-issued ID and apply for a state medical marijuana card.
- Patients can obtain medical marijuana from compassion centers without a medical marijuana card but could then be prosecuted for possession of marijuana.
- Patients should be aware that concomitant use of other medications such as opiates and benzodiazepines should be avoided as it could lead to somnolence and respiratory suppression.
- Patients should store medical marijuana away from children given the risk of toxic ingestions.

SUGGESTED READINGS

Available at ExpertConsult.com

RELATED CONTENT

Pain Management in Chronic Pain
Chemotherapy-Induced Nausea and Vomiting

AUTHORS: **ANJULIKA CHAWLA, M.D.,** and **SETH CLARK, M.D., M.P.H.**

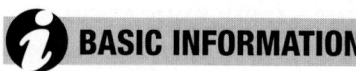

BASIC INFORMATION

DEFINITIONS

- **Classic Meigs syndrome:** A triad characterized by the presence of ascites and pleural effusion (usually right-sided) in association with a benign fibroma or fibroma-like ovarian tumor (thecoma, granulosa cell tumor, or Brenner tumor).
- **Nonclassic Meigs syndrome:** Characterized by ascites and pleural effusion in conjunction with a benign ovarian, fallopian tube, or broad ligament tumor that is not included in the definition of classic Meigs syndrome.
- **Pseudo-Meigs syndrome:** Characterized by both ascites and pleural effusion but caused by a pelvic or abdominal tumor, either benign or malignant, not included in either classic Meigs or nonclassic Meigs syndrome, such as leiomyomas, struma ovarii, mucinous cystadenoma, teratoma, and malignancies that are metastatic to the ovary (particularly colorectal cancer).
- **Pseudo-pseudo Meigs (Tjalma) syndrome:** Characterized by the triad of ascites, pleural effusion, and an elevated CA-125 (Cancer antigen 125) in a patient with systemic lupus erythematosus.

ICD-10CM CODES

C56.9	Malignant neoplasm of unspecified ovary
D27.9	Benign neoplasm of unspecified ovary
D28.2	Benign neoplasm of uterine tubes and ligaments
D28.7	Benign neoplasm of other specified female genital organs
J91.8	Pleural effusion in other conditions classified elsewhere
R18.0	Malignant ascites
R18.8	Other ascites

EPIDEMIOLOGY & DEMOGRAPHICS

- Occurs in 1% to 2% of ovarian fibromas (associated with approximately 0.004% of ovarian tumors)
- <1% progress to malignancy
- Incidence begins to increase in the 30s. Most frequently encountered in postmenopausal women (average age 50 yr)

PHYSICAL FINDINGS & CLINICAL PRESENTATION

- Abdominal bloating/increased girth
- Intermittent pelvic pain (intermittent torsion)
- Weight gain or loss
- Pelvic mass on bimanual examination
- Acute pelvic/abdominal tenderness
- Fluid wave
- Shifting dullness
- "Puddle sign" (physical exam maneuver)
- Hyperresonance or flatness to chest percussion, absence of tactile and vocal fremitus
- Absent or loud bronchial breath sounds, rales, mediastinal displacement, tracheal shift

ETIOLOGY

- Unknown
- Hypothesized to be due to "edematous" fibromas (or other benign ovarian solid tumors) in excess of 10 cm that may stimulate the peritoneal lining to produce peritoneal fluid
- Alternative theory of large fibroma with narrow stalk has inadequate lymphatic drainage; when coupled with intermittent torsion, results in backflow transudation into the peritoneal cavity
- Pleural effusion likely arises from passage of accumulated peritoneal ascites to the right pleural cavity via lymphatics (overloaded thoracic duct) or abdominal pleural commutation (i.e., foramen of Bochdalek)
    1. Fluid accumulation may be due to substances like vascular endothelial growth factor (VEGF) that raise capillary permeability

DIAGNOSIS

DIFFERENTIAL DIAGNOSIS

- Ovarian malignancy
- Various gynecologic disorders:
    1. Uterus: Endometrial tumor, sarcoma, leiomyoma ("pseudo-Meigs syndrome")
    2. Fallopian tube: Hydrosalpinx, granulomatous salpingitis, fallopian tube malignancy
    3. Ovary: Benign, serous, mucinous, endometrioid, clear cell, Brenner tumor, granulosa, stromal, dysgerminoma, fibroma, metastatic tumor
- Nongynecologic causes of abdominopelvic ascites:
    1. Portal vein obstruction
    2. Inferior vena cava obstruction
    3. Hypoproteinemia
    4. Thoracic duct obstruction
    5. Tuberculosis
    6. Amyloidosis
    7. Pancreatitis
    8. Gastrointestinal/genitourinary neoplasm
    9. Ovarian hyperstimulation
    10. Pleural effusion
    11. Congestive heart failure
    12. Collagen-vascular disease
    13. Cirrhosis

WORKUP

- Clinical condition characterized by ovarian mass, ascites, and predominantly right-sided pleural effusion
- History of early satiety, weight loss with increased abdominal girth, bloating, intermittent abdominal pain, dyspnea, and nonproductive cough

LABORATORY TESTS

- Complete blood count to rule out inflammatory process
- Tumor markers (CA-125, hCG, AFP, CEA, LDH) to evaluate gynecologic malignancy
- Chemical and liver function testing profile to evaluate metabolic or hepatic involvement
- Arterial blood gases if respiratory compromise

IMAGING STUDIES

- Pelvic sonography (color-flow Doppler evaluation of adnexal mass) initially to evaluate pelvic pathology (CT scan or MRI to further delineate neoplastic lesions)
- Chest x-ray to confirm pleural effusion

Procedures

- Paracentesis/thoracentesis will usually show a transudate

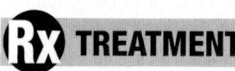

TREATMENT

NONPHARMACOLOGIC THERAPY

- Informed consent and proper preparation of patient for possible staging laparotomy (total abdominal hysterectomy and bilateral salpingo-oophorectomy, possible omentectomy, possible bowel resection, and possible pelvic/periaortic lymphadenectomy)
    1. Can consider unilateral salpingo-oophorectomy in reproductive-age women, whereas total hysterectomy is preferred in postmenopausal women
- Bowel prep if considering pelvic malignancy

ACUTE GENERAL TREATMENT

Depending on clinical presentation, size of pelvic mass, amount of ascites, and pleural effusion:

- If pelvic mass <10 cm with minimal ascites/ pleural effusion: Consider diagnostic laparoscopy (possible exploratory laparotomy) and salpingo-oophorectomy with removal of ovarian fibroma (tumor).
- If pelvic mass >10 cm with moderate/large amount ascites/pleural effusion: Consider pleurocentesis if respiratory compromise (cytology: AFB) and exploratory laparotomy with salpingo-oophorectomy and removal of ovarian tumor.
- Treat pelvic malignancy, gastrointestinal, or genitourinary tumor as indicated.

CHRONIC TREATMENT

- Resolution of ascites and pleural effusion after removal of ovarian tumor
- Routine gynecologic follow-up for benign ovarian tumor

DISPOSITION

Dramatic resolution of ascites and effusion within weeks of resection of pelvic mass is seen. Excellent progress and complete survival are expected. Recurrence rate is low.

REFERRAL

- To gynecologic oncologist for evaluation and treatment, especially if malignancy considered or encountered
- To pulmonologist for management of pleural effusion

SUGGESTED READING

Available at ExpertConsult.com

AUTHORS: **NIMA R. PATEL, M.D., M.S.,** and **TERRI Q. HUYNH, M.D.**

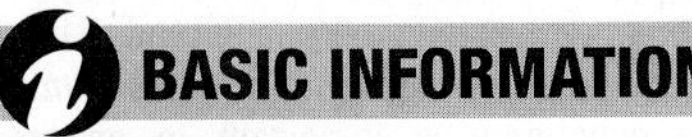

BASIC INFORMATION

DEFINITION

Melanoma is a skin neoplasm arising from the malignant degeneration of melanocytes. It is classically subdivided in four types:

1. Superficial spreading melanoma (70%)
2. Nodular melanoma (15% to 20%)
3. Lentigo maligna melanoma (5% to 10%) (Fig. 1)
4. Acral lentiginous melanoma (7% to 10%)

SYNONYMS

Malignant melanoma
Cutaneous malignant melanoma

ICD-10CM CODES

C43.9	Malignant melanoma of skin, unspecified
C43.30	Malignant melanoma of unspecified part of face
C43.31	Malignant melanoma of nose
C43.4	Malignant melanoma of scalp and neck
C43.51	Malignant melanoma of anal skin
C43.52	Malignant melanoma of skin of breast
C43.59	Malignant melanoma of other part of trunk
C43.8	Malignant melanoma of overlapping sites of skin
D03.8	Melanoma in situ of other sites
D03.9	Melanoma in situ, unspecified

EPIDEMIOLOGY & DEMOGRAPHICS

- In 2018, there were an estimated 91,270 new cases and 9,320 deaths in the U.S.; the estimated lifetime risk of development of melanoma is 1 in 50.
- Melanoma is much more common in whites (17.2 per 100,000 white men) than in African Americans (1 per 100,000 African American men). Increased risk of developing melanomas is found in patients with fair skin, red hair, light eyes, abundance of freckles, atypical moles or large amount of moles (>50). A personal history of any skin cancer or a family history of melanoma also increases the risk.
- Melanoma is the leading cause of death from skin cancer. Although it represents <10% of all skin-cancers, it accounts for at least 70% of deaths related to skin cancer.
- The median age at diagnosis is 53 yr.
- Superficial spreading melanoma occurs most often in young adults on sun-exposed areas.
- Acral lentiginous melanoma is most often found in Asian Americans and African Americans and is unrelated to sun exposure.
- 8% to 10% of melanomas arise in people with a family history of the disease.

PHYSICAL FINDINGS & CLINICAL PRESENTATION

Variable depending on the subtype of melanoma:

- Superficial spreading melanoma is most often found on the lower legs, arms, and upper back. It may have a combination of many colors or may be uniformly brown or black.
- Nodular melanoma can be found anywhere on the body, but it most frequently occurs on the trunk on sun-exposed areas. It has a dark-brown or red-brown appearance and can be dome shaped (Fig. 2) or pedunculated. Lesions are frequently misdiagnosed because they may resemble a blood blister or hemangioma and may also be amelanotic.
- Lentigo maligna melanoma is generally found in older adults in areas continually exposed to the sun and frequently arising from lentigo maligna (Hutchinson's freckle) or melanoma in situ. It might have a complex pattern and variable shape; color is more uniform than in superficial spreading melanoma.
- Acral lentiginous melanoma frequently occurs on soles, subungual mucous membranes, and palms (sole of the foot is the most prevalent site). Unlike other types of melanoma, it has a similar incidence in all ethnic groups.
- The warning signs that the lesion may be a melanoma can be summarized with the ABCDE mnemonic (Table 1):
  - **A:** Asymmetry (e.g., lesion is bisected and halves are not identical)
  - **B:** Border irregularity (uneven, ragged border) (Fig. E3)
  - **C:** Color variegation (presence of various shades of pigmentation)
  - **D:** Diameter enlargement (>6 mm)
  - **E:** Evolving (mole changing in size, shape, or color, or mole that differs visibly from surrounding moles ["ugly duckling" sign])

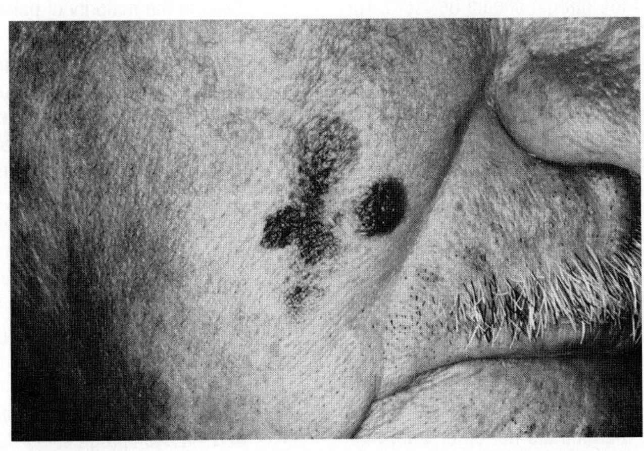

FIG. 1 Lentigo maligna melanoma. (From James WD, et al.: *Andrews' diseases of the skin: clinical dermatology*, ed 12, Philadelphia, 2016, Elsevier.)

ETIOLOGY

- Ultraviolet light is the most important cause of malignant melanoma.
- There is a modest increase in melanoma risk in patients with small nondysplastic nevi and a much greater risk in those with dysplastic lesions.
- The *CDKN2A* gene, residing at the *9p21* locus, is often deleted in patients with familial melanoma.
- A mutated signal transduction molecule, v-raf murine sarcoma viral oncogene homolog B (BRAF), has been identified in 40% to 60% of patients with melanoma.

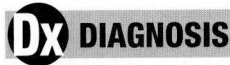

DIAGNOSIS

DIFFERENTIAL DIAGNOSIS

- Dysplastic nevi
- Solar lentigo
- Vascular lesions
- Blue nevus
- Basal cell carcinoma
- Seborrheic keratosis

WORKUP

- Dermoscopy (use of an instrument that shines polarized light on skin surfaces and magnifies skin lesions) can increase the accuracy in diagnosing melanoma by 10% to 27%.
- Any suspicious lesion (Fig. E4) should be biopsied. Perform excisional biopsy with elliptical excision that includes 1 to 2 mm of normal skin surrounding the lesion and extends to the subcutaneous tissue; incisional punch biopsy is sometimes necessary in surgically sensitive areas (e.g., digits, nose). It is essential that the size of the specimen be adequate to determine the histologic depth of penetration, which is known as the Breslow depth.
- Sentinel lymph node excision (SLNE) is the most important staging and potentially therapeutic procedure for patients with melanoma. It should be considered in patients with intermediate (1 to 4 mm) melanomas or high-risk skin tumors to obtain information regarding a patient's subclinical lymph node status with minimal morbidity. The National Comprehensive Cancer Network (NCCN) recommends that SLNE be discussed with and offered to patients classified as stage IB or II, and should be considered for patients with stage IA melanoma and "adverse" features that might portend a higher risk of sentinel node involvement (e.g., Clark level IV or V, tumor thickness of 0.75 mm or more, lymphovascular invasion, positive deep margins). SLNE involves the use of radiologic lymphoscintigraphy to map lymphatic drainage from the site of the primary melanoma to the first

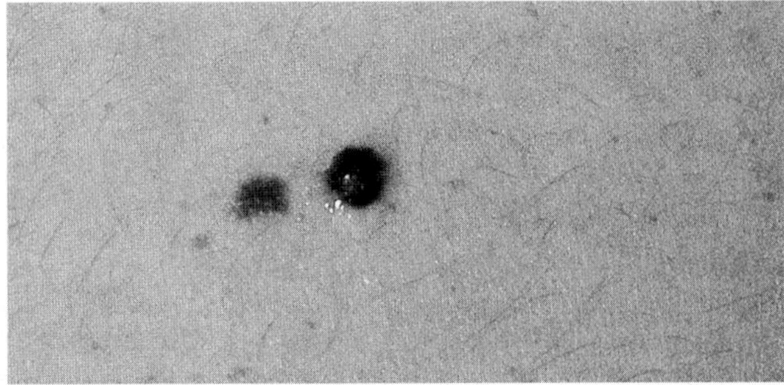

FIG. 2 Malignant melanoma (MM). This small, black papule was noted on this 10-year-old male with fair skin and red hair; excision confirmed a nodular MM. (From Paller AS, Mancini AJ: *Hurwitz clinical pediatric dermatology, a textbook of skin disorders of childhood and adolescence*, ed 5, Philadelphia, 2016, Elsevier.)

TABLE 1 Clinical Features (ABCDE Signs) of Malignant Melanoma

	Clinical Feature*	Comment
A	Asymmetry	The two halves of the lesion are not alike
B	Border irregularity	Borders notched, scalloped, irregular
C	Color changes	Especially blue, red, black, white
D	Diameter >6 mm	Size of a pencil eraser; not applicable to congenital nevi, which are often >6 mm early in their evolution
E	Enlargement	Evolutionary change in the lesion

*Original text (Paller, 2016) includes important discussion of features that may be more specific to pediatric melanoma.
From Paller AS, Mancini AJ: *Hurwitz clinical pediatric dermatology, a textbook of skin disorders of childhood and adolescence*, ed 5, Philadelphia, 2016, Elsevier.

sentinel lymph node in the region. When properly performed, if the sentinel node is negative the remaining lymph nodes in the region will not have metastases in more than 98% of cases. If the sentinel nodes are negative, no additional regional surgery is recommended. The staging of intermediate thickness (1.2-3.5 mm) primary melanomas, according to the results of sentinel node biopsy, provides important prognostic information and identifies patients with nodal metastases whose survival can be prolonged by immediate lymphadenectomy.

- The staging system for melanoma adapted by the American Joint Committee on Cancer (AJCC) can be found in Table 2.

LABORATORY TESTS

The pathology report should indicate the following:

- Tumor thickness (Breslow microstage).
- Tumor depth: The depth of invasion is the most important histologic prognostic parameter in evaluating the primary tumor.
- Mitotic rate: Tabulated as mitoses per square millimeter in the dermal part of the tumor in which most mitoses are identified.
- Radial growth rates versus vertical growth rate: Radial growth phase describes the growth of melanoma within the epidermis and along the dermal-epidermal junction.
- Tumor infiltrating lymphocytes have a strong predictive value in vertical growth phase melanomas and are defined as brisk, nonbrisk, or absent.
- Histologic regression: Characterized by the absence of melanoma in the epidermis and dermis flanked on one or both sides by melanoma.
- Reverse-transcription polymerase chain reaction assay for tyrosine messenger RNA is a useful marker for the presence of melanoma cells. It is performed on sentinel lymph node biopsy and is useful for detection of submicroscopic metastases.

Rx TREATMENT

- Initial excision of the melanoma
- Re-excision of the involved area after histologic diagnosis:
  1. The margins of re-excision depend on the Breslow depth. For melanoma in situ with Breslow depth ≤2.0 mm, recommended surgical margin is 1 cm. If Breslow depth is ≤2.0 mm, margin should be 2 cm. For melanoma in situ, margin should be 5 mm.
  2. Low-risk or intermediate-risk tumors require excision of 1 to 3 cm.
  3. Melanomas of moderate thickness (0.9-2.0 mm) can be excised safely with 2-cm margins.
  4. A 1-cm margin of excision for melanoma with a poor prognosis (as defined by a tumor thickness ≥2 mm) is associated with a significantly greater risk of regional recurrence than is a 3-cm margin, but with a similar overall survival rate. Randomized clinical trials have also shown that radical surgery with 2-cm excision margins did not differ from that with 4-cm margins for survival in patients with cutaneous melanoma >2 mm thick.
- Lymph node dissection: Recommended in all patients with enlarged lymph nodes. Lymph node evaluation is important in patients with melanoma 1 mm in depth because it determines the overall prognosis and need for therapeutic lymph node dissection or adjuvant treatment.
  1. Elective lymph node dissection remains controversial.
  2. It is indicated with positive sentinel node. It may be considered in those with a primary melanoma between 1 and 4 mm thick (especially in patients >60 yr).
- Adjuvant therapy:
  1. Interferon alfa-2b and Peginterferon alfa-2b have been previosuly used for the adjuvant treatment resected stage III melanoma despite modest benefits.
  2. Ipilimumab, an antibody that blocks cytotoxic T-lymphocyte–associated antigen 4 (CTLA-4), improves survival in stage III high-risk resected melanoma but is associated with significant immune adverse events.
  3. Immune checkpoint PD-1 (programmed death receptor-1) antibodies nivolumab and pembrolizumab have demonstrated superiority to ipilimumab in patients with resected high-risk stage III melanoma; currently only nivolumab is approved in this setting.
- Advanced disease:
  1. The use of immune checkpoint inhibitors has improved overall survival in patients with previously treated or untreated metastatic melanoma irrespective of BRAF mutation status. Monotherapy with the PD-1 inhibitors nivolumab or pembrolizumab has been approved for the treatment of metastatic melanoma in treatment-naïve patients and also in cases of progression after initial therapy with ipilimumab.
  2. Combination immunotherapy with the use of nivolumab and ipilimumab in previously untreated patients with unresectable or metastatic melanoma has been shown to be more effective than ipilimumab alone as first-line treatment in high-risk patients though severe immune toxicity is seen in the majority of patients.
  3. In patients who carry the V600E *BRAF* mutation, the current approach involves the use of oral BRAF inhibitors in combination with oral selective MEK inhibitors, with resultant improved rates of overall and progression-free survival in patients with previously untreated melanoma. Three such combination regimens (vemurafenib plus cobimetinib; dabrafenib plus trametinib; and encorafenib plus binimetinib) are approved by the FDA for use in this setting. Targeted therapy is useful in patients with rapidly growing melanoma with *BRAF* mutations, but resistance appears in almost all patients, and median progression-free survival is 15 to 18 mo. Interestingly, the majority of patients with melanoma CNS metastases

TABLE 2 The TNM Classification for Melanoma Adapted by the American Joint Committee on Cancer (AJCC, eighth edition)

T classification	Thickness	Ulceration status/mitoses
T_{is} (in situ)	n/a	n/a
T_1	<1.0 mm	Unknown or unspecified
T_{1a}	<0.8 mm	Without ulceration
T_{1b}	<0.8 mm 0.8-1.0 mm	With ulceration Without ulceration
T_2	>1.0-2.0 mm	Unknown or unspecified
T_{2a}	>1.0-2.0 mm	Without ulceration
T_{2b}	>1.0-2.0 mm	With ulceration
T_3	>2.0-4.0 mm	Unknown or unspecified
T_{3a}	>2.0-4.0 mm	Without ulceration
T_{3b}	>2.0-4.0 mm	With ulceration
T_4	>4.0 mm	Unknown or unspecified
T_{4a}	>4.0 mm	Without ulceration
T_{4b}	>4.0 mm	With ulceration
Regional nodes (N)	**Number of nodes**	**Presence of in-transit, satellite and/or microsatellite metastases**
N_0	0	None
N_1	One tumor-involved node or any number of in-transit, satellite, and/or microsatellite metastases with no tumor-involved nodes	
N_{1a}	One clinically occult (sentinel biopsy detected)	No
N_{1b}	One clinically detected	No
N_{1c}	No regional node	Yes
N_2	2 or 3 tumor-involved nodes or any number of in-transit, satellite, and/or microsatellite metastases with one tumor-involved node	
N_{2a}	2 or 3 clinically occult (sentinel biopsy detected)	No
N_{2b}	2 or 3, at least one clinically detected	No
N_{2c}	One clinically occult or clinically detected	yes
N_3	4 or more tumor-involved nodes or any number of in-transit, satellite, and/or microsatellite metastases with 2 or more tumor-involved nodes, or any number of matted nodes without or with in-transit, satellite, and/or microsatellite metastases	
N_{3a}	4 or more clinically occult (sentinel biopsy detected)	No
N_{3b}	4 or more, at least one of which was clinically detected, or the presence of any number of matted nodes	No
N_{3c}	2 or more clinically occult or clinically detected and/or presence of any number of matted nodes	Yes
M category	**Anatomic site**	**LDH level**
M_0	No distant metastases	n/a
M_1	Evidence of distant metastases	
M_{1a}	Distant metastasis to skin, soft tissue including muscle, and/or nonregional lymph node	$M_{1a}(0)$: Normal $M_{1a}(1)$: Elevated
M_{1b}	Distant metastasis to lung with or without M1a sites of disease	$M_{1b}(0)$: Normal $M_{1b}(1)$: Elevated
M_{1c}	Distant metastasis to non-CNS visceral sites with or without M1a or M1b sites of disease	$M_{1c}(0)$: Normal $M_{1c}(1)$: Elevated
M_{1d}	Distant metastasis to CNS with or without M_{1a}, M_{1b}, or M_{1c} sites of disease	$M_{1d}(0)$: Normal $M_{1d}(1)$: Elevated

CNS, Central nervous system; *LDH*, lactic dehydrogenase; *TNM*, tumor, nodes, metastases.

in this setting have similar response rates in the CNS as systemically.

- Patients with a history of melanoma should be followed up with skin examinations every 6 mo or sooner if patient detects any new lesions; the assessments usually consist of medical history, physical examination, laboratory values, and chest radiograph.

DISPOSITION

- Prognosis varies with the stage of the melanoma. The 5-yr survival related to thickness is as follows: <0.76 mm, 99% survival; 0.6 to 1.49 mm, 85%; 1.5 to 2.49 mm, 84%; 2.5 to 3.9 mm, 70%; >4 mm, 44%.
- The 5-yr survival in patients with distant metastasis was historically <10% but is improving with current therapeutic options and is now >20%.
- Treatment of advanced disease consists (in addition to surgical excision and lymph node dissection) of chemotherapy, immunotherapy, and radiation therapy. Nivolumab combined with ipilimumab has shown clinically meaningful activity in melanoma metastatic to the brain (see Tawbi HA, et al. in Suggested Readings).

SUGGESTED READINGS

Available at ExpertConsult.com

RELATED CONTENT

Melanoma (Patient Information)

AUTHOR: **BHARTI RATHORE, M.D.**

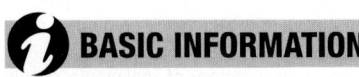

BASIC INFORMATION

DEFINITION

Ménière disease is a syndrome characterized by recurrent vertigo with fluctuating hearing loss, tinnitus, and fullness in the ear.

SYNONYMS

Endolymphatic hydrops
Lermoyez syndrome
Idiopathic endolymphatic hydrops

ICD-10CM CODES

H81.09 Ménière disease, unspecified ear
H81.01 Meniere disease, right ear
H81.02 Meniere disease, left ear
H81.03 Meniere disease, bilateral

EPIDEMIOLOGY & DEMOGRAPHICS

INCIDENCE (IN U.S.): Approximately 190/100,000 persons
PREDOMINANT SEX: Female:male ratio of 1.3:1
PEAK INCIDENCE: Fourth to sixth decade of life

PHYSICAL FINDINGS & CLINICAL PRESENTATION

- Hearing may be unilaterally decreased.
- Pallor, sweating, and nausea may occur during a severe attack.
- Usually the patient develops a sensation of fullness and pressure along with decreased hearing and tinnitus in a single ear.
- The patient typically experiences severe vertigo, which peaks within minutes, then slowly subsides over hours.
- May see spontaneous nystagmus on examination.
- Persistent sense of disequilibrium for days is typical after an acute episode.
- May have vestibulopathy demonstrable with a positive head thrust test.

ETIOLOGY

- Unknown; viral, autoimmune, and genetic causes have been suggested.
- Endolymphatic hydrops is the postmortem histologic hallmark. Endolymphatic hydrops may create cytochemical changes that disturb endolymphatic fluid homeostasis, leading to spiral ganglion cell death.

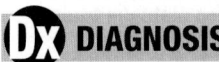

DIAGNOSIS

Proposed guidelines by the American Academy of Otolaryngology-Head and Neck Surgery (AAO-HNS) for diagnosis of Ménière disease:

DIFFERENTIAL DIAGNOSIS

- Acoustic neuroma
- Migrainous vertigo
- Multiple sclerosis
- Autoimmune inner ear syndrome
- Otitis media
- Vertebrobasilar disease
- Labyrinthitis

WORKUP

- Diagnosis is primarily made by history, although further diagnostic tests may help support the diagnosis. Guidelines to define Ménière disease are described in Table 1.
- Audiogram may show sensorineural hearing loss with lower frequencies primarily affected. Hearing loss may recover either partially or completely after an attack. Recurrent attacks may lead to a persistent and progressive sensorineural hearing loss.
- Electronystagmography may show peripheral vestibular deficit.
- Both vestibular-evoked myogenic potential (VEMP) studies and electrocochleography (ECoG) have low sensitivity and specificity for Ménière disease and are not clinically useful.

LABORATORY TESTS

No laboratory serologic test is specific for Ménière disease. A thyroid panel, glucose, hemoglobin A1C, antinuclear antibodies, urinalysis, chemistry panel, rapid plasma reagin, Lyme disease antibodies, and allergy testing can be ordered to screen for other disorders such as thyroid or autoimmune diseases, diabetes, otorenal syndrome, syphilis, Lyme disease, and allergy-mediated Ménière disease.

TABLE 1 Guidelines to Define Ménière Disease

Definition	Symptoms
Certain Ménière disease	Histopathologic confirmation
Definite Ménière disease	≥2 definitive spontaneous episodes of vertigo 20 min to 12 hours Audiometrically documented low- to medium-frequency sensorineural hearing loss in one ear, defining the affected ear on at least one occasion before, during, or after one of the episodes of vertigo Fluctuating aural symptoms (hearing, tinnitus, or fullness) in the affected ear Not better accounted for by another vestibular diagnosis
Probable Ménière disease	One definite episode of vertigo Audiometrically documented hearing loss on at least one occasion Tinnitus or aural fullness in the treated ear Other causes excluded
Possible Ménière disease	Episodic vertigo without documented hearing loss, or sensorineural hearing loss (SNHL) fluctuating or fixed, with disequilibrium but nonepisodic Other causes excluded

IMAGING STUDIES

- MRI to rule out acoustic neuroma or other retrocochlear lesion, especially if cerebellar or CNS dysfunction is present.
- Recent efforts have shown a role for MRI with intratympanic gadolinium.

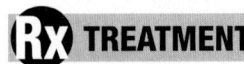

TREATMENT

NONPHARMACOLOGIC THERAPY

Limit activity during attacks.

ACUTE GENERAL Rx

- Prochlorperazine 5 to 10 mg PO q6h or 25 mg PO bid
- Promethazine 12.5 to 25 mg PO q4 to 6h
- Diazepam 5 to 10 mg IV/PO for acute attack
- Meclizine 25 mg q6h
- Scopolamine patch

CHRONIC Rx

- Diuretics such as furosemide, hydrochlorothiazide, or acetazolamide.
- Lifestyle modification recommendations include salt restriction and avoidance of caffeine.
- For refractory cases, intratympanic gentamicin injections to the affected ear; endolymphatic sac surgery.

DISPOSITION

- Patients are usually followed by an otoneurologist or ENT specialist.
- Usual course of disease consists of alternating attacks and remissions.
- Majority of patients can be managed medically. Of all patients, 10% to 30% will undergo surgical intervention for persistent incapacitating vertigo.

REFERRAL

To an otolaryngologist for surgical intervention if attacks persist despite medical therapy

SUGGESTED READINGS

Available at ExpertConsult.com

RELATED CONTENT

Ménière Disease (Patient Information)

AUTHORS: **KATHERINE KOSTROUN, B.S., JOSEPH S. KASS, M.D., J.D.,** and **SHARON S. HARTMAN POLENSEK, M.D., PH.D.**

BASIC INFORMATION

DEFINITION

Meningiomas are generally slow-growing tumors arising from arachnoid cells of the arachnoid villi; 90% are benign.

ICD-10CM CODE

D32.0 Benign neoplasm of cerebral meninges

EPIDEMIOLOGY & DEMOGRAPHICS

INCIDENCE: 6/100,000 persons/yr; Most common primary type of central nervous system tumor.

PREDOMINANT SEX AND AGE: Female/male ratio of almost 3:1 in the brain and up to 6:1 in the spinal cord; 1:1 in childhood

PEAK INCIDENCE: Males: Sixth decade, females: Seventh decade, incidence increases with age; rare in childhood

RISK FACTORS: Ionizing radiation results in increased incidence and a shorter latency period. Neurofibromatosis type 2 (NF2) is an autosomal dominant genetic disorder that predisposes to multiple intracranial tumors. Approximately half of all individuals with NF2 have meningiomas, most of which are intracranial. Studies have suggested a link between hormonal factors and development of meningioma. At present, there is no conclusive evidence to support a causal relationship with cell phone usage and subsequent development of meningioma.

GENETICS: Meningiomas may be isolated or found in association with other genetic diseases, such as NF2 and familial meningioma. Approximately half of meningiomas have allelic losses involving the *NF2* and *DAL-1* genes. Allelic losses of chromosomes 1p, 2p, 6q, 9q, 10q, 14q, 17p, and 18q may be associated with histologic progression.

PHYSICAL FINDINGS & CLINICAL PRESENTATION

- Neurologic symptoms vary with location and size (see Table 1); meningiomas can arise from the dura at any site, although they most commonly occur within the skull and at sites of dural reflection (i.e., the cerebral convexities and the falx). Other less common locations include the sphenoid wing, olfactory groove, and optic nerve sheath.
- The presence of focal symptoms such as vision loss, hearing loss, or mental status change depend on the site of origin and the time course of growth.
- Most common presentation is with a focal or generalized seizure or gradually worsening neurologic deficit. Seizures are present preoperatively in 30% to 40%.
- Typically are slow growing and asymptomatic; many meningiomas are asymptomatic and/or discovered incidentally on a neuroimaging study or at autopsy.

ETIOLOGY

- Meningiomas are thought to arise from a multistep progression of genetic changes.
- Mutations of the *NF2* gene on chromosome 22 are found in patients with neurofibromatosis type 2 and >50% of sporadic meningiomas. This gene is thought to act as a tumor suppressor gene; the protein product, merlin, is also involved in cytoskeletal organization.
- *DAL-1*, located on chromosome 18p, is another tumor suppressor gene that has been identified in a subset of the approximately 40% of sporadic meningiomas with neither the *NF2* gene mutations nor allelic loss of chromosome 22q.
- Cranial radiation may be responsible for some cases following an appropriate latency period from 10 to 20 years. Meningiomas that result from radiation are generally more aggressive.
- The link with steroid hormones and their receptors is suggested by the increase in growth rate and/or development of meningiomas during pregnancy, increased incidence in women who use postmenopausal hormones, and in association with breast carcinomas.

DIAGNOSIS

DIFFERENTIAL DIAGNOSIS

Other well-circumscribed intracranial tumors that involve the dura or subdural space:

- Acoustic schwannoma (typically at the pontocerebellar junction)
- Ependymoma, lipoma, and metastases within spinal cord
- Metastatic disease from lymphoma/adenocarcinoma
- Inflammatory disease such as sarcoidosis and Wegener granulomatosis
- Infections such as tuberculosis

WORKUP

Imaging studies with CT or MRI, followed by surgical removal with histologic confirmation

LABORATORY TESTS

According to the World Health Organization (WHO) classification, there are nine benign histologic variants (account for 90% of all meningiomas) and four variants associated with increased recurrence and rates of metastasis. Ninety percent of meningiomas are classified as benign meningiomas or WHO grade I.

IMAGING STUDIES

- Cranial CT scanning or MRI can detect and determine the extent of meningiomas (Fig. 1). CT can show hyperostosis and/or intratumoral calcifications. MRI with contrast (Fig. 2) is the imaging modality of choice to demonstrate the dural origin of the tumor in most cases, with the characteristic "tail" sign that tracks along the dura outside brain parenchyma.
- On nonenhanced scans, meningiomas are typically isodense or slightly hyperdense to brain and are homogeneous in appearance. They show homogeneous contrast enhancement; gadolinium can facilitate imaging of smaller additional lesions that are missed on unenhanced images.
- Indistinct margins, marked edema, mushroomlike projections from tumor, brain parenchymal infiltration, and heterogeneous enhancement are suggestive of more aggressive behavior.
- Positron emission tomography (PET) scan may help in predicting the aggressiveness of the tumor and the potential for recurrence, but it is not used routinely.

TREATMENT

Primary management depends on signs or symptoms, age of patient, and location and size of tumor. Observation may be appropriate if tumors are discovered incidentally and/or if growth is indolent and unlikely to cause symptoms.

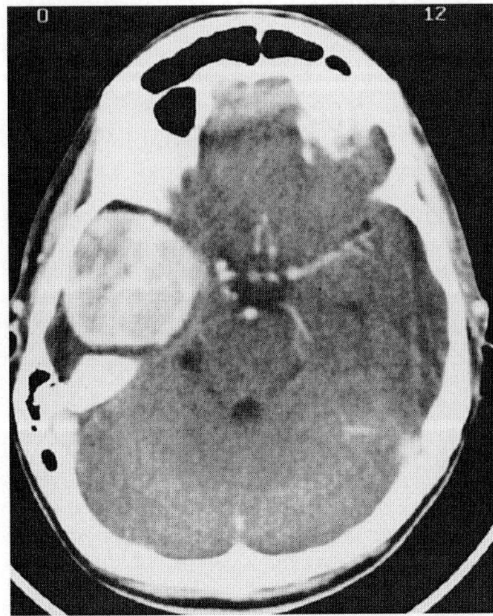

FIG. 1 Contrast-enhanced computed tomography scan demonstrates a large contrast-enhancing right sphenoid wing meningioma. (From Specht N [ed]: *Practical guide to diagnostic imaging,* St Louis, 1998, Mosby.)

TABLE 1 Locations and Presentations of Meningiomas

Location	Presenting Manifestation
Parasagittal	Urinary incontinence, dementia, gradual paraparesis, seizures
Lateral convexity	Variable depending on structures compressed, including slow hemiparesis, speech abnormalities
Olfactory groove	Anosmia, visual disturbance, dementia, Foster-Kennedy syndrome
Suprasellar	Hormonal failure, bitemporal hemianopsia, optic atrophy
Sphenoid ridge	Extraocular nerve paresis, exostoses, proptosis, seizures

From Goetz CG, Pappert EJ: *Textbook of clinical neurology,* Philadelphia, 1999, Saunders.

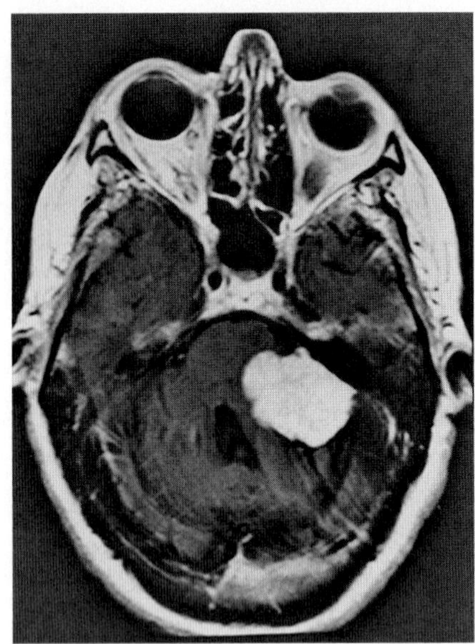

FIG. 2 Magnetic resonance imaging picture of a posterior fossa meningioma, demonstrated an extra-axial homogeneously contrast-enhanced mass arising from the tentorium and compressing the cerebellar hemisphere. (From Goetz CG, Pappert EJ: *Textbook of clinical neurology,* Philadelphia, 1999, Saunders.)

PHARMACOLOGIC THERAPY

- Although a variety of chemotherapeutic agents have been studied, such as hydroxyurea, there is no established effective systemic therapy.
- Inhibition of hormone receptors, such as progesterone, estrogen, and androgen, has failed to demonstrate clinical benefit.
- Treatment with molecularly targeted approaches, such as angiogenesis inhibition, is currently under way.

NONPHARMACOLOGIC THERAPY

- The mainstay of treatment for meningiomas remains surgical removal. Complete resection is usually attempted, when feasible. After total excision, recurrence rates of 0% to 20% have been observed, while 20% to 50% of patients recur within 5 yr of a subtotal resection.
- Active surveillance to monitor for tumor recurrence is important.
- Radiation therapy is the only validated form of adjuvant therapy and may be beneficial in patients with incomplete resections or inoperable tumors. Stereotactic radiosurgery can provide local control with more limited toxicity.

ACUTE GENERAL Rx

- For lesions that cause significant mass effect, steroids are sometimes used to decrease brain edema.
- Anticonvulsants are used if the patient presents with seizures.

CHRONIC Rx

- Prophylactic use of anticonvulsants is not recommended in patients without a history of seizures.
- There is limited data on the efficacy of traditional chemotherapy, and the evidence is largely anecdotal. The most extensively evaluated agents are hydroxyurea, mifepristone (RU486), and interferon alfa-2b. Recently, somatostatin analogs have been evaluated in multicenter clinical trials.

DISPOSITION

- Estimated surgical mortality is 7%. Significant morbidity and mortality can be observed in meningiomas with otherwise favorable pathology secondary to unfavorable location (e.g., skull base).
- Long-term outcome varies based on pathology, tumor grade, location, and completeness of resection.
- Most incidentally discovered meningiomas remain asymptomatic and have a slow rate of growth. Calcified tumors may be less likely to progress than noncalcified ones.
- Meningiomas may recur after surgical resection or progress to a higher grade. Risk factors for recurrence include multiple allelic chromosomal losses, local brain invasion, high rate of mitosis, and highly anaplastic features.

REFERRAL

- Neurosurgical consultation for all cases
- Neurology, radiation oncology, and oncology consults depending on presence of other sequelae or in the setting of recurrence

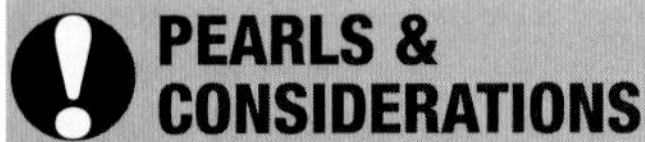

PEARLS & CONSIDERATIONS

COMMENTS

- Many meningiomas are discovered incidentally; most are benign and remain asymptomatic. A first follow-up MRI should be performed 3 to 6 mo after the tumor is identified to rule out an atypical meningioma with rapid growth.
- "Dural tail," which is the thickening of the dura adjacent to the mass, is a classic finding on neuroimaging studies.
- Individuals with neurofibromatosis type 2 are at high risk to develop meningiomas.

PATIENT & FAMILY EDUCATION

Meningioma mommas: meningiomamommas.org
Meningioma Support and Patient Information Group
National Brain Tumor Society
Meningioma Online Support Group: brainstrust.org/meningioma.htm

SUGGESTED READINGS

Available at ExpertConsult.com

RELATED CONTENT

Meningioma (Patient Information)

AUTHORS: **DANYELLE EVANS, M.D., JOSEPH S. KASS, M.D., J.D.,** and **NICOLE J. ULLRICH, M.D., PH.D.**

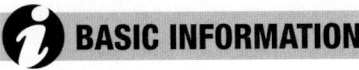

BASIC INFORMATION

DEFINITION

Bacterial meningitis is an inflammation of meninges with increased intracranial pressure, and pleocytosis or increased WBCs in cerebrospinal fluid (CSF) secondary to bacteria in the pia-subarachnoid space and ventricles, leading to neurologic sequelae and abnormalities.

SYNONYMS

Spinal meningitis
Bacterial meningitis

ICD-10CM CODES

G00.9	Bacterial meningitis, unspecified
G00.8	Other bacterial meningitis
G01	Meningitis in bacterial diseases classified elsewhere

EPIDEMIOLOGY & DEMOGRAPHICS

INCIDENCE (IN U.S.): 1.3 to 2.0 cases/100,000 persons; 1.2 million cases per year in the world; 135,000 deaths annually worldwide. The rate of bacterial meningitis declined dramatically in the U.S. starting in the early 1990s with the introduction of the *Haemophilus influenzae* type b (Hib) vaccine and in 2000 with the introduction of the conjugate pneumococcal vaccine.
PREDOMINANT SEX: Male = female
PREDOMINANT AGE: All ages, neonate to geriatric

PHYSICAL FINDINGS & CLINICAL PRESENTATION

- Fever
- Headache
- Neck stiffness, nuchal rigidity, meningismus
- Altered mental state, lethargy
- Vomiting, nausea
- Photophobia
- Seizures
- Coma; lethargy, stupor
- Rash: Petechial and purpuric lesions (Fig. E1) associated with meningococcal infection, purpura fulminans
- Myalgia
- Cranial nerve abnormality (unilateral)
- Papilledema
- Dilated, nonreactive pupil(s)
- Posturing: Decorticate/decerebrate
- Physical examination findings of Kernig sign and Brudzinski sign (Fig. E2) in adults with meningitis are often seen later in the course of disease and may not be helpful in determining early meningeal inflammation

ETIOLOGY

The bacterial etiology of meningitis depends on the age of the patient. *Neisseria meningitidis* is now more common than *Haemophilus influenzae* as a cause of bacterial meningitis in children as well as adults, and streptococci (*streptococcus pneumoniae*) are still common causes of community-acquired bacterial meningitis. *H. influenzae* is the cause of >30% of cases of meningitis (usually in infants and children <6 yr of age). It is associated with sinusitis, otitis media.

- Neonates: Group B streptococcus, gram-negative rods such as *E. coli, Listeria monocytogenes*
- Infants ≥1 mo and <3 mo: Group B streptococci (40%), gram-negative rods (30%), *Streptococcus pneumoniae* (14%), and *Neisseria meningitidis* (12%)
- Infants ≥3 mo and <3 yr:
  1. *S. pneumoniae* (45%)
  2. *N. meningitidis* (34%)
  3. *S. agalactiae* (group B streptococci) (11%)
  4. *H. influenzae*
  5. *E. coli*
- Ages ≥3 yr and <10 yr:
  1. *S. pneumoniae* (47%)
  2. *N. meningitidis* (32%)
- Ages ≥10 yr and <19 yr
  1. *N. meningitidis* (55%)
  2. S. pneumoniae
- Adults: *S. pneumoniae, N. meningitidis,* and *streptococcus agalactiae* (third most common cause in adults).
- *L. monocytogenes* is uncommon in the general population but is often seen in older adults and in those with cell-mediated immune deficiencies.
- People with HIV/AIDS are at increased risk for invasive meningococcal disease (IMD).

DIAGNOSIS

Diagnostic approach is based on patient presentation and physical examination (Fig. 3). Lumbar puncture should be performed as soon as possible. Key elements to diagnosis are CSF evaluation and CT scan or MRI if the patient is in a coma or has focal neurologic deficits, pupillary abnormalities, or papilledema. Table 1 describes tests of CSF in patients with suspected CNS infection.

DIFFERENTIAL DIAGNOSIS (BOX E1)

- Endocarditis, bacteremia
- Intracranial tumor
- Lyme disease
- Brain abscess
- Partially treated bacterial meningitis
- Medications
- SLE
- Seizures
- Acute mononucleosis
- Other infectious meningitides
- Neuroleptic malignant syndrome
- Subdural empyema
- Subarachnoid hemorrhage (Table 2)
- Rocky Mountain spotted fever

WORKUP

CSF examination (Table 3):
- Opening pressure >100 to 200 mm Hg
- WBC usually >1000/mm^3
- Neutrophilic predominance: >80%
- Gram stain of CSF: Positive in 60% to 90% of patients
- CSF protein: >50 mg/dl
- CSF glucose: <40 mg/dl
- Culture: Positive in 65% to 90% of cases
- Multiplex PCR assay for detection of *S. pneumoniae, H. influenca, N. meningitidis,* and *L. monocytogenes* offer 100% sensitivity and 98% specificity.

LABORATORY TESTS

Blood culturing, WBC with differential, and CSF examination (see "Workup")

IMAGING STUDIES

- Guidelines from the Infectious Society of America recommend CT of brain before lumbar puncture in patients presenting with:
  1. A high clinical suspicion for subarachnoid hemorrhage
  2. New focal neurologic deficit
  3. Papilledema
  4. Seizures within a week
  5. Altered mental status
  6. History of central nervous system disease (e.g., tumor, stroke)
  7. Immunodeficiency
  8. Age 60 or older

TREATMENT

Empiric therapy is necessary with IV antibiotic treatment if patient has purulent CSF fluid at time of lumbar puncture, is asplenic, or has signs of DIC/sepsis pending gram stain and culture results. Try to obtain blood and CSF cultures before starting antimicrobial therapy, but do not delay therapy if obtaining them is not possible. If CT scan is indicated (see "Imaging Studies" for indications) it should not delay empiric antibiotic therapy. Therapy after gram stain pending cultures is recommended for the following:

- Neonates: Ampicillin: 200 to 400 mg/kg per day divided q6 to 8 hr plus gentamicin: 7.5 mg/kg IV in three divided doses plus a third-generation cephalosporin: cefotaxime or ceftriaxone
- 1 to 23 mo: Vancomycin: 60 mg/kg per day IV (maximum up to 4 g/day) divided in four doses plus third-generation cephalosporin: Ceftriaxone: 100 mg/kg (maximum dose 4 g/day) in one or two divided doses or cefotaxime: 300 mg/kg per day IV (maximum dose of 12 g/day) in three or four divided doses
- Children: Vancomycin: 60 mg/kg per day IV (maximum dose 4 g/day) in four divided doses plus third-generation cephalosporin: Ceftriaxone 100 mg/kg per day IV (maximum 4 g/day) or cefotaxime: 300 mg/kg IV (maximum dose of 12 g/day) in three or four divided doses
- Adults: Vancomycin: 15 to 20 mg/kg IV every 8 to 12 hours plus third-generation cephalosporin: Ceftriaxone: 2 g IV q12 hours or cefotaxime: 2 g IV q4 to 6 hr. For adults over 50 yr of age also add ampicillin 2 g IV every 4 hr to cover *Listeria*
- Immunocompromised patients: Vancomycin *plus* ampicillin *plus* either cefepime 2 g IV every 8 hr to cover *Pseudomonas* or meropenem 2 g IV q8 hr for adults, which also covers *Pseudomonas*

Use of corticosteroids in adults:
1. Dexamethasone 0.15 mg/kg q6h for first 4 days of therapy should be used for adults in developed countries with known or suspected bacterial meningitis. Decreased mortality and neurologic sequelae are seen with adjunct therapy. The benefit of dexamethasone is less clear in developing countries with high HIV prevalence and malnutrition or with delayed clinical presentations.

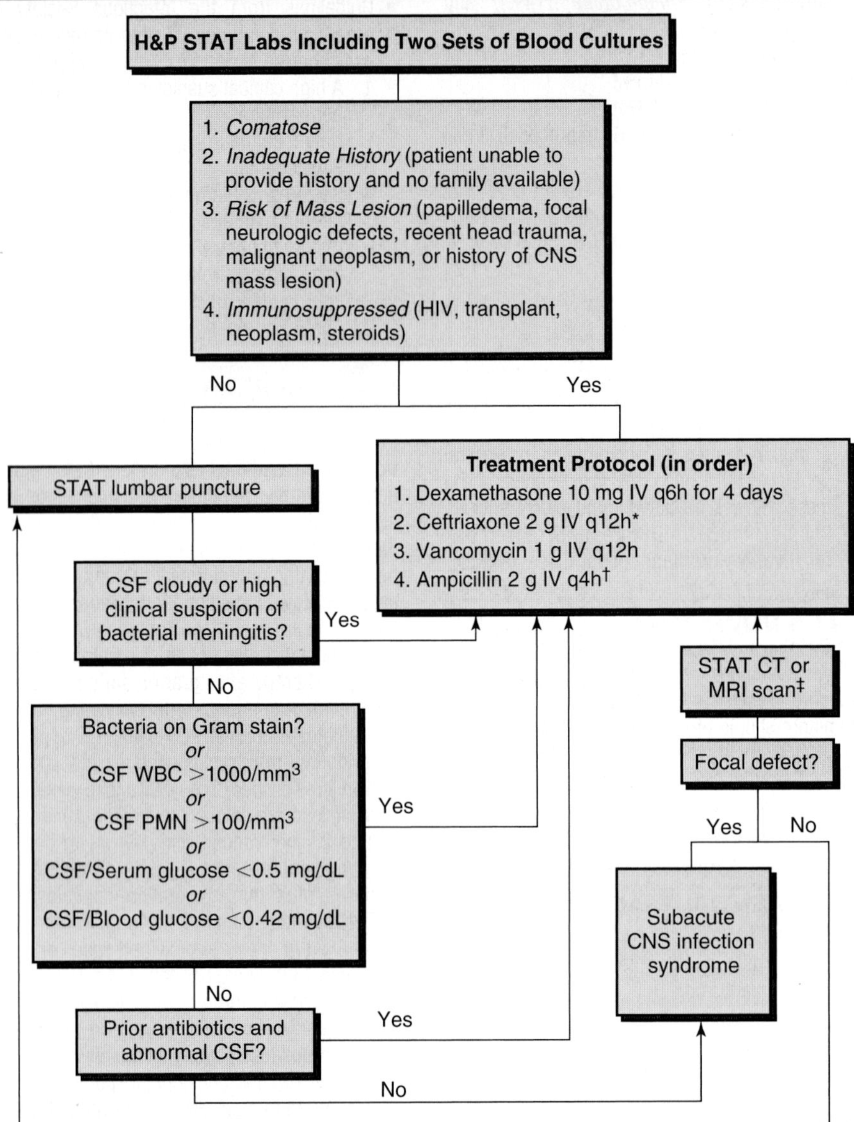

FIG. 3 Algorithm for management of adult patients with acute meningitis syndrome. *For severe cephalosporin allergy, consider meropenem or moxifloxacin. †Ampicillin is indicated if there is a history of alcoholism, organ transplant, malignancy, pregnancy, or age older than 50 years. For penicillin-allergic patients, an alternative is trimethoprim-sulfamethoxazole. ‡Consider magnetic resonance imaging *(MRI)* if the patient is known or suspected to have human immunodeficiency virus *(HIV),* if it can be obtained rapidly. *CNS,* Central nervous system; *CSF,* cerebrospinal fluid; *CT,* computed tomography; *H&P,* history and physical examination; *PMN,* polymorphonuclear leukocyte; *WBC,* white blood cell. (From Vincent JL et al: *Textbook of critical care,* ed 6, Philadelphia, 2011, Saunders.)

2. Dexamethasone also benefits children with Hib meningitis if given at the same time or before the first dose of the antibiotic: 0.15 mg/kg per dose q6 hr for 2 to 4 d. The use and benefit of corticosteroids in suspected or pneumococcal or meningococcal meningitis to prevent neurologic sequelae is not as clear and should be individualized after analysis of risk and benefits.

DISPOSITION

Bacterial meningitis is a reportable disease that needs to be reported to local health authorities. Droplet precautions should be used for first 24 hr of therapy for suspected or confirmed *N. meningitidis* infection.

REFERRAL

- To a neurologist if persistent neurologic sequelae develop after bacterial meningitis
- To an infectious disease consultant if a patient has recurrent bacterial meningitis; such patients deserve a workup for an anatomic (CSF dural leak) or immunologic defect (complement defect, hyposplenism, immunoglobulin deficiency)

TABLE 1 Tests of Cerebrospinal Fluid in Patients with Suspected Central Nervous System Infection

Routine Tests
White blood cell count with differential
Red blood cell count[a]
Glucose concentration[b]
Protein concentration
Gram stain
Bacterial culture
Selected Specific Tests Based on Clinical Suspicion
Viral culture[c]
Smears and culture for acid-fast bacilli
Venereal Disease Research Laboratory (VDRL)
India ink preparation
Cryptococcal polysaccharide antigen
Fungal culture
Antibody tests (IgM or IgG, or both)[d]
Nucleic acid amplification tests (e.g., polymerase chain reaction)[e]
Cytology[f]
Flow cytometry

[a]Should be checked in the first and last tubes; in patients with a traumatic tap, there should be a decrease in the number of red blood cells with continued flow of cerebrospinal fluid (CSF). See text for the formula for determining whether the numbers of CSF red blood cells and white blood cells are consistent with a traumatic tap.
[b]Compare with serum glucose drawn just before lumbar puncture.
[c]Yield of viral culture may be low.
[d]May be useful for specific causes of meningitis and encephalitis.
[e]Most useful for specific viral causes of encephalitis and causes of chronic meningitis.
[f]In patients with suspected malignancy.
From Bennett JE, Dolin R, Blaser MJ: *Mandell, Douglas, and Bennett's principles and practice of infectious diseases*, ed 8, Philadelphia, 2015, Saunders.

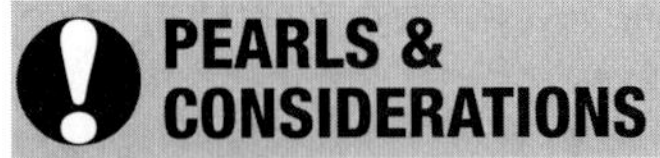

PEARLS & CONSIDERATIONS

COMMENTS

- Nosocomial bacterial meningitis may result from invasive procedures (e.g., placement of ventricular catheters, lumbar puncture, craniotomy, spinal anesthesia). Treatment of this different spectrum of microorganisms requires empirical antimicrobial therapy with vancomycin plus either cefepime, ceftazidime, or meropenem. In cases of basilar skull fracture, effective empirical antimicrobial therapy consists of vancomycin plus a third-generation cephalosporin.
- False-positive elevations of CSF where blood cell counts can be found after traumatic lumbar puncture or in patients with intracerebral or subarachnoid hemorrhage in which RBCs and WBCs are introduced into the

TABLE 2 Acute Bacterial Meningitis and Subarachnoid Hemorrhage

Finding	Frequency (%)
Acute Bacterial Meningitis	
Neck stiffness	84
Fever	66-97
Altered mental status	55-95
Kernig or Brudzinski sign	61
Focal neurologic signs	9-37
Seizures	5-28
Petechial rash	3-52
Subarachnoid Hemorrhage	
Neck stiffness	21-86
Seizures	7-32
Altered mental status	29-64
Focal neurologic findings	10-36
Fever	6
Preretinal hemorrhage	4

Diagnostic standard: For *meningitis*, cerebrospinal fluid pleocytosis and microbiologic or postmortem data supporting bacterial meningitis; for *subarachnoid hemorrhage*, computed tomography or lumbar puncture.
From McGee, S: *Evidence-based physical diagnosis*, ed 4, Philadelphia, 2018, Elsevier.

TABLE 3 Typical Cerebrospinal Fluid Findings in Patients with Selected Infectious Causes of Meningitis

Cause of Meningitis	White Blood Cell Count (cells/mm^3)	Primary Cell Type	Glucose (mg/dl)	Protein (mg/dl)
Viral	50-1000	Mononuclear[a]	>45	<200
Bacterial	1000-5000[b]	Neutrophilic[c]	<40[d]	100-500
Tuberculous	50-300	Mononuclear[e]	<45	50-300
Cryptococcal	20-500[f]	Mononuclear	<40	>45

[a]May be neutrophilic early in presentation.
[b]Range from <100 to >10,000 cells/mm^3.
[c]About 10% of patients have cerebrospinal fluid lymphocyte predominance.
[d]Should always be compared with a simultaneous serum glucose; ratio of CSF to serum glucose is ≤0.4 in most cases.
[e]May see a "therapeutic paradox," in which a mononuclear predominance becomes neutrophilic during antituberculous therapy.
[f]More than 75% of patients with acquired immunodeficiency syndrome have <20 cells/mm^3.
From Bennett JE, Dolin R, Blaser MJ: *Mandell, Douglas, and Bennett's principles and practice of infectious diseases*, ed 8, Philadelphia, 2015, Saunders.

subarachnoid space. In those instances, the following formula should be used as a correction factor for the true WBC count in the presence of CSF RBCs:

$$\text{Adjusted WBC in CSF} = \text{Actual WBC in CSF} - \frac{\text{WBC in blood} \times \text{RBC in CSF blood}}{\text{RBC in blood}}$$

In the previous equation, the amount being subtracted is the predicted CSF WBC that would occur if all the CSF WBCs were the result of blood contamination.[1]

[1]Bennett JE et al: *Mandell, Douglas and Bennett's principles and practice of infectious diseases*, ed 8, Philadelphia, 2015, Saunders, p 1093.

- Prevention of meningitis can be achieved through chemoprophylaxis of close contacts (household members and anyone exposed to oral secretions).
- Effective medications are rifampin 10 mg/kg PO bid for 2 days or ceftriaxone 250 mg IM single dose in patients older than age 12; 125 mg IM if age 12 or younger.
- Ciprofloxacin 500 mg for prevention of *Neisseria* meningitis can be given to patients older than 18 yr who cannot tolerate rifampin to eradicate pharyngeal colonization.
- Menactra: A protein-conjugate vaccine against serogroup A, C, Y, W-135 capsular polysaccharides is available for adults (up to 55 yr) and children older than 2 yr.
- Two new vaccines for *Neisseria* meningitis serogroup B (MenB) are now available: Bexsero and Trumenba.
- Children with cochlear implants are at increased risk of developing bacterial meningitis.
- Patients on eculizumab (Soliris) are at high risk for invasive meningococcal disease and should receive Menactra and a MenB vaccine and may need lifelong antibiotic prophylaxis as well.

SUGGESTED READINGS

Available at ExpertConsult.com

RELATED CONTENT

Meningitis (Patient Information)
Meningitis, Viral (Related Key Topic)
Meningitis, Fungal (Related Key Topic)

AUTHOR: **GLENN G. FORT, M.D., M.P.H.**

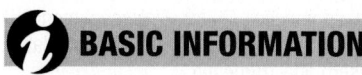

BASIC INFORMATION

DEFINITION

Viral meningitis is an acute febrile illness with signs and symptoms of meningeal irritation, usually with a lymphocytic pleocytosis of the cerebrospinal fluid (CSF) and negative CSF bacterial stains and cultures.

SYNONYMS

Aseptic meningitis
Viral meningitis

ICD-10CM CODES
A87.8 Other viral meningitis
A87.9 Viral meningitis, unspecified

EPIDEMIOLOGY & DEMOGRAPHICS (TABLE 1)

INCIDENCE (IN U.S.): 11 cases/100,000 persons. Leads to 26,000 to 42,000 hospitalizations a yr

PREDOMINANT SEX: Male = female

GENETICS: Those with abnormal humoral immunity and agammaglobulinemia have associated difficulty with viral clearance.

PHYSICAL FINDINGS & CLINICAL PRESENTATION

- Fever
- Headache
- Nuchal rigidity
- Photophobia
- Myalgias
- Vomiting
- Rash

ETIOLOGY

- Enterovirus: 85% to 95% of all cases. Most common are coxsackie viruses and echoviruses
- Parechoviruses
- Mumps virus
- Measles
- Arboviruses from mosquitoes: EEE, West Nile, St Louis
- Herpes: HSV-1, HSV-2, VZV, HHV-6, and HHV-7
- Acute HIV
- Lymphocytic choriomeningitis virus
- Adenovirus
- CMV and EBV
- Other arthropod-borne viruses: Powassan virus
- Influenza A and B virus
- Box E1 summarizes etiologic agents, factors, and diseases associated with aseptic meningitis

DIAGNOSIS

The diagnostic approach is similar to that for bacterial meningitis (see "Meningitis, Bacterial"); the foremost need is to rule out bacterial meningitis with CSF evaluation. Presentation may be similar to that of meningitis with bacterial involvement.

DIFFERENTIAL DIAGNOSIS

- Bacterial meningitis
- Meningitis secondary to Lyme disease, TB, syphilis, amebiasis, leptospirosis
- Rickettsial illnesses: Rocky Mountain spotted fever
- Migraine headache
- Medications
- SLE
- Acute mononucleosis/Epstein-Barr virus
- Seizures
- Carcinomatous meningitis

WORKUP

CSF examination:

- Usually shows pleocytosis
- Lymphocytic predominance (neutrophils in early stages)
- Opening pressure: 200 to 250 mm Hg H_2O (≤250 mm/H_2O)
- WBC: 100 to 1000 mm^3
- Increased CSF protein (<200 mg/dl)
- Slightly decreased or normal CSF glucose (>45 mg/dl)
- Negative gram stain, cultures, CIE, latex agglutination
- Viral cultures or serologic testing may be diagnostic
- Polymerase chain reaction for HSV or enterovirus (which could shorten duration of antibiotic treatment and hospitalization if bacterial meningitis was suspected)
- Antibody detection in CSF for diagnosis of West Nile virus meningitis

LABORATORY TESTS

CBC with differential, blood culturing, and CSF examination (see "Workup")

IMAGING STUDIES

CT scan or MRI: If cerebral edema, focal neurologic findings develop

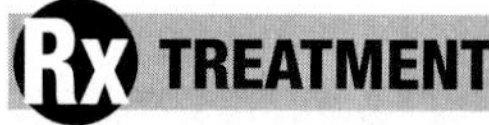

TREATMENT

- No specific antiviral therapy for most viruses. Treatment is supportive unless HSV is detected, which would be treated with IV acyclovir: 10 mg/kg q8h in adults for 14 to 21 days. Up to 20 mg/kg q8h in children >12 yr.
- Empiric antibiotics may be given until CSF cultures exclude bacterial meningitis.

DISPOSITION

Viral meningitis is almost always an uncomplicated illness that will resolve; however, relapsing headache, myalgia, and weakness may occur for 2 to 3 wk after onset of symptoms.

PEARLS & CONSIDERATIONS

- Enteroviruses are the most common cause of viral meningitis and are transmitted by fecal-oral route and less commonly by the respiratory route. They are more common in summer and fall months. From 2000 to 2005, the most common serotypes were coxsackie viruses A9, B5, and B1 and echoviruses 6, 9, 13, 18, and 30.
- Herpes simplex type 2 (HSV-2) can be a cause of a primary episode of meningitis and also be a cause of recurrent episodes of lymphocytic meningitis. HSV-2 meningitis presents most often without a history of genital herpes or genital symptoms. Recurrent aseptic meningitis, also known as Mollaret disease, is predominantly caused by HSV-2 infection.

TABLE 1 Epidemiology of Acute Viral Meningitis

Epidemiologic Factors*				
Season	**Patient's Age (yr)**	**Patient's Sex**	**Risk Factor**	**Suggested Viral Agent**
Summer-fall	Infant	—	Infected mother	Coxsackievirus B
	1-15	—	Swimming pools, closed communities	Enteroviruses
			Geographic area: California, southeastern United States	California serogroup virus
Winter	1-15	—	School exposure	Varicella virus, measles virus
		Male:female 3:1		Mumps virus
	16-21	—	College exposure	Measles virus
		Male:female 3:1		Mumps virus
				Epstein-Barr virus (mononucleosis)
	Any	—	Mice, rats, hamsters	Lymphocytic choriomeningitis virus
	Adults	—	Varicella-zoster	Varicella-zoster virus
Any	Any	—	Immunocompromise	Adenovirus
		—	Acquired immunodeficiency syndrome	Human immunodeficiency virus

*Epidemiologic factors are suggestive but should not be used to exclude diagnoses in individual cases.
From Gorbach SI: *Infectious diseases*, ed 2, Philadelphia, 1998, Saunders.

SUGGESTED READINGS
Available at ExpertConsult.com

RELATED CONTENT

Meningitis (Patient Information)
Meningitis Bacterial (Related Key Topic)

AUTHOR: **GLENN G. FORT, M.D., M.P.H.**

BASIC INFORMATION

DEFINITION

Menopause is the permanent cessation of menstrual periods for 1 yr after age 40 yr or permanent cessation of ovulation after lost ovarian activity. It is the reproductive stage of life marked by waxing and waning estrogen levels followed by decreasing ovarian function. Primary ovarian insufficiency (previously also referred to as premature ovarian failure) and no menstrual periods may also occur because of depletion of ovarian follicles before the age of 40 yr.

SYNONYMS

Change of life
Climacteric ovarian failure

ICD-10CM CODES	
Z78.0	Asymptomatic menopausal state
N95.1	Menopausal and female climacteric states
N95.8	Other specified menopausal and perimenopausal disorders
E28.310	Symptomatic premature menopause
E28.319	Asymptomatic premature menopause

EPIDEMIOLOGY & DEMOGRAPHICS

- Average age of menopause in the United States is 51 yr.
- Age at which menopause occurs is primarily genetically determined.
- Smokers experience menopause an average of 1.5 yr earlier than nonsmokers.
- More than one third of a woman's life may be spent after menopause.
- Onset of perimenopause is usually in a woman's mid- to late-40s.
- Approximately 4000 women begin menopause each day.

PHYSICAL FINDINGS & CLINICAL PRESENTATION

- Atrophic vaginitis, which can cause burning, itching, bleeding, dyspareunia
- Either complete cessation of menses or a period of irregular cycles and diminished or heavier bleeding
- Osteoporosis
- Osteopenia/psychological dysfunction:
  1. Anxiety
  2. Depression
  3. Insomnia
  4. Nervousness
  5. Irritability
  6. Inability to concentrate
- Sexual changes, decreased libido, dyspareunia
- Urinary incontinence
- Menopausal vasomotor symptoms (VMS, hot flashes, flushes), night sweats, cardiovascular disease, coronary artery disease, atherosclerosis, headaches, tiredness, and lethargy.

A study from the University of Pennsylvania noted that the median duration of moderate-to-severe hot flashes is 10.2 yr but that the length of hot flashes was largely dictated by how early these began in the perimenopause.

ETIOLOGY

- The most common etiology: Physiologic, caused by depleted granulosa and theca cells that fail to react to endogenous gonadotropins, producing less estrogen; decreased negative feedback in the hypothalamic pituitary access, increased follicle-stimulating hormone (FSH), and increased luteinizing hormone (LH), which leads to stromal cells that continue to produce androgens as a result of the LH stimulation
- Surgical castration
- Family history of early menopause, cigarette smoking, blindness, abnormal chromosomal karyotype (Turner syndrome, gonadal dysgenesis), precocious puberty, and left-handedness

Dx DIAGNOSIS

DIFFERENTIAL DIAGNOSIS

- Asherman syndrome
- Hypothalamic dysfunction
- Hypothyroidism
- Pituitary tumors
- Adrenal abnormalities
- Ovarian abnormalities
- Polycystic ovarian syndrome
- Pregnancy
- Ovarian neoplasm
- Tuberculosis of the endometrium

WORKUP

- If the clinical picture is highly suggestive of menopause, estrogen can be prescribed. If all symptoms resolve, then a diagnosis essentially has been made. Before estrogen is prescribed, however, a complete history and physical examination are needed. If a patient has an estrogen-dependent malignancy, unexplained abnormal uterine bleeding, a history of thrombophlebitis, or acute liver disease, estrogen therapy is contraindicated.
- Progesterone challenge test: Medroxyprogesterone 10 to 20 mg PO or progesterone 100 mg IM to induce withdrawal bleeding. If no withdrawal bleeding is obtained, a hypoestrogenic state is assumed to be present. This test is increasingly controversial, even if very commonly performed.
- Physical examination, height, weight, blood pressure, breast examination, and pelvic examination are needed.
- Assess risk for coronary artery disease, osteoporosis, cigarette smoking, personal history, history of breast cancer, liver disease, active coagulation disorder, or any unexplained vaginal bleeding.

LABORATORY TESTS

- FSH, LH, and estrogen levels: Markedly elevated FSH and markedly depressed estrogen level constitute laboratory diagnosis of ovarian failure; LH only if polycystic ovarian disease is to be ruled out in a younger patient. It is not necessary to obtain an FSH if the patient fulfills the clinical criteria for menopause. Similarly, since estradiol levels vary during the menstrual cycle, estradiol levels are rarely necessary or informative.
- TSH to rule out thyroid dysfunction and prolactin level if patient has symptoms of galactorrhea and if suspicion of pituitary adenoma exists
- A general chemistry profile to check for any systemic diseases
- Pap smear per standard guidelines, endometrial biopsy, or dilation and curettage in patients who have had irregular periods or intermenstrual or postmenopausal bleeding
- Mammogram as recommended by American Congress of Obstetricians and Gynecologists.

IMAGING STUDIES

- Per standard protocols, CT scan or MRI of sella if pituitary tumor is suspected
- Bone density studies if high-risk condition for osteoporosis exists
- Pelvic ultrasound to check endometrial stripe as determined by clinical history

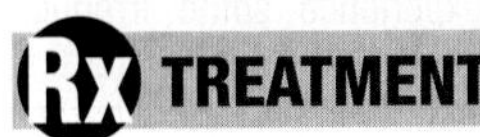

Rx TREATMENT

NONPHARMACOLOGIC THERAPY

- A balanced diet: Low in fat, with total fat intake being <30% of calories; total calories sufficient to maintain body weight or produce weight loss if that is desired
- Avoidance of smoking and excessive alcohol or caffeine intake
- Exercise: Weight-bearing exercise for osteoporosis prevention
- Kegel exercises for strengthening the pelvic floor
- Adequate calcium intake: 1500 mg elemental calcium qd is necessary to maintain zero calcium balance in postmenopausal women
- Change in the ambient temperature (may ameliorate hot flashes and reduce night sweats)
- Vitamin E
- Avoidance of caffeine, alcohol, and spicy foods if they trigger hot flashes
- Vaginal lubricants to help with the dyspareunia attributable to vaginal dryness (e.g., Replens, K-Y Jelly, or Gyne-Moistrin cream)

ACUTE GENERAL Rx

Vasomotor symptoms are best managed with systemic hormone therapy given in the lowest dose and for the shortest period possible. Estrogen replacement in symptomatic patients can be administered in a variety of forms, including oral estrogen and transdermal estrogen patch. The lowest effective dose should be prescribed.

- Examples of oral estrogen include:
  1. Conjugated estrogens: Start with 0.3 mg qd and increase to 1.25 mg qd depending on symptoms.

2. Estradiol: Start with 0.5 mg qd and increase to 2 mg qd.
3. Esterified estrogens: Start with 0.3 to 1.25 mg qd.
4. Estropipate: Start with 0.625 to 2.5 mg qd.
5. Esterified estrogen/testosterone combination: Give 1.25 mg and methyltestosterone 2.5 mg (Estratest) and esterified estrogen 0.625 mg and methyltestosterone 1.25 mg (Estratest HS [half-strength]). May improve sexual enjoyment and libido.

- If the patient has had a hysterectomy for benign disease, estrogen alone is sufficient. In patients who have an intact uterus, progestin is critical to prevent endometrial hyperplasia associated with unopposed estrogen, which is protective against endometrial cancer. Progestins can be prescribed as continual daily dose or cyclic fashion. Most commonly prescribed progestins include medroxyprogesterone acetate 2.5 mg, 5 mg, and 10 mg; Prometrium 100 mg, 200 mg, and 400 mg; and Aygestin 5 mg. Continuous hormone replacement therapy is preferred because after time the patient should be amenorrheic. Patients should be counseled that they may experience some irregular spotting for the first 6 to 9 mo after starting hormone replacement therapy. Cyclic therapy will cause withdrawal bleeding.
- Combination oral preparations FemHRT, Prefest, Prempro, Activella, Premphase are commonly used. However, the U.S. Preventive Services Task Force recommends against the use of combined estrogen and progestin for the prevention of chronic conditions such as cardiovascular disease in postmenopausal women.
- The combination of conjugated estrogen and bazedoxifene is approved for the treatment of moderate to severe vasomotor symptoms associated with menopause and also for prevention of postmenopausal osteoporosis in women with an intact uterus.
- Transdermal patches can be either estradiol (Estraderm, Vivelle, FemPatch) 0.025 to 0.1 mg applied twice weekly or Climara 0.025 to 0.1 mg used once a wk. With these preparations, progesterone should be used in a similar fashion. Apply CombiPatch twice weekly (combination estrogen and progesterone) or Climara Pro once per wk (one patch).
- Vaginal creams can be used; these should be reserved for local therapy of atrophic vaginitis. Minimal systemic absorption does occur; however, blood levels are unpredictable. Usual dose 0.5 to 2 g intravaginally daily, cyclically 3 wk on 1 wk off. When symptoms improve, once to twice weekly is adequate maintenance.
- Vagifem estradiol vaginal tablets. Initial dosage: One Vagifem tablet, inserted vaginally, qd for 2 wk. Maintenance dose: One Vagifem tablet, inserted vaginally, twice weekly.
- Femring vaginal ring delivering the equivalent of 0.5 mg/day inserted every 3 mo or Estring 0.0075 mg/day.
- EstroGel 0.06% (estradiol gel) One Pump (1.25 g/day) applied to one arm from wrist to shoulder.
- The FDA contraindications to menopause hormone therapy include the following diseases and disorders: active liver disease; current, past, or suspected breast cancer; active or recent anterior thromboembolic disease (angina, myocardial infarction); known or suspected estrogen-sensitive malignant conditions; known hypersensitivity to the active substance of the therapy or to any of the excipients; porphyria cutanea tarda; previous idiopathic or current venous thromboembolism; undiagnosed genital bleeding; untreated hypertension; untreated endometrial hyperplasia.
- For women in whom estrogen is contraindicated or for those who do not wish to take estrogen, the following regimens can be used:
    1. Serotonin reuptake inhibitors.
    2. Depo-Provera 150 mg IM every month (may be helpful in alleviating hot flashes).
    3. Clonidine 0.05 to 0.15 mg PO qd (questionable efficacy) or transdermal clonidine patch.
    4. Bellergal-S (questionable efficacy).
- Tibolone significantly improves vasomotor symptoms, libido, and vaginal lubrication. Not available in the U.S.

CHRONIC Rx

Hormone replacement therapy should be used only for the short term unless benefits outweigh the risks of long-term use. As a result of the results of the Women's Health Initiative (WHI), the FDA has instituted a "black box" warning on postmenopausal hormone replacement products suggesting that the lowest dose should be used for the shortest period of time. This necessitates a considered and nuanced counseling session with patients contemplating hormone replacement prior to the initiation of therapy and then on a periodic basis after that, usually at least a yearly basis.

DISPOSITION

If treated, the patient should have resolution of her symptoms and reduced incidence of osteoporosis. Lifelong medical supervision is necessary to monitor adequacy of treatment and prevention of complications. This should include regular Pap smears in accordance with American Society for Colposcopy and Cervical Pathology (ASCCP) guidelines until the age of 65, pelvic examinations, breast examinations, mammography, and endometrial sampling of any type of abnormal bleeding. If untreated, the vasomotor symptoms will eventually dissipate; however, this may take several years in a small percentage of women. Some women who are in their 80s have experienced hot flashes. Urogenital atrophy will continue to worsen. Osteoporosis and coronary artery disease risks will increase with every passing year.

REFERRAL

Most menopausal women are managed by their gynecologists. However, this condition can be managed adequately by the patient's primary care physician who has an interest in treating menopausal women.

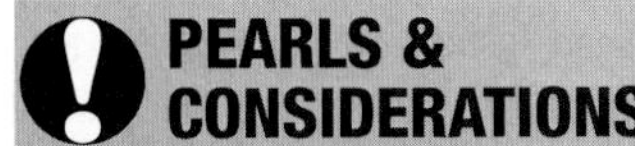

PEARLS & CONSIDERATIONS

COMMENTS

- Short-term risks of hormone replacement therapy (HT) include an eighteenfold increased rise for cholecystitis, three-and-a-half-fold risk of a thrombocardiac event in the first year, and possible increased risk of stroke and myocardial infarction.
- Results of the WHI study found that for every 10,000 women taking HT (combination of both estrogen and progesterone) for 1 yr (10,000 person-yr), seven more would have coronary events, eight would have more strokes, eight would have more pulmonary emboli, and eight would have earlier breast cancer than would 10,000 women taking placebo. Benefits of HT were six fewer cases of colorectal cancer and five fewer hip fractures per 10,000 women.
- HT should not be initiated or continued for the primary or secondary prevention of coronary heart disease.
- Estrogen-replacement therapy should only be prescribed for patients with sufficient menopausal symptoms that impact the patient's quality of life.
- Interestingly, women who start hormone therapy early in menopause may have cardiac and other benefits. A recent trial showed that oral estradiol therapy was associated with less progression of subclinical atherosclerosis (measured as change in carotid-artery intima media thickness [CIMT]) than with placebo when therapy was initiated within 6 yr after menopause but not when it was initiated 10 or more yr after menopause. Estradiol had no significant effect on cardiac CT measures of atherosclerosis in either postmenopause stratum.[1]

SUGGESTED READINGS

Available at ExpertConsult.com

RELATED CONTENT

Menopause (Patient Information)
Hot Flashes (Related Key Topic)
Osteoporosis (Related Key Topic)

AUTHOR: **ELIZABETH ZADZIELSKI, M.D., M.B.A., N.C.M.P.**

[1] Hodis HN, et al.: Vascular effects of early versus late postmenopausal treatment with estradiol, *N Engl J Med* 374:1221-1231, 2016.

BASIC INFORMATION

DEFINITION

Mesenteric venous thrombosis (MVT) is a thrombotic occlusion of the mesenteric venous system involving major trunks or smaller branches and can lead to intestinal infarction in its acute form.

SYNONYM

MVT

ICD-10CM CODES
K55.0 Acute vascular disorders of intestine
K55.1 Chronic vascular disorders of intestine

EPIDEMIOLOGY & DEMOGRAPHICS

Between 5% and 15% of patients with acute mesenteric ischemia has MVT. MVT is slightly more common in men than women. The typical age of occurrence is 50 to 60 yr. Table 1 summarizes the incidence of ischemic bowel disease.

PHYSICAL FINDINGS & CLINICAL PRESENTATION

Acute MVT:
- Symptoms: Abdominal pain in 90% of patients, typically out of proportion to the physical findings. Nausea and vomiting occur in 50% and gastrointestinal (GI) bleeding occurs in 50% (occult) and 15% (gross).
- Physical findings:
  1. Early: Abdominal tenderness, decreased bowel sounds, abdominal distention
  2. Later: Guarding and rebound tenderness, fever, septic shock

Subacute MVT:
- Symptoms: Nonspecific abdominal pain for weeks or months
- Physical findings: None

Chronic MVT:
- Symptoms: Typically asymptomatic, tends to present with complications of portal hypertension (hemorrhage from bleeding varices, ascites) due to concomitant portal vein or splenic vein thrombosis.
- Physical findings: None other than signs of portal hypertension if the portal/splenic veins are also involved.

ETIOLOGY & PATHOGENESIS

Hypercoagulable states:
- Personal or family history of thrombophilia or personal history of thromboembolism
- Neoplasms
- Antithrombin III, protein C, protein S deficiencies or activated protein C resistance
- Lupus anticoagulant (antiphospholipid antibody syndrome)
- Factor V Leiden or prothrombin G20210A mutations
- Oral contraceptive use, pregnancy
- Myeloproliferative disorders (polycythemia vera, essential thrombocytosis)
- Paroxysmal nocturnal hemoglobinuria

TABLE 1 Incidence of Ischemic Bowel Diseases

Disease	Incidence (%)*
Superior mesenteric artery (SMA) embolism: • The SMA is susceptible to embolism because of large vessel caliber and a narrow angle of departure from the aorta. • The proximal SMA is most commonly obstructed within 6-8 cm of the aorta	50
Nonocclusive ischemia	25
SMA thrombosis	20
Mesenteric venous thrombosis	5

*Percentage of all cases of acute mesenteric ischemia.
From Adams JG et al: *Emergency medicine, clinical essentials,* ed 2, Philadelphia, 2013, Elsevier.

BOX 1 Factors Associated with Mesenteric Venous Thrombosis

Hypercoagulable states
- Polycythemia vera
- Sickle cell disease
- Antithrombin III deficiency
- Protein C or S deficiency
- Malignancy
- Myeloproliferative disorders
- Estrogen therapy, oral contraceptive pills
- Pregnancy

Inflammatory conditions
- Pancreatitis
- Diverticulitis
- Appendicitis
- Cholangitis

Trauma
- Operative venous injury
- Postsplenectomy
- Blunt or abdominal trauma
- Miscellaneous
- Congestive heart failure
- Renal failure

Decompression sickness

Portal hypertension. From Marx JA et al: *Rosen's emergency medicine*, ed 8, Philadelphia, 2014, Saunders.

Portal hypertension:
- Cirrhosis

Inflammation:
- Pancreatitis
- Peritonitis (e.g., appendicitis, diverticulitis, perforated viscus)
- Inflammatory bowel disease
- Pelvic or intraabdominal abscess
- Intraabdominal cancer

Postoperative state or trauma:
- Blunt abdominal trauma
- Postoperative states (abdominal surgery)
- Box 1 summarizes factors associated with mesenteric venous thrombosis

Thrombosis may begin in small mesenteric branches (e.g., in hypercoagulable states) and propagate to the major venous mesenteric trunks or begin in large veins (e.g., in cirrhosis, intraabdominal cancer, surgery) and extend distally. If collateral drainage is inadequate, the intestine becomes congested, edematous, cyanotic, and hemorrhagic and eventually may infarct.

DIAGNOSIS

DIFFERENTIAL DIAGNOSIS

All other causes of abdominal pain (e.g., peritonitis, intestinal obstruction, pancreatitis, peptic ulcer disease, gastritis, inflammatory bowel disease, perforated viscus) are also to be considered in the differential diagnosis.

WORKUP

Laboratory tests and imaging studies

LABORATORY TESTS

- Complete blood count: Leukocytosis
- Electrolytes: Metabolic acidosis (lactic) indicates bowel infarction
- Tests for hypercoagulable states

IMAGING STUDIES

- Computed tomography (CT) with and without oral and IV contrast (Fig. 1) is a good initial screening study due to widespread availability and the ability to detect sequelae of MVT (such as intestinal ischemia or infarction).
- If regular CT does not demonstrate MVT and the clinical suspicion is high, computed tomographic angiography (CTA) is another imaging modality with higher sensitivity but more use of contrast material. Use of two-phase imaging improves sensitivity for venous thrombosis.
- Magnetic resonance angiography/venography (MRA/MRV) can also be used; it avoids the risk of radiation and contrast material but takes longer and may be limited due to motion artifact.

TREATMENT

- Acute and subacute MVT: Anticoagulation with unfractionated heparin or low-molecular-weight heparin with eventual transition to a vitamin K antagonist or novel oral anticoagulant for 3 to 6 mo, or longer if a hypercoagulable state has been identified. When medical treatment is unsuccessful, options include transhepatic and percutaneous mechanical thrombectomy, intravascular catheter-directed thrombolysis, and open intraarterial thrombolysis.
- Intravenous fluid administration (due to relative hypovolemia from bowel wall edema), bowel rest and decompression if ileus forms.

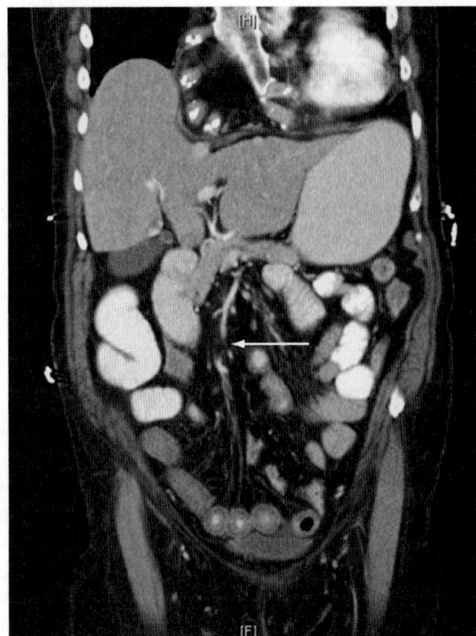

FIG. 1 Computed tomography after administration of oral and intravenous contrast in a patient with an embolism to the superior mesenteric artery and ischemia of the small bowel and right colon. The arrow points to the embolus in the superior mesenteric artery. (From Vincent JL et al: *Textbook of critical care*, ed 7, Philadelphia, 2017, Elsevier.)

- Consider prophylactic antibiotics to reduce the incidence of bacterial translocation.
- Laparotomy if intestinal infarction is suspected.

CHRONIC MVT

- Anticoagulation should be considered but is a decision specific to each individual patient.
- If anticoagulation is pursued, ensure potential bleeding complications (esophageal varices) have been identified and treated.
- If varices are present, initiate beta blockade, similar to cirrhosis-related portal hypertension.

PROGNOSIS

- Mortality rate of acute MVT: With prompt diagnosis and anticoagulation, 10% to 20%. The presence of intestinal infarction is a poor prognostic sign for overall mortality.
- Recurrence rate: 15% to 25%.

SUGGESTED READING

Available at ExpertConsult.com

RELATED CONTENT

Acute Mesenteric Ischemia (Related Key Topic)

AUTHOR: **DAVID J. LUCIER JR., M.D., M.B.A., M.P.H., C.P.P.S.**

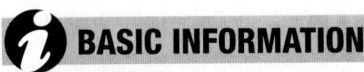

BASIC INFORMATION

DEFINITION

Malignant mesothelioma is a neoplasm originating from the mesothelial surfaces of the pleural (80%) or peritoneal cavities (20%).The three major histologic subtypes are epithelial (most common), sarcomatous, and mixed (epithelial/sarcomatous).

SYNONYM

Malignant mesothelioma

ICD-10CM CODES

C45.0 Mesothelioma of pleura
C45.1 Mesothelioma of peritoneum
C45.2 Mesothelioma of pericardium
C45.7 Mesothelioma of other sites
C45.9 Mesothelioma, unspecified

EPIDEMIOLOGY & DEMOGRAPHICS

- Associated with asbestos exposure (all fiber types) and has a latency of 20 to 40 yr.
- About 2000 to 3000 new cases are diagnosed in the U.S. annually.
- More common in men (5:1) as a result of workplace asbestos exposure; however, even family members of workers exposed to asbestos have a higher risk due to cleaning of contaminated clothes.
- Incidence in the U.S. has leveled off due to lack of asbestos use and mining.
- Incidence of mesothelioma increases with age; median age at presentation is >70 yr.
- More than 8 million persons in the U.S. are currently at risk for mesothelioma because of prior asbestos exposure.

PHYSICAL FINDINGS & CLINICAL PRESENTATION

- Dyspnea
- Nonpleuritic chest pain
- Fever, weight loss, sweats, fatigue, loss of appetite
- Dysphagia, superior vena cava syndrome, Horner's syndrome in advanced stages
- Auscultation may reveal unilateral loss of breath sounds
- Dullness on percussion may be present

ETIOLOGY

- Asbestos exposure (>70% of patients)
- Other reported potentially causal factors include prior radiation therapy and extravasated thorotrast, zeolite, and erionite fibers

DIAGNOSIS

DIFFERENTIAL DIAGNOSIS

Metastatic adenocarcinomas (from lung, breast, ovary, kidney, stomach, prostate)

WORKUP

- Staging evaluation (Box 1) includes complete history (including occupational history), physical examination, and testing to determine potential operability (CT, bone scan, pulmonary function tests [PFTs])
- Thoracoscopy, pleuroscopy, and open-lung biopsy are useful in obtaining adequate tissue samples for diagnosis
- Pulmonary function tests
- PET-CT scan is performed only in patients considered candidates for surgery to determine resectability
- Staging: The TNM system categorizes mesothelioma in stages I to IV similar to that used for non–small cell lung cancer

LABORATORY TESTS

- Diagnostic thoracentesis is generally insufficient for diagnosis because pleural effusions may only reveal atypical mesothelial cells.
- Immunohistochemistry is useful to distinguish adenocarcinoma from epithelial malignant mesothelioma (mesotheliomas are generally carcinoembryonic antigen negative and cytokeratin positive).
- Thrombocytosis and anemia may be found on initial laboratory evaluation.
- Serum osteopontin levels (when available) can also be used to distinguish persons with exposure to asbestos who do not have cancer from those with exposure to asbestos who have pleural mesothelioma.

IMAGING STUDIES

- Chest radiographs may reveal pleural plaques (Fig. E1) or calcifications in the diaphragm.
- CT scans of the chest and abdomen, bone scan, and PET scan are used to assess the stage of disease.

BOX 1 International Mesothelioma Interest Group (IMIG) Staging System

T: Primary Tumor and Extent

T_1
a. Tumor limited to ipsilateral parietal pleura, including mediastinal and diaphragmatic pleura; no involvement of the visceral pleura
b. Tumor involving the ipsilateral parietal pleura, including mediastinal and diaphragmatic pleura; scattered foci or tumor also involving the visceral pleura

T_2 Tumor involving each of the ipsilateral pleural surfaces (parietal, mediastinal, diaphragmatic pleura); scattered foci or tumor also involving the visceral pleura
a. Involvement of diaphragmatic muscle
b. Confluent visceral pleura (including the fissures) or extension of tumor from visceral pleura into the underlying pulmonary parenchyma

T_3 Locally advanced but potentially resectable tumor; tumor involving all the ipsilateral pleural surfaces (parietal, mediastinal, diaphragmatic, and visceral pleura) with at least one of the following features:
a. Involvement of the endothoracic fascia
b. Extension into mediastinal fat
c. Solitary, complete resectable focus or tumor extending into the soft tissues of the chest wall
d. Nontransmural involvement of the pericardium

T_4 Locally advanced, technically nonresectable tumor; tumor involving all the ipsilateral pleural surfaces (parietal, mediastinal, diaphragmatic, and visceral pleura) with at least one of the following features:
a. Diffuse extension or multifocal mass of tumor in the chest wall, with or without associated rib destruction
b. Direct transdiaphragmatic extension of the tumor to the peritoneum
c. Direct extension of tumor to the contralateral pleura
d. Direct extension of tumor to one or more mediastinal organs
e. Direct extension of tumor into the spine
f. Tumor extending through the internal surface of the pericardium with or without a pericardial effusion or tumor involving the myocardium

N: Lymph Nodes

N_x Regional lymph nodes cannot be assessed
N_0 No regional lymph node metastases
N_1 Metastases in ipsilateral bronchopulmonary or hilar lymph nodes
N_2 Metastases in the subcarinal or the ipsilateral mediastinal lymph nodes, including the ipsilateral internal mammary nodes
N_3 Metastases in contralateral mediastinal, contralateral internal mammary, ipsilateral, or contralateral supraclavicular scalene lymph nodes

M: Metastases

M_x Presence of distant metastases cannot be assessed
M_0 No (known) metastasis
M_1 Distant metastasis present

Stage Grouping

I.
a. $T_{1a}N_0M_0$
b. $T_{1b}N_0M_0$
II. $T_2N_0M_0$
III. Any T_3M_0, any N_1M_0, any N_2M_0
IV. Any T_4, any N_3, any M_1

From Sellke FW, del Nido PJ, Swanson SJ: *Sabiston & Spencer surgery of the chest*, ed 9, Philadelphia, 2016, Elsevier.

BOX 2 Therapeutic Options for Malignant Pleural Mesothelioma

Single-Modality Therapy
- Debulking surgery (pleurectomy/decortication or extrapleural pneumonectomy)
- Radiation (external beam, brachytherapy)
- Chemotherapy (single- or double-agent approach: doxorubicin, cyclophosphamide, cisplatinum; gemcitabine, pemetrexed, and cisplatin)

Multimodality Therapy
- Surgery and adjuvant radiation
- Surgery and adjuvant chemotherapy
- Surgery and adjuvant chemoradiotherapy

Innovative Therapies Under Investigation
- Intracavitary lavage with hyperthermic chemotherapy
- Photodynamic therapy
- Gene therapy
- Angiogenesis
- Immunogenic therapy

From Sellke FW, del Nido PJ, Swanson SJ: *Sabiston & Spencer surgery of the chest*, ed 9, Philadelphia, 2016, Elsevier.

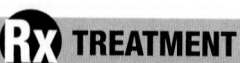

TREATMENT

GENERAL Rx

- Box 2 summarizes therapeutic options for malignant pleural mesothelioma.
- Operable patient (epithelial type, no positive nodes, confined to pleura, adequate PFTs): The two surgical techniques for therapeutic intervention are decortication (pleurectomy) and extrapleural pneumonectomy. Postoperative chemotherapy with cisplatin and pemetrexed and subsequent external-beam radiation are used with limited success.
- Inoperable patient (elderly patient, extensive disease, sarcomatous or mixed histology type, poor PFTs): Chemotherapy is administered to improve survival; supportive care is a standard option. Combined modality therapies (radiation therapy, chemotherapy, and biologics) have also been used to reduce both local and distant recurrences. First-line chemotherapy options include the combination of cisplatin and pemetrexed with or without additional bevacizumab (antiangiogenic agent).
- Patients with progressive cancer after initial chemotherapy can often be treated with single-agent chemotherapy such as gemcitabine or vinorelbine.
- Recent data have shown improvement in survival with use of immune checkpoint inhibitors targeting the programmed death-1 (PD-1) pathway such as pembrolizumab and nivolumab.
- Intrapleural instillation of cisplatin or biologics (e.g., interferons, interleukin-2) is generally limited to very early disease because it can only penetrate a very limited depth of the tumor and there is a propensity of the pleural space to become progressively obliterated with advancing disease.
- Radiation therapy is often used for palliation of local chest pain.
- Obliteration of the pleural space (pleurodesis) with instillation of talc or tetracycline into the pleural cavity is done in the treatment of recurrent symptomatic pleural effusions.
- Several biomarkers have been evaluated extensively in mesothelioma management. Serum mesothelin is not sensitive or specific for diagnostic purposes, but serial measurements during chemotherapy can be useful as a monitoring tool. Recent data reveal that plasma fibulin-3 levels can distinguish healthy persons with exposure to asbestos from patients with mesothelioma. In conjunction with effusion fibulin-3 levels, plasma fibulin-3 levels can further differentiate mesothelioma effusions from other malignant and benign effusions.

DISPOSITION

The overall prognosis of malignant mesothelioma is dismal, with a median survival of 6 to 8 mo. Survival is better for patients with the epithelial form, although overall median survival is approximately still 1 yr.

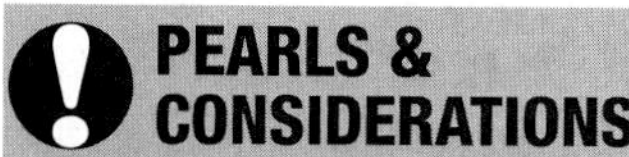

PEARLS & CONSIDERATIONS

- Patients with early disease should be referred to treatment centers specializing in multidisciplinary therapy before attempts are made to obliterate the pleural space with pleurodesis.
- Patients with advanced or resected disease should be treated with appropriate combination chemotherapy as listed previously.

SUGGESTED READINGS

Available at ExpertConsult.com

RELATED CONTENT

Mesothelioma (Patient Information)
Asbestosis (Related Key Topic)

AUTHOR: **BHARTI RATHORE, M.D.**

BASIC INFORMATION

DEFINITION

An accidental or intentional ingestion of 1 g per kg methanol or ethylene glycol is considered lethal, although even small amounts can be toxic. Inhalational and dermal exposures rarely cause toxicity.

SYNONYMS

Toxic alcohols
Moonshine
Wood alcohol
Antifreeze

ICD-10CM CODES

T51.8	Toxic effect of alcohols
T51.1X1	Toxic effect of methanol
T51.1X2	Toxic effect of methanol, intentional self-harm
T52.8X1	Ethylene glycol poisoning

EPIDEMIOLOGY & DEMOGRAPHICS

INCIDENCE:

- In 2016, the American Association of Poison Control Centers reported 6,508 single-exposure cases of ethylene glycol poisoning and 1,853 of methanol poisoning.
- Most cases are reported in adults and predominantly in men.
- Accidental exposure is common in children, while alcoholism, polysubstance abuse, depression, and suicide are seen in adults.
- Suicide attempts involving toxic alcohols frequently involve the ingestion of multiple substances.
- Outbreaks or epidemic poisoning with methanol is frequently the result of bootleg distillation or counterfeit alcohol.

PHYSICAL FINDINGS & CLINICAL PRESENTATION

- Clinical manifestations depend on the quantity of ingestion, duration of time since ingestion, and whether co-ingestion of other substances occurs.
- Early ingestion of either substance causes CNS depression, nausea, and vomiting; inebriation can mimic ethanol ingestion. Late effects include progressive CNS dysfunction, including seizure and coma, as well as respiratory and cardiopulmonary failure.
- Visual symptoms ranging from blurry or snowy vision to complete visual loss and findings of papillary edema and, later, optic atrophy, fixed and dilated pupils, retinal hyperemia, and a Parkinson-like syndrome are indicative of methanol poisoning. Other CNS effects are hemorrhage and white matter lesions in the putamen, subcortical structures, brainstem, and cerebellum.
- Oliguria, hematuria, calcium oxalate crystalluria, tetany, cranial nerve palsy, and acute kidney injury suggest ethylene glycol toxicity.
- Abdominal pain may result from exposure to either substance, while methanol can cause acute pancreatitis.
- Kussmaul respirations (rapid, labored breathing) may be evident with severe acidosis.

PATHOPHYSIOLOGY

- Toxicity of these alcohols is related to their metabolites rather than the parent compound.
- Lethal dose for methanol is >15 to 30 ml and >1 to 1.5 ml/kg for ethylene glycol.
- Sequential metabolism by alcohol and aldehyde dehydrogenases converts methanol to formaldehyde and then formic acid, while ethylene glycol is converted to glycoaldehyde, glycolic acid, and then oxalate.
- Fig. E1 depicts the pathways involved in methanol metabolism.
- While methanol metabolites primarily cause retinal injury, ethylene glycol metabolites produce renal tubular injury and calcium oxalate stones.
    1. Formaldehyde binds to tissue proteins and is likely the major toxin in methanol poisoning involving necrosis of retinal and optic neurons and the basal ganglia (putamen). Formic acid, the acid produced in the largest quantity, inhibits cytochrome oxidase, preventing oxygen utilization by mitochondria and causing further organ dysfunction. Leukotriene has been implicated in the inflammation and neurotoxicity characteristic of acute methanol poisoning.
    2. Glycoaldehyde may be the major nephrotoxin, while glycolic acid is the acid produced in the largest quantity in ethylene glycol poisoning, with a small quantity converted to oxalic acid by lactate dehydrogenase. Oxalate then forms calcium oxalate crystals, which are deposited in the renal parenchyma, cerebral blood vessels, and meninges, causing hypocalcemic tetany.

DIAGNOSIS

DIFFERENTIAL DIAGNOSIS

- Other causes of a high anion gap metabolic acidosis include lactic acidosis, diabetic and alcoholic ketoacidosis, kidney failure (acute and chronic), early toluene toxicity, and salicylate intoxication. Of note, L-lactate may be elevated in methanol toxicity due to cytochrome oxidase inhibition by formic acid and an increase of the NADH:NAD^+ ratio that is driven by methanol metabolism.
- Elevated plasma osmolal gap may be encountered in ethyl alcohol or isopropyl alcohol ingestion.

EVALUATION AND WORKUP

- Diagnosis depends on history, clinical presentation, and laboratory abnormalities.
- High anion gap metabolic acidosis (AG >12 mEq/L) with elevated plasma osmolal gap (>10 mOsm/kg; usually >25 mOsm/Kg) in an appropriate clinical setting should raise the suspicion of methanol or ethylene glycol ingestion.
- In either intoxication, an osmolal gap will initially be positive, but as the parent compound is converted to its metabolites, the osmolal gap will normalize and the serum anion gap will increase.
- Serum methanol and ethylene glycol levels are elevated in their respective ingestions.
- Acute kidney injury, hypocalcemia with prolonged QT interval, and calcium oxalate crystalluria are seen with ethylene glycol toxicity.
- Metabolic acidosis in the absence of acute kidney injury suggests methanol toxicity; that is, ethylene glycol is more often associated with acute kidney injury.
- Wood's lamp uses ultraviolet light to detect urinary presence of fluorescein, which is contained in some ethylene glycol preparations. Fluorescence lacks sensitivity and specificity. Therefore, fluorescence is not considered a reliable clinical tool.

LABORATORY TESTS

- Calculation of the anion gap and serum osmolal gap
    1. Anion gap determination: Electrolytes and albumin
    2. Osmolal gap determination: Measured and calculated serum osmolalities (sodium, BUN, glucose, ± ethanol)
- Arterial blood gas analysis, lactate, calcium, and creatine kinase
- Creatinine and urinalysis to evaluate presence of tubular injury and calcium oxalate crystals
- ECG to evaluate QT interval
- Toxicology screen with quantification: Acetaminophen, salicylate, ethanol, methanol, ethylene glycol, and isopropyl alcohol

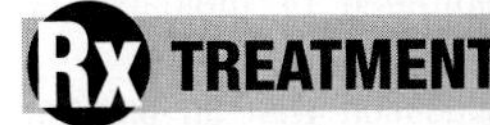

TREATMENT

High index of suspicion and immediate recognition with early treatment remain crucial to reduce mortality. Box 1 describes common commercial products that may contain ethylene glycol.

NONPHARMACOLOGIC THERAPY

- Cardiorespiratory support as required
- Rapid (within 60 minutes) gastric decontamination (charcoal and/or gastric lavage). Later intervention is not beneficial due to rapid and complete invasion (methanol).
- Induction of vomiting is contraindicated even in conscious patients given the risks of development of central nervous system depression in these patients.

BOX 1 Common Commercial Products That May Contain Ethylene Glycol

Paints and lacquers
Polishes and detergents
Inks
Cosmetics
Hydraulic brake fluids
Solar collector fluids
Car wash fluids

Data from Kruse JA: Methanol, ethylene glycol, and related intoxications. In Carlson RW, Geheb MA (eds): *Principles and practice of medical intensive care*, Philadelphia, 1993, Saunders.

ACUTE GENERAL Rx

- Principles of therapy include prevention of formation of toxic metabolites, correction of acidosis, and toxin removal.
- Intravenous isotonic fluids can facilitate urinary excretion of volatile alcohol and its metabolites; when acidosis is present (pH <7.3), isotonic bicarbonate should be used because reversal of acidosis helps prevent end-organ damage from toxic metabolites (target pH: 7.35-7.45).
- Ethanol, a competitive substrate, and fomepizole (4-methylpyrazole or 4-MP), a competitive inhibitor of alcohol dehydrogenase, prevent formation of toxic metabolites of ethylene glycol and methanol.
- Fomepizole is preferred over ethanol given the increased incidence of GI and CNS adverse events with ethanol administration, greater inhibition of alcohol dehydrogenase, and easier administration. Cost and availability of fomepizole may influence the decision to administer this agent vs. ethanol.
- Ethanol: Dosing:
  1. Target ethanol concentration is 100-200 mg/dl and requires close monitoring.
  2. Loading dose: 800 mg/kg in a 10% solution of 5% dextrose in water will raise serum ethanol by 100 mg/dl.
  3. Maintenance dose: Infusion of 80-160 mg/kg/hr based on blood concentrations.
  4. Comment on dosing adjustment in patients receiving concomitant dialysis.
- Fomepizole: Indications for use
  1. Plasma concentration of methanol or ethylene glycol >20 mg/dl OR
  2. Documented ingestion with an osmolal gap >10 mOsm/kg OR
  3. Suspected ingestion with at least two of the following criteria:
     a. Arterial pH <7.3
     b. Serum bicarbonate <20 mEq/L
     c. Osmolal gap >10 mOsm/L
     d. Urinary oxalate crystals in the case of ethylene glycol toxicity
- Fomepizole (4-methylpyrazole): Dosing:
  1. Loading dose: 15 mg/kg body weight
  2. Maintenance dose: 10 mg/kg body weight every 12 hr for 4 doses, then 15 mg/kg every 12 hr (if blood levels do not reach goal by 48 hours)
  3. During hemodialysis: Add 1-1.5 mg/kg/hr, or repeat loading dose every 4 hr
- The half-lives of ethylene glycol and methanol increase with ethanol or fomepizole.
- The half-life of methanol metabolism during treatment with fomepizole is as much as 87 hr. Treatment with fomepizole alone is not recommended, and hemodialysis should be considered to prevent a prolonged requirement for intensive care.
- In contrast, the observed half-life of ethylene glycol with use of fomepizole is only around 17 hours. Ethylene glycol poisoning (even with levels greater than 50 mg/dl) in patients without kidney injury or acidosis can be managed with fomepizole alone, and without hemodialysis.
- Hemodialysis is indicated for likely or confirmed methanol poisoning in the setting of any of the following: New vision or neurologic deficit (particularly seizure or coma); metabolic acidosis or acidemia with pH ≤7.15; elevated anion gap >24 mmol/L; methanol concentration >70 mg/dl (or 21.8 mmol/L) in the context of fomepizole, or >50 mg/dl (or 15.6 mmol/L) in the absence of an ADH blocker.
- Hemodialysis is indicated for likely or confirmed ethylene glycol poisoning in the setting of any of the following: Acute kidney injury; anion gap metabolic acidosis; EG level >50mg/dl (see above regarding use of fomepizole when elevated levels without acidosis or acute kidney injury are present).
- Hemodialysis also should be considered in patients with poisoning and electrolyte imbalances refractory to pharmacologic treatments, or hemodynamic instability.
- Average duration of dialysis in studies was 8.4 ± 3.2 hr.
  1. Treatment with medications and/or hemodialysis is continued until the methanol or ethylene glycol concentration is <20 mg/dl.
  2. Intermittent hemodialysis is the preferred modality of dialysis, as continuous renal replacement therapy (CRRT) alone is ineffective in achieving rapid clearance of methanol and ethylene glycol. In the treatment of a mass outbreak of methanol poisoning, acidemia correction was faster with intermittent hemodialysis than CRRT.
  3. CRRT is an acceptable alternative when intermittent hemodialysis is not available.
  4. If blood concentration levels are not available, start by conducting an 8-hr intermittent hemodialysis session followed by 18 hr of continuous renal replacement therapy; adjust therapy afterward as clinically indicated.
  5. Do not use heparin with dialysis, as heparin may increase the risk of cerebral hemorrhage.

ADJUNCTIVE Rx

- In ethylene glycol poisoning, thiamine (100 mg IV q6h) and pyridoxine (100 mg IV daily) may decrease oxalic acid formation and direct metabolism to less toxic metabolites.
- In methanol poisoning, folinic acid doses (50 mg IV every 6 hr) may increase formic acid metabolism to CO_2 and H_2O. Correct electrolyte abnormalities (hypocalcemia, etc.).
- Treat seizures.

DISPOSITION

Transfer to a hospital with an intensive care unit and hemodialysis capabilities should be carried out early in the course of intoxication.

REFERRAL

- Regional poison center (toxicologist) and nephrology recommended to avoid treatment delays
- Ophthalmology for patients with visual symptoms
- Psychiatry if depression and suicidal ideation are present
- Detoxification centers for patients with substance abuse

PROGNOSIS

- Coma or seizures at presentation and prolonged severe acidosis correlate with increased mortality
- High osmolal gap and high anion gap acidosis associated with high mortality
- Hyperglycemia may correlate with worse prognosis in methanol poisoning

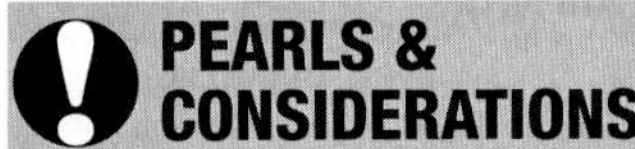

- Profound plasma osmolal gap or anion gap metabolic acidosis should raise suspicion for ethylene glycol and/or methanol ingestion. A high index of suspicion and early treatment are crucial to reducing mortality. The metabolites of methanol and ethylene glycol produce the clinical toxidrome.
- Complaints of visual blurring, central scotomata, and blindness are consistent with methanol poisoning.
- Calcium oxalate crystalluria, oliguria, hematuria, and acute kidney injury are consistent with ethylene glycol poisoning.
- Fomepizole is preferred to ethanol due to complications associated with ethanol use.
- Emergent hemodialysis is indicated with end organ damage and/or severe metabolic acidosis.
- Elevated osmolal gap and anion gap metabolic acidosis may occur rarely with other toxic alcohols such as diethylene glycol and propylene glycol.

SUGGESTED READINGS

Available at ExpertConsult.com

RELATED CONTENT

Algorithm for the management of acute poisoning (Algorithm, Section III)

AUTHOR: **NIKOLAS HARBORD, M.D.**

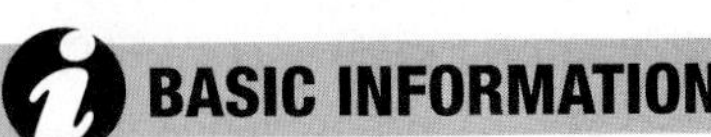

BASIC INFORMATION

DEFINITION

Methicillin-resistant *Staphylococcus aureus* (MRSA) is a common bacterial pathogen with resistance to many antibiotics. It is defined as an *S. aureus* that shows a minimum inhibitory concentration (MIC) of greater than or equal to 4 mcg/ml to oxacillin. There are two types of MRSA:

- HA-MRSA: Hospital-acquired MRSA, usually multidrug resistant
- CA-MRSA: Community-acquired MRSA; an emerging pathogen, usually acquired outside of the hospital setting; resistance may differ from HA-MRSA and is generally susceptible to more antibiotics than HA-MRSA

SYNONYMS

Multidrug-resistant *Staphylococcus aureus*
Oxacillin-resistant *Staphylococcus aureus*

ICD-10CM CODES

A41.02	Sepsis due to Methicillin resistant *Staphylococcus aureus*
A49.02	Methicillin resistant *Staphylococcus aureus* infection, unspecified site
B95.62	Methicillin resistant *Staphylococcus aureus* infection as the cause of diseases classified elsewhere
J15.212	Pneumonia due to Methicillin resistant *Staphylococcus aureus*
Z22.322	Carrier or suspected carrier of Methicillin resistant *Staphylococcus aureus*
Z86.14	Personal history of Methicillin resistant *Staphylococcus aureus* infection

EPIDEMIOLOGY & DEMOGRAPHICS

INCIDENCE: 1:3000

PEAK INCIDENCE: Occurs year round; may peak during summer and fall months for CA-MRSA

PREVALENCE: The national rate of MRSA colonization or infection is 46.3 per 10,000 inpatients. Hospital prevalence rate of MRSA is as high as 60% in hospitals, which means that 60% of *S. aureus* strains in that hospital will be MRSA.

PREDOMINANT SEX AND AGE: All ages and both sexes

RISK FACTORS:

- HA-MRSA: Hospitalization, invasive medical device, residing in long-term nursing facility
- CA-MRSA: Initially seen in young men engaged in athletic activities and in gyms, prisons, military barracks, etc., but has now spread to the entire age spectrum including neonates and the elderly

PHYSICAL FINDINGS & CLINICAL PRESENTATION

- CA-MRSA: Can present with skin infection, associated with opening in the skin; red bump, pustule, or boil; erythema, swelling; edema, often fluctuant and very painful
- HA-MRSA: Bacteremia; infection associated with intravenous device
  1. Catheters: Pneumonia
  2. Skin: Cellulitis
  3. Bone: Osteomyelitis
  4. Endocarditis
  5. Abscesses: Skin or organ
  6. Pneumonia: Nosocomial

ETIOLOGY

- CA-MRSA: The most prevalent strain in the US on pulse field electrophoresis (PFGE) is called USA 300.
  1. CA-MRSA: Common cause of skin and soft tissue infections seen in the emergency room. It can, however, also cause necrotizing pneumonia, sepsis, osteomyelitis, etc.
  2. Virulence factors particular to CA-MRSA: Panton-Valentine leukocidin (PVL) toxin, alpha-hemolysin toxin, phenol soluble modulins, etc., that enhance ability to cause infection
- HA-MRSA: Most strains on PFGE are USA 100 or USA 200 and tend to have multidrug resistance. Patients with HA-MRSA infection have higher mortality and morbidity than patients with a methicillin-sensitive *S. aureus* (MSSA) infection.
- By definition, all MRSA strains carry the *mecA* gene, which confers resistance to all beta-lactam antibiotics, including cephalosporins and carbapenems.

Dx DIAGNOSIS

LABORATORY TESTS

- Rapid detection methods for MRSA:
  1. Rapid culture methods: Chromogenic agar, which uses a culture media that changes color if *Staphylococcus aureus* is present and then has antibiotics incorporated into media that only allows MRSA strains to grow. This allows for early detection of MRSA in 24 to 48 hr
  2. Molecular methods that target gene sequences of the bacteria: PCR and gene probe hybridization. Examples include IDI-MRSA, Genotype MRSA direct and Gene Expert MRSA assay. The sensitivity and specificity of these assays compared to traditional cultures range from 90% to 98% and from 91% to 99%, respectively
- PFGE usually done only for epidemiologic or outbreak purposes

IMAGING STUDIES

- Radiographs or computed tomography scan of suspected organ
- Echocardiogram: All adult patients with *S. aureus* bacteremia should undergo echocardiography

Rx TREATMENT

- CA-MRSA: Oral antibiotics that may be effective include trimethoprim-sulfamethoxazole, doxycycline, minocycline, or clindamycin; linezolid and tedizolid are other options but are very expensive.
- HA-MRSA: Intravenous antibiotics, vancomycin, linezolid, tedizolid, daptomycin, tigecycline

ACUTE GENERAL Rx

- Trimethoprim-sulfamethoxazole, one double-strength tablet PO bid, is useful in cases of CA-MRSA since 95% of community-acquired MRSA strains are susceptible to it in vitro. Other agents that can be used for CA-MRSA include:
  1. Clindamycin: 300 to 450 mg q6 to 8h also inhibits toxin production. If strain tests sensitive to clindamycin but resistant to erythromycin, then a D test must be done to ensure there will not be inducible resistance while on therapy with the clindamycin.
  2. Doxycycline: 100 mg PO q12h and minocycline also have some activity against MRSA.
  3. Rifampin: Never used alone but can be used with one of the other oral agents
- Vancomycin 15 to 20 mg/kg IV q8 to 12h is the mainstay of parenteral therapy for MRSA infections. There is an increasing concern of MRSA strains developing tolerance to vancomycin, requiring higher doses to achieve eradication. True vancomycin resistant strains (MIC ≥32 mg/L) remain rare. Vancomycin trough levels of at least 15 to 20 mcg/ml are recommended to treat MRSA infections.
- Linezolid 600 mg PO or IV bid is a synthetic oxazolidinone FDA-approved for MRSA skin and soft tissue infections and pneumonia. It has been shown to be more effective than vancomycin for MRSA pneumonia. A similar agent, tedizolid (200 mg IV or PO for 6 days), was recently approved for skin and soft tissue infections. These agents are much more expensive than vancomycin.
- Daptomycin: 4 mg/kg/day to 6 mg/kg/day IV is approved for skin and soft tissue infections, bacteremia, and right-sided endocarditis but should not be used for pneumonia as it is inactivated by pulmonary surfactant.
- Tigecycline: 100 mg IV load, then 50 mg IV q12h, is approved for MRSA skin and soft tissue infections and intraabdominal abscess.
- Ceftaroline is a fifth-generation cephalosporin, also effective against MRSA but only skin and soft tissue infections, not pneumonia: 600 mg IV q12h.
- Newer glycopeptide agents: Dalbavancin (1000 mg IV followed by 500 mg IV a week later for complicated skin and soft tissue infections) and telavancin (10 mg/kg IV daily for 7-14 days) to treat skin infections or pneumonia; these are expensive alternatives to vancomycin.

CHRONIC Rx

- Patients with MRSA colonization may have reexposure or may be unable to eradicate colonized state.
- Oral agents used to attempt eradication of colonization are rifampin, tetracycline, and minocycline.

SUGGESTED READINGS

Available at ExpertConsult.com

RELATED CONTENT

Methicillin-Resistant *Staphylococcus aureus* (Patient Information)

AUTHOR: **GLENN G. FORT, M.D., M.P.H.**

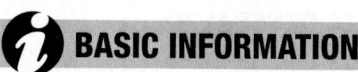

BASIC INFORMATION

DEFINITION

Microangiopathic hemolytic anemia (MAHA) is used to describe any nonautoimmune hemolytic anemia that results in red blood cell fragmentation associated with small vessel disease. Several diseases, including thrombotic thrombocytopenic purpura (TTP), disseminated intravascular coagulation (DIC), hemolytic-uremic syndrome (HUS), HELLP syndrome (hemolysis, elevated liver enzymes, and low platelets) of pregnancy, and malignant hypertension, are associated with MAHA.

SYNONYMS

MAHA
Thrombotic microangiopathy (TMA)
Mechanical hemolytic anemias
Nonautoimmune hemolytic anemias
Fragmentation hemolytic anemia

ICD-10CM CODE
D59.4 Other non-autoimmune hemolytic anemias

EPIDEMIOLOGY & DEMOGRAPHICS

- TTP:
  1. Increased incidence in women and African Americans.
- Typical HUS:
  1. Associated with *E. coli* 0157:H7 in 80% of cases.
  2. Person-person transmission is implicated.
  3. Children are more commonly affected than adults.
- Atypical HUS:
  1. Diarrhea is not a presenting feature.
  2. Adults are more commonly affected.
- DIC:
  1. Always secondary to underlying causes, including sepsis, trauma, malignancy, surgery, or obstetrical complications.
  2. DIC can occur in about 20% of acute leukemias.
- HELLP syndrome:
  1. Occurs in 10% to 20% of pregnancies with preeclampsia.
  2. Develops between 28 and 36 weeks of gestation.
  3. Can also present after delivery of fetus in 30% cases.
- Malignant hypertension:
  1. MAHA complicates about 25% of malignant hypertension cases.

PHYSICAL FINDINGS & CLINICAL PRESENTATION

- Mucosal pallor
- Fatigue
- Acute onset of generalized weakness
- Jaundiced skin
- Icteric sclera
- Dark-colored urine

ETIOLOGY

TTP	Idiopathic or familial deficiency of ADAMTS13 Acquired antibodies against ADAMTS13
Typical HUS	Shiga toxin–producing enterohemorrhagic *E. coli* 0157:H7
Atypical HUS	Inherited disorders of complement regulation
DIC	Secondary to multiple causes resulting in subendothelial tissue factor exposure and subsequent activation of coagulation cascade
HELLP syndrome	Mechanism not clearly identified, but endothelial injury from hypertension associated with preeclampsia has been implicated
Malignant hypertension	Endothelial damage

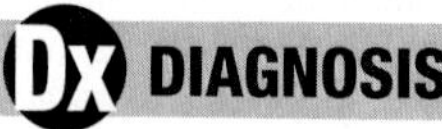

DIAGNOSIS

Pathognomonic findings in MAHA include anemia consistent with an intravascular hemolytic picture, including schistocytes (Fig. 1) on peripheral blood smear, elevated lactate dehydrogenase (LDH), increased indirect bilirubin, decreased serum haptoglobin, increased urinary urobilinogen, along with an elevated reticulocyte count and negative Coombs test.

DIFFERENTIAL DIAGNOSIS

- Immune-mediated hemolysis (positive Coombs test):
  1. Autoimmune hemolytic anemia
  2. Paroxysmal nocturnal hemoglobinuria
  3. Cold agglutinin disease
- Infections affecting red blood count (RBC):
  1. Malaria
  2. Babesiosis
  3. Bartonellosis
- Hemolysis due to mechanical stress or oxidative injury:
  1. G6PD deficiency
  2. Runner's anemia or march hemoglobinuria
- Extravascular hemolysis:
  1. Intrinsic RBC defects
  2. Liver disease
  3. Hypersplenism

WORKUP

- Peripheral blood smear showing schistocytes.
- Laboratory workup including CBC, liver function tests, LDH, haptoglobin, reticulocyte count, Coombs test, and urine analysis.
- MAHA and thrombocytopenia are sufficient to make a diagnosis of TTP or HUS; the classic "pentad" of fever, neurologic abnormalities, and renal failure is no longer necessary.
- In DIC, activated partial thromboplastin time and prothrombin time are prolonged, along with decreased fibrinogen levels and increased fibrin degradation products (including D-dimer).
- Blood pressure is greater than 180/120 mm Hg in malignant hypertension and usually associated with acute kidney injury (including hematuria and proteinuria).
- Additional specific tests:
  1. ADAMTS13 activity assay: Decreased activity is associated with idiopathic TTP, and ADAMTS13-directed antibodies are associated with secondary TTP.
  2. Stool culture for shiga toxin–producing *E. coli* in typical HUS.
  3. Although gold standard, renal biopsy is often not required for diagnosis of malignant hypertension.

TREATMENT

If specific etiology of MAHA is not readily identified, plasma exchange therapy should be instituted immediately, in presence of thrombocytopenia and appropriate clinical picture.

- TTP:
  1. Emergent plasma exchange (PEX) to remove unusually large von Willebrand factor (vWF) multimers and autoantibodies directed against ADAMTS13.
  2. Platelet transfusions reserved only for bleeding patients.
  3. If needed, PEX can be increased from once a day to twice daily, along with concomitant use of corticosteroids.
  4. Patients nonresponsive to PEX can be treated with second-line rituximab with or without cyclophosphamide.
- Typical HUS:
  1. Supportive care, including hemodialysis, for severe acute kidney injury and hypertension management.
- Atypical HUS:
  1. Eculizumab has been shown to be more effective than PEX.

FIG. 1 Peripheral blood smear depicting schistocytes or fragmented red blood count.

- DIC:
  1. Treatment of underlying cause corrects the coagulopathy.
  2. Supportive care, including hemodynamic support and antimicrobial therapy, as indicated.
  3. Activated protein C (APC) is FDA-approved for DIC complicated by sepsis.
- HELLP syndrome:
  1. Emergent delivery of fetus if more than 34 weeks into gestation, preferably vaginal delivery.
  2. If less than 34 weeks' gestation, corticosteroids are recommended for expediting fetal lung maturation and delivery, but not beneficial to the mother.
- Malignant hypertension:
  1. Control blood pressure with medical therapy as indicated.
  2. Care should be taken to avoid rapid lowering of systolic blood pressure, which can lead to ischemia or hyperperfusion syndrome.

MONITORING & FOLLOW-UP

Serial laboratory monitoring of CBC, LDH, and presence of schistocytes on peripheral smear is required to asses MAHA disease activity.

- TTP:
  1. Idiopathic TTP has a relapse rate of 18%, which can happen up to 10 yr from initial presentation.
  2. Serial measurements of ADAMTS13 activity may have predictive value in assessing risk of relapse.
- Typical HUS:
  1. Full recovery of renal function, baseline neurologic status, and resolution of diarrhea.
- DIC:
  1. With adequate management of underlying cause, coagulopathy associated with DIC is reversible.
- HELLP syndrome:
  1. MAHA, thrombocytopenia, and liver injury is resolved within 48 hours after fetal delivery.
  2. Patients should be monitored for at least 2 days, with laboratory workup including CBC, LDH, and liver function.
- Malignant hypertension:
  1. Early adequate blood pressure control can reverse acute kidney injury.
  2. Patients can be discharged from the hospital after achieving adequate blood pressure control on an oral regimen.

PROGNOSIS

TTP:

- If untreated, TTP has a high mortality rate of 90%.
- With PEX, mortality rate in idiopathic TTP is 15% and up to 59% in nonidiopathic TTP.

Typical HUS:

- Typical HUS has a mortality rate of 5%, and younger children have better prognosis compared with adults.
- Central nervous system involvement or other extrarenal manifestations portend poor outcomes.

Atypical HUS:

- Mortality ranges between 15% and 25%.
- Adults have poor prognosis compared with children.
- At 1-yr mark, about 25% of all patients have chronic renal failure.

DIC:

- Prognosis of DIC depends on the severity of coagulopathy and underlying condition.
- DIC has been shown to be an independent predictor of mortality in sepsis and trauma, increasing the risk of death by a factor of 1.5 to 2.

HELLP:

- Increased risk of preeclampsia in future pregnancies.
- Recurrence of HELLP with subsequent pregnancies is about 5%.

Malignant hypertension:

- 10-yr overall survival is approximately 50%.
- MAHA in malignant hypertension predicts an increased likelihood of need for future hemodialysis.

REFERRAL

- Hematologist
- Nephrologist
- Neurologist
- Obstetrician

PEARLS & CONSIDERATIONS

- MAHA is not an individual clinical entity by itself, but rather includes many causes with different pathologic mechanisms, with a common phenomenon of small-vessel disease causing intravascular hemolysis.
- Presence of anemia with schistocytes and thrombocytopenia are key features in recognizing MAHA.
- If the etiology of MAHA is not readily apparent on initial evaluation, PEX must be immediately instituted for presumed TTP because it has a very high mortality rate of 90% if untreated.

SUGGESTED READING

Available at ExpertConsult.com

RELATED CONTENT

Disseminated Intravascular Coagulation (Related Key Topic)
HELLP Syndrome (Related Key Topic)
Hemolytic-Uremic Syndrome (Related Key Topic)
Thrombotic Thrombocytopenic Purpura (Related Key Topic)

AUTHOR: **SHIVA KUMAR R. MUKKAMALLA, M.D., M.P.H.**

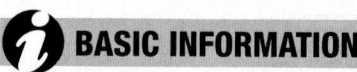

BASIC INFORMATION

DEFINITION

Microsporidiosis is an infection caused by single-celled protozoan intracellular spore-forming organisms called microsporidia. Recent evidence suggests a relationship between microsporidia and fungi. Infections occur more commonly in patients with HIV/AIDS, travelers, children, organ transplant recipients, contact lens wearers, and the elderly.

SYNONYMS

Enterocytozoon bieneusi infection
Encephalitozoon species infection

ICD-10CM CODES
B60.8 Microsporidiosis
A07.8 Microsporidiosis, intestinal
H16.8 Keratitis, microsporidia

EPIDEMIOLOGY & DEMOGRAPHICS

Microsporidia are a phylum of ubiquitous protists that exist worldwide in the environment and can infect vertebrate and invertebrate hosts, entering via ingestion or inhalation of spores and by direct contact through broken skin or lesions in the eyes.

PREVALENCE: Prevalence in immunocompetent persons is unclear, with rates varying from 5% to 45% in recent studies of stool from healthy human subjects.

In the postantiretroviral therapy era, prevalence rates have decreased; however, in a study of asymptomatic HIV patients, 15% had evidence of microsporidia on small bowel biopsy.

RISK FACTORS: Infections such as a non-bloody watery diarrhea and keratoconjunctivitis in contact lens wearers can occur in normal hosts, but immunocompromised hosts such as AIDS patients, organ transplant recipients, and bone marrow graft recipients are at greater risk for more severe disease, other organ involvement, and disseminated infection. Patients living with AIDS who have CD4 counts <200 should be advised to avoid untreated water and undercooked meat or seafood.

ETIOLOGY

- There are 1200 species of Microsporidia, but only 14 infect humans from seven different genuses. The four most common species to cause human disease are:
  1. *Enterocytozoon bieneusi*
  2. *Encephalitozoon intestinalis*
  3. *Encephalitozoon cuniculi*
  4. *Encephalitozoon hellem*
- These genotypes that infect humans have been identified in domestic, farm, and wild animals and thus may be a form of zoonotic disease.

PHYSICAL FINDINGS & CLINICAL PRESENTATION

Each species of microsporidia has different reported infections:

- *Enterocytozoon bieneusi* can cause diarrhea, wasting syndrome, cholangitis, rhinitis, or bronchitis.
- *Encephalitozoon intestinalis* can cause diarrhea, intestinal perforation, cholangitis, nephritis, keratoconjunctivitis, and disseminated infection.
- *Encephalitozoon cuniculi* can cause hepatitis, peritonitis, encephalitis, urethritis, prostatitis, nephritis, sinusitis, keratoconjunctivitis, cystitis, cellulitis, and disseminated infection.
- *Encephalitozoon hellem* can cause keratoconjunctivitis, sinusitis, pneumonitis, nephritis, prostatitis, urethritis, cystitis, and disseminated infection.

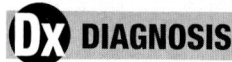

DIAGNOSIS

DIFFERENTIAL DIAGNOSIS

- Other causes of watery non-bloody diarrhea: *Norovirus, Giardia, Cryptosporidia, Cyclospora*, and *Isospora belli*
- Other causes of keratoconjunctivitis: Herpetic keratoconjunctivitis and acanthamoeba keratitis

WORKUP

Consists of the microscopic detection of microsporidia spores (1-2 mcm in diameter) in stool, body fluids, or tissue samples

LABORATORY TESTS

- Modified trichrome stain with light microscopy can be used on stool, urine, mucus, or tissues. Spores stain pink against a blue-green background.
- Fluorescent techniques: Calcofluor white stain, Uvitex 2B, and Fungi-Fluor kit
- Indirect immunofluorescence
- Serology: Detects IgM and IgG antibodies
- For exact speciation: PCR

Rx TREATMENT

ACUTE GENERAL Rx

Treatment will depend on organism and site involved.

- There is no available therapy currently for *E. bieneusi*; however, immune restoration through initiation of antiretroviral therapy (ART) has been shown to resolve symptoms in AIDS patients. ART should be offered as a part of initial management where applicable.
- Intestinal or disseminated infection caused by microsporidia other than *E. bieneusi* and *V. corneae*: Albendazole 400 mg PO bid for 2 to 4 weeks depending on level of immunosuppression. Children: 15 mg/kg/day PO in divided doses. For disseminated disease (especially *Trachipleistophora* or *Anncaliia* infections), consider the addition of itraconazole.
- Keratoconjunctivitis: Topical fumagillin 70 mcg/ml eye drops (2 drops every 2 hours for 4 days, then 2 drops 4 times a day). If associated with intestinal disease, add albendazole 400 mg PO bid for 2 to 4 weeks depending on degree of immunosuppression.

CHRONIC Rx

- Antimotility agents are useful to control diarrhea.
- Recurrence or relapse may occur with ongoing immunosuppression; therefore, consider chronic maintenance therapy until CD4 counts remain >200 for 6 months in those living with HIV.

REFERRAL

- Infectious diseases physician for antiretroviral therapy if positive for HIV/AIDS
- Ophthalmologist if keratoconjunctivitis is suspected

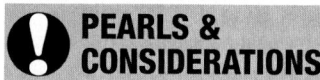

PEARLS & CONSIDERATIONS

COMMENTS

- Microsporidia infections occur particularly in HIV-positive patients with CD4+ cell counts <50/ml.
- Microsporidia spores can remain active in the environment for prolonged periods of time (e.g., months).

SUGGESTED READINGS
Available at ExpertConsult.com

AUTHORS: **PHILIP A. CHAN, M.D., M.S.,** and **GLENN G. FORT, M.D., M.P.H.**

M

Diseases and Disorders

BASIC INFORMATION

DEFINITION

Migraine headaches are recurrent severe headaches that either are preceded by a focal neurologic symptom (migraine with aura), occur independently without preceding focal neurologic symptoms (migraine without aura), or have atypical presentations (migraine variants). The migraine aura (Box 1) typically is characterized by visual or sensory symptoms that develop over 5 to 60 min. If the aura includes unilateral motor weakness, the migraine is referred to as hemiplegic. In migraine with and without aura, the headache is typically moderate to severe, unilateral, pulsatile, made worse with head movement, and associated with nausea and vomiting, photophobia, and phonophobia. Migraines that occur ≥15 days every month for ≥3 mo are known as chronic; otherwise, they are referred to as episodic. Table 1 summarizes criteria for migraine.

ICD-10CM CODES

G43.909	Migraine, unspecified, not intractable, without status migrainosus
G43.1	Migraine with aura (classical migraine)
G43.0	Migraine without aura (common migraine)
G43.2	Status migrainosus
G43.3	Complicated migraine

EPIDEMIOLOGY & DEMOGRAPHICS

INCIDENCE: Increases from infancy, peaks during the third decade of life, then decreases

PREVALENCE (IN U.S.): Migraine is very common, affecting 1 in 6 people in the U.S. It is the fourth or fifth most common reason for an emergency room visit and the seventh leading cause of time spent disabled worldwide.

AGE: Peak prevalence between ages of 18 and 49

PREDOMINANT SEX: Female:male ratio of 3:1

GENETICS:

- Familial predisposition: More than 50% of migraine sufferers have an affected family member
- Autosomal-dominant transmission for some rare migraine variants (familial hemiplegic migraine, cerebral autosomal-dominant arteriopathy with subcortical infarcts and leukoencephalopathy [CADASIL]); familial hemiplegic migraines have been associated with calcium channelopathy, sodium channelopathy, and Na^+/K^+-ATPase dysfunction.

BOX 1 Auras of Migraine

Sensory phenomena
- Special senses
  - Visual, olfactory, auditory, gustatory
- Paresthesias, especially lips and hand

Motor deficits
- Hemiparesis, hemiplegia

Neuropsychologic changes

Aphasia

Perceptual impairment, especially for size, shape, and time

Emotional and behavioral
- Anxiety, depression, irritability, (rarely) hyperactivity

From Kaufman DM, Geyer HL, Milstein MJ: *Kaufman's clinical neurology for psychiatrists*, ed 8, Philadelphia, 2017, Elsevier.

PHYSICAL FINDINGS & CLINICAL PRESENTATION

- Normal between episodes
- Normal for migraine without aura.
- Focal motor or sensory abnormalities possible for migraine with aura or migraine variants.
- Common aura types include scintillating scotoma, bright zigzags (fortifications), and other visual distortions such as macropsia or micropsia (enlargement or shrinkage of objects) that often cross visual fields. Homonymous visual disturbance, sensory phenomena such as hemibody paresthesia, speech disturbances, or hemiparesis (familial or sporadic hemiplegic migraine) also can occur independently or associated with visual symptoms.

ETIOLOGY

The pathophysiology of migraines is not clearly understood, although the primary neuronal event results in a trigeminovascular reflex causing neurogenic inflammation. Calcitonin-gene related peptide (CGRP) is released by the trigeminal ganglion and binds receptors around meningeal vessels leading to inflammation. Serotonin, substance P, and nitric oxide also play a role, but the exact mechanism is unknown. Cortical spreading depressions also likely are responsible for the aura.

DIAGNOSIS

Migraine without aura:

- Five attacks fulfilling criteria
- Headache attacks lasting 4 to 72 hr
- Headache has at least two of the following characteristics:
  1. Unilateral location
  2. Pulsating quality
  3. Moderate or severe pain intensity
  4. Aggravation or causing avoidance of routine physical activity
- At least one of the following during headache:
  1. Nausea and/or vomiting
  2. Photophobia and phonophobia

Migraine with typical aura:

- At least two attacks
- Aura consisting of at least one of the following, but no motor weakness:
  1. Fully reversible visual symptoms, including positive and/or negative features
  2. Fully reversible sensory symptoms, including positive and/or negative features
  3. Fully reversible dysphasic speech disturbance
- At least two of the following:
  1. Homonymous visual symptoms and/or unilateral sensory symptoms
  2. At least one aura symptom develops gradually over >5 min and/or different aura symptoms occur in succession over >5 min
  3. Each symptom lasts between 5 and 60 min.
- A migraine occurring during or within 60 min of the aura

DIFFERENTIAL DIAGNOSIS

- A diagnosis of migraine is possible only after five recurrent episodes.
- The first or the worst headache should always be investigated, and the differential includes headaches from all secondary causes.
- Headache red flags can be remembered by the mnemonic SSNOOP5:
  1. S: Systemic symptoms of fever, weight loss
  2. S: Secondary risk factors of immunosuppression from any cause, cancer
  3. N: Neurologic deficits, altered consciousness
  4. O: Onset is sudden, abrupt, split second thunderclap
  5. O: Older, age >50 for new-onset headache should be worked up for giant cell arteritis
  6. P: Pattern: change in headache pattern
  7. P: Pregnancy
  8. P: Positional or postural
  9. P: Papilledema
  10. P: Precipitation with Valsalva maneuver or exertion
- Section II describes the differential diagnosis of headaches. Table 1 compares tension-type and migraine headaches.
- Useful mnemonic for migraine is POUND: Pulsatile, One day in duration, Unilateral, Nausea/vomiting, Disabling.

WORKUP

- In general, no additional investigation is needed with recurrent, typical attacks with usual age of onset, family history, and a normal physical examination.

TABLE 1 Comparison of Tension-Type and Migraine Headaches

	Tension-Type	Migraine
Location	Bilateral	Hemicranial*
Nature	Dull ache	Throbbing*
Severity	Slight–moderate	Moderate–severe
Associated symptoms	None	Nausea, hyperacusis, photophobia
Behavior	Continues working	Seeks seclusion
Effect of alcohol	Reduces headache	Worsens headache

*In approximately half of patients, at least at onset

From Kaufman DM, Geyer HL, Milstein MJ: *Kaufman's clinical neurology for psychiatrists*, ed 8, Philadelphia, 2017, Elsevier.

- If there is an unusual presentation, headache with red flags, and/or unexpected findings on examination, investigation for other causes is required.

LABORATORY TESTS

Lumbar puncture for history of abrupt-onset headaches and uncertain diagnosis of migraine

IMAGING STUDIES

- Imaging should be done in patients with any of the red flags for secondary headache such as described by the SSNOOP5 mnemonic (see "Differential Diagnosis" above).
- MRI brain with and without contrast is the imaging modality of choice for almost all headache types, although CT head without contrast may be used in the acute setting to evaluate for subarachnoid hemorrhage or other causes of acute intracranial hemorrhage.

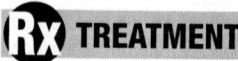

TREATMENT

Consider the use of a headache log/diary to identify triggers of headaches, record efficacy of treatments, and track history of headaches.

NONPHARMACOLOGIC THERAPY

- Avoid any identifiable provoking factors: Caffeine, tobacco, and alcohol may trigger attacks, as may dietary or other environmental precipitants (less common).
- Avoid emotional stressors and minimize variations in daily routine with regular sleep, meals, and exercise.
- Relaxation training, behavioral therapy, and biofeedback. Trials have shown that among young persons with chronic migraine, the use of cognitive behavior therapy (CBT) plus amitriptyline results in greater reductions in days with headaches and migraine-related disability compared with use of headache education plus amitriptyline.
- Trials in patients with migraine without aura have shown that acupuncture may be associated with long-term reduction in migraine recurrence.[1]

ACUTE ANALGESIC Rx

- Many oral agents are ineffective because of poor absorption from migraine-induced gastric stasis. Non-oral route of administration should be selected in patients with severe nausea or vomiting.
- NSAIDs such as ketorolac, ibuprofen, and naproxen, or combination analgesics, may be used first line for mild migraine headaches.
- Barbiturate-containing compounds are potentially addictive and promote medication overuse headaches.
- Opioids are not effective for treating patients with migraine headaches and should not be used.

ACUTE ABORTIVE Rx

- Triptans (SC, PO, and intranasal) are the drug class of choice for abortive therapy. Meta-analysis suggests that 10 mg rizatriptan, 40 mg eletriptan, and 12.5 mg almotriptan are most effective. Sumatriptan may also be given, especially in combination with naproxen. Early administration improves effectiveness. Triptans are relatively contraindicated in heart disease and hemiplegic migraine.
- IV antiemetics (prochlorperazine, metoclopramide, chlorpromazine) may be used in addition to triptans. Acute dystonic reactions, QT prolongation, and akathisia are rare side effects. These are generally not used as monotherapy.
- Ergotamine, ergotamine combinations (PO/PR), and dihydroergotamine (DHE 45) (SC, IV, IM, intranasal) have well-documented efficacy against migraines. DHE is usually administered in combination with an antiemetic drug (Table 2) but cannot be given within 24 hours of a triptan.
- IV dexamethasone may be used to prevent recurrence but should not be used frequently due to risk for toxicity.
- Greater and lesser occipital nerve blocks may also be performed to alleviate pain in the acute setting. These injections may be combined with auriculotemporal, supraorbital, and supratrochlear nerve block to achieve anesthesia in the area of perceived pain.

PROPHYLAXIS Rx

- Prophylactic treatment is generally indicated when headaches occur more than once a week or when symptomatic treatments are contraindicated or not effective. They are most effective when initiated during a headache-free period. All prophylaxis should be maintained for at least 3 mo before deeming the medication a failure.
- Well-established options for prophylactic treatment include β-blockers (propranolol, timolol, atenolol, metoprolol), tricyclic antidepressants (amitriptyline, nortriptyline), and the antiepileptic drugs topiramate and sodium divalproate (valproic acid).
- CGRP monoclonal antibodies: A new class of injectable drugs that target the CGRP molecule or its receptor have been approved recently. There are currently three FDA-approved drugs in this class–erenumab (Aimovig), fremanezumab (Ajovy), and galcanezumab (Emgality), with more under study. These drugs can be used first line for episodic and chronic migraine.
- Less-established options include calcium channel blockers, selective norepinephrine serotonin reuptake inhibitors, memantine, and other antiepileptic medications.
- Supraorbital transcutaneous electrical stimulation has been approved by the FDA for prophylaxis of episodic migraine and is widely available with a prescription in Europe and North America.
- The FDA has approved injection of onabotulinum toxin A (Botox) for prevention of headaches in adult patients with chronic migraines only (≥15 headache days/mo for ≥3 mo).
- Surgical treatment for migraine using nerve decompression has been recently advocated but remains highly controversial, with poorly established results. This should be pursued only in collaboration with a headache specialist.

DISPOSITION

With advancing age, many patients will have sustained reduction in frequency of migraine headaches.

REFERRAL

To neurologist if uncertain about diagnosis or treatment not effective

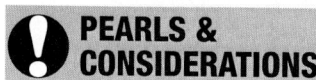

PEARLS & CONSIDERATIONS

- Migraines that change in character or headaches that are different from the patient's typical ones need to be reevaluated.
- Avoid use of narcotics, barbiturates, and benzodiazepines because they are habit-forming. Narcotics and barbiturates also promote medical overuse headaches.
- Long-term use of analgesic medications can result in medication overuse or rebound headaches.
- Migraine with aura is associated with excess stroke and thromboembolism risk and a relative contraindication to the use of combined oral contraceptives in women.

SUGGESTED READINGS

Available at ExpertConsult.com

RELATED CONTENT

Migraine Headache (Patient Information)

AUTHORS: **COREY GOLDSMITH, M.D.,** and **JOSEPH S. KASS, M.D., J.D.**

[1] Zhao L et al: The long-term effect of acupuncture for migraine prophylaxis: a randomized clinical trial, *JAMA Intern Med* 177(4):508–515, 2017.

TABLE 2 Abortive and Analgesic Therapy for Migraine*

Drug	Route	Dose
Triptans (Serotonin Agonists)		
Sumatriptan	Subcutaneous	6 mg, repeat in 2 hr (max 2 doses/day)
Sumatriptan	Oral	25 mg, 50 mg, 100 mg, repeat in 2 hr (max 200 mg/day)
Sumatriptan	Nasal spray	5 mg, 20 mg, repeat in 2 hr (max 40 mg/day)
Zolmitriptan	Oral	1.25, 2.5 mg, 5 mg, repeat in 2 hr (max 10 mg/day)
Zolmitriptan	Nasal spray	5 mg, repeat in 2 hr (max 10 mg/day)
Zolmitriptan	Orally disintegrating tab	2.5, 5 mg, repeat in 2 hr (max 10 mg/day)
Naratriptan	Oral	1 mg, 2.5 mg, repeat in 4 hr (max 5 mg/day)
Rizatriptan	Oral	5 mg, 10 mg, repeat in 2 hr (max 30 mg/day)
Almotriptan	Oral	6.25 mg, 12.5 mg, may repeat in 2 hr (max 25 mg/day)
Eletriptan	Oral	20 mg, 40 mg, may repeat in 2 hr (max 80 mg/day)
Frovatriptan	Oral	2.5 mg, may repeat in 2 hr (max 7.5 mg/day); may also be used for mini prophylaxis
Ergotamine Preparations		
Ergotamine and caffeine	Oral	2 tablets, may repeat 1 tab q30 min (max 6/day)
Ergotamine and caffeine	Rectal	1 suppository, repeat in 1 hr (max 2/day)
Ergotamine	Sublingual	1 tablet, repeat in 1 hr (max 2/day)
Dihydroergotamine	Intramuscular	0.5-1.0 mg, repeat twice at 1-hr intervals (max 3 mg/attack)
	Subcutaneous	
	Intravenous	
	Nasal spray	
Isometheptene+ dichloralphenazone+ acetaminophen	Oral	1 to 2 capsules, repeat in 4 hr (max 8/day)
Nonsteroidal Antiinflammatory Drugs		
Acetaminophen+ (should not be used alone)	Oral	2 tablets, repeat in 6 hr (max 8/day aspirin+caffeine)
Naproxen	Oral	550-750 mg, repeat in 1 hr (max 3 times/wk)
Meclofenamate	Oral	100-200 mg, repeat in 1 hr (max 3 times/wk)
Flurbiprofen	Oral	50-100 mg, repeat in 1 hr (max 3 times/wk)
Ibuprofen	Oral	200-300 mg, repeat in 1 hr (max 3 times/wk)
Antiemetics		
Promethazine	Oral	50-125 mg
	Intramuscular	No clear benefit in migraine, may be used
Prochlorperazine	Oral	1-25 mg
	Rectal	2.5-25 mg (suppository)
	Intramuscular/IV	5-10 mg, good evidence for strong benefit
Chlorpromazine	Oral	10-25 mg
	Rectal	50-100 mg (suppository)
	Intravenous	Up to 35 mg, use with monitoring, some evidence for good benefit
Trimethobenzamide	Oral	250 mg
	Rectal	200 mg
Metoclopramide	Oral	5-10 mg
	Intramuscular	10 mg
	Intravenous	5-10 mg
Dimenhydrinate	Oral	50 mg

*For side effects and contraindications, consult the manufacturer's drug insert before prescribing any of these drugs.
Modified from Wiederholt WC: *Neurology for non-neurologists*, ed 4, Philadelphia, 2000, Saunders.

BASIC INFORMATION

DEFINITION

Significant cognitive impairment in the absence of dementia with preserved activities of daily living (ADLs). Mild cognitive impairment (MCI) is an intermediate state between normal cognitive function and dementia. The main distinctions between MCI and mild dementia are that in the latter, more than one cognitive domain is invariably involved and substantial interference with daily life is evident.[1]

SYNONYMS

Mild neurocognitive disorder
MCI

ICD-10CM CODE

G31.84 Mild cognitive impairment, so stated

EPIDEMIOLOGY & DEMOGRAPHICS

INCIDENCE:

- 12 to 15 cases per 1000 person-yr age ≥65
- 51 to 77 cases per 1000 person-yr age ≥75

PEAK INCIDENCE: In the elderly

PREVALENCE: 15% to 25% in those older than age 70

PREDOMINANT SEX AND AGE: Male, age ≥75

GENETICS: *APOE4* genotype

- Various pathways result in amyloid accumulation and deposition in pre-Alzheimer's presenting as MCI.

RISK FACTORS: Male sex, age, lower socioeconomic status, lower educational level

CLINICAL PRESENTATION

- Subjective memory problems, preferably corroborated by another person.
- Preserved functional status (ADLs).
- Normal general thinking and reasoning skills.
- Subtypes of MCI include amnestic (mainly involves memory loss) vs. nonamnestic with involvement of other cognitive domains (single domain vs. multiple domains).
- Domains affected in MCI include memory, visuospatial skills, language, attention, and executive function.
- Olfactory dysfunction may be associated with amnestic MCI and progression to Alzheimer's dementia.

ETIOLOGY

Neurodegenerative, vascular, traumatic, depression, or due to underlying medical condition

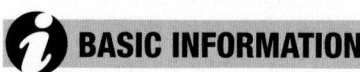

DIAGNOSIS

DIFFERENTIAL DIAGNOSIS

- Delirium
- Dementia
- Depression
- "Reversible" cognitive impairment:
  1. Medication related (anticholinergics)
  2. Hypothyroidism
  3. Vitamin B_{12} deficiency
- Reversible CNS conditions:
  1. Subdural hematoma
  2. Normal pressure hydrocephalus
  3. Metastatic disease

WORKUP

History:

- Focus on cognitive deficits and impairment.
- Review all medications that may impact cognition (i.e., anticholinergics).
- Rule out depression and delirium.
- Perform functional assessment.
- Additional history from family members or caregivers is important.

Physical exam:

- Check blood pressure
- Neurologic exam to rule out reversible CNS causes of cognitive impairment
- Gait and balance assessment

Cognitive function testing:

- Brief mental status testing using MOCA (Montreal Cognitive Assessment) or SLUMS (Saint Louis University Mental Status) for office screening followed by neuropsychological testing if appropriate for specific deficits in cognitive domains. MOCA may be a better tool in identifying and following MCI with higher sensitivity to monitor cognitive decline in longitudinal monitoring.

LABORATORY TESTS

- Complete blood count
- Comprehensive metabolic profile
- TSH
- Vitamin B_{12}

IMAGING STUDIES

- CT imaging can detect most reversible CNS conditions leading to cognitive impairment.
- MRI further evaluates vascular, infectious, neoplastic, and inflammatory conditions.

Rx TREATMENT

- There is insufficient evidence to recommend use of cholinesterase inhibitors for MCI. They are not approved for treating MCI, have shown little efficacy in altering progression to dementia, and can have significant side effects.
- Consider treatment with these medications only if memory complaints appear to be affecting day-to-day quality of life in individual patients or in amnestic subtypes of MCI after risk-versus-benefit discussion with patient and family.

NONPHARMACOLOGIC THERAPY

- Role of cognitive rehabilitation to target specific deficits
- Caregiver education and counseling
- Physical and mental exercises to maintain cognition should be recommended

COMPLEMENTARY & ALTERNATIVE MEDICINE

No clear indications for antioxidants, and studies in humans are inconclusive.

DISPOSITION

- Progression to Alzheimer's at the rate of 5% to 15% per yr.
  1. Risk factors for progression to dementia include presence of vascular risk factors, significant cognitive impairment, depression, and presence of extrapyramidal signs.
- Mortality of those with MCI is twice that of those without MCI.
- Two- to threefold increase in risk of nursing home placement in those with MCI.

REFERRAL

Consider referral to a memory specialist if more than just memory is involved or for further evaluation of specific deficits.

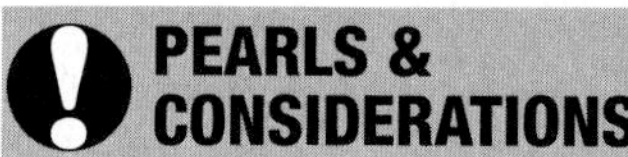

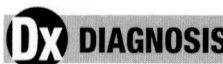

PEARLS & CONSIDERATIONS

COMMENTS

- Patients with MCI usually report short-term memory concerns such as misplacing things, not remembering names of people, word-finding difficulties, forgetting day-to-day tasks, not being able to read a book, or not being able to follow a conversation.
- MCI becomes clinically relevant when quality of life is affected such as problems making financial decisions and problems with personal day-to-day interactions.
- Depression should be ruled out prior to making a diagnosis of MCI since it is highly prevalent in the elderly.
- Anticholinergic medication use should be evaluated carefully prior to making a diagnosis of MCI.

PREVENTION

Patients with MCI should be counseled on strategies to prevent progression to dementia. They should remain physically and mentally active, have a well-balanced diet, continue activities that are socially engaging, reduce stress in their lives, and aggressively pursue treatment of vascular risk factors.

PATIENT & FAMILY EDUCATION

- Patients with MCI typically have poor retention and rapid loss of newly learned information.
- For additional information for patients, families, and clinicians: Alzheimer's Association (www.alzheimers.org).

SUGGESTED READINGS

Available at ExpertConsult.com

AUTHORS: **BIRJU B. PATEL, M.D.,** and **N. WILSON HOLLAND, M.D.**

---

[1]Knopman DS, Petersen RC: Mild cognitive impairment and mild dementia: a clinical perspective, *Mayo Clin Proc* 89:1452, 2014.

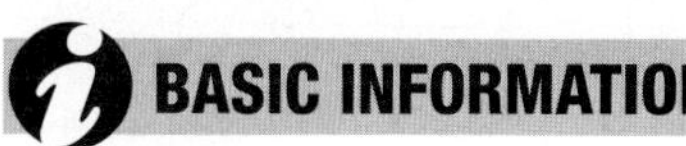

BASIC INFORMATION

DEFINITION

Mitral regurgitation (MR) is retrograde blood flow into the left atrium resulting from an incompetent mitral valve. This condition may cause left ventricular (LV) failure as well as increased left atrial and pulmonary pressures leading to pulmonary hypertension and right-sided heart failure.

SYNONYMS

Mitral insufficiency
MR

ICD-10CM CODES

I34.0 Nonrheumatic mitral (valve) insufficiency
I05.1 Rheumatic mitral insufficiency
I05.9 Mitral valve disease, unspecified
I05.2 Rheumatic mitral stenosis with insufficiency
Q23.3 Congenital mitral insufficiency

EPIDEMIOLOGY & DEMOGRAPHICS

The incidence of MR has increased over the past 30 yr. However, this may be due to increasing availability of echocardiography leading to MR diagnosis rather than to an actual increase in the prevalence of this condition.

PHYSICAL FINDINGS & CLINICAL PRESENTATION

- Holosystolic, high-pitched, "blowing" murmur at apex with radiation to base, left axilla, or back. There is a poor correlation between the intensity of the systolic murmur and the degree of regurgitation. However, an early diastolic to mid-diastolic rumble (pseudo-mitral stenosis) suggests severe MR.
- The murmur of acute MR (e.g., from papillary muscle rupture) can be very soft or inaudible due to a large regurgitant volume entering a noncompliant left atrium. This causes an acute rise in left atrial pressure and thus a lack of significant gradient for an audible murmur.
- Hyperdynamic apex, sometimes with palpable LV lift and apical thrill.
- Diminished S1, reflecting failure of valve leaflets to coapt completely; widely split S2 (decreased LV ejection time results in early A2); and presence of an S3.
- Many patients with mild to moderate MR will remain asymptomatic without evidence of hemodynamic compromise for years until LV remodeling occurs.
- Symptomatic patients with MR generally present with the following:
  1. Symptoms suggestive of heart failure (fatigue, dyspnea, orthopnea, paroxysmal nocturnal dyspnea, edema)
  2. Hemoptysis (caused by pulmonary hypertension)
  3. Atrial fibrillation

ETIOLOGY

Primary MR:
- Idiopathic myxomatous degeneration of the mitral valve, mitral valve prolapse (most common cause of MR in industrialized countries)
- Papillary muscle dysfunction or rupture (typically as a result of an inferior wall myocardial infarction)
- Ruptured chordae tendineae
- Infective endocarditis
- Calcified mitral valve annulus
- Rheumatic valvulitis (may be combined with mitral stenosis; common in developing countries)
- Systemic lupus erythematosus (Libman-Sacks endocarditis)
- Drugs: Fenfluramine, dexfenfluramine, pergolide, cabergoline
- Congenital cleft valve
- Ischemic mitral regurgitation due to papillary muscle dysfunction from multivessel CAD

Secondary MR:
- Hypertrophic cardiomyopathy
- LV dilation (e.g., secondary to dilated cardiomyopathy)

DIAGNOSIS

DIFFERENTIAL DIAGNOSIS

- Hypertrophic cardiomyopathy
- Tricuspid regurgitation
- Aortic stenosis
- Aortic sclerosis
- Ventricular septal defect
- Atrial septal defect

WORKUP

- Diagnostic workup consists of echocardiography, ECG, and chest radiograph; cardiac catheterization is sometimes needed to confirm severity of the disease.
- Tables 1 and 2 summarize stages of chronic primary and chronic secondary mitral regurgitation.
- Recent studies suggest that in patients with severe asymptomatic MR, normal LV function and elevations of brain natriuretic peptide (BNP) >105 pg/ml have an independent and additive prognostic value that may identify high-risk patients and aid in the selection of patients for early surgery.

IMAGING STUDIES

- Echocardiography (Fig. 1): Dilated left atrium, hyperdynamic left ventricle (erratic motion of the leaflet is seen in patients with ruptured chordae tendineae); color flow Doppler will show evidence of MR. The most important aspect of the echocardiographic examination is the quantification of the severity of MR (Table 3); LV systolic performance, estimated right ventricular (RV) systolic pressure vena contracta width >0.7 cm, regurgitant volume >60 ml, regurgitant orifice area >0.40 cm2 by PISA (proximal isovelocity surface area), and systolic pulmonary vein flow reversal are all echocardiographic criteria of severe MR.
- Chest x-ray:
  1. Left atrial enlargement, LV enlargement
  2. Possible pulmonary congestion, although most often normal
- ECG:
  1. Left atrial enlargement
  2. LV hypertrophy
  3. Atrial fibrillation
- Cardiac catheterization: To confirm severity of MR, or to rule out presence of coronary artery disease in patients being evaluated for surgical replacement
- Can consider cardiac MRI in cases where echocardiography is limited or LV function/dimensions are borderline, or when clinical condition and echocardiographic findings are discordant.

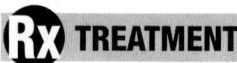

TREATMENT

NONPHARMACOLOGIC THERAPY

- Salt restriction
- Surgical repair or replacement (see the following)

ACUTE GENERAL Rx

- Medical: Medical therapy is primarily directed toward treatment of the source or its complications (e.g., atrial fibrillation, ischemic heart disease, infective endocarditis, hypertension, and heart failure).
  1. The utility of afterload reduction to decrease the regurgitant fraction and increase cardiac output depends upon the etiology of MR. In acute MR, intravenous nitroprusside has shown some utility. Long-term use of oral afterload reducers (e.g., ACE inhibitors or angiotensin receptor blockers), while they do not slow the progression of mitral regurgitation, should be implemented when other indications such as hypertension and LV dysfunction are present.
  2. Control ventricular response in atrial fibrillation with rapid ventricular response when present. Use anticoagulants if atrial fibrillation occurs, which of note is not considered valvular, and novel anticoagulation agents may be used for stroke prophylaxis.
  3. Diuresis and achieving a euvolemic state may significantly decrease the degree of functional MR caused by volume overload and heart failure.
- Surgery: Surgery is the only definitive treatment for MR. Although no randomized trial of mitral valve repair vs. replacement exists, repair is favored over replacement in degenerative mitral valve disease due to its lower perioperative risk, improved event-free survival, freedom from complications of prosthetic valves, and better postoperative LV function. It is a class I indication in patients with the following diagnoses (Fig. 2):
  1. Acute severe MR
  2. Symptomatic patients with severe primary MR despite optimal medical therapy and LVEF >30%, LV dilation, severe MR by echo criteria
  3. Asymptomatic patients with severe MR but with evidence of declining LV function (EF <60% but >30%) or progressive dilation (LV at end-systole >40 mm)

TABLE 1 Stages of Chronic Primary Mitral Regurgitation

Grade	Definition	Valve Anatomy	Valve Hemodynamics*	Hemodynamic Consequences	Symptoms
A	**At risk for MR**	Mild mitral valve prolapse with normal coaptation Mild valve thickening and leaflet restriction	No MR jet or small central jet area <20% LA on Doppler Small vena contracta <0.3 cm	None	None
B	**Progressive MR**	Severe mitral valve prolapse with normal coaptation Rheumatic valve changes with leaflet restriction and loss of central coaptation Previous IE	Central jet MR 20%-40% LA or late systolic eccentric jet MR Vena contracta <0.7 cm Regurgitant volume <60 ml Regurgitant fraction <50% ERO <0.40 cm^2 Angiographic grade 1-2+	Mild LA enlargement No LV enlargement Normal pulmonary pressure	None
C	**Asymptomatic severe MR**	Severe mitral valve prolapse with loss of coaptation or flail leaflet Rheumatic valve changes with leaflet restriction and loss of central coaptation Previous IE Thickening of leaflets with radiation heart disease	Central jet MR >40% LA or holosystolic eccentric jet MR Vena contracta ≥0.7 cm Regurgitant volume ≥60 ml Regurgitant fraction ≥50% ERO ≥0.40 cm^2 Angiographic grade 3-4+	Moderate or severe LA enlargement LV enlargement Pulmonary hypertension may be present at rest or with exercise C1: LVEF >60% and LVESD <40 mm C2: LVEF ≤60% and LVESD ≥40 mm	None
D	**Symptomatic severe MR**	Severe mitral valve prolapse with loss of coaptation or flail leaflet Rheumatic valve changes with leaflet restriction and loss of central coaptation Previous IE Thickening of leaflets with radiation heart disease	Central jet MR >40% LA or holosystolic eccentric jet MR Vena contracta ≥0.7 cm Regurgitant volume ≥60 ml Regurgitant fraction ≥50% ERO ≥0.40 cm^2 Angiographic grade 3-4+	Moderate or severe LA enlargement LV enlargement Pulmonary hypertension present	Decreased exercise tolerance Exertional dyspnea

ERO, Effective regurgitant orifice; *IE*, infective endocarditis; *LA*, left atrium; *LVEF*, left ventricular ejection fraction; *LVESD*, left ventricular end-systolic dimension; *MR*, mitral regurgitation.

*Several valve hemodynamic criteria are provided for assessment of MR severity, but not all criteria for each category will be present in each patient. Classification of MR severity as mild, moderate, or severe depends on data quality and integration of these parameters in conjunction with other clinical evidence.

From Nishimura RA, Otto CM, Bonow RO et al: 2014 AHA/ACCF guideline for the management of patients with valvular heart disease: a report of the American College of Cardiology Foundation/American Heart Association Task Force on Practice Guidelines, *J Am Coll Cardiol* 63:e57, 2014.

From Mann DL, Zipes DP, Libby P, Bonow RO: *Braunwald's heart disease*, ed 10, Philadelphia, 2015. Elsevier.

TABLE 2 Stages of Chronic Secondary Mitral Regurgitation

Grade	Definition	Valve Anatomy	Valve Hemodynamics*	Associated Cardiac Findings	Symptoms
A	At risk of MR	Normal valve leaflets, chords, and annulus in a patient with coronary disease or a cardiomyopathy	No MR jet or small central jet area <20% LA on Doppler Small vena contracta <0.30 cm	Normal or mildly dilated LV size with fixed (infarction) or inducible (ischemia) regional wall motion abnormalities Primary myocardial disease with LV dilation and systolic dysfunction	Symptoms due to coronary ischemia or HF may be present that respond to revascularization and appropriate medical therapy
B	Progressive MR	Regional wall motion abnormalities with mild tethering of mitral leaflet Annular dilation with mild loss of central coaptation of the mitral leaflets	ERO <0.20 cm^2[†] Regurgitant volume <30 ml Regurgitant fraction <50%	Regional wall motion abnormalities with reduced LV systolic function LV dilation and systolic dysfunction due to primary myocardial disease	Symptoms due to coronary ischemia or HF may be present that respond to revascularization and appropriate medical therapy
C	Asymptomatic severe MR	Regional wall motion abnormalities and/or LV dilation with severe tethering of mitral leaflet Annular dilation with severe loss of central coaptation of the mitral leaflets	ERO ≥0.20 cm^2[†] Regurgitant volume ≥30 ml Regurgitant fraction ≥50%	Regional wall motion abnormalities with reduced LV systolic function LV dilation and systolic dysfunction due to primary myocardial disease	Symptoms due to coronary ischemia or HF may be present that respond to revascularization and appropriate medical therapy
D	Symptomatic severe MR	Regional wall motion abnormalities and/or LV dilation with severe tethering of mitral leaflet Annular dilation with severe loss of central coaptation of the mitral leaflets	ERO ≥0.20 cm^2[†] Regurgitant volume ≥30 ml Regurgitant fraction ≥50%	Regional wall motion abnormalities with reduced LV systolic function LV dilation and systolic dysfunction due to primary myocardial disease	HF symptoms due to MR persist even after revascularization and optimization of medical therapy Decreased exercise tolerance Exertional dyspnea

ERO, Effective regurgitant orifice; *HF*, heart failure; *LA*, left atrium; *MR*, mitral regurgitation.

*Several valve hemodynamic criteria are provided for assessment of MR severity, but not all criteria for each category will be present in each patient. Categorization of MR severity as mild, moderate, or severe depends on data quality and integration of these parameters in conjunction with other clinical evidence.

†The measurement of the proximal isovelocity surface area by two-dimensional TTE in patients with secondary MR underestimates the true ERO because of the crescentic shape of the proximal convergence.

From Nishimura RA, Otto CM, Bonow RO et al: 2014 AHA/ACCF guideline for the management of patients with valvular heart disease: a report of the American College of Cardiology Foundation/American Heart Association Task Force on Practice Guidelines, *J Am Coll Cardiol* 63:e57, 2014.

From Mann DL, Zipes DP, Libby P, Bonow RO: *Braunwald's heart disease*, ed 10, Philadelphia, 2015. Elsevier.

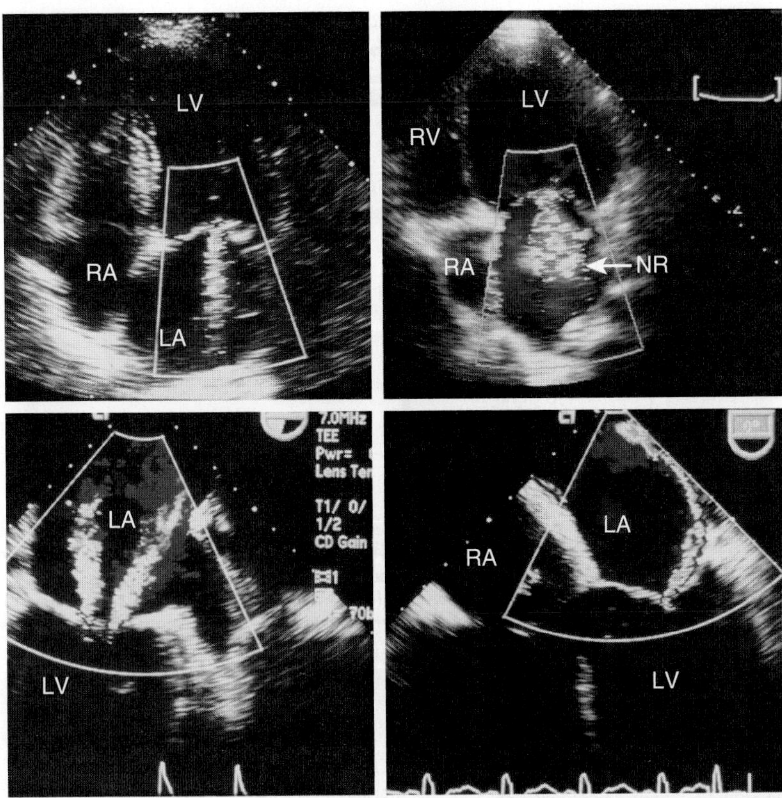

FIG. 1 Mitral regurgitation. Four panels depicting varying degrees of mitral regurgitation; the two *top panels* are apical four-chamber transthoracic views showing, on the *left,* mild mitral regurgitation and, on the *right,* moderate to severe mitral regurgitation. On the *left,* note the relatively narrow jet directed from the tips of the mitral valve toward the posterior left atrial wall. On the right, note the larger jet, filling approximately 40% of the left atrial cavity. The two *bottom panels* are transesophageal echocardiograms. On the *left,* note the mitral regurgitation occurring in two discrete jets and, on the *right,* the highly eccentric jet, which courses along the extreme lateral wall of the left atrium. *LA,* Left atrium; *LV,* left ventricle; *RA,* right atrium; *RV,* right ventricle. (From Zipes DP, et al. [eds]: *Braunwald's heart disease,* ed 7, Philadelphia, 2005, Saunders.)

TABLE 3 Mitral Regurgitation Severity*

	I (Mild)	II (Moderate)	III (Moderate)	IV (Severe)
MR = jet (%LA)	<15	15-30	35-50	>50
Spectral Doppler	Faint	—	—	Dense
Vena contracta	<3 mm	—	—	≥7 mm
Pulmonary vein flow	S > D	Normal to systolic blunting	Systolic blunting	Systolic reversal
RV (ml)	<30	30-44	45-59	≥60
ERO (cm2)	<0.2	0.2-0.29	0.3-0.39	≥0.40
PISA	Small	—	—	Large

D, Antegrade flow in diastole; *ERO,* effective regurgitant orifice; *%LA,* percentage of left atrial area encompassed by the *MR* jet with color flow Doppler; *MR,* mitral regurgitation; *PISA,* proximal isovelocity surface area; *RV,* regurgitant volume; *S,* antegrade flow in systole.

*For some parameters, the observation is valid at the extremes of MR severity and there may be marked overlap in intermediate (grades II, III) MR. In these instances, no value is presented.

From Zipes DP, et al. (eds): *Braunwald's heart disease,* ed 7, Philadelphia, 2005, Saunders and the 2017 American Society of Echocardiography Guidelines.

4. Concomitant mitral valve repair or MVR is indicated in patients with chronic severe primary MR undergoing cardiac surgery for other indications

- Surgery is a class IIa (reasonable) recommendation in:
  1. Severe MR with new-onset atrial fibrillation, even if asymptomatic.
  2. Asymptomatic severe MR with pulmonary hypertension (≥50 mm Hg at rest or ≥60 mm Hg during exercise).
  3. Asymptomatic severe MR secondary to flail leaflet.
  4. A recent study of early surgical intervention for severe MR secondary to a flail leaflet in patients with asymptomatic disease shows greater long-term survival and reduced rates of heart failure when compared with medical therapy alone.
     a. Asymptomatic severe MR with preserved LVEF (>60%) and size (<40 mm in end-systole) in whom the likelihood of successful repair without residual MR is >95% and operative mortality is <1%.
- Surgery is a class IIb recommendation in symptomatic patients (NYHA class III-IV) with severe MR with severe LV dysfunction or dilatation (LVEF <30% or LV at end-systole >55 mm, respectively) in whom LV dysfunction is not the primary cause for the MR as well as functional MR where it is secondary to LV dysfunction.
- Quantitative grading of MR is a powerful predictor of the clinical outcome of asymptomatic MR. In general, patients with regurgitant orifice areas of ≥40 mm^2 should be considered for prompt surgery, whereas those with orifices between 20 and 39 mm^2 can be followed closely.
- Percutaneous mitral valve repair methods are currently being investigated. The MitraClip device is FDA-approved for use in patients with significant symptomatic degenerative MR (>3+) who are too high risk for surgery. The device is a catheter-delivered clip that grasps and approximates the edges of the mitral leaflets at the origin of the regurgitant jet. Early data had not demonstrated a significant efficacy in MR reduction compared with surgical replacement; however, in a recent trial investigators compared guideline-directed medical therapy (GDMT) alone versus transcatheter mitral repair with mitraclip plus GDMT in patients with severe MR who were not surgical candidates. After 24 mo heart failure hospitalizations were 36% in the dense group versus 68% in the other group. Device therapy also improved symptoms and quality of life and decreased all-cause mortality (29% in device vs. 46% in the GDMT-only group[1]).
- Ischemic MR has been a source of controversy as to whether moderate or greater MR should be fixed at the time of revascularization with CABG. Based on the 2015 CT surgery guidelines, mitral valve repair can be considered at the time of CABG in moderate MR or for other cardiac surgery such as aortic valve replacement (class IIb); mitral valve repair is reasonable for severe MR (class IIa) in the presence of a basal aneurysm or dyskinesis, significant leaflet tethering due to wall motion abnormalities, and moderate to severe LV remodeling (LV end diastolic diameter >65 mm).

DISPOSITION

Prognosis is generally good unless there is significant impairment of left ventricular function or significantly elevated pulmonary artery pressures. Most patients remain asymptomatic for many years (average interval from diagnosis to onset of symptoms is 16 yr). In patients with chronic severe MR, MR is commonly progressive, with onset of other symptoms or left ventricular dysfunction within 6 to 10 yr. However surgery should be advised well before the onset of symptoms in case of worsening LVEF and LV

[1] Stone GW, et al.: Transcatheter mitral-valve repair in patients with heart failure, *N Engl J Med* 379:2307–18, 2018.

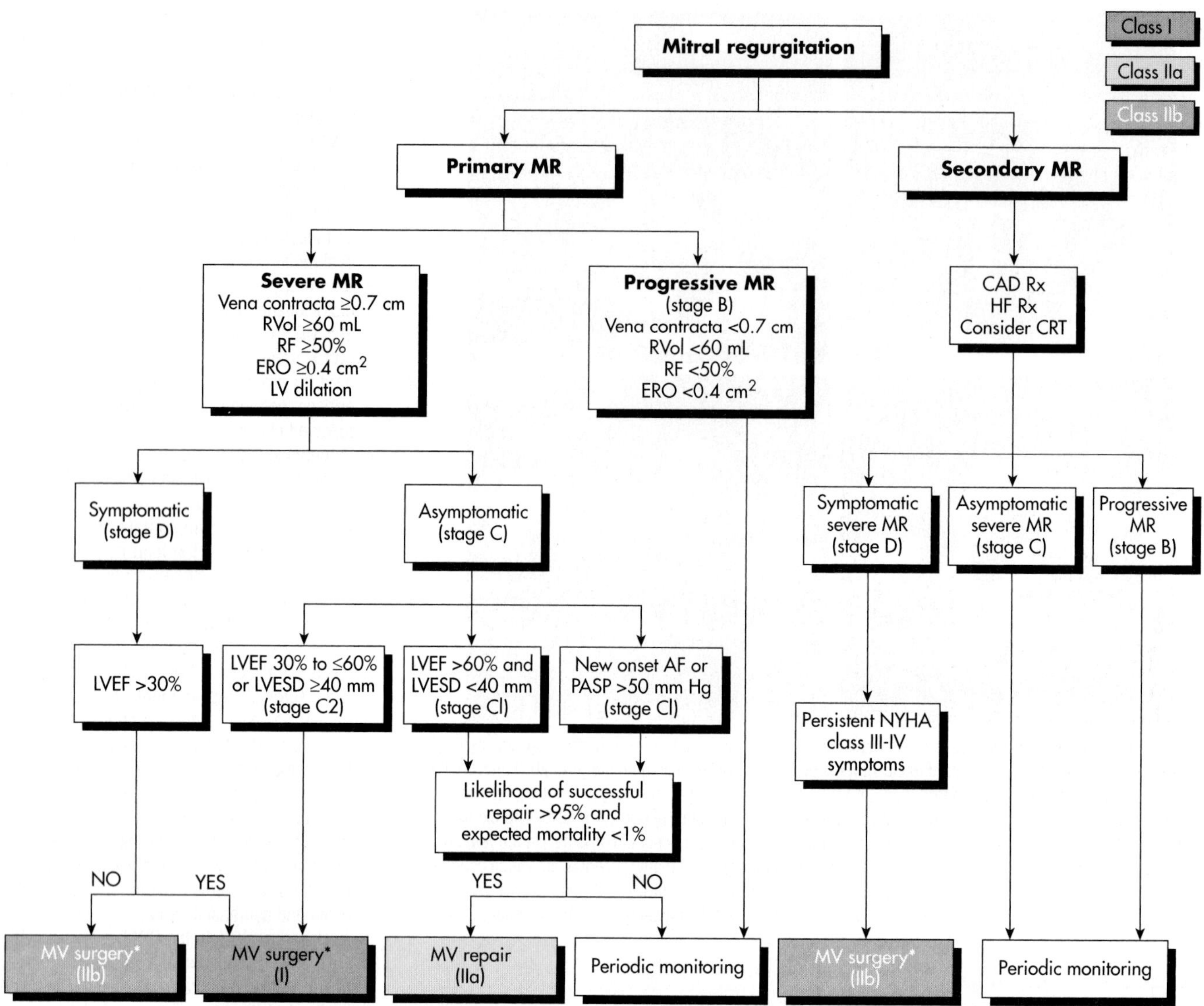

FIG. 2 Indications for surgery for MR. *Mitral valve repair is preferred over MVR when possible. *AF,* Atrial fibrillation; *CAD,* coronary artery disease; *CRT,* cardiac resynchronization therapy; *ERO,* effective regurgitant orifice; *HF,* heart failure; *LV,* left ventricular; *LVEF,* left ventricular ejection fraction; *LVESD,* left ventricular end-systolic dimension; *MR,* mitral regurgitation; *MV,* mitral valve; *MVR,* mitral valve replacement; *NYHA,* New York Heart Association; *PASP,* pulmonary artery systolic pressure; *RF,* regurgitant fraction; *RVol,* regurgitant volume; and *Rx,* therapy. (From Nishimura RA, et al.: ACC/AHA focused update of valvular heart disease guideline, *J Am Coll Cardiol* 70(2):254–289, 2017. http://www.onlinejacc.org/content/accj/70/2/252.full.pdf.)

systolic dimensions and presence of pulmonary hypertension or atrial fibrillation, all of which are poor prognostic signs.

REFERRAL

- Surgical referral in selected patients (see "Acute General Rx"). Emergency surgery is usually necessary in patients with acute MR caused by ruptured papillary muscle or chordae tendineae after myocardial infarction.
- Mitral valve repair can also be accomplished with percutaneous implantation of a MitraClip device in patients who are too high risk for surgery. The role of percutaneous repair of functional MR is still under active investigation.

PEARLS & CONSIDERATIONS

COMMENTS

- Although vasodilators and other agents should be used to treat hypertension in patients with severe mitral regurgitation, there is no evidence that they will delay the need for eventual valve surgery, which is the definitive treatment for severe MR.
- In 2007, the AHA guidelines for prevention of infectious endocarditis were revised and routine antibiotic prophylaxis to undergo dental or other invasive procedures is no longer recommended, unless the patient has had prior endocarditis.

SUGGESTED READINGS

Available at ExpertConsult.com

RELATED CONTENT

Mitral Regurgitation (Patient Information)

AUTHOR: **UYEN T. LAM, M.D.**

BASIC INFORMATION

DEFINITION

Mitral stenosis is a narrowing of the mitral valve orifice that prevents proper opening during diastole and obstruction of blood flow from the left atrium to the left ventricle. Due to thickening of the leaflets there is restricted movement. The cross section of a normal orifice measures 4 to 6 cm^2. Symptoms usually develop with exercise when the orifice measures <2.5 cm^2, and symptoms may develop at rest when the orifice is <1.5 cm^2.

SYNONYM

MS

ICD-10CM CODES

I05.0 Rheumatic mitral stenosis
I05.2 Rheumatic mitral stenosis with insufficiency
I34.2 Nonrheumatic mitral (valve) stenosis
Q23.2 Congenital mitral stenosis

EPIDEMIOLOGY & DEMOGRAPHICS

- The predominant cause of mitral stenosis is rheumatic heart disease; however, the occurrence of mitral valve stenosis has decreased worldwide over the past 30 yr (particularly in developed countries) as a result of declining incidence of rheumatic fever due to appropriate antibiotic use.
- Rheumatic heart disease has a predilection for the mitral valve, aortic valve, and to some extent the tricuspid valve.
- The incidence of MS is higher in women (2:1 female-to-male ratio).
- There is high prevalence of rheumatic heart disease in developing countries.
- Outbreaks of rheumatic fever in the U.S. are due to increased virulence of a streptococcal strain or enhanced immigration from where rheumatic heart disease is prevalent.

PHYSICAL FINDINGS & CLINICAL PRESENTATION

- Dyspnea is the most common symptom, along with fatigue and decreased exercise capacity. These symptoms occur due to an inability to increase cardiac output, especially with exercise, and elevated pulmonary capillary wedge pressures, with resultant increase in pulmonary artery pressures. Stages of mitral stenosis are summarized in Table 1.
- "Mitral facies" which are pinkish-purple patches on the cheek due to low cardiac output and vasoconstriction, usually indicate severe MS.
- Paroxysmal nocturnal dyspnea (PND) and orthopnea secondary to elevated left atrial pressure may occur.
- Acute pulmonary edema may occur after an increase in flow across the mitral valve secondary to an increase in cardiac output or heart rate (exertion, tachyarrhythmias, fever, anemia, etc.).
- Pulmonary hypertension that results from chronically elevated pulmonary capillary wedge pressures can lead to right ventricular (RV) dysfunction and signs and symptoms of right heart failure (hepatomegaly, pulsatile liver, peripheral edema, ascites).
- The left ventricle is typically "protected" in mitral stenosis and exists in a low-pressure state; however, MS often coexists with mitral regurgitation and occasionally with aortic valve dysfunction, both of which can cause left ventricular dysfunction.
- Hemoptysis can be present secondary to rupture of thin-walled dilated bronchial veins due to an abrupt increase in left atrial pressure.
- Systemic embolic events are caused by left atrial thrombi. These are associated with atrial fibrillation 80% of the time, since mitral stenosis leads to left atrial enlargement, which is a predisposing factor for atrial arrhythmias.
- Atrial fibrillation is more prevalent in patients with more severe MS, increasing age, and other valvular abnormalities.
- Chest pain can be caused by RV pressure overload and/or concomitant coronary artery disease in up to 15% of patients.
- Loud first heart sound (S1) caused by delayed valve closure preceded by an opening snap and rapid rising left ventricular (LV) pressure.
- A low-pitched rumbling diastolic murmur is heard best at the apex. The intensity of the murmur is not related to the severity of the stenosis, but the duration is holodiastolic in severe MS.
- An opening snap (OS) caused by tensing of the valve leaflets after the cusps have opened completely. The OS follows S2 by 0.03 to 0.14 sec, and the shorter the S2-OS interval, the more severe the MS, due to the increasing left atrial pressures.
- Prominent A wave on the pulmonary capillary wedge pressure tracing. This is analogous to the prominent A wave seen in systemic venous pressure tracings with tricuspid stenosis.
- A diastolic thrill may be palpable at the apex, especially with the patient in the left lateral recumbent position.
- A left parasternal heave secondary to RV hypertrophy and pulmonary hypertension.
- An accentuated P2 and/or a soft, early diastolic decrescendo murmur (Graham Steell murmur) caused by pulmonary regurgitation may be present in patients with pulmonary hypertension (not specific for mitral stenosis).
- Hoarseness due to the enlargement of the left atrium compressing the recurrent laryngeal nerve.
- Straightening of the left heart border seen on chest radiography indicative of left atrial enlargement.
- Fig. 1 shows schematic representations of LV, aortic, and left atrial (LA) pressures, showing normal relationships and alterations with mild and severe MS.

ETIOLOGY

- Rheumatic fever (RF) is the predominant cause of MS. RF causes thickening of the leaflet tips, commissure fusion, and chordal shortening and fusion. This leads to the classic doming of the leaflets in diastole due to fusion of the leaflet tips at the commissures.

TABLE 1 Stages of Mitral Stenosis

Stage	Definition	Valve Anatomy	Valve Hemodynamics	Hemodynamic Consequences	Symptoms
A	**At risk for MS**	Mild valve doming during diastole	Normal transmitral flow velocity	None	None
B	**Progressive MS**	Rheumatic valve changes with commissural fusion and diastolic doming of the mitral valve leaflets Planimetered MVA >1.5 cm^2	Increased transmitral flow velocities MVA >1.5 cm^2 Diastolic pressure half-time <150 msec	Mild to moderate LA enlargement Normal pulmonary pressure at rest	None
C	**Asymptomatic severe MS**	Rheumatic valve changes with commissural fusion and diastolic doming of the mitral valve leaflets Planimetered MVA ≤1.5 cm^2 (MVA ≤1 cm^2 with very severe MS)	MVA ≤1.5 cm^2 (MVA ≤1 cm^2 with very severe MS) Diastolic pressure half-time ≥150 msec (Diastolic pressure half-time ≥220 msec with very severe MS)	Severe LA enlargement Elevated PASP >30 mm Hg	None
D	**Symptomatic severe MS**	Rheumatic valve changes with commissural fusion and diastolic doming of the mitral valve leaflets Planimetered MVA ≤1.5 cm^2	MVA ≤1.5 cm^2 (MVA ≤1 cm^2 with very severe MS) Diastolic pressure half-time ≥150 msec (Diastolic pressure half-time ≥220 msec with very severe MS)	Severe LA enlargement Elevated PASP >30 mm Hg	Decreased exercise tolerance Exertional dyspnea

The transmitral mean pressure gradient should be obtained to determine the full hemodynamic effect of the MS and usually is >5 to 10 mm Hg in severe MS; however, because of the variability of the mean pressure gradient with heart rate and forward flow, it has not been included in the criteria for severity. *LA*, Left atrium; *MS*, mitral stenosis; *MVA*, mitral valve area; *PASP*, pulmonary artery systolic pressure.
From Mann DL et al: *Braunwald's heart disease*, ed 10, Philadelphia, 2015, Elsevier.

Rheumatic fever involves the leaflet tips first with progression toward the annulus. This is opposite of mitral annular calcification, which typically starts in the annulus and proceeds out to the leaflet tips, leading to mitral stenosis in severe cases.
- Congenital defect (parachute valve) has the usual two mitral leaflets, but the chordae, instead of diverging to insert into two papillary muscles, converge into one major papillary muscle, which allows little mobility of the leaflets, as in cor triatriatum (heart with three atria), in which there is a thin membrane that obstructs the pulmonary vein flow and simulates mitral stenosis.
- Rare causes are severe mitral annular calcification usually seen in end-stage renal disease patients, endomyocardial fibroelastosis, malignant carcinoid syndrome, systemic lupus erythematosus, Whipple disease, Fabry disease, rheumatoid arthritis, and MDMA use.
- Atrial septal defect in association with rheumatic mitral stenosis is termed Lutembacher syndrome.
- Medications: Ergot alkaloids (methysergide and ergotamine).

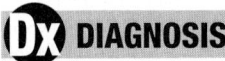

DIAGNOSIS

DIFFERENTIAL DIAGNOSIS

- Left atrial myxoma
- Ball valve thrombus
- Other valvular abnormalities (e.g., tricuspid stenosis, mitral regurgitation)
- Atrial septal defect

WORKUP

Physical examination and echocardiography

IMAGING STUDIES

- Echocardiography (Fig. 2):
  1. Two-dimensional echocardiogram can measure valve area by direct planimetry or calculate it by the Doppler pressure half-time method (this may be inaccurate in patients with concomitant diastolic dysfunction, atrial septal defects, or aortic insufficiency, and those who recently have undergone mitral valvuloplasty), or the continuity equation can be used to calculate the valve area. It also can be measured using the proximal isovelocity surface area method. A valve area ≤ 1.5 cm^2 is consistent with severe MS (and ≤ 1.0 cm^2 with very severe MS). The transmitral gradient can also be calculated. A mean gradient of >10 mm Hg indicates severe MS, a gradient of 5 to 10 mm Hg is consistent with moderate MS, and 0 to 5 mm Hg is consistent with mild MS or no MS.
  2. M-Mode echocardiography will also show a markedly diminished E-to-F slope of the anterior mitral valve leaflet during diastole. There can be loss of the "A-wave" due to increased left atrial pressure or the presence of associated atrial fibrillation. There is also fusion of the commissures, resulting in "doming" of the leaflets during diastole.

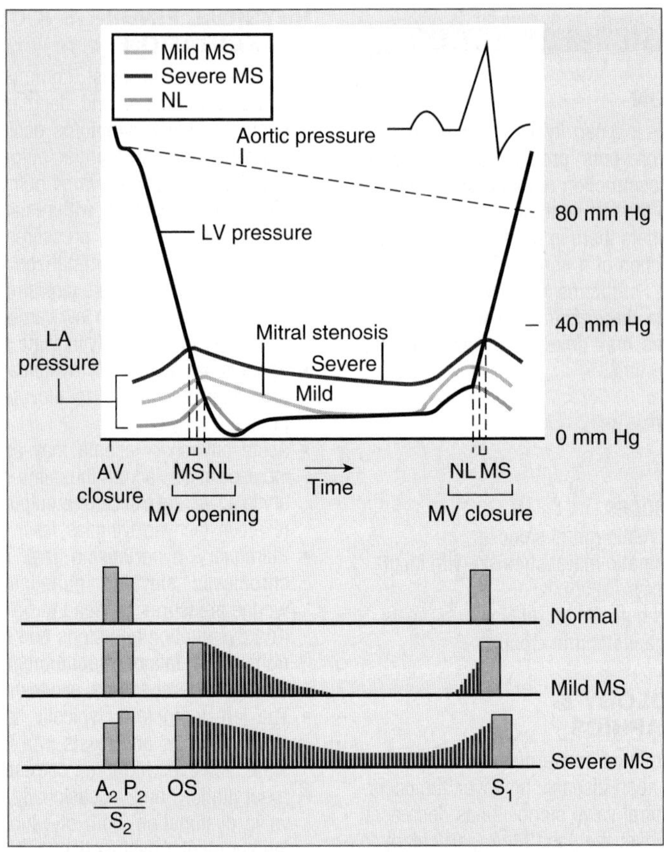

FIG. 1 Schematic representation of left ventricular *(LV)*, aortic, and left atrial *(LA)* pressures, showing normal relationships and alterations with mild and severe mitral stenosis *(MS)*. Corresponding classic auscultatory signs of MS are shown at the bottom. The higher left atrial v wave of severe MS causes earlier pressure crossover and earlier mitral valve *(MV)* opening, leading to a shorter time interval between aortic valve *(AV)* closure and the opening snap *(OS)*. The higher left atrial end-diastolic pressure with severe MS also results in later closure of the mitral valve. With severe MS, the diastolic rumble becomes longer and there is accentuation of the pulmonic component *(P_2)* of the second heart sound *(S_2)* in relation to the aortic component *(A_2)*. *NL*, Normal limits. (From Bonow RO: *Heart disease,* 9th ed, Philadelphia, 2012, Saunders.)

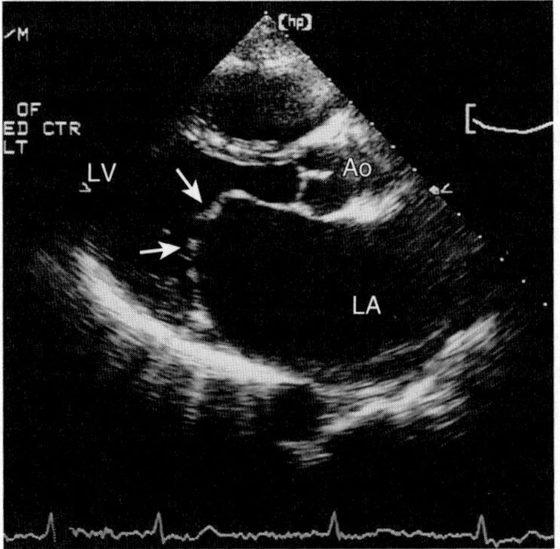

FIG. 2 Mitral stenosis. Parasternal long-axis view of a patient with mitral stenosis and a pliable noncalcified mitral valve leaflet. Note the "doming" motion of the mitral valve leaflets *(arrows)*. Valves with these morphologic features are excellent candidates for percutaneous balloon valvotomy. *Ao,* Aorta; *LA,* left atrium; *LV,* left ventricle. (From Zipes DP et al [eds]: *Braunwald's heart disease,* ed 7, Philadelphia, 2005, Saunders.)

  3. Grading of leaflet thickness, mobility, calcification, and subvalvular thickening (Wilkins score) with a score of 0 to 4 for each characteristic can predict hemodynamic results and outcome of balloon mitral valvuloplasty (a low score of less than 8 is favorable for balloon valvuloplasty and a high score is unfavorable). A score above 8 would favor a surgical approach. In addition, mitral regurgitation

that is greater than mild would preclude a balloon mitral valvuloplasty procedure.

4. Doppler echocardiography can be used to assess for pulmonary hypertension and to give an estimate of the pulmonary artery systolic pressure at rest and with exercise.
5. Patients with known mitral stenosis: A follow-up echocardiography is recommended to assess for pulmonary artery pressures and valve gradient (very severe MS with mitral valve area <1.0 cm^2 every year, severe MS with mitral valve area ≤1.5 cm^2 every 1 to 2 yr, and progressive MS with mitral valve area >1.5 cm^2 every 3 to 5 yr).

- Chest radiograph:
  1. Straightening of the left cardiac border caused by enlarged left atrium
  2. Left atrial enlargement on lateral chest radiograph
  3. Prominence of pulmonary arteries that indicates pulmonary hypertension
  4. Possible pulmonary congestion and edema (Kerley B lines)
- ECG:
  1. RV hypertrophy; right axis deviation caused by pulmonary hypertension
  2. Left atrial enlargement (broad, biphasic P waves in lead V1 and duration of P-waves >0.11 sec in lead II). This is termed "P-mitrale."
  3. Atrial fibrillation
- Cardiac catheterization:
  1. Allows the measurement of pulmonary artery pressure and transmitral pressure gradients at rest or with exercise (supine biking or raising weights with arms while lying supine).
  2. Allows the measurement of transmitral flow and calculation of the valve area.
  3. Is not routinely recommended for the evaluation of MS but is useful when the echocardiographic findings are nondiagnostic or discrepant with the clinical scenario.
  4. Cardiac catheterization in addition to echocardiography can be used to monitor the hemodynamics during a balloon mitral valvuloplasty procedure.

TABLE 2 Approaches to Mechanical Relief of Mitral Stenosis

Approach	Advantages	Disadvantages
Closed surgical valvotomy	Inexpensive Relatively simple Good hemodynamic results in selected patients Good long-term outcome	No direct visualization of valve Only feasible with flexible, noncalcified valves Contraindicated with MR grade higher than 2+ Surgical procedure with general anesthesia
Open surgical valvotomy	Visualization of valve allows directed valvotomy Concurrent annuloplasty for MR is feasible	Best results with flexible, noncalcified valves Surgical procedure with general anesthesia
Valve replacement	Feasible in all patients regardless of extent of valve calcification or severity of MR	Surgical procedure with general anesthesia Effect of loss of annular-papillary muscle continuity on LV function Prosthetic valve Chronic anticoagulation
Balloon mitral valvotomy	Percutaneous approach Local anesthesia Good hemodynamic results in selected patients Good long-term outcome	No direct visualization of valve Only feasible with flexible noncalcified valves Contraindicated with MR grade higher than 2+

LV, Left ventricle; *MR*, mitral regurgitation.
From Mann DL et al: *Braunwald's heart disease*, ed 10, Philadelphia, 2015, Elsevier.

Rx TREATMENT

NONPHARMACOLOGIC THERAPY

Decrease level of activity in symptomatic patients, and salt restriction if pulmonary congestion is present.

ACUTE GENERAL Rx

- Medical:
  1. Anticoagulation for the prevention of systemic embolic events in patients with MS and:
     a. Atrial fibrillation: In patients with atrial fibrillation and rheumatic mitral stenosis, anticoagulation with a vitamin K antagonist is indicated
     b. Prior embolic event
     c. Documented left atrial thrombus or left atrial appendage thrombus
  2. Ventricular rate control (to increase diastolic filling period) with beta-blockers, non-dihydropyridine calcium channel blockers, or digitalis and aggressive treatment of tachyarrhythmias.
  3. Treat congestive heart failure with loop diuretics and sodium restriction.
  4. Antibiotic prophylaxis to prevent recurrent rheumatic fever is usually not indicated unless presence of high-risk features such as prior endocarditis, prosthetic heart valves, valvulopathy of the transplanted heart, and certain cases of cyanotic congenital heart disease.
  5. Physical activity and exercise. Patients with mild MS in sinus rhythm with a peak pulmonary artery pressure <50 mm Hg can participate in all competitive sports. Patients with moderate MS and in sinus rhythm or atrial fibrillation with a peak pulmonary artery pressure of <50 mm Hg can participate in low to moderate static and dynamic sports. Patients in sinus rhythm with severe MS should not participate in any competitive sports. Patients in atrial fibrillation with any degree of MS and on anticoagulation should avoid all competitive sports.
  6. Pregnancy in females with advanced MS may be poorly tolerated due to the hemodynamic changes such as increased cardiac output occurring in pregnancy. Mild to moderate MS may be tolerated in pregnancy with medical therapy alone.
- Table 2 summarizes approaches to mechanical relief of mitral stenosis.
- Percutaneous mitral balloon commissurotomy (PMBC) is the therapy of choice for symptomatic patients with severe MS (valve area ≤1.5 cm^2) with a favorable valvuloplasty score, minimal or no mitral regurgitation, and no left atrial thrombus. PMBC is reasonable for asymptomatic patients with very severe MS (mitral valve area ≤1.0 cm^2) and favorable valve morphology in the absence of left atrial thrombus or moderate to severe MR (class IIa indication). PMBC is also considered the procedure of choice in pregnant women with rheumatic MS and in NYHA class III to IV heart failure and/or unresponsive to adequate medical treatment. In addition, it may be considered for severely symptomatic (NYHA class III/IV) patients with very severe MS (mitral valve area ≤1.5 cm^2) who are not candidates for surgery or are at high risk for surgery, even if they have suboptimal valve anatomy (class IIb indication). Regular follow-up is needed after PMBC because restenosis may reoccur. Repeat intervention can be performed as long as valve anatomy remains favorable; however, there is usually more fibrosis and deformation of the valve with subsequent procedures. The approximate frequency of repeat intervention is 10% at 7 yr.
- Mitral valve surgery is indicated for patients with moderate to severe symptomatic MS when PMBC is not available or is contraindicated (valvuloplasty score greater than or equal to 8) or the valve is calcified, when MR is more than mild, when left atrial thrombus is present, and when the surgical risk is acceptable. The surgical approaches include closed mitral valvotomy, open valvotomy and repair (preferred), and mitral valve replacement when repair is not possible.

DISPOSITION

- Prognosis is generally good except in patients with chronic pulmonary hypertension.
- Operative mortality rates for mitral valve replacement are 1% to 5% at most institutions.

SUGGESTED READING

Available at ExpertConsult.com

RELATED CONTENT

Mitral Stenosis (Patient Information)

AUTHORS: **ROBERT VAZQUEZ, M.D.,** and **ARAVIND RAO KOKKIRALA, M.D., FACC**

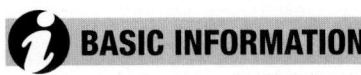

BASIC INFORMATION

DEFINITION

Mitral valve prolapse (MVP) is the bulging of one or both of the mitral valve leaflets ≥2 mm above the annular plane into the left atrium during systole. MVP syndrome refers to a constellation of MVP and associated symptoms (e.g., autonomic dysfunction, palpitations) or other physical abnormalities (e.g., pectus excavatum). Table 1 describes a classification of mitral valve prolapse.

SYNONYMS

MVP
Mitral click murmur syndrome
Barlow's syndrome

ICD-10CM CODES

I34.1 Nonrheumatic mitral (valve) prolapse
I34.0 Nonrheumatic mitral (valve) insufficiency

EPIDEMIOLOGY & DEMOGRAPHICS

- MVP can be found by echocardiogram in 1% to 2.4% of the general population, with some studies suggesting that it is more common in women than in men.
- Increased incidence is seen with autoimmune thyroid disorders, Ehlers-Danlos syndrome, Marfan syndrome, osteogenesis imperfecta, pseudoxanthoma elasticum, pectus excavatum, anorexia nervosa, and bulimia.
- Compared to men, women with MVP have less posterior prolapse (22% vs. 31%), less flail (2% vs. 8%), more leaflet thickening (32% vs. 28%), and less frequent severe mitral regurgitation (MR) (10% vs. 23%).

TABLE 1 Classification of Mitral Valve Prolapse

Mitral Valve Prolapse Syndrome

- Younger age (20-50 yr)
- Predominantly female
- Click or click-murmur on physical examination
- Thin leaflets with systolic displacement on echocardiography
- Associated with low blood pressure, orthostatic hypotension, palpitations
- Benign long-term course

Myxomatous Mitral Valve Disease

- Older age (40-70 yr)
- Predominantly male
- Thickened, redundant valve leaflets
- Mitral regurgitation on physical exam and echocardiography
- High likelihood of progressive disease requiring mitral valve surgery

Secondary Mitral Valve Prolapse

- Marfan syndrome
- Hypertrophic cardiomyopathy
- Ehlers-Danlos syndrome
- Other connective tissue diseases

Modified from Otto CM: *Valvular heart disease*, ed 2, Philadelphia, 2004, Saunders, p. 369.

- Although MVP is more common in women than men, men more often develop severe regurgitation requiring surgical intervention.

PHYSICAL FINDINGS & CLINICAL PRESENTATION

- Mid to late systolic click, heard best at the apex. Midsystolic click is caused by degeneration of the valve resulting in an abnormal ratio between the length of the mitral apparatus and left ventricle (LV) during contraction. When the valve prolapses, it gets caught by the subvalvular structures, causing an abrupt halt that creates the click.
- If regurgitation is present, a crescendo mid to late systolic murmur may be heard that worsens with standing and Valsalva maneuver.
- Timing of click within the cardiac cycle varies with loading conditions within the left ventricle (i.e., may occur earlier with standing or Valsalva and later with squatting or expiration).
- May be associated with small anteroposterior chest diameter, scoliosis, pectus excavatum, or low BMI.
- Most patients with MVP are asymptomatic; symptoms if present consist primarily of chest pain, palpitations, fatigue, dyspnea, and anxiety.
- Neurologic abnormalities (e.g., transient ischemic attack [TIA] or stroke) are rare.
- A spectrum of arrhythmias, mainly paroxysmal supraventricular tachycardia and atrial and ventricular premature beats, etc. is also observed with mitral valve prolapse. There is also an increased association with Wolff-Parkinson-White syndrome and QT prolongation.

ETIOLOGY

- Myxomatous degeneration of connective tissue within mitral valve, usually involving multiple leaflet segments (e.g., Barlow disease). In contrast, fibroelastic deficiency of single leaflet segment develops in elderly patients.
- Congenital deformity of mitral valve and supportive structures.
- Secondary to other disorders of connective tissue such as Ehlers-Danlos, Marfan, or pseudoxanthoma elasticum; association with other connective tissue disorders suggests MVP result of defective embryogenesis in cells of mesenchymal origin.

DIAGNOSIS

DIFFERENTIAL DIAGNOSIS

- Other valvular abnormalities (especially mitral regurgitation [MR])
- Anxiety or panic disorders
- Pulmonary embolism
- Atypical chest pain

WORKUP

- Medical history and physical examination, with increased suspicion in patients with other findings of connective tissue disorder.
- Two- or three-dimensional echocardiography in patients with a systolic click or murmur on careful auscultation.
- Cardiac MRI is an emerging tool for the evaluation and diagnosis of MVP but has not yet been independently validated. However, MRI should be considered because it may be helpful in accurately quantifying the amount of mitral regurgitation when present. ECG is most often normal but may show nonspecific ST-T wave changes, prolonged QT interval, prominent Q waves, or early repolarization with J-point elevation in young patients.

IMAGING STUDIES

Echocardiography (Fig. 1) shows one or more leaflets prolapsing >2 mm into the left atrium during systole in a long axis view. Mitral leaflets may be thickened (>5 mm) with myxomatous degeneration. MR is typically present but may only occur during late systole or with exertion. If moderate or severe MR is present findings of dilated left atrium, LV dilation and/or dysfunction, and elevated estimated RV systolic pressures may also be present. There is an increased incidence of secundum-type atrial septal defects (ASDs) in patients with MVP, which may also be identified with echocardiography.

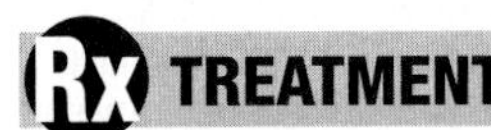

TREATMENT

NONPHARMACOLOGIC THERAPY

Avoidance of stimulants (e.g., caffeine, nicotine) in patients with palpitations. Sometimes

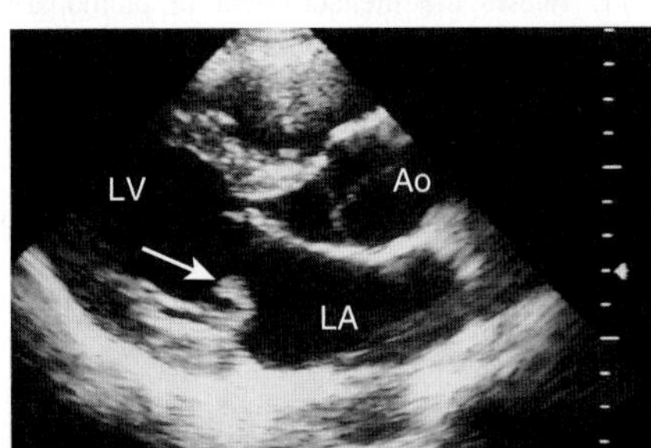

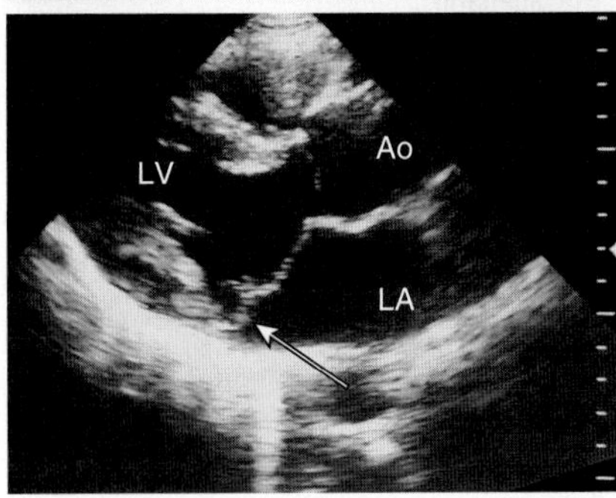

FIG. 1 Mitral valve prolapse. Parasternal long-axis view in diastole *(top)* and systole *(bottom)* in a patient with mitral valve prolapse and myxomatous changes. In the *upper panel,* note the open mitral valve and the diffuse thickening of the posterior mitral valve leaflet *(arrow)*. The *lower panel* was recorded in systole. Note that both leaflets prolapse behind the plane of the mitral valve annulus. The prolapse of the posterior leaflet is somewhat more prominent *(arrow)*. *Ao,* Aorta; *LA,* left atrium; *LV,* left ventricle. (From Zipes DP et al [eds]: *Braunwald's heart disease,* ed 7, Philadelphia, 2005, Saunders.)

TABLE 2 Predictors of Clinical Outcome in Mitral Valve Prolapse

Predictor	Survival	Valve Surgery	Arrhythmias or Sudden Death	Endocarditis
Age	+++	+++	–	–
Gender	++	++	–	–
Leaflet thickness or redundancy	+++	+++	++++	++++
Severity of mitral regurgitation	++++	++++	++++	++++
Systolic click	+	–	–	–
Left ventricular dilation	+	++++	++	–
Left atrial dilation	–	++	+	–

Symbols indicate the relative predictive value of each variable for the listed clinical outcomes on a scale of no predictive value (–) to strongly predictive (++++).
From Bonow RO et al: *Braunwald's heart disease: a textbook of cardiovascular medicine*, Philadelphia, 2012, Saunders.

reassurance is sufficient to reduce the severity of symptoms in many patients.

ACUTE GENERAL Rx

β-blockers may be used in symptomatic patients (e.g., palpitations, chest pain) to decrease the heart rate and contractility, thus potentially decreasing the stretch on the prolapsing valve leaflets.

CHRONIC Rx

Monitoring for complications:

- Mitral regurgitation (most common complication); on rare occasion may occur acutely due to rupture of chordae tendineae.
- Routine echocardiographic monitoring is indicated at the following intervals with patients with evidence of mitral regurgitation:
  1. Stage B with mild regurgitation: Every 3 to 5 yr.
  2. Stage B with moderate regurgitation: Every 1 to 2 yr.
  3. Stage C1 (asymptomatic severe MR without LV dysfunction): Every 6 to 12 mo.
- Bacterial endocarditis (risk is three to eight times that of the general population); higher risk in patients with concomitant regurgitation. However, routine antibiotic prophylaxis is not recommended.
- TIA or stroke caused by embolic phenomena (from fibrin and platelet thrombi) in patients with thickened leaflets; risk in young patients is <0.05% per yr. If present, aspirin (75 mg to 325 mg) is indicated for secondary prevention.
- Cardiac arrhythmias with the vast majority being supraventricular and benign.
- Sudden death (rare); most often associated with acute flail leaflets or caused by ventricular arrhythmias associated with other structural heart disease.
- The incidence of complications of MVP is very low (<1% per yr). Mitral leaflet thickness is ≤0.5 mm, young patients <45 yr, and in the absence of mitral systolic murmur or MR on Doppler echocardiography. Table 2 lists variables that are predictors of favorable clinical outcome in mitral valve prolapse.
- Risk factors that predict higher risk of complications are presence of moderate to severe MR, LV ejection fraction <50%, LA dimension >40 mm, age >50 yr.

SURGICAL REFERRAL

Surgical referral may be necessary in patients who develop progressive MR with surgical indications as per guidelines for valvular heart disease (see topic on mitral regurgitation).

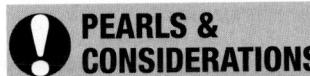

PEARLS & CONSIDERATIONS

COMMENTS

- Recent studies suggest that the prevalence of MVP and its propensity to cause symptoms and serious complications have been overestimated in the past.
- The relationship between MVP syndrome and sudden cardiac death is unclear. The best evidence suggests that there is only a slight risk in subsets of patients with MVP who have severe MR, severe valvular deformity, complex ventricular arrhythmias, QT prolongation, and a history of syncope.
- Asymptomatic patients with MVP and mild or no MR can be evaluated clinically every 3 to 5 yr. High-risk patients (those with symptoms, arrhythmias, or significant regurgitation) should undergo a follow-up examination once a yr.
- In 2007, the AHA guidelines for prevention of infectious endocarditis were revised and prophylactic antibiotics are no longer recommended for patients with MVP without previous endocarditis.

PATIENT & FAMILY EDUCATION

www.themitralvalve.org

SUGGESTED READING

Available at ExpertConsult.com

RELATED CONTENT

Mitral Valve Prolapse (Patient Information)

AUTHOR: **UYEN T. LAM, M.D.**

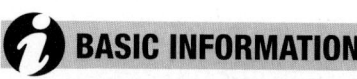

BASIC INFORMATION

DEFINITION

Molar pregnancy (hydatidiform mole) is a premalignant gestational disorder and is included in the spectrum of disorders characterized as gestational trophoblastic disease. Molar pregnancies are classified as complete or partial based on morphologic and pathologic examination. Both complete and partial molar pregnancies have an abnormal placenta with enlargement and swelling of the chorionic villi and hyperplasia of the villous trophoblastic cells. Most molar pregnancies are complete and are characterized by generalized hydropic villous changes with no fetal tissue. Partial moles are characterized by a mixture of large hydropic villi and normal placental tissue and often have fetal tissue present. Gestational trophoblastic disease (GTD) comprises a spectrum of neoplastic conditions derived from the placenta. Whereas hydatidiform moles, gestational choriocarcinoma, and placental site trophoblastic tumor (PSTT) are histologic diagnoses, postmolar GTN is defined by clinical and laboratory criteria. The disease entities included in GTD have a wide variation in behavior, but GTN specifically refers to those with the potential for tissue invasion and metastases.

The risk of malignant sequelae (gestational trophoblastic neoplasia) for a complete mole is 6% to 32% and for a partial mole is less than 5%.

SYNONYM

Hydatidiform mole

ICD-10CM CODES

O01.0 Classical hydatidiform mole
O01.1 Incomplete and partial hydatidiform mole
O01.9 Hydatidiform mole, unspecified

EPIDEMIOLOGY & DEMOGRAPHICS

INCIDENCE: 1/1500 pregnancies in the U.S.
PREDOMINANT SEX AND AGE: Females of reproductive age, highest rates at extremes of reproductive ages
RISK FACTORS:
- Extremes of reproductive age (<21 and >40 years)
- Previous molar pregnancy
- History of spontaneous abortion
- Use of combined oral contraceptives

PHYSICAL FINDINGS & CLINICAL PRESENTATION

Complete molar pregnancy:
- 80% to 90% present with vaginal bleeding at 6 to 16 weeks' gestational age
- 28% with uterine enlargement greater than expected for gestational age
- 8% with hyperemesis gravidarum
- 1% with pregnancy-induced hypertension in the first or second trimester
- 15% to 25% with bilateral theca lutein cysts
- 15% will have a beta hCG >100,000 mIU/ml
- <10% with anemia

Partial molar pregnancy:
- 90% present with an incomplete or missed abortion
- 75% present with vaginal bleeding
- <10% will have a beta hCG of >100,000 mIU/ml

ETIOLOGY

Complete molar pregnancy:
- Fertilization of an oocyte with absent or inactive maternal chromosomes and duplication of paternal chromosomes (85% to 90% are 46, XX) or fertilization of an empty oocyte with 2 sperm (46, XY or XX).
- Diffuse villous enlargement and trophoblastic proliferation (Fig. E1) with no development of a fetus.

Partial molar pregnancy:
- Fertilization of a normal oocyte with two sperm (usually 69, XXY or 69, XXX)
- Focal villous edema and trophoblastic proliferation with identifiable fetus

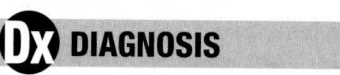

DIAGNOSIS

DIFFERENTIAL DIAGNOSIS

Complete mole, partial mole (Table 1), ectopic pregnancy, abortion (incomplete or spontaneous), normal intrauterine pregnancy

WORKUP

- Pelvic exam to evaluate for uterine size and bleeding
- Blood pressure to assess for gestational hypertension or preeclampsia (systolic blood pressure >140 or diastolic blood pressure >90)
- Fig. 2 describes an algorithm for the diagnosis and management of molar pregnancy

LABORATORY TESTS

- Quantitative beta human chorionic growth hormone (beta hCG); significantly elevated levels >100,000 will raise suspicion for molar pregnancy
- Complete blood count (CBC) to assess for acute anemia from vaginal bleeding
- Comprehensive metabolic panel to evaluate for renal or liver disease
- TSH to evaluate for hyperthyroidism
- Urinalysis for proteinuria to evaluate for preeclampsia
- Type and screen to evaluate Rh status and to prepare for surgery

IMAGING STUDIES

- Pelvic ultrasound (Figs. E3 and E4):
  1. Complete moles in the first trimester will demonstrate a complex, echogenic, intrauterine mass containing many small cystic spaces that are secondary to swollen chorionic villi and no identifiable fetus. This is the classic "snowstorm" appearance (Fig. 5).
  2. Partial mole will show a thickened, hydropic placenta with fetal parts.
  3. Baseline chest x-ray to use for comparison if malignant trophoblastic disease develops

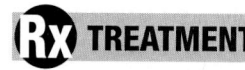

TREATMENT

NONPHARMACOLOGIC THERAPY

Surgical uterine evacuation with dilatation and curettage (D&C) is the mainstay of management of a molar pregnancy, either partial or complete. Tables 2 and 3 summarize the management of hydatidiform moles.

ACUTE GENERAL Rx

D&C, Rh immune globulin if Rh negative

CHRONIC Rx & DISPOSITION

If pathology results are consistent with complete or partial mole, patients must be followed to evaluate for trophoblastic neoplasia. 15% to 20% of complete moles and 1% to 5% of partial moles can develop into trophoblastic neoplasia. Quantitative beta hCG should be followed weekly until three consecutive results show normal levels. After that, check quantitative beta hCG every month for a total of 6 mo. Patients should remain on reliable contraception during this time to prevent confusion from a rising beta hCG in the case of a new pregnancy.

TABLE 1 Features of Partial and Complete Hydatidiform Moles

Feature	Partial Mole	Complete Mole
Karyotype	69,XXX or –,XXY	46,XX or –,XY
Pathology		
Fetus	Often present	Absent
Amnion, fetal RBC	Usually present	Absent
Villous edema	Variable, focal	Diffuse
Clinical Presentation		
Diagnosis	Missed abortion	Molar gestation
Uterine size	Small for dates	50% large for dates
Theca-lutein cysts	Rare	25%–30%
Postmolar GTN	2.5%–7.5%	6.8%–20%

GTN, Gestational trophoblastic neoplasia; *RBC*, red blood cell.
From Disaia PJ et al: *Clinical gynecologic oncology*, ed 9, Philadelphia, 2017, Elsevier.

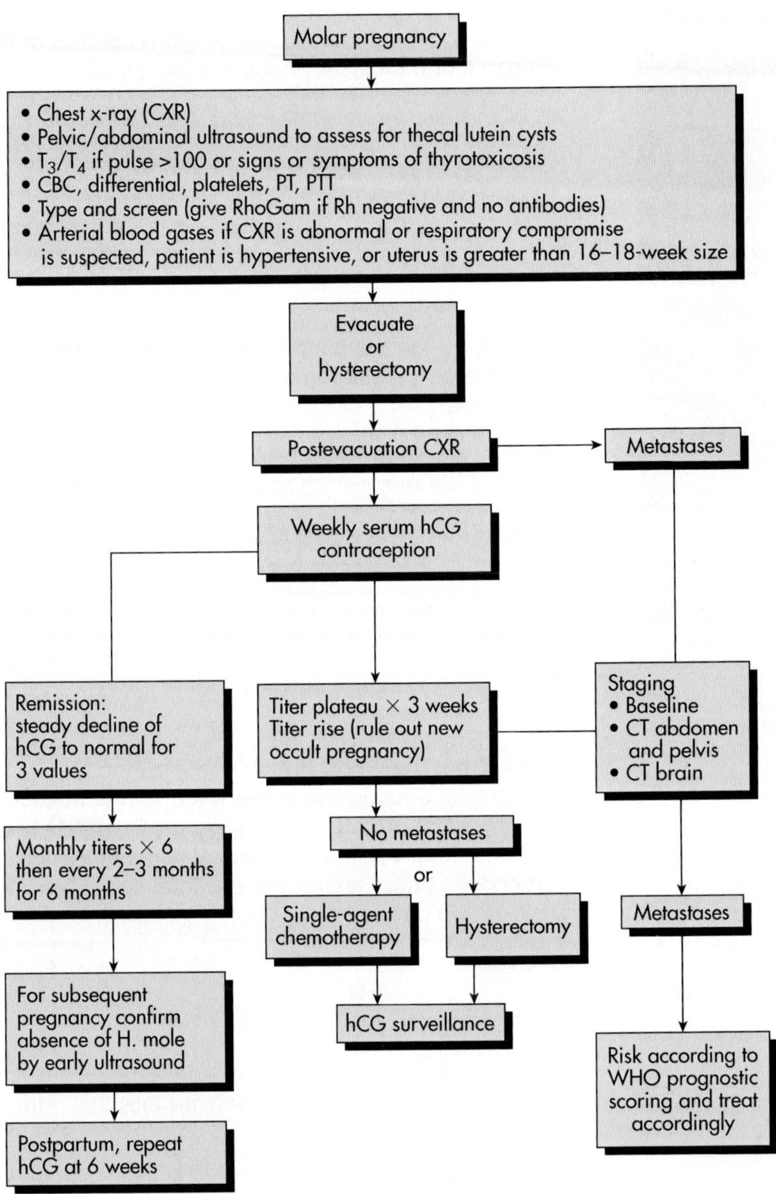

FIG. 2 Algorithm for the management of molar pregnancy. (From Gabbe SG: *Obstetrics*, ed 6, Philadelphia, 2012, WB Saunders.)

Specific criteria by beta hCG have been established by FIGO for diagnosis of postmolar gestational trophoblastic disease (see Tables 4 through 6).

REFERRAL

- If there is concern for a molar pregnancy, the patient should be managed by a gynecologist for uterine evacuation and follow-up.
- If there is a plateau or rise of the beta hCG during follow-up, the patient should be referred to a gynecologic oncologist for treatment with either further surgery or prophylactic chemotherapy.

SUGGESTED READINGS

Available at ExpertConsult.com

RELATED CONTENT

Spontaneous Miscarriage (Related Key Topic)
Vaginal Bleeding During Pregnancy (Related Key Topic)

AUTHORS: **SHIVANI SHAH, M.D.,** and **PATRICIA W. LO, M.D.**

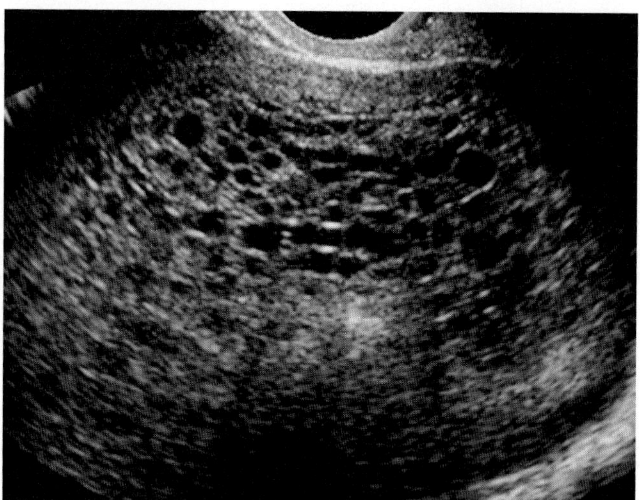

FIG. 5 Complete molar pregnancy: Classic appearance. Transabdominal scan shows a vesicular echogenic mass distending the endometrium. The mass is filled with innumerable uniformly distributed cystic spaces that corresponded to hydropic chorionic villi at pathology. (From Rumack CM et al: *Diagnostic ultrasound*, ed 4, Philadelphia, 2011, Mosby.)

TABLE 2 Management of Hydatidiform Mole

Evacuation: Suction D&E (or hysterectomy in selected patients)

Postevacuation quantitative hCG level and chest radiography

Monitor quantitative hCG levels every 1-2 weeks until three normal values or criteria for GTN

After hCG level is normal for three values, then monitor hCG levels every 1-3 mo for 6 mo

Initiate chemotherapy for GTN using indications listed in Table 3:

1. Plateaued or rising hCG values
2. Histologic diagnosis of choriocarcinoma, invasive mole, or placental site trophoblastic tumor
3. Persistent hCG >6 mo after evacuation
4. Metastatic disease

D&E, Suction dilation and evacuation; *GTN,* gestational trophoblastic neoplasia; *hCG,* human chorionic gonadotropin.
From Disaia PJ et al: *Clinical gynecologic oncology*, ed 9, Philadelphia, 2017, Elsevier.

TABLE 3 Diagnosis and Evaluation of Gestational Trophoblastic Neoplasia

Diagnosis of GTN

After molar evacuation: Four values or more of plateaued hCG (±10%) over at least 3 weeks: days 1, 7, 14, and 21

After molar evacuation: A rise of hCG of 10% or greater for three values or more over at least 2 weeks: days 1, 7, and 14

After molar evacuation: Persistence of hCG beyond 6 mo

The histologic diagnosis of choriocarcinoma, invasive mole, or PSTT

Metastatic disease without established primary site with elevated hCG (pregnancy has been excluded)

Evaluation of GTN

Complete physical and pelvic examination; baseline hematologic, renal, and hepatic functions

Baseline quantitative hCG level

Chest radiograph or CT scan of chest

Brain MRI

CT or MRI scan of abdomen and pelvis

CT, Computed tomography; *GTN,* gestational trophoblastic neoplasia; *hCG,* human chorionic gonadotropin; *MRI,* magnetic resonance imaging; *PSTT,* placental site trophoblastic tumor.
From Disaia PJ et al: *Clinical gynecologic oncology*, ed 9, Philadelphia, 2017, Elsevier.

TABLE 4 The 2002 Criteria for the Diagnosis of Post Hydatidiform Mole Trophoblastic Neoplasia

HCG-level plateau of 4 values ±10% recorded over a 3-week duration (days 1, 7, 14, and 21)

An hCG-level increase of more than 10% of 3 values recorded over a 2-week duration (days 1, 7, and 14)

Persistence of detectable hCG for more than 6 months after molar evacuation

TABLE 5 International Federation of Gynecology and Obstetrics Staging of Gestational Trophoblastic Neoplasia

Stage I	Disease confined to the uterus
Stage II	GTN extends outside the uterus but is limited to the genital structures (adnexa, vagina, broad ligament)
Stage III	GTN extends to the lungs with or without genital tract involvement
Stage IV	All other metastatic sites

Kohorn EI: The new FIGO 2000 staging and risk factor scoring system for gestational trophoblastic disease: description and critical assessment, *Int J Gynecol Cancer* 2001;11:73–77.

TABLE 6 The World Health Organization (WHO) Prognostic Scoring System Is Used for the Medical Management of Patients with Partial, Complete Moles and Choriocarcinomas. Individual scores for each prognostic factor are added up. Total score 0-6 = low risk; >7 = high risk.

Figo Scoring	0	1	2	4
Age	<40	≥ 40	-	-
Antecedent pregnancy	Mole	Abortion	Term	-
Interval months from index pregnancy	<4	4-<7	7-<13	≥13
Pretreatment serum HCG (IU/L)	<103	103-<104	104-<105	≥105
Large tumor size (including uterus) cm	<3	3-<5	≥5	-
Site of metastases	Lung	Spleen, kidney	Gastrointestinal	Liver, brain
Previous failed chemotherapy	-	-	Single drug	2 or more drugs

BASIC INFORMATION

DEFINITION

Molluscum contagiosum is a poxvirus infection characterized by discrete skin lesions with central umbilication.

SYNONYM

MC

ICD-10CM CODE

B08.1 Molluscum contagiosum

EPIDEMIOLOGY & DEMOGRAPHICS

- Molluscum contagiosum spreads by autoinoculation, scratching, or touching a lesion.
- It usually occurs in young children. It is also common in sexually active adults and patients with HIV infection.
- Incubation period varies between 4 and 8 wk.
- Spontaneous resolution in immunocompetent patients can occur after several months.

PHYSICAL FINDINGS & CLINICAL PRESENTATION

- The individual lesion appears initially as a small (2-3 mm), flesh-colored, firm, smooth-surfaced papule with subsequent central umbilication. Lesions are frequently grouped (Fig. 1). The size of each lesion generally varies from 2 to 6 mm in diameter.
- Typical distribution in children involves the face, extremities, and trunk. Mucous membranes are spared.
- Distribution in adults generally involves pubic and genital areas (Fig. E2).
- Erythema and scaling at the periphery of the lesions may be present as a result of scratching or hypersensitivity reaction.
- Lesions are not present on the palms and soles.

ETIOLOGY

Viral infection of epithelial cells caused by a poxvirus, molluscum contagiosum

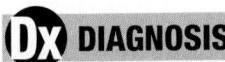

DIAGNOSIS

Diagnosis is usually established by the clinical appearance of the lesions (distribution and central umbilication). A magnifying lens can be used to observe the central umbilication. If necessary, the diagnosis can be confirmed by removing a typical lesion with a curette and examining the content on a slide after adding potassium hydroxide and gentle heating. Staining with toluidine blue will identify viral inclusions.

DIFFERENTIAL DIAGNOSIS

- Verruca plana (flat warts): No central umbilication, not dome shaped, irregular surface, can involve palms and soles
- Herpes simplex: Lesions become rapidly umbilicated
- Varicella: Blisters and vesicles are present
- Folliculitis: No central umbilication, presence of hair piercing the pustule or papule
- Cutaneous cryptococcosis in AIDS patients: Budding yeasts will be present on cytologic examination of the lesions
- Basal cell carcinoma: Multiple lesions are absent
- Cellulitis

WORKUP

Careful examination of the papules

LABORATORY TESTS

Generally not indicated in children. Screening for other sexually transmitted diseases is recommended in all cases of genital molluscum contagiosum.

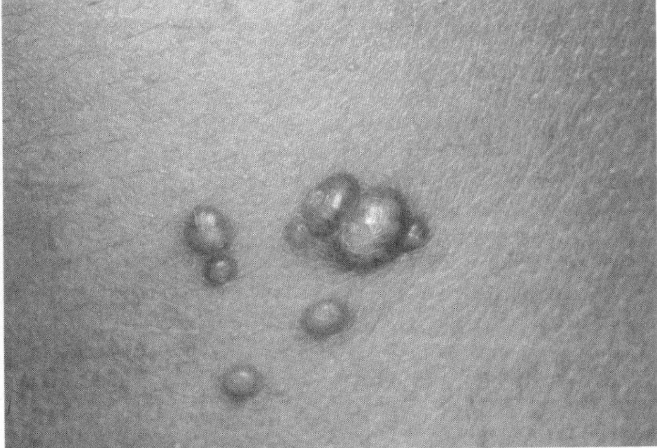

FIG. 1 Grouped molluscum. (From Kliegman RM et al: *Nelson textbook of pediatrics,* ed 19, Philadelphia, 2011, Saunders.)

TREATMENT

GENERAL THERAPY

- Therapy is individualized depending on number of lesions, immune status, and patient's age and preference.
- Observation for spontaneous resolution is reasonable in patients with few, small, nonirritated, and nonspreading lesions. Genital lesions should be treated in all sexually active patients.
- Liquid nitrogen cryotherapy.
- Carbon dioxide laser.
- Curettage after pretreatment of the area with combination prilocaine 2.5% with lidocaine 2.5% cream (EMLA) for anesthesia is useful for treatment of a few lesions. Curettage should be avoided in cosmetically sensitive areas because scarring may develop.
- Treatments with liquid nitrogen therapy in combination with curettage are effective in older patients who do not object to some discomfort.
- Application of cantharidin 0.7% to individual lesions covered with clear tape will result in blistering over 24 hr and possible clearing without scarring. This medication should be avoided on facial lesions.
- Other treatment measures include use of imiquimod cream or tretinoin 0.025% gel or 0.1% cream at bedtime, daily use of salicylic acid (Occlusal) at bedtime, and use of laser therapy.
- Trichloroacetic acid peel generally repeated every 2 wk for several weeks is useful in immunocompromised patients with extensive lesions.

DISPOSITION

Most patients respond well to the therapeutic modalities listed previously. Spontaneous resolution can occur after 6 to 9 mo in some immunocompetent patients.

REFERRAL

To dermatology when diagnosis is in doubt or in patients with extensive lesions

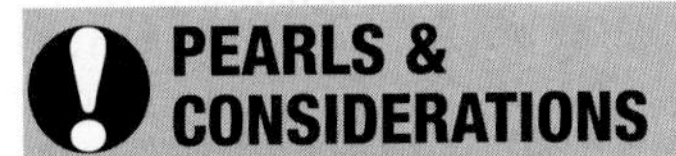

PEARLS & CONSIDERATIONS

COMMENTS

Genital molluscum contagiosum in children may be indicative of sexual abuse.

RELATED CONTENT

Molluscum Contagiosum (Patient Information)

AUTHOR: **FRED F. FERRI, M.D.**

BASIC INFORMATION

DEFINITION

MGUS is a premalignant disorder characterized by the clonal expansion of plasma cells or lymphoplasmacytic cells. It is typically detected incidentally when patients undergo testing with serum or urine protein electrophoresis. The term "monoclonal gammopathy of undetermined significance" (MGUS) is defined by the presence of a serum monoclonal (M) protein less than 3 g/dl and clonal plasma cells less than 10% in the bone marrow. In addition, there must be no evidence of end organ dysfunction such as renal insufficiency, anemia, hypercalcemia, or bony lesions on skeletal surveys (Table 1).

SYNONYMS

MGUS
Non-IgM MGUS
IgM MGUS
Light chain MGUS

ICD-10CM CODE
D47.2 Monoclonal gammopathy of undetermined significance (MGUS)

EPIDEMIOLOGY & DEMOGRAPHICS

INCIDENCE: In the U.S., the estimated age-adjusted incidence of MGUS is higher in men than in women. The annual incidence of MGUS in men is 120 per 100,000 at age 50 yr and increases to 530 per 100,000 at age 80 yr, whereas the incidence for women is 60 per 100,000 at age 50 yr and 370 per 100,000 at age 80 yr.

PREVALENCE: MGUS is associated with increasing age; approximately 1.5% of persons older than 50 yr and 3.0% of persons older than 70 yr have an elevated M protein level without end organ dysfunction. Studies have shown that at clinical diagnosis, MGUS is most likely to have been present undetected for a median duration of more than 10 yr. The prevalence of MGUS is also higher in African Americans. In one study, there was an almost threefold increase in prevalence among the African American population compared with the Caucasian population (8.6% vs. 3.6%).

PREDOMINANT SEX AND AGE: The median age at diagnosis is about 70 yr. Prevalence is higher in men than in women at any given age.

RISK FACTORS: Race (African American), older age, male sex, or exposure to pesticides. Environmental and/or genetic defects play an important role, since the risk of MGUS in relatives of multiple myeloma or MGUS patients is increased twofold to threefold when compared to the general population. The cumulative risk of progression into multiple myeloma or related disorders is approximately 1% per yr. A variety of disorders (Table 2) are also associated with monoclonal gammopathy.

PHYSICAL FINDINGS & CLINICAL PRESENTATION

- MGUS typically is detected after a routine blood test reveals an elevated total protein concentration and is a common finding in medical practice.
- Patients are asymptomatic.
- Physical exam is normal.

ETIOLOGY

- The mechanism is unknown, and most cases are sporadic. The causes of malignant transformation of MGUS into multiple myeloma is still not well understood. Genetic predisposition, cytokine release, and bone marrow angiogenesis may play a role in the progression of MGUS into multiple myeloma.
- Characterized by a rearrangement of immunoglobulin genes resulting in the production of a monoclonal protein.

Dx DIAGNOSIS

DIFFERENTIAL DIAGNOSIS

- Smoldering myeloma (Table E3)
- Multiple myeloma
- Waldenström's agammaglobulinemia
- Secondary monoclonal gammopathies
  1. Chronic liver disease
  2. Rheumatologic diseases
  3. Chronic myelomonocytic leukemia
  4. Chronic neutrophilic leukemia
  5. Lichen myxedematosus
- Pyoderma gangrenosum
- AL amyloidosis
- Idiopathic Bence Jones proteinuria

LABORATORY TESTS

- Protein studies with serum free light chain assay
- Serum protein electrophoresis (Fig. E1)
  1. IgG most common, followed by IgM and IgA
- 24-hour urine protein excretion and urine electrophoresis
- Serum and urine immunofixation
- Determination of serum free light chain ratio (kappa and lambda free light chains)
- Hemoglobin
- Serum calcium and creatinine
- Examination of the bone marrow aspirate only when clinically indicated. It is not necessary in MGUS patients with low risk fractures (no end organ damage. I8g gammopathy less than 1.5 g/dl, normal serum free light chain ratio)

IMAGING STUDIES

- Skeletal survey
- Bone mineral density resting at baseline (MGUS is associated with increased risk of osteoporosis)

Rx TREATMENT

- Risk stratification
  1. Low risk: Serum M protein <1.5 g/dl, IgG subtype, normal genetics, free light chain ratio between 0.26 and 1.65. Absolute risk of progression (ARP) at 20 yr is 5%.
  2. Low-intermediate risk: Any 1 factor abnormal. ARP at 20 yr is 21%.
  3. High-intermediate risk: Any 2 factors abnormal. ARP at 20 yr is 37%.
  4. High risk: More than 3 factors abnormal. ARP at 20 yr is 58%.
- Follow-up by risk category
  1. Patients with MGUS should be tested again within 4 to 6 mo from the time of first diagnosis to exclude evolving multiple myeloma. Those with low-risk MGUS can be followed up every 1 to 2 yr, whereas those with intermediate- or high-risk MGUS need to be followed up at least annually for life or until they develop a life-expectancy-threatening condition.
- Reevaluation consists of:
  1. Serum protein electrophoresis
  2. 24-hour urine protein excretion
  3. Serum free light chain assessment
     a. Complete blood count
     b. Serum creatinine and calcium
     c. Careful history and physical examination to look for signs and symptoms known to evolve from MGUS

DISPOSITION

- Risk of myeloma at 25 yr is 30%
- Annual risk of transformation to myeloma depends on type of M protein:
  1. Immunoglobulin MGUS: 1% per yr
  2. Light-chain MGUS: 0.3% per yr
- Risk of infection (bacterial and viral) is twofold compared with healthy controls
- Increased risk of mortality from bacterial infections
- Patients with high M protein concentrations and abnormal free light-chain ratios have excess risk for malignant transformation or development of AL amyloidosis

REFERRAL

To hematologist/oncologist for evaluation

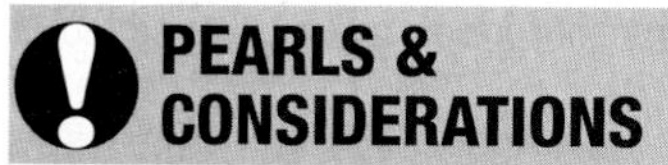

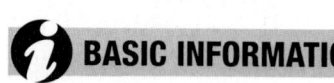

PEARLS & CONSIDERATIONS

- Approximately 55% of 70-yr-old patients diagnosed as having MGUS have had the condition for more than 10 yr.
- Most patients with MGUS should be monitored every 6 to 12 mo for signs and symptoms of progression.
- There is no indicated treatment.

SUGGESTED READINGS
Available at ExpertConsult.com

AUTHORS: **JORGE J. CASTILLO, M.D.**, and **IRENE M. GHOBRIAL, M.D.**

TABLE 1 Disease Definitions for the Monoclonal Gammopathies: MGUS and Related Disorders

Type of Monoclonal Gammopathy	Premalignancy with a Low Risk of Progression (1%-2% per year)	Premalignancy with a High Risk of Progression (10% per year)	Malignancy
IgG and IgA (non-IgM) monoclonal gammopathies*	**Non-IgM MGUS** All 3 criteria must be met: Serum monoclonal protein <3 g/dl Clonal bone marrow plasma cells <10%, and Absence of end-organ damage such as hypercalcemia, renal insufficiency, anemia, and bone lesions (CRAB) that can be attributed to the plasma cell proliferative disorder	**Smoldering multiple myeloma** Both criteria must be met: Serum monoclonal protein (IgG or IgA) ≥3 g/dl and/or clonal bone marrow plasma-cells ≥10%, and Absence of end-organ damage such as lytic bone lesions, anemia, hypercalcemia, or renal failure that can be attributed to a plasma cell proliferative disorder	**Multiple myeloma** All 3 criteria must be met except as noted: Clonal bone marrow plasma cells ≥10% Presence of serum and/or urinary monoclonal protein (except in patients with true nonsecretory multiple myeloma), and Evidence of end-organ damage that can be attributed to the underlying plasma cell proliferative disorder, specifically Hypercalcemia: Serum calcium >11.5 mg/dl or Renal insufficiency: Serum creatinine >2 mg/dl or estimated creatinine clearance <40 ml/min Anemia: Normochromic, normocytic with a hemoglobin value of >2 g/dl below the lower limit of normal or a hemoglobin value <10 g/dl Bone lesions: Lytic lesions or severe osteopenia attributed to a plasma cell proliferative disorder or pathologic fractures
IgM monoclonal gammopathies	**IgM MGUS**† All 3 criteria must be met: Serum IgM monoclonal protein of any level Normal bone marrow and absence of end-organ damage such as anemia, constitutional symptoms, hyperviscosity, lymphadenopathy, or hepatosplenomegaly that can be attributed to the underlying lymphoproliferative disorder	**Smoldering Waldenström's macroglobulinemia** Both criteria must be met: Serum IgM monoclonal protein of any level and/or bone marrow lymphoplasmacytic infiltration of any level, and No evidence of anemia, constitutional symptoms, hyperviscosity, lymphadenopathy, or hepatosplenomegaly that can be attributed to the underlying lymphoproliferative disorder	**Waldenström's macroglobulinemia** All criteria must be met: IgM monoclonal gammopathy of any level, and any level of bone marrow lymphoplasmacytic infiltration (usually intratrabecular) by small lymphocytes that exhibit plasmacytoid or plasma cell differentiation and a typical immunophenotype (e.g., surface IgM^+, $CD5^{+/-}$, CD10–, $CD19^+$, $CD20^+$, CD23–) that satisfactorily excludes other lymphoproliferative disorders including chronic lymphocytic leukemia and mantle cell lymphoma Evidence of anemia, constitutional symptoms, hyperviscosity, lymphadenopathy, or hepatosplenomegaly that can be attributed to the underlying lymphoproliferative disorder. Presence of the MYD88 L265P mutation **IgM myeloma** All criteria must be met: Symptomatic monoclonal plasma cell proliferative disorder characterized by a serum IgM monoclonal protein regardless of size Presence of 10% plasma cells on bone marrow biopsy Presence of lytic bone lesions related to the underlying plasma cell disorder and/or translocation t(11;14) on fluorescence in situ hybridization
Light-chain monoclonal gammopathies	**Light-chain MGUS** All criteria must be met: Abnormal FLC ratio (<0.26 or >1.65) Increased level of the appropriate involved light-chain (increased kappa FLC in patients with ratio >1.65 and increased lambda FLC in patients with ratio <0.26) No immunoglobulin heavy-chain expression on immunofixation Clonal bone marrow plasma cells <10%, and Absence of end-organ damage such as hypercalcemia, renal insufficiency, anemia, and bone lesions (CRAB) that can be attributed to the plasma cell proliferative disorder	**Idiopathic Bence Jones proteinuria** All criteria must be met:Urinary monoclonal protein on urine protein electrophoresis ≥500 mg/24 h and/or clonal bone marrow plasma cells ≥10% No immunoglobulin heavy-chain expression on immunofixation Absence of end-organ damage such as hypercalcemia, renal insufficiency, anemia, and bone lesions (CRAB) that can be attributed to the plasma cell proliferative disorder	**Light-chain multiple myeloma**† Same as multiple myeloma except no evidence of immunoglobulin heavy-chain expression

FLC, Free light chain; *MGUS,* monoclonal gammopathy of undetermined significance.

*Occasionally patients with IgD and IgE monoclonal gammopathies have been described and will be considered to be part of this category as well.

†Note that conventionally IgM MGUS is considered a subtype of MGUS, and similarly light-chain multiple myeloma is considered as a subtype of multiple myeloma. Unless specifically distinguished, when the terms MGUS and multiple myeloma are used in general, they include IgM MGUS and light-chain multiple myeloma, respectively.

Modified from Rajkumar SV, et al.: Advances in the diagnosis, classification, risk stratification, and management of monoclonal gammopathy of undetermined significance: implications for recategorizing disease entities in the presence of evolving scientific evidence, *Mayo Clin Proc* 85(10):945-948, 2010.

TABLE 2 Diseases Associated With Monoclonal Gammopathy

Plasma cell and related disorders	MGUS Solitary plasmacytoma: Bone Soft tissue Multiple myeloma Waldenström's macroglobulinemia Primary amyloidosis	
Lymphoid disorders	Non-Hodgkin's lymphoma	Monoclonal protein observed in CLL (>20% of cases with IgM, ≈50% with IgG, light chains also observed), extranodal marginal zone lymphomas (>30% of cases and correlated with BM involvement), follicular, mantle cell, and diffuse large B-cell lymphomas also reported with serum M proteins as has AITL
	Hodgkin's lymphoma	Rare but reported
	Castleman disease	<2% with monoclonal gammopathy
Other hematologic disorders	Acquired von Willebrand disease	IVIG more effective than factor concentrate in increasing factor VIII coagulant and VWF levels
	Gaucher disease	Observed in 25% in one study; M protein declined after splenectomy
	Pernicious anemia, pure RBC aplasia, hereditary spherocytosis, MPD, MDS	
Connective tissue disorders	SLE	IgG, IgM, and IgA have been observed, no difference in disease activity or outcome
	Inclusion body myositis	80% with IgG M protein
	Polymyositis, RA, scleroderma	
Neurologic disorders	POEMS syndrome	Most have M-protein of λ light chain
	Peripheral neuropathy	Most common is IgM followed by IgG and IgA In half, IgM protein binds to myelin-associated glycoprotein Size of M protein not correlated with severity of neuropathy Some benefit from plasma exchange for those with IgG and IgA Fludarabine and rituximab with some benefit for IgM
	Myasthenia gravis, ALS, Alzheimer's disease	
Dermatologic disorders	Schnitzler syndrome	Neutrophilic urticarial dermatitis, monoclonal IgM protein, and two of: lymphadenopathy, fever, hepatosplenomegaly, joint pain, increased ESR, increased neutrophils, or abnormal bone imaging
	Scleredema	
	Pyoderma gangrenosum	Frequently an IgA protein
Infections	HIV	Both IgG and IgM M proteins observed
	HCV	M protein present in up to 10% of patients
Immunosuppression	Renal transplant	In children CMV infection associated with M protein
	Liver and heart transplant	Most patients with posttransplant lymphoproliferative disorders have M proteins
	BM transplant	Observed in both autologous and allogeneic transplants Appearance of M protein correlated with GVHD

AITL, Angioimmunoblastic T-cell lymphoma; *ALS,* amyotrophic lateral sclerosis; *BM,* bone marrow; *CLL,* chronic lymphocytic leukemia; *CMV,* cytomegalovirus; *ESR,* erythrocyte sedimentation rate; *GVHD,* graft-versus-host disease; *HCV,* hepatitis C virus; *HIV,* human immunodeficiency virus; *Ig,* immunoglobulin; *IVIG,* intravenous immunoglobulin; *MGUS,* monoclonal gammopathy of uncertain significance; *MDS,* myelodysplastic syndrome; *MPD,* myeloproliferative disorder; *POEMS,* polyneuropathy, organomegaly, endocrinopathy, monoclonal gammopathy, and skin changes; *RA,* rheumatoid arthritis; *RBC,* red blood cell; *SLE,* systemic lupus erythematosus; *VWF,* von Willebrand factor.

From Hoffman R, et al.: *Hematology: basic principles and practice*, ed 7, Philadelphia, 2018, Elsevier.

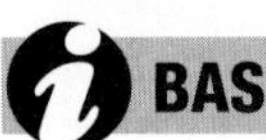

BASIC INFORMATION

DEFINITION

Mononucleosis is a symptomatic infection most commonly caused by Epstein-Barr virus (EBV) and characterized by fever, tonsillar pharyngitis, and lymphadenopathy.

SYNONYMS

IM
Infectious mononucleosis (IM)
EBV
Kissing disease

ICD-10CM CODES

B27	Infections mononucleosis
B27.0	Gamma herpesviral mononucleosis
B27.1	Cytomegaloviral mononucleosis
B27.8	Other infectious mononucleosis
B27.9	Infectious mononucleosis

EPIDEMIOLOGY & DEMOGRAPHICS

INCIDENCE (IN U.S.): 500 cases/100,000 persons/yr. Worldwide, approximately 95% of adults are infected with EBV at some point in life.

PREDOMINANT SEX: Incidence is the same, but occurs earlier in females.

PREDOMINANT AGE: Most common between the ages of 15 and 24 yr.

PHYSICAL FINDINGS & CLINICAL PRESENTATION

- Following an incubation period of 1 to 2 mo, a prodrome may occur, with fever, chills, malaise, and anorexia for several days. This is followed by the classic triad, which includes pharyngitis, fever, and adenopathy. Pharyngitis (Fig. E1) is typically the most severe symptom. Tonsillitis with marked tonsillar exudates is common.
- Lymphadenopathy can be diffuse, but most commonly occurs in both the anterior and posterior triangles of the neck.
- Splenomegaly may occur, most commonly during the second week of illness.
- Rash (Fig. E2) is uncommon but will occur in nearly all patients who receive ampicillin or amoxicillin.
- At times, IM can present as fever and adenopathy without pharyngitis. Although complications may be severe, they are uncommon and tend to resolve completely.
- Involvement of the hematologic, pulmonary, cardiac, or nervous system may occur.
- Splenic rupture is rare; incidence of <1%.
- IM is usually a self-limited illness, but symptoms of malaise and fatigue may last months before resolving.
- Children are at the highest risk of airway obstruction. This is the most common cause of hospitalization from IM.
- Box 1 and Table E1 summarize the features of IM in immunocompetent patients.

ETIOLOGY

The most common cause of IM is primary infection with EBV. Cytomegalovirus (CMV) can cause a similar disease syndrome, but CMV infection often occurs in infancy or early childhood and is minimally symptomatic. Primary EBV infection during childhood also often causes few or no symptoms; persistent fatigue and recurrent/persistent fevers are the most common reasons parents bring symptomatic children to medical care. Infection during childhood is more common in lower socioeconomic groups. The frequency of IM in late adolescence is attributed to the onset of social contact between the sexes. Close personal contact is usually necessary for transmission. Transfer via saliva while kissing may be responsible for many cases. EBV can persist in the oropharynx of patients with IM for up to 18 months. Transmission may also occur sexually as EBV can be isolated in cervical epithelial cells and male seminal fluid and can also be transmitted by blood transfusion.

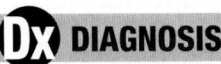

DIAGNOSIS

DIFFERENTIAL DIAGNOSIS

- Heterophile-negative IM caused by cytomegalovirus (CMV)
- Bacterial and viral causes of pharyngitis
- Toxoplasmosis
- Acute retroviral syndrome of HIV, lymphoma

WORKUP

Initial testing consists of heterophile antibody (monospot) and CBC with differential. Fig. 3 illustrates the serologic evaluation of patients with clinical symptoms of acute IM and atypical lymphocytosis.

LABORATORY TESTS

- A heterophile antibody test is the best initial test for diagnosis of EBV infection (sensitivity of 71% to 90% for diagnosing IM). However, the test has a 25% false negative rate in the first week of illness.
- Increased white blood count (WBC) is common, with a relative lymphocytosis and neutropenia. Atypical lymphocytes (Fig. E4) are the hallmark of IM, but are not pathognomonic. Mild thrombocytopenia is common. A falling hematocrit may signal splenic rupture or severe immune-mediated hemolytic anemia. Elevated hepatocellular enzymes and cryoglobulins occur in many cases. Heterophile antibody, as measured by the monospot test, may be positive at presentation, or may appear later in the course of illness. A negative test should be repeated if clinical suspicion is high; negative results are common in patients symptomatic for <2 wk and children <4 yr. If this test remains negative for 8 wk,

BOX 1 Summary of Features of Infectious Mononucleosis (IM) in Immunocompetent Patients

Epstein-Barr Virus (Human Herpesvirus-4)

Pathophysiology
- Virus enters through oropharyngeal epithelial and lymphoid cells.
- Virus attaches to CD21 on B cells.
- Viral antigens—viral capsid antigen (VCA), early antigen (EA), Epstein-Barr nuclear antigen (EBNA)—are produced and elicit antibody production.

Humoral Immune Response
- Immunoglobulin (Ig)M against VCA rises during incubation and prodrome, falls over few weeks to months.
- IgG against VCA rises during incubation, decreases during convalescence, remains detectable for life.
- Antibodies to EA rise 2-3 weeks after onset of illness, then fall.
- Antibodies to EBNA rise during convalescence, detectable for life.

Cellular Immune Response
- T cells activated during second week of illness.
- CD8-positive cytotoxic T cells kill infected B cells.
- Natural killer cells kill infected B cells.
- Some resting memory B cells remain latently infected.

Clinical Features
- 2- to 5-week incubation period
- Vague onset of symptoms
- Fever, sore throat, lymphadenopathy
- Adolescents, young adults more often symptomatic than younger children

Laboratory Features
- Leukocytosis with absolute lymphocytosis and atypical lymphocytes
- Transient monocytosis
- Relative and absolute neutropenia early on
- Mild thrombocytopenia in half of cases
- Hemolytic anemia in 1%-3% of cases, often with anti-I specificity
- Elevated transaminases in 85%-100% of cases, but clinical jaundice rare
- Spot test is simple, rapid, specific, based on agglutination of horse red blood cells (RBCs)
- Heterophil antibody (HA) test is based on differential absorption of IM-specific HA by beef RBC stroma and guinea pig kidney

From McPherson RA, Pincus MR: *Henry's clinical diagnosis and management by laboratory methods*, ed 23, Philadelphia, 2017, Elsevier.

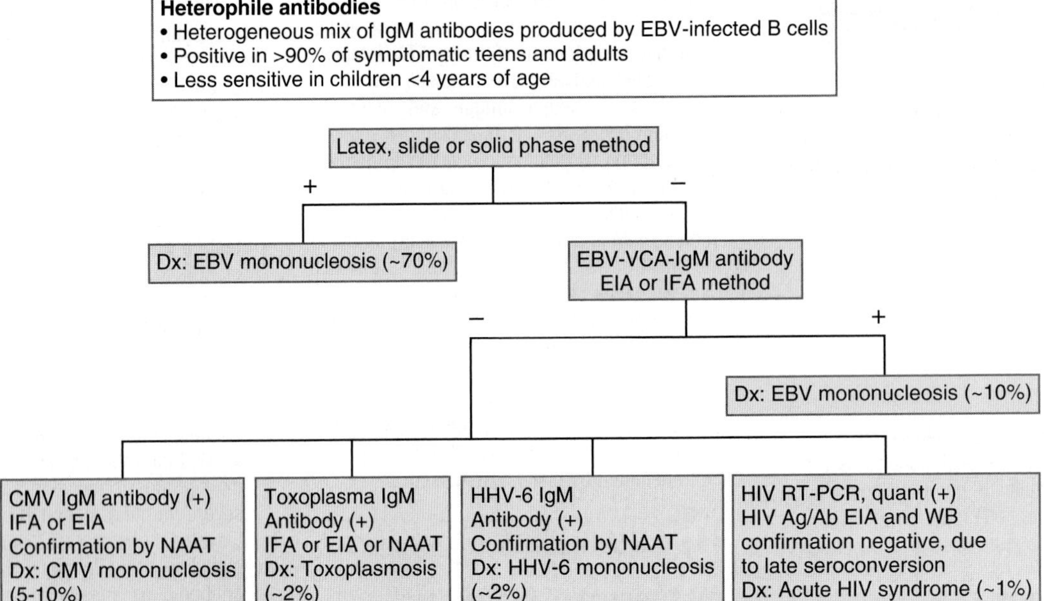

FIG. 3 Serologic evaluation of patients with clinical symptoms of acute infectious mononucleosis and atypical lymphocytosis. *CMV*, Cytomegalovirus; *Dx*, diagnosis; *EBV*, Epstein-Barr virus; *EIA*, enzyme immunoassay; *HHV-6*, human herpesvirus 6; *HIV*, human immunodeficiency virus; *IFA*, immunofluorescent assay; *IgM*, immunoglobulin M; *NAAT*, nucleic acid amplification testing; *quant*, quantitative; *RT-PCR*, reverse transcriptase polymerase chain reaction; *VCA*, viral capsid antigen. (From McPherson RA, Pincus MR: *Henry's clinical diagnosis and management by laboratory methods*, ed 23, Philadelphia, 2017, Elsevier.)

alternative diagnoses should be considered. The monospot usually remains positive for 3 to 6 mo but can last >1 yr.
- In addition to the heterophile antibody, virus-specific antibodies may result in response to IM. Determination of these EBV-specific antibodies is rarely necessary to diagnose IM, although early diagnosis in monospot-negative cases may be made by isolating IgM to the viral capsid antigen, which is usually positive during the acute illness and disappears after 4 to 6 wk.

IMAGING STUDIES

Chest x-ray may rarely show infiltrates. An elevated left hemidiaphragm may occur in cases of splenic rupture.

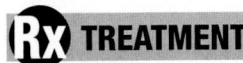

Rx TREATMENT

NONPHARMACOLOGIC THERAPY

- Supportive rest is advocated by some, but effect on outcome is not clear.
- Splenectomy if rupture occurs; transfusions for severe anemia or thrombocytopenia

GENERAL Rx

- Pharmacologic therapy, including corticosteroids, is not indicated in mild illness.
- The use of steroids (Fig. E5) has not been shown to have sustained clinical benefit, but should be considered in patients who have severe thrombocytopenia or hemolytic anemia, or impending airway obstruction as a result of enlarged tonsils.
- There is no role for antiviral agents such as acyclovir in the management of IM.

CHRONIC Rx

A rare, chronic form of IM with persistent organ infection and inflammation has been described. This should not be confused with chronic fatigue syndrome, which is unrelated to EBV.

DISPOSITION

Eventual resolution of all symptoms is the rule.

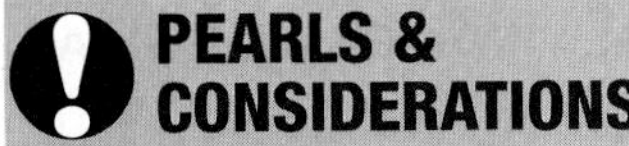

PEARLS & CONSIDERATIONS

COMMENTS

- Contact sports should be avoided during the first month of illness because splenic rupture can occur during this time, even in the absence of clinically detectable splenomegaly.
- Between 30% and 75% of college freshmen are seronegative for EBV. Each year nearly 20% of susceptible persons become infected and up to 50% of these persons develop IM.

SUGGESTED READINGS

Available at ExpertConsult.com

RELATED CONTENT

Mononucleosis (Patient Information)
Epstein-Barr Virus Infection (Related Key Topic)

AUTHORS: **NATHANIEL P. GOODRICH, M.D.,** and **RUSSELL J. MCCULLOH, M.D.**

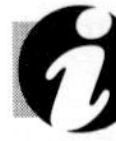

BASIC INFORMATION

DEFINITION

Mucormycosis is a fungal infection by Zygomycetes fungi and includes species in the order Mucorales (*Rhizopus* sp., *Rhizomucor, Cunninghamella, Apophysomyces, Saksenaea, Absidia, Syncephalastrum, Cokeromyces, Mortierella*) and in the order Entomophthorales (*Conidiobolus* and *Basidiobolus*).

SYNONYM

Zygomycosis

ICD-10CM CODES

B46.5 Mucormycosis, unspecified
B46.1 Rhinocerebral mucormycosis
B46.0 Pulmonary mucormycosis
B46.3 Cutaneous mucormycosis
B46.4 Disseminated mucormycosis

EPIDEMIOLOGY & DEMOGRAPHICS

- Mucormycosis is the third most frequent cause of invasive fungal infections in immunocompromised hosts. These fungi are ubiquitous in nature and can be found in soil and decaying vegetation. Infection is seen in association with underlying conditions, including diabetes mellitus especially with ketoacidosis, hematologic malignancies, stem cell or solid organ transplants, severe burns or trauma, treatment with deferoxamine or iron overload states, steroid treatment, immunodeficiency states (e.g., AIDS), injection drug use, and malnutrition. Immunocompetent hosts may become infected in tropical climates.
- The fungus gains entry to the body most commonly through the respiratory tract. The spores are deposited in the nasal turbinates and may be inhaled into the pulmonary alveoli. In cases of cutaneous mucormycosis, the spores are introduced directly into the skin lesion.
- After a tornado with winds >200 mph struck Joplin, Missouri, in May 2011, there were 13 confirmed cases of mucormycosis *(Apophysomyces trapeziformis),* including five deaths. While two patients had diabetes, none were immunocompromised. It was felt that the fungus entered through wounds sustained during the tornado. Wooden splinters were found in four patients.

PHYSICAL FINDINGS & CLINICAL PRESENTATION

- Rhinocerebral-rhinoorbital-paranasal syndrome (Fig. E1) is the most common presentation, which presents with fever, facial and orbital pain, headache, diplopia, loss of vision, facial or orbital cellulitis, facial anesthesia, cranial nerve dysfunction, black nasal discharge, epistaxis, and seizure. Physical findings in this situation include proptosis; chemosis; nasal, palatal, or pharyngeal necrotic ulcerations; and retinal infarction. Thrombosis of the cavernous sinus or internal carotid artery may occur. This form of mucormycosis is found most commonly in diabetics, primarily in the presence of acidosis, and in patients with leukemia and neutropenia. Isolated CNS mucormycosis may result from hematogenous spread (can occur with injection drug users).
- Pulmonary mucormycosis can present with pneumonia, lung abscess, pulmonary infarction, pleurisy, pleural effusion, hemoptysis, chills, and fever. This form of mucormycosis is found most commonly in immunocompromised neutropenic hosts after chemotherapy for hematologic malignancies.
- Gastrointestinal zygomycosis presents with abdominal pain, diarrhea, gastrointestinal hemorrhage, ulcers, peritonitis, and bowel infarction. This form of mucormycosis is found most commonly in patients with extreme malnutrition and is believed to arise from ingestion of spores of the fungi.
- Cutaneous zygomycosis presents as nodular lesions (hematogenous seeding) or a wound infection. It primarily involves the epidermis and dermis after use of occlusive dressings that have not been properly sterilized.
- Cardiac mucormycosis is a form of endocarditis.
- Septic arthritis and osteomyelitis.
- Brain abscess occurs most often from extension of the fungus from the nose or paranasal sinuses through adjacent bones in severely debilitated patients.
- Disseminated zygomycosis (rare but uniformly fatal).
- Physical findings depend on the location of the infection.

ETIOLOGY & PATHOGENESIS

The cause of mucormycosis is infection by a fungus of the Zygomycetes class (see "Definition"). Rhizopus and mucor species are the most common causes. Normal host defenses include leukocytes and pulmonary macrophages. Quantitative (e.g., neutropenia) or qualitative (e.g., diabetes mellitus or steroid treatment) disruption in the host defenses predisposes the patient to infection. Patients treated with deferoxamine for iron-overload states are also at risk.

Dx DIAGNOSIS

A high index of suspicion is critical since mucormycosis infection is acute and rapidly faster if untreated. The hallmark of mucormycosis is infarction and necrosis of host tissues that result from invasion of the vasculature by the fungal elements. Black eschars and discharges should be closely evaluated. Diagnosis depends on the demonstration of the organism in the tissue of a biopsy specimen.

DIFFERENTIAL DIAGNOSIS

- Infection of the sites described previously by other organisms (bacterial [including tuberculosis and leprosy], viral, fungal, or protozoan)
- Noninfectious tissue necrosis (e.g., neoplasia, vasculitis, degenerative) of the sites described previously

WORKUP

- Biopsy of infected tissue with direct-light microscopy examination establishes the diagnosis within minutes of the biopsy in the case of nasopharyngeal infection. Fungal hyphae are broad (5- to 15-micron diameter) and irregularly branched and have rare septations, in contrast to molds such as *Aspergillus,* which are narrower, have regular branching, and have many septations.
- Bronchoalveolar lavage or bronchoscopy with biopsy for smear, culture, and histologic examination.
- Radiographs and other imaging studies such as CT of symptomatic sites may be required before infection is suspected and tissue specimens are obtained.
- It should be noted that serum tests that measure fungal cell wall components, such as the 1, 3-beta D glucan assay and the Aspergillus galactomannan assay used to diagnosis other invasive fungal diseases, will be negative in mucormycosis, as mucormycocis agents lack these cell wall components.

Rx TREATMENT

Aggressive correction of underlying disease (e.g., hyperglycemia, high steroid doses, use of immunosuppressive drugs) should be undertaken.

Standard therapy consists of aggressive surgical debridement of involved tissues and antifungal therapy. For invasive mucormycosis recommended treatment is with a lipid formulation of amphotericin B that allows higher doses with less nephrotoxicity. The start dose is 5 mg/kg of liposomal amphotericin B or amphotericin B lipid complex. Doses as high as 10 mg/kg have also been used. Weeks of therapy are usually required.

Traditional amphotericin B given IV at a daily dose of 1.0 to 1.5 mg/kg infused over 2 to 4 hr daily for a total of 1 to 4 g can also still be used, but is associated with significant nephrotoxicity and adverse reactions such as fever, chills, myalgias, vomiting, and electrolyte disturbances.

- Other antifungals do not appear to be effective except posaconazole, which may serve as an oral step-down therapy after amphotericin B at a dose of 400 mg bid with a fatty meal. Isavuconazole is another agent with efficacy in mucormycosis that, like posaconazole, comes in IV and oral formulation and can serve to transition patient from IV to po.
- Some studies suggest that caspofungin with amphotericin B may be synergistic for *Rhizopus oryzae* infections only.
- The role of colony-stimulating factors remains unclear, beyond that of increasing the neutrophil count in patients with neutropenia.
- Hyperbaric oxygen has been used in some patients but its utility in therapy is still not clear.

PROGNOSIS

- Sinus infection with no underlying disease: 75% survival
- Sinus infection with diabetes: 60% survival
- Sinus infection with renal disease: 25% survival

SUGGESTED READINGS

Available at ExpertConsult.com

AUTHOR: **GLENN G. FORT, M.D., M.P.H.**

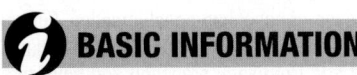

BASIC INFORMATION

DEFINITION

Multifocal atrial tachycardia (MAT) is a supraventricular tachyarrhythmia (rate greater than 100 beats/min) with P waves having at least three or more different morphologies and irregular P-P, P-R, and R-R intervals. MAT is differentiated from atrial fibrillation by discrete P wave depolarizations and an isoelectric baseline between P waves.

SYNONYMS

MAT
Chaotic atrial rhythm
Chronic atrial tachycardia
Repetitive multifocal paroxysmal atrial tachycardia
Multifocal ectopic atrial tachycardia
The term *wandering pacemaker* is used for a similar arrhythmia associated with a normal or slow heart rate (<100 beats/min).

ICD-10CM CODE
I47.1 Supraventricular tachycardia

EPIDEMIOLOGY & DEMOGRAPHICS

Estimated prevalence in hospitalized patients of 0.05% to 0.32%. Average age is 70s. Usually associated with underlying pulmonary disease with right atrial electromechanical delay. Chronic obstructive pulmonary disease (COPD) is present in approximately 55% of patients with MAT. It may also be seen in patients with valvular heart disease, pulmonary hypertension, and hypomagnesemia.

PHYSICAL FINDINGS & CLINICAL PRESENTATION

Symptoms:
- Palpitation
- Lightheadedness
- Syncope
- Symptoms of the underlying pulmonary disease
- Physical findings associated with the underlying pulmonary disease

ETIOLOGY

- Exact mechanism unknown
- Potentially caused by right atrial distention such as in pulmonary hypertension due to underlying lung disease
- Exacerbated by underlying pulmonary disease (COPD, hypoxia, pulmonary embolism, pneumonia), cardiac disease, hypercarbia, acidosis, electrolyte disturbances

Dx DIAGNOSIS

DIFFERENTIAL DIAGNOSIS

- Atrial fibrillation (up to 55% of patients with MAT will develop atrial fibrillation)
- Atrial flutter with variable AV conduction
- Sinus tachycardia
- Paroxysmal atrial tachycardia
- Sinus tachycardia with premature atrial or ventricular contractions

WORKUP

- ECG (Fig. 1)
- Chest x-ray
- Pulmonary function tests
- Electrolytes
- Arterial blood gases

Rx TREATMENT

- Correction and/or improvement in the underlying pulmonary or metabolic dysfunction if possible
- Avoid drugs such as theophylline, isoproterenol, etc.
- Electrolyte repletion, especially magnesium and potassium, to normal levels.
- Intravenous magnesium infusion may occasionally be helpful in patients with normal magnesium levels.
- Calcium channel blockers—verapamil may be effective acutely and chronically and is often used as first line in patients with preserved LV function.
- β-blockers are typically contraindicated by obstructive lung disease or acute heart failure.
- If the arrhythmia is asymptomatic, it can be left untreated.
- Direct current cardioversion is ineffective.
- No significant role for antiarrhythmics or catheter ablation.
- Anticoagulation is not indicated, although some recent studies have linked frequent atrial ectopy on ambulatory monitoring with stroke risk.
- In extreme cases of refractory MAT in symptomatic patients who cannot tolerate medical therapy or in MAT resistant to medical therapy, AV nodal ablation with pacemaker implantation has been performed.
- Table E1 summarizes the treatment of multifocal atrial tachycardia.

SUGGESTED READINGS
Available at ExpertConsult.com

AUTHORS: **BARRY FINE, M.D., PH.D.,** and **JOHN WYLIE, M.D., F.A.C.C.**

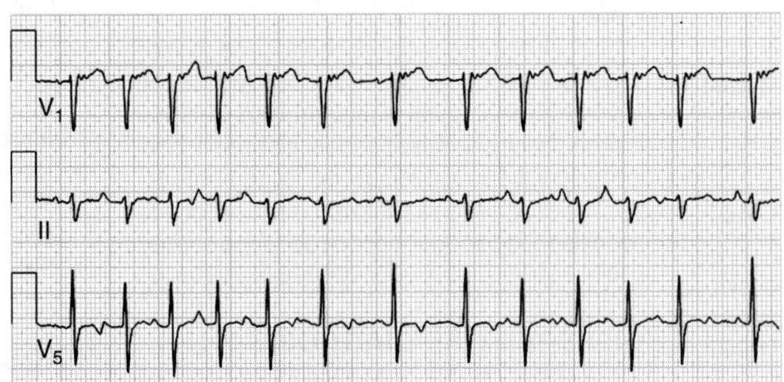

FIG. 1 Multifocal atrial tachycardia. This three-lead rhythm strip (leads V_1, II, and V_5) shows an irregularly irregular narrow QRS complex rhythm. However, unlike AF, each QRS complex is preceded by discrete P waves. There are at least three different P wave morphologies and PR intervals, consistent with MAT. (From Olshansky B et al: *Arrhythmia essentials*, ed 2, Philadelphia, 2017, Elsevier.)

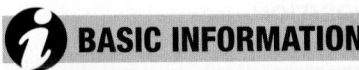

BASIC INFORMATION

DEFINITION

Multiple endocrine neoplasia (MEN) refers to a group of heritable genetic syndromes characterized by the development of specific groups of tumors of the endocrine glands.

SYNONYMS

MEN I: Wermer syndrome
MEN IIA: Sipple Syndrome

ICD-10CM CODES

E31.2	Multiple endocrine neoplasia [MEN] syndromes
E31.20	Multiple endocrine neoplasia [MEN] syndrome, unspecified
E31.21	Multiple endocrine neoplasia [MEN] syndrome type I
E31.22	Multiple endocrine neoplasia [MEN] syndrome type IIA
E31.23	Multiple endocrine neoplasia [MEN] syndrome type IIB

EPIDEMIOLOGY & DEMOGRAPHICS

INCIDENCE:
- MEN I: 25 in 10,000
- MEN II: 1 in 30,000

PEAK INCIDENCE: N/A
PREVALENCE:
- MEN I: 1/30,000
- MEN II: 1/35,000 (predominantly MEN IIA)

PREDOMINANT SEX & AGE: N/A
GENETICS:
- MEN I: Autosomal-dominant mutation in MEN1 tumor-suppressor gene
- MEN IIA and MEN IIB: Autosomal-dominant mutations in RET proto-oncogene

RISK FACTORS: Family history of MEN syndrome, although it can also occur sporadically

PHYSICAL FINDINGS & CLINICAL PRESENTATION

- Patients may present due to screening or may present with a MEN-associated tumor. Tumors are found incidentally due to biochemical abnormalities or to symptoms.
- MEN I (PPP [pituitary, pancreas, parathyroid])
  1. Diagnostic criteria generally include two MEN-associated tumors, one tumor in a patient with a family history, or positive genetic testing.
  2. Primary hyperparathyroidism (parathyroid adenoma or hyperplasia) is the most common manifestation and can cause hypercalcemia (urolithiasis, GI disturbance, bone pain, neuropsychiatric disturbances).
  3. Pancreatic neuroendocrine tumors cause symptoms related to their secretory properties.
     a. Gastrinoma: Peptic ulcers, diarrhea, esophageal symptoms (see Gastrinoma)
     b. Insulinoma: Hypoglycemic symptoms upon fasting and after exercise (see Insulinoma)
     c. Glucagonoma: Necrolytic migratory erythema (a blistering skin lesion), diabetes/glucose intolerance, weight loss
     d. VIPoma: Diarrhea, hypokalemia, decreased gastric acid
     e. Nonfunctioning tumors can metastasize, a frequent cause of death in MEN I
  4. Pituitary tumors may cause compressive symptoms, such as visual field defects or hypopituitarism (see "Pituitary Adenoma"). Hormonal secretion may also cause symptoms.
     a. Prolactinoma (most common pituitary tumor in MEN I): Menstrual irregularities, sexual dysfunction, gynecomastia, and/or galactorrhea (see "Prolactinoma").
     b. Somatotroph adenomas (producing growth hormone): Gigantism or acromegaly (frontal bossing, increased shoe/hat size, hyperglycemia, hyperhidrosis) depending on patient age (see "Acromegaly").
     c. Corticotroph adenomas (producing adrenocorticotropic hormone): Cushingoid features such as weight gain, moon facies, hyperglycemia, bone loss, and proximal muscle weakness (see "Cushing's Disease and Syndrome").
     d. Nonfunctioning (nonsecretory) tumors
  5. Other manifestations: Collagenomas, angiofibromas, meningiomas, lipomas
- MEN IIA:
  1. Medullary thyroid carcinoma (MTC) is a tumor of the thyroid's calcitonin-secreting C cells. It can present with a neck mass, as well as flushing and diarrhea due to elevated calcitonin levels.
  2. Primary hyperparathyroidism: See MEN I. Less aggressive in MEN IIA.
  3. Pheochromocytoma is an adrenal tumor producing catecholamines.
- MEN IIB:
  1. Medullary thyroid carcinoma (MTC)
  2. Pheochromocytoma
  3. Oral mucosal neuromas

ETIOLOGY

Tumor development facilitated by the previously described genetic mutations (Table E1).

DIAGNOSIS

DIFFERENTIAL DIAGNOSIS

Tumors associated with MEN may occur sporadically.

WORKUP

- MEN I:
  1. Genetic testing: Offered to patients meeting MEN I clinical criteria or to patients in whom there is high suspicion, as well as to first-degree relatives of MEN I patients
  2. Hyperparathyroidism screening: Parathyroid hormone (PTH) and calcium annually
  3. Pancreatic tumor screening: Annual pancreas imaging (endoscopic ultrasonography, CT, or MRI) and annual biochemical testing (glucose, gastrin, vasoactive intestinal peptide [VIP], glucagon, insulin, pancreatic polypeptide, chromogranin A)
  4. Pituitary tumor screening: Insulin-like growth factor 1 (IGF-1) and prolactin annually and pituitary MRI every 3 to 5 yr
  5. Carcinoid tumor screening: Chest CT or MRI every 2 yr
- MEN IIA:
  1. Genetic testing: At-risk members of families with known RET mutations should undergo screening for the specific mutation. Patients with MTC should have genetic testing of the tumor and genetic testing based on results. Cutaneous lichen amyloidosis (a skin finding) should prompt testing; Hirschsprung disease may also prompt testing.
  2. Hyperparathyroidism screening: PTH and calcium annually
  3. Pheochromocytoma: Plasma catecholamines and metanephrines annually for screening, age to begin depending on specific mutation; CT and MRI may localize; I-123 and PET also helpful
  4. MTC screening: Depends on risk category; physical exam, neck ultrasound, and calcitonin level yearly; carcinoembryonic antigen may also be indicated
- MEN IIB:
  1. Genetic testing: See MEN IIA
  2. Pheochromocytoma: See MEN IIA
  3. MTC screening: Although there may be a role for monitoring, prophylactic thyroidectomy is typically performed early

LABORATORY TESTS

See Workup.

IMAGING STUDIES

See Workup.

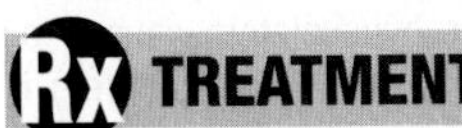

TREATMENT

No therapy to reverse the underlying cause. Treatment (both medical and surgical) focuses on tumor prevention and management.

NONPHARMACOLOGIC THERAPY

- MEN I:
  1. Hyperparathyroidism may be treated surgically with subtotal or total parathyroidectomy, or parathyroidectomy with gland reimplantation at an alternate site.
  2. Pituitary tumors may be surgically excised via transsphenoidal approach; notably, medical therapy is first-line for prolactinoma.
  3. Pancreatic tumor treatment is extremely variable. Gastrinoma is frequently complicated by duodenal metastases, which are difficult to treat surgically. Ulcers caused by gastrinoma may require endoscopic or surgical management. Surgery is preferred for insulinoma, VIPoma, and glucagonoma. Nonfunctioning tumors may be treated surgically depending on tumor

size and location. Conservative management for insulinoma may involve frequent carbohydrate intake.

- MEN IIA:
  1. MTC is generally treated surgically. Prophylactic thyroidectomy is considered based on genetic mutation. Almost all children with MEN IIA will require thyroidectomy (screening as previously described). Patients should undergo ultrasound and total thyroidectomy with cervical lymph node dissection. Extent of further neck dissection depends on metastases and may be guided by calcitonin levels. A more palliative surgical approach is considered in the setting of advanced disease.
  2. Hyperparathyroidism: Resection of only enlarged glands with intraoperative PTH monitoring is preferred.
  3. Pheochromocytoma is treated surgically. Unilateral adrenalectomy is preferred, although many patients will develop a contralateral pheochromocytoma. Preoperative blood pressure control is key. If present, pheochromocytoma must be removed before thyroidectomy.
- MEN IIB:
  1. MTC: Prophylactic thyroidectomy offered in childhood.
  2. Pheochromocytoma: See MEN IIA.

ACUTE GENERAL Rx

- MEN I:
  1. Hyperparathyroidism causes hypercalcemia that may be treated with IV hydration, diuretics, and bisphosphonates. Early vitamin D repletion prevents bone destruction postoperatively.
  2. Gastrinoma may lead to peptic ulcers requiring IV proton-pump inhibitor (PPI).
  3. Supportive care (glucose for hypoglycemia caused by insulinoma; fluids and electrolytes for hypovolemia caused by diarrhea from VIPoma or gastrinoma) is required.
- MEN IIA:
  1. Hyperparathyroidism: See MEN I.
  2. Pheochromocytoma: Preoperative blood pressure control is key; alpha blockers are first-line. Phenoxybenzamine irreversibly blocks alpha adrenergic receptors; doxazosin is also first-line. Calcium channel blockers and then beta-blockers can be added if needed.
- MEN IIB:
  1. Pheochromocytoma: See MEN IIA.

CHRONIC Rx

- MEN I:
  1. Hyperparathyroidism may be amenable to agonists of the calcium-sensing receptor (cinacalcet), although surgery is preferred.
  2. Pancreatic tumors may benefit from medical therapy.
     a. Gastrinoma: PPI or H2 antagonists
     b. Insulinoma: Diazoxide or somatostatin agonists (such as octreotide)
     c. Glucagonoma and VIPoma: Somatostatin agonists
  3. Pituitary tumors may be treated medically although surgical treatment is first-line with the exception of prolactinoma (for which medical therapy is first-line). Radiation therapy and/or medical therapy are considered in cases of incomplete resection or regrowth.
     a. Prolactinoma: Dopamine agonists (bromocriptine or cabergoline)
     b. Somatotroph adenoma: Somatostatin or dopamine agonists, growth hormone receptor antagonists
     c. Corticotroph adenoma: Antiadrenal agents, adrenal enzyme blocker (such as ketoconazole), somatostatin or dopamine agonists, glucocorticoid receptor blockers
  4. MEN II A:
     a. Hyperparathyroidism: See MEN I.
     b. MTC: Tyrosine kinase inhibitors and chemotherapy may help treat metastatic disease. After thyroidectomy, levothyroxine is indicated (TSH suppression not required).

COMPLEMENTARY & ALTERNATIVE MEDICINE

MEN is unlikely to be amenable to this.

DISPOSITION

Most workup can be done as an outpatient (multidisciplinary team); inpatient stays may be required due to acute complications or for surgical procedures.

REFERRAL

Patients with MEN should be followed by a multispecialty team, including endocrinologists, endocrine surgeons, and genetic counselors.

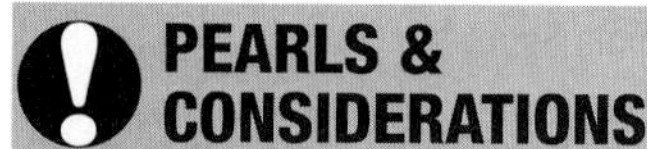

PEARLS & CONSIDERATIONS

COMMENTS

MEN is a group of genetic syndromes that requires close monitoring and intervention to prevent and treat tumor development, as well as genetic counseling of patients and family members.

PREVENTION

Prevention focuses on screening for MEN in persons at risk and early identification of MEN-associated tumors.

PATIENT/FAMILY EDUCATION

- American Multiple Endocrine Neoplasia Support: http://www.amensupport.org/
- Association for Multiple Endocrine Neoplasia Disorders: http://www.amend.org.uk/

SUGGESTED READINGS

Available at ExpertConsult.com

RELATED CONTENT

Acromegaly (Related Key Topic)
Cushing's Disease and Syndrome (Related Key Topic)
Gastrinoma (Related Key Topic)
Hyperparathyroidism (Related Key Topic)
Insulinoma (Related Key Topic)
Pheochromocytoma (Related Key Topic)
Pituitary Adenoma (Related Key Topic)
Prolactinoma (Related Key Topic)
Thyroid Carcinoma (Related Key Topic)

AUTHORS: **HARIKRASHNA B. BHATT, M.D.,** and **SHIVANG U. DANAK, M.D.**

BASIC INFORMATION

DEFINITION

Multiple myeloma (MM) is a plasma cell neoplasm characterized by clonal proliferation of malignant plasma cells in the bone marrow, monoclonal protein in the blood or urine, and associated end-organ dysfunction. Diagnostic criteria for the diagnosis of MM require the following:

- Presence of ≥20% plasma cells on examination of the bone marrow (or biopsy of a tissue with monoclonal plasma cells).
- Monoclonal protein in the serum or urine. Occasional patients without detectable monoclonal protein are considered to have nonsecretory myeloma.
- Evidence of end-organ damage (**c**alcium elevation, **r**enal insufficiency, **a**nemia, or **b**one lesions [CRAB criteria]).

SYNONYM

MM

ICD-10CM CODES

C90.00	Multiple myeloma not having achieved remission
C90.01	Multiple myeloma in remission
C90.02	Multiple myeloma in relapse

EPIDEMIOLOGY & DEMOGRAPHICS

ANNUAL INCIDENCE:

- Five cases/100,000 persons (blacks affected twice as frequently as whites, males more than females)
- MM accounts for 10% of all hematologic cancers and is the most common primary bone malignancy.
- More than 30,770 new cases and 12,770 deaths occurred in 2018 in the U.S.

PREDOMINANT AGE: The peak incidence is in the seventh decade at a median age of 70 yr.

PHYSICAL FINDINGS & CLINICAL PRESENTATION

The patient usually comes to medical attention because of one or more of the following:

- Bone pain (58%) commonly in the back and thorax or pathologic fractures (30%) caused by osteolytic lesions
- Anemia from bone marrow infiltration by plasma cells
- Recurrent infections as a result of impaired neutrophil function and deficiency of normal immunoglobulins (humoral deficiency)
- Nausea and vomiting caused by constipation and uremia
- Delirium resulting from hypercalcemia
- Neurologic complications, such as spinal cord or nerve root compression, blurred vision from hyperviscosity
- Purpura, epistaxis from thrombocytopenia
- Paresthesias, weight loss, generalized weakness

DIAGNOSIS

DIFFERENTIAL DIAGNOSIS

- Metastatic carcinoma to bone marrow
- Lymphoma, non-Hodgkin's
- Bone neoplasms (e.g., sarcoma)
- Monoclonal gammopathy of undetermined significance
- Primary amyloidosis
- Waldenström's macroglobulinemia
- Table 1 compares diagnostic criteria for multiple myeloma, myeloma variants, and MGUS

LABORATORY TESTS

- The evaluation of patients with multiple myeloma is summarized in Table 2.
- Normochromic, normocytic anemia; rouleaux formation on peripheral smear (Fig. 1)
- Hypercalcemia is present in 15% of patients at diagnosis.
- Elevated blood urea nitrogen, creatinine, uric acid, and total protein
- Urine protein immunoelectrophoresis: Proteinuria from overproduction and secretion of free monoclonal kappa or lambda chains (Bence Jones protein)
- Serum protein immunoelectrophoresis: Monoclonal spike (M spike) on protein immunoelectrophoresis in approximately 75% of patients (Fig. 2); decreased levels of normal immunoglobulins (Ig)
  1. The increased immunoglobulins are generally IgG (70%) and IgA (20%).

TABLE 1 Diagnostic Criteria for Multiple Myeloma, Myeloma Variants, and Monoclonal Gammopathy of Unknown Significance

Monoclonal Gammopathy of Undetermined Significance (MGUS) or Monoclonal Gammopathy, Unattributed/Unassociated (MG[u])
M protein in serum <30 g/L
Bone marrow clonal plasma cells <10%
No evidence of other B-cell proliferative disorders
No myeloma-related organ or tissue impairment (no end-organ damage, including bone lesions)
Asymptomatic Myeloma (Smoldering Myeloma)
M protein in serum >30 g/L and/or
Bone marrow clonal plasma cell ≥10% to 60%
No related organ or tissue impairment (no end-organ damage, including bone lesions) or symptoms
Symptomatic Multiple Myeloma (MM)
M protein in serum and/or urine[a]
Bone marrow (clonal) plasma cells[a] or plasmacytoma
Related organ or tissue impairment (end-organ damage, including bone lesions)
Solitary Plasmacytoma of Bone
No M protein in serum and/or urine[b]
Single area of bone destruction caused by clonal plasma cells
Bone marrow not consistent with MM
Normal skeletal survey (and MRI of spine and pelvis if done)
No related organ or tissue impairment (no end-organ damage other than solitary bone lesion)[b]
Nonsecretory Myeloma
No M protein in serum and/or urine with immunofixation
Bone marrow clonal plasmacytosis ≥10% or plasmacytoma
Related organ or tissue impairment (end-organ damage, including bone lesions)
Extramedullary Plasmacytoma
No M protein in serum and/or urine[c]
Extramedullary tumor of clonal plasma cells
Normal bone marrow
Normal skeletal survey
No related organ or tissue impairment (end-organ damage including bone lesions)
Multiple Solitary Plasmacytomas (Recurrent or Not)
No M protein in serum and/or urine[d]
More than one localized area of bone destruction or extramedullary tumor of clonal plasma cells that may be recurrent
Normal bone marrow
Normal skeletal survey and MRI of spine and pelvis if done
No related organ or tissue impairment (no end-organ damage other than the localized bone lesions)
Myeloma-Related Organ or Tissue Impairment (End-Organ Damage)
Calcium levels increased: Serum calcium >0–25 mmol/L above the upper limit of normal or >2–75 mmol/L
Renal insufficiency: Creatinine >173 mmol/L
Anemia: Hemoglobin 2 g/dl below the lower limit of normal or hemoglobin <10 g/dl
Bone lesions: Lytic lesions or osteoporosis with compression fractures (MRI or CT may clarify)
Other: Symptomatic hyperviscosity, amyloidosis, recurrent bacterial infections (more than two episodes in 12 mo)

CT, Computed tomography; *MRI*, magnetic resonance imaging.
[a]If flow cytometry is performed, most plasma cells (>90%) will show a neoplastic phenotype.
[b]A small M component may sometimes be present.
[c]A small M component may sometimes be present.
[d]A small M component may sometimes be present.
From Hoffman R, et al.: *Hematology, basic principles and practice,* ed 7, Philadelphia, 2018, Elsevier.

TABLE 2 Evaluation of Patients With Multiple Myeloma

Evaluation for Diagnosis

Evaluation for Monoclonal Protein

Serum protein electrophoresis, immunofixation
Quantitative immunoglobulin by nephelometric method
24-hour urine collection for electrophoresis and Bence Jones protein assessment and immunofixation
Serum free light chain and ratio

Evaluation for Clonal Plasma Cells

Bone marrow aspirate and biopsy for
Histology
Clonality by immunostaining or flow cytometry by κ/λ staining
Fine-needle aspiration of plasmacytoma if indicated

Evaluation for End-Organ Damage

Hemogram to detect anemia
Chemistry panel for renal function and calcium
Radiologic evaluation: Skeletal survey
PET-CT or MRI as indicated for bone lesions or extramedullary disease

Evaluation for Risk Stratification

β_2-Microglobulin and serum albumin for ISS stage
Cytogenetics and fluorescence in situ hybridization on bone marrow sample
LDH
C-reactive protein

Other Investigations for Selected Patients

Abdominal fat pad or rectal biopsy for amyloid
Solitary lytic lesion biopsy
Serum viscosity if IgM component or high IgA levels or serum M component >7 g/dl
Immunofixation for IgD or IgE in select cases

CT, Computed tomography; *Ig,* immunoglobulin; *ISS,* International Staging System; *LDH,* lactate dehydrogenase; *MRI,* magnetic resonance imaging; *PET,* positron emission tomography.
From Hoffman R, et al.: *Hematology, basic principles and practice,* ed 7, Philadelphia, 2018, Elsevier.

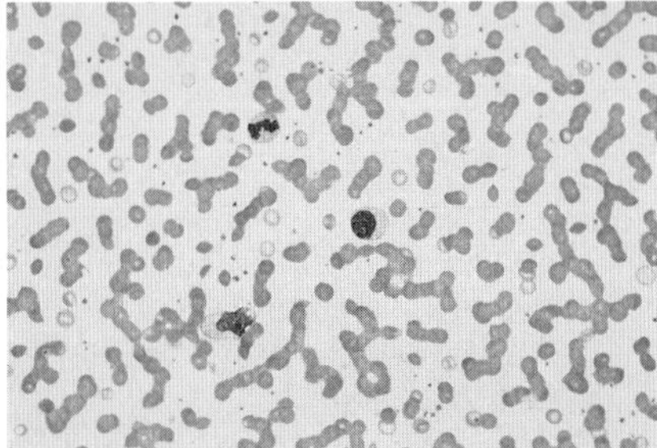

FIG. 1 Increased rouleaux formation is seen in this blood smear from a patient with a large M protein. Marked rouleaux formation is often a clue to the diagnosis of a plasma cell neoplasm but may also be observed in other conditions (Wright-Giemsa stain). (From Jaffe ES, et al.: *Hematopathology,* Philadelphia, 2011, Saunders.)

2. Approximately 5% to 10% of patients have only increased light chains in the urine by electrophoresis (light chain MM).
3. A small percentage (<2%) of patients have nonsecretory MM (no increase in immunoglobulins and no light chains in the urine) but have other evidence of the disease (e.g., positive bone marrow examination).

- Elevated serum free light chains (kappa or lambda types) with abnormally elevated or decreased kappa:lambda ratios suggestive of the presence of monoclonal light chain proteins.
- Hyponatremia, increased serum viscosity (more common with production of IgM)
- Bone marrow examination demonstrates nests or sheets of plasma cells, which comprise >20% of the bone marrow
- Serum beta-2 microglobulin is useful for prognosis because levels >8 mg/L indicate high tumor mass and aggressive disease.
- Elevated serum lactate dehydrogenase at diagnosis defines a subgroup of myeloma patients with very poor prognosis.
- Nearly all patients with MM present with abnormal chromosomes (Table 3) identified by fluorescence in situ hybridization (FISH). High-risk patients (<25% of patients at diagnosis) are those with any of the following: Deletion 17p, translocation 4:14, translocation 14:16, deletion 13q, or cytogenetic hypodiploidy.

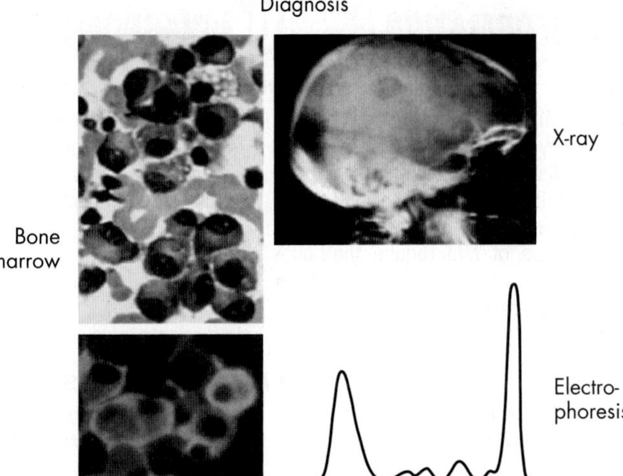

FIG. 2 Common diagnostic features in multiple myeloma. Light chain–restricted plasma cells in a bone marrow aspirate; multiple lytic lesions in a skull radiograph; large monoclonal spike in the g-globulin area in serum electrophoresis. (From Hoffman R, et al.: *Hematology, basic principles and practice,* ed 5, Philadelphia, 2009, Churchill Livingstone.)

TABLE 3 Recurrent Cytogenetic Changes in Myeloma

Chromosomal Abnormality	Patients (%)	Genes Involved
Common Cytogenetic Alterations		
Hyperdiploidy	50–60	Unclear
Hypodiploid	20	Unclear
Pseudodiploid	15	Unclear
del(17p)	8	p53
t(4:14)	15	*FGFR3, MMSET*
t(11;14)	20	Cyclin D1
t(14;16)	3	*c-MAF*
t(14;20)	1	*MAFB*
t(6p25 or 6p21;14)	1	*IRF4* or *CCND3*
t(8;14)	5	*c-Myc*
t(9;14)	<1%	*PAX5*
del(13 or 13q)	50%	Unclear
Recently Identified Alterations		
1q+	35%	
1p–	30%	
5q+	50%	
12p–	10%	

From Hoffman R, et al.: *Hematology, basic principles and practice,* ed 7, Philadelphia, 2018, Elsevier.

IMAGING STUDIES

Imaging modalities for disease assessment in myeloma are summarized in Table 4. Radiograph films of painful areas often demonstrate punched-out lytic lesions or osteoporosis (Fig. 2). CT can identify rib involvement not evident on plain films and differentiate it from osteoporotic and traumatic fractures (Fig. 3). MRI is the preferred technique for suspected spinal compression or soft tissue plasmacytomas. Bone scans may not be useful because MM lesions are not blastic.

STAGING

Table 5 describes the Revised International Staging System (R-ISS) for multiple myeloma that incorporates traditional laboratory parameters alongside high-risk chromosomal abnormalities detected by fluorescence in-situ hybridization (FISH) techniques on bone marrow samples. This system provides important prognostic assessment and classifies patients into three risk groups (high, intermediate, and standard). Risk stratification in multiple myeloma is summarized in Tables 6 and 7.

Rx TREATMENT

NONPHARMACOLOGIC THERAPY

Prevention of renal failure with adequate hydration and avoidance of nephrotoxic agents and dye contrast studies.

ACUTE GENERAL Rx

- Treatment strategy is initially related to the determination of transplant-eligible patients.
- All transplant-eligible patients should be considered for approximately 12 weeks of

TABLE 4 Imaging Modalities for Disease Assessment in Myeloma

	Use	Sensitivity/Specificity	False-Negatives	False-Positives
Bone scan	• For diagnostic screening, except for multiple myeloma	Varies	• Pure osteolytic lesions	• Trauma • Inflammation • Benign tumor • Healing
X-ray	• Can clarify nonspecific findings on bone scan • Assesses risk of fracture • Possible follow-up of tumor response, but evidence of response takes considerable time to appear	Low sensitivity	• Low disease burden • Osteopenia	• Trauma • Inflammation • Benign tumor • Healing
CT	• For anatomic detail in axial skeleton • Possible follow-up of tumor response, but role is still undefined	High sensitivity	• Low disease burden	• Trauma • Inflammation • Benign tumor • Healing
MRI	• Detection of spinal cord compression • Can help distinguish benign from malignant vertebral compression fracture • Possible follow-up of tumor response, but role is still undefined	High sensitivity and specificity	• Lesion only in cortex	• Edema
PET scan	• May eventually become first-line screening test for bone metastases • Possible follow-up of tumor response, but role is still undefined	High specificity	• Lesion only in cortex	• After chemotherapy
Bone density	• Measure osteoporosis • Response to bisphosphonates	High specificity and sensitivity		• Age-related Osteoporosis

CT, Computed tomography; *MRI*, magnetic resonance imaging; *PET*, positron emission tomography.
From Hoffman R et al: *Hematology, basic principles and practice*, ed 7, Philadelphia, 2018, Elsevier.

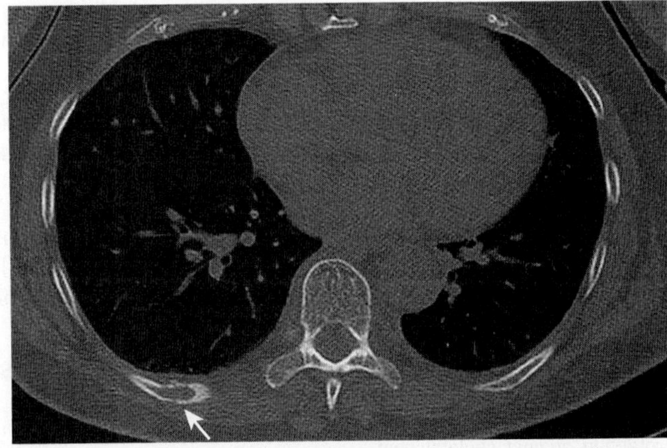

FIG. 3 Rib involvement in multiple myeloma *(arrow)*. There is thinning of the cortex and enlargement of a circumscribed area of the rib. Soft tissue Hounsfield units are noted within the lesion. In contrast to osteoporotic or traumatic fractures of the rib, no callus formation is seen. In a whole-body examination, every single rib must be screened by scrolling through it posteriorly to anteriorly. (From Pope TL, et al.: *Musculoskeletal imaging*, ed 2, Philadelphia, 2015, Saunders.)

TABLE 5 Revised International Staging System (R-ISS) for Multiple Myeloma Staging System

Stage	Criteria
I	ALL of the following: • Serum β-2 microglobulin <3.5 mg/L • Serum albumin >3.5 mg/dl • no high-risk chromosomal abnormalities by FISH • Normal LDH level
II	• Fitting neither stage I nor III
III	• Serum β-2 microglobulin >5.5 mg/L *AND* Either elevated LDH OR high-risk chromosomal abnormalities by FISH [(del 17(p) and/or translocation t(14;16) and/or translocation t(4;14)]

induction chemotherapy with triplet regimens such as the VRD regimen (bortezomib, lenalidomide, and dexamethasone) or the CyBorD regimen (cyclophosphamide, bortezomib, and dexamethasone). Upon demonstration of at least a very good partial response, these patients can undergo stem cell mobilization and collection.

- All patients with high-risk features (high R-ISS stage, poor cytogenetics) should be offered autologous stem cell transplant (ASCT) subsequently, provided they have adequate cardiac, pulmonary, and hepatic function. Currently, ASCT can be safely performed in most centers in fit patients up to age 75 yr. The duration of median improved survival with single ASCT is estimated to be 12 months.
- Patients should be offered maintenance chemotherapy with either lenalidomide or bortezomib after recovery from ASCT for at least 2 yr but potentially indefinitely.
- Induction chemotherapy in patients ineligible for transplantation (age >75 yr, high comorbidity index, poor performance status) can be identical to that offered transplant-eligible patients. Alternatively, less aggressive regimens (doublet regimens or single agents) can be recommended, including the following:
  1. Lenalidomide and dexamethasone (RD)
  2. Bortezomib and dexamethasone (VD)
- Therapy for relapsed and refractory myeloma can include second- or third-generation proteasome inhibitors (carfilzomib and ixazomib), immunomodulatory drugs (thalidomide, pomalidomide), and steroids. The monoclonal antibodies elotuzumab (targeting signaling lymphocytic activation molecule F7 [SLAMF7]) and daratumumab (targeting the CD38 antigen) have both shown improved responses and survival in relapsed or refractory multiple myeloma and are useful options in this setting. The histone deacetylase inhibitor panobinostat is also approved in this setting.
- If the relapse occurs more than 6 months after conventional therapy is stopped, the initial chemotherapy regimen can be reinstituted.
- ASCT can be considered as salvage therapy in patients who had stem cells cryopreserved early in the course of the disease.
- Approximately 15% of patients with newly diagnosed MM are recognized incidentally and present without significant symptoms (asymptomatic MM, formerly known as smoldering myeloma). The rate of progression of

TABLE 6 Risk Stratification in Multiple Myeloma

Investigations Recommended for Risk Stratification
Serum albumin and β_2-microglobulin to determine ISS stage
Bone marrow examination for t(4;14), t(14;16), and del(17p) on identified PCs by FISH
LDH
Immunoglobulin type: IgA
Histology: Plasmablastic disease or plasma cell leukemia
Additional Investigations for Risk Stratification
Cytogenetics
Gene expression profiling
Labeling index
MRI/PET scan
DNA copy number alteration by CGH/SNP array

CGH/SNP, Comparative genomic hybridization/single-nucleotide polymorphism; *FISH,* fluorescence in situ hybridization; *IgA,* immunoglobulin A; *ISS,* International Staging System; *LDH,* lactate dehydrogenase; *MRI,* magnetic resonance imaging; *PET,* positron emission tomography.

From Hoffman R, et al.: *Hematology, basic principles and practice*, ed 7, Philadelphia, 2018, Elsevier.

smoldering MM to symptomatic disease is 10% per yr for the initial 5 yr, decreasing to 5% for the next 5 yr, and decreasing further to 1.5% per yr thereafter. Observation alone is reasonable in these patients because no survival advantage has been demonstrated by treating them.

- An exception to this may be in high-risk smoldering myeloma patients. A recent trial has shown that early treatment with lenalidomide plus dexamethasone in patients with high-risk smoldering myeloma delays progression to active disease and increases overall survival.

CHRONIC Rx

- Promptly diagnose and treat infections. Common bacterial agents are *Streptococcus pneumoniae* and *Haemophilus influenzae.* Prophylactic therapy against *Pneumocystis jiroveci* with trimethoprim-sulfamethoxazole must be considered in patients receiving chemotherapy and high-dose corticosteroid regimens. Vaccinate against *S. pneumoniae,* influenza, and *H. influenzae.*

TABLE 7 Standard Risk Factors for Multiple Myeloma and the Revised International Staging System

Prognostic Factor	Criteria
ISS stage	
I	Serum β_2-microglobulin <3.5 mg/L, serum albumin ≥3.5 g/dl
II	Not ISS stage I or III
III	Serum β_2-microglobulin ≥5.5 mg/L
CA by iFISH	
High risk	Presence of del(17p) and/or translocation t(4;14) and/or translocation t(14;16)
Standard risk	No high-risk CA
LDH	
Normal	Serum LDH below the upper limit of normal
High	Serum LDH above the upper limit of normal
A New Model for Risk Stratification for MM	
R-ISS stage	
I	ISS stage I and standard-risk CA by iFISH and normal LDH
II	Not R-ISS stage I or III
III	ISS stage III and either high-risk CA by iFISH or high LDH

CA, Chromosomal abnormalities; *iFISH,* interphase fluorescence in situ hybridization; *ISS,* International Staging System; *LDH,* lactate dehydrogenase; *MM,* multiple myeloma; *R-ISS,* revised International Staging System.

From Greipp PR, et al.: International staging system for multiple myeloma. *J Clin Oncol* 23:3412, 2005. In Hoffman R, et al.: *Hematology, basic principles and practice*, ed 7, Philadelphia, 2018, Elsevier.

- Hypercalcemia is aggressively treated with IV fluids, bisphosphonates, and corticosteroids. Monthly infusions of the bisphosphonate pamidronate or zoledronate provide significant protection against skeletal complications and improve the quality of life of patients with advanced MM. The RANK-ligand inhibitor denosumab is effective in the treatment of hypercalcemia in this setting and in cases in which bisphosphonates are contraindicated (e.g., renal failure).
- Control pain with analgesics; radiation therapy to treat painful bone lesions or cord compression. Perform surgical stabilization of pathologic fractures. Consider vertebroplasty or kyphoplasty for selected vertebral lesions.
- Anemia is treated with erythropoietin.

DISPOSITION

- In patients presenting at an age <60 yr, the 10-yr survival is approximately 30%. The median length of survival after diagnosis is now 7 to 8 yr. Prognosis is better in asymptomatic patients with indolent or smoldering myeloma. Median survival time is approximately 10 yr in persons with no lytic bone lesions and a serum myeloma protein concentration <3 g/dl. Adverse outcome is associated with increased levels of beta-2 microglobulin, low levels of serum albumin, circulating plasma cells, plasmablastic features in bone marrow, increased plasma cell labeling index, poor cytogenetics (t (4;14) or t (14;16) translocation, deletion 17p).
- Tandem transplantation (two successive ASCT) improves survival among patients with MM who do not have a very good partial response after undergoing a single transplantation.
- Recent trials reveal that among patients with newly diagnosed myeloma, survival in recipients of a hematopoietic stem cell autograft followed by a stem cell allograft from an HLA-identical sibling is superior to that in recipients of tandem stem cell autografts.

REFERRAL

To hematologist for management of disease, and bone marrow transplant (BMT) specialist for transplantation options and management.

SUGGESTED READINGS

Available at ExpertConsult.com

RELATED CONTENT

Multiple Myeloma (Patient Information)

AUTHOR: **BHARTI RATHORE, M.D.**

BASIC INFORMATION

DEFINITION

Multiple sclerosis (MS) is a chronic predominantly autoimmune demyelinating disease of the central nervous system (CNS) characterized by subacute neurologic deficits correlating with CNS lesions separated in time and space, excluding other possible disease.

Subtypes include:

- **Relapsing-remitting MS (RRMS)** (82%): Relapses followed by complete or near-complete recovery, 50% to 85% of which later transition to SPMS
- **Secondary progressive MS (SPMS):** Progression of disability with few or no relapses
- **Primary progressive MS (PPMS)** (18%): Progression from the onset, rare relapses
- Progressive relapsing or relapsing progressive courses can be incorporated into PPMS or SPMS, respectively.
- Relapses are defined as a subacute onset of neurologic dysfunction that lasts for at least 24 hr due to inflammatory demyelination.

Classic rare MS variants include:

- **Marburg variant:** MRI reveals a tumor-like lesion with notable edema in one cerebral hemisphere. Pathology shows severe inflammation with necrosis: Typically acute onset with a fulminant, often malignant, course. May also involve peripheral nerves.
- **Balo concentric sclerosis:** Neuroimaging and pathology show alternating rings of myelination and demyelination resembling an onion bulb macroscopically and microscopically.
- **Schilder diffuse sclerosis:** Childhood onset with one to two large confluent lesions. Some cases were later found to be due to metabolic defects, and many have thus abandoned this disorder.

Neuromyelitis optica spectrum disorder (NMOSD): NMOSD is a distinct demyelinating disease with unique pathophysiology, treatment, and prognosis. Unlike MS, NMOSD usually involves extensive portions of the optic nerves and spinal cord (typically three or more spinal segments). Other areas of the CNS may also be involved, including the area postrema (presenting with intractable hiccups or nausea/vomiting), the brainstem, or the cerebral cortex. Additionally, patients may present with symptomatic narcolepsy. The lesions look very different on MRI than typical MS demyelinating lesions. The majority of patients are aquaporin-4 receptor Ab positive (NMO-IgG positive) while some are antibody negative or are myelin oligodendrocyte glycoprotein Ab positive (MOG-IgG positive), which has a better prognosis. The actual diagnostic criteria for NMOSD vary depending on the patient's aquaporin-4 receptor antibody status. Prognosis is typically worse than MS, and this condition does not respond to MS-specific therapies. Steroids, plasma exchange, rituximab, mycophenolate mofetil, and azathioprine are among the treatments that may be used.

SYNONYMS

MS
Disseminated sclerosis

ICD-10CM CODE

G35 Multiple sclerosis

EPIDEMIOLOGY & DEMOGRAPHICS

PEAK INCIDENCE: 20 to 40 yr in two thirds of patients; it is the most common permanently disabling disorder of the central nervous system in young adults; mean age of onset is 30 yr, range is infancy to 70 yr.

PREVALENCE: More common in people raised in northern latitudes and in certain genetic clusters. Prevalence per 10,000 varies from 20 in southern Europe to 150 to 180 in Canada, northern United States, and northern Europe; and <10 in Asia, Central America, and most of Africa.

PREDOMINANT SEX & AGE: Female/male ratio is 2 to 3:1.

GENETICS: Frequency of MS in dizygotic twins and siblings is 3% to 5%, and 20% to 40% in monozygotic twins. Most common associations include human leukocyte antigen classes I and II *(DRB1*1501, DQA1*0102, DQB1*0602)*, (*DRB1*0405-DQA1*0301-DQB1*0302* in Mediterranean population). A notable epigenetic interaction between vitamin D and the main MS-linked HLA-DRB1*1501 allele has been elucidated.

PHYSICAL FINDINGS & CLINICAL PRESENTATION

Findings depend on the location of the CNS lesion(s) and may include the following:

- Common: Nonspecific complaints such as fatigue, blurred vision, diplopia, vertigo, falls, hemiparesis, paraparesis, monoparesis, numbness, paresthesias, ataxia, cognitive deficits, depression, sexual dysfunction, and urinary dysfunction
- Visual abnormalities: Horizontal nystagmus, visual field defects, ***Marcus Gunn pupil*** (i.e., relative afferent papillary defect—normal direct and consensual light reflexes; however, when swinging flashlight from one eye to the other, direct light causes dilatation of pupil of affected eye), ***internuclear ophthalmoplegia*** (paresis of the adducting eye on conjugate lateral gaze with horizontal nystagmus of the abducting eye) (Fig. 1)
- Corticospinal tract(s) involvement: Leads to upper motor neuron signs such as spasticity, hyperreflexia, clonus, extensor plantar responses, and upper motor neuron pattern of weakness
- Sensory loss: May include partial or full dermatomal loss of pain and temperature, loss of vibration (common) and position sense, or a thoracic band of sensory loss
- Ataxia: Intention tremor, dysmetria, dysdiadochokinesis, titubation, inability to tandem gait
- Bladder dysfunction: Detrusor hyperreflexia (urge incontinence), flaccidity (neurogenic bladder), and dyssynergia (bladder contracts against a closed sphincter)
- ***Lhermitte* sign:** Flexion of the neck elicits an electrical sensation extending down the spine and occasionally into the extremities
- ***Uhthoff* phenomenon:** Transient worsening of preexisting symptoms with small elevations in body temperature (e.g., during exercise or warm bathing)

ETIOLOGY

Remains unknown but multifactorial with evidence for autoimmunity (autoreactive T and B cells), environmental factors, and genetics (Mendelian and epigenetic). Environmental risk factors during childhood include certain viruses (e.g., Epstein-Barr virus and human herpes virus 6), low UV exposure, and month of birth (higher in spring). Other risk factors include low vitamin D level and smoking.

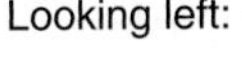

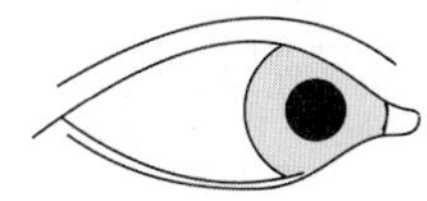

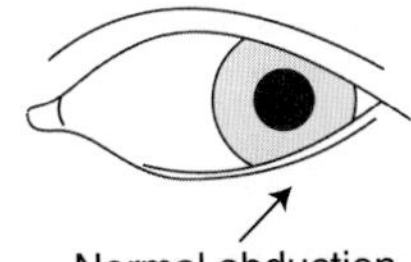

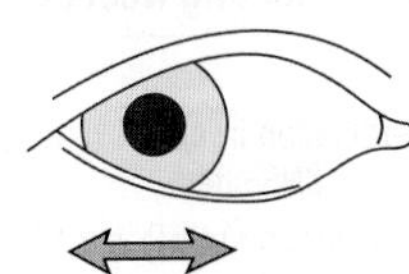

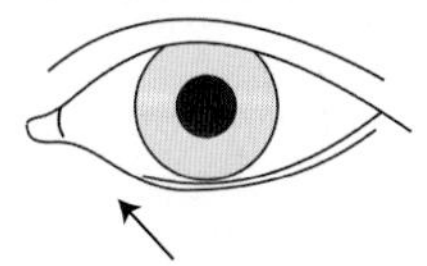

FIG. 1 Internuclear ophthalmoplegia. When the patient in the figure looks to the left (*top* row), both eyes move normally, but when the patient looks to the right (*bottom* row), the left eye fails to adduct ("weak" medial rectus) and the contralateral eye develops a jerk nystagmus. The finding is named for the side with weak adduction (i.e., in this example, a *left* internuclear ophthalmoplegia), and the lesion is in the *ipsilateral* medial longitudinal fasciculus (i.e., *left* medial longitudinal fasciculus in this example). See the text. (From McGee S: *Evidence-based physical diagnosis*, ed 4, Philadelphia, 2018, Elsevier.)

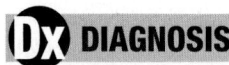

DIAGNOSIS

- MS: Based on revised 2017 McDonald criteria (Table 1)
- RRMS: See Table 1
- PPMS: Insidious progression of disability for at least 1 yr with a positive CSF and MRI evidence of >1 brain or >2 spinal cord MS-like lesions.

DIFFERENTIAL DIAGNOSIS (TABLE 2)

- Autoimmune: Acute disseminated encephalomyelitis (ADEM), postvaccination encephalomyelitis, neuromyelitis optica spectrum disorder
- Degenerative: Subacute combined degeneration of the cord (vitamin B_{12} deficiency), amyotrophic lateral sclerosis, primary lateral sclerosis
- Infections: Lyme disease, neurosyphilis, HIV, tropical spastic paraparesis, progressive multifocal leukoencephalopathy, Whipple disease
- Inflammatory: Systemic lupus erythematosus, vasculitis, sarcoidosis, Sjögren's disease, Behçet's disease, celiac disease
- Inherited metabolic disorders: Leukodystrophies
- Mitochondrial: Leber hereditary optic neuropathy, mitochondrial encephalopathy, lactic acidosis, and strokelike episodes (MELAS)
- Neoplasms: CNS lymphoma, metastases
- Vascular: Subcortical infarcts, Binswanger disease

WORKUP

- Lumbar puncture for cases that are atypical and to evaluate for mimics of MS. Typical CSF abnormalities may include increased protein (less than 100 mg/dl), mild elevation of mononuclear white blood cells, and increased IgG synthesis rate. 70% of clinically definite MS (CDMS) have elevated CSF immunoglobulin (Ig) G index, and 90% have CSF oligoclonal bands. (Serum for a serum protein electrophoresis needs to be sent to lab simultaneously with CSF for both tests.) False-positive results with IgG index and rarely with positive OCBs can be seen in CNS infections, parainfections, vasculitis, and CNS lymphoma.
- Serum: Complete blood count, chemistry panel, liver function tests, vitamin B_{12}, 25-OH vitamin D_3.
- Consider in the proper clinical setting: Neuromyelitis optica IgG, ANA, ACE (a test with low specificity and sensitivity for sarcoidosis) TSH, free T_4, very-long-chain fatty acids, arylsulfatase A.
- Consider optical coherence tomography or evoked potentials (visual, somatosensory, and brain stem auditory evoked response).

TABLE 2 Conditions That Can Be Mistaken for Multiple Sclerosis and Other Diseases of Myelin

Vascular Disease
Small-vessel cerebrovascular disease
Vasculitis
CADASIL
Antiphospholipid antibody syndrome
Structural Lesions
Craniocervical junction, posterior fossa, or spinal tumors
Cervical spondylosis or disc herniation
Chiari malformation or syrinx
Degenerative Diseases
Hereditary myelopathy
Spinocerebellar degeneration
Infections
HTLV-1 infection
HIV myelopathy or HIV-related cerebritis
Neuroborreliosis (e.g., Lyme disease) JC virus/progressive multifocal leukoencephalopathy
Neurosyphilis
Other Inflammatory Conditions
Systemic lupus erythematosus
Sjögren's syndrome
Sarcoidosis
Monofocal or Monophasic Demyelinating Syndromes
Neuromyelitis optica spectrum disorder
Acute disseminated encephalomyelitis
Other Conditions
Hashimoto thyroiditis with or without encephalopathy
Nonspecific MRI abnormalities related to migraine, aging, or trauma

CADASIL, Cerebral autosomal dominant arteriopathy with subcortical infarcts and leukoencephalopathy; *HIV,* human immunodeficiency virus; *HTLV,* human T-cell lymphotropic virus; *MRI,* magnetic resonance imaging.
From Goldman L, Schafer AI: *Goldman's Cecil Medicine*, ed 24, Philadelphia, 2012, Saunders.

TABLE 1 Summary of Revised 2017 McDonald Criteria for Diagnosis of Multiple Sclerosis

RRMS/Clinical Attacks	Clinical Lesions	Paraclinical Testing Needed
2	2	None
2	1	MRI dissemination in space *or* a second clinical attack at a different CNS site
1	2	MRI dissemination in time *or* CSF-specific oligoclonal bands
1	1	1. Additional clinical attack at a different CNS site *or* MRI dissemination in space 2. MRI dissemination in time *or* CSF-specific oligoclonal bands

Evidence of clinical lesions by physical examination or evoked potentials. *CNS,* Central nervous system; *CSF,* cerebrospinal fluid; *MRI dissemination in space:* ≥1 T2 lesions in 2 of the 4 typical areas for MS lesions—periventricular, juxtacortical, infratentorial, or spinal cord; *MRI dissemination in time:* a new lesion at follow-up MRI at any time, or presence of both an enhancing and nonenhancing lesion at any time; *RRMS,* relapsing-remitting multiple sclerosis.

IMAGING STUDIES

Brain MRI with and without gadolinium is recommended in all cases. Fig. 2 illustrates imaging features of MS. MRI with and without contrast of the cervical (Fig. E3) and thoracic spine can be helpful. MRI assesses acute and chronic lesions as well as atrophy. A normal MRI of the brain does not conclusively exclude early MS but makes it extremely unlikely.

Rx TREATMENT

NONPHARMACOLOGIC THERAPY

Patient education regarding disease characteristics, treatment options, risks and benefits of treatment, and prognosis. Often patients need intermittent rest periods on a daily basis and when physically active, and avoid exposure to heat, which typically worsens symptoms (not the disease).

Recommend physical therapy for new or worsening weakness, incoordination, or spasticity.

ACUTE GENERAL Rx

Relapses: High-dose IV methylprednisolone (3-5 days of 1 g/day), often followed by a 7- to 10-day prednisone or methylprednisolone taper. High-dose corticosteroids do not alter the long-term course of disease. May consider plasmapheresis for refractory cases.

CHRONIC Rx

- The vast majority of FDA-approved therapies are only for relapsing MS; the FDA-approved ocrelizumab is the first medication for primary progressive MS.
- Disease-modifying injection therapy includes interferon beta-1a (IM Avonex, IM Plegridy, SC Rebif), interferon beta-1b (SC Betaseron, SC Extavia), and glatiramer acetate (SC Copaxone). Common side effects for interferons include flulike symptoms, depression, liver toxicity, and leukopenia; CBC and LFTs (initially q1mo, then q3mo). Common side effects for glatiramer acetate include injection site reactions and benign chest tightness; no serum studies are needed. Daclizumab (Zinbryta), a monoclonal antibody to a subunit of IL-2, is a monthly subcutaneous injection for patients with active disease who have failed at least two MS therapies. Because of its serious side effects, the medication is distributed through a restricted access program. Some of the serious side effects include autoimmune conditions such as autoimmune hepatitis, leading to fulminant liver injury and death, as well as autoimmune skin condition, autoimmune colitis, and diffuse lymphadenopathy.
- Disease-modifying oral therapy: Consider baseline pregnancy test and infectious tests for all oral therapies, although not required by the FDA, such as VZV Ab, Lyme Ab, TB test, JC virus Ab, hepatitis Ab panel. Also

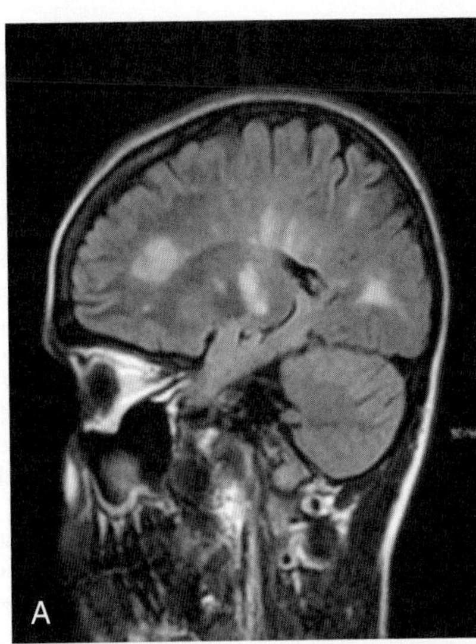

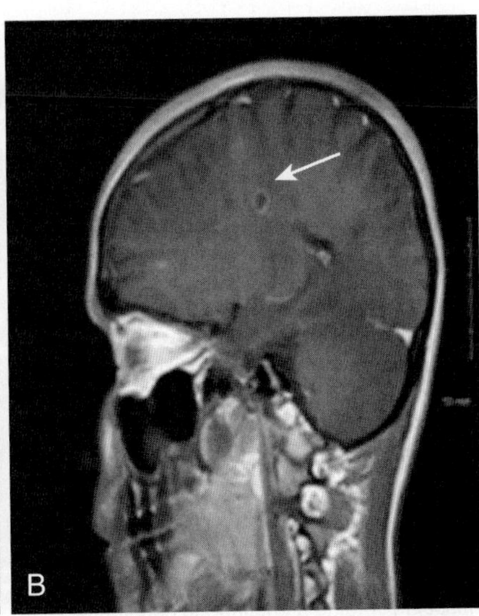

FIG. 2 Multiple sclerosis. A, Sagittal fluid-attenuated inversion recovery (FLAIR) image magnetic resonance scan shows multiple lesions in corpus callosum, "Dawson's fingers" (periventricular fingerlike lesions oriented toward the ventricles), along with ovoid and punctuate lesions in the deep white matter. **B,** Gadolinium-enhanced scan shows an enhancing lesion *(arrow)*.

review general risk of infections (hx UTIs, kidney stones, smoking, diabetes, bronchitis, disability, pulmonary function, and age). Typically monthly CBC and liver function tests for 6 mo then q3mo; pregnancy test.

1. Fingolimod (Gilenya), a sphingosine-1-phosphate receptor modulator and lymphocyte sequester. Possible side effects: Liver toxicity, bradycardia with first dose (requiring cardiac monitoring and ECG for at least 8 hr after administration of first dose), arrhythmia, pancytopenia, macular edema (ophthalmologic exam at baseline, at 3 mo, and thereafter for those with hx DM or uveitis), and reduced pulmonary function. Obtain VZV serology.
2. Teriflunomide (Aubagio), reversible inhibitor of pyrimidine synthesis (enzyme dihydroorotate dehydrogenase). Possible side effects: Diarrhea, abnormal liver function tests, nausea, and hair loss; pregnancy category X. Men should not impregnate their partners while on teriflunomide. Serum levels can be measured, and drug can be eliminated by charcoal or cholestyramine. Obtain TB test.
3. Dimethyl fumarate (Tecfidera), mechanism includes inhibition of transcription of NF-KB. Frequent side effects include nausea, abdominal discomfort, and flushing—especially during the first month—and rarely leukopenia.

- Disease-modifying IV therapy:
  1. Natalizumab (Tysabri) is a monoclonal humanized Ab that binds integrin-α4 interfering with binding to VCAM-1. It has been associated with a *higher* risk of progressive multifocal leukoencephalopathy (JC virus) than other immunomodulatory therapies. Test for JC virus Ab at least annually because conversion to a positive antibody occurs at increased frequency while on this drug. If positive, PML is still rare, but risk increases with increased length of therapy (>2 yr), history of chemotherapy, and concomitant immunosuppressants.
  2. Alemtuzumab (Lemtrada): An anti-CD52 humanized monoclonal antibody and second-line therapy for patients who have failed at least two FDA-approved MS therapies. The medication is delivered in two treatment courses. After an initial series of five daily infusions, the medication is administered 1 yr later for 3 days. Serious side effects include the development of autoimmune conditions (34% developed autoimmune thyroid disorders), infusion reactions, and certain cancers. The medication is only available through a restricted access program.
  3. Ocrelizumab (Ocrevus): A first-line therapy that is a humanized monoclonal antibody to CD20+ B cells. This is the only drug approved not only for relapsing forms of MS but also for primary progressive MS. Infections are the most common side effects.
- Symptomatic therapy:
  1. Dalfampridine (Ampyra) is a potassium channel blocker recently approved to improve walking speed in patients with MS. This medication is contraindicated in patients with epilepsy.
  2. Treat spasticity with baclofen or tizanidine. Onabotulinum toxin type A injection for focal intractable spasticity. Intrathecal baclofen pump for generalized intractable spasticity. Acute worsening may be due to infections such as UTI, injury, recent surgery, or colder temperatures.
  3. Treat urge incontinence with anticholinergic/muscarinic therapy such as oxybutynin, tolterodine, or solifenacin. Treat urinary retention with tamsulosin. In both cases, rule out a bladder infection.
  4. Treat dysesthesias with gabapentin or pregabalin.
  5. Fatigue: Consider amantadine 100 mg bid, modafinil, or a stimulant.
  6. Tremor: Conazepam, propranolol, or gabapentin.
  7. Depression and anxiety are common. Consider referring to both a counselor and psychiatrist.

DISPOSITION

Most patients have complete or near-complete recovery weeks to months after a relapse. Typically, 2 relapses occur in RRMS patient per yr (75% will have >1 relapse). Although the rate of disease progression is highly variable, there is higher risk of greater long-term disability with higher relapse rate during the first 2-5 yr, poor recovery from initial relapses, older age of onset, involvement of multiple systems, male sex, African American, and primary progressive disease.

REFERRAL

- Referral to neurologist is highly recommended. Referral to MS specialist should be considered in cases of poor response to therapy and/or if there is concern about complications of therapies.
- Consider referrals for physical, speech, and occupational therapy.
- Consider referral to urology if bladder-sphincter dyssynergia is possible or if not responsive to treatment.

PEARLS & CONSIDERATIONS

- Clinically isolated syndrome (CIS): Isolated demyelinating event and assessing risk of CDMS 1) in optic neuritis, if brain MRI is completely normal, there is 20% to 25% chance of CDMS over 15 yr. 2) In CIS, if there are >1 T2 hyperintensity on brain MRI, there is 84% risk, and if there are >2 Gd + lesions there is a 96% risk of CDMS over 18 mo.
- Pseudorelapses may occur with heat, fever, or infections (urinary tract infections common in patients with MS).
- Headache, fever, altered mental status, elevated CSF WBCs, or recurrent relapses over days to weeks raises concern for CNS infection or ADEM.

SUGGESTED READINGS

Available at ExpertConsult.com

RELATED CONTENT

Multiple Sclerosis (Patient Information)

AUTHORS: **COREY GOLDSMITH, M.D.,** and **ALEXANDRA DEGENHARDT, M.D., M.M.SC.**

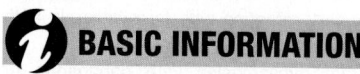

BASIC INFORMATION

DEFINITION

Mushroom poisoning is intoxication resulting from ingestion of poisonous mushrooms.

ICD-10CM CODE

T62.0X1A Toxic effect of ingested mushrooms, accidental (unintentional), initial encounter

EPIDEMIOLOGY & DEMOGRAPHICS

- 5% of all mushrooms are poisonous. Distinction between poisonous and edible mushrooms may be difficult even by experienced persons.
- Common poisonous species include *Amanita, Russula, Gyromitra,* and *Omphalotus* (see Table E1). *Amanita phalloides*, colloquially known as the "death cap," belongs to the *Phalloideae* section of the *Amanita* family of mushrooms and is responsible for most deaths following ingestion of foraged mushrooms worldwide.
- Identification of syndromes is more important than knowing the associated species (Table 2).

PHYSICAL FINDINGS & CLINICAL PRESENTATION

- *Russula* causes confusion, delirium, visual disturbance, tachycardia, and diarrhea within a few hours of ingestion. Prognosis: Spontaneous recovery (mortality rate >1%).
- *Amanita* and *Gyromitra* intoxication begins with symptoms of gastroenteritis (nausea, vomiting, diarrhea, and abdominal cramps) approximately 10 hr after ingestion. *Amanita* then causes cardiomyopathy and hepatic and renal failure. *Gyromitra* produces jaundice and seizures. Both mushrooms are associated with a 50% mortality rate.
- *Omphalotus* causes symptoms of gastroenteritis that subside spontaneously within 24 hr.

ETIOLOGY

- *Amanita* contains cytotoxic substances and isoxazoles that are gamma-aminobutyric acid neurotransmitter analogs. Amatoxins, consisting of alpha-, beta-, and gamma-amanitin, account for >90% of deaths related to mushroom poisoning. The amatins are heat stable and not inactivated by cooking.
- *Gyromitra* contains a pyridoxine antagonist that disrupts the gastrointestinal mucosa and causes hemolysis.
- *Russula* contains a cholinergic substance.

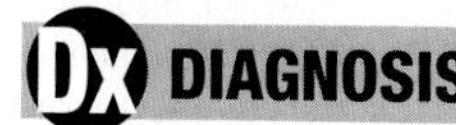

DIAGNOSIS

DIFFERENTIAL DIAGNOSIS

- Food poisoning
- Overdose of prescription or illegal drug
- Other intoxications
- See topic on specific organ failure (e.g., renal or hepatic failure) for differential diagnosis of those conditions

WORKUP

- History
- Inspection and identification of suspected mushrooms
- Mushroom or gastric content analysis (by thin-layer chromatography or radioimmunoassay)

Rx TREATMENT

- Gastric lavage.
- Repeated administration of activated charcoal.
- Penicillin G or silibinin can be used for *Amanita* mushroom intoxication. Silibinin interferes with hepatic uptake of alpha-amanitine. IV silibinin is not currently available in the U.S. Where available, it is given at a rate of 5 mg/kg IV over 1 hr, followed by 20 mg/kg/day. An oral form of silibinin is available in health food stores as an extract from milk thistle called silymarin. Dose is 1 g PO qid. IV benzyl penicillin reduces hepatocyte uptake of amatoxin.
- Supportive care as needed (may require respiratory assistance, hemodialysis, or emergency liver transplantation) in the event of irreversible fulminant liver failure.
- In patients with severe *Amanita* poisoning, early contact with the nearest liver transplant center is recommended.

SUGGESTED READING

Available at ExpertConsult.com

RELATED CONTENT

Mushroom Poisoning (Patient Information)

AUTHOR: **FRED F. FERRI, M.D.**

TABLE 2 Mushroom Poisoning Syndromes

Syndrome	Commonly Implicated Mushrooms	Toxins
Short Incubation		
Delirium, restlessness	*Amanita muscaria, Amanita pantherina*	Ibotenic acid, muscimol
Parasympathetic hyperactivity	*Inocybe* spp., *Clitocybe* spp., *Boletus* spp.	Muscarine
Hallucinations, somnolence, dysphoria	*Psilocybe* spp., *Panaeolus* spp., *Conocybe* spp.	Psilocybin
Disulfiram reaction	*Coprinus atramentarius*	Coprine
Gastroenteritis	Many	Various uncharacterized irritants
Long Incubation		
Gastroenteritis, hepatorenal failure	*Amanita phalloides, Amanita virosa,* and other *Amanita; Galerina, Cortinarius,* and *Lepiota* spp.	Cyclopeptides (i.e., amatoxins, phallotoxins)
Gastroenteritis, muscle cramping, hepatic failure, hemolysis, seizures, coma	*Gyromitra* spp.	Gyromitrin
Gastroenteritis, acute renal failure (temporary)	*Amanita smithiana*	Allenic norleucine
Gastroenteritis, acute renal failure (often irreversible)	*Cortinarius* spp.	Orellanine

From Bennett JE et al: *Mandell, Douglas, and Bennett's principles and practice of infectious diseases*, ed 8, Philadelphia, 2015, WB Saunders.

BASIC INFORMATION

DEFINITION

Myasthenia gravis (MG) is an autoimmune disorder affecting postsynaptic neuromuscular transmission, most commonly mediated by antibodies directed against the nicotinic acetylcholine receptor (AChR) of the neuromuscular junction. Anti-AChR antibodies cause a decrease in functional postsynaptic ACh receptors, resulting in fatigable weakness. A small percentage of MG patients lack AChR antibodies, and a subset of these patients possess antibodies against muscle-specific tyrosine kinase (MuSK), impacting both pre- and postsynaptic function of the neuromuscular junction.

SYNONYM

MG

ICD-10CM CODES

G70.00	Myasthenia gravis without (acute) exacerbation
G70.01	Myasthenia gravis with (acute) exacerbation
P94.0	Transient neonatal myasthenia gravis

EPIDEMIOLOGY & DEMOGRAPHICS

INCIDENCE (IN U.S.): 8 to 10 cases annually per 1 million persons. It is the most common disorder of neuromuscular junction transmission.

PEAK INCIDENCE: Female, second to third decades; male, sixth to eighth decades

PREVALENCE (IN U.S.): 150 to 250 cases per 1 million

PREDOMINANT SEX: Females are affected more often than males (3:2) in adults; they are equally affected in the elderly.

GENETICS: Increased frequency of HLA-B8, DR3

PHYSICAL FINDINGS & CLINICAL PRESENTATION

- The hallmark of MG is weakness worsened with exercise and improved with rest.
- Generalized weakness involving proximal muscles, diaphragm, and neck extensors is common.
- Weakness is confined to eyelids and extraocular muscles in approximately 15% of patients (Fig. 1).
- Bulbar symptoms of ptosis, diplopia, dysarthria, and dysphagia are common.
- Reflexes, sensation, and coordination are normal.

ETIOLOGY

Antibody-mediated decrease in nicotinic AChR in the postsynaptic neuromuscular junction resulting in defective neuromuscular transmission and subsequent muscle weakness and fatigue. Early-onset MG is associated with *HLA-DR3, HLA-B8,* and non-*HLA* genes. Late-onset MG is associated with *HLA-DR2, HLA-B27,* and *HLA-DRB1.* MuSK antibodies have been recognized since 2001 and present with a similar syndrome to AchR MG although they may have more bulbar weakness, proximal muscle atrophy, and either lack of or paradoxical response to pyridostigmine.

Dx DIAGNOSIS

DIFFERENTIAL DIAGNOSIS

Lambert-Eaton myasthenic syndrome, botulism, medication-induced myasthenia, chronic progressive external ophthalmoplegia, congenital myasthenic syndromes, thyroid disease, basilar meningitis, intracranial mass lesion with cranial neuropathy, Miller-Fisher variant of Guillain-Barré syndrome

WORKUP

- Edrophonium (Tensilon) test (Fig. 2): Useful in MG patients with ocular symptoms. Cardiac monitoring and atropine ready at the bedside are essential. Patients with MG may also have a positive ice pack test (Fig. E3).
- Repetitive nerve stimulation: Successive stimulation shows decrement of muscle action potential in clinically weak muscle; may be negative in up to 50%.
- Single-fiber electromyography: Highly sensitive; abnormal in up to 95% of patients.
- Serum AChR antibodies found in up to 90% of patients.
- A subset of patients with seronegative MG may have MuSK antibodies.

ADDITIONAL TESTS

- Forced vital capacity (FVC) is the most useful test for assessing neuromuscular respiratory status. Patients with an FVC of <20 ml/kg are at high risk of respiratory failure and should be monitored in an ICU setting. Although the decision of when to intubate is a clinical one, FVC falling below 10 to 15 ml/kg generally requires intubation.
- CT scan with contrast of anterior chest to look for thymoma or residual thymic tissue. 10% of patients with MG have a thymoma and the prevalence increases with age.
- Thyroid-stimulating hormone, free T_4 to rule out thyroid disease.

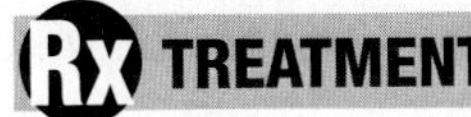

TREATMENT

NONPHARMACOLOGIC THERAPY

- Patient education to facilitate recognition of worsening symptoms and impress need for medical evaluation at onset of clinical deterioration
- Avoidance of selected drugs (Box 1) known to provoke exacerbations of MG (beta-blockers, aminoglycoside and quinolone antibiotics, penicillamine, interferons, class I antiarrhythmics [procainamide, quinidine, etc.])
- Prompt treatment of infections, diet modification, and speech evaluation with dysphagia

ACUTE GENERAL Rx

- Symptomatic treatment with acetylcholinesterase inhibitors:
  1. Pyridostigmine 30 to 60 mg PO q4 to 6h initially; onset of effects is 30 min, duration 4 hr. May be titrated up to 120 mg every 4 hr. GI upset is not uncommon with higher doses and may respond to hyoscyamine.
- Immunosuppressive treatment with corticosteroids and azathioprine is first line treatment:
  1. Prednisone initiated at 10 to 20 mg qd titrated by 5-mg increments to effect or dose of 1 mg/kg/day with improvement in 2 to 4 wk and maximal response by 3 to 6 mo.
  2. Azathioprine initiated at 50 mg qd titrated to 2 to 3 mg/kg/day with clinical effect in 6 to 12 mo. Azathioprine is not recommended in patients with no thiopurine methyltransferase activity.

BOX 1 Drugs That May Increase Weakness in Myasthenia Gravis

Neuromuscular-blocking agents
Selected antibiotics
- Aminoglycosides, particularly gentamycin
- Macrolides, particularly erythromycin and azithromycin

Selected cardiovascular agents
- Beta-blockers
- Calcium channel blockers
- Procainamide

Quinidine
Quinine
Corticosteroids
Magnesium salts
- Antacids, laxatives, intravenous tocolytics

Iodinated contrast agents
D-Penicillamine

From Vincent JL et al: *Textbook of critical care*, ed 7, Philadelphia, 2017, Elsevier.

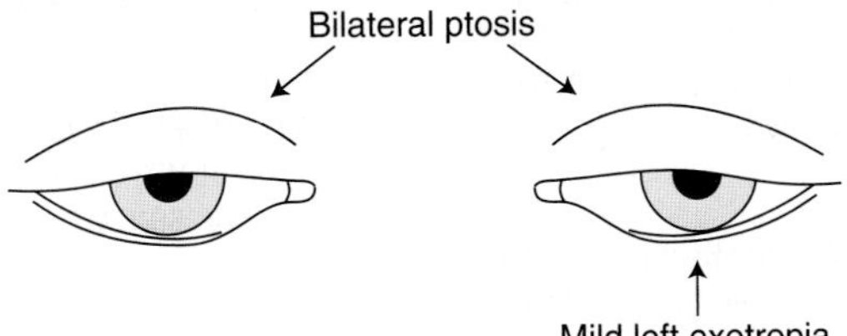

FIG. 1 Myasthenia gravis. Myasthenia gravis may mimic any ocular disorder causing diplopia, although most often it mimics weakness of the superior rectus muscle or medial rectus muscle (i.e., difficulty with sustained elevation or adduction of the eye, respectively). Clues to the diagnosis of myasthenia gravis are associated ptosis, fluctuating course, and normal pupils. (From McGee S: *Evidence-based physical diagnosis*, ed 4, Philadelphia, 2018, Elsevier.)

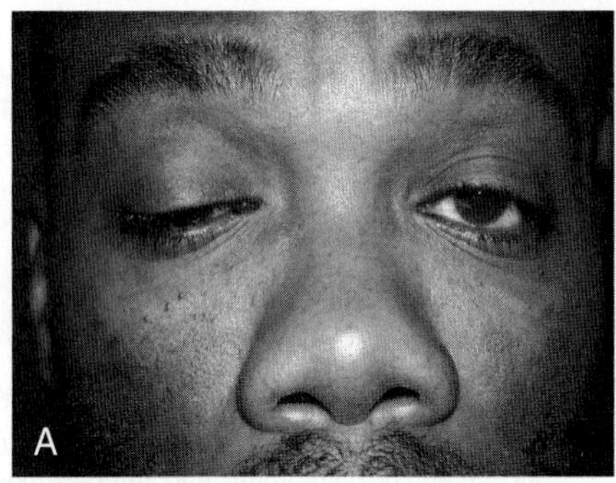

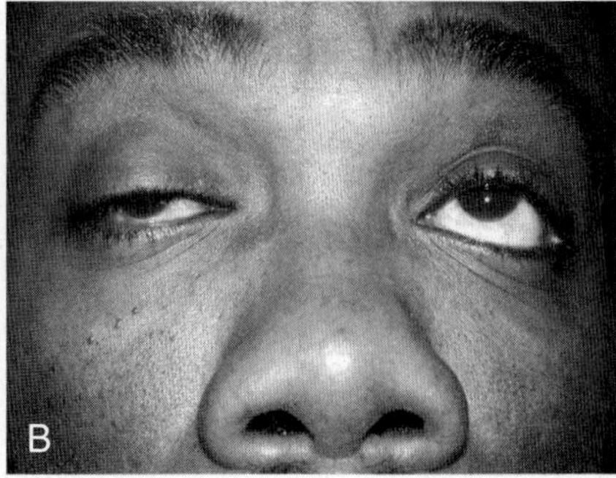

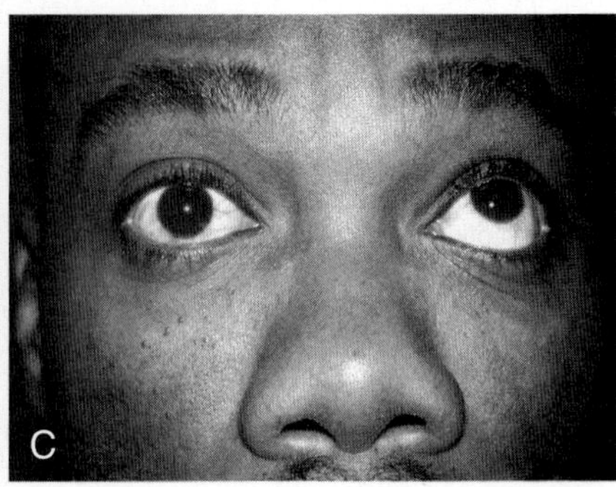

FIG. 2 Positive edrophonium test in myasthenia gravis. A, Asymmetric ptosis in the primary position. **B,** Defective upgaze. **C,** Following injection of edrophonium, there is marked bilateral improvement of ptosis and modest improvement of left upgaze. (From Kanski JJ et al: *Clinical ophthalmology: a systematic approach,* ed 7, Philadelphia, 2010, Saunders.)

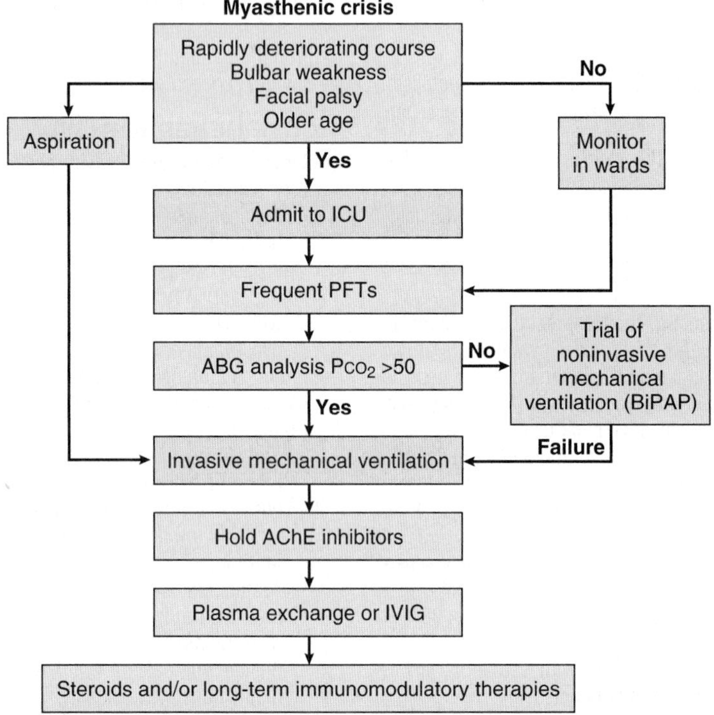

FIG. 4 Clinical flowchart for the management of myasthenic crisis. *ABG,* Arterial blood gas; *AChE,* acetyl cholinesterase; *BiPAP,* bilevel positive airway pressure; *ICU,* intensive care unit; *IVIG,* intravenous immunoglobulin; *PFTs,* pulmonary function tests. (From Parrillo JE, Dellinger RP: *Critical care medicine, principles of diagnosis and management in the adult,* ed 4, Philadelphia, 2014, Elsevier.)

- Alternative secondary agents:
  1. Eculizumab, a first-in-class compliment inhibitor, is FDA-approved for adult patients who are acetylcholine-antibody positive and continue to suffer from severe symptoms despite current immunotherapy use.
  2. Cyclosporine initiated at 5 mg/kg/day with clinical effect within 1 to 2 mo.
  3. Mycophenolate mofetil 500 mg twice a day titrated to 2 g/day with clinical effect in 3 to 6 mo, but can be up to 12 mo.
  4. Rituximab.
- Plasmapheresis and IV immunoglobulin are short-term options for immunotherapy during an exacerbation. There is no significant difference in efficacy between IVIG and plasmapheresis.
- Mechanical ventilation is lifesaving in setting of a myasthenic crisis. Consider elective intubation if forced vital capacity <10 to 15 ml/kg.
- Fig. 4 illustrates a flowchart for the management of myasthenic crisis.

SURGICAL Rx

- In thymomatous MG, thymectomy is indicated in all patients. If the tumor cannot be surgically resected, chemotherapy can be considered for prevention of local invasion and symptom relief.
- For nonthymomatous autoimmune MG, thymectomy may improve clinical outcomes and reduce the need for steroids over a 3-yr period. Surgical referral should be considered in patients under 60 without significant medical comorbidities.
- MUSK myasthenia is not associated with thymic pathology.

DISPOSITION

Course of disease is highly variable. Mortality rate has decreased from 75% to 4.5% over the past four decades.

REFERRAL

Referral to a general neurologist or neuromuscular specialist is appropriate.
Surgical referral for thymectomy in selected cases (see "Surgical Rx")

PEARLS & CONSIDERATIONS

- Sustained upward or lateral gaze and arm abduction for 120 sec may be necessary to elicit subtle signs on examination.
- Myasthenic patients can worsen rapidly and warrant careful observation during an exacerbation or when ill.

SUGGESTED READINGS

Available at ExpertConsult.com

RELATED CONTENT

Myasthenia Gravis (Patient Information)

AUTHORS: **RADHIKA SAMPAT, D.O., COREY GOLDSMITH, M.D.,** and **TAYLOR HARRISON, M.D.**

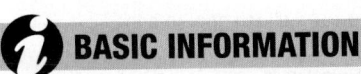

BASIC INFORMATION

DEFINITION

Myelodysplastic syndromes (MDS) are a group of acquired clonal disorders affecting hematopoietic stem cells and are characterized by altered differentiation and proliferation. Patients present with peripheral blood cytopenias and morphologic abnormalities but have a hypercellular bone marrow upon examination. The increased marrow cellularity reflects ineffective hematopoiesis with inadequate maturation resulting in cytopenias.

CLASSIFICATION

- In 1982, the French-American-British (FAB) classification included refractory anemia (RA), refractory anemia with ringed sideroblasts (RARS), refractory anemia with excess blasts (RAEB), chronic myelomonocytic leukemia (CMML), and refractory anemia with excess blasts in transformation (RAEB-T).
- In 1999, the World Health Organization (WHO) modified the FAB by incorporating newer morphologic insights and cytogenetic findings. It reduced the blast percentage for the diagnosis of acute myeloid leukemia (AML) to 20%, added refractory cytopenia with multilineage dysplasia (RCMD), refined refractory anemia with excessive blasts into types 1 and 2 (RAEB-1, RAEB-2), and added unclassified MDS, and MDS associated with isolated del(5q).
- In 2008, the WHO further modified the classification by subcategorizing MDS into six different categories. (Table 1).

SYNONYMS

MDS
Preleukemia

ICD-10CM CODES

D46.9 Myelodysplastic syndrome, unspecified
D46.C Myelodysplastic syndrome with isolated del(5q) chromosomal abnormality
D46.Z Other myelodysplastic syndromes

EPIDEMIOLOGY & DEMOGRAPHICS

INCIDENCE (IN U.S.): Approximately five new cases/100,000 persons per yr. An estimated 30,000 new cases are diagnosed annually in the U.S.

PREDOMINANT AGE: More common in elderly patients; median age >65 yr

PHYSICAL FINDINGS & CLINICAL PRESENTATION

- Patients often present with fatigue due to anemia and also with thrombocytopenia and leukopenia.
- Skin pallor, mucosal bleeding, and ecchymosis may be present.
- Fever, infection, and dyspnea are common.

ETIOLOGY

Exposure to radiation, chemotherapeutic agents, benzene, or other organic compounds is associated with myelodysplasia. Table 2 describes predisposing factors and epidemiologic associations of patients with MDS. Up to 40 genes that affect specific functional pathways are mutated in MDS, with 90% of patients having at least one mutation and a median of two to three mutations detected per patient. The most common mutations occur in genes involved in RNA splicing (*SF3B1, SRSF2, U2AF1,* and *ZRSR2*), epigenetic modification (*TET2, ASXL1,* and *DNMT3A*), regulators of signal transduction (*NRAS* and *JAK2*), and transcription factors (*RUNX1* and *TP53*).

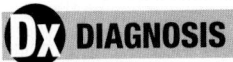

DIAGNOSIS

DIFFERENTIAL DIAGNOSIS

- Hereditary dysplasias (e.g., Fanconi anemia, Diamond-Blackfan syndrome)
- Vitamin B_{12}/folate deficiency
- Exposure to toxins (drugs, alcohol, chemotherapy)
- Renal failure
- Irradiation
- Autoimmune disease
- Paroxysmal nocturnal hemoglobinuria

TABLE 1 2008 World Health Organization Classification of the Adult Myelodysplastic Syndromes

Refractory Cytopenia with Unilineage Dysplasia	
Dysplasia	≥10% of cells from a single lineage
Blasts	<5% in marrow; <1% in peripheral blood; no Auer rods
Notes	Includes refractory anemia (RA), refractory neutropenia, refractory thrombocytopenia; RA is by far the most common subtype
Refractory Anemia with Ring Sideroblasts	
Dysplasia	Isolated erythroid dysplasia
Blasts	<5% in marrow; <1% in peripheral blood; no Auer rods
Notes	≥15% of erythroid precursors are ring sideroblasts
	Frequently associated with SF3B1 mutations
MDS with Isolated del(5q)	
Dysplasia	Normal or increased megakaryocytes with hypolobated nuclei
Blasts	<20% (though usually much less)
Notes	del(5q31) must be sole chromosomal abnormality
Refractory Cytopenia with Multilineage Dysplasia	
Dysplasia	≥10% of cells from two or more myeloid lineages
Blasts	<5% in marrow; <1% in peripheral blood; no Auer rods
Notes	Peripheral monocyte count must be $<1 \times 10^9$/L; ring sideroblasts may be present
Refractory Anemia with Excess Blasts	
Dysplasia	No specific requirement
Blasts	RAEB-1: 5%–9% in marrow, <5% in peripheral blood, AND no Auer rods
	RAEB-2: 10%–19% in marrow, 5%–19% in peripheral blood, OR Auer rods
Notes	Old designation of RAEB-t (20%–30% blasts) now considered AML
Unclassifiable MDS	
Dysplasia	Minimal, or not meeting criteria for another subtype
Blasts	<5% in marrow; <1% in peripheral blood; no Auer rods
Notes	In presence of *clonal cytogenetic finding* considered diagnostic of MDS

Note: Excludes refractory cytopenias of childhood. MDS/myeloproliferative neoplasms such as chronic myelomonocytic leukemia and RARS with thrombocytosis are classified separately.*AML*, Acute myeloid leukemia; *MDS*, myelodysplastic syndrome; *RAEB*, refractory anemia with excess blast.

From Hoffman R et al: *Hematology, basic principles and practice*, ed 7, Philadelphia, 2018, Elsevier.

TABLE 2 Predisposing Factors and Epidemiologic Associations of Patients with Myelodysplastic Syndrome

Heritable

Constitutional Genetic Disorders

Trisomy 8 mosaicism
Familial monosomy 7
Down syndrome (trisomy 21)
Neurofibromatosis 1
Germ cell tumors [embryonal dysgenesis del(12p)]

Congenital Neutropenia

Kostmann syndrome
Shwachman-Diamond syndrome

DNA Repair Deficiencies

Fanconi anemia
Ataxia-telangiectasia
Bloom syndrome
Xeroderma pigmentosum
Pharmacogenomic polymorphisms (GSTq1-null)

Acquired

Senescence

Mutagen Exposure

Alkylator therapy (chlorambucil, cyclophosphamide, melphalan, N-mustards)
Topoisomerase II inhibitors (anthracyclines)
β Emitters (32p)
Autologous stem cell transplantation
Environmental/occupational (benzene)
Tobacco
Aplastic anemia
Paroxysmal nocturnal hemoglobinuria

From Hoffman R et al: *Hematology, basic principles and practice*, ed 7, Philadelphia, 2018, Churchill Livingstone.

WORKUP

Diagnostic workup includes laboratory evaluation and bone marrow examination (Fig. E1). Cytogenetic analysis (Box E1) by conventional metaphase karyotyping or by MDS FISH assessment should be performed in patients with MDS. Genes recurrently mutated in myelodysplastic syndrome are summarized in Table 3. Physical examination, medical history, and laboratory tests aiding in diagnosis of MDS are described in Table 4. Key features of the major myelodysplastic syndromes are summarized in Table 5.

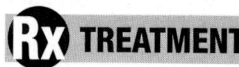

TREATMENT

NONPHARMACOLOGIC THERAPY

- Packed red blood cell transfusions in patients with severe symptomatic anemia
- Platelet transfusions in patients with severe thrombocytopenia or those with bleeding episodes

ACUTE GENERAL Rx

- The initial focus of MDS therapy involves stratification of patients into low-, intermediate-, and high-risk states using well-defined and validated risk stratification systems. The original International Prognostic Scoring System (IPSS), which incorporated cytopenias, cytogenetics, and blast percentage, is still clinically used. The revised IPSS (IPSS-R) has been created from an evaluation of more than 7000 patients and utilizes a five-tier risk grouping that accounts for the degree of cytopenias and bone marrow blast percentage and has 15 cytogenetic subtypes.
- Low-risk patients are treated with supportive care or growth factors.
- Poor-risk patients are treated with hypomethylating agents along with supportive care.
- Appropriate patients are offered allogeneic stem cell transplantation as a potentially curative option, with high-volume centers treating patients <80 yr old.
- Erythropoietin (10,000-40,000 units/week) or pegylated erythropoietin (200-500 mg every 1-3 weeks) is used in patients with symptomatic anemia. Responses with increase in hemoglobin and decreased transfusion requirements are achieved typically in patients who have serum erythropoietin levels <500 U/L and adequate iron stores.
- DNA methyltransferase inhibitors: Azacitidine, a pyrimidine nucleoside analogue of cytidine, has been shown to improve the quality of life for patients and to prolong overall survival. Decitabine, another nucleoside analogue, has also been FDA approved for patients with MDS. These agents may also be useful in preventing the transition of MDS to AML.

TABLE 3 Genes Recurrently Mutated in Myelodysplastic Syndrome

Gene	Frequency (%)	Notes
Splicing Factors		
SF3B1	20–30	Strong association with RARS
SRSF2	10–15 (MDS) 40 (CMML)	Enriched in CMML
U2AF1	5–12	Association with del(20q)
Epigenetic Modifiers		
TET2	20–30 (MDS) 40–50 (CMML)	Enriched in CMML Mutually exclusive with IDH
DNMT3A	8–13	
ASXL1	10–20 (MDS) 30–40 (CMML)	Enriched in CMML
EZH2	5–10 (MDS) 20–30 (CMML)	Enriched in CMML May be functionally involved in 7q–
IDH1/2	<5	More frequent in AML
ATRX	Rare	Associated with acquired thalassemia
Transcription Factors		
RUNX1	10–15	Can be somatic or germline
GATA2	Rare	Mostly germline
ETV6	<5	Can be somatic or germline
TP53	10–12	Association with complex karyotype, therapy-related disease
Kinases and Receptors		
JAK2	<5	Enriched in RARS-T
NRAS	5–10	Seen in progression to AML
CBL	<5	Enriched in JMML
PTPN11	<5	More common in JMML
BRAF	Rare	Also seen in hairy cell leukemia
Cohesin Complex		
STAG2	5–10	Cohesin class mutations enriched in high-risk MDS and secondary AML.
RAD21	<5	
SMC3	<2	
SMC1A	<2	
GCPR Complex		
GNAS	Rare	Mutations recently described in wide range of hematologic malignancies, including MDS.
GNB1	Rare	

AML, Acute myeloid leukemia; *CMML*, chronic myelomonocytic leukemia; *GCPR*, G-coupled protein receptor; *IDH*, isocitrate dehdryogenase; *JMML*, juvenile myelomonocytic leukemia; *MDS*, myelodysplastic syndrome; *RARS*, refractory anemia with ring sideroblasts; *RARS-T*, RARS with thrombocytosis.
From Hoffman R, et al.: *Hematology, basic principles and practice*, ed 7, Philadelphia, 2018, Elsevier.

TABLE 4 Physical Examination, Medical History, and Laboratory Tests Aiding in Diagnosis of Myelodysplastic Syndrome

Medical History
- Duration of symptoms
- History of blood disease
- History of exposure to occupational toxins or cytotoxic agents
- Medication history
- Alcohol intake
- Comorbid conditions

Physical Examination
- Pallor
- Petechiae
- Purpura
- Bruising
- Tachypnea
- Signs of infection
- Splenomegaly

Laboratory Testing
- Complete blood count with a manual differential
- Reticulocyte count
- Vitamin B_{12} and folate levels
- Consider methylmalonic acid and red blood cell folate levels
- Iron, total iron-binding capacity, and ferritin level
- Thyroid-stimulating hormone level
- Lactate dehydrogenase
- Antinuclear antibody
- Coombs test and haptoglobin
- Serum erythropoietin level
- Human leukocyte antigen (histocompatibility antigens) typing in appropriate patients
- Paroxysmal nocturnal hemoglobinuria screen

Bone Marrow Testing
- Hematopathology
- Percentage of blasts on 200 cell aspirate differential
- Presence or absence of Auer rods
- Percentage of cellularity of bone marrow biopsy
- Iron stain on aspirate (ringed sideroblasts)
- Iron stain on biopsy (storage)
- Dysplastic features (% and number of dysplastic lineages)
- Cytogenetics (karyotype of 20 metaphase cells)
- Fluorescent in situ hybridization
- Flow cytometry (not useful for quantitation)

From Hoffman R, et al.: *Hematology, basic principles and practice*, ed 7, Philadelphia, 2018, Churchill Livingstone.

- Immunomodulators: Lenalidomide, a novel analogue of thalidomide, has demonstrated hematologic activity in patients with low-rise MDS who have no response to erythropoietin or who are unlikely to benefit from conventional therapy. Lenalidomide can also reduce transfusion requirements and reverse cytologic and cytogenetic abnormalities in patients who have MDS with the 5q31 deletion.
- Results of chemotherapy are generally disappointing. Combination chemotherapy regimens (e.g., cytarabine plus doxorubicin) that are used to treat AMLs generally induce a complete response in only a minority of patients, and the average duration of response is <1 yr.
- The use of myeloid growth factors (granulocyte colony-stimulating factor [G-CSF], granulocyte-macrophage colony-stimulating factor [GM-CSF]) is reserved for patients with severe neutropenias and high infection risk. Additionally, these provide a synergistic effect when used in combination with erythropoietin in terms of improvement in the hemoglobin levels.

CHRONIC Rx

Monitor for infections, bleeding, and complications of anemia. Supportive measures include PRBC transfusions and erythropoietin for anemia and antibiotics to treat opportunistic infections. Iron overload from frequent transfusions (>100 PRBC units) requires iron chelation therapy.

DISPOSITION

- The 5-yr overall survival is approximately 30%. Median overall survival rates are best for patients with refractory anemia (56 months), refractory anemia with ring sideroblasts (48 months), and deletion 5q subtype (32 months).The International Prognostic Scoring System (IPSS) for MDS is summarized in Tables 6 and 7. Table 8 describes survival based on IPSS.
- Long-term remission rates in young patients with allogeneic stem cell transplantation approach 40% to 50%.
- The risk of transformation to AML varies with the percentage of blasts in the bone marrow.

REFERRAL

- Hematology referral for all patients
- Bone marrow transplant evaluation for stem cell transplant eligibility as a potentially curative modality

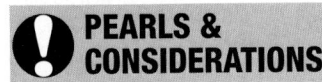

PEARLS & CONSIDERATIONS

COMMENTS

- Somatic point mutations in *TP53, EZH2, ETV6, RUNX1,* and *ASXL1* are predictors of poor overall survival in patients with MDS independent of established risk factors. Patients with cytogenetic abnormalities associated

TABLE 5 Diagnostic Criteria for Myelodysplastic Syndrome

A. Presence of at Least One Unexplained Cytopenia for at Least 6 Months[a]

Hemoglobin <11 g/dl, *or*

Absolute neutrophil count $<1.5 \times 10^9$/L, *or*

Platelet count $<100 \times 10^9$/L

***plus* B. Presence of One or More MDS-Qualifying Criteria:**

>10% dysplasia in one or more hematopoietic lineage, *or*

5%–19% blasts in bone marrow, *or*

MDS-defining cytogenetic abnormality, such as:

t(1;3)(p36.3;q21.1)	t(2;11)(p21;q23)	inv(3)(q21;q26.2)
t(3;21)(q26.2;q22.1)	−5 or del(5q)	t(6;9)(p23;q34)
−7 or del(7q)		del(9q)
del(11q)	t(11;16)(q23;p13.3)	del(12p) or t(12p)
−13 or del(13q)	i(17q) or del(17p)	idic(X)(q13)

***plus* C. Exclusion of Alternative Diagnoses**

AML (i.e., <20% blasts, and no t(8;21), inv(16), t(16;16), t(15;17), or erythroleukemia) or *ALL*

Other hematologic diseases (aplastic anemia, PNH, LGL, lymphoma, myelofibrosis and other MPN)

Viral infections (HIV, EBV, parvovirus)

Nutritional deficiencies (iron, copper, B_{12}, folate)

Medications (methotrexate, azathioprine, isoniazid, cytotoxic chemotherapy)

Alcohol or other toxins

Autoimmune diseases (SLE, Felty syndrome, ITP, autoimmune hemolytic anemia)

Congenital disorders (Diamond-Blackfan anemia, Shwachman-Diamond syndrome, Fanconi anemia, and others)

ALL, Acute lymphoblastic leukemia; *AML*, acute myeloid leukemia; *EBV*, Epstein-Barr virus; *HIV*, human immunodeficiency virus; *ITP*, immune thrombocytopenic purpura; *LGL*, large granular lymphocyte leukemia; *MDS*, myelodysplastic syndrome; *MPN*, myeloproliferative neoplasm; *PNH*, paroxysmal nocturnal hemoglobinuria; *SLE*, systemic lupus erythematosus.

[a]Diagnosis can be made earlier than 6 months if no other cause is apparent for cytopenias, or there are excess blasts or an MDS-defining cytogenetic abnormality

From Hoffman R, et al.: *Hematology, basic principles and practice*, ed 7, Philadelphia, 2018, Elsevier.

TABLE 6 1997 International Prognostic Scoring System for Myelodysplastic Syndromes (IPSS)

	Score			
Variable	**0**	**0.5**	**1**	**1.5**
Marrow blasts (%)	<5	5–10	–	11–20
Karyotype	Good	Intermediate	Poor	–
Cytopenias	0–1	2–3	–	–

From Hoffman R, et al.: *Hematology, basic principles and practice*, ed 7, Philadelphia, 2018, Elsevier.

TABLE 7 2012 Revised International Prognostic Scoring System for Myelodysplastic Syndrome (IPSS-R)

Cytogenetic Risk	Included Karyotypic Abnormalities
Very good	del(11q), −Y
Good	Normal, del(20q), del(5q) alone or +1 other abnormality, del(12p)
Intermediate	+8, del(7q), i(17q), +19, +21 Any other single or double abnormality Two or more independent clones
Poor	der(3q), −7, double with del(7q), complex with exactly 3 abnormalities
Very poor	Complex with >3 abnormalities

Scoring Table

Parameter	***Category/Score***				
Cytogenetic risk	**Very good** 0	**Good** 1	**Intermediate** 2	**Poor** 3	**Very poor** 4
Marrow blasts (%)	≤2 0	3–4 1	5–10 2	>10 3	
Hemoglobin (g/dl)	≥10 0	8–9.9 1	<8 1.5		
Platelet count (× 10^9/L)	≥100 0	50–99 0.5	<50 1		
Neutrophil count (× 10^9/L)	≥0.8 0	<0.8 0.5			

IPSS-R Risk Group	Total Score	% of Patients	Median Survival (Years)	25% With AML (Years)
Very low	≤1.5	19	8.8	NR
Low	2–3	38	5.3	10.8
Intermediate	3.5–4.5	20	3	3.2
High	5–6	13	1.6	1.4
Very high	>6	10	0.8	0.73

AML, Acute myeloid leukemia; *NR,* not reached.
From Hoffman R, et al.: *Hematology, basic principles and practice,* ed 7, Philadelphia, 2018, Elsevier.

TABLE 8 Survival Based on International Prognostic Scoring System for Myelodysplastic Syndromes (Percent)

IPSS Risk Group	# Patients	2 Years	5 Years	10 Years	15 Years
Low	267 (33%)	85	55	28	20
Intermediate-1	314 (38%	70	35	17	12
Intermediate-2	179 (22%)	30	8	0	–
High	56 (7%)	5	0	–	–

From Hoffman R, et al.: *Hematology, basic principles and practice,* ed 7, Philadelphia, 2018, Elsevier.

with poor prognosis should be considered for allogeneic stem cell transplantation.

- Many younger patients who respond to immunosuppressive therapy with drugs such as antithymocyte globulin and cyclosporine have clonal expansions of cytotoxic CD8+ T cells that suppress normal hematopoiesis, as well as expansion of CD4+ helper T-cell subsets that promote and sustain autoimmunity.
- Nearly 50% of the deaths that result from MDS are the result of cytopenias associated with bone marrow failure.

SUGGESTED READINGS

Available at ExpertConsult.com

RELATED CONTENT

Myelodysplastic Syndrome (Patient Information)

AUTHOR: **RITESH RATHORE, M.D.**

BASIC INFORMATION

DEFINITION

Myocardial infarction (MI) is a clinical syndrome characterized by symptoms of myocardial ischemia, persistent electrocardiographic (ECG) changes, and release of biomarkers of myocardial necrosis resulting from an insufficient supply of oxygenated blood to an area of the heart. MI may be classified as ST-segment elevation MI (STEMI) and non–ST-segment elevation MI (NSTEMI) depending on the ECG findings on MI presentation. Acute coronary syndrome (ACS) refers to acute myocardial ischemia without myocardial necrosis (unstable angina) or myocardial infarction (NSTEMI or STEMI). According to the European Society of Cardiology/American College of Cardiology guidelines, the following criteria for acute evolving or recent MI (NSTEMI and STEMI) satisfies the diagnosis:

- Detection of the rise and/or fall of cardiac biomarker values (preferably cardiac troponin [cTn]) with at least one value above the 99th percentile upper reference limit and with at least one of the following:
  1. Symptoms of ischemia
  2. Development of pathologic Q waves in the ECG
  3. Imaging evidence of new loss of viable myocardium or a new regional wall motion abnormality
  4. Identification of an intracoronary thrombus by angiography or autopsy pathologic findings of acute MI
  5. Electrocardiogram criteria:
     a. STEMI:
        (1) New, or presumed new, significant ST-T changes or new left bundle branch block (LBBB)
        (2) New ST elevation at the J-point in at least 2 contiguous leads of ≥2 mm (0.2 mV) in men or ≥1.5 mm (0.15 mV) in women in leads V2 to V3 and/or of ≥1 mm (0.1 mV) in another contiguous chest leads or the upper limb leads
     b. NSTEMI:
        (1) New ST-segment depression ≥0.5 mV (0.5 mm) and T-wave abnormalities

New generation troponin assays are extremely sensitive to small changes in serum troponin levels at the cost of diagnostic specificity for MI related to plaque rupture or erosion.

Universal classification of acute MI:

- Type 1: Spontaneous MI related to ischemia due to a primary coronary event such as plaque erosion and/or rupture, fissuring, or dissection.
- Type 2: MI secondary to ischemia, other than coronary artery disease, due to either increased oxygen demand or decreased supply (e.g., coronary endothelial dysfunction, coronary artery spasm, coronary embolism, anemia, arrhythmias, respiratory failure, hypertension with/without left ventricular hypertrophy (LVH), or hypotension). Also in critically ill patients or in patients undergoing major noncardiac surgery, elevated values of cardiac biomarkers may appear due to the direct toxic effects of endogenous or exogenous high circulating catecholamine levels.
- Type 3: Sudden unexpected cardiac death, including cardiac arrest, often with symptoms suggestive of myocardial ischemia, accompanied by presumed new ST elevation, new left bundle branch block, or evidence of fresh thrombus in a coronary artery by angiography and/or at autopsy, or death occurring before blood samples could be obtained or at a time before the appearance of cardiac biomarkers in the blood.
- Type 4a: MI associated with percutaneous coronary intervention. Elevation of cTN >5× percentile of upper reference limit (URL) in patients with normal baseline value, or a rise of cTN >20% if the baseline values are stable and are stable or falling. In addition to either symptoms of ischemia, new ischemic ECG changes or new LBBB, or angiographic loss of a patent coronary artery, persistent slow or no-flow, or embolization, or imaging of new wall motion abnormality.
- Type 4b: MI associated with stent thrombosis as documented by angiography or at autopsy in the setting of myocardial ischemia and with a rise/fall of cardiac biomarker values.
- Type 5: MI associated with coronary artery bypass grafting. Elevation of cardiac biomarker values >10× 99% URL in patients with normal baseline cTn values, in addition to either new pathological Q waves or new LBBB, or new native coronary artery occlusion or imaging of new abnormal wall motion abnormality.

SYNONYMS

MI
Myocardial infarction
ST-elevation MI
Heart attack
Acute myocardial infarction
AMI
Coronary thrombosis
Coronary occlusion

ICD-10CM CODES

I21.01	ST elevation (STEMI) myocardial infarction involving left main coronary artery
I21.02	ST elevation (STEMI) myocardial infarction involving left anterior descending coronary artery
I21.09	ST elevation (STEMI) myocardial infarction involving other coronary artery of anterior wall
I21.11	ST elevation (STEMI) myocardial infarction involving right coronary artery
I21.19	ST elevation (STEMI) myocardial infarction involving another coronary artery of inferior wall
I21.21	ST elevation (STEMI) myocardial infarction involving left circumflex coronary artery
I21.29	ST elevation (STEMI) myocardial infarction involving other sites
I21.3	ST elevation (STEMI) myocardial infarction of unspecified site
I21.4	Non-ST elevation (NSTEMI) myocardial infarction
I22.0	Subsequent ST elevation (STEMI) myocardial infarction of anterior wall
I22.1	Subsequent ST elevation (STEMI) myocardial infarction of inferior wall
I22.2	Subsequent non-ST elevation (NSTEMI) myocardial infarction
I22.8	Subsequent ST elevation (STEMI) myocardial infarction of other sites
I22.9	Subsequent ST elevation (STEMI) myocardial infarction of unspecified site

EPIDEMIOLOGY & DEMOGRAPHICS

INCIDENCE/PREVALENCE (IN U.S.):

- According to data from National Health and Nutrition Examination Survey (NHANES) 2009 to 2012 (National Heart, Lung, and Blood Institute [NHLBI] tabulation), the overall prevalence for MI is 2.8% in U.S. adults ≥20 years of age. MI prevalence is 4.0% for men and 1.8% for women.
- In 2013 in the U.S., coronary heart disease alone caused ≈1 of every 7 deaths. In 2013, 370,213 Americans died of coronary heart disease. Each year, an estimated 660,000 Americans have a new coronary attack (defined as first hospitalized myocardial infarction or coronary heart disease death), and 305,000 have a recurrent attack. It is estimated that an additional 160,000 silent myocardial infarctions occur each year. Approximately every 34 seconds, one American has a coronary event, and approximately every 1 minute 24 seconds, an American will die of one.
- Community incidence rates as well as mortality rates from STEMI have declined over the past decade, whereas those for NSTEMI have increased. At present, STEMI comprises approximately 30% to 40% of MI presentations. In-hospital mortality (approximately 5% to 6%) and 1-year mortality (approximately 7% to 18%). The most common cause of death in adults over the age of 40 is myocardial infarction. A heart attack takes the life of >1,500,000 people each year in the United States.
- Modifiable risk factors such as hypertension, diabetes, and cigarette smoking have recently declined, although hyperlipidemia has shown no significant change, and obesity has steadily increased.
- Tobacco use remains the second-leading cause of total deaths and disability. The percentage of adults who reported current cigarette use declined from 24.1% in 1998 to 15.5% in 2016. Still, almost one-third of coronary heart disease deaths are attributable to smoking and exposure to secondhand smoke. Patients with first acute MI were found to have an almost threefold increase in cigarette smoking from 2002 to 2009. Cigarette smoking is associated with endothelial dysfunction, prothrombotic defects, and increased oxidative stress.
- It is more prevalent in males between the ages of 45 and 65 years old; there is no predominant sex differential after the age of 65.

- Women comprised 30% of STEMI patients. They experience more lethal and severe first acute MIs than men regardless of comorbidity, previous angina, or age. Studies have suggested that women are less likely to receive reperfusion therapy, have longer reperfusion times, are often given the standard of care treatment within 24 hours of presentation, and have higher risk of bleeding with antithrombotic therapy.
- At least one fourth of all MIs are clinically unrecognized. Approximately 23% of patients with STEMI in the U.S. have diabetes mellitus, and three quarters of all deaths among patients with diabetes mellitus are related to coronary artery disease. Diabetes mellitus is associated with higher short- and long-term mortality after STEMI. In the CRUSADE (Can Rapid risk stratification of Unstable angina patients Suppress ADverse outcomes with Early implementation of the ACC/AHA guidelines) trial, 7% of eligible patients did not receive reperfusion therapy. The most important factor for not providing reperfusion therapy in eligible patients was increasing age.

PHYSICAL FINDINGS & CLINICAL PRESENTATION

The clinical presentation of myocardial infarction is usually based on a history of substernal pressure type chest pain radiated to the neck, lower jaw, left arm, or mid-back lasting 20 min or more that is not completely relieved by sublingual nitroglycerin. The pain may not be severe. Some patients may present with atypical symptoms such as nausea/vomiting, shortness of breath, fatigue, palpitations, and diaphoresis. The elderly in particular may present with dizziness, or syncope. The patients who tend to present with atypical symptoms are more likely to be women, diabetic patients, or elderly patients and less frequently receive reperfusion therapy and other evidence-based therapies than patients with a typical chest pain presentation. Records show that up to 30% of patients with STEMI present with atypical symptoms.

Physical findings:

- Skin may be diaphoretic and exhibit pallor (because of decreased oxygen).
- Rales may be present at the bases of lungs (indicative of heart failure [HF]).
- Cardiac auscultation may reveal an apical systolic murmur caused by mitral regurgitation from papillary muscle dysfunction; S_3 or S_4 may also be present.
- Up to 10% of patients may present with acute pulmonary edema and/or cardiogenic shock.
- Physical examination may be completely normal.

ETIOLOGY

- Coronary atherosclerosis and plaque rupture
- Coronary artery spasm
- Coronary embolism (caused by infective endocarditis, rheumatic heart disease, intracavitary thrombus, atrial fibrillation)
- Periarteritis and other coronary artery inflammatory diseases
- Dissection into coronary arteries (aneurysmal or iatrogenic or spontaneous)
- Anomalous origin of coronary artery especially interarterial (aorta and pulmonary artery) course of coronary artery
- MI with normal coronaries: More frequent in younger patients and cocaine addicts. The risk of acute MI is increased by a factor of 24 during the 60 min after the use of cocaine in persons who are otherwise at relatively low risk. Most patients with cocaine-related MI are young, nonwhite, male cigarette smokers without other risk factors for coronary heart disease and who have a history of repeated cocaine use. Blood and urine toxicology screen for cocaine is recommended in all young patients who present with acute MI.
- Hypercoagulable states, increased blood viscosity (polycythemia vera and autoimmune diseases such as systemic lupus, antiphospholipid syndrome)

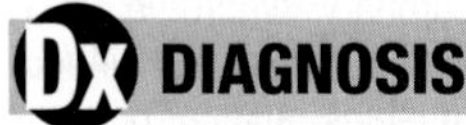

Dx DIAGNOSIS

DIFFERENTIAL DIAGNOSIS

The various causes of myocardial ischemia are described along with the differential diagnosis of chest pain.

LABORATORY TESTS

- Electrocardiogram (Fig. 1): A 12-lead ECG should be performed and shown to an experienced emergency physician within 10 min of emergency department (ED) arrival for all patients with chest discomfort (or anginal equivalent) or other symptoms suggestive of MI. Table 1 describes ECG findings in myocardial infarction. If the initial ECG is not diagnostic for MI but the patient remains symptomatic and there is a high clinical suspicion for MI, serial ECGs at 5- to 10-minute intervals or continuous 12-lead ST-segment monitoring should be performed to detect the potential development of ST deviation. In patients with inferior STEMI, right-sided ECG leads should

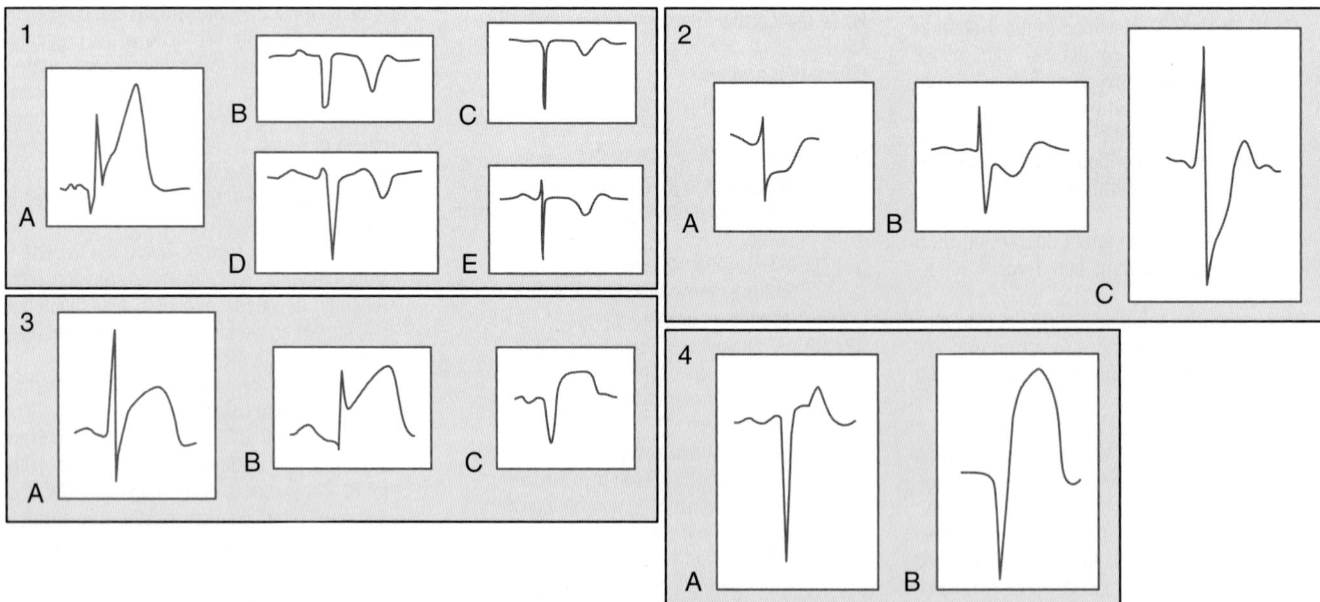

FIG. 1 Electrocardiographic findings of acute myocardial infarction (AMI). 1, T-wave abnormalities of AMI. *A,* Prominent "hyperacute" T wave. *B-E,* T-wave inversions of non-ST-segment elevation MI (NSTEMI). **2,** ST-segment depression. *A,* Flat. *B,* Downsloping. *C,* Upsloping. **3,** ST-segment elevation. *A,* Convex ST-segment elevation. *B,* Obliquely straight ST-segment elevation. *C,* Convex ST-segment elevation. **4,** Pathologic Q waves. *A,* Pathologic Q wave of completed myocardial infarction. *B,* Simultaneous ST-segment elevation with pathologic Q wave 2 hours into the course of ST-segment elevation MI (STEMI). (From Vincent JL, et al.: *Textbook of critical care,* ed 6, Philadelphia, 2011, Saunders.)

be obtained to look for ST elevation suggestive of right ventricular (RV) infarction. The joint ESC/ACCF/AHA committee for the definition of MI established the definition for the diagnosis of ST-elevation MI, which is considered to be present when there is an ST-segment elevation in two contiguous leads, ≥2 mm for men and ≥1.5 mm for women in precordial leads and/or ≥1 mm in limb leads. ST-segment elevation is measured at 0.08 sec after the J point (the junction between the end of the QRS and the beginning of the ST segment). In addition, ST depression in >2 precordial leads (V1–V4) may indicate transmural posterior injury; multilead ST depression with coexistent ST elevation in lead aVR has been described in patients with left main or proximal left anterior descending artery involvement.

- New or presumably new LBBB at presentation occurs infrequently, may interfere with ST-elevation analysis, and should not be considered diagnostic of acute myocardial infarction (MI) in isolation.
- Diagnosing new STEMI in patients with old left bundle branch block could be challenging. Sgarbossa and colleagues, emphasized that concordant 1 mm ST-segment elevation in any lead with a positive QRS deflection or discordant ST-segment elevation >5 mm in any lead with negative QRS deflection suggest STEMI.
- New ST- segment depression ≥0.5 mV (0.5 mm) and T-wave abnormalities suggests NSTEMI. ECG findings alone, without laboratory results, are sufficient to diagnose STEMI; therefore, treatment should not be delayed until biomarkers are available.
- Cardiac troponin levels: Cardiac-specific troponin T (cTnT) and cardiac-specific troponin I (cTnI) are generally indicative of myocardial injury with increases in serum levels of >99th percentile of a normal reference population. Detection of a rise and fall pattern of the measurements is essential to the diagnosis of AMI. The rise may occur relatively early after muscle damage (3 to 6 hours), peak at 12 to 16 hours, and may be present for several days after MI (up to 7 days for cTnI and more than 14 days for cTnT). Earlier peaking and rapid decline of cardiac enzymes may present in light of successful revascularization (Fig. 2). cTnT or cTnI tests can be falsely positive for myocardial infarction in patients with renal failure, heart failure, myocarditis, aortic dissection, and pulmonary embolism. Recently, highly sensitive troponin assays (hs-cTnI, hs-cTnT) have also been developed to facilitate an early diagnosis of AMI. Most patients can be diagnosed with AMI within the first 2 to 3 hours of presentation. However, an initial negative high-sensitivity troponin at the time of presentation is not sensitive enough to completely rule out AMI. MI can be excluded in most patients by 6 hours of presentation, and guidelines suggest serial samples be obtained every 3 to 6 hours after an initial sample if there is a high degree of suspicion for AMI.
- Troponin is the preferred marker for the diagnosis of myocardial necrosis. A single high-sensitivity assay for cardiac troponin (hs-CTnT) concentration below the limit of detection in combination with a nonischemic ECG may successfully rule out an MI in patients presenting to EDs with possible emergency acute coronary syndrome.[1] Because troponins need 7 to 14 days to be cleared by the kidneys, they are not sensitive enough to detect a recurrent MI within days from the initial MI. CK-MB isoenzyme can be useful in such circumstances (Fig. 2).
- CK-MB isoenzyme is also a useful marker for MI if troponin levels are not available. It is released in the circulation in amounts that correlate with the size of the infarct. An increased CK-MB value for the diagnosis of MI is defined as a measurement above the 99th percentile

TABLE 1 Leads Showing Abnormal Electrocardiographic Findings in Myocardial Infarction

	Limb Leads	Precordial Leads
Lateral	I, aVL	V5, V6
Anterior		V1, V2, V3
Anterolateral	I, aVL	V2-V6
Diaphragmatic	II, III, aVF	
Posterior		V1-V3*

*None of the leads is oriented toward the posterior surface of the heart. Therefore, in posterior infarction, changes that would have been present in the posterior surface leads will be seen in the anterior leads as a mirror image (e.g., tall and slightly wide R waves in V1 and V2, comparable to abnormal Q waves, and tall and wide, symmetric T waves in V1 and V2).
aVF, Augmented vector foot; *aVL*, augmented vector left.
From Park MK: *Park's pediatric cardiology for practitioners,* ed 6, Philadelphia, 2014, Elsevier.

[1] Pickering JW, et al.: Rapid rule-out of acute myocardial infarction with a single high-sensitivity cardiac troponin T measurement below the limit of detection: a collaborative meta-analysis, *Ann Intern Med* 166:715-724, 2017.

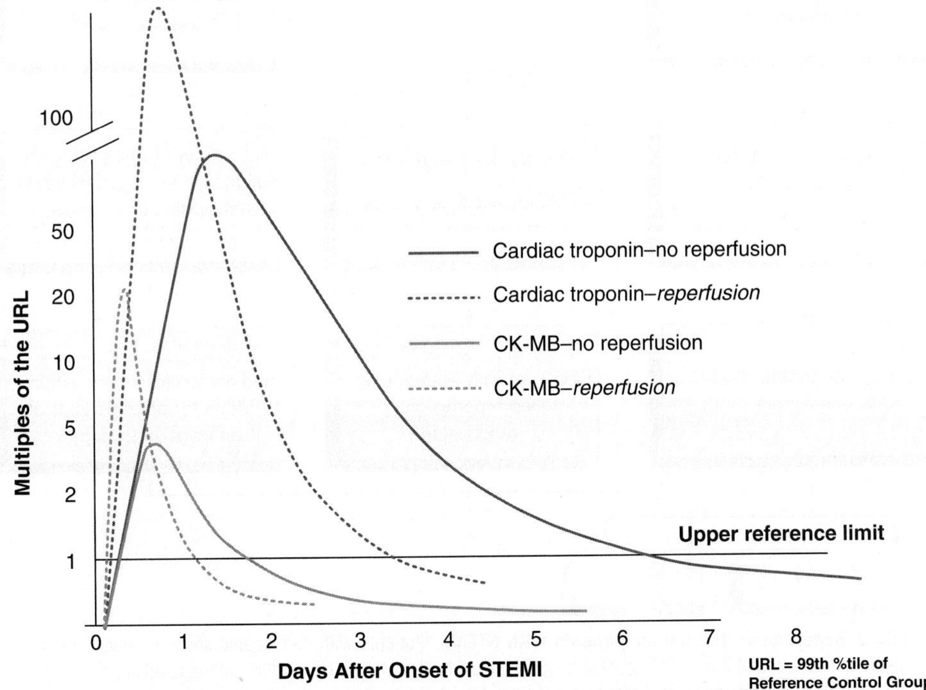

FIG. 2 Trends of Troponin and CK-MB following revascularization in MI. *CK-MB*, Creatine kinase-MB; *STEMI*, ST-segment elevation myocardial infarction; *URL*, upper reference limit. (Modified from Shapiro BP, Jaffe AS: Cardio biomarkers. In: Murphy JG, Lloyd MA (eds): *Mayo Clinic cardiology: concise textbook,* ed 3, Rochester, MN, 2007, Mayo Clinic Scientific Press, and New York, 2007, Informa Healthcare USA. Used with permission of Mayo Foundation for Medical Education and Research.)

of the upper reference limit. CK-MB can be detected within 3 to 8 hours of the onset of chest pain, peak at 12 to 24 hours, and return to baseline levels within 24 to 48 hours.

IMAGING STUDIES

Imaging studies such as a high-quality portable chest x-ray, transthoracic echocardiography, and a contrast chest CT scan should be used to differentiate MI from aortic dissection, pulmonary embolism, and other intrathoracic causes of chest pain (i.e., pneumonia and pneumothorax) in patients for whom this distinction is initially unclear, or to assess for complications of AMI such as pulmonary edema. Transthoracic echocardiography may provide evidence of focal wall motion abnormalities and facilitate triage in patients with ECG findings that are difficult to interpret.

RISK ASSESSMENT

For STEMI patients, TIMI (Thrombolysis in Myocardial Infarction) risk index, TIMI risk score (30-day outcomes), and GRACE (Global Registry of Acute Coronary Events) risk score (6-month outcomes) are commonly available risk assessment models. In the TIMI risk score for STEMI, the mean 30-day mortality was 6.7%. It is composed of eight baseline variables. The risk score showed a >40-fold graded increase in mortality, with scores ranging from 0 to >8 (P <0.0001); 30-day mortality was 0.1% among patients with a score of 0, 2.25 with a score of 5, and >8.8% among patients with a score of 8 or greater. The higher the score, the higher the 30-day mortality rate. The variables are divided between historical, exam, and presentation:

Historical:
- Age 65 to 74 (2 points), >75 (3 points),
- Diabetes/HTN or angina (1 point).

Exam:
- SBP <100 mm Hg (3 points),
- Heart rate >100 bpm (2 points),
- Killip 2 to 4 (2 points),
- Weight <67 kg (1 point).

Presentation:
- Anterior ST elevation or LBBB (1 point),
- Time to reperfusion >4 hours (1 point).

For NSTEMI patients, TIMI risk score (14-day outcomes) and GRACE (Global Registry of Acute Coronary Events) risk score (in hospital outcomes) are available.
- Age ≥65 yr.
- Presence of ≥3 risk factors for CAD.
- Known CAD (coronary artery stenosis ≥50%).
- Aspirin use in the past 7 days.
- ≥2 episodes of angina within 24 hours.
- ST changes ≥0.05 mV.
- Positive cardiac enzymes.

In TIMI score for the NSTEMI patients, each variable scores one point. The risk score of 6-7 carries estimated major acute coronary event (MACE) rate of 41% during 14 days of post-MI. Risk assessment is a continuous process that should be repeated throughout hospitalization and at time of discharge.

Rx TREATMENT

NONPHARMACOLOGIC THERAPY

- Limit patient's activity: Bed rest with bedside commode for the initial 12 to 24 hours. If the patient remains stable, gradually increase.[1]
- Diet: Nothing by mouth until stable, then clear liquids as tolerated to advance gradually to a diet tailored to the patient's comorbidities (i.e., diabetes, hypertension, heart failure, hyperlipidemia, renal failure, chronic obstructive pulmonary disease [COPD], etc.).
- Patient education to decrease the risk of subsequent cardiac events, counseling on smoking cessation, dietary restrictions, regular exercise, and medication compliance should be initiated when the patient is medically stable.

ACUTE GENERAL Rx

- Fig. 3 shows a treatment algorithm for STEMI. Assessment and treatment algorithm for

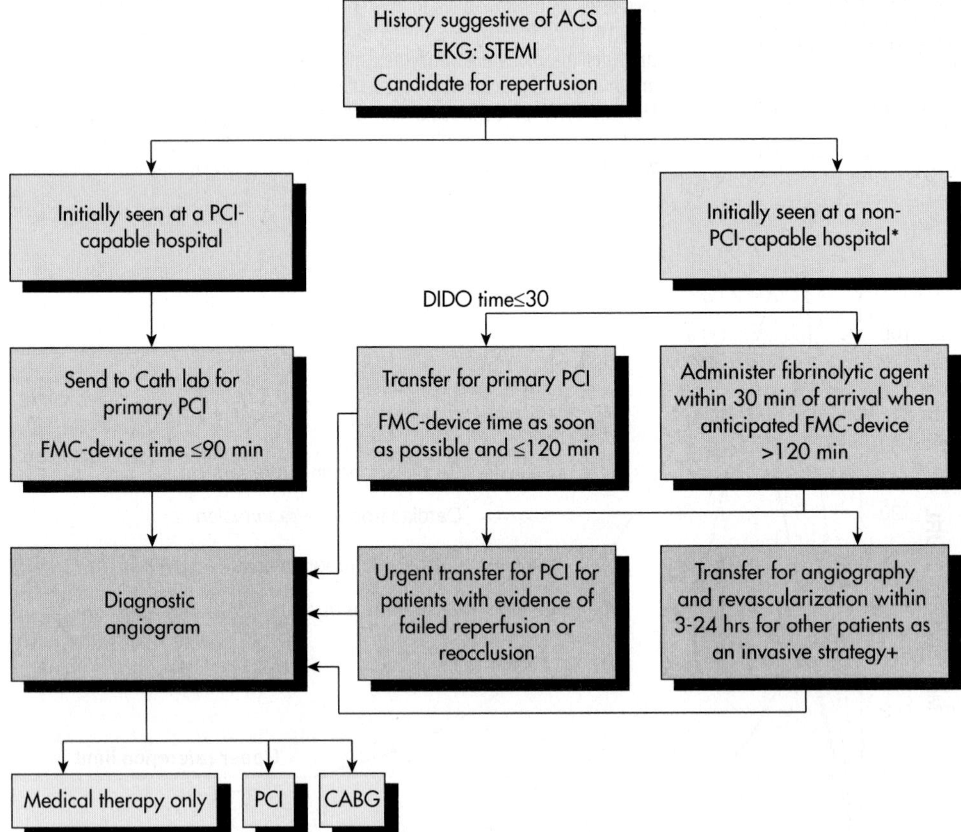

FIG. 3 Reperfusion therapy for patients with STEMI. *Patients with cardiogenic shock or severe heart failure initially seen at a non–PCI-capable hospital should be transferred for cardiac catheterization and revascularization as soon as possible, irrespective of time delay from MI onset. +Angiography and revascularization should not be performed within the first 2 to 3 hours after administration of fibrinolytic therapy. *ACS,* Acute coronary syndrome; *CABG,* coronary artery bypass graft; *Cath,* catheterization; *DIDO,* door-in to door-out; *EKG,* electrocardiogram; *FMC,* first medical contact; *MI,* myocardial infarction; *PCI,* percutaneous coronary intervention; *STEMI,* ST-elevation myocardial infarction. (Modified from O'Gara PT, et al.: 2013 ACCF/AHA guideline for the management of ST-elevation myocardial infarction, *JACC* 61(4): e78-e140, 2013.)

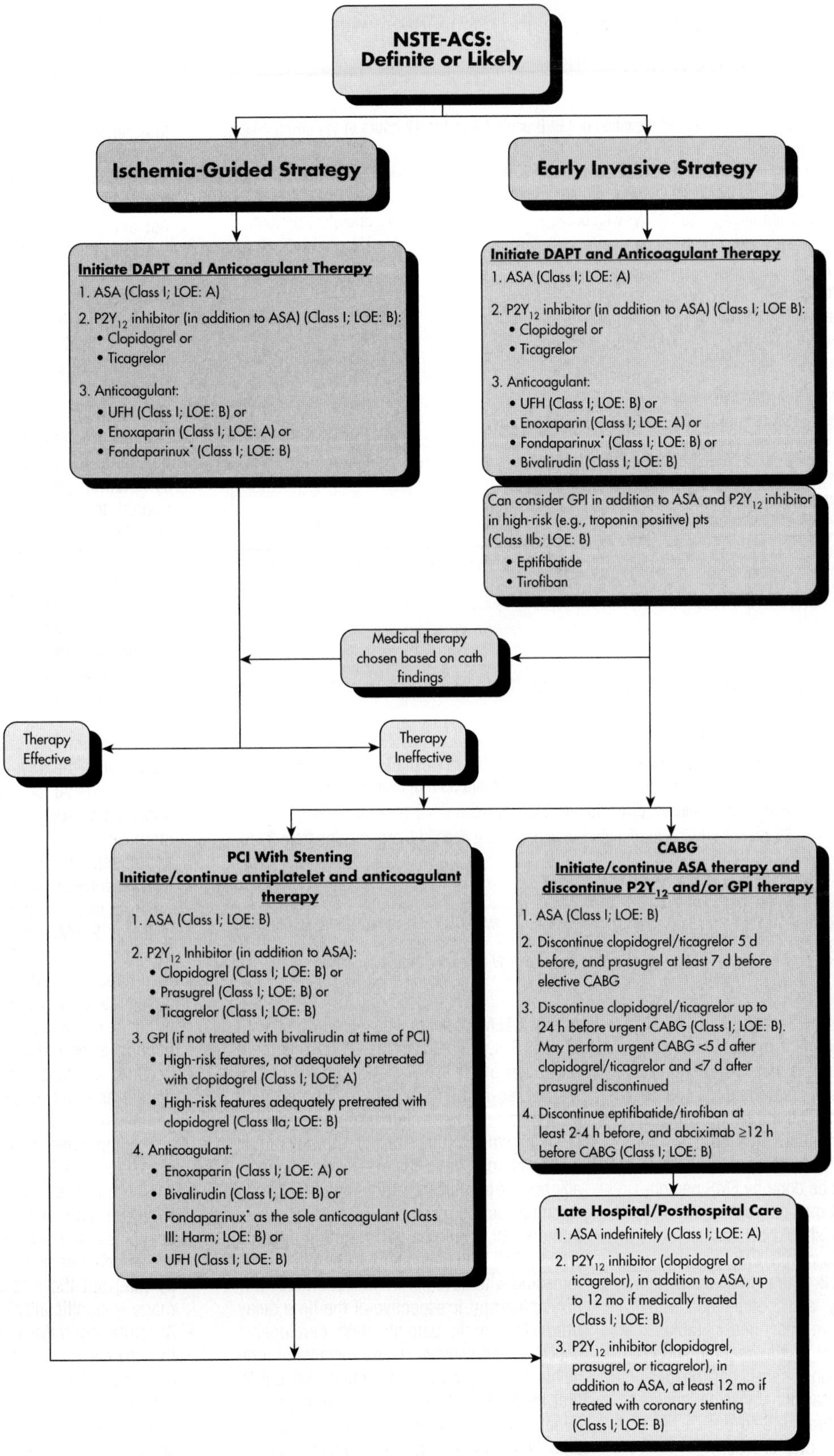

FIG. 4 Management algorithm for definite or likely NSTE-ACS. *In patients who have been treated with fondaparinux (as upfront therapy) who are undergoing PCI, an additional anticoagulant with anti-IIa activity should be administered at the time of PCI because of the risk of catheter thrombosis. *ACS,* Acute coronary syndrome; *ASA,* aspirin; *CABG,* coronary artery bypass graft; *cath,* catheter; *DAPT,* dual antiplatelet therapy; *GPI,* glycoprotein IIb/IIIa inhibitor; *LOE,* level of evidence; *NSTE-ACS,* non–ST-elevation acute coronary syndrome; *PCI,* percutaneous coronary intervention; *pts,* patients; *UFH,* unfractionated heparin. (From Amsterdam EA, et al.: 2014 AHA/ACC guideline for the management of patients with non-ST-elevation acute coronary syndromes: a report of the American College of Cardiology/American Heart Association Task Force on Practice Guidelines, *JACC* 64:2645-2687, 2014.)

TABLE 2 Indications for Primary Angioplasty and Comparison with Fibrinolytic Therapy

Indications

Alternative recanalization strategy for ST segment elevation or LBBB acute MI within 12 hours of symptom onset (or >12 hours if symptoms persist)

Cardiogenic shock developing within 36 hours of ST segment elevation/Q wave acute MI or LBBB acute MI in patients >75 yr old who can be revascularized within 18 hours of shock onset

Recommended only at centers performing >200 PCI/yr with backup cardiac surgery and for operators performing <75 PCI/yr

Advantages of Primary PCI

Higher initial recanalization rates

Reduced risk of intracerebral hemorrhage

Less residual stenosis; less recurrent ischemia or infarction

Usefulness when fibrinolysis contraindicated

Improvement in outcomes with cardiogenic shock

Disadvantages of Primary PCI (Compared with Fibrinolytic Therapy)

Access, advantages restricted to high-volume centers, operators

Longer average time to treatment

Greater dependence on operators for results

Higher system complexity, costs

LBBB, Left bundle branch block; *MI,* myocardial infarction; *PCI,* percutaneous coronary intervention (includes balloon angioplasty, stenting).
From Goldman L, Schafer AI: *Goldman's Cecil medicine,* ed 24, Philadelphia, 2012, Saunders.

TABLE 3 Dosing Regimens of Commonly Used Thrombolytic Agents

Thrombolytic Agents	Dosing Regimen
t-PA (alteplase)	15 mg bolus IV, followed by 0.75 mg/kg body weight (not to exceed 50 mg) over 30 min, followed by 0.5 mg/kg (not to exceed 35 mg) over 60 min
r-PA (reteplase)	Two 10-U IV boluses, given 30 min apart
TNK–t-PA (tenecteplase)	Single bolus IV 0.5 mg/kg (dose rounded to the nearest 5 mg, ranging from 30 to 50 mg)
Streptokinase	1.5 million U IV over 60 min

IV, Intravenous; *PA,* plasminogen activator; *r-PA,* reteplase plasminogen activator; *TNK–t-PA,* tenecteplase tissue plasminogen activator; *t-PA,* alteplase plasminogen activator; *U,* units.
From Andreoli TE, et al.: *Andreoli and Carpenter's Cecil essentials of medicine,* ed 8, Philadelphia, 2010, Saunders.

non-ST-segment MI is described in Fig. 4. Rationale of the treatment of a patient with STEMI is based on "time is muscle." Therefore, all communities should create and maintain a regional system of STEMI care that includes assessment and continuous quality improvement of EMS and hospital-based activities. A 12-lead ECG must be done by EMS personnel at the site of first medical contact (FMC).

- Reperfusion therapy should be administered to all eligible patients with STEMI with symptom onset within 12 hours. Indications for primary angioplasty and comparison with fibrinolytic therapy are described in Table 2. Primary PCI (Fig. E5) is the recommended method of reperfusion when it can be performed in a timely fashion by experienced operators with an ideal FMC-to-device time system goal of 90 minutes or less.
- In the absence of contraindications, fibrinolytic therapy (Table 3) should be administered to patients with STEMI at non-PCI-capable hospitals when the anticipated FMC-to-device time at a PCI-capable hospital exceeds 120 minutes because of unavoidable delays. It should be administered within 30 minutes of hospital arrival.
- Among STEMI patients who were treated with fibrinolytics, patients with >50% ST-segment resolution on EKG were at much lower risk for cardiac-related mortality compared with those with <50% resolution at 30 days.
- PCI is superior to thrombolytic therapy and is the standard of care. It is effective and generally results in more favorable outcomes than thrombolytic therapy.
- Primary PCI should be performed in patients with STEMI and persistent ischemic symptoms and who have contraindications to fibrinolytic therapy, irrespective of the time delay from FMC, or in patients with cardiogenic shock or acute severe HF irrespective of time delay from myocardial infarction (MI) onset, first medical contact to balloon time is <90 minutes or door to balloon/door to needle time is <1 hour, symptoms onset was >3 hours ago and when diagnosis of STEMI in doubt. Coronary stents (drug-eluting or bare-metal) are useful in patients with STEMI.
- The question of culprit vessel vs. complete revascularization during PCI has been brought up since the stent technology was applied to the management of STEMI. The most recent clinical trials (CuLPRIT, PRAMI and DANAMI3-PRIMULTI [FFR-driven revascularization]) appear to favor complete revascularization in the setting of STEMI. However, CULPRIT-SHOCK trial showed culprit vessel only PCI associated with 9.5% absolute reduction in the rate of death or renal replacement therapy at 30 days compared to multivessel PCI in acute MI patients with cardiogenic shock. One-year outcomes did not show significant difference in mortality between two groups. Korea Acute Myocardial Infarction-National Institutes of Health (KAMIR-NIH) Registry data showed better outcomes with multivessel PCI in cardiogenic shock patients compared to culprit vessel-only PCI. Thus, multivessel PCI should be reserved for few selective patients.
- For patients presenting to a non–PCI-capable hospital, rapid assessment should be done of (1) the time from onset of symptoms, (2) the risk of complications related to STEMI, (3) the risk of bleeding with fibrinolysis, (4) the presence of shock or severe HF, and (5) the time required for transfer to a PCI-capable hospital and a decision about administration of fibrinolytic therapy reached. Because the effectiveness of thrombolytics is time dependent, these agents should ideally be administered either in the field or within 30 min of the patient's arrival to the emergency department (door-to-needle time).
- Fibrinolytic therapy: If tissue plasminogen activator (t-PA) or reteplase is used, anticoagulants, such as heparin, are given to increase the likelihood of patency in the infarct-related artery for 48 hr and preferably for the duration of the index hospitalization, up to 8 days. In patients receiving fibrinolysis for STEMI, treatment with enoxaparin is superior to treatment with unfractionated heparin for 48 hr but is associated with an increase in major bleeding episodes. In patients receiving streptokinase or APSAC, heparin after thrombolysis is not indicated because it does not offer any additional benefit and can result in increased bleeding complications. Tenecteplase and reteplase are comparable with accelerated infusion recombinant t-PA in terms of efficacy and safety but are more convenient because they are administered by bolus injection. Lanoplase and heparin bolus plus infusion are as effective as tPA with regard to mortality rate, but the rate of intracranial hemorrhage is significantly higher.
- Absolute contraindications to thrombolytic therapy (Table 4) include history of intracranial hemorrhage, known intracranial malignant neoplasm or arteriovenous malformation, ischemic stroke within 3 mo (except acute ischemic stroke within 4.5 hours), suspected aortic dissection, active bleeding or bleeding diathesis (except menses), significant closed head or facial trauma within 3 mo, intracranial or intraspinal surgery within 2 mo, or severe uncontrolled hypertension (unresponsive to therapy). For streptokinase, this applies to prior treatment within 6 mo.

TABLE 4 Contraindications to Thrombolytic Therapy in Acute Myocardial Infarction

Absolute

Suspected aortic dissection
Active bleeding*
Any prior cerebral hemorrhage
Intracranial neoplasm
Cerebral aneurysm or arteriovenous malformation
Ischemic cerebrovascular accident within 3 mo

Relative

Bleeding diathesis, coagulopathy, or anticoagulant use
Major surgery within 3 wk
Puncture of a noncompressible vessel, internal bleeding, or head or major body trauma within previous 2 wk
Nonhemorrhagic stroke or gastrointestinal hemorrhage within 6 mo
Proliferative retinopathy
Active peptic ulcer disease
History of chronic, severe, poorly controlled hypertension
Severe uncontrolled hypertension on presentation (systolic blood pressure >180 mm Hg or diastolic blood pressure >110 mm Hg)
Traumatic or prolonged (>10 min) cardiopulmonary resuscitation
Pregnancy

*Does not include menstrual bleeding.
From Andreoli TE, et al.: *Andreoli and Carpenter's Cecil essentials of medicine*, ed 8, Philadelphia, 2010, Saunders.

- Relative contraindications: History of chronic severe, poorly controlled hypertension, SBP >180 mm Hg, DBP >110 mm Hg, history of prior ischemic stroke more than 3 mo, dementia, known intracranial pathology, traumatic or prolonged CPR (>10 min), major surgery <3 wk, recent internal bleeding within 2 to 4 wk, noncompressible vascular punctures, pregnancy, active peptic ulcer, oral anticoagulant therapy. After the administration of thrombolytics, immediate transfer to a PCI-capable facility is advisable without waiting for lytic results.
- Transfer to a PCI-capable hospital: Immediate transfer for STEMI patients who develop cardiogenic shock or acute severe HF, irrespective of the time delay from MI onset. Urgent transfer if the patient demonstrates evidence of failed reperfusion or reocclusion after fibrinolytic therapy.
- Coronary angiography should not be performed within the first 2 to 3 hours after administration of fibrinolytic therapy.
- Coronary artery bypass graft (CABG): Urgent CABG is indicated in patients with STEMI and coronary anatomy not amenable to PCI who have ongoing or recurrent ischemia, cardiogenic shock, severe HF, or other high-risk features. CABG is recommended in patients with STEMI at time of operative repair of mechanical defects.
- Therapeutic hypothermia should be started as soon as possible in comatose patients with STEMI and out-of-hospital cardiac arrest caused by ventricular fibrillation (VF) or pulseless ventricular tachycardia, including patients who undergo primary PCI.
- Immediate angiography and PCI when indicated should be performed in resuscitated out-of-hospital patients.
- The use of mechanical circulatory support is reasonable in patients with STEMI who are hemodynamically unstable and require urgent CABG.
- For NSTEMI patients, immediate invasive strategy (within 2 hours) recommended in patients with refractory angina, signs or symptoms of congestive heart failure or new or worsening ischemic mitral regurgitation, hemodynamic instability, recurrent angina or ischemia at rest or with low level activities despite intensive medical therapy and sustained ventricular tachycardia or ventricular fibrillation.
- Early invasive strategy (<24 hours) for NSTEMI patients recommended if GRACE risk for more than 140, dynamic ST changes on EKG and temporal change in troponin levels.
- NSTEMI patient with low-risk TIMI score (0 or 1) and/or low GRACE score (<109) and/or troponin-negative female patients can benefit from ischemia-guided strategy. Fibrinolytic therapy is contraindicated in NSTEMI patients.
- Medical therapy should be initiated immediately in the emergency department for all MI patients. This includes:
  1. Routine measures
     a. Oxygen: Supplemental oxygen should be administered to patients with arterial oxygen desaturation (SaO_2 less than 90%). No benefit has been demonstrated to supplemental oxygen in patients with normal SaO_2.
     b. Nitroglycerin: Increase oxygen supply by reducing coronary vasospasm and decrease oxygen consumption by reducing ventricular preload. Patients with ongoing ischemic discomfort should receive sublingual nitroglycerin every 5 min for a total of three doses, after which an assessment should be made about the need for intravenous nitroglycerin. Intravenous nitroglycerin is indicated for relief of ongoing ischemic discomfort, control of hypertension, or management of pulmonary congestion. Nitrates should not be administered to patients whose systolic blood pressure is <90 mm Hg or ≥30 mm Hg below baseline or severe bradycardia (<50 beats/min), tachycardia (>100 beats/min), or suspected RV infarction. Nitrates should not be administered to patients who have received a phosphodiesterase inhibitor for erectile dysfunction within the last 24 hours (48 hours for tadalafil).
     c. Adequate analgesia: Morphine sulfate 2 to 4 mg IV initially with increments of 2 to 8 mg IV at 5- to 10-min intervals can be given for severe pain unrelieved by nitroglycerin. Morphine can reduce the catecholamine surge caused by anxiety and pain, particularly in patients with anterior myocardial infarctions, which in turn can reduce heart rate and pulmonary capillary wedge pressure (PCWP), the increased cardiac workload and oxygen demand, leading to decreased ischemia and pulmonary congestion. Hypotension from morphine can be treated with careful IV hydration with saline solution. If sinus bradycardia accompanies hypotension, use atropine (0.5 to 1.0 mg IV q5min prn to a total dose of 2.5 mg). Respiratory depression caused by morphine can be reversed with naloxone 0.8 mg. Morphine sulfate and nitroglycerine should be avoided in patients with RV involvement who usually present with bradycardia and hypotension. Pain management in these cases should be provided preferentially with meperidine 25 to 50 mg intravenously q 4h, in combination with phenergan 12.5 mg to prevent nausea and/or vomiting. Blood pressure support with normal saline solution is of critical importance to maintain adequate hemodynamics until optimal revascularization is accomplished.
     d. Aspirin 162 to 325 mg PO should be crushed and chewed to enhance drug absorption and delivery. It should be given as soon as possible and continued indefinitely, at 81 mg daily. Depending on the clinical and ECG findings, if the patient is suspected to have a coronary anatomy that needs CABG rather than PCI, aspirin should be continued. P2Y12 receptor antagonists should be avoided (except Cangrelor) because they increase the perioperative bleeding risk; on-pump surgery should be deferred for at least 24 hours after clopidogrel and ticagrelor. Off-pump surgery might be considered within 24 hours of clopidogrel or ticagrelor if the benefits of revascularization outweigh the risk of bleeding. However, if the coronary artery disease is likely to benefit from PCI alone, then a loading dose of clopidogrel 600 or 300 mg or ticagrelor 180 mg PO or prasugrel

60 mg should be given as early as possible and no later than 1 hour after PCI. P2Y12 receptor antagonist should be continued for at least 1 yr after acute coronary syndrome or after primary PCI (Fig. 6). Prasugrel showed significant net clinical benefit (MACE vs. bleeding complications) only in patients with MI who underwent revascularization. It shouldn't be given for non-revascularized patients. Ticagrelor or Clopidogrel can be given in patients with MI with or without catheter-based revascularization. Cangrelor is the newest direct-acting P2Y12 platelet receptor inhibitor. It has a similar chemical structure to ATP, with a half-life of 3 to 6 min. It is given IV as a bolus plus 120 min of infusion at the time of primary PCI in patients who are naïve to P2Y12 receptor antagonists. It was approved by the FDA in 2015 after the CHAMPION PHOENIX trial. Clopidogrel and prasugrel should be started after its infusion is finished. The ticagrelor loading dose can be given during the infusion. Considering rapid onset action and clearance, Cangrelor can be started in the emergency room at the time of high-risk acute myocardial infarction diagnosis irrespective surgical or catheter-based revascularization.

2. In patients receiving fibrinolytics only or balloon angioplasty without stent, P2Y12 antagonists can be given for as little as 14 days. Clopidogrel is recommended for post-fibrinolytic patients.
3. Unfractionated heparin (UFH) is recommended in all patients with NSTEMI and STEMI (fibrinolysis or invasive revascularization). UFH infusion should not exceed more than 48 hours after PCI or fibrinolysis in the absence of an ongoing indication due to risk of heparin-induced thrombocytopenia. NSTEMI patients who underwent ischemia-guided therapy, low molecular weight heparin (LMWH) showed better MACE outcomes compared with UFH. The benefit was not significant in revascularized patients. Bivalirudin was associated with lower MACE and bleeding events in STEMI patients compared with UFH. However, it increased the risk of stent thrombosis. In NSTEMI patients who are undergoing PCI, LMWH, Bivalirudin, and UFH are acceptable.
4. Beta-adrenergic blocking agents should generally be given to all patients who do not exhibit evidence of shock. Beta-blockers are useful to reduce myocardial oxygen consumption and prevent tachyarrhythmias. Early IV beta blockage (in the initial 24 hr) followed by institution of an oral maintenance regimen is also effective in reducing recurrent infarction and ischemia. Oral beta-blockers should be initiated in the first 24 hours in patients with MI who do not have any of the following: signs of HF, evidence of a low-output state, sinus tachycardia, increased risk for cardiogenic shock, or other contraindications for its use (bradycardia, PR interval more than 0.24 seconds, second- or third-degree heart block, active asthma, or reactive airways disease).
   They should be continued during and after hospitalization for all patients with MI and with no contraindications to their use for at least 2 yr. Patients with initial contraindications to the use of beta-blockers in the first 24 hours after MI should be reevaluated to determine their subsequent eligibility. It is reasonable to administer intravenous beta-blockers at the time of presentation to patients with MI and no contraindications to their use who are hypertensive or have ongoing ischemia.
5. In patients with acute MI, treatment with drug-eluting stents is associated with decreased 2-yr mortality rates and a reduction in the need for repeated revascularization procedures compared with treatment including bare-metal stents.
6. Gp IIb/IIIa inhibitors in the era of DAPT therapy and primary PCI have failed to show benefit with "upstream" treatment. Abciximab might be useful in the presence of large thrombus burden during primary PCI. For patients receiving bivalirudin as the primary anticoagulant, routine adjunctive use of GP IIb/IIIa inhibitors is not recommended but may be considered as adjunctive or "bail-out" therapy in selected cases. In patients with acute coronary syndrome with high-risk features and not adequately pretreated with P2Y12 inhibitors, it is useful to administer GP IIb/IIIa inhibitors at the time of PCI.

CHRONIC Rx

- Discharge medications in all patients with MI (unless contraindicated) should include anti-ischemic medications (e.g., nitroglycerin, beta-blocker), lipid-lowering agents, and antiplatelet therapy (aspirin and/or P2Y12 antagonists).
- Aspirin, 81 mg PO daily, but should be continued indefinitely unless not tolerated (e.g., GI bleed). In MI patients, Clopidogrel 75 mg PO daily; ticagrelor, 90 mg bid, or prasugrel, 10 mg PO daily, can be combined with aspirin and should be continued without interruption for a minimum of 12 mo after drug-eluting stent placement; however, aspirin should be continued indefinitely. In cases of high bleeding risk or significant overt bleeding, consider discontinuation of P2Y12 inhibitor after 6 mo (Fig. 6). Combining P2Y12 antagonists with aspirin reduces risk for repeat myocardial infarction and stent thrombosis. If there is an elective surgical intervention pending, it is recommended to defer the surgery until completion of the full course of the P2Y12 antagonist treatment.
- Angiotensin-converting enzyme inhibitors (ACEIs) should be started within the first 24 hours of MI to all patients having MI with anterior infarction, pulmonary congestion, or LV EF <40%, in the absence of hypotension. They reduce LV dysfunction and dilation and slow the progression to HF during and after acute MI. Angiotensin receptor blockers (ARBs) should be given to patients who have indication but are intolerant of ACEIs. IV formulations of ACEIs should not be given within the first 24 hours of STEMI due to risk of hypotension. ARBs offer no advantage over ACEIs and should be considered only in patients who are intolerant to ACEIs.
  1. Commonly used ACEIs are ramipril 2.5 mg PO bid, captopril 12.5 mg PO bid, enalapril 2.5 mg PO bid, and lisinopril 2.5 to 5 mg PO qd initially, with subsequent titration as needed. Ramipril is associated with a lower mortality rate than most ACEIs.
  2. ACEIs may be stopped in patients without complications and no evidence of LV dysfunction after 6 to 8 wk.
  3. ACEIs should be continued indefinitely in patients with impaired LV function (EF <40%) or clinical HF.
- Long-term aldosterone antagonist therapy should be prescribed for post-MI patients without significant renal dysfunction (creatinine ≤2.5 mg/dl in men and ≤2.0 mg/dl in women) or hyperkalemia who are already taking an ACEI, a beta-blocker, and have LV EF <40% with symptomatic HF or diabetes.
- High-intensity statins (Atorvastatin 40 to 80 mg or Rosuvastatin 20 to 40 mg) should be started as early as possible in all patients with MI regardless of lipid panel, not only for their lipid-lowering effects, but also their anti-inflammatory properties (JUPITER trial), which can stabilize the ruptured plaque. Atorvastatin 80 mg can be used (PROVE IT-TIMI 22 and MIRACL trials). IMPROVE-IT trial showed adding Ezetimibe to statin treatment could decrease recurrent MI and ischemic stroke in MI patients. FDA also approved two PCSK9 (Proprotein convertase subtilisin/kexin type 9) inhibitors (Alirocumab and Evolocumab) for heterozygous familial hypercholesterolemia patients who are receiving maximally tolerated statins or patients with clinical atherosclerotic cardiovascular disease who require lowering LDL levels. A fasting lipid panel should be checked during the first 24 hours of hospital course, and the intensive therapy can be stepped down if appropriate.
- ACC/AHA 2013 lipid management guidelines recommend high-intensity statin for recurrent ASCVD events without aiming for LDL goals. However, recent clinical data suggest that the lower the LDL in MI patients, the fewer the MACE events. In general LDL <50 to 70 mg/dl carries the lowest risk of recurrent MACE events.
- In diabetic patients, HbA1c goal should be aimed at below or around 7.0% to reduce micro- and macrovascular complications. Oral hypoglycemic agents GLP1 (Glucagon like peptide) agonist (Liraglutide) and SGLT2 (sodium-glucose

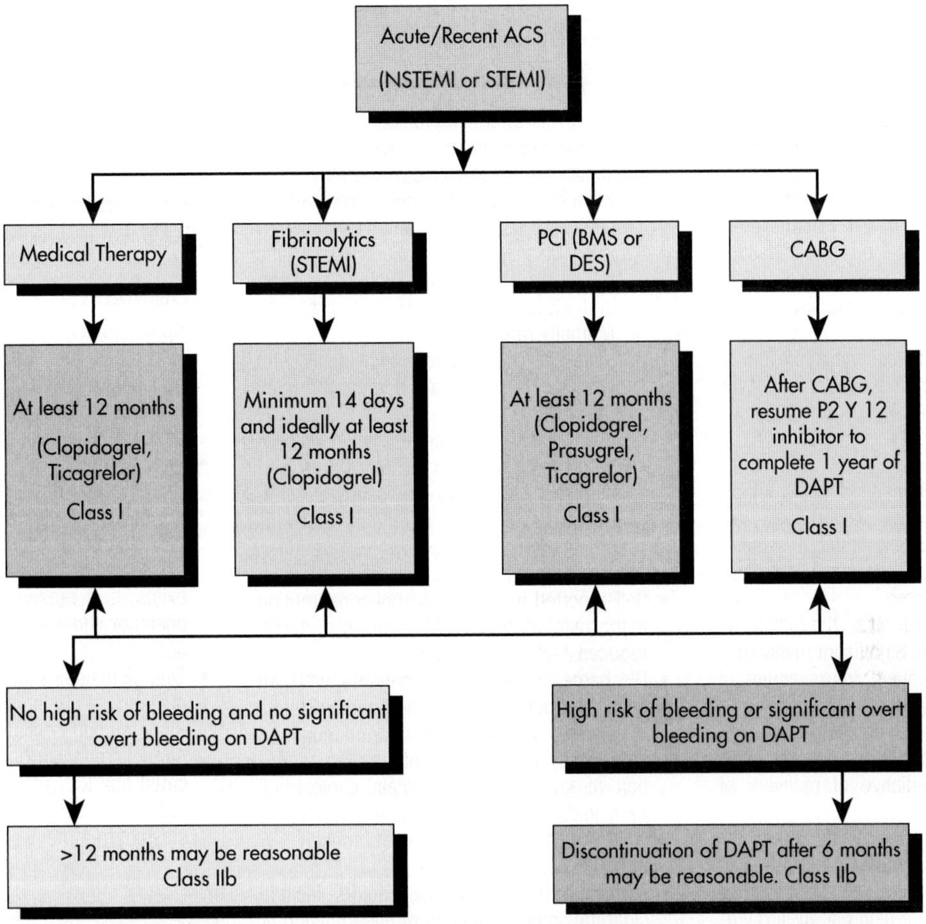

Acute/Recent ACS (NSTEMI or STEMI)

Medical Therapy → At least 12 months (Clopidogrel, Ticagrelor) Class I

Fibrinolytics (STEMI) → Minimum 14 days and ideally at least 12 months (Clopidogrel) Class I

PCI (BMS or DES) → At least 12 months (Clopidogrel, Prasugrel, Ticagrelor) Class I

CABG → After CABG, resume P2 Y 12 inhibitor to complete 1 year of DAPT Class I

No high risk of bleeding and no significant overt bleeding on DAPT → >12 months may be reasonable Class IIb

High risk of bleeding or significant overt bleeding on DAPT → Discontinuation of DAPT after 6 months may be reasonable. Class IIb

FIG. 6 Treatment algorithm for duration of P2Y12 inhibitor therapy in patients with recent ACS (NSTE-ACS or STEMI). *ACS,* Acute coronary syndrome; *BMS,* bare metal stent; *CABG,* coronary artery bypass graft surgery; *DAPT,* dual antiplatelet therapy; *DES,* drug-eluting stent; *NSTE-ACS,* non–ST-elevation acute coronary syndrome; *NSTEMI,* non-ST-segment elevation myocardial infarction; *PCI,* percutaneous coronary intervention; *STEMI,* ST-elevation myocardial infarction. (Modified from Levine GN, et al.: 2016 ACC/AHA guideline focused update on duration of dual antiplatelet therapy in patients with coronary artery disease: a report of the American College of Cardiology/American Heart Association Task Force on Clinical Practice Guidelines, *JACC* 68:1082-1115, 2016.)

cotransporter) inhibitor (Empagliflozin) showed significant mortality benefit in type 2 diabetic patients with history of CAD.

- ACC/ AHA 2017 hypertension guidelines recommend initiation of blood pressure (BP)-lowering medications in patients with clinical CVD and an average SBP ≥130 mm Hg or a DBP ≥80 mm Hg for goal BP of <130/80.

COMPLICATIONS OF MI

Cardiogenic shock: Emergent revascularization with either PCI or CABG is the recommended treatment.

Sustained ventricular tachycardia: Implantable cardioverter-defibrillator therapy (ICD) is indicated before discharge in patients who develop sustained ventricular tachycardia/ventricular fibrillation more than 48 hours after STEMI, provided the arrhythmia is not due to transient or reversible ischemia, reinfarction, or metabolic abnormalities.

Pacing in MI: Temporary pacing is indicated for symptomatic bradyarrhythmias unresponsive to medical treatment and after revascularization. AV block and bradyarrhythmias in the setting of inferior wall MI are usually transient, will not require long-term pacing, and usually resolve within 2 to 4 wk of the event. On the contrary, AV block and bradyarrhythmias or new LBBB in the presence of an anterior wall MI is usually a sign of severe disruption of the bundle of His and often requires a permanent pacemaker.

Pericarditis after MI: Post-MI pericarditis can occur early after MI. Dressler syndrome is an autoimmune inflammatory reaction to myocardial antigen after myocardial infarction. Symptoms of pericarditis usually occur 2 to 3 wk after myocardial infarction. Aspirin is recommended for treatment of pericarditis after MI. Glucocorticoids and nonsteroidal anti-inflammatory drugs are potentially harmful for treatment of pericarditis after STEMI.

Severe mitral regurgitation from papillary muscle rupture (1%), interventricular septum rupture (0.2%), and free wall rupture (1% to 3%) are the three major mechanical complications that can occur after acute myocardial infarction. Echocardiogram is helpful in diagnosing papillary muscle rupture, ventricular septal rupture, and free wall rupture. Right heart catheterization is needed to show "step-up" in oxygen saturation at the level of right ventricle. Emergent surgical repair is the treatment of choice for ventricular free wall rupture, intraventricular septum rupture, and papillary muscle rupture.

EVALUATION OF POST-MI PATIENTS

- Noninvasive testing for ischemia should be performed before discharge to assess the presence and extent of inducible ischemia in patients with STEMI who have not had coronary angiography and do not have high-risk clinical features for which coronary angiography would be warranted. It might be considered before discharge to evaluate the functional significance of a noninfarct artery stenosis previously identified at angiography and/or before discharge to guide the postdischarge exercise prescription.
- Assessment of LV function: LV ejection fraction should be measured in all patients with STEMI. Echocardiography to rule out presence of mural thrombi in patients suspected of having an extensive infarction (more common with anterior wall MI); contrast echocardiography is added if mural thrombus is suspected.

1. Assessment of risk for sudden cardiac death: Patients with an initially reduced LV ejection fraction, <40%, who are possible candidates for implantable cardioverter-defibrillator therapy should undergo reevaluation of LV ejection fraction at 90 days (or 42 days if no revascularization was performed). ICD is recommended when LVEF remains <35% in the presence of NYHA class II or III heart failure, or in patients with LVEF <30% regardless of symptoms, if the life expectancy is > 1 yr.

- Cardiac rehabilitation/secondary prevention programs are recommended for patients with STEMI.

DISPOSITION

The prognosis after MI depends on multiple factors:

- New bundle branch block, Mobitz II second-degree block, and third-degree heart block adversely affect outcome.
- Size of infarct: The larger it is, the higher the post-MI mortality rate. Significant myocardial stunning with subsequent improvement of ventricular function occurs in most patients after anterior MI. A lower level of creatine kinase, an estimate of the extent of necrosis, is independently predictive of recovery of function.
- Site of infarct: Inferior wall MI carries a better prognosis than anterior wall MI; however, patients with inferior wall MI and right ventricular involvement have a high risk for arrhythmic complications and cardiogenic shock.
- Ejection fraction after MI: The lower the LV ejection fraction, the higher the mortality rate after MI. The risk of death is higher in the first 30 days after MI among patients with LV dysfunction, HF, or both.
- Presence of post-MI angina indicates a high mortality rate.
- Performance on low-level exercise test: The presence of ST-segment changes during the test is a predictor of high mortality rate during the first year.
- Presence of pericarditis during the acute phase of MI increases mortality rate at 1 yr.
- Type A behavior (competitive drive, ambitiousness, hostility) is associated with a lower mortality rate after symptomatic MI.
- The Killip classification is an independent predictor of all-cause 30-day mortality:
    1. Killip class I includes individuals with no clinical signs of HF. Mortality rate is 6%.
    2. Killip class II includes individuals with rales or crackles in the lungs, S_3 gallop, and elevated jugular venous pressure. Mortality rate is 17%.
    3. Killip class III describes individuals with frank acute pulmonary edema. Mortality rate is 38%.
    4. Killip class IV describes individuals in cardiogenic shock or hypotension (measured as systolic blood pressure <90 mm Hg) and evidence of peripheral vasoconstriction (oliguria, cyanosis, or sweating). Mortality rate is 67%.
- Self-reported moderate alcohol consumption in the year before acute MI is associated with reduced 1-yr mortality rate.
- Discharge medication in patients with MI should include lipid-lowering agents. Statins may also lower vascular inflammation and damage by mechanisms other than reduction of low-density lipoprotein cholesterol. Early initiation of statin treatment in patients with acute MI is associated with reduced 1-yr mortality rate.
- Additional poor prognostic factors include cigarette smoking, history of hypertension or prior MI, presence of ST-segment depression in acute MI, older age, diabetes mellitus, and female sex (especially women >50 yr). Lammintausta and Fonarow reported that single men and women who live alone have a 60% to 70% greater risk of a heart attack. Furthermore, the study showed >160% increase in the risk of sudden death in these groups when compared to people who are married or live with family.
- Renal disease, even mild, as assessed by the estimated glomerular filtration rate, is a major risk factor for cardiovascular complications after MI.
- Although black patients with MI have worse outcomes than their white counterparts, these differences did not persist after adjustment for patient factors and site of care.

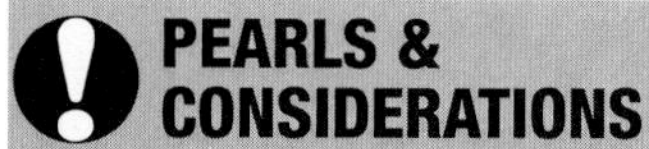

COMMENTS

- Approximately 1.5 million patients undergo PCI in the United States each year. Depending on local practices and the diagnostic criteria used, 5% to 30% of these patients have evidence of a periprocedural MI.
- The 12-lead ECG has low sensitivity for the detection of MI if the culprit lesion is in the left circumflex artery (LCX). If the initial 12-lead ECG is not diagnostic and high clinical suspicion for acute coronary syndrome exists, it is reasonable to obtain additional posterior chest leads (V_7 to V_9) to detect LCX occlusion.
- Triad of hypotension, elevated jugular venous pressure, and clear lungs are suggestive of RV infarction in patients with inferior AMI. Administration of nitroglycerin is contraindicated due to hypotension. IV fluids, inotropic support, and early reperfusion are the mainstays of treatment.

SUGGESTED READINGS

Available at ExpertConsult.com

RELATED CONTENT

Heart Attack (Patient Information)
Acute Coronary Syndrome (Related Key Topic)
Angina Pectoris (Related Key Topic)
Coronary Artery Disease (Related Key Topic)

AUTHOR: **MAHESWARA SATYA GANGADHARA RAO GOLLA, M.D.**

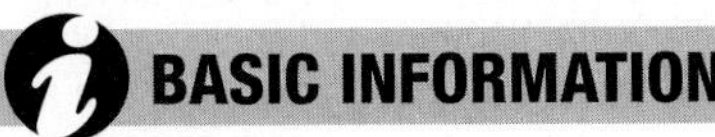

BASIC INFORMATION

DEFINITION

Myocarditis broadly refers to inflammation of the heart muscle (myocardium). This may result from exposure to discrete external antigens such as viruses, bacteria, parasites, and drugs or from internal triggers such as autoimmune conditions. When cardiac dysfunction ensues, it is then commonly defined as inflammatory cardiomyopathy.

ICD-10CM CODES

I40.0	Infective myocarditis
I40.1	Isolated myocarditis
I40.8	Other acute myocarditis
I40.9	Acute myocarditis, unspecified
A39.52	Meningococcal myocarditis
B26.82	Mumps myocarditis
B33.22	Viral myocarditis
B58.81	Toxoplasma myocarditis
D86.85	Sarcoid myocarditis
I01.2	Acute rheumatic myocarditis
I09.0	Rheumatic myocarditis
I41	Myocarditis in diseases classified elsewhere
I51.4	Myocarditis, unspecified

EPIDEMIOLOGY & DEMOGRAPHICS

- The incidence of focal myocarditis reported at autopsy is 1% to 9% in asymptomatic patients and 50% in patients infected with HIV.
- Myocarditis is the third leading cause of sudden unexpected death (as high as 8% to 9%) in young adults <40 yr of age, especially in cases of idiopathic dilated cardiomyopathy, where myocarditis may account for 10% to 40% of the cases overall.

PHYSICAL FINDINGS & CLINICAL PRESENTATION

- The most common presentations in patients are dyspnea (72%), chest pain (32%), and arrhythmias (18%), which include sinus tachycardia as well as atrial and ventricular premature contractions.
- Chest pain, especially pleuritic and positional, presents when the pericardium is involved.
- Persistent tachycardia out of proportion to fever.
- Bradyarrhythmia and new-onset unexplained heart block may also occur both in infectious (e.g., Lyme disease) and in immune-mediated forms of myocarditis.
- Faint S_1, S_3, and S_4 gallops on auscultation are important signs of impaired ventricular function.
- Murmur of functional mitral regurgitation and functional tricuspid regurgitation caused by severe left ventricular and right ventricular dilation.
- Pericardial friction rub if associated with pericarditis as in the clinical syndrome of myopericarditis.
- Patients may present with a history of a recent flulike syndrome or nonspecific viral prodrome (fever, arthralgias, malaise, fatigue); children often have a more fulminant presentation than adults. Difficulty breathing is the most common presentation of pediatric myocarditis.
- Congestive heart failure (CHF) symptoms that usually manifest with fatigue and decreased exercise capacity.
- If myocarditis is severe and diffuse and rapid in evolution, it can present with acute CHF symptoms leading to cardiogenic shock and death.
- Signs of biventricular failure (hypotension, hepatomegaly, peripheral edema, distention of neck veins, S_3 sounds, and pulmonary edema).
- Presyncope or syncope secondary to ventricular arrhythmias.
- Sudden cardiac death from ventricular tachycardia/ventricular fibrillation mediated by inflammation and/or a scar, which sets up a reentry-mediated pathway for ventricular arrhythmias.
- Acute coronary syndrome, which can occur due to local coronary spasm and inflammation and can present on ECG as acute injury pattern or ischemic changes.

ETIOLOGY

- Infection
  1. Viral (adenovirus, parvovirus B19, hepatitis C virus [HCV], Coxsackie B virus, cytomegalovirus, enterovirus, poliovirus, mumps, HIV, and Epstein-Barr virus, etc.). Viruses are the most common cause of myocarditis in developed countries. In the 1980s and 1990s, enteroviruses were frequently associated with myocarditis and dilated cardiomyopathy. In the past 10 yr, however, other viruses such as adenovirus, HCV, parvovirus B19, and herpesvirus 6 (HH6) have emerged as the significant pathogens (Box E1).
  2. Bacterial (*Staphylococcus aureus, Clostridium perfringens,* diphtheria, mycoplasma, and any severe bacterial infection).
  3. Mycotic (*Candida, Mucor, Aspergillus, Blastomyces, Histoplasma*).
  4. Parasitic (*Trypanosoma cruzi*—most common worldwide, *Trichinella, Echinococcus, Amoeba, Toxoplasma*).
  5. *Rickettsia rickettsii.*
  6. Spirochetal (*Borrelia burgdorferi*–Lyme carditis).
- Rheumatic fever
- Systemic lupus erythematosus
- Granulomatosis with polyangiitis (Wegener granulomatosis)
- Giant cell arteritis and Takayasu arteritis
- Drugs (e.g., cocaine, emetine, doxorubicin, sulfonamides, isoniazid, methyldopa, amphotericin B, tetracycline, phenylbutazone, lithium, 5-fluorouracil, phenothiazines, interferon-alfa, nivolumab, ipilimumab, tricyclic antidepressants, cyclophosphamides, smallpox vaccination)
- Toxins (carbon monoxide, ethanol, diphtheria toxin, lead, arsenicals)
- Systemic and collagen-vascular disease (scleroderma, sarcoidosis, celiac disease, Sjögren's syndrome, Kawasaki syndrome, etc.)
- Celiac disease: Two reports from Italy suggest that celiac disease, which is often clinically unsuspected, accounts for as many as 5% of patients with autoimmune myocarditis or idiopathic DCM
- Radiation
- Postpartum status
- Post–stem cell transplantation
- Hypersensitivity reactions from insect bites, such as bee and wasp bites; from snake bites; and from tetanus toxoid

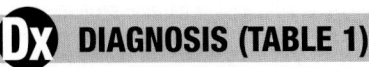

DIAGNOSIS (TABLE 1)

DIFFERENTIAL DIAGNOSIS

- Ischemic cardiomyopathy and other, nonischemic cardiomyopathies
- Acute coronary syndromes
- Valvulopathies
- Infiltrative diseases of the myocardium, such as sarcoidosis, amyloidosis, hemochromatosis, and Chagas disease.

The differential diagnosis of chest pain is described in Section II.

WORKUP

- Medical history: The clinical presentation of myocarditis is nonspecific and can consist of fatigue, palpitations, dyspnea, precordial discomfort, and myalgias.
- Diagnostic workup includes chest x-ray examination, ECG, laboratory evaluation, echocardiogram, cardiac catheterization, cardiac MRI with late gadolinium enhancement, and endomyocardial biopsy (in selected patients on the basis of the likelihood of finding specific treatable disorders such as giant cell myocarditis). Of note, endomyocardial biopsy has a sensitivity of only 10% to 35% using standard histologic criteria. This is due to variability in interpretation and sampling error.

LABORATORY TESTS

- Elevated cardiac troponin is suggestive of myocarditis in patients with clinically suspected myocarditis. Troponin I specificity is 89%; sensitivity is 34% to 53%. A normal level does not rule out the diagnosis.
- Increased creatine kinase (CK) (with elevated MB fraction, lactate dehydrogenase), and aspartate aminotransferase from myocardial necrosis.
- Elevation of cardiac troponin I or T is more common than CK-MB elevation in patients with biopsy-proven myocarditis.
- The elevations of cardiac troponin I were correlated with a short duration (typically less than 1 mo) of CHF symptoms, indicating that the majority of myocardial necrosis occurs early in the disease course.
- Persistent elevations of cardiac biomarkers are indicative of ongoing myocardial necrosis.

TABLE 1 Expanded Criteria for Diagnosis of Myocarditis

Suggestive of myocarditis:	2 positive categories
Compatible with myocarditis:	3 positive categories
High probability of being myocarditis:	all 4 categories positive

(Any matching feature in category = positive for category)

Category I: Clinical Symptoms

- Clinical heart failure
- Fever
- Viral prodrome
- Fatigue
- Dyspnea on exertion
- Chest pain
- Palpitations
- Presyncope or syncope

Category II: Evidence of Cardiac Structural or Functional Perturbation *in the Absence* of Regional Coronary Ischemia

- Echocardiography evidence
- Regional wall motion abnormalities
- Cardiac dilation
- Regional cardiac hypertrophy
- Troponin release
- High sensitivity (>0.1 ng/ml)
- Positive indium In 111 antimyosin scintigraphy
- Normal coronary angiography *or*
- Absence of reversible ischemia by coronary distribution on perfusion scan

Category III: Cardiac Magnetic Resonance Imaging

- Increased myocardial T2 signal on inversion recovery sequence
- Delayed contrast enhancement after gadolinium-DTPA infusion

Category IV: Myocardial Biopsy—Pathologic or Molecular Analysis

- Pathology findings compatible with Dallas criteria
- Presence of viral genome by polymerase chain reaction or in situ hybridization

DTPA, Diethylenetriamine penta-acetic acid.
From Bonow RO, et al.: *Heart disease,* 9th ed, Philadelphia, 2012, Saunders.

- BNP or NT-proBNP is recommended if patient has heart failure symptoms.
- Increased erythrocyte sedimentation rate (nonspecific but may be of value in following the progress of the disease and the response to therapy).
- Increased white blood cell count, again, nonspecific (increased eosinophils if parasitic infection).
- Viral titers (acute and convalescent).
- Cold agglutinin titer, antistreptolysin O titer, blood cultures.
- Lyme disease antibody titer.
- RPR, VDRL.
- Histology on endomyocardial biopsy may reveal histiocytic and mononuclear cellular infiltrates, fulfilling the Dallas criteria, which were developed by a panel of cardiac pathologists as a working standard to define the disease; active myocarditis is defined as "an inflammatory infiltrate of the myocardium with necrosis and/or degeneration of adjacent myocytes not typical of the ischemic damage associated with coronary artery disease."

IMAGING STUDIES

- Chest x-ray: Enlargement of cardiac silhouette with or without pulmonary congestion may be present.
- ECG: May be normal or show nonspecific findings. Sinus tachycardia with nonspecific ST-T wave changes unless there is concomitant pericarditis in which the ECG changes are more specific; intraventricular conduction defects and bundle branch blocks are uncommon in typical viral myocarditis but are common manifestations in cardiac sarcoid and idiopathic giant cell myocarditis. The presence of Q waves or left bundle branch block was associated with higher rates of death or transplantation in some patients.
  1. Lyme disease and diphtheria can cause varying degrees of heart block.
  2. Changes mimicking acute myocardial infarction (regional ST elevations and Q waves) can occur with focal necrosis from myocarditis.
- Echocardiogram:
  1. The most useful test in detecting decreased ventricular function in suspected myocarditis even when subclinical.
  2. Acute severe myocarditis is associated with systolic dysfunction with decreased ejection fraction.
  3. Dilated and hypokinetic chambers.
  4. The systolic dysfunction is generally global but may be regional or segmental as in the case of focal myocarditis.
  5. Exercise-induced wall motion abnormalities may also be seen. This is usually due to microvascular dysfunction.
  6. Abnormal tissue Doppler signal can provide additional evidence for the presence of myocarditis.
  7. The echocardiogram can also be helpful with diagnosing coexisting pericardial involvement.
  8. The spheroid dysfunctional ventricle in acute myocarditis tends to remodel to the more normal elliptical shape over several months.
- Cardiac catheterization and angiography:
  1. To rule out coronary artery disease and valvular disease. Coronary angiography is most commonly normal with evidence of minimal or no coronary artery disease.
  2. A right ventricular endomyocardial biopsy can confirm the diagnosis, although a negative biopsy result does not exclude myocarditis owing to the low sensitivity of this test. Recent studies have shown that myocardial biopsy may be unnecessary because immunosuppression therapy based on biopsy results is generally ineffective. However, if idiopathic giant cell myocarditis is suspected, biopsy can confirm this diagnosis, and immunosuppression therapy is often helpful in this patient cohort.
- Cardiac MRI (Fig. E1):
  1. Can be used to detect myocardial edema and myocyte injury in myocarditis.
  2. Increased focal or global signal intensity can be used to calculate an edema ratio. Edema in the absence of necrosis or scar represents reversible injury and thus can predict functional recovery.
  3. Late gadolinium enhancement (LGE) and the presence of increased focal and global myocardial contrast enhancement relative to skeletal muscle.
  4. Any combination of two of the above has a sensitivity and specificity of 76% and 96%, with 85% diagnostic accuracy, and is probably the gold standard for diagnosis of myocarditis, as opposed to routine biopsy.
  5. Cardiac MRI has demonstrated that myocarditis tends to start as a focal process and becomes a more global process over time, with the extent of myocardial enhancement correlating with clinical status and left ventricular function.
  6. Some viral pathogens have focal involvement of the myocardium. Parvovirus B19 involves the subepicardial lateral wall of the left ventricle. HHV6 and especially the combination of HHV6/parvovirus B19 tend to involve the septum and present with more acute and chronic heart failure symptoms.
  7. The pattern of LGE is different from that in ischemic cardiomyopathy. LGE in myocarditis tends to involve the epicardium with variable extension into the midmyocardium and sparing of the endocardium. This is in contrast to ischemic injury, which involves endocardium first with extension outward.
- Indium-111-labeled antimyosin antibody scintigraphy is positive in myocarditis with a sensitivity of up to 65%.

Rx TREATMENT

NONPHARMACOLOGIC THERAPY

- Supportive care is the first line of therapy for patients with myocarditis.
- Restrict physical activity (to decrease cardiac work). Bed rest is advisable during viremia.

- Avoid heavy use of alcohol.
- Nonsteroidal antiinflammatory drugs (NSAIDs) should be avoided in patients with HF generally, given the risk of HF exacerbation and possible risk of increased mortality. NSAIDs in the lowest required dose are reserved for patients with perimyocarditis in whom LV function is clearly normal and who have prominent chest pain from pericarditis.

ACUTE GENERAL Rx

- Treat underlying cause (e.g., use specific antibiotics for bacterial infection).
- Treat congestive heart failure (CHF) with diuretics, angiotensin-converting enzyme inhibitors (ACE inhibitors), and salt restriction. A beta-blocker may be added once clinical stability has been achieved. Digoxin should be used with caution and only at low doses.
- Patients who are left with an LVEF ≤35% despite optimal medical therapy for 3 to 9 mo, and who have good functional status with prognosis >1 yr, will benefit from primary prevention therapy with implantable cardioverter-defibrillator (ICD) implantation as in patients with ischemic cardiomyopathy and other nonischemic cardiomyopathies.
- Antiarrhythmics if needed for ventricular arrhythmias. When antiarrhythmic therapy is necessary, options include amiodarone, dofetilide, and, in patients without class IV HF, cautious use of beta-blockers or calcium channel blockers. ICD implantation for secondary prevention in patients who have life-threatening ventricular arrhythmias and have good functional status with prognosis >1 yr.
- Complete heart block and/or symptomatic bradycardia are indications for pacing during the acute phase of myocarditis but are usually transient, so temporary pacing is sufficient.
- In patients with chronic CHF from myocarditis, only ACE inhibitors, beta-blockers, and possibly aldosterone receptor antagonists will decrease their mortality in the long term (as with all CHF etiologies).
- Anticoagulation is indicated in patients with evidence of systemic embolism or presence of acute left ventricular thrombus. Standard criteria for anticoagulation for atrial fibrillation should also be applied. Heart failure and/or low EF with normal sinus rhythm are generally not indications for anticoagulation.
- Inotropes or mechanical assist devices such as intraaortic balloon pumps, Impella device, and left ventricular assist device (LVAD) if severe heart failure or if cardiogenic shock persists despite medical therapy.
- Cardiac transplantation in patients with chronic or acute fulminant myocarditis with intractable cardiomyopathy and persistent CHF.
- Corticosteroid use is contraindicated in early infectious myocarditis; it may be justified in only selected patients with intractable CHF, severe systemic toxicity, and severe life-threatening arrhythmias.
- Immunosuppressive drugs (prednisone with cyclosporine/Cytoxan or azathioprine) do not have any significant effect on the prognosis of myocarditis and should not be used in the routine treatment of patients with myocarditis. Immunosuppression may have a role in the treatment of myocarditis from systemic autoimmune disease (e.g., lupus, scleroderma); in idiopathic giant cell myocarditis, sarcoidosis, or myocarditis caused by hypersensitivity reactions; or in severe hemodynamic compromise.
- Observational data suggest that patients with giant cell myocarditis treated with certain immunosuppressive regimes have improved survival compared with patients who do not receive immunosuppressive treatment.
- In patients with ongoing viral genomic expression, preliminary data suggest that treatment with interferons may improve both symptoms and left ventricular function when compared with standard heart failure therapy.
  - IV immunoglobulins have been studied, but because of lack of efficacy data, at present there is no indication for their use except in some pediatric cases or those refractory to immunosuppressive therapy.
- Improved cardiac function and arrhythmias have been reported in patients with celiac disease and myocarditis or DCM following a gluten-free diet with or without immunosuppressive therapy, but controlled data are lacking.
- A treatment algorithm for patients with myocarditis is described in Fig. 2.

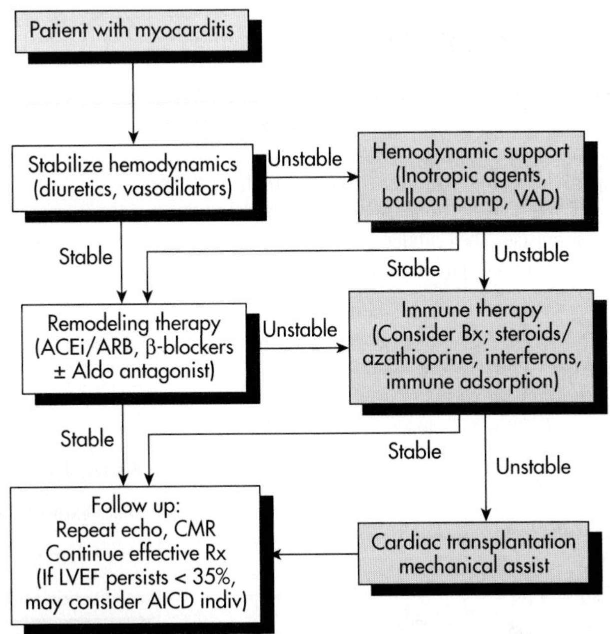

FIG. 2 Treatment algorithms for patients with myocarditis, depending on hemodynamic stability and response to general supportive and remodeling treatment regimen at each step. All patients should have aggressive support and appropriate follow-up. Immune therapy at present is still mainly to support those who have failed to improve spontaneously. *ACEi*, Angiotensin-converting enzyme inhibitors; *AICD*, automatic implantable cardioverter-defibrillator; *Aldo*, aldosterone; *ARB*, angiotensin receptor blockers; *Bx*, biopsy; *CMR*, cardiac magnetic resonance; *indiv*, based on individual assessment of risk versus benefit; *LVEF*, left ventricular ejection fraction; *VAD*, ventricular assist device. (From Bonow RO et al: *Heart disease*, ed 9, Philadelphia, 2012, Saunders.)

DISPOSITION

- Most patients with acute myocarditis and mild cardiac involvement have a partial or a full clinical recovery. In some cases, however, the process may continue subclinically with eventual progression to a cardiomyopathy. Therefore all patients with myocarditis should be followed up at least initially at intervals of 1 to 3 mo. Of those with advanced cardiac dysfunction, one third will have residual cardiac dysfunction, and 25% may progress to cardiac transplantation or death.
- Prognosis is best for patients with fulminant lymphocytic myocarditis (severe hemodynamic compromise, rapid onset of symptoms, or high fever). These patients tend to have complete recovery with total resolution of myocarditis on repeat biopsy.
- In contrast, patients with giant cell myocarditis have an extremely poor prognosis with a median survival of <6 mo, and most require cardiac transplantation.
- The American Heart Association recommends 3 to 6 mo abstinence from competitive sports after myocarditis.

REFERRAL

Consider heart transplant if intractable CHF develops.

SUGGESTED READINGS

Available at ExpertConsult.com

RELATED CONTENT

Myocarditis (Patient Information)

AUTHORS: **HANNAH CHAUDRY, M.D.,** and **ARAVIND RAO KOKKIRALA, M.D. F.A.C.C.**

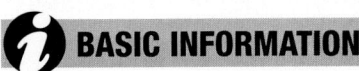

BASIC INFORMATION

DEFINITION

- Myofascial pain syndrome is myalgia characterized by trigger point.
- Trigger point: Trigger points are discrete, focal, hyperirritable spots located in a taut band of skeletal muscle. They produce pain locally and in a referred pattern. Muscle involvement is asymmetric and focal.

SYNONYMS

Chronic myofascial pain
CMP

ICD-10CM CODE

M79.1 Myalgia, myofascial pain syndrome

EPIDEMIOLOGY & DEMOGRAPHICS

Myofascial pain syndrome is a common painful muscle disorder which can affect any sex at any age. About 85% of the general population at some point suffers from it during their lifetime. It also coexists with other chronic pain conditions.

PHYSICAL FINDINGS & CLINICAL PRESENTATION

- Regional body pain and stiffness; often muscles responsible for body posture are affected. Neck, upper back, and lower back muscles are commonly involved. The most commonly affected muscles are trapezius, scalene, infraspinatus, subscapularis, levator scapulae, piriformis, tensor fasciae latae, iliopsoas, gluteus, and quadratus lumborum. Pain is present at rest and with muscle movement
- Table 1 lists some distinguishing features of myofascial pain and fibromyalgia
- Limited range of motion and pain-related weakness of affected muscle
- Twitch response: Brisk contraction of a taut band of skeletal muscle fibers elicited by snapping palpation of a trigger point in that band producing a taut band
- One or more trigger points asymmetrical location
- Referred pain from a trigger point to a zone of reference, but not following dermatomal distribution
- Resolution of the symptoms with lidocaine injection of the trigger point

ETIOLOGY

- Etiology is unknown. There are several proposed histopathologic mechanisms to account for the development of trigger points, but they are lacking scientific evidence. Most researchers agree that acute trauma or repetitive microtrauma may lead to the development of a trigger point.
- Fig. 1 lists causes of myofascial pain and dysfunction.
- Lack of exercise, prolonged poor posture, vitamin deficiencies, sleep disturbances, and joint problems may all predispose to the development of microtrauma.

TABLE 1 Distinguishing Features of Myofascial Pain and Fibromyalgia

	Myofascial Pain	Fibromyalgia
Age distribution	20-40 yr	20-50 yr
Gender distribution	Mainly women	Mainly women
Distribution of pain	Localized; usually unilateral	Generalized; bilaterally symmetric
Tender points	Few	Multiple
Trigger points	Uncommon	Common
Fatigue	Localized muscle fatigue	Generalized fatigue
Sleep disturbance	Common	Common

From Firestein GS, et al.: *Kelley's textbook of rheumatology*, ed 9, Philadelphia, 2013, Saunders.

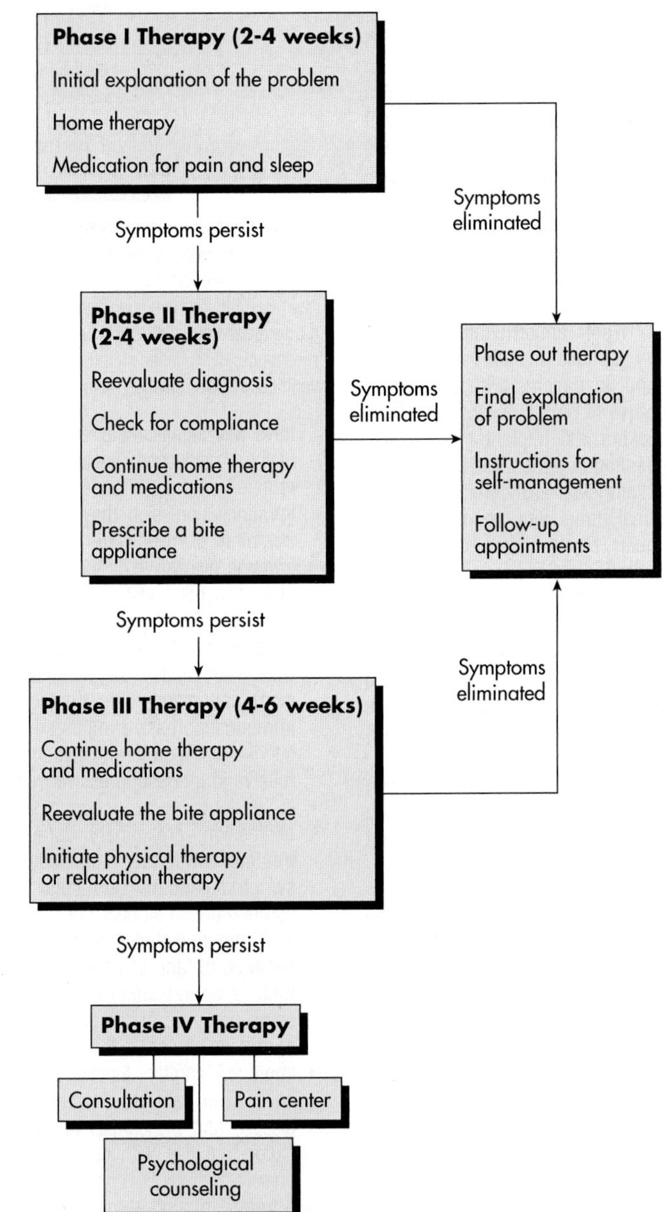

FIG. 1 Management of myofascial pain and dysfunction. Treatments are divided into four phases. If the symptoms are eliminated in any of the first three phases, the ongoing therapy is gradually phased out, and the patient is instructed in continued self-management of the condition. (Modified from Laskin DM, Block S: Diagnosis and treatment of myofacial pain-dysfunction [MPD] syndrome, *J Prosthet Dent* 56:75–84, 1986.)

DIAGNOSIS

A detailed physical examination and clinical presentation usually make the diagnosis of myofascial pain syndrome.

DIFFERENTIAL DIAGNOSIS

- Fibromyalgia
- Polymyositis
- Migraine
- Tension headache
- Muscle strain
- Bursitis and tendinitis
- Radiculopathies

WORKUP

Not indicated usually, treatment can be started on clinical grounds alone.

LABORATORY TESTS

Generally not indicated, except to exclude other causes of myalgia.

IMAGING STUDIES

Generally not indicated in clear-cut cases of myofascial pain syndrome. Indicated only to exclude other causes of pain (e.g., referred pain).

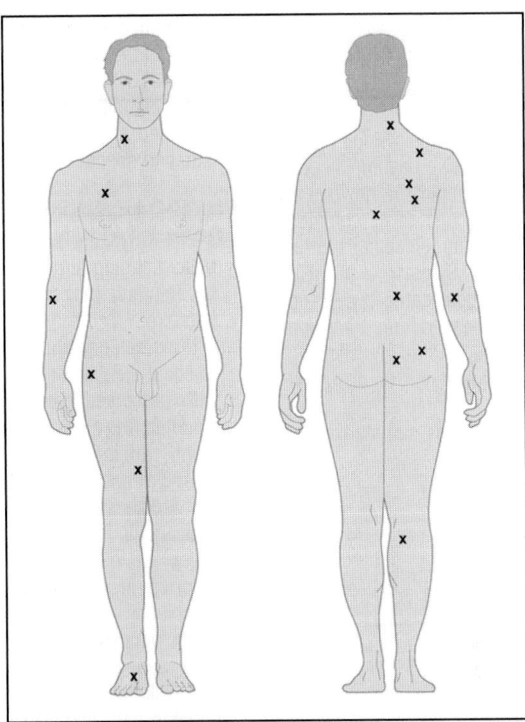

FIG. 2 Most frequent locations of myofascial trigger points. (Adapted from Rachlin E, Rachlin I: *Myofascial pain and fibromyalgia: trigger point management*, ed 2, St Louis, 2002, Mosby.)

TREATMENT

- Spray and stretch therapy: Involves passive stretching of the affected muscle. Position patient for maximum decrease in muscle tension, identify trigger points, and mark them. Apply vapocoolant spray over entire length of the affected muscle. Passively stretch muscle by applying gentle pressure.
- Physical therapy: TENS unit, ultrasound, massage therapy, myofascial release technique.
- Invasive technique: Trigger point injection with 1% lidocaine is the most commonly used technique.
- NSAIDs and muscle relaxants: Short-term use.
- Fig. 2 shows the management of myofascial pain and dysfunction.

REFERRAL

An interventional pain management referral is made if trigger point injection is indicated. To physical therapist for increasing ROM and massage therapy.

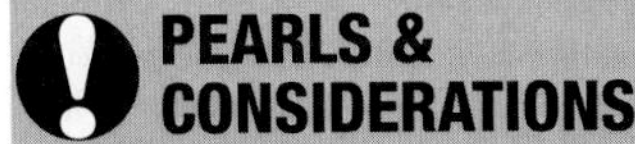

PEARLS & CONSIDERATIONS

- Trigger point is commonly misdiagnosed as tender point, which is characteristic finding of fibromyalgia
- Tender point: Characterized as non-palpable nodule with symmetric and multiple locations. Tender points are located close to muscle attachment, usually not associated with specific muscle activity. Lacking twitch response and relief of symptoms with localized lidocaine injection.

SUGGESTED READINGS

Available at ExpertConsult.com

AUTHORS: **UZMA NASIR, M.D.,** and **SYEDA M. SAYEED, M.D.**

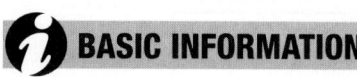

DEFINITION

Narcolepsy is a chronic neurologic sleep disorder characterized by excessive daytime sleepiness and dysregulation of rapid eye movement (REM) sleep. It is the second most common cause of disabling daytime sleepiness after obstructive sleep apnea. Symptoms of REM sleep dysregulation include cataplexy, sleep paralysis, and hallucinations during transition between wake and sleep. Difficulty sleeping with either frequent awakenings or disrupted sleep may also occur. An international classification of sleep disorders is summarized in Table 1.

SYNONYMS

Hypersomnia of central origin
Narcolepsy with cataplexy
Narcolepsy-cataplexy syndrome
Narcolepsy with hypocretin deficiency
Gélineau syndrome

ICD-10CM CODES
G47.419 Narcolepsy without cataplexy
G47.411 Narcolepsy with cataplexy

EPIDEMIOLOGY & DEMOGRAPHICS

INCIDENCE: 0.74/100,000 persons/yr
PREVALENCE: 1 in 2,000 people
PREDOMINANT SEX: Males and females are equally affected.
AGE OF ONSET: Peak 15 to 30 yr (range, 10-55 yr)
GENETICS:
- Associated with human leukocyte antigen (HLA) subtypes, specifically, *DQB1*0602,* which is present in 95% of patients with cataplexy and 96% of patients with hypocretin deficiency.
- Risk of narcolepsy increases 20 to 40 times if a family member is affected.
- Monozygotic twin concordance rate is 17% to 36%, thus indicating an incomplete penetrance and suggesting an environmental factor in the disease process.

RISK FACTORS: Anesthesia, head injury, history of meningitis or encephalitis, family history of narcolepsy, tumor, vascular malformations, stroke, and obesity.

PHYSICAL FINDINGS & CLINICAL PRESENTATION

- Overwhelming urge to sleep with chronic hypersomnia may occur during the day.
- Cataplexy occurs in 60% to 100% of patients with narcolepsy and is reported as a partial or complete loss of voluntary muscle control with preserved consciousness that is precipitated by a strong emotion, more commonly with laughter. This is the most specific symptom and is considered pathognomonic for narcolepsy.
- Hypnagogic (wake to sleep) or hypnopompic (sleep to wake) hallucinations have been reported in 60% to 80% of patients with narcolepsy.
- Sleep paralysis, defined as loss of muscle tone during the transition between sleep and wakefulness, occurs in 60% to 80% of patients with narcolepsy. It may occur with hallucinations and can be interrupted by sensory stimuli.
- Only about one third of patients will have all four symptoms of narcolepsy: Chronic daytime sleepiness, cataplexy, hypnagogic hallucinations, and sleep paralysis.
- Fragmented sleep is seen in 60% to 80% of narcolepsy patients and can often be mistaken for insomnia or other intrinsic sleep disorder.
- Other symptoms that have been reported in narcolepsy include automatic behavior or semipurposeful movements in 40% of patients and memory disturbance in 50% of patients.

ETIOLOGY

The loss of hypocretin/orexin signaling, genetic factors, and brain lesions are presently identified factors in the development of narcolepsy. May be a manifestation of neuromyelitis optica spectrum disorder.

HYPOCRETIN/OREXIN:
- Loss of hypocretin-1 and hypocretin-2 (also known as orexin-A and orexin-B) producing neurons in the lateral hypothalamus.
- Human cerebrospinal fluid (CSF) levels of hypocretin-1 are low to undetectable in narcoleptics with cataplexy.
- Narcolepsy without cataplexy may have a different cause because CSF hypocretin levels are usually normal in these patients, so there may be a completely separate mechanism in these patients, or it may result from less extensive loss of hypocretin neurons or impaired signaling.

SECONDARY ETIOLOGIES:
- Central nervous system lesions including tumors, vascular malformations, and strokes have all been reported to cause secondary narcolepsy.
- Direct injury to the hypocretin neurons or their projections is the most likely cause of secondary narcolepsy due to central nervous system lesions.
- Narcolepsy has been reported in genetic syndromes, including Prader-Willi syndrome and Niemann-Pick disease type C, as well as neuromyelitis optica spectrum disorder and paraneoplastic syndromes.

TABLE 1 International Classification of Sleep Disorders: Definitions and Pathophysiology

Condition	Diagnostic Criteria*	Pathophysiology
Type 1 narcolepsy	Presence of two or more of the following: cataplexy, positive MSLT, and low CSF hypocretin-1	Hypocretin deficiency 98% HLA-DQB1*06:02
Type 2 narcolepsy	Positive MSLT; most often with no or unclear cataplexy	Unknown, heterogenous ~16% Hypocretin deficiency ~40% HLA-DQB1*0602
Secondary narcolepsy	As above, but due to neurologic conditions	With or without hypocretin deficiency, various disorders
Idiopathic hypersomnia	No cataplexy, no SOREMPs during the MSLT	Unknown, likely heterogeneous

CSF, Cerebrospinal fluid.
*Abnormal Multiple Sleep Latency Test (MSLT): Sleep latency ≤8 min, ≥2sleep-onset REM periods (SOREMPs), including a nocturnal SOREMP. For details, see *International Classification of Sleep Disorders,* third edition. (American Academy of Sleep Medicine: *International classification of sleep disorders,* ed 3, Darien, IL, 2014, American Academy of Sleep Medicine.)
From Kryger M, Roth T, Dement WC: *Principles and practice of sleep medicine,* ed 6, Philadelphia, 2017, Elsevier.

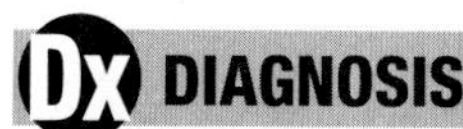

DIFFERENTIAL DIAGNOSIS

Excessive daytime somnolence:
- Autism
- Autosomal dominant cerebellar ataxia, deafness, and narcolepsy
- Behaviorally induced insufficient sleep syndrome
- Central or obstructive sleep apnea (sleep-disordered breathing)
- Circadian rhythm disorder
- Depression
- Diencephalic lesions
- Drug or alcohol abuse
- Hypothyroidism
- Idiopathic hypersomnia with long or short sleep time
- Inadequate sleep hygiene
- Insufficient sleep
- Increased intracranial pressure

Insomnia:
- Kleine-Levin syndrome
- Medication effect
- Menstrual-related hypersomnia
- Posttraumatic narcolepsy
- Seizures
- Sleep fragmentation (multiple causes)

Cataplexy:
- Seizures
- Periodic paralysis
- Cardiovascular insufficiency
- Psychogenic (multiple causes)
- Lesions of the hypothalamus or brain stem

WORKUP

- Because persistent sleepiness can occur with many conditions, it is important to rule out other sleep disorders.

- Narcolepsy is often diagnosed by clinical history. The Epworth Sleepiness Scale is very useful in determining the degree of excessive daytime sleepiness (Table 2).
- The diagnosis of narcolepsy can be made without the need for further testing if there is a clear history of cataplexy in the setting of excessive daytime somnolence. Sleep laboratory testing or possibly laboratory testing is required if cataplexy does not exist, if a diagnosis needs to be confirmed, or if concerns exist for another sleep disorder.
- The medical history should include questions regarding severity of daytime hypersomnia while also evaluating for sleep-disordered breathing, transient muscle weakness triggered by emotion, hallucinations while falling asleep or upon awakening, and inability to move after awakening. The clinical evaluation should also address symptoms of seizures and paraneoplastic disorders while also asking about previous stroke or genetic disorders. A detailed family history is imperative. Hypothalamic dysfunction such as unexplained weight gain, endocrine abnormalities, circadian dysrhythmias, and autonomic nervous system problems may provide useful insight.
- A thorough examination including a detailed neurologic examination should be performed.
- Nocturnal polysomnography followed by a multiple sleep latency test (MSLT) remains the gold standard for the diagnosis of narcolepsy. A drug screen should also be performed to rule out pharmacologic modulations of sleep.

LABORATORY TESTS

HLA subtyping and CSF hypocretin/orexin levels may be attempted in suspected cases of narcolepsy. For a fee, CSF hypocretin/orexin analysis can be performed at the Center for Narcolepsy at Stanford University (med.stanford.edu/psychiatry/narcolepsy). CSF hypocretin levels below 110 pg/ml are indicative of narcolepsy, but normal or high CSF hypocretin levels do not exclude the diagnosis.

Rx TREATMENT

Narcolepsy can be treated with a combination of behavioral and pharmacologic approaches. Examples of initial treatment packages for adults are summarized in Table 3.

NONPHARMACOLOGIC THERAPY

Avoidance of over-the-counter drugs and illicit drugs, optimal sleep hygiene and scheduled daily naps, and psychosocial support can be used for symptoms of excessive daytime somnolence. However, nonpharmacologic therapy is typically not sufficient for treatment of narcolepsy alone but is often used as adjunct therapy with medications.

PHARMACOLOGIC THERAPY (TABLE 4)

For excessive daytime somnolence:

- Sodium oxybate: A central nervous system depressant that can be used for the treatment of cataplexy and REM-related symptoms

TABLE 2 Epworth Sleepiness Scale

How likely are you to doze off or fall asleep in the following situations, in contrast to just feeling tired? This refers to your usual way of life in recent time. Even if you have not done some of these things recently, try to work out how they would have affected you. Use the following scale to choose the most appropriate number for each situation.

0 = would never doze
1 = slight chance of dozing
2 = moderate chance of dozing
3 = high chance of dozing

Situation	Chance of Dozing
Sitting and reading	
Watching TV	
Sitting and inactive in a public place (theater or meeting)	
As a passenger in a car for an hour without a break	
Lying down to rest in the afternoon when circumstances permit	
Sitting and talking to someone	
Sitting quietly after lunch (without alcohol)	
In a car, while stopped for a few minutes in traffic	
Total	

From Johns MW: A new method for measuring daytime sleepiness: the Epworth Sleepiness Scale, *Sleep* 14:540-545, 1991.

TABLE 3 Examples of Initial Treatment Packages for Adults

General Measures

Avoid shifts in sleep schedule.
Avoid heavy meals and alcohol intake.
Regular timing of nocturnal sleep: 10:30 PM to 7 AM
Naps: Strategically timed naps if possible (e.g., 15 minutes at lunchtime, 15 minutes at 5:30 PM)

Medications for Sleepiness

The effects of stimulant medications vary widely among patients. The dosing and timing of medications should be individualized to optimize performance. Additional doses, as needed, may be suggested for periods of anticipated sleepiness.

Modafinil* 100-200 mg (taken when waking up in the morning) and 100-200 mg at lunchtime *or*

Sodium oxybate† at bedtime: Dosage must start low at 2.25 g taken twice while in bed (at bedtime and 2.5-4 hr after bedtime); increase to total dosage of 5-6 g within 2-4 wk. This initial dose is usually ineffective, so increase to 3 g at bedtime and 3 g approximately 2.5-4 hr after bedtime if tolerated. Depending on response, dosage can be increased to as high as 9 g total nightly dose. Do not increase above 9 g because of risk of serious side effects during sleep. It may take more than 2 mo for daytime symptoms to improve, and cataplexy may improve faster than excessive daytime sleepiness. If the patient is already taking a daytime stimulant, it may be possible to reduce the stimulant dose or to discontinue it once a therapeutic dosage of sodium oxybate has been reached.

Methylphenidate 5 mg (3 or 4 tablets; 10 mg when waking up; 5 mg 30 minutes before lunch; 5 mg near 3 PM; better action is always obtained if the drug is taken on an empty stomach) or 20 mg SR in the morning (on an empty stomach)

If Persistent Difficulties

Modafinil 200 mg in the morning and 200 mg at lunch (total daily dosage, 400 mg) *or*
Add sodium oxybate (GHB) at bedtime: Dosage must start low as indicated above.
Methylphenidate (SR): 20 mg in the morning; 5 mg after noon nap; 5 mg at 4 PM *or*
Possibly (more in teenagers) atomoxetine: Start at 0.5 mg/kg within 1 wk to appropriate dosage of 1-1.2 mg/kg taken in the morning

If No Response

Dextroamphetamine sulfate: 15 mg on awakening; 5 mg after noon nap; 5 mg at 3:30 or 4 PM (or 15 mg at awakening and 15 mg after noon nap)

Medications for Cataplexy‡

Sodium oxybate (see above)
Venlafaxine 150-300 mg
Fluoxetine 20-60 mg
Duloxetine 60 mg

If No Response

Clomipramine 75-125 mg, *or*
Viloxazine 150-200 mg, *or*
Imipramine 75-125 mg

SR, Sustained-release tablet.
*Modafinil works best in naive subjects. It should be the drug of first choice in children and adults.
†Response to sodium oxybate is slow.
‡Medications may be taken in the evening near bedtime (sodium oxybate, clomipramine, imipramine), only in the morning (fluoxetine), or in the morning and at lunchtime (viloxazine, venlafaxine). The only medications specifically approved for use in narcolepsy by the Food and Drug Administration are modafinil and sodium oxybate.
From Kryger M, Roth T, Dement WC: *Principles and practice of sleep medicine*, ed 6, Philadelphia, 2017, Elsevier.

TABLE 4 Narcolepsy Drugs Currently Available

Drug	Usual Dosage* (All Drugs Administered Orally)
Treatment of EDS	
Stimulants†	
Modafinil	100-400 mg/day
Sodium oxybate	6-9 g/day (divided in two doses)
Methylphenidate	10-60 mg/day
Atomoxetine	10-25 mg/day
Dextroamphetamine	5-60 mg/day
Methamphetamine	20-25 mg/day
Treatment of Auxiliary Effects (e.g., Cataplexy)	
Sodium oxybate (gamma-hydroxybutyrate)	6-9 g/day (divided in two doses)
Antidepressants‡	
Without Atropinic Side Effects	
Venlafaxine XR	75-300 mg/day
Fluoxetine	20-60 mg/day
Viloxazine	50-200 mg/day
Duloxetine	60 mg/day
With Atropinic Side Effects	
Protriptyline	2.5-20 mg/day
Imipramine	25-200 mg/day
Clomipramine	25-200 mg/day
Desipramine	25-200 mg/day

*On occasion, depending on clinical response, the dose may be outside the usual dosage range.

†Most stimulants should be administered in divided doses, commonly in the morning and at lunchtime. This is recommended for amphetamines and modafinil. Methylphenidate has a fast elimination rate, so the slow-release (SR) formula may be helpful in the morning (e.g., 20 mg SR). If it is administered by 5-mg increments, the usual timing of methylphenidate administration is every 3 to 4 hr until 3 PM.

From Kryger M, Roth T, Dement WC: *Principles and practice of sleep medicine*, ed 6, Philadelphia, 2017, Elsevier.

- Modafinil 200 to 600 mg PO every morning or divided bid
- Armodafinil 150 or 250 mg PO as a single dose in the morning
- Methylphenidate 5 to 15 mg PO bid to tid
- Methylphenidate SR 18 to 54 mg PO every morning or divided bid
- Dextroamphetamine 10 to 60 mg PO qd
- Eldepryl 5 mg PO bid

For cataplexy:

- Sodium oxybate: A central nervous system depressant that can be used for the treatment of cataplexy and REM-related symptoms
- Fluoxetine 20 mg PO qd initially
- Sertraline 25 mg PO qd initially
- Venlafaxine 25 mg PO qd initially
- Clomipramine 25 mg/day initially
- Protriptyline 5 mg tid initially
- Imipramine 25 to 50 mg/day initially
- Desipramine 10 mg bid initially

DISPOSITION

This is a chronic sleep disorder that may worsen for the first few years and then persist for life.

REFERRAL

Because of the complexity of this disorder and its ever-changing management and treatment, patients should be referred to centers or programs with highly trained sleep specialists with expertise caring for these patients, especially if sodium oxybate (Xyrem) therapy is needed.

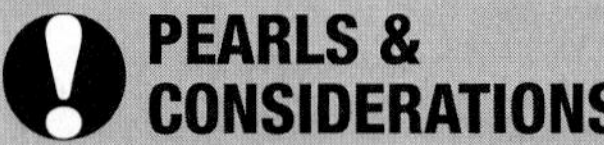

PEARLS & CONSIDERATIONS

Many narcoleptics report the onset of symptoms beginning in childhood to early adulthood, with a long delay of actual diagnosis on the order of 10 to 15 yr. Typically, excessive daytime sleepiness is the initial symptom, followed by REM dysregulation (e.g., cataplexy, sleep paralysis, hypnagogic hallucinations). Patients with narcolepsy also have higher than expected incidence of other sleep disorders, including obstructive sleep apnea, periodic limb movements of sleep, and REM sleep behavior disorder.

COMMENTS

Narcolepsy is a rare disorder that is underdiagnosed. The average time from onset of symptoms to diagnosis is 5 to 15 yr. Cataplexy is specific for narcolepsy, but other symptoms of REM dysregulation, including sleep paralysis and hypnagogic or hypnopompic hallucinations, can occur even in normal patients. Sleep-onset REM or REM periods on an MSLT may occur as a result of sleep deprivation or withdrawal from REM-suppressing drugs.

SUGGESTED READINGS

Available at ExpertConsult.com

RELATED CONTENT

Narcolepsy (Patient Information)

AUTHOR: **DON HAYES JR., M.D., M.S., M.ED.**

BASIC INFORMATION

DEFINITION

Necrotizing fasciitis (NF) is a rapidly spreading bacterial infection of the deep fascia, with associated inflammation, leading to necrosis of subcutaneous tissue planes. This infection can occur in wounds from trauma or surgical wounds or can be spontaneous or idiopathic. There are two clinical types, both of which carry a high rate of morbidity and mortality.

SYNONYMS

NF
Soft tissue gangrene
Flesh-eating bacteria
Fournier's gangrene
Hemolytic streptococcal gangrene

ICD-10CM CODE
M72.6 Necrotizing fasciitis

EPIDEMIOLOGY & DEMOGRAPHICS

PREDOMINANT SEX: Male > female.
PREDOMINANT AGE: 6 to 50 yr; less common in children.

EPIDEMIOLOGY

Invasive group A *Streptococcus* infection occurs at a rate of 3.5 cases per 100,000 persons, with a case fatality rate of around 24%.

PHYSICAL FINDINGS & CLINICAL PRESENTATION

CLINICAL TYPES OF NECROTIZING FASCIITIS:

- Type I: Necrotizing fasciitis: At least one anaerobic species is isolated in conjunction with one or more facultative anaerobic species, such as streptococci (not group A), *and* members of the Enterobacteriaceae (Gram negative rods)
- Anaerobic bacteria, most commonly *Bacteroides* or *Peptostreptococcus* spp.
- Enterobacteriaceae: *Escherichia coli*, *Klebsiella* spp., *Proteus* spp., *Enterobacter* spp.
- Usually associated with diabetes or peripheral vascular disease
- Example of type I: Fournier gangrene of the perineum
- Type II: Necrotizing fasciitis: Group A *Streptococcus* is isolated alone or in combination with other bacteria, most likely *Staphylococcus aureus.* Also known as hemolytic streptococcal gangrene
  1. Example of type II: Invasive group A *Streptococcus*, associated with virulence factors type 1 and type 3 M protein

EXAMPLES OF NECROTIZING FASCIITIS:

- Fournier gangrene: Aggressive type I infection of the perineum usually caused by penetration of the gastrointestinal or urethral mucosa by enteric organisms. It can rapidly spread to involve the scrotum, penis, and abdominal wall or gluteal muscles, causing gangrene.
- Clostridial cellulitis: Caused by *Clostridium perfringens* associated with local trauma or surgery and crepitus caused by gas production; generally noted in the skin, with deeper tissues generally spared.

PHYSICAL FINDINGS

Minor skin trauma, toxic-appearing patient:

- Open skin wound
- Severe pain at injury or surgical site
- Fever, confusion, weakness, diarrhea
- Early skin erythema, quickly spreading in hours to days
- Skin redness changes to purple discoloration
- Gangrenous skin changes may develop
- Loosening of skin and subcutaneous skin in association with deep fascial necrosis (Fig. 1). "Woody" induration and crepitus of involved area are characteristics
- Muscle involvement, thrombosis of blood vessels, and myonecrosis may develop
- Bullae and gas formation at site

ETIOLOGY

- NF usually arises from skin damage or trauma. Risk is increased with presence of comorbidities (DM, cancer, liver disease, immunosuppression)
- Polymicrobial: Mixture of anaerobes and aerobic enteric gram-negative rods
- Group A streptococci *(S. pyogenes)*
- *S. aureus*
- *C. perfringens*
- *Bacteroides fragilis*
- *Vibrio vulnificus*
- Methicillin-resistant *S. aureus* (MRSA), especially community-acquired MRSA

DIAGNOSIS

DIFFERENTIAL DIAGNOSIS

- Cellulitis.
- Pyomyositis.
- Gas gangrene.
- A classification of necrotizing skin, soft-tissue, and muscle infections is described in Table 1.

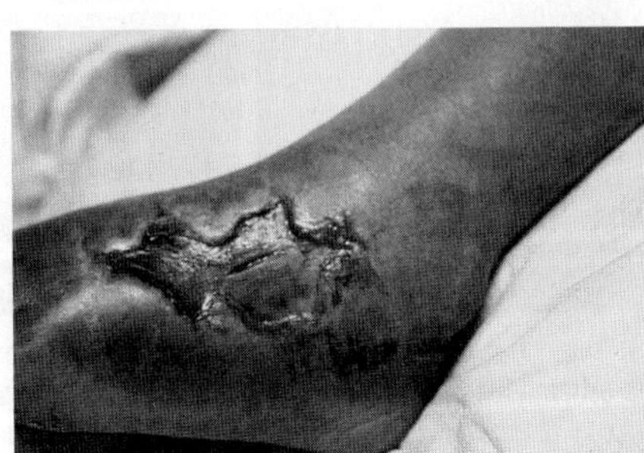

FIG. 1 Necrotizing fasciitis. The so-called flesh-eating bacteria, group A β-hemolytic Streptococcus, can cause significant tissue destruction rapidly. This 32-year-old woman had pain, erythema, and swelling of the foot followed by necrotic ulceration over a week. There was no history of trauma. (Courtesy Roger Bitar, MD. From White GM, Cox NH [eds]: *Diseases of the skin, a color atlas and text,* ed 2, St Louis, 2006, Mosby.)

WORKUP

- Diagnosis of necrotizing fasciitis generally requires incision and probing. In patients with necrotizing fasciitis, there is no resistance to probing subcutaneously, and there is fascial plane involvement.
- Laboratory tests:
  1. The laboratory risk indicator for necrotizing fasciitis (LRINEC) consists of the following 6 variables. When present the reported positive predictive value is 92%: Complete blood cell count (CBC) with differential (leukocytosis [WBC >15,000], anemia [Hb <13.5]), elevated CRP (≥15 mg/dl), hyponatremia (sodium <135 mEq/L), elevated creatinine (>1.6 mg/dl), hyperglycemia (glucose >180 mg/dl).
  2. Cultures of skin, soft tissue, or debrided tissue, aerobically and anaerobically. Blood cultures are positive in 60% of patients with type II infections and 20% with type I infections.
- Imaging:
  1. Radiographs may show subcutaneous gas in fascial planes (Fig. 2).
  2. Computed tomography (CT) or magnetic resonance imaging (MRI) may be helpful because they can detect gas in the tissues. MRI with contrast is more sensitive than CT.

TREATMENT

- Aggressive surgical debridement of involved necrotic tissues is essential *as soon as possible* to reduce mortality.
- Fasciotomies of extremities may be necessary.
- Immediate start of empiric antibiotics:
  1. Type I: Vancomycin, daptomycin, or linezolid plus piperacillin/tazobactam; a carbapenem (such as imipenem, meropenem, or doripenem); and third-generation cephalosporin + metronidazole or a fluroquinolone plus metronidazole (ceftriaxone) are reasonable choices pending cultures. Empiric clindamycin may also be added to suppress toxin production by staphylococci and streptococci. It is important to always have anaerobic coverage. Use the highest dosages possible for age and CrCl.
  2. Type II: For group A *Streptococcus*, give intravenous (IV) penicillin G, 4 million U q4h in patients who weigh >60 kg with clindamycin, 600 to 900 mg IV q8h.
     a. Clindamycin has the added effect of suppressing toxin production. If MRSA is suspected, add vancomycin, daptomycin, or linezolid.
- Intravenous gammaglobulin (IVIG): 1 g/kg on day 1 and 0.5 g/kg on days 2 and 3 neutralizes circulating streptococcal toxins and has been shown beneficial in severe forms of invasive group A streptococcal infections, although data are not definitive.

TABLE 1 Classification of Necrotizing Skin, Soft-Tissue, and Muscle Infections

Disease	Bacteriology	Comments
Necrotizing Cellulitis		
Clostridial cellulitis	*Clostridium perfringens*	Local trauma, recent surgery; fascial/deep muscle spared
Nonclostridial cellulitis	Mixed: *Escherichia coli, Enterobacter, Peptostreptococcus* spp., *Bacteroides fragilis*	Diabetes mellitus predisposes; produces foul odor
Meleney synergistic gangrene	*Staphylococcus aureus,* microaerophilic streptococci	Rare infection; postoperative; slowly expanding, indolent, ulceration in superficial fascia
Synergistic necrotizing cellulitis	Mixed aerobic and anaerobic, including *B. fragilis, Peptostreptococcus* spp.	Diabetes mellitus predisposes; variant of necrotizing fasciitis type I; involves skin, muscle, fat, and fascia
Necrotizing Fasciitis		
Type I	Mixed aerobic and anaerobic; staphylococci, *B. fragilis, E. coli,* group A streptococci, *Peptostreptococcus* spp., *Prevotella, Porphyromonas* spp., *Clostridium* spp.	Usually requires a breach in the mucous membrane layer either through surgery or penetrating injuries or from chronic medical conditions such as diabetes, peripheral vascular disease, malignancy, and anal fissures
Type II	Group A streptococci	Increasing in frequency and severity since 1985; very high mortality; often begins at site of nonpenetrating minor trauma such as a bruise or muscle strain but often no identified precursor Predisposing factors: Blunt/penetrating trauma, varicella (chickenpox), lintravenous drug abuse, surgical procedures, childbirth, nonsteroidal antiinflammatory drug use
Myonecrosis		
Clostridial myonecrosis	*Clostridium* spp.	Predisposing factors: Deep/penetrating injury, bowel and biliary tract surgery, improperly performed abortion and retained placenta, prolonged rupture of the membranes, and intrauterine fetal demise or missed abortion in postpartum patients. Recurrent gas gangrene occurs at sites of previous gas gangrene.
Streptococcal myonecrosis	Streptococci	
Special Type of Necrotizing Soft-Tissue Infection		
Fournier gangrene	Polymicrobial, with *E. coli* the predominant aerobe and *Bacteroides* the predominant anaerobe. Other microflora: *Proteus, Staphylococcus, Enterococcus,* aerobic and anaerobic *Streptococcus, Pseudomonas, Klebsiella,* and *Clostridium*	Necrosis of the scrotum or perineum that starts with scrotal pain and erythema and rapidly spreads onto anterior abdominal wall and gluteal muscle. It is more often seen in diabetics and can be associated with trauma.

From Vincent JL, et al.: *Textbook of critical care,* ed 6, Philadelphia, 2011, Saunders.

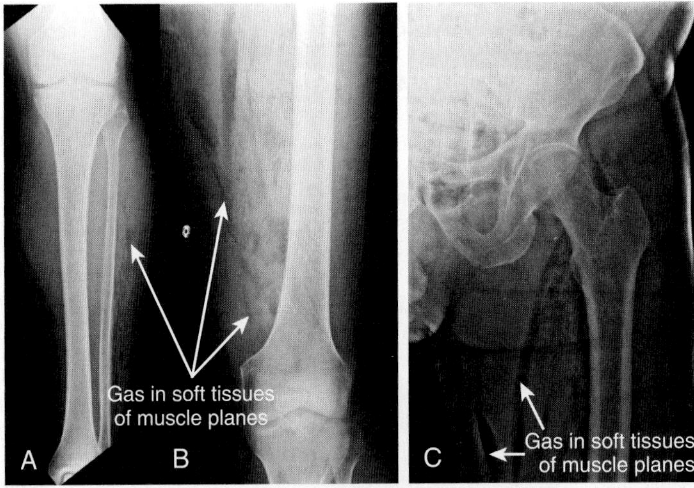

FIG. 2 Necrotizing fasciitis. This 71-year-old man with aplastic anemia presented with fevers to 38.9° C (102.02° F), leg weakness, and extreme leg pain. Initially, the patient was thought to have neuropathic pain and weakness, possibly indicating spinal disease such as epidural abscess. He rapidly developed crepitus of his legs. Radiographs of the patient's legs were obtained, followed by noncontrast CT. **A,** Anterior-posterior (AP) tibia and fibula. **B,** AP femur. **C,** AP hip. Air is seen dissecting in muscle planes of the legs. On radiograph, air appears black. Given the wide distribution of air, a focal abscess is unlikely, and necrotizing fasciitis with gas-producing organisms should be suspected. (From Broder JS: *Diagnostic imaging for the emergency physician,* Philadelphia, 2011, Saunders.)

- For *Vibrio vulnificus* use doxycycline plus ceftazidime; for *Aeromonas hydrophila* use doxycycline plus ciprofloxacin.
- Hyperbaric oxygen evaluation as an adjunct to surgery and IV antibiotics.

SUGGESTED READINGS

Available at ExpertConsult.com

AUTHOR: **GLENN G. FORT, M.D., M.P.H.**

BASIC INFORMATION

DEFINITION

Nephrotic syndrome is characterized by heavy proteinuria (usually defined as >3.5 g/24 hr), hypoalbuminemia, hyperlipidemia, lipiduria, and edema. Nephrotic-range proteinuria can have many causes that share a common mechanism of glomerular injury leading to proteinuria, with proteinuria constituted primarily as albuminuria due to glomerular damage. Patients with this degree of proteinuria may not have other features of the syndrome.

ICD-10CM CODES

N04.9	Nephrotic syndrome with unspecified morphologic changes
N04.0	Nephrotic syndrome with minor glomerular abnormality
N04.1	Nephrotic syndrome with focal and segmental glomerular lesions
N04.2	Nephrotic syndrome with diffuse membranous glomerulonephritis
N04.3	Nephrotic syndrome with diffuse mesangial proliferative glomerulonephritis
N04.4	Nephrotic syndrome with diffuse endocapillary proliferative glomerulonephritis
N04.5	Nephrotic syndrome with diffuse mesangiocapillary glomerulonephritis
N04.6	Nephrotic syndrome with dense deposit disease
N04.7	Nephrotic syndrome with diffuse crescentic glomerulonephritis
N04.8	Nephrotic syndrome with other morphologic changes

EPIDEMIOLOGY & DEMOGRAPHICS

- Among children (especially <6 yr of age), the most common causes of nephrotic syndrome are:
  1. Minimal change disease (MCD) (75% of pediatric cases)
  2. Focal and segmental glomerulosclerosis (FSGS) (7% to 20% of cases)
- Among adults, FSGS is the most common primary cause of nephrotic-range proteinuria. Membranous nephropathy is the second most common primary cause of nephrotic syndrome. FSGS is more common in persons of African ancestry, and membranous nephropathy is seen more commonly in Caucasians. Overall, diabetic nephropathy remains the most common cause of nephrotic-range proteinuria.

PHYSICAL FINDINGS & CLINICAL PRESENTATION

- Patients usually present with severe lower extremity, periorbital edema, and weight gain.
- Ascites and anasarca may occur.
- Hypercoagulability (i.e., pulmonary embolism and risk of infection (i.e., pneumococcal infection) are potential clinical manifestations.
- Pediatric patients are at risk for infections due to urinary immunoglobulin loss.

ETIOLOGY

Glomerular diseases can be thought of as diseases affecting one of five elements that comprise the renal corpuscle: endothelium, basement membrane, podocyte, mesangium, or parietal epithelium. In general, disorders that involve the endothelium and/or mesangial compartment activate inflammatory mediators. Disorders that exclusively affect the basement membrane or podocyte generally have a noninflammatory pathology. Structural integrity abnormalities in each of these cases lead to a breach of the normal mechanisms that prevent abnormal filtration, leading to proteinuria as primarily albuminuria, the hallmark of glomerular disease.

Traditionally, the clinical correlate to this pathological schema has been a subdivision of patients into those with a nephrotic versus nephritic presentation. Disorders that are considered "nephritic" have subnephrotic proteinuria and low glomerular filtration rates. "Nephrotic" disorders have greater proteinuria and more robust glomerular filtration rates. While generally true, this schema may cause diagnostic confusion because nephritic disease may present with nephrotic-range proteinuria, *especially earlier in the disease course before glomerular filtration is substantially reduced.* It is better to categorize these diseases with a noninflammatory urine sediment (proteinuria alone with no casts or cellular elements) versus an inflammatory sediment (i.e., RBC casts and/or dysmorphic RBCs in conjunction with proteinuria).

Fig. 1 details this breakdown. In this chapter, we focus on primary diseases that present with a noninflammatory sediment (namely, minimal change disease, focal segmental glomerulosclerosis, membranous nephropathy, and amyloidosis) and on primary disorder with inflammatory sediment often with nephrotic-range proteinuria, membranoproliferative glomerulonephritis (MPGN). The evaluation of "nephritic syndrome" is noted by worsening GFR in the setting of proteinuria and hematuria as detailed elsewhere. Important points regarding the most common etiologies of nephrotic syndrome are detailed in the following text (Table 1).

- MCD has a bland urine sediment with abrupt onset of disease and abrupt remission. Proteinuria may exceed 20 grams daily. Nonsteroidal anti-inflammatory drug (NSAID) use, lithium use, viral infections, and lymphomas are associated with secondary forms of MCD.
- FSGS, primary or secondary: Primary FSGS denotes an idiopathic cause that typically manifests with heavy proteinuria and nephrotic syndrome, and requires immunosuppressive therapy. FSGS is more prevalent in persons of African ancestry. Secondary FSGS is caused by a known etiology, including heroin use, sickle cell disease, scarring of any kind from prior injury, obesity, low nephron mass, HIV, etc. Most cases of

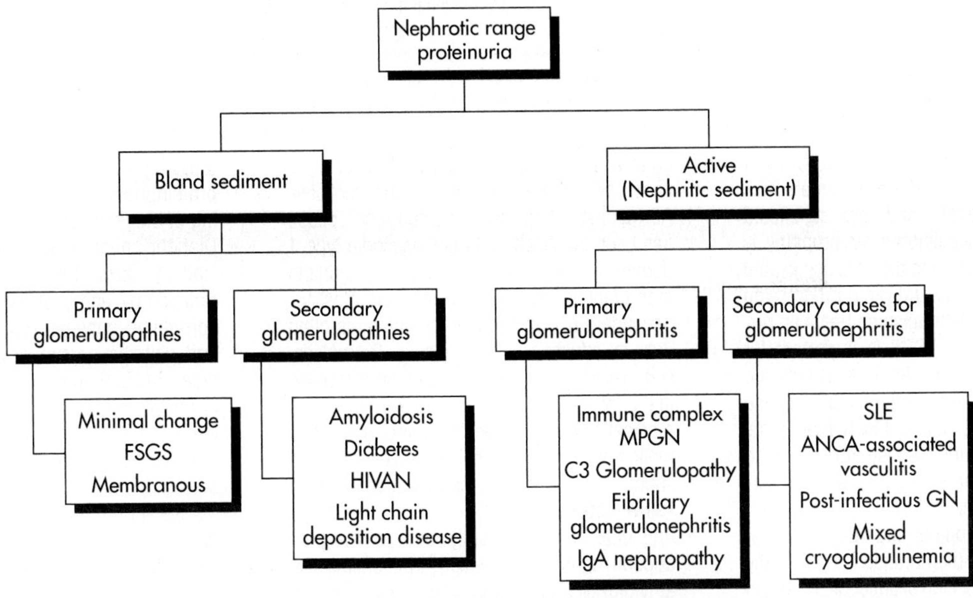

FIG. 1 An approach to nephrotic-range proteinuria.

TABLE 1 Important Clinical, Serological, and Pathological Features of Selected Diseases Causing Nephrotic Syndrome

Disease	Important Clinical Features	Serological Features	Pathological Features
Minimal change disease	Rapid onset with heavy proteinuria and rapid remission with therapy. True steroid resistance is rare and should prompt repeat biopsy to rule out FSGS.	Complements are normal.	Light microscopy (LM) shows completely normal kidney architecture. Immunofluorescence microscopy: Normal. Electron microscopy (EM): Diffuse podocyte effacement.
Primary FSGS	Often heavier proteinuria and low serum albumin and edema. Tip lesion subtype and collapsing FSGS often have more explosive onset. Sediment usually bland, but RBCs can be seen. Usually no cellular casts.	Complements are normal.	LM: Only one glomerulus need show features of FSGS to make diagnosis. Immunofluorescence microscopy: Often devoid of immunoglobulin, although IgM can be seen. EM: Often has diffuse podocyte effacement.
Secondary FSGS	Proteinuria is often subnephrotic, or if nephrotic, serum albumin levels are maintained. Minimal edema.	HIV and parvovirus infection can cause phenotype identical to idiopathic collapsing FSGS.	LM: Often shows evidence of glomerulomegaly. EM: Foot process effacement is less diffuse.
Primary membranous nephropathy	Often seen in older Caucasian patients. More likely than other forms of nephrotic syndrome to be associated with thrombotic complications Sediment: Bland. RBCs can be found, although RBC casts are usually found.	Serum antiphospholipase A2 receptor antibodies are found in 70% of patients with idiopathic primary membranous nephropathy. Antineutral endopeptidase antibodies are found in a minority of others.	LM: Characterized by thickening of the GBM; "spikes" can be seen on silver stain. Immunofluorescence microscopy: C3 and IgG noted in granular pattern. Newer techniques stain for antiphospholipase A2 receptor antibody in situ. EM: Associated with subepithelial deposits.
Secondary membranous nephropathy	Associated with **malignancy,** lupus, syphilis, hepatitis B and C, medications (gold, captopril, penicillamine, etc.).	Notable for the absence of antiphospholipase A2 antibodies. ANA, hepatitis B, HCV serologies are helpful. RPR can be sent in context of appropriate history.	Morphology is exactly the same except when examined by EM. On high power, one sees both subendothelial and mesangial deposits in addition to classic subepithelial deposits.
Amyloidosis	Often found with massive proteinuria. Kidney size is enlarged. Bland sediment.	UPEP, SPEP, serum free light chains may be positive. The UPEP will show glomerular proteinuria, which can help differentiate from myeloma kidney.	LM: Often notable for nodular pattern. Diagnosis can be made by staining using Congo red or thioflavin T. Immunofluorescence microscopy: Antibody use can differentiate AA from AL amyloid. EM: Shows characteristic random 10-nm fibrils.
Diabetes	Often associated with nephrotic-range proteinuria in the setting of retinopathy. Kidney sizes are preserved.	No specific serologic tests are positive.	LM: Nodular pattern often seen, thickened GBM.
MPGN	Often associated with nephrotic-range proteinuria with a "nephritic" sediment. RBC casts often seen along with dysmorphic RBC.	C3 and C4 are often low in immune complex MPGN. Immune complex GN warrants checking SPEP and UPEP, as gammopathy is associated with MPGN. Hepatitis B, HCV, ANA, and cryoglobulins are also warranted. C3 alone is low in dense deposit disease and C3 glomerulonephritis, which may prompt specific tests for complement dysregulation.	The key point here is to look at the IF. If immunofluorescence shows both immunoglobulin and complement deposition, the diagnosis is immune complex MGPN. If only complement, the diagnosis is most likely C3 glomerulopathy (either dense deposit disease or C3 glomerulonephritis).

ANA; Anti-nuclear antibody; *FSGS;* focal and segmental glomerulosclerosis; *GBM;* glomerular basement membrane; *GN;* glomerulonephritis; *HCV;* hepatitis C virus; *Ig;* immunoglobulin; *MPGN;* membranoproliferative glomerulonephritis; *RBC,* red blood cell; *RPR;* rapid plasma reagin; *SPEP;* serum protein electrophoresis; *UPEP;* urine protein electrophoresis.

secondary FSGS are associated with lower levels of proteinuria (often subnephrotic), higher albumin levels, and less significant edema (e.g., HIV-associated nephropathy is an important exception in that it is associated with heavy proteinuria and rapid progression when untreated). Distinguishing between primary and secondary FSGS is important for therapy (see following text). It should be noted that prior kidney injury can produce morphological features of FSGS over time. Essentially, proteinuric disease attributable to secondary FSGS can be seen in any progressive kidney disease.

- Membranous nephropathy may be primary or secondary. Primary membranous nephropathy is due to in situ deposition of antibodies directed against a glomerular antigen (in 70% or more cases, the epitope is identified as phospholipase A2 receptor). A second, less-common epitope has been identified as thrombospondin type-1 domain-containing 7A (THSD7A). Proteinuria in membranous nephropathy may be massive. Secondary membranous nephropathy is often due to infection (e.g., hepatitis B, malaria, schistosomiasis, syphilis), autoimmune disease (e.g., systemic lupus erythematosus [SLE]), medications (e.g., D-penicillamine, gold), and malignancies. Distinguishing between the two subtypes is important for management (see following text).
- Amyloidosis is frequently due to overproduction of immunoglobulin light chains (AL amyloid) or a chronic inflammatory state (AA amyloid). Kidney size is often enlarged, and proteinuria may be massive. Congo red staining of amyloid establishes the diagnosis.
- Diabetic nephropathy is often characterized by slowly progressive proteinuria with retinopathy and preserved kidney size. The correlation between retinopathy, proteinuria, and diabetic nephropathy is very strong in type 1 diabetic patients, and kidney biopsies are usually not done. The relationship is less strong in type 2 diabetes, and absence of retinopathy does not preclude a diagnosis of diabetic nephropathy.
- Membranoproliferative glomerulonephritis (MPGN) is usually from immune complex deposition with complement, or activation of the alternate complement system without

immune complex formation (e.g., C3 glomerulopathy). Prior classification schema involving types 1, 2, and 3 MGPN are now deemed obsolete after better understanding of the pathophysiology of this morphology. Common immune complex causes are from infections (e.g., hepatitis C), autoimmune disorders (e.g., SLE), or dysproteinemias (e.g., monoclonal gammopathies). Distinguishing between these possibilities guides therapy. The urine is associated with heavy proteinuria. Urinary sediment often contains dysmorphic erythrocytes and erythrocyte casts, and is also associated with heavy proteinuria.

Dx DIAGNOSIS

DIFFERENTIAL DIAGNOSIS

- Other states that present with edema (CHF, cirrhosis, protein-losing enteropathy, severe malnutrition)
- Glomerulonephritis from disorders commonly associated with inflammatory urinary sediment and glomerular inflammation.
- Mimickers of glomerulonephritis (malignant HTN, preeclampsia, antiphospholipid syndrome)

WORKUP

- Evaluation includes determining the rate of change of serum creatinine, quantification of proteinuria by 24-hr collection, and manual of the urinary sediment examination.
- Bland urinary sediment and proteinuria >3.5 g/24 hr should prompt nephrology consultation.
- Serologic tests of use may be urine and serum electrophoresis, human immune HIV, hepatitis B surface antigen, hepatitis C virus (HCV) antibody, and antinuclear antibody (ANA). As urinary sediment examination is not 100% sensitive in ruling out an inflammatory process, C3 and C4 can be checked, as complement levels are often low in many inflammatory glomerulonephritides and often low in MPGN. Low complement levels may change the nature of the differential diagnosis before kidney biopsy. Depending on practice patterns, these tests are used selectively before or (in some cases) after biopsy to better define an etiology.
- A newer serological test available to clinicians commercially is an antiphospholipase A2 receptor antibody (anti-PLA2r) titer. This test is associated with the development of primary membranous nephropathy but *not* secondary membranous nephropathy. If present, primary membranous nephropathy can suggest a potential diagnosis, determine the need for immunosuppressive therapy (as opposed to merely treating the underlying disease with secondary membranous nephropathy), and potentially allows the practitioner to establish a baseline titer value prior to therapy (to monitor efficacy). As titers correlate with disease activity and usually decrease well before a decrement in proteinuria, using this commercially available test may allow for a decrease in the intensity of immunosuppression and potential side effects. These tests, along with targeted therapy (i.e., rituximab), may soon result in more patient-tailored rather than generic immunosuppressive protocols. Ultimately, given that clinical acumen cannot reliably distinguish between various etiologies, a kidney biopsy is usually required, except in very young children where there is a very high likelihood of MCD, or in adults if contraindications are present (coagulopathy).
- Patients should also have a renal ultrasound to document the presence of two kidneys before kidney biopsy is attempted and kidney size is documented.

TABLE 2 Important Definitions in Dealing with Treatment of Primary Nephrotic Syndrome

	Adults	Children
Definition		
Complete Remission	Reduction in proteinuria to <0.3 g/24 hours	<4 mg/m^2/hr on at least 3 occasions within 7 days and serum albumin >3.5 g/dl
Partial Remission	Reduction in proteinuria between 0.3 g/24 hours and 3.5 g daily with ≥50% decrease in proteinuria from baseline	Disappearance of edema, increase in serum albumin >3.5 g/dl, and persistent proteinuria >4 mg mg/m^2/hr or >100 mg mg/m^2/hr
Relapse*	Increase in proteinuria to >3.5 g daily after one month of complete or partial remission	Urine dipstick 3+ or proteinuria >40 mg/m^2/hr occurring on 3 days within 1 week
Steroid Dependent*	Two consecutive relapses occurring during therapy or within 14 days of completing therapy	Two relapses of proteinuria within 14 days after stopping or during alternate-day steroid therapy
Steroid Resistant*	Persistence of proteinuria without significant reduction despite prednisone therapy at 1 mg/kg for 16 wk	Persistence of proteinuria despite prednisone therapy at 60 mg/m^2 for 4 wk

*These definitions only truly apply to diseases such as minimal change disease and FSGS.
Adapted from Cattran DC, et al.: Cyclosporine in idiopathic glomerular disease associated with the nephrotic syndrome: workshop recommendations, *Kidney Int* 72(12):1429-1447, 2007, and *KDIGO clinical practice guidelines for glomerulonephritis.*

Rx TREATMENT

NONIMMUNOSUPPRESSIVE THERAPY

- Control of proteinuria is key to mitigating risk of progression. Almost all trials of nondiabetic chronic kidney disease demonstrate that reducing proteinuria improves renal survival. Angiotensin–converting-enzyme inhibitors or angiotensin II receptor blockers should be used at maximally tolerated doses, except in MCD, where it is not usually given due to complete response. Dual angiotensin–converting-enzyme inhibitor and angiotensin II receptor blocker therapy is generally not recommended due to increased risks of hyperkalemia and elevating the serum creatinine. Non-dihydropyridine calcium channel blockers (verapamil and diltiazem) can be used to in lieu of angiotensin-converting enzyme inhibitors, angiotensin II receptor blockers when the latter are contraindicated.
- For proteinuria >1 gram per day, target blood pressure is <125/75 mm Hg.
- With the exception of MCD, patients with nephrotic-range proteinuria and hyperlipidemia should be treated with HMG CoA synthetase inhibitors (statins).
- Although some patients with nephrotic syndrome are hypercoagulable (particularly patients with membranous nephropathy), the role of prophylactic anticoagulation is not well-defined and controversial. For patients with membranous nephropathy and serum albumin levels <2.0 g/dl, anticoagulation should be considered if bleeding risk is low.
- Low sodium diet (<2 gram per day) with diuretics.
- Diuretic resistance is common due to gut wall edema and hypoalbuminemia. More bioavailable diuretics (bumetanide, torsemide) may increase urine output better than furosemide, along with thiazide diuretics.
- To prevent "diuretic braking," most loop diuretics should be dosed at least on a twice-daily basis (with the exception of torsemide, which can be given once daily).

IMMUNOSUPPRESSIVE THERAPY

In general, immunosuppressive therapy is dictated by the identified disorder. Important terms in dealing with the management of nephrotic-range proteinuria due to primary glomerular diseases are listed in Table 2. First-line therapies for each disease are highlighted in the following.

- MCD: First-line therapy in adults is prednisone (1 mg/kg per day to a maximum of 80 mg per day) for a minimum of 4 wk and maximum of 16 wk. Steroids are tapered over 6 mo for favorable responses. Second-line options include cyclophosphamide and/or cyclosporine. Newer, randomized, controlled trial data from children (not adults) have suggested an impressive record for rituximab in steroid-dependent patients unable to be weaned off steroids without inducing relapse and frequently relapsing MCD. Consequently, rituximab may become a reasonable option for patients who do not respond to conventional therapy.

- FSGS: Primary FSGS is often treated with high-dose prednisone (maximum, 80 mg daily in adults) for 6 mo. Alternative regimens include low-dose prednisone with cyclosporine. Mycophenolate mofetil (MMF) has also been used with success in primary FSGS. Newer therapies that have been tried in pilot settings have included exogenous adrenocorticotropic hormone (ACTH) as well as abatacept. While efficacious in some patients, randomized, controlled trials have not verified these initial results. Therefore, these treatments cannot be recommended as initial therapy currently. A new, randomized, controlled trial aims to examine whether a novel agent that blocks endothelin-1 and angiotensin II receptors (RE-021) has efficacy in treatment of primary FSGS. Treatment of secondary FSGS is based on arresting the underlying cause and nonspecific therapy with blockade of the renin-angiotensin-aldosterone system. Immunosuppression is avoided.
- Membranous nephropathy: Suggested first-line therapy for primary membranous nephropathy involves the intravenous methylprednisolone and oral cyclophosphamide (chlorambucil). Alternative therapy includes low-dose prednisone with cyclosporine or tacrolimus alone for at least one year. Rituximab may become more commonly used as first-line therapy in the coming years. A novel therapy that can be used is a synthetic depot formulation of ACTH. ACTH may exert effects on the podocyte independent of stimulation of endogenous cortisol production. Given conflicting reports from the U.S. and Europe, exogenous ACTH can be viewed as a last-line resort when all other options have failed, but it is not the standard of care. Therapy for secondary membranous nephropathy is directed at treating the underlying cause (malignancy, SLE, etc.).
- Treatment of amyloidosis, diabetes, and immune complex MPGN is directed at the underlying disorder. In rapidly progressive HCV-related MPGN, immunosuppressive therapy with rituximab or glucocorticoids and cyclophosphamide can be administered during HCV therapy.
- More recently, reclassification of MPGN has shown that some forms of MPGN are caused by alternative complement cascade activation (C3 glomerulonephritis). There is renewed interest in exploiting medications (e.g., eculizumab) that target the end product of this pathway (membrane attack complex). Prior non-targeted approaches (e.g., steroids) for MPGN have been largely unsuccessful except in selected pediatric cases.

REFERRAL

Nephrology consultation is recommended for all cases of nephrotic syndrome.

PEARLS & CONSIDERATIONS

- Proteinuria >2 gram per day generally implies glomerular disease unless multiple myeloma is present. The urine protein electropheresis defines the type(s) of proteins excreted: albumin, immunoglobulins, and tubular.
- Massive proteinuria (>20 g per day) is rarely seen with inflammatory diseases and generally indicates MCD, FSGS, membranous nephropathy, or amyloidosis.
- Partial remissions and steroid resistance are rarely seen in primary minimal change disease. These circumstances mandate reexamination of the cause of nephrotic syndrome because repeat biopsy in these cases often demonstrates FSGS.
- Quantification of proteinuria should be done with a 24-hr urine collection with evaluation of urinary creatinine excretion to document validity of the collection. Spot collections have not been validated for heavy proteinuria or patients with rapidly changing creatinine values. A "spot" urine protein-to-creatinine ratio taken from the 24-hr collection defines the relationship between spot and "true" collections to monitor response to therapy.
- Most noninflammatory processes progress slowly. If a sediment without red blood cell casts is detected with a rapidly increasing serum creatinine and heavy proteinuria, the differential is relatively narrow:
  1. MCD and acute interstitial nephritis, as occurs with nonsteroidal anti-inflammatory drug administration
  2. Nephrotic syndrome associated with acute tubular necrosis from hypovolemia
  3. Bilateral renal vein thrombosis superimposed on nephrotic syndrome
  4. Myeloma cast nephropathy
  5. Collapsing FSGS/HIV-associated nephropathy

SUGGESTED READINGS

Available at ExpertConsult.com

RELATED CONTENT

Nephrotic Syndrome (Patient Information)

AUTHORS: **ALISON GRAZIOLI, M.D.,** and **SANJEEV R. SHAH, M.D.**

BASIC INFORMATION

DEFINITION

The American Psychiatric Association's *Diagnostic and Statistical Manual of Mental Disorders,* 5th edition (DSM-5), includes delirium and major and mild neurocognitive disorders, as well as their subtypes, under the grouping *neurocognitive disorders.*

The core features of neurocognitive disorders (NCDs) are deficits in cognitive function. The cognitive dysfunction is acquired rather than developmental and thus represents a decline from a previously attained level of functioning. The NCDs are subtyped according to known or presumed etiologic/pathologic entities underlying the decline. The subtypes may be distinguished by clinical characteristics such as time course, physical examination, and cognitive domains affected. It is possible for more than one NCD to be identified in a given patient at a given time.

In major and mild NCDs, the cognitive deficits are present in one or more cognitive domains. The initial evidence is based on concern brought forth by the patient, a knowledgeable informant, or the clinician and is often supported by performance on objective standardized assessments such as neuropsychological testing. In major NCDs, the deficits interfere with independence in everyday activity, whereas in minor NCDs, the impairment is more modest and does not interfere with capacity for independence in everyday activity.

In the DSM-5, *delirium* is subsumed under the category *neurocognitive disorders.* Although it shares the core feature of acquired deficit in cognitive function, it is discussed as a distinct entity from major and minor neurocognitive disorders and is discussed separately in this text. The DSM-IV term *dementia* is subsumed under the entity *major neurocognitive disorder* in the DSM-5, and the DSM-IV term *amnestic disorder* and its subtypes are subsumed under the category *major neurocognitive disorder due to another medical condition* in the DSM-5.

Some of the more commonly seen NCDs include major or mild NCD due to Alzheimer's disease, major or mild vascular NCD, and major or mild NCD due to Lewy body disease.

ICD-10CM CODES:

F02.81 Major or mild neurocognitive disorder, with behavior disturbance

F02.80 Major or mild neurocognitive disorder, without behavior disturbance

DSM-5 CODES:

294.10 Major or mild neurocognitive disorder, without behavior disturbance

294.11 Major or mild neurocognitive disorder, with behavior disturbance

EPIDEMIOLOGY & DEMOGRAPHICS

The prevalence varies depending on the etiology of the neurocognitive disorder and age of the patient. Among patients >60 yr, the prevalence tends to increase sharply for the most common neurocognitive disorders. Overall prevalence estimates for major NCDs are approximately 1% to 2% at 65 yr old and as high as 30% at 85 yr. Mild NCD prevalence is variable, ranging from 2%-10% at age 65 and 5% to 25% at age 85. The strongest risk factor for major and mild NCD is age. Female gender is associated with a higher prevalence in major and mild NCD due to Alzheimer's disease.

PHYSICAL FINDINGS & CLINICAL PRESENTATION

Neurocognitive domains that are affected in NCDs include:

- Complex attention, including sustained attention, divided attention, selective attention, and processing speed.
- Executive functioning, such as planning, decision making, working memory, and mental flexibility.
- Learning and memory, including immediate memory, recent memory.
- Language expression and reception, including word recall, grammar, and syntax.
- Perceptual motor skills, including visual construction, praxis, and gnosis.
- Social cognition, including recognition of emotions.

Associated physical findings, time course of illness, and response to treatment depend on etiology of the NCD. Mood disturbance, psychosis, and behavior disturbances are recognized as common neuropsychiatric symptoms associated with NCDs. Mood symptoms are common early in the course of NCDs due to Alzheimer's disease, NCD with Lewy bodies, and vascular NCD. Psychoses, including delusions and paranoia, may present across the spectrum of illness but are more common in mild to moderate stages of NCD with Lewy bodies and in moderate to severe stages of NCD due to Alzheimer's disease. Psychosis, agitation, and other behavioral disturbances lead to increased rate of hospitalization, early admission to assisted living environments or nursing homes, and increased level of caregiver depression and distress. Apathy manifests early in the course of NCDs and is the most common neuropsychiatric symptom of NCD due to Alzheimer's disease across the spectrum of the disease.

ASSOCIATED SIGNS AND SYMPTOMS BY ETIOLOGY

(For each etiology, the criteria are met for major or mild neurocognitive disorder.)

- **Major or mild neurocognitive disorder due to Alzheimer's disease:** Insidious onset and gradual progression, occasionally with brief plateaus. Impairment in memory, learning, and executive function are prominent early in the disease. In moderate to severe disease, language deficits manifest and problematic behaviors, including agitation, combativeness, and psychosis, may arise. Apathy, agitation, and psychosis are often more distressing to caregivers than the cognitive deficits.
- **Major or mild frontotemporal neurocognitive disorder:** Behavior and language variants are characterized by progressive development of personality changes, behavior changes including disinhibition, and/or language impairment. Patients with behavior variant may present with impaired insight, socially inappropriate behaviors, apathy, hyperorality, or compulsive behaviors. Learning and memory dysfunction may be spared in the early stages.
- **Major or mild neurocognitive disorder with Lewy bodies:** Cognitive decline occurs prior to or within 1 yr of the onset of parkinsonism motor symptoms. Recurrent, well-formed, and detailed visual hallucinations and fluctuating cognition that can resemble delirium are core features. Mood disturbances, autonomic dysfunction, and REM sleep disorder are suggestive of this diagnosis. Patients with major or mild neurocognitive disorder with Lewy bodies are sensitive to neuroleptics, which can often worsen symptoms and should be used with caution. Individuals with major or mild neurocognitive disorder with Lewy bodies are typically functionally more impaired than would be expected for their cognitive deficits because of the motor and autonomic impairments.
- **Major or mild neurocognitive disorder due to Parkinson's disease:** Parkinson's disease onset precedes the onset of major neurocognitive decline by at least 1 yr. Apathy, depression, hallucinations, and REM sleep disorder are suggestive of this diagnosis. The atypical parkinsonian syndrome progressive supranuclear palsy presents with early postural instability and retropulsion, supranuclear gaze palsy, and early cognitive impairment with depression, apathy, and anxiety. Corticobasal degeneration is a progressive asymmetric movement disorder with attentional deficits, slow processing speed, extreme rigidity, aphasia, apraxia, and alien-limb syndrome.
- **Major or mild vascular neurocognitive disorder:** The onset of cognitive decline is temporally related to one or more cerebrovascular events. The diagnosis is supported by neuroimaging evidence of parenchymal injury, including large vessel infarcts or hemorrhages, two or more lacunar infarcts outside the brainstem, or confluent white matter lesions attributed to cerebrovascular disease. Patients typically present with decline in processing speed, complex attention, and executive dysfunction. Stepwise and/or fluctuating decline is described. Prominent depression, apathy, and personality changes are common.
- **Major or mild neurocognitive disorder due to traumatic brain injury:** This NCD presents immediately after the occurrence of or can be attributed to a traumatic brain injury that causes loss of consciousness, posttraumatic amnesia, disorientation, or

neurologic signs such as seizure or hemiparesis. Cognitive presentation may be variable but may include difficulty with complex attention, executive dysfunction, or deficits in learning and memory. Associated findings include disturbances in emotional function and personality change. The features of major or mild NCD due to TBI vary by age of patient and specifics of the injury as well as other factors, such as premorbid functioning of the patient.

- **Substance/medication-induced major or mild neurocognitive disorder:** An NCD that persists beyond the duration of intoxication and acute withdrawal from a substance. NCD due to alcohol frequently manifests with memory, learning, and executive impairments. Wernicke syndrome is an acute neurologic disorder caused by thiamine deficiency manifesting with a clinic triad of encephalopathy, oculomotor dysfunction, and gait ataxia. Korsakoff syndrome is a late manifestation of Wernicke syndrome manifesting with dense anterograde amnesia and confabulation. MRI may show mammillary body atrophy. Major or mild NCD may be induced by medication or combinations of medications, including those with sedating and pain-ameliorating properties and those with anticholinergic properties. Particular attention should be paid to review of medications in any patient with major or mild NCD, especially those in the geriatric population.
- **Major or mild neurocognitive disorder due to HIV infection:** Neurocognitive deficits may show a subcortical pattern with prominent impairment of executive function with slowed processing speed and difficulty with learning new information.
- **Major or mild neurocognitive disorder due to Prion disease:** Neurocognitive deficits occur rapidly, typically over 6 mo. In some variants, prominent psychiatric symptoms such as depression and anxiety may occur prior to neurocognitive deficits. Ataxia, myoclonus, chorea, and a prominent startle reflex are typically present.
- **Major or mild neurocognitive disorder due to Huntington disease:** Early prominent changes in processing speed, organization, and planning rather than learning and memory are common. Behavior changes, changes in mood, anxiety, obsessive-compulsive symptoms, irritability, and apathy often precede motor symptoms.
- **Major or mild neurocognitive disorder due to another medical condition:** Many medical conditions can cause NCDs. Examples include structural brain lesions such as primary or secondary brain tumors, subdural hematomas or those seen in normal pressure hydrocephalus, hypoxia, infectious causes, endocrine conditions, immune disorders, and metabolic conditions. The temporal association between the onset or exacerbation of the medical condition and the development of the cognitive deficit supports the diagnosis.

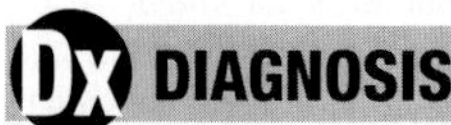

DIAGNOSIS

DIFFERENTIAL DIAGNOSIS

Etiology is assessed by a detailed history from the patient, family members, or other informants, complete physical examination, and ancillary tests, including neuropsychological testing and imaging studies.

LABORATORY TESTS & IMAGING STUDIES

- Detailed physical examination and neuropsychological testing and neuroimaging are indicated. In some cases, serology and lab testing, including B12 and TSH levels, are useful or diagnostic. Biomarkers and genetic screening tests are diagnostic in some cases. Particular attention should be paid to rule out underlying medical causes of the major or mild NCD.
- Alzheimer's disease: Detailed history and physical examination including neuropsychological testing often points to the diagnosis. MRI may show hippocampal and temporoparietal cortical atrophy. PET scan may reveal hypometabolism in temporoparietal regions. Cerebrospinal fluid biomarkers include elevated total tau and phosphorylated tau levels with reduced amyloid beta-42. Amyloid PET scanning may have diagnostic value. *APOE* testing may detect APOE4, a risk factor for development of Alzheimer's disease. For early onset, autosomal dominant inheritance mutation in *APP, PSEN1,* or *PSEN2* may be detected.
- Frontotemporal disorder: In cases with early-onset behavior or language disorders, an MRI or CT scan may show atrophy in frontal lobes and/or corresponding parts of anterior or inferior temporal lobes either bilaterally or asymmetrically. Functional imaging may show hypoperfusion in the corresponding regions. In familial cases, genetic mutations in genes encoding the microtubule-associated protein tau and the granulin gene may confirm the diagnosis.
- Lewy body disease: Sleep study may help to confirm a diagnosis of REM sleep behavior disorder. Nuclear medicine testing including SPECT or PET may show low striatal dopamine transporter uptake.
- Parkinson's disease: Abnormal dopamine transporter scans are supportive of the diagnosis.
- Vascular disorder: Neurologic assessment often reveals a history of stroke or TIA. MRI or CT scan may show significant parenchymal injury attributed to cerebrovascular disease.
- TBI: May be associated with abnormal CT or MRI scan showing petechial hemorrhages, subdural or subarachnoid hemorrhage, or evidence of contusion.
- Prion disease: May be suspected in patients with appropriate clinical presentation, including rapidly progressive course. MRI may show gray matter hyperintensities in the subcortical region, particularly in the putamen and head of caudate nuclei. EEG reveals periodic synchronous biphasic or triphasic sharp waves complexes. CSF biomarkers including 14-3-3, tau, S100 protein, or neuron-specific enolase is suggestive, though not diagnostic.
- Huntington disease: Genetic testing for trinucleotide CAG repeat expansion in the gene that encodes Huntington protein on chromosome 4 is diagnostic.

Rx TREATMENT

- Initial treatment is directed to the underlying etiology.
- Treatment of memory disturbance may be indicated in some causes of major or mild NCDs, such as those caused by Alzheimer's disease.
- Treatment both acutely and chronically is often supportive and aimed at ameliorating behavior and other neuropsychiatric disturbances that may be present.
- Behavioral treatments should be considered first line for most behavior manifestations. Pharmacologic treatments for behavior disturbance have a limited role in improving overall quality of life for most causes of major or minor NCD, although they may have short-term efficacy in acute circumstances.
- Pharmacologic and cognitive behavior treatment may be helpful for associated psychiatric symptoms such as mood disorders, psychosis, and anxiety.
- Patient safety, including risks associated with driving, wandering, and cooking, should be addressed early in the course of the illness.
- Family education and support may help reduce the need for a skilled nursing facility and reduce caregiver stress and burnout.
- Cognitive rehabilitation to promote recovery may be helpful.
- Supervised living may ensure appropriate long-term care in late stages of progressive illness.

SUGGESTED READINGS

Available at ExpertConsult.com

RELATED CONTENT

Alzheimer's Disease (Related Key Topic)
Delirium (Related Key Topic)
Human Immunodeficiency Virus (Related Key Topic)
Huntington Disease (Related Key Topic)
Parkinson's Disease (Related Key Topic)
Progressive Supranuclear Palsy (Related Key Topic)
Traumatic Brain Injury (TBI) (Related Key Topic)
Wernicke Syndrome (Related Key Topic)

AUTHOR: **MICHAEL FRIEDMAN, M.D.**

BASIC INFORMATION

DEFINITION

Neurofibromatosis (NF) is an autosomal-dominant disorder affecting bone, the nervous system, soft tissue, and skin. There are three major subtypes of NF disorders: NF type 1 (NF1), NF type 2 (NF2), and schwannomatosis (SWN). SWN has only recently been recognized as a distinct disorder; currently very little is known about it.

SYNONYMS

NF1: von Recklinghausen disease, peripheral NF
NF2: Bilateral acoustic neurofibromatosis, central NF

ICD-10CM CODES
Q85.00 Neurofibromatosis, unspecified
Q85.01 Neurofibromatosis, type 1
Q85.02 Neurofibromatosis, type 2

EPIDEMIOLOGY & DEMOGRAPHICS

- Incidence of NF1 (one case/3000 live births), NF2 (one case/25,000 live births).
- Prevalence of NF1 (one case/5000 persons), NF2 (one case/210,000 persons).
- NF1 and NF2 are autosomal dominant; approximately 50% of cases have no family history.
- The two disorders affect approximately 100,000 people in the U.S.
- Affects males and females equally.
- NF1 may be associated with optic gliomas, astrocytomas, spinal neurofibromas, pheochromocytomas, and chronic myeloid leukemia.
- NF2 may be associated with meningiomas, spinal schwannomas, and cataracts.
- For SWN, the incidence is one per 30,000 persons, and the disease is mostly sporadic in nature.

PHYSICAL FINDINGS & CLINICAL PRESENTATION

- Common features of NF1 include:
  1. Café-au-lait macules (100% of children by age 2 yr).
     a. Hyperpigmented skin lesions (Fig. 1) occurring anywhere on the body except the face, palms, and soles.
     b. Appear early in life and increase in size and number during puberty.
     c. Are focal or diffuse.
  2. Axillary and inguinal freckling (70%).
  3. Multiple neurofibromas (Fig. 2) can be soft or firm; three subtypes:
     a. Cutaneous: Circumscribed, not specific for NF1.
     b. Subcutaneous: Circumscribed, not specific for NF1.
     c. Plexiform: Noncircumscribed, thick and irregular; can cause disfigurement of supportive structures and specific for NF1.
  4. Lisch nodule (small hamartoma of the iris) found in >90% of adult cases.
  5. Visual defects possibly related to optic gliomas (2% to 5%).
  6. Neurodevelopment problems such as learning disability and mental retardation (30% to 40%).
  7. Skeletal disorders, including long bone dysplasia, pseudoarthrosis, scoliosis, short stature, and decreased bone mineral density.
- Common features of NF2 include:
  1. Hearing loss and tinnitus related to bilateral acoustic neuromas (>90% of adults).
  2. Cataracts (81%).
  3. Headache (may be due to intracranial meningiomas, which are present in 80% of patients).
  4. Unsteady gait.
  5. Cutaneous and subcutaneous neurofibromas but fewer than in NF1.
  6. Café-au-lait macules (1%) (Fig. 3).
- Common features of SWN include painful multiple schwannomas of the spinal (74%), peripheral (89%), or cranial nerves *except* the vestibular nerve (9%).

ETIOLOGY

- NF1 is caused by DNA mutations located on the long arm of chromosome 17 responsible for encoding the protein neurofibromin.
- NF2 is caused by DNA mutations located in the middle of the long arm of chromosome 22 responsible for encoding the protein merlin, which is a potent inhibitor of glioma growth.
- Both proteins are speculated to act as tumor suppressors.
- The etiology of SWN remains unclear; however, most cases are attributed to mutations on chromosome 22, which inactivate two distinct tumor-suppressor genes.

Dx DIAGNOSIS

- NF1 is diagnosed if the person has two or more of the following features:
  1. Six or more café-au-lait macules >5 mm in prepubertal patients and >15 mm in postpubertal patients
  2. Two or more neurofibromas of any type or one plexiform neurofibroma
  3. Axillary or inguinal freckling
  4. Optic glioma
  5. Two or more Lisch nodules (iris hamartomas)
  6. Sphenoid wing dysplasia or cortical thinning of long bones, with or without pseudoarthrosis
  7. A first-degree relative (parent, sibling, or child) with NF1 based on the previous criteria
- NF2 is diagnosed if the person has either of the following two criteria:
  1. Bilateral eighth nerve masses seen by appropriate imaging studies (e.g., CT, MRI)
  2. A first-degree relative with NF2 and either a unilateral eighth nerve mass or two of the following: neurofibroma, meningioma, glioma, schwannoma, or juvenile posterior subcapsular lenticular opacity
- SWN is diagnosed in an individual >30 yr having either of the following two criteria:
  1. Two nonintradermal schwannomas, no vestibular tumor found on MRI scan, no NF2 mutation
  2. One nonvestibular schwannoma and a first-degree relative fitting the above criteria

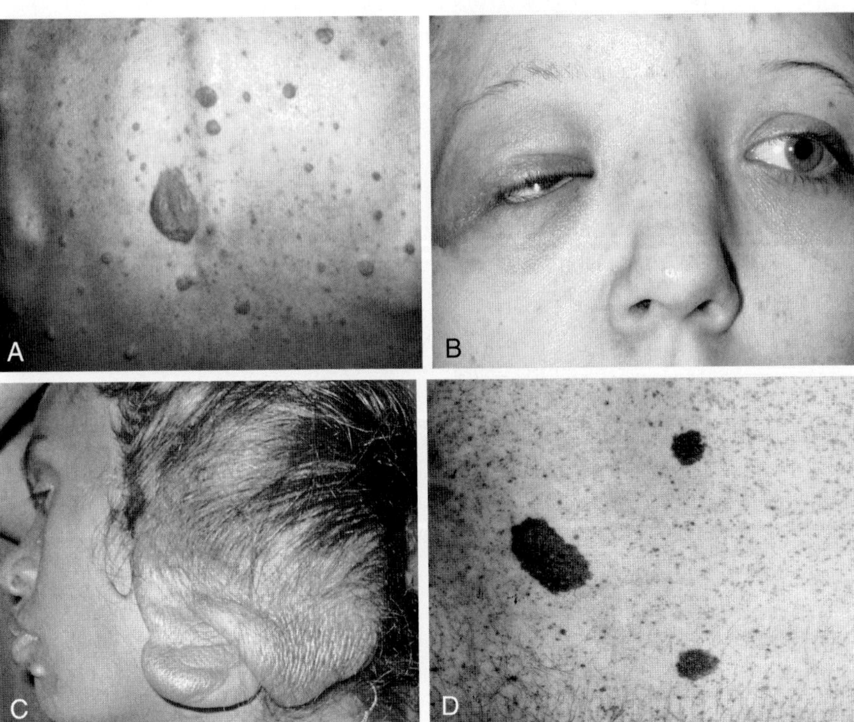

FIG. 1 Systemic features of NF1. A, Discrete neurofibromas. **B,** Nodular plexiform neurofibroma of the eyelid. **C,** Elephantiasis nervosa. **D,** Cafe-au-lait spots. (Courtesy S. Kumar Puri; From Kanski JJ, Bowling B: *Clinical ophthalmology, a systematic approach,* ed 7, Philadelphia, 2010, Saunders.)

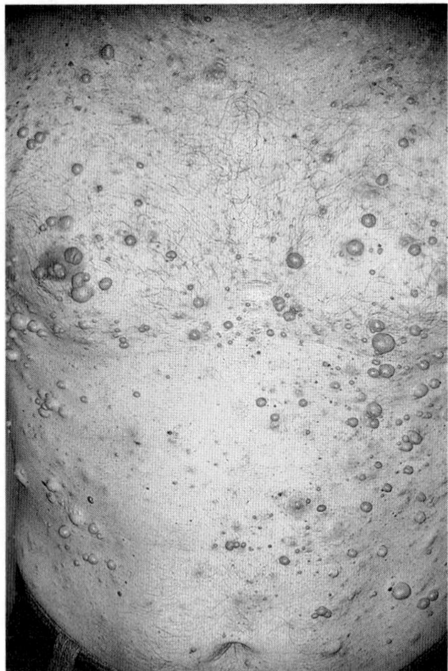

FIG. 2 Multiple neurofibromas are present in this individual. (From Callen JP et al: *Dermatological signs of systemic disease*, ed 5, Philadelphia, 2017, Elsevier.)

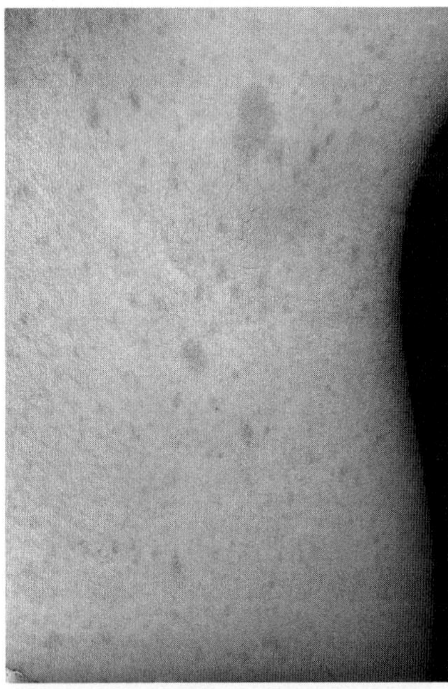

FIG. 3 A café-au-lait spot and multiple freckles (Crowe sign) in the axillary vault is seen in this patient with neurofibromatosis. (From Callen JP et al: *Dermatological signs of systemic disease*, ed 5, Philadelphia, 2017, Elsevier.)

DIFFERENTIAL DIAGNOSIS

- Abdominal NF
- Myxoid lipoma
- Nodular fasciitis
- Fibrous histiocytoma
- Segmental NF

WORKUP

The diagnosis of NF is usually self-evident. Workup is dictated by clinical symptoms in NF1 and usually includes MRI evaluation of the head and spine in NF2 and SWN. In fact, if NF2 is suspected but no vestibular nerve schwannomas are found, the diagnosis points to SWN.

LABORATORY TESTS

- Genetic testing is possible in individuals who desire prenatal diagnosis for NF1. There is no single standard test and multiple tests are required. Results can only tell if an individual is affected but cannot predict the severity of the disease due to variable expression.
- In NF2, linkage analysis testing provides a >99% certainty the individual has NF2.

IMAGING STUDIES

- MRI with gadolinium is the imaging study of choice in both NF1 and NF2 patients. MRI increases detection of optic gliomas, tumors of the spine, acoustic neuromas, and "bright spots" believed to represent hamartomas.
- MRI of the spine is recommended in all patients diagnosed with NF2 to exclude intramedullary tumors.

OTHER TESTS

- Wood lamp examination may be useful in patients with very pale skin for visualizing café-au-lait spots.
- Slit-lamp examination is recommended for children >6 yr to confirm the presence of Lisch nodules and subcapsular opacity.

Rx TREATMENT

Treatment is directed primarily at symptoms and complications of NF1 and NF2. As for SWN, resection should be reserved for tumors that are symptomatic or threaten to cause spinal cord compression.

NONPHARMACOLOGIC THERAPY

- Counseling addressing prognosis and genetic, psychological, and social issues.
- Hearing testing and speech pathology evaluation.

ACUTE GENERAL Rx

- Surgery is usually not done on skin tumors unless cosmetically requested or if suspicion of malignant transformation exists.
- Surgery may be indicated for spinal or cranial neurofibromas, gliomas, or meningiomas.
- Acoustic neuromas can be treated by surgical excision.

CHRONIC Rx

- Radiation may be indicated in optic nerve gliomas and patients whose central nervous system tumors show radiographic progression.
- Stereotactic radiosurgery with a gamma knife may be an alternative approach to surgery for acoustic neuromas.
- Bevacizumab continues to be studied as a treatment option for NF2 meningiomas (which express VEGF).

DISPOSITION

- Prognosis varies according to the severity of involvement.
- There is no cure for NF.

REFERRAL

A multidisciplinary team of consultants is needed in patients with NF, including neurosurgeon, otolaryngologist, dermatologist, neurologist, audiologist, speech pathologist, geneticist, and neuropsychologist.

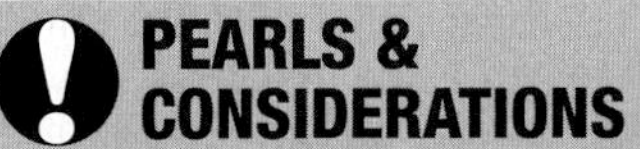

PEARLS & CONSIDERATIONS

- Friedrich Daniel von Recklinghausen first reported his cases in 1882, although there had been similar accounts dating back to the 1600s.
- A high SPRED1 mutation detection rate has been identified in NF1 mutation-negative families with an autosomal dominant phenotype of CALMs with or without freckling and no other NF1 features.

COMMENTS

For additional information and patient resources, refer to the National Neurofibromatosis Foundation (www.nf.org) or Neurofibromatosis Inc. (www.nfinc.org).

SUGGESTED READINGS

Available at ExpertConsult.com

RELATED CONTENT

Neurofibromatosis Type 1 (Patient Information)
Neurofibromatosis Type 2 (Patient Information)

AUTHORS: **CRAIG BLAKENEY, M.D.**, and **MARK F. BRADY, M.D., M.P.H., M.M.S.**

BASIC INFORMATION

DEFINITION

Neuroleptic malignant syndrome (NMS) is a disorder characterized by hyperthermia, muscular rigidity, autonomic dysfunction, and depressed/fluctuating levels of arousal that evolve over 24 to 72 hr. This occurs as an idiosyncratic adverse reaction to medications that affect the central dopaminergic system, usually D2 receptors blockade.

SYNONYM

NMS

ICD-10CM CODE

G21.0 Malignant neuroleptic syndrome

EPIDEMIOLOGY & DEMOGRAPHICS

INCIDENCE (IN U.S.): 0.02% to 0.2% annual incidence in psychiatric population

PREDOMINANT SEX: More than two thirds of patients are male.

PREDOMINANT AGE: Young and middle-aged adults

PREDISPOSING FACTORS: History of intake of dopamine antagonists, e.g., antipsychotics

PHYSICAL FINDINGS & CLINICAL PRESENTATION

- Syndrome typically begins abruptly while the patient is taking therapeutic (not toxic) dosages of neuroleptics and reaches maximum severity within 72 hr
- Severe muscle rigidity (hypertonia, cogwheeling, or "lead pipe" rigidity)
- Hyperthermia (38.6° to 42.3° C [101.48° to 108.14° F], usually <40° C [104° F])
- Autonomic symptoms: Diaphoresis, dysphagia, sialorrhea, skin pallor, urinary incontinence
- Tachycardia, tachypnea
- Labile blood pressure (hypertension or postural hypotension)
- Agitation, catatonia, fluctuating consciousness, obtundation

ETIOLOGY

- Exact etiology is unknown, but it has been suggested that sudden and marked dopamine receptor blockade in nigrostriatal, hypothalamic, mesolimbic, and mesocortical pathways leads to clinical manifestations seen in NMS.
- Neuroleptic drugs have different potencies for inducing NMS:
  1. Typical neuroleptics:
     a. High potency: Haloperidol
     b. Medium potency: Chlorpromazine, fluphenazine
     c. Low potency: Levomepromazine, loxapine
  2. Atypical neuroleptics:
     a. Low potency: Risperidone, olanzapine, clozapine, quetiapine

DIAGNOSIS

DIFFERENTIAL DIAGNOSIS

- Infectious: Encephalitis, meningitis, brain abscess, rabies, tetanus, sepsis
- Endocrine: Pheochromocytoma, thyrotoxicosis
- Toxic: Substances of abuse (ecstasy, phencyclidine), heavy metals (lead, arsenic), lithium, salicylates
- Pharmacologic: Serotonin syndrome, malignant hyperthermia, drug withdrawal, or overdose
- Environmental: Heatstroke, spider envenomation
- Neuropsychiatric: Catatonia, acute psychosis with agitation, status epilepticus
- Table E1 summarizes the differential diagnosis of neuroleptic malignant syndrome

WORKUP

A careful and thorough drug history should be obtained. There is a significant overlap in the features of NMS and serotonin syndrome. The major difference is the presence of hyperreflexia and myoclonus with serotonin syndrome.

LABORATORY TESTS

- Elevated creatine phosphokinase (CPK) (sensitivity 0.71)
- Urinary myoglobin
- Leukocytosis, usually 10,000 to 40,000/mm3
- Electrolytes and renal function
- Blood gases
- Drug levels

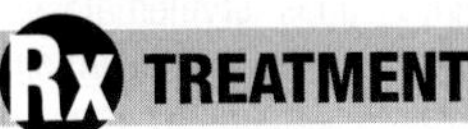

TREATMENT

NONPHARMACOLOGIC THERAPY

- Stop all neuroleptic drugs and reinstitute any recently discontinued dopaminergic agonists.
- Remember that metoclopramide is also an antidopaminergic drug that must be discontinued and avoided.
- Respiratory and nutritional support as required.
- Careful fluid balance monitoring with adequate hydration (intravenous in severe cases).
- Active cooling (cooling blanket and antipyretics).
- Skilled nursing care is necessary to prevent decubitus ulcers in bed-confined patients.

ACUTE GENERAL Rx

- Bromocriptine, a dopamine receptor agonist, is the mainstay of therapy for patients with NMS. Initial doses of 2.5 to 10 mg are given IV q8h and are increased by 5 mg/day until clinical improvement is seen. The drug should be continued for at least 10 days after the syndrome has been controlled and then tapered slowly.
- Dantrolene, which blocks calcium efflux from the sarcoplasmic reticulum of skeletal muscles, inhibits the excessive muscle contractions that generate myoglobinemia. Initially, patients can be given 0.25 mg/kg IV q6-12h, followed by a maintenance dose up to 3 mg/kg/day. After 2 to 3 days, patients may be given the drug orally (25 to 600 mg/day in divided doses). Oral dantrolene therapy (50 to 600 mg/day) may be continued for several days afterward.
- Amantadine, an NMDA receptor antagonist with possible dopaminergic properties, can be administered orally at doses of 100 to 200 mg PO bid for moderate to severe cases. As an adjunctive treatment, it has been shown to reduce mortality in comparison to supportive therapy alone.
- IV benzodiazepines (e.g., diazepam 2 to 10 mg, with total daily dose of 10 to 60 mg) to relax muscles and control agitation.
- Electroconvulsive therapy with neuromuscular blockage may be beneficial in pharmacologically refractory cases. Succinylcholine should not be used because it may cause hyperkalemia and cardiac arrhythmias in patients with rhabdomyolysis or dysautonomia.

CHRONIC Rx

- Respiratory care, nutritional support, and physical therapy may be required in more severe cases.
- Appropriate therapy would be required in patients with persistent neuropsychiatric sequelae of NMS (e.g., antidepressants for depression, cognitive behavioral therapy for cognitive deficits, rehabilitation for contractures).

DISPOSITION

- Mortality rate is currently 5% to 10% despite therapeutic measures. Serious sequelae may occur in a further 20%. Complete recovery occurs in >70% of patients.
- Rhabdomyolysis is the most common complication. Other complications include acute kidney injury, respiratory failure, pneumonia, and sepsis.
- Causes of death include cardiac arrhythmias, myocardial infarction, renal failure secondary to rhabdomyolysis, seizures, pulmonary edema, and bronchopneumonia.
- Factors adversely affecting mortality are increased age, acute respiratory failure, renal failure, and core temperature >104° F (40° C).
- Patients should be monitored closely for future complications of pharmacologic therapy.

REFERRAL

If the patient's condition is critical, it is preferable to treat the patient in a medical/neurologic ICU.

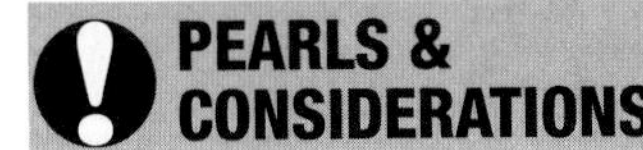

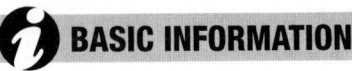

PEARLS & CONSIDERATIONS

COMMENTS

- Early detection and diagnosis lead to a more favorable outcome. Refer to recent consensus diagnostic criteria as a guide. Treatment is a medical emergency.
- Sudden withdrawal from dopaminergic agents (such as those used in Parkinson's disease) may lead to "levodopa withdrawal syndrome" that presents with similar clinical manifestations.
- Patients with dementia with Lewy bodies have increased susceptibility to neuroleptic malignant syndrome.

SUGGESTED READING

Available at ExpertConsult.com

AUTHORS: **CHLOE MANDER NUNNELEY, M.D., JOSEPH S. KASS, M.D., J.D,** and **FARIHA ZAHEER, M.D.**

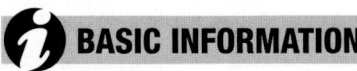

DEFINITION

Neuropathic pain is not itself a disease but rather a symptom that is associated with multiple different diseases. Thus, it is not enough to define its presence without searching for a cause. It is defined as the sensation derived from the abnormal discharges of impaired or injured neural structures in either the peripheral or central nervous system. Descriptors include:

- Hyperesthesia: Heightened sensitivity to nonpainful stimuli (e.g., light touch)
- Hyperalgesia: Heightened sensitivity to painful stimuli (e.g., pinprick), or reduced threshold to feel pain
- Allodynia: Pain provoked by a stimulus that is not normally painful

SYNONYM

Neuralgia

ICD-10CM CODES

G58.0	Intercostal neuropathy
G58.7	Mononeuritis multiplex
G58.8	Other specified mononeuropathies
G58.9	Mononeuropathy, unspecified
G60.0	Hereditary sensory and motor neuropathy
G61.9	Inflammatory polyneuropathy, unspecified
G62.0	Drug-induced polyneuropathy
G62.1	Alcoholic polyneuropathy
G62.9	Polyneuropathy, unspecified
G63.2	Diabetic polyneuropathy
G63.5	Polyneuropathy in systemic connective tissue disease
G63.8	Polyneuropathy in other diseases classified elsewhere

EPIDEMIOLOGY & DEMOGRAPHICS

- Estimates of the prevalence of neuropathic pain in the general population range from 1.6% to 8.2%.
- Demographics vary widely depending on etiology, for example:
  1. Postherpetic neuralgia: Affects elderly, pain seen in almost 100% of cases
  2. AIDS: 30% of patients affected
  3. Diabetes mellitus: 20% to 24% affected (prevalence rates vary, increasing with longer disease duration)
  4. Fabry disease: Affects mostly children, pain in 81% to 90% of patients

PHYSICAL FINDINGS & CLINICAL PRESENTATION

- History: Localize the disease with questions
  1. Quality (description) of neuropathic pain: Burning, hot or cold, "icy hot," "pins and needles," stinging, lancinating, sharp, shooting
  2. Distribution of symptoms may aid in localization (i.e., "stocking-glove" symptoms in generalized neuropathy, numbness in a peripheral nerve territory in focal neuropathy)
  3. Generalized small fiber neuropathy: Dysesthesias without numbness common, but many etiologies (e.g., diabetes) cause both small and large fiber dysfunction
  4. Large fiber neuropathy (LFPN): Coexisting numbness, hyporeflexia, or weakness may be seen, usually worse distally
  5. Nerve root: Coexisting neck or low back pain that radiates along a specific dermatome; most common cause is structural compression
  6. Spinal cord symptoms: Coexisting spasticity, bowel or bladder involvement, sensory level
  7. Prior history of thalamic stroke in central thalamic pain syndrome (Dejerine-Roussy syndrome)
  8. Family history may suggest a genetic cause
- Examination: See Table 1. Table 2 describes joint involvement in neuropathic arthropathy. Fig. 1 illustrates a diagnostic approach to neuropathic pain. Fig. 2 shows a neuropathic ankle.

ETIOLOGY & LABORATORY EVALUATION (TABLE 3)

- Metabolic: Diabetes mellitus; malnutrition and alcoholism; vitamin B_{12} deficiency; thiamine deficiency; porphyria; Fabry's disease
- Inflammatory: Autoimmune diseases (systemic vasculitides, systemic lupus erythematosus, Sjögren's syndrome, etc.), acute inflammatory demyelinating polyneuropathy (classically presents with ascending weakness and numbness, although pain is also a common feature), chronic inflammatory demyelinating polyneuropathy, sarcoidosis, multiple sclerosis
- Infiltrative: Amyloidosis, paraproteinemias (e.g., monoclonal gammopathy of uncertain significance [MGUS] associated neuropathy)
- Infectious: Postviral (brachial neuritis), HIV/AIDS, HSV, varicella-zoster virus (VZV; postherpetic neuralgia), Lyme disease, leprosy (thickened nerves and skin lesions), syphilis
- Neoplastic and paraneoplastic-carcinomatous infiltration of nerve/nerve root, anti-Hu
- Drugs/toxins: History of exposure to alcohol, chemotherapeutic agents (paclitaxel, vincristine), isoniazid, metronidazole, or heavy metals (thallium, arsenic)

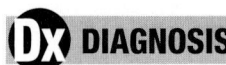

LABORATORY TESTS

- Fasting blood glucose (FBG)
- 2-hour oral glucose tolerance test (OGTT)
- Vitamin B_{12} level
- If B_{12} level normal: Serum methylmalonic acid and homocysteine levels
- Serum erythrocyte sedimentation rate (ESR), ANA, SS-A and SS-B, c-ANCA, p-ANCA
- RPR or FTA-ABS
- Serum ACE level (sarcoid)
- HIV antibody
- SPEP, UPEP, immunofixation
- Urine and stool protoporphyrins, if porphyria is suspected clinically

TABLE 1 Examination

Exam Finding	Localization
Pinprick/temperature loss alone	Small fibers only
Pinprick/temperature loss + vibratory/proprioceptive loss	Small and large fibers
Sensory loss and motor dysfunction worse distally than proximal	Large fiber neuropathy
Sensory loss and motor dysfunction along single nerve distribution	Single nerve
Sensory loss and motor dysfunction along multiple single nerves	Multiple mononeuropathies (i.e., mononeuropathy multiplex)
Motor and sensory loss involving multiple nerves belonging to specific region of brachial or lumbar plexus	Plexopathy
Sensory loss along dermatome with multiple myotomal muscles affected	Nerve root lesion
Asymmetric sensory loss without weakness and pseudoathetosis	Dorsal root ganglion
Vibratory/proprioceptive loss without pinprick/temperature loss	Dorsal column dysfunction (from compressive lesion, B_{12} deficiency, or tabes dorsalis from neurosyphilis)
Sensory level with weakness below the level of lesion and long tract signs (spasticity/Babinski sign)	Spinal cord lesion
Hemisensory hyperalgesia	Contralateral thalamus

TABLE 2 Joint Involvement in Neuropathic Arthropathy

Disease	Site of Involvement
Diabetes mellitus	Midtarsal, metatarsophalangeal, tarsometatarsal
Syringomyelia	Shoulder, elbow, wrist
Amyloidosis	Knee, ankle
Congenital sensory neuropathy	Knee, ankle, intertarsal, metatarsophalangeal
Tabes dorsalis	Knee, hip, ankle
Leprosy	Tarsal, tarsometatarsal

From Hochberg MC, et al.: *Rheumatology,* ed 5, St Louis, 2011, Mosby.

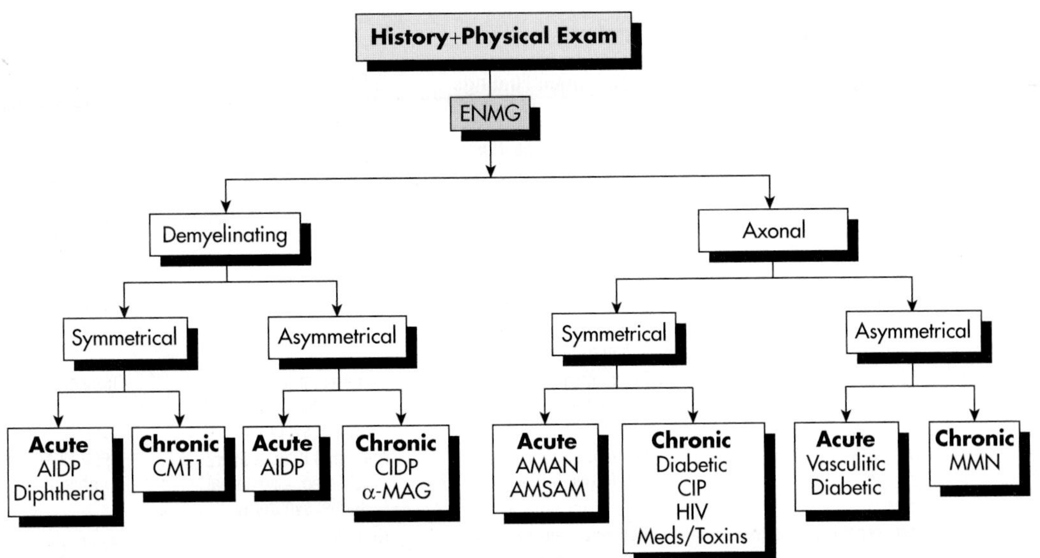

FIG. 1 A systematic approach to evaluate neuropathy. The diseases listed are examples of neuropathies associated with specific neurophysiologic and clinical findings. Diabetic distal, predominantly sensory neuropathies are manifested as chronic axonal neuropathies; acute asymmetric neuropathies can also occur with diabetes. Most neuropathies caused by toxins or by side effects of medication are chronic, symmetric axonal neuropathies. AIDP, AMAN, and AMSAN are subtypes of Guillain-Barré syndrome. These and other examples are discussed in more detail in the text. *AIDP,* Acute inflammatory demyelinating polyradiculoneuropathy; *AMAN,* acute motor axonal neuropathy; *AMSAN,* acute motor and sensory axonal neuropathy; *CIDP,* chronic inflammatory polyradiculoneuropathy; *CIP,* chronic illness polyneuropathy; *CMT1,* Charcot-Marie-Tooth disease type 1, a genetic disorder; *ENMG,* electroneuromyography; *HIV,* human immunodeficiency virus–related neuropathy; *α-MAG,* anti-myelin-associated glycoprotein; *MMN,* multifocal motor neuropathy. (From Goldman L, Schafer AI: *Goldman's Cecil medicine,* ed 24, Philadelphia, 2012, Saunders.)

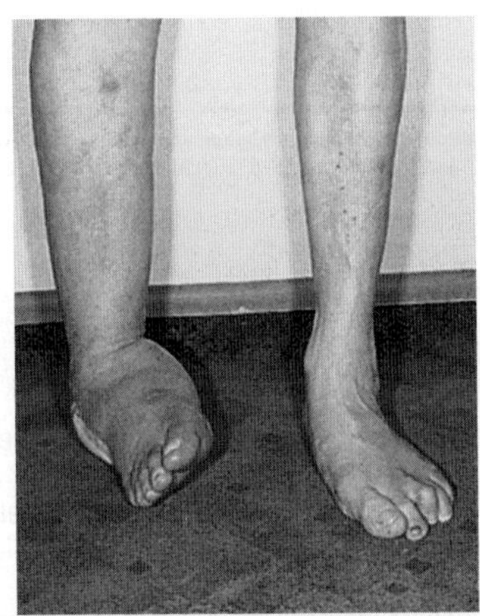

FIG. 2 Neuropathic ankle. Marked instability of the subtalar and midtarsal joints is seen with collapse on weight bearing. (From Hochberg MC, et al.: *Rheumatology,* ed 5, St Louis, 2011, Mosby.)

- Hu antibody: Can be seen in both small cell and non–small cell lung cancers, may be positive without evidence of lung cancer
- Lumbar puncture: Protein elevation, oligoclonal bands, CSF/serum IgG index

ELECTROPHYSIOLOGY STUDIES

- Electrophysiologic testing (electromyography with nerve conduction studies): May be normal in small fiber neuropathies or CNS lesion, but is often abnormal in large fiber neuropathies
- Quantitative sensory testing: Abnormal in small and large fiber neuropathy
- Evoked potentials (only if suspicion for spinal cord lesion)

PATHOLOGY STUDIES

- Nerve biopsy is occasionally useful in selected cases, particularly when vasculitis, sarcoidosis, or amyloid neuropathy are in the differential.
- Skin biopsy for intraepidermal nerve fiber (IENF) density may be useful for small fiber neuropathy when other studies are normal.
- Rectal or abdominal fat pad biopsy may show amyloid deposition in systemic amyloidosis.

IMAGING STUDIES

- MRI (with and without contrast):
  1. Of the brain to exclude thalamic pathology if symptoms and signs are consistent with thalamic lesion (hemibody pain)
  2. Of the spinal cord and nerve roots to exclude structural, inflammatory, neoplastic, or infectious causes
  3. Of the lumbar spine to evaluate for arachnoiditis
- If MRI cannot be performed, consider:
  1. CT of the brain for thalamic pathology
  2. CT myelography of the spinal cord to evaluate for structural/neoplastic disease, but only if clinical signs of spinal or nerve root compromise are present

Rx TREATMENT

NONPHARMACOLOGIC THERAPY

- Counseling should be initiated at the beginning of therapy to address psychological issues exacerbating physiologic pain.
- Physical therapy: Especially in cases of chronic neck and low back pain.

ACUTE GENERAL Rx

- Treatment of the underlying cause if possible will help slow or prevent worsening.
- Medications may reduce or alleviate pain but do not affect numbness.
- Antidepressants:
  1. Tricyclic antidepressants (TCAs): Nortriptyline preferred over amitriptyline (fewer anticholinergic side effects with nortriptyline). Begin 25 mg PO qd in adults, or 10 mg qd in elderly. Increase dose by 25 mg every week as tolerated until usual maximal effective dose of 150 mg/day.
  2. Duloxetine: Begin 30 mg daily, increase to 60 to 120 mg daily. Duloxetine is effective in diabetic neuropathy, post-herpetic neuropathy, and chemotherapy-induced painful peripheral neuropathy.
- Antiepileptics:
  1. Gabapentin: Begin 300 mg PO qd, advance to 300 mg PO tid by the end of the first week. Effective dose: Higher than 1600 mg/day. Max dose: 1200 mg PO tid.
  2. Carbamazepine: For trigeminal neuralgia. Begin 400 mg PO bid, increase to tid if necessary. Side effects and drug levels help to determine optimal dosing. Risk of aplastic anemia and hyponatremia (monitor CBC and chemistries). Risk of Stevens-Johnson syndrome, especially in Asian population (check HLA before starting).
  3. Oxcarbazepine: Better tolerated than carbamazepine. Start 150 mg PO bid and gradually increase to a dose of 600 mg bid. Maximum dose is 1200 mg bid.

TABLE 3 Clinical Presentation and Laboratory Findings

Neuropathy Type	Predisposition	Examination Findings	EMG/NCS	Laboratory Analysis
Idiopathic small fiber PN	Age >50	Strength: Normal Reflexes: Normal Pos/vib: Normal Pain/temp: Decreased distally	Normal	Serum studies: Normal Skin biopsy: Abnormal Sudomotor studies: Abnormal
Diabetic PN	Long-standing disease Family history	Strength normal to reduced, sensation reduced distally	Abnormal	Abnormal glucose tolerance High fasting glucose
Inherited PN	Family history	Pes cavus, hammer toes, reduced reflexes, sensation reduced distally	Abnormal	Genetic studies may be abnormal, other studies normal
Familial amyloid PN	Family history	Pain/temp loss, reduced reflexes, orthostasis	Abnormal if large fibers affected; also carpal tunnel syndrome	Transthyretin genetic study
Acquired amyloid PN	Monoclonal gammopathy	Pain/temp loss, reduced reflexes, orthostasis	Abnormal if large fibers affected; also carpal tunnel syndrome	SPEP, UPEP, immunofixation abnormal
Fabry disease	Age, renal failure, strokes	Normal; possible reduced pain/temp sensation	Normal	α-Galactosidase levels in cultured fibroblasts
PN + mixed connective tissue disease	History of lupus, rheumatoid arthritis, Sjögren's syndrome	Reduced reflexes and distal sensation	Abnormal	ANA, RF, SS-A/SS-B may be abnormal
Peripheral nerve vasculitis	Asymmetric disease	Multiple peripheral nerves involved	Abnormal	ANA, RF, SS-A/SS-B, ANCA, cryoglobulins may be abnormal
Paraneoplastic neuropathy	Lung cancer risk factors, chemical exposures	Asymmetric sensory loss, pseudoathetosis, relatively preserved strength	Abnormal	Anti-Hu
Sarcoidosis	Pulmonary sarcoid	Multiple mononeuropathies	Abnormal	Abnormal biopsy, elevated serum ACE, CXR abnormal
Arsenic	Pesticides, copper smelting	Reduced reflexes and distal sensation	Abnormal	Elevated arsenic in plasma, urine, and hair
HIV	Promiscuity, unprotected sex, IV drug abuse, blood transfusion	Variable, but most often reduced reflexes and distal sensation	Abnormal if large fibers involved	HIV antibody

ACE, Angiotensin-converting enzyme; *ANA*, antibody to nuclear antigens; *ANCA*, antineutrophil cytoplasmic antibodies; *CXR*, chest x-ray; *EMG*, electromyography; *HIV*, human immunodeficiency virus; *IV*, intravenous; *NCS*, nerve conduction studies; *PN*, polyneuropathy; *Pos*, position sensation; *RF*, rheumatoid factor; *SPEP*, serum protein electrophoresis; *SS-A*, Sjögren's syndrome A; *SS-B*, Sjögren's syndrome B; *Temp*, temperature sensation; *UPEP*, urine protein electrophoresis; *Vib*, vibration sensation.
Adapted from Mendell JR, Sahenk Z: Painful sensory neuropathy, *N Engl J Med* 348(13):1243, 2003.

4. Pregabalin: Begin 50 mg PO tid, increase slowly to 100 to 200 mg PO tid.

- Analgesics: When first-line agents are ineffective. While effective, the use of opioids is associated with substantial adverse effects as well as novel pain syndromes. Chronic use of opioids leads to tolerance and escalation of dose:
  1. Tramadol: 150 mg/day (50 mg tid), increase by 50 mg/wk, max 200 to 400 mg/day.
  2. Morphine (oral): 15 to 30 mg q8h, max 90 to 360 mg/day.
  3. Oxycodone: 20 mg q12h, increase by 10 mg/wk, max 40 to 160 mg/day.
  4. Fentanyl patch: 25 to 100 mcg transdermally q3 days.
- Topical anesthetics:
  1. 5% lidocaine patch, apply to area of pain, max three patches every 12 hr.
  2. Capsaicin is inconsistent in its ability to relieve pain and may exacerbate it.
- Procedural/surgical: This option is considered mostly when the patient suffers from pain secondary to spinal cord or cauda equina injury. Studies are limited and benefit is not completely established. Procedures should be considered only when all other therapeutic modalities have failed. In addition, the patient should be cautioned that surgical procedures may not result in pain relief and may be associated with significant morbidity and even mortality.
  1. Dorsal root rhizotomy.
  2. Nerve blocks.
  3. Spinal cord stimulator.

DISPOSITION

Prognosis depends on multiple factors, including:

- Etiology of pain
- Treatment of any underlying condition
- Initiation of appropriate (often multiple) therapeutic modalities
- Patient compliance with prescribed regimen

Most care is accomplished in the outpatient setting, except when surgery is required.

REFERRAL

- Pain clinic
- Neurology
- Psychiatry
- Psychology
- Physiatry
- Anesthesiology (nerve blocks)
- Neurosurgery if considering surgical management

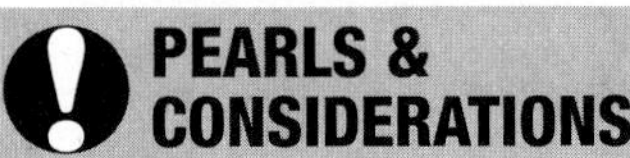

PEARLS & CONSIDERATIONS

- Factitious disorder and malingering frequently manifest with pain complaints. These are diagnoses of exclusion and require negative evaluation for organic etiologies before diagnosis is made.
- Peripheral neuropathy in diabetics increases the risk of foot ulceration by sevenfold. Abnormal results in monofilament testing and vibratory perception (alone or in combination with the appearance of the feet, ulceration, and ankle reflexes) are the most helpful sign for the detection of LFPN.

SUGGESTED READINGS

Available at ExpertConsult.com

AUTHORS: **JOSEPH S. KASS, M.D., J.D., GAVIN BROWN, M.D.,** and **COREY GOLDSMITH, M.D.**

BASIC INFORMATION

DEFINITION

An unprovoked seizure is a seizure that occurs without triggers or precipitating factors. In contrast, an acute symptomatic seizure occurs in the setting of an insult to the brain (infectious, toxic, etc.). The presentation of a new seizure can vary greatly depending on the type (focal or generalized), progression, and severity.

SYNONYM

Convulsions

ICD-10CM CODES

G40.10	Localization-related (focal) (partial) symptomatic epilepsy and epileptic syndromes with simple partial seizures, not intractable
G40.001	Localization-related (focal) (partial) idiopathic epilepsy and epileptic syndromes with seizures of localized onset, not intractable, with status epilepticus
G40.009	Localization-related (focal) (partial) idiopathic epilepsy and epileptic syndromes with seizures of localized onset, not intractable, without status epilepticus
G40.101	Localization-related (focal) (partial) symptomatic epilepsy and epileptic syndromes with simple partial seizures, not intractable, with status epilepticus
G40.109	Localization-related (focal) (partial) symptomatic epilepsy and epileptic syndromes with simple partial seizures, not intractable, without status epilepticus
G40.201	Localization-related (focal) (partial) symptomatic epilepsy and epileptic syndromes with complex partial seizures, not intractable, with status epilepticus
G40.209	Localization-related (focal) (partial) symptomatic epilepsy and epileptic syndromes with complex partial seizures, not intractable, without status epilepticus
G40.301	Generalized idiopathic epilepsy and epileptic syndromes, not intractable, with status epilepticus
G40.309	Generalized idiopathic epilepsy and epileptic syndromes, not intractable, without status epilepticus
G40.A01	Absence epileptic syndrome, not intractable, with status epilepticus
G40.A09	Absence epileptic syndrome, not intractable, without status epilepticus
G40.401	Other generalized epilepsy and epileptic syndromes, not intractable, with status epilepticus
G40.409	Other generalized epilepsy and epileptic syndromes, not intractable, without status epilepticus
G40.501	Epileptic seizures related to external causes, not intractable, with status epilepticus
G40.509	Epileptic seizures related to external causes, not intractable, without status epilepticus
G40.4	Other generalized epilepsy and epileptic syndromes
G40.909	Epilepsy, unspecified, not intractable, without status epilepticus

EPIDEMIOLOGY & DEMOGRAPHICS

INCIDENCE: 29 to 39 per 100,000 per yr for acute symptomatic seizures. 23 to 61 per 100,000 person-yr for unprovoked seizures. Approximately 8% to 10% of the population will experience a seizure during their lifetime; however, less than 3% go on to develop epilepsy.

PREVALENCE: 5 to 8.4 cases per 1000 persons.

PREDOMINANT SEX AND AGE: Males younger than 12 mo and older than 65 yr

RISK FACTORS:
- Age of onset
- Family history of epilepsy
- Excessive sleep deprivation, use of alcohol, or illicit drugs
- History of head trauma, diseases of the brain, brain surgeries, and strokes
- History of congenital cerebral anomalies or developmental delay

GENETICS

Although some new onset seizures are related to specific genes, most are not.

PHYSICAL FINDINGS & CLINICAL PRESENTATION

- Patients with generalized seizures will typically have normal physical exams. Patients with focal seizures due to persistent structural CNS damage may have exam findings consistent with the location of the lesion.
- A generalized seizure may start without warning and can typically last from 30 to 120 seconds, during which the patient will be unconscious and may have increased rigidity and/or jerking of the whole body, or staring spells. Cyanosis (especially of the lips and face) can result from temporary airway compromise due to muscle spasms. Tonic-clonic seizures can cause injuries, tongue biting, and bladder incontinence. Patients are usually unaware of the seizure afterwards. A postictal state characterized by confusion, lethargy, headaches, or drowsiness may result and can last from minutes to hours depending on the severity of the seizure.
- A complex partial seizure may be associated with an aura (itself a simple partial seizure) and lasts between 30 and 120 seconds. The patient may be aware (simple partial seizure) or have impaired consciousness (complex partial seizures). Motor or nonmotor symptoms may predominate in focal seizures, including jerking of one limb, automatisms, head turning, auditory hallucinations, or feelings of derealization. A focal seizure may progress to a generalized seizure, which usually involves the head and eye turning to one side. Postictal weakness may result after focal seizures and can last for hours but usually resolves within 1 day. Persistent neurological deficits beyond this time may indicate other causes and should be investigated.

ETIOLOGY

- New, unprovoked seizures are often idiopathic
- Acute symptomatic seizures can be due to cerebral abnormalities (e.g., infections/abscesses, subarachnoid hemorrhages, ischemic strokes, tumors, arteriovenous malformations, venous malformations) or systemic causes (e.g., electrolyte abnormalities, hypoglycemia, hyperthyroidism, drug intoxication or withdrawal)

Dx DIAGNOSIS

DIFFERENTIAL DIAGNOSIS

- Syncope
- Transient ischemic attacks
- Migraines
- Sleep disorders
- Paroxysmal movement disorders
- Panic attacks, hallucinations, and other psychiatric disorders

WORKUP

- Ambulatory 30-min EEG if patient fully recovers after seizure within 30 to 60 min. May be delayed if treatment does not depend on EEG result.
- Consider inpatient continuous EEG if patient does not fully recover within 60 min or for recurrent seizures.
- ECG.

LABORATORY TESTS

Comprehensive metabolic panel and urine drug screen

IMAGING STUDIES

- Acutely, CT of the head with and without contrast to evaluate for hemorrhage and space-occupying lesions
- Brain MRI with and without contrast with epilepsy protocol in patients with recurrent seizures, in consultation with a neurologist

Rx TREATMENT

- Provoked seizures do not need long-term treatment.
- The choice of treatment depends largely on seizure type and etiology. Antiepileptics may be thought of as narrow- or wide-spectrum drugs. Treatment with wide-spectrum antiepileptics is advisable in generalized seizures or those of unknown type, whereas partial seizures are better controlled with narrow-spectrum antiepileptics.
- Narrow-spectrum drugs include carbamazepine, oxcarbazepine, gabapentin, pregabalin, lacosamide, and phenytoin. Wide-spectrum drugs include valproate, topiramate, zonisamide, lamotrigine, and levetiracetam.
- In patients with significant comorbidities, the use of antiepileptics with limited drug interactions is advised (lamotrigine, levetiracetam, lacosamide).
- Older patients may benefit from lamotrigine, levetiracetam, or gabapentin due to a lower risk of adverse events.

NONPHARMACOLOGIC THERAPY

None

ACUTE GENERAL RX

- Patients with a first unprovoked seizure who have a normal EEG, imaging, lab values, and physical exam do not require treatment with antiepileptic drugs but may be offered therapy because the use of an antiepileptic drug after a first unprovoked seizure in an adult reduces the absolute risk of seizure recurrence at 2 yr by 35%. However, there is no difference at 3 yr.
- For generalized seizures: **Levetiracetam** initial dose of 500 mg bid. If recurrent seizures, increase by 500 mg every 1 to 2 wk until maximum dose of 1500 mg bid is reached.
- For partial seizures: **Oxcarbazepine** initial dose 300 mg bid, increase by 300mg/day every 3 days to 600 mg bid. If recurrent seizures, continue to titrate by 300 mg/day every 3 days to 1200 mg bid.

CHRONIC RX

Patients with two or more unprovoked seizures, or those with one seizure and an abnormal workup consistent with epilepsy findings, should be continued on antiepileptic drugs. Patients electing antiepileptic therapy after first unprovoked seizure with negative workup may be weaned off antiepileptic drug if seizure-free after 2 yr.

COMPLEMENTARY AND ALTERNATIVE MEDICINE

Not applicable

DISPOSITION

- Patients should avoid swimming unobserved, bathing alone, working at heights, using heavy machinery, or other activities that may be high-risk in the event of a seizure.
- Discontinue driving until seizures are well controlled and in accordance with state laws.

REFERRAL

Patients may be referred to a neurologist.

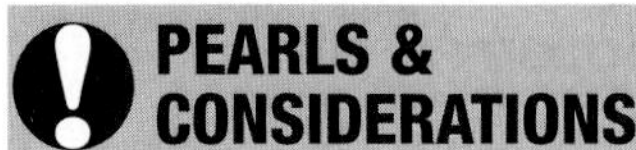

PEARLS & CONSIDERATIONS

COMMENTS

- Driving: Physicians should be aware of the law in their jurisdiction about driving after a seizure. Although a few U.S. states require physicians to notify the state government authority that issues driver's licenses, most do not impose such an obligation on physicians. However, states do require patients to self-report and abstain from driving until seizure-free for a specified period of time, depending on the state.
- Recurrence risk: Greatest recurrence risk in an adult with a first unprovoked seizure is within the first 2 yr and is between 21% and 45%. The recurrence risk is lower in patients treated with an antiepileptic drug and higher in patients with a brain MRI abnormality causing the seizure or an EEG showing epileptiform activity.

PREVENTION

Patients with recurrent seizures should be extensively counseled on avoiding seizure triggers such as sleep deprivation, alcohol or drug use, stress, and exposure to excessive flashing lights. Such patients may need dose titration of antiepileptic drug and referral to a neurologist.

PATIENT/FAMILY EDUCATION

- Physicians should inform patients with first-time seizures that they are subject to state law restrictions on driving after a seizure. Physicians should also counsel patients with epilepsy about not swimming unattended, not climbing heights, and taking showers rather than baths (because of the risk of drowning in a bathtub during a generalized seizure). Physicians should counsel women of childbearing potential about effects of antiepileptic drugs on both oral contraceptive efficacy and on a developing fetus. They should recommend supplemental folic acid for such women if they are taking antiepileptic drugs. They should also recommend that women plan pregnancy if they are on antiepileptic drugs to minimize adverse effects on the pregnancy. All such counseling should be documented in the medical record.
- A diagnosis of epilepsy has significant medical, social, and emotional consequences. Patient information on seizures and locating support groups can be found at the Epilepsy Foundation website: http://www.epilepsy.com.

SUGGESTED READINGS

Available at ExpertConsult.com

RELATED CONTENT

Absence Seizures (Related Key Topic)
Febrile Seizures (Related Key Topic)
Seizures, Generalized Tonic-Clinic (Related Key Topic)
Partial Seizures (Related Key Topic)
Status Epilepticus (Related Key Topic)

AUTHORS: **SUDAD KAZZAZ, M.D., JOSEPH S. KASS, M.D., J.D.,** and **COREY GOLDSMITH, M.D.**

BASIC INFORMATION

DEFINITION

- *Nonalcoholic fatty liver disease* (NAFLD) is a spectrum of diseases based on histopathologic findings and representing a morphologic rather than a clinical diagnosis. It is liver disease occurring in patients who do not abuse alcohol and manifesting histologically by mononuclear cells and/or polymorphonuclear cells, hepatocyte ballooning, and spotty necrosis. *Nonalcoholic steatohepatitis* (NASH) is a subset of NAFLD. Patients with NASH have progressive disease that can result in fibrosis and cirrhosis. A diagnosis of NAFLD is contingent on the following factors:
  1. Alcohol consumption in amounts less than those considered hepatotoxic.
  2. Absence of serologic evidence of other hepatic diseases or disorders.
  3. Liver biopsy showing predominant macrovesicular steatosis or steatohepatitis.
- NAFL is defined as ≥ 5% hepatic steatosis without evidence of hepatocellular injury or fibrosis.
- NASH is ≥ 5% hepartic fibrosis with inflammation and hepatocellular injury with or without fibrosis.
- *NASH cirrhosis* is the presence of cirrhosis with current or past evidence of steatosis.

SYNONYMS

Nonalcoholic steatohepatitis (NASH)
NAFLD
Fatty liver hepatitis
Diabetes hepatitis
Alcohol-like liver disease
Laënnec disease

ICD-10CM CODE

K76.0 Fatty (change of) liver, not elsewhere classified

EPIDEMIOLOGY & DEMOGRAPHICS

- NAFLD affects 30% to 40% of the adult general population in the U.S.
- Increased prevalence in obese persons (57% to 74%), type 2 diabetes mellitus, and hyperlipidemia (primarily hypertriglyceridemia).
- Most common cause of abnormal liver test results in adults in the United States (accounts for up to 90% of cases of asymptomatic ALT elevations).
- NAFLD is more prevalent in men than women.
- NAFLD is more prevalent in the Hispanic population.
- Approximately 20% of patients with NAFLD have NASH, and 10% to 30% of patients with NASH have NASH cirrhosis.

PHYSICAL FINDINGS & CLINICAL PRESENTATION

- Most patients are asymptomatic.
- Patients may report a sensation of fullness or discomfort on the right side of the upper abdomen.
- Nonspecific complaints of fatigue or malaise may be reported.
- Hepatomegaly (Table 1) is generally the only positive finding on physical examination.
- Acanthosis nigricans may be found in children.

ETIOLOGY

- Metabolic syndrome and insulin resistance are the most reproducible factors in the development of NAFLD and accumulation of triglycerides within the liver. High baseline and continuously increasing fasting insulin levels are independent determinants for future development of NAFLD. The transition from NAFLD to NASH is poorly understood; there may be a genetic component. The presence of the I48M variant of PNPLA3 increases risk for and severity of NAFLD.

TABLE 1 Symptoms, Signs, and Laboratory Features of Nonalcoholic Fatty Liver Disease

Symptoms	Signs	Laboratory Features
Common		
None (48%-100% of patients)	Hepatomegaly	2- to 4-fold elevation of serum ALT and AST levels AST/ALT ratio <1 in most patients Serum alkaline phosphatase level slightly elevated in one third of patients Normal serum bilirubin, serum albumin, and prothrombin time Elevated serum ferritin level
Uncommon		
Vague right upper quadrant pain Fatigue Malaise	Splenomegaly Spider telangiectasias Palmar erythema Ascites	Low-titer (<1:320) antinuclear antibodies

ALT, Alanine aminotransferase; *AST,* aspartate aminotransferase.
From Feldman M, Friedman LS, Brandt LJ: *Sleisenger and Fordtran's gastrointestinal and liver disease,* ed 10, Philadelphia, 2016, Elsevier.

BOX 1 Causes of Fatty Liver Disease

Acquired Metabolic Disorders
Diabetes mellitus
Dyslipidemia
Kwashiorkor and marasmus
Obesity
Rapid weight loss
Starvation

Cytotoxic and Cytostatic Drugs
L-Asparaginase
Azacitidine
Bleomycin
Cisplatin
5-Fluorouracil
Methotrexate
Tetracyclines (inhibit mitochondrial beta oxidation)

Other Drugs and Toxins
Amiodarone
Camphor
Chloroform
Cocaine
Ethanol
Ethyl bromide
Estrogens
Glucocorticoids
Griseofulvin
HAART (zidovudine, stavudine, didanosine)
Lycopodium serratum (Jin Bu Huan, an herbal supplement)
Nifedipine
Nitrofurantoin
NSAIDs (piroxicam, ibuprofen, indomethacin, sulindac)
Tamoxifen
Valproic acid

Metals
Antimony
Barium salts
Chromates
Mercury
Phosphorus
Rare earth metals of low atomic number
Thallium compounds
Uranium compounds

Inborn Errors of Metabolism
Abetalipoproteinemia
Familial hepatosteatosis
Galactosemia
Glycogen storage disease
Hereditary fructose intolerance
Homocystinuria
Systemic carnitine deficiency
Tyrosinemia
Weber-Christian syndrome
Wilson disease

Surgical Procedures
Biliopancreatic diversion
Extensive small bowel resection
Jejunoileal bypass

Miscellaneous Conditions
Industrial exposure to petrochemicals
IBD
Jejunal diverticulosis with bacterial overgrowth
Partial lipodystrophy
TPN

HAART, Highly active antiretroviral therapy; *IBD,* inflammatory bowel disease; *NSAIDs,* nonsteroidal antiinflammatory drugs; *TPN,* total parenteral nutrition.
From Feldman M, Friedman LS, Brandt LJ: *Sleisenger and Fordtran's gastrointestinal and liver disease,* ed 10, Philadelphia, 2016, Elsevier.

 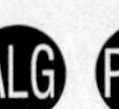 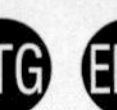

TABLE 2 NAFLD Activity Score on a Liver Biopsy Specimen

Steatosis	
5%	1
5%-33%	2
33%-66%	3
Ballooning	
None	0
Few	1
Many	2
Lobular Inflammation	
Mild	1
Moderate	2
Severe	3
Total Score	
0-2	Likely not NASH
3-4	Intermediate
5-8	Likely NASH

NAFLD, Nonalcoholic fatty liver disease; *NASH*, nonalcoholic steatohepatitis.
From Feldman M, Friedman LS, Brandt LJ: *Sleisenger and Fordtran's gastrointestinal and liver disease*, ed 10, Philadelphia, 2016, Elsevier.

Genetic polymorphism (TM6SF2) also increases NAFLD risk.

- Risk factors are obesity (especially truncal obesity), diabetes mellitus, hyperlipidemia.

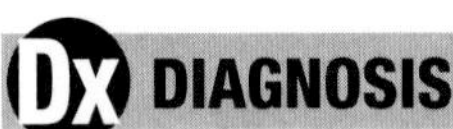

DIAGNOSIS

DIFFERENTIAL DIAGNOSIS

- Alcohol-induced liver disease (a daily alcohol intake of 20 g in females and 30 g in males [three 12-oz beers or 12 oz of wine] may be enough to cause alcohol-induced liver disease).
- Viral hepatitis.
- Autoimmune hepatitis.
- Toxin- or drug-induced liver disease.
- Box 1 summarizes the various causes of fatty liver disease.

WORKUP

Diagnosis is usually suspected on the basis of hepatomegaly, asymptomatic elevations of transaminases, or "fatty liver" on sonogram of abdomen in obese patients with little or no alcohol use. Fig. E1 describes an algorithm for the diagnostic approach to NAFLD. Transient elastography is a noninvasive imaging modality that can be used to screen for the development of hepatic fibrosis. In obese patients newer "XL" FibroScan machines are more accurate. Liver biopsy can confirm diagnosis and provide prognostic information. It should be considered in patients with suspected advanced liver fibrosis (presence of obesity or type 2 diabetes, AST/ALT ratio 1, age 45 yr). NAFLD activity score on liver biopsy is described in Table 2.

LABORATORY TESTS

- Elevated ALT, AST: AST/ALT ratio is usually <1, but can increase as fibrosis advances. In advanced fibrosis AST to ALT ratio is >1 and platelet count is low.
- Negative serology for infectious hepatitis; generally normal GGTP and serum alkaline phosphatase.
- Hyperlipidemia (primarily hypertriglyceridemia) may be present.
- Elevated glucose levels may be present.
- Prolonged prothrombin time, hypoalbuminemia, and elevated bilirubin may be present in advanced stages.
- Elevated serum ferritin and increased transferrin saturation may be found in up to 10% of patients; however, hepatic iron index and hepatic iron level are normal.
- Antismooth muscle antibodies and antinuclear antibodies at low titer are not uncommon.

IMAGING STUDIES

- Ultrasound generally reveals diffuse increase in echogenicity as compared with that of the kidneys; CT scan reveals diffuse low-density hepatic parenchyma. The sensitivity of ultrasound and CT scan for detection of fat in liver is over 90% if hepatic steatosis exceeds 33%.
- Occasionally patients may have focal rather than diffuse steatosis, which may be misinterpreted as a liver mass on ultrasound or CT (Fig. E2); use of MRI in these cases will identify focal fatty infiltration.
- Ultrasound elastography (Fibroscan) can also be used to evaluate hepatic fibrosis and to further stratify patients.

Rx TREATMENT

NONPHARMACOLOGIC THERAPY

- Weight reduction in all obese patients. The American Gastroenterological Association recommends that the initial target weight loss be 10% of baseline weight at a rate of 1 to 2 lb (0.45 to 0.90 kg) per week.
- Increase physical activity. Vigorous and moderate exercise are equally effective in reducing intrahepatic triglyceride content, the effect being largely mediated by weight loss.
- Alcohol has a deleterious effect on NAFLD and should be avoided.

GENERAL Rx

- There are no drugs currently approved by FDA for NAFLD. Medications to control hyperlipidemia (e.g., fenofibrates for elevated triglycerides) and hyperglycemia (e.g., pioglitazone, insulin, metformin) can lead to improvement in abnormal liver test results.
- A 3-yr trial with pioglitazone (30 mg/day), an insulin-sensitizing thiazolidinedione, revealed that pioglitazone treatment was associated with long-term metabolic and histologic improvement in patients with prediabetes or type 2 diabetes mellitus and NASH. These results suggest that that NASH progression may be halted and the natural history of the disease may be modified with the use of pioglitazone in patients with prediabetes or type 2 diabetes mellitus.[1]

DISPOSITION

- Patients with pure steatosis on liver biopsy generally have a relatively benign course.
- The presence of steatohepatitis or advanced fibrosis on liver biopsy is associated with a worse prognosis.

REFERRAL

- Liver transplantation should be considered in patients with decompensated, end-stage disease; however, in these patients there may be a recurrence of NAFLD posttransplantation.

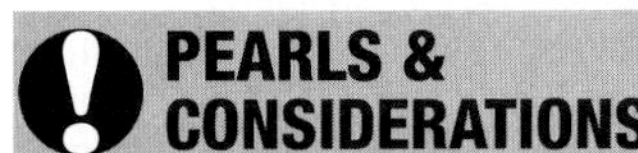

PEARLS & CONSIDERATIONS

COMMENTS

- NAFLD is closely associated with metabolic disorders, even in nonobese, nondiabetic subjects. It can be considered an early predictor of metabolic disorders, particularly in the normal-weight population. The presence of metabolic syndrome is a strong predictor of NAFLD.
- NAFLD is associated with an increased risk of incident cardiovascular disease that is independent of the risk conferred by traditional risk factors and components of the metabolic syndrome.
- 10% of patients with NASH have progression to advanced fibrosis. Most common in patients older than 50, ALT > twice normal, BMI >28, triglycerides >150 mg/dl.
- Statins are not contraindicated in patients with NASH and should be considered in hypercholesterolemic patients.

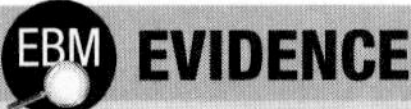

EVIDENCE

Available at ExpertConsult.com

SUGGESTED READINGS

Available at ExpertConsult.com

RELATED CONTENT

Fatty Liver (Patient Information)

AUTHOR: **FRED F. FERRI, M.D.**

[1] Cusi K, et al.: Long-term pioglitazone treatment for patients with nonalcoholic steatohepatitis and prediabetes or type 2 diabetes mellitus: a randomized trial, *Ann Intern Med* 165:305-315, 2016.

BASIC INFORMATION

DEFINITION

Nonallergic rhinitis (NAR) is characterized by chronic episodic or perennial symptoms of rhinitis (congestion, rhinorrhea, and postnasal drainage) that are not the result of IgE-mediated events. It is a heterogeneous group of diseases classified as inflammatory (infectious rhinosinusitis, rhinitis with eosinophilia syndrome) or noninflammatory (including but not limited to gustatory rhinitis, atrophic rhinitis, rhinitis medicamentosa, hormone-induced rhinitis, rhinitis in the elderly, rhinitis associated with systemic disease). Vasomotor rhinitis has previously been used interchangeably with NAR but is being phased out, as the term is too narrow with regard to the multiple mechanisms of action associated with NAR.

SYNONYMS

Chronic nonallergic rhinitis
Idiopathic rhinitis
Intrinsic rhinitis
NAR
Nonallergic-noninfectious chronic rhinitis
Vasomotor rhinitis

ICD-10CM CODES

J30.0 Vasomotor rhinitis
J31.0 Chronic rhinitis NOS (atrophic, granulomatous, hypertrophic, obstructive rhinitis)

EPIDEMIOLOGY & DEMOGRAPHICS

- Nonallergic rhinitis affects approximately 17 to 22 million individuals in the U.S.
- Approximately 50% of patients presenting with rhinitis may have NAR alone or a "mixed form."
  1. "Mixed nonallergic/allergic rhinitis" may occur in up to an additional 22 million Americans.
- Nonallergic rhinitis typically presents in adulthood with 70% of patients presenting after 20 yr of age. Onset of allergic rhinitis usually occurs in childhood.
- Risk factors for nonallergic rhinitis include female sex and age of >40 yr.
- May have genetic component in those individuals whose parents have allergic rhinitis.
- Medications that can cause chronic nasal symptoms are summarized in Table 1.
- Table 2 describes occupations with increased prevalence of work-related rhinitis.

PHYSICAL FINDINGS & CLINICAL PRESENTATION

- Physical exam can be completely unremarkable.
- Swollen erythematous turbinates or pale/violaceous swollen turbinates can both be seen in NAR patients.
- Clear or mucoid nasal secretions.
- Nasal crusting, anosmia (loss of smell), and foul odor from the nares are indicative of atrophic rhinitis.
- Clinical presentation: Can be nonspecific but usually consists of nasal congestions and/or rhinorrhea with often associated postnasal drip, sneezing, and throat clearing. Other allergic symptoms including nasal and palatal pruritus, sneezing, and conjunctival symptoms are typically absent.

ETIOLOGY

- NAR is composed of a heterogeneous group of diseases without a clear unifying theory of pathogenesis. In general, inflammatory NAR involves elevated numbers of immune cells (eosinophils, mast cells, neutrophils) leading to mediator release and inflammatory changes. For noninflammatory NAR, it is postulated that an abnormality in the autonomic nervous system is present with increased concentrations of intranasal neuropeptides. These are often triggered by perfumes, strong odors, changes in climate, and smoke. Specific subtypes likely have unique pathophysiologies:
  1. Infectious rhinosinusitis: Viral, bacterial, or fungal infections. Typically occurs following an acute viral infection.
  2. Nonallergic rhinitis with eosinophilia syndrome (NARES): Unknown etiology.
  3. Gustatory rhinitis: Abnormal vagally mediated rhinitis after ingestion of any food.
  4. Atrophic rhinitis: Unknown etiology but bacterial infection is thought to be involved.
  5. Rhinitis medicamentosa: Rebound nasal congestion from prolonged use of decongestant/vasoconstrictor agents (phenylephrine, oxymetazoline). Can also occur from cocaine, α-receptor antagonist, or phosphodiesterase-5-selective inhibitors.
  6. Hormone-induced rhinitis: Pregnancy-associated, menstrual cycle–associated, and oral contraceptive–related hormonal changes.
  7. Rhinitis associated with systemic disease: Severe hypothyroidism, diabetes mellitus.

DIAGNOSIS

DIFFERENTIAL DIAGNOSIS

- Allergic rhinitis (sensitivity to pollens, indoor allergens, occupational allergens)
- Systemic diseases with nasal manifestations (e.g., systemic lupus erythematosus, granulomatous disease, GERD)
- Mechanical obstruction (e.g., deviated septum, nasal polyps, nasal neoplasms, foreign bodies)
- Cerebral spinal fluid (CSF) leak from head trauma, postoperative complication from sinus surgery, or spontaneous leak
- Local allergic rhinitis
- Chronic rhinosinusitis
- Box 1 summarizes the differential diagnosis in chronic rhinitis

WORKUP

- A detailed history and physical examination can be helpful to determine if diagnostic testing is necessary. Most cases can be empirically treated without further testing.
- Distinguishing NAR from allergic rhinitis or other forms of rhinitis can be difficult, but a detailed history (lack of allergic symptoms such as sneezing, nasal pruritus) can be helpful. Questionnaires, including the Cincinnati Irritant Index Scale, have proven useful in differentiating NAR from allergic rhinitis.
  1. Because allergic rhinitis cannot be definitively ruled out with history alone, skin testing or assessment for serum-specific IgE should be considered. Adding to the diagnostic complexity, many individuals have a "mixed form" of rhinitis including both allergic and nonallergic types.
- Although not typically performed in a clinical setting, examination of nasal smears for the presence of neutrophils and eosinophils may be helpful.
- Anterior rhinoscopy or nasal endoscopy may be necessary to rule out nasal polyps or anatomic deformity, which may contribute to chronic rhinorrhea.

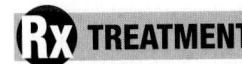

TREATMENT

NONPHARMACOLOGIC THERAPY

- Identification and avoidance of specific triggers (e.g., smoke/smog, specific foods, perfumes, strong odors, occupational irritants) may provide relief.
- Discontinuing any medication/drugs that could be contributing, including topical decongestants/vasoconstrictors, oral

TABLE 1 Medications Associated with Chronic Nasal Symptoms

Category	Example(s)
Antihypertensives	Angiotensin-converting enzyme inhibitors
	β-Adrenergic blockers
	Amiloride
	Prazocin
	Hydralazine
Psychotropics	Risperidone
	Chlorpromazine
	Amitriptyline
Phosphodiesterase-5 inhibitors	Sildenafil
	Tadalafil
	Vardenafil
Nonsteroidal antiinflammatory drugs	Ibuprofen
Others	Gabapentin

From Adkinson NF et al: *Middleton's allergy principles and practice*, ed 8, Philadelphia, 2014, Elsevier.

TABLE 2 Occupations with Increased Prevalence of Work-Related Rhinitis

Category	Occupation	Likely Trigger
Irritant	Drywall installer	Gypsum dust
	Makeup artist	Cosmetic power, perfume
Corrosive	Janitor	Ammonia
	Chemistry technician	Hydrochloric acid
Immunologic		
Immunoglobulin E	Baker	Grain flour
	Furrier	Animal dander
	Livestock breeder	Animal dander
	Veterinarian	Animal dander
	Food-processing worker	Foodstuffs
	Pharmacist	Medication powders
Low-molecular-weight substances	Boat builder	Anhydrides

From Adkinson NF et al: *Middleton's allergy principles and practice*, ed 8, Philadelphia, 2014, Elsevier.

contraceptives (OCPs), cocaine, and alcohol (Table 1).
- Daily nasal lavage and over-the-counter nasal saline sprays have been shown to improve symptoms.
- Surgical intervention (turbinectomy, vidian nerve resection) can be considered if medical measures fail, but surgery has not proved to be efficacious and involves the risk of complications.

ACUTE AND CHRONIC Rx

- Second-generation antihistamines have not been shown to be beneficial in nonallergic rhinitis. Although first-generation antihistamines may improve rhinorrhea due to their anticholinergic properties, topical therapies including intranasal antihistamines (azelastine, olopatadine), intranasal steroids (fluticasone propionate, triamcinolone, mometasone), and intranasal anticholinergics (ipratropium bromide) have been shown to be most beneficial.
- Treatments should be individualized to the underlying pathophysiology.
  1. *Vasomotor rhinitis:* Initial therapy typically involves intranasal steroids with the addition of an intranasal antihistamine or intranasal ipratropium bromide if symptoms are not well controlled. A combination intranasal steroid and intranasal antihistamine is now available that may be more convenient.
  2. *Infectious rhinosinusitis:* Supportive care and intranasal saline spray. May take up to 6 to 8 wk to improve after resolution of acute infection.
  3. *Nonallergic rhinitis with eosinophilia syndrome (NARES):* Topical nasal corticosteroids.
  4. *Gustatory rhinitis*: Preprandial intranasal ipratropium bromide.
  5. *Atrophic rhinitis:* Frequent irrigation with nasal saline, antibiotics to treat potential underlying bacterial infection; debridement and possible surgical intervention to reduce nasal cavity size can be considered.
  6. *Rhinitis medicamentosa:* Discontinuation of offending agent (topical decongestant/vasoconstrictor agent, cocaine, α-receptor antagonist or phosphodiesterase-5-selective inhibitors). Patient may require short course of nasal or oral corticosteroids during withdrawal process.
  7. *Hormone-induced rhinitis:* Typically resolves with delivery if during pregnancy. Consider discontinuing OCP if offending agent. Nasal saline spray alone can be efficacious.
  8. *Rhinitis associated with systemic disease:* Optimally managing the underlying condition.
  9. *Rhinitis in the elderly:* Intranasal ipratropium bromide.
- Several studies have shown that repeated administration of topical capsaicin has a long-term beneficial effect on symptoms in patients with idiopathic rhinitis.
- Alternative treatments: Silver nitrate, and acupuncture.

BOX 1 Differential Diagnosis in Chronic Rhinitis

- Concha bullosa
- Nasal septal deviation
- Adenoidal enlargement
- Nasal polyps
- Nasal cancer
- Nasal foreign body

From Adkinson NF et al: *Middleton's allergy principles and practice*, ed 8, Philadelphia, 2014, Elsevier.

DISPOSITION

Most patients experience mild to moderate symptomatic relief with avoidance of triggers and appropriate use of medications. Up to 52% of patients with NAR report worsening symptoms at 3- to 7-yr follow-ups. Periodic reevaluations should be performed, as there is evidence supporting increase in comorbidities (asthma, allergic rhinitis, conjunctivitis) with length of NAR diagnosis.

REFERRAL

Referral to allergist and/or ENT may be appropriate when severe symptoms are unresponsive to therapy and/or diagnosis is uncertain.

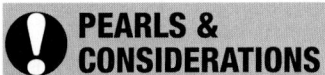

COMMENTS

- Nonallergic rhinitis symptoms are nonspecific, and a specific trigger is often never identified. Compared to allergic rhinitis, patients typically lack symptoms of sneezing, nasal pruritus, and conjunctival symptoms.
- Second-generation oral antihistamines are typically not efficacious, and the treatment of nonallergic rhinitis should be individualized based on its underlying pathophysiology.

SUGGESTED READINGS

Available at ExpertConsult.com

RELATED CONTENT

Allergic Rhinitis (Patient Information)
Allergic Rhinitis (Related Key Topic)

AUTHOR: **SHYAM JOSHI, M.D.**

BASIC INFORMATION

DEFINITION

Non-Hodgkin's lymphoma (NHL) is a heterogeneous group of malignancies of the lymphoreticular system. There are approximately 60 different NHL subtypes. The WHO classification of lymphomas is summarized in Table 1 and Fig. 1

SYNONYMS

NHL
Non-Hodgkin's lymphoma

ICD-10CM CODES

C85.90 Non-Hodgkin's lymphoma, unspecified, unspecified site
C85.91 Non-Hodgkin's lymphoma, unspecified, lymph nodes of head, face, and neck
C85.92 Non-Hodgkin's lymphoma, unspecified, intrathoracic lymph nodes
C85.93 Non-Hodgkin's lymphoma, unspecified, intra-abdominal lymph nodes
C85.94 Non-Hodgkin's lymphoma, unspecified, lymph nodes of axilla and upper limb
C85.95 Non-Hodgkin's lymphoma, unspecified, lymph nodes of inguinal region and lower limb
C85.96 Non-Hodgkin's lymphoma, unspecified, intrapelvic lymph nodes
C85.97 Non-Hodgkin's lymphoma, unspecified, spleen
C85.98 Non-Hodgkin's lymphoma, unspecified, lymph nodes of multiple sites
C85.99 Non-Hodgkin's lymphoma, unspecified, extranodal and solid organ sites

EPIDEMIOLOGY

- Sixth most common neoplasm in the U.S. (>70,000 new cases annually). Incidence increases with age; majority of patients are above 60 yr of age.
- In the U.S. and Europe, diffuse large B-cell lymphoma (DLBCL) is the most common subtype (30% of the cases), and follicular lymphoma (FL) is the second most common subtype (25% of the cases).
- In patients with HIV, NHL is the most common tumor (followed by Kaposi sarcoma). DLBCL accounts for 80% to 90% of the cases of HIV-associated NHL.

PHYSICAL FINDINGS & CLINICAL PRESENTATION

- Patients often present with lymphadenopathy.
- Approximately one third of the NHL involve extranodal sites, which can result in unusual presentations (e.g., gastrointestinal tract involvement can simulate peptic ulcer disease).
- Presence of B symptoms like unexplained weight loss, fever, fatigue, and night sweats

TABLE 1 World Health Organization Classification of Lymphomas[a]

Mature B-Cell Neoplasms

Chronic Lymphocytic Leukemia/Small Lymphocytic Lymphoma

- B-cell prolymphocytic leukemia
- Splenic B-cell marginal zone lymphoma
- Hairy cell leukemia
- *Splenic B-cell lymphoma/leukemia, unclassifiable*
- *Splenic diffuse red pulp small B-cell lymphoma*
- *Hairy cell leukemia-variant*
- Lymphoplasmacytic lymphoma
- Waldenström macroglobulinemia
- Heavy chain diseases
- Alpha heavy chain disease
- Gamma heavy chain disease
- Mu heavy chain disease

Plasma Cell Myeloma

- Solitary plasmacytoma of bone
- Extraosseous plasmacytoma

Extranodal Marginal Zone Lymphoma of Mucosa-Associated Lymphoid Tissue (MALT Lymphoma)

- Nodal marginal zone lymphoma
- *Pediatric nodal marginal zone lymphoma*

Follicular Lymphoma

- *Pediatric-type follicular lymphoma*
- Primary cutaneous follicle center lymphoma

Mantle Cell Lymphoma

Diffuse Large B-Cell Lymphoma (DLBCL), NOS

- T-cell/histiocyte–rich large B-cell lymphoma
- Primary DLBCL of the CNS
- Primary cutaneous DLBCL, leg type
- EBV-positive DLBCL
- DLBCL associated with chronic inflammation
- Lymphomatoid granulomatosis
- Primary mediastinal (thymic) large B-cell lymphoma
- Intravascular large B-cell lymphoma
- ALK-positive large B-cell lymphoma
- Plasmablastic lymphoma
- HHV8-positive diffuse large B-cell lymphoma and primary effusion lymphoma
- Burkitt lymphoma
- High grade B-cell lymphomas, with *MYC* and *BCL2* and/or *BCL6* rearrangements
- B-cell lymphoma unclassifiable, with features intermediate between diffuse large B-cell lymphoma and classic Hodgkin's lymphoma

Mature T-Cell and NK-Cell Neoplasms

- T-cell prolymphocytic leukemia
- T-cell large granular lymphocytic leukemia
- *Chronic lymphoproliferative disorder of NK-cells*
- Aggressive NK leukemia
- Systemic EBV-positive T-cell lymphoma of childhood
- Hydroa vacciniforme-like lymphoma
- Adult T-cell leukemia/lymphoma
- Extranodal NK/T-cell lymphoma, nasal type
- Enteropathy-associated T-cell lymphoma
- Monomorphic epitheliotropic intestinal T-cell lymphoma
- Hepatosplenic T-cell lymphoma
- Subcutaneous panniculitis-like T-cell lymphoma

Mycosis Fungoides

- Sézary syndrome
- Primary cutaneous CD30-positive T-cell lymphoproliferative disorders
- Lymphoid papulosis
- Primary cutaneous anaplastic large cell lymphoma
- Primary cutaneous gamma-delta T-cell lymphoma
- Primary cutaneous CD8-positive aggressive epidermotropic cytotoxic T-cell lymphoma
- Primary cutaneous CD4-positive small/medium T-cell lymphoproliferative disease

Peripheral T-Cell Lymphoma, NOS

Angioimmunoblastic T-Cell Lymphoma

Anaplastic Large Cell Lymphoma, ALK-Positive

- Anaplastic large cell lymphoma, ALK-negative

Hodgkin's Lymphoma

Nodular Lymphocyte Predominant Hodgkin's Lymphoma

Classic Hodgkin's Lymphoma

Nodular Sclerosis Hodgkin's Lymphoma

- Lymphocyte-rich classic Hodgkin's lymphoma
- Mixed cellularity classic Hodgkin's lymphoma
- Lymphocyte-depleted classic Hodgkin's lymphoma

ALK, Anaplastic lymphoma kinase; *CNS*, central nervous system; *EBV*, Epstein-Barr virus; *HHV-8*, human herpesvirus-8; *NK*, natural killer; *NOS*, not otherwise specified.
[a]Most common entities are underlined. Provisional entities are in italics. Some rare entities or variants are omitted.
From Hoffman R, et al.: *Hematology, basic principles and practice*, ed 7, Philadelphia, 2018, Elsevier.

 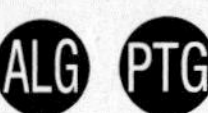

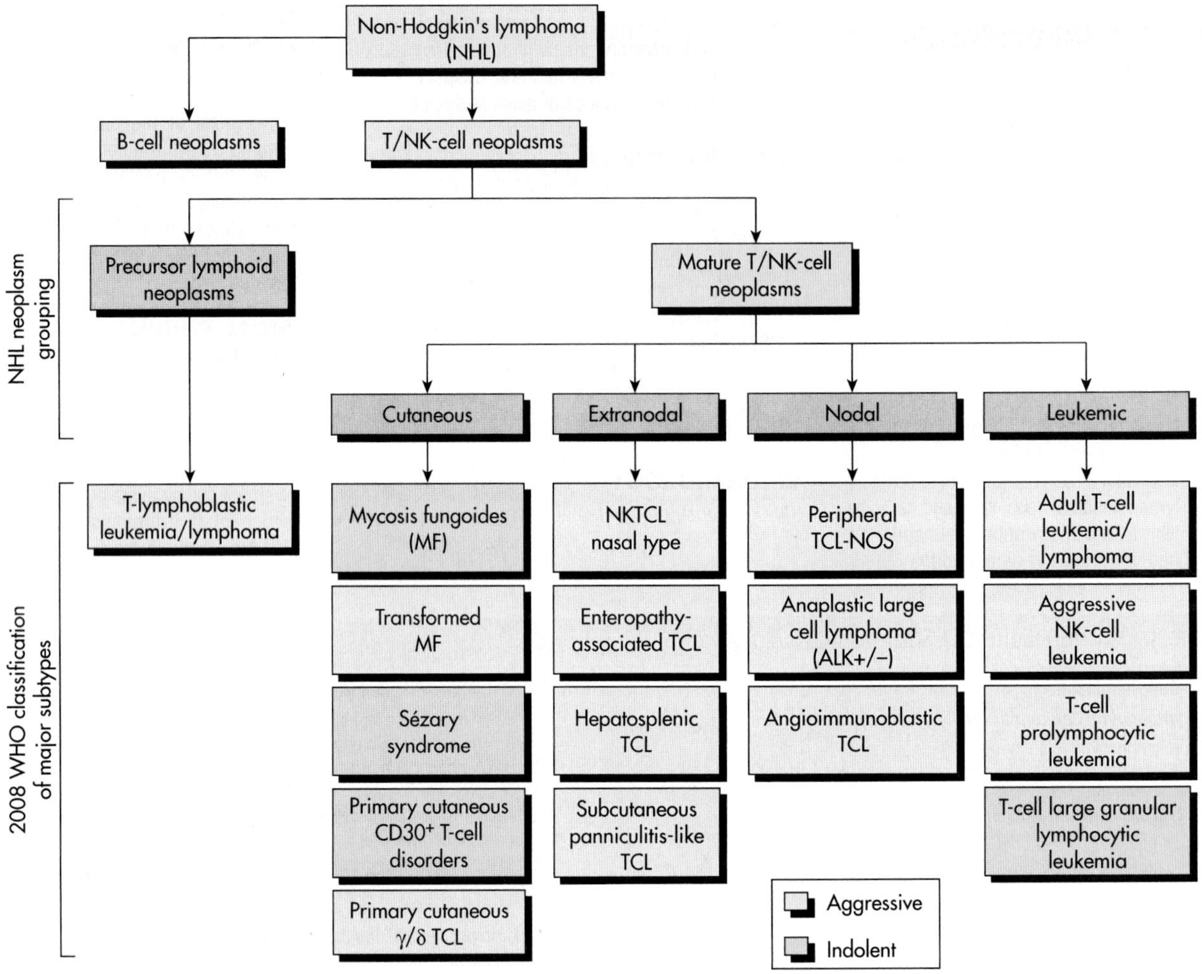

Non-Hodgkin's lymphoma (NHL)
B-cell neoplasms
T/NK-cell neoplasms
NHL neoplasm grouping
Precursor lymphoid neoplasms
Mature T/NK-cell neoplasms
Cutaneous
Extranodal
Nodal
Leukemic
2008 WHO classification of major subtypes
T-lymphoblastic leukemia/lymphoma
Mycosis fungoides (MF)
Transformed MF
Sézary syndrome
Primary cutaneous CD30+ T-cell disorders
Primary cutaneous γ/δ TCL
NKTCL nasal type
Enteropathy-associated TCL
Hepatosplenic TCL
Subcutaneous panniculitis-like TCL
Peripheral TCL-NOS
Anaplastic large cell lymphoma (ALK+/−)
Angioimmunoblastic TCL
Adult T-cell leukemia/ lymphoma
Aggressive NK-cell leukemia
T-cell prolymphocytic leukemia
T-cell large granular lymphocytic leukemia
Aggressive
Indolent

FIG. 1 World Health Organization (WHO) classification of the mature T-cell neoplasms. *NK,* Natural killer; *NKTCL,* nasal NK/T-cell lymphoma; *NOS,* not otherwise specified; *TCL,* T-cell lymphoma. (From Hoffman R, et al.: *Hematology, basic principles and practice,* ed 7, Philadelphia, 2018, Elsevier.)

are seen typically in aggressive or highly aggressive lymphomas.

- Aggressive lymphomas have acute or subacute presentation with increasing size of the mass and B symptoms.
- Indolent lymphomas have a more chronic course, with asymptomatic lymphadenopathy and/or slowly progressive cytopenias.
- Hepatomegaly and splenomegaly may be present.
- Cough, dyspnea with bulky mediastinal involvement.

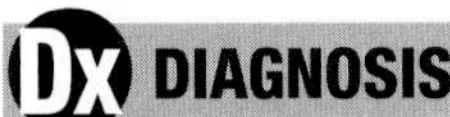

DIAGNOSIS

DIFFERENTIAL DIAGNOSIS

- Hodgkin's lymphoma
- Viral infections
- Metastatic carcinoma
- Autoimmune conditions
- Sarcoidosis

WORKUP

Initial laboratory evaluation may be entirely normal. Elevated LDH may be seen in aggressive lymphoma or in indolent lymphoma with high disease bulk. In cases of highly aggressive NHL (e.g., Burkitt lymphoma), spontaneous tumor lysis syndrome (TLS) may be seen, but rarely; it is characterized by hyperkalemia, hyperuricemia, hypocalcemia, hyperphosphatemia, and acidosis. TLS can be life threatening and is considered a medical emergency. Acute management includes aggressive IV fluid repletion and rasburicase. Proper staging of NHL includes the following:

- A thorough history and physical examination.
- Excisional or incisional surgical biopsy is preferred. Image-guided core needle biopsies may be acceptable in patients without peripheral adenopathy. Fine needle aspirates are not adequate for precise lymphoma subclassification. Laparoscopic lymph node biopsy or mediastinoscopy can be used on an outpatient basis for most patients with intraabdominal or mediastinal lymphoma, respectively.
- Tissue biopsy with histologic, immunophenotypic, and genetic studies interpretation.
- Routine laboratory evaluation (complete blood count, flow cytometry in selected circumstances, ESR, urinalysis, LDH, blood urea nitrogen, creatinine, serum calcium, uric acid, liver function tests, serum protein electrophoresis).
- HIV and hepatitis B testing.
- Bone marrow evaluation (aspirate and biopsy) (Fig. E2).
- CT scan of chest, abdomen, and pelvis with IV contrast, if possible.
- Fluorine-18 fluorodeoxyglucose (FDG) positron emission tomography (PET) integrated with CT has emerged as a powerful tool for staging, response evaluation, and post-treatment surveillance in patients with aggressive subtypes of NHL.
- Depending on the histopathology, the results of the previous studies, and the planned therapy, some other tests may be performed.
- Lumbar puncture is needed in some patients with aggressive NHL, and most patients with HIV-associated NHL, to evaluate for CNS involvement by lymphoma.

CLASSIFICATION: For clinical approach, NHL is subdivided lymphomas into indolent, aggressive, and highly aggressive disease.

STAGING: The Ann Arbor staging system with Cotswold modification is described in Table 2. Histopathology has greater therapeutic implications in NHL than in Hodgkin's lymphoma. Fig. 3 illustrates a diagnostic algorithm outlining the steps in classification of B-cell lymphomas composed of cells of small to intermediate size.

TABLE 2 Ann Arbor Staging System for Lymphomas

Stage*	Cotswold Modification of Ann Arbor Classification
I	Involvement of a single lymph node region or lymphoid structure
II	Involvement of two or more lymph node regions on the same side of the diaphragm (the mediastinum is considered a single site, whereas the hilar lymph nodes are considered bilaterally); the number of anatomic sites should be indicated by a subscript (e.g., II_3)
III	Involvement of lymph node regions on both sides of the diaphragm: III_1 (with or without involvement of splenic hilar, celiac, or portal nodes) and III_2 (with involvement of para-aortic, iliac, and mesenteric nodes)
IV	Involvement of one or more extranodal sites in addition to a site for which the designation E has been used

*All cases are subclassified to indicate the absence (A) or presence (B) of the systemic symptoms of significant fever (>38.0° C [100.4° F]), night sweats, and unexplained weight loss exceeding 10% of normal body weight within the previous 6 months. The clinical stage (CS) denotes the stage as determined by all diagnostic examinations and a single diagnostic biopsy only. In the Ann Arbor classification, the term pathologic stage (PS) is used if a second biopsy of any kind has been obtained, whether negative or positive. In the Cotswold modification, the PS is determined by laparotomy; X designates bulky disease (widening of the mediastinum by >one third or the presence of a nodal mass >10 cm), and E designates involvement of a single extranodal site that is contiguous or proximal to the known nodal site.

From Hoffmann R, et al.: *Hematology: basic principles and practice*, ed 5, Philadelphia, 2009, Churchill Livingstone.

DIAGNOSTIC ALGORITHM: B CELL NEOPLASMS OF SMALL TO INTERMEDIATE CELL SIZE

Step 1: Confirm B cell lineage (CD19, CD20, and/or CD79a)
AND
Assess for clonality (kappa, lambda, smig negative*).

Step 2: Evaluate expression of CD5 and CD10.

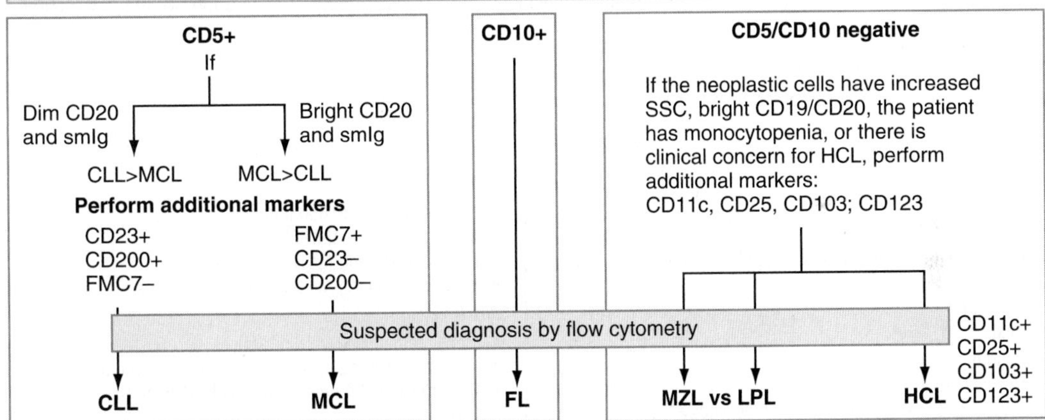

Step 3: Confirm the suspected diagnosis with additional data

CLL	MCL	FL	MZL vs LPL	HCL
Clinical and laboratory correlation need >5000 abnormal cells/µl or disease related sequelae to distinguish MBL and CLL	Cyclin D1 over-expression by IHC or a t(11;14) is required to confirm the diagnosis of MCL	Morphology Note: Typically, CD38 is low to absent while BCL2 is over-expressed in FL. These features help distinguish FL from BL	Morphology between MZL and LPL may overlap To distinguish: 1. Lab data- A large IgM monoclonal spike would favor LPL 2. Clinical data- Waldenstrom's would favor LPL	Flow cytometry allows for definitive diagnosis BRAF V600E mutation positive but not needed for diagnosis.

FIG. 3 This diagnostic algorithm outlines the steps in classification of B-cell lymphomas composed of cells of small to intermediate size. *BL,* Burkitt lymphoma; *CLL,* chronic lymphocytic leukemia; *FL,* follicular lymphoma; *HCL,* hairy cell leukemia; *IgM,* immunoglobulin M; *IHC,* immunohistochemistry; *LPL,* lymphoplasmacytic lymphoma; *MBL,* monoclonal B cell lymphocytosis; *MCL,* mantle cell lymphoma; *MZL,* marginal zone lymphoma; *Smlg,* surface immunoglobulin; *SSC,* scleroderma and systemic sclerosis. (From McPherson RA, Pincus MR: *Henry's clinical diagnosis and management by laboratory methods*, ed 23, Philadelphia, 2017, Elsevier.)

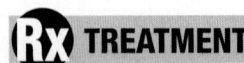

TREATMENT

ACUTE GENERAL Rx

The therapeutic regimen varies with specific lymphoma subtype and pathologic stage. Following are the commonly used therapeutic modalities:

INDOLENT NHL:

- Deferment of therapy and careful observation in asymptomatic patients with low volume disease.
- Local radiotherapy for stage I disease.
- Rituximab, an anti-CD20 monoclonal antibody, with or without chemotherapy is used in patients with symptomatic or progressive disease.
- The addition of rituximab to chemotherapy is generally well tolerated and has increased response and survival rates in NHL patients. Patients who received rituximab, cyclophosphamide, doxorubicin, vincristine, and prednisone (R-CHOP) had higher response rates (96% vs. 90%) with a better 2-yr overall survival rate (95% vs. 90%) than patients who received CHOP without rituximab. Similarly, patients who received rituximab, cyclophosphamide, vincristine, and prednisone (R-CVP) had higher response rates (81% vs. 57%) and better overall survival at 4 yr (83% vs. 77%) than patients who were treated with CVP without rituximab.
- In a recent phase III noninferiority study, the combination of bendamustine and rituximab was associated with better progression-free survival rates than R-CHOP (70 vs. 31 months) with fewer toxic effects. Subset analyses showed better progression-free survival in patients with follicular lymphoma, mantle cell lymphoma, and lymphoplasmacytic lymphoma.
- Maintenance rituximab after rituximab-containing regimens has been associated with a better progression-free survival at 3 yr (75% vs. 58%) than observation alone without a difference in overall survival.
- The combination of obinutuzumab and chemotherapy followed by obinutuzumab maintenance was approved by the FDA in previously untreated patients with follicular lymphoma based on a randomized study, in which obinutuzumab and chemotherapy were associated with longer median progression-free survival than rituximab and chemotherapy.
- The combination of obinutuzumab and bendamustine followed by obinutuzumab maintenance was approved by the FDA for the treatment of patients with rituximab-refractory follicular lymphoma.
- The oral BTK inhibitor ibrutinib is FDA-approved for the treatment of patients with relapsed mantle cell lymphoma, lymphoplasmacytic lymphoma, and marginal zone lymphoma. Acalabrutinib, a second-generation BTK inhibitor, has also been approved for relapsed mantle cell lymphoma.
- The oral PI3K inhibitors idelalisib and copanlisib, as well as the novel anti-CD20 monoclonal antibody obinutuzumab, have been FDA-approved for the treatment of relapsed follicular lymphoma.
- The proteasome inhibitor bortezomib and the immunomodulating agent lenalidomide are FDA-approved for the treatment of relapsed mantle cell lymphoma.
- *H. pylori*-associated gastric marginal zone lymphoma can be treated with a course of antibiotics. For persistent cases after eradication or *H. pylori*-negative cases, radiotherapy is highly effective.
- Splenic marginal zone lymphoma is typically treated with rituximab or splenectomy. Chemoimmunotherapy or ibrutinib may be appropriate in relapsed disease.

TABLE 3 Chemotherapy Regimens in Indolent Lymphomas

BR (Every 28 Days)

- Bendamustine 120 mg/m^2 days 1 and 2
- Rituximab 375 mg/m^2 IV day 1

CVP-R (Every 21 Days)

- Cyclophosphamide 750 mg/m^2 IV on day 1
- Vincristine 1.4 mg/m^2, up to a maximal dose of 2 mg IV, on day 1
- Prednisone 40 mg/m^2 daily PO days 1-5
- Rituximab 375 mg/m^2 IV day 1[32]

R-CHOP (Every 21 Days)

- Cyclophosphamide 750 mg/m^2 IV on day 1
- Doxorubicin 50 mg/m^2 IV on day 1
- Vincristine 1.4 mg/m^2, up to a maximal dose of 2 mg IV, on day 1
- Prednisone 100 mg daily orally on days 1-5
- Rituximab 375 mg/m^2 IV on day 1 of each therapy cycle[33] or by alternate schedule[34]

CNOP (Every 21 Days)

- Cyclophosphamide 750 mg/m^2 IV on day 1
- Mitoxantrone 10 mg/m^2 IV on day 1
- Vincristine 1.4 mg/m^2, up to a maximal dose of 2 mg IV, on day 1
- Prednisone 50 mg/m^2 daily orally on days 1-5

R-CHVP-IFN (Every 28 Days for 6 Months, Then Every 2 Months for 6 Months).[35]

- Cyclophosphamide 600 mg/m^2
- Doxorubicin 25 mg/m^2
- Etoposide 100 mg/m^2 on day 1 (replaces original teniposide 60 mg/m^2 on day 1)
- Prednisolone 40 mg/m^2 on days 1-5
- Interferon-α 5-3 times a week
- Patients being treated with R-CHVP also received 375 mg/m^2 of rituximab IV on day 1 of each therapy cycle for 6 cycles

FMD (Every 28 Days)

- Fludarabine 25 mg/m^2 IV on day 1-3
- Mitoxantrone 10 mg/m^2 IV on day 1
- Dexamethasone 20 mg/day PO days 1-5
- Patients being treated with R-FMD also received 375 mg/m^2 of rituximab IV on day 1 of each therapy cycle

ProMACE-MOPP

- Cycles repeated every 28 days

Day 1

- Cyclophosphamide 650 mg/m^2 IV
- Doxorubicin 25 mg/m^2 IV
- Etoposide 120 mg/m^2 IV
- Prednisone 60 mg/m^2 orally daily days 1-14

Day 8

- Mechlorethamine 6 mg/m^2 IV
- Vincristine 1.4 mg/m^2 (maximum 2 mg) IV on day 8
- Procarbazine 100 mg/m^2 orally daily days 8-14

Day 15

- Methotrexate 500 mg/m^2 IV on day 15 with leucovorin 50 mg/m^2 orally every 6 hours for four doses beginning 24 hours after methotrexate

R-Hyper-CVAD (Every 21 Days)[36]

Cycles 1, 3, 5 and 7

- Rituximab 375 mg/m^2 IV on day 1
- Cyclophosphamide (with mesna) 300 mg/m^2 IV over 3 hours every 12 hours on days 2-4 (total 6 doses)
- Vincristine 1.4 mg/m^2 (maximum 2 mg) IV on days 5 and 12
- Doxorubicin 16.6 mg/m^2 IV by continuous infusion on days 5-7
- Dexamethasone 40 mg/day PO/IV on days 2–5 and days 12-15

Cycles 2,4, 6 and 8

- Rituximab 375 mg/m^2 IV on day 1
- Methotrexate 200 mg/m^2 IV over 2 hours, followed by 800 mg/m^2 IV continuous infusion over 22 hours on day 2
- Leucovorin 50 mg PO starting 12 hours after completion of methotrexate infusion, followed by 15 mg PO every 6 hours for 8 dosed until the methotrexate level is less than 0.1 μM/L
- Cytarabine 3000 mg/m^2 IV over 2 hours every 12 hours on days 3 and 4 (4 doses total)

Rituximab Monotherapy

Rituximab 375 mg/m^2 weekly for 4 weeks

NOTE: Reference endnotes retained from the source.
IV, Intravenous; *PO*, by mouth.
From Hoffman R, et al.: *Hematology, basic principles and practice*, ed 7, Philadelphia, 2018, Elsevier.

- Stem cell transplantation (autologous or allogeneic) may confer long-term disease control in multiple relapsed or refractory disease.
- Table 3 summarizes chemotherapy regimens in indolent lymphomas.

AGGRESSIVE NHL: The most common aggressive NHL is DLBCL. The addition of rituximab against CD20 B-cell lymphoma to the CHOP regimen (R-CHOP) increased the complete response rate and prolonged overall survival in patients with DLBCL, based on randomized controlled trials, without clinically significant increase in toxicity. R-CHOP has shown to be safe and effective in patients with HIV-associated NHL with CD4+ counts >50 cells/mm^3.

Most common regimens used in DLBCL include:

- Three cycles of R-CHOP followed by involved-field radiotherapy or 6 cycles of R-CHOP alone are appropriate approaches in patients with localized DLBCL.
- 6 cycles of R-CHOP with or without radiotherapy are appropriate in patients with advanced-stage DLBCL.
- For patients with double-hit lymphomas (defined as harboring rearrangement of MYC, BCL-2, and/or BCL-6), who have poorer outcomes to R-CHOP than regular DLBCL, the use of R-EPOCH (infusional etoposide, doxorubicin, and vincristine, along with cyclophosphamide, prednisone, and rituximab) might also be effective.
- Granulocyte-colony stimulating factor (e.g., filgrastim, MYC) may be effective in reducing the risk of febrile neutropenia in patients over 65 yr with aggressive lymphoma undergoing chemotherapy.
- Treatment with high-dose chemotherapy and autologous bone marrow transplant: Compared with conventional chemotherapy, increases overall survival in patients with chemotherapy-sensitive relapsed DLBCL.
- Chimeric antigen receptor T-cell therapy was recently approved for patients with relapsed or refractory diffuse large B-cell lymphoma after two prior lines of chemotherapy.
- Combination chemotherapy regimens for NHL are described in Table 4.

TABLE 4 Combination Chemotherapy Regimens for Non-Hodgkin's Lymphoma

Regimen	Dose	Days of Administration	Frequency
R-bendamustine			**Every 28 days**
Bendamustine	90 mg/m_2 IV	1-2	
Rituximab	375 mg/m_2 IV	1	
R-CHOP			**Every 21 days**
Cyclophosphamide	750 mg/m_2 IV	1	
Doxorubicin	50 mg/m_2 IV	1	
Vincristine	1.4 mg/m_2 IV	1	
Prednisone, fixed dose	100 mg PO	1-5	
Rituximab	375 mg/m_2 IV	1	
R-CVP			**Every 21 days**
Cyclophosphamide	1000 mg/m_2 IV	1	
Vincristine	1.4 mg/m_2 IV	1	
Prednisone, fixed dose	100 mg PO	1-5	
Rituximab	375 mg/m_2 IV	1	

IV, Intravenous; *PO,* by mouth.
Adapted from Goldman L, Schafer AI: *Goldman's Cecil medicine,* ed 24, Philadelphia, 2012, Saunders.

HIGHLY AGGRESSIVE NHL: The most common high-grade NHL subtype is Burkitt lymphoma (BL). BL affects younger patients than DLBCL and is common in HIV-infected individuals. Regimens more intensive than R-CHOP are needed to cure patients with high-grade NHL. The most commonly used multi-agent regimens include hyperCVAD, CODOX-M/IVAC, and dose-adjusted EPOCH, usually in combination with rituximab. The 5-yr survival approximates 75%.

DISPOSITION

- Patients with indolent NHL in the rituximab era experience long survival despite the lack of curative potential of chemoimmunotherapy. Patients with aggressive NHL may achieve a cure with chemoimmunotherapy.
- Complete remission occurs in 50% to 60% of patients with aggressive NHL. Prognostic factors include the lymphoma subtype, age of patient, and extent of disease. Table E5 describes the International Prognostic Index for aggressive lymphomas.
- Patients who present with HIV-related NHL and low CD4+ cell count have a poor prognosis (median duration of survival is 15-34 mo). Despite therapeutic advances, the management of HIV-associated lymphomas is challenging due to potential pharmacologic interactions and increased risk of infectious complications. It is important to optimize the CD4 cell count during treatment. Referral to an HIV oncologist is recommended.

SUGGESTED READINGS

Available at ExpertConsult.com

RELATED CONTENT

Non-Hodgkin's Lymphoma (Patient Information)

AUTHORS: **JORGE J. CASTILLO, M.D.,** and **ANN S. LACASCE, M.D., M.M.SC.**

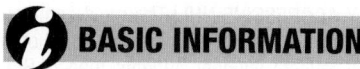

BASIC INFORMATION

DEFINITION

Obesity refers to having an excess amount of body fat in relation to lean body mass, or a body mass index (BMI) of ≥30 kg/m^2. Overweight is defined as BMI of 25 to 29.9 kg/m^2, and morbid obesity refers to adults with a BMI ≥40 kg/m^2. BMI is used as a surrogate measure of obesity. Abdominal obesity is defined as waist circumference >102 cm (40 inches) in men and >88 cm (35 inches) in women.

ICD-10CM CODES

E66.9	Obesity, unspecified
E66.01	Morbid (severe) obesity due to excess calories
E66.09	Other obesity due to excess calories
E66.1	Drug-induced obesity
E66.2	Morbid (severe) obesity with alveolar hypoventilation
E66.8	Other obesity
099.210	Obesity complicating pregnancy, unspecified trimester
099.211	Obesity complicating pregnancy, first trimester
099.212	Obesity complicating pregnancy, second trimester
099.213	Obesity complicating pregnancy, third trimester
099.214	Obesity complicating childbirth
099.215	Obesity complicating the puerperium

EPIDEMIOLOGY & DEMOGRAPHICS

- The World Health Organization first recognized obesity as a worldwide epidemic in 1997. As of 2005, 1.6 billion adults worldwide were classified as overweight, 400 million of whom were obese. It is predicted that the combination of overweight and obesity will soon eclipse public health issues such as malnutrition and infectious diseases as the most significant cause of poor health.
- Worldwide, data from the Global Burden of Disease Study from 1980 to 2013 indicate the prevalence of adult obesity has increased from 28.8% to 36.9% in men and 29.8% to 38% in women. The prevalence of childhood and adolescent obesity has also substantially increased.
- Based on U.S. NHANES data from 2011 to 2012, the prevalence of abdominal obesity was 54%. It is estimated that by 2020, 2 in every 5 adults and 1 in every 4 children in the U.S. will be categorized as obese.
- The present cost of obesity in the U.S. population is estimated at $100 billion annually. Approximately two thirds of people living in the United States are overweight, which is the highest percentage in the world (Marie Ng, 2014).
- For persons with a BMI ≥30 kg/m^2, all-cause mortality is increased by 50% to 100% above that of persons with BMI in the range of 20 to 25 kg/m^2.
- Obesity is an independent risk factor for cardiovascular disease (CVD), type 2 diabetes, hypertension, cancer (particularly colon, prostate, breast, and gynecologic malignancies), sleep apnea, degenerative joint disease, thromboembolic disorders, digestive tract diseases (gallstones), and dermatologic disorders.
- Significant morbidity and risk of death are projected to begin in young adulthood, resulting in >100,000 excess cases of CHD by 2035, even with the most modest projection of future obesity.
- When children enter kindergarten, 12.4% are obese, and another 14.9% are overweight. Data show that incident obesity between the ages of 5 and 14 yr is more likely to have occurred at younger ages.[1]
- Obesity in adolescence is significantly associated with increased risk of incident severe obesity in adulthood, with variations by sex and race/ethnicity. Overweight or obese adults who were obese as children have increased risk of type 2 DM, dyslipidemia, hypertension, and carotid artery atherosclerosis.
- Obesity is a major preventable cause of death and disability in the U.S. (the other is tobacco).
- Extensive data indicate that weight loss can reverse or arrest the harmful effects of obesity.
- In 2013 nearly 180,000 bariatric surgery procedures were performed in the U.S. Of these procedures 42% were laparoscopic sleeve gastrectomy, 34% were Roux-en-Y gastric bypass, and 15% were laparoscopic adjustable gastric banding.

PHYSICAL FINDINGS & CLINICAL PRESENTATION

- Physical examination should assess the degree and distribution of body fat, signs of secondary causes of obesity, and obesity-related comorbidities.
- Increased waist circumference is apparent. Excess abdominal fat is clinically defined as a waist circumference >40 inches (>102 cm) in men and >35 inches (>88 cm) in women (in Asian men and women, >36 inches and >33 inches, respectively). Central obesity is a risk factor for mortality even among individuals with normal BMIs.
- Symptoms associated with hypertension, coronary artery disease (CAD), and diabetes (e.g., polyuria, polydipsia, acanthosis nigricans, retinopathy, and neuropathy) may be present.
- Obesity is associated with cardiac hypertrophy, diastolic dysfunction, and decreased aortic compliance, which are independent predictors of cardiovascular risk.
- Joint pain and swelling are associated with degenerative joint disease secondary to obesity.
- The physical exam and ECG often underestimate the presence and extent of cardiac dysfunction in obese patients. Jugular venous distention and hepatojugular reflux may not be seen and heart sounds are frequently distant.
- A large quantity of fluid is present in the interstitial space of adipose tissue, as the interstitial space is ~10% of the tissue wet weight. This excess fluid in this compartment, if redistributed into the circulation, can have negative repercussions in obese individuals with heart failure. Obese individuals have higher cardiac output and a lower total peripheral resistance than do lean individuals, and obesity is associated with persistence of elevated cardiac filling pressure during exercise.
- Obesity predisposes to heart failure through several different mechanisms: increased total blood volume, increased cardiac output, LVH, left ventricular diastolic dysfunction, and adipositas cordis (excessive epicardial fat and fatty infiltration of the myocardium).

ETIOLOGY

- The pathophysiology of obesity is complex and poorly understood, but includes social, nutritional, physiologic, psychological, and genetic factors.
- Environmental factors such as a sedentary lifestyle and chronic ingestion of excess calories can cause obesity.
- Obesity may be related to genetic factors, which are thought to be polygenic. Genetic studies with adopted children have demonstrated that they have similar BMIs to their biologic parents but not their adoptive parents. Twin studies also demonstrate a genetic influence on BMI.
- Secondary causes of obesity can result from medications (antipsychotics, steroids, and protease inhibitors being common ones) and neuroendocrine disorders (like Cushing's syndrome and hypothyroidism).

Dx DIAGNOSIS

- BMI will establish the diagnosis of obesity. BMI is defined as the adult's weight in kilograms divided by the square of his or her height—and is closely correlated with total body fat content.
- BMI values can categorize patients into three classes of obesity:
  1. Class I (mild): BMI of 30.0 to 34.9 kg/m^2
  2. Class II (moderate): BMI of 35.0 to 39.9 kg/m^2
  3. Class III (severe): BMI of ≥40 kg/m^2
- Although BMI is commonly used to define obesity, it is not a highly accurate indicator of body fat composition in children, who are undergoing rapid changes in height, or in bodybuilders or athletes who have large amounts of muscle tissue.
- Waist circumference or waist-hip ratio is indicative of visceral adipose tissue/intraabdominal fat, which may be more deleterious than overall overweight or obesity.

---

[1] Cunningham SA, et al.: Incidence of childhood obesity in the United States, *N Engl J Med*, 370:403-411, 2014.

DIFFERENTIAL DIAGNOSIS

It is important to evaluate obese patients for secondary medical causes of obesity. Hypothalamic disorders, hypothyroidism, Cushing's syndrome, insulinoma, depression, and drugs (corticosteroids, antidepressants, second-generation antipsychotics, sulfonylureas, and HIV protease inhibitors) can cause obesity. In children, certain genetic conditions, such as Prader-Willi syndrome, are associated with obesity.

WORKUP

History should be obtained regarding weight change, family history of obesity, and eating and exercise behavior. Assessment for eating disorders and depression should be made. Attention should be directed to the use of nutritional supplements, over-the-counter medications, hormones, diuretics, and laxatives. The workup of an obese patient typically requires laboratory work to assess for risks and complications as well as to rule out underlying causative medical conditions. Fig. E1 describes the evaluation of patients with suspected endocrine cause of obesity.

LABORATORY TESTS

- Obese patients should be assessed for medical consequences of their obesity by screening for metabolic syndrome. This includes measurement of fasting lipid profile, blood pressure, and waist circumference and screening for diabetes or prediabetes (oral glucose tolerance test, fasting glucose, or hemoglobin A1C).
- Polycythemia might warrant screening for sleep apnea. Liver function tests should be obtained to screen for hepatic steatosis.
- In the proper clinical setting, thyroid function studies and dexamethasone suppression testing will exclude hypothyroidism and Cushing's syndrome as underlying causes of obesity. If insulinoma is suspected, the patient will need to undergo a 72-hr fast to confirm hypoglycemia with inappropriate insulin secretion.
- Obesity is associated with changes in the ECG, including a reduction in voltage and nonspecific ST-T changes that may interfere with diagnosis of left ventricular hypertrophy (LVH) or CAD.

IMAGING STUDIES

- Several methods are available for determining or calculating total body fat but offer no significant advantage over the BMI. These include measurement of total body water, total body potassium, bioelectrical impedance, and dual-energy x-ray absorptiometry.
- Buoyancy testing is an accurate method for determining total body fat composition.

OTHER STUDIES

Obesity increases the risk of obstructive sleep apnea, which, in turn, increases the risks of hypertension, cardiac arrhythmias, CVD, stroke, and heart failure. Therefore one should have a low threshold to screen obese patients for obstructive sleep apnea via sleep study/polysomnography.

TABLE 1 Weight-Loss Treatment Guidelines from the National Heart, Lung, and Blood Institute*

	BMI				
Treatment	**25.0-26.9**	**27.0-29.9**	**30.0-34.9**	**35.0-39.9**	**>40.0**
Diet, physical activity, behavioral therapy, or all three	Yes	Yes	Yes	Yes	Yes
Pharmacotherapy†		In patients with obesity-related diseases	Yes	Yes	Yes
Surgery‡				In patients with obesity-related diseases	Yes

*Data are from www.nhlbi.nih.gov/guidelines/obesity/ob_home.htm. These guidelines are generally consistent with those from the American Heart Association, the American Medical Association, the American Diabetic Association, the Obesity Society (Practical Guide), the American Diabetes Association, the American Academy of Family Physicians, the American College of Sports Medicine, and the American Cancer Society. *BMI* denotes body mass index, calculated as the weight in kilograms divided by the square of the height in meters.

†Pharmacotherapy should be considered only in patients who are not able to achieve adequate weight loss with available conventional lifestyle modifications and who have no absolute contraindications for drug therapy.

‡Bariatric surgery should be considered only in patients who are unable to lose weight with available conventional therapy and who have no absolute contraindications for surgery.

Rx TREATMENT

The National Heart, Lung, and Blood Institute (NHLBI) developed guidelines for selecting treatment strategies for overweight and obese patients based on BMI and comorbidities. They recommend a combination of dietary management, physical activity management, and behavior therapy for anyone with a BMI ≥25 or with a high-risk waist circumference and two or more obesity-associated comorbidities. Pharmacotherapy should be considered for patients with a BMI ≥30 or ≥27 with comorbidities.

Bariatric surgery is indicated for patients with a BMI ≥35 with comorbidities and for any patient with a BMI ≥40 (Table 1).

NONPHARMACOLOGIC THERAPY

- The cornerstones for weight management and reduction are calorie restriction, exercise, and behavioral modification. Assessment of patient's willingness to make changes must be evaluated, as treatment is more likely to succeed in motivated patients.
- The NHLBI guidelines recommend an initial diet to produce a calorie deficit of 500 to 1000 kcal/day. This has been shown to reduce total body weight by an average of 8% over 3 to 12 mo.
- These guidelines recommend the use of a food diary to focus on dietary substitutes.
- Thirty minutes of moderate-intensity activity on 5 or more days of the week results in health benefits for obese individuals. Moreover, several studies indicate that 60 to 80 min of moderate to vigorous physical activity may provide additional benefit.
- Increased physical activity without caloric restriction (minimal or no weight loss) can reduce abdominal (visceral) adipose tissue and improve insulin resistance.
- The key features of the standard behavioral modification program include goal setting, self-monitoring, stimulus control (modification of one's environment to enhance behaviors that will support weight management), cognitive restructuring (increased awareness of perceptions of oneself and one's weight), and prevention of relapse (weight regain).
- Mammalian sleep is closely integrated with the regulation of energy balance. Trials have shown that the amount of human sleep contributes to the maintenance of fat-free body mass at times of decreased energy intake. Lack of sufficient sleep may compromise the efficacy of typical dietary interventions for weight loss and related metabolic risk reduction.

ACUTE GENERAL Rx

- According to the NHLBI *Guidelines on the Identification, Evaluation, and Treatment of Overweight and Obesity in Adults* and the U.S. Food and Drug Administration (FDA), pharmacotherapy is indicated for:
  1. Obese patients with a BMI ≥30.
  2. Overweight patients with a BMI of ≥27 and concomitant obesity-related risk factors or diseases, such as hypertension, diabetes, or dyslipidemia.
- Pharmacologic treatment options include:
  1. Gastrointestinal lipase inhibitors: Orlistat is the only drug available for long-term treatment of obesity. It blocks the digestion and absorption of ingested dietary fat. It is a reversible inhibitor of pancreatic, gastric, and carboxyl ester lipases and phospholipase A2, which are required for the hydrolysis of dietary fat in the gastrointestinal tract. Side effects include flatulence, fecal incontinence, cramps, and oily spotting. There can also be impairment of absorption of fat-soluble vitamins (A, D, E, K) and beta-carotene. Oxalate-associated acute kidney injury and rare severe liver injury have also been reported.
  2. C serotonin agonists: Lorcaserin is a selective serotonin agonist that acts centrally to reduce appetite, aiding weight

loss. Adverse effects include headache, upper respiratory infections, dizziness, and nausea. While there is little evidence of serotonin-associated cardiac valvular disease or pulmonary hypertension (as seen with nonselective serotonergic agonists fenfluramine and dexfenfluramine), long-term data is currently limited.

3. Sympathomimetic medications: Phentermine and diethylpropion are currently approved for short-term treatment of obesity. They reduce food intake by causing early satiety. Side effects include increased blood pressure and increased pulse. They are Schedule IV drugs with a potential for abuse. Other sympathomimetic drugs that have been removed from the market due to concerns about cardiovascular safety are sibutramine, phenylpropanolamine, and ephedrine.
4. Antidepressants: While not FDA-approved for treatment of obesity alone, bupropion and fluoxetine are antidepressants that have been associated with modest weight loss. The FDA has recently approved a fixed-dose combination of bupropion with the opioid receptor antagonist naltrexone. It is called Contrave and approved for use as an adjunct to diet and exercise in patients with BMI ≥30 kg/m^2 or a BMI ≥27 kg/m^2 and one or more weight-related comorbidities (e.g., diabetes, hypertension, dyslipidemia).
5. Antiepileptic drugs: Zonisamide and topiramate (also used in migraine therapy) have been associated with weight loss in clinical trials but are not currently FDA-approved for treatment of obesity alone.
6. Diabetes drugs: While not FDA-approved for treatment of obesity alone, metformin, pramlintide (synthetic human amylin), and glucagon-like polypeptide-1 agonists (GLP-1) (exenatide) have been associated with weight loss in the treatment of individuals with diabetes. The GLP-1 receptor agonist liraglutide (Victoza) is now FDA approved at a higher dose as Saxenda for chronic weight management in adults with BMI ≥30 or a BMI ≥27 with a weight-related comorbidity such as hypertension, dyslipidemia, or diabetes.

CHRONIC Rx

- According to the NHLBI guidelines, surgical intervention is an option for selected patients with clinically severe obesity (a BMI ≥40 or a BMI ≥35 with comorbid conditions), when patients are at high risk for obesity-associated morbidity or death, and when less invasive methods of weight loss have failed. Box 1 summarizes patient requirements for bariatric surgery.
- Eligible patients should also be at an acceptable risk for surgery, well informed, and motivated.
- Bariatric surgery for weight loss falls into one of three general categories:
- Restrictive surgeries limit the amount of food the stomach can hold and slow the rate of gastric emptying. These include vertical banded gastroplasty and laparoscopic adjustable silicone gastric banding LAGB. Band slippage is the most common LAGB complication. Other potential complications include port or tubing malfunction, stomal obstruction, band erosion, pouch dilatation, and port infection. Gastric necrosis of the stomach wall is a rarer late complication that results from ischemia caused by a combination of gastric prolapse—the part of the stomach below the band herniates up through the device —and pressure from the band. Complications of bariatric surgery are summarized in Box 2.
- Gastric bypass has better outcomes than gastric band procedures for long-term weight loss, type 2 diabetes control and remission, hypertension, and hyperlipidemia. These procedures have benefits that include lower perioperative mortality rate, a quicker recovery period, and no malabsorption issues. However, they are not as effective as gastric bypass for weight reduction and comorbidity improvement.
  1. Malabsorptive surgeries reduce nutrient absorption by shortening the length of small intestine. These include jejunoileal bypass and the duodenal switch operation (DS).
  2. Restrictive malabsorptive bypass procedures combine the elements of gastric restriction and selective malabsorption. These include Roux-en-Y gastric bypass (considered the gold standard because of its high level of effectiveness and durability) and biliopancreatic diversion. These procedures have higher rates of comorbidity improvement than restrictive surgeries, but can be complicated by malabsorption and nutritional deficiencies.
- Compared with usual care, bariatric surgery is associated with reduced number of cardiovascular deaths and lower incidence of cardiovascular events in obese adults. A study on bariatric surgery patients demonstrated a significant reduction in long-term cardiovascular events. Ten-year follow-up estimated relative risk reductions ranging from 18% to 79% according to the Framingham risk score and 8% to 62% with the PROCAM risk score.
- A long-term observational study of obese patients with type 2 diabetes showed that bariatric surgery was associated with higher diabetes remission rates and fewer complications than usual care (Sjostrom et al., 2014). Remission of type 2 DM occurs in 60% to 80% of patients 2 yr after surgery and persists in about 30% of patients 15 yr after Roux-en-Y gastric bypass.
- Liposuction is removal of fat by aspiration after injection of physiologic saline. This

BOX 1 Patient Requirements for Bariatric Surgery

1. Patients with a BMI of 40 kg/m^2 or greater are potential candidates for bariatric surgery.
2. Patients with a BMI of 35 to 40 kg/m^2 with significant obesity-related comorbidity are also potential candidates for bariatric surgery.
3. Patients with a history of dieting.
4. Patients with no recent substance abuse.
5. Patients should be evaluated by a multidisciplinary team that includes a dietician and psychologic evaluation before surgery.

BMI, Body mass index.
From Cameron JL, Cameron AM: *Current surgical therapy*, ed 12, Philadelphia, 2017, Elsevier.

BOX 2 Complications of Bariatric Surgery

Complications Common to All Bariatric Procedures

Early (Up to 30 Days After Surgery)
Venous thromboembolic disease
Bleeding
Anastomotic leaks
Wound infections
Persistent nausea/vomiting, dehydration
Regional abdominal organ trauma
Incisional and internal hernias
Bowel obstruction
Atelectasis
Pneumonia
Cardiac dysrhythmias
Urinary tract infection
Death

Late (Beyond 30 Days After Surgery)
Incisional and internal hernias
Bowel obstruction from adhesions
Nutritional deficiencies
Anastomotic strictures and marginal ulcers or erosions
Cholelithiasis
Anemia
Persistence or recurrence of obstructive sleep apnea
Need for body contouring
Regaining weight

Procedure-Unique Complications/Adverse Effects

Roux-en-Y Gastric Bypass
Dumping syndrome

Laparoscopic Adjustable Gastric Banding
Band slippage or erosion
Port or device malfunction

Vertical Sleeve Gastrectomy
Refractory reflux

Biliopancreatic Diversion
Loose, foul-smelling stools
Protein-calorie malnutrition

(From Kryger M, Roth T, Dement WC: *Principles and practice of sleep medicine*, ed 6, Philadelphia, 2017, Elsevier)

technique reduces the subcutaneous fat but has failed to improve insulin sensitivity or risk factors for CHD.

- The Maestro Rechargeable System is a subcutaneously implanted device recently FDA approved for weight loss in adults with a BMI of 40 to 45 or with a BMI of ≥35 and at least one obesity-related comorbidity. It utilizes high-frequency electrical pulses to block vagus nerve signals between the brain and stomach. It is less effective than bariatric surgery for weight loss. The list price for the Maestro system is exceeds $15,000.
- The AspireAssist device is FDA approved for weight loss in adults ≥22 yr old with a BMI of 35 to 55. It requires the insertion of a PEG tube endoscopically and pulled through a percutaneous incision. Thirty minutes after a meal, the patient attaches a connector to it and drains a portion of their stomach content into a toilet. The tube is then flushed with potable water. The connector stops working after 115 cycles (6 wk) and is replaced at a follow-up appointment. Estimated cost for procedure and follow-ups are $13,000 for the first year.

DISPOSITION

- The incidence of venous thromboembolism in the upper tertile of BMI was 2.42 times that of the lowest BMI tertile. Obese patients have a higher incidence of postoperative thromboembolic events when undergoing noncardiac surgery.
- Obesity may be associated with higher rates of postoperative pulmonary complications and poor wound healing.
- Weight-stable obese subjects have an increased risk of arrhythmias and sudden death even in the absence of cardiac dysfunction.
- Obesity and the cardiac autonomic nervous system are intrinsically related. A 10% increase in body weight is associated with a decline in parasympathetic tone accompanied by a rise in mean heart rate. Conversely, a 10% weight loss in severely obese patients is associated with significant improvement in autonomic nervous system cardiac modulation, including decreased heart rate and increased heart rate variability.
- Postmortem Determinants of Atherosclerosis in Youth (PDAY) study data provided convincing evidence that obesity in adolescents and young adults accelerates the progression of atherosclerosis decades before the appearance of clinical manifestations.
- Obesity accelerates the progression of native coronary atherosclerosis and after coronary artery bypass grafting.
- In older adults, obesity is associated with protection against hip fracture, but this protective effect on bone status does not offset the extensive array of potential adverse effects on conditions common in the older population.

REFERRAL

- Obesity is commonly seen in the primary care setting. If pharmacologic therapy is considered, consultation with physicians specializing in obesity and experienced with the use of the drug is recommended. In addition, consultation with nutritionists and behavioral therapists is helpful. A consultation with general surgery is indicated in patients being considered for surgical intervention.

PEARLS & CONSIDERATIONS

COMMENTS

- Enhanced weight-loss counseling helps about one third of obese patients achieve long-term, clinically meaningful weight loss. Adults can lose 1-2 lb (0.45-0.9 kg per week by consuming 500-1000 fewer calories per day.
- The NHLBI launched the Obesity Education Initiative in January 1991. The overall purpose of the initiative is to help reduce the prevalence of overweight along with the prevalence of physical inactivity to reduce the risk of CHD and overall morbidity and mortality rates from CHD.
- The American Medical Association, in association with the Robert Wood Johnson Foundation and the U.S. Department of Health and Human Services, produced a primer for the assessment and management of adult obesity. The primer consists of 10 booklets that offer practical recommendations for addressing adult obesity in the primary care setting and is available free of charge at: http://www.amaassn.org/ama/pub/physician-resources.
- A recent study on BMI and all-cause mortality in a large prospective study suggests that optimal BMI range is between 20 and 24.9 (Patel AV, 2014).
- Recent research indicates that brown adipose tissue represents a natural target for the modulation of energy expenditure. The presence of brown adipose tissue in humans may be quantified with the use of ^{18}F-FDG PET-CT. The amount of brown adipose tissue is inversely correlated with BMI, suggesting a potential role of brown adipose tissue in adult human metabolism.
- Obesity, glucose intolerance, and hypertension in childhood are strongly associated with increased rates of premature death from endogenous causes in this population.
- Recent trials have shown that among persons living in a controlled setting, calories alone account for the increase in fat. Protein affected energy expenditure and storage of lean body mass, but not body fat storage.
- There have been no evidence-based studies supporting combination medical therapy for weight loss.
- Data are lacking for the role of pharmacotherapy and bariatric surgery in the elderly population.

PREVENTION

- Prevention of overweight and obesity involves both increasing physical activity and dietary modification to reduce caloric intake.
- There is compelling evidence that prevention of weight regain in formerly obese individuals requires 60 to 90 min of moderate-intensity activity or lesser amounts of vigorous intensity activity.
- Moderate-intensity activity of approximately 45 to 60 min per day, or 1.7 physical activity level (PAL), is required to prevent the transition to overweight or obesity. For children, even more activity time is recommended.
- Clinicians can help guide patients to develop personalized eating plans and help them recognize the contributions of fat, concentrated carbohydrates, and large portion sizes.
- Clinicians must work with patients to modify other risk factors such as tobacco use, high glycemic intake, and elevated blood pressure to prevent the long-term chronic disease sequelae of obesity.
- Regular screening of body weight and BMI measurements at routine office visits can help identify early weight gain.
- Among obese adolescents, the most rapid weight gain occurs between 2 and 6 yr of age. Most children who are obese at that age are obese in adolescence.[2]

PATIENT & FAMILY EDUCATION

Information can be obtained on the American Obesity Association website (http://www.obesity.org) and the American Medical Association website (http://www.ama-assn.org).

SUGGESTED READINGS

Available at ExpertConsult.com

RELATED CONTENT

Obesity, Female (Patient Information)
Obesity, Male (Patient Information)
Obesity, Child (Patient Information)

AUTHOR: **FRED F. FERRI, M.D.**

[2] Geserick M, et al.: Acceleration of BMI in early childhood and risk of sustained obesity, *N Engl J Med* 379:303-12, 2018.

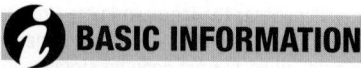

BASIC INFORMATION

DEFINITION

The obesity-hypoventilation syndrome (OHS), also known as Pickwickian syndrome, is conventionally defined as a combination of obesity (body mass index [BMI] ≥30 kg/m^2) and daytime hypercapnia ($PaCO_2$ ≥45 mm Hg in arterial blood gas analysis) in the absence of other causes for hypoventilation. This syndrome is often accompanied by obstructive sleep apnea (apnea-hypopnea index [AHI] ≥5 events/hour) or nonobstructive sleep hypoventilation (AHI <5, $PaCO_2$ >55 mm of Hg for more than 10 min or an increase in the $PaCO_2$ >10 mm of Hg compared with daytime $PaCO_2$, to a value >50 mm of Hg for >10 min during sleep). The hypercapnia stems from low tidal volumes and from inappropriate central respiratory response to hypoxemia and elevated PCO_2 levels.

SYNONYMS

Pickwickian syndrome
OHS
Extreme obesity with alveolar hypoventilation
Obesity alveolar hypoventilation syndrome

ICD-10CM CODES

E66.2	Obesity hypoventilation syndrome (OHS)
278.03	Obesity hypoventilation syndrome (OHS)

EPIDEMIOLOGY & DEMOGRAPHICS

PREVALENCE: The worldwide prevalence of obesity more than doubled in the last 30 yr and has become a global epidemic. In 2014, the World Health Organization estimated that more than 600 million adults were obese. A Centers for Disease Control report in 2015 estimated the prevalence of obesity among U.S. adults during 2011 to 2014 at 36.5%. The obesity epidemic is likely to increase the prevalence of myriad complications such as OHS. The prevalence of OHS in the general population is estimated to be 0.6%, and 8% to 20% in patients evaluated for sleep breathing disorders at sleep clinic centers.

PREDOMINANT SEX & AGE: Male gender and 50-60 yr of age

RISK FACTORS:
- Male gender
- 50-60 yr of age
- Morbidly obese (BMI ≥40 kg/m ^{2})
- Severe OSA (≥30 obstructive respiratory events/hour of sleep)
- Increased waist-hip ratio
- Neck circumference >45 cm

PHYSICAL FINDINGS & CLINICAL PRESENTATION

Most of the OHS symptoms are similar to OSA:
- Excessive daytime somnolence
- Fatigue
- Disorientation
- Loss of concentration
- Change in mood
- Amnesia
- Morning headache

Symptoms and signs most common in OHS compared with OSA:
- Injected sclera (probably related to high PCO_2 leading to cerebral vasodilation)
- Anasarca, dyspnea on exertion, signs of circulatory congestion, and cor pulmonale on cardiac and hepatic exam

ETIOLOGY

- Etiology of hypoventilation in obese patients depends on many factors.
- Three hypotheses for chronic hypoventilation are widely accepted (Fig. E1): the increase in mechanical load on respiratory muscles from obesity; leptin resistance inhibiting central respiratory drive causing worsening hypoventilation; and decreased response to elevated PCO_2 levels in OSA.
- Often subclinical OHS becomes clinical with external triggers such as sedative medications, overdiuresis, and other systemic disease.

DIAGNOSIS

DIFFERENTIAL DIAGNOSIS

- Anemia
- Heart failure with excessive diuresis
- Liver failure
- Stroke
- Central sleep apnea
- OSA
- Circadian rhythm disorder
- Drug or alcohol abuse
- Depression
- Hypothyroidism
- Sedative medication
- Metabolic abnormalities (e.g., hypo- or hypernatremia, hypercalcemia)
- Neuromuscular disease
- Pulmonary and lung disease
- Restless legs syndrome

WORKUP

- Detailed history and physical examination are helpful to identify patients who are at high risk for OHS. Fig. 2 illustrates a decision tree to screen for obesity-hypoventilation syndrome. Diagnostic features of obesity-hypoventilation syndrome are summarized in Box E1. Physiologic differences between eucapnic morbidly obese patients and those with obesity-hypoventilation syndrome are summarized in Box 2.
- Screen for OHS in men or women with BMI ≥30 or with sleep breathing disorder.
- The Epworth Sleepiness Scale (ESS) and the Stanford Sleepiness Scale (SSS) are the most commonly used scales for daytime sleepiness.
- If OSA is suspected, screen with STOP-BANG questionnaire (**s**noring, **t**iredness, **o**bserved apnea, blood **p**ressure, **B**MI, **a**ge >50, **n**eck circumference >16 inches, and **g**ender).
- Overnight polysomnography to confirm whether AHI >5
- Assess daytime oxygen saturation (SpO_2) levels to assess blood oxygenation level and serum bicarbonate level to assess carbon dioxide retention.
- If SpO_2 <90% on room air, serum bicarbonate >27 mEq/L, and BMI >30 with underlying sleep breathing disorder, consider obtaining an arterial blood gas to diagnose OHS.
- Consider forced vital capacity (FVC) and negative inspiratory force (NIF) if any suspicion of neuromuscular disease.
- ECG and echocardiogram are helpful to assess structural changes of the heart and pulmonary hypertension.

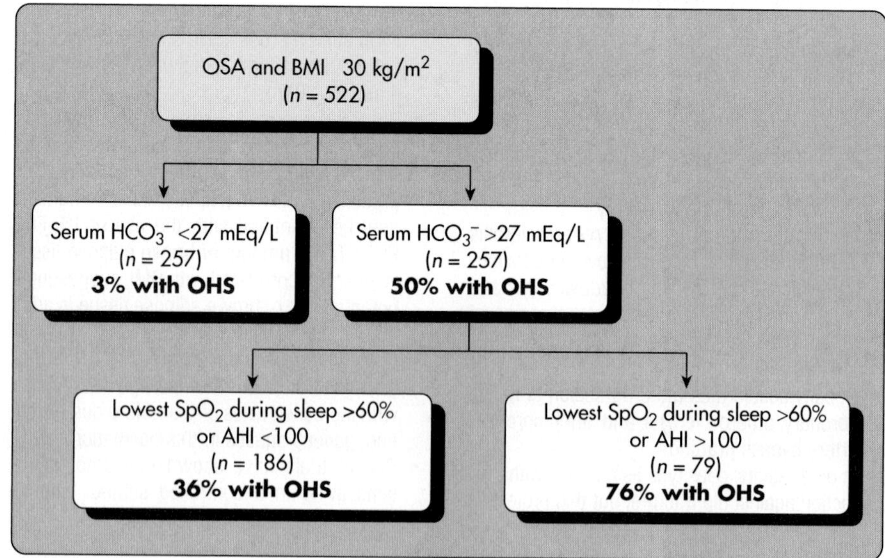

FIG. 2 Decision tree to screen for obesity-hypoventilation syndrome *(OHS)* based on observation in 522 obese patients with OSA (BMI ≥30 kg/$m^2$and AHI ≥5). Among those with a venous serum bicarbonate level above 27 mEq/L, OHS was present in 50% of patients. Very severe OSA (AHI >100 events/hour or SpO_2 nadir during sleep <60%) increased the prevalence of OHS to 76%. *AHI,* Apnea-hypopnea index; *BMI,* body mass index; *OSA,* obstructive sleep apnea; *SpO_2,* the saturation of arterial blood with oxygen as measured by pulse oximetry. (From Kryger M, Roth T, Dement WC: *Principles and Practice of sleep medicine*, ed 6, Philadelphia, 2017, Elsevier.)

BOX 2 Physiologic Differences Between Eucapnic Morbidly Obese Patients and Those with Obesity-Hypoventilation Syndrome

	Eucapnic Morbid Obesity	Obesity-Hypoventilation Syndrome
Waist:hip ratio	↑	↑↑
FEV_1/FVC	Normal	Normal/↓
Total lung capacity	Normal	Slight ↓
Functional residual capacity	↓	↓
Vital capacity	Normal or ↓	↓↓
Expiratory reserve volume	↓	↓↓
Work of breathing	↑	↑↑
Hypercapnic/hypoxic ventilatory drive	Normal	↓
Inspiratory muscle strength	Normal	↓

FEV_1, Forced expiratory volume in first second; *FVC,* forced vital capacity.
From Kryger M, Roth T, Dement WC: *Principles and Practice of sleep medicine,* ed 6, Philadelphia, 2017, Elsevier.

- Polysomnography with continuous positive airway pressure (CPAP) titration can guide the physician to choose appropriate settings for positive airway pressure.
- Avoid medications that decrease respiratory drive and worsen ventilation.

LABORATORY TESTS

- Arterial blood gas (ABG) analysis on room air is the gold standard test to diagnose OHS in appropriate clinical setting.
- Venous blood gases (VBG), end-tidal carbon dioxide, arterialized capillary blood gases, and transcutaneous carbon dioxide monitoring can be used as alternatives to ABG to assess hypoventilation and carbon dioxide retention.
- Serum bicarbonate (>27 mEq/L) can be used as a great screening tool for OHS in an appropriate clinical setting. In a patient with normal kidney function, respiratory acidosis from OHS is usually compensated by retaining serum bicarbonate.
- Several studies showed serum bicarbonate level <27 mEq/L carries 97% negative predictive value for excluding a diagnosis of OHS in patients diagnosed as obese with OSA and normal renal function.
- Sleep hypoventilation can be measured by continuous end-tidal or transcutaneous carbon dioxide level measurement.

IMAGING STUDIES

- Echocardiogram will be helpful to assesses structural changes of the heart and pulmonary hypertension.
- Consider chest x-ray if any suspicion of pneumonia, COPD, or any lung disease.
- Consider CT chest or bronchoscopy if clinical condition warrants.

Rx TREATMENT

Four types of therapies available for both acute and chronic therapies for OHS: positive airway (PAP) therapy, supplemental nasal oxygen, bariatric surgery, and oral respiratory stimulants.

NONPHARMACOLOGIC THERAPY

Positive airway therapy:

- Two types of PAP therapy available: CPAP and bilevel PAP (BiPAP). PAP therapy is considered first line for OHS.
- Short-term (≤3 weeks of PAP use) benefits of PAP: Improvement in $PaCO_2$ and PaO_2 levels and sleep breathing disorder.
- Long-term benefits of PAP (≥4 weeks of PAP use): Improvement in $PaCO_2$ and PaO_2 levels, lung volumes, central respiratory drive to carbon dioxide, and possible lowering of mortality.
- BiPAP recommend in patients who failed CPAP therapy (AHI ≥5 or a mean nocturnal oxygen saturation <90% on CPAP therapy) or who are intolerant to high PAP.

Oxygen therapy:

- Approximately 40% of patients with OHS on PAP therapy were at risk of hypoxemia during sleep. It can be controlled with supplemental oxygen as low as possible. However, inadvertent administration of excess oxygen might decrease minute ventilation significantly, which results in hypercapnia and respiratory acidosis.

Bariatric surgery:

- Bariatric surgery is indicated in all patients with a BMI ≥40 or with BMI ≥35 with obesity-related comorbid conditions. Recent studies showed significant improvement in PaO_2, $PaCO_2$, FEV_1, and FVC after bariatric surgery. After successful surgery, 14% of OHS patients may need PAP.

Tracheostomy:

- Reserved for patients who are not tolerant to PAP therapy.

ACUTE Rx

- Two respiratory stimulants currently available: Medroxyprogesterone acetate and acetazolamide.
- Medroxyprogesterone acetate stimulates respiratory center in hypothalamus. Clinical data showed neutral effect on $PaCO_2$ level.
- Acetazolamide increases bicarbonate excretion by the kidneys and causes metabolic acidosis, which increases respiratory drive. Acetazolamide has been shown to improve respiratory drive and decrease $PaCO_2$ level. However, clinical data are limited.

REFERRAL

Sleep specialist referral in case of diagnostic uncertainty and/or for patients not responding to positive airway therapy.

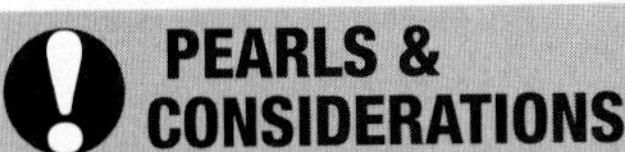

PEARLS & CONSIDERATIONS

- It is impossible to differentiate OHS from OSA based on clinical presentation alone.
- If SpO_2 <90% on room air, serum bicarbonate (>27 mEq/L), and BMI of >30 with underlying SBD, get an ABG to diagnose OHS.
- Positive airway therapy is a very effective treatment of choice for OHS.

PREVENTION

- Avoid sedative medications.
- Avoid overdiuresis in heart failure patients.
- Avoid alcohol intake.

PATIENT/FAMILY EDUCATION

- Weight loss.
- Avoid sedative medication.
- Avoid alcohol intake and recreational drug use.
- Daily use of positive airway therapy for sleep.

SUGGESTED READING

Available at ExpertConsult.com

RELATED CONTENT

Sleep Apnea (Related Key Topic)
Obesity (Related Key Topic)

AUTHOR: **MAHESWARA SATYA GANGADHARA RAO GOLLA, M.D.**

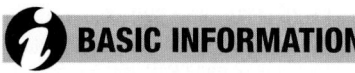

BASIC INFORMATION

DEFINITION

Obsessive-compulsive disorder (OCD) is characterized by obsessions (recurrent and persistent thoughts, urges, or images experienced as intrusive and unwanted) and/or compulsions (repetitive behaviors or mental acts performed in response to obsessions, or according to rules that must be applied rigidly) that are time-consuming (e.g., >1 hr/day) or cause marked impairment or distress. The symptoms are usually, but not always, perceived as excessive and unreasonable.

SYNONYM

OCD

ICD-10CM CODES

F42 Obsessive-compulsive disorder

F60.5 Obsessive-compulsive personality disorder

DSM-5 CODES

300.3 Obsessive-compulsive disorder

301.4 Obsessive-compulsive personality disorder

EPIDEMIOLOGY & DEMOGRAPHICS

PEAK INCIDENCE: Mean age at onset is 19.5 yr.

12-MONTH PREVALENCE: 1.2% of adults in the U.S., international prevalence estimates are similar (1.1% to 1.8%).

PREDOMINANT SEX: Slightly more common among females than males in adulthood, although males are more commonly affected in childhood.

PREDOMINANT AGE:

- Modal age of onset for females is between 20 and 29 yr.
- Modal age of onset for males is between 6 and 15 yr.

DISEASE COURSE:

- Condition is chronic with waxing and waning pattern.
- Symptoms typically worsen with stress.
- 15% show progressive deterioration, whereas 5% show an episodic course with little impairment between episodes.

GENETICS:

- OCD is a multifactorial familial condition that involves both polygenic and environmental risk factors.
- Rate of concordance is higher in monozygotic (57%) compared with dizygotic (27%) twins.
- Rate of disorder is also much higher in first-degree relatives of individuals with OCD and Tourette's disorder (8.2%) than in the general population (2%).

PHYSICAL FINDINGS & CLINICAL PRESENTATION

- Persistent and recurrent intrusive and ego-dystonic obsessive ideas, thoughts, urges, or images that are perceived as alien and beyond one's control.
- Frequent experiencing of obsessions related to contamination (e.g., when using the telephone), excessive doubt (e.g., was the door locked?), organization (the need for a particular order), violent impulses (e.g., to yell obscenities in church), or intrusive sexual imagery.
- Compulsive behaviors (e.g., repeated hand washing, checking, rearranging) or mental rituals (e.g., counting, repeating phrases) meant to temporarily ameliorate anxiety caused by obsessions.
- Obsessions and compulsions are almost always accompanied by high anxiety and subjective distress. Both are usually, but not always, seen as excessive and unreasonable.

ETIOLOGY

- Strong evidence of cortico-striato-thalamo-cortical circuit dysfunction.
- OCD onset may be temporally associated with infectious illness of CNS (e.g., Von Economo encephalitis, Sydenham's chorea).
- OCD may follow head trauma or other premorbid neurologic condition, including birth hypoxia and Tourette's syndrome.
- Serotonergic, dopaminergic, and glutamatergic systems believed important in some ritualistic instinctual behaviors, with dysfunction of these pathways possibly giving rise to OCD.

Dx DIAGNOSIS

DIFFERENTIAL DIAGNOSIS

- Obsessive-compulsive personality disorder (OCPD) is a maladaptive personality style defined by excessive rigidity, need for order and control, preoccupation with details, and excessive perfectionism. Unlike OCD, OCPD is ego-syntonic.
- Other psychiatric disorders in which obsessive or intrusive thoughts occur (e.g., body dysmorphic disorder, eating disorders, hypochondriasis, phobias, posttraumatic stress disorder).
- Impulse control disorders (e.g., trichotillomania [hair-pulling disorder], excoriation [skin-picking] disorder, pathologic gambling disorder, compulsive shopping, kleptomania, paraphilias/sexual compulsions).
- Neurologic disorders with repetitive behaviors (e.g., Tourette's syndrome, Sydenham's chorea, torticollis, autism).
- Delusions or psychosis, which may be mistaken for obsessive thoughts; unlike OCD, these individuals do not believe their obsessions are unreal and may likely meet criteria for another psychotic spectrum disorder that fully accounts for the obsessions (e.g., schizophrenia).

WORKUP

- Careful history leading to diagnosis.
- In adolescents and children: Psychological testing to reveal learning disabilities.
- Screen for presence of past or current tic disorder, and ascertain degree of insight (good or fair, poor, absent/delusional) into OCD beliefs.

Rx TREATMENT

NONPHARMACOLOGIC THERAPY

- Cognitive-behavioral therapy (CBT), comprising exposure/response prevention with or without cognitive reappraisal, is successful in up to 70% of patients. Best results are found for contamination obsessions and washing compulsions.
- Barriers to CBT include lack of availability/access, intense time requirements, and patient motivation to engage in treatment (e.g., anxiety resulting from exposure exercises).

GENERAL Rx

- Antidepressants with serotonin reuptake blockade, including clomipramine, fluvoxamine, fluoxetine, paroxetine, sertraline, citalopram, and escitalopram; optimal dosages are typically at the high end of the prescription range. Risk/benefit/alternatives discussion is crucial (e.g., dose-related risk of QT interval prolongation with serotonin reuptake inhibitors in general and clomipramine, citalopram, and escitalopram in particular).
- Benzodiazepines (e.g., clonazepam) have limited efficacy in OCD.
- Most experience some symptom relief with treatment, but even after adequate treatment trials, 40% to 60% of patients endorse significant residual symptoms.
- Likely indefinite treatment. Relapse is common if medications are discontinued.
- Recent studies suggest that combination CBT and pharmacotherapy yields superior outcomes. More severe symptoms warrant combination therapy.
- Patients who do not respond to first-line treatments and those with comorbid psychosis and/or tic disorders may benefit from augmentation with a first- or second-generation antipsychotic medication (e.g., haloperidol, olanzapine, risperidone).
- Neurosurgical intervention (e.g., cingulotomy, deep brain stimulation) is reserved for the most severely symptomatic and treatment-resistant cases.

DISPOSITION

- Most mild to moderate cases can be managed on a regular outpatient basis. Treatment should typically start with SSRI monotherapy with regular follow-up to assess treatment response and side-effect management. Dose should be increased to maximum tolerated.
- Patient and family education may help improve medical adherence and support.

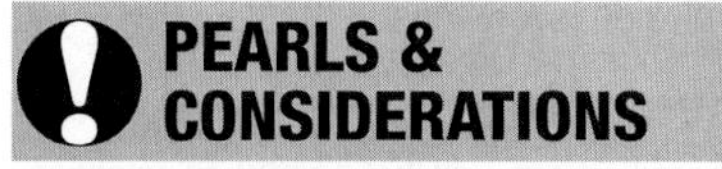

PEARLS & CONSIDERATIONS

Patients with OCD typically have insight regarding the irrationality of their obsessions and compulsions but lack the ability to control them. This may cause intense shame and avoidance of medical care unless patient education and support are provided. Screen for OCD, especially among patients who present with "depression" or "anxiety."

SUGGESTED READINGS

Available at ExpertConsult.com

RELATED CONTENT

Obsessive-Compulsive Disorder (OCD) (Patient Information)

AUTHOR: **AGUSTIN G. YIP, M.D., PH.D.**

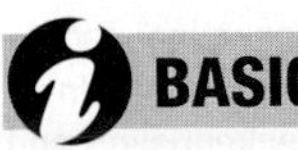

BASIC INFORMATION

DEFINITION

Excessive use of an opioid, either derived from the opium poppy or semi- or fully synthetic, resulting in respiratory depression, central nervous system depression, and/or death

SYNONYMS

Opiate overdose
Heroin overdose
Narcotic overdose
Opioid poisoning

ICD-10CM CODES

T40.0X1	Poisoning by opium, accidental (unintentional)
T40.0X2	Poisoning by opium, intentional self-harm
T40.0X3	Poisoning by opium, assault
T40.0X4	Poisoning by opium, undetermined
T40.0X5	Adverse effect of opium
T40.1X	Poisoning by heroin
T40.4	Poisoning by other synthetic narcotics

EPIDEMIOLOGY & DEMOGRAPHICS

INCIDENCE: Drug overdose deaths and opioid-involved deaths continue to increase in the U.S. The majority of drug overdose deaths (more than six out of ten) involve an opioid. Ninety-one Americans die every day from an opioid overdose.

PREVALENCE: From 2000 to 2015 more than half a million Americans died from drug overdoses. Since 1999, the number of overdose deaths involving opioids (including prescription opioids and heroin) quadrupled. Among 70,237 fatal drug overdoses in the U.S. in 2017, prescription opioids were involved in 2422. The amount of prescription opioids sold in the U.S. nearly quadrupled, yet there has not been an overall change in the amount of pain that Americans report.

PREDOMINANT SEX AND AGE: The "typical" heroin death involves experienced users in their 20s to 30s using coingestants with a male predilection.

RISK FACTORS: The majority of drug-overdose deaths are unintentional or accidental (74%). The following increase risk for opioid overdose:
- Opioid dependence, in particular following reduced tolerance (following detoxification, release from incarceration, cessation of treatment)
- Injecting opioids
- Using prescription opioids, in particular taking higher doses
- Using opioids in combination with other sedating substances
- Using opioids and having comorbidities such as HIV, liver or lung disease, or suffering from depression
- Household members of people in possession of opioids (including prescription opioids)

The highest drug-induced mortality is associated with the following factors: 40 to 49 yr of age, male gender, non-Hispanic whites, and living in the South, all of which account for approximately 38.2% of drug-induced deaths in the U.S.

PHYSICAL FINDINGS & CLINICAL PRESENTATION

Patients with opioid overdose classically present with the triad of altered mental status, pinpoint pupils, and respiratory depression. Patients may be apneic or with low respiratory rate and tidal volumes. Respiratory depression becomes profound enough to cause anoxia, leading to death. Little to no response will be elicited from painful stimuli. Look for clinical clues, such as "track marks" or darkening along the length of veins from injection drug use that may suggest opioid overdose. The use of coingestants, which is exceedingly common in opioid overdose, can alter the classic exam findings one may expect. For example, use of sympathomimetics like cocaine can cause pupillary dilation. Respiratory rate <12 breaths/min is most sensitive for predicting response to naloxone. Once the patient is hemodynamically stable, examine for other sequelae of drug use, including pulmonary rales suggestive of aspiration pneumonia or murmurs and skin lesions associated with endocarditis in IV drug abusers.

ETIOLOGY

N/A

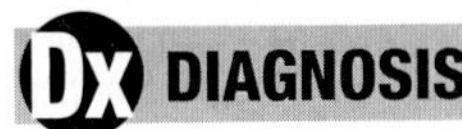

DIAGNOSIS

DIFFERENTIAL DIAGNOSIS

- Hypoglycemia
- Alcohol or sedative overdose
- Postictal state
- Infectious or metabolic encephalopathy
- Clonidine overdose
- Phenothiazine overdose
- Organophosphate exposure

WORKUP

Opioid overdose requires little workup if the patient's altered mental status can be completely attributed to the overdose (i.e., by full recovery with naloxone). However, if the patient remains altered or with significant respiratory compromise after adequate treatment, continue appropriate workup. Obtain an ECG in the following scenarios: use of methadone, oxycodone, loperamide or a coingestant tricyclic antidepressant to screen for QTc prolongation; coingestion of a sympathomimetic to rule out arrhythmias.

LABORATORY TESTS

- Serum glucose should be quickly obtained as with any resuscitation.
- Urine drug screen is not routinely required unless the history or physical exam raises suspicion for coingestants that would alter management.
- Tylenol and aspirin levels in intentional overdoses or when used in a combination formulation with an opioid.

IMAGING STUDIES

Not required unless guided by your physical exam and/or response to therapy:
- Computed tomography of the head and cervical spine for suspected trauma
- Chest x-ray if signs of aspiration
- Echocardiogram if concerned for endocarditis

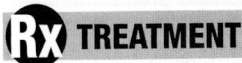

TREATMENT

The principal goals of treatment for opioid overdose are support of ventilation and reversal of the drug.

NONPHARMACOLOGIC THERAPY

Support the airway and breathing. For apneic or bradypneic patients, use bag-valve-mask ventilation.

ACUTE GENERAL Rx

Administer naloxone, a short-acting opioid antagonist, as soon as possible. Intravenous is the preferred route; however, in November 2015 Narcan Nasal Spray became the first FDA-approved non-injectable naloxone product for the treatment of opioid overdose. Higher concentration intranasal naloxone 2 mg/ml seems to have efficacy similar to IM naloxone for reversal of opioid overdose. Via the IV route, onset of action is within 1 to 2 minutes. Dosing is as follows:
- For most adult patients, 0.4 to 1.2 mg should yield recovery of consciousness.
- For patients in cardiac arrest, 2 mg is the starting dose.
- Younger than 5 yr or body weight 20 kg or less: 0.1 mg/kg administered by IV push, intraosseous (IO) push, or by endotracheal tube (ETT).
- 5 yr and older or body weight more than 20 kg: 2 mg administered by IV push, IO, or ETT.

Prepare for adverse effects of acute withdrawal, including agitation, nausea, vomiting, piloerection, diarrhea, lacrimation, yawning, and rhinorrhea after naloxone administration to chronic opioid users, especially with higher doses. Naloxone continues to block binding of additional opioids to the receptor for 20 to 90 minutes.

CHRONIC Rx

- Naloxone autoinjectors and nasal sprays are available in some states and intended for buddy administration. Patients can buy these formulations over-the-counter in some states, whereas others require a prescription. Check your state's legislature for continual updates on this matter.
- A 2016 nonrandomized study demonstrated that patients prescribed opioids plus naloxone had 47% fewer opioid-related emergency department visits within 6 months than those not prescribed naloxone.

REFERRAL

Patients can be offered referral to drug rehabilitation services. Otherwise, follow up with the primary care physician is appropriate.

SUGGESTED READINGS

Available at ExpertConsult.com

RELATED CONTENT

Drug Abuse (Related Key Topic)
Opioid Use Disorder (Related Key Topic)

AUTHORS: **AMANDA BOX, M.D., M.S.,** and **MARK F. BRADY, M.D. M.P.H., M.M.S.**

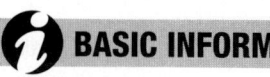

BASIC INFORMATION

DEFINITION

- Opioid use disorder is defined as a cluster of cognitive, behavioral, and physiologic symptoms in which the individual continues use of opiates despite significant opiate-induced problems. Opiate use disorder is a chronic, relapsing disorder characterized by repeated self-administration that usually results in opiate tolerance, withdrawal, and compulsive drug use. Tolerance is the need to increase dose to achieve the same effect. Dependence may occur with or without the physiologic symptoms of tolerance and withdrawal.
- There are four stages of addiction:
  1. Stage I, acute drug effects: Rewarding effects of drug result from neurobiologic changes in response to the acute drug use. Duration varies from hours to days.
  2. Stage II, transformation to addiction: Associated with changes in neuronal function that accumulate with repeated administration and diminish over days or weeks after discontinuation of drug use.
  3. Stage III, relapse after extended periods of abstinence: Precipitated by an incubation of cue-induced craving (people, places, and things as triggers) and priming (relapse precipitated by drug exposure).
  4. Stage IV, end-stage addiction: Vulnerability to relapse endures for years and results from prolonged changes at the cellular level.
- Pseudoaddiction: Undertreatment of pain resulting in "opiate-seeking" behaviors such as "doctor shopping" and multiple emergency department visits. These behaviors disappear with adequate treatment of pain.

SYNONYMS

Opioid dependence
OUD (opioid use disorder)
Opiate addiction
Opiate abuse
Narcotic addiction
Narcotic abuse
Substance use disorder

ICD-10CM CODES

F11.10	Opioid abuse, uncomplicated
F11.120	Opioid abuse with intoxication, uncomplicated
F11.121	Opioid abuse with intoxication delirium
F11.122	Opioid abuse with intoxication with perceptual disturbance
F11.129	Opioid abuse with intoxication, unspecified
F11.14	Opioid abuse with opioid-induced mood disorder
F11.150	Opioid abuse with opioid-induced psychotic disorder with delusions
F11.151	Opioid abuse with opioid-induced psychotic disorder with hallucinations
F11.159	Opioid abuse with opioid-induced psychotic disorder, unspecified
F11.181	Opioid abuse with opioid-induced sexual dysfunction
F11.182	Opioid abuse with opioid-induced sleep disorder
F11.188	Opioid abuse with other opioid-induced disorder
F11.19	Opioid abuse with unspecified opioid-induced disorder

EPIDEMIOLOGY & DEMOGRAPHICS

INCIDENCE: It is estimated that more than 2.5 million Americans have an opioid use disorder.

PREVALENCE:

- In 2014, U.S. retail pharmacies dispensed 245 million prescriptions for opioid pain relievers.
- In 2014, 10.3 million persons reported using prescription opioids nonmedically.
- In the U.S., 400,000 persons have used heroin in the past month, and 4 million have reported nonmedical use of prescription pain relievers.
- Emergency department visits involving misuse or abuse of prescription opioids increased 153% between 2004 and 2011.
- Admissions to substance-abuse treatment programs linked to prescription opioids more than quadrupled between 2002 and 2012.
- The percentage of eighth-, tenth-, and twelfth-graders who have used heroin has more than doubled since the late 1990s. This increase has largely been attributed to decreased price and increased purity in the last decade.
- In 2015, 33,000 Americans died of opioid-related overdose—quadrupling the rates from 1999.
- In March and October 2015, the Drug Enforcement Administration and Centers for Disease Control and Prevention issued nationwide alerts identifying fentanyl, particularly illicitly manufactured fentanyl, as a threat to public health and safety. Illicitly manufactured fentanyl is pharmacologically similar to pharmaceutical fentanyl but is unlawfully produced in clandestine laboratories and obtained via illicit drug markets; it also includes fentanyl analogs. Fentanyl is a synthetic opioid 50 to 100 times more potent than morphine and approved for the management of surgical/postoperative pain, severe chronic pain, and breakthrough cancer pain.
- In the U.S., approximately 10 million adults are prescribed long-term opioid therapy (LTOT) for chronic pain despite inadequate evidence of long-term benefit and growing evidence of harm.

PREDOMINANT SEX: Males abuse opioids more commonly than females, with a male:female ratio of 3:1 for heroin and 1.5:1 for prescription opiates.

PEAK INCIDENCE: The majority of new abusers of opiates are <26 yr.

RISK FACTORS:

- Family history
- Prior history of addiction
- Psychiatric disorders

GENETICS:

- Genetic epidemiologic studies suggest a high degree of heritable vulnerability for opioid dependence.
- Gene polymorphism for dopamine receptor/transporters, opioid receptors, serotonin receptors/transporters, proenkephalin, and catechol-*O*-methyltransferase all appear to be associated with vulnerability to opioid dependence. Future interventions for opiate dependence may include medications identified through genetic research.

PHYSICAL FINDINGS & CLINICAL PRESENTATION

- Physical examination is often noncontributory.
- Small-sized pupils may be the only observable sign of use because only mild tolerance develops for miosis.
- Scars or tracks from chronic IV use may be visible over the veins of the arms, hands, ankles, neck, and breasts.
- Inflamed nasal mucosa or respiratory wheezing may be apparent in patients who are snorting heroin or OxyContin.
- Patients in withdrawal may have more dramatic findings such as tachycardia, hypertension, fever, piloerection (goose flesh), mydriasis, lacrimation, central nervous system (CNS) arousal, irritability, and repeated yawning. In patients with sympathetic overactivity and panic attacks, use of CNS stimulants, such as amphetamines or cocaine, should also be ruled out.
- Although gastrointestinal symptoms of nausea, vomiting, and abdominal pain are common in opioid withdrawal, other causes such as gastroenteritis, pancreatitis, peptic ulcer disease, and intestinal obstruction need to be ruled out.
- The history may provide relevant information in making the diagnosis. Significant findings may include:
  1. A long history of opioid self-administration, typically by the IV or intranasal route but sometimes through smoking as well.
  2. Polysubstance use. Intoxication by drugs other than narcotics (e.g., benzodiazepines, barbiturates) should be ruled out in unconscious patients.
  3. A high incidence of nonopioid-related psychiatric disorders (>80%).
  4. History of problems at work, school, or relationships associated with drug use.
  5. History of legal problems associated with drug use, such as arrest for possession, robbery, or prostitution.
  6. History of interpersonal violence (as perpetrator or victim).
  7. History of physical problems such as skin infections, phlebitis, endocarditis, or liver diseases attributable to acetaminophen toxicity (Vicodin/Percocet) or viral hepatitis. Hepatitis C is the most prevalent blood-borne pathogen. It is present in approximately 90% of opiate-dependent people and is often spread by sharing IV drug paraphernalia or snorting devices. There is also a higher incidence of HIV infection.

ETIOLOGY

Opioid use disorder is a biopsychosocial disorder. Pharmacologic, social, genetic, and psychodynamic factors interact to influence abusive

TABLE 1 Cage-Aid

1. Have you ever tried to **C**ut down on your alcohol or drug use?
2. Do you get **A**nnoyed when people comment about your drinking or drug use?
3. Do you feel **G**uilty about things you have done while drinking or using drugs?
4. Do you need an **E**ye-opener to get started in the morning?

Two or more questions answered in the affirmative require further assessment. *AID*, adapted to include drugs.
From Bowman S, Eiserman J, Beletsky, L, Stancliff S: Reducing the health consequences of opioid addiction in primary care, *Am J Med* 126, 565-571, 2013.

TABLE 2 Drug Abuse Screening Test (DAST-10)

1. Have you used drugs other than those required for medical reasons?
2. Do you abuse more than one drug at a time?
3. Are you unable to stop using drugs when you want to?
4. Have you ever had blackouts or flashbacks as a result of drug use?
5. Do you ever feel bad or guilty about your drug use?
6. Does your spouse (or parents) ever complain about your involvement with drugs?
7. Have you neglected your family because of your use of drugs?
8. Have you engaged in illegal activities in order to obtain drugs?
9. Have you ever experienced withdrawal symptoms (felt sick) when you stopped taking drugs?
10. Have you had medical problems as a result of your drug use (e.g., memory loss, hepatitis, convulsions, bleeding)?

Two or more questions answered in the affirmative require further assessment.
From Bowman S, Eiserman J, Beletsky L, Stancliff S: Reducing the health consequences of opioid addiction in primary care, *Am J Med* (2013) 126, 565-571.

behaviors. Pharmacologic factors are especially prominent in opiate addiction because these drugs are strong reinforcing agents because of their euphoric effects and their ability to reduce anxiety and increase self-esteem and the patient's subjective feelings of improved ability to cope with daily challenges.

Dx DIAGNOSIS

DIFFERENTIAL DIAGNOSIS

- Psychiatric disorders (e.g., anxiety, depression, bipolar disorder).
- Acute medical illness (e.g., hypoglycemia, seizure disorder, sepsis, renal or hepatic insufficiency) may mimic opiate withdrawal symptoms.

WORKUP

The history is the most important part of the workup. Useful screening tools are the CAGE-AID (Table 1), the DAST-10 (Table 2), and the CRAFFT (Table 3). The CAGE-AID has a sensitivity of 70% and a specificity of 85% when two questions are answered in the affirmative. The DAST-10

TABLE 3 CRAFFT Screening Tool for Adolescents

1. Have you ever ridden in a **C**ar driven by someone (including yourself) who was high or had been using alcohol or drugs?
2. Do you ever use alcohol or drugs to **R**elax, feel better about yourself, or fit in?
3. Do you ever use alcohol or drugs while you are by yourself **A**lone?
4. Do you ever **F**orget things you did while using alcohol or drugs?
5. Do your **F**amily or Friends ever tell you that you should cut down on your drinking or drug use?
6. Have you ever gotten into **T**rouble while you were using alcohol or drugs?

Two or more questions answered in the affirmative require further assessment.
From Bowman S, Eiserman J, Beletsky L, Stancliff S: Reducing the health consequences of opioid addiction in primary care, *Am J Med* 126, 565-571, 2013.

can discriminate between current users versus former users. The CRAFFT is a useful screening tool for adolescents. A CRAFFT score of 2 or higher is optimal for identifying any problem (sensitivity 76%, specificity 94%), any disorder (sensitivity 80%, specificity 86%), and drug dependence (sensitivity 92%, specificity 80%).

- Observation of opioid withdrawal is indicative of opioid addiction.
- Observation of purposeful behaviors such as complaints and manipulations directed at getting more drugs and anxiety during withdrawal is suggestive of opioid addiction.
- Screen blood and urine for opioid metabolites.
- Screen for communicable diseases: HIV, hepatitis B and hepatitis C, tuberculosis.
- Screen for endocarditis in patients with newly diagnosed murmurs.

LABORATORY TESTS

- Urine and serum toxicology screen
- Complete blood count
- Chemistries (alanine aminotransferase, aspartate aminotransferase, serum creatinine): Elevated liver function test (LFT) results may be from viral hepatitis or acetaminophen toxicity
- Hepatitis screen: If hepatitis C antibody positive, follow up with hepatitis C polymerase chain reaction (viral load) even in patients with normal LFTs
- HIV
- PPD

IMAGING STUDIES

Generally not helpful in routine diagnosis and treatment. Consider echocardiography in patients with heart murmurs and liver sonography or CT scan in patients with elevated LFTs or who are positive for hepatitis C or B (increased risk of hepatocellular carcinoma).

Rx TREATMENT

NONPHARMACOLOGIC THERAPY

- Brief counseling interventions during a visit with their primary care physician or OB/GYN have proved efficacious in motivating patients for treatment.
- Therapeutic communities (residential).
- 12-step or other self-help groups (e.g., Alcoholics Anonymous, Narcotics Anonymous).
- Relapse prevention (counseling).
- Opioid prevention education (Table 4).

TABLE 4 Basic Components of Opioid Overdose Prevention Education Curriculum

1. Know the signs of an opioid overdose (e.g., unresponsive, limp, slow, shallow breathing, pale or clammy, finger nails or lips turning blue, gurgling)
2. Call 911
3. Administer rescue breathing
4. Administer naloxone if no response and Emergency Medical Services have not yet arrived
5. Stay with the person until help arrives

From Bowman S, Eiserman J, Beletsky, L, Stancliff S: Reducing the health consequences of opioid addiction in primary care, *Am J Med* 126, 565-571, 2013.

ACUTE Rx

- Medical withdrawal (not overdosed). Opioid withdrawal alone is not recommended for treatment of opioid use disorder in most patients because of increased risk of overdose death and infectious disease (e.g., HIV through IV drug use) following detoxification.
- Short- (30 days) or long-term (30 to 180 days) protocols.
- Buprenorphine (opioid partial agonist) or methadone (opioid agonist) is initiated in tapering doses.
- Clonidine 0.1 mg bid to tid can be used to minimize autonomic symptoms (sweating) and craving.
- Nonsteroidal antiinflammatory drugs for body and muscle aches.
- The anticholinergic dicyclomine can be used to minimize gastrointestinal hyperactivity.
- Nonbenzodiazepine hypnotics, low-dose atypical antipsychotics (e.g., quetiapine), or low-dose tricyclic antidepressants are effective for promoting adequate sleep.
- Psychosocial supports tailored to patient needs should be offered as an adjunct to medical treatment.

CHRONIC Rx

Opioid antagonist treatment:

- Buprenorphine/naloxone is the preferred first-line treatment. Methadone is an alternative in certain populations.
- Naltrexone: Does not stabilize neuronal circuitry like partial or full opioid agonists and generally results in poor outcomes, much like Antabuse for alcohol.
- Opioid partial agonist therapy: Buprenorphine (Suboxone, Bunavail).
- Opioid agonist therapy: Methadone.

NOTE: Buprenorphine and methadone are both metabolized by the cytochrome P450 3a4 and 2d6 I isoenzyme pathways. Prescribers should be aware of multiple possible drug interactions. Methadone and buprenorphine produce similar improvements during opioid withdrawal, although buprenorphine is associated with less sedation and respiratory depression. To avoid precipitating more intense withdrawal, buprenorphine should be initiated 12 to 18 hours after the last administration of opioids in patients who misuse shorter-acting opioids (48 hours in patients who are receiving long-acting drugs such as methadone), with initial doses of 4 to 8 mg.[1]

PATIENT SELECTION FOR BUPRENORPHINE OR METHADONE

- Appropriate patients for buprenorphine office-based treatment:
  1. Patients interested (highly motivated) in treatment
  2. Have no major contraindications (see following)
  3. Can be expected to be reasonably compliant with treatment
  4. Understand the benefits and risks of buprenorphine treatment
  5. Willing to follow safety precautions
- Less likely to be appropriate for office-based treatment:
  1. Have comorbid dependence on benzodiazepines or other CNS depressants (including ethylene alcohol)
  2. Have significant untreated psychiatric comorbidities
  3. Have active or chronic suicidal or homicidal ideation or attempts
  4. Have multiple previous treatments with frequent relapses
  5. Have poor response to previous treatment with buprenorphine
  6. Have significant medical complications (e.g., hepatic insufficiency, bacterial endocarditis, active tuberculosis)
- Methadone maintenance: Narcotic treatment program (clinic setting) indications:
  1. Evidence of opiate addiction >1 yr
  2. Two failed previous treatment attempts
  3. Patients not appropriate for office-based treatment
  4. Eligible without active "use" if prior methadone maintenance patient within previous 2 mo
  5. Pregnancy

DISPOSITION

- Opioid addiction is a chronic, relapsing disease.
- High rate of relapse after "detox."
- Relapse potential after medically supervised withdrawal from methadone:
  1. 90% after 1 yr stable in treatment
  2. 80% after 3 yr stable in treatment
  3. 70% after 5 yr stable in treatment
- Postmarketing surveillance indicates that the diversion and abuse of prescription opioid medications increased between 2002 and 2010 and plateaued or decreased between 2011 and 2013. These findings suggest that the U.S. may be making some progress in controlling the abuse of opioid analgesics.[2]

[1] Schuckit MA: Treatment of opioid-use disorders, *N Engl J Med* 375:357-368, 2016.

TABLE 5 Organizations Providing Referral Information for Patients

Organization	Resources/Website
Substance Abuse and Mental Health Services Administration (SAMHSA)	Opioid treatment program directory: http://dpt2.samhsa.gov/treatment/
Physicians who provide buprenorphine	Buprenorphine physician and treatment program locator: http://buprenorphine.samhsa.gov/bwns_locator/
Pain Action	Chronic pain management materials for patients: www.painaction.org
Substance abuse treatment facilities	Substance Abuse treatment facility locator: http://dasis3.samhsa.gov/
Harm Reduction Coalition	Local risk reduction resources and programs, overdose prevention education, and naloxone prescribing information: http://www.harmreduction.org/
Narcotics Anonymous (NA)	General information and meeting information for NA, a 12-step program modeled after Alcoholics Anonymous: www.na.org

From Bowman S, Eiserman J, Beletsky, L, Stancliff S: Reducing the health consequences of opioid addiction in primary care, *Am J Med* 126, 565-571, 2013.

REFERRAL

Refer to addiction medicine specialist or narcotic treatment program when the neurobiologic disease of opioid addiction is identified.

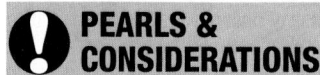

PEARLS & CONSIDERATIONS

COMMENTS

- Methadone maintenance is the gold standard for the pregnant opioid-addicted patient regardless of the duration of the addiction or prior treatment attempts. Detoxification is contraindicated during pregnancy.
- Breastfeeding is encouraged in mothers on methadone maintenance. The American Academy of Pediatrics statement regarding "Transfer of Drugs and Other Chemicals into Human Milk" has placed methadone into the "usually compatible with breastfeeding" group based on the assumption that maternal urine is monitored to detect use of illicit drugs. The U.S. Department of Health and Human Services also recommends that mothers on methadone be encouraged to breastfeed.
- When a physician identifies a patient as a "drug seeker," it is imperative that the physician avoid abruptly stopping the opioid prescription because this will often result in the patient's buying the drugs illegally. These patients should be counseled and referred for treatment.
- Patients on methadone or buprenorphine who have pain resulting from an acute injury will need pain medication in addition to their daily dose of methadone or buprenorphine. They will require higher than usual doses of pain medications because of opioid receptor blockade attributable to their methadone or buprenorphine use.
- Opioid-dependent patients have a lower pain threshold resulting from hyperalgesia caused by the long-term use of opioids.

[2] Dart RC, et al.: Trends in opioid analgesic abuse and mortality in the United States, *N Engl J Med* 372:241-248, 2015.

PREVENTION

Education is the hallmark of prevention:

- School drug prevention education programs.
- Educate children about their family medical history, including diseases of addiction.
- Address childhood psychiatric disorders to prevent self-medicating.

Opioid overdose:

- Naloxone (Narcan) is a competitive mu-opioid receptor antagonist in the brain and is effective for opioid overdose. It is available for IM/IV and intranasal administration. It begins to reverse respiratory depression, sedation, and hypotension 2 to 5 min after IM administration and 1 to 2 min after IV administration.

PATIENT & FAMILY EDUCATION

- Stigma of addictions and treatment often interferes with good treatment.
- Family needs to be educated so they can support the patient's efforts.
- Encourage family meeting with addiction specialist, counselor.
- Recommend support groups for family members. Table 5 identifies organizations providing referral information for patients. Recommendations for integrating risk reduction strategies for addressing opioid misuse in the primary care setting are summarized in Table E6.

SUGGESTED READINGS

Available at ExpertConsult.com

RELATED CONTENT

Drug Abuse (Patient Information)
Opioid Overdose (Related Key Topic)

AUTHOR: **FRED F. FERRI, M.D.**

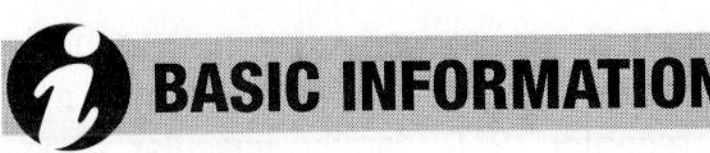

BASIC INFORMATION

DEFINITION

Optic neuritis is an inflammation of the optic nerve resulting in impaired visual function.

SYNONYMS

Optic papillitis
Retrobulbar neuritis

ICD-10CM CODES

H46.9 Unspecified optic neuritis
H46.8 Other optic neuritis

EPIDEMIOLOGY & DEMOGRAPHICS

INCIDENCE (IN U.S.): 1 to 5/100,000 person(s) per yr; rates vary according to incidence of multiple sclerosis (MS). Optic neuritis affects 1% to 5% of patients with neurosarcoid.
PREVALENCE (IN U.S.): Common in patients with MS
PREDOMINANT SEX: Female:male ratio: 1.8:1
PEAK INCIDENCE: 20 to 49 yr, mean 30
GENETICS: Unknown. If due to MS, it is more common in patients with certain HLA blood types and in monozygotic twins of affected siblings.

PHYSICAL FINDINGS & CLINICAL PRESENTATION

- Presentation with acute or subacute (days) visual loss, often accompanied by periocular tenderness that worsens with eye movements.
- **Marcus Gunn pupil** (relative afferent pupillary defect [RAPD]): Direct and consensual response is normal; however, when flashlight is swung from eye to eye, the affected eye's pupil dilates to direct light.
- Decreased visual acuity.
- Unilateral visual field abnormalities—often a central scotoma (Fig. E1).
- Color desaturation; red is most often affected.
- Normal fundus examination in 66% cases; disc edema is noted in 33%. Other abnormalities include uveitis or periphlebitis. In neurosarcoid, the optic nerve head may exhibit a lumpy appearance suggestive of granulomatous infiltration, and there may be associated vitritis (Fig. E2).
- May have movement or light-induced phosphenes (flashes of light lasting 1 to 2 sec).
- Uhthoff phenomenon (benign exercise- or heat-induced deterioration of vision) is seen in some. Vision may also worsen in bright sunlight.
- Over time the optic disc may atrophy and become pale.

ETIOLOGY

An inflammatory response associated with an infection or autoimmune disease (such as collagen vascular disease, granulomatous disease, MS, or neuromyelitis optica).

Dx DIAGNOSIS

Diagnosis is clinically established in a young patient with acute onset of monocular vision loss associated with retroorbital pain associated with eye movements and presence of RAPD. Absence of other orbital or ocular pathology is based on clinical examination.

DIFFERENTIAL DIAGNOSIS

For optic neuritis
- Inflammatory: MS, neuromyelitis optica spectrum disorder (NMOSD), sarcoidosis, lupus, Sjögren's, Behçet's, postinfectious, postvaccination, neuroretinitis, acute disseminated encephalomyelitis, paraneoplastic, autoimmune optic neuropathy
- Infectious: Syphilis, TB, Lyme disease, *Bartonella,* HIV, CMV, herpes, helminths, chickenpox, Q fever, periorbital infections, *Toxocara* sp.
- Ischemic: Anterior and posterior ischemic optic neuropathies, diabetic papillopathy, branch or central retinal artery or vein occlusion
- Drugs and toxins: Arsenic, methanol, ethambutol, cyclosporine, etc.
- Mitochondrial: Leber hereditary optic neuropathy, other mitochondrial

WORKUP

A thorough neurologic examination; dilated ophthalmoscopy

LABORATORY TESTS

Acute optic neuritis is a clinical diagnosis based on presentation with classical features: acute, painful unilateral loss of vision associated with RAPD in a young person with no other apparent causes such as trauma. In atypical cases additional studies may be considered.
- CBC, ANA, ACE, ESR
- Consider HIV Ab, Lyme titer, RPR, other autoimmune or infectious causes
- Bilateral or recurrent ON: NMO IgG, MOG IgG, paraneoplastic CRMP-5-IgG

IMAGING STUDIES

- Contrast-enhanced MRI of the brain is performed to assess the risk of developing MS. Often enhancement of the optic nerve is seen. MRI orbits with thin sections of fat-suppressed sequences may be needed if the patient demonstrates atypical features.
- Consider using optical coherence tomography to follow optic nerve atrophy objectively longitudinally.

Rx TREATMENT

NONPHARMACOLOGIC THERAPY

Assure patient that in most cases there is near complete recovery of vision.

ACUTE Rx

Treat if the visual loss is severe or if there is an abnormal MRI (higher risk of MS). Treatment is with methylprednisolone (MP) 250 mg IV every 6 hr (or 1 g IV daily) for 3 days followed by an oral prednisone taper of 11 days.

CHRONIC Rx

Depends on underlying cause. Disease-modifying treatment when increased risk of developing MS or neuromyelitis optica spectrum disorder. See topic "Multiple Sclerosis."

DISPOSITION

Most often vision is worst at the end of week 1, followed by recovery over months. In the Optic Neuritis Treatment Trial (ONTT), 90% had 20/40 or better vision at 1 yr and 3% had 20/200 or worse. Of initial 20/200 or worse cases, only 5% remained in that group at 6 mo.

REFERRAL

- To neurologist for other neurologic signs and to assess risk of developing MS. In ONTT (Optic Neuritis Treatment Trial), risk of MS >15 yr was 72% with ≥1 lesion(s) on MRI, and 25% with a normal MRI
- To ophthalmologist when atypical features or slowly progressive; urgently when other ocular pathology is present or if vision worsens or does not improve after several wk, or pain is severe

PEARLS & CONSIDERATIONS

- Bilateral optic neuritis suggests a systemic inflammatory disorder, infection, NMOSD, or paraneoplastic, but can also occur in MS.
- Acute bilateral loss of vision with a severe headache or diplopia should raise concern for pituitary apoplexy and/or giant cell arteritis.

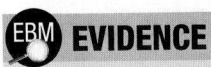

EBM EVIDENCE

Available at ExpertConsult.com

RELATED CONTENT

Idiopathic Intracranial Hypertension (Related Key Topic)
Multiple Sclerosis (Related Key Topic)

AUTHORS: **SACHIN KEDAR, M.B.B.S., M.D.,** and **COREY COLDSMITH, M.D.**

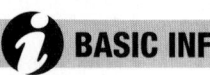

BASIC INFORMATION

DEFINITION

Oral cancers refer to malignant transformation of the oral tissues usually preceded by a process of sequential dysplastic changes leading to the development of squamous carcinoma. Oral squamous cell cancers (OSCC) include oral cavity cancers (lip, floor of mouth, buccal mucosa, anterior tongue, gingivae, hard palate, retromolar trigone), oropharynx cancers (base of tongue, tonsils, soft palate, pharyngeal walls), and hypopharynx cancers (pyriform sinus, postcricoid area, posterior pharyngeal wall).

SYNONYMS

Head and neck cancer
Oral malignant neoplasm
OSCC

ICD-10CM CODES

C01	Malignant neoplasm of base of tongue
C03	Malignant neoplasm of gum
C04	Malignant neoplasm of floor of mouth
C05	Malignant neoplasm of palate
C06	Malignant neoplasm of other and unspecified parts of mouth
C09	Malignant neoplasm of tonsil
C10	Malignant neoplasm of oropharynx
C11	Malignant neoplasm of nasopharynx
C12	Malignant neoplasm of piriform sinus
C13	Malignant neoplasm of hypopharynx
C14	Malignant neoplasm of other and ill-defined sites of lip, oral cavity and larynx
C14.0	Malignant neoplasm of pharynx, unspecified
C14.2	Malignant neoplasm of Waldeyer's ring
C14.8	Malignant neoplasm of overlapping sites of lip, oral cavity and pharynx

EPIDEMIOLOGY & DEMOGRAPHICS

INCIDENCE & PREVALENCE: OSCC comprise the sixth most common cancer in the world. An estimated 530,000 cases are diagnosed annually around the globe, and the rates have been rising, particularly in young people and among minorities. It is estimated that in 2018, approximately 51,540 new cases and 10,030 deaths will occur in the U.S. The incidence of oral cancers linked to alcohol and tobacco use has been declining in the U.S., whereas those linked to human papillomavirus (HPV), primarily HPV type 16, are on the rise, especially for cancers located in the tonsils and base of tongue. In developed countries across the world, HPV is increasingly implicated in the growing incidence of oral cancer. In Asian countries where chewing betel nut is customary, oral cancer accounts for up to 40% of cancers in some regions. Squamous cell carcinoma is the most common malignancy that occurs in the oral cavity. Minor salivary gland cancers, lymphomas, and sarcomas are less common.

PREDOMINANT SEX & AGE: The ratio of oral cancer in males:females is 2.5:1 in the U.S. Black males have a higher early incidence in the 50- to 60-yr age group, but with increasing age, white men predominate.

GENETICS: The genes that are critically altered in OSCC include *TP53*, the retinoblastoma family, *p16* and cyclin *D1*. The *TP53*, *CCND1*, and *CDKN2A* genes are established cancer genes in HPV-negative cancers. *TP53* and the genes encoding the Rb family are established cancer genes in HPV-positive cancers. Signaling pathways that are involved in the pathogenesis of oral cancers include that of the human epidermal receptor (HER) family, vascular endothelial growth factor (VEGF) receptor, and signal transducer and activator of transcription 3 (STAT 3). The tumor suppressor gene *TP53* is frequently mutated in HPV-negative tumors.

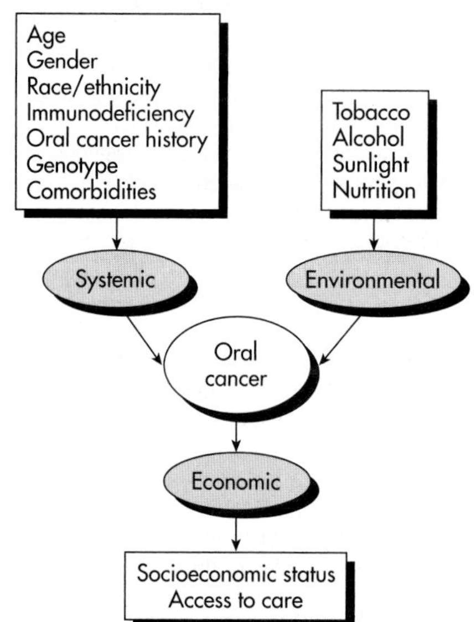

FIG. 1 Risk model for oral cancer. Oral cancer is a multifactorial disease process that includes systemic, environmental, and economic effects. The interplay of these variables ultimately leads to the incidence of this disease. The multifactorial nature of oral cancer should be addressed in the assessment of a patient's risk. (From Jones DL, Rankin KV: Oral cancer and associated risk factors. In Cappelli D, Mobley C [eds]: *Prevention in clinical oral health care,* St. Louis, 2008, Elsevier, pp 68–77.)

RISK FACTORS (FIG. 1): The following factors are implicated in the development of oral cancer:

- Tobacco use
- HPV infection (primarily types 16 and 18)
- Alcohol
- Immune deficiency
- Radiation
- Betel nut consumption
- Solar radiation

PHYSICAL FINDINGS & CLINICAL PRESENTATION

- Specific patient complaints may include the following: oral ulcers or mass, choking, difficulty breathing, dysphagia, odynophagia, voice hoarseness, globus sensation, otalgia, ear or nose stuffiness, hemoptysis, trismus, neck mass, and pain in the head/neck region.
- Generalized symptoms and signs may include weight loss, fatigue, anorexia, altered mood, and sleep.
- Clinically, oral cancers can present as:
  1. Erythroplakia (flat red patch); can mimic inflammatory or traumatic lesions
  2. Leukoplakia (white patch; Fig. 2)
  3. Raised lesion
  4. Ulcerated lesion
  5. Warty lesion or growth

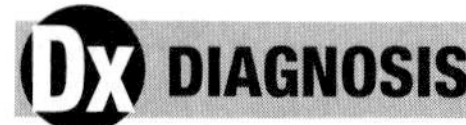

DIAGNOSIS

DIFFERENTIAL DIAGNOSIS

- Oral leukoplakia
- Invasive fungal infections

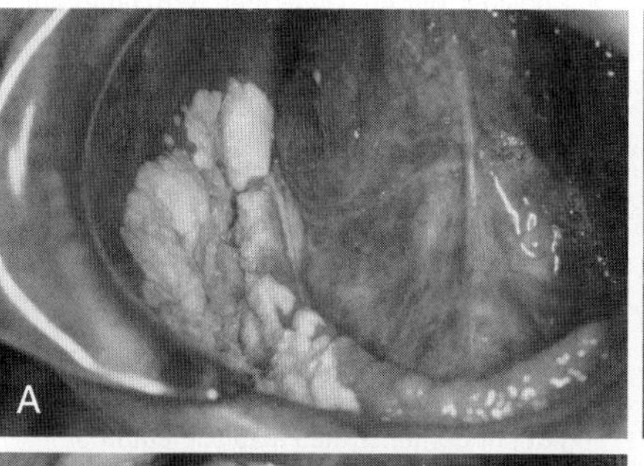

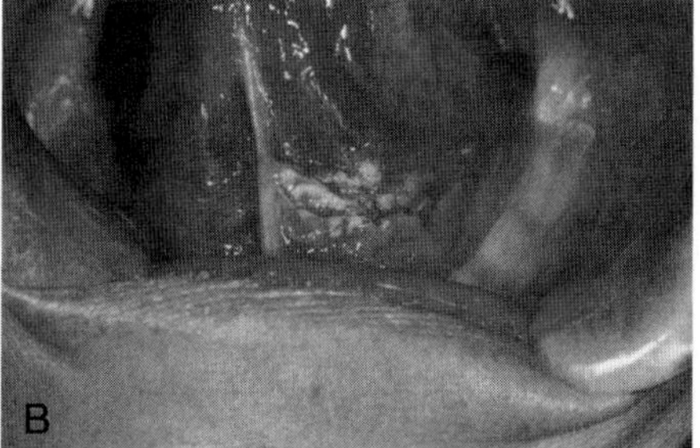

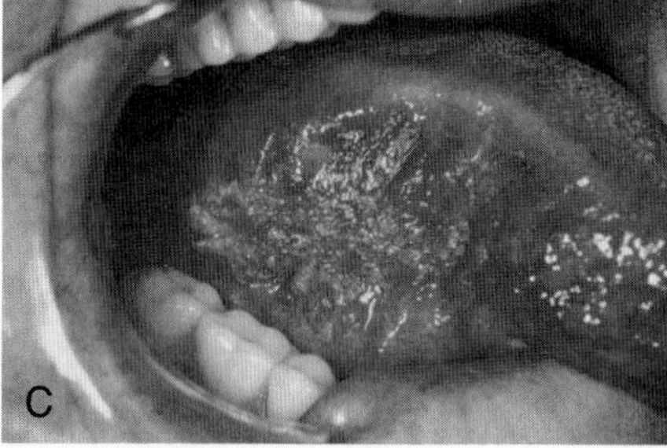

FIG. 2 Squamous cell carcinoma of the oral mucosa. A, Leukoplakia. **B,** Invasive carcinoma of the floor of the mouth. **C,** Invasive carcinoma of the tongue. (Courtesy G. Putnam. In White GM, Cox NH [eds]: *Diseases of the skin: a color atlas and text,* ed 2, St Louis, 2006, Mosby.)

- Chancre of early syphilis and gumma of tertiary syphilis
- Chronic ulcer
- Metastatic or locally invading cancers from sinuses or other sites of the body

PATIENT WORKUP

- Primary workup includes either biopsy or fine-needle aspiration (FNA) of the presenting lesion or suspected neck lymph node for histopathologic analysis. HPV assessment with p16 immunohistochemical staining and confirmatory in situ hybridization (ISH) testing is performed when indicated for oropharynx primary tumors.
- Detailed examination of the oral cavity, pharynx, larynx, neck, ears, nose, and cranial nerves should be performed.
- Laryngoscopy and examination under anesthesia are commonly performed.
- Pretreatment evaluation of tumor size, the extent of invasion, and the presence or absence of regional lymph node metastases is critical for planning treatment.
- Laboratory workup can include complete blood count, complete chemistry panel, and thyroid function.
- Staging workup includes CT or MRI imaging of the head and neck and a chest x-ray. If locoregional or advanced disease is a consideration, a PET scan is typically completed.
- The TNM system is used for staging of OSCC and is subdivided according to primary tumor sites: (1) lip and oral cavity, (2) pharynx.

Rx TREATMENT

- Surgery, radiation therapy, and chemotherapy are treatment modalities involved in the treatment plan for OSCC.
- The use of supportive and special therapeutic modalities such as nutritional therapy including feeding gastrostomy, speech and swallowing therapy, reconstructive surgery, and speech prosthesis is required often.
- For treatment purposes OSCC are classified as early (T1 or T2 lesions), locoregional (T3-4 or any N), or metastatic (M1) stages. Site-specific TNM staging is done as per the primary tumor site (e.g., oral cavity, oropharynx, hypopharynx, etc.)
- After staging completion, the initial treatment considerations include:
  1. Determination of primary tumor resectability (resectable vs. unresectable)
  2. Management of neck nodes
  3. Intent of radiation therapy (curative vs. palliative)
  4. Need for organ preservation
  5. Need for reconstructive surgery
  6. Need for chemotherapy
  7. HPV status of tumor
- Localized tumors (stage I or II) can be approached by initial surgical resection or definitive radiotherapy. Loco-regionally advanced tumors (stage III and localized IV) that are resectable are typically approached by upfront surgery followed by adjuvant radiation and/or chemotherapy. Unresectable patients are typically treated with definitive chemotherapy and radiotherapy. Patients with distant metastatic disease are treated with systemic chemotherapy, while locally recurrent tumors can be approached with either surgery or chemotherapy or both.
- Surgery is typically associated with less long-term morbidity than radiation therapy. Surgical therapy traditionally involved wide-exposure approaches (mandibulotomy, transpharyngeal access). Newer surgical techniques allow tumor resection through the mouth. Recently, transoral robotic surgery (TORS) has been developed to improve access to oropharyngeal squamous cell carcinomas with excellent oncologic outcomes.
  1. Acute surgical complications can include infection, bleeding, aspiration, wound breakdown, fistula, and flap loss.
  2. Surgical procedures can cause functional deficits in speech and swallowing, but these adverse effects can be minimized by appropriate reconstruction and prostheses.
- Definitive radiation therapy is reserved for patients who cannot tolerate surgery or for whom surgical resection would result in particularly severe functional impairment.
  1. Radiation therapy can include external beam radiation and brachytherapy.
  2. Radiation therapy side effects include mucositis, radiation dermatitis, loss of taste, dysphagia, dental caries and decay, and xerostomia.
  3. Late complications can include skin/soft tissue atrophy and fibrosis, osteoradionecrosis, and trismus.
- Systemic chemotherapy can be administered alone or in combination with radiotherapy, depending on the disease stage. Agents typically used include cisplatin, carboplatin, 5-fluorouracil, taxanes, and the epidermal growth factor receptor (EGFR) antibody cetuximab.
- For locally advanced OSCC, the combination of cisplatin and radiotherapy is the regimen of choice. In selected patients with large primary tumors or bulky nodal disease, neoadjuvant chemotherapy may be utilized prior to chemoradiotherapy administration.
- For metastatic or recurrent OSCC, combination chemotherapy regimens in combination with the EGFR antibody cetuximab have been shown to improve overall survival. More recently, the PD-1 immune checkpoint inhibitors nivolumab and pembrolizumab have been shown to improve overall survival outcomes in patients who have received prior chemotherapy.
- The negative predictive value of post-treatment PET imaging in patients with locally advanced cancer who have been treated with chemoradiotherapy is 98% to 99%.

DISPOSITION

- Prognosis depends on the staging and resectability of the primary tumor as well as on patient performance status.
- Tumor HPV status is a strong and independent prognostic factor for survival among patients with base of tongue and oropharyngeal cancer.

REFERRAL

Referral to multidisciplinary head and neck cancer team consisting of ENT or head/neck surgeon, radiation oncologist, and medical oncologist.

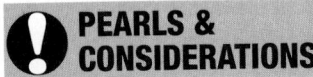

PEARLS & CONSIDERATIONS

COMMENTS

- Oral and pharyngeal cancer is the sixth most common cancer globally.
- Biopsy with HPV-status assessment is the key for accurate diagnosis.
- Posttreatment rehabilitation and surveillance is important.

PREVENTION

- Encourage patients to stop using any type of tobacco and drinking alcohol.
- Examine oral cavities at annual checkups and work up suspicious lesions.

SUGGESTED READINGS

Available at ExpertConsult.com

RELATED CONTENT

Mouth Cancer (Patient Information)

AUTHOR: **RITESH RATHORE, M.D.**

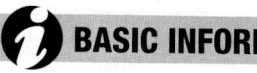

BASIC INFORMATION

DEFINITION

Oral hairy leukoplakia (OHL) is a painless, white, nonremovable, plaquelike lesion typically located on the lateral aspect of the tongue.

SYNONYMS

Oral hairy leukoplakia
OHL

ICD-10CM CODE
K13.3 Hairy leukoplakia

EPIDEMIOLOGY & DEMOGRAPHICS

INCIDENCE AND PREVALENCE: Epstein-Barr virus (EBV) is implicated in the etiology of OHL, and the incidence of EBV seroprevalence is high in individuals who are HIV seropositive. However, OHL occurs in only 25% of these cases but may also occur in other immunosuppressed individuals, for example, organ transplant recipients.

RISK FACTORS: OHL is usually found in HIV-seropositive individuals (median CD4 count is 468/ml) but may also be identified in smokers and other immunocompromised patients such as transplant recipients (particularly renal) and patients taking steroids. Diagnosing OHL is an indication to institute a workup to evaluate and manage HIV disease.

PHYSICAL FINDINGS & CLINICAL PRESENTATION

- Varying morphology and appearance, which may change daily.
- May be unilateral or bilateral.
- White plaques can be small with fine, vertical corrugations on the lateral margin of the tongue (Fig. 1). The plaques from OHL are adherent to the tongue surface (in contrast to candidal plaques, which may be easily scraped off).
- Irregular surface; may have prominent folds or projection, occasionally markedly resembling hairs.
- May spread to cover the entire dorsal surface or spread onto the ventral surface of the tongue where the lesions usually appear flat.
- Rarely, lesions can manifest on the soft palate, buccal mucosa, or posterior oropharynx.
- Usually asymptomatic, but some patients have mouth pain, soreness, or a burning sensation; impaired taste, or difficulty eating; others complain of its unsightly appearance.
- OHL may rarely progress to oral squamous cell carcinoma, particularly in smokers, which has a poor prognosis.

ETIOLOGY

EBV is implicated in its etiology, and OHL is a result of replication EBV in the epithelium of keratinized cells. OHL differs from most EBV-related diseases in that infection is predominantly lytic, with abundant virus production resulting in cell lysis, rather than latent.

DIAGNOSIS

DIFFERENTIAL DIAGNOSIS

- *Candida albicans*
- Lichen planus
- Idiopathic leukoplakia
- White sponge nevus
- Dysplasia
- Squamous cell carcinoma

WORKUP

Requires physical examination and evaluation of HIV disease

LABORATORY TESTS

The *provisional* diagnosis is clinical and based on:

- Visual inspection
- Inability to scrape the lesion off the tongue with a blade
- Failure to respond to antifungal therapy

The *presumptive* diagnosis requires biopsy and histologic demonstration of:

- Epithelial hyperplasia with hairs
- Absence of inflammatory cell infiltrate

The *definitive* diagnosis requires:

- In situ hybridization of histologic or cytologic specimens revealing EBV DNA *or*
- Electron microscopy of specimens revealing herpes-like particles
- Measurement of the DNA content in cells of oral leukoplakia may be used to predict the risk of oral carcinoma

NOTE: Specimens obtained from lesions may demonstrate hyphae of *Candida albicans,* which may coexist and potentiate EBV-induced OHL.

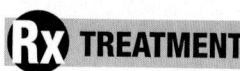

TREATMENT

NONPHARMACOLOGIC THERAPY

OHL is usually asymptomatic and requires no specific therapy. It may resolve spontaneously and is generally benign in HIV-seropositive patients.

ACUTE GENERAL Rx

- Antiretroviral therapy (ART) has considerably changed the frequency of oral lesions caused by opportunistic infections in HIV-seropositive individuals.
- Topical retinoids (0.1% vitamin A) may improve the appearance of OHL-affected oral surfaces through their dekeratinizing and immunomodulation effects; however, they are expensive, and prolonged use may result in a burning sensation over the treated area.
- Topical podophyllin resin 25% solution has been reported to induce resolution.
- Surgical excision and cryotherapy may help, but the lesions may recur.
- High-dose acyclovir 800 mg five times per day, valacyclovir 1000 mg tid, famciclovir 500 mg tid, ganciclovir 1000 mg tid, or foscarnet 40 mg/kg IV tid will cause lesions to resolve but only temporarily.

REFERRAL

Referral to ENT or oral surgeon for biopsy of tongue to confirm diagnosis

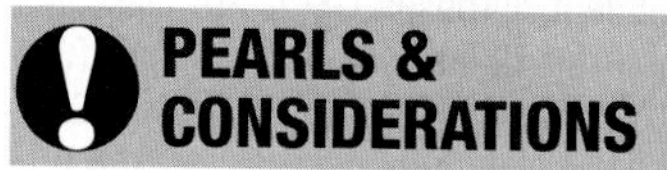

PEARLS & CONSIDERATIONS

- OHL may be the presenting sign of patients infected with HIV who are unaware of their status.
- The incidence has decreased significantly in the era of antiretroviral therapy.

RELATED CONTENT

Acquired Immunodeficiency Syndrome (Related Key Topic)
Oral Hairy Leukoplakia (Patient Information)
Epstein-Barr Virus Infection (Related Key Topic)
Human Immunodeficiency Virus (Related Key Topic)

AUTHOR: **SAJEEV HANDA, M.D., S.F.H.M.**

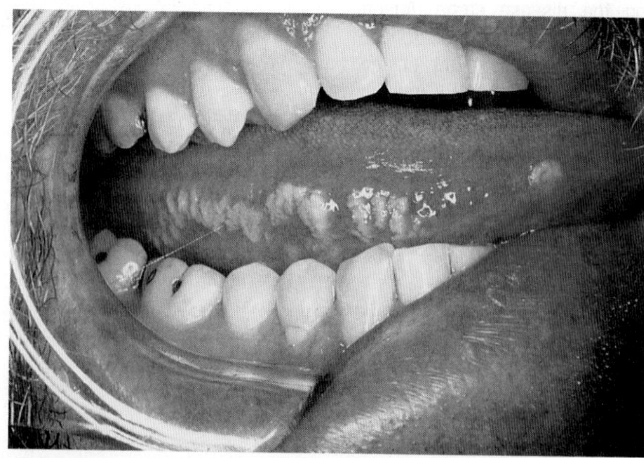

FIG. 1 Oral hairy leukoplakia. (From Callen JP et al: *Dermatological signs of systemic disease*, ed 5, Philadelphia, 2017, Elsevier.)

BASIC INFORMATION

DEFINITION

Orchitis is an inflammatory process (usually infectious) involving the testicles. Infection may be viral or bacterial and can be associated with infection of other male sex organs (prostate, epididymis, or bladder) or lower urogenital tract or sexually transmitted diseases often via hematogenous spread. Common causes are:

- Viral: Mumps—20% postpubertal; coxsackie B virus
- Bacterial: Pyogenic via spread from involving epididymis; bacteria include *Escherichia coli, Klebsiella pneumoniae, P. aeruginosa, Staphylococcus, Streptococcus* or *Rickettsia, Brucella* spp.
- Other:
  1. Viral—HIV-associated, CMV
  2. Fungi
     a. Cryptococcosis
     b. Histoplasmosis
     c. *Candida*
     d. Blastomycosis
     e. Syphilis
  3. *Mycobacterium tuberculosis and M. leprae*
  4. Parasitic causes: Toxoplasmosis, filariasis, schistosomiasis
- Table 1 describes a classification of epididymitis and orchitis based on etiology.

SYNONYMS

Epididymo-orchitis
Testicular infection
Testicular inflammation

ICD-10CM CODES

N45.9	Orchitis, epididymitis, and epididymo-orchitis without abscess
A54.1	Gonococcal orchitis
A56.1	Chlamydial orchitis
N51.1	Mumps orchitis

EPIDEMIOLOGY & DEMOGRAPHICS

PREDOMINANT SEX: Male

PREDOMINANT ORGANISM: The leading cause of viral orchitis is mumps. The mumps virus rarely causes orchitis in prepubertal males but involves one or both testicles in nearly 30% of postpubertal males.

PHYSICAL FINDINGS & CLINICAL PRESENTATION

- Testicular pain, unilateral or bilateral swelling
- May have associated epididymitis, prostatitis, fever, scrotal edema, erythema, cellulitis
- Inguinal lymphadenopathy
- Acute hydrocele (bacterial)
- Rare development: Abscess formation, pyocele of scrotum, testicular infarction
- Spermatic cord tenderness may be present
- Granulomatous

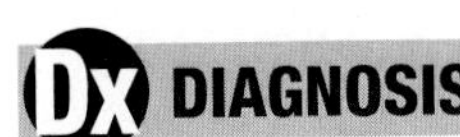

DIAGNOSIS

Clinical presentation as described previously with possible history of acute viral illness or concomitant epididymitis

DIFFERENTIAL DIAGNOSIS

- Epididymo-orchitis-gonococcal
- Autoimmune disease
- Vasculitis
- Epididymitis
- Mumps, with or without parotitis
- Neoplasm
- Hematoma
- Spermatic cord torsion

LABORATORY TESTS

- CBC with differential
- Urinalysis
- Viral titer—mumps. Mumps IgM will be detectable after 5 days of onset of clinical mumps and remain positive for up to 4 weeks. A reverse-transcriptase PCR (RT-PCR) on serum or buccal or oral swab is another option.
- Urine culture for mumps virus
- Ultrasound of testicle to rule out abscess

IMAGING STUDIES

Ultrasound if abscess suspected

TREATMENT

- Dependent on cause.
- Viral (mumps): Observation; bed rest, ice packs, analgesics, and a scrotal sling for support may provide some relief of discomfort that accompanies mumps orchitis.
- Bacterial: Empiric antibiotic treatment with parenteral antibiotic treatment until pathogen identified: Ceftriaxone (250 mg IM once) plus doxycycline (100 mg PO bid for 10 days), in men <35 yr old to cover *Neisseria gonorrhoeae* and *Chlamydia trachomatis*. In homosexual men or men >35 yr old: Levofloxacin 500 to 750 mg IV/PO qd for 10 to 14 days *or* ampicillin-sulbactam *or* third-generation cephalosporin or piperacillin/tazobactam.
- Surgery for abscess, pyogenic process.

DISPOSITION

Follow-up for evidence of recurrence, hypogonadism, and infertility may be needed with bilateral orchitis.

REFERRAL

- To a urologist if surgical drainage is needed
- To an endocrinologist if hypogonadism develops
- To a fertility specialist if infertility develops

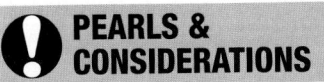

PEARLS & CONSIDERATIONS

Consider tuberculous orchitis if symptoms fail to respond to standard antibacterial therapy, even in the absence of chest radiographic evidence of pulmonary tuberculosis.

SUGGESTED READINGS

Available at ExpertConsult.com

RELATED CONTENT

Orchitis (Patient Information)
Epididymitis (Related Key Topic)
Mumps (Related Key Topic)

AUTHOR: **GLENN G. FORT, M.D., M.P.H.**

TABLE 1 Classification of Epididymitis and Orchitis

Acute Epididymitis or Epididymo-orchitis	Granulomatous Epididymitis or Orchitis	Viral Orchitis
Neisseria gonorrhoeae	*Mycobacterium tuberculosis*	Mumps
Chlamydia trachomatis	*Treponema pallidum*	Enteroviruses
Escherichia coli		
Streptococcus pneumoniae	*Brucella* spp.	
Klebsiella spp.	Sarcoid	
Salmonella spp.	Fungal	
Other urinary tract pathogens	Parasitic	
Idiopathic	Idiopathic	

From Cohen J, Powderly WG: *Infectious diseases*, ed 2, St Louis, 2004, Mosby.

BASIC INFORMATION

DEFINITION

Orthostatic hypotension (OH) is defined as the presence of at least one of the following: a decrease in systolic blood pressure by ≥20 mm Hg or a decrease in diastolic blood pressure by ≥10 mm Hg within 3 min of standing. It is a physical sign that requires further investigation to discern its underlying etiology. Recent studies have shown that blood pressure measurements within 1 min might be more useful in predicting fractures, falls, and other adverse events and for most patients, assessment within 1 min of standing rather than waiting for 3 min may be sufficient.[1]

SYNONYMS

Postural hypotension
OH

ICD-10CM CODE
I95.1 Orthostatic hypotension

EPIDEMIOLOGY & DEMOGRAPHICS

- The incidence of OH is increased in older people and in those with diseases associated with autonomic dysfunction (e.g., Parkinson disease, diabetes mellitus).
- OH may cause up to 30% of all syncopal events in the elderly, and OH is associated with an increased risk of heart failure among those aged 45 to 55 yr and an increased risk of cardiovascular disease and all-cause mortality among those aged 55 yr and older.
- There is an association between orthostatic hypotension and cognitive dysfunction among older adults.

PHYSICAL FINDINGS & CLINICAL PRESENTATION

- Symptoms may include dizziness, lightheadedness, syncope, visual and auditory disturbances, weakness, diaphoresis, pallor, and nausea. OH may also be asymptomatic, especially in older hypertensive patients.
- Associated with increased autonomic activity during meals (from increased splanchnic blood flow), exercise, and hot weather.
- Supine and nocturnal hypertension in patients with OH may indicate an underlying autonomic dysfunction.

ETIOLOGY

- The assumption of an upright posture results in the pooling of approximately 500 ml of blood in the lower extremities due to gravity and decreased venous return, decreased cardiac output, and decreased arterial pressure. The consequent increase in sympathetic tone due to increased carotid baroreceptor activity causes arterial and venous constriction as well as positive inotropic and chronotropic effects, thereby limiting the fall in upright blood pressure. Peripheral vasoconstriction is also mediated by increased activity of the renin-angiotensin system and decreased activity of atrial natriuretic factor.
- Impairment of the baroreceptor reflex, as in central or peripheral autonomic dysfunction and aging, may cause OH because decreased blood pressure cannot be counteracted by the aforementioned regulatory mechanisms.

Dx DIAGNOSIS

DIFFERENTIAL DIAGNOSIS

Common:

- Medications: Antihypertensives, antidepressants (tricyclics), antipsychotics (phenothiazines), alcohol, narcotics, barbiturates, insulin, nitrates, PDE-5 inhibitors, alpha-adrenergic antagonists
- Reduced intravascular volume (hemorrhage, dehydration, hyperglycemia, hypoalbuminemia)
- Postprandial effect (especially in the elderly)
- Vasovagal syncope
- Deconditioning
- Central autonomic dysfunction (Parkinson's disease)
- Peripheral autonomic dysfunction (diabetes mellitus, Guillain-Barré syndrome)

Uncommon:

- Central autonomic dysfunction (Shy-Drager syndrome)
- Postganglionic autonomic dysfunction: Impaired norepinephrine release
- Autoimmune autonomic dysfunction: Nicotinic acetylcholine receptor autoantibodies
- Paraneoplastic autonomic dysfunction: Anti-Hu antibodies (in small-cell lung cancer)
- Postural tachycardia syndrome (POTS): Usually occurs in young women; an abnormally large increase in heart rate is observed in the upright position, caused by increased venous pooling from autonomic dysfunction of the lower extremities, but blood pressure is not affected because of an excess of plasma norepinephrine
- Impaired cardiac output (myocardial infarction, aortic stenosis, arrhythmias)
- Cerebrovascular accident
- Adrenal insufficiency
- Deconditioning
- Carotid sinus hypersensitivity
- Anxiety, panic attacks
- Seizures
- Sepsis
- Idiopathic

WORKUP

- Measure supine blood pressure after the patient has been resting comfortably. The duration of time that the patient should spend supine and standing when measuring orthostatic hypotension is controversial. Limited evidence supports having the patient remain supine for 5 to 10 min before obtaining the supine blood pressure, followed by blood pressure measurement within 1 min of standing and again after 3 min of standing. The blood pressure cuff must be held at the level of the right atrium; holding the cuff below this level will result in a 5 to 10 mm Hg underestimation of blood pressure.
- Thorough neurologic examination should be performed.
- Rule out treatable causes (e.g., medications, volume depletion).

LABORATORY TESTS

- Hemoglobin and hematocrit
- Consider when treatable causes of OH have been ruled out:
  1. Blood pressure and heart rate monitoring with a tilt table test
  2. Plasma norepinephrine measurements (to distinguish postganglionic from preganglionic autonomic dysfunction)
  3. Other methods, which use the Valsalva maneuver or measure sweating as indirect means of evaluating the autonomic nervous system

IMAGING STUDIES

None

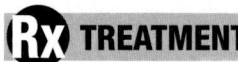

Rx TREATMENT

NONPHARMACOLOGIC THERAPY

- Patient education (leg crossing, prolonged sitting before first standing in the morning, avoid excessive straining and hot baths)
- High-salt diet (e.g., bouillon cubes); caution if history of heart failure
- Liberal fluid intake
- Take needed antihypertensive medications at different times of the day
- Raise the head of the bed at night
- Compression stockings (to include splanchnic circulation)
- Multiple low-carbohydrate meals to avoid postprandial OH
- Avoid large carbohydrate loads and excess alcohol consumption

ACUTE GENERAL Rx

- Correction of volume status and impairment of cerebral perfusion
- Review medication list and attempt to eliminate those potentially contributing to OH

CHRONIC Rx

- Fludrocortisone: 0.1 mg/day (may combine with an alpha-1 agonist to lower the dose of each); monitor for electrolyte disturbances and supine hypertension
- Midodrine (alpha-1 agonist): 10 mg three times a day; monitor for supine hypertension
- Erythropoietin (consider if anemic)
- Caffeine (for postprandial hypotension)
- Table 1 summarizes management of orthostatic hypotension in older adults

OTHER TREATMENTS

- Pyridostigmine (enhances renal sodium reabsorption): 0.2 to 0.6 mg/day (not FDA-approved for this indication)

[1]Juraschek SP, et al.: Associated of history of dizziness and long-term adverse outcomes with early vs. later orthostatic hypotension assessment times in middle-aged adults, *JAMA Intern Med* 2017.

TABLE 1 Management of Orthostatic Hypotension in Older Adults

Identify and treat correctable causes.

Reduce or eliminate drugs causing orthostatic hypotension.

Avoid situations that may exacerbate orthostatic hypotension.

- Standing motionless
- Prolonged recumbency
- Large meals
- Hot weather
- Hot showers
- Straining at stool or with voiding
- Isometric exercise
- Ingesting alcohol
- Hyperventilation
- Dehydration

Raise the head of the bed to a 5- to 20-degree angle.

Wear waist-high, custom-fitted, elastic stockings and an abdominal binder.

Participate in physical conditioning exercises.

Participate in controlled postural exercises using the tilt table.

Avoid diuretics and eat salt-containing fluids (unless congestive heart failure is present).

Drug therapy

- Caffeine
- Fludrocortisone
- Midodrine
- Desmopressin
- Erythropoietin

From Fillit HM: *Brocklehurst's textbook of geriatric medicine and gerontology*, ed 8, Philadelphia, 2017, Elsevier.

- Octreotide: 300 to 600 mg/day (not FDA-approved for this indication)
- Indomethacin (prostaglandin inhibitor)
- DDAVP (experimental)
- Droxidopa (used for patients with autonomic dysfunction to increase the availability of norepinephrine) has been FDA approved for treatment of adults with symptomatic neurogenic orthostatic hypotension caused by primary autonomic failure or nondiabetic autonomic neuropathy

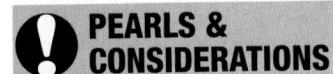

PEARLS & CONSIDERATIONS

COMMENTS

- The presence of OH should always trigger a search for an underlying etiology.
- OH is diagnosed by observing changes in blood pressure, not heart rate.
- Volume depletion should cause an increased heart rate on standing; a lack of heart rate response in this setting suggests autonomic dysfunction.
- Pharmacotherapy with mineralocorticoids may require concomitant potassium replenishment and monitoring for hypertension.
- Evidence to support the efficacy of pharmacologic interventions to treat OH, including midodrine, is limited.
- The etiology of OH is often multifactorial in older patients, but increased susceptibility to volume depletion due to decreased baroreceptor reflexes frequently contributes. Chronic vitamin D deficiency is associated with the development of OH.
- Intensive blood pressure control did not increase injurious falls compared with controls among community-dwelling older adults participating in the Systolic Blood Pressure Intervention Trial (SPRINT).
- The physical examination of patients with dizziness, gait disturbance, and/or falls should include an assessment for OH. OH is an independent predictor of unexplained falls in older adults.
- Because OH may be asymptomatic, physical examination of those at risk must include assessment of blood pressure in both the supine and upright positions.

SUGGESTED READINGS

Available at ExpertConsult.com

AUTHOR: **TIMOTHY W. FARRELL, M.D., AGSF.**

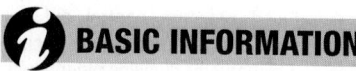

BASIC INFORMATION

DEFINITION

Osteoarthritis (OA) is a progressive disease of the joint representing failed repair of joint damage. Intraarticular stresses that lead to joint damage may be initiated by abnormalities in articular cartilage, subchondral bone, ligaments, menisci, periarticular muscles, peripheral nerves, or synovium. The result is the breakdown of cartilage and bone, leading to symptoms of pain, stiffness, and functional disability. As an illness, it encompasses a symptom complex of pain, aching, discomfort, stiffness, and sleep disturbance that results in functional limitation, physical disability, and reduced health-related quality of life. It also has a significant economic burden (up to 2.5% of the gross domestic product [GDP] in the U.S.). The American College of Rheumatology Classification criteria for osteoarthritis is described in Table 1.

SYNONYMS

Degenerative joint disease (DJD)
DJD
Arthrosis
OA

ICD-10CM CODES

M15.1 Heberden nodes (with arthropathy)
M15.2 Bouchard nodes (with arthropathy)
M15.3 Secondary multiple arthritis
M15.4 Erosive OA
M15.8 Other polyosteoarthritis
M15.9 Polyarthrosis, unspecified
M17 Gonarthrosis (arthrosis of knee)
M18 Arthrosis of first metacarpal joint
M19 Other arthrosis
M19.8 Other specified arthrosis
M19.9 Arthrosis, unspecified

EPIDEMIOLOGY & DEMOGRAPHICS

PREVALENCE: Affects more than 30 million individuals in the U.S. Approximately 10% of men and 18% of women over the age of 60 yr are affected.

PREDOMINANT SEX: Prior to age 50, there is almost no gender discrepancy. After age 50, there is increased incidence of OA in females compared to males.

PREDOMINANT AGE: Occurs more frequently after 50 yr of age, but it is increasingly being recognized that OA may occur as early as 30 yr of age.

GENETICS: 39% to 65% heritability rate in twin studies of women who have generalized OA, concordance rate of 0.64 in monozygotic twins. In genome-wide association studies, 11 candidate loci have been identified, but all with a very small effect size (1.11-1.2).

RISK FACTORS: Osteoarthritis is considered predominantly a mechanical non-inflammatory form of arthritis. Osteoarthritis is thought to be the result of hostile biomechanics on an already susceptible joint. Risk factors may be classified as either local or systemic. Local or biomechanical factors include obesity leading to increased load on the articular cartilage, mechanical environment of the joint (includes deformities like pes planus, genu varus and valgus, proprioception at the joint), local joint activity/occupation (textile worker leading to hand OA, high-impact runners leading to knee OA), and muscle weakness (quadriceps weakness leading to knee OA). Other deformities, such as femoro-acetabular impingement and limb length inequality, can confer significant risk of developing end-stage osteoarthritis. Systemic risk factors include nutritional factors such as antioxidant and vitamin D deficiency, hormonal status, high bone mineral density, and genetics (candidate genes being evaluated include IGF-1 gene, cartilage oligomeric protein gene, vitamin D receptor gene). That said, there is no concrete evidence showing that preventing the disease or reducing disease progression can be achieved by supplemental vitamin D, antioxidants, or estrogen. Obesity also increases the susceptibility of developing osteoarthritis via systemic adipokines.

PHYSICAL FINDINGS & CLINICAL PRESENTATION

- Similar symptoms in most forms: Pain generally with activity, stiffness, or gelling (generally short-lived and morning stiffness lasting less than 30 minutes), crepitus
- Loss of function in joints (e.g., loss of dexterity in patients with hand osteoarthritis, with or without significant pain)
- Joint tenderness, swelling
- Crepitus with motion
- Bouchard and Heberden nodes (bony enlargement of the proximal interphalangeal [PIP] and distal interphalangeal [DIP] joints of the hand, respectively) (Fig. 1)
- Pain with range of motion

ETIOLOGY

Osteoarthritis is most often primary or idiopathic and can be monoarticular, oligoarticular, or polyarticular. Secondary OA is due to an identifiable condition such as trauma, mechanical abnormalities, or congenital disorders. Risk factors for osteoarthritis are summarized in Table 2.

TABLE 1 American College of Rheumatology Classification Criteria for Osteoarthritis

Hip	Knee (Clinical Criteria)	Hand
Pain in the hip and two of the following: ESR <20 mm/hr Radiographic joint space narrowing Radiographic osteophytes	Pain in the knee and five of the following: Age >50 <30 min morning stiffness Crepitus Bony enlargement Bony tenderness No synovial warmth	Pain, aching, and stiffness in the hand and three of the following: Fewer than three MCP joints swollen Hard tissue enlargement of two or more DIP joints Hard tissue enlargement of two or more of the following joints: second and third DIP, second and third PIP, both CMC joints Deformity of at least one of the following joints: second and third DIP, second and third PIP, both CMC joints

CMC, Carpometacarpal; *DIP,* distal interphalangeal; *ESR,* erythrocyte sedimentation rate; *MCP,* metacarpophalangeal joint; *PIP,* proximal interphalangeal.

Modified from [1]Altman R, Alarcon G, Appelrouth D, et al.: The American College of Rheumatology criteria for the classification and reporting of osteoarthritis of the hand., *Arthritis Rheum* 331601-1610, 1990; [2]Altman R, Alarcon G, Appelrouth D, et al.: The American College of Rheumatology criteria for the classification and reporting of osteoarthritis of the hip, *Arthritis Rheum* 34:505–514, 1991; [3]Altman R, Asch E, Bloch D, et al.: Development of criteria for the classification and reporting of osteoarthritis. Classification of osteoarthritis of the knee, *Arthritis Rheum* 29:1039–1049, 1986. In: Fillit HM: *Brocklehurst's textbook of geriatric medicine and gerontology,* ed 8, Philadelphia, 2017, Elsevier.

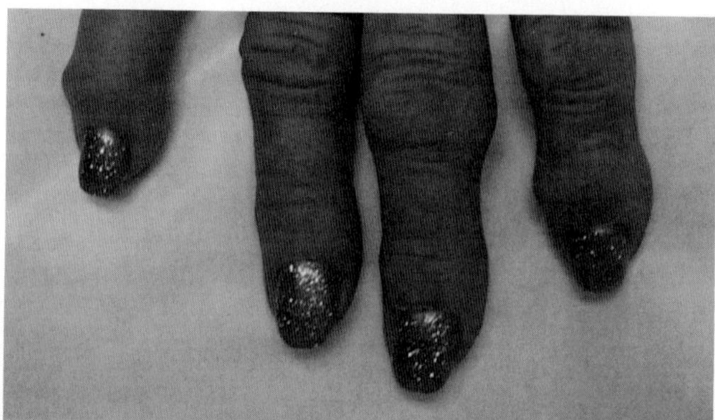

FIG. 1 The fingers of a patient with primary nodal osteoarthritis of the hands demonstrating Heberden and Bouchard nodes. (Heberden nodes: posterior lateral swelling of the distal interphalangeal joints. Bouchard nodes: posterior lateral swelling of the proximal interphalangeal joints) (From Fillit HM: *Brocklehurst's textbook of geriatric medicine and gerontology,* ed 8, Philadelphia, 2017, Elsevier.)

TABLE 2 Risk Factors for Osteoarthritis

Host Factors		Environmental Factors	
Genetic factors	Familial clustering has also been found at the hip and knee	Biomechanics	Repetitive ergonomic and biomechanical demands may create joint stresses leading to OA Hemiparesis associated with reduction of expression of OA in the affected limb and overexpression in the remaining functional limb Chopstick use associated with OA of the IP joint of the thumb, second and third MCP, and PIP joints
Age	The strongest identifiable risk factor	Trauma	Injuries to the joint, such as dislocations, fractures, ligament ruptures, and meniscal tears
Gender	The age association is strongest in women: possibly a hormonal influence Hand OA has a peak incidence in menopausal women		
Hormones	Controversial Hand OA has a peak in menopausal women; however, the Chingford and Framingham studies suggested estrogen has protective effect		
Bone mineral density	Negative relationship between bone mineral density and OA at some sites		
BMI	Obesity is strongly associated with the incidence of knee OA Hand OA likely to be related to biomechanical factors		
Joint alignment	Varus deformity of the knee is associated with progressive OA, as is varus/valgus ligamentous instability at the knee joint Developmental problems leading to altered joint biomechanics such as congenital dysplasias		

BMI, Body mass index; *IP*, interphalangeal; *MCP*, metacarpophalangeal joint; *OA*, osteoarthritis; *PIP*, proximal interphalangeal.
Modified from Fillit HM: *Brocklehurst's textbook of geriatric medicine and gerontology*, ed 8, Philadelphia, 2017, Elsevier.

Inflammatory arthritis, crystal deposition diseases, metabolic disorders, Paget disease of bone, and osteonecrosis may also contribute to the development of secondary OA.

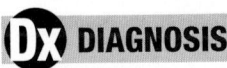

DIAGNOSIS

DIFFERENTIAL DIAGNOSIS

- Bursitis,tendinitis
- Infectious arthritis
- Crystal arthropathies like calcium pyrophosphate arthropathy
- Inflammatory arthritis such as rheumatoid arthritis (Fig. E2), seronegative arthritis

WORKUP

- No specific laboratory test exists for osteoarthritis, and investigations are not always needed for the diagnosis of osteoarthritis.
- Rheumatoid factor, erythrocyte sedimentation rate, complete blood count, and antinuclear antibody tests may be required if inflammatory component is suggested by history and are normal in patients with osteoarthritis.
- Arthrocentesis of swollen joints: Synovial fluid examination is noninflammatory in character (clear, viscous fluid with normal white cell count).

IMAGING STUDIES

- Plain x-ray of the involved joints is the first step and usually of high diagnostic value.
- Radiographic evaluation (Fig. E3) reveals:
  1. Joint space narrowing
  2. Subchondral sclerosis
  3. New bone formation in the form of osteophytes
- MRI can detect other sources of pain such as synovial thickening, effusions, bone marrow edema, bony attrition, and periarticular lesions.
- Musculoskeletal ultrasound (MSKUS) is emerging as an alternative modality to identify joint damage, presence of osteophytes, effusions, and noninflammatory synovial proliferation identified using Doppler studies.

Rx TREATMENT

- Optimal use of both pharmacologic and nonpharmacologic measures (Fig. 4) yields best outcome
- Education and reassurance

NONPHARMACOLOGIC THERAPY

HAND OA:

- Joint protection techniques
- Assistive devices
- Thermal modalities
- Trapeziometacarpal splints

HIP AND KNEE OA:

- Weight loss for overweight patients is probably the most crucial therapy.
- Pedometer step-count of more than 10,000 steps per day has been shown to prevent osteoarthritis.
- Physical therapy includes closed-chain quadriceps strengthening, aerobics, aquatics, and resistance exercises.
- Medial wedge insoles for valgus deformities at the knee.
- Subtalar strapped lateral insoles for varus knees.
- Patellar taping.
- Hinged and unhinged knee braces, offloader knee braces.
- Assistive devices such as canes or walkers.
- Thermal agents.
- Tai chi.

ACUTE GENERAL Rx/ PHARMACOLOGIC Rx

- Hot or cold fomentation.
- Topical applications of capsaicin.
- Topical application of NSAIDs like diclofenac.
- Oral acetaminophen recommended for mild pain.
- Oral NSAIDs definitely more effective than oral acetaminophen. Must consider side effects of NSAIDs, including GI bleeding, cardiovascular toxicity, and renal toxicity. All NSAIDs can increase myocardial infarction risk. Topical NSAIDs are safer than oral NSAIDs.
- Duloxetine if previous initial treatment fails.
- Opioid analgesics including tramadol are recommended only for severe pain that is unresponsive to other treatment modalities.
- Arthrocentesis of the involved joint, followed by intraarticular steroid injection, has been shown to provide short-term relief of symptoms. Clinical studies demonstrate the safety of this approach with regard to the joint.
- Nutritional supplements such as glucosamine and chondroitin are unproven. Most trials indicate that neither glucosamine sulfate nor glucosamine hydrochloride reduces pain compared with placebo in knee or hip osteoarthritis. A recent trial did however show modest long-term benefit for physical function with glucosamine sulfate.[1]

[1]Gregori D, et al.: Association of pharmacological treatments with long-term pain control in patients with knee osteoarthritis: a systematic review and meta-analysis, *JAMA* 320:2564–2579, 2018.

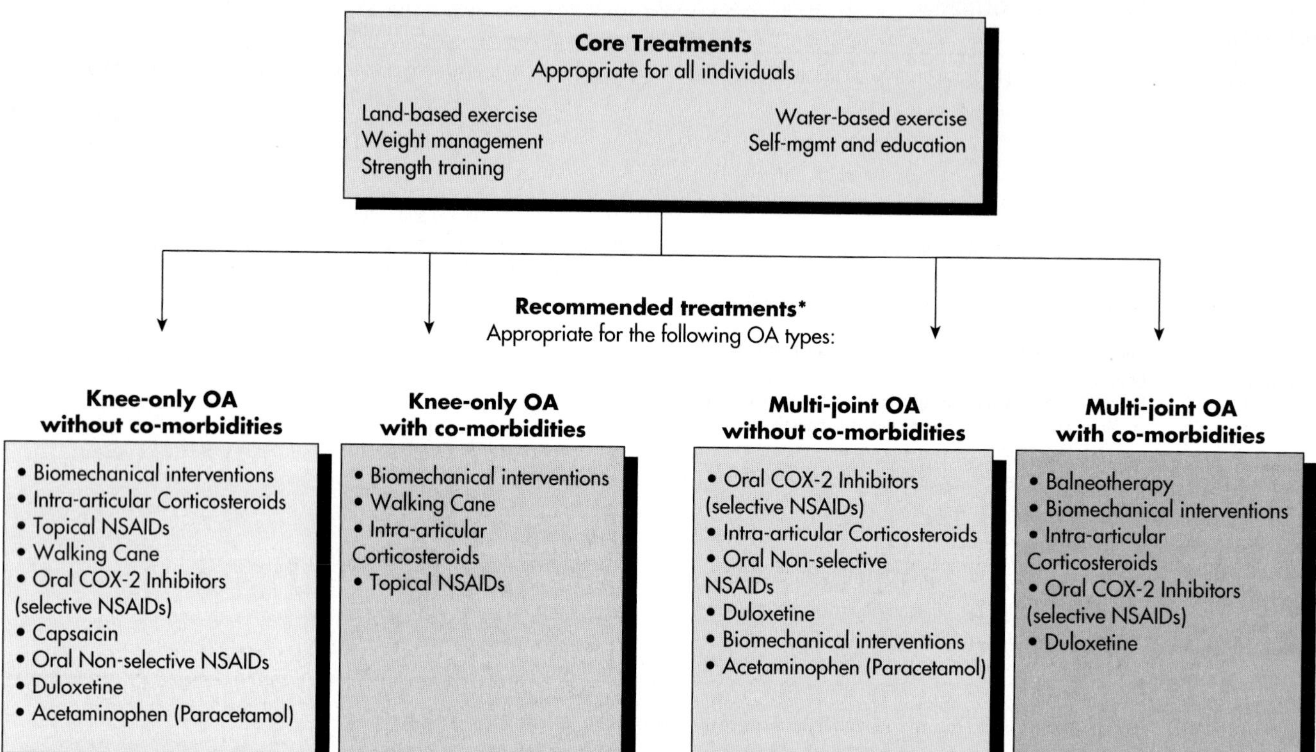

FIG. 4 Appropriate treatments summary. *COX-2,* Cyclooxygenase-2; *NSAID,* nonsteroidal antiinflammatory drug; *OA,* osteoarthritis; *OARSI,* Osteoarthritis Research Society International. (From McAlindon TE, et al.: OARSI guidelines for the non-surgical management of knee osteoarthritis, *Osteoarthritis Cartilage* 22:363-388, 2014.)

- Use of intraarticular hyaluronan injection is controversial. Most trials have shown that hyaluronic acid injections are only minimally better than sham injections in improving pain and function in patients with knee DJD. Positive trials could possibly be influenced by the pharmaceutical industry.

DISPOSITION

Progression of OA is not always inevitable, and the prognosis is variable depending on the site and extent of the disease.

REFERRAL

Surgical consultation for patients not responding to nonpharmacologic and pharmacologic management. Rheumatology referral could be sought for local injections.

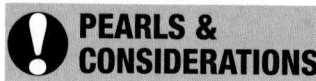

PEARLS & CONSIDERATIONS

COMMENTS

Surgical intervention is generally helpful in degenerative joint disease. Arthroplasty, arthrodesis, and realignment osteotomy are the most common procedures performed. Arthroscopic debridement of the knee appears to be of questionable value. In patients needing hip arthroplasty, resurfacing hip arthroplasty (in which the femoral head is resurfaced with a cap and the neck is preserved) is increasingly popular among younger patients because it results in more hip movement and allows total hip arthroplasty later in the patient's life if necessary.

SUGGESTED READINGS

Available at ExpertConsult.com

RELATED CONTENT

Osteoarthritis (Patient Information)
Osteoarthritis of the Knee (Patient Information)

AUTHOR: **DEEPAN DALAL, M.D., M.P.H.**

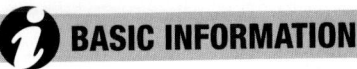

BASIC INFORMATION

DEFINITION

Osteomyelitis is an acute or chronic infection of the bone secondary to the hematogenous or contiguous source of infection or direct traumatic inoculation, which is usually bacterial.

SYNONYM

Bone infection

ICD-10CM CODES	
M86	Osteomyelitis
M86.0	Acute hematogenous osteomyelitis
M86.1	Other acute osteomyelitis
M86.2	Subacute osteomyelitis
M86.3	Chronic multifocal osteomyelitis
M86.6	Other chronic osteomyelitis
M86.9	Osteomyelitis, unspecified

EPIDEMIOLOGY & DEMOGRAPHICS

PREDOMINANT SEX: Male > female
PREDOMINANT AGE: All ages

PHYSICAL FINDINGS & CLINICAL PRESENTATION

HEMATOGENOUS OSTEOMYELITIS:

- Usually occurs in tibia/fibula (children)
- Localized inflammation: Often secondary to trauma with accompanying hematoma or cellulitis
- Abrupt fever
- Lethargy
- Irritability
- Pain in involved bone

VERTEBRAL OSTEOMYELITIS:

- Usually hematogenous
- Fever: 50%
- Localized pain/tenderness. Back pain is the most common initial symptom (86% of cases)
- Neurologic defects: Motor/sensory (sensory loss, weakness, radiculopathy)

CONTIGUOUS OSTEOMYELITIS:

- Direct inoculation
- Associated with trauma, fractures, surgical fixation
- Chronic infection of skin/soft tissue
- Fever, drainage from surgical site

CHRONIC OSTEOMYELITIS:

- Bone pain
- Sinus tract drainage, nonhealing ulcer
- Chronic low-grade fever
- Chronic localized pain

ETIOLOGY

- *Staphylococcus aureus*
- MRSA: Methicillin-resistant *S. aureus*
- *Pseudomonas aeruginosa*
- Enterobacteriaceae
- *Streptococcus pyogenes*
- Enterococcus
- Mycobacteria
- Fungi
- Coagulase-negative staphylococci
- *Salmonella* (in sickle cell disease)

Dx DIAGNOSIS

DIFFERENTIAL DIAGNOSIS

- Gaucher disease
- Bone infarction
- Charcot joint
- Fracture

WORKUP

- ESR, C-reactive protein: Nondiagnostic but if significantly elevated they increase the pretest probability of osteomyelitis and can be useful in monitoring therapeutic response
- Blood culturing, CRC with differential
- Bone culture. A culture of a biopsy specimen has a significantly higher overall diagnostic yield than does a blood culture. Bone samples should be cultured for aerobic and anaerobic bacteria and for fungi
- Pathologic evaluation of bone biopsy for acute/chronic changes consistent with necrosis or acute inflammation
- PCR analysis of specimens obtained by means of biopsy or puncture may be useful for organisms that are difficult to identify (anaerobic bacteria, *Bartonella* sp., *Kingella kingae*); however, broad-range PCR has suboptimal sensitivity and specificity due to contamination and may not provide sufficient information on the susceptibility of the microorganisms to antibiotics

IMAGING STUDIES

- Bone radiograph examination: Initial study but not sensitive in early osteomyelitis as may not show changes for as much as 2 wks
- MRI with and without contrast (Fig. 1): Most accurate imaging study. CT only if patient has contraindication to MRI
- Triple-phase technetium-99m bone scan (Fig. 2) when MRI is unavailable or contraindicated. Typically positive within a few days after onset of symptoms but accuracy is lower than that of MRI
- Gallium scan (Ga-67) scintigraphy with single-photon emission CT (SPECT) has

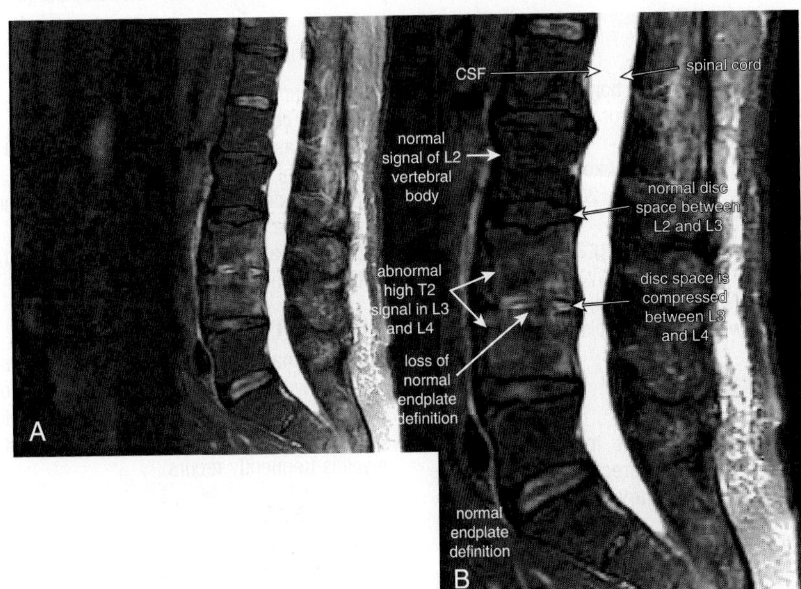

FIG. 1 Osteomyelitis and discitis of L3 and L4. A, T2-weighted fast spin–echo magnetic resonance imaging without contrast demonstrates typical findings of vertebral osteomyelitis and discitis. **B,** Close-up. The inferior endplate of L3 and the superior endplate of L4 are abnormal and ill-defined. The L3 and L4 vertebral bodies show a high T2 signal, indicating an abnormally high fluid content. In comparison, L2 shows a normal marrow signal and appears dark gray due to a normal fat signal. *CSF,* Cerebrospinal fluid. (From Broder JS: *Diagnostic imaging for the emergency physician,* Philadelphia, 2011, Saunders.)

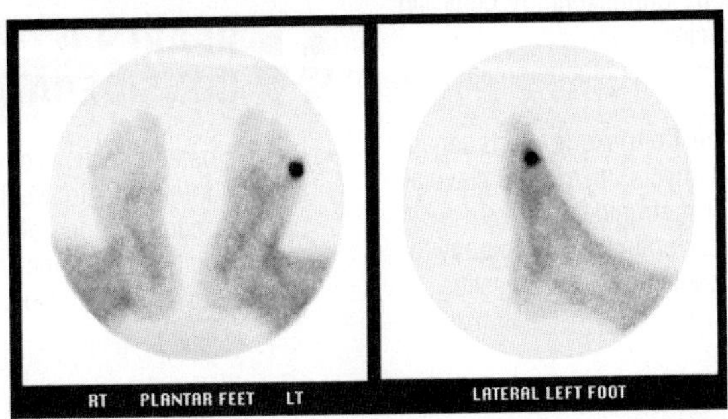

FIG. 2 Osteomyelitis. Intense accumulation of Tc-99m white blood cells in proximal phalanx of fifth digit of left foot at 4 hours after injection. (From Specht N [ed]: *Practical guide to diagnostic imaging,* St Louis, 1998, Mosby.)

TABLE 1 Antimicrobial Therapy for Selected Microorganisms in Chronic Osteomyelitis in Adults

Microorganism	First Choice*	Alternative Choice
Methicillin/oxacillin/nafcillin-sensitive staphylococci	Nafcillin sodium or oxacillin sodium 1.5-2 g IV q4-for 4-6 wk *or* cefazolin 1-2 g IV q8h for 4-6 wk	Vancomycin 15 mg/kg IV q12h for 4-6 wk
Methicillin/oxacillin/nafcillin-resistant staphylococci (MRSA)	Vancomycin† 15 mg/kg IV q12h for 4-6 wk *or* daptomycin 6 mg/kg IV q24h	Linezolid 600 mg PO/IV q12h *or* levofloxacin† 500-750 mg PO/IV daily, plus rifampin 600-900 mg PO for 6 wk if susceptible to both drugs
Penicillin-sensitive streptococci	Aqueous penicillin G 20 × 10^6 U/24 hr IV either continuously or in six equally divided daily doses *or* ceftriaxone 1-2 g IV q24h *or* cefazolin 1-2 g IV q8h for 4-6 wk	Vancomycin 15 mg/kg IV q12h for 4-6 wk
Enterococci	Aqueous crystalline penicillin G 20 × 10^6 U/24 hr IV either continuously or in six equally divided daily doses *or* ampicillin sodium 12 g/24 hr IV either continuously or in six equally divided daily doses; the addition of gentamicin sulfate 1 mg/kg IV or IM q8h for 1-2 wk is *optional*	Vancomycin† 15 mg/kg IV q12h; the addition of gentamicin sulfate 1 mg/kg IV or IM q8h for 1-2 wk is *optional*
Enterobacteriaceae	Ceftriaxone 1-2 g IV q24h for 4-6 wk or ertapenem 1 g IV q24h	Ciprofloxacin 500-750 mg PO q12h for 4-6 wk or levofloxacin 500-750 mg PO q24h
Pseudomonas aeruginosa	Cefepime 2 g IV q12h, meropenem 1 g IV q8h, or imipenem 500 mg IV q6h for 4-6 wk	Ciprofloxacin 750 mg PO q12h for 4-6 wk or ceftazidime 2 g IV q8h

IM, Intramuscular; *IV*, intravenous; *MRSA*, methicillin-resistant *Staphylococcus aureus; PO*, by mouth.
*Antimicrobial selection should be based on in vitro sensitivity data, as well as allergies, intolerances, and drug interactions in individual patients.
†Doses shown are based on normal renal and hepatic function and may need to be adjusted or serum levels monitored (vancomycin).

higher accuracy than bone scan but is less sensitive for detection of epidural abscess in vertebral osteomyelitis
- Indium-111–labeled leukocyte scintigraphy scan; low sensitivity (<20%) for vertebral osteomyelitis
- Positron emission tomography (PET) scanning with ^{18}F-fluorodeoxyglucose has high accuracy (similar to MRI) and is useful in patients with metallic implants

Rx TREATMENT

- Surgical debridement in biopsy-positive cases will guide direction for antibiotic therapy. This will vary with type of osteomyelitis. Duration of therapy is usually 4 to 6 wk for acute osteomyelitis; chronic osteomyelitis may need a longer course of medication
- Orthopedic hardware should be removed if possible
- *S. aureus:* Cefazolin IV, nafcillin IV, vancomycin IV (in patient allergic to penicillin)
- *S. aureus* (methicillin resistant): Vancomycin IV, linezolid, daptomycin, or
- *Streptococcus* spp.: Ceftriaxone, IV penicillin G in sensitive species
- *P. aeruginosa:* Cefepime, imipenem/cilastatin, or meropenem
- Enterobacteriaceae: Ceftriaxone or ertapenem
- Anaerobes: Clindamycin, ticarcillin clavulanate, cefotetan, or metronidazole
- Table 1 summarizes antimicrobial therapy for selected microorganisms in osteomyelitis
- Hyperbaric oxygen therapy: May be useful in chronic osteomyelitis
- Wound-assisted vacuum device may help closure of wound
- Surgical debridement of all devitalized bone and tissue
- Immobilization of affected bone (plaster, traction) if bone is unstable

DISPOSITION

Acute hematogenous osteomyelitis usually resolves without recurrence or long-term complications, but contiguous focus osteomyelitis, bone infections from open fractures, or osteomyelitis frequently recurs.

REFERRAL

- To an orthopedic surgeon if chronic osteomyelitis with need for bone debridement, bone grafting, or stabilization of infected tissue adjacent to a bone fracture
- To an infectious disease specialist for appropriate treatment for difficult-to-treat or recalcitrant infections
- To a hyperbaric oxygen chamber service for nonhealing, chronic osteomyelitis

PEARLS & CONSIDERATIONS

- Chronic osteomyelitis is one of the most challenging infections to treat; the high failure rate is a consequence of poor vascular supply, nondistensible bone tissue, and limited penetration of bone tissue.
- Parenteral antibiotics are usually chosen initially, but oral fluoroquinolones have good bone penetration and may be used in stable patients. A recent trial comparing oral versus IV antibiotics for bone and joint infections found that oral antibiotic therapy is not inferior to IV antibiotic therapy when used during the first 6 wk for complex orthopedic infections.[1]
- The optimal duration of therapy for vertebral osteomyelitis is unclear. Trials comparing 6 weeks to 12 wk of antibiotic treatment in pyogenic vertebral osteomyelitis showed similar cure rates (91%) in both groups.

SUGGESTED READINGS

Available at ExpertConsult.com

RELATED CONTENT

Osteomyelitis (Patient Information)

AUTHORS: **GLENN G. FORT, M.D., M.P.H.**, and **TANYA ALI, M.D.**

[1]Li HK, et al.: Oral versus intravenous antibiotics for bone and joint infection, *N Engl J Med* 380(5): 425–436, 2019.

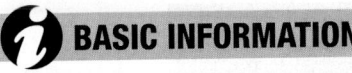

BASIC INFORMATION

DEFINITION

Osteoporosis is a skeletal disorder characterized by a progressive loss of bone mass and a decline in bone quality that results in increased bone fragility and a higher fracture risk. The various types are as follows:

PRIMARY OSTEOPOROSIS: Affects 80% of women and 60% of men with osteoporosis.

- Idiopathic osteoporosis: Unknown pathogenesis; may occur in children and young adults.
- Type I osteoporosis (postmenopausal women): Characterized by accelerated and disproportionate trabecular bone loss and associated with vertebral body and distal forearm fractures due to estrogen deficiency.
- Type II osteoporosis (involutional): Occurs in both men and women aged >70 yr; characterized by both trabecular and cortical bone loss and associated with fractures of the hip, long bone, and vertebrae.

SECONDARY OSTEOPOROSIS: Affects 20% of women and 40% of men with osteoporosis; osteoporosis that exists as a common feature of another disease process, heritable disorder of connective tissue, or drug side effect (see "Differential Diagnosis")

ICD-10CM CODES

M81.0	Age-related osteoporosis without current pathological fracture
M81.4	Drug-induced osteoporosis
M81.5	Idiopathic osteoporosis
M81.6	Localized osteoporosis

EPIDEMIOLOGY & DEMOGRAPHICS

PREVALENCE (IN U.S.):

- Affects more than 10 million people in the U.S.
- Annual incidence of osteoporotic fractures exceeds 1.5 million in the U.S. (70% women)
- Twice as common in women
- Results: Institutionalization, death, and costs in excess of $17 billion annually

RISK FACTORS:

- Advanced age
- Previous low-trauma fracture
- Long-term glucocorticoid use
- Low body weight (<58 kg)
- Family history of hip fracture
- Tobacco use
- Excess alcohol use
- Primary ovarian insufficiency–related estrogen deficiency
- Chronic disease states; e.g., diabetes mellitus, androgen deficiency, inflammatory bowel disease, hyperthyroidism, hypercortisolism

PHYSICAL FINDINGS & CLINICAL PRESENTATION

- Most commonly silent with no signs and symptoms.
- Insidious and progressive development of dorsal kyphosis ***(dowager's hump),*** loss of height, and skeletal pain typically associated with fracture; reduced gait speed or grip strength; other physical findings related to other conditions with associated increased risk for osteoporosis such as nodular thyroid, hepatic enlargement, jaundice, cushingoid features (see "Risk Factors").

ETIOLOGY

Normal bone turnover involves balance between process of bone resorption and bone formation. Osteoclasts resorb bone, and osteoblasts secrete bone matrix for building bone. In postmenopausal women, rate of bone turnover increases after loss of ovarian function, leading to progressive bone loss.

Clinical risk factors used in the World Health Organization Fracture Risk Assessment Tool (WHO FRAX) 10-yr fracture risk calculator are summarized in Table 1.

Dx DIAGNOSIS

DIFFERENTIAL DIAGNOSIS

- Malignancy (multiple myeloma, lymphoma, leukemia, metastatic carcinoma)
- Primary hyperparathyroidism
- Osteomalacia
- Paget's disease
- Osteogenesis imperfecta: Types I, III, and IV

WORKUP

- History and physical examination, with appropriate evaluation for identified risk factors and secondary causes. Investigations for secondary osteoporosis are summarized in Box E1.
- WHO guidelines for the diagnosis of osteoporosis are based on bone mineral density (BMD) measurements of the hip or spine in g/cm^2 and are reported as a T score.
  1. Dual-energy x-ray absorptiometry (DEXA) is the gold standard for screening and monitoring changes in BMD due to excellent precision, widespread availability, low cost, and minimal radiation exposure.
  2. DEXA (Fig. 1) is indicated in all women 65 yr and older and in postmenopausal women younger than 65 yr of age who are at risk for fracture (e.g., weight <127 lbs, parental history of hip fracture, use of medications that cause bone loss, current smoking, excessive alcohol use (>2 drinks per day), rheumatoid arthritis, or presence of diseases that cause bone loss). Causes of erroneous bone mineral density measures by DEXA in the lumbar spine are summarized in Table 2.
  3. Use of FRAX calculator (https://shelf.ac.uk/FRAX/) is proposed by the U.S. Preventive Services Task Force (USPSTF) to determine the need for screening in women between the ages of 50 and 64. If the FRAX 10-yr major osteoporotic risk is greater than or equal to 9.3%, the USPSTF recommends screening with DEXA scan.
  4. Currently, routine testing in men for osteoporosis is not recommended unless there are clinical manifestations of low bone mass.
  5. Quantitative ultrasound can be used as an adjunctive tool to predict risk of fracture in both men and women. It is cheaper than DEXA and has no radiation. However, at this point, additional research and trials are needed to establish its utility in diagnosis and management of osteoporosis.
- Recommendations as to when to repeat bone density testing should be based on initial T scores (Fig. 2). Data from the Study of Osteoporotic Fractures indicates that in women with normal bone density or mild osteopenia, repeat testing might not be necessary for another 10 to 15 yr. For women with moderate osteopenia, a screening interval of 3 to 5 yr may be appropriate. For women with advanced bone loss/osteoporosis, testing every 1-2 yr is recommended.

LABORATORY TESTS

- Biochemical profile to evaluate renal and hepatic function, primary hyperparathyroidism, and malnutrition.
- CBC: For nutritional status and myeloma.
- TSH to rule out the presence of hyperthyroidism.
- 24-hour urinary calcium levels and 26-hydroxyvitamin D level may be helpful in evaluating for secondary causes of osteoporosis.
- May consider celiac panel and serum protein electrophoresis. Biochemical markers of bone remodeling may be useful to predict rate of bone loss and/or follow therapy response. Specific biochemical markers are followed (e.g., 3-mo interval) to document normalization as a response to therapy.
  1. High-turnover osteoporosis: High levels of resorption markers (lysyl pyridinoline, deoxy lysyl pyridinoline, n-telopeptide of collagen cross-links, C-telopeptide of collagen cross-links) and formation markers (osteocalcin and bone-specific alkaline phosphatase); accelerated bone loss responding best to antiresorptive therapy.

TABLE 1 1994 WHO Criteria for the Diagnosis of Osteoporosis Based on the Measurement of Bone Density and T Score Equivalent Cut Points

Diagnostic Category	Standard Deviations Below the Young-Adult Mean	T Score
Normal	≤1 SD	Equal to or better than −1
Osteopenia (low bone mass)	Between 1 and 2.5 SD	Between −1 and −2.5
Osteoporosis	≥2.5 SD	Equal to or poorer than −2.5
Severe (established) osteoporosis	≥2.5 SD + a fragility fracture	Equal to or poorer than −2.5 + a fragility fracture

SD; Standard deviation; *WHO,* World Health Organization. From Hochberg MC et al: *Rheumatology,* ed 5, St Louis, 2011, Mosby.

 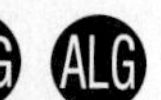

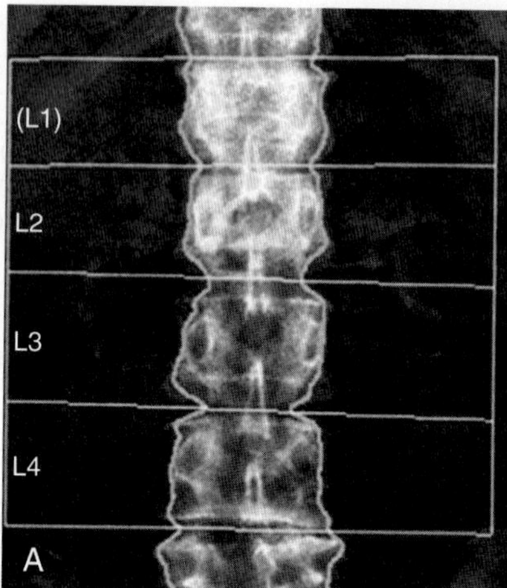

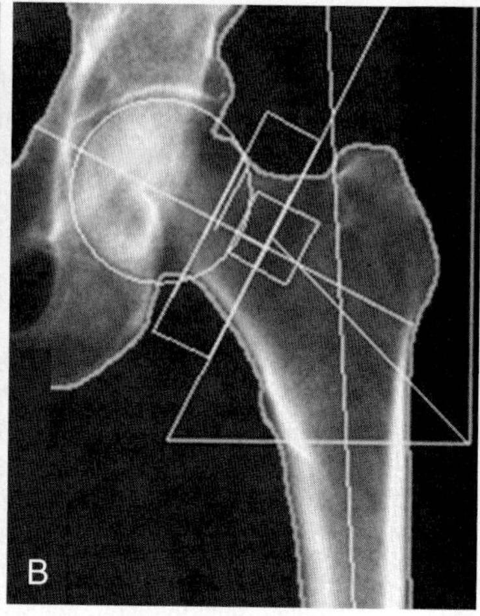

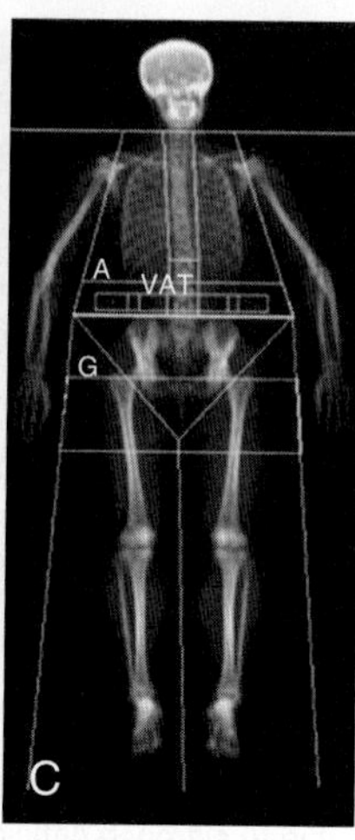

FIG. 1 Dual-energy x-ray absorptiometry (DEXA) provides "areal" bone mineral density (BMD) (g/cm^2) and is currently the gold standard for diagnosis of osteoporosis by bone densitometry (World Health Organization definition T score −2.5 or below) in **(A)** posteroanterior lumbar spine *(L1-4)* or **(B)** hip (femoral neck or total). **C,** DEXA of the whole body can provide information on total and regional BMD and body composition (fat and muscle mass). Recent additional parameters measured are android *A*/gynoid *G* ratio and visceral adipose tissue *(VAT)*. (From Pope TL, et al.: *Musculoskeletal imaging,* ed 2, Philadelphia, 2014, Saunders.)

TABLE 2 Causes of Erroneous Bone Mineral Density Measures by DEXA in the Lumbar Spine

Overestimation of Bone Mineral Density
Extraneous calcification (lymph nodes, aorta)
Degenerative disk and spine disease (osteophytes)
Ankylosing spondylitis
Vertebral fracture
Sclerotic metastases
Vertebral hemangioma
Overlying metal artifacts (navel rings)
Surgical interventions (metallic rods, spinal fusion)
Vertebroplasty
Paget disease
Treatment with strontium ranelate
Underestimation of Bone Mineral Density
Laminectomy

DEXA; Dual-energy x-ray absoptiometry. From Pope TL, et al.: *Musculoskeletal imaging,* ed 2, Philadelphia, 2014, Saunders.

2. Low-normal-turnover osteoporosis: Normal or low levels of the markers of resorption and formation (see "high-turnover osteoporosis" listed previously); no accelerated bone loss; responds best to drugs that enhance bone formation.

IMAGING STUDIES

- BMD determination (see "Workup") should be performed on all women with determined risk factors and/or associated secondary causes; criteria for diagnosis of osteoporosis based on measurement of bone density and T score equivalent cut points are summarized in Table 1.
  1. Normal: BMD <1 SD of the young adult reference mean
  2. Osteopenia: BMD 1 to 2.5 SD below the young adult reference mean
  3. Osteoporosis: BMD >2.5 SD below the young adult reference mean
- For patient undergoing treatment: The frequency of BMD monitoring is controversial and many experts recommend that clinicians should not monitor BMD during the initial 5-yr drug treatment period because no studies have proven that such monitoring improves fracture outcomes.
- X-ray exam of appropriate part of skeleton (Figs. E3 and E4) to evaluate clinical osteoporotic fracture only.

Rx TREATMENT

- Osteoporosis based on DEXA measurements of BMD
- History of hip and vertebral fracture
- Osteopenia on DEXA + 10-yr FRAX score of greater than or equal to 3% at hip or greater than or equal to 20% of major osteoporotic fracture

NONPHARMACOLOGIC THERAPY

Prevention:

- Identification and minimization of risk factors
- Appropriate diagnosis and treatment of secondary causes
- Behavioral modification: Proper nutrition, physical activity, fracture prevention strategies

ACUTE GENERAL Rx

- Vitamin D supplement: 600 IU/day for persons 19 to 70 yr of age and 800 IU/day for persons 71 yr and older.
- Calcium supplement: The recommended dietary intake of calcium for women 19 to 50 years of age and men 19 to 70 years of age is 1000 mg/day; women older than age 50 and men older than age 70 require 1200 mg/day. Calcium intake above 2500 mg/day (2000 mg/day in persons >50 years of age) should be avoided. Consumption of calcium-rich foods and beverages is the preferred approach to ensuring adequate calcium intake.[1]
- Oral bisphosphonates (alendronate, risedronate): Decrease bone resorption by attenuating osteoclast activity. They are first-line therapy for the treatment of most patients with osteoporosis, with proven efficacy to reduce fracture risk. The bisphosphonates differ in binding affinity, dose frequency, and route of administration. To facilitate absorption, most oral bisphosphonates are taken on an empty stomach with a full glass of water. Patients are instructed to remain in a sitting or standing position for 30 to 60 min. Risks include gastroesophageal reflux disease, esophagitis, jaw necrosis, and atypical femur fracture. Zoledronic acid: A bisphosphonate given by IV infusion over at least 15 min, 5 mg once/yr. It is contraindicated in patients with acute renal failure.
- Biologic agents: Denosumab is a human monoclonal antibody that inhibits osteoclast formation and prevents resorption for treatment of postmenopausal osteoporosis. Dosage is 60 mg subcutaneously every 6 mon. Romosozumab is a monoclonal antibody that in recent trials increased bone formation and decreased bone resorption by binding to sclerostin.
- Teriparatide is a recombinant human parathyroid hormone used for postmenopausal women with osteoporosis who are at high risk for fracture, especially vertebral fractures. It is also used in men with primary or hypogonadal osteoporosis who are at high risk of fracture. It is administered by injection 20 mcg qd SC into the thigh or abdominal wall. Use for >2 yr is not recommended. It stimulates bone formation and reduces the risk of fracture but may increase the risk

[1] Bauer DC: Calcium supplements and fracture prevention, *N Engl J Med* 369:1537-1543, 2013.

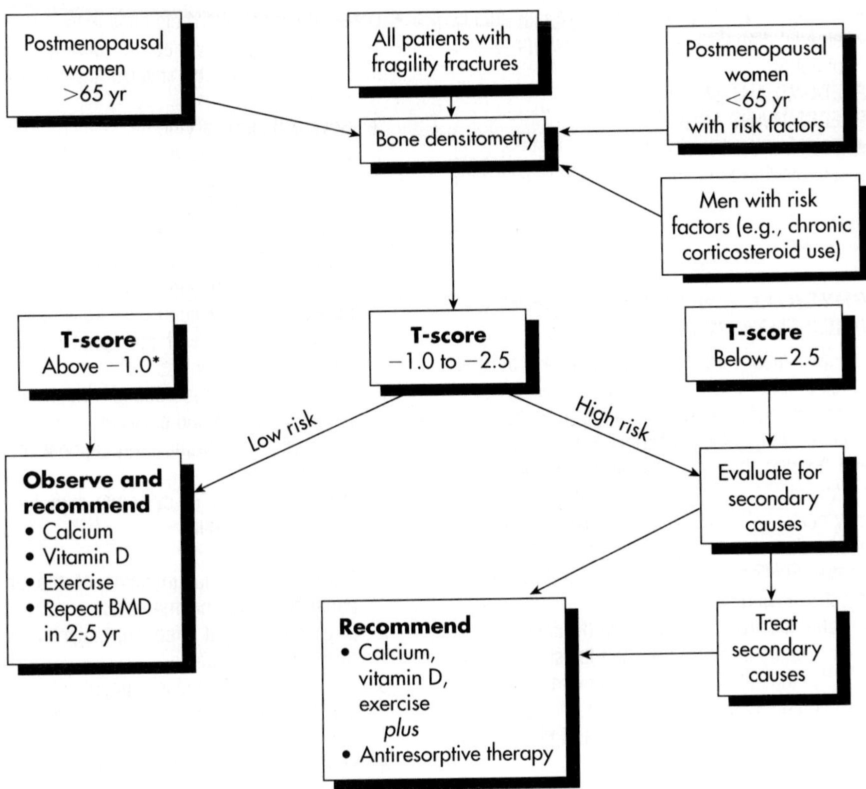

*Patients with fragility fractures and a T-score above −1.0 should be evaluated for other causes of pathologic fracture.

FIG. 2 Diagnosis and management of osteoporosis.

of stroke in older women with osteoporosis. Common side effects include headaches, myalgia, hypercalcemia, and hypercalciuria. Trials involving abaloparatide, a selective activator of the parathyroid hormone type 1 receptor have also shown reduced risk of new vertebral and nonvertebral fractures in postmenopausal women with osteoporosis.

- Estrogen prescription drugs or raloxifene should not be prescribed to treat women with osteoporosis.

CHRONIC Rx

- Lifelong attention to behavior modification issues (nutrition, physical activity, fracture prevention strategies) and compliance with pharmacologic intervention. Recommendations include weight-bearing and muscle-strengthening exercises, smoking cessation, reduced alcohol intake, and adoption of fall prevention strategies.
- There is little evidence to guide physicians about long-term bisphosphonate therapy. The decision to continue drug therapy beyond 5 yr should reflect reassessment of risk and benefit. Evidence is accumulating that the risk of atypical fracture of the femur increases after 5 yr of bisphosphonate use. It is reasonable to consider a drug holiday in post-menopausal women who are not at high fracture risk after 3 yr (IV) to 5 yr (oral) of biphosphonate therapy. Continued treatment may be advisable in those at highest risk.
- Continuing need to eliminate high-risk factors when possible and to optimally manage secondary causes of osteoporosis.

DISPOSITION

Goals for diagnosis and treatment include identification of women at risk; initiation of preventive measures for all women lifelong; institution of treatment modalities that will result in a decrease in fracture risk; and reduction of morbidity, mortality, and unnecessary institutionalization, thereby improving quality of independent life and productivity. Table E3 summarizes the effect of major treatment options on the risk of vertebral, nonvertebral, and hip fractures.

REFERRAL

- To reproductive endocrinologist, medical endocrinologist, gynecologist, or rheumatologist if unfamiliar with diagnosis and management of osteoporosis
- If multidisciplinary management is required, to other specialties depending on presence of acute fracture and/or secondary associated disorders

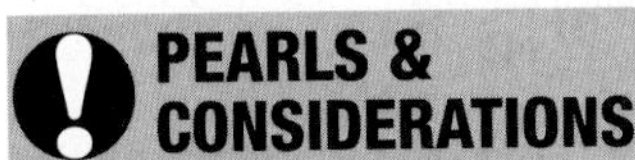

PEARLS & CONSIDERATIONS

COMMENTS

- Osteonecrosis of the jaw is a known complication of high-dose IV bisphosphonate therapy for cancer; however, there is considerable debate on whether low-dose bisphosphonates used for osteoporosis can also cause this disorder. Evidence for this is inconclusive.
- Long-term use (>10 yr) of bisphosphonates has been reported to increase risk of atypical subtrochanteric or femoral shaft fractures in several uncontrolled case series. Prodromal symptoms of thigh pain, lack of trauma prior to the procedure, and specific radiologic characteristics (cortical thickening) have been reported. The evidence remains inconclusive. Patients can be reassured that short or intermediate use of bisphosphonates does not increase the risk of atypical femoral fractures. Current strategies should include considering a 12-mo interruption in therapy after 5 yr in patients who are clinically stable and considering teriparatide treatment in individuals who experience an atypical fracture while receiving bisphosphonate therapy.
- Increased risk of esophageal cancer and atrial fibrillation have been reported as possible adverse effects of bisphosphonate therapy.

SUGGESTED READINGS

Available at ExpertConsult.com

RELATED CONTENT

Osteoporosis (Patient Information)
Bisphosphonate-Related Osteonecrosis of Jaw (Related Key Topic)
Vertebral Compression Fractures (Related Key Topic)

AUTHORS: **DENNIS M. WEPPNER, M.D.,** and **PATRICIA W. LO, M.D.**

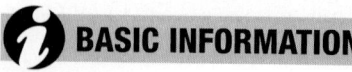

BASIC INFORMATION

DEFINITION

Otitis externa refers to a variety of conditions causing inflammation and/or infection of the external auditory canal (and/or auricle and tympanic membrane). There are six subgroups of otitis externa:

1. Acute localized otitis externa (furunculosis)
2. Acute diffuse bacterial otitis externa (i.e., "swimmer's ear")
3. Chronic otitis externa
4. Eczematous otitis externa
5. Fungal otitis externa (otomycosis)
6. Invasive or necrotizing (malignant) otitis externa

SYNONYMS

See "Definition."

ICD-10CM CODES

H60.90	Unspecified otitis externa, unspecified ear
H60.2	Malignant otitis externa
H60.3	Other infective otitis externa
H60.5	Acute otitis externa, non-infective
H60.8	Other otitis externa

EPIDEMIOLOGY & DEMOGRAPHICS

INCIDENCE (IN U.S.):

- Among the most common disorders
- An estimated 10% of people develop external otitis during their lifetime
- Affects 3% to 10% of patients seeking otologic care

PREVALENCE (IN U.S.):

- Diffuse otitis externa is most often seen in swimmers and in hot, humid climates, conditions that lead to water retention in the ear canal. In the U.S., 44% of AOE-related healthcare visits occur June to August.
- Necrotizing otitis externa is more common in elderly, diabetics, and immunocompromised patients.

PREDOMINANT SEX: None

PREDOMINANT AGE:

- Occurs at all ages, however incidence is highest during childhood and decreases with age
- Necrotizing otitis externa: Typically occurs in elderly: Mean age >65 yr

PHYSICAL FINDINGS & CLINICAL PRESENTATION

The two most common symptoms are otalgia, ranging from pruritus to severe pain exacerbated by motion (e.g., chewing), and otorrhea. Patients may also experience aural fullness and hearing loss as a result of swelling with occlusion of the canal. More intense symptoms may occur with bacterial otitis externa, with or without fever, and lymphadenopathy (anterior to tragus). Findings unique to specific forms of the infection include:

- Acute localized otitis externa (furunculosis):
  1. Occurs from infected hair follicles, usually in the outer third of the ear canal, forming pustules and furuncles
  2. Furuncles are superficial and pointing or deep and diffuse
- Impetigo:
  1. In contrast to furunculosis, this is a superficial spreading infection of the ear canal that may also involve the concha and the auricle
  2. Begins as a small blister that ruptures, releasing straw-colored fluid that dries as a golden crust
- Erysipelas:
  1. Caused by group A *Streptococcus*
  2. May involve the concha and canal
  3. May involve the dermis and deeper tissues
  4. Area of cellulitis, often with severe pain
  5. Fever, chills, malaise
  6. Regional adenopathy
- Eczematous or seborrheic otitis externa:
  1. Stems from a variety of dermatologic problems that can involve the external auditory canal
  2. Severe itching, erythema, scaling, crusting (Fig. 1), and fissuring possible
- Acute diffuse otitis externa (swimmer's ear):
  1. Begins with itching and a feeling of pressure and fullness in the ear that becomes increasingly tender and painful
  2. Mild erythema and edema of the external auditory canal, which may cause narrowing and occlusion of the canal (Fig. 2), leading to hearing loss
  3. Minimal serous secretions, which may become profuse and purulent
  4. Tympanic membrane may appear dull and infected
  5. Usually absence of systemic symptoms such as fever, chills
- Otomycosis:
  1. Chronic superficial infection of the ear canal and tympanic membrane
  2. In primary fungal infection, major symptom is intense itching
  3. In secondary infection (fungal infection superimposed on bacterial infection), major symptom is pain
  4. Fungal growth of variety of colors
- Chronic otitis externa:
  1. Dry and atrophic canal
  2. Typically lack of cerumen
  3. Itching, often severe, and mild discomfort rather than pain
  4. Occasionally mucopurulent discharge
  5. With time, thickening of the walls of the canal, causing narrowing of the lumen
- Necrotizing otitis externa (also known as malignant otitis externa). Typically seen in older patients with diabetes or in patients who are immunocompromised.
  1. Redness, swelling, and tenderness of the ear canal
  2. Classic finding of granulation tissue on the floor of the canal and the bone–cartilage junction
  3. Small ulceration of necrotic soft tissue at bone–cartilage junction
  4. Most common symptoms: Pain (often severe) and otorrhea
  5. Lessening of purulent drainage as infection advances
  6. As the infection advances, osteomyelitis of the base of the skull and temporomandibular joint osteomyelitis can develop
  7. Facial nerve palsy often the first and only cranial nerve defect
  8. Possible involvement of other cranial nerves

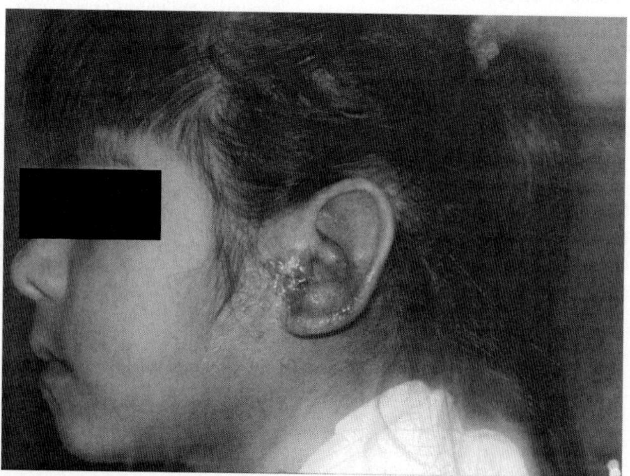

FIG. 1 Patient with acute otitis externa, with purulent drainage from the ear canal and mild edema and erythema of the pinna. (From Cherry JD et al: *Feigin and Cherry's pediatric infectious diseases*, ed 8, Philadelphia, 2019, Elsevier.)

ETIOLOGY

- Box 1 summarizes common pathogens in otitis externa
- Acute localized otitis externa: *Staphylococcus aureus*
- Impetigo:
  1. *S. aureus* including MRSA
  2. *Streptococcus pyogenes*
- Erysipelas: *S. pyogenes*

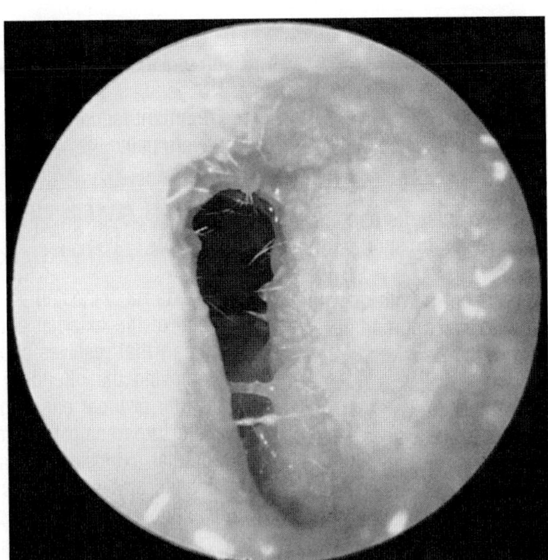

FIG. 2 Acute otitis externa. (From Swartz MH: *Textbook of physical diagnosis, history and examination*, ed 7, Philadelphia, 2014, Elsevier.)

BOX 1 Common Pathogens in Otitis Externa

Gram-Negative Organisms
Pseudomonas aeruginosa
Pseudomonas spp. Nov. "otitidis"
Proteus mirabilis
Serratia marcescens

Gram-Positive Organisms
Staphylococcus aureus
Staphylococcus epidermidis
Corynebacterium auris
Enterococcus faecalis

Fungi and Yeasts
Aspergillus fumigatus
Candida albicans
Candida parapsilosis

From Cherry JD et al: *Feigin and Cherry's pediatric infectious diseases*, ed 8, Philadelphia, 2019, Elsevier.

- Eczematous otitis externa:
  1. Seborrheic dermatitis
  2. Atopic dermatitis
  3. Psoriasis
  4. Neurodermatitis
  5. Lupus erythematosus
- Acute diffuse otitis externa:
  1. Swimming
  2. Hot, humid climates
  3. Tightly fitting hearing aids
  4. Use of ear plugs
  5. *Pseudomonas aeruginosa*
  6. *S. aureus* including MRSA
- Otomycosis:
  1. Prolonged use of topical antibiotics and steroid preparations
  2. Uncontrolled diabetes mellitus can contribute to risk
  3. *Aspergillus* (80% to 90%)
  4. *Candida*
- Chronic otitis externa: Persistent low-grade infection and inflammation
- Necrotizing otitis externa (NOE):
  1. Complication of persistent otitis externa
  2. Extends through Santorini's fissures, small apertures at the bone-cartilage junction of the canal, into the mastoid and along the base of the skull
  3. *P. aeruginosa*

Dx DIAGNOSIS

DIFFERENTIAL DIAGNOSIS

- Acute otitis media
- Bullous myringitis
- Mastoiditis
- Foreign bodies
- Neoplasms
- Contact dermatitis
- Eczema
- Ramsey-Hunt syndrome
- Seborrhea
- Otomycosis
- Referred pain

WORKUP

Thorough history and physical examination

LABORATORY TESTS

- Cultures from the canal are usually not necessary unless the condition does not respond to treatment.
- Leukocyte count normal or mildly elevated.
- Erythrocyte sedimentation rate is often quite elevated in malignant otitis externa.

IMAGING STUDIES

- CT scan is the best technique for defining bone involvement and extent of disease in malignant otitis externa.
- MRI is slightly more sensitive in evaluation of soft tissue changes and intracranial extension of infection.
- Gallium scans are more specific than bone scans in diagnosing NOE.
- Follow-up scans are helpful in determining efficacy of treatment.

NOTE: Expert opinion supports history and physical examination as the best means of diagnosis. Persistent pain that is constant and severe should raise the question of NOE (particularly in the elderly, diabetics, and immunocompromised patients).

Rx TREATMENT

NONPHARMACOLOGIC THERAPY

- Cleansing and debridement of the ear canal with cotton swabs and hydrogen peroxide or other antiseptic solution allows a more thorough examination of the ear.
- If the canal lumen is edematous and too narrow to allow adequate cleansing, a cotton wick or gauze strip inserted into the canal serves as a conduit for topical medications to be drawn into the canal. Usually remove wick after 2 days.
- Local heat is useful in treating deep furunculosis.
- Incision and drainage is indicated in treatment of superficial pointing furunculosis.

ACUTE GENERAL Rx

Topical medications:

- An acidifying agent such as 2% acetic acid (Vosol) inhibits growth of bacteria and fungi.
- Topical antibiotics (in the form of otic or ophthalmic solutions) or antifungals, often in combination with an acidifying agent and a steroid preparation. Direct application of topical agents to the infected site is a key element in the treatment of external otitis regardless of severity. Proper installation of eardrops entails tilting the head toward the opposite shoulder, pulling the superior aspect of the auricle upward, and filling the ear canal with drops. In young children, the earlobe should be pulled downward to fill the canal.
- The ideal antibiotic regimen should have coverage against the most common pathogens, *S. aureus* and *P. aeruginosa.*
- Side effect profile can also influence choice of treatment. Ototoxicity is the most important concern with aminoglycoside drugs, including neomycin, tobramycin, and gentamicin. Aminoglycosides are a significant potential source for iatrogenic hearing loss and balance dysfunction, particularly in the presence of tympanic membrane perforation. Allergic contact dermatitis is commonly associated with neomycin when used for prolonged courses. Topical fluoroquinolones can cause local irritation.
- The following are some of the available preparations:
  1. Neomycin otic solutions and suspensions:
     a. With polymyxin-B-hydrocortisone (Cortisporin)
     b. With hydrocortisone-thonzonium (Coly-Mycin S)
  2. Polymyxin-B-hydrocortisone (Otobiotic)
  3. Quinolone otic solutions:
     a. Ofloxacin 0.3% solution (Floxin Otic)
     b. Ciprofloxacin 0.3% with hydrocortisone (Cipro HC)

4. Quinolone ophthalmic solutions:
   a. Ofloxacin 0.3% (Ocuflox)
   b. Ciprofloxacin 0.3% (Ciloxan)
5. Aminoglycoside ophthalmic solutions:
   a. Gentamicin sulfate 0.3% (Garamycin)
   b. Tobramycin sulfate 0.3% (Tobrex)
   c. Tobramycin 0.3% and dexamethasone 0.1% (TobraDex)
6. Chloramphenicol 0.5% otic solution or 0.25% ophthalmic solution (Chloromycetin)
7. Gentian violet (methylrosaniline chloride 1%, 2%)
8. Antifungals:
   a. Amphotericin B 3% (Fungizone lotion)
   b. Clotrimazole 1% solution (Lotrimin)
   c. Tolnaftate 1% (Tinactin)

- Topical preparations should be applied qid (bid for quinolones, antifungals), generally for 3 days after cessation of symptoms (average 10-14 days total)

Systemic antibiotics:

- Reserved for when the infection has spread beyond the ear canal
- Treatment usually for 10 days with ciprofloxacin 750 mg q12h or ofloxacin 400 mg q12h, or with antistaphylococcal agent (e.g., dicloxacillin or cephalexin 500 mg q6h). Use Bactrim or clindamycin when MRSA suspected or cultured at one DS twice a day instead of cephalexin or dicloxacillin. For malignant otitis externa (due to Pseudomonas aeruginosa in >90% of cases), effective agents are meropenem 1 g IV q8h or ciprofloxacin 400 mg IV q12h or 750 mg PO q12h or cefepime 2 g q12h.

Treatment for NOE:

- Requires prolonged therapy up to 3 mo; whether to use oral parenteral therapy is based on clinical judgment
- Oral quinolones, ciprofloxacin 750 mg q12h or ofloxacin 400 mg q12h may be appropriate initial therapy or used to shorten the course of IV therapy
- Intravenous antipseudomonals with or without aminoglycosides are also appropriate
- Local debridement

Pain control:

- May require NSAIDs or opioids
- Topical corticosteroids to reduce swelling and inflammation

CHRONIC Rx

- Patients prone to recurrent infections should try to identify and avoid precipitants to infection.
- Swimmers should try tight-fitting ear plugs or tight-fitting bathing caps and remove all excess water from the ears after swimming.
- Treat underlying systemic diseases and dermatologic conditions that predispose to infection.
- Hearing aids should be removed nightly and regularly cleaned.

DISPOSITION

Inadequate treatment of otitis externa may lead to NOE and mastoiditis.

REFERRAL

To an otolaryngologist:

- NOE
- Treatment failure
- Severe pain

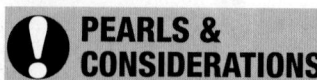

PEARLS & CONSIDERATIONS

Otitis externa varies in severity from a mild irritation of the external acoustic canal (swimmer's ear) that resolves spontaneously by simply removing the offending agent (stay out of freshwater or wear ear plugs when swimming) to a life-threatening infection with the risk of intracranial extension, gram-negative bacterial meningitis, and severe neurologic impairment with multiple cranial neuropathy. Do not miss severe malignant otitis externa in patients who are diabetic or immunocompromised.

SUGGESTED READINGS

Available at ExpertConsult.com

RELATED CONTENT

Otitis Externa (Patient Information)

AUTHOR: **DIANE KOCOVSKY, APRN.**

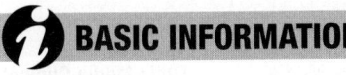

BASIC INFORMATION

DEFINITION

Acute otitis media (AOM) is defined by acute signs of illness and signs and symptoms of middle ear inflammation resulting in moderate to severe bulging of the tympanic membrane (TM) or new onset of otorrhea not due to acute otitis externa.

SYNONYMS

Acute suppurative otitis media
Purulent otitis media
Acute otitis media
AOM

ICD-10CM CODES
H65.0 Acute serous otitis media
H65.1 Other acute nonsuppurative otitis media
H65.9 Nonsuppurative otitis media, unspecified
H65.2 Chronic serous otitis media
H65.3 Chronic mucoid otitis media
H65.6 Other chronic nonsuppurative otitis media
H66.0 Acute suppurative otitis media
H66.4 Suppurative otitis media, unspecified
H66.9 Otitis media, unspecified
H66.1 Chronic tubotympanic suppurative otitis media
H66.2 Chronic atticoantral suppurative otitis media

EPIDEMIOLOGY & DEMOGRAPHICS

INCIDENCE (IN U.S.):
- Affects patients of all ages but is largely a disease of infants and young children.
- Affects approximately 80% of all children by age 5 yr.
- Occurs three or more times in one third of all children by age 3 yr.
- Costs associated with otitis media exceed $5 billion, with 40% of the costs occurring from patients ages 1 to 3.
- One of the most common indications for antibiotic prescription among children.
- Antibiotics prescribed to treat AOM increased adverse events (vomiting, diarrhea, or rash) by 8%.

PEAK INCIDENCE:
- AOM occurs at all ages but is most prevalent between 6 and 24 months of age
- Second peak at the time of school entry between ages 4 and 6 yr
- Fall, winter, early spring (coincident with peak respiratory virus prevalence in the community)

PREDOMINANT SEX: Males

PREDOMINANT AGE:
- 47% to 60% of all children have their first episode of otitis media during their first yr of life and 62% by their fifth birthday.
- Incidence of infection declines with age; seen infrequently in adults.

GENETICS: Familial disposition:
- Native Americans
- Eskimos
- Australian aborigines
- Those with a strong family history
- Immune globulin G (IgG) or subclass deficiencies

Congenital infection: High incidence in children born with cleft palates and other craniofacial abnormalities

Other risk factors:
- Day care attendance
- Limited or lack of breastfeeding
- Tobacco smoke exposure
- Pacifier use

PHYSICAL FINDINGS & CLINICAL PRESENTATION

- Moderate to severe bulging of the tympanic membrane
- Fluid in the middle ear along with signs and symptoms of local inflammation
  1. Erythema with diminished light reflex (Fig. E1)
- As infection progresses, middle ear exudation occurs (exudative phase); the exudate rapidly changes from serous to purulent (suppurative phase).
  1. Retraction and poor motility of the tympanic membrane, which then becomes bulging and convex
- At any time during the suppurative phase the tympanic membrane may rupture, releasing the middle ear contents (otorrhea).
- Erythema of the tympanic membrane without other abnormalities is not a diagnostic criterion for acute otitis media (AOM) because it may occur with any inflammation of the upper respiratory tract, crying, or nose blowing.
- Symptoms:
  1. Rapid- or recent-onset otalgia, ranging from slight discomfort to severe, spreading to the temporal region
  2. Ear stuffiness and hearing loss may precede or follow otalgia
  3. Otorrhea if tympanic membrane has ruptured
  4. Vertigo, nystagmus, tinnitus, fever, lethargy, irritability, nausea, vomiting, anorexia
  5. Table 1 summarizes symptom scoring systems designed to aid in diagnosis
- After an episode of AOM:
  1. Persistence of effusion for weeks or months (called secretory, serous, or nonsuppurative otitis media)
  2. Fever and otalgia usually absent
  3. Hearing loss possible (10 to 50 dB, with predominant involvement of the low frequencies)

ETIOLOGY

- Most common etiologic factor is a viral upper respiratory tract infection, which causes inflammation and dysfunction of the eustachian tube and transient aspiration of nasopharyngeal secretions into the middle ear (Fig. 2). Bacterial colonization from the nasopharynx in conjunction with eustachian tube dysfunction leads to infection.
- May occasionally develop as a result of hematogenous spread or by direct invasion from the nasopharynx.
- Conjugated pneumococcal vaccination of children has resulted in decreases in *Streptococcus pneumoniae* causing AOM.
- Most common bacterial pathogens:
  1. *S. pneumoniae* causes approximately 50% of cases and is the least likely of the major pathogens to resolve without treatment.
  2. *Haemophilus influenzae* causes more than 45% of cases.
  3. *Moraxella catarrhalis* causes 10% to 15% of cases.
  4. Of increasing importance, infection caused by penicillin-nonsusceptible *S. pneumoniae* (MIC >0.1 mg/ml), ranging from 8% to 34%. About 50% of PNSSP isolates are penicillin-intermediate (MIC 0.1 to 2.0 mg/ml).
  5. Group A streptococci is associated with higher rates of TM perforation than AOM caused by other pathogens.
- Viral pathogens:
  1. Respiratory syncytial virus
  2. Rhinovirus
  3. Adenovirus
  4. Influenza
- Others:
  1. Mycoplasma pneumoniae
  2. Chlamydia trachomatis
  3. Streptococcus pyogenes (Latin America)

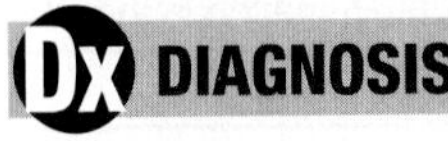

DIAGNOSIS

DIFFERENTIAL DIAGNOSIS

- Otitis externa
- Otitis media with effusion (OME)
- Referred pain
  1. Mouth
  2. Nasopharynx
  3. Tonsils
  4. Other parts of the upper respiratory tract
- Section II describes the differential diagnosis of earache

WORKUP

Thorough otoscopic examination. AOM is a visual diagnosis based on viewing the tympanic membrane. Adequate visualization of the tympanic membrane may require removal of cerumen and debris.
- Tympanometry
  1. Measures compliance of the tympanic membrane and middle ear pressure
  2. Detects the presence of fluid
- Acoustic reflectometry
  1. Measures sound waves reflected from the middle ear
  2. Useful in infants >3 mo
  3. Increased reflected sound correlated with the presence of effusion
  4. Tympanometry and acoustic reflectometry are useful in detection of middle ear effusion but do not provide information regarding infection/inflammation

LABORATORY TESTS

- Tympanocentesis
  1. Not necessary in most cases because the microbiology of middle ear effusions has been shown to be quite consistent

TABLE 1 Acute Otitis Media Symptom Scoring Systems Designed to Aid in Diagnosis

3-Item Otitis Media Score (OM-3)	Ear Treatment Group Symptom Questionnaire (ETG-5)	Acute Otitis Media Faces Scale (AOM-FS)	Otoscopic Severity Scale (OS-8)	Acute Otitis Media Severity of Symptom Scale (AOM-SOS)	Otitis Media Clinical Severity Index (OM-CSI) 30-Point Scale[a]	Otitis Media Clinical Severity Index (OM-CSI) 10-Point Scale[a]
Physical suffering	Ear pain	Seven facial expressions ranging from no problem to extreme problem	Eight categories of TM inflammation[b]	Ear pain	Ear pain	Ear pain
Emotional distress	Fever			Ear tugging	Fever	Fever
Limitation of activities	Irritability			Irritability	Irritability	Irritability
	Appetite			Decreased play	Fever at examination	Fever at examination
	Sleep quality			Decreased appetite	TM erythema	TM erythema
				Difficulty sleeping	TM mobility	TM mobility
				Fever	TM position	TM position
					Effusion color	Effusion color
					Otorrhea	Otorrhea

TM, Tympanic membrane.

[a]The 30-point scale used a 2- to 5-point Likert scale and the 10-point scale used a 2- to 3-point Likert scale.

[b]0 = normal; 1 = erythema only; 2 = erythema, air-fluid level, clear fluid; 3 = erythema, complete effusion, no opacification; 4 = erythema, opacification with air-fluid level or air bubbles, no bulging; 5 = erythema, complete effusion, opacification, no bulging; 6 = erythema, bulging rounded doughnut appearance of the tympanic membrane; 7 = erythema, bulging, complete effusion and opacification with bulla formation.

From Cherry JD et al: *Feigin and Cherry's pediatric infectious diseases*, ed 8, Philadelphia, 2019, Elsevier.

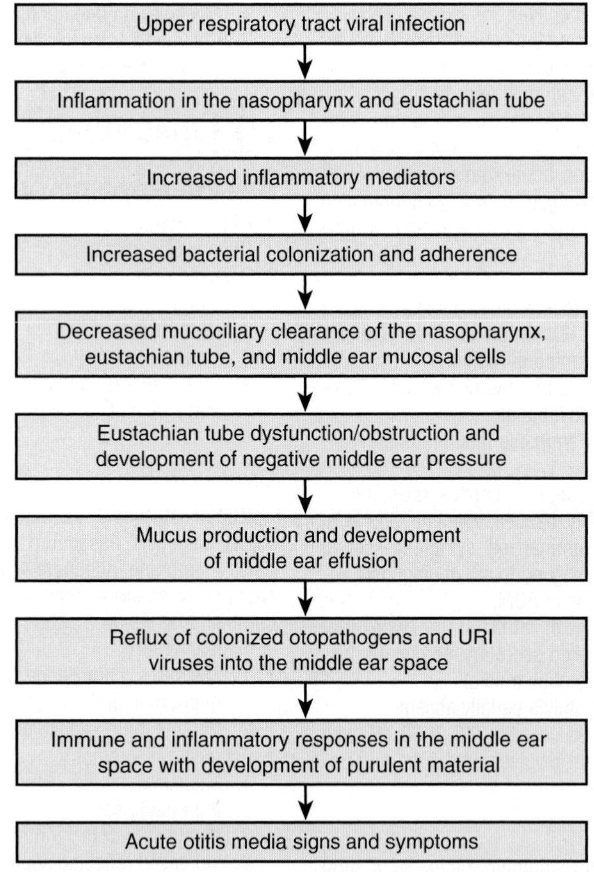

FIG. 2 Pathogenesis of virus-induced acute otitis media. *URI,* Upper respiratory infection. (From Cherry JD, et al.: *Feigin and Cherry's pediatric infectious diseases*, ed 8, Philadelphia, 2019, Elsevier.)

2. May be indicated in:
   a. Highly toxic patients
   b. Patients who do not respond to treatment in 48 to 72 hr
   c. Immunocompromised patients

- Cultures of the nasopharynx: Sensitive but not specific
- Blood counts (generally not necessary): Usually show a leukocytosis with polymorphonuclear elevation
- Plain mastoid radiographs: Generally not indicated; will reveal haziness in the periantral cells that may extend to entire mastoid
- CT or MRI may be indicated if serious complications suspected (meningitis, brain abscess, severe mastoiditis)

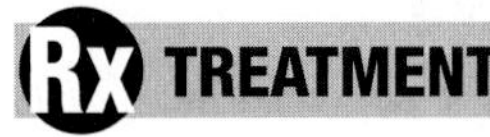

TREATMENT

ACUTE GENERAL Rx

Hydration, avoidance of irritants (e.g., tobacco smoke), nasal systemic decongestants, cool mist humidifier, and oral ibuprofen or acetaminophen. Topical procaine or lidocaine preparations (if available) are an alternative to oral analgesics for children ≥2 yr but should not be used in children with tympanic membrane perforation.

Antimicrobials:

NOTE: Most uncomplicated cases of AOM resolve spontaneously, without complications. Studies have demonstrated limited therapeutic benefit from antibiotic therapy. Watchful waiting is appropriate for children who look well, can be comforted with supportive care, and are old enough to easily evaluate. Children <24 mo with bilateral AOM should receive antibiotic therapy. Children with severe signs or symptoms (moderate or severe otalgia or otalgia for ≥48 hr or temperature ≥39°C) should also receive antibiotic therapy. When opting to use antibiotic therapy:

- Amoxicillin remains the drug of choice for first-line treatment of uncomplicated AOM despite increasing prevalence of drug-resistant *S. pneumoniae.*
- Treatment failure is defined by lack of clinical improvement of signs or symptoms after 3 days of therapy.

- With treatment failure, in the absence of an identified etiologic pathogen, therapy should be redirected to cover:
  1. Drug-resistant *S. pneumoniae*
  2. β-lactamase–producing strains of *H. influenzae* and *M. catarrhalis*
- Agents fulfilling these criteria include amoxicillin/clavulanate, second-generation (e.g., cefuroxime axetil, cefaclor) or third-generation cephalosporins (e.g., oral cefdinir or cefpodoxime or IM ceftriaxone). Do not use cefaclor, cefixime, loracarbef, and ceftibuten given limited activity against pneumococci.
- Cross-resistance between TMP/SX and macrolides and the β-lactams exists; therefore patients who do not respond to amoxicillin are more likely to have infections resistant to TMP/SMX and macrolides.
- Fluoroquinolones are not indicated as first- or second-line therapy for AOM and should be avoided in young children due to risks of musculoskeletal effects and limited dosing guidance.
- Treatment should be modified according to cultures and sensitivities when available.
- Generally treatment course is 10 days for children <2 yr and those with severe symptoms, 7 days for children age 2 to 5 yr, and 5 to 7 days for children ≥6 yr.
- Follow-up should be tailored to clinical improvement and concern for neurocognitive development delays in at-risk children. Standard follow-up of all cases is no longer required.
- Antibiotic prophylaxis to reduce the frequency of AOM episodes in children with recurrent AOM is not recommended.

NOTE: Effusions may persist for 8 wk or longer in many cases of adequately treated otitis media.

SURGICAL Rx

- No evidence to support the routine use of myringotomy, but in severe cases it provides prompt pain relief and accelerates resolution of infection.
- Purulent secretions retained in the middle ear can lead to increased pressure that may lead to spread of infection to contiguous areas. Myringotomy to decompress the middle ear is sometimes necessary to avoid complications.
- Complications include mastoiditis, facial nerve paralysis, labyrinthitis, meningitis, and brain abscess.
- Other procedures used for drainage of the middle ear include insertion of a ventilation tube and/or simple.
- There is no role for mastoidectomy in treating children with uncomplicated CSOM.

CHRONIC Rx

- Myringotomy and tympanostomy tube placement for persistent or recurrent middle ear effusion unresponsive to medical therapy for ≥3 mo if bilateral or ≥6 mo if unilateral.
- Adenoidectomy, with or without tonsillectomy, often advocated for treatment of recurrent otitis media, although indications for this procedure are controversial.
- Long-term complications include tympanic membrane perforations, cholesteatoma, tympanosclerosis, ossicular necrosis, toxic or suppurative labyrinthitis, hearing loss, and intracranial suppuration.

DISPOSITION

Patients can be treated at home as outpatients with the rare exception of patients with evidence of local suppurative complications (e.g., meningitis, acute mastoiditis, brain abscess, cavernous sinus, or lateral vein thrombosis).

REFERRAL

- To otorhinolaryngologist if:
  1. Medical treatment failure
  2. Diagnosis uncertain: Adults with one or more episodes of otitis media should be referred for ear-nose-throat evaluation to rule out underlying process (e.g., malignancy)
  3. Any of the above-mentioned acute and chronic complications

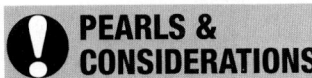

PEARLS & CONSIDERATIONS

COMMENTS

- Otoscopic findings are critical for accurate AOM diagnosis. AOM microbiology has changed with use of pneumococcal conjugate vaccine (PCV13). Antibiotics are modestly more effective than no treatment but cause adverse effects in 4% to 10% of children. Most antibiotics have comparable clinical success.

Prevention:

- Multiple component conjugate vaccines have helped decrease recurrent episodes of AOM
- Breastfeed and bottle-feed infants in an upright position
- Avoidance of irritants (e.g., tobacco smoke)

SUGGESTED READINGS

Available at ExpertConsult.com

AUTHORS: **DIANE KOCOVSKY APRN,** and **RUSSELL J. MCCULLOH, M.D.**

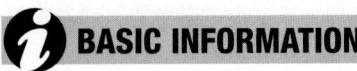

BASIC INFORMATION

DEFINITION

Ovarian cancer is not one disease but a constellation of distinct cancer subtypes, some of which originate outside of the ovary. 90% of tumors are epithelial ovarian cancers, 5% are gram cell tumors, and 5% are sex cord-stromal tumors. A classification of ovarian epithelial tumors is summarized in Table 1.

SYNONYMS

Epithelial ovarian cancer
Germ cell tumor
Sex cord stromal tumor
Ovarian tumor of low malignant potential

ICD-10CM CODES
C56.9 Malignant neoplasm of unspecified ovary
C56.1 Malignant neoplasm of right ovary
C56.2 Malignant neoplasm of left ovary

EPIDEMIOLOGY & DEMOGRAPHICS

INCIDENCE: 12.9 to 15.1 cases/100,000 persons; ~25,000 new cases annually. Lifetime risk for developing ovarian cancer is 1.3%. It is the leading cause of gynecologic cancer-related deaths.

PREVALENCE: It is most commonly diagnosed in those 55 to 64 yr of age.

RISK FACTORS:

- Low parity
- Delayed childbearing
- Smoking
- Polycystic ovary syndrome
- Endometriosis
- Use of talc on the perineum (unlikely)
- High-fat diet
- Fertility drugs (unlikely)
- Lynch II syndrome (nonpolyposis colon cancer, endometrial cancer, breast cancer, and ovarian cancer clusters in first- and second-degree relatives)
- Breast-ovarian familial cancer syndrome
- Site-specific familial ovarian cancer
- The **strongest** risk factors are advancing age and family history of ovarian and breast cancer
- Factors that **decrease** the risk of ovarian cancer include previous pregnancy, oral contraceptive pill use, hysterectomy, tubal ligation, or salpingectomy

GENETICS: The greatest risk factors of ovarian cancer are a family history and associated genetic syndromes. Familial susceptibility has been shown with the *BRCA1* gene located on 17q12 to 21. This correlates with breast-ovarian cancer syndrome. There are other genetic mutations associated with ovarian malignancies, but more than 90% of inherited ovarian malignancies are associated with *BRCA* mutations. *BRCA* mutations interact with and affect DNA repair proteins.

Genetic counseling is recommended for certain patients, including those with:

- Epithelial ovarian cancer at any age
- Breast cancer diagnosed at age 45 yr or younger
- Breast cancer with two distinct and sequential primaries, the first one diagnosed at age 50 yr or younger
- Breast cancer that is triple-negative and diagnosed at age 60 yr or younger
- Breast cancer at any age, with at least one close relative diagnosed at age 50 yr or younger
- Breast cancer diagnosed at any age, with two or more close relatives with breast cancer; one close relative with epithelial ovarian cancer; or two close relatives with pancreatic cancer or aggressive prostate cancer
- Breast cancer, with a close male relative at any age who has breast cancer
- Breast cancer and Ashkenazi Jewish ancestry
- A family with a known deleterious *BRCA1* or *BRCA2* mutation

PHYSICAL FINDINGS & CLINICAL PRESENTATION

- 60% present with advanced disease
- Abdominal fullness, early satiety, dyspepsia
- Pelvic pain, back pain, constipation
- Pelvic or abdominal mass
- Lymphadenopathy (inguinal)
- Sister Mary Joseph nodule (umbilical mass)

ETIOLOGY

- Can be inherited as site-specific familial ovarian cancer (two or more first-degree relatives have ovarian cancer)
- Breast-ovarian cancer syndrome (clusters of breast and ovarian cancer among first- and second-degree relatives)
- Lynch syndrome
- No family history and unknown etiology in the majority of ovarian cancer cases

TABLE 1 Classification of Ovarian Epithelial Tumors

Terminology	Notes
Serous Tumors	Most common epithelial tumor group
Adenocarcinoma	More than 85% involve the ovarian surface or adjacent structures Includes low (≈10%) and high (≈90%) grade carcinomas
Noninvasive low-grade serous carcinoma (LGSC)	Grade 1, synonymous with micropapillary/cribriform borderline
Borderline	Can be intracystic or involve the ovarian surface
Benign	Includes adenofibroma
Mucinous Tumors	Include intestinal (common) and müllerian (less common) types
Adenocarcinoma	Includes borderline tumors with "intraepithelial carcinoma"
Borderline	
Benign	
With mural nodules	
Endometrioid Tumors	
Adenocarcinoma	High-grade carcinomas overlap with high-grade serous carcinomas (HGSCs)
Carcinosarcoma	
Adenosarcoma	
Borderline	Also known as *proliferative cystadenoma/adenofibroma;* including squamous morules
Benign	
Clear Cell Tumors	
Adenocarcinoma	Papillary and adenofibromatous types
Borderline	Occur in adenofibromas
Benign	Very rare
Transitional Cell Tumors	
Malignant	Includes malignant Brenner tumors and the rare transitional cell carcinoma
Borderline	Typically proliferating Brenner tumors
Benign	Usually Brenner tumors
Squamous Cell Tumors	
Malignant	Rare squamous carcinomas with or without a coexisting teratoma
Benign	Epidermoid cysts
Mixed Epithelial Tumors	
Malignant	Commonly a mixture of high-grade serous and endometrioid (high-grade müllerian)
Borderline and benign	Overlap with serous and müllerian mucinous tumors, also called "seromucinous borderline tumors"
Benign	
Undifferentiated or Unclassified	

Modified from the World Health Organization.
From Crum CP, et al.: *Diagnostic gynecologic and obstetric pathology*, ed 3, Philadelphia, 2018, Elsevier.

TABLE 2 International Federation of Gynecology and Obstetrics (FIGO) Classification of Ovarian Carcinoma

Stage	Description
Stage I	Growth limited to the ovaries:
	Stage I_A: Growth limited to one ovary, no ascites and no tumor present on the external surface; capsule intact
	Stage I_B: Growth limited to both ovaries, no ascites and no tumor present on the external surface; capsule intact
	Stage I_C: Stage 1_A or 1_B where there is tumor on the surface of either ovary; or with ruptured capsules or with ascites containing malignant cells or positive peritoneal washings. Surgical spillage of a malignant cyst upgrades the patient to I_C, although it is unlikely that this event affects prognosis.
Stage II	Growth involving one or both ovaries with pelvic extension:
	Stage II_A: Extension and/or metastases to the uterus and tubes
	Stage II_B: Extension to other pelvic tissues
	Stage II_C: Stage II_A or II_B with tumor on the surface of either ovary or positive peritoneal washings or malignant ascites
Stage III	Growth involving one or both ovaries with peritoneal implants outside the pelvis or positive retroperitoneal or inguinal lymph nodes:
	Stage III_A: Microscopic seeding of abdominal peritoneal surfaces
	Stage III_B: Macroscopic disease outside the pelvis less than 2 cm in diameter
	Stage III_C: Abdominal implants greater than 2 cm and/or positive nodes
Stage IV	Growth involving one or both ovaries with distant metastases including parenchymal (but not superficial) liver metastases and pleural effusions containing malignant cells

From Symonds EM, Symonds IM: *Essential obstetrics and gynaecology*, ed 4, London, 2004, Churchill Livingstone.

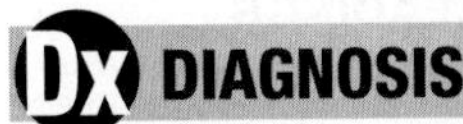

DIAGNOSIS

DIFFERENTIAL DIAGNOSIS

- Primary peritoneal cancer mesothelioma
- Benign ovarian tumor
- Functional ovarian cyst
- Endometriosis
- Ovarian torsion
- Pelvic kidney
- Pedunculated uterine fibroid
- Primary cancer from breast, gastrointestinal tract, or other pelvic organ metastasized to the ovary

WORKUP

- Definitive diagnosis made at laparotomy; epithelial ovarian cancer most common type of ovarian cancer (90% of ovarian cancer)
- Careful physical and history, including family history
- Exclusion of nongynecologic etiologies
- Observation of small cystic masses in premenopausal women for regression for 2 mo
- FIGO classification of ovarian carcinoma is described in Table 2
- Referral to specialists who have extensive training and experience in treating ovarian cancer significantly increases survival after an ovarian cancer diagnosis

LABORATORY TESTS

- Complete blood count.
- Chemistry profile including liver tests and calcium (to evaluate for paraneoplastic syndrome).
- CA-125 or lysophosphatidic acid level. Use of these tests for annual screening is controversial, and most experts warn against universal screening with this marker. Only about 50% of early-stage ovarian cancers will be associated with elevated CA-125. Additionally, false elevations may occur with uterine leiomyoma, endometriosis, pregnancy, and intraabdominal infections. The PLCO cancer screening trial revealed that annual screening based on CA-125 and vaginal ultrasound is ineffective, and diagnostic follow-up of false positives resulted in 15% serious complication rate.
- Consider: Human chorionic gonadotropin, inhibin, alpha-fetoprotein, neuron-specific enolase, and lactate dehydrogenase in patients at risk for germ cell tumors.
- A panel of three serum biomarkers (apolipoprotein A-1 [ApoA-1], transthyretin [TTR], and transferrin [TF]) has been reported useful in distinguishing normal samples from early-stage ovarian cancer with a sensitivity of 84% and normal samples from late-stage ovarian cancer with a sensitivity of 97%.
- *BRCA1/2* testing is recommended for all women with ovarian cancer.

IMAGING STUDIES

- Ultrasound
- Chest x-ray
- CT or MRI of abdomen and pelvis help evaluate extent of disease (Fig. E1)
- Mammogram

Rx TREATMENT

NONPHARMACOLOGIC THERAPY

Virtually all cases of ovarian cancer involve surgical exploration. This includes:

- Abdominal cytology
- Total abdominal hysterectomy and bilateral salpingo-oophorectomy (except in early stages in which fertility preservation is an issue)
- Omentectomy
- Diaphragm sampling
- Selective lymphadenectomy (pelvic and paraaortic nodes)
- Primary cytoreduction with a goal of residual tumor diameter <<2 cm
- Bowel surgery, splenectomy if needed to obtain optimal (<<2 cm) cytoreduction
- Conventional treatment includes surgical debulking (cytoreduction) followed by chemotherapy. However, patients with low-grade, well-differentiated stage I ovarian cancer do not benefit from adjuvant chemotherapy

ACUTE GENERAL Rx

- Optimal cytoreduction (debulking) is generally followed by chemotherapy (except in some early-stage disease [stage I without high-risk features is treated with surgery alone]).
- Cisplatin-based combination chemotherapy is used for stage II or greater, 6-mo treatment. Compared with IV paclitaxel plus cisplatin, IV paclitaxel plus intraperitoneal cisplatin and paclitaxel improves survival rates in patients with optimally debulked stage III ovarian cancer.
- Chemotherapy regimens continue to change as research continues. Bevacizumab, a humanized antivascular endothelial growth factor monoclonal antibody, has been shown to be effective in improving progression-free survival in women with ovarian cancer. Trials using bevacizumab during and up to 10 mo after carboplatin and paclitaxel chemotherapy have shown prolongation of the median progression-free survival by about 4 mo in patients with advanced epithelial ovarian cancer.
- PARP inhibitors are up-and-coming chemotherapeutic agents that have been used for maintenance therapy and have been shown to improve progression-free survival among patients with platinum-sensitive high-grade serous cancers. PARP inhibitors work by pharmacologically inhibiting the enzyme poly (ADP-ribose) polymerase. Three PARP inhibitors are currently FDA approved for different indications. Olaparib, an oral polymerase inhibitor, was approved in 2014 and has shown antitumor activity in patients with high-grade serous ovarian cancer with or without *BRCA1* and *BRCA2* germline mutations. Rucaparib was approved in 2016 to treat high-grade serous cancers with *BRCA1* and *BRCA2* germline or somatic mutations. Lastly, Niraparib was approved in 2017 for use in high-grade serous cancers with or without *BRCA1* and *BRCA2* mutations.
- Second-look surgery when chemotherapy is complete generally is no longer recommended because this has not been shown to improve survival.

- In most cases, neoadjuvant (presurgical) chemotherapy has no advantage over postsurgical initiation of chemotherapy. However, some trials have shown that neoadjuvant chemotherapy followed by interval debulking surgery is not inferior to debulking surgery followed by chemotherapy as a treatment option for patients with bulky stage IIIC or IV ovarian carcinoma. Complete resection of all macroscopic disease, whether performed as primary treatment or after neoadjuvant chemotherapy, remains the objective whenever cytoreductive surgery is performed.

CHRONIC Rx

- If CA-125 elevated, may have recurrent disease
- Physical and pelvic examinations every 3 mo for 2 yr, every 4 mo during third yr, then every 6 mo
- Routine monitoring of CA-125 at every visit does not improve survival and should be reserved for addressing specific clinical concerns
- Yearly Pap smear

DISPOSITION

- Overall 5-yr survival rates remain low because of the preponderance of late-stage disease:
    1. Stage I and II: 80% to 100%
    2. Stage III: 15% to 20%
    3. Stage IV: 5%
- Younger patients (<50 yr) in all stages have a considerably better 5-yr survival than older patients (40% vs. 15%).
- Among women with high-grade serous ovarian cancer, *BRCA2* mutation, but not *BRCA1* deficiency, is associated with improved survival, improved chemotherapy response, and genome instability compared with *BRCA* wild-type.
- Among patients with invasive epithelial ovarian cancer (EOC), having a germline mutation in *BRCA1* or *BRCA2* is associated with improved 5-yr overall survival. *BRCA2* carriers have the best prognosis.

COMMENTS

- The U.S. Preventive Services Task Force has concluded that current evidence does not show any mortality benefit to routine screening for ovarian cancer with transvaginal ultrasonography or single-threshold serum CA-125 testing and that the harms of such screening are at least moderate. This recommendation applies to asymptomatic women who are not known to have a high-risk hereditary cancer syndrome.
- Oral contraceptives reduce the risk of ovarian cancer by 40% to 50%. The greatest risk reduction is present after ≥15 yr of oral contraceptive use.
- Patients at high risk for developing ovarian cancer (*BRCA1/BRCA2* gene mutation, hereditary nonpolyposis colorectal cancer syndrome) should consider prophylactic salpingo-oophorectomy after childbearing is complete. Prophylactic bilateral salpingo-oophorectomy reduces ovarian cancer by 80%. It is recommended by age 35 to 40 yr for *BRCA1* carriers and by age 45 for *BRCA2* carriers. If surgery is declined, the National Comprehensive Cancer Network guidelines recommend intensive surveillance with pelvic and abdominal sonogram and serum CA-125 every 6 mo starting at age 35 or 10 yr earlier than cancer diagnosis in family member.

SUGGESTED READINGS

Available at ExpertConsult.com

RELATED CONTENT

Ovarian Cancer (Patient Information)
Ovarian Neoplasm, Benign (Related Key Topic)

AUTHOR: **BETH LEOPOLD, M.D.**

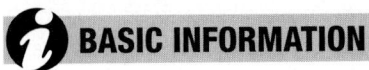

BASIC INFORMATION

DEFINITION

Benign ovarian neoplasms are often clinically indistinguishable from their malignant counterparts. Therefore, all persistent adnexal masses must be considered malignant until proven otherwise. Nonneoplastic tumors include:

- Germinal inclusion cyst
- Follicle cyst
- Corpus luteum cyst
- Pregnancy luteoma
- Theca lutein cysts
- Sclerocystic ovaries
- Endometrioma

Neoplastic tumors derived from coelomic epithelium include:

- Cystic tumors: Serous cystadenoma, mucinous cystadenoma, mixed forms
- Tumors with stromal overgrowth: Fibroma, adenofibroma, Brenner tumor

Tumors derived from germ cells are dermoids (benign cystic teratomas).

ICD-10CM CODES

D27.9 Benign neoplasm of unspecified ovary
D27.0 Benign neoplasm of right ovary
D27.1 Benign neoplasm of left ovary

EPIDEMIOLOGY & DEMOGRAPHICS

- **Reproductive years:**
  1. Most common benign ovarian neoplasms: Serous cystadenoma and benign cystic teratoma
  2. Most common adnexal mass: Functional cyst
  3. Risk of malignancy increases after age 40 yr.
- **Infants:** Adnexal masses are usually follicular cysts attributable to maternal hormone stimulation that regress during first few months of life.
- **Childhood:**
  1. Adnexal masses are rare
  2. 9% to 11% malignant
  3. Almost always dysgerminomas or teratomas (germ cell origin)
  4. Frequency of malignancy is inversely correlated with age
- **Adolescence:**
  1. Most common adnexal mass is a functional cyst.
  2. Most common neoplastic ovarian tumor is a benign cystic teratoma.
  3. Solid/cystic adnexal tumors are rare and almost always dysgerminomas or malignant teratomas.

PHYSICAL FINDINGS & CLINICAL PRESENTATION

- Usually asymptomatic
- Pelvic pain or pressure
- Dyspareunia
- Abdominal pain ranging from mild to severe peritoneal irritation
- Increasing abdominal girth or distention
- Adnexal mass of pelvic examination
- Children: Abdominal or rectal mass, early-onset puberty

ETIOLOGY

- Physiologic
- Endometriosis
- Unknown

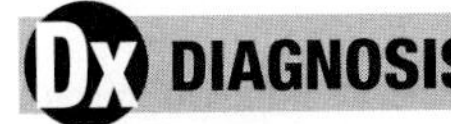

DIAGNOSIS

DIFFERENTIAL DIAGNOSIS

- Ovarian torsion
- Endometrioma
- Uterine fibroid
- Ectopic pregnancy
- Tubo-ovarian abscess
- Paratubal or paraovarian cyst
- Hydrosalpinx
- Malignancy: Ovary, fallopian tube, colon
- Diverticular abscess, diverticulitis
- Appendiceal abscess, appendicitis (especially in children)
- Urethral diverticulum
- Nerve sheath tumors
- Distended bladder
- Pelvic kidney
- Retroperitoneal cyst or neoplasm

WORKUP

- Complete history and physical examination
- Pelvic or rectovaginal examination to reveal firm, irregular, mobile mass
- Pelvic ultrasound
- Laparoscopy or laparotomy to establish diagnosis

LABORATORY TESTS

- Pregnancy test
- Serum tumor markers:
  1. Cancer antigen 125 (CA-125)
  2. Alpha-fetoprotein (endodermal sinus tumor, immature teratoma)
  3. Beta-human chorionic gonadotropin
  4. Lactate dehydrogenase (dysgerminoma)

IMAGING STUDIES

Ultrasound (Fig. 1):

- May differentiate adnexal mass from other pelvic masses
- Features that increase risk of malignancy include solid component, papillae, multiple septations or solitary thick septa, ascites, matted bowel, bilaterality, irregular borders
- CT scan with contrast
- Colonoscopy or barium enema, if symptomatic

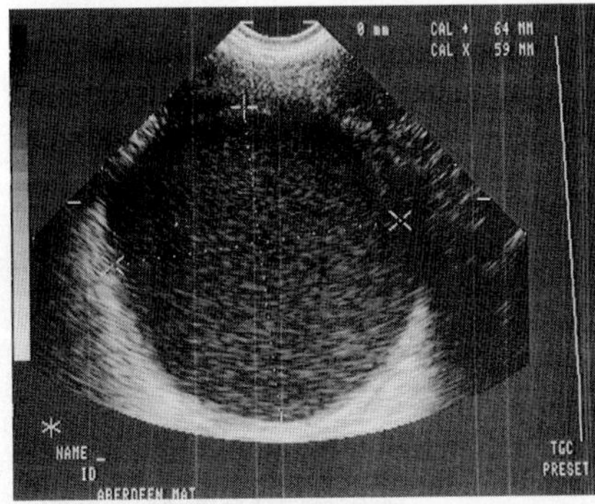

FIG. 1 Ultrasonogram reveals a cyst 6.5 cm across, which was found at laparotomy to be an endometrioma full of altered blood, the so-called chocolate cyst. This may cause cyclical or chronic pelvic pain. (From Greer IA et al: *Mosby's color atlas and text of obstetrics and gynecology,* London, 2000, Harcourt.)

TREATMENT

NONPHARMACOLOGIC THERAPY

Repeat pelvic examination, typically with transvaginal pelvic ultrasound, for premenopausal women in 4 to 6 wk to rule out persistent cyst.

ACUTE GENERAL Rx

Indications for surgery:

- Postmenopausal or premenarchal palpable adnexal mass
- Adnexal mass with suspicious ultrasound features
- Adnexal mass greater than 10 cm
- Suspected torsion or rupture

CHRONIC Rx

- Depends on diagnosis
- Possible suppression of formation of new cysts by oral contraceptives

DISPOSITION

- Depends on diagnosis
- One study showed that all malignant masses demonstrated growth within 7 mo. Expert opinion recommends limiting observation of stable masses without solid components to 1 yr and with solid components to 2 yr

REFERRAL

- If malignancy suspected
- If surgery required

SUGGESTED READING

Available at ExpertConsult.com

RELATED CONTENT

Ovarian Cysts (Patient Information)
Ovarian Cancer (Related Key Topic)

AUTHOR: **BETH LEOPOLD, M.D.**

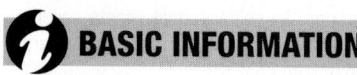

BASIC INFORMATION

DEFINITION

Paget disease of bone is a focal disorder of chaotic bone remodeling with increased osteoblastic and osteoclastic activity that results in disorganized woven and lamellar bone in one or more skeletal sites. The end result is bone of poor quality that is enlarged, hypervascular, and susceptible to deformation and fracture.

SYNONYM

Osteitis deformans

ICD-10CM CODES	
M88.9	Osteitis deformans of unspecified bone
M88.0	Osteitis deformans of skull
M88.1	Osteitis deformans of vertebrae
M88.869	Osteitis deformans of unspecified lower leg
M88.89	Osteitis deformans of multiple sites
M90.60	Osteitis deformans in neoplastic diseases, unspecified site
M90.679	Osteitis deformans in neoplastic diseases, unspecified ankle and foot
M90.68	Osteitis deformans in neoplastic diseases, other site
M90.69	Osteitis deformans in neoplastic diseases, multiple sites

EPIDEMIOLOGY & DEMOGRAPHICS

Epidemiologic data suggest an origin of Paget disease in Great Britain spreading to other areas by English colonists beginning in the seventeenth century. Highest prevalence occurs in Eastern and Western Europe and in those who have emigrated to New Zealand, Australia, South Africa, and North America. Paget is rarely seen in Japanese, Chinese, Asian Indians, sub-Saharan Africans, and Middle Eastern Arabs.

Most commonly diagnosed in those aged >50 yr and rare before 40 yr.

Prevalence estimates of up to 3% of population aged >50 yr and up to 10% in those aged >90 yr.

PREDOMINANT SEX: Variable preponderance of males

PREDOMINANT AGE: Middle or advanced yr

FAMILIAL INCIDENCE: Common, family history positive in up to 40% of cases

PHYSICAL FINDINGS & CLINICAL PRESENTATION

- Most common sites of involvement: Pelvis (70%), lumbar spine (53%), sacrum, femur (55%), skull (42%), tibia (30%) (Fig. E1), humerus, scapula.
- Uncommon: Hand, foot, fibula.
- Lesions in one (monostotic) or more bones (polyostotic).
- Gradual progression of disease in affected bone(s) with rare appearance at new site(s).
- Many patients are asymptomatic, but up to 40% of patients who come to medical attention present with bone pain.
- Symptoms and signs include bone and articular pain often related to secondary arthritis, bone deformities and enlargement, increased warmth over pagetic bone, skull enlargement, nerve entrapment or compression syndromes, cranial nerve deficits especially deafness, spinal cord compression and vascular steal syndromes, fissure fractures, fractures, and neoplastic degeneration.

ETIOLOGY

Etiology remains unknown. Extensive epidemiologic and laboratory data are in keeping with potential role of paramyxoviral infection of osteoclasts in a genetically susceptible individual with or without documented genetic mutations.

Dx DIAGNOSIS

Diagnosis is often suspected in asymptomatic patients with isolated elevation of alkaline phosphatase without evidence of liver disease.

DIFFERENTIAL DIAGNOSIS

- Osteosclerosis
- Hyperphosphatasia
- Familial expansile osteolysis
- Fibrous dysplasia
- Skeletal neoplasm (primary or metastatic)
- Osteomalacia with secondary hyperparathyroidism

LABORATORY TESTS

- Increase in serum alkaline phosphatase or bone-specific alkaline phosphatase
- Increase in urine NTx/creatinine ratio or plasma CTx
- Bone biopsy is rarely needed but may be necessary in selected cases to rule out sarcomatous degeneration or metastatic disease

IMAGING STUDIES (FIG. E2)

Bone scintigraphy is the most sensitive test for delineating the extent and site of pagetic lesions but nonspecific in that areas of uptake may be related to arthritis or metastatic lesions. Radiographs (Fig. 3) will further delineate characteristic pagetic changes (thickening of cortical bone, coarsened tradecular markings, distortion and expansion of involved bone).

Rx TREATMENT

Indications for therapy include extensive or symptomatic disease; neurologic complications; involvement of weight-bearing bones, skull, vertebrae, and other areas of critical involvement, for example, in proximity to joints; and prevention of excess bleeding from an orthopedic procedure on pagetic bone.

NONPHARMACOLOGIC THERAPY

- Optimization of calcium and vitamin D intake and appropriate guidance regarding ambulatory needs.
- Orthopedic stabilization may be required for patients with pseudofractures.

SPECIFIC THERAPY

Bisphosphonates are the mainstay of therapy and include oral alendronate or risedronate and intravenous pamidronate or zoledronic acid. A one time dose of zoledronic acid (5mg IV) may be effective in controlling symptoms for over 3 yr.

- SC salmon calcitonin when bisphosphonates are not tolerated or are contraindicated as in those with GFR of <35 ml/min
- Acetaminophen, aspirin, and nonsteroidal drugs for relief of pain

DISPOSITION

- Without treatment, progression of disease is common.
- With treatment, remissions of varying duration in most patients. Bisphosphonates can normalize bone turnover in a high proportion of patients, but evidence that long-term suppression of bone turnover prevents complications or improves the clinical outcome is currently inconclusive.
- Careful and regular clinical and biochemical follow-up at 3- to 6-month intervals with necessity of retreatment in patients with continued pagetic activity or reactivation.
- With first ever intravenous dose of pamidronate or zoledronic acid, patients may experience a flulike syndrome for several days that may be prevented with acetaminophen.

SUGGESTED READINGS

Available at ExpertConsult.com

RELATED CONTENT

Paget Disease of Bone (Patient Information)

AUTHOR: **JOSEPH R. TUCCI, M.D., F.A.C.P., F.A.C.E.**

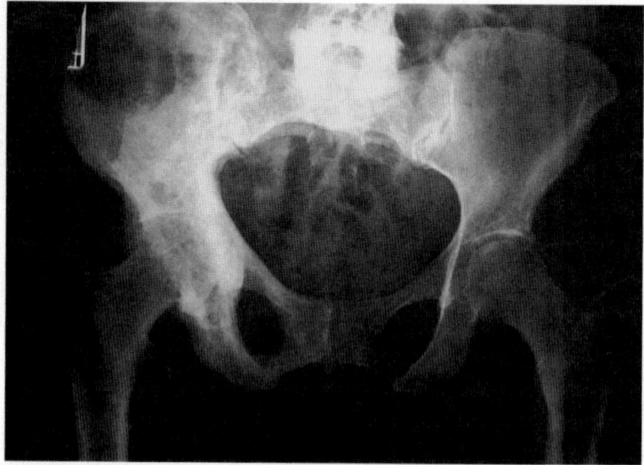

FIG. 3 Paget disease of the bone. Frontal radiograph of the pelvis shows marked prominence of the trabeculae in the right ilium, ischium, and pubic bones, with small lytic areas identified as compatible with the later stages of Paget disease. (From Specht N [ed]: *Practical guide to diagnostic imaging,* St Louis, 1998, Mosby.)

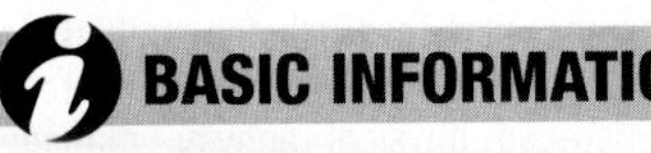

BASIC INFORMATION

DEFINITION

Paget disease of the breast is a malignant disease that presents itself as a scaly, sore, eroding, bleeding ulcer of the nipple. It represents an extension of a ductal adenocarcinoma of the breast. Microscopically, typical large clear cells (Paget cells) with pale and abundant cytoplasm and hyperchromatic nuclei with prominent nucleoli are found in the epidermal layer. Paget disease is more often associated with primary invasive or in situ carcinoma of the breast.

ICD-10CM CODES

C50.0	Malignant neoplasm of nipple and areola
C50.011	Malignant neoplasm of nipple and areola, right female breast
C50.012	Malignant neoplasm of nipple and areola, left female breast
C50.019	Malignant neoplasm of nipple and areola, unspecified female breast
C50.021	Malignant neoplasm of nipple and areola, right male breast
C50.022	Malignant neoplasm of nipple and areola, left male breast
C50.029	Malignant neoplasm of nipple and areola, unspecified male breast

EPIDEMIOLOGY & DEMOGRAPHICS

- Not common
- Found in one in 100 to 200 breast cancer patients

PHYSICAL FINDINGS & CLINICAL PRESENTATION

- Variable; most often reveals an erythematous, irregularly bordered plaque that starts on the nipple and spreads to the areola.
- Itching or burning nipple and/or reported lump. Itching/burning may occur before lesion.
- Very minimal scaly lesion that may bleed when scales are lifted.
- Typical ulcer located on nipple with serous fluid weeping or small amount of bleeding coming from it (Fig. 1) Bloody discharge may also occasionally occur.
- Palpable carcinoma in the breast of some patients.
- 21% with no palpable mass will have suspicious finding on mammogram.

ETIOLOGY

- Exact origin unknown
- Possibly migration of either in situ or invasive carcinoma cells in breast to nipple skin to produce Paget disease

Dx DIAGNOSIS

DIFFERENTIAL DIAGNOSIS

- Chronic dermatitis
- Florid papillomatosis of the nipple or nipple adenoma
- Eczema
- Skin cancer

WORKUP

- Clinically apparent
- Careful breast examination with diagnosis in mind
- Palpable mass or mammographic lesions in 60% to 70% of patients

LABORATORY TESTS

Biopsy of nipple lesion

IMAGING STUDIES

Mammograms to search for possible primary carcinoma

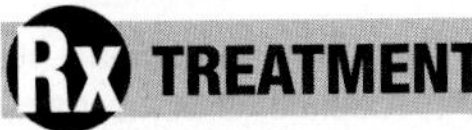

TREATMENT

NONPHARMACOLOGIC THERAPY

- Paget disease without palpable mass and negative mammogram:
  1 Consideration of wide excision of nipple with or without radiation
  2 Mastectomy is also an option
- Paget disease with palpable mass or abnormal mammogram findings:
  1. Mastectomy
  2. Breast conservation surgery and whole breast radiation

Presence of underlying in situ or invasive carcinoma in mastectomy specimen of majority of patients

ACUTE GENERAL Rx

Systemic adjuvant therapy depending on extent of invasive carcinoma found

DISPOSITION

- Parallel prognosis to that of breast cancer patient without Paget disease
- Prognosis is better in those without palpable mass
- Regular follow-up as in other invasive or in situ carcinoma patients

REFERRAL

At outset, all suspicious nipple lesions should be referred for evaluation and treatment.

SUGGESTED READING

Available at ExpertConsult.com

RELATED CONTENT

Paget Disease of the Breast (Patient Information)
Breast Cancer (Related Key Topic)

AUTHORS: **GINA RANIERI, D.O.,** and **ANTHONY SCISCIONE, D.O.**

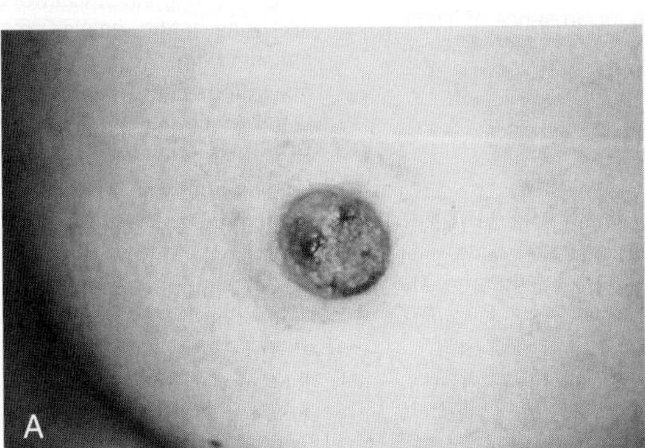

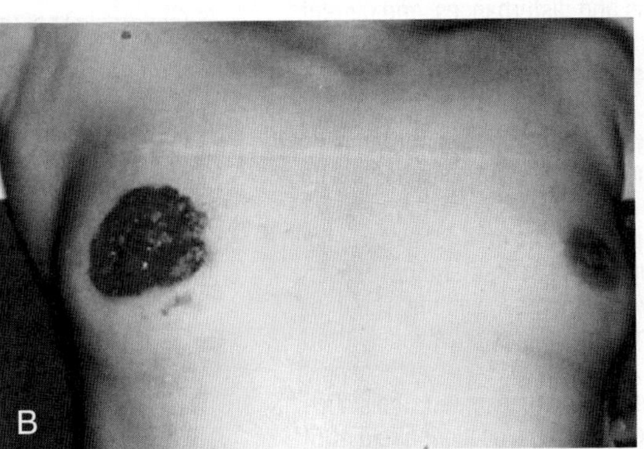

FIG. 1 **A** and **B,** Paget disease of the nipple. (Courtesy Sehwan Han, M.D.)

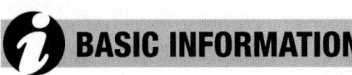

BASIC INFORMATION

DEFINITION

Chronic pain is pain that persists for longer than the expected time frame (typically >3 mo) or that is associated with progressive, nonmalignant disease. Pain is an unpleasant sensory and emotional experience associated with actual or potential tissue damage or described in terms of such damage. The perception of pain is influenced by physiologic, psychological, and social factors.

SYNONYMS

Chronic pain management
Nonmalignant chronic pain
Pain management

ICD-10CM CODES

G89.4	Chronic pain syndrome
G89.29	Other chronic pain
G89.21	Chronic pain due to trauma
G89.22	Chronic post-thoracotomy pain
G89.28	Other chronic postprocedural pain
G89.3	Neoplasm-related pain (acute) (chronic)

EPIDEMIOLOGY & DEMOGRAPHICS

Estimates of the prevalence of chronic pain in the United States vary widely. A 2011 report from the Institute of Medicine, *Relieving Pain in America*, estimates that 116 million adults live with chronic pain at a cost of almost $635 billion per yr. Chronic pain is the third leading cause of physical impairment in the United States. Patients with chronic pain may also experience mood changes, depression, sleep disturbances, fatigue, and decreased overall physical functioning.

CLINICAL PRESENTATION

- History: Comprehensive patient assessment, including history of present illness (cause of pain, location, timing, characteristics, exacerbating/relieving factors, triggers), past therapies (pharmacologic and nonpharmacologic and outcomes of these therapies), medical history, family and social history, psychiatric history (including history of depression, anxiety, abuse, and/or other psychological disorders), substance use history, allergies, sleep patterns and disturbances, and current medications. Social supports, coping mechanisms, and spirituality can also help guide development of a treatment plan.
- Pain assessment should be performed at each visit; includes pain intensity (1 to 10), response to medication, and attributes of pain. Standardized templates for both initial and follow-up pain assessment have been developed by various organizations. The Brief Pain Inventory is an example of a widely used assessment tool. In addition, a functional assessment should be performed. Tools such as the Functional Ability Questionnaire (FAQ5) can guide the clinician in determining a patient's functional status. Lastly, consider assessment of a patient's risk for substance abuse.
- Physical examination: Directed at systems affected by pain (often musculoskeletal) and neurologic examination.
- Look for contributing factors (e.g., comorbidities, lifestyle factors) and barriers to effective care (e.g., behavioral, social, insurance). Increasing evidence points to a relation between obesity and chronic pain.

ETIOLOGY

Mechanisms of chronic pain can be divided into three broad categories:

- Nociceptive—pain arising from damage to peripheral tissue from injury or inflammatory, mechanical, or metabolic causes
- Neuropathic—peripheral nerve impairment
- Central—central disturbance in pain processing

Dx DIAGNOSIS

DIFFERENTIAL DIAGNOSIS

- Depends on etiology:
  1. Nociceptive—osteoarthritis, rheumatoid arthritis, postsurgical pain, posttraumatic, cancer pain
  2. Neuropathic—postherpetic neuralgia, diabetic neuropathy, nerve root compression
  3. Central—fibromyalgia, irritable bowel syndrome, chronic headache, phantom limb
- Many chronic pain syndromes may involve one or more of the previously named mechanisms.
- Depression and anxiety disorders can be both a cause and a result of chronic pain, so temporal association of these disorders is important.

WORKUP

- Workup should be directed at identifying the source of pain. Identification of the mechanism of pain will guide the development of an appropriate treatment plan.
- Laboratory testing, imaging studies, and/or electromyographic studies should be used when etiology of chronic pain is unknown or unclear, when comorbidities are suspected, and as the history and physical examination direct.
- Consider use of random urine drug screens or other tests to screen for presence of illegal drugs, unreported prescribed medications, or alcohol use.

Rx TREATMENT

- Studies increasingly support the application of a multidisciplinary, biopsychosocial approach that addresses the multiple facets of pain and includes the patient's perspective and goals.
- Therapeutic goal is the reduction of pain (elimination of chronic pain is generally unlikely and providers need to discuss these limitations with patients at outset).
- A written care plan that includes methods to address the patient's personal goals, improve sleep, increase physical activity, manage stress, and reduce pain.

NONPHARMACOLOGIC THERAPY

- Exercise (recommended for all patients and tailored to individual abilities and needs)
- Modalities: Heat therapy, cold therapy, transcutaneous electrical nerve stimulation (TENS) units, manipulative therapy, cognitive behavioral therapy, psychological counseling, and physical therapy
- Electrostimulation therapy: TENS units
- Behavioral therapies: Cognitive behavioral therapy, hypnosis, biofeedback, relaxation therapy
- Music therapy (in conjunction with other types of therapy)
- Surgery (rarely considered a first-line therapy for chronic pain)

GENERAL PHARMACOLOGIC Rx

- Short-acting antiinflammatory and analgesic medications (e.g., acetaminophen/NSAIDs/opioids). Avoid use of NSAIDs in patients with hypertension, CHF, or any type of CKD. These medications should be considered first-line therapy for all patients without contraindications
- Topical analgesics (lidocaine, NSAIDs, capsaicin)
- Trigger point or joint injections (immediate anesthetic plus long-acting corticosteroids)
- Epidural steroid injections
- Nerve blocks
- Antidepressants (tricyclic and selective serotonin reuptake inhibitors)
- Anticonvulsant medications (e.g., carbamazepine, valproic acid, gabapentin, pregabalin); particularly helpful for neuropathic conditions
- Implantable methods, epidural and intrathecal drug delivery systems, dorsal column stimulators
- Treatment of insomnia and sleep disorders to reduce pain with standard sleep-inducing agents (trazodone, antihistamines)
- Many patients may require combination drug therapy (CDT) for adequate control of pain, with appropriate attention given to interactions and side effects

OPIOID THERAPY

- Although a mainstay of treatment over the past two decades, limited evidence is available demonstrating the efficacy of both immediate- and long-acting opioid preparations. Some patients with severe chronic pain syndromes may still benefit from this form of treatment. Full opioid agonists are generally the drug of choice for severe chronic cancer pain.
- Opioids are rarely beneficial in the treatment of inflammatory or mechanical pain and are not indicated for treatment of headaches.
- The Centers for Disease Control and Prevention has published detailed guidelines for prescribing opioids for chronic pain in light of rising rates of opioid addiction and overdose. The guidelines include when and with whom to use opioid therapy, opioid selection, dosing, duration, and follow-up,

along with assessment of the risks, benefits, and discontinuation of therapy.

- Current recommendations include aiming for daily opioid doses of <50 MME/day to limit the risk of overdose and side effects, prescribing naloxone to patients receiving daily doses >50 MME/day, and avoiding doses >90 MME/day, or referral to a pain management specialist for close monitoring.
- Sustained-release opioids (used for moderate to severe pain that has failed other therapeutic interventions): Oxycodone, morphine SR, methadone (use with caution), or fentanyl patch; short-acting opioids can be used in conjunction with these agents for management of breakthrough pain. Conversion to a long-acting opioid should be based on an equianalgesic conversion. Table E1 compares morphine milligram equivalent doses for commonly prescribed opioids. (http://www.acpinternist.org/archives/2008/01/extra/pain_charts.pdf).
- Table 2 provides guidelines for opioid dose selection, conservative initial starting doses for opioid-naïve individuals, and conversion ratios for opioid rotation in patients on chronic opioids. Titration of these medications should not exceed the equivalent of 100 mg morphine/day to avoid risk of overdose. Box E1 summarizes CDC recommendations for prescribing opioids for chronic pain outside of active cancer and palliative and end-of-life care. Box E2 summarizes the interpretation of recommendation categories and evidence types.

MEDICAL MARIJUANA

- Limited studies on efficacy, side effects, or outcomes for use in CNCP
- Some small RCTs show benefit of low-dose cannabinoids for chronic neuropathic pain

COMPLEMENTARY & ALTERNATIVE MEDICINE

Acupuncture and massage (evidence-based for some indications). Acupuncture is most likely to benefit patients with low back pain, neck pain, chronic idiopathic or tension headache, migraine, and knee osteoarthritis. Recent evidence has demonstrated the benefit of modalities such as yoga, tai chi, and music therapies. Supplements, although popular, do not have substantial evidence to recommend for or against their use.

REFERRAL

- Pain medicine specialist or multidisciplinary pain clinic: Useful when primary therapies fail, in patients with complex pain conditions, in patients requiring a high daily MME, or for invasive therapies
- Consider referral to an addiction specialist if patient has a history of substance abuse or addiction
- Psychiatry/psychological services for counseling, if needed

PEARLS & CONSIDERATIONS

- Patient consent should be obtained in the form of a written treatment agreement before initiating treatment. This agreement should outline the goals of therapy, use of a single provider or treatment team and a single pharmacy, limitations on dose and number of prescribed medications, prohibition on use with alcohol or sedating medications, keeping medication safe and secure, prohibition on selling or sharing medication, limitations on refills, compliance with all components of the treatment plan, the role of drug screening, and consequences of nonadherence.
- Follow-up assessment should occur every 1 to 6 mo and include a complete pain assessment (see earlier), review of the type of long-acting analgesic used and dosage, use of breakthrough analgesics, side effects and their management, use of nonpharmacologic therapies, and adjunct medication use.

COMMENTS

- Medication dependence and addiction should not be confused. Most patients receiving chronic opioid therapy can become dependent on these medications for pain relief but opioid addiction does not occur. Patients exhibiting signs of addiction often will seek escalating doses of medication, request refills of prescriptions earlier than planned, and engage in drug-seeking activities (e.g., emergency department visits between prescriptions, seeking multiple prescriptions).
- Side effects need not preclude use of opioid medications and should be anticipated. Antiemetics can aid in controlling nausea. Constipation can be managed with stool softeners and laxatives.
- The emphasis of comprehensive pain management for noncancer-related chronic pain has led to a fourfold increase in prescribing of opioid medications in the United States. This increase in opiate use has also led to a rise in the misuse and abuse of these medications. Providers should proceed with caution before initiating pain management with opiate medications and should familiarize themselves with processes and tools for pain assessment and medication management. Forty-two states have developed prescription drug monitoring programs (PDMPs) to assist providers in identifying issues of abuse, polypharmacy, and misuse of controlled substances.

PATIENT & FAMILY EDUCATION

National Pain Foundation (http://www.painconnection.org)

American Pain Foundation (http://www.painfoundation.org)

National Institutes of Health (http://www.nih.gov)

SUGGESTED READINGS

Available at ExpertConsult.com

RELATED CONTENT

Pain Medications (Patient Information)

AUTHOR: **ANNGENE ANTHONY, M.D., M.P.H., F.A.A.F.P.**

P

Diseases and Disorders

TABLE 2 Guidelines for Opioid Dose Selection, Conservative Initial Starting Doses for Opioid-Naïve Individuals, and Conversion Ratios for Opioid Rotation in Patients on Chronic Opioids

Opioid Naïve	Morphine SR	Codeine	Oxycodone	Hydrocodone	Hydromorphone	Methadone	Fentanyl	Oxymorphone
Initial dose and range in opioid-naive patient (starting dose range for repeated dosing)*	15 mg (15-30 mg q 8-12h)	30 mg (15-60 mg q 4-6h)	5 mg (5-15 mg q 4-6h)	5 mg (5-10 mg q 4-6h)	2 mg (2-4 mg q 4-6h)	2.5 mg q 6-12h	NA	5 mg q 4-6h
Opioid Tolerant Converting from:	**Morphine PO**	**Codeine**	**Oxycodone**	**Hydrocodone**	**Hydromorphone**	**Methadone**	**Fentanyl**	**Oxymorphone**
Morphine IM 10 mg (the gold standard for opioid comparisons)	20-30 mg	60-90 mg†	5 mg	5-10 mg q 4-6h	2 mg	2.5 mg	25-μg patch/72 hr	5 mg (the gold standard for opioid comparisons)
Morphine SR 30 mg PO q 8-12h, 60-90 mg/24h		30-90 mg q 4h	3-45 mg/24 hr oxycodone, approx 50% of morphine dose	30-45 mg/24 hr	12-18 mg/24 hr	24-hr dose morphine 30-90 mg 4:1 conversion 90-300 mg 8:1 conversion >300 mg 12:1	25-mcg patch/72 hr	5 mg q 12h ER
Codeine 30-60 mg q 4h	15-30 mg q 3-4h		5-7.5 mg q 4h	5-10 mg q 4h	12 mg/24 hr	2.5 mg q 8-12h	12.5-μg patch/72 hr	2.5-5 mg q 4-6h IR
Oxycodone 5 mg q 3-4h	10 mg	30-60 mg q 3-4h		5-10 mg q 4h	12 mg/24 hr	2.5 mg q 8-12h	25-μg patch/72 hr	5 mg q 4-6h IR
Hydrocodone 10 mg q 3-4h	15 mg	30-60 mg q 3-4h	5 mg q 3-4h		12 mg/24 hr		12.5-μg patch/72 hr	2.5-5 mg q 4-6h IR
Hydromorphone 2 mg q 4h	10 mg		5 mg	5-10 mg q 4h		2.5 mg q 8-12h	25-μg patch/72 hr	5 mg q 4-6h IR
Methadone 5 mg q 8h	20 mg SR q 8h		10 mg q 3-4h		4 mg q 4-6h		25-μg patch/72 hr	5 mg q 12h ER
Fentanyl 25 μg/hr patch	90 mg morphine per 24 hr (1 μg to 4 mg morphine)					5 mg q 8-12h		5 mg q12h ER
Oxymorphone ER 5 mg q 12h	15 mg SR q 12h		5 mg q 8-12h	10 mg q 4-6h	12 mg/24 hr	5 mg q 8-12h	25-μg patch/72 hr	

NOTE: Recommended starting doses are low and should be titrated upward slowly to minimize adverse effects. Limitations of equianalgesic tables exist because they are based on single-dose studies in opioid-naïve individuals. Convert opioid 1 to morphine equivalents and calculate dose of opioid 2 according to conversion ratio then reduce the calculated dose for opioid 2 by 1/3 to 1/2 to ensure safety of the 24-hr total daily dose. Rescue dose is 10% to 20% of daily opioid dose given every 3 to 4 hr as needed. Titration upward for unrelieved pain should be by 25% to 30% of the current 24-hr dose, adjusted by daily amount of rescue medications needed over a several-week period. Equivalent or equianalgesic doses for the different opioid preparations vary in different publications. *ER,* Extended release; *IR,* immediate release.

*Conservative low equianalgesic starting doses for opioid-naïve individuals adapted from published recommendations.

†Doses above 1.5 mg/kg not recommended because of increase in side effects.

From Hochberg MC, et al.: *Rheumatology,* ed 5, St Louis, 2011, Mosby.

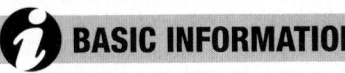

BASIC INFORMATION

DEFINITION

Pancreatic cancer is an adenocarcinoma derived from pancreatic duct epithelium.

ICD-10CM CODES
C25.9 Malignant neoplasm of pancreas, unspecified
C25.0 Malignant neoplasm of head of pancreas
C25.1 Malignant neoplasm of body of pancreas
C25.2 Malignant neoplasm of tail of pancreas
C25.3 Malignant neoplasm of pancreatic duct

EPIDEMIOLOGY & DEMOGRAPHICS

INCIDENCE: In the U.S., it is estimated that there will be 55,440 new cases and 44,330 deaths in 2018. It is the fourth leading cause of cancer-related death in the U.S. The majority of patients present with advanced disease, and less than 20% of patients present with potentially resectable tumors.
PREDOMINANT SEX: Male:female ratio of 2:1
PREDOMINANT AGE: Median age at diagnosis is 71 yr.

PHYSICAL FINDINGS & CLINICAL PRESENTATION

Presenting symptoms are generally related to location:

- Jaundice (60% to 70% of pancreatic cancers are located in the head of the pancreas).
- Abdominal pain: Generally dull upper abdominal pain or vague abdominal discomfort.
- Weight loss.
- Anorexia/change in taste, asthenia.
- Nausea.
- Uncommonly: Depression, gastrointestinal bleeding, acute pancreatitis (from obstruction of the pancreatic duct), back pain.
- Trousseau syndrome (hypercoagulability in the setting of malignancy) may be initial presentation in some patients.
- Table 1 summarizes demographic features and presenting symptoms in pancreatic cancer patients.

Physical findings:

- Icterus
- Cachexia, temporal wasting
- Ascites, peripheral lymphadenopathy, hepatomegaly
- Excoriations from scratching pruritic skin

ETIOLOGY

Unknown, but several conditions have been associated with pancreatic cancer:

- Smoking
- Alcoholism
- Genetics: 5% to 10% of patients have a family history of the disease
- Genetic syndromes and associated genes: Hereditary pancreatitis (*PRSS1, SPINK1*), Peutz-Jeghers syndrome (*STK11[LKB1]*), familial atypical multiple mole and melanoma syndrome (*p16*), hereditary breast and ovarian cancer syndromes (*BRCA1, BRCA2, PALB2*), ataxia telangiectasia (*ATM*), Li-Fraumeni syndrome (*P53*)
- Gallstones
- Diabetes mellitus (present in at least 50% of patients with pancreatic cancer)
- Chronic pancreatitis
- Diet rich in animal fat
- Occupational exposure: Oil refining, paper manufacturing, chemical industry
- Overweight or obesity during early adulthood is associated with a greater risk of pancreatic cancer and a younger age of disease onset. Obesity at an older age is associated with a lower overall survival in patients with pancreatic cancer
- There are four major driver genes for pancreatic cancer: *KRAS, CDKN2A, TP53*, and *SMAD4. KRAS* mutation and alterations in *CDKN2A* are early events in pancreatic cancer tumorigenesis.

Dx DIAGNOSIS

DIFFERENTIAL DIAGNOSIS

- Common duct cholelithiasis
- Cholangiocarcinoma
- Common duct stricture
- Sclerosing cholangitis
- Primary biliary cirrhosis
- Autoimmune pancreatitis
- Drug-induced cholestasis (e.g., phenothiazines)
- Other pancreatic tumors (islet cell tumor, cystadenocarcinoma, epidermoid carcinoma, sarcomas, lymphomas)

WORKUP

Initial laboratory testing includes complete blood count, serum chemistries. The bile duct antigen CA 19-9 is not used as a screening test but can be utilized as a modality for detecting recurrence and for therapeutic monitoring in patients undergoing therapy.

Routine Laboratory Tests	% Abnormal
Alkaline phosphatase	80
Bilirubin	55
Total protein	15
Amylase	15
Hemoglobin	60

IMAGING STUDIES

- Multidetector helical CT (Fig. E1) with IV administration of contrast is the imaging procedure of choice for initial evaluation.
- Endoscopic ultrasonography (Fig. E2) is useful when the diagnosis is strongly suspected and tissue is required for diagnostic purposes. Fine-needle aspiration biopsy combined with endoscopic ultrasonography is the preferred modality for evaluation of cystic or mass lesions to determine malignancy.
- Endoscopic retrograde cholangiopancreatography (ERCP, Fig. E3) is useful in patients with jaundice needing an endoscopic stent to relieve obstruction.
- PET scans are of limited value in pancreatic cancer and are not part of standard management.

Noninvasive Imaging	% Abnormal
Abdominal ultrasonography	60
Abdominal CT scan (with contrast) (Fig. E4)	90
Abdominal MRI scan Invasive Imaging	90
ERCP	90
CT scan or ultrasonography-guided needle aspiration cytology	90-95

STAGING

2018 AJCC EIGHT EDITION STAGING SYSTEM FOR PANCREATIC CANCER

PRIMARY TUMOR (T):

T_X Primary tumor cannot be assessed
T_0 No evidence of primary tumor
T_1 Tumor <2 cm
T_2 Tumor >2 cm and <4 cm

TABLE 1 Demographic Features and Presenting Symptoms and Signs in Patients with Unresectable (Palliated) and Resectable (Resected) Pancreatic Cancer

	Palliated (*N* = 256)	Resected (*N* = 512)
Demographic Features		
Age, average (yr)	64.0	65.8
Men/women	57%/43%	55%/45%
Race	91% white	91% white
Symptoms and Signs (%)		
Abdominal pain	64	36*
Jaundice	57	72*
Weight loss	48	43
Nausea/vomiting	30	18*
Back pain	26	2*

*P = 0.001 vs. palliated group.
From Feldman M, Friedman LS, Brandt LJ: *Sleisenger and Fordtran's gastrointestinal and liver disease*, ed 10, Philadelphia, 2016, Elsevier.

T_3 Tumor >4 cm
T_4 Tumor involves celiac axis or superior mesenteric artery (unresectable primary)

LYMPH NODES (N):

N_0 No regional lymph nodes
N_1 metastasis in 1-3 regional lymph nodes
N_2 metastasis in >4 regional lymph nodes

DISTANT METASTASES (M):

M_X Presence of distant metastasis cannot be assessed
M_0 No distant metastasis
M_1 Distant metastasis

STAGING GROUPS:

I_A	T_1, N_0, M_0
I_B	T_2, N_0, M_0
II_A	T_3, N_0, M_0
II_B	T_{1-3}, N_1, M_0
III	T_{1-3}, N_2, M_0 T_4, any N, M_0
IV	Any T, any N, M_1

Rx TREATMENT

Treatment sequencing strategies are summarized in Fig. 5 and Table 2.

SURGERY FOR RESECTABLE DISEASE

Curative cephalic pancreaticoduodenectomy (Whipple procedure) for tumors in the head and neck of the pancreas is appropriate for only 10% to 20% of patients whose lesion is <5 cm, solitary, and without locoregional invasion. Surgical mortality rate can be up to 5%. Tumors in the body or tail of the pancreas are removed by means of a distal pancreatectomy, which often includes a splenectomy. Due to the complexity of surgery and risk for significant morbidity and mortality, current guidelines recommend that pancreatic resections be carried out in centers that perform at least 15 to 20 cases annually. In addition, a recent review concluded that high-volume institutions are associated with higher negative-margin status and higher 5-yr survival rates, and that patients are more likely to receive multimodality therapy at these centers.

ADJUVANT THERAPY

Adjuvant chemotherapy has been demonstrated to improve postoperative survival in multiple randomized trials and is considered the standard of care in patients with resected cancers.

- The use of single agent 5-fluorouracil (5-FU) or gemcitabine is associated with median survival in the 20-24-month range and reserved for patients with older age or borderline status.
- The combination of gemcitabine and capecitabine is superior to gemcitabine alone in the adjuvant setting, with median overall survival in the 28-month range.
- Most recently, the use of a triplet chemotherapy combination regimen (FOLFIRNOX; 5-FU, oxaliplatin, and irinotecan) in this setting strikingly improves outcomes with median overall survival reported at 54 months.

The use of adjuvant radiotherapy in this setting is controversial and is best limited to patients with poor risk features, margin-positive surgery, or with multiple nodal or extranodal tumor involvement. An emerging strategy is the use of neoadjuvant preoperative chemotherapy combined with radiotherapy in patients with resectable pancreatic cancer. Palliative therapeutic ERCP with metal or plastic stents is performed for biliary decompression.

RECURRENT/METASTATIC DISEASE

In patients with metastatic disease, accepted approaches can include the administration of gemcitabine alone. More recently, a combination therapy regimen consisting of 5-fluorouracil, leucovorin, irinotecan, and oxaliplatin (FOLFIRINOX) offers increased median survival when compared with gemcitabine (11.1 mo versus 6.8 mo) but at the cost of increased toxicity. A second trial revealed that the combination of nab-paclitaxel plus gemcitabine significantly improved overall survival, but rates of peripheral neuropathy and myelosuppression were increased. Liposomal irinotecan in combination with infusional 5-fluorouracil is now also approved in this setting.

- Poor survival outcomes are seen in patients with poor performance status, significant weight loss, and with liver metastases.
- Combined chemotherapy and radiotherapy can be utilized in the case of patients with locally advanced but unresectable cases and confers a modest improvement in median overall survival.

DISPOSITION

- Adjuvant postoperative chemotherapy has a significant survival benefit in patients with resected pancreatic cancer.

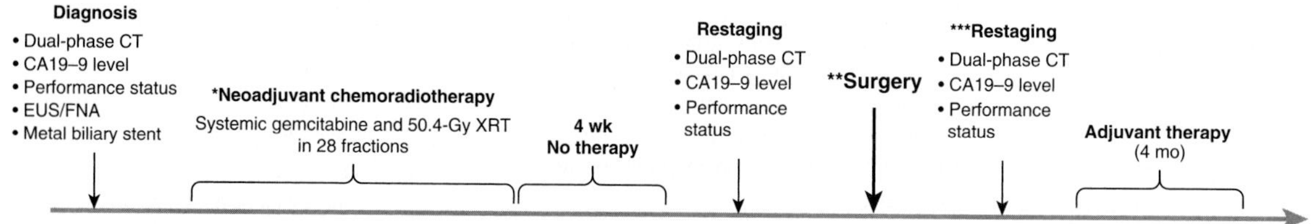

*Systemic therapy alone (FOLFIRINOX, gem-nab) is being considered by many clinicians because of the efficacy of these regimens in advanced disease and the challenges of delivering FOLFIRINOX in the adjuvant setting after such a large operation.
**Surgery is typically performed in the fifth week after the completion of XRT.
***Patients are restaged during postop week six if their recovery has been uncomplicated; however, there is no need to restage if recovery is complicated and the patient is not a suitable candidate to receive further systemic therapy.

A

Diagnosis
• Dual-phase CT
• CA19–9 level
• Performance status
• EUS/FNA
• Metal biliary stent
Neoadjuvant chemotherapy (2 mo)
Restaging
• Dual-phase CT
• CA19–9 level
• Performance status
Neoadjuvant chemoradiotherapy
Systemic gemcitabine and 50.4-Gy XRT in 28 fractions
4 wk No therapy
Restaging
• Dual-phase CT
• CA19–9 level
• Performance status
Surgery
Restaging
• Dual-phase CT
• CA19-9 level
• Performance status
*Adjuvant therapy (4 mo)

*The benefit of further postoperative/adjuvant systemic therapy after a more prolonged induction phase is being questioned, especially in those patients of advanced age or when postoperative recovery is slow.

B

FIG. 5 Schematic representation of treatment sequencing in **(A)** resectable and **(B)** borderline resectable pancreatic cancer (PC). *CA19-9*, Cancer antigen 19-9; *CT*, computed tomography; *EUS*, endoscopic ultrasound scan; *FNA*, fine-needle aspiration; *FOLFIRINOX*, 5-fluorouracil, leucovorin, irinotecan, and oxaliplatin; *gem-nab*, gemcitabine/nab-paclitaxel; *XRT*, external radiotherapy. (From Cameron JL, Cameron AM: *Current surgical therapy*, ed 12, Philadelphia, 2017, Elsevier.)

TABLE 2 Comparison of Treatment Sequencing Strategies for Patients with Pancreatic Cancer (outside of a clinical trial)

Stage	NCCN	MCW
Resectable	• Surgery • Restaging • Adjuvant therapy (+/− chemoradiotherapy; 6 months)	• Neoadjuvant chemoradiotherapy (5.5 wk)* • Restaging • Surgery • Restaging • Adjuvant therapy (4 months)
Borderline resectable	• Neoadjuvant therapy (regimen not specified) • Restaging • Surgery • Restaging • Consider adjuvant therapy	• Neoadjuvant chemotherapy (2 mo) • Restaging • Neoadjuvant chemoradiotherapy (5.5 wk) • Restaging • Surgery • Restaging • Adjuvant therapy (4 months)
Locally advanced	• Chemotherapy • Restaging • Chemoradiotherapy in selected patients	• Chemotherapy (minimum 4 months) • Restaging • Chemoradiotherapy • Restaging • Surgery in highly selected patients
Metastatic	• Systemic therapy • Clinical trial	• Systemic therapy • Clinical trial

NOTE: Clinical trials are preferred in all patients with pancreatic cancer (regardless of stage of disease) who have a performance status acceptable for treatment.

FOLFIRINOX, 5-fluorouracil, leucovorin, irinotecan, and oxaliplatin; *gem-nab*, gemcitabine/nab-paclitaxel; *MCW*, Medical College of Wisconsin; *NCCN*, National Comprehensive Cancer Network.

*Systemic therapy alone (FOLFIRINOX, gem-nab) is being considered by many clinicians because of the efficacy of these regimens in advanced disease and the challenges of delivering FOLFIRINOX in the adjuvant setting after such a large operation.

From Cameron JL, Cameron AM: *Current surgical therapy*, ed 12, Philadelphia, 2017, Elsevier.

- Adjuvant chemotherapy with FOLFIRINOX regimen significantly delays the development of recurrent disease after complete resection of pancreatic cancer. Median survival in this setting is approximately 54 months.
- Pancreatic cancer is usually diagnosed at an advanced stage and is resistant to therapy. Median survival for locally unresectable disease is about 14 to 16 months, while the median survival for metastatic disease is 10 to 12 months.

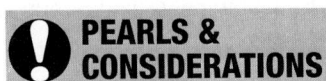

PEARLS & CONSIDERATIONS

COMMENTS

- The U.S. Preventive Services Task Force (USPSTF) recommends against routine screening for pancreatic cancer in asymptomatic adults by abdominal palpation, ultrasonography, or serologic markers. The USPSTF found no evidence that screening for pancreatic cancer is effective in reducing mortality rates. There is potential for significant harm because of the low prevalence of pancreatic cancer, limited accuracy of available screening tests, invasive nature of diagnostic tests, and poor outcome of treatment. Alcohol consumption, specifically liquor consumption of three or more drinks per day, increases pancreatic cancer mortality independent of smoking.
- Patients should be referred for pancreatic cancer surgery to high-volume medical centers that perform at least 15 to 20 cases a yr.
- Adjuvant chemotherapy with either a single-agent or doublet regimen for 6 months has been shown to improve survival and should be recommended in all patients with a maintained performance status after surgical resection. The role of radiotherapy in the adjuvant setting is best restricted to patients who have a high risk for locoregional recurrence.

SUGGESTED READINGS

Available at ExpertConsult.com

RELATED CONTENT

Pancreatic Cancer (Patient Information)

AUTHOR: **RITESH RATHORE, M.D.**

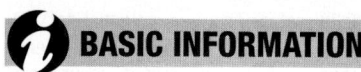

BASIC INFORMATION

DEFINITION

- Acute pancreatitis is an inflammatory process of the pancreas with intrapancreatic activation of enzymes that may also involve peripancreatic tissue and/or remote organ systems. The diagnosis of acute pancreatitis requires at least 2 of the following criteria: serum amylase or lipase ≥3 times normal, abdominal pain consistent with pancreatitis, and radiographic findings (CT or MRI) of acute pancreatitis.
- Commonly used scoring systems for acute pancreatitis are described in Table 1.

The **Revised Atlanta Criteria**[1] use early prognostic signs, organ failure, and local complications to define disease severity:

1. **Mild pancreatitis:** No organ failure, no local or systemic complications, pancreatitis typically resolves in first week
2. **Moderate pancreatitis:** Transient organ failure (≤48 hours) *or* local complications (e.g., pancreatic necrosis, peripancreatic fluid collections, peripancreatic necrosis) *or* exacerbation of comorbid disease
3. **Severe pancreatitis:** Persistent organ failure (>48 hours)

The **BALI Score**[2] evaluates only four variables:

1. BUN ≥25 mg/dl
2. Age ≥65 yr
3. LDH ≥300 U/L
4. Interleukin-6 level ≥300 pg/ml

These measurements are taken at admission and at 48 hours. Mortality is >25% for a score of 3 and exceeds 50% with a score of 4.

Severe acute pancreatitis (SAP) is diagnosed by the presence of any of the following four criteria:

1. Organ failure with one or more of the following: shock (systolic blood pressure <90 mm Hg), pulmonary insufficiency (Pao_2 ≤60 mm Hg), renal failure (serum creatinine >2 mg/dl after rehydration), and gastrointestinal bleeding (>500 ml/24 hr)
2. Local complications such as necrosis, pseudocyst, or abscess
3. At least three of Ranson criteria (see tables at end) *or*
4. At least eight of the Acute Physiology and Chronic Health Evaluation II (APACHE II) criteria

ICD-10CM CODES

K85.0 Idiopathic acute pancreatitis
K85.1 Biliary acute pancreatitis
K85.2 Alcohol induced acute pancreatitis
K 85.3 Drug induced pancreatitis
K85.6 Other acute pancreatitis
K85.9 Acute pancreatitis, unspecified

EPIDEMIOLOGY & DEMOGRAPHICS

- The incidence of pancreatitis is increasing in the U.S. Admissions for acute pancreatitis have increased dramatically, and acute pancreatitis was the number-one GI-related cause for admission across U.S. hospitals in 2012. There are >270,000 cases of acute pancreatitis reported annually in the United States, with nearly 40% due to gallstone disease (most common cause) and 30% due to alcohol.
- Incidence in urban areas is twice that of rural areas (20/100,000 persons in urban areas).
- 20% of patients have necrotizing pancreatitis; the remainder have interstitial, or edematous, pancreatitis.
- Drugs are responsible for less than 5% of all cases of acute pancreatitis.

PHYSICAL FINDINGS & CLINICAL PRESENTATION

- Epigastric tenderness and guarding, often radiating to the back; pain usually developing suddenly, reaching peak intensity within 10 to 30 min, severe and lasting several hours without relief. Rarely, some patients can have painless severe pancreatitis
- Nausea and vomiting (up to 90% of cases)
- Hypoactive bowel sounds (from ileus)
- Tachycardia, shock (from decreased intravascular volume)
- Confusion (from metabolic disturbances)
- Fever (SIRS response or infection when pancreatic necrosis is present)
- Decreased breath sounds (pleural effusions) or rales (atelectasis, acute respiratory distress syndrome [ARDS])
- Jaundice (from obstruction or compression of biliary tract)
- Ascites (from tear in pancreatic duct, leaking pseudocyst)
- Palpable abdominal mass (pseudocyst, phlegmon, abscess, carcinoma)
- Evidence of hypocalcemia (Chvostek sign, Trousseau sign)
- Evidence of retroperitoneal bleeding (hemorrhagic pancreatitis):
  1. Ecchymosis around the umbilicus **(Cullen sign)**
  2. Ecchymosis involving the flanks **(Grey Turner sign)**
- Tender subcutaneous nodules (caused by subcutaneous fat necrosis)

ETIOLOGY

- In >90% of cases: Biliary tract disease (calculi or sludge) or alcohol, most common after 5 to 10 yr of heavy drinking

TABLE 1 Commonly Used Scoring Systems: Advantages and Disadvantages

System	Scoring	Advantages	Disadvantages
Ranson criteria on admission: 1. Age >55 yr 2. WBC >16 × 10^9/L 3. LDH >350 U/L 4. AST >250 U/L 5. Glucose >200 mg/dl During initial 48 hr: 1. Hgb falls below 10 mg/dl 2. BUN rises by >5 mg/dl 3. Ca <8 mg/dl 4. Pao_2 <60 mm Hg 5. Base deficit >4 mEq/L 6. Fluid sequestration >6 L	One point for each factor listed; score >3 indicates SAP	Well known, relatively easy to calculate	Requires 48 hr to complete evaluation
APACHE II*	Score >8 predicts SAP	Can be calculated within 24 hr of admission	Requires large dataset for processing
BISAP 1. BUN >25 mg/dl 2. Altered mental status 3. Presence of SIRS 4. Age >60 yr 5. Pleural effusions	One point for each factor listed; score >3 indicates SAP	Ease of use, available within 24 hr of admission	Significantly lower sensitivity than either Ranson's or APACHE II; results in greater likelihood of missing severe AP
CTSI	Based on radiographic data	Excellent predictor of local complications; can show infected pancreatic necrosis	Requires 72 to 96 hr, making it a poor test for guiding decisions at admission

APACHE, Acute Physiology and Chronic Health Evaluation; *AST*, aspartate aminotransferase; *BISAP*, Bedside Index for Severity in Acute Pancreatitis; *BUN*, blood urea nitrogen; *Ca*, serum calcium; *CTSI*, Computed Tomography Severity Index; *Hgb*, hemoglobin; *LDH*, lactate dehydrogenase; *SAP*, severe acute pancreatitis; *SIRS*, systemic inflammatory response syndrome; *WBC*, white blood cell count.

*Based on diverse variables, including age, physiology, and long-term health; equation available at www.sfar.org/scores2/apache22.html#calcul. Adding body mass index (BMI) to APACHE II (the APACHE 0 score) increases discrimination (1 point added for BMI 26-30; 2 points for BMI >30).

From Cameron JL, Cameron AM: *Current surgical therapy*, ed 10, Philadelphia, 2011, Saunders.

[1] Banks PA, et al.: Acute Pancreatitis Classification Working Group: classification of acute pancreatitis-2012: revision of the Atlanta classification and definitions by international consensus, *Gut* 62(1):102-111, 2013.

[2] Spitzer AL, et al.: Applying Ockham's razor to pancreatitis prognostication: a four-variable predictive model, *Ann Surg* 243(3):380-388, 2006.

P

Diseases and Disorders

I

- Hypertriglyceridemia (usually >1000 mg/dl) from any cause
- Drugs (e.g., thiazides, furosemide, corticosteroids, tetracycline, estrogens, valproic acid, metronidazole, azathioprine, methyldopa, pentamidine, ethacrynic acid, procainamide, amiodarone, sulindac, nitrofurantoin, angiotensin-converting enzyme inhibitors, danazol, cimetidine, piroxicam, gold, ranitidine, sulfasalazine, isoniazid, acetaminophen, cisplatin, didanosine, opiates, erythromycin, metformin, GLP-1 receptor agonists, incretin mimetics)
- Abdominal trauma
- Surgery
- Endoscopic retrograde cholangiopancreatography (ERCP), especially with manipulation of the pancreatic duct
- Infections (predominantly viral)
- Peptic ulcer (penetrating duodenal ulcer)
- Pancreas divisum (congenital failure to fuse of dorsal or ventral pancreas)
- Idiopathic
- Pregnancy
- Vascular (vasculitis, ischemic)
- Hypercalcemia
- Pancreatic carcinoma (primary or metastatic)
- Renal failure
- Hereditary pancreatitis, such as in patients with cystic fibrosis
- IgG4 disease
- Occupational exposure to chemicals: Methanol, cobalt, zinc, mercuric chloride, creosol, lead, organophosphates, chlorinated naphthalenes
- Others: Scorpion venom, obstruction at ampulla region (neoplasm, duodenal diverticula, Crohn disease, rarely celiac disease), hypotensive shock, autoimmune pancreatitis

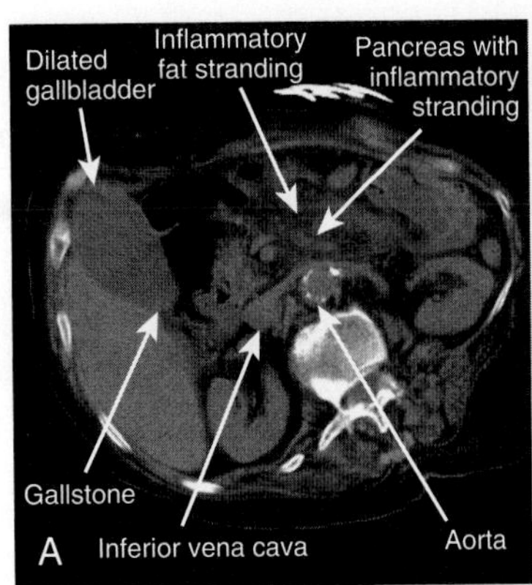

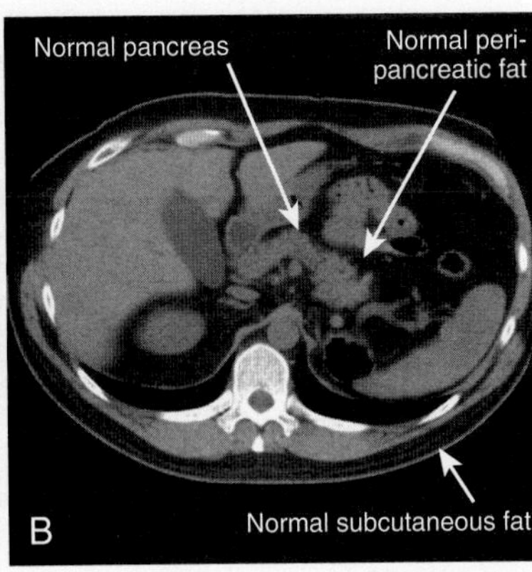

FIG. 1 Gallstone pancreatitis and normal pancreas for comparison, axial computed tomography without contrast. A, Gallstone pancreatitis CT. A dilated gallbladder is visible with a hyperdense dependent lesion consistent with a gallstone. The region of the pancreas shows significant inflammatory stranding. In this patient, the pancreas lies just anterior to the left renal vein, which can be seen crossing anterior to the aorta and entering the inferior vena cava. **B,** A normal pancreas is visible. This pancreas is surrounded by uninflamed fat, which is dark (nearly black). Compare this normal fat with normal subcutaneous fat. (From Broder JS: *Diagnostic imaging for the emergency physician,* Philadelphia, 2011, Saunders.)

Dx DIAGNOSIS

DIFFERENTIAL DIAGNOSIS

- PUD
- Acute cholangitis, biliary colic
- High intestinal obstruction
- Early acute appendicitis
- DKA
- Pneumonia (basilar)
- Myocardial infarction (inferior wall)
- Renal colic
- Ruptured or dissecting aortic aneurysm
- Mesenteric ischemia

LABORATORY TESTS

Pancreatic enzymes:

Amylase is increased, usually elevated in the initial 3 to 5 days of acute pancreatitis. Isoamylase determinations (separation of pancreatic cell isoenzyme components of amylase) are useful in excluding occasional cases of salivary hyperamylasemia. The use of isoamylase rather than total serum amylase reduces the risk of erroneously diagnosing pancreatitis and is preferred by some as initial biochemical test in patients suspected of having acute pancreatitis.

Urinary amylase determinations are useful to diagnose acute pancreatitis in patients with lipemic serum, to rule out elevated serum amylase caused by macroamylasemia, and to diagnose acute pancreatitis in patients whose serum amylase is normal.

Serum lipase levels are elevated in acute pancreatitis; the elevation is less transient than serum amylase and more sensitive in patients with alcoholic pancreatitis. Concomitant evaluation of serum amylase and lipase increases diagnostic accuracy of acute pancreatitis. Elevated serum trypsin levels are diagnostic of pancreatitis (in absence of renal failure).

Serum C-reactive protein is an excellent laboratory marker of severity; a level >150 mg/dl at 48 hr is associated with severe pancreatitis.

Rapid measurement of urinary trypsinogen-2 (if available) is useful in the emergency department as a screening test for acute pancreatitis in patients with abdominal pain; a negative dipstick test for urinary trypsinogen-2 rules out acute pancreatitis with a high degree of probability, whereas a positive test indicates need for further evaluation.

Interleukin-6 level: Worse prognosis with level ≥300 pg/ml.

ADDITIONAL TESTS

- Complete blood count: Reveals leukocytosis; hematocrit (Hct) may be initially increased as a result of hemoconcentration; decreased Hct may indicate hemorrhage or hemolysis.
- Blood urea nitrogen (BUN) is increased because of dehydration. Serial BUN measurements are the most valuable lab test for predicting mortality during the initial 48 hr.
- Elevation of serum glucose in a previously normal patient correlates with the degree of pancreatic malfunction and may be related to increased release of glycogen, catecholamines, and glucocorticoid release and decreased insulin release.
- Liver profile: Aspartate aminotransferase (AST) and lactate dehydrogenase (LDH) are increased as a result of tissue necrosis; bilirubin and alkaline phosphatase may be increased from common bile duct obstruction. A threefold or greater rise in serum alanine aminotransferase concentrations is an excellent indicator (95% probability) of biliary pancreatitis.
- Serum calcium is decreased as a result of saponification, precipitation, and decreased parathyroid hormone response.
- Arterial blood gases: Pao_2 may be decreased as a result of ARDS, pleural effusion(s); pH may be decreased as a result of lactic acidosis, respiratory acidosis, and renal insufficiency.
- Serum electrolytes: Potassium may be increased from acidosis or renal insufficiency; sodium may be increased from dehydration.

IMAGING STUDIES

- Abdominal plain films are useful initially to distinguish other conditions that may mimic pancreatitis (perforated viscus). They may reveal localized ileus (sentinel loop), pancreatic calcifications (chronic pancreatitis), blurring of left psoas shadow, dilation of transverse colon, calcified gallstones.
- Chest x-ray may reveal elevation of one or both diaphragms, pleural effusions, basilar infiltrates, or plate-like atelectasis.
- Abdominal ultrasonography is useful in detecting gallstones (sensitivity of 60%-70% for detecting stones associated with pancreatitis). Its availability and noninvasive nature make it the initial imaging study of choice; its major limitation is the presence of distended bowel loops overlying the pancreas.
- CT scan (Fig. 1) is less sensitive than ultrasound in identifying gallstones and exposes the patient to risk of contrast-induced nephropathy. It is, however, superior to ultrasonography in identifying pancreatitis and defining its extent, and it also plays a role in diagnosing pseudocysts (they appear as

TABLE 2 Computed Tomography (CT) Severity Index Score for Pancreatitis*

Grade†	CT Findings	Score
A	Normal pancreas	0
B	Focal or diffuse enlargement of the pancreas, contour irregularities, heterogeneous attenuation, no peripancreatic inflammation	1
C	Grade B plus peripancreatic inflammation	2
D	Grade C plus a single fluid collection	3
E	Grade C plus multiple fluid collections or gas	4
Percent Necrosis Present on CT		
0		
<33		
33-50		
>50		

*Severity Index Score = Grade score + Percent necrosis score. Maximum score = 10; severe disease = 6 or higher.
†Severity of the acute inflammatory process.
From Adams JG et al: *Emergency medicine, clinical essentials,* ed 2, Philadelphia, 2013, Elsevier.

a well-defined area surrounded by a high-density capsule); gastrointestinal fistulization or infection of a pseudocyst can also be identified by the presence of gas within the pseudocyst. Sequential contrast-enhanced CT is useful for detection of pancreatic necrosis. The severity of pancreatitis can also be graded by CT scan (Table 2). (A = normal pancreas, B = enlarged pancreas [1 point], C = pancreatic and/or peripancreatic inflammation [2 points], D = single peripancreatic collection [3 points], E = at least two peripancreatic collections and/or retroperitoneal air [4 points]. Percentage of pancreatic necrosis <30% [2 points], 30% to 50% [4 points], >50% [6 points]. The CT severity index is calculated by adding grade points to points assigned for percentage of necrosis.)

- Magnetic resonance cholangiopancreatography (MRCP) has >90% sensitivity for choledocholithiasis and can identify other anatomic abnormalities.
- Endoscopic ultrasonography (EUS) is a minimally invasive test that provides high-resolution imaging of the pancreas. It is useful to identify anatomic abnormalities of the pancreas and has good sensitivity and specificity for small gallstones (≤5 mm).
- ERCP indications: Useful to perform biliary sphincterotomy and stone removal in the presence of a retained bile duct stone seen on imaging. The role and timing of ERCP in patients with acute biliary pancreatitis has been controversial. Guidelines from the American College of Gastroenterology suggest that urgent ERCP (within 24 hr of admission) is indicated in patients with biliary pancreatitis who have concurrent acute cholangitis, but it is not needed in most patients who do not have evidence of ongoing biliary obstruction.[3,4,5]

[3] Fogel EL, Sherman S: ERCP for gallstone pancreatitis, *N Engl J Med* 370:150-157, 2014.
[4] Tenner S, et al.: American College of Gastroenterology guidelines: management of acute pancreatitis, *Am J Gastroenterol* 108:1400-1415, 2013.
[5] Bakker OJ, et al.: Early versus on-demand nasogastric tube feeding in acute pancreatitis, *N Engl J Med* 371:1983-1993, 2014.

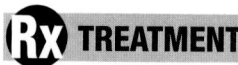

Rx TREATMENT

NONPHARMACOLOGIC THERAPY

- Bowel rest with avoidance of liquids or solids during the acute illness. Limited data suggest that early feeding in patients with acute pancreatitis does not seem to increase adverse events and, for patients with mild to moderate pancreatitis, may reduce length of hospital stay.[1]
- Avoidance of alcohol and any drugs associated with pancreatitis.

ACUTE GENERAL Rx

GENERAL MEASURES:

- Assess severity of pancreatitis (see Table 1).
- An algorithm for the management of acute pancreatitis is described in Fig. 2.
- Maintain adequate intravascular volume with vigorous IV hydration. Aggressive fluid resuscitation (250-500 ml/hr) with isotonic crystalloids is critical in managing acute pancreatitis, unless cardiac or renal disease precludes it.
- Patient should remain NPO until clinically improved, stable, and hungry. Enteral feedings are preferred over total parenteral nutrition if supplemental nutrition is necessary. Enteral nutrition reduces mortality, multiple organ failure, systemic infections, and operative interventions more than total parenteral nutrition does in patients with acute pancreatitis. Parenteral nutrition may be necessary in patients who do not tolerate enteral feeding or in whom an adequate infusion rate cannot be reached within 2 to 4 days. Early (within 24-48 hr of admission) enteral feeding through a nasogastric (NG) feeding tube has limited evidence to support this strategy. A recent trial did not show superiority of early NG tube feeding, as compared with oral diet after 72 hours, in reducing the rate of infection or death in patients with acute pancreatitis at high risk for complications.

[1] Vaughn VM, et al.: Early versus delayed feeding in patients with acute pancreatitis, a systematic review, *Ann Intern Med* 166:883-892, 2017.

- Nasogastric suction is useful only in severe pancreatitis to decompress the abdomen in patients with ileus.
- Control pain: IV hydromorphone or fentanyl. Meperidine and morphine are also commonly used narcotics for pain control, although morphine has been shown to increase sphincter of Oddi pressure and has delayed metabolite clearance in patients with concomitant renal failure.
- Correct metabolic abnormalities (e.g., replace calcium and magnesium as necessary).
- Prophylactic antibiotics are not recommended, regardless of the severity or presence of pancreatic necrosis.
- An algorithm for the management of acute pancreatitis at various stages is described in Fig. 2.

SPECIFIC MEASURES:

- Pancreatic or peripancreatic infection develops in 30% of patients with pancreatic necrosis. The use of antibiotics is justified if the patient has evidence of septicemia, pancreatic abscess, or pancreatitis caused by biliary calculi with concomitant cholangitis. Their use should generally be limited to 5 to 7 days to prevent development of fungal superinfection. Appropriate empiric antibiotic therapy should penetrate pancreatic necrosis. Options include a carbapenem alone (due to anaerobic coverage) or a quinolone, ceftazidime, or cefepime, combined with an enteric anaerobic agent such as metronidazole. CT-guided fine-needle aspiration (FNA) can be performed to culture the infected necrosis and tailor antibiotic therapy. If sampling of infected necrosis occurs and is sterile, antibiotics should be discontinued.
- Surgical therapy has a limited role in acute pancreatitis; it is indicated in the following:
  1. Gallstone-induced pancreatitis: Cholecystectomy when acute pancreatitis subsides. However, randomized trials have shown that patients with mild gallstone pancreatitis can undergo cholecystectomy safely during the first 48 hr of hospitalization.
  2. Perforated peptic ulcer.
  3. Necrotizing pancreatitis with infected necrotic tissue is associated with an elevated rate of complications and increased risk of death. Traditional treatment has been open necrosectomy; surgical necrosectomy induces a proinflammatory response and is associated with a high complication rate. Recent trials have shown that a step-up approach consisting of percutaneous drainage followed, if necessary, by minimally invasive retroperitoneal necrosectomy may have a lower rate of complications and death. Endoscopic transgastric necrosectomy, a form of natural orifice transluminal endoscopic surgery, has been shown in recent trials to be effective in reducing the proinflammatory response as well as reducing complications.

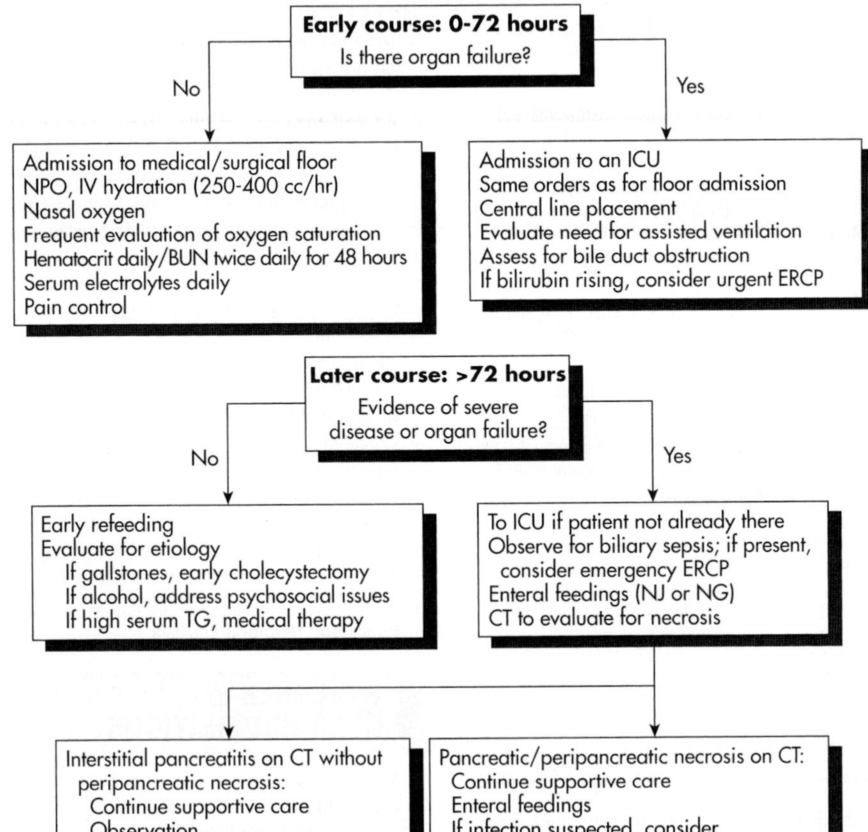

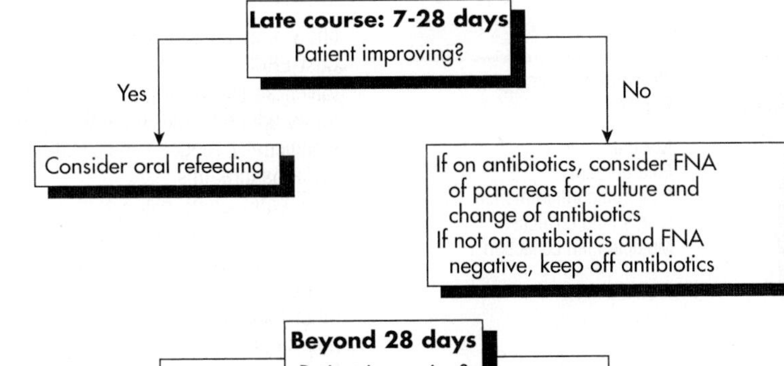

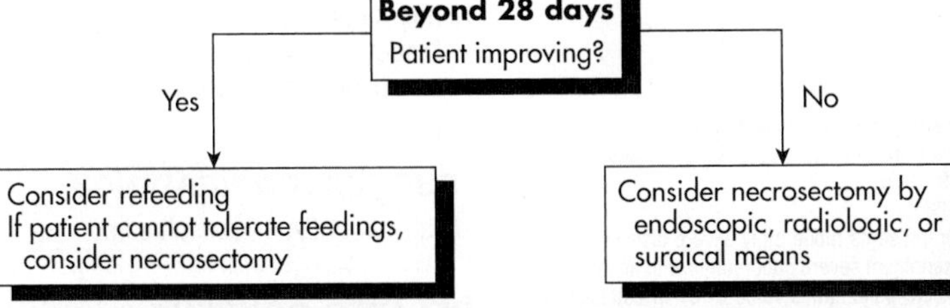

FIG. 2 Algorithm for the management of acute pancreatitis at various stages in its course. *NJ*, Nasojejunal. (From Feldman M, Friedman LS, Brandt LJ: *Sleisenger and Fordtran's gastrointestinal and liver disease*, ed 10, Philadelphia, 2016, Elsevier.)

- Identification and treatment of complications:
  1. **Pseudocyst:** Round or spheroid collection of fluid, tissue, pancreatic enzymes, and blood.
     a. Diagnosed by CT scan or sonography.
     b. Treatment: Pancreatic pseudocysts can be drained surgically or endoscopically. The endoscopic approach is preferable when the patient's anatomy is suitable and an experienced endoscopist is available. CT scan or ultrasound-guided percutaneous drainage (with a pigtail catheter left in place for continuous drainage) can be used, but the recurrence rate is high; the conservative approach is to reevaluate the pseudocyst (with CT scan or sonography) after 6 to 7 wk and surgically drain it if the pseudocyst has not decreased in size.
     c. Generally, pseudocysts <5 cm in diameter are reabsorbed without intervention, whereas those >5 cm require surgical intervention after the wall has matured.
  2. **Phlegmon:** Represents pancreatic edema. It can be diagnosed by CT scan or sonography. Treatment is supportive as it usually resolves spontaneously.
  3. **Pancreatic abscess:** Diagnosed by CT scan (presence of air in the retroperitoneum); Gram staining and cultures of fluid obtained from guided percutaneous aspiration usually identify bacterial organism. Therapy is surgical (or catheter) drainage and IV antibiotics (carbapenem is the drug of choice).
  4. **Pancreatic ascites:** Usually caused by leaking of pseudocyst or tear in pancreatic duct. Paracentesis reveals very high amylase and lipase levels in the pancreatic fluid; ERCP may demonstrate the lesion. Treatment is surgical correction if exudative ascites from severe pancreatitis does not resolve spontaneously.
  5. **Abdominal compartment syndrome:** Caused by intraabdominal leakage of fluids from volume resuscitation or ascites. Diagnosed with sustained intraabdominal pressure >20 mm Hg with new-onset organ failure.
  6. Gastrointestinal bleeding: Caused by alcoholic gastritis, bleeding varices, stress ulceration, or disseminated intravascular coagulation (DIC).
  7. Renal failure: Caused by hypovolemia, resulting in oliguria or anuria, cortical or tubular necrosis (shock, DIC), or thrombosis of renal artery or vein.
  8. Hypoxia: Caused by ARDS, pleural effusion, or atelectasis.
  9. Vascular: Splenic, portal, or superior mesenteric vein thrombosis; pseudoaneurysm.

THERAPY OF UNCOMMON FORMS OF PANCREATITIS

- **Autoimmune pancreatitis (AIP):** Fibroinflammatory disease characterized by an IgG4 lymphoplasmacytic infiltrate. It is a variant of chronic pancreatitis and has been associated with other autoimmune disorders (e.g., primary sclerosing cholangitis, Sjögren's syndrome). The inflammatory process is generally responsive to corticosteroid therapy. Older men aged 60 to 70 yr are primarily affected. Patients present with abdominal pain, weight loss, anorexia, and obstructive jaundice. Immunoglobulin G_4 levels are elevated. Radiographically on CT, the pancreas is diffusely enlarged, with a characteristic smooth, capsule-like rim ("sausage pancreas"). Features of type 1 and type 2 autoimmune pancreatitis are summarized in Table 3. Type II autoimmune hepatitis (idiopathic duct-centric chronic pancreatitis) is associated with inflammatory bowel disease and not related to IgG4 cell deposition.

TABLE 3 Features of Type 1 and Type 2 Autoimmune Pancreatitis

Feature	Type 1	Type 2
Histology	Lymphoplasmacytic infiltration Dense periductal infiltrate without damage to ductal epithelium Storiform fibrosis Obliterative phlebitis Abundant (>10 cells/HPF) IgG4-positive cells Fibroinflammatory process may extend to peripancreatic region	Periductal lymphoplasmacytic and neutrophilic infiltration Destruction of the duct epithelium by neutrophils (granulocytic epithelial lesion, or GEL) Obliterative phlebitis is rare No IgG4-positive cells
Average age at presentation	60-70 years	40-50, but may present in young adults and even children
Gender predominance	Male	Equal
Usual clinical presentations	Obstructive jaundice (75%) Acute pancreatitis (15%)	Obstructive jaundice (50%) Acute pancreatitis (33%)
Pancreatic imaging	Diffuse pancreatic enlargement (40%) Focal pancreatic enlargement (60%)	Diffuse pancreatic enlargement (15%) Focal pancreatic enlargement (85%)
IgG4	Level elevated in serum (≈2/3 of patients) Positive in staining of involved tissues	Not associated
Other organ involvement	Biliary strictures Pseudotumors Kidney Lung Others Retroperitoneal fibrosis Sialoadenitis	Not associated
Associated diseases	See above (other organ involvement)	IBD
Long-term outcome	Frequent relapses	Rare or no relapse

IgG4, Immunoglobulin G, subclass 4.
From Feldman M, Friedman LS, Brandt LJ: *Sleisenger and Fordtran's gastrointestinal and liver disease*, ed 10, Philadelphia, 2016, Elsevier.

TABLE 4 Prognostic Criteria for Acute Pancreatitis

Ranson Criteria*	Simplified Glasgow Criteria†	Computed Tomography Criteria‡
On admission: Age >55 yr	*Within 48 hr of admission:*	Normal
WBC >16,000/μL	Age >55 yr	Enlargement
AST >250 U/L LDH >350 U/L	WBC >15,000/μL	Pancreatic inflammation
Glucose >200 mg/dl	LDH >600 U/L	Single fluid collection
48 hr after admission:	Glucose >180 mg/dl	Multiple fluid collection
Hematocrit decrease by >10	Albumin <3.2 g/dl	
BUN increase by >5 mg/dl	Ca^{2+} <8 mg/dl	
Ca^{2+} <8 mg/dl	Arterial Po_2 <60 mm Hg	
Arterial Po_2 <60 mm Hg	BUN >45 mg/dl	
Base deficit >4 mEq/L		
Fluid sequestration >6 L		

AST, Aspartate aminotransferase; *BUN,* blood urea nitrogen; *LDH,* lactate dehydrogenase; *WBC,* white blood cells.
*Three or more Ranson's criteria predict a complicated clinical course. Data from Ranson JH et al: Prognostic signs and nonoperative peritoneal lavage in acute pancreatitis, *Surg Gynecol Obstet,* 143:209-219, 1976.
†Data from Blamey SL et al: Prognostic factors in acute pancreatitis, *Gut* 25:1340, 1984.
‡Grades A and B represent mild disease with no risk of infection or death. Grade C represents moderately severe disease with a minimal likelihood of infection and essentially no risk of mortality. Grades D and E represent severe pancreatitis with an infection rate of 30% to 50% and mortality rate of 15%. Data from Balthazar EJ et al: Acute pancreatitis value of CT in establishing prognosis, *Radiology,* 174:331, 1990.
From Goldman L, Ausiello D (eds): *Cecil textbook of medicine,* ed 24, Philadelphia, 2012, Saunders.

- **Hypertriglyceridemic pancreatitis (HTGP):** IV insulin therapy is the cornerstone of immediate treatment, with supplemental IV glucose infusion if the serum glucose levels are not elevated. IV heparin was previously used as well, but its effectiveness has come into question. Antihyperlipidemic agents (fibrates) should be initiated as adjuvant therapy as soon as possible for long-term control. Beneficial results have been reported with early (within 48 hr) initiation of apheresis with therapeutic plasma exchange when there is concomitant hypocalcemia, lactic acidosis, or other signs of organ dysfunction.

DISPOSITION

Prognosis varies with the severity of pancreatitis; overall mortality rate in acute pancreatitis is 5% to 10%. Prognostic criteria for acute pancreatitis are described in Table 4.

REFERRAL

- Hospitalization is indicated in moderate to severe cases of pancreatitis.
- Surgical consultation is needed in suspected gallstone pancreatitis, perforated peptic ulcer, or presence of necrotic or infected foci. Acute pancreatitis can generally be attributed to gallstones when patients have both abnormal liver enzymes and gallstones (or sludge) on imaging. Such patients should consider cholecystectomy prior to discharge to prevent recurrent pancreatitis.
- Gastroenterology consultation in severe or recurrent pancreatitis, when ERCP is needed for gallstone pancreatitis, or when the cause of pancreatitis is unclear.
- Consider intensive care unit transfer for patients who require aggressive fluid resuscitation and are at risk of volume overload from cardiac or renal causes. Similarly, consider transfer for patients with developing ARDS, patients with abdominal compartment syndrome (with surgical consultation), and those who require apheresis.

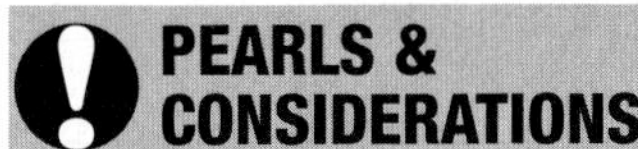

PEARLS & CONSIDERATIONS

- Acute pancreatitis is the most common major complication of ERCP. NSAIDs are potent inhibitors of phospholipase A_2, cyclooxygenase, and neutrophil-endothelial interactions, which play an important role in the pathogenesis of acute pancreatitis. Preliminary trials show that among patients at high risk for post-ERCP pancreatitis, rectal indomethacin (given as two 50-mg indomethacin suppositories administered immediately after ERCP) significantly reduced the incidence of post-ERCP pancreatitis.
- Pancreatic stent placement decreases the risk of post-ERCP pancreatitis.
- Statins reduce risk for pancreatitis in adults. Fibrates do not affect risk for pancreatitis other than in patients with hypertriglyceridemia-induced pancreatitis.
- Diabetes mellitus may develop from extensive pancreatic necrosis.

SUGGESTED READINGS

Available at ExpertConsult.com

RELATED CONTENT

Acute Pancreatitis (Patient Information)

AUTHOR: **DAVID J. LUCIER JR., M.D., M.B.A., M. P.H., C.P.P.S.**

BASIC INFORMATION

DEFINITION

Chronic pancreatitis is a recurrent or persistent inflammatory process of the pancreas characterized by chronic pain and by pancreatic exocrine and/or endocrine insufficiency. It is classified anatomically as either large-duct disease or small-duct (minimal change) disease.

ICD-10CM CODES

K86.1 Other chronic pancreatitis
K86.0 Alcohol-induced chronic pancreatitis

EPIDEMIOLOGY & DEMOGRAPHICS

- Chronic pancreatitis occurs in approximately five to 10 per 100,000 persons in industrialized countries.
- Average age at diagnosis is 35 to 55 yr; male:female ratio is 5:1.

PHYSICAL FINDINGS & CLINICAL PRESENTATION

- Persistent or recurrent epigastric and left upper quadrant pain that may radiate to the back
- Tenderness over the pancreas, muscle guarding
- Significant weight loss
- Bulky, foul-smelling stools, greasy in appearance
- Epigastric mass (10% of patients)
- Jaundice (5%-10% of patients)

ETIOLOGY

- Chronic alcoholism (most common cause)
- Obstruction (ampullary stenosis, tumor, trauma [with pancreatic duct stricture], pancreas divisum, annular pancreas)
- Tobacco
- Recurrent pancreatitis
- Vascular disease/ischemia
- Hypertriglyceridemia
- Chronic kidney disease
- Hereditary pancreatitis
- Severe malnutrition
- Idiopathic
- Untreated hyperparathyroidism (hypercalcemia)
- Mutations of the cystic fibrosis transmembrane conductance regulator *(CFTR)* gene and the TF genotype
- Other genetic mutations (Cationic trypsinogen gene, chymotrypsinogen C gene, calcium-sensing receptor gene, claudin-2 gene, serine protease inhibitor, Kazal type 1 gene)
- ***Autoimmune pancreatitis (AIP):*** (5% of chronic pancreatitis cases): Presents clinically with jaundice (63% of patients) and abdominal pain (35%). CT may reveal diffusely enlarged pancreas, enhanced peripheral rim of hypoattenuation "halo," and low-attenuation mass in head of pancreas. Laboratory values reveal elevated serum immunoglobulin (Ig) G4, elevated serum Ig or gamma-globulin level, presence of antilactoferrin antibody (ALA), anticarbonic anhydrase (ACA) II level, anti-smooth-muscle antibody (ASMA), or antinuclear antibody (ANA)
- ***Sclerosing pancreatitis:*** A form of chronic pancreatitis characterized by infrequent attacks of abdominal pain, irregular narrowing of the pancreatic duct, and swelling of the pancreatic parenchyma; patients have high levels of serum immunoglobulins (IgG4). Chronic sclerosing pancreatitis is also known as *autoimmune pancreatitis*

DIAGNOSIS

DIFFERENTIAL DIAGNOSIS

- Pancreatic cancer
- Peptic ulcer disease
- Cholelithiasis with biliary obstruction
- Malabsorption from other etiologies
- Recurrent acute pancreatitis
- Renal insufficiency
- Intestinal ischemia or infarction
- Other: Crohn's disease, gastroparesis, inflammatory bowel disease

WORKUP

Medical history with focus on alcohol use, laboratory tests, diagnostic imaging. Table 1 summarizes available diagnostic tests for chronic pancreatitis.

LABORATORY TESTS

- Serum amylase and lipase may be elevated (normal amylase levels, however, do not exclude the diagnosis).
- Hyperglycemia, glycosuria, hyperbilirubinemia, and elevated serum alkaline phosphatase may also be present.
- 72-hr fecal fat determination (rarely performed) reveals excess fecal fat. Fecal elastase test requires only 20 g of stool.
- Secretin stimulation test is the best test for diagnosing pancreatic exocrine insufficiency. Pancreatic secretory function tests are summarized in Table 2.
- Lipid panel: Significantly elevated triglycerides can cause pancreatitis.
- Serum calcium: Hyperparathyroidism is a rare cause of chronic pancreatitis.
- Elevated levels of serum IgG4 are found in sclerosing pancreatitis and AIP.
- Elevated serum Ig or gamma-globulin level, presence of ALA, ACA II level, ASMA, or ANA in AIP.

IMAGING STUDIES

- Plain abdominal radiographs may reveal pancreatic calcifications in 25% of patients (95% specific for chronic pancreatitis).
- Ultrasound of abdomen may reveal duct dilation, pseudocyst, calcification, and presence of ascites.
- Contrast-enhanced CT scan of abdomen is the initial modality of choice. It is useful to detect calcifications (Fig. 1), evaluate for ductal dilation (Fig. E2), AIP, and rule out pancreatic cancer. CT in AIP reveals narrowed main pancreatic duct and a homogenous "sausage-shaped" pancreas.
- Endoscopic retrograde cholangiopancreatography (ERCP) (Fig. E3) had been traditionally used to evaluate for the presence of dilated ducts, strictures, pseudocysts, and intraductal stones. However, for the evaluation of pancreatic parenchyma and duct system newer, less invasive modalities such as magnetic resonance cholangiopancreatography and endoscopic ultrasonography (EUS) are preferred. EUS (Fig. E4) has a sensitivity of 97% and a specificity of 60% for chronic pancreatitis and a very low complication rate. The diagnosis of chronic pancreatitis on EUS is summarized in Table 3. Fine-needle aspiration biopsy combined with EUS is the preferred modality for evaluation of cystic or mass lesions to determine malignancy.

TABLE 1 Available Diagnostic Tests for Chronic Pancreatitis*

Tests of Pancreatic Structure	Tests of Pancreatic Function
EUS	Direct hormonal stimulation (with pancreatic stimulation by secretin or CCK or both): Using oroduodenal tube† Using endoscopy†
MRI with MRCP, with or without secretin stimulation	Fecal elastase
CT	Serum trypsinogen (trypsin)
ERCP	Fecal chymotrypsin
Abdominal US	Fecal fat
Plain abdominal film	Blood glucose level

*Tests are listed in estimated order of decreasing sensitivity for each category.
†See text for explanations.
From Feldman M, Friedman LS, Brandt LJ: *Sleisenger and Fordtran's gastrointestinal and liver disease*, ed 10, Philadelphia, 2016, Elsevier.

TREATMENT

NONPHARMACOLOGIC THERAPY

- Avoidance of alcohol and tobacco
- Frequent, small-volume, low-fat meals

ACUTE GENERAL Rx

- Avoidance of narcotics if possible (simple analgesics or NSAIDs can be used). Fig. 5 describes an approach to the patient with painful chronic pancreatitis. Management of chronic pancreatitis focuses on treatment of symptoms.
- Treatment of steatorrhea with pancreatic supplements (e.g., Pancrease, Creon, pancrelipase titrated prn based on the amount of steatorrhea and patient's weight loss). Enzyme products for the treatment of chronic pancreatitis are summarized in Table 4. All non–enteric-coated enzymes should be used with acid-suppressing medications. Proton pump inhibitors and H_2 blockers reduce inactivation of the enzymes from gastric acid.
- Antioxidants (vitamin A, selenium, vitamin E) may be helpful for pain control in chronic pancreatitis.
- Percutaneous or via EUS celiac plexus blockade with corticosteroids or neurolysis with ethanol may provide temporary pain relief.

TABLE 2 Pancreatic Secretory Function Tests

Test	Description	Advantages	Disadvantages	Clinical Indications
Direct				
Secretin	Measurements of volume and HCO_3- secretion into the duodenum after IV secretin	Provide the most sensitive and specific measurements of exocrine pancreatic function	Require duodenal intubation and IV administration of hormones; not widely available	Detection of mild, moderate, or severe exocrine pancreatic dysfunction
CCK	Measurements of duodenal outputs of amylase, trypsin, chymotrypsin, and/or lipase after IV CCK			
Secretin and CCK	Measurements of volume, HCO_3-, and enzymes after IV secretin and CCK			
Indirect (Requiring Duodenal Intubation)				
Lundh test meal	Measurement of duodenal trypsin concentration after oral ingestion of a test meal	Does not require IV administration of hormones	Requires duodenal intubation, a test meal, and normal anatomy, including small intestinal mucosa; not widely available	Detection of moderate or severe exocrine pancreatic dysfunction when a direct test cannot be done (e.g., due to limited availability)
Indirect (Tubeless)				
Fecal fat	Measurement of fat in the stool after ingesting meals with a known amount of fat	Provides a quantitative measurement of steatorrhea	Requires sufficient dietary fat intake and collection of stool; only detects severe pancreatic dysfunction	Detection of severe exocrine pancreatic dysfunction and steatorrhea
Fecal chymotrypsin Fecal elastase 1	Measurement of chymotrypsin or elastase 1 in the stool	Do not require IVs, tubes, or administration of oral substrates	Insensitive for detecting mild or moderate dysfunction	Detection of severe exocrine pancreatic dysfunction
NBT-PABA Fluorescein dilaurate	Oral ingestion of NBT-PABA or fluorescein dilaurate with a meal, followed by measurements of PABA or fluorescein in serum or urine	Provide simple measurements for severe pancreatic dysfunction	Do not detect mild or moderate dysfunction; results may be abnormal in patients with small intestinal mucosal disease	Detection of severe exocrine pancreatic dysfunction

NBT-PABA, *N*-benzoyl-L-tyrosyl-*p*-aminobenzoic acid.
From Feldman M, Friedman LS, Brandt LJ: *Sleisenger and Fordtran's gastrointestinal and liver disease*, ed 10, Philadelphia, 2016, Elsevier.

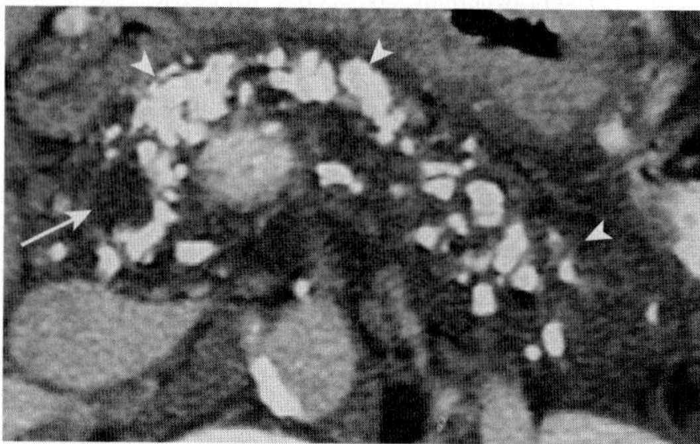

FIG. 1 Chronic pancreatitis: Calcifications. Numerous coarse calcifications are seen throughout the pancreas (*arrowheads*) in this patient with recurrent alcoholic pancreatitis. The common bile duct (*arrow*) is mildly dilated because of a benign stricture in the pancreatic head. (Webb WR et al: *Fundamentals of body CT*, ed 4, Philadelphia, 2015, WB Saunders.)

- Treatment of complications (e.g., type 1 diabetes mellitus).
- Autoimmune pancreatitis (AIP): Glucocorticoid therapy in patients with AIP and sclerosing pancreatitis can induce clinical remission and significantly decrease serum concentrations of IgG4, immune complexes, and the IgG4 subclass of immune complexes. Starting dose of oral prednisolone is 0.6 to 1.0 mg/kg/day tapered over 3 mo. Recurrent AIP is treated with glucocorticoids and immunomodulators (azathioprine, mycophenolate, mercaptopurine) or rituximab.

CHRONIC Rx

- Surgical intervention may be necessary to eliminate biliary tract disease and improve flow of bile into the duodenum by eliminating obstruction of pancreatic duct.
- ERCP with endoscopic sphincterectomy and stone extraction is useful in selected patients.
- Transduodenal sphincteroplasty or pancreaticojejunostomy in selected patients. Surgery should also be considered in patients with intractable pain.
- Percutaneous or EUS-guided celiac plexus blockade using glucocorticoids is effective in providing short-term pain relief in nearly half of patients.

DISPOSITION

- Long-term survival is poor (50% of patients die within 10 yr from chronic pancreatitis or malignancy).
- Prognosis is best in patients with recurrent acute pancreatitis resulting from cholelithiasis, hyperparathyroidism, or stenosis of the sphincter of Oddi.

REFERRAL

Gastrointestinal referral for ERCP, surgical referral in selected patients (see "Chronic Rx")

RELATED CONTENT

Chronic Pancreatitis (Patient Information)
Malabsorption (Related Key Topic)
Pancreatitis, Acute (Related Key Topic)

AUTHOR: **FRED F. FERRI, M.D.**

TABLE 3 Diagnosis of Chronic Pancreatitis on Endoscopic Ultrasound (EUS)

Standard EUS Grading System		Rosemont Criteria for EUS Diagnosis	
Parenchymal abnormalities	Hyperechoic foci Hyperechoic strands Lobularity of contour Cysts	Major features	Hyperechoic foci with shadowing (major A) Main pancreatic duct calculi (major A) Lobularity with honeycombing (major B)
Ductal abnormalities	Main duct dilatation Main duct irregularity Hyperechoic ductal walls Visible side branches Calcification	Minor features	Lobularity without honeycombing Hyperechoic foci without shadowing Stranding Cysts Irregular main pancreatic duct contour Main pancreatic duct dilatation Hyperechoic duct margin Dilated side branches

In the standard EUS grading system, each finding counts equally, and the score is the total number of findings. In the Rosemont system, the diagnostic strata are as follows:

Most consistent with chronic pancreatitis	One major A feature and ≥3 minor features *or* One major A feature and major B feature *or* Two major A features
Suggestive of chronic pancreatitis	One major A feature and <3 minor features *or* One major B feature and ≥3 minor features *or* ≥5 minor features
Indeterminate for chronic pancreatitis	Three to four minor features *or* One major B feature with <3 minor features
Normal	≤2 minor features

From Feldman M, Friedman LS, Brandt LJ: *Sleisenger and Fordtran's gastrointestinal and liver disease*, ed 10, Philadelphia, 2016, Elsevier.

 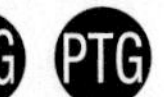

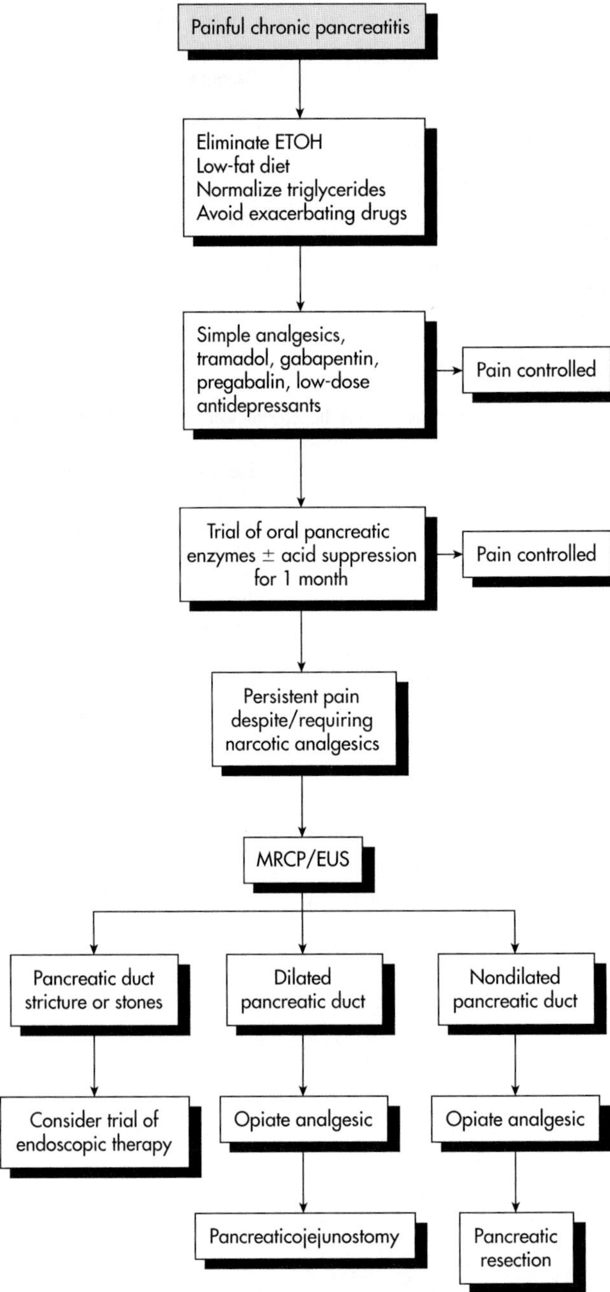

FIG. 5 Approach to the patient with painful chronic pancreatitis. *ETOH,* Alcohol; *EUS,* endoscopic ultrasound; *MRCP,* magnetic resonance cholangiopancreatography. (From Goldman L, Ausiello D [eds]: *Cecil textbook of medicine,* ed 24, Philadelphia, 2012, Saunders.)

TABLE 4 Enzyme Products for the Treatment of Chronic Pancreatitis

Product	Formulation	Lipase Content per Pill or Capsule (USP units)
Creon	Enteric-coated capsule	3000; 6000; 12,000; 24,000; 36,000
Zenpep	Enteric-coated capsule	3000; 5000; 10,000; 15,000; 20,000; 25,000
Pancreaze	Enteric-coated capsule	4200; 10,500; 16,800; 21,000
Ultresa	Enteric-coated capsule	13,800; 20,700; 23,000
Pertzye	Enteric-coated with bicarbonate	8000; 16,000
Viokase	Non–enteric-coated tablet*	10,440; 20,880

The total dose of lipase per meal should be titrated based on response but usually requires at least 60,000 and usually 90,000 USP units (30,000 international units) of lipase per meal and one half that amount with snacks. The dose should be split equally during the meal and immediately after the meal.

*Non–enteric-coated agents require cotreatment with an H2RA or PPI to avoid denaturation of the enzymes by gastric acid.

From Feldman M, Friedman LS, Brandt LJ: *Sleisenger and Fordtran's gastrointestinal and liver disease*, ed 10, Philadelphia, 2016, Elsevier.

BASIC INFORMATION

DEFINITION

- A **panic attack** is a relatively brief, sudden episode of intense fear or apprehension, often associated with a sense of impending doom and various uncomfortable and disquieting physical symptoms. Panic attacks may be uncued ("out of the blue") or cued (i.e., triggered by a particular object or situation). Panic attacks may be present in a variety of different anxiety-related disorders (e.g., phobias, social anxiety, obsessive-compulsive disorder). Table 1 describes criteria for diagnosis of panic attack.
- **Panic disorder** is diagnosed after at least two uncued panic attacks have occurred followed by at least 1 mo (or more) of significant concern about future attacks, worry about their implications, or a major change in behavior related to these attacks. The criteria for diagnosis of panic disorder are summarized in Table 2. **Agoraphobia** is anxiety about, and avoidance of, places or situations in which the ability to escape is perceived to be limited or embarrassing or in which help might not be available in the event of having a panic attack.

SYNONYMS

Anxiety attacks
Fear attacks
Ataque de nervios

ICD-10CM CODES
F41.0 Panic disorder
F40.0 Agoraphobia
DSM-5 CODES
300.01 Panic disorder
300.22 Agoraphobia

EPIDEMIOLOGY & DEMOGRAPHICS

INCIDENCE (IN U.S.): 1% 1-mo incidence of panic attacks

TABLE 1 Criteria for Diagnosis of a Panic Attack

A discrete period of intense fear or discomfort, in which ≥4 of the following symptoms developed abruptly and reached a peak within 10 min:

- Palpitations, pounding heart, or accelerated heart rate
- Sweating
- Trembling or shaking
- Sensations of shortness of breath or being smothered
- Feeling of choking
- Chest pain or discomfort
- Nausea or abdominal distress
- Feeling dizzy, unsteady, light-headed, or faint
- Derealization (feelings of unreality) or depersonalization (being detached from oneself)
- Fear of losing control or going crazy
- Paresthesias (numbness or tingling sensations)
- Chills or hot flashes

From Kliegman RM, et al.: *Nelson essentials of pediatrics,* ed 5, Philadelphia, 2006, Saunders.

PREVALENCE (IN U.S.):

- 15% to 20% lifetime prevalence of one or more panic attacks.
- Panic disorder is much more uncommon, with a lifetime prevalence of 1.5% to 3.5%; chronicity of condition reflected by a similar 1-yr prevalence rate of 1% to 2%.
- Agoraphobia is relatively rare; 0.3% to 1% lifetime prevalence; 30% to 50% of patients diagnosed with panic disorder also have agoraphobia.
- Lower rates of panic disorder are reported among Latinos, African Americans, Caribbean blacks, and Asian Americans (DSM-5).
- Lower estimates for Asian, African, and Latin American countries (0.1% to 0.8%) (DSM-5).

PEAK INCIDENCE:

- Chronic condition with a waxing and waning course.
- Bimodal incidence peaks noted, with the first peak between ages 15 and 24 yr and second peak between ages 35 and 44 yr.

PREDOMINANT SEX:

- Women more commonly affected (>85% of clinical population).
- Panic disorder twice as common in women.
- Panic disorder with agoraphobia three times as common in women.

PREDOMINANT AGE:

- Age of onset is typically late adolescence to mid-30s. Onset earlier in males (24 yr) than females (28 yr).
- Onset after age 45 yr is rare and should raise suspicion of different etiology.

GENETICS:

- Risk of developing panic disorder in first-degree relatives of individuals with panic disorder is four to seven times that of general population.
- Findings in twin studies: Approximately 60% of contributing factors to panic are genetic.

PHYSICAL FINDINGS & CLINICAL PRESENTATION

Panic disorder:

- Present either with a panic attack or with fear and anxiety related to anticipation of a future panic attack or its implications.
- Typical presentation: Unexpected, untriggered periods of intense anxiety and fear with associated physiologic changes (e.g., palpitations, sweating, tremulousness, shortness of breath, chest pain, gastrointestinal distress, faintness, derealization, paresthesia). This is accompanied by associated fears of dying, heart attack, stroke, passing out, losing control, or losing one's mind. Panic attacks are often described as "the most terrifying" episode an individual has experienced.

TABLE 2 Criteria for Diagnosis of Panic Disorder

1. Recurrent unexpected panic attacks with associated worry or behavior change
2. Not due to effects of a drug, medication, or medical condition

- Emergency or physician visits often occasioned by physical symptoms such as chest pain, dizziness, or difficulty breathing. Thirty percent of patients presenting with chest pain have panic disorder.
- In a recent study of 1327 patients reporting noncardiac chest pain, 77.1% had visited the emergency department.
- Patients reporting a fear of dying from a panic attack tend to have more symptomatic panic attacks and agoraphobia.

Agoraphobia:

- Rare complaints to physician. May manifest in missed office visits or tardiness. Patients may request home visits or telephone care.
- Activities usually self-limited by avoiding public situations where the patient believes he or she might experience a panic attack and would be unable to exit readily, such as the following:
  1. Crowded public areas (stores, public transportation, flying, church)
  2. Individual interactions (hairdresser, dentist, neighborhood meetings)
  3. Driving (especially if alone, far from home, over bridges, through tunnels, on highways, or on isolated roads)
- On exposure to or anticipation of exposure to feared situations, significant anxiety occurs. Anxiety may generate somatic symptoms that trigger a full-blown panic attack. Patients believe that escape from these situations reduces the alarming symptoms, thus reinforcing future avoidance. In actuality, symptom relief stems from adrenaline breaking down in the body after approximately 20 minutes.

ETIOLOGY

Hypotheses (NOTE: There are sufficient data to support each model. Models are not mutually exclusive.):

- Central dyscontrol of autonomic arousal (typically localized to the locus ceruleus); similar symptoms may be chemically induced with yohimbine, caffeine, or cholecystokinin.
- Cognitive overreaction (i.e., "catastrophic misinterpretation") to relatively mild or benign physiologic cues that then triggers a genuine autonomic cascade and further misinterpretations.
- Dysfunction of a central suffocation alarm mechanism; some signs of compensated respiratory alkalosis. Can be experimentally induced with sodium lactate or carbon dioxide.

RISK FACTORS

- Temperamental: Negative affect and anxiety sensitivity are risk factors for the onset of panic attacks. Severe separation anxiety in childhood may precede the panic disorder.
- Environmental: Sexual and physical abuse in childhood is common in panic disorder. Most panic sufferers are able to identify a coalescence of stressors preceding their first panic attack.
- Genetic and physiological: Although the exact genes are unknown, it is believed that multiple genes contribute to the vulnerability to panic attacks.

Panic Disorder, with or without Agoraphobia PTG

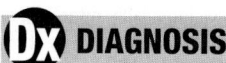

DIAGNOSIS

DIFFERENTIAL DIAGNOSIS

Medical conditions:

- Endocrinopathies:
  1. Hyperthyroidism
  2. Hyperparathyroidism
  3. Pheochromocytoma
  4. Carcinoid tumor
- Cardiac and respiratory diseases:
  1. Arrhythmias
  2. Myocardial infarction
  3. Chronic obstructive pulmonary disease
  4. Asthma
  5. Mitral valve prolapse
- Metabolic:
  1. Hypoglycemia
  2. Electrolyte imbalances
  3. Porphyria
- Seizure disorders
- Psychiatric disorders (NOTE: Panic attacks are common in a variety of psychiatric disorders. Panic disorder could be conceptualized as a phobia of the somatic sensations or situations that have become paired with panic attacks.)
  1. Phobias (e.g., specific phobia or social phobia). Note that fear of going on a plane because of crashing would be a specific phobia, whereas fear of going on a plane because one is then trapped and worries about panic is more suggestive of panic disorder with agoraphobia
  2. Obsessive-compulsive disorder (cued by exposure to the object of the obsession)
  3. Posttraumatic stress disorder (cued by recall of a stressor)
  4. Generalized anxiety disorder (cued by excessive worry)
- Therapeutic (theophylline, steroids) and recreational (cocaine, amphetamine, caffeine, diet pills) drugs and drug withdrawal (alcohol, cannabis, barbiturates, benzodiazepines)

WORKUP

- Emergency presentation: Cardiac, respiratory, or neurologic symptoms
- History and physical examination to rule out a concomitant medical or substance-related condition

NOTE: Panic disorder and agoraphobia are not diagnoses of exclusion, but exclusion of other conditions is usually required.

LABORATORY TESTS

- Thyroid profile
- Electrolyte measures, including calcium
- Toxicology screen
- ECG
- Acute cases: Possible monitoring and cardiac enzymes to rule out arrhythmia or ischemia

IMAGING STUDIES

- For temporal lobe dysfunction (e.g., temporal lesions or as ictal or interictal manifestation of temporal lobe seizures): Brain CT scan or MRI or an electroencephalogram in some patients
- Holter monitor to rule out occult or episodic arrhythmias
- Chest x-ray, arterial blood gases, or pulmonary function tests if respiratory compromise suspected

Rx TREATMENT

NONPHARMACOLOGIC THERAPY

- Cognitive-behavioral therapy (CBT), in particular Panic Controlled Treatment, is generally very effective, with strongest results for cognitive restructuring (i.e., challenging catastrophic misinterpretations of somatic symptoms), in vivo or imaginal exposures (i.e., exposure to panic triggers in a controlled graded hierarchical fashion from least to most difficult with the goal of habituation and extinction of the fear response), and interoceptive exposures (i.e., repeated recreation and management of feared somatic sensations via activities such as chair spinning, straw breathing, and hyperventilation).
- CBT effect sizes are equal to or larger than for pharmacotherapy, attrition rates are lower, and relapse rates are lower. Treatment may take several sessions spread over weeks and may require referral to a behavioral specialist. CBT has been shown to be the most effective intervention for panic disorder with or without agoraphobia across treatment sites.
- A recent dismantling study of cognitive-behavioral therapy components for panic disorder suggests that interoceptive exposure and a face-to-face setting were associated with better treatment efficacy whereas muscle relaxation and virtual reality exposure were associated with significantly lower efficacy.

ACUTE GENERAL Rx

- Benzodiazepines, particularly alprazolam: Highly effective in the acute setting, although long-term use is contraindicated for effective outcome.
- Low-dose alprazolam for patients with rare panic attacks and asymptomatic periods (0.25-0.5 mg PO or sublingually prn).
- Start patient on selective serotonin reuptake inhibitor (SSRI) or similar agent and taper patient off benzodiazepine by wk 2 to 3.

CHRONIC Rx

- Preferred pharmacologic agents: Antidepressants with a significant serotonin reuptake inhibitory action. Generally start at low dose and titrate upward. Minimum treatment duration is 6 to 8 mo, but many patients need to take medications indefinitely
  1. SSRIs: Paroxetine (10-60 mg/day), sertraline (50-200 mg/day), citalopram (20-60 mg/day), escitalopram (5-30 mg/day), and fluoxetine (5-60 mg/day)
  2. Imipramine (100-300 mg/day)
  3. Venlafaxine (75-225 mg/day)
- Combination CBT plus SSRI has shown good long-term effects and is somewhat better than antidepressants or CBT alone. Combination CBT plus benzodiazepine does not provide any added benefit and may undermine CBT (interoceptive and in vivo exposures may be less effective if the benzodiazepine is completely controlling the anxiety).

DISPOSITION

- Typical course is chronic but with significant waxing and waning (common to have long periods of remission).
- Presence of agoraphobia associated with a more chronic course.
- Findings with long-term follow-up studies: 6 to 10 yr after treatment some 30% are in remission, 40% to 50% have improved with residual symptoms, and the remainder are either unchanged or worse.

REFERRAL

- If patients do not respond to an SSRI.
- Cognitive-behavioral therapy is the preferred treatment.

PEARLS & CONSIDERATIONS

- Patient and family education is an important first step in the management of panic disorder. Education provides more adaptive explanations for the benign somatic sensations paired with panic. Presentation of genetic information and explanation of the benign nature of the physiology of each of the symptoms the patient experiences serve as a good start to allay fears and reduce stigma.
- Resumption of avoided activities or situations is a positive prognostic sign and may promote further therapeutic gains.
- The therapist's adherence to the treatment protocol and the therapeutic alliance established during the first session predict a better outcome for the long-term success of CBT for panic disorder with or without agoraphobia.

SUGGESTED READINGS

Available at ExpertConsult.com

RELATED CONTENT

Panic Disorder (Patient Information)

AUTHOR: **JEFFREY P. WINCZE, PH.D.**

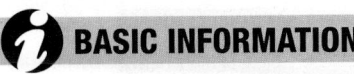

BASIC INFORMATION

DEFINITION

Panniculitis refers to inflammation of subcutaneous fat. Most cases are found in association with a systemic disease. Panniculitis can be separated into groups based on histopathologic characteristics. Panniculitis is classified into lobular or septal panniculitis based on whether the inflammation is seen in the fat lobules or septae, respectively. It can be further classified based on whether the inflammation is found with or without vasculitis (Table 1) and by predominant cell type. A classification of the subtypes of panniculitis is summarized in Box 1.

ICD-10CM CODES

M79.3	Unspecified panniculitis
M5400	Panniculitis affecting regions of neck and back, site unspecified
M5401	Panniculitis affecting regions of neck and back, occipito-atlanto-axial region
M5402	Panniculitis affecting regions of neck and back, cervical region
M54.03	Panniculitis affecting regions of neck and back, cervicothoracic region
M54.04	Panniculitis affecting regions of neck and back, thoracic region
M54.05	Panniculitis affecting regions of neck and back, thoracolumbar region
M54.06	Panniculitis affecting regions of neck and back, lumbar region
M54.07	Panniculitis affecting regions of neck and back, lumbosacral region
M54.08	Panniculitis affecting regions of neck and back, sacral and sacrococcygeal region
M54.09	Panniculitis affecting regions, neck and back, multiple sites in spine

EPIDEMIOLOGY & DEMOGRAPHICS

The epidemiology of the various panniculitides varies with each disease process. The most common panniculitis is erythema nodosum (refer to topic "Erythema Nodosum"). Another common panniculitis seen in the clinical setting is lipodermatosclerosis (LDS), which is usually seen in young, overweight females with associated venous insufficiency.

PHYSICAL FINDINGS & CLINICAL PRESENTATION

- Skin lesions can appear as nonspecific areas of erythema or erythematous nodules and/or plaques. The nodules can be palpated beneath the dermis. Ulceration, atrophy, and sclerosis can be associated clinical features of these lesions.
- The lesions are frequently painful and tender to palpation.
- Associated constitutional symptoms such as low-grade fevers, malaise, fatigue, myalgias, and arthralgias may be present.
- These skin findings usually are found on the lower limbs; however, the location of these lesions can vary with each specific panniculitis, that is, erythema nodosum is found on the pretibial areas of the lower extremities (Fig. 1), erythema induratum occurs on the calf, and lupus panniculitis occurs on the upper arms, shoulders, and face.
- Skin findings tend to evolve as the types of inflammatory cells change over the course of a few days.

ETIOLOGY

Panniculitis can be either primary/idiopathic or secondary. Common secondary etiologies can be classified into the following broad categories:

- Infections: Bacterial (streptococci), mycobacterial, fungal, parasitic, and viral.
- Inflammatory/connective tissue disease: Erythema nodosum, erythema induratum, lipodermatosclerosis, lupus panniculitis, cutaneous polyarteritis nodosa, dermatomyositis-associated panniculitis.
- Malignancy: Subcutaneous panniculitis-like type T-cell lymphoma.
- Pancreatic disease: Pancreatic panniculitis, which is associated with pancreatitis or pancreatic carcinoma.
- Immunodeficiency states: Alpha-1 antitrypsin deficiency panniculitis, which is associated with pulmonary and hepatic disease.
- Trauma: Cold panniculitis (due to exposure to the cold), traumatic panniculitis, and factitial panniculitis (due to injection of medication or foreign substances into the subcutaneous fat).
- Deposition: Calciphylaxis, gout.

Panniculitis can be a sign of an underlying systemic disease. Lupus panniculitis can occur alone or may present before or after the onset of either discoid lupus erythematosus or systemic lupus erythematosus.

DIAGNOSIS

DIFFERENTIAL DIAGNOSIS

- The skin lesions of panniculitis need to be distinguished from other skin lesions that may manifest similarly, such as insect bites, thrombophlebitis, and cellulitis.
- Disorders affecting the deep dermis or fascia (i.e., plaque morphea, eosinophilic fasciitis), benign or malignant tumors manifesting as subcutaneous nodules, and nodules with deep bruising may have similar clinical findings and be difficult to distinguish from panniculitis.

WORKUP

- Diagnosis of panniculitis depends on a thorough history and physical examination, evaluation of patient's risk factors, skin lesion appearance and distribution, as well as any associated clinical findings.
- If the diagnosis is unclear or needs to be confirmed, a deep skin biopsy should be performed. The preferred biopsy is an excisional biopsy, but a large 6- to 8-mm punch biopsy may be sufficient.

Although the above often establishes a diagnosis, there are times when it is difficult to accurately diagnose a specific panniculitis. Different forms of panniculitides have similar clinical findings while others are rare, complicating the presentation. Biopsy specimens may be too superficial to assess for the involvement of the subcutaneous fat or to assess for the presence of vasculitis. Inflammation of the subcutaneous fat is a changing process, with varying histologic findings as well as physical characteristics of skin lesions based on the stage of evolution. Cellular infiltrates may not be confined to one location in the subcutaneous fat, and may overlap between septa and lobules (Fig. 2).

TABLE 1 Classification of Panniculitis

I. Without prominent vasculitis
  A. Septal inflammation
    1. Lymphocytic and mixed: Erythema nodosum and variants.
    2. Granulomatous: Palisaded granulomatous diseases, sarcoidosis, subcutaneous infection: tuberculosis, syphilis.
    3. Sclerotic: Scleroderma, eosinophilic fasciitis, lipodermatosclerosis, toxins.
  B. Lobular inflammation
    1. Neutrophilic: Infection, ruptured folliculitis and cysts, pancreatic fat necrosis.
    2. Lymphocytic: Lupus panniculitis, post-steroid panniculitis, lymphoma/leukemia.
    3. Macrophagic: Histiocytic cytophagic panniculitis.
    4. Granulomatous: Erythema induratum/nodular vasculitis, palisaded granulomatous diseases, sarcoidosis, Crohn's disease.
    5. Mixed inflammation with many foam cells: α1-antitrypsin deficiency, traumatic fat necrosis.
    6. Eosinophilic: Eosinophilic panniculitis, arthropod bites, parasites.
    7. Enzymatic fat necrosis: Pancreatic enzyme panniculitis.
    8. Crystal deposits: Scleredema neonatorum, subcutaneous fat necrosis of the newborn, gout, oxalosis.
    9. Embryonic fat pattern: Lipoatrophy, lipodystrophy.
II. With prominent vasculitis (septal or lobular)
  A. Neutrophilic: Leukocytoclastic vasculitis, subcutaneous polyarteritis nodosa, thrombophlebitis, ENL.
  B. Lymphocytic: Nodular vasculitis, perniosis, angiocentric lymphomas.
  C. Granulomatous: Nodular vasculitis/erythema induratum, ENL, granulomatosis with polyangiitis, Churg-Strauss allergic granulomatosis.
III. Mixed patterns

ENL, Erythema nodosum leprosum.
From Lee L, Werth V: The skin and rheumatic diseases: panniculitis, In Firestein G et al [eds]: *Kelley's textbook of rheumatology,* ed 9, Philadelphia, 2013, Elsevier Saunders, p. 611.

BOX 1 Classification of the Subtypes of Panniculitis

Erythema nodosum
Infection
  Bacterial
  Mycobacterial (erythema induratum of Bazin)
  Fungal
Enzymatic disorders
  α1-Antitrypsin disease
  Pancreatic disease
Poststeroid
Malignant panniculitis
  Cytophagic histiocytic panniculitis
  Subcutaneous panniculitis-like T-cell lymphoma
  Edematous, scarring vasculitic panniculitis (hydroa-like lymphoma)
Lipoatrophic panniculitis
  Associated with autoimmune disorders: Systemic lupus erythematosus, deep morphea, juvenile dermatomyositis (usually subclinical), polyarteritis nodosa
  Lipophagic panniculitis of childhood
  Atrophic connective tissue panniculitis of the ankles
  Recurrent lobular panniculitis
Physical agents
  Cold panniculitis (popsicle, equestrian)
  Injections, including factitial
  Blunt trauma
Subcutaneous fat necrosis of the newborn
Sclerema neonatorum
Selected syndromes
  H syndrome
  CANDLE syndrome

CANDLE, Chronic atypical neutrophilic dermatosis with lipodystrophy and elevated temperature.
From Paller AS, Mancini, AJ: *Hurwitz clinical pediatric dermatology, a textbook of skin disorders of childhood and adolescence*, ed 5, 2016, Elsevier.

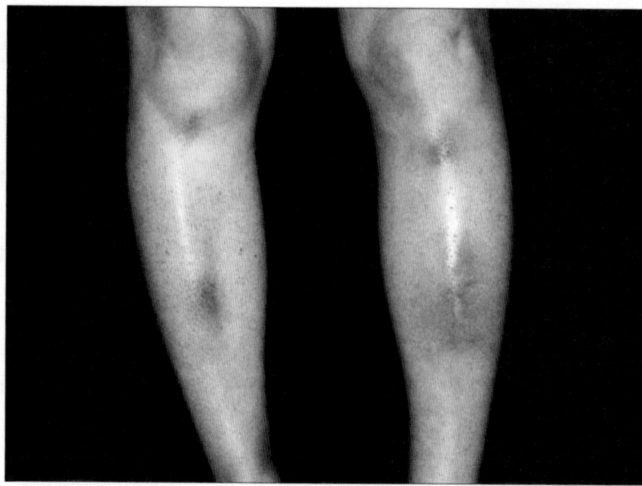

FIG. 1 Erythema nodosum secondary to acute sarcoidosis. (From Hochberg MC et al: *Rheumatology,* ed 5, St Louis, 2011, Mosby.)

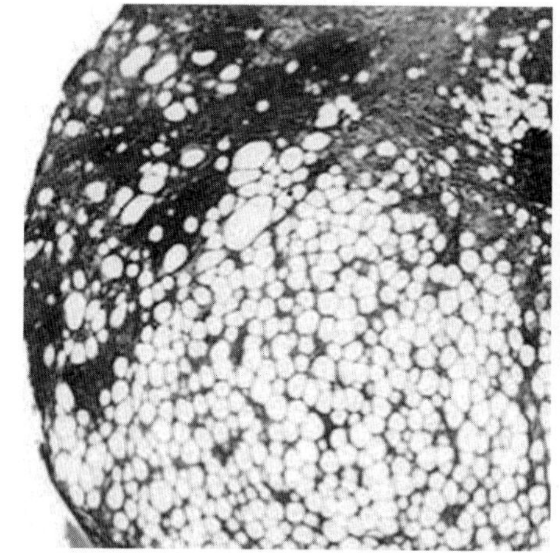

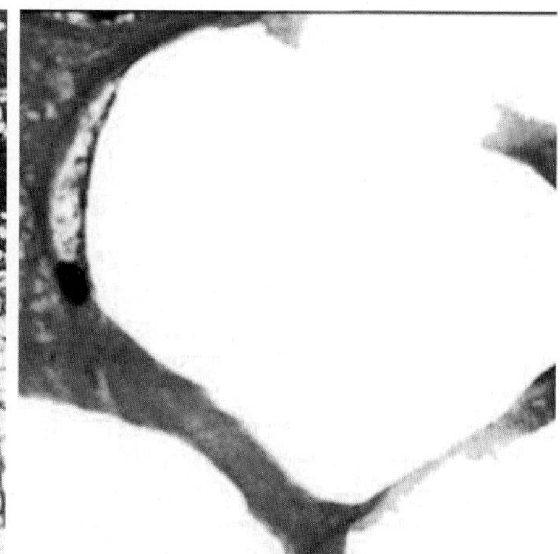

FIG. 2 Mixed lobular and septal panniculitis. (From Callen JP, Requena L: Cutaneous vasculitis and panniculitis, In Hochberg MC et al [eds]: *Rheumatology,* ed 6, Philadelphia, 2015, Elsevier Mosby, p 1350.)

LABORATORY TESTS

Depending on the suspected underlying disorder, the following workup may be considered:

- Throat swab for rapid streptococcal screen, ASO titer, CBC, PPD, chest radiograph, tissue cultures, and histologic stains for organisms
- Amylase, lipase
- Serum alpha-1 antitrypsin level
- ESR, CRP
- Laboratory evaluation for possible connective tissue disease
- Further special studies of biopsy sample if malignancy is suspected

IMAGING STUDIES

- Chest radiography.
- Ankle-brachial index for assessment of peripheral vascular disease.
- Further imaging based on clinical suspicion of disease (i.e., CT scan of abdomen for pancreatitis).

Rx TREATMENT

Treatment of panniculitis is toward treatment of the underlying etiology. Any suspected medications should be discontinued. Appropriate antibiotics to treat underlying infections should be prescribed.

NONPHARMACOLOGIC THERAPY

- Leg elevation, bed rest
- Support stockings

ACUTE GENERAL Rx

- Nonsteroidal antiinflammatory medications (NSAIDs)
- Oral corticosteroids

CHRONIC Rx

- Oral potassium iodide (300-900 mg per day)
- Oral corticosteroids
- Colchicine
- Hydroxychloroquine
- Immunosuppressive medications

REFERRAL

- Dermatology for biopsy of skin lesions
- Specific specialists based on underlying etiology

SUGGESTED READING

Available at ExpertConsult.com

RELATED CONTENT

Erythema Nodosum (Related Key Topic)

AUTHOR: **JOANNE SZCZYGIEL CUNHA, M.D.**

BASIC INFORMATION

DEFINITION

Paraneoplastic syndromes are a large group of disorders caused by either an abnormal immune response to a malignancy or by hormonal or other soluble factors produced by these malignancies. They often affect areas of the body away from the site of the original tumor or metastases, which is in contrast with syndromes that are direct complications of tumor invasion, compression, or metastasis (e.g., superior vena cava syndrome). Findings and symptoms are specific to each syndrome. Paraneoplastic syndromes affect multiple organ systems and remain a challenging diagnostic entity.

ICD-10CM CODES

G13.0	Paraneoplastic neuromyopathy and neuropathy
G13.1	Other systemic atrophy primarily affecting central nervous system in neoplastic disease
E83.5	Disorders of calcium metabolism
GE73.1	Lambert-Eaton syndrome in neoplastic disease
GE73.3	Myasthenic syndromes in other diseases classified elsewhere
E22.2	Syndrome of inappropriate secretion of antidiuretic hormone

EPIDEMIOLOGY & DEMOGRAPHICS

- Paraneoplastic syndromes may affect as many as 8% of cancer patients.
- See Table 1 for epidemiology of each syndrome.

PHYSICAL FINDINGS & CLINICAL PRESENTATION

Hypercalcemia of malignancy
- Nausea/vomiting
- Constipation
- Abdominal pain
- Anorexia
- Hypertension
- Fatigue
- Altered mental status (from confusion to coma)
- Depression/anxiety
- Polyuria
- Acute kidney injury
- Bone pain

SIADH
- Headache
- Weakness
- Anorexia
- Nausea, vomiting
- Memory impairment, irritability, restlessness, seizures
- Obtundation or coma may be seen with hyponatremia <125 mEq/L

Cushing's syndrome
- Muscle weakness
- Rapid weight gain
- Centripetal fat distribution, progressing to obesity; limbs are often spared or wasted
- Characteristic "moon facies" due to accumulation of fat deposition in the cheeks
- Skin atrophy, easy bruising, and purple abdominal striae due to skin fragility
- Hyperpigmentation, notably in sun-exposed areas
- Menstrual irregularity, mild hirsutism in women
- Hypertension
- Depression, anxiety, irritability

Limbic encephalitis (LE)
- Insidious mood or psychiatric changes; hallucinations
- Short-term memory loss
- Hyperthermia or somnolence if hypothalamic involvement
- Seizures occur in up to half of patients

Paraneoplastic thrombocytosis
- Thrombosis
- Nausea, vomiting
- Paresthesias, visual disturbances, headache

Paraneoplastic erythrocytosis
- Erythroderma
- Post-shower (aquagenic) pruritus
- Plethora

Paraneoplastic cerebellar degeneration (PCD)
- May develop prodrome of dizziness, nausea, vomiting
- Ataxia
- Diplopia
- Dysphagia, dysarthria

Paraneoplastic glomerulonephritis
- Renal failure: Oliguric or anuric
- Malaise
- Nausea, vomiting

Lambert-Eaton myasthenic syndrome (LEMS)
- Gradual onset of symmetric proximal muscle weakness and fatiguability; lower extremity involvement is more common
- Hyporeflexia
- Mild bulbar dysfunction, although respiratory failure can occur late in the disease process
- Dysautonomia, especially erectile dysfunction

Myasthenia gravis (MG)
- Ocular symptoms: Ptosis and diplopia
- Weakness of facial muscles, notably with fatigable chewing
- Weakness of neck extensor and flexor muscles; proximal and distal extremities may also be involved
- May progress to involve muscles of respiration and respiratory crisis

Opsoclonus myoclonus syndrome (OMS)
- Truncal ataxia and unsteady gait
- Involuntary and conjugate gaze rapid eye movements (opsoclonus)
- Muscle twitching (myoclonus)
- Other symptoms: Irritability, sleep disturbance, dysarthria or mutism

Stiff-person syndrome (Table 2)

Paraneoplastic dermatologic and rheumatologic syndromes
- Acanthosis nigricans
- Dermatomyositis (DM)
- Necrolytic migratory erythema
- Hypertrophic osteoarthropathy
- Leukocytoclastic vasculitis
- Paraneoplastic pemphigus (PNP)

TABLE 1 Epidemiology of Each Paraneoplastic Syndrome

Condition	Prevalence	Risk Factors
Hypercalcemia of malignancy	Up to 20% of all cancer patients	Squamous cell cancers (lung, head, and neck), breast, kidney, bladder, and ovarian cancers, lymphoma
Syndrome of inappropriate antidiuretic hormone (SIADH)	Up to 2% of all cancer patients Found in 10%-45% of SCLC patients	SCLC
Cushing's syndrome	Approximately 2% of all cancer patients (50% of these are SCLC)	SCLC Pituitary adenoma, benign and malignant adrenal tumors, carcinoid tumors
Limbic encephalitis (LE)	Less than 1%	SCLC Testicular germ cell tumor Breast cancer Ovarian teratoma
Paraneoplastic cerebellar degeneration	Less than 1%	SCLC Hodgkin's lymphoma Breast cancer
Lambert-Eaton myasthenic syndrome (LEMS)	3% of SCLC patients	SCLC, prostate cancer, lymphoma
Paraneoplastic thrombocytosis	5%-20% of patients with solid tumors	Lung, colorectal, mesothelioma
Paraneoplastic erythrocytosis	4% of patients	Renal cell carcinoma, hepatocellular carcinoma
Paraneoplastic glomerulonephritis	2%-4% of patients	Hodgkin's lymphoma, thymoma, prostate cancer
Myasthenia gravis (MG)	15% of thymoma patients	Thymoma
Opsoclonus myoclonus syndrome (OMS)	Less than 1%	SCLC, breast cancer, ovarian teratoma in adults; neuroblastoma in children

SCLC, Small cell lung cancer.

TABLE 2 Paraneoplastic Syndromes

Syndrome	Tumor	Associated Antibodies
Cerebellar degeneration	SCLC Gynecologic Breast Lymphoma Thymoma	Anti-Hu Anti-Yo Anti-Ri Anti-CV2
Limbic encephalitis	SCLC Testes Breast Ovarian teratoma Thymoma	Anti-Hu Anti-Ma Anti-Amphiphysin Anti-NMDA receptor Anti-VGKC Anti-GAD
Lambert–Eaton myasthenic syndrome	SCLC	Anti-VGCC
Sensory neuronopathy	SCLC	Anti-Hu
Stiff-person syndrome	SCLC Breast Thymoma	Anti-GAD Anti-Amphiphysin
Opsoclonus-myoclonus	Neuroblastoma SCLC Gynecologic Breast	Anti-Ri
Dermatomyositis/ polymyositis	Ovary Pancreas Stomach Colorectal Non-Hodgkin's lymphoma	No associated antibody

GAD, Glutamic acid decarboxylase; *NMDA, N*-methyl-D-aspartate; *SCLC,* small cell lung cancer; *VGCC,* voltage-gated calcium channel; *VGKC,* voltage-gated potassium channel.
From Kaufman DM, Geyer HL, Milstein MJ: *Kaufman's clinical neurology for psychiatrists,* ed 8, Philadelphia, 2017, Elsevier.

TABLE 3 Hypercalcemia of Malignancy

Cancer	Frequency (%)	Mechanism
Lung	35	PTHrP Local osteolysis
Breast	25	PTHrP Local osteolysis
Head and neck	6	PTHrP
Renal	3	PTHrP Local osteolysis
Multiple myeloma	15	PTHrP (rare) Local osteolysis 1,25-Dihydroxyvitamin D
Prostate	7	Local osteolysis
Lymphoma	15	1,25-Dihydroxyvitamin D PTHrP

PTHrP, Parathyroid hormone related protein.
From Skorecki, K et al.: *Brenner and Rector's the kidney,* ed 10, Philadelphia, 2016, Elsevier.

- Polymyalgia rheumatica (PMR)
- Sweet syndrome (acute febrile neutrophilic dermatosis)
- Sign of Leser-Trélat (explosive onset of multiple seborrheic keratoses)

ETIOLOGY

Paraneoplastic endocrine syndromes (PES) are due to ectopic production of bioactive substances (e.g., hormones or peptides) that lead to metabolic derangements:

- **Hypercalcemia of malignancy:**
  1. *Humoral hypercalcemia of malignancy (HHM):* Due to production of parathyroid hormone-related peptide (PTHrP). Accounts for 80% of hypercalcemia of malignancy cases. Most common in lung (Table 3) and breast cancer (also seen in renal, bladder, and ovarian cancer).
  2. *Other etiologies of hypercalcemia of malignancy:* 1,25-dihydroxyvitamin D production from increased 1α-hydroxylase activity causes hypercalcemia in most Hodgkin and some non-Hodgkin lymphomas. Tumors can also produce ectopic parathyroid hormone (PTH).
  3. *Osteolytic activity:* 20% of hypercalcemia of malignancy cases. Tumor cells produce local factors that stimulate osteoclast activation, resulting in increased bone resorption.
- **SIADH:** Ectopic production of antidiuretic hormone (ADH) (arginine vasopressin, atrial natriuretic peptide) by tumor cells leads to inappropriately concentrated urine and natriuresis.
- **Cushing's syndrome:** Ectopic ACTH promotes excess production of cortisol and other glucocorticoids from the adrenal glands, which do not respond to normal HPA feedback.
- **Paraneoplastic erythrocytosis**: Mediated by inappropriate production of erythropoietin (EPO) and is associated most commonly with renal cell carcinoma and hepatocellular carcinoma.
- **Paraneoplastic thrombocytosis**: Overproduction of inflammatory cytokines, especially IL-6, which induces thrombopoietin (TPO) mRNA expression and protein synthesis in the liver. Unlike secondary (reactive) thrombocytosis, TPO levels are not elevated.
- **Paraneoplastic glomerulonephritis**: Acute renal failure in the setting of newly diagnosed malignancy that is not explained by direct tumor involvement of the kidneys or genitourinary system. Diseases include minimal change disease, rapidly progressive glomerulonephritis, focal segmental glomerulonephritis, IgA nephropathy, and membranous nephropathy.
- **Paraneoplastic neurologic syndromes (PNS):** Due to immune cross-reactivity between tumor cells and components of the nervous system. Tumor-directed antibodies (onconeural antibodies) are produced by the patient in response to a developing cancer. These onconeural antibodies and associated onconeural antigen-specific T lymphocytes attack components of the nervous system because of antigenic similarity (molecular mimicry). Diagnostic criteria for paraneoplastic neurologic syndromes is summarized in Table 4.
- **LE, PCD, LEMS, MG, OMS:** Cross-reactive autoantibodies against various components of the central and peripheral nervous system.

Dx DIAGNOSIS

DIFFERENTIAL DIAGNOSIS

- **Hypercalcemia of malignancy:** Primary hyperparathyroidism, familial hypocalciuric hypercalcemia, excess calcium intake, vitamin D toxicity, chronic granulomatous disorders, thiazide diuretics. It is important to differentiate between HHM and osteolytic causes of malignancy-associated hypercalcemia because prognosis and response to treatment differ.
- **SIADH:** Hypovolemic hyponatremia, volume overload, reset osmostat, adrenal insufficiency, hypothyroidism, psychogenic polydipsia.
- **Cushing's syndrome:** Excess glucocorticoid administration, pituitary adenoma, benign or malignant adrenal tumors.
- **Paraneoplastic thrombocytosis**: Reactive thrombocytosis from iron deficiency anemia, infection, inflammation, essential thrombocythemia.
- **Paraneoplastic erythrocytosis**: Polycythemia vera, secondary polycythemia from smoking, high-affinity hemoglobinopathies, or chronic hypoxia (e.g., obstructive sleep apnea).
- **Paraneoplastic glomerulonephritis**: Renal failure from intrinsic injury from nephrotoxic agents (e.g., chemotherapy), postrenal failure from bladder obstruction, or rarely direct metastatic invasion from a primary tumor.
- **LE, PCD, LEMS, MG, OMS:** Multiple sclerosis, stroke, meningitis, encephalitis, neurodegenerative diseases

TABLE 4 Diagnostic Criteria for Paraneoplastic Neurologic Syndromes

Definite Praneoplastic Neurologic Syndromes

- A classical syndrome and cancer that develops within 5 years of the diagnosis of the neurologic disorder
- A nonclassical syndrome that resolves significantly after cancer treatment without concomitant immunotherapy provided that the syndrome is not susceptible to spontaneous remission
- A nonclassical syndrome with onconeural antibodies (well characterized or not) and cancer that develops within 5 years of the diagnosis of the neurologic disorder
- A neurologic syndrome (classical or not) with well-characterized onconeural antibodies (anti-Hu, Yo, CV2, Ri, Ma2, or amphiphysin) and no cancer

Possible Paraneoplastic Neurologic Syndromes

- A classical syndrome, no onconeural antibodies, no cancer, but at high risk to have an underlying tumor
- A neurologic syndrome (classical or not) with partially characterized onconeural antibodies and no cancer
- A nonclassical syndrome, no onconeural antibodies, and cancer present within 2 years of diagnosis

From Swaiman, KF et al.: *Swaiman's pediatric neurology: principles and practice*, ed 6, Philadelphia, 2017, Elsevier.

BOX 1 Evaluation and Diagnosis of Paraneoplastic Syndromes

- Characterize abnormality; obtain laboratory studies, imaging, and biopsy as necessary.
- Carefully elicit any additional symptoms and signs.
- Eliminate common causes.
- If there is no obvious etiology, consider a paraneoplastic syndrome.
- If signs and symptoms are consistent with a paraneoplastic syndrome, undertake a search for an unknown primary cancer or recurrence or progression of a known primary tumor.
- Screening should include a careful physical examination with breast, gynecologic, and prostate evaluations; basic hematology, chemistry, and urine studies; chest radiograph; and mammography.
- Computed tomography (CT) of the chest, abdomen and pelvis, or positron emission tomography/CT is indicated if there are any suspicious symptoms, signs, or laboratory abnormalities. Antibody testing for paraneoplastic neurologic syndromes and/or skin biopsy should be performed as indicated.
- Consider treatment of cancer and/or appropriate palliative treatment, including immunosuppressive therapy for paraneoplastic symptoms when possible.

WORKUP

- History and physical examination. Box 1 summarizes the evaluation and diagnosis of paraneoplastic syndromes.
- Age-appropriate cancer screening
- Chest-abdomen-pelvis CT; PET in the paraneoplastic neurologic syndromes (PNS)
- EEG, EMG

LABORATORY TESTS

Hypercalcemia of malignancy

- Serum calcium and albumin levels to measure corrected calcium (HHM more common when serum Ca^{2+} >13 mg/dl)
- Ionized serum calcium
- PTH (low to normal)
- PTHrP (elevated)
- $1,25(OH)_2D$ levels (if the above values are inconclusive)

SIADH

- Serum (corrected for glucose) and urine sodium (serum sodium <135 mEq/L or urine sodium >40 mEq/L)
- Serum and urine osmolality (serum osm <280 mOsm/kg of water and/or urine osm >100 mOsm/kg of water)

Cushing's syndrome

- Initial testing: Low-dose dexamethasone suppression test, late-night salivary cortisol, 24-hour urinary free cortisol excretion
- Once diagnosis is confirmed: High-dose dexamethasone suppression tests can help to distinguish Cushing's syndrome (pituitary hypersecretion of ACTH) from patients with ectopic ACTH production
- Potassium and glucose should be monitored closely due to increased risk of hypokalemia and hyperglycemia
- **LE:** Anti-Hu, Anti-Ma2, Anti-CRMP5, Anti-LGI1, Anti-AMPAR, Anti-mGluR5, CSF analysis, Anti-NMDAR, Anti-GABA-AR, Anti-GABA-BR
- **PCD:** Anti-Yo, Anti-Tr Anti-Hu, Anti-Ma, Anti-Ri, Anti-CV2, Anti-VGCC, Anti-mGluR1, CSF analysis
- **LEMS:** Anti-VGCC (P/Q), CSF analysis
- **MG:** Anti-AchR, Anti-MuSk, CSF analysis
- **Paraneoplastic thrombocytosis**: CBC, liver panel, iron panel, *JAK2* mutation, *CALR* mutation, *MPL* mutation
- **Paraneoplastic erythrocytosis**: CBC, EPO level, *JAK2* mutation, peripheral blood smear
- **Paraneoplastic glomerulonephritis**: BMP, urinalysis, urine protein to creatinine ratio, 24-hour urine protein collection, urine sediment analysis

IMAGING STUDIES

- **Hypercalcemia of malignancy:** CT imaging to evaluate for breast lesion, lung mass, or lymphadenopathy
- **SIADH:** CT imaging to evaluate for brain or lung mass
- **Cushing's syndrome:** CT scan, MRI, or octreotide scan
- **LE, PCD, LEMS, MG:** CT chest, FDG-PET scan, MRI
- **Paraneoplastic erythrocytosis**: CT renal mass protocol or renal ultrasound to evaluate for renal cell carcinoma

Rx TREATMENT

NONPHARMACOLOGIC THERAPY

Hypercalcemia of malignancy

- Treatment of underlying malignancy, either surgical resection or chemotherapy/radiation of identified tumors
- Fluid resuscitation, typically with initial 1 L bolus of isotonic saline followed by 200 to 300 ml/hr to achieve euvolemia, followed by maintenance hydration

SIADH

- Surgical resection of identified tumors
- Fluid restriction
- Maintain adequate dietary protein and salt intake

Cushing's syndrome

- Surgical resection of identified tumors

LE, PCD, LEMS, MG

- IVIG
- Plasma exchange

ACUTE GENERAL Rx

Hypercalcemia of malignancy

- Aggressive fluid hydration with normal saline (0.9%) to promote renal calcium excretion
- Bisphosphonates, either pamidronate or zoledronic acid intravenous infusions (treatment side effects are renal dysfunction and osteonecrosis of the jaw)
- Calcitonin weight-based dosing, although tachyphylaxis occurs after 48 hours of administration
- Corticosteroids in cases of myeloma and lymphoma
- Hemodialysis in severe cases

SIADH

- If patient develops seizure or obtundation in cases of severe hyponatremia, then sodium replacement with hypertonic saline (3%) is indicated
- Sodium should not be corrected at a rate faster than 8 mEq/L in any 24-hour period to decrease chances of osmotic demyelination syndrome. Desmopressin, free water, and/or nephrology consultation may be required for an overly rapid correction.

Cushing's syndrome

- Diuretics and antihypertensive agents for blood pressure and volume status management

CHRONIC Rx

- Chronic treatment is centered on treatment of the underlying malignancy
- **Hypercalcemia of malignancy**
  1. Bisphosphonate therapy every 4 weeks in cases of bone metastasis
  2. Chronic calcitonin use can be considered
  3. Denosumab, a monoclonal antibody that inhibits osteoclastic bone resorption by blocking RANKL from binding to osteoclastic

RANK receptors, can be used in patients refractory to bisphosphonate therapy

- **SIADH**
  1. Demeclocycline and vasopressin receptor antagonists (vaptans: Conivaptan and tolvaptan, although tolvaptan should not be used for longer than 30 days and should be avoided in patients with liver disease)
  2. Cessation of any possible causative medications
  3. Oral salt tablets if dietary salt intake insufficient
- **Cushing's syndrome:** Inhibition of adrenal enzymes with ketoconazole, mitotane, metyrapone
- **LE/PCD:** Glucocorticoids, cyclophosphamide, rituximab
- **LEMS:** Pyridostigmine, azathioprine, glucocorticoids
- **MG:** Pyridostigmine, azathioprine, cyclosporine, mycophenolate, rituximab
- **Paraneoplastic thrombocytosis**: Consider prophylactic low-molecular-weight heparin or aspirin if no contraindications exist

DISPOSITION

Specific to each condition; however, humoral hypercalcemia of malignancy carries a poor overall prognosis with 30-day mortality of 50%.

REFERRAL

Oncology, endocrinology, neurology, nephrology

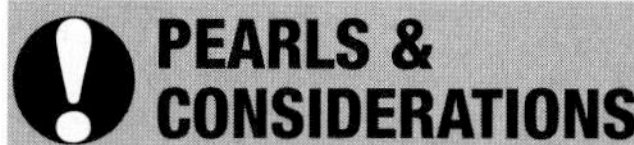

PEARLS & CONSIDERATIONS

COMMENTS

- Signs or symptoms of a paraneoplastic syndrome may manifest prior to the identification of a malignancy.
- If paraneoplastic syndrome is suspected, a thorough workup for a tumor is indicated.
- With treatment of the primary tumor, the clinical effects of hypercalcemia of malignancy, SIADH, and Cushing's syndrome may improve or resolve.
- Neurologic paraneoplastic syndromes can have long-term effects due to permanent CNS or PNS damage. Tumor detection can also be difficult as these immune-mediated syndromes may also be keeping the tumor in check.
- New neurologic deficits after starting a checkpoint inhibitor (e.g., PD-1 inhibitor) may indicate drug-induced autoimmunity rather than a paraneoplastic syndrome.

PREVENTION

- Smoking cessation
- Age-appropriate cancer screening

PATIENT & FAMILY EDUCATION

In conditions with autoimmune etiology (LE, PCD, LEMS, MG, OMS), symptoms may not improve even if the tumor is identified and treated, as damage to the nervous system may be sustained or permanent.

SUGGESTED READINGS

Available at ExpertConsult.com

AUTHORS: **BRIANNA R. BAKOW, M.D.,** and **JOHN L. REAGAN, M.D.**

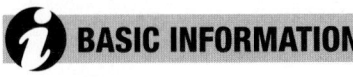

BASIC INFORMATION

DEFINITION

Idiopathic Parkinson disease (PD) is a progressive neurodegenerative disorder characterized clinically by rigidity, tremor, postural instability, and slowness of movement (bradykinesia).

SYNONYMS

PD
Paralysis agitans

ICD-10CM CODES

G20	Parkinson's disease
G21.11	Neuroleptic induced parkinsonism
G21.1	Other drug-induced secondary parkinsonism
G21.2	Secondary parkinsonism due to other external agents
G21.3	Postencephalitic parkinsonism
G21.4	Vascular parkinsonism
G21.8	Other secondary parkinsonism
G21.9	Secondary parkinsonism, unspecified

EPIDEMIOLOGY & DEMOGRAPHICS

PREVALENCE:

- Affects more than 1 million people in North America. It is the second most common neurodegenerative disease worldwide.
- In age group <40 yr, <5/100,000 are affected.
- In those aged >70 yr, 700/100,000 are affected.
- Highest incidence in whites, lowest incidence in Asians and African Americans.

PHYSICAL FINDINGS & CLINICAL PRESENTATION

- Tremor (Fig. E1)—typically a resting tremor with a frequency of 4 to 6 Hz that is often first noted in the hand as a pill-rolling tremor (thumb and forefinger). Can also involve the leg and lip. Tremor improves with purposeful movement. Usually starts asymmetrically.
- Rigidity—increased muscle tone that persists throughout the range of passive movement of a joint. Rigidity, like resting tremor, is usually asymmetric at onset.
- Akinesia/bradykinesia—slowness in initiating movement and decrement with repeated movements.
- Postural instability—tested by "pull test." Ask patient to stand in place with back to examiner. Examiner pulls patient back by the shoulders, and proper response would be to take no steps back or very few steps back without falling. Retropulsion is a positive test, as is falling straight back. Postural instability is not usually severe early on. If falls and postural reflexes are greatly impaired early on, then consider other disorders, such as progressive supranuclear palsy.
- Masked facies (hypomimia)—face seems expressionless, giving the appearance of depression. Decreased blink; often there is excess drooling.
- Gait disturbance.
- Stooped posture, decreased arm swing.
- Difficulty initiating the first step; small shuffling steps that increase in speed (festinating gait). Steps become progressively faster and shorter while the trunk inclines further forward.
- Other complaints and findings early on include handwriting becoming smaller (micrographia), and voice becoming softer and often "gruffer" (hypophonia).

ETIOLOGY

- Unknown.
- Most cases are sporadic. Age is the most common risk factor, although a combination of both environmental and genetic factors likely contributes to disease expression. Rare familial forms with at least seven different genes have been identified; these include the parkin gene, a significant cause of early-onset autosomal recessive PD, and *LRRK2*, the most common cause of familial and sporadic parkinsonism.

Dx DIAGNOSIS

A clinical diagnosis can be made based on a comprehensive history and physical examination. The four cardinal signs used to diagnose PD are (mnemonic = TRAP):

1. **T**remor (resting, typically 4-6 Hz)
2. **R**igidity, of the cogwheel type
3. **A**kinesia/bradykinesia—slowing and decrement of movement
4. **P**ostural instability—failure of postural "righting" reflexes leading to poor balance and falls

Bradykinesia plus at least one other sign are necessary, but all four cardinal signs do not need to be present to make a presumptive diagnosis of PD and begin treatment.

DIFFERENTIAL DIAGNOSIS

- Multiple system atrophy—distinguishing features include early autonomic dysfunction (including urinary incontinence, orthostatic hypotension, and erectile dysfunction), parkinsonism, cerebellar signs, and normal cognition.
- Dementia with Lewy bodies—parkinsonism with concomitant dementia: Patients often have early hallucinations and fluctuations in level of alertness and mental status.
- Corticobasal syndrome—often begins asymmetrically with apraxia, cortical sensory loss in one limb, and sometimes, alien limb phenomenon.
- Progressive supranuclear palsy—tends to have axial rigidity greater than appendicular (limb) rigidity. These patients have early and severe postural instability. Hallmark is supranuclear gaze palsy that usually involves vertical gaze (especially downward) before horizontal.
- Essential tremor—bilateral postural and action tremor.
- Secondary (acquired) parkinsonism (Box 1):
  1. Iatrogenic—any of the neuroleptics and antipsychotics. The high-potency D_2-blocker neuroleptics are most likely to cause parkinsonism. Quetiapine is an atypi-

BOX 1 Causes of Parkinsonism

Primary Parkinsonism

- Parkinson disease (idiopathic/sporadic parkinsonism)

Secondary Parkinsonism

- Drug-induced parkinsonism
  - Neuroleptic drugs
  - Calcium blocker cinnarizine
- Vascular parkinsonism (pseudoparkinsonism)
  - Multi-infarct states
  - Single basal ganglia/thalamic infarct
  - Binswanger disease
- Multisystem degenerative diseases
  - Progressive supranuclear palsy
  - Multiple system atrophy (striatonigral type)
  - Corticobasal degeneration
  - Alzheimer's disease
  - Wilson disease (young-onset parkinsonism)
  - Dementia with Lewy bodies
  - Neurofibrillary tangle parkinsonism
- Toxins
  - MPTP
  - Manganese
- Familial parkinsonism
- Postinfectious parkinsonism
  - Creutzfeldt-Jakob disease
  - AIDS
  - Postencephalitis (encephalitis lethargica)
- Miscellaneous causes
  - Hydrocephalus
  - Posttraumatic
  - Tumors
- Metabolic causes (postanoxic)

AIDS, Acquired immunodeficiency syndrome; *MPTP,* 1-methyl-4-phenyl-1,2,2,6-tetrahydropyridine.
From Fillit HM: *Brocklehurst's textbook of geriatric medicine and gerontology,* ed 8, Philadelphia, 2017, Elsevier.

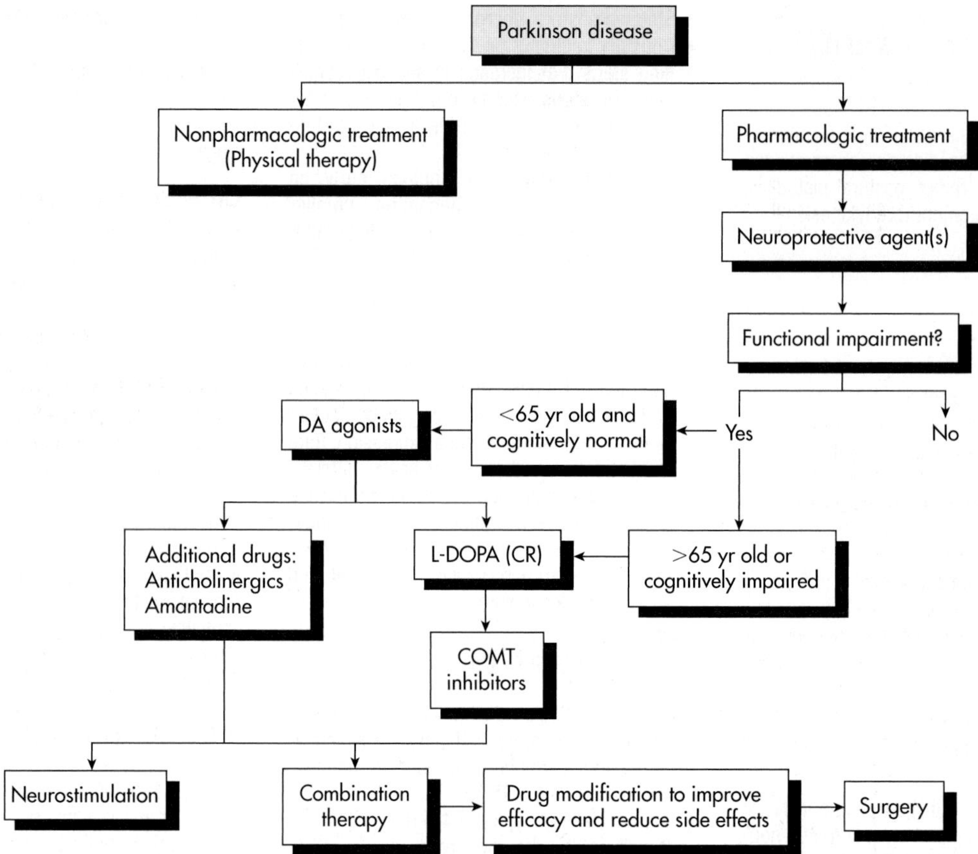

FIG. 2 Diagrammatic representation of a therapeutic approach to patients with parkinsonism. *COMT,* Catechol-O-methyl transferase; *CR,* controlled release; *DA,* dopamine. (Modified from Goldman L, Ausiello D [eds]: *Cecil textbook of medicine,* ed 24, Philadelphia, 2012, Saunders.)

cal antipsychotic with lower risk of parkinsonism. Metoclopramide can also cause parkinsonism. Abuse of methamphetamine has been recently linked to risk of PD.

2. Postinfectious parkinsonism—von Economo encephalitis.
3. Dementia pugilistica—parkinsonism and dementia after repeated head trauma.
4. Toxins (e.g., MPTP, manganese, carbon monoxide).
5. Cerebrovascular disease "vascular parkinsonism" (basal ganglia infarcts); often lower limbs (especially gait) affected more than upper extremities.

WORKUP

- Identification of clinical signs and symptoms associated with PD (see "Physical Findings"), and elimination of conditions that may mimic it with a comprehensive history and physical examination.
- Routine genetic testing is not recommended.

IMAGING STUDIES

Computed tomographic (CT) scan has almost no role in investigations. Magnetic resonance imaging (MRI) of the head may sometimes distinguish between idiopathic PD and other conditions that present with signs of parkinsonism (see "Differential Diagnosis").

Dopamine transporter imaging (DaTScan with [^{123}I]β-CIT SPECT) evaluates the level of dopamine in the striatum and can be used to confirm parkinsonism in atypical cases. DaTScan is approved to distinguish essential tremor from parkinsonism but cannot distinguish between different causes of parkinsonism. Interpretation can be tricky, and routine use is not recommended at this time.

Rx TREATMENT

NONPHARMACOLOGIC THERAPY

- Physical therapy, patient education and reassurance, treatment of associated conditions (e.g., depression) are important. A safe, practical, and reasonable exercise regimen must be encouraged, individualized to the patient's access to resources and motivation. Recent trials reveal that t'ai chi training is effective in reducing balance impairment and falls and improving functional capacity.
- Avoidance of drugs that can induce or worsen parkinsonism: Neuroleptics (especially high potency), certain antiemetics (prochlorperazine, trimethobenzamide), metoclopramide, nonselective MAO inhibitors (may induce hypertensive crisis), reserpine, methyldopa.

ACUTE GENERAL Rx

- There continues to be controversy whether levodopa or dopamine agonists should be the initial treatment. In younger patients, agonists may be favored; in patients >65 yr, levodopa is typically the preferred initial therapy.
- It is appropriate to initiate pharmacotherapy when required by symptoms; prior practice of waiting for limitation of ADLs is now outdated. Fig. 2 describes an approach to patients with parkinsonism.
- Motor complications do develop during the course of the disease and likely reflect the combination of disease progression together with the side effects of dopaminergic medications.

CHRONIC Rx

- Levodopa therapy:
  1. The most efficacious treatment and cornerstone of symptomatic therapy—should be used with a peripheral dopa decarboxylase inhibitor (carbidopa) to minimize side effects (nausea, lightheadedness, postural hypotension). The combination of the two drugs is marketed under the trade name Sinemet. Levodopa therapy has been found to reduce morbidity and mortality in PD patients.

2. Usual starting dose is 25/100 mg (carbidopa/levodopa) tid 1 hr before (or after) meals.
3. Controlled-release (Sinemet CR) and extended-release (Rytary) preparations are also available, but their use should be supervised by a neurologist.
4. Stalevo (combination Sinemet and entacapone, a COMT inhibitor). Useful for patients with motor fluctuations (wearing off); has no role in treating early patients with PD.
5. Duopa (carbidopa/levodopa), administered via a 16-hour infusion to the jejunum through either a nasojejunal tube (short-term) or PEG-J tube (long-term), is used for treating motor fluctuations in patients with advanced PD.

- Dopamine receptor agonists (ropinirole and pramipexole) are not as potent as levodopa, but they are often used as initial treatment in younger patients to attempt to delay the onset of complications (dyskinesias, motor fluctuations) associated with levodopa therapy. These medications are more expensive than levodopa. In general, they cause more side effects than levodopa, including nausea, vomiting, light-headedness, peripheral edema, confusion, and somnolence. They can also cause impulse control behaviors such as hypersexuality, binge eating, and compulsive shopping and gambling. Presence of these must be assessed at each visit as the appearance of these side effects is often under-reported and their consequences can be severe.
  1. Ropinirole: Initial dose is 0.25 mg tid but must be titrated over the course of 4 weeks to 1 mg tid and then may be increased by 1.5 mg/week to a maximum of 24 mg/day. An extended-release formulation is also available.
  2. Pramipexole: Initial dose is 0.125 mg tid but must be titrated over the course of weeks to 1.5 to 4.5 mg/day in three doses. An extended-release formulation is also available.
- MAO-B inhibitors can be used as monotherapy early in the disease or as adjunctive therapy in later stages; they have been shown to have milder symptomatic benefit than dopamine agonists or levodopa. They are well tolerated and easy to titrate. Concurrent use of stimulants and sympathomimetics should be avoided. Certain food restrictions may apply.
  1. Rasagiline: Initial dose is 0.5 mg qd, then 1 mg daily. The ADAGIO study suggests that 1 mg rasagiline may have disease-modifying benefits, but results must be interpreted with caution.
  2. Selegiline: Usual dose, 5 mg bid with breakfast and lunch. Has amphetamine byproduct so has mild stimulant-like effects, which can be beneficial in some patients.
  3. Safinamide: FDA approved as add-on therapy for carbidopa-levodopa that reduces "off time" and increases "on time" with fewer dyskinesias. Starting dose is 50 mg daily for 2 weeks, which can be increased if needed to 100 mg daily.
- Amantadine (unclear mechanism of action, but reported to modulate the dopamine and glutamate systems in the CNS) can be used alone early in the disease. Later in the disease, it is especially useful in the treatment of dyskinesias. Dosage is 100 mg tid (titrate q week from 100 mg qd). Must adjust for elderly and renal impairment. The most notable side effect, especially in the elderly, is confusion. An extended-release version is now FDA approved for the treatment of dyskinesia.
- Anticholinergic agents are only helpful in treating tremor but may be more effective than levodopa for tremor in some circumstances. They can also be used to treat drooling in patients with PD. Potential side effects include constipation, urinary retention, memory impairment, and hallucinations. They should be avoided in the elderly.
  1. Trihexyphenidyl: Initial dose, 1 mg PO tid
  2. Benztropine: Usual dose, 0.5 to 1 mg qd or bid
- Treatment of nonmotor symptoms: Nonmotor symptoms such as depression, anxiety, irritability, dementia, psychosis, urinary and sexual dysfunction, sleep disturbances such as REM behavior disorder, decreased sense of smell, and impulsive behavior among others often cause a great deal of distress for patients and caretakers alike. Treatable symptoms should be addressed pharmacologically using medications appropriate for elderly patients sensitive to antidopaminergic medications. In addition, two medications are specifically indicated for nonmotor symptoms associated with PD.
- Psychosis: Pimavanserin (Nuplazid) is FDA approved for the treatment of Parkinson disease psychosis and has been shown effective for the treatment of hallucinations and delusions associated with Parkinson disease psychosis. The medication is an inverse agonist of 5-HT2A and 5-HT2C receptors without any evidence of dopamine blockade.
- Parkinson disease dementia: Rivastigmine (Exelon), a cholinesterase inhibitor available both orally and transdermally as a patch (with few GI side effects), is approved to treat not only Alzheimer's disease but also Parkinson disease dementia.

SURGICAL OPTIONS

- Pallidal (globus pallidus interna) and subthalamic deep-brain stimulation (subthalamic nucleus) are currently the surgical options of choice for patients with advanced PD; similar improvement in motor function and adverse effects have been reported after either procedure. Compared with ablative procedures, DBS has the advantage of being reversible and adjustable. Thalamic DBS may be useful for refractory tremor. It improves the cardinal motor symptoms, extends medication "on" time, and reduces motor fluctuations during the day. In general, patients are likely to benefit from this therapy if they show a clear response to levodopa. Therefore, when considering DBS, patients should be evaluated for motor response to levodopa by stopping levodopa overnight and evaluating motor response before and after a dose of levodopa.
- Surgery is often limited to patients with disabling, medically refractory problems, and patients must still have a good response to L-dopa to undergo surgery. Yet for many patients, earlier stimulation might provide an improved motor benefit before disability from other symptoms has occurred and should be considered at an earlier stage of PD. DBS results in decreased dyskinesias, fluctuations, rigidity, and tremor.

DISPOSITION

PD usually follows a slowly progressive course leading to disability over the course of several years. However, every patient will progress individually, and patients should be reassured that this diagnosis does not, by definition, result in being either wheelchair- or bed-bound.

REFERRAL

- Neurology consultation is recommended at initial diagnosis of PD.
- Exercise is important for all patients with PD.
- Participation in outpatient physical therapy program is recommended for patients with moderate to advanced disease.

PEARLS & CONSIDERATIONS

- Asymmetry of symptoms at onset is typical of PD and therefore very useful in distinguishing PD from other causes of parkinsonism.
- Although resting tremor is a common presenting symptom, up to 25% of patients with idiopathic PD do not have classic resting tremor.

SUGGESTED READINGS

Available at ExpertConsult.com

RELATED CONTENT

Parkinson Disease (Patient Information)

AUTHORS: **COREY GOLDSMITH, M.D., JOSEPH S. KASS, M.D., J.D.,** and **U. SHIVRAJ SOHUR, M.D., PH.D.**

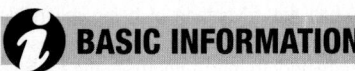

DEFINITION

Partial seizures are characterized by focal cortical discharges that provoke seizure symptoms related to the area of the brain involved. Simple partial seizures do not cause impairment of consciousness. However, partial seizures can evolve into complex partial and/or tonic clonic seizures. In the revised International League Against Epilepsy (ILAE) classification of seizures, the name "partial seizures" has been replaced with "focal seizures."

SYNONYMS

Focal seizures
Simple partial seizures
Seizures, partial

ICD-10CM CODES

G40.0	Localization-related (focal) (partial) idiopathic epilepsy and epileptic syndromes with seizures of localized onset
G40.109	Localization-related (focal) (partial) symptomatic epilepsy and epileptic syndromes with simple partial seizures, not intractable, without status epilepticus

EPIDEMIOLOGY & DEMOGRAPHICS

INCIDENCE: 30 to 50 cases per 100,000 person per yr
PREVALENCE: 5 to 8 cases per 1000 persons
PREDOMINANT SEX AND AGE: No gender preference

PHYSICAL FINDINGS & CLINICAL PRESENTATION

- Patients with partial seizures usually have normal physical and neurologic examinations unless the focal seizures are due to a structural abnormality such as a stroke, where the patient will have a neurologic exam consistent with the area of CNS structural damage.
- During partial seizures the patients are conscious, but they may have an alteration of awareness. However, if there is spread of the epileptic focus causing secondary generalization, the patient will then lose consciousness. A focal seizure can evolve into a generalized tonic clonic seizure. Clues to this progression include a subjective aura before the onset of convulsion, unilateral shaking, and head turning to one side (versive head turning).
- Patients with partial seizures can experience postictal weakness/paralysis that usually resolves within 24 hr (Todd paralysis). However, focal neurologic deficits may also be indicative of a new structural brain lesion.
- Manifestations of complex partial seizures may include automatisms (semipurposeful behaviors) such as fumbling of fingers or lip smacking.

ETIOLOGY

- Seizures in general are a cardinal sign of cortical neurologic injury.
- The etiology of partial seizures can be either genetic or due to a neurologic injury.
- Frequent causes of partial seizures are tumors, stroke, CNS infections (neurocysticercosis among others), arteriovenous malformations (AVMs), cavernous malformations, traumatic brain injury, cortical dysplasia, and structural abnormalities.

Dx DIAGNOSIS

DIFFERENTIAL DIAGNOSIS

- Transient ischemic attack.
- Movement disorders.
- Psychogenic nonepileptic spells.
- Migraines.
- The differential diagnosis of nonepileptic events is summarized in Table 1. Table 2 summarizes clinical characteristics that help distinguish epileptic from nonepileptic events.

WORKUP

EEG. Ambulatory EEG and/or video EEG recommended for patients with diagnostic uncertainty

LABORATORY TESTS

Routine blood workup (CBC, CMP, glucose, electrolytes) may be considered in appropriate clinical situations.

IMAGING STUDIES

- In the acute setting, a CT scan of the head is high yield to rule out space-occupying lesions.
- MRI of the brain with a defined epilepsy protocol should be performed in all patients with recurrent seizures.

Rx TREATMENT

- Almost all antiepileptic drugs are approved for partial seizures, either in monotherapy or in adjunct. Carbamazepine traditionally has been the standard initial drug treatment for partial seizures. However, newer antiepileptic drugs have better side effect profiles.
- Lamotrigine, levetiracetam, and oxcarbazepine are effective and well-tolerated antiepileptic drugs for treating partial seizures.
- Eslicarbazepine is indicated for the treatment of partial-onset seizures as monotherapy or adjunctive therapy. The recommended initial dose of eslicarbazepine is 400 mg once daily. Increase the dose in weekly increments of 200 mg, based on clinical response and tolerability, to a recommended maintenance dose of 800 to 1600 mg once daily.
- Lacosamide is indicated as monotherapy or adjunctive therapy in patients with partial-onset seizures. The initial recommended dose is 50 mg twice daily; increase at weekly intervals by 50 mg twice daily, up to a recommended maintenance dose of 100 to 200 mg twice daily.
- Patients who continue to have seizures despite a trial of two antiepileptic drugs and adequate doses should be referred for evaluation for epilepsy surgery. Surgical treatments (e.g., temporal lobectomy in mesial temporal sclerosis) may be indicated in refractory cases of partial seizures.

GENERAL Rx

- After a first unprovoked seizure with normal examination, imaging, and EEG, no treatment may be necessary, although patients may elect to undergo treatment.
- According to a recent joint American Academy of Neurology and American Epilepsy Society evidence-based guideline on the management of a first unprovoked seizure in adults, there is strong evidence that the risk of a second seizure is highest in the first 2 yr and ranges from 21% to 45%. This risk is higher for patients with prior brain insults such a traumatic brain injury or stroke or those with epileptiform abnormalities on EEG. Significant brain imaging abnormalities and nocturnal seizures also indicate a more elevated risk of recurrent seizures. Chronic treatment with antiepileptic drugs is indicated for more than two unprovoked seizures or in patients with one seizure with abnormal workup. However, moderate evidence supports

TABLE 1 Differential Diagnosis of Nonepileptic Events

General Medical Conditions
- Transient ischemic attack (TIA)
- Complicated migraine
- Syncope
- Hypoglycemia
- Parasomnia (e.g., rapid eye movement [REM], behavior disorder, or night terrors)
- Narcolepsy
- Myoclonus (from metabolic disturbance)

Psychiatric Causes
- Conversion disorder
- Somatic symptom disorder
- Dissociative disorder
- Panic disorder (simulating partial seizures)

Volitional Deception
- Factitious disorder (goal is to maintain the sick role)
- Malingering (goal is to obtain secondary gain, e.g., disability income)

From Stern TA et al: *Massachusetts General Hospital handbook of general hospital psychiatry,* ed 7, Philadelphia, 2018, Elsevier.

TABLE 2 Clinical Characteristics That Help Distinguish Epileptic From Nonepileptic Events

	Epileptic Seizures	Nonepileptic Seizures/Events
Onset	Sudden onset and offset	Often gradual
Duration	Often <3 minutes	Variable
Perception	May experience olfactory, gustatory, visual hallucination; déjà vu; derealization	May experience auditory hallucinations; paranoia
Eyes during event	Open	Closed
Incontinence	Common	Rare
Awareness	Often impaired; can stay aware during some focal seizures	Variable; may be responsive during parts of the event
Recall of event	None or limited (e.g. aura)	Usually intact
Ictal EEG	Almost always abnormal	Unchanged from baseline
Inter-ictal EEG	Normal or abnormal	Often normal
Tongue bite	Lateral tongue	None or tip of tongue
Injury	May be present	Rarely present (suggestive of serious psychopathology)
Incontinence	May be present	Rare
Post-ictal state	Confusion or drowsiness is common	Rare
Prolactin	Elevated; or normal	Normal; rarely elevated from baseline

From Stern TA et al: *Massachusetts General Hospital handbook of general hospital psychiatry*, ed 7, Philadelphia, 2018, Elsevier.

advising the patient that immediate antiepileptic therapy, compared with delaying treatment until a second unprovoked seizure, is likely to reduce the risk of a seizure recurrence in the next 2 yr. Furthermore, the risk of adverse events with antiepileptic drugs ranges from 7% to 31%, with most of these adverse events being mild and reversible. Thus, the practice guideline suggests that under certain circumstances, adults with one provoked seizure even without high-risk EEG or MRI findings can be treated with antiepileptic drugs because, at least over the next 2 yr, the risk of a recurrent seizure is reduced. Although there is no strong evidence that such treatment improves quality of life, even one seizure can have negative consequences on social and occupational functioning such as driving, making treatment an attractive option for many.

- Recurrent seizures and seizures with abnormal studies require treatment in the form of medicines, consideration of surgery, or with approved medical devices.

DISPOSITION

- Response to treatment often depends on the etiology of the partial seizures.
- 47% of patients become seizure free with monotherapy and 67% with polytherapy.
- Patients who do not respond to two drugs should be referred to an epilepsy center for consideration of surgical treatment.
- No driving until seizure free in accordance with local laws and regulations.
- Patients should avoid situations that may cause injuries or accidents in the event of a seizure, such as climbing ladders, swimming unsupervised, or taking baths (rather than showers).
- Many antiepileptic drugs also affect vitamin D absorption or metabolism, prompting attention to patients' bone health.
- All patients with epilepsy are at higher risk for depression and should be screened.

REFERRAL

Patients with epilepsy and seizures should be referred for a consultation by a neurologist, preferably one with a special interest in epilepsy.

PEARLS & CONSIDERATIONS

COMMENTS

- Successful treatment depends on the correct choice of antiepileptic drugs based on patient's gender and comorbidities.
- Valproic acid should be avoided in girls and women with childbearing potential due to the risk of teratogenicity.
- All women of childbearing age taking antiepileptic drugs should take folic acid supplementation (1-4 mg/day) for the prevention of neural tube defects. Many antiepileptic drugs interact with oral contraception.

PREVENTION

- Sleep deprivation and alcohol consumption should be avoided.
- Drug compliance is compulsory to prevent seizure recurrence.

PATIENT & FAMILY EDUCATION

- Patient education and information can be obtained at the Epilepsy Foundation: www.epilepsyfoundation.org.
- Patients should be counseled on general seizure precautions such as swimming, bathing, and heights.

SUGGESTED READING

Available at ExpertConsult.com

RELATED CONTENT

Partial Motor Seizures (Patient Information)

AUTHORS: **PATRICIO SEBASTIAN ESPINOSA, M.D., M.P.H.**, and **COREY GOLDSMITH, M.D.**

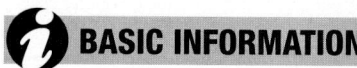

BASIC INFORMATION

DEFINITION

Pediculosis is lice infestation. Human beings can be infested with three kinds of lice: *Pediculus capitis* (head louse, Fig. 1), *Pediculus corporis* (body louse), and *Phthirus pubis* (pubic, or crab, louse). Lice feed on human blood and deposit their eggs (nits) on the hair shafts (head lice and pubic lice) and along the seams of clothing (body lice). Nits generally hatch within 7 to 10 days. Lice are obligate human parasites and cannot survive away from their hosts for longer than 7 to 10 days. Fig. 2 illustrates the life cycle of the head louse.

SYNONYM

Lice

ICD-10CM CODES

B85.2	Pediculosis, unspecified
B85.0	Pediculosis due to *Pediculus humanus capitis*
B85.1	Pediculosis due to *Pediculus humanus corporis*
B85.4	Mixed pediculosis and phthiriasis
Z20.7	Contact with and (suspected) exposure to pediculosis, acariasis and other infestations

EPIDEMIOLOGY & DEMOGRAPHICS

- There are 6 to 12 million cases of head lice in the United States yearly. The estimated annual direct and indirect cost of head lice infestation in the United States is $1 billion.
- Lice infestation of the scalp is most common in children (girls affected more often than boys).
- Infestation of the eyelashes is most frequently seen in children and may indicate sexual abuse.
- The chance of acquiring pubic lice from one sexual exposure with an infested partner is >90% (most contagious STI known).
- Body lice are most common in conditions of poor hygiene.

PHYSICAL FINDINGS & CLINICAL PRESENTATION

- Pruritus with excoriation may be caused by hypersensitivity reaction, inflammation from saliva, and fecal material from the lice.
- Nits can be identified by examining hair shafts (Fig.E3).
- The presence of nits on clothes is indicative of body lice.
- Lymphadenopathy may be present (cervical adenopathy with head lice, inguinal lymphadenopathy with pubic lice).
- Head lice are most frequently found in the back of the head and neck, behind the ears.
- Scratching can result in pustules and crusting.
- Pubic lice may affect the hair around the anus.

ETIOLOGY

Lice are transmitted by close personal contact or use of contaminated objects (e.g., combs, clothing, bed linen, hats).

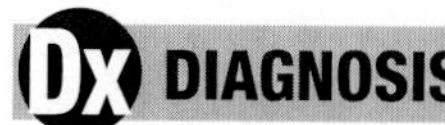

DIAGNOSIS

DIFFERENTIAL DIAGNOSIS

- Seborrheic dermatitis
- Scabies
- Eczema
- Other: Pilar casts, trichonodosis (knotted hair), monilethrix
- Table 1 describes the differential diagnosis of nits

WORKUP

Diagnosis is made by seeing the lice (Fig. 4) or their nits. Combing hair with a fine-toothed comb is recommended because visual inspection of the hair and scalp may miss more than 50% of infestations.

LABORATORY TESTS

Wood's light examination is useful to screen a large number of children: live nits fluoresce, empty nits have a gray fluorescence, and nits with unborn lice reveal white fluorescence.

Rx TREATMENT

NONPHARMACOLOGIC THERAPY

- Patients with body lice should discard infested clothes and improve their hygiene. Items that cannot be washed can be sealed in a plastic bag for 48 hours.
- Combing out nits is a widely recommended but unproven adjunctive therapy.
- Personal items such as combs and brushes should be soaked in hot water for 15 to 30 min. Clothing and bed linens should be washed in hot water (>130° F; 54.4° C) and then dried for at least 10 min at the hottest setting.
- Close contacts and household members should also be examined for the presence of lice.

ACUTE GENERAL Rx

The following products are available for treatment of lice:

- Permethrin: Available over the counter (1% permethrin [Nix]) or by prescription (5% permethrin [Elimite]); should be applied to the hair and scalp and rinsed out after 10 min. A repeat application 7 days later is generally not necessary in patients with head lice. It can be applied to clean, dry hair and left on overnight (8-14 hours) under a shower cap. Resistance to permethrin is now widespread.
- Malathion, an organophosphate, is effective in head lice. It is available by prescription. Use should be avoided in children ≤2 yr. It is not commonly used because of its objectionable odor, fear of flammability, and prolonged application time (8-12 hours).
- Spinosad (Natroba) is a newer FDA-approved product for head lice. It is a topical suspension applied to dry hair for 10 min, then rinsed. It may be repeated 7 days later if necessary. It is more effective than permethrin but also much more expensive. It is safe in pregnancy (category B—no evidence of risk in humans).
- Benzyl alcohol lotion, 5% (Ulesfia) can be used for treatment of head lice in patients >6 mo old. The lotion is applied to dry hair and left on for 10 min. Treatment must be repeated after 7 days because the drug is not ovicidal.
- Eyelash infestation can be treated with the application of petroleum jelly rubbed into the eyelashes three times a day for 5 to 7 days. The application of baby shampoo to

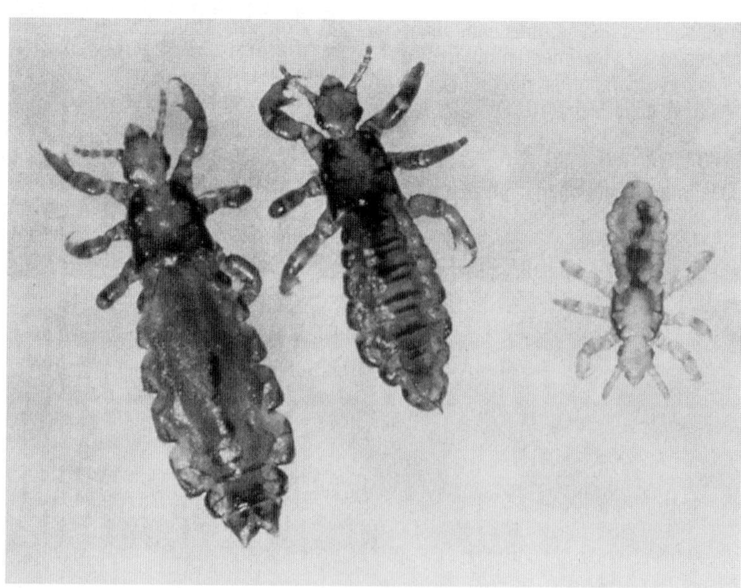

FIG. 1 Head louse family. From left to right: female, male, and nymph. (With permission from Taplin D, Meinking TL: Infestations. In Schachner LA, Hansen RC [eds]: *Pediatric dermatology*, ed 4, Edinburgh, 2011, Mosby, pp 1141–80; Bolognia JL et al: *Dermatology*, ed 4, Philadelphia, 2018, Elsevier.)

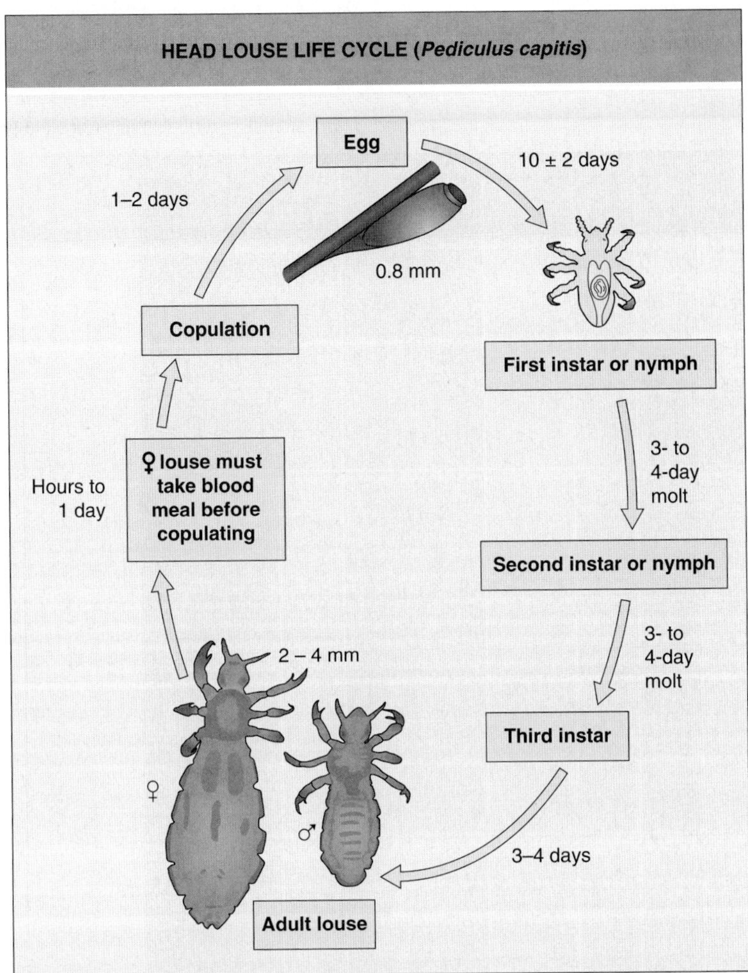

FIG. 2 Head louse life cycle (*Pediculus capitis*). (From Bolognia JL et al: *Dermatology*, ed 4, Philadelphia, 2018, Elsevier.)

the eyelashes and brows three or four times a day for 5 days is also effective. The use of fluorescein drops applied to the lids and eyelashes is also toxic to lice.

- In patients who have previously not responded to treatment or in whom resistance with 1% permethrin cream rinse occurs, a 10-day course of trimethoprim-sulfamethoxazole (TMP-SMX) 8 mg/kg/day in divided doses is an effective treatment for head lice infestation, especially for eyelash infestations with *Phthirus pubis.*
- Ivermectin, an antiparasitic drug, given as an oral dose of 400 mcg/kg of body weight on days 1 and 8, is effective for head lice resistant to other treatments (currently not FDA approved for pediculosis). Ivermectin 0.5% lotion is FDA approved as a single-use topical treatment for head lice in patients 6 mo or older. Cost is more than $200 for 4 oz.
- Fig. 5 summarizes treatments for head lice.

PEARLS & CONSIDERATIONS

COMMENTS

- Patients with pubic lice should notify their sexual contacts. Sex partners within the last month should be treated.
- Parents of patients should also be educated that head lice infestation (unlike body lice) does not indicate poor hygiene.

TABLE 1 Differential Diagnosis of Nits

Diagnosis	Comment
Nits	Firmly adherent to hair shaft; not easily removed with fingers
Seborrheic dermatitis (dandruff)	Diffuse scalp scaling; scales occasionally adhere to hair but easy to remove; scalp erythema may be present
Hair casts	Keratin protein that encircles hair shaft; easily removed
Piedra	Fungal infection of hair; firm nodules attached to hair shafts, white or black in color
Psoriasis	Thick silvery scales, often present overlying red plaques on the scalp
Hair products	Hairspray, mousse, gel

From Paller AS, Mancini, AJ: *Hurwitz clinical pediatric dermatology, a textbook of skin disorders of childhood and adolescence*, ed 5, Philadelphia, 2016, Elsevier.

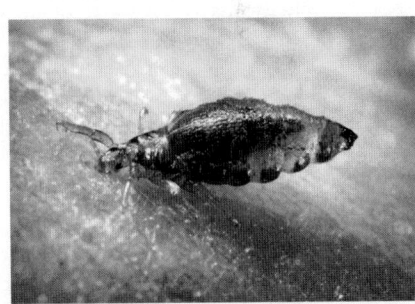

FIG. 4 Body louse, *Pediculus humanus* var. *corporis*, as it was obtaining a blood meal from human host. (Courtesy Public Health Image Library, Centers for Disease Control and Prevention. From Vincent JL et al: *Textbook of critical care,* ed 6, Philadelphia, 2011, Saunders.)

SUGGESTED READINGS

Available at ExpertConsult.com

RELATED CONTENT

Lice (Patient Information)

AUTHOR: **FRED F. FERRI, M.D.**

TREATMENTS FOR HEAD LICE

Treatment	Group	Administration on days 1 and 8	Concerns	Efficacy & resistance
Pyrethrins (0.33%) synergized with piperonyl butoxide (4%), various formulations*	Natural botanicals	Topical application for 10 minutes to dry hair	Allergic reactions in individuals with sensitivity to chrysanthemums, ragweed, and related plants	Poor–fair; resistance common
Permethrin cream rinse or lotion (1%)*	Synthetic pyrethroid	Topical application for 10 minutes to clean, dry hair	None	Poor–fair; resistance common
Permethrin cream (5%)†	Synthetic pyrethroid	Topical overnight application to clean, dry hair	Allergic contact dermatitis in individuals with sensitivity to formaldehyde	Poor–fair; resistance common
Lindane shampoo (1%)	Organochlorine	Topical application for 4 minutes to clean, dry hair, then add water to lather and rinse	Potential CNS toxicity; not recommended for infants, children, breastfeeding mothers or pregnant women (category C)	Poor; resistance common
Carbaryl shampoo (0.5%)	Carbamate cholinesterase inhibitor	Topical application for 8–12 hours	Possible carcinogen	Poor–fair; resistance common (not approved in the U.S.)
Benzyl alcohol lotion (5%)§	Alcohol	Topical application for 10 minutes to dry hair	Potential skin irritation	Good; no resistance noted to date
Dimethicone (4%)	Silicone oil	Topical application for 15 minutes or overnight	None	Good
Spinosad cream rinse (0.9%)§	Bacterial fermentation product	Topical application for 10 minutes to dry hair	None	Good; no resistance noted to date
Malathion lotion or gel (0.5%)‡	Organophosphate cholinesterase inhibitor	Topical application for 8–12 hours to dry hair (Ovide® and gel products with isopropyl alcohol base are effective at 20 minutes)	Flammable isopropyl alcohol base; burning or stinging at sites of eroded skin	Excellent (in U.S.); resistance noted in Europe and Australia, but to date not in U.S.
Ivermectin solution (0.5%)§	Avermectin	Topical application for 10 minutes to dry hair	Potential skin and eye irritation	Excellent; no resistance noted to date
Oral ivermectin (available as 3 mg tablets)		Oral dose of 200–400 mcg/kg	Potential CNS toxicity; not recommended for children weighing <33 pounds (15 kg), breastfeeding mothers or pregnant women (category C)	

*Over-the-counter products.
†Approved for individuals ≥2 months of age; pregnancy category B.
‡Approved for individuals ≥6 years of age; pregnancy category B.
§Approved for individuals ≥6 months of age; pregnancy category B.

FIG. 5 Treatments for head lice. In general, treatments should be given on two separate occasions, 1 week apart. However, the FDA-approved regimen for treatment of head lice with 0.5% ivermectin solution is a single application. Airallé ® is an FDA-cleared medical device that uses hot air to treat head lice via dehydration of their eggs and, to a lesser degree, hatched lice. Abametapir 0.74% lotion, an ovicidal metalloprotease inhibitor, has been shown in phase 3 clinical trials to have efficacy in the treatment of head lice. *CNS,* Central nervous system; *FDA,* U.S. Food and Drug Administration. (Bolognia JL et al: *Dermatology*, ed 4, Philadelphia, 2018, Elsevier.)

BASIC INFORMATION

DEFINITION

Pelvic abscess is an acute or chronic infection, most commonly involving the pelvic viscera. Treatment requires directed therapy including broad-spectrum antimicrobials and, if medical therapy fails, surgical intervention. There are four categories based on etiologic factors:

- Ascending infection, spreading from cervix through endometrial cavity to adnexa, forming a tuboovarian complex
- Infection occurring in the puerperium, which spreads to the adnexa from the endometrium or myometrium by a hematogenous or lymphatic route
- Abscess complicating pelvic surgery
- Involvement of the pelvic viscera as a result of spread from contiguous organs, such as appendicitis or diverticulitis

SYNONYMS

Tuboovarian abscess (TOA)
Vaginal cuff abscess

ICD-10CM CODES	
N70.93	Salpingitis and oophoritis, unspecified
N70.0	Acute salpingitis and oophoritis
N70.1	Chronic salpingitis and oophoritis
K63.0	Abscess of intestine
K65.1	Peritoneal abscess
K68.11	Postprocedural retroperitoneal abscess
K68.12	Psoas muscle abscess
K68.19	Other retroperitoneal abscess

EPIDEMIOLOGY & DEMOGRAPHICS

INCIDENCE:

- 34% of hospitalized patients with pelvic inflammatory disease
- 1% to 2% of patients undergoing hysterectomy, most with vaginal approach
- Peak incidence third to fourth decade

RISK FACTORS: Same risk factors as for pelvic inflammatory disease, although in 30% to 50% of patients there is no prior history of salpingitis before abscess forms.

PHYSICAL FINDINGS & CLINICAL PRESENTATION

- Abdominal or pelvic pain (90%)
- Fever or chills (50%)
- Abnormal bleeding (21%)
- Vaginal discharge (28%)
- Nausea (26%)
- Up to 60% to 80% present in the absence of fever or leukocytosis; absence of these findings should not exclude diagnosis

ETIOLOGY

- Mixed flora of anaerobes, aerobes, and facultative anaerobes, such as *Escherichia coli, Bacteroides fragilis, Prevotella* spp., aerobic streptococci, and *Peptococcus* and *Peptostreptococcus* spp.
- *Neisseria gonorrhoeae* and *Chlamydia* are the major etiologic bacteria in cervicitis and salpingitis but are rarely found in abscess cavity cultures.
- In elderly patients consider diverticular disease.

Dx DIAGNOSIS

DIFFERENTIAL DIAGNOSIS

- Pelvic neoplasms, such as ovarian tumors and leiomyomas.
- Ovarian torsion.
- Inflammatory masses involving adjacent bowel or omentum, such as ruptured appendicitis or diverticulitis.
- Pelvic hematomas, as may occur after cesarean section or hysterectomy.
- Section III describes the diagnostic approach to patients with a pelvic mass; the differential diagnosis of pelvic mass is described in Section II.
- The differential diagnosis of pelvic pain is described in Section II.
- Pelvic ultrasound or CT scan: Commonly used to characterize anatomic abnormalities such as a pelvic mass and to assess for suitability for possible drainage by interventional radiology techniques. Can also be used to follow response to treatment and to assess for resolution of abscess.
- Most common cause of preventable death: Physician delay in diagnosis.

LABORATORY TESTS

- CBC with differential
- Aerobic as well as anaerobic cultures of cervix, blood, urine, sputum, peritoneal cavity (if entered), and abscess cavity before starting antibiotics
- Pregnancy test in patients of reproductive age

IMAGING STUDIES

- Sonogram: Noninvasive, inexpensive study to confirm diagnosis, estimate size of abscess, and monitor response to therapy; sensitivity >90%
- CT scan: Used for both diagnosis and therapy (CT-guided drainage) (Fig. E1)
  1. Useful where sonogram provides insufficient information, as with intraabdominal abscesses
  2. Success rate with CT-guided abscess drainage: Unilocular, 90%; multilocular, 40%

Rx TREATMENT

Major concerns:

- Desire for future fertility
- Likelihood of rupture of abscess, with resulting peritonitis, septic shock, and morbid sequelae

ACUTE GENERAL Rx

- Clinical quandary is whether patient requires immediate laparoscopic surgery (uncertain diagnosis or suspicion of rupture) or management with IV antibiotics, reserving surgery for those with inadequate clinical response (e.g., 48-72 hr of therapy, with persistent fever or leukocytosis, increasing size of mass, or suspicion of rupture)
- Surgery indicated in poor response to medical therapy. Early surgery may be needed in those with large adnexal masses (>8 cm), or in immunocompromised patients
- Antibiotic combinations:
  1. Clindamycin 900 mg IV q8h or metronidazole 500 mg IV q6-8h plus gentamicin either 5 to 7 mg/kg q24h or 1.5 mg/kg q8h
  2. Alternatives: Ampicillin-sulbactam 3 g IV q6h or cefoxitin 2 g IV q6h or cefotetan 2 g IV q12h plus doxycycline 100 mg IV q12h
- During medical management, high index of suspicion for acute rupture, such as acute worsening of abdominal pain or new-onset tachycardia and hypotension, mandating immediate surgical intervention after patient stabilization
- Surgical options:
  1. Laparoscopy with drainage and irrigation
  2. CT-guided drainage (interventional radiology)
  3. Transvaginal colpotomy (abscess must be midline, dissect rectovaginal septum, and be adherent to vaginal fornix)
  4. Laparotomy, including total abdominal hysterectomy with bilateral salpingo-oophorectomy or unilateral salpingo-oophorectomy
  5. Evidence of ruptured tuboovarian abscess is a surgical emergency

DISPOSITION

- Of patients treated with medical therapy, response in 75%, with a 50% pregnancy rate. Pregnancy rate decreases with recurrent episodes.
- No response in 30% to 40%; can be treated with either CT-guided drainage or surgical intervention, keeping in mind that unilateral adnexectomy may give equal chance of cure versus hysterectomy, yet preserve reproductive potential.

REFERRAL

If patient has a tuboovarian abscess, refer to gynecologist.

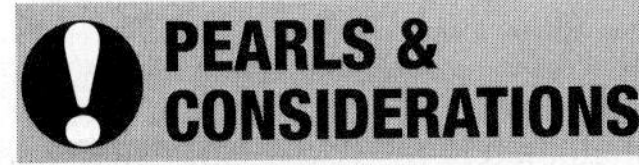

PEARLS & CONSIDERATIONS

COMMENTS

If *Actinomyces* species is isolated from culture, treatment with penicillin is required for an extended period (6 wk-3 mo).

SUGGESTED READING

Available at ExpertConsult.com

RELATED CONTENT

Pelvic Abscess (Patient Information)
Pelvic Inflammatory Disease (Related Key Topic)

AUTHOR: **ANTHONY SCISCIONE, D.O.**

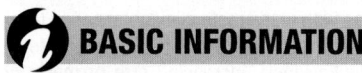

BASIC INFORMATION

DEFINITION

Pelvic inflammatory disease (PID) is infection and inflammation of the upper female genital tract (including uterus, fallopian tubes, ovaries, and/or pelvic peritoneum) unrelated to pregnancy or surgical intervention. PID can be classified as acute (≤30 days duration), subclinical, or chronic (>30 days duration).

SYNONYMS

PID
Salpingitis
Oophoritis
Adnexitis
Pyosalpinx
Tubo-ovarian abscess
TOA

ICD-10CM CODES

A18.17	Tuberculous female pelvic inflammatory disease
A52.76	Syphilitic pelvic inflammatory disease
A54.2	Gonococcal pelviperitonitis and other gonococcal genitourinary infections
A54.24	Gonococcal female pelvic inflammatory disease
A56.1	Chlamydial infection of pelviperitoneum and other genitourinary organs
A56.11	Chlamydial female pelvic inflammatory disease
N70	Salpingitis and oophoritis
N70.0	Acute salpingitis and oophoritis
N70.01	Acute salpingitis
N70.02	Acute oophoritis
N70.03	Acute salpingitis and oophoritis
N70.1	Chronic salpingitis and oophoritis
N70.11	Chronic salpingitis
N70.12	Chronic oophoritis
N70.13	Chronic salpingitis and oophoritis
N70.9	Salpingitis and oophoritis, unspecified
N70.91	Salpingitis, unspecified
N70.92	Oophoritis, unspecified
N70.93	Salpingitis and oophoritis, unspecified
N71	Inflammatory disease of uterus, except cervix
N71.0	Acute inflammatory disease of uterus
N71.1	Chronic inflammatory disease of uterus
N71.9	Inflammatory disease of uterus, unspecified
N73.0	Other female pelvic inflammatory diseases
N73.8	Other specified female pelvic inflammatory diseases
N74	Female pelvic inflammatory disorders in diseases classified elsewhere

EPIDEMIOLOGY & DEMOGRAPHICS

INCIDENCE/PREVALENCE: Pelvic inflammatory disease is most often diagnosed in young, sexually active women. The incidence of PID is difficult to ascertain given its broad diagnostic criteria, its propensity to be missed as a diagnosis, and the challenges with follow-up due to patients seeking urgent or emergent care for this condition. The Centers for Disease Control and Prevention estimates 1 million new cases of PID are diagnosed yearly. The incidence may be rising given recent sharp increases in STDs associated with PID in the United States. PID has long-term health risks for women including recurrent infection, chronic pelvic pain, pelvic adhesive disease, and tubal disease resulting in ectopic pregnancy and infertility.

RISK FACTORS:
- Sexually active adolescent and young women
- Previous episode of PID
- Prior chlamydial infection
- Multiple or new sexual partners within past 12 months
- Sexual partner diagnosed with sexually transmitted infection (STI)
- Non-use of barrier contraception

CLINICAL PRESENTATION

- Lower abdominal pain
- Abnormal vaginal discharge
- Abnormal uterine bleeding
- Postcoital bleeding
- Dysuria
- Dyspareunia
- Fever
- Nausea and vomiting (suggestive of peritonitis)

PHYSICAL FINDINGS

- Fever
- Abdominal tenderness
- Abnormal vaginal discharge
- Cervical friability
- Cervical motion tenderness
- Adnexal tenderness
- Adnexal mass
- Right upper quadrant tenderness (perihepatitis): 5% of PID cases

NOTE: Women with PID may be asymptomatic and/or have a benign physical examination.

ETIOLOGY

Pelvic inflammatory disease occurs as a result of ascending infection from the lower genital tract. Infections are often polymicrobial, and although gonorrheal and chlamydial infections are commonly implicated in the development of PID, fewer than 50% of women test positive for these organisms. This is likely due in part to increased STI screening efforts. PID may also arise in the setting of organisms associated with normal vaginal flora such as:
- *Bacteroides fragilis*
- *Escherichia coli and other enteric gram-negative rods*
- *Gardnerella vaginalis*
- *Haemophilus influenzae*

Rarer infectious causes include the following: *Mycoplasma hominis, Ureaplasma urealyticum, Mycoplasma genitalium* (a concern due to antibiotic resistance), *Mycobacterium tuberculosis* (an important cause in developing countries), and cytomegalovirus (CMV).

Dx DIAGNOSIS

Diagnosis of PID is made when a patient has clinical or pathologic evidence of upper genital tract infection and inflammation. Although no single test or measure reliably diagnoses the spectrum of disorders that comprise PID:
- Providers should maintain a low threshold for diagnosis and treatment of PID given significant long-term health risks associated with the disease, especially if untreated.
- Definitive criteria for diagnosis of PID include:
  1. Laparoscopic abnormalities consistent with PID
  2. Histopathologic evidence of endometritis in women with clinical suspicion for PID
  3. Transvaginal sonography or other imaging techniques showing thickened, fluid-filled tubes, with or without free pelvic fluid or tubo-ovarian complex
- The CDC suggests that women with risk factors, abdominal or pelvic pain, and any pelvic tenderness (cervical, uterine, and/or adnexal) be treated for PID.

DIFFERENTIAL DIAGNOSIS

- Appendicitis
- Ectopic pregnancy
- Intrauterine/other pregnancy
- Ovarian cyst
- Adnexal torsion
- Endometriosis
- Urinary tract infection (cystitis or pyelonephritis)

WORKUP

- History—as in risk factors and clinical presentation, previously
- Physical examination—as in physical findings, previously

LABORATORY TESTS

- Wet mount: Clue cells, increased white cells
- Gram stain of endocervical exudate: >30 polymorphonuclear cells per high-power field correlates with chlamydial or gonococcal infection
- Endocervical cultures for *N. gonorrhoeae* and *C. trachomatis*
- Fallopian tube aspirate or peritoneal exudate culture if laparoscopy performed
- WBC: Leukocytosis
- Elevated acute phase reactants: ESR >15 mm/hr, C-reactive protein
- HCG to rule out intrauterine or ectopic pregnancy
- HIV, with consideration for other STI screening such as RPR, HBsAg, Hep C Ab (HIV increases incidence of TOA)

IMAGING STUDIES

Ultrasonography is commonly used to assess for PID and can be used to determine inpatient vs. outpatient treatment by presence or absence of TOA. Findings include:
- Thick-walled adnexal mass with heterogenous or cystic contents suggestive of abscess
- Dilated fallopian tubes (note that normal fallopian tubes are rarely identified on ultrasonography)

- "Cogwheel sign" indicating thickened fallopian tube walls
- Heterogenous fluid within the endometrium

CT scan or MRI may be useful to better characterize adnexal masses and/or rule out other pathology such as appendicitis or renal calculus. Choice of imaging modality will depend on clinical suspicion, logistical access, and associated cost.

PROCEDURES

Endometrial biopsy that reveals endometritis may support a diagnosis of PID. Laparoscopy has been utilized as a gold standard for diagnosing PID, but due to the invasive nature of this procedure and the risks, and costs associated, it is rarely indicated as a diagnostic tool.

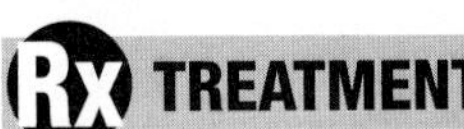

TREATMENT

Primary management of PID is medical, with broad-spectrum antibiotics administered in an outpatient setting. Inpatient treatment should be initiated when:

- Surgical emergency is not excluded
- Tubo-ovarian abscess is present
- Patient is unable or unwilling to complete outpatient treatment (including medication regimen and clinical follow-up)
- Outpatient treatment fails to improve symptoms in 48 to 72 hours
- Pregnancy, immunodeficiency, or other complicating medical condition exists

Evidence-based guidelines recommended by the CDC for acute PID are as follows:

INPATIENT REGIMENS: Recommended parenteral regimens

- Cefotetan 2 g IV q12h *PLUS* Doxycycline 100 mg PO or IV q12h OR
- Cefoxitin 2 g IV q6h *PLUS* Doxycycline 100 mg PO or IV q12h
  OR
- Clindamycin 900 mg IV q8h *PLUS* Gentamicin loading dose IV or IM (2 mg/kg of body weight), followed by a maintenance dose (1.5 mg/kg) q8h. Single daily dosing (3-5 mg/kg) can be substituted.

Alternative parenteral regimen

- Ampicillin/sulbactam 3 g IV q6h *PLUS* Doxycycline 100 mg PO or IV q12h

When clinical improvement is apparent based on symptoms, physical exam, and laboratory criteria, antibiotics may be transitioned from IV to PO with doxycycline PO or clindamycin PO (depending on the regimen selected) administered to complete 14 days of total antibiotic therapy. If a patient does not improve despite use of a recommended antibiotic regimen, further workup and potential procedural intervention are warranted.

OUTPATIENT REGIMENS: Recommended intramuscular/oral regimens

- Ceftriaxone 250 mg IM in a single dose *PLUS* Doxycycline 100 mg PO bid for 14 days
  WITH or WITHOUT Metronidazole 500 mg PO bid for 14 days
  OR
- Cefoxitin 2 g IM in a single dose and Probenecid, 1 g PO administered concurrently in a single dose *PLUS* Doxycycline 100 mg PO bid for 14 days
  WITH or WITHOUT Metronidazole 500 mg PO bid for 14 days
  OR
- Other third-generation cephalosporin (Ceftizoxime or Cefotaxime) *PLUS* Doxycycline 100 mg orally bid for 14 days
  WITH or WITHOUT Metronidazole 500 mg orally twice a day for 14 days

Alternative intramuscular/oral regimen

- Azithromycin 1 g PO once weekly for 2 weeks PLUS Ceftriaxone 250 mg IM in a single dose

TREATMENT CONSIDERATIONS

- Antimicrobials should include coverage against *N. gonorrhoeae* and *C. trachomatis* even if these organisms are not identified on culture.
- Due to increasing antibiotic resistance of *N. gonorrhoeae*, fluoroquinolones should be avoided in the treatment of PID. If gonorrhea is isolated in a woman with PID, addition of azithromycin 1 g orally one time should be considered in treatment.
- Women should avoid sexual activity until they and their sexual partners have been adequately treated and symptoms have resolved.
- TOA may require drainage, which may be accomplished by interventional radiology via aspiration or placement of a drain, or by a gynecologist via vaginal or laparoscopic means. Recurrent/persistent TOAs may be managed by total abdominal hysterectomy with bilateral salpingo-oophorectomy after acute treatment of infection.
- Treatment of PID in women with intrauterine devices (IUDs) does not include/require removal of the device unless there is no clinical improvement after 48 to 72 hours of treatment with an approved regimen. IUDs rarely serve as a source for PID, especially greater than 3 weeks after insertion.
- Sexual partners of patients diagnosed with PID or other STIs should be evaluated and treated appropriately. In the setting of PID, treat all sexual partners within 60 days of onset of symptoms. Some states allow for expedited partner therapy (EPT), such that a woman's provider is able to supply her with enough medication to treat herself and her partner(s).
- Treatment of chronic PID may be aimed at a different spectrum of microbes and should be tailored appropriately.

DISPOSITION

- Given the risk of reinfection, all women should be retested for gonorrhea and chlamydia 3 to 6 months after treatment.
- Follow-up includes confirmation of partner treatment, education on use of barrier contraception, and risks of PID and long-term sequelae, including:
  1. Recurrent PID.
  2. Chronic pelvic pain.
  3. Fallopian tubal damage that leads to infertility and/or ectopic pregnancy.
  4. Fitz-Hugh-Curtis syndrome.
  5. Potential risk for cancer: Limited studies have suggested a small association between PID and ovarian, endometrial, and colon cancer.

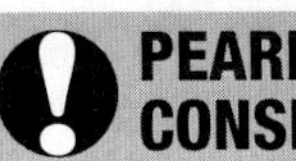

PEARLS & CONSIDERATIONS

COMMENTS

- Maintain a low threshold for the diagnosis and treatment of PID given the risks for progression to severe infection and to significant and chronic medical and reproductive complications.
- Most patients are candidates for outpatient therapy, but inpatient hospitalization is recommended in select cases.
- Use only CDC-recommended treatment regimens unless contraindicated due to severe patient allergy; in such cases, check local susceptibilities of suspected pathogen.
- Offer HIV and other STI screening to all women with suspected or diagnosed PID.
- IUDs may be retained unless women have failed to improve with 48 to 72 hours of treatment.
- Treat sexual partners of women with PID, with EPT if possible.
- Counsel patients on abstinence until they and their partners have completed treatment.
- Test for reinfection with gonorrhea and chlamydia 3 to 6 months after treatment.

PREVENTION

Women aged <25 yr and/or participating in high-risk sexual behavior should be screened annually for chlamydia; studies have shown such screening to reduce cases of PID by >50%. The importance of minimizing partner exposures and using barrier contraception (either alone or in conjunction with another method) should also be emphasized.

SUGGESTED READINGS

Available at ExpertConsult.com

RELATED CONTENT

Pelvic Inflammatory Disease (Patient Information)
Chlamydia Genital Infections (Related Key Topic)
Gonorrhea (Related Key Topic)
Pelvic Abscess (Related Key Topic)

AUTHOR: **GRETCHEN MAKAI, M.D.**

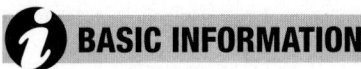

BASIC INFORMATION

DEFINITION

Pelvic organ prolapse (POP) refers to descent of vaginal tissue into the vaginal canal. It results from injury to or weakness in the connective tissue and muscles of the pelvic floor. Modern definitions of POP describe anterior and posterior vaginal wall defects as well as apical defects in pelvic floor connective tissue. Synonyms include terms such as cystocele, rectocele, uterine prolapse, enterocele, and vaginal vault prolapse. Descriptions of this condition as a "dropped bladder," "dropped uterus," or defect in other pelvic organs should be avoided. These types of descriptions do not accurately reflect the pathophysiology of POP and often create confusion and unnecessary stress for patients. Table 1 describes the various types of POP affecting each vaginal compartment with corresponding ICD-10 codes.

SYNONYMS

Vaginal prolapse
Uterine prolapse
Genital prolapse
Uterine descensus
POP
Pelvic floor disorder
PFD

ICD-10CM CODES

N81.4 Uterovaginal prolapse, unspecified
N81.5 Vaginal enterocele
N81.6 Rectocele
N81.I8 Other female genital prolapse
N81.2 Incomplete uterovaginal prolapse
N81.82 Incompetence or weakening of pubocervical tissue

EPIDEMIOLOGY & DEMOGRAPHICS

INCIDENCE AND PREVALENCE: Recent estimates of overall prevalence reveal a rate of 3% to 4% based on objective criteria and physical examination. Prevalence estimates based on nonobjective criteria are often higher. Prevalence increases with age, parity, and BMI. Exact prevalence estimates are difficult to determine due to varying definitions of POP and various diagnostic criteria. POP is common and carries a high burden of disease negatively affecting overall quality of life. The lifetime risk of undergoing surgery due to POP is estimated to be 12%. Annual direct health care costs are high, and repeat operations are common.

GENETICS: Data suggest a heritable component to POP. No specific genes or genetic factors outside of specific connective tissue diseases have been identified. For example, the risk of POP is increased in women with Marfan syndrome and Ehlers-Danlos syndrome. Because POP is multifactorial and has a long latency, risk estimates based on genetics or family history are difficult to quantify. In general, a genetic susceptibility exists in certain families, which is then affected by external factors to increase an individual woman's risk of POP.

RISK FACTORS: POP has a long latency and is multifactorial. Multiple risk factors have been identified. Some are modifiable, suggesting POP may be preventable. However, many risk factors are not modifiable. Below is a list of the most common risk factors for POP:

- Vaginal childbirth
- Labor
- Pregnancy
- Age
- Chronic obstructive pulmonary disease (COPD) and chronic coughing
- Smoking
- Chronic constipation
- Chronic heavy lifting
- Chronic steroid use
- Connective tissue diseases (Marfan syndrome, Ehlers-Danlos syndrome)
- Pelvic surgery (including hysterectomy)
- Menopause
- Family history
- Caucasian and Hispanic race

ETIOLOGY

- The cause of pelvic organ prolapse is usually multifactorial, but pregnancy is the most commonly associated risk factor.
- Muscle injury (levator ani) and connective tissue damage (pubocervical fascia) cause failure of pelvic floor support.
- Increased intraabdominal pressure results in strain on pelvic floor support structures.
- Injury to pelvic floor muscles or connective tissue supports results in uncompensated forces on pelvic floor, resulting in further injury to pelvic floor support structures.
    1. Acute (traumatic) injury to pelvic floor support can result from vaginal delivery, labor, or surgery.
    2. Chronic injury or strain on pelvic floor connective tissue and muscle can result from conditions such as COPD with chronic coughing or chronic constipation.
    3. Neurologic injury from acute or chronic strain on pelvic floor can result in denervation and subsequent muscular atrophy.
    4. Diseases or medications that weaken connective tissue (Marfan syndrome, corticosteroids) can predispose to injury.
    5. Hypoestrogenism may weaken pelvic floor tissue and impair ability to heal from injury.
- With injury to pelvic floor support structures, vaginal tissue becomes subjected to the forces from intraabdominal pressure and will stretch and become displaced downward and out through the vaginal opening, resulting in clinical symptoms.

PHYSICAL FINDINGS AND CLINICAL PRESENTATION

- Bulge symptoms
    1. Vaginal pressure
    2. Protrusion from vagina (Fig. E1)
- Urinary symptoms (mainly from obstruction)
    1. Urinary hesitancy
    2. Urinary frequency or urgency
    3. Manual reduction of prolapse to complete urination
    4. Incomplete emptying
    5. Weak urinary stream
- Bowel symptoms
    1. Incomplete defecation
    2. Altered rectal sensation (urgency, lack of sensation)
    3. Splinting of vagina/perineum to defecate
- Sexual symptoms
    1. Dyspareunia
    2. Difficulty with vaginal penetration
- Other
    1. Vaginal bleeding from excoriated vaginal epithelium from chronic exteriorization
    2. Incarcerated prolapse with inability to be manually reduced

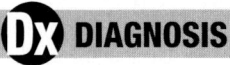

DIAGNOSIS

WORKUP

- Elicit specific symptoms.
- Perform detailed pelvic exam. Examine anterior, posterior, and apical segments of vagina independently.
- POP is dynamic and may not appear the same at various time points or exam conditions.
- Exam is done in standard lithotomy position, and POP is assessed with Valsalva during exam.
    1. If symptoms are out of proportion to findings, repeat exam in standing position.
- Describe exam findings objectively (Boxes 1, 2, and 3).
    1. Quantitatively with POP-Q.
    2. Descriptively with Baden-Walker halfway systems.
- Urinary symptoms should be evaluated separately.
    1. POP is associated with urinary incontinence but *does not cause* urinary incontinence.
- Evaluate post void residual urine volume in advanced POP (stages 3 and stage 4).
    1. Bladder ultrasound or catheterization at time of exam.

TABLE 1 Types of Genital Prolapse

Original Position of Organs	Prolapse	Symptoms (in addition to the general symptoms of discomfort, dragging, the feeling of a "lump," and, rarely, coital problems)
Anterior	Urethrocele Cystocele	Urinary symptoms (stress incontinence, urinary frequency)
Central	Cervix/uterus: 1st, 2nd, and 3rd degree Procidentia	Bleeding and/or discharge from ulceration in association with procidentia
Posterior	Rectocele Enterocele	Bowel symptoms, particularly the feeling of incomplete evacuation and sometimes having to press the posterior wall backward to pass stool

P

Diseases and Disorders

BOX 1 Points of Reference for POP-Q

Point	Description	Range of Values
Aa	3 cm above the hymen on anterior vaginal wall roughly corresponds with the urethrovesical junction.	−3 cm to +3 cm
Ba	The lowest extent of the segment of vagina between point Aa and the apex of the vagina. Unlike point Aa, it is not fixed but will be the same as Aa if point Aa is the most protruding point. In maximal prolapse, it will be the same as point C.	−3 cm to + tvl
C	Most distal edge of cervix (vaginal cuff if uterus/cervix absent).	
D	Posterior fornix (n/a if hysterectomy).	
Ap	3 cm above the hymen on posterior vaginal wall.	−3 cm to +3 cm
Bp	The lowest extent of the segment of vagina between point Ap and the apex of the vagina. Unlike point Ap, it is not fixed but will be the same as Ap if point Ap is the most protruding point. In maximal prolapse it will be the same as point D.	−3 cm to + tvl
GH (Genital Hiatus)	From urethral meatus to inferior hymenal ring.	
PB (Perineal Body)	From inferior hymenal ring to middle of anal orifice.	
TVL	Total Vaginal Length without stretch or Valsalva.	

Key Points: Measure position of six points with respect to the position of the hymen. Points above the hymen (inside) are negative, points below the hymen are positive, and points at the hymen are 0.
Modified from Pemberton J (ed): *The pelvic floor,* Philadelphia, 2002, WB Saunders; and Bump RC et al: *Am J Obstet Gynecol* 175(1):13, 1996.

BOX 2 POP-Q Examination and Staging

Stage 0	No prolapse
Stage I	Leading edge ≥1 cm above hymenal ring
Stage II	Leading edge ≤1 cm above hymenal ring but ≤1 cm below hymenal ring
Stage III	Most distal point is >1 cm but < (TVL -2) cm below the hymenal ring
Stage IV	Leading edge ≥ (TVL-2) cm below hymenal ring

BOX 3 Baden Walker Halfway System

Grade 0	Normal position for each respective site
Grade 1	Descent halfway to the hymen
Grade 2	Descent to the hymen
Grade 3	Descent halfway past the hymen
Grade 4	Maximum possible descent for each site

LABORATORY TESTS

Not indicated for routine evaluation of POP. Urine testing may be indicated based on presence or absence of urinary tract symptoms.

IMAGING STUDIES

- Not indicated for routine evaluation of POP. Imaging studies for other gynecologic or urologic conditions may be indicated.
- Pelvic ultrasound may be considered in the *absence of POP* in patients with specific symptoms (i.e., pelvic pressure) (Fig. E2).

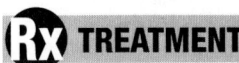

Rx TREATMENT

NONPHARMACOLOGIC THERAPY

Primary prevention:

- Diagnosis and treatment of chronic cough
- Correction of constipation
- Weight control, nutrition, and smoking cessation counseling
- Pelvic muscle exercises
- Proper management of vaginal apex at time of hysterectomy in patients without POP
- McCall culdoplasty to prevent vaginal vault prolapse
- Cesarean delivery NOT indicated for prevention of POP
- Untreated urinary retention, even if asymptomatic, can cause bladder infection, reflux, and renal damage

ACUTE GENERAL TREATMENT

TREATMENT OPTIONS:

- Expectant management is appropriate, except in cases of incomplete bladder emptying associated with POP.
- Pessaries:
  1. Support device
  2. Silicone, not latex
  3. Various shapes and sizes exist
  4. Use the simplest and smallest pessary that works
  5. 85% of women can be fitted successfully with a pessary
     a. Includes sexually active women
  6. Self-care can be learned by the majority of women
     a. Usually remove and clean once per month; otherwise, office visit every 3 months for cleaning and exam
  7. Pessary use associated with higher risk of UTI
  8. Small vaginal erosions and very mild bleeding or spotting are common side effects
     a. First episode of vaginal bleeding needs evaluation in postmenopausal patients
  9. Neglected pessary can cause vaginitis, odor, severe vaginal erosion/bleeding, and fistula
  10. Vaginal estrogen may prevent or treat erosions and minimize risk of vaginitis and UTI

CHRONIC Rx

- Surgery:
  1. Goals of surgery are to eliminate vaginal bulge and improve associated symptoms.
     a. Most reliable symptom resolution is elimination of bulge/protrusion.
     b. Resolution of bladder and bowel symptoms is not routinely associated with surgical correction of POP.
  2. Evaluate and treat all defects present on exam.
     a. Combination defects are the most common presentation.
     b. 60% of patients present with multiple defects.
     c. Anterior and apical combination is most common.
  3. There are multiple ways to classify operations for POP (Table 2).
  4. Obliterative vs. reconstructive procedures:
     a. Obliterative procedures remove the vaginal tissue and close off the genital hiatus.
     b. High success rates with low morbidity.
     c. Option for women who are willing to forgo future vaginal intercourse.
     d. Associated with high rates of postoperative incontinence; most surgeons offer anti-incontinence procedure at the same setting.
  5. Reconstructive procedures:
     a. Restore normal functional anatomy.
     b. Subdivided into restorative or compensatory procedures:
        (1) Restorative procedures use normal anatomic relationships and structures.
        (2) Compensatory procedures utilize nonanatomic relationships and may or may not use synthetic meshes and graphs.
  6. Table 3 categorizes various common procedures for POP.
  7. Hysterectomy alone does not treat POP.
     a. Often performed concomitantly with POP repair as necessary step to expose critical anatomy.
  8. Choice of operation should be tailored to patient's presenting problems, lifestyle, and goals for the surgery.

TABLE 2 Surgical Approach to Pelvic Organ Prolapse

POP-Q Site	Vaginal	Abdominal
Aa	Anterior repair	Retropubic urethropexy
Urethra	Bladder neck suspension sling	
Ba	Anterior repair	Wedge colpectomy
Bladder	Paravaginal repair	Paravaginal repair
	Colpocleisis	Abdominal sacrocolpopexy
C	Uterosacral ligament suspension	Abdominal hysterectomy
Cervix/cuff	Iliococcygeus suspension	Uterosacral ligament suspension
	Sacrospinous fixation	Abdominal sacral colpopexy
	Manchester operation	Uterine suspension
	Hysteropexy	
	Vaginal hysterectomy	
	Colpocleisis	
D	McCall culdoplasty	Halban culdoplasty
Cul-de-sac		Moschkowitz culdoplasty
Ap	Rectovaginal plication (posterior repair)	Colpoperineopexy
	Site-specific repairs	

POP-Q, Pelvic Organ Prolapse Quantification System.
From Wein AJ et al: *Campbell-Walsh urology,* ed 11, Philadelphia, 2016, Elsevier.

TABLE 3 Procedures for POP

Classification		Procedure	Compartment(s)
Obliterative		Le Fort colpocleisis	All
		Total colpocleisis	All
Reconstructive	Restorative	Uterosacral ligament suspension	Apex
		Hysteropexy	Apex
		Paravaginal defect repair	Anterior
		Anterior colporrhaphy	Anterior
		Posterior colporrhaphy	Posterior
		Defect-directed posterior repair	Posterior
		Perineorrhaphy	Posterior
	Compensatory		
	Mesh	Sacral colpopexy	All
		Sacral hysteropexy	Apex
		Transvaginal mesh	All
	Nonmesh	Sacrospinous ligament suspension	Apex
		Ileococcygeus suspension	Apex
		Enterocele repair	Posterior

9. For symptomatic women who desire childbearing: Management with pessaries or pelvic muscle exercises is recommended; if surgical correction is required, uterosacral ligament hysteropexy is the preferred method.
   a. Patients should be counseled that repair will likely break down with subsequent pregnancy.
10. Women without stress incontinence undergoing vaginal surgery for POP are at risk for postoperative urinary incontinence.
11. Use of a prophylactic midurethral sling inserted during vaginal prolapse surgery has been shown to result in a lower rate of urinary incontinence at 3 and 12 months, but also in a higher rate of adverse events (UTIs, major bleeding complications, incomplete bladder emptying).
12. Abdominal mesh-based repairs and anterior vaginal mesh repairs have superior durability but higher risk and potential for unique complications.
13. Mesh erosion rates have been reported up to 10%, with similar incidence between biologic and synthetic graft. However, synthetic graft erosion often requires surgical revision.

DISPOSITION

- Surgical success rates range between 70% and 95%.
- Up to 30% of patients may require a second operation for POP.
- Untreated POP does not necessarily worsen.

REFERRAL

- To a urogynecologist/gynecologist if surgical intervention is needed or for complex cases involving bladder dysfunction.
- Treating physicians should have special training with synthetic mesh products, if they are used.

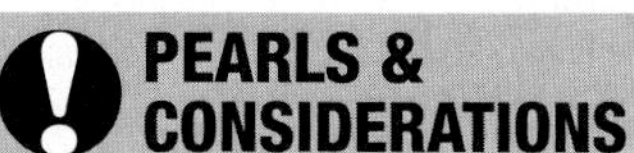

PEARLS & CONSIDERATIONS

- POP rarely, if ever, causes pain.
- Stage of POP does not dictate treatment or prognosis.
- Treatment for POP is based on symptoms and patient bother.
- Options for most patients are no treatment, pessary, or surgery.

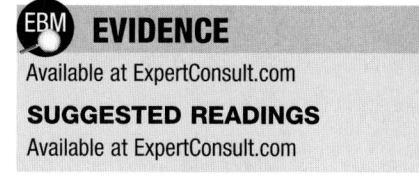

EVIDENCE

Available at ExpertConsult.com

SUGGESTED READINGS

Available at ExpertConsult.com

RELATED CONTENT

Pelvic Organ Prolapse (Patient Information)
Uterine Prolapse (Patient Information)
Incontinence, Urinary (Related Key Topic)

AUTHORS: **SHIVANI SHAH, M.D.,** and **MATTHEW J. FAGAN, M.D., F.A.C.O.G.**

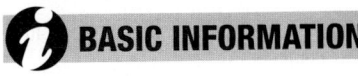

BASIC INFORMATION

DEFINITION

Peptic ulcer disease (PUD) is an ulceration in the stomach or duodenum resulting from an imbalance between mucosal protective factors and various mucosal damaging mechanisms (see "Etiology").

SYNONYMS

PUD
Duodenal ulcer (DU)
Gastric ulcer (GU)

ICD-10CM CODES

K25.3	Acute gastric ulcer without hemorrhage or perforation
K25.7	Chronic gastric ulcer without hemorrhage or perforation
K26.3	Acute duodenal ulcer without hemorrhage or perforation
K26.7	Chronic duodenal ulcer without hemorrhage or perforation
K27.0	Acute peptic ulcer, site unspecified, with hemorrhage
K27.1	Acute peptic ulcer, site unspecified, with perforation
K27.2	Acute peptic ulcer, site unspecified, with both hemorrhage and perforation
K27.3	Acute peptic ulcer, site unspecified, without hemorrhage or perforation
K27.4	Chronic or unspecified peptic ulcer, site unspecified, with hemorrhage
K27.5	Chronic or unspecified peptic ulcer, site unspecified, with perforation
K27.6	Chronic or unspecified peptic ulcer, site unspecified, with both hemorrhage and perforation
K27.7	Chronic peptic ulcer, site unspecified, without hemorrhage or perforation
K27.9	Peptic ulcer, site unspecified, unspecified as acute or chronic, without hemorrhage or perforation
P78.82	Peptic ulcer of newborn
Z87.11	Personal history of peptic ulcer disease

EPIDEMIOLOGY & DEMOGRAPHICS

- Incidence: 250,000 to 500,000 (200,000 to 400,000 duodenal; 50,000 to 100,000 gastric) annually; duodenal ulcer/gastric ulcer ratio is 4:1.
- Anatomic location: <90% of duodenal ulcers occur in the first portion of the duodenum; gastric ulcers occur most frequently in the lesser curvature near the incisura angularis.

PHYSICAL FINDINGS & CLINICAL PRESENTATION

- Epigastric pain is the most frequently reported symptom of PUD. The pain is typically improved with food or antacids and worsened by fasting.
- Physical examination is often unremarkable.
- Patient may have epigastric tenderness, tachycardia, pallor, hypotension (from acute or chronic blood loss), nausea and vomiting (if pyloric channel is obstructed), board-like abdomen and rebound tenderness (if perforated), and hematemesis or melena (with a bleeding ulcer). Box 1 describes key symptoms and signs of peptic ulcer.

ETIOLOGY

Often multifactorial. The following are common mucosal damaging factors:

- *Helicobacter pylori* infection. *H. pylori* is the major cause of PUD. It is found in more than 70% of patients with duodenal ulcers and gastric ulcers in the United States. Rates are much higher (>90%) in other parts of the world. Eradication of *H. pylori* markedly reduces peptic ulcer recurrence.
- Medications (NSAIDs, glucocorticoids). Risk factors for development of NSAID-related ulcers are described in Table 1.
- Incompetent pylorus or lower esophageal sphincter.
- Bile acids.
- Impaired proximal duodenal bicarbonate secretion.
- Decreased blood flow to gastric mucosa.
- Acid secreted by parietal cells and pepsin secreted as pepsinogen by chief cells.
- Cigarette smoking.
- Alcohol.

BOX 1 Key Symptoms and Signs of Peptic Ulcer

Uncomplicated Ulcer
No symptoms ("silent ulcer" in up to 40% of cases)
Epigastric pain
Pain may radiate to the back, thorax, other parts of abdomen (cephalad most likely, caudad least likely)
Pain may be nocturnal (most specific), "painful hunger" relieved by food, or continuous (least specific)
Nausea
Vomiting
Heartburn (mimics or associated with gastroesophageal reflux)

Complicated Ulcer
Acute perforation
Severe abdominal pain
Shock
Abdominal boardlike rigidity (and rebound and other signs of peritoneal irritation)
Free intraperitoneal air
Hemorrhage
Hematemesis and/or melena
Hemodynamic changes, anemia
Previous history of ulcer symptoms (80%)
Gastric outlet obstruction
Satiation, inability to ingest food, eructation
Nausea, vomiting (and related disturbances)
Weight loss

From Goldman L, Schafer AI: *Goldman's Cecil medicine*, ed 24, Philadelphia, 2012, Saunders.

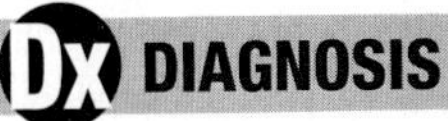

DIAGNOSIS

DIFFERENTIAL DIAGNOSIS

- Gastroesophageal reflux disease
- Cholelithiasis syndrome
- Pancreatitis
- Gastritis
- Nonulcer dyspepsia
- Neoplasm (gastric carcinoma, lymphoma, pancreatic carcinoma)
- Angina pectoris, myocardial infarction, pericarditis
- Dissecting aneurysm
- Other: High small-bowel obstruction, pneumonia, subphrenic abscess, early appendicitis

WORKUP

Comprehensive history and physical exam to exclude other diagnoses. Diagnostic modalities include endoscopy or upper GI series. Endoscopy is preferred and remains the gold standard for diagnosis of PUD. The presence of a mucosal break ≥5 mm in the stomach or duodenum confirms the diagnosis.

TABLE 1 Risk Factors for Development of NSAID-Related Ulcers

Definite
Advanced age
History of ulcer
Concomitant corticosteroid therapy
Concomitant anticoagulation therapy
High doses of NSAIDs
Serious systemic disorders

Possible
Concomitant infection with *Helicobacter pylori*
Cigarette smoking
Consumption of alcohol

NSAIDs, Nonsteroidal antiinflammatory drugs.
From Andreoli TE et al: *Andreoli and Carpenter's Cecil essentials of medicine,* ed 8, Philadelphia, 2010, Saunders.

LABORATORY TESTS

- Routine laboratory evaluation is usually unremarkable.
- Anemia may be present in patients with significant GI bleeding.
- *H. pylori* testing by endoscopic biopsy, urea breath test or stool antigen test (*H. pylori* stool antigen) is recommended:
  1. The urea breath test documents active infection (sensitivity and specificity >90%). The patient ingests a small amount of urea labeled with carbon 13 or carbon 14. If urease is present (produced by the organism), the urea is hydrolyzed and the patient exhales labeled carbon dioxide that is then collected and measured. Use of proton pump inhibitors (PPI) within 2 wk of the urea breath test may interfere with test results.
  2. Stool antigen test is an ELISA that identifies *H. pylori* antigen in a stool specimen through a polyclonal anti–*H. pylori* antibody. It is as accurate as the urea breath test for diagnosis of active infection and follow-up evaluation of patients treated for *H. pylori.* A negative result on the stool antigen test 6 wk after completion of therapy identifies patients in whom eradication of *H. pylori* was successful.
  3. Serologic testing for antibodies to *H. pylori* is easy and inexpensive; however, the presence of antibodies demonstrates previous but not necessarily current infection. Antibodies to *H. pylori* can remain elevated for months to years after infection has cleared; therefore antibody levels must be interpreted in light of the patient's symptoms and other test results (e.g., PUD seen on upper GI series).
  4. Histologic evaluation of endoscopic biopsy samples is considered by many the gold standard for accurate diagnosis of *H. pylori* infection. However, detection of *H. pylori* depends on the site and number of biopsy samples, the method of staining, and experience of the pathologist.
- Additional laboratory evaluation is indicated only in specific cases (e.g., amylase level in suspected pancreatitis, serum gastrin level in suspected Zollinger-Ellison [ZE] syndrome).

IMAGING STUDIES

- Conventional upper GI barium studies identify approximately 70% to 80% of PUD; accuracy can be increased to approximately 90% by using double contrast.
- Abdominal CT is helpful when suspecting perforating peptic ulcer disease (sensitivity >95%).

Rx TREATMENT

NONPHARMACOLOGIC THERAPY

- Stop smoking; smoking increases the risk of PUD, decreases the healing rate, and increases the frequency of recurrence.
- Avoid NSAIDs and alcohol.
- Special diets have been proved unrelated to ulcer development and healing; however, avoid foods that cause symptoms.

ACUTE GENERAL Rx

Eradication of *H. pylori,* when present, can be accomplished with various regimens (see "*Helicobacter pylori* Infection")

PUD patients testing negative for *H. pylori* should be treated with antisecretory agents:

- H_2 receptor antagonists (H_2RAs): Ranitidine, famotidine, and nizatidine are all effective; they are usually given in split dose or at nighttime.
- PPIs: Can also induce rapid healing; they are usually given 30 min before meals.

Antacids and sucralfate are also effective agents for the treatment and prevention of PUD.

CHRONIC Rx

Maintenance therapy in peptic ulcer patients is indicated in the following situations:

- Persistent smokers
- Recurrent ulcerations
- Long-term treatment with NSAIDs, glucocorticoids
- Elderly or debilitated patients
- Aggressive or complicated ulcer disease (e.g., perforation, hemorrhage)
- Asymptomatic bleeders

DISPOSITION

- The recurrence rate for untreated PUD is ~60% (>70% in smokers). Treatment decreases the recurrence rate by nearly 30%.
- Patients with recurrent ulcers should be re-treated for an additional 8 wk and then placed on maintenance therapy with H_2RAs, PPIs, sucralfate, or antacids.
- An ulcer is considered refractory to treatment if healing is not evident after 8 wk for duodenal ulcers and 12 wk for gastric ulcers. In these patients maximum acid inhibition (e.g., esomeprazole 40 mg bid) is preferred over continued therapy with standard antiulcer therapy.
- Eradication of *H. pylori* (when present) is indicated in all patients. A negative stool antigen test for *H. pylori* 6 wk after treatment accurately confirms cure of *H. pylori* infection with reasonable sensitivity in initially seropositive healthy subjects.
- Screening for ZE syndrome should also be considered in patients with multiple recurrent ulcers; in patients with ZE, the serum gastrin level is >1000 pg/ml and the basal acid output is usually >15 mEq/hr.
- Surgery for refractory ulcers is now only rarely performed; it consists of highly selective vagotomy for duodenal ulcers or ulcer removal with antrectomy or hemigastrectomy without vagotomy for gastric ulcers.

REFERRAL

- GI referral for patients requiring endoscopy
- Surgical referral for patients with nonhealing ulcers despite appropriate medical therapy

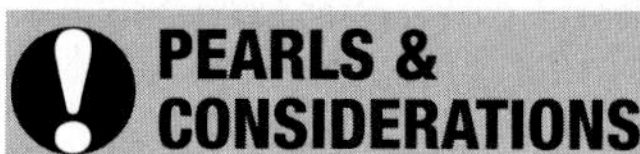

PEARLS & CONSIDERATIONS

COMMENTS

- Patients with gastric ulcers should generally have repeat endoscopy after 8 to 12 wk of antisecretory therapy to document healing and test exfoliative cytology for gastric carcinoma. Patients with duodenal ulcers and those with low risk gastric ulcers, such as young patients on NSAIDs, generally do not require endoscopic surveillance.
- After endoscopic treatment of bleeding peptic ulcers, bleeding recurs in up to 20% of patients. PPI administration intravenously by continuous infusion substantially reduces the risk of recurrent bleeding. High-dose IV esomeprazole (80 mg IV bolus followed by 8 mg/hr infusion over 72 hr) given after successful endoscopic therapy to patients with high-risk peptic ulcer bleeding has been reported to reduce recurrent bleeding at 72 hr and to maintain sustained clinical benefits for up to 30 days.
- Among low-dose aspirin recipients who had peptic ulcer bleeding, continuous aspirin therapy may increase the risk for recurrent bleeding.

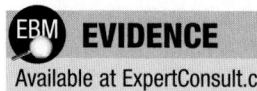

EVIDENCE

Available at ExpertConsult.com

RELATED CONTENT

Peptic Ulcer (Patient Information)
Helicobacter pylori Infection (Related Key Topic)

AUTHOR: **FRED F. FERRI, M.D.**

BASIC INFORMATION

DEFINITION

Acute pericarditis is the inflammation (or infiltration) of the pericardium. It is characterized by at least two of the following four criteria: (1) chest pain, (2) specific electrocardiographic changes, (3) pericardial friction rub, or (4) pathognomonic pericardial friction rub.

ICD-10CM CODES

I30.0	Acute nonspecific idiopathic pericarditis
I30.1	Infectious pericarditis
I30.8	Other forms of acute pericarditis
I30.9	Acute pericarditis, unspecified
I301.0	Chronic adhesive pericarditis
I31.1	Chronic constrictive pericarditis
I31.3	Pericardial effusion (non-inflammatory)
I31.9	Diseases of pericardium, unspecified (tamponade)
I31.2	Hemopericardium

EPIDEMIOLOGY & DEMOGRAPHICS

- Most common form of pericardial disease worldwide.
  It is diagnosed in 0.1% to 0.2% of hospitalized patients and is responsible for 5% of patients admitted for nonischemic chest pain.

PHYSICAL FINDINGS & CLINICAL PRESENTATION

- Chest pain: Characteristically sharp, pleuritic, positional (due to rubbing of inflamed pericardial layers). It is improved by sitting up and leaning forward.
- A triphasic, scratchy sound best heard at the lower left sternal border with patient sitting up and leaning forward is considered pathognomonic. Unlike pleural friction rub, the rub of pericarditis is not affected by respiration.
- Pericardial effusion: Beck triad (hypotension, elevated jugular venous pressure, and muffled heart sounds) suggests pericardial tamponade.

ETIOLOGY

- Etiology is dichotomized into infectious and noninfectious causes.
- In developed countries, virus is the most common cause of pericarditis. However, a lot of cases are categorized as idiopathic due to lack of established etiology. Tuberculosis accounts for 80% to 90% of pericarditis in developing countries.
- Other infectious agents include HIV, fungus, parasites, and bacteria.
- Noninfectious causes include neoplasm (7% to 13%), systemic autoimmune syndromes (3% to 4%), and perimyocardial infarction (Dressler syndrome, typically 2 weeks after MI).
- Drug-induced: Procainamide, hydralazine, phenytoin, isoniazid, rifampin, doxorubicin, mesalamine, adalimumab.
- Metabolic: Uremia, myxedema, anorexia nervosa.
- Posttraumatic: Postpericardiotomy, post pacemaker lead placement, post catheter ablation, post CPR.

DIAGNOSIS

DIFFERENTIAL DIAGNOSIS

- Angina pectoris and acute coronary syndrome
- Myopericarditis/perimyocarditis
- Dissecting aortic aneurysm
- Pulmonary causes: Embolism, infarction, pneumothorax, pneumonia with pleurisy
- Gastrointestinal causes: Hepatitis, cholecystitis, GERD, esophageal spasm or rupture
- Musculoskeletal strain

WORKUP (TABLE 1)

Diagnosis of pericarditis requires at least two of the four following clinical criteria:

- Typical pleuritic chest pain
- Pericardial friction rub
- Suggestive ECG changes (ST segment elevation, PR depression)
- New or worsening pericardial effusion

LABORATORY TESTS

Laboratory tests may help elucidate the underlying cause and are adjunctive to the clinical criteria.

- Inflammatory markers: Erythrocyte sedimentation rate, C-reactive protein (CRP), and complete blood count with differential are elevated in pericarditis.
- Basic metabolic profile.
- Cardiac biomarkers (troponin I and T) when elevated indicate involvement of the myocardium (i.e., myopericarditis).

The following tests may be useful when specific etiologies of pericarditis are suspected:

- HIV
- PPD
- Antinuclear antibody, rheumatoid factor
- Routine viral studies are not indicated since they are low yield

PERICARDIAL SAMPLING

Indications for echocardiogram or pericardiocentesis are:

- Tamponade physiology.
- Moderate to large pericardial effusion with symptoms, or refractory to medical therapy.

TABLE 1 Diagnostic Pathway and Sequence of Performance in Acute Pericarditis

Diagnostic Measure	Characteristic Findings
Obligatory	
Auscultation	Pericardial rub (monophasic, biphasic, or triphasic)
ECG*	*Stage I:* Anterior and inferior concave ST segment elevation. PR segment deviations opposite to P wave polarity
	Early stage II: All ST junctions return to the baseline. PR segments deviated
	Late stage II: T waves progressively flatten and invert
	Stage III: Generalized T-wave inversions in most or all leads
	Stage IV: ECG returns to prepericarditis state
Echocardiography	Effusion types B to D (Horowitz)
	Signs of tamponade
Blood analyses	Erythrocyte sedimentation rate, C-reactive protein, lactate dehydrogenase, leukocytes (inflammation markers)
	Troponin I,† CK-MB (markers of myocardial involvement)
Chest radiograph	Ranging from normal to "water bottle" shape of the heart shadow
	Performed primarily to reveal pulmonary or mediastinal pathology
Mandatory in Tamponade, Optional in Large/Recurrent Effusions or if Previous Tests Inconclusive in Small Effusions	
Pericardiocentesis/drainage	Polymerase chain reaction and histochemistry for etiopathogenetic classification of infection or neoplasia
Optional or if Previous Tests Inconclusive	
CT	Effusions, pericardium, and epicardium
MRI	Effusions, pericardium, and epicardium
Pericardioscopy, pericardial/epicardial biopsy	Establishing the specific etiology

*Typical lead involvement: I, II, aVL, aVF, and V3-V6. The ST segment is always depressed in aVR, frequently in V1, and occasionally in V2. Stage IV may not occur, and there are permanent T-wave inversions and flattenings. If an ECG is first recorded in stage III, pericarditis cannot be differentiated by ECG from diffuse myocardial injury, "biventricular strain," or myocarditis. ECG in early repolarization is very similar to stage I. Unlike stage I, this ECG does not acutely evolve, and J-point elevations are usually accompanied by a slur, oscillation, or notch at the end of the QRS just before and including the J point (best seen with tall R and T waves—large in an early repolarization pattern). Pericarditis is likely if, in lead V6, the J point is greater than 25% of the height of the T-wave apex (using the PR segment as a baseline).

†A rise in cardiac muscle troponin I (cTnI) is detected in 32.2% of patients, more frequently in younger, male patients, with ST segment elevation and pericardial effusion at presentation. An increase beyond 1.5 ng/ml is uncommon (7.6%) and associated with CK-MB elevation. cTnI increase and is not a negative prognostic marker for the incidence of recurrences, constrictive pericarditis, cardiac tamponade, or residual left ventricular dysfunction.

CK-MB, Creatine kinase-MB; *CT,* computed tomography; *ECG,* electrocardiogram; *MRI,* magnetic resonance imaging.

From Vincent JL, Abraham E, Moore FA, et al.: *Textbook of critical care*, ed 7, Philadelphia, 2017, Elsevier.

- Suspicion of a neoplastic, bacterial, or tuberculous process.
- Evidence of constrictive or effusive-constrictive pericarditis.
- Pericardiocentesis (Fig. E1) is for diagnostic and therapeutic purposes. The pericardial fluid should be analyzed for RBC, WBC, gram stain, culture, cytology, glucose, pH, LDH, and protein. In select cases, consider checking triglyceride or PCR for tuberculosis.
- Pericardial biopsy may be helpful in recurrent pericardial effusion with an elusive diagnosis and when malignancy or tuberculosis is suspected.

IMAGING STUDIES

- ECG (Fig. 2): Changes in the ECG reflect inflammation of the epicardium, since the parietal pericardium is electrically inert. The ECG changes are staged as follows:
  1. Stage I (Acute phase): Hours to few days. PR-segment depression (PR elevation in aVR) and diffuse concave ST-segment elevations, which can be distinguished from acute MI by the lack of reciprocal changes and the absence of Q waves.
  2. Stage II (Intermediate phase): Seen in first week with return of PR and ST segments to baseline.
  3. Stage III (Intermediate): T-wave inversion in leads previously showing ST-segment elevation.
  4. Stage IV (Late phase): Normalization of the ECG or indefinite persistence of T-wave inversions.
- Echocardiogram is required to evaluate for pericardial effusion (present in 50% to 60% of patients) (Fig. 3). It is also important for the diagnosis of tamponade and constrictive pericarditis.
- Chest x-ray: Done primarily to rule out abnormalities of the mediastinum or lung fields that may cause chest pain. Cardiac silhouette may appear enlarged in patients with pericardial effusion if ≥200 ml of fluid has accumulated (Fig. 4). Calcifications around the heart may be seen with chronic constrictive pericarditis.
- Computed tomography: Evaluation of associated pleuropulmonary and extra thoracic diseases and pericardial calcifications.
- MRI (Fig. 5) may be useful in patients with chronic constrictive pericarditis and when malignancy is suspected.

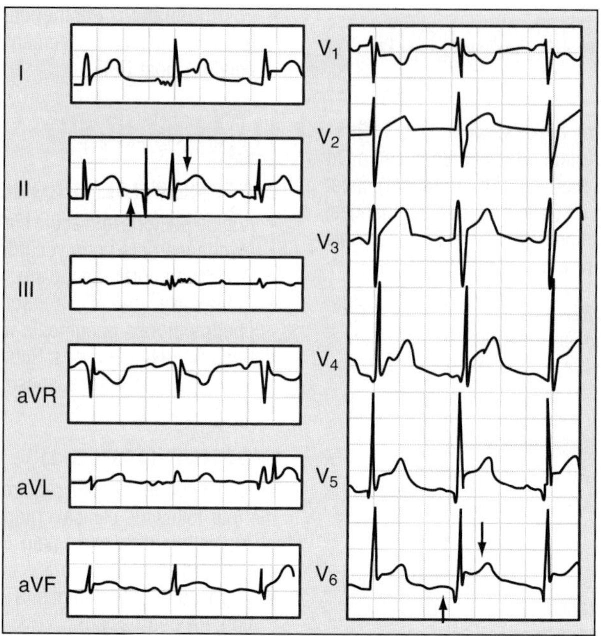

FIG. 2 Typical electrocardiographic changes in acute pericarditis: PR depression (*small arrow*) and concave ST-segment elevation (*large arrow*). *aVF,* Augmented vector foot; *aVL,* augmented vector left; *aVR,* augmented vector right. (From Vincent JL, et al.: *Textbook of critical care*, ed 7, Philadelphia, 2017, Elsevier.)

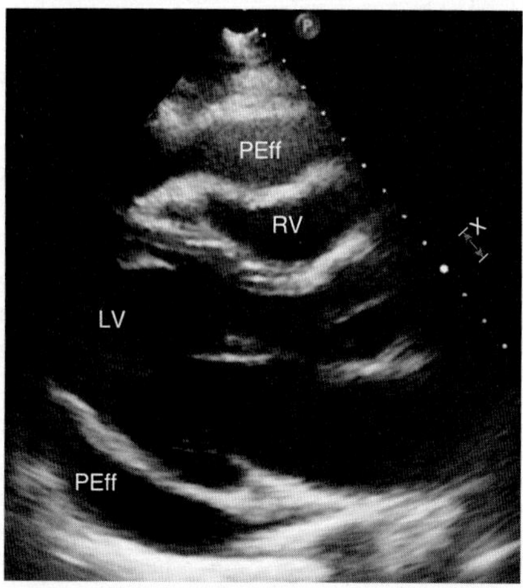

FIG. 3 Bedside echocardiogram showing pericardial effusion compressing the right ventricle during diastole, consistent with cardiac tamponade. *LV,* Left ventricle; *PEff,* pericardial effusion; *RV,* right ventricle.

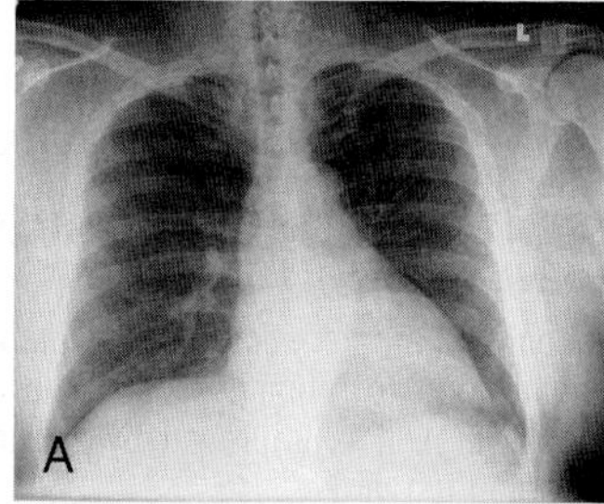

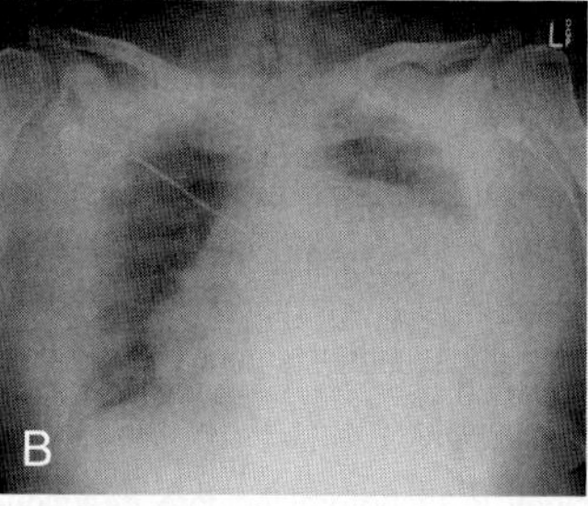

FIG. 4 Chest x-ray. A, Patient's chest radiograph 1 year before presentation with cardiac tamponade. **B,** Same patient's chest radiograph on presentation to the emergency department with cardiac tamponade. (From Adams JG, et al.: *Emergency medicine, clinical essentials,* ed 2, Philadelphia, 2013, Elsevier.)

Rx TREATMENT

NONPHARMACOLOGIC THERAPY

- Physical activity restriction until pain abates and normalization of CRP, ECG, and echo.
- Athletes should avoid competitive activity for 3 months, whereas nonathletes can resume activities after remission (expert consensus).
- Patient education regarding potential complications: e.g., cardiac tamponade, recurrent pericarditis (which can occur in up to one third of patients), and chronic constrictive pericarditis.

ACUTE GENERAL Rx

- High-dose aspirin (650-1000 mg tid) or NSAIDs (e.g., ibuprofen 600-800 mg tid, indomethacin 50 mg tid) for a month. NSAIDs should be avoided in patients with recent MI, CHF, acute renal failure, and upper GI bleed.
- Colchicine 0.5 to 0.6 mg bid for 3 months should be used as adjunctive therapy. Current evidence (COPE, CORE, CORP, ICAP, CORP-2 trials) supports the effectiveness of colchicine in symptomatic relief and prevention of recurrent pericarditis.
- Corticosteroids should be used only as second-line treatment. They are associated with severe adverse effects, more hospitalizations, and higher rates of recurrences.
- Low- to moderate-dose (0.25-0.5 mg/kg/day) systemic steroid therapy for a month, followed by taper, is restricted to patients with rheumatologic disease, failure, or contraindication to NSAID/colchicine.
- Immunosuppressors such as azathioprine, intravenous immunoglobulins, and a biological agent such as Anakinra are treatment options for patients with refractory recurrent pericarditis.

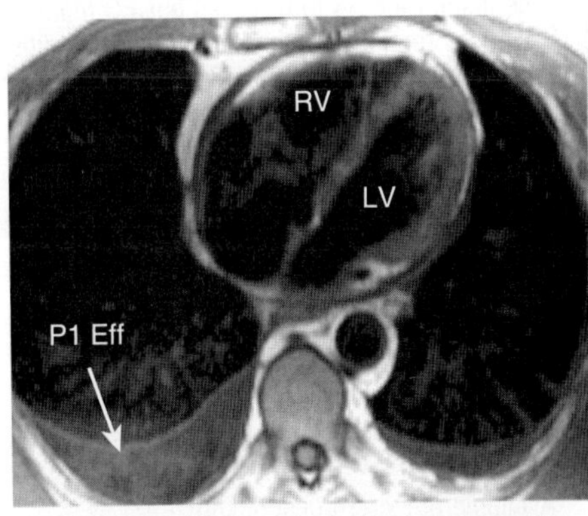

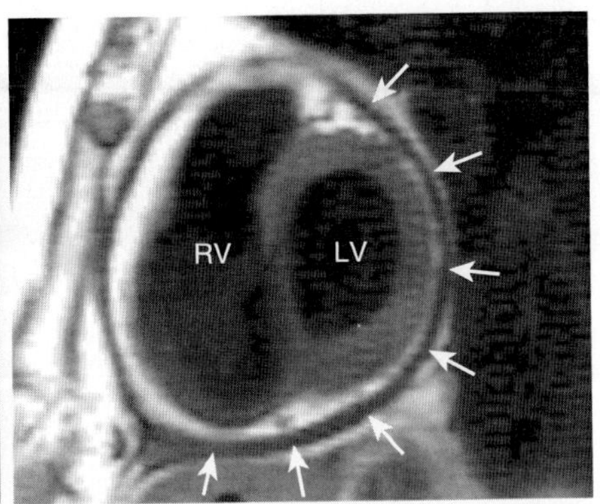

FIG. 5 Cardiovascular magnetic resonance in a patient with constrictive pericarditis. On the *right* is a basal short-axis view of the ventricles showing a thickened pericardium encasing the heart (*arrows*). On the *left* is a transaxial view, again showing the thickened pericardium, particularly over the right heart, but also a pleural effusion (*Pl Eff*). *LV,* Left ventricle; *RV,* right ventricle. (From Zipes DP, et al. [eds]: *Braunwald's heart disease,* ed 7, Philadelphia, 2005, Saunders.)

- Pericardiectomy and pericardiotomy at specialized centers are reserved for recurrent cardiac tamponade or refractory pericarditis.
- Avoidance of anticoagulants (increased risk of hemopericardium).

TREATMENT OF UNDERLYING CAUSE:

- Bacterial pericarditis: Systemic antibiotics and drainage of pericardium
- Collagen vascular disease: Prednisone
- Uremic: Dialysis

POTENTIAL COMPLICATIONS FROM PERICARDITIS:

- **Chronic constrictive pericarditis:** Occurs in <1% of patients with acute idiopathic pericarditis.
  1. Physical examination: Signs of right heart failure—hepatomegaly, splenomegaly, ascites, pedal edema, scrotal edema, possible anasarca, jugular venous pressure, Kussmaul sign (paradoxical increase in jugular venous pressure during inspiration), pericardial knock (early diastolic filling sound heard 0.06-0.1 sec after S2), and clear lungs.
  2. ECG: Low QRS voltage, nonspecific ST-segment changes, biatrial enlargement.
  3. Chest radiograph: Mild alveolar edema, pleural effusions, biatrial enlargement, pericardial calcification (seen in tuberculous pericarditis).
  4. Echocardiography: May show thickened pericardium (>4 mm), >25% mitral and >50% tricuspid valve inflow variation with respiration, interventricular septal bounce, and mitral annulus reversus (medial e' velocity> lateral e' velocity) suggest constrictive pericarditis.[1]
  5. Hemodynamics: Elevation of right-sided filling pressures, equalization of diastolic pressures, as well as prominent "x" and rapid "y" descent in the atrial tracing are seen in constrictive pericarditis. Right ventricular pressure tracing typically shows a "dip and plateau" (square root sign) that is due to the unimpeded early filling of the RV with an abrupt halt to the late diastolic filling by the stiff pericardium. Discordance of right ventricular and left ventricular systolic pressures during respiration is also suggestive of constrictive pericarditis.
  6. Therapy: Complex surgical stripping or removal of both layers of the constricting pericardium improves the functional class in majority of late survivors, but has high operative mortality.[2]
- **Cardiac tamponade:** Occurs in 5% to 15% of patients with idiopathic pericarditis, but in up to 60% of those with neoplastic, tuberculous, or purulent pericarditis.
  1. Signs and symptoms: Dyspnea, orthopnea, chest pain, fatigue.
  2. Physical examination: Beck triad (distended neck veins, distant heart sounds, hypotension), reduced apical impulse, diaphoresis, tachypnea, tachycardia, narrowed pulse pressure, or pulsus paradoxus (decrease in systolic blood pressure ≥10 mm Hg during inspiration; most specific sign).
  3. ECG: Decreased amplitude of the QRS complex, electrical alternans (occurs more frequently with large neoplastic effusions).
  4. Chest x-ray: Cardiomegaly ("water-bottle" configuration of the cardiac silhouette may be seen) with clear lungs.
  5. Echocardiography (Table 2): Pericardial effusion, >25% mitral and >50% tricuspid valve inflow variation with respiration, paradoxical motion of interventricular septum, diastolic right or left atrium collapse, diastolic right ventricular collapse (pathognomonic).
  6. Hemodynamics: Equalization of diastolic pressures within chambers of the heart, elevation of right atrial pressure with a prominent "x" but no significant "y" descent. Table 3 summarizes hemodynamics in cardiac tamponade and constrictive pericarditis.
  7. Therapy: Cardiac tamponade is a life-threatening condition usually requiring emergent pericardiocentesis. Avoid drugs (diuretics, nitrates) or therapies (high PEEP) that reduce the preload, as volume repletion may be required. In patients with recurrent effusions (e.g., neoplasms), placement of a percutaneous drainage catheter or pericardial window may be necessary.
- **Effusive-constrictive pericarditis:** Uncommon syndrome characterized by concomitant tamponade caused by tense pericardial effusion and constriction caused by the visceral pericardium.
  1. Signs and symptoms of both tamponade and or constriction. Pulsus paradoxus is present but Kussmaul sign and pericardial knock are typically absent.
  2. Echocardiography: Low sensitivity to distinguish effusive-constrictive pericarditis from other types.
  3. Cardiac catheterization: Before drainage, "y" descent is usually less prominent than expected and right atrial "v" wave persists. After drainage, may continue to have elevated right atrial and pulmonary wedge pressures.
  4. Therapy: Extensive epicardiectomy (with disruption of the visceral layer of pericardium) is the procedure of choice in symptomatic patients.
- **Myopericarditis**: Myocarditis and pericarditis may coexist in 20% to 30% of patients presenting with pericarditis. The laboratory hallmark is the elevation of cardiac enzymes. Overall, myopericarditis has a good prognosis with very low rates of morbidity, mortality, and heart failure.

DISPOSITION

- Complete resolution of pain and other signs and symptoms during the initial 3 wk of therapy occurs in 70% to 90% of cases.
- Admission is highly recommended if any of the following poor prognostic features (high risk factors) is present: Fever >38° C (100.4° F), subacute onset, large pericardial effusion/tamponade, failure to respond to 1 wk of outpatient treatment.
- The following are considered moderate risk factors but should also prompt admission: myopericarditis, trauma, immunosuppression, oral anticoagulant therapy.
- Recurrent pericarditis occurs after 4 to 6 weeks of a symptom-free interval after a first episode of pericarditis. Incidence is reported as 10% to 15% and increases to 50% in patients who are not on colchicine.

[1] Welch TD, Ling LH, Espinosa RE, et al.: Echocardiographic diagnosis of constrictive pericarditis, *Circ Cardiovasc Imaging* 7(3):526–534, 2014.

[2] Vustarini N, Chen C, Mazine A, et al.: Pericardiectomy for constrictive pericarditis: 20 years of experience at the Montreal Heart Institute, *Ann Thorac Surg* 100(1):107–113, 2015.

TABLE 2 Hemodynamic and Echocardiographic Features of Constrictive Pericarditis Versus Restrictive Cardiomyopathy

	Constriction	Restriction
Prominent *y* descent in venous pressure	Present	Variable
Paradoxical pulse	≈ ⅓ of cases	Absent
Pericardial knock	Present	Absent
Equal right- and left-sided filling pressure	Present	Left at least 3-5 mm Hg > right
Filling pressure >25 mm Hg	Rare	Common
Pulmonary artery systolic pressure >60 mm Hg	No	Common
"Square root" sign	Present	Variable
Respiratory variation in left-right pressure/flow	Exaggerated	Normal
Ventricular wall thickness	Normal	Usually increased
Pericardial thickness	Increased	Normal
Atrial size	Possible left atrial enlargement	Biatrial enlargement
Septal "bounce"	Present	Absent
Tissue Doppler E′ velocity	Increased	Reduced
Speckle tracking	Normal longitudinal, decreased circumferential restoration	Decreased longitudinal, normal circumferential restoration

From Mann DL, Zipes DP, Libby P, Bonow RO: *Braunwald's heart disease*, ed 10, Philadelphia, 2015, Elsevier.

TABLE 3 Hemodynamics in Cardiac Tamponade and Constrictive Pericarditis

	Tamponade	Constriction
Paradoxical pulse	Usually present	Present in ≈ ⅓
Equal left/right-sided filling pressure	Present	Present
Systemic venous wave morphology	Absent *y* descent	Prominent *y* descent (M or W shape)
Inspiratory change in systemic venous pressure	Decrease (normal)	Increase or no change (Kussmaul sign)
"Square root" sign in ventricular pressure	Absent	Present

From Mann DL, Zipes DP, Libby P, Bonow RO: *Braunwald's heart disease*, ed 10, Philadelphia, 2015, Elsevier.

- Incessant pericarditis is defined as pericarditis lasting for >4 to 6 weeks but <3 months without remission, while chronic pericarditis is pericarditis lasting for >3 months.
- In patients with pericardial effusion after cardiac surgery, use of NSAIDs is not recommended because they have not been shown to reduce the size of the effusions or prevent late cardiac tamponade. The COPPS trial suggested that prophylactic colchicine may reduce the risk of developing a postpericardiotomy pericarditis.

SUGGESTED READINGS

Available at ExpertConsult.com

RELATED CONTENT

Pericarditis (Patient Information)
Cardiac Tamponade (Related Key Topic)

AUTHOR: **MAXWELL EYRAM AFARI, M.D.**

BASIC INFORMATION

DEFINITION

A disorder characterized by periodic episodes of involuntary repetitive limb movements during sleep, causing sleep disturbances that are not due to a primary sleep disorder. They consist of triple flexion movements of the legs that repeat in 5 to 90 second cycles during sleep.

SYNONYMS

PLMD
Periodic leg movements of sleep (PLMS)
Nocturnal myoclonus

ICD-10CM CODE

G47.61 Periodic limb movement disorder

EPIDEMIOLOGY & DEMOGRAPHICS

INCIDENCE: Unknown
PEAK INCIDENCE: None
PREVALENCE: 5% to 8%
PREDOMINANT SEX AND AGE: Prevalence is higher in females and increases with age
GENETICS: Unknown, but may share autosomal dominant inheritance pattern if concurrent with restless leg syndrome.
RISK FACTORS:
- Female sex
- Musculoskeletal disease, heart disease, obstructive sleep apnea, cataplexy, psychiatric disorders
- Shift work
- Snoring
- Stress
- Restless leg syndrome

PHYSICAL FINDINGS & CLINICAL PRESENTATION

- Patients may complain of excessive daytime sleepiness, fatigue, and unrestful sleep.
- During an episode of periodic limb movements, the patient may experience repetitive dorsiflexion of the ankle and extension of the big toe, but other movements may occur, such as kicking. These movements last up to 5 seconds and may recur every 5 to 90 seconds, with the total episode lasting minutes to an hour. The movements are typically involuntary, and the patient is unaware of their occurrence, in contrast to those of restless leg syndrome (RLS).
- Neurologic examination is usually normal but may reveal an associated neuropathy or myelopathy.

ETIOLOGY

The exact etiology is unknown. It is hypothesized that PLMD may share a common pathophysiology with restless leg syndrome, which involves iron metabolism and dopaminergic pathways in the brain.

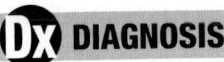

DIAGNOSIS

DIFFERENTIAL DIAGNOSIS

- Restless leg syndrome
- Neuroleptic-induced akathisia
- Positional discomfort
- Nocturnal leg cramps

WORKUP

In addition to a history of excessive daytime sleepiness or sleep disturbance, the diagnosis of PLMD requires a polysomnographic study to exclude other sleep disorders and to document the periodic limb movements resulting in sleep disturbances (Table 1). During the study, the movements must occur in a series of at least four, recurring every 5 to 90 seconds, each with a duration of 0.5 to 5 seconds.

LABORATORY TEST(S)

- No laboratory tests are required to diagnose PLMD.
- A CBC, iron panel, and BMP may be ordered if RLS is suspected.

IMAGING STUDIES

Imaging studies are not required for diagnosis of PLMD.

TREATMENT

- The treatment of PLMD is the same as that for RLS.
- Patients with periodic limb movements only, without sleep disturbances, may not require treatment.
- Calcium channel ligands such as gabapentin or pregabalin are effective and do not worsen symptoms with long-term use.
- Dopaminergic agonists such as pramipexole or ropinirole have been shown to decrease PLMS, but long-term use may be associated with worsening of symptoms (augmentation).
- Iron replacement should be started in case of iron deficiency, and the cause of iron-deficiency investigated.

NONPHARMACOLOGIC THERAPY

- Follow good sleep hygiene.
- Minimize shift work.
- Avoid caffeine, alcohol, nicotine.

ACUTE GENERAL Rx

- Treatment is indicated when PLMD is suspected and causing significant sleep fragmentation
- For calcium channel ligands: Gabapentin initial dose of 100 to 300 mg/day before bedtime, with therapeutic range of 300 to 2400 mg/day. Pregabalin initial dose of 50 to 75 mg/day, with therapeutic range of 75 to 450 mg/day
- For dopamine agonists: Pramipexole initial dose of 0.125 mg before bedtime, with a therapeutic range of 0.125 to 0.75 mg/day. Ropinirole initial dose of 0.25 mg/day, with a therapeutic range of 0.25 to 4 mg/day

CHRONIC Rx

For patients treated with dopamine agonists, close monitoring is recommended to screen for augmentation of symptoms.

COMPLEMENTARY AND ALTERNATIVE MEDICINE

None

REFERRAL

Refer to neurologist if diagnosis is uncertain or an underlying disorder is suspected.

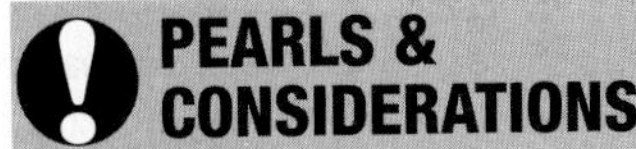

PEARLS & CONSIDERATIONS

COMMENTS

- Periodic limb movements disorder is a diagnosis of exclusion. PLMS occur during many sleep disorders and do not support a diagnosis of PLMD until all possible underlying causes are excluded.
- Certain medications such as antihistamines, dopamine receptor blockers, selective serotonin reuptake inhibitors, and stimulants may worsen PLMS and should be avoided if possible.

PREVENTION: As mentioned in nonpharmacologic therapy

PATIENT/FAMILY EDUCATION

Patient information on PLMD and other sleep disorders can be found at the National Sleep Foundation website: www.sleepfoundation.org

SUGGESTED READINGS

Available at ExpertConsult.com

RELATED CONTENT

Restless Legs Syndrome (Related Key Topic)

AUTHORS: **SUDAD KAZZAZ, M.D.,** and **COREY GOLDSMITH, M.D.**

TABLE 1 Recording and Scoring of Periodic Leg Movements According to the Guidelines of the World Association of Sleep Medicine/International Restless Legs Syndrome Study Group (WASM/IRLSSG)[1] and the American Academy of Sleep Medicine (AASM)[2,3]

Feature/Component	WASM/IRLSSG	AASM
Recording of Leg Movements		
Electrodes	Surface electrodes	Surface electrodes
Electrode positioning	Tibialis anterior muscles	Tibialis anterior muscles
	Placed longitudinal, symmetrically around the middle, 2-3 cm apart or one third of length of anterior tibialis muscle, whichever is shorter	Placed longitudinal, symmetrically around the middle, 2-3 cm apart or one third of length of anterior tibialis muscle, whichever is shorter
Combined recording of left and right legs	Bilateral recordings are required. Use of two channels, one for each leg, is strongly recommended for all studies and is required for research	Both legs should be monitored for the presence of leg movements. Use of separate channels for each leg is strongly preferred
	Clinical applications may, however, combine the electrodes from both legs into one recorded channel, although this practice is discouraged	Combining electrodes from the two legs to give one recorded channel may suffice for some clinical settings, although this strategy may reduce the number of detected leg movements
Sampling rate	≥200 Hz in clinical studies	≥200 Hz
	≥400 Hz in research studies	500 Hz desirable
Filter	10-100 Hz in clinical studies	10-100 Hz
	10-200 Hz in research studies	Use of 60-Hz (notch) filters should be avoided.
Impedance	≤10 KΩ in clinical studies	<10 KΩ
	≤5 KΩ in research studies	<5 KΩ preferred
Definition of Leg Movement		
Onset	EMG increase ≥8 μV	EMG increase ≥8 μV
	above the resting baseline	above the resting baseline
Offset	EMG decrease to <2 μV	EMG decrease to ≤2 μV
	above the resting level	above the resting level
	for ≥0.5 s	for ≥0.5 s
Duration	Time between onset and offset, 0.5-10 s	Time between onset and offset, 0.5-10 s
Baseline	Resting EMG	Stable resting EMG
	Relaxed muscle	Relaxed muscle
	Absolute signal amplitude, 4-6 μV peak to peak	Absolute signal amplitude, ≤10 μV peak to peak
	Calibration: Relaxed anterior tibialis lasting: ≤10 μV in clinical setting ≤6 μV in research setting	
	Special criteria for events during wake time: If EMG >6-10 μV for ≥15 s, then new increased baseline is defined as average amplitude during this period	
Scoring of Periodic Leg Movements (PLMs)		
Intermovement interval (IMI)	Onset-to-onset: 5-90 s	Onset-to-onset: 5-90 s
Number of leg movements	≥4 (Leg movements lasting <0.5 s or >10 s are disregarded)	≥4
IMI >90 s	PLM series ends	PLM series ends
IMI <5 s	PLM series goes on; leg movement with IMI <5 s is disregarded	*Not specified*
Sleep-wake	All leg movements form PLM series For PLMS, only those during sleep are counted	Only leg movements during sleep form PLM series
Bilateral leg movements	Offset-to-onset <0.5 s	Onset-to-onset <5 s
Respiratory-related leg movements (RRLMs)	Excluded from PLM series	Excluded from PLMS series
RRLM definition	Any leg movement occurring within:	Any leg movement occurring within:
	±0.5 s around the ending of an apnea/hypopnea event	0.5 s before the start to 0.5 s after the end of an apnea or hypopnea, respiratory effort–related arousal, or sleep-disordered breathing event

EMG, Electromyogram; *PLMS*, periodic leg movements during sleep.

[1]Zucconi M et al: The official World Association of Sleep Medicine (WASM) standards for recording and scoring periodic leg movements in sleep (PLMS) and wakefulness (PLMW) developed in collaboration with a task force from the International Restless Legs Syndrome Study Group (IRLSSG), *Sleep Med* 7:175–83, 2006.

[2]Berry R et al: *The AASM manual for the scoring of sleep and associated events: rules, terminology and technical specifications, version 2.0.3,* Darien, IL, 2014, American Academy of Sleep Medicine. Available at: <www.aasmnet.org>.

[3]Berry R et al: The AASM manual for the scoring of sleep and associated events: rules, terminology and technical specifications, version 2.0. Darien, IL, 2012, American Academy of Sleep Medicine.

From Kryger M et al: *Principles and practice of sleep medicine*, ed 6, Philadelphia, 2017, Elsevier.

BASIC INFORMATION

DEFINITION

Peripheral artery disease (PAD) refers to atherosclerotic, inflammatory, occlusive, and aneurysmal diseases involving the abdominal aorta and its branch arteries. (This topic focuses on lower-extremity PAD.)

SYNONYMS

PAD
Peripheral vascular disease (PVD)
Arteriosclerosis obliterans
Atherosclerotic occlusive disease
Atherosclerosis of the extremities
Peripheral arterial stenosis
Vaso-occlusive disease of the legs
Chronic critical limb ischemia

ICD-10CM CODES

I70	Atherosclerosis
I70.2	Atherosclerosis of native arteries of the extremities
I70.21	Atherosclerosis of native arteries of extremities with intermittent claudication
I70.22	Atherosclerosis of native arteries of extremities with rest pain
I70.3	Atherosclerosis of unspecified type of bypass graft(s) of the extremities
I73	Other specified peripheral vascular diseases
I73.8	Other specified peripheral vascular diseases
I73.9	Peripheral vascular disease, unspecified
I79	Disorders of arteries, arterioles, and capillaries in diseases classified elsewhere

EPIDEMIOLOGY & DEMOGRAPHICS

- There are >202 million patients afflicted with PAD globally; it affects approximately 8.5 million Americans above the age of 40.
- The prevalence is nearly equal in men and women. It increases with age, from 5.28% in those aged 40 to 49 yr to 18.83% in those aged 70 to 79 yr. However, symptoms of claudication are more likely to be present in males with PAD (50%) vs. women with PAD (25%).
- As per the PARTNERS study, the prevalence of PAD in patients >70 yr or 50 to 69 yr with history of smoking or diabetes was 29%.
- Risk factors that increase risk of PAD according to a 2013 meta-analysis of 112,027 studied patients include:
  1. Smoking (odds ratio 2.72)
  2. Diabetes (odds ratio 1.88)
  3. Hypertension (odds ratio 1.55)
  4. Hypercholesterolemia (odds ratio 1.19)
- Smoking is three times more likely to lead to PAD than CAD. Conversely, the association of HTN and hyperlipidemia with PAD is lower than that with CAD and cerebrovascular disease.
- Patients at increased risk of PAD include those aged greater than 65 yr, those aged 50 to 64 yr with risk factors of atherosclerosis, those aged less than 50 yr with diabetes and an additional risk factor, as well as those individuals with known atherosclerotic disease in another vascular bed.
- Black race/ethnicity has greater prevalence according to NHANES data (odds ratio 2.83).
- Patients with newly diagnosed PAD are six times more likely to die within the next 10 yr when compared with patients without PAD.
- The total annual costs associated with the hospitalization of patients with PAD in the U.S. exceed $21 billion, and account for ~13% of all Medicare Part A and B expenditures.

PHYSICAL FINDINGS & CLINICAL PRESENTATION

- Peripheral artery disease may present in a variety of ways:
  1. 20% to 50%: Asymptomatic
  2. 10% to 35%: Intermittent claudication (IC), defined as aching pain, cramping, weakness, numbness, or heaviness of the leg induced by exercise, relieved by rest
  3. 1% to 2%: Critical limb ischemia (CLI), defined as chronic (>2 wk) rest pain, or tissue loss with nonhealing ulceration, necrosis, or gangrene (Fig. 1)
  4. 40% to 50%: Atypical symptoms involving the calf, thigh, or buttock
  5. Acute limb ischemia (ALI) will be present in 14 per 100,000 individuals in the general population. It is defined as acute (<2 wk) onset of symptoms due to severe poor perfusion of the extremities, and further categorized into the following:
     a. Viable: No sensory or muscle weakness with audible Doppler pulses
     b. Threatened: Mild to moderate sensory or motor loss; inaudible arterial Doppler
     c. Irreversible: Severe sensory loss and muscle weakness; inaudible arterial Doppler
- Physical findings include:
  1. Diminished pulses and/or cool skin temperature of lower extremities
  2. Bruits heard over the distal aorta, iliac, or femoral arteries
  3. Change in skin color:
     a. Dependent rubor in critical limb ischemia
     b. Livedo reticularis, or a mottled reticulated vascular pattern that appears lacelike
  4. Trophic changes of hair loss, brittle nails, and muscle atrophy

ETIOLOGY

PAD is primarily the result of atherosclerotic narrowing of the arterial lumen that results in impaired blood flow to the lower-extremity tissues. Fig. 2 illustrates the pathophysiology of intermittent claudication.

Symptoms initially manifest with exercise as metabolic demands increase. Critical limb ischemia (CLI) may develop gradually from progressive atherosclerosis or in a subacute fashion from multisegmental atherothrombosis or atheroembolization. In contrast, acute limb ischemia (ALI) is marked by a sudden onset of symptoms (<2 wk) due to poor perfusion of the extremities.

Dx DIAGNOSIS

DIFFERENTIAL DIAGNOSIS

- Vasculitis
- Musculoskeletal disorder
- Spinal stenosis or nerve root compression (neurogenic or pseudoclaudication)
- Peripheral neuropathy
- Reflex sympathetic dystrophy
- Raynaud's phenomenon
- Compartment syndrome
- Deep venous thrombosis
- Popliteal entrapment syndrome
- Direct vascular injury

WORKUP

- Thorough history, including symptoms regarding walking impairment, claudication, ischemic rest pain, or nonhealing wounds in patients ≥70 yr or those ≥50 yr with a history of smoking and/or diabetes.
- Careful physical examinations include:
  1. Measurement of blood pressure in both arms; pressure difference of >15-20 mm Hg is abnormal and suggestive of subclavian artery stenosis
  2. Palpation and recording of carotid pulses, upstroke, amplitude, and presence of bruits
  3. Auscultation and palpation of abdomen for bruits, aortic pulsation, and diameter
  4. Palpation of brachial, radial, ulnar, femoral, popliteal, dorsalis pedis, and posterior tibial pulses. Pulse intensity should be recorded as follows: 0, absent; 1+, diminished; 2+, normal; 3+, bounding
  5. Auscultation of femoral arteries for the presence of bruits
  6. Extremities should be inspected for color, temperature, integrity of the skin, hair loss, and hypertrophic nails
- Classification/staging system for PAD:
  1. Fontaine's staging system (Table 1):
     a. I: Asymptomatic
     b. IIa: Mild claudication
     c. IIb: Moderate-severe claudication
     d. III: Ischemic rest pain
     e. IV: Ulceration or gangrene
- Resting ankle-brachial index (ABI) is the first-line noninvasive test to establish a diagnosis of PAD in individuals with symptoms or signs suggestive of disease (individuals with one or more of the following exertional leg symptoms: nonhealing wounds, age >65 yr, or age >50 yr with smoking or diabetes history).
- ABI of each leg is calculated by dividing the highest dorsalis pedis or posterior tibial systolic blood pressure by the highest systolic brachial pressure obtained from either the right or left arm.
  1. Noncompressible/calcified: >1.40
  2. Normal: 1.00 to 1.40 at rest
  3. Borderline: 0.91 to 0.99 at rest
  4. Abnormal: ≤0.90

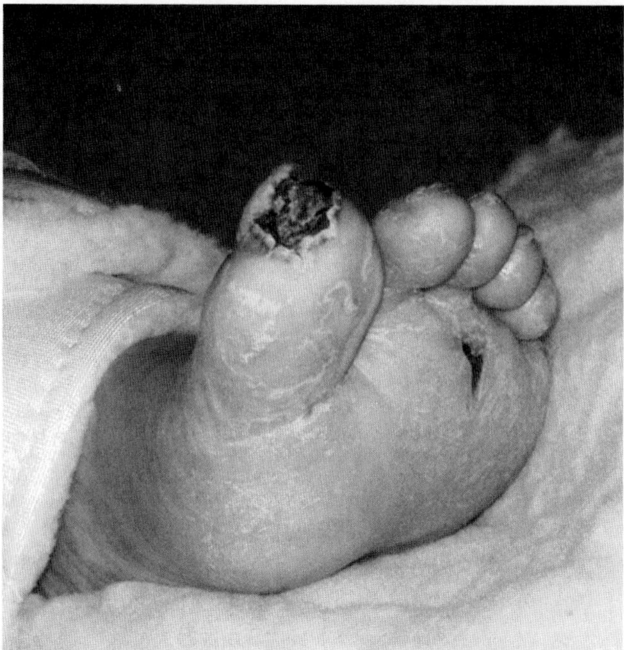

FIG. 1 Ulceration and gangrene of the foot representative of critical limb ischemia in a patient with peripheral artery disease. (From Hoffman R, et al.: *Hematology, basic principles and practice,* ed 7, Philadelphia, 2018, Elsevier.)

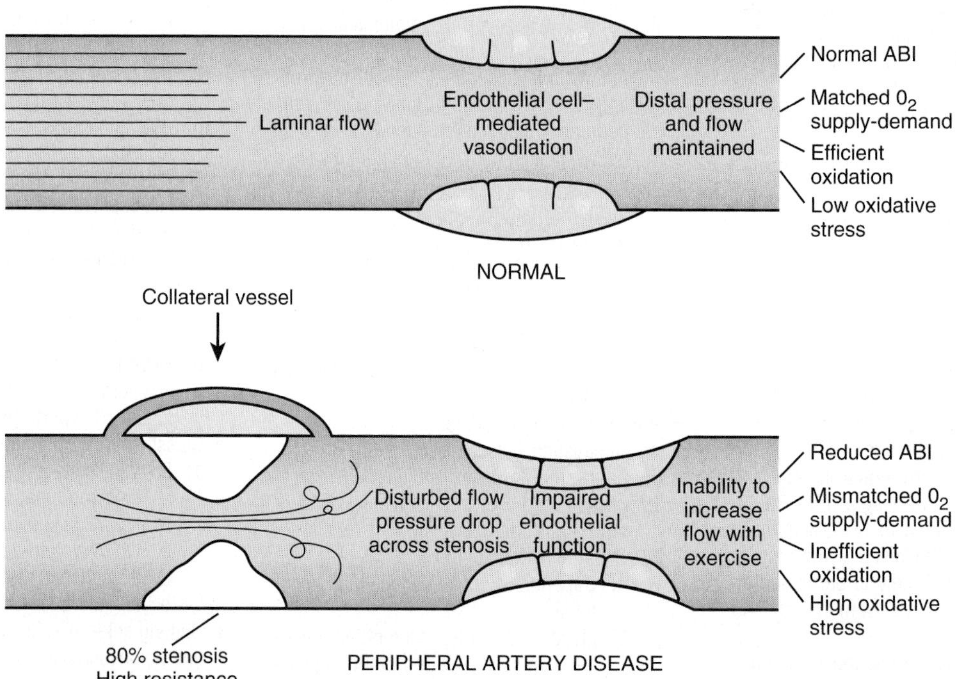

FIG. 2 Pathophysiology of intermittent claudication. In healthy arteries *(top),* flow is laminar and endothelial function is normal; therefore blood flow and oxygen delivery match muscle metabolic demand at rest and during exercise. Muscle metabolism is efficient and results in low oxidative stress. In contrast, in peripheral artery disease *(PAD) (bottom),* arterial stenosis results in disturbed flow, and the loss of kinetic energy results in a drop in pressure across the stenosis. Collateral vessels have high resistance and only partially compensate for the arterial stenosis. In addition, endothelial function is impaired, thereby resulting in further loss of vascular function. These changes limit the blood flow response to exercise and result in a mismatch of oxygen delivery to muscle metabolic demand. Changes in skeletal muscle metabolism further compromise the efficient generation of high-energy phosphates. Oxidant stress, the result of inefficient oxidation, further impairs endothelial function and muscle metabolism. *ABI,* Ankle-brachial index. (From the text *Anatomie, physiologie, pathologie des vaisseaux lymphatiques* by PC Sappey [1874], courtesy Harvard Medical Library, Francis A. Countway Library of Medicine, in Hiatt WR, Brass EP: Pathophysiology of intermittent claudication. In Creager MA, et al. [eds]: *Vascular medicine. A companion to Braunwald's heart disease,* ed 2, Philadelphia, 2013, Elsevier.)

- ABI should be measured in both legs in all new patients (Fig. 3).
- Exercise ABI is recommended if resting ABI is borderline or normal (>0.9) and symptoms of claudication are suggestive.
- Toe-brachial index should be used in patients suspected of PAD with ABI of >1.4. A TBI of <0.70 is abnormal and diagnostic of PAD. TBI may be used to assess perfusion in patients with suspected CLI.
- Routine screening for lower-extremity PAD in the absence of risk factors, history, signs, or symptoms is not recommended.
- PAD is recognized as a risk factor for abdominal aortic aneurysm (AAA), and in observational studies the prevalence of AAA was higher in patients with symptomatic PAD.

LABORATORY TESTS

Laboratory tests can help identify risk factors or other potential causative etiologies. These include lipid profile, hemoglobin A1C, d-dimer, and CRP/ESR.

TABLE 1 Fontaine Classification of Peripheral Artery Disease

Stage	Symptoms
I	Asymptomatic
II	Intermittent claudication
IIa	Pain free, claudication walking >200 m
IIb	Pain free, claudication walking <200 m
III	Rest and nocturnal pain
IV	Necrosis, gangrene

From Bonow RO, et al.: *Braunwald's heart disease: a textbook of cardiovascular medicine*, ed 9, Philadelphia, 2012, Saunders.

PHYSIOLOGIC TESTING AND IMAGING STUDIES

- Rest or exercise pulse volume recordings (PVRs) and segmental limb pressures are also useful. PVRs measure volume of limb flow per pulse in different segments of the limb (e.g., thigh, calf, ankle, metatarsal, and toes). They help to assess the location and severity of the lesion with alterations in the pulse volume contour and amplitude indicating proximal arterial obstruction.
- Duplex ultrasound (DUS) incorporates anatomic and physiologic evaluation by combining 2D ultrasound to visualize arterial segments and pulse wave Doppler to sample blood flow velocities at specific locations in the arterial lumen.
- Conventional contrast angiography remains the gold standard, but duplex ultrasonography, computed tomography angiography (CTA), and magnetic resonance angiography (MRA) have largely replaced catheter-based angiography in anatomic assessment for revascularization. Contrast angiography (Fig. 4) is now reserved for patients with PAD who are being considered for endovascular revascularization. It allows assessment of translesional pressure gradients prior to percutaneous intervention.
- Carotid intima-media thickness and brachial artery flow-mediated dilation have shown promise but have not been widely applied.

Rx TREATMENT

The treatment goal in patients with PAD is to focus on cardiovascular risk factor reduction to decrease morbidity and mortality as well as to improve limb-related symptoms. There are also medical and surgical approaches to management of limb-related symptoms. Fig. 5 illustrates an approach to a patient with PAD. ACCF/AHA guidelines for medical management of patients with peripheral artery disease are summarized in Table 2.

MEDICAL THERAPY

LOWERING CARDIOVASCULAR RISK FACTORS, MORBIDITY, AND MORTALITY:

- Smoking cessation or avoidance of secondhand smoke should be emphasized in patients with PAD at each visit with assistance of behavioral and pharmacologic treatment (Class I).
- Proper foot care, including use of appropriate footwear, chiropody/podiatric medicine, daily foot inspection, skin cleansing, and use of topical moisturizing creams, should be encouraged, and skin lesions and ulcerations should be addressed urgently in all patients with diabetes and lower-extremity PAD (Class I).
- A foot infection should be suspected in patients presenting with local pain, periwound erythema, edema, or discharge; these patients should undergo prompt diagnosis and treatment with an interdisciplinary care team to avoid amputation.
- Antiplatelet therapy is indicated to reduce risk of myocardial infarction, stroke, and vascular death in individuals with symptomatic PAD with either aspirin (75 to 325 mg) or clopidogrel (75 mg) (Class I) and in asymptomatic patients (Class IIa). Uncertain benefit has been observed with combination aspirin and clopidogrel therapy (Class IIb). Limited data on use of newer P2Y12 receptor antagonists in PAD. In the EUCLID trial, ticagrelor was not shown to be superior to clopidogrel for the reduction of cardiovascular events, with major bleeding being similar in the two groups. Uncertain benefit with vorapaxar (Class IIb).
- Warfarin is not indicated except in select postsurgical bypass conditions.
- Lipid-lowering therapy in patients with lower limb PAD has been shown to help slow disease progression, alleviate symptoms, and improve walking distance. The 2013 ACC/AHA Guideline on the Treatment of Blood Cholesterol recommends that patients with atherosclerotic PAD receive moderate- to high-dose statin therapy in order to lower risk of cardiovascular events regardless of baseline cholesterol values. Prior guidelines have recommended goal LDL cholesterol of <100 mg/dl and possibly <70 mg/dl in high-risk patients.
- Management of hypertension should be in accordance with current HTN guidelines. Ramipril use has been reported to improve walking ability and quality of life in PAD patients with intermittent claudication.
- Control of blood sugar in diabetic patients with PAD is recommended (hemoglobin A1C goal <6.5), although studies have failed to demonstrate a beneficial effect on intensive insulin therapy in lowering risk of PAD. Annual influenza vaccination reduces CV event rates in patients with PAD (Class I).

How to Perform and Calculate the ABI

Partners Program ABI Interpretation
Above 0.90—Normal
0.71-0.90—Mild Obstruction
0.41-0.70—Moderate Obstruction
0.00-0.40—Severe Obstruction

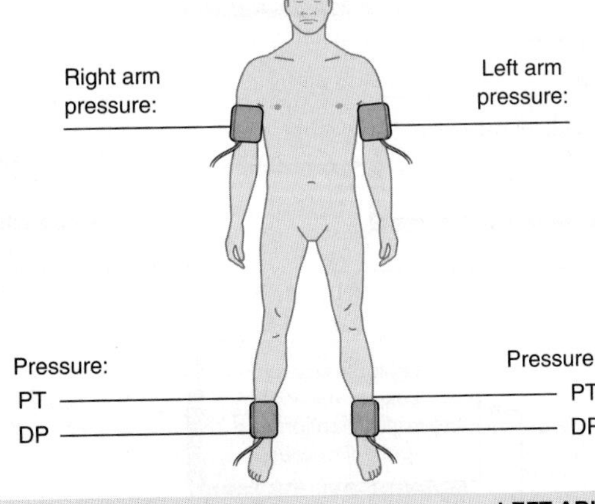

RIGHT ABI

Higher right ankle pressure / Higher arm pressure = mm Hg / mm Hg = ______

LEFT ABI

Higher left ankle pressure / Higher arm pressure = mm Hg / mm Hg = ______

EXAMPLE

Higher ankle pressure / Higher arm pressure = 92 mm Hg / 164 mm Hg = 0.56 See ABI Chart

FIG. 3 Performing pressure measurements and calculating the ankle-brachial index *(ABI)*. To calculate the ABI, systolic pressures are determined in both arms and both ankles with the use of a handheld Doppler instrument. The highest readings for the dorsalis pedis *(DP)* and posterior tibial *(PT)* arteries are used to calculate the index. (From Goldman L, Schafer AI: *Goldman's Cecil medicine*, ed 24, Philadelphia, 2012, Saunders.)

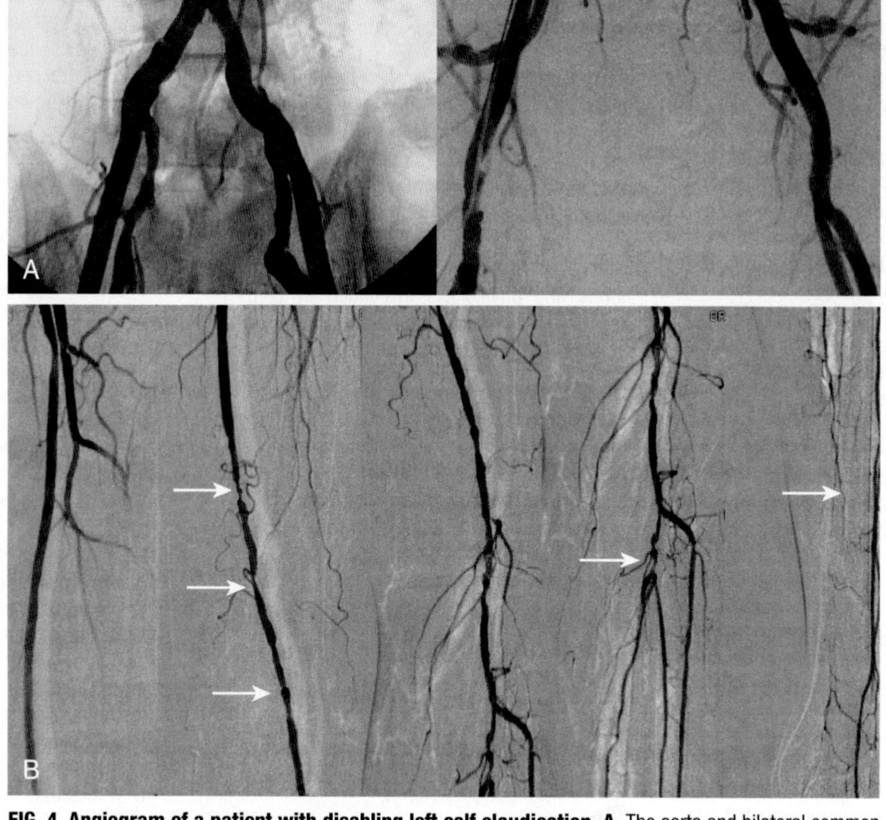

FIG. 4 Angiogram of a patient with disabling left calf claudication. A, The aorta and bilateral common iliac arteries are patent. **B,** The left superficial femoral artery has multiple stenotic lesions *(arrows).* There is a significant stenosis of the left tibioperoneal trunk and left posterior tibial artery *(arrows).* (From Zipes DP, et al. [eds]: *Braunwald's heart disease,* ed 7, Philadelphia, 2005, Saunders.)

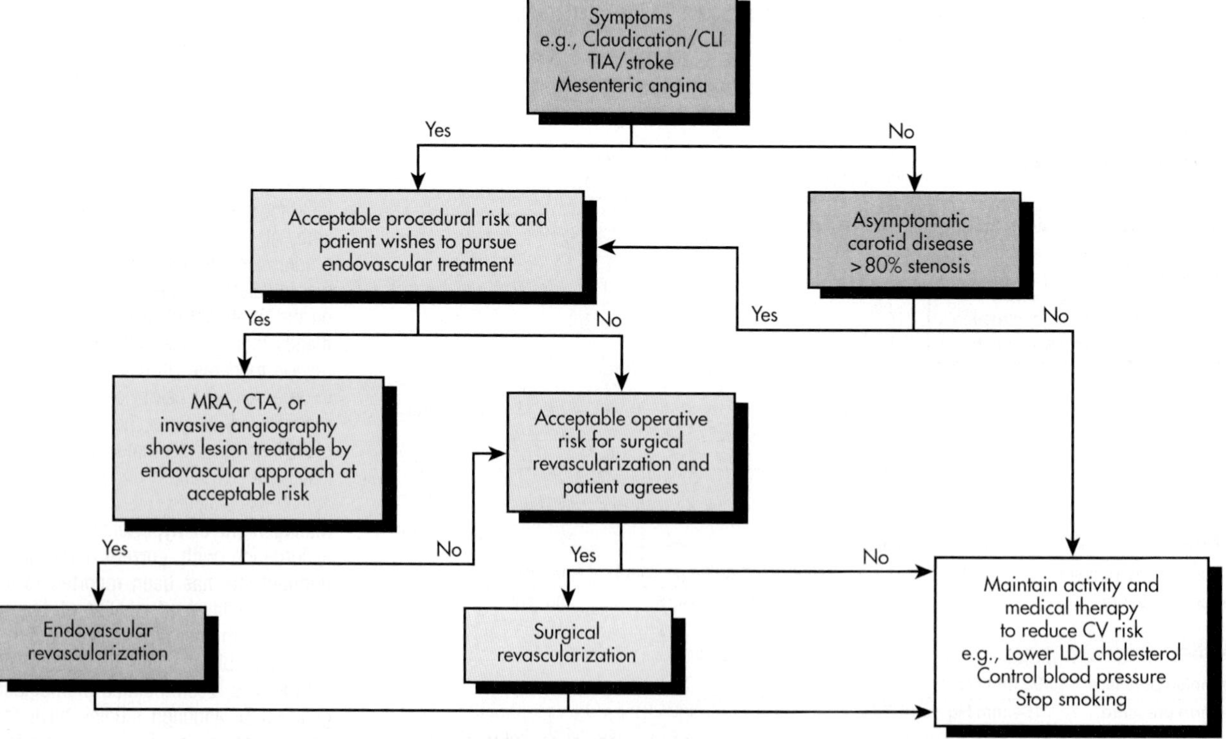

FIG. 5 Approach to a patient with peripheral artery disease *(PAD).* This strategy is based on assessment of the risk for adverse events with and without treatment by taking into consideration procedural or operative risks and the patient's informed decision to proceed with revascularization. *CLI,* Critical limb ischemia; *CTA,* CT angiography; *CV,* cardiovascular; *LDL,* low-density lipoprotein; *MRA,* MR angiography; *TIA,* transient ischemic attack. (From Mann DL, et al.: *Braunwald's heart disease,* ed 10, Philadelphia, 2015, Elsevier.)

TABLE 2 ACCF/AHA Guidelines for Medical Management of Patients With Peripheral Artery Disease

Class	Indication	Level of Evidence
I	1. Treatment with a hydroxymethylglutaryl–coenzyme A reductase inhibitor (statin) medication is indicated for all patients with PAD to achieve a target low-density lipoprotein (LDL) cholesterol level of <100 mg/dl.	B
	2. Antihypertensive therapy should be administered to hypertensive patients with lower extremity PAD to achieve a goal of <140 mm Hg systolic over 90 mm Hg diastolic (individuals without diabetes) or <130 mm Hg systolic over 80 mm Hg diastolic (individuals with diabetes and those with chronic renal disease) to reduce the risk for MI, stroke, congestive heart failure, and cardiovascular death.	A
	3. Patients who smoke cigarettes should be assisted by counseling and developing a plan for quitting that may include pharmacotherapy and/or referral to a smoking cessation program.	A
	4. In the absence of contraindications or other compelling clinical indications, one or more of the following pharmacologic therapies should be offered: varenicline, bupropion, and nicotine replacement therapy.	A
	5. Antiplatelet therapy is indicated to reduce the risk for MI, stroke, and vascular death in individuals with symptomatic atherosclerotic lower extremity PAD, including those with intermittent claudication or critical limb ischemia (CLI), previous lower extremity revascularization (endovascular or surgical), or previous amputation for lower extremity ischemia.	A
	6. Proper foot care, including the use of appropriate footwear, chiropody/podiatric medicine, daily foot inspection, skin cleansing, and topical moisturizing creams, should be encouraged, and skin lesions and ulcerations should be addressed urgently in all patients with diabetes and lower extremity PAD.	B
	7. A program of supervised exercise training is recommended as an initial treatment modality for patients with intermittent claudication.	A
	8. Cilostazol (100 mg orally 2 times per day) is indicated as an effective therapy to improve symptoms and increase walking distance in patients with lower extremity PAD and intermittent claudication (in the absence of heart failure).	A
IIa	1. Treatment with a statin medication to achieve a target LDL cholesterol level of <70 mg/dl is reasonable for patients with lower extremity PAD at very high risk for ischemic events.	B
	2. The use of angiotensin-converting enzyme (ACE) inhibitors is reasonable for symptomatic patients with lower extremity PAD to reduce the risk for adverse cardiovascular events.	B
	3. Treatment of diabetes in individuals with lower extremity PAD by administration of glucose control therapies to reduce hemoglobin A1c to <7% can effectively reduce microvascular complications and potentially improve cardiovascular outcomes.	C
	4. Antiplatelet therapy can reduce the risk for MI, stroke, or vascular death in asymptomatic individuals with an ABI of ≤0.90.	C
IIb	1. ACE inhibitors may be considered for patients with asymptomatic lower extremity PAD to reduce the risk for adverse cardiovascular events.	C
	2. The usefulness of antiplatelet therapy to reduce the risk for MI, stroke, or vascular death in asymptomatic individuals with a borderline abnormal ABI, defined as 0.91-0.99, is not well established.	A
	3. The combination of aspirin and clopidogrel may be considered to reduce the risk for cardiovascular events in patients with symptomatic atherosclerotic lower extremity PAD, including those with intermittent claudication or CLI, previous lower extremity revascularization (endovascular or surgical), or previous amputation for lower extremity ischemia, who do not have an increased risk for bleeding and who have a high perceived cardiovascular risk.	B
	4. The usefulness of unsupervised exercise programs is not well established as an effective initial treatment modality for patients with intermittent claudication.	B
	5. Pentoxifylline (400 mg 3 times per day) may be considered as a second-line alternative therapy to cilostazol to improve walking distance in patients with intermittent claudication.	A
	6. Parenteral administration of prostaglandin E_1 or iloprost for 7-28 days may be considered to reduce ischemic pain and facilitate ulcer healing in patients with CLI, but its efficacy is likely to be limited to a small percentage of patients.	A
III	1. In the absence of any other proven indication for warfarin, its addition to antiplatelet therapy to reduce the risk for adverse cardiovascular ischemic events in individuals with atherosclerotic lower extremity PAD has no benefit and is potentially harmful because of an increased risk for major bleeding.	B
	2. Oral vasodilator prostaglandins such as beraprost and iloprost are not effective medications to improve walking distance in patients with intermittent claudication.	A
	3. Vitamin E is not recommended for the treatment of patients with intermittent claudication.	C
	4. Chelation (e.g., ethylenediaminetetraacetic acid) is not indicated for the treatment of intermittent claudication and may have harmful adverse effects.	A
	5. Parenteral administration of pentoxifylline is not useful for the treatment of CLI.	B
	6. Oral iloprost is not an effective therapy to reduce the risk for amputation or death in patients with CLI.	B

ABI, Ankle-brachial index; *ACCF*, American College of Cardiology Foundation; *AHA*, American Heart Association; *MI*, myocardial infarction; *PAD*, peripheral artery disease.
From Mann DL, et al.: *Braunwald's heart disease*, ed 10, Philadelphia, 2015, Elsevier.

TREATMENT OF CLAUDICATION:

- Exercise therapy: Supervised exercise-training may be as beneficial as stent revascularization in symptomatic improvement. Patients should be prescribed exercise for a minimum of 30 to 45 min, in sessions performed at least three times per wk for a minimum of 12 wk (Class I).

1. Pharmacologic therapy:
   a. Cilostazol (100 mg bid) is indicated as effective therapy for enabling pain-free and maximal walking distance (Class 1). It is a phosphodiesterase (PDE-3) inhibitor that reduces platelet aggregation and causes vasodilatation. It may have an added benefit of reducing restenosis and repeat revascularization following endovascular therapy. Cilostazol is contraindicated in patients with systolic heart failure.
   b. Pentoxifylline is no longer considered effective in treatment of claudication (Class III).

REVASCULARIZATION

In general, there is no difference in clinical outcomes in percutaneous vs. surgical revascularization in iliac and femoropopliteal disease except for the higher morbidity with surgery and greater re-interventions in the percutaneous approach.

- The 2016 ACC/AHA guidelines on PAD have recommended revascularization as a reasonable treatment option for the patient with lifestyle-limiting claudication with inadequate response to guideline-directed medical therapy. The following approach is discussed:
  1. Considerations in percutaneous/endovascular treatment:
     a. In patients with a vocational- or lifestyle-limiting disability due to claudication or limb ischemia from either significant aortoiliac or femoropopliteal disease despite optimal medical therapy when clinical features suggest a reasonable likelihood of symptomatic improvement with endovascular intervention.
     b. Endovascular intervention is not indicated as prophylactic therapy in an asymptomatic patient with lower-extremity PAD.
     c. Durability of endovascular intervention is greater in iliac artery than in the femoropopliteal segment.
  2. Considerations in surgical revascularization:
     a. Individuals with claudication symptoms who have a significant functional disability that is vocational or lifestyle limiting. These patients need to also be unresponsive to exercise or pharmacotherapy and should have a reasonable likelihood of symptomatic improvement with an acceptable surgical risk and technical factors favoring surgical vs endovascular approach.
     b. Autogenous vein graft is superior to prosthetic graft if surgical revascularization is performed (Class I).
     c. Iliac or femoropopliteal disease with long segments; multifocal segments; long segment occlusions; and eccentric, calcified stenosis, which are less amenable to percutaneous interventions.
     d. Surgical intervention is not indicated to prevent progression to limb-threatening ischemia in patients with intermittent claudication as generally claudication does not progress to severe ischemia.
  3. Revascularization for acute limb ischemia (Table 3)
     a. Management approach is dependent on whether affected limb is viable, threatened, or irreversible. Initial management will depend on the absence of sensation and movement. If absent, then urgent surgery should be considered.
     b. Heparin should be given to all patients with ALI; direct thrombin inhibitor is used if patient has history of HIT.

TABLE 3 ACCF/AHA Guidelines for Management of Acute Limb Ischemia

Class	Indication	Level of Evidence
I	Patients with acute limb ischemia and a salvageable extremity should undergo an emergency evaluation that defines the anatomic level of occlusion and leads to prompt endovascular or surgical revascularization.	B
	Catheter-based thrombolysis is an effective and beneficial therapy and is indicated for patients with acute limb ischemia (Rutherford categories I and IIa) of <14 days' duration.	A
IIa	Mechanical thrombectomy devices can be used as adjunctive therapy for acute limb ischemia secondary to peripheral arterial occlusion.	B
IIb	Catheter-based thrombolysis or thrombectomy may be considered for patients with acute limb ischemia (Rutherford category IIb) of >14 days' duration.	B
III	Patients with acute limb ischemia and a nonviable extremity should not undergo an evaluation to define the vascular anatomy or efforts to attempt revascularization.	B

ACCF, American College of Cardiology Foundation; *AHA,* American Heart Association.
From Mann DL, et al.: *Braunwald's heart disease,* ed 10, Philadelphia, 2015, Elsevier.

  4. (cont.)
     a. Catheter-based thrombolysis is effective in ALI with salvageable limb.
     b. Amputation should be performed in patients with irreversible damage.

DISPOSITION

Risk factors for atherosclerosis should be assessed, and appropriate modification instituted. Focus should be placed on smoking cessation, dietary adjustment, and pharmacotherapy for dyslipidemia, hyperglycemia, and hypertension. All patients with PAD should receive aspirin therapy unless contraindicated. Revascularization should be considered for refractory lifestyle-limiting symptoms.

- More than 1 in 6 patients with peripheral arterial disease who undergo peripheral arterial revascularization have unplanned readmission within 30 days with high associated mortality risks and costs. Procedure- and patient-related factors were the primary reasons for readmission.[1]

REFERRAL

Consultation with vascular medicine, vascular surgery, interventional cardiology, or other physicians with expertise in PAD is recommended in patients with rest pain, functional disability from pain, ABI <0.90 at rest, or any physical signs of limb ischemia or gangrene.

PEARLS & CONSIDERATIONS

COMMENTS

- PAD is a highly prevalent disease process that remains underdiagnosed and undertreated.
- Patients with PAD are at markedly higher risk of future coronary, cerebrovascular, and other vascular events.
- Medical treatment is aimed mainly at cardiovascular risk factor modification, except for cilostazol.
- Studies of the natural history of claudication show the relative safety of initial conservative treatment of PAD in the absence of critical limb ischemia.
- When PAD limits a patient's ability to walk and exercise, revascularization should be considered.
- Exercise training is an important and often neglected treatment strategy that has proven beneficial in improving functional status, reducing symptoms, and improving quality of life. Exercise capacity alone is the strongest predictor of mortality in patients with PAD.
- Surgical intervention should be considered in patients who meet the criteria for intervention but have lesions that are not amenable to PTA/stenting or in older patients with a low surgical risk. Advances in endovascular therapy have broadened the range of revascularization options for refractory claudication and critical and acute limb ischemia in patients with multiple comorbidities.

PREVENTION

Cardiovascular disease is the major cause of death in patients with intermittent claudication. Therefore, the treatment of claudication is directed not only at improving walking distance but also at reducing cardiovascular risk.

PATIENT & FAMILY EDUCATION

The following organizations offer more information about PAD:

- American College of Cardiology (http://www.acc.org)
- Vascular Disease Foundation (http://www.vdf.org)

SUGGESTED READINGS

Available at ExpertConsult.com

RELATED CONTENT

Peripheral Arterial Disease (Patient Information)

AUTHORS: **SONIA R. SAMTANI, M.D.,** and **PRANAV M. PATEL, M.D., F.A.C.C., F.A.H.A., F.S.C.A.I.**

[1] Secemsky EA, et al.: Readmissions after revascularization procedures for peripheral arterial disease, *Ann Int Med* 168:93-99, 2018..

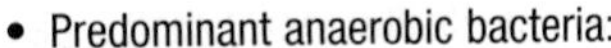

BASIC INFORMATION

DEFINITION

A perirectal abscess is a localized inflammatory process that can be associated with infections of soft tissue and anal glands based on anatomic location. Perianal and perirectal abscesses may be simple or complex, causing suppuration. Infections in these spaces may be classified as superficial perianal or perirectal with involvement in the following anatomic spaces: ischiorectal, intersphincteric, perianal, and supralevator. The Parks classification of anorectal abscess is subdivided into intersphincteric, transsphincteric, suprasphincteric, and extrasphincteric abscess (Fig. 1).

SYNONYMS:

Rectal abscess
Perianal abscess
Anorectal abscess

ICD-10CM CODES
K61.0 Anal abscess
K61.1 Rectal abscess

EPIDEMIOLOGY & DEMOGRAPHICS

INCIDENCE (IN U.S.): Commonly encountered
PREDOMINANT SEX: Male > female
PREDOMINANT AGE: All ages
PEAK INCIDENCE: Not seasonal; common
GENETICS: None known

PHYSICAL FINDINGS & CLINICAL PRESENTATION

- Localized perirectal or anal pain—often worsened with movement or straining
- Perirectal erythema or cellulitis
- Perirectal mass by inspection or palpation
- Fever and signs of sepsis with deep abscess
- Urinary retention

ETIOLOGY

- Polymicrobial aerobic and anaerobic bacteria involving one of the anatomic spaces (see "Definition"), often associated with localized trauma
- Microbiology: Most bacteria are polymicrobial, mixed enteric, and skin flora
- Predominant anaerobic bacteria:
  1. *Bacteroides fragilis*
  2. *Peptostreptococcus* spp.
  3. *Prevotella* spp.
  4. *Porphyromonas* spp.
  5. *Clostridium* spp.
  6. *Fusobacterium* spp.
- Predominant aerobic bacteria:
  1. *Staphylococcus aureus*
  2. *Streptococcus* spp.
  3. *Escherichia coli*
  4. *Enterococcus* spp.

DIAGNOSIS

Many patients will have predisposing underlying conditions including:
- Malignancy or leukemia
- Immune deficiency
- Diabetes mellitus
- Recent surgery
- Steroid therapy

DIFFERENTIAL DIAGNOSIS

- Neutropenic enterocolitis
- Crohn disease (inflammatory bowel disease)
- Pilonidal disease
- Hidradenitis suppurativa
- Tuberculosis or actinomycosis; Chagas disease
- Cancerous lesions
- Chronic anal fistula
- Rectovaginal fistula
- Proctitis—often STD-associated, including syphilis, gonococcal, chlamydia, chancroid, condylomata acuminata
- AIDS-associated: Kaposi sarcoma, lymphoma, CMV

WORKUP

- Examination of rectal, perirectal/perineal areas
- Rule out necrotic process and crepitance suggesting deep tissue involvement
- Local aerobic and anaerobic culture
- Blood cultures if toxic, febrile, or compromised
- Possible sigmoidoscopy

IMAGING STUDIES

Usually not indicated unless extensive disease is suspected. CT has a sensitivity of 77% and is relatively poor in detecting a perirectal abscess in immunocompromised patients.

TREATMENT

ACUTE GENERAL Rx

- Incision and drainage of abscess
- Debridement of necrotic tissue
- Rule out need for fistulectomy
- Local wound care—packing
- Sitz baths
- Antibiotic treatment: Directed toward coverage for mixed skin and enteric flora

OUTPATIENT—ORAL:
- Trimethoprim/sulfamethoxazole DS bid or ciprofloxacin 500 mg bid or levofloxacin 500 mg q24h plus metronidazole 500 mg q8h x 7 to 10 days
- Amoxicillin/clavulanic acid 875 to 1000 mg 1 tabs bid
- Clindamycin 150 to 300 mg PO q6 to 8h ± ciprofloxacin

INPATIENT—INTRAVENOUS:
- Piperacillin/tazobactam 3.375 g IV q6 to 8h
- Ampicillin/sulbactam 1.5 to 3 g IV q6h
- Cefotetan 1 to 2 g IV q8h
- Imipenem or meropenem 500 to 1000 mg IV q8h

DISPOSITION

Follow-up with a general surgeon or infectious disease physician is often warranted.

REFERRAL

- General surgeon or colorectal surgeon for drainage.
- AIDS specialist may be needed for perirectal complications of HIV infection.
- Gastroenterologist follow-up may be warranted in Crohn disease with perirectal fistula and other complications.
- Endoscopic ultrasound–guided perirectal abscess drainage is a recently described promising alternative treatment.

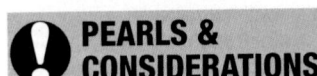

PEARLS & CONSIDERATIONS

Perirectal abscess may be a presenting manifestation of type 2 diabetes mellitus in older adults. Check the blood sugar in patients to exclude the possibility of undiagnosed diabetes mellitus.

SUGGESTED READINGS

Available at ExpertConsult.com

RELATED CONTENT

Perirectal Abscess (Patient Information)

AUTHOR: **GLENN G. FORT, M.D., M.P.H.**

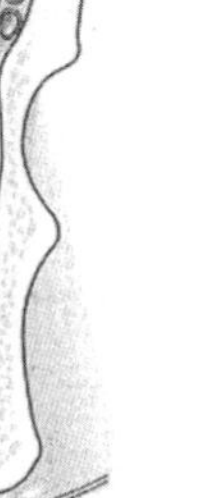

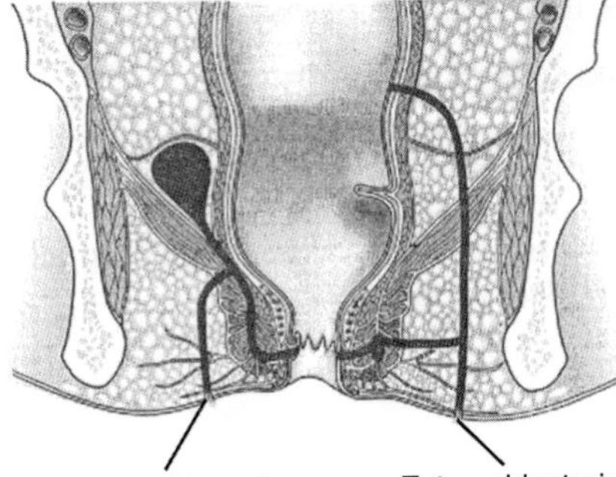

FIG. 1 Parks classification of anorectal abscess. (From Cameron JL, Cameron AM: *Current surgical therapy*, ed 10, Philadelphia, 2011, Saunders.)

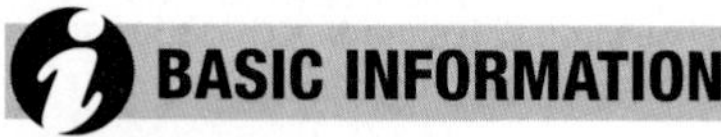

BASIC INFORMATION

DEFINITION

Peritonitis refers to the acute onset of severe abdominal pain caused by peritoneal inflammation.

Secondary peritonitis is peritonitis stemming from another condition; commonly a defect in an abdominal viscus.

SYNONYMS

Acute abdomen
Surgical abdomen

ICD-10CM CODES	
K65.0	Generalized (acute) peritonitis
K65.8	Other peritonitis
K65.9	Peritonitis, unspecified
A18.31	Tuberculous peritonitis
A54.85	Gonococcal peritonitis
A74.81	Chlamydial peritonitis
K35.2	Acute appendicitis with generalized peritonitis
K35.3	Acute appendicitis with localized peritonitis
K65.2	Spontaneous bacterial peritonitis
N73.3	Female acute pelvic peritonitis
N73.4	Female chronic pelvic peritonitis
N73.5	Female pelvic peritonitis, unspecified
P78.1	Other neonatal peritonitis

EPIDEMIOLOGY & DEMOGRAPHICS

Common presentation as a result of diverse etiologies; for example, 5% to 10% of the population has acute appendicitis at some point in their lives.

PHYSICAL FINDINGS & CLINICAL PRESENTATION

- Acute abdominal pain
- Abdominal distention and ascites
- Abdominal rigidity, rebound, and guarding
- Fever, chills
- Exacerbation with movement
- Anorexia, nausea, and vomiting
- Constipation
- Decreased bowel sounds
- Hypotension and tachycardia
- Tachypnea, dyspnea

ETIOLOGY

- Acute perforation peritonitis: Gastrointestinal perforation, intestinal ischemia, pelvic peritonitis, and other forms
- Microbiology: Most common is gram-negative bacteria (*Escherichia coli, Enterobacter, Klebsiella, Proteus*), gram-positive bacteria (enterococci, streptococci, staphylococci), anaerobic bacteria (*Bacteroides, Clostridium*), and fungi
- Postoperative peritonitis: Anastomotic leak, accidental perforation, and devascularization
- Posttraumatic peritonitis: After blunt or penetrating abdominal trauma

Dx DIAGNOSIS

DIFFERENTIAL DIAGNOSIS

- Postoperative: Abscess, sepsis, bowel obstruction, injury to internal organs
- Gastrointestinal: Perforated viscus, appendicitis, inflammatory bowel disease, infectious colitis, diverticulitis, acute cholecystitis, peptic ulcer perforation, pancreatitis, bowel obstruction
- Gynecologic: Ruptured ectopic pregnancy, pelvic inflammatory disease, ruptured hemorrhagic ovarian cyst, ovarian torsion, degenerating leiomyoma
- Urologic: Nephrolithiasis, interstitial cystitis
- Miscellaneous: Abdominal trauma, penetrating wounds, infections caused by intraperitoneal dialysis

WORKUP

- Acute peritonitis is mainly a clinical diagnosis based on patient history and physical examination.
- Laboratory and imaging studies (see "Laboratory Tests") assist in determining the need for and type of intervention.
- If patient is hemodynamically unstable, immediate diagnostic laparotomy should be performed in lieu of adjuvant diagnostic studies.

LABORATORY TESTS

- Complete blood count: Leukocytosis, left shift, anemia
- SMA7: Electrolyte imbalances, kidney dysfunction
- Liver function tests: Ascites from liver disease, cholelithiasis
- Amylase: Pancreatitis
- Blood cultures: Bacteremia, sepsis
- Peritoneal cultures: Infectious etiology
- Blood gas: Respiratory versus metabolic acidosis
- Ascitic fluid analysis: Exudate versus transudate, culture
- Urinalysis and culture: Urinary tract infection
- Cervical cultures for gonorrhea and *Chlamydia*
- Urine/serum human chorionic gonadotropin

IMAGING STUDIES

- Abdominal series: Free air from perforation, small or large bowel dilation from obstruction, identification of fecalith
- Chest x-ray examination: Elevated diaphragm, pneumonia
- Pelvic/abdominal ultrasound: Abscess formation, abdominal mass, intrauterine versus ectopic pregnancy, identify free fluid suggestive of hemorrhage or ascites
- CT: Mass, ascites

Rx TREATMENT

NONPHARMACOLOGIC THERAPY

- IV hydration to correct dehydration, hypovolemia
- Blood transfusion to correct anemia from hemorrhage
- Nasogastric decompression, especially if obstruction is present
- Oxygen: Intubation if necessary
- Bed rest

ACUTE GENERAL Rx

- Surgery to correct underlying pathology, such as controlling hemorrhage, correcting perforation, draining abscess
- Broad-spectrum antibiotics to cover both gram-negative aerobic and gram-negative anaerobic bacteria:
  1. Mild-moderate disease: Piperacillin-tazobactam 3.375 g IV q6h or 4.5 g IV q8h *or* ticarcillin-clavulanate 3.1 g IV q6h. Alternative agents are ciprofloxacin 400 mg IV q12h or levofloxacin 750 mg IV q24h *plus* metronidazole 1 g IV q12h.
  2. Severe life-threatening disease: Imipenem 500 mg IV q6h or meropenem 1 g IV q8h. Alternative agents are ampicillin *plus* metronidazole *plus* ciprofloxacin.
- Pain control: Morphine or meperidine as needed (hold until diagnosis confirmed)

DISPOSITION

Depends on etiology of peritonitis, age of patient, coexisting medical disease, and duration of process before presentation

REFERRAL

Surgical consultation is required in all cases of acute peritonitis.

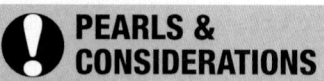

PEARLS & CONSIDERATIONS

Computed tomographic scan guides therapeutic approach and should be considered as the primary imaging study if available. As with forms of sepsis, early administration of broad spectrum antibiotics, fluid resuscitation, and rapidly obtaining anatomic source control (when appropriate) will lead to improved outcomes.

AUTHOR: **MATTHEW K. HOFFMAN, M.D., M.P.H., F.A.C.O.G.**

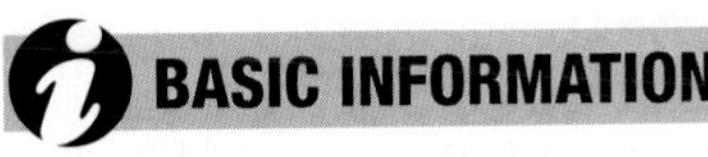

BASIC INFORMATION

DEFINITION

Peritonsillar abscess is an acute infection located between the capsule of the palatine tonsil and the superior constrictor muscle of the pharynx.

SYNONYMS

Quinsy
PTA

ICD-10CM CODE

J36 Peritonsillar abscess

EPIDEMIOLOGY & DEMOGRAPHICS

INCIDENCE (IN U.S.): 30:100,000/yr for ages 5 to 59. For adolescents, the incidence is 40:100,000/yr. It is the most common deep infection of the head and neck in children and adolescents, accounting for at least 50% of cases.
PEAK INCIDENCE: Bimodal frequency during the year, with highest occurrence from November to December and April to May.
PREVALENCE: 45,000 cases/yr in the United States
PREDOMINANT SEX: Male > female
PREDOMINANT AGE: Highest incidence is adults aged 20 to 40 yr
RISK FACTORS: Smoking, periodontal disease, oropharyngeal or dental infection, male gender

PHYSICAL FINDINGS & CLINICAL PRESENTATION

- There is often a delay of 2 to 5 days between abscess formation and local and systemic symptoms
- Sore throat, which may be severe and unilateral (Table 1)
- Dysphagia and odynophagia
- Otalgia on the side of abscess
- Foul-smelling breath
- Facial swelling
- Drooling
- Headache
- Fever
- Trismus: The examination of the pharynx can be limited by trismus
- Hoarseness, muffled voice (also called "hot potato voice")
- Tender submandibular and anterior cervical lymph nodes
- Tonsillar hypertrophy with likely peritonsillar edema
- Contralateral deflection of the uvula: The distinguishing feature of peritonsillar abscess is inferior medial displacement of the infected tonsil with contralateral deviation of the uvula (Fig. 1)
- Stridor

ETIOLOGY

- Peritonsillar abscess is usually a complication of tonsillitis or acute bacterial pharyngitis caused by blockage of salivary ducts. Tonsillitis → peritonsillar cellulitis → peritonsillar abscess.
- Group A β-hemolytic *Streptococcus* is the most common bacterial cause, accounting for 15% to 30% of cases in children and 5% to 10% of cases in adults.
- Less common aerobic causes are *Staphylococcus aureus, Haemophilus influenzae, Neisseria* species.
- The most common anaerobic organism is *Fusobacterium.*

Dx DIAGNOSIS

DIFFERENTIAL DIAGNOSIS

- Hypertrophic tonsillitis
- Infectious mononucleosis
- Peritonsillar cellulitis
- Retropharyngeal abscess
- Epiglottitis
- Dental abscess (retromolar)
- Lymphoma
- Ludwig angina
- Tubercular granuloma
- Cervical adenitis
- Diphtheria
- Foreign body
- Neoplasm

WORKUP

- Based on history and physical exam. Aspiration of pus established diagnosis of peritonsillar abscess
- Consider additional testing if presentation is less clear.

LABORATORY TESTS

- Consider rapid strep antigen testing and/or pharyngeal culture and sensitivity.
- Aspiration of the abscess for culture and sensitivity (see "Treatment" for role of aspiration in tx)
- Consider lab testing for mononucleosis (patients with peritonsillar abscess have a 20% incidence of mononucleosis)

IMAGING STUDIES

- Consider ultrasound, CT scan (Fig. 2), or MRI to help differentiate abscess from cellulitis or mass when diagnosis is unclear.
- Intraoral ultrasound may improve diagnosis and aspiration of PTA compared with visual inspection in adult patients.
- MRI provides better soft-tissue differentiation than CT.

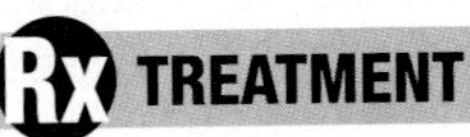

Rx TREATMENT

NONPHARMACOLOGIC THERAPY

Drainage of the abscess by needle aspiration or by surgical incision and drainage. Intraoral ultrasound-guided needle aspiration is a useful adjunct in the presence of trismus

ACUTE GENERAL Rx

- Aspiration or surgical drainage AND antibiotics for 10 to 14 days

TABLE 1 Clinical Differentiation of Common Conditions Arising as Sore Throat

Feature	Viral Pharyngitis	Bacterial Tonsillitis	Peritonsillar Abscess	Epiglottitis
Tonsillar Enlargement	Usual	Rare	None	None
Tonsillar Exudates	Occasional (mononucleosis)	Usual	Often	None
Tonsillar Asymmetry	None	None	Usual	None
Trismus (Inability to Open Jaw)	None	None	Usual	None
Cervical Adenopathy	Occasional	Usual (tender)	Usual (tender)	None
Tender Larynx	Rare	None	None	Usual

From Goldman L, Schafer AI: *Goldman's Cecil Medicine*, ed 24, Philadelphia, 2012, Saunders.

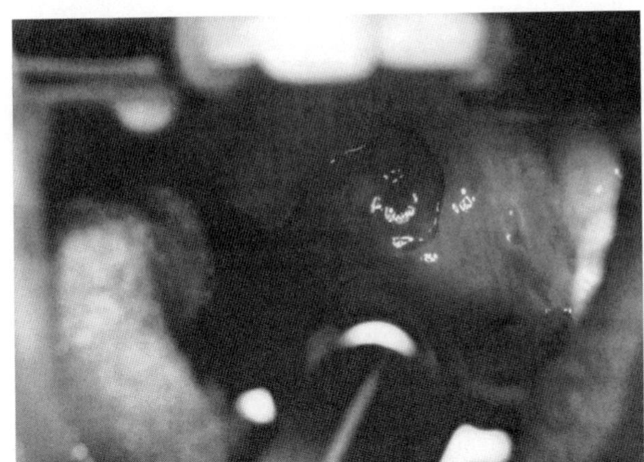

FIG. 1 Peritonsillar abscess with uvular displacement to the right. (From Marx JA et al: *Rosen's emergency medicine*, ed 8, Philadelphia, 2014, WB Saunders.)

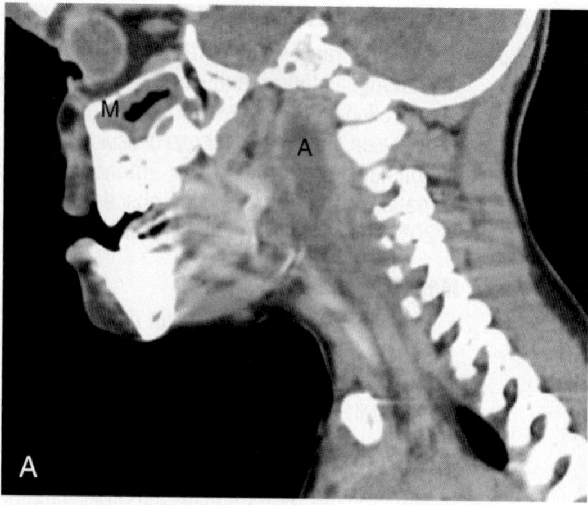

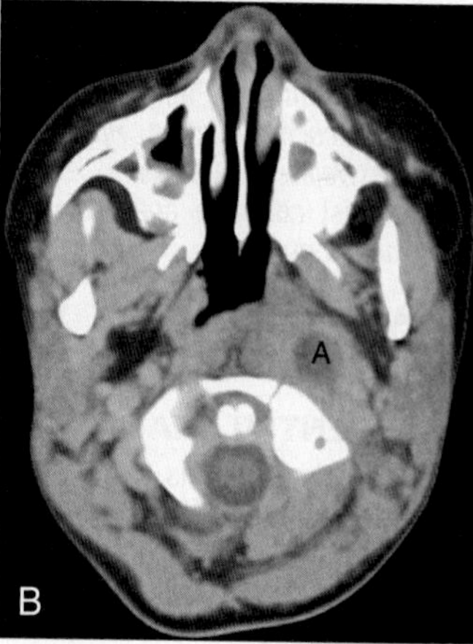

FIG. 2 Computed tomography of parapharyngeal abscess in a 3-year-old child. A, Sagittal section demonstrating parapharyngeal abscess *(A)* and mucosal swelling *(M)* in the maxillary sinus. **B,** Coronal section of parapharyngeal abscess *(A)*. (From Kliegman RM et al: *Nelson textbook of pediatrics*, ed 19, Philadelphia, 2011, Saunders.)

- Initial antibiotics should cover group A *Streptococcus* and anaerobes
- Intravenous
  1. Piperacillin/tazobactam or ticarcillin/clavulanate. If penicillin allergic, use IV clindamycin (600-900 mg IV q8h)
  2. Ampicillin-sulbactam 3 g q6h
  3. Penicillin G 10 million units q6h AND metronidazole 500 mg q6h (may use clindamycin 900 mg q8h if penicillin allergic)
- OR oral
  1. Amoxicillin-clavulanic acid 875 mg twice daily
  2. Penicillin VK 500 mg 4 times daily AND metronidazole 500 mg 4 times daily
  3. Clindamycin 600 mg twice daily or 300 mg 4 times daily
- Selection of antibiotics should be guided by culture and sensitivity of the organism. Consulting local antimicrobial guidelines for resistance profiles is also advisable for empiric coverage before culture results are available

CHRONIC Rx

- Tonsillectomy can be considered 3 to 6 mo after diagnosis of peritonsillar abscess with or without the diagnosis of recurrent tonsillitis.
- Though rare, in adults and children with an acute case of peritonsillar abscess and a history of recurrent pharyngitis or previous peritonsillar abscess, a specialist may recommend a *quinsy or hot tonsillectomy*, an immediate removal of the tonsils after starting IV antibiotics.

DISPOSITION

- Successful treatment is defined by symptomatic improvement in sore throat, fever, and/or tonsillar swelling within 24 hr of intervention.
- Treatment failure is defined by lack of symptomatic improvement or worsening despite 24 hr of antimicrobial therapy (with or without surgical drainage).

REFERRAL

- Consider ENT or diagnostic radiology for drainage of abscess.
- Consider ENT for tonsillectomy if criteria are met.

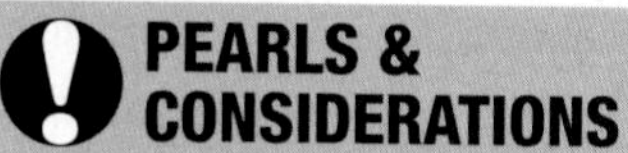

PEARLS & CONSIDERATIONS

COMMENTS

- Risk for a recurrence is immediate (within 4 days) and long term (2 to 3 yr).
- Most recurrences occur shortly after the initial presentation, suggesting continued infection rather than recurrence.
- Overall recurrence rate is 10% to 15%.
- Supportive treatment for pain control and hydration. Newer reports suggest a single dose of dexamethasone (10 mg) administered following needle aspiration will reduce pain at 24 hours as compared with placebo (see "Suggested Readings").

PREVENTION

- Adequate treatment of peritonsillar abscess.
- Up to 30% of patients with peritonsillar abscess meet criteria for tonsillectomy.

PATIENT/FAMILY EDUCATION

Advise family members to call with any trouble breathing, swallowing, or talking.

SUGGESTED READINGS

Available at ExpertConsult.com

AUTHORS: **PETER J. SELL, D.O.**, and **AMITY RUBEOR, D.O., C.A.Q.S.M.**

BASIC INFORMATION

DEFINITION

Pertussis is a prolonged bacterial infection of the upper respiratory tract characterized by paroxysms of an intense cough.

SYNONYM

Whooping cough

ICD-10CM CODES

A37.90	Whooping cough, unspecified species without pneumonia
A37.00	Whooping cough due to Bordetella pertussis without pneumonia
A37.01	Whooping cough due to Bordetella pertussis with pneumonia
A37.10	Whooping cough due to Bordetella parapertussis without pneumonia
A37.11	Whooping cough due to Bordetella parapertussis with pneumonia
A37.80	Whooping cough due to other Bordetella species without pneumonia
A37.81	Whooping cough due to other Bordetella species with pneumonia
A37.90	Whooping cough, unspecified species without pneumonia
A37.91	Whooping cough, unspecified species with pneumonia

EPIDEMIOLOGY

INCIDENCE (IN U.S.): Case reports from 2016 were 15,737, including seven deaths. This represents a decrease in the number of case reports compared with each of the 3 previous years. The reported rates were 20,762 and 32,971 in 2015 and 2014, respectively. In 2012, there were 48,277 cases reported, which is the highest rate reported since 1955. The highest incidence, in 2016, was among infants <6 months (85.5/100,000), with a second peak in adolescents 11 to 19 yr of age (13.9/100,000).

PEAK INCIDENCE:
- Childhood
- Usually affects children aged <1 yr
- Increasing infections seen in adolescence

PREDOMINANT AGE:
- 50% in children aged <1 yr.
- 20% in children aged >15 yr.
- Classically an infection of infants and young children, pertussis is often overlooked as a cause of chronic cough in adults. However, a resurgence of pertussis has been observed in recent years, with nearly 50% of all cases identified in adolescents and adults, likely due to waning immunity and decreased effectiveness of acellular vaccines in early childhood compared to older, whole-cell-derived vaccines.

PHYSICAL FINDINGS & CLINICAL PRESENTATION

- Infection is characterized by three phases: Catarrhal, paroxysmal, and convalescent
- Catarrhal phase: Usually begins with a 1- to 2-wk prodrome that resembles a common cold. This phase may be mild or absent in adolescents and adults given partial immunity from prior immunization
- After this initial phase, increased production of mucus occurs. Excessive lacrimation and conjunctival infection should heighten the suspicion for pertussis
- Paroxysmal phase: Increased mucus production is followed by an intense, paroxysmal cough, ending with gasps and an inspiratory whoop
- In some children, apnea, cyanosis, and anoxia are noted; posttussive gagging and vomiting are characteristic of pertussis
- Cases can be severe and life-threatening in young infants, particularly children <6 months old
- When prolonged, frank exhaustion and even apnea occur. The paroxysmal phase lasts from 2 wk to 2 mo
- Convalescent phase: Lasts over 2 months and is characterized by cough of decreasing severity
- See Box 1 for complications of pertussis

ETIOLOGY

Bordetella pertussis, a gram-negative rod that adheres to human cilia and respiratory epithelia

DIAGNOSIS

DIFFERENTIAL DIAGNOSIS

- Croup
- Epiglottitis
- Foreign body aspiration
- Bacterial pneumonia
- Viral pneumonia

WORKUP

Pertussis is often overlooked as a cause of chronic cough, especially in adolescents and adults. The presence of posttussive emesis and/or inspiratory whoop increases the likelihood of pertussis but only modestly. Therefore, clinicians must use their overall impression in pursuing the diagnosis.

- Enzyme-linked immunosorbent assay for detection of antibody to pertussis. Polymerase chain reaction (PCR) is the most sensitive method for rapid detection of pertussis. PCR testing should be used only to confirm a diagnosis in persons with signs and symptoms consistent with pertussis. PCR testing sensitivity declines and is unlikely to be positive after 1 mo of infection. PCR testing after 5 days of treatment with antibiotics can cause false-negative results and is generally not recommended.
- Blood cultures in hospitalized patients.
- Chest x-ray.
- Culture of bacteria, usually from nasopharynx by aspiration or by swabbing the posterior nasopharynx with a polyester-tipped, rayon-tipped, or nylon-flocked swab.
- Immunofluorescent staining of nasopharyngeal secretions.
- Serologic tests for immunoglobulin G (IgG) or A (IgA) are available. A twofold increase between acute and convalescent sera is considered proof of seroconversion. A single elevated IgG or IgA titer is considered diagnostic when no acute serum is available. Can be useful for diagnosis later in illness.

BOX 1 Pertussis Complications

- Periorbital edema
- Subconjunctival hemorrhage
- Petechiae
- Epistaxis
- Hemoptysis
- Subcutaneous emphysema
- Pneumothorax
- Pneumomediastinum
- Diaphragmatic rupture
- Umbilical and inguinal hernias
- Rectal prolapse

From Marx J, et al.: Rosen's emergency medicine: concepts and clinical practice, ed 7, Philadelphia, 2010, Mosby.

LABORATORY TESTS

Complete blood count, which usually demonstrates marked lymphocytosis:
- Up to 18,000 white blood cells
- 70% to 80% lymphocytes

IMAGING STUDIES

Chest x-ray examination is of value if secondary bacterial pneumonia is suspected.

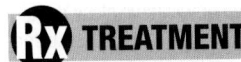

TREATMENT

ACUTE GENERAL Rx

- Intensive supportive care:
  1. Adequate hydration
  2. Control of secretions
  3. Maintenance of airway
- Antibiotics (Table 1) are indicated, even though their ability to alter the course of the disease is controversial.
  1. Azithromycin 500 mg on day 1, followed by 250 mg for days 2 to 5. Erythromycin 50 mg/kg/day for 14 days. Recent literature reports indicate that a 7-day treatment regimen may be as effective as a 14-day course of erythromycin. TMP/SMX 320/1600 mg per day in divided doses can be used in patients with allergy or intolerance to macrolides.
  2. Although unproved, dexamethasone 1 mg/kg/day in four doses for severe, life-threatening paroxysms.
  3. Ceftriaxone 75 mg/kg/day in two doses for broad coverage of secondary bacterial pneumonias.
  4. Close observation of infants <6 mo old as risk for apnea is high in this age group.
- Vaccination is successful in preventing the disease: Universal vaccination is advised for all children and adults. Children are recommended to receive the five-dose DTaP series at months 2, 4, 6, and 15 to 18, and at 4 to 6 yr of age.

TABLE 1 Recommended Antimicrobial Treatment and Postexposure Prophylaxis for Pertussis, by Age Group

	Primary Agents		Alternate Agent*	
Age Group	**Azithromycin**	**Erythromycin**	**Clarithromycin**	**TMP-SMZ**
<1 mo	Recommended agent. 10 mg/kg/day in a single dose for 5 days (only limited safety data available)	Not preferred. Erythromycin is substantially associated with infantile hypertrophic pyloric stenosis. Use if azithromycin is unavailable; 40-50 mg/kg/day in 4 divided doses for 14 days	Not recommended (safety data unavailable)	Contraindicated for infants aged <2 mo (risk for kernicterus)
1-5 mo	10 mg/kg/day in a single dose for 5 days	40-50 mg/kg/day in four divided doses for 14 days	15 mg/kg/day in two divided doses for 7 days	Contraindicated at age <2 mo. For infants aged ≥2 mo: TMP 8 mg/kg/day plus SMZ 40 mg/kg/day in two divided doses for 14 days
Infants aged ≥6 mo and children	10 mg/kg in a single dose on day 1 (maximum 500 mg), then 5 mg/kg/day (maximum 250 mg) on days 2-5	40 mg/kg/day (maximum 1-2 g/day) in four divided doses for 14 days	15 mg/kg/day in 2 divided doses (maximum 1 g/day) for 7 days	TMP 8 mg/kg/day plus SMZ 40 mg/kg/day in two divided doses for 14 days
Adolescents and adults	500 mg in a single dose on day 1 then 250 mg/day on days 2-5	2 g/day in four divided doses for 14 days	1 g/day in two divided doses for 7 days	TMP 320 mg/day, SMZ 1600 mg/day in two divided doses for 14 days

*Trimethoprim-sulfamethoxazole (TMP-SMZ) can be used as an alternative agent to macrolides in patients aged ≥2 mo who are allergic to macrolides, who cannot tolerate macrolides, or who are infected with a rare, macrolide-resistant strain of *Bordetella pertussis.*

SMZ, sulfamethoxazole; *TMZ,* trimethoprim.

From Centers for Disease Control and Prevention: Recommended antimicrobial agents for treatment and postexposure prophylaxis of pertussis: 2005 CDC guidelines, *MMWR Morbid Mortal Wkly Rep* 54:1-16, 2005.

- The Advisory Committee on Immunization Practices (ACIP) updated Tdap recommendations to include a single dose of Tdap vaccine in place of routine Td for adults age 19 to 64 yr and a single-dose Tdap for adults 65 yr and older who have or will have close contact with an infant (<12 mo). The ACIP also recommends that all pregnant women receive a dose of Tdap with every pregnancy, preferably during weeks 27 to 36 of gestation.
- Azithromycin, clarithromycin, or erythromycin is recommended for all household contacts and should be given to all persons at high risk of severe disease from pertussis and who were in contact with a pertussis case within 21 days of cough onset: TMP/SMX in two oral doses per day for those intolerant to macrolides.

DISPOSITION

Close attention to accepted vaccination schedules is the best prevention.

REFERRAL

To intensive care setting for life-threatening infections:

- Pulmonologist
- Infectious disease specialist

PEARLS & CONSIDERATIONS

- The diagnosis of pertussis in a young child is easily recognized, but in adults pertussis can be a subtle diagnosis and is often missed. The tip-off is often a persistent, hacking, and productive cough with minor or no fever in a previously healthy person that lasts <2 wk.
- Approximately 11% of pertussis cases in the pediatric population are attributable to vaccine refusal, dispelling the myth that herd immunity protects children whose parents refuse pertussis vaccine.

SUGGESTED READINGS

Available at ExpertConsult.com

RELATED CONTENT

Pertussis (Patient Information)

AUTHOR: **RUSSELL J. MCCULLOH, M.D.**

BASIC INFORMATION

DEFINITION

- A hamartomatous polyp is a benign intestinal growth that may contain all components of the intestinal mucosa. In Peutz-Jeghers syndrome (PJS), hamartomas are found primarily in the small bowel but can also be present in the colon and stomach. In gastrointestinal polyposis, multiple such polyps coexist within the intestinal tract, and associated manifestations are usually also present.
- Juvenile polyps are benign polyps composed of cystic dilations of glandular structures within the fibroblastic stroma of the lamina propria. They may cause bleeding or intussusception.
- Commonly recognized syndromes are Peutz-Jeghers syndrome, juvenile polyposis syndrome, Cowden disease, Bannayan-Ruvalcaba-Riley syndrome, and Cronkhite-Canada syndrome. Other, lesser known inherited hamartomatous polyposis syndromes are hereditary mixed polyposis syndrome, intestinal ganglioneuromatosis and neurofibromatosis (variant of von Recklinghausen syndrome), Devon family syndrome, basal cell nevus syndrome, and tuberous sclerosis (may involve gastrointestinal tract). Table 1 describes general features of some inherited colorectal cancer syndromes.

ICD-10CM CODE

D12.6 Colon, unspecified (adenomatosis of colon, hereditary polyposis)

EPIDEMIOLOGY

- The incidence of PJS is 1 in 200,000.
- Colonic adenomas, the precursors of nearly all colorectal cancers, are found in nearly 40% of patients by age 60 yr.
- 25% of men and 15% of women who undergo colonoscopy are found to have one or more adenomas.
- Detection of any adenoma in patients <60 yr confers an increased risk of colorectal cancer (by a factor of 2.6) in their first-degree relatives.

PHYSICAL FINDINGS & CLINICAL PRESENTATION

PEUTZ-JEGHERS SYNDROME:

- Transmission: Autosomal dominant with incomplete penetrance. The syndrome is caused in the majority of patients by a germline mutation of the *STK11/LKB1* tumor suppression gene on chromosome 19P13.
- Disease expression:
  1. Stomach, small and large intestinal hamartomas with bands of smooth muscle in the lamina propria
  2. Pigmented lesions around mouth (lips and buccal mucosa [Fig. 2]), nose, hands, feet, genitals, and perineal areas
  3. Ovarian tumors
  4. Sertoli cell testicular tumors
  5. Airway polyps
  6. Pancreatic cancer
  7. Breast cancer
  8. Urinary tract polyps
- Cumulative lifetime cancer risk:
  1. Colon cancer: 39%
  2. Stomach cancer: 29%
  3. Small intestine cancer: 13%
  4. Pancreatic cancer: 36%
  5. Breast cancer: 54%
  6. Ovarian cancer: 10%
  7. Sertoli cell tumor: 9%
  8. Overall cancer risk: 93%
- Clinical manifestation:
  1. Gastrointestinal, small-bowel obstruction, intussusception, gastrointestinal bleeding
  2. See chapters on relevant malignancies for their signs and symptoms

DIAGNOSIS: The diagnosis of PJS is made with any of four major criteria:

1. Two or more histologically confirmed PJS polyps
2. Any number of PJS polyps and a family history of PJS
3. Characteristic mucocutaneous pigmentation and a family history of PJS, or
4. Any number of PJS polyps and characteristic mucocutaneous pigmentation

JUVENILE POLYPOSIS SYNDROME:

- Transmission: Autosomal dominant
- Disease expression:
  1. Solitary juvenile polyps numbering 10 or more in the rectum or throughout the gastrointestinal tract; the polyps are smooth and covered with normal epithelium
  2. Various congenital abnormalities coexist in 20%
- Cumulative cancer risk is increased (may be as high as 50%)
- Clinical manifestation:
  1. Intestinal obstruction
  2. Intussusception
  3. Gastrointestinal bleeding

COWDEN DISEASE:

- Transmission: Autosomal dominant, rare
- Disease expression:
  1. Juvenile intestinal polyposis
  2. Orocutaneous hamartomas
  3. Fibrocystic breast disease and breast cancer
  4. Goiter and thyroid cancer
  5. Facial tricholemmomas (papules) in 83%
- Cumulative cancer risk:
  1. Gastrointestinal: Same as general population
  2. Thyroid: 3% to 10%
  3. Breast: 25% to 50%

BANNAYAN-RUVALCABA-RILEY SYNDROME:

- Transmission: Autosomal dominant, rare
- Disease expression:
  1. Juvenile intestinal polyposis
  2. Macrocephaly
  3. Developmental delay
  4. Penile pigmented spots
  5. Cumulative cancer risk unknown

TABLE 1 General Features of Some Inherited Colorectal Cancer Syndromes

Syndrome	Polyp Histology	Polyp Distribution	Age of Onset	Risk of Colon Cancer	Genetic Lesion	Clinical Manifestations	Associated Lesions
Familial adenomatous polyposis (Fig. 1)	Adenoma	Large intestine, duodenum	16 yr (range, 8-34 yr)	100%	5q (*APC* gene)	Rectal bleeding, abdominal pain, bowel obstruction	Desmoids, CHRPE
Peutz-Jeghers syndrome	Hamartoma	Large and small intestine	First decade	Slightly above average	19p (*STK11* gene)	Possible rectal bleeding, abdominal pain, intussusception	Orocutaneous melanin pigment spots, other tumors
MUTYH-associated polyposis	Adenoma	Large intestine, duodenum	45-50 yr (range, 13-60 yr)	75% (range, 50%-100%)	1p (*MYH* gene)	Rectal bleeding, abdominal pain, bowel obstruction	CHRPE, osteomas
Juvenile polyposis	Hamartoma (rarely adenoma)	Large and small intestine	First decade	≈9%	*PTEN, SMAD4, BMPR1*	Possible rectal bleeding, abdominal pain, intussusception	Pulmonary AVMs
Hereditary nonpolyposis colon cancer	Adenoma	Large intestine	40 yr (range, 18-65 yr)	30%	Mismatch repair genes+*	Rectal bleeding, abdominal pain, bowel obstruction	Other tumors (e.g., ovary, uterus, pancreas, stomach)

AVM, Arteriovenous malformation; *CHRPE,* congenital hypertrophy of the retinal pigment epithelium; *MUTYH,* mutY homolog (*Escherichia coli*).
*Including *hMSH2, hMSH3, hMSH6, hMLH1, hPMS1,* and *hPMS2.*
From Goldman L, Schafer AI: *Goldman's Cecil medicine,* ed 24, Philadelphia, 2012, Saunders.

 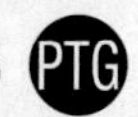

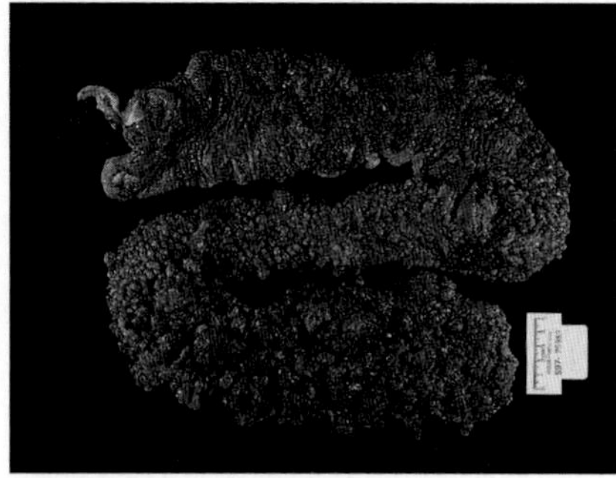

FIG. 1 Familial adenomatous polyposis. This disorder is marked by the development of hundreds of large bowel adenomas, as seen in this segment of large bowel, which is covered with adenomas of various sizes. It usually arises in the second and third decades. (From Skarin AT: *Atlas of diagnostic oncology*, 4th ed, St Louis, 2010, Mosby, 2010.)

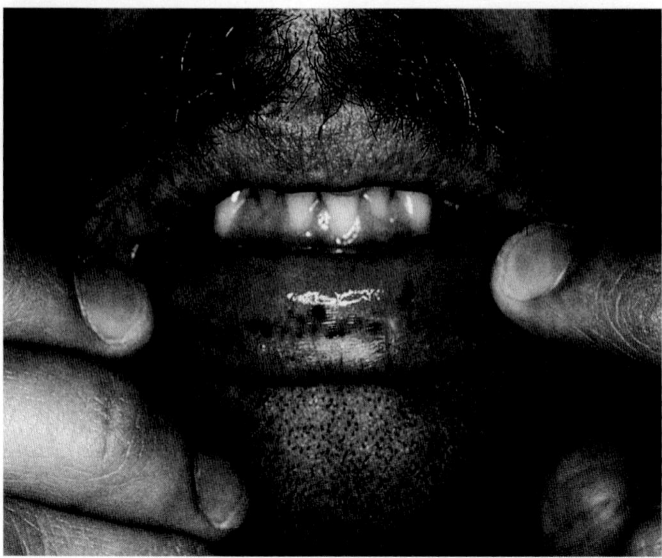

FIG. 2 Peutz-Jeghers syndrome, macular pigmentation of lower lip. (James WD et al: *Andrews' diseases of the skin,* ed 12, Philadelphia, 2016, WB Saunders.)

CRONKHITE-CANADA SYNDROME:

- Transmission: Acquired
- Age of onset: Midlife
- Disease expression:
  1. Diffuse gastrointestinal juvenile polyposis (50% to 95% of cases)
  2. Chronic diarrhea and protein-losing enteropathy (the entire intestinal mucosa may be inflamed), which leads to abdominal pain, weight loss, and various complications of malnutrition
  3. Dystrophic nails
  4. Alopecia
  5. Hyperpigmentation
- Cumulative cancer risk: Same as the average population

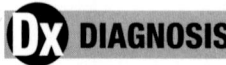

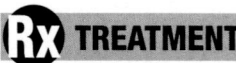

DIAGNOSIS

Diagnosis is suggested in many cases by family history and confirmed by colonoscopy and physical findings described previously.

TREATMENT

GENERAL Rx/SURVEILLANCE

Peutz-Jeghers syndrome:

- Colonoscopies with polypectomies and upper endoscopy every 2 to 3 yr beginning in teen yr
- MRI or endoscopic ultrasound of the pancreas every 1 to 2 yr beginning at age 30
- Screening for breast cancer, testicular cancer, possibly ovarian cancer
- Surveillance of small bowel with capsule endoscopy or CT or magnetic resonance enterography every 2 to 3 yr starting at age 8 to 10 yr

Juvenile polyposis syndrome:

- Colonoscopies with polypectomies and upper endoscopy every 2 to 3 yr beginning at age 15
- Total colectomy if numerous polyps
- Esophagogastroscopies and polypectomies

Cowden disease:

- Rigorous breast cancer screening or prophylactic simple bilateral mastectomy with reconstruction

Cronkhite-Canada syndrome:

- Progressive malabsorption syndrome is the hallmark of this syndrome, and no specific treatment exists. Enteral or parenteral feeding is the cornerstone of management and can result in remission.
- Other syndromes:
  1. Serrated polyposis syndrome: Colonoscopy yearly
  2. PTEN hamartoma tumor syndrome: Colonoscopy every 5 yr beginning at age 35

DISPOSITION

- The screening of first-degree relatives of patients with colonic adenomas detected before 60 yr of age is controversial. Some recommend beginning colonoscopic screening at age 40 yr or 10 yr younger than the age at diagnosis of the youngest person in the family with an adenoma.
- Recommended interval between colonoscopies from the U.S. Consensus Guidelines for Colonoscopic Surveillance after Polypectomy are as follows:
  1. 10 yr for small, rectal hyperplastic polyps
  2. 5 to 10 yr for one to two low-risk adenomas (tubular adenomas <1 cm)
  3. 3 yr for low-risk adenomas or any high-risk adenoma (large [≥1 cm] or histologically advanced adenomas [tubulovillous or villous adenomas or villous adenomas and those with high-grade dysplasia])
  4. <3 yr for presence of >10 adenomas
  5. 2 to 6 mo for inadequately removed adenomas

RELATED CONTENT

Peutz-Jeghers Syndrome (Patient Information)
Colorectal Cancer (Related Key Topic)
Familial Adenomatous Polyposis and Gardner Syndrome (Related Key Topic)
Lynch Syndrome (Related Key Topic)

AUTHOR: **FRED F. FERRI, M.D.**

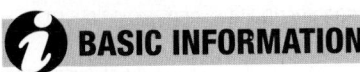

BASIC INFORMATION

DEFINITION

Inflammation of the pharynx or tonsils

SYNONYMS

Sore throat
Group A streptococci (GAS)
Pharyngitis
Tonsillitis
GABHS

ICD-10CM CODES

J02.9 Acute pharyngitis, unspecified
J03.0 Acute tonsillitis
J03.9 Acute tonsillitis, unspecified
J04.0 Acute laryngitis

EPIDEMIOLOGY & DEMOGRAPHICS

Acute pharyngitis accounts for 1.3% of outpatient visits to health care providers in the United States and is diagnosed in 2 million persons in the outpatient setting each year in the United States.

PEAK INCIDENCE: Late winter/early spring (GAS infections)

PREDOMINANT SEX: Females = males

PREDOMINANT AGE:

- All ages affected
- Streptococcal pharyngitis most common among school-age children (5-15 yr of age). GAS are responsible for 5% to 15% of cases of pharyngitis in adults and 20% to 30% of cases in children (5-15 yr of age).

PHYSICAL FINDINGS & CLINICAL PRESENTATION

- Pharynx:
  1. May appear normal to severely erythematous (Fig. 1)
  2. Tonsillar hypertrophy and exudates commonly seen but do not indicate etiology
- Viral infection:
  1. Rhinorrhea
  2. Conjunctivitis
  3. Cough
- Bacterial infection, especially GAS:
  1. High fever
  2. Systemic signs of infection
- Herpes simplex or enterovirus infection: Vesicles
- Streptococcal infection:
  1. Rare complications:
     a. Scarlet fever
     b. Rheumatic fever
     c. Acute glomerulonephritis
  2. Extension of infection: Tonsillar, parapharyngeal, or retropharyngeal abscess presenting with severe pain, high fever, trismus
- Streptococcal tonsillitis is manifested as acute onset of fever, headache, neck pain, odynophagia, sore throat, otalgia, red tongue with enlargement of papillae, sore throat, red swollen uvula, and tender anterior cervical adenitis.

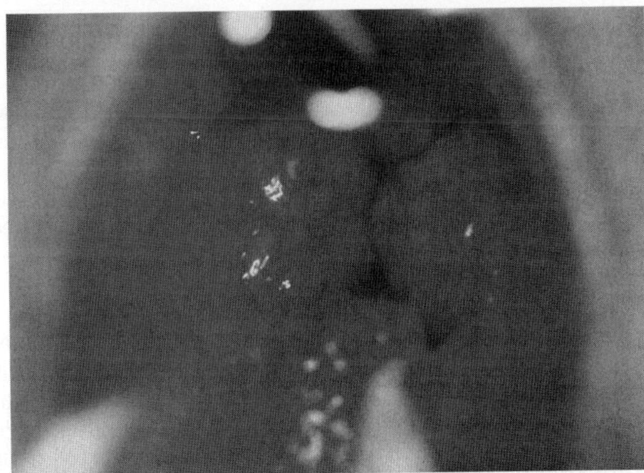

FIG. 1 Bilateral tonsillopharyngitis. (From Marx JA et al: *Rosen's emergency medicine*, ed 8, Philadelphia, 2014, Elsevier.)

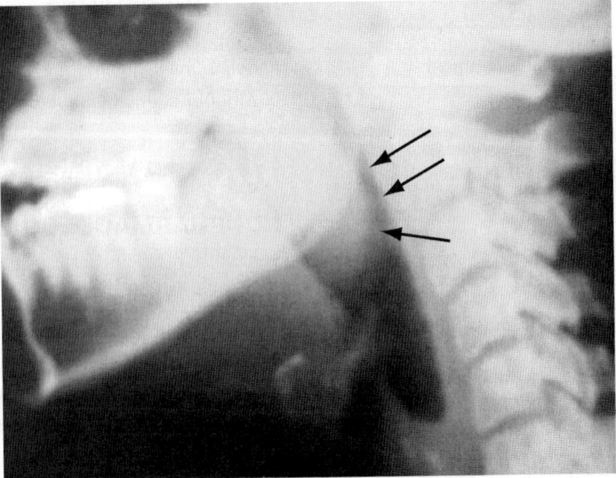

FIG. 2 Lingual tonsillitis. Notice the scalloped appearance of the lingual tonsil on the anterior surface of the vallecula (*arrows*) with a normal epiglottis and aryepiglottic fold. (From Marx JA et al: *Rosen's emergency medicine*, ed 8, Philadelphia, 2014, Elsevier.)

- Peritonsillar abscess (accumulation of pus between the tonsil and its capsule) is the most common complication of acute tonsillitis. Clinical signs include deformed posterior pharynx, medial displacement of the uvula, trismus, and muffled voice (hot-potato voice).
- Lingual tonsillitis is a rarely diagnosed cause of pharyngitis that predominantly occurs in patients who have had palatine tonsils removed. The lingual tonsils are located below the inferior pole of the palatine tonsils and anterior to the vallecula at the base of the tongue. The lymphoid tissue may enlarge after tonsillectomy and repeated infections. Patients have a sore throat that worsens with movement of the tongue. Physical findings often include a normal-appearing pharynx and hyperemia. Lateral soft tissue neck films reveal a normal-appearing epiglottis and a scalloped appearance of the lingual tonsil (Fig. 2).
- Table 1 describes seven danger signs in patients with sore throat.

TABLE 1 Seven Danger Signs in Patients with Sore Throat

1. Persistence of symptoms longer than 1 wk without improvement
2. Respiratory difficulty, particularly stridor
3. Difficulty in handling secretions
4. Difficulty in swallowing
5. Severe pain in the absence of erythema
6. A palpable mass
7. Blood, even in small amounts, in the pharynx or ear

From Andreoli TE et al: *Andreoli and Carpenter's Cecil essentials of medicine*, ed 8, Philadelphia, 2010, Saunders.

ETIOLOGY

- Viruses:
  1. Respiratory syncytial virus
  2. Influenza A and B
  3. Epstein-Barr virus
  4. Adenovirus
  5. Herpes simplex
- Bacteria:
  1. GAS: *Streptococcus pyogenes*. β-Hemolytic GAS are the most common cause of acute tonsillitis.
  2. *Neisseria gonorrhoeae*
  3. Fusobacterium necrophorum (10% of pharyngitis): Highest incidence in patients aged 15 to 30 yr

BOX 1 Centor Criteria for Determining Group A Beta-Hemolytic Streptococcal Pharyngitis

- Tonsillar exudates
- Tender anterior lymphadenopathy or lymphadenitis
- Absence of cough
- History of fever

From Marx JA et al: *Rosen's emergency medicine*, ed 8, Philadelphia, 2014, Elsevier.

BOX 2 Centor Criteria Scoring for Determining Testing and Treatment for Group A Beta-Hemolytic Streptococcal Pharyngitis

Centor Score	Testing and Treatment
0-1	None
2-3	Treatment based on results of rapid streptococcal test results
4	Treat without testing

From Marx JA et al: *Rosen's emergency medicine*, ed 8, Philadelphia, 2014, Elsevier.

- Other organisms:
  1. *Mycoplasma pneumoniae*
  2. *Chlamydophila pneumoniae*
  3. *Arcanobacterium haemolyticum*

Dx DIAGNOSIS

DIFFERENTIAL DIAGNOSIS

- Sore throat associated with granulocytopenia, thyroiditis
- Tonsillar hypertrophy associated with lymphoma
- Section II describes the differential diagnosis of sore throat.

WORKUP

The Centor criteria (Boxes 1 and 2) to identify patients at risk for GAS consists of (1) fever subjective or measured >38.1° C (100.5° F), (2) absence of cough, (3) tonsillar exudates, (4) tender anterior cervical lymphadenopathy. Patients with ≤1 criteria are at low risk and do not need additional testing. The McIsaac criteria adds one point for ages 3 to 14 and subtracts one point for ages ≥45 yr.

- Rapid streptococcal antigen test (culture should be performed if rapid test negative)
- Throat swab for culture to exclude *S. pyogenes, N. gonorrhoeae* (requires specific transport medium) in selected cases

LABORATORY TESTS

- Bloodwork is only rarely necessary
- Complete blood count with differential
  1. May help support diagnosis of bacterial infection when diagnosis is unclear
  2. Streptococcal infection suggested by leukocytosis >15,000/mm^3
- Viral cultures, serologic studies rarely needed
- Monospot if diagnosis is unclear

IMAGING STUDIES

Seldom indicated. If necessary to distinguish between tonsillitis and peritonsillar abscess, CT or MRI of the neck can be done.

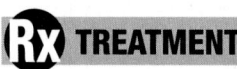

TREATMENT

NONPHARMACOLOGIC THERAPY

- Fluids
- Salt water gargles

ACUTE GENERAL Rx

- Analgesics: Aspirin (adults) or acetaminophen or ibuprofen (adults and children). Clinical trials have shown that corticosteroids can hasten pain relief in patients with sore throat. Single dose oral dexamethasone (10 mg in adults, 0.6 ms/kg for children) was the most common intervention and resulted in pain resolution approximately 11 hours sooner than placebo.[1] Prescribing corticosteroids in all cases of sore throat is not indicated and should be considered only in cases of severe sore throat.
- If streptococcal infection proven or suspected:
  1. Amoxicillin 500 mg bid or penicillin V 500 mg PO bid for 10 days or benzathine penicillin 1.2 million U IM once (adults). Children: Penicillin V 250 mg bid or tid
  2. Azithromycin 500 mg on day 1 then 250 mg on days 2 through 5 or erythromycin 500 mg PO bid or 250 mg qid for 10 days if penicillin allergic
- If gonococcal infection proven or suspected: Ceftriaxone 250 mg IM once.
- Amoxicillin 500 mg tid for 10 days is the primary antibiotic treatment of streptococcal tonsillitis. Cephalosporins are also effective. Macrolides or clindamycin or can be used in penicillin-allergic patients.
- Treatment of peritonsillar abscess is drainage through needle or incision.
- Avoid quinolones, sulfonamides, and tetracyclines due to treatment failures.

[1] Sadehira B et al: Corticosteroids for treatment of sore throat: systematic review and meta-analysis of randomized trials, *BMJ* 358:3887, 2017.

CHRONIC Rx

- Recurrent streptococcal infections are common and may represent reinfection from other household members, including pets.
- There is no conclusive evidence from randomized clinical trials that tonsillectomy is superior to antibiotic therapy for recurrent tonsillitis in adults.
- Tonsillopharyngitis is generally managed in an outpatient setting with follow-up arranged in 1 to 2 wk. Admission to the hospital is indicated for local suppurative complications (peritonsillar abscess; lateral pharyngeal or posterior pharyngeal abscess; impending airway closure; or inability to swallow food, medications, or water).

REFERRAL

- To otolaryngologist:
  1. If peritonsillar or other abscess is suspected
  2. If tonsillar hypertrophy persists

SUGGESTED READINGS

Available at ExpertConsult.com

RELATED CONTENT

Sore Throat (Patient Information)
Strep Throat (Patient Information)
Tonsillitis (Patient Information)

AUTHOR: **GLENN G. FORT, M.D., M.P.H.**

BASIC INFORMATION

DEFINITION

Pheochromocytomas are catecholamine-producing tumors that originate from the chromaffin cells of the adrenergic system. While they generally secrete both norepinephrine and epinephrine, norepinephrine is usually the predominant amine.

SYNONYM

Paraganglioma

ICD-10CM CODES

C74.9 Malignant neoplasm of adrenal gland, unspecified
C75.9 Malignant neoplasm of endocrine gland, unspecified
E27.5 Adrenomedullary hyperfunction

EPIDEMIOLOGY & DEMOGRAPHICS

- Incidence: 0.05% of population; peak incidence in 30s and 40s.
- Approximately 25% of patients with apparently sporadic pheochromocytoma may be carriers of mutations.
- Approximately 25% of pheochromocytomas are familial and associated with genetic disorders (Table 1). Pheochromocytoma is a feature of two disorders with an autosomal-dominant pattern of inheritance:
  1. Multiple endocrine neoplasia (MEN) type 2
  2. Von Hippel-Lindau disease: Angioma of the retina, hemangioblastoma of the central nervous system, renal cell carcinoma, pancreatic cysts, and epididymal cystoadenoma
- Pheochromocytomas occur in 5% of patients with neurofibromatosis type 1.

PHYSICAL FINDINGS & CLINICAL PRESENTATION

- Hypertension: Can be sustained (55%) or paroxysmal (45%).
- Headache (80%): Usually paroxysmal in nature and described as "pounding" and severe.
- Palpitations (70%): Can be present with or without tachycardia.
- Hyperhidrosis (60%): Most evident during paroxysmal attacks of hypertension.
- Physical examination may be entirely normal if done in a symptom-free interval; during a paroxysm the patient may demonstrate marked increase in both systolic and diastolic pressure, profuse sweating, visual disturbances (caused by hypertensive retinopathy), dilated pupils (from catecholamine excess), paresthesias in the lower extremities (caused by severe vasoconstriction), tremor, and tachycardia.
- Orthostatic hypotension is common among patients with pheochromocytoma due to reduction of blood volume and desensitization of adrenergic receptors by the chronic excess of catecholamines.

ETIOLOGY

- Catecholamine-producing tumors that are usually located in the adrenal medulla.
- Specific mutations of the RET protooncogene cause familial predisposition to pheochromocytoma in MEN 2.
- Mutations in the von Hippel-Lindau tumor suppressor gene (*VHL* gene) cause familial disposition to pheochromocytoma in von Hippel-Lindau disease.
- Recently identified genes for succinate dehydrogenase subunit D *(SDHD)* and succinate dehydrogenase subunit B *(SDHB)* predispose carriers to pheochromocytoma and globus tumors.

DIAGNOSIS

DIFFERENTIAL DIAGNOSIS

- Anxiety disorder
- Thyrotoxicosis
- Amphetamine or cocaine abuse
- Carcinoid
- Essential hypertension

WORKUP

Laboratory evaluation and imaging studies to locate the neoplasm (Fig. 1). Anatomic and functional imaging studies that can be used to localize pheochromocytomas are summarized in Table E2. Misdiagnosis of pheochromocytoma is common. Correct interpretation of biochemical tests and imaging is crucial to a correct diagnosis.

LABORATORY TESTS

- Although there is no consensus on the best test, plasma-free metanephrines have been suggested as the test of first choice for excluding the tumor. Elevated plasma concentrations of normetanephrine or metanephrine have a sensitivity of up to 100%, but the specificity is markedly lower (85%).
- 24-hr urine collection will also show increased metanephrines (90% sensitivity, 95% specificity); the accuracy of the 24-hr urinary levels for metanephrines can be improved by indexing urinary metanephrine levels by urine creatinine levels.

IMAGING STUDIES

- Abdominal CT scan (Fig. E2) with and without contrast (88% sensitivity) is useful in locating pheochromocytomas >0.5 inch in diameter (90% to 95% accurate).

TABLE 1 Autosomal Dominant Syndromes Associated with Pheochromocytoma and Paraganglioma

Syndrome	Gene	Gene Locus	Protein Product	Protein Function	Gene Mechanism	Typical Tumor Location
SDHD (familial paraganglioma type 1)*	*SDHD*	11q23	SDH D subunit	ATP production	Tumor suppressor	Skull base and neck; occasionally adrenal medulla, mediastinum, abdomen, pelvis
Familial paraganglioma type 2*	*SDHAF2*	11q13.1	Flavination cofactor	ATP production	Tumor suppressor	Skull base and neck; occasionally abdomen and pelvis
SDHC (familial paraganglioma type 3)	*SDHC*	1q21	SDH C subunit	ATP production	Tumor suppressor	Skull base and neck
SDHB (familial paraganglioma type 4)	*SDHB*	1p36.1-35	SDH B subunit	ATP production	Tumor suppressor	Abdomen, pelvis and mediastinum; rarely adrenal medulla, skull base, and neck
MEN1	*MEN1*	11q13	Menin	Transcription regulation	Tumor suppressor	Adrenal medulla
MEN2A and MEN2B	*RET*	10q11.2	RET	Tyrosine kinase receptor	Protooncogene	Adrenal medulla, bilaterally
Neurofibromatosis type 1	*NF1*	17q11.2	Neurofibromin	GTP hydrolysis	Tumor suppressor	Adrenal-periadrenal
von Hippel-Lindau disease	*VHL*	3p25-26	VHL	Transcription elongation suppression	Tumor suppressor	Adrenal medulla, bilaterally; occasionally paraganglioma
Familial pheochromocytoma	*FP/TMEM127*	2q11	Transmembrane protein	Regulation of the mTORC1 signaling complex	Tumor suppressor	Adrenal medulla

ATP, Adenosine triphosphate; *GTP,* guanosine triphosphate; *MEN,* multiple endocrine neoplasia; *mTORC1,* mammalian target of rapamycin complex 1; *RET,* "rearranged during transfection" proto-oncogene; *SDH,* succinate dehydrogenase; *VHL,* von Hippel–Lindau disease.
*Associated with maternal imprinting.
From Melmed S: *Williams textbook of endocrinology,* ed 12, Philadelphia, 2011, Saunders, Elsevier.

- MRI with contrast: Pheochromocytomas demonstrate a distinctive MRI appearance (up to 100% sensitivity); MRI may become the diagnostic imaging modality of choice.
- Scintigraphy with 131 or 1-123 I-MIBG (up to 100% sensitivity) (Fig. E2): This norepinephrine analog localizes in adrenergic tissue; it is particularly useful in locating extraadrenal pheochromocytomas.
- 6-[^{18}F]Fluorodopamine positron emission tomography is reserved for cases in which clinical symptoms and signs suggest pheochromocytoma, and results of biochemical tests are positive but conventional imaging studies cannot locate the tumor. It is also used for identification of metastatic disease.

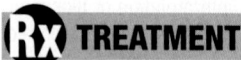

TREATMENT

GENERAL Rx

Laparoscopic adrenalectomy (surgical resection for both benign and malignant disease):

- Preoperative stabilization with combination of alpha-adrenergic blocking agents (phenoxybenzamine, prazosin, doxazosin, or terazosin), beta-blocker, and liberal fluid and salt intake starting 10 to 14 days before surgery. Beta-blockers should be avoided until patients receive adequate alpha-adrenergic blockade for several days to avoid hypertensive crisis due to unopposed alpha stimulation. Amlodipine or verapamil can be added to beta-blockers if blood pressure control is still inadequate. Table E3 describes orally administered drugs to treat pheochromocytoma.
- Hypertensive crisis preoperatively and intraoperatively can be controlled with nitroprusside. Table E4 summarizes intravenously administered drugs used to treat pheochromocytoma.

PEARLS & CONSIDERATIONS

COMMENTS

- Obtaining a detailed family history is important because 25% of pheochromocytomas are familial.
- Screening for pheochromocytoma should be considered in patients with any of the following:
  1. Malignant hypertension
  2. Poor response to antihypertensive therapy
  3. Paradoxical hypertensive response
  4. Hypertension during induction of anesthesia, parturition, surgery, or thyrotropin-releasing hormone testing
  5. Hypertension associated with imipramine or desipramine
  6. Neurofibromatosis (increased incidence of pheochromocytoma)
- All patients with pheochromocytoma should be screened for MEN-2 and von Hippel-Lindau disease with the pentagastrin test, serum parathyroid hormone, ophthalmoscopy, MRI of the brain, CT scan of the kidneys and pancreas, and ultrasonography of the testes.
- In patients with pheochromocytoma, routine analysis for mutations of *RET, VHL, SDHD,* and *SDHB* is indicated to identify pheochromocytoma-associated syndromes.

SUGGESTED READINGS

Available at ExpertConsult.com

RELATED CONTENT

Pheochromocytoma (Patient Information)
Hypertension (Related Key Topic)

AUTHORS: **BRETT PATRICK, M.D., MARK F. BRADY, M.D., M.P.H., M.M.S,** and **FRED F. FERRI, M.D.**

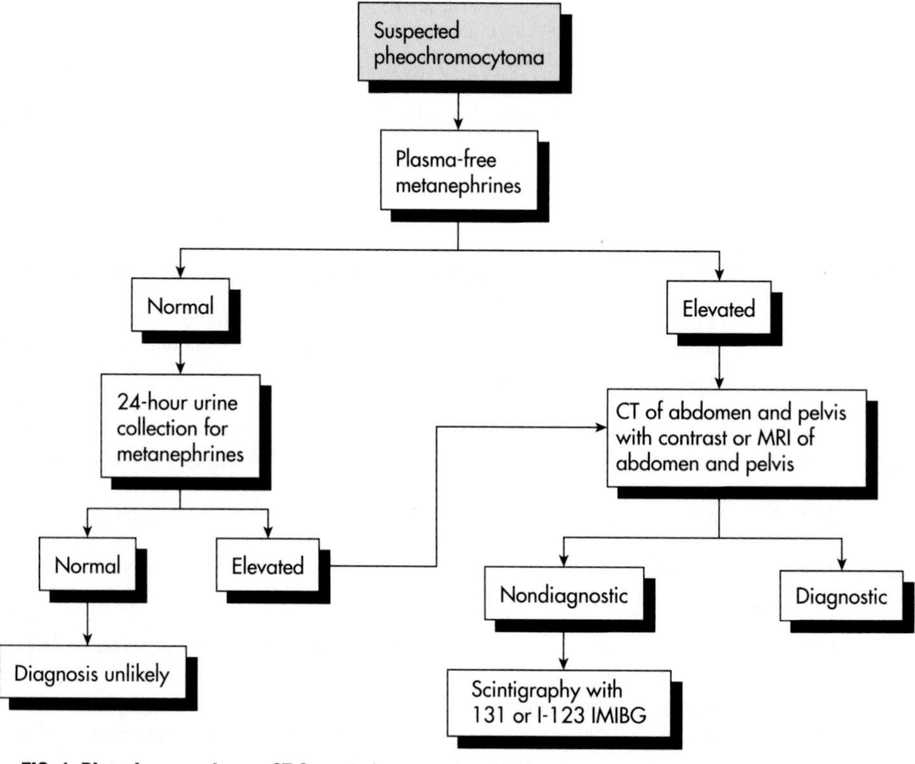

FIG. 1 Pheochromocytoma. *CT,* Computed tomography; *IMIBG,* iodine metaiodobenzylguanidine; *MRI,* magnetic resonance imaging.

BASIC INFORMATION

DEFINITION

From the Latin words *pilus,* meaning "hair," and *nidus,* meaning "nest."

A *pilonidal sinus* is a short tract extending from the skin surface that contains hair and skin debris. It is most commonly found in the intergluteal fold sacrococcygeal region, but it can also occur in the interdigital area, umbilicus, chest wall, and scalp. An *acute pilonidal abscess* consists of pus and a wall of edematous fat. A chronic *pilonidal cyst* develops from a chronic abscess of long duration as a thin and flat lining of epithelium grows into the cavity from the skin surface.

SYNONYMS

Jeep disease: During World War II, many soldiers developed pilonidal cysts thought to be caused by hours of riding on Jeeps
Pilonidal sinus
Pilonidal cyst

ICD-10CM CODES

L05	Pilonidal cyst
L05.0	Pilonidal cyst with abscess
L05.9	Pilonidal cysts without abscess

EPIDEMIOLOGY & DEMOGRAPHICS

INCIDENCE: 26 cases per 100,000 persons
PREDOMINANT SEX: Males are more commonly affected than females (2.2:1).
AVERAGE AGE OF PRESENTATION: 21 yr
RISK FACTORS:
- Male sex
- Local trauma or irritation
- Family predisposition
- Obesity
- Sedentary lifestyle
- Occupation requiring prolonged sitting or excessive exposure to hair (barbers)
- Local hirsutism
- Poor hygiene
- Increased sweat activity

PHYSICAL FINDINGS & CLINICAL PRESENTATION

- Asymptomatic pits or pores in the natal cleft (Fig. E1)
- Tenderness after physical activity or prolonged sitting
- Acute pilonidal abscess presents as a hot, tender, fluctuant swelling just lateral to the midline over the sacrum that may exude pus through the midline pit
- Acute pilonidal abscess in 20% of patients with pilonidal disease
- Chronic pilonidal may have recurrent pain and drainage
- Chronic pilonidal abscess in 80% of patients with pilonidal disease
- Infrequently, systemic reaction: Occasionally fever, leukocytosis, and malaise

ETIOLOGY

- Currently believed to be acquired rather than congenital.
- Drilling of hair shed from the perineum or the head into sebaceous or hair follicles in the natal cleft.
- Drilling is facilitated by the friction of the natal cleft.
- Subsequent infection by skin organisms leads to pilonidal abscess.

Dx DIAGNOSIS

DIFFERENTIAL DIAGNOSIS

- Perianal abscess arising from the posterior midline crypt
- Hidradenitis suppurativa
- Skin abscess: Furuncle or carbuncle
- Folliculitis
- Anorectal fistula
- Anal complication of Crohn disease
- Case report of squamous cell carcinoma arising from neglected chronic pilonidal sinuses

WORKUP

- Diagnosis is based on history and physical examination.
- Midline pits present behind the anus overlying the sacrum and coccyx.
- Broken hairs are often seen extruding from the midline pits.
- Insert probe in pilonidal sinus in path away from the anus.
- Complicated anal fistula may be angulating posteriorly before passing into a retrorectal abscess, but thorough examination of the anal cavity usually discloses point of origin.

Rx TREATMENT

NONPHARMACOLOGIC THERAPY

Prevention of exacerbations:
- Local hygiene.
- Avoidance of prolonged sitting position.
- Weight reduction.
- Early in the infection, sitz baths may decrease pain and decrease the chance that a cyst may develop into an abscess.
- Treatment of an asymptomatic sinus is not indicated.

Treatment of acute abscess
- Procedure of choice for first-episode acute abscess: Simple incision and drainage in an outpatient setting. Box E1 describes surgical options for the treatment of pilonidal sinus.
- Cure rate of about 50% within 5 weeks; recurrence rate 20% to 55%.
- Antibiotics: Generally not indicated, except for the treatment of cellulitis or in patients with immunosuppression, high risk of endocarditis, MRSA, or underlying systemic disease.
- First-generation cephalosporin plus metronidazole is the antibiotic regimen of choice.

TREATMENT OF CHRONIC OR RECURRENT DISEASE

Elective treatment of pilonidal disease:
- Minimal surgery:
  1. Remove hair from midline pits and shave buttocks.
  2. May use a fine wire brush with local anesthesia to clear the pits and any lateral openings of granulation tissue and hair (Fig. E2).
  3. Keep area clean.
- Fistulotomy and curettage:
  1. Used when minimal surgery does not control episodes of suppuration.
  2. Pass probe to outline the pilonidal sinus and open tract surgically.
  3. Curette granulation tissue at the base of the sinus and excise edges of the skin.
  4. Keep open granulating wound meticulously clean and allow to heal.
  5. If complete healing does not take place, use a skin graft or advancement flap to close the defect.
- Marsupialization:
  1. This is the treatment of choice for chronic pilonidal disease.
  2. Wide excision of the pilonidal area is performed, including all affected skin and subcutaneous tissues down to the presacral fascia.
  3. Wound is left open, allowed to marsupialize, or closed as a primary procedure.
  4. Give antibiotics for 24 hr (particularly those directed against *Staphylococcus* and *Bacteroides* species).
- Other procedures:
  1. Excision and primary closure or closure with skin grafts or flaps: Z-plasty, V-Y advancement flap, rhomboid flap, gluteus maximus myocutaneous flap
  2. Bascom procedure (follicle removal and lateral drainage)
  3. Recurrence rate for excision (most definitive procedure): 1% to 6%
  4. Incidence of squamous cell carcinoma in a chronic, recurrent pilonidal sinus is rare (<1%)

REFERRAL

- Emergency department for incision and drainage for an acute abscess
- General surgeon for elective treatment or management of chronic or recurrent disease

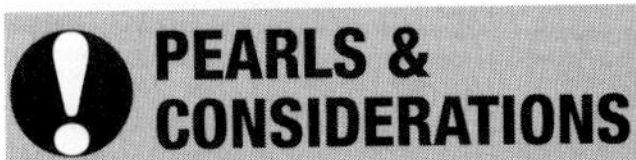

PEARLS & CONSIDERATIONS

COMMENTS

Because of significant associated morbidity, the elective surgical procedures outlined are performed only after the potential risks versus benefits are carefully weighed by a general or colorectal surgeon.

RELATED CONTENT

Pilonidal Cyst (Patient Information)

AUTHOR: **MARIA E. SOLER, M.D., M.P.H., M.B.A.**

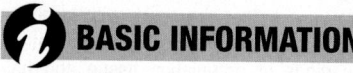

BASIC INFORMATION

DEFINITION

Pinworms are a noninvasive infestation of the intestinal tract by *Enterobius vermicularis,* a helminth of the nematode family. It is a small (1 cm in length), white, thread-like roundworm that typically inhabits the cecum, appendix, and adjacent areas of the ileum and ascending colon.

SYNONYMS

Enterobiasis
Oxyuriasis

ICD-10CM CODE
B80 Enterobiasis

EPIDEMIOLOGY & DEMOGRAPHICS

- Most common intestinal nematode; approximately 30,000 cases annually in the United States.
- Worldwide distribution, but most common in temperate climates.
- The prevalence of pinworm infection is lowest in infants and reaches highest infection rate in school-age children (ages 5-14 yr).
- Eggs are infective within 6 hr of oviposition and may remain so for 20 days.
- Clusters are found in families, institutionalized persons, and homosexual men.

PHYSICAL FINDINGS & CLINICAL PRESENTATION

- Most infested persons are asymptomatic.
- Perianal itching is the most common reported symptom, with scratching leading to excoriation and sometimes secondary infection.
- The vagina may become infested with pinworms.
- Rarely insomnia, irritability, anorexia, and weight loss are described.
- Granulomas have been described in various organs resulting from worms wandering outside the intestines and dying there.

ETIOLOGY & PATHOGENESIS

- *E. vermicularis* is highly prevalent throughout the world, particularly in countries of the temperate zone. Human beings are the only host for this worm. Infestation is by fecal-oral route; ingested eggs hatch in the stomach and the larvae migrate to the colon, where they mature. Gravid female worms containing an average of 10,000 ova migrate to the perianal skin at night, lay their eggs there, and die. The eggs embryonate within 6 hr and cause itching; scratching causes egg deposition under fingernails, from which they can contaminate food or lead to autoreinfection. Ova may also be airborne and collect in dust that may be on the floor or on furniture.
- *E. vermicularis* may be transmitted between sexual partners, especially those engaging in oral-anal sex.

DIAGNOSIS

DIFFERENTIAL DIAGNOSIS

- Perianal itching related to poor hygiene
- Hemorrhoidal disease and anal fissures
- Perineal yeast/fungal infections

  Section II describes the causes of pruritus ani.

WORKUP

Identification of adult worms or eggs. *E. vermicularis* ova are ovoid but flattened on one side and measure approximately 56 × 27 micrometers (Fig. 1). The eggs can be identified on transparent tape (Fig. 2) placed on the perianal skin on awakening. (NOTE: Five consecutive negative tests rule out the diagnosis.) A single examination detects 50% of infections, three examinations detect 90%, and five examinations detect 99%.

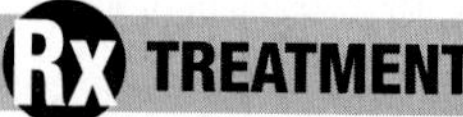

TREATMENT

- Single dose of mebendazole (100 mg) with a repeat dose given after 2 wk results in cure rates of 90% to 100%.
- Single dose of albendazole (400 mg) with a second dose given 2 wk later is also highly effective.
- Pyrantel pamoate (11 mg/kg up to 1 g) can prevent against *E. vermicularis.* It is available as a suspension and has minimal toxicity (mild transient gastrointestinal symptoms, headache, drowsiness). A repeat dose after 2 wk is recommended because of the frequency of reinfection and autoinfection.
- Other infected family members, classmates, or residents of long-term care facilities should be treated at the same time as the index case.

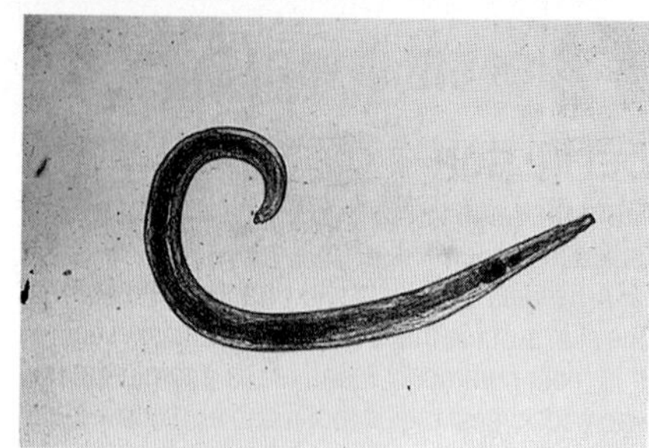

FIG. 1 Adult male pinworm, Enterobius vermicularis, with curved posterior end; note prominent esophageal bulb (4x). (From McPherson RA, Pincus MR: *Henry's clinical diagnosis and management by laboratory methods,* ed 23, Philadelphia, 2017, Elsevier.)

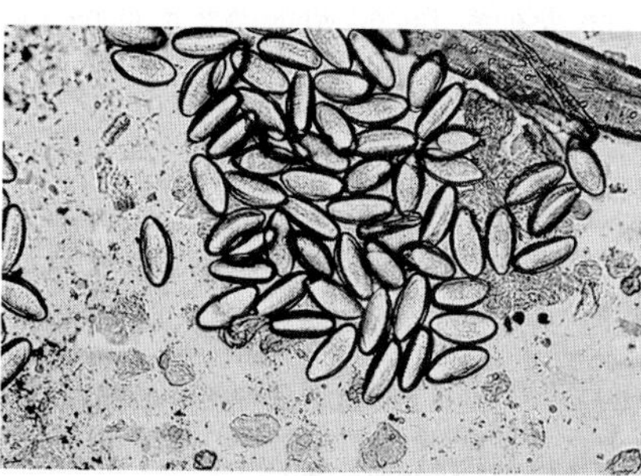

FIG. 2 Numerous eggs of Enterobius vermicularis as seen on a cellophane tape preparation (400x). (From McPherson RA, Pincus MR: *Henry's clinical diagnosis and management by laboratory methods,* ed 23, Philadelphia, 2017, Elsevier.)

PEARLS & CONSIDERATIONS

- Eosinophilia is not observed in most cases because tissue invasion does not occur.
- Good hand hygiene is the most effective method of prevention.
- Frequent changing of underclothes, bed clothes, and bed sheets is helpful to decrease risk of autoinfection.
- Personal hygiene and cleanliness are crucial. Fingernails should be cut short and scrubbed frequently.

RELATED CONTENT

Pinworms (Patient Information)

AUTHOR: **FRED F. FERRI, M.D.**

BASIC INFORMATION

DEFINITION

Pituitary adenoma is a benign neoplasm of the anterior lobe of the pituitary that causes symptoms, either by excess secretion of hormones or by a local mass effect as the tumor impinges on other, nearby structures (e.g., optic chiasm, hypothalamus, pituitary stalk). Pituitary adenomas are classified by their size, function, and features that characterize their appearance. Microadenomas are <10 mm in size, macroadenomas are ≥10 mm in size, and giant adenomas are ≥40 mm in size.

- *Nonsecretory pituitary adenomas* are those in which the neoplasm is a space-occupying lesion whose secretory products do not cause a specific disease state.

Endocrine manifestations of secretory adenomas include:

- *Acromegaly,* a disease state characterized by a pituitary adenoma that secretes growth hormone (GH)
- Galactorrhea, which is the result of a *prolactinoma* that secretes prolactin (PRL)
- *Cushing's disease,* a disease state of hypersecretion of adrenocorticotropic hormone (ACTH)
- *Hyperthyroidism due to a thyrotropin-secreting pituitary adenomas,* which secrete primarily thyroid-stimulating hormone (TSH).

ICD-10CM CODE
D35.2 Benign neoplasm of pituitary gland

EPIDEMIOLOGY & DEMOGRAPHICS

CLASSIFICATION (BY HORMONE SECRETED):

- PRL only: 35%
- No hormone: 30%
- GH only: 20%
- PRL and GH: 7%
- ACTH: 7%
- Luteinizing hormone (LH), follicle-stimulating hormone (FSH), TSH: 1%

PREVALENCE/INCIDENCE:

- Pituitary adenomas: Up to 10% to 15% of all intracranial neoplasms; 3% to 27% at autopsy series
- Prolactinomas: Up to 20% in women with unexplained primary or secondary amenorrhea
- GH-secreting pituitary adenoma: 50 to 60 cases per 1 million persons. They account for 8% to 16% of pituitary tumors
- Thyrotropin-secreting pituitary adenoma: 1% of pituitary adenomas with a slight female/male predominance of 1.7:1
- Corticotropin-secreting pituitary adenomas: Female/male predominance of 8:1 but overall uncommon diagnosis, accounting for 2% to 6% of adenomas

PHYSICAL FINDINGS & CLINICAL PRESENTATION

PROLACTINOMAS:

- Females:
  1. Galactorrhea
  2. Amenorrhea
  3. Oligomenorrhea with anovulation
  4. Infertility
  5. Estrogen deficiency and associated osteopenia
  6. Decreased vaginal lubrication
- Males:
  1. Large tumors more common as a result of delayed diagnosis
  2. Possible impotence, decreased libido, or hypogonadism
  3. Galactorrhea rare because males lack the estrogen-dependent breast growth and differentiation

GH-SECRETING PITUITARY ADENOMA: ACROMEGALY:

- Coarse facial features.
- Oily skin.
- Prognathism.
- Carpal tunnel syndrome.
- Osteoarthritis.
- History of increased hat, glove, or shoe size.
- Decreased exercise capacity.
- Visual field deficits.
- Diabetes mellitus.

CORTICOTROPIN-SECRETING PITUITARY ADENOMA: CUSHING'S DISEASE:

- Usually present when the tumor is small (1 to 2 mm)
- 50% of the tumors are <<5 mm
- Other symptoms:
  1. Truncal obesity
  2. Round facies (moon face)
  3. Dorsocervical fat accumulation (buffalo hump)
  4. Hirsutism
  5. Acne
  6. Menstrual disorders
  7. Hypertension
  8. Striae
  9. Bruising
  10. Thin skin
  11. Hyperglycemia

THYROTROPIN-SECRETING PITUITARY ADENOMA:

- In males, larger, more invasive, and more rapidly growing tumors that present later in life
- Other symptoms: Thyrotoxicosis, goiter, visual impairment

NONSECRETORY PITUITARY ADENOMAS (ENDOCRINE INACTIVE PITUITARY ADENOMA):

- Usually large at the time of diagnosis.
- Symptoms:
  1. Bitemporal hemianopsia as a result of compression of the optic chiasm
  2. Hypopituitarism from compression of the pituitary gland
  3. Hypogonadism in men and in premenopausal women
  4. Cranial nerve deficits caused by extension into the cavernous sinus
  5. Hydrocephalus from extension into the third ventricle, compressing the foramen of Monro
  6. Diabetes insipidus resulting from compression of the hypothalamus or pituitary stalk (a rare complication)

ETIOLOGY

Benign neoplasms of epithelial origin linked to genetic mutations of MEN1, Gs-Alpha, and AIP

DIAGNOSIS

DIFFERENTIAL DIAGNOSIS

PROLACTINOMA:

- Pregnancy
- Postpartum puerperium
- Primary hypothyroidism
- Breast disease
- Breast stimulation
- Drug ingestion (especially phenothiazines, antidepressants, haloperidol, methyldopa, reserpine, opiates, amphetamines, and cimetidine).
- Chronic renal failure
- Liver disease
- Polycystic ovarian disease
- Chest wall disorders
- Spinal cord lesions
- Previous cranial irradiation

ACROMEGALY: Ectopic production of GH-releasing hormone from a carcinoid or other neuroendocrine tumor

CUSHING'S DISEASE:

- Diseases that cause ectopic sources of ACTH overproduction (including small-cell carcinoma of the lung, bronchial carcinoid, intestinal carcinoid, pancreatic islet cell tumor, medullary thyroid carcinoma, or pheochromocytoma)
- Adrenal adenomas, adrenal carcinoma
- Nelson syndrome

THYROTROPIN-SECRETING PITUITARY ADENOMAS: Primary hypothyroidism

NONSECRETORY PITUITARY ADENOMA: Nonneoplastic mass lesions of various etiologies (e.g., infectious, granulomatous)

WORKUP

Pituitary adenomas should be identified at an early stage so that effective treatment can be implemented.

Screening tests for functional pituitary adenomas are described in Table 1.

PROLACTINOMA: First step: Measurement of basal PRL levels (practitioners should be aware of discriminatory values in their own institutions).

- Elevated PRL levels are correlated with tumor size.
- Level >200 ng/ml indicates likely prolactinoma, with levels of 100 to 200 ng/ml being equivocal and possibly associated with medications or other sources.
- Basal PRL levels between 20 and 100 suggest a microadenoma but can be due to common medications (estrogen, antidepressants, meotoclopramide, alomet, and others) or recent breast stimulation.
- Basal level <<20 ng/ml is usually considered normal. Each laboratory should develop its own normative values, however, and practitioner should refer to these values.
- Threshold level for obtaining imaging such as MRI should be developed by individual providers depending on the level of specificity and sensitivity desired.

ACROMEGALY:

- First screening tests are the measurement of the serum insulin-like growth factor I level, postprandial serum GH, and TRH stimulation test.

TABLE 1 Screening Tests for Functional Pituitary Adenomas

Disorder	Test	Comments
Acromegaly	IGF1 OGTT with GH obtained at 0, 30, and 60 min	Interpret IGF1 relative to age- and gender-matched controls. Normal subjects should suppress GH to <1 μg/L.
Prolactinoma	Serum PRL level	A level >500 μg/L is pathognomonic for macroprolactinoma. If >200 μg/L, prolactinoma is likely.*
Cushing's disease	24-hr UFC Nighttime salivary cortisol dexamethasone (1 mg) at 11 PM and fasting plasma cortisol measured at 8 AM ACTH assay	Ensure that urine collection is total and accurate by measuring urinary creatinine. Free salivary cortisol reflects circadian rhythm, and elevated levels may indicate Cushing's disease. Normal subjects suppress to <1.8 μg/dl. Distinguishes adrenal adenoma from ectopic ACTH or Cushing's disease.
TSH-secreting tumor	TSH measurement Free T_4 by dialysis Total T_3	If T_4 or T_3 is elevated and TSH is measurable or elevated, a TSH-secreting tumor may be present.

ACTH, Adrenocorticotropic hormone; *GH*, growth hormone; *IGF1*, insulin-like growth factor type 1; *OGTT*, oral glucose tolerance test; *PRL*, prolactin; *T3*, triiodothyronine; *T4*, thyroxine; *TSH*, thyroid-stimulating hormone; *UFC*, urinary free cortisol.
*Risperidone may result in prolactin levels >200 μg/L.
From Melmed S et al: *Williams textbook of endocrinology*, ed 12, Philadelphia, 2011, WB Saunders.

- Follow with an oral glucose tolerance test.
- Failure to suppress serum GH to <2 ng/ml with an oral load of 100 g glucose is considered conclusive.
- A GH-releasing hormone level >300 ng/ml is indicative of an ectopic source of GH.

CUSHING'S DISEASE:

- Measurement of late-night salivary cortisol level is the best screening test.
- Normal or slightly elevated corticotropin levels ranging from 20 to 200 pg/ml; normal is 10 to 50 pg/ml (normative data should be developed by each institution for its population).
- Level <<10 pg/ml usually indicates an autonomously secreting adrenal tumor.
- Level >>200 pg/ml suggests an ectopic corticotropin-secreting neoplasm.
- Cushing's disease can be assessed by absence of cortisol suppression with the low-dose dexamethasone test but with the presence of cortisol suppression after the high-dose test. As a method to distinguish Cushing's disease from an ectopic source of ACTH, this test is robust.
- 24-hr urine collection should demonstrate an increased level of cortisol excretion.

THYROTROPIN-SECRETING PITUITARY ADENOMA:

- Highly sensitive thyrotropin assays, which evaluate the presence of thyrotoxicosis, are one way to detect a thyrotropin-secreting tumor.
- Free alpha subunit is secreted by >80% of tumors, with the ratio of the alpha subunit to thyrotropin <1.
- With central resistance to thyroid hormone, ratio is <1, and the sella is normal.
- Laboratory tests show elevated serum levels of both T_3 and T_4.

NONSECRETORY PITUITARY ADENOMA:

- Visual field testing
- Assessment of the pituitary and organ function to determine if there is hypopituitarism or hypersecretion of hormones (even if the effects of hypersecretion are subclinical)
- TRH to provoke secretion of FSH, LH, and LH-beta-subunit; will not elicit response in normal persons
- Exclusion of Klinefelter syndrome in patient with longstanding primary hypogonadism, elevated gonadotropin levels, and enlargement of the sella

IMAGING STUDIES

Study of choice: MRI of the pituitary (Fig. E1) and hypothalamus. If an MRI shows the tumor impinging on the optic chiasm, then formal visual field testing is indicated.

- When evaluating Cushing's disease, small size at the onset of symptoms noted.
- MRI, in this case, only 60% sensitive at best and may yield false-positive results.
- CT scan only when MRI is unavailable or is otherwise contraindicated.

Rx TREATMENT

NONPHARMACOLOGIC THERAPY

SURGERY:

- Selective transsphenoidal resection of the adenoma (Table 2) is the treatment of choice for acromegaly, Cushing's disease, and thyrotropin-secreting pituitary adenomas, all of which tend to be microadenomas at the time of onset of symptoms.
- Macroadenomas, such as the nonsecretory pituitary adenoma, may also be surgically removed, but risk of recurrence is greater with these tumors and adjunctive therapy such as irradiation may also be necessary.
- Bilateral adrenalectomy has been performed in patients with Cushing's disease after failure of other therapies; complications requiring lifelong hormone replacement or Nelson syndrome (rapid enlargement of pituitary tumor due to adrenal resection) may occur.

TABLE 2 Transsphenoidal Pituitary Surgery

Primary Indications
General
Visual tract or central nervous system compression arising from within sella
Relief of compressive hypopituitarism by presenting, residual, or recurrent tumor tissue
Tumor recurrence after surgery or irradiation
Pituitary hemorrhage
Cerebrospinal fluid leak
Resistance to medical therapy
Intolerance of medical therapy
Personal choice
Desire for immediate pregnancy with macroadenoma
Requirement for diagnostic tissue histology
Specific
Acromegaly
Cushing's disease
Clinically nonfunctioning macroadenoma
Prolactinoma
Nelson syndrome
TSH-secreting adenoma
Side Effects
Transient
Diabetes insipidus
Cerebrospinal fluid leak and rhinorrhea
Inappropriate ADH secretion
Arachnoiditis
Meningitis
Postoperative psychosis
Local hematoma
Arterial wall damage
Epistaxis
Local abscess
Pulmonary embolism
Narcolepsy
Permanent (up to 10%)
Diabetes insipidus
Total or partial hypopituitarism
Visual loss
Inappropriate ADH secretion
Vascular occlusion
CNS damage: oculomotor palsy, hemiparesis, encephalopathy
Nasal septum perforation
Surgery-Related Mortality (up to 1%)
Brain, hypothalamic
Vascular damage
Postoperative meningitis
Cerebrospinal fluid leak
Pneumocephalus
Acute cardiopulmonary disease
Anesthesia-related
Seizure

ADH, Antidiuretic hormone; *CNS*, central nervous system; *TSH*, thyroid-stimulating hormone.
From Melmed S et al: *Williams textbook of endocrinology*, ed 12, Philadelphia, 2011, WB Saunders.

RADIOTHERAPY:

- Radiotherapy is used primarily as adjuvant treatment. It is reserved for patients who have not responded to surgical treatment and who still have symptoms of the adenoma.
- Used with varying degrees of success in all the different pituitary adenomas.

- Radiotherapy complications include long-term hypopituitarism (40% of patients) and secondary neoplasms (1.5% of patients).

ACUTE GENERAL Rx

PROLACTINOMA:

- For prolactinomas, initial therapy is generally dopamine agonists. Bromocriptine, a dopamine analogue, is generally given orally in divided doses of 1.5 to 10 mg. Cabergoline is given once or twice weekly. It is better tolerated and more effective than bromocriptine for tumor shrinkage but more expensive.
- Side effects include orthostatic hypotension, nausea, and dizziness; avoided by beginning with low-dose therapy.
- Other compounds include pergolide mesylate, a long-acting ergot derivative with dopaminergic properties, as well as other nonergot derivatives.

ACROMEGALY:

- Somatostatin analogues: Octreotide, lanreotide administered as monthly injections.
- Cabergoline or bromocriptine can also be used. They have modest activity but can be administered orally and are less expensive than somatostatin analogues.
- Pegvisomant can also be used to normalize IGF-1 levels.

CUSHING'S DISEASE:

- Ketoconazole, which inhibits the cytochrome P-450 enzymes involved in steroid biosynthesis, is effective in managing mild to moderate disease in daily oral doses of 600 to 1200 mg.
- Metyrapone and aminoglutethimide can be used to control hypersecretion of cortisol but are generally used when preparing a patient for surgery or while waiting for a response to radiotherapy.

THYROTROPIN-SECRETING PITUITARY ADENOMA:

- Ablative therapy with either radioactive iodide or surgery is indicated.
- Treatment directed to the thyroid alone may accelerate growth of the pituitary adenoma.
- Octreotide has been shown to be effective in doses similar to those used for acromegaly.

NONSECRETORY PITUITARY ADENOMA:

- There is no role for medical therapy at this time.
- Surgery and radiotherapy may be indicated. An algorithm for the management of nonfunctioning pituitary adenomas is described in Fig. 2.

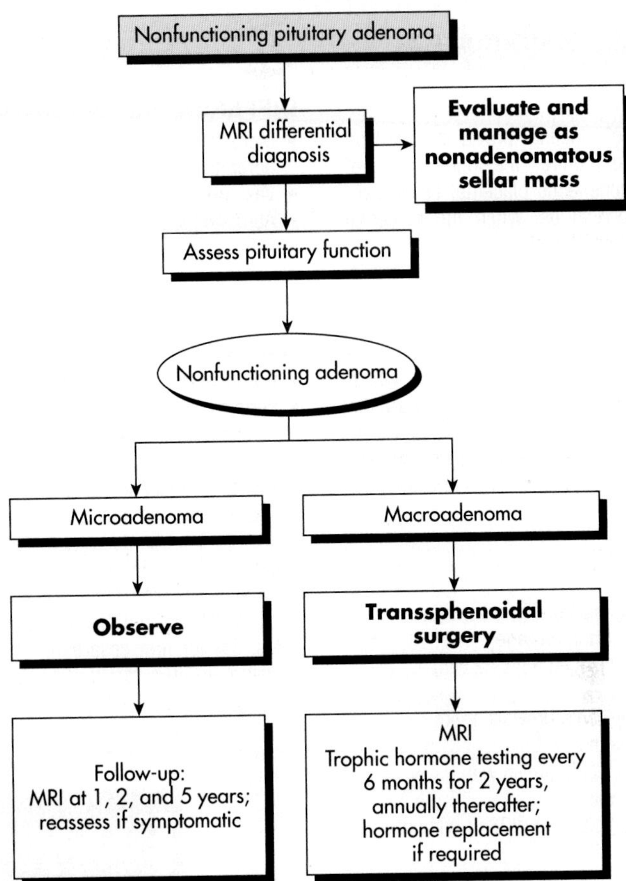

FIG. 2 Management of nonfunctioning pituitary adenomas. Skilled interpretation of magnetic resonance images is crucial to diagnosing a nonadenomatous mass such as a meningioma, aneurysm, or other sellar lesion. (From Melmed S et al: *Williams textbook of endocrinology*, ed 12, Philadelphia, 2011, WB Saunders.)

CHRONIC Rx

For all pituitary adenomas:

- Careful follow-up is important. Patients undergoing transsphenoidal microsurgical resection should be seen in 4 to 6 wk to ensure that the adenoma has been completely removed and that the endocrine hypersecretion is resolved.
- If there is good clinical response, patient should be monitored yearly for recurrence and to follow the level of the hypersecreted hormone.
- Patients who have undergone irradiation should have close follow-up with backup medical therapy because response to radiotherapy may be delayed; incidence of hypopituitarism also increases with time.
- Surgical resection is not indicated in pituitary incidentalomas that are microadenomas since only 10% will experience tumor growth.

SUGGESTED READINGS

Available at ExpertConsult.com

RELATED CONTENT

Evaluation of Suspected Pituitary Tumor (Algorithm, Section III)
Pituitary Adenoma (Patient Information)
Acromegaly (Related Key Topic)
Amenorrhea (Related Key Topic)
Cushing's Disease and Syndrome (Related Key Topic)
Galactorrhea (Related Key Topic)
Prolactinoma (Related Key Topic)

AUTHORS: **MATTHEW K. HOFFMAN, M.D., M.P.H., F.A.C.O.G.**

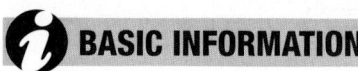

BASIC INFORMATION

DEFINITION

The diagnosis of placenta previa is based on sonography and requires the identification of echogenic homogeneous placental tissue over the internal cervical os. When the placental edge is <2 cm from the internal os, the placenta is called "low-lying." The historic terms "marginal" and "partial" for characterizing a placenta previa are no longer used.

One hypothesis is that the lower uterine cavity contains more vascularized decidua, which promotes implantation of trophoblast toward the cervical os. Another hypothesis is that a particularly large placental surface area increases the probability that the placenta will implant over the cervical os.

ICD-10CM CODES

044	Placenta previa
044.0	Complete placenta previa NOS or without hemorrhage
044.1	Complete placenta previa with hemorrhage
044.2	Partial placenta previa without hemorrhage
044.3	Partial placenta previa with hemorrhage
044.4	Low-lying placenta NOS or without hemorrhage
044.5	Low-lying placenta with hemorrhage

EPIDEMIOLOGY & DEMOGRAPHICS

INCIDENCE: The pooled prevalence of major placenta previa was 4.3 cases per 1000 pregnancies. Prevalence was highest among Asian studies (12.2 per 1000) and lower among studies from Europe (3.6 per 1000), North America (2.9 per 1000), and sub-Saharan Africa (2.7 per 1000).

RISK FACTORS:

- Previous placenta previa (recurs in 4% to 8% of subsequent pregnancies)
- Previous cesarean delivery (increases incidence by 47% to 60%)
- Multiparity
- Multiple gestation (increases prevalence by 40%)
- Smoking and cocaine use
- Previous intrauterine surgical procedure or Asherman syndrome
- Abnormal or large placenta

PHYSICAL FINDINGS & CLINICAL PRESENTATION

The classic presentation of placenta previa is painless vaginal bleeding, usually in the second or third trimester. Ten percent to 20% of women present with uterine contractions, pain, and bleeding. On physical examination, the uterus is soft and pain free. The fetus is often in breech, transverse lie, or high. Fetal distress is usually not present.

DIAGNOSIS

DIFFERENTIAL DIAGNOSIS

- Morbidly adherent placenta (accreta, increta, percreta)
- Vasa previa
- Abruptio placentae
- Vaginal or cervical trauma
- Labor
- Local malignancy

WORKUP

- Do *not* perform a digital vaginal examination.
- Perform a speculum examination in a hospital setting to exclude any local bleeding.
- Perform a transvaginal ultrasonography to assess for placental location.
- Exclude the presence of placenta previa-accreta in patients with a history of cesarean sections. In a prospective study, the frequency of placenta accreta increased with an increasing number of cesarean deliveries: 3% for first cesarean, 11% for second cesarean, 40% for third cesarean, 61% for fourth cesarean, and up to 67% for fifth or more cesarean sections.

LABORATORY TESTS

- A complete blood count can be used to monitor hemoglobin and hematocrit.
- A Kleihauer-Betke preparation of maternal blood in all Rh-negative women and Rh-immune globulin when indicated

IMAGING STUDIES

- The simplest and safest method of placental localization is transabdominal sonography with confirmatory imaging by transvaginal ultrasonography (TVUS). Transabdominal ultrasonography alone is inaccurate in the diagnosis of placenta previa and should be used only as a screening tool. TVUS (Fig. 1) has become the gold standard for the diagnosis of placenta previa. It is safe even in the presence of active bleeding.
- MRI has also been effective in detecting placenta previa, although sonography remains the preferred method due to lower cost, widespread availability, and well-established accuracy.

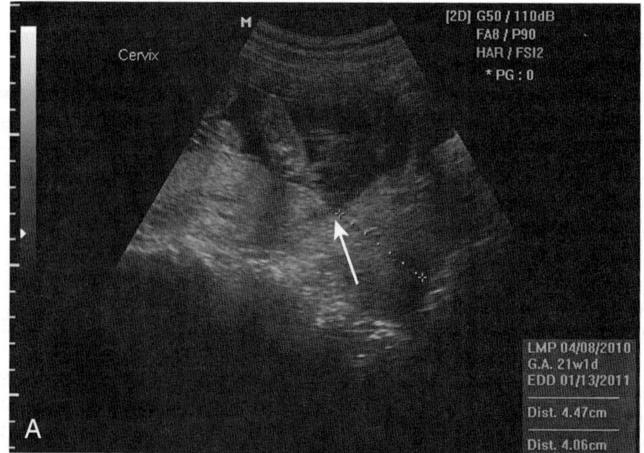

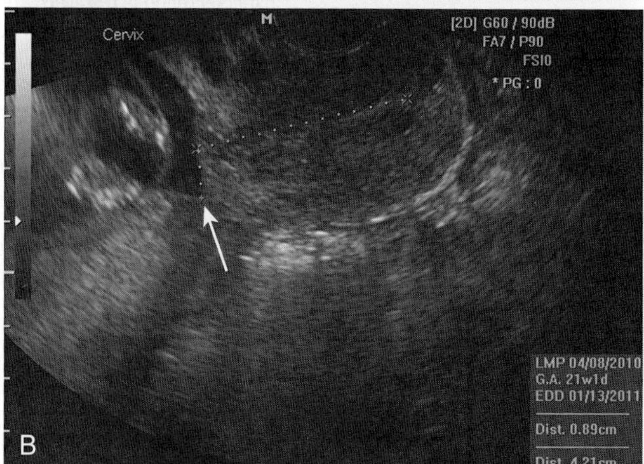

FIG. 1 Transabdominal ultrasonography and transvaginal ultrasonography of marginal placenta previa. *Arrows* identify placental edge. (Courtesy K. Francois. From Gabbe SG: *Obstetrics*, ed 6, Philadelphia, 2012, WB Saunders.)

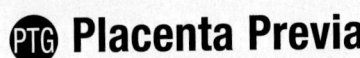

Rx TREATMENT

MANAGEMENT OF ASYMPTOMATIC PLACENTA PREVIA

- Avoid sexual activity, digital exams, and extraneous exercise.
- Review bleeding precautions and anticipatory guidance, including the need for cesarean section and the risk for hysterectomy early in pregnancy.

Sequential assessment of placental location:

- At 32 weeks, follow-up is indicated:
  1. If the placental edge is ≥2 cm from the internal os, placenta previa has resolved and no further assessment is required.
  2. If the placental edge is over or <2 cm from the internal os, placenta previa persists and repeat at 36 weeks is indicated.
- At 36 weeks:
  1. If the placental edge is ≥2 cm, the patient is consented for vaginal delivery.
  2. If the placental edge is over the internal os, cesarean delivery is scheduled.

Timing of delivery:

- Cesarean delivery at 36+0 to 37+6 weeks in pregnancies with uncomplicated placenta previa.

MANAGEMENT OF SYMPTOMATIC PLACENTA PREVIA

- Initial assessment for signs of maternal hemodynamic compromise or hemorrhagic shock; large-bore IV access with crystalloid fluid resuscitation.
- Assess fetal status and gestational age by sonogram and continuous fetal heart rate monitoring.
- Cross-matched blood should be made available during bleeding episodes.
- Tocolytic therapy should not be administered in an actively bleeding patients.
- Magnesium sulfate therapy for fetal neuroprotection should be considered in those with symptomatic preterm (less than 32 weeks) placenta previa if the decision has been made to likely deliver the patient within 24 hours. Emergent delivery should not be delayed to administer magnesium.
- Cesarean delivery is indicated for active labor, nonreassuring fetal heart rate tracing, active bleeding with hemodynamic instability, and significant bleeding after 34 weeks' gestation.

Expectant management after a resolved bleed:

- Antenatal corticosteroid should be administered to symptomatic women between 23+0 and 36+6 weeks of gestation to enhance fetal pulmonary maturity.
- Correct anemia.
- Administer anti-D immune globulin to D-negative women.

DISPOSITION

Inpatient versus outpatient: Consider discharge for women whose bleeding has stopped for 24 hours and live in close proximity to the hospital, demonstrate compliance with medical management, can maintain bed rest, understand bleeding precautions, and have an adult companion available for transport 24 hours a day.

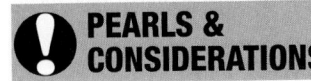

PEARLS & CONSIDERATIONS

COMMENTS

- Placenta previa is diagnosed by TVUS, with repeat assessment at 32 and 36 weeks when indicated.
- Asymptomatic placenta previa can be managed expectantly with a planned cesarean delivery at 36+0 to 37+6 weeks.
- Symptomatic placenta previa is managed by assessing hemodynamic stability, considering steroids for fetal lung maturity, magnesium sulfate for fetal neuroprotection when indicated, and cesarean delivery.

SUGGESTED READING

Available at ExpertConsult.com

RELATED CONTENT

Placenta Previa (Patient Information)
Vaginal Bleeding During Pregnancy (Related Key Topic)

AUTHOR: **HELEN B. GOMEZ, M.D.**

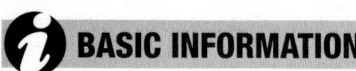

BASIC INFORMATION

DEFINITION

Pleural effusion is the pathologic accumulation of fluid in the pleural space, with a wide range of etiologies.

SYNONYMS

Hydrothorax
Hemothorax
Chylothorax
Empyema

ICD-10CM CODES

J90	Pleural effusion
J91.8	Pleural effusion in other conditions classified elsewhere

PHYSICAL FINDINGS & CLINICAL PRESENTATION

- Subjective symptoms include dyspnea, cough, fatigue, fever, chest pain. Box 1 summarizes signs and symptoms of pleural effusion.
- Physical examination findings include dullness to percussion, decreased tactile fremitus, and decreased breath sounds.
- Bedside transthoracic ultrasound can be helpful to identify characteristics of pleural effusion, including:
  1. Size, location, and laterality
  2. Presence of loculations, pleural adhesions, or implants
  3. Safe site for thoracentesis
  4. Underlying lung parenchymal pathology (e.g., pulmonary edema, consolidation, pneumothorax)

ETIOLOGY

Caused by a number of factors, including increased capillary permeability, increased vascular hydrostatic pressure, decreased vascular oncotic pressure, inflammation of the pleurae, traumatic/iatrogenic causes, and/or obstruction of normal pleural fluid efflux. Box 2 summarizes causes of pleural effusion.

BOX 1 Signs and Symptoms of Effusion

Dyspnea
Cough (dry, nonproductive)
Chest pain (pleuritic or nonpleuritic)
Chest wall discomfort
Decreased breath sounds
Dullness to percussion
Egophony, tactile fremitus
Pleural friction rub

Disease-specific signs and symptoms may include:
Orthopnea
Paroxysmal nocturnal dyspnea
Fever
Night sweats

From Adams JG et al: *Emergency medicine, clinical essentials*, ed 2, Philadelphia, 2013, Elsevier.

Dx DIAGNOSIS

DIFFERENTIAL DIAGNOSIS

Transudate (pleural to serum LDH ratio <0.6 or total protein ratio <0.5)

- Congestive heart failure
- Cirrhosis (hepatic hydrothorax)
- Chronic renal insufficiency

BOX 2 Causes of Pleural Effusions

Transudates
Atelectasis (early)
Congestive heart failure
Cirrhosis
Glomerulonephritis
Hypoalbuminemia
Myxedema
Nephrotic syndrome
Peritoneal dialysis
Pulmonary embolism
Superior vena cava syndrome

Exudates
Infectious
Bacterial infection
Bronchiectasis
Fungal infection
Lung abscess
Parasitic infection
Traumatic hemothorax
Tuberculosis
Viral illness

Malignancies
Lymphoma
Mesothelioma
Primary lung cancer
Pulmonary metastasis

Connective Tissue Disease
Rheumatoid arthritis
Systemic lupus erythematosus

Abdominal/Gastrointestinal
Esophageal rupture
Pancreatic disorders
Subphrenic abscess

Other
Atelectasis (chronic)
Chylothorax
Drug reactions (amiodarone)
Postpartum state
Pulmonary infarction or embolism
Uremia

From Adams JG et al: *Emergency medicine, clinical essentials*, ed 2, Philadelphia, 2013, Elsevier.

- Hypoalbuminemia
- Constrictive pericarditis
- Superior vena cava obstruction
- Urinothorax

Exudate (defined as pleural to serum LDH ratio ≥0.6 or total protein ratio ≥0.5)

- Malignancy (secondary to metastatic cancer or primary; e.g., mesothelioma)
- Infection
  1. Uncomplicated parapneumonic effusion (pH >7.2)
  2. Complicated parapneumonic effusion (pH ≤7.2)
  3. Tuberculous effusion
  4. Viral pleurisy
- Pulmonary embolism
- Hemothorax
- Chylothorax
- Esophageal perforation
- Pleuropancreatic fistula
- Connective tissue disease

WORKUP

The Light criteria for classification of pleural effusions is summarized in Box 3. Fig. 1 illustrates a diagnostic algorithm for pleural effusions.

LABORATORY TESTS

See Table 1.

IMAGING STUDIES

Chest radiography (Fig. 2)**:** Blunting of the costophrenic angle, ipsilateral atelectasis, contralateral shift of the mediastinum with large effusions, elevated hemidiaphragm with subpulmonic effusions, "spine sign" on lateral chest x-ray, may be free-flowing or fixed on lateral decubitus film depending on etiology.

Ultrasonography: Can demonstrate size/location of effusion relative to chest wall, lung, and diaphragm. Can be used to assess for loculations, septations/adhesions, and parietal/visceral pleural implants.

Computed tomography: Useful to identify loculated effusions and to assess underlying lung parenchyma to aid in establishing a diagnosis. In empyema, can demonstrate heterogeneity and gas bubbles.

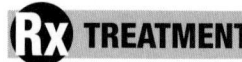

TREATMENT

See Table 2.

BOX 3 Light Criteria for Classification of Pleural Effusions

In 1972, Light et al developed the currently accepted benchmark for classifying pleural fluid, as follows:
Pleural fluid protein to serum protein ratio >0.5:1
Pleural fluid lactate dehydrogenase (LDH) to serum LDH ratio >0.6:1
Pleural fluid LDH greater than two thirds the upper limit of normal for serum LDH (a cutoff value of 200 IU/L was used previously)
Pleural fluid is classified as an exudate if it meets any of the aforementioned criteria. Conversely, if all three characteristics are absent, the fluid is classified as a transudate. These researchers achieved a diagnostic sensitivity of 99% and a specificity of 98% for classification of an exudate.

From Adams JG et al: *Emergency medicine, clinical essentials*, ed 2, Philadelphia, 2013, Elsevier.

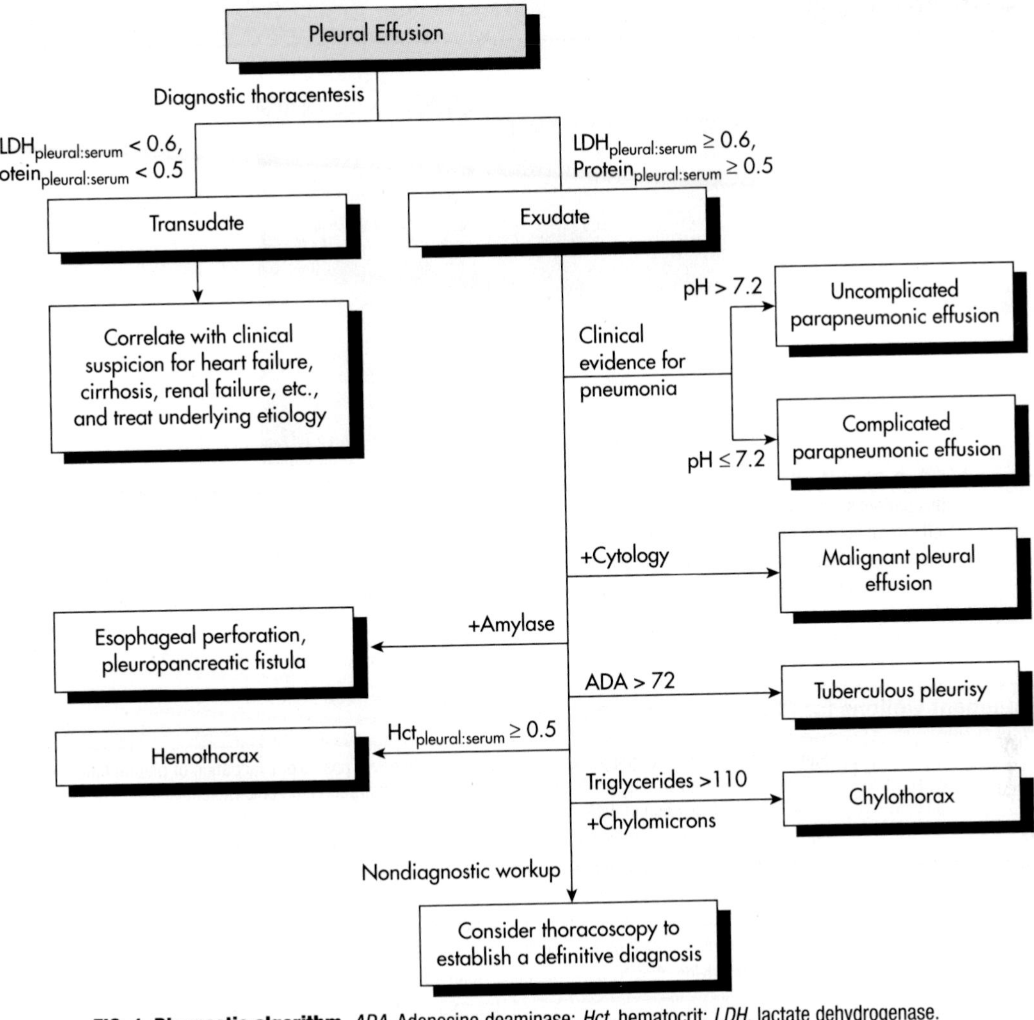

FIG. 1 Diagnostic algorithm. *ADA,* Adenosine deaminase; *Hct,* hematocrit; *LDH,* lactate dehydrogenase.

TABLE 1 Selected Laboratory Tests Used to Diagnose Pleural Effusion

Test	Diagnostic Utility	Comments
Adenosine deaminase (ADA)	>40 IU/L suggestive of tuberculous pleurisy	Values >72 IU/L highly specific for tuberculosis, with improved yield with pleural biopsy and PCR
Albumin	Pleural: Serum albumin ratio <0.83 more consistent with transudate	Can be used to corroborate mixed findings from LDH and protein ratios
Amylase	Esophageal perforation, pancreatitis	
Cell count	**Lymphocyte** predominance suggestive of tuberculosis, lymphoma, other pleural malignancy, pulmonary embolism **Neutrophil** predominant effusions seen with bacterial infection, occasionally with malignancy (20%)	Helpful in distinguishing causes of exudative effusions
Chylomicrons	Positive finding adds to specificity of triglycerides for establishing chylothorax	Consider thoracic duct defect (due to malignancy, trauma or iatrogenic)
Creatinine	Pleural:serum creatinine >1 suggests urinothorax	
Culture	Positive findings used to narrow therapy	Should be sent from every suspected parapneumonic effusion to guide antimicrobial selection
Cytology	Sensitivity for malignancy of ~65%	Modest increment in diagnostic yield with up to three serial samples
Glucose	<60 mg/dl suggests complicated parapneumonic effusion, malignancy, tuberculous pleurisy or rheumatoid effusion	
Hematocrit	Pleural fluid hematocrit >50% peripheral blood hematocrit consistent with hemothorax	Pleural fluid with relatively low hematocrit can appear bloody on gross exam, does not necessarily represent hemothorax
Lactate dehydrogenase (LDH)	Pleural to serum LDH ratio >0.6 or pleural LDH >2/3 the upper limit of normal serum LDH suggests exudate	
NT-proBNP	>1500 pg/ml suggests heart failure even if effusion meets criteria for exudate	Chronic pleural effusions related to heart failure in patients on diuretic therapy may appear exudative
pH	≤7.2 with clinical suspicion highly suggestive of complicated parapneumonic effusion	Can also have low pH with malignant pleural effusions and esophageal perforation
Triglycerides	Triglycerides >110mg/dl seen with chylothorax	Absent triglycerides w/high suspicion for chylothorax can be confirmed with pleural chylomicrons

LDH, lactate dehydrongenase; *NT-proBNP,* N-terminal pro b-type natriuretic peptide; *PCR,* polymerase chain reaction.

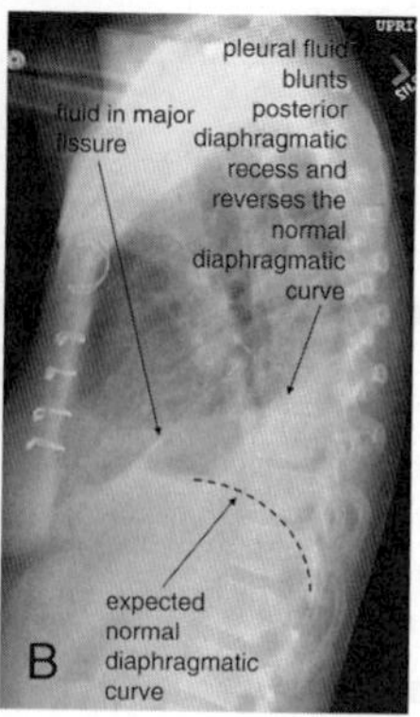

FIG. 2 Pleural effusions. A, Posterior-anterior upright view in which a pleural effusion is most evident on this patient's left side. Both costophrenic angles are blunted. The pleural effusion forms a meniscus against the left lateral chest wall. **B,** Lateral upright view shows two meniscus densities, suggesting bilateral pleural effusions. The posterior diaphragmatic recess is filled with pleural fluid, which forms a meniscus with the posterior chest wall. (From Broder JS: *Diagnostic imaging for the emergency physician*, Philadelphia, 2011, Saunders.)

TABLE 2 Treatment Options for Pleural Effusion

Thoracentesis	Site selection should be guided by ultrasonography whenever possible; evacuation of pleural fluid can be limited when the lung cannot fully re-expand, including central airway obstruction, chronic atelectasis, and the presence of extensive pleural adhesions; aspiration in these circumstances can lead to pneumothorax ex vacuo
Tube thoracostomy	Consider when ongoing drainage will be needed, especially for empyema or hemothorax
Indwelling tunneled pleural catheter	A cuffed pleural drainage catheter tunneled through subcutaneous tissue, drained regularly on an outpatient basis, most commonly used to manage malignant pleural effusions
Pleurodesis	Instillation of a chemical irritant under direct thoracoscopic visualization (e.g., talc poudrage) or via tube thoracostomy to adhere the visceral and parietal pleurae
Pharmacotherapy	Based on underlying etiology (e.g., diuretics, antimicrobials, chemotherapy)

REFERRAL

Negative diagnostic workup after initial pleural fluid sampling should be followed by referral to a pulmonologist for further evaluation (including consideration for thoracoscopy for pleural biopsy).

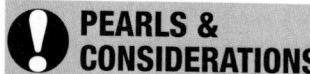

PEARLS & CONSIDERATIONS

- One-time drainage of pleural effusions alone is seldom a definitive therapy. Early identification of the underlying etiology of new effusions should be pursued.
- Managing patients with malignant pleural effusion can be challenging. A recent trial showed that, among patients with malignant pleural effusion, outpatient administration of talc via an indwelling tunneled pleural catheter resulted in a higher rate of pleurodesis than placement of a tunneled catheter alone.[1]
- In patients with malignant pleural effusion near the end of life, simple thoracentesis, repeated as needed, is a reasonable strategy.

[1] Bhatnagar R et al: Outpatient talc administration by indwelling pleural catheter for malignant effusion, *NEJM* 378:1313–1322, 2018.

SUGGESTED READINGS

Available at ExpertConsult.com

RELATED CONTENT

Empyema (Related Key Topic)
Heart Failure (Related Key Topic)
Lung Neoplasms, Primary (Related Key Topic)

AUTHOR: **VIVEK MURTHY, M.D.**

BASIC INFORMATION

DEFINITION

Pleurisy refers to the inflammation of the parietal pleura. This inflammation results in pleuritic chest pain that is characteristically worsened with respiration or movement.

SYNONYM

Pleuritis

ICD-10CM CODE

R09.1 Pleurisy

EPIDEMIOLOGY & DEMOGRAPHICS

INCIDENCE: One of the most common causes of pleuritic chest pain is viral pleurisy. However, there are a variety of disorders that may result in pleurisy. Infectious diseases, rheumatologic disorders, thromboembolic events, and trauma may all lead to pleural inflammation. Therefore, the incidence of pleurisy varies in accordance with the underlying etiology.

PHYSICAL FINDINGS & CLINICAL PRESENTATION

- The defining characteristic of pleurisy is chest pain that worsens with respiration, coughing, or sneezing.
- Pleuritic chest pain is typically described as sharp or stabbing. However, pleuritic chest pain may also be described as dull pain, burning pain, or a "catch" while breathing.
- Movements of the trunk or chest wall may exacerbate pain. Patients with pleurisy may locate the position of minimal discomfort and remain still in that position.
- Dyspnea may be associated with pleurisy.
- Physical exam may be remarkable for a pleural friction rub.
- Decreased breath sounds, rales, or egophony may be appreciated if pneumonia is the underlying etiology of the patient's pleurisy.

ETIOLOGY

- Pleurisy is caused by inflammation of the parietal pleura. The visceral pleura is not innervated by nociceptors. However, injury or inflammation at the periphery of the lung parenchyma often results in inflammation of the overlying parietal pleura. The parietal pleura, which lines the rib cage and the lateral portion of each hemidiaphragm, is innervated by intercostal nerves; therefore pain is localized to the cutaneous distribution of those nerves (over the chest wall). The parietal pleura of the central diaphragm is innervated by fibers that travel with the phrenic nerve; therefore pain associated with inflammation in this area is referred to the ipsilateral shoulder or neck.
- Various underlying etiologies may result in pleurisy, including the following:
  1. Thromboembolism (pulmonary embolism)
  2. Viral infection (coxsackieviruses, respiratory syncytial virus [RSV], cytomegalovirus [CMV], adenovirus, Epstein-Barr virus [EBV], parainfluenza, influenza)
  3. Bacterial infection (pneumonia or tuberculous pleuritis)
  4. Fungal infection (coccidioidomycosis, histoplasmosis)
  5. Rheumatologic disease (rheumatoid arthritis, systemic lupus erythematosus [SLE])
  6. Medications
  7. Malignancy of the lung or pleura
  8. Trauma (rib fracture)
  9. Hereditary (familial Mediterranean fever, sickle cell disease)

Dx DIAGNOSIS

DIFFERENTIAL DIAGNOSIS

- Cardiac: Myocardial infarction, ischemia, pericarditis
- Intraabdominal process: Pancreatitis, cholecystitis
- Thromboembolic: Pulmonary embolism, infarction of lung parenchyma
- Traumatic/mechanical: Rib fracture or pneumothorax
- Viral infection: Viral infections may lead to epidemic pleurodynia (also known as Bornholm disease). Implicated viruses include coxsackieviruses, RSV, CMV, adenovirus, EBV, parainfluenza, influenza. Of note, viral pleurisy is a diagnosis of exclusion
- Bacterial infection: Pneumonia or tuberculous pleurisy
- Fungal infection: Coccidioidomycosis, histoplasmosis
- Rheumatologic disease: Rheumatoid arthritis, SLE
- Medications: Drug-induced lupus
- Hereditary causes: Familial Mediterranean fever, sickle cell disease
- Malignancy: Malignancy affecting the lung or pleura
- Uremia

WORKUP

- A thorough history and physical exam of all patients presenting with pleuritic chest pain should be taken. The time course of the patient's symptoms can provide valuable diagnostic clues. Acute onset of symptoms is suggestive of traumatic injuries, spontaneous pneumothorax, pulmonary embolism, or myocardial infarction. Subacute onset of symptoms suggests a potential infectious, rheumatologic, or medication-induced cause. Viral pleurisy is often associated with prodromal symptoms of upper respiratory infection. Chronic or recurrent symptoms suggest a potential malignant, tuberculous, or hereditary cause.
- Chest x-ray to evaluate for pneumonia, pneumothorax, or pleural effusion.
- ECG to evaluate for infarction, ischemia, or pericarditis.
- Evaluation for pulmonary embolism should be undertaken if clinical suspicion exists.

LABORATORY TESTS

- Laboratory testing varies based on suspected underlying etiology. Consider CBC, Chem 7, and D-Dimer testing depending on clinical presentation.
- If a pleural effusion is present, diagnostic thoracentesis may provide valuable diagnostic clues to the underlying etiology.

IMAGING STUDIES

- Chest x-ray
- ECG
- CT chest in selected patients

Rx TREATMENT

- Treatment of pleurisy consists of pain control as well as treating the underlying condition.
- NSAIDs are the preferred first-line agent to control pain associated with pleurisy. Human studies have been limited to trials using indomethacin for pain control, although an NSAID class effect is presumed.
- Indomethacin 50 mg orally up to three times a day has been found to be effective in relieving pain and is associated with an improvement in mechanical lung function.

AUTHOR: **CHAKRAVARTHY REDDY, M.D.**

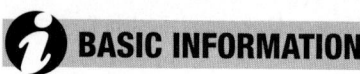

BASIC INFORMATION

DEFINITION

Pneumonia is defined as inflammation of the pulmonary parenchyma caused by an infectious agent (in this case, bacteria). It can be further categorized as community-acquired or health care-associated. The definition of community-acquired pneumonia (CAP), traditionally referred to alveolar infection that develops in the outpatient setting or within 48 hours of admission, now includes patients previously categorized as having health care-associated pneumonia (HCAP) since the microbiology and treatment is similar. Hospital-acquired pneumonia (HAP) is pneumonia occurring ≥48 hours after hospital admission and not incubating at the time of admission.

SYNONYMS

Community-acquired pneumonia
CAP

ICD-10CM CODES

J15.9	Unspecified bacterial pneumonia
J15.9	Unspecified bacterial pneumonia
J13	Pneumonia due to *Streptococcus pneumoniae*
J15.1	Pneumonia due to *Pseudomonas*
J15.20	Pneumonia due to staphylococcus, unspecified
J15.0	Pneumonia due to *Klebsiella pneumoniae*
J14	Pneumonia due to *Haemophilus influenzae*
J15.211	Pneumonia due to methicillin-susceptible *Staphylococcus aureus*
J15.212	Pneumonia due to methicillin-resistant *Staphylococcus aureus*
J15.6	Pneumonia due to other aerobic Gram-negative bacteria
J15.7	Pneumonia due to *Mycoplasma pneumoniae*

EPIDEMIOLOGY & DEMOGRAPHICS

- The annual incidence of pneumonia in the U.S. is 24.8 cases per 10,000 adults, with the highest rates among adults between 65 and 79 years of age (63 cases per 10,000 adults) and those 80 years or older (164.3 cases per 10,000 adults). Health care expenditures for CAP exceed $10 billion annually.
- Hospitalization rate for pneumonia is 15% to 20%. Incidence is highest among the oldest adults.
- In 2014, the eighth leading cause of mortality in the U.S. reported by the National Center for Health Statistics was influenza and pneumonia together.
- Globally, *Streptococcus pneumoniae* (pneumococcus) is the most common pathogen causing community-acquired pneumonia.

PHYSICAL FINDINGS & CLINICAL PRESENTATION

- Fever, tachypnea, chills, tachycardia, cough; pleurisy in the case of pleural effusion.
- Presentation varies with the cause of pneumonia, the patient's age, and the clinical situation:
  1. Patients with streptococcal pneumonia usually present with high fever, chills, atypical chest pain, cough, and copious production of rusty-appearing purulent sputum. Pleurisy in the setting of parapneumonic effusions can also occur. Potential complications include bacteremia, empyema, and distant infections (e.g., meningitis).
  2. *Mycoplasma pneumoniae:* Insidious onset; headache; dry, paroxysmal cough that is worse at night; myalgias; malaise; sore throat; extrapulmonary manifestations (e.g., erythema multiforme, aseptic meningitis, urticaria, erythema nodosum) may be present.
  3. *Chlamydia pneumoniae:* Persistent, nonproductive cough, low-grade fever, headache, sore throat.
  4. *Legionella pneumophila:* High fever, mild cough, mental status change, myalgias, diarrhea, respiratory failure.
  5. MRSA pneumonia: Often preceded by influenza, may present with shock and respiratory failure.
  6. Elderly or immunocompromised hosts with pneumonia may initially present with only minimal symptoms (e.g., low-grade fever, confusion); respiratory and nonrespiratory symptoms are less commonly reported by older patients with pneumonia.
  7. In general, auscultation of patients with pneumonia reveals crackles and diminished breath sounds.
  8. Dullness on percussion may be an indication that pleural effusion is present.
  9. The clinical impression of pneumonia has an overall sensitivity of 70% to 90%; specificity ranges from 40% to 70%.

ETIOLOGY

- Table 1 summarizes common pathogens causing CAP.
- *Streptococcus pneumoniae* (5% to 15% of hospitalized CAP cases): Incidence has been declining due to widespread use of pneumococcal vaccination and reduced rate of cigarette smoking
- *Haemophilus influenzae* (3% to 10% of CAP cases).
- *L. pneumophila* (1% to 5% of adult pneumonias) (2% to 8% of CAP cases).
- *Klebsiella pneumoniae, Pseudomonas aeruginosa, Escherichia coli*
- *Staphylococcus aureus* (3% to 5% of CAP cases).
- Atypical organisms such as *Mycoplasma pneumoniae, Chlamydia pneumoniae,* and *Legionella pneumophila* implicated in up to 40% of cases of CAP.
- Influenza infection is one of the important predisposing factors to *S. pneumoniae* and *S. aureus* pneumonia; gram-negative organisms cause >80% of nosocomial pneumonias.
- Predisposing factors (Table 2 and Table 3):
  1. Chronic obstructive pulmonary disease: *H. influenzae, S. pneumoniae, Legionella, Moraxella catarrhalis*
  2. Seizures: aspiration pneumonia
  3. Compromised hosts: *Legionella, gram-negative organisms*
  4. Alcoholism: *K. pneumoniae, S. pneumoniae, H. influenzae*
  5. HIV: *S. pneumoniae*
  6. IV drug addicts with right-sided bacterial endocarditis: *S. aureus*
  7. Older patient with comorbid diseases: *C. pneumoniae*

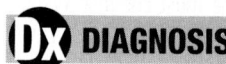

DIAGNOSIS

DIFFERENTIAL DIAGNOSIS

- Viral pneumonias: Viral pneumonias/pneumonitis are on the rise. Several viruses alone or in combination can cause pneumonias in adults. Influenza is the predominant virus, but respiratory syncytial virus (RSV), parainfluenza viruses, adenoviruses, rhinoviruses, coronaviruses, and human metapneumovirus are all possible etiologies. The diagnosis is based on clinical suspicion, negative bacterial workup, and/or respiratory cultures, serologies, or rapid PCR testing
- Exacerbation of chronic bronchitis
- Pulmonary embolism or infarction
- Lung neoplasm
- Bronchiolitis
- Sarcoidosis
- Hypersensitivity pneumonitis
- Pulmonary edema
- Drug-induced lung injury
- Fungal pneumonias
- Parasitic pneumonias
- Atypical pneumonia
- Tuberculosis

WORKUP

Diagnostic testing for CAP is summarized in Table 4. Useful tools for assessing severity of illness are the *CURB-65* (see "Disposition") and *Pneumonia Severity Index* (Fig. 1 and Box 1). Poor prognostic indicators are hypotension (SBP <90 or DBP <60), respiratory rate >30/min, fever (>40° C; 104° F), or hypothermia (<35° C; 95° F). None of these indices is as valuable as clinical judgment.

LABORATORY TESTS

- Complete blood count with differential; white blood cell count is elevated, usually with left shift or the presence of bandemia.
- Blood cultures (hospitalized patients only): Positive in approximately 20% of cases of pneumococcal pneumonia.
- Pneumococcal urinary antigen test can be used to detect the C-polysaccharide antigen

TABLE 1 Common Pathogens Causing Community-Acquired Pneumonia

Inpatient, with No Cardiopulmonary Disease or Modifying Factors

Streptococcus pneumoniae, Haemophilus influenzae, Mycoplasma pneumoniae, Chlamydophila pneumoniae, mixed infection (bacteria plus atypical pathogen), viruses (including influenza), *Legionella* spp., and others (*Mycobacterium tuberculosis,* endemic fungi, *Pneumocystis jirovecii*)

Inpatient, with Cardiopulmonary Disease and/or Modifying Factors

All of the above, but drug-resistant *S. pneumoniae* (DRSP) and enteric gram-negative organisms are more of a concern

Severe Community-Acquired Pneumonia, with No Risks for *Pseudomonas Aeruginosa*

S. pneumoniae (including DRSP), *Legionella* spp., *H. influenzae,* enteric gram-negative bacilli, *Staphylococcus aureus* (including methicillin-resistant *S. aureus*), *M. pneumoniae,* respiratory viruses (including influenza), others (*C. pneumoniae, M. tuberculosis,* endemic fungi)

Severe CAP, with Risks for *P. Aeruginosa*

All of the pathogens above plus *P. aeruginosa*

From Vincent JL et al: *Textbook of critical care,* ed 7, Philadelphia, 2017, Elsevier.

TABLE 2 Risk Factors for Developing Severe Community-Acquired Pneumonia

Advanced age
Comorbid illness (e.g., chronic respiratory illness, cardiovascular disease, diabetes mellitus, neurologic illness, renal insufficiency, malignancy)
Cigarette smoking
Alcohol abuse
Absence of antibiotic therapy before hospitalization
Failure to contain infection to its initial site of entry
Immune suppression
Genetic polymorphisms in the immune response

From Vincent JL et al: *Textbook of critical care,* ed 7, Philadelphia, 2017, Elsevier.

TABLE 3 Clinical Associations with Specific Pathogens

Condition	Commonly Encountered Pathogens
Alcoholism	*Streptococcus pneumoniae* (including penicillin-resistant), anaerobes, gram-negative bacilli (possibly *Klebsiella pneumoniae),* tuberculosis
Chronic obstructive pulmonary disease/current or former smoker	*S. pneumoniae, Haemophilus influenzae, Moraxella catarrhalis*
Residence in nursing home	*S. pneumoniae,* gram-negative bacilli, *H. influenzae, Staphylococcus aureus, Chlamydophila pneumoniae;* consider *M. tuberculosis* Consider anaerobes, but these are less common
Poor dental hygiene	Anaerobes
Bat exposure	*Histoplasma capsulatum*
Bird exposure	*Chlamydophila psittaci, Cryptococcus neoformans, H. capsulatum*
Rabbit exposure	*Francisella tularensis*
Travel to southwestern United States	*Coccidioidomycosis;* hantavirus in selected areas
Exposure to farm animals or parturient cats	*Coxiella burnetii* (Q fever)
Postinfluenza pneumonia	*S. pneumoniae, S. aureus* (including the community-acquired strain of methicillin-resistant *S. aureus*), *H. influenzae*
Structural disease of the lung (e.g., bronchiectasis, cystic fibrosis)	*Pseudomonas aeruginosa, Pseudomonas cepacia,* or *S. aureus*
Sickle cell disease, asplenia	Pneumococcus, *H. influenzae*
Suspected bioterrorism	Anthrax, tularemia, plague
Travel to Asia	Severe acute respiratory syndrome, tuberculosis, melioidosis

From Vincent JL et al: *Textbook of critical care,* ed 7, Philadelphia, 2017, Elsevier.

of *S. pneumoniae* (70% sensitivity). It is a useful tool in the treatment of hospitalized adult patients with CAP.

- When suspecting *Legionella,* a respiratory specimen culture on special media and/or a urinary antigen should be requested.
- Serologic testing for HIV in selected patients.
- Serum electrolytes (hyponatremia in suspected *Legionella* pneumonia), BUN, creatinine.
- Serum procalcitonin level: May be helpful to distinguish pneumonia from heart failure in patients presenting to the emergency department with acute dyspnea. The procalcitonin level is significantly higher in patients with pneumonia than in those without.[1] However, recent trials regarding procalcitonin-guided use of antibiotics for lower respiratory tract infections did not result in less use of antibiotics than did usual care among patients with suspected lower respiratory tract infection.[2]
- Pulse oximetry or arterial blood gases: Hypoxemia with partial pressure of oxygen <60 mm Hg while the patient is breathing room air, a standard criterion for hospital admission.
- Fig. 2 illustrates an algorithm for the diagnosis and treatment of nosocomial pneumonia.

IMAGING STUDIES

Chest x-ray (PA and lateral) (Fig. 3): Findings vary with the stage and type of pneumonia and the hydration of the patient:

- Classically, pneumococcal pneumonia presents with a segmental lobe infiltrate.
- Diffuse infiltrates on chest x-ray can be seen with *L. pneumophila* (Fig. 4), *M. pneumoniae,* viral pneumonias, *P. jirovecii (carinii),* miliary tuberculosis, aspiration, aspergillosis.
- An initial chest x-ray is also useful to rule out the presence of any complications (pneumothorax, empyema, abscesses).

Rx TREATMENT

NONPHARMACOLOGIC THERAPY

- Avoidance of tobacco use
- Oxygen to maintain partial oxygen pressure in arterial blood >60 mm Hg or oxygen saturation >88% in COPD patients and >92% in non-COPD patients
- IV hydration, correction of dehydration
- Assisted ventilation in patients with significant respiratory failure

ACUTE GENERAL Rx

- Antibiotic therapy should be based on clinical, radiographic, and laboratory evaluation. Empiric therapy regimens for severe community-acquired pneumonia are summarized in Table 5.
- Macrolides (azithromycin or clarithromycin) or doxycycline is recommended for empiric outpatient treatment of CAP as long as the patient has not received antibiotics within the past 3 months and does not reside in a community in which the prevalence of macrolide resistance is high. Fig. 5 summarizes empiric therapy for CAP. The treatment of choice in suspected *Legionella* pneumonia is either a quinolone (e.g., moxifloxacin) or a macrolide (e.g., azithromycin) antibiotic. A beta-lactam antibiotic is usually added to macrolides.

[1] Alba GA et al: Diagnostic and prognostic utility of procalcitonin in patients presenting to the emergency department with dyspnea, *Am J Med* 129:96, 2016.
[2] Huang DT et al: Procalcitonin-guided use of antibiotics for lower respiratory tract infection, *N Engl J Med* 379:236-49, 2018.

TABLE 4 Diagnostic Testing for Community-Acquired Pneumonia

Test	Sensitivity	Specificity	Comment
Chest radiograph	65%-85%	85%-95%	Computed tomography is more sensitive to infiltrates. Recommended for all patients.
Computed tomography	Gold standard	Not infection specific	Should not be performed routinely but helpful to identify cavitation and loculated pleural fluid. Recommended in the evaluation of nonresponding patients.
Blood cultures	10%-20%	High when positive	Usually shows pneumococcus (in 50%-80% of positive samples) and defines antibiotic susceptibility. Recommended in patients with severe CAP, particularly if not on antibiotic therapy at the time of testing.
Sputum Gram stain	40%-100% depending on criteria	0%-100% depending on criteria	Can correlate with sputum culture to define predominant organism and can be used to identify unsuspected pathogens. Recommended if sputum culture is obtained. May not be able to narrow empiric therapy choices.
Sputum culture			Use if suspect drug-resistant or unusual pathogen, but a positive result cannot differentiate colonization from infection. Obtain via tracheal aspirate in all intubated patients.
Oximetry or arterial blood gas			Define both severity of infection and need for oxygen; if hypercarbia is suspected, a blood gas sample is needed. Recommended in severe community-acquired pneumonia.
Serologic testing for *Legionella, Chlamydophila pneumoniae, Mycobacterium pneumoniae*, viruses			Accurate, but usually requires acute and convalescent titers collected 4 to 6 weeks apart. Not routinely recommended.
Legionella urinary antigen	50%-80%		Specific to serogroup 1, but the best acute diagnostic test for *Legionella*.
Pneumococcal urinary antigen	70%-100%	80%	False positives if recent pneumococcal infection. Can increase sensitivity with concentrated urine.
Serum procalcitonin			Not a routine test, but if performed, should be measured with the highly sensitive Kryptor assay. May help guide duration of therapy and need for ICU admission.

From Vincent JL et al: *Textbook of critical care*, ed 7, Philadelphia, 2017, Elsevier.

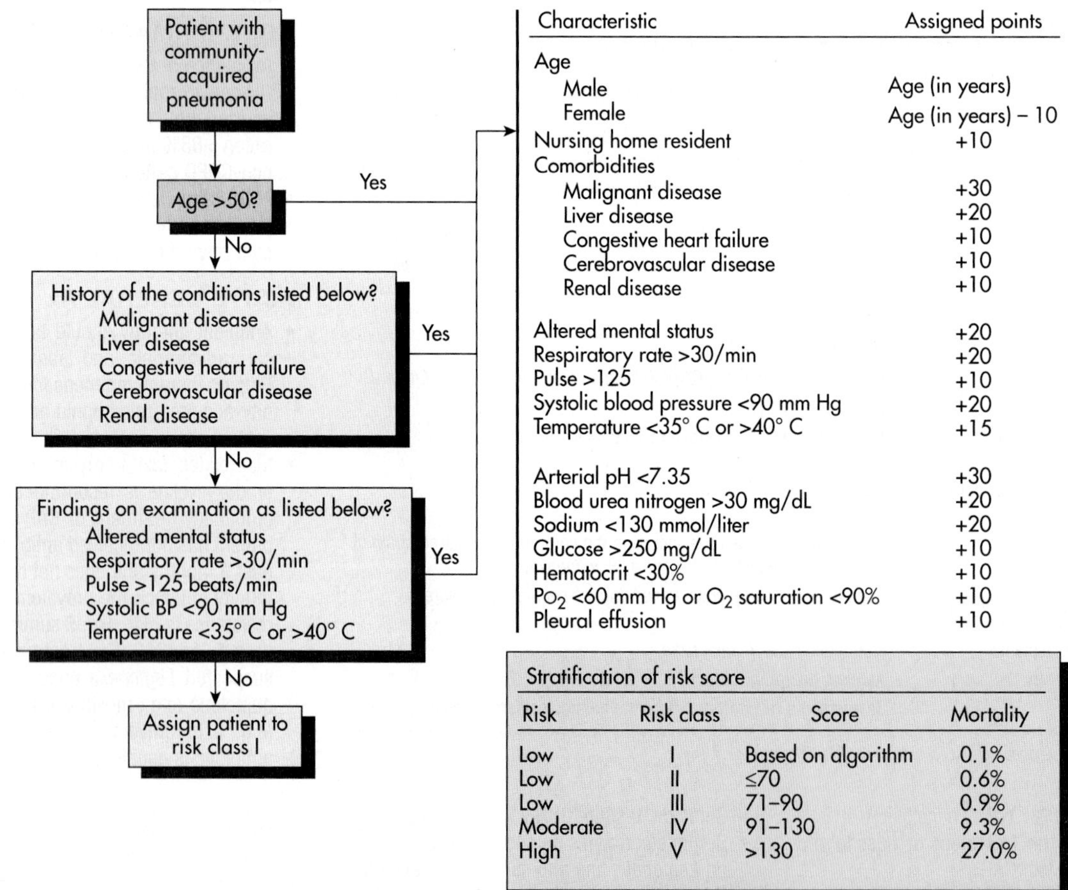

FIG. 1 The pneumonia severity index. *BP,* Blood pressure; O_2, oxygen; Po_2, partial pressure of oxygen. (From Sellke FW et al: *Sabiston & Spencer surgery of the chest*, ed 9, 2016, Elsevier.)

BOX 1 Severe Pneumonia: Diagnostic Criteria[1]

Major Criteria
Invasive mechanical ventilation
Use of vasopressors to maintain blood pressure

Minor Criteria
Respiratory rate ≥30 breaths/min
Multilobar infiltrates
New-onset confusion/disorientation
Uremia (BUN >20 mg/dl)
Leukopenia (WBC count <4000 cells/μL)
Pao_2/Fio_2 ratio ≥250
Thrombocytopenia (platelet count <100,000 cells/μL)
Hypothermia (core temperature <36°C; 96.8° F)
Hypotension requiring aggressive fluid resuscitation

ATS/IDSA, American Thoracic Society/Infectious Diseases Society of America; *BUN,* blood urea nitrogen; *WBC,* white blood cell.
[1]According to ATS/IDSA 2007 guidelines.
From Parrillo JE, Dellinger RP: *Critical care medicine: principles of diagnosis and management in the adult,* ed 4, Philadelphia, 2014, Saunders.

- In the hospital setting, patients admitted to the general ward can be treated empirically with a second- or third-generation cephalosporin (ceftriaxone, cefotaxime, or cefuroxime) plus a macrolide (azithromycin or clarithromycin) or doxycycline. An antipseudomonal quinolone (levofloxacin or moxifloxacin) can be substituted in place of the macrolide or doxycycline.
- Empiric therapy in ICU patients: IV beta-lactam (ceftriaxone, cefotaxime, ampicillin-sulbactam) plus an IV quinolone (levofloxacin, moxifloxacin) or IV azithromycin.
- In hospitalized patients at risk for *P. aeruginosa* infection, empiric treatment should consist of an antipseudomonal beta-lactam (meropenem, doripenem, imipenem, or piperacillin-tazobactam) with or without a second antipseudomonal agent such as an aminoglycoside or an antipseudomonal quinolone.
- In patients with suspected methicillin-resistant *S. aureus,* vancomycin or linezolid is effective.
- Corticosteroids: A meta-analysis published in 2015 by Siemieniuk et al showed that in hospitalized adults with CAP, systemic corticosteroid therapy may reduce mortality, the need for mechanical ventilation, and length of hospital stay. Based on those results and several other supportive studies, corticosteroids (i.e., methylprednisolone 0.5 mg/kg IV q12h for 5 days) are recommended by several experts in hospitalized adult patients presenting with severe CAP, as long as no major contraindications for steroid usage are present.
- Adjunctive treatment with corticosteroids improves initial clinical response and reduces length of hospital stay but does not offset mortality or clinical failure and increases readmission rate in hospitalized patients with CAP.
- Duration of treatment ranges from 5 to 14 days. Trials have shown that in adults hospitalized with community-acquired pneumonia, stopping antibiotic treatment after 5 days in clinically stable patients is reasonable and noninferior to usual care. Hematogenous *Staphylococcus* infection, abscesses, and cavitary lesions might require prolonged antibiotic therapy, sometimes until radiological resolution is documented.

CHRONIC Rx

Parapneumonic effusion and empyema can be managed with chest tube placement for drainage. Instillation of fibrinolytic agents (streptokinase, urokinase, or, more commonly, tissue plasminogen activator [TP]) along with DNase (i.e., dornase alfa) twice a day via chest tube may facilitate the drainage of effusions not responding to chest tube drainage alone. A thoracoscopic debridement or a surgical decortication may be necessary in resistant cases.

DISPOSITION

- Risk factors for a poor outcome from CAP are summarized in Table E6.
- Indications for hospital admission are:
  1. Hypoxemia (oxygen saturation <90% while patient is breathing room air)
  2. Hemodynamic instability
  3. Inability to tolerate medications
  4. Active coexisting condition requiring hospitalization. A criterion often used to determine hospital admission is known as the "CURB-65": **C**onfusion, B**U**N >19.6 mg/dl, **R**espiratory rate >30 breaths/min, systolic **B**P <90 mg Hg, and diastolic BP ≤60 mm Hg, age ≥**65.** Patients are generally admitted to the hospital if they fulfill 2 or more criteria and to the ICU if they have 3 or more criteria

PEARLS & CONSIDERATIONS

COMMENTS

- Use of gastric acid suppressive therapy (H_2 receptor antagonists, proton pump inhibitors [PPIs]) has been reported to increase the risk of CAP. It has been reported that PPI therapy started within the previous 30 days is associated with a risk for CAP, whereas longer-term current use is not. Recent studies have failed to confirm increased risk of CAP with PPI use and have shown that risk of CAP is higher during 30 days before PPI prescription than during the 30 days after PPI prescription.[3]
- Causes of slowly resolving or nonresolving pneumonia:
  1. Difficult to treat infections: Viral pneumonia, *Legionella,* pneumococci or staphylococci with impaired host response, tuberculosis, fungi
  2. Neoplasm: Lung, lymphoma, metastasis
  3. Congestive heart failure
  4. Pulmonary embolism
  5. Immunologic or idiopathic: Wegener granulomatosis, pulmonary eosinophilic syndromes, systemic lupus erythematosus
  6. Drug toxicity (e.g., amiodarone)
- If patients with pneumonia don't improve within a reasonable time frame, repeat films should be taken promptly. In those with complete clinical recovery, it is reasonable to wait 6 to 8 weeks before repeating the imaging study to document clearing of the infiltrate. The benefit of routine radiography after pneumonia has been questioned due to the low 1-yr incidence of lung cancer. Opponents propose a selective approach limiting follow-up chest x-ray to middle-aged and older adults.
- Prevention: Older adults should receive sequentially the 23-valent pneumococcal polysaccharides vaccine (PPSV23) and the pneumococcal conjugated vaccine (PCV13). The ACIP recommends giving the PCV13 first to be followed after a year by the PPSV23. This recommendation includes patients younger than 65 years with some defined risk factors (end-stage renal disease, sickle cell disease, congenital or acquired asplenia, HIV infection, congenital or acquired immunodeficiency, nephrotic syndrome, leukemia, lymphoma, Hodgkin's disease, generalized malignancy, iatrogenic immunosuppression, solid organ transplant, multiple myeloma, CSF leak, cochlear implant).
- Prevention: During the influenza season, patients should also receive influenza vaccination.

SUGGESTED READINGS

Available at ExpertConsult.com

RELATED CONTENT

Bacterial Pneumonia (Patient Information)
Aspiration Pneumonia (Related Key Topic)
Pneumonia, Mycoplasma (Related Key Topic)
Pneumonia, Viral (Related Key Topic)
Legionnaires' Disease (Related Key Topic)

AUTHOR: **JORGE MERCADO, M.D.**

[3]Othman F et al: Community acquired pneumonia incidence before and after proton pump inhibitor prescription, *BMJ* 355:i5813, 2016.

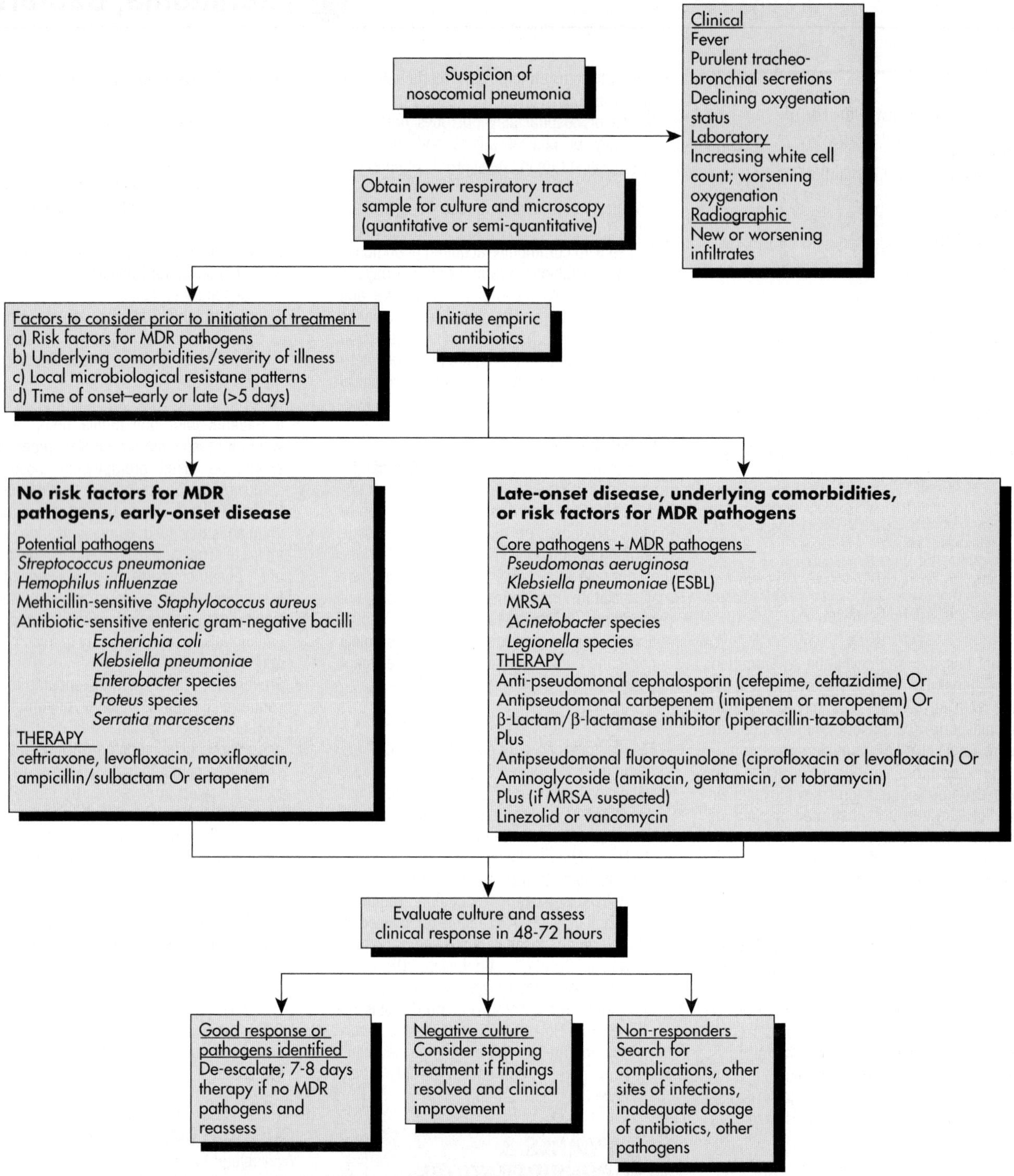

Suspicion of nosocomial pneumonia

Clinical
Fever
Purulent tracheobronchial secretions
Declining oxygenation status
Laboratory
Increasing white cell count; worsening oxygenation
Radiographic
New or worsening infiltrates

Obtain lower respiratory tract sample for culture and microscopy (quantitative or semi-quantitative)

Factors to consider prior to initiation of treatment
a) Risk factors for MDR pathogens
b) Underlying comorbidities/severity of illness
c) Local microbiological resistane patterns
d) Time of onset–early or late (>5 days)

Initiate empiric antibiotics

No risk factors for MDR pathogens, early-onset disease

Potential pathogens
Streptococcus pneumoniae
Hemophilus influenzae
Methicillin-sensitive *Staphylococcus aureus*
Antibiotic-sensitive enteric gram-negative bacilli
Escherichia coli
Klebsiella pneumoniae
Enterobacter species
Proteus species
Serratia marcescens
THERAPY
ceftriaxone, levofloxacin, moxifloxacin, ampicillin/sulbactam Or ertapenem

Late-onset disease, underlying comorbidities, or risk factors for MDR pathogens

Core pathogens + MDR pathogens
Pseudomonas aeruginosa
Klebsiella pneumoniae (ESBL)
MRSA
Acinetobacter species
Legionella species
THERAPY
Anti-pseudomonal cephalosporin (cefepime, ceftazidime) Or
Antipseudomonal carbepenem (imipenem or meropenem) Or
β-Lactam/β-lactamase inhibitor (piperacillin-tazobactam)
Plus
Antipseudomonal fluoroquinolone (ciprofloxacin or levofloxacin) Or
Aminoglycoside (amikacin, gentamicin, or tobramycin)
Plus (if MRSA suspected)
Linezolid or vancomycin

Evaluate culture and assess clinical response in 48-72 hours

Good response or pathogens identified
De-escalate; 7-8 days therapy if no MDR pathogens and reassess

Negative culture
Consider stopping treatment if findings resolved and clinical improvement

Non-responders
Search for complications, other sites of infections, inadequate dosage of antibiotics, other pathogens

FIG. 2 A suggested algorithm for the diagnosis and treatment of nosocomial pneumonia. (From Parrillo JE, Dellinger RP: *Critical care medicine, principles of diagnosis and management in the adult*, ed 4, Philadelphia, 2014, Elsevier.)

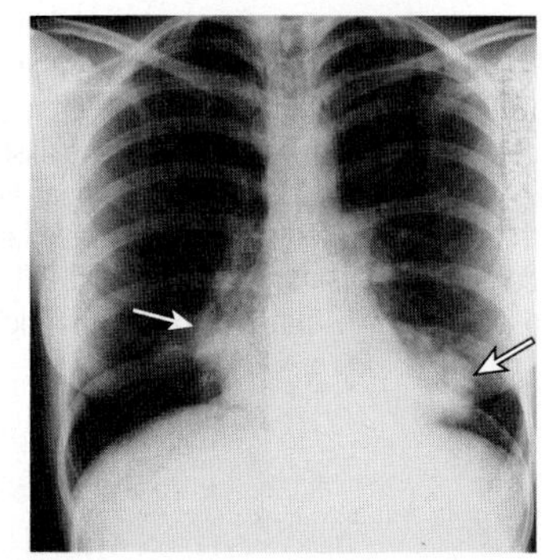

FIG. 3 *Streptococcus pneumoniae* pneumonia, bilateral lower zone consolidation (*arrows*). Although pneumococcal pneumonia is typically unifocal, multifocal involvement is not uncommon. (From Grainger RG et al: *Grainger and Allison's diagnostic radiology*, ed 4, London, 2001, Harcourt.)

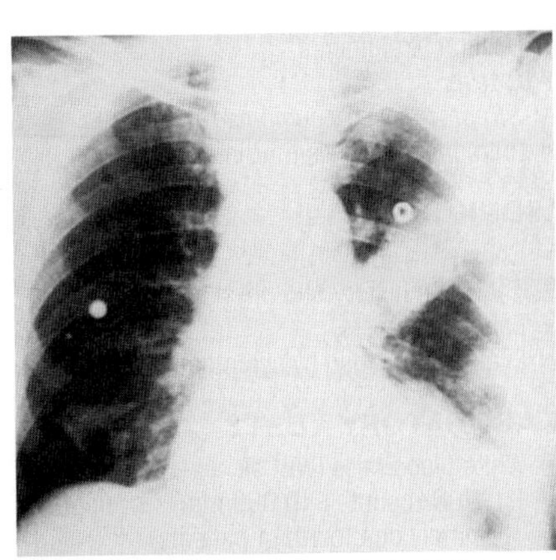

FIG. 4 Multilobar involvement occurring with *Legionella pneumophila* pneumonia. (From Mason RJ: *Murray & Nadel's textbook of respiratory medicine*, ed 5, Philadelphia, 2010, Saunders.)

TABLE 5 Empiric Therapy Regimens for Severe Community-Acquired Pneumonia

No Pseudomonal Risk Factors
Selected beta-lactam (cefotaxime, ceftriaxone)
plus
Intravenously administered macrolide *or* quinolone (moxifloxacin or levofloxacin*)
Pseudomonal Risk Factors Present
Selected antipseudomonal beta-lactam (cefepime, piperacillin/tazobactam, imipenem, meropenem)
plus
Ciprofloxacin
or
Selected antipseudomonal beta-lactam
plus
Aminoglycoside
plus
Intravenously administered macrolide or antipneumococcal quinolone (moxifloxacin or levofloxacin*)

NOTE: Although routine methicillin-resistant *Staphylococcus aureus* (MRSA) coverage is NOT recommended for all severe community-acquired pneumonia, consider community-acquired MRSA, especially after influenza and with bilateral necrotizing pneumonia, and if suspected, treat by adding either linezolid or the combination of vancomycin and clindamycin.

*For patients with normal renal function, the recommended dose of levofloxacin is 750 mg daily.

From Vincent JL et al: *Textbook of critical care*, ed 7, Philadelphia, 2017, Elsevier.

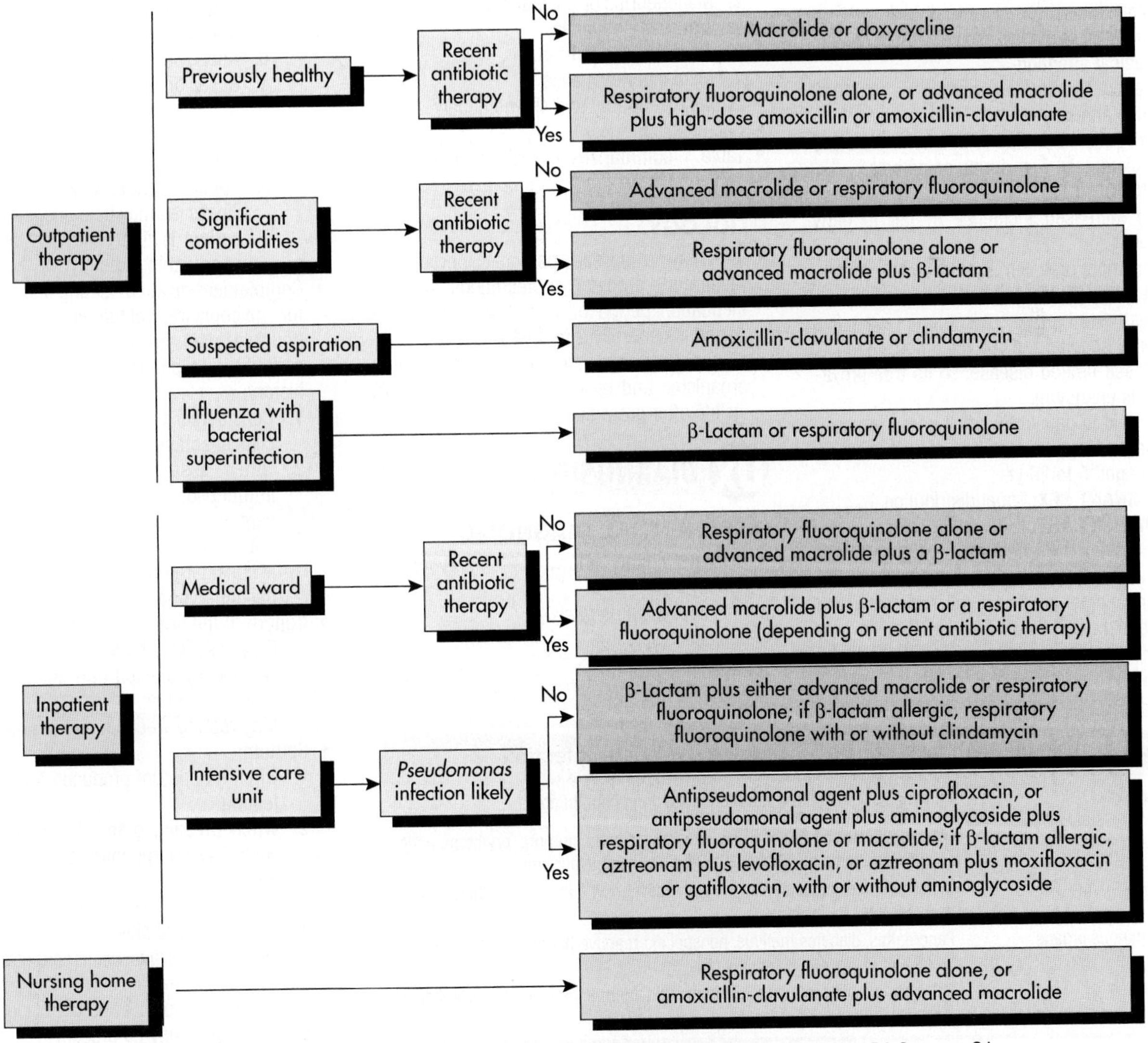

- Outpatient therapy
  - Previously healthy → Recent antibiotic therapy
    - No → Macrolide or doxycycline
    - Yes → Respiratory fluoroquinolone alone, or advanced macrolide plus high-dose amoxicillin or amoxicillin-clavulanate
  - Significant comorbidities → Recent antibiotic therapy
    - No → Advanced macrolide or respiratory fluoroquinolone
    - Yes → Respiratory fluoroquinolone alone or advanced macrolide plus β-lactam
  - Suspected aspiration → Amoxicillin-clavulanate or clindamycin
  - Influenza with bacterial superinfection → β-Lactam or respiratory fluoroquinolone
- Inpatient therapy
  - Medical ward → Recent antibiotic therapy
    - No → Respiratory fluoroquinolone alone or advanced macrolide plus a β-lactam
    - Yes → Advanced macrolide plus β-lactam or a respiratory fluoroquinolone (depending on recent antibiotic therapy)
  - Intensive care unit → *Pseudomonas* infection likely
    - No → β-Lactam plus either advanced macrolide or respiratory fluoroquinolone; if β-lactam allergic, respiratory fluoroquinolone with or without clindamycin
    - Yes → Antipseudomonal agent plus ciprofloxacin, or antipseudomonal agent plus aminoglycoside plus respiratory fluoroquinolone or macrolide; if β-lactam allergic, aztreonam plus levofloxacin, or aztreonam plus moxifloxacin or gatifloxacin, with or without aminoglycoside
- Nursing home therapy → Respiratory fluoroquinolone alone, or amoxicillin-clavulanate plus advanced macrolide

FIG. 5 Empiric therapy for community-acquired pneumonia. (From Sellke FW, del Nido PJ, Swanson SJ: *Sabiston & Spencer surgery of the chest*, ed 9, Philadelphia, 2016, Elsevier.)

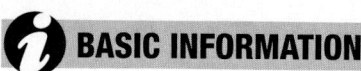

DEFINITION

Mycoplasma pneumonia is an infection of the lung parenchyma caused by a small rod-shaped bacterium, *Mycoplasma pneumoniae.*

SYNONYMS

Primary atypical pneumonia
Eaton pneumonia
Walking pneumonia

ICD-10CM CODE
J15.7 Pneumonia due to *Mycoplasma pneumoniae*

EPIDEMIOLOGY & DEMOGRAPHICS

INCIDENCE (IN U.S.):

- It is a frequent cause of community-acquired pneumonia (CAP), accounting for up to 37% of CAP in patients treated as outpatients and 10% of pneumonia in persons requiring hospitalization. CDC estimates 2 million cases a year with 100,000 pneumonia-related hospitalizations.
- Many cases probably resolve without coming to medical attention.
- Incidence is estimated at one case per 1000 persons annually.
- Incidence is estimated to at least triple every (approximately) 5 yr during epidemics.

PEAK INCIDENCE:

- Some increased incidence in fall to early winter.
- Seems more prevalent in temperate climates.

PREVALENCE (IN U.S.):

- Estimated to be present in one in every five patients hospitalized for pneumonia (generally a self-limited disease, so its true prevalence is unknown).
- Estimated to cause 7% of all cases of pneumonia and approximately half the cases in those aged 5 to 20 yr.

PREDOMINANT SEX: Equal distribution
PREDOMINANT AGE:

- Most commonly affected: School-age children and young adults (ages 5-20 yr).
- Occurs in older adults as well, especially with household exposure to a young child.
- More severe infections in affected elderly patients.

GENETICS: Familial disposition:

- None known.
- May be more severe in patients with sickle cell anemia.
- Neonatal infection: Severe respiratory distress, sometimes requiring intubation, attributed to this disease in infants.

PHYSICAL FINDINGS & CLINICAL PRESENTATION

- Nonexudative pharyngitis (common)
- Headache, otalgia common
- Fever may be mild or not present
- Rhonchi or rales without evidence of consolidation (common) in lower lung zones
- Associated with bullous myringitis (nonspecific finding; perhaps no more frequently than in other pneumonias)
- Skin rashes in up to one fourth of patients:
  1. Morbilliform
  2. Urticaria
  3. Erythema nodosum (unusual)
  4. Erythema multiforme (unusual)
  5. Stevens-Johnson syndrome (rare)
- Muscle tenderness (<50% of the patients)
- On examination (and confirmed with testing)
  1. Mononeuritis or polyneuritis
  2. Transverse myelitis
  3. Cranial nerve palsies
  4. Meningoencephalitis
- Lymphadenopathy and splenomegaly
- Conjunctivitis
- Table 1 summarizes the clinical manifestations of *Mycoplasma pneumoniae*

ETIOLOGY

- Infection is spread person-to-person via respiratory droplets or secretions with an incubation period of 1 to 4 wk. Incubation period is generally 2 to 3 wk.
- Mycoplasma are the smallest free-living organisms and lack a cell wall and are not visible after gram staining.

Dx DIAGNOSIS

DIFFERENTIAL DIAGNOSIS

- *Chlamydia* (now known as *Chlamydophila*) *pneumoniae*
- *Chlamydophila psittaci*
- *Legionella* spp
- *Coxiella burnetii*
- Several viral agents
- Q fever
- *Streptococcus pneumoniae*
- Pulmonary embolism or infarction

WORKUP

- Chest x-ray (Fig. 1).
- Thorough history and physical examination.
- Laboratory tests.
- Evaluation guided by symptoms and findings.

LABORATORY TESTS

- White blood cells (WBCs):
  1. WBC count $>10,000/mm^3$ in approximately one fourth of patients
  2. Differential count nonspecific
  3. Leukopenia rare
- Cold agglutinins:
  1. Detected in approximately 50% to 70% of all patients within 1 to 2 weeks after infection; highest in children with yield decreasing with age. Since neither sensitive nor specific, the use of cold agglutinins has come into question
  2. Also may be found in:
     a. Lymphoproliferative diseases
     b. Influenza
     c. Mononucleosis
     d. Adenovirus infections
     e. Occasionally, Legionnaires' disease
  3. Titers typically >1:64:
     a. May be detectable with bedside testing
     b. Appear between days 5 and 10 of the illness (so may be demonstrable when patient is first examined) and disappear within 1 mo
- Complement fixation testing assay specific for mycoplasma antigens of paired sera (fourfold rise) or a single titer ≥1:32 in patients with pneumonia and a compatible history:
  1. Considered diagnostic in the appropriate clinical setting
  2. Other assays include enzyme-linked immunosorbent assay (ELISA), antigen capture-enzyme immunoassay, and polymerase chain reaction (PCR); if available, is considered diagnostic test of choice on nasopharyngeal samples
- Culture of the organism from specimens
  1. Only truly specific test for infection
  2. Technically difficult and done reliably by few laboratories
  3. May require weeks to get results
- Sputum:
  1. Often no sputum produced for laboratory testing
  2. When present, gram-stained specimens show polymorphonuclear cells without organisms
- Infection occasionally complicated by pancreatitis or glomerulitis
- Disseminated intravascular coagulation is a rare complication
- Electrocardiographic evidence of pericarditis or myocarditis may be present

TABLE 1 Clinical Manifestations of *Mycoplasma Pneumoniae* Infection

Respiratory tract	Pharyngitis, laryngitis, acute bronchitis, bronchopneumonia
Skin and mucosa	Maculopapular and vesicular exanthema, urticaria, purpura, erythema nodosum, erythema multiforme, Stevens-Johnson syndrome
Central nervous system	Meningitis, meningoencephalitis, acute psychosis, cerebellitis, Guillain-Barré syndrome*
Parenchymatous organs	Pancreatitis, diabetes mellitus, nonspecific reactive hepatitis, subacute thyroiditis*
Miscellaneous	Hemorrhagic bullous myringitis, hemolytic anemia, pericarditis, thromboembolism*

*Some association remains uncertain.
From Cohen J, Powderly WG: *Infectious diseases,* ed 2, St Louis, 2004, Mosby.

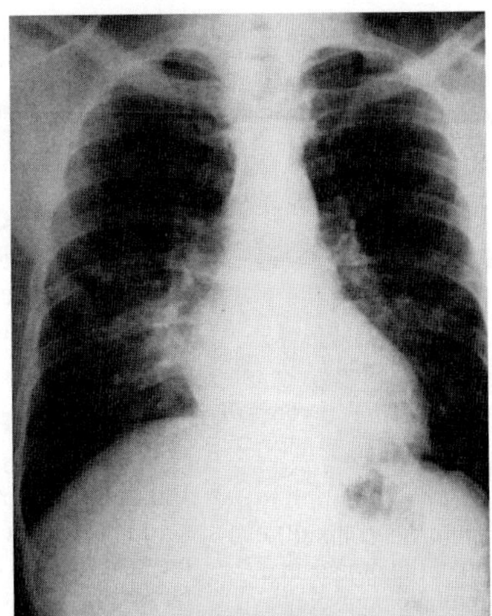

FIG. 1 Radiographic findings in *Mycoplasma pneumoniae* pneumonia are nonspecific. Bilateral bronchopneumonia occurred in this patient. (From Mason RJ, et al.: *Murray and Nadel's textbook of respiratory medicine*, ed 5, Philadelphia, 2010, Saunders.)

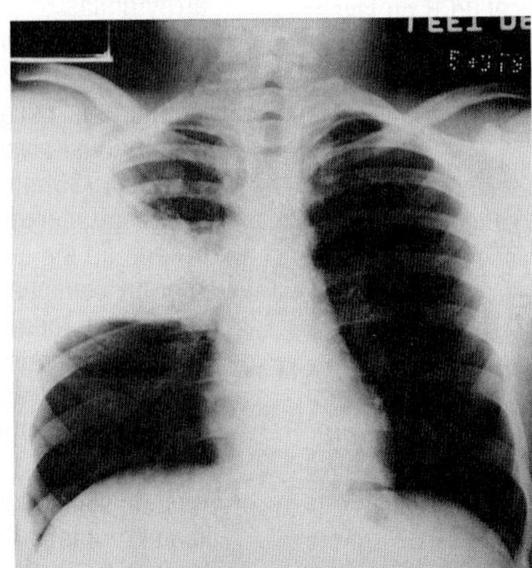

FIG. 2 Localized airspace opacification resulting from *Mycoplasma pneumoniae*. (From Specht N [ed]: *Practical guide to diagnostic imaging,* St Louis, 1998, Mosby.)

IMAGING STUDIES

- Predilection for lower lobe involvement (upper lobes involved in less than a fourth), with radiographic abnormalities frequently out of proportion to those on physical examination (Fig. 2).
- Small pleural effusions in approximately 30% of patients.
- Large effusions: Rare.
- Infiltrates: Patchy, unilateral, and with a segmental distribution, although multilobar involvement may be seen.
- Evidence of hilar adenopathy on chest radiographs in 20% to 25%.
- Rare cases reported:
  1. Associated lung abscess.
  2. Residual pneumatoceles.
  3. Lobar collapse.
  4. Hyperlucent lung syndrome.

Rx TREATMENT

ACUTE GENERAL Rx

- Therapy: Azithromycin 500 mg qd × 3 or 500 mg initially, then 250 mg daily for 4 days for adults. For children: 10 mg/kg in one dose on first day, then 5 mg/kg in one dose for 4 days or clarithromycin: 500 mg bid for 10 days in adults, 15 mg/kg per day in two divided doses for 10 days in children. Alternatives include erythromycin (500 mg qid) for adults or 30 to 40 mg/kg per day in four divided doses in children or doxycycline: 2 to 4 mg/kg per day in one or two divided doses for 10 days, maximum daily dose: 100 to 200 mg, but this agent cannot be used in young children or women of childbearing age. Respiratory fluoroquinolones such as Levaquin or moxifloxacin are alternative agents for treatment in adults but should not be used in young children.
- Therapy shortens the duration and severity of symptoms and may hasten radiographic clearing, but the disease is self-limiting.
- Macrolide resistance is becoming a concern, starting in Asia in 2000s and then spread to Europe and North America. One study showed resistance of 5% to 13% in France and U.S.

CHRONIC Rx

- Effective antimicrobial therapy does not eliminate the organism from the respiratory secretions, which may be positive for weeks.
- Serum antibody response does not necessarily provide lifelong immunity.
- Chronic symptoms do not occur, although clinical relapses may occur 7 to 10 days after the initial response and may be associated with new areas of infiltration.

DISPOSITION

- Clinical improvement is almost universal within 10 days.
- Infiltrates generally clear within 5 to 8 wk.
- Rare deaths are likely attributable to underlying medical diseases.
- Person-to-person spread can be minimized by avoiding open coughing, especially in enclosed areas. Azithromycin prophylaxis can prevent infection in close contacts of patients.

REFERRAL

- Not responding to treatment
- Severe infection
- Severe extrapulmonary manifestations
- Multilobe involvement accompanied by respiratory embarrassment (very rare)

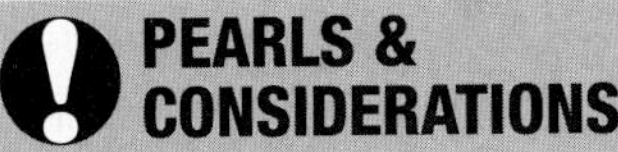

PEARLS & CONSIDERATIONS

COMMENTS

- Outbreaks occur in military recruits, group homes, nursing homes, and in the community. Between 2006 and 2013, the CDC investigated 17 sporadic cases, clusters, and local outbreaks in the U.S.
- Infection control: In the hospital these patients should be on droplet precautions.
- X-ray resolution complete by 8 wk in approximately 90% of patients.

SUGGESTED READINGS

Available at ExpertConsult.com

RELATED CONTENT

Mycoplasma Pneumonia (Patient Information)
Pneumonia, Bacterial (Related Key Topic)

AUTHOR: **GLENN G. FORT, M.D., M.P.H.**

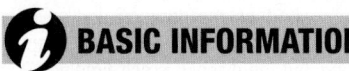

BASIC INFORMATION

DEFINITION

Pneumocystis jiroveci pneumonia (PJP) is a respiratory infection caused by the fungal pathogen *P. jiroveci* (formerly known as *P. carinii*).

SYNONYMS

Pneumocystis jiroveci pneumonia
PCP
PJP

ICD-10CM CODE
B59 Pneumocystosis

EPIDEMIOLOGY & DEMOGRAPHICS

INCIDENCE (IN U.S.):

- Approximately 95% of cases occur in HIV-infected individuals with CD4 counts <200/mm^3 who are not on prophylaxis.
- Also seen in other immunocompromised patients with severe cell-mediated immune deficiency (congenital T-cell deficiency, acute leukemia, lymphoma, bone marrow or organ transplant deficiency).
- May be associated with prednisone use (usually higher than 20 mg/day), usually in conjunction with a second immune-modulating agent.
- Rituximab use has been associated with PJP in HIV-negative patients, most of whom have hematologic cancers.

PEAK INCIDENCE: Age 20 to 40 yr (parallel to AIDS epidemic)

PREDOMINANT SEX: Equal incidence when adjusted for HIV status

PREDOMINANT AGE: 20 to 40 yr

GENETICS: Neonatal infection:

- Most frequent opportunistic infection among HIV-infected children
- Neonatal occurrence unusual

PHYSICAL FINDINGS & CLINICAL PRESENTATION

- Fever, cough, shortness of breath present in almost all cases. May be subacute or insidious in HIV patients; acute onset with rapid progression seen in non–HIV-immunocompromised patients
- Lungs frequently clear to auscultation, although rales occasionally present
- Cyanosis and pronounced tachypnea in severe cases
- Hemoptysis is unusual. Spontaneous pneumothorax is possible

ETIOLOGY

- *P. jiroveci* (formerly *P. carinii*) reclassified as a fungal organism (previously classified as a protozoan) (Fig. E1)
- Reactivation of dormant infection
- Extrapulmonary involvement rare but possible

DIAGNOSIS

DIFFERENTIAL DIAGNOSIS

- Other opportunistic respiratory infections:
    1. Tuberculosis
    2. Histoplasmosis
    3. Cryptococcosis
    4. Mycobacterium avium complex (MAC)
- Nonopportunistic infections:
    1. Bacterial pneumonia
    2. Viral pneumonia
    3. Mycoplasma pneumonia
    4. Legionella
- Occurs almost exclusively in the setting of profound depression of cellular immunity.

WORKUP

- Chest x-ray (Fig. 2) or chest CT (Fig. E3).
- Arterial blood gases.
- Because *Pneumocystis* cannot be cultured, diagnosis relies on detection of the organism by cytologic stains, direct immunofluorescent antibody test, or PCR.
- Sputum examination for cysts of PJP and to exclude other pathogens.
- Bronchoscopy with bronchoalveolar lavage or lung biopsy for diagnosis if sputum examination is negative or equivocal. PCR on lavage is very sensitive but less specific.
- Serum beta-D glucan has good negative predictive performance (very sensitive, less specific).
- Fig. 4 describes an algorithm for the diagnostic evaluation and management of patients with suspected *Pneumocystis* pneumonia.

LABORATORY TESTS

- Arterial blood gas monitoring
- Elevated lactate dehydrogenase in majority of cases
- HIV antibody test and CD4 cell count if cause of underlying immune deficiency state is unclear
- Beta-D-glucan testing may be positive (92% sensitivity, 86% specificity)

IMAGING STUDIES

PJP may appear as diffuse, unilateral, bilateral, or interstitial infiltrates on chest x-ray. CT with mixed alveolar-interstitial patterns, often with sparing of the periphery. Pneumatoceles, which may cause pneumothorax, are common.

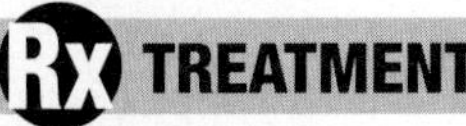

TREATMENT

NONPHARMACOLOGIC THERAPY

- Supplemental oxygen
- Ventilation support if needed
- Prompt chest tube placement if pneumothorax develops

ACUTE GENERAL Rx

For confirmed or suspected PJP:

- Trimethoprim-sulfamethoxazole (15-20 mg/kg trimethoprim and 75-100 mg/kg sulfamethoxazole qd) PO or IV per day divided and given q6 to 8h.
- Pentamidine (4 mg/kg IV qd) (severe cases with a contraindication to trimethoprim/sulfamethoxazole). Careful monitoring is required, can cause nephrotoxicity, numerous electrolyte disturbances, and cardiac arrhythmias.
- Either regimen with prednisone (40 mg PO bid):
    1. If arterial oxygen pressure <70 mm Hg.
    2. If arterial-alveolar oxygen pressure difference >35 mm Hg.
    3. Dose tapered to 20 mg bid after 5 days and 20 mg qd after 10 days.
- Therapy continued for three weeks.
- Alternative therapies available for patients unable to tolerate conventional therapy:
    1. Dapsone/trimethoprim
    2. Clindamycin/primaquine
    3. Atovaquone
- Table 1 summarizes causes of deterioration in an HIV-infected patient receiving treatment for PJP.

CHRONIC Rx

- After completion of therapy, prophylaxis should be maintained with trimethoprim-sulfamethoxazole (one single-strength tablet PO qd or double-strength three times weekly)

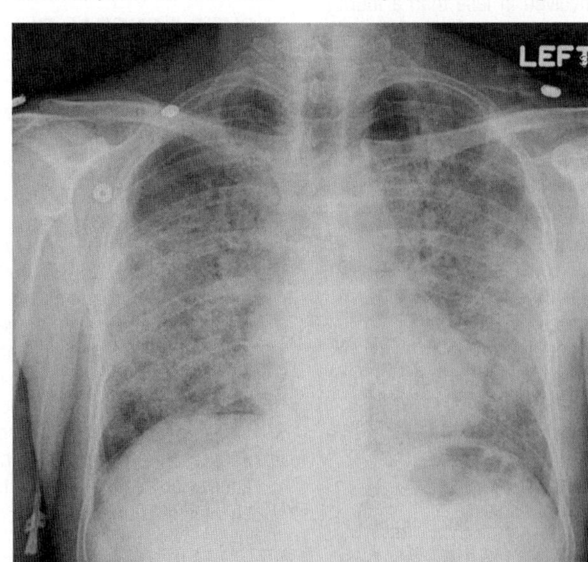

FIG. 2 Chest radiograph showing diffuse interstitial infiltrate in a patient with *Pneumocystis jiroveci* pneumonia. (From Firestein GS et al [eds]: *Kelly's textbook of rheumatology,* ed 9, Philadelphia, 2013, Saunders.)

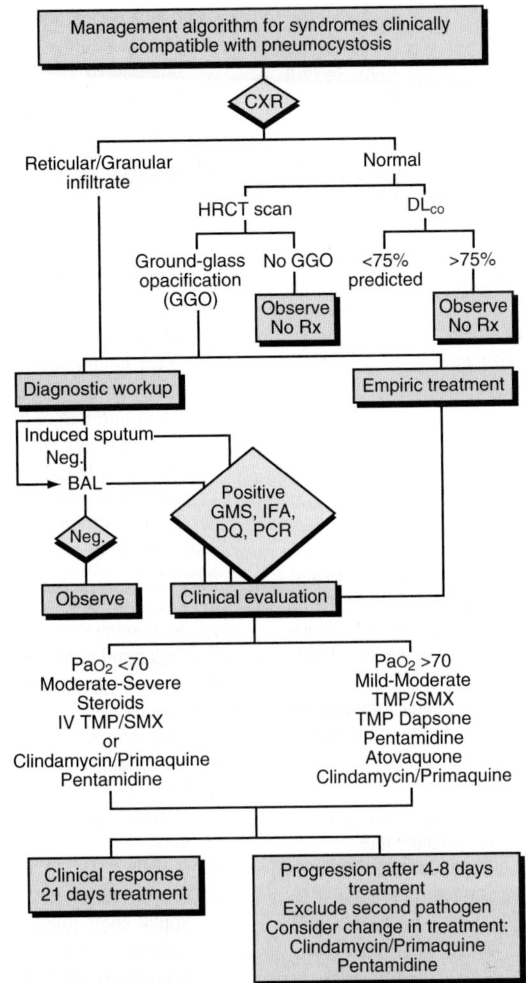

FIG. 4 Algorithm for the diagnostic evaluation and management of patients with suspected *Pneumocystis* pneumonia. *BAL*, Bronchoalveolar lavage; *CXR*, chest x-ray; *DL_{CO}*, single-breath diffusing capacity for carbon monoxide; *DQ*, Diff-Quik (stain); *GGO*, ground-glass opacities; *GMS*, Gomori methenamine silver (stain); *HRCT*, high-resolution computed tomography; *IFA*, immunofluorescent antibody (stain); *IV*, intravenous; *PCR*, polymerase chain reaction; *Rx*, treatment; *TMP/SMX*, trimethoprim-sulfamethoxazole. (Bennett JE et al: *Mandell, Douglas, and Bennett's principles and practice of infectious diseases*, ed 8, Philadelphia, 2015, WB Saunders.)

TABLE 1 Causes of Deterioration in an HIV-Infected Person Receiving Treatment for PJP

Etiology	Explanation
Severe Progressive PCP	
Iatrogenic	Pulmonary edema due to IV fluid overload when giving TMP-SMX IRIS following early initiation of ART
Side effects of therapy	Anemia (e.g., caused by TMP-SMX), methemoglobinemia (e.g., caused by dapsone, primaquine)
Inadequate therapy	Incorrect dosage or route of administration Adjuvant glucocorticoids not given for treatment of moderate or severe PCP
Postbronchoscopy	Sedation Pneumothorax
Pneumothorax	Spontaneous Associated with intubation and positive pressure ventilation
Copathology in lung	Bacterial infection Pulmonary Kaposi sarcoma Intercurrent pulmonary embolism
Wrong diagnosis	Empiric diagnosis of PCP, and correct diagnosis is another pathology (e.g., bacterial pneumonia)

ART, Antiretroviral therapy; *HIV*, human immunodeficiency virus; *IRIS*, immune reconstitution inflammatory syndrome; *IV*, intravenous; *PJP*, *Pneumocystis jiroveci* pneumonia; *TMP-SMX*, trimethoprim-sulfamethoxazole.
Bennett JE et al: *Mandell, Douglas, and Bennett's principles and practice of infectious diseases*, ed 8, Philadelphia, 2015, WB Saunders.

until the CD4 cell count is >200 for three months.
- Patients intolerant of this therapy should be treated with dapsone (100 mg PO qd) or atovaquone (1500 mg PO qd).
- Inhaled pentamidine (300 mg monthly by standardized nebulizer) is less effective and is reserved for patients intolerant to other forms of prophylaxis.

DISPOSITION

After completion of therapy, long-term ambulatory follow-up is mandatory to provide secondary prevention of PJP (see "Chronic Rx" previously) and management of the underlying immunodeficiency syndrome.

REFERRAL

- To pulmonologist for bronchoscopy if diagnosis cannot be confirmed by sputum examination.
- To an infectious disease specialist if case is severe or difficult to manage and to evaluate underlying immune deficiency.

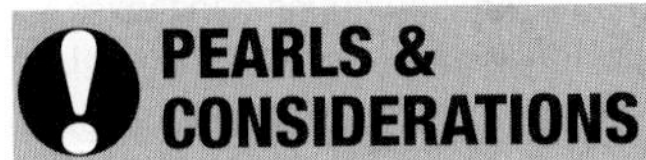

PEARLS & CONSIDERATIONS

COMMENTS

- All patients, especially those with severe infection or intolerant of conventional therapy, should be followed by a physician experienced in the management of PJP and, if appropriate, in the long-term management of HIV infection or other underlying disease.
- Severe and life-threatening hypoglycemia may occur 1 or 2 weeks after start of IV pentamidine. Monitor closely and advise the patient of symptoms of hypoglycemia.

RELATED CONTENT

Pneumocystis Pneumonia (Patient Information)
Acquired Immunodeficiency Syndrome (Related Key Topic)

AUTHOR: **SEBASTIAN KURZ, M.D.**

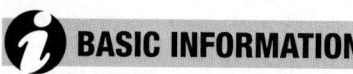

DEFINITION

Viral pneumonia is a lung infection caused by any of a large number of viral pathogens. The most important viruses are discussed in this chapter.

SYNONYMS

Viral pneumonia
Nonbacterial pneumonia

ICD-10CM CODES
J12.9 Viral pneumonia, unspecified
J12.89 Other viral pneumonia

EPIDEMIOLOGY & DEMOGRAPHICS

INCIDENCE (IN U.S.):

- Influenza virus:
  1. 10% to 20% of population in temperate zones infected during 1 to 2 mo epidemics occurring yearly during winter months.
  2. Up to 50% infected during pandemics.
  3. Secondary bacterial pneumonia develops in a small percentage of infected persons.
- Incidence of other important viral pathogens that cause pneumonia can vary widely depending on setting, geography, and testing modalities. With the more widespread use of rapid molecular testing of respiratory secretions, an increase in the detection of viral pathogens has been observed. However, drawing conclusions as to causality of the identified virus to the actual pneumonia remains challenging because respiratory viruses remain detectable for several weeks after initial infection, and the pneumonia may be due to secondary bacterial infection.

PEAK INCIDENCE:

- Influenza:
  1. Winter months for influenza A
  2. Year round for influenza B
  3. Peak of pneumonia seen weeks into the outbreak of infection
- Respiratory syncytial virus (RSV) and parainfluenza virus:
  1. Winter and spring
- Adenovirus:
  1. Endemic (military)
- Varicella:
  1. Spring in temperate zones
- Measles:
  1. Year round
- Cytomegalovirus (CMV):
  1. Year round
- Human metapneumovirus:
  1. Winter months

PREVALENCE (IN U.S.):

- Often related to immune status of the population or presence of an epidemic
- Normal hosts (estimates):
  1. 86% of cases of pneumonia resulting in hospitalization in American adults
  2. 16% of pediatric pneumonias managed as outpatients
  3. 49% of hospitalized infants with pneumonia
- Important problem in hosts with impaired immunity

PREDOMINANT SEX:

- Equal predominance.
- Male sex may predispose to more severe respiratory disease in RSV infection.

PREDOMINANT AGE:

- Influenza:
  1. Overall incidence greatest at age 5 yr
  2. Lower incidence with increasing age
  3. The most serious sequelae in those with chronic medical illnesses, especially cardiopulmonary disease
  4. Hospitalizations greatest in infants and adults aged >64 yr
- RSV and parainfluenza virus:
  1. Young children (as the major cause of pneumonia)
  2. Occurs throughout life
- Adenoviruses:
  1. Young children
  2. Adults, primarily military recruits
- Varicella:
  1. Approximately 16% of adults (not infected in childhood) who contract chickenpox
  2. Acute varicella during pregnancy more likely to be complicated by severe pneumonia
  3. 90% of reported varicella pneumonia cases are in adults (highest incidence ages 20 to 60 yr)
- Measles:
  1. Young adults and older children who received a single vaccination (5% failure rate)
  2. Measles during pregnancy more likely to be complicated by pneumonia
  3. Underlying cardiopulmonary diseases and immunosuppression predispose to serious pneumonia complicating measles
  4. Before availability of measles vaccine, 90% of pneumonias in those <10 yr
  5. Currently more than one third of patients >14 yr in the U.S.
  6. 3% to 50% of measles cases are complicated by pneumonia
- CMV:
  1. Neonatal through adult
  2. Immunosuppression is key predisposing factor
- Human metapneumovirus:
  1. Children: Peak incidence 11 mo
  2. Increasingly detected in adults (bronchitis, COPD exacerbation, pneumonia)
  3. Frequent cause of lower respiratory tract infection (LRTI) in lung transplant recipients

GENETICS: Familial disposition:

- Close contact, not genetics, is important in acquisition
- Congenital anomalies and immunosuppression worsen course of RSV pneumonia

Congenital infection:

- CMV is the most common intrauterine infection in the U.S.
- Pneumonia occurs occasionally in infants with symptomatic congenital infection

Neonatal infection:

- Severe RSV pneumonia
- Adenovirus pneumonia
  1. 5% to 20% mortality rate
  2. Can lead to residual restrictive or obstructive functional abnormalities
- "Varicella neonatorum"
  1. Disseminated visceral disease including pneumonia
  2. May develop in neonates whose mothers develop peripartum chickenpox
- CMV pneumonia
  1. Generally fatal
  2. Associated with severe cerebral damage in this population

PHYSICAL FINDINGS & CLINICAL PRESENTATION

- Influenza:
  1. Fever, cough, or sore throat (referred to as influenza-like illness [ILI])
  2. Uncomfortable or lethargic appearance
  3. Prominent dry cough (rarely hemoptysis)
  4. Flushed integument and erythematous mucous membranes
  5. Rales or rhonchi
- RSV, parainfluenza, and human metapneumovirus:
  1. Fever
  2. Tachypnea
  3. Prolonged expiration
  4. Wheezes and rales
- Adenoviruses:
  1. Hoarseness
  2. Pharyngitis
  3. Tachypnea
  4. Cervical adenitis
- Measles:
  1. Conjunctivitis
  2. Rhinorrhea
  3. Koplik spots (white lesions on the buccal mucosa)
  4. Exanthem (maculopapular rash that starts on the head, then moves down to rest of body)
  5. Pneumonitis
     a. May occur as a complication in 3% to 4% of adolescents and young adults
     b. Coincident with rash
     c. May also develop after apparent recovery from measles
  6. Fever
  7. Dry cough
- Varicella:
  1. Fever
  2. Maculopapular or vesicular rash (all lesions at the same stage)
     a. Becomes encrusted
     b. Pneumonia typical 1 to 6 days after rash appears
     c. Pneumonia (Fig. 1) accompanied by cough and occasionally hemoptysis
  3. Few auscultatory abnormalities noted on examination of the lungs
- CMV:
  1. Fever
  2. Paroxysmal cough
  3. Occasional hemoptysis
  4. Diffuse adenopathy when pneumonia occurs after transfusion

ETIOLOGY

Viral infection can lead to pneumonia in both immunocompetent and immunocompromised hosts.

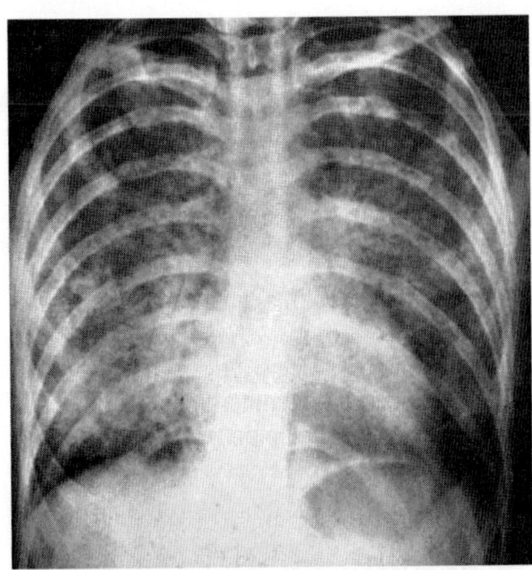

FIG. 1 This chest radiograph demonstrates bilateral nodular and interstitial pneumonia characteristic of varicella pneumonia. The patient, a 27-year-old gravida 6, para 2, abortus 3, was exposed to varicella infection in her two children. Characteristic skin vesicles of varicella occurred several days before the development of pulmonary symptoms. She required endotracheal intubation and mechanical ventilation for 6 days. She was treated with intravenous acyclovir and ceftazidime for possible superimposed infection. The patient recovered fully and delivered a healthy infant at term. (From Gabbe SG: *Obstetrics*, ed 6, Philadelphia, 2012, Saunders.)

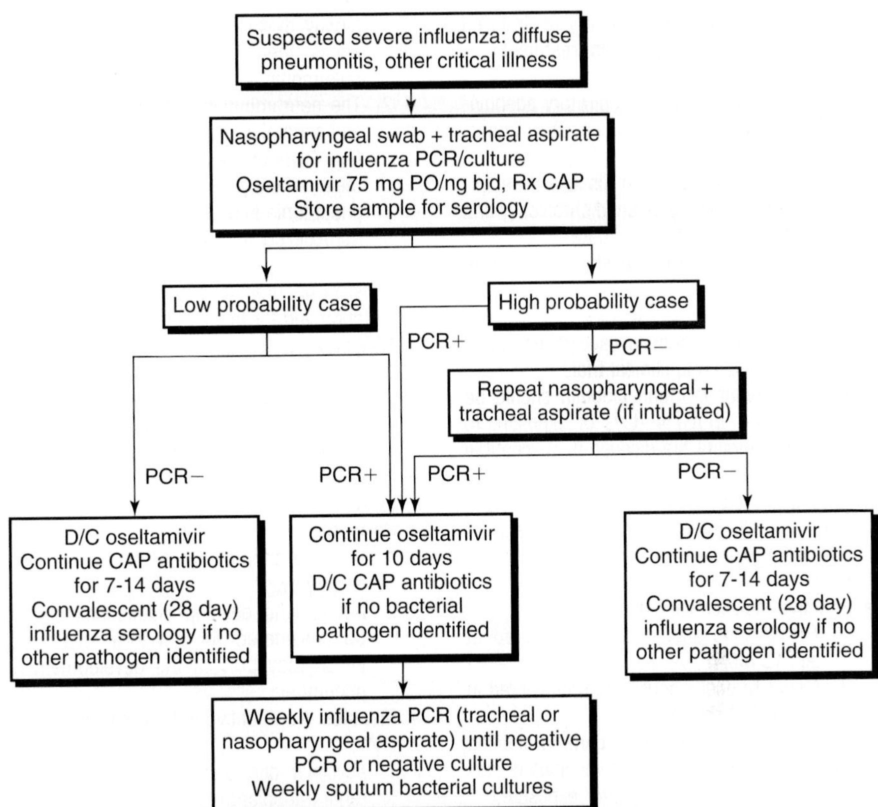

FIG. 2 Suggested algorithm in the workup and management of suspected severe influenza pneumonia in the critical care unit. *CAP,* Community-acquired pneumonia; *D/C,* discontinue; *PCR,* polymerase chain reaction; *PO,* by mouth; *Rx,* prescription. (From Vincent JL et al: *Textbook of critical care,* ed 6, Philadelphia, 2011, Saunders.)

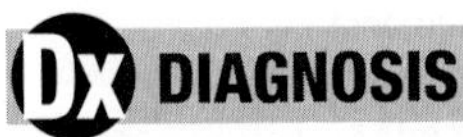

Dx DIAGNOSIS

DIFFERENTIAL DIAGNOSIS

- Bacterial pneumonia, which frequently complicates (i.e., can follow or be simultaneous with) viral pneumonia
- Other causes of atypical pneumonia:
  1. *Mycoplasma* spp.
  2. *Chlamydia* spp.
  3. *Coxiella* spp.
  4. Legionnaires' disease

  In certain patient populations (e.g., immunocompromised), consider fungal infections, tuberculosis, or atypical mycobacterium.
- Acute respiratory distress syndrome (ARDS)
- Physical findings and associated hypoxemia confused with pulmonary emboli

WORKUP

- Information about the current prevalent strain of influenza virus can be obtained from local health departments or from the Centers for Disease Control and Prevention.
- Influenza and other viruses may be cultured from respiratory secretions during the initial few days of the illness (special media and techniques necessary).
- Respiratory viral panels that use PCR-based assays to test for a variety of viruses are extremely sensitive and are becoming the test of choice.
- Rapid flu tests have a 50% sensitivity in diagnosing influenza (a negative test does not mean the patient does not have influenza).
- Measles and adenovirus pneumonia are usually diagnosed clinically and can be confirmed with serology.
- CMV may be grown in culture or PCR amplified from bronchoalveolar lavage samples. An algorithm for the workup and management of suspected severe influenza pneumonia in the critical care unit is described in Fig. 2. Open lung biopsy is required for a definite diagnosis of CMV pneumonia.

LABORATORY TESTS

- Sputum Gram stain (usually produced in scanty amounts) typically shows few polymorphonuclear leukocytes and few bacteria.
- White blood cell count may vary from leukopenic to modest elevation, usually without a leftward shift.
- Disseminated intravascular coagulation occasionally complicates adenovirus type 7 pneumonia.
- Multinucleated giant cells on Tzanck preparation of an unroofed vesicular lesion are useful in diagnosing varicella in a patient with an infiltrate (also found in herpes simplex).
- Severe immunosuppression is associated with symptomatic CMV pneumonia (usually reactivation of latent infection or in previously seronegative recipients from the donor).
- Hypoxemia may be profound.
- Cultures may be helpful in identifying superinfecting bacterial pathogens.
- When they occur, parapneumonic pleural effusions are exudative.

IMAGING STUDIES

- Chest radiographs may demonstrate a spectrum of findings from ill-defined, patchy, or generalized interstitial infiltrates, which can be associated with ARDS.
- A localized dense alveolar infiltrate suggests a superimposed bacterial pneumonia.
- Small calcified nodules may develop as a radiographic residual of varicella pneumonia.

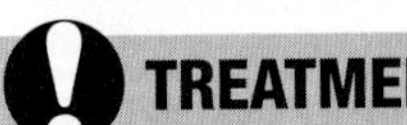

TREATMENT

NONPHARMACOLOGIC THERAPY

General:
- Measures to diminish person-to-person transmission
- Modified bed rest
- Maintenance of adequate hydration
- Possible ventilation support for severe pneumonia or ARDS

Influenza:
- Yearly prophylactic strain-specific influenza vaccination can be given to prevent infection.
- Live, attenuated influenza vaccines administered by nose drops as effective as injected inactivated viral vaccines.

RSV:
- Isolation techniques are important in limiting spread of RSV infections.

- Immunoglobulins with a high RSV-neutralizing antibody titer are beneficial in treatment.

Adenoviruses:
- Intestinal inoculation of respiratory adenoviruses has been used to successfully immunize military recruits.
- Although they produce no disease in recipients, the viruses may be shed chronically and may infect others at a later date.
- These vaccines are not available for civilian populations.

Varicella:
- Live, attenuated varicella vaccine has been successfully used in clinical trials.
- Varicella-zoster immune globulin should be administered within 4 days of exposure to prevent or modify the disease in susceptible persons.
- Nonimmunized persons exposed to varicella are potentially infectious between 10 and 21 days after exposure.

Measles:
- Effective measles vaccine is available.
    1. The vaccine should be administered at age 15 mo.
    2. A second dose should be administered at the time of school entry.
- Live, attenuated vaccine or gamma-globulin can prevent measles in unvaccinated persons if administered early after exposure.
- Vitamin A given PO for 2 days reduces morbidity and mortality rates from measles in exposed children.

ACUTE GENERAL Rx

- **General:** Administer appropriate antibiotics for bacterial superinfections.
- **Influenza:**
    1. Amantadine and rimantadine for influenza A (not active against influenza B). Early use can speed recovery from small airway dysfunction, but whether it influences the development or course of pneumonia is uncertain.
    2. The neuraminidase inhibitors oseltamivir and zanamivir are effective if given in the first 48 hours of symptoms of influenza; their efficacy in established influenza pneumonia is unclear.
    3. Aerosolized ribavirin or amantadine may have a role in treating severe influenza pneumonia, but they have not been approved for this indication.
- **RSV and parainfluenza**:
    1. Ribavirin aerosol may be effective for severe RSV pneumonia.
    2. There is no approved antiviral therapy for parainfluenza virus pneumonia.
- **Adenoviruses:** No effective agent; some case reports of cidofovir use but unproved.
- **Varicella:**
    1. Varicella pneumonia can be treated with IV acyclovir.
    2. Adults who develop chickenpox should be considered for acyclovir treatment, which may prevent the development of pneumonia.
- **Measles:** No effective antimeasles agent.
- **CMV:**
    1. Acyclovir can prevent CMV infection in renal transplant recipients.
    2. Ganciclovir and foscarnet, with or without CMV hyperimmune globulin, show promise in the treatment of serious CMV infection, including pneumonia, in compromised hosts.
- Human metapneumovirus:
    1. No specific treatment available

DISPOSITION

- Supportive therapy is useful.
- Death is possible during acute illness.
- Residual functional abnormalities may be persistent or develop into or predispose to chronic respiratory diseases in later life.
- Morbidity and mortality rates after most viral pneumonias are increased by bacterial superinfection.

REFERRAL

- Uncertainty about the diagnosis in a compromised host.
- Symptoms or findings are progressive.
- Severe respiratory compromise, diffuse infiltrates, or the development of ARDS.

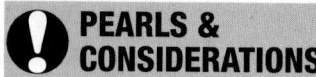

COMMENTS

- Influenza spreads by close contact and by small droplets transmitted by cough.
- RSV is effectively transmitted by fomites and by direct contact (little by aerosol).
- Varicella is transmitted by direct contact or by aerosol.
- Of the three major forms of parainfluenza viruses (types 1 to 3), type 3 is the most common cause of viral pneumonia; types 1 and 2 primarily cause laryngotracheitis.
- Human metapneumovirus is a recently identified common cause of upper respiratory infections and pneumonia.

RELATED CONTENT

Viral Pneumonia (Patient Information)
Cytomegalovirus Infection (Related Key Topic)
Influenza (Related Key Topic)
Varicella (Related Key Topic)

AUTHOR: **SEBASTIAN KURZ, M.D.**

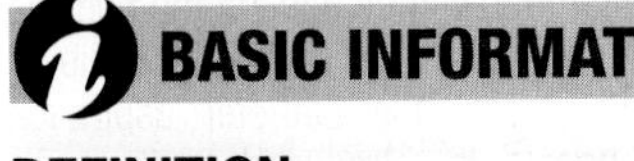

BASIC INFORMATION

DEFINITION

A spontaneous pneumothorax (SP) is defined as air in the pleural space, collapsing the lung without a precipitating event. This can be primary SP (otherwise healthy people without any obvious underlying lung disease) or secondary SP (with underlying lung disease).

SYNONYMS

Primary spontaneous pneumothorax (PSP)
Secondary spontaneous pneumothorax (SSP)
SP
PSP
SSP

ICD-10CM CODES	
J93.0	Spontaneous tension pneumothorax
J93.11	Primary spontaneous pneumothorax
J93.12	Secondary spontaneous pneumothorax
J93.81	Chronic pneumothorax
J93.83	Other pneumothorax
J93.9	Pneumothorax, unspecified
J95.811	Postprocedural pneumothorax
P25.1	Pneumothorax originating in the perinatal period
S27.0XXA	Traumatic pneumothorax, initial encounter
S27.0XXD	Traumatic pneumothorax, subsequent encounter
S27.0XXS	Traumatic pneumothorax, sequela

EPIDEMIOLOGY & DEMOGRAPHICS

- Approximately 20,000 new cases of SP occur each year in the United States.
- SP is more common in men than women (6:1).
- Incidence of primary SP is 7.4 per 100,000 in men and 1.2 per 100,000 in women.
- Incidence of secondary SP is 6.3 per 100,000 in men and 2.0 per 100,000 in women.
- SP is commonly seen in tall, thin young men aged 20 to 40 yr.
- Risk factors include smoking, family history, Marfan syndrome, homocystinuria, and thoracic endometriosis.
- Anorexia nervosa is thought to be a risk factor due to pulmonary parenchymal consequences of malnutrition.

PHYSICAL FINDINGS & CLINICAL PRESENTATION

- Sudden onset of pleuritic chest pain (90%), usually at rest and no relationship between the onset of pneumothorax and physical activity, which often becomes dull after a few hours.
- Pain is usually unilateral and can be sharp and agonizing and associated with considerable apprehension.
- Dyspnea (80%), which often resolves within 24 hr, despite persistence of pneumothorax.
- Cough (10%).
- Asymptomatic (5%); may take up to 7 days to come to medical attention.
- Tachycardia.
- Hypoxemia.
- Hypercapnia is rare because the alveolar ventilation is maintained by the contralateral lung.
- Decreased chest excursion on the affected side (Fig. 1).
- Diminished breath sounds.
- Subcutaneous emphysema may be present.
- Hyperresonance on percussion.

ETIOLOGY

- In primary SP, rupture of small blebs and bullae, usually located near the apex of the upper lobes, is a common cause.
- In secondary SP, chronic obstructive pulmonary disease is the most common cause, but it can also be associated with pneumonia, bronchogenic carcinoma, mesothelioma, sarcoidosis, tuberculosis, cystic fibrosis, and many other lung diseases. Causes of secondary spontaneous pneumothorax are summarized in Box 1.

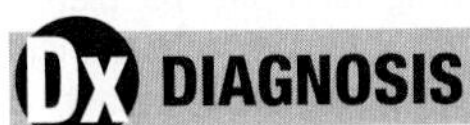

DIAGNOSIS

Established by the chest x-ray (Fig. 2)

DIFFERENTIAL DIAGNOSIS

- Pleurisy
- Pulmonary embolism
- Myocardial infarction
- Pericarditis
- Asthma
- Pneumonia

WORKUP

CXR

LABORATORY TESTS

Arterial blood gases may show hypoxemia and hypocapnia as a result of hyperventilation.

IMAGING STUDIES

- SP is usually confirmed by upright CXR:
  1. A white visceral pleural line. The absence of vessel markings peripheral to this line helps differentiate from mimicking conditions such as an overlying skin fold. A lateral width of 1 cm corresponds to 27% pneumothorax, and 2 cm occupies 49% of the hemithorax.
  2. The left lateral decubitus position is the most sensitive and the supine position the least sensitive. Inspiratory and expiratory films have equal sensitivities.
  3. As little as 50 ml of air can be detected on upright film.
- Tension pneumothorax (Fig. 3) is a medical emergency and should be suspected when the patient is hemodynamically unstable or with contralateral tracheal and mediastinal deviation and ipsilateral flattening or inversion of the diaphragm on the CXR (Fig. 4).
- CT scan is considered acceptable for a patient with recurrent pneumothorax or persistent air leak, and for planning surgery.
- Lung ultrasound has emerged as a rapid and accurate screening tool for pneumothorax. The lung point sign, a sonographic

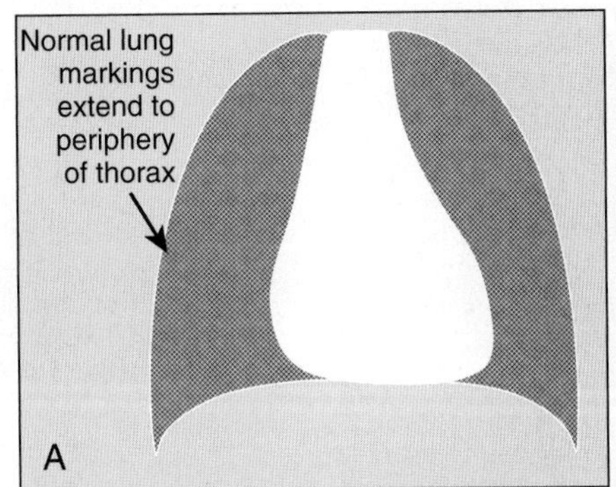

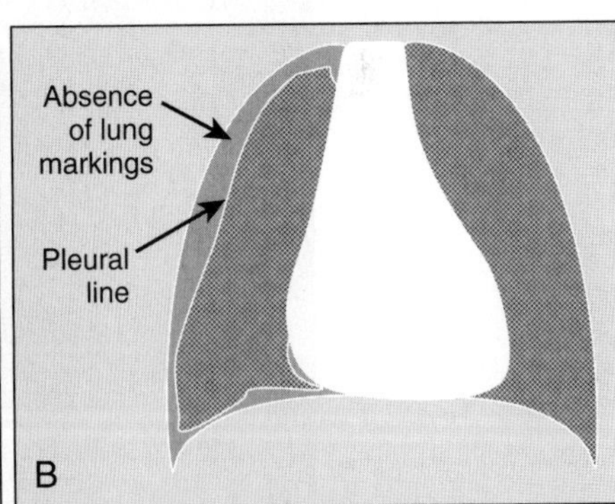

FIG. 1 Pneumothorax. A, Schematic of normal lung. **B,** Schematic of pneumothorax. Pneumothoraces can range in size from tiny to massive. Because of the variability in their size and location, pneumothoraces can be difficult to detect on chest x-ray. For example, a pneumothorax that is anterior or posterior rather than lateral may be hidden on frontal chest x-ray, particularly one taken in the supine position. An upright chest x-ray should be obtained if possible. An expiratory film is thought to be more sensitive, because the lung and thorax decrease in size during expiration, but air trapped in the pleural space remains the same size and thus appears relatively larger. Subtle pneumothoraces may not be visible on chest x-ray. In some cases, subcutaneous air may be the only visible clue to underlying lung injury. CT is extremely sensitive for pneumothorax, although controversy remains over the proper management of pneumothoraces seen only on CT. Ultrasound is also thought to be more sensitive than chest x-ray for detection of pneumothorax, although, again, the management of pneumothorax seen only on ultrasound is uncertain because this is a relatively newly described method of detection. The chest x-ray findings of pneumothorax include a lack of the normal lung markings, which should be visible to the periphery of the chest wall. Sometimes a line marking the boundary of the lung and visceral pleura is visible, although this can be confused with ribs and with the medial margin of the scapula. Depending on the degree of pneumothorax and lung collapse, the lung parenchyma may appear denser than the opposite side. In extreme cases of tension pneumothorax, the pressure exerted by the air in the pleural space may begin to displace other structures, including the diaphragm and mediastinum. In tension pneumothorax, the hyperinflated hemithorax may also have abnormally positioned ribs, with a position more horizontal than usual. (From Broder JS: *Diagnostic imaging for the emergency physician,* Philadelphia, 2011, Saunders.)

 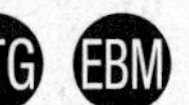

BOX 1 Causes of Secondary Spontaneous Pneumothorax

Airway Disease
Chronic obstructive pulmonary disease
Asthma
Cystic fibrosis

Infections
Necrotizing bacterial pneumonia, lung abscess
Pneumocystis jiroveci pneumonia
Tuberculosis

Interstitial Lung Disease
Sarcoidosis
Idiopathic pulmonary fibrosis
Lymphangiomyomatosis
Tuberous sclerosis
Pneumoconioses

Neoplasms
Primary lung cancers
Pulmonary or pleural metastases

Miscellaneous
Connective tissue diseases
Pulmonary infarction
Endometriosis, catamenial pneumothorax

From Marx JA et al: *Rosen's emergency medicine*, ed 8, Philadelphia, 2014, Elsevier.

representation of the point of the chest wall where the pleural layers readhere, is 100% specific to confirm the diagnosis.[1]

Rx TREATMENT

INITIAL MANAGEMENT

- 100% oxygen administration reduces the partial pressure of nitrogen in pleural capillaries, consequently quadrupling the rate of pneumothorax absorption, and should be administered to all patients with pneumothorax.
- Further treatment is based on the size of the pneumothorax.
  1. If the pneumothorax is small (<2 cm between lung and chest wall on CXR) and the patient is asymptomatic, the patient can be treated with observation alone. Repeat imaging should be performed to ensure stability/resorption of the pneumothorax.
  2. If the pneumothorax is large (>2 cm), or if the patient is symptomatic with chest pain and dyspnea, initial management should focus on removing air from the pleural space. Needle aspiration is the treatment of choice in the clinically stable patient.

[1]Aspler A et al: Double-lung point sign in traumatic pneumothorax, *Am J Emerg Med* 32:819, 2014.

- Needle aspiration can be done at the bedside using a large-bore angiocatheter needle or commercially available catheter aspiration kit. The needle is introduced in the second intercostal space midclavicular line. The catheter is left in place and attached to a three-way stopcock and a large syringe. Air is aspirated until resistance is met or the patient experiences significant coughing. Repeat CXR is done immediately after aspiration and again in 4 to 24 hours to document reexpansion of the lung. If the pneumothorax fails to resolve with aspiration, repeated aspiration is reasonable for primary spontaneous pneumothorax.
- If there is improvement but not complete resolution of pneumothorax after the aspiration, the catheter can be attached to a Heimlich (one-way) valve to allow further lung expansion. Some stable patients can be discharged home with this device in place if close follow-up monitoring can be obtained. Chest tube insertion has been recommended for patients with primary SP who are unsuccessful in controlling symptoms by simple aspiration or catheter aspiration. Most patients can be managed with small chest tubes (<12 Fr). The chest tube can be connected to a water seal device, with or without suction, and left

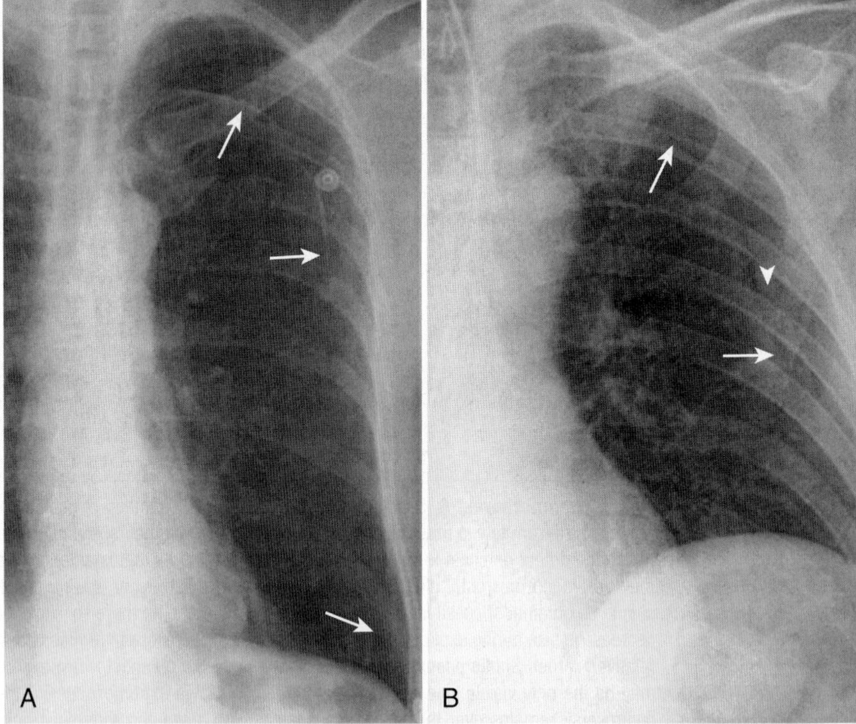

FIG. 2 A, Chest radiograph of a pneumothorax. The pleural line has lucency on either side, representing air in the pleural space on one side of the line and air in the lung on the other. The line is sharply demarcated and can be traced along its course (*lower arrow*). No blood vessels can be seen beyond the superior (*upper arrow*) and lateral (*middle arrow*) extent of the line. **B,** Chest radiograph of a skinfold (*arrows*) that could be mistaken for a pneumothorax. The border is more of an edge, with lucency on only one side. The edge is poorly defined and cannot be followed continuously (*lower arrow*). Blood vessels can be traced beyond the border of the fold (*arrowhead*). (Courtesy Michael B. Gotway, MD, Scottsdale Medical Imaging, and the Department of Radiology, University of California, San Francisco. From Mason RJ et al: *Murray & Nadel's textbook of respiratory medicine*, ed 5, Philadelphia, 2010, Saunders.)

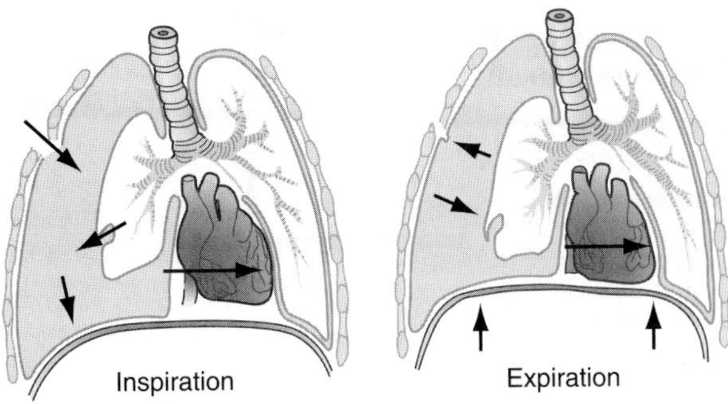

FIG. 3 Tension pneumothorax with total collapse of the right lung and shift of mediastinal structures to the left. Air is forced into the pleural space during inspiration and cannot escape during expiration. (From Marx JA et al: *Rosen's emergency medicine,* ed 8, Philadelphia, 2014, Elsevier.)

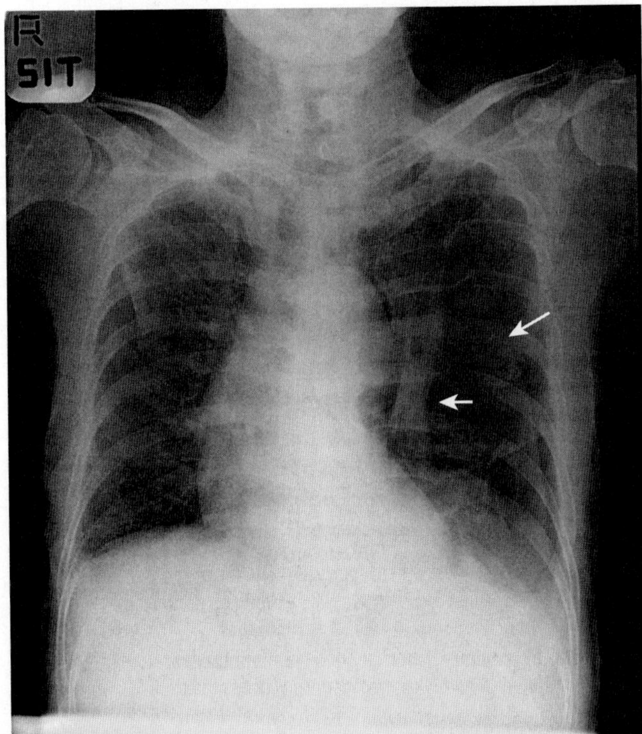

FIG. 4 Chest radiograph showing left pneumothorax with shift of the mediastinum and trachea to the right side (*white arrows*). The left lung is not completely collapsed, suggesting the presence of a loculated tension pneumothorax. (From Siu Wa Chan S: Tension pneumothorax managed without immediate needle decompression, *Am J Emerg Med* 36[3]:242–245, 2009.)

in position until the pneumothorax has resolved.

- An algorithmic approach to the treatment of primary spontaneous pneumothorax is outlined in Fig. 5.

PREVENTION

- Approximately 25% to 50% of patients with primary SP with have a recurrence within 5 yr. Recurrence rate is higher in patients with secondary spontaneous pneumothorax.
- Prevention of spontaneous pneumothorax is surgical intervention or instillation of sclerosing agents through a chest tube.
- Indication for the surgical intervention is second ipsilateral SP, first contralateral SP, simultaneous bilateral SP, persistent air leak (>5 to 7 days), failure of lung reexpansion by the chest tube, and professions at risk (e.g., pilots, divers).
- The current recommended surgical approach is the use of video-assisted thoracoscopy (VATS) with bullectomy and pleurodesis. Surgical chemical pleurodesis is best achieved with sterile talc. The overall recurrence rate is estimated at <5% after VATS.
- Instillation of a sclerosing agent through a chest tube: Doxycycline and talc slurry are the preferred agents; minocycline is considered to be an acceptable agent. The recurrence rates for the instillation of sclerosing agents (minocycline 5 mg/kg in 50 ml of normal saline or doxycycline 500 mg in 50 ml of normal saline) are higher than for VATS-guided therapy (<25%). Therefore this mode of therapy should be reserved for patients who are poor surgical candidates.

DISPOSITION

- Smoking cessation should be advised.
- Death from primary SP is uncommon. In patients with secondary SP and chronic obstructive pulmonary disease, mortality rates range from 1% to 16%.

REFERRAL

A pulmonary specialist and surgical consultation are recommended.

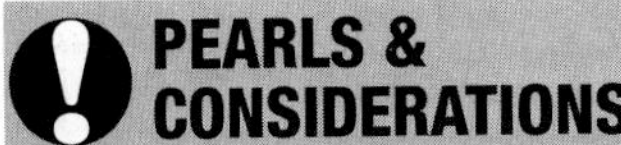

PEARLS & CONSIDERATIONS

- The rate of pleural air absorption is approximately 1.25% of the volume of the hemithorax per day. Therefore the interval for complete resolution of pneumothorax with observation can be estimated.
- Catamenial pneumothorax is a rare condition characterized by recurrent SP coinciding with the onset of menses. It usually affects the right lung and is believed to be caused by endometriosis with involvement of the diaphragm and/or pleura. It is believed to be hormonally related, and treatment is aimed at endometrial suppression.
- Air travel should be avoided until complete resolution of pneumothorax.
- Scuba diving is contraindicated. It may be considered on a case by case basis in patients who have had surgical pleurectomy.

COMMENTS

Patients with AIDS and *Pneumocystis jiroveci* infection have a high incidence of SP. Treatment typically requires chest tube placement and either thoracoscopy or open thoracotomy.

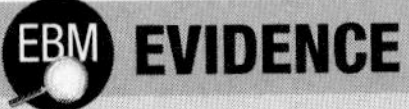

EVIDENCE

Available at ExpertConsult.com

SUGGESTED READINGS

Available at ExpertConsult.com

RELATED CONTENT

Pneumothorax (Patient Information)

AUTHOR: **HISASHI TSUKADA, M.D., PH.D.**

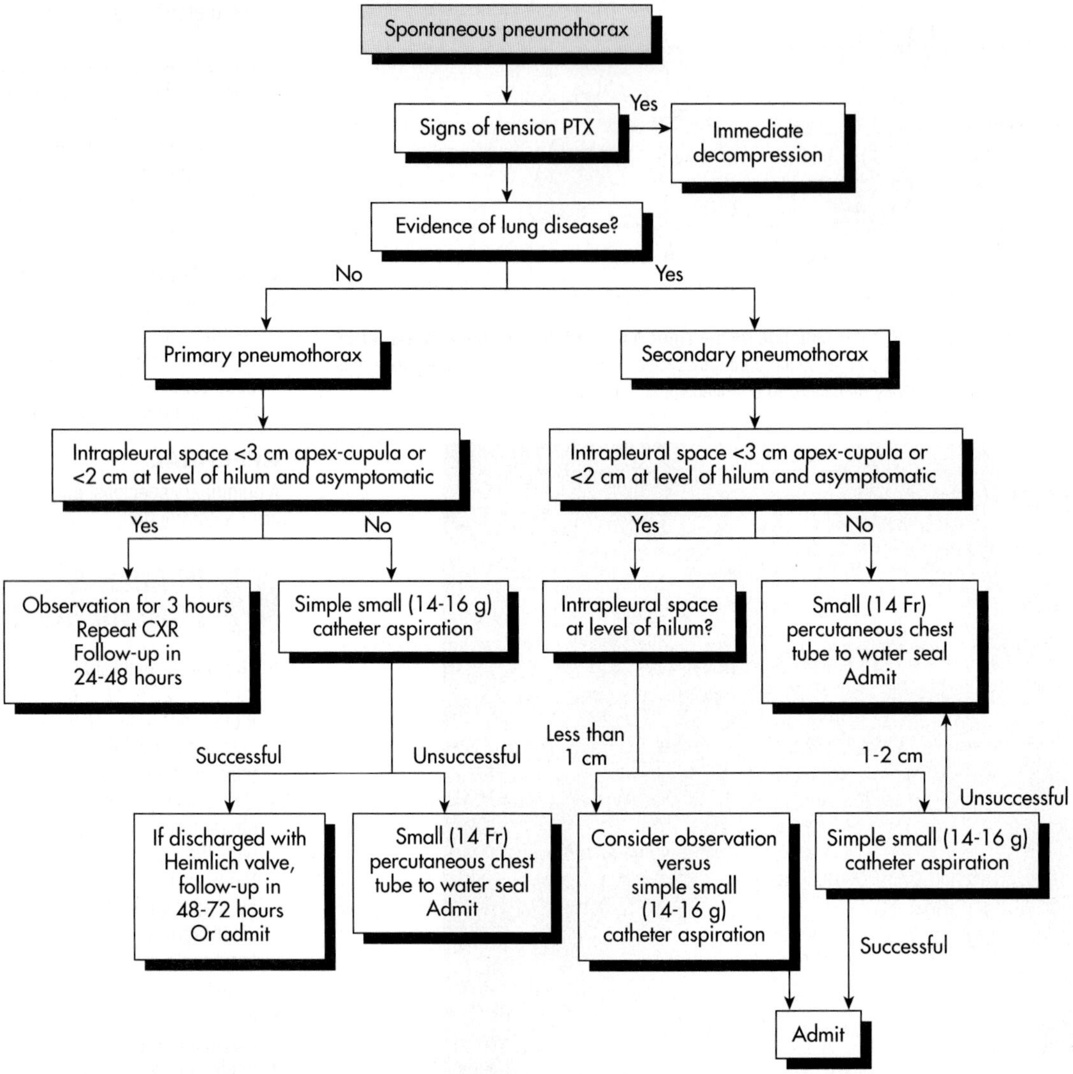

Spontaneous pneumothorax
Signs of tension PTX
Yes
Immediate decompression
Evidence of lung disease?
No
Yes
Primary pneumothorax
Secondary pneumothorax
Intrapleural space <3 cm apex-cupula or <2 cm at level of hilum and asymptomatic
Yes
No
Observation for 3 hours
Repeat CXR
Follow-up in 24-48 hours
Simple small (14-16 g) catheter aspiration
Successful
Unsuccessful
If discharged with Heimlich valve, follow-up in 48-72 hours
Or admit
Small (14 Fr) percutaneous chest tube to water seal
Admit
Intrapleural space <3 cm apex-cupula or <2 cm at level of hilum and asymptomatic
Yes
No
Intrapleural space at level of hilum?
Small (14 Fr) percutaneous chest tube to water seal
Admit
Less than 1 cm
1-2 cm
Consider observation versus simple small (14-16 g) catheter aspiration
Simple small (14-16 g) catheter aspiration
Unsuccessful
Successful
Admit

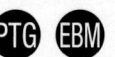

FIG. 5 Algorithmic approach to the treatment of primary spontaneous pneumothorax. *CXR*, Chest radiograph; *PTX*, pneumothorax. (From Adams JG et al: *Emergency medicine: clinical essentials,* ed 2, Philadelphia, 2013, Elsevier.)

BASIC INFORMATION

DEFINITION

Polycystic ovary syndrome (PCOS) is characterized by an accumulation of incompletely developed follicles in the ovaries due to anovulation and associated with ovarian androgen production. In its complete form, it is associated with polycystic ovaries, amenorrhea, hirsutism, and obesity. Criteria for PCOS according to published definitions are described in Table 1.

SYNONYMS

Polycystic ovarian syndrome
Stein-Leventhal syndrome
PCOS

ICD-10CM CODE
E28.2 Polycystic ovarian syndrome

EPIDEMIOLOGY & DEMOGRAPHICS

- 6% to 25% of reproductive-age women (most common endocrine disorder in this population).
- Symptoms usually begin around the time of menarche, and the diagnosis is often made during adolescence or young adulthood.
- Increased risk of endometrial and ovarian cancers.
- PCOS is the most common cause of anovulatory infertility

PHYSICAL FINDINGS & CLINICAL PRESENTATION

- Oligomenorrhea or amenorrhea
- Dysfunctional uterine bleeding
- Infertility
- Hirsutism
- Acne, alopecia, acanthosis nigricans (Fig. E1)
- Obesity (40% only), predominantly abdominal obesity
- Insulin resistance (type 2 diabetes mellitus)
- Hypertension

ETIOLOGY & PATHOGENESIS

Elevated serum luteinizing hormone (LH) concentrations and an increased serum LH/follicle-stimulating hormone (FSH) ratio result either from an increased gonadotropin-releasing hormone hypothalamic secretion or less likely from a primary pituitary abnormality. This results in dysregulation of androgen secretion and increased intraovarian androgen, the effect of which in the ovary is follicular atresia, maturation arrest, polycystic ovaries, and anovulation. Hyperinsulinemia is a contributing factor to ovarian hyperandrogenism, independent of LH excess. A role for insulin growth factor (IGF) receptors has been postulated for the association of PCOS and diabetes. Fig. E2 illustrates the pathologic mechanisms in PCOS.

Dx DIAGNOSIS

The diagnosis of PCOS excludes secondary causes (androgen-producing neoplasm, hyperprolactinemia, adult-onset congenital adrenal hyperplasia).
Clinical:
- The symptoms, signs, and biochemical features of PCOS vary greatly among women and may change over time.
- PCOS is the most common cause of chronic anovulation with estrogen present. A positive progesterone withdrawal test establishes the presence of estrogen. Medroxyprogesterone (Provera) 10 mg qd is administered for 5 days and bleeding occurs if estrogen is present.
- The presence of oligomenorrhea, hirsutism, obesity, and documented polycystic ovaries establishes the diagnosis.

DIFFERENTIAL DIAGNOSIS

Causes of amenorrhea:
- Primary (unusual in PCOS):
  1. Genetic disorder (Turner syndrome)
  2. Anatomic abnormality (e.g., imperforate hymen)
- Secondary:
  1. Pregnancy
  2. Functional (cause unknown, anorexia nervosa, stress, excessive exercise, hyperthyroidism, less commonly hypothyroidism, adrenal dysfunction, pituitary dysfunction, severe systemic illness, drugs such as oral contraceptives, estrogens, or dopamine agonists)
  3. Abnormalities of the genital tract (uterine tumor, endometrial scarring, ovarian tumor)

LABORATORY TESTS

- Glucose tolerance test at the initial presentation and every 2 yr thereafter (rule out diabetes mellitus). Impaired glucose tolerance is very common, occurring in approximately 30% of women with PCOS
- Fasting lipid panel (rule out dyslipidemia), alanine aminotransferase, aspartate aminotransferase (rule out hepatic steatosis)
- Elevated LH/FSH ratio >2.5
- Prolactin level elevation in 25%
- Elevated androgens (testosterone [free and total levels], DHEA-S) (rule out androgen-secreting tumor)
- Other: Thyroid-stimulating hormone (rule out hypothyroidism), 17-hydroxyprogesterone (rule out congenital adrenal hyperplasia), 24-hr urine for cortisol and creatinine (rule out Cushing's syndrome)
- TSH
- Table 2 summarizes laboratory testing to exclude other causes of ovulatory dysfunction and hyperandrogenism

IMAGING STUDIES

Pelvic ultrasound (Fig. E3) reveals the presence of twofold to fivefold ovarian enlargement with a thickened tunica albuginea, thecal hyperplasia, and 20 or more subcapsular follicles from 1 to 15 mm in diameter. It is important to note that having polycystic ovaries alone does not make the diagnosis of PCOS because 20% of women with polycystic ovaries have no symptoms.

TABLE 1 Criteria for Polycystic Ovary Syndrome According to Published Definitions

	NICHD/NIH/1990	Rotterdam 2003	AE-PCOS/2009
Diagnostic criteria	Requires simultaneous presence of: • Clinical and/or biochemical hyperandrogenism • Menstrual dysfunction	Requires the presence of at least two criteria: • Clinical and/or biochemical hyperandrogenism • Ovulatory dysfunction • PCOM	Requires the presence of: • Hyperandrogenism and/or hyperandrogenemia • Ovarian dysfunction: Oligoovulation or anovulation and/or polycystic ovaries
Exclusion criteria	Congenital adrenal hyperplasia, androgen-secreting tumors, Cushing's syndrome, and hyperprolactinemia	Congenital adrenal hyperplasia, androgen-secreting tumors, and Cushing's syndrome	21-hydroxylase-deficient nonclassic adrenal hyperplasia, androgen-secreting neoplasms, androgenic–anabolic drug use or abuse, the hyperandrogenic-insulin resistance-acanthosis nigricans syndrome, thyroid dysfunction, and hyperprolactinemia
Clinical traits	Hirsutism, acne, and alopecia	Hirsutism, acne, and androgenic alopecia	Hirsutism
PCOM	Not included	At least one ovary showing either: • Twelve or more follicles of 2-9 mm in diameter • Ovarian volume, 10 ml	At least one ovary showing either: • Twelve or more follicles of 2-9 mm in diameter • Ovarian volume, 10 ml

AE-PCOS, Androgen Excess and PCOS Society; *NICHD/NIH,* National Institute for Child Health and Human Development/National Institutes of Health; *PCOM,* polycystic ovarian morphology.
From Fielding JR et al: *Gynecologic imaging,* Philadelphia, 2011, Saunders.

TABLE 2 Laboratory Testing to Exclude Other Causes of Ovulatory Dysfunction and Hyperandrogenism

Lab	Evaluation for:	Comment
Total and/or bioavailable testosterone	Androgen-secreting tumor	Measure if there are symptoms concerning for an androgen-secreting tumor or if biochemical evidence of hyperandrogenism is needed to make the diagnosis of polycystic ovary syndrome. Rapid progression or a total testosterone >200 ng/dl should prompt a workup for an androgen-secreting tumor.
Dehydroepiandrosterone sulfate	Androgen-secreting tumor	Measure if there are symptoms concerning for an androgen-secreting tumor. Although modest elevations in dehydroepiandrosterone sulfate can be seen in polycystic ovary syndrome, rapid progression or greater elevations should prompt a workup for an adrenal androgen-secreting tumor.
Morning 17-hydroxyprogesterone	Late-onset congenital adrenal hyperplasia	This disorder is caused by a partial adrenal enzyme defect that leads to impaired cortisol production, compensatory elevation in adrenocorticotropic hormone, and subsequent excess androgen production. Symptoms may mimic polycystic ovary syndrome. Normal values <200 ng/dl. If higher than this, adrenocorticotropic hormone stimulation test recommended.
24-hour urine for cortisol and creatinine; dexamethasone suppression test; salivary cortisol	Cushing's syndrome	Consider ruling out Cushing's syndrome in women with an abrupt change in menstrual pattern, later-onset hirsutism, or other evidence of cortisol excess such as hypertension, facial plethora, supraclavicular fullness, hyperpigmented striae, and fragile skin.
Prolactin	Hyperprolactinemia	May be accompanied by galactorrhea. Consider ruling this out in all women with irregular menstrual cycles.
Thyroid function studies	Hyperthyroidism or hypothyroidism	Consider ruling out thyroid dysfunction in all women with irregular menstrual cycles.

From Setji TL, Brown AJ: Polycystic ovary syndrome: update on diagnosis and treatment, *Am J Med* 127:912-919, 2014.

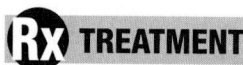

TREATMENT

The goal is to interrupt the self-perpetuating abnormal hormone cycle:

- Reduction of ovarian androgen secretion by laparoscopic ovarian wedge resection. Laparoscopic ovarian surgery (laparoscopic ovarian drilling [LOD]) is a useful alternative that does not trigger ovarian hyperstimulation.
- Reduction of ovarian androgen secretion by using oral contraceptives or LH-releasing hormone (LHRH) analogs.
- Weight reduction for all obese women with PCOS. Loss of abdominal fat seems to be crucial to restore ovulation.
- FSH stimulation with clomiphene HMG or pulsatile LHRH.
- Urofollitropin (pure FSH) administration.
- Metformin improves ovulation, insulin sensitivity, and possibly hyperandrogenemia.

Choice of treatment:

- The management of hirsutism without risking pregnancy includes oral contraceptives, glucocorticoids, LHRH analogs, or spironolactone (an antiandrogen). Finasteride and flutamide may be similarly effective in reducing hirsutism as spironolactone.
- Pregnancy can be achieved with clomiphene (alone or with glucocorticoids, human chorionic gonadotropin, or bromocriptine), HMG, urofollitropin, pulsatile LHRH, or ovarian wedge resection. Metformin may also induce ovulation. Recent trials comparing the aromatase inhibitor letrozole to clomiphene for infertility have shown higher live-birth and ovulation among infertile women with PCOS treated with letrozole. When considering in vitro fertilization (IVF), the transfer of fresh embryos is generally preferred over the transfer of frozen embryos; however, a recent trial among infertile women with PCOS undergoing IVF revealed that frozen-embryo transfer is associated with a higher rate of live birth, a lower risk of the ovarian hyperstimulation syndrome, and a higher risk of preeclampsia after the first transfer than with fresh-embryo transfer.[1]
- Psychological screening for depression is recommended. Women with PCOS are fourfold more likely to have abnormal depression scores.
- Table 3 describes a mnemonic for assessment and management of PCOS.

DISPOSITION

- Table 4 summarizes metabolic complications in PCOS.

SUGGESTED READINGS

Available at ExpertConsult.com

RELATED CONTENT

Polycystic Ovarian Syndrome (Patient Information)
Amenorrhea (Related Key Topic)
Dysfunctional Uterine Bleeding (Related Key Topic)

AUTHOR: **FRED F. FERRI, M.D.**

[1] Chen ZJ et al: Fresh versus frozen embryos for infertility in the polycystic ovary syndrome, *N Engl J Med* 375:523–533, 2016.4

TABLE 3 MY PCOS: Mnemonic for Assessment and Management of Polycystic Ovary Syndrome (PCOS)

	Assessment	Management
Metabolic	2-hour glucose tolerance test with 75 grams oral glucose, measuring serum glucose at time 0 and 120 min. Lipid profile Liver function tests (if other risk factors for nonalcoholic fatty liver disease)	Lifestyle intervention: Diet, exercise, and weight loss (if overweight or obese) Metformin for abnormal glucose tolerance not controlled with lifestyle Statin therapy if patient meets criteria (Adult Treatment Panel-III or American College of Cardiology/American Heart Association guidelines)
Cycle control	Ask about menstrual pattern; normal cycle length is 28 days (range 21-35)	If amenorrhea for 3 months or more, induce withdrawal bleed with progesterone (after negative pregnancy test) Hormonal therapy Examples: • Estrogen-containing oral contraceptives (monthly cycling, seasonal cycling, continuous use) • Vaginal ring • Patch • Progestin-only pill (smokers, hypertension) • Progestin-eluting intrauterine device (Mirena) • Progesterone prn to induce withdrawal bleeding (medroxyprogesterone acetate 10 mg daily for 10-14 days, micronized progesterone 400 mg daily for 10-14 days) • Metformin (second-line therapy)
Psychosocial	Screen for depression, disordered eating Affirm that polycystic ovary syndrome is an important medical issue; provide nonjudgmental support Discuss stress management Reinforce self-care behaviors	Mental health referral and/or antidepressant therapy may be warranted if depression or disordered eating is identified
Cosmetic	Ferriman-Gallwey score as guide to assess hirsutism Evaluate for acne and male pattern hair loss Serum androgen levels if uncertain about degree of hirsutism or atypical symptoms	Estrogen-containing hormonal contraception Antiandrogens such as spironolactone or finasteride. Teratogenic; only use with contraception) Cyproterone acetate (not available in the U.S.) Eflornithine hydrochloride 13.9% cream Laser or electrolysis Topical treatment for acne Minoxidil 2.5% or 5% for male pattern hair loss
Ovulation and fertility	Counsel that fertility is reduced in polycystic ovary syndrome, but patients typically not infertile Assess fertility goals	If subfertility is an issue, consider referral to Reproductive Endocrine for possible clomiphene citrate therapy Metformin has limited role
Sleep apnea	Screen for sleep apnea: Daytime somnolence, morning headache, reflux symptoms, snoring, observed interrupted breathing	Refer for sleep study Continuous positive airway pressure therapy recommended if sleep apnea diagnosed

PCOS, Polycystic ovary syndrome.
From Setji TL, Brown AJ: Polycystic ovary syndrome: Update on diagnosis and treatment, *Am J Med* 127:912–919, 2014.

TABLE 4 Metabolic Complications in Polycystic Ovary Syndrome

Abnormal glucose tolerance (impaired glucose tolerance or type 2 diabetes)	30% of obese polycystic ovary syndrome women have impaired glucose tolerance, and 10% have type 2 diabetes by age 40. In thin women with polycystic ovary syndrome, 10% have impaired glucose tolerance, and 1.5% have type 2 diabetes.
Obesity	Prevalence of obesity varies considerably in women with polycystic ovary syndrome. Previously, prevalence rates of obesity were estimated based on populations of women with polycystic ovary syndrome seeking care. A recent study comparing patients presenting for care in a polycystic ovary syndrome clinic with an unselected population evaluated during a preemployment physical suggests that obesity and overweight may not be more common in polycystic ovary syndrome. In that study, 63.7% of polycystic ovary syndrome clinic patients were obese, compared with 28% of unselected women with polycystic ovary syndrome identified during screening, and 28% of nonpolycystic ovary syndrome controls. Polycystic ovary syndrome symptoms, including hyperandrogenism and oligo-ovulation, are exacerbated by obesity.
Metabolic syndrome	33%-50% of U.S. women with polycystic ovary syndrome have metabolic syndrome compared to only 12% in a similarly aged National Health and Nutrition Examination Survey population. In contrast, only 8.2% of women with polycystic ovary syndrome in Italy met criteria for metabolic syndrome. Thus, metabolic syndrome varies by geographic location, a finding likely related to different body mass index, though other causes including genetics and diet could also be playing a part.
High blood pressure	Data have been conflicting, but a large Kaiser Permanente study demonstrated that hypertension or elevated blood pressure was more than twice as common in women with polycystic ovary syndrome (27% vs. 12%).
Dyslipidemia	Dyslipidemia is more prevalent in women with polycystic ovary syndrome compared to controls (15% vs. 6%). In a meta-analysis, triglyceride values were 26 mg/dl higher (95% CI 17-35), low-density lipoprotein cholesterol was 12 mg/dl higher (95% CI 10-16), and high-density lipoprotein-cholesterol was 6 mg/dl lower (95% CI 4-9) in women with polycystic ovary syndrome compared with controls. Women with polycystic ovary syndrome also have higher concentrations and proportions of small, dense low-density lipoprotein cholesterol.
Nonalcoholic fatty liver disease and nonalcoholic steatohepatitis	Nonalcoholic fatty liver disease and nonalcoholic steatohepatitis have recently been recognized as a potential complication in women with polycystic ovary syndrome. Prevalence of fatty liver disease in polycystic ovary syndrome women has been estimated to be 15%-55%, depending on the diagnostic parameter used (level of serum alanine aminotransferase or ultrasound). Individuals that may be at higher risk of nonalcoholic fatty liver disease including nonalcoholic steatohepatitis include those with metabolic syndrome, insulin resistance, and possibly hyperandrogenemia.
Cardiovascular disease	Many studies demonstrate abnormal surrogate markers of cardiovascular disease in women with polycystic ovary syndrome. However, data regarding cardiovascular disease risk are conflicting with some studies suggesting an increased risk in women with polycystic ovary syndrome, whereas other studies have not found this difference in cardiovascular risk. While it is important to recognize and treat cardiovascular risk factors in this population, further research of cardiovascular risk and complications is still needed to clarify the long-term risk.

CI, Confidence interval.
From Setji TL, Brown AJ: Polycystic ovary syndrome: update on diagnosis and treatment, *Am J Med* 127:912–919, 201

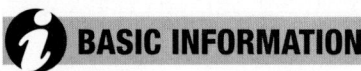

BASIC INFORMATION

DEFINITION

Polycythemia vera is a clonal disorder of aberrant myeloid/erythroid stem cells resulting in erythropoietin-independent proliferation of erythrocytes.

SYNONYMS

PV
Primary polycythemia

ICD-10CM CODE
D45 Polycythemia vera

EPIDEMIOLOGY & DEMOGRAPHICS

INCIDENCE:
- 1 case per 100,000 persons.
- Occurs most commonly in patients ages 50 to 75 yr.
- Mean age at onset is 60 yr; men are affected more often than are women.

PHYSICAL FINDINGS & CLINICAL PRESENTATION

Polycythemia vera has a latent, proliferative, and spent phase. The patient generally comes to medical attention because of symptoms associated with increased blood volume and viscosity or impaired platelet function:
- Impaired cerebral circulation resulting in headache, vertigo, blurred vision, dizziness, transient ischemic attack, cerebrovascular accident
- Fatigue, poor exercise tolerance
- Pruritus, particularly after bathing (caused by overproduction of histamine)
- Bleeding: Epistaxis, upper gastrointestinal bleeding (increased incidence of peptic ulcer disease)
- Abdominal discomfort from splenomegaly; hepatomegaly may be present
- Hyperuricemia may result in nephrolithiasis and gouty arthritis
- Up to 40% of patients experience arterial or venous thrombosis during the course of their disease. Cerebral and splanchnic thrombotic events occur commonly and can be presenting events.

The physical examination may reveal:
- Facial plethora, congestion of oral mucosa, ruddy complexion
- Enlargement and tortuosity of retinal veins
- Erythromelalgia—painful redness, swelling, and warmth of the skin of the hands and feet
- Splenomegaly (found in >75% of patients)

DIAGNOSIS

DIFFERENTIAL DIAGNOSIS

Smoking:
- Polycythemia is caused by increased carboxyhemoglobin, resulting in left shift in the hemoglobin (Hgb) dissociation curve.
- Laboratory evaluation shows increased hematocrit (Hct), RBC mass, erythropoietin level, and carboxyhemoglobin.
- Splenomegaly is not present on physical examination.

Hypoxemia (secondary polycythemia):
- Living for prolonged periods at high altitudes, pulmonary fibrosis, congenital cardiac lesions with right-to-left shunts.
- Laboratory evaluation shows decreased arterial oxygen saturation and elevated erythropoietin level.
- Splenomegaly is not present on physical examination.

Erythropoietin-producing states:
- Renal cell carcinoma, hepatoma, cerebral hemangioma, uterine fibroids, polycystic kidneys.
- The erythropoietin level is elevated in these patients, and the arterial oxygen saturation is normal.
- Splenomegaly may be present with metastatic neoplasms.

Stress polycythemia (Gaisböck syndrome, relative polycythemia):
- Laboratory evaluation demonstrates normal RBC mass, arterial oxygen saturation, and erythropoietin level; plasma volume is decreased.
- Splenomegaly is not present on physical examination.

Hemoglobinopathies associated with high oxygen affinity:
- An abnormal oxyhemoglobin-dissociation curve (P50) is present.

WORKUP

PV is suspected when the hemoglobin level exceeds 18.5 g/dl in men or 16.5 g/dl in women after secondary causes have been excluded. A single, acquired point mutation in the Janus kinase 2 *(JAK2)* gene is detected in approximately 99% of patients with polycythemia vera and can be used for diagnostic purposes. The exon 14 JAK2V617F mutation is seen in 97% cases and the remainder 3% of JAK2 mutations are spread across exons 12, 13, and 14. Testing for the *JAK2 V617F* mutation with polymerase chain reaction assay is routine. In patients with high hematocrit (>52% in men or >48% in women) and in the absence of coexisting secondary erythrocytosis, the presence of a *JAK2* mutation is sufficient for the diagnosis of polycythemia vera.

The World Health Organization diagnostic criteria for polycythemia vera are described in Table 1.

LABORATORY TESTS

- Elevated RBC count (>6 million/mm^3), elevated Hgb (>18.5 g/dl in men, >16.5 g/dl in women), elevated Hct (<54% in men, <49% in women)
- Increased white blood cell count (often with basophilia; basophilia is a strong predictor of PV instead of a reactive state); thrombocytosis is found in the majority of patients
- Elevated leukocyte alkaline phosphatase, serum vitamin B_{12}, and uric acid levels were used previously but have been supplanted by molecular testing
- Low serum erythropoietin level
- Peripheral blood smear: May reveal basophils or immature myeloid forms
- Bone marrow aspiration revealing RBC hyperplasia (Fig. E1) and absent iron stores

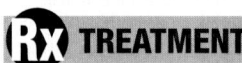

TREATMENT

NONPHARMACOLOGIC THERAPY

Phlebotomy to keep Hct >45% in men and >42% in women is the mainstay of therapy. Phlebotomy, however, has no effect on the development of myelofibrosis.

ACUTE GENERAL Rx

- Add aspirin in patients younger than 60 yr without prior thromboembolic event.
- Hydroxyurea can be used in conjunction with phlebotomy in patients older than 60 years to decrease the incidence of thrombotic events.
- Interferon-alpha-2b is effective in controlling RBC values without significant side effects.
- Box 1 describes an algorithm for management of patients with polycythemia vera.
- Ruxolitinib, a Janus kinase (JAK) 1 and 2 inhibitor, is superior to standard therapy in controlling the hematocrit, reducing the spleen volume and improving symptoms associated with polycythemia vera.

CHRONIC Rx

- Patient education regarding need for lifelong monitoring and treatment.

TABLE 1 World Health Organization 2008 Diagnostic Criteria for Polycythemia Vera

Major Criteria

1. Hemoglobin (Hgb) >18.5 g/dl (men), >16.5 (women); *or* Hgb or hematocrit (Hct) >99% reference range for age, sex, or altitude of residence; *or* Hgb >17 g/dl (men), >15 g/dl (women) if associated with a sustained increase of ≥2 g/dl from baseline that cannot be attributed to correction of iron deficiency; *or* elevated red cell mass (>25% above mean normal predicted value)
2. Presence of *JAK2 V617F* or similar mutation

Minor Criteria

1. Bone marrow trilineage myeloproliferation
2. Subnormal serum erythropoietin level
3. Endogenous erythroid colony formation in vitro

Either both major criteria and one minor criterion *or* the first major criterion and two minor criteria must be met for diagnosis of polycythemia vera.

From Andreoli TE et al: *Andreoli and Carpenter's Cecil essentials of medicine,* ed 8, Philadelphia, 2010, Saunders.

BOX 1 Algorithm for Management of Patients With Polycythemia Vera

Low-Risk Young Patients (Age <60 Yr) and No History of Thrombosis, Platelet Count <1.5 × 10^6 mm^{-3}

Phlebotomy + low-dose aspirin (81 mg/day) to maintain hematocrit lower than 45%. Aspirin should not be used in patients with histories of a hemorrhagic episode or with extreme thrombocytosis (>1.5 × 10^6 mm^{-3}) or acquired von Willebrand's syndrome.

↓

Thrombosis or hemorrhage
Systemic symptoms
Severe pruritus refractory to histamine antagonists
Painful splenomegaly

↓

Hydroxyurea 15-20 mg/kg (unless age <40 yr, pregnant, intolerant to hydroxyurea; consider pegylated interferon [IFN])

↓

Pegylated IFN 45-180 μg/wk or IFN-α (3 × 10^6 units three times a week; alter dose depending on response and toxicity) or ruxolitinib 10 mg twice daily and titrate dose depending on the response. →

In a patient with a prior thrombosis or a history of bleeding due to acquired von Willebrand's syndrome, normalization of platelet numbers is necessary. If platelet control is inadequate or the patient cannot tolerate interferon, one option is the use of anagrelide. In this case, supplemental phlebotomy is required to maintain hematocrit lower than 45%, and the use of hydroxyurea should be considered, especially if the patient continues to have thrombotic episodes.

↓

If the patient has increasing splenomegaly, systemic symptoms, or repeated thromboses despite adequate dose of hydroxyurea (2-3 g/day) or if unable to tolerate hydroxyurea, start ruxolitinib 10 mg twice daily and titrate up or down based on hematologic parameters.

For patients unable to tolerate ruxolitinib or resistant to it, start low doses of busulphan or melphalan, which should be administered until the blood counts are normalized. Therapy should be then discontinued because patients frequently enjoy drug-free prolonged remissions lasting months. Therapy should be reinstituted only at the time the blood counts begin to be elevated again. Such therapy with alkylating agents should be rarely used in young patients. It should be mentioned that the sequential use of hydroxyurea and alkylating agents may be associated with an increased risk of leukemia. Supplemental phlebotomy may be required.

Painful splenomegaly

↓

Patients should be treated with ruxolitinib
If unable to tolerate or insufficient response
Splenectomy + continued systemic therapy

↓

High-risk patients (age >60 years), previous thrombosis, platelet count >1.5 × 10^6 mm^{-3}
Phlebotomy to hematocrit of 45%
Aspirin (81 mg/day) to be given only in patients with platelet counts <1.5 × 10^6 mm^{-2}
Myelosuppressive therapy with hydroxyurea 30 mg/kg orally for 1 week
Then 15-20 mg/kg

↓

If patient continues to have thrombotic episodes and has extreme thrombocytosis or cannot tolerate hydroxyurea

Consider pegylated IFN 45-180 μg/week, anagrelide, or ruxolitinib 10 mg twice daily, or add intermittent busulphan or melphalan (in older patients).

If on busulphan or melphalan, stop when blood counts are normalized or platelet count is lower than 300,000 mm^{-3}.

Occasional supplemental phlebotomy if hematocrit is >45%; when patient relapses (patient is symptomatic), initiate busulphan therapy again at same dose.

Patient Age >70 Yr

Phlebotomy + low-dose aspirin + hydroxyurea

↓

No response or poor compliance
Ruxolitinib, melphalan, or busulfan.

From Hoffman R et al: *Hematology, basic principles and practice,* ed 7, Philadelphia, 2018, Elsevier.

- Adjunctive therapy: Treatment of pruritus with antihistamines, control of significant hyperuricemia with allopurinol, reduction of gastric hyperacidity with antacids of H_2 blockers, low-dose aspirin to treat vasomotor symptoms in patients without bleeding diathesis. Low-dose aspirin can safely prevent thrombotic complications in patients with polycythemia vera and should be given to all patients in absence of contraindications.

DISPOSITION

- The median survival time without treatment is 6 to 18 mo after diagnosis; phlebotomy extends the average survival time to 12 yr.
- Patients with polycythemia vera with a hematocrit <45% have a significantly lower rate of cardiovascular death and major thrombosis than those with hematocrit of 45% to 50%.
- Prognosis is worse in patients >60 yr and those with a history of thrombosis.

SUGGESTED READINGS

Available at ExpertConsult.com

RELATED CONTENT

Polycythemia Vera (Patient Information)

AUTHOR: **BHARTI RATHORE, M.D.**

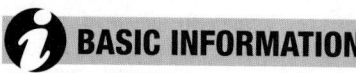

BASIC INFORMATION

DEFINITION

Polymyalgia rheumatica (PMR) is an inflammatory condition characterized by neck, shoulder, and pelvic girdle muscle pain and stiffness, which is worse in the morning, and primarily affects the elderly. PMR can occur alone or in conjunction with giant cell arteritis (GCA).

SYNONYMS

Anarthritic rheumatoid syndrome
PMR

ICD-10CM CODE

M35.3 Polymyalgia rheumatica

EPIDEMIOLOGY & DEMOGRAPHICS

INCIDENCE/PREVALENCE: In the U.S., incidence is 52.5 cases per 100,000; increases with advancing age. Prevalence is 0.5% to 0.7%. Scandinavian and Northern European populations have higher incidence.
PREDOMINANT SEX: Female:male ratio of 2:1.
PREDOMINANT AGE: Almost exclusively occurs above age 50, with peak incidence between seventh and eighth decades.

PHYSICAL FINDINGS & CLINICAL PRESENTATION

- Patients with PMR often have symptoms for 1 to 3 mo before a diagnosis is made.
- Onset of symmetric muscle aching and stiffness, worse in the morning. Stiffness recurs with periods of inactivity.
- Neck, shoulders, lower back, hips, thighs, and occasionally trunk and arms are involved. Shoulders are usually affected first.
- Constitutional symptoms of fatigue, malaise, weight loss, loss of appetite, and low-grade fever may accompany pain and stiffness.
- Physical exam may reveal limited range of motion of shoulder (most common), cervical spine, and hips. May have subdeltoid and subacromial bursitis and peripheral joint synovitis. Motor exam is normal, although can be limited by pain.
- High-spiking fevers, night sweats, visual disturbances, headaches, or jaw claudication should raise suspicion of giant cell arteritis and be further evaluated.

ETIOLOGY

The cause is unknown, but both PMR and GCA are associated with HLA-DR4 haplotype. High levels of IL-6 are associated with increased disease activity.

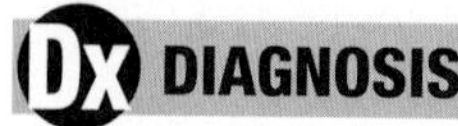

DIAGNOSIS

DIFFERENTIAL DIAGNOSIS

See Box 1.

WORKUP

- Initial laboratory evaluation: ESR, CRP, CBC, CPK.
- ESR >40 in majority of patients. CRP elevation may be more common than high ESR.
- CBC may show a normocytic anemia and thrombocytosis.
- CPK is normal. Antibodies (ANA, RF, CCP) are typically negative.
- An algorithm for diagnosing polymyalgia rheumatica without giant cell arteritis (GCA) is described in Fig. E1, and Table 1 describes classification criteria for PMR.
- Use of ultrasonography or MRI of the shoulders and hips may identify bursitis or bicipital tenosynovitis, features of the 2012 PMR classification of criteria, which increase sensitivity and specificity.

Rx TREATMENT

TREATMENT

- Prednisone 15 to 20 mg/day, with dramatic improvement usually within 3 days, but up to one third of patients may have an incomplete response at 4 weeks.
- Dose adjustment may be necessary for weight, symptom severity, and comorbidities (e.g., diabetes mellitus, hypertension, or heart failure).
- If symptoms persist after 1 week, increase dose by 5 mg. Ongoing symptoms require consideration of alternative diagnosis.
- If nighttime symptoms are bothersome, can try divided dose of prednisone.
- Initial prednisone dose should be maintained for 4 to 8 weeks. Steroid dose is then tapered every 2 to 4 weeks as tolerated to minimum amount required to remain symptom free. When dose reaches 10 mg/day, taper slowly, usually by 1 mg/month.
- Flares are typical during tapering, can manage by increasing prednisone by 10% to 20%. Most require treatment for 1 to 2 yr with steroids.
- Monitor both clinical response and ESR and CRP intermittently.
- Gastroprotection should be considered, and attention should be paid to bone health, with calcium and vitamin D supplementation started early. Consider prophylactic bisphosphonates if indicated.
- Routine use of adjunctive therapy is not recommended, but certain cases (refractory disease, high-risk steroid use) can consider methotrexate. TNFi has not been shown to have benefit. It has been found more recently that tocilizumab (IL6i) may be beneficial in patients with contraindications to methotrexate use, and was recently approved to treat GCA.

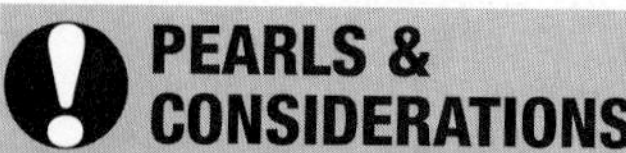

PEARLS & CONSIDERATIONS

Patients with PMR should be monitored closely for the development of GCA. Patients who have incomplete response to prednisone or have an evolving pattern of pain and swelling should be re-evaluated for the possibility of a different diagnosis such as rheumatoid arthritis.

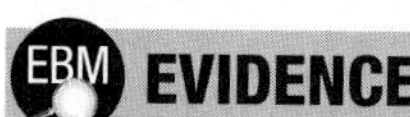

EVIDENCE

Available at ExpertConsult.com

SUGGESTED READINGS

Available at ExpertConsult.com

RELATED CONTENT

Polymyalgia Rheumatica (PMR) (Patient Information)
Giant Cell Arteritis (Related Key Topic)
Vasculitis, Systemic (Related Key Topic)

AUTHOR: **DAPHNE SCARAMANGAS-PLUMLEY, M.D.**

BOX 1 Differential Diagnosis of Polymyalgia Rheumatica

- Rheumatoid arthritis
- Rotator cuff syndrome
- Osteoarthritis of shoulder and hip joints
- Fibromyalgia
- Polymyositis/dermatomyositis
- Spondyloarthritis
- Systemic lupus erythematosus
- Vasculitides
- Paraneoplastic myalgias
- Infection-associated myalgias
- RS3PE (remitting seronegative symmetric synovitis and pitting edema)
- Parkinson's disease
- Hypothyroidism

TABLE 1 2012 European League Against Rheumatism/American College of Rheumatology Classification Criteria for Polymyalgia Rheumatica*

Criteria	Points With Ultrasonography	Points Without Ultrasonography
1. Morning stiffness duration >45 min	2	2
2. Hip pain or limited range of movement	1	1
3. Absence of rheumatoid factor or anticitrullinated protein antibody	2	2
4. Absence of other joint involvement	1	1
5. ≥1 shoulder with subdeltoid bursitis and/or biceps tenosynovitis and/or glenohumeral synovitis (either posterior or axillary) and ≥1 hip with synovitis and/or trochanteric bursitis	1	—
6. Both shoulders with subdeltoid bursitis, biceps tenosynovitis, or glenohumeral synovitis	1	—

*Score ≥4 without ultrasonography or ≥5 with ultrasonography is categorized as polymyalgia rheumatica.

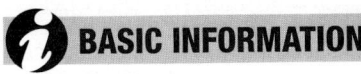

BASIC INFORMATION

DEFINITION

Clinically significant portal hypertension is defined as a portal vein pressure >10 mm Hg, most commonly attributable to liver disease.

ICD-10CM CODE
K76.6 Portal hypertension

EPIDEMIOLOGY & DEMOGRAPHICS

- Incidence of portal hypertension is not known.
- Cirrhosis is the most common cause of portal hypertension in the United States.
- Portal hypertension is developed by >90% of patients with cirrhosis.
- Alcoholic and viral liver diseases are the most common causes of cirrhosis and portal hypertension in the United States.
- Schistosomiasis is the main cause of portal hypertension outside the United States.
- Esophageal varices may appear when portal vein pressure rises to >10 mm Hg.
- Variceal hemorrhage is the most serious complication of portal hypertension and may occur when portal pressures rise >12 mm Hg.

PHYSICAL FINDINGS & CLINICAL PRESENTATION

- Jaundice
- Ascites (Fig. 1)
- Spider angiomata
- Testicular atrophy
- Gynecomastia
- Palmar erythema
- Dupuytren contracture
- Asterixis (with advanced liver failure)
- Irritability, encephalopathy
- Splenomegaly
- Dilated veins in the anterior abdominal wall
- Venous pattern on the flanks
- Caput medusae (tortuous collateral veins around the umbilicus)
- Hemorrhoids
- Hematemesis
- Melena
- Pruritus

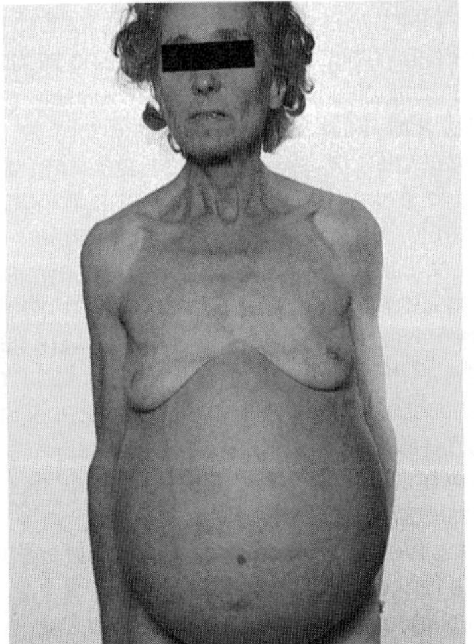

FIG. 1 Ascites secondary to portal hypertension. Note the dilated collateral vein running up the right side of the abdomen. (From Forbes A et al [eds]: *Atlas of clinical gastroenterology,* ed 3, Oxford, 2005, Mosby.)

ETIOLOGY

Pathophysiologically caused by:

- Conditions resulting in an increased resistance to flow:
  1. **Prehepatic** (e.g., portal vein thrombosis, splenic vein thrombosis, congenital stenosis).
  2. **Hepatic** (e.g., cirrhosis, alcoholic liver disease, primary biliary cirrhosis, schistosomiasis).
  3. **Posthepatic** (e.g., Budd-Chiari syndrome, constrictive pericarditis, inferior vena cava obstruction, cor pulmonale, tricuspid regurgitation).
- Conditions leading to increase in portal blood flow:
  1. Splanchnic arterial vasodilation accompanying portal hypertension, mediated by local release of nitric oxide.
  2. Arterial-portal venous fistulae.

Table 1 describes the pathophysiologic changes in portal hypertension and Table 2 summarizes the etiologies of portal hypertension.

DIAGNOSIS

- The diagnosis of portal hypertension is made on clinical grounds after a comprehensive history and physical examination.
- Noninvasive and invasive procedures confirm diagnosis and determine the severity of portal hypertension.

DIFFERENTIAL DIAGNOSIS

- Ascites from infection, neoplasm, or other inflammatory processes
- Obesity
- Abdominal organomegaly

WORKUP

The workup of portal hypertension includes blood tests and noninvasive imaging studies to determine if the cause of portal hypertension is prehepatic, hepatic, or posthepatic. Ascitic fluid analysis is a key part of the diagnosis.

LABORATORY TESTS

- Complete blood count with platelets
- Liver function tests with serum albumin
- Prothrombin and partial thromboplastin times
- Hepatitis B surface antigen and antibody
- Hepatitis C antibody
- In selected cases: Iron, total iron-binding capacity, and ferritin; antinuclear antibody, anti–smooth muscle antibodies, antimitochondrial antibody, ceruloplasmin, alpha-1 antitrypsin
- Ascitic fluid analysis: A serum-ascites albumin gradient ≥1.1 mg/dl suggests portal hypertension. Polymorphonuclear cells ≥250 cells/ml or positive Gram stain or culture suggest complicating spontaneous bacterial peritonitis (SBP)

IMAGING STUDIES

- Duplex-Doppler ultrasound is effective in screening for portal hypertension.
- Less commonly, CT/MRI/MRA scanning (Figs. 2 and E3) or liver-spleen nuclear medicine scanning can be used if the results from ultrasound are equivocal.
- Upper endoscopy is the most reliable test documenting the presence of esophageal varices.

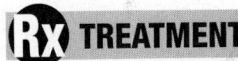

TREATMENT

The treatment of portal hypertension is complex and involves measures to reduce the hypertension directly, minimize volume overload, correct underlying disorders, and prevent complications (most notably SBP and variceal bleeding).

TABLE 1 Pathophysiologic Changes in Portal Hypertension

Pathophysiologic Change	Specifics
Hepatic resistance	Passive, mechanical component: 60%-70%
	Active, dynamic component: 30%-40%
Portal hypertension	
Shunts	
Splanchnic vasodilation	
Increased portal inflow	
Decrease in effective circulating volume; redistribution total blood volume	
Increase in endogenous vasopressors (RAA, SNS, VP)	Increase in endothelin-1
	Angiotensin II
	Norepinephrine
	Vasopressin
	PGF-2 alpha
Decrease in NO, CO	

CO, carbon monoxide; *NO,* nitrogen monoxide; *PGF,* prostaglandin; *RAA,* renin-angiotensin-aldosterone; *SNS,* sympathetic nervous system; *VP,* vasopressin. From Vincent JL et al: *Textbook of critical care,* ed 7, Philadelphia, 2017, Elsevier.

TABLE 2 Etiology of Portal Hypertension Grouped by Location of Insult

Site of Increased Resistance	Condition	FHVP	WHVP	HVGP	SPP
Presinusoidal (extrahepatic)	Extrahepatic portal, splenic, or mesenteric vein thrombosis	Normal	Normal	Normal	Increased
Presinusoidal (intrahepatic)	Early primary biliary cirrhosis	Normal	Normal/raised (?)	Normal/raised (?)	Increased
Presinusoidal (intrahepatic)	PSC	Normal	Normal/raised (?)	Normal/raised (?)	Increased
Presinusoidal (intrahepatic)	Sarcoid	Normal	Normal/raised (?)	Normal/raised (?)	Increased
Presinusoidal (intrahepatic)	Schistosomiasis	Normal	Normal/raised (?)	Normal/raised (?)	Increased
Presinusoidal (intrahepatic)	Congestive heart failure	Normal	Normal/raised (?)	Normal/raised (?)	Increased
Presinusoidal (intrahepatic)	Noncirrhotic portal fibrosis	Normal	Normal/raised (?)	Normal/raised (?)	Increased
Intrahepatic sinusoidal	Cirrhosis (any etiology)	Normal	Increased	Increased	Increased
Intrahepatic sinusoidal	Alcoholic hepatitis	Normal	Increased	Increased	Increased
Intrahepatic sinusoidal	Fulminant liver failure (any etiology)	Normal	Increased	Increased	Increased
Extrahepatic postsinusoidal hypertension	Budd-Chiari syndrome	Increased	Increased	Normal	Increased
Extrahepatic postsinusoidal hypertension	Constrictive pericarditis	Increased	Increased	Normal	Increased
Extrahepatic postsinusoidal hypertension	Inferior vena cava obstruction	Increased	Increased	Normal	Increased
Extrahepatic postsinusoidal hypertension	Congenital inferior vena cava web	Increased	Increased	Normal	Increased
Extrahepatic postsinusoidal hypertension	Right heart failure	Increased	Increased	Normal	Increased

FHVP, Free hepatic venous pressure; *HVPG,* hepatic venous pressure gradient; *PSC,* primary sclerosing cholangitis; *SPP,* systolic pulse pressure; *WHVP,* wedged hepatic venous pressure.
From Vincent JL et al: *Textbook of critical care*, ed 7, Philadelphia, 2017, Elsevier.

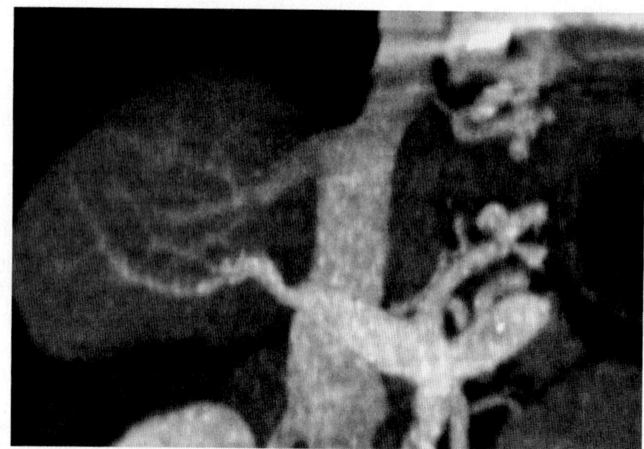

FIG. 2 Magnetic resonance angiography showing portal hypertension with collaterals. The shrunken liver and collateral are obvious. (From Forbes A et al [eds]: *Atlas of clinical gastroenterology,* ed 3, St Louis, 2005, Mosby.)

NONPHARMACOLOGIC THERAPY

Dietary sodium restriction to generally 2000 mg/day forms the basis of therapy to limit fluid overload.

ACUTE GENERAL Rx

- For tense ascites, serial large-volume paracentesis (LVP) is generally recommended. The use of albumin infusion (8 to 10 g/L of ascites fluid removed) during LVP >5 L has been shown to reduce the incidence of postparacentesis circulatory dysfunction, although its use remains somewhat controversial.
- IV diuretics, typically furosemide and spironolactone, are used to achieve natriuresis and net negative salt and water balance. Renal function and serum electrolytes are monitored frequently, with transition to an oral regimen for long-term therapy.
- SBP is treated with IV antibiotics directed against enteric bacteria.
- Acute variceal hemorrhage is treated with crystalloid and blood product resuscitation, IV octreotide, terlipressin/vasopressin or somatostatin, and urgent upper endoscopy, often with sclerotherapy or band ligation. Patients with acute variceal hemorrhage should receive empiric antibiotic therapy for SBP.
- Traditionally, a transjugular intrahepatic portosystemic shunt (TIPS) or surgical shunt placement may be considered in patients not responding to above measures. However, recent data show *early* TIPS placement improved outcomes in acute variceal hemorrhage. Table 3 summarizes indications, contraindications, and complications of the TIPS procedure.
- Table 4 compares treatment modalities for portal hypertension.

CHRONIC Rx

- Dietary sodium restriction in combination with diuretics: The typical ratio of furosemide 40 mg to spironolactone 100 mg retains normal serum potassium levels in most patients.
- Nonselective beta-blockers (propranolol and nadolol) in dosages sufficient to reduce the resting heart rate by 25% have been shown to be effective in primary prophylaxis for first-time variceal bleeding and for preventing recurrent variceal bleeding. Dosages are usually given bid and decreased if heart rate falls to <55 beats/min or systolic blood pressure drops to <90 mm Hg. The addition of a long-acting nitrate (e.g., isosorbide-5-mononitrate) has been shown to improve portal hemodynamics. Findings of a prospective trial of beta-blockers to prevent the formation of varices were negative. The combination of beta-blockade plus endoscopic esophageal variceal banding is superior to either intervention alone.
- Intermittent LVP may be needed in "diuretic resistant" patients.
- Patients with prior SBP merit lifelong antibiotics for secondary prevention.
- Abstinence from alcohol or treatment for hepatitis B or hepatitis C. Vaccination for hepatitis A and B as appropriate.
- Hepatic transplantation is an option in selected patients.

TABLE 3 Indications, Contraindications, and Complications of the TIPS Procedure

Indications	Relative Contraindications	Contraindications	Acute Complications	Chronic Complications
Upper GI bleeding	Pulmonary hypertension	Right-sided heart failure	Neck hematoma	Congestive heart failure
Ascites	Severe liver failure	Biliary tract obstruction	Arrhythmia	Portal vein thrombosis
Hepatic hydrothorax	Portal vein thrombosis	Uncontrolled infection	Stent displacement	Progressive liver failure
	Multiple hepatic cysts	Chronic recurrent disabling hepatic encephalopathy	Hemolysis	Chronic recurrent encephalopathy
		Hepatocellular carcinoma involving hepatic veins	Bilhemia	Stent dysfunction
			Hepatic vein obstruction	TIPSitis
			Shunt thrombosis	
			Hemoperitoneum	
			Hemobilia	
			Liver ischemia	
			Cardiac failure	
			Sepsis	

GI, Gastrointestinal; *TIPS*, transjugular intrahepatic portosystemic shunt. From Vincent JL et al: *Textbook of critical care*, ed 7, Philadelphia, 2017, Elsevier.

TABLE 4 Comparison of Treatment Modalities

Treatment Modality	No (%), N = 77	Age, Yr (Mean)	Female %	Initial Meld (Mean, Range)	Child-Pugh Score (N = 74)	Ascites Size	Death (No, %) (N = 44)	Days from Presentation Until Death or End of Study
Medical management	64/77 (83%)	52	23/64 (36%)	16 (4-46)	A = 1 B = 31	None: 6 Small: 34 Moderate: 16 Large: 8	40/64 (63%)	321 ± 463
TIPS	8/77 (10%)	56	5/8 (63%)	12 (7-28)	A = 0 B = 5 C = 2	None: 1 Small: 3 Moderate: 3 Large: 1	4/8 (50%)	845 ± 407
Transplant	5/77 (7%)	54	0	21 (10-40)	A = 1 B = 1 C = 1	Large: 1	0	1896 ± 1752

TIPS, Transjugular intrahepatic portosystemic shunt. From Vincent JL et al: *Textbook of critical care*, ed 7, Philadelphia, 2017, Elsevier.

DISPOSITION

- The most common complication associated with portal hypertension is variceal bleeding. The risk of bleeding from varices is approximately 15% at 1 yr.
- Development of the hepatorenal syndrome (HRS) is associated with high near-term mortality. In particular, HRS may complicate SBP, which emphasizes the importance of making the diagnosis of SBP and instituting appropriate prophylaxis.

REFERRAL

Consultation with a gastroenterologist is recommended in all patients with portal hypertension to screen for esophageal varices.

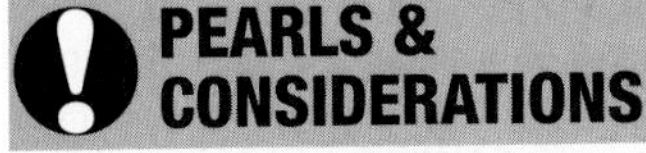

PEARLS & CONSIDERATIONS

Splanchnic arterial vasodilation is increasingly recognized as an important component of the pathophysiology of portal hypertension and ascites. There may be vasodilation in other capillary beds as well; of note, pulmonary arteriolar vasodilation can create a significant shunt fraction and resultant hypoxemia in the absence of chest radiograph or CT chest evidence of parenchymal disease. The diagnosis is suspected when otherwise unexplained hypoxia arises in a patient with cirrhosis, along with platypnea (dyspnea worse when sitting upright) and orthodeoxia (desaturation with upright posture). The diagnosis is confirmed by echocardiography with agitated saline, in which there is delayed appearance of bubbles in the left heart after injection into a peripheral vein.

COMMENTS

Portal hypertension and its complications carry significant morbidity and mortality rates. Emphasize ethanol abstinence, provide vaccinations and prophylactic therapy where indicated, and consider early referral to a specialist for assistance with management and consideration for hepatic transplantation.

SUGGESTED READING

Available at ExpertConsult.com

AUTHOR: **FRED F. FERRI, M.D.**

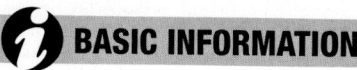

BASIC INFORMATION

DEFINITION

Portal vein thrombosis (PVT) is thrombotic occlusion of the portal vein. The thrombus can also involve segments of the mesenteric veins and/or the splenic vein.

SYNONYMS

Pylethrombosis
PVT

ICD 10CM CODE

I81 Portal vein thrombosis

EPIDEMIOLOGY & DEMOGRAPHICS

- Occurs with equal frequency in children (peak age: 6 yr) and adults (peak age: 40 yr)
- Occurs in 8% to 25% of patients with decompensated cirrhosis

PHYSICAL FINDINGS & CLINICAL PRESENTATION

- Acute PVT may present with sudden onset of fever and abdominal pain (when there is mesenteric extension).
- Upper gastrointestinal hemorrhage (hematemesis and/or melena) caused by esophageal varices.

ETIOLOGY & PATHOPHYSIOLOGY

In children: Umbilical sepsis (pathophysiology unknown). In adults:

- Hypercoagulable states:
  1. Antiphospholipid syndrome
  2. Neoplasm (common cause)
  3. Paroxysmal nocturnal hemoglobinuria
  4. Myeloproliferative diseases
  5. Oral contraceptives
  6. Polycythemia vera
  7. Pregnancy
  8. Protein S or C deficiency
  9. Sickle cell disease
  10. Thrombocytosis
- Inflammatory diseases:
  1. Crohn disease
  2. Pancreatitis
  3. Ulcerative colitis
- Complications of medical intervention:
  1. Ambulatory dialysis
  2. Chemoembolization
  3. Liver transplantation
  4. Partial hepatectomy
  5. Sclerotherapy
  6. Splenectomy
  7. Transjugular intrahepatic portosystemic shunt
- Infections:
  1. Appendicitis
  2. Diverticulitis
  3. Cholecystitis
- Miscellaneous:
  1. Cirrhosis (common cause)
  2. Bladder cancer

Pathophysiology: PVT results in portal hypertension, leading to esophageal and gastrointestinal varices. The liver sustained by the hepatic artery maintains normal function.

DIAGNOSIS

DIFFERENTIAL DIAGNOSIS

Causes of upper gastrointestinal hemorrhage and abdominal pain are described in Section II.

WORKUP

- Abdominal ultrasound with Doppler (Fig. 1) or MRI may show the PVT. Abdominal ultrasound color Doppler imaging has a 98% negative predictive value and is considered the imaging modality of choice in diagnosing PVT.
- Determination of underlying cirrhosis of the liver should be the foremost step. It is crucial to differentiate acute from chronic PVT because chronic PVT does not require treatment.
- Esophagogastroscopy typically shows esophageal varices.
- Laboratory evaluation for hypercoagulable state is not cost-effective in patients with cirrhosis.

TREATMENT

- Anticoagulation data on thrombolytic therapy are inconclusive and there is no formal recommendation for or against anticoagulation in acute PVT. However, anticoagulation is generally recommended for patients with extension of PVT into the superior mesenteric vein to prevent intestinal infarction. In patients with chronic PVT and concomitant cirrhosis, long-term anticoagulation is generally not recommended.
- Variceal sclerotherapy or banding.
- Surgical mesocaval or splenorenal shunt.
- The roles of thrombolysis and transjugular intrahepatic portosystemic shunt continue to evolve.

REFERRAL

- To surgeon to rule out intestinal infarction
- To gastroenterologist

SUGGESTED READING

Available at ExpertConsult.com

AUTHOR: **FRED F. FERRI, M.D.**

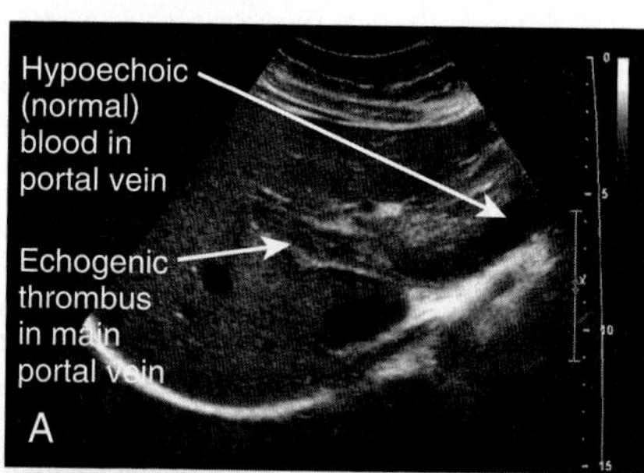

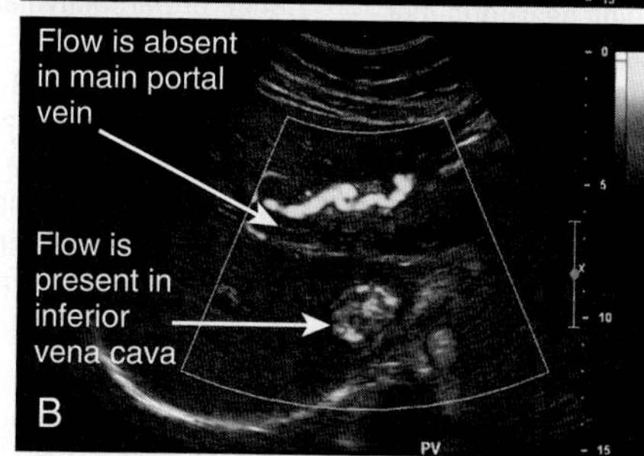

FIG. 1 Portal vein thrombosis: Ultrasound. This 22-year-old female, 2 months postpartum, presented with 1 week of right upper quadrant pain. Ultrasound was performed to evaluate for suspected cholecystitis or symptomatic cholelithiasis. Instead, portal vein thrombosis was discovered. The postpartum state is a risk factor for this condition. Hypercoagulable states and inflammatory or neoplastic abdominal conditions, including pancreatitis and abdominal malignancies, also can result in portal vein thrombosis. **A,** Ultrasound gray scale image showing thrombus in the main portal vein. **B,** Doppler ultrasound showing no flow within the portal vein. (From Broder JS: *Diagnostic imaging for the emergency physician,* Philadelphia, 2011, Saunders.)

BASIC INFORMATION

DEFINITION

Postconcussive syndrome (PCS) refers to nonspecific neurologic, cognitive, and psychological symptoms that result from traumatic brain injury (TBI) and persist beyond the expected recovery period. There is no consensus regarding the duration of symptoms to make the diagnosis, but symptoms usually manifest or significantly worsen within a few days following head trauma and persist for weeks to months. PCS can also follow moderate and severe brain injury, although it is more commonly associated with mild brain injury or concussion. Concussion is an acute trauma-induced alteration of mental function lasting <24 hours, with or without preceding loss of consciousness.

SYNONYMS

PCS
Postconcussion syndrome
Posttraumatic nervous instability or brain injury
Postcontusion syndrome or encephalopathy
Status post commotio cerebri

ICD-10CM CODE

F07.81 Postconcussional syndrome

EPIDEMIOLOGY & DEMOGRAPHICS

- Incidence is approximately 27 cases per 100,000 persons/yr.
- From 30% to 80% of patients with mild to moderate brain injury will experience some symptoms of PCS.
- Usually reported in the young, ages 20 to 30 yr old.
- Risk factors include female sex, low socioeconomic status, anxiety sensitivity, previous TBI, severe bodily injury from TBI, headaches, and unsettled court cases.

PHYSICAL FINDINGS & CLINICAL PRESENTATION

- Symptoms start within a few days to weeks after the head injury and usually persist after 3 months. 15% of patients will have persistent symptoms 1 yr later.
- At least three of the following symptoms after TBI are required to meet ICD-10 criteria:
  1. Headache (usually of fronto-occipital location and showing characteristics of tension or migraine headache). The International Headache Society suggests that coding and attribution of headaches with characteristics of primary headaches but in the setting of an inciting event should be attributed to the event, unless there was a known history of the headache and the inciting event was seen as aggravating/initiating the preexisting migraine/tension headache.
  2. Fatigue
  3. Dizziness and/or vertigo
  4. Impaired memory
  5. Difficulty in concentrating
  6. Insomnia
  7. Irritability
  8. Lowered tolerance of stress, emotion, or alcohol
- Other associated symptoms: Noise sensitivity, neck pain, nondermatomal paresthesias, interference with social role functioning.
- Focal neurologic deficits are typically absent on examination.

ETIOLOGY

- The inciting TBI may occur as a result of events such as falls, motor vehicle accidents, military injuries, and contact sports.
- The primary injury triggers a slew of pathophysiological changes at the cellular level secondary to the axonal stretching and injury, leading to alterations in membrane and intracellular physiology, thereby affecting neurotransmission. These changes are believed to be a factor in determining whether the outcome will be an apparent normal recovery or persistent postconcussion symptoms.
- Postmortem findings reveal diffuse axonal injury as the primary pathologic finding, along with small petechial hemorrhages and local edema.
- A psychogenic origin has been suggested by a number of empiric and clinical observations; however, limitations in methodology and differing definitions preclude firm conclusions. Prior history of anxiety is a strong risk factor for occurrence of PCS.

DIAGNOSIS

A careful history, a nonfocal neurologic examination, and normal neurologic testing will usually establish the diagnosis.

DIFFERENTIAL DIAGNOSIS

- Headache (dissection of the vertebral artery, occipital neuralgia)
- Epidural hematoma
- Subdural hematoma
- Skull fracture
- Cervical spine disk disease
- Whiplash
- Cerebrovascular accident
- Depression
- Anxiety

WORKUP

To exclude other causes of neurologic symptoms after TBI:

- Normal results of electroencephalography
- Normal evoked potentials
- Neuropsychological testing, which often reveals difficulties in concentration, memory, language, and executive function

LABORATORY TESTS

Various biomarkers in blood and cerebrospinal fluid and genetic testing have been proposed and studied in patients with TBI, but these tests are not specific and are not routinely used.

IMAGING STUDIES

- There is no imaging modality to diagnose PCS. PCS is primarily a clinical diagnosis. The American College of Emergency Physicians' clinical policy regarding neuroimaging in adults with mild traumatic brain injury is summarized in Box 1.
- 10% of CT scans of the head following mild TBI are abnormal, showing mild subarachnoid hemorrhage, subdural hemorrhage, or contusions.
- MRI of the head after a mild traumatic brain injury (mTBI) is abnormal in 30% of patients

BOX 1 American College of Emergency Physicians' Clinical Policy Regarding Neuroimaging in Adults with Mild Traumatic Brain Injury

A noncontrast head CT is indicated (level one recommendation) in adults with LOC or posttraumatic amnesia only if at least one of the following is present:

- Headache
- Vomiting
- Age older than 60 yr
- Drug or alcohol intoxication
- Deficits in short-term memory
- Physical evidence of trauma above the clavicle
- Posttraumatic seizure
- GCS score below 15
- Focal neurologic deficit
- Coagulopathy

A noncontrast head CT should be considered (level two recommendation) in head trauma patients with no LOC or posttraumatic amnesia if any of the following is present:

- Focal neurologic deficit
- Vomiting
- Severe headache
- Age 65 yr or older
- Physical signs of a basilar skull fracture
- GCS score below 15
- Coagulopathy
- A dangerous mechanism (e.g., ejection from motor vehicle, pedestrian struck, fall of more than 3 feet or 5 stairs)

CT, Computed tomography; *GCS*, Glasgow Coma Scale; *LOC*, loss of consciousness.
From Marx J, et al.: *Rosen's emergency medicine: concepts and clinical practice*, ed 7, Philadelphia, 2010, Mosby.

with normal CT scans and may show irregular brain contours or old cerebral contusions.

- Recent improvements in imaging modalities, including diffuse tensor imaging (DTI) and susceptibility weighted imaging (SWI) in MRI, functional MRI (fMRI), and metabolic imaging such as magnetic resonance spectroscopy (MRS), positron emission tomography (PET), and single-photon emission computed tomography (SPECT) imaging, appear to be promising in elucidating the underlying pathophysiology of TBI and PCS, although they have not found a major role in clinical practice yet.
- None of the imaging modalities have been able to predict the occurrence of PCS in patients with mild TBI.

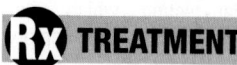

TREATMENT

PCS must be recognized as a physiologic and psychological problem and treated accordingly. Treatment should be individualized to target the patient's particular symptoms and is typically completed on an outpatient basis. Some symptoms may be refractory to treatment.

NONPHARMACOLOGIC Rx

- Early reassurance and patient education are major components of treatment. Explanation of symptoms and expectations, combined with early follow-up with reassurance, may hasten resolution of symptoms.
- Graduated physical activity is preferred over prolonged cognitive and physical rest. Light aerobic activity that avoids risk for reinjury has been shown beneficial in mitigating refractory concussion symptoms. Physical and occupational therapy may be beneficial.
- Cognitive behavioral therapy may be effective in treating symptoms.
- Avoidance of alcohol, narcotics, and sleep deprivation.

PHARMACOLOGIC THERAPY

- Supportive symptomatic care may include the use of nonnarcotic analgesics and antiemetics.
- Amitriptyline has been widely used for posttraumatic tension-type headaches as well as for nonspecific symptoms such as irritability, dizziness, insomnia, and depression.
- Posttraumatic migraine-type headaches can be treated with a trial of propranolol or amitriptyline alone or in combination.
- Depression can be treated with selective serotonin reuptake inhibitors but may not respond as well when compared with patients without PCS who have depression.

DISPOSITION

- Most patients improve after mild TBI without any residual deficits within 3 mo.
- Although good improvement is typically seen within the first 6 mo, patients can continue to show improvement for up to 12 to 18 mo.
- Patients with very severe brain injuries (low Glasgow Coma Scale [GCS] score) and prolonged anterograde amnesia are at increased risk of development of some degree of permanent cognitive and personality disturbance.
- Predictors for the development of persistent PCS include:
  1. Female sex
  2. Ongoing litigation (conflicting studies)
  3. Low socioeconomic status
  4. Prior headaches
  5. Prior TBI
  6. Prior psychiatric illnesses, particularly anxiety

REFERRAL

Early consultations with psychologists, psychiatrists, neurologists, and rehabilitation specialists in an outpatient setting may be beneficial.

PEARLS & CONSIDERATIONS

- PCS starts within a few days after the injury.
- Recognizing depression and treating pain symptoms early in the course may help prevent the development of persistent PCS (>1 yr).
- The severity of the trauma does not clearly predict the risk of PCS.
- The severity of brain injury is usually documented by initial GCS score, duration of loss of consciousness, and duration of amnesia; however, there is a move toward tests of function, such as neuropsychological testing or fMRI.

COMMENTS

- Attempts to determine how much of a role psychological and/or neurologic factors play in the PCS are important but very difficult.
- No medication at hospital discharge has been proved to change the natural course of the disease.
- Engaging in physical activity within 7 days after concussion is associated with a lower rate of persistent postconcussive symptoms.

SUGGESTED READINGS

Available at ExpertConsult.com

RELATED CONTENT

Post-concussion Syndrome (Patient Information)
Concussion (Related Key Topic)
Traumatic Brain Injury (Related Key Topic)

AUTHORS: **CHLOE MANDER NUNNELEY, M.D., JOSEPH S. KASS, M.D., J.D.,** and **PRASHANTH KRISHNAMOHAN, M.B.B.S, M.D.**

BASIC INFORMATION

DEFINITION

Postherpetic neuralgia (PHN) is a pain syndrome that results as a complication of herpes zoster (HZ). HZ, also known as shingles, is a painful vesicular eruption in a dermatomal distribution. HZ is caused by the reactivation of varicella zoster virus (VZV) in someone with a known history of varicella. PHN is pain and/or dysesthesia that persist for 3 or more months at the site of resolved HZ.

ICD-10CM CODE

B02.29 Other postherpetic nervous system involvement

EPIDEMIOLOGY & DEMOGRAPHICS

INCIDENCE: PHN occurs in approximately 9% to 34% of HZ patients. It is the most frequent chronic complication of herpes zoster and the most common neuropathic pain disorder resulting from infection. In one study, approximately 60% of patients with HZ developed PHN at age 60 yr, and 75% developed PHN at age 70 yr. In another study, the incidence of PHN at 9 yr post-HZ eruption was 21%.

PEAK INCIDENCE: Unknown

PREDOMINANT SEX AND AGE:

- PHN occurs equally in males and females.
- The likelihood of developing PHN significantly increases with advancing age.

GENETICS: Family history of HZ is considered a risk factor for HZ, with higher risk if multiple family members have had HZ.

RISK FACTORS:

- Advanced age
- Greater severity of HZ prodromal pain
- Greater severity of pain during acute HZ eruption
- Location—specifically ophthalmic (V1) location and brachial plexus
- Severe immunosuppression

PHYSICAL FINDINGS & CLINICAL PRESENTATION

- HZ typically presents as a painful vesicular eruption in a dermatomal distribution. Rarely, HZ can occur subclinically with dermatomal pain in the absence of a rash.
- PHN is pain that continues for 3 months at the dermatomal site of the resolved HZ. The pain may be described as burning, stabbing, shooting, or shock-like.
- Patients may note an amplified response to stimuli at the site of PHN, with increased pain response (hyperalgesia), pain to typically non-noxious stimuli (allodynia), or focal changes in autonomic function (e.g., increased sweating).
- Physical examination should include a comparison of sensory function in the affected dermatome with that on the contralateral side.

ETIOLOGY

PHN is associated with damage and scarring to the dorsal root ganglion secondary to inflammation related to active herpes zoster infection.

Dx DIAGNOSIS

DIFFERENTIAL DIAGNOSIS

Zoster sine herpete (subclinical HZ without skin eruption)

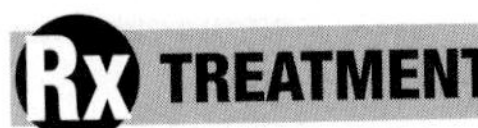

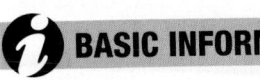

TREATMENT

ACUTE GENERAL Rx

- Administration of acyclovir or valacyclovir within 72 hours of HZ onset is thought to help reduce the likelihood of developing PNH. However, one Cochrane review paper found no difference with acyclovir administration.
- A single published study supports the use of amitriptyline (25 mg daily) as an adjunct to an antiviral agent in acute HZ to decrease the incidence of PHN and the pain associated with subsequent PHN.
- A suggestive noncontrolled study with co-administration of valacyclovir and gabapentin during acute HZ reduced the incidence of PHN as well.
- Corticosteroids do NOT prevent PHN.

CHRONIC Rx

TOPICAL TREATMENTS:

- Lidocaine 5% patches may be used for mild pain.
- Capsaicin 0.075% cream (although little reported efficacy) 5 times per day.
- Capsaicin 8% patch has greater efficacy, but overall analgesia may be minimal at best, with one third of patients unable to tolerate the agent due to burning, stinging, and erythema. However, a single 60-minute treatment with high concentration capsaicin patch was found in one study to reduce PHN for up to 12 weeks regardless of concomitant systemic neuropathic pain medication use.

ORAL TREATMENTS: First line:

- Gabapentinoids (gabapentin, pregabalin) are the only FDA-approved oral therapy for PHN and are some of the most commonly used first-line therapies for chronic PHN pain. Gabapentin may be administered in the immediate-release or extended-release formulation. Dosing includes gabapentin 300 mg 3 times a day (titrating up to max 3600 mg/day) and pregabalin 75 mg nightly (titrating up to 300 mg twice daily).
- Tricyclic antidepressants such as amitriptyline (25 mg/day, increased by 25 mg every night to a maximum of 75 mg/night), desipramine (10-25 mg/day, increased by 25 mg/day every 3 days as needed to a maximum of 150 mg/day), and nortriptyline (10-25 mg/day, increased by 25 mg/day weekly as needed to maximum of 75 mg day) are other first line treatments. These medications have a delayed onset of action and may not work as well in patients with certain types of pain, such as burning pain or allodynia. They have a considerable side effect profile. Their use in elderly patients should be carefully considered. A recent study showed the combination of gabapentin and nortriptyline was more efficacious than either drug as monotherapy for neuropathic pain.

Second line:

- Opiates (e.g., controlled-release oxycodone): Side effects, the possibility of misuse, and the potential for abuse must be weighed.

Other modalities:

- Dorsal root entry zone (DREZ) lesions have been used with an improvement rate of 20% in long-term studies.
- For recalcitrant cases, epidural corticosteroids and nerve blocks, botulinum toxin, and cryotherapy.
- Fig. 1 describes a treatment algorithm for HZ and PHN.

COMPLEMENTARY AND ALTERNATIVE MEDICINE:

- Acupuncture:
    1. Studies on acupuncture and PHN pain have had varying results; however, the only randomized, controlled study showed no significant difference in pain reduction between control and treatment groups.

REFERRAL

For complicated cases, dermatology, neurology, and/or pain management input can be helpful.

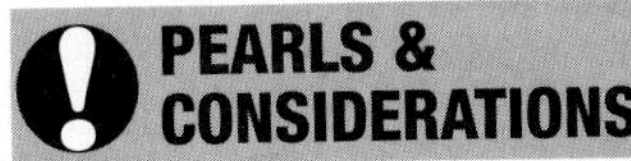

PEARLS & CONSIDERATIONS

COMMENTS

- Careful consideration of treatment side effects and drug interactions is needed.
- The natural history of PHN is slow resolution, and most individuals respond to medical therapy. However, a subtype of patients may develop severe, long-lasting pain that is recalcitrant to medical therapy.
- In a questionnaire study of 385 adults age >65 yr with persistent acute pain, the mean duration of PHN was 3.3 yr.

PREVENTION

- Vaccination:
    1. A non-live VZV vaccine (Shingrix®) is approved by the FDA for individuals age 50 and older. It is administered as two shots spaced 2 months apart and is 97% effective against shingles in people ages 50 to 69, and 91% effective against PHN in people 50 and older. It is more effective than the live attenuated VZV vaccine (zostvax).
    2. The CDC recommends that those who received Zostavax be revaccinated with Shingrix.

PATIENT/FAMILY EDUCATION

- The only well-documented means of preventing PHN is the prevention of herpes zoster through vaccination.

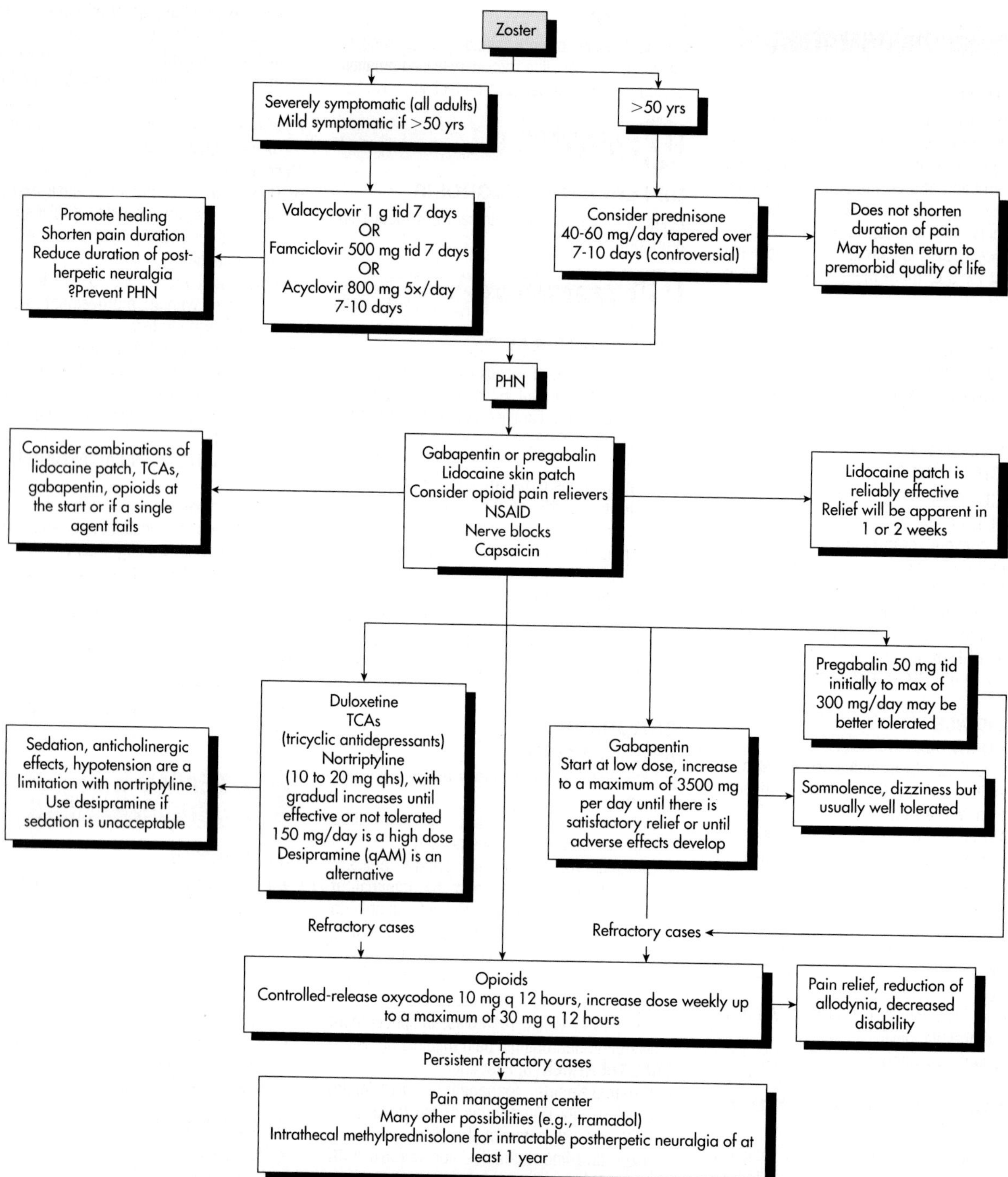

FIG. 1 Treatment of herpes zoster and postherpetic neuralgia. *NSAID,* Nonsteroidal antiinflammatory drug; *PHN,* postherpetic neuralgia. (Modified from Habif TA: *Clinical dermatology,* ed 6, St Louis, 2016, Elsevier.)

- Patients should understand both the benefits and the potential adverse effects of treatment.
  1. They should be informed that pain relief will likely not be immediate.
  2. Frequent reassessment may be needed, and drug doses should be increased as necessary.

SUGGESTED READING

Available at ExpertConsult.com

RELATED CONTENT

Herpes Zoster (Related Key Topic)

AUTHOR: **LISA K. PAPPAS-TAFFER, M.D.**

BASIC INFORMATION

DEFINITION

Major or minor depressive episodes that are severe enough to affect activities of daily living and occur most commonly within 1 to 3 wk after delivery, but can also present up to 12 mo postpartum.

SYNONYMS

Spectrum of disease presentation
Postpartum blues
Postpartum depression
Postpartum psychosis

ICD-10CM CODES

F53	Includes postpartum depression and postpartum psychosis
090.6	Includes postpartum blues, postpartum dysphoria and sadness

EPIDEMIOLOGY & DEMOGRAPHICS

INCIDENCE: Approximately 800,000 women who deliver in the U.S. or 20% of all live births are affected by postpartum depression annually.
PREVALENCE: Perinatal depression affects approximately 10% to 15% of women.
GENETICS: A family history of mood disorders is a risk factor for postpartum depression.
RISK FACTORS: Risk factors include depression or anxiety during pregnancy, traumatic birth experiences, stressful life events during pregnancy or the postpartum period, infant NICU admission or preterm delivery, poor social support, history of depression, and problems with breastfeeding.

PHYSICAL FINDINGS & CLINICAL PRESENTATION

Patients present with depressed or irritable mood, decreased interest in activities, appetite and sleep changes, weight changes, decreased energy, excessive guilt or feelings of worthlessness, psychomotor agitation or retardation, and possibly suicidal/homicidal ideation. The diagnosis of major depressive episode requires that symptoms be present nearly every day for 2 wk and that the woman experiences a decline from a previous level of functioning.

ETIOLOGY

The decline in reproductive hormones following delivery is believed to contribute to the development of postpartum depression in some women. In addition, women with a history of depression, premenstrual syndrome or dysphoric disorder, stressful life events, and a family history of mood disorders have an increased risk of both depression and postpartum depression.

DIAGNOSIS

DIFFERENTIAL DIAGNOSIS

- Hyperthyroid
- Hypothyroid
- Postpartum blues: Syndrome involving symptoms of depression, anxiety, or anger that usually occurs 2 to 3 days after delivery and resolves within a few days to 1 to 2 weeks postpartum without treatment.
- Postpartum psychosis: Usually occurs between 1 to 2 wk post-delivery and is characterized by extreme disorganization of thought, hallucinations, and bizarre behavior. It requires rapid intervention, as there is a real risk of suicide or infanticide
- Bipolar disorder

WORKUP

- History and physical examination
- Screening all postpartum women with a screening instrument such as the Edinburgh Postnatal Depression Scale (specific to the postpartum period and takes less than 5 min to complete) or the Patient Health Questionnaire 9
- In any patient with postpartum depression, screening for bipolar disorder

LABORATORY TESTS

Thyroid screening tests (if high suspicion for thyroid disorder)

TREATMENT

NONPHARMACOLOGIC THERAPY

- Psychotherapy: Studies have shown psychotherapy to be equally effective to fluoxetine.

ACUTE GENERAL Rx

- Therapy with a selective serotonin reuptake inhibitor should be considered as first-line treatment because of low risk of toxic effects with overdose and ease of dosing. However, if the patient has had good success with another medication in the past, then it is appropriate to restart that medication. Start at half the recommended dose and increase after 4 days, with gradual up-titration until therapeutic effects are seen.
- A single medication is favored over multiple medications in order to decrease exposure to the fetus/neonate.
- Sertraline is the first-line selective serotonin reuptake inhibitor recommended for breastfeeding mothers secondary to existing evidence suggesting little risk for infants. There is, however, no evidence of adverse infant effects from mothers taking sertraline, paroxetine, or fluvoxamine. Fluoxetine may be present in higher levels in breast milk and breastfed infants.
- Tricyclic antidepressants do not appear to pass in significant amounts into breastfeeding infants and their use appears to be safe. Data regarding atypical antidepressants and breastfeeding are limited.
- The FDA recently approved an IV infusion of the drug brexanolone (Zulresso). It is administered as a single 60-hour IV drip and is currently only available to patients through a restricted distribution program at certified health care facilities.

CHRONIC Rx

- Medical therapy should be continued until at least 6 mo after remission.
- Long-term therapy should be considered for women with a history of three or more episodes of depression.

DISPOSITION

- Without treatment, the duration of postpartum depression averages 7 mo.
- Fifteen percent to 85% of women will experience at least one relapse after completing medical therapy.

REFERRAL

- Consider referral to psychiatrist if a patient demonstrates no improvement after 6 wk of drug therapy or experiences a relapse.
- Prompt or urgent referral to psychiatrist is indicated if a patient has signs/symptoms of postpartum psychosis, bipolar disorder, or expresses suicidal/homicidal ideation.

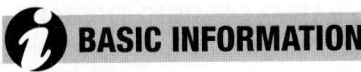

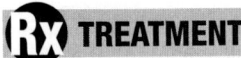

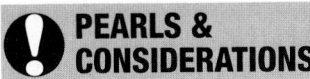

PEARLS & CONSIDERATIONS

COMMENTS

- Depression and anxiety both during and after pregnancy can have negative effects not only on the mother but also on her fetus, new baby, and family. Low birth weight, decreased fetal growth, increased NICU admission rates, increased neonate crying, and decreased developmental scores have been seen with these disorders when untreated. In addition, depression is associated with increased smoking, alcohol, and drug use, which can have negative effects on the infant and family. These factors should be taken into account when counseling women about medical therapy.
- Selective serotonin reuptake inhibitors do pass through breast milk but are present in very small quantities compared with the transplacental exposure infants receive in utero. Adverse infant effects are extremely rare; however, long-term data are lacking.

PREVENTION

In a patient with a history of postpartum depression, recurrence risk is approximately 25%. These patients should be screened for depression both during and after pregnancy. It is reasonable to initiate prophylactic therapy in patients with a history of depression, and they should have close postpartum follow-up for early identification of depressive episodes.

PATIENT/FAMILY EDUCATION

- National Women's Health Information Center: www.womenshealth.gov
- Postpartum Support International: www.postpartum.net
- Centers for Disease Control and Prevention: www.cdc.gov/reproductivehealth/depression/

SUGGESTED READINGS

Available at ExpertConsult.com

RELATED CONTENT

Depression, Major (Related Key Topic)

AUTHOR: **JHENETTE LAUDER, M.D.**

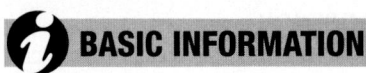

BASIC INFORMATION

DEFINITION

Postpartum hemorrhage (PPH) is classically defined as estimated blood loss >500 ml after a vaginal birth or >1000 ml after a cesarean section. Primary PPH is hemorrhage within the first 24 hr after delivery. Secondary PPH is hemorrhage after 24 hr and within 6 to 12 wk.

SYNONYMS

Obstetric hemorrhage
PPH

ICD-10CM CODES

- 072.1 Other immediate postpartum hemorrhage
- 072.2 Delayed and secondary postpartum hemorrhage

EPIDEMIOLOGY & DEMOGRAPHICS

INCIDENCE: 3% to 5% of obstetric patients will experience postpartum hemorrhage. Postpartum hemorrhage is the cause of one fourth of maternal deaths worldwide and 12% of maternal deaths in the U.S.

PREDOMINANT SEX AND AGE: Female of reproductive age

RISK FACTORS: Prolonged labor, augmented labor, rapid labor, history of PPH, episiotomy, retained placenta/membranes, lacerations, preeclampsia, multiple gestation, macrosomic infant, operative delivery, chorioamnionitis, bleeding dyscrasia

PHYSICAL FINDINGS & CLINICAL PRESENTATION (TABLE 1)

- Bleeding is generally brisk at time of delivery.
- Examination findings include boggy uterus with continued passage of clot or blood with fundal pressure.
- Objective findings can also include hypotension, tachycardia, and oliguria with substantial blood loss.

ETIOLOGY

- Primary: Uterine atony (>80%), retained placenta, coagulopathies, lacerations
- Secondary: Subinvolution of placental site, retained products, infection, coagulopathies

Dx DIAGNOSIS

WORKUP

- Bladder should be emptied
- Bimanual examination to evaluate for atony; massage if it is present
- Examination to verify that no lacerations are present, including cervical examination with necessary lighting and retractors
- Ultrasonography at bedside to evaluate for retained tissue or clot
- Examination to verify that placenta is intact

LABORATORY TESTS

Significant hemorrhage can lead to disseminated intravascular coagulation (DIC). If DIC is suspected, complete blood count and coagulation panels should be ordered. Similarly, if coagulopathy is suspected, evaluation of clotting factors should be ordered.

IMAGING STUDIES

Ultrasonography can be used to scan for retained products, including clot or placenta. It can be performed to assess the need for more invasive measures, such as instrumentation or a manual sweep.

Rx TREATMENT

The most effective strategy for the prevention of postpartum hemorrhage is active management of the third stage of labor (AMTSL). Medical management with uterotonics is generally the first line of treatment:

- Oxytocin (IV, 10-40 units diluted into IV solution, or 10 units IM); often given prophylactically immediately after delivery (preferred)
- Methergine (IM, 0.2 mg)
- Hemabate (IM, 0.25 mg)
- Misoprostol (400-800 mcg sublingually, buccally, or rectally)

Other medical management:

- Tranexamic acid (IV, 1 g)

NONPHARMACOLOGIC THERAPY

Secondary management includes the following:

- Controlled cord traction (Brandt-Andrews maneuver)
- Uterine massage after delivery of placenta
- Packing with gauze, Foley catheter, or tamponade balloon
- Uterine curettage for suspected retained products
- Uterine artery embolization
- Ensure adequate IV access
- Surgical management with laparotomy:
  1. Hypogastric artery ligation
  2. Bilateral uterine artery ligation (O'Leary sutures)
  3. B-lynch sutures
  4. Hysterectomy

ACUTE GENERAL Rx

- Uterotonics, surgical management, embolization, blood transfusion. Fig. 1 outlines the management of postpartum hemorrhage.
- Table 2 describes therapeutic response to initial fluid resuscitation. Dosing regimen for oxytocic drugs is summarized in Table 3. Blood product replacement is described in Box 1.

TABLE 1 Presentation of Symptoms in Postpartum Hemorrhage

% Blood loss (ml)	Systolic blood pressure (mm Hg)	Signs and symptoms
10-15 (500-1000)	Normal	Tachycardia, palpitations, dizziness
15-25 (1000-1500)	Low-normal	Tachycardia, weakness, diaphoresis
25-35 (1500-2000)	70-80	Restlessness, pallor, oliguria
35-45 (2000-3000)	50-70	Collapse, air hunger, anuria

From Vincent JL et al: *Textbook of critical care,* ed 6, Philadelphia, 2011, WB Saunders.

TABLE 2 Therapeutic Response to Initial Fluid Resuscitation

Response	Description	Follow-up treatment
Rapid response	<20% of blood volume lost	No additional fluids or blood are needed.
Transient response	20%-40% of blood volume lost; responds to initial fluid bolus but later has worsening vital signs	Continue fluids and consider blood transfusions.
Minimal or no response	Ongoing severe hemorrhage with >40% blood volume lost	Continue aggressive fluid and blood product replacements.

From Vincent JL et al: *Textbook of critical care,* ed 6, Philadelphia, 2011, WB Saunders.

TABLE 3 Dosing Regimens for Oxytocic Drugs

Drugs	Regimens
Oxytocin (Pitocin)	5-unit IV bolus
	Add 20–40 units oxytocin to 1 L of fluids.
	10 units intramyometrially
Methylergonovine (Methergine)	0.2 mg IM every 2–4 h
Ergonovine maleate (Ergotrate)	100-125 μg IM or intramyometrially every 2-4 h
	200-250 μg IM
	Total dose 1.25 mg
Carboprost (Hemabate)	250 μg IM or intramyometrially every 15-90 min
	Total dose 2 mg
Misoprostol	800 μg PR or 800 μg of sublingual misoprostol

IM, intramuscular; *IV,* intravenous; *PR,* per rectum.
From Vincent JL et al: *Textbook of critical care,* ed 7, Philadelphia, 2017, Elsevier.

CHRONIC Rx

For anemia: Ferrous sulfate supplementation to support new red blood cell production

DISPOSITION

- The patient should be closely watched for at least 24 hr after a postpartum hemorrhage. Vital signs should be monitored for evidence of hemodynamic stability and appropriate response to anemia. Serial laboratory tests can be performed in the setting of concern for ongoing bleeding.
- Morbidity can include shock, acute respiratory distress syndrome, Sheehan syndrome, thromboembolic disease, and loss of fertility.

REFERRAL

During the course of a postpartum hemorrhage, the anesthesiology department and blood bank should be notified, and adequate nursing should be available. Early considerations should be made to notify obstetricians. If bleeding is brisk or estimated blood loss is considerable, preparation should be made for transfusion of blood products, including drawing blood for typing and notifying the blood bank.

SUGGESTED READINGS

Available at ExpertConsult.com

AUTHOR: **LEO HAN, M.D., M.P.H.**

BOX 1 Blood Product Replacement

Crossmatched blood
Type-specific or "saline crossmatched" blood
Compatible ABO and Rh blood types
Rh-negative blood is preferable.
Warm the blood, if possible, especially if the rate of infusion is >100 ml/min or if the total volume transfused is high; cold blood is associated with an increased incidence of arrhythmias and paradoxic hypotension.
Administer calcium if blood is transfused rapidly at >100 ml/min because of binding of calcium by anticoagulants in banked blood.
Give 6–10 units fresh frozen plasma (FFP) for every 10 units of packed red blood cell (PRBC) transfusions.
Give 10–12 units of platelets if the platelet count decreases to <50 × 10^9/L.
Cryoprecipitate can be given to replace fibrinogen in addition to the FFP.
Consider 60–120 μg/kg intravenous bolus injection of recombinant activated factor VII (rFVIIa).

From Vincent JL et al: *Textbook of critical care*, ed 7, Philadelphia, 2017, Elsevier.

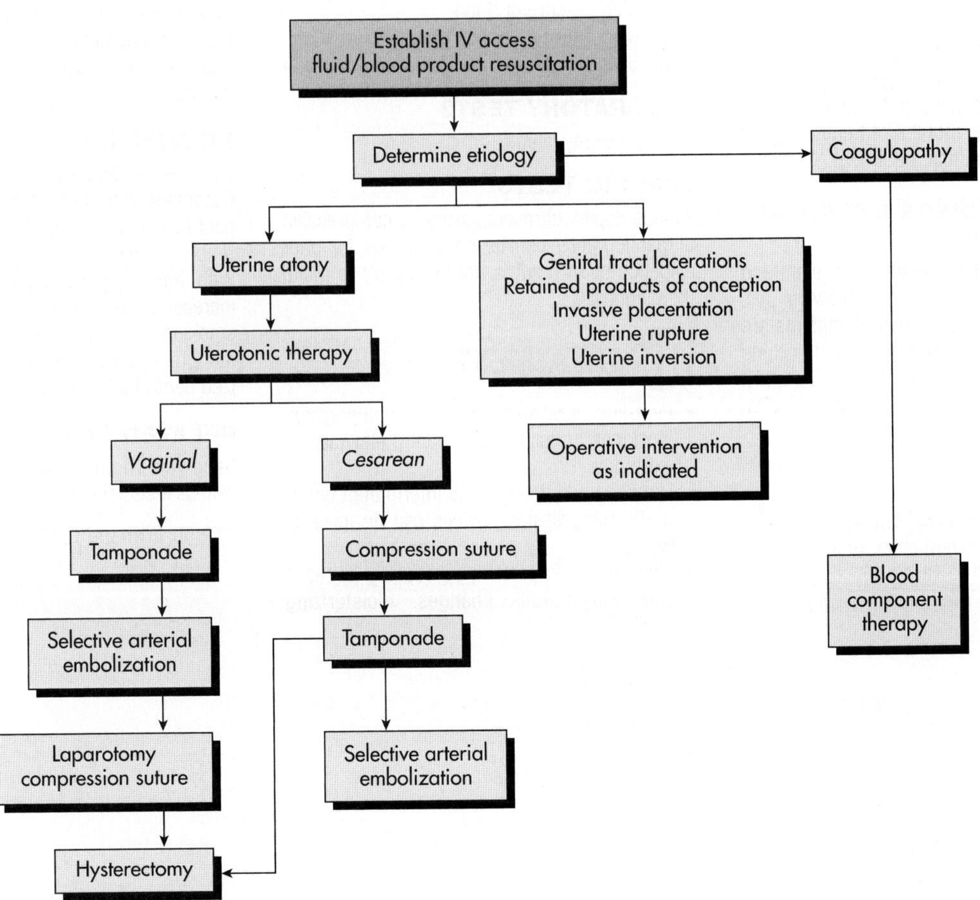

FIG. 1 Management of postpartum hemorrhage. (From Gabbe SG: *Obstetrics*, ed 6, Philadelphia, 2012, WB Saunders.)

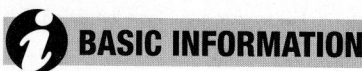

BASIC INFORMATION

DEFINITION

Postthrombotic syndrome (PTS) is a delayed complication of deep vein thrombosis (DVT) that leads to signs and symptoms of venous insufficiency.

SYNONYMS

Postphlebitic syndrome
Chronic venous insufficiency
PTS

ICD-10CM CODES

I87.001	Postthrombotic syndrome without complications of right lower extremity
I87.002	Postthrombotic syndrome without complications of left lower extremity
I87.003	Postthrombotic syndrome without complications of bilateral lower extremities

EPIDEMIOLOGY & DEMOGRAPHICS

INCIDENCE: 23% to 60% of people with DVT will experience postthrombotic syndrome, often within 2 yr of onset of DVT.
PREVALENCE: Unknown
PREDOMINANT SEX: Slightly female predominance
RISK FACTORS: Symptomatic DVT, postoperative DVT, recurrent DVT, underlying primary venous insufficiency, younger age, obesity, presence of varicose veins, proximal DVT, residual thrombus after 6 months of treatment, and inadequate antithrombotic treatment

PHYSICAL FINDINGS & CLINICAL PRESENTATION

Symptoms can be intermittent or constant and often appear weeks to months following DVT, but can occur up to years later. Symptoms are generally progressive over time and include edema in the extremity, pain in the extremity, changes in skin pigmentation, ulceration (Fig. E1), and venous dilation.

ETIOLOGY

Venous insufficiency results from chronic venous hypertension due to obstruction from thrombus and to reflux related to valvular incompetence. Inflammatory cytokines such as interleukin-6 are thought to play a role.

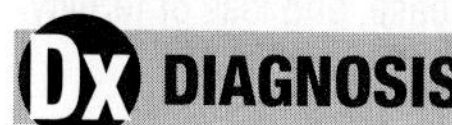

DIAGNOSIS

DIFFERENTIAL DIAGNOSIS

DVT, primary venous insufficiency, Baker cyst, tumor, lymphedema, lipedema, and injury to extremity

WORKUP

Clinical diagnosis based on history of DVT and signs and symptoms of chronic venous insufficiency. The Villalta scale can be used in cases when the diagnosis is uncertain. It is the most widely used scoring system for both diagnosing postthrombotic syndrome (PTS) and assessing its severity.

- Entails five patient symptoms (pain, leg cramps, heaviness in extremity, paresthesia, and pruritus) and six physical signs (pretibial edema, skin induration, hyperpigmentation, pain with calf compression, venous ectasia, and redness).
- Scored on a scale of 0 to 3 (0 = none, 1 = mild, 2 = moderate, 3 = severe).
- Total score ranges from 0 to 33; a score ≥5 is consistent with a diagnosis of PTS.
  1. PTS can also be diagnosed if a venous ulcer is present independent of total score.
- Severity is assessed based on score:
  1. Mild = score of 5 to 9
  2. Moderate = score of 10 to 14
  3. Severe = score of 15 to 33

LABORATORY TESTS

None presently used

IMAGING TESTS

Venous duplex ultrasonography or compression ultrasonography can be done to look for prior evidence of DVT but is not necessary to make the diagnosis.

Rx TREATMENT

- First-line treatment includes compression stockings, regular exercise, and elevation of extremity.
- Lymphedema therapy and intermittent pneumatic compression devices can be used as well.
- Skin care is important, particularly in cases with eczematous changes. Moisturizing lotions can be used in conjunction with mild potency corticosteroids.
- Diuretics have a limited role but can decrease edema in some patients.
- Endovascular recanalization can be considered for cases that are refractory to treatment and where pain control is difficult. There are no randomized controlled trials to evaluate endovascular repair.
- Surgical repair is generally reserved for severe cases and for those with nonhealing ulcers. Surgical options include angioplasty, venous bypass, or endophlebectomy.

DISPOSITION

- Chronic venous insufficiency can impair quality of life and is often a chronic condition.
- Early treatment with anticoagulation may decrease the risk of postthrombotic syndrome.
- Early use of compression stockings can reduce symptoms of venous insufficiency and halt progression.

REFERRAL

Lymphedema clinic, interventional radiology, and vascular surgery

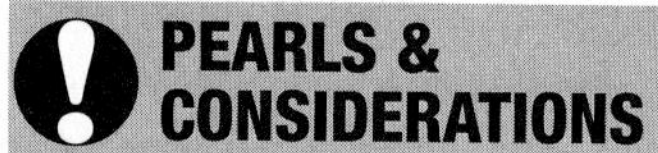

PEARLS & CONSIDERATIONS

COMMENTS

Compression stockings have the most evidence both for preventing postthrombotic syndrome and for treatment once the syndrome has developed.

PREVENTION

There is evidence both for and against early treatment with thrombolytic drugs to prevent postthrombotic syndrome. Reducing the recurrence of DVT is the best way to prevent PTS. With each subsequent DVT the risk of PTS increases. Periodic leg elevation, weight loss, smoking cessation, and regular exercise are all thought to prevent PTS; however, no randomized controlled trial has been done to evaluate.

RELATED CONTENT

Deep Vein Thrombosis (Related Key Topic)
Venous Insufficiency, Chronic (Related Key Topic)

AUTHOR: **LYNN DADO, M.D.**

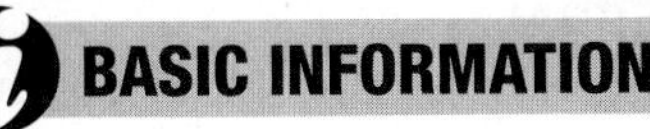

BASIC INFORMATION

DEFINITION

Posttraumatic stress disorder (PTSD) develops in some people after witnessing or experiencing a traumatic event that involves actual or threatened injury to self or others. Symptoms continue longer than a month after the event or may have delayed onset and include intrusive thoughts, nightmares, flashbacks, avoidance of things associated with the trauma, hypervigilance, sleep disturbance, and negative changes in mood and cognition. These symptoms cause distress and a decline in interpersonal, social, and occupational functioning. People with PTSD may feel numb or irritable, may be easily startled or frightened, and sometimes isolate themselves from others. They are at risk for comorbid psychiatric illness, substance abuse, and suicide.

SYNONYMS

PTSD
Soldier's heart
Effort syndrome
Shell shock
Concentration camp syndrome

ICD-10CM CODES

F43.10	Post-traumatic stress disorder, unspecified
F43.11	Post-traumatic stress disorder, acute
F43.12	Post-traumatic stress disorder, chronic

DSM-5 CODES

309.81	Posttraumatic stress disorder
309.89	Other specified trauma and related disorder
309.9	Unspecified trauma and stressor-related disorder

EPIDEMIOLOGY & DEMOGRAPHICS

INCIDENCE: Fewer than 10% of individuals who have experienced a traumatic event will develop PTSD; however, there is considerable variability in prevalence rates associated with specific trauma types.

PREVALENCE (IN U.S.):
- 12-mo prevalence in the U.S. 3% to 6%. Estimated lifetime prevalence 7.8% to 12.3%.
- Prevalence among high-risk populations (e.g., combat veterans or victims of violent crimes) up to 58%.
- Comorbidity is common: Depression, anxiety, substance use, personality disorders, and somatic symptom disorder.
- Factors most associated with development are previous traumatic experience and subsequent life stress and perceived lack of social support.

PREDOMINANT AGE AND SEX:
- No predisposing age factors.
- Twice as many women as men are affected (prevalence 10% to 14% for women and 5% to 6% for men). More than 50% of cases in women are related to sexual assault.

GENETICS: Several studies, including twin studies, have demonstrated genetic factors associated with increased risk of developing PTSD after trauma exposure.

PHYSICAL FINDINGS & CLINICAL PRESENTATION

Core symptom clusters include intrusion, avoidance, negative mood and cognition, hyperarousal, and sometimes dissociative symptoms. Individuals present with different variations of these symptoms. Symptoms must occur for >1 mo and result in significant distress and functional impairment.

Key PTSD symptoms:
- Distressing memories or dreams of the event. Note: Children older than 6 yr may express this symptom in repetitive play
- Flashbacks
- Intense distress after reminders of the event
- Avoidance due to trauma-related thoughts or feelings
- Persistent negative trauma-related emotions
- Feeling detached
- Aggressive or reckless behavior
- Hypervigilance
- Problems with concentration or sleep
- Depersonalization

ETIOLOGY

- Common types of trauma: Violent personal assault, natural disaster, military combat, rape, motor vehicle accident, childhood abuse and neglect, critical illness or hospitalization in ICU, severe physical injury, diagnosis of life-threatening illness.
- Risk factors: Previous trauma, initial severity of reaction to event, psychiatric history, traumatic brain injury, childhood abuse or neglect, poor social support, gender, age.
- Interpersonal violence is more likely to cause PTSD than events such as motor vehicle accidents or natural disasters.
- Severity of physical injury is a weaker predictor of PTSD than the psychological distress; stress duration and social support are factors, among others.
- Proposed mechanisms include activation of the amygdala, disruption of prefrontal cortex modulation of the amygdala, and excessive stress-induced HPA and alpha-1 receptor activation.

Dx DIAGNOSIS

Diagnosis is made when the stressor is consistent with DSM-5 definition, with symptoms of re-experiencing, avoidance, negative mood and cognition, and arousal and reactivity. The symptoms must be present for >1 mo, must cause impairment in functioning, and must not be attributable to substance use or other medical conditions. Subtypes include dissociative (PTSD criteria and depersonalization or derealization) and delayed onset (PTSD criteria starting at least six months after the event).

Definition of stressor:
- Exposure to death, threatened death, actual or threatened serious injury, or actual or threatened sexual violence with directly experiencing the event, witnessing the event occur to others, or learning that a close relative or close friend was exposed to trauma. If the event involved actual or threatened death, it must have been violent or accidental.
- Repeated or extreme indirect exposure to aversive details of the event(s), usually in the course of professional duties (e.g., first responders collecting body parts; professionals repeatedly exposed to details of child abuse).

DIFFERENTIAL DIAGNOSIS

- Adjustment disorders: Precipitating stress is less catastrophic and psychological reaction is less specific
- Mood disorder: Depression or bipolar
- Anxiety disorders
- Somatic symptom or conversion disorder (functional neurological symptom disorder)
- Psychotic disorder
- Traumatic brain injury

WORKUP

- Validated self-report questionnaires and structured diagnostic instruments include the Posttraumatic Diagnostic Scale and Clinician Administered PTSD Scale (CAPS).
- Although numerous potential biomarkers have been identified and are under investigation, at this time evidence is not conclusive. To date, laboratory and imaging are not clinically useful.
- Primary care PTSD (PC-PTSD) screen recommended by the Veterans' Administration.
- "Yes" answer to three of four of the following questions is a positive screen. In your life, have you ever had any experience that was so frightening, horrible, or upsetting that, in the past month, you:
    1. Have had nightmares about it or thought about it when you did not want to?
    2. Tried hard not to think about it or went out of your way to avoid situations that reminded you of it?
    3. Were constantly on guard, watchful, or easily startled?
    4. Felt numb or detached from others, activities, or your surroundings?

Rx TREATMENT

- According to the most recent International Society for the Study of Traumatic Stress (ISTSS) treatment guidelines, cognitive-behavioral therapy approaches, including prolonged exposure (PE) and cognitive processing therapy (CPT), have the greatest empirical support to date among psychotherapy approaches.
- Prolonged exposure (PE) includes psychoeducation on the stress response, imaginal exposure focused on recounting trauma memories, and in vivo exposure focusing on reducing avoidance of anxiety-provoking situations associated with the trauma.

- CPT includes written exposure to the trauma memory combined with cognitive therapy.
- A recent clinical trial found that brief written exposure therapy intervention was noninferior to standard CPT and had fewer dropouts.
- Group therapy. Current standards recommend individual therapy as first-line. A growing number of studies have demonstrated efficacy of cognitive behavioral therapy (CBT) in a group format, although results are mixed, with some studies finding individual therapy to be superior.
- Eye movement desensitization reprocessing (EMDR) is considered an evidence-based treatment for PTSD in treatment guidelines, demonstrating comparable efficacy to traditional CBT approaches in clinical trials. However, to date it is unclear whether it offers advantages over, or operates through distinct mechanisms from, traditional CBT approaches. Evidence supporting the efficacy of the eye movements and parallel stimulation component is limited.
- A growing number of studies have demonstrated efficacy of CBT approaches for PTSD delivered through novel formats, including exposure therapy integrating virtual reality technology and Internet- and telephone-delivered CBT, although more research is needed to ascertain whether these approaches are comparable to traditional formats.
- Couples therapy when appropriate.

MEDICATIONS

There is no definitive cure for PTSD, and individuals have varying responses to different medications. Sertraline and paroxetine, both SSRIs, are the only FDA-approved medications for PTSD. Other medication use is off-label with differing levels of evidence to support use. Medications are used to target symptoms and the physiologic changes associated with PTSD and with psychiatric disorders that are frequently comorbid with PTSD. According to ISTSS treatment guidelines, SSRIs and SNRIs are currently considered the first-line pharmacologic treatments for PTSD, and it is recommended that they be prescribed for duration of at least 8 to 12 wk, with some studies demonstrating maximum benefit reached as late as 36 wk.

- SSRIs: Sertraline, paroxetine, fluoxetine.
- SNRIs: Venlafaxine, duloxetine.
- Other antidepressants: Mirtazapine has shown efficacy in small randomized trials.
- Alpha-adrenergic receptor blockers: Prazosin has demonstrated efficacy in reducing nightmares.
- Atypical antipsychotics (e.g., risperidone, quetiapine, olanzapine) have demonstrated efficacy as augmenting agents for individuals with partial response to SSRIs and may be particularly beneficial for individuals with paranoia, extreme anxiety, or angry outbursts.
- Transcranial magnetic stimulation (TMS) is being evaluated as a possible effective treatment modality.
- Ketamine: Recent clinical trials of intravenous ketamine infusion showed PTSD and depression symptom reduction, although more research is needed.
- *N*-methyl-D-aspartate (NMDA) agonists and partial agonists have shown some efficacy in early clinical trials, although more research is needed.
- Recent efforts are underway to examine the efficacy of pharmacologic interventions in preventing development of PTSD early after exposure to trauma, though more research is needed.

ACUTE GENERAL Rx

- Immediate postincident debriefing may worsen outcome.
- Benzodiazepines are not currently recommended as monotherapy for the treatment of PTSD, as there is no evidence that they reduce reexperiencing and avoidance/numbing symptoms.
- Beta-adrenergic blockers may be helpful if given within hours after the trauma to disrupt the physiologic stress response, although more research is needed.
- Sedating antidepressants or sleep aids may be helpful for initial insomnia.

DISPOSITION

- Recovery rates are highest in the first 12 mo after onset.
- Average duration of symptoms is 36 mo for those who undergo treatment and 64 mo for those never treated.
- 50% chance of remission at 2 yr; 50% have chronic symptoms.
- Predictors of chronic course include previous trauma, premorbid psychiatric function, panic reaction at time of event, prolonged terror, or dissociation at time of event.

REFERRAL

Because early intervention improves outcome, refer to a specialist as soon as diagnosis made.

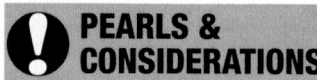

PEARLS & CONSIDERATIONS

- PTSD is associated with increased occurrence of suicidal ideation and attempts.
- PTSD can be associated with aggressive and violent behavior.
- Traumatic medical experiences such as being in the ICU, myocardial infarction, or an emergent cesarean section can cause PTSD.
- Individuals with PTSD frequently present with comorbid psychiatric disorders, including substance abuse, major depression, anxiety disorders, and personality disorders.
- Among combat veterans of recent wars, there is a 41% co-occurrence with mild TBI.
- PTSD may vary culturally and present as culturally specific syndromes and idioms of distress.
- Treatment can be effective even if it begins years after the traumatic event occurred.
- Cannabis is available from medical dispensaries in many states for treating PTSD, yet its efficacy in treating PTSD symptoms remains uncertain. Current evidence is insufficient to draw conclusions about the benefits and harms of plant-based cannabis preparations in patients with PTSD, but several ongoing studies may soon provide answers.[1]

SUGGESTED READINGS

Available at ExpertConsult.com

RELATED CONTENT

Posttraumatic Stress Disorder (PTSD) (Patient Information)

AUTHOR: **CATHERINE D'AVANZATO, PH.D.**

[1] O'Neil MF, et al.: Benefits and harms of plant-based cannabis for prosttraumatic stress disorder, *Ann Int Med* 167:332-340, 2017.

BASIC INFORMATION

DEFINITION

Preeclampsia involves the presence of hypertension with other associated comorbidities in a pregnant woman. In 2013, the American College of Obstetrics and Gynecology (ACOG) Task Force on Hypertension in Pregnancy revised the criteria, making preeclampsia a hypertensive disorder and one where the presence of proteinuria was no longer needed to make the diagnosis. The task force reinforced the importance of hypertension as a necessary condition and deemphasized proteinuria. In the absence of proteinuria, thrombocytopenia, new development of renal insufficiency, impaired liver function, pulmonary edema, new-onset cerebral or visual symptoms could substitute as criteria.

Additionally, the task force emphasized the categories employed in prior ACOG bulletins:

- Preeclampsia: Hypertension with or without proteinuria, but with the presence of one of the previously mentioned comorbidities
- Preeclampsia with severe features (Table 1)
- Chronic hypertension: Hypertension predating pregnancy or present at <20 wk gestation
- Gestational hypertension: Hypertension in pregnancy after 20 wk without proteinuria or any of the previously mentioned comorbidities
- Chronic hypertension with superimposed preeclampsia: The presence of chronic hypertension with sudden increase in blood pressure or escalation of medication when previously well controlled or with development of new onset of signs or symptoms meeting criteria for severe preeclampsia. Table 1 summarizes the criteria for the diagnosis of severe preeclampsia
- Atypical preeclampsia: Onset prior to 20 wk; onset after 48 hr postpartum; gestational proteinuria with symptoms of preeclampsia, hemolysis, thrombocytopenia, or elevated liver enzymes

SYNONYMS

Pregnancy-induced hypertension
Toxemia of pregnancy

ICD-10CM CODES

011.1	Pre-existing hypertension with pre-eclampsia, first trimester
011.2	Pre-existing hypertension with pre-eclampsia, second trimester
011.3	Pre-existing hypertension with pre-eclampsia, third trimester
011.9	Pre-existing hypertension with pre-eclampsia, unspecified trimester
014.00	Mild to moderate pre-eclampsia, unspecified trimester
014.02	Mild to moderate pre-eclampsia, second trimester
014.03	Mild to moderate pre-eclampsia, third trimester
014.10	Severe pre-eclampsia, unspecified trimester
014.12	Severe pre-eclampsia, second trimester
014.13	Severe pre-eclampsia, third trimester
014.90	Unspecified pre-eclampsia, unspecified trimester
014.92	Unspecified pre-eclampsia, second trimester
014.93	Unspecified pre-eclampsia, third trimester

EPIDEMIOLOGY & DEMOGRAPHICS

INCIDENCE: 2% to 7% in primigravidas, up to more than 50% in multigravidas with risk factors

RISK FACTORS: See Table 2.

GENETICS: Positive correlation with maternal and paternal family history

PHYSICAL FINDINGS & CLINICAL PRESENTATION

- Preeclampsia typically presents with hypertension and proteinuria, most commonly in the third trimester of pregnancy.
- May be asymptomatic.
- Generalized swelling or nondependent edema, possibly manifested by rapid weight gain (>4 lb/wk), even in the absence of edema, is common but is nonspecific and is seen in many normal pregnancies.
- Auscultation of pulmonary rales.
- Right upper quadrant pain (HELLP syndrome [hemolysis, elevated liver enzymes, and low platelet count] or subcapsular liver hematoma).
- Hyperreflexia or clonus.
- Vaginal bleeding (placental abruption).
- Chronic fetal compromise manifested by intrauterine growth restriction or acute fetal compromise manifested by nonreassuring fetal testing.
- Wide range of symptoms attributable to multiorgan system dysfunction, involving hepatic, hematologic, renal, pulmonary, and central nervous systems.
- Possibility of severe disease despite "normal" blood pressure readings, so a high index of suspicion must be maintained in high-risk situations.

ETIOLOGY

- Exact etiology is unknown.
- Theories:
  1. Imbalance between thromboxane A_2 (vasoconstrictor and platelet aggregator) and prostacyclin (vasodilator)
  2. Abnormal trophoblastic invasion of spiral arteries
  3. Increased sensitivity to angiotensin II by the muscular walls of the arteries
  4. Excess circulating soluble FMS-like tyrosine kinase 1 (*sFlt1*), which binds placental growth factor (PIGF) and vascular endothelial growth factor (VEGF), may have a pathogenic role
- Potential secondary effects of the metabolic, inflammatory endothelial alternatives in preeclampsia are described in Table 3.

Dx DIAGNOSIS

DIFFERENTIAL DIAGNOSIS

- Acute fatty liver of pregnancy
- Appendicitis
- Diabetic ketoacidosis
- Gallbladder disease
- Gastroenteritis
- Glomerulonephritis
- Hemolytic-uremic syndrome
- Hepatic encephalopathy
- Hyperemesis gravidarum
- Idiopathic thrombocytopenia
- Thrombotic thrombocytopenic purpura
- Nephrolithiasis
- Pyelonephritis
- Peptic ulcer disease
- Systemic lupus erythematosus
- Viral hepatitis
- Medications or medication withdrawal

TABLE 1 Criteria for the Diagnosis of Preeclampsia with Severe Features

In patients with preeclampsia, **preeclampsia with severe features** can be diagnosed if any one of the following criteria is present:

Blood pressure ≥160 mm Hg systolic or ≥110 mm Hg diastolic on two separate occasions at least 4 hr apart

Serum creatinine >1.1 mg/dl or a doubling of the serum creatinine

New onset of cerebral or visual disturbances

Pulmonary edema

Hepatocellular injury (serum transaminases at least twice normal) or severe persistent right upper quadrant or epigastric pain

Thrombocytopenia <100,000

TABLE 2 Risk Factors for Preeclampsia

- Nulliparity
- Age >40 years
- Pregnancy with assisted reproduction
- Interpregnancy interval >7 years
- Family history of preeclampsia
- Woman born small for gestational age
- Obesity/gestational diabetes
- Multifetal gestation
- Preeclampsia in a previous pregnancy
- Poor outcome in a previous pregnancy
- Fetal growth restriction, placental abruption, fetal death
- Preexisting medical-genetic conditions
- Chronic hypertension
- Renal disease
- Type 1 (insulin-dependent) diabetes mellitus
- Antiphospholipid antibody syndrome

From Gabbe SG et al: *Obstetrics,* ed 7, 2016, Philadelphia, Elsevier.

WORKUP

Hypertension:
- Two blood pressure measurements at least 4 hr apart, with the patient sitting or semi-reclining with the back supported, with an absolute pressure ≥140 mm Hg systolic or ≥90 mm Hg diastolic.
- A single blood pressure ≥160 mm Hg systolic or ≥110 mm Hg diastolic.

Hypertension can thus be confirmed in a brief period to allow for immediate treatment of the blood pressure.

Proteinuria:
- ≥300 mg per 24-hr urine collection
- Protein/creatinine ratio ≥0.3
- +1 on dipstick ONLY IF OTHER METHODS NOT AVAILABLE
- In the absence of proteinuria, preeclampsia may be diagnosed with new onset of hypertension and one of the following:
  1. Platelet count less than 100,000/ml
  2. New-onset, progressive renal insufficiency, serum creatinine concentrations greater than 1.1 mg/dl, or doubling of serum Cr levels in the absence of other renal disease
  3. Elevated serum liver transaminases to twice the normal concentration
  4. Pulmonary edema
  5. New-onset cerebral or visual symptoms
- Because of the insidious nature of the disease with potential for multiple organ involvement, as well as its prevalence, complete evaluation for preeclampsia in any pregnant patient presenting with central nervous system derangement or gastrointestinal symptoms after 20 wk of gestation
- Evaluation for associated conditions such as disseminated intravascular coagulation, hepatic dysfunction, or subcapsular hematoma
- Fig. 1 outlines a management plan for patients with severe preeclampsia

TABLE 3 Potential Secondary Effects of the Metabolic, Inflammatory Endothelial Alternatives in Preeclampsia

CVS	Increased peripheral resistance leading to hypertension; increased vascular permeability and reduced maternal plasma volume.
Lungs	Laryngeal and pulmonary edema.
Renal	Glomerular damage leading to proteinuria, hypoproteinemia, and reduced oncotic pressure, which further exacerbates the hypovolemia. May develop acute renal failure ± cortical necrosis.
Clotting	Hypercoagulability, with increased fibrin formation and increased fibrinolysis (i.e., disseminated intravascular coagulation).
Liver	HELLP syndrome hepatic rupture.
CNS	Thrombosis and fibrinoid necrosis of the cerebral arterioles. Eclampsia (convulsions), cerebral hemorrhage, and cerebral edema.
Fetus	Impaired uteroplacental circulation, potentially leading to FGR, hypoxemia, and intrauterine death.

CVS, Cardiovascular system; *CNS,* central nervous system; *FGR,* fetal growth restriction; *HELLP,* hemolysis, elevated liver enzymes, low platelets.
From Drife J, Magowan B: *Clinical obstetrics and gynecology,* Philadelphia, 2004, WB Saunders.

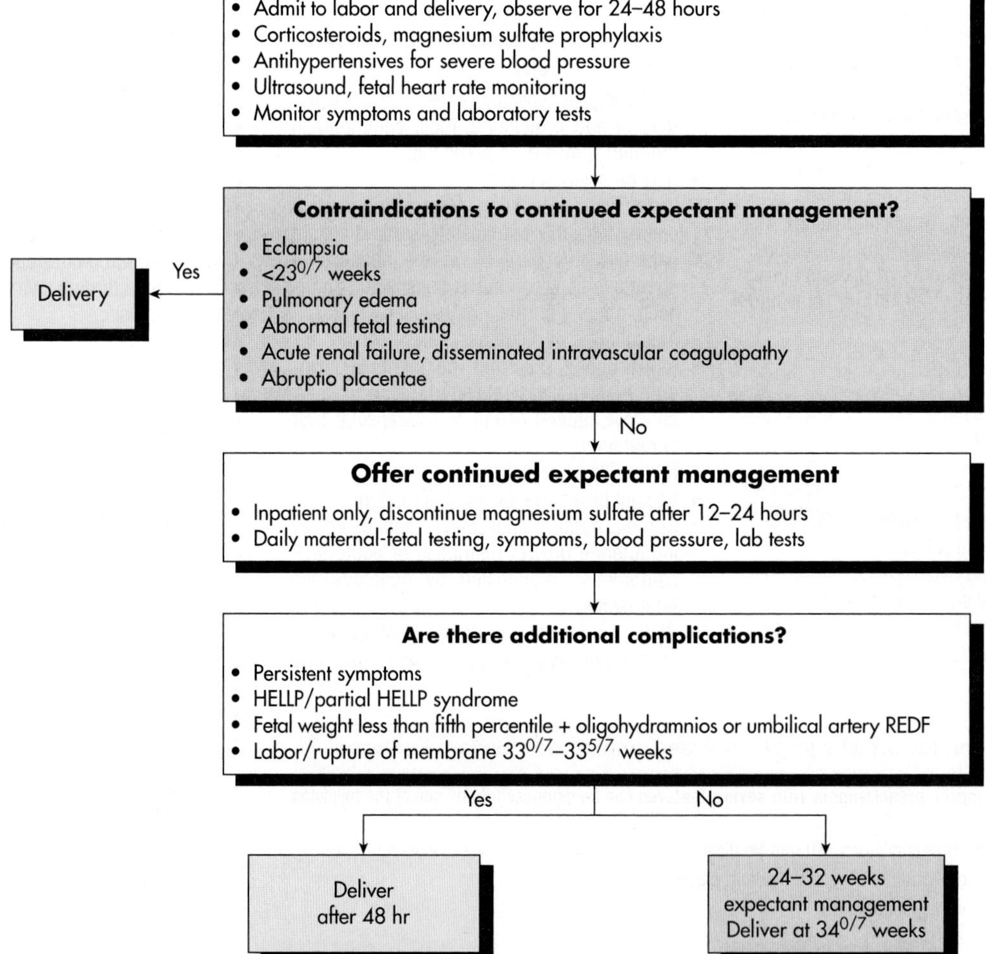

FIG. 1 Management plan for patients with preeclampsia with severe features before 34 weeks' gestation. *HELLP,* hemolysis, elevated liver enzymes, and low platelets; *REDF,* reversed end-diastolic flow. (From Gabbe, SG et al: *Obstetrics: Normal and problem pregnancies,* ed 7, Philadelphia, 2017, Elsevier.)

LABORATORY TESTS

- High-risk patients: Baseline assessment of renal function (24-hr urine collection for protein and creatinine clearance), complete blood count, serum creatinine, liver function tests (LFTs), and uric acid should be obtained at the first prenatal visit.
- Complete blood count (hemoglobin, hematocrit, platelets) may show signs of volume contraction or HELLP syndrome.
- LFTs (aspartate aminotransferase, alanine aminotransferase, lactate dehydrogenase) are useful in evaluation for HELLP syndrome or to exclude important differentials.
- Hyperuricemia or increased creatinine may indicate decreasing renal function.
- Prothrombin time, partial thromboplastin time, and fibrinogen should be checked to rule out disseminated intravascular coagulation.
- Peripheral smear may demonstrate microangiopathic hemolytic anemia.
- Complement levels can be used to differentiate from an acute exacerbation of a collagen-vascular disease.
- The ratio of soluble FMS-like tyrosine kinase 1 (sFlt-1) to placental growth factor (PIGF) is elevated in pregnant women before the clinical onset of preeclampsia. Increased levels of sFlt1 and reduced levels of PIGF predict subsequent development of preeclampsia. An sFlt-1:PIGR ratio of 38 or lower can be used to predict the short-term absence of preeclampsia in women in whom the syndrome is suspected clinically.[1]

IMAGING STUDIES

- CT or MRI scan of head if atypical presentation of eclampsia or preeclampsia with atypical cerebral symptoms, possibility of intracerebral bleed, or prolonged postictal state
- Sonogram of fetus to evaluate for intrauterine growth restriction amniotic fluid, placenta
- Sonogram of maternal liver if subcapsular hematoma suspected

Rx TREATMENT

ACUTE GENERAL Rx

Delivery is the treatment of choice and the only cure for the disease. This must be taken in the context of the gestational age of the fetus, severity of the preeclampsia, and the likelihood of a successful induction and reliability of patient.

- For preeclampsia with severe features, administer magnesium sulfate 4 to 6 g IV loading dose, with 2 g/hr maintenance (adjust dosage for renal insufficiency), or phenytoin at 10 to 15 mg/kg loading dose, then 200 mg IV q8h starting 12 hr after loading dose if a contraindication to magnesium sulfate, such as myasthenia gravis.
- Treat BP >160 mm Hg systolic or >110 mm Hg diastolic either with hydralazine 5 to 10 mg IV, then 10 mg, then 20 mg every 20 minutes; or with labetalol hydrochloride 20, 40, 80, 80 mg IV, escalating dosage every 10 min; or with nifedipine 10, 20, 20 mg orally every 20 min for acute blood pressure control. If maximum dose of one medication is reached, add an additional medication to reach goal of BP 140-150/90-100 mm Hg.
- Continuous fetal monitoring.
- Epidural is anesthesia of choice for pain management in labor or cesarean section.
- All patients undergoing induction of labor or cesarean section should receive antiseizure medications (magnesium sulfate) if disease with severe features, for delivery and 24 hr postpartum.

CHRONIC Rx

- Preeclampsia without severe features <37 wk: Close observation for worsening maternal or fetal condition, with delivery at 37 wk. If 24 to 36 wk, consider antenatal corticosteroids. If severe features develop or there is evidence of fetal compromise, earlier delivery would be appropriate.
- Preeclampsia with severe features: Delivery in the presence of maternal or fetal compromise, labor, or 34 wk; at 24 to 34 wk consider steroids with very close monitoring, and at <24 wk consider termination of pregnancy. Risks of expectant management include severe worsening of disease, eclampsia, abruptio placenta, stillbirth, HELLP syndrome, ICU admission, and pulmonary edema.
- Contraindications to expectant management include eclampsia, HELLP syndrome, pulmonary edema, DIC, abruptio placenta, uncontrollable severe hypertension, fetal demise, and nonreassuring fetal status.
- Labetalol, hydralazine, and nifedipine are the drugs of choice for long-term blood-pressure control during pregnancy.

DISPOSITION

Preeclampsia is a progressive and unpredictable disease process; a course of expectancy should be managed with caution. Up to 20% of patients who have seizures are normotensive.

The reoccurrence rate for preeclampsia in a subsequent pregnancy is approximately 20%, and higher in cases with a second trimester presentation or complications. This risk may be decreased with the use of low-dose aspirin.

REFERRAL

Obstetric management is indicated because of the insidious nature of the disease, with transfer of all cases <34 wk to a facility with appropriate maternal and neonatal care facilities.

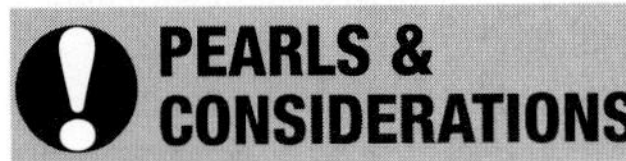

PEARLS & CONSIDERATIONS

COMMENTS

- Low-dose aspirin, beginning as early as the second trimester, decreases the risk of preeclampsia, preterm birth, and intrauterine growth retardation in women who are at high risk of preeclampsia. The American College of Obstetricians and Gynecologists (ACOG) and the U.S. Preventive Services Task Force (USPSTF) recommend the use of low-dose aspirin as preventive medication starting after 12 wk of gestation (ideally before 16 weeks) in women who are at high risk for preeclampsia (previous preeclampsia, multifetal gestation, chronic hypertension, type 1 or 2 diabetes, renal disease, or autoimmune disease).
- The use of low-dose aspirin, 150 mg/day started at 11 to 14 wk gestation, has been demonstrated to decrease the incidence of preterm preeclampsia in a selected high-risk population.[2] In the U.S., low-dose aspirin is available as an 81 mg tablet. U.S. clinicians who recommend aspirin for preeclampsia prevention should consider prescribing two 81 mg tablets daily.
- Although the absolute risk of end-stage renal disease (ESRD) in women who have had preeclampsia is low, preeclampsia is a marker for an increased risk of subsequent ESRD.
- The development of preeclampsia may be one of the earliest identifiable risk markers for potential future cardiovascular disease in women. It has been shown that women who develop preeclampsia have a higher incidence of cardiovascular risk factors including components of the metabolic syndrome within 1 yr of delivery.

SUGGESTED READINGS

Available at ExpertConsult.com

RELATED CONTENT

Preeclampsia (Patient Information)
Eclampsia (Related Key Topic)
Hypertension (Related Key Topic)

AUTHOR: **PHILIP A. SHLOSSMAN, M.D.**

[1] Zeisler H et al: Predictive value of the sFlt-1:PIGF ratio in women with suspected preeclampsia, *N Engl J Med* 374:13-22, 2016.

[2] Rolnick DL et al: Aspirin versus placebo in pregnancies at high risk for preterm preeclampsia, *N Engl J Med* 377:613-622, 2017.

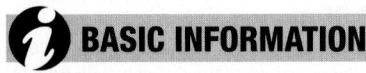

BASIC INFORMATION

DEFINITION

Premature rupture of membranes (PROM) is defined as rupture of membranes at term before the onset of labor.

SYNONYMS

Preterm premature rupture of membranes (prior to 37 weeks)
PROM

ICD-10CM CODES

042	Premature rupture of membranes
042.113	Preterm premature rupture of membranes

EPIDEMIOLOGY & DEMOGRAPHICS

INCIDENCE: Affects approximately 8% of all pregnancies

RISK FACTORS: Intraamniotic infection, low socioeconomic status, second- and third-trimester bleeding, low body mass index, nutritional deficiencies, connective tissue disorders, maternal cigarette use, cervical conization or cerclage, short cervix, pulmonary disease in pregnancy, uterine overdistention, amniocentesis, prior history of PROM, prior history of preterm delivery

PHYSICAL FINDINGS & CLINICAL PRESENTATION

Patients will classically present complaining of leakage or gush of fluid from the vagina. Patients may also present with contractions and vaginal bleeding. Additional symptoms can include fever, chills, or abdominal pain if there is concurrent infection. Ultrasound will often demonstrate oligohydramnios.

ETIOLOGY

Premature rupture of membranes at term may occur due to physiologic changes in addition to uterine contractions causing shearing forces. Although there are many risk factors for PROM, it often occurs in the absence of any known risk factor.

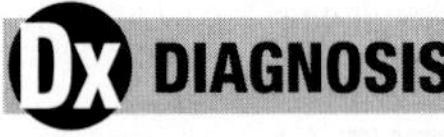

DIAGNOSIS

DIFFERENTIAL DIAGNOSIS

Differential diagnosis includes leakage of urine or vaginal discharge.

WORKUP

Sterile speculum examination demonstrating pooling of fluid in posterior fornix, visualization of fluid coming out of the cervix during Valsalva maneuver, basic vaginal pH, and characteristic ferning pattern of vaginal fluid that is dried on a microscope. Table 1 summarizes bedside testing for premature rupture of membranes.

Care should be taken to avoid any procedure that may introduce infection, so digital examination should be avoided unless patient is in active labor or delivery is imminently planned. This is of particular importance in preterm PROM.

LABORATORY TESTS

- pH test: Sample vaginal fluid from posterior fornix. Normal vaginal pH is 4.5 to 6.0. pH of amniotic fluid is 7.1 to 7.3. False-positive test can occur in presence of blood or semen, antiseptic or bacterial vaginosis.
- Microscopy: Visualization of ferning of vaginal fluid allowed to dry on the microscope slide. False-positive test can occur if cervical mucus is sampled.
- Commercially available tests: AmniSure and other tests are available and demonstrate good sensitivity and specificity; however, per the American College of Obstetrics and Gynecology, these should be considered ancillary to standard evaluation.

IMAGING STUDIES

- Abdominal ultrasound: Evaluation of amniotic fluid volume either by maximum vertical pocket or amniotic fluid index. Oligohydramnios or low fluid volume in itself should not be considered diagnostic of PROM.
- Amniotic fluid dye test: This is considered the gold standard in diagnosis of PROM, used in clinical scenario of suspected preterm PROM with equivocal testing. Indigo carmine dye is injected via ultrasound guidance into the amniotic sac, and diagnosis made if blue dye passes into vagina.

Rx TREATMENT

NONPHARMACOLOGIC THERAPY

All patients with PROM should have prompt evaluation of gestational age, fetal well-being via NST monitoring, and fetal presentation. In a patient with evidence of intraamniotic infection or fetal distress, prompt delivery is recommended. Close monitoring and consideration of delivery is recommended if there is concern for placental abruption. Collect swab for evaluation of GBS status and gonorrhea/chlamydia.

ACUTE GENERAL Rx

Term PROM:

- At 37.0 weeks' gestation or more, delivery is recommended for all women with ruptured membranes. Induction of labor has been shown to decrease time to delivery, risk of chorioamnionitis, endometritis, and NICU admissions, with no increase in rate of operative delivery.
- A period of expectant management can be offered in select patients who decline induction and have been appropriately counseled.
- Routine induction agents may be used. The most researched agents for induction in setting of PROM include oxytocin and prostaglandins. Oxytocin has been shown to be associated with lower rates of chorioamnionitis. Infection is also a concern with mechanical methods of cervical ripening, such as Foley balloon.
- GBS prophylaxis should be provided in GBS-positive individuals or individuals with GBS-unknown status and concurrent risk factors.

Preterm PROM:

- 34 weeks or above: Clinician should proceed toward delivery as in term patients. Administration of betamethasone for fetal lung maturity as indicated by Antenatal Late Preterm Steroids trial.
- 24 to 34 weeks:
  1. Administration of betamethasone for fetal lung maturity.
  2. Administration of prophylactic antibiotics to prolong latency period, consisting of 7-day course of parenteral and oral therapy. Current guidelines recommend ampicillin or amoxicillin and erythromycin.
  3. Expectant management until 34 weeks, unless fetal lung maturity is demonstrated between 32 to 34 weeks.
  4. Magnesium sulfate administration if delivery is imminent and <32 weeks.
  GBS prophylaxis in setting of GBS unknown/GBS positive if delivery is expected.

CHRONIC Rx

Hospitalization with expectant management is recommended for all patients with preterm PROM. Ongoing maternal and fetal surveillance in a hospital setting allows for quick recognition of infection, labor, or fetal compromise secondary to cord compression.

DISPOSITION

- Most women with preterm PROM will proceed to deliver within one week despite medical interventions. Latency period is generally longer when PROM occurs at an earlier gestational age.
- Clinical chorioamnionitis develops in 13% to 16% of preterm PROM. This risk is increased with earlier PROM as well as with an increase in the number of digital vaginal examinations. Complications of preterm PROM are related mostly to complications of prematurity, and

TABLE 1 Bedside Testing for Premature Rupture of Membranes

Method	Result
Nitrazine	Amniotic fluid (pH >6.5) will turn nitrazine paper blue; normal vaginal secretions (pH <5.5) will leave nitrazine paper yellow.
Ferning	Amniotic fluid crystallizes.
Smear combustion	Amniotic fluid, when flamed, turns white and crystallizes. Vaginal secretions caramelize and turn brown.

From Marx J, et al.: *Rosen's emergency medicine: concepts and clinical practice*, ed 7, Philadelphia, 2010, Mosby.

decrease with increasing gestational age at time of delivery. The most common complications include respiratory distress, neonatal infection, intraventricular hemorrhage, and necrotizing enterocolitis.
- There is a 1% to 2% risk of antenatal demise in the setting of preterm PROM.

REFERRAL

Consultation with an Ob-Gyn or maternal fetal medicine specialist is recommended in the setting of preterm PROM.

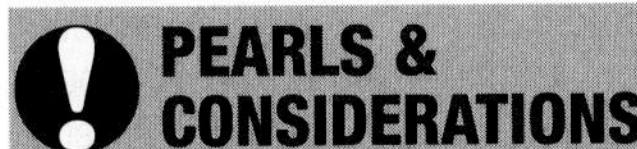

PEARLS & CONSIDERATIONS

PREVENTION

Patients with a history of preterm delivery (with or without PROM) may benefit from administration of progesterone supplementation in future singleton pregnancy starting at 16 to 24 weeks to prevent preterm delivery.

SUGGESTED READINGS

Available at ExpertConsult.com

RELATED CONTENT

Abruptio Placentae (Related Key Topic)
Premature Labor (Related Key Topic)

AUTHOR: **GHAMAR BITAR, M.D.**

BASIC INFORMATION

DEFINITION

Premenstrual syndrome (PMS) consists of various somatic and physical complaints that develop during the luteal phase of the menstrual cycle and that are of sufficient severity to interfere with daily functioning and/or interpersonal relationships. The symptoms resolve shortly after the onset of menses.

SYNONYM

PMS

ICD-10CM CODE
N94.3 Premenstrual tension syndrome

EPIDEMIOLOGY & DEMOGRAPHICS

- Premenstrual disorders affect about 12% of reproductive-age women, although as many as 80% of women will report at least one somatic or affective symptom during their luteal phase (Table 1).
- Severe cases of premenstrual dysphoric disorder (PMDD), which is more of a psychiatric diagnosis, occur in approximately 1.3% to 5.3% of women.
- The prevalence of PMS is not associated with age, race, or socioeconomic status.
- Those seeking treatment for PMS are usually in their 30s or 40s.
- Based on some identical twinning studies, a genetic component is thought to exist, but no genes have been identified.
- The natural history of PMS has not been clearly elucidated.

PHYSICAL FINDINGS & CLINICAL PRESENTATION

- Diverse and potentially disabling symptoms. Table 1 summarizes common symptoms of PMS
- Associated with multiple psychological, physical, and behavioral symptoms
- Most frequent reason for seeking treatment: Emotional symptoms
- Most common emotional symptoms: Depression, irritability, anxiety, labile moods, anger, crying easily, sadness, extreme sensitivity, nervous tension
- Most common physical symptoms: Headache, bloating, cramps, breast tenderness, migraines, fatigue, weight gain, aches and pains, palpitations
- Most common behavior symptom: Food cravings
- Other behavioral symptoms: Increased appetite, increased alcohol intake, decreased motivation, decreased efficiency, avoidance of activities, staying home, sleep changes, libido changes, forgetfulness, decreased concentration

ETIOLOGY

- Etiology is poorly understood. The syndrome is thought to result from steroid hormone effects on serotonin, ϒ-aminobutyric acid, dopamine systems, and the renin-aldosterone system, thus causing some of the bloating symptoms.
- Because of the multifactorial, multiorgan nature of PMS, a single etiologic cause is unlikely.

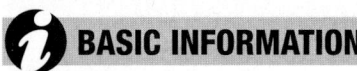

DIAGNOSIS

DIFFERENTIAL DIAGNOSIS

- A diagnosis of exclusion, so other medical or psychological disorders should be ruled out.
- Common disorders to rule out: Depression or anxiety, anemia, migraines, endometriosis, thyroid disease.

WORKUP

- History.
- Physical examination.
- Laboratory studies to rule out alternative diagnosis.
- If no alternative diagnosis, confirm by either history of regular menses, basal body temperature charting, or elevated luteal progesterone that patient is ovulatory.
  1. If she is not ovulating, it is not PMS.
  2. A prospective questionnaire given over two menstrual cycles has been found to be the most accurate way to assess the presence of PMS or PMDD. If symptoms are not occurring only in the luteal phase, it is not PMS, and further investigation is needed.
     a. If symptoms occur in the follicular phase, patient has premenstrual exacerbation of another condition.
     b. If symptoms do not occur in the follicular phase, diagnosis of PMS is confirmed.

LABORATORY TESTS

- None available to specifically confirm the diagnosis of PMS
- Thyroid function tests to rule out thyroid disease

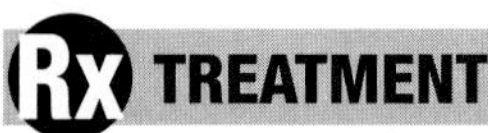

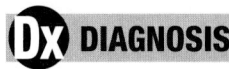

TREATMENT

NONPHARMACOLOGIC THERAPY

- Individualization of the treatment plan to maximize therapeutic response. Fig. E1 describes a summary of treatment approaches to PMS.
- Psychosocial intervention:
  1. Education
  2. Stress management
  3. Environmental changes
  4. Adequate rest and sleep
  5. Regular exercise
- Nutritional recommendations:
  1. Regularly eaten, well-balanced meals
  2. Adequate amounts of protein, fiber, and complex carbohydrates; low fat
  3. Avoidance of foods that are high in salt and simple sugars; may promote water retention, weight gain, and physical discomfort
  4. Avoidance of alcohol and illicit drugs; may worsen emotional lability
  5. Calcium supplementation (1000 mg/day for women 19 to 50 yr, 1300 mg/day for girls 14 to 18 yr) to reduce the physical and emotional symptoms
  6. The data are mixed regarding the benefits of vitamin D supplementation in reducing PMS symptoms, so more studies are needed
  7. Pyridoxine (vitamin B_6) 80 mg qd to improve depression, fatigue, and irritability has been suggested in small studies

ACUTE GENERAL Rx

Suppression of ovulation:

- Oral contraceptives: One pill per day; continuous use associated with better treatment effect
- Progestin-only oral contraceptive: One pill per day
- Oral micronized progesterone: 100 mg every morning and 200 mg every evening on days 17 through 28 of menstrual cycle
- Progestin suppository: 200 to 400 mg bid on days 17 through 28 of menstrual cycle
- Medroxyprogesterone: 150 mg IM q3mo
- Levonorgestrel implants: Surgical insertion every 5 yr

TABLE 1 Common Symptoms of Cyclic Premenstrual Syndrome

Somatic Symptoms	
Abdominal bloating	Constipation or diarrhea
Acne	Headache
Alcohol intolerance	Peripheral edema
Breast engorgement and tenderness	Weight gain
Clumsiness	
Emotional and Mental Symptoms	
Anxiety	Insomnia
Change in libido	Irritability
Depression	Lethargy
Fatigue	Mood swings
Food cravings (especially salt and sugar)	Panic attacks
Hostility	Paranoia
Inability to concentrate	Violence toward self and others
Increased appetite	Withdrawal from others

From Goldman L, Schafer AI: *Goldman's Cecil medicine*, ed 24, Philadelphia, 2012, WB Saunders.

- Transdermal estradiol: One or two 100-μg patches every 3 days
- Danazol: 100 to 200 mg/day (ovulation not suppressed at this dose); has significant side-effect profile
- Gonadotropin-releasing hormone (GnRH) agonists: Daily by intranasal spray or monthly by depot injection; profound hypoestrogenism, concerns for osteoporosis and vasomotor symptoms

Suppression of physical symptoms:

- Spironolactone: 25 to 50 mg bid on days 14 through 28 of menstrual cycle—need a reliable form of birth control
- Mefenamic acid
  1. For fluid retention: 250 mg tid on days 24 through 28 of cycle
  2. For pain: 500 mg tid on days 19 through 28 of cycle
- Bromocriptine: 5 mg/day on days 10 through 26 of cycle
- Naproxen: 550 mg bid on days 17 through 28 of cycle, Naprosyn-500 mg bid on days 17 through 28 of cycle

Suppression of psychological symptoms:

- SSRI, or serotonergic antidepressants, are first-line treatment for PMS/PMDD, treating mostly the psychological aspects but also some physical aspects.
- Sertraline, paroxetine, fluoxetine, citalopram, escitalopram.
- In 2013 the *Cochrane Reviews* reported a statistically significant benefit over placebo when taken either continuously or in the luteal phase.
- Serotonin-norepinephrine reuptake inhibitors (SNRI) such as venlafaxine; use is off-label, but onset of action is quick and has been found to be helpful.
- Seroquel: Smaller studies.
- Wellbutrin: Not as effective as the other options.

CHRONIC Rx

- Therapy is largely trial and error, with the goal of providing effective treatment with the safest therapy. Provider should initially attempt to ameliorate the most pronounced symptom(s).
- Limited evidence exists that acupuncture and/or acupressure may ameliorate some symptoms associated with PMS and improve quality of life. More studies are needed to determine if this option is as good as or better than conventional therapies such as treatment with an SSRI.
- For severe intractable PMS: Bilateral oophorectomy; give trial of GnRH therapy or danazol before surgery (bilateral oophorectomy should be exceedingly rare).
- Estrogen replacement therapy recommended postoperatively to reduce the risk of osteoporosis, heart disease, and genitourinary atrophy.

DISPOSITION

Improved symptoms in 90% of women over time

REFERRAL

- For counseling with a psychologist or psychiatrist if underlying psychiatric disorder is discovered (cognitive-behavioral therapy)
- To a gynecologist if surgical therapy is contemplated

SUGGESTED READINGS

Available at ExpertConsult.com

RELATED CONTENT

Premenstrual Syndrome (Patient Information)
Dysmenorrhea (Related Key Topic)
Premenstrual Dysphoric Disorder (Related Key Topic)

AUTHOR: **ADRIENNE B. NEITHARDT, M.D.**

BASIC INFORMATION

DEFINITION

The 2016 National Pressure Ulcer Advisory Panel (NPUAP) defines pressure injury (previously pressure ulcer) as a localized area of damage to the skin and/or underlying soft tissue over a bony prominence related to a medical or other device. This occurs as a result of intense or prolonged pressure or pressure in combination with shear. The tolerance of soft tissue for pressure and shear may also be affected by microclimate, nutrition, perfusion, co-morbidities, and condition of the soft tissue. Common sites include the sacrum, ischium, and calcaneus among others. This revised nomenclature allows for the recognition of lesser degrees of skin damage that are not necessarily associated with pressure ulcers.

SYNONYMS

Decubitus ulcers
Pressure sores
Bedsores
Pressure ulcers
Pressure-induced skin injury
Pressure-induced soft tissue injury

ICD-10CM CODES

L89	Pressure ulcers
Subcategories of codes determined by stage and location of ulcer	
L89.153	Example: Stage 3 ulcer of sacral area
L98.491	Non-pressure chronic ulcer of skin of other sites limited to breakdown of skin
L98.492	Non-pressure chronic ulcer of skin of other sites with fat layer exposed
L98.493	Non-pressure chronic ulcer of skin of other sites with necrosis of muscle
L98.494	Non-pressure chronic ulcer of skin of other sites with necrosis of bone
L98.499	Non-pressure chronic ulcer of skin of other sites with unspecified severity

EPIDEMIOLOGY & DEMOGRAPHICS

- The incidence of pressure injury varies by clinical setting. It is a recognizable indicator of the quality of healthcare in both Canada and the U.S.
- An estimated 2.5 million cases of pressure injuries are treated each year in acute care facilities across the U.S.
- Pressure injuries resulted in 28,500 documented deaths globally in 2013, more than double from 13,700 deaths in 1990.
- Development of pressure injury results in increased hospital length of stay by 7 to 10 days. These patients are three times more likely to be discharged to long-term care facilities.
- Although there is consensus that pressure injuries may not entirely be unavoidable, they certainly can be prevented in most instances.
- In the U.S., the Centers for Medicare and Medicaid (CMS) does not provide any reimbursement to hospitals for treatment of stage 3 and 4 pressure injuries acquired during hospitalization.
- Patients who develop pressure injuries tend to be older patients (mean age of 71 yr), debilitated, and immobile and have multiple medical problems, including dementia, diabetes, urinary or fecal incontinence, and nutritional deficiencies. A cohort study observed that pressure injuries occurred in 36% of older patients with hip fracture.
- Occurs in all health care settings including hospitals, nursing homes, and residential homes. The reported rates upon admission to a nursing home range from 10% to 35%. The incidence rate is highest in institutions with lower staffing levels of registered nurses and certified nursing assistants, reflecting the importance of healthcare resources rather than medical decision-making.
- Associated with impaired quality of life and significant morbidity and mortality. One-yr mortality rate approaches 40%. Emotional and psychological trauma often accompany pressure injury, leading to more significant reduction in overall well-being and quality of life.
- Significant pain occurs in two thirds of patients with stage 2 or greater pressure injury.

CLINICAL PRESENTATION

There are a number of staging systems that have been developed and utilized to describe the stages of pressure injury. The most commonly used system is that from the National Pressure Ulcer Advisory Panel (NPUAP). The European Pressure Ulcer Advisory Panel (EPUAP) recommends similar staging except for the presence of suspected deep tissue injury and unstageable ulcers. The staging of the wound should be based according to the extent or depth of injury.

The NPUAP 2016 guidelines (Fig. 1) described the staging system as follows:

- **Stage 1 pressure injury: nonblanchable erythema of intact skin**
  1. Skin is intact with a localized area of nonblanchable erythema, which may appear differently in patients with darkly pigmented skin color. The presence of blanchable erythema or changes in sensation, temperature, or firmness may precede visual changes. Color changes do not include purple or maroon discoloration; these may indicate deep tissue pressure injury.
- **Stage 2 pressure injury: partial-thickness skin loss with exposed dermis**
  1. The wound bed is viable, pink or red, moist, and may also present as an intact or ruptured serum-filled blister. Adipose (fat) is not visible, and deeper tissues are not visible. Granulation tissue, slough, and eschar are not present. These injuries commonly result from adverse microclimate and shear in the skin over the pelvis and on the heel. This stage should not be used to describe moisture-associated skin damage, including incontinence-associated dermatitis, intertriginous dermatitis, medical adhesive–related skin injury, or traumatic wounds (skin tears, burns, abrasions).
- **Stage 3 pressure injury: full-thickness skin loss**
  1. At this stage there is full-thickness loss of skin with adipose tissue visible in the ulcer; granulation tissue and epibole (rolled wound edges) are often present. Slough and/or eschar may be visible. The depth of tissue damage varies by

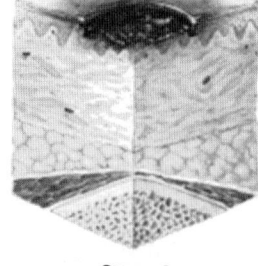

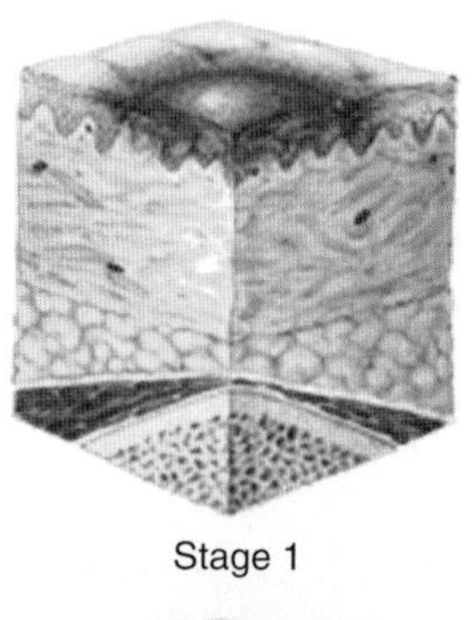
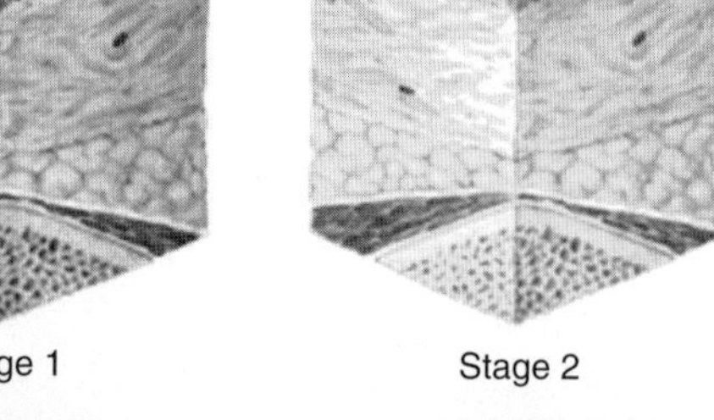

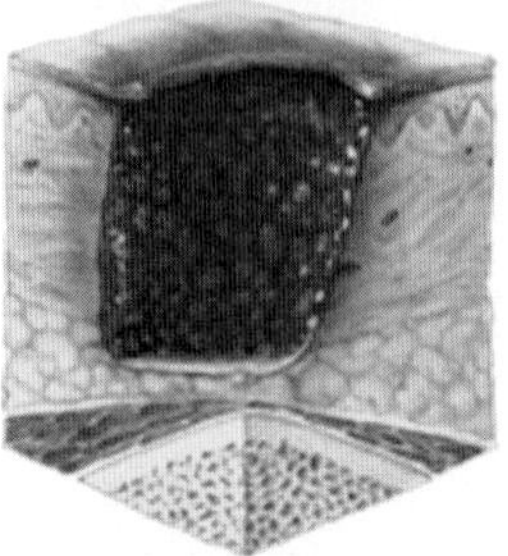
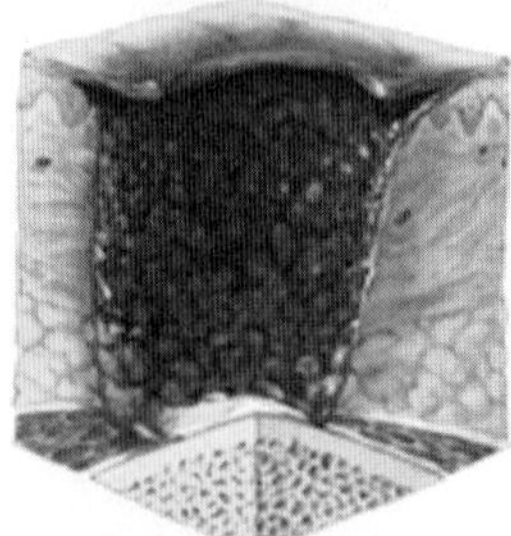

FIG. 1 Staging of pressure ulcers. (Used with permission of the National Pressure Ulcer Advisory Panel. (From Marx JA, et al.: *Rosen's emergency medicine*, ed 8, Philadelphia, 2014, Elsevier.)

anatomical location; areas of significant adiposity can develop deep wounds. Undermining and tunneling may occur. Fascia, muscle, tendon, ligament, cartilage, and/or bone are not exposed. If slough or eschar obscures the extent of tissue loss, this is an unstageable pressure injury. The depth of a stage 3 pressure injury varies by anatomic location.

- **Stage 4 pressure injury: full-thickness skin and tissue loss**
  1. At this stage there is full-thickness skin and tissue loss with exposed or directly palpable fascia, muscle, tendon, ligament, cartilage, or bone in the ulcer. Slough and/or eschar may be visible. Epibole (rolled edges), undermining, and/or tunneling often occur. Depth varies by anatomical location. If slough or eschar obscures the extent of tissue loss, this is an unstageable pressure injury. The extent of stage 4 ulcers is often underestimated due to undermining and fistula formation. A relatively small superficial defect may mask extensive tissue necrosis.
- **Unstageable pressure injury: obscured full-thickness skin and tissue loss**
  1. Unstageable pressure injury is full-thickness skin and tissue loss in which the extent of tissue damage within the ulcer cannot be confirmed because it is obscured by slough or eschar. If slough or eschar is removed, a stage 3 or stage 4 pressure injury will be revealed. Stable eschar (i.e., dry, adherent, intact without erythema or fluctuance) on the heel or ischemic limb should not be softened or removed.
- **Suspected deep tissue injury: Persistent nonblanchable deep red, maroon, or purple discoloration**
  1. Deep tissue pressure injury consists of intact or non-intact skin with a localized area of persistent nonblanchable deep red, maroon, or purple discoloration, or with epidermal separation revealing a dark wound bed or blood-filled blister. Pain and temperature changes often precede skin color changes. Discoloration may appear differently in darkly pigmented skin. This injury results from intense and/or prolonged pressure and shear forces at the bone-muscle interface. The wound may evolve rapidly to reveal the actual extent of tissue injury, or it may resolve without tissue loss. If necrotic tissue, subcutaneous tissue, granulation tissue, fascia, muscle, or other underlying structures are visible, a full-thickness pressure injury is present (unstageable, stage 3 or stage 4). Deep tissue pressure injury should not be used to describe vascular, traumatic, neuropathic, or dermatologic conditions.
- **Medical device–related pressure injury**
  1. Medical device–related pressure injuries result from the use of devices designed and applied for diagnostic or therapeutic purposes. The resultant pressure injury generally conforms to the pattern or shape of the device. The injury should be classified using the staging system.
- **Mucosal membrane pressure injury**
  1. Mucosal membrane pressure injury is found on mucous membranes with a history of a medical device in use at the location of the injury. Due to the anatomy of the tissue, these ulcers cannot be staged.

PATHOGENESIS

The development of a pressure injury is a complex interaction of external forces and host-specific factors. These forces include pressure, friction, shearing, and moisture. Pressure applied to the skin in excess of the arteriolar pressure of 32 mm Hg prevents the delivery of oxygen and nutrients to tissues, leading to tissue hypoxia, accumulation of metabolic waste products, and free radical generation. The most commonly affected sites include the sacrum, heels, and buttocks. The tolerance of soft tissue for pressure and shear may also be affected by immobility, microclimate factors, nutrition, perfusion, incontinence, comorbidities (including sensory perception disorders), and the condition of the soft tissue. Body mass index (BMI) has an important role in the risk for pressure injury. Underweight (BMI <19 kg/m^2) and morbidly obese (BMI >40 kg/m^2) patients are at high risk for pressure injury formation. Diseases that affect tissue perfusion such as peripheral vascular disease, diabetes mellitus, and heart failure pose a heightened risk for pressure injury development. However, it is important to note that patients with poor arterial flow in addition to liver failure, sepsis, and acute respiratory distress syndrome may be presenting with acute skin failure (ASF) rather than pressure injury. Unlike pressure injury, ASF is not considered preventable. Kennedy Terminal Ulcer (KTU) has also been described in the literature as an unavoidable skin breakdown or skin failure that occurs as part of the dying process. There have been no studies differentiating KTUs from ASF at this time.

Complications of untreated pressure injury include cellulitis, abscess formation, sinus tract formation, heterotopic calcification, systemic amyloidosis from chronic inflammation, and squamous cell cancer, particularly in a nonhealing pressure injury.

Dx DIAGNOSIS

DIFFERENTIAL DIAGNOSIS

- Venous insufficiency ulcers
- Arterio-occlusive ulcers
- Diabetic ulcers
- Neuropathic ulcers
- Skin cancer
- Cellulitis and erysipelas
- Skin abscess
- Kennedy terminal ulcers (KTU)
- Acute skin failure (ASF)
- Incontinence-associated dermatitis (IAD)
- Perineal dermatitis

WORKUP

- A thorough physical examination of the identified areas of skin damage and of a minimum of 4 cm of periwound tissue should be performed.
- These areas should be evaluated for their length, width, and depth and for the presence of sinus tracts, undermining, tunneling, fistulas, exudate, and necrotic tissue as well as any evidence for healing such as the formation of granulation tissue.
- Adequate documentation is a must.
- Additionally, it is equally important to rule out infection, as this would impair wound healing. Cellulitis, abscess, and osteomyelitis should be ruled out.

LABORATORY TESTS

- Directed at identifying causes, risk factors, and/or any complications arising from the pressure injury (e.g., abscess or osteomyelitis).
- Cultures of wound bed are not believed to be helpful and should be avoided. Deep tissue biopsy is the gold standard to rule out osteomyelitis.
- Useful markers for nutritional status include prealbumin, albumin, transferrin, lymphocyte count, and total cholesterol level.
- Complete blood count may be obtained if systemic infection is suspected.

IMAGING STUDIES

- Ultrasound is not proven to be effective.
- Plain radiographs, MRI, and triple-phase bone scan may help identify osteomyelitis when clinically suspected.
  1. A comparison study of 44 patients scheduled for open biopsy did not show MRI to have superior diagnostic benefit over plain radiography.

Rx PREVENTION & TREATMENT

- Conduct a structured and individualized risk assessment on a regular basis, especially when the clinical condition changes.
- Identify high-risk patients using standardized risk assessment scales and risk prediction tools (e.g., Braden and Norton in the U.S., Waterlow scale in the U.K., Cubbin and Jackson scale for ICU patients).
- Use of prophylactic dressings in high-risk patients is being studied in small randomized pilot studies in the U.S. and Australia. Focus is on the prevention of shearing and pressure injury to the sacrum and heels. Foam and silicone dressings show initial promise; it is too early to generalize results. Practice meticulous skin inspection and good skin care for at-risk patients.
- Focus on controlling the microclimate (moisture and temperature).
  1. Minimize prolonged skin exposure to moisture, urine, or stool.
  2. Treat dry, cracked skin.
- Use repositioning and pressure-reducing devices (e.g., foam mattresses, air-fluidized beds, low–air loss beds, pillows, gel pads, or foam wedges when in bed or in a chair).
  1. Patient repositioning (based on individual tissue tolerance): To date, there are no randomized trials available to identify

whether repositioning makes a difference in the healing rates or the optimal repositioning approaches utilized to prevent pressure injuries. Results from multiple studies have shown inconsistent results. Pilot studies continue in acute care hospitals, rehabilitation facilities, nursing homes, and in homebound populations. Additional areas of investigation include critical care, spinal cord injury, and surgical patients.

2. Bed surface:
    a. Two randomized controlled trials (RCTs) found that use of air-fluidized beds contributed to the healing of a greater number of pressure injuries after 15 days compared with standard care.
    b. A systematic review revealed no differences in rate of pressure injury healing with the use of either alternating-pressure mattresses or low air-loss beds compared with standard care.
3. Support surface:
    a. The first meta-analysis of support surfaces and pressure injury prevention concluded with moderate certainty that powered active air surfaces and powered hybrid air surfaces probably reduce the incidence of pressure injuries by 58% and 78% when compared to standard hospital surfaces.
    b. There is low certainty that nonpowered reactive surfaces reduce pressure injuries.
    c. Pressure-relieving overlays: One RCT demonstrated that a viscoelastic pad on the operating table significantly reduced incidence of postoperative pressure injuries compared with a standard operating table.
    d. Use adequate support surfaces while in bed or in a chair to prevent "bottoming out" (defined as less than 1 inch between patient and support surface; measured by putting hand under support surface and feeling thickness to patient).
4. Foam alternatives:
    a. Forty-one RCTs demonstrated that patients lying on standard hospital mattresses are more likely to develop pressure injuries than those patients lying on higher-specification foam mattresses.

- Recent systematic review of pressure injury prevention strategies showed poor methodology in most studies. Use of support surfaces, repositioning, optimized nutrition, and sacral skin moisturizing was most appropriate.
- The 2016 NPUAP consensus statement identified risk factors in specific situations that may lead to the development of unavoidable pressure injuries. These include the following: impaired tissue oxygenation, cardiovascular instability, hypovolemia, sepsis, anasarca, peripheral vascular disease, sensory impairment, immobility, end-of-life skin failure, multi-organ failure.

NON-PHARMACOLOGIC THERAPY

- Pressure injuries should be cleaned at each dressing change.
- Avoid agents that are cytotoxic to epithelial cells (e.g., iodine, iodophor, sodium hypochlorite, hydrogen peroxide, acetic acid, alcohol).
- Wound irrigation should not exceed 15 psi and is best done with an 18-gauge angiocatheter. Necrotic tissue should be debrided quickly because it delays wound healing and increases risk of infection.
- Do not debride hard, dry, stable eschar on heels or ischemic limbs.
- No single dressing or product is superior; keep wound bed moist and protect it from urine/stool. Silver dressings (thought to be antimicrobial), topical phenytoin, and growth factors should be limited to difficult-to-heal wounds, chronic ulcers, and extensive burns given their extra cost and limited scientific validation. Reduce pressure by using foam mattress, dynamic support surface (e.g., low–air loss bed), and frequent repositioning (e.g., every 2 hours or, in case of poor perfusion, more frequently).
- Hyperbaric oxygen therapy when used for some wounds provided temporary benefit. There have been no studies specifically looking at treatment of pressure injuries. Moreover, serious adverse events such as pneumothorax and seizures.
- The data on the efficacy of ultrasound as wound therapy is limited. Similarly RCTs on electromagnetic therapy found no evidence of benefit on wound healing.
- Use of topical agents such as phenytoin, becaplermin gel, sucralfate, and medicinal honey showed limited evidence for the healing of stage 2 ulcers.
- Negative-pressure wound therapy (NPWT) may be useful for wounds that have significant drainage. They help improve healing by promoting angiogenesis, improving tissue perfusion, and decreasing bacterial count. Calcium alginate and foam dressings may also be beneficial for such wounds. Randomized studies have not identified any significant differences to quantitative wound healing; however, it provided some level of patient and provider comfort.
- Although controlling poor nutrition has been shown to be beneficial, a recent large investigation demonstrated that feeding tubes did not prevent or heal pressure injuries, but increased the risk for their development.
- Minimize or promptly remove urinary and/or fecal contamination.
- Use standardized assessment tools to monitor wound healing on a weekly basis. Examples include the Pressure Sore Status Tool (PSST), Pressure Ulcer Scale for Healing (PUSH), Wound Healing Scale, and the Sessing Scale. The PUSH tool in conjunction with the NPUAP staging system is the most readily applied tool.
- No RCTs have compared debridement versus no debridement in the treatment of pressure injuries.
    1. Thirty-two RCTs have compared different debridement agents, but there is insufficient evidence to promote the use of one particular agent.
    2. One RCT demonstrated pressure injuries treated with collagenase healed significantly more quickly than those treated with hydrocolloid.
    3. One RCT comparing honey-treated dressings with dressings soaked with saline showed faster healing times with the honey-treated group.
    4. A meta-analysis and one RCT found significant benefit in rates of healing with use of hydrocolloid dressings versus traditional saline gauze dressings but not over other forms such as hydrogels, foam dressings, or collagenase.
- No benefit was found with nutritional and vitamin supplementation for those without known nutritional deficiencies. There is inconclusive evidence for use of vitamin C and zinc to promote wound healing. There are limited data for enteral or parenteral nutrition for patients whose oral intake is inadequate.
- There are insufficient data to recommend for the use of anabolic steroids such as oxandrolone therapy to promote weight gain and repletion of protein stores.

ACUTE GENERAL Rx

- Management of pressure injury is directed by its staging.
- The cornerstone of therapy involves the use of appropriate wound dressings, pressure-reducing devices, treatment of infection, debridement, and surgical consultation when appropriate.
- Traditional bedside debridement provides excellent results in reducing the surface area for a majority of the wounds. Sharp debridement can effectively remove devitalized tissue and is a proven significant component to advancing wound closure.
- All pressure injuries are colonized with bacteria. Clinically evident infections should be assessed with culture and treated appropriately with topical and systemic antibiotics.
- Adjunctive therapies such as negative pressure wound therapy, therapeutic ultrasound, hyperbaric oxygen, topical oxygen, and application of growth factors to the wound are continually being investigated.
- A randomized controlled trial in 2017 showed significant reduction in stage 2 to 4 pressure injuries using anode and cathode high-voltage electrical stimulation.
- Pain medications are necessary if pressure injuries are present. One study found that excruciating pain was more prevalent in nursing home residents with pressure injuries. Local factors that may be contributing to pain such as ischemia, infection, or breakdown of surrounding skin should be properly addressed.

CHRONIC Rx

- Continue vigilance with pressure reduction because pressure injuries can recur with minimal trauma.
- There are no randomized trials available to identify whether repositioning makes a difference in the healing rates of pressure injuries or what the optimal repositioning regimen should be.
- Consider radiologic evaluation for infected ulcer bed, occult osteomyelitis, or abscess.

COMPLEMENTARY & ALTERNATIVE MEDICINE

- Vitamin C, zinc, and multivitamin supplements may be beneficial for patients with nutritional deficiencies. However, their efficacy has not been conclusively demonstrated.
- Anabolic steroids are sometimes recommended in patients with weight loss and protein depletion. However, the evidence is not conclusive as of yet.

DISPOSITION

- When systematic risk assessments are done and preventive measures are followed, most pressure injuries can be prevented. Most injuries heal when appropriate management strategies are followed.
- Stage 4 pressure injuries in high-risk patients (e.g., paraplegics) can take months to years to heal.

REFERRAL

- Physical and occupational therapists to help improve bed and chair mobility, as well as basic activities of daily living
- Wounds with necrotic tissue need referral to providers trained in sharp debridement
- Role of plastic surgeons for operative repair for large stage 3 or 4 pressure injuries that do not respond to optimal care
- To a specialty wound care center for nonhealing complex pressure injuries

PEARLS & CONSIDERATIONS

COMMENTS

- Up to 10% of older persons will have a pressure injury.
- Because 70% of pressure injuries occur in older persons, the approach should be similar to other multifactorial geriatric syndromes with an interprofessional team approach.
- Identify and reduce all modifiable risk factors for pressure injuries.
- Treat the pain associated with pressure injuries.
- Proper skin care, use of support surfaces, mobilization, and nutritional support are integral for prevention and treatment. Of these, pressure redistribution is the most important factor for prevention.
- Effective prevention practices consist of timely wound reassessments, regular communication with team members, patient and caregiver empowerment, and utilization of clinical decision support tools for the health care providers.
- Clinical studies have not revealed that any one dressing product is superior to another.
- Nonhealing pressure injuries require assessment for debridement, infection, abscess, and/or referral to a wound center.

PATIENT & FAMILY EDUCATION

- Educate patient and family members on the risk factors for pressure injury formation.
- Encourage mobility and adequate nutritional intake as well as avoidance of bed rest.
- There is a need for patient involvement and education during periods of care transition and service changes by health care providers.

RELATED CONTENT

Bed Sores (Patient Information)

SUGGESTED READINGS

Available at ExpertConsult.com

AUTHORS: **MARY-BETH WELESKO, M.S., A.P.R.N.-B.C., W.C.C.,** and **NOELLE MARIE JAVIER, M.D.**

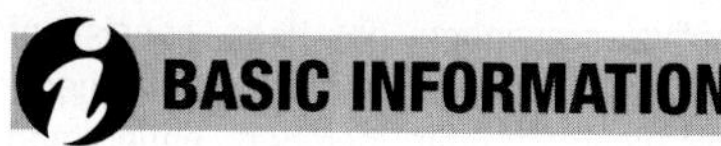

BASIC INFORMATION

DEFINITION

Preterm labor is defined as regular contractions that result in cervical dilation or effacement prior to 37 wk gestation. Preterm birth is one that occurs after 20 wk gestation and before the completion of 37 wk gestational age.

SYNONYM

Premature labor

ICD-10CM CODES

060.0	Preterm labor without delivery
060.1	Preterm spontaneous labor with preterm delivery
060.2	Preterm spontaneous labor with term delivery

EPIDEMIOLOGY & DEMOGRAPHICS

INCIDENCE: The incidence of preterm births in the U.S. increased from 9.5% in 1981 to 12.7% in 2006 before falling gradually to 11.4% by 2013. The increase since 1981 is attributed to improvements in pregnancy dating by ultrasound, increased use of assisted reproductive technology, and increased preterm induction or preterm operative delivery for maternal or fetal indications. Between 40% and 45% of these births follow spontaneous preterm labor; either the remaining preterm births result from preterm premature rupture of membranes (PPROM), or they occur secondary to intentional delivery for maternal or fetal indications.

PREDOMINANT AGE AND RACIAL DIFFERENCES: Pregnant women at the extremes of reproductive age (<17 yr and >35 yr) are at greatest risk. Black race is one of the most significant risk factors with the rate of preterm birth averaging 18.4% between 2005 and 2007 compared to 10.8% among Asian Americans and 11.6% in white women. The disparity between African American and other ethnic American races persists after adjusting for income, education, and other medical risk factors.

GENETICS: A genetic component has been suggested. Women with sisters who have had preterm births and women with grandparents who were born preterm may be at increased risk for having preterm deliveries themselves. Single-nucleotide polymorphisms have also been associated with preterm labor.

RISK FACTORS: Risk factors for premature labor include a prior preterm delivery, intrauterine infection, systemic or genital tract infections, periodontal disease, interpregnancy interval (<6 mo), short cervical length (<25 to 30 mm), low pre-pregnancy body mass index (BMI) (<19.8 kg/m^2), age (<17 yr or >35 yr), a history of elective pregnancy termination, history of prior stillbirth, African-American ethnicity, vaginal bleeding, polyhydramnios or oligohydramnios, multiple gestation, structural abnormalities of the uterus, history of cervical cone biopsy or loop electrocautery excision, in vitro fertilization or ovulation induction, tobacco use, heavy alcohol consumption, cocaine use, heroin use, and psychological or social stress. The strongest historic risk factor for preterm birth is a previous birth between 16 and 36 wk gestation.

PHYSICAL FINDINGS & CLINICAL PRESENTATION

Presenting symptoms include increased pelvic pressure, abdominal cramping or contractions, increased vaginal discharge, vaginal spotting, or leakage of fluid.

ETIOLOGY

Causes of premature labor are varied and often difficult to determine. Premature labor may be secondary to infection, systemic illness, trauma, anatomic abnormalities (i.e., uterine anomaly), or a combination of factors. It is thought that cervical ripening is the most common first step to premature labor or delivery. Subsequently, decidual-membrane activation occurs followed by contractions (Box 1).

Dx DIAGNOSIS

DIFFERENTIAL DIAGNOSIS

The differential diagnosis for preterm labor should include preterm rupture of membranes, preterm contractions (contractions before 37 wk gestation that do not result in cervical change), and abdominal pain or cramping secondary to other medical conditions. There are many medical conditions that may cause preterm contractions or premature labor. Treating some of these underlying conditions may improve the prognosis for stopping the preterm labor. Possible medical conditions include:

- Infection
  1. Chorioamnionitis
  2. Genital tract infections, including bacterial vaginosis, gonorrhea, chlamydia
  3. Urinary tract infections, including pyelonephritis, cystitis, or asymptomatic bacteriuria
  4. Gastroenteritis
- Trauma
- Placental abruption
- Illicit drug use
- Preterm premature rupture of membranes
- Appendicitis
- Nephrolithiasis
- Pancreatitis
- Cholelithiasis

WORKUP

- History and physical exam to rule out trauma, abuse, other causes of abdominal pain, and infection
- Fetal heart rate monitoring and tocometry to determine fetal status and contraction frequency
- Speculum exam to visually assess the cervix and assess for rupture of membranes, bleeding, infection, or advanced cervical dilation
  1. If the patient is <35 wk gestation, a Fetal Fibronectin (FFN) test should be collected prior to performing a digital exam or transvaginal ultrasound. A FFN test can help predict preterm delivery if the patient has a cervical length on transvaginal ultrasound of <30 mm.
- Digital exam in the unruptured patient with normal placentation to determine cervical dilation and effacement, and fetal station

LABORATORY TESTS

- CBC
- Urine analysis and culture
- Urine toxicology screen
- Collect tests for GBS, gonorrhea, and *Chlamydia*

BOX 1 Factors Linked to Preterm Labor

Demographic and Psychosocial
- Extremes of age (>40 yr, teenagers)
- Lower socioeconomic status
- Tobacco use
- Cocaine abuse
- Prolonged standing (occupation)
- Psychosocial stressors

Reproductive and Gynecologic
- Prior preterm delivery
- Diethylstilbestrol exposure
- Multiple gestations
- Anatomic endometrial cavity anomalies
- Cervical incompetence
- Low pregnancy weight gain
- First-trimester vaginal bleeding
- Placental abruption or previa

Surgical
- Prior reproductive organ surgery
- Prior paraendometrial surgery other than genitourinary (appendectomy)

Infectious
- Urinary tract infections
- Nonuterine infections
- Genital tract infections (bacterial vaginosis)

From Marx JA et al: *Rosen's emergency medicine: concepts and clinical practice,* ed 7, Philadelphia, 2010, Elsevier.

- Perform a wet prep for yeast, bacterial vaginosis, and *Trichomonas*
- Fetal fibronectin swab
- Consider PT, PTT, INR, CMP, amylase, and lipase
- Amniocentesis may be performed if an intraamniotic infection is suspected

IMAGING STUDIES

A formal ultrasound is indicated to determine estimated fetal weight, fetal presentation, amniotic fluid volume, placental location and appearance, and cervical length.

The diagnosis of preterm labor is confirmed in the presence or regular contractions if the patient is >3 cm dilated, ≥80% effaced, or <2 cm cervical length by cervical ultrasonography. Diagnosis may also be confirmed if the patient is <3 cm dilated or <80% effaced or 2–3 cm cervical length if FFN is positive or if cervical change is documented over time.

Rx TREATMENT

Patients with premature labor should be delivered promptly when an intraamniotic infection is suspected or when they have cervical dilation >5 cm, a persistently nonreassuring fetal heart rate tracing, intrauterine growth restriction, or vaginal bleeding concerning for placental abruption.

NONPHARMACOLOGIC THERAPY

- Smoking cessation
- Bedrest, activity restriction, and pelvic rest are often recommended, but there are insufficient data to support this practice.

ACUTE GENERAL Rx

- Antenatal administration of corticosteroids between 24 wk and 33 6/7 wk gestation is recommended for women at risk of preterm delivery to prevent neonatal respiratory distress syndrome and decrease the incidence of intraventricular hemorrhage and necrotizing enterocolitis.

BOX 2 Commonly Used Tocolytic Agents

Magnesium sulfate
- 4-6 g IV bolus over 30 min
- 2-4 g/hr IV infusion

Terbutaline
- 5-10 mg PO q4-6h
- 0.25-0.5 mg SC q30 min-6 h
- 10-80 μg/min IV

Ritodrine[1]
- 10 mg PO q2-4 h
- 5-10 mg IM q2-4 h
- 50-350 μg/min IV

Isoxsuprine
- 20 mg PO q4-6 h
- 0.05-0.5 mg/min IV

[1]Ritodrine is currently discontinued in the U.S. *IV*, Intravenously; *PO*, orally; *SC*, subcutaneously.
From Marx JA et al: *Rosen's emergency medicine: concepts and clinical practice,* ed 7, Philadelphia, 2010, Elsevier.

- Numerous tocolytic agents have been used in an attempt to inhibit contractions (Box 2). Although efficacy is unclear, they can be utilized during an observation period in an effort to prolong gestation for administration of steroids or to transfer the mother to a facility capable of caring for preterm infants. This, of course, assumes there are no maternal or fetal medical contraindications to use of tocolytic drugs and no indications for rapid delivery. The most commonly used tocolytics are beta-mimetics (terbutaline), magnesium sulfate, calcium channel blockers (nifedipine), or prostaglandin synthetase inhibitors (indomethacin, ketorolac, sulindac). Table E1 summarizes side effect profiles of tocolytic agents.
- Routine antibiotic use has failed to show benefit in the absence of a known infection. But all mothers in preterm labor (without a documented negative group B strep culture) should be given antibiotics to prevent neonatal GBS infection.
- Intravenous magnesium sulfate has been shown to decrease cerebral palsy in children exposed antenatally with premature labor or premature rupture of the membranes.

PROPHYLACTIC OR CHRONIC Rx

- Patients with a history of prior spontaneous preterm birth may be candidates for prophylactic use of 17 alpha-hydroxyprogesterone caproate between 16 wk and 36 wk gestation.
- Patients with a history of preterm birth and short cervix may also be candidates for prophylactic or rescue cerclage.
- There is no evidence supporting the use of maintenance tocolytic therapy.

REFERRAL

- Women who present in preterm labor should be referred to an obstetrician and transferred to a facility with a neonatal intensive care unit.
- For women who present for prenatal care with a history of preterm delivery, early referral to an obstetrician is also recommended.

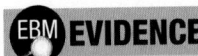

EVIDENCE

Available at ExpertConsult.com

SUGGESTED READINGS

Available at ExpertConsult.com

RELATED CONTENT

Abruptio Placentae (Related Key Topic)
Breech Birth (Related Key Topic)

AUTHOR: **ELIZABETH SHY, M.D.**

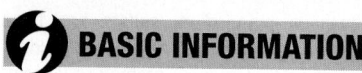

DEFINITION

Primary biliary cholangitis (PBC), previously known as primary biliary cirrhosis is a chronic, variably progressive cholestatic liver disease most often affecting middle-aged women and characterized by autoimmune destruction of intralobular bile ducts leading to portal inflammation, hepatic cell necrosis, fibrosis, cirrhosis and, ultimately, liver failure.

SYNONYMS

PBC
Primary biliary cirrhosis
Biliary cirrhosis
Nonsuppurative destructive cholangitis
Autoimmune cholangiopathy (AIC)

ICD-10CM CODE
K74.3 Primary biliary cholangitis

EPIDEMIOLOGY & DEMOGRAPHICS

INCIDENCE:

- Annual incidence rates range from 3.3 to 58 cases per million.
- PBC accounts for up to 2% of deaths from cirrhosis worldwide.

PREVALENCE: Prevalence is greatest in North America and Northern Europe and varies tremendously by time and geographic areas, ranging globally from 2.7 to 492 cases per million. Disease burden seems to be increasing, which may be a result of better detection rather than true rise in disease incidence.

PREDOMINANT SEX: Female to male ratio of 9:1.

PREDOMINANT AGE: Onset typically occurs between the ages of 30 and 65 yr and is uncommon before age 25 yr.

PREDOMINANT RACE: Most often described in Caucasians but PBC affects all races.

GENETICS:

- Pathogenesis is unknown, but it is thought to be in the setting of environmental influences and genetic predisposition.
- There are no clearly identified genetic factors associated with PBC; however, there is a clear familial occurrence. Prevalence among familial clustering of PBC is approximately 3% to 9% in the United States, Brazil, Japan, and Europe. The concordance rate among monozygotic twins is 63%.
- Up to 73% of patients with PBC have at least one other extrahepatic autoimmune disorder such as thyroiditis, Sjögren's syndrome, rheumatoid arthritis, cutaneous scleroderma (which can include CREST syndrome), systemic lupus erythematosus, pernicious anemia, celiac disease, autoimmune thrombocytopenia purpura, autoimmune diabetes mellitus, and/or other autoimmune diseases.
- A variant form of PBC exists as an overlap syndrome with autoimmune hepatitis (AIH).
- PBC is closely associated with a greater risk of hepatocellular carcinoma as well as an overall greater risk of cancer.

ETIOLOGY

- Although the cause of PBC remains unknown, it is believed to require both a genetic susceptibility as well as an environmental trigger ultimately leading to the modification of mitochondrial proteins triggering a persistent T lymphocyte–mediated attack on intralobular bile ducts.
- PBC is associated most strongly with HLA alleles DRA, DRB1, DPB1, DQB1, BTNL2 and c6orf10. PBC is also associated with ORMDL3, CD80, STAT1/STAT4, IL12A, NF-κB and RPL3/SYNGR1. However, there is variation across ethnic groups.
- Possible environmental triggers include infectious agents, cigarette smoking, environmental pollutants, radiation, urinary tract infections, reproductive hormone replacement, prior pregnancy, toxic waste sites (particularly exposure to halogenated hydrocarbons), electrophilic drugs, and xenobiotics found in food additives and cosmetics.
- The enzyme complex subunit PDC-E2 is an autoantigen that plays a major role in the early pathogenesis of PBC. Patients with PBC have a tenfold increased concentration of PDC-E2 specific cytotoxic $CD8^+$ lymphocytes in their livers compared to their blood, and antimitochondrial antibodies (AMAs), which are the serologic hallmark of this disease, react to the PDC-E2 subunit leading to a strong inflammatory response. In addition, biliary epithelial cells handle PDC-E2 in a unique way that exposes them to immune-mediated attack. Future therapies may be specific immunomodulation directed at these peptides.
- In addition, secondary damage to hepatocytes results from the chronic accumulation of bile acids.

PHYSICAL FINDINGS & CLINICAL PRESENTATION

Clinical stages:

- Asymptomatic
- Symptomatic
- Cirrhotic
- Hepatic failure

Symptoms:

- 50% to 65% of patients may be asymptomatic; 50% of patients develop symptoms in five yr, 80% in 10 yr, and 95% in 20 yr.
- Fatigue (20% to 85% of patients) and pruritus (40% to 80% of patients) are the usual presenting symptoms and are independent of disease severity.
- Fatigue can be chronic and correlate with daytime somnolence and autonomic dysfunction.
- Pruritus is worse at night, with constricting, coarse garments, and in association with dry skin and hot, humid weather. The cause is unknown but elevated histamine, bile salt concentration, endogenous opioids, lysophosphatidic acid, and female steroid hormones and their metabolites have been discussed as potential causes. Pruritus may first occur during pregnancy but is distinguished from pruritus of pregnancy because it persists into the postpartum period and beyond.
- Symptoms include jaundice (10% to 60%), unexplained right upper quadrant pain (10%), manifestations of portal hypertension, dyslipidemia (76% to 96%), xanthomas (15% to 50%), osteoporosis (20% to 44%), Sjögren's syndrome (4% to 73%), rheumatoid arthritis (2% to 6%), systemic lupus erythematosus (up to 4%), celiac disease (up to 6%), and thyroid disorders (6% to 24%) with the most common being Hashimoto thyroiditis.
- Other symptoms can include steatorrhea, fat-soluble vitamin deficiencies, and anemia.

Physical examination:

- Variable: Findings depend on stage of disease at time of presentation; patients at the early stage may be completely unaffected.
- Excoriations may be present due to extensive scratching from pruritus and can be severe enough to cause bleeding.
- Hepatomegaly and splenomegaly can worsen with disease progression.
- Xanthomas and jaundice generally appear in advanced disease. Kayser-Fleischer rings are rare and result from copper retention. Hyperpigmentation of the skin due to melanin deposition may also occur.
- Late physical findings mirror those of cirrhosis: Spider nevi, caput medusae, temporal and proximal limb wasting, ascites, palmar erythema, digital clubbing, gynecomastia, and edema.

Dx DIAGNOSIS

The diagnosis of PBC can be established when two of the following three criteria are met.

- Positive serum AMA, titer >1:40 or PBC-specific anti-nuclear antibody reactivity
- Biochemical evidence of cholestasis (mainly alkaline phosphatase elevation [ALP] ≥ 1.5 times the upper limit of normal [ULN])
- Characteristic liver histology demonstrating nonsuppurative destruction of small to medium-sized interlobular biliary ducts

DIFFERENTIAL DIAGNOSIS

- Drug-induced cholestasis (common medications: phenothiazines, anabolic steroids, some antibiotics as TMP-SMX, oxacillin, and ampicillin)
- PBC-AIH overlap syndrome; reported in 2% to 20% of patients initially diagnosed with PBC. Transition from stable PBC to AIH and vice versa also seen
- Other etiologies of chronic liver disease and cirrhosis, such as alcoholic cirrhosis, chronic viral hepatitis, primary sclerosing cholangitis, AIH, sarcoidosis, hepatic amyloidosis, chemical/toxin-induced cirrhosis, other hereditary or familial disorders (e.g., cystic fibrosis, α-1-antitrypsin deficiency)
- Biliary obstruction
- Secondary biliary cirrhosis or secondary sclerosing cholangitis

WORKUP

History, physical examination, laboratory evaluation, liver biopsy

LABORATORY TESTS

- AMAs found in 90% to 95% of patients with PBC and are 98% specific.
- Antinuclear antibodies (ANAs) and AMAs found in 53% of patients. In approximately 5% to 10% of patients, AMAs are absent (AMA-negative PBC). Nearly all patients have ANA or AMAs, or both.
- Cholestatic pattern of liver biochemical markers; markedly increased ALP (of hepatic origin). ALP levels along with bilirubin levels correlate with the risk of liver transplantation or death.
- γ-Glutamyl transpeptidase is increased (indicate biliary origin of ALP)
- Serum IgM levels are increased (lower in AMA-negative PBC).
- Bilirubin level is normal early on and increases with disease progression (direct and indirect). Increased serum bilirubin level is a poor prognostic indicator.
- Aminotransferase level may be normal and, if increased, is rarely more than 5 x ULN.
- Markedly increased serum lipids in more than 50% of patients is largely due to increased lipoprotein X (LpX). Total cholesterol may surpass 1000 mg/dl (with increased xanthomas rather than xanthelasmas). In the early stages of PBC, patients can have relatively higher HDL in comparison to LDL and VLDL. This rise in HDL might explain the lack of increased risk for cardiovascular disease. However, cardiovascular risk may still exist due to other risk factors (e.g., family history and metabolic syndrome).
- Percutaneous liver biopsy confirms or rules out the diagnosis, allows staging, but is not essential to make the diagnosis or to initiate medical therapy in patients with typical liver chemistry and positive AMA test.
- Histology is not uniform, so histologic stage is based on the most advanced lesion present.
  1. Stage I: Nonsuppurative cholangitis indicated by lymphocytic infiltration of small bile ducts with or without epithelioid granulomas or plasma cells, limited to portal areas
  2. Stage II: Extension of inflammatory cells to periportal parenchyma, ductular proliferation
  3. Stage III: Bridging necrosis or fibrous septa linking portal triads
  4. Stage IV: Frank cirrhosis with regenerative nodules

IMAGING STUDIES

If history, physical examination, blood tests, and liver biopsy are all consistent with PBC neither imaging nor cholangiography is necessary (Fig. 1).

PROGNOSIS

- Median survival is 7.5 to 16 yr in untreated patients but is getting longer with earlier diagnosis and initiation of treatment. Table 1 summarizes time course of histologic progression to a higher stage in patients with PBC.
- Eighty percent of patients progress one stage within 3 years, and 31% of patients progress from stage I to stage IV within 4 years.
- Neither presence nor total titer level of AMAs predicts survival, disease progression, or response to therapy.
- Prognostic laboratory measures: Serum bilirubin is the best predictor of survival and the most heavily weighted factor in prognostic models. Box 1 summarizes independent predictors of survival in patients with PBC.
- Response to ursodeoxycholic acid (UDCA) therapy can be prognostic, with approximately 40% of patients failing to respond. There are multiple biochemical response criteria that, if met after 1 yr of treatment with UDCA, are associated with improved clinical outcomes. Three of these criteria are Barcelona (decrease in ALP level of at least 40% or to the reference range), Paris I (ALP <3 x ULN, AST <2 x ULN and bilirubin within normal limits), and Paris II (ALP <1.5 x ULN, ALT <1.5 x ULN and bilirubin within normal limits). Similarly, the Mayo Risk score, a predictor of short-term survival probability in non-transplanted patients. (www.mayoclinic.org/girst/mayomodel1.html), can also reliably predict life expectancy when calculated after 6 months of UDCA therapy.

Poorer prognosis is associated with jaundice, advanced histologic stage, elevated bilirubin or ALP, low albumin, hepatocellular carcinoma, non-response to UDCA, and esophageal varices.

Rx TREATMENT

- Treatment is according to the clinical stage of the disease.
- Asymptomatic stage:
  - Follow liver function tests every 3 mo.
  - Once ALP is elevated up to 1.5 x ULN, begin UDCA at 13 to 15 mg/kg/day in two to four divided doses regardless of histologic stage.
    1. Side effects may include headaches, dizziness, diarrhea or constipation, dyspepsia, nausea, weight gain, back pain, and upper respiratory infections.
    2. Watch for interactions with fibric acid derivatives, bile acid sequestrants,

TABLE 1 Time Course of Histologic Progression to a Higher Stage in Patients with PBC

Histologic Progression*	Initial Histologic Stage 1	2	3
1 year	41	43	35
2 years	62	62	50

*Percent of patients in whom the histologic stage increases at 1 year and 2 years.

From Feldman M et al: *Sleisenger and Fortran's gastrointestinal and liver disease*, ed 10, Philadelphia, 2016, Elsevier.

FIG. 1 Primary biliary cholangitis demonstrated by endoscopic retrograde cholangiopancreatography. (From Berk RN, Ferrucci Jr JT, Leopold GR: *Radiology of the gallbladder and bile ducts: diagnosis and intervention*, Philadelphia, 1983, Saunders.)

BOX 1 Independent Predictors of Survival in Patients with PBC in Various Clinical Studies

Clinical
Age
Ascites
Edema
Hepatomegaly
Variceal bleeding

Laboratory
Serum albumin level
Serum alkaline phosphatase level
Serum bilirubin level
Prothrombin time

Liver Histology
Cholestasis
Cirrhosis
Fibrosis
Mallory's hyaline

PBC, Primary biliary cholangitis.
From Feldman M et al: *Sleisenger and Fortran's gastrointestinal and liver disease*, ed 10, Philadelphia, 2016, Elsevier.

estrogen derivatives, as well as aluminum hydroxide, which may interfere with the therapeutic effect or serum concentration of UDCA.

3. Efficacy is best if started during stage I or II disease but should be started at any stage of disease. Lifelong therapy is currently recommended.

- Treatment also includes treatment of associated conditions such as fatigue, pruritus, osteoporosis, hypercholesterolemia, malabsorption, fat-soluble vitamin deficiencies, anemia, hypothyroidism, and any complications of cirrhosis.

ACUTE GENERAL Rx

- Symptomatic stage: Goals of treatment are resolution of symptoms such as pruritus, treatment of chronic cholestatic complications, and delay of liver failure.
- Obeticholic acid has recently been approved as a second line treatment for PBC.
  1. It is a farnesoid X receptor agonist and is used in combination with UDCA for patients who have an inadequate response to UDCA or as monotherapy for patients who are UDCA non-responders.
  2. It is initially dosed at 5 mg once daily and can be increased to 10 mg once daily after three months if there has been an inadequate decrease in bilirubin and/or ALP.
  3. The most common adverse event noted is pruritus and therefore this drug may not be ideal for patients with that symptom.
- Prednisone, azathioprine, colchicine, methotrexate, fibrates, penicillamine, cyclosporine, silymarin, and mycophenolate mofetil are no longer used because of limited efficacy and/or significant toxicity.
- For the pruritus of PBC, cholestyramine resin (4 to 16 g/day) reduces pruritus in most patients but must be given at least 4 hrs before UDCA to avoid reducing the efficacy of that drug. Antihistamines at bedtime help nighttime symptoms. Rifampin (150 to 300 mg bid), oral opiate antagonists such as naltrexone (12.5 to 50 mg daily) and sertraline (75 to 100 mg daily) can be used for pruritus refractory to bile acid sequestrants. Table 2 summarizes treatment recommendations for pruritus in PBC. Intractable pruritus can be an indication for liver transplantation.
- Newer agents that are being investigated for pruritus include ileal bile acid transporter inhibitors and fibrates.

CHRONIC Rx

- Liver function tests should be checked every 3 to 6 mo.
- Management of sicca syndrome: Artificial tears can be used initially for dry eyes. Saliva substitutes can be used for xerostomia and dysphagia; pilocarpine or cevimeline can be used for refractory cases. Moisturizers can be given for vaginal dryness.
- Treatment/Prevention of osteopenia/osteoporosis: Patients with PBC should be given 1000 to 1200 mg calcium daily in divided doses and 1000 IU of vitamin D daily in the diet and as supplements if needed. Weight-bearing exercises are also recommended. Bone densitometry should be done at time of diagnosis, after a fragility fracture, in patients with cirrhosis, prior to transplant, or in patients receiving steroids more than 3 months. It should then be performed every 2 to 4 yr. Alendronate (70 mg weekly) or other bisphosphonates should be considered if patients have osteopenia in the absence of acid reflux or known varices.
- Hyperlipidemia is common in patients with PBC. However, there is no elevated risk of cardiovascular disease. Statins are safe and effective in patients who may need treatment even if liver chemistry is abnormal.
- Vitamin A, K, and E deficiencies can be clinically important in advanced cases and respond to oral replacement.
- Upper endoscopy to assess for varices is indicated every 1 to 3 yr in patients with cirrhosis or Mayo risk score >4.1. Nonselective beta-blockers or endoscopic banding can be considered for prevention of variceal hemorrhage.
- Regular screening for hepatocellular carcinoma with ultrasound and α-fetoprotein every 6 mo is recommended for patients with cirrhosis.
- Liver transplantation is the only effective treatment for patients with liver failure, and approximately 25% of PBC patients ultimately need a liver transplant. Indications for transplantation include hepatic decompensation (encephalopathy, recurrent variceal bleeding, intractable ascites and spontaneous bacterial peritonitis), hepatocellular carcinoma fulfilling Milan criteria (see "Hepatocellular Carcinoma"), and intractable pruritus. Liver transplant should also be considered with a Mayo risk score >7.8, MELD score >12, and bilirubin ≥ 6 mg/dl.
- The outcome of liver transplantation for patients with PBC is more favorable than that of nearly all other liver disease categories. The survival rates at one year are now up to 90% to 95%. Although recurrent disease may develop in 11% to 42% of patients after liver transplantation within a median of 47 mo, patient and graft survival is usually not affected.

DISPOSITION

Definitive treatment requires liver transplantation. Among untreated patients transplant-free survival is 79%, 59%, and 32% at 5, 10, and 15 yr, respectively.

REFERRAL

Gastroenterology and/or hepatology for treatment, evaluation for liver transplantation, and management of portal hypertension.

SUGGESTED READINGS

Available at ExpertConsult.com

RELATED CONTENT

Primary Biliary Cirrhosis (PBC) (Patient Information)

AUTHORS: **JEANETTE G. SMITH, M.D.**, and **DINA IBRAHIM, M.D.**

TABLE 2 Current Recommendations for Treatment of Pruritus in Primary Biliary Cholangitis

Approach	Drug	Mechanism of Action	Dose	Adverse Effects	Comments
First line	Cholestyramine	Bile acid resin	4-16 g/day	Unpleasant taste, bloating, constipation, and diarrhea	Morning dose preferred; separate at least 3 hr from other drugs
	Colesevelam	Bile acid resin	3.75 g/day in two or three divided doses	As above (but less frequent), headache, myalgia	Separate at least 3 hr from other drugs
Second line	Rifampicin (rifampin)	Pregnane X receptor (PXR) agonist and enzyme inducer	150-600 mg/day	Hepatitis, liver failure, hemolysis	150 mg/day when serum bilirubin level <3 mg/dl; 300 mg/day when serum bilirubin level >3 mg/dl; regular monitoring of blood count and liver biochemistry
Third line	Naltrexone	Opiate mu receptor antagonist	50 mg/day	Opioid withdrawal–like reaction—abdominal pain, high blood pressure, tachycardia, goose bumps, nightmares	Start at 12.5 mg/day; increase gradually; regular monitoring of liver biochemistry
Fourth line	Sertraline	Serotonin reuptake inhibitor (SSRI)	100 mg/day	Nausea, dizziness, diarrhea, visual hallucinations, increased fatigue	Start at 25 mg/day; increase gradually

From Fillit HM: *Brocklehurst's textbook of geriatric medicine and gerontology*, ed 8, 2017, Elsevier.

BASIC INFORMATION

DEFINITION

Primary chest wall tumors are a heterogeneous group of rare neoplasms originating from soft tissue, bone, or cartilage of chest wall. Approximately 50% to 80% of chest wall tumors are malignant; approximately 55% arise from bone cartilage and 45% from soft tissue. Chondrosarcomas are the most common primary chest wall sarcoma. The most common soft-tissue primary malignant tumors are fibrosarcomas and malignant fibrous histiocytomas. The most common benign chest wall tumors are osteochondroma, chondroma, and fibrous dysplasia.

ICD-10CM CODES

R22	Localized swelling, mass and lump of skin, and subcutaneous tissue
R22.2	Localized swelling, mass and lump, trunk
C41	Malignant neoplasm of bone and articular cartilage of other unspecified sites
C49.9	Malignant neoplasm of connective and soft tissue, unspecified

EPIDEMIOLOGY & DEMOGRAPHICS

INCIDENCE:

- 1% to 2% of all new cancer diagnosed and 5% of all thoracic neoplasm.
- More common in the elderly.
- Ewing sarcoma and rhabdomyosarcoma are the most common tumors in children.
- Chondrosarcoma, lymphoma, or solitary plasmacytoma are more frequently seen in the adult.

PHYSICAL FINDINGS & CLINICAL PRESENTATION

- Palpable enlarging mass over the chest wall or pain.
- Soft tissue masses are usually painless but skeletal lesions can be painful from periosteal invasion.
- Weakness and atrophy of upper extremities can be found from compression of a tumor on the brachial plexus.
- Patients with malignant neoplasms are typically older than patients with benign tumors (60 vs. 42 yrs) and have larger tumors (9 vs. 7 cm).

ETIOLOGY

- Most primary chest wall tumors arise sporadically.
- Risk factors: previous radiation treatment, chronic lymphedema, or exposure to chemicals.
- Genetic predispositions: Neurofibromatosis type 1 or familial retinoblastoma.

DIAGNOSIS

DIFFERENTIAL DIAGNOSIS

- Bone tumors
  1. Benign: Fibrous dysplasia, osteochondroma, chondroma, Langerhans cell/histiocytosis/eosinophillic granuloma, aneurysmal bone cyst, osteoid osteoma, osteoblastoma, and giant cell tumor
  2. Malignant: Chondrosarcoma, Ewing sarcoma, osteosarcoma, and solitary plasmacytoma
- Soft tissues
  1. Benign: Lipomas, lipoblastoma, fibroma, fibromatosis, hemangiomas, benign peripheral nerve sheath tumors, and mesenchymal hamartomas
  2. Malignant: Malignant fibrous histiocytoma, synovial sarcomas, rhabdomyosarcoma, fibrosarcoma, and metastatic disease

IMAGING STUDIES

- Chest x-rays (CXR) can reveal sclerotic or lytic bone lesions.
- Chest CT to assess the extent of size, location, and structure involvement such as soft tissue, bone, pleura, or mediastinal area. It is also a good test to evaluate lung metastasis.
- MRI is now a preferred imaging modality to assess primary chest wall tumors. It provides better-detailed information on soft tissue, vascular, and nerve involvement and extension to the spine or thoracic inlet. Malignant tumors usually appear dark on T1-weighted MRI and bright on T-weighted MRI images.

BIOPSY

- Excisional biopsy is preferred for lesions less than 2 cm, thought to be benign and possible for primary closure.
- Incisional biopsy should be considered for lesions larger than 2 cm. A minimum of 1 cm^3 is recommended.
- Fine-needle aspiration biopsy can give high diagnostic accuracy with ancillary techniques such as immunohistochemical stain or cytogenetic analysis.
- Core needle biopsy can be used for deep lesions under the guidance of imaging modalities.

LABORATORY TEST

Cytogenetic analysis is widely used to increase diagnostic accuracy and is sometimes helpful for making the therapeutic decision.

TREATMENT

- Surgical resection and reconstruction are the main principles of treatment.
- Systemic treatment and radiation are often combined with surgery as adjuvant or neoadjuvant treatment for malignant disease.
- Isolated plasmacytoma can be treated with chemotherapy or radiation (see "Multiple Myeloma").
- Metastatic or locally advanced soft tissue sarcomas: systemic treatment with cytotoxic agent ± platelet-derived growth factor receptor-α (PDGFRα)-blocking antibody (olaratumab) or tyrosine kinase inhibitor (Pazopanib).

FOLLOW UP

- Evaluation for rehabilitation (OT, PT). Continue until maximal function is achieved
- H&P every 3 to 6 mo for 2 to 3 y, then every 6 mo for next 2 yr, then annually.
- Imaging of chest and other known sites of metastatic disease.
- Consider obtaining postoperative baseline and periodic imaging of primary site based on estimated risk of locoregional recurrence.

SUGGESTED READINGS

Available at ExpertConsult.com

RELATED TOPICS

Sarcoma

AUTHOR: **PATAN GULTAWATVICHAI, M.D.**

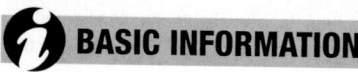

BASIC INFORMATION

DEFINITION

- Women younger than 40 yr of age with amenorrhea, oligomenorrhea, or dysfunctional uterine bleeding for 4 mo or more along with follicle stimulating hormone (FSH) levels in the menopausal range meet diagnostic criteria for primary ovarian insufficiency.
- Menopause younger than the age of 40 yr.

SYNONYMS

POI
Hypergonadotropic hypogonadism
Premature ovarian failure
Premature menopause
Gonadal dysgenesis

ICD-10CM CODES

E28.3	Primary ovarian failure
E28.9	Ovarian dysfunction, unspecified
E28.310	Symptomatic premature menopause
E28.39	Other primary ovarian failure

EPIDEMIOLOGY & DEMOGRAPHICS

INCIDENCE: Affects 1% to 4% of the female population in the U.S.
PREDOMINANT AGE: 1:250 incident cases by age 35 and 1:100 by age 40

PHYSICAL FINDINGS & CLINICAL PRESENTATION

- The most common presentation is disturbance in menstrual pattern due to intermittent ovarian function.
- Between 5% and 30% of affected women have another affected female relative.
- Between 10% and 30% of affected women already have a concurrent autoimmune condition, the most common of which is hypothyroidism.
- Symptoms of estrogen deficiency include hot flashes, night sweats, poor concentration, drying of the vagina, and infertility.
- Physical exam may reveal stigmata of an autoimmune condition such as vitiligo, thyroid enlargement, or Turner syndrome (webbed neck, short stature, and high-arched palate).

ETIOLOGY (SEE TABLE 1)

Idiopathic in 95% of cases

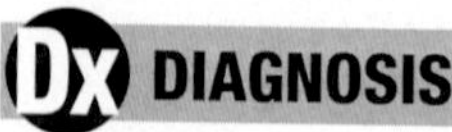

DIAGNOSIS

DIFFERENTIAL DIAGNOSIS

- Pregnancy.
- Causes of secondary amenorrhea include eating disorder, exercise, drugs, sarcoidosis, polycystic ovarian disease, hypothalamic amenorrhea, hyperprolactinemia/prolactinoma, and Cushing's disease.

WORKUP

- After pregnancy is ruled out, the initial evaluation should include the measurement of serum prolactin, FSH, and thyrotropin (TSH) levels.
- If the FSH level is in the menopausal range (>40 µIU/ml by radioimmunoassay), the test should be repeated in 1 mo along with a serum estradiol measurement to confirm the diagnosis of primary ovarian insufficiency.

LABORATORY TESTS

Once a diagnosis of premature ovarian failure is made, other evaluations include:

- Autoimmune disorders, adrenal insufficiency (seen in 3% of cases): Serum anti-adrenal and anti-21 hydroxylase antibodies should be measured.
- Hypothyroidism: Serum TSH, T_4, and anti-TPO antibodies.
- All cases should be screened for osteoporosis by DXA for bone mineral density.
- A karyotype analysis should be performed for all patients to look for chromosomal defects including Turner variant or deletions of the X chromosome.
- Permutations for the fragile X syndrome (*FMR1* gene) should be checked for as well.

IMAGING STUDIES

Pelvic ultrasound has no proven benefit in the management of these patients.

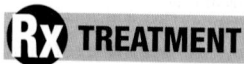

TREATMENT

NONPHARMACOLOGIC THERAPY

Counseling or patient support group should be offered to all women with low self-esteem and depression due to the psychological scar left by the diagnosis.

ACUTE GENERAL Rx

- Physiologic estrogen and progestin replacement is reasonable in the cases of young women until they reach the age of natural menopause.
- A dose of 100 mcg of estradiol per day, administered by transdermal patch, achieves average estradiol level observed in normal menstruating women and effectively treats symptoms.
- Cyclic medroxyprogesterone at a dose of 10 mg per day for 12 days each month is the preferred progestin to provide protection against endometrial cancer.
- Pregnancy may occur while a woman is taking estrogen and progesterone therapy and the therapy should be stopped immediately if the pregnancy test is found to be positive.

CHRONIC Rx

- Intake of 1200 mg of elemental calcium and 800 units of vitamin D_3 per day should be encouraged to prevent bone loss. A serum 25-hydroxyvitamin D level of 30 ng per ml or higher should be maintained.
- Patients with positive tests for adrenal antibodies should be evaluated annually for adrenal insufficiency by corticotropin stimulation test.
- Patients who wish to avoid pregnancy should use a barrier method or an IUD.
- Options for parenthood include adoption, foster parenthood, egg donation, and embryo donation.

DISPOSITION

Women with the known diagnosis should be encouraged to maintain a lifestyle that optimizes bone and cardiovascular health, including regular weight-bearing exercises, adequate intake of calcium (1200 mg daily) and vitamin D (800 IU daily), healthy diet to prevent obesity, and screening for cardiovascular risk factors.

REFERRAL

Referral to gynecologist and reproductive endocrinologist may be helpful in patients who decide to pursue parenthood.

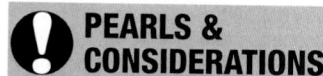

PEARLS & CONSIDERATIONS

COMMENTS

- Common etiologies should be ruled out, including chromosomal abnormalities, fragile X premutations, and autoimmune causes.
- Management directed at symptom resolution and bone protection primarily, but should include psychosocial support for women facing this devastating diagnosis.

PREVENTION

Early diagnosis of primary ovarian insufficiency important for osteoporosis prevention and possibly prevention of coronary artery disease.

PATIENT & FAMILY EDUCATION

www.pofsupport.org
poi.nichd.nih.gov

RELATED CONTENT

Amenorrhea (Related Key Topic)

TABLE 1 Mechanisms and Causes of Primary Ovarian Insufficiency

Accelerated Follicular Depletion

Genetic: Turner syndrome, fragile X premutations, galactosemia
Toxic: Chemotherapy, radiation, infections such as mumps or cytomegalovirus
Autoimmune: Polyglandular failure, hypothyroidism, Addison disease, vitiligo, myasthenia gravis

Abnormal Follicular Stimulation

Gonadotropin receptor function: Follicle stimulating hormone/luteinizing hormone receptor mutation
Enzyme defects: Aromatase deficiency, luteinized follicles

SUGGESTED READING

Available at ExpertConsult.com

AUTHOR: **FRED F. FERRI, M.D.**

BASIC INFORMATION

DEFINITION

Primary sclerosing cholangitis (PSC) is an autoimmune fibroinflammatory disease predominantly affecting the large bile ducts. It is characterized by segmental fibrosing and inflammation of intrahepatic and extrahepatic bile ducts complicated by recurrent cholangitis, cholangiocarcinoma (CCA), cirrhosis, and portal hypertension.

SYNONYMS

Chronic obliterative cholangitis
Fibrosing cholangitis
Stenosing cholangitis
PSC

ICD-10CM CODES
K83.0 Cholangitis
K83.0 Disease of biliary tract, unspecified

EPIDEMIOLOGY & DEMOGRAPHICS

- The incidence and prevalence of PSC are 0.9 to 1.3 cases per 100,000 persons per yr and 8.5 to 16.2 cases per 100,000 persons, respectively.
- About 65% of patients with PSC are men.
- Mean age of presentation is 30 to 40.
- Over 80% of patients with PSC also have inflammatory bowel disease (IBD). 4% to 5% of patients with ulcerative colitis (UC) will develop PSC. A PSC-IBD phenotype may be present which carries a higher risk of colon cancer and is characterized by mild pancolitis, rectal sparing, and backwash ileitis. PSC is an independent risk factor for developing colon cancer in patients with IBD.
- PSC can coexist with other autoimmune liver diseases. Autoimmune hepatitis (AIH) and PSC overlap syndrome can be seen and is more common in young adults and children.
- Cholangiocarcinoma is present in 1% to 2% of PSC patients at diagnosis and should be considered a premalignant disease. The lifetime risk is 5% to 10%.
- Box 1 summarizes a classification of and diseases associated with sclerosing cholangitis.
- The median survival from time of diagnosis is 10 to 15 yr without liver transplantation.

PHYSICAL FINDINGS & CLINICAL PRESENTATION

- Many patients are asymptomatic (up to 50%) at the time of diagnosis with normal physical examination findings. However, many patients will have abnormal liver tests and a known diagnosis of IBD.
- More than 75% of asymptomatic patients develop symptoms, the most common of which are nonspecific pruritus, abdominal pain, and fatigue. Physical findings of symptomatic patients may reveal jaundice, skin excoriation and hyperpigmentation from scratching, hepatosplenomegaly, and xanthelasma. Other symptoms include steatorrhea and weight loss, which are concerning for advanced PSC, sepsis, or mechanical obstruction (i.e., cholangitis), and malignancy (i.e., cholangiocarcinoma).
- Patients can also present with advanced liver disease and decompensated cirrhosis (i.e., ascites, spontaneous bacterial peritonitis, hepatic encephalopathy, and variceal hemorrhage) or hepatic failure. In patients with cirrhosis, physical findings may reveal a shrunken nodular liver and evidence of portal hypertension.

ETIOLOGY

- The cause of PSC is unknown, but the most likely mechanism is immunologic priming in a genetically susceptible patient causing phenotypic expression of PSC.
- Genetic and immunologic factors are supported by reports of familial occurrence of this disorder and increased frequency of HLA B8 and DR3. Genome-wide association studies have discovered novel loci associated with PSC, but the functional aspects of these genes are still unknown.
- Portosystemic inflammation caused by translocation of the gut microbiota is an increasing area of research. The close association with UC and PSC may be secondary to gut-activated T lymphocytes in IBD causing portal inflammation because of overlapping adhesion molecules in the gut and liver. Furthermore, intestinal dysbiosis in PSC has also been seen and remains an area of ongoing research.
- Dysregulated inflammatory cytokine production by cholangiocytes is also more recently suggested to be playing a role in the pathogenesis of PSC.

Dx DIAGNOSIS

Diagnosis is based on characteristic cholangiographic findings in combination with clinical, biochemical, and in some cases histologic features. It is increasingly common to diagnose PSC based on imaging with magnetic resonance cholangiopancreatography (MRCP). Liver biopsy is now rarely used to diagnose disease. Table 1 describes staging of PSC. Work is being done to enable a diagnosis to be made based on biomarkers such as microRNA and fecal microbiota profiles.

DIFFERENTIAL DIAGNOSIS

- IgG4-associated cholangitis (IAC)
- Surgical biliary trauma
- Ischemic cholangitis, recurrent pyogenic cholangitis, recurrent pancreatitis
- Choledocholithiasis, cholangiocarcinoma
- Intraarterial chemotherapy (5-FU/floxuridine)
- Diffuse intrahepatic metastasis, sarcoidosis, or amyloidosis
- AIDS-related, eosinophilic, or mast cell cholangiopathy
- Histiocytosis X, graft-versus-host disease
- Hepatic inflammatory pseudotumor, portal hypertensive biliopathy

WORKUP

History, physical examination, laboratory evaluation, and imaging studies (MRCP). Liver biopsy is generally not necessary for diagnosis

LABORATORY TESTS

- Serum biochemical tests usually indicate cholestasis with predominant elevation in the serum alkaline phosphatase (3-10 times the upper limit of normal for more than 6 months). However, this value can vary and be normal during the disease course. Serum aminotransferase levels are elevated in the majority of patients (2-3 times the upper limits of normal). Serum bilirubin is usually normal at the time of diagnosis unless the patient has advanced stricturing disease; an initial elevation of bilirubin at diagnosis may be related to worse prognosis.
- A wide range of autoantibodies can be detected in patients with PSC; however, they are nonspecific for PSC, including the perinuclear antineutrophil cytoplasmic antibody (pANCA), autoantibodies such as antinuclear antibody (ANA), and anti-smooth muscle antibody (ASMA).
  1. Anti-mitochondrial antibody (AMA), which is characteristic of primary biliary cholangitis (PBC), is *NOT* found in PSC and can be helpful in excluding PSC.
  2. Serum IgG levels are useful in the diagnosis of PSC-AIH overlap syndrome (more common in pediatric patients) and IAC with autoimmune pancreatitis.
  3. In particular, elevated levels of IgG4 are found in 10% to 20% of PSC patients, with a subset of these patients displaying features of autoimmune pancreatitis. PSC patients with elevated IgG4 tend to have worse outcomes and seem to respond to corticosteroid therapy; hence, IgG4 levels should be checked at least once in all patients with PSC.

IMAGING STUDIES

- Cholangiography (Fig. E1), with magnetic resonance cholangiopancreatography (MRCP) or endoscopic retrograde cholangiopancreatography (ERCP), is considered to be the gold standard for the diagnosis of PSC. Characteristic findings reveal segmental fibrosis of bile ducts with saccular dilatation of normal intervening areas resulting in a "beads-on-a-string" appearance.
- MRCP has an overall diagnostic accuracy rate of 90%. It is the first imaging modality of choice when PSC is suspected because ERCP can be associated with increased rates of serious complications (i.e., pancreatitis and cholangitis) in patients with PSC.
- Liver biopsy is not necessary for the diagnosis of PSC in patients with typical cholangiographic findings. Biopsies are subject to sample variation, and typical "onion skin"–type periductal fibrosis is rare. Liver biopsy may help in the diagnosis of PSC-AIH overlap syndrome, small-duct PSC (normal cholangiogram), or IAC.

BOX 1 Classification of and Diseases Associated with Sclerosing Cholangitis

Primary Sclerosing Cholangitis

Principal Disease Associations

Inflammatory bowel disease
- Crohn colitis or ileocolitis
- Ulcerative colitis

Other Disease Associations

Systemic diseases with fibrosis
- Inflammatory pseudotumor
- Mediastinal fibrosis
- Peyronie disease
- Pseudotumor of the orbit
- Retroperitoneal fibrosis
- Riedel's thyroiditis

Autoimmune or collagen vascular disorders
- Autoimmune hemolytic anemia
- Celiac disease
- Chronic sclerosing sialoadenitis
- Membranous nephropathy
- PSS
- Rapidly progressive glomerulonephritis
- RA
- Sjögren's syndrome
- SLE
- Type 1 diabetes mellitus

Alloimmune diseases
- Hepatic allograft rejection
- Hepatic graft-versus-host disease after bone marrow transplantation

Infiltrative diseases
- Hypereosinophilic syndrome
- Histiocytosis X
- Sarcoidosis
- Systemic mastocytosis

Immunodeficiency
- Congenital immunodeficiency
  - Combined immunodeficiency
  - Dysgammaglobulinemia
  - X-lined agammaglobulinemia
- Acquired immunodeficiency
  - AIDS
  - Angioimmunoblastic lymphadenopathy
  - Opportunistic infections (e.g., cryptosporidiosis, cytomegalovirus, microsporidiosis)
  - Selective IgA deficiency

Secondary Sclerosing Cholangitis

Obstructive

Autoimmune pancreatitis
Biliary parasites
Caroli disease
Choledocholithiasis
Chronic pancreatitis
Congenital abnormalities
- CF
- Choledochal cyst

Fungal infection
Recurrent pyogenic cholangitis
Surgical stricture

Toxic

Intra-arterial floxuridine (FUDR)
Intraductal formaldehyde or hypertonic saline (echinococcal cyst treatment)

Ischemic

Hepatic allograft arterial occlusion
Paroxysmal nocturnal hemoglobinuria
Toxic vasculitis (FUDR)
Vascular trauma

Neoplastic

Cholangiocarcinoma
Hepatocellular carcinoma
Lymphoma
Metastatic cancer

AIDS, Acquired immunodeficiency syndrome; *FUDR*, 5-fluorouracil deoxyribonucleoside; *Ig*, immunoglobulin.
From Feldman M et al: *Sleisenger and Fordtran's gastrointestinal and liver disease*, ed 10, Philadelphia, 2016, Elsevier.

TABLE 1 Staging of Primary Sclerosing Cholangitis

Stage	Description
I—Portal	Portal edema, inflammation, ductal proliferation; abnormalities do not extend beyond the limiting plate
II—Periportal	Periportal fibrosis with or without inflammation extending beyond the limiting plate
III—Septal	Septal fibrosis, bridging necrosis, or both
IV—Cirrhotic	Biliary cirrhosis

From Cameron JL, Cameron AM: *Current surgical therapy*, ed 10, Philadelphia, 2011, Saunders.

- Noninvasive measurements of liver elastography including MR elastography are promising methods for evaluating for cirrhosis but have not yet been validated in this patient cohort.

Rx TREATMENT

- No medical therapy has been established to be effective in halting the disease progression of PSC. Liver transplantation is indicated in patients with decompensated cirrhosis, hilar cholangiocarcinoma, and in those with recurrent bacterial cholangitis.
- Ursodeoxycholic acid (UDCA) has shown variable benefit in randomized controlled trials.
- Although biochemical improvement has been seen with UDCA, there has been no proven benefit on survival.
- In two trials, high-dose UDCA (28-30 mg/kg/day) was associated with colorectal dysplasia, liver transplantation, and varices. Therefore, high-dose UDCA is *NOT* universally recommended as medical therapy in patients with PSC. A trial of medium- or low-dose UDCA ~20 mg/kg/day is used by some clinicians, since some trials have shown biochemical response.
- Oral vancomycin may show clinical and biochemical response in pediatric patients, but no randomized clinical trial has been performed.
- The use of corticosteroids and other immunosuppressive agents is not recommended in patients with PSC alone; however, it is recommended in patients with PSC-AIH overlap syndrome or elevated IgG4.
- Use of tumor necrosis factor inhibitors has been ineffective in PSC. Other monoclonal antibody therapies targeting lymphocyte trafficking, tyrosine kinase signaling, and liver fibrosis are being studied. Furthermore, other targets for treatment are ongoing and aimed at bile acid synthesis and mast cell inhibition.
- Bile acid–based therapeutic approaches are currently in clinical trials, including peroxisome proliferator-activated receptor agonists and farnesoid X receptor agonists.
- Management of PSC patients is aimed at symptom relief and management of

complications from PSC (i.e., obstruction/strictures, cirrhosis, portal hypertension).

ACUTE GENERAL Rx

- With mild pruritus, skin emollients and antihistamines are recommended as the first-line treatment.
- With moderate or severe pruritus, bile acid sequestrants (i.e., cholestyramine 16 g/day) are the preferred choice for the initial management of pruritus. Alternative agents for pruritus refractory to bile acid sequestrants include rifampicin 150 to 300 mg twice daily, naltrexone 50 mg daily, sertraline 75 to 100 mg daily, or phenobarbital 90 mg at bedtime.
- Patients who present with increasing serum bilirubin and/or worsening pruritus, progressive bile duct dilation on imaging studies, or cholangitis need to be evaluated for dominant strictures with imaging. A dominant stricture is a stenosis <1.5 mm in the common bile duct or <1 mm in the hepatic duct.
- ERCP with brushings, cytology, and fluorescent in situ hybridization (FISH) is recommended to evaluate dominant strictures for cholangiocarcinoma, which is found in 15% to 20% of cases. Once malignancy is excluded, balloon dilation with or without stenting is recommended to treat symptoms. Routine stenting is not required, but short-term stenting may be helpful in patients with severe stricture. If ERCP is unsuccessful, percutaneous cholangiopancreatography with stenting should be considered.
- In noncirrhotic patients with dominant strictures refractory to endoscopic or percutaneous management, surgery should be considered, although this may complicate future liver transplantation surgery.
- Antibiotic usage is recommended in patients with dominant strictures/obstructions both acutely and for long-term prophylaxis in patients with recurrent cholangitis.

CHRONIC Rx

- Avoidance of alcohol and vaccination against hepatitis A and B is advised.
- Patients with PSC are at risk for osteoporosis and osteopenia.
  1. The pathophysiology of bone loss is poorly understood but likely multifactorial. Impaired absorption of fat-soluble vitamins, such as vitamins D and K, and possible impairment of osteoblasts by bilirubin may be contributing factors. The risk of osteoporosis appears to be independent of cumulative corticosteroid exposure.
  2. DEXA scan should be performed at diagnosis and should be repeated in 2 to 4 yr.
  3. Calcium (1000-1500 mg) and vitamin D 600 to 800 IU daily are recommended for patients with osteopenia, and the addition of bisphosphonate is recommended in patients with osteoporosis.
- Patients with newly diagnosed PSC should have a full colonoscopy with biopsies to exclude concurrent IBD and for surveillance of colorectal cancer. In patients with IBD, continued surveillance colonoscopy with biopsies, or chromoendoscopy, at 1- to 2-yr intervals is recommended. In patients without IBD, a suggested 3- to 5-yr surveillance interval has been recommended due to an increased risk of colorectal cancer.
- Cholangiocarcinoma (CCA) development is common in PSC. PSC patients with biochemical or symptomatic deterioration should be evaluated for CCA. Surveillance for CCA with annual MRCP and CA19-9 has been recommended by some experts. Abnormal values should prompt further investigation of dominant strictures with ERCP. Although CA19-9 may detect CCA, even high levels (>129 U/ml) may lack specificity since one-third of patients did not have CCA after 30 months of follow-up. These differences may in part be due to genotypic differences in *FUT2/3* alleles that affect expression of CA19-9.
- Annual transabdominal ultrasound is recommended due to the increased risk of gallbladder malignancy. If masses or polyps >8 mm are detected, cholecystectomy should be performed.
- Patients with cirrhosis are recommended to have gastroesophageal variceal and hepatocellular carcinoma (HCC) surveillance at regular intervals.
- With advanced disease, fat-soluble vitamin deficiencies such as A, E, and D should be assessed.
- In cases of HCC and CCA, depending on underlying liver disease, resection versus liver transplantation would be required.

DISPOSITION

Liver transplantation is the only effective treatment for patients with end-stage liver disease, portal hypertension, liver failure, and recurrent or intractable bacterial cholangitis. Survival is excellent, with 90% and 80% survival rates at 1 and 5 yr, respectively. The recurrence of PSC after transplant is reportedly 5% to 20%. Transplant referral is warranted when MELD exceeds 14 or greater, or with worsening cholangitis or intractable pruritus.

REFERRAL

Gastroenterology and/or hepatology for treatment of PSC, management of its complications, surveillance of associated malignancy, and evaluation for liver transplantation.

PEARLS & CONSIDERATIONS

- Management of PSC targets symptom relief, complications of PSC, cirrhosis, early carcinoma detection, and timely referral for liver transplantation.
- High-dose UDCA is not universally recommended for treatment of PSC.
- Patients are at increased risk for the development of colorectal cancer, gallbladder cancer, and cholangiocarcinoma and need surveillance.
- Patients with PSC and ulcerative colitis have more common right-sided colon involvement and greater risk of pouchitis after colectomy with an ileal pouch-anal anastomosis.
- In patients with cirrhosis, surveillance for gastroesophageal varices and HCC is recommended.
- Liver transplant remains the only definitive therapy for complications of PSC.

SUGGESTED READINGS

Available at ExpertConsult.com

RELATED CONTENT

Ulcerative Colitis (Related Key Topic)

AUTHORS: **MANIDA WUNGJIRANIRUN, M.D.,** and **AMANDA PRESSMAN, M.D.**

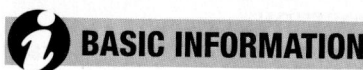

DEFINITION

Prolactinomas are monoclonal tumors that secrete prolactin.

ICD-10CM CODES
D35.2 Benign neoplasm of pituitary gland
E22.8 Other hyperfunction of pituitary gland

EPIDEMIOLOGY & DEMOGRAPHICS

INCIDENCE: Most common pituitary tumor; nearly 30% of all pituitary adenomas secrete enough prolactin to cause hyperprolactinemia.
PREDOMINANT SEX: Microadenomas are more common in women; macroadenomas are found more frequently in men.

PHYSICAL FINDINGS & CLINICAL PRESENTATION

- Men: Decreased facial and body hair, infertility, small testicles; may also have decreased libido, erectile dysfunction, and delayed puberty (caused by decreased testosterone as a result of inhibition of gonadotropin secretion).
- Women: Physical examination may be normal; history may reveal amenorrhea, galactorrhea (Fig. E1), oligomenorrhea, and anovulation.
- Both sexes: Visual field defects and headache may occur depending on size of tumor and its expansion.

ETIOLOGY

Prolactin-secreting pituitary adenomas: Microadenomas (<10 mm diameter) or macroadenomas (>10 mm diameter). No risk factors have been identified for sporadic prolactinomas. Rarely prolactinomas can be part of multiple endocrine neoplasia (MEN) type 1 syndrome.

Dx DIAGNOSIS

DIFFERENTIAL DIAGNOSIS

Secretion of prolactin is under tonic inhibitory control by hypothalamic dopamine. Hyperprolactinemia may be caused by the following:

- Drugs: Risperidone, phenothiazines, methyldopa, reserpine, monoamine oxidase inhibitors, androgens, progesterone, cimetidine, tricyclic antidepressants, haloperidol, meprobamate, chlordiazepoxide, estrogens, narcotics, metoclopramide, verapamil, amoxapine, cocaine, oral contraceptives
- Hepatic cirrhosis, renal failure, primary hypothyroidism
- Ectopic prolactin-secreting tumors (hypernephroma, bronchogenic carcinoma)
- Infiltrating diseases of the pituitary (sarcoidosis, histiocytosis)
- Head trauma, chest wall injury, spinal cord injury
- Polycystic ovary disease, pregnancy, nipple stimulation
- Idiopathic hyperprolactinemia, stress, exercise

WORKUP

- The diagnosis of prolactinoma is established by demonstration of an elevated serum prolactin level (after exclusion of other causes of hyperprolactinemia) and radiographic evidence of a pituitary adenoma.
  1. Normal mean prolactin levels are 8 ng/ml in women and 5 ng/ml in men.
  2. Prolactin levels >100 ng/ml are suspicious for prolactinomas. Most macroprolactinomas raise prolactin levels >250 ng/ml and levels >500 ng/ml are virtually diagnostic of macroprolactinomas.
  3. Prolactin levels can vary with time of day, stress, sleep cycle, and meals. More accurate measurements can be obtained 2 to 3 hr after awakening, preprandially, and when patient is not distressed.
  4. Serial measurements are recommended in patients with mild prolactin elevations.
- TSH, free T_4, BUN, Creat, ALT, AST are useful tests. Pregnancy test in all women of childbearing age.
- All patients with prolactinomas should undergo visual field testing. Serial evaluation is recommended, particularly during pregnancy in patients with macroadenomas.

IMAGING STUDIES

- MRI with gadolinium enhancement is the procedure of choice in the radiographic evaluation of pituitary disease.
- In absence of MRI, a radiographic diagnosis is best accomplished with a high-resolution CT scanner and special coronal cuts through the pituitary region.

Rx TREATMENT

NONPHARMACOLOGIC THERAPY

Pregnancy and breastfeeding should be avoided because they can encourage tumor growth.

ACUTE GENERAL Rx

- Management of prolactinomas depends on their size and encroachment on the optic chiasm and other vital structures, the presence or absence of gonadal dysfunction, and the patient's desires regarding fertility. Patients with microprolactinomas without symptoms of hypogonadism do not require treatment. Fig. 2 describes a management algorithm for prolactinomas. Women with hypogonadism related to a microadenoma who do not desire fertility can be treated with a combined oral contraceptive.
- Medical therapy is preferred when fertility is an important consideration. Prolactinomas are treated with the dopamine agonists (DA) bromocriptine and cabergoline.
  1. Bromocriptine: Initial dose is 0.625 mg at bedtime for the first week. After 1 wk, add morning dose of 1.25 mg. Gradually increase dose by 1.25 mg/wk until dose of 5 to 10 mg/day is achieved. Bromocriptine decreases size of the tumor and generally lowers the prolactin level into the normal range when the initial serum prolactin is <500 ng/ml. Side effects of bromocriptine are nausea, constipation, dizziness, and nasal stuffiness. Bromocriptine appears to be safe during pregnancy.
  2. Cabergoline is a longer-acting dopamine agonist that is more expensive but may be more effective and better tolerated than bromocriptine; initial dose is 0.25 mg twice weekly.
  3. After therapy is initiated, MRI should be repeated in 1 yr for microprolactinomas if the prolactin level normalizes. For macroprolactinomas, MRI is repeated after 2 mo and every 6 to 12 mo until stable on serial studies.
- Transsphenoidal resection: Option in an infertile patient who cannot tolerate bromocriptine or cabergoline or when medical therapy is ineffective. The success rate depends on the location of the tumor (entirely intrasellar), experience of the neurosurgeon, and size of the tumor (<10 mm in diameter); the recurrence rate may reach 80% within 5 yr. Possible complications of transsphenoidal surgery vary with experience and skill of the neurosurgeon and tumor anatomy and include transient diabetes insipidus, hypopituitarism, cerebrospinal fluid rhinorrhea, and infections (meningitis, wound infection).
- Pituitary irradiation is useful as adjunctive therapy of macroadenomas (>10 mm in diameter) and in patients with persistent hypersecretion after surgery. Potential complications include cranial nerve damage, radionecrosis, and cognitive abnormalities.
- Stereotactic radiosurgery (gamma knife) has become popular as a modality in the treatment of prolactinomas. A high dose of ionizing radiation is delivered to the tumor through multiple ports. Its advantage is minimal irradiation to surrounding tissues. Proximity of the tumor to the optic chiasm limits this therapeutic modality.

CHRONIC Rx

- Patients on medical therapy require periodic measurement of prolactin levels. An attempt to reduce the dose of bromocriptine or cabergoline can be made after the prolactin level has been normal for 2 yr. An MRI scan of the pituitary should be obtained to rule out tumor enlargement within 6 mo of initiation of tapering regimen.
- Evaluation and monitoring of pituitary function are recommended after transsphenoidal surgery.

DISPOSITION

- Transsphenoidal surgery will result in a cure in nearly 50% to 75% of patients with microadenomas and 10% to 20% of patients with macroadenomas.
- Nearly 20% of microprolactinomas resolve during long-term dopamine agonist treatment.

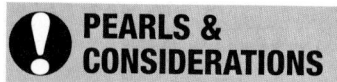

COMMENTS

- Patients must be monitored for several years after surgery because up to 50% of

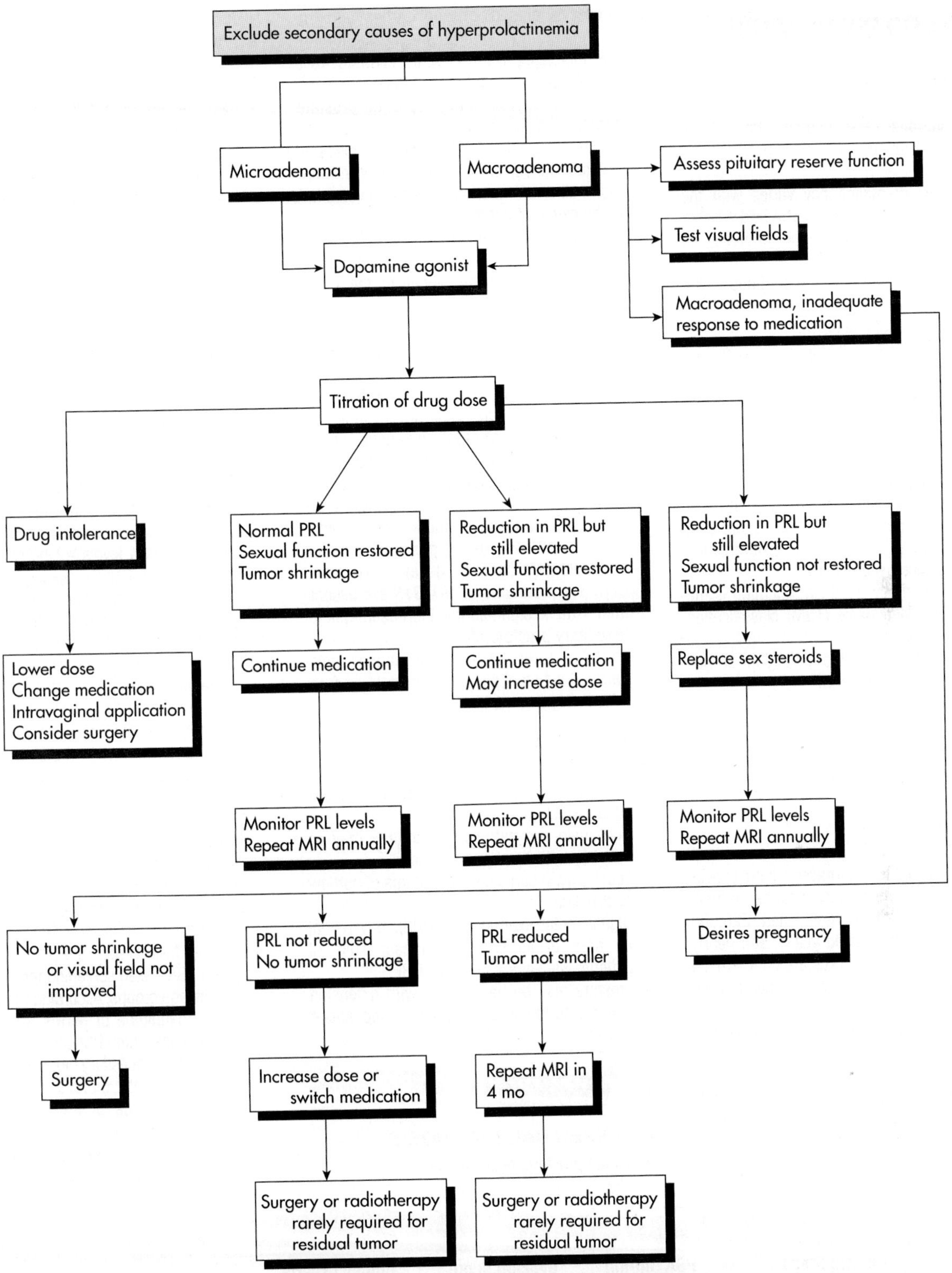

Exclude secondary causes of hyperprolactinemia

Microadenoma

Macroadenoma

Assess pituitary reserve function

Test visual fields

Macroadenoma, inadequate response to medication

Dopamine agonist

Titration of drug dose

Drug intolerance

Lower dose
Change medication
Intravaginal application
Consider surgery

Normal PRL
Sexual function restored
Tumor shrinkage

Continue medication

Monitor PRL levels
Repeat MRI annually

Reduction in PRL but still elevated
Sexual function restored
Tumor shrinkage

Continue medication
May increase dose

Monitor PRL levels
Repeat MRI annually

Reduction in PRL but still elevated
Sexual function not restored
Tumor shrinkage

Replace sex steroids

Monitor PRL levels
Repeat MRI annually

No tumor shrinkage or visual field not improved

Surgery

PRL not reduced
No tumor shrinkage

Increase dose or switch medication

Surgery or radiotherapy rarely required for residual tumor

PRL reduced
Tumor not smaller

Repeat MRI in 4 mo

Surgery or radiotherapy rarely required for residual tumor

Desires pregnancy

FIG. 2 Prolactinoma management. After secondary causes of hyperprolactinemia have been excluded, subsequent management decisions are based on clinical imaging and biochemical criteria. *MRI,* Magnetic resonance imaging; *PRL,* prolactin. (Modified from Larsen PR, et al.: *Williams textbook of endocrinology,* ed 11, Philadelphia, 2008, Saunders.)

microadenomas and nearly 90% of macroadenomas can recur.

- Pituitary microadenomas are found in 10.9% of autopsies, and 44% of these microadenomas are prolactinomas.

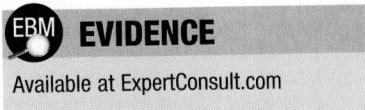

EVIDENCE

Available at ExpertConsult.com

SUGGESTED READING

Available at ExpertConsult.com

RELATED CONTENT

Prolactinoma (Patient Information)
Pituitary Adenoma (Related Key Topic)

AUTHOR: **FRED F. FERRI, M.D.**

BASIC INFORMATION

DEFINITION & CLASSIFICATION

Prostate cancer is a neoplasm involving the prostate. Various classifications have been developed to evaluate malignancy potential and prognosis.

- The degree of malignancy varies with the stage:
  1. Stage A: Confined to the prostate, no nodule palpable.
  2. Stage B: Palpable nodule confined to the gland.
  3. Stage C: Local extension.
  4. Stage D: Regional lymph nodes or distant metastases.
- In the Gleason classification (Box E1 and Fig. E1), two histologic patterns are independently assigned numbers 1 to 5 (best to least differentiated). These numbers are added to give a total tumor score between 2 and 10. Prognosis is best for highly differentiated tumors (e.g., Gleason score 2-4) compared with most poorly differentiated tumors (Gleason score 7-10).
- Another commonly used classification is the Tumor-Node-Metastasis (TNM) classification of prostate cancer.
- Table 1 summarizes the definition of risk groups and biopsy criteria.

ICD-10CM CODES

C61 Malignant neoplasm of prostate

D07.5 Carcinoma in situ of prostate

EPIDEMIOLOGY & DEMOGRAPHICS

- Prostate cancer has surpassed lung cancer as the most common nonskin cancer in men.
- In the United States, more than 220,000 new cases are diagnosed yearly, and nearly 30,000 males die from prostate cancer each year (second leading cause of death from cancer in U.S. men).
- Incidence of prostate cancer increases with age: Uncommon <50 yr; 80% of new cases are diagnosed in patients aged ≥65 yr. Widespread prostate-specific antigen (PSA) testing has doubled the incidence of prostate cancer and the lifetime risk for prostate cancer to approximately 16%. Prostate cancer is also diagnosed earlier, and the incidence of clinically "silent" T1 tumors has increased from 17% in 1989 to 48% in 2001 since the advent of PSA screening. Currently, approximately 80% of prostate cancer cases are diagnosed as localized disease and only 4% as metastatic disease.
- Prostate cancer is found at autopsy in more than half of U.S. men older than 50 years but is the cause of death in only 3%.
- Average age at time of diagnosis is 72 yr.
- Blacks in the United States have the highest incidence of prostate cancer in the world (one in every nine males).
- Incidence is low in Asians.
- Approximately 9% of all prostate cancers may be familial. Obesity is a risk factor for prostate cancer. High-fat, low-fiber diet increases risk. High insulin levels may also increase the risk of prostate cancer. Dietary supplementation with vitamin E has been reported to significantly increase the risk of prostate cancer among healthy men. Linkage studies have implicated chromosome 17p21-22 as a possible location of a prostate-cancer susceptibility gene. Germline mutations in *HOXB13* are associated with a significantly increased risk of hereditary prostate cancer.
- Mortality rates of prostate cancer have declined substantially in the past 15 yr from 34% in 1990 to <20% currently.

PHYSICAL FINDINGS & CLINICAL PRESENTATION

- Generally silent disease until it reaches advanced stages.
- Bone pain and pathologic fractures may be initial symptoms of prostate cancer.
- Local growth can cause symptoms of outflow obstruction.
- Digital rectal examination (DRE) may reveal an area of increased firmness; 10% of patients will have a negative DRE.
- Prostate may be hard, fixed, with extension of tumor to the seminal vesicles in advanced stages.

Dx DIAGNOSIS

DIFFERENTIAL DIAGNOSIS

- Benign prostatic hypertrophy
- Prostatitis
- Prostate stones

LABORATORY TESTS

- Measurement of PSA is controversial in early diagnosis of prostate cancer. PSA screening is associated with psychological harm, and its potential benefits remain uncertain. In asymptomatic men with no history of prostate cancer, screening using PSA does not reduce all-cause mortality or death from prostate cancer. Normal PSA is found in >20% of patients with prostate cancer, whereas only 20% of men with PSA levels between 4 ng/ml and 10 ng/ml have prostate cancer. Most guidelines encourage a shared decision-making approach between patient and physician regarding PSA testing. Available evidence favors clinician discussion of the pros and cons of PSA screening with average-risk men aged 65 to 69 yr. Only men who express a definite preference for screening should have PSA testing. Rather than widespread annual PSA screening, a reasonable approach may be to focus on high-risk men (those with PSA levels ≥2 ng/ml at age 60). The American Cancer Society recommends offering the PSA test and DRE yearly to men aged ≥50 yr who have a life expectancy of at least 10 yr. Earlier testing, starting at age 40 to 45 yr, is recommended for men at high risk (e.g., blacks, men with family history of prostate cancer). An isolated elevation in PSA level should be confirmed several weeks later before proceeding with further testing, including prostate biopsy. Screening for prostate cancer in men aged ≥75 yr is controversial and generally not recommended. The American College of Physicians (ACP) recommends that clinicians should not screen for prostate cancer using the PSA in average-risk men under age 50, men over age 69, or men with a life expectancy of <10 to 15 yr. The U.S. Preventive Services Task Force (USPSTF) recommends against PSA-based screening for prostate cancer in all age groups. According to the USPSTF:
  1. The magnitude of harms from screening (e.g., falsely high PSA levels, psychological effects, unnecessary biopsies, overdiagnosis of indolent tumors) is "at least small."
  2. The magnitude of treatment-associated harms (i.e., adverse effects of surgery, radiation, and hormonal therapy) is "at least moderate."

TABLE 1 Definition of Risk Groups

Risk Group	Clinical Stage	PSA (ng/ml)	Gleason Score	Biopsy Criteria
Low	T_{1a} or T_{1c}	<10	2-6	Unilateral or <50% of core involved
Intermediate	T_{1b}, T_{1c}, or T_{2a}	<10	3 + 4 = 7	Bilateral
High	T_{1b}, T_{1c}, T_{2b}, or T_3	10-20	4 + 3 = 7	>50% of core involved or perineural invasion or ductal differentiation
Very high	T_4	>20	8-10	Lymphovascular invasion or neuroendocrine differentiation

From Wein AJ et al: *Campbell-Walsh urology*, ed 11, Philadelphia, 2016, Elsevier.

3. The 10-yr mortality benefit of PSA-based prostate cancer screening is "small to none."
4. The overall balance of benefits and harms results in "moderate certainty that PSA-based screening has no net benefit."

- Free PSA: The use of serum free PSA for prostate screening has been proposed by some urologists as a means to decrease unwarranted biopsies without missing a significant number of prostate cancers. This approach is based on the higher free PSA in men with benign prostatic hyperplasia and the higher protein-bound PSA levels in men with prostate cancer. For example, in men with total PSA levels of 4 to 10 ng/ml, the cancer probability is 0.25, but if the percentage of free PSA is ≤17%, the probability of cancer increases to 0.45.
- PSA velocity: The rate of increase of serum PSA over time (PSA velocity) can aid in the diagnosis of prostate cancer. A yearly PSA velocity >0.75 ng/ml increases the likelihood of later malignancy when total PSA is still within normal range. Proper interpretation of PSA velocity requires at least three PSA measurements over an 18-month period because most PSA variations are physiologic. Recent trials have cast a doubt on the value of PSA velocity by showing that adding PSA velocity as a trigger for biopsy did not improve predictive accuracy beyond that of using PSA threshold values alone.
- Age-adjusted PSA: There is evidence that the current threshold of 4.0 ng/ml is inadequate for younger men, because in a recent study 22% of men with PSA levels between 2.6 and 4.0 were found to have prostate cancer. The concept of age-related cutoffs remains controversial. Lowering the upper limit of normal for PSA would improve sensitivity but decrease specificity.
- Prostatic acid phosphatase can be used for evaluation of nonlocalized disease.
- Prostate cancer gene 3 (*PCA3*) is overexpressed in prostate cancer cell, and high levels are suggestive of prostate cancer. Measurement of *PCA3* in urine specimens collected after digital exams is helpful to make decisions about prostate biopsy in men with elevated PSA.
- Transrectal biopsy and fine-needle aspiration of prostate can confirm the diagnosis. Indications for biopsy include an abnormal PSA level, an abnormal DRE, or a previous biopsy specimen that showed prostatic intraepithelial neoplasia or prostatic atypia. The number of cores taken is patient specific, typically including a minimum of 10 cores. Prostate volume negatively affects cancer detection rate (23% in glands >50 cm^3, 38% in glands <50 cm^3).

IMAGING STUDIES

- Bone scan is useful to evaluate bone metastasis (present or eventually develops in almost 80% of patients). However, according to the American Urological Association (AUA), the routine use of bone scanning is not required for staging of prostate cancer in asymptomatic men with clinically localized cancer if the PSA level is ≤20 ng/ml.
- CT scan, MRI, and transrectal ultrasonography may be useful in selected patients to assess extent of prostate cancer. High-resolution MRI with magnetic nanoparticles has been used for the detection of small and otherwise undetectable lymph node metastases in patients with prostate cancer. However, according to the AUA, transrectal ultrasonography adds little to the combination of PSA and DRE. Similarly, CT and MRI imaging are generally not indicated for cancer staging in men with clinically localized cancer and PSA <25 ng/ml. With regard to pelvic lymph node dissection in staging, the AUA states that it may not be required in patients with PSA levels <10 ng/ml and when PSA level is <20 ng/ml and the Gleason score is <6.

Rx TREATMENT

NONPHARMACOLOGIC THERAPY

Watchful waiting is reasonable in selected patients with early-stage (T-IA) and projected life expectancy <10 yr or in patients with focal and moderately differentiated carcinoma.

ACUTE GENERAL Rx

- Therapeutic approach varies with the following:
  1. Stage of the tumor.
  2. Patient's life expectancy.
  3. General medical condition.
  4. Patient's treatment preference (e.g., patient may be opposed to orchiectomy).
- The optimal treatment of clinically localized prostate cancer is unclear. It is important to remember that all forms of treatment have potential adverse effects. Management requires careful consideration of the potential benefits and harms of intervention, the patient's age, health status, and individual preferences. Table 2 summarizes recommended treatment based on risk group and life expectancy.
  1. Radical prostatectomy is generally performed in patients with localized prostate cancer and life expectancy >10 yr. Radical prostatectomy reduces disease-specific mortality, overall mortality, and the risks of metastasis and local progression. The absolute reduction in the risk of death after 10 yr is small, but the reductions in the risks of metastasis and local tumor progression are substantial. A 29 yr follow-up comparing radical prostatectomy with watchful waiting showed that men with clinically detected, localized prostate cancer and a long life expectancy benefited from radical prostatectomy with a mean 2.9 yr of life gained. Postoperative complications of radical prostatectomy include urinary incontinence (10% to 20% depending on degree of neurovascular bundle and urethral preservation, patient age, and correct mucosal apposition) and erectile dysfunction (percentage >50% and varies with patient age, preoperative erectile dysfunction, stage of

TABLE 2 Recommended Treatment

Risk Group	Life Expectancy (Years)	Recommended Treatment
Low	0-5	AS, HT
	5-10	AS, RT, HT, O
	>10	RP, RT, AS, O
Intermediate*	0-5	AS, HT, RT, O
	5-10	RT, HT, RP, O
	>10	RP, RT, O, HT
High*	0-5	AS, RT + HT, O
	5-10	RT + HT, HT, RP, O
	>10	RT + HT, RP + RT + HT, HT
Very high*	0-5	AS, RT + HT, O
	5-10	H, RT + HT, ST
	>10	RT + HT, RP + RT + HT, HT, ST, IT

AS, active surveillance; *HT,* hormone therapy; *IT,* investigational multimodal therapy; *O,* others; *RP,* radical prostatectomy; *RT,* radiation therapy; *ST,* systemic therapy.
*If there is more than a 20% probability of positive lymph nodes, AS, HT, ST + HT.
From Wein AJ, et al.: *Campbell-Walsh urology*, ed 11, Philadelphia, 2016, Elsevier.

tumor at time of surgery, and preservation of neurovascular bundle). Lower complication rates occur in hospitals that perform a large number of prostatectomies. Fewer men will have postsurgical erectile dysfunction after unilateral or bilateral nerve-sparing surgery. In men undergoing prostatectomy, robotic-assisted laparoscopic surgery represents an alternative to open retropubic radical prostatectomy. Despite advertisements that suggest that there are fewer complications after robotic surgery, data show that sexual dysfunction occurs postoperatively in about 88% of patients who have undergone robotic-assisted or conventional prostatectomy and that incontinence problems are more prevalent (33%) with robotic surgery than with open retropubic radical prostatectomy (RPP) (27%). Trials have shown that prostatectomy is preferred over "watchful waiting" in patients with localized prostate cancer detected by PSA if the PSA level is >10 ng/ml. In this subgroup, the 10-year mortality is 48.4% with prostatectomy versus 61.6% with watchful waiting. In men who have low-risk disease (PSA level <10 mcg/L, stage <T2a, Gleason score ≤3 + 3), and <6% risk for prostate cancer–specific death at 15 yr, watchful waiting (WW) and active surveillance (AS) are reasonable and underutilized options.

2. Radiation therapy (external-beam irradiation or brachytherapy with implantation of radioactive pellets [iodine-125 or palladium-103 seeds] into the prostate gland) represents an alternative in patients with localized prostate cancer, especially poor surgical candidates or patients with a high-grade malignancy. The efficacy of brachytherapy is comparable to external radiation. In patients receiving external-beam radiation, a total dose of 79.2 Gy (high dose) compared with a total dose of 70.2 Gy (conventional dose) has been reported to lower the risk of recurrence without increased risk of morbidity and mortality. Newer radiation treatments such as intensity-modulated radiation therapy (IMRT) and proton therapy are becoming increasingly popular and replacing the older technique of conformal radiation therapy over the past 10 years. Trials have shown that among patients with nonmetastatic prostate cancer, the use of IMRT compared with conformal therapy is associated with less gastrointestinal morbidity and fewer hip fractures but more erectile dysfunction; IMRT compared with proton therapy is associated with less GI morbidity. Patients with localized prostate cancer and high risk for extraprostatic disease and disease recurrence (e.g., Gleason score ≤7 with multiple positive biopsy cores and clinical stage T1b-T2b) may benefit (increased overall survival) with the addition of 6 mo of androgen suppression therapy to radiation therapy.
3. Watchful waiting is reasonable in patients who are too old or too ill to survive longer than 10 yr. If the cancer progresses to the point where it becomes symptomatic, palliation can be attempted with several methods. Conservative management is also reasonable for patients with Gleason score of 2 to 4 because these patients do not have a shortened life expectancy and treatment is associated with long-term side effects. Watchful waiting also appears to be safe in older men with less-aggressive disease. Individual preferences play a central role in the decision whether to treat or to pursue active surveillance.

- Patients with advanced disease and projected life expectancy <10 yr are candidates for radiation therapy and hormonal therapy (diethylstilbestrol, luteinizing hormone–releasing hormone analogues, antiandrogens, bilateral orchiectomy).
- Recommended treatment of patients with regional metastatic prostate cancer with projected life expectancy ≥10 yr includes radiation therapy and hormonal therapy.
- Prostate cancer is an androgen-receptor-dependent disease, and the blocking of androgen-receptor signaling is an effective treatment modality. Table 3 summarizes major circulating androgens. Androgen deprivation therapy (ADT) is the mainstay of treatment for metastatic prostate cancer. Adverse effects of ADT include decreased libido, impotence, hot flashes, osteopenia with increased fracture risk, metabolic alterations, and changes in mood and cognition. Adjuvant treatment with luteinizing hormone-releasing hormone (LHRH) agonists (goserelin, leuprolide, or triptorelin) plus antiandrogens (flutamide, bicalutamide, or nilutamide), when started simultaneously with external-beam radiation, improves local control and survival in patients with locally advanced prostate cancer. Pamidronate inhibits osteoclast-mediated bone resorption and prevents bone loss in the hip and lumbar spine in men receiving treatment for prostate cancer. Gonadotropin-releasing hormone (GnRH) receptor antagonists can be used for rapid medical castration of men with advanced prostate cancer. Degarelix is an injectable GnRH agonist useful to suppress testosterone in patients with prostate cancer who are not good candidates for LHRH agonists and refuse surgical castration. Assessment of bone density and treatment with once-weekly oral alendronate can prevent and improve the bone loss that occurs in men receiving ADT for prostate cancer.
- Docetaxel plus prednisone or docetaxel plus estramustine can be used in metastatic hormone–refractory prostate cancer. Newer treatments for hormone-refractory prostate cancer (castration-resistant cancer) include immunotherapy with sipuleucel and cabazitaxel, a microtubule inhibitor that interferes with cell mitosis and replication. Both agents can prolong survival but adverse effects can be severe and both agents are very expensive. Abiraterone is an oral agent that blocks biosynthesis of androgens by inhibiting CYP17, an enzyme required for androgen biosynthesis. It has been FDA approved for oral treatment, in combination with prednisone, of metastatic castration-resistant prostate cancer in patients previously treated with docetaxel.
- Enzalutamide is a newer nonsteroidal antiandrogen. Trials have shown it to be highly effective in extending survival in patients with metastatic castration-resistant prostate cancer. It can be used sequentially with other agents such as docetaxel, abiraterone, cabazitaxel, and immunotherapy. Radium-223, an alpha emitter, selectively targets bone metastases and has been found effective in improving survival in men with castration-resistant prostate cancer and bone metastases.
- The poly(adenosine diphosphate [ADP]-ribose) polymerase (PARP) inhibitor has shown a high response rate in patients whose prostate cancers were no longer responding to standard treatments and who had defects in DNA-repair genes.

CHRONIC Rx

- Patients should be monitored at 3- to 6-mo intervals with clinical examination and PSA for the first year, then every 6 mo for the second year, then yearly if stable. For patients who have undergone radical prostatectomy, a

TABLE 3 Major Circulating Androgens

Source	Androgen	Amount Produced/Day (mg)	Relative Potency	Relative Potency/Amount Produced
Testes	Testosterone	6.6	100	15.2
Testes and peripheral tissues	Dihydrotestosterone	0.3	160-190	533-633
Adrenal glands	Androstenedione	1.4	39	27.9
Adrenal glands	Dehydroepiandrosterone	29	15	0.5

From Wein AJ, et al.: *Campbell-Walsh urology*, ed 11, Philadelphia, 2016, Elsevier.

TABLE 4 Common Pain Syndromes in Metastatic Castration-Resistant Prostate Cancer

Pain Syndrome	Initial Management	Other Therapeutic Alternatives
Localized bone pain	Pharmacologic pain management Localized radiotherapy (special attention to weight-bearing areas, lytic metastasis, and extremities)	Surgical stabilization of pathologic fractures or extensive bone erosions Epidural metastasis and cord compression should be evaluated in all patients with focal back pain Radiopharmaceuticals should be considered if local radiation therapy fails
Diffuse bone pain	Pharmacologic pain management "Multispot" or wide-field radiotherapy Radiopharmaceuticals	Corticosteroids Bisphosphonates or RANK ligand inhibitors Calcitonin Chemotherapy
Epidural metastasis and cord compression	High-dose corticosteroids Radiation therapy Surgical decompression and stabilization are indicated in high-grade epidural compressions, extensive bone involvement, or recurrence after irradiation.	Pharmacologic pain management Physical therapy for recovery of neurologic function
Nerve plexopathies caused by direct tumor extension or previous therapy (rare)	Pharmacologic pain management Radiation therapy (if not previously used) Neurolytic procedures (nerve blocks)	Tricyclic antidepressants (amitriptyline) Anticonvulsants (gabapentin, pregabalin)
Miscellaneous neurogenic causes: Postherpetic neuralgia, peripheral neuropathies	Complete neurologic evaluation Pharmacologic pain management Discontinuation of neurotoxic drugs: Docetaxel, platinum compounds	Tricyclic antidepressants (amitriptyline) Anticonvulsants (gabapentin, pregabalin)
Other uncommon pain syndromes: Extensive skull metastasis with cranial nerve/skull base involvement, extensive painful liver metastasis, or pelvic masses	Radiation therapy Pharmacologic pain management Corticosteroids (cranial nerve involvement)	Chemotherapy Intrathecal chemotherapy may ameliorate symptoms of meningeal involvement

RANK, receptor activator of nuclear factor-κB.
From Wein AJ, et al.: *Campbell-Walsh urology*, ed 11, Philadelphia, 2016, Elsevier.

rising PSA level suggests evidence of residual or recurrent prostate cancer. A recent study revealed that if the PSA level remains undetectable 3 to 5 years after radical prostatectomy, the probability of biochemical recurrence is extremely low and it is reasonable to stop PSA monitoring.[1] Salvage radiotherapy may potentially cure patients with disease recurrence after radical prostatectomy. Recent trials have shown that addition of 24 months of antiandrogen therapy with daily bicalutamide to salvage radiation therapy results in significantly higher rates of long-term overall survival and lower incidences of metastatic prostate cancer and death from prostate cancer than radiation therapy plus placebo.[2]

- Chest radiography and bone scan should be performed yearly or sooner if patient develops symptoms.

DISPOSITION

- Prognosis varies with the stage of the disease and the Gleason classification (see "Definition"). For patients between ages 65 and 69 yr at diagnosis and a Gleason score of 2 to 4, the probability of dying from prostate cancer 15 yr after diagnosis is 0.06 and that of dying from other causes is 0.56. If the Gleason score is 7 to 10, the probability of dying from prostate cancer increases to 0.72 and from other causes varies from 0.25 to 0.36.
- The ploidy of the tumor also has prognostic value; prognosis is better with diploid tumor cells and worse with aneuploid tumor cells.
- For grade 1 tumors, the extended 10-yr, disease-specific survival is similar for patients with prostatectomy (94%), radiotherapy (90%), and conservative management (93%); survival rate is better with surgery than with radiotherapy or conservative management in patients with grade 2 or 3 localized prostate cancer.
- Expression of the gene *EZH2* has been identified as an important factor in the determination of the aggressiveness of prostate cancer. A recent study revealed that expression of the *EZH2* gene may be a better predictor of clinical failure than Gleason score, tumor stage, or surgical margin status. Testing for EZH2 protein in prostate cancer tissue may be useful to determine prognosis and direct treatment.
- Preoperative PSA level and PSA velocity have prognostic significance. Men whose PSA level increases by >2.0 mcg/ml during the year before the diagnosis of cancer may have a relatively high risk of death from prostate cancer despite undergoing radical prostatectomy.
- Extraprostatic disease is detected at radical prostatectomy in 38% to 52% of patients and is associated with a risk of disease recurrence, progression, and death. In these patients, adjuvant radiotherapy results in significantly reduced risk of PSA relapse and disease recurrence; however, the improvements in metastases-free survival and overall survival are not statistically significant. Table 4 summarizes common pain syndromes in metastatic castration-resistant prostate cancer.
- The Prostate Cancer Prevention trial revealed that the use of 5-alpha-reductase inhibitors lowers the incidence of prostate cancer but also increases the incidence of high-grade tumors (Gleason score >7). It is possible that these agents delay diagnosis of prostate cancer by lowering PSA levels and decreasing prostate size. The tradeoff inherent in using 5-alpha-reductase inhibitors for prostate cancer prevention is risk of one additional high-grade cancer in order to avert three or four lower-grade cancers. Based on these results, the FDA's Oncologic Drugs Advisory Committee

[1] Matsumoto K, et al.: Determining when to stop prostate specific antigen monitoring after radical prostatectomy: the role of ultrasensitive prostate specific antigen, *J Urol* 197:655, 2017.
[2] Shirley WV, et al.: Radiation with or without antiandrogen therapy in recurrent prostate cancer, *N Engl J Med* 376:417-428, 2017.

concluded that finasteride and dutasteride do not have a favorable risk-benefit profile for chemoprevention of prostate cancer in healthy men.

- Patients undergoing prostatectomy are more likely to have urinary incontinence than those undergoing radiotherapy at 2 years and 5 years. However, at 15 years there are no significant relative differences in disease-specific functional outcomes among men undergoing prostatectomy or radiotherapy.
- Bone health is a significant concern in men with prostate cancer. Trials involving biphosphonates and denosumab reveal that both improve bone mineral density (BMD) in men with non-metastatic prostate cancer receiving androgen deprivation therapy. Denosumab has also been shown to reduce the risk of vertebral fractures.

SUGGESTED READINGS

Available at ExpertConsult.com

RELATED CONTENT

Prostate Cancer (Patient Information)

AUTHOR: **FRED F. FERRI, M.D.**

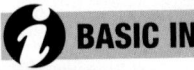

BASIC INFORMATION

DEFINITION

Prostatitis refers to inflammation of the prostate gland. There are four major categories (Table 1):
1. Acute bacterial prostatitis (type I)
2. Chronic bacterial prostatitis (type II)
3. Chronic prostatitis/pelvic pain syndrome (CP/CPPS) (type III): Subdivided into type IIIA (inflammatory) and IIIB (noninflammatory)
4. Asymptomatic inflammatory prostatitis (type IV)

ICD-10CM CODES

N41.0 Acute prostatitis
N41.1 Chronic prostatitis

EPIDEMIOLOGY & DEMOGRAPHICS

- 50% of men will have symptoms of prostatitis in their lifetime.
- Prostatitis accounts for >8% of visits to urologists and 1% of visits to primary care physicians.
- The prevalence of chronic bacterial prostatitis is 5% to 10%.
- CP/CPPS is the most common of the clinically defined prostatitis syndromes, with prevalence ranging from 9% to 12% of men.
- Acute bacterial prostatitis accounts for 10% of all cases of prostatitis.

PHYSICAL FINDINGS & CLINICAL PRESENTATION

- Acute bacterial prostatitis:
  1. Sudden or rapidly progressive onset of:
     a. Dysuria.
     b. Frequency.
     c. Urgency.
     d. Nocturia.
     e. Perineal pain that may radiate to the back, rectum, or penis.
  2. Hematuria or a purulent urethral discharge may occur.
  3. Occasionally urinary retention complicates the course.
  4. Fever, chills, and signs of sepsis can also be part of the clinical picture.
  5. On rectal examination the prostate is typically tender.
- Chronic bacterial prostatitis:
  1. Characterized by positive culture of expressed prostatic secretions. May cause symptoms such as suprapubic, low back, or perineal pain; mild urgency, frequency, and dysuria with urination; and possibly recurrent urinary tract infections.
  2. May be asymptomatic when the infection is confined to the prostate.
  3. May present as an increase in severity of baseline symptoms of benign prostatic hypertrophy (BPH).
  4. When cystitis is also present, urinary frequency, urgency, and burning may be reported.
  5. Hematuria may be a presenting complaint.
  6. In elderly men, new onset of urinary incontinence may be noted.
- CP/CPPS:
  1. Presents similarly with pain in the pelvic region lasting >3 mo. Symptoms also can include pain in the suprapubic region, low back, penis, testes, or scrotum.
  2. The symptoms can be of variable severity and may include lower urinary tract symptoms, sexual dysfunction, and reduced quality of life.

ETIOLOGY

- Acute bacterial prostatitis:
  1. Acute, usually gram-negative infection of the prostate gland. *E. coli* is the most commonly isolated organism.
     a. Generally associated with cystitis.
     b. Results from the ascent of bacteria into the urethra.
  2. Occasionally the route of infection is hematogenous or a lymphatogenous spread of rectal bacteria.
  3. Consider *Neisseria gonorrhoeae* or *Chlamydia trachomatis* in young patients (age <35 yr) with risk of sexually transmitted disease (STD).
- Chronic bacterial prostatitis:
  1. Often asymptomatic. *E. coli* is the most commonly isolated organism.
  2. Exacerbation of symptoms of BPH caused by the same mechanism as in acute bacterial prostatitis.
- CP/CPPS:
  1. Type IIIA: Refers to symptoms of prostatic inflammation associated with the presence of white blood cells in prostatic secretions with no identifiable bacterial organism.
  2. *Chlamydia* infection may be etiologically implicated in some cases.
  3. Type IIIB: Refers to symptoms of prostatic inflammation with no or few white blood cells in the prostatic secretion. Its cause is multifactorial (Fig. 1).

DIAGNOSIS

DIFFERENTIAL DIAGNOSIS

- BPH with lower urinary tract symptoms
- Prostate cancer
- Interstitial cystitis/bladder pain syndrome
- Pelvic floor dysfunction
- Bladder cancer
- Urolithiasis
- UTI
- Proctitis

WORKUP

- Rectal examination:
  1. Tender prostate most suggestive of acute bacterial prostatitis
  2. Enlarged prostate common in chronic bacterial prostatitis
  3. Normal prostate is consistent with chronic bacterial prostatitis and CP/CPPS
- Expression of prostatic secretions by prostate massage is contraindicated in acute bacterial prostatitis but is appropriate in the other three situations.

LABORATORY TESTS

- Urinalysis.
- Urine culture and sensitivity.
- Bacterial localization studies can be performed but are cumbersome and impractical in most clinical settings.
- Cell count and culture of expressed prostatic secretions.
- Prostate-specific antigen (PSA) is not used to diagnose prostatitis and is not recommended unless a nodule is present on digital examination. A rapid rise over baseline should raise the possibility of prostatitis even in

TABLE 1 Classification System for the Prostatitis Syndromes

Traditional	National Institutes of Health	Description
Acute bacterial prostatitis	Category I	Acute infection of the prostate gland
Chronic bacterial prostatitis	Category II	Chronic infection of the prostate gland
N/A	Category III Chronic pelvic pain syndrome (CPPS)	Chronic genitourinary pain in the absence of uropathogenic bacteria localized to the prostate gland employing standard methodology
Nonbacterial prostatitis	Category IIIA Inflammatory CPPS	Significant number of white blood cells in expressed prostatic secretions, postprostatic massage urine sediment (VB3), or semen
Prostatodynia	Category IIIB Noninflammatory CPPS	Insignificant number of white blood cells in expressed prostatic secretions, postprostatic massage urine sediment (VB3), or semen
N/A	Category IV Asymptomatic inflammatory prostatitis (AIP)	White blood cells (and/or bacteria) in expressed prostatic secretions, postprostatic massage urine sediment (VB3), semen, or histologic specimens of prostate gland

From Wein AJ et al: *Campbell-Walsh urology*, ed 11, Philadelphia, 2016, Elsevier.

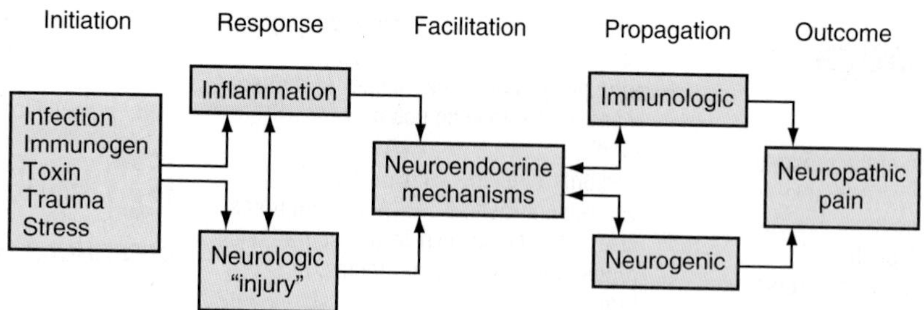

FIG. 1 The cause and pathogenesis of chronic prostatitis/chronic pelvic pain syndrome (category III chronic pelvic pain syndrome) appears to involve a pluricausal, multifactorial mechanism. An initiating stimulus, such as infection, reflux of some toxic or immunogenic urine substance, or perineal or pelvic trauma, starts a cascade of events in an anatomically or genetically susceptible man, resulting in a local response of inflammation or neurogenic injury or both. Further interrelated immunologic, neuropathic, endocrinologic, and psychologic mechanisms propagate or sustain the chronicity of the initial (or ongoing) event. The final outcome is the clinical manifestation of chronic perineal or pelvic pain and associated symptoms with local and central neuropathic mechanisms involving areas outside the prostate or pelvic area. (From Wein AJ et al: *Campbell-Walsh urology*, ed 11, Philadelphia, 2016, Elsevier.)

BOX 1 Suggested Therapies for Chronic Prostatitis and Chronic Pelvic Pain Syndrome (National Institutes of Health Category III)

Recommended
1. α-Blocker therapy as part of a multimodal treatment strategy for newly diagnosed, α-blocker–naive patients who have voiding symptoms
2. Antimicrobial therapy trial for selected newly diagnosed, antimicrobial-naive patients
3. Selected phytotherapies: Cernilton and quercetin
4. Multimodal therapy directed by clinical phenotype
5. Directed physiotherapy. Although level 1 evidence is not available, evidence from multiple weak trials and vast clinical experience strongly suggests benefit for selected patients

Not Recommended
1. α-Blocker monotherapy, particularly in patients previously treated with α-blockers
2. Antiinflammatory monotherapy
3. Antimicrobial therapy as primary therapy, particularly for patients in whom treatment with antibiotics has previously failed
4. 5α-Reductase inhibitor monotherapy; can be considered in older patients with coexisting benign prostatic hyperplasia
5. Most minimally invasive therapies such as transurethral needle ablation (TUNA), laser therapies
6. Invasive surgical therapies such as transurethral resection of the prostate (TURP) and radical prostatectomy

Requiring Further Evaluation
1. Low-intensity shock wave treatment
2. Acupuncture
3. Biofeedback
4. Invasive neuromodulation (e.g., pudendal nerve modulation)
5. Electromagnetic stimulation
6. Botulinum toxin A injection
7. Medical therapies including mepartricin, muscle relaxants, neuromodulators, and immunomodulators

Modified from Nickel JC et al: Male chronic pelvic pain syndrome (CPPS). In Chapple C, Abrams P (eds): *Male lower urinary tract symptoms (LUTS). An International Consultation on Male LUTS, Fukuoka, Japan, Sept 30–Oct 4, 2012*, Montreal, 2013, Société Internationale d'Urologie.
From Wein AJ et al: *Campbell-Walsh urology*, ed 11, Philadelphia, 2016, Elsevier.

the absence of symptoms. In such cases, a follow-up PSA after treatment of prostatitis is appropriate.
- Complete blood count and blood cultures if fever, chills, or signs of sepsis exist.

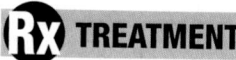

Rx TREATMENT

- Acute bacterial prostatitis:
  1. Uncomplicated (with risk of STD, age <35 yr): Ceftriaxone 250 mg IM × 1 dose *or* cefixime 400 mg PO × 1 *then* doxycycline 100 mg bid × 10 days.
  2. Uncomplicated with low risk of STD: Levofloxacin 500 mg qd or ciprofloxacin 500 mg bid × 10 to 14 days.
- Chronic bacterial prostatitis:
  1. First-line choice is a quinolone (ciprofloxacin or levofloxacin) for 4 wk.
  2. Trimethoprim-sulfamethoxazole (TMP-SMX) is second-line choice for 1 to 3 mo if the organism is sensitive. Tissue penetration for TMP-SMX is not as good as quinolones, and there is evidence of increasing uropathogenic resistance.
- CP/CPPS:
  1. Suggested therapies for CP/CPPS are summarized in Box 1.

SUGGESTED READINGS

Available at ExpertConsult.com

RELATED CONTENT

Prostatitis (Patient Information)

AUTHOR: **FRED F. FERRI, M.D.**

BASIC INFORMATION

DEFINITION

Calcium pyrophosphate dihydrate crystal deposition (CPPD) disease refers to the precipitation of calcium pyrophosphate dihydrate (CPP) in connective tissues that may be asymptomatic or may be associated with several clinical syndromes, including acute and chronic arthritis. CPP was formerly abbreviated and commonly referred to as "CPPD," but the abbreviation is now reserved for "CPP deposition." Alternative names representing specific clinical or radiographic features of CPPD disease include pseudogout, chondrocalcinosis, and pyrophosphate arthropathy.

Pseudogout/acute CPP crystal arthritis is used to describe acute attacks of CPP crystal-induced arthritis that clinically resembles the arthritis that is commonly encountered in gout. The term *acute CPP crystal arthritis* is now preferred in place of *pseudogout*.

Chondrocalcinosis (CC) refers to radiographic calcification in hyaline cartilage and/or fibrocartilage and does not confirm the diagnosis of CPP-related arthritis as it can be present in other types of crystal deposition diseases or be asymptomatic.

Pyrophosphate arthropathy is the term used for a chronic structural arthropathy related to CPPD deposition.

SYNONYMS

Calcium pyrophosphate dihydrate crystal deposition disease
CPP crystal deposition disease
CPPD
CC
Chondrocalcinosis
Pyrophosphate arthropathy

ICD-10CM CODES
M11.2 Other chondrocalcinosis
M11.9 Crystal arthropathy, unspecified
M11.8 Other specified crystal arthropathies
M11.1 Familial chondrocalcinosis

EPIDEMIOLOGY & DEMOGRAPHICS

PREVALENCE:
- The epidemiology of CPPD crystal deposition is described in Table 1.
- Most linked with advancing age (average age of 72)

GENETICS: Familial forms
- Associated with *ANKH* (ankylosis human) gene, which functions to transport inorganic pyrophosphate (PPi) out of cells. Familial mutations can increase extracellular PPi levels and lead to onset of CPPD disease in the third or fourth decade of life.

PHYSICAL FINDINGS & CLINICAL PRESENTATION

- *Acute CPP crystal arthritis/pseudogout*: Monoarticular attacks most commonly involve the knee and wrist but can be polyarticular. Patients, especially the elderly, can have systemic manifestations such as fever and altered mental status. Situations that may trigger acute CPPD crystal arthritis are described in Box E1
- Asymptomatic disease ("asymptomatic CPPD")
- Pseudogout (acute CPP crystal arthritis)
- Pseudo-RA (chronic CPP crystal inflammatory arthritis): Symmetric polyarthritis
- Pseudo-OA, with or without superimposed acute attacks (OA with CPPD)
- Pseudo-neuropathic joint disease
- Crowned-dens syndrome caused by crystal deposition in the ligamentum flavum of the cervical spine either asymptomatic or causing acute neck pain
- Pseudo-polymyalgia rheumatica (pseudo-PMR): Pain and stiffness in the neck and shoulder girdle mimicking PMR

ETIOLOGY

- Idiopathic
- Familial
- Trauma
- Hemochromatosis
- Metabolic and endocrine disorders: Hyperparathyroidism, hypophosphatasia, hemochromatosis, hypomagnesemia, Gitelman syndrome, gout, ochronosis, acromegaly, Wilson disease, familial hypocalciuric hypercalcemia, X-linked hypophosphatemic rickets

TABLE 1 Epidemiology of Calcium Pyrophosphate Dihydrate Crystal Deposition

Age Association	Rises with Age
Sex distribution	(F:M) 1:1
Chondrocalcinosis prevalence	8.1% (age range 63 to 93)
Pyrophosphate arthropathy prevalence	3.4% (age range 40 to 89)
Geography	Appears ubiquitous
Genetic associations	Mutations of *ANKH* gene on chromosome 5p (CCAL2) and unknown genes on chromosome 8q (CCAL1)

From Hochberg MC et al: *Rheumatology*, ed 5, St Louis, 2011, Mosby.

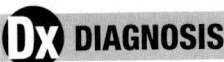

DIAGNOSIS

DIFFERENTIAL DIAGNOSIS

- Gouty arthritis
- Septic arthritis
- RA
- Spondyloarthritis (ReA, PsA)
- PMR

Table 2 describes metabolic diseases predisposing to CPPD disposition. Section II describes the differential diagnosis of acute monoarticular and oligoarticular arthritis and crystal-induced arthritides. An algorithm for evaluation and treatment of CPPD is shown in Fig. 1.

LABORATORY TESTS

- Arthrocentesis with presence of weakly positive birefringent rhomboid-shaped crystals by compensated polarized light microscopy (Fig. E2)
- Synovial fluid should always be analyzed for cell count with differential, crystals, Gram stain, and culture because acute CPP crystal arthritis/pseudogout and septic arthritis can coexist.
- Evaluate for possible metabolic cause, especially in younger patients aged <55 yr or patients with florid polyarticular disease. Box 2 describes screening blood tests for metabolic diseases associated with CPPD crystal deposition.

IMAGING STUDIES

- Plain radiographs often reveal CC located parallel to subchondral bone.
    1. Classic locations for CC (Fig. E3) include knee menisci (Fig. E4), wrist triangular fibrocartilage, symphysis pubis, and glenoid and acetabular labra.
- Musculoskeletal ultrasound can detect deposition of CPP crystals within the hyaline cartilage and/or fibrocartilage. In contrast to urate crystal deposits in gout, CPP crystals often deposit within the substance of the hyaline cartilage and fibrocartilage, providing a means to distinguish CPP from urate deposition that occurs on the surface of the hyaline cartilage as seen in gout (Fig. E5).

TABLE 2 Metabolic Diseases Predisposing to Calcium Pyrophosphate Dihydrate Deposition

	CC	Pseudogout	Chronic PA
Hemochromatosis	Yes	Yes	Yes
Hyperparathyroidism	Yes	Yes	No
Hypophosphatasia	Yes	Yes	No
Hypomagnesemia	Yes	Yes	No
Gout	Possibly	Possibly	No
Acromegaly	Possibly	No	No
Ochronosis	Yes	Yes	No
Familial hypocalciuric hypercalcemia	Possibly	No	No
X-linked hypophosphatemic rickets	Possibly	Possibly	Possibly

CC, Chondrocalcinosis; *PA*, pyrophosphate arthropathy.

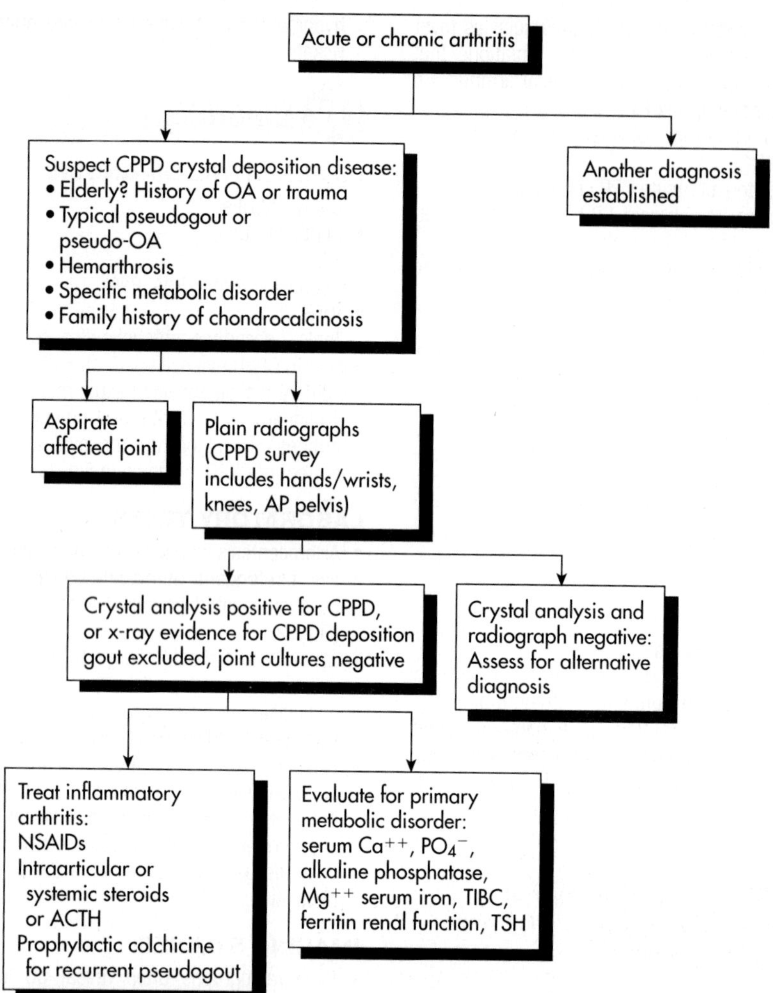

FIG. 1 Algorithm for evaluation and treatment of calcium pyrophosphate dihydrate disease. *ACTH,* Adrenocorticotropic hormone; *AP,* anteroposterior; *CPPD,* calcium pyrophosphate deposition; *NSAIDs,* nonsteroidal antiinflammatory drugs; *OA,* osteoarthritis; *TIBC,* total iron-binding capacity; *TSH,* thyroid-stimulating hormone. (From Harris ED et al: *Kelley's textbook of rheumatology,* ed 7, Philadelphia, 2005, Saunders.)

BOX 2 Screening Blood Tests for Metabolic Diseases Associated with Calcium Pyrophosphate Dihydrate Crystal Deposition

Calcium
Alkaline phosphatase
Magnesium
Ferritin, iron, transferrin
Liver function
Thyroid-stimulating hormone

From Hochberg MC et al: *Rheumatology,* ed 5, St Louis, 2011, Mosby.

Rx TREATMENT

NONPHARMACOLOGIC THERAPY

General measures such as immobilization of inflamed joint

ACUTE GENERAL Rx

- Monoarticular pseudogout:
    1. Aspiration followed by intraarticular corticosteroid injection (often superior to systemic treatment in the elderly)
- Polyarticular pseudogout:
    1. Oral corticosteroids, colchicine, or NSAIDs, if not contraindicated.

CHRONIC GENERAL Rx

Prophylaxis: Daily low-dose colchicine 0.6 mg twice daily or once daily as tolerated

- Pseudo-RA or refractory disease: Hydroxychloroquine or methotrexate
- Anakinra (Interleukin-1 receptor antagonist): Treatment and prophylaxis of polyarticular acute CPP crystal arthritis unresponsive to oral corticosteroids
- Treat underlying metabolic disease

DISPOSITION

Structural joint damage may occasionally occur, requiring arthroplasty in rare cases.

REFERRAL

Rheumatology

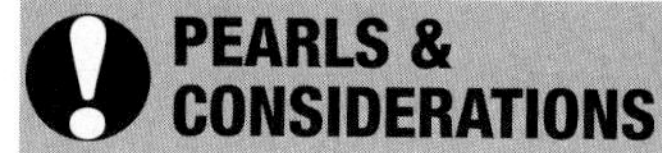

PEARLS & CONSIDERATIONS

COMMENTS

Acute CPP crystal arthritis/pseudogout attacks have been reported to occur in the setting of surgical procedures, diuresis, bisphosphonate administration, and hyaluronate joint injections.

SUGGESTED READINGS

Available at ExpertConsult.com

RELATED CONTENT

Pseudogout (Patient Information)
Gout (Related Key Topic)

AUTHORS: **NICOLE B. YANG, M.D.,** and **ANTHONY M. REGINATO, PH.D., M.D.**

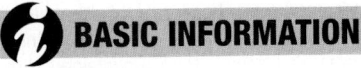

BASIC INFORMATION

DEFINITION

Psoriasis is a chronic skin disorder characterized by excessive proliferation of keratinocytes, resulting in the formation of thickened scaly plaques, itching, and inflammatory changes of the epidermis and dermis. Psoriasis is also associated with cardiovascular, metabolic, and neuropsychiatric effects. The various forms of psoriasis include plaque (most common), guttate, erythrodermic, pustular, inverse, and arthritis variants.

ICD-10CM CODES

L40	Psoriasis
L40.4	Guttate psoriasis
L40.1	Generalized pustular psoriasis
L40.8	Other psoriasis
L40.9	Psoriasis unspecified
L40.54	Psoriatic juvenile arthropathy
L40.0	Psoriasis vulgaris

EPIDEMIOLOGY & DEMOGRAPHICS

- Psoriasis affects 2% to 4% of the world's population. Most patients have limited psoriasis involving <5% of their body surface.
- There is a strong association between psoriasis and human leukocyte antigens (HLAs) B13, B17, and B27 (pustular psoriasis).
- Peak age of onset is bimodal (age 30 to 39 yr and at age 60 yr). Mean age at diagnosis is 34 yr.
- Men and women are affected equally. Approximately 20% of patients with psoriasis also have psoriatic arthritis. Median time from development of joint symptoms to diagnosis of psoriatic arthritis is 5 yr. Nail psoriasis affects over 50% of patients with psoriasis and can occur with any of the subtypes.

PHYSICAL FINDINGS & CLINICAL PRESENTATION

- Approximately 85% of patients with psoriasis have mild-to-moderate disease.
- The primary psoriatic lesion is an erythematous papule topped by a loosely adherent scale. Scraping the scale results in several bleeding points *(Auspitz sign)*.
- Chronic plaque psoriasis generally manifests with symmetric, sharply demarcated, erythematous, silver-scaled patches affecting primarily the intergluteal folds, elbows, scalp, fingernails, toenails, and knees (Figs. E1 and 2). This form accounts for 80% of psoriasis cases. Psoriasis may also involve the forehead, particularly contiguous to the scalp (Fig. 3).
- Psoriasis can also develop at the site of any physical trauma (sunburn, scratching). This is known as *Koebner phenomenon.*
- Nail involvement is common (pitting of the nail plate), resulting in hyperkeratosis, onychodystrophy with onycholysis (Fig. E4).
- Pruritus is variable; soreness and bleeding may occur.
- Joint involvement can result in sacroiliitis and spondylitis.
- Guttate psoriasis is generally preceded by streptococcal pharyngitis and manifests with multiple droplike lesions on the extremities and the trunk.
- Erythrodermic psoriasis is characterized by widespread cutaneous erythema and scaling.
- Pustular psoriasis manifests with widespread pustules. Localized forms may affect palms and soles.
- Inverse psoriasis is characterized by red and sharply demarcated thinner patches involving intertriginous areas (axillae, inguinal areas).
- Adverse effect on psychological and social functioning, with affected persons often feeling stigmatized.

ETIOLOGY

- Unknown, but there is a strong genetic component and high heritability. There are at least nine chromosomal loci with linkage to psoriasis. These loci are called psoriasis susceptibility 1 through 9 (PSORS1-PSORS9). PSORS1 locus in the major histocompatibility complex (MHC) region on chromosome 6 is considered the most important susceptibility locus and is believed to account for 35% to 50% of the heritability of the disease.
- Familial clustering (genetic transmission with a dominant mode with variable penetrants).
- One third of persons affected have a positive family history.
- A high prevalence of celiac disease has been noted in patients with psoriasis.

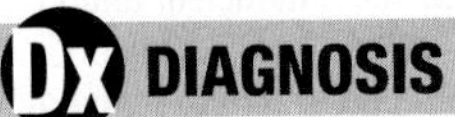

DIAGNOSIS

DIFFERENTIAL DIAGNOSIS

- Contact dermatitis
- Atopic dermatitis
- Stasis dermatitis
- Tinea
- Nummular dermatitis
- Candidiasis
- Mycosis fungoides, Sezary syndrome
- Cutaneous systemic lupus erythematosus
- Secondary and tertiary syphilis
- Drug eruption

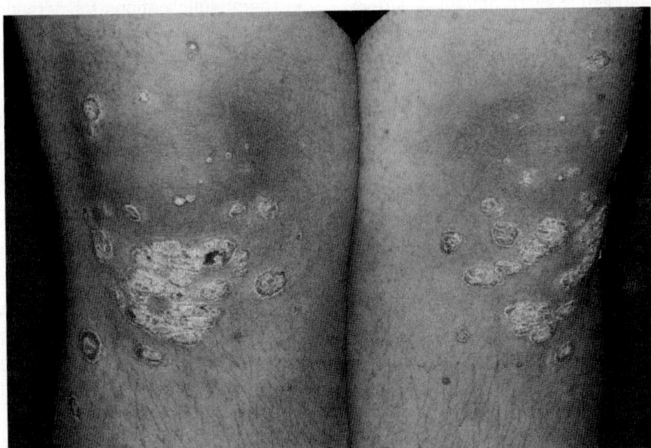

FIG. 2 Typical plaques of psoriasis with thick, micaceous scale overlying erythema. (From Paller AS, Mancini AJ: *Hurwitz clinical pediatric dermatology, a textbook of skin disorders of childhood and adolescence,* ed 5, 2016, Elsevier.)

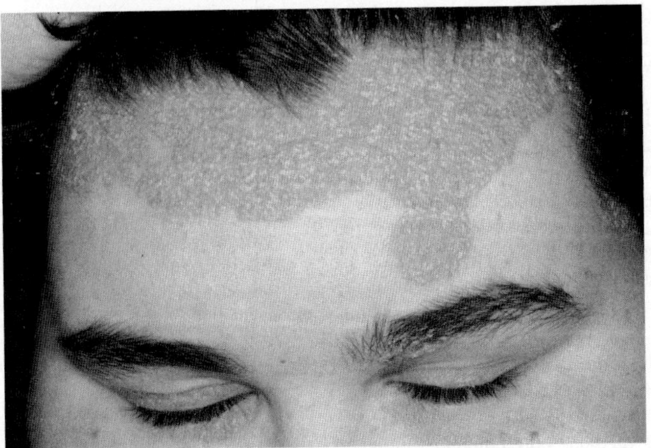

FIG. 3 Psoriasis often involves the forehead, particularly contiguous to the scalp. Note the eyelid and brow involvement. Given the yellowish scaling, this has been called "sebopsoriasis." (From Paller AS, Mancini AJ: *Hurwitz clinical pediatric dermatology, a textbook of skin disorders of childhood and adolescence,* ed 5, 2016, Elsevier.)

- Dermatomyositis (DM)
- Lupus erythematosus (LE)
- Seborrheic dermatitis
- Pityriasis rosea
- Lichen planus
- Pityriasis rubra pilaris

WORKUP

- Diagnosis is clinical. Blood work is rarely needed. A rapid plasma regain test is useful when ruling out syphilis. Antinuclear antibody (ANA) and anti-Ro and anti-La antibodies are helpful in ruling out subacute cutaneous lupus.
- Skin biopsy is rarely necessary.

LABORATORY TESTS

Generally not necessary for diagnosis

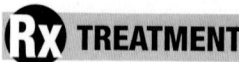

TREATMENT

NONPHARMACOLOGIC THERAPY

- Sunbathing generally leads to improvement.
- Eliminate triggering factors (e.g., stress, certain medications [e.g., lithium, beta-blockers, antimalarials]). Severe emotional stress tends to aggravate psoriasis.
- Patients with psoriasis benefit from a daily bath in warm water followed by application of a cream or ointment moisturizer. Regular use of an emollient moisturizer limits evaporation of water from the skin and allows the stratum corneum to rehydrate itself.
- Psoralen and ultraviolet A (PUVA) therapy (see "General Rx").
- Local hyperthermia has been used successfully to clear psoriatic plaques, but relapse is common.
- Occlusive treatment with surgical tape or dressings is effective as monotherapy or in combination with topical medications.
- Avoidance of tobacco. Smoking tobacco may worsen psoriasis.

GENERAL Rx

Therapeutic options vary according to the extent of disease. Approximately 70% to 80% of all patients can be treated adequately with topical therapy.

- Patients with limited disease (<20% of the body) can be treated with the following:
  1. Topical steroids: Disadvantages are brief remissions, expense, and decreased effect with continued use. Salicylic acid can be compounded by pharmacist in concentrations of 2% to 10% and used in combination with a corticosteroid to decrease the amount of scale.
  2. Calcipotriene: A vitamin D analogue effective for moderate plaque psoriasis. Adults should comb the hair, apply solution to the lesions, and rub it in, avoiding uninvolved skin. Disadvantages include its cost and potential burning and skin irritation. It should not be used concurrently with salicylic acid because calcipotriene is inactivated by the acidic nature of salicylic acid. Taclonex ointment and Enstilar aerosol foam formulation are a combination of calcipotriene and the high-potency corticosteroid betamethasone dipropionate. They are well tolerated and more effective than either agent used alone but also much more expensive.
  3. Tar products (Estar, liquor carbonis detergens [LCD], Psorigel) can be used overnight and are most effective when combined with ultraviolet B (UVB) light (Goeckerman regimen).
  4. Anthralin: Useful for chronic plaques; can result in purple-brown staining; best used with UVB light.
  5. Retinoids such as tazarotene 0.05%, 0.1% cream or gel, are effective in thinning plaques but are expensive and can cause irritation.
  6. Other useful measures include tape or occlusive dressing, UVB and lubricating agents, and interlesional steroids.
- Therapeutic options for persons with generalized disease (affecting >20% of the body) and for those with inadequate response to topical agents:
  1. UVB light exposure three times a week: This therapy does not require administration of a systemic drug (unlike psoralen plus ultraviolet A [PUVA]), but to be effective, it requires removal of scale with keratolytic agents and emollients.
  2. Oral PUVA administered two to three times weekly is effective for generalized disease. It is often considered in patients for whom narrow-band UVB therapy is ineffective. However, many PUVA treatments are required, necessitating frequent office visits, and it may be associated with phototoxicity, such as erythema and blistering, and increased risk of skin cancer.
- Systemic treatments include methotrexate 25 mg/wk for severe psoriasis. Etretinate (a synthetic retinoid) is most effective for palmar-plantar pustular psoriasis. Dose is 0.5 to 1 mg/kg/day. It can cause liver enzyme and lipid abnormalities and is teratogenic.
- Apremilast is a phosphodiesterase type-4 inhibitor used in moderate to severe plaque psoriasis. Side effects include diarrhea, nausea, headache, and worsening depression.
- Cyclosporine is also effective in severe psoriasis; however, relapses are common.
- Chronic plaque psoriasis may be treated with alefacept, a recombinant protein that selectively targets T lymphocytes. Treatment with alefacept for 12 wk (0.025, 0.075, or 0.150 mg/kg of body weight IV weekly) may result in significant improvement. Some patients also demonstrate a sustained clinical response after the cessation of treatment. This medication is very expensive (a 12-wk course can cost >$8000).
- Biologic therapies are now routinely used when traditional systemic agents are ineffective or poorly tolerated. Screening for tuberculosis is necessary before initiating treatment with these agents. Active, serious infection is a contraindication to the use of biologics.
- Tumor necrosis factor (TNF) inhibitors (adalimumab [Humira], etanercept [Enbrel], infliximab [Remicade]): Trials revealed a reduction in severity of plaque psoriasis. Efalizumab, a humanized monoclonal antibody that inhibits the activation of T cells, has also been reported to produce significant improvement in plaque psoriasis treatment period. Adalimumab has been reported to be effective for joint and skin manifestations of psoriasis.
- Newer biologic agents in patients with moderate to severe plaque psoriasis are ustekinumab (Stelera; an interleukin-12 and interleukin-23 blocker), brodalumab (Siliq), ixekizumab (Talz), secukinumab (Cosentix) anti–interleukin-17 receptor antagonists, and guselkumab (Tremfya), and tildrakizumab (Ilumya) interleukin-23 blockers. Cost is a limiting factor with all these agents.

DISPOSITION

The course of psoriasis is chronic, and the disease may be refractory to treatment.

REFERRAL

- Dermatology referral is recommended in all patients with generalized disease.
- Hospital admission may be necessary for severe diffuse or poorly responsive psoriasis. The Goeckerman regimen combines daily application of tar with UVB exposure and can result in prolonged remissions.

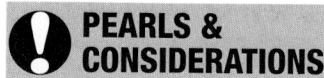

PEARLS & CONSIDERATIONS

COMMENTS

Psoriasis is more emotionally than physically disabling for most patients. Counseling may be indicated, particularly when it affects younger patients.

SUGGESTED READINGS

Available at ExpertConsult.com

RELATED CONTENT

Psoriasis (Patient Information)
Psoriatic Arthritis (Related Key Topic)

AUTHOR: **FRED F. FERRI, M.D.**

BASIC INFORMATION

DEFINITION

Psoriatic arthritis (PsA) is an inflammatory arthropathy, often included in a class of disorders called the *seronegative spondyloarthropathies (SpA),* a family of diseases characterized by inflammation of the spine, peripheral joints, and entheses (sites of insertion of tendon into bone). Both the Moll and Wright and CASPAR classification criteria are described in Table 1.

ICD-10CM CODES
L40.5+ Arthropathic psoriasis
L40.54 Psoriatic juvenile arthropathy
L40.52 Psoriatic arthritis mutilans

EPIDEMIOLOGY & DEMOGRAPHICS

INCIDENCE: 6 per 100,000 per yr
PREVALENCE: One to two per 1000 in the general population. Variable estimates of 4% to 30% of patients with underlying psoriasis
PREDOMINANT SEX: Equal male-to-female distribution
PREDOMINANT AGE: Symptom onset generally between age 30 to 55

PHYSICAL FINDINGS & CLINICAL PRESENTATION

- Psoriasis precedes arthritis in 67% of cases by an average of 8 to 10 yr.
- Arthritis precedes psoriasis or occurs concomitantly in 33% of patients.
- Arthritis, dactylitis, spondylitis, and enthesitis are main features.
- On examination, about 15% of patients will have psoriasis without prior diagnosis of skin disease.
- Arthritis is inflammatory, commonly characterized by prolonged morning stiffness, improvement with activity, joint erythema, warmth, or swelling.
- There are five classically described patterns of joint involvement (Box 1).
- Some patients may present with more than one pattern, and patterns can evolve over time. The distal interphalangeal (DIP) joints and spine are each affected in 40% to 50% of cases. It is rare to have spondyloarthritis alone, and it usually occurs with peripheral involvement.
- Dactylitis, also known as "sausage digit," refers to diffuse swelling of a finger or toe; it is fairly common and occurs in approximately 30% to 40% of patients during the disease course. It is associated with increased risk of radiographic joint damage.
- Enthesitis commonly occurs at the Achilles and plantar fascia, and swelling and tenderness may be seen on exam. Subclinical disease may be evident by ultrasonography examination.
- Dystrophic changes of the nails (pitting, onycholysis, leukonychia) may occur in association with joint inflammation in involved digits.
- Spondyloarthritis may include sacroiliitis, but is generally less likely to cause fusion to the extent seen in ankylosing spondylitis. More common to have asymmetric sacroiliac joint involvement.
- Ocular inflammation including conjunctivitis and uveitis can be seen.

ETIOLOGY

Remains unknown, but felt to be interplay of genetics and environmental factors

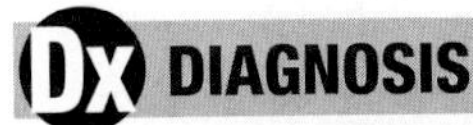

DIAGNOSIS

DIFFERENTIAL DIAGNOSIS

- Rheumatoid arthritis (RA)
- Erosive osteoarthritis
- Crystalline arthritis, including gout and pseudogout
- Other seronegative spondyloarthropathies, which includes reactive arthritis, enteropathic arthritis, and ankylosing spondylitis (also see differential diagnosis of SpA in Section III)

WORKUP

- Diagnosis is generally made on clinical grounds based on history, exam, and radiographic findings given lack of specific lab findings. An algorithm for the diagnosis of psoriatic arthritis is described in Fig. 1.
- Early diagnosis can be difficult to establish when the joint symptoms develop before skin and nail findings.

LABORATORY TESTS

- No specific diagnostic lab tests.
- Acute phase reactants such as ESR and CRP may be elevated, although less commonly than in patients with rheumatoid arthritis.
- Anemia of chronic disease may be seen.
- Rheumatoid factor (RF) and anti-CCP are generally negative, but can be present in up to 15% of patients.
- *HLA-B27* is significantly more common in patients with axial inflammation.
- Arthrocentesis generally demonstrates inflammatory synovial fluid without crystals.

IMAGING STUDIES

Radiographic findings (Fig. E2) of involved joints may include soft tissue swelling, joint space narrowing, subluxation, erosive changes, and new bone formation (periostitis, fusion). As opposed to RA, see more asymmetric joint involvement and DIP joint changes.

BOX 1 Subtypes of Psoriatic Arthritis

- Distal interphalangeal joint–predominant arthritis (10%) (Fig. 3).
- Symmetric polyarthritis–predominant arthritis (5%-20%).
- Asymmetric oligoarthritis or monoarthritis (70%-80%).
- Axial disease–predominant (spondylitis and/or sacroiliitis) (5%-20%).
- Arthritis mutilans (rare).

From Hochberg MC, et al.: *Rheumatology,* ed 5, St Louis, 2011, Mosby.

TABLE 1 Classifications of Psoriatic Arthritis

	Classification Criteria for Psoriatic Arthritis (Caspar)*		
Moll and Wright	**Points**	**Category**	**Description**
Presence of psoriasis and: An inflammatory arthritis (peripheral arthritis and/or sacroiliitis or spondylitis) The (usual) absence of serologic tests for rheumatoid factor	2	Current psoriasis or personal or family history of psoriasis	Psoriatic skin or scalp disease confirmed by dermatologist or rheumatologist; history of psoriasis from patient, family physician, dermatologist, rheumatologist, or other qualified practitioner; patient-reported history of psoriasis in first- or second-degree relative
	1	Psoriatic nail dystrophy on current physical examination	Includes onycholysis, pitting, and hyperkeratosis
	1	Negative for rheumatoid factor	Enzyme-linked immunosorbent assay or nephelometry preferred (no latex) using local laboratory reference range
	1	Current dactylitis or history of dactylitis documented by a rheumatologist	Swelling of entire digit
	1	Radiographic evidence of juxtaarticular new bone formation	Ill-defined ossification near joint margins excluding osteophyte formation on plain radiographs of hand or foot

*Psoriatic arthritis is diagnosed when ≥3 points are assigned in the presence of inflammatory articular disease (joint, spine, or entheseal).
From Hochberg MC, et al.: *Rheumatology,* ed 5, St Louis, 2011, Mosby.

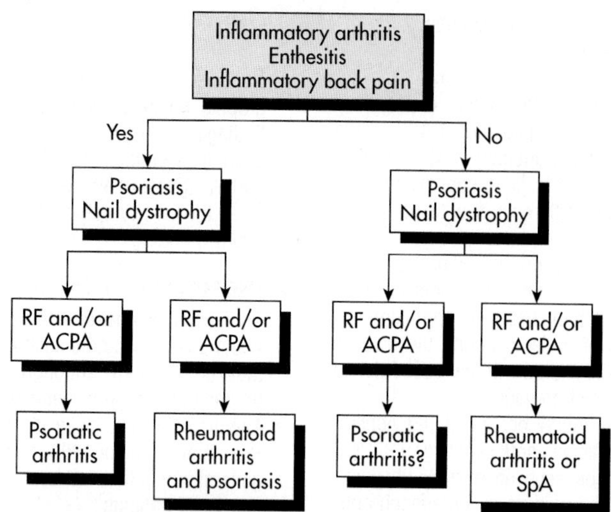

FIG. 1 Algorithm to be used in the diagnosis of individual patients presenting with possible psoriatic arthritis. Some patients may present with typical articular manifestations of psoriatic arthritis but in the absence of skin or nail disease. They can be diagnosed as having definite psoriatic arthritis only when psoriasis subsequently develops. *ACPA,* Anticitrullinated protein antibody; *RF,* rheumatoid factor; *SpA,* spondyloarthropathy. (From Firestein GS, et al.: *Kelly's textbook of rheumatology,* ed 9, Philadelphia, 2013, Saunders.)

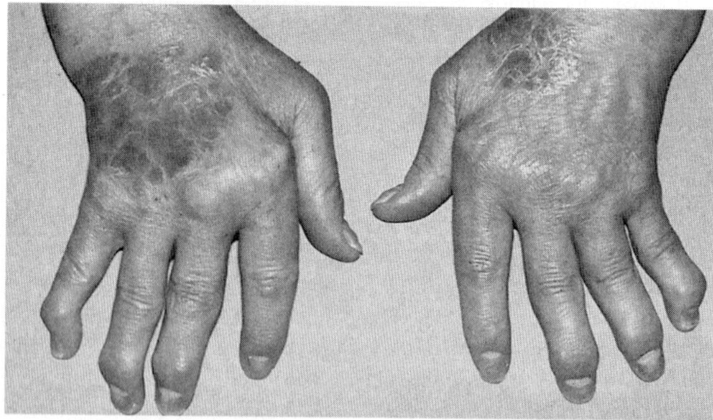

FIG. 3 The hands of a woman with symmetric polyarthritis. Initially this was indistinguishable from rheumatoid disease, but note the distal interphalangeal joint involvement, which is uncommon in rheumatoid arthritis, as well as the skin psoriasis. (From Klippel J, et al. [eds]: *Primary care rheumatology,* London, 1999, Mosby.)

- Severe digital erosive change with adjacent heterotopic bone formation may give rise to "pencil in cup" deformity. Can see whittling of the phalanges.
- With axial involvement can see sacroiliac joint changes (sclerosis, erosions, pseudowidening, ankylosis) and bridging vertebral syndesmophytes.
- Musculoskeletal ultrasonography can be used in the evaluation of enthesitis or arthritis.
- MRI may be helpful in further evaluation of sacroiliac and spinal involvement.

Rx TREATMENT

PHARMACOLOGIC THERAPY

The choice of therapeutic agent depends on the type of clinical manifestations, as not all agents are effective for all manifestations. For example, enthesis and spinal involvement are not responsive to traditional oral disease-modifying agents such as methotrexate or leflunomide but are responsive to tumor necrosis factor (TNF) blocking agents.

- NSAIDs may be used for mild or limited disease.
- Intra-articular corticosteroid injections can be used as adjunctive rx for involved joints.
- Oral glucocorticoids should generally be avoided, given increased risk for development of erythrodermic or pustular psoriasis.
- In patients with active peripheral joint disease, elevated acute phase reactants, or evidence of changes on imaging, traditional DMARDs such as methotrexate, sulfasalazine, and leflunomide should be considered early on, though data supporting their use is limited.
- Apremilast is an oral phosphodiesterase 4 (PDE 4) inhibitor, and is safe to use, especially in those with multiple comorbidities. Can also be beneficial for enthesitis and dactylitis.
- In patients with peripheral arthritis who fail to respond to traditional DMARDs, escalation of therapy should be considered. All five TNF inhibitors are FDA-approved to treat psoriatic arthritis (etanercept, infliximab, adalimumab, golimumab, certolizumab pegol). In those resistant to a TNFi, a second TNFi can be tried. If adequate response is still not achieved, a different mechanism of action such as IL-17 blockade can be tried.
- Secukinumab, an IL-17 inhibitor, is approved to treat psoriasis, PsA, and AS. Ixekizumab, an anti-IL-17 monoclonal antibody, can also be used to treat psoriasis and PsA. Brodalumab, an anti-IL17RA monoclonal antibody, treats psoriasis alone currently.
- Ustekinumab is a human IgG monoclonal antibody that binds to the p40 subunit of interleukin (IL)-12 and -23 and is approved to treat psoriasis, psoriatic arthritis, and Crohn.
- More recently abatacept (selective T-cell costimulation modulator) was approved to treat PsA, but has shown limited efficacy in treatment of psoriasis. Tofacitinib (oral Janus kinase inhibitor) has also been approved.
- In patients with predominantly axial disease not responsive to NSAIDs, TNFi or IL17i can be tried. For e• nthesitis/dactylitis TNFi, IL17i, IL12/23, and apremilast can be considered.

REFERRAL

Rheumatology, dermatology

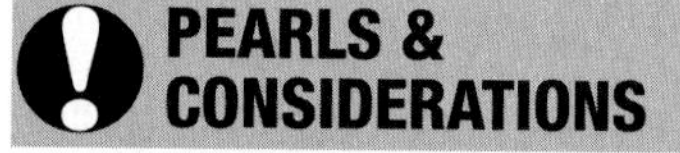

PEARLS & CONSIDERATIONS

- Patients frequently have a positive family history of psoriasis or psoriatic arthritis.
- Severity of skin psoriasis and activity of inflammatory arthritis can be discordant.

SUGGESTED READINGS

Available at ExpertConsult.com

RELATED CONTENT

Psoriatic Arthritis (Patient Information)

AUTHOR: **DAPHNE SCARAMANGAS-PLUMLEY, M.D.**

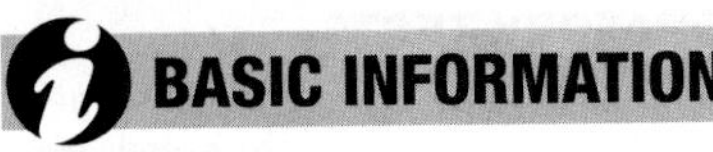

BASIC INFORMATION

DEFINITION

Psychosis is a state in which external reality is distorted by delusions and/or hallucinations (a delusion is a fixed false idiosyncratic belief; a hallucination is a false auditory, visual, olfactory, tactile, or taste perception).

Psychosis is a key finding in many mental illnesses, such as brief psychotic disorder, delusional disorder, schizoaffective disorder, schizophrenia, schizophreniform disorder, or shared psychotic disorder. Psychosis can also present as part of the evolution of a mood disorder (depression and bipolar disorder), a sign of an underlying medical condition, or a manifestation of a toxic state, i.e., abuse of substances or withdrawal state.

ICD-10CM CODES

F09	Unspecified organic or symptomatic mental disorder
F10.5	Psychotic disorder due to psychoactive substance use
F05	Delirium not induced by alcohol and other psychoactive substances
F06.0	Organic hallucinosis
F32.3	Major depressive disorder, single episode, severe with psychotic features
F30.2 and F31.2	Manic episode with psychosis and bipolar affective disorder with psychosis

DSM-5 CODES
Depends on specific diagnosis

EPIDEMIOLOGY & DEMOGRAPHICS

1-year prevalence: 4.5 per 1000. The (demographics of) psychosis depends on the underlying disorder.

PHYSICAL FINDINGS & CLINICAL PRESENTATION

History:

- Past and current medical history important to identify potential medical etiologies
- Medication use
- Use of illicit substances or alcohol
- Identification of functional and social impairment
- Behavior that is odd or unpredictable; patient may be acting based on misinterpretation of their reality or false perceptions (delusions or hallucinations)

Examination:

- Examine for symptoms of:
  1. Mood disorder: Delusions or hallucinations are usually congruent with the mood (e.g., auditory hallucinations in a depressed patient may tell the patient what a terrible person he is)
  2. Altered or disorganized thought pattern: Usually reflected in disorganized speech (including word salad, thought blocking, rhyming, clang associations) or disorganized behavior
  3. Lack of insight into problems
  4. Signs of Parkinson's disease, dementia

ETIOLOGY

- Involves an interaction among:
  1. Dopaminergic overactivity (particularly in the mesolimbic, nigrostriatal, and mesocortical systems)
  2. Environmental, social, or childhood factors
  3. Genetic predisposition

Dx DIAGNOSIS

WORKUP

- Evaluate for potential confounding factors
- Underlying mental disorder: Schizophrenia, major depression, brief psychotic disorder, delusional disorder, schizoaffective disorder, schizophreniform disorder
- Underlying personality disorder: Borderline, paranoid, schizoid, schizotypal
- Underlying medical conditions: Infections ranging from UTIs to HIV/AIDS, Parkinson's disease, Huntington disease, leprosy, malaria, sarcoidosis, systemic lupus erythematosus, prion disease, hypoglycemia, postpartum state, cerebrovascular event, temporal lobe epilepsy, brain neoplasm
- Medications: Systemic steroids, anticonvulsants, antiparkinsonian medications, some chemotherapy, scopolamine
- Underlying dementia: Alzheimer's disease, Lewy body dementia, vascular dementia
- Illicit drugs (usually with chronic use; can be caused by intoxication or withdrawal): LSD, PCP, cocaine, gamma-hydroxybutyrate (GHB; withdrawal), alcohol, amphetamines, and marijuana. New substances of abuse (e.g., "bath salts," synthetic cannabinoids) may not be detected by current toxicology panels
- Traumatic brain injury
- Intensive care unit stay: Hypoxia, decreased cardiac output, infection, medications, sleep deprivation, alteration of diurnal cycle, sensory deprivation or overload, pain
- Emotional stress

LABORATORY TESTS

Consider checking chemistry panel (calcium), complete blood count, UA, liver function tests, cortisol, HIV, rapid plasma reagin, thyroid-stimulating hormone, toxicology screen, lumbar puncture (LP).

IMAGING STUDIES

Consider chest x-ray (rule out sarcoid), electroencephalography, head CT or MRI

Rx TREATMENT

NONPHARMACOLOGIC THERAPY

- Cognitive-behavioral therapy.
- Social and behavioral skills training.
- Training for self-management of disease
- Aforementioned strategies favored over psychoanalytic techniques given the relative inability for abstract thought and lack of insight in psychotic patients
- Family intervention, including education and strategies to reduce emotional expression
- Counseling for substance abuse

ACUTE GENERAL Rx

- Antipsychotics (first or second generation equally effective but different in side effect profile) consider combining with anticholinergics like benztropine to reduce motor side effects if such arise; low doses should control first episode. Use with caution in elderly patients because adverse effects limit effectiveness. Second-generation antipsychotics are also useful starting with low doses. Alternative formulations are available; e.g., rapid injectable form or oral disintegrating tablets. Obtain baseline lab work including lipid profile, glucose/A1c, CBC.
- Benzodiazepines if agitation is severe.
- Discontinue offending medication if present.

CHRONIC Rx

Second-generation antipsychotics may reduce the incidence of tardive dyskinesia but may increase incidence of metabolic disorders compared with first-generation antipsychotics. Multicenter trials showed similar efficacy between first and second generation. Consider economic factors, including insurance formulary, when selecting a maintenance regimen.

DISPOSITION

Prognosis varies according to etiology of psychosis. In general, the more severe and longer the psychotic episode, the worse the prognosis.

REFERRAL

Patient should be admitted for acute stabilization if actively psychotic to prevent harm to self and others as well as ensure administration of medications.

PEARLS & CONSIDERATIONS

- Delusions and/or hallucinations are hallmarks of psychosis.
- Rule out medical or drug causes of psychosis.
- Antipsychotics are the mainstay of acute and chronic treatment.
- Consider alternatives to antipsychotics in elderly or intellectually disabled patients (see "Nonpharmacologic Therapy").

SUGGESTED READINGS

Available at ExpertConsult.com

RELATED CONTENT

Psychosis (Patient Information)
Delirium (Related Key Topic)

AUTHORS: **ARNALDO A. BERGES, M.D.,** and **RICHARD J. GOLDBERG, M.D., M.S.**

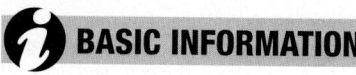

BASIC INFORMATION

DEFINITION

Acute cardiogenic pulmonary edema (ACPE) is a clinically observed consequence of increased capillary leakage of fluid into the interstitial space in the pulmonary vasculature, resulting in the constellation of clinical signs and symptoms of decreased gaseous exchange in the alveoli.

SYNONYMS

Cardiogenic pulmonary edema (CPE)
Acute cardiogenic pulmonary edema (ACPE)
Acute decompensated heart failure (ADHF) with pulmonary edema
Acute diastolic heart failure with pulmonary edema
Acute systolic heart failure with pulmonary edema

ICD-10CM CODES

I50.1	Left ventricular failure
J68.1	Pulmonary edema due to chemicals, gases, fumes and vapors
J81.0	Acute pulmonary edema
J81.1	Chronic pulmonary edema

EPIDEMIOLOGY & DEMOGRAPHICS

- The prevalence of heart failure (HF) is estimated around 6.5 million people and is expected to increase to 8 million by the year 2030.
- In 2012, 1.7 million HF-related visits to the U.S. physician offices, and half a million emergency department visits were reported.
- Within 30 days, 25% to 30% of these patients are readmitted with recurrent ADHF.
- In-hospital mortality rate is 10% to 20%, particularly when associated with acute MI.

CLINICAL PRESENTATION

- Altered mental status
- Dyspnea (exertional or at rest, paroxysmal nocturnal dyspnea, orthopnea)
- Cough and wheezing (cardiac asthma)
- Diaphoresis, cold and clammy skin
- Perioral and peripheral cyanosis
- Pink, frothy sputum

PHYSICAL EXAMINATION FINDINGS

- Hypertension (in cardiogenic shock could be hypotensive)
- Tachycardia
- Elevated jugular venous pressure with hepatojugular reflex
- Bilateral pulmonary rales/decreased or absent air entry
- S3 gallop/S4 and or laterally displaced apex
- Abdominal distention/ascites
- Peripheral edema
- Weight gain

ETIOLOGY

Common causes of acute pulmonary edema include the following:

- Acute myocardial infarction
- Poor dietary compliance or medication nonadherence
- Atrial and ventricular arrhythmias
- Valvular heart disease (mitral, aortic, tricuspid, and pulmonary valve disease)
- Renal and liver disease
- Endocrine (thyrotoxicosis, obesity, metabolic syndrome, diabetes)
- Toxin mediated (cocaine, alcohol, chemotherapy agents, ephedra)
- Peripartum cardiomyopathy/heart failure of pregnancy
- Infections (myopericarditis, endocarditis, HIV, Chagas)
- Uncontrolled hypertension
- Structural heart disease (ventricular septal defect, infiltrative heart disease, hypertrophic cardiomyopathy)
- Pulmonary embolism
- Box 1 summarizes common causes of cardiogenic and noncardiogenic pulmonary edema

Dx DIAGNOSIS

DIFFERENTIAL DIAGNOSIS

- Noncardiogenic pulmonary edema (see Fig. E1 and Table 1)
- Viral pneumonitis and other pulmonary infections
- Pulmonary embolism
- Exacerbation of asthma/chronic obstructive pulmonary disease
- High altitude pulmonary edema (HAPE)
- Sarcoidosis
- Pulmonary fibrosis
- Lymphangitic carcinomatosis

BOX 1 Common Causes of Cardiogenic and Noncardiogenic Pulmonary Edema

Cardiogenic Pulmonary Edema
- Acute exacerbation of heart failure
- Acute valve dysfunction (e.g., mitral valve chordae tendineae rupture)
- Arrhythmia/myocardial infarction
- Hypertensive crisis
- Fluid overload following aggressive volume resuscitation (e.g., postoperative)
- Ventricular septal rupture
- Pericardial tamponade

Noncardiogenic Pulmonary Edema
- Direct lung injury
  - Pneumonia
  - Gastric aspiration
  - Toxic inhalation
  - Negative pressure related (e.g., strangulation)
- Indirect causes of lung injury
  - Sepsis
  - Trauma
  - Pancreatitis
  - Multiple blood transfusions
  - Burn injury

From Vincent JL et al: *Textbook of critical care*, ed 7, Philadelphia, 2017, Elsevier.

LABORATORY TESTS

- Arterial blood gases (ABGs): Respiratory and metabolic acidosis, decreased Pa_{O_2}, increased Pa_{CO_2}, low pH. (NOTE: The patient may initially show respiratory alkalosis as a result of hyperventilation in attempts to maintain Pa_{O_2}.)
- BNP and NT-pro BNP add diagnostic value to the history and physical examination as evidenced in the Breathing Not Properly (BNP) study.
- Cardiac biomarkers: Troponin T or I if suspicion for acute coronary syndrome.
- Basic metabolic profile: Assess for electrolyte abnormalities; renal failure can dictate diuretic choice.
- Complete blood count: Anemia can trigger acute pulmonary edema.
- Glucose, Hb A1C, fasting lipid profile, TSH for risk stratification.
- Urinalysis and urine toxicology if indicated.

IMAGING STUDIES

- ECG: May elucidate the specific cause of the pulmonary edema. Causes may include ischemia/infarct, arrhythmias, LV hypertrophy, atrial enlargement.
- Chest x-ray (Fig. 2):
  1. Bilateral interstitial and alveolar infiltrates.
  2. Cephalization of the pulmonary vessels.
  3. Kerley B lines; fluffy perihilar infiltrates.
  4. Pleural effusions.
  5. Enlarged cardiac silhouette.
- Echocardiogram:
  1. Assess left and right ventricular systolic/diastolic function.
  2. Structural abnormalities (VSD, LV rupture).
  3. Evaluate valvular abnormalities.
  4. Engorged inferior vena cava (IVC) and IVC plethora, based on bedside ultrasound, suggests elevated filling pressures.
- Computed tomography of the chest; sometimes this is required to differentiate between cardiogenic and noncardiogenic pulmonary edema.
- Right heart catheterization (RHC): Is useful for diagnosis (differentiate between different causes of shock) and to guide tailored therapy (inotrope and pressor infusion) in cardiogenic shock. In cardiogenic shock, pulmonary artery diastolic pressure and pulmonary capillary wedge pressure are elevated. In patients with acute decompensated heart failure, pulmonary artery catheters failed to demonstrate survival benefit but rather caused adverse events in the ESCAPE Trial.

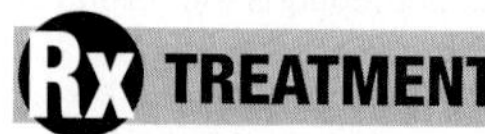

Rx TREATMENT

ACUTE GENERAL Rx (FIG. 3)

Nonpharmacologic treatment:

- Heart failure teaching.
- Sodium restriction. Restriction in patients with ACC/AHA class C and D heart failure is controversial with conflicting data.
- Fluid restriction (1.5 to 2 L), especially in patients with hyponatremia.

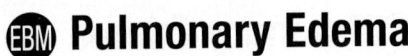

TABLE 1 Distinguishing Cardiogenic and Noncardiogenic Pulmonary Edema

	History	Exam	Labs	Imaging	Pulmonary Artery Catheter
Cardiogenic	Heart disease Renal disease Uncontrolled HTN Edema Orthopnea Recent administration of IV fluids or blood products	Heart failure exam findings: Distended neck veins S3 heart sound Dependent edema Elevated blood pressure Cool extremities	*↑BNP >1200 pg/ml ↑Creatinine (in setting of volume overload) †↑Troponin	CXR: CMG Pleural effusions ‡Kerley B lines TEE: ↓LVEF Diastolic filling defect Severe mitral or aortic valvular disease Pericardial effusion with tamponade VSD	PCWP >18 mm Hg Prominent V-waves (mitral regurgitation) Elevation and equilibration of right atrial pressure, pulmonary artery diastolic and PCWP (tamponade physiology) CVP >12 mm Hg
Noncardiogenic	Sepsis Aspiration event Trauma (long bone fractures) Burn injury Pancreatitis Multiple transfusions	Signs of active infection Extensive burn injury Evidence of trauma (absence of heart failure exam findings)	↑WBC *BNP <200 pg/ml	CXR: Diffuse central and peripheral infiltrates Normal heart size No or minimal pleural effusions TEE: Normal LV and valvular function No evidence of volume overload	PCWP <18 mm Hg CVP <12 mm Hg

BNP, Brain natriuretic peptide; *CVP*, central venous pressure; *CXR*, chest x-ray; *HTN*, hypertension; *IV*, intravenous; *LVEF*, left ventricle ejection fraction; *PCWP*, pulmonary capillary wedge pressure; *S3*, third heart sound; *TEE*, transesophageal echocardiogram; *VSD*, ventricular septal defect; *WBC*, white blood count.
From Vincent JL et al: *Textbook of critical care*, ed 7, Philadelphia, 2017, Elsevier.

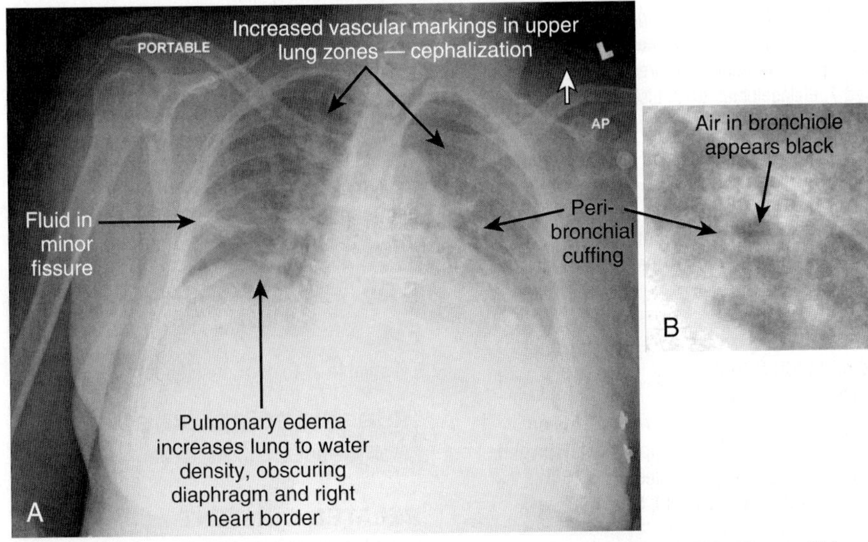

FIG. 2 Pulmonary edema. A, Anterior-posterior chest x-ray. **B,** Close-up from **A.** This 53-year-old female with end-stage renal disease missed dialysis and presented to the emergency department. Her examination demonstrated bilateral rales. Her x-ray shows mild cardiomegaly, bilateral interstitial opacities, and cephalization of the pulmonary vascular markings. The minor fissure appears thickened. These findings are consistent with pulmonary edema. In addition, peribronchial cuffing is present. As discussed elsewhere, this is a nonspecific thickening of the bronchial wall that can occur from edema in the setting of heart failure, asthma, viral illness, or even infections such as pertussis. The thickened wall appears white, whereas the air-filled bronchiole appears black and has a circular short-axis cross section. (From Broder JS: *Diagnostic imaging for the emergency physician,* Philadelphia, 2011, Saunders.)

- Risk factor modification (blood pressure control).
- Oxygen supplementation if signs of hypoxia.
- Noninvasive ventilation (continuous positive airway pressure [CPAP]) or bilevel noninvasive positive-pressure ventilation [NPPV]) reduces dyspnea and may reduce the need for endotracheal intubation. They improve oxygenation and lower carbon dioxide. Positive pressure ventilation (invasive or noninvasive) decreases preload and afterload and reduces the work of breathing, while positive end expiratory pressure improves oxygenation.

Pharmacologic-preload and afterload reducers:

- Loop diuretics are the cornerstone of the treatment of volume overload. Furosemide, torsemide, or bumetanid are initiated at a low dose and then increased to achieve desired urine output. There is no difference in symptoms or kidney function whether the diuretic is given as a bolus versus continuous infusion (DOSE trial; NEJM March 3, 2011).
- Nitrates: Particularly useful if the patient has concomitant chest pain or is hypertensive.
  1. Nitroglycerin: 0.4 to 0.8 mg SL or nitroglycerin spray may be given immediately on arrival and repeated every 5 min up to three times if the patient remains symptomatic and blood pressure remains stable.
  2. 2% nitroglycerin ointment: 1 to 3 inches out of the tube applied continuously; absorption may be erratic.
  3. IV nitroglycerin for refractory chest pain or and hypertension: Start at 0.2 to 0.4 mcg/kg/min.
- Nitroprusside is useful for afterload reduction in severe hypertension, acute mitral regurgitation, or acute aortic regurgitation.
  1. Start at low-dose 0.5 μg/kg/min with an arterial line in place.
  2. Monitor for cyanide toxicity.
- ACE inhibitors, angiotensin II receptor blockers, aldosterone antagonist, and sacubitril-valsartan are vasodilators with long-term mortality benefit in patients with heart failure with reduced ejection fraction.
- Ultrafiltration/aquapheresis if diuretic resistant.

Pharmacologic-vasopressors:

- Patients with profound hypotension benefit from vasopressors.
  1. Norepinephrine: It is a powerful vasoconstrictor with small inotropic effect.
  2. Dopamine: Low doses (0.5 to 3 μg/kg/min) increase blood flow to coronary, renal, and cerebral beds. Intermediate doses (3 to 10 μg/kg/min) increase cardiac contractility. High doses (10 to 20 μg/kg/min) have a pressor effect. However, in clinical trials, low-dose dopamine failed to demonstrate improved diuresis or renal function when added to a diuretic and was associated with more arrhythmias in cardiogenic shock patients. It should be used only in rare circumstances of diuretic-resistant patients under the care of a cardiologist.

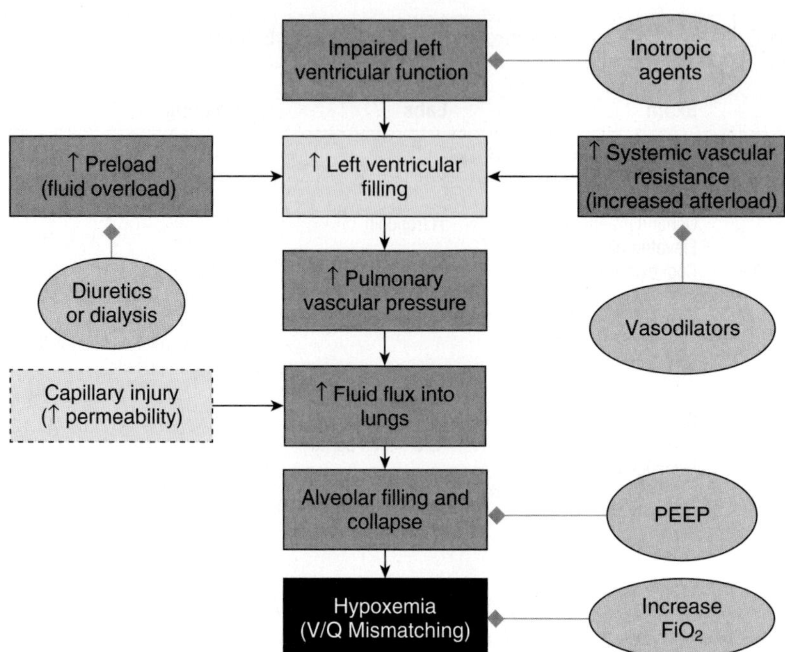

FIG. 3 Acute management of pulmonary edema. This schematic represents basic mechanisms distinguishing cardiogenic and noncardiogenic pulmonary edema and the contributing factors *(blue boxes)* that ultimately lead to impaired gas exchange *(black box)*. The *green circles* represent treatments that are available in the intensive care unit setting to reduce pulmonary edema or to mitigate its adverse consequences. *FiO_2*, fraction of inspired oxygen; *PEEP*, post end-expiratory pressure; *V/Q*, ventilation/perfusion. (From Vincent JL et al: *Textbook of critical care*, ed 7, Philadelphia, 2017, Elsevier.)

Pharmacologic-inotropes:

- Dobutamine: Potent inotrope, mild chronotropic effects. Dose ranges from 2.5 to 20 mcg/kg/min.
- Phosphodiesterase inhibitors (amrinone, milrinone, and enoximone [not available in U.S.]) may be useful in refractory cases. Milrinone may be associated with increased hypotension and new atrial arrhythmias with increased mortality in patients with ischemia.

Mechanical support:

- Intraaortic balloon pump (IABP): Decreases afterload, increases coronary blood flow. The IABP-SHOCK II trial failed to demonstrate reduction in all-cause mortality in patients with cardiogenic shock.
- Impella: Axial-flow pump on a pigtail catheter that crosses the aortic valve and unloads the left ventricle. Compared with the IABP, it is associated with improvement in hemodynamics.
- Tandem heart device: Oxygenated blood is pumped from the left atrium into the femoral artery. It can provide 3.5 to 4.5 L/min of cardiac output.
- Extracorporeal membrane oxygenation (ECMO): Destination therapy or bridge to transplant.

DISPOSITION

Admit to ICU/CCU if:

- Need for intubation.
- Signs and symptoms of hypoperfusion.
- SpO_2 <90% despite supplemental oxygen.
- Use of accessory muscles/RR >25/min.
- Heart rate <40 or >130, SBP <90.

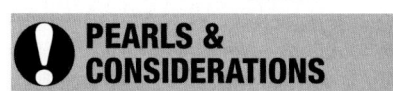

PEARLS & CONSIDERATIONS

COMMENTS

Accumulated evidence still favors the use of noninvasive ventilation, especially CPAP, in patients with ACPE, especially as this therapy reduces dyspnea and helps correct metabolic abnormalities more rapidly than standard oxygen therapy. The role of morphine in the treatment of ACPE has come into question.

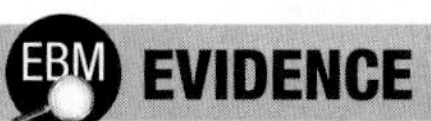

EVIDENCE

Available at ExpertConsult.com

SUGGESTED READINGS

Available at ExpertConsult.com

RELATED CONTENT

Heart Failure (Related Key Topic)

AUTHORS: **MAXWELL EYRAM AFARI, M.D.,** and **GEMINI YESODHARAN, M.D.**

BASIC INFORMATION

DEFINITION

Pulmonary embolism (PE) refers to the lodging of a thrombus or other embolic material from a distant site in the pulmonary circulation. A classification of acute pulmonary embolism is described in Table 1.

SYNONYMS

Pulmonary thromboembolism
PE

ICD-10CM CODES

I26	Pulmonary embolism
I26.01	Septic pulmonary embolism with acute cor pulmonale
126.09	Other pulmonary embolism with acute cor pulmonale
126.90	Septic pulmonary embolism without acute cor pulmonale
126.99	Other pulmonary embolism without acute cor pulmonale
127.82	Chronic pulmonary embolism
Z86.711	Personal history of pulmonary embolism

EPIDEMIOLOGY & DEMOGRAPHICS

- 650,000 cases of PE occur in the U.S. each year (increased incidence in women and with advanced age); annually, as many as 100,000 people in the U.S. die from acute PE, and the diagnosis is often not made until after autopsy. The incidence of PE is increasing with the increasing use of spiral CT scans, with a lower severity of illness and lower mortality, suggesting the increase is caused by earlier diagnosis.
- More than 90% of pulmonary emboli originate in the deep venous system of the lower extremities.
- Pulmonary thromboembolism is associated with >200,000 hospitalizations. 8% to 10% of victims of PE die within the first hour.

PHYSICAL FINDINGS & CLINICAL PRESENTATION

- Most common symptom: Dyspnea (82% to 85%)
- Tachypnea (30% to 60%)
- Cough (30% to 40%)
- Wheezing (20%)
- Chest pain: May be nonpleuritic or pleuritic (infarction) (40% to 49%)
- Syncope (massive PE) (10% to 14%)
- Fever, diaphoresis, apprehension
- Hemoptysis (2%)
- Evidence of DVT may be present (e.g., swelling and tenderness of extremities)
- Cardiac examination may reveal: Tachycardia (23%), increased pulmonic component of S2, murmur of tricuspid insufficiency, right ventricular heave, right-sided S3
- Pulmonary examination: May demonstrate rales, localized wheezing, friction rub

ETIOLOGY

- Thrombus, fat, or other foreign material
- Risk factors for PE:
    1. Prolonged immobilization, reduced mobility
    2. Postoperative state, major surgery
    3. Trauma to lower extremities, immobilizer, or cast
    4. Estrogen-containing birth control pills, hormone replacement therapy
    5. Prior history of DVT or PE
    6. CHF
    7. Pregnancy and early puerperium
    8. Visceral cancer (lung, pancreas, alimentary and genitourinary tracts)
    9. Spinal cord injury
    10. Advanced age
    11. Obesity
    12. Hematologic disease (e.g., factor V Leiden mutation, antithrombin III deficiency, protein C deficiency, protein S deficiency, lupus anticoagulant, polycythemia vera, dysfibrinogenemia, paroxysmal nocturnal hemoglobinuria, acquired protein C resistance without factor V Leiden, G20210A prothrombin mutation)
    13. COPD, diabetes mellitus, acute medical illness
    14. Prolonged air travel
    15. Central venous catheterization
    16. Autoimmune diseases (SLE, IBD, RA)

TABLE 1 Classification of Acute Pulmonary Embolism

Category (Frequency)	Presentation	Therapy
Massive PE (5%-10%)	Systolic blood pressure <90 mm Hg or poor tissue perfusion or multisystem organ failure plus extensive thrombosis, such as "saddle" PE or right or left main pulmonary artery thrombus	Anticoagulation (usually starting with intravenous UFH), plus consider advanced therapy: Systemic thrombolysis, pharmacomechanical catheter-directed therapy, surgical embolectomy, or inferior vena cava (IVC) filter.
Submassive PE (20%-25%)	Hemodynamically stable but moderate or severe right ventricular dysfunction or enlargement, coupled with biomarker elevation indicative of right ventricular microinfarction and/or right ventricular pressure overload	Anticoagulation usually with intravenous UFH until decision made regarding implementation of advanced therapy; controversy centers on this group. For systemic thrombolysis, reducing the rate of cardiovascular collapse and death must be balanced against the increased rate of hemorrhagic stroke. For patients at low bleeding risk with severe right ventricular dysfunction, consider same interventions as for massive PE.
Small to moderate PE (70%)	Normal hemodynamics and normal right ventricular size and function	Anticoagulation with parenteral therapy as a bridge to warfarin or, alternatively, with oral rivaroxaban regimen as monotherapy.

PE, Pulmonary embolism; *UFH,* unfractionated heparin.
From Mann DL, et al.: *Braunwald's heart disease,* ed 10, Philadelphia, 2015. Elsevier.

DIAGNOSIS

DIFFERENTIAL DIAGNOSIS

- Myocardial infarction
- Pericarditis
- Pneumonia
- Pneumothorax
- Chest wall pain
- GI abnormalities (e.g., peptic ulcer, esophageal rupture, gastritis)
- CHF
- Pleuritis
- Anxiety disorder with hyperventilation
- Pericardial tamponade
- Dissection of aorta
- Asthma

WORKUP

- Recent guidelines from the Clinical Guidelines Committee of the American College of Physicians for the Evaluation of Patients with Suspected Acute Pulmonary Embolism recommend the following:[1]
    1. Use of validated clinical prediction rules to estimate pretest probability in patients in whom acute PG is being considered.
    2. Not obtaining a D-dimer measurement or imaging studies in patients with low pretest probability of PE and who meet all pulmonary embolism rule-out criteria.
    3. Obtaining a high-sensitivity D-dimer measurement as the initial diagnostic test in patients who have an intermediate pretest probability of PE or in patients with low pretest probability of PE who do not meet all pulmonary embolism rule-out criteria. Clinicians should not use imaging studies as the initial test in patients who have a low or intermediate pretest probability of PE.
    4. Use age-adjusted D-dimer thresholds (age × 10 ng/ml rather than a generic 500 ng/ml) in patients older than 50 yr to determine whether imaging is warranted.
    5. Clinicians should not obtain any imaging studies in patients with a D-dimer level below the age-adjusted cutoff.

[1] Raja AS, et al.: Evaluation of patients with suspected acute pulmonary embolism: best practice advice from the Clinical Guidelines Committee of the American College of Physicians, *Ann Intern Med* 163:701-711, 2015.

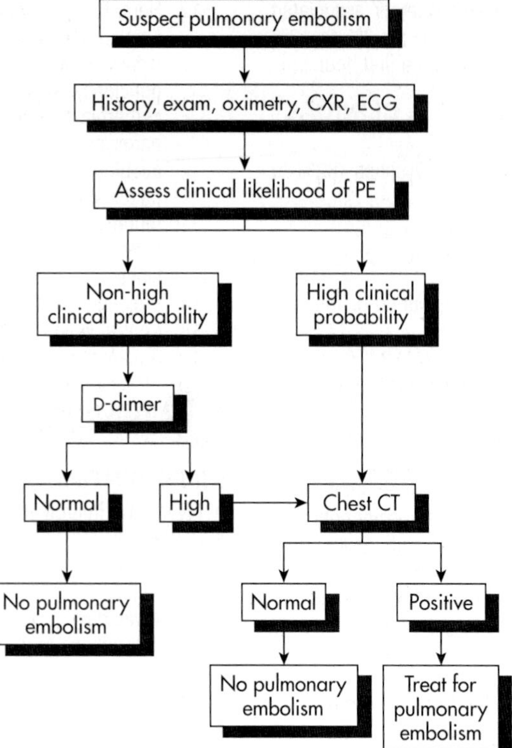

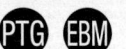

FIG. 1 Integrated diagnostic approach. *CT,* Computed tomography; *CXR,* chest x-ray [examination]; *ECG,* electrocardiogram; *PE,* pulmonary embolism. (From Mann DL, et al.: *Braunwald's heart disease*, ed 10, Philadelphia, 2015. Elsevier.)

TABLE 2 Wells Score for Pulmonary Embolism*

Characteristic	Points
Risk Factors	
Previous pulmonary embolism or deep venous thrombosis	1.5
Immobilization or surgery in the previous 4 wk	1.5
Cancer	1
Clinical Findings	
Hemoptysis	1
Heart rate >100/min	1.5
Clinical signs of deep venous thrombosis	3
Other	
Alternative diagnosis is less likely than pulmonary embolism	3

Interpretation of total score: 0-1 point, low probability; 2-6 points, moderate probability; 7 or more points, high probability.

*Wells PS, et al.: Derivation of a simple clinical model to categorize patients probability of pulmonary embolism: increasing the models utility with the SimpliRED D-dimer, *Thromb Haemost* 83:416–420, 2000.

From McGee S: *Evidence-based physical diagnosis*, ed 4, Philadelphia, 2018, Elsevier.

TABLE 3 Revised Geneva Score for Pulmonary Embolism*

Characteristic	Points
Risk Factors	
Age >65 yr	1
Previous pulmonary embolism or deep venous thrombosis	3
Surgery (under general anesthesia) or fracture (of lower limbs) within 1 mo	2
Cancer (active or considered cured <1 yr)	2
Clinical Findings	
Unilateral leg pain	3
Hemoptysis	2
Heart Rate	
75-94 beats/min	3
≥95 beats/min	5
Pain on palpation of lower-limb deep veins and unilateral edema	4

Interpretation of total score: 0-3 points, low probability; 4-10 points, moderate probability; ≥11 points, high probability.

*Le Gal G, et al.: Prediction of pulmonary embolism in the emergency department: the revised Geneva score, *Ann Intern Med* 144:165–171, 2006.

From McGee S: *Evidence-based physical diagnosis*, ed 4, Philadelphia, 2018, Elsevier.

6. CTPA should be obtained in patients with high pretest probability of PE. Ventilation-perfusion scans should be reserved for patients who have a contraindication to CTPA or if CTPA is not available.
7. A D-dimer measurement should not be obtained in patients with a high pretest probability of PE.

- Clinical assessment alone is insufficient to diagnose or rule out PE. It is also important to remember that no single noninvasive test has both high sensitivity and high specificity for PE. Consequently, in addition to clinical assessment, most patients require an imaging test to diagnose PE. An integrated diagnostic approach to PE is illustrated in Fig. 1. The Wells prediction rules (Table 2) and the revised Geneva score (Table 3) can be used to estimate the probability of PE. In the Wells prediction rules, each of the following findings is assigned a score:
  1. Clinical signs/symptoms of deep vein thrombosis (score = 3.0).
  2. No alternate diagnosis as likely or more likely than PE (score = 3.0).
  3. Heart rate >100/min (score = 1.5).
  4. Immobilization or surgery in last 4 weeks (score = 1.5).
  5. Previous history of DVT or PE (score = 1.5).
  6. Hemoptysis (score = 1.0).
  7. Cancer actively treated within last 6 months (score = 1.0).
- The probability of PE is high if total score is >6, moderate if 2-6; and low if <2.
- The modified Wells score divides PE as likely (>4 points) or unlikely (<4 points).
- A low clinical probability of PE in association with a normal plasma D-dimer measurement essentially rules out PE, and further imaging is not needed. If clinical probability is intermediate or high, and/or the D-dimer measurement is abnormal, further workup with imaging is needed.
- CT pulmonary angiography (CTPA) (see Fig. 2) is an excellent diagnostic modality (83% sensitivity and 96% specificity).
- V/Q scan is reserved for patients with clinically significant contrast allergies or renal insufficiency, or when CTPA is not available.
- Pulmonary angiogram (gold standard) can confirm the diagnosis in equivocal cases, but is rarely used.
- Serial compressive duplex ultrasonography of lower extremities can be used in patients with "low-probability" lung scan and high clinical suspicion (see "Imaging Studies"). It is useful if positive; negative results do not exclude PE.

LABORATORY TESTS

- ABGs may reveal hypoxemia and respiratory alkalosis (decreased Pa_{O_2} and Pa_{CO_2} and increased pH); normal results do not rule out PE.
- Alveolar-arteriolar (A-a) oxygen gradient, a measure of the difference in oxygen concentration between alveoli and arterial blood, may be elevated. However, a normal A-a gradient does not rule out PE.
- High-sensitivity plasma D-dimer measurement: D-dimer assays by ELISA detect the presence of plasmin-mediated degradation products of fibrin that contain cross-linked D fragments in the whole blood or plasma. A normal plasma D-dimer level is useful to exclude PE in patients with a low pretest probability of PE. However, it cannot be used to "rule in" the diagnosis because it increases with many other disorders (e.g., metastatic cancer, trauma, sepsis, postoperative state). Plasma D-dimer can also be used in conjunction with lower-extremity compression ultrasonography in patients with indeterminate V/Q and spiral CT scans. Absence of DVT and presence of a normal D-dimer level

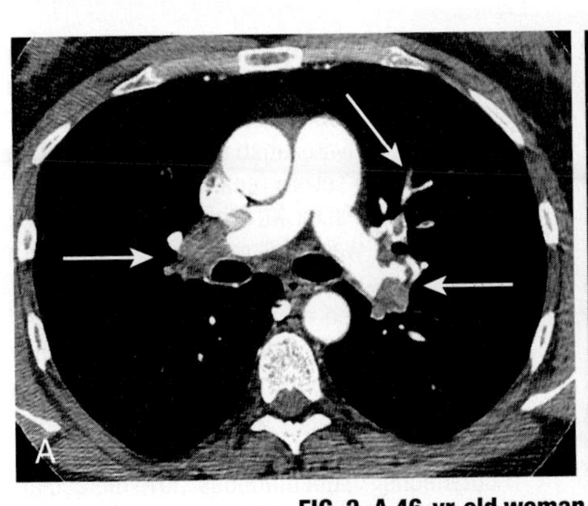

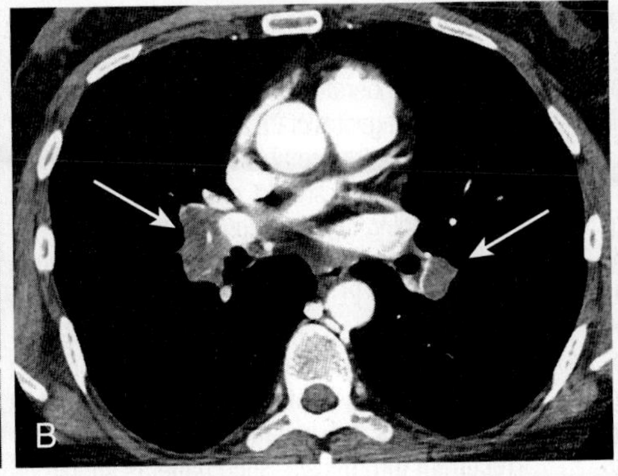

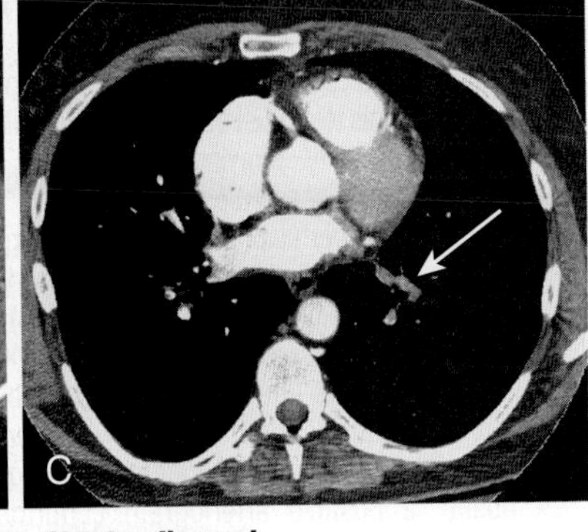

FIG. 2 A 46-yr-old woman presented with acute shortness of breath and hypoxia. Chest radiograph was normal. A, Chest computed tomography shows a low-attenuation filling defect in left and right main pulmonary arteries *(arrows)* and left upper lobe segmental artery *(arrow)*, representing massive pulmonary embolism. Emboli extend to left and right interlobar arteries *(arrows)*, as well as a left lower lobe segmental artery *(arrow)*, seen in **B** and **C,** respectively. (From Vincent JL, et al.: *Textbook of critical care*, ed 6, Philadelphia, 2011, Saunders.)

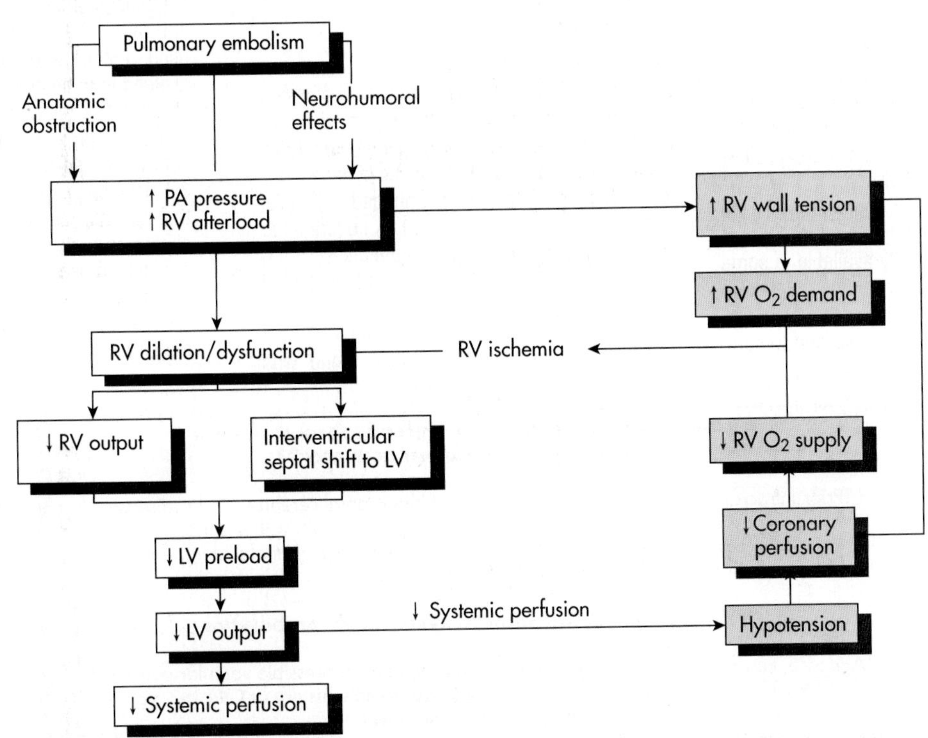

FIG. 3 Pathophysiology of right ventricular dysfunction and its deleterious effects of causing decreased systemic arterial pressure, decreased coronary perfusion, and deteriorating ventricular function. *LV,* Left ventricle/ventricular; *PA,* pulmonary artery; *RV,* right ventricle/ventricular. (From Mann DL, et al.: *Braunwald's heart disease*, ed 10, Philadelphia, 2015. Elsevier.)

in these settings generally rules out clinically significant PE.

- Elevated cardiac troponin levels also occur in patients with PE because of right ventricular dilation and myocardial injury; therefore, PE should be considered in the differential diagnosis of all patients presenting with chest pain or dyspnea and elevated cardiac troponin levels.
- Elevated serum BNP levels in patients with acute PE may reflect RV overload. The pathophysiology of RV dysfunction in PE is illustrated in Fig. 3.
- ECG is abnormal in 85% of patients with acute PE. Frequent abnormalities are sinus tachycardia; nonspecific ST-segment or T-wave changes; S-1, Q-3, T-3 pattern (10% of patients); S-1, S-2, S-3 pattern; T-wave inversion in V_1 to V_6; acute RBBB; new-onset atrial fibrillation; ST segment depression in lead II; right ventricular strain. A right ventricular strain pattern on ECG in patients with PE and normal blood pressure is associated with adverse short-term outcome and adds incremental prognostic value to echocardiographic evidence of right ventricular function.

IMAGING STUDIES

- Chest x-ray may be normal; suggestive findings include elevated diaphragm, pleural effusion, dilation of pulmonary artery, infiltrate or consolidation, abrupt vessel cut-off, oligemia distal to the PE (*Westermark sign*), or atelectasis. A wedge-shaped consolidation in the middle and lower lobes is suggestive of a pulmonary infarction and is known as *Hampton's hump*.
- CT angiography is an accurate, noninvasive tool in the diagnosis of PE at the main, lobar, and segmental pulmonary artery levels. A major advantage of CT angiography over standard pulmonary angiography is its ability to diagnose intrathoracic disease other than PE that may account for the patient's clinical picture. It is also less invasive, less costly, and

more widely available. Its major shortcoming is its poor sensitivity for subsegmental emboli.

- V/Q Lung scan (in patient with normal chest x-ray examination): This test must be interpreted within the pretest probability of having a PE.
  1. A normal lung scan rules out PE.
  2. A ventilation-perfusion mismatch is suggestive of PE, and a lung scan interpretation of high probability is confirmatory (Fig. E4).
  3. If the clinical suspicion of PE is high and the lung scan is interpreted as low probability, moderate probability, or indeterminate, a pulmonary arteriogram is diagnostic; a positive arteriogram confirms diagnosis; a positive compressive duplex ultrasonography for DVT obviates the need for an arteriogram, because treatment with IV anticoagulants is indicated in these patients; the overall sensitivity of compressive ultrasonography for DVT in patients with PE is 29%, specificity 97%; adding ultrasonography in patients with a nondiagnostic lung scan prevents 9% of angiographies; however, this improvement in efficacy is achieved at the cost of unnecessary anticoagulant therapy in 26% of patients who have false-positive ultrasonography results.
- Angiography: Pulmonary angiography is the historic gold standard; however, it is invasive, expensive, and not readily available in some clinical settings. False-positive pulmonary angiograms may result from mediastinal disorders such as radiation fibrosis and tumors.
- Gadolinium-enhanced magnetic resonance angiography (MRA/MRV) of the pulmonary arteries has a moderate sensitivity and high specificity for the diagnosis of PE at experienced centers, but obtaining acceptable images is technically challenging and should only be performed if other imaging tests are contraindicated.
- Echocardiography: Useful for identifying patients with PE who may have poor prognosis. Moderate or severe hypokinesis, persistent pulmonary hypertension, patent foramen ovale, and free-floating right heart thrombus are markers for increased risk of death or recurrent thrombosis. Such patients should be considered for thrombolysis or embolectomy.

Rx TREATMENT

NONPHARMACOLOGIC THERAPY

Correction of risk factors (see "Etiology") to prevent future PE.

ACUTE GENERAL Rx

Patients with acute PE should be initially stratified according to risk (Table 1) so that higher-risk therapies (e.g., thrombolysis, embolectomy) are offered to patients with the greatest chance of benefit.

- Anticoagulants are recommended as initial therapy in patients with small to moderate PE.
- Oral rivaroxaban, a factor Xa inhibitor (15 mg bid for 3 wk, then 20 mg/d), has been studied as a treatment for DVT and for PE, without prior parenteral therapy. For both DVT and PE, treatment with rivaroxaban alone was noninferior to treatment with LMWH followed by a vitamin K antagonist with regard to the endpoint of recurrent venous thromboembolism. Use of rivaroxaban should be avoided in patients with severe renal failure.
- Apixaban, a Factor Xa inhibitor (10 mg twice a day for a week, followed by 5 mg twice a day), is also approved for the treatment of acute PE based on the data in the AMPLIFY and AMPLIFY-EXT trials, in which apixaban met its noninferiority mark in terms of efficacy and improved safety compared to warfarin.
- Unfractionated heparin (UFH) (IV or subcutaneous), subcutaneous low-molecular-weight heparin (LMWH), or subcutaneous fondaparinux can be used for the initial treatment for at least 5 days when used with warfarin or dabigatran. If IV unfractionated heparin is used, a bolus dose (80 U/kg) followed by a weight-based (18 U/kg/hr) continuous infusion to achieve therapeutic anti-factor Xa (or aPTT) levels should be used. LMWH and fondaparinux should be avoided in patients with severe renal failure.
- Thrombolytic agents (urokinase, tPA, streptokinase): Provide rapid resolution of clots with increased risk of major bleeding (up to 3% incidence of intracranial hemorrhage); thrombolytic agents are the treatment of choice in patients with massive PE who are hemodynamically unstable and with no contraindication to their use. Fig. 5 illustrates the approach to "high-risk" submassive pulmonary embolus with right ventricular injury.

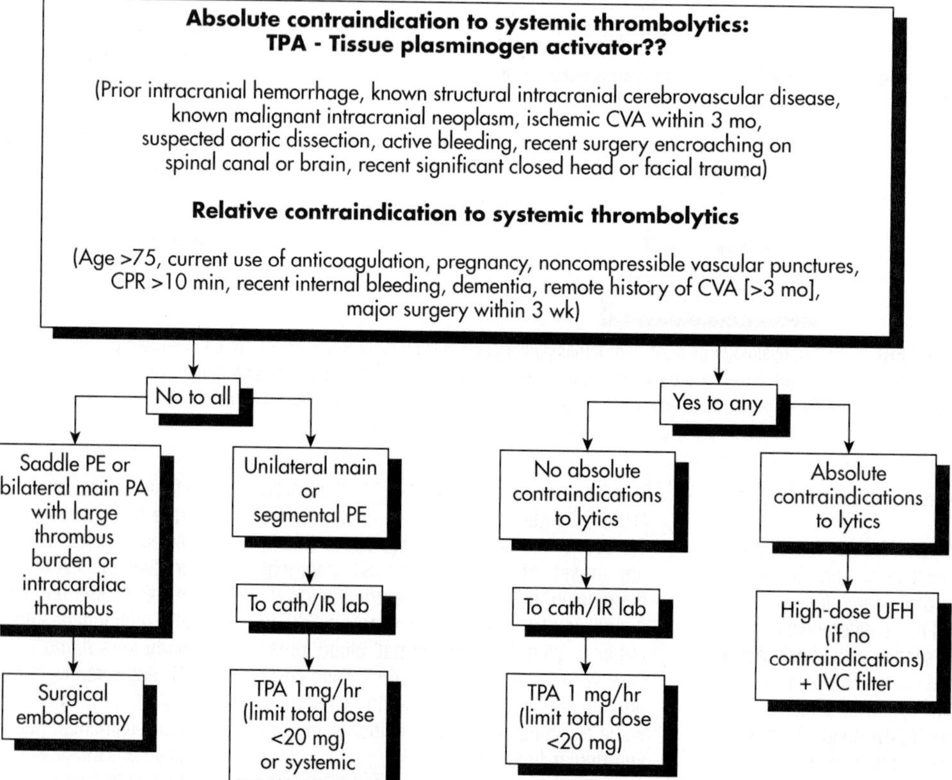

FIG. 5 "High-risk" submassive pulmonary embolus with right ventricular injury algorithm. *CPR,* Cardiopulmonary resuscitation; *CVA,* cerebrovascular accident; *IR,* interventional radiology; *IVC,* intravenous cholangiography; *PA,* pulmonary artery; *PE,* pulmonary embolism; *UFH,* unfractionated heparin. (From Parrillo JE, Dellinger RP: *Critical care medicine, principles of diagnosis and management in the adult,* ed 4, Philadelphia, 2014, Elsevier.)

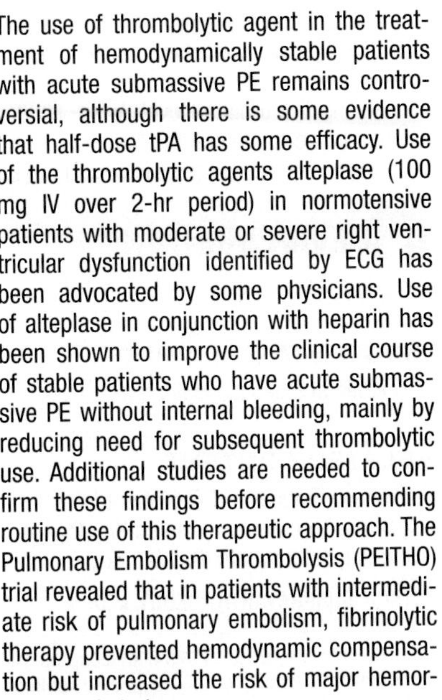

The use of thrombolytic agent in the treatment of hemodynamically stable patients with acute submassive PE remains controversial, although there is some evidence that half-dose tPA has some efficacy. Use of the thrombolytic agents alteplase (100 mg IV over 2-hr period) in normotensive patients with moderate or severe right ventricular dysfunction identified by ECG has been advocated by some physicians. Use of alteplase in conjunction with heparin has been shown to improve the clinical course of stable patients who have acute submassive PE without internal bleeding, mainly by reducing need for subsequent thrombolytic use. Additional studies are needed to confirm these findings before recommending routine use of this therapeutic approach. The Pulmonary Embolism Thrombolysis (PEITHO) trial revealed that in patients with intermediate risk of pulmonary embolism, fibrinolytic therapy prevented hemodynamic compensation but increased the risk of major hemorrhage and stroke.

- Long-term treatment for PE not associated with malignancy can be carried out with warfarin therapy or rivaroxaban.
- For PE associated with malignancy, LMWH is recommended for long-term therapy.
- For PE occurring in the setting of a reversible risk factor, anticoagulation should be continued for 3 mo. For patients with an unprovoked PE, longer-term anticoagulation should be considered, and indefinite long-term anticoagulation should be used in patients with recurrent unprovoked PE. Important factors to consider in the decision to extend anticoagulation include the patient's risk of bleeding and patient preferences after an informed discussion of risks and benefits.
- If thrombolytics and anticoagulants are contraindicated (e.g., GI bleeding, recent CNS surgery, recent trauma) or if the patient continues to have recurrent PE despite anticoagulation therapy, vena caval interruption is indicated by transvenous placement of an inferior vena caval filter.
- IVC filters are also strongly associated with reduced in-hospital fatality rate in stable patients who received thrombolytic therapy. It seems prudent to consider a vena cava filter in patients with PE who are receiving thrombolytic therapy.
- Acute pulmonary artery surgical embolectomy or catheter-based thrombectomy may be indicated in a patient with massive PE who cannot receive thrombolytic therapy. Pulmonary embolectomy is also recommended for those whose critical status does not allow sufficient time for thrombolytic therapy to be effective and for those who remain unstable after receiving fibrinolysis.

CHRONIC Rx

- Elimination of risk factors (see "Etiology").
- Patients with unprovoked DVT/PE have a high rate of recurrent VTE. Longer durations of chronic anticoagulation after unprovoked DVT/PE result in lower rates of recurrent DVT/PE while on anticoagulation, but benefits are lost once anticoagulation is halted. The use of indefinite anticoagulation in selected individuals with apparently unprovoked DVT/PE must be weighed against ongoing bleeding risk and other factors.
- Aspirin (100 mg daily) is superior to placebo in preventing recurrence of venous thromboembolism in patients with a first-ever unprovoked venous thromboembolism (VTE) who had already completed 6 to 18 mos of oral anticoagulation. This suggests that aspirin could be offered as an alternative to oral anticoagulants for prevention of recurrent VTE in patients who refuse to or cannot continue oral anticoagulant therapy but who have a high risk of recurrent VTE.
- Trials involving extending the treatment time of the novel oral anticoagulants (rivaroxaban, dabigatran, and apixaban) all showed superior efficacy and reduced morbidity compared to placebo as well as similar rate of major bleeding (though increased all bleeding).

DISPOSITION

- Mortality can be reduced to <10% by rapid and effective treatment. Stratification of risk of death associated with PE and severity-adjusted treatment is described in Table 4. Indicators of poor prognosis include hemodynamic instability/hypotension, signs of RV dysfunction, elevated BNP, elevated troponin, thrombus burden, coexisting DVT, and right ventricular thrombus. The Pulmonary Embolism Severity Index (PESI) is summarized in Table 5.
- Mortality from recurrent pulmonary emboli is 8% with effective treatment and >30% in patients with untreated pulmonary emboli.

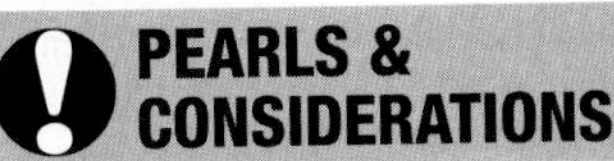

PEARLS & CONSIDERATIONS

COMMENTS

- Use of clinical prediction rules in association with D-dimer testing may reduce the use of unnecessary imaging in patients in whom PE is unlikely.
- Massive PE (PE associated with hypotension, shock, or circulatory arrest) remains the clearest situation in which thrombolytics should be employed. Submassive PE (PE associated with right ventricular dysfunction or injury but without hypotension) remains an area of controversy with regards to thrombolytic use.
- A recent prospective study revealed that suspected pulmonary embolism in pregnant patients can be ruled out by using a pregnancy-adapted YEARS diagnostic algorithm across all trimesters of pregnancy. The three following criteria from the YEARS algorithm were used: (1) clinical signs of deep-vein thrombosis, (2) hemoptysis, (3) pulmonary

TABLE 4 Stratification of Risk of Death Associated with Pulmonary Embolism and Severity-Adjusted Treatment*

	Risk Factor			
Early Risk of Death	**Shock or Hypotension (on Clinical Examination)**	**Right Ventricular Dysfunction (on Echocardiography or Multidetector CT)**	**Myocardial Injury (on Cardiac Troponin Testing)**	**Recommended Treatment**
High	Present	Present†	NA‡	Unfractionated heparin plus thrombolysis or embolectomy
Intermediate§	Absent	Present	Present	Low-molecular-weight heparin or fondaparinux; as a rule, no early thrombolysis; monitor clinical status and right ventricular function
Low	Absent	Absent	Absent	Low-molecular-weight heparin or fondaparinux; consider outpatient treatment

*Adapted with modifications from the 2008 Guidelines on the Diagnosis and Management of Acute Pulmonary Embolism of the European Society of Cardiology. NA denotes not applicable.
†If RV function is normal on echocardiography, or if a CT scan shows no RV dilatation in a patient with hemodynamic compromise and clinically suspected pulmonary embolism, an alternative diagnosis should be sought.
‡Troponin test results do not influence risk assessment or treatment in hemodynamically compromised patients with acute pulmonary embolism.
§Although it has been suggested that normotensive patients with both RV dysfunction and myocardial injury have a higher risk of death than those with only one of these risk factors, there is currently no definitive proof that they should receive more aggressive treatment.
CT, Computed tomography; *RV,* right ventricle.
From Konstantinides S: Acute pulmonary embolism, *N Engl J Med* 359:2804-2813, 2008.

TABLE 5 Original and Simplified Pulmonary Embolism Severity Index (PESI)

Variable	Original PESI	Simplified PESI
Age	Age, in yr	1 (if age >80 yr)
Male sex	+10	—
History of cancer	+30	1
History of heart failure	+10	1 for either or both of these items
History of chronic lung disease	+10	
Pulse >110 beats/min	+20	1
Systolic blood pressure <100 mm Hg	+30	1
Respiratory rate >30 breaths/min	+20	—
Temperature <36°C	+20	—
Altered mental status	+60	—
Arterial oxyhemoglobin saturation (SaO_2) <90%	+20	1
30-DAY MORTALITY RISK STRATA (BASED ON THE SUM OF POINTS)		
LOW-RISK PESI	**LOW-RISK sPESI**	
Class I: <65 Points (event rate 95% CI, 0-1.6)	**0 Points** (event rate 95% CI, 0-2.1)	
Class II: 66-85 Points (event rate 95% CI, 1.7-3.5)		
HIGH-RISK PESI	**HIGH-RISK sPESI**	
Class III: 86-105 Points (event rate 95% CI, 3.2-7.1)	**≥1 Point** (event rate 95% CI, 8.5-13.2)	
Class IV: 106-125 Points (event rate 95% CI, 4.0-11.4)		
Class V: >125 Points (event rate 95% CI, 10.0-24.5)		

CI, Confidence interval; *sPESI*, Simplified Pulmonary Embolism Severity Index.
From Vincent JL, et al.: *Textbook of critical care*, ed 7, Philadelphia, 2017, Elsevier.

embolism as the most likely diagnosis. A D-dimer level was also obtained. PE was ruled out if none of the three criteria were met and the D-dimer level was <1000 mg/ml or if one or more of the three criteria were met and the D-dimer level was <500 mg/ml.[2]

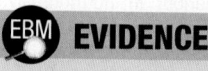

EVIDENCE

Available at ExpertConsult.com

SUGGESTED READINGS

Available at ExpertConsult.com

RELATED CONTENT

Pulmonary Embolism (PE) (Patient Information)
Deep Vein Thrombosis (Related Key Topic)
Hypercoagulable State (Related Key Topic)

AUTHOR: **CHAKRAVARTHY REDDY, M.D.**

[2] van der Pol LM, et al.: Pregnancy-adapted YEARS algorithm for diagnosis of suspected pulmonary embolism, *N Engl J Med* 380(12):1139–1149, 2019.

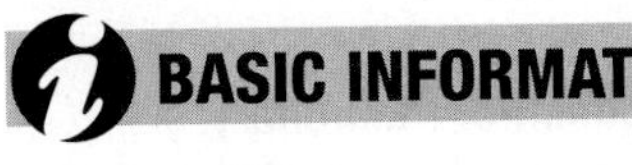

BASIC INFORMATION

DEFINITION

Pulmonary hypertension (PH) is defined as the presence of an elevated mean pulmonary arterial pressure (PAP) ≥25 mm Hg at rest. Pulmonary hypertension is classified into five major groups: pulmonary arterial hypertension (Group 1), pulmonary hypertension due to left heart disease (Group 2), pulmonary hypertension due to lung disease (Group 3), pulmonary hypertension due to chronic thromboembolic disease (Group 4), and miscellaneous (Group 5).

Pulmonary arterial hypertension (PAH) is a syndrome defined as mean pulmonary pressure ≥25 mm Hg with pulmonary capillary wedge pressure <15 mm Hg and a pulmonary vascular resistance ≥3 Wood units on right heart catheterization. Idiopathic pulmonary arterial hypertension (IPAH) is diagnosed when PAH is present without any apparent cause. It is a highly morbid disease characterized by progressive obliteration of precapillary arterioles. Pulmonary hypertension from lung disease is covered under the separate topic "Cor Pulmonale."

SYNONYMS

PH
Pulmonary arterial hypertension
Idiopathic pulmonary arterial hypertension
IPAH
Associated pulmonary arterial hypertension
PAHA, also known as secondary pulmonary hypertension
Heritable pulmonary arterial hypertension
HPAH
Group I pulmonary hypertension

ICD-10CM CODES
I27.0 Primary pulmonary hypertension
I27.2 Other secondary pulmonary hypertension

EPIDEMIOLOGY & DEMOGRAPHICS

- IPAH is rare, occurring in one to two cases per 1 million people per yr, with an overall prevalence estimated at 15 to 50 per 1 million.
- IPAH is more common in women than men (3:1), usually presenting in the third to fourth decades of life.
- In adults the most common cause of pulmonary hypertension is due to left-sided heart disease (Group 2).
- Prevalence of secondary PAH could range from 8% to 12% in cases of scleroderma, 0.5% of HIV, 23% to 53% of mixed connective tissue disorders, and 1% to 4% cases of systemic lupus erythematosus.

PHYSICAL FINDINGS & CLINICAL PRESENTATION

- Insidious, may go undetected for years
- Exertional dyspnea most common presenting symptom (60%)
- Fatigue and weakness
- Syncope, classically exertion-related or after a warm shower with peripheral vasodilation
- Chest pain
- Hoarse voice from compression of recurrent laryngeal nerve by an enlarged pulmonary artery (Ortner syndrome)
- Loud P2 component of the second heart sound and paradoxical splitting of second heart sound
- Right-sided S4
- Jugular venous distention
- Abdominal distention and ascites
- Prominent parasternal (right ventricular [RV]) impulse
- Holosystolic tricuspid regurgitation murmur heard best along the left fourth parasternal line that increases in intensity with inspiration
- Peripheral edema
- Features of the physical exam pertinent to the evaluation of pulmonary hypertension are summarized in Table 1

ETIOLOGY

- The etiology of IPAH is unknown. APAH (associated PAH) has several known risk factors: connective tissue disorders such as systemic sclerosis, portal hypertension and liver cirrhosis, appetite-suppressant drugs (e.g., fenfluramine), and infections, including schistosomiasis and HIV disease. High altitude, schistosomiasis, and HIV disease are common causes of PH worldwide; however, pulmonary venous hypertension from left ventricular failure and PH related to COPD are more common causes of PH in developed nations.
- Several genetic abnormalities have been associated with HPAH (heritable PAH), many of which are mutations in the genes that code for members of the tumor growth factor-beta family of receptors (BMPR-II, ALK-1, endoglin) on chromosome 2q33. A recent study has identified the association of a novel gene, *KCNK3,* with familial and idiopathic pulmonary arterial hypertension.
- Heritable PAH is an autosomal-dominant disease with variable penetrance, affecting only about 10% to 20% of carriers.
- Several factors play a role in the pathogenesis of PAH, including a genetic predisposition, endothelial cell dysfunction, abnormalities in vasomotor control, thrombotic obliteration of the vascular lumen, and vascular remodeling through cell proliferation and matrix production.
- SSRI use in late pregnancy is associated with increased persistent PAH in newborns.
- The updated clinical classification of pulmonary hypertension is described in Table 2.

Dx DIAGNOSIS

- PAH is a hemodynamic diagnosis involving the detection of elevated pressure in the pulmonary arteries and elevated pulmonary vascular resistance in the pulmonary vascular bed, occurring in the absence of significant pulmonary venous hypertension; characterization of this abnormality determines its etiology.
- Right-sided heart catheterization must be performed in all patients suspected of having PAH to establish the diagnosis and to assess pulmonary hemodynamics including reactivity response to vasodilators.
- One of the most challenging differential diagnoses of IPAH is heart failure with preserved EF (HFpEF). In such patients, the PCWP may be at the higher limit of normal at rest. Exercise or fluid challenge at the time of right heart catheterization can result in disproportionate rise in PCWP, which favors group 2 pulmonary hypertension.
- IPAH is a diagnosis of exclusion; causes that lead to groups 2–5 pulmonary hypertension must be ruled out. TTE, HR-CT, PFT, and V/Q scan must be performed before the diagnosis of IPAH is established and treatment started.

DIFFERENTIAL DIAGNOSIS

The differential diagnosis is as listed under "Etiology." Table 3 summarizes distinguishing pulmonary arterial hypertension from heart failure with preserved ejection fraction.

EVALUATION

- Consists of establishing the diagnosis and etiology.
- Echocardiography with Doppler technique can provide a noninvasive but limited estimation of systolic PAP. Common findings include tricuspid regurgitation, right heart enlargement, abnormal movement of septum and, rarely, pericardial effusion. However, the diagnosis of PH cannot be established by echocardiography alone, as echocardiography can overestimate or underestimate PAP.
- ECG shows RV enlargement, strain pattern, and right axis deviation.
- Chest radiograph (Fig. 1) shows enlarged central pulmonary arteries and right heart enlargement. Chest radiography is abnormal in 90% of patients at diagnosis.
- A normal chest radiograph does not rule out the diagnosis. High-resolution computed tomography (CT) (Fig. E2) can assist in the evaluation for emphysema or interstitial lung disease. Ventilation-perfusion lung scan has high sensitivity for chronic thromboembolic disease. The diagnosis can be confirmed by pulmonary angiography, which has high specificity. Pulmonary angiography is also useful in identifying patients who can benefit from pulmonary endarterectomy (PEA).
- Cardiac magnetic resonance imaging (CMR) can provide accurate noninvasive evaluation of the right ventricular size, morphology, and function.
- Pulmonary function tests may show obstructive (airway disease) and/or restrictive disease (parenchymal disease) depending on etiology. Diffusion capacity of carbon monoxide in the lung is reduced due to pulmonary vascular destruction in PAH.

TABLE 1 Features of the Physical Examination Pertinent to the Evaluation of Pulmonary Hypertension

Sign	Implication
PHYSICAL SIGNS THAT REFLECT THE SEVERITY OF PULMONARY HYPERTENSION	
Accentuated pulmonary component of S_2 (audible at the apex in >90%)	High pulmonary pressure that increases force of pulmonic valve closure
Early systolic click	Sudden interruption of opening of the pulmonary valve into a high-pressure artery
Midsystolic ejection murmur	Turbulent transvalvular pulmonary outflow
Left parasternal lift	High right ventricular pressure and hypertrophy present
Right ventricular S_4 (in 38%)	High right ventricular pressure and hypertrophy present
Increased jugular A wave	Poor right ventricular compliance
PHYSICAL SIGNS THAT SUGGEST MODERATE TO SEVERE PULMONARY HYPERTENSION	
Moderate to severe pulmonary hypertension	
Holosystolic murmur that increases with inspiration	Tricuspid regurgitation
Increased jugular V waves	
Pulsatile liver	
Diastolic murmur	Pulmonary regurgitation
Hepatojugular reflux	High central venous pressure
Advanced pulmonary hypertension with right ventricular failure	
Right ventricular S_3 (in 23%)	Right ventricular dysfunction
Distention of jugular veins	Right ventricular dysfunction or tricuspid regurgitation, or both
Hepatomegaly	Right ventricular dysfunction or tricuspid regurgitation, or both
Peripheral edema (in 32%)	
Ascites	
Low blood pressure, diminished pulse pressure, cool extremities	Reduced cardiac output, peripheral vasoconstriction
PHYSICAL SIGNS THAT SUGGEST A POSSIBLE UNDERLYING CAUSE FOR OR ASSOCIATIONS WITH PULMONARY HYPERTENSION	
Central cyanosis	Abnormal ventilation-perfusion ratio, intrapulmonary shunt, hypoxemia, pulmonary-to-systemic shunt
Clubbing	Congenital heart disease, pulmonary venopathy
Cardiac auscultatory findings, including systolic murmurs, diastolic murmurs, opening snap, and gallop	Congenital or acquired heart or valvular disease
Rales, dullness, or decreased breath sounds	Pulmonary congestion or effusion, or both
Fine rales, accessory muscle use, wheezing, protracted expiration, productive cough	Pulmonary parenchymal disease
Obesity, kyphoscoliosis, enlarged tonsils	Possible substrate for disordered ventilation
Sclerodactyly, arthritis, telangiectasia, Raynaud phenomenon, rash	Connective tissue disorder
Peripheral venous insufficiency or obstruction	Possible venous thrombosis
Venous stasis ulcers	Possible sickle cell disease
Pulmonary vascular bruits	Chronic thromboembolic pulmonary hypertension
Splenomegaly, spider angiomas, palmar erythema, icterus, caput medusae, ascites	Portal hypertension

From McLaughlin VV, et al.: ACCF/AHA 2009 expert consensus document on pulmonary hypertension: a report of the American College of Cardiology Foundation Task Force on Expert Consensus Documents and the American Heart Association developed in collaboration with the American College of Chest Physicians; American Thoracic Society, Inc., and the Pulmonary Hypertension Association, *J Am Coll Cardiol* 53:1573, 2009; In Mann DL et al: *Braunwald's heart disease,* ed 11, Philadelphia, 2019, Elsevier.

TABLE 2 Updated Clinical Classification of Pulmonary Hypertension

Group 1
Pulmonary arterial hypertension
Idiopathic pulmonary arterial hypertension
Heritable
BMPR2
ALK1, endoglin (with or without hereditary hemorrhagic telangiectasia)
Unknown
Drug- and toxin-induced
Associated with:
Connective tissue diseases
HIV infection
Portal hypertension
Congenital heart diseases
Schistosomiasis
Chronic hemolytic anemia
Persistent pulmonary hypertension of the newborn
Pulmonary veno-occlusive disease with left to right shunts and/or pulmonary capillary hemangiomatosis
Group 2
Pulmonary hypertension owing to left heart disease
Systolic dysfunction
Diastolic dysfunction
Valvular disease
Group 3
Pulmonary hypertension owing to lung diseases and/or hypoxia
Chronic obstructive pulmonary disease
Interstitial lung disease
Other pulmonary diseases with mixed restrictive and obstructive pattern
Sleep-disordered breathing
Alveolar hypoventilation disorders
Chronic exposure to high altitude
Developmental abnormalities
Group 4
Chronic thromboembolic pulmonary hypertension
Group 5
Pulmonary hypertension with unclear multifactorial mechanisms
Hematologic disorders: Myeloproliferative disorders, splenectomy
Systemic disorders: Sarcoidosis, pulmonary Langerhans cell histiocytosis: Lymphangioleiomyomatosis, neurofibromatosis, vasculitis
Metabolic disorders: Glycogen storage disease, Gaucher's disease, thyroid disorders
Others: Tumoral obstruction, fibrosing mediastinitis, chronic renal failure on dialysis

ALK1, Activin receptor-like kinase type 1; *BMPR2,* bone morphogenetic protein receptor type 2; *HIV,* human immunodeficiency virus.

From Simonneau G, et al.: Updated clinical classification of pulmonary hypertension, *J Am Coll Cardiol* 54:S43-S54, 2009.

- In asymptomatic patients the severity of pulmonary arterial hypertension (PAH) disease should be evaluated in a systematic and consistent manner, using a combination of World Health Organization (WHO) functional class (FC), exercise capacity, and echocardiographic, laboratory, and hemodynamic variables to inform therapeutic decisions.
- Right heart catheterization is required to assess pulmonary hemodynamics, exclude shunts and left heart disease, and perform acute vasoreactivity response testing.
- Symptomatic patients with PAH, in the absence of contraindications, should undergo acute vasoreactivity testing using a short-acting agent at a center with experience in the performance and interpretation of vasoreactivity testing.
- Screening for the presence of PAH with Doppler echocardiography is warranted in individuals with a known predisposing genetic mutation or first-degree relative with IPAH, connective tissue diseases (especially scleroderma), congenital heart disease with left-to-right shunt, or portal hypertension undergoing evaluation for orthotopic liver transplantation.
- Determining the degree of functional impairment, as assessed by the WHO functional classification system (Classes I-IV) and the 6-min walk test (6MWT), is a useful way to monitor disease progression and assess response to treatment.
- The longitudinal evaluation of patients with pulmonary arterial hypertension is summarized in Table 4.

LABORATORY TESTS

- Complete blood count is usually normal in PAH but may show secondary polycythemia.
- Arterial blood gases show low PO_2 and oxygen saturation.
- Overnight oximetry and/or sleep study to rule out sleep apnea or hypopnea.
- Other blood tests: Antinuclear antibody (ANA), antineutrophil cytoplasmic antibodies (ANCA), anti-Scl-70, anticentromere, ribonucleoprotein antibody levels, and rheumatoid factor (RF) to screen for underlying connective tissue disease, HIV serology, liver function tests, and antiphospholipid antibodies.
- Brain natriuretic peptide (BNP) level can provide prognostic information, with elevation in BNP level being associated with increased mortality.
- Ventilation-perfusion lung scan has high sensitivity for chronic thromboembolic PAH. The diagnosis should be confirmed by pulmonary angiography, which has high specificity.

TABLE 3 Distinguishing Pulmonary Arterial Hypertension from Heart Failure with Preserved Ejection Fraction

Characteristic	PAH More Likely	HFpEF More Likely
Age	Younger	Older
Comorbid conditions—DM, HTN, CAD, obesity (metabolic syndrome)	Often absent	Often multiple present
Symptoms—PND, orthopnea	Often absent	Often present
Cardiac examination	RV heave, loud P_2, TR murmur	Sustained LV impulse, LS4
CXR	Clear lung fields	Pulmonary vascular congestion, pleural effusions, pulmonary edema
Chest CT	Often clear lungs	Mosaic perfusion pattern, ground-glass opacities consistent with chronic interstitial edema
ECG	RAD, RVE	LAE, LVE, atrial fibrillation, no RAD
Natriuretic peptides	Often elevated	Often elevated
Echo—LAE, LVH	Absent	Often present
Echo—diastolic dysfunction	Grade 1 common	Grade 2, 3 common
Echo—right ventricle	Often enlarged, may share the apex	Often normal, mildly enlarged
Echo—pericardial effusion	Sometimes	Rare

CAD, Coronary artery disease; *CXR,* chest x-ray; *DM,* diabetes mellitus; *Echo,* echocardiography; *HTN,* hypertension; *LAE,* left atrial enlargement; *LS4,* left-sided fourth heart sound; *LV,* left ventricular; *LVE,* left ventricular enlargement; *LVH,* left ventricular hypertrophy; *PND,* paroxysmal nocturnal dyspnea; *RAD,* right-axis deviation; *RV,* right ventricular; *RVE,* right ventricular enlargement; *TR,* tricuspid regurgitation.

From Mann DL, et al.: *Braunwald's heart disease,* ed 10, Philadelphia, 2015, Elsevier.

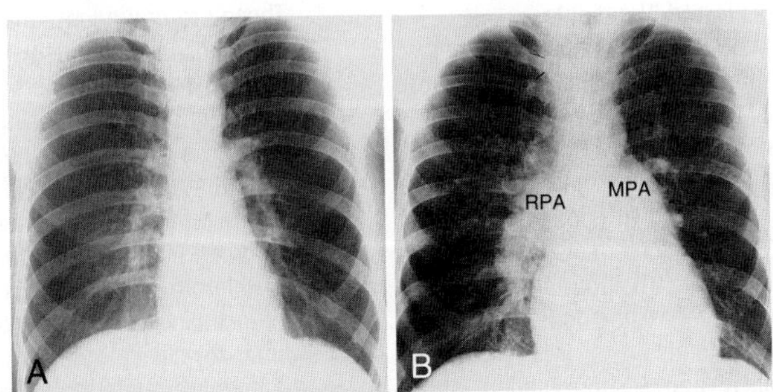

FIG. 1 Progressive pulmonary arterial hypertension. This patient initially presented with a relatively normal chest radiograph **(A).** However, several years later **(B)** there is increasing heart size and marked dilation of the main pulmonary artery *(MPA)* and right pulmonary artery *(RPA).* Rapid tapering of the arteries as they proceed peripherally is suggestive of pulmonary hypertension and is sometimes referred to as pruning. (From Mettler FA [ed]: *Primary care radiology,* Philadelphia, 2000, WB Saunders.)

Rx TREATMENT (FIG. 3)

- Most of the evidence in management of PAH is limited to IPAH/HPAH. There is some evidence in treatment of APAH associated with connective tissue disease, especially scleroderma, and congenital heart disease. The recommendations for treating PAH associated with other causes are limited to case studies and expert opinions.
- There is some evidence for the use of advanced therapies for sarcoidosis-associated PH. The heterogeneity of sarcoid-associated PH complicates the interpretation.

GENERAL MEASURES AND TREATMENT:

- Patients should be encouraged to remain active within symptom limits and avoid excessive physical activity.
- PAH is a contraindication to pregnancy as it carries a 30% to 50% mortality risk.
- PAH patients have a higher risk of death from infections and should be vaccinated against influenza and pneumococcal pneumonia.
- Although there are no randomized data to suggest that long-term O_2 therapy is beneficial, oxygen administration has shown to reduce PVR. Ambulatory O_2 may be considered for exercise-induced desaturations.
- Diuretics (e.g., furosemide 40-80 mg qd) improve dyspnea by reducing preload and peripheral edema. Avoid excessive diuresis in patients who are preload dependent.
- Digoxin has been used in patients with IPAH with inconclusive benefits. It can be considered in patients who develop atrial tachyarrhythmia. There is no conclusive data regarding the use of beta-blockers, ACE inhibitors, or ARB in IPAH unless required by comorbidities such as concurrent hypertension or cardiomyopathy.
- Evidence for the use of oral anticoagulation with warfarin for IPAH is derived mostly from retrospective single-center experience. Data from RCT and registries remain heterogeneous and inconclusive. A large multicenter observational longitudinal registry of patients with IPAH (REVEAL Registry) assessed the effect of warfarin treatment on survival and found no benefit; it also found poorer survival in patients with PAH associated with systemic sclerosis. Generally, patients with IPAH who are undergoing IV prostaglandin therapy are anticoagulated if there are no

TABLE 4 Longitudinal Evaluation of Patients with Pulmonary Arterial Hypertension*

	Low Risk	High Risk
Clinical course	Stable; no increase in symptoms and/or decompensation	Unstable; increase in symptoms and/or decompensation
Physical examination	No evidence of right-sided heart failure	Signs of right-sided heart failure
Functional class†	I/II	IV
6MW distance†	>400 m	<300 m
Echocardiogram	RV size/function normal	RV enlargement/dysfunction
Hemodynamics	RAP normal CI normal	RAP high CI low
BNP	Nearly normal/remaining stable or decreasing	Elevated/increasing
Treatment	Oral therapy	Intravenous prostacyclin and/or combination treatment
Frequency of evaluation	Every 3-6 mo‡	Every 1-3 mo
FC assessment	Every clinic visit	Every clinic visit
6MW distance	Every clinic visit	Every clinic visit
Echocardiogram§	Yearly or center dependent	Every 6-12 mo or center dependent
BNP¶	Center dependent	Center dependent
RHC	Clinical deterioration and center dependent	Every 6-12 mo or clinical deterioration

CI, Cardiac index; *FC*, functional class; *RAP*, right atrial pressure; *6MW*, 6-minute walk.
*For patients in the high-risk category, consider referral to a PAH specialty center for consideration of advanced therapies, clinical trials, and/or lung transplantation.
†The frequency of follow-up evaluation for patients in functional class III and/or 6MW distance between 300 and 400 m would depend on a composite of detailed assessments of the other clinical and objective characteristics listed.
‡For patients who remain stable with established therapy, follow-up assessments can be performed by referring physicians or PH specialty centers.
§Echocardiographic measurement of pulmonary artery systolic pressure is an estimation only, and it is strongly advised that its evaluation not be relied on as the sole parameter to make therapeutic decisions.
¶The usefulness of serial BNP levels to guide management in individual patients has not been established.
From McLaughlin VV, et al.: ACCF/AHA 2009 expert consensus document on pulmonary hypertension. A report of the American College of Cardiology Foundation Task Force on Expert Consensus Documents and the American Heart Association developed in collaboration with the American College of Chest Physicians; American Thoracic Society, Inc.; and the Pulmonary Hypertension Association, *J Am Coll Cardiol* 53:1573, 2009.
From Mann DL, et al.: *Braunwald's heart disease*, ed 10, Philadelphia, 2015, Elsevier.

contraindications to anticoagulation, as they are at high risk for catheter-related thrombosis. There are no data regarding the role of novel oral anticoagulants in IPAH.

- Iron deficiency with or without anemia is common and is associated with reduced exercise capacity; it should be closely monitored and replenished as needed.

CHRONIC Rx

Calcium channel blocker (CCB):

- Acute vasoreactivity response testing should be done in all patients at the time of right heart catheterization. Epoprostenol, adenosine, or nitric oxide is generally used to assess the response. A positive response is a fall in mean PAP of ≥10 mm Hg to a value of <40 mm Hg, with increased or unchanged cardiac output. Fewer than 10% of patients are responders in IPAH, and they are the only patients who can be safely treated with this type of therapy. Acute vasoreactivity study is not recommended for patients in groups 2-5.
- The positive responders may benefit from treatment with calcium channel blockers (diltiazem, amlodipine, or nifedipine). Verapamil is not recommended because of its negative inotropic effects. All patients should be reassessed in 6 to 8 wk to demonstrate sustained benefit from the calcium channel blocker.
- CCBs should not be used empirically to treat PAH in the absence of demonstrated acute vasoreactivity because of potential severe side effects.
- If patients do not show an adequate response, additional PAH therapy should be started.

PROSTANOIDS

- These synthetic prostacyclin analogues act as potent vasodilators of pulmonary arteries and inhibitors of platelet aggregation. They all have shown improvement in symptoms, exercise capacity including 6MWD, and hemodynamics. They are ideal for WHO functional class III and IV patients.
  1. Epoprostenol: IV formulation with very short half-life (3-5 min). It is the only drug that has shown to improve mortality. It requires long-term IV access with associated risks of infection and thrombosis. Rapid tachyphylaxis with dose escalation is seen. Common side effects include jaw pain, abdominal cramping, and diarrhea. Limited evidence exists for use in secondary PAH patients.
  2. Treprostinil: IV and SQ formulation with longer half-life. Main disadvantage is pain at SQ pump site (no long-term evidence for IV formulation). Treprostinil is also available as a nebulized inhaled solution.
  3. Iloprost: Aerosolized formulation with short half-life requiring 6 to 8 treatments/day. Oral and IV forms are also available. Well tolerated, with flushing and jaw pain being the most frequent side effects.
  4. Beraprost: PO formulation. Not approved in the U.S.

RIOCIGUAT: GUANYLATE CYCLASE STIMULATORS

Guanylate cyclase stimulators enhance cGMP production and in preclinical studies show antiproliferative and antiremodeling properties in animal models. These oral agents are useful for class II and III patients and have shown favorable results on exercise capacity, hemodynamics (decrease in PVR), WHO functional class, and time to clinical worsening without any mortality benefit. Recently, it has shown improvement in 6MWD and reduction in PVR in patients with group IV pulmonary hypertension. The most serious side effect is syncope.

Endothelin receptor antagonists (ERAs): Activation of the endothelin system results in vasoconstriction of the pulmonary vascular smooth muscles. These oral pulmonary vasodilators require monthly liver function tests, and often the response is delayed by weeks. Thus, it is not an ideal starting therapy for WHO class IV patients. It is effective in class II and III patients and improves symptoms, exercise capacity, and hemodynamics without any improvement in mortality.

- Bosentan is an oral nonselective endothelin A and B receptor blocker, whereas sitaxsentan and ambrisentan are oral selective endothelin A receptor blockers. Ambrisentran does not require monitoring of liver function tests.
- ERAs have been shown to cause improvement in exercise capacity, WHO functional class, hemodynamic and echocardiographic variables without affecting mortality.
- Macitentan is a nonselective endothelin receptor antagonist that showed significant reduction in composite end point of death in patients with IPAH. It has no liver toxicity but can cause reduction in hemoglobin.

- **Phosphodiesterase (PDE-5) inhibitors:**
  1. These are oral agents that act by inhibiting phosphodiesterase type 5 enzyme (PDE-5), resulting in increased concentration of nitric oxide causing vasodilatation through the cGMP/NO pathway. In addition, they exert antiproliferative effects. Highly effective in WHO class II patients, both in IPAH and scleroderma-associated PAH. Improve symptoms, exercise capacity including 6MWD, hemodynamics, and time to clinical worsening. Most side effects are related to vasodilation including headache, flushing, and epistaxis.
  2. Sildenafil is administered as 20 mg PO tid. Tadalafil dose is 40 mg once daily. They are also used as combination ther-

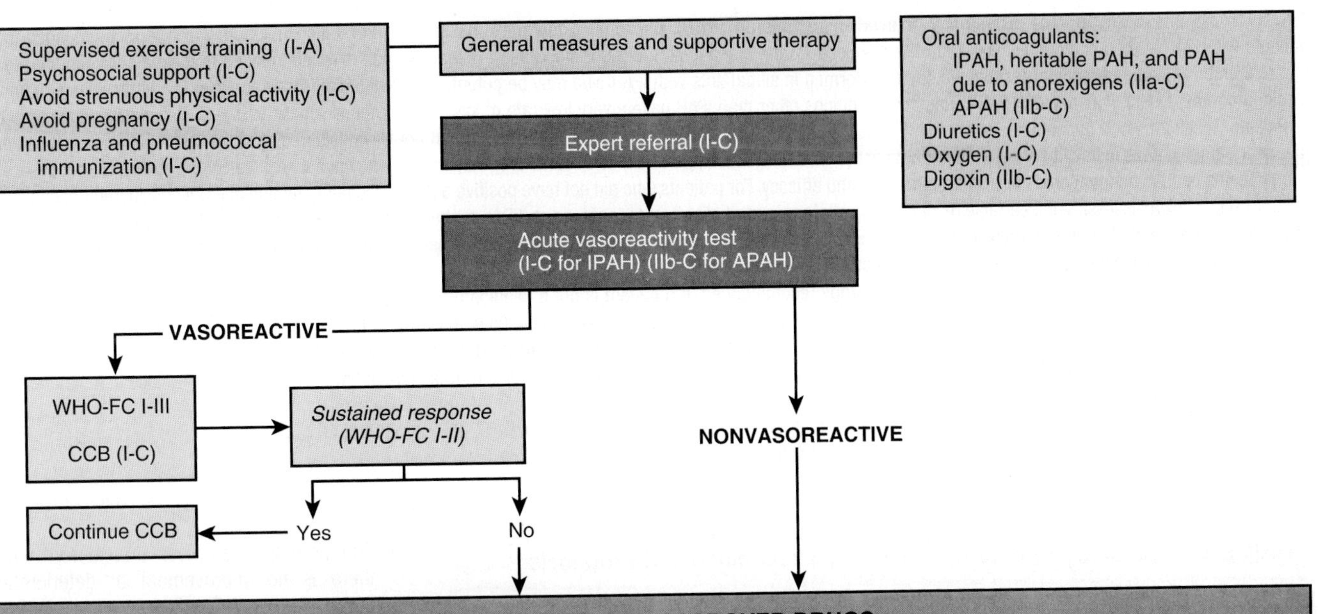

INITIAL THERAPY WITH PAH-APPROVED DRUGS

RED: Morbidity and mortality as primary endpoint in randomized controlled study or reduction in all-cause mortality (prospectively defined)
* Level of evidence is based on the WHO-FC of most of the patients in the studies
† Approved only, in the United States (treprostinil inhaled), in New Zealand (iloprost IV), in Japan and S. Korea (beraprost)
‡ Drugs under regulatory approval

Recommendation	Evidence*	WHO-FC II	WHO-FC III	WHO-FC IV
I	A or B	Ambrisentan, Bosentan Macitentan‡ Riociguat‡ Sildenafil Tadalafil	Ambrisentan, Bosentan, Epoprostenol IV Iloprost inhaled Macitentan‡ Riociguat‡ Sildenafil Tadalafil Treprostinil SC, inhaled†	Epoprostenol IV
IIa	C		Iloprost IV† Treprostinil IN	Ambrisentan, bosentan Iloprost inhaled, and IV† Macitentan‡ Riociguat‡ Sildenafil, tadalafil Treprostinil SC, IV, inhaled†
IIb	B		Beraprost†	
	C		Initial combination therapy	Initial combination therapy

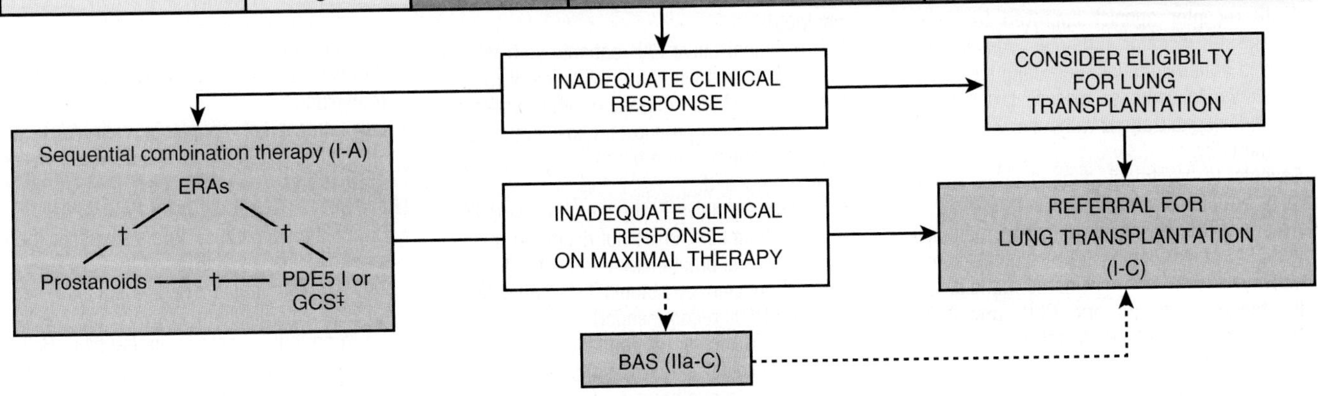

FIG. 3 Treatment algorithm for pulmonary arterial hypertension *(PAH)*. Background therapies include warfarin anticoagulation, which is recommended in all patients with IPAH and no contraindication. Diuretics are used for the management of right-sided heart failure. Oxygen is recommended to maintain oxygen saturation higher than 90%. Acute vasodilator testing should be performed in all patients with IPAH who may be potential candidates for long-term therapy with calcium channel–blocking agents (CCBs). Patients with PAH caused by conditions other than IPAH have a very low rate of long-term responsiveness to oral CCBs, and the value of acute vasodilator testing in such patients needs to be individualized. Patients with IPAH in whom CCB therapy would not be considered, such as those with right-sided heart failure or hemodynamic instability, should not undergo acute vasodilator testing. CCBs are indicated only for patients who have a positive acute vasodilator response, and such patients need to be monitored closely for both safety and efficacy. For patients who did not have positive acute vasodilatory testing and are considered to be at lower risk based on clinical assessment (see Table 5), oral therapy with an endothelin receptor antagonist (ERA) or phosphodiesterase-5 inhibitor (PDE5 I) would be the first line of therapy recommended. If an oral regimen is not appropriate, consideration of the other treatments would need to be based on the patient's profile, side effects, and risk associated with each therapy. For patients who are considered high risk based on clinical assessment (Table 5), continuous treatment with an intravenous prostacyclin (epoprostenol or treprostinil) would be the first line of therapy recommended. If a patient is not a candidate for continuous intravenous treatment, consideration of the other therapies would have to be based on the patient's profile and the side effects and risk associated with each treatment. Epoprostenol improves exercise capacity, hemodynamics, and survival in patients with IPAH and is the preferred treatment option for the most critically ill patients. Combination therapy should be considered when patients are not responding adequately to initial monotherapy. *APAH,* Associated PAH; *BAS,* balloon atrial septostomy; *GCS,* guanylate cyclase stimulators; *WHO FC,* World Health Organization functional class.
(From Galiè N, et al.: Updated treatment algorithm of pulmonary arterial hypertension, *J Am Coll Cardiol* 62[25 Suppl]:D60, 2013.)
(From Mann DL, et al.: *Braunwald's heart disease*, ed 10, Philadelphia, 2015, Elsevier.)

TABLE 5 Pulmonary Arterial Hypertension: Determinants of Prognosis*

Determinants of Risk	Lower Risk (Good Prognosis)	Higher Risk (Poor Prognosis)
Clinical evidence of RV failure	No	Yes
Progression of symptoms	Gradual	Rapid
WHO class†	II, III	IV
6MW distance‡	Longer (>400 m)	Shorter (<300 m)
CPET	Peak V_{O_2} >10.4 ml/kg/min	Peak V_{O_2} <10.4 ml/kg/min
Echocardiography	Minimal RV dysfunction	Pericardial effusion, significant RV enlargement/dysfunction, right atrial enlargement
Hemodynamics	RAP <10 mm Hg, CI >2.5 L/min/m^2	RAP >20 mm Hg, CI <2.0 L/min/m^2
BNP§	Minimally elevated	Significantly elevated

BNP, Brain natriuretic peptide; *CI,* cardiac index; *CPET,* cardiopulmonary exercise testing; *peak V_{O_2},* average peak oxygen uptake during exercise; *RAP,* right atrial pressure; *RV,* right ventricular.
*Most data available pertain to IPAH, with little data available for other forms of PAH. One should not rely on any single factor to make risk predictions.
†The WHO class is the functional classification for PAH and is a modification of the NHYA functional class.
‡6MW distance is also influenced by age, sex, and height.
§Because data regarding the influence of BNP on prognosis are currently limited and many factors, including renal function, weight, age, and sex, may influence BNP, absolute numbers are not given for this variable.
From McLaughlin VV, et al.: ACCF/AHA 2009 expert consensus document on pulmonary hypertension. A report of the American College of Cardiology Foundation Task Force on Expert Consensus Documents and the American Heart Association developed in collaboration with the American College of Chest Physicians; American Thoracic Society, Inc.; and the Pulmonary Hypertension Association, *J Am Coll Cardiol* 53:1573, 2009. In Mann DL et al: *Braunwald's heart disease*, ed 10, Philadelphia, 2015, Elsevier.

apy with epoprosternol and endothelin receptor antagonists.

- **Prostacyclin agonists:**
  1. Selexipag is an oral selective prostacyclin IP receptor agonist approved for PAH. The IP receptor promotes vasodilation and antiproliferation. Selexipag has been shown to decrease disease progression and hospitalizations without any effect on mortality.

Caveats to treatment depending on WHO class of symptoms are as follows:

- According to consensus definition, patients with PAH who demonstrate acute vasoreactivity should be considered candidates for therapy with an oral CCB, except in the case of right heart failure or other contraindications.
- CCBs should not be used empirically to treat PAH in the absence of demonstrated acute vasoreactivity, as described previously.
- For treatment-naive PAH patients with WHO functional class (FC) II or III symptoms who are not candidates for, or who have failed CCB therapy, monotherapy should be initiated with an approved ERA, phosphodiesterase-5 (PDE5) inhibitor, or the soluble guanylate cyclase stimulator riociguat.
- For treatment-naive PAH patients with WHO FC III symptoms who have evidence of rapid progression of their disease or other markers of a poor clinical prognosis, consideration of initial treatment with a parenteral prostanoid is recommended.
- For treatment-naive PAH patients in WHO FC IV who are unable, or do not desire, to manage parenteral prostanoid therapy, treatment with an inhaled prostanoid in combination with an ERA is recommended.
- For WHO FC III or IV PAH patients with unacceptable clinical status despite established PAH-specific monotherapy, addition of a second class of PAH therapy to improve exercise capacity is recommended. Such patients should be evaluated at centers with expertise in the evaluation and treatment of complex patients with PAH.
- Combination therapies: Considered when there is no improvement or deterioration on monotherapy. The FDA has approved the use of ambrisentan and tadalafil together as the first two-drug regimen for PAH. Starting dose is 5 mg for ambrisentan and 20 mg for tadalafil once daily.
- Bosentan + inhaled iloprost (STEP trial) showed some benefit over monotherapy.
- IV epoprostenol + oral bosentan (BREATH-2 trial) did not show much difference.
- IV epoprostenol + oral sildenafil (PACES trial) showed benefit over monotherapy.

INVASIVE Rx

Lung transplantation and heart-lung transplantation are other options in patients with end-stage class IV disease.

- Atrial septostomy may be performed as a bridge to transplant. It involves creation of an interatrial communication, resulting in right-to-left shunt, which decreases right-sided pressure and increases LV preload and cardiac output. The defect can be closed at the time of transplantation. Atrial septostomy is recommended for individuals with a room air SaO_2 >90% who have severe right-sided heart failure (with refractory ascites) despite maximal diuretic therapy, or who have signs of impaired systemic blood flow (such as syncope) from reduced left heart filling.
- Extracorporeal membrane oxygenation (ECMO) is also commonly used as a bridge to transplant.
- Lung transplant recipients with IPAH had survival rates of 73% at 1 yr, 55% at 3 yr, and 45% at 5 yr.

TREATMENT OF SECONDARY PAH, APAH:

- Directed toward cause. Some situations merit mention:
  1. PAH with uncorrected congenital heart disease: Eisenmenger syndrome. Medical treatment generally ineffective. Heart-lung transplantation required in most patients. PH may persist after surgical correction of congenital heart disease, and pulmonary vasodilators can be effective therapies in this patient population.
  2. PAH with scleroderma: Selective pulmonary vasodilators are effective.

3. PAH with lung disease or hypoxia: Oxygen therapy, for hypoxemia, CPAP (for OSA), control of primary disease process.
4. PAH with chronic thromboembolic disease: Pulmonary endarterectomy is curative; may consider pulmonary vasodilators after anticoagulation (for at least 3 mo and if endarterectomy is not an option) if continued symptoms and elevation in PVR and transpulmonary gradient.
5. PAH with HIV: Control of viral load by antiretroviral therapy.

FOLLOW-UP

Regular follow-up at 3- to 6-mo intervals with clinical assessment: WHO class and 6MWT, 6 to 12 mo objective assessment of RV function by ECG and BNP levels. TTE should be performed every 6–12 mo after initiation of therapy and right cardiac catheterization should be performed annually after changes in therapy.

DISPOSITION

- The 6MWT is predictive of survival in patients with idiopathic PAH. A baseline 6MWT <250 m is associated with a 50% risk of death at 2 yr. Drop in O_2 saturation >10% during the test increases mortality risk 2.9 times over a median follow-up of 26 mo.
- Cardiopulmonary exercise testing (CPET) is also performed, during which gaseous exchange and ventilation are continuously measured during incremental exercise. A peak oxygen uptake (pVO_2) of <10 ml/kg/min independently predicts a worse prognosis.
- A BNP level ≥350 pg/ml at baseline evaluation is associated with a 25% risk of death at 2 yr.
- WHO class II and III patients with PAH have a mean survival of 3.5 yr.
- WHO class IV patients have a mean survival of 6 mo.
- As per the REVEAL (Registry to Evaluate Early and Long-term Pulmonary Arterial Hypertension Disease Management) risk score, poor prognostic signs include:

1. Signs of RV failure.
2. WHO functional class III or IV.
3. Walk a distance of <165 meters in 6-min walk test.
4. Peak V02 <10 ml/min/kg in cardiopulmonary testing.
5. Elevated BNP levels >180 pg/ml.
6. Presence of pericardial effusion.
7. TAPSE [tricuspid annular plane systolic excursion] <2 cm on echo of right ventricle.
8. Right atrial pressure >20 mm Hg or pulmonary vascular resistance of >32 Wood units on right heart catheterization.
9. Increased heart rate >92 or BP <109 mm Hg.
10. Male gender >60 yr of age.
11. Concomitant renal dysfunction with estimated glomerular filtration rate ≤30/ml/min/m.
12. Diffusion capacity of lung for carbon monoxide (DLCO) <33%.

REFERRAL

If the diagnosis of IPAH/HPAH is suspected, a consultation with a pulmonary specialist is recommended. PHA may require disease-specific consultations. Advanced cases need to be transferred to transplant centers.

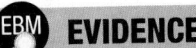

PEARLS & CONSIDERATIONS

- The exertional dyspnea of PAH is typically described by patients as being relentlessly progressive over several months to a year, often out of proportion to, or in the absence of, underlying heart or lung disease.
- Over 20% of patients in the Registry to Evaluate Early and Long-term PAH Disease Management had symptoms for more than 2 yr before PAH was recognized. Consideration of the diagnosis of PAH in the differential diagnosis of unexplained dyspnea, especially in younger individuals, is essential.
- Chest x-ray may reveal evidence of interstitial fluid or fibrosis within the lungs in cases of secondary PH. IPAH is not associated with infiltrates on chest radiograph.

COMMENTS

- RV systolic pressure (RVSP) as estimated by echocardiography is not a good indicator of the presence of PAH because RVSP increases with age and body mass index. Athletically conditioned men also have a higher resting RVSP. Thus, these measurements can be misleading.
- Abrupt development of pulmonary edema during acute vasodilator testing suggests pulmonary venoocclusive disease or pulmonary capillary hemangiomatosis and is a contraindication to long-term vasodilator treatment.
- In advanced PAH, heart rate increase is the main compensatory mechanism and reflects increased sympathetic tone. A higher heart rate at rest is an important marker of prognosis and should be assessed at frequent intervals after initiation of treatment for PAH.

FUTURE DIRECTIONS

- Serotonin receptor modulators, platelet-derived growth factor, and Rho kinase inhibitors.
- Gene analysis to identify genes that determine individual disease susceptibility and help identify targeted therapy.

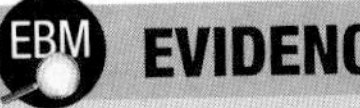

EVIDENCE

Available at ExpertConsult.com

SUGGESTED READINGS

Available at ExpertConsult.com

RELATED CONTENT

Pulmonary Hypertension (Patient Information)

AUTHOR: **WAJIH A. SYED, M.D.**

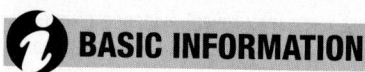

BASIC INFORMATION

DEFINITION

Pulseless electrical activity (PEA) is defined as the presence of organized cardiac electrical activity without sufficient mechanical contraction to produce a palpable pulse.

SYNONYM

Electromechanical dissociation (EMD)

ICD-10CM CODES

I46.9 Cardiac arrest, cause unspecified
I49.9 Cardiac arrhythmia, unspecified

EPIDEMIOLOGY & DEMOGRAPHICS

- Accounts for about 35% of cardiac arrest cases.
- Increasingly recognized as the cause of sudden cardiac death in patients with implantable cardioverter-defibrillators.

PHYSICAL FINDINGS & CLINICAL PRESENTATION

PRIMARY PEA:
- Organized electrical activity (not VT/VF)
- No detectable pulse

SECONDARY PEA: As in primary PEA and may also have:
- Bradycardia: Drug overdose, elevated vagal tone
- Tachycardia: Hypovolemia, massive PE
- Elevated JVP and no pulse with CPR: Cardiac tamponade, massive PE, tension pneumothorax
- Absent unilateral breath sounds and tracheal deviation: Tension pneumothorax
- Cyanosis: Hypoxia

ETIOLOGY

PRIMARY PEA: Myocardial electromechanical uncoupling secondary to advanced heart muscle disease

SECONDARY PEA: Related to changes in the loading conditions of the heart, ischemia, and/or myocardial depressants. Current guidelines suggest using the 5Hs and 5Ts as diagnostic tools when determining the etiology:
- **H**ypovolemia
- **H**ypoxia
- **H**ypothermia
- **H**ypo-/hyperkalemia
- **H**ydrogen ions (acidosis)
- **T**ension pneumothorax
- **T**amponade
- **T**hrombosis in the lungs (pulmonary embolism)
- **T**hrombosis in the heart (ACS)
- **T**oxins: β-blockers, calcium channel blockers, digoxin, tricyclic antidepressants, benzodiazepines, opioids

DIAGNOSIS

WORKUP

- Stabilizing patient and workup to establish etiology should proceed simultaneously.
- History, physical examination, laboratory tests, imaging studies (refer to 5Hs/5Ts).

LABORATORY TESTS

- CBC, potassium, magnesium, CK-MB, troponin, toxicology screen
- Arterial blood gas
- ECG (Fig. 1):
  1. Low voltage: Tamponade
  2. Right heart strain (S1-Q3-T3 pattern, right axis deviation): PE, pneumothorax
  3. Arrhythmias: MI, metabolic abnormalities, drug effects
  4. ST changes, Q waves: MI

IMAGING STUDIES

- Chest radiograph: Rule out pneumothorax, aortic dissection (widened mediastinum).
- Echocardiogram: Rule out tamponade, ischemia (LV contractility, wall motion), valve dysfunction, tumors, and clots. May help diagnose aortic dissection and PE and assess intravascular volume status.
- Abdominal radiograph or ultrasound: Rule out ruptured abdominal aortic aneurysm.

TREATMENT

Identifying and treating a reversible cause is critical.

Physiologic parameters can help monitor quality of CPR and detect the return of spontaneous circulation (ROSC). Suggested methods include quantitative waveform capnography, arterial relaxation diastolic pressure, arterial pressure monitoring, or central venous oxygen saturation.

NONPHARMACOLOGIC THERAPY

- Activate emergency response service.
- Begin CPR; ensure high quality, minimize interruptions. Perform CPR for 2 min between pauses to assess rhythm and circulation.
- Attach cardiac monitor/defibrillator.
- Obtain IV/intraosseous (IO) access.
- Consider advanced airway placement.
- Confirm absence of blood flow with Doppler ultrasound, arterial line, or bedside echocardiogram.

ACUTE GENERAL Rx

- Treat specific cause if known.
- Give 100% oxygen.
- Epinephrine 1 mg IV push/IO, q3 to 5min.
- Give normal saline (20 ml) bolus after peripheral IV administration of medication to improve its distribution.
- Medication can be given via endotracheal tube if IV/IO access cannot be obtained; IV/IO routes preferred because they provide more predictable drug delivery and pharmacologic effects. Give 2 to 2.5× the IV dose in 10 ml of sterile water.
- If rhythm changes to VF or pulseless VT:
  1. Defibrillate.
  2. For refractory VF or pulseless VT consider amiodarone.
- If achieve ROSC, initiate postcardiac arrest care.

DISPOSITION

Of hospitalized patients who develop PEA, <15% survive to discharge. Survival rates much lower in patients with prehospital PEA. Survivors often have poor neurologic outcomes.

REFERRAL

As needed for underlying condition

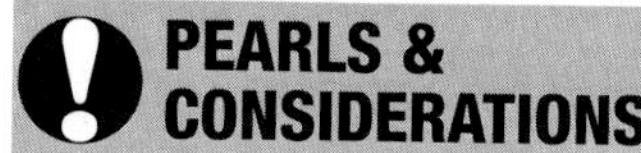

PEARLS & CONSIDERATIONS

- The benefit of epinephrine in PEA resuscitation is uncertain; it may be associated with worse neurologic outcomes and increased long-term mortality. However, the 2015 American Heart Association guidelines support its continued use.
- Targeted temperature management (32° to 36° C [89.6° to 96.8° F] for 24 hr) may improve neurologic outcomes and reduce mortality in comatose cardiac arrest survivors; however, the evidence for therapeutic hypothermia in PEA is based on nonrandomized trials and its role continues to be evaluated. The current AHA guidelines published in 2015 recommend therapeutic hypothermia for all cardiac arrest patients with contraindications.
- Termination of resuscitation guidelines exist for out-of-hospital cardiac arrest. Similar guidelines for in-hospital cardiac arrest are not available; termination of resuscitation is based on multiple patient factors.
- Prognosis may be guided by testing, but no single exam finding or test is definitive; a multimodal approach is needed. Delay testing for at least 72 hr after ROSC. In addition to neurologic examination (corneal and pupillary reflexes, motor response), testing may include median nerve somatosensory-evoked potentials, EEG, biomarkers, and neuroimaging. Prognostication is more difficult in patients treated with hypothermia; wait >72 hr after return to normothermia before attempting to predict outcome.

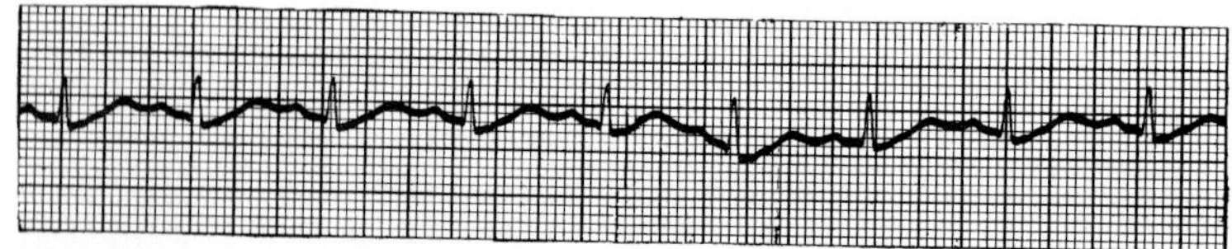

FIG. 1 Sinus rhythm with pulseless electrical activity (PEA). Although the electrocardiogram showed sinus rhythm, the patient had no pulse or blood pressure. In this case the PEA was a result of depressed myocardial function after a cardiac arrest. (From Goldberg AL: *Clinical electrocardiography,* ed 5, St Louis, 1994, Mosby.)

SUGGESTED READINGS

Available at ExpertConsult.com

AUTHOR: **NATHAN RIDDELL, M.D.**

P

Diseases and Disorders

BASIC INFORMATION

DEFINITION

Ascending infection of a bacterial pathogen that infects the renal pelvis and kidney. It primarily presents as a urinary tract infection (UTI) characterized by painful urination (dysuria) with associated flank pain/tenderness, nausea, vomiting, and/or fever. The elderly may also present with failure-to-thrive, unexplained anorexia, other organ system decompensation, or generalized deterioration.

CONSISTS OF TWO GROUPS:

Uncomplicated: Can be treated as an outpatient with oral antibiotics.

Complicated: Inpatient treatment with intravenous antibiotics is required. Hospitalization is indicated for persistent vomiting, progression of uncomplicated UTI, suspected sepsis, immunosuppression, or urinary tract obstruction. This is a potentially life-threatening infection that can lead to renal parenchymal damage. Timely diagnosis and management can significantly impact patient outcomes.

- Acute pyelonephritis
- Pyonephrosis
- Renal carbuncle
- Lobar nephronia
- Acute bacterial nephritis

ICD-10CM CODES

N10	Acute tubulo-interstitial nephritis
N11	Chronic tubulo-interstitial nephritis
N11.0	Nonobstructive reflux-associated chronic pyelonephritis
N11.1	Chronic obstructive pyelonephritis
N11.8	Other chronic tubulo-interstitial nephritis
N11.9	Chronic tubulo-interstitial nephritis, unspecified
N12	Tubulo-interstitial nephritis, not specified as acute or chronic
N20.9	Calculus pyelonephritis

Use additional code (B95-B97) to identify infectious agent.

EPIDEMIOLOGY & DEMOGRAPHICS

INCIDENCE: Pyelonephritis is extremely common in the U.S. (450,000 cases per yr), with highest incidence in the summer. Pyelonephritis is responsible for 9.1% to 31% of severe sepsis cases annually, depending on geographic area. Mortality averages 16.1% annually, ranging from 5% for ages <25 yr to 43% for ages >64 yr.

PREDOMINANT SEX: Women are five times more likely to be hospitalized than men until age 65 yr. Afterward, in males, the difference in prevalence narrows. Risk factors associated with pyelonephritis in healthy women are sexual intercourse (three or more times weekly over the previous 30 days), a new sex partner in the past yr use of spermicide, UTI in the past 12 months, mother with a history of UTI, diabetes mellitus, and urinary incontinence. Urinary tract obstruction is the most important risk factor for a complicated UTI.

PREDOMINANT AGE: Trimodal distribution described in females

- Girls, age 0 to 4 yr
- Women, age 15 to 35 yr, especially if sexually active
- Gradual increase in frequency after age 50 yr, with peak incidence at 80 yr
- Bimodal distribution in males
- Boys, age 0 to 4 yr
- Gradual increase after age 35 yr with peak incidence at 85 yr

GENETICS: Congenital urologic structural disorders associated with vesicoureteral reflux predispose to infections at an early age (<5 yr), and may produce renal scarring in most males and some females. Pyelonephritis may produce an Ask-Upmark kidney (segmental renal hypoplasia) which is found more often in young females with severe hypertension.

PHYSICAL FINDINGS & CLINICAL PRESENTATION

Diagnosis established by clinical presentation, history, and physical examination.

Diagnosis is suspected in cases of lower urinary tract symptoms (e.g., urinary frequency, urgency, and dysuria) accompanied by any of the following:

- Fever, rigors, chills (fever may not be present in the elderly or immunosuppressed)
- Flank pain
- Hematuria: gross hematuria is rare with acute pyelonephritis and raises suspicion for acute cystitis, papillary necrosis, or lower genitourinary malignancy
- Toxic appearance
- Nausea and vomiting
- Headache
- Diarrhea

Physical examination may elicit costovertebral angle tenderness with exquisite flank pain. Flank pain is a nearly universal finding, and its absence suggests an alternative diagnosis. Patients presenting with nephrolithiasis/ureterolithiasis usually do not present with costovertebral angle tenderness. Usually, abdominal or suprapubic tenderness is present.

ETIOLOGY

Ascending infections from intestinal bacteria that colonize the perineum and vulva in women account for most infections. Less commonly, bacteria, viruses, or fungal pathogens may produce hematogenously induced pyelonephritis.

- Gram-negative bacilli cause 95% of cases (e.g., *E. coli* and *Klebsiella* species).
- Less common gram-negative bacteria may produce infection, particularly after urinary tract instrumentation (e.g., *Enterobacter, Serratia,* and *Proteus mirabilis, Pseudomonas*, among others).
- Resistant gram-negative organisms or fungi such as *Candida* may colonize indwelling catheters.
- Gram-positive organisms such as enterococci and rarely, *Staphylococcus saprophyticus*.
- *Staphylococcus aureus* indicates hematogenous spread to the kidneys.
- Viruses generally are limited to the lower urinary tract.
- Urea-splitting organisms generate alkaline urine, which fosters production of staghorn calculi. These stones may grow to large size and cause infection, obstruction, or both.

In the elderly, *E. coli* is less common (60%). Diabetics develop infections from *Klebsiella* species, *Enterobacteriaceae*, *Clostridia* species, or *Candida* species.

During the past decade, community-acquired bacteria (particularly *E. coli*) that produce extended-spectrum beta-lactamases have emerged as a cause of acute pyelonephritis worldwide. The most common risk factors for these uropathogens include frequent visits to health care centers, recent use of antimicrobials (e.g., cephalosporins and fluoroquinolones), older age, immunosuppression, recurrent pyelonephritis, nephrolithiasis, and comorbid conditions such as diabetes mellitus and recurrent UTIs.

Dx DIAGNOSIS

DIFFERENTIAL DIAGNOSIS

Differential diagnosis includes any of the following:

- Abdominal abscess
- Acute abdomen
- Appendicitis
- Basilar pleural process
- Diverticulitis
- Endometriosis
- Herpes zoster
- Lower rib fracture
- Metastatic disease
- Musculoskeletal disorders
- Nephrolithiasis
- Pancreatitis
- Papillary necrosis
- Pelvic inflammatory disease
- Prostatitis
- Pulmonary infarctions
- Renal corticomedullary necrosis
- Renal vein thrombosis
- Retroperitoneal hemorrhage or abscess
- Splenic abscess or infarct
- Urinary tract obstruction
- Vascular pathology

WORKUP

Evaluation includes prostate health assessment in older males.

URINALYSIS

Conducted on a clean-catch voided or catheterized specimen, if unable to void or cooperate. Dipstick and microscopic examination must be performed on a fresh specimen for preservation of formed elements (e.g., cells, casts, and microorganisms). Most cases demonstrate pyuria and positive leukocyte esterase in association with positive blood reaction and microhematuria. Leukocyte casts are generally of renal origin, but may be absent.

URINE CULTURE

Historically, clean, midstream cultures are obtained from all patients suspected of having acute pyelonephritis to guide antibiotic therapy. However, a clean-catch specimen may not be necessary because recent evidence demonstrates no significant difference in the number of contaminated or unreliable culture results when collected with or without preparatory cleansing. Obtain a catheterized urine sample if the patient is unable to void, is uncooperative, or has a change in mental status. There is no difference in colony counts or organisms between catheterized and midstream voiding samples.

More than 95% of acute pyelonephritis cases exhibit more than 10^5 colony-forming units of a single bacterium per ml of urine. However, it is important to obtain an accurate history regarding the timing of culture acquisition and prior antibiotic administration. A negative culture with classic clinical and radiological findings does not rule-out acute pyelonephritis as proven in a prospective study in which only 23.5% of 196 patients with clinical and radiological evidence of acute pyelonephritis demonstrated positive urine cultures. A urine gram stain may aid in the choice of empiric antimicrobial therapy pending urine culture. If gram-positive cocci are seen, one should consider *Enterococcus* species or *Staphylococcus saprophyticus* as causative.

Posttreatment urinalysis and culture are unnecessary if symptomatic improvement occurs, but these studies should be obtained if symptomatic improvement does not occur within 2 to 3 days of antibiotic treatment, or symptoms recur within 2 weeks of treatment. Urinary tract imaging is recommended in these cases.

BLOOD CULTURES

Cultures are obtained from hospitalized patients, but may not be routinely required in uncomplicated cases. Approximately 15% to 30% of patients with acute pyelonephritis are bacteremic. The elderly and individuals with complicated acute pyelonephritis are more likely to develop bacteremia and sepsis.

Urine cultures yield a causative organism in nearly all cases of acute pyelonephritis. Therefore, a positive blood culture may be diagnostically redundant. However, in unclear cases, or when an alternative diagnosis to acute pyelonephritis is considered, endometriosis, intraabdominal or psoas abscess, or cholangitis, blood cultures should be obtained.

RADIOLOGY

Most uncomplicated cases of acute pyelonephritis do not require imaging studies, unless symptoms do not improve or recurrence occurs or patient has prolonged fever (>72 hours) or persistent bacteremia. Abdominal radiographs (i.e., kidney, ureter, and bladder x-ray [KUB]) are of limited use in acute pyelonephritis, unless staghorn calculi are present. Retrograde or antegrade pyelography may be helpful in severe obstruction that is not demonstrated noninvasively. Voiding cystourethrography demonstrates vesicoureteral reflux and is generally performed routinely only in children.

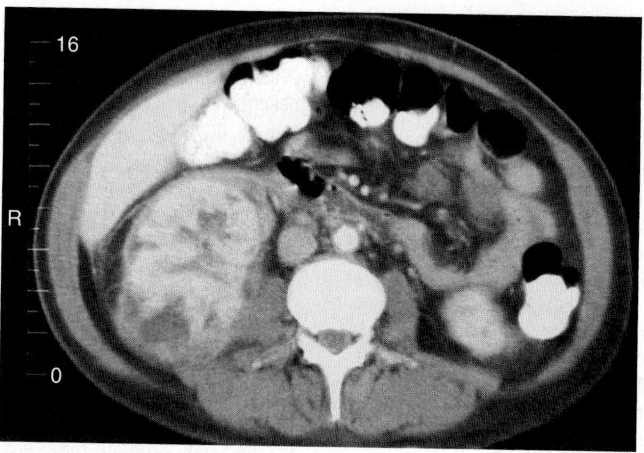

FIG. 1 Acute pyelonephritis: Contrast material–enhanced computed tomographic (CT) scan. The heterogeneous CT nephrogram shows the diffuse involvement of the right kidney. Stranding and some fluid are visible in the perinephric space with thickening of Gerota fascia. (From Skorecki K et al: *Brenner & Rector's the Kidney*, ed 10, Philadelphia, 2016, Elsevier.)

Recommendations for radiologic tests:

- Healthy patients with uncomplicated pyelonephritis typically do not require radiologic workup when therapeutic responses occur within 72 hours of antibiotic therapy.
- If no response to therapy occurs within 72 hours, abdominal CT is the study of choice.
- Diabetics and immunocompromised patients should undergo precontrast and postcontrast abdominal and pelvic CT scans (Fig. 1) within 24 hours of diagnosis when response to therapy is not prompt.
- Ultrasound (Fig. 2) is reserved for patients in whom exposure to contrast or radiation is considered hazardous. There is a high false-negative rate for renal abscess with ultrasound. In a prospective study of acute pyelonephritis of 213 patients submitted for CT/NMR study, 50 patients (23.5%) had a renal abscess, yet only two were detected by ultrasound.
- All other adults with complicated cases (i.e., history of stones or other urologic conditions, prior urologic surgery, repeated episodes of pyelonephritis) should be evaluated early by CT.
- Helical CT detects calculi with high sensitivity.
- Urologic imaging studies should be conducted in all young men and boys.

Although the risk of contrast nephropathy has declined substantially, exert caution during contrast administration to patients with chronic kidney disease or taking metformin. When evaluating kidney function, base diagnostic decision making on eGFR, not serum creatinine, especially in the elderly. Patients with acute pyelonephritis and acutely elevated baseline serum creatinine may warrant CT imaging as part of an evaluation to rule out obstruction. If the risk of radiocontrast administration outweighs benefits, consider retrograde or antegrade pyelography.

The purpose of imaging is to identify underlying structural abnormalities, such as occult obstruction from a stone or abscess, and serious complications such as emphysematous pyelonephritis. In a prospective study of 213 patients with acute pyelonephritis, no differences occurred in frequency of fever, leukocytosis, C-reactive protein, pyuria, urine cultures, and duration of symptoms before hospitalization for positive or negative CT. Thus, systematic CT or magnetic resonance imaging is not required to exclude an anatomical abnormality, as noted previously, and such an abnormality cannot be predicted based on clinical, biochemical, or culture parameters. Emphysematous pyelonephritis is a necrotizing infection that produces intraparenchymal kidney gas identifiable by renal imaging that is associated with high mortality. Risk factors include diabetes mellitus and/or urinary tract obstruction. Gas-forming bacteria, most commonly *E. coli*, produce gas that is usually restricted within Gerota's fascia. If gas is localized to the kidney, mortality is 60%. If gas spreads to the perinephric space, mortality is 80%. In emphysematous pyelitis, the mortality is 20%. This must be differentiated from a renal abscess that can also be associated with a gas collection. With drainage and antibiotic treatment, a renal abscess has a favorable prognosis.

LABORATORY TESTS

A basic metabolic profile and CBC with differential count are needed on all patients with suspected acute pyelonephritis to estimate renal function. If the diagnosis is in doubt, other laboratory tests may be appropriate to clarify the differential diagnosis (e.g., lipase, transaminase, and β-HCG levels).

Rx TREATMENT

ACUTE GENERAL Rx

UNCOMPLICATED ACUTE PYELONEPHRITIS: Close outpatient follow-up is possible with minimal gastrointestinal symptoms, and an ability to maintain fluid intake and oral medications. Prompt antibiotic therapy prevents progression of infection and must be initiated following acquisition of appropriate cultures. Begin empiric therapy based on risk of adverse effects, local community bacterial profiles, and

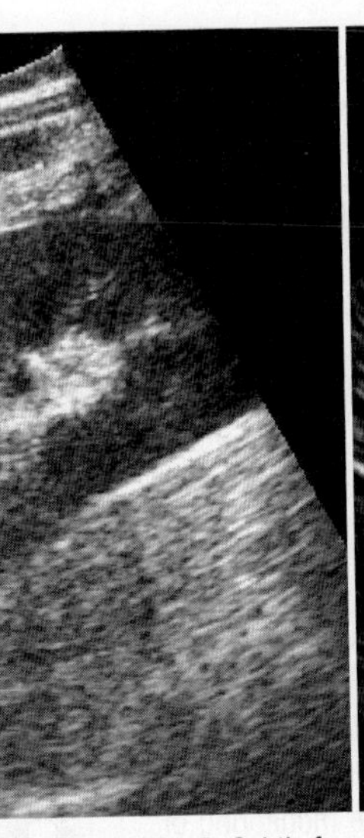
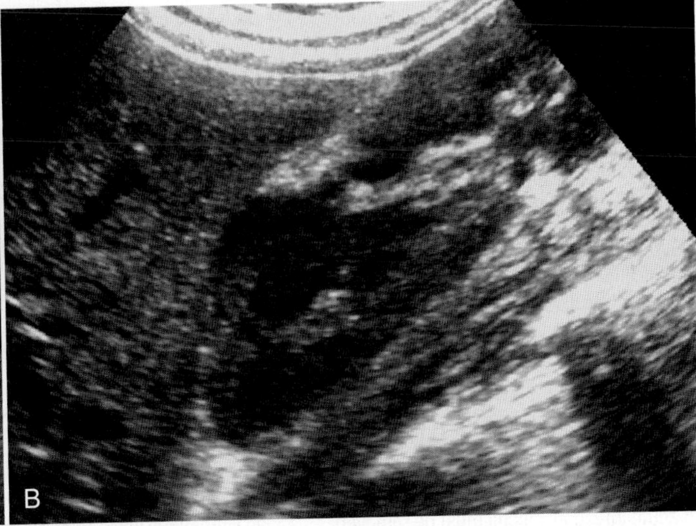

FIG. 2 Acute pyelonephritis. A, Subtle focal increased echogenic areas are seen in the anterior cortex of the right kidney. **B,** Single focal hypoechoic area is seen in the upper pole of the kidney in another patient. (From Rumack CM et al: *Diagnostic ultrasound*, ed 4, Philadelphia, 2011, Elsevier.)

resistance rates. Antibiotics are revised after urine culture results are available.

The concept of requiring long-term treatment of acute pyelonephritis has been questioned. Women with acute pyelonephritis were randomized to oral treatment with ciprofloxacin 500 mg twice daily for 7 days or 14 days, and 27% of these patients experienced bacteremia from *E. coli*. No differences in the cure rates were found (87% and 96%, respectively).

Outpatient regimens:

- Fluoroquinolones are preferred in communities where local prevalence of resistant *E. coli* is ≤10%.
- Ciprofloxacin 500 mg by mouth twice daily or a single, 1000-mg dose in the extended-release form by mouth daily for 7 days.
- Levofloxacin 750 mg by mouth daily for 5 days.
- The initial dose may be administered intravenously (ciprofloxacin 400 mg or levofloxacin 500 mg).
- When a fluoroquinolone is contraindicated, alternative treatment with trimethoprim/sulfamethoxazole 160/800 mg PO twice daily for 10 to 14 days may be administered if the pathogen is susceptible. Recent data suggest that stopping treatment at 7 days may be equally effective.

Because of the high prevalence of resistance to oral beta-lactam antibiotics and trimethoprim/sulfamethoxazole, these agents usually are reserved for cases where susceptibility results are known, but additional factors (e.g., allergy history, potential drug-drug interactions, drug availability) may require empiric treatment with these agents before susceptibility results are known. For such cases, a long-acting, broad-spectrum parenteral drug (e.g., ceftriaxone 1 gram or gentamicin 5 mg/kg) may be administered as a one-time dose or longer until sensitivities of the organism are known. If the local prevalence of fluoroquinolone resistance to *E. coli* exceeds 10%, an initial intravenous dose of ceftriaxone or gentamicin is recommended, followed by an oral fluoroquinolone regimen.

Significant clinical improvement during appropriate empiric antibiotic therapy should occur within 48 to 72 hours. If improvement does not occur, a complication of acute pyelonephritis or an alternative diagnosis such as an abscess, emphysematous pyelonephritis, or an obstructing calculus should be considered. Any unexpected change in the clinical picture warrants immediate investigation with CT or MRI, with potential for surgical intervention.

COMPLICATED ACUTE PYELONEPHRITIS: Hospitalization is indicated for the following reasons:

- Toxic patients
- Complicated infections
- Diabetes or otherwise immunosuppressed
- Suspected bacteremia

Inpatient care includes supportive care, monitoring of culture results, adjustment of antibiotic regimen, and intravenous volume repletion as required. Intravenous antibiotics are continued until defervescence, and clinical improvement occurs, with subsequent conversion to an oral antibiotic regimen for a total duration of 10 to 14 days.

- Intravenous antibiotic options for more toxic patients pending cultures include ceftriaxone (1 to 2 g once daily), IV ciprofloxacin (400 mg every 12 hours) or IV levofloxacin (500 to 750 mg IV once daily), piperacillin/tazobactam (3.375 g IV every 6 hours) or carbapenems such as meropenem or imipenem (500 mg IV every 6 to 8 hours).
- Ceftazidime 1 to 2 g IV every 8 hours, piperacillin/tazobactam, and carbapenems are optimal choices for *Pseudomonas* due to this organism's increasing ciprofloxacin resistance.
- Aminoglycosides (2 mg/kg IV loading dose followed by 1 mg/kg IV every 8 to 12 hours, adjusted for kidney function) are potentially nephrotoxic, and are used only when there is no better alternative. Vancomycin 1 g IV every 12 hours, linezolid 600 mg IV or PO every 12 hours, or daptomycin 4 to 6 mg/kg IV daily for gram-positive cocci (e.g., enterococci, staphylococci).
- Ampicillin 1 to 2 g IV every 4 to 6 hours for ampicillin-sensitive enterococci with aminoglycoside for synergy. Urinary obstruction is promptly drained by nephrostomy tube. Surgical drainage of abscess formation(s).
- Pregnant females with acute pyelonephritis are hospitalized and treated initially with a second- or third-generation cephalosporin.

RENAL ABSCESSES (RENAL CARBUNCLES)

Cortical abscesses historically required surgical drainage; however, using current antibiotics is commonly sufficient for cure.

- Semisynthetic penicillin, cephalosporin, fluoroquinolone, or vancomycin, with guidance from culture and sensitivity results.
    1. Parenteral therapy for 10 to 14 days followed by oral therapy for 2 to 4 wk.
    2. Fever should resolve in 5 to 6 days and pain within 24 hours.
    3. If no clinical response within 48 hours, percutaneous or open drainage should be considered. More extreme measures are sometimes needed including enucleation or nephrectomy.

CORTICOMEDULLARY ABSCESSES

- Parenteral therapy for at least 48 hours is typically successful.
- May require incision and drainage and possibly nephrectomy.
- If clinical defervescence occurs, intravenous antibiotic treatment may be switched to complete a 2-wk course of oral antibiotic therapy.

PERINEPHRIC ABSCESSES

- Serious complication with mortality in the 25% to 50% range.

- Requires early recognition, surgical drainage, and parenteral antibiotics (not adequate alone) to reduce mortality.
- Initial antibiotic therapy should include an aminoglycoside and an antistaphylococcal agent.
  1. If *Pseudomonas* species grow in culture or is suspected, add an antipseudomonal beta-lactam antibiotic to the aminoglycoside.
  2. For enterococcus, an aminoglycoside and ampicillin are recommended.
- Reported with tuberculosis or fungi as rare causes.
- Nephrectomy may be considered with clinical deterioration despite aggressive therapy.

CALCULI-RELATED INFECTIONS

Organisms may survive within calculi making these cases especially problematic.

- With acute infection, calculi must be removed immediately using cystoscopy or open surgical procedure.
  1. Surgical observation is not recommended as mortality is 28% with observation versus 7.2% in surgical treated group.
- In staghorn calculi, it is optimal to remove the entire stone (as remaining fragments are still infected and may recur).
  1. Urease inhibitors are effective at reducing stone formation.
     a. Limited by long-term toxicity with neurosensory, hematologic, and dermatologic adverse side effects.

RENAL PAPILLARY NECROSIS

- Admission for parenteral antibiotics:
  1. Initial therapy should cover *E. coli*, *Enterobacter*, *Proteus*, and *Klebsiella* species pending culture results.
  2. For more serious infections, also cover *Pseudomonas* and *Enterococcus.*
  3. Empiric therapy agent options include:
     a. Aminoglycosides
     b. Cefotaxime
     c. Ceftriaxone
     d. Ceftazidime
     e. Cefepime
     f. Piperacillin-tazobactam
     g. Imipenem-cilastatin
     h. Meropenem
     i. Ciprofloxacin
  4. Continue parenteral therapy until fever and clinical symptoms defervesce (typically 14 days).

CHRONIC Rx

- Repair underlying structural problems, especially when kidney function is compromised.
  1. Reflux
  2. Obstruction
  3. Suspect nephrolithiasis
- Avoid urinary catheters.

DISPOSITION

- If pyelonephritis is uncomplicated with no significant GI symptoms, it can be treated on an outpatient basis with close monitoring of therapeutic response(s) in 48 to 72 hours.
- If pyelonephritis is complicated and symptoms persist for >48 to 72 hours, or any of the following exist, admission is warranted: significant GI symptoms that preclude oral therapy, pregnancy, urinary tract obstruction, suspected renal or perinephric abscess, bacterial sepsis, diabetes or other immunocompromised states, recurrent or refractory pyelonephritis, or infection with unusual or antibiotic-resistant microorganism.
- If sepsis is present, consider intensive care unit care.
- Acute pyelonephritis may be fatal when complications develop, such as emphysematous pyelonephritis (20% to 80% mortality rate), perinephric abscess (20% to 50% mortality rate), or sepsis syndrome (>25% overall mortality rate).
- Acute deterioration or nonresponse to conventional therapy may be due to a complication, resistant organism, or unrecognized comorbidity.
- Diabetic patients with acute pyelonephritis are prone to bacteremia, longer hospital stays, and greater mortality. Diabetics should be considered complicated patients.
- Patients >65 yr of age experience greater mortality, septic shock, bedridden status, and immunosuppression. In males, mortality is also increased with the use of antibiotics in the previous month.

REFERRAL

- General surgery or urology for suspected abscess
- Infectious disease for resistant organisms and poor response to routine antibiotic therapy as outlined
- Urology to correct underlying urologic problems (e.g., reflux and hydronephrosis)
- Nephrology consult if renal dysfunction is present or for nephrolithiasis workup
- Critical care medicine, if patient requires ICU admission

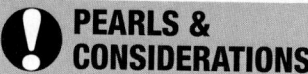

PEARLS & CONSIDERATIONS

- Consider acute pyelonephritis in anyone with urinary symptoms, flank pain, and fever.
- Obtain a urinalysis and culture before starting empiric antibiotic therapy, and adjust treatment, pending antibiotic sensitivity testing.
- Evaluate clinical response in 48 to 72 hours during outpatient therapy. If no or delayed improvement, continue evaluation to rule out urinary tract obstruction.
- Urology consultation in all cases of urinary tract obstruction or detection of urinary tract gas (e.g., emphysematous pyelonephritis).
- Treat all diabetics as complicated acute pyelonephritis.

SUGGESTED READINGS

Available at ExpertConsult.com

RELATED CONTENT

Pyelonephritis (Patient Information)

AUTHORS: **JAMES P. REICHART, M.D.,** and **NELSON KOPYT, D.O.**

BASIC INFORMATION

DEFINITION

Radial tunnel syndrome describes a form of compression neuropathy of the posterior interosseous nerve, a branch of the radial nerve, which presents mainly as pain over the dorso-radial aspect of the forearm (Fig. 1). The radial tunnel is formed by the capitellum posteriorly, the brachioradialis and the extensor carpi radialis longus and brevis muscles anterolaterally, and the brachialis muscle and biceps tendon medially. The posterior interosseous nerve supplies the supinator and extensor muscles of the forearm, including the extensor carpi ulnaris, extensor digitorum, extensor digiti minimi, extensor indicis, extensor pollicis longus and brevis muscles, and abductor pollicis longus.

There is some controversy as to whether radial tunnel syndrome is a distinct entity or a variation of posterior interosseous nerve (PIN) syndrome. Patients may be found to have radial tunnel syndrome in the presence of forearm pain and localized tenderness over the radial nerve without weakness.

SYNONYM

Radial pronator syndrome

ICD-10CM CODE

G56.30 Lesion of radial nerve, unspecified upper limb.

EPIDEMIOLOGY & DEMOGRAPHICS

INCIDENCE: Rare, annual incidence is <0.03%

PEAK INCIDENCE: Unknown

PREDOMINANT SEX & AGE: Peak between age 30 and 50, likely slight female predominance, studies range from a female:male ratio of 1:1 to 6:1

GENETICS: Unknown

RISK FACTORS: Trauma and heavy manual labor, especially those who perform forearm extensions in pronation or supination

PHYSICAL FINDINGS & CLINICAL PRESENTATION

Patients with radial tunnel syndrome present with pain in the proximal forearm, which is often exacerbated by activities that involve repetitive forearm pronation, wrist extension, and elbow extension. Pain is usually felt over lateral epicondyle of the humerus radiating distally toward radial styloid and thumb with maximum pain 3 to 5 cm distal to the lateral epicondyle.

Physical examination shows localized tenderness over the radial nerve distal to the lateral epicondyle. Pain is worsened with forearm pronation, wrist flexion, and elbow extension. The finding of localized forearm pain with extension of the third digit against resistance is thought to be specific for radial tunnel syndrome. The finding of weakness in the distribution of the radial nerve suggests diagnosis of PIN syndrome.

ETIOLOGY

- Localized compression sometimes related to repetitive movements or work-force injury; but often idiopathic
- Rarely, space occupying lesions, such as lipomas or ganglions

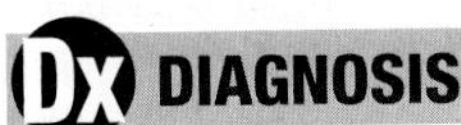

DIAGNOSIS

DIFFERENTIAL DIAGNOSIS

- Lateral epicondylitis, which may often co-occur
- Posterior interosseous nerve syndrome

WORKUP

Anesthetic injection into the radial tunnel, which should provide pain relief, and can then serve as a marker for correct injection location for corticosteroids

LABORATORY TESTS

N/A

IMAGING STUDIES

- No role for electromyogram (EMG)/nerve conduction velocity (NCV) large myelinated fibers of PIN remain normal (no weakness)
- MRI usually negative and has a limited role. Can be helpful in ruling out lipoma/ganglion as cause of compression, or rarely show denervation/edema within supinator/extensor.

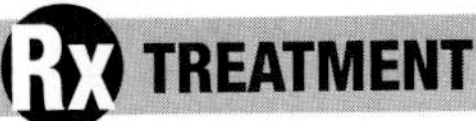

TREATMENT

ACUTE GENERAL Rx

- Wrist splinting, generally at nighttime
- NSAIDs
- Corticosteroid injection

CHRONIC Rx

Activity modification

DISPOSITION

- Conservative treatment and steroid injection results in about 60% of patients being pain free at 2 yr
- Radial tunnel release surgery has a patient satisfaction rate of about 40%

REFERRAL

Surgical referral for radial tunnel release surgery—if conservative measures fail

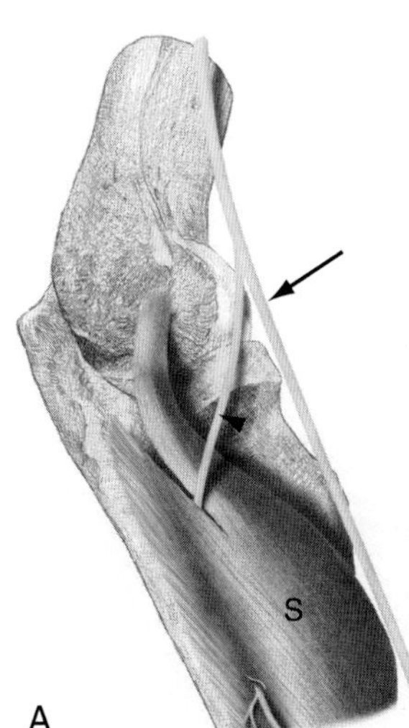

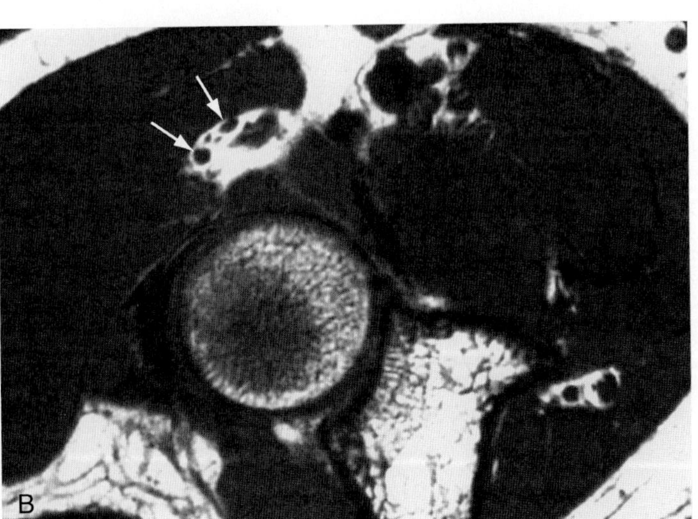

FIG. 1 Normal anatomy of the radial nerve in the elbow area. A, Lateral illustration. The radial nerve courses distally in the anterior aspect of the elbow and arm. At the level of the elbow joint it divides into two branches: the superficial sensory branch *(arrow)* and the deep motor branch or posterior interosseous nerve *(arrowhead)*. The posterior interosseous nerve penetrates the supinator muscle *(S)* between the superficial and the deep layers (the arcade of Fröhse). **B,** Axial T1-weighted magnetic resonance image. (From Pope TL et al: *Musculoskeletal imaging*, ed 2, Philadelphia, 2015, Elsevier.)

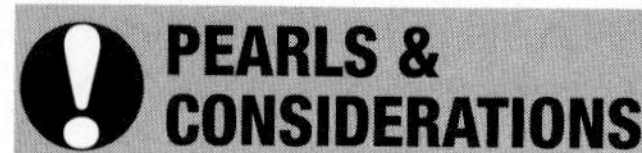

PEARLS & CONSIDERATIONS

COMMENTS

Radial tunnel syndrome coexists with lateral epicondylitis in about 5% of patients. In lateral epicondylitis, pain is directly over lateral epicondyle rather than more distal, as in radial tunnel syndrome.

PREVENTION

Activity modification and avoidance of forearm pronation, wrist flexion, and elbow extension

SUGGESTED READINGS

Available at ExpertConsult.com

RELATED CONTENT

Epicondylitis
Pronator Syndrome

AUTHOR: **JAN M. KARCZEWSKI, M.D.**

BASIC INFORMATION

DEFINITION

Ramsay Hunt syndrome is a localized herpes zoster infection involving the seventh nerve and geniculate ganglia, resulting in hearing loss, vertigo, and facial nerve palsy.

SYNONYMS

Herpes zoster oticus
Geniculate herpes
Herpetic geniculate ganglionitis

ICD-10CM CODE
B02.21 Postherpetic geniculate ganglionitis

EPIDEMIOLOGY & DEMOGRAPHICS

PREDOMINANT SEX: Equal sex distribution
PREDOMINANT AGE:
- Increasingly common with advancing age
- Rare in childhood

PHYSICAL FINDINGS & CLINICAL PRESENTATION

- Characteristic vesicles:
  1. On pinna
  2. In external auditory canal (Fig. 1)
  3. In distribution of the facial nerve and, occasionally, adjacent cranial nerves
- Facial paralysis on the involved side
- Auditory symptoms include mild to severe tinnitus, deafness, vertigo, and nystagmus.

ETIOLOGY

- Reactivation of dormant infection with varicella-zoster virus after primary varicella.
- Herpetic inflammation of the geniculate ganglion is thought to be the cause of this syndrome.

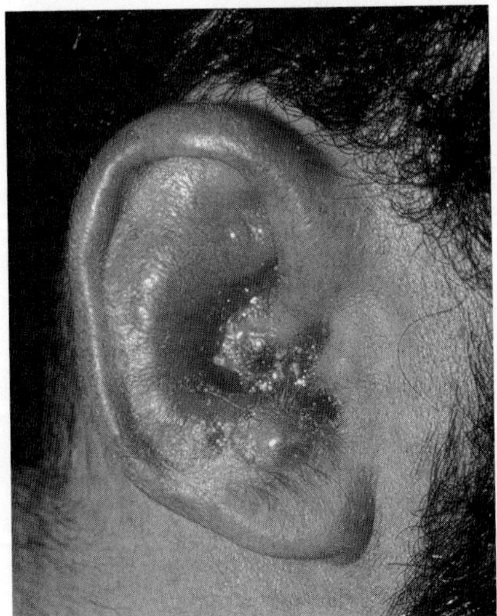

FIG. 1 Herpes zoster of the geniculate ganglion resulting in vesicles on the ear (as shown here) and tympanic membrane occurs in Ramsay Hunt syndrome. Both seventh and eighth cranial nerve functions may be affected. (From White GM, Cox NH [eds]: *Diseases of the skin: color atlas and text*, ed 2, St Louis, 2006, Mosby.)

DIAGNOSIS

- Usually made by recognition of the clinical features detailed previously
- Viral culture and/or microscopic examination of specimens taken from active vesicles

DIFFERENTIAL DIAGNOSIS

- Herpes simplex
- External otitis
- Impetigo
- Enteroviral infection
- Guillain-Barre syndrome
- Bell palsy of other etiologies, such as Lyme disease
- Acoustic neuroma (before appearance of skin lesions)

The differential diagnosis of headache and facial pain is described in Section II.

WORKUP

If the diagnosis is in doubt, confirm varicella-zoster virus infection.

LABORATORY TESTS

- Generally not necessary
- Viral culture of specimens of vesicular fluid and scrapings of the vesicle base
- Tzanck preparation, which may reveal multinucleated giant cells
- Direct immunofluorescent staining of scrapings

IMAGING STUDIES

MRI may demonstrate enhancement of the facial and vestibulocochlear nerves before appearance of vesicles.

TREATMENT

ACUTE GENERAL Rx

- Use of corticosteroids is controversial.
- Acyclovir (800 mg PO five times qd for 10 days), famciclovir (500 mg tid for 7 days), or valacyclovir (1 g q8h for 7 days) may hasten healing.
- Use of prednisone (60 mg PO qd for 7 days or on a tapering regimen, 40 mg PO for 2 days, 30 mg for 7 days, followed by tapering course) is recommended by some authors, but its use remains controversial.
- Analgesics should be used as indicated.

CHRONIC Rx

- Duloxetine and amitriptyline are effective in postherpetic pain.
- Other agents for postherpetic pain include gabapentin and pregabalin.
- Narcotic analgesics may occasionally be necessary.

DISPOSITION

Recurrences are unusual.

REFERRAL

To otolaryngologist: Patients with persistent facial paralysis for potential surgical decompression of the facial nerve

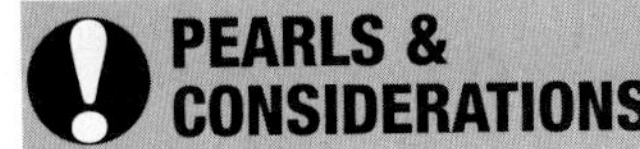

PEARLS & CONSIDERATIONS

COMMENTS

Immunodeficiency states, particularly HIV infection, should be considered in:
- Younger patients
- Severe cases
- Patients with a history of specific risk behavior

SUGGESTED READINGS

Available at ExpertConsult.com

RELATED CONTENT

Ramsay Hunt Syndrome (Patient Information)
Herpes Zoster (Related Key Topic)

AUTHOR: **GLENN G. FORT, M.D., M.P.H.**

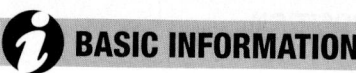

BASIC INFORMATION

DEFINITION

Raynaud's phenomenon (RP) is a vasospastic disorder that causes an exaggerated response to cold temperatures and/or emotional stress, resulting in episodic digital ischemia. It presents as a cold-induced, symmetric, sharply demarcated white or blue discoloration of the distal fingers or toes, followed by erythema at a variable time after rewarming.

SYNONYMS

Primary Raynaud's phenomenon or Raynaud's disease
Secondary Raynaud's phenomenon
RP

ICD-10CM CODES

I73.0 Raynaud's syndrome
I73.00 Raynaud's syndrome without gangrene
I73.01 Raynaud's syndrome with gangrene

EPIDEMIOLOGY & DEMOGRAPHICS

- RP is classified clinically into primary or secondary forms and affects approximately 3% to 5% of the general population, 15% of children younger than 12 yr, and less than 1% of adults older than 60 yr.
- Occurs more commonly in colder climates.
- Primary RP usually occurs between the ages of 12 and 25 yr.
- It is more likely to affect women than men (4:1).
- 5% to 15% of patients with primary Raynaud's phenomenon develop a secondary cause later in the course of the disease (mostly a connective tissue disorder).
- Secondary RP tends to begin after age 35 to 40 yr.
- Secondary RP occurs in more than 90% of patients with scleroderma and in approximately 30% of patients with systemic lupus erythematosus or Sjögren's syndrome.

PHYSICAL FINDINGS & CLINICAL PRESENTATION

- The typical manifestation of RP is the biphasic color response of the digits to cold exposure and rewarming, which may or may not be accompanied by pain. RP most often affects the hand (Fig. 1).
  1. White (pallor) or blue (cyanotic) discoloration of the digit(s) resulting from vasospasm on cold or vibration exposure.
  2. Red (rubor) with or without pain and paresthesia when vasospasm resolves and blood returns to the digit.
- Color changes can sometimes be induced by placing the hand in an ice bath, although this is not recommended as a diagnostic maneuver because responses may be inconsistent even in patients with definite RP.
- Color changes are well delineated, symmetric, and usually bilateral, involving the fingers and toes. The index, middle, and ring fingers are commonly involved and the thumb infrequently; however, if the thumb is involved, that suggests secondary causes of RP.
- Fingertips are most often involved, but feet, ears, nose, tongue, and nipples can also be affected.
- Patients with RP may exhibit a violaceous or reticular pattern of skin of arms and legs, sometimes with regular, unbroken circles (livedo reticularis).
- Duration of attacks can range from seconds to hours and averages 15 to 20 min.
- Chronic skin changes resulting from repeated attacks may include skin thickening and brittle nails. Ulcerations and, rarely, gangrene may occur.
- Physical examination should also include examination for symptoms associated with autoimmune disease, such as fever, rash, arthritis, dry eyes, dry mouth, myalgias, or cardiopulmonary abnormalities.

ETIOLOGY

- Primary RP can also be called idiopathic Raynaud's phenomenon, primary Raynaud's syndrome, or Raynaud's disease. It occurs in the absence of any associated disease.
- With primary RP, the possibility that another first-degree family member is affected is reported as approximately 25%.
- Secondary RP is associated with an underlying pathologic condition or disorder, use of certain drugs, or related occupation. Secondary causes of Raynaud's phenomenon are summarized in Box 1.

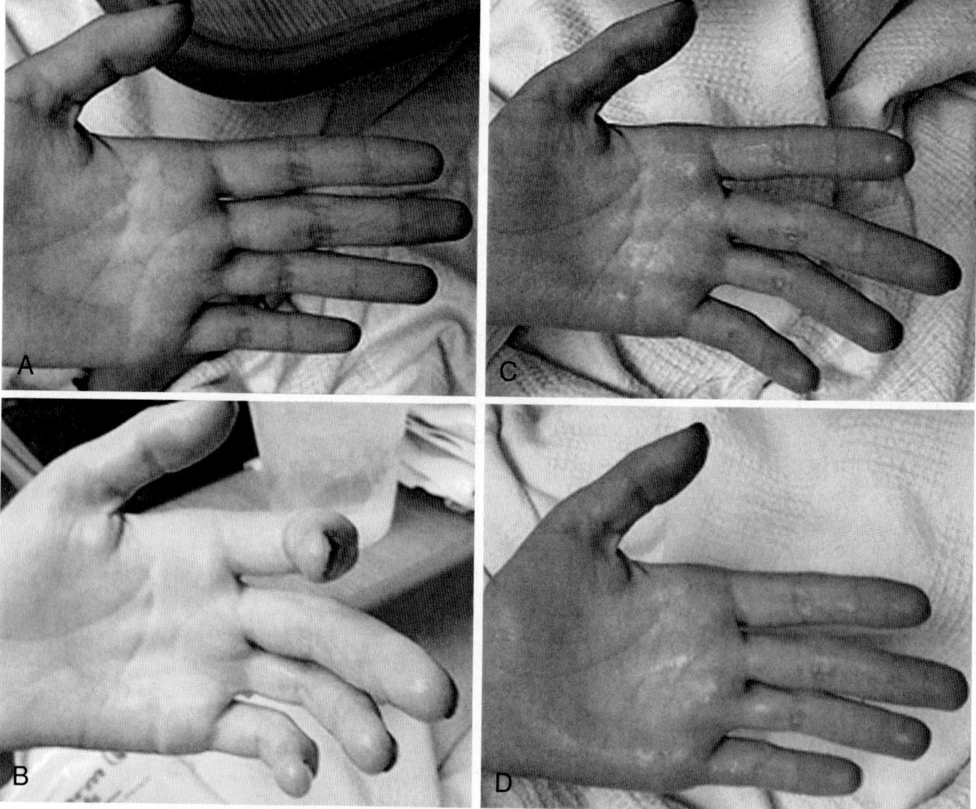

FIG. 1 Raynaud's phenomenon in a patient with Ehlers-Danlos syndrome to illustrate the color changes associated with stressful stimuli. **A,** Normal-appearing hand. **B,** After cold stimuli, the pallor from vasoconstriction can be seen. **C,** After 30 seconds, the hyperemic red appears in fingers with blood reperfusion. **D,** Hand after 3 minutes exposed to stimuli. (From Cameron JL, Cameron AM: *Current surgical therapy*, ed 12, Philadelphia, 2017, Elsevier.)

BOX 1 Secondary Causes of Raynaud's Phenomenon

Rheumatologic
Systemic sclerosis (CREST syndrome)
Sjögren's syndrome
Systemic lupus erythematosus
Ehlers-Danlos syndrome
Rheumatoid arthritis
Dermatomyositis
Polymyositis
Mixed connective tissue disease

Autoimmune
Reiter syndrome
Vasculitis (polyarteritis nodosa, Henoch-Schönlein purpura)
Antiphospholipid syndrome
Primary pulmonary hypertension

Endocrine
Hypothyroidism
Pheochromocytoma
Carcinoid

Infectious
Hepatitis B and C infection
Mycoplasma pneumonia

Medications
Cyclosporine
Ergotamine
Beta-blockers
Cytotoxic (bleomycin, cisplatin, vinblastine)
Bromocriptine
Nicotine
Cocaine
Sulfasalazine
Interferon-alpha and interferon-beta
Clonidine
Sympathomimetics
Estrogen in oral contraceptives
Caffeine

Occlusive Vascular
Arteriosclerosis
Vascular trauma (hypothenar hammer syndrome)
Buerger disease
Thoracic outlet syndrome
Thromboembolism

Hematologic Proliferative
Leukemia
Lymphoma
Polycythemia vera
Multiple myeloma
Disseminated intravascular coagulation
Cryoglobulinemia
Cold agglutinin disease

Neurologic
Migraines
Carpal tunnel syndrome
Polyneuropathy

Environmental
Emotional stress
Frostbite
Repetitive trauma or injuries to hand

Malignancy
Lung, stomach, small bowel
Paraneoplastic syndrome
Neurofibromatosis

From Cameron JL, Cameron AM: *Current surgical therapy*, ed 12, Philadelphia, 2017, Elsevier.

Dx DIAGNOSIS

Clinical criteria:
- Definite RP: Repeated episodes of biphasic color change on cold exposure
- Possible RP: Uniphasic color changes plus numbness or paresthesia on cold exposure
- No RP: No color change on cold exposure

The suggested criteria for primary RP are:
- Symmetric attacks
- Absence of tissue necrosis, ulceration, gangrene, or peripheral vascular disease
- Absence of a secondary cause on the basis of a patient's history and general physical examination
- Negative nail-fold capillary examination
- Negative test for antinuclear antibody (ANA)
- Normal erythrocyte sedimentation rate (ESR)

Secondary RP is suggested by the following findings:
- Onset of symptoms after age 30 yr
- Male gender
- Episodes that are painful, asymmetric, or associated with ischemic skin lesions
- Clinical features suggestive of a connective-tissue disease
- Elevated specific autoantibody tests and ESR
- Evidence of microvascular disease on microscopy of nail-fold capillaries
- It is critical to differentiate primary and secondary RP since management is significantly different for the two conditions. Table 1 summarizes characteristics of primary and secondary Raynaud's phenomenon

DIFFERENTIAL DIAGNOSIS

- Neurogenic thoracic outlet syndrome or carpal tunnel syndrome
- Frostbite or cold weather injury
- Medication reaction (ergotamine, chemotherapeutic agents)
- Atherosclerosis, thromboembolic disease
- Buerger disease, embolic disease
- Acrocyanosis
- Livedo reticularis
- Injury from repetitive motion

WORKUP

- Fig. 2 describes an approach to diagnosis of Raynaud's phenomenon. Once the diagnosis of RP is established, differentiating primary from secondary is helpful in treatment and prognosis.
- Patients who are younger when their symptoms occur, have a normal history and physical examination and normal nail-fold capillaries, and have no history of digital ischemic lesions can be considered as having primary RP. These patients can be monitored clinically without any further testing.
- If a secondary cause of RP is suspected, appropriate laboratory testing is recommended (see "Laboratory Tests"). Secondary RP has associated abnormal nail-fold microscopy.

LABORATORY TESTS

- CBC, serum electrolytes, blood urea nitrogen, creatinine, ESR, ANAs, VDRL antibody test, rheumatoid factor, and urinalysis should be included in the initial evaluation.
- If the history, physical examination, and initial laboratory tests suggest a possible secondary

TABLE 1 Characteristics of Primary and Secondary Raynaud's Phenomenon

Characteristic	Primary	Secondary
Age	Younger (<30 years)	Older (>30 years)
Gender preference	Female	Male (depending on secondary cause)
Incidence	Most common	Less common
Familial predisposition	Yes	Yes
Combination with other disease	No, idiopathic	Associated with systemic disease
Vascular defect	Functional dysregulation of autonomic nervous system	Structural changes in connective tissue or vessels
Associated signs	None	Arthritis, sclerodactyly, cardiopulmonary abnormality, rash
Frequency	Precipitated by stimuli	Periodic and stimuli trigger
Severity of symptoms	Long history of mild attacks	Severe and disabling pain
Distribution	Symmetric	Asymmetric
Duration	Self-limited	Need for additional treatment (pharmacologic, surgery)
Critical complications	None	Ischemia and ulcers
Capillaroscopy	Normal (symmetric, thin, and uniform)	Abnormal (dilated, irregular, elongated, and tortuous vessel)
Vascular examination	Normal pulses	Abnormal pulses
Erythrocyte sedimentation rate	Normal	Elevated
Serologic studies	Negative	Antinuclear antibody, autoantibodies
C-reactive protein	Normal	Elevated

From Cameron JL, Cameron AM: *Current surgical therapy*, ed 12, Philadelphia, 2017, Elsevier.

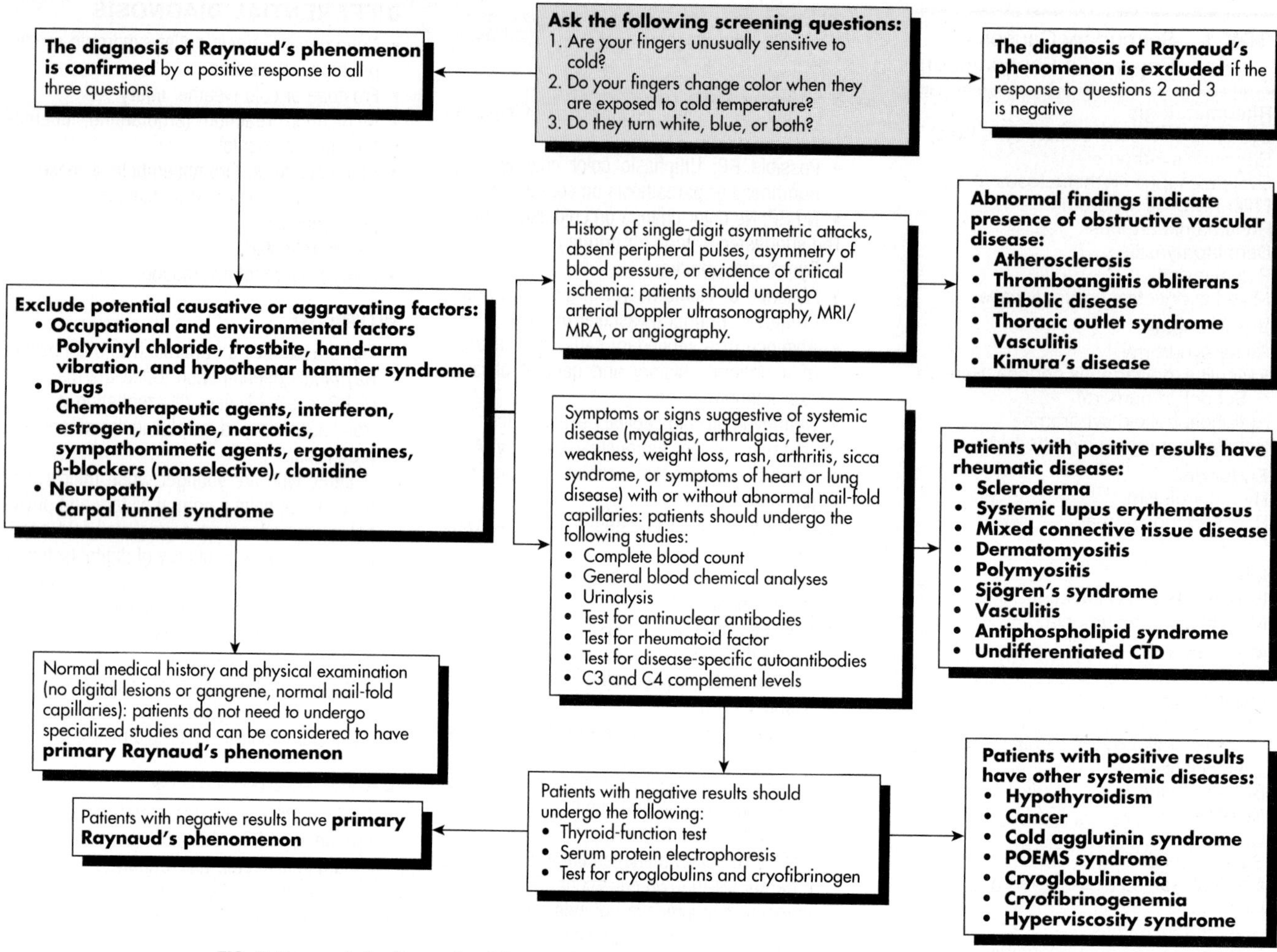

FIG. 2 Approach to diagnosis of Raynaud's phenomenon. *CTD,* Connective tissue disease; *MRA,* magnetic resonance angiography; *MRI,* magnetic resonance imaging; *POEMS,* polyneuropathy, organomegaly, endocrinopathy, monoclonal gammopathy, and skin changes. (From Firestein GS et al [eds]: *Kelly's textbook of rheumatology,* ed 9, Philadelphia, 2013, Saunders.)

cause, specific serologic testing (e.g., anticentromere antibodies, anti-Scl 70, cryoglobulins, complement testing, and serum protein electrophoresis) may be indicated.

- Noninvasive vascular testing includes finger systolic blood pressures, segmental blood pressure measurements, cold recovery time (measure vasoconstrictor and vasodilator responses of finger to cold), fingertip thermography, and laser Doppler with thermal challenge (measures relative change in skin blood flow with ambient warming).

IMAGING STUDIES

- The diagnosis of RP should not be made on the basis of laboratory tests, and imaging studies should not replace a good history and physical examination.
- Duplex ultrasound can image the palmar arch and digital arteries for patency.
- Magnetic resonance angiography is useful for imaging larger arteries.
- Contrast angiography is the gold standard for arterial imaging.
- Nail-fold capillary microscopy can differentiate primary from secondary RP.
- Videomicroscopy and thermography are also useful for diagnosis of RP.

Rx TREATMENT

NONPHARMACOLOGIC THERAPY

- Avoid drugs that may precipitate RP (see "Etiology").
- Avoid cold exposure and sudden temperature shifts. Use warm gloves, hats, and garments during the winter months or before going into cold environments (e.g., air-conditioned rooms).
- Avoid stressful situations, and use relaxation techniques in preventing RP attacks.

ACUTE GENERAL Rx

- Acute measures to terminate an attack include rotating the arms in a windmill pattern, placing the hands under warm water or in a warm body fold such as the axilla, and the swing-arm maneuver.
- Medications are indicated in the treatment of RP if there are signs of critical ischemia or if the quality of life of the patient is affected to the degree that activities of normal living are no longer possible and preventive techniques do not work.

CHRONIC Rx

- Dihydropyridine calcium channel blockers (e.g., nifedipine, amlodipine, felodipine, nisoldipine, isradipine) are the most effective pharmacologic treatment for RP and are the drugs of choice. Amlodipine or nifedipine are commonly used.
- Amlodipine dosage ranges from 2.5 to 10 mg/day. Nifedipine is most often prescribed at a dose of 10 to 20 mg 30 min before cold exposure. If symptoms occur with long duration, nifedipine XL 30 to 180 mg PO qd is often effective.
- When calcium channel blockers do not appropriately control symptoms, phosphodiesterase inhibitors (cilostazol, pentoxifylline, and sildenafil) can be added or substituted. Sildenafil can be started at a dosage of 20 mg/day. Angiotensin 2 receptor antagonists (losartan), and selective serotonin reuptake inhibitors (fluoxetine) have also been used with some limited success.

- Some potential therapeutic options include direct vasodilators such as nitroprusside, hydralazine, papaverine, minoxidil, niacin, and griseofulvin. Topical 1% nitroglycerin or topical l-arginine, ethyl nicotinate, hexyl nicotinate, thurfyl salicylate may also be useful, particularly if low blood pressure is a concern.
- Alpha receptor antagonists such as prazosin and phenoxybenzamine have also shown some effectiveness in treating RP.
- The prostaglandins, including inhaled iloprost, IV epoprostenol, alprostadil, and tadalafil, may be promising in severe RP. However, additional experience and controlled studies are needed.
- Antioxidants like zinc gluconate have been used to decrease tissue damage.
- *N*-Acetylcysteine and probucol have been shown to lead to improvement in RP.
- Anticoagulation with IV unfractionated heparin or subcutaneous low-molecular-weight heparin and addition of aspirin can be considered during the acute phase of a severe ischemic event. Aspirin (81 mg/day) therapy can be considered in all patients with secondary RP with a history of ischemic ulcers or thrombotic events; however, caution should be exercised because aspirin can theoretically worsen vasospasm by the inhibition of prostacyclin. Long-term anticoagulation with heparin or warfarin is not recommended unless there is evidence of a hypercoagulable state.
- Bypass surgery can be performed for severe RP associated with reconstructible arterial occlusive disease.
- Sympathectomy is available for unreconstructible occlusive disease or pure vasospastic disease refractory to medical treatment.
- Microsurgical revascularization of the hand and digital reconstruction may improve digital vascular perfusion and heal digital ulcers when proximal arterial occlusion is associated with digital vasospasm.
- Ischemic digital lesions should be treated with topical antibiotics and daily cleansing with soap and water. Digits that progress to dry gangrene should be permitted to undergo autoamputation. Surgical amputation is limited for intractable pain or deep tissue infection.

DISPOSITION

The prognosis of patients with RP depends on the etiology.

- Primary RP is fairly benign, usually remaining stable and controlled with nonpharmacologic medical treatment.
- Remission of primary RP can occur spontaneously.
- Patients with secondary RP, specifically those with scleroderma, CREST syndrome, or thromboangiitis obliterans, may develop severe ischemic digits with ulceration, gangrene, and autoamputation.
- Box 2 summarizes features suggestive of progression of Raynaud's phenomenon.

REFERRAL

- Rheumatology consult is indicated if secondary collagen vascular disease is diagnosed.
- Vascular surgery consult is indicated if ulcers, gangrene, or threatened digit loss is noted.

PEARLS & CONSIDERATIONS

- Most patients with RP can be managed by a primary care provider.
- It is important to differentiate primary from secondary forms. Secondary forms may become manifest as far out as 10 yr from the diagnosis of RP. It is important to take immediate action during an attack, and patients are encouraged to:
  1. Keep warm
  2. Not use tobacco products
  3. Avoid aggravating medications
  4. Control stress
  5. Exercise
  6. Follow up with a physician

BOX 2 Features Suggestive of Progression of Raynaud's Phenomenon

Clinical
- Older age at onset (>35 yr)
- Recurrence of chilblains as adult
- Vasospasm all year round
- Asymmetric attacks
- Sclerodactyly
- Digital ulceration
- Finger pulp pitting scars

Laboratory
- Increased inflammatory markers
- Detection of autoantibodies
- Increased von Willebrand factor antigen

Nail fold microscopy
- Abnormal vessels

From Hochberg MC et al: *Rheumatology*, ed 5, St Louis, 2011, Mosby.

SUGGESTED READINGS

Available at ExpertConsult.com

RELATED CONTENT

Raynaud's Phenomenon (Patient Information)

AUTHOR: **FRED F. FERRI, M.D.**

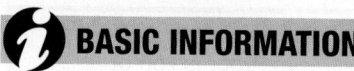

BASIC INFORMATION

DEFINITION

Reiter syndrome is one of the seronegative spondyloarthropathies, so called because serum rheumatoid factor is not present in these forms of inflammatory arthritis. Its characteristic clinical trial consists of urethritis, conjunctivitis, and arthritis. Hans Reiter was a Nazi war criminal and many believe that he should no longer be given name recognition to designate this syndrome. There is an international consensus that the term *reactive arthritis* (ReA) should replace the name "Reiter syndrome" to describe this constellation of signs and symptoms. Unfortunately, the original name is still associated with the syndrome. Reiter syndrome is an asymmetric polyarthritis that affects mainly the lower extremities and is associated with one or more of the following:

- Urethritis
- Cervicitis
- Dysentery
- Inflammatory eye disease
- Mucocutaneous lesions

SYNONYMS

Reiter's disease
Reactive arthritis
Seronegative spondyloarthropathy

ICD-10CM CODE
M02.30 Reiter disease, unspecified site

EPIDEMIOLOGY & DEMOGRAPHICS

INCIDENCE (IN U.S.): 0.0035% annually of men ≤50 yr
PEAK INCIDENCE: Most common in the third decade
PREDOMINANT SEX: Male
PREDOMINANT AGE: 20 to 40 yr
GENETICS: Familial disposition: Strongly associated with HLA-B27 (63% to 96%)

PHYSICAL FINDINGS & CLINICAL PRESENTATION

- Polyarthritis:
  1. Affecting the knee and ankle
  2. Commonly asymmetric
- Heel pain and Achilles tendinitis, especially at the insertion of the Achilles tendon
- Plantar fasciitis
- Large effusions
- Dactylitis, or "sausage toe"
- Urethritis
- Uveitis or conjunctivitis; uveitis can progress to blindness without treatment
- Keratoderma blennorrhagicum, circinate balanitis:
  1. Hyperkeratotic lesions on soles of the feet (Fig. E1), toes, penis (Fig. E2), hands
  2. Closely resembles psoriasis
- Aortic regurgitation similar to that seen in ankylosing spondylitis

ETIOLOGY

- Epidemic Reiter syndrome after outbreaks of dysentery has been well described.
- Genetically susceptible HLA-B27 individuals are at risk for developing Reiter syndrome after infection with certain pathogens:
  1. *Salmonella*
  2. *Shigella*
  3. *Yersinia enterocolitica*
  4. *Chlamydia trachomatis*
- Symptom complex indistinguishable from Reiter syndrome has been described in association with HIV infection.

Dx DIAGNOSIS

DIFFERENTIAL DIAGNOSIS

- Ankylosing spondylitis
- Psoriatic arthritis
- Rheumatoid arthritis
- Gonococcal arthritis-tenosynovitis
- Rheumatic fever
- Serum sickness
- Gout
- Chronic mucocutaneous candidiasis

WORKUP

- X-ray examination of affected joints
- Synovial fluid examination and culture
- Careful examination of eyes and skin
- Cultures for gonococcus (urethral, cervical, stool)

LABORATORY TESTS

- Elevated but nonspecific erythrocyte sedimentation rate
- No specific laboratory tests to diagnose Reiter syndrome
- Do not use HLA-B27 testing as a diagnostic tool

IMAGING STUDIES

Plain radiographs:

- Juxtaarticular osteopenia of affected joints
- Erosions and joint space narrowing in more advanced disease
- Periostitis and reactive new bone formation at the insertions of the Achilles tendon and the plantar fascia
- Sacroiliitis:
  1. Unilateral or bilateral
  2. Indistinguishable from ankylosing spondylitis
- Vertebral bridging osteophytes

Rx TREATMENT

NONPHARMACOLOGIC THERAPY

Physical therapy to maintain range of motion of the spine and other joints

ACUTE GENERAL Rx

- Flares treated with nonsteroidal antiinflammatory drugs such as indomethacin (25-50 mg PO tid). Refractory cases can be treated with methotrexate or infliximab.
- Mucocutaneous lesions are visually self-limited and clear with topical corticosteroids. Acitretin or cyclosporine can be used for refractory skin lesions.
- Enteric or urethral infection should be treated with appropriate antibiotic coverage.
- Uveitis should be treated with steroid eye drops in consultation with an ophthalmologist.
- Achilles tendinitis and plantar fasciitis should be treated with injections of methylprednisolone (40-80 mg).
- Sulfasalazine (500-1000 mg PO bid, then titrate up to maximum 3 g/day) may be effective.
- Careful monitoring for the following is essential:
  1. Gastrointestinal toxicity
  2. Hypersensitivity
  3. Bone marrow suppression
- Persistent and uncontrolled disease should be managed with cytotoxic drugs (methotrexate, azathioprine) in consultation with a rheumatologist.
- The role of tumor necrosis factor alpha inhibitors in therapy is evolving, but agents such as etanercept for 6 mo or infliximab have been shown to be helpful in small studies.

CHRONIC Rx

Chronic disease is best managed by a team approach with the collaboration of a rheumatologist or other experienced physician and physical therapist.

DISPOSITION

- Recurrences are frequent, even with treatment.
- Long-term sequelae:
  1. Persistent polyarthritis
  2. Chronic back pain
  3. Heel pain
  4. Progressive iridocyclitis
  5. Aortic regurgitation

REFERRAL

- To ophthalmologist if uveitis is suspected
- To rheumatologist if arthritis and tendinitis fail to improve rapidly after a course of nonsteroidal antiinflammatory drugs

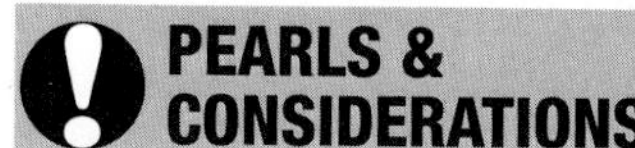

PEARLS & CONSIDERATIONS

COMMENTS

- Infection with HIV is associated with particularly severe cases of Reiter syndrome.
- HIV testing is recommended, especially if risk factors such as unprotected sexual activity or IV drug use are identified.
- The role of antibiotics seems useful in *Chlamydia*-triggered arthritis, but the role of antibiotics in arthritis triggered by enteric pathogens is less clear.

SUGGESTED READINGS

Available at ExpertConsult.com

RELATED CONTENT

Reiter Syndrome (Patient Information)

AUTHOR: **GLENN G. FORT, M.D., M.P.H.**

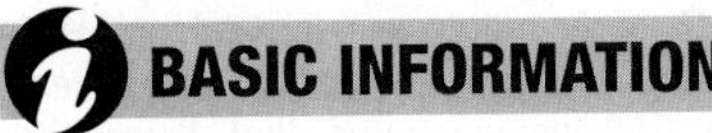

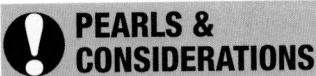

BASIC INFORMATION

DEFINITION

Renal abscess and perinephric abscess are purulent complications of an underlying urinary infection of the ascending tract with an obstructed pyelonephritis. Predisposing factors include diabetes and renal stones. There is lobar necrosis with renal abscess and perirenal fat necrosis in perinephric abscess.

SYNONYMS

Intrarenal abscess
Perinephric abscess
Kidney abscess

ICD-10CM CODE

N15.1 Renal and perinephric abscess

EPIDEMIOLOGY & DEMOGRAPHICS

INCIDENCE: Ranges from 1 to 10 per 10,000 hospital admissions
PREDOMINANT SEX AND AGE: In one study median age was 59.8 yr
RISK FACTORS: Diabetes and renal stones

PHYSICAL FINDINGS & CLINICAL PRESENTATION

- Symptoms include fever, flank pain, abdominal pain, and urinary frequency or dysuria.
- At times renal abscess can present insidiously in the elderly or persons with diabetes.

ETIOLOGY

These infections may be a complication of a urinary tract infection that ascends to the upper tract, usually due to gram-negative bacteria, or a complication of a bacteremia with hematogenous seeding to the kidney, usually secondary to a *Staphylococcus aureus* infection.

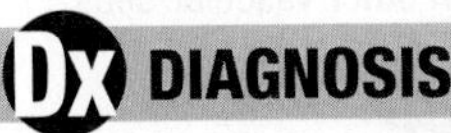

DIAGNOSIS

DIFFERENTIAL DIAGNOSIS

- Acute pyelonephritis with papillary necrosis
- Acute lobar nephronia: Acute nonsuppurative renal infection
- Renal cell carcinoma
- Malakoplakia: Rare granulomatous inflammatory disease seen with *Escherichia coli* infection
- Emphysematous pyelonephritis: Gas formation within the renal parenchyma caused by infection by facultative anaerobes or *Candida* spp.

WORKUP

Combination of laboratory tests and imaging

LABORATORY TESTS

- Blood cultures, urine cultures, urinalysis, and CBC are basic tests.
- Elevated ESR or C-reactive protein may be marker for a deep-seated infection.

IMAGING STUDIES

- Ultrasound may show thick-walled fluid-filled cavity in renal parenchyma. A perinephric abscess is confined to the perinephric space by Gerota fascia.
- CT with contrast (Fig. E1) is preferred over ultrasound for the diagnosis.
- MRI and nuclear scans are of limited value.

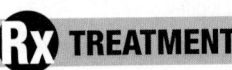

TREATMENT

Antibiotic therapy and, when necessary, interventional radiology or surgical drainage procedure

NONPHARMACOLOGIC THERAPY

- Therapy for a renal abscess greater than 5 cm in diameter should be percutaneous drainage by CT- or US-guided therapy along with intravenous antibiotics.
- A perinephric abscess should be drained percutaneously with CT or US guidance.
- At times a nephrectomy may be required for severe cases, usually in diabetic patients.

ACUTE GENERAL Rx

A renal abscess less than 5 cm in diameter can be treated successfully with targeted intravenous therapy (92% success rate for abscess 3-5 cm in diameter). Antibiotic choices are based on culture results but initially should target gram-negative bacteria unless infection is secondary to staphylococcal bacteremia. Empiric antibiotic therapy in geographic areas where fluoroquinolone resistance rates are <10% consists of ciprofloxacin 400 mg IV loading dose. In areas with high fluoroquinolone resistance rates, ceftriaxone 1 g IV is appropriate. If perinephric abscess is associated with staphylococcal bacteremia, give IV nafcillin if methicillin-susceptible *Staphylococcus aureus* (MSSA) or vancomycin 1 g IV q12h if methicillin-resistant *S. aureus*.

CHRONIC Rx

Antibiotic therapy generally continues for 2 to 3 weeks, some of which can be completed with oral therapy.

DISPOSITION

Antibiotics such as trimethoprim-sulfamethoxazole and quinolone antibiotics penetrate well in the kidney and are ideal oral agents for therapy.

REFERRAL

Interventional radiology, urologic surgeon, and infectious diseases consult

PEARLS & CONSIDERATIONS

COMMENTS

This diagnosis should be considered in patients who are being treated for pyelonephritis with appropriate antibiotics and fail to respond clinically after 5 days.

PREVENTION

Early and targeted therapy for urinary tract infections, especially in diabetic patients

SUGGESTED READINGS

Available at ExpertConsult.com

RELATED CONTENT

Pyelonephritis (Related Key Topic)
Urinary Tract Infection (Related Key Topic)

AUTHOR: **GLENN G. FORT, M.D., M.P.H.**

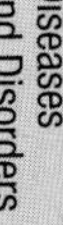

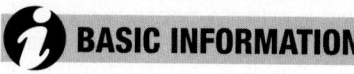

BASIC INFORMATION

DEFINITION

Renal artery stenosis (RAS) is the progressive narrowing of the renal artery, which is most commonly due to atherosclerosis or fibromuscular dysplasia (FMD). RAS is an important, potentially reversible cause of hypertension, ischemic nephropathy, and destabilizing cardiac syndromes. RAS increases the risk of renal artery occlusion via progression of the severity of the stenosis.

SYNONYMS

Fibromuscular disease
FMD
RAS
Renovascular disease

ICD-10CM CODES

I70.1	Atherosclerosis of renal artery
I15.0	Renovascular hypertension
I77.9	Disorder of arteries and arterioles, unspecified
Q27.1	Congenital renal artery stenosis

EPIDEMIOLOGY & DEMOGRAPHICS

- RAS:
  1. Atherosclerotic RAS (ARAS) accounts for about 90% of cases. True prevalence is unknown.
     a. General population autopsy studies: 10%, 27% over 50 yr; hypertensive patients: 0.2% to 5%.
     b. In the general population >65 yr of age, the prevalence is 6.8% by Doppler ultrasound (5.5% of women, 9.1% of men, 6.7% of African Americans, and 6.9% of Caucasians). Of those with ARAS, 12% had bilateral disease.
     c. In patients with malignant hypertension, the prevalence is 43% in Caucasians and 7% in African Americans. In patients with mild hypertension, the prevalence is <1%.
     d. In patients with peripheral artery disease, the prevalence is 22% to 59%.
  2. FMD accounts for approximately 10% of chronic RAS. It is typically seen in women (90%). FMD was previously thought to be a disease of the young and healthy with few risk factors, but recent data suggest an average age of diagnosis of 54 yr, and 26% have bilateral disease.

ETIOLOGY

- Atherosclerosis: Atherosclerotic renal artery stenosis is a process similar to atherosclerosis in other vascular beds with similar risk factors: family history, smoking, diabetes, hypertension, and hyperlipidemia. ARAS most often involves the ostium and proximal third of the main renal artery.
- Fibromuscular dysplasia (FMD) (Fig. 1): Etiology unknown. Classified into three categories based on the layer of arterial wall affected: medial (>90%), intimal (<10%), adventitial (<1%). FMD typically involves the distal main renal artery and intrarenal branches.

PATHOGENESIS

- Pathogenesis of fibromuscular dysplasia is unknown. Fibromuscular dysplasia involves abnormal constrictions and dilations of the renal artery, leading to a typical "string of beads" finding on angiography.
- The pathogenesis of atherosclerotic RAS is similar to that of atherosclerosis in other vascular beds.
- The pathogenesis of renovascular hypertension is related to the neurohormonal cascade resulting from renal ischemia. The macula densa of the kidney senses a decreased systemic blood pressure caused by the reduced blood flow through the stenotic artery. Renal hypoperfusion or ischemia produces an increase in plasma renin that converts angiotensin I to angiotensin II, producing vasoconstriction and aldosterone secretion, sodium retention, and potassium wasting. Hypertension results and can be self-sustaining, even in the case of unilateral RAS, because of hypertensive damage to the contralateral kidney.
- The pathogenesis of ischemic nephropathy is a topic of current debate. Whether renal dysfunction develops purely from persistent ischemia related to progressively narrowed vessels or from repetitive small ischemic insults and upregulation of inflammatory mediators is yet to be fully elucidated.
- "Flash" or sudden-onset pulmonary edema, a manifestation usually seen in bilateral ARAS, results from sodium and water retention as well as upregulation of the sympathetic nervous system.

NATURAL HISTORY

- RAS caused by fibromuscular dysplasia rarely causes renal artery occlusion or ischemic nephropathy.
- ARAS rarely progresses to total occlusion. One study of serial ultrasounds of patients with RAS demonstrated that those with >60% stenosis progressed to total occlusion in 1 yr in only 5% of cases; an additional 11% progressed after 2 yr.

PHYSICAL FINDINGS & CLINICAL PRESENTATION

Progressive RAS:

- Renal artery stenosis should be considered in any white female aged <30 yr with hypertension not attributed to any other cause, or in any patient aged >50 yr with new-onset refractory hypertension, or with stable hypertension that has abruptly and significantly worsened.
- RAS most often presents as a clinically asymptomatic finding. Manifestations can include renovascular hypertension, ischemic nephropathy, or flash pulmonary edema.
- Flash pulmonary edema in the absence of cardiac disease most often indicates severe bilateral renal artery stenosis.
- Renovascular hypertension should be considered if blood pressure control remains suboptimal on a medication regimen that includes 3 maximally dosed medications, including a diuretic.
- Ischemic nephropathy should be considered if kidney function is rapidly deteriorating or parenchymal sizes are decreasing on serial imaging, particularly with bilateral disease.
- Acute elevation of serum creatinine (>30%) after starting angiotensin–converting-enzyme inhibitors (ACEIs) or angiotensin type 1 receptor blockers (ARBs) may be seen in bilateral disease.
- A bruit heard in either upper quadrant on abdominal auscultation may suggest RAS. Patients with atherosclerotic RAS will often have bruits heard in other vascular beds.

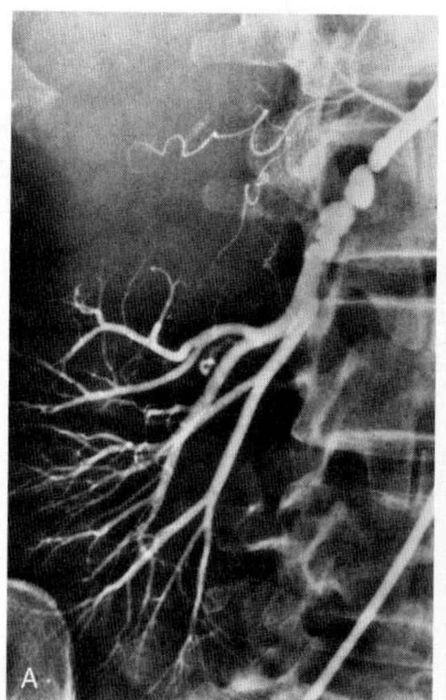

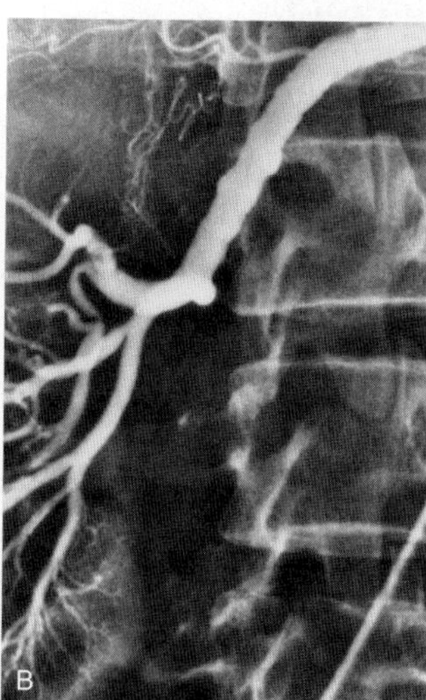

FIG. 1 Fibromuscular dysplasia. A, Selective renal arteriogram illustrating the beaded appearance of fibromuscular dysplasia with multiple webs characteristic of medial fibroplasia in a 39-yr-old woman. **B,** Selective injection of the same renal artery after technically successful percutaneous transluminal renal angioplasty. (Courtesy Michael McKusick, M.D., Mayo Clinic, Rochester, Minnesota. From Floege J et al: *Comprehensive Clinical Nephrology*, ed 4, Philadelphia, 2010, Saunders.)

Dx DIAGNOSIS

SCREENING

American College of Cardiology and American Heart Association (ACC/AHA) guidelines for identification of patients who should be screened for RAS:

- Onset of hypertension at age <30 yr or severe hypertension at age >55 yr
- Clinical findings that suggest secondary hypertension as opposed to essential hypertension in the absence of a more likely cause of secondary hypertension such as pheochromocytoma
- Malignant hypertension: Hypertension with coexistent evidence of acute end-organ damage (acute renal failure, acute decompensated heart failure, new visual or neurologic disturbance, and/or advanced retinopathy)
- Accelerated hypertension: Sudden and persistent worsening of previously controlled hypertension
- Resistant hypertension: Full doses of a 3-drug regimen that includes a diuretic
- Sudden unexplained pulmonary edema
- New azotemia or acute kidney injury following initiation of an ACEI or ARB
- Unexplained atrophic kidney or variation in size of both kidneys by >1.5 cm, smaller kidney likely affected by RAS

Consider screening when renal asymmetry is noted with kidney lengths differing by ≥1.5 cm

LABORATORY TESTS

- Basic chemistry panel including sodium, potassium, blood urea nitrogen, and serum creatinine.
- Urinalysis.
- Renal vein renin sampling helps determine whether one or both kidneys are overproducing renin in cases of suspected renovascular hypertension (RVH). A positive result has strong predictive value. However, 50% of patients with no evidence for lateralization can still respond to unilateral intervention. This procedure is rarely performed except in specialized hypertension centers.

IMAGING STUDIES

Renal Duplex Doppler ultrasonography, CT angiography, and magnetic resonance angiography (MRA) are effective diagnostic screening methods. The choice of imaging modality will depend on the availability of the diagnostic tool, the experience and local accuracy of each modality, patient characteristics including body size, renal function, and contrast allergy, and the presence of prior stents.

RENAL DOPPLER ULTRASOUND:

- Renal Doppler is a noninvasive, inexpensive screening study, and it can determine whether a stenosis of >60% is present.
- Abnormal results in RAS:
  1. Peak systolic velocity (PSV) >250 cm/sec
  2. Peak diastolic velocity >150 cm/sec
  3. Renal-to-aortic ratio (RAR) >3.5
  4. Acceleration time >100 msec
  5. Exact definitions of a positive renal Doppler for RAS will vary by institution
- Compared to renal angiography, Doppler studies have shown varied performance, with a sensitivity of 84% to 98% and a specificity of 62% to 99%.
- Limitations include high user variability. Valid test performance requires technicians who perform a high volume of these tests to reduce user error. If significant user variability exists at certain institutions, renal Doppler may be excluded from diagnostic algorithm. Patients with a large body habitus may have limited imaging results. It is not as sensitive or specific as MR or CT methods. Detection of RAS is limited to identifying whether stenosis of 60% to 99% is present.
- Duplex Doppler is a good modality for monitoring patency after a stent has been placed.

MAGNETIC RESONANCE ANGIOGRAPHY:

- MRA provides good visualization of both main and accessory renal arteries. The test has high sensitivity (90% to 100%) and a specificity of 76% to 94%. It is superior to renal Doppler ultrasonography and equivalent to CT angiography.
- Benefits include the lack of exposure to iodine contrast or radiation.
- Limitations include claustrophobia, high cost, and inability to image within a previously placed metallic stent. In addition, gadolinium exposure is relatively contraindicated in CKD patients with an estimated glomerular filtration rate (GFR) <30 ml/min per 1.73 m^2 due to the risk of inducing nephrogenic systemic fibrosis.

COMPUTED TOMOGRAPHY ANGIOGRAPHY:

- CT angiography is rapid and effective. When compared with angiography, CT has a sensitivity of 59% to 96% and a specificity of 82% to 99%. It is superior to renal Doppler and equivalent to MRA. Contrast uptake in kidneys can also be used to estimate viability of affected kidneys.
- CT has good spatial resolution and can detect restenosis through metal stents.
- CTA can be used more easily than MRA in obese or claustrophobic patients.
- Limitations include radiation exposure and potentially nephrotoxic, iodinated radiocontrast medium exposure to CKD patients. Heavily calcified arteries may appear narrower than in actuality.

DIRECT ANGIOGRAPHY:

- IV digital subtraction angiography (DSA) has an 88% sensitivity and 90% specificity. It is the gold standard for anatomic diagnosis of RAS. It is not a first-line screening tool, but it is recommended after a positive noninvasive test. DSA is also used for patients with a high clinical suspicion for RAS and inconclusive noninvasive tests and in whom the decision has already been made that correction of stenosis will produce clinical benefit. DSA allows for angioplasty with stenting during the same procedure. Renal fractional flow reserve at the time of DSA can evaluate the severity of RAS during maximal vasodilatation.
- This modality is reserved for patients with a high likelihood of intervention.
- Limitations include its invasive nature, requiring intraaortic catheterization that may lead to aortic and renal artery trauma with possible dissection, rupture, thrombosis, or embolization.
- Procedure requires a skilled interventionalist (radiologist, cardiologist, or vascular surgeon) knowledgeable in RAS.
- Procedure requires iodinated contrast and must be used cautiously with CKD. Carbon dioxide contrast imaging and limiting image acquisition number reduce kidney injury risk.

NUCLEAR RENOGRAPHY (WITHOUT CAPTOPRIL):

A noninvasive test conducted when renal atrophy is present to document differential kidney function. This can be useful when determining whether to revascularize an atrophic kidney or to remove it in renovascular hypertension. Atrophic kidneys with <20% differential renal function are unlikely contributors to ongoing worsening kidney function but may still contribute to renovascular hypertension.

Rx TREATMENT

ACUTE GENERAL Rx

The treatment of renal artery stenosis must be targeted to the clinical presentation:

- Asymptomatic RAS requires no treatment.
- Patients with chronic hypertension in the setting of incidentally discovered RAS require only antihypertensive medical therapy.
- Patients in whom RVH is suspected should be initially treated with antihypertensive therapy, specifically medications that block the renin-angiotensin-aldosterone system. As discussed below, failure to control blood pressure on an aggressive regimen represents a reason to consider renal revascularization.
- Patients with ischemic nephropathy should be considered for intervention only if the renal function is rapidly declining or flash pulmonary edema develops in the setting of bilateral renal artery stenosis.

PHARMACOLOGIC THERAPY

- Because of the activation of the renin-angiotensin-aldosterone system in RAS, ACEIs or ARBs are recommended and well tolerated (92%) for the treatment of RVH. Kidney function should be monitored carefully when initiating or titrating these medications, particularly when bilateral RAS (78% tolerability) or unilateral stenosis with solitary kidney is present to avoid precipitating AKI.
- Diuretics should be considered in patients with congestive heart failure or flash pulmonary edema.
- Antiplatelet therapy and statin therapy in patients with atherosclerotic RAS.

NONPHARMACOLOGIC THERAPY

- If either blood pressure cannot be controlled by medications alone, flash pulmonary edema occurs, or there is rapid decline in renal function, referral for renal angiography, angioplasty, and stenting may be indicated.

- Angioplasty without stenting is insufficient for atherosclerotic lesions due to a high failure rate of adequate dilation of the artery or a high rate of restenosis.
- Occasionally a kidney that has lost its function due to RAS may cause refractory hypertension. This situation would be discovered only by renal vein renin sampling in a patient with unilateral renal atrophy. In such cases, nephrectomy of the atrophied kidney may be the best method to control blood pressure.
- Rarely is renal artery bypass required.
- If RAS is suspected as the cause of flash pulmonary edema or rapidly declining kidney function, bilateral disease is likely, and, if confirmed by angiography, both renal arteries should be stented.
- Hypertension is rarely cured with revascularization in patients with atherosclerotic RAS due to high background essential hypertension. The goal of intervention is to gain control of blood pressure and reduce the number of blood pressure medications.
- The ACC/AHA guidelines for clinical indications of renal artery revascularization in the presence of significant stenosis include:
  1. Accelerated, resistant, or malignant hypertension (class IIa)
  2. Hypertension with unilateral small kidney (class IIa)
  3. Hypertension with intolerance to medication (class IIa)
  4. Treatment of cardiac destabilization syndromes such as unexplained heart failure exacerbations or episodes of flash pulmonary edema (class I) and refractory or unstable angina (class IIa)
  5. Progressive chronic kidney disease with bilateral RAS or RAS associated with a solitary functioning kidney (class IIa)
- Many patients who meet these criteria will not demonstrate a beneficial response to renal revascularization. Careful selection of patients for angiography and intervention must be made.
- Multiple, randomized, controlled trials (e.g., ASTRAL, CORAL, DRASTIC, and STAR) have not shown benefit to percutaneous therapy compared to medical therapy, with end points of blood pressure control, renal function, and cardiovascular events. However, these trials did have several inherent limitations.
  1. DRASTIC trial was a small angioplasty-only trial that demonstrated no difference in blood pressure, but it did show decrease in daily doses of antihypertensive drugs and number of drugs in the intervention group. Crossover was high from the medication arm to the intervention arm.
  2. The ASTRAL trial was a moderate-sized trial of stenting versus medication in RAS that showed no difference in blood pressure control or in the number of antihypertensive medications required to achieve blood pressure control. RAS severity was only moderate in the study population, decreasing the likelihood of finding a positive result.
  3. CORAL is a large, prospective, multicenter trial comparing stenting versus medication in severe RAS (>60% stenosis). This study confirms that with atherosclerotic renal artery stenosis and hypertension, clinical outcomes are not improved by stenting and that renal artery stenting is futile in general. RAS severity was moderate in many patients and may have diluted the beneficial effects of intervention on those with severe RAS.
  4. Follow-up of the CORAL population at 3 yr failed to show any difference in blood pressure control, change in GFR, end-stage renal disease, or death with stenting vs. medical therapy.
- With these limitations in mind, there is no prospective, randomized, controlled trial that has shown a benefit in any subgroup of patients with renal artery stenosis of revascularization over medical management. Therefore it is recommended that the decision to refer a patient for revascularization be made by specialists who are practiced and skilled in handling hypertension and renal artery stenosis.

FIBROMUSCULAR DYSPLASIA

- Medical therapy should include an ACEI or ARB to control blood pressure unless severe bilateral disease is present (rare).
- RVH from fibromuscular dysplasia (FMD) is often cured by renal artery revascularization because many younger patients do not have background essential hypertension.
- In most cases, patients should be referred for renal artery angioplasty regardless of whether blood pressure can be controlled medically.
- Stenting is not appropriate in patients with FMD because angioplasty alone usually yields a durable result. In addition, recurrence of FMD is common, and the presence of stents may hinder additional interventions.
- Renal artery bypass may be necessary in patients whose FMD recurs multiple times or in whom angioplasty failed to yield an improvement in blood pressure.

DISPOSITION & REFERRAL

- Patients with uncontrolled hypertension on multiple agents should be referred for management by a hypertension specialist.
- Percutaneous intervention for atherosclerotic RAS must be reserved for selected patients until further data are available.

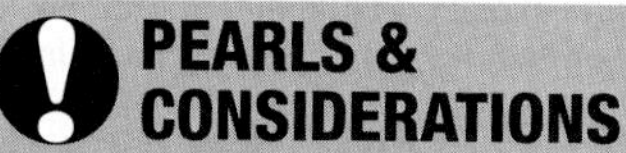

PEARLS & CONSIDERATIONS

- Renal artery stenosis is most commonly an incidental finding and clinically silent.
- Renal artery stenosis may present as hypertension, renal dysfunction, or both, or flash pulmonary edema.
- Stenting is inappropriate for most patients with RAS. Consideration should be made only in high-risk patients and after consultation with a specialist in the field.
- The modality for the type of imaging should depend on the expertise of the institution.

SUGGESTED READINGS

Available at ExpertConsult.com

RELATED CONTENT

Renal Artery Stenosis (Patient Information)
Hypertension (Related Key Topic)

AUTHOR: **JAMES F. SIMON, M.D.**

BASIC INFORMATION

DEFINITION

Renal cell carcinoma (RCC) is a primary carcinoma originating in the renal parenchyma from the malignant transformation of proximal renal tubular epithelial cells. The majority of renal cell cancers are of clear cell type; papillary tumors comprise 15%, and chromophobe cancers comprise 10%.

SYNONYMS

Hypernephroma
RCC
Renal cell adenocarcinoma

ICD-10CM CODES

C64.9 Malignant neoplasm of kidney, except renal pelvis
C64.1 Malignant neoplasm of right kidney, except renal pelvis
C64.2 Malignant neoplasm of left kidney, except renal pelvis
C64.9 Malignant neoplasm of unspecified kidney, except renal pelvis
C65.9 Malignant neoplasm of renal pelvis

EPIDEMIOLOGY & DEMOGRAPHICS

INCIDENCE: In 2018, an estimated 65,340 new cases and 14,970 deaths were expected in the U.S. Two percent of cases of renal cancer are associated with inherited syndromes.

PREDOMINANT SEX: Male:female ratio is approximately 2:1.

PREDOMINANT AGE: Peak incidence is at age 50 to 70 yr.

PHYSICAL FINDINGS & CLINICAL PRESENTATION

Patients are often asymptomatic until they have advanced disease. Paraneoplastic syndromes such as hypercalcemia, erythrocytosis, anemia, and hepatic dysfunction may occur with renal cell carcinoma. The classic triad of flank pain, hematuria, and a palpable abdominal mass currently represents an unusual presentation. Current presenting findings in RCC include:

Hematuria	50% to 60%
Elevated erythrocyte sedimentation rate	50% to 60%
Abdominal mass	25% to 45%
Anemia	20% to 40%
Flank pain	35% to 40%
Hypertension	20% to 40%
Weight loss	30% to 35%
Fever	5% to 15%
Hepatic dysfunction	10% to 15%
Classic triad (hematuria, abdominal mass, flank pain)	5% to 10%
Hypercalcemia	3% to 6%
Erythrocytosis	3% to 4%
Varicocele	2% to 3%

ETIOLOGY

Hereditary forms:
- Familial renal carcinoma
- Renal carcinoma associated with Von Hippel-Lindau disease
- Hereditary papillary renal cell carcinoma

Risk factors:
- Cigarette smoking
- Obesity
- Phenacetin-containing analgesics
- Asbestos, lead, Thorotrast, and chromium exposure
- Gasoline and other petroleum products
- Role of the *VHL* gene on chromosome 3

DIAGNOSIS

DIFFERENTIAL DIAGNOSIS

- Transitional cell carcinomas of the renal pelvis (8% of all renal cancers)
- Wilms tumor
- Other primary renal carcinomas and sarcomas
- Renal cysts
- Retroperitoneal tumors

WORKUP

LABORATORY TESTS:

- Urinalysis: Hematuria
- Complete blood count: Anemia or erythrocytosis
- Chemistry panel: Renal failure and electrolyte issues, including hypercalcemia
- Liver function tests: Hepatic dysfunction with elevated alkaline phosphatase, prolonged prothrombin time, and hypoalbuminemia

IMAGING STUDIES

Nearly 50% of renal cancers are now detected because a renal mass is incidentally detected on radiographic evaluation.

- Renal ultrasound
- Abdominal CT scan with contrast (Figs. E1 and 2); CT-guided biopsy is generally not necessary for diagnosis of solid masses >4 cm (high likelihood of cancer)
- MRI
- Renal arteriogram
- Intravenous pyelography

STAGING

See Table 1.

COMMON SITES OF METASTASES

Lung	50% to 60%
Bone	30% to 40%
Regional nodes	15% to 30%
Main renal vein	15% to 20%
Perirenal fat	10% to 20%
Adrenal (ipsilateral)	10% to 15%
Vena cava	10% to 15%
Brain	10% to 15%
Adjacent organs (colon, pancreas)	10%
Kidney (contralateral)	2%

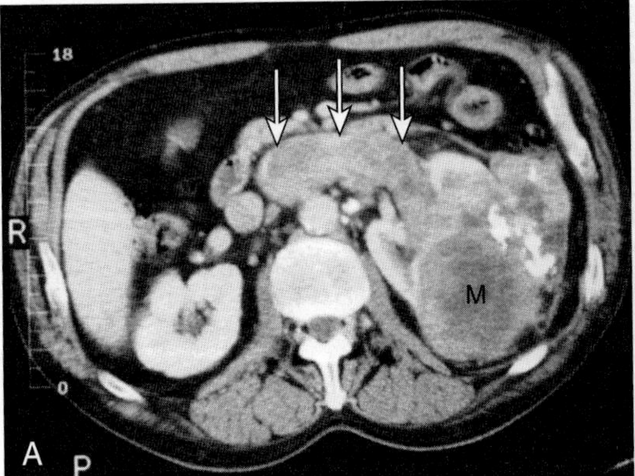

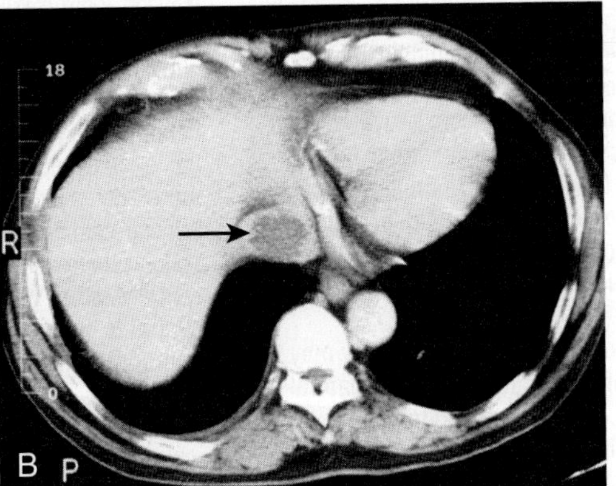

FIG. 2 Renal cell carcinoma. In this patient, the computed tomography scan at the midportion of the kidneys **(A)** demonstrates a large left renal mass (*M*) that extends into the renal vein and into the inferior vena cava (*arrows*). **B,** An image at the level of the base of the heart shows that the tumor thrombus (*arrow*) extends into the right atrium. (From Mettler FA Jr: *Essentials of radiology,* ed 3, Philadelphia, 2014, Saunders.)

TABLE 1 TNM Staging of Renal Cell Carcinomas as per the AJCC eighth edition

T Stage	Description
T_x	Tumor cannot be assessed
T_1: Tumor ≤7 cm, limited to kidney	T_{1a}: Tumor <4 cm T_{1b}: Tumor ≥4 cm to ≤7 cm
T_2: Tumor >7 cm, limited to kidney	T_{2a}: Tumor >7 cm but ≤10 cm T_{2b}: Tumor >10 cm
T_3: Tumor extending into major veins or perinephric tissue but not into ipsilateral adrenal gland or beyond Gerota fascia	T_{3a}: Tumor extends to renal vein/branches or invades perirenal and/or renal sinus fat T_{3b}: Tumor extends into IVC below diaphragm T_{3c}: Tumor extends into IVC above diaphragm or wall of IVC
T_4	Tumor invades beyond Gerota fascia (including contiguous extension into ipsilateral adrenal gland)
N stage	**Description**
N_x	Regional nodes cannot be assessed
N_1	No regional nodes involved
N_2	Metastasis in regional node(s)
M stage	**Description**
M_0	No distant metastases
M_1	Distant metastasis present
Stage	**TNM grouping**
I	$T_1N_0M_0$
II	$T_2N_0M_0$
III	$T_3N_0M_0$ or $T_{1-3}N_1M_0$
IV	$T_4N_{any}M_{any}$ or $T_{any}N_{any}M_1$

AJCC, American Joint Committee on Cancer; *IVC,* intravenous cholangiography; *TNM,* tumor, node, metastases.

Rx TREATMENT

- Surgery:
  1. Surgical nephrectomy (open procedure or laparoscopic approach) is the only effective management for stages I, II, and some stage III tumors. Although radical nephrectomy had long been the standard treatment, retrospective studies have shown that partial rather than radical nephrectomy is associated with improved survival and is appropriate for patients with renal cell neoplasms <4 cm that are not adjacent to the renal pelvis or invading the vena cava.
  2. Laparoscopic robotic-assisted nephrectomy has been adopted in multiple centers, primarily for nephron-sparing surgery in the case of tumors <4 cm. Advantages include less blood loss, minimal effects on renal function, and similar oncologic outcomes. Disadvantages include increased costs and limitations in tumor size and locations eligible for robotic surgery.
  3. Various forms of partial nephrectomy may be available for patients with bilateral cancers or with a solitary kidney.
  4. Cytoreductive nephrectomy in patients with metastatic RCC before immunotherapy improved survival in patients compared with immunotherapy alone on the basis of randomized trials data. However, recent results from the randomized Clinical Trial to Assess the Importance of Nephrectomy (CARMENA) demonstrated no benefit for intermediate- and poor-risk patients in the setting of modern tyrosine kinase inhibitor (sunitinib) therapy. Additional trials data are awaited to assess the role of nephrectomy in favorable risk patients and with the use of neoadjuvant tyrosine kinase inhibitor therapy.
- Angioinfarction, cryoablation, or radiotherapy (for palliation).
- Chemotherapy: In patients with unresectable disease, therapy with the tyrosine kinase inhibitors axitinib, sunitinib, pazopanib, and sorafenib and also mTOR kinase inhibitors such as everolimus and temsirolimus can be used as first-line therapy or sequential therapy. Typically, patients are offered sequential therapy with either of these agents until maximum response duration or onset of major toxicity from each agent. The majority of responses with these agents are typically either partial or stable disease, and relapse is the norm.
- Immunotherapy: High-dose interleukin-2 therapy may achieve a 15% response rate, which is often durable and associated with long-term survival in highly selected patients with excellent performance status. The severe toxicities associated with this therapy and the requirement for specialized treatment centers have put limits on the use of this approach.
- Checkpoint inhibitors: The PD-1 inhibitors nivolumab and pembrolizumab have demonstrated efficacy in patients previously treated with targeted therapies. Recent data with the use of combination immunotherapy (PD-1 inhibitor plus CTLA-4 inhibitor) demonstrated a survival benefit when used in first-line therapy in comparison to targeted therapy.
- Cabozantinib, an inhibitor of the c-met oncogene, has also shown improved survival in patients with relapsed metastatic renal carcinoma.

PROGNOSIS

The 5-year survival rate among patients with kidney cancer has increased from 57% in 1987 to 1989 to 74% in 2006 to 2012. The prognosis of surgically treated patients is shown in the following:

TNM Stage	5-yr Survival (%)
I	95
II	88
III (renal vein or vena cava)	50-60
III (nodal involvement)	15-25
IV	5-20

REFERRAL

- To urologist for staging and surgery
- To medical oncologist if metastatic disease is present

CLINICAL PEARLS

- Patients should be considered for nephron-sparing surgery in case of smaller tumors (<4 cm).
- Laparoscopic robotic-assisted surgery is utilized for standard nephron-sparing surgery routinely; it is utilized for central tumors and tumors >4 cm in some experienced centers.
- Adjuvant therapy utilizing tyrosine kinase inhibitors has showed mixed results when used in the postresection setting and is not approved for use in this setting. An intergroup study showed no survival benefit, whereas a smaller study limited to high-risk patients showed a progression-free survival benefit.
- High-dose interleukin-2 can lead to long-term remissions in 10% to 15% of carefully selected patients.

SUGGESTED READINGS

Available at ExpertConsult.com

RELATED CONTENT

Kidney Cancer (Patient Information)

AUTHOR: **BHARTI RATHORE, M.D.**

BASIC INFORMATION

DEFINITION

Renal tubular acidosis (RTA) is a group of chronic diseases characterized by hyperchloremic metabolic acidosis (HCMA) produced by inability of the renal tubules to either excrete hydrogen ion (H^+) or retain bicarbonate ion (HCO_3^-). Factors differentiating types of RTA are described in Table 1. Four main types of RTA are described:

- Type 1 (classic, distal RTA): Abnormality in distal tubule hydrogen secretion, resulting in hypokalemic HCMA
- Type 2 (proximal RTA): Decreased proximal tubule bicarbonate reabsorption, resulting in hypokalemic HCMA
- Type 3 (mixed RTA): Rare autosomal recessive disorder with features of distal and proximal RTA
- Type 4 (hyporeninemic, hypoaldosteronism RTA): Aldosterone deficiency or a disease of the cortical collecting duct characterized by decreased distal sodium reabsorption and decreased distal tubule acidification hyperkalemic HCMA

SYNONYM

Renal tubular acidosis (RTA)

ICD-10CM CODE
N25.89 Other disorders resulting from impaired renal tubular function

EPIDEMIOLOGY & DEMOGRAPHICS

RTA type 4 affects primarily adults, whereas RTA types 1 and 2 are more frequent in children.

PHYSICAL FINDINGS & CLINICAL PRESENTATION

- Examination may be normal.
- Reduced skin turgor may be present from polyuria and dehydration.
- Muscle weakness and aches, paralysis, and cardiac arrhythmias from hypokalemia may occur.
- Low back pain and bone pain may be present in patients with abnormalities of calcium and phosphorus metabolism (RTA type 2).
- Failure to thrive or delayed growth in children.
- Some patients may present with sensorineural deafness in RTA type 1 (H^+-ATPase mutations).

ETIOLOGY

- Type 1 RTA inherited as a primary disorder with mutation of the basolateral chloride-bicarbonate exchanger (*SLC4A1* gene) or apical proton-ATPase (H^+-ATPase). Acquired causes: Autoimmune disorders (SLE, Sjögren's syndrome); primary biliary cirrhosis and other liver diseases; medications (amphotericin, NSAIDs, lithium carbonate, ifosfamide); genetic disorders (Ehlers-Danlos syndrome, Marfan syndrome, hereditary elliptocytosis); toxins (toluene); disorders with nephrocalcinosis (primary hyperparathyroidism, vitamin D intoxication, idiopathic hypercalciuria); and tubulointerstitial disease (renal transplantation, renal medullary cystic disease, obstructive uropathy, chronic urinary tract infections, and analgesic nephropathy).
- Type 2 RTA includes inherited disorders such as proximal tubule cell sodium bicarbonate co-transporter (NBCe1) defect, carbonic anhydrase type 2 deficiency, and Fanconi syndrome (caused by cystinosis, Wilson disease, hereditary fructose intolerance, Lowe syndrome, Fanconi-Bickel syndrome, Dent disease, tyrosinemia, galactosemia). Acquired causes include primary hyperparathyroidism, multiple myeloma, amyloidosis, light chain deposit diseases, heavy metals (copper, lead, mercury, and cadmium), chronic rejection of a transplanted kidney, and medications (acetazolamide, topiramate, outdated tetracycline, ifosfamide, zidovudine, didanosine, aminoglycosides).
- Type 3 RTA: Rare inherited recessive disorder with carbonic anhydrase (CA) 2 deficiency, drugs (topiramate).
- Type 4 RTA includes inherited disorders such as pseudohypoaldosteronism type 1 or type 2 (Gordon syndrome). Acquired causes include diabetes mellitus, HIV/AIDS, sickle cell disease, obstructive uropathy, lupus, amyloidosis, adrenal insufficiency, kidney transplant rejection, drugs (spironolactone, eplerenone, amiloride, angiotensin–converting-enzyme [ACE] inhibitors, angiotensin-receptor blockers [ARBs], trimethoprim, pentamidine, heparin, NSAIDs, and calcineurin inhibitors [cyclosporine, tacrolimus]).

DIAGNOSIS

DIFFERENTIAL DIAGNOSIS: EXTRARENAL ORIGIN

- Diarrhea with significant bicarbonate loss
- External loss of biliary and pancreatic secretions
- Gastrointestinal-urinary diversion procedures (e.g., ureterosigmoidostomy, ileal conduit)
- Respiratory acidosis
- Drugs: Calcium chloride, magnesium sulfate, cholestyramine

WORKUP

Detection of HCMA by serum electrolyte and arterial blood gas (ABG) analysis followed by evaluation of potential causes (see "Etiology"). Fig. 1 describes an approach to the patient with RTA.

LABORATORY TESTS

- ABG reveals metabolic acidosis.
- Anion gap is normal.
- Serum potassium is low in RTA types 1 and 2, normal in type 3, and high in type 4.
- First-morning urine pH is >5.5 in RTA type I, <5.5 in types 2 and 3, and <5.5 (low mineralocorticoid secretion) or >5.5 (collecting duct abnormality) in RTA type 4.
- Urinary anion gap (UAG) is an indirect evaluation of urinary ammonium excretion, which differentiates renal from extrarenal causes of normal anion gap metabolic acidosis (e.g., diarrhea). UAG is 0 or positive in all types of RTA.
- $UAG = U_{(Na + K)} - U_{Cl}$.
- UAG is valid only if U_{Na} >20 mEq/L and urine pH <6.5.
- Urine osmolar gap (UOG) is an independent surrogate of urinary ammonium concentration and is not affected by the presence of other nonreabsorbable anions (e.g., keto acids, 5-oxoproline/pyroglutamic acid, bicarbonate, or hippurate).
- Calculated U_{NH4^+} = 0.5 (measured Uosm − calculated Uosm [2 (Na + K) + Urine Urea (mg/dl/2.8) + glucose (mg/dl/18]).
- Calculated urine ammonium ≥75 mEq/L denotes intact renal tubular function and supports an extrarenal origin of HCMA.
- Calculated urine ammonium ≤25 mEq/L denotes inappropriately low concentration.

TABLE 1 Contrasting Features and Diagnostic Studies in Renal Tubular Acidosis

	Types of Renal Tubular Acidosis		
Finding	**Proximal (Type 2)**	**Classical Distal (Type 1)**	**Generalized Distal Dysfunction (Type 4)**
Plasma potassium	Low	Low	High
Urine pH during metabolic acidosis (ABG pH <7.3)	<5.5	>5.5	<5.5 or >5.5
Urine net charge	Positive	Positive	Positive
Fanconi's lesion	Present	Absent	Absent
Fractional bicarbonate excretion	10%-15%	2%-5%	5%-10%
Urine-Blood PCO_2	Normal	Low	Low
H^+-ATPase defect		Low	
HCO_3–/Cl– transporter defect		High	
Amphotericin B		Normal	
Response to therapy	Least responsive	Responsive	Less responsive
Associated features	Fanconi's syndrome	Nephrocalcinosis/ hypergammaglobulinemia	Chronic kidney disease

ATPase, Adenosine triphosphatase; (U – B) PCO_2, urine–blood CO_2 tension difference, <30 is low.
Modified from DuBose TD: Disorders of acid-base balance. In *Brenner and Rector's the kidney,* ed 9, Philadelphia, 2011, WB Saunders.

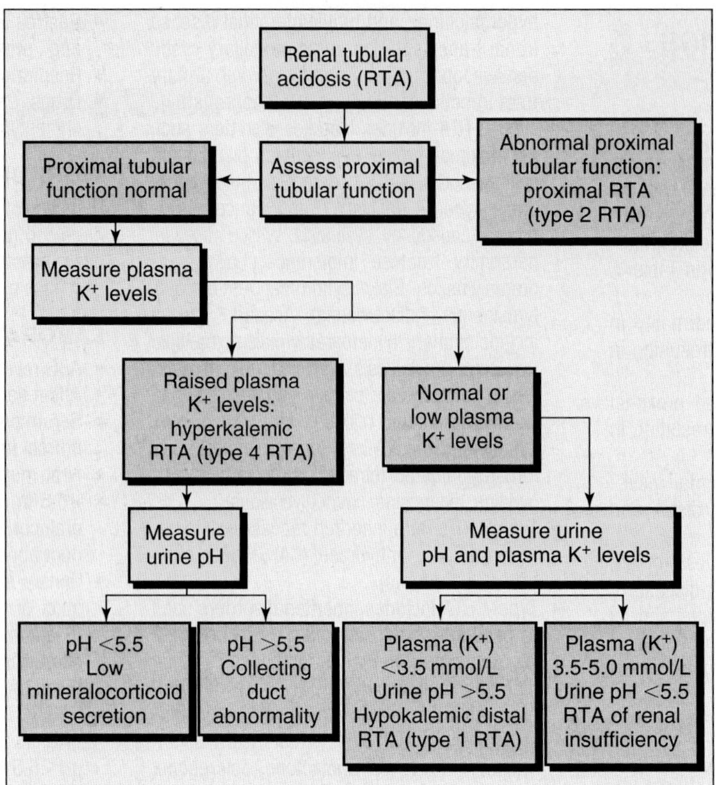

FIG. 1 Approach to the patient with renal tubular acidosis. (From Floege J et al: *Comprehensive clinical nephrology,* ed 4, Philadelphia, 2010, WB Saunders.)

- UOG cannot be used if there are other neutral substances in the urine (e.g., mannitol, alcohols) or during a urinary tract infection urease-producing bacteria.
- Additional studies include urine and serum calcium concentrations.
- Parathyroid hormone measurement when primary hyperparathyroidism is suspected (type 2 RTA).

IMAGING STUDIES

- Plain abdominal radiographs for evaluation of nephrocalcinosis
- Kidney ultrasound to determine kidney sizes or presence of stones
- Noncontrast-enhanced CT scan in patients with nephrocalcinosis or nephrolithiasis

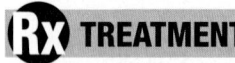

TREATMENT

ACUTE GENERAL Rx

- Types 1 and 2 are treated with oral sodium bicarbonate (1–2 mEq/kg/day in RTA type I, 2–4 mEq/kg/day in RTA type 2) titrated to correct metabolic acidosis (serum bicarbonate >22 mEq/L).
- Potassium supplementation is required for hypokalemic patients.
- Type 4 RTA can be treated with diuretics to lower elevated potassium levels and with sodium bicarbonate to correct significant acidosis. Fludrocortisone 0.1–0.3 mg/day can be used to correct mineralocorticoid deficiency.

CHRONIC Rx

- Monitor potassium levels in RTA type 4.
- Monitor for bone disease (osteomalacia) in RTA type 2.
- Monitor for nephrolithiasis and nephrocalcinosis in RTA type I.

DISPOSITION

- Prognosis varies with the associated conditions (see "Etiology").
- Untreated distal RTA may result in hypocalcemia, hypophosphatemia, nephrolithiasis, and nephrocalcinosis.

PEARLS & CONSIDERATIONS

- Non-anion gap metabolic acidosis: Check for urine ammonium (urine anion and osmolar gaps) to differentiate nonrenal vs. renal causes of HCMA.
- Examine serum potassium to differentiate between RTA Types 1 or 2 vs. Type 4.
- In Type 4 hyperkalemic RTA, carefully review medication list and rule out urinary obstruction, especially in elderly males.

COMMENTS

Patient education material can be obtained from the National Kidney and Urologic Diseases Information Clearinghouse, Box NKUDIC, Bethesda, MD 20893.

SUGGESTED READING

Available at ExpertConsult.com

AUTHORS: **JIAN LI, M.D., PH.D.,** and **BAHA AL-ABID, M.D.**

BASIC INFORMATION

DEFINITION

Renal vein thrombosis (RVT) is the thrombotic occlusion of one or both renal veins.

ICD-10CM CODE
I82.3 Embolism and thrombosis of renal vein

EPIDEMIOLOGY & DEMOGRAPHICS

- Incidence unknown; probably an underdiagnosed condition
- May occur at any age with no gender preference
- Epidemiology tied to the underlying cause

PHYSICAL FINDINGS & CLINICAL PRESENTATION

Acute bilateral renal vein thrombosis:
- Back and bilateral flank pain
- Acute renal failure

Acute unilateral renal vein thrombosis:
- Flank pain
- Decline in renal function
- Hematuria
- Increase in the amount of proteinuria if associated with nephrotic syndrome

Chronic unilateral renal vein thrombosis:
- May be silent
- Pulmonary emboli and hemolysis
- Back pain
- Deep vein thrombosis in lower extremities
- Edema
- Glycosuria
- Hyperchloremic acidosis
- Left varicocele (if the left renal vein is thrombosed)
- Dilated abdominal veins

ETIOLOGY & PATHOGENESIS

- Nephrotic syndrome, especially when the serum albumin is <2 g/dl
- Extrinsic compression by a tumor or retroperitoneal mass
- Invasion of the renal vein or inferior vena cava by tumor (almost always renal cell cancer)
- Trauma
- Other hypercoagulable states
- Severe dehydration

NOTE: For unknown reasons, diabetic nephropathy is not commonly associated with renal vein thrombosis even if the nephrotic syndrome is present.

Controversy has existed regarding whether the renal vein thrombosis association with nephrotic syndrome is a complication of nephrotic syndrome or whether renal vein thrombosis occurring in the setting of increased renal vein pressure (e.g., with congestive heart failure, constrictive pericarditis, or extrinsic compression) can independently cause proteinuria. Current evidence is that renal vein thrombosis does not cause nephrotic syndrome.

DIAGNOSIS

DIFFERENTIAL DIAGNOSIS

The diagnosis of renal vein thrombosis does not include any differential consideration. The differential diagnosis is that of proteinuria. Renal vein thrombosis should be considered if proteinuria worsens or if renal function worsens in a patient with glomerulonephritis. Renal vein thrombosis should also be considered in patients with pulmonary emboli and no lower-extremity deep vein thrombosis.

WORKUP

Clinical suspicion (see "Differential Diagnosis") and imaging studies.

IMAGING STUDIES

- Abdominal ultrasound with Doppler (Fig. E1)
- Abdominal MRI or CT with contrast (Fig. 2) in the absence of significant renal failure
- Renal arteriography (delayed films during venous phase)
- Selective renal vein venography
- Renal biopsy may be indicated if evidence of nephritis is present (e.g., active urinary sediment)

TREATMENT

- Anticoagulation with heparin or low-molecular-weight heparin as a bridge to coumadin in acute renal vein thrombosis to prevent pulmonary emboli and in attempt to improve renal function and decrease proteinuria.
- Note that patients with nephrotic syndrome can be resistant to heparin because of antithrombin III deficiency.
- Direct thrombin and factor Xa inhibitors have not been studied in patients with nephrotic syndrome–related RVT. However, there are case reports of their effectiveness in patients who have contraindications or refuse warfarin or low-molecular-weight heparin.
- Thrombolytic therapy or surgical thrombectomy has also been reported to be effective.
- The value of anticoagulation in chronic renal vein thrombosis is dubious. The exception is in nephrotic patients with membranous glomerulonephritis with profound hypoalbuminemia, where prolonged prophylactic anticoagulation may be of benefit even if renal vein thrombosis has not been documented.

PROGNOSIS

Probable worsening of the underlying nephropathy by acute renal vein thrombosis; the effect of chronic renal vein thrombosis is unclear.

AUTHOR: **DAVID J. LUCIER JR., M.D., M.B.A., M.P.H., C.P.P.S.**

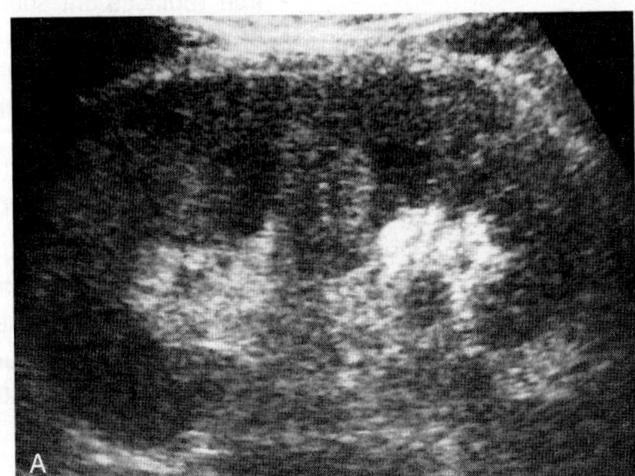

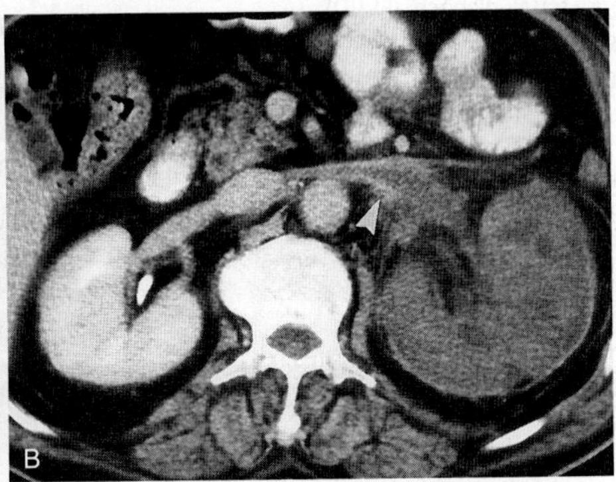

FIG. 2 Renal vein thrombosis. A, Sagittal sonogram demonstrates a diffusely enlarged, edematous left kidney with loss of corticomedullary differentiation. **B,** Confirmatory contrast-enhanced computed tomography shows a large, poorly perfused left kidney and thrombus in the left renal vein *(arrowhead)*. (From Rumack CM et al: *Diagnostic ultrasound*, ed 4, Philadelphia, 2011, Elsevier.)

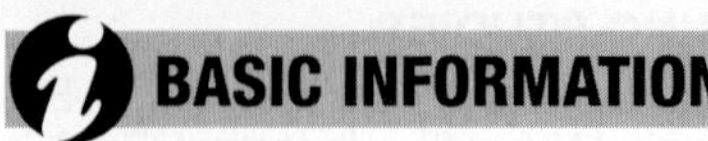

BASIC INFORMATION

DEFINITION

Restless legs syndrome (RLS) is an awake phenomenon consisting of an urge to move legs, usually associated with feeling of discomfort in legs. Symptoms typically are present only at rest and at least partially improve with movement. Additionally, symptoms are usually worse at night. RLS can result in sleep disturbance with associated executive dysfunction and depression.

SYNONYMS

RLS
Wittmaack-Ekbom syndrome

ICD-10CM CODE

G25.81 Restless legs syndrome

EPIDEMIOLOGY & DEMOGRAPHICS

PREVALENCE: Average prevalence rate is 1% to 29%. Prevalence estimates in Europe are around 10%, and 0.1% to 12% in East Asian population.
PEAK PREVALENCE: 10% in persons aged 30 to 79 and 19% in persons aged 80 or above.
PREDOMINANT SEX: Early-onset RLS is more common in females, with 2:1 female/male ratio.
PREDOMINANT AGE: Prevalence of RLS increases with age, and it is more commonly seen in the elderly population.
GENETICS: Genetic basis of RLS has been reported, particularly in early-onset RLS.

- Autosomal dominant disorder
- Common among first-degree relatives
- RLS associated with certain sequences in chromosome 6p, 12q, 14q, 9p, 20p, 2p, 16p
- These include polymorphisms in the genes *BTBD9*, *MEIS1*, *PTPRD*, *MAP2K5*, *SKOR1*, and *TOX3*

RISK FACTORS: Diabetes mellitus (most consistent risk factor for RLS), iron deficiency anemia (IDA), end-stage renal disease (ESRD) requiring hemodialysis, pregnancy, rheumatoid arthritis, Parkinson's disease, neuropathy, and myelopathy

CLASSIFICATION

- Primary RLS is without any obvious cause, with no associated disorder.
- Secondary RLS results from other medical conditions; the most frequently found associations are pregnancy, IDA, ESRD, and Parkinson disease.

PHYSICAL FINDINGS & CLINICAL PRESENTATION

- Wide spectrum of severity of clinical manifestations has been reported in RLS.
- Most common symptom is unpleasant sensations in legs ("dysesthesias"), reported as discomfort or "creepy-crawling" sensations, mostly bilateral. Arms are occasionally involved.
- There is an extreme urge to move legs, and relief is sustained as long as the movement continues.
- Symptoms are worse at night or evening. Best sleep is usually early in the morning.

ETIOLOGY

The exact etiology remains unknown. Pharmacologic, pathologic, physiologic, and imaging studies have implicated dopaminergic pathways, brain iron metabolism, and endogenous opioid pathways.

Dx DIAGNOSIS

DIFFERENTIAL DIAGNOSIS

- Periodic limb movement disorder (PLMD)
- Nocturnal leg cramps
- Painful peripheral neuropathy
- Akathisia
- Positional discomfort
- Volitional movements, foot tapping, leg rocking

WORKUP

- Diagnosis of RLS is based on established clinical criteria (Table 1) and normal neurologic examination
- Testing is done to determine possible cause of secondary RLS. All patients with RLS should be screened for iron deficiency because iron supplementation in patients with iron deficiency may resolve the symptoms
- Polysomnography to document periodic limb movements during sleep
- Leg activity monitors to determine limb movements during sleep, but they are unable to distinguish periodic limb movements from periodic movements associated with sleep apnea
- Nerve conduction studies and electromyography for associated peripheral neuropathy

LABORATORY TESTS

- Iron status: Serum ferritin, total iron binding capacity, percent saturation
- CBC for anemia in case of iron deficiency
- Metabolic panel: Blood urea nitrogen and serum creatinine for renal insufficiency

IMAGING STUDIES

No imaging studies are required for diagnosis for RLS.

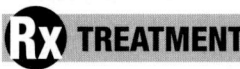

TREATMENT

Treatment options (Table 2) for RLS include:

- Anticonvulsants, such as gabapentin, have been shown to be effective in multiple studies. Gabapentin enacarbil and pregabalin (1) would now be considered first-line agents in the treatment on RLS. These agents do not cause iatrogenic worsening (augmentation) of RLS with long-term treatment. Limited case reports support use of lamotrigine and topiramate in patients who are intolerant to other agents.
- Dopaminergic agents such as levodopa and dopamine agonists help to ameliorate RLS symptoms, decrease periodic limb movements, and improve sleep. Dopamine agonists, pramipexole and ropinirole, can be first-line agents in the treatment of RLS but often cause augmentation of RLS with long-term treatment.
- Rotigotine patch (Neupro) is also effective and FDA-approved for moderate to severe RLS.
- Opiates, mostly methadone, are generally reserved as last line of treatment.
- Iron replacement should be started in case of iron deficiency. Iron supplements are indicated even with low-normal ferritin levels (<45 ng/ml). Sometimes IV iron replacement is used.

NONPHARMACOLOGIC THERAPY

- Avoidance of caffeine, alcohol, nicotine, and medications that exacerbate RLS (selective serotonin reuptake inhibitors, dopamine blocking agents, stimulants)
- Physical and mental activity
- Good sleep hygiene

ACUTE GENERAL Rx

Once the diagnosis of RLS is considered based on clinical criteria as mentioned in Table 1 and causes impairment of quality of life, an anticonvulsant (gabapentin enacarbil or pregabalin) or dopamine agonist (bromocriptine, pramipexole, or ropinirole) should be started at low dose and then gradually tapered depending on tolerance. Dopaminergic medications have the potential to

TABLE 1 Diagnostic Criteria for Restless Legs Syndrome

Minimal Criteria

- Desire to move the legs usually associated with paresthesias
- Motor restlessness, as characterized by floor pacing, leg rubbing, stretching, and flexing
- Worse at rest, with relief by activity
- Worse at night

Additional Criteria

- Sleep disturbances, as difficulty in sleep onset and maintaining sleep, daytime fatigue, or somnolence
- Involuntary movements, as periodic limb or leg movements in sleep and periodic or aperiodic limb movements while awake
- Neurologic examination is normal in idiopathic restless legs syndrome
- Clinical course may begin at any age but most severe in middle and older age
- Family history suggests autosomal dominant mode of inheritance in 1/3 of the cases

From Stiansy K, et al.: Clinical symptomatology and treatment of restless leg syndrome and periodic limb movement disorder, *Sleep Med Rev* 6(4):253-265, 2002.

TABLE 2 Management of Restless Legs Syndrome LS/WED

Agent and Daily Dosage	Side Effects	Countermeasures
Step 1: $\alpha 2\delta$ Agents First-line treatment, particularly if sleep disturbance, pain, or anxiety is present		
Gabapentin enacarbil, 300-600 mg Pregabalin, 50-450 mg* Gabapentin, 100-1800 mg*	Dizziness	Reduce dose and add alternate medication class as needed. If fall risk, then discontinue and change to alternate medication class.
	Somnolence, daytime fatigue	Reduce dose and add alternate medication class as needed. If significant, discontinue and change to alternate medication class.
	Tolerance	Discontinue, take drug holiday with return to medication. Switch to alternate medication class.
	Weight gain	Reduce dose and add alternate medication class as needed. If significant, discontinue and change to alternate medication class.
Step 2: Dopamine Agonists Alternative first-line treatment if depression is present and dose kept low.		
Pramipexole, 0.125-0.5 mg* (0.75 mg in Europe) Ropinirole, 0.5-4.0 mg* Rotigotine, 1-3 mg/24 h	Nausea and orthostatic hypotension	Slowly increase dosage or use domperidone if available (10-30 mg).
	Insomnia	Add or switch to $\alpha 2\delta$ agent. Use a small dose of benzodiazepines in association with dopamine agonists.
	Daytime fatigue and somnolence	Reduce dosage or discontinue dopamine agonists.
	Compulsive or impulsive behavior	Reduce dose and add alternate medication class as needed. If significant, discontinue and change to alternate medication class.
	Tolerance	Discontinue and switch to longer-acting dopamine agonist or alternate medication class.
	Augmentation	Discontinue and switch to alternate medication class or longer-acting dopamine agonist.
Step 3: Dopamine Precursors Useful for intermittent treatment, such as twice a week		
Levodopa-benserazide or levodopa-carbidopa (regular or slow release), 100/25 or 200/50 mg†	Same as for dopamine agonists	See countermeasures for dopamine agonists.
	Morning rebound or augmentation of restless legs syndrome in early evening	Use small extra dose of levodopa during daytime or reduce dosage or combine levodopa with dopamine agonists or benzodiazepines or discontinue levodopa (if severe and persistent).
	Augmentation	Do not use daily. Discontinue and switch to dopamine agonists or a nondopamine medication.
Benzodiazepines Useful for sleep promotion		
Clonazepam, 0.5-2.0 mg‡ Temazepam, 15-30 mg‡ Nitrazepam, 5-10 mg*	Daytime somnolence	Reduce dosage.
	Tolerance	Take drug holiday for 2 wk then return to lower dosage.
Opiates Second-line treatment		
Oxycodone-naloxone, 10/5 to 40/20 mg/day Methadone, 2.5-20 mg Oxycodone, 5-40 mg	Constipation	Use for symptom treatment.
	Dependency	Take a drug holiday. Discontinue and switch to alternate medication.
Oral Iron Always consider if serum iron ≤75 mcg/L *or* transferrin saturation ≤17%		
Ferrous sulfate, 650 mg (325 mg with vitamin C, 100 mg twice a day)	Constipation, stomach upset and pain	Reduce dose, discontinue, take with food.
	Diarrhea, nausea, vomiting	Reduce dose, discontinue, take with food.

*One hour before onset of symptoms in the evening or 1-2 hours before bedtime if symptoms are not present in the evening.
†Considered most appropriate for PRN dosing not more than 3 times a week rather than daily use.
‡Before bedtime usually to promote sleep with restless legs syndrome.
From Kryger M, et al.: *Principles and practice of sleep medicine*, ed 6, Philadelphia, 2017, Elsevier.

cause iatrogenic worsening (augmentation) of RLS with long-term treatment.

REFERRAL

Refer to neurologist if diagnosis is uncertain or an underlying disorder is suspected.

SUGGESTED READINGS

Available at ExpertConsult.com

RELATED CONTENT

Restless Legs Syndrome (Patient Information)

AUTHORS: **FARIHA ZAHEER, M.D.,** and **COREY GOLDSMITH, M.D.**

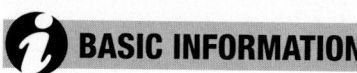

DEFINITION

Retropharyngeal abscess is a soft tissue infection of the throat that involves retropharyngeal space and that primarily affects children. The anatomic boundaries of the retropharyngeal space are the buccopharyngeal fascia (middle layer of the deep cervical fascia) anteriorly and the alar fascia (deep layer of the deep cervical fascia) posteriorly. The space begins at the skull base superiorly and ends inferiorly where the two fasciae fuse at the level between the first and second thoracic vertebrae.

ICD-10CM CODE
J39.0 Retropharyngeal and parapharyngeal abscess

EPIDEMIOLOGY & DEMOGRAPHICS

Retropharyngeal abscess occurs most commonly in children between the ages of 2 and 4 yr, analogous to suppurative cervical adenitis. 70% of cases are in patients under the age of 6, and 50% are in patients under the age of 3. This represents the peak age group for numerous viral upper respiratory tract infections and their attendant complications, acute otitis media and sinusitis. Retropharyngeal space infection is less common in older children and adults because the lymph nodes generally atrophy by puberty.

PHYSICAL FINDINGS & CLINICAL PRESENTATION

- The onset of a retropharyngeal infection may be insidious, with little more than fever, irritability, drooling, a muffled voice (dysphonia), or possibly nuchal rigidity.
- The acute symptoms relate to pressure and inflammation produced by the abscess on either the airway or the upper digestive tract and pharynx. The patient may have intense dysphagia, drooling, and odynophagia, or there may be some element of respiratory distress from edema and inflammation of the airway (stridor, tachypnea, or both).
- Unwillingness to move the neck because of discomfort is often a prominent presenting feature and should lead to consideration of retropharyngeal abscess if the child is febrile and irritable.
- Extension of the neck is usually affected more than flexion. This causes the patient to hold his or her neck stiffly or to present with torticollis.
- Trismus is unusual.
- On physical examination it may be possible to appreciate midline or unilateral swelling of the posterior pharyngeal wall. The mass may be fluctuant to the examining finger, and care must be taken to avoid rupture of the abscess into the upper airway.

Complications are numerous and could be fatal; these include airway obstruction, septicemia, thrombosis of the internal jugular vein, carotid artery rupture, and acute necrotizing mediastinitis. Aspiration with resultant pneumonia may complicate retropharyngeal abscess if rupture of the abscess occurs and empties into the airway. Infection can spread from one space in the neck to another.

The most dreaded complication is jugular vein suppurative thrombophlebitis (Lemierre's syndrome), in which the vessels of the carotid sheath become infected, leading to bacteremia and spread of infection to the lungs, brain, and mediastinum.

ETIOLOGY

- The retropharyngeal space comprises two chains of lymph nodes that drain the nasopharynx, adenoids, posterior paranasal sinuses, middle ear, and eustachian tube. Accordingly, suppurative infections in these areas may provide the seeds for infection for retropharyngeal abscess.
- The predominant bacterial species are *Streptococcus pyogenes* (group A *Streptococcus*), *Staphylococcus aureus,* and respiratory anaerobes (including *Fusobacteria, Prevotella,* and *Veillonella* species). *Haemophilus* species are also occasionally found.
- In young children, infection usually reaches this space by lymphatic spread from a septic focus in the pharynx or sinuses.
- In adults, infection may reach the retropharyngeal space from either local or distant sites. Penetrating trauma (e.g., from chicken bones or iatrogenic) is the usual source of local spread. More distant sources of infection include odontogenic sepsis and peritonsillar abscess (now a rare cause).

Dx DIAGNOSIS

DIFFERENTIAL DIAGNOSIS

- Cervical osteomyelitis
- Pott disease
- Meningitis
- Calcific tendonitis of the long muscle of the neck
- Differentiating features of deep neck infections are summarized in Table 1

LABORATORY STUDIES

- CBC with differential.
- Blood cultures may be considered in refractory cases or for severe symptoms.

IMAGING STUDIES

- A lateral neck film should be obtained and can be helpful in delineating the presence of a retropharyngeal abscess and may demonstrate cervical lordosis; the retropharyngeal space is considered widened and pathologic if it is greater than 7 mm at C2 or 14 mm at C6 (Fig. E1).
  1. There must be attention to technical issues when performing the study, especially in children. The film should be a perfect lateral, and the child must keep the neck in extension during inspiration to avoid a false thickening of the retropharyngeal space. Crying, particularly in infants, may also cause false thickening of the retropharyngeal space.
- CXR should be considered to evaluate for mediastinitis or aspiration pneumonia.
- A CT scan of the neck is useful for patients with moderate or high suspicion of having a deep neck space abscess. It is the most useful imaging modality to identify abscesses in the retropharyngeal space, but it is not perfect. Both the sensitivity and specificity of the CT scan in predicting the presence of drainable purulent material are quite variable from study to study, ranging between 68% and 100%.
  1. The CT scan provides more information than the plain radiograph because it can generally differentiate between retropharyngeal cellulitis and retropharyngeal abscess and can demonstrate extension of the retropharyngeal abscess to

TABLE 1 Differentiating Features of Deep Neck Infections

Space	Clinical Features*
Submandibular space (Ludwig angina)	Woody submental induration, protruding swollen/necrotic tongue, no trismus, rotted lower molars commonly present
Lateral pharyngeal space (anterior)	Fever, toxicity, trismus, neck swelling
Lateral pharyngeal space (posterior)	No trismus, no swelling (unless ipsilateral parotid is involved), cranial nerve IX-XII palsies, Horner syndrome, carotid artery erosion
Retropharyngeal space (retropharynx)	Neck stiffness, decreased neck range of motion, soft-tissue bulging of posterior pharyngeal wall, sore throat, dysphagia, dyspnea
Retropharyngeal space ("danger space")	Mediastinal or pleural involvement
Retropharyngeal space (prevertebral)	Neck stiffness, decreased neck range of motion, cervical instability, possible spread along length of vertebral column
Jugular vein septic thrombophlebitis (Lemierre syndrome)	Sore throat, swollen tender neck, dyspnea, chest pain, septic arthritis

*Fever and signs of systemic toxicity are common to all.
From Vincent JL et al: *Textbook of critical care*, ed 7, Philadelphia, 2017, Elsevier.

TABLE 2 Therapeutic Options for Deep Neck Infections

Syndrome	Likely Flora	Therapeutic Options*
Submandibular space infection (community acquired)	Anaerobes, streptococci, *Staphylococcus aureus*	Ampicillin-sulbactam (3 g IV q 6 h) Ceftriaxone (1-2 g IV q 24 h) *plus* clindamycin (300-900 mg IV q 8 h) *or* metronidazole (500 mg IV q 6 h) Ertapenem (1 g IV q day)
Submandibular space infection (hospital/ICU acquired)	*Pseudomonas aeruginosa,* methicillin-resistant *S. aureus* (MRSA), anaerobes	Imipenem (500 mg IV q 6 h) *or* piperacillin-tazobactam (3.375 g IV q 8 h by continuous infusion) *plus* vancomycin (1 g IV q 12 h)
Retropharyngeal space infection	Anaerobes, streptococci, *S. aureus*	Ampicillin-sulbactam (3 g IV q 6 h) Ceftriaxone (1-2 g IV q 24 h) *plus* clindamycin (300-900 mg IV q 8 h) *or* metronidazole (500 mg IV q 6 h) Ertapenem (1 g IV q day)
Lateral pharyngeal space infection	Anaerobes, streptococci, *S. aureus*	Ampicillin-sulbactam (3 g IV q 6 h) Ceftriaxone (1-2 g IV q 24 h) *plus* clindamycin (300-900 mg IV q 8 h) *or* metronidazole (500 mg IV q 6 h) Ertapenem (1 g IV q day)
Internal jugular vein septic thrombophlebitis	*Fusobacterium necrophorum*	Metronidazole (500 mg IV q 6 h) Clindamycin (300-900 mg IV q 8 h) Ampicillin-sulbactam (3 g IV q 6 h)

*Antibiotic choices listed are examples, because for most infections, multiple different antibiotics are effective; individual choice will be influenced by patient factors (e.g., allergies, concurrent medications), local hospital bacterial resistance rates, and microbiological culture results.

ICU, Intensive care unit; *IV,* Intravenous.

From Vincent JL et al: *Textbook of critical care,* ed 7, Philadelphia, 2017, Elsevier.

contiguous spaces in the neck. Findings on CT common to both cellulitis and abscess are a low-density core, soft tissue swelling, obliterated fat planes, and mass effect. Findings on CT scan that are indicative of abscess are "complete rim enhancement" and scalloping of the abscess borders (Fig. E2). The abscess may be seen as a mass impinging on the posterior pharyngeal wall.

- MRI of the neck is rarely used for diagnosis, especially in the pediatric population because of the longer time to acquire the study and the need for sedation in the younger population. T2-weighted images may identify and localize areas of pus for drainage or aspiration. Gadolinium enhancement is important to accurately define the soft tissue component. It also can be useful for distinguishing inflammatory from congenital or neoplastic lesions. Magnetic resonance angiography can be helpful for imaging vascular lesions, such as jugular thrombophlebitis.

Rx TREATMENT

ACUTE GENERAL & CHRONIC Rx

- When the CT findings suggest cellulitis or phlegmon, a trial of IV antibiotic therapy without drainage is initiated, and the child is monitored as an inpatient for 48 hr. If the child is clinically improved, consider discharge home with a course of oral antibiotics. If the clinical course is not improved or is worse, a repeat CT scan should be obtained, and surgical drainage or prolonged IV antibiotic therapy may be warranted. Some investigators also support a trial of IV antibiotic therapy alone when small abscesses are identified by CT scans, as long as the airway is not compromised.
  1. Ampicillin-sulbactam (300 mg/kg/day IV divided q6h) or clindamycin (25-40 mg/kg/day IV divided q8h) are effective antimicrobial selections. In adults, ampicillin-sulbactam 3 g IV q6h or clindamycin 600 mg IV q8h. Antibiotics should be adjusted as culture data become available, and oral therapy is continued to complete at least a 14-day course. Therapeutic options for deep neck infections are summarized in Table 2.
- Surgical intervention has historically played a prominent role in the management of retropharyngeal abscess in conjunction with antibiotic therapy. Prompt surgical drainage is indicated when there is a large hypodense area suggestive of an abscess or when a patient has not responded to parenteral therapy alone.

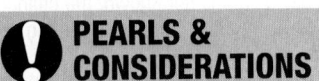

PEARLS & CONSIDERATIONS

PREVENTION

The complications of deep neck infection in any space are numerous and potentially fatal. Early diagnosis, with prompt and appropriate management, is key to avoiding these complications.

SUGGESTED READING

Available at ExpertConsult.com

AUTHOR: **LOUIS INSALACO, M.D.**

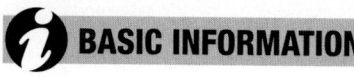

BASIC INFORMATION

DEFINITION

Rhesus (Rh) incompatibility is a clinical scenario where discordance of the maternal and fetal Rh type leads to the development of maternal Rh sensitization and hemolytic disease of the neonate. Individuals whose RBCs express the Rh D antigen are classified as Rh-positive, whereas those whose RBCs do not express the antigen are classified as Rh-negative.

ICD-10CM CODES

O36.0910	Maternal care for other rhesus isoimmunization, first trimester, not applicable or unspecified
T80.4	Rh incompatibility reaction
T80.4	Unspecified complication following infusion, transfusion, and therapeutic injection

EPIDEMIOLOGY & DEMOGRAPHICS

INCIDENCE:

- The absence of the D antigen (Rh negative blood type) occurs in 15% of whites, 7% of blacks, and less than 1% of the Native American and Asian populations. If the father's blood type is not known, the chance that an Rh− pregnant woman is bearing an Rh+ fetus is approximately 60%.
- Of those pregnancies complicated by Rh incompatibility, the risk of maternal isoimmunization to the D antigen is approximately 8% for each ABO-compatible pregnancy if no prophylaxis is given.
- Maternal-fetal ABO incompatibility is somewhat protective against Rh isoimmunization.

GENETICS: Five major loci determine Rh status: C, D, E, c, e. The presence of the D antigen results in an Rh+ individual, while its absence results in an Rh− individual. Of Rh+ fathers, 45% are homozygotes, and 55% are heterozygotes. For homozygous Rh+ fathers, the probability of an Rh+ offspring is 100%. The probability for heterozygotes is approximately 50%.

RISK FACTORS:

- RhD-negative woman
- Antepartum: Fetal-to-maternal transfusion
- Intrapartum: Fetal-to-maternal transfusion, spontaneous abortion, ectopic pregnancy, abruptio placentae, abdominal trauma, chorionic villus sampling, amniocentesis, percutaneous umbilical blood sampling (PUBS), external cephalic version, manual removal of the placenta, therapeutic abortion, autologous blood product administration
- Maternal history of hydrops or sensitization to RhD

ETIOLOGY

The initial response to D antigen exposure is production of immunoglobulin (Ig) M that does not cross the placenta. With a repeated exposure, IgG is produced. Hemolysis in the fetus results once maternal IgG is present in the fetal circulation by crossing the placenta. This may result in a spectrum of hemolytic disease in the newborn, resulting in antepartum or neonatal death or neurologic damage to the fetus because of hyperbilirubinemia and kernicterus.

Dx DIAGNOSIS

LABORATORY TESTS

ABO and Rh blood type and an antibody screen as part of the initial prenatal profile.

- If antibody screen negative:
  1. Repeat antibody screen at 28 weeks of gestation.
  2. Obtain neonatal blood type after delivery.
  3. If Rh incompatibility is confirmed by the neonatal blood type, a Kleihauer-Betke/flow cytometry or rosette test should be performed to determine the amount of fetomaternal transfusion in the following high-risk circumstances: abruptio placentae, placenta previa, cesarean delivery, intrauterine manipulation, manual removal of the placenta.
- If anti-D antibody screen is positive:
  1. Maternal indirect Coombs test is needed to determine antibody titer.
  2. Determine paternal Rh status and zygosity.
  3. If father is heterozygous, PUBS or amniotic fluid is needed to determine fetal Rh status.

IMAGING STUDIES

Ultrasound evaluation may show subcutaneous edema, ascites, pleural effusion, pericardial effusion, or hepatomegaly. It can diagnose hydrops fetalis, but it cannot predict it.

Doppler ultrasound of middle cerebral artery can predict moderate to severe anemia.

Rx TREATMENT

PREVENTION OF D-ISOIMMUNIZATION

- 50 mcg of D immunoglobulin: After spontaneous or induced abortion or ectopic pregnancy <13 weeks' gestation.
- 300 mcg of D immunoglobulin (protects against 30 ml of fetal blood).
  1. After spontaneous or induced abortion >13 weeks' gestation, amniocentesis, chorionic villous sampling, PUBS, external cephalic version, or other intrauterine manipulation.
  2. As antepartum prophylaxis at 28 weeks' gestation. Maternal anti-D prophylaxis does not cause hemolysis in the fetus or newborn.
  3. At 40 weeks' gestation or at delivery if the neonate is D- or Du-positive.
  4. If Kleihauer-Betke or rosette test confirms >30 ml of fetal red blood in maternal circulation, additional D immunoglobulin is indicated. Confirm adequacy of therapy by a maternal indirect Coombs test 48 to 72 hr after Rh immunoglobulin is given.

MANAGEMENT OF D-ISOIMMUNIZED PREGNANCIES

- Serial amniocentesis for assessment of amount of fetal bilirubin in fluid (OD_{450}) after 25 weeks' gestation with interpretation of the Delta OD_{450} according to criteria established by Liley.
- PUBS if ultrasonographic evidence of hydrops, rising zone II Delta OD_{450} values on amniocentesis, or maternal history of a severely affected child.
- Intrauterine exchange transfusion if severe anemia is documented remote from term.
- Initiation of steroids for lung maturation at 28 weeks in severely affected pregnancies with delivery at lung maturity.
- Delivery as soon as lung maturation is achieved in mild to moderately affected pregnancies.

Fig. 1 shows an algorithm for clinical management of a patient with red cell sensitization in the first affected pregnancy and Fig. 2 shows an algorithm for clinical management of a patient with red cell sensitization and a previously affected fetus or infant.

DISPOSITION

Survival of nonhydropic infants is 90%. Of infants with hydrops, 82% survive.

REFERRAL

Refer all Rh isoimmunized pregnancies to a tertiary care center before 18 to 20 weeks of gestation.

SUGGESTED READINGS

Available at ExpertConsult.com

AUTHOR: **BHARTI RATHORE, M.D.**

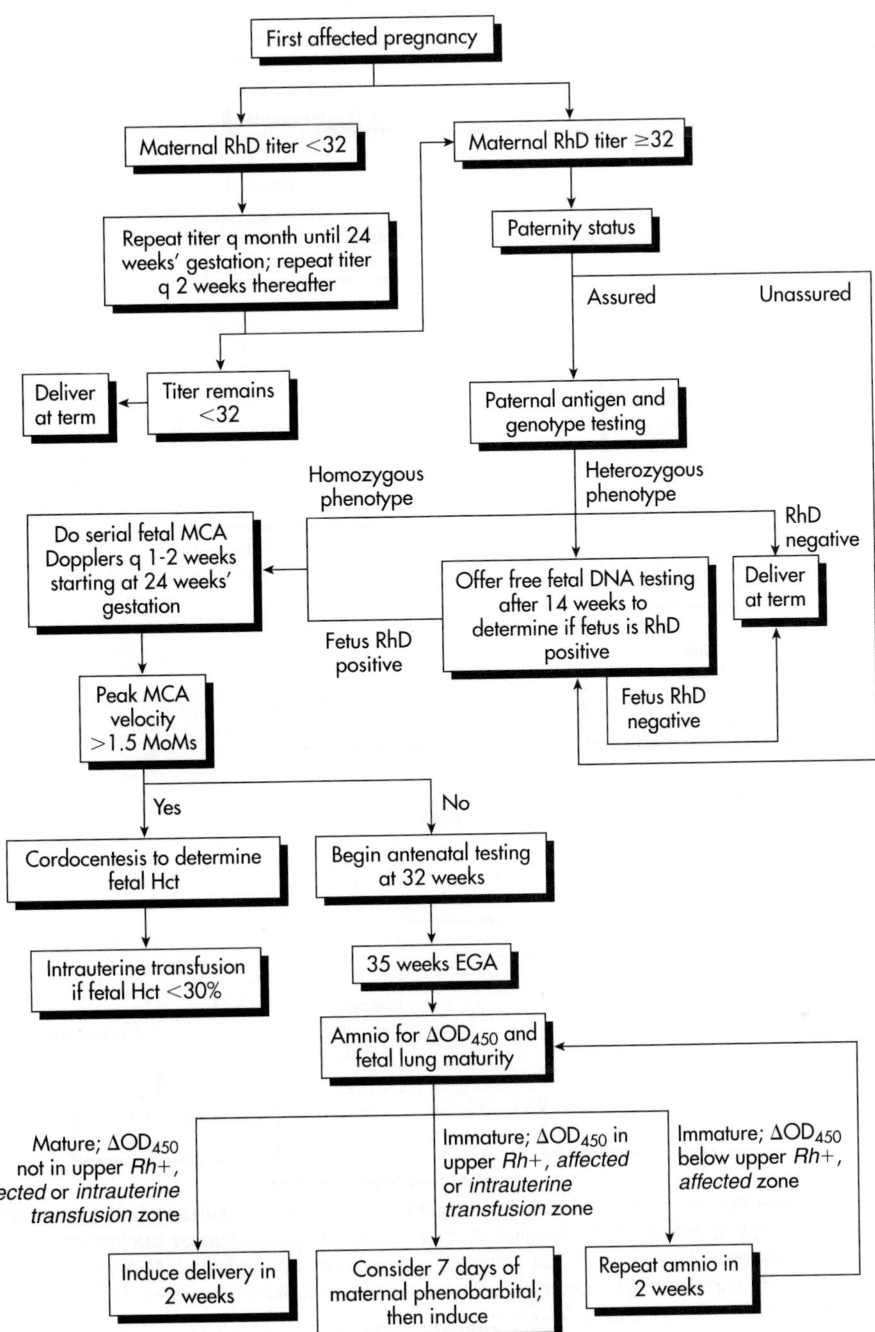

FIG. 1 Algorithm for clinical management of a patient with red cell sensitization in the first affected pregnancy. ΔOD_{450}, Deviation of optical density of amniotic fluid by spectrophotometer at 450nm; *DNA*, deoxyribonucleic acid; *EGA*, estimated gestational age; *Hct*, hematocrit; *MCA*, middle cerebral artery; *MoMs*, multiples of the median; *Rh+*, Rhesus positive; *RhD*, Rhesus D antigen. (From Gabbe SG: *Obstetrics*, ed 6, Philadelphia, 2012, Saunders.)

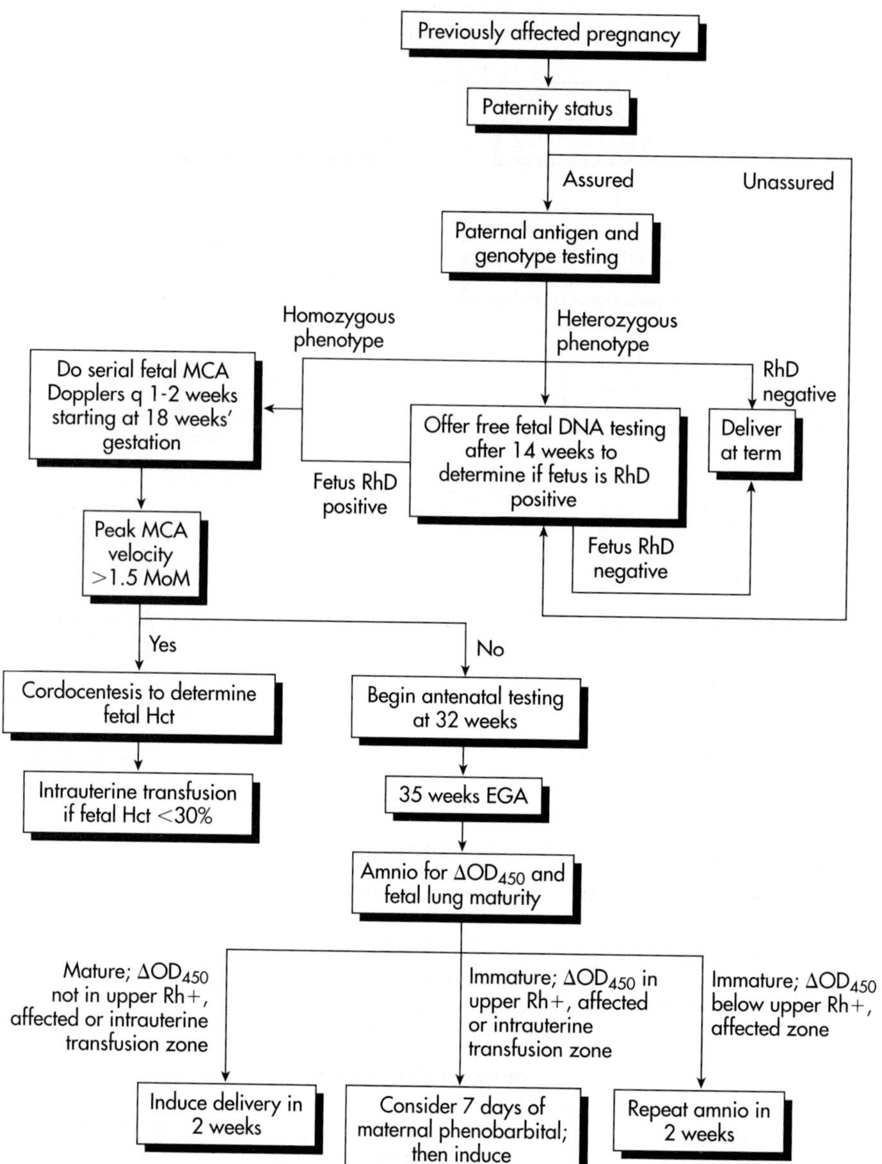

FIG. 2 Algorithm for clinical management of a patient with red cell sensitization and a previously affected fetus or infant. *OD450,* Deviation of optical density of amniotic fluid by spectrophotometer at 450nm; *DNA,* deoxyribonucleic acid; *EGA,* estimated gestational age; *Hct,* hematocrit; *MCA,* middle cerebral artery; *MoMs,* multiples of the median; *Rh+,* Rhesus positive; *RhD,* Rhesus D antigen. (From Gabbe SG: *Obstetrics,* 6 ed, Philadelphia, 2012, Saunders.)

BASIC INFORMATION

DEFINITION

Rhabdomyolysis is a syndrome characterized by striated muscle lysis with resulting muscle damage and leakage of intracellular contents into the circulation. The presentation may range from asymptomatic elevation of creatine kinase (CK) to severe muscle injury with irreversible kidney failure. In general, five- to tenfold elevations of CK levels, muscle pain, and myoglobinuria in an appropriate clinical setting (see below) are sufficient criteria for the diagnosis of rhabdomyolysis. Acute renal injury occurs from a combination of factors, including volume depletion, tubular obstruction, direct heme-induced proximal tubular cell injury, and associated renal vasoconstriction.

ICD-10CM CODES

M62.82	Rhabdomyolysis (idiopathic)
T79.6	Traumatic ischemia of muscle
M62.89	Other specified disorders of muscle

EPIDEMIOLOGY & DEMOGRAPHICS

PREDOMINANT AGE: Incidence of 1 in 10,000 in the U.S.

- Rare in children. Increased risk with advanced age, i.e., >80 yr.
- Reported incidence of AKI with rhabdomyolysis is 10% to 55%.
- 7% to 10% of cases of AKI are due to rhabdomyolysis.

MORTALITY RATE: 5% to 8%. Prognosis is better in the absence of AKI.

ONSET: Evidence is limited regarding the onset of physical exertion-induced rhabdomyolysis. Exercise levels exceeding usual exercise tolerance levels for individuals are commonly causative. Extracellular volume depletion and vasoconstriction are common predisposing features. Patients with risk factors (e.g., metabolic myopathies, advanced age) develop symptoms associated with rhabdomyolysis within 2 to 6 hr after activity. Patients without such risk factors generally become symptomatic 12 to 36 hr after muscle injury. The presence of concurrent electrolyte abnormalities such as hypokalemia, hyponatremia, hypernatremia, hypomagnesemia, hypophosphatemia, and hypocalcemia increases the risk for rhabdomyolysis.

CK levels rise within 2 to 12 hr of the onset of muscle injury, peak generally by 24 to 72 hr, and decline within 3 to 5 days after cessation of muscle injury. Peak CK concentrations may predict development of renal injury. In patients with rhabdomyolysis secondary to malignant hyperthermia, CK concentrations peak approximately 14 hr after an acute episode.

Cholesterol-lowering therapy with HMG-CoA synthetase inhibitors (statins) in association with clinical rhabdomyolysis is reported in less than 0.1% of cases, although myalgia is a frequent complaint. Among the statins, pravastatin has been reported to have a lower risk of rhabdomyolysis, presumably due to its lower lipid solubility. The average duration of statin therapy before the onset of myopathy is 6 mo. Symptom resolution with normalization of serum CK concentrations occurs in days to weeks following drug discontinuation. The average time for onset of rhabdomyolysis after addition of fibrate to statin therapy is 32 days.

PHYSICAL FINDINGS & CLINICAL PRESENTATION

- Classic triad: (1) muscle pain, (2) weakness, and (3) dark urine from myoglobinuria
- Muscle tenderness is present only 50% of the time
- Muscle swelling
- Muscular rigidity
- Fever
- Altered consciousness
- In statin-induced rhabdomyolysis, fatigue (74%) is nearly as common as muscle pain (88%)
- Oliguria or anuria in the presence of kidney injury

ETIOLOGY

Causes can be divided into three categories:

- Traumatic or muscle compression:
  1. High-current electrical injury
  2. Crush injury and compartment syndrome
  3. Tourniquet and limb ischemia
  4. Reperfusion after revascularization procedures for ischemia
  5. Extensive surgical (spinal) dissection, bariatric surgery
- Nontraumatic exertional:
  1. Exercise: More than 10 genetically predisposing mutations are associated with exertional rhabdomyolysis
  2. Sickle cell trait, rarely; usually additional predisposing factors are involved (e.g., BMI >30 kg/m^2, tobacco use, statin use, antipsychotic use, high altitude)
  3. Heat stroke
  4. Metabolic myopathies
  5. Malignant hyperthermia and neuroleptic malignant syndrome
  6. Seizure activity
- Nontraumatic, nonexertional:
  1. Drug-induced (statins alone, combination of statins with fibrates, or erythromycin, simvastatin and amiodarone, amphetamines, haloperidol)
  2. Alcoholism
  3. Hypothyroidism
  4. Infectious and inflammatory myositis

Table 1 summarizes the various causes of rhabdomyolysis.

DIAGNOSIS

DIFFERENTIAL DIAGNOSIS

"Creatine Kinase Elevation" in Section IV describes a clinical algorithm for the evaluation of CK elevation.

LABORATORY TESTS

- Creatine kinase: Usually CK is 5 to 10 times the upper limit of normal and typically peaks 24 to 72 hours after the initial insult (Fig. 1). Levels >15,000 IU/L are more likely to be associated with renal injury. However, in patients with concomitant risk factors such as hypokalemia or volume depletion, CK levels as low as 5000 U/L have been associated with AKI.
- Myoglobin: Excreted in urine with visible changes in urine ("port wine") at levels >100 to 300 mg/dl. Myoglobinuria can be suspected by a positive urine dipstick test for blood and minimal or no microhematuria. Due to its more rapid hepatic metabolism, myoglobin lacks sensitivity in detecting rhabdomyolysis. Therefore, serum and/or urine myoglobin measurement is not recommended to establish diagnosis. Blood urea nitrogen and creatinine help monitor the severity of AKI.
- Potassium, calcium, phosphorus, and uric levels are released from damaged muscle, and levels should be monitored.
- Calcium: Hypocalcemia from influx and deposition of calcium phosphate in damaged muscle tissue. Hypercalcemia may follow resolution of rhabdomyolysis from subsequent release of muscle-sequestered calcium back into the circulation and increased gastrointestinal calcium absorption from enhanced vitamin D production.
- Anion gap metabolic acidosis may occur from release of organic acids and phosphates from damaged muscle.
- Urinalysis: Myoglobin is detected as blood on dipstick, but erythrocytes are absent on microscopy. Presence of pigmented tubular casts establishes acute tubular necrosis.

TABLE 1 Causes of Rhabdomyolysis

Muscle injury/ischemia	Trauma, pressure necrosis, electric shock, burns, acute vascular disease
Myofiber exhaustion	Seizures, excessive exercise, heat exhaustion
Toxins	Alcohol, cocaine, heroin, amphetamines, ecstasy, phencyclidine, snakebite
Drugs	Statins, fibrates, zidovudine, neuroleptic malignant syndrome, azathioprine, theophylline, lithium, diuretics
Electrolyte disorders	Hypophosphatemia, hypokalemia, excess water shifts (hyperosmolality)
Infections	Viral (influenza, HIV, coxsackievirus, Epstein-Barr virus), bacterial (*Legionella, Francisella, Streptococcus pneumoniae, Salmonella, Staphylococcus aureus)*
Familial	McArdle disease, carnitine palmitoyl transferase deficiency, malignant hyperthermia
Other	Hypothyroidism, polymyositis, dermatomyositis

From Floege J et al: *Comprehensive clinical nephrology,* ed 4, Philadelphia, 2010, Saunders.

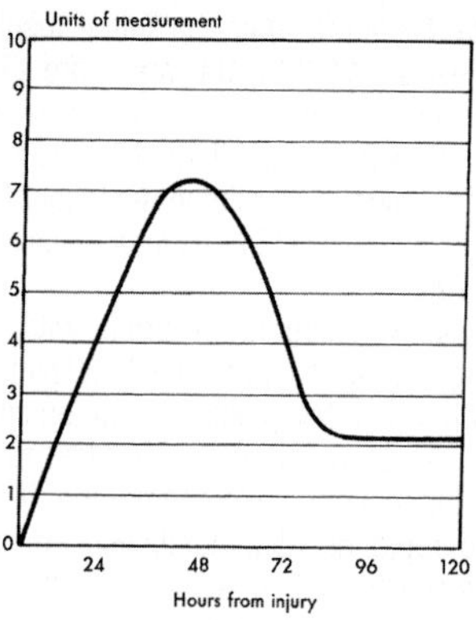

FIG. 1 Typical creatine kinase elimination curve.

- Unlike most other causes of acute tubular necrosis, rhabdomyolysis may result in a fractional excretion of sodium (FENa) of <1% due to renal vasoconstriction.
- Box 1 summarizes laboratory abnormalities observed with rhabdomyolysis.

BOX 1 Laboratory Abnormalities Observed with Rhabdomyolysis

Potassium
Elevated
Risk for acute kidney injury

Bicarbonate
Decreased (20 mEq/L)
Metabolic acidosis

Uric Acid
Elevated (>7 mg/dl)
Marker of acute renal failure

Sodium
Usually normal
Can decrease with mannitol therapy
Use serum osmolality values as a guide

Phosphate
Elevated
Risk for precipitation of calcium phosphate
May need phosphate binders if phosphate >7 mg/dl

Creatine Kinase
Elevated
Associated with creatine kinase level of 15 to 75,000

Blood Urea Nitrogen
Elevated (>20 mg/dl)

Creatinine
Elevated

Calcium
Initially low
Rebound phase may demonstrate hypercalcemia

Liver Function Tests
Occasionally elevated
Serum aspartate transaminase, lactate dehydrogenase, aldolase, muscle enzyme levels elevated

Troponin
Normal
Suspect myocardial damage as a cause (or effect) if elevated
7% false-positive rate for troponin I

Anion Gap
Sometimes elevated
May predict acute kidney injury

Prothrombin Time, Partial Thromboplastin Time, D-Dimer
Disseminated intravascular coagulation in up to 30% of severe cases
Associated with greater mortality

From Adams JG et al: *Emergency medicine, clinical essentials,* ed 2, Philadelphia, 2013, Elsevier.

Rx TREATMENT

ACUTE GENERAL Rx

- Identify precipitating factor(s) and discontinuation of drugs or toxins that might be a contributing factor.
- Early, aggressive, high-volume IV fluid replacement with normal saline. Extracellular fluid volume loading and diuresis reduce the risk for renal damage by elimination of urate and phosphate that can precipitate in the kidneys. Fig. 2 describes a treatment algorithm for rhabdomyolysis.
- Fasciotomy is indicated in compartment syndrome for preservation of muscle and nerve function.
- Initiate volume repletion with normal saline at a rate of 200 to 1000 ml/hour depending on the clinical circumstances and severity of muscle damage. Titrate to maintain a urine output of at least 200 ml/hr. Consider treatment with mannitol (up to 200 g/day with cumulative dose up to 800 g) to GFR, diuresis, and scavenge free radicals. Typically, a 20% mannitol infusion at a dose of 0.5 g/kg is given over a 15-min period followed by an infusion at 0.1 g/kg/hour. Discontinue mannitol and volume resuscitation if diuresis (>20 ml/hr) is not established. Maintain volume repletion until myoglobinuria stops (negative urine dipstick blood test) or plasma CK levels decrease to <5000 U/L.
- Correct hypocalcemia if symptomatic or hyperkalemia is severe enough to produce electrocardiographic changes.
- Treatment of all electrolyte imbalances.
- Urine alkalinization: Maintain urine pH at 6 to 7 pH units and serum pH at ~7.50. This recommendation is controversial but appears helpful in research models when administered early in the course of rhabdomyolysis. Urine alkalinization may prevent renal tubular myoglobin precipitation and reduce lipid peroxidation, reactive oxygen species formation, and myoglobin-induced vasoconstriction. However, early volume resuscitation and expansion is the most important treatment.
- Initiation of renal replacement therapy is guided by the severity of renal injury and electrolyte imbalances. The use of continuous renal replacement therapy or high-flux membranes to enhance myoglobin clearance has not been validated.

DISPOSITION

Early diagnosis and management are required to avoid AKI that occurs in 30% of cases. Rhabdomyolysis accounts for 7% to 10% of all cases of AKI in the U.S.

REFERRAL

Renal consultation and surgical consultation if compartment syndrome develops

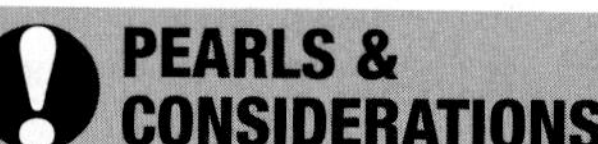

PEARLS & CONSIDERATIONS

COMMENTS

- Statin-induced rhabdomyolysis occurs 12 times more frequently when statins are combined with fibrates than when used alone.
- Short-term, high-dose glucocorticoid steroid administration (500-1000 mg methylprednisolone) has been used for treatment of alcohol-induced rhabdomyolysis, refractory to volume repletion. This treatment may be efficacious in cases of severe rhabdomyolysis by retarding secondary leukocyte inflammatory muscle injury.

SUGGESTED READINGS

Available at ExpertConsult.com

RELATED CONTENT

Rhabdomyolysis (Patient Information)
Statin-Induced Muscle Syndrome (Related Key Topic)

AUTHOR: **HESHAM SHABAN, M.D.**

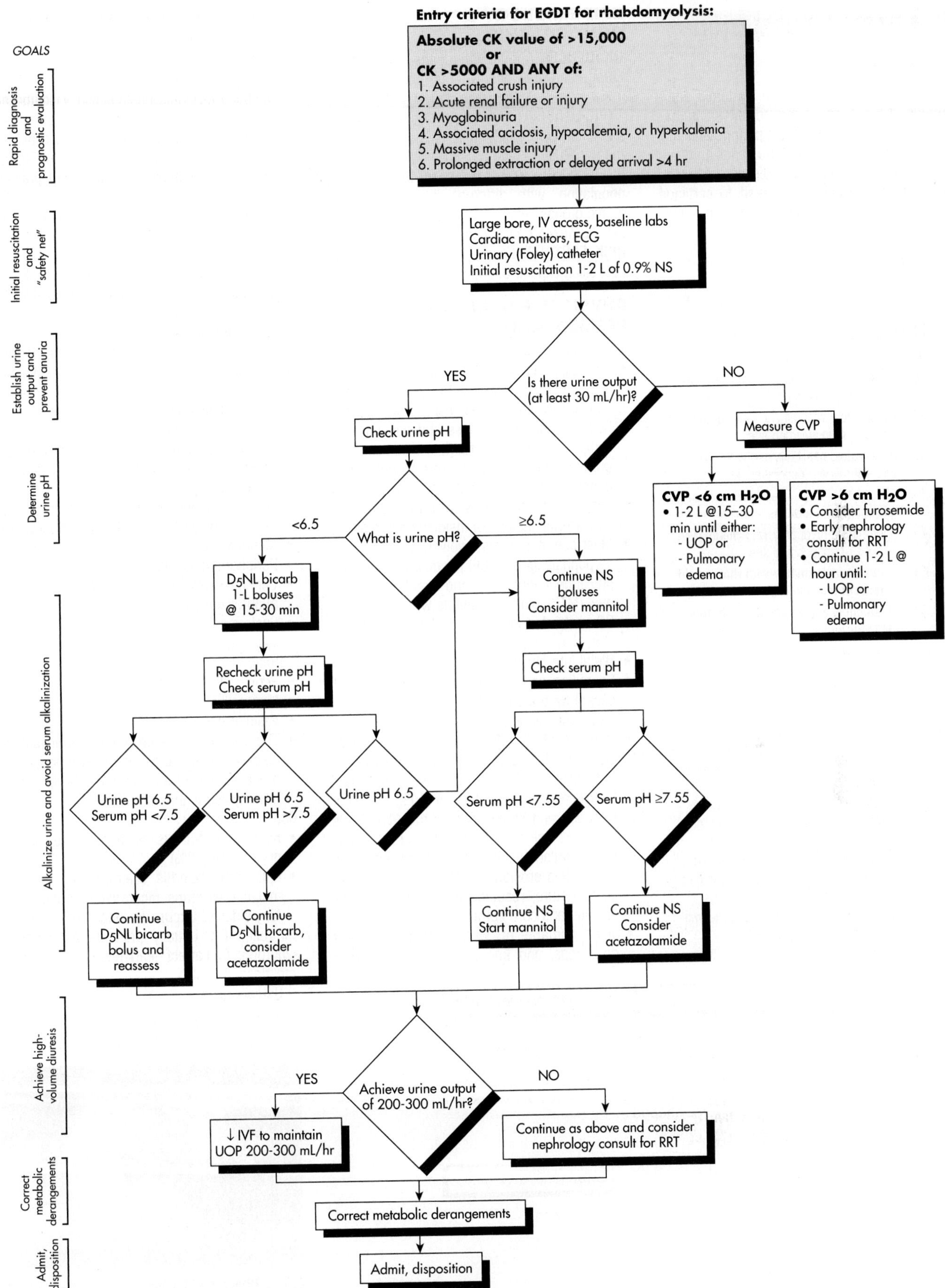

FIG. 2 Early goal-directed therapy for rhabdomyolysis. *CK*, Creatine kinase; *CVP*, central venous pressure; *D5NL bicarb*, 5% dextrose in normal sodium bicarbonate solution; *EGDT*, early goal-directed therapy; *IV*, intravenous; *IVF*, intravenous fluid; *NS*, normal saline; *RRT*, renal replacement therapy; *UOP*, urinary output. (From Adams JG et al: *Emergency medicine, clinical essentials*, 2nd ed, Philadelphia, Elsevier 2013.)

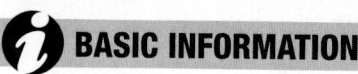

BASIC INFORMATION

DEFINITION

Rheumatoid arthritis (RA) is a systemic autoimmune disease characterized by inflammatory polyarthritis which affects peripheral joints, especially the small joints of the hands and feet. It is a chronic, progressive disease in which untreated inflammation may lead to cartilage and bone erosions and joint destruction resulting in functional impairment.

SYNONYM

RA

ICD-10CM CODES

M06.9	Rheumatoid arthritis, unspecified
M05.10	Rheumatoid lung disease with rheumatoid arthritis of unspecified site
M05.20	Rheumatoid vasculitis with rheumatoid arthritis of unspecified site
M05.30	Rheumatoid heart disease with rheumatoid arthritis of unspecified site
M05.39	Rheumatoid heart disease with rheumatoid arthritis of multiple sites
M05.40	Rheumatoid myopathy with rheumatoid arthritis of unspecified site
M05.49	Rheumatoid myopathy with rheumatoid arthritis of multiple sites
M05.50	Rheumatoid polyneuropathy with rheumatoid arthritis of unspecified site
M05.59	Rheumatoid polyneuropathy with rheumatoid arthritis of multiple sites
M05.60	Rheumatoid arthritis of unspecified site with involvement of other organs and systems
M05.69	Rheumatoid arthritis of multiple sites with involvement of other organs and systems
M05.70	Rheumatoid arthritis with rheumatoid factor of unspecified site without organ or systems involvement
M05.79	Rheumatoid arthritis with rheumatoid factor of multiple sites without organ or systems involvement
M05.80	Other rheumatoid arthritis with rheumatoid factor of unspecified site

EPIDEMIOLOGY & DEMOGRAPHICS

INCIDENCE: Annual incidence in northern Europe and the United States 0.15 to 0.60 per 1000

TYPICAL AGE AT DIAGNOSIS: Usually fourth or fifth decade. Steadily increases with age until the mid-70s

PREVALENCE: 0.5% to 1.0% of the worldwide population, with different rates in different ethnic groups

PREDOMINANT SEX: Females > males (2-3:1)

RISK FACTORS: Female gender, age, tobacco use, silica exposure, and obesity

PHYSICAL FINDINGS & CLINICAL PRESENTATION

Initial presentation:

- Pain, swelling, warmth in one or more peripheral joints, frequently with symmetric small joint involvement, often associated with >1 hour of morning stiffness and constitutional symptoms such as fatigue, malaise, low-grade fevers, and weight loss occurring over a period of weeks to months. A subset of patients can also present with acute-onset polyarthritis instead of insidious symptoms.
- Most common joints involved include metacarpophalangeal (MCP) joints, proximal interphalangeal (PIP) joints, and metatarsophalangeal (MTP) joints, as well as wrists.
- Other affected joints involved include elbows, shoulders, hips, knees, and ankles.
- Distal interphalangeal (DIP) joints are spared.
- Sacroiliac and vertebral joints are spared, except for the C1 and C2 articulations.

Chronic longstanding disease:

- "Swan-neck" (DIP flexion and PIP hyperextension), "boutonniere" (DIP hyperextension and PIP flexion), and "Z-thumb" (MCP flexion and IP hyperextension) deformities (Fig. 1), ulnar deviation and subluxation of the MCP joints (Fig. 2) as well as radial deviation of the wrists.
- C1-C2 (atlantoaxial) inflammation can lead to odontoid erosion and transverse ligament laxity/rupture, resulting in atlantoaxial subluxation and cord compression.
- Joint damage of wrists, elbows, shoulders, hips, and knees can lead to severe osteoarthritis, necessitating joint surgery and/or replacement.

Extraarticular manifestations:

- Secondary Sjögren's syndrome (~35%): Immune-mediated inflammation of lacrimal and salivary glands, resulting in dry mouth (xerostomia) and eyes (keratoconjunctivitis sicca).
- Rheumatoid nodules (25%): Nontender, firm nodules on extensor surfaces and pressure points, usually in rheumatoid factor positive (RF+) disease. Histopathology demonstrates palisading histiocytes surrounding a central area of fibrinoid necrosis.
- Felty syndrome: RA with splenomegaly and leukopenia. Most patients are positive for HLA-DR4 and RF.

Pulmonary disease:

- Pleural disease (exudative effusions, pleuritis)
- Interstitial lung disease (up to 10% clinically significant)
- Bronchiolitis obliterans
- Cryptogenic organizing pneumonia
- Pulmonary nodules: A combination of RA and pneumoconiosis is called Caplan syndrome

Neuromuscular:

- Entrapment neuropathy (carpal tunnel, tarsal tunnel, cubital tunnel most commonly involved)
- Mononeuritis multiplex
- Peripheral neuropathy
- Cervical myelopathy and cord compression in atlantoaxial subluxation
- Pachymeningitis (rare)

Vasculitis.

Cardiac disease:

- Pericarditis (most common)
- Myocarditis
- Valvular nodules
- There is an increased risk of cardiovascular disease compared to the general population, probably due to accelerated atherosclerosis from systemic inflammation

Ocular disease:

- Keratoconjunctivitis sicca (dry eye, without dry mouth) (10%)
- Episcleritis, scleritis, scleral thinning, scleromalacia perforans, ulcerative keratitis

Amyloidosis: Occurs in longstanding, poorly controlled RA. Usually presents as nephrotic syndrome. Can affect heart, kidney, liver, spleen, intestines, and skin.

Osteoporosis

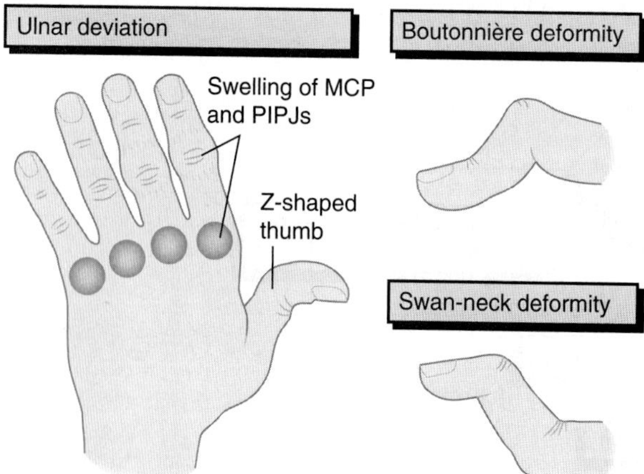

FIG. 1 Characteristic hand deformities in rheumatoid arthritis. *MCP,* Metacarpophalanges; *PIPJs,* proximal interphalangeal joints. (From Ballinger A: *Kumar & Clark's essentials of clinical medicine,* ed 6, Edinburgh, 2012, Saunders.)

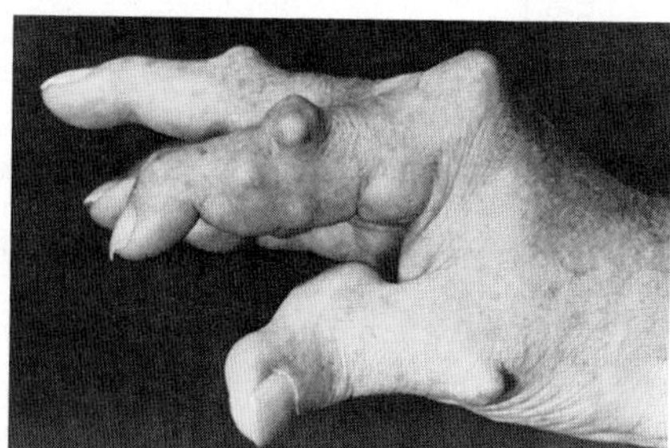

FIG. 2 Rheumatoid arthritis. Hand of a 60-year-old man with seropositive rheumatoid arthritis. There are fixed deformities and gross rheumatoid nodules. (From Canoso JJ: *Rheumatology in primary care,* Philadelphia, 1997, Saunders.)

ETIOLOGY

The exact cause of RA remains unknown despite extensive research. It is likely that a combination of genetic, hormonal, and environmental factors lead to aberrant immune activation and inflammatory response in the joint. A common genetic background plays a role in susceptibility to disease, as twins and first-degree relatives of RA patients are at increased risk of developing the disease compared to the general population. Patients with HLA-DR4, DR1, and DR14 alleles have increased susceptibility to RA; in particular, one amino acid sequence in the DR β chain, known as the shared epitope, is overrepresented in these patients. Other identified genetic associations include polymorphisms in *PTPN22, PADI4, CTLA4, TRAF1-C5, STAT4, TNFAIP3*. Epigenetic factors are also likely to be involved. Multiple environmental factors have also been implicated as possible etiologic factors, including cigarette smoking, silica exposure, and low socioeconomic class. Infectious agents such as *P. gingivalis*, Epstein-Barr virus, and parvovirus B19 have also been reported as possible triggers.

Stages of disease development presumably include:

- Initiation of the innate immune response through toll-like receptor (TLR) activation by a stimulating signal.
- Perpetuation of inflammatory response through activation of the adaptive immune system. There is migration of inflammatory cells (autoreactive B and T cells, monocytes) into the joint space, activation of macrophage-like and fibroblast-like synoviocytes, and development of a "synovial pannus," a thickened synovial membrane.
- The pannus releases proinflammatory cytokines (TNF-α, IL-1, IL-6, IL-15, IL-17, IL-18) as well as proteases, which erode cartilage and bone. Bone erosions are caused mainly by osteoclasts, which express the receptor activator of NF-κB (RANK). TNF-α, IL-1, IL-6, and IL-17 promote the expression of RANK ligand (RANKL) on T cells and fibroblast-like synoviocytes, thus creating a positive feedback loop. IL-6 and TNF-α act synergistically to increase vascular endothelial growth factor levels, which in turn stimulate angiogenesis, thereby maintaining pannus formation. B-cell differentiation is also promoted by IL-6, leading to the production of autoantibodies.
- Many of the new "biologic" disease-modifying antirheumatic drugs (DMARDs) are engineered to target these cytokines (see "Treatment" section).

TABLE 1 Factors Useful for Differentiating Early Rheumatoid Arthritis from Osteoarthritis

	Rheumatoid Arthritis	Osteoarthritis
Age at onset	Childhood and adults, peak incidence in 50s	Increases with age
Predisposing factors	Susceptibility epitopes (HLA-DR4, HLA-DR1, HLA-DR14)	Trauma
	Polymorphisms, epigenetic factors, infectious agents	Congenital abnormalities (e.g., shallow acetabulum)
	Smoking, silica exposure	
Early symptoms	Morning stiffness, pain, swelling	Pain increases through the day and with use
Joints involved	Wrists, MCP, PIP, and MTP joints; DIP joints are almost never involved.	DIP joints (Heberden nodes), PIP joints (Bouchard nodes), carpometacarpal joints, weight-bearing joints (hips, knees)
Physical findings	Soft tissue swelling, warmth	Bony osteophytes, minimal soft tissue swelling early on, crepitus
Radiologic findings	Periarticular osteopenia, marginal erosions	Subchondral sclerosis, osteophytes
Laboratory findings	Increased CRP, RF, and anti-CCP antibody, anemia, thrombocytosis	Normal

anti-CCP, anticitrullinated protein; *CRP-RF,* C-reactive protein-rheumatoid factor; *DIP,* distal interphalangeal joint; *MCP,* metacarpophalangeal joint; *MTP,* metatarsophalangeal joint; *PIP,* proximal interphalangeal joint.

Dx DIAGNOSIS

The American College of Rheumatology (ACR) and the European League against Rheumatism (EULAR) developed new classification criteria for RA in 2010. These are based on a point system where patients with score ≥6/10 are considered to have "definite RA." Four variables constitute the new criteria:

- The number and size of involved joints (0 to 5 points, with higher scores for a larger number of small joints affected).
- Levels of rheumatoid factor (RF) and anti-cyclic citrullinated peptide (CCP) antibody (0 to 3 points, with a higher score for a high-titer positive RF or anti-CCP).
- Elevated erythrocyte sedimentation rate (ESR) or C-reactive protein (CRP) (1 point).
- Symptom duration ≥6 wk (1 point).

DIFFERENTIAL DIAGNOSIS

- Infectious causes: Parvovirus B19, hepatitis B, hepatitis C, poststreptococcal reactive arthritis, acute rheumatic fever
- Connective tissue diseases: Systemic lupus erythematosus, scleroderma, mixed connective tissue disease, Sjögren's syndrome
- Seronegative spondyloarthropathies
- Calcium pyrophosphate deposition (CPPD or "pseudo-RA")
- Polyarticular gout
- Polymyalgia rheumatica
- Remitting seronegative symmetric synovitis with pitting edema (RS3PE) can resemble seronegative RA in elderly patients
- Hemochromatosis
- Paraneoplastic syndrome
- Osteoarthritis, a degenerative arthritis that lacks prolonged morning stiffness and that usually lacks synovitis, should not be confused with RA (see Table 1)

LABORATORY TESTS

- RF (sensitivity ~60%; specificity ~80%). False positives are seen with hepatitis C, subacute bacterial endocarditis, primary biliary cirrhosis, sarcoidosis, malignancy, Sjögren's syndrome, SLE, and increasing age.
- Anti-CCP antibodies. Sensitivity is similar to RF, but it is more specific for RA than RF (up to 95% to 98%).
- The presence of either RF or anti-CCP ("seropositive RA") is associated with more severe disease, more extraarticular manifestations, and worse prognosis.
- Elevated ESR and/or CRP. Will decline with treatment; thus can be used to monitor disease activity along with physical examination and clinical presentation.
- CBC with differential. Possible anemia of chronic disease (through production of the iron-regulating hormone, hepcidin) and thrombocytosis.
- Hypoalbuminemia and hypergammaglobulinemia.
- ANA is present is 20% to 30% of patients. However, complement will usually be normal or increased, in contrast to patients with systemic lupus erythematosus. Many patients will have secondary Sjögren's syndrome (positive ANA with negative SSA and SSB).
- Inflammatory synovial fluid with >2000 PMNs. Of note, patients with RA have an increased risk of developing septic arthritis. Hence, synovial fluid with white blood cells >50,000 cells/mm^3 is concerning for an infectious process and must always be ruled out.

IMAGING STUDIES

Plain radiography:

- Early changes include soft tissue swelling, symmetrical joint space narrowing, and periarticular osteopenia.
- Later changes include periarticular erosions and deformities. This reflects cartilage and bone destruction secondary to pannus formation (Fig. 3).
- Radiographs of hands and feet should be obtained at disease onset and repeated to monitor disease progression and to ensure that adequate treatment is achieved.

MRI and musculoskeletal US:

- Are more sensitive for detecting erosive disease and joint effusions/synovitis.

Rx TREATMENT

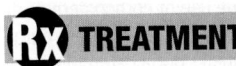

- Early identification and treatment of RA with DMARDs is crucial. More than half of patients have radiographic joint damage within 2 yr of disease onset, but early aggressive treatment with DMARDs and/or biologic agents is associated with decreased progression

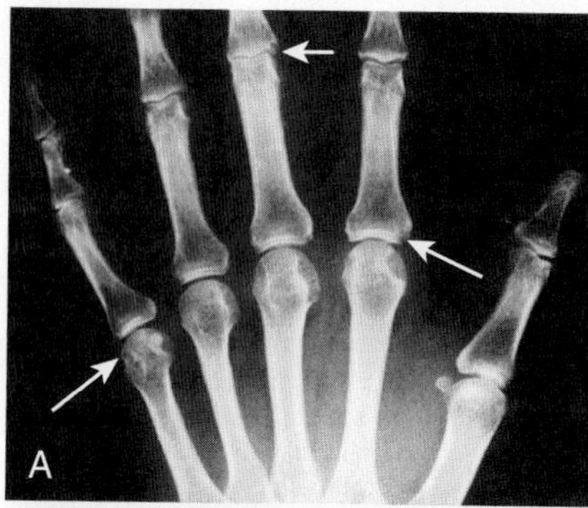

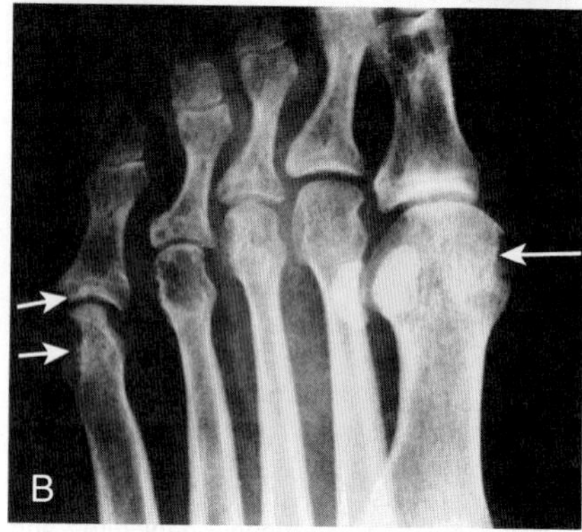

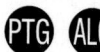

FIG. 3 Rheumatoid arthritis. A, Periarticular osteopenia and marginal erosions in metacarpophalangeal joints and a proximal interphalangeal joint *(arrows)*. **B,** In the same patient, marginal erosions at metatarsal heads *(arrows)*. (From Canoso JJ: *Rheumatology in primary care*, Philadelphia, 1997, Saunders.)

of synovitis and bone erosions, and with decreased disability. Fig. 4 describes the American College of Rheumatology recommendations for treatment of rheumatoid arthritis. Goal of therapy is to "treat to a target" of low disease activity or remission.

- There are several tools to measure disease activity and define remission in rheumatoid arthritis, including (but not limited to) the following: Clinical Disease Activity Index (CDAI), Simplified Disease Activity Index (SDAI), Disease Activity Score (DAS) 28, Routine Assessment of Patient Index Data 3 (RAPID3), Stanford Health Assessment Questionnaire (HAQ), and Patient Activity Scale (PAS).

ACUTE GENERAL Rx

- NSAIDs: Can be used initially to relieve pain and mild inflammation, or used later in the disease course for additional control of mild pain. NSAIDs are not disease modifying.
- Corticosteroids: Oral or intraarticular, frequently used initially to reduce inflammation rapidly until oral DMARD treatments take effect. They may also be used during acute flares or in low doses for additional control of inflammation. The use of corticosteroids at the lowest dose possible and shortest duration is recommended. Corticosteroids have many side effects, including but not limited to weight gain, increased risk of diabetes, osteoporosis, cataract formation, peptic ulcer disease (especially when used in combination with NSAIDs), and avascular necrosis.
- Smoking has an additive detrimental effect in RA patients (two-fold excess mortality risk).

CHRONIC Rx

- DMARDs: Can be classified into "nonbiologic" and "biologic" treatments.
  1. Nonbiologic DMARDs: Most commonly used agents are methotrexate (MTX), hydroxychloroquine (HCQ), sulfasalazine (SSZ), and leflunomide (LEF). Most of these are associated with potential toxicity and require close monitoring. They are also slow-acting drugs that require >8 wk to become fully effective.
  2. MTX is the most commonly used DMARD worldwide for the treatment of RA. It is effective as monotherapy in only 30% of patients with RA.
  3. "Triple therapy"—MTX, HCQ, and SSZ—has been shown to be superior to MTX alone.
- Biologic DMARDs: Newer biologically engineered therapies, which target cytokines and cells involved in the RA inflammatory response. Major side effects include an increased risk of severe infection, most notably reactivation of tuberculosis with anti-TNF agents. A negative PPD or interferon γ-release assay is a prerequisite to initiate therapy. Biologic DMARDs are most effective when used in combination with a nonbiologic DMARD, usually MTX.
- The five approved tumor necrosis factor α inhibitors (TNFI) include infliximab, etanercept, adalimumab, certolizumab pegol, and golimumab.
- Abatacept (CTLA-4Ig) is a recombinant protein that prevents costimulatory binding of antigen presenting cell to T cell, preventing T cell activation.
- Tocilizumab (anti–IL-6) is a monoclonal antibody against the IL-6 receptor.
- Sarilumab is another IL-6 inhibitor monoclonal antibody, approved by the FDA in 2017 for treatment of RA, and can be used as monotherapy or in combination with MTX or other conventional DMARDs.
- Tofacitinib (JAK3 inhibitor) inhibits the JAK-STAT intracellular signaling pathway, thus preventing the production of inflammatory mediators. The first oral biologic DMARD, it can be used as monotherapy or in combination with MTX. Baricitinib, an oral, once-daily Janus kinase (JAK1 and JAK2) inhibitor, has been approved by the FDA in May 2018 for treatment of moderate to severe RA in patients who did not respond adequately to one or more TNFIs. A dose of 2 mg was approved, with concerns that higher doses had increased adverse events.
- Rituximab (anti-CD20) is a monoclonal antibody against the CD20 antigen on B lymphocytes.
- Biosimilars are beginning to be available. These molecules are highly similar, but not identical, to the original drugs. Legal disputes have delayed the widespread adoption of these drugs in the US, but they are likely to be of increasing prevalence in the future.
- Treatment recommendations in RA patient with high-risk comorbidities:
  1. TNFI should be avoided in patients with congestive heart failure, as it can worsen the condition.
  2. In patients with hepatitis B, immunosuppressive therapy can be safely prescribed along with concomitant antiviral therapy.
  3. Treatment of hepatitis C patients with RA should be done following standard guidelines in collaboration with gastroenterology/hepatology. Immunosuppressive therapy can be used safely in conjunction with antiviral therapy; avoidance of DMARDs such as MTX and LEF should be taken into consideration.
  4. In patients with a history of skin cancer, DMARDs are recommended over the use of biologics. For patients with previously treated lymphoproliferative disorders, use of rituximab should be considered first, as well as combination DMARDs and non-TNF biologics. One should avoid TNFI, as there is an increased risk of lymphoma with these agents. Recommendations for treatment of patients with previously treated solid organ malignancy are the same as for patients without the condition.

Immunization, cardiovascular disease prevention (smoking cessation, blood pressure control, cholesterol control), and osteoporosis prevention (with calcium and vitamin D supplementation and bisphosphonate therapy) should be addressed in all RA patients.

DISPOSITION

- Remissions and exacerbations are common, but condition is chronically progressive in the majority of cases.
- Joint degeneration and deformity often lead to disability. Joint replacement is indicated for patients with severe joint damage whose symptoms are poorly controlled by medical management. The ACR published guidelines in 2017 concerning the perioperative management of antirheumatic medications in patients undergoing elective total hip or total knee arthroplasty.
- Early and aggressive diagnosis and treatment are crucial in preventing or slowing joint destruction.

REFERRAL

- Early referral to rheumatologist
- Orthopedic consultation for corrective surgery

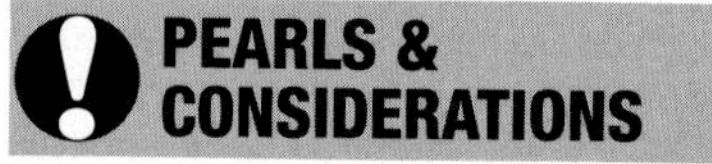

PEARLS & CONSIDERATIONS

RA sometimes develops acutely in the postpartum patient; conversely, as high as 75% of pregnant RA patients will experience remission during pregnancy.

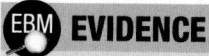

EVIDENCE

Available at ExpertConsult.com

SUGGESTED READINGS

Available at ExpertConsult.com

RELATED CONTENT

Rheumatoid Arthritis (Patient Information)

AUTHOR: **EDITH GARNEAU, M.D., M.S.**

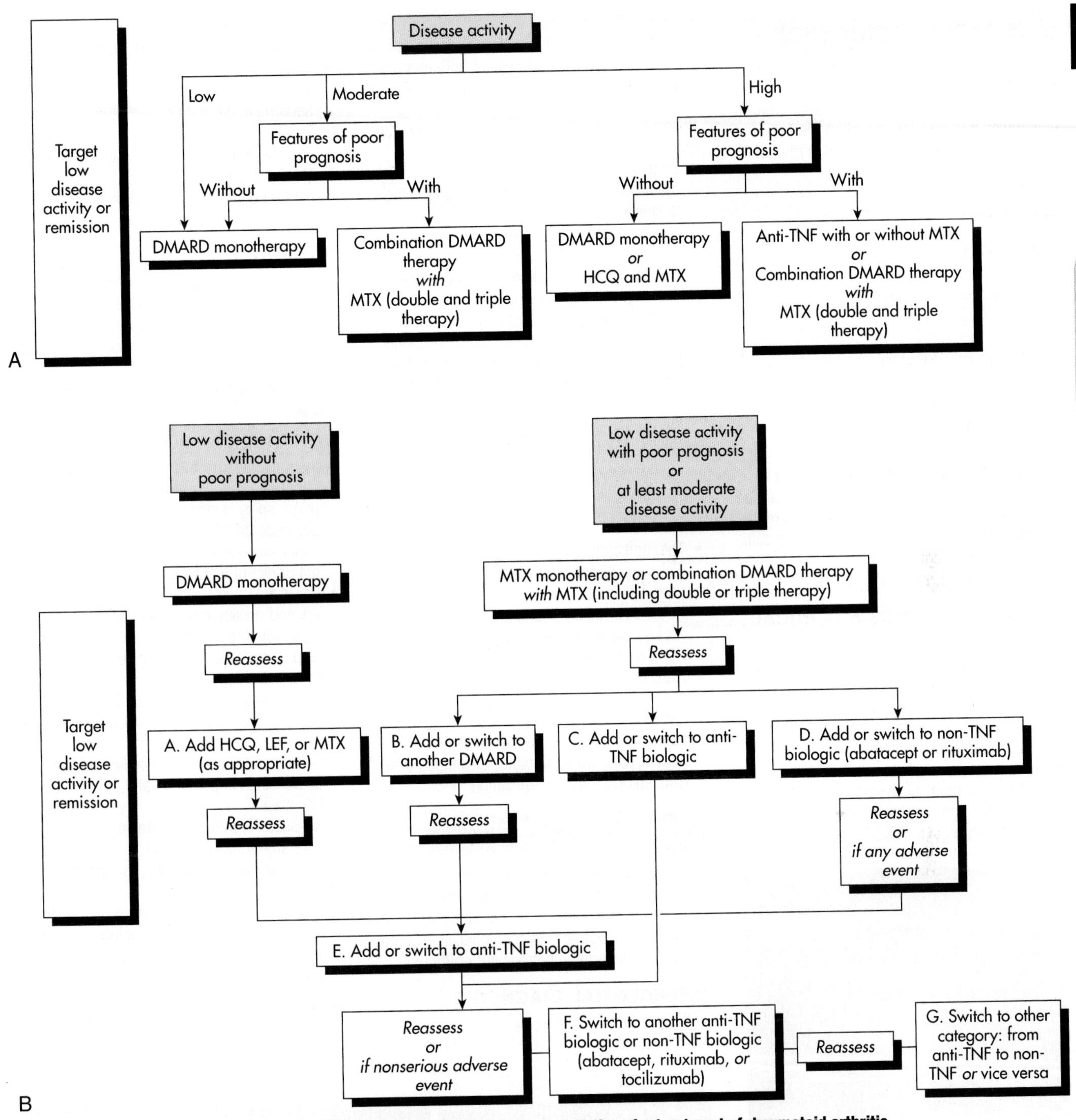

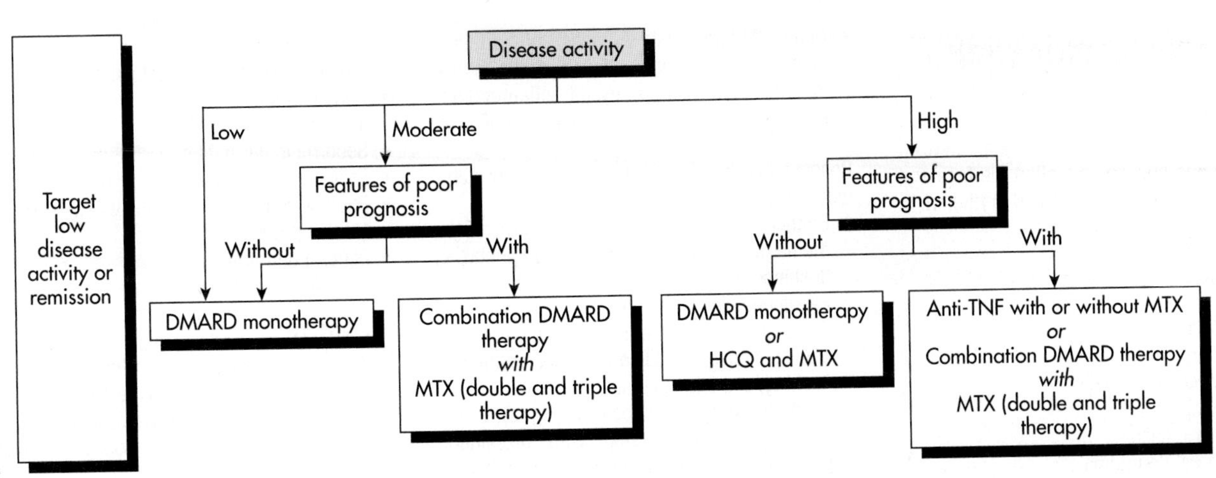

A
Target low disease activity or remission
Disease activity
Low
Moderate
High
Features of poor prognosis
Without
With
DMARD monotherapy
Combination DMARD therapy with MTX (double and triple therapy)
Features of poor prognosis
Without
With
DMARD monotherapy or HCQ and MTX
Anti-TNF with or without MTX or Combination DMARD therapy with MTX (double and triple therapy)
B
Target low disease activity or remission
Low disease activity without poor prognosis
DMARD monotherapy
Reassess
Low disease activity with poor prognosis or at least moderate disease activity
MTX monotherapy or combination DMARD therapy with MTX (including double or triple therapy)
Reassess
A. Add HCQ, LEF, or MTX (as appropriate)
B. Add or switch to another DMARD
C. Add or switch to anti-TNF biologic
D. Add or switch to non-TNF biologic (abatacept or rituximab)
Reassess
Reassess
Reassess or if any adverse event
E. Add or switch to anti-TNF biologic
Reassess or if nonserious adverse event
F. Switch to another anti-TNF biologic or non-TNF biologic (abatacept, rituximab, or tocilizumab)
Reassess
G. Switch to other category: from anti-TNF to non-TNF or vice versa

FIG. 4 American College of Rheumatology recommendations for treatment of rheumatoid arthritis. **A,** Early disease. **B,** Established disease. *DMARD*, Disease-modifying antirheumatic drug; *HCQ*, hydroxychloroquine; *LEF*, leflunomide; *MTX*, methotrexate; *TNF*, tumor necrosis factor. (From Firestein GS, et al. [eds]: *Kelly's textbook of rheumatology*, ed 9, Philadelphia, 2013, Saunders.)

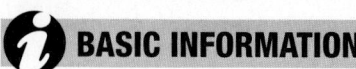

BASIC INFORMATION

DEFINITION

Rosacea is a chronic skin disorder characterized by papules and pustules affecting the face and often associated with flushing and erythema.

SYNONYM

Acne rosacea

ICD-10CM CODES

L71	Rosacea
L71.9	Rosacea unspecified
L71.1	Rhinophyma
L71.8	Other rosacea
L71.0	Perioral dermatitis

EPIDEMIOLOGY & DEMOGRAPHICS

- Rosacea occurs in 1 in 20 Americans
- Onset often between ages 30 and 50 yr
- More common in people of Celtic origin; however, this disease may be overlooked in nonwhites because skin pigmentation results in atypical presentation
- Female:male ratio of 3:1

PHYSICAL FINDINGS & CLINICAL PRESENTATION

- Facial erythema, presence of papules, pustules, and telangiectasia (Fig. 1).
- Excessive facial warmth and redness are the predominant presenting symptoms.
- Itching is generally absent.
- Comedones are absent (unlike acne).
- Women are more likely to show symptoms on the chin and cheeks, whereas in men the nose is commonly involved.
- Ocular findings (mild dryness and irritation with blepharitis, conjunctival injection, burning, stinging, tearing, eyelid inflammation, swelling, and redness) are present in 50% of patients.

Rosacea can be classified into four major subtypes (Table E1):

1. Erythematotelangiectatic (vascular): Erythema in central part of face, telangiectasia, flushing
2. Papulopustular (inflammatory): Presence of dome-shaped erythematous papules and small pustules, in addition to facial erythema, flushing, and telangiectasia
3. Phymatosis/glandular rosacea (Fig. 2): Presence of thickened skin with prominent pores that may affect the nose (rhinophyma) (Fig. 3), chin (gnathophyma), forehead (metophyma), eyelids (blepharophyma), and ears (otophyma)
4. Ocular: Conjunctival injection, sensation of foreign body in the eye, telangiectasia and erythema of lid margins, scaling

ETIOLOGY

- The pathophysiology of rosacea is incompletely understood but believed to involve the vasculature.
- Hot drinks, alcohol, and sun exposure may accentuate the erythema by causing vasodilation of the skin.
- Flare-ups may also result from reactions to medications (e.g., simvastatin, angiotensin-converting enzyme inhibitors, vasodilators, fluorinated corticosteroids), stress, extreme heat or cold, wind, humidity, strenuous exercise, spicy drinks, menstruation.

Dx DIAGNOSIS

The presence of at least one of the following primary features in a central distribution of the face is generally sufficient to diagnose rosacea: papules and pustules, telengiectasia, flushing (transient erythema), nontransient erythema.

DIFFERENTIAL DIAGNOSIS

- Drug eruption
- Acne vulgaris
- Contact dermatitis
- Systemic lupus erythematosus
- Carcinoid flush
- Idiopathic facial flushing
- Seborrheic dermatitis
- Facial sarcoidosis
- Photodermatitis
- Mastocytosis
- Perioral dermatitis
- Granulomas of the skin

WORKUP

Diagnosis is based on clinical findings. Distinguishing features between acne and rosacea are the presence of telangiectasia and deep diffuse erythema and absence of comedones in rosacea.

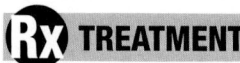

TREATMENT

NONPHARMACOLOGIC THERAPY

- Instruct patients to keep a diary to identify stimuli and triggers that exacerbate rosacea (e.g., spicy foods, drugs, cosmetics) and avoid identified triggers.
- Avoid alcohol, excessive sun exposure, and hot drinks of any type.
- Use of mild, nondrying soap or soap-free cleansers and nonoily moisturizers is recommended; local skin irritants should be avoided. General recommendations for skin care in patients with rosacea are summarized in Table 2.
- Sunscreens are an important component of therapy and should be applied each morning.
- Daily circular massage for several minutes of the central portion of the face is helpful in decreasing lymphedema and inflammation in this area.
- Reassure patient that rosacea is completely unrelated to poor hygiene.
- Vascular laser surgery is effective for telangiectasia.
- Surgical options are available for telangiectasia and rhinophyma and include dermabrasion, laser ablation, heated scalpel, electrocautery, and radiofrequency electrosurgery.

GENERAL Rx

- Several classes of drugs are used in treatment of rosacea, including the metronidazole

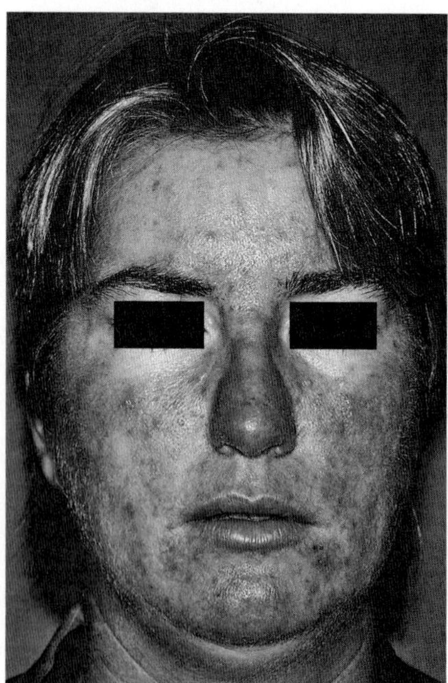

FIG. 1 Papulopustular rosacea. (Courtesy Curt Samlaska, M.D. From James WD et al: *Andrews' diseases of the skin*, ed 12, Philadelphia, 2016, Elsevier.)

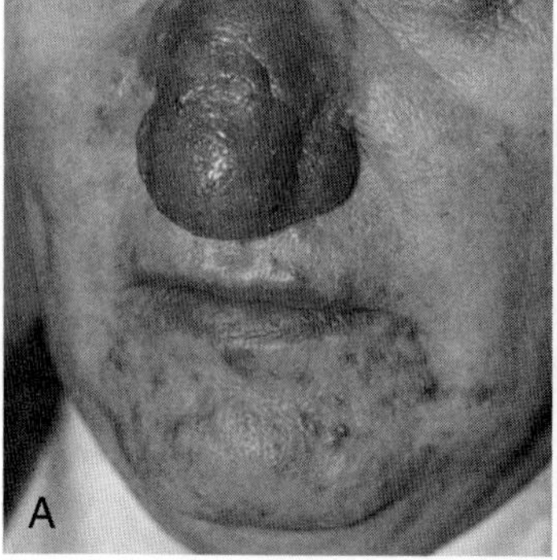

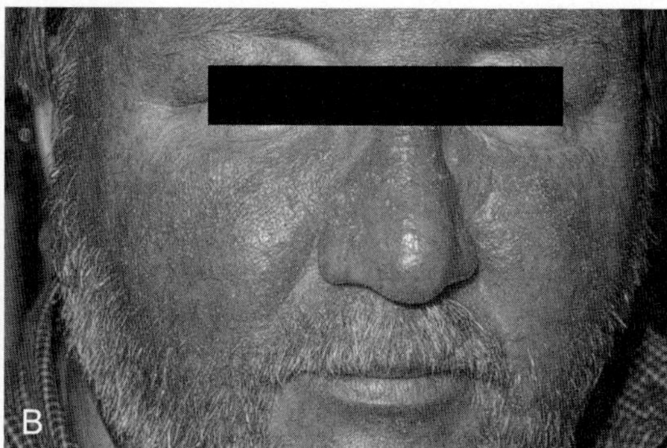

FIG. 2 Severe rosacea. A, Note the scattered papules on the face and the confluent involvement of the nose. Alcohol ingestion is not related to this appearance. **B,** Note the severe inflammation with confluent redness and significant edema. (From White GM, Cox NH [eds]: *Diseases of the skin: a color atlas and text,* ed 2, St Louis, 2006, Mosby.)

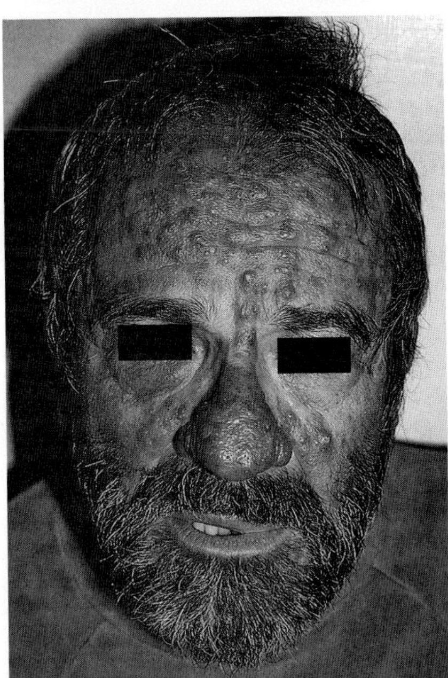

FIG. 3 Glandular rosacea. (From James WD et al: *Andrews' diseases of the skin*, ed 12, Philadelphia, 2016, Elsevier.)

TABLE 2 General Recommendations for Facial Skin Care and Education in Patients With Rosacea

Facial Skin Care

- Wash with lukewarm water and use soap-free cleansers that are pH balanced.
- Cleansers are applied gently with fingertips.
- Use sunscreens with both UVA and UVB protection and an SPF ≥30.
- Sunscreens containing the inorganic filters titanium dioxide and/or zinc oxide are usually well tolerated.
- Use cosmetics and sunscreens that contain protective silicones.
- Water-soluble facial powder containing inert green pigment helps to neutralize the perception of erythema.
- Moisturizers containing humectants (e.g., glycerin) and occlusives (e.g., petrolatum) help to repair the epidermal barrier.
- Avoid astringents, toners, and abrasive exfoliators.
- Avoid cosmetics that contain alcohol, menthols, camphor, witch hazel, fragrance, peppermint, and eucalyptus oil.
- Avoid waterproof cosmetics and heavy foundations that are difficult to remove without irritating solvents or physical scrubbing.
- Avoid procedures such as glycolic peels or dermabrasion.

Patient Education

- Reassure the patient about the benign nature of the disorder and the rarity of rhinophyma, particularly in women.
- Emphasize the chronicity of the disease and the likelihood of exacerbations.
- Direct patients to information websites such as those of the National Rosacea Society (www.rosacea.org) or the American Academy of Dermatology (www.aad.org).
- Advise to avoid recognized triggers.
- Explain the importance of compliance with topical regimens.
- Educate on the importance of sun avoidance.

SPF, Sun protective factor; *UVA,* ultraviolet A; *UVB,* ultraviolet B.
Adapted from Del Rosso JQ, Baum EW: Comprehensive medical management of rosacea: an interim study report and literature review, *J Clin Aesthet Dermatol* 1:20–25, 2008; Powell FC: Rosacea, *N Engl J Med* 352:793–803, 2005; and Pelle MT et al: Rosacea: II. Therapy, *J Am Acad Dermatol* 51:499-512, 2004; In From Bolognia J: *Dermatology*, ed 4, 2018, Elsevier.

family, the tetracycline family, ivermectin cream, and azelaic acid.

- Vascular rosacea: Topical therapy with metronidazole aqueous gel (MetroGel) applied bid is effective as initial therapy for mild cases. A new 1% formulation of metronidazole (Noritate) applied daily may improve patient compliance. Clindamycin lotion (Cleocin), sulfacetamide, or erythromycin 2% solution may also be effective. Brimonidine (Mirvaso) is a selective alpha$_2$-adrenergic receptor agonist FDA-approved as a gel preparation for topical treatment of adults with persistent facial erythema of rosacea. Oxymetazoline (Rhofane) 1% cream is also an FDA-approved selecting alpha1a-adrenergic receptor agonist for topical treatment of persistent facial erythema in adults. Neither brimonidine or oxymetazoline are indicated for the treatment of inflammatory lesions of rosacea.
- Pustular and ocular rosacea: Systemic antibiotics (doxycycline 100 mg qd or tetracycline 250 mg qid until symptoms diminish, then taper off). Minocycline 50 to 100 mg qd should be used only in resistant cases because this medication is expensive. Oral metronidazole (200 mg qd to bid) for 4 to 6 wk is also effective. A 1% cream formulation of the antiparasitic drug ivermectin (Soolantra) is effective for papulopustular rosacea with minimal adverse effects. After 3 months of therapy, it will produce clearing of rosacea lesions in up to 80% of patients with moderate to severe symptoms. Its mechanism of action is unknown, but it may be due to the combination of its antiinflammatory effects and its antiparasitic effects on the Demodex mite, which may contribute to the symptoms of rosacea. Cost may be a limiting factor ($320 for one 30-g tube).
- Isotretinoin (Accutane) 0.5 to 1 mg/kg/day in two divided doses for 15 to 20 wk can be used for refractory papular and pustular rosacea; use of retinoids may, however, worsen erythema and telangiectasis.
- Erythema and flushing may respond to low-dose clonidine (0.05 mg bid).
- Treatment of phymatous rosacea: Oral tetracyclines, oral isotretinoin, ablative/pulsed dye laser therapy, electrosurgery.
- Treatment of ocular rosacea: Topical or oral tetracyclines, artificial tears, and/or lid cleansing for eyelid hygiene. Medical and surgical therapies for rosacea are summarized in Table E3.

DISPOSITION

- Rosacea is often resistant to initial treatment and recurrent. Periods of remission and relapse are common.
- The progression of rosacea is variable. Typical stages include:
  1. Facial flushing
  2. Erythema and/or edema and ocular symptoms
  3. Papules and pustules
  4. Rhinophyma

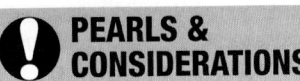

PEARLS & CONSIDERATIONS

COMMENTS

- The course of the disease is typically chronic, with remissions and relapses.
- Patients with resistant cases may have *Demodex folliculorum* mite infestation or tinea infection (diagnosis can be confirmed with potassium hydroxide examination); the role of *D. folliculorum* in rosacea is unclear. These mites can sometimes be found in large numbers in the lesions; however, their numbers do not generally decline with treatment.
- Rosacea can result in emotional and social stigmas, especially because many people associate rosacea and rhinophyma with alcohol abuse.
- Early consultation with an ophthalmologist is recommended in patients with suspected ocular involvement.

SUGGESTED READINGS

Available at ExpertConsult.com

RELATED CONTENT

Rosacea (Patient Information)

AUTHOR: **FRED F. FERRI, M.D.**

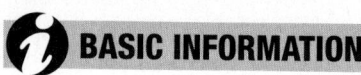

DEFINITION

Salmonellosis is an infection caused by one of several serotypes of a gram-negative bacillus of the genus *Salmonella.* Salmonella infection can be typhoidal (serotype Typhi or Paratyphi) or nontyphoidal. Current *Salmonella* nomenclature is described in Table 1.

SYNONYMS

Typhoid fever
Paratyphoid fever
Enteric fever

ICD-10CM CODES

A02.0 *Salmonella* enteritis
A02.1 *Salmonella* sepsis
A02.2 Localized *Salmonella* infections
A02.8 Other specified *Salmonella* infections
A0.9 *Salmonella* infection, unspecified

EPIDEMIOLOGY & DEMOGRAPHICS

INCIDENCE (IN U.S.):

- Epidemiologically, the clinical syndromes are divided into those that cause a typhoidal type of infection (systemic illness with fever and abdominal pain) such as *Salmonella typhi* and those that do not: nontyphoidal *Salmonella* infections (gastroenteritis) such as *S. enteritidis, S. newport,* and *S. typhimurium.*
- Estimated 1 million cases/yr of nontyphoidal salmonellosis in the United States (leading cause of foodborne illness in the U.S.). In 2017 an outbreak occurred linked to live poultry in backyard flocks with over 960 cases in 48 states caused by several different *Salmonella* bacteria.
- Largest outbreak of gastroenteritis syndrome (nontyphoidal): 200,000 who ingested contaminated milk.
- Approximately 500 cases of *Salmonella typhi* infection are reported each yr, of which nearly 80% is associated with foreign travel.

PEAK INCIDENCE: Summer and fall

PREDOMINANT AGE:

- <20 yr old
- >70 yr old
- Highest rates of infection in infants, especially neonates

GENETICS:

Neonatal Infection:

- Highly susceptible to infection with nontyphoidal *Salmonella*

PHYSICAL FINDINGS & CLINICAL PRESENTATION

- Infections:
  1. Localized to GI tract (gastroenteritis)
  2. Systemic (typhoid fever)
  3. Localized outside of GI tract
- Gastroenteritis:
  1. Incubation period: 12 to 48 hr
  2. Nausea, vomiting
  3. Diarrhea, abdominal cramps
  4. Fever
  5. Bacteremia: Occurs mostly in the immunocompromised host or those with underlying conditions, including HIV infection
  6. Self-limited illness lasting 3 or 4 days
  7. Colonization of GI tract persistent for months, especially in those treated with antibiotics
- **Typhoid fever:**
  1. Incubation period of few days to several wk
  2. Prolonged fever, often with a stepwise-increasing temperature pattern
  3. Myalgias
  4. Headache, cough, sore throat
  5. Malaise, anorexia
  6. Abdominal pain
  7. Hepatosplenomegaly
  8. Diarrhea or constipation early in the course of illness
  9. Rose spots (faint, maculopapular, blanching lesions) sometimes seen on chest or abdomen
- Untreated disease:
  1. Fever lasting 1 to 2 mo
  2. Main complication: GI bleeding caused by perforation from ulceration of Peyer's patches in the ileum
  3. Rare complications:
     a. Mental status changes
     b. Shock
  4. Relapse rate of approximately 10%
- Infections outside GI tract:
  1. Can occur in virtually any location
  2. Usually occur in patients with underlying diseases
  3. Endocarditis, endovascular infections are caused by seeding of atherosclerotic plaques or aneurysms
  4. Hepatic or splenic abscesses in patients with underlying disease in these organs
  5. Urinary tract infections in patients with renal TB or schistosomiasis
  6. *Salmonellae* are a frequent cause of gram-negative meningitis in neonates
  7. Osteomyelitis in children with hemoglobinopathies (particularly sickle cell disease)

ETIOLOGY

- More than 2000 serotypes of *Salmonella* exist, but only a few cause disease in humans. Host factors and conditions predisposing to the development of systemic disease with nontyphoidal *Salmonella* strains are described in Table 2 and Table 3.
- Raw produce is an increasingly recognized vehicle for salmonellosis. In 2008 there was a large outbreak due to contaminated jalapeno and Serrano peppers with *Salmonella Saintpaul* involving 1500 persons, of whom 21% were hospitalized and 2 died. In 2009 there was an outbreak associated with contaminated peanut butter and peanuts. In 2017 there was an outbreak associated with papaya.
- Some found only in humans are the cause of enteric fever:
  1. *S. typhi*
  2. *S. paratyphi*
- Some responsible for gastroenteritis and frequently isolated from raw meat and poultry and uncooked or undercooked eggs:
  1. *S. typhimurium*
  2. *S. enteritidis*
- *S. choleraesuis* is a prototype organism that causes extraintestinal nontyphoidal disease.
- Transmission generally via ingestion of contaminated food or drink.
- Outbreaks of gastroenteritis related to contaminated poultry, meat, and dairy products are common.
- Typhoid fever is a systemic illness caused by serotypes exclusive to humans:
  1. Acquisition by ingestion of food or water contaminated by other humans.
  2. Most cases in the United States are:
     a. Acquired during foreign travel: 80% of cases.
     b. Acquired by ingestion of food prepared by chronic carriers, many of whom have acquired the organism outside of the United States.

TABLE 1 *Salmonella* Nomenclature

Traditional Usage	Formal Name	CDC Designation
S. typhi	*S. enterica** subsp. enterica ser. Typhi	*S.* ser. Typhi
S. dublin	*S. enterica* subsp. enterica ser. Dublin	*S.* ser. Dublin
S. typhimurium	*S. enterica* subsp. enterica ser. Typhimurium	*S.* ser. Typhimurium
S. choleraesuis	*S. enterica* subsp. enterica ser. Choleraesuis	*S.* ser. Choleraesuis
S. marina	*S. enterica* subsp. houtenae ser. Marina	*S.* ser. Marina

CDC, Centers for Disease Control and Prevention; *ser.,* serovar; *subsp.,* subspecies.
*Some authorities prefer *S. choleraesuis* or *S. enteritidis* rather than *S. enterica* to describe the species.
From Kliegman RM et al: *Nelson textbook of pediatrics,* ed 19, Philadelphia, 2011, Saunders.

TABLE 2 Host Factors and Conditions Predisposing to the Development of Systemic Disease with Nontyphoidal *Salmonella* Strains

Neonates and young infants (≤3 mo of age)
HIV/AIDS
Other immunodeficiencies and chronic granulomatous disease
Immunosuppressive and corticosteroid therapies
Malignancies, especially leukemia and lymphoma
Hemolytic anemia, including sickle cell disease, malaria, and bartonellosis
Collagen vascular disease
Inflammatory bowel disease
Achlorhydria or use of antacid medications
Impaired intestinal motility
Schistosomiasis, malaria
Malnutrition

From Kliegman RM et al: *Nelson textbook of pediatrics,* ed 19, Philadelphia, 2011, Saunders.

TABLE 3 Susceptibility to *Salmonella* spp. Infection

Patient Group at Risk	Mechanism
Newborn	Achlorhydria, rapid gastric emptying
	Poorly developed cell-mediated immunity
	Complement deficiency
	Immunoglobulin deficiency in premature infants
Sickle-cell anemia	Reticuloendothelial system overload owing to hemolysis
	Functional asplenia
	Tissue infarcts
	Defective opsonization
Neutropenia (congenital or acquired)	Polymorphonuclear neutrophils needed for killing
Chronic granulomatous disease	Defective killing by polymorphonuclear neutrophils
Defects of immune system IL-12/interferon-γ axis	Defective signaling resulting in failure to activate macrophages and recurrent/persistent infection by nontyphoid *Salmonella*
Acquired immunodeficiency syndrome	Low CD4
	Effects of malnutrition on cell-mediated immunity
	Survival of organisms in macrophages (owing to *Salmonella* genes *PhoP/PhoQ, spvA-D, R*)
Organ transplantation, immunosuppression	Defective cell-mediated immunity
Gastrectomy	Loss of stomach acid barrier
Malaria	Reticuloendothelial overload during hemolysis
	Abnormal complement levels
	Abnormal macrophage function
Bartonellosis (verruga peruana)	Reticuloendothelial overload during hemolysis
Schistosomiasis	*Salmonella* sequestered in schistosomes protected from host defenses and antibiotics

From Cherry JD et al: *Feigin and Cherry's textbook of pediatric infectious diseases*, ed 8, Philadelphia, 2019, Elsevier.

TABLE 4 Treatment of *Salmonella* Gastroenteritis in Children

Organism and Indication	Dose and Duration of Treatment
Salmonella infections in infants <3 mo of age or immunocompromised persons (in addition to appropriate treatment for underlying disorder)	Cefotaxime 100-200 mg/kg/day every 6 hr for 5-14 days *or* Ceftriaxone 75 mg/kg/day once daily for 7 days *or* Ampicillin 100 mg/kg/day every 6 hr for 7 days *or* Cefixime 15 mg/kg/day for 7-10 days

From Kliegman RM et al: *Nelson textbook of pediatrics*, ed 19, Philadelphia, 2011, Saunders.

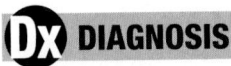

DIAGNOSIS

DIFFERENTIAL DIAGNOSIS

- Other causes of prolonged fever:
  1. Malaria
  2. TB
  3. Brucellosis
  4. Amebic liver abscess
- Other causes of gastroenteritis:
  1. Bacterial: *Shigella, Yersinia, Campylobacter* spp
  2. Viral: Norwalk virus, rotavirus
  3. Parasitic: *Entamoeba histolytica, Giardia lamblia*
  4. Toxic: *Enterotoxigenic E. coli, Clostridium difficile*

WORKUP

- Typhoid fever:
  1. Cultures of blood, stool, urine; repeat if initially negative.
  2. Blood cultures are more likely to be positive early in the course of illness.
  3. Stool and urine cultures are more commonly positive in the second and third wk of illness.
  4. Highest yield with bone marrow biopsy cultures: 90% positive.
  5. Serology using Widal test is helpful in retrospect, showing a fourfold increase in convalescent titers.
- Gastroenteritis: Stool cultures.
- Extraintestinal localized infection:
  1. Blood cultures.
  2. Cultures from the site of infection.

LABORATORY TESTS

- Neutropenia is common.
- Transaminitis is possible.
- Culture to grow organism: Blood, body fluids, biopsy specimens.

IMAGING STUDIES

- Not routinely indicated.
- Radiographs of bone may be suggestive of osteomyelitis (particularly in patients with sickle cell disease and bone infarctions).
- CT scan or sonogram of abdomen:
  1. May reveal hepatic or splenic abscesses or pleural involvement.
  2. May reveal aortic aneurysm.

Rx TREATMENT

NONPHARMACOLOGIC THERAPY

Adequate hydration and electrolyte replacement in people with diarrhea.

ACUTE GENERAL Rx

Treatment decisions must consider the severity of infection and the risk for extraintestinal disease.

- Typhoid fever:
  1. Levofloxacin 750 mg PO/IV q24h or ciprofloxacin 500 mg PO bid or 400 mg IV bid for 7 to 10 days. Should not be used as first line in patients from South Asia due to resistance unless known to be susceptible.
  2. Ceftriaxone 2 g IV qd for 7 to 14 days or cefixime (20-30 mg/kg/day orally divided into q12h dosing for 7-14 days).
  3. Another alternative agent: Azithromycin (1 g orally then 500 mg daily for 5-7 days)
  4. Children: See Table 4. In general, quinolones are avoided in children unless a multidrug-resistant strain is involved due to concerns of possible cartilage damage. Another alternative for children: Azithromycin (10-20 mg/kg to 1 g maximum once daily for 5-7 days)
  5. If tests show susceptibility, can also use amoxicillin or trimethoprim/sulfamethoxazole in adults and children (Table 5)
  6. Dexamethasone 3 mg IV initially, followed by 1 mg IV q6h for eight doses for patients with shock or mental status changes
- Gastroenteritis:
  1. Usually not indicated for gastroenteritis alone because this illness usually self-limited
  2. Treatment may prolong the carrier state and is discouraged for healthy patients <50 yr of age who have relatively mild disease
  3. Prophylactic treatment for patients who are at high risk of developing complications from bacteremia (see Table 4):
     a. Neonates
     b. Patients with hemoglobinopathies
     c. Patients with atherosclerosis
     d. Patients with aneurysms
     e. Patients with prosthetic devices
     f. Immunocompromised patients

CHRONIC Rx

- Carrier states are possible in those with typhoid fever.
- More common in people >60 yr of age and in people with gallstones.
- Usual site of colonization is the gallbladder.
- Treatment should be considered for those with persistently positive stool cultures and for food handlers.
- Suggested regimens for eradication of carrier state:
  1. Ciprofloxacin 500 mg PO bid for 4 wk.
  2. SMX/TMP 1 to 2 DS tabs PO bid for 6 wk (if susceptible).
  3. Amoxicillin 2 g PO q8h for 6 wk (if susceptible).
- Cholecystectomy may be required in carriers with gallstones who fail medical therapy,

TABLE 5 Antibiotics Commonly Used in the Treatment of *Salmonella* Infections

Drug	Dose	Comments
Ciprofloxacin	20-30 mg/kg per day in 2 doses PO or IV	First-line therapy[a]
Ceftriaxone	75-100 mg/kg per day in 1 or 2 doses IM or IV	First-line therapy
Cefotaxime	100-300 mg/kg per day in 3–4 doses IM or IV	First-line therapy
Cefixime	20-30 mg/kg per day in 1 or 2 doses PO	Alternative therapy
Azithromycin	10 mg/kg per day in 1 dose PO	Alternative therapy
Chloramphenicol	50-100 mg/kg per day in 4 doses PO	High frequency of resistance; use only for susceptible strains
Ampicillin	200-400 mg/kg per day in 4 doses PO, IM, or IV	High frequency of resistance; use only for susceptible strains
TMP-SMX	10 mg/kg per day TMP, 50 mg/kg per day SMX in 2 doses PO or IV	High frequency of resistance; use only for susceptible strains

TMP-SMX, Trimethoprim-sulfamethoxazole.
[a]Not approved by the US Food and Drug Administration in children <18 yr; current expert opinion agrees in recommending this agent as an effective therapy for regions with susceptible *Salmonella* strains and especially for severe infections.
From Cherry JD et al: *Feigin and Cherry's textbook of pediatric infectious diseases*, ed 8, Philadelphia, 2019, Elsevier.

but this is rarely indicated for nontyphoidal salmonellosis currently.
- Prolonged course of oral therapy or lifetime suppression for patients with AIDS who have chronic infection.

DISPOSITION

- Typhoid fever:
  1. Treated patients usually respond to therapy; small percentage of chronic carriers.
  2. Untreated patients may have serious complications.
- Gastroenteritis:
  1. Usually self-limited.
  2. May be recurrent or persistent in AIDS patients.

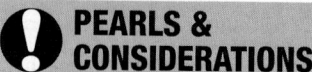

PEARLS & CONSIDERATIONS

COMMENTS

- Fluoroquinolones remain the most reliably effective class of antibiotics for empiric therapy despite increasing resistance. They should not be used in children or pregnant women.
- Infections should be reported to local health departments.
- Other recent outbreaks in the U.S. have been traced back to raw tomatoes, peanut butter, pet turtles, and frozen pot pies.
- Vaccine is available for *Salmonella typhi*: Oral live weakened vaccine (four doses, one every other day) for age >6 yr and lasts for 5 yr or one dose of inactivated injectable vaccine for persons >2 yr old that lasts for 2 yr, but neither vaccine is greater than 75% effective.

SUGGESTED READINGS

Available at ExpertConsult.com

RELATED CONTENT

Salmonellosis (Patient Information)
Typhoid Fever (Related Key Topic)

AUTHOR: **GLENN G. FORT, M.D., M.P.H.**

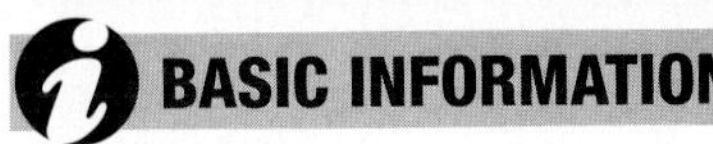

DEFINITION

Sarcoidosis is a chronic multisystem granulomatous disease characterized histologically by the presence of nonspecific, noncaseating granulomas.

SYNONYM

Boeck sarcoid

ICD-10CM CODES

D86	Sarcoidosis
D86.0	Sarcoidosis of lung
D86.1	Sarcoidosis of lymph nodes
D86.2	Sarcoidosis of lung with sarcoidosis of lymph nodes
D86.3	Sarcoidosis of skin
D86.8	Sarcoidosis of other and combined sites
D86.9	Sarcoidosis, unspecified

EPIDEMIOLOGY & DEMOGRAPHICS

INCIDENCE (IN U.S.): Incidence is 11 in 100,000 in whites and 35 in 100,000 in blacks; presents most commonly in the winter and early spring. (The adjusted annual incidence among black Americans is roughly three times higher than among white Americans [35.5 cases/100,000, as compared with 10.9/100,000] and is likely more chronic and fatal in black Americans.)

PREDOMINANT SEX: Increased incidence in females

PREDOMINANT AGE: 20 to 40 yr

GENETICS: Familial clustering has been described. Having a first-degree relative with sarcoidosis increases the risk for disease fivefold (ACCESS study). There have been reports of association between sarcoidosis and gene products, specifically HLA class II antigens, encoded by HLA-DRB1 and DQB1 alleles.

PHYSICAL FINDINGS & CLINICAL PRESENTATION

- Clinical manifestations often vary with the stage of the disease and degree of organ involvement. Patients may be asymptomatic, but a chest radiograph may demonstrate findings consistent with sarcoidosis (see "Imaging Studies"). Nearly 50% of patients with sarcoidosis are diagnosed by incidental findings on chest radiograph. Lung involvement occurs in >90% of patients with sarcoidosis.
- Frequent manifestations:
  1. Pulmonary manifestations: Dry, nonproductive cough; dyspnea; chest discomfort.
  2. Constitutional symptoms: Fatigue, weight loss, anorexia, malaise, night sweats.
  3. Visual disturbances: Blurred vision, ocular discomfort, conjunctivitis, iritis, uveitis (65% of patients).
  4. Dermatologic manifestations (30% of patients): Erythema nodosum (10% of patients), macules, papules, subcutaneous nodules, hyperpigmentation, lupus pernio (indurated violaceous lesions on the nose, lips, ears, and cheeks that can erode into underlying cartilage and bone) (Fig. E1).
  5. Myocardial disturbances, arrhythmias, cardiomyopathy, various conduction abnormalities, and pericardial effusion. Cardiac sarcoidosis is much more common than clinically appreciated and is found in up to 25% of patients in the U.S.
  6. Splenomegaly, hepatomegaly.
  7. Rheumatologic manifestations: Arthralgias have been reported in up to 40% of patients. It typically affects the ankles but can also involve the knees, wrists, and small joints of the hands and feet.
  8. **Löfgren syndrome,** consisting of triad of arthritis, erythema nodosum, and bilateral hilar adenopathy, occurs in 9% to 34% of patients. Fever is frequently present.
  9. Neurologic and other manifestations: Cranial nerve palsies, diabetes insipidus, meningeal involvement, parotid enlargement, hypothalamic and pituitary lesions, peripheral adenopathy. Neurosarcoidosis is detected in up to 25% of patients and can occur in the absence of apparent disease elsewhere. The presence of anterior uveitis, parotiditis, fevers, and facial nerve palsy is known as **Heerfordt syndrome.**

ETIOLOGY & PATHOGENESIS

A cardinal feature of sarcoidosis is the presence of CD4+ T cells that interact with antigen-presenting cells to initiate the formation and maintenance of granulomas. Multiple lines of evidence suggest that sarcoidosis may result from the interaction of multiple genes with environmental exposures or infection.

GENETIC PREDISPOSITION TO SARCOIDOSIS

Various HLA antigens have been implicated in diverse patient populations. Familial predisposition has been reported dating back to 1923, with a wide percentage of variability of affected relatives (0.4% to 21%) and heterogeneity based on genetic background. A more recent study was published by the ACCESS (A Case Controlled Etiologic Survey of Sarcoidosis) study group, which confirmed increased risk for family members with an odds ratio of 4.6 for all relatives. Absolute risk, however, for a family member to be affected was less than 1%. This study also showed a higher risk in white versus African American siblings and parents.

IMMUNOPATHOGENESIS OF SARCOIDOSIS: Numerous chemokines and cytokines have been implicated in the development and/or resolution of the disease. In sarcoidosis, the alveolitis seen at disease presentation represents an increase in primarily lymphocytic cellularity, predominated by CD4 cells. Presence of increased neutrophils in the bronchoalveolar lavage of patients with sarcoidosis has been associated with persistence of disease, with spontaneous remission noted in 36% of patients with elevated neutrophil counts. Other interstitial lung diseases in which neutrophils have been associated with worse outcomes include interstitial pulmonary fibrosis hypersensitivity pneumonitis.

Dx DIAGNOSIS

DIFFERENTIAL DIAGNOSIS

- Tuberculosis
- Lymphoma
- Hodgkin's disease
- Metastases
- Pneumoconioses
- Enlarged pulmonary arteries
- Infectious mononucleosis
- Lymphangitic carcinomatosis
- Idiopathic hemosiderosis
- Alveolar cell carcinoma
- Pulmonary eosinophilia
- Hypersensitivity pneumonitis
- Fibrosing alveolitis
- Collagen disorders
- Parasitic infection

Section II describes the differential diagnosis of granulomatous lung disease and a classification of granulomatous disorders.

WORKUP

- No pathognomonic diagnostic test exists for sarcoidosis, so the diagnosis remains one of exclusion. Workup is aimed at excluding critical organ involvement, determining extent and severity of disease, and excluding other disease. The presence of noncaseating granulomas does not establish the diagnosis, because conditions such as tuberculosis and malignancies, among others, can cause granulomas. A complete neurologic and ophthalmologic examination is mandatory. A complete occupational and environmental exposure history is recommended.
- Initial laboratory evaluation should include complete blood count, serum chemistries (alanine aminotransferase, aspartate aminotransferase, alkaline phosphatase, electrolytes, blood urea nitrogen, creatinine, serum calcium), urinalysis, 24-hour urinary excretion of calcium, CRP, ESR, and tuberculin skin test.
- Chest radiograph and ECG should also be obtained in all patients with sarcoidosis.
- Pulmonary function testing: Spirometry, diffusion capacity of carbon monoxide–single breath.
- Biopsy should be done on accessible tissues suspected of sarcoid involvement (conjunctiva, skin, lymph nodes); bronchoscopy with transbronchial biopsy (85% diagnostic yield) is often performed in patients without any readily accessible site. Endobronchial ultrasound-guided fine-needle aspiration of intrathoracic lymph nodes also has high diagnostic yield and makes use of mediastinoscopy usually unnecessary. Among patients with suspected Stage I/II pulmonary sarcoidosis undergoing tissue confirmation, the use of endosonographic nodal aspiration compared with bronchoscopic biopsy resulted in greater diagnostic yield.

LABORATORY TESTS

Laboratory abnormalities:

- Hypergammaglobulinemia, anemia, leukopenia may be present.
- Liver function test abnormalities are common, e.g., elevated alkaline phosphatase.
- Hypercalcemia (11% of patients), hypercalciuria (40% of patients; attributable to increased gastrointestinal absorption, abnormal vitamin D metabolism, and increased calcitriol production by sarcoid granuloma).
- Angiotensin-converting enzyme: Elevated in approximately 75% of patients with untreated sarcoidosis; nonspecific and poor sensitivity; generally not useful as a diagnostic tool or in following the course of the disease.
- Serum adenosine deaminase (ADA); serum amyloid A (SAA) elevated but nonspecific.

IMAGING STUDIES

- Chest radiograph (Fig. 2): Pulmonary sarcoidosis is classified based on radiographic pattern. Adenopathy of the hilar and paratracheal nodes is a frequent finding. Parenchymal changes may also be present, depending on the stage of the disease (stage 0, normal radiograph; stage I, bilateral hilar adenopathy; stage II, stage I plus pulmonary infiltrate; stage III, pulmonary infiltrate without adenopathy; stage IV, advanced fibrosis with evidence of "honeycombing," hilar retraction, bullae, cysts, and emphysema).
- Pulmonary function tests (spirometry and diffusing capacity of the lung for carbon dioxide): May be normal or may reveal a restrictive ventilatory defect with reduced forced vital capacity, reduced DLCO, or both. Endobronchial sarcoidosis may exhibit obstructive physiology, depending on severity.
- For patients without apparent lung involvement, ^{18}F-fluorodeoxyglucose positron emission tomography (FDG-PET) is useful in identifying sites for diagnostic biopsy.
- CT imaging, more specifically high-resolution CT, may help detect early parenchymal abnormalities. It is indicated when the chest radiograph is atypical for sarcoidosis.
- FDG-PET and MRI with gadolinium are useful in patients with suspected cardiac and neurologic involvement.
- Gallium-67 scan: Represents an older testing modality. It will localize in areas of granulomatous infiltrates; however, it is not specific and not necessary. The "panda" sign (localization in the lacrimal and salivary glands, giving a "panda" appearance to the face) is suggestive of sarcoidosis.
- Bronchoscopy: Flexible bronchoscopy and bronchoalveolar lavage (BAL) with transbronchial biopsy (showing noncaseating granulomas) are traditional methods for the minimally invasive diagnosis of sarcoidosis. With hilar adenopathy, endobronchial ultrasound (EBUS) is the preferred method for lymph node sampling. BAL may show predominantly lymphocytosis, elevated ADA levels, and elevated CD4:CD8 ratio (4:1).
- Mediastinoscopy: Rarely used nowadays for lymph node sampling and diagnosis.

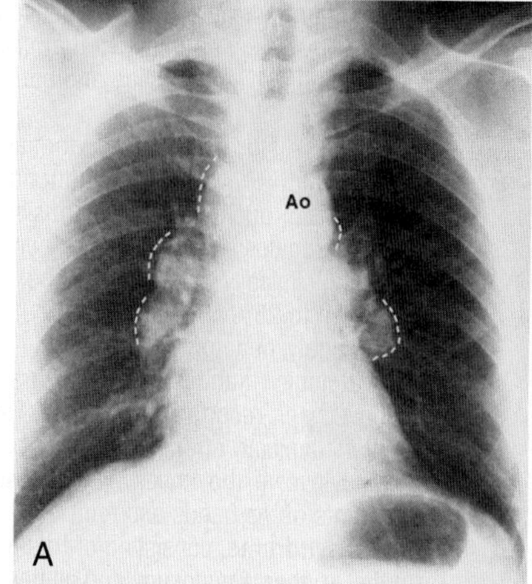

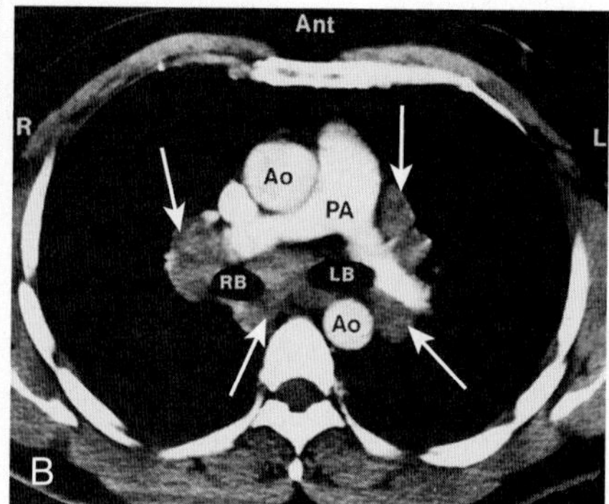

FIG. 2 Sarcoid. Marked lymphadenopathy *(dotted lines)* is seen in the region of both hila in the right paratracheal region **(A).** The transverse contrast-enhanced CT scan of the upper chest **(B)** clearly shows the ascending and descending aorta *(Ao)* as well as the pulmonary artery *(PA)* and superior vena cava. The right and left mainstem bronchus area is also seen. The *arrows* indicate the extensive lymphadenopathy. *LB,* Left bronchus; *RB,* right bronchus. (From Mettler FA [ed]: *Primary care radiology,* Philadelphia, 2000, Saunders.)

TABLE 1 Indications for Use of Corticosteroids in Sarcoidosis

Disorder	Treatment
Iridocyclitis	Corticosteroid eye drops; local subconjunctival deposit of cortisone
Posterior uveitis	Oral prednisone
Pulmonary involvement	Steroids rarely recommended for stage I; typically used if infiltrate remains static or worsens over 3-mo period or the patient is symptomatic
Upper airway obstruction	Rare indication for intravenous steroids
Lupus pernio	Oral prednisone shrinks the disfiguring lesions
Hypercalcemia	Responds well to corticosteroids
Cardiac involvement	Corticosteroids usually recommended if patient has arrhythmias or conduction disturbances
Central nervous system involvement	Response is best in patients with acute symptoms
Lacrimal/salivary gland involvement	Corticosteroids recommended for disordered function, not gland swelling
Bone cysts	Corticosteroids recommended if symptomatic

From Andreoli TE (ed): *Cecil essentials of medicine,* ed 8, Philadelphia, 2010, Saunders.

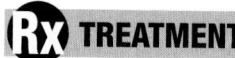

TREATMENT

GENERAL Rx

- Many patients with sarcoidosis will not require any treatment. In general, treatment should be instituted when organ function is threatened. Corticosteroids (Table 1) are the mainstay of therapy when treatment is required (e.g., prednisone 40 mg qd for 8 to 12 wk with gradual tapering of the dose to 10 mg qod over 8 to 12 mo); corticosteroids should be considered in patients with severe symptoms (e.g., dyspnea, chest pain); hypercalcemia; ocular, central nervous system, or cardiac involvement; or progressive pulmonary disease. Patients with interstitial lung disease benefit from oral steroid therapy for 6 to 24 mo.
- A lack of benefit from steroid therapy may be due to the presence of irreversible fibrotic disease. Patients with progressive disease refractory to corticosteroids may be treated with methotrexate 7.5 to 15 mg once per week or another immunosuppressant such as azathioprine or mycophenolate mofetil.
- Methotrexate, at a dose of 7.5 to 10 mg per week, has been demonstrated to be relatively safe and can also be used as a steroid-sparing agent. Additional agents that have been used with limited clinical experience include pentoxifylline, infliximab, cyclosporine, minocycline, and leflunomide.
- Immunomodulators: Etanercept has not been found to be useful in sarcoidosis. Infliximab has been used with some benefits in cutaneous, pulmonary, and neurologic disease.
- NSAIDs are useful for musculoskeletal symptoms and erythema nodosum.
- Pulmonary rehabilitation in patients with significant respiratory insufficiency. Consider liver and lung transplantation in patients unresponsive to conventional treatment.
- Pulmonary hypertension is a dreaded complication of advanced pulmonary sarcoidosis. The prognosis for patients with sarcoidosis-associated pulmonary hypertension is not known.

DISPOSITION

- The majority of patients with sarcoidosis have spontaneous remission within 2 yr and do not require treatment. Their course can be followed by periodic clinical evaluation, chest radiographs, and pulmonary function tests.
- Blacks have increased rates of pulmonary involvement, a worse long-term prognosis, and more frequent relapses.
- Up to one third of patients have unrelenting disease, leading to clinically significant organ impairment. Adverse prognostic factors in sarcoidosis include age of onset >40 yr, cardiac involvement, neurosarcoidosis, progressive pulmonary fibrosis, chronic hypercalcemia, chronic uveitis, involvement of nasal mucosa, nephrocalcinosis, and presence of cystic bone lesions and lupus pernio.
- Prognosis for Loeffler syndrome is good with remittance within 16 wk in most patients. Symptoms can generally be controlled with NSAIDs. Low-dose glucocorticoids, hydroxychloroquine, and colchicine are also effective.

REFERRAL

Ophthalmologic examination is indicated in all patients with suspected sarcoidosis because ocular findings (iridocyclitis, uveitis, conjunctivitis, and keratopathy) are found in ≥25% of documented cases.

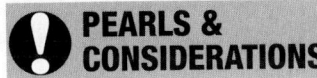

PEARLS & CONSIDERATIONS

COMMENTS

- Serial spirometry and measurement of DLCO can be useful in following response to therapy and disease progression.
- Approximately 15% to 20% of patients with lung involvement advance to irreversible lung impairment (bronchiectasis, cavitation, progressive fibrosis, pneumothorax, and respiratory failure). Death from pulmonary failure occurs in 5% to 7% of patients with sarcoidosis.
- Newer treatment approaches are aimed at targeting mechanisms involving CD4 type 1 helper T cells.
- The diagnosis of sarcoidosis should be reconsidered in the presence of atypical manifestations or persistent/progressive disease despite appropriate therapy.
- Diagnostic biopsy may not be necessary in most patients presenting with asymptomatic bilateral lymphadenopathy (with no other evidence of malignancy), in those with Lofgren syndrome, or in those with Heerfordt syndrome.

SUGGESTED READINGS

Available at ExpertConsult.com

RELATED CONTENT

Sarcoidosis (Patient Information)

AUTHOR: **IMRANA QAWI, M.D.**

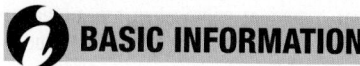

BASIC INFORMATION

DEFINITION

Scabies is a contagious disease caused by the mite *Sarcoptes scabiei.*

ICD-10CM CODE
B86 Scabies

EPIDEMIOLOGY & DEMOGRAPHICS

- Scabies is generally acquired by sleeping with or in the bedding of infested individuals.
- It is generally associated with poor living conditions and is also common in hospitals and nursing homes.

PHYSICAL FINDINGS & CLINICAL PRESENTATION

- Primary lesions are caused when the female mite burrows within the stratum corneum, laying eggs within the tract she leaves behind; burrows (linear or serpiginous tracts, see Fig. 1) end with a minute papule or vesicle.
- Primary lesions (Fig. 2) are most commonly found in the web spaces of the hands, wrists, buttocks, scrotum, penis, breasts, axillae, and knees. They are often confused with eczema (Fig. E3).
- Secondary lesions result from scratching or infection.
- Intense pruritus, especially nocturnal, is common; it is caused by an acquired sensitivity to the mite or fecal pellets and is usually noted 1 to 4 wk after the primary infestation.
- Examination of the skin may reveal burrows, tiny vesicles, excoriations, inflammatory papules.
- Widespread and crusted lesions (Norwegian or crusted scabies) may be seen in elderly and immunocompromised patients (Fig. 4). Pruritus may be mild or absent due to impaired host immune response.
- Table 1 summarizes the different presenting forms of scabies.

ETIOLOGY

- Human scabies is caused by the mite *S. scabiei,* var. *hominis* (Fig. 5). After impregnation on the skin surface, the gravid female burrows in the stratum corneum within 30 min and gradually extends the tract along the boundary with the stratum granulosum depositing 10 to 25 oval eggs in a 4- to 5-wk period. The eggs hatch in 3 to 5 days, and larvae move to the skin surface and mature in 2 to 3 wk, resuming the cycle.
- Clinical manifestations result from a delayed type IV hypersensitivity reaction to the mite, eggs, saliva, or scybala.

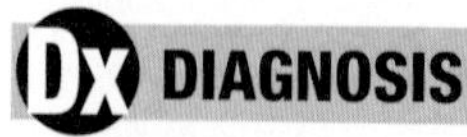

DIAGNOSIS

DIFFERENTIAL DIAGNOSIS

- Pediculosis
- Atopic dermatitis
- Flea bites
- Seborrheic dermatitis
- Dermatitis herpetiformis
- Contact dermatitis
- Nummular eczema
- Syphilis
- Other insect infestation

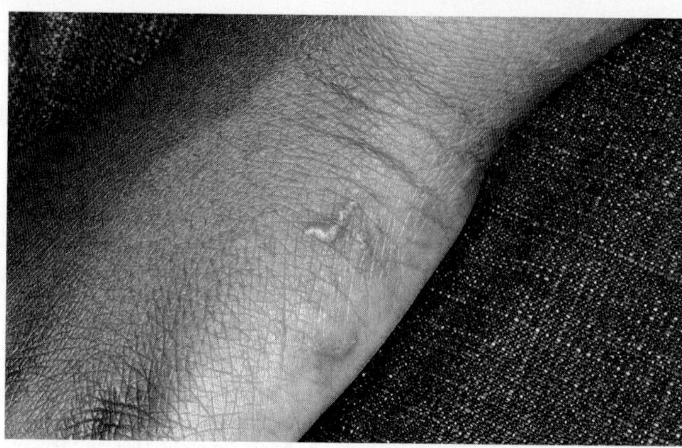

FIG. 1 Scabies. Curvilinear burrow of the lateral hand. (From Paller AS, Mancini AJ: *Hurwitz clinical pediatric dermatology, a textbook of skin disorders of childhood and adolescence*, ed 5, Philadelphia, 2016, Elsevier.)

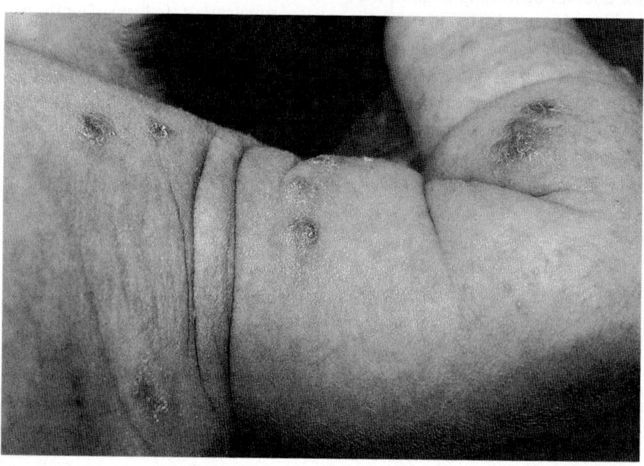

FIG. 2 Scabies nodules. Early scabies nodules developing at sites of crusting; these lesions persisted long after adequate therapy for the infestation. (From Paller AS, Mancini AJ: *Hurwitz clinical pediatric dermatology, a textbook of skin disorders of childhood and adolescence*, ed 5, Philadelphia, 2016, Elsevier.)

WORKUP

Diagnosis is made on the clinical presentation and on the demonstration of mites, eggs, or mite feces.

LABORATORY TESTS

- Microscopic demonstration of the organism, feces, or eggs: A drop of mineral oil may be placed over the suspected lesion before removal (Box 1); the scrapings are transferred directly to a glass slide; a drop of potassium hydroxide is added and a cover slip is applied.
- Skin biopsy is rarely necessary to make the diagnosis.

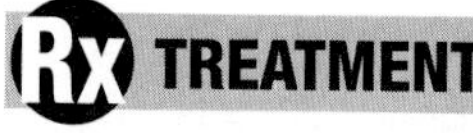

TREATMENT

NONPHARMACOLOGIC THERAPY

Clothing, underwear, and towels used in the 48 hours before treatment must be laundered.

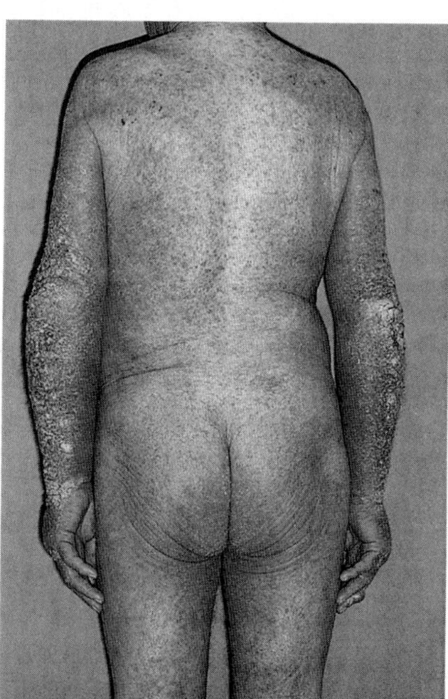

FIG. 4 Norwegian scabies. (From Swartz MH: *Textbook of physical diagnosis,* 7 ed, Philadelphia, 2014, Saunders, 2014.)

TABLE 1 Different Presenting Forms of Scabies

Presenting Forms of Scabies	Specific High-Risk Populations	Clinical Manifestations	Limited Differential Diagnoses
Classic scabies (scabies vulgaris)	Infants and children; sexually active adults; men who have sex with men	Intense generalized pruritus, worse at night; inflammatory pruritic papules localized to finger webs, flexor aspects of wrists, elbows, axillae, buttocks, genitalia, female breasts; lesions and pruritus spare the face, head, and neck; secondary lesions include eczematization, excoriation, impetigo	Dermatitis herpetiformis, drug reactions, eczema, pediculosis corporis, lichen planus, pityriasis rosea
Scalp scabies	Infants and children; institutionalized older adults; AIDS patients; patients with preexisting crusted scabies	Atypical crusted papular lesions of the scalp, face, palms, and soles	Dermatomyositis, ringworm, seborrheic dermatitis
Crusted scabies (Norwegian scabies, scabies norvegica, scabies crustosa)	Institutionalized older adults; institutionalized developmentally disabled (Down syndrome); homeless, especially HIV-positive; all immunocompromised patients, particularly those with AIDS or positive for HIV or HTLV-1; transplant recipients; patients on prolonged systemic corticosteroids and chemotherapy	Psoriasiform hyperkeratotic papular lesions of the scalp, face, neck, hands, feet, with extensive nail involvement; eczematization and impetigo common	Contact dermatitis, drug reactions, eczema, erythroderma, ichthyosis, psoriasis
Nodular scabies	Sexually active adults; men who have sex with men; HIV-positive men > HIV-positive women	Violaceous pruritic nodules localized to male genitalia, groin, axillae, representing hypersensitivity reaction to mite antigens	Acropustulosis, atopic dermatitis, Darier disease, lupus erythematosus, lymphomatoid papulosis, papular urticaria, necrotizing vasculitis, secondary syphilis

AIDS, Acquired immunodeficiency syndrome; *HIV*, human immunodeficiency virus; *HTLV-1*, human T cell lymphotropic virus type 1.
From Bennett JE et al: *Mandell, Douglas, and Bennett's principles and practice of infectious diseases*, ed 8, Philadelphia, 2015, WB Saunders.

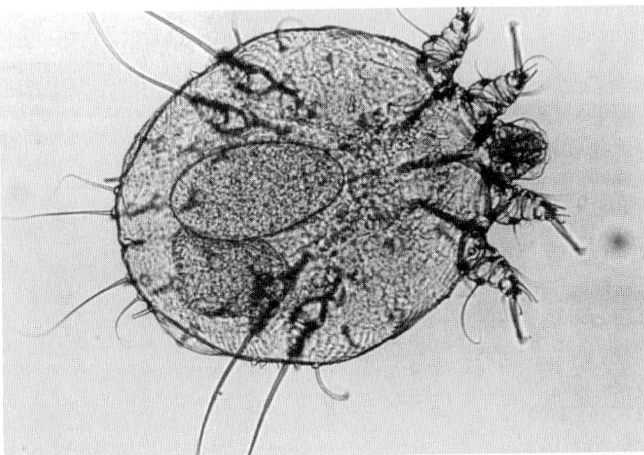

FIG. 5 Scabies mite. Note the eggs within the body of the mite. (Live scabies mite, ×40 magnification.) (From Paller AS, Mancini AJ: *Hurwitz clinical pediatric dermatology, a textbook of skin disorders of childhood and adolescence*, ed 5, Philadelphia, 2016, Elsevier.)

BOX 1 Performing a Mineral-Oil Examination for Scabies

1. Apply a drop of mineral oil to the lesion(s) to be scraped.
2. Scrape through the lesion with a number 15 scalpel blade (a small amount of bleeding is expected with appropriately deep scrapings).
3. Smear contents of scraping on a clean glass slide.
4. Add a few more drops of mineral oil.
5. Place cover slip over oil and examine under microscope at low power.

Criteria for a positive mineral oil examination:

Scabies mite
or
Ova (eggs)
or
Scybala (feces)

From Paller AS, Mancini AJ: *Hurwitz clinical pediatric dermatology, a textbook of skin disorders of childhood and adolescence*, ed 5, Philadelphia, 2016, Elsevier.

ACUTE GENERAL Rx

- Permethrin 5% cream is usually effective with one treatment; it should be massaged into the skin from head to soles of feet and applied under fingernails and toenails (it's best if applied in the evening and left overnight to maximize exposure); remove 8 to 14 hr later by washing. Repeat in 1 to 2 wk. Permethrin is safe for children >2 mo old.
- A single dose (150 to 200 μg/kg in 6-mg tablets) of ivermectin, an antihelmintic agent, is also effective for the treatment of scabies. It is the best treatment for generalized crusted scabies. Three to seven doses of ivermectin given on days 1, 2, 8, 9, 15, 22, and 28 may be needed for crusted scabies.
- Pruritus generally abates 24 to 48 hr after treatment but can last up to 2 wk; oral antihistamines are effective in decreasing postscabietic pruritus.
- Topical corticosteroid creams may hasten the resolution of secondary eczematous dermatitis.
- If the patient is a resident of an extended care facility, it is important to educate the patients, staff, family, and frequent visitors about scabies and the need to have full cooperation in treatment. Scabicide should be applied to all patients, staff, and frequent visitors, whether symptomatic or not; symptomatic family members of staff and visitors should also receive treatment.
- Table 2 summarizes currently recommended treatment for scabies.

TABLE 2 Currently Recommended Treatment for Scabies

Scabicides	FDA Approved?	Pregnancy Category*	Dosing Schedule	Safety Profile	Contraindications
5% Permethrin cream (Actin, Nix, Elimite)	Yes	B	Apply from neck down; wash off after 8-14 hr; good residual activity, but second application recommended after 1 wk	Excellent; itching and stinging on application	Prior allergic reactions; infants <2 mo of age; breastfeeding
1% Lindane lotion or cream	Yes	B	Apply 30-60 ml from neck down; wash off after 8-12 hr; no residual activity; increasing drug resistance	Potential for central nervous system toxicity from organochloride poisoning, usually manifesting as seizures, with overapplication and ingestions	Preexisting seizure disorder; infants and children <6 mo of age; pregnancy; breastfeeding
10% Crotamiton cream or lotion (Eurax)	Yes	C	Apply from neck down on two consecutive nights; wash off 24 hr after second application	Excellent; not very effective; exacerbates pruritus	None
2%-10% Sulfur in petrolatum ointments	No	C	Apply for 2-3 days, then wash	Excellent; not very effective	Preexisting sulfur allergy
10%-25% Benzoyl benzoate lotion	No	None	Two applications for 24 hr with 1-day to 1-wk interval	Irritant; exacerbates pruritus; can induce contact irritant dermatitis and pruritic cutaneous xerosis	Preexisting eczema
0.5% Malathion lotion (Ovide), 1% malathion shampoo (unavailable in the U.S.)	No	B	95% ovicidal; rapid (5 min) killing; good residual activity; increasing drug resistance	Flammable 78% isopropyl alcohol vehicle stings eyes, skin, mucosa; increasing drug resistance; organophosphate poisoning risk with overapplication and ingestions	Infants and children <6 mo of age; pregnancy; breastfeeding
Ivermectin (Stromectol)	Yes	C	200 μg/kg single PO dose, may be repeated in 14-15 days; not ovicidal, second dose on day 14 or 15 highly recommended; recommended for endemic or epidemic scabies in institutions and refugee camps	Excellent; may cause nausea and vomiting; take on empty stomach with water	Safety in pregnancy uncertain; probably safe during breastfeeding; not recommended for children younger than 5 yr of age or weighing <15 kg

*U.S. Food and Drug Administration (FDA) safety in pregnancy categories: A, safety established; B, presumed safe; C, uncertain safety; D, unsafe; X, highly unsafe.
FDA, U.S. Food and Drug Administration; *PO*, by mouth.
From Bennett JE et al: *Mandell, Douglas, and Bennett's principles and practice of infectious diseases*, ed 8, Philadelphia, 2015, WB Saunders.

DISPOSITION

Refractory cases usually are seen with immunocompromised hosts or patients with underlying skin diseases. ***Norwegian scabies*** refers to a highly contagious variant often found in institutions caring for physically and mentally disabled individuals.

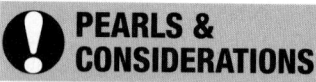

PEARLS & CONSIDERATIONS

COMMENTS

- Lindane is potentially neurotoxic and should not be used on infants or pregnant women (permethrin is safe in pregnancy and infants over 2 mo old).
- Sexual partners should be notified and treated.

SUGGESTED READINGS

Available at ExpertConsult.com

RELATED CONTENT

Scabies (Patient Information)

AUTHOR: **FRED F. FERRI, M.D.**

BASIC INFORMATION

DEFINITION

Schizophrenia is a disorder that causes significant distortions in thinking, perception, speech, and behavior. Characteristics include psychosis, apathy, social withdrawal, and cognitive impairment, which result in significant social impairment.

SYNONYM

Dementia praecox

ICD-10CM CODES
F20 Schizophrenia
F20.0 Paranoid schizophrenia
F20.1 Hebephrenic schizophrenia
F20.2 Catatonic schizophrenia
F20.3 Undifferentiated schizophrenia
F20.5 Residual schizophrenia
F20.6 Simple schizophrenia
F20.8 Other schizophrenia
F20.9 Schizophrenia, unspecified
DSM-5 CODE
295.90

EPIDEMIOLOGY & DEMOGRAPHICS

INCIDENCE: 0.2 per 1000

PREVALENCE: 0.5%; lifetime prevalence risk, 0.4%

PREDOMINANT SEX: Males have a more severe illness with earlier onset. Prevalence in males approximately 1.4 times higher.

PREDOMINANT AGE:
- Age of onset of psychotic symptoms is the early 20s for males and the late 20s for females.
- Age of onset of negative symptoms is usually earlier (i.e., the mid-teenage yrs).

PEAK INCIDENCE: Between ages of 16 and 30 yr

GENETICS:
- Genetics accounts for 70% of risk; the remaining 30% associated with other factors such as urban environments, migration, or cannabis use.
- First-degree relatives have a 10 times greater chance of becoming schizophrenic.
- Discordant rates among identical twins are higher than expected with the simple inheritance pattern.
- Associations with several chromosomes have been described, but none has been replicated.
- Evidence exists that triple nucleotide repeat expansion (e.g., such as that seen with Huntington disease) may play a role in the inheritance of the disease.

PHYSICAL FINDINGS & CLINICAL PRESENTATION

- Schizophrenia is best defined as a dementing illness that begins early in life and that progresses slowly throughout the lifetime.
- Frequent structural brain imaging findings include the enlargement of the ventricular system, a loss of brain volume and cortical gray matter, and an alteration of the white matter tracts.
- The initial "negative" symptoms of adolescence (prodromal phase)—cognitive decline, social withdrawal and awkwardness, loss of motivation and pleasure, and loss of emotional expressiveness—begin after a period of normal development.
- During early adulthood, positive symptoms of psychosis and thought disturbance occur; psychotic symptoms then wax and wane throughout life. Treatment ameliorates positive symptoms, but generally does little for negative ones.
- The condition is also accompanied by cognitive impairment, including problems with attention and concentration, psychomotor speed, learning, memory, and executive functions (e.g., abstract thinking, problem solving, planning).
- Social and occupational dysfunction can be profound.

ETIOLOGY

- The basic determination of whether this is a degenerative or developmental condition has not been made.
- The major hypothesis is that abnormality of the mesocortical pathways produces the hypofrontality and the negative symptoms. This occurs along with a compensatory hyperactivation of the mesolimbic pathways, which produces the positive symptoms of psychosis.

DIAGNOSIS

DIFFERENTIAL DIAGNOSIS

- Schizophrenia is diagnosed when an individual has experienced at least 6 mo (1 mo if using ICD-10 criteria) of hallucinations, delusions, thought disorders, catatonia, or negative symptoms (e.g., avolition, anhedonia, social isolation, affective flattening).
- Any medical condition, medicine, or substance that can affect brain homeostasis can cause psychosis; this is distinguished from schizophrenia by a relatively brief course and an alteration in mental status that suggests an underlying delirium.
- Other neurologic conditions that have psychosis as the initial presentation (e.g., Huntington disease) need to be ruled out.
- Mood disorders with psychosis: These are indistinguishable from schizophrenia cross-sectionally but have a longitudinal course that includes full recovery.
- Delusional disorder involves non- bizarre delusions and lacks the thought disturbance, hallucinations, and negative symptoms of schizophrenia.
- Autism in the adult has an early age of onset and lacks significant hallucinations or delusions.

WORKUP

- History and physical examination to help determine whether the psychosis is primary or secondary.
- Neurologic examination to uncover the soft neurologic signs (e.g., clumsiness, cortical thumb, loss of fine motor movements) that are common with schizophrenia.

LABORATORY TESTS

- No laboratory tests are specific.
- Laboratory examinations (e.g., chemistry profile, blood count, sedimentation rate, toxicology screen, and urinalysis) are geared toward excluding a primary medical condition or toxic state. Note that new common drugs of abuse may not be detectable with regular screening tests.

IMAGING STUDIES

- CT or MRI of the brain during the initial workup; repeated if the course of the illness varies from what is expected.
- EEG may reveal slowing when psychosis is the result of an encephalopathy. Findings can be similar as a result of common medication use for treatment of psychosis.

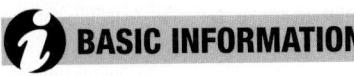

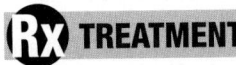

TREATMENT

NONPHARMACOLOGIC THERAPY

- Significant social support is required by most schizophrenic patients, but available support services are grossly inadequate. Schizophrenic patients constitute nearly one third of all homeless individuals and approximately 5% of the incarcerated population. They usually require help with basic social, occupational, and interaction skills.
- Family stress can precipitate relapse and re-hospitalization. Family interventions can reduce morbidity.
- Cognitive behavioral therapy can reduce the severity of both psychotic and negative symptoms.
- Illness management training for patients can increase medication adherence and reduce symptom distress.
- Integrated treatment that includes assertive community treatment, family involvement programs, and social skills training reduces the severity of both psychotic and negative symptoms, reduces comorbid substance misuse, reduces hospital days, increases adherence to treatment, and increases satisfaction with treatment.

ACUTE GENERAL Rx

- Acute psychosis is usually adequately controlled with antipsychotic agents.
- Few differences in effectiveness exist between first-generation antipsychotics (e.g., haloperidol, perphenazine, fluphenazine, chlorpromazine) and second-generation antipsychotics (e.g., risperidone, olanzapine, quetiapine, ziprasidone, aripiprazole, clozapine, lurasidone) for nonrefractory patients. First-generation antipsychotics are slightly more likely than second-generation antipsychotics to cause a parkinsonian state and eventual tardive dyskinesia (rate of tardive dyskinesia, 15% to 30%). Antiparkinsonian drugs (e.g., benztropine, amantadine) are used to ameliorate the parkinsonism. Risperidone has been shown to be superior to haloperidol for the prevention of acute psychotic relapse.

- Sedatives (i.e., benzodiazepines and, to a lesser degree, barbiturates) can be used transiently if a patient is in an agitated state.

CHRONIC Rx

- Relapse prevention is a major goal of treatment. Noncompliance is common and leads to high relapse rates. Antipsychotic agents usually must be continued at the same doses that controlled psychosis. For noncompliant patients, long-acting injectable preparations given biweekly, monthly, or every 3 mo can be used.
- Most patients frequently switch among antipsychotics; there is considerable individual variability with regard to antipsychotic response and vulnerability to specific adverse effects.
- Clozapine is more effective than other agents for treatment-refractory patients. However, it requires monitoring to prevent life-threatening adverse effects. Olanzapine may also be more effective than less expensive first-generation drugs but has substantial adverse metabolic effects. Lurasidone is a newer second-generation antipsychotic that appears to be better tolerated, but longer-term studies are needed.
- Neurocognitive improvement associated with antipsychotic treatment among patients with schizophrenia is small and does not differ between first-generation and second-generation antipsychotics.
- Antiparkinsonian agents may also need to be continued for the long term.
- Tardive dyskinesia (i.e., choreoathetoid movements of the muscles of tongue and face and occasionally of other muscle groups) can occur in as many as 30% of patients with the long-term use of neuroleptics.
- The negative symptoms of schizophrenia can resemble depression. In addition, depressive disorders may occur in schizophrenic patients. Antidepressant treatment of the negative symptoms is usually not effective. However, antidepressants can improve the symptoms of a comorbid depressive episode.
- Mood stabilizers (e.g., lithium, valproate, carbamazepine) are of little use unless the patient has a comorbid impulse control disorder.
- Substance abuse is a major problem for more than a third of schizophrenic patients. More than half of these patients smoke cigarettes. Unfortunately, these individuals do poorly in traditional substance abuse treatment programs. Specialized "dual-diagnosis" programs with highly structured aftercare are required.
- Specific antipsychotic medications have been associated with weight gain (i.e., olanzapine and clozapine) and QT prolongation. Hyperlipidemia and diabetes mellitus are associated with second-generation antipsychotics, and hyperprolactinemia is associated with first-generation antipsychotics. (Risperidone, a second-generation antipsychotic, can also produce hyperprolactinemia.) Clozapine is associated with agranulocytosis and a decrease in intestinal motility. Metabolic status and weight should be screened before the start of treatment and at regular intervals.
- Patients with schizophrenia have a higher lifetime incidence of suicide, with 20% attempting on one or more occasions and 5% to 6% completing suicide. Comorbid use of substances and hopelessness are associated risk factors. Clozapine has shown the ability to decrease the incidence of suicidal attempts in schizophrenia patients.
- Several first and second generation antipsychotics are available in long-acting injectable preparations that may be helpful in addressing issues of poor compliance or difficulty when treatment needs to be supervised. Current preparation can be given in intervals that range between every 2 to every 3 mo. Consider economic factor and importance of regular checks when using long-acting injectables.

DISPOSITION

- The positive symptoms of as many as 20% to 30% of schizophrenic patients do not respond to available treatments. A much higher fraction of patients experience relapse as a result of poor compliance.
- Negative symptoms are responsible for the 50% to 70% of patients in whom deterioration in occupational and social function continues.
- Approximately 10% of schizophrenic patients will complete suicide.
- The course of the illness is most strongly predicted by the level of social development attained at the onset of psychosis.
- Schizophrenic patients die 12 to 15 yr sooner than the average population, mostly as a result of physical causes related to a lack of access to health care or as a result of health risk factors (e.g., smoking, obesity).

REFERRAL

- If hospitalization is required
- If patient is noncompliant
- If patient is resistant to treatment

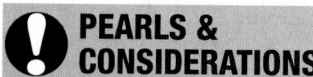

PEARLS & CONSIDERATIONS

- Rule out delirium caused by medical conditions, medications, or substance abuse before diagnosing an individual's psychotic behavior as schizophrenia.
- All antipsychotic medications have high discontinuation rates in chronic schizophrenia treatment. Olanzapine and clozapine may be more effective than other antipsychotics for chronic treatment, but they have significant side effects.
- Significant social support is required for most patients with schizophrenia. Nonpharmacologic therapy should be used in conjunction with pharmacotherapy.

SUGGESTED READINGS

Available at ExpertConsult.com

RELATED CONTENT

Schizophrenia (Patient Information)

AUTHOR: **ARNALDO A. BERGES, M.D.**

BASIC INFORMATION

DEFINITION

Sciatica refers to the neuralgia following the sciatic nerve down the leg along its distribution. Sciatica usually occurs unilaterally. Pain is described as sharp or aching, and it typically radiates from the buttock down the leg posteriorly, laterally, or anteriorly depending on the level of nerve root compression.

SYNONYMS

Bilateral sciatica
Deep gluteal syndrome
Gout of the hip
Ischiagra
Left-sided sciatica
Low back pain with left sciatica
Low back pain with right sciatica
Low back pain—sciatica
Lumbago with sciatica
Lumbar nerve root pain
Lumbar radiculopathy (LBP)—sciatica
Neuropathy—sciatic nerve
Right-sided sciatica
Sciatic nerve dysfunction
Sciatic neuritis

ICD-10CM CODES:

M54.30	Sciatica, unspecified side
M54.31	Sciatica, right side
M54.32	Sciatica, left side
M54.40	Lumbago with sciatica, unspecified side
M54.41	Lumbago with sciatica, right side
M54.42	Lumbago with sciatica, left side
M54.5	Low back pain
M54.9	Dorsalgia, unspecified
M62.838	Other muscle spasm
G57.00	Lesion of sciatic nerve, unspecified lower limb
G57.01	Lesion of sciatic nerve, right lower limb lesion
G57.02	Lesion of sciatic nerve, left lower limb

EPIDEMIOLOGY & DEMOGRAPHICS

INCIDENCE: Very few studies have determined the incidence of sciatica. However, 5% to 10% of patients with low back pain have sciatica. The highest incidence recorded is 40%.

PEAK INCIDENCE: Age 30 to 64 yr

PREVALENCE: Annual prevalence of disc-related sciatica in the general population is estimated at 2.2%.

RISK FACTORS:

- Increasing risk with height
- Smoking
- Diabetes
- Obesity
- Prolonged sitting and sedentary lifestyle
- Occupational factors:
  1. Strenuous physical activity (e.g., frequent lifting while bending and twisting)
  2. Driving

PHYSICAL FINDINGS & CLINICAL PRESENTATION

- Unilateral leg pain greater than low back pain
- Pain radiating to foot or toes
- Numbness and paresthesia in the same distribution
- Straight leg raising test induces more leg pain
- Localized neurology limited to one nerve root

ETIOLOGY

- Sciatica is usually caused by disc herniation at the L4-L5 and L5-S1 level, less commonly at the L3-L4 level
- Other causes include lumbar spinal stenosis, facet joint osteoarthritis or other arthropathies, spinal cord infection or tumor, sacroiliac joint dysfunction, degenerative disc disease, or isthmic spondylolisthesis

DIAGNOSIS

DIFFERENTIAL DIAGNOSIS

- Nonspecific low back pain
- Piriformis syndrome
- Muscular problems (sprain, spasm)
- Vascular problems (claudication, compartment syndrome)
- Chronic edema
- Box 1 summarizes the differential diagnosis for low back pain

WORKUP

History taking and the physical examination are important steps in the evaluation of sciatica. Historical clues to the cause of low back pain are summarized in Table 1. Red flags that may indicate cauda equina or spinal infection mandate emergent workup. Fig. 1 summarizes an algorithm for the management of low back pain.

HISTORY TAKING:

- Severity of pain
- Duration
- Influence of coughing, movement, or rest
- Complaints of radiating pain in the leg following a dermatomal pattern
- Low back pain, less severe than leg pain
- Pain generally radiates below the knee, into the foot
- Dermatome maps used to locate origin of the pain
- Sensory symptoms

PHYSICAL EXAMINATION: Neurological testing

- Myotomes
- Reflexes (L4-S3)
- Sensations (dermatomes; see Fig. 2)

LUMBAR MOBILITY ASSESSMENT: Neural tension tests (preferable seated position)

- Straight leg raise test
- Reversed straight leg raise test
- Bragard test
- Crossed straight leg raise test
- Slump test
- Femoral nerve tension test

BOX 1 Differential Diagnosis for Low Back Pain

Localized and Common
Uncomplicated musculoskeletal back pain
Intervertebral disk herniation
Spinal stenosis
Spondylolisthesis
Osteoarthritis
Fracture

Localized and Uncommon

Infection
Spondylitis
Epidural abscess
Diskitis
Herpes zoster

Malignancy
Metastatic
Breast
Lung
Prostate
Kidney, thyroid, colon (less common)
Primary
Multiple myeloma
Lymphoma
Leukemia
Primary cord or extradural tumors
Osteoid osteoma
Other primary bone tumors

Pediatric
Spondylolisthesis, spondylolysis
Severe scoliosis
Scheuermann disease

Rheumatologic
Ankylosing spondylitis
Psoriatic arthritis
Polymyalgia rheumatica
Reiter syndrome

Vascular
Arteriovenous malformation of spinal cord
Epidural hematoma

Life-Threatening Referred Pain
Abdominal aortic aneurysm

Gastrointestinal System
Biliary pathology
Pancreatitis
Peptic ulcer disease
Diverticulitis

Genitourinary System
Renal colic
Pyelonephritis
Prostatitis
Cystitis

Gynecologic System
Menstrual cramps
Spontaneous abortion
Labor
Ectopic pregnancy
Pelvic inflammatory disease
Endometriosis
Ovarian cyst
Ovarian torsion

Hematologic System
Sickle cell crisis

Functional
Somatization disorder
Depression
Fibrositis
Malingering

From Marx JA et al: *Rosen's emergency medicine*, ed 8, Philadelphia, 2014, Elsevier.

TABLE 1 Historical Clues to the Cause of Low Back Pain

Questions for Patient	Potential Diagnosis
Does the back pain radiate down past the knees?	Radiculopathy and likely a herniated disk
Is the pain worse with walking and better with bending forward and sitting?	Spinal stenosis
Do you have morning back stiffness that improves with exercise?	Ankylosing spondylitis
Are you older than 50 yr?	Osteoporotic fracture, spinal malignancy
Has there been any recent history of blunt trauma?	Fracture
Do you take long-term corticosteroids?	Fracture, spinal infection
Do you have a history of cancer?	Spinal metastatic malignancy
Does your pain persist at rest?	Spinal malignancy, spinal infection
Has there been persistent pain for longer than 6 weeks?	Spinal malignancy
Has there been unexplained weight loss?	Spinal malignancy
Is the pain worse at night?	Spinal malignancy, spinal infection
Are you immunocompromised (e.g., HIV infection, alcoholism, diabetes)?	Spinal infection
Have you had fevers or chills?	Spinal infection
Do you have pain, weakness, or numbness in both legs?	Cauda equina syndrome
Do you have bladder or bowel control problems?	Cauda equina syndrome

HIV, Human immunodeficiency virus.
From Walls RM et al: *Rosen's emergency medicine: concepts and clinical practice*, ed 9, Philadelphia, 2018, Elsevier.

Major maneuvers:
- Lumbar lateral bending
- Hip flexion
- Lasegue test
- Bechterew test
- Fajersztajn test
- Knee extension

Minor maneuvers:
- Cervical flexion
- Spinal flexion
- Hip internal rotation
- Hip adduction
- Great toe dorsiflexion
- Increased intrathecal/intradiscal pressure

LABORATORY TESTS

No laboratory tests specifically identify sciatica; it is a clinical diagnosis.
- Occasionally laboratory tests such as complete blood count (CBC) may suggest infection, anemia due to certain cancers, or other unusual causes of sciatica.
- Elevated erythrocyte sedimentation rate may suggest inflammation somewhere in the body.
- Urinalysis may suggest a kidney stone if there is blood in the urine, or infection if bacteria and white blood cells are present in the urine.

IMAGING STUDIES

- If pain does not resolve on its own, computed tomography (CT) or magnetic resonance imaging (MRI) scans of spine can be ordered to evaluate for other causes
- If patient has a history of cancer, HIV infection, or IV drug use, or has been taking steroids over a period of time, imaging or bone scan are recommended
- Electromyography (EMG)
- X-ray of spine may be examined for compression of nerve due to bone overgrowth

Rx TREATMENT

Treatment for sciatica is activity modification and pain medication.
- Prescription-strength nonsteroidal antiinflammatory drugs, such as meloxicam and diclofenac
- Analgesics, such as acetaminophen
- Muscle relaxants, such as cyclobenzaprine and tizanidine
- Corticosteroids
- Nerve pain medication (e.g., gabapentin)
- If pain is severe and not relieved by previous measures, then narcotic medications may be prescribed for a short period

NONPHARMACOLOGIC THERAPY

- Back surgery may be recommended if the pain continues and the CT and MRI indicate an anatomic problem with disc or bone and all other methods of treatment do not work
- Ice or heat on affected area for 20 min every 2 hr
- Physical therapy
- Acupuncture, relaxation techniques
- Epidural injections
- Exercise therapy, including walking, yoga, Pilates
- Reducing pressure on the nerve root
- Bed rest is not recommended

ACUTE GENERAL Rx

- Acetaminophen for mild pain.
- Prescription-strength nonsteroidal antiinflammatory drugs, such as meloxicam and diclofenac for moderate pain. Muscle relaxants, such as cyclobenzaprine and tizanidine are frequently used but efficacy is questionable. They are contraindicated in elderly patients.
- Gabapentin or pregabalin are frequently prescribed, but trials have failed to show reduced intensity of leg pain or improved outcomes.

CHRONIC Rx

If pain is severe and not relieved by previous measures, then narcotic medications may be considered for a short period, although the medical community is increasingly turning away from long-term opioids due to the associated morbidity and mortality

COMPLEMENTARY AND ALTERNATIVE MEDICINE

- Acupuncture
- Spinal manipulation/chiropractic treatment techniques
- Physical therapy

DISPOSITION

Outpatient workup and assessment, including:
- Checking for red flags that may indicate malignancies, osteoporotic fractures, infection, or cauda equina syndrome
- Taking a history to determine localization, severity, loss of strength, sensation, duration, course, influence of coughing, rest or movement
- Physical examination, including straight leg raising test
- Imaging or laboratory diagnostic testing if red flags are present
- Prescribe medication as needed

REFERRAL

- Orthopedic surgeon
- Pain management
- Physical therapist
- Refer to neurosurgeon immediately in cases of cauda equina syndrome or acute severe paresis or progressive paresis (within a few days)
- Refer to neurologist, neurosurgeon, or orthopedic surgeon for consideration of surgery in cases of intractable radicular pain (not responding to morphine) or if pain does not diminish after 6 to 8 wk of conservative care

PEARLS & CONSIDERATIONS

COMMENTS

- Most people recover fully from sciatica and often without treatment, but it can potentially cause nerve damage. Important to seek immediate medical attention with loss of feeling in affected leg, weakness in affected leg, or loss of bowel or bladder function, as this could indicate cauda equina or epidural abscess.
- Sciatica does have a tendency to recur.
- Bed rest is not recommended.

PREVENTION

- Exercise regularly.
- Maintain proper posture when you sit.
- Use good body mechanics.

SUGGESTED READINGS

Available at ExpertConsult.com

RELATED CONTENT

Lumbar Disk Syndrome (Related Key Topic)
Piriformis Syndrome (Related Key Topic)

AUTHORS: **CYRIL PATRA, M.P.H.,** and **MARK F. BRADY, M.D., M.P.H., M.M.S.**

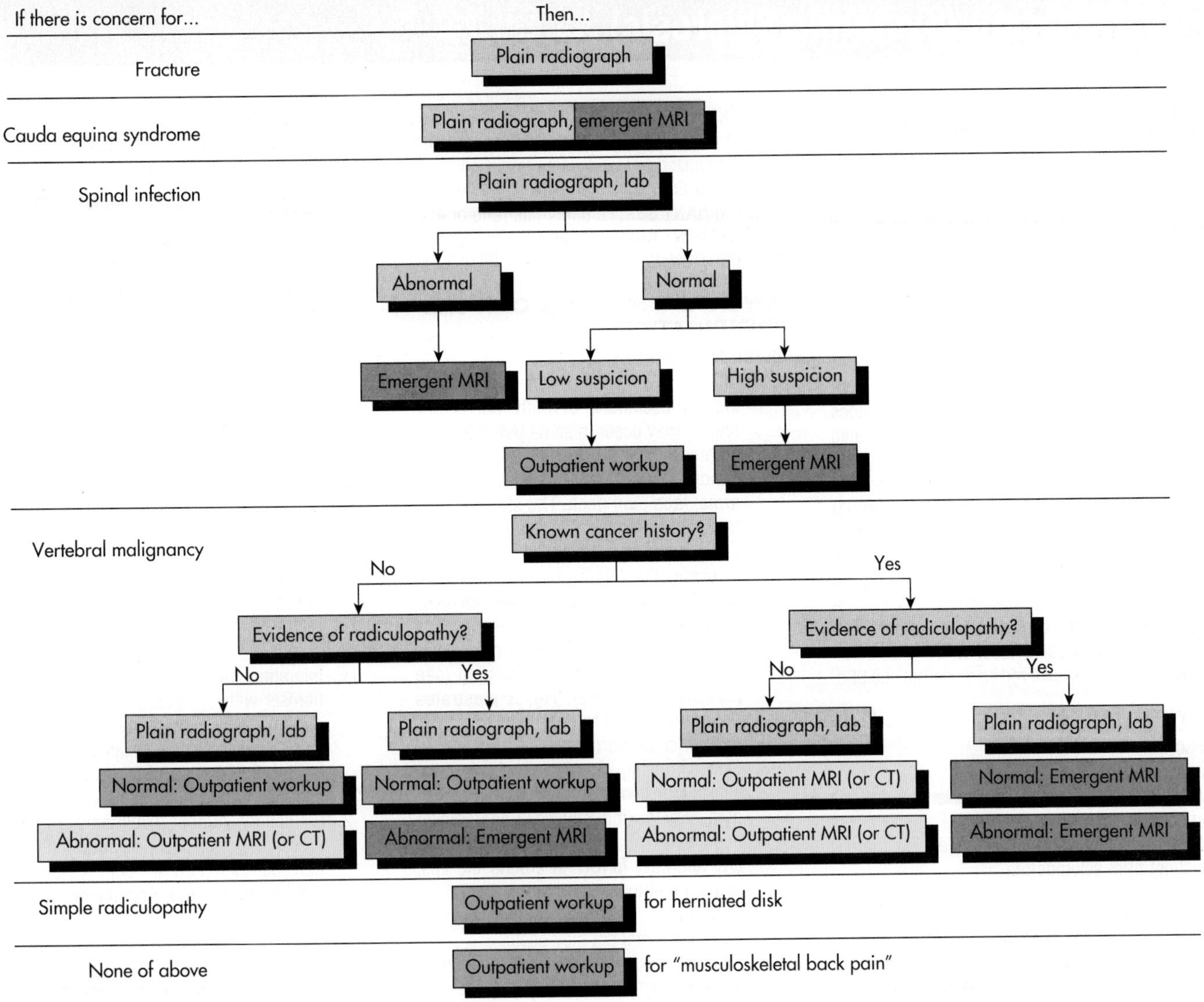

If there is concern for...	Then...
Fracture	Plain radiograph
Cauda equina syndrome	Plain radiograph, emergent MRI
Spinal infection	Plain radiograph, lab → Abnormal → Emergent MRI; Normal → Low suspicion → Outpatient workup; Normal → High suspicion → Emergent MRI
Vertebral malignancy	Known cancer history? No → Evidence of radiculopathy? No → Plain radiograph, lab; Normal: Outpatient workup; Abnormal: Outpatient MRI (or CT). Yes → Plain radiograph, lab; Normal: Outpatient workup; Abnormal: Emergent MRI. Known cancer history? Yes → Evidence of radiculopathy? No → Plain radiograph, lab; Normal: Outpatient MRI (or CT); Abnormal: Outpatient MRI (or CT). Yes → Plain radiograph, lab; Normal: Emergent MRI; Abnormal: Emergent MRI
Simple radiculopathy	Outpatient workup for herniated disk
None of above	Outpatient workup for "musculoskeletal back pain"

FIG. 1 Algorithm for management of low back pain. The patient's history may be concerning for more than one red flag diagnosis. *CT,* Computed tomography; *MRI,* magnetic resonance imaging. (From Marx JA et al: *Rosen's emergency medicine*, ed 8, Philadelphia, 2014, Elsevier.)

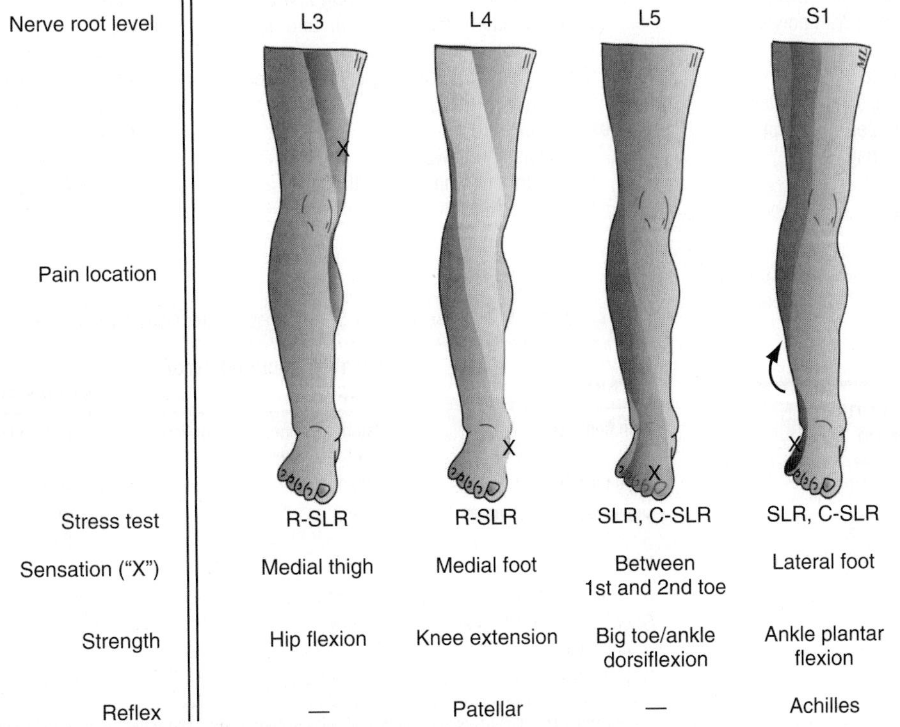

Nerve root level
L3
L4
L5
S1
Pain location
X
Stress test
R-SLR
R-SLR
SLR, C-SLR
SLR, C-SLR
Sensation ("X")
Medial thigh
Medial foot
Between 1st and 2nd toe
Lateral foot
Strength
Hip flexion
Knee extension
Big toe/ankle dorsiflexion
Ankle plantar flexion
Reflex
—
Patellar
—
Achilles

FIG. 2 Physical examination findings for L3-S1 radiculopathy. The *X* marks the ideal location to test for sensation for each nerve root. *C-SLR,* Crossed straight leg raise; *R-SLR,* reverse straight leg raise; *SLR,* straight leg raise. (From Marx JA et al: *Rosen's emergency medicine*, ed 8, Philadelphia, 2014, Elsevier.)

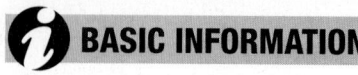

BASIC INFORMATION

DEFINITION

Scleroderma or systemic sclerosis (SSc) is a term used to describe a connective tissue disorder that is characterized by thickening and fibrosis of the skin. Scleroderma is divided into two forms: localized scleroderma and systemic sclerosis. Systemic sclerosis is a multiorgan disease characterized by fibrosis and vasculopathy. Skin thickening without any organ involvement is known as localized scleroderma and includes three subset conditions (see Box 1). Systemic sclerosis includes skin fibrosis along with variable severe involvement of diverse internal organs. It is further divided into two major subgroups: (1) limited cutaneous SSc (lcSSc), which involves skin thickening of the face, neck, and distal to the elbows and knees; and (2) diffuse cutaneous SSc (dcSSc), which affects the skin in a more generalized distribution including the proximal and distal extremities, face, neck, and trunk. Table 1 compares localized scleroderma and SSc.

SYNONYMS

SSc
Systemic sclerosis
Morphea applies to localized scleroderma that affects only the skin
Scleredema is a disease of the skin that is distinct from scleroderma

ICD-10CM CODES

M34.0	Progressive systemic sclerosis
M34.1	CREST syndrome
M34.2	Systemic sclerosis induced by drug and chemical
M34.81	Systemic sclerosis with lung involvement
M34.82	Systemic sclerosis with myopathy
M34.83	Systemic sclerosis with polyneuropathy
M34.89	Other systemic sclerosis
M34.9	Systemic sclerosis, unspecified
L94.0	Localized scleroderma (morphea)
L94.1	Linear scleroderma

EPIDEMIOLOGY & DEMOGRAPHICS

Incidence and prevalence of SSc varies between studies due to variations between geographic regions and time periods.

INCIDENCE: There are an estimated 19 cases per 1 million persons/yr, but many mild cases go unrecognized.
PREVALENCE: 276 cases per 1 million persons
PREDOMINANT SEX: Female/male ratio of 4:1
PREDOMINANT AGE: 30 to 50 yr
DISTRIBUTION: Worldwide

PHYSICAL FINDINGS & CLINICAL PRESENTATION

PHYSICAL FINDINGS:

- Skin:
  1. Initial presentation of puffy hands and fingers may occur in some patients.
  2. Tightening of the skin begins on the hands and then progresses to the forearms, face, and neck. The skin is shiny, taut, and sometimes red, with loss of creases and hair. Skin thickening involving the fingers or toes is known as sclerodactyly (Fig. 1). Skin involvement in scleroderma is classified as lcSSc or dcSSc, depending on the distribution of the skin thickening (see previously) (Fig. E2). Fig. 3 illustrates the method used to quantify skin thickness in scleroderma.
  3. Skin tightening may limit movement by causing flexion contractures of the fingers, wrists, and elbows. Perioral skin tightening (Fig. E4) results in decreased oral aperture, furrowing around the lips, and dry membranes.
  4. Pigmentary skin changes (hypo- or hyperpigmentation) may occur.
  5. Telangiectasias (dilated capillaries) may be seen on face, hands, mucous membranes (Fig. E4), and trunk.
  6. Subcutaneous calcinosis.
  7. In dsSSc patients, the skin fibrosis can soften to normal skin (occurring 2 yr after onset of skin manifestation), and joint mobility can improve.
  8. Skin atrophy and thinning can also occur in the late stages of SSc.
- Musculoskeletal:
  1. Arthralgias and swelling
  2. Symmetric inflammatory arthritis
  3. Myalgias
  4. Myopathy
  5. Tendon friction rubs (physical exam finding of a palpable rub felt over tendon sheaths—fingers, wrists, elbows, knees, and/or ankles)
- Gastrointestinal involvement:
  1. Esophageal dysmotility with heartburn
  2. Esophageal stricture with dysphagia and odynophagia
  3. Delayed gastric emptying
  4. Gastrointestinal bleeding from mucosal telangiectasias, gastric antral vascular ectasias, or gastritis
  5. Small bowel dysmotility with abdominal cramps, bloating, and diarrhea
  6. Colon dysmotility with constipation
  7. Intestinal bacterial overgrowth resulting in irregular bowel movements (diarrhea alternating with constipation)
  8. Pseudo-obstruction (functional ileus)
  9. Primary biliary cirrhosis (see "Primary Biliary Cirrhosis" in Section I)
- Pulmonary:
  1. Interstitial lung disease (ILD): Pulmonary fibrosis with symptoms of dyspnea and nonproductive cough as well as fine inspiratory crackles on examination. Seen in both lcSSc and dcSSC, but it is more common and severe in dcSSC.
  2. Pulmonary arterial hypertension (PAH): Presenting with dyspnea and/or fatigue. Can be identified in both lcSSc and dcSSc, but it is more commonly seen in lcSSc.
- Cardiac:
  1. Pericarditis or pericardial effusion
  2. Myositis or myocardial fibrosis that can lead to congestive heart failure or arrhythmias
  3. Left or right systolic or diastolic dysfunction
- Renal:
  1. Rapidly progressive renal failure also known as scleroderma renal crisis (SRC): New-onset hypertension, anemia with schistocytes on peripheral blood smear, thrombocytopenia and renal insufficiency with active urinary sediment and proteinuria

BOX 1 Classification of Scleroderma

I. Localized scleroderma
   A. Morphea
   B. Linear scleroderma
   C. Scleroderma en coup de sabre
II. Systemic sclerosis
   A. Limited cutaneous systemic sclerosis
   B. Diffuse cutaneous systemic sclerosis

From Hochberg MC, et al.: *Rheumatology,* ed 5, St Louis, 2011, Mosby.

TABLE 1 Comparison of Localized Scleroderma and Systemic Sclerosis

Feature	Localized Scleroderma/ Morphea	Systemic Sclerosis
Skin findings	Patches or linear distribution of thickened skin	Sclerodactyly ± proximal skin thickening
Raynaud's phenomenon	Absent	Present
Digital ischemic changes	Absent	Usually present (digital pitting scars or ulcers, loss of fingerpad substance)
Internal organ disease	Absent	Present
Antinuclear antibody	Positive in ≥50% of cases	Positive in ≥85% of cases
Scleroderma-specific autoantibodies*	Negative	Positive in 60% of cases
Biopsy—histologic findings	Dermal fibrosis	Dermal fibrosis

*Scleroderma-specific antibodies include antibodies to centromere, topoisomerase-1 (Scl 70), and RNA polymerase III.
From Hochberg MC, et al.: *Rheumatology,* ed 5, St Louis, 2011, Mosby.

- Vascular:
  1. Raynaud phenomenon (RP): Vasospasm of the fingers with exposure to cold, resulting in color changes of the digits along with numbness/tingling and pain or discomfort.
  2. Complications of this vascular involvement include digital pitted scars or ulcers, nonreversible ischemic changes with impending tissue loss, dry gangrene, and auto-amputation.
  3. Nailfold capillary abnormalities: Seen with nailfold capillaroscopy, including capillary dilatation, avascularity, or "drop out" of capillaries.
- Other organ involvement:
  1. Hypothyroidism
  2. Erectile dysfunction
  3. Sjögren syndrome
  4. Entrapment neuropathies
  5. Depression

CLINICAL PRESENTATION:

- Raynaud's phenomenon: Initial complaint in 70% of patients (NOTE: The prevalence of Raynaud's phenomenon is 5% to 10% in the general population; most cases do not progress to scleroderma)
- Finger or hand swelling that is sometimes associated with carpal tunnel syndrome
- Arthralgias/arthritis
- Internal organ involvement
- LcSSc (previously known as CREST syndrome):
  1. Calcinosis, Raynaud's phenomenon, Esophageal dysmotility, Sclerodactyly telangiectasias—skin fibrosis is limited to the distal extremities. This acronym is now considered obsolete by many because it does not accurately reflect the burden of internal organ involvement.

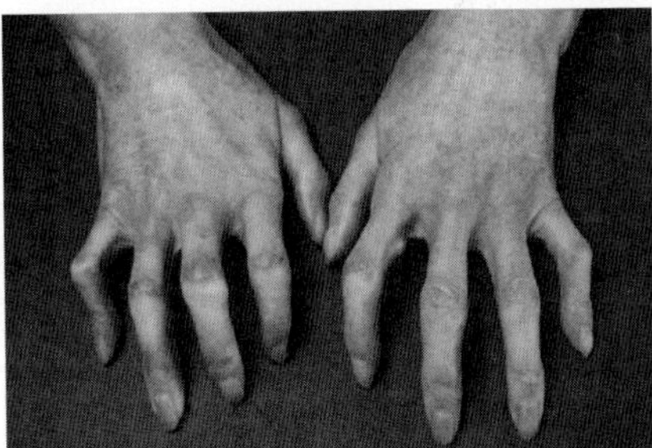

FIG. 1 Sclerodactyly in a patient with systemic sclerosis. (From Hochberg MC et al: *Rheumatology*, ed 5, St Louis, 2011, Mosby.)

ETIOLOGY

The etiology of this condition is unknown, but genetic and environmental factors (infectious agents, occupational exposures, drugs) contribute to the manifestation of the disease. Genetic profiles show clustering of different alleles according to the subtype of SSc.

Pathologically, small- and medium-sized arteries become injured, leading to fibrin deposition and ultimately luminal occlusion, causing chronic tissue hypoxia. There is also an abnormal selection of fibroblasts and aberrant control of connective tissue synthesis by fibroblasts and other cells. This fibrosis occurs in different organs, causing dysfunction and eventual failure. Although there are characteristic autoantibodies detected, it is not clear that they directly participate in the pathogenesis of the disease.

Dx DIAGNOSIS

The American College of Rheumatology (ACR) and European League Against Rheumatism (EULAR) have created criteria as a guide in diagnosing and classifying SSc. These include a scoring system for both clinical and laboratory findings (sclerodactyly, fingertip lesions, telangiectasias, abnormal nailfold capillaries, Raynaud's phenomenon, PAH/ILD, and SSc-related autoantibodies).

DIFFERENTIAL DIAGNOSIS

DERMATOLOGIC:

- Scleredema
- Amyloidosis
- Porphyria cutanea tarda
- Eosinophilic fasciitis
- Reflex sympathetic dystrophy
- Nephrogenic systemic fibrosis

SYSTEMIC:

- Idiopathic pulmonary fibrosis
- Primary pulmonary hypertension
- Primary biliary cirrhosis
- Cardiomyopathies
- Gastrointestinal dysmotility problems
- Systemic lupus erythematosus and overlap syndromes

WORKUP

Laboratory tests and imaging studies

LABORATORY TESTS

- Antinuclear antibodies (ANA): Nucleolar (more common), homogeneous, or speckled patterns.
- Rheumatoid factor positive in 20% of patients.
- Routine biochemistry tests may indicate specific organ involvement (e.g., liver, kidney, muscle).

The following extractable nuclear antigens are either present or absent in SSc:

- Anticentromere antibodies: Generally positive in one third of patients with lcSSc
- Anti-Scl-70 antibody: Positive in 40% of patients with dcSSc and has an increased risk of developing ILD
- Anti-RNA polymerase III antibody: Portends a worse prognosis and extensive skin fibrosis and increases risk of developing SRC
- Autoantibodies against ribonucleoprotein (anti-RNP): Positive in 20% of patients
- Negative antibody to native DNA
- Negative anti-smooth muscle antibody
- Table 2 summarizes autoantigens and autoantibodies in scleroderma

IMAGING AND OTHER STUDIES

- Arthritis: Joint radiographs
- Gastrointestinal:
  1. Endoscopy (diagnostic procedure of choice; may be therapeutic)
  2. Cine-esophagography (in rare circumstances)
  3. Barium swallow (occasionally indicated)
  4. Esophageal manometry (almost never necessary)
- Pulmonary:
  1. Chest x-ray
  2. Pulmonary function tests (especially single-breath diffusion capacity for carbon monoxide)
  3. Thoracic high-resolution computed tomography (HRCT) scan
  4. Bronchoscopy with biopsy
  5. Bronchoalveolar lavage
- Cardiac:
  1. ECG
  2. Ambulatory (Holter) ECG monitoring
  3. Echocardiography
  4. Cardiac catheterization
- Kidney: Renal biopsy
- Skin: Skin biopsy
- Vascular: Nailfold capillaroscopy

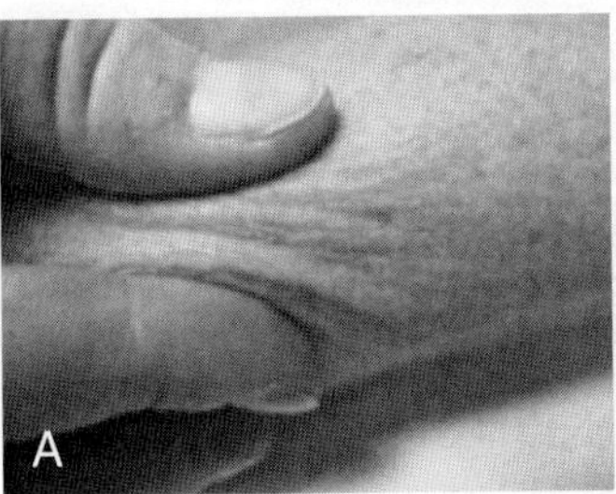

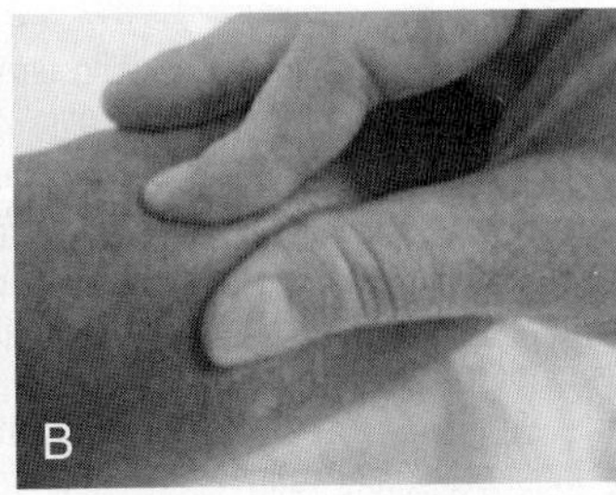

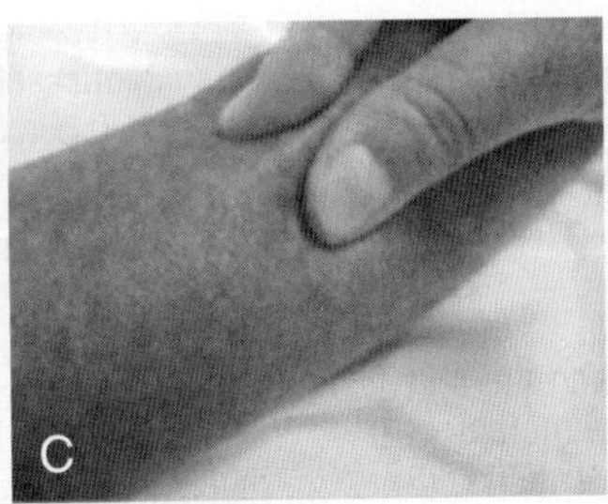

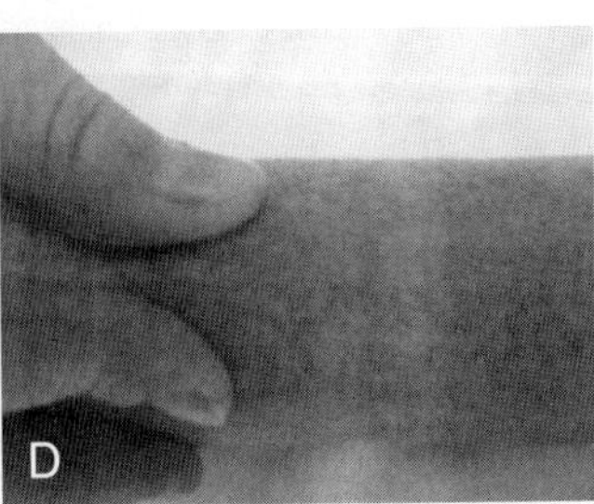

FIG. 3 Method used to semi-quantify skin thickness in scleroderma. The modified Rodnan skin score is obtained by clinical palpation of 17 different body areas (fingers, hands, forearms, upper arms, chest, abdomen, thighs, lower legs, and feet) and subjective averaging of the thickness of each specific site: 0 = normal **(A)**; 1 = mild **(B)**; 2 = moderate **(C)**; and 3 = severe **(D)**. The maximum score is 51. (From Firestein GS et al: *Kelly's textbook of rheumatology*, ed 9, Philadelphia, 2013, Saunders.)

 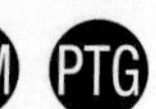

TABLE 2 Autoantigens and Autoantibodies in Scleroderma

Autoantigen	Molecular Structure	Autoantibody Frequency
Scl-70	100-kD native and 70-kD degradation product; DNA topoisomerase I	75% in diffuse scleroderma; 20%-59% in all patients; 13% in CREST
Centromere	Proteins 17, 80, and 140 kD; localized at inner and outer kinetochore plates	57%-82% in CREST; 8% in diffuse form
RNA Pol I	RNA Pol I complex of subunit proteins, 210-211 kD	4%-30% in scleroderma; 13% in diffuse form
RNA Pol II	Transcripts mRNA	4%
RNA Pol III	Transcripts 5S rRNA, tRNA	23% in scleroderma; 45% in diffuse form; 6% in CREST
Fibrillarin	Protein 34 kD, component of U3 RNP particle	6%-8%; 5% in diffuse form; 10% in CREST
U1nRNP	Spliceosome complex	2%-5% in all patients; 24% in PM/scleroderma overlap
PM-Scl	Complex of 11 proteins, 110-120 kD	4%-11%; 24% in PM/scleroderma overlap
Ku	DNA-binding protein	1%-14% in scleroderma; 26%-55% in PM/scleroderma overlap
Th/To	Protein 40 kD, complexes with 7S and 8S RNAs	1%-13% in scleroderma; 1%-11% in diffuse form; 8%-19% in CREST; up to 3% in PM/scleroderma overlap
NOR-90	Protein 90 kD, human upstream binding factor, localized in nucleolus organizer region	Rare

CREST, calcinosis, Raynaud's phenomenon, esophageal dysfunction, sclerodactyly, and telangiectasia; *DNA,* deoxyribonucleic acid; *mRNA,* messenger RNA; *PM,* polymyositis; *RNA,* ribonucleic acid; *RNP,* ribonucleoprotein; *rRNA,* ribosomal RNA; *tRNA,* transfer RNA. From McPherson RA, Pincus MR: *Henry's clinical diagnosis and management by laboratory methods*, ed 23, Philadelphia, 2017, Elsevier.

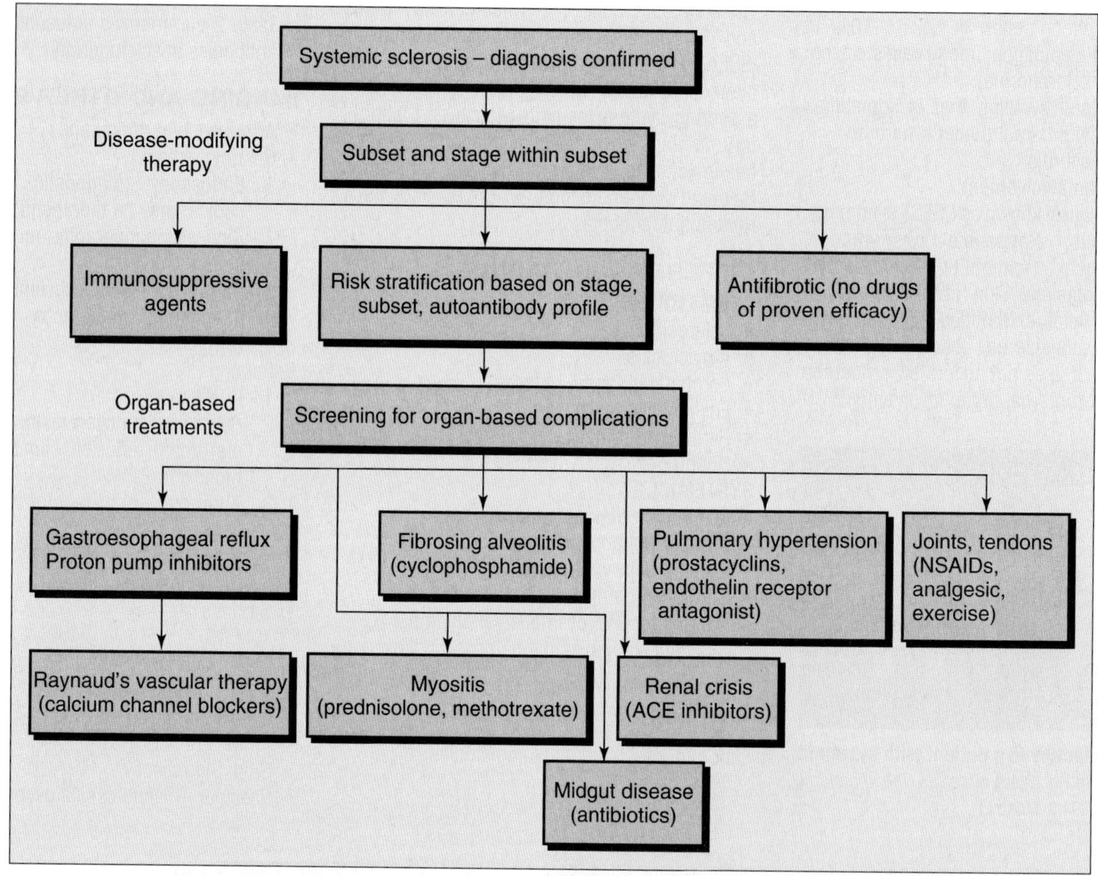

FIG. 5 Management strategies in systemic sclerosis. *ACE,* Angiotensin-converting enzyme; *NSAIDs,* nonsteroidal antiinflammatory drugs. (From Hochberg MC, et al.: *Rheumatology,* ed 5, St Louis, 2011, Mosby.)

Rx TREATMENT

Currently, there is no disease-modifying therapy available for SSc. Generally, the internal organ involvement of the disease is treatable. Fig. 5 illustrates management strategies in SSc. Immunosuppressive agents are used in individual patients. Prednisone should be used with extreme caution, especially in doses >20 mg/day. Table 3 summarizes current recommendations for treatment of scleroderma.

- Raynaud's phenomenon:
  1. Keep hands and body warm
  2. Avoid smoking
  3. Calcium channel blockers (i.e., long-acting dihydropyridines)
  4. Peripheral α1-adrenergic blockers
  5. Angiotensin II receptor blockers
  6. Pentoxifylline
  7. Phosphodiesterase inhibitors
  8. Stellate ganglion blockades
  9. Digital sympathectomy
- Arthralgias: NSAIDs or low-dose corticosteroids (5-10 mg of prednisone per day)
- Myositis: Methotrexate or azathioprine with low-dose corticosteroids
- Skin: For extensive skin fibrosis, immunomodulatory drugs have been used, such as methotrexate, mycophenolate mofetil, and cyclophosphamide, but have not been proved to be beneficial

TABLE 3 Current Recommendations for Treatment of Scleroderma

Manifestation	Primary Therapy	Alternative/Second-Line Therapy
Raynaud's phenomenon	Vasodilators (CCB) Antiplatelet	PDE5 inhibitors, prostacyclin, endothelin antagonists
Hypertensive renal disease	ACE inhibitors	ARBs, CCB, prostacyclin, renal transplant (wait at least 24 mo)
GI involvement	**Upper GI** Dental/periodontal care, lifestyle modifications, proton pump inhibitors, prokinetics	EGD to treat stenosis and/or GAVE
	Lower GI Probiotics, rotational antibiotics	Total parenteral nutrition
Skin	Mycophenolate mofetil, cyclophosphamide	IVIG, ATG, research trial (severe cases)
Interstitial lung disease	Cyclophosphamide, mycophenolate mofetil, azathioprine	Research trial
Pulmonary arterial hypertension	PDE5 inhibitors, endothelin antagonists, prostacyclin	Combination therapy, atrioseptostomy, lung transplant, research trial
Cardiac involvement	Heart failure therapy, diuretics, CCB	Immunosuppression (myocardial inflammation)
Joints	Prednisone, methotrexate, TNF inhibitors	IVIG (if contractures and rubs are present), PT/OT
Muscles	Prednisone, methotrexate, azathioprine	IVIG
Psychosocial	Antidepressants, pain control, sleep control	Support group

ACE, Angiotensin-converting enzyme; *ARBs*, angiotensin receptor blockers; *ATG*, antithymocyte globulin; *CCB*, calcium channel blockers; *EGD*, esophagogastroduodenoscopy; *GAVE*, gastric antral vascular ectasia; *GI*, gastrointestinal; *IVIG*, intravenous immunoglobulin; *PDE5*, phosphodiesterase-5 inhibitor; *PT/OT*, physical therapy/occupational therapy; *TNF*, tumor necrosis factor.
From Firestein GS, et al.: *Kelly's textbook of rheumatology*, ed 9, Philadelphia, 2013, Saunders.

- Esophageal reflux:
  1. H_2-receptor blockers
  2. Proton pump inhibitors
- Interstitial lung disease:
  1. Cyclophosphamide for symptomatic scleroderma-related ILD
  2. Mycophenolate mofetil and rituximab have been reported to be beneficial but are still being studied in clinical trials
  3. Lung transplantation for patients with advanced pulmonary involvement
- Pulmonary hypertension:
  1. Oxygen
  2. Diuretics (with caution)
  3. Prostacyclins (epoprostenol, iloprost, treprostinil)
  4. Endothelin-1 receptor inhibitors (bosentan, ambrisentan)
- Phosphodiesterase 5 inhibitors (sildenafil, tadalafil)
- Renal involvement:
  1. Angiotensin-converting enzyme inhibitors
  2. Dialysis
  3. Renal transplantation

REFERRAL

Rheumatology consultation is indicated. Consider pulmonary, cardiology, or gastrointestinal consultations depending on organ involvement.

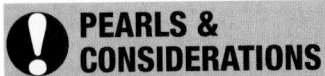

PEARLS & CONSIDERATIONS

COMMENTS

A recent trial of autologous hematopoietic stem cell therapy (HSCT) versus monthly cyclophosphamide in patients with early diffuse cutaneous systemic sclerosis showed better long-term event-free survival and overall survival at a median follow-up of approximately 6 yr and clinically meaningful improvements in objective and patient-reported outcome measures at 2 yr with HSCT. However, there was greater treatment-related mortality.

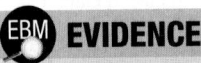

EVIDENCE

Available at ExpertConsult.com

SUGGESTED READINGS

Available at ExpertConsult.com

RELATED CONTENT

Scleroderma (Patient Information)

AUTHOR: **JOANNE SZCZYGIEL CUNHA, M.D.**

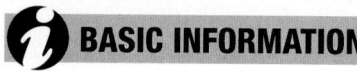

BASIC INFORMATION

DEFINITION

Scoliosis is a three-dimensional spine deformity characterized by lateral and rotational curvature of the spine. Scoliosis may be classified as either structural (fixed, nonflexible) or nonstructural (flexible, correctable, and secondary to nonspinal pathology). Scoliosis is often detected on physical examination (Adam's forward bend test) and confirmed radiographically.

ICD-10CM CODES

M41	Scoliosis
M41.0	Infantile idiopathic scoliosis
M41.1	Juvenile idiopathic scoliosis
M41.3	Thoracogenic scoliosis
M41.20	Other idiopathic scoliosis, site unspecified
M41.80	Other forms of scoliosis, site unspecified
Q67.5	Congenital deformity of spine
M41.40	Neuromuscular scoliosis, site unspecified

EPIDEMIOLOGY & DEMOGRAPHICS (IDIOPATHIC FORM)

PREDOMINANT SEX: The incidence of scoliosis is the same in males and females; however, females have up to a tenfold greater risk of curve progression. Females are roughly seven times as likely to require orthopedic surgical intervention for idiopathic scoliosis.

PREVALENCE: 1.5% to 3% of adolescents

PREDOMINANT AGE:

- Onset variable
- Most curves found in adolescents (age ≥11 yr)

PHYSICAL FINDINGS & CLINICAL PRESENTATION

- Record patient age (in years plus months) and height.
- Perform neurologic examination to rule out neuromuscular disease.
- Inspect the shoulders and iliac crests to determine if they are level.
- Palpate the spinous processes to determine their alignment.
- Have the patient bend forward at the waist to approximately 45 degrees with the arms hanging free (Adams' position); observe from the back to detect whether one side of the back appears higher than the other (Fig. 1).

ETIOLOGY

- 90% unknown, usually referred to as *idiopathic* (genetic)
- Congenital spine deformity
- Neuromuscular disease
- Leg-length inequality
- Local inflammation or infection
- Acute pain (disk disease)
- Chronic degenerative disk disease with asymmetric disk narrowing

Curves of an idiopathic nature or those accompanying congenital deformity or neuromuscular disease are associated with structural changes. The nonstructural types (leg-length discrepancy, muscle spasm, inflammation, or acute pain) disappear when the offending disorder is corrected.

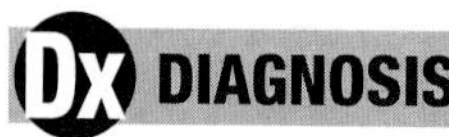

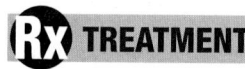

DIAGNOSIS

WORKUP

- Curvatures associated with congenital spine abnormalities, neuromuscular disease, and other less common forms of scoliosis can usually be identified by history or associated radiographic or physical findings.
- The diagnosis of scoliosis is suspected on the basis of physical examination and confirmed by radiography performed while the patient is in a standing position. Physical examination with the Adams' forward bend test and scoliometer measurement can identify scoliosis, and the radiologic testing for Cobb angle measurement can confirm the diagnosis. The Cobb angle is measured on a thoraco-lumbar radiograph and is defined as the intersecting angle between lines drawn from the two vertebrae with the greatest amount of tilt. The Risser grade measures ossification of the iliac apophysis. It consists of 5 grades ranging from 25% ossification in grade 1 to full ossification of the apophysis in grade 5. Lower Risser scores are associated with higher spinal growth potential. Patients with Risser scores of 0 or 1 are at greatest risk of scoliosis curve progression. Scoliosis screening is described in Fig. 2.

IMAGING STUDIES

- There is high potential for repeated radiation exposure in adolescents evaluated for scoliosis. Therefore, if you suspect this diagnosis, order radiographs, which include a coronal PA image of the entire spine, from the base of the skull to the iliac crests, as well as a full-length lateral view of the spine. Use breast and gonadal shielding whenever possible. If you are referring to a specialist that will be unable to view the images obtained, instruct the patient's family to bring a printed copy to their visit.
- Diagnosis of idiopathic scoliosis is confirmed by a Cobb angle greater than 10 degrees as measured on a radiograph.
- Severity of the curve is measured in degrees, usually by the Cobb method (Fig. 3).
- MRI is usually not indicated unless there is pain, a neurologic deficit, or a left thoracic curve (which is often associated with an underlying spinal disorder).

TREATMENT

ACUTE GENERAL Rx

- Treatment or correction of cause if curve is nonstructural.
- Early detection is key in treating genetic (idiopathic) curve.
- Regular observation for curves <20 degrees.
- Bracing for idiopathic curves of 25 to 45 degrees in patients with an immature skeleton (Risser score 0-2) to prevent progression.
- Surgery for idiopathic curves >45 degrees in patients with an immature skeleton.

DISPOSITION

- The larger the curve at detection, the greater the chance of progression.
- Progression is more common in young children who are beginning their growth spurt.
- Curves in females are more likely to progress.
- Curves <20 degrees will improve spontaneously >50% of the time.
- Failure to diagnose and treat these curves may allow progressive deformity, pain, and cardiopulmonary compromise to develop.
- Spinal deformities >50 degrees in adults may progress and eventually become painful or compromise pulmonary function.
- There is no difference in the rate of back pain in the general population and patients with adolescent idiopathic scoliosis.

REFERRAL

Refer for orthopedic consultation if structural curve >20 degrees is present or if structural curve <20 degrees progresses 5 degrees or more upon follow-up evaluation.

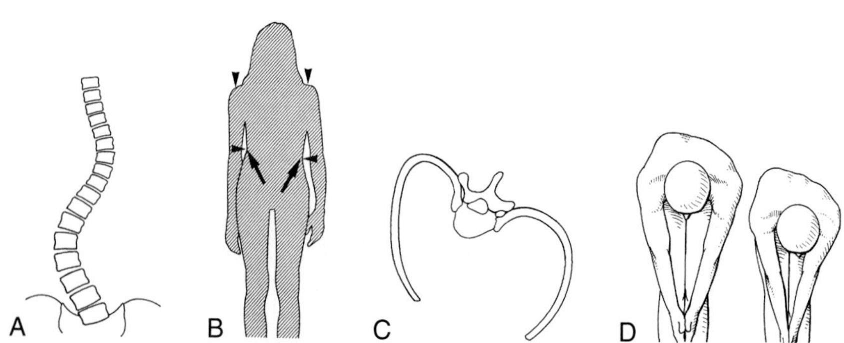

FIG. 1 Structural changes in idiopathic scoliosis. A, As curvature increases, alterations in body configuration develop in both the primary and compensatory curve regions. **B,** Asymmetries of shoulder height, waistline, and the elbow-to-flank distance are common findings. **C,** Vertebral rotation and associated posterior displacement of the ribs on the convex side of the curve are responsible for the characteristic deformity of the chest wall in scoliosis patients. **D,** In the school screening examination for scoliosis, the patient bends forward at the waist. Rib asymmetry of even a small degree is obvious.

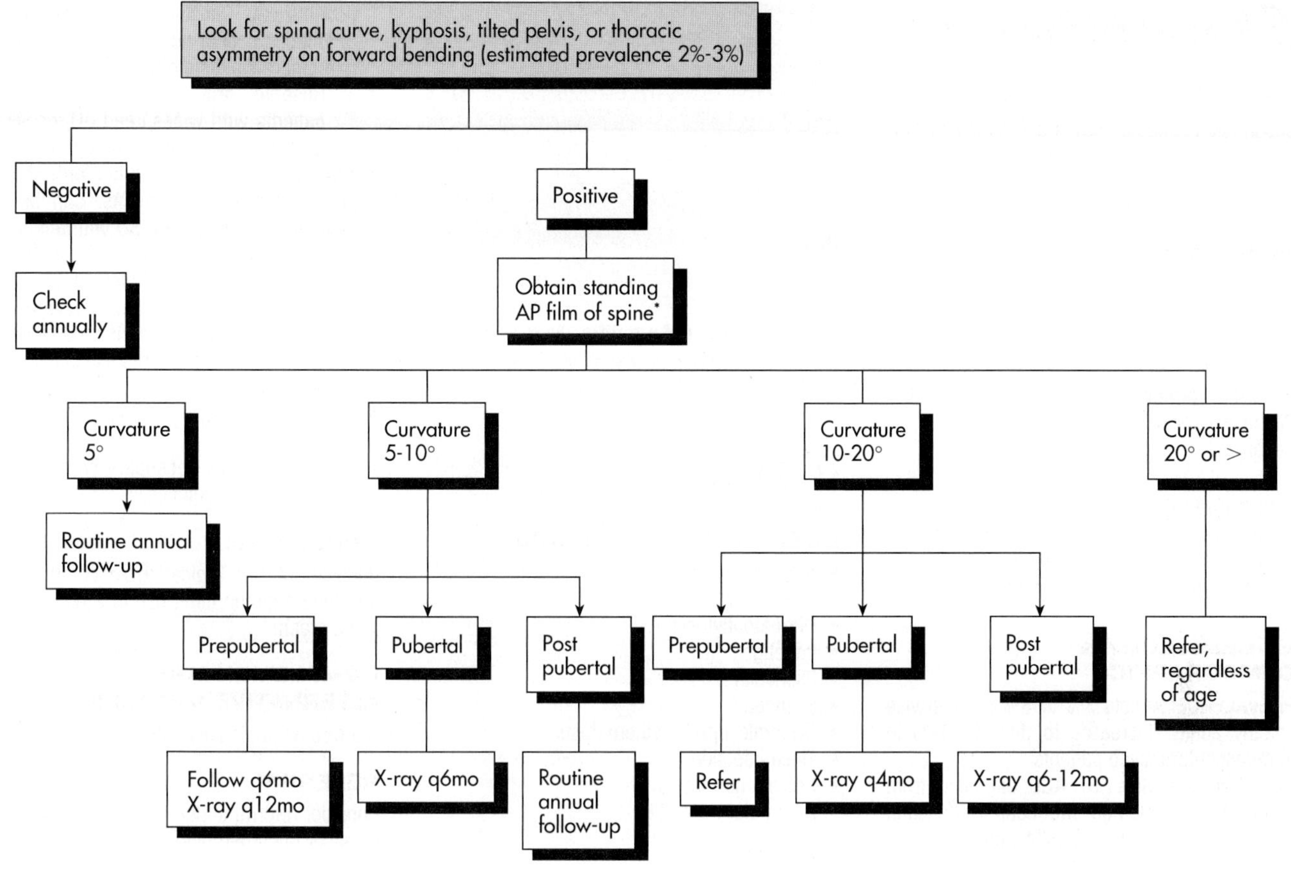

*Cobb method of angle measurement.

1. Find the lowest vertebra whose bottom tilts toward concavity of curve.
2. Erect a perpendicular line from extension of bottom surface.
3. Find highest vertebra as in #1 and erect perpendicular from extension of top surface.
4. Measure intersecting angle = angle of scoliosis.

FIG. 2 Scoliosis screening and follow-up. *AP,* Anteroposterior.

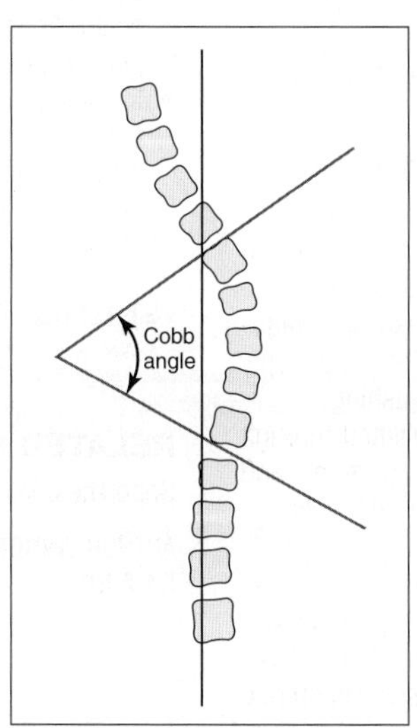

FIG. 3 Cobb angle. This is measured using the superior and inferior end plates of the most tilted vertebrae at the end of each curve. (From Tschudy MM, Arcara KM: *The Harriet Lane handbook,* ed 19, Philadelphia, 2012, Mosby.)

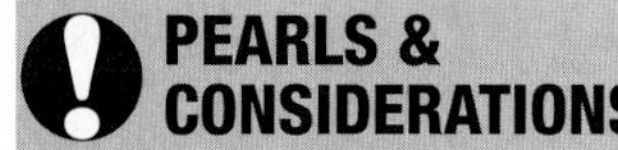

PEARLS & CONSIDERATIONS

COMMENTS

- Congenital scoliosis has a high incidence of cardiac and urinary tract abnormalities.
- Bracing is not intended to completely straighten the idiopathic curve. It may improve the curvature, but is mainly used to stabilize and prevent progression.
- The initial Cobb angle magnitude (≥25 degrees) is the most important predictor of long-term curve progression.

SUGGESTED READINGS

Available at ExpertConsult.com

RELATED CONTENT

Scoliosis (Patient Information)

AUTHOR: **GREGORY ELIA, M.D.**

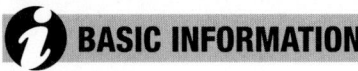

BASIC INFORMATION

DEFINITION

Seborrheic dermatitis (SD) is a common, inflammatory skin condition characterized by a mild to severe rash with scaling and erythema that occurs in areas of the skin rich in sebaceous glands.

SYNONYMS

SD
Dandruff
Cradle cap (Fig. E1)
Sebopsoriasis
Seborrheic eczema
Pityriasis capitis
Seborrhea

ICD-10CM CODES
L21.9 Seborrheic dermatitis, unspecified
L21.1 Seborrheic infantile dermatitis
L21.8 Other seborrheic dermatitis

EPIDEMIOLOGY & DEMOGRAPHICS

PREVALENCE: Affects 3% to 5% of otherwise healthy adults; increases to 34% to 83% in immunocompromised patients

PREDOMINANT SEX AND AGE: Can occur from infancy through old age, with peak incidence in adolescents and young adults and increasing again after age 50 yr. More common in men than women.

RISK FACTORS: More common in patients with HIV/AIDS, Parkinson's disease, other neurologic disorders, mood disorders, chronic alcoholic pancreatitis, hepatitis, cancer, and genetic disorders (e.g., Down syndrome). Recent evidence linking obesity and metabolic syndrome with an increased occurrence of SD. Occurs more often during winter season and during periods of increased stress.

PHYSICAL FINDINGS & CLINICAL PRESENTATION

- Mild, greasy scaling of the scalp and nasolabial folds (Fig. 2); postauricular skin, beard area, eyebrows, trunk, and sometimes the central face. Blepharitis, otitis externa, and coexisting acne vulgaris or pityriasis may also be present. Itching and stinging of lesions can occur. Increased occurrence during times of stress or sleep deprivation.
- The scale often has a yellow, greasy appearance.

ETIOLOGY

- Fungal infections of the *Malassezia* species have been associated with SD, and the skin changes are thought to result from an inflammatory response to Malassezia yeast.
- Altered immune function may play a role. Patients with SD may show upregulation of interferon (IFN)-α, expressed interleukin-6 (IL-6), expressed IL-1β, and IL-4.

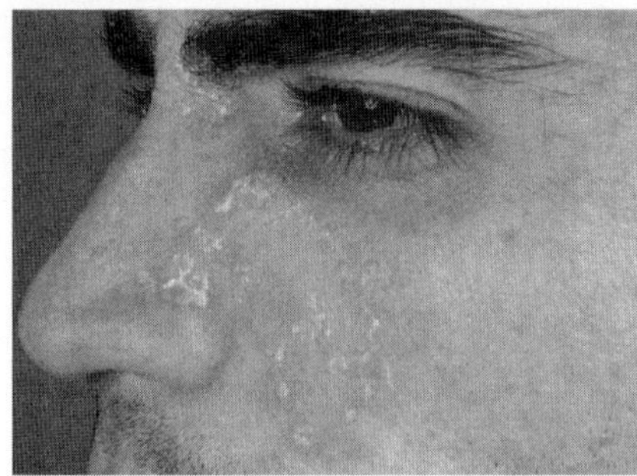

FIG. 2 Seborrheic dermatitis. (From Swartz MH: *Textbook of physical diagnosis,* ed 7, Philadelphia, 2014, Saunders, 2014.)

DIAGNOSIS

DIFFERENTIAL DIAGNOSIS

- Atopic dermatitis
- Candidiasis
- Dermatophytosis
- Impetigo
- Psoriasis
- Rosacea
- Systemic lupus erythematosus
- Tinea infection
- Contact dermatitis
- Nummular dermatitis

WORKUP

- Diagnosis usually based on clinical identification of lesions (distribution and appearance).
- Skin biopsies can be performed, if warranted, to distinguish SD from similar disorders.

LABORATORY TESTS

- Microscopic examination with special stains can be used to determine whether yeast cells are present in keratinocytes.
- Biopsy can demonstrate parakeratosis in the epidermis, plugged follicular ostia, and spongiosis.
- HIV testing.

TREATMENT

NONPHARMACOLOGIC THERAPY

- Patient education that SD is a chronic condition and treatment is aimed at resolving lesions but does not prevent recurrence.
- General recommendations: wash skin regularly, soften and remove scales, and apply moisturizing emollients after washing.
- Scale removal can be accomplished through the application of mineral or olive oil and removed with a comb or brush after 1 hr.

ACUTE GENERAL Rx

- Antifungals (e.g., Nizoral, selenium sulfide, ketoconazole [the most evidence for effectiveness among antifungals], ciclopirox, fluconazole). Considered first-line therapy. Shampoos should be kept on the skin for 5 min before washing off.
  1. Reserve oral antifungal therapy for patients with widespread SD, or SD that is refractory to topical therapy.
- Topical steroids: can be in the form of shampoos, creams, or ointments. Can be used alone or in more severe SD with antifungals. Desonide and momestasone display the lowest recurrence rates and highest clearance.
- Calcineurin inhibitors (e.g., tacrolimus ointment, pimecrolimus cream): good when face and ears are affected. Limit use due to potential side effects.
- Keratolytics (e.g., tar, salicylic acid, zinc pyrithione).
- Treatment of any secondary bacterial infection with oral antibiotics.

CHRONIC Rx

Recalcitrant SD: Topical azole combined with desonide regimen (limit use to 2 wk), pimecrolimus cream

COMPLEMENTARY & ALTERNATIVE MEDICINE

Tea tree oil (melaleuca oil)

REFERRAL

Consider referral to dermatology for recalcitrant cases or uncertain diagnosis

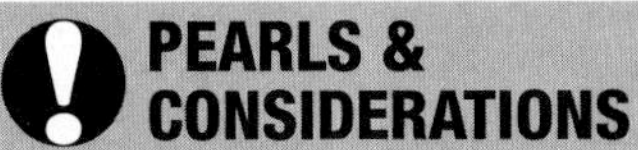

PEARLS & CONSIDERATIONS

- Use a combination of topical steroids and antifungal cream for severe SD.
- Limit use of steroids to 2-wk course of treatment due to risk of cutaneous atrophy and telangiectasias.
- SD of the scalp can be treated with an antifungal (e.g., 2% ketoconazole) or keratolytic shampoo. Limit use of antifungal shampoos to twice a week to prevent drying of the scalp. Alternate the use of antifungal shampoos with a moisturizing shampoo.
- In patients with widespread SD, consider testing for HIV infection. In patients with HIV/AIDS, the severity of sebhorreic dermatitis is inversely correlated with the CDs counts.

SUGGESTED READING

Available at ExpertConsult.com

RELATED CONTENT

Seborrheic Dermatitis (Patient Information)

AUTHOR: **ANNGENE ANTHONY, M.D., M.P.H., F.A.A.F.P.**

BASIC INFORMATION

DEFINITION

Tonic clonic seizures are characterized by sudden loss of consciousness, muscle contraction (tonic phase), followed by rhythmic jerking activity (clonic phase).

SYNONYMS

Bilateral tonic-clonic seizures
Convulsive seizures
Grand mal seizures
Generalized tonic clonic seizures

ICD-10CM CODES
G40.6 Grand mal seizures, unspecified
G41.0 Grand mal status epilepticus

EPIDEMIOLOGY & DEMOGRAPHICS

INCIDENCE: 30 to 50 cases per 100,000 person-yr (epilepsy incidence)
PEAK INCIDENCE: Not applicable
PREVALENCE: 5 to 8 cases per 1000 persons (epilepsy incidence)
PREDOMINANT SEX AND AGE: No gender preference

PHYSICAL FINDINGS & CLINICAL PRESENTATION

- Patients with tonic clonic seizures usually have normal physical and neurologic examinations.
- During the seizures, the patients are unresponsive and can have violent postures with severe repetitive muscle contractions (Fig. 1).
- After the seizure, the patients are usually lethargic and confused.
- Tonic clonic seizures are associated with injuries, bladder incontinence, and tongue biting.
- Any warning or aura before onset of the seizure or focal postictal weakness (Todd's paralysis) may point toward a focal neurologic lesion.

ETIOLOGY

- Seizures are a cardinal sign of cortical neurologic injury. Generalized seizures include both hemispheres of the brain at onset. However, seizures can start focally and then quickly generalize across both hemispheres of the brain and be almost identical to primary generalized seizures. Any warning or aura symptoms before the generalized seizure starts would point to a focal onset.
- The etiology of seizures can be genetic or due to an acquired injury to the brain.

DIAGNOSIS

DIFFERENTIAL DIAGNOSIS

- Convulsive syncope
- Psychogenic nonepileptic spells, conversion disorder, somatic symptom disorder, dissociative disorder
- EPI
- TIA
- Vertigo
- Factitious disorder
- Malingering
- Myoclonus (from metabolic disturbance)

WORKUP

- EEG (Fig. 2). An EEG can help confirm the presence of epilepsy but cannot be used to exclude the diagnosis.
- Ambulatory EEG and/or video EEG recommended for patients with diagnostic uncertainty.
- MRI of the brain.

LABORATORY TESTS

- Routine blood workup (CBC, CMP, glucose, electrolytes)
- Urine drug screen
- Lumbar puncture is recommended in patients with suspicion of meningitis

IMAGING STUDIES

- Neurodiagnostic imaging studies such as CT of the head or, preferably, MRI of the brain should be performed in all patients with first unprovoked seizure.
- CT scans of the head should be avoided in children due to unnecessary exposure to radiation and the low yield of the test. CT scans of the head are reserved for neurologic emergencies and are adjusted for weight in children.

TREATMENT

- The immediate management of a seizure focuses on stabilization of the patient with focus on the airway and vital signs and rapid identification and correction of reversible causes.
- Seizures lasting >5 minutes or multiple seizures without return to baseline in between should be treated as status epilepticus.
- Treatment is based on the type and etiology of seizures (i.e., metabolic disturbance, infectious, etc.). Provoked seizures likely do not need long-term treatment.
- Multiple antiepileptic medication choices are available. Choice depends on side effect profile as well as whether the seizure started focally or is secondary to an idiopathic generalized epilepsy syndrome.

NONPHARMACOLOGIC THERAPY

Not applicable

GENERAL Rx

- First unprovoked seizure with normal imaging, EEG, and laboratory workup requires no treatment.
- Recurrent seizures and seizures with abnormal studies require treatment depending on the etiology.
- Primary generalized epilepsies:
  1. Levetiracetam (Keppra): Initial dose 250 to 500 bid, maximum dose 1500 mg bid.
  2. Lamotrigine (Lamictal): Initial dose 25 mg daily and increase slowly to goal dose 150-250 mg daily (depends on combination of other medications).
  3. Topiramate (Topamax): Initial dose 25 mg bid and increase to usual dose of 100 to 200 mg bid.
  4. Perampanel (Fycompa): Initial dose of 2 mg once daily at bedtime, increments of 2 mg once daily at weekly intervals to a recommended maintenance dose of 8 to 12 mg (adjunctive treatment in patients with epilepsy 12 yr of age and older).
  5. Valproic acid (Depakote): Initial dose: 10 to 15 mg/kg/day (divided bid), maximum dose 60 mg/kg/day. Valproic acid should be avoided in girls and women with childbearing potential due to the risk of teratogenicity.
- Focal epilepsies with secondary generalization: Almost all antiepileptic drugs are approved for partial seizures, either in monotherapy or in adjunct. Carbamazepine, oxcarbazepine, eslicarbazepine, lamotrigine, levetiracetam, or lacosamide are all possibilities among others.

CHRONIC Rx

According to a recent joint American Academy of Neurology and American Epilepsy Society evidence-based guideline on the management of a first unprovoked seizure in adults, there is strong evidence that the risk of a second seizure is highest in the first 2 yr and ranges from 21% to 45%. This risk is higher for patients with prior brain insults such a traumatic brain injury or stroke or those with epileptiform abnormalities on EEG. Significant brain imaging abnormalities and nocturnal seizures also indicate a more elevated risk of recurrent seizures. Chronic treatment with antiepileptic drugs is indicated for ≥2 unprovoked seizures or in patients with one seizure with abnormal workup. However, moderate evidence supports advising the patient that immediate antiepileptic therapy, compared with delaying treatment until a second unprovoked seizure, is likely to reduce the risk of a seizure recurrence in the next 2 yr. Furthermore, the risk of adverse events with antiepileptics ranges from 7% to 31%, with most of these adverse events being mild and reversible. Thus, the practice guideline suggests that under certain circumstances adults with one provoked seizure, even without high-risk EEG or MRI findings, can be treated with antiepileptic drugs because at least in the next 2 yr the risk of a recurrent seizure is reduced. Although there is no strong evidence that such treatment improves quality of life, even one seizure can have negative consequences on social and occupational functioning such as driving, making treatment an attractive option for many.

COMPLEMENTARY & ALTERNATIVE MEDICINE

Not applicable

DISPOSITION

- Patients should avoid situations that may cause injuries or accidents in the event of a seizure, such as climbing ladders, swimming unsupervised, or taking baths (rather than showers).
- No driving until seizure-free in accordance with local laws and regulations.

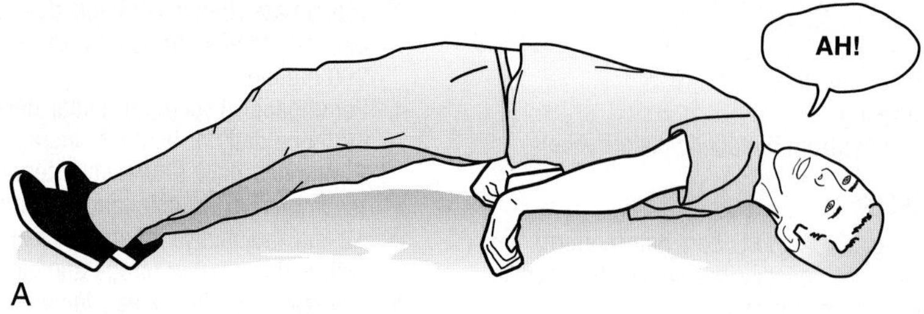

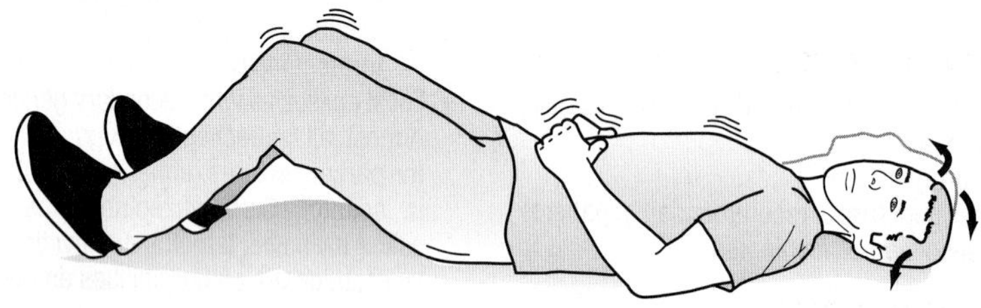

FIG. 1 **A,** This man in the tonic phase of a tonic-clonic seizure arches his torso and extends his arms and legs. He assumes this position because of the relatively greater strength of the extensor muscles compared to the flexor muscles. Simultaneous diaphragm, chest wall, and laryngeal muscle contractions force air through his tightened larynx to produce the shrill "epileptic cry." During this phase, he may also bite his tongue and lose control of his urine. **B,** In the clonic phase, his head, neck, and legs contract symmetrically and forcefully for about 10 to 20 seconds. Saliva, aerated and often blood-tinged from tongue lacerations, froths from his mouth. His pupils dilate, and he sweats profusely. Finally, his muscular contractions lose strength. The seizure usually ends with stertorous breathing. In the immediate postictal period, he remains unresponsive. Before regaining consciousness, he may pass through a state of confusion and agitation. (From Kaufman DM et al: *Kaufman's clinical neurology for psychiatrists*, ed 8, Philadelphia, 2017, Elsevier.)

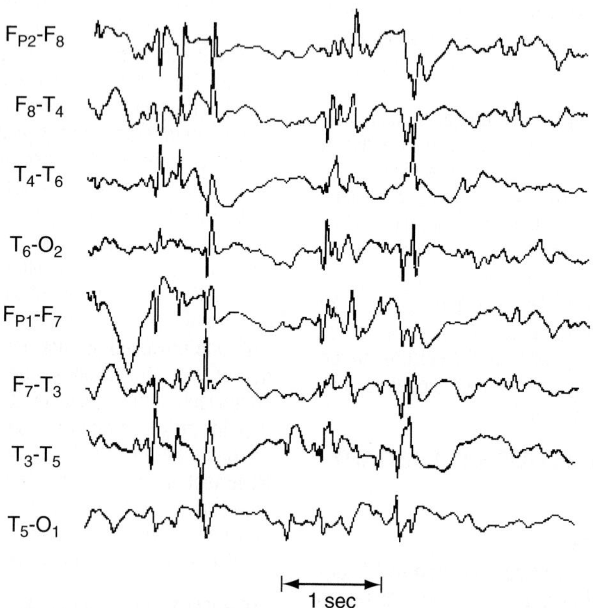

FIG. 2 During a tonic-clonic seizure, the EEG ideally shows paroxysms of spikes, polyspikes, and occasional slow waves in all channels; however, muscle artifact can obscure this pattern. Even during interictal periods, the EEG contains multiple bursts of generalized spikes in the background. In contrast to occasional temporal lobe spikes, this pattern confirms a diagnosis of epilepsy in patients with seizures. (From Kaufman DM et al: *Kaufman's clinical neurology for psychiatrists*, ed 8, Philadelphia, 2017, Elsevier.)

REFERRAL

Patients with epilepsy and seizures should be referred for a consultation by a neurologist, preferably one with epilepsy training.

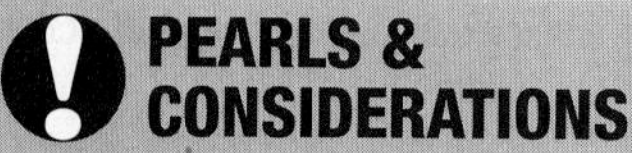

PEARLS & CONSIDERATIONS

COMMENTS

- It is crucial to understand that tonic clonic seizures can occur in variety of acute neurologic diseases.
- Successful treatment depends on the correct choice of antiepileptic drugs based on the type (partial onset versus generalized onset) and etiology of the seizures.
- All women of childbearing age taking antiepileptic drugs should take folic acid supplementation (1-4 mg/day) for the prevention of neural tube defects.
- Many antiepileptic drugs also affect vitamin D absorption or metabolism, prompting attention to patients' bone health.

PREVENTION

Sleep deprivation and alcohol consumption should be avoided.

PATIENT & FAMILY EDUCATION

Patients with ongoing seizures are forbidden to drive; check your state regulations and laws regarding driving and epilepsy.

SUGGESTED READING

Available at ExpertConsult.com

RELATED CONTENT

Generalized Tonic-Clonic Seizures (Patient Information)
Status Epilepticus (Related Key Topic)

AUTHORS: **PATRICIO SEBASTIAN ESPINOSA, M.D., M.P.H., JOSEPH S. KASS, M.D., J.D.,** and **COREY GOLDSMITH, M.D.**

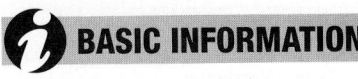

BASIC INFORMATION

DEFINITION

Sepsis is an exaggerated inflammatory response to an infectious stimulus. It is usually caused by generalized bacterial or fungal infection and characterized by evidence of infection, fever or hypothermia, hypotension, and evidence of end-organ compromise. The Sepsis Definitions Task Force in 2016 updated definitions for sepsis and septic shock. A major change in the definitions is the elimination of mention of SIRS*. According to the new definitions, sepsis is now defined as evidence of infection plus life-threatening organ dysfunction, clinically codified by an acute change in 2 points or greater in the SOFA score (Table 1). The new clinical criteria for septic shock include sepsis with fluid, unresponsive hypotension, serum lactate level greater than 2 mmol/L, and the need for vasopressors to maintain mean arterial pressure of 65 mm Hg or greater.[1,2]

SYNONYMS

Septicemia
Sepsis syndrome
Severe sepsis
Systemic inflammatory response syndrome
Septic shock

*SIRS (Systemic Inflammatory Response Syndrome): Variables in SIRS criteria include respiratory rate (breaths/min), white blood cell count (10^9/L), hands (%), heart rate (beats/min), temperature (°C), and arterial carbon dioxide tension (mm Hg). Score range is 0-4.

[1]Abraham E: New definitions for sepsis and septic shock: continuing evolution but with much still to be done, *JAMA* 315(8):757-759, 2016.

[2]Shankar-Hari M et al: Developing a new definition and assessing new clinical criteria for septic shock: for the Third International Consensus Definitions for Sepsis and Septic Shock (Sepsis-3), *JAMA* 315(8):775-787, 2016.

ICD-10CM CODES

A41.9	Sepsis, unspecified organism
A41.50	Gram-negative sepsis, unspecified
A41.2	Sepsis due to unspecified *Staphylococcus*
A41.4	Sepsis due to anaerobes
A41.51	Sepsis due to *Escherichia coli* [E. coli]
A41.52	Sepsis due to Pseudomonas
A54.86	Gonococcal sepsis
B37.7	Candidal sepsis
A32.7	Listerial sepsis
A40.0	Sepsis due to streptococcus, group A
A40.1	Sepsis due to streptococcus, group B
A40.3	Sepsis due to Streptococcus pneumoniae
A40.8	Other streptococcal sepsis
A40.9	Streptococcal sepsis, unspecified
A41.01	Sepsis due to Methicillin susceptible *Staphylococcus aureus*
A41.02	Sepsis due to Methicillin resistant *Staphylococcus aureus*

EPIDEMIOLOGY & DEMOGRAPHICS

INCIDENCE (IN U.S.):
- Sepsis occurs in 6% of hospitalized patients; approximately half require ICU admission.
- More than 1 million cases of sepsis occur each yr in the U.S. 15% of sepsis patients die in the hospital; 6% are discharged to hospice.

PREDOMINANT SEX: Males are slightly more commonly affected than females.

PREDOMINANT AGE:
- Neonatal period.
- Patients >65 yr of age account for 60% of all cases of sepsis.

GENETICS:
- Familial disposition: A great variety of congenital immunodeficiency states and other inherited disorders may predispose to septicemia.
- Neonatal infection: Incidence is high in neonatal period.

PHYSICAL FINDINGS & CLINICAL PRESENTATION

- Fever or hypothermia
- Hypotension
- Tachycardia
- Tachypnea
- Altered mental status
- Bleeding diathesis
- Skin rashes
- Symptoms that reflect primary site of infection: urinary tract, GI tract, CNS, respiratory tract
- Table 2 describes some clinical signs and symptoms of sepsis

ETIOLOGY

- Disseminated infection with a great variety of bacteria:
  1. Gram-negative bacteria:
     a. *Escherichia coli*
     b. *Klebsiella* spp.
     c. *Pseudomonas aeruginosa*
     d. *Proteus* spp.
     e. *Neisseria meningitides*
  2. Gram-positive bacteria:
     a. *Staphylococcus aureus* (including MRSA)
     b. *Streptococcus* spp.
     c. *Enterococcus* spp.
- Less common infections:
  1. Fungal
  2. Viral
  3. Rickettsial
  4. Parasitic
- Sepsis is a complex dysregulation of both inflammation and coagulation. There is activation of coagulation, inflammatory cytokines, complement, and kinin cascades with release of a variety of vasoactive endogenous mediators

TABLE 1 The Sequential Organ Failure Assessment (SOFA) Score[2]

Score	0	1	2	3	4
Respiration					
PaO_2/FiO_2, mm Hg	>400	≤400	≤300	≤200 With respiratory support	≤100
Coagulation					
Platelets × $10^3/mm^3$	>150	≤150	≤100	≤50	≤20
Liver					
Bilirubin, mg/dL (μmol/L)	<1.2 (<20)	1.2–1.9 (20–32)	2.0–5.9 (33–101)	6.0–11.9 (102–204)	>12.0 (>204)
Cardiovascular					
Hypotension	No hypotension	MAP <70 mm Hg	Dopamine ≤5 or dobutamine (any dose)*	Dopamine >5 or epinephrine ≤0.1 or norepinephrine ≤0.1*	Dopamine >15 or epinephrine >0.1 or norepinephrine >0.1*
Central Nervous System					
Glasgow coma score	15	13–14	10–12	6–9	<6
Renal					
Creatinine, mg/dL (μmol/L) OR urine output	<1.2 (<110)	1.2–1.9 (110– 170)	2.0–3.4 (171–299)	3.5–4.9 (300–440) <500 ml/d	>5.0 (>440) <200 ml/d

*Adrenergic agents administered for at least 1 hour (doses given are in mcg/kg per minute).
From Ronco C, et al.: *Critical care nephrology,* ed 3, Philadelphia, 2019, Elsevier.

TABLE 2 Clinical Signs and Symptoms of Sepsis

Infection	General	Inflammatory	Hemodynamic	Tissue Perfusion
Documented or suspected	Temperature >38° C (100.4° F) or <36° C (96.8° F) Heart rate >90 beats/min Respiratory rate ≥20 breaths/min Altered mental status Hyperglycemia Third spacing of fluid	WBC count <4000 or >12,000 cells/mcL or ≥10% bands	Hypotension: systolic blood pressure <90 mm Hg MAP <70 mm Hg SVo_2 >70 CI >3.5 L/min/m^2	Hypoxemia: (Pao_2/Fio_2 <300) Acute oliguria (urine output <0.5 ml/kg/hr) Coagulopathy Abnormal liver function tests Platelet count <100,000 cells/μL Lactic acidosis Skin mottling

CI, Cardiac index; *MAP*, mean arterial pressure; *SVo_2*, mixed venous oxygen saturation; *WBC*, white blood cell.
From Cameron JL, Cameron AM: *Current surgical therapy*, ed 10, Philadelphia, 2011, Saunders.

- Predisposing host factors:
  1. General medical condition
  2. Extremes of age
  3. Immunosuppressive therapy
  4. Recent surgery
  5. Granulocytopenia
  6. Hyposplenism
  7. Diabetes
  8. Instrumentation

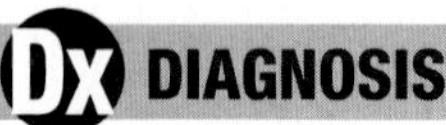

DIAGNOSIS

DIFFERENTIAL DIAGNOSIS

- Cardiogenic shock
- Acute pancreatitis
- Pulmonary embolism
- Systemic vasculitis
- Toxic ingestion
- Exposure-induced hypothermia
- Fulminant hepatic failure
- Collagen-vascular diseases

WORKUP

- Evaluation should focus on identifying a specific pathogen and localizing the site of primary infection.
- Hemodynamic, metabolic, coagulation disorders should be carefully characterized.
- Intensive monitoring.

LABORATORY TESTS

- Cultures of blood and examination and culture of sputum, urine, wound drainage, stool, and CSF, depending on the presenting signs and symptoms for each patient.
- CBC with differential, coagulation profile
- Routine chemistries, LFTs
- ABGs, lactic acid level
- Procalcitonin can be useful as a serum marker of bacterial infection as a cause of the sepsis, and has been shown to improve survival and facilitate earlier discontinuation of antibiotics
- Urinalysis

IMAGING STUDIES

- Chest x-ray
- Other radiographic and radioisotope procedures according to suspected site of primary infection

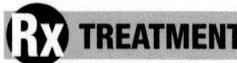

TREATMENT

NONPHARMACOLOGIC THERAPY

- Tissue oxygenation: Mixed venous oxygen saturation maintained >70% if possible; early mechanical ventilation with low tidal volume (6 ml/kg predicted body weight) to protect lung parenchyma from overstretching and "volutrauma." Recommended plateau pressure for sepsis-related ARDS is ≤30 cm H_2O.
- Focal infection should be drained if possible, and potentially infected catheters should be removed.

ACUTE GENERAL Rx

- Blood pressure support, rapid IV fluid resuscitation and vasopressors (Fig. 1), if needed, with the goal of reestablishing a mean arterial blood pressure >65 mm Hg; reduction in blood lactate and improved mixed venous oxygen saturation >70% within 6 hr of recognition of septic shock is associated with improved survival. If possible, measure vena cava oxygen saturation ($ScvO_2$) to assess adequacy of resuscitation. If the $ScvO_2$ is <70%, consider packed red blood cell transfusion to achieve Hct >30%. Start inotropic agents if $ScvO_2$ is <70% despite transfusion and adequate fluid resuscitation.
  1. IV hydration; crystalloids are as effective as colloids as resuscitation fluids. Use the fluid challenge technique to evaluate the effect (and safety) of fluid administration. For sepsis-induced hypoperfusion, give 30 ml/kg of IV crystalloids within 3 hours, with additional fluid based on frequent reassessment using dynamic variables (e.g., passive leg raise test or pulse or stroke volume variations induced by mechanical ventilation) rather than previous guidelines using target-specific values of central venous pressure. Fluid administration should be discontinued when the response to fluids is no longer beneficial. Most patients need 4 to 6 L of fluid in the first 6 hours. Trials have shown that resuscitation with balanced crystalloids or albumin compared with other fluids seems to be associated with reduced mortality, and that albumin replacement in addition to crystalloids alone does not improve the rate of survival at 28 and 90 days.
  2. Therapy with vasopressors if mean arterial blood pressure of >65 mm Hg cannot be maintained by hydration alone. Use norepinephrine as a first-choice vasopressor and target a mean arterial pressure (MAP) of 65 mm Hg.
- Correction of acidosis by improving the tissue perfusion, not by giving bicarbonate.
  1. Mechanical ventilation as needed.
- Antibiotics:
  1. Directed at the most likely sources of infection. Table 3 describes initial antibiotic recommendations for septic patients.
  2. Should generally provide broad coverage of gram-positive and gram-negative bacteria (or fungi if clinically indicated).
  3. Antibiotics should be administered within 1 hr of the diagnosis of septic shock—this is a medical emergency.
- The role of corticosteroids in the acute management of septicemia has long been debated. Previous trials had shown that corticosteroid therapy improved hemodynamic outcomes in patients with severe septic shock. Patients with relative adrenal insufficiency may benefit from low-dose therapy with hydrocortisone (200 mg IV by continuous infusion for 7 days). Recent trials, however, revealed that hydrocortisone did not improve survival or reversal of shock, either overall or in patients who did not have a response to corticotropin, although hydrocortisone hastened reversal of shock in patients in whom shock was reversed. Until definitive data are available, the decision to administer corticosteroids for septic shock should be based on the individual patient's severity of illness versus risk of corticosteroid administration. Current evidence and guidelines support limiting the use of IV hydrocortisone for patients with septic shock to these instances with fluid resuscitation and vasopressor therapy are inadequate to restore hemodynamic stability.[1] A recent meta-analysis revealed that although 28 day mortality is lower with corticosteroids in adult patients with sepsis, that effect does not persist at 90 days.[2] The corticotropin (ACTH) stimulation test is not helpful and should not be used to determine the need for corticosteroid in these patients.
- Blood transfusion: A lower hemoglobin threshold is preferred. Trials have shown that among patients with septic shock, mortality at 90 days and rates of ischemic events and use of life support is similar among those assigned to blood transfusion at a higher hemoglobin threshold (hemoglobin level of 9 g/dl or less) and those assigned to blood

[1] Yende S, Thompson T: Evaluating glucocorticoids for sepsis. Time to change course, *JAMA* 316(17):1769–1770, 2016.
[2] Fang F, et al.: Association of corticosteroid treatment with outcomes in adult patients with sepsis: a systematic review and meta-analysis, *JAMA Intern Med* 179(2):213–223, 2019.

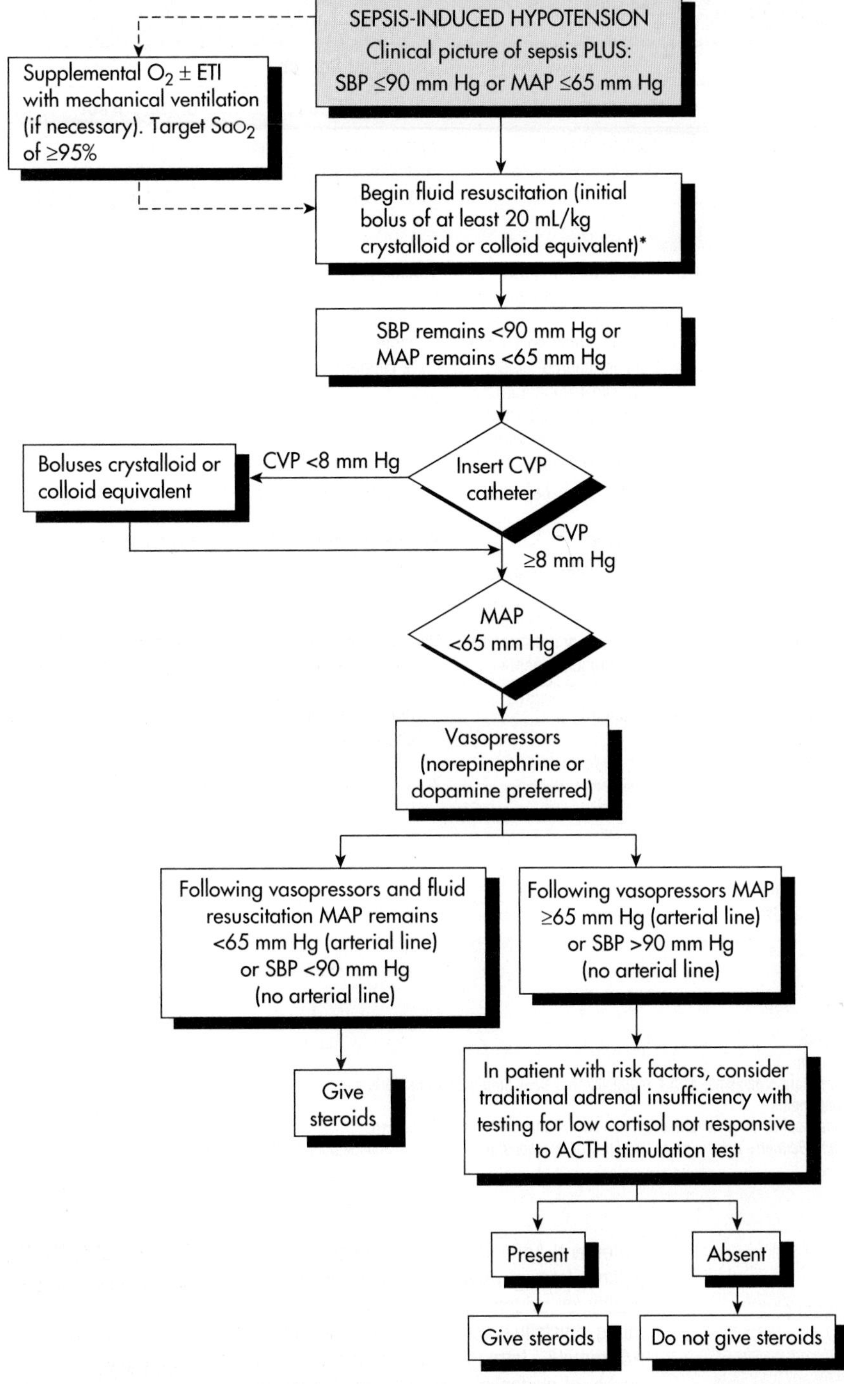

FIG. 1 Algorithm for management of severe sepsis/septic shock. *CVP*, Central venous pressure; *ETI*, endotracheal intubation; *MAP*, mean arterial pressure; *SBP*, systolic blood pressure. (From Parrillo JE, Dellinger RP: *Critical care medicine: principles of diagnosis and management in the adult*, ed 4, Philadelphia, 2014, Elsevier.)

transfusion at a lower threshold (hemoglobin level of 7 g/dl or less).

CHRONIC Rx

- Adjust antibiotic therapy on the basis of culture results.
- In general, continue antibiotic therapy for a minimum of 7 to 10 days.
- Infection source control (e.g., removal of catheter/device suspected to be infected).
- If hyperglycemia develops during treatment, start continuous insulin IV infusion, maintain blood glucose in the 110 to 180 mg/dl level, and avoid insulin-induced hypoglycemia.

DISPOSITION

- All patients with sepsis should be hospitalized and given access to intensive monitoring and nursing care.
- Among adults with suspected infection admitted to an ICU, an increase in SOFA score of 2 or more has greater prognostic accuracy for in-hospital mortality than SIRS criteria or the qSOFA score (quick SOFA).[3]

[3] Raith EP, et al.: Prognostic accuracy of the SOFA score, SIRS criteria, and qSOFA score for in-hospital mortality among adults with suspected infection admitted to the intensive care unit, *JAMA* 310(3):290–300, 2016.

TABLE 3 Empirical Antibiotic Options for Patients with Severe Sepsis or Septic Shock

	Suspected Source				
	Lung	**Abdomen**	**Skin/Soft Tissue**	**Urinary Tract**	**Source Uncertain**
Major Community-Acquired Pathogens	*Streptococcus pneumoniae* Haemophilus influenzae Legionella *Chlamydia pneumoniae*	*Escherichia coli* *Bacteroides fragilis*	*Streptococcus pyogenes* Staphylococcus aureus Polymicrobial	*E. coli* Klebsiella species Enterobacter species Proteus spp. Enterococci	
Empirical Antibiotic Therapy	Moxifloxacin *or* levofloxacin *or* azithromycin *plus* cefotaxime *or* ceftazidime *or* cefepime *or* piperacillin-tazobactam	Imipenem *or* meropenem *or* doripenem *or* piperacillin-tazobactam ± aminoglycoside If biliary source: piperacillin-tazobactam, ampicillin-sulbactam, *or* ceftriaxone with metronidazole	Vancomycin *or* daptomycin *plus either* imipenem *or* meropenem *or* piperacillin-tazobactam; ± clindamycin (see text)	Ciprofloxacin *or* levofloxacin (if gram-positive cocci, use ampicillin *or* vancomycin ± gentamicin)	Vancomycin *plus either* doripenem *or* ertapenem *or* imipenem *or* meropenem
Major Commensal or Nosocomial Microorganisms	Aerobic gram-negative bacilli	Aerobic gram-negative rods Anaerobes *Candida* spp.	*Staphylococcus aureus* (? MRSA) Aerobic gram-negative rods	Aerobic gram-negative rods Enterococci	Consider MDRO if in area of high prevalence. Consider echinocandin if neutropenic or indwelling intravascular catheter
Empirical Antibiotic Therapy	Imipenem *or* meropenem *or* doripenem *or* cefepime (if *Acinetobacter baumannii* or carbapenem-resistant *Klebsiella* in ICU, add colistin)	Imipenem *or* meropenem ± aminoglycoside (consider echinocandin)	Vancomycin *or* daptomycin *plus* imipenem-cilastatin *or* meropenem *or* cefepime, ± clindamycin	Vancomycin *plus* imipenem *or* meropenem *or* cefepime	Cefepime *plus* vancomycin ± caspofungin

Dosages for intravenous administration (normal renal function):
- Imipenem-cilastatin, 0.5-1.0g q6-8h
- Meropenem, 1-2g q8h
- Doripenem, 0.5g q8h
- Piperacillin-tazobactam, 3.375g q4h or 4.5g q6h
- Vancomycin, load 25-30mg/kg, then 15-20 q8-12h
- Cefepime, 1-2g q8h
- Levofloxacin, 750mg q24h
- Ciprofloxacin, 400 mg q8-12hr
- Moxifloxacin, 400mg qd
- Ceftriaxone, 2g q24h
- Caspofungin, 70mg, followed by 50mg q24h
- Colistin: loading dose = 5mg/kg body weight.

ICU, Intensive care unit; *MDRO*, multidrug-resistant organisms; *MRSA*, methicillin-resistant *Staphylococcus aureus.*
For MDRO, resistance usually includes carbapenems.
Carbapenems are less susceptible to extended-spectrum β-lactamases; base choice on local resistance pattern.
From Bennett JE, et al.: *Mandell, Douglas, and Bennett's principles and practice of infectious diseases,* ed 8, Philadelphia, 2015, WB Saunders.

REFERRAL

- To infectious diseases expert
- To physician experienced in critical care

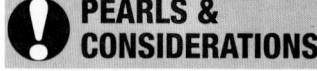

PEARLS & CONSIDERATIONS

COMMENTS

- Mortality rises quickly if antibiotic therapy is not instituted promptly (preferably within 1 hr of onset of shock) and metabolic derangements are not treated aggressively.
- The Surviving Sepsis Campaign hour-1 bundle 2018 update recommends: Measure lactate level. Re-measure if initial lactate is >2 mmol/L. [weak recommendation, low quality of evidence] Obtain blood cultures prior to administration of antibiotics. [best practice statement] Administer broad spectrum antibiotics. [strong recommendation, moderate quality of evidence] Rapidly administer 30 ml/kg crystalloid for hypotension or lactate ≥4 mmol/L [strong recommendation, low quality of evidence] and apply vasopressors if patient is hypotensive during or after fluid resuscitation to maintain MAP ≥65 mm Hg. [strong recommendation, moderate quality of evidence]
- Recent trials have shown that early, goal-directed therapy (EGDT) does not result in better outcomes than usual care and is associated with higher hospitalization costs across a broad range of patient and hospital characteristics.[4]

[4] The PRISM Investigators: Early, goal-directed therapy for septic shock–a patient-level meta-analysis, *N Engl J Med* 376:2223–2234, 2017.

SUGGESTED READINGS

Available at ExpertConsult.com

AUTHORS: **GLENN G. FORT, M.D., M.P.H.,** and **FRED F. FERRI, M.D.**

BASIC INFORMATION

DEFINITION

Septic arthritis is a highly destructive form of joint disease most often caused by hematogenous spread of organisms from a distant site of infection. Direct penetration of the joint as a result of trauma or surgery and spread from adjacent osteomyelitis may also cause bacterial arthritis. Any joint in the body may be affected.

SYNONYMS

Infectious arthritis
Bacterial arthritis
Pyogenic arthritis

ICD-10CM CODE

M00.9 Pyogenic arthritis, unspecified

EPIDEMIOLOGY & DEMOGRAPHICS

INCIDENCE (IN U.S.): Between 2 and 6 cases per 100,000 people per yr
PREVALENCE (IN U.S.): Unknown
PREDOMINANT SEX: Gonococcal arthritis in females
PREDOMINANT AGE: Gonococcal arthritis in sexually active adults
PEAK INCIDENCE:

- Gonococcal arthritis: Young adults
- Other bacterial causes: All ages

PHYSICAL FINDINGS & CLINICAL PRESENTATION

- Hallmark: Acute onset of monoarticular joint pain, erythema, heat, and immobility
- Limited range of motion of the joint
- Effusion, with varying degrees of erythema and increased warmth around the joint
- Single joint affected in 80% to 90% of cases of nongonococcal arthritis
- Gonococcal dermatitis-arthritis syndrome:
  1. Typical pattern is a migratory polyarthritis or tenosynovitis
  2. Small pustules on the trunk or extremities
- Febrile patient at presentation
- Most commonly affected joints in adult: Knee and hip, but any joint may be involved; in children—hip.

ETIOLOGY

- Bacteria spread from another locus of infection.
  1. Highly vascular synovium is invaded by hematogenously spread bacteria.
  2. WBC enzymes cause necrosis of synovium, cartilage, and bone.
  3. Extensive joint destruction is rapid if infection is not treated with appropriate IV antibiotics and drainage of necrotic material.
- Predisposing factors: Rheumatoid arthritis, prosthetic joints, advanced age, immunodeficiency (HIV, DM, immunosuppressive drugs), gout, sexual activity (gonococcal arthritis), skin infections, cutaneous ulcers (contiguous spread), recent joint surgery, recent intraarticular infection. Fig. E1 illustrates routes by which bacteria can reach the joint.
- The most common nongonococcal organisms are staphylococci (40%), streptococci (28%), and gram-negative bacilli (19%). Less common are mycobacteria (8%), gram-negative cocci (3%), anaerobes (1%), and gram-positive bacilli (1%).
- Staphylococci (*S. aureus* and coagulase-negative staphylococcal species) account for >50% of prosthetic-hip and prosthetic-knee infections. *S. aureus* is very common in patients with rheumatoid arthritis.

DIAGNOSIS

DIFFERENTIAL DIAGNOSIS

- Gout
- Pseudogout
- Trauma
- Hemarthrosis
- Rheumatic fever
- Adult or juvenile rheumatoid arthritis
- Spondyloarthropathies such as reactive arthritis (Reiter syndrome)
- Osteomyelitis
- Viral arthritides
- Septic bursitis
- Lyme disease caused by *Borrelia burgdorferi*

WORKUP

- Joint aspiration, gram stain, and culture of the synovial fluid. Fig. 2 describes an algorithm for synovial fluid analysis in septic arthritis.
- Immediate arthrocentesis before other studies are undertaken or antibiotics instituted. Synovial fluid should be evaluated at bedside and then sent for lab evaluation.

LABORATORY TESTS

- Joint fluid analysis:
  1. Synovial fluid leukocyte count is usually elevated >50,000 cells/mm^3 with > 80% polymorphonuclear cells.
  2. Counts are highly variable, with similar findings in gout, pseudogout, or rheumatoid arthritis. Lower WBC counts can occur in joint replacement, disseminated gonococcal disease, and peripheral leukopenia.
  3. Synovial fluid glucose or protein is not helpful because results are not specific for septic arthritis. The differential diagnosis of synovial fluid abnormalities is described in Section IV.
  4. PCR testing: Useful for detection of uncommon organisms (e.g., Lyme disease).
  5. Crystal analysis: Septic arthritis can coexist with crystal arthropathy; therefore, the presence of crystals does not preclude a diagnosis of septic arthritis.
- Blood cultures: Positive in 25% to 50% of patients with septic arthritis.
- Culture of possible extraarticular sources of infection.
- Elevated peripheral WBC count, ESR (nonspecific), C-reactive protein (CRP) (nonspecific). When elevated, ESR and CRP may be useful to monitor therapeutic response.
- If gonococcus is suspected, perform nucleic acid amplification tests (NAATs) on synovial fluid.

IMAGING STUDIES

- Radiograph of the affected joint (Fig. E3): Useful to rule out osteomyelitis, fractures, chondrocalcinosis, or inflammatory arthritis.
- MRI: Findings that suggest an acute intraarticular infection include the combination of bony erosions with marrow edema.
- CT scan: Useful for early diagnosis of infections of the spine, hips, and sternoclavicular and sacroiliac joints.
- Ultrasound: Can be useful for detecting effusions in joints that are more difficult to examine (e.g., hip).

TREATMENT

NONPHARMACOLOGIC THERAPY

- Affected joints aspirated daily to remove necrotic material and to follow serial WBC counts and cultures.
- If no resolution with IV antibiotics and closed drainage: Open debridement and lavage, particularly in nongonococcal infections.
- Prevention of contractures:
  1. After acute stage of inflammation, range-of-motion exercises of the affected joint.
  2. Physical therapy helpful.

ACUTE GENERAL Rx

- IV antibiotics immediately after joint aspiration and gram stain of the synovial fluid. Empiric antibiotic therapy (Table E1) is based on organism found on gram stain of synovial fluid:
  1. Gram-positive cocci: Vancomycin: 15 to 20 mg/kg IV q8 to 12h. Keep trough levels at 15 to 20 mcg/ml. Alternatives include daptomycin and linezolid.
  2. Gram-negative cocci: Ceftriaxone: 1 to 2 g IV q day in adults (children: 50 to 100 mg/kg IV q day). Alternative includes cefotaxime.
  3. Gram-negative rods: Ceftriaxone, cefepime: 1 to 2 g IV q8 to 12 h in adults (children: 100-150 mg/kg/day divided in q8h dosing), piperacillin-tazobactam: 3.375 g IV to 4.5 g IV q6h. Aztreonam or fluoroquinolones can be used in patients with allergy to penicillin or cephalosporins.
  4. Negative gram stain: Vancomycin plus either cefepime or a carbapenem such as meropenem: 1 g IV q8h in adults (children: 60 mg/kg/day divided in q8h dosing) or ertapenem.

SUGGESTED READINGS

Available at ExpertConsult.com

RELATED CONTENT

Septic Arthritis (Patient Information)

AUTHOR: **GLENN G. FORT, M.D., M.P.H.**

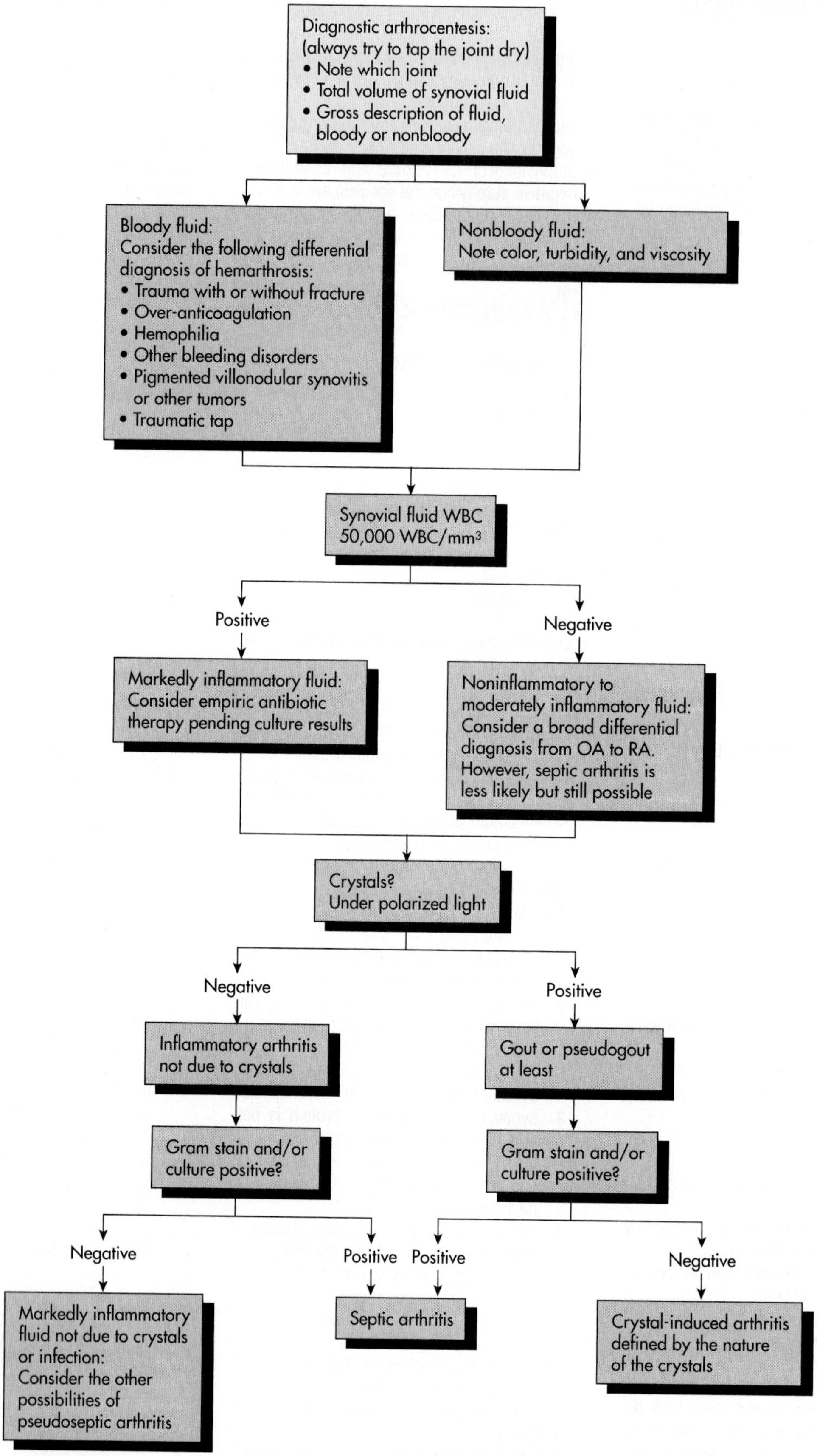

Diagnostic arthrocentesis:
(always try to tap the joint dry)
- Note which joint
- Total volume of synovial fluid
- Gross description of fluid, bloody or nonbloody

Bloody fluid:
Consider the following differential diagnosis of hemarthrosis:
- Trauma with or without fracture
- Over-anticoagulation
- Hemophilia
- Other bleeding disorders
- Pigmented villonodular synovitis or other tumors
- Traumatic tap

Nonbloody fluid:
Note color, turbidity, and viscosity

Synovial fluid WBC
50,000 WBC/mm^3

Positive

Markedly inflammatory fluid:
Consider empiric antibiotic therapy pending culture results

Negative

Noninflammatory to moderately inflammatory fluid:
Consider a broad differential diagnosis from OA to RA.
However, septic arthritis is less likely but still possible

Crystals?
Under polarized light

Negative

Inflammatory arthritis not due to crystals

Gram stain and/or culture positive?

Positive

Gout or pseudogout at least

Gram stain and/or culture positive?

Negative

Markedly inflammatory fluid not due to crystals or infection:
Consider the other possibilities of pseudoseptic arthritis

Positive Positive

Septic arthritis

Negative

Crystal-induced arthritis defined by the nature of the crystals

FIG. 2 Algorithm for synovial fluid analysis in septic arthritis. *OA,* osteoarthritis; *RA,* rheumatoid arthritis; *WBC,* white blood cell count. (From Harris ED et al: *Kelley's textbook of rheumatology,* ed 7, Philadelphia, 2005, Saunders.)

BASIC INFORMATION

DEFINITION

Serotonin syndrome (SS) is a potentially life-threatening condition resulting from excessive serotonergic stimulation of 5-HT_{1A} and 5-HT_{2A} receptors in the CNS and PNS. SS is a drug-induced disorder that is classically characterized by mental status changes, neuromuscular hyperactivity, and autonomic dysfunction.

SYNONYMS

SS
Hyperserotonemia
Serotonergic syndrome
Serotonin toxicity

ICD-10CM CODES

Y49	Adverse effects due to psychotropic drugs
Y49.0	Adverse effects due to tricyclic and tetracyclic antidepressants
Y49.1	Adverse effects due to monoamino-oxidase-inhibitor antidepressants
Y49.2	Adverse effects due to other and unspecified antidepressants
Y49.3	Adverse effects due to phenothiazine antipsychotics and neuroleptics
G25.89	Other specified extrapyramidal and movement disorders

EPIDEMIOLOGY & DEMOGRAPHICS

- The incidence of SS is not known.
- SS is seen in all age groups.
- SS classically occurs in patients receiving two or more serotonergic drugs, but it can also occur with monotherapy—selective serotonin reuptake inhibitor (SSRI) monotherapy has an incidence of 0.5 to 0.9 cases of SS per 1000 patient-mo. Although there is an FDA alert, it has been argued that there is a lack of sufficient evidence showing that SSRIs and triptans cause serious SS.
- Concomitant use of an SSRI with a monoamine oxidase inhibitor (MAOI) poses the greatest risk of developing SS.
- Combination of SSRIs with other serotonergic drugs (e.g., tryptophan, illicit drugs like cocaine and MDMA, "Ecstasy") or drugs with serotonergic properties (e.g., methylene blue, lithium, meperidine, triptans, linezolid) may also lead to SS.

PHYSICAL FINDINGS & CLINICAL PRESENTATION

- Findings of clonus with hyperreflexia in the setting of recent (<5 wk) use of serotonergic agents strongly suggest the diagnosis of SS.
- Symptoms can manifest within minutes to hours after starting a new psychopharmacologic treatment, increasing the dose of a serotonergic drug, or administering a second serotonergic drug.
- Clonus (inducible, spontaneous, and ocular) is the key finding in establishing a diagnosis of SS.
- Classic triad of clinical features:
  1. Neuromuscular excitation: Hyperreflexia, myoclonus, muscle rigidity, tremor.
  2. Autonomic nervous system excitation: Nausea/vomiting, diarrhea, hypertension, tachycardia, diaphoresis, fever >38° C (100° F) to severe hyperthermia.
  3. Altered mental status: Anxiety, agitation, confusion, coma.

ETIOLOGY

- Hyperstimulation of the brain stem and spinal cord serotonin receptors leading to the neuromuscular and autonomic symptoms.
- Psychopharmacologic drugs—in particular, fluoxetine and sertraline co-administered with MAOI (e.g., tranylcypromine and phenelzine)—have been cited as a common cause of SS. Triptans (serotonin-receptor agonists used in the treatment of migraines) may also precipitate the SS when used in combination with SSRIs and serotonin-norepinephrine reuptake inhibitors (SNRIs). Box 1 describes classes of medications that produce SS.

BOX 1 Classes of Medications That Produce Serotonin Syndrome in Psychiatric Patients

Selective serotonin reuptake inhibitors
Monoamine oxidase inhibitors
Atypical antipsychotics
Heterocyclic antidepressants
Trazodone
Dual-uptake inhibitors
Psychostimulants
Buspirone
Mood stabilizers
Analgesics
Antiemetics
Cough suppressants
Dietary supplements
Linezolide

From Goldman L, Schafer AI: *Goldman-Cecil medicine*, ed 24, Philadelphia, 2012, Saunders.

DIAGNOSIS

- SS is a clinical diagnosis. There are no specific laboratory tests for SS. A high index of suspicion along with a detailed medication history is the mainstay of diagnosis.
- Diagnostic criteria: Most accurate is Hunter Serotonin Toxicity Criteria (sensitivity 84%, specificity 97%, confirmation by toxicologist). Sternbach's diagnostic criteria (Table 1) are also commonly used.
- To fulfill Hunter criteria a patient must have consumed a serotonergic drug and have one of the following:
  1. Spontaneous clonus.
  2. Inducible clonus plus agitation or diaphoresis.
  3. Ocular clonus plus agitation or diaphoresis.
  4. Tremor and hyperreflexia.
  5. Temperature >38° C (100° F) plus hypertonia plus ocular clonus or inducible clonus.

DIFFERENTIAL DIAGNOSIS

- Neuroleptic malignant syndrome (NMS), substance abuse (e.g., cocaine, amphetamines), anticholinergic toxicity, thyroid storm, infection (e.g., meningitis, encephalitis), alcohol and opioid withdrawal.
- Classic features in differentiation of NMS from SS are that SS develops over 24 hr, involves neuromuscular hyperactivity (hyperreflexia, myoclonus), and begins to resolve within 24 hr with appropriate therapy, whereas NMS develops gradually over days to weeks, involves sluggish neuromuscular response, and resolves over an average period of 1 wk to 10 days.

WORKUP

- Because SS is a clinical diagnosis, there is no laboratory test that confirms the diagnosis, and serum serotonin concentration

TABLE 1 Criteria to Determine Serotonin Syndrome and Toxicity

Sternbach diagnostic criteria for serotonin syndrome	1. Recent addition or increase of proserotonergic medication 2. At least three of the following: 1. Agitation 2. Ataxia 3. Diaphoresis 4. Diarrhea 5. Hyperreflexia 6. Hyperthermia 7. Mental status changes 8. Myoclonus 9. Shivering 10. Tremor 3. Neuroleptic agent not added or dose increased before the onset of symptoms 4. Diagnosis of infections, withdrawal, and other poisoning or metabolic disruptions excluded
Hunter criteria for serotonin toxicity (context of serotonergic medications)	1. If patient has spontaneous clonus, serotonin toxicity present 2. If no spontaneous clonus, one of the following needed for a diagnosis of serotonin toxicity: 1. Inducible clonus *and* agitation *or* diaphoresis 2. Ocular clonus *and* agitation *or* diaphoresis 3. Tremor *and* hyperreflexia 4. Temperature >38° C *and* ocular clonus *or* inducible clonus

From Adams JG, et al.: *Emergency medicine, clinical essentials*, ed 2, Philadelphia, 2013, Elsevier.

does not correlate with the clinical picture. Other causes are described in "Differential Diagnosis." Thus, all patients should have blood tests and diagnostic imaging studies to rule out infectious, toxic, and metabolic causes.
- Additional laboratory tests are performed to exclude complicating features of SS (e.g., renal failure secondary to rhabdomyolysis).

LABORATORY TESTS

- CBC with differential when considering sepsis
- Urine and blood cultures
- Electrolytes, BUN, and creatinine to rule out acidosis and renal failure
- Blood and urine toxicology screen, including acetaminophen and salicylate levels if overdose was intentional
- Thyroid function tests
- Creatine-phosphokinase (CPK) with isoenzymes
- ECG because ventricular rhythm disturbance is a potentially fatal complication
- CSF studies to rule out meningitis

IMAGING STUDIES

Imaging studies are not specific in the diagnosis of SS and are only ordered to exclude other causes with similar clinical presentations as SS.

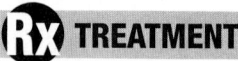

TREATMENT

- Once a diagnosis of SS is established, consultation with a medical toxicologist, clinical pharmacologist, and/or poison control center should be sought
- Management includes:
  1. Discontinue use of all potential precipitating drugs
  2. Provide supportive management
  3. Control agitation
  4. Administer serotonin antagonists
  5. Control autonomic instability
  6. Control hyperthermia
  7. Reassess the need to resume the use of the serotonergic agent once the symptoms have resolved

NONPHARMACOLOGIC THERAPY

- Discontinuation of the drug is the mainstay of therapy.
- Treatment is supportive: Maintaining oxygenation and blood pressure and monitoring respiratory status. Hypotensive patients may require both IV fluids and vasopressor therapy.
- Patients who are severely hyperthermic with temperatures >41° C (106° F) should be given IV sedation, paralyzed, and intubated. Cooling blankets can be used for patients with mild to moderate hyperthermia. There is no role for acetaminophen here.
- Intubation is recommended for patients unable to protect their airways as a result of mental status changes or seizures.

ACUTE GENERAL Rx

- Benzodiazepines for control of agitation are preferred to physical restraints.
  1. Lorazepam 1 to 2 mg IV every 30 min has been used effectively in treating agitation, muscle rigidity, myoclonus, and seizure complications.
  2. Diazepam is an alternative choice.
- Blood pressure management with short-acting agents such as esmolol and nitroprusside.
- Serotonin antagonists should be titrated to clinical effectiveness in patients for whom nonpharmacologic therapy and benzodiazepines are not achieving adequate response, although substantial and rigorous data are lacking.
  1. Cyproheptadine 4 mg tablet or 2 mg/5 ml syrup is given 12 mg initially followed by 2 mg every 2 hr until therapeutic response is achieved in adults (up to 32 mg/day); children ages 7 to 14 should receive 4 mg every 6 hr (up to 16 mg/day), children ages 2 to 6 should receive 2 mg every 6 hr (up to 12 mg/day), and children younger than 2 yr should receive a maximum of 0.25 mg/kg/day as 0.06 mg/kg every 6 hr.
  2. Atypical antipsychotic agents with serotonin antagonist properties (e.g., olanzapine 10 mg SL) have been tried with some success.
  3. Chlorpromazine 50 to 100 mg IM may be considered in severe cases, but intravenous fluid loading is essential to prevent hypotension.

CHRONIC Rx

For patients not requiring hospital admission, cyproheptadine and lorazepam can be given in an oral dose on a prn basis with close follow-up.

DISPOSITION

- SS is a potentially life-threatening condition if not recognized early, although it does exist on a spectrum.
- Prompt diagnosis and withdrawal of the medication result in improvement of symptoms within 24 hr.
- Seizures, rhabdomyolysis, hyperthermia, ventricular arrhythmia, respiratory arrest, and coma are all complicating features of SS.

REFERRAL

All cases of SS secondary to psychotropic medications should be referred to a psychiatrist.

PREVENTION

Modify prescription practices by avoiding multidrug regimens.

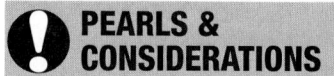

PEARLS & CONSIDERATIONS

The combined use of SSRIs and MAOIs is contraindicated.

COMMENTS

- The use of SSRIs and other serotonergic agents is not an absolute contraindication; however, prompt withdrawal of the medication is recommended if any symptoms suggesting SS occur.
- SS is usually found in patients being treated for depression, bipolar disorders, obsessive-compulsive disorder, attention-deficit disorder, and Parkinson's disease.

SUGGESTED READINGS

Available at ExpertConsult.com

AUTHORS: **MICHAEL AUSTIN, D.O.,** and **MARK F. BRADY, M.D., M.P.H., M.M.S.**

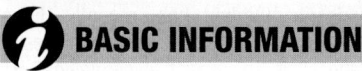

DEFINITION

A sexual dysfunction in a woman is any disorder that interferes with female sexuality and that causes marked distress to that person. These disorders are generally categorized into five types:

- Hypoactive sexual desire disorder (most common)
- Sexual arousal disorder
- Orgasmic disorders
- Sexual pain disorders (including dyspareunia, vaginismus, and vulvodynia)
- Anxiety about sexual performance

Female sexual dysfunction is also further categorized as lifelong (primary) or acquired (secondary), situational (e.g., current partner) or generalized (all partners and settings).

SYNONYMS

Female sexual dysfunction
Hypoactive sexual desire disorder
HSDD

ICD-10CM CODES	
R37	Sexual dysfunction, unspecified
F52.0	Hypoactive Sexual Desire Disorder
F52.31	Female orgasmic disorder
N94.1	Dyspareunia
N94.81	Vulvodynia

EPIDEMIOLOGY & DEMOGRAPHICS

INCIDENCE: According to the National Health and Social Life Survey, in 1999, ~20% to 50% of women reported some form of sexual dysfunction during their lifetimes. One third of women reported a decrease in sexual interest, and one fourth reported an inability to achieve orgasm.

PREVALENCE (TABLE 1): A more recent survey of women 18 yr of age and older found an age-adjusted prevalence of any sexual problem to be ~43%.

PREDOMINANT AGE: Sexually related personal distress was more common in middle-aged women (aged 45-64) than in younger or older women.

RISK FACTORS:

- Correlates of distressing sexual problems include poor self-assessed health, low education level, depression, anxiety, thyroid conditions, and urinary incontinence.
- Higher insomnia scores and shorter sleep duration are associated with decreased sexual function.
- Obesity and overweight body status have been associated with lower sexual satisfaction and desire.
- Comorbid conditions such as arthritis, diabetes mellitus, hypertension, malignancy, neuromuscular disorders, renal failure, and gynecologic (e.g., chronic pelvic pain) and dermatologic conditions (e.g., lichen sclerosis, psoriasis) can contribute to sexual dysfunction.
- Aging is associated with decreased sexual responsiveness, sexual activity, and libido.
- Decreased hormonal levels associated with menopause can cause decreased vaginal lubrication and dyspareunia.

PHYSICAL FINDINGS & CLINICAL PRESENTATION

- History:
  1. Important to obtain the patient's definition of the dysfunction, including its onset and duration; to determine whether the dysfunction is situational or global; and to determine whether more than one dysfunction exists and the interrelationship among the dysfunctions. Dysfunction is diagnosed if the symptoms are causing distress to the patient
- Related medical and gynecologic conditions (including prior gynecologic surgery)
- Psychosocial factors, including sexual abuse, sexual orientation, depression and anxiety, status of current relationships and sexual activity, personal and family beliefs about sexuality
- Current medications including OTC and herbal preparations; alcohol, tobacco, and drug use; and birth control method, substance use/misuse
- Physical examination:
  1. The gynecologic examination can aid in identifying signs of decreased estrogen and androgen levels, infection, endometriosis, pelvic floor dysfunction, and systemic disease
  2. Other body systems as indicated (e.g., cardiovascular, thyroid)

ETIOLOGY

- Chronic medical conditions (e.g., diabetes, coronary vascular disease, arthritis, urinary incontinence)
- Medication induced (e.g., antihypertensives, narcotics, hormonal preparations, anti-histamines, amphetamines, psychotrophic medications). SSRIs are the most common medications linked to sexual dysfunction
- Gynecologic conditions (e.g., cystitis, posthysterectomy, gynecologic cancers, breast cancer [femininity/self-image issues; chemotherapy effects], postpregnancy, postmenopausal). Premenopausal BSO is associated with a higher risk of HSDD
- Psychosocial (e.g., religion, taboos, identity conflicts, guilt, relationship problems, abuse, rape, life stressors)
- Fig. E1 illustrates the four phases of the human sexual response as postulated by Masters and Johnson

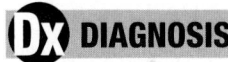

DIFFERENTIAL DIAGNOSIS

- Depression
- Psychosocial stressors
- Medical disease (e.g., thyroid dysfunction)
- Menopausal status can be assessed using STRAW + 10 tool

TABLE 1 Prevalence and Definition of Female Sexual Dysfunctions

	Prevalence*	Definition†
Hypoactive sexual desire/low libido	9%-60%	Diminished feelings of sexual interest or desire, absence of sexual thoughts, and/or lack of receptivity to sexual activity‡
Sexual arousal disorder/sex not pleasurable	5%-51%	**Genital Female Sexual Arousal Disorder (GFSAD)**: Disruption of clitoral erection, vaginal vasocongestion, vaginal lubrication
Difficulty with genital lubrication	8%-60%	**Psychological Female Sexual Arousal Disorder (PFSAD):** Absent or markedly diminished feelings of excitement or pleasure in response to sexual stimuli **Mixed Female Sexual Arousal Disorder:** GFSAD and PFSAD
Persistent genital arousal disorder	~1%	Persistent, recurrent, intrusive, and/or distressing sensations of genital arousal not related to sexual stimulation and that do not resolve after orgasm
Female orgasmic disorder	7%-65%	Lack of experience of orgasm or diminished orgasm intensity despite high sexual arousal after a period of sufficient sexual stimulation and arousal
Sexual pain disorders	4%-42%	**Dyspareunia**: Persistent/recurrent pain with attempted/complete vaginal entry with a penis, finger, or other object **Vaginismus:** Vaginal spasm or pain in response to penetration with a penis, finger, or other object despite a desire for penetration to occur‡
Anxiety about sexual performance	6%-16%	N/A

*Laumann et al, 1999; Nicolosi et al, 2005, 2006a, 2006b; Shifren et al, 2008; West et al, 2008; Witting et al, 2008; Garvey et al, 2009.
†Waldinger et al, 2009; Basson et al, 2010b.
‡The term *vaginismus* is no longer preferred, as it includes significant semantic baggage as a psychological disorder.

LABORATORY TESTS

- Cervical cultures and vaginal swabs for infectious disease
- Cervical cancer screening as per current guidelines
- Appropriate laboratory tests if comorbid or chronic disease is suspected
- Measurement of prolactin, thyroid function tests, estrogen, progesterone, LH, testosterone, and sex hormone binding globulin is indicated only if a hormonal etiology is suspected from history

IMAGING STUDIES

Appropriate imaging studies if comorbid or chronic disease is suspected

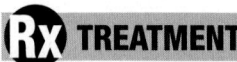

TREATMENT

NONPHARMACOLOGIC THERAPY

- Treat genital arousal and pelvic pain symptoms before addressing HSDD
- Education including a discussion of normal sexual behavior
- Stress management
- Behavioral therapy (e.g., cognitive-behavioral therapy) and mindfulness-based interventions can treat low sexual desire and arousal disorders
- Counseling (individual or couples) for relationship issues
- Activities to enhance stimulation and eliminate routine
- Distraction techniques
- Noncoital behavior
- Position changes (e.g., female astride)
- Lubricants (e.g., nonpetroleum based). There are several over-the-counter lubricants and massage oils, some of which are hypoallergenic, that can be safely applied to female genitalia
- Physical therapy may be useful for patients with pelvic floor dysfunction and pain

ACUTE GENERAL Rx

NSAIDs before intercourse for sexual pain disorders

CHRONIC Rx

- Treat underlying medical, gynecologic, or psychological conditions.
- Reduce comorbidities, including weight loss.
- Increase physical activity (associated with increased satisfaction and sexual engagement).
- For medication-induced conditions, decrease dose or change medication.
- For postmenopausal women or those with hypoestrogenism, try estrogen replacement therapy with or without progesterone. Local vaginal estrogen therapy is preferred over systemic therapy. Transdermal estradiol is superior to oral estradiol for improving sexual function because oral estradiol increases circulating sex hormone-binding globulin (SHBG) and lowers free testosterone, thus effecting libido adversely. Estrogen replacement is associated with improvements in dyspareunia and vaginal dryness.
- For postmenopausal vaginal and/or vulvar atrophy, ospemifene has been associated with improved sexual function.
- Transdermal testosterone therapy: Results show increase in satisfying sexual activity and sexual desire. Must weigh risks (hirsutism, acne, virilization, and cardiovascular complications) vs. benefits of use. Monitoring of testosterone levels to avoid supraphysiologic therapy is recommended.
- Sildenafil (evidence from RCTs for use in patients with neurodegenerative disease and antidepressant-induced FSD after traditional therapy has failed). Data are conflicting. Phosphodiesterase inhibitors may increase blood flow to the genitalia but generally appear to have little benefit in treating arousal disorders. Sildenafil has been helpful in patients with SSRI-induced sexual dysfunction.
- Bupropion 300 to 400 mg/day was shown to increase sexual arousal and orgasm completion in a recent trial. In addition, adjunctive treatment with bupropion significantly improved key aspects of sexual function in women with SSRI-induced sexual dysfunction.
- Flibanserin (Addyi) has recently been approved to treat hypoactive sexual desire disorder. It is an agonist at serotonin 5-HT receptors and an antagonist at 5-HT_{2A} receptors. Its mechanism of action in treating HSDD is unknown. The recommended dose is 100 mg once daily at bed time. Side effects include hypotension, syncope, and CNS depression. Consumption of alcohol increases risk of side effects and is contraindicated. It is mostly effective with approximately 10% of women reporting "much" or "very much" improvement in HSDD symptoms.
- Table E2 summarizes investigational pharmacotherapy for women's sexual dysfunctions.

REFERRAL

- Gynecologic referral for conditions that may be amenable to surgical therapy (e.g., pelvic floor disorders)
- Psychological referral for conditions (e.g., depression, abuse) that may benefit from counseling or psychotherapy
- Social services referrals for active abuse issues

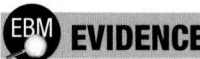

EVIDENCE

Available at ExpertConsult.com Evidence

SUGGESTED READINGS

Available at ExpertConsult.com

RELATED CONTENT

Female Sexual Dysfunction (Patient Information)
Hypoactive Sexual Desire Disorder (Related Key Topic)

AUTHOR: **ANNGENE ANTHONY, M.D., M.P.H., F.A.A.F.P.**

BASIC INFORMATION

DEFINITION

- Shift work refers to nonstandard work schedules, including permanent or intermittent night work, early morning work, and rotating schedules.
- Shift work disorder (SWD) is defined as the development of sleep disturbances and impairment of waking alertness and performance that some, but not all, individuals experience when adapting to shift work.

SYNONYM

Circadian rhythm sleep disorder of shift work type

SWD

ICD-10CM CODE

G47.26. Circadian rhythm sleep disorder, shift work type

EPIDEMIOLOGY & DEMOGRAPHICS

- The disorder is caused by the patient working at a time when his/her circadian rhythm is trying to initiate and maintain sleep.
- It is not known why some people are more resilient to the effects of shift work than others.
- Most people will have some difficulty tolerating shift work and may benefit from the same interventions as those with more significant problems associated with SWD.

INCIDENCE: Not known

PEAK INCIDENCE: Not known

PREVALENCE:

- Prevalence of SWD is difficult to estimate because the boundary between a "normal response" to night work, and a diagnosable disorder is not sharp.
- Approximately 16% to 20% of the total work force is engaged in night-shift work. Survey data suggest that 5% to 10% of all shift workers experience clinically significant problems that would warrant a diagnosis of SWD.

PREDOMINANT SEX AND AGE: More prevalent in shift workers aged above 50 yr and worsens with passage of time if the work hours persist.

GENETICS: No known genetic contribution to SWD.

RISK FACTORS: SWD is more likely in shift workers who have a morning-type disposition, sleep need greater than 8 hours, or strong competing social and/or personal demands (e.g., child rearing).

PHYSICAL FINDINGS & CLINICAL PRESENTATION

- Diagnosis is based on history of the patient working outside 8:00 AM to 6:00 PM daytime window on a regular basis.
- Sleep logs and actigraphy (devices that estimate sleep/wake schedule based on movement) can be helpful, but are not required for the diagnosis.

ETIOLOGY

SWD is understood to be a circadian rhythm disorder primarily caused by exogenously determined alterations in the timing of sleep and wakefulness rather than disturbances of the endogenous circadian rhythm itself.

DIAGNOSIS

Diagnostic criteria include persistent sleep disruption that leads to excessive sleepiness or difficulty sleeping or both. The sleep disturbance causes clinically significant distress or impairment and problems occur as a result of shift work schedule. Diagnostic criteria for SWD are summarized in Table 1.

DIFFERENTIAL DIAGNOSIS

- Normal variations in sleep with shift work (e.g., short-term or mild difficulties adjusting to new shift)
- Insomnia disorder (sleep problems not specifically linked to shift work)
- Other circadian rhythm disorder (e.g., jet lag, free running disorder)
- Sleep apnea (a common comorbidity that can make shift work more difficult)

WORKUP

- Ideally, SWD is assessed by clinical interview, supplemented with sleep logs and actigraphy. Actigraphy is the estimation of sleep and wake times based on movement. Several medical-grade devices are available that have been validated in relation to polysomagraphy (the gold-standard for sleep assessment).
- Clinical interview should address difficulties with performance during night shift, problems sleeping during the day, and assess other sleep, psychiatric, and medical conditions that can co-occur with SWD and exacerbate symptoms (see Differential Diagnosis above).

LABORATORY TEST

Polysomnography (i.e., a comprehensive, in-lab sleep study) is usually not necessary in diagnosis or treatment of SWD, but may be helpful for ruling out other sleep disorders with overlapping symptoms.

TREATMENT

SWD requires behavioral changes to minimize impact of scheduling on sleep and circadian biology. Pharmacological interventions must be carefully timed in order to be most beneficial. Table 2 summarizes clinical guidelines for assessment and management of SWD.

NONPHARMACOLOGIC THERAPY

- Planned naps before night shifts improve performance without compromising sleep after shift has ended. Planned naps during shifts can also be helpful when feasible, but workers can be impaired immediately after awakening.

TABLE 1 Diagnostic Criteria for Shift Work Disorder

***International Classification of Sleep Disorders* (ICSD3) Criteria: General Criteria for Any Circadian Rhythm Sleep-Wake Disorder**

A. A chronic or recurrent pattern of sleep-wake rhythm disruption due primarily to alteration of the endogenous circadian timing system or misalignment between the endogenous circadian rhythm and the sleep-wake schedule desired or required by the person's physical environment or social/work schedules.

B. The circadian rhythm disruption leads to insomnia symptoms, excessive sleepiness, or both.

C. The sleep and wake disturbances cause clinically significant distress or impairment in mental, physical, social, occupational, educational, or other important areas of functioning.

Specific Criteria for Circadian Rhythm Sleep-Wake Disorder, Shift Work Disorder (ICD-9-CM code: 327.36)*

A. There is a report of insomnia and/or excessive sleepiness, accompanied by a reduction of total sleep time, which is associated with a recurring work schedule that overlaps the usual time for sleep.

B. The symptoms have been present and associated with the shift work schedule for at least 3 months.

C. Sleep log and actigraphy monitoring (whenever possible and preferably with concurrent light exposure measurement) for at least 14 days (work and free days) demonstrate a disturbed sleep and wake pattern.

D. The sleep and/or wake disturbance are not better explained by another current sleep disorder, medical or neurologic disorder, mental disorder, medication use, poor sleep hygiene, or substance use disorder.

Diagnostic and Statistical Manual of Mental Disorders, Fifth Edition: DSM-5*: Diagnostic Criteria for Circadian Rhythm Sleep Disorder (307.45)

A. A persistent or recurrent pattern of sleep disruption that is due primarily to an alteration of the circadian system or to a misalignment between the endogenous circadian rhythm and the sleep-wake schedule required by the person's physical environment or social or professional schedule.

B. The sleep disruption leads to excessive sleepiness or insomnia, or both.

C. The sleep disturbance causes clinically significant distress or impairment in social, occupational, and other important areas of functioning.

Specify Type:

Shift work type: Insomnia during the major sleep period and/or excessive sleepiness (including inadvertent sleep) during the major awake period associated with a shift work schedule (i.e., recurring unconventional work hours).

*ICD-10CM code: G47.26 circadian rhythm sleep-wake disorder, shift work type.

ICD-9-CM: International Classification of Diseases, Ninth Revision, Clinical Modification.

From Kryger M et al: *Principles and practice of sleep medicine*, ed 6, Philadelphia, 2017, Elsevier.

TABLE 2 Clinical Guidelines for Assessment and Management of Shift Work Disorder

Assessment

I. Determine circadian misalignment (sleep diaries and actigraphy with concurrent light exposure).
II. Assess sleep disturbance.
  A. Determine difficulty falling asleep, staying asleep, or having nonrestorative sleep (both during daytime and nighttime sleeps).
  B. Measure degree of alertness.
  C. Assess falling asleep during inappropriate circumstances or times (using Epworth Sleepiness Scale [ESS]), with special attention to drowsy driving.
  D. Determine important job-related factors: Duration of commute after shift, number of consecutive shifts, type of shift, time between shifts.
III. Determine impact on social and domestic responsibilities.[1]

Management[2]

I. Shift workers should have regular physical examinations with attention to psychological (e.g., depression), gastrointestinal, cardiovascular, and potential cancer risks associated with shift work.[2]
  A. Sleep-related comorbidity: Determine risk of sleep-disordered breathing, restless legs syndrome, or other potential sleep disorder.
  B. Other comorbidity: Identify medical or psychiatric disorders that may contribute to the symptoms of insomnia or excessive sleepiness.
II. Determine if removal from shift work is appropriate or practically feasible. If patient meets criteria for a diagnosis of shift work disorder, cessation of the shift work schedule should be the first option discussed with the patient.
III. Determine patient-specific therapeutic approach.
  A. Circadian adaptation
    1. Consider individual difference factors (e.g., age, phase preference).
    2. Consider compromise phase position (e.g., partial phase delay using bright light during first half of night and increased darkness during daytime).
    3. *Night workers*: On days off, adopt a late sleep schedule (i.e., bedtime of 3:00 to 4:00 AM).
  B. Symptom management
    1. Insomnia
      a. Good sleep behaviors
        i. Target inappropriate sleep behaviors and encourage use of eye mask, ear plugs, and light-blocking shades during daytime sleep.
      b. Sleep maintenance a primary concern
        i. Consider intermediate-acting hypnotic (half-life of 5 to 8 hours).
        ii. Consider melatonin treatment for daytime sleep (~3 mg).
      c. Sleep initiation problems
        i. Consider short-acting hypnotic.
      d. Sleep problems on days off
        i. Consider fixed sleep-wake schedule and consider anchor sleep.
        ii. Excessive sleepiness (i.e., ESS score <10)
    2. Address sleep disturbance if present.
      a. Consider wake-enhancing medication before shift (e.g., modafinil, armodafinil) or off-label stimulants (e.g., amphetamine, methylphenidate).
      b. Prophylactic nap before work shift is recommended.
      c. Judicious use of brief to moderate-length naps (30 to 60 min), with recognition of risk of sleep inertia (consider prenap caffeine to reduce sleep inertia).
      d. Consider combined treatment strategies during the work shift (alerting medications, bright light, anchor sleep and naps).
IV. Address additional work, social, and domestic factors.
  A. Social/family/psychological: Improve balance between family/social, work, and sleep time and treat psychosocial stress, depression, or marital discord if present,[1] educate patient's family regarding shift worker's need of protected time for sleep.
  B. Health and safety: Promote improved healthy eating habits with respect to regularity and timing relative to the major sleep period (not within 2 to 4 hours of bedtime), reduce inappropriate substance use, increase exercise at appropriate times (not within 2 to 4 hours of bedtime), educate on risks of drowsy driving and critical times of performance vulnerability.
  C. Work-related: Reduce number of consecutive shifts (<4),[1] reduce shift duration (<12 hours), use clockwise rotation,[3] ensure adequate time between shifts (>11 hours),[1] move heavy workload outside circadian nadir (4:00 to 7:00 AM), address commute time (longer = greater accident risk), move to day or evening shift,[4] consider incorporation of a shift work awareness program.[5]

[1]Knauth P, Hornberger S: Preventive and compensatory measures for shift workers, *Soc Occup Med* 53:109–116, 2003.
[2]Costa G: Guidelines for the medical surveillance of shift workers, *Scand J Work Environ Health* 24(Suppl. 3):151–155, 1998.
[3]Monk TH: What can the chronobiologist do to help the shift worker? *J Biol Rhythms* 15:86–94, 2000.
[4]Pilcher JJ et al: Differential effects of permanent and rotating shifts on self-report sleep length: a meta-analytic review, *Sleep* 23:155–163, 2000.
[5]Monk TH, Folkard S: *Making shift work tolerable*, Boca Raton, 1992, CRC Press.
From Kryger M et al: *Principles and practice of sleep medicine*, ed 6, Philadelphia, 2017, Elsevier.

- Bright light during night shift work improves alertness. Both short- and long-duration light exposure has been shown to be helpful relative to normal lighting.
- Bright light should be avoided in the morning when feasible to protect daytime sleep. Darkened glasses can be helpful provided that they do not compromise driving ability (if shift worker must drive home after shift).
- Daytime sleep environment should be protected from both light and noise. Sleep masks, black-out curtains, ear plugs, and noise machines can be helpful.
- Circadian adaptation during jet travel is illustrated in Fig. 1.

ACUTE GENERAL Rx

- Wake-promoting medications such as modafinil/armodafinil, caffeine, and amphetamine have been shown to improve performance during the night shift. Modafinil and caffeine have established safety records and are generally considered as first-line treatments. Ideally, medications would be administered at times and doses where daytime sleep after the shift work is not affected.
- Hypnotic medications can be helpful for promoting daytime sleep after night shift work. Carryover sedation must be evaluated to ensure performance during night shift work is not impaired. Specific agents that have been tested include triazolam, temazepam, and zopiclone. Evidence is stronger for promoting sleep during day than improving waking performance during night shift work.
- Melatonin administered before daytime sleep (after night shift work) has been shown to be effective. Melatonin is not regulated by the FDA, and so it is important to avoid brands with poor performance in independent laboratory tests. Fig. 2 illustrates using light and melatonin to phase shift the internal biologic time.

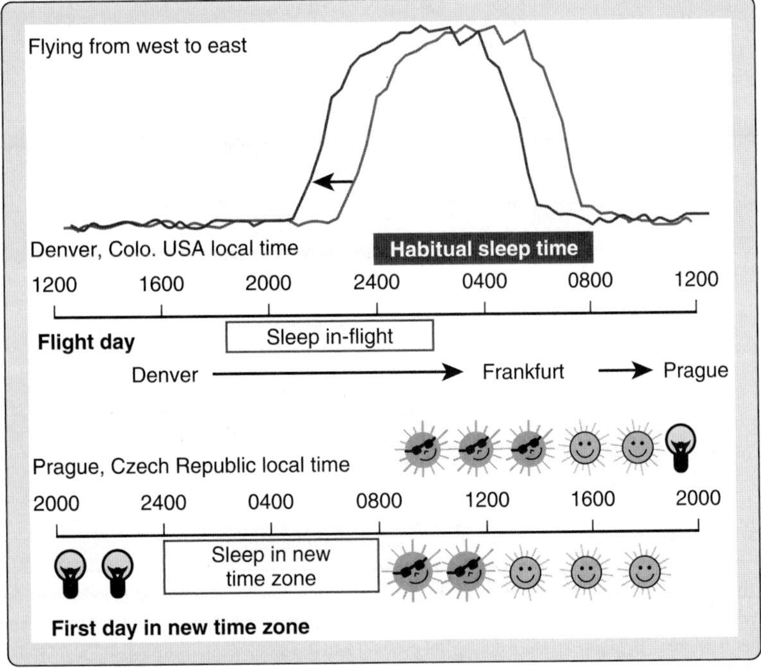

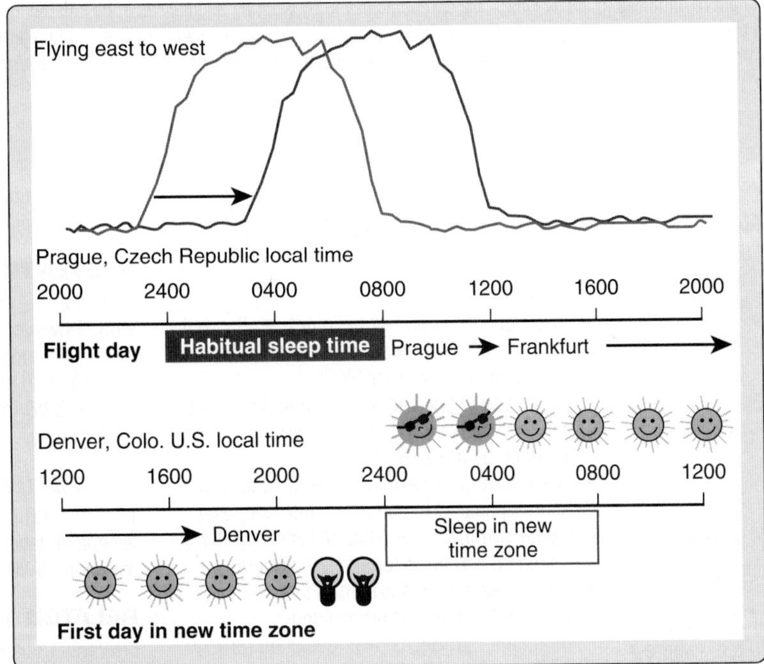

FIG. 1 Circadian adaptation during jet travel. *Top:* When traveling eastward, the jet traveler needs to advance the timing of his or her sleep schedule as well as the phase of the internal circadian clock so that both occur earlier. In the current example of a trip from Denver, Colorado, to Prague, Czech Republic, the primary plane flight to Frankfurt (*long black arrows*) occurs during the beginning of the biologic night, when endogenous melatonin levels are high (*green line; top panel*). The traveler should sleep as much as possible on the plane flight to reduce the negative impact of sleep deprivation during jet travel. Exogenous melatonin taken shortly after boarding the plane may help the traveler fall asleep earlier than normal when endogenous melatonin levels are low. In this example, the traveler spends several hours in Frankfurt before the flight connection to Prague. Light exposure during most of the biologic night will induce a westward phase delay, opposite to what is needed for an eastward shift; accordingly, the traveler should avoid exposure to bright light (*sun with sunglasses*) and wear an eye mask or sunglasses until after the habitual time of awakening in the home time zone. Subsequent exposure to bright light (*sun without sunglasses and light bulb*) will facilitate the eastward phase advance of the traveler's circadian clock (*red line; top panel*). Sleep timing should be consistent with the local time zone in Prague, and melatonin may again help phase shift the clock and promote sleep onset if taken when endogenous melatonin levels are low. The next day, the traveler should at first continue to avoid exposure to bright light. Each day, the time of exposure to bright light can be moved earlier by 1 to 2 hours per day. *Bottom:* When traveling westward, the jet traveler needs to delay the timing of his or her sleep schedule as well as the phase of the internal circadian clock (*green line; bottom panel*) so that both occur later. In the example of a trip from Prague to Denver, plane flights occur across the biologic day when endogenous melatonin levels are low, and the traveler should remain awake for much of the trip, assuming that sleep was adequate before travel. Caffeine and/or a nap can help to support subsequent wakefulness. Exposure to bright light should occur across the entire plane flight and until just before bedtime in the new time zone, to facilitate a westward phase delay (*red line; bottom panel*). (From Kryger M et al: *Principles and practice of sleep medicine*, ed 6, Philadelphia, 2017, Elsevier.)

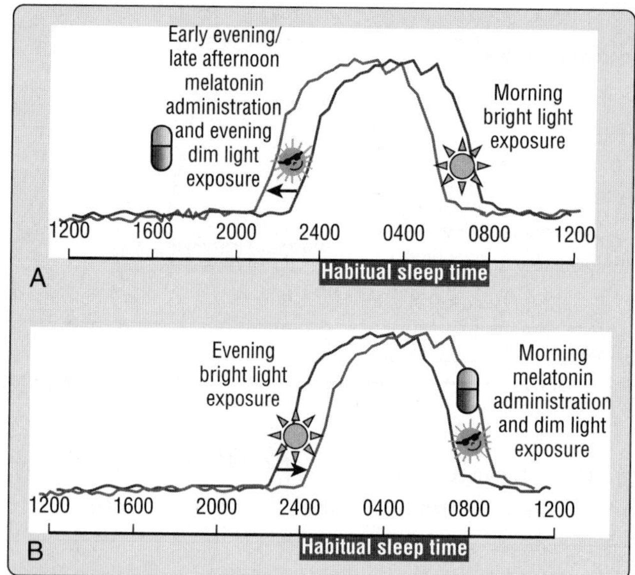

FIG. 2 Using light and melatonin to phase shift the internal biologic time. A, When the traveler is entrained to local time, light exposure during the morning and melatonin ingestion in the afternoon will induce an eastward phase advance shift of the internal circadian clock. *Red line* shows initial melatonin rhythm and *green line* shows advanced melatonin rhythm after treatment. **B,** Light exposure during the evening and melatonin administration in the morning will induce a westward phase delay shift of the internal circadian clock. *Red line* shows initial melatonin rhythm and *green line* shows delayed melatonin rhythm after treatment. Adjustment to eastward travel should include exposure to dim light or darkness in the evening. This can be achieved by wearing sunglasses if the sun has not set and by turning down the lights in the house. Adjustment to westward travel should include exposure to dim light or darkness in the morning. Administration of melatonin when the jet traveler is required to be awake (e.g., for work or driving) should be avoided, because melatonin has been reported to impair performance. (From Kryger M et al: *Principles and practice of sleep medicine*, ed 6, Philadelphia, 2017, Elsevier.)

CHRONIC Rx

Patients with chronic difficulty adapting to shift work despite adequate treatment may need to find other work. Many shift work jobs can be dangerous if completed by individuals who are impaired by sleepiness.

COMPLEMENTARY AND ALTERNATIVE MEDICINE

No evidence-based recommendations currently available.

REFERRAL

- Sleep medicine specialists in pulmonology, neurology, or psychiatry generally have expertise to treat SWD.
- Psychologists specializing in behavioral sleep medicine can be consulted (where available).

PEARLS & CONSIDERATIONS

COMMENTS

- Most people who work night shifts will experience difficulties and can benefit from treatment strategies for SWD.
- All shift workers should be educated about dangers associated with working while impaired by sleep deprivation.
- Co-occurring sleep disorders, especially sleep apnea, are common and can exacerbate symptoms of SWD. All shift workers should be screened for sleep disorders.
- When possible, inconsistent shifts and rotating schedules should be avoided.
- Treatment strategies are designed around delaying circadian rhythms as much as possible, then providing countermeasures for fatigue during shift, and protecting or promoting sleep during the day.

PREVENTION

SWD can be prevented by avoiding night shift work. However, many essential services require night shift workers. Early detection and treatment for mild SWD is essential. Those with more severe SWD may need to consider working earlier shifts.

PATIENT/FAMILY EDUCATION

The National Sleep Foundation (sleepfoundation.org) provides high-quality information on SWD and ways to manage symptoms.

RELATED TOPIC

Insomnia (Related Key Topic)

AUTHOR: **JARED D. MINKEL, PH.D.**

BASIC INFORMATION

DEFINITION

Shigellosis is an inflammatory disease of the bowel caused by one of four species of *Shigella.* It is the third most common cause of diarrhea in the United States after *Salmonella* and *Campylobacter* and the most common cause of bacillary dysentery in the United States.

SYNONYM

Bacillary dysentery

ICD-10CM CODES

A03.9 Shigellosis, unspecified
A03.0 Shigellosis due to Shigella dysenteriae
A03.1 Shigellosis due to Shigella flexneri
A03.2 Shigellosis due to Shigella boydii
A03.3 Shigellosis due to Shigella sonnei
A03.8 Other shigellosis

EPIDEMIOLOGY & DEMOGRAPHICS

INCIDENCE (IN U.S.): 6.59 cases per 100,000 population with approximately 450,000 cases/yr
PREDOMINANT SEX: Male homosexuals are at increased risk.
PREDOMINANT AGE: Shigellosis predominantly affects children (Box 1), with 28 cases per 100,000 population in children <4 yr old and 25.67 cases per 100,000 population in children aged 4 to 11.
PEAK INCIDENCE: Summer
GENETICS: Neonatal infection: Rare but severe

PHYSICAL FINDINGS & CLINICAL PRESENTATION

- Possibly asymptomatic, but incubation period can range from 1 to 7 days with an average of 3 days
- Mild illness that is usually self-limited, resolving in a few days
- High fever
- Watery diarrhea. Dysentery (abdominal cramps, tenesmus, and numerous, small-volume stools with blood, mucus, and pus)
- Descending intestinal tract illness, reflecting infection of small bowel first and then the colon
- Severe disease is more common in children and elderly and outside of the U.S.

BOX 1 Risk Factors for Severe Disease

Infants, and adults >50 yr
Children who are not breastfed
Children recovering from measles
Patients with HIV
Malnourished children and adults
Any patient who develops dehydration, unconsciousness, hypothermia, or hyperthermia, or has a history of convulsion with first seen

From Cherry JD et al: *Feigin and Cherry's pediatric infectious diseases*, ed 8, Philadelphia, 2019, Elsevier.

- Complications of severe illness (Box 2):
  1. Seizures
  2. Megacolon
  3. Intestinal perforation
  4. Death
- Extraintestinal manifestations are uncommon (reactive arthritis in up to 3% of patients)
- Bacteremia is more common in children; in adults it has been described in patients with AIDS, the elderly, and diabetics
- Hemolytic-uremic syndrome (HUS): Can be caused by *S. dysenteriae*
- Reactive arthritis, sometimes as part of Reiter syndrome following *S. flexneri* infection

ETIOLOGY

- *Shigella:* Gram-negative rod bacteria that are less susceptible to stomach acid and thus as few as 10 to 100 bacteria can cause disease. The bacteria invade colonic tissue and cause inflammation.
  1. *S. flexneri*
  2. *S. dysenteriae*
  3. *S. sonnei*
  4. *S. boydii*
- *S. sonnei* is the most commonly isolated species in the United States (over 75% of cases), and it usually causes a mild, watery diarrhea.
- Direct person-to-person transmission by consumption of contaminated food or water is thought to be the most common route. Outbreaks among men who have sex with men have occurred because of direct or indirect oral-anal contact.
- Contaminated food or water may transmit disease.
- Outbreaks have occurred in day care centers, a community wading pool frequented by toddlers, and residential institutions.

DIAGNOSIS

DIFFERENTIAL DIAGNOSIS

- May mimic other bacterial gastroenteritis, such as *Clostridium difficile, Salmonella, Campylobacter*, and *Yersinia.*
- Dysentery can also be caused by *Entamoeba histolytica.*
- Bloody diarrhea may resemble disease caused by invasive *E. coli* (IEC).
- Hemolytic-uremic syndrome caused by enterohemorrhagic *E. coli* (0157:H7).

LABORATORY TESTS

- The diagnosis is established by bacterial stool culture.
- Stool should be cultured from fresh samples, because the yield is increased by processing the specimen soon after passage. The best yield is from the mucoid part of the stool.
- Serology is available but rarely useful.
- Polymerase chain reaction (PCR) is available but due to cost used mainly for outbreak investigations.
- Fecal leukocyte preparation may show WBCs.
- Total WBCs may be low, normal, or high. Leukemoid reactions can occur in children.
- Blood cultures should be obtained in patients with severe disease or sepsis syndromes.

IMAGING STUDIES

Abdominal radiographs may suggest megacolon or perforation in rare, severe cases.

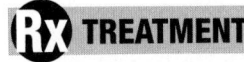

TREATMENT

NONPHARMACOLOGIC THERAPY

- Adequate hydration
- Electrolyte replacement

BOX 2 Complications of Shigellosis

Abdominal
- Persistent diarrhea
- Postdysenteric irritable bowel syndrome
- Ileus, toxic megacolon, intestinal perforation
- Protein-losing enteropathy, malnutrition
- Surgical complications: Intestinal perforation and obstruction, appendicitis, intraabdominal abscesses

Neurologic
- Seizures
- Headache, lethargy, disorientation, hallucinations
- Coma
- Severe toxin encephalopathy or ekiri syndrome

Bacteremia
- In malnourished children, young infants, and HIV-AIDS patients

Hemolytic-Uremic Syndrome
- Only with *Shigella dysenteriae* serotype 1

Urogenital
- Vulvovaginitis, urinary tract infections

Other
- Conjunctivitis, keratitis, corneal ulcers
- Reactive arthritis
- Reiter syndrome
- Hepatitis
- Myocarditis

From Cherry JD et al: *Feigin and Cherry's pediatric infectious diseases*, ed 8, Philadelphia, 2019, Elsevier.

ACUTE GENERAL Rx

Antibiotics recommended in all patients with positive stool cultures, severe illness, immunocompromised status:

- To shorten course of illness.
- To limit transmission of illness.
- For adults: Pending susceptibilities, ciprofloxacin 750 mg PO bid for 3 days or levofloxacin 500 to 750 mg q day for 3 days should be used. An alternative is azithromycin 500 mg q day for 3 days.
- For children: IV ceftriaxone (50 mg/kg/day) for 5 days in cases of severe disease. For oral therapy, can use cefixime: 8 mg/kg/day as single daily dose or divided q12h vfor 5 days *or* azithromycin: 10 mg/kg/day in a single daily dose for 3 days. A short course of an oral quinolone can also be used safely although they are not approved for children.

DISPOSITION

- Most disease is self-limited and resolves without treatment.
- Severe illness may be fatal.

REFERRAL

For severe illness or complications

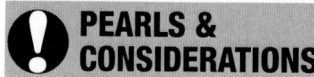

PEARLS & CONSIDERATIONS

COMMENTS

- Shigella is one cause of "gay bowel syndrome."
- Illness is worsened by agents that decrease intestinal motility.
- Food handlers, child care providers, and health care workers should have a negative stool culture documented following treatment.

SUGGESTED READINGS

Available at ExpertConsult.com

RELATED CONTENT

Shigellosis (Patient Information)

AUTHOR: **GLENN G. FORT, M.D., M.P.H.**

BASIC INFORMATION

DEFINITION

Short bowel syndrome (SBS) is a malabsorption syndrome that results from extensive small intestinal resection or congenital causes (Table 1).

SYNONYMS

Short bowel
SBS

ICD-10CM CODE

K91.2 Postsurgical malabsorption, not elsewhere classified

EPIDEMIOLOGY & DEMOGRAPHICS

- Parallels Crohn disease (see "Crohn Disease" in Section I), which is the most common cause of the syndrome in adults.
- In children, two thirds of short bowels are related to congenital abnormalities (intestinal atresia, gastroschisis, volvulus, aganglionosis) and one third are related to necrotizing enterocolitis.
- Prevalence: 10,000 to 20,000 cases are estimated to exist in the U.S.

PHYSICAL FINDINGS & CLINICAL PRESENTATION

- Diarrhea and steatorrhea
- Weight loss
- Anemia related to iron or vitamin B_{12} absorption
- Bleeding diathesis related to vitamin K malabsorption
- Osteoporosis/osteomalacia related to vitamin D and calcium malabsorption
- Hyponatremia, hypokalemia
- Hypovolemia
- Other macronutrient or micronutrient deficiency states

ETIOLOGY

- Extensive bowel resection for treatment of the conditions mentioned previously (see "Epidemiology"). SBS typically does not occur until less than 200 cm of healthy small intestine remains. Risk for SBS is decreased if colon is intact.
- Congenital.
- Box 1 summarizes causes of short bowel syndrome.

The human intestine is 3 to 8 m in length. Removal of up to half of the small intestine produces no disruption in nutrient absorption, and most patients can maintain nutritional balance on oral feeding if they have more than 100 cm (3 ft) of jejunum. Similarly, 100 cm of intact jejunum can maintain a normal water, sodium, and potassium balance under normal circumstances. The presence of an intact colon can compensate for some small intestine loss.

Site-specific functions (Fig. 1):

- Calcium, magnesium, phosphorus, iron, and vitamins are absorbed in the duodenum and proximal jejunum.
- Vitamin B_{12} and bile acids are absorbed in the ileum. The resection of more than 60 cm of ileum results in vitamin B_{12} malabsorption. The loss of more than 100 cm results in fat malabsorption (from the loss of bile acids).
- The loss of gastrointestinal endocrine hormones can affect intestinal motility.
- Intestinal bacterial overgrowth may also occur, especially if the ileocecal valve is lost.

BOX 1 Causes of Short Bowel Syndrome (SBS) and Intestinal Failure in Adults and Children

Adults
Catastrophic vascular accidents:
Superior mesenteric arterial embolism
Superior mesenteric arterial thrombosis
Superior mesenteric venous thrombosis
Chronic intestinal pseudo-obstruction
Intestinal resection for tumor or trauma
Midgut volvulus
Multiple intestinal resections for Crohn disease
Radiation enteritis
Refractory sprue
Scleroderma and mixed connective tissue disease

Children
Congenital villus atrophy
Extensive aganglionosis
Gastroschisis
Jejunal or ileal atresia
*Necrotizing enterocolitis

*Functional SBS can also occur in conditions associated with severe malabsorption and intact bowel length.
From Feldman M et al: *Sleisenger and Fordtran's gastrointestinal and liver disease*, ed 10, Philadelphia, 2016, Elsevier.

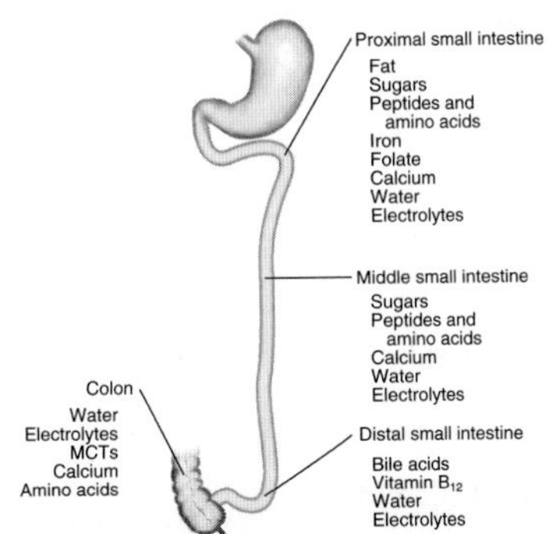

FIG. 1 Specific areas of absorption of dietary constituents and secretions in the small intestine and colon. Macronutrients and micronutrients are absorbed predominantly in the proximal jejunum. Bile acids and vitamin B_{12} (cobalamin) are absorbed only in the ileum. Electrolytes and water are absorbed in both the small and large intestine. Medium-chain triglycerides *(MCTs)*, calcium, and some amino acids can be absorbed in the colon. (From Feldman M et al: *Sleisenger and Fordtran's gastrointestinal and liver disease*, ed 10, Philadelphia, 2016, Elsevier.)

- Macronutrient requirements in patients with short bowel syndrome are summarized in Table 2.

DIAGNOSIS

Presence of macronutrient and/or micronutrient loss in a patient with a known history of bowel resection. Daily stromal or fecal losses of electrolytes, minerals, and trace elements in SBS are summarized in Table 1.

DIFFERENTIAL DIAGNOSIS

Because the history of significant bowel resection is typically known, there is no differential diagnosis. If that history is not known, all causes of weight loss, malabsorption, and diarrhea must be considered.

TREATMENT

Extensive small bowel resection with colectomy (<100 cm of jejunum):

- Rx: Long-term total parenteral nutrition (TPN). Some patients can switch to oral intake after 1 to 2 yr of TPN. In jejunostomy patients, excessive fluid loss can be reduced with H_2 blockers, proton pump inhibitors, or octreotide. Micronutrients are supplemented.

Extensive small bowel resection with partial colectomy (usually patients with Crohn disease):

- Rx: Oral intake alone is possible in all patients with >100 cm of jejunum. In addition to vitamin B_{12} deficiency, these patients often have diarrhea. Consider lactose malabsorption and bacterial overgrowth treated, respectively, with lactose restriction and antibiotics (tetracycline 250 mg tid or metronidazole 500 mg tid for 2 wk). Nonspecific antidiarrheal agents may also be indicated (e.g., Imodium or codeine). The patient must be monitored for micronutrient losses.
- Table 3 and Fig. 2 summarize management strategies for SBS. Intestinal transplantation is performed mostly in children at selective centers.
- Therapeutic agents used to decrease intestinal transit and diarrheal volume are summarized in Table E4.
- FDA-approved medications for SBS in patients receiving nutritional support are:
  1. Recombinant growth hormone somatropin (Zorbtive): Effective in increasing weight and reducing parenteral nutrition volume. These effects do not persist when the drug is stopped.
  2. Teduglutide (Gattex), a recombinant DNA analog of glucagon-like peptide-2. It promotes mucosal growth in the small bowel through stimulation of crypt cell proliferation and inhibition of enterocyte apoptosis. This drug may have to be continued indefinitely for effects to persist.

COMPLICATIONS

- Oxalate kidney stones
- Cholesterol gallstones
- D-Lactic acidosis

TABLE 1 Daily Stomal or Fecal Losses of Electrolytes, Minerals, and Trace Elements in Severe Short Bowel Syndrome*

Component	Amount Lost
Sodium	90-100 mEq/L
Potassium	10-20 mEq/L
Calcium	772 (591-950) mg/day
Magnesium	328 (263-419) mg/day
Iron	11 (7-15) mg/day
Zinc	12 (10-14) mg/day
Copper	1.5 (0.5-2.3) mg/day

*For sodium and potassium, the average concentration per liter of stomal effluent is given. Values for minerals and trace elements are mean 24-hour losses, with the range in parentheses.
From Feldman M et al: *Sleisenger and Fordtran's gastrointestinal and liver disease*, ed 10, Philadelphia, 2016, Elsevier.

TABLE 2 Macronutrient Requirements in Patients with Short Bowel Syndrome

Colon Present	Colon Absent
Carbohydrate	
Complex carbohydrates/starches	Variable types
30-35 kcal/kg per day	30-35 kcal/kg per day
Soluble fiber	
Fat	
MCT/LCT	LCT
20%-30% of caloric intake	20%-30% of caloric intake
Protein	
Intact protein	Intact protein
1.0-1.5 g/kg per day	1.0-1.5 g/kg per day

LCT, Long-chain triglycerides; *MCT*, medium-chain triglycerides.
From Feldman M et al: *Sleisenger and Fordtran's gastrointestinal and liver disease*, ed 10, Philadelphia, 2016, Elsevier.

TABLE 3 Management Strategies for Short Bowel Syndrome

1. Acute phase
   a. Treat postoperative complications
   b. Maintain full support via the parenteral route
   c. Initiate low-rate trophic enteral feeds
   d. Document amount and site of remaining bowel and underlying disease
2. Early adaptation (up to 1 yr postsurgery)
   a. Increase enteral nutrition to tolerance; supplement with glutamine
   b. Achieve permanent parenteral access, if indicated
   c. Maximize antiperistaltic agents
   d. Octreotide for high-output ostomy or fistula
   e. Dietary counseling
   f. Clinical trials of trophic growth factors
3. Long-term adaptation (>1 yr postsurgery)
   a. Recruit bypassed bowel
   b. Bowel-lengthening procedure (Bianchi or STEP)
   c. Monitor for development of TPN-associated complications, and refer for transplant before recurrent sepsis, thrombosis, or end-stage liver disease

STEP, Serial transverse enteroplasty; *TPN*, total parenteral nutrition.
From Cameron JL, Cameron AM: *Current surgical therapy*, ed 10, Philadelphia, 2011, Saunders.

PROGNOSIS

- Directly dependent on the extent of the bowel resection and in the case of Crohn disease by the underlying illness.
- Whether the colon remains in continuity with the small bowel is an important factor in the patient's ability to adapt after significant small bowel resection.

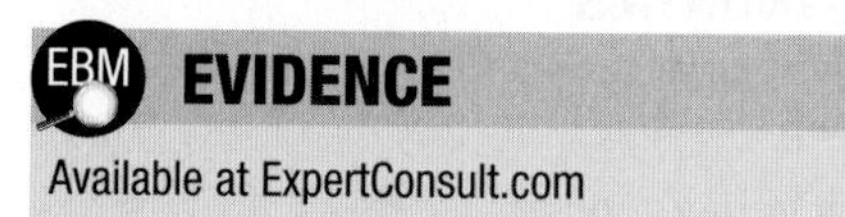

EVIDENCE

Available at ExpertConsult.com

RELATED CONTENT

Short Bowel Syndrome (Patient Information)
Malabsorption (Related Key Topic)

AUTHOR: **FRED F. FERRI, M.D.**

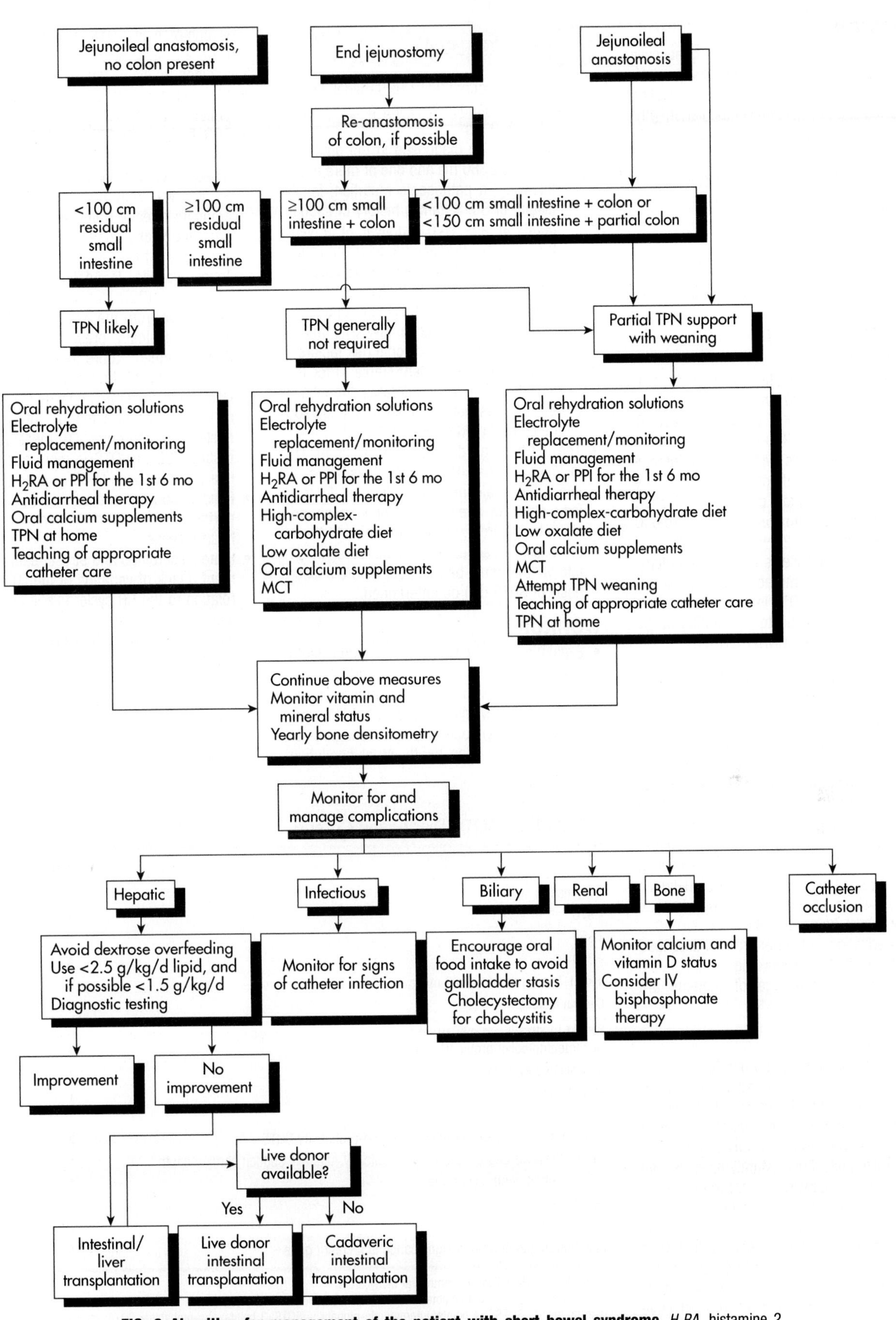

FIG. 2 Algorithm for management of the patient with short bowel syndrome. *H_2RA,* histamine 2 receptor antagonist; *IV,* intravenous; *MCT,* medium-chain triglycerides; *PPI,* proton pump inhibitor; *TPN,* total parenteral nutrition. (From Feldman M et al: *Sleisenger and Fordtran's gastrointestinal and liver disease,* ed 10, Philadelphia, 2016, Elsevier.)

DEFINITION

Short QT syndrome (SQTS) is a genetically inherited disorder of cardiac repolarization characterized by a severely shortened QT interval on the ECG, leading to atrial and ventricular arrhythmias and sudden cardiac death in affected individuals. This is a primary electrical disorder and patients have structurally normal hearts.

SYNONYM

SQTS

ICD-10CM CODE

I45.89 Other specified conduction disorders

EPIDEMIOLOGY AND DEMOGRAPHICS

- The disease is a relative new entity, first documented in 2000. In most (but not all) cases of SQTS, the QT or QTc (correct QT interval) has been <360 ms; however, there are many individuals with that QT interval who are clinically unaffected. Although poorly defined, the estimated prevalence of short QTc ≤340 ms is estimated to be 5 in 10,000 in persons less than 21 yr of age.
- Genetics: The disease is genetically heterogeneous and transmitted in an autosomal dominant fashion. SQT1 is the most common variant described, due to a mutation in the cardiac ion channel KCNH2(HERG).

PHYSICAL FINDINGS AND CLINICAL PRESENTATION

- Seen across all age groups, though most patients are children or young adults.
- Syncope and cardiac arrest are the most common presenting features. Syncope is likely due to ventricular arrhythmias. Sudden death can happen with exercise as well as at rest. Cardiac arrest is often the first manifestation of the disease with a peak incidence in the first year of life and second peak between 20 and 40 yr of age; overall risk cardiac arrest is 40% before age 41.
- Atrial fibrillation and flutter are well described as being part of the syndrome.
- A significant percentage of patients are asymptomatic.

ETIOLOGY

- Cardiac repolarization abnormality.
- A total of 22 different mutations have been found in 9 different genes, 15 in single families. At present, the chance of finding a causative mutation in a family with SQTS is approximately 20%. Mutations cause an increase in net outward current from either a reduction in inward depolarizing currents INa or ICa or augmentation of outward repolarizing currents I to I K1, I K-ATP, I ACh, I Kr or I Ks as well as defects in Cl/HCO_3 exchanger. The resultant shortening of the action potential causes a shortening of the effective refractory period, with subsequent increased susceptibility of both atrial and ventricular muscle to premature depolarizations that lead to AF and VF.
- Acquired causes—see "Differential Diagnosis."

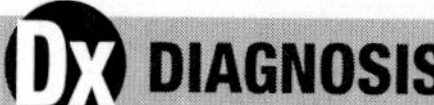

DIAGNOSIS

- Per the most recent 2013 HRS guidelines:
  1. SQTS is diagnosed in the presence of a QTc ≤330 ms.
  2. SQTS can be diagnosed in the presence of a QTc ≤360 ms and one or more of the following: a pathogenic mutation, family history of SQTS, family history of sudden death at age ≤40, survival of a ventricular tachycardia/ventricular fibrillation episode in the absence of heart disease.
  3. Notably, more recent studies suggest the use of somewhat more liberal cutoffs of 340 ms as standalone and 370 ms in combination with additional risk factors.
- A proposed scoring system (Table 1) for the diagnosis of SQTS incorporates the above criteria but has not yet been fully endorsed by the current guidelines.
- The differential diagnosis of a short QT includes various conditions such as hyperkalemia, hypercalcemia, acidosis, digitalis toxicity, effect of acetylcholine or epinephrine, sinus tachycardia, or hyperthermia. All these are possible causes of an acquired short QT interval that must be ruled out before a diagnosis of SQTS can be entertained.

WORKUP

- Evaluation of any survivor of sudden death starts with a detailed history and physical examination, with particular emphasis on family history. Many patients with SQTS have unexplained syncope or palpitations prior to resuscitated sudden death. Atrial fibrillation is common in SQTS patients and a family history of lone AF should also be sought, in addition to resuscitated VF arrest.
- Physical examination is mostly normal in patients with SQTS.
- ECG findings in SQTS include not only an abnormally short QT interval (usually <360 msec), but usually also a short or even absent ST interval, with the T-wave appearing to emanate directly from the S-wave. T-waves are usually any combination of tall, narrow, and symmetric, with a prolonged Tpeak-Tend ratio (Fig. 1). Additionally, PQ-segment depression (PQD), defined as 0.05-mV PQ depression from the isoelectric TP segment, is more typically present in patients with SQTS. Another feature to look for is the lack of adaptation of the QT interval to the heart rate (diminished rate dependence) as a result of which the corrected QT interval can be misleading; therefore, QT measurement on resting ECG in SQTS is more accurate with heart rate as close to 60 as possible.
- Echocardiogram and cardiac MRI should be performed to confirm a lack of structural heart disease.
- Holter recordings and stress tests can document a lack of variation of the QT interval in relation to the RR cycle; this is an important aspect of establishing the diagnosis. The QT interval shortens only slightly with increasing heart rates, so the QT and QTc values approach normal levels during faster heart rates. The QT fails to lengthen at slower heart rates.
- At electrophysiology study, the atrial and ventricular refractory periods are usually

TABLE 1 SQTS Diagnostic Criteria

	Points
QTc, msec	
<370	1
<350	2
<330	3
Jpoint-Tpeak interval <120 msec	1
Clinical history	
History of sudden cardiac arrest	2
Documented polymorphic VT or VF	2
Unexplained syncope	1
Atrial fibrillation	1
Family history	
First- or second-degree relative with high-probability SQTS	2
First- or second-degree relative with autopsy-negative sudden cardiac death	1
Sudden infant death syndrome	1
Genotype	
Genotype positive	2
Mutation of undetermined significance in a culprit gene	1

VF, ventricular fibrillation; *VT*, ventricular tachycardia.

A minimum of 1 point must be obtained in the electrocardiographic section in order to obtain additional points.

High-probability SQTS: ≥4 points; intermediate-probability SQTS: 3 points; low-probability SQTS: ≤2 points. Electrocardiogram: Must be recorded in the absence of modifiers known to shorten the QT. Jpoint-Tpeak interval must be measured in the precordial lead with the greatest amplitude T-wave. Clinical history: Events must occur in the absence of an identifiable etiology, including structural heart disease. Points can only be received for 1 of cardiac arrest, documented polymorphic VT, or unexplained syncope. Family history: Points can only be received once in this section.

Adapted from Gollob MH, Redpath CJ, Roberts JD: The short QT syndrome: proposed diagnostic criteria, *J Am Coll Cardiol* 57(7):802-812, 2011.

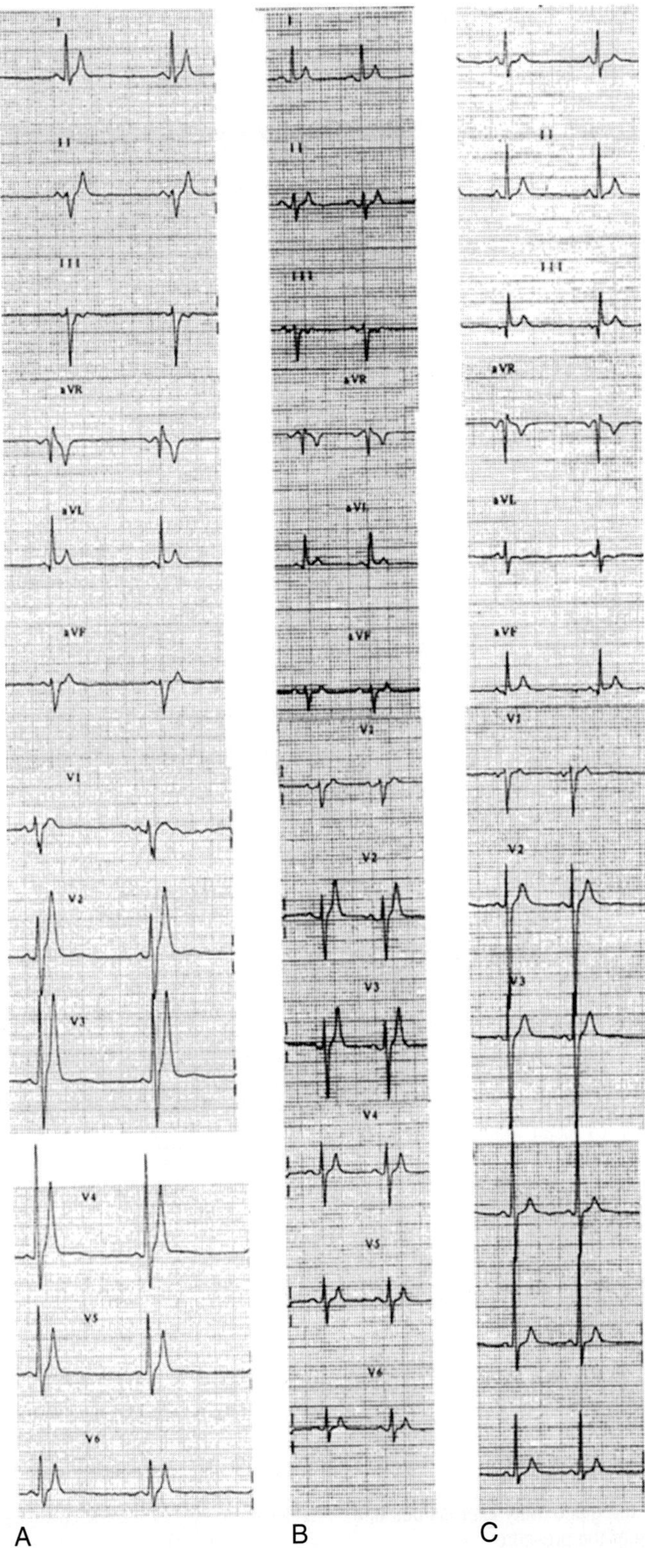

FIG. 1 Twelve-lead electrocardiogram (25 mm/s paper speed) of family 1 patients. A, Patient 1 (IV, 3): sinus rhythm, heart rate 52 beats per minute (bpm); left-axis deviation, QT 280 msec. **B,** Patient 2 (IV, 2): sinus rhythm, heart rate 96 bpm; left-axis deviation, QT 220 msec. **C,** Patient 3 (V, 1): sinus rhythm with mean heart rate 92 bpm, QT 260 msec. (Adapted with permission from Gaita F et al: Short QT syndrome: a familial cause of death, *Circulation* 108:965-970, 2003.)

very short (140-200 msec at a CL of 400-600 msec). Sustained atrial fibrillation or flutter with rapid ventricular rates is often induced with programmed stimulation in the atrium. The inducibility of VF in SQTS patients at EPS is about 60%. EPS has a role in adding to the diagnosis by demonstrating short A and V refractory periods (also seen in other channelopathies such as Brugada syndrome), but given its low sensitivity, it cannot be used for risk stratification.

LABORATORY TESTS

Genetic testing is recommended for all patients in whom a diagnosis of SQTS is suspected. This is especially true if they have a clinical or family history of syncope or sudden death.

Rx TREATMENT

- There is no significant clinical data on how to approach patients with an isolated short QT interval but no family or clinical history or genotype criterion (low and intermediate probability of SQTS). Risk stratification of these patients is not possible at this time; however, they should be referred to an electrophysiologist with expertise on this topic for comprehensive testing, including genetic testing.
- Patients with QT <330 msec and one criterion from clinical/family history or genetic testing fall in the high probability category of SQTS and hence a higher-risk subgroup for sudden cardiac death. An ICD implant is recommended in this group for secondary and possibly also primary prevention against sudden cardiac death.
- SQTS is a highly lethal disease, and survivors of cardiac arrest are at high risk for subsequent events. ICD implantation is strongly recommended in this group.
- A peculiar issue in patients with SQTS implanted with an ICD is double counting of peaked T-waves that are closely coupled to the QRS complex. This often leads to inappropriate ICD shocks. Most ICDs have programming modifications that can be turned on to get around this problem.
- Pharmacologic therapy is usually only advised in patients with multiple and frequent appropriate ICD shocks.
- However, medications may be the mainstay of therapy in patients in whom an ICD cannot be implanted for various reasons, including in children in whom technical challenges are significant.
- While many drugs, such as flecainide, sotalol, ibutilide, hydroquinone, and amiodarone, have been used in an attempt to increase the QT interval, most of the available data favor hydroquinidine as the drug of choice across all forms of the SQTS.

REFERRAL

Consultation with an electrophysiologist is strongly recommended if SQTS is suspected.

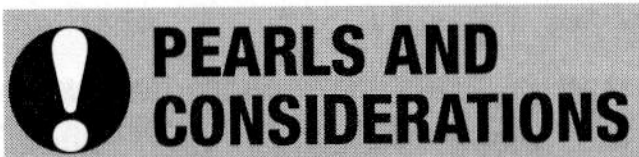

PEARLS AND CONSIDERATIONS

- SQTS is a rare genetic syndrome causing arrhythmias and sudden death.
- Should be suspected in patients with QT interval <370 msec presenting with syncope, sudden cardiac death, or atrial fibrillation and a family history of the same.

SUGGESTED READINGS

Available at ExpertConsult.com

AUTHOR: **SIMON GRINGUT, M.D.**

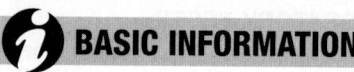

DEFINITION

Sialadenitis is an inflammation of one or multiple salivary glands. It may present as acute or chronic disease with multiple potential etiologies. This section focuses mainly on the workup and management of acute sialadenitis.

ICD-10CM CODE
K11.20 Sialadenitis, unspecified

EPIDEMIOLOGY & DEMOGRAPHICS

INCIDENCE:
- Accounts for approximately 0.01% to 0.02% of hospital admissions.
- 30% to 40% of affected patients are postoperative patients.
- Parotid gland is most frequently affected, followed by the submandibular glands (Fig. E1).

PREDOMINANT SEX AND AGE

- Affects men and women equally.
- Patients are usually in the sixth and seventh decades of life.

PHYSICAL FINDINGS & CLINICAL PRESENTATION

- Pain and swelling of the affected salivary gland
- Increased pain with meals
- Erythema and localized tenderness at the duct opening
- Massage may express purulent discharge from duct orifice
- Induration and pitting of the skin, with involvement of the masseteric and submandibular spatial planes in severe cases

ETIOLOGY

- Ductal obstruction is generally from salivary stasis and increased salivary viscosity as a result of dehydration, medication-induced xerostomia, or poor dental hygiene. This predisposes patients to retrograde migration of bacteria, which can then lead to suppurative sialadenitis.
- Acute suppurative sialadenitis is a bacterial infection of the salivary gland. Most frequent infecting organisms are *Staphylococcus aureus* (50% to 90% of cases), streptococcal species, *Haemophilus influenzae,* and *E. coli*; more recently, anaerobic infections have been increasing in prevalence.
- Recent surgery, Sjögren's syndrome, diabetes mellitus, hypothyroidism, renal failure, trauma, radiation therapy, chemotherapy, dehydration, and chronic illness are predisposing factors.
- Mumps is the most common cause of nonsuppurative acute sialadenitis. Majority of cases (>80%) occur in children younger than 15 yr.

Dx DIAGNOSIS

DIFFERENTIAL DIAGNOSIS

- Salivary gland neoplasm
- Ductal stricture
- Sialolithiasis
- Decreased salivary secretion as a result of medications (e.g., amitriptyline, diphenhydramine, anticholinergics)
- Dental infections
- Lymphoma
- Cervical adenitis
- Infected branchial cleft or sebaceous cysts

WORKUP

- Generally not necessary. Fig. E2 describes a diagnostic algorithm.
- Ultrasound or CT scan in patients not responding to medical treatment.

LABORATORY TESTS

- Generally not indicated.
- Complete blood count with differential to possibly reveal leukocytosis with left shift.
- Mumps antibodies if there is clinical suspicion.
- Culture of purulent drainage from salivary duct opening or percutaneously should be obtained to provide useful information in tailoring antibiotic therapy if the patient is not responding to empiric therapy.

IMAGING STUDIES

- Ultrasound or CT scan may be needed in patients with no improvement or clinical worsening after 48 to 72 hours of medical therapy. This can provide information on the presence of a drainable collection.
- Sialography should not be performed during the acute phase, as it can worsen symptoms.
- MRI is also of little utility in acute sialadenitis.

Rx TREATMENT

Nonpharmacologic therapy—these interventions are crucial in expediting resolution of symptoms.
- Massage of the gland: May express pus and relieve some of the pressure
- Hydration with intravenous fluid or aggressive oral hydration along with electrolyte repletion
- Warm compresses
- Oral cavity irrigations
- Administration of sialagogues such as lemon drops or vitamin C lozenges

ACUTE GENERAL Rx

- Amoxicillin-clavulanate 500 to 875 mg bid or cefuroxime 250 to 500 mg bid should be given for 10 days. Clindamycin is an alternative choice in patients allergic to penicillin.
- In patients coming from nursing homes or in cases of nosocomial infections, consider empiric treatment with vancomycin given the prevalence of methicillin-resistant *S. aureus.*
- IV antibiotics (e.g., cefoxitin, nafcillin) can be given in severe cases.
- Patients generally improve with 48 to 72 hours of medical treatment. If there is no improvement, consider imaging with CT or ultrasound.
- Surgical drainage is indicated for the rare cases that are refractory to medical management and that are found to have an abscess on CT or ultrasound.

DISPOSITION

Complete recovery unless the patient has underlying obstruction (e.g., ductal stricture, tumor, or stone)

REFERRAL

- To ear-nose-throat specialist for cases refractory to appropriate medical therapy
- For salivary gland incision and drainage, which may be necessary in resistant cases

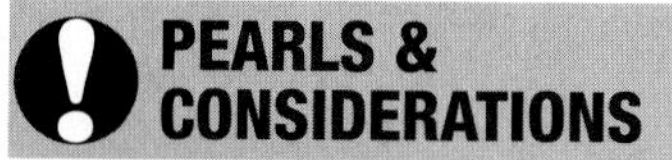

COMMENTS

Prevention of dehydration will decrease the risk of sialadenitis.

SUGGESTED READINGS
Available at ExpertConsult.com

RELATED CONTENT

Salivary Gland Inflammation (Patient Information)
Sialolithiasis (Related Key Topic)
Salivary Gland Neoplasm (Related Key Topic)

AUTHOR: **LOUIS INSALACO, M.D.**

BASIC INFORMATION

DEFINITION

Sialolithiasis is the existence of hardened intraluminal deposits in the ductal system of a salivary gland.

SYNONYMS

Salivary gland stone
Salivary calculus

ICD-10CM CODE

K11.5 Sialolithiasis

EPIDEMIOLOGY & DEMOGRAPHICS

Affects patients mostly in the fifth to eighth decades and occurs most commonly in the submandibular gland (80%); less than 20% of occurrences are located in a parotid gland.

PHYSICAL FINDINGS & CLINICAL PRESENTATION

- Symptoms: Colicky postprandial pain and swelling of a salivary gland. Tends to have a remitting/relapsing course.
- Signs: Swelling and tenderness of a salivary gland. The stone may be felt with bimanual palpation of the floor of the mouth or inner cheek.

ETIOLOGY

- The cause is unknown. Contributing factors include saliva stagnation, sialadenitis (inflammation of a salivary gland), ductal inflammation, or injury (Fig. 1).
- Gout is a known cause of salivary gland calculi.
- Salivary calculus composition is mainly calcium phosphate and carbonate, often combined with small proportions of magnesium, zinc, ammonium salts, and organic materials or debris.

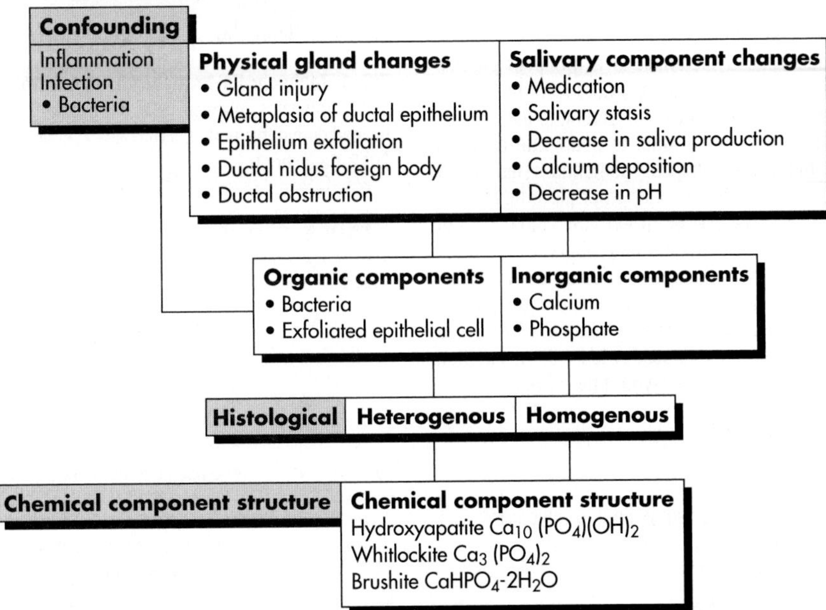

FIG. 1 Algorithm of clinical findings and pathogenesis of sialolithiasis. (From Lee LT, Wong YK: Sialolithiasis in minor salivary glands, *J Oral Maxillofac Surg*, 2010.)

DIAGNOSIS

DIFFERENTIAL DIAGNOSIS

- Lymphadenitis
- Salivary gland tumor
- Salivary gland bacterial (*Staphylococcus* or *Streptococcus*), viral (mumps), or fungal infection (sialadenitis)
- Noninfectious salivary gland inflammation (e.g., Sjögren's syndrome, sarcoidosis, lymphoma)
- Salivary duct stricture
- Dental abscess

IMAGING STUDIES

- X-ray: 90% of submandibular stones are radiopaque and will show up on x-ray. 90% of parotid stones are radiolucent and will not show up on x-ray.
- Non–contrast-enhanced computed tomography is very useful in detecting nearly all salivary stones.
- Ultrasound can detect 90% of salivary stones >2 mm.
- Sialography has a 95% to 100% sensitivity in detecting stones, although it is more invasive than the above options and requires contrast injection into the affected duct.

TREATMENT

- Nonsurgical management is usually the first-line treatment.
  1. Warm compresses, gland massages, sialogogues (lemon wedges, sour candies), IV or oral hydration.
  2. Antibiotics if associated bacterial sialadenitis is present.
- Surgical treatment:
  1. The surgical approach depends on the location of the stone. Submandibular stones in the distal aspect of the duct that are palpable may be excised transorally under local anesthesia. More proximal stones may require removal of the submandibular gland. Sialoendoscopy is a newer technique where a rigid endoscope and specialized instruments and/or lasers are used to visualize and remove the stones. Stones in the parotid duct also may be accessible via the transoral approach or may require parotidectomy. Sialoendoscopy is also an option for parotid stones.
  2. Extracorporeal shock wave lithotripsy is an alternative technique that breaks up the stones into smaller fragments that can be secreted naturally through the duct.

REFERRAL

To otorhinolaryngologist

SUGGESTED READINGS

Available at ExpertConsult.com

RELATED CONTENT

Salivary Gland Stones (Patient Information)
Sialadenitis (Related Key Topic)

AUTHOR: **LOUIS INSALACO, M.D.**

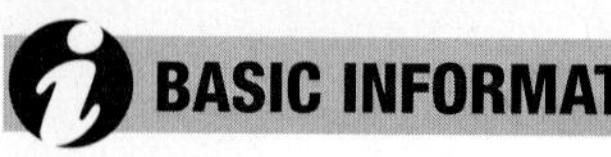

BASIC INFORMATION

DEFINITION

Sinus node dysfunction is a group of cardiac rhythm disturbances characterized by abnormalities of the sinus node leading to the inability of the SA node to react to heart rate changes to meet physiological demands. This entity includes (1) chronic, inappropriate bradycardia; (2) sinus pauses or arrest; (3) sinoatrial exit block; and (4) alternating sinus bradycardia with paroxysmal supraventricular tachyarrhythmias (frequently atrial fibrillation) known as tachycardia-bradycardia syndrome. When sinus node dysfunction is associated with symptoms, it is called sick sinus syndrome (SSS).

SYNONYMS

Sinus pause
Sinus arrest
Inappropriate persistent sinus bradycardia
Tachycardia-bradycardia syndrome
Sinoatrial exit block
SSS
Bradycardia-tachycardia syndrome

ICD-10CM CODE
I49.5 Sick sinus syndrome

EPIDEMIOLOGY & DEMOGRAPHICS

- In children: Associated with congenital and acquired heart disease, particularly after cardiac surgery.
- In adults: It is primarily a disease of the elderly secondary to progressive idiopathic degenerative disease. A modern population study has suggested that white race, increased BMI, prolonged baseline QRS or right bundle branch block, elevated N-terminal pro-B-type natriuretic peptide, HTN, or other cardiovascular diseases are associated with increased incidence of sick sinus syndrome. With an aging population, the annual incidence of SSS is projected to increase significantly.

PHYSICAL FINDINGS & CLINICAL PRESENTATION

- Fatigue, light-headedness, syncope, presyncope, palpitations. Other manifestations include dyspnea on exertion and worsening angina.
  1. Usually symptoms are progressive; however, abrupt symptoms are not uncommon (i.e., syncope).
- Physical examination may be normal or reveal abnormalities (e.g., irregular heart rhythm, signs of congestive heart failure, heart murmurs or gallop sounds) associated with the underlying heart disease.

ETIOLOGY

- Sinus node fibrosis is the primary etiology, which may also affect the atrioventricular node, the His bundle, or its branches. Polypharmacy should be considered and obtaining an accurate medicine list is essential.
  1. Common medications include beta blockers, non-dihydropyridine calcium channel blockers, digoxin, and antiarrhythmic medications.
- Additional etiologies include acute coronary syndromes, diseases of the SA nodal artery, inflammatory and infiltrative diseases such as hemochromatosis, amyloidosis, sarcoidosis, collagen vascular diseases (SLE and scleroderma), epicardial and pericardial diseases, trauma following cardiac surgery, hypothyroidism, hypothermia, hypoxia, sepsis, muscular dystrophies (e.g., myotonic dystrophy, Friedreich ataxia), infectious etiologies such as Lyme disease, increased intracranial pressure.
  1. The sinus node artery arises from right coronary artery in 55% to 60% of people and the left circumflex artery in 40%.

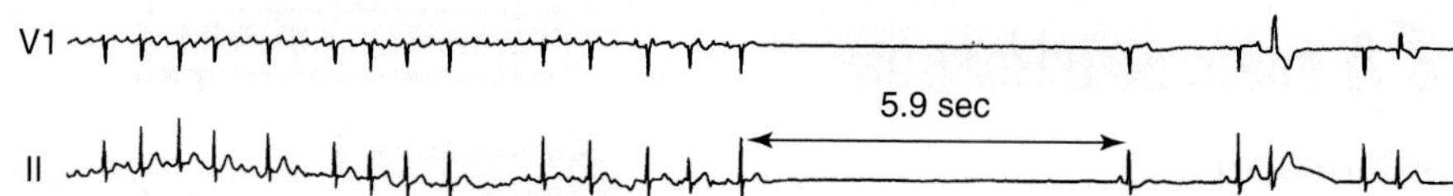

FIG. 1 Tachycardia-bradycardia syndrome. Two surface ECG leads show atrial fibrillation that spontaneously terminates followed by a 5.9-second pause before sinus rhythm resumes. The patient became lightheaded during this period. (From Issa Z, et al.: *Clinical arrhythmology and electrophysiology,* ed 2, Philadelphia, 2012, Saunders.)

TABLE 1 Indications for Permanent Pacing in Sinus Node Dysfunction

Class	Indications
I	• Sinus node dysfunction with documented symptomatic bradycardia or sinus pauses that produce symptoms • Symptomatic sinus bradycardia that is iatrogenic and will occur as a consequence of essential long-term therapy of a type and dose of drugs for which there are no acceptable alternatives • Symptomatic chronotropic incompetence
IIa	• Sinus node dysfunction, occurring spontaneously or as a result of necessary drug therapy, with a heart rate of less than 40 beats/min when a clear association between significant symptoms consistent with bradycardia has not been documented • Unexplained syncope when sinus abnormalities are observed or provoked with electrophysiologic study
IIb	• A chronic heart rate of less than 40 beats/min, while awake, in the minimally symptomatic patient
III	• Sinus node dysfunction in asymptomatic patients, including those in whom substantial sinus bradycardia (heart rate of less than 40 beats/min) is a consequence of long-term drug treatment • Sinus node dysfunction in which symptoms suggestive of bradycardia are clearly documented as not associated with a slow heart rate • Symptomatic bradycardia associated with nonessential drug therapy

ACC, American College of Cardiology; *AHA,* American Heart Association; *HRS,* Heart Rhythm Society.
Adapted from ACC/AHA/HRS 2008 revised guidelines with 2012 update

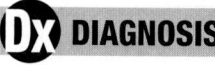

DIAGNOSIS

DIFFERENTIAL DIAGNOSIS

- Bradycardia: Atrioventricular block
- Tachycardia: Atrial fibrillation or atrial flutter, sinus tachycardia
- Medication toxicity
- Carotid sinus hypersensitivity
- Metabolic abnormality (e.g., hyperkalemia in acute kidney injury)

WORKUP

- ECG (Fig. 1)
- Ambulatory cardiac rhythm monitoring
- 24-hour ambulatory ECG (Holter) with diary to correlate symptoms to findings:
  1. Event recorder or an implantable loop recorder if symptoms are less frequent.
  2. Establishment of diagnosis is more effective with longer-term recording (at least 2-4 weeks) compared with 24-hour ambulatory ECG.
  3. Exercise stress testing to evaluate the severity of chronotropic incompetence.
  4. The term *chronotropic incompetence* is felt to represent the inability to augment heart rates appropriately in response to exercise or activities of daily living.
- Electrophysiologic testing, including sinus node recovery time and sinoatrial conduction time

Rx TREATMENT

- Permanent pacemaker placement is primarily indicated if bradycardia is symptomatic and a reversible etiology is not identified. Indications for permanent pacemaker in sinus node dysfunction are described in Table 1.
- In tachycardia-bradycardia syndrome, drug treatment is indicated for tachycardia, primarily with AV node blocking agents, after placement of the permanent pacemaker.

SUGGESTED READINGS

Available at www.expertconsult.com

AUTHORS: **MAX WEISS, M.D., RYAN WATSON, M.D., AMANDA C. DORAN, M.D., PH.D., and DANIEL R. FRISCH, M.D.**

BASIC INFORMATION

DEFINITION

- Sickle cell disease (SCD) is a hemoglobin disorder in which the substitution of valine for glutamic acid at position six of the beta globin chain yields a variant hemoglobin, hemoglobin S. When hemoglobin S is not bound to oxygen (deoxy HgbS) it can polymerize into long strands, deforming red blood cells (RBCs) into a characteristic sickle shape. Chronic RBC membrane damage from this process locks cells into the sickle shape. These abnormal cells can obstruct the microcirculation because of abnormal adherence to vascular endothelium, causing painful crises, which are the hallmark of sickle cell disease.
- Patients with SCD include those who are homozygous for sickle cell hemoglobin (HbSS), also called sickle cell anemia (SCA), and those with one sickle hemoglobin gene inherited with other hemoglobin abnormalities, notably beta thalassemia (Hgb S/β^0 or Hgb S/β^+ thalassemia) and hemoglobin C (HbSC).

SYNONYMS

Sickle cell anemia
SCA
SCD
Hemoglobin S disease

ICD-10CM CODES

D57.1	Sickle-cell disease without crisis
D57.20	Sickle-cell/Hb-C disease without crisis
D57.211	Sickle-cell/Hb-C disease with acute chest syndrome
D57.212	Sickle-cell/Hb-C disease with splenic sequestration
D57.219	Sickle-cell/Hb-C disease with crisis, unspecified
D57.3	Sickle-cell trait
D57.40	Sickle-cell thalassemia without crisis
D57.411	Sickle-cell thalassemia with acute chest syndrome
D57.412	Sickle-cell thalassemia with splenic sequestration
D57.419	Sickle-cell thalassemia with crisis, unspecified
D57.80	Other sickle-cell disorders without crisis
D57.811	Other sickle-cell disorders with acute chest syndrome
D57.812	Other sickle-cell disorders with splenic sequestration
D57.819	Other sickle-cell disorders with crisis, unspecified

EPIDEMIOLOGY & DEMOGRAPHICS

- Sickle cell disease is an autosomal-recessive disorder. In African Americans, the incidence of sickle cell anemia at birth is 1 in 600 and the incidence of all genotypes of sickle cell disease is 1 in 300. Approximately 90,000 people in the U.S. have sickle cell disease.
- Sickle cell trait occurs in approximately 300 million people worldwide, with the highest prevalence of approximately 30% to 40% in sub-Saharan Africa, but also in the southern Mediterranean region (usually as Hgb S/β^0 or Hgb S/β^+), parts of the Middle East, and India. In the U.S., it is found in nearly 10% of black Americans.
- An estimated 2000 babies are born with sickle cell disease in the U.S. each yr, and worldwide 275,000 infants are born with the disease annually.
- There is no predominant sex.

PHYSICAL FINDINGS & CLINICAL PRESENTATION

- Physical examination is variable depending on the degree of anemia and presence of acute vaso-occlusive syndromes, as well as acute pulmonary, neurologic, cardiovascular, genitourinary, and musculoskeletal complications. Table 1 summarizes organ damage seen in sickle cell disease.
- A study of the prevalence of pain sickle cell patients found that patients complained of pain on 55% of days surveyed; another study showed 40% to 80%. Chronic pain may be due to avascular necrosis of joints and is sometimes poorly explained.
- There is no clinical laboratory finding that is pathognomonic of painful crisis of sickle cell disease. The diagnosis of a painful episode is made solely on the basis of the medical history and physical examination. Elevated total bilirubin and lactate dehydrogenase (LDH) are sometimes seen with crisis due to increased hemolysis. However, hemolytic anemia is typical for sickle cell disease at baseline. "Aplastic crisis" refers to crisis presenting with severe anemia and low reticulocyte count, usually caused by B19 parvovirus infection.
- Bones are the most common site of pain. Dactylitis, or hand-foot syndrome (acute, painful swelling of the hands and feet), is the first manifestation of sickle cell disease in many infants. Irritability and refusal to walk are other common symptoms. After infancy, musculoskeletal pain can be symmetric, asymmetric, or migratory, and it may or may not be associated with swelling, low-grade fever, redness, or warmth.
- In both children and adults, sickle vaso-occlusive episodes are difficult to distinguish from osteomyelitis, septic arthritis, synovitis, rheumatic fever, or gout.
- Cholecystitis should be considered when abdominal pain is present because this is common in patients with chronic hemolysis. In general, localizing symptoms for infection (e.g., urinary symptoms) should be evaluated because these can trigger sickle crisis. Whereas patients with severe sickle cell disease have splenic atrophy in adulthood, patients with milder disease (e.g., Hgb S/C) may have splenic infarct pain in adulthood.
- The acute chest syndrome is a potentially life-threatening complication of sickle cell disease that manifests with chest pain, fever, wheezing, tachypnea, and cough. Chest radiograph may reveal pulmonary infiltrates. Causes include infection (*Mycoplasma, Chlamydia,* viruses), infarction, and fat embolism, but often no cause is identified.
- Musculoskeletal and skin abnormalities seen in sickle cell anemia include leg ulcers (particularly on the malleoli) and limb-girdle deformities caused by avascular necrosis of the femoral and humeral heads. Osteonecrosis of the heads of the femur and humerus is found in nearly 50% of adults with Hgb S/S sickle cell disease.
- Endocrine abnormalities include delayed sexual maturation and late physical maturation, especially evident in boys.
- Neurologic abnormalities on examination may include seizures and altered mental status. Strokes occur in about 10% of children and adults with sickle cell anemia and approximately 35% of children with sickle cell anemia have cerebrovascular disease.
- Infections, particularly involving *Salmonella, Staphylococcus aureus, Mycoplasma,* and *Streptococcus,* are relatively common. Catheter-associated bacteremia should be considered if a vascular access device is present; these may present without fever.
- Severe splenomegaly as a result of sequestration often occurs in children before splenic atrophy.

TABLE 1 Organ Damage Seen in Sickle Cell Disease

Organ or System	Injury
Skin	Stasis ulcer
Central nervous system	Cerebrovascular accident
Eye	Retinal hemorrhage, retinopathy
Cardiac	Congestive heart failure
Pulmonary	Intrapulmonary shunting, embolism, infarct, infection
Vascular	Occlusive phenomenon at any site
Liver	Hepatic infarct, hepatitis resulting from transfusion, hepatic sequestration, intrahepatic cholestasis
Gallbladder	Increased incidence of bilirubin gallstones caused by hemolysis
Spleen	Acute sequestration
Urinary	Hyposthenuria, hematuria
Genital	Decreased fertility, impotence, priapism
Skeletal	Bone infarcts, osteomyelitis, aseptic necrosis
Placenta	Insufficiency with fetal wastage
Leukocytes	Relative immunodeficiency
Erythrocytes	Chronic hemolysis

From Marx J et al: *Rosen's emergency medicine: concepts and clinical practice*, ed 7, Philadelphia, 2010, Mosby.

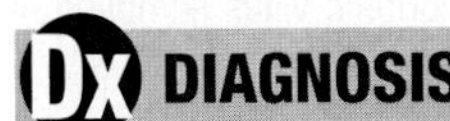
DIAGNOSIS

DIFFERENTIAL DIAGNOSIS

- Thalassemia
- Other hemolytic anemias
- The differential diagnosis of patients presenting with a painful crisis is discussed in "Physical Findings"

TABLE 2 Baseline Evaluations to Consider

	Tests
Blood tests	CBC with differential
	Reticulocyte count
	Hemoglobin HPLC or electrophoresis
	LDH
	Renal function tests
	Liver function tests
	Mineral panel
	Serum iron, ferritin, TIBC
	Vitamin D level
	Hepatitis B sAg
	Hepatitis C antibody
	RBC alloantibody screen
	RBC typing
	D-dimer[a]
	C-reactive protein[a]
	Brain natriuretic peptide
Urine and kidney tests	Urinalysis
	Renal ultrasonography[b]
Radiology	MRI or MRA brain (adults)[c] or transcranial Doppler ultrasonography starting at age 2 yr (children)
	Chest radiography[d]
	Hip or shoulder radiograph or MRI (or both)[c]
	Bone density in teenagers and adults
Cardiology and pulmonary	Echocardiogram
Neurocognitive	Neurocognitive testing[d]

CBC, Complete blood count; *HPLC*, high performance liquid chromatography; *LDH*, lactate dehydrogenase; *MRA*, magnetic resonance angiography; *MRI*, magnetic resonance imaging; *RBC*, red blood cell; *sAg*, surface antigen; *TIBC*, total iron-binding capacity.
[a]Consider following as surrogate markers after initiation of disease-modifying intervention.
[b]If hematuria with red blood cells in urine.
[c]As clinically indicated.
[d]If the patient has poor school performance, an abnormal memory, or abnormal MRI findings.
From Hoffman R et al: *Hematology, basic principles and practice*, ed 7, Philadelphia, 2018, Elsevier.

WORKUP (TABLE 2)

- Screening of all newborns regardless of racial background is performed in the U.S. Screening can be performed with sodium metabisulfite reduction test (Sickledex test).
- Hemoglobin electrophoresis will also confirm the diagnosis and is useful to identify hemoglobin variants such as fetal hemoglobin and hemoglobin C.
- Patients will have evidence of hemolysis (elevated reticulocyte count, low haptoglobin, variable elevation of LDH and total bilirubin).
- Chest x-ray often reveals typical vertebral body changes ("fish mouth" vertebrae) caused by chronic vaso-occlusive injury to vertebral bodies.
- For prenatal diagnosis, initial step is identification of parenteral globin gene mutation by DNA-based testing. If positive, then DNA-based testing of chorionic villus sampling or amniotic fluid cells is performed.

LABORATORY TESTS

- Anemia (resulting from chronic hemolysis), reticulocytosis, leukocytosis, and thrombocytosis are common. Hgb S/β^0 and Hgb S/β^+ thalassemia will have microcytosis; Hgb S/C is also typically microcytic. Hgb S/C may have normal or near-normal hematocrit, but will have characteristic changes on peripheral smear (target cells).
- Elevations of bilirubin and lactate dehydrogenase are also common, as is low haptoglobin, consistent with chronic hemolysis.
- Peripheral blood smear may reveal sickle cells, target cells, poikilocytosis, and hypochromia (Fig. 1).
- Elevated blood urea nitrogen and creatinine may be present in patients presenting acutely with dehydration or chronically with progressive renal insufficiency.
- Urinalysis may reveal hematuria and proteinuria. Patients with SCD should be screened for microalbuminuria and proteinuria with spot urine testing by 10 yr of age.

IMAGING STUDIES

- Chest x-ray or non-contrast chest CT scan to evaluate acute and chronic lung changes is helpful.
- Routine skeletal imaging is rarely helpful in acute crisis and should usually be reserved for pain that is not consistent with transient acute crisis.
- MRI or bone scan is useful to address chronic avascular necrosis or, in the acute setting osteomyelitis.
- CT scan or MRI of brain is not indicated in asymptomatic adults and children with SCD but is often needed in patients with neurologic complications such as transient ischemic attack, cerebrovascular accident, seizures, or altered mental status.
- Transcranial Doppler ultrasonography (TCD) is used to identify children with sickle cell anemia who are at risk for stroke. There should be an annual screening starting at age 2 until age 16. Patients determined to be at risk (transcranial Doppler velocity ≥200 cm/s) should be enrolled in long-term transfusion programs. These are effective in reducing risk of stroke by >90%. In adults, magnetic resonance angiography (MRA) can be used instead of TCD to identify those at risk for stroke.
- Doppler echocardiography should be performed in patients with unexplained respiratory symptoms to evaluate for pulmonary hypertension, with right heart catheterization performed if abnormal. Screening for vasculopathy is done by estimating the tricuspid regurgitant jet velocity (TRV). Elevated values are predictive of early mortality. The prevalence of pulmonary hypertension when right heart catheterization is performed is approximately 6% in adults with sickle cell disease.

Rx TREATMENT

NONPHARMACOLOGIC THERAPY

- Patients should be instructed to avoid conditions that may precipitate sickling crisis, such as extremes of cold and heat and dehydration.
- Maintain adequate hydration (PO or IV).
- Correct hypoxia when present.

ACUTE GENERAL Rx

- Initiate aggressive IV or oral hydration; most patients in crisis have evidence of dehydration.
- Aggressively diagnose and treat suspected infections such as urinary infection, respiratory infections, or catheter-associated line infections. Table 3 summarizes bacteria and viruses that most frequently cause serious infection in patients with sickle cell disease.
- Provide pain relief during the vaso-occlusive crisis (Table 4). Most patients will have a treatment history that can guide dosing. Opiate management is complicated by high levels of tolerance in patients often treated over many yrs. Patient-controlled analgesic pumps are often helpful; caution should be used when employing continuous infusions, which are usually not necessary or helpful. Morphine and hydromorphone are most commonly used. Meperidine is rarely used now and generally discouraged because of neurologic side effects, although some patients state a preference for it.
- Oral diphenhydramine (Benadryl) is used to control pruritus, which is commonly associated with opiate analgesics; preferred to IV therapy in guidelines.

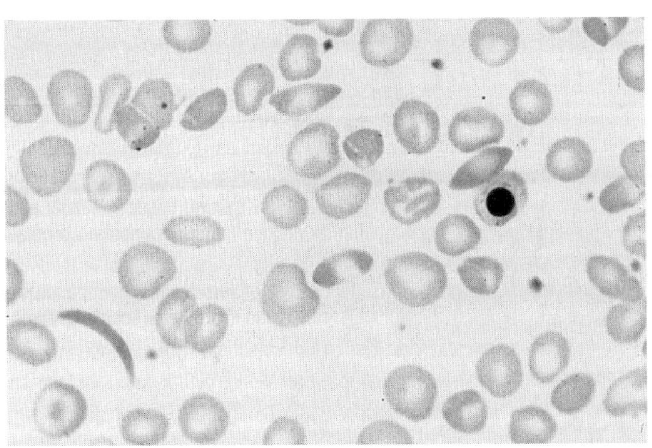

FIG. 1 Photomicrograph of a blood film. Sickle cell anemia (homozygosity for hemoglobin S). Shown are a sickle cell, boat-shaped cells, a nucleated red cell, and target cells. (From Bain BJ et al: *Dacie and Lewis practical haematology*, ed 12, Philadelphia, 2017, Elsevier.)

TABLE 3 Bacteria and Viruses That Most Frequently Cause Serious Infection in Patients with Sickle Cell Disease

Microorganism	Type of Infection	Comments
Streptococcus pneumoniae	Septicemia	Common despite prophylactic penicillin and pneumococcal vaccine
	Meningitis	Less frequent than in yrs past
	Pneumonia	Rarely documented except in infants and young children
	Septic arthritis	Uncommon
Haemophilus influenzae type b	Septicemia	
Meningitis		
Pneumonia	Much less common in recent yrs because of immunization with conjugate vaccine	
Salmonella species	Osteomyelitis	
Septicemia	Most common cause of bone and joint infection	
Escherichia coli and other gram-negative enteric pathogens	Septicemia	
Urinary tract infection		
Osteomyelitis	Focus sometimes not apparent	
Staphylococcus aureus	Osteomyelitis	Uncommon
Mycoplasma pneumoniae	Pneumonia	Pleural effusions; multilobe involvement
Chlamydia pneumoniae	Pneumonia	
Parvovirus B19	Bone marrow suppression (aplastic crisis)	High fever common; rash and other organ involvement infrequent
Hepatitis viruses (A, B, and C)	Hepatitis	Marked hyperbilirubinemia

Data from Buchanan GR, Glader BE: Benign course of extreme hyperbilirubinemia in sickle cell anemia: analysis of six cases, *J Pediatr* 91:21, 1977. (From Hoffman R et al: *Hematology, basic principles and practice*, ed 7, Philadelphia, 2018, Elsevier.)

- Incentive spirometry is helpful to reduce the risk of acute chest syndrome.
- Follow oxygenation in patients presenting with chest pain or respiratory symptoms; assess for evolving acute chest syndrome if oxygenation deteriorates.
- Urology evaluation for priapism.

CHRONIC Rx

- Hydroxyurea increases hemoglobin F levels and reduces the incidence of vaso-occlusive complications. It is helpful in patients with Hgb S/S and S/β^0 thalassemia; its value in other variants is less certain. A study of hydroxyurea with 17.5 yr of follow-up showed evidence of improved survival and no safety signals. There is strong evidence to support use of hydroxyurea therapy in children 9 mo and older to decrease the frequency of vasoocclusive crises and acute chest syndrome. Hydroxyurea therapy is also strongly recommended for adults with three or more vaso-occlusive crises during any 12-month period, with SCD pain or chronic anemia interfering with daily activities, or with severe or recurrent episodes of acute chest syndrome. Recommended starting doses are 15 mg/kg/day in adults, 5 to 10 mg/kg/day in patients with renal disease, and 20 mg/kg/day in children. It should be stopped in pregnancy and contraception counseling should be given to patients taking it. Guidelines for dose adjustments and monitoring are available (https://www.nhlbi.nih.gov/sites/www.nhlbi.nih.gov/files/sickle-cell-disease-report%20020816.pdf)
- Pharmaceutical grade L-glutamine is approved to decrease crisis symptoms in patients with Hgb S/S and Hgb S/β^0 thalassemia; benefits include decrease in acute crisis episodes, reduced hospitalization, and decrease in episodes of acute chest syndrome. Dosing is 5 to 15 g daily twice daily, taken with food or 8 oz of cold or room-temperature fluid. Constipation, nausea, headache, and abdominal discomfort were common side effects, occurring in about 15% to 20% of patients. It may work with or without concomitant use of hydroxyurea. Caution may be warranted in prescribing L-glutamine to patients with clinically significant renal or hepatic dysfunction.
- Replace folic acid (1 mg PO qd) due to loss from increased utilization of folic acid stores from to chronic hemolysis. Sickle cell patients also often have mineral and vitamin deficiencies (calcium, zinc, and vitamins A, C, D, and E) and may need vitamin and nutritional supplementation.
- Chronic pain management represents an enduring challenge, made more difficult by the current opiate addiction and overdose epidemic. In one study, patients reported pain 55% of days. Review of guidelines for safe opiate prescribing is strongly recommended and management with pain management specialists is also strongly recommended.
- Indications for transfusion in sickle cell disease are described in Table 5. Urgent exchange transfusion for acute chest syndrome with progressive hypoxia (arterial oxygen saturation <90%) or multiorgan failure may be lifesaving. Simple transfusion may be adequate in milder cases with a target Hgb of 10 g/dl. Transfusion therapy is appropriate for patients with stroke or at high risk by transcranial Doppler study (see above) if possible. Transfusion has shown benefit in children with silent infarcts by MRI in preventing progression. Transfusion to Hgb 10 g/dl is recommended in anemic patients undergoing general anesthesia to reduce crisis and respiratory complications after surgery. Patients on chronic transfusion therapy should receive RBC matched at C, E, and K antigens to avoid alloimmunization. Transfusion is not recommended for asymptomatic anemia. Serum ferritin level should be monitored quarterly. Iron overload due to blood transfusions (transfusional hemosiderosis) can be treated with chelating agents (deferoxamine [SC infusion], deferasirox [PO], and deferiprone [PO]).
- Annual screening for proteinuria is recommended. Angiotensin-converting enzyme inhibitor therapy should be started for microalbuminuria in adults with SCD to prevent

TABLE 4 Recommended Dose and Interval of Analgesics Necessary to Obtain Adequate Pain Control in Patients with Sickle Cell Disease

	Dose/Rate	Comments
Severe to Moderate Pain		
Morphine	Parenteral: 0.1-0.15 mg/kg every 3-4 h Recommended maximum single dose, 10 mg PO: 0.3-0.6 mg/kg every 4 h	Drug of choice for pain; lower doses in elderly adults and infants and in patients with liver failure or impaired ventilation
Meperidine	Parenteral: 0.75-1.5 mg/kg every 2-4 h Recommended maximum dose, 100 mg PO: 1.5 mg/kg every 4 h	Increased incidence of seizures; avoid in patients with renal or neurologic disease and those who receive MAOIs
Hydromorphone	Parenteral: 0.01-0.02 mg/kg every 3-4 h PO: 0.04-0.06 mg/kg every 4 h	
Oxycodone	PO: 0.15 mg/kg/dose every 4 h	
Ketorolac	IM: Adults: 30 or 60 mg initial dose followed by 15-30 mg; children: 1 mg/kg load followed by 0.5 mg/kg every 6 h	Equal efficacy to 6 mg MS; helps narcotic-sparing effect; not to exceed 5 days; maximum, 150 mg first day, 120 mg maximum on subsequent days; may cause gastric irritation
Butorphanol	Parenteral: Adults: 2 mg every 3-4 h	Agonist–antagonist; can precipitate withdrawal if given to patients who are being treated with agonists
Mild Pain		
Codeine	PO: 0.5-1 mg/kg every 4 h Maximum dose, 60 mg	Mild to moderate pain not relieved by aspirin or acetaminophen; can cause nausea and vomiting
Aspirin	PO: Adults: 0.3-6 mg every 4-6 h; children: 10 mg/kg every 4 h	Often given with a narcotic to enhance analgesia; can cause gastric irritation; avoid in febrile children
Acetaminophen	PO: Adults: 0.3-0.6 g every 4 h; children: 10 mg/kg	Often given with a narcotic to enhance analgesia
Ibuprofen	PO: Adults: 300-400 mg every 4 h; children: 5-10 mg/kg every 6-8 h	Can cause gastric irritation
Naproxen	PO: Adults: 500 mg/dose initially and then 250 every 8-12 h; children: 10 mg/kg/day (5 mg/kg every 12 h)	Long duration of action; can cause gastric irritation
Indomethacin	PO: Adults: 25 mg every 8 h; children: 1-3 mg/kg/day given 3 or 4 times	Contraindicated in psychiatric, neurologic, renal diseases; high incidence of gastric irritation; useful in gout

IM, Intramuscular; *MAOI*, monoamine oxidase inhibitor; *MS*, morphine sulphate; *PO*, oral.
Adapted from Charache S et al: Effect of hydroxyurea on the frequency of painful crises in sickle cell anemia: Investigators of the Multicenter Study of Hydroxyurea in Sickle Cell Anemia, *N Engl J Med* 332:1317, 1995
In Hoffman R et al: *Hematology, basic principles and practice*, ed 7, Philadelphia, 2018, Elsevier.

TABLE 5 Indications for Transfusion in Sickle Cell Disease

	Duration	Consensus	Method	Goal*
Stroke, acute	Single	+	Ex	HbS <30%
Stroke, ongoing care	Chronic	+	Either	HbS <30%
High-velocity transcranial Doppler	Chronic	+	Either	HbS <30%
ACS, initial episode	Single	+	Dir > Ex	Hgb 10
ACS, recurrent	6-12 mo	+	Either	
Pulmonary hypertension	Chronic	+	Either	
Multiorgan failure	Single	+	Ex	
Major surgery	Single	+	Dir	Hgb 10
Acute anemia	Single	+	Dir	
Recurrent spleen sequestration	Chronic	+		
Sepsis/meningitis	Single	+	Dir	
Severe chronic pain	6-12 mo	+		
Congestive heart failure	Chronic	+		
Silent infarct with abnormal neuropsychology	Chronic	–		
Pregnancy		–		
Anemia/renal failure	Chronic	–		
Leg ulcers	6-12 mo	–		
Severe growth delay		–		
Severe eye disease		–		
Priapism		–		

ACS, Acute chest syndrome; *Dir*, direct; *Ex*, exchange; *Hb*, hemoglobin type; *Hgb*, hemoglobin concentration; +, consensus reached; –, consensus not reached.
*Goal of transfusion if a consensus has been reached.
From Fuhrman BP et al: *Pediatric critical care*, ed 4, Philadelphia, 2011, Saunders.

progression of renal injury. Progressive renal injury may cause worsening anemia and responds to erythropoietin.

- Annual retinopathy screening should be performed beginning at age 10, especially for patients with Hgb S/C variant, in whom proliferative retinopathy occurs in about 30% to 50%. It is less common in Hgb S/S and other variants.
- Gene therapy for patients with sickle cell disease represents a novel approach. Clinical trials with lentiviral vector-mediated addition of an antisickling β-globin gene into autologous hematopoietic stem cells are ongoing with encouraging early results in terms of reduction of sickle cell crises and correction of the biologic hallmarks of the disease.
- Allogeneic stem cell transplantation can be curative in young patients with symptomatic sickle cell disease.
- A recent phase 2 trial for the prevention of pain crises in sickle cell disease involving crizanlizumab, an antibody against the adhesion molecule p-selectin, revealed a significantly lower rate of sickle cell–related pain crisis than placebo and was associated with a low incidence of adverse events.[2]
- Penicillin V 125 mg PO bid should be administered by age 2 mo and increased to 250 mg bid by age 3 yr. Penicillin prophylaxis can be

TABLE 6 Disease-Modifying Treatments to Consider[a]

Robust clinical data	Penicillin prophylaxis
	Streptococcus pneumoniae vaccination
	Hydroxyurea
	Chronic exchange transfusion
	Iron chelation for chronic iron overload[b]
Limited clinical data	Daily multivitamin without iron or folate supplementation *and* vitamin D replacement[c]
	Haemophilus influenzae vaccination
	Influenza vaccination
	Erythropoietin
	Phlebotomy
Experimental	Hb F reactivation with decitabine, histone deacetylase inhibitors, or imids
	Erythropoietin for chronic relative reticulocytopenia
	Nutritional supplements and antioxidants (e.g., glutamine, zinc, multivitamins)
	N-acetylcysteine

Hb F, Fetal hemoglobin.
[a]See text for specific indications and limitations.
[b]Best data from thalassemia patient experience.
[c]Risks minimal; therefore, it is generally done.
From Hoffman R et al: *Hematology, basic principles and practice*, ed 7, Philadelphia, 2018, Elsevier.

discontinued after age 5 yr except in children who have had splenectomy.
- Table 6 summarizes disease-modifying treatments to consider.

REFERRAL

- Hospitalization for pain crisis unresponsive to oral analgesics, or involving fever, respiratory symptoms, or vomiting and diarrhea.
- Optimal management requires coordination with hematology, blood banking, pain management, and psychosocial counseling and support.
- Referral for patients with organ-specific complications, notably pulmonary hypertension, acute/chronic kidney disease, and ophthalmologic complications.
- Referral to an ophthalmologist for an annual dilated retinal examination beginning at 10 yr of age.

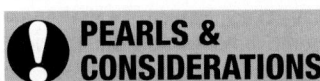

PEARLS & CONSIDERATIONS

COMMENTS

- The average life span of individuals with sickle cell trait is similar to that of the general population. It may be associated with hematuria, often painless, and rhabdomyolysis under extreme conditions. Chronic pain and acute pain are not typical of sickle cell trait. It is also associated with a higher incidence of renal medullary cancer.
- Regular immunizations, especially pneumococcal vaccination, are recommended. The prophylactic administration of penicillin soon after birth and the timely administration of pneumococcal and *Haemophilus influenzae* type b vaccines have resulted in a significant decline in the incidence of these infections. The heptavalent conjugated pneumococcal vaccine (Prevnar) should be administered from 2 mo of age. The 23-valent unconjugated pneumococcal vaccine (Pneumovax) is given from age 2 yr and can be boosted once 3 yr later. Influenza vaccination can be given after 6 mo of age.
- Pulmonary hypertension is a complication of chronic hemolysis and is associated with a high risk of death. It can be detected by Doppler echocardiography in more than 30% of adult patients with sickle cell disease. Cardiac catheterization will confirm the diagnosis. It is resistant to hydroxyurea therapy.

SUGGESTED READINGS

Available at ExpertConsult.com

RELATED CONTENT

Sickle Cell Anemia (Patient Information)

AUTHOR: **BHARTI RATHORE, M.D.**

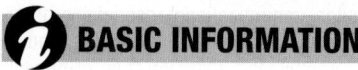

BASIC INFORMATION

DEFINITION

Silicosis is a spectrum of lung disease attributable to the inhalation of silica (silicon dioxide) in crystalline form.

SYNONYM

Pneumoconiosis caused by silica

ICD-10CM CODE

J62.8 Pneumoconiosis due to other dust containing silica

EPIDEMIOLOGY & DEMOGRAPHICS

- Occupational disease affecting men and women involved in gathering, milling, processing, or using silica-containing rock or sand. Jobs that can lead to silicosis are described in Box 1.
- According to the Occupational Safety and Health Administration (OSHA), an estimated 200,000 miners and 1.7 million others have experienced an occupational exposure to silica.
- African Americans have a seven times greater rate of developing silicosis compared to whites at the same level of exposure. The annual number of silicosis deaths declined 40% from 185 in 1999 to 111 in 2013, but the decline appears to have leveled off during 2010 to 2013, according to the Centers for Disease Control and Prevention.

PHYSICAL FINDINGS & CLINICAL PRESENTATION

- There are three patterns of silicosis: acute, chronic, and accelerated. The chronic form can be further subdivided in chronic simple silicosis and chronic complicated silicosis (progressive massive fibrosis).
- Acute silicosis is also known as silicoproteinosis. Develops several weeks to <5 yr after silica exposure. Presents with rapid onset of cough, weight loss, fatigue, and pleuritic chest pain.
- Chronic silicosis is the most common clinical presentation, and onset occurs after decades of repeated exposure. It has two types:
  1. Simple silicosis, which may be asymptomatic, with the only manifestation being an abnormal chest radiograph. Latency period is 10 to 20 yr and progression to massive fibrosis is rare.
  2. Progressive massive fibrosis characterized by radiographic progression and resulting fibrosis.
- Accelerated silicosis may have an initial asymptomatic phase followed by rapidly increasing frequency of symptoms parallel with worsening radiographic abnormalities. Develops <10 yr after initial high-level exposure.

BOX 1 Jobs That Can Lead to Silicosis

Mining: Surface or underground mining (tunneling)
Milling: Ground silica for abrasives and filler
Quarrying
Sandblasting (e.g., of buildings, preparing steel for painting)
Pottery; ceramic or clay work
Grinding, polishing using silica wheels
Stone work
Foundry work: Grinding, molding, chipping
Refractory brick work
Glass making: To polish and as an abrasive
Boiler work: Cleaning boilers
Manufacture of abrasives

From Goldman L, Schafer AI: *Goldman's Cecil medicine,* ed 24, Philadelphia, 2012, Saunders.

ETIOLOGY

- Silica particles are ingested by alveolar macrophages, which in turn release oxidants causing cell injury and cell death, attract fibroblasts, and activate lymphocytes, increasing immunoglobulins in the alveolar space.
- Hyperplasia of alveolar epithelial cells occurs.
- Collagen accumulates in the interstitium.
- Neutrophils also accumulate and secrete proteolytic enzymes, which leads to tissue destruction and emphysema.
- Silica dust may be carcinogenic (not proven).
- Exposure to silicosis predisposes to tuberculosis.
- Some patients develop rheumatoid silicotic pulmonary nodules and may have arthritic symptoms of rheumatoid arthritis (Caplan syndrome). Scleroderma has also been associated with silicosis.

DIAGNOSIS

DIFFERENTIAL DIAGNOSIS

- Other pneumoconiosis, berylliosis, hard metal disease, asbestosis
- Sarcoidosis
- Tuberculosis
- Interstitial lung disease
- Hypersensitivity pneumonitis
- Lung cancer
- Langerhans cell granulomatosis (histiocytosis X)
- Granulomatous pulmonary vasculitis

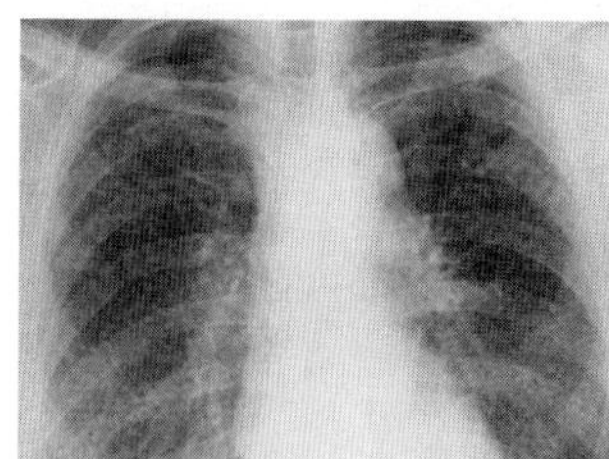

FIG. 1 Simple silicosis. There are multiple small (2- to 4-mm) nodules distributed throughout the lungs with an upper lobe predominance. (From McLoud TC: *Thoracic radiology: the requisites,* St Louis, 1998, Mosby.)

WORKUP

- History of occupational exposure
- Chest radiograph (Fig. 1)

Acute silicosis:

- Chest radiograph demonstrates bilateral, diffuse ground-glass opacities.
- Chest CT demonstrates diffuse nodular and patchy consolidative opacities with enlargement of hilar lymph nodes.
- Milky and lipoproteinaceous effluent is seen on bronchoalveolar lavage (BAL).
- Lung biopsy is not necessary in the setting of a definite exposure history.
- Exclusion of other causes like pulmonary edema, alveolar hemorrhage, and pulmonary alveolar proteinosis is necessary.

Chronic silicosis:

- Chest radiograph demonstrates multiple small, rounded opacities (<10 cm in diameter) distributed in the upper lung zones.
- Progressive massive fibrosis (PMF) refers to coalescence of the nodules of chronic silicosis with calcified hilar adenopathy.
- Pulmonary function tests (PFT) show mixed obstructive and restrictive defect.
- High resolution CT scan (HRCT), bronchoscopy, and lung biopsies have limited diagnostic role unless atypical radiographic features are noted.

Accelerated silicosis:

- Radiographic pattern is that of simple silicosis, although development of radiographic abnormalities is more rapid. This has greater risk for PMF.

TREATMENT

- Treatment is symptomatic (supplemental O_2 for hypoxemia, bronchodilators, antibiotics for infections).
- Prevention (industrial hygiene).
- Smoking cessation.
- Vaccination against influenza and pneumococcus.
- Whole-lung lavage may have a role in acute silicoproteinosis.
- Treatment of associated tuberculosis if present.
- Consider lung transplant for patients who develop chronic respiratory failure.
- Once patients progress to fibrosis, no therapies can alter the course of the disease.

ASSOCIATED COMPLICATIONS

Silicosis is associated with increased risk of mycobacterial infections, including tuberculosis, chronic necrotizing aspergillosis, lung cancer, rheumatic disorders, and chronic airflow obstruction.

RELATED CONTENT

Silicosis (Patient Information)

AUTHORS: **JAVERYAH SAFI, M.D.,** and **SAMAAN RAFEQ, M.D.**

BASIC INFORMATION

DEFINITION

Sinusitis is inflammation of the mucous membranes lining one or more of the paranasal sinuses. The various presentations are:

- Acute sinusitis: Infection lasting <4 wk, with complete resolution of symptoms.
- Subacute infection: Lasts from 4 to 12 wk, with complete resolution of symptoms.
- Recurrent acute infection: Episodes of acute infection lasting <30 days, with resolution of symptoms, which recur at intervals at least 10 days apart.
- Chronic sinusitis: Inflammation of the paranasal sinuses and nasal cavities lasting >12 wk, with persistent upper respiratory symptoms. It accounts for 1% to 2% of total physician encounters.
- Acute bacterial sinusitis superimposed on chronic sinusitis: New symptoms that occur in patients with residual symptoms from prior infection(s). With treatment, the new symptoms resolve but the residual ones do not.

SYNONYM

Rhinosinusitis: Sinusitis is almost always accompanied by inflammation of the nasal mucosa; thus it is now the preferred term.

ICD-10CM CODES

J32.9	Chronic sinusitis, unspecified
J01.90	Acute sinusitis, unspecified
J01.00	Acute maxillary sinusitis, unspecified
J01.01	Acute recurrent maxillary sinusitis
J01.10	Acute frontal sinusitis, unspecified
J01.11	Acute recurrent frontal sinusitis
J01.20	Acute ethmoidal sinusitis, unspecified
J01.21	Acute recurrent ethmoidal sinusitis
J01.30	Acute sphenoidal sinusitis, unspecified
J01.31	Acute recurrent sphenoidal sinusitis
J01.80	Other acute sinusitis
J01.81	Other acute recurrent sinusitis
J01.91	Acute recurrent sinusitis, unspecified
J32.0	Chronic maxillary sinusitis
J32.1	Chronic frontal sinusitis
J32.2	Chronic ethmoidal sinusitis
J32.3	Chronic sphenoidal sinusitis
J32.8	Other chronic sinusitis

EPIDEMIOLOGY & DEMOGRAPHICS

INCIDENCE (IN U.S.): Seems to correlate with the incidence of upper respiratory tract infections and higher in women than men; 30 million cases a yr in the U.S.

PEAK INCIDENCE:

- Fall, winter, spring: September through March
- In adults: Greatest incidence between 45 and 74 yr of age
- Approximately 6% to 7% of children presenting with respiratory symptoms have acute sinusitis

PHYSICAL FINDINGS & CLINICAL PRESENTATION

- Patients often give a history of a recent upper respiratory illness with some improvement, then a relapse.
- Mucopurulent secretions in the nasal passage:
  1. Purulent nasal and postnasal discharge lasting 7 to 10 days
  2. Facial tightness, pressure, or pain
  3. Nasal obstruction
  4. Headache
  5. Decreased sense of smell
  6. Purulent pharyngeal secretions, brought up with cough, often worse at night
- Erythema, swelling, and tenderness over the infected sinus in a small proportion of patients:
  1. Diagnosis cannot be excluded by the absence of such findings.
  2. These findings are not common, and do not correlate with number of positive sinus aspirates.
- Intermittent low-grade fever in about half of adults with acute bacterial sinusitis.
- Toothache is a common complaint when the maxillary sinus is involved.
- Periorbital cellulitis and excessive tearing with ethmoid sinusitis:
  1. Orbital extension of infection: Chemosis, proptosis, impaired extraocular movements
- Characteristics of acute sinusitis in children with upper respiratory tract infections:
  1. Persistence of symptoms
  2. Cough
  3. Bad breath
- Symptoms of chronic sinusitis (may or may not be present):
  1. Nasal or postnasal discharge
  2. Fever
  3. Facial pain or pressure
  4. Headache
- Nosocomial sinusitis is typically seen in patients with nasogastric tubes or nasotracheal intubation.

ETIOLOGY

- Each of the four paranasal sinuses is connected to the nasal cavity by narrow tubes (ostia), 1 to 3 mm in diameter; these drain directly into the nose through the turbinates. The sinuses are lined with a ciliated mucous membrane (mucoperiosteum).
- Acute viral infection:
  1. Infection with the common cold or influenza
  2. Mucosal edema and sinus inflammation
  3. Decreased drainage of thick secretions/obstruction of the sinus ostia
  4. Subsequent entrapment of bacteria
     a. Multiplication of bacteria
     b. Secondary bacterial infection
- Other predisposing factors:
  1. Tumors
  2. Polyps
  3. Foreign bodies
  4. Congenital choanal atresia
  5. Other entities that cause obstruction of sinus drainage
  6. Allergies
  7. Asthma
- Dental infections lead to maxillary sinusitis.
- Viruses recovered alone or in combination with bacteria (in 16% of cases):
  1. Rhinovirus
  2. Coronavirus
  3. Adenovirus
  4. Parainfluenza virus
  5. Respiratory syncytial virus
- The principal bacterial pathogens in sinusitis are *Streptococcus pneumoniae*, nontypable *Haemophilus influenzae,* and *Moraxella catarrhalis.*
- In the remainder of cases *Streptococcus pyogenes, Staphylococcus aureus,* beta-hemolytic streptococci, and mixed anaerobic infections (*Peptostreptococcus, Fusobacterium, Bacteroides, Prevotella* spp.) are found.
- Infection is polymicrobial in about one third of cases.
- Anaerobic infections are seen more often in cases of chronic sinusitis and in cases associated with dental infection; anaerobes are unlikely pathogens in sinusitis in children.
- Fungal pathogens are isolated with increasing frequency in immunocompromised patients but remain uncommon pathogens in the paranasal sinuses. Fungal pathogens include *Phaeohyphomycosis, Aspergillus, Pseudallescheria, Sporothrix,* and *Zygomycetes* spp.
- Nosocomial infections: Occur in patients with nasogastric tubes, nasotracheal intubation, cystic fibrosis, and immunocompromised state.
  1. *S. aureus* (including MRSA)
  2. *Pseudomonas aeruginosa*
  3. *Klebsiella pneumoniae*
  4. *Enterobacter* spp.
  5. *Proteus mirabilis*
- Organisms typically isolated in chronic sinusitis:
  1. *S. aureus*
  2. *S. pneumoniae*
  3. *H. influenzae*
  4. *P. aeruginosa*
  5. Anaerobes

DIAGNOSIS

DIFFERENTIAL DIAGNOSIS

- Temporomandibular joint disease
- Migraine headache
- Cluster headache
- Dental infection
- Trigeminal neuralgia
- Allergic rhinitis
- Drugs (cocaine, decongestant overuse)
- Gastroesophageal reflux disease
- Wegener granulomatosis
- Cystic fibrosis

WORKUP

- The diagnosis is generally based on clinical signs and symptoms (purulent rhinorrhea and facial pain). Radiologic tests and cultures are not recommended initially and should be considered only when treatment is ineffective and sinusitis persists.

- In the normal healthy host, the paranasal sinuses should be sterile. Although the contiguous structures are colonized with bacteria and likely contaminate the sinuses, the mucociliary lining functions to remove these bacteria.
- Gold standard for diagnosis: Recovery of bacteria in high-density $\geq 10^4$ colony-forming units/ml from a paranasal sinus, in the setting of a patient with history of upper respiratory infection and symptoms persisting for 7 to 10 days. Sinus aspiration is the best method for obtaining cultures; however, it must be performed by an otorhinolaryngologist and is not practical for the primary care practitioner. Therefore, most diagnoses are based on the clinical history and presentation, possibly supported by radiologic evaluations.
  1. Overall, standard radiographs are of limited use in diagnosis, although negative films are strong evidence against the diagnosis
  2. CT scans:
     a. Much more sensitive than plain radiographs in detecting acute changes and disease in the sinuses
     b. Recommended for patients requiring surgical intervention, including sinus aspiration; it is a useful adjunct to guide therapy
  3. Transillumination:
     a. Used for diagnosis of frontal and maxillary sinusitis
     b. Absence of light transmission indicates that sinus is filled with fluid
     c. Dullness (decreased light transmission) is less helpful in diagnosing infection
  4. Endoscopy:
     a. Used to visualize secretions coming from the ostia of infected sinuses
     b. Culture collection via endoscopy often contaminated by nasal flora; not nearly as good as sinus puncture
  5. Sinus puncture:
     a. Gold standard for collecting sinus cultures
     b. Generally reserved for treatment failures, suspected intracranial extension, and nosocomial sinusitis

Rx TREATMENT

NONPHARMACOLOGIC THERAPY

To help promote sinus drainage:

- Air humidification with vaporizers (for steam) or humidifiers (for a cool mist)
- Application of hot, wet towel over the face
- Sipping hot beverages
- Hydration

ACUTE GENERAL Rx

- Sinus drainage:
  1. Nasal vasoconstrictors, such as phenylephrine nose drops, 0.25% or 0.5%
  2. Topical decongestants should not be used for more than a few days because of the risk of rebound congestion
  3. Systemic decongestants
  4. Corticosteroids: Nasal or systemic corticosteroids, such as nasal beclomethasone. Oral corticosteroids combined with antibiotics may be associated with modest benefit for short-term relief of symptoms in adults with severe symptoms of acute sinusitis compared with antibiotics alone. Oral corticosteroids as monotherapy are not associated with improved clinical outcomes in adults with clinically diagnosed acute sinusitis[1]
  5. Nasal irrigation, with hypertonic or normal saline (saline may act as a mild vasoconstrictor of nasal blood flow)
  6. Use of antihistamines has no proven benefit, and the drying effect on the mucous membranes may cause crusting, which blocks the ostia, thus interfering with sinus drainage
- Analgesics, antipyretics

Antimicrobial therapy:

- Most cases of acute sinusitis have a viral cause and will resolve within 2 wk without antibiotics.
- Current treatment recommendations favor symptomatic treatment for those with mild symptoms. 85% of persons have a reduction or resolution of symptoms within 7 to 15 days without antibiotic therapy. Physicians grossly overprescribe antibiotics for presumed bacterial sinusitis despite a much higher prevalence of viral infections.
- Antibiotics should not be prescribed for mild to moderate sinusitis within the first week of illness. They should be reserved for those with persistent symptoms for more than 10 days, high fever and purulent nasal discharge or facial pain lasting for at least 3 consecutive days, or worsening symptoms after a typical viral illness lasting >5 days that had initially improved ("double sickening").
- Antibiotic therapy is usually empiric, targeting the common pathogens:
  1. First-line antibiotics in children include amoxicillin or amoxicillin/clavulanate. For adults amoxicillin/clavulanate or doxycycline is first-line agent, with quinolones (levofloxacin or moxifloxacin) reserved as second-line agents unless patient is penicillin allergic.
  2. Second-line antibiotics include the newer macrolides: clarithromycin, and oral cephalosporins: cefuroxime axetil, cefprozil, cefaclor, loracarbef, but high rate of resistance of *S. pneumoniae* is a concern with these agents as is *H. influenzae* resistance with TMP-SMX and azithromycin such that they should no longer be used as first-line agents.
  3. For patients with uncomplicated acute sinusitis, the less expensive first-line agents appear to be as effective as the costlier second-line agents.
- Hospitalization and IV antibiotics may be required for more severe infection and those with suspected intracranial complications. Broader-spectrum antibiotic coverage may be indicated in severe cases, to cover for MRSA, *Pseudomonas*, and fungal pathogens.
- Duration of therapy generally 5 to 7 days in adults rather than 10 to 14 days as recommended in the past.
  1. Optimal duration of treatment in children varies from 10 to 28 days.

Surgery:

- Surgical drainage indicated
  1. If intracranial or orbital complications suspected
  2. Many cases of frontal and sphenoid sinusitis
  3. Chronic sinusitis recalcitrant to medical therapy
- Surgical debridement imperative in the treatment of fungal sinusitis

Complications:

- Untreated, sinusitis may lead to a number of serious, life-threatening complications.
- Intracranial complications include meningitis, brain abscess, and epidural and subdural empyema.
- Intracranial sequelae are more common with frontal and ethmoid infections.
- Extracranial complications include orbital cellulitis, blindness, orbital abscess, osteomyelitis.
- Extracranial sequelae are more commonly seen with ethmoid sinusitis.

CHRONIC Rx

- Chronic sinusitis: Evidence supports daily high-volume saline irrigation with topical corticosteroid therapy as a first-line therapy for chronic sinusitis. A short course of systemic corticosteroids (1-3 wk), short course of doxycycline (3 wk), or a leukotriene antagonist may be considered in patients with nasal polyps. A prolonged course (3 mo) of macrolide antibiotic may be considered for patients without polyps.
- Surgical intervention may be necessary in nonresponders

REFERRAL

- To infectious disease specialist if failure to respond to initial therapy
- To otorhinolaryngologist for:
  1. Failure to respond to therapy
  2. Suspected fungal infection
  3. Suspected intracranial or orbital complications

SUGGESTED READINGS

Available at ExpertConsult.com

RELATED CONTENT

Sinusitis (Patient Information)

AUTHOR: **GLENN G. FORT, M.D., M.P.H.**

[1]Venekamp RP et al: Systemic corticosteroid therapy for acute sinusitis, *JAMA* 313(12):1258–1259, 2015.

BASIC INFORMATION

DEFINITION

Sjögren syndrome (SS) is a chronic autoimmune disorder that targets exocrine glands. It is characterized by lymphocytic and plasma cell infiltration and destruction of salivary and lacrimal gland, resulting predominantly in dry eyes and dry mouth, but it can affect other organ systems as well.

Primary and secondary forms have been described:

- Primary: Dry mouth (xerostomia) and dry eyes (xerophthalmia) develop as isolated entities. Is immunogenetically associated with HLA-DRB1*0301 and DRB1*1501 and serologically associated with antibodies to Ro/SS-A and La/SS-B.
- Secondary: Associated with other autoimmune connective tissue diseases. The immunogenetic and serologic findings are usually those of the accompanying disease (e.g., HLA-DR4 if associated with RA).

SYNONYMS

SS
Sicca syndrome
Keratoconjunctivitis sicca
Sicca complex
Dry eye syndrome/dysfunctional tear syndrome

ICD-10CM CODES

M35.00	Sicca syndrome, unspecified
M35.01	Sicca syndrome with keratoconjunctivitis
M35.02	Sicca syndrome with lung involvement
M35.03	Sicca syndrome with myopathy
M35.04	Sicca syndrome with tubulo-interstitial nephropathy
M35.09	Sicca syndrome with other organ involvement

EPIDEMIOLOGY & DEMOGRAPHICS

INCIDENCE: 4 per 100,000; of these cases, 70% had primary SS.

PREVALENCE: Prevalence is 0.2% to 2.7% of population; secondary SS is also common and can affect up to 19% of patients with systemic lupus erythematosus (SLE) and 26% to 31% of rheumatoid arthritis (RA) and scleroderma patients.

PREDOMINANT SEX: Female:male ratio is approximately 10:1.

PREDOMINANT AGE: Peak incidence is in the fourth and fifth decade, but SS can occur in all ages.

RISK FACTOR: Seen in all races/ethnicities, but more common in Caucasians.

PHYSICAL FINDINGS & CLINICAL PRESENTATION

SS is the most common autoimmune disease and should be considered in any patient with unexplained symptoms and a positive antinuclear antibody.

2016 American College of Rheumatology/ European League Against Rheumatism classification criteria for primary SS: A score of >4 when the weights from the criteria are summed:

- Labial salivary gland with focal lymphocytic sialadenitis and focus of >1 foci/4 mm^2—score 3
- Anti-SSA/Ro positive—score 3
- Ocular staining score >5 in at least one eye—score 1
- Schirmer's test <5 mm/5 min in at least one eye—score 1
- Unstimulated whole saliva flow rate <0.1 ml/min—score 1

  Diagnosis of SS based on the prior diagnostic criteria was presence of at least two of three objective diagnostic tests below:

  1. Positive serum levels of anti-SS-A/Ro and/or anti-SS-B/La or a positive rheumatoid factor and antinuclear antibody (ANA) titer of at least 1:320.
  2. Salivary gland biopsy exhibiting focal sites of inflammation. One or more sites of inflammation per 4 mm^2 are considered to be positive.
  3. Keratoconjunctivitis sicca with ocular staining score of three or more (the dissipation rate of a specialized dye that is applied to the tear film that bathes the surface of the eye; a score of three or more is considered to be positive).
- Dry mouth with dry lips (cheilosis), erythema of tongue and other mucosal surfaces, carious teeth
- Dry eyes (conjunctival injection, corneal ulceration, blurred vision, decreased luster, enlargement of lacrimal glands, and irregularity of the corneal light reflex)
- Salivary gland enlargement and dysfunction, with subsequent difficulty in chewing and swallowing food and in speaking without frequent water intake, thickened saliva, and burning sensation in mouth
- Extra-glandular involvement occurs in 50% of patients. There are multiple systemic manifestations associated with SS, which include the following:
  1. Fever/fatigue
  2. Leukocytoclastic vasculitis may be present
  3. Skin ulceration, photosensitivity, Raynaud's phenomenon, and allergic drug eruptions
  4. Dyspareunia and pruritus can occur secondary to vaginal dryness
  5. Pulmonary involvement includes interstitial lung disease (e.g., NSIP), chronic obstructive pulmonary disease, lymphocytic interstitial pneumonitis (LIP), usual interstitial pneumonitis (UIP), fibrosis, and xerotrachea
  6. Gastrointestinal conditions such as celiac disease, esophageal dysmotility, type I autoimmune hepatitis, primary biliary cirrhosis, and pancreatitis can occur
  7. Renal manifestations include type 1 renal tubular acidosis, Fanconi syndrome, glomerulonephritis, and interstitial nephritis
  8. Neurologic involvement including peripheral neuropathy and trigeminal neuropathy
  9. Musculoskeletal symptoms including arthralgias and polymyopathy
  10. Hematologic conditions such as lymphoma and pancytopenia. Nearly 5% of patients develop B-cell lymphoma
  11. RA and other connective tissue diseases are present in secondary SS
  12. Autoimmune thyroiditis may be observed in patients with SS
  13. Pregnancy: Patients with anti-SSA antibodies have an increased risk of delivering a fetus with skin rashes or complete heart block

ETIOLOGY

Sjögren syndrome is an autoimmune disorder of unclear etiology. It is associated with certain HLA-DQ and HLA-DR alleles. It has been postulated that viral agents (e.g., hepatitis C and Epstein-Barr virus) may trigger the clinical manifestations. The pathogenesis involves a complex interplay of several factors, including genetic and epigenetic controls of immune homeostasis and gene expression, age, gender, and environmental insults.

Over 90% of the infiltrating cells are CD4+ T lymphocytes with memory phenotype (70%) and B lymphocytes (20%). The remaining 10% are an admixture of plasma cells, CD8+ T lymphocytes, T regulatory cells, natural killer cells, and dendritic cells.

Dx DIAGNOSIS

DIFFERENTIAL DIAGNOSIS

- Medication-related dryness (e.g., anticholinergics, antihistamines, diuretics)
- Age-related exocrine gland dysfunction
- Mouth breathing
- Anxiety
- HIV infection
- Hepatitis C infection
- Diabetes mellitus
- Chronic sialadenitis
- Acromegaly
- Type V hyperlipidemia
- Graft-versus-host disease
- Other: Sarcoidosis, primary salivary hypofunction, radiation injury, amyloidosis
- IgG4-related disease
- Ocular herpetic lesions, blepharitis, corneal abrasions, contact lens irritation
- Vitamin A deficiency
- An algorithm for the diagnosis of SS is provided in Fig. 1

WORKUP

Workup involves ocular and oral examination and laboratory and radiographic testing to demonstrate the following criteria for diagnosis of primary and secondary SS.

 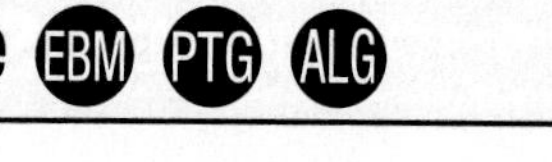

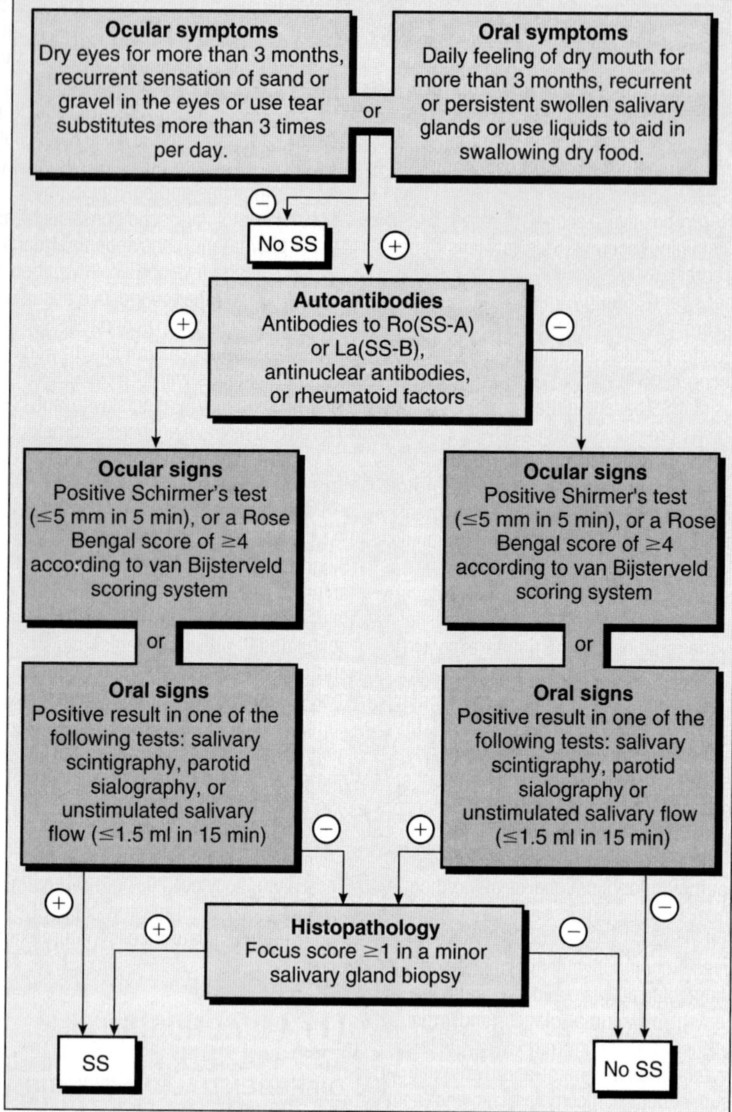

FIG. 1 Suggested algorithm for the diagnosis of Sjögren syndrome. Exclusion criteria include hepatitis C or human immunodeficiency virus infection, sarcoidosis, graft-versus-host disease, preexisting lymphoma, previous head or neck irradiation, and use of anticholinergic drugs. (From Hochberg MC et al: *Rheumatology,* ed 5, St Louis, 2011, Mosby.)

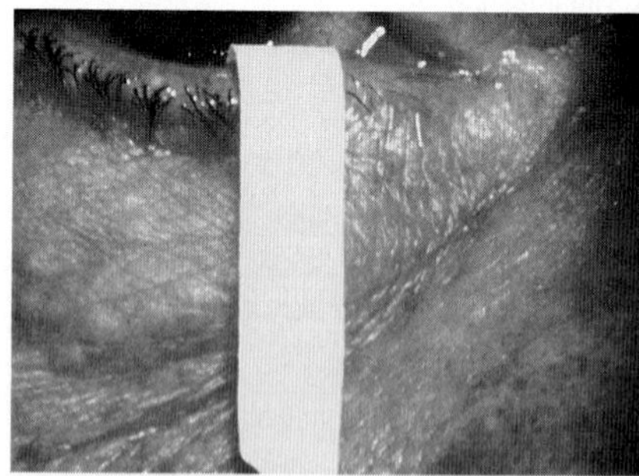

FIG. 2 Schirmer test in a patient with Sjögren syndrome. Wetting of less than 5 mm/5 min of the filter paper strip is shown. (From Hochberg MC et al: *Rheumatology,* ed 5, St Louis, 2011, Mosby.)

PRIMARY:

- Symptoms and objective signs of ocular dryness:
  1. Schirmer test (Fig. 2): <5 mm wetting per 5 min. There is a 15% false-positive and false-negative rate.
  2. Zone-quick diagnostic threads: A sterile cotton thread with pH indicator, phenol red. Yellow turns to red in contact with tears
  3. Positive Rose Bengal or fluorescein staining of cornea and conjunctiva to demonstrate keratoconjunctivitis sicca
  4. Tear breakup time and tear osmolality measured after instillation of fluorescein
- Symptoms and objective signs of dry mouth:
  1. Decreased parotid flow using Lashley cups or other methods
  2. Abnormal biopsy result of minor salivary gland (focus score >1 based on average of four assessable lobules)
  3. Sialometry (sensitivity 56%, specificity 81%): Assessment of rate of saliva production in which collection of ≤1.5 ml after two expectorations 15 min apart is considered positive
- Evidence of systemic autoimmune disorder:
  1. Elevated rheumatoid factor (70% to 90% of patients)
  2. Elevated titer of ANA >1:320 (80% of patients)
  3. Presence of anti-SS-A (Ro) (>60% of patients) or anti-SS-B (La) antibodies (40% of patients)

SECONDARY:

- Characteristic signs and symptoms of SS
- Clinical features sufficient to allow a diagnosis of RA, SLE, polymyositis, or scleroderma

LABORATORY TESTS

- Positive ANA (80% of patients) with autoantibodies anti-SS-A and anti-SS-B may be present.
- Additional laboratory abnormalities may include elevated erythrocyte sedimentation rate, anemia, leukopenia, thrombocytopenia, abnormal liver function studies, elevated serum $beta_2$ microglobulin levels, rheumatoid factor (50% to 60%), hypergammaglobulinemia, antibodies to double-stranded DNA (in cases with proteinuria), depressed C3 and C4, and the presence of cryoglobulins (30% of patients).
- A definite diagnosis of SS can be made with a salivary gland biopsy (gold standard) showing focal lymphocytic sialadenitis with focus score of 1 per 4 mm^2 of glandular tissue.
- Salivary gland ultrasound can be done to characterize changes in salivary gland parenchyma (sensitivity 75%, specificity 78%). Diseased gland shows hypoechoic areas with convex borders.
- MRI of the gland shows inhomogeneous parenchyma. Finding correlates with biopsy of the gland.

Rx TREATMENT

NONPHARMACOLOGIC THERAPY

- Adequate fluid replacement. Ameliorate skin dryness by gently blotting dry after bathing, leaving a small amount of moisture, and then applying a moisturizer
- Increased environmental moisture by using humidifiers
- Proper oral hygiene (daily topical fluoride use, antimicrobial mouth rinses, and stabilization of oral cavity pH) to reduce the incidence of caries
- Sugar-free chewing gum and sour lemon lozenges to stimulate salivary secretion
- Periodic dental and ophthalmologic evaluations to screen for complications
- Reduce caffeine intake and smoking

GENERAL Rx

- Use artificial tears frequently.
- The muscarinic agonist pilocarpine (5 mg PO qid) is useful to improve dryness.
- Cyclosporine 0.05% ophthalmic emulsion may also be useful for dry eyes.
- Cevimeline, a cholinergic agent with muscarinic agonist activity, 30 mg PO tid is effective for the treatment of dry mouth in patients with SS.

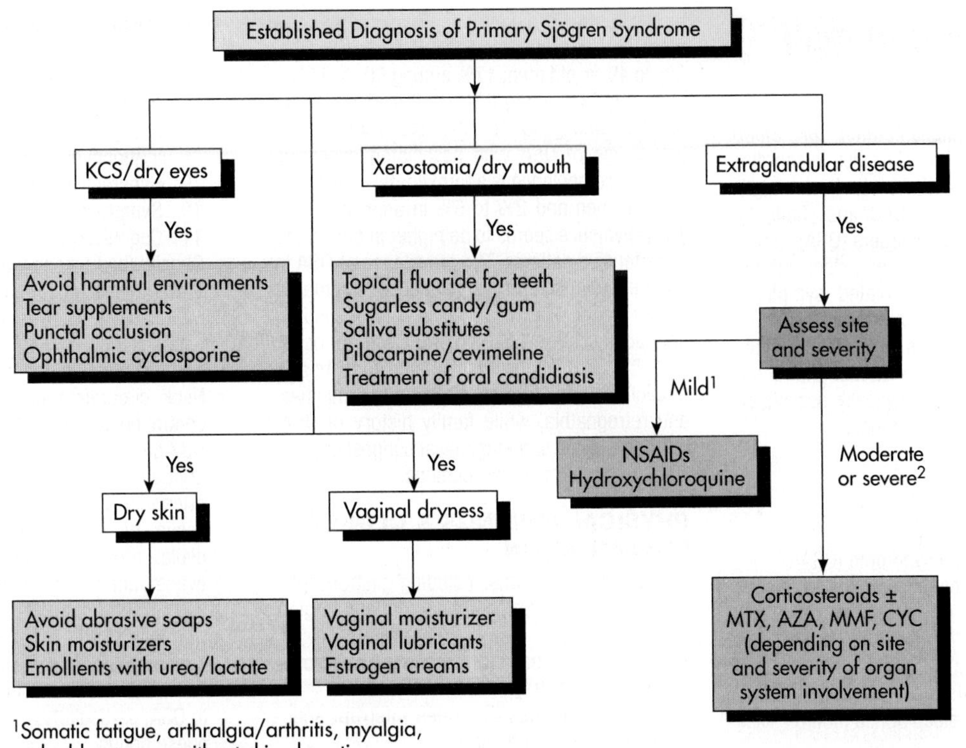

FIG. 3 Treatment algorithm for Sjögren syndrome. The treatment of Sjögren syndrome usually requires a multidisciplinary approach involving rheumatologists, ophthalmologists, dentists/oral surgeons, otolaryngologists, and other subspecialists, depending on the extent of extra-glandular disease. In all cases, it is prudent to minimize the use of medications that can exacerbate the symptoms of dryness, such as antihistamines, antidepressants, muscle relaxers, and other drugs with anticholinergic properties. The treatment of extra-glandular disease is individualized according to the site and severity of organ system involvement. The approaches indicated in the algorithm for the treatment of extra-glandular disease are not supported by evidence from randomized, controlled trials, but rather from expert opinion based on retrospective case series and clinical experience. *AZA,* Azathioprine; *CNS,* central nervous system; *CYC,* cyclophosphamide; *KCS,* keratoconjunctivitis sicca; *LIP,* lymphocytic interstitial pneumonitis; *MMF,* mycophenolate mofetil; *MTX,* methotrexate; *NSAIDs,* nonsteroidal antiinflammatory drugs; *NSIP,* nonspecific interstitial pneumonitis; *PNS,* peripheral nervous system. (From Firestein GS et al: *Kelly's textbook of rheumatology,* ed 9, Philadelphia, 2013, Saunders.)

- Hydroxychloroquine alone or in conjunction with methotrexate may be useful for arthralgias and cutaneous manifestations.
- Oral cyclosporine only improves the symptoms of subjective dryness.
- Tumor necrosis factor (TNF) antagonists have not shown benefit in short-duration placebo-controlled trials.
- Rituximab (RTX) has shown some improvement in oral dry mouth symptoms, relieving marked salivary and lacrimal gland swelling in a retrospective review and showing possible reduced fatigue in a randomized clinical trial.
- Propionic acid gel can be used for vaginal dryness.
- Systemic manifestations are treated according to symptoms and complications.
- Cyclophosphamide, azathioprine, and mycophenolate mofetil are generally reserved for life-threatening extra-glandular manifestations.
- Fig. 3 describes a treatment algorithm for Sjögren syndrome.

REFERRAL

- Rheumatology referral is generally indicated.
- Referral should be made to an oncologist when lymphoma is suspected.

PEARLS & CONSIDERATIONS

COMMENTS

- Unusual presentations of SS may occur in association with polymyalgia rheumatica, chronic fatigue syndrome, fever of unknown origin, and inflammatory myositis.
- The most serious complication of primary SS is the development of non-Hodgkin's lymphoma and other lymphoproliferative disorders, which occur at a 10- to 44-fold increased rate as compared to age-matched controls.
- The presence of parotid gland enlargement, rheumatoid factor, low C4, cryoglobulinemia, lymphopenia, and higher levels of disease activity as measured by EULAR Sjögren Syndrome Disease Activity Index (ESSDAI) predicts a higher lymphoma risk.

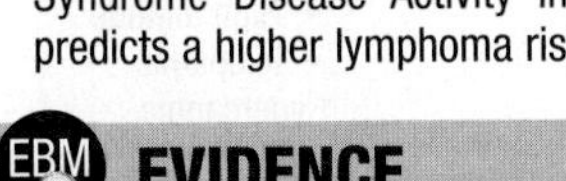

EVIDENCE

Available at ExpertConsult.com

SUGGESTED READINGS

Available at ExpertConsult.com

RELATED CONTENT

Sjögren Syndrome (Patient Information)

AUTHOR: **PIEUSHA MALHOTRA, M.D., M.P.H.**

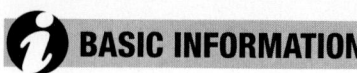

DEFINITION

The *International Classification of Sleep Disorders, Third Edition,* classifies sleep-disordered breathing disorders into five categories: central sleep apnea syndrome (Table 1), obstructive sleep apnea disorders (OSA), sleep-related hypoventilation disorders, sleep-related hypoxemia disorder, and isolated symptoms and normal variants. The American Academy of *Sleep Medicine* defines OSA as repetitive episodes of upper airway obstruction that occur during sleep and that are typically associated with oxyhemoglobin desaturations.

SYNONYMS

Sleep apnea syndrome
Sleep-disordered breathing
Obstructive sleep apnea syndrome (OSA)
Obstructive sleep apnea–hypopnea syndrome

ICD-10CM CODES

G47.30	Sleep apnea, unspecified
G47.31	Primary central sleep apnea
G47.33	Obstructive sleep apnea (adult) (pediatric)
G47.37	Central sleep apnea in conditions classified elsewhere
G47.39	Other sleep apnea
P28.3	Primary sleep apnea of newborn

EPIDEMIOLOGY & DEMOGRAPHICS

OSA is a common disease in the U.S. Data from the Wisconsin Cohort Study indicated that the current prevalence of moderate to severe sleep-disordered breathing (apnea-hypopnea index, measured as events/hour, ≥15) is 10% among 30- to 49-yr-old men; 17% among 50- to 70-yr-old men; 3% among 30- to 49-yr-old women; and 9% among 50- to 70-yr-old women.[1] The prevalence of OSA with associated excessive daytime somnolence is approximately 3% to 7% in adult men and 2% to 5% in adult women.[2] The prevalence seems to be higher in obese and hypertensive patients. The prevalence of OSA in the general pediatric population is estimated to be 1% to 6%. However, in obese children and adolescents, OSAH is reported to occur in 19% to 61%. Risk factors include obesity, craniofacial and upper airway abnormalities, and retrognathia, while family history of OSA, current tobacco smoking, nasal congestion, and diabetes are clinical associations.

PHYSICAL FINDINGS & CLINICAL PRESENTATION

- Nocturnal symptoms, including gastroesophageal reflux symptoms, nocturia, and angina pectoris
- Snoring (potentially loud, habitual, and bothersome to others)
- Witnessed apneas that often interrupt snoring and end with a snort
- Gasping, choking, or smothering sensations that arouse the patient from sleep
- Restless sleep associated with frequent arousals
- Daytime symptoms:
  1. Nonrestorative sleep
  2. Not feeling refreshed upon awakening
  3. Morning headache
  4. Dry mouth or throat upon awakening
  5. Excessive daytime sleepiness, typically during quiet activities
  6. Daytime fatigue or tiredness
  7. Problems with memory, concentration, and cognitive function, especially with executive functioning
  8. Easily angered, short tempered, and inattentive
  9. Hyperactivity in children
  10. Symptoms of fibromyalgia
  11. Cognitive decline (older population)
- Obesity (body mass index >30 kg/m^2)
- Insulin resistance or type 2 diabetes mellitus
- Mood swings, irritability, anxiety, and/or depression
- Decreased libido and/or impotence
- Neck circumference (surrogate marker for central obesity) of >43 cm (17 in) in men and >37 cm (15 in) in women
- Erythematous oropharynx because of snoring
- Adenotonsillar hypertrophy, excessive soft tissue, high-arched hard palate, pendulous uvula, prominent tongue, large degree of overjet, and retrognathia or micrognathia can be present
- Narrowing of lateral airway walls is independent predictor of OSA in men but not women
- Craniofacial skeletal abnormalities can lead to OSA, particularly among children and nonobese adults
- Systemic hypertension (HTN)
- Pulmonary HTN
- Family history of OSA increases risk with each additional close family member further increasing odds
- Table 2 summarizes clinical characteristics of patients with sleep apnea

ETIOLOGY

- Narrowing of upper airway as a result of obesity or increased peripharyngeal fat deposition, retrognathia and/or micrognathia, adenotonsillar hypertrophy, macroglossia, or neuromuscular weakness (Fig. 1)
- Upper airway muscular weakness as a result of neuromuscular disorders, primary CNS disorders (e.g., stroke), or metabolic disorders
- Other diseases associated with the development of OSAH (e.g., hypothyroidism, acromegaly)
- Fig. 2 illustrates the pathophysiologic consequences of OSA

Dx DIAGNOSIS

DIFFERENTIAL DIAGNOSIS

- Anemia
- Anxiety or panic disorder
- Behaviorally induced insufficient sleep syndrome
- Cardiac or heart disease
- Central sleep apnea
- Circadian rhythm disorder
- Depression
- Drug or alcohol abuse
- Gastroesophageal reflux
- Hypothyroidism
- Idiopathic hypersomnia with long or short sleep time
- Inadequate sleep hygiene

TABLE 1 Pathophysiologic Classification of Central Sleep Apneas

Physiologic	Pathologic
• Sleep transition • Phasic REM	Nonhypercapnic • Medical condition related 1. Congestive heart failure 2. Poststroke 3. ESRD 4. PAH 5. Atrial fibrillation • High altitude • Idiopathic Hypercapnic • Congenital central hypoventilation syndrome • Primary chronic alveolar hypoventilation syndromes • Other CNS disorders associated with CSA 1. Encephalitis, tumors, strokes 2. Anatomic abnormalities 3. Neurodegenerative disorders • Muscular and PNS disorders associated with CSA (selected examples) 1. Muscular dystrophies 2. Acid maltase deficiency 3. Charcot-Marie-Tooth disease and other neuropathies 4. Postpolio syndrome 5. Myasthenia gravis Disintegrative (e.g., brainstem injury, opioid induced) CSA with OSA or upper airway disorders (including treatment emergent CSA)

CNS, Central nervous system; *CSA,* central sleep apnea; *ESRD,* end-stage renal disease; *OSA,* obstructive sleep apnea; *PAH,* pulmonary arterial hypertension, *PNS,* peripheral nervous system; *REM,* rapid eye movements.
From Kryger M et al: *Principles and practice of sleep medicine,* ed 6, Philadelphia, 2017, Elsevier.

- Insomnia
- Medication effect
- Narcolepsy
- Nocturnal asthma
- Nocturnal gastroesophageal reflux
- Nocturnal seizures
- Obesity-hypoventilation syndrome
- Parasomnias
- Parkinson's disease
- Periodic limb movement disorder
- Primary snoring
- Pulmonary or lung disease
- Restless legs syndrome
- Shift work sleep disorder
- Sleep fragmentation (multiple causes)

TABLE 2 Clinical Characteristics of Patients with Sleep Apnea

Central		
Nonhypercapnic	**Hypercapnic**	**Obstructive**
Insomnia	Daytime sleepiness Morning headache	Daytime sleepiness
Mild intermittent snoring	Snoring	Prominent snoring
Awakenings (choking, dyspnea)	Respiratory failure	Witnessed apneas, gasping
Normal body habitus	Normal or obese Polycythemia Cor pulmonale	Commonly obese Upper airway narrowing

From Kryger M et al: *Principles and practice of sleep medicine*, ed 6, Philadelphia, 2017, Elsevier.

WORKUP

- Evaluation should include questions about snoring, witnessed apneas, gasping or choking episodes, restless sleep, and excessive daytime sleepiness. Fig. 3 describes the Epworth Sleepiness Scale, an instrument that evaluates the likelihood of dozing in eight different situations in the preceding 30 days.
- Mood swings and personality changes should be addressed.
- Job performance and difficulty driving or previous motor vehicle accidents related to excessive daytime sleepiness should be discussed.
- Additional concerns include morning dry mouth/throat, morning headaches, alcohol intake, weight gain, mood or personality changes.
- A thorough drug history should be performed that includes the use of narcotics, muscle relaxants, and sedatives.
- A family history should target the presence of OSA.
- Physical exam is frequently normal in patients with OSA except for the presence of obesity, enlarged neck circumference, and possibly HTN.
- OSAH is confirmed by nocturnal polysomnography (PSG), which is the gold standard for diagnosis (Fig. 4). The PSG should be performed during the patient's typical sleeping hours; it should include all in all stages of sleep in the supine position. A growing trend is evaluating patients with home testing rather than in-lab polysomnography, although this is not yet approved for routine pediatric testing.
- The severity of the OSA is determined by the apnea-hypopnea index (AHI) (Table 3), which is derived from the total number of apneas and hypopneas divided by the total sleep time.
- Recommended severity cutoff levels for the AHI in adult patients are as follows:
  1. Mild: 5 to 15 respiratory events per hour (with symptoms)
  2. Moderate: 15 to 30 respiratory events per hour
  3. Severe: >30 respiratory events per hour

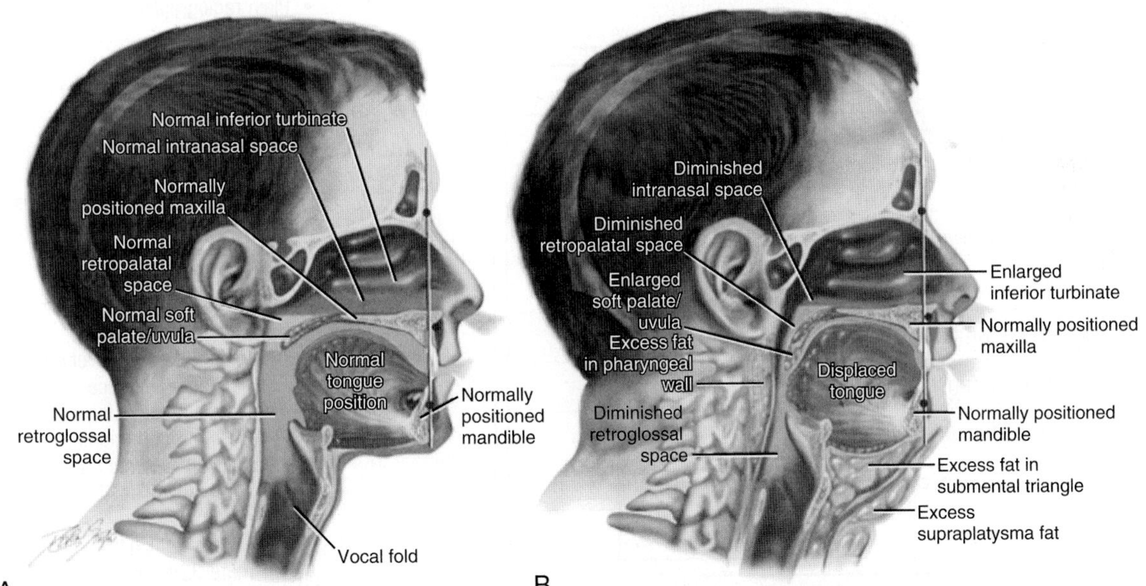

FIG. 1 Normal and abnormal airway anatomy. A, This illustrated midline sagittal cross section of the head and neck depicts the normal upper airway and maxillofacial spaces and anatomy of a healthy, normal-weight 20-year-old man. The patient has a normal upper and lower facial skeleton and normal soft tissue indicators (soft palate, tongue, tonsils, and adenoids), without any compromise of the intranasal cavity. **B,** With increasing age and weight gain, the same individual, 3 decades later, has an elevated body mass index. Although the anatomy of the upper and lower facial skeleton remains fixed without any changes, fatty tissue consisting of adipose cells has expanded and infiltrated the crevices and space in the upper airway. Particularly compromised are the retropharyngeal and the lateral pharyngeal tissues, the soft palate, and the floor of the mouth, culminating in restricted airflow. At age 20 yr, the patient had normal upper airway space (the intranasal, retropalatal, and the retroglossal sites were all well visualized and with appropriate space for air flow to proceed smoothly and unimpeded). At age 50 yr, he has developed obstructive sleep apnea: The normal airspace *(green)* is severely compromised because of restriction of the upper airway, intranasal space, and retropalatal and the retroglossal spaces. A *perfect storm* indeed. (From Posnick JC: *Orthognathic surgery: principles and practice*, St. Louis, 2014, Elsevier, 992–1058.)

Pathophysiologic consequences of obstructive sleep apnea

- Hypoxemia
- Hypercapnia
- Intrathoracic pressure fluctuations
- Reoxygenation
- Arousals

→

Possible intermediate CV disease mechanisms

- Sympathetic activation
  - Vasoconstriction
  - Acute tachycardia
  - Acute BP elevations
  - ↓ CV variability
- ↑ LV wall stress
- ↑ Afterload
- Acute diastolic dysfunction
- Left atrial stretch
- Left atrial enlargement
- Insulin resistance
- Hyperleptinemia
- Hypercoagulability
- Systemic inflammation
- Oxidative stress
- Endothelial dysfunction

→

CV disease associations and risks

- Hypertension
- Diastolic dysfunction
- Systolic dysfunction
- Sinus pause or arrest
- Atrioventricular block
- Atrial fibrillation
- Ventricular ectopy
- Nocturnal angina
- Coronary artery disease
- Cerebrovascular disease
- Sudden cardiac death

FIG. 2 The pathophysiologic consequences of obstructive sleep apnea disorders (OSA) may acutely and chronically elicit multiple intermediate cardiovascular *(CV)* disease mechanisms, which may promote the association of OSA with a number of cardiovascular conditions and diseases. *BP,* Blood pressure; *LV,* left ventricular. (From Mann DL et al: *Braunwald's heart disease,* ed 10, Philadelphia, 2015, Elsevier.)

Epworth Sleepiness Scale

Situation	Score
Sitting and reading	
Watching TV	
Sitting inactive in public place	
Passenger in car	
Lying down to rest in afternoon	
Sitting talking to someone	
Sitting after lunch without alcohol	
In a car, stopped for minutes in traffic	
Total (normal #10)	

Dozing
0 = Never
1 = Slight chance
2 = Moderate chance
3 = High chance

FIG. 3 The Epworth Sleepiness Scale. This instrument asks patients about their likelihood of dozing in eight different situations over the past month. (From Mason RJ et al: *Murray and Nadel's textbook of respiratory medicine,* ed 5, Philadelphia, 2010, WB Saunders.)

- In children, the thresholds for severity of OSA are lower compared to adults.
- Criteria for the treatment of mild OSAH often require symptoms, including excessive daytime sleepiness, cardiovascular disease, HTN, and mood swings.
- In certain patients, portable sleep studies or pulse oximetry may be an effective alternative to PSG for evaluation of OSA.

LABORATORY TESTS

- Arterial blood gas testing should be performed if a patient has suspected pulmonary HTN or cor pulmonale to rule out daytime hypoxemia and/or hypercapnia.
- Thyroid studies should be obtained if thyroid dysfunction is suspected.
- Fasting glucose level is recommended because OSA increases risk of diabetes mellitus independent of other risk factors.
- Complete blood count is helpful to look for anemia; iron studies if anemia is detected and ferritin level if concomitant restless legs syndrome is present.
- Pulmonary function testing if lung disease is suspected or to assess severity of neuromuscular disease in that patient population.
- 12-lead electrocardiogram (ECG) or echocardiogram is indicated if cardiac dysfunction is suspected.

IMAGING STUDIES

- Plain radiography of the neck can be helpful to assess the soft tissues of patients with anatomic abnormalities.
- Chest x-ray if lung disease is suspected.

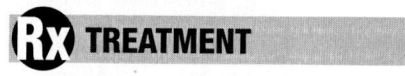

TREATMENT

Fig. 5 illustrates medical therapies for obstructive sleep apnea stratified by mechanisms targeted.

NONPHARMACOLOGIC THERAPY

- Behavioral modifications:
  1. Weight loss in overweight and obese patients. Evidence exists that weight loss is effective for reducing the severity of OSA, and if significant, it may potentially allow some patients to discontinue continuous positive airway pressure (CPAP) therapy.
  2. 10% weight gain predicted an approximate 32% increase in the AHI and sixfold increase in the odds of developing moderate to severe sleep disordered breathing.
  3. 10% weight loss predicted a 26% decrease in the AHI.
  4. Weight loss with bariatric surgery may improve OSA in some patients, but its definitive role remains unclear. In a recent trial in obese patients with OSA, bariatric surgery compared with conventional weight loss therapy did not statistically reduce AHI despite major differences in weight loss.
  5. Exercise without weight loss may improve OSA.

FIG. 4 Central and obstructive sleep apnea. The relationship between airflow and respiratory effort in central and obstructive apnea. During central apnea, cessation of airflow occurs without associated ventilatory effort. Respiratory effort is present during an obstructive apnea. (From Wellman A, White DP: Central sleep apnea and periodic breathing. In Kryger M, Dement W [eds]: *Principles and practice of sleep medicine,* ed 5, Philadelphia, 2011, Saunders, 1140–1152.)

TABLE 3 Definitions*

Events

Apnea: Cessation of breathing lasting 10 seconds or longer. Obstructive—continued respiratory effort with paradoxical motion of rib cage and abdomen; central—absent respiratory effort.

Hypopnea: Different definitions used. Two alternative definitions are part of the scoring criteria advanced by the American Academy of Sleep Medicine:

1. Score a hypopnea if all of the following are present:
   a. Nasal pressure signal excursions; drop ≥30% of baseline for at least 10 seconds.
   b. There is a ≥4% desaturation from pre-event baseline.
   c. At least 90% of the event's duration must meet the amplitude reduction of criteria for hypopnea.
2. Score a hypopnea if all of the following are present:
   a. Nasal pressure signal excursions; drop ≥50% of baseline for at least 10 seconds.
   b. There is a ≥3% desaturation from pre-event baseline *or* the event is associated with an arousal. (The latter does not require a desaturation.)
   c. At least 90% of the event's duration must meet the amplitude reduction of criteria for hypopnea.
3. *Respiratory Effort–Related Arousal (RERA)*: Pattern of progressively more negative esophageal pressure terminated by a sudden change in pressure to a less negative level and an arousal; events last 10 seconds or longer.

Metrics of Severity

Apnea-Hypopnea Index: Average number of apneas plus hypopneas per hour of sleep.
Respiratory Disturbance Index: Average number of apneas plus hypopneas plus RERAs per hour of sleep.

Consensus Definitions of Severity

Normal: <5 episodes/hr
Mild sleep apnea: ≥5 and <15 episodes/hr
Moderate sleep apnea: ≥15 and <30 episodes/hr
Severe sleep apnea: ≥30 episodes/hr

Concept of Sleep Apnea Syndrome

Sleep-disordered breathing with complaint of excessive sleepiness

*See also American Academy of Sleep Medicine.
From Mason RJ et al: *Murray and Nadel's textbook of respiratory medicine,* ed 5, Philadelphia, 2010, WB Saunders.

6. Avoid alcohol for 4 to 6 hours before bedtime.
7. Avoid narcotics, muscle relaxants, and sedating medications.
8. Sleep hygiene training, especially avoidance of sleep deprivation.
9. Avoid or reduce supine sleeping positions.
10. Avoid medications that may worsen OSA.

- Medical treatment:
  1. CPAP is the primary therapy for OSA. It delivers a constant airway pressure that serves as a pneumatic splint relieving upper airway obstruction.
  2. Other methods of delivering positive pressure include:
     a. Bilevel positive airway pressure (BiPAP), which delivers predetermined inspiratory and expiratory airway pressures.
     b. Auto-titrating positive airway pressure (APAP), which increases or decreases the level of pressure in response to change in airflow, vibratory snoring, or changes in circuit pressure.
  3. Oral appliances constructed by a reputable and qualified dentist may be effective for the treatment of mild OSA in certain patients, especially those with retrognathia. Mandibular advancement devices (MADs) are a good alternative to CPAP in patients who are unable to tolerate CPAP. Trials have shown that although CPAP is more effective than MADs in reducing AHI (4.5 vs 11 events/h, respectively), self-reported adherence with use of MADs is higher (6.5 vs 5.2 h/night for CPAP use). Important health outcomes were similar after 1 month of optimal MAD and CPAP treatment in patients with moderate-severe OSAH, which may be explained by the greater efficacy of CPAP being offset by inferior compliance relative to MAD, resulting in similar effectiveness. There was no overall difference between MADs and CPAP with respect to improvement in blood pressure, daytime sleepiness, or quality of life.
  4. Optimal treatment of allergic rhinitis should be pursued, including nasal irrigation and direct antiinflammatory therapies.
  5. Symptoms of excessive daytime sleepiness that linger despite good compliance to CPAP may require further investigation or medical therapy with stimulants.
  6. Patients should be considered for surgery if multiple attempts at CPAP therapy have failed and if an oral appliance is not an option. If the patient opts for surgery, ensure that it is performed by a reputable and qualified otolaryngologist and is based on the location of airway collapse.
- Surgical treatment:
  1. Surgery is done to correct specific anatomic areas of narrowing: nasal, pharyngeal, and tongue base/hypopharynx.
  2. Adenotonsillectomy is often curative for children with OSA.
  3. Nasal septoplasty/turbinectomy should be considered for patients with nasoseptal deformities.
  4. Uvulopalatopharyngoplasty, which involves resection of the uvula and soft palate, is effective for a small number of patients. Predicting which patients will benefit from this surgical treatment is difficult.
  5. Palatal implant surgery and distraction osteogenesis maxillary expansion (DOME) for high-arched palates are other surgical options.
  6. Hypoglossal nerve stimulation (by surgical placement of an implant in the upper chest) helps recruit lingual muscles, reduce pharyngeal collapsibility, and decrease upper airway resistance.
  7. Tracheostomy is typically reserved for patients with very severe OSA who failed medical therapy or who have cor pulmonale.

DISPOSITION

- The short-term prognosis for excessive daytime sleepiness and snoring is good to excellent with the regular use of CPAP, but no studies have been performed to address the long-term effects in a large population of patients.
- Residual symptoms of excessive daytime sleepiness can occur in some patients with OSA despite regular CPAP use. This has led the FDA to approve modafinil for the management of residual sleepiness.

REFERRAL

- Highly trained sleep specialists with expertise in caring for patients with OSA are recommended, especially for complex cases.

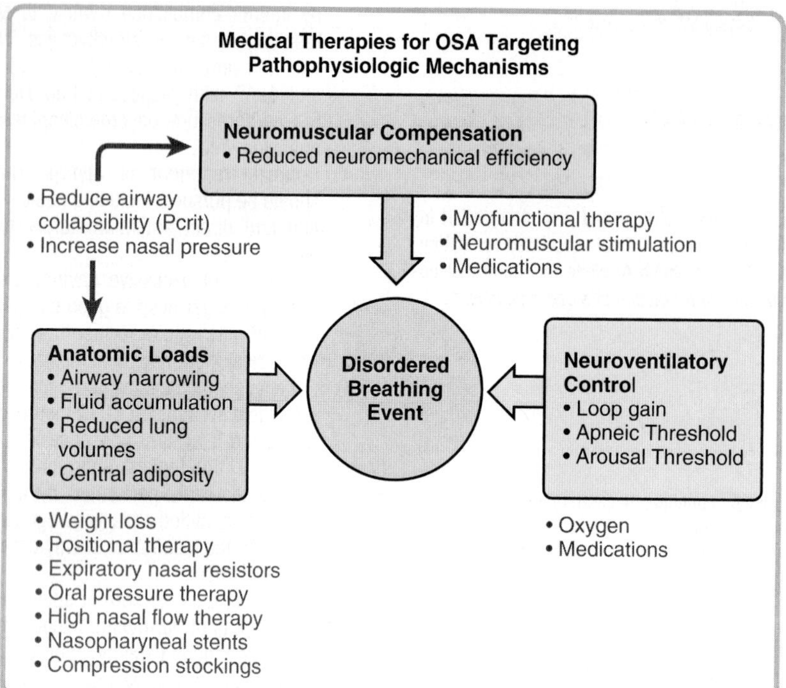

FIG. 5 Medical therapies for obstructive sleep apnea *(OSA)*, stratified by mechanisms targeted. Certain therapies can be considered on the basis of the pathophysiologic mechanisms targeted. OSA is thought to occur as a consequence of increases in anatomic loads on the upper airway, impairments in neuromuscular compensation, or alterations in neuroventilatory control. Traditional therapies such as continuous positive airway pressure (CPAP) use nasal pressure to overcome anatomic loads. By contrast, upper airway surgery or weight loss results in reduced airway collapsibility (Pcrit). Other therapies that may relieve anatomic loads on the upper airway include positional therapy, use of expiratory nasal resistors, oral pressure therapy, nasopharyngeal stenting, and application of compression stockings. Therapies that address impairments in neuromuscular function include myofunctional therapies, use of certain medications, and neuromuscular stimulation. Therapies that may affect neuroventilatory control include use of medications to increase the arousal threshold and supplemental oxygen, which can affect loop gain. (From Kryger M et al: *Principles and practice of sleep medicine,* ed 6, Philadelphia, 2017, Elsevier.)

- Surgical referral to otolaryngology should be considered for children with adenotonsillar hypertrophy and for adults who are unresponsive to weight loss and CPAP therapy.
- Referral to a qualified dentist for treatment with an oral appliance may be useful for certain patients with mild OSA.

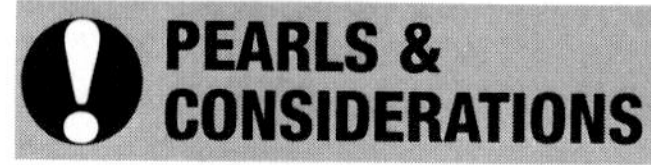

PEARLS & CONSIDERATIONS

- OSAH is a common disorder that is underrecognized and underdiagnosed, so the identification of risk factors is crucial for making the correct diagnosis.
- The prevalence of OSA increases among women after menopause.
- The single most effective therapy for OSA is CPAP administered by nasal or facial masks or other interfaces if required.
- Patients with OSA are more vulnerable than healthy persons to the effects of alcohol consumption and sleep restriction with regard to various driving performance variables.
- OSA is a risk factor for systemic and pulmonary HTN, stroke, atrial fibrillation, and coronary artery disease. In patients with untreated HTN and OSA, the use of CPAP results in small but statistically significant reductions in blood pressure. Therapy with CPAP has not been shown to prevent cardiovascular events in patients with moderate-to-severe obstructive sleep apnea and established cardiovascular disease.
- OSA may also be an independent risk factor for peptic ulcer bleeding.
- Ethnic differences may exist for some populations, with South Asians having a higher prevalence and risk for cardiovascular side effects.

SUGGESTED READINGS

Available at ExpertConsult.com

RELATED CONTENT

Sleep Apnea (Patient Information)

AUTHORS: **GRACE REBECCA PAUL, M.B.B.S., M.D.,** and **DON HAYES JR., M.D., M.S., M.ED.**

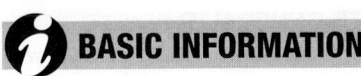

BASIC INFORMATION

DEFINITION

Small bowel bacterial overgrowth (SIBO) is the presence of excessive native and/or nonnative bacteria in the small intestine (bacterial count >10^5/ml per jejunal aspirate) causing chronic diarrhea and malabsorption.

SYNONYMS

Bacterial overgrowth syndrome
SIBO

ICD-10CM CODES

K90.4	Malabsorption due to intolerance, NEC
K90.89	Other intestinal malabsorption

EPIDEMIOLOGY & DEMOGRAPHICS

PREVALENCE: The prevalence of SIBO is varied based on the population studied and the diagnostic tests used. It has shown to be prevalent in up to 12.5% to 20% of the healthy population using glucose and lactulose breath test.

PREDOMINANT SEX AND AGE: SIBO affects predominantly the elderly population or those with recent UGI surgery, including bariatric surgery. The elderly population has decreased gastric secretion and hypomotility due to age-associated decline as well as increased use of motility-altering medications.

RISK FACTORS:

- Advanced age is a known risk factor as there is thought to be an age-associated decline in GI motility.
- Patients with irritable bowel syndrome have a higher prevalence of SIBO compared to the general population. Initial studies have shown up to 65% to 80% of IBS patients with confirmed SIBO with an abnormal lactulose breath test.
- Other risk factors include UGI tract surgery, inflammatory bowel disease, chronic pancreatitis, immunodeficiency, liver disease, and obesity.

PHYSICAL FINDINGS & CLINICAL PRESENTATION

- Patients will present with nonspecific findings, which include abdominal distention, bloating, and/or pain. Other common symptoms include diarrhea and subsequent weight loss and weakness. Pathophysiology of symptoms and clinical consequences of SIBO are summarized in Table 1.
- The severity of symptoms reflects the extent of bacterial overgrowth.
- Severe malabsorption can present as symptoms secondary to vitamin deficiencies. Fat-soluble vitamin deficiencies can present as night blindness (vitamin A), osteomalacia and hypocalcemia (vitamin D), or prolonged bleeding (vitamin K). Bacterial overgrowth can affect vitamin B_{12} absorption in the ileum leading to neuropathies with sensory ataxia.

ETIOLOGY

Disorders that disrupt protective mechanisms against bacterial burden predispose patients to SIBO. Box 1 summarizes diseases and disorders linked to SIBO based on pathophysiology.

- Patients with structural or anatomical abnormalities are at greater risk. These include patients with small bowel diverticula, small intestinal strictures, surgical blind loops, ileocecal resections, or gastric resections (increasing common cause of SIBO).
- Motility disorders predispose to SIBO because of the ineffective clearance of bacteria from the proximal bowel into the colon. Examples of this include gastroparesis and small bowel dysmotility, both suggestive of poorly controlled diabetes. Long-standing celiac disease can also interfere with small bowel motility.
- It is thought that recent antibiotic use as well as antacid medication can alter the normal bacterial flora in the small intestine, contributing to SIBO.

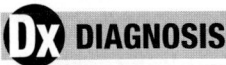

DIAGNOSIS

DIFFERENTIAL DIAGNOSIS

- Celiac disease
- Chronic pancreatitis
- Inflammatory bowel disease
- Irritable bowel syndrome
- Tropical sprue
- Whipple disease
- Lactose intolerance

WORKUP

Diagnostic testing should include workup for diarrhea, anemia, and malabsorption. While endoscopy with jejunal aspirate and culture was a diagnostic tool of choice, its role is limited because of low specificity. While hydrogen breath tests have their limitations as well, they are noninvasive and easy to perform.

LABORATORY TESTS

- Breath tests have become more commonplace in diagnosing SIBO. Typically fermenting bacteria reside in the colon. In SIBO, fermenting bacteria is present in the small intestine as well. A carbohydrate test dose (typically lactulose or glucose) is given and its byproduct (hydrogen) is measured as it is excreted in the breath. In SIBO, exhaled hydrogen concentrations rise early.
- Standard anemia workup is essential. CBC may suggest macrocytic anemia secondary to B_{12} deficiency.
- Nutritional status should be evaluated with albumin levels.
- Stool evaluation can aid in the diagnosis as well. An increase in fecal fat may be suggestive of SIBO. Stool WBC, culture, ova, and parasites should be ordered as well to rule out other infectious etiology.

TABLE 1 Pathophysiology of Symptoms and Clinical Consequences in Small Bowel Bacterial Overgrowth

Process	Mechanisms of Action	Clinical Consequences
Mucosal injury induced by bacteria and/or their toxins or products	Loss of brush-border enzymes	Carbohydrate maldigestion
	Injury to epithelial barrier leading to enhanced intestinal permeability	Protein-losing enteropathy; bacterial translocation and portal and systemic endotoxemia
	Inflammatory response generating inflammatory cytokines	Liver injury and inflammation, systemic inflammatory responses
Luminal competition with the host for nutrients	Consumption of dietary protein	Hypoproteinemia, edema
	Consumption of vitamin B_{12}	B_{12} deficiency, megaloblastic anemia, neurologic symptoms
	Consumption of thiamine	Thiamine deficiency
	Consumption of nicotinamide	Nicotinamide deficiency
Bacterial metabolism	Fermentation of unabsorbed carbohydrates	Bloating, distension, flatulence
	Deconjugation of primary bile acids	Diarrhea due to the effects of deconjugated bile acids in the colon; depletion of the bile acid pool leading to fat and fat-soluble vitamin malabsorption
	Synthesis of vitamin K	Interference with dosing of vitamin K antagonists (e.g., warfarin)
	Synthesis of folate	High serum folate levels
	Synthesis of D-lactic acid	D-lactic acidosis
	Synthesis of alcohol	Liver injury
	Synthesis of acetaldehyde	Liver injury

From Feldman Metal: *Sleisenger and Fordtran's gastrointestinal and liver disease*, ed 10, Philadelphia, 2016, Elsevier.

BOX 1 Diseases and Disorders Linked to Small Bowel Bacterial Overgrowth (SIBO) Based on Pathophysiology

Dysmotility
Acromegaly
Amyloidosis
Chronic opiate use
Diabetic autonomic neuropathy
Gastroparesis
Hypothyroidism
Idiopathic intestinal pseudo-obstruction
Long-standing use of motility-suppressing drugs
Myotonic muscular dystrophy
Systemic sclerosis/scleroderma

Altered Anatomy
Blind loops
Gastrocolic or jejunocolic fistula
Ileocecal valve resection
Small intestinal diverticulosis
Strictures (Crohn disease, radiation, surgery)
Surgically induced alterations in anatomy (Billroth II gastrectomy, end-to-side anastomosis)

Hypochlorhydria
Long-term acid suppression (?)
Postsurgical

Immune Deficiency
Acquired immune deficiency (e.g., AIDS, severe malnutrition)
Inherited immune deficiencies

Multifactorial Causes
Advanced age
Celiac disease
Chronic pancreatitis
Crohn disease
Cystic fibrosis
End-stage kidney disease
Intestinal failure
Liver disease
Radiation enteropathy
Tropical sprue

Unclear or Undefined Relationship to SIBO
Erosive esophagitis
Interstitial cystitis
IBS
Parkinson's disease
Restless legs syndrome
Rosacea
Severe obesity

From Feldman M et al: *Sleisenger and Fordtran's gastrointestinal and liver disease*, ed 10, Philadelphia, 2016, Elsevier.

IMAGING STUDIES

- Endoscopic evaluation of the small intestine can be useful in finding structural and motility causes of bacterial overgrowth such as diverticula and strictures. Small bowel biopsy may aid in the diagnosis of celiac disease as well.
- Jejunal aspirate cultures via endoscopy are considered a standard of diagnosis. Aspirate cultures that exceed 10^5 organisms/ml suggest the presence of SIBO.
- There are several limitations to jejunal aspirate cultures. Bacterial overgrowth is not uniform and may be in inaccessible areas to endoscopist and can easily be missed. Contamination from oropharyngeal flora can lead to false-positive tests. Also endoscopy is an invasive test and other methods of testing such as a breath test may be a more practical initial approach.

Rx TREATMENT

The goal is to treat the underlying cause and treat the bacterial overgrowth with antibiotic therapy.

NONPHARMACOLOGIC THERAPY

Structural disorders such as strictures, fistula, and diverticula may require surgical intervention.

ACUTE GENERAL Rx

- 7- to 10-day course of antibiotic therapy with rifaximin, amoxicillin-clavulanate, or metronidazole and ciprofloxacin has been shown to be beneficial.
- Nutritional support with vitamin replacement and dietary modification (lactose-free diet).

CHRONIC Rx

- Recurrence is common after antibiotic therapy. These patients may require subsequent courses of antibiotic therapy.
- Avoid using antacid medication.
- Avoid drugs that reduce GI motility (opioids).
- Consider lactose-free diet if the response to antimicrobial agents is incomplete.

DISPOSITION

Prognosis is dependent on underlying cause of SIBO. Although recurrence rate is high, antibiotic therapy remains the mainstay of therapy often requiring repeated courses if the underlying condition cannot be resolved.

REFERRAL

- Gastroenterology consultation for small bowel evaluation.
- Surgical consultation with an underlying structural disorder.

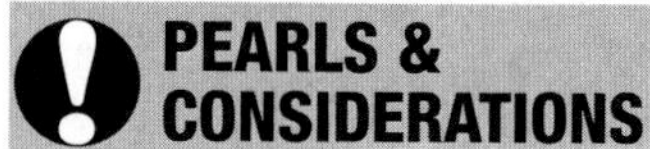

COMMENTS

- SIBO is due to a disruption of protective mechanisms against bacterial burden
- Look for risk factors including UGI tract surgery, structural disorders, IBD, IBS, and disorders decreasing GI motility.
- Diagnosis can be made with hydrogen breath test or endoscopic jejunal aspirate culture.
- Treatment is with antibiotics.
- The combination of vitamin B_{12} deficiency (due to bacterial consumption) and an elevated serum folate level (due to bacterial production) is suggestive of SIBO.
- SIBO can contribute to symptoms of IBS or IBD.

SUGGESTED READINGS

Available at ExpertConsult.com

RELATED CONTENT

Small Intestinal Bacterial Overgrowth (Patient Information)
Irritable Bowel Syndrome (Related Key Topic)
Malabsorption (Related Key Topic)

AUTHOR: **GEORGE CHOLANKERIL, M.D.**

BASIC INFORMATION

DEFINITION

- Small bowel obstruction can be **functional** (as a result of intrinsic abnormal intestinal pathology) or **mechanical** (which may occur acutely or may be chronic).
- Mechanical obstruction means the blockage of the intestinal lumen, preventing the passage of luminal contents through the gut tube.
- Mechanical obstruction may be either:
  1. **Simple obstruction**: In which the lumen may be *partially* or *completely blocked* but with intact intestinal blood flow *OR*
  2. **Strangulated obstruction:**
     a. This is a surgical emergency.
     b. Usually the obstruction is complete; blood flow to the obstructed segment is cut off; and tissue necrosis, gangrene, and perforation may occur.

ICD-10CM CODES

K56.6	Other and unspecified intestinal obstruction
K56.9	Ileus, unspecified
K56.5	Intestinal adhesions (bands) with obstruction
K56.4	Other impaction of intestine
K56.3	Gallstone ileus
K56.2	Volvulus
K5.1	Intussusception
K56	Paralytic ileus and intestinal obstruction

EPIDEMIOLOGY & DEMOGRAPHICS

- The most frequently encountered surgical disorder of the small intestines is mechanical small bowel obstruction (SBO). This is a common surgical emergency.
- 75% of all cases of small bowel obstruction are due to intraabdominal adhesion related to prior abdominal surgery, such as appendectomy, colorectal surgery, and gynecologic procedures.

PREDOMINANT SEX AND AGE: None

RISK FACTORS

- Previous abdominal or pelvic surgery—most important risk factor for mechanical SBO in the U.S.
- Hernia (abdominal wall or groin)
- Prior abdominal irradiation
- Bowel neoplasm
- Foreign-body ingestion
- Parasitic infestation
- Gallstones
- Inflammatory/ischemic stricture

PHYSICAL FINDINGS & CLINICAL PRESENTATION

PHYSICAL FINDINGS: These may include:

- Dehydration (manifested by tachycardia, decreased urine output, orthostatic hypotension, dry mucus membrane)
- Abdominal distention, especially in distal bowel obstruction
- Hyperactive bowel sounds (an early occurrence)
- Hyperresonance or tympany to abdominal percussion
- High-pitched "tinkling" sound on auscultation of the abdomen
- Hypoactive bowel sounds (late finding)
- Hernia
- Rectal examination may reveal:
  1. Blood (suggestive of neoplasm or strangulation)
  2. Masses (may suggest obturator hernia)
  3. Fecal impaction

CLINICAL PRESENTATION: There are four key symptoms: abdominal pain, vomiting, distention, and constipation.

- Abdominal pain (abrupt onset):
  1. Often crampy; intermittent
  2. Constant pain (that is, change in pain's character) signifies serious complication
- Nausea
- Vomiting (bilious vomiting seen in proximal obstructions)
- Diarrhea (early finding)
- Constipation (a late finding)
- Obstipation (inability to pass gas)
- Fever, tachycardia, and peritoneal signs (these late findings may be seen with strangulation or intestinal ischemia)
- It is important to perform serial abdominal examinations to detect changes early

ETIOLOGY

- Postoperative adhesions (may cause acute obstruction usually within one month of surgery; or chronic obstructions can occur yrs later)
- Incarcerated inguinal hernia
- Malignant tumor
- IBD
- Gallstone ileus
- Stricture
- Cystic fibrosis
- Volvulus
- In children consider pyloric stenosis, intussusception, congenital atresia

Dx DIAGNOSIS

DIFFERENTIAL DIAGNOSIS

- Paralytic ileus
- Pseudo-obstruction
- Acute cholangitis
- Cholecystitis
- Gastroenteritis
- Inflammatory bowel disease
- Diverticulitis
- Endometriosis
- Mesenteric ischemia
- Pancreatitis
- Dysmenorrhea
- Ovarian torsion

WORKUP

During the initial evaluation of patients with suspected SBO, the primary objectives are to gauge the degree of metabolic derangement and volume depletion and to assess the need for and expediency of surgery. As with many surgical conditions, determining the correct diagnosis and management strategy hinges on a focused yet thorough history and physical examination.

LABORATORY TESTS

- Laboratory abnormalities are not diagnostic of bowel obstruction but instead may indicate complications of obstruction. Essential laboratory tests include:
  1. Basic metabolic panel (hyponatremia, hypokalemia)
  2. CBC: Hemoconcentration, leukocytosis
  3. Urinalysis
  4. Serum amylase: May be elevated
  5. LDH
  6. Hepatic panel
  7. Check serum lactate, blood cultures, ABG in patients with signs such as fever, hypotension, or change in mental status
  8. Type and cross-match (in anticipation of possible surgical intervention)

IMAGING STUDIES

- Image to confirm diagnosis, identify the location of the obstruction, and access the type of obstruction.
- Imaging also helps identify complications (perforation, necrosis, etc.) and possible cause of the obstruction.
- Initial radiographic evaluation begins with plain x-ray films of the abdomen (supine and upright) and an upright chest radiograph. An upright chest radiograph is of paramount importance to inspect for pneumoperitoneum and also for evidence of aspiration in a patient with a history of vomiting. A supine and upright plain abdominal x-ray in patients with suspected small bowel obstruction may show:
  1. Ladder-like pattern of dilated small bowel loops with air-fluid levels (Fig. 1) indicating small bowel obstruction
  2. Accumulation of air and fluid proximal and clearance of fluid and air distal to the post of obstruction
- Enteroclysis (a fluoroscopic x-ray of the small intestine) is useful in detecting obstruction and can distinguish partial from complete blockage and adhesions from metastases.
- CT scan is the study of choice if the patient has fever, tachycardia, abdominal pain, and leukocytosis. It can reveal the etiology of the obstruction: abscess, inflammatory process, extra-luminal pathology, and/or metastases.
- CT can elucidate the cause, such as the presence of a mass (Fig. 2) or a hernia with subsequent obstruction (Fig. 3). In addition, CT has high sensitivity for detecting strangulation and pneumoperitoneum indicative of a perforation and is particularly useful in the early postoperative setting to rule out ischemia, intraabdominal abscess, or morbidity as the underlying cause. It is also useful in patients with a history of malignancy to differentiate potentially recurrent disease from adhesions (Fig. 4).
- CT enterography, in which intraluminal distention is achieved with administration of large volumes of oral contrast such as water-methylcellulose solution, can be useful. This modality is most often used to diagnose patients with Crohn disease–related strictures, and its benefit is high-resolution imaging of the bowel wall; however, it is

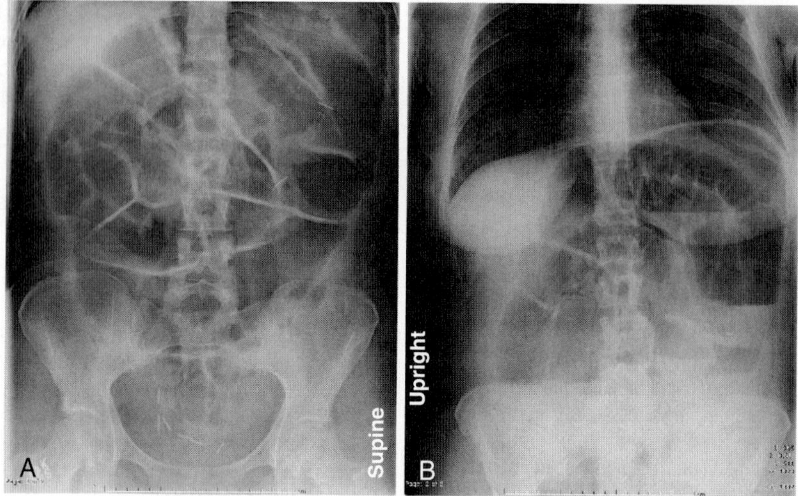

FIG. 1 A, Supine film showing dilated loops of small bowel in a patient with small bowel obstruction. **B,** Upright abdominal film revealing multiple air-fluid levels and small bowel dilation, consistent with a diagnosis of small bowel obstruction. (From Marx J: *Rosen's emergency medicine: concepts and clinical practice*, ed 6, Philadelphia, 2006, Saunders.)

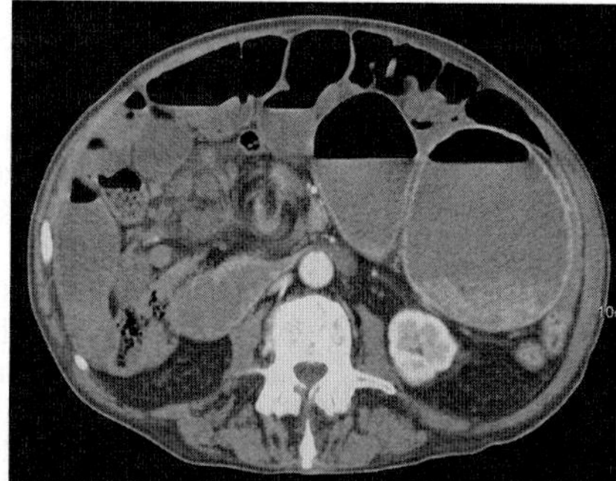

FIG. 2 Computed tomography scan of small bowel volvulus with notable mesenteric torsion. (From Cameron JL, Cameron AM: *Current surgical therapy*, ed 10, Philadelphia, 2011, Saunders.)

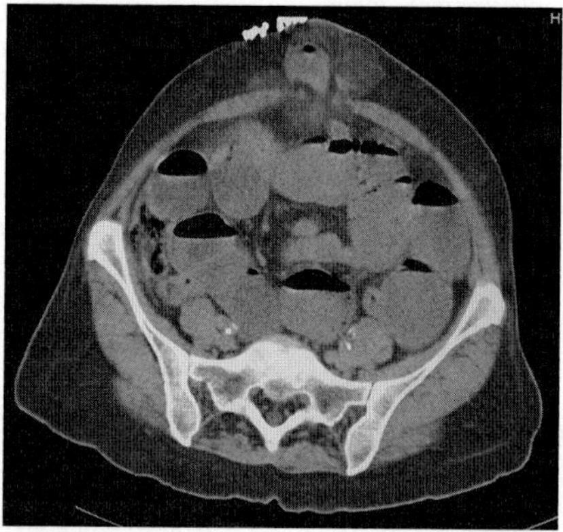

FIG. 3 Computed tomography scan of complete small bowel obstruction due to incisional hernia. (From Cameron IL, Cameron AM: *Current surgical therapy*, ed 10, Philadelphia, 2011, Saunders.)

impractical in the patient with gastrointestinal (GI) distress who is nauseated and vomiting.

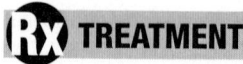

TREATMENT

EMERGENCY ROOM CARE

- Vigorous fluid resuscitation and correction of electrolyte disorders underpin the initial therapeutic goals of both nonoperative and preoperative management strategies. Placing a Foley catheter to measure urinary output, establishing adequate intravenous access, and reassessing hemodynamic and electrolyte status are all essential in the initial management.
- Initial treatment consists of:
  1. Designate the patients nothing by mouth ("NPO")
  2. Fluid resuscitation (with isotonic Ringer or normal saline solution)
  3. Bowel decompression (via nasogastric [NG] tube placement): A standard NG tube provides symptomatic relief, prevents added gas and fluid accumulation proximally, and enables the serial assessment of antegrade fluid movement
  4. Correction of metabolic and electrolyte abnormalities
  5. Pain management
  6. Antiemetic administration
  7. Surgical consultation: Must be done early
  8. Antibiotic administration

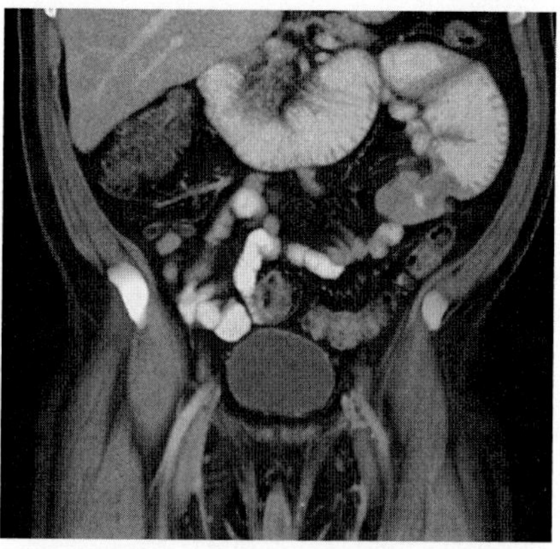

FIG. 4 Coronal image of computed tomography scan showing mass in proximal small bowel with decompressed loops of small bowel distal to obstruction. (From Cameron JL, Cameron AM: *Current surgical therapy*, ed 10, Philadelphia, 2011, Saunders.)

NONSURGICAL INPATIENT CARE

- Continue NG suction.
- Provide adequate fluid.

Patients with low-grade partial SBOs are prone to spontaneous resolution with conservative interventions such as bowel rest, NG decompression, and appropriate fluid resuscitation. For partial or simple obstructions resolution usually occurs within 72 hr.

SURGICAL CARE

More than 25% of inpatients admitted because of SBO will require an operation. Patients with complete or high-grade partial SBO are most likely to need surgery, with less than 20% successfully managed nonoperatively. Surgery is indicated in:

- Strangulated obstruction (which is a surgical emergency)
- Patients with signs of necrosis or perforation (require prompt surgery)
- Simple complete obstruction: After failed nonoperative care

AUTHOR: **DANIEL K. ASIEDU, M.D., PH.D., F.A.C.P.**

BASIC INFORMATION

DEFINITION

A rash, similar to the erythema migrans (EM) rash of Lyme disease, and flulike illness associated with the bite of the lone star tick (*Amblyomma americanum)* in eastern, southeastern, and south-central United States.

SYNONYMS

Master disease
Southern Lyme disease

ICD-10CM CODE
A93.8 Other specified arthropod-borne viral fevers

EPIDEMIOLOGY & DEMOGRAPHICS

INCIDENCE: Unknown as not a reportable disease in the United States
PEAK INCIDENCE: As it is temporally associated with tick bites, occurs more often in spring and summer
RISK FACTORS: Activities that lead humans to enter wooded areas where the ticks reside, such as hiking, lawn care, hunting, and walking in the woods.

PHYSICAL FINDINGS & CLINICAL PRESENTATION

- The rash of STARI is an expanding erythematous lesion (Fig. 1) with irregular borders and central clearing that develops around the site of the lone star tick bite. Usually appears within 7 days of the bite and can expand to a diameter of 8 cm or more. It is described as being similar to erythema migrans rash of Lyme disease.
- Other associated symptoms include headache, fatigue, generalized achiness, and/or nausea similar to Lyme disease but without clinical progression or complications.

ETIOLOGY

The cause of STARI remains unknown. At one point a putative causative organism, *Borrelia lonestari,* was identified but it has never been isolated from a human patient. The organism has been isolated in lone star ticks (Fig. 2) and deer.

DIAGNOSIS

DIFFERENTIAL DIAGNOSIS

Lyme disease: Caused by the bite of the *Ixodes scapularis* tick and also causes a similar rash called erythema migrans. Causative organism is *Borrelia burgdorferi.*

WORKUP

Diagnosis should be considered in a patient from geographic areas that harbor the lone star tick and have a compatible rash, clinical syndrome, and a recent tick bite.

LABORATORY TESTS

- There is no definitive serology test for STARI.
- The ELISA for Lyme disease may be equivocal or weakly positive in patients with STARI but the Lyme Western blot test and Lyme C6 peptide assay will be negative.

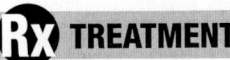

TREATMENT

Doxycycline 100 mg orally twice a day for 10 days has been shown to produce rapid resolution of symptoms. This is also the antibiotic used for Lyme disease. For patients allergic to doxycycline or pregnant women or small children, amoxicillin can be used. Adults: 500 mg po 3 times a day.

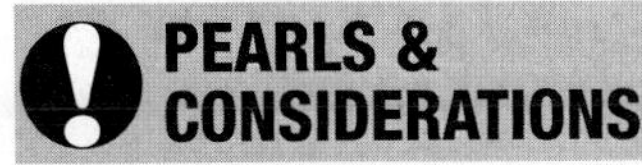

PEARLS & CONSIDERATIONS

COMMENTS

A study by Wormser et al. looked at the differences between STARI and Lyme disease:

- Patients with STARI were more likely to recall tick bite than patients with Lyme disease.
- The time period from tick bite to onset of skin lesion was shorter in STARI (average of 6 days).
- STARI patients with an erythema migrans rash were less likely to have other symptoms than were Lyme disease patients with erythema migrans rash.
- STARI patients were less likely to have multiple skin lesions, had lesions that were smaller in size than Lyme patients (6–10 cm for STARI vs 6–28 cm for Lyme disease), and had lesions that were more circular and with more central clearing.
- With antibiotic therapy, patients with STARI had resolution of symptoms faster than patients with Lyme disease.

PREVENTION

Insect repellants can be useful in preventing attachment of the tick. Examples include DEET, picaridin, oil of lemon eucalyptus (OLE) or PMD, and the synthetic version of OLE.

RELATED TOPICS

Lyme Disease (Related Key Topic)
Ehrlichiosis and Anaplasmosis (Related Key Topic)
Babesiosis (Related Key Topic)
Rocky Mountain Spotted Fever (Related Key Topic)

AUTHOR: **GLENN G. FORT, M.D., M.P.H.**

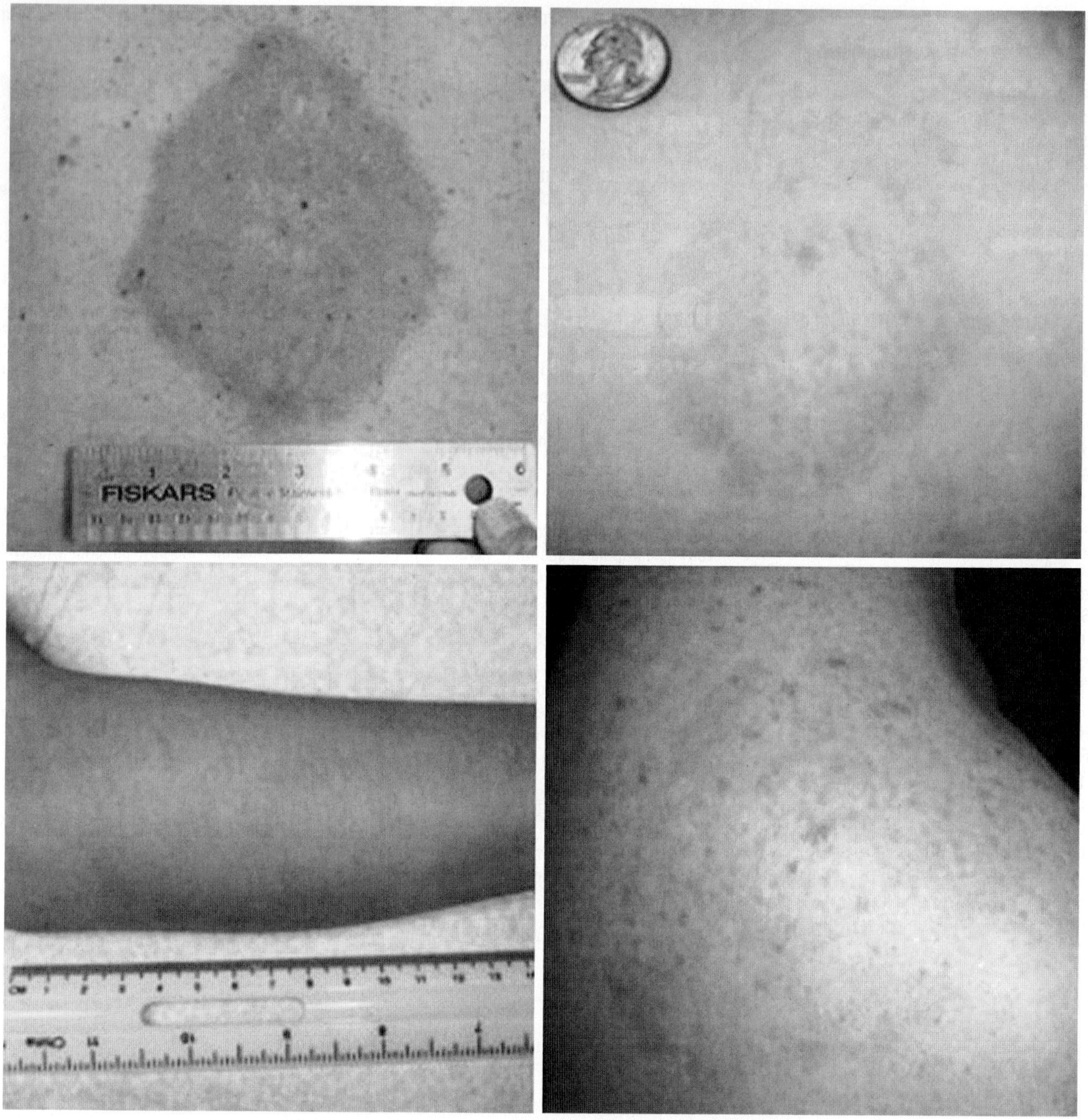

FIG. 1 Rash commonly seen with southern tick-associated rash illness.

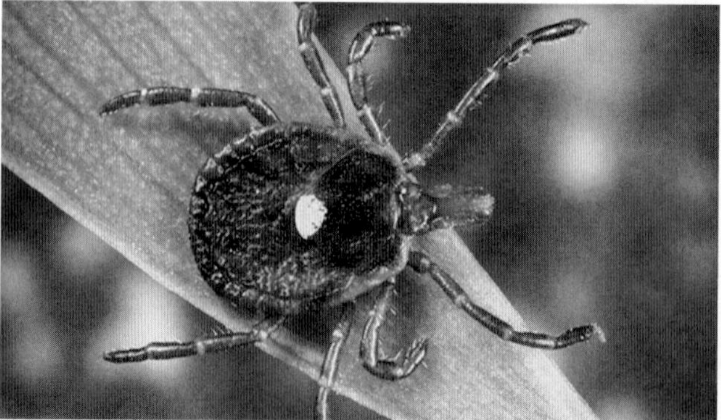

FIG. 2 Tick vector for southern tick-associated rash illness.

BASIC INFORMATION

DEFINITION

Spinal cord compression is characterized by direct compression of the spinal cord within the spinal canal. This may result in loss of neurologic function from compression of the spinal cord in the cervical, thoracic, and upper lumbar spinal canal. Note that compression may also occur at the cauda equina in the lower lumbar spinal canal, which is anatomically below the level of the spinal cord. Fig. 1 illustrates a schematic demarcation of principal dermatomes shown as distinct segments. Depending on the underlying etiology, symptoms may develop gradually or acutely and may result in complete or incomplete deficits. Neurologic deficits related to compression of the cord itself are referred to as myelopathy, while deficits cause by compression on nerve roots are described as radiculopathy.

- Signs and symptoms of myelopathy:
  1. Upper motor neuron signs (Hoffman sign, inverted radial reflex, Babinski sign, spasticity, hyperreflexia, clonus) in chronic cases
  2. Weakness
  3. Sensory deficits
  4. Clumsiness, difficult ambulation, ataxic gait (secondary to loss of proprioception in legs)
- Signs and symptoms of radiculopathy:
  1. Lower motor neuron signs (hyporeflexia, hypotonicity, fasciculations, muscle atrophy)
  2. Weakness
  3. Sensory deficits

Incomplete spinal cord lesions may classically present in distinct syndromic patterns (Table 1), for example, as follows:

- Anterior cord syndrome
- Central cord syndrome
- Cauda equina syndrome (not a true example of spinal cord compression but rather of cauda equina compression, affecting lower motor neurons in lumbosacral nerve roots)
- Conus medullaris syndrome
- Brown-Séquard syndrome

SYNONYMS

Central cord syndrome
Anterior cord syndrome
Brown-Séquard syndrome
Acute spinal cord compression
Cauda equina syndrome
Conus medullary syndrome

ICD-10CM CODES

S14.13XX	Anterior cord syndrome
G83.81	Brown-Séquard syndrome
G83.4	Cauda equina syndrome
S14.12XX	Central cord syndrome
G95.81	Conus medullaris syndrome

EPIDEMIOLOGY AND DEMOGRAPHICS

Dependent on etiology of cord compression

DEGENERATIVE SPINE DISORDERS

May affect the cervical, thoracic, and/or lumbar spine. Underlying pathology involves changes in keratin sulfate-to-chondroitin sulfate ratio in intervertebral disks with aging. This leads to a cascade of secondary events, including loss of disk height, disk herniation, spondylosis, increased intersegmental motion, formation of osteophytes, ligamentum flavum hypertrophy, and arthrosis of the facet joints. Compression of the nerve roots and/or spinal cord may result.

Spinal cord and nerve root compression from degenerative conditions are more common with increasing age, although any age group may be affected. Specific epidemiology and demographics are dependent on the type of degenerative changes.

TUMOR

Epidemiology dependent entirely on tumor type. Malignant tumors in the spine are most commonly metastatic disease, although primary musculoskeletal tumors are possible. The spine is the third-most common site for tumor metastases, after the lung and liver. Common metastatic lesions to the spine include lung cancer, breast cancer, prostate cancer, cancer of the GI tract, multiple myeloma, and lymphoma.

INFECTION

Diskitis/osteomyelitis may progress to epidural abscess, causing spinal cord or cauda equina compression. If not adequately addressed in a timely manner, this may result in permanent neurologic deficit. Epidural abscess incidence is approximately 0.2 to 3.0 per 10,000 hospital admissions. *Staphylococcus aureus* is the most common offending organism. Risk factors include increasing age, diabetes mellitus, end-stage renal disease, chronic hepatitis/cirrhosis, known endocarditis, immunocompromise, and IV drug abuse.

SPINAL CORD INJURY

Occurred most commonly in males with a mean age of 37 yr in 2010. Alcohol plays a major role in at least 25% of SCI.

INCIDENCE: 12,400 new cases/yr in 2010 in the U.S.

PREVALENCE: 250,000 persons in 2005 in the U.S.

COST (IN U.S.): >$5 billion/yr

RISK FACTORS: Underlying spinal disease can predispose to SCI:

- Inflammatory spondyloarthropathies, especially ankylosing spondylitis
- Diffuse idiopathic skeletal hyperostosis (DISH)
- Congenital spinal disorders
- Preexisting spinal canal stenosis or compromise
- Atlantoaxial instability
- Osteoporosis
- Rheumatoid arthritis (cervical spine)

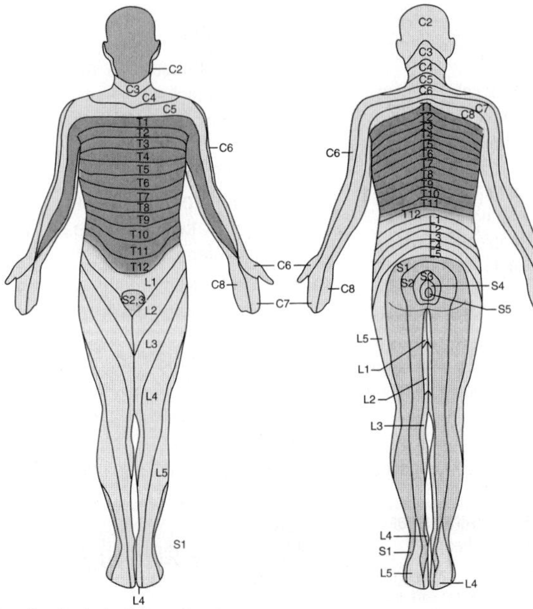

PHYSICAL FINDINGS & CLINICAL PRESENTATION

Clinical features reflect the amount of spinal cord involvement:

- Weakness, sensory changes (dependent on level of compression/lesion/injury).
- Myelopathy if cord involvement, radiculopathy if nerve root involvement (may involve both).

Levels of principal dermatomes

C5	Clavicles	T10	Level of umbilicus
C5,6,7	Lateral parts of upper limbs	T12	Inguinal or groin regions
C8, T1	Medial sides of upper limbs	L1,2,3,4	Anterior and inner surfaces of lower limbs
C6	Thumb	L4,5 S1	Foot
C6,7,8	Hand	L4	Medial side of great toe
C8	Ring and little fingers	S1,2, L5	Posterior and outer surfaces of lower limbs
T4	Level of nipples	S1	Lateral margin of foot and little toe
		S2,3,4	Perineum

FIG. 1 Schematic demarcation of levels of principal dermatomes shown as distinct segments. There is actually considerable overlap between any two adjacent dermatomes. (From Goldman L, Schafer AI: *Goldman's Cecil medicine,* ed 24, Philadelphia, 2011, Saunders.)

TABLE 1 Spinal Cord Syndromes

Syndrome	Sensory	Motor	Sphincter Involvement
Central cord syndrome	Variable	Upper extremity weakness, distal > proximal	Variable
Brown-Séquard syndrome	Ipsilateral position and vibration sense loss Contralateral pain and temperature sensation loss	Motor loss ipsilateral to cord lesion	Variable
Anterior cord syndrome	Loss of pin and touch sensation Vibration, position sense preserved	Motor loss or weakness below cord level	Variable
Transverse cord syndrome—complete	Loss of sensation below level of cord injury	Loss of voluntary motor function below cord level	Sphincter control lost
Cauda equina syndrome	Saddle anesthesia may be present, or sensory loss may range from patchy to complete transverse pattern	Weakness may be of lower motor neuron type	Sphincter control impaired

From Marx JA et al: *Rosen's emergency medicine*, ed 8, Philadelphia, 2014, WB Saunders.

TABLE 2 Physical Examination Findings Associated with Vertebral Fractures and Spinal Cord Injuries

Injury	Physical Examination Area	Associated Findings
Vertebral fracture	Spine	Tenderness of the neck and/or back. Examine the entire spine because vertebral fractures may occur in multiples.
	Neurologic	See "Spinal cord injury" below.
	Chest	*Thoracic spine fractures:* Check for chest tenderness, unequal breath sounds, and arrhythmia, which are suggestive of an associated intrathoracic injury or myocardial contusion.
	Abdomen/pelvis	*Thoracolumbar and lumbar spine fractures:* Check for abdominal or pelvic tenderness. A transverse area of ecchymosis on the lower abdominal wall (seat belt sign) increases the chance of an abdominopelvic injury.
	Extremity	*Thoracolumbar and lumbar spine fractures*: Check for calcaneal tenderness because 10% of calcaneal fractures are associated with a low thoracic or lumbar fracture. Mechanistically, these areas are fractured as a result of axial loading.
Spinal cord injury	Neurologic, motor (anterior column)	Assess motor function on a scale of 0 to 5. The *motor level* is defined as the most caudal segment with at least 3/5 strength. Injuries to the first eight cervical segments result in tetraplegia (previously known as quadriplegia); lesions below the T1 level result in paraplegia.
	Neurologic, sensory (spinothalamic tract)	Assess sensory function via pinprick and light touch on the following scale: 0 = absent; 1 = impaired; 2 = normal. The *sensory level* is defined as the most caudal segment of the spinal cord with normal sensory function. The highest intact sensory level should be marked on the patient's spine to monitor for progression.
	Neurologic, sensory (dorsal column)	Assess vibratory sensory function on a scale of 0 to 2 by using a tuning fork over bony prominences. Assess position sense (proprioception) by flexing and extending the great toe.
	Neurology, deep tendon reflex	On a scale of 0 to 4, assess the deep tendon reflexes in the upper (biceps, triceps) and lower (patellar, Achilles) extremities.
	Anogenital	Assess rectal tone, sacral sensation, signs of urinary or fecal retention or incontinence, and priapism. Also check the anogenital reflexes. An *anal wink* (S2-S4) is present if the anal sphincter contracts in response to stroking the perianal skin area. The *bulbocavernosus reflex* (S3-S4) is elicited by squeezing the glans penis or clitoris (or pulling on an inserted Foley catheter), which results in reflexive contraction of the anal sphincter.
	Head-to-toe examination	A spinal cord injury may mask a patient's ability to perceive and localize pain. Imaging of high-risk areas, such as the abdomen, and areas of bruising or swelling may be required to exclude occult injuries.

From Adams JG et al: *Emergency medicine, clinical essentials,* ed 2, Philadelphia, 2013, Elsevier.

- ***Central cord syndrome (most common incomplete spinal cord injury):*** Motor impairment greater in upper than in lower extremities, variable degree of sensory loss below the injury level. Weakness and poor hand dexterity are especially common. Classically occurs after mild trauma including cervical hyperextension in the setting of preexisting cervical spondylosis.
- ***Anterior cord syndrome (worst prognosis of incomplete spinal cord injury):*** Affects the anterior or ventral 2/3 of the spinal cord, sparing the dorsal columns. May be caused by a vascular injury to the anterior spinal artery or by a flexion/compression injury. Impairment usually is worse in the lower extremities than upper extremities. Physical manifestations include motor, pain, and temperature loss below the lesion. Proprioception and vibratory sense may be preserved as dorsal columns are preserved.
- ***Brown-Séquard syndrome:*** Rare in isolation. Caused by injury to either half of the spinal cord and resulting in the loss of motor function, position, vibration, and light touch on the side of injury as well as loss of pain and temperature sense on the contralateral side.
- ***Conus medullaris syndrome:*** Results in variable motor loss in the lower extremities with loss of bowel and bladder function. In general, more bowel and bladder is affected earlier than motor.
- ***Cauda equina syndrome:*** Low back pain, weakness in bilateral lower extremities, saddle anesthesia, and loss of voluntary bladder and/or bowel control, often presenting as bladder retention and/or bowel incontinence.

ETIOLOGY

- Trauma (most SCIs result from high-speed motor vehicle accidents, falls, sports injuries, or violence)
- Tumor
- Infection (e.g., epidural abscess)
- Inflammatory processes
- Degenerative disk disease with associated spinal stenosis
- Acute disk herniation
- Cystic abnormalities
- Ankylosing spondylitis, DISH. Patients with underlying DISH or ankylosing spondylitis are at high risk of SCI with otherwise relatively minor fractures of the spine
- Table 2 summarizes physical examination findings associated with vertebral fractures and spinal cord injuries

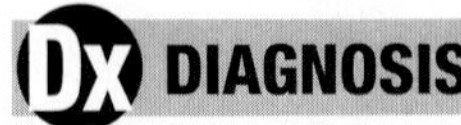

DIAGNOSIS

DIFFERENTIAL DIAGNOSIS

See "Etiology."

WORKUP

- Signs and symptoms of spinal cord or cauda equina compression often indicate urgent surgical conditions and thus require urgent imaging and early referral for assessment by a spine specialist.

- In cases of acute trauma in which spinal cord injury is suspected, patient should undergo full trauma evaluation following advanced trauma life support protocol in emergency room setting. With suspected injury to the cervical spine, the patient should be immobilized in a hard cervical collar or in-line traction at all times during evaluation. Log-roll precautions may be indicated as well to immobilize the spine during acute injury evaluation.
- Inflammatory labs will usually be elevated both in cases of trauma and infectious processes. Laboratory tests ordered should be specific to the suspected etiology or differential diagnosis for spinal cord compression.

IMAGING STUDIES

- Signs and symptoms of spinal cord compression in most cases will mandate advanced imaging, often including CT and CT myelogram and/or MRI.
- Plain x-rays may be helpful; however, normal plain films do not negate the need for further advanced imaging in the setting of signs and symptoms of spinal cord compression or spinal cord injury.
- In the trauma setting, after primary and secondary surveys, fine-cut helical CT scans with axial, coronal, and sagittal reconstructions have replaced plain cervical radiographs in most trauma centers as the initial evaluation of choice in detecting fractures of the cervical spine.
- Detection of injury to any part of the spine during trauma evaluation mandates full imaging evaluation of the entire spine, as noncontiguous injuries are common.
- While CT scan is excellent at imaging bony structures and detecting fractures, MRI provides more detailed imaging of the soft-tissue structures, including neural structures, discoligamentous structures, the posterior ligamentous complex, and paraspinal soft tissues. MRI is very sensitive for detecting ligamentous injury, spinal cord edema, spinal cord compression from soft-tissue structures, epidural hematoma, diskitis, osteomyelitis, and epidural abscess. Of note, gadolinium contrast may increase the sensitivity of the MRI study for the detection of tumors or infections.

Rx TREATMENT

- Depending on the etiology of spinal cord compression as well as the specific signs and symptoms during physical examination and history-taking, urgent surgical decompression and/or stabilization may be indicated. Referral to a spine specialist is indicated in most cases of spinal cord compression.
- Corticosteroids: Controversial in cases of acute spinal cord injury. Methylprednisolone was thought to reduce the amount of secondary injury that occurs after SCI and was previously used in many trauma centers. However, current evidence is insufficient to support corticosteroids for this use, and most spine trauma centers no longer utilize steroids in cases of acute spinal cord injury.
- Vasopressors: Current evidence supports the use of vasopressors in cases of spinal cord injury to maintain spinal cord perfusion and to prevent ischemic damage to the cord. The ideal mean arterial pressure and duration of treatment are yet to be defined. Both the treatment modality and the injury itself mandate admission to ICU level of care in most cases for close monitoring.

DISPOSITION

Indicators regarding prognosis:

- Patients with acute traumatic SCI need monitoring in the ICU and evaluation for potential life-threatening complications, including cardiovascular instability and respiratory failure.
- In general, the greater the distal motor and sensory sparing, the greater the expected recovery.
- In most cases of spinal cord compression and/or spinal cord injury, the primary goal of surgical decompression and/or stabilization should be to spare the remaining functional levels and to prevent worsening of the injury. Return of function should not be guaranteed.
- Prophylaxis against deep vein thrombosis and pulmonary embolism should always be provided. In acute injuries to the spine or postoperatively, this may consist of mechanical prophylaxis including TEDs and SCDs. Pharmacologic deep vein thrombosis/pulmonary embolism prophylaxis is often held initially to prevent development of epidural hematoma.

REFERRAL

Signs and symptoms of spinal cord or cauda equina compression often indicate urgent surgical conditions and thus require urgent imaging and early referral for assessment by a spine specialist.

SUGGESTED READINGS

Available at ExpertConsult.com

RELATED CONTENT

Spinal Stenosis (Patient Information)
Lumbar Disk Syndrome (Related Key Topic)
Spinal Epidural Abscess (Related Key Topic)
Spinal Stenosis, Lumbar (Related Key Topic)

AUTHORS: **DANIEL BRIAN CARLIN REID, M.D., M.P.H.,** and **SHYAM A. PATEL, M.D.**

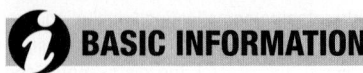

BASIC INFORMATION

DEFINITION

A spinal epidural abscess (SEA) is a focal suppurative infection occurring in the spinal epidural space.

SYNONYM

SEA

ICD-10CM CODE
G06.1 Intraspinal abscess and granuloma

EPIDEMIOLOGY & DEMOGRAPHICS

INCIDENCE (IN U.S.):

- 2 to 25 cases/100,000 hospitalized patients/yr
- May be increasing over the past 3 decades

PREDOMINANT AGE

- Median age of onset approximately 50 yr (35 yr in intravenous drug users)
- Peak incidence in seventh and eighth decades of life

PHYSICAL FINDINGS & CLINICAL PRESENTATION

- The presentation of SEA can be nonspecific.
- Fever, malaise, and back pain are the most consistent early symptoms.
- Pain is often focal. It may initially be mild but can progress to become severe.
- As the disease progresses, root pain can occur, followed by motor weakness, sensory changes, bladder and bowel dysfunction, and paralysis.
- Physical findings may be limited to fever or spinal tenderness.
- The evolution to neurologic deficits can occur as quickly as a few hours, or over weeks to months.
- Once paralysis occurs, it may quickly become irreversible without the appropriate intervention.

ETIOLOGY

- SEA most commonly results from hematogenous dissemination.
- Pyogenic bacteria account for the majority of cases in the U.S. Immigrants from TB-endemic areas may present with tuberculous SEAs. Fungi and parasites can also cause this condition. The most common causative organism is *Staphylococcus aureus.* Gram-negative bacilli and anaerobes may be seen if the infection has a urinary or GI source.
- Most posterior SEAs are thought to originate from distant focus (e.g., skin and soft tissue infections), while anterior SEAs are commonly associated with diskitis or vertebral osteomyelitis. No source was found in approximately one third of cases.
- Associated predisposing conditions include diabetes mellitus, alcoholism, cancer, AIDS, and chronic renal failure, or following epidural anesthesia, spinal surgery or trauma, prolonged epidural catheter placement, paraspinal glucocorticoid or analgesic injections, acupuncture, or IV drug use. No predisposing condition is found in approximately 20% of patients.
- Damage to the spinal cord can be caused by direct compression of the spinal cord, vascular compromise, bacterial toxins, and inflammation.

Dx DIAGNOSIS

DIFFERENTIAL DIAGNOSIS

- Herniated disk
- Vertebral osteomyelitis and diskitis
- Metastatic tumors
- Meningitis

LABORATORY TESTS

- WBC may be normal or elevated.
- ESR and C-reactive proteins are usually elevated.
- Blood cultures are positive in approximately 60% of patients with SEA and should be obtained prior to starting antibiotics.
- CSF cultures are positive in 19%, but lumbar puncture is unnecessary, and may be contraindicated.
- Once imaging is done, CT-guided aspiration or open biopsy should be done to determine causative organism. Abscess content culture is positive in 90% of patients.

IMAGING STUDIES

- MRI with gadolinium is the imaging modality of choice (Fig. 1); CT scan with contrast may

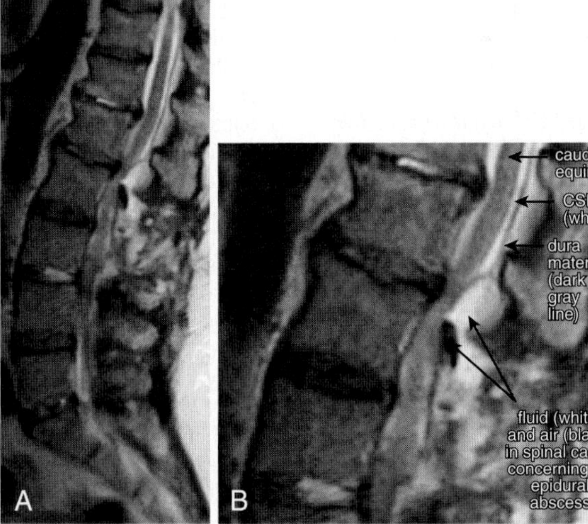

FIG. 1 Same patient as in Fig. 2, in whom noncontrast computed tomography showed air in the spinal canal, concerning for epidural abscess. Magnetic resonance imaging (MRI) of the lumbar spine without contrast was performed, as the patient was in acute renal failure. **A,** This T_2-weighted sagittal MRI provides useful information even without gadolinium contrast. **B,** Close-up. On T_2-weighted MRI sequences, fluid including cerebrospinal fluid *(CSF)* appears white. Fat-containing tissues such as bone marrow and the spinal cord or cauda equina appear dark gray. Calcified bone appears nearly black due to an absence of resonating protons. Air appears completely black for the same reason. The midline sagittal image shows the cauda equina to be impinged upon by an epidural fluid collection containing air—an epidural abscess. The dura mater is visible as a thin, dark gray line parallel to the spinal cord. It is indented in the region of the epidural abscess. (From Broder JS: *Diagnostic imaging for the emergency physician*, Philadelphia, 2011, Saunders.)

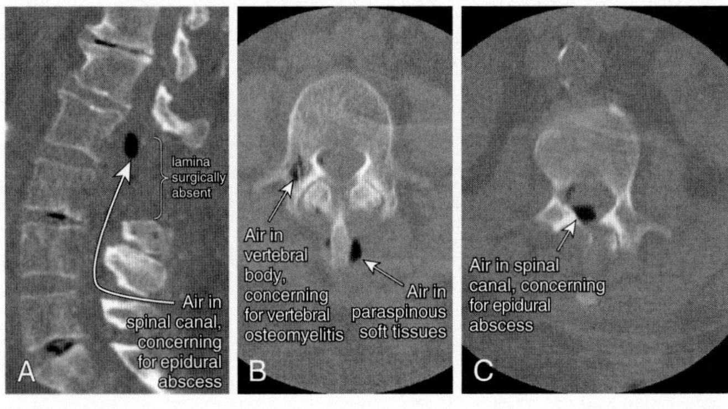

FIG. 2 This 67-year-old female presented with delirium and fever. Three months prior, she had undergone lumbar laminectomy, and her wound had been treated with a wound VAC dressing. Magnetic resonance imaging was not initially available, so noncontrast computed tomography (CT) was performed. Noncontrast CT is excellent at delineating air, which appears black on bone windows. **A,** The midsagittal view demonstrates air *(black)* in the spinal canal at the L2 and L3 levels. On the axial views **(B, C),** air is visible in the spinal canal, in paraspinal soft tissues, and within the vertebral body. These findings are concerning for a paraspinal infection that has developed into an epidural abscess with vertebral osteomyelitis. (From Broder JS: *Diagnostic imaging for the emergency physician*, Philadelphia, 2011, Saunders.)

show the abscess (Fig. 2) but is less sensitive than MRI.

- CT with myelography is more sensitive for cord compression.

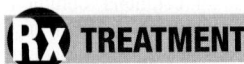

TREATMENT

NONPHARMACOLOGIC THERAPY

- Surgical decompression is the mainstay of treatment. Decompression within the first 24 hr has been related to an improved prognosis.
- Nonsurgical treatment is effective in some patients, but failure rate may be excessive. This approach should not be considered and should only be attempted in the absence of signs of compressive myelopathy and with very careful follow-up.

ACUTE GENERAL Rx

- In addition to surgery, antibiotics directed at the most likely organism should be initiated. Fig. 3 describes an algorithm for the management of patients with SEA.
- If the organism is unknown, broad coverage against staphylococci, streptococci, and gram-negative bacilli should be initiated. Empiric antimicrobial intravenous therapy typically includes vancomycin (loading dose: 25-30 mg/kg, then 15-20 mg/kg q 8-12 hr, aiming for trough levels of 15-20) plus an antipseudomonal cephalosporin such as piperacillin/tazobactam at high dose (4.5 g IV q 6 hr) or carbapenem such as meropenem (1-2 g IV q 8 hr) or imipenem. The regimen can be adjusted according to culture results. Therapy should continue for at least 4 to 6 wk.

CHRONIC Rx

Neurologic deficits may remain despite aggressive treatment.

DISPOSITION

Irreversible paralysis and death can occur in up to 25% of patients.

REFERRAL

All cases should be referred to a neurosurgeon and an infectious disease specialist.

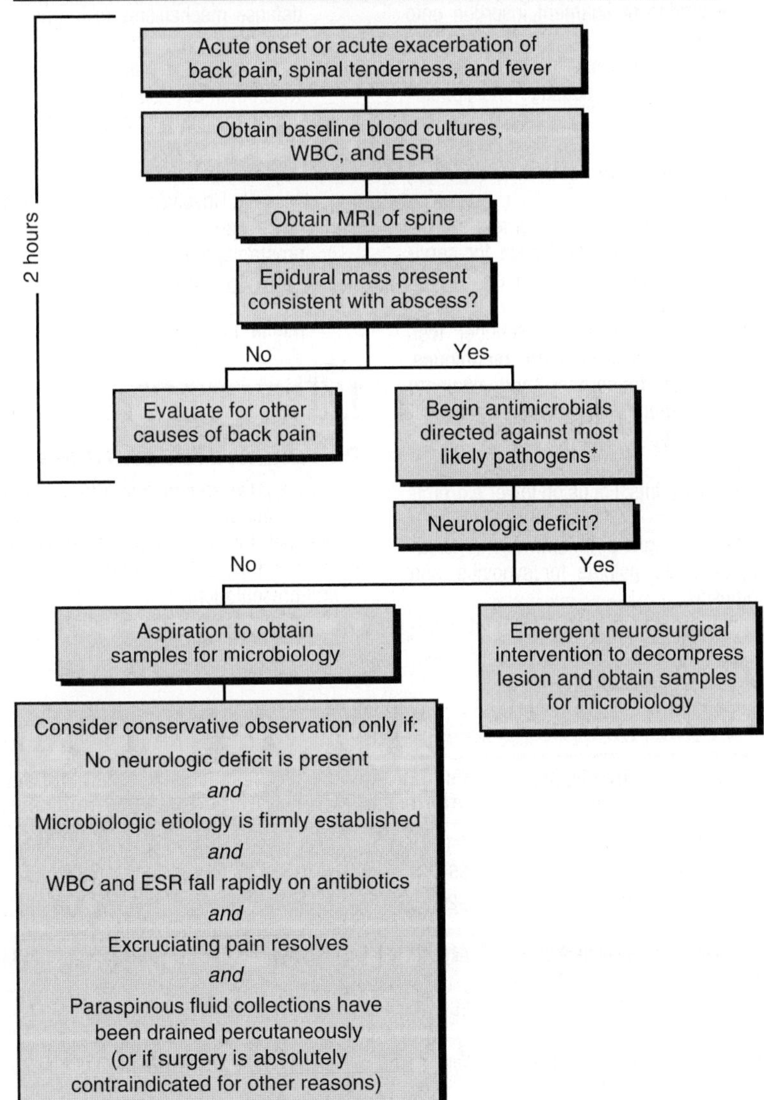

FIG. 3 Algorithm for the management of patients with spinal epidural abscess syndrome. If magnetic resonance imaging *(MRI)* cannot be performed, myelography, high-contrast computed tomography (CT), or CT-myelography may be an acceptable alternative to localize an epidural abscess. *If abscess drainage can be performed promptly, antimicrobial drugs may be withheld until specimens for microbial analysis are obtained. *ESR,* Erythrocyte sedimentation rate; *WBC,* white blood cell. (From Vincent JL et al: *Textbook of critical care,* ed 6, Philadelphia, 2011, Saunders.)

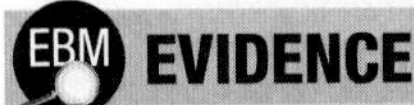

PEARLS & CONSIDERATIONS

- Follow-up imaging with MRI is not necessary unless patient develops new neurologic signs or symptoms, has poor clinical response, or has persistent elevation of inflammatory markers.
- It is critically important to recognize this process early; the prognosis is generally excellent if treatment is initiated while symptoms are localized and before evidence of myelopathy develops.
- The likelihood of success postsurgery is low in patients who have developed complete paralysis for longer than 36 hours.

SUGGESTED READINGS

Available at ExpertConsult.com

EBM EVIDENCE

Available at ExpertConsult.com

AUTHOR: **GLENN G. FORT, M.D., M.P.H.**

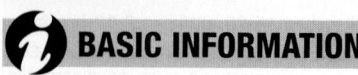

BASIC INFORMATION

DEFINITION

Spondyloarthropathies (SpAs) are a group of interrelated systemic autoinflammatory conditions that are serologically negative for rheumatoid factor, connected by an underlying genetic risk with similar patterns of inflammation. This group encompasses ankylosing spondylitis, psoriatic arthritis, reactive arthritis, enteropathic arthritis, and undifferentiated spondyloarthritis (Table 1). SpAs are broadly classified by axial versus peripheral joint involvement, with or without radiographic progression.

SYNONYMS

Spondyloarthritis
Spondylopathy
Spondylitis
Spondylosis
SPAs

ICD-10CM Codes

M46.80 Other specified inflammatory spondylopathies, unspecified site
M46.82 Other specified inflammatory spondylopathies, cervical region
M46.83 Other specified inflammatory spondylopathies, cervicothoracic region
M46.86 Other specified inflammatory spondylopathies, lumbar region
M46.87 Other specified inflammatory spondylopathies, lumbosacral region
M46.89 Other specified inflammatory spondylopathies, multiple sites
M46.81 Other specified inflammatory spondylopathies, occipito-atlanto-axial region
M46.88 Other specified inflammatory spondylopathies, sacrococcygeal region
M46.84 Other specified inflammatory spondylopathies, thoracic region
M46.85 Other specified inflammatory spondylopathies, thoracolumbar region

EPIDEMIOLOGY & DEMOGRAPHICS

PREVALENCE: Worldwide prevalence of SpA is 0.2% to 1.6%, with over 1% of the U.S. population affected. Varies regionally with prevalence of HLA-B27.

PREDOMINANT SEX AND AGE: Males younger than age 45 yr are predominately affected.
Patients older than 45 yr may present with chronic and severe disease due to delay in diagnosis.

GENETICS: Association with the *HLA-B27* allele is the strongest known genetic risk factor.

RISK FACTORS: *HLA-B27* allele,* male sex,* smoking,* ethnic background, family history of SpA, and certain infections (*Associated with more severe disease)

PHYSICAL FINDINGS & CLINICAL PRESENTATION

- History:
  1. Inflammatory low back pain may be the primary presenting symptom
     a. Pain and stiffness in low back or buttocks that is worst in the morning, may awaken the patient from sleep, and is improved with exercise
     b. Morning stiffness lasting longer than 1 hour
     c. Improvement with NSAIDs
     d. Sensitivity up to 90% and positive likelihood ratio up to 2.2 for axial SpA
  2. Symptoms of systemic and peripheral inflammation are additional clues that should be elicited in a comprehensive review of systems.
     a. Uveitis: Painful ocular inflammation
     b. Psoriasis: Chronic skin inflammation with red patches and silvery scales
     c. Inflammatory bowel disease: Crohn disease and ulcerative colitis
     d. Synovitis: Inflammation of the synovial membrane, only in synovial joints
     e. Enthesitis: Inflammation at the site of tendon or ligament insertion onto bone
     f. Dactylitis: Tenosynovitis of the digits causing classic sausage-like appearance
- Physical exam:
  1. Axial joints: Spine and sacroiliac (SI) joints.
  2. Inspect curvature, palpate for tenderness, and evaluate range of motion for cervical, thoracic, and lumbar spine. Measure degree of axial involvement with occiput wall, thoracic expansion, Schober test, and lumbar side-bending techniques. Palpate for tenderness and evaluate range of motion of the SI joints. Test for sacroiliitis with Patrick and Gaenslen tests.
  3. Peripheral joints: Focus on lower extremities.
  4. Inspect for signs of inflammation, including dactylitis, palpate for synovitis, and enthesitis.
  5. Evaluate for systemic involvement manifesting as anterior uveitis and psoriasis.
     a. Slit lamp is necessary to diagnose anterior uveitis.
     b. Full skin exam is critical to detect occult psoriasis.
- Musculoskeletal manifestations commonly affect weight-bearing joints with high mechanical stress; thus, it is particularly important to examine the lumbar spine, SI joints, and lower extremities.
- Degree of axial involvement can be measured via specialized exam techniques, which are used to track disease activity and response to treatment over time.

ETIOLOGY

- Genetic:
  1. The *HLA-B27* allele has a strong association with SpA, through mechanisms not fully understood.
- Environmental:
  1. Microbial infections, disruptions in barrier defense mechanisms (skin and intestinal mucosa), and mechanical articular stressors may trigger an inflammatory response, which then develops into signs and symptoms specific to each type of SpA.
- Autoinflammatory:
  1. Key components of the inflammatory cascade involved in the pathogenesis of SpA are TNF, IL-12, IL-17, IL-23, and prostaglandins. Success in treatment with targeted therapies to each of these molecules has helped us understand their role in the etiology of SpA.

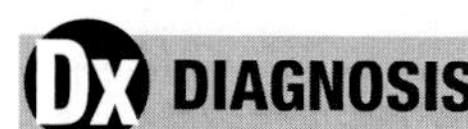

DIAGNOSIS

DIFFERENTIAL DIAGNOSIS

- Seronegative rheumatoid arthritis (peripheral presentation)
- Degenerative disc disease (axial presentation)
- Inflammatory osteoarthritis (axial or peripheral presentation)
- Hypertrophic osteoarthropathy (peripheral presentation)

TABLE 1 Comparison of Ankylosing Spondylitis and Related Disorders

Feature	Ankylosing spondylitis	Psoriatic arthritis	Reactive arthritis	Enteropathic arthropathy
Sex (male:female)	2–3:1	1:1	1:1	1:1
Age of onset	<40 yr	35–55 yr	20–40 yr	Any age
Sacroiliitis or spondylitis (%)	100	~20	~40	<20
Symmetry of sacroiliitis	Symmetrical	Asymmetrical	Asymmetrical	Symmetrical
Peripheral arthritis (%)	~25	95	90	5–20
Distribution	Axial and lower limbs	Variable	Lower limbs	Variable
HLA-B27 positivity (%)	85–95	25–60*	30–70	7–70†
Uveitis	0–40	~20	~50	<15

*60% when spondylitis is present.
†70% when spondylitis is present.
From Hochberg M et al: *Rheumatology*, ed 7, Philadelphia, 2019, Elsevier.

WORKUP

- Young patients, particularly men younger than 45 yr, with chronic inflammatory low back pain responsive to NSAIDs should be screened.
- Patients with psoriasis, inflammatory bowel disease, or recent gastrointestinal or genitourinary infections presenting with new-onset low back or peripheral joint pain should also be screened.
- Screening begins with a comprehensive history and physical exam.
- HLA-B27 testing and imaging of SI joints and/or lumbar spine are indicated based on clinical suspicion.

LABORATORY TESTS

- HLA-B27:
  1. Negative test does not rule out SpA.
  2. Sensitivity: 95% for ankylosing spondylitis, 80% for reactive arthritis, 70% for psoriatic arthritis, and 50% for enteropathic arthritis
- Elevated ESR and CRP, anemia of chronic disease, leukocytosis, and thrombocytosis may reflect active inflammation. A normal CRP or ESR does not rule out spondyloarthropathies.
- Testing for rheumatoid arthritis is negative (rheumatoid factor, cyclic-citrullinated peptide antibodies).
- Synovial fluid is inflammatory and nonspecific, with WBC >2,000/mm^2.

IMAGING STUDIES

- **X-Ray:** SI joints and lumbar spine
  1. May not detect early inflammation
  2. 20% to 80% have nonradiographic disease at time of presentation
  3. May show signs of structural damage such as erosions, syndesmophytes, sclerosis, and ankylosis in chronic axial disease
- **MRI:** SI joints and lumbar spine
  1. Subchondral bone marrow edema in early disease
  2. Useful when x-ray and clinical findings are nondiagnostic but clinician's suspicion for axial SpA remains high

Rx TREATMENT

Improvement in symptoms, preservation of function, and prevention of structural damage can be achieved through a multidisciplinary approach.

NONPHARMACOLOGIC THERAPY

- Physical and occupational therapies improve functional outcomes
- Surgery:
  1. Joint replacements (high-impact joints such as hips)
  2. Spinal wedge osteotomy (advanced axial disease)
  3. Colectomy (advanced enteropathic arthritis)

ACUTE GENERAL Rx

- NSAIDs are first-line.
- Avoid steroids in psoriatic arthritis due to risk of life-threatening pustular psoriasis and erythroderma.

CHRONIC Rx

- **NSAIDs**:
  1. Up to 35% of patients may achieve remission.
  2. Best response in early disease.
  3. Continuous dosing may prevent radiographic progression of axial disease.
- **DMARDs:** Effective for peripheral involvement only, not effective in axial disease
  1. Methotrexate, leflunomide, sulfasalazine
- **TNF inhibitors:** NSAID or DMARD failure
  1. Infliximab, adalimumab, golimumab, etanercept, certolizumab pegol
- **IL-17 and IL-12/23 inhibitors:** 2nd TNF inhibitor failure
  1. Recent studies show similar efficacy compared to TNF inhibitors.
  2. Ustekinumab (IL-12/23 inhibitor) and secukinumab (IL-17 inhibitor) are effective in psoriatic arthritis.
  3. Only ustekinumab is effective in enteropathic arthritis.

COMPLEMENTARY AND ALTERNATIVE MEDICINE

- Strong clinical trials are lacking.
- Small studies have shown pilates, tai chi, deep tissue massage, and hydroelectric therapy are beneficial in axial SpA.

DISPOSITION

- Function and mobility may be limited in advanced axial disease.
- Psoriatic arthritis is an independent risk factor for cardiovascular disease.

REFERRAL

Rheumatology, dermatology, ophthalmology, gastroenterology, infectious disease

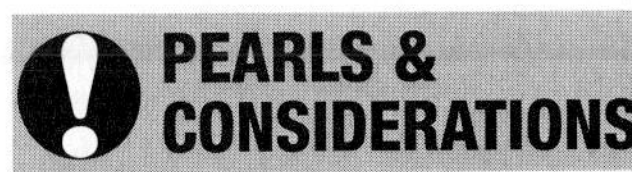

COMMENTS

Young men with chronic inflammatory low back pain deserve referral to a rheumatologist. HLA-B27 positivity is not required for diagnosis if strong clinical features are present. MRI may be needed to detect early axial disease. Track axial disease activity with clinical scoring systems and physical exam measurements. Traditional DMARDs are not effective in axial disease.

PREVENTION

High index of suspicion and prompt referral allows for early diagnosis. Early treatment with treat-to-target approach may prevent symptomatic and radiographic progression.

PATIENT/FAMILY EDUCATION

Smoking cessation is key. Discuss with family the implications of strong genetic component. Educate patients with psoriasis and inflammatory bowel disease about symptoms of inflammatory low back or peripheral joint pain to monitor for development of SpA in these high-risk individuals.

RELATED TOPICS

Ankylosing Spondylitis (Related Key Topic)
Psoriatic Arthritis (Related Key Topic)
Reactive Arthritis (Related Key Topic)
Enteropathic Arthritis (Related Key Topic)
Reiter Syndrome (Reactive Arthritis) (Related Key Topic)

AUTHOR: **MATTHEW J. WHITE, D.O.**

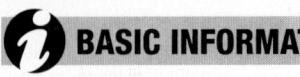

BASIC INFORMATION

DEFINITION

Spontaneous abortion is fetal loss before week 20 of pregnancy, calculated from the patient's last menstrual period, or the delivery of a fetus weighing <500 g. Early loss is before menstrual week 12, whereas late loss refers to losses from weeks 12 to 20.

Spontaneous abortion can also be classified as incomplete (partial passage of fetal tissue through partially dilated cervix), complete (spontaneous passage of all fetal tissue), threatened (uterine bleeding without cervical dilation or passage of tissue), inevitable (bleeding with cervical dilation without passage of fetal tissue), or missed abortion (intrauterine fetal demise without passage of tissue).

Recurrent spontaneous abortion involves three or more spontaneous pregnancy losses before week 20. It affects approximately 1% of couples attempting to conceive. However, in actual practice, most reproductive experts consider two spontaneous pregnancy losses sufficient to initiate an evaluation for habitual or recurrent spontaneous abortion, since the risk of another loss is similar at this point, and the emotional stress is high. As many as 5% of couples and probably even a higher proportion of couples in which the woman is over the age of 35 are affected by two or more consecutive spontaneous abortions.

SYNONYMS

Spontaneous miscarriage
Miscarriage
Spontaneous pregnancy loss

ICD-10CM CODES

O03.9	Complete or unspecified spontaneous abortion without complication
O03.89	Complete or unspecified spontaneous abortion with other complications

EPIDEMIOLOGY & DEMOGRAPHICS

INCIDENCE: 10% to 20% of clinically recognized pregnancies; 80% of miscarriages occur in the first trimester. Recurrent miscarriage occurs in <1% of couples attempting to have children.

ETIOLOGY

In a general overview, the etiology can be classified in terms of maternal (environmental) and fetal (genetic) factors, with the majority of miscarriages being related to genetic or chromosomal causes.

GENETICS

- Fetal chromosomal aneuploidy and polyploidy account for the overwhelming majority of first-trimester losses.
- Autosomal trisomy accounts for the majority of abnormalities, followed by monosomy X, tetraploidy, and, lastly, structural chromosomal abnormalities.
- The incidence of trisomy increases as maternal age increases.

MATERNAL CAUSES

- Uterine anomalies: Mullerian abnormalities such as unicornuate, bicornuate, or septated uterus are associated with increased miscarriage risk, although rates vary in different studies. A septated uterus is most highly associated with recurrent loss and can be surgically corrected and thus is important to diagnose. Other intrauterine pathologies such as synechiae, leiomyomas, or prior DES exposure are important to rule out also.
- Incompetent cervix (iatrogenic or congenital, associated with 20% of mid-trimester losses).
- Antiphospholipid antibody syndrome.
- Uncontrolled diabetes mellitus.
- Rare or controversial causes include HLA associations between mother and father; infections such as tuberculosis, *Chlamydia,* and *Ureaplasma;* smoking and alcohol use; irradiation; progesterone deficiency; and environmental toxins. Most of the literature is observational in nature, which may skew risk factor data.
- With two or more spontaneous miscarriages, a karyotype can be performed on the products of conception to evaluate for aneuploidy, which may be associated with a balanced translocation in one of the parents, and which has a substantially increased risk for abortion (depending on the actual type of translocation); if the pregnancy is carried to term, it has a 3% to 5% risk for an unbalanced karyotype. In patients with habitual abortion, evaluation for anatomic defects such as uterine septum and for antiphospholipid syndrome (lupus anticoagulant, beta 2 glycoprotein IgG/IgM, and anticardiolipin antibody IgG/IgM) should also be obtained.

RISK FACTORS

- Vaginal bleeding, especially >3 d, carries with it a 15% to 20% chance of miscarriage
- Advancing maternal age
- 2 or more prior miscarriages
- Significant underlying maternal health issues such as uncontrolled diabetes, thyroid disease, or other endocrine disturbances
- Illicit substance use
- Obesity
- Alcohol, smoking, and excessive caffeine intake
- Use of fluconazole in pregnancy is associated with a statistically significant increased risk of spontaneous miscarriage

PHYSICAL FINDINGS & CLINICAL PRESENTATION

- Profuse bleeding and cramping have a higher association with miscarriage than bleeding without cramping, which is more consistent with a threatened miscarriage.
- Cervical dilation with history or finding of fetal tissue at cervical os may be present.
- In cases of missed abortion, uterine size may be smaller than menstrual dating, in contrast to molar gestation, where size may be greater than dates.
- The presence of nausea and vomiting in early pregnancy is associated with a reduced risk for pregnancy loss.

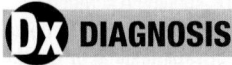

DIAGNOSIS

DIFFERENTIAL DIAGNOSIS

- Normal pregnancy
- Hydatidiform molar gestation
- Ectopic pregnancy
- Dysfunctional uterine bleeding
- Pathologic endometrial or cervical lesions

WORKUP

- All patients with bleeding in the first trimester should have an evaluation for possible ectopic pregnancy.
- If there are three early, prior pregnancy losses, a workup and treatment for recurrent miscarriage should begin before next conception. If there is a strong history for second-trimester loss, consideration for cerclage should be given if the history is consistent with incompetent cervix (e.g., painless cervical dilation).
- Most providers will initiate an evaluation for couples who have had 2 previous losses.
- One unexplained fetal loss beyond 10 weeks or 1 birth before 34 weeks because of preeclampsia should prompt an evaluation for antiphospholipid antibody syndrome.

LABORATORY TESTS

- Type and antibody screen are used to evaluate the need for Rh immune globulin.
- Recurrent pregnancy loss: During the preconception period in patients with recurrent pregnancy loss, hemoglobin A_{1c}, TSH, prolactin, anticardiolipin antibody, lupus anticoagulant, 20210A beta 2 glycoprotein antibodies, karyotyping, and anatomic evaluation with hysterosalpingography, or saline ultrasonography to assess for uterine septum. With increasing age, oocyte quality is a factor, and some practitioners will perform day 3 of the menstrual cycle FSH and anti-müllerian hormone to assess for diminished ovarian reserve. Progesterone level <5 mg/dl suggests nonviable gestation vs. >25 mg/dl, which suggests a good prognosis.

IMAGING STUDIES

Transvaginal sonogram (preferred) (Figs. 1–3) can be used with menstrual dating and serum quantitative human chorionic gonadotropin to document pregnancy location, fetal heart presence, gestational sac size, and adnexal pathology.

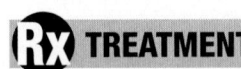

TREATMENT

NONPHARMACOLOGIC THERAPY

Depending on the patient's clinical status, desire to continue the pregnancy, and certainty of the diagnosis, expectant management can be considered. In pregnancies <6 wk or >14 wk, complete expulsion of fetal tissue usually occurs, and surgical intervention such as D&C can be avoided.

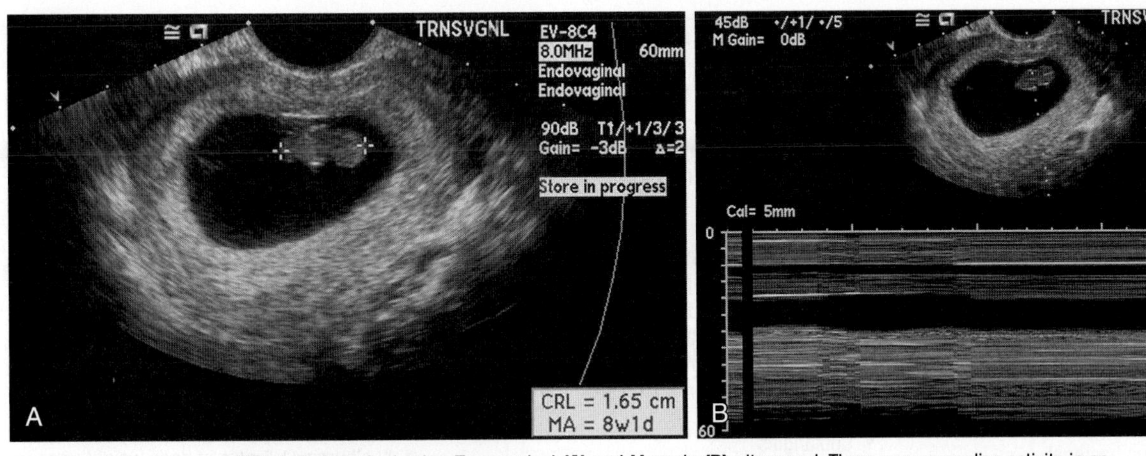

FIG. 1 Embryonic demise. Transvaginal **(A)** and M-mode **(B)** ultrasound. There was no cardiac activity in an embryo measuring more than the threshold of 5 mm. (From Fielding JR et al: *Gynecologic imaging*, Philadelphia, 2011, Saunders.)

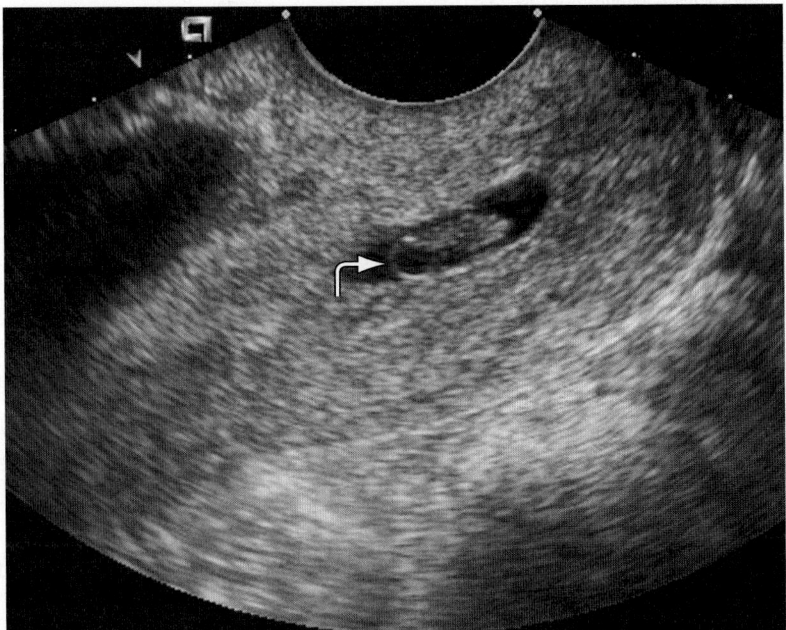

FIG. 2 Inevitable abortion. Transvaginal ultrasonography shows a sac in the cervical canal, past the internal os. The embryo *(curved arrow)* was nonviable. (From Fielding JR et al: *Gynecologic imaging*, Philadelphia, 2011, Saunders.)

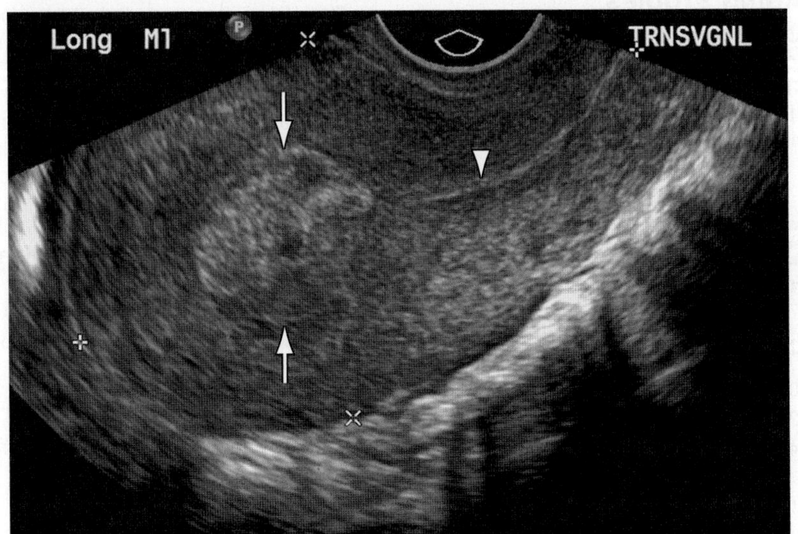

FIG. 3 Incomplete abortion. Transvaginal ultrasonography shows an echogenic mass *(arrows)* in the fundal endometrial cavity. The lower-segment endometrium *(arrowhead)* is normal. (From Fielding JR et al: *Gynecologic imaging*, Philadelphia, 2011, Saunders.)

ACUTE GENERAL Rx

- Incomplete miscarriage between 6 and 14 wk can be associated with great blood loss; these patients should undergo D&C.
- In cases of missed abortion, if fetal demise has occurred >6 wk before or gestational age is >14 wk, there is an increased risk of hypofibrinogenemia with disseminated intravascular coagulation. Thus D&C or manual vacuum aspiration should be performed early in the disease course. Consider use of misoprostol (Cytotec) in appropriate cases where the patient wishes to avoid surgery.
- There is evidence that a surgical approach leads to quicker resolution of the pregnancy event with fewer visits being required.
- Rh-negative patients should be given RhoGAM 50 mcg IM to prevent Rh isoimmunization.

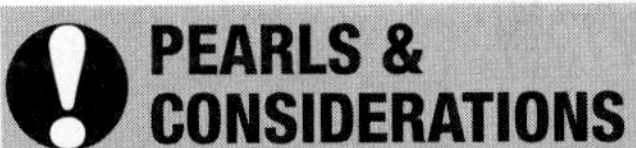

PEARLS & CONSIDERATIONS

Spontaneous pregnancy loss is recommended as a replacement for the term *abortion* and to acknowledge the emotional aspects of losing a pregnancy.

SUGGESTED READINGS

Available at ExpertConsult.com

RELATED CONTENT

Miscarriage (Patient Information)

AUTHOR: **ADRIENNE B. NEITHARDT, M.D.**

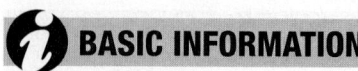

BASIC INFORMATION

DEFINITION

Spontaneous bacterial peritonitis (SBP) is an inflammatory reaction of the peritoneum secondary to the presence of bacteria or other microorganisms. More specifically, SBP is defined as an ascitic fluid infection without an evident intraabdominal surgically treatable source occurring primarily in patients with advanced cirrhosis of the liver.

SYNONYMS

Primary peritonitis
SBP
Peritonitis, spontaneous bacterial

ICD-10CM CODE

K65.2 Spontaneous bacterial peritonitis

EPIDEMIOLOGY & DEMOGRAPHICS

PREVALENCE: The prevalence of SBP in cirrhotic patients admitted to the hospital has been estimated at 10% to 30%.

PREDOMINANT SEX: Males are affected more often than females.

PHYSICAL FINDINGS & CLINICAL PRESENTATION

- Acute fever with accompanying abdominal pain/ascites, nausea, vomiting, diarrhea.
- In cirrhotic patients, presentation may be subtle with a low-grade temperature (100° F; 37.8° C) with or without abdominal abnormalities.
- In patients with ascites, a heightened degree of awareness is necessary for detection.
- Jaundice and encephalopathy.
- Deterioration of mental status and/or renal function.
- Table 1 summarizes symptoms and signs of ascetic fluid infection.

ETIOLOGY

- *Escherichia coli*
- *Klebsiella pneumoniae*
- *Streptococcus pneumoniae*
- *Streptococcus* and *Enterococcus* spp.
- *Staphylococcus aureus*
- Anaerobic pathogens: *Bacteroides, Clostridium* organisms
- Other: Fungal, mycobacterial, viral

DIAGNOSIS

The diagnosis of SBP is established by a positive ascitic fluid bacterial culture and an elevated ascitic fluid absolute polymorphonuclear leukocyte count (≥250 cells/mm^3).

DIFFERENTIAL DIAGNOSIS

- Appendicitis (in children)
- Perforated peptic ulcer
- Secondary bacterial peritonitis
- Peritoneal abscess
- Splenic, hepatic, or pancreatic abscess
- Cholecystitis
- Cholangitis

WORKUP

Paracentesis and ascitic fluid analysis will confirm diagnosis (see "Laboratory Tests").

LABORATORY TESTS

Ascitic fluid analysis reveals the following:

- Cell count with an absolute polymorphonuclear cell count >250/mm^3
- Presence of bacteria on gram stain
- pH <7.31
- Lactic acid >32 mg/dl
- Protein <1 g/dl
- Glucose >50 mg/dl
- Lactate dehydrogenase <225 mU/ml
- Positive culture of peritoneal fluid
- Measurement of the serum/ascites/albumin gradient: The serum/ascites/albumin gradient indirectly measures portal pressure. The albumin concentration of ascitic fluid and serum must be obtained on the same day. The ascitic fluid value is subtracted from the serum value to obtain the gradient. If the difference (not a ratio) is >1.1 g/dl, the patient has portal hypertension, with 97% accuracy. If the difference is <1.1 g/dl, portal hypertension is not present. The majority of patients with SBP have portal hypertension as a result of cirrhosis

IMAGING STUDIES

- Abdominal ultrasound: If there is clinical difficulty in performing paracentesis
- CT scan: To rule out secondary peritonitis (if indicated) and to exclude abscess, mass

TABLE 1 Symptoms and Signs of Ascitic Fluid Infection

	Frequency (%)				
Symptom or Sign	**SBP**	**Bacterascites**	**CNNA**	**Secondary Peritonitis**	**Polymicrobial Bacterascites**
Fever	68	57	50	33	10
Abdominal pain	49	32	72	67	10
Abdominal tenderness	39	32	44	50	10
Rebound tenderness	10	5	0	17	0
Altered mental status	54	50	61	33	0

CNNA, Culture-negative neutrocytic ascites.
From Feldman M et al: *Sleisenger and Fordtran's gastrointestinal and liver disease,* ed 10, Philadelphia, 2016, Elsevier.

TREATMENT

ACUTE GENERAL Rx

- Cefotaxime (2 g IV q8h) or ceftriaxone (2 g IV q24h). Alternative agents include ticarcillin-clavulanate, piperacillin-tazobactam, cefoxitin, and meropenem. Continue therapy for 5 to 7 days. Repeat diagnostic paracentesis can be done at day 2. Repeat paracentesis at 48 hr will demonstrate a significant decrease in polymorphonuclear count in patients with SBP. If ascites PMN count decreases by at least 25% at day 2, IV therapy can be switched to PO (levofloxacin 500-750 mg qd) to complete 7 days of therapy if organisms are susceptible.
- IV albumin (1.5 g/kg of body weight upon initial diagnosis and 1 g/kg of albumin on day 3) if BUN >30 mg/dl, serum creatinine >1 mg/dl, bilirubin >4 mg/dl.

PROPHYLAXIS

- Ciprofloxacin 500 mg PO qd or levofloxacin 250 mg PO qd.
- Alternative therapy: TMP-SMX one double-strength tablet PO qd.
- Rifaximin 1200 mg a day was shown in a recent study to be superior to norfloxacin.
- Prophylaxis should be continued until disappearance of ascites or until liver transplantation.

DISPOSITION

The overall mortality rate from an episode of SBP is 20%, and following an episode, the 1-yr mortality rate approaches 70%. Patients that develop SBP should be considered for liver transplantation.

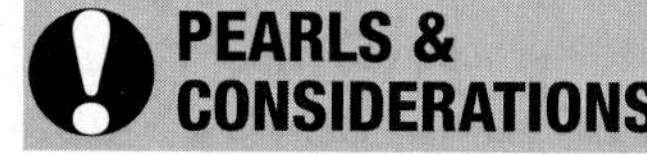

PEARLS & CONSIDERATIONS

COMMENTS

- Renal failure is a major cause of morbidity in cirrhotic patients with SBP. The use of IV albumin (1.5 g/kg at the time of diagnosis and 1 g/kg on day 3) may lower the rate of renal failure and mortality in patients with SBP.
- The criteria for the diagnosis of SBP require that abdominal paracentesis be performed and ascitic fluid be analyzed before a diagnosis of SBP can be made.
- Culturing ascitic fluid as if it were blood (with bedside inoculation of at least 10 ml of ascitic fluid directly into blood culture bottles at the bedside) has been shown to significantly increase the culture positivity of the ascitic fluid in the 80% to 100% range.
- Avoid therapeutic paracenteses during active infection.
- Positive blood cultures in an individual with ascites require exclusion of a peritoneal source by paracentesis.
- Follow-up paracentesis is indicated only in selected cases (worsening clinical status, nosocomial SBP, infection with atypical organism, recent β-lactam exposure).

SUGGESTED READINGS

Available at ExpertConsult.com

AUTHOR: **GLENN G. FORT, M.D., M.P.H.**

BASIC INFORMATION

DEFINITION

Squamous cell carcinoma (SCC) is a malignant neoplasm of keratinocytes.

SYNONYMS

SCC
Skin cancer

ICD-10CM CODES

C44.5	Malignant neoplasm of skin of trunk
C44.4	Malignant neoplasm of skin of scalp and neck
D04	Carcinoma in situ of skin
C44.9	Malignant neoplasm of skin, unspecified
C44.0	Malignant neoplasm of skin of lip
C44.2	Malignant neoplasm of skin of ear and external auricular canal
C44.3	Malignant neoplasm of skin of other and unspecified parts of skin
C44.02	Squamous cell carcinoma of skin of lip
C44.121	Squamous cell carcinoma of skin of unspecified eyelid, including canthus
C44.122	Squamous cell carcinoma of skin of right eyelid, including canthus
C44.129	Squamous cell carcinoma of skin of left eyelid, including canthus
C44.221	Squamous cell carcinoma of skin of unspecified ear and external auricular canal
C44.222	Squamous cell carcinoma of skin of right ear and external auricular canal
C44.229	Squamous cell carcinoma of skin of left ear and external auricular canal
C44.320	Squamous cell carcinoma of skin of unspecified parts of face
C44.321	Squamous cell carcinoma of skin of nose
C44.329	Squamous cell carcinoma of skin of other parts of face
C44.42	Squamous cell carcinoma of skin of scalp and neck
C44.520	Squamous cell carcinoma of anal skin
C44.521	Squamous cell carcinoma of skin of breast
C44.529	Squamous cell carcinoma of skin of other part of trunk
C44.621	Squamous cell carcinoma of skin of unspecified upper limb, including shoulder
C44.622	Squamous cell carcinoma of skin of right upper limb, including shoulder
C44.629	Squamous cell carcinoma of skin of left upper limb, including shoulder
C44.721	Squamous cell carcinoma of skin of unspecified lower limb, including hip
C44.722	Squamous cell carcinoma of skin of right lower limb, including hip
C44.729	Squamous cell carcinoma of skin of left lower limb, including hip
C44.82	Squamous cell carcinoma of overlapping sites of skin

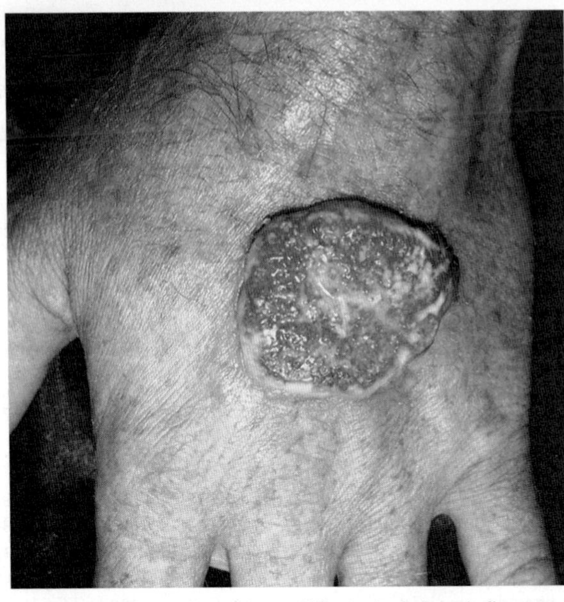

FIG. 1 Squamous cell carcinoma. (From James WD et al: *Andrews' diseases of the skin*, ed 12, Philadelphia, 2016, Elsevier.)

EPIDEMIOLOGY & DEMOGRAPHICS

- SCC is the second most common cutaneous malignancy, comprising 20% of all cases of nonmelanoma skin cancer.
- Incidence is highest in lower latitudes (e.g., southern U.S., Australia).
- Male:female ratio is 2:1.
- Incidence increases with age and sun exposure.
- In black patients, SCC are 20% more common than basal cell carcinomas (BCC).
- Average age at diagnosis is 66 yr.

PHYSICAL FINDINGS & CLINICAL PRESENTATION

- SCC frequently begins at the site of actinic keratosis and commonly affects the scalp, neck region, back of hands (Fig. 1), superior surface of the pinna, and the lip (Fig. 2). On the lower lip, SCC often develops on actinic cheilitis. A history of smoking is a significant predisposing factor.
- Bowen disease refers to SCC in situ.
- SCC lesions may have a scaly, erythematous macule or plaque.
- Telangiectasia, central ulceration may also be present. The ulcer may be superficial and hidden by a crust. Removal of the crust may reveal a well-defined papillary base.
- Most SCCs present as exophytic lesions that grow over a period of months.
- Although most SCCs are relatively slow growing and nonaggressive, some (2% to 5%) can exhibit rapid growth and metastases. Aggressive tumors are more common in immunocompromised patients and when arising from scars, burns, or prior injury (Marjolin's ulcer). Presence of SCC on ears, lips, or size >2 cm are high-risk features of SCC.

ETIOLOGY

Risk factors include ultraviolet B radiation, immunosuppression (kidney transplant recipients have a significantly increased risk), arsenic exposure, HPV infection, medications (azathioprine, sorafenib, tumor necrosis factor [TNF] inhibitors), discoid LE, erosive lichen planus, chronic ulcers, prior radiation exposure, and tobacco abuse.

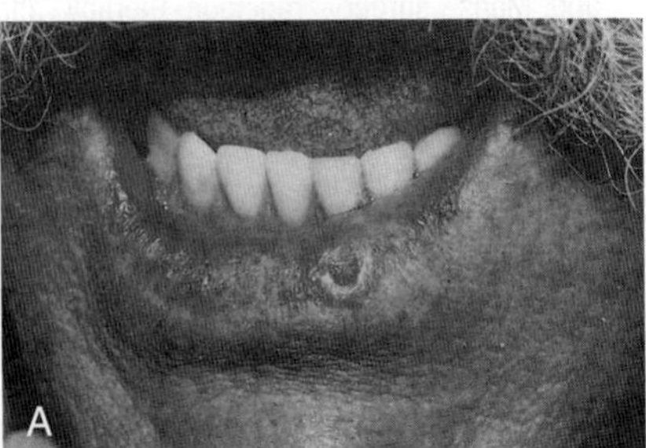

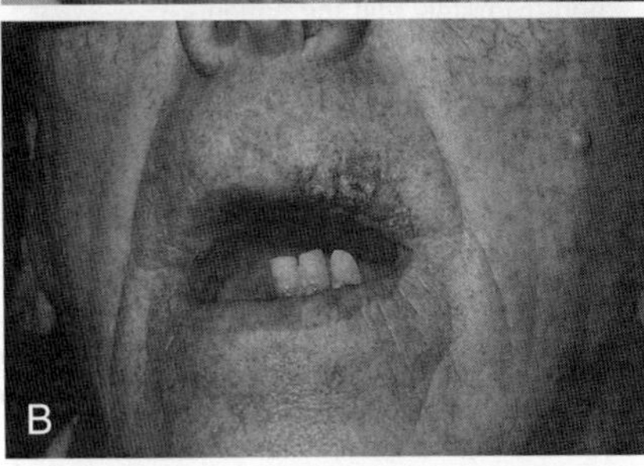

FIG. 2 Squamous cell carcinoma of the lip. The lower lip **(A)** is a relatively commonly affected site. Smoking is a risk factor for this site, and the prognosis is poorer compared to similar-sized lesions at other sun-exposed sites. Treatment is usually by wedge excision or with radiotherapy. By contrast, the upper lip margin **(B)** is a relatively uncommon site. The chronic trauma from the patient's only three teeth may have been relevant. (From White GM, Cox NH [eds]: *Diseases of the skin, a color atlas and text,* ed 2, St Louis, 2006, Mosby.)

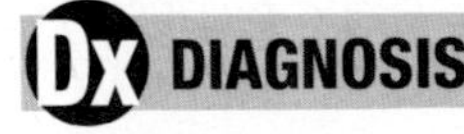

DIAGNOSIS

DIFFERENTIAL DIAGNOSIS

- Keratoacanthomas
- Actinic keratosis

- Amelanotic melanoma
- Basal cell carcinoma
- Benign tumors
- Healing traumatic wounds
- Spindle cell tumors
- Warts

WORKUP

Diagnosis is made by full-thickness skin biopsy (incisional or excisional).

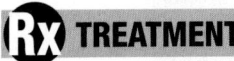

TREATMENT

ACUTE GENERAL Rx

- Electrodesiccation and curettage for small SCCs (<2 mm in diameter), superficial tumors, and lesions located in extremity and trunk.
- Tumors thinner than 4 mm can be managed by simple local removal.
- Lesions 4 to 8 mm thick or those with deep dermal invasion should be excised.
- Tumors penetrating the dermis can be treated with several modalities, including excision and Mohs' surgery, radiation therapy, and chemotherapy. Mohs' surgery is commonly used for lesions on the face.
- Metastatic SCC can be treated with cryotherapy and combination of chemotherapy using 13-*cis*-retinoic acid and interferon-alpha 2A.
- In a recent phase 1 study of PD-1 blockade with cemiplimab among patients with advanced cutaneous squamous cell carcinoma, cemiplimab induced a response in approximately half the patients.[1]

DISPOSITION

- Survival is related to size, location, degree of differentiation, immunologic status of the patient, depth of invasion, and presence of metastases. Risk factors for metastasis include lesions on the lip or ear, increasing lesion depth, and poor cell differentiation. Table 1 summarizes risk factors for metastasis of invasive squamous cell carcinoma.
- Patients whose tumors penetrate through the dermis or exceed 8 mm in thickness are at risk of tumor recurrence.
- The most common metastatic locations are regional lymph nodes, liver, and lung.
- Tumors on the scalp, forehead, ears, nose, and lips also carry a higher risk.
- The rate of SCC metastasis from all skin sites ranges from 0.5% to 5.2%.
- SCCs originating in the lip and pinna metastasize in 10% to 20% of cases.
- 5-yr survival for metastatic SCC is 34%.

TABLE 1 Risk Factors for Metastasis of Invasive Squamous Cell Carcinoma

Risk Factors
Tumor thickness: >2 mm (high risk: tumor thickness >6 mm)
Diameter: >2 cm
Location: Ear, lips, and mucosae, including tongue, vulva, and penis (perineural growth may be an additional risk factor in these locations)
Arising within a scar (e.g., burn, radiation)
Histopathologic features: Poorly differentiated or undifferentiated, acantholytic,* developing within Bowen disease
Immunosuppression

*Recently questioned Ogawa T et al: Acantholytic squamous cell carcinoma is usually associated with hair follicles, not acantholytic actinic keratosis, and is not "high risk": diagnosis, management, and clinical outcomes in a series of 115 cases, *J Am Acad Dermatol* 76:327–333, 2017.

Based in part on Brantsch KD et al: Analysis of risk factors determining prognosis of cutaneous squamous-cell carcinoma: a prospective study, *Lancet Oncol* 9:713–720, 2008.

REFERRAL

Oncology referral for metastatic SCC

PEARLS & CONSIDERATIONS

COMMENTS

- SCC arising in areas of prior radiation, thermal injury, and areas of chronic ulcers or chronic draining sinuses are more aggressive and have a higher frequency of metastasis than those originating in actinic damaged skin.
- Oral retinoids may be useful as a preventive strategy in patients with immunosuppression.
- Nicotinamide (500 mg bid, available over the counter) mitigates some of the deleterious effects of UV radiation and has been reported to lower the incidence of nonmelanoma skin cancer (NMSCO) by 23%.[2]

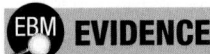

EVIDENCE

Available at ExpertConsult.com

RELATED CONTENT

Squamous Cell Carcinoma (Patient Information)

AUTHOR: **FRED F. FERRI, M.D.**

[1] Migden MR et al: PD-1 blockade with cemiplimab in advanced cutaneous squamous-cell carcinoma, *N Engl J Med* 379:341-51, 2018.

[2] Chen AC et al: A phase 3 randomized trial of nicotinamide for skin cancer chemoprevention, *N Engl J Med* 373:1618, 2015.

BASIC INFORMATION

DEFINITION

Statin-induced muscle syndromes (SIMS) include myopathy, myalgia, myositis, and rhabdomyolysis. Definitions for these syndromes are inconsistent in the medical literature.

- Myopathy: A general term defined as any disease of muscles.
- Myalgia: Muscle weakness or pain without serum creatinine kinase elevation.
- Myositis: Muscle weakness or pain with an increased serum creatinine kinase level.
- Rhabdomyolysis: Muscle weakness or pain and a marked serum creatinine kinase level usually greater than 10 times the upper limit of normal and serum creatinine elevation as well as signs of brown urine and elevated urine myoglobin. A rare **immune-mediated necrotizing myopathy (IMNM)**, also known as **statin-associated autoimmune myopathy**, has also been associated with the use of statins with symptoms persisting after discontinuation of the drug. This condition presents with symmetric proximal arm and leg weakness and severe elevations of muscle enzymes.

SYNONYMS

SIMS
Statin-induced myopathies
Statin-induced myositis
Statin-induced myalgias
Statin-induced rhabdomyolysis
Statin-associated autoimmune myopathy

ICD-10CM CODES

M60.9	Myositis, unspecified
M62.82	Rhabdomyolysis
G72.2	Myopathy due to other toxic agents
G72.9	Myopathy, unspecified
G72.81	Critical illness myopathy
G72.89	Other specified myopathies
M60.89	Other myositis, multiple sites

EPIDEMIOLOGY & DEMOGRAPHICS

INCIDENCE: Risk of statin-induced rhabdomyolysis is 1.2 per 10,000 persons/yr. Rhabdomyolysis risk of death is 0.15 deaths per 1 million prescriptions. SIMS most commonly occur in people aged 51 to 75, which may reflect the pattern of statin use. Statin-associated autoimmune myopathy occurs in an estimated 2 or 3 of every 100,000 patients treated with statins.

PEAK INCIDENCE: Patients on high-dose statins have a 0.9% incidence of statin-induced rhabdomyolysis.

PREVALENCE: The prevalence of statin-induced myalgias is about 1% to 5%, similar to placebo in clinical trials, although observational studies have suggested a prevalence of 10% or higher. Statins may cause elevated transaminases (ALT, AST) at a prevalence of 0.5% to 2.0% and rhabdomyolysis ~0.08%.

PREDOMINANT SEX AND AGE: The mean age of hospitalized patients with statin-induced myopathy or rhabdomyolysis was 64 yr old and was slightly more common in women (56%).

GENETICS: Interpatient variability exists in the activity of the *CYP3A4* gene for the metabolism of simvastatin, atorvastatin, and lovastatin. Homozygous carriers of *CYP2D6* (poor metabolizers) had a higher rate of discontinuation of simvastatin due to muscle syndromes compared with the *CYP2D6* wild-type genotype; patients taking atorvastatin and having a muscle event were more likely to have the CYP2D6*4 allele. *SLCO1B1* polymorphisms encode for the organic anion transport of statins into the liver cells. The variant C allele may increase the risk of the *SLCO1B1* statin–induced myopathy. Simvastatin-induced myopathy is more likely to be associated with *SLO1B1* genotype and not *ABCB1* genotype. A statin-associated autoimmune myopathy has shown a link to class II HLA allele DRB1*11:01 in the development of anti-HMG coA reductase antibodies, leading to an increase in expression of the antibodies in the muscles of patients exposed to statins. Deficiencies in ubiquinone (coenzyme Q10) may exist in patients with a mutation in the *COQ2* gene. The *EYS* gene can affect neuromuscular tissue and may have a role.

RISK FACTORS: Small body frame; age over 80 yr; women, particularly frail elderly women; patients taking multiple drugs, especially gemfibrozil, niacin, cyclosporine, itraconazole, ketoconazole, erythromycin, clarithromycin, verapamil, amiodarone; renal or liver impairment; pharmacogenetic variability; hypothyroidism; excessive alcohol intake; vigorous exercise; severe infections; excessive grapefruit juice ingestion; inherited defects of muscle metabolism such as carnitine palmityl transferase II deficiency, McArdle disease, and myoadenylate deaminase deficiency; acquired myopathies such as postpoliomyelitis syndrome; lipophilic statins (simvastatin, atorvastatin, lovastatin); multiple conditions such as diabetes; renal impairment, and prior elevated CK; and drugs of abuse (amphetamines, heroin, cocaine, phencyclidine).

PHYSICAL FINDINGS & CLINICAL PRESENTATION

- Myopathy can occur at any time, although it is more common within the first 4 weeks of therapy; statin-associated necrotizing myopathy may occur after months of using statins
- Proximal generalized muscle aches, body aches, and pains, and may be mild or severe
- Dark-colored urine
- Muscle cramps, spasms, tenderness, or stiffness
- Unusually tired or weak
- Nocturnal cramping
- Tendon pain

ETIOLOGY

- History of current statin use.
- May be explained by one of three deficiencies of end products of the 3-hydroxy-3-methylglutaryl-coA reductase pathway: cell signaling and apoptosis, mitochondrial function and ubiquinone concentrations, and cholesterol concentrations and cell membrane integrity.
- The risk may be enhanced by drug interactions that interfere with hepatic metabolism and gut wall transport of interacting medications and by pharmacodynamic effects.
- Underlying metabolic muscle disorder may predispose a patient to develop myopathy.
- Patients with statin-associated autoimmune myopathy have been found to have anti-HMG-CoA reductase antibodies even prior to exposure to statin therapy.

DIAGNOSIS

DIFFERENTIAL DIAGNOSIS

Bursitis, tendinitis, radiculopathy, osteoarthritis, muscle strain, myofascial pain, hypothyroidism, proton pump inhibitor–induced polymyositis, viral illness, polymyositis, idiopathic inflammatory myositis, and polymyalgia rheumatica

WORKUP

Workup consists of a thorough history, including exercise history, urine color, medication history, and physical exam to palpate tenderness and obtain blood tests to evaluate muscle and kidney damage.

LABORATORY TESTS

If severe myopathy or rhabdomyolysis is suspected:

- Elevated CPK, positive serum myoglobin, elevated BUN, serum creatinine, AST, ALT, LDH, and potassium
- Urine creatinine, positive casts, and hemoglobin in urine with absence of red blood cells
- Consider electrocardiogram and assessment of calcium, phosphate, and uric acid

If mild to moderate myopathy is suspected:

- Monitor TSH and CPK levels; CPK may only be elevated when sudden severe myopathy occurs.
- If the patient has brown or dark urine or elevated CPK, monitor BUN and serum creatinine.
- In statin-associated autoimmune myopathy, the creatine kinase level is usually ≥10 times the upper limit of normal. In these patients, muscle biopsy specimens will be positive for autoantibodies against HMG-CoA reductase and may have necrosis.

IMAGING STUDIES

- Not recommended.
- In statin-associated autoimmune myopathy, electromyography shows small-amplitude motor-unit potentials with increased spontaneous activity characteristic of an active myopathic process. Muscle edema is evident on MRI.[1]
- Statin Intolerance Tool:
  1. The American College of Cardiology has created a tool to assess statin muscle symptoms and to guide clinicians that can be of value: http://tools.acc.org/statinintolerance/#!/

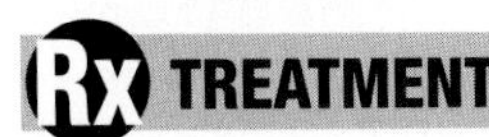

TREATMENT

NONPHARMACOLOGIC THERAPY

- Treatment of rhabdomyolysis is generally supportive in nature (see "Rhabdomyolysis" topic).

[1] Mammen AL: Statin-associated autoimmune myopathy, *N Engl J Med* 374:664–669, 2016.

 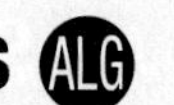

ACUTE GENERAL Rx

- Stop statin therapy immediately if muscle symptoms occur. Check history, potential drug-drug interactions, CPK, TSH, renal function, hepatic function, and urinalysis.
- If patients have suspected rhabdomyolysis, they should be hospitalized and treated with supportive therapy and monitoring of complications.
- If CPK <10× the upper limit of normal without symptoms, continue statin therapy at the same or lower dosage.
- If CPK <10× the upper limit of normal with intolerable symptoms, discontinue statin.
- If CPK >10× the upper limit of normal, discontinue statin.

Box E1 describes recommendations of the National Lipid Association Statin Safety Assessment Task Force regarding statin and muscle safety.

CHRONIC Rx

- After stopping the statin and symptom or CPK resolution, which may take up to 4 months, consider the same statin at a lower dosage or a different statin at an equivalent or lower dosage.
- When restarting therapy, consider statins such as low-dose rosuvastatin; pravastatin; and alternate-day dosing of rosuvastatin or atorvastatin.
- If patient had rhabdomyolysis secondary to statin therapy, consider nonstatin treatments.
- If the patient develops myopathy after a second trial of therapy, statin treatment should be permanently discontinued and nonstatin cholesterol-lowering therapy initiated.
- For IMNM (statin-associated autoimmune myopathy and idiopathic inflammatory myositis), immunosuppressive therapy with prednisone (1 mg per kilogram of body weight per day) and at least one agent (methotrexate, azathioprine, or mycophenolate mofetil) have been used. In resistant cases, IV immune globulin or another agent such as rituximab may be added.

INTEGRATIVE MEDICINE

- The effect of coenzyme Q10 on reducing or preventing SIMS remains controversial. Given its safety, coenzyme Q10 can be recommended if the actions listed under "Chronic Rx" are insufficient to continue the use of the statin and if the muscle symptoms have been limited to myalgias. Use coenzyme Q10 with caution in patients taking warfarin, as its anticoagulant effect may be decreased.
- A 2015 meta-analysis of observational studies reported that vitamin D levels were lower in patients with statin-induced myalgias than in individuals who did not have these symptoms.
- In a study of 282 patients with vitamin D levels less than 32 ng/ml and with myalgia-myositis from statins, vitamin D supplementation (median 50,000 IU D3/week) for 6 months improved symptoms and statin tolerance in 74% to 85% of patients; another study showed that replacement of vitamin D in patients with low-serum vitamin D may be able to maintain or restart previously failed statin therapy.

DISPOSITION

- Usually resolves within 1 wk up to 4 mo after discontinuing statin therapy.
- Once the patient has a full recovery, an alternative statin can be tried.
- Statins should not be restarted in IMNM or idiopathic inflammatory myositis.

REFERRAL

If rhabdomyolysis is suspected, immediate referral for hospitalization is suggested.

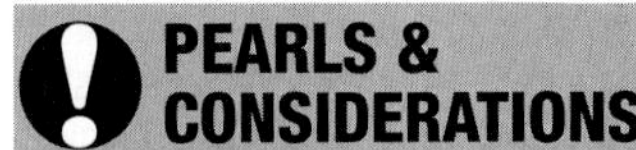

PEARLS & CONSIDERATIONS

COMMENTS

SIMS are usually mild and will resolve within a few wk after discontinuing statin therapy. However, such syndromes may progress to rhabdomyolysis.

PREVENTION

- Follow the 2013 AHA/ACC treatment guidelines and the 2017 ACC focused update on nonstatin therapies for LDL cholesterol and limit the concomitant use of fibrates with statins.
- Discontinue statin therapy prior to and during surgical procedures.
- If patient requires a short-term therapy with an interacting medication such as an azole antifungal, temporarily discontinue statin therapy until interacting therapy is completed.
- If statin–fibric acid therapy is warranted, fenofibrate is preferred over gemfibrozil to decrease risk of myopathy.
- Baseline liver function testing before initiation of statin therapy and only if clinically indicated thereafter.

PATIENT & FAMILY EDUCATION

- Inform patients to promptly report muscle weakness, unexpected muscle pain, or brownish urine.
- Ensure that the pharmacist and/or primary care physician checks for drug-drug interactions with every new prescription, including those from dentists and physicians from other specialties.
- Coenzyme Q10 may lessen milder muscle symptoms from statins, but patients should inform their physician and pharmacist if they decide to use this supplement.
- A recent clinical trial comparing lipid-lowering efficacy for two nonstatin therapies, ezetimibe and evolocumab, among patients with statin intolerance revealed that evolocumab resulted in a significantly greater reduction in LDL-C levels after 24 weeks. Further studies are needed to assess long-term efficacy and safety.

SUGGESTED READINGS

Available at ExpertConsult.com

RELATED CONTENT

Rhabdomyolysis (Related Key Topic)

AUTHORS: **LISA COHEN, PHARM.D.,** and **ANNE L. HUME, PHARM.D.**

BASIC INFORMATION

DEFINITION

Status epilepticus is a medical neurologic emergency. It is historically defined as 30 min of continuous seizure activity or two or more seizures without full recovery of consciousness between seizures. However, in practice a continuous seizure that lasts >5 min is treated as status epilepticus.

SYNONYMS

Convulsive status epilepticus
Nonconvulsive status epilepticus

ICD-10CM CODES

G41	Status epilepticus
G40.301	Generalized idiopathic epilepsy and epileptic syndromes, not intractable, with status epilepticus

EPIDEMIOLOGY & DEMOGRAPHICS

INCIDENCE: 40 to 100 cases per 100,000 persons

PEAK INCIDENCE: It is most common among children younger than 1 yr and adults older than 60 yr.

PREDOMINANT SEX AND AGE: No gender preference

PHYSICAL FINDINGS & CLINICAL PRESENTATION

- Patients can present with repetitive tonic clonic movements of the body (convulsive status epilepticus); other patients are comatose and nonresponsive (nonconvulsive status epilepticus).
- Patients may also present with lethargy, intermittent confusion, and involuntary movements.

ETIOLOGY

- Status epilepticus can be the result of an acute neurologic injury, such as stroke, meningitis, brain tumor, etc. Table 1 summarizes causes of status epilepticus in adults presenting in the community.
- In patients with epilepsy, abrupt discontinuation of antiepileptic drugs can result in status epilepticus.

DIAGNOSIS

DIFFERENTIAL DIAGNOSIS

- Convulsive syncope
- Encephalopathies: Metabolic, infectious, toxic, etc.
- Nonepileptic spells

WORKUP

- ABCs
- ICU admission
- Emergent electroencephalogram (EEG)
- Continuous video EEG in refractory cases
- Table 2 describes a suggested timetable for emergency diagnosis and treatment of status epilepticus. A treatment approach is summarized in Table 3 and Fig. 1

LABORATORY TESTS

- Routine blood workup (CBC, CMP, glucose, electrolytes)
- Urine drug screen
- Lumbar puncture and CSF analysis in patients with suspected infectious meningitis or encephalitis or suspected autoimmune or paraneoplastic encephalitis

TABLE 1 Causes of Status Epilepticus in Adults Presenting from the Community

Previous Seizures	No Previous Seizures
Common	
Subtherapeutic anticonvulsant	Ethanol-related
Ethanol-related	Drug toxicity
Intractable epilepsy	CNS infection
	Head trauma
	CNS tumor
Less Common	
CNS infection	Metabolic aberration
Metabolic aberration	Stroke
Drug toxicity	
Stroke	
CNS tumor	
Head trauma	

CNS, Central nervous system.
From Vincent JL et al: *Textbook of critical care*, ed 7, Philadelphia, 2017, Elsevier.

IMAGING STUDIES

- Immediate CT scan of the head
- MRI of the brain with and without contrast should be performed once the patient is in a stable condition

TREATMENT

- Patients with continuous seizure activity over 3 min need intravenous lorazepam 0.1 mg/kg at 2 mg/min (or diazepam 0.2 mg/kg at 5 mg/min only when lorazepam is not available).
- In the absence of intravenous access, intramuscular administration of midazolam 10 mg in an adult is a superior alternative.
- Failure of response to lorazepam or midazolam is referred to as established status epilepticus and should be followed by second-line therapy of intravenous fosphenytoin 20 mg/kg (PE) at a rate not greater than 150 mg/min, phenytoin 20 mg/kg IV at up to 50 mg/min as tolerated, intravenous valproic acid 40 mg/kg IV, or intravenous levetiracetam 60 mg/kg IV. Vital signs should be monitored during the infusion.
- If seizures continue, an additional infusion of intravenous valproate, levetiracetam, lacosamide, or brivaracetam or continuous infusions of phenobarbital, midazolam, and propofol are alternatives. Many of these drugs remain under investigation, and superiority of any one agent is not established. Treatment alternatives for refractory and super-refractory status epilepticus are summarized in Table 4.

TABLE 2 Suggested Timetable for Emergency Diagnosis and Treatment of Status Epilepticus

Time	Exam/Intervention	Testing
Initial presentation: 0 min	Airway, breathing, circulation, IV access, monitoring	Glucose, oxygenation via pulse oximetry ± blood gas analysis
Primary survey: 5 min	Neurologic exam Administer antiepileptic drugs Lorazepam, 0.1 mg/kg IV Phenobarbital, 20 mg/kg IV Normal saline maintenance IV Reduce fever	Electrolytes, renal and liver function, ammonia, anticonvulsant levels, toxicology, complete blood cell count, urinalysis
Secondary survey: 15-30 min	Evaluate treatment results Second-line antiepileptic drug if seizure persists Fosphenytoin, 20 mg/kg IV, or phenytoin, 20 mg/kg IV	Patient-specific: Cranial imaging (CT vs. MRI), lumbar puncture, EEG, ECG
Status epilepticus: >30 min	Intubation and mechanical ventilation	
Refractory status epilepticus: >60 min	Titrate antiepileptic drug to burst suppression Pentobarbital, 10 mg/kg IV given over 30 min, then 5 mg/kg every hour for 3 doses, then 1 mg/kg/h; titrate to effect Midazolam, 0.15 mg/kg IV, then 1-2 μg/kg/min, titrate to effect Phenobarbital, 5-10 mg/kg IV every 20 minutes to achieve burst suppression, then every 12 hours Evaluate need for vasopressors	Continuous EEG Neurologic consultation Consider anesthesia consultation for treatment with inhaled anesthetic

CT, Computed tomography; *ECG*, electrocardiogram; *EEG*, electroencephalogram; *IV*, intravenous; *MRI*, magnetic resonance imaging.
From Vincent JL et al: *Textbook of critical care*, ed 7, Philadelphia, 2017, Elsevier.

TABLE 3 Treatment Approach to Status Epilepticus

1. Appropriate critical care treatment should be provided as soon as possible and simultaneously with emergent initial therapy for seizures. Treatment should be escalated quickly until seizures are controlled.

1a. Critical care treatment (dictated by clinical circumstances):
   a. Intubation for airway protection and mechanical ventilation
   b. Vital sign monitoring
   c. Peripheral IV access
   d. Treatment of hypotension with vasopressors
   e. Finger stick blood glucose
   f. Nutrient resuscitation (thiamine before dextrose)
   g. Hypertension may be related to ongoing seizure activity, and termination of status epilepticus often substantially corrects it. Additionally, many agents used to terminate status epilepticus can produce hypotension.

1b. Emergent initial therapy with benzodiazepines
   a. Lorazepam 0.1 mg/kg up to 4 mg per dose, may repeat after 5-10 min
   b. Midazolam 0.2 mg/kg IM/IV up to 10 mg
   c. Diazepam 0.15 mg/kg up to 10 mg per dose, may repeat after 5 min

2. Urgent control therapy—antiseizure drugs available in IV formulations
   a. Fosphenytoin/phenytoin 20 mg PE/kg IV, may repeat bolus of 5 mg/kg IV
   b. Valproic acid 20-40 mg/kg IV, may repeat bolus of 20 mg/kg IV
   c. Levetiracetam 1000-3000 mg IV
   d. Phenobarbital 20 mg/kg IV, may repeat bolus of 5-10 mg/kg
   e. Lacosamide 200-400 mg IV
   f. Midazolam bolus 0.2 mg/kg IV, followed by 0.05-2 mg/kg/h continuous infusion

3. Refractory therapy–continuous infusion of antiseizure drugs, titrated to either seizure cessation, suppression-burst, or complete suppression on cEEG
   a. Midazolam bolus 0.2 mg/kg IV, followed by 0.05-2 mg/kg/h continuous infusion
   b. Propofol bolus 1-2 mg/kg, followed by 20 mcg/kg/min continuous infusion, titrate up to 30-200 mcg/kg/min
   c. Pentobarbital 5-15 mg/kg, may repeat bolus of 5-10 mg/kg, followed by 0.5-5 mg/kg/h continuous infusion

4. Treat complications

   Complications of status epilepticus are numerous and can involve multiple organ systems. In particular, convulsive status epilepticus is associated with cardiac complications such as hypertension and tachycardia, as well as rhabdomyolysis and hyperthermia. Respiratory complications, including respiratory failure, hypoxia, and neurogenic pulmonary edema, may be seen. Status epilepticus is associated with neuronal damage and cerebral edema with increased intracranial pressure, which may require intracranial pressure monitoring and aggressive treatment with hypertonic agents.

From Vincent JL et al: *Textbook of critical care*, ed 7, Philadelphia, 2017, Elsevier.

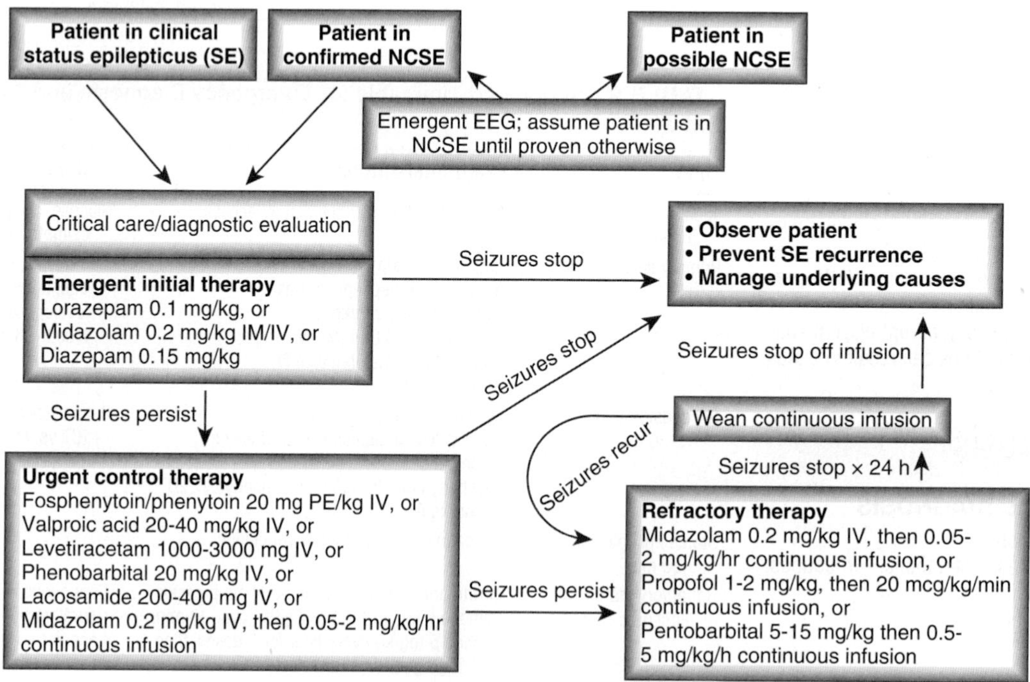

FIG. 1 Management algorithm for status epilepticus. *EEG;* Electroencephalogram; *IM,* intramuscular; *IV,* intravenous; *NCSE,* nonconvulsive status epilepticus; *SE,* status epilepticus. (From Vincent JL et al: *Textbook of critical care*, ed 7, Philadelphia, 2017, Elsevier.)

TABLE 4 Treatment Alternatives for Refractory and Super-Refractory Status Epilepticus

	Comments	Adverse Events
Thiopental	Metabolized to pentobarbital	Hypotension Respiratory depression Cardiac depression
Ketamine	Mechanism of action particularly well-suited to treat refractory and super-refractory SE (NMDA receptor antagonist)	High intracranial pressure Hypotension Hallucinations
Inhaled anesthetics	High rate of complications Needs closed system (gas recovery)	Hypotension Infection Paralytic ileus
Ketogenic diet	Relatively safe (no respiratory and cardiocirculatory instability) Slow onset of action Requires skilled dietician	Gastroesophageal reflux Constipation Acidosis Hypertriglyceridemia
Lidocaine	Minor respiratory depression compared with other drugs	Cardiocirculatory instability Possible induction of seizures
Hypothermia	Only transitory control (cannot be a prolonged therapy)	Hypotension Cardiovascular instability Impaired coagulation (bleeding risks)
Resective surgery	Long-term treatment of seizures Not all patients are eligible	Surgical risks

NMDA, N-methyl-D-aspartate; *SE,* status epilepticus.
From Swaiman KF et al: *Swaiman's pediatric neurology, principles and practice*, ed 6, Philadelphia, 2017, Elsevier. See original table for references.

NONPHARMACOLOGIC THERAPY

None

GENERAL Rx

It is important to find out the etiology of the status epilepticus (e.g., metabolic disturbance, infection). The appropriate treatment/understanding of the underlying cause of the status epilepticus will impact successful treatment.

CHRONIC Rx

- Chronic treatment of status epilepticus depends on underlying etiology.
- Patient with status epilepticus due to epilepsy will need chronic treatment.

COMPLEMENTARY & ALTERNATIVE MEDICINE

Not applicable

DISPOSITION

- Response to treatment depends on the etiology of the status epilepticus.
- When there is no CNS injury as a cause or result of the status epilepticus, the prognosis is good.
- No driving until seizure freedom in accordance with local laws and regulations.

REFERRAL

Status epilepticus is a neurologic emergency; therefore immediate inpatient neurologic consultation is warranted.

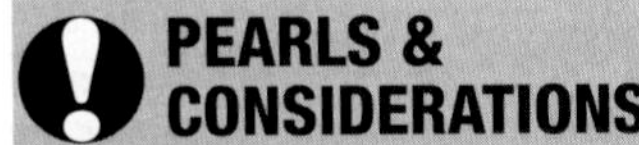

PEARLS & CONSIDERATIONS

COMMENTS

- Status epilepticus is a medical emergency that carries a high risk of mortality. Mortality among patients who present in status epilepticus is 15% to 22%. Among those who survive, functional ability will decline in 25% of cases.
- Continuous video EEG is crucial in the treatment of these patients because some of them may not be clinically seizing (convulsing) but electrographically they may still have subclinical repetitive seizures or subclinical status epilepticus.

PREVENTION

Medication compliance is crucial in patients with epilepsy.

PATIENT & FAMILY EDUCATION

- Patients with epilepsy have normal lives.
- The goal of treatment is no seizures and no side effects to medications.
- Patient education and information can be obtained at the Epilepsy Foundation: www.epilepsyfoundation.org
- Pregnant women with epilepsy should visit the Antiepileptic Drug Pregnancy Registry website for information and assistance: www.massgeneral.org/aed
- Patients with ongoing seizures are forbidden from driving; check state regulations and laws regarding driving and epilepsy.

AUTHORS: **PATRICIO SEBASTIAN ESPINOSA, M.D., M.P.H.,** and **COREY GOLDSMITH, M.D.**

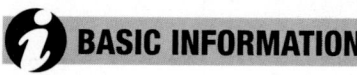

BASIC INFORMATION

DEFINITION

Stomatitis is inflammation involving the oral mucous membranes. Mucositis is inflammation and ulceration of the mucous membranes. It is most commonly seen in the mouth but can occur anywhere in the GI, genitourinary (GU), or respiratory tract. It is most often due to side effects of chemotherapy or radiation therapy (Fig. 1) in cancer patients.

SYNONYM

Heterogeneous grouping of unrelated illnesses, each with its own designation(s)

ICD-10CM CODES	
K12	Stomatitis and related lesions
K12.1	Other forms of stomatitis
K13.0	Other and unspecified lesions of oral mucosa
K12.0	Recurrent oral aphthae
B37.0	Candidal stomatitis
A69.0	Necrotizing ulcerative stomatitis
B08.4	Enteroviral vesicular stomatitis with exanthem
B08.61	Bovine stomatitis
B37.0	Candidal stomatitis
K12.30	Oral mucositis (ulcerative), unspecified
K12.31	Oral mucositis (ulcerative) due to antineoplastic therapy
K12.32	Oral mucositis (ulcerative) due to other drugs
K12.33	Oral mucositis (ulcerative) due to radiation
K12.39	Other oral mucositis (ulcerative)

PHYSICAL FINDINGS & CLINICAL PRESENTATION

WHITE LESIONS:

- Candidiasis (thrush)
- Caused by yeast infection *(Candida albicans)*
- Examination: White, curdlike material (Fig. E2) that, when wiped off, leaves a raw, bleeding surface
- Epidemiology: Seen in the very young and the very old, those with immunodeficiency (AIDS, cancer), persons with diabetes, and patients treated with antibacterial agents
- Other:
  1. Leukoedema: Filmy opalescent-appearing mucosa, which can be reverted to normal appearance by stretching. This condition is benign
  2. White sponge nevus: Thick, white corrugated folds involving the buccal mucosa. Appears in childhood as an autosomal dominant trait. Benign condition
  3. Darier disease (keratosis follicularis): White papules on the gingivae, alveolar mucosa, and dorsal tongue. Skin lesions also present (erythematous papules). Inherited as an autosomal dominant trait
  4. Chemical injury: White sloughing mucosa
  5. Nicotine stomatitis: Whitened palate with red papules
  6. Lichen planus: Linear, reticular, slightly raised striae on buccal mucosa. Skin is involved by pruritic violaceous papules on forearms and inner thighs
  7. Discoid lupus erythematosus: Lesion resembles lichen planus
  8. Leukoplakia: White lesions that cannot be scraped off; 20% are premalignant epithelial dysplasia or squamous cell carcinoma
  9. Hairy leukoplakia: Shaggy white surface that cannot be wiped off; seen in HIV infection, caused by Epstein-Barr virus

RED LESIONS:

- Candidiasis may present with red lesions instead of the more frequent white. Median rhomboid glossitis is a chronic variant
- Benign migratory glossitis (geographic tongue): Area of atrophic depapillated mucosa surrounded by a keratotic border. Benign lesion, no treatment required
- Hemangiomas
- Histoplasmosis: Ill-defined, irregular patch with a granulomatous surface, sometimes ulcerated
- Allergy
- Anemia: Atrophic reddened glossal mucosa seen with pernicious anemia
- Erythroplakia: Red patch usually caused by epithelial dysplasia or squamous cell carcinoma
- Burning tongue (glossopyrosis): Normal examination; sometimes associated with denture trauma, anemia, diabetes, vitamin B_{12} deficiency, psychogenic problems

DARK LESIONS (BROWN, BLUE, BLACK):

- Coated tongue: Accumulation of keratin; harmless condition that can be treated by scraping
- Melanotic lesions: Freckles, lentigines, lentigo, melanoma, Peutz-Jeghers syndrome, Addison disease
- Varices
- Kaposi sarcoma: Red or purple macules that enlarge to form tumors; seen in patients with AIDS

RAISED LESIONS:

- Papilloma
- Verruca vulgaris
- Condyloma acuminatum
- Fibroma
- Epulis
- Pyogenic granuloma
- Mucocele
- Retention cyst

BLISTERS:

- Primary herpetic gingivostomatitis (Fig. E3)
- Caused by herpes simplex virus type 1 or, less frequently, type 2

COURSE: Day 1: malaise, fever, headache, sore throat, cervical lymphadenopathy; days 2 and 3: appearance of vesicles that develop into painful ulcers of 2 to 4 mm in diameter; duration of up to 2 wk

- Recurrent intraoral herpes: Rare; recurrences typically involve only the keratinized epithelium (lips). Table 1 summarizes distinctions between aphthous and herpetic oral ulcers
- Pemphigus and pemphigoid
- Hand-foot-mouth disease: Caused by coxsackievirus group A
- Erythema multiforme
- Herpangina: Caused by echovirus
- Traumatic ulcer
- Primary syphilis
- Perlèche (or angular cheilitis)

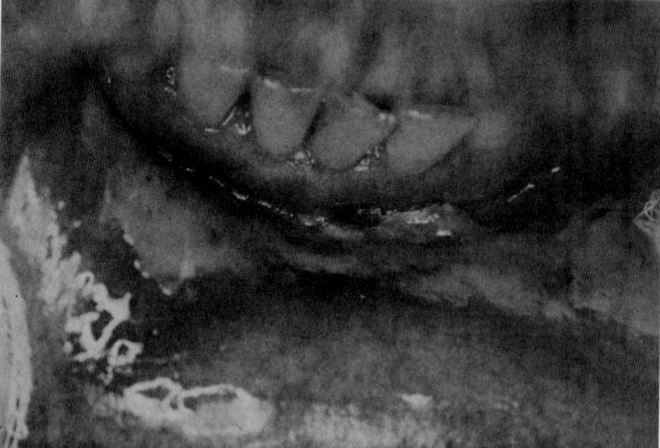

FIG. 1 Oral mucositis caused by radiation therapy. (From Keefe ZDM, Logan R: Oral complications of cancer and its treatment. In Walsh TD et al [eds]: *Palliative medicine,* Philadelphia, 2008, Saunders.)

TABLE 1 Distinctions between Aphthous and Herpetic Oral Ulcers

Condition	Mucosa	Location
Aphthous ulcers	Unkeratinized	Lateral tongue, floor of the mouth, labial and buccal mucosa, soft palate, pharynx
Herpetic ulcers	Keratinized	Gingiva, hard palate, dorsal tongue

From Feldman M et al: *Sleisenger and Fordtran's gastrointestinal and liver disease*, ed 10, Philadelphia, 2016, Elsevier.

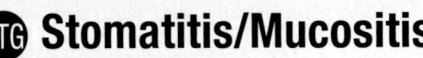

- Recurrent aphthous stomatitis (canker sores): Most common oral mucosa lesion; may be associated with many systemic diseases
- Behçet's syndrome (aphthous ulcers, uveitis, genital ulcerations, arthritis, and aseptic meningitis)
- Reiter syndrome (conjunctivitis, urethritis, and arthritis with occasional oral ulcerations)
- Unknown cause

COURSE: Solitary or multiple painful ulcers may develop simultaneously and heal over 10 to 14 days. The size of the lesions and the frequency of recurrences are variable.

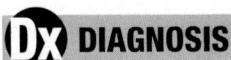

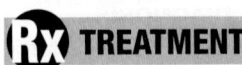

DIAGNOSIS

WORKUP

- White lesions: Candidiasis (thrush) diagnosis—ovoid yeast and hyphae seen in scrapings treated with KOH culture
- Blisters:
  1. Exfoliative cytology
  2. Viral culture
  3. Immunofluorescence for herpes antigen

TREATMENT

White lesions: Candidiasis (thrush) treatment:
- Topical with nystatin or clotrimazole
- Systemic with ketoconazole or fluconazole

Blisters:
- Supportive
- Consider acyclovir

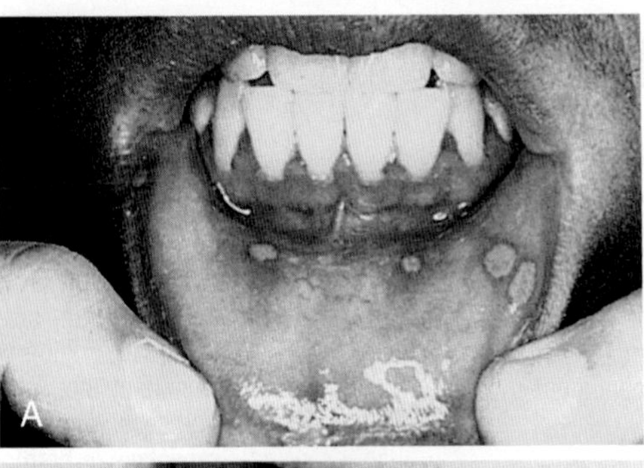

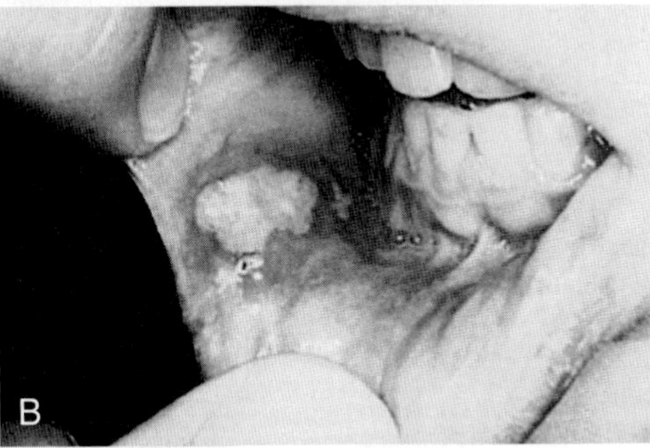

FIG. 4 A, Multiple minor aphthous ulcers. **B,** A major aphthous ulcer. (From Feldman M et al: *Sleisenger and Fordtran's gastrointestinal and liver disease,* ed 10, Philadelphia, 2016, Elsevier.)

Recurrent intraoral herpes/aphthous ulcerations (Fig. 4): Topical corticosteroids (dexamethasone ointment applied to the identified ulcer tid) or systemic steroids for severe cases.

RELATED CONTENT

Stomatitis (Patient Information)

AUTHOR: **FRED F. FERRI, M.D.**

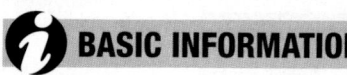

BASIC INFORMATION

DEFINITION

Ischemic stroke is the sudden onset of a focal neurologic deficit as a result of cerebral ischemia resulting in cell death. The purpose of this chapter is to help the provider make decisions about the management of the acute stroke patient within the first several hours of symptoms; this is the crucial time for definitive treatment interventions.

SYNONYMS

Stroke
Brain attack
Cerebrovascular accident (this is a nonspecific term and should not be used)

ICD-10CM CODES

I63	Cerebral infarction
I63.3	Cerebral infarction due to thrombosis of cerebral arteries
I63.4	Cerebral infarction due to embolism of cerebral arteries
I63.5	Cerebral infarction due to unspecified occlusion or stenosis of cerebral arteries
I63.6	Cerebral infarction due to cerebral venous thrombosis, nonpyogenic
I63.8	Other cerebral infarction
I63.9	Cerebral infarction, unspecified
I67.89	Other cerebrovascular disease

EPIDEMIOLOGY & DEMOGRAPHICS

INCIDENCE:
- ~795,000 new or recurrent strokes occur each yr in the U.S.
- Stroke is the number five cause of death (165,000 deaths every yr) and the leading cause of long-term disability in the U.S.

PREVALENCE: There are ~4.5 million stroke survivors in the U.S.

RISK FACTORS: Hypertension, dyslipidemia, diabetes mellitus, and smoking are the four major modifiable risk factors. Other risk factors include age, gender, atrial fibrillation (most common cause of cardioembolic stroke), mechanical heart valve, patent foramen ovale, recent myocardial infarction, metabolic syndrome, carotid artery stenosis, vertebral artery stenosis, intracranial artery stenosis, hypercoagulable states, subclinical atrial tachyarrhythmias without clinical atrial fibrillation, sickle cell disease, and obesity.

GENETICS: Multifactorial

PHYSICAL FINDINGS & CLINICAL PRESENTATION

When a patient presents with an acute ischemic stroke acutely, the most important considerations are determination of the time the patient was last known normal, the etiology (ischemic or hemorrhagic), and the severity, because these aspects will determine acute treatment. The time last known normal was when the patient was last seen normal (by themselves or by someone else). If they awoke with the deficits, the time last seen normal was when they went to bed.

Clinical presentation varies with the artery and region of CNS affected. Clinical presentation cannot reliably distinguish between hemorrhagic and ischemic causes, and so imaging must be done. Below is a noncomprehensive list of common stroke syndrome presentations based on the cerebral vascular territory affected. Please note that this list is not comprehensive and that all findings for a particular syndrome may not be listed here.

- Large- to medium-sized arteries:
  1. Dominant middle cerebral artery (MCA): Dominant face and arm > leg weakness and sensory loss with aphasia (expressive, receptive, or both); possible hemianopia
  2. Nondominant middle cerebral artery (MCA): Nondominant face and arm > leg weakness and sensory loss with hemineglect; possible hemianopia
  3. Anterior cerebral artery (ACA): Contralateral leg weakness and sensory loss
  4. Internal carotid artery: Combination of contralateral MCA and ACA
  5. Basilar artery: Typically an acute loss of consciousness preceded by vertigo, nausea, vomiting, and diplopia; quadriparesis or quadriplegia may be seen, including "locked-in" syndrome
  6. Posterior cerebral artery: Unilateral hemianopia; blindness with anosognosia (Anton syndrome) if bilateral
  7. Posterior inferior cerebellar artery: Lateral medullary (Wallenberg) syndrome—ipsilesional loss of pinprick and temperature on the face and contralateral loss of pinprick and temperature on the body; ipsilesional Horner syndrome and ipsilesional palatal weakness with resulting dysphagia, dysarthria. Also with vertigo, nystagmus, ataxia.
- **Small arteries: Lacunar syndromes;** no cortical signs are present in lacunar syndromes.
  1. Pure motor hemiparesis: Typically due to an ischemic lesion in either the internal capsule or pons.
  2. Pure sensory stroke: Typically due to an ischemic lesion of the thalamus.
  3. Ataxic hemiparesis: Ataxia out of proportion to the hemiparesis; typically due to an ischemic lesion of either the internal capsule or pons.
  4. Sensorimotor stroke: Typically due to ischemic lesion involving both the thalamus and internal capsule.
  5. Dysarthria–clumsy hand syndrome: Multiple localizations possible but typically the pons; facial weakness, dysarthria, and mild clumsiness and weakness of the hand.

ETIOLOGY

Etiologies include atherosclerosis, cardioembolism, artery-to-artery embolism, small-vessel lipohyalinosis, arteritis, arterial dissection, and vasospasm.

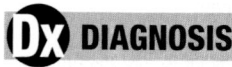

DIAGNOSIS

DIFFERENTIAL DIAGNOSIS

The differential diagnosis of acute ischemic stroke includes hemorrhagic stroke (intracerebral hemorrhage), subarachnoid or subdural hemorrhage, seizure with postictal paralysis, migraine with hemiparesis or other aura, syncope, hypoglycemia, hypertensive encephalopathy, and conversion disorder.

LABORATORY TESTS

- Immediate (Box 1): CBC, metabolic panel that includes blood glucose and renal function,

BOX 1 Immediate Diagnostic Studies: Evaluation of a Patient with Suspected Acute Ischemic Stroke

All Patients
Noncontrast brain computed tomographic scan (magnetic resonance imaging, if available)
Blood glucose level[1]
Serum electrolyte and renal function tests
Electrocardiography
Markers of cardiac ischemia
Complete blood count, including platelet count[2]
Prothrombin time/international normalized ratio
Activated partial thromboplastin time
Oxygen saturation

Selected Patients
CT angiogram head and neck or MR angiogram head and neck
CT or MR perfusion
Hepatic function tests
Toxicology screen
Blood alcohol level
Pregnancy test
Arterial blood gas tests (if hypoxia is suspected)
Chest radiography (if lung disease is suspected)
Lumbar puncture (if subarachnoid hemorrhage is suspected and computed tomography scan is negative for blood)
Electroencephalogram (if seizures are suspected)

[1] Only test recommended before initiation of IV rtPA.
[2] Although it is desirable to know the results of these tests before giving a patient tissue plasminogen activator, thrombolytic therapy should not be delayed while awaiting the results unless (1) there is clinical suspicion of a bleeding abnormality or thrombocytopenia; (2) the patient has received heparin or warfarin; or (3) the patient's use of anticoagulants is not known.
From Christensen H et al: Abnormalities on ECG and telemetry predict stroke outcome at 3 months, *J Neurol Sci* 234:99–103, 2005.

TABLE 1 National Institutes of Health Stroke Scale

1A. Level of Consciousness (LOC)	1B. LOC Questions	1C. LOC Commands
0 = Alert 1 = Not alert, but arousable 2 = Not alert, obtunded 3 = Coma	Ask the month and his/her age. 0 = Answers both correctly 1 = Answers one correctly 2 = Answers neither correctly	Open and close the eyes. Open and close the nonparetic hand. 0 = Performs both tasks correctly 1 = Performs one task correctly 2 = Performs neither task correctly
2. Best Gaze (Horizontal)	**3. Visual Fields**	**4. Facial Palsy**
0 = Normal 1 = Partial gaze palsy 2 = Forced deviation or total gaze paresis	0 = No visual loss 1 = Partial hemianopia 2 = Complete hemianopia 3 = Bilateral hemianopia	0 = Normal 1 = Minor paralysis 2 = Partial paralysis (total or near total paralysis of lower face) 3 = Complete paralysis of upper and lower face
5. Motor Arm	**6. Motor Leg**	**7. Limb Ataxia**
Right Arm extended with palms down 90 degrees (if sitting) or 45 degrees (if supine) for 10 s 0 = No drift 1 = Drift; limb drifts down from position and does not hit bed or support in 10 s 2 = Some effort against gravity 3 = No effort against gravity 4 = No movement **Left**	**Right** Leg extended at 30 degrees, always tested supine for 5 s 0 = No drift 1 = Drift; limb drifts down from position and does not hit bed or support in 5 s 2 = Some effort against gravity 3 = No effort against gravity 4 = No movement **Left**	The finger-nose-finger and heel-shin tests 0 = Absent 1 = Present in one limb 2 = Present in two limbs
8. Sensory	**9. Best Language**	**10. Dysarthria**
To Pinprick or Noxious Stimuli 0 = Normal 1 = Mild to moderate sensory loss 2 = Severe to total sensory loss	0 = No aphasia, normal 1 = Mild-to-moderate aphasia 2 = Severe aphasia 3 = Mute, global aphasia, coma	0 = Normal 1 = Mild-to-moderate 2 = Severe (including mute/anarthric due to aphasia) Do not score if intubated.
11. Extinction and Inattention	**Total Score:**	
0 = No abnormality 1 = Present 2 = Profound (two modalities)		

From Vincent JL et al: *Textbook of critical care*, ed 7, Philadelphia, 2017, Elsevier.

PT/INR, aPTT, troponin I, and urinalysis. Blood glucose is the only test required before initiation of IV tPA

- National Institutes of Health Stroke Scale (Table 1): A brief, focused neurologic examination aimed at providing a numeric estimate of the severity of stroke; can be performed by any health care provider trained in its use; may increase the likelihood of the correct assessment of stroke
- ECG and telemetry monitoring
- Echocardiogram to look for potential cardiogenic source of embolism, infective endocarditis, and intracardiac shunts

IMAGING STUDIES

- Immediate (Fig. 1): Computed tomography (CT) of the head without contrast to rule out hemorrhage.
- CT angiogram of the head and neck is necessary acutely in selected patients if deficits are severe to assess whether there is a thrombus that is amenable to intervention as well as CT head perfusion to assess for the degree of salvageable tissue (Table 2).
- MRI of the brain with stroke protocol to assess the extent of stroke (because CT typically will not show an ischemic stroke for several hours), but it is rarely needed in the hyperacute setting to determine appropriateness of reperfusion strategy.

Cross reference: See "Transient Ischemic Attack" for general workup, which is identical to that for ischemic stroke.

Rx TREATMENT

NONPHARMACOLOGIC THERAPY

GENERAL CONSIDERATIONS:

- Airway and breathing should be maintained.
- Supplemental oxygen should be provided to keep the oxygen saturation at ≥92%.
- Pneumatic compression devices or pharmacologic means should be applied to help prevent deep venous thrombosis.
- Avoid any and all oral intake until swallowing is evaluated and found to be unimpaired; this helps to avoid aspiration pneumonia.
- Early mobilization for rehabilitation is desirable.
- Consider neurosurgical intervention for craniectomy in select cases. Typical cases in which craniectomy may be performed include cerebellar ischemia with compression of the brain stem and/or the fourth ventricle as well as large middle cerebral artery ischemia. Available evidence suggests that it may be better to perform early hemicraniectomy (<48 hr) to achieve better outcomes in malignant hemispheric strokes. Decompressive hemicraniectomy has shown good benefit in terms of mortality but not much benefit in terms of disability and functional outcomes.

ACUTE GENERAL Rx

INTRAVENOUS THROMBOLYSIS:

- IV t-PA, or alteplase, is the only medical therapy approved by the U.S. FDA for the treatment of acute ischemic stroke.
- The time window for administration is generally accepted to be within 4.5 hours of symptom onset, although the FDA indication is still within 3 hours. The American Heart Association/American Stroke Association recommends a t-PA administration window of up to 4.5 hours with certain additional exclusion criteria when compared to the 3-hour administration.
- There are strict criteria for the administration of IV t-PA (see Table 3).
- The protocol is weight based, with 90 mg being the maximum allowable dose.
- The risk of brain hemorrhage with IV t-PA is about 6% in stroke patients.
- Endovascular intervention is useful only for large, accessible thrombi. Therefore, if a stroke patient is a candidate for IV t-PA, treatment with IV t-PA should be started and then the patient should be assessed for possible endovascular therapy.

IMMEDIATE CATHETER CEREBRAL ANGIOGRAPHY FOR ENDOVASCULAR INTERVENTION

(Figs. E2 and E3): Methods available:

- The American Heart Association/American Stroke Association 2018 guidelines now recommend mechanical thrombectomy with a stent-retriever device for highly selected patients who present with large vessel occlusion (LVO) up to 16 hours after last known normal and suggest that it is reasonable up to 24 hours.
  1. IV tPA should be administered in this group if eligible.
  2. All patients should be assessed with CT angiogram head and neck or MRA head and neck for possible LVO if they have an NIHSS of ≥6 or suspicion of a large vessel stroke.
  3. In selected patients with acute ischemic stroke within 6 to 24 hours of last known normal who have LVO on noninvasive angiogram, obtaining a CT perfusion, DW-MRI, or perfusion is recommended to aid in patient selection for mechanical thrombectomy.

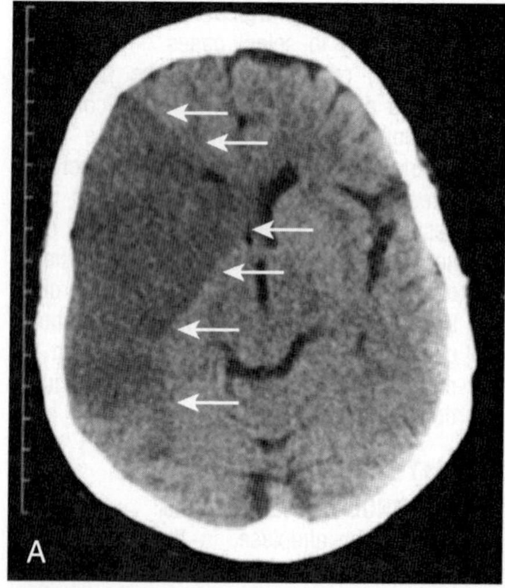

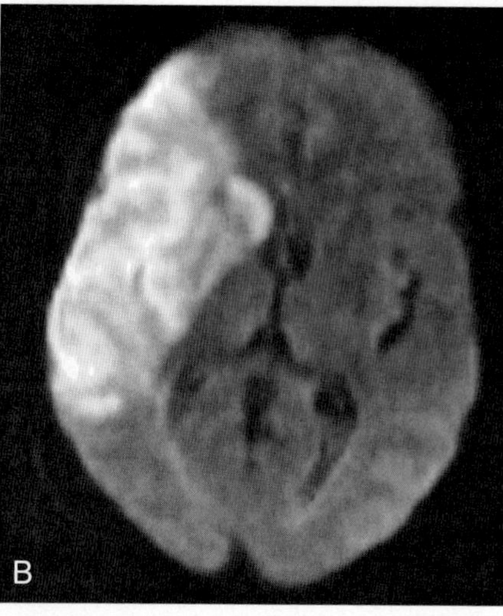

FIG. 1 Large right middle cerebral artery infarct on an unenhanced computed tomographic scan **(A)** and a diffusion-weighted magnetic resonance image **(B)**. There is a mass effect, and this patient is at risk for cerebral herniation syndromes.

TABLE 2 Imaging Modalities for Stroke

Imaging Modality	Advantage	Disadvantage
Cerebral catheter angiography	• Allows for the definitive assessment of cerebral circulation (gold standard) • Allows for the deployment of intra-arterial thrombolysis and thrombectomy devices if a thrombus is found • Allows for the assessment of collateral circulation	• Invasive (significant risks) • High cost • Not available at all facilities
Doppler studies	• Noninvasive • May be performed at the patient's bedside	• Can be limited by the patient's body habitus • Operator dependent
Magnetic resonance angiography	• Excellent view of the large arteries of the neck and brain • No contrast material needed	• Cannot be performed in patients who are critically ill, who are unable to tolerate supine positioning, who have a pacemaker or other ferromagnetic hardware, or who are claustrophobic
Magnetic resonance perfusion	• Assesses cerebral hemodynamics • May show ischemic penumbra (i.e., the area of the brain that may be saved by timely intervention)	• Not commonly available • Not well standardized
CT angiography	• Excellent view of the large arteries of the neck and brain • Similar to magnetic resonance angiography with regard to resolution	• Requires intravenous contrast
CT perfusion	• Assesses cerebral hemodynamics • May show ischemic penumbra (i.e., the area of the brain that may be saved by timely intervention)	• Challenging to interpret in some cases • Not routinely available at many facilities • Requires intravenous contrast

- Adult patients should receive mechanical thrombectomy with a stent retriever if they present within 6 hours of last known normal with a causative LVO (especially of the internal carotid artery or MCA segment 1 [M1] but reasonable in the setting of a causative MCA segment 2 or 3 [M2/3] or other large vessel cerebral artery) if they were relatively independent before the stroke and have an NIHSS score of ≥6 and an ASPECTS score of ≥6. Treatment needs to be able to be initiated (groin puncture) within 6 hours of symptom onset.
- Patients should receive mechanical thrombectomy with a stent retriever if treatment can be initiated within 16 hours (and possibly up to 24 hours) of last known normal with a large anterior circulation LVO and they meet the DAWN or DEFUSE-3 criteria (a defined mismatch between clinical severity and/or infarct volume compared to the penumbra [tissue at risk]). The number needed to treat to improve functional outcomes is only 2.8, and so patients should be aggressively evaluated for possible treatment.
- Complications can ensue from the endovascular procedure itself, including an intracerebral hemorrhage rate that is similar to that associated with IV t-PA. A recent meta-analysis revealed that among patients with acute ischemic stroke, endovascular therapy with mechanical thrombectomy versus standard medical care with t-PA was associated with improved functional outcomes and higher rates of angiographic revascularization, but no significant difference in symptomatic intracranial hemorrhage or all-cause mortality at 90 days.[1]
- Endovascular intervention is typically available only at comprehensive stroke centers.

HYPERTENSION: Elevated blood pressure is common during acute stroke, and it often subsides without specific therapy. In general, hypertension is not treated acutely unless it is extremely high (e.g., >220 mm Hg systolic blood pressure); there is evidence of hypertension-induced organ damage; or thrombolysis is being considered, in which case the blood pressure needs to come down (if it can be safely accomplished) to <185/110 mm Hg. It is risky to decrease blood pressure dramatically and quickly in the presence of acute ischemic stroke as it can cause an extension of the infarcted tissue into the ischemic penumbra. A 15% to 25% decrease over the first 24 hours is recommended.

HYPOTENSION: The presence of systemic hypotension in acute ischemic stroke portends a poor outcome. The cause should be sought, and volume depletion should be corrected with normal saline. Cardiac arrhythmias should be treated. Induced hypertension with vasopressor agents may be useful for select cases with an ischemic penumbra that is at risk, but caution is strongly advised.

HYPOGLYCEMIA: Hypoglycemia can mimic stroke. Prompt assessment of serum glucose level and replacement as necessary are important.

HYPERGLYCEMIA: The presence of hyperglycemia worsens ischemic stroke outcome. Hyperglycemia should be managed aggressively.

FEVER: Fever is harmful during acute stroke. Ascertaining and addressing the cause while lowering an elevated temperature is strongly advised.

ANTIPLATELET THERAPY: Oral, rectal, or feeding tube administration of aspirin (325 mg/day) within 48 hours of stroke onset is advised to decrease the likelihood of a repeat ischemic stroke. Other oral antiplatelet regimens approved for secondary stroke prophylaxis (e.g., clopidogrel, aspirin plus extended-release dipyridamole) may also be used. Patients who have received t-PA cannot be given antithrombotic or anticoagulant agents within the first 24 hr after administration. In patients with acute ischemic stroke and atrial fibrillation, full dose anticoagulation

[1] Badhiwala JH et al: Endovascular thrombectomy for acute ischemic stroke: a meta-analysis, *JAMA* 314(17):1832–1843, 2015.

TABLE 3 Eligibility Criteria for Acute Thrombolysis in Acute Ischemic Stroke

Eligibility Criteria

- Diagnosis of ischemic stroke causing measurable neurological deficit
- The neurological signs should not be minor and isolated. Caution should be exercised in treating a patient with major deficits
- Onset of symptoms <4.5 hours before beginning treatment
- The neurologic signs should not be clearing spontaneously
- The symptoms of stroke should not be suggestive of subarachnoid hemorrhage
- The patient or family members should understand the potential risks and benefits from treatment

Contraindications for Thrombolysis

- Evidence of intracranial hemorrhage on CT
- Head trauma or prior stroke in previous 3 months
- Myocardial infarction in the previous 3 months
- Gastrointestinal or urinary tract hemorrhage in previous 21 days
- Arterial puncture at a noncompressible site in the previous 7 days
- Major surgery in the previous 14 days
- History of previous intracranial hemorrhage
- Elevated blood pressure (systolic >185 mm Hg and diastolic >110 mm Hg)
- Evidence of active bleeding or acute trauma (fracture) on examination
- Taking an oral anticoagulant or, if taking anticoagulant, INR ≥1.7 is a contraindication
- If receiving heparin in previous 48 hours, aPTT must be in normal range
- Platelet count ≤100,000 mm^3
- Blood glucose concentration ≥50 mg/dl (2.7 mmol/L)
- Seizure with postictal residual neurologic impairments
- CT shows a multilobar infarction (hypodensity >⅓ cerebral hemisphere)

aPTT, Activated partial thromboplastin time; *CT*, computed tomography; *INR*, international normalized ratio.
From Hoffman R et al: *Hematology, basic principles and practice*, ed 7, Philadelphia, 2018, Elsevier.

with heparin infusion or low molecular weight heparin should be avoided in the acute setting, as this could potentially harm the patient by causing symptomatic intracranial hemorrhage, and there is very little evidence to suggest any benefit. However, chronic anticoagulation is indicated after the acute period has passed.

DISPOSITION

Patients with acute ischemic stroke should be cared for in a stroke unit or an intensive care unit. Nurses with skills in stroke care and telemetry monitoring should be routine. Once the patient is stable and the workup is complete, rehabilitation should be arranged.

REFERRAL

Patients with acute ischemic stroke should be transported to a hospital in which providers are skilled in stroke care. Depending on the severity and duration of symptoms, the patient may qualify for immediate endovascular intervention at a comprehensive stroke center, even if he or she is not a candidate for IV TPA. If complications from brain edema develop, further evaluation by a neurosurgeon may be helpful during the acute phase.

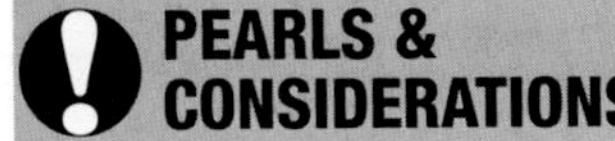

PEARLS & CONSIDERATIONS

PREVENTION

- The prevention of acute ischemic stroke depends on the aggressive management of risk factors in individual patients.
- Cross reference: Stroke, secondary prevention.
- Paroxysmal atrial fibrillation is common in patients with cryptogenic stroke. A recent study found that noninvasive ambulatory ECG monitoring for 30 days significantly improved the detection of atrial fibrillation by a factor of >5 and nearly doubled the rate of anticoagulant treatment compared to the standard practice of short-duration ECG monitoring.

PATIENT & FAMILY EDUCATION

Patients and families need to be taught about ways to reduce the risk for recurrent stroke, including lifestyle modifications. Education about rehabilitation goals, when appropriate, should also be accomplished.

SUGGESTED READINGS

Available at ExpertConsult.com

RELATED CONTENT

Stroke (Patient Information)
Stroke, Secondary Prevention (Related Key Topic)
Transient Ischemic Attack (Related Key Topic)
Atrial Fibrillation (Related Key Topic)

AUTHORS: **COREY GOLDSMITH, M.D.,** and **PRASHANTH KRISHNAMOHAN, M.B.B.S., M.D.**

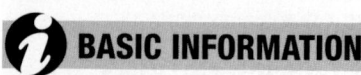

DEFINITION

Hemorrhagic stroke is the sudden onset of a focal neurologic deficit caused by hemorrhage into or around the brain.

SYNONYMS

Intracerebral hemorrhage (ICH)
Intracranial hemorrhage
Cerebrovascular attack (this is a nonspecific term and should not be used)
The term *subarachnoid hemorrhage* refers to a specific location for hemorrhage, which commonly occurs as a result of a ruptured aneurysm. Please see "Subarachnoid Hemorrhage" for additional information.

ICD-10CM CODES

I61 Intracerebral hemorrhage
I61.0 Intracerebral hemorrhage in hemisphere, subcortical
I61.1 Intracerebral hemorrhage in hemisphere, cortical
I61.2 Intracerebral hemorrhage in hemisphere, unspecified
I61.3 Intracerebral hemorrhage in brainstem
I61.4 Intracerebral hemorrhage in cerebellum
I61.5 Intracerebral hemorrhage, intraventricular
I61.6 Intracerebral hemorrhage, multiple localized
I61.9 Nontraumatic intracerebral hemorrhage, unspecified

EPIDEMIOLOGY & DEMOGRAPHICS

INCIDENCE: There are approximately 795,000 new or recurrent strokes per yr in the U.S., of which approximately 10% are hemorrhagic.[1]

RISK FACTORS:
- Hypertension
- Anticoagulant use
- Thrombolysis
- Alcoholism
- Illicit drug use (e.g., cocaine)
- Cerebral amyloid angiopathy
- Increased age
- African American race
- Low cholesterol, LDL, and triglycerides
- Minuscule increase in absolute risk from antiplatelet therapy
- Questionable effect of chronic kidney disease and selective use of serotonin reuptake inhibitors

GENETICS: Multifactorial

PHYSICAL FINDINGS & CLINICAL PRESENTATION

The presentation varies with the region of the brain that is affected. Table 1 summarizes correlation between levels of brain function and clinical signs. There is no clinical way to distinguish between a primary cerebral hemorrhage and an ischemic stroke; therefore imaging is required. Imaging can also help determine if the diagnosis is ischemic stroke with hemorrhagic conversion versus primary hemorrhage.

The following are common locations for hypertensive hemorrhage:
- Basal ganglia
- Cerebellum
- Pons

Lobar hemorrhage in an older adult is likely due to amyloid angiopathy.

A systematic, detailed examination is necessary when approaching a comatose patient (Box 1). The ICH score is a widely used grading scale to estimate mortality based on CT scan results. Parameters used to calculate the ICH score include Glasgow Coma Scale (GCS) (0 to 2 points) at presentation, patient age ≥80 (1 point), ICH volume ≥30 ml (1 point), presence of intraventricular blood (1 point), and infratentorial origin of blood (1 point). Scores range from 0 to 6, with a score of 0 conferring 0% mortality and a score of 6 with estimated 100% mortality.

ETIOLOGY

- Rupture of vessels
- Aneurysm
- Arteriovenous malformation
- Brain tumor
- Amyloid angiopathy

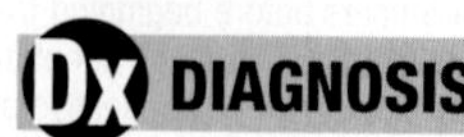

DIFFERENTIAL DIAGNOSIS

- Ischemic stroke
- Seizure with postictal paralysis
- Syncope
- Migraine with hemiparesis
- Conversion disorder

LABORATORY TESTS

- CBC, metabolic panel including blood glucose and renal function, PT/INR, aPTT, urinalysis, and toxicology screens
- ECG and telemetry monitoring

IMAGING STUDIES

- Immediate: CT scanning of the head without contrast is highly sensitive for hemorrhage (Fig. 1).
- CT or MR angiogram to rule out an underlying vascular malformation. CT spot sign on the CTA has been shown to be a reliable early predictor of hematoma expansion.

TABLE 1 Correlation between Levels of Brain Function and Clinical Signs

Structure	Function	Clinical Sign
Cerebral cortex	Conscious behavior	Speech (including any sounds) Purposeful movement Spontaneous To command To pain
Brainstem activating and sensory pathways (reticular activating system)	Sleep-wake cycle	Eye opening Spontaneous To command To path
Brainstem motor pathways	Reflex limb movements	Flexor posturing (decorticate) Extensor posturing (decerebrate)
Midbrain CN III	Innervation of ciliary muscle and certain extraocular muscles	Pupillary reactivity
Pontomesencephalic MLF	Connects pontine gaze center with CN III nucleus	Internuclear ophthalmoplegia
Upper pons		
CN V	Facial and corneal	Corneal reflex-sensory
CN VIII	Facial muscle innervation	Corneal reflex-motor response Blink Grimace
Lower pons		
CN VIII (vestibular portion) connects by brainstem pathways with CN III, IV, VI	Reflex eye movements	Doll's eyes Caloric responses
Pontomedullary junction pressure	Spontaneous breathing Maintained blood pressure	Breathing and blood pressure do not require mechanical or chemical support
Spinal cord	Primitive protective responses	Deep tendon reflexes Babinski response

CN, Cranial, nerve; *MLF,* medial longitudinal fasciculus.
Parrillo JE, Dellinger RP: *Critical care medicine, principles of diagnosis and management in the adult,* ed 4, Philadelphia, 2014, Elsevier.

[1] Chatterjee S et al: New oral anticoagulants and the risk of intracranial hemorrhage: traditional and Bayesian meta-analysis and mixed treatment comparison of randomized trials of new oral anticoagulants in atrial fibrillation, *JAMA Neurol* 70(12):1486–1490, 2013.

BOX 1 Neurologic Profile: A Modified Glasgow Coma Scale

Verbal Response
Oriented speech
Confused conversation
Inappropriate speech
Incomprehensible speech
No speech

Eye Opening
Spontaneous
Response to verbal stimuli
Response to noxious stimuli
None

Motor Response
Obeys
Localizes
Withdraws (flexion)
Abnormal flexion
None

Pupillary Reaction
Present
Absent

Spontaneous Eye Movement
Orienting
Roving conjugate
Roving disconjugate
Miscellaneous abnormal movements
None

Oculocephalic Response
Normal (unpredictable)
Full
Minimal
None

Oculovestibular Response
Normal (nystagmus)
Tonic conjugate
Minimal or disconjugate
None

Deep Tendon Reflexes
Normal
Increased
Absent

From Parrillo JE, Dellinger RP: *Critical care medicine, principles of diagnosis and management in the adult,* ed 4, Philadelphia, 2014, Elsevier.

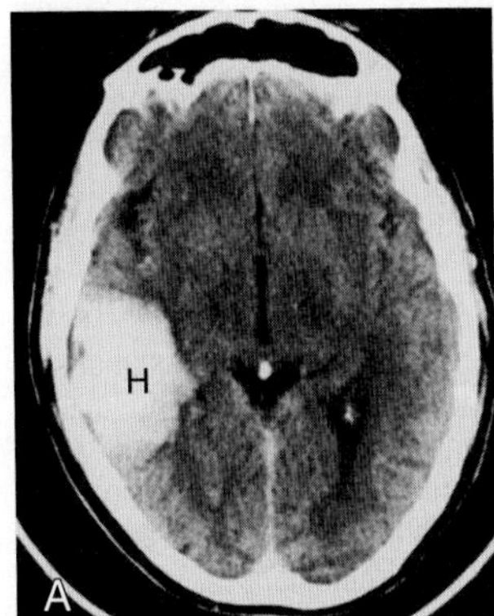

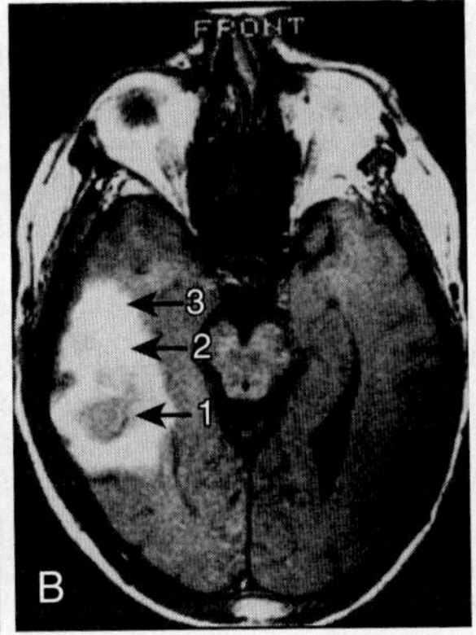

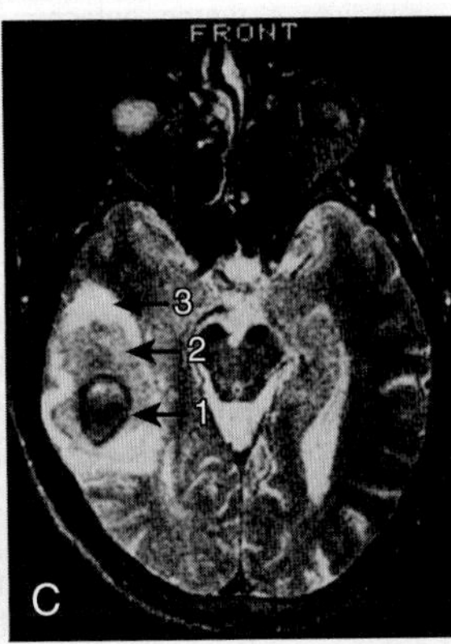

FIG. 1 Hemorrhage. Axial computed tomography image **(A)** demonstrates a large area of acute hemorrhage *(H)* in right temporal lobe. T_1-weighted **(B)** and T_2-weighted **(C)** magnetic resonance imaging scans demonstrate the hemorrhage in various stages of breakdown. Center of lesion is dark on T_1- and T_2-weighted images, indicating oxyhemoglobin *(1).* Intermediate zone is bright on T_1-weighted image and gray on T_2-weighted image, indicating intracellular methemoglobin *(2).* Outer rim is bright on both T_1- and T_2-weighted images, indicating extracellular methemoglobin *(3).* (From Vincent JL et al: *Textbook of critical care,* ed 6, Philadelphia, 2011, Saunders.)

- MRI of the brain with a gradient echo sequence is also highly sensitive for hemorrhage, including intracerebral microhemorrhages that may not be visible with computed tomography scanning. MRI may also help to identify underlying brain tumors or vascular malformations, especially if the bleeding occurs at atypical sites. In the acute setting the MRI may show only the hematoma, but repeat MRI approximately 6 weeks after initial hemorrhage may help exclude these other etiologies.

Rx TREATMENT

NONPHARMACOLOGIC THERAPY

- Urgent neurosurgical evaluation is needed in many cases either for evacuation of the hematoma or for relieving raised intracranial pressure by procedures such as EVD placement or decompressive surgeries.
- Surgery should be performed promptly for cases of cerebellar hemorrhage of >3 cm when the patient is deteriorating clinically, showing brain stem edema or hydrocephalus.
- Surgery for lobar or deep brain clots may be considered for select cases, although the level of evidence for efficacy is not high. Currently, guidelines recommend standard craniotomy for patients with lobar clots >30 ml within 1 cm of the cerebral cortex.
- Recent innovative surgical techniques, such as instillation of thrombolytic agents for intraventricular hemorrhage and minimally invasive surgery for hematoma evacuation, appear to be promising. Clinical trials are currently in progress to assess whether these approaches improve mortality and neurologic outcomes.

ACUTE GENERAL Rx

The cornerstones of medical management of acute intracerebral hemorrhage include:

- Control of hypertension
- Correction of coagulopathy
- Management of elevated intracranial pressure
- Treatment of seizures

HYPERTENSION (BOX 2): Blood pressure should be quickly lowered by 15% and then gradually and safely brought to the individual patient's target range. In theory, this may diminish the expansion of the hematoma. More aggressive control of systolic blood pressure (SBP) to 140 or less in the acute setting has been shown to be safe in clinical trials (INTERACT2 trial) with nonsignificant improvement in outcomes compared to less aggressive BP control (target SBP <180 mm Hg). ATACH 2 studied aggressive blood pressure lowering in patients randomized within 4.5 hr of symptom onset. Patients were randomized to aggressive blood pressure lowering to a target SBP of 110 to 139 mm Hg compared to standard blood pressure lowering to target SBP of 179 to 140 mm Hg. The trial was stopped early because there was no difference in neurological outcome or death, but patients in the aggressive blood pressure lowering arm suffered more kidney injury. Evidence suggests that a more sustained BP control with continuous IV medications might be more beneficial than using intermittent medications resulting in significant BP variability. The most recent guidelines, published in 2015, state that for ICH patients presenting with SBP between 150 and 220 mm Hg and without contraindication to acute BP treatment, acute lowering of SBP to 140 mm Hg is safe and can be effective for improving functional outcome. For ICH patients presenting with SBP >220 mm Hg, it may be reasonable to consider aggressive reduction of BP with a continuous intravenous infusion and frequent BP monitoring.

CORRECTION OF COAGULOPATHY:

- Early hematoma expansion has been associated with poor outcome.
- Protamine sulfate is used to treat cases of heparin-induced intracerebral hemorrhage. Protamine dosage is 1 mg IV for every 100 units of heparin administered in the previous 2 to 3 hours (maximum dose is 50 mg).
- Prothrombin concentrate complex (PCC) is now recommended for reversal of warfarin-associated ICH. FFP may also be used for this purpose, although it carries the disadvantage of administering more volume, potentially leading to complications such as pulmonary edema and slightly longer times to reversal of coagulopathy compared to PCC. Vitamin K should be administered IV along with flash-frozen plasma (FFP)/PCC for sustained effects. Routine use of recombinant factor VII concentrates is not recommended due to insufficient evidence and concern for increased risk of thromboembolic events.
- Idarucizumab (Praxbind) is a humanized monoclonal antibody fragment that can be used for urgent reversal of the anticoagulant effect of the direct thrombin inhibitor dabigatran (Pradaxa).

BOX 2 Suggested Recommended Guidelines for the Treatment of Elevated Blood Pressure in Patients with Spontaneous Intracerebral Hemorrhage

1. SBP of >200 mm Hg or MAP of >150 mm Hg: Consider the aggressive reduction of BP with continuous intravenous infusion, with BP monitoring every 5 min.
2. SBP of >180 mm Hg or MAP of >130 mm Hg with evidence or suspicion of elevated ICP: Consider ICP monitor and reducing BP with intermittent or continuous intravenous medications to keep cerebral perfusion pressure >60 to 80 mm Hg.
3. SBP of >180 mm Hg or MAP of >130 mm Hg without evidence or suspicion of elevated ICP: Consider a modest reduction of BP (e.g., MAP of 110 mm Hg or target blood pressure of 160/90 mm Hg) with intermittent or continuous intravenous medications, and clinically reexamine the patient every 15 min.

BP, Blood pressure; *ICP,* intracranial pressure; *MAP,* mean arterial pressure; *SBP,* systolic blood pressure.
Modified from Broderick J et al: Guidelines for the management of spontaneous intracerebral hemorrhage in adults: 2007 update, *Stroke* 38:2001–2023, 2007.

- Andexanet alfa, a recombinant modified human factor X2 decoy protein has been effective for reversion of the anticoagulant effect of apixaban (Eliquis), rivaroxaban (Xarelto), and edoxaban (Savaysa).
- Recommendations for thrombolytic-associated intracerebral hemorrhage treatment include the consideration of the infusion of platelets and cryoprecipitate.
- Hemostatic therapy has not been shown convincingly to improve outcomes, despite reducing hematoma expansion. Efforts are under way to identify patients at high risk of early hematoma expansion by using clinical and radiographic information to determine who may benefit from more aggressive hemostatic intervention.
- Platelet transfusion for patients experiencing ICH while on aspiring appears to result in worse outcomes than no platelet transfusion according to the PATCH trial. The odds of death or dependence at 3 mo were significantly higher in the transfused group as compared to the nontransfused group.

ELEVATED INTRACRANIAL PRESSURE: This condition should be treated with a graded approach, which may include the elevation of the head of the bed, analgesia/sedation, hyperventilation, and osmotic therapy. In patients clinically suspected to have elevated ICP or with GCS <8, invasive monitoring of the ICP may be required. If conservative treatment fails to control ICP, EVD placement or other decompressive procedures like craniotomy should be pursued.

SEIZURES: If seizures occur, they should be treated aggressively, including with intravenous medications, if needed. Although widely practiced, routine use of prophylactic antiepileptic medications is not recommended. Continuous EEG monitoring should be employed in patients with suspected seizures or unexplained low levels of consciousness.

SUPPORTIVE TREATMENT:
- Hyperglycemia: A high blood glucose level predicts a worse outcome. Markedly elevated glucose levels should be lowered to <200 mg/dl.
- Antipyretics should be administered for fever in addition to searching for a cause of the fever.
- Care should be taken to avoid hypoxia. Airway and ventilatory management should happen early and concurrently with the primary management of ICH.
- Pneumatic compression devices should be applied to help prevent deep venous thrombosis. Chemical DVT prophylaxis can be started after 48 to 72 hours in most situations once the bleed has been determined to be stable.
- Early mobilization for rehabilitation is desirable.

DISPOSITION

For large hemorrhages or unstable patients, immediate referral to a stroke center

REFERRAL

Patients with hemorrhagic stroke should be transported to a hospital where providers are skilled in the treatment of stroke and cerebrovascular diseases including the availability of neurosurgery services and neurocritical care. Depending on the severity and duration of symptoms, the patient may require neurosurgical intervention.

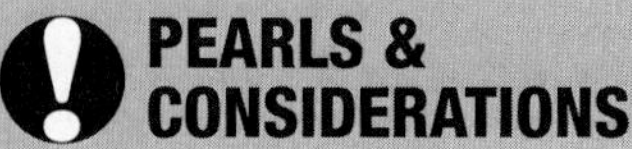

PEARLS & CONSIDERATIONS

- Outcomes are inversely correlated with hemorrhage size.
- Specific reversal agents may be useful for warfarin-, heparin-, DOAC-, or thrombolysis-associated hemorrhage.
- No procoagulant medications have yet been shown to be safe and effective for the mitigation of spontaneous intracerebral hemorrhage in placebo-controlled trials.

PREVENTION

- Prevention depends on the aggressive management of risk factors in individual patients, including hypertension, smoking, alcohol use, and cocaine use.
- Direct oral anticoagulants (DOACs) dabigatran, apixaban, rivaroxaban, and edoxaban are uniformly associated with an overall reduced risk of iatrogenic ICH when used for stroke prevention in atrial fibrillation when compared to warfarin. Any of the currently available DOACs can be considered first line for patients at high risk for ICH.

PATIENT & FAMILY EDUCATION

Patients and families need to understand that most patients will not soon achieve functional independence and that rehabilitation will be a long process. Education about avoiding antithrombotic agents should be stressed as appropriate for individual circumstances.

SUGGESTED READINGS

Available at ExpertConsult.com

RELATED CONTENT

Stroke (Patient Information)

AUTHORS: **A. BASIT KHAN, M.D., COREY GOLDSMITH, M.D.,** and **PRASHANTH KRISHNAMOHAN, M.B.B.S., M.D.**

BASIC INFORMATION

DEFINITION

Secondary prevention of stroke involves preventing the recurrence of a cerebral vascular ischemic or hemorrhagic stroke after a primary event (including transient ischemic attack) and early rehabilitation.

SYNONYMS

Brain attack
Stroke
Cerebral thrombosis
Cerebral hemorrhage
Brain infarct

ICD-10CM CODES

I65.2	Occlusion and stenosis of carotid artery
I65.0	Occlusion and stenosis of vertebral artery
I65.9	Occlusion and stenosis of unspecified precerebral artery
I66	Occlusion and stenosis of cerebral artery, not resulting in cerebral infarction
I65.1	Occlusion and stenosis of basilar artery

EPIDEMIOLOGY

Stroke is the fifth leading cause of death in the U.S. and the leading cause of disability. Each yr, there are a total of 795,000 strokes, of which 185,000 are recurrent strokes. Thus, secondary prevention of ischemic stroke remains good treatment strategy. Secondary prevention is specifically targeted toward modifiable risk factors.

RISK FACTORS: Age is the most important nonmodifiable risk factor. Modifiable risk factors include hypertension, hyperlipidemia, cigarette smoking, excessive alcohol consumption, physical inactivity, obesity (i.e., a body mass index of >25 kg/m^2), obstructive sleep apnea, illegal drug use (amphetamines, cocaine), and diabetes mellitus.

GENETICS: Multifactorial and strong family correlation if idiopathic strokes occur in parents <65 yr old.

PHYSICAL FINDINGS & CLINICAL PRESENTATION

- Stroke can have a varied presentation. Typically, the individual has a sudden definable loss of motor, sensory, visual, or cognitive functions that have a clear time of onset and that are noticed by others or by the individuals themselves.
- Physical findings such as weakness and/or numbness in one limb or on one side of the body, facial droop, visual field loss, or the inability to understand or communicate with others raises one's suspicion of a stroke event.

ETIOLOGY

- Strokes are broadly divided into ischemic or hemorrhagic (i.e., intraparenchymal or subarachnoid hemorrhage). It is impossible to distinguish ischemic from hemorrhagic intracerebral hemorrhage by history alone; therefore imaging is required to confirm stroke subtype.
- Ischemic strokes can be caused by large-vessel atherosclerosis, cardioembolism due to atrial fibrillation or cardiomyopathy, or small vessel disease such as lacunar stroke. Rare causes such as recreational drug use (e.g., cocaine abuse); arterial dissection; and hypercoagulable states need to be considered when ischemic stroke occurs in younger individuals.
- The most common cause of intracerebral hemorrhage is uncontrolled hypertension. Older patients with lobar hemorrhages likely have amyloid angiopathy as the cause of their hemorrhagic stroke. Spontaneous rupture of a brain aneurysm causes subarachnoid hemorrhage.

DIAGNOSIS

DIFFERENTIAL DIAGNOSIS

- Seizure and postictal states
- Brain tumor
- Complicated migraine
- Hypoglycemia
- Psychogenic disorder

WORKUP

- Blood glucose level HBA1c
- APTT, PT/INR, CBC, and CMP
- Fasting lipid panel
- Hypercoagulability tests for young stroke patients with no obvious risk factors

IMAGING STUDIES

- Computed tomography scanning of the head without contrast can differentiate between ischemic and hemorrhagic stroke. MRI of the brain is a more specific and prognostic study.
- Carotid ultrasound and transcranial Doppler are used to detect large-vessel extracranial carotid atherosclerosis but are not useful for visualizing the intracranial vasculature or the posterior circulation. Magnetic resonance angiography (MRA) and computed tomography angiography (CTA) of the head and neck provide imaging of the entire extracranial and intracranial vascular supplying both the anterior and posterior circulations. MRA can be performed without contrast, whereas CTA requires iodinated contrast and may be inappropriate for patients with renal dysfunction.
- Echocardiogram to look for structural abnormalities that could be the source of cardioembolism.
- Heart rhythm monitoring to detect atrial fibrillation. It is rare for an isolated ECG to detect paroxysmal atrial fibrillation that may be the source of the ischemic stroke or TIA. It can even be missed under 24 hr of telemetry in many patients. If a high index of suspicion for a cardioembolic source exists, working with a cardiologist to place a monitoring device should be considered because many cases of paroxysmal atrial fibrillation require more prolonged monitoring for detection.

TREATMENT

The secondary prevention of stroke is targeted toward modifiable risk factors. These include lifestyle modifications such as appropriate diet, exercise, weight loss, and smoking cessation, avoidance of heavy alcohol use, and risk factor modification as listed in the following.

ANTIPLATELET OR ANTICOAGULANT CHOICE: All patients with noncardioembolic ischemic stroke or transient ischemic attack (TIA) should be on aspirin (50 to 325 mg/day), a combination of aspirin and extended-release dipyridamole, or clopidogrel. Long-term treatment with a combination of clopidogrel and aspirin in secondary stroke prevention when no other pressing medical conditions require their use is no longer recommended due to increased mortality from intracerebral hemorrhage. In some circumstances, short-term treatment with the combination of clopidogrel and aspirin is reasonable in the first 30 to 90 days. Ticagrelor and prasugrel are not indicated for stroke prevention. Ticagrelor failed to show benefit for secondary stroke prevention compared with aspirin. Prasugrel is contraindicated in patients with a history of stroke or TIA. If a patient is already on an antiplatelet drug at the time of stroke or TIA, then consideration of switching to another agent is reasonable, although a holistic approach that includes assessment of compliance with the antiplatelet agent and the extent other risk factors have been controlled is recommended.

PREVENTING STROKE IN SPECIFIC CONDITIONS

- Cardioembolic strokes as a result of nonvalvular atrial fibrillation (AF): All patients with a ischemic stroke secondary to nonvalvular atrial fibrillation would have a CHA2DS2-VASc score of >2, and therefore anticoagulation is recommended. Two first-line drug therapies can be recommended: direct oral anticoagulants (DOACs) such as apixiban, dabigatran, endoxiban, and rivoroxiban; and warfarin with an international normalized ratio (INR) between 2.0 and 3.0. DOACs have been shown to result in a lower rate of intracerebral hemorrhage. Although more expensive than warfarin, DOACs do not require monitoring, do not have the dietary issues associated with warfarin, and have fewer drug-drug interactions. However, patients on enzyme-inducing medications such as phenytoin or HIV patients on protease inhibitors cannot use DOACs. Warfarin is still preferred in patients with marked renal impairment (see specific information available from the FDA about renal impairment and dosing for each DOAC) and in patients with mechanical heart valves or valvular causes of atrial fibrillation. Reversible therapies for some of the DOACs have recently been made available. A patients on a DOAC experiencing a recurrent stroke should only receive tissue plasminogen activator (t-PA) if the patient has been off the medication for at least 48 hr. For patients on warfarin, an INR of less than 1.7 allows for administration of t-PA. There is no evidence that aspirin monotherapy is helpful in reducing cardioembolic events. The Active-A trial suggested that a combination of aspirin and clopidogrel is slightly better than aspirin alone for those unable to tolerate warfarin, but patients on dual therapy experienced an increased risk of hemorrhagic complications. Because dual-antiplatelet therapy and DOACs have similar rates of bleeding complications but different levels of efficacy for prevention of cardioembolic stroke, the use of aspirin/clopidogrel dual therapy instead of a DOAC is almost never indicated. Furthermore, apixiban and aspirin monotherapies have been shown to have similar rates of bleeding. Thus, patients at risk of bleeding who previously were put on aspirin rather than warfarin could now be prescribed apixiban and experience the same bleeding risk but with actual benefit in terms of stroke risk reduction.

- Cardioembolic strokes as a result of a prosthetic metallic valve: Anticoagulant therapy with warfarin is recommended with a goal INR between 2.5 and 3.5.
- Strokes as a result of large-vessel extracranial atherosclerosis (i.e., symptomatic carotid stenosis): For patients with recent TIA or ischemic stroke and ipsilateral severe (70% to 99%) carotid artery stenosis, carotid endarterectomy (CEA) or carotid stenting is recommended, preferably within 14 days of the event if no contraindication. For patients with recent TIA or ischemic stroke and ipsilateral moderate (50% to 69%) carotid stenosis, intervention is recommended on a case-by-case basis only if the surgeon's perioperative morbidity and mortality rate is <6%.When the degree of stenosis is <50%, there is no indication for CEA. Carotid stenting can be an alternative to CEA in patients with low or average risk of periprocedural complications. In older patients (>70), CEA is associated with better outcomes.
- Symptomatic intracranial atherosclerosis (i.e., cavernous carotid stenosis, basilar stenosis): The symptomatic intracranial artery stenosis stenting trial (SAMMPRIS) demonstrated superiority of aggressive medical management of intracranial atherosclerosis compared with angioplasty and stenting for secondary stroke prevention. Therefore the use of aspirin plus clopidrogel 75 mg daily for 90 days is reasonable in addition to modifiable risk factor management, including high-intensity statin and SBP <140. There is no advantage to using warfarin over aspirin.
- Patent foramen ovale (PFO): The American Academy of Neurology's 2016 guidelines recommend medical therapy with antiplatelets for stroke patients with PFO though recent trials (CLOSE and REDUCE trials) suggest a benefit for PFO closure devices especially in the setting of an atrial septal aneurysm or large inter-atrial shunt.
- Intracerebral hemorrhage: For immediate management, please refer to the chapter on intracerebral hemorrhage. Anticoagulation or antiplatelet agents should be held for 3 to 4 weeks and can be restarted if there is a compelling indication such as nonvalvular atrial fibrillation. The American Stroke Association/American Heart Association 2014 guideline recommends avoiding long-term anticoagulation (e.g., warfarin, heparin) after spontaneous lobar intracerebral hemorrhage, but antiplatelet therapy (e.g., aspirin, clopidogrel, Aggrenox) may be considered in all cases of intracerebral hemorrhage where there is a definite indication. Consider a neurology consultation in these cases.
- Antiplatelet therapy is recommended in cases of cryptogenic strokes. A consultation with a neurologist should be considered for young stroke patients and for patients with no obvious cause or with stroke from unusual causes (e.g., hypercoagulable states, dissections).

PREVENTING LONG-TERM COMPLICATIONS AFTER A STROKE

- Evaluation by a physical, occupational, and speech therapist will reduce the long-term disability that can follow a stroke event. The American Stroke Association 2014 guideline recommends a multidisciplinary approach to rehabilitation. Studies have shown an improved survival and recovery. Home-based rehabilitation can be considered after discussion with the rehabilitation specialist.
- Depression rates are high after an ischemic stroke and patients should be screened.

RISK FACTOR MODIFICATION

- Hypertension: Antihypertensive treatment is recommended for both the prevention of recurrent stroke and the prevention of other vascular events in persons who have had an ischemic stroke or a TIA. Absolute target blood pressure level and reduction should be individualized, but a target of <140/90 is reasonable. Blood pressure should be lowered gradually over the first several days after an ischemic stroke to prevent cerebral hypoperfusion and extension of stroke. After a hemorrhagic stroke, blood pressure should be lowered quickly. Lifestyle modifications as listed previously should be included as part of a comprehensive antihypertension treatment plan.
- Diabetes: The goal for the hemoglobin A_{1c} level should be <7%. For type 2 diabetics, diet and exercise can prove very beneficial. Type 1 diabetics can also benefit from diet and compliance with their insulin regimen. Uncontrolled hyperglycemia can lead to acceleration of both intracranial and extracranial arteriosclerosis. Always consider consulting a diabetic educator.
- Hyperlipidemia: For patients with ischemic stroke or TIA with elevated cholesterol levels, statin agents are recommended. The SPARCL study demonstrated that, compared with patients taking placebo, patients taking atorvastatin 80 mg daily experienced a statistically significant reduction in the risk of experiencing a recurrent ischemic stroke.
- Cigarette smoking: Absolute cessation is required. Try to offer pharmacologic therapy or counseling services to the patient. Secondhand tobacco exposure is just as dangerous, so inquire about secondhand exposure.
- Obesity: Weight reduction may be considered for all overweight ischemic stroke and TIA patients to maintain the goal of a body mass index of between 18.5 and 24.9 kg/m^2 and a waist circumference of <35 in for women and <40 in for men.
- Excessive alcohol consumption: Patients with ischemic stroke or TIA who are heavy drinkers should eliminate or reduce their consumption of alcohol. Light to moderate levels of no more than two drinks per day for men and one drink per day for nonpregnant women may be considered.
- Obstructive sleep apnea: A sleep study should be considered due to high prevalence of obstructive sleep apnea in this population and improvement in outcomes.

DISPOSITION

Secondary stroke prevention is a multifaceted approach of lifestyle modification and pharmacologic intervention that is aimed at preventing or limiting disability.

REFERRAL

For complicated recurrent strokes, a referral to a neurologist who specializes in stroke is recommended.

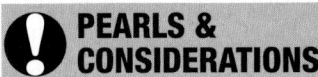

PEARLS & CONSIDERATIONS

The modification of risk factors is the best preventive measure for stroke. Lifestyle modification is a very important aspect of secondary stroke prevention. Always consider the patient's ability to afford the therapy and prescribed follow-up tests. Experience teaches us that patients sometimes will not let us know about their ability to afford therapies unless we inquire.

PREVENTION

Prevention is the goal of treatment, and compliance is the most important factor. Review risk factor reduction and pharmacologic therapy as previously discussed.

PATIENT/FAMILY EDUCATION

More information can be obtained from the following sources:

- American Heart Association, National Center, 7272 Greenville Avenue, Dallas, TX 75231
- American Stroke Association, 1-888-4-STROKE or 1-888-478-7653
- H.O.P.E. for Stroke, 250 Duck Pond Drive, Wantagh, NY 11793, 516-804-8495

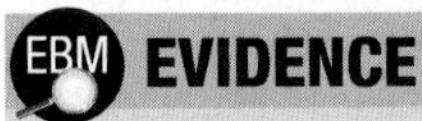

EVIDENCE

Available at ExpertConsult.com

SUGGESTED READINGS

Available at ExpertConsult.com

RELATED CONTENT

Stroke (Patient Information)
Transient Ischemic Attack (Related Key Topic)

AUTHORS: **JOSEPH S. KASS, M.D., J.D.,** and **COREY GOLDSMITH, M.D.**

BASIC INFORMATION

DEFINITION

Subarachnoid hemorrhage (SAH) is defined as hemorrhage into the subarachnoid space surrounding the brain. This can be either nontraumatic (typically due to cerebral aneurysm rupture) or traumatic in nature. Here we will focus upon nontraumatic subarachnoid hemorrhage. Box 1 describes the Hunt and Hess clinical classification of patients presenting with aneurysmal SAH.

SYNONYMS

Subarachnoid bleed
SAH

ICD-10CM CODES

I60	Subarachnoid hemorrhage
I60.1	Subarachnoid hemorrhage from middle cerebral artery
I60.2	Subarachnoid hemorrhage from anterior communicating artery
I60.3	Subarachnoid hemorrhage from posterior communicating artery
I60.4	Subarachnoid hemorrhage from basilar artery
I60.5	Subarachnoid hemorrhage from vertebral artery
I60.7	Subarachnoid hemorrhage from intracranial artery, unspecified

EPIDEMIOLOGY & DEMOGRAPHICS

INCIDENCE: Nontraumatic: 6 to 8 cases/100,000 persons per yr

PREDOMINANT SEX: Women aged >55 yr were found to have a 25% greater risk of developing SAH compared with men of the same age.

PREDOMINANT AGE: The mean age at onset is 55 yr.

PEAK INCIDENCE: Most aneurysmal SAH occurs in people who are between the ages of 55 and 60 yr.

GENETICS:

- First-degree relatives have a 5 to 12 times greater risk of developing SAH compared with the general population.
- Autosomal dominant polycystic kidney disease is known to be associated with cerebral aneurysms in 8% of cases; screening is recommended in families with this condition in which one family member has experienced a ruptured aneurysm.
- Collagen vascular diseases such as Marfan syndrome, Ehler Danlos syndrome have also been implicated in the formation of aneurysms.

RISK FACTORS: Although genetics seem to play a factor in SAH, lifestyle factors are more important for determining overall risk. These risk factors include smoking, hypertension, oral contraception, pregnancy, and amphetamine/cocaine use.

BOX 1 Hunt and Hess Clinical Classification of Subarachnoid Hemorrhage

I	Asymptomatic or mild headache and neck stiffness
II	Moderate to severe headache and neck stiffness ± cranial nerve palsy
III	Mild focal deficit, lethargy, or confusion
IV	Stupor, moderate to severe hemiparesis
V	Deep coma, extensor posturing

From Vincent JL et al: *Textbook of critical care,* ed 6, Philadelphia, 2011, Saunders.

PHYSICAL FINDINGS & CLINICAL PRESENTATION

- The primary symptom is a sudden, severe headache in 97% of cases. This is classically described as the "worst headache of my life" and reaches maximal intensity within 1 min—the so-called thunderclap headache. This headache may be associated with nausea/vomiting, neck pain, seizure, or complete loss of consciousness.
- 30% to 60% of patients report a history of headaches during the weeks preceding the actual hemorrhage event. These are most likely sentinel bleeds that represent microhemorrhages.
- Altered mental status and coma may result from the direct effect (hemorrhagic mass effect), but more likely is the result of acutely increased intracranial pressure.
- A posterior communicating artery aneurysm may present as oculomotor (cranial nerve III) palsy, typically involving the pupillary fibers, even in a nonruptured setting.
- Table 1 describes the World Federation of Neurologic Surgeons clinical classification of SAH.

ETIOLOGY

- A ruptured saccular (berry) aneurysm is the most common cause of spontaneous SAH (75% to 80% of spontaneous SAH).
- Idiopathic SAH, also known as angiogram-negative SAH, accounts for 5% to 20% of spontaneous SAH. In these cases, no angiographic cause of the hemorrhage is found. This entity is also known as benign perimesencephalic SAH and is thought to occur due to rupture of venous plexus in the cisterns surrounding the brain stem.
- Other causes of spontaneous SAH include arteriovenous malformations, bleeding into preexisting tumors, vasculitis, and rarely reversible cerebral vasoconstriction syndrome, cerebral venous sinus thrombosis, or intracranial cerebral artery dissection.
- Cocaine abuse, sickle cell anemia, coagulopathies, and pituitary apoplexy can also result in SAH.
- Trauma.

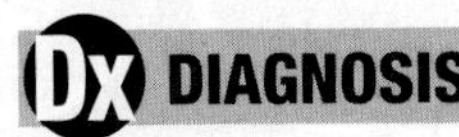

DIAGNOSIS

DIFFERENTIAL DIAGNOSIS

- Intracerebral hemorrhage as a result of spontaneous rupture of intracerebral arteries or arterioles (rather than arteries passing through the subarachnoid space) due to hypertension or amyloid angiopathy, as well as trauma, intratumoral bleed, ischemic stroke with hemorrhagic conversion, cerebral venous sinus hemorrhage associated with venous sinus thrombosis, mycotic aneurysm rupture.
- Other causes: Thunderclap headaches due to reversible cerebral vasoconstriction syndrome (often with recurrent thunderclap headaches), migraine headache, sexual headache, cough headache, exertional headache, secondary causes including, but not limited to, pituitary apoplexy or acute hydrocephalus.

WORKUP

IMAGING STUDIES:

- Computed tomography (CT) of the head (Fig. 1) shows hemorrhage in more than 95% of cases, especially during the acute phase (i.e., 24-48 hr) after the onset of bleeding. Box 2 describes the Fisher grade of SAH on initial CT (Fisher III being associated with highest risk of vasospasm). About 3% to 5% of SAH may be missed on initial CT of the head. MRI brain, specifically FLAIR sequence, is helpful in detecting subarachnoid blood if clinically suspected.
- Lumbar puncture should be performed in all cases of suspected SAH with "normal CT of the head" between 6 and 12 hours after the onset of the headache for highest yield. The following suggest SAH:
    1. An RBC count of more than $100,000/m^3$ in tubes 1 AND 4. This is to differentiate from a traumatic tap in which there will be a drop in RBC count from tube 1 to 4.
    2. Presence of xanthochromia or bilirubin in the cerebrospinal fluid.
    3. SAH can also be excluded by the following two criteria: CSF RBC count $<2000 \times 10^6$/L and no xanthochromia.
- CT angiogram of the brain (Fig. 2).

TABLE 1 World Federation of Neurologic Surgeons Clinical Classification of Subarachnoid Hemorrhage

Grade	Glasgow Coma Scale	Motor Deficits
I	15	Absent
II	13-14	Absent
III	13-14	Present
IV	7-12	Present or absent
V	3-6	Present or absent

From Vincent JL et al: *Textbook of critical care,* ed 6, Philadelphia, 2011, Saunders.

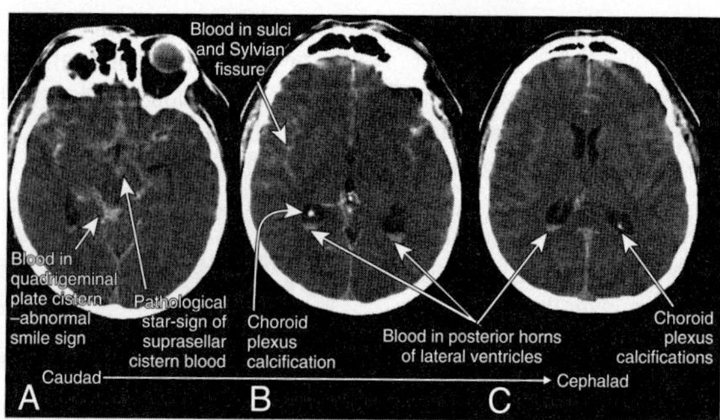

FIG. 1 Subarachnoid hemorrhage (SAH), noncontrast CT, brain windows. Acute SAH appears white on noncontrast computed tomography (CT) brain windows. **A** through **C,** nonconsecutive axial slices, progressing from caudad to cephalad. In this case of diffuse SAH, note the presence of subarachnoid blood filling the sulci, as well as extending into the cisterns, Sylvian fissures, and even lateral ventricles. In **A,** blood *(white)* fills the suprasellar cistern. This star-shaped structure is normally filled with CSF *(black)*. The quadrigeminal plate cistern is normally a smile-shaped black crescent, filled with CSF, but in this case is filled with blood. Extremely bright calcifications in the choroid plexus of the posterior horns of the lateral ventricles are common, normal findings—do not mistake these for hemorrhage. Note their similarity in density to bone of the calvarium. (From Broder JS: *Diagnostic imaging for the emergency physician,* Philadelphia, 2011, Saunders.)

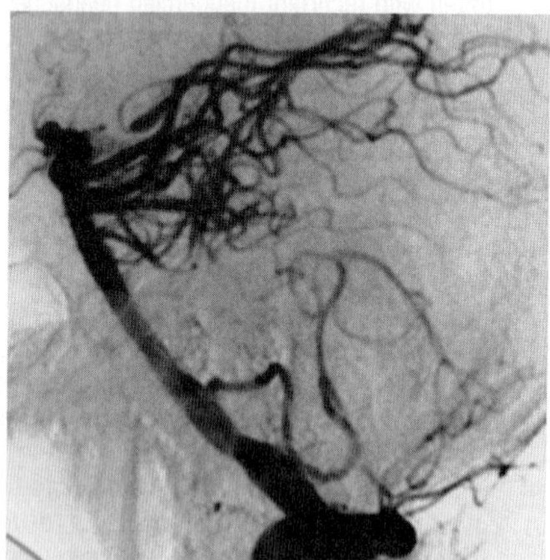

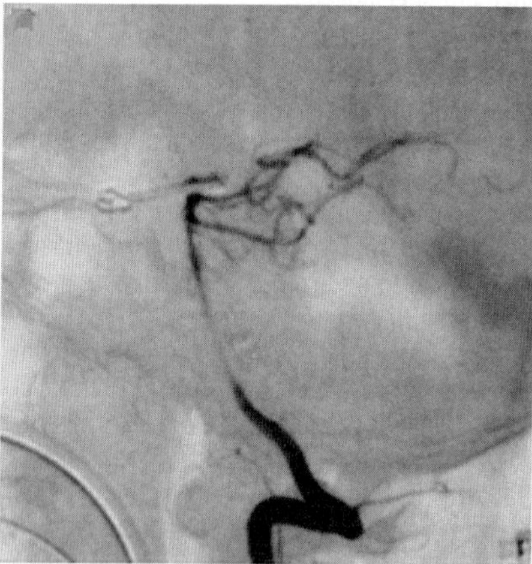

FIG. 2 Baseline angiogram obtained shortly after subarachnoid hemorrhage *(left)* and repeat angiogram obtained 7 days later *(right)* showing severe vasospasm of basilar artery, with reduced distal flow. (From Vincent JL et al: *Textbook of critical care*, ed 7, Philadelphia, 2017, Elsevier.)

BOX 2 Fisher Grade of Subarachnoid Hemorrhage on Initial Computed Tomography

1	No blood detected
2	Diffuse or vertical layers <1 mm thick
3	Localized subarachnoid clot and/or vertical layers ≥1 mm thick
4	Intraparenchymal or intraventricular clot with diffuse or no SAH
Modified Fisher CT Rating Scale	
1	Minimal or diffuse thin SAH without IVH
2	Minimal or thin SAH with IVH
3	Thick cisternal clot without IVH
4	Thick cisternal clot with IVH

CT, Computed tomography; *IVH,* intraventricular hemorrhage; *SAH,* subarachnoid hemorrhage.
From Vincent JL et al: *Textbook of critical care,* ed 6, Philadelphia, 2011, Saunders.

- Digital subtraction angiography with 3D processing when indicated is the gold standard for diagnosis of etiology in subarachnoid hemorrhage.

LABORATORY TESTS

- Basic laboratory values, including CBC, chemistry panel, prothrombin time, partial thromboplastin time, and platelet count.
- Serum troponin to evaluate for severe cardiac stress; elevated troponins indicate cardiac ischemia secondary to catecholamine surge and is associated with poor outcome.
- Patients with SAH are prone to developing cerebral salt wasting, resulting in hyponatremia. Sodium levels should be monitored frequently.

Rx TREATMENT

NONPHARMACOLOGIC THERAPY

- Airway, breathing, and circulation
- Once stabilized, good neurologic exam
- Cerebrospinal fluid drainage may be required for patients who develop hydrocephalus and increased intracranial pressure. It is also recommended for patients with Hunt and Hess grade 3 or higher.

ACUTE GENERAL Rx

- Critical care management: Initial management strategies are geared toward stabilizing the patient and preventing re-hemorrhage and hydrocephalus. Re-hemorrhage is associated with very high mortality rates.
- Blood pressure control: Tight blood pressure control is paramount before securing the aneurysm to protect against re-rupture. Blood pressure control can be achieved with the use of antihypertensive infusions such as intravenous nicardipine. A systolic blood pressure of less than 140 mm Hg is recommended. Placement of arterial line is recommended. After securing of the aneurysm, liberalization of blood pressure parameters is the standard.
- Pain control: Using short-acting and less-sedating medications (e.g., codeine, low-dose morphine).
- Seizures occur in about 3% of patients during the acute phase; use of prophylactic antiepileptics is controversial and not recommended, but patients presenting with seizures should be treated appropriately with anticonvulsants.
- Vasospasm: Cerebral vasospasm is a morbid complication leading to cerebral ischemia, disability, and death after SAH. It typically develops between day 4 and 14 (but may occur up to day 21) after the hemorrhage, and it reaches a peak on day 6 to 8. Treatment strategies include:
  1. Current medical therapy for vasospasm focuses upon hypertension, with typical mean arterial pressure goals of 90 to 100 (after aneurysm is secured) and with euvolemia instead of hypervolemia, as the latter was found to lead to significant cardiopulmonary and hemodynamic complications. "Triple H" therapy—*H*ypertension, *H*ypervolemia, and *H*emodilution—was originally employed to maintain cerebral perfusion, but it has fallen out of favor due to its many complications. Rather, nimodipine (60 mg q4h or 30 mg q2h if blood pressure is low) has been shown to improve outcomes if it is administered between days 4 and 21 after the hemorrhage, even if it does not significantly reduce the amount of vasospasm detected on angiography.
  2. Statins are no longer recommended for vasospasm prevention.
  3. Intraarterial therapies such as intraarterial calcium channel blockers and balloon angioplasty may be employed as needed.
- In cases of aneurysmal SAH, treatment focuses on occlusion/exclusion of the aneurysm to prevent rebleeding. The most common treatment methods are:
  1. Microsurgical clipping: Performed through a craniotomy by placing a clip around the neck of the aneurysm.
  2. Endovascular coiling (Fig. 3): Performed via digital subtraction angiography; it consists of deploying platinum coils inside the aneurysm or stents in the

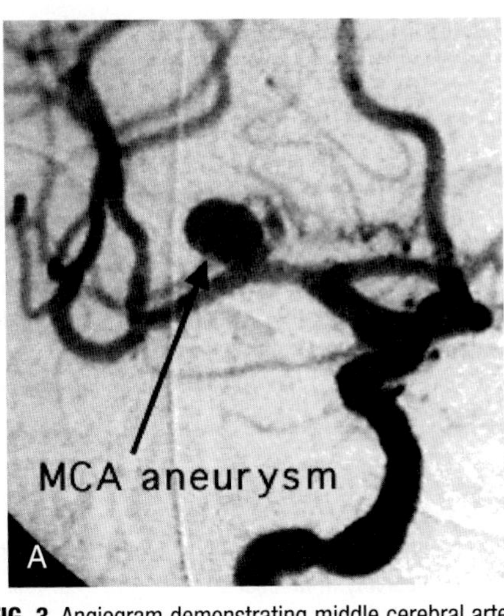

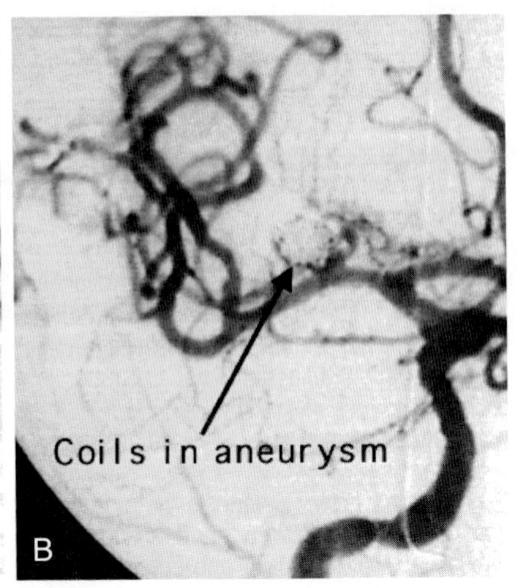

FIG. 3 Angiogram demonstrating middle cerebral artery aneurysm before **(A)** and after placement of detachable coils to thrombose the aneurysm **(B).** (From Vincent JL et al: *Textbook of critical care*, ed 7, Philadelphia, 2017, Elsevier.)

parent artery to cause thrombosis of the aneurysmal sac. Most aneurysms are currently treated endovascularly. Stentlike devices called flow diverters (Pipeline) are now also being used.

CHRONIC Rx

- Management of reversible risk factors mentioned above (smoking, hypertension, drug use)
- Management of neurologic disability through physical therapy and rehabilitation

DISPOSITION

- SAH is often associated with a poor outcome with a death rate between 30% and 40%; 10% to 15% of patients die before they reach the hospital.
- Almost half of those who survive hospitalization have cognitive impairments or disability that affect their lifestyles.

REFERRAL

Patients should be managed in a cerebrovascular center that maintains capacity to perform open surgical and endovascular procedures, with a critical care unit experienced in caring for neurosurgical patients.

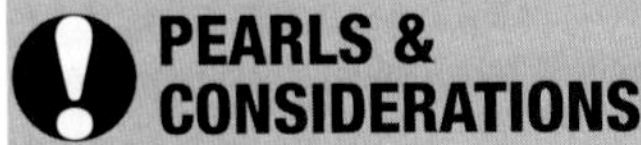

PEARLS & CONSIDERATIONS

COMMENTS

- "Thunderclap" headaches should be considered SAH until proven otherwise and evaluated by CT of the head with/without LP. MRI FLAIR sequence is also a helpful modality.
- All SAH should be managed in a critical care setting (preferably neurocritical care unit) with neurosurgical care available.
- Measures to prevent rebleeding include adequate control of blood pressure and aneurysm treatment with the use of coiling or clipping.

PREVENTION

Controlling some of the modifiable risk factors, especially smoking and blood pressure, may help to decrease the risk of aneurysmal rupture.

PATIENT & FAMILY EDUCATION

- SAH is a devastating condition, with most survivors developing significant neurologic or cognitive deficits. A good support system and an adequate physical and cognitive rehabilitation program may prove useful to survivors.
- Screening may be useful for patients with two or three first-degree relatives with SAH.

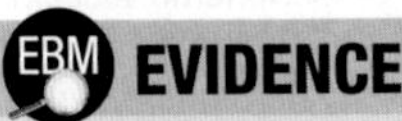

EVIDENCE

Available at ExpertConsult.com

SUGGESTED READINGS

Available at ExpertConsult.com

RELATED CONTENT

Subarachnoid Hemorrhage (Patient Information)

AUTHORS: **FARHAN A. MIRZA, M.D.,** and **JUSTIN F. FRASER, M.D.**

BASIC INFORMATION

DEFINITION

Subclavian steal syndrome is an occlusion or severe stenosis of the proximal subclavian artery leading to decreased antegrade flow or retrograde flow in the ipsilateral vertebral artery and neurologic symptoms referable to the posterior circulation.

SYNONYM

Proximal subclavian (or innominate) artery stenosis or occlusion

ICD-10CM CODE

G45.8 Other transient cerebral ischemic attacks and related syndromes

EPIDEMIOLOGY & DEMOGRAPHICS

- Similar to that of other manifestations of atherosclerosis (coronary artery disease, cerebrovascular disease, or peripheral vascular disease)
- Affects middle-aged persons (men somewhat younger than women on average) with arteriosclerotic risk factors, including family history, smoking, diabetes mellitus, hyperlipidemia, hypertension, and sedentary lifestyle

PHYSICAL FINDINGS & CLINICAL PRESENTATION

Symptoms:

- Many patients are asymptomatic.
- Upper-extremity ischemic symptoms: Fatigue, exercise-related aching, coolness, numbness of the involved upper extremity.
- Neurologic symptoms are reported by 25% of patients with known unilateral subclavian steal. These include brief spells of:
  1. Vertigo
  2. Diplopia
  3. Decreased vision
  4. Oscillopsia
  5. Gait unsteadiness

These spells are only occasionally provoked by exercising the ischemic upper extremity (classic subclavian steal). Left subclavian steal is more common than right, but the latter is more serious.

- Posterior circulation stroke related to subclavian steal is rare.
- Innominate artery stenosis can cause decreased right carotid artery flow and cerebrovascular symptoms of the anterior cerebral circulation, but this is uncommon.

Physical findings:

- Delayed and smaller volume pulse (wrist or antecubital) in the affected upper extremity
- Lower blood pressure in the affected upper extremity
- Supraclavicular bruit

NOTE: Inflating a blood pressure cuff will increase the bruit if it originates from a vertebral artery stenosis and decrease the bruit if it originates from a subclavian artery stenosis.

ETIOLOGY & PATHOGENESIS

Etiology:

- Atherosclerosis
- Arteritis (Takayasu disease and temporal arteritis)
- Embolism to the subclavian or innominate artery
- Cervical rib
- Long-term use of a crutch
- Occupational (baseball pitchers and cricket bowlers)

Pathogenesis: The vertebral artery originates from the subclavian artery. For subclavian steal to occur, the occlusion must be proximal to the takeoff of the vertebral artery. On the right side, only a small distance separates the bifurcation of the innominate artery and the takeoff of the vertebral artery, explaining why the condition occurs less commonly on the right side. Occlusion of the innominate artery must affect right carotid artery flow.

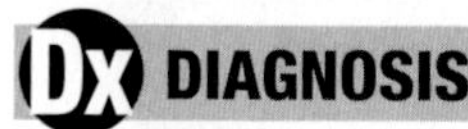

DIAGNOSIS

The carotid arteries should be evaluated at least noninvasively in all cases.

DIFFERENTIAL DIAGNOSIS

- Posterior circulation transient ischemic attack or stroke
- Upper-extremity ischemia:
  1. Distal subclavian artery stenosis or occlusion
  2. Raynaud's syndrome
  3. Thoracic outlet syndrome

WORKUP

- Noninvasive upper-extremity arterial flow studies
- Doppler sonography of the vertebral, subclavian, and innominate arteries
- Arteriography, magnetic resonance arteriogram (Fig. 1)

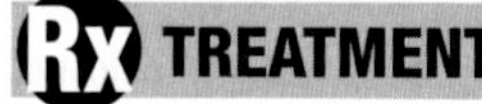

TREATMENT

- In most patients the disease is benign and requires no treatment other than atherosclerosis risk factor modification and aspirin. Symptoms tend to improve over time as collateral circulation develops.
- Vascular surgical reconstruction requires a thoracotomy; it may be indicated in innominate artery stenosis or when upper-extremity ischemia is incapacitating.

AUTHOR: **FRED F. FERRI, M.D.**

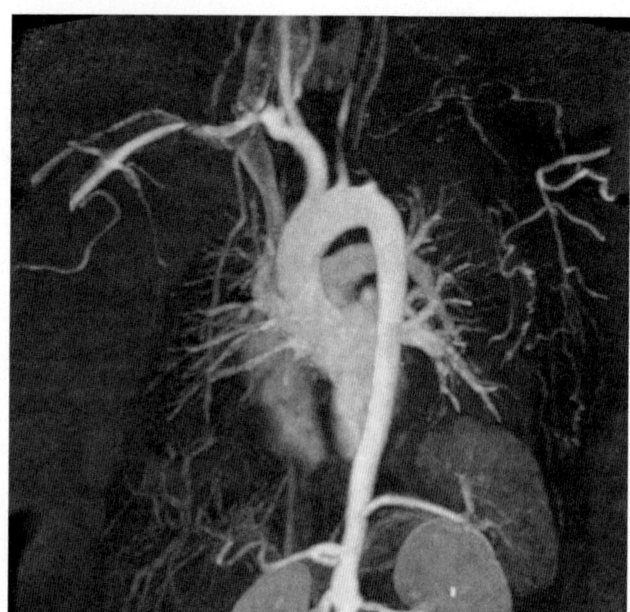

FIG. 1 Magnetic resonance arteriogram demonstrating diffuse moderate stenosis of the proximal left common carotid and proximal occlusion of the left subclavian artery coming off the aortic arch with development of an extensive collateral network. (From Hochberg MC et al: *Rheumatology,* ed 5, St Louis, 2011, Mosby.)

BASIC INFORMATION

DEFINITION

A subdural hematoma (SDH) is a collection of blood or blood products between the brain and dura mater. Subdural hematomas can be acute (ASDH) or chronic (CSDH) and vary significantly in presentation and treatment.

SYNONYM

Subdural hemorrhage

ICD-10CM CODES

S06.5 Traumatic subdural hemorrhage
I62.03 Chronic subdural hematoma
I62.01 Acute subdural hematoma

EPIDEMIOLOGY & DEMOGRAPHICS

INCIDENCE:
- The exact incidence of ASDH is unknown, but it is commonly seen in patients with head injury.
- CSDH is most common in the elderly with an estimated incidence of 1.72 to 13.1 per 100,000.

PREVALENCE: Unknown

PREDOMINANT AGE AND SEX:
- Peak incidence of CSDH is in the eighth decade and is notably higher in males.
- ASDHs usually present in the trauma setting and can happen in all age groups. In particular, shaken baby syndrome can be associated with SDH in the infant population.

RISK FACTORS:
- Trauma and antithrombotic therapy are the most common risk factors for ASDH and CSDH.
- Brain atrophy secondary to advanced age and alcoholism are common risk factors, especially with the coagulopathy/thrombocytopenia seen in chronic alcoholics.
- Intracranial hypotension associated with CSF shunts or leaks is uncommon but can result in acute or chronic SDH.

PHYSICAL FINDINGS & CLINICAL PRESENTATION

Symptoms vary on the basis of acuity, size, and location. Acute traumatic SDHs are often seen in traumatic brain injury patients, and their Glasgow Coma Scale may vary according to the extent of brain injury, size of hematoma, and associated compression. When associated with a midline shift (i.e., >5 mm), they can cause signs of cerebral herniation (e.g., ipsilateral pupil dilation, contralateral weakness) requiring prompt surgical evacuation.

- Patients with CSDH may present with diverse nonspecific symptoms such as headaches, confusion, gait disturbance, incontinence, aphasia, hemiparesis, TIA-like symptoms, and seizures.

ETIOLOGY

SDH is usually the result of shearing and tearing of a bridging vein between the brain parenchyma and the dura mater. Other causes of bleeding into the subdural space include contusion, extension of parenchymal hemorrhage. In the setting of spontaneous SDH, other vascular abnormalities, such as AV malformation, aneurysm, and dural AV fistula, should be kept in mind.

DIAGNOSIS

DIFFERENTIAL DIAGNOSIS

CSF hygromas, abscesses, and tumor infiltrations

WORKUP

- Clinical assessment: Patient history, including medications, specifically anticoagulants/antiplatelets; alcohol abuse; recent trauma; cancer; and recent bacterial infections
- Neurologic examination: Glasgow Coma Scale, cranial nerves, motor/sensory exam CT head

LABORATORY TESTS

Assessment of the patient's coagulation status including CBC with platelet count, prothrombin time, partial thromboplastin time and liver function test (especially with a history of alcoholism or liver failure)

IMAGING STUDIES

CT head (Fig. 1): Demonstrates the classic crescentic collection between the brain and inner table. For comatose and trauma patients, include a cervical spine CT scan. ASDH is usually hyperdense, whereas a CSDH is usually hypodense on noncontrast CT. Contrast is only needed if there are concerns about tumor or infection.

TREATMENT

- Correction of underlying coagulopathy, if present (e.g., warfarin/ASA/clopidogrel reversal).
- Admission for monitoring in the setting of acute SDH.
- The majority of SDH can be managed without surgery in awake patients with normal neurologic examinations.

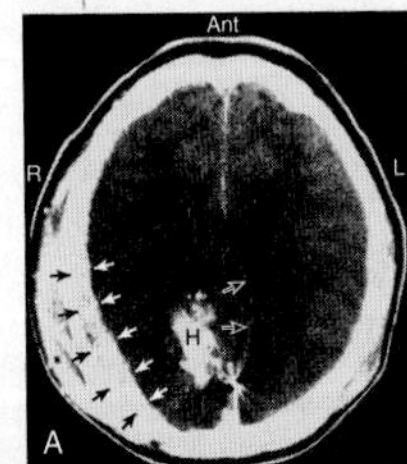

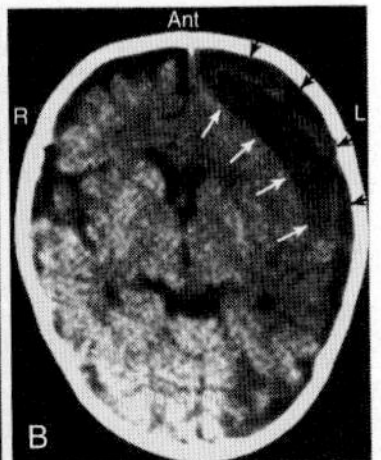

FIG. 1 A, Noncontrast computed tomography scan of an acute subdural hematoma shows a crescentic area of increased density in the right posterior parietal region between the brain and the skull *(black and white arrows).* An area of intraparenchymal hemorrhage *(H)* is also seen. **B,** A chronic subdural hematoma for a different patient is shown. There is an area of decreased density in the left frontoparietal region *(arrows)* that effaces the sulci, compresses the anterior horn of the left lateral ventricle, and shifts the midline somewhat to the right. (From Mettler FA [ed]: *Primary care radiology,* Philadelphia, 2000, Saunders.)

- Medical management of CSDH using antifibrinolytic therapy with tranexamic acid 650 mg per day is showing promising results. Studies will continue to evaluate its efficacy as a medical therapy for SDH.
- Seizure prophylaxis with phenytoin or levetiracetam for seven days should be considered in almost all cases, as there is underlying injury to the brain tissue associated with acute subdural hematoma. The irritative effects of blood products on the brain can also contribute to seizures, in both acute and chronic subdural hematomas. If seizures do occur, video EEG monitoring should be instituted and aggressive treatment undertaken.

NONPHARMACOLOGIC THERAPY

Surgical treatment is indicated in:
- ASDHs measuring >10 mm in thickness with a midline shift >5 mm on CT scan and a compromised neurologic status (Glasgow Coma Scale <9, pupillary asymmetry or fixation) should be immediately evacuated.
- In CSDH with a mass effect, a clear change in the neurologic examination from baseline, and/or enlargement of the hematoma size, evacuation via craniotomy or burr hole should be considered.

DISPOSITION

Depending on the size and location of the SDH and the examination of the patient, observation can range from the ICU to outpatient management. When observation of the patient is considered, clinical examinations should be serially performed. Patient baseline and follow-up clinical examinations are more important than CT scan findings.

REFERRAL

Neurosurgical and operative consultation should be made available.

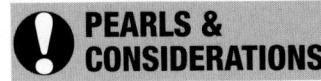

PEARLS & CONSIDERATIONS

COMMENTS

- Many elderly patients have small CSDHs or hygromas. Unless these are associated with seizures or clinical or radiographic progression, they are usually not emergent and usually do not require neurosurgical intervention. Recurrence after surgical management for CSDH is common.
- SDHs in elderly patients can have a mixed hyperdense and hypodense appearance on noncontrast CT scan; this finding is suggestive of subdural membranes and chronic components.

PATIENT & FAMILY EDUCATION

Individuals with SDHs are at higher risk for seizure, so surveillance is important.

RELATED CONTENT

Subdural Hematoma (Patient Information)

AUTHORS: **FARHAN A. MIRZA, M.D.,** and **JUSTIN F. FRASER, M.D.**

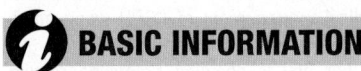

BASIC INFORMATION

DEFINITION

A localized accumulation of infected fluid, often encapsulated, located under the diaphragm and may also involve the liver and spleen

SYNONYMS

Subdiaphragmatic abscess
Infradiaphragmatic abscess

ICD-10CM CODES

K65.1	Peritoneal abscess
K68.11	Postprocedural retroperitoneal abscess

EPIDEMIOLOGY & DEMOGRAPHICS

INCIDENCE: Not well known but intra-abdominal abscess occurs in 1% to 2% of all cases of abdominal surgery. It increases to 10% to 30% in cases with preoperative perforation of a hollow viscus, spillage of fecal material into peritoneum, or intestinal ischemia.

RISK FACTORS:
- Abdominal surgery, especially with accidental viscus perforation
- Peptic ulcer perforation
- Appendiceal perforation
- Diverticulitis with perforation
- Mesenteric ischemia with bowel infarction
- Abdominal trauma especially penetrating trauma
- Foreign body ingestion with subsequent viscus perforation

PHYSICAL FINDINGS & CLINICAL PRESENTATION

- Constitutional symptoms include:
  1. Fever, malaise or chills
  2. Cough, increased respiratory rate with shallow or grunting respiration
  3. Shoulder-tip pain on affected side (referred pain)
- Physical findings can include:
  1. Dullness to percussion on affected side
  2. Diminished or absent breath sounds on affected side
  3. Tenderness over the 8th to 11th ribs

ETIOLOGY

Infection is usually polymicrobial: Aerobic gram-negative rods, most commonly *Escherichia coli*, *Klebsiella* species, *Enterobacter* species, and *Pseudomonas aeruginosa*, and gram-positive cocci: *Streptococcus viridians*, enterococci and *Staphylococcus aureus*, and anaerobes (found in 60% to 70% of cases) such as *Bacteroides fragilis* and *Clostridia* species.

Dx DIAGNOSIS

DIFFERENTIAL DIAGNOSIS

- Liver abscess
- Subhepatic abscess
- Lesser sac abscess
- Empyema of the lung
- Diaphragmatic hernia

WORKUP

Should be started in patients with recent abdominal surgery (weeks to months) with the constitutional symptoms and physical findings mentioned above

LABORATORY TEST(S)

- CBC with differential may show an elevated WBC with left shift
- Blood cultures may be positive in up to 50% of the cases
- Gram stain and culture, aerobically and anaerobically, of any aspiration procedure

IMAGING STUDIES

- Plain x-ray films can suggest the location of the abscess in about 50% of the cases and can demonstrate elevation of the hemidiaphragm and/or subphrenic air-fluid level
- Ultrasonography and CT (Fig. 1) are more sensitive
- Other options include leukocyte tagged with gallium 67 and indium 111 scans and MRI

Rx TREATMENT

Includes source control with either percutaneous drainage or surgery and intravenous antibiotics:
- Percutaneous drainage via interventional radiology:
  1. Percutaneous drainage with catheter placement remains the preferred treatment despite the fact that the subphrenic location can be problematic for imaging-guided percutaneous drainage.
  2. Approaches include subcostal approach or intercostal approach. The intercostal approach is associated with a higher risk for pleural complications, but these tend to be minor.
  3. Radiographic modalities used include ultrasonography, CT, and fluoroscopy.
  4. Complications of drainage procedures can include pleural effusion, pneumothorax, or empyema.
- Surgery: May be required in recurrence of abscess or due to multiple abscesses not amenable to percutaneous drainage procedure
- Antibiotics: Broad-spectrum antibiotics should be used to cover Gram-negative rods, Gram-positive bacteria, and anaerobes until cultures are resulted and should be continued at least 4–7 days after adequate drainage procedure. Examples include:
  1. Piperacillin/tazobactam 3.375 g IV q6h or 4.5 g IV q8h
  2. Meropenem 1 g IV q8h or imipenem 0.5–1 g IV q6h
  3. Ciprofloxacin IV 400 mg IV q12h plus IV metronidazole 500 mg IV q8h for penicillin allergic patients

REFERRAL

- Interventional radiology
- General surgery
- Infectious diseases

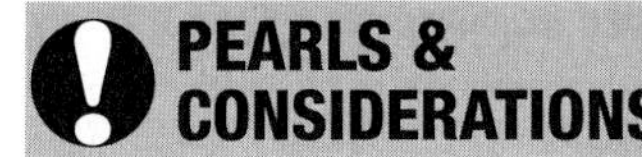

PEARLS & CONSIDERATIONS

COMMENTS

Success of percutaneous drainage procedures is greater than 85%, and recurrence rates are about 1% to 10%.

SUGGESTED READINGS

Available at ExpertConsult.com

RELATED TOPICS

Peritonitis

AUTHOR: **GLENN G. FORT, M.D., M.P.H.**

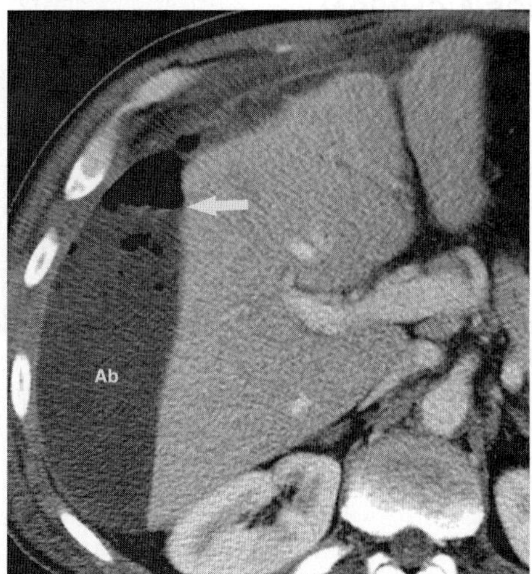

FIG. 1 Subphrenic abscess. A postoperative abscess *(Ab)* is seen as a fluid collection between the diaphragm and the liver. Mass impression on the liver is evidence of fluid loculation. An air–fluid level *(arrow)* is evident, caused by gas-producing *Escherichia coli.* This abscess was successfully treated using percutaneous catheter drainage guided by computed tomography. (From Webb WR, et al.: *Fundamentals of body CT*, ed 4, Philadelphia, 2015, Saunders.)

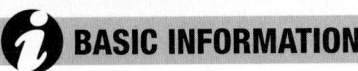

BASIC INFORMATION

DEFINITION

The recurrent use of alcohol and/or drugs that causes clinically and functionally significant impairment, such as health problems, disability, and failure to meet major responsibilities at work, school, or home.

SYNONYMS

Drug use
Addiction
Substance abuse

ICD-10CM CODE
F10-F19 Defined by specific substance
DSM-5
Depends on specific substance of abuse

EPIDEMIOLOGY & DEMOGRAPHICS

Genetic factors have a major influence on progression of substance use to dependence, whereas environmental factors unique to the individual play an important role in exposure and initial use of substances.

INCIDENCE: Peak period of both alcohol and illicit drug use disorders occurs in late adolescence and early adulthood, with a substantial reduction in substance use disorders after age 26 yr.

PREVALENCE: The lifetime prevalence of alcohol use disorders is approximately 8%, and prevalence of illicit drug use disorders is 2% to 3%.

PREDOMINANT SEX AND AGE: Substance abuse in general is more common among males than among females (1.3 times more).

GENETICS: Multiple biological mechanisms are involved in tolerance, craving, anxiety, dysphoria, executive cognitive function, and reward. Genome's role in neuroadaptation to drugs and the ways in which genetic variations and environmental exposures cause vulnerability to addictions are still under investigation. Addictive drugs induce adaptive changes in gene expression in brain reward regions, causing tolerance and habit formation with craving and negative affect. A specific effect of the μ-opioid receptor polymorphism (*OPRM1*; Asn40Asp) Asp40 to predict favorable naltrexone treatment response in alcoholism was recently replicated.

RISK FACTORS: Offspring of substance abusers were at twofold increased risk for any substance use disorder and a threefold risk for alcohol and marijuana abuse or dependence compared with offspring of control parents. Individuals who develop substance use disorders in adolescence are more likely to have those symptoms persist into adulthood.

Common risk factors are:

- Family history of addiction
- Being male
- Having another mental health disorder
- Peer pressure
- Lack of family involvement
- Taking a highly addictive drug

PHYSICAL FINDINGS & CLINICAL PRESENTATION

Physical and behavioral symptoms are helpful to determine drug use. Bloodshot or glazed eyes, dilated or constricted pupils, abrupt weight changes, bruises, infections, and track marks are common physical signs. Behavioral changes occur as individual becomes more dependent on the drug. Increased aggression or irritability, sudden changes in social network, dramatic changes in habits and/or priorities, involvement in criminal activity, and financial problems are commonly observed.

ETIOLOGY

Theories are categorized into three main subgroups: social, psychological, and biological. There has been an emphasis on the role of personality, age of starting drug abuse, and hereditary and genetic factors. Some studies identified family as the most important and crucial risk factor for drug abuse in the youth (lack of a safe and warm environment at home, weak attachment between children and the parents, role modeling of the parents, loss of a parent, and lack of supervision). Peer pressure is also a strong risk factor. Although there is no general agreement on the gateway effect of drugs such as cannabis, poverty, neighborhood, living in poor and polluted suburbs, and low level of leisure facilities have been identified as impacting factors.

Dx DIAGNOSIS

DIFFERENTIAL DIAGNOSIS

Use a motivational interviewing style and evidence-based interventions; identify and treat co-occurring medical and psychiatric conditions.

WORKUP

Screening and assessment tools are available. CAGE (Cutdown, Guilty, Annoyed, Eyeopener) and AUDIT (Alcohol Use Disorders Identification Test) are commonly used for alcohol use disorder, and DAST (Drug Abuse Screening Test) is for drugs. CIWA-Ar (revised Clinical Institute Withdrawal Assessment for Alcohol scale assessment) and COWS (Clinical Opiate Withdrawal Scale) are used to assess the severity of alcohol and opioid withdrawal symptoms consequently.

LABORATORY TESTS

Blood alcohol levels, breathalyzer test results, urine drug screens, and, less commonly, hair and saliva analysis can be used to assess patients for possible alcohol and other drug use. Chemicals and their metabolites can be detected in the samples for limited times. Therefore, tests should be chosen and timed carefully.

IMAGING STUDIES

Imaging techniques such as positron emission tomography (PET), functional magnetic resonance imaging (fMRI), and electroencephalography (EEG) have been used to investigate these behaviors in drug-addicted human populations. However, there is no current therapeutic use or monitoring the outcome.

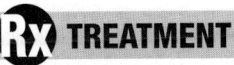

TREATMENT

Multiple treatment options for substance use disorders exist that can help individuals reach treatment goals. No single treatment is right for everyone. Treatment options should be discussed with patients and families to help them decide which ones are best for the patients' conditions. The outcomes of self-change efforts and treatment experiences should be reviewed frequently.

NONPHARMACOLOGIC THERAPY

Talk therapy has been shown to teach skills to avoid relapse, to reduce harmful substance use, and to improve health and quality of life. Cognitive behavioral therapy for substance use disorders and 12-step facilitation and motivational enhancement therapy are commonly used techniques. Peer support by Alcoholics Anonymous, Narcotics Anonymous, and SMART Recovery are also helpful.

ACUTE GENERAL Rx

Inpatient medically supervised withdrawal may be necessary for patients with symptoms of at least moderate alcohol withdrawal and patients with histories of severe withdrawal seizures. Benzodiazepine use disorder also requires inpatient admission, or taper in outpatient settings should be closely monitored. Comfort medications (clonidine, dicyclomine, loperamide, ibuprofen) are useful in management of opioid withdrawal symptoms. Buprenorphine can be used for both withdrawal and long-term maintenance treatment. Antipsychotics (i.e., haloperidol) may be considered for agitation, hallucinations, and other behavioral disturbances.

CHRONIC Rx

Acamprosate, disulfiram, naltrexone (oral or injectable), and topiramate are the medications that are commonly used for alcoholism treatment. Benzodiazepines should be avoided due to their own risk of addiction, and risk of triggering alcohol relapses. Because these are chronic conditions, the length of the treatment will depend on the individual treatment plan and the patient's success in achieving goals. Maintenance programs with methadone and buprenorphine may be continued for yrs.

COMPLEMENTARY AND ALTERNATIVE MEDICINE

The top three therapies—religious healing, relaxation techniques, and meditation—are commonly used techniques. Neurofeedback and acupuncture were also reported as supportive.

DISPOSITION

Because of the nature of this chronic/relapsing condition, individuals should be referred to and monitored at outpatient drug and/or alcohol treatment centers. Other health conditions and co-occurring psychiatric disorder treatment can be provided at general mental health clinics. Drug rehabilitation may require a controlled environment, such as those in sober houses and long-term recovery clinics. Alcoholics Anonymous (AA) programs are also effective in providing peer support.

REFERRAL

https://findtreatment.samhsa.gov/

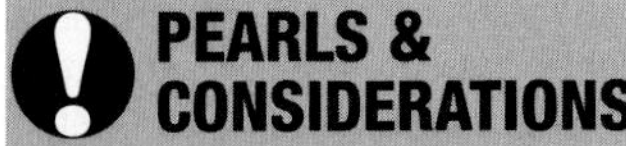

PEARLS & CONSIDERATIONS

COMMENTS

Goals of substance use disorder treatment:

- Stop the harmful use of addictive substances.
- Improve health and wellness.
- Live a self-directed life.
- Strive to reach full potential.
- Improve quality of life.

PREVENTION

Efforts typically focus on children and teens. Besides national recognition of substance use prevention, family-based, school-based, and community prevention programs focus on changing community conditions or policies so that the availability of substances is reduced.

PATIENT/FAMILY EDUCATION

Individuals are provided information to understand the many aspects of what substance abuse is; warning signs of addiction; information about how alcohol and specific drugs affect the mind and body; and the consequences of addiction. Family therapy and education play important roles in the change process.

SUGGESTED READINGS

Available at ExpertConsult.com

RELATED TOPICS

Alcohol Abuse (Related Key Topic)
Drug Abuse (Related Key Topic)
Hallucinogenic Overdose (Related Key Topic)
Opioid Overdose (Related Key Topic)
Opioid Use Disorder (Related Key Topic)
Synthetic Cannabinoids (Related Key Topic)

AUTHOR: **TAHIR TELLIOGLU, M.D.**

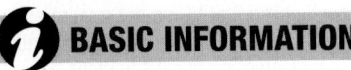

BASIC INFORMATION

DEFINITION

Superior vena cava (SVC) syndrome is a set of symptoms that results when a mediastinal mass compresses the SVC or the veins that drain into it, resulting in obstruction of blood flow from the head, neck, upper torso, or extremities to the right atrium.

SYNONYM

SVC

ICD-10CM CODES

I87.1	Compression of vein
S25.20XA	Unspecified injury of superior vena cava, initial encounter
S25.29XA	Other specified injury of superior vena cava, initial encounter

EPIDEMIOLOGY & DEMOGRAPHICS

- SVC syndrome occurs in 15,000 persons in the U.S. every yr.
- More than 50% of patients present with SVC on presentation of malignancy.
- Mirrors lung cancer (especially small cell carcinoma) and lymphoma (see "Lung Neoplasm" and "Lymphoma" in Section I).

PHYSICAL FINDINGS & CLINICAL PRESENTATION

The pathophysiology of the syndrome involves increased pressure in the venous system draining into the SVC producing edema of the head, neck, and upper extremities. Symptoms develop over a period of 2 weeks in one third of patients and include:

- Shortness of breath
- Chest pain
- Cough

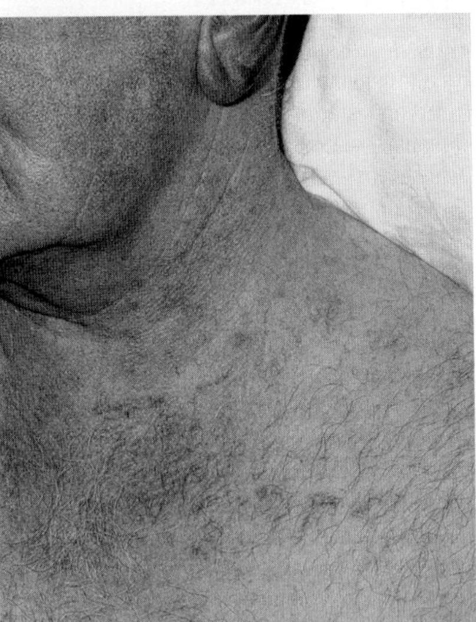

FIG. 1 Superior vena cava obstruction causing dilated veins and plethora of the upper trunk and neck in a patient with bronchial carcinoma. Patients with superior vena cava obstruction are occasionally referred to dermatologists with suspected contact allergy (eyelid swelling) or angioedema (facial or hand swelling). (From White GM, Cox NH [eds]: *Diseases of the skin, a color atlas and text*, ed 2, St Louis, 2006, Mosby.)

- Dysphagia, hoarseness, stridor
- Headache
- Syncope
- Visual trouble

Signs:

- Chest wall vein distention (Fig. 1)
- Neck vein distention
- Facial edema, facial plethora
- Upper-extremity swelling
- Cyanosis

ETIOLOGY

- Lung cancer (65% of all cases, of which half are small cell lung cancer)
- Lymphoma (15%)
- Thymoma
- Tuberculosis
- Goiter
- Aortic aneurysm (arteriosclerotic or syphilitic)
- SVC thrombosis:
  1. Primary: Associated with a central venous catheter
  2. Secondary: Complication of SVC syndrome associated with one of the above-mentioned causes
- Inflammatory process, fibrosing mediastinitis
- Fig. 2 illustrates the anatomy of superior vena cava syndrome. Table 1 summarizes common malignancies associated with SVC syndrome in adults.

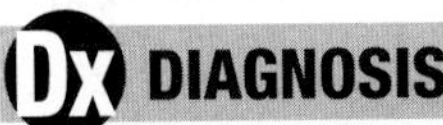

DIAGNOSIS

Diagnostic imaging (Fig. 3): CT scan of the chest with contrast is the most useful diagnostic study. MRI is usually adequate to establish the

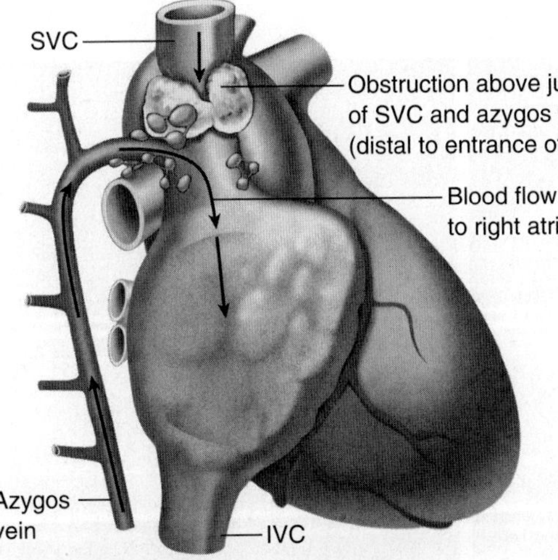

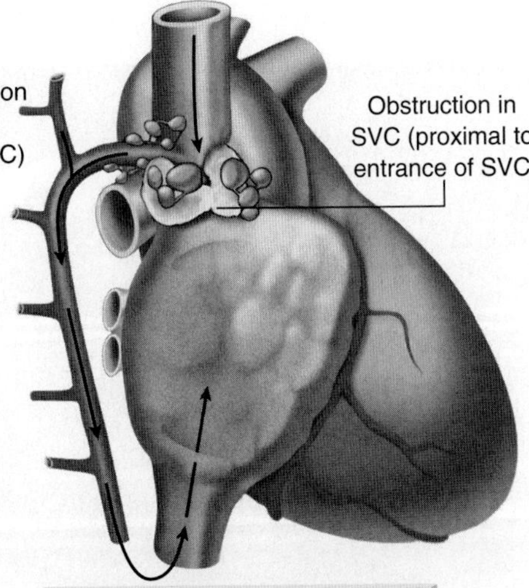

FIG. 2 Anatomy of superior vena cava *(SVC)* syndrome. Lymph nodes may obstruct blood return above the entrance of the azygos vein **(A)**, resulting in edema of the face, neck, and arms and distended veins in the neck and arms and over the upper chest. Obstruction below the return of the azygos vein **(B)** results in retrograde flow through the azygos through collateral veins to the inferior vena cava *(IVC)*, with all the symptoms and signs in **A** plus dilation of the veins over the abdomen as well. (Modified from Skatin AT [ed]: *Atlas of diagnostic oncology*, ed 3, Philadelphia, 2003, Elsevier.)

diagnosis of SVC obstruction and to assist in the differential diagnosis of probable cause.

DIFFERENTIAL DIAGNOSIS

The syndrome is characteristic enough to exclude other diagnoses. The differential diagnosis concerns the underlying etiologies listed previously.

WORKUP

- Chest radiograph (mediastinal widening, pleural effusion)
- Chest CT with contrast or MRI (in patient who cannot tolerate contrast medium) usually confirms the diagnosis
- Venography: Rarely needed. Warranted only when an intervention (e.g., stent or surgery) is planned
- Percutaneous needle biopsy, endobronchial ultrasound-guided needle biopsy, or mediastinoscopy are usually the initial diagnostic modalities used to establish a histologic diagnosis

Rx TREATMENT

- Tissue diagnosis is usually needed before commencing therapy. EBUS is now considered the first step in evaluation. Mediastinoscopy would be considered if EBUS is non-diagnostic or there is high clinical suspicion for lymphoma.
- Management is guided by the severity of the symptoms and the underlying etiology.
- Most patients with SVC do not require emergency intervention. Emergency empiric radiation is indicated in critical situations such as respiratory failure or central nervous system signs associated with increased intracranial pressure.
- Treatment of the underlying malignancy:
  1. Radiotherapy: The majority of tumors causing SVC syndrome are sensitive to radiotherapy
  2. Systemic chemotherapy
- Anticoagulant or fibrinolytic therapy in patients who do not respond to cancer treatment within a week or if an obstructing thrombus has been documented.
- Loop diuretics are often used, but their effect is limited.
- Upright positioning and fluid restriction until collateral channels develop and allow for clinical regression are useful modalities for SVC syndrome secondary to benign disease.
- Steroids (dexamethasone 4 mg q6h) may be useful in reducing the tumor burden in lymphoma and thymoma after definitive diagnosis is made.
- Percutaneous self-expandable stents that can be placed under local anesthesia with radiologic manipulation are useful in the treatment of SVC syndrome to bypass the obstruction, especially in cases associated with malignant tumors.
- Surgical bypass grafting is infrequently used to treat SVC syndrome.

TABLE 1 Malignancies Associated with Superior Vena Cava (SVC) Syndrome in Adults*

Neoplastic Diagnosis	Percentage of SVC	Percentage of Disease-Associated SVC
Lung cancer, stage 3B or 4:	48-81	
Small cell lung cancer		15-45
Squamous cell cancer		20-25
Adenocarcinoma		5-25
Large cell carcinoma		4-30
Lymphoma:	2-21	
Diffuse large cell lymphoma		64
Lymphoblastic lymphoma		33
Breast cancer	11	

*Includes lung cancer, lymphomas, and metastases from other solid tumors. 75% to 85% of patients with SVC have neoplastic disease.
From Zipes DP et al (eds): *Braunwald's heart disease*, ed 7, Philadelphia, 2005, Saunders.

REFERRAL

To a thoracic surgeon, pulmonary specialist, or oncologist

AUTHOR: **GAETANE MICHAUD, M.D.**

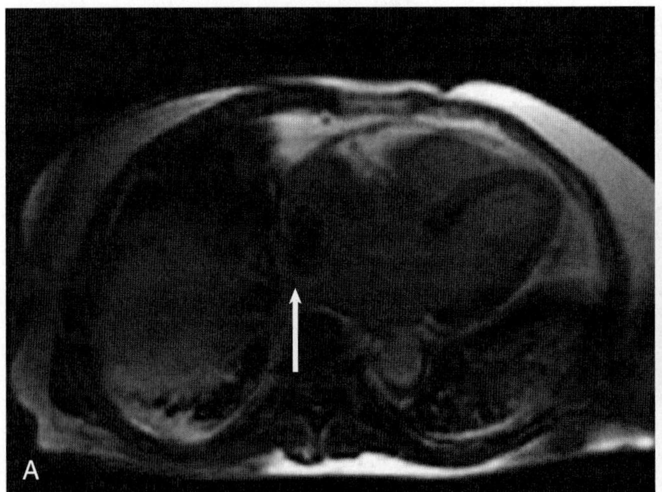

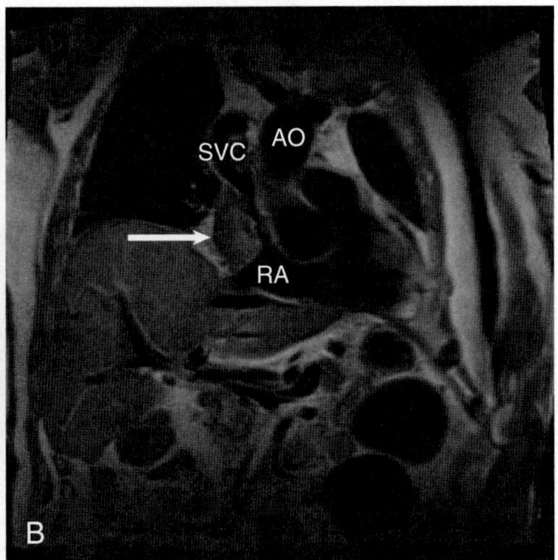

FIG. 3 Superior vena cava *(SVC)* obstruction. A, Fast imaging with steady-state precession (FISP) showing a large irregular right atrial mass extending into the SVC *(arrow)*. **B,** Dark blood image showing almost complete obstruction of the SVC from a right atrial mass in a patient with a mediastinal mass and neck and facial swelling *(arrow)*. *AO*, Aorta; *RA*, right atrium. (From Mann DL et al: *Braunwald's heart disease*, ed 10, Philadelphia, 2015. Elsevier.)

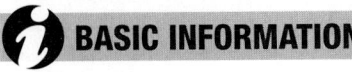

BASIC INFORMATION

DEFINITION

Supraventricular tachycardia (SVT) is a group of rapid regular tachyarrhythmia. There are three major categories of SVT:

1. Atrial tachycardia (AT): An arrhythmia that originates from the atrium and does not involve the AV node. This is usually a focal arrhythmia. In some cases, the underlying mechanism may be a reentry circuit, either a small circuit (microreentry) or a large circuit (macroreentry)
2. AV nodal reentrant tachycardia (AVNRT)
3. AV reentrant tachycardia (AVRT) (Fig. 1)

The latter two are reentrant arrhythmia that always involve the AV node as part of the circuit (Fig. 1).

Other forms of arrhythmia that involve the atria, such as atrial fibrillation and atrial flutter, have distinct electrocardiographic features and are covered in separate chapters. Rare forms of SVT such as inappropriate sinus tachycardia, sinus mode reentry tachycardia, and junctional tachycardia are beyond the scope of this chapter.

SYNONYMS

SVT
Paroxysmal supraventricular tachycardia
PSVT

ICD-10CM CODE
I47.1 Supraventricular tachycardia

EPIDEMIOLOGY & DEMOGRAPHICS

SVT is most commonly diagnosed between the ages of 12 and 30. SVT occurs most commonly in patients with no prior cardiac conditions. AVNRT is the most common type of SVT in both genders and in all ages. It occurs most commonly in young women. AVRT is the second most common SVT, and it is typically diagnosed in younger patients as compared to the age of patients with AVNRT. AT is more commonly associated with structural heart disease.

PHYSICAL FINDINGS & CLINICAL PRESENTATION

- Patients may be either symptomatic or asymptomatic.
- Patient may be aware of "fast" regular heartbeat (but sometimes complain of irregular heartbeat: palpitations); may complain of weakness, dyspnea, dizziness, chest pain, presyncope or, rarely, syncope.
- Patients with AVNRT may complain of neck pounding during the episode due to simultaneous contraction of the atria and ventricles with closed AV valves and hence sharp increase in atrial and neck-jugular venous pressure.
- In some cases the episodes can be triggered by physical activity or psychological stress, but in others there may not be an obvious trigger. In patients with AVNRT, sometimes the arrhythmia is reproducibly initiated when bending forward to pick up an item from the floor.
- Hemodynamic status during the arrhythmia may vary and depend on the patient's comorbidities and presence of underlying structural heart disease. Usually, patients are hemodynamically stable.
- Physical examination is most commonly normal and unrevealing, except rapid regular heart rate and occasionally hypotension. In patients with AVNRT sharp tall jugular vein A waves may be seen when the right atrium contracts against a closed tricuspid valve.

ETIOLOGY (SEE FIG. 1)

- AVNRT: Dual electrical pathways within the AV node. In typical AVNRT the anterograde limb conducts slowly (slow pathway) and the retrograde limb has fast conduction properties (fast pathway), and vice versa in atypical AVNRT.
- AVRT is accessory pathway mediated, either orthodromic (antegrade through the AV node and retrograde through the accessory pathway) or, much less commonly, antidromic (antegrade through the accessory pathway and retrograde through the AV node). In the case of antidromic tachycardia, the QRS will be wide and fully preexcited. In some patients, the presence of accessory pathway is not evident on the baseline ECG (concealed accessory pathway), while in others it is manifest in the baseline ECG, presenting the typical features of the Wolff-Parkinson-White (WPW) syndrome.
- Paroxysmal atrial tachycardia and multifocal atrial tachycardia: abnormal automaticity of atrial tissue or triggered activity. In some cases (especially in patients who underwent previous cardiac surgery such as valve replacement or ASD closure), the underlying mechanism is macroreentrant AT.

Dx DIAGNOSIS AND DIFFERENTIAL DIAGNOSIS

The diagnosis of SVT relies principally on the 12-lead ECG. Every patient suspected of having an episode of SVT should have a 12-lead ECG done immediately. Typically patients with SVT will present with a narrow complex QRS tachycardia with a ventricular rate faster than 100 beats per minute (bpm) and typically faster than 130-150 bpm.

- P wave morphology can be useful in discriminating rhythms. P waves with a similar axis to the sinus node can be atrial tachycardias and sinus tachycardias. P waves with retrograde depolarization of the atria (seen as inverted in the inferior leads) can be seen in AVNRT, AVRT, and atrial tachycardia. Sawtooth P waves are indicative of classical counterclockwise typical type I flutter, and an absence of P waves with irregular R-R intervals points to atrial fibrillation. Variable (>3) morphologies of P wave are suggestive of multifocal atrial tachycardia. Wide QRS complex (>0.12 sec) with initial slurring (delta wave) during sinus rhythm and short PR (<0.12 sec) is characteristic of Wolff-Parkinson-White syndrome.

In typical AVNRT, due to the small size of the circuit within the AV node and the fast retrograde conduction, there is simultaneous depolarization of the ventricles and atria, thus making the P wave "buried" in the QRS and therefore not visible or inscribed very close to the QRS at the final part of the QRS complex, and sometimes creating a "pseudo terminal S wave" usually seen in leads II, III, and aVF and "pseudo terminal R waves" at the end of the QRS in V1 and avR (Fig. 1).

In orthodromic AVRT, the P wave is usually visible close after the QRS due to the rapid conduction properties of the accessory pathway (short RP tachycardia). In AT, the P wave is usually noticed farther away after the QRS (long RP tachycardia) (Fig. 1).

Other diagnostic maneuvers that may assist in the differential diagnosis are vagal maneuvers (such as carotid sinus massage) or giving intravenous AV nodal blocking agents such as adenosine or verapamil) to produce AV nodal conduction block. This will terminate reentrant arrhythmia dependent on the AV node—AVNRT and AVRT—but not AT, which will continue, albeit with nonconducted P waves.

Other arrhythmias that present with narrow complex tachycardia like PSVT are:

- Fascicular VT
- Junctional tachycardias
- Artifact such as with Parkinson's disease

SVT can conduct with bundle branch block (BBB) and wide QRS either due to preexisting BBB on the baseline ECG or due to aberrant conduction (rapid rate–dependent BBB). When a patient presents with wide QRS tachycardia, VT must be excluded first. Features to distinguish SVT from ventricular tachycardia are outlined in Table 1.

WORKUP

- Electrocardiography
- Echocardiography to exclude structural heart disease
- Thyroid function tests
- Complete blood count to exclude anemia or infection as an underlying trigger for the event
- In most cases the workup will be negative, with no underlying cardiac or systemic pathology and no clear triggers for an acute episode
- Holter or event monitor to document the arrhythmias if they are paroxysmal and not documented yet

TABLE 1 Features That May Differentiate Ventricular Tachycardia from Supraventricular Tachycardia with Aberrancy

Helpful Features	Implications
Positive QRS concordance	Diagnostic of VT
Presence of AV dissociation, capture beats, or fusion beats	Diagnostic of VT
Atypical RBBB (monophasic R, QR, RS, or triphasic QRS in V_1; R:S ratio <1, QS or QR, monophasic R in V_6)	Suggests VT
Atypical LBBB (R >30 min or R to S [nadir or notch] >60 min in V_1 or V_2; R:S ratio <1, QS or QR in V_6)	Suggests VT
Shift of axis from baseline	Suggests VT
History of CAD	Suggests VT
QRS during tachycardia identical to QRS during sinus rhythm	Suggests SVT
Termination with adenosine	Suggests SVT

AV, Atrioventricular; *CAD,* coronary artery disease; *LBBB,* left bundle branch block; *RBBB,* right bundle branch block; *SVT,* supraventricular tachycardia; *VT,* ventricular tachycardia.
Stambler BS et al: Etripamil nasal spray for rapid conversion of supraventricular tachycardia to sinus rhythm, *J Am Coll Cardiol* 72:489–497, 2018.

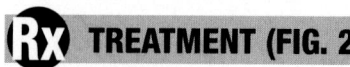

Rx TREATMENT (FIG. 2)

NONPHARMACOLOGIC THERAPY

Acute termination: If the patient is hemodynamically unstable, prompt synchronized cardioversion with an external defibrillator using 50 to 100 J should be performed.

If the patient is stable, Valsalva maneuver in the supine position is the most effective way to terminate most types of SVT; carotid sinus massage (after excluding occlusive carotid disease and murmurs over the carotid arteries) is also commonly used to elicit vagal efferent impulses. These are effective in terminating AVRT, AVNRT, and may occasionally terminate some types of atrial tachycardia, but in the case of sinus tachycardia, atrial flutter, and atrial fibrillation, they only transiently slow down AV conduction without terminating the actual tachycardia.

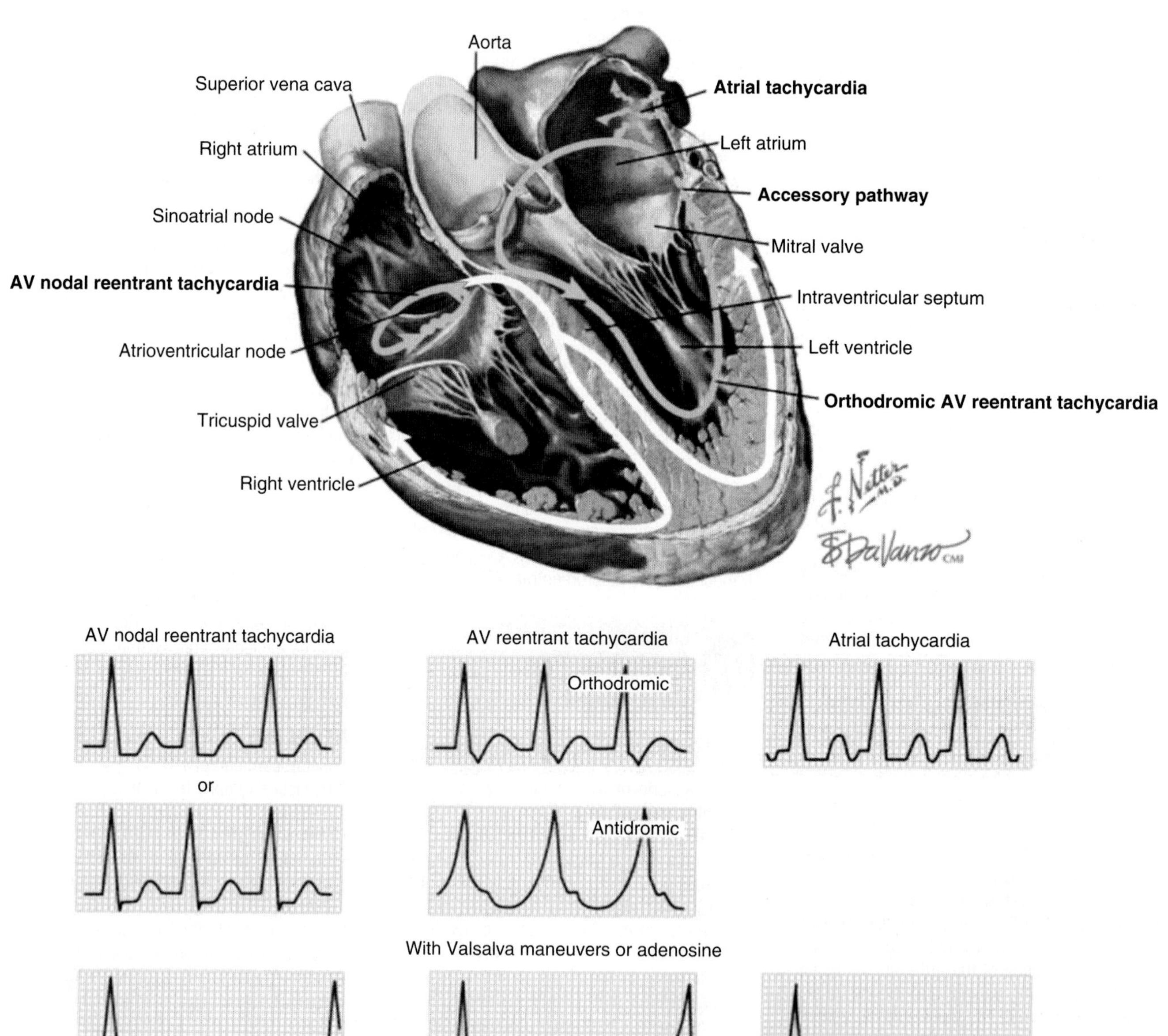

FIG. 1 Typical electrocardiographic recordings and anatomic representation of the common supraventricular tachycardias. *AV,* Atrioventricular. (From Runge MS et al [eds]: *Netter's cardiology,* ed 2, Philadelphia, 2010, Saunders. Adapted from Delacretaz E: Clinical practice: supraventricular tachycardia, *N Engl J Med* 354:1039–1051, 2006.)

PHARMACOLOGIC THERAPY

- Adenosine is useful to terminate acutely orthodromic AVRT and AVNRT and can uncover the underlying rhythm in paroxysmal atrial tachycardia (Fig. E3); it is the first choice of therapy for treatment of almost all episodes of SVT unresponsive to vagal maneuvers. The dose is 6 mg given as a rapid IV bolus; tachycardia is usually terminated within a few seconds. If this fails, one may repeat with 12 mg IV bolus. Contraindications are second- or third-degree atrioventricular block; WPW with atrial fibrillation; sick sinus syndrome; and chronic use of drugs such as dipyridamole, theophylline, or aminophylline; and heart transplant. Adenosine may cause bronchospasm in asthmatics.
- Verapamil 5 to 10 mg IV is given over 5 min; if no effect, may repeat in 30 min.
  1. Verapamil should be used cautiously in patients with SVT associated with hypotension.
  2. Slow injection of calcium chloride (10 ml of a 10% solution given over 5–8 min before verapamil administration) decreases the hypotensive effect without compromising its antiarrhythmic effect.
- Metoprolol (IV 5 mg/2 min up to 15 mg) or esmolol (500 μg/kg IV bolus, then 50 μg/kg/min) may be effective in the treatment of SVT.
- IV digoxin (0.75 to 1 mg slow IV loading in increments of 0.25 mg over several hours) is rarely used in SVT but may tried if other agents are not effective.
  1. Digoxin, beta-blockers, and calcium-channel blockers should be avoided in patients with pre-excitation syndrome and antidromic AVRT or preexcited atrial fibrillation to avoid increased conduction through the accessory pathway.
- Recently a new rapidly acting intranasal calcium-channel blocker—etripamil—was reported to be effective in rapid conversion of SVT to sinus rhythm. This may prove in the future to be an important treatment modality but is not yet available for routine clinical use.[1]

CHRONIC TREATMENT

The goal is prevention of recurrent episodes. In patients with infrequent and minimally symptomatic episodes without preexcitation, it is optional to provide treatment only during acute episodes. In patients with recurrent symptomatic episodes, regular treatment with beta-blockers or nondihydropyridines calcium channel blockers can be tried; if these fail, class Ic antiarrhythmics are an option. It is also possible to treat patients who have infrequent symptomatic episodes with a "pill-in-the-pocket" strategy with either beta-blockers or other antiarrhythmics. Patients who fail antiarrhythmic therapy, develop side effects due to medications, or refuse medical therapy should be referred for catheter ablation. This is a highly effective mode of treatment with low risk of complications. Recent studies show that ablation therapy is highly effective, safe, and associated with a very low recurrence rate[2,3]

[2]Katritsis DG et al: Catheter ablation vs. antiarrhythmic drug therapy in patients with symptomatic atrioventricular nodal re-entrant tachycardia: a randomized, controlled trial, *Europace* 19:602–6, 2017.
[3]Brachmann J et al: Long-term symptom improvement and patient satisfaction following catheter ablation of supraventricular tachycardia: insights from the German ablation registry, *Eur Heart J* 38:1317–1326, 2017.

DISPOSITION

Most patients respond well with resolution of the SVT upon treatment (see "Acute General Rx"). Some patients may need chronic AV blocking agents for recurrence.

REFERRAL

Radiofrequency ablation (RFA) is the procedure of choice in symptomatic patients who are refractory to medical therapy especially in AVRT, AVNRT, and atrial flutter. RFA has high efficacy rates (single procedure success is 93.2%), low all-cause mortality (0.1%), and low adverse events (2.9%). Despite high reported success rates, RFA appears to be underused in clinical practice.

SUGGESTED READINGS

Available at ExpertConsult.com

RELATED CONTENT

Supraventricular Tachycardia (Patient Information)

AUTHORS: **MOTI HAIM, M.D.,** and **YUVAL KONSTANTINO, M.D.**

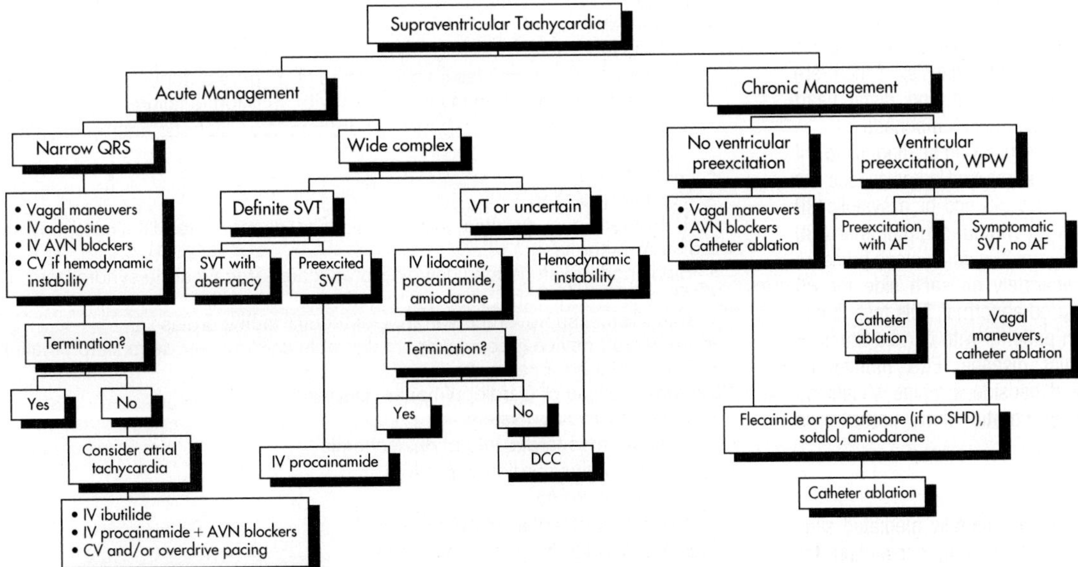

FIG. 2 Supraventricular tachycardia. *AF,* Atrial fibrillation; *AVN,* atrioventricular node; *CV,* cardioversion; *IV,* intravenous; *DCC,* direct current cardioversion; *SHD,* structural heart disease (no overt evidence of myocardial, valvular, congenital or coronary heart disease); *SVT,* supraventricular tachycardia; *VT,* ventricular tachycardia; *WPW,* Wolff-Parkinson-White. (From Olshansky B et al: *Arrhythmia essentials,* ed 2, Philadelphia, 2017, Elsevier.)

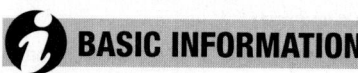

BASIC INFORMATION

DEFINITION

Syncope is the transient loss of consciousness with spontaneous recovery that results from an acute global reduction in cerebral blood flow. There are 3 major types: neurocardiogenic, orthostatic, and cardiac. Syncope is a symptom, and the goal is to distinguish lethal causes from benign causes of transient loss of consciousness.

ICD-10CM CODE
R55 Syncope and collapse

EPIDEMIOLOGY & DEMOGRAPHICS

- Syncope accounts for 3% to 5% of emergency department visits.
- 30% of the adult population will experience at least one syncopal episode during their lifetimes.
- Incidence of syncope is highest in elderly men and young women.
- 15% of children and adolescents experience syncope; fewer than 5% have cardiac causes.

PHYSICAL FINDINGS & CLINICAL PRESENTATION

- Blood pressure: If low, consider orthostatic hypotension; if unequal in both arms (difference >20 mm Hg), consider subclavian steal or dissecting aneurysm. (NOTE: Blood pressure [BP] and heart rate should be recorded in the supine and standing positions, waiting at least 5 minutes between each position.) If there is a drop in BP but no change in heart rate (HR), the patient may be taking a beta-blocker or may have an autonomic neuropathy.
- Pulse: If patient has tachycardia, bradycardia, or irregular rhythm, consider arrhythmia.
- Heart: If there are murmurs present, consider syncope attributable to left ventricular outflow obstruction (aortic stenosis or idiopathic hypertrophic subaortic stenosis); if there are jugular venous distention and distal heart sounds, consider cardiac tamponade.
- Carotid sinus pressure: Can be diagnostic if it reproduces symptoms and other causes are excluded; a pause >3 sec or a systolic BP drop >50 mm Hg without symptoms or <30 mm Hg with symptoms when sinus pressure is applied separately on each side for <5 sec is considered abnormal. This test should be avoided in patients with carotid bruits or cerebrovascular disease. ECG monitoring, IV access, and bedside atropine should be available when carotid sinus pressure is applied.

ETIOLOGY

- Neurocardiogenic or neurally mediated syncope: most common type, accounting for two-thirds of cases. It includes vasovagal, situational, carotid hypersensitivity, and post-exertional syncope (Box 1).
  1. Psychophysiologic (emotional upset, panic disorders, hysteria, hyperventilation)
  2. Visceral reflex (micturition, defecation, food ingestion, coughing, ventricular contraction, glossopharyngeal neuralgia)
  3. Carotid sinus pressure
  4. Reduction of venous return caused by Valsalva maneuver
  5. Postural tachycardia syndrome (POTS)
- Orthostatic hypotension (10% of cases):
  1. Hypovolemia
  2. Vasodilator medications
  3. Autonomic neuropathy (diabetes, amyloid, Parkinson's disease, multisystem atrophy)
  4. Pheochromocytoma
  5. Carcinoid syndrome
- Cardiac (10% to 20%):
  1. Reduced cardiac output
     a. Left ventricular outflow obstruction (aortic stenosis, hypertrophic cardiomyopathy)
     b. Obstruction to pulmonary flow (pulmonary embolism, pulmonic stenosis, primary pulmonary hypertension)
     c. Myocardial infarct with pump failure
     d. Cardiac tamponade
     e. Mitral stenosis
     f. Reduction of venous return (atrial myxoma, valve thrombus)
     g. Beta-blocker therapy
  2. Arrhythmias or asystole:
     a. Extreme tachycardia (>160-180 beats/min)
     b. Severe bradycardia (<30-40 beats/min)
     c. Sick sinus syndrome
     d. Atrioventricular block (second or third degree)
     e. Ventricular tachycardia or fibrillation
     f. Long QT syndrome
     g. Pacemaker malfunction
     h. Psychotropic medications and beta-blockers (Table 1)

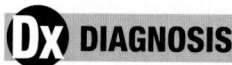

DIAGNOSIS

DIFFERENTIAL DIAGNOSIS

- Seizure (see "Workup").
- Vertebrobasilar transient ischemic attack (TIA) usually manifests as diplopia, vertigo, or ataxia but not loss of consciousness. Isolated episodes of transient loss of consciousness (TLOC, Fig. 1) without accompanying neurologic symptoms are unlikely to be TIAs.
- Recreational drugs or alcohol.
- Functional causes such as somatoform disorders.

BOX 1 Causes of Syncope

Reflex Syncopal Syndromes
- Vasovagal faint (common faint)
- Carotid sinus syncope
- Situational faint
  1. Acute hemorrhage
  2. Cough, sneeze
  3. Gastrointestinal stimulation (swallow, defecation, visceral pain)
  4. Micturition (postmicturition)
  5. Postexercise
  6. Pain, anxiety
- Glossopharyngeal and trigeminal neuralgia

Orthostatic
- Aging
- Antihypertensives
- Autonomic failure
  1. Primary autonomic failure syndromes (e.g., pure autonomic failure, multiple system atrophy, Parkinson disease with autonomic failure)
  2. Secondary autonomic failure syndromes (e.g., diabetic neuropathy, amyloid neuropathy)
- Medications
- Volume depletion
  1. Hemorrhage, diarrhea, Addison disease, diuretics, febrile illness, hot weather

Cardiac Arrhythmias
- Sinus node dysfunction (including bradycardia-tachycardia syndrome)
- Atrioventricular conduction system disease
- Paroxysmal supraventricular and ventricular tachycardias
- Implanted device (pacemaker, implantable cardioverter defibrillator) malfunction
- Drug-induced proarrhythmias

Structural Cardiac or Cardiopulmonary Disease
- Cardiac valvular disease
  1. Acute myocardial infarction, ischemia
  2. Obstructive cardiomyopathy
  3. Atrial myxoma
  4. Acute aortic dissection
  5. Pericardial disease, tamponade
  6. Pulmonary embolus, pulmonary hypertension

Cerebrovascular
- Vascular steal syndromes

Multifactorial

Fillit HM: *Brocklehurst's textbook of geriatric medicine and gerontology*, ed 8, Philadelphia, 2017, Elsevier.

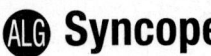

TABLE 1 Drugs That Can Cause or Contribute to Syncope

Drug	Mechanism
Diuretics	Volume depletion
Vasodilators • Angiotensin-converting enzyme inhibitors • Calcium channel blockers • Hydralazine • Nitrates • α-Adrenergic blockers • Prazosin	Reduction in systemic vascular resistance and venodilation
Other antihypertensive drugs • α-Methyldopa • Clonidine • Guanethidine • Hexamethonium • Labetalol • Mecamylamine • Phenoxybenzamine	Centrally acting antihypertensives
Drugs associated with torsades de pointes • Amiodarone • Disopyramide • Encainide • Flecainide • Quinidine • Procainamide • Solatol	Ventricular tachycardia associated with a prolonged QT interval
Digoxin	Cardiac arrhythmias
Psychoactive drugs • Tricyclic antidepressants • Phenothiazines • Monamine oxidase inhibitors • Barbiturates	Central nervous system effects causing hypotension; cardiac arrhythmias
Alcohol	Central nervous system effects causing hypotension; cardiac arrhythmias

Fillit HM: *Brocklehurst's textbook of geriatric medicine and gerontology*, ed 8, Philadelphia, 2017, Elsevier.

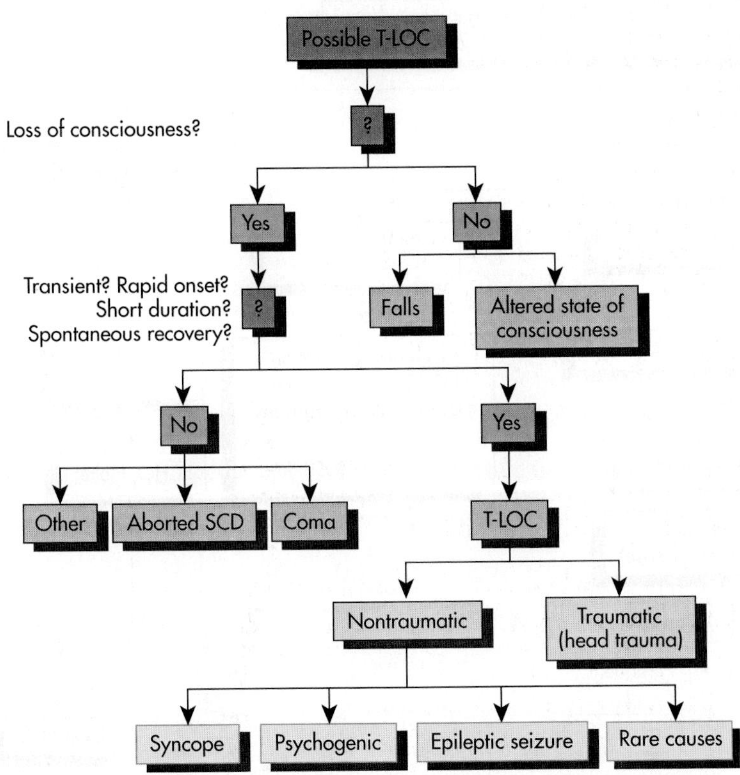

FIG. 1 Approach to the evaluation of patients with transient loss of consciousness *(T-LOC)*. *SCD,* sudden cardiac death. (From Mann DL, et al.: *Braunwald's heart disease*, ed 10, Philadelphia, 2015. Elsevier.)

- Sleep disorders, such as sleep attacks and narcolepsy, are also in the differential for TLOC.
- Head trauma.

WORKUP

The history is crucial to diagnosing the cause of syncope and may suggest a diagnosis that can be evaluated with directed testing. History is also important to determine other etiologies for TLOC, such as seizure.

- Sudden LOC: Consider cardiac arrhythmias.
- Gradual LOC: Consider orthostatic hypotension, vasodepressor syncope, hypoglycemia.
- History of aura before LOC or prolonged confusion (>1 min), amnesia, or lethargy after LOC suggests seizure rather than syncope.
- Patient's activity at the time of syncope:
  1. Micturition, coughing, defecation: Consider syncope caused by decreased venous return.
  2. Turning head or while shaving: Consider carotid sinus syndrome.
  3. Physical exertion in a patient with murmur: Consider aortic stenosis.
  4. Arm exercise: Consider subclavian steal syndrome.
  5. Assuming an upright position: Consider orthostatic hypotension.
- Associated events:
  1. Chest pain: Consider myocardial infarction, pulmonary embolism.
  2. Palpitations: Consider arrhythmias or POTS.
  3. Incontinence (urine or fecal) and tongue biting are associated with seizure or syncope.
  4. Brief, transient shaking after LOC may represent myoclonus from global cerebral hypoperfusion and not seizures. However, sustained tonic/clonic muscle action is more suggestive of seizure.
  5. Focal neurologic symptoms or signs point to a neurologic event such as a seizure with residual deficits (e.g., Todd paralysis) or cerebral ischemic injury.
  6. Psychologic stress: Syncope may be vasovagal.
  7. Multiple nonspecific symptoms (fatigue, diffuse weakness, headache, "brain fog," exercise intolerance) can be seen in POTS as well as in psychophysiologic or functional causes.
- Review current medications, particularly antihypertensive and psychotropic drugs.
- Carotid sinus massage (CSM) may be reasonable in patients older than 40 with syncope of unknown origin and possibly due to vasovagal mechanism. It is contraindicated in patients with carotid disease.
- Table 2 differentiates syncope caused by neutrally mediated hypotension, arrhythmias, seizures, and psychogenic causes.
- Fig. 2 illustrates an approach to the evaluation of syncope.

LABORATORY TESTS

Routine blood tests rarely yield diagnostically useful information and should be done only if they are specifically suggested by the results

TABLE 2 Differentiation of Syncope Caused by Neurally Mediated Hypotension, Arrhythmias, Seizures, and Psychogenic Causes

	Neurally Mediated Hypotension	Arrhythmias	Seizures	Psychogenic
Demographics and clinical setting	Female > male sex Younger age (<55 yr) More episodes (>2) Standing, warm room, emotional upset	Male > female sex Older age (>54 yr) Fewer episodes (<3) During exertion or supine Family history of sudden death	Younger age (<45 yr) Any setting	Female > male sex Occurs in the presence of others Younger age (<40 yr) Many episodes (often many episodes in a day) No identifiable trigger
Premonitory symptoms	Longer duration (>5 sec) Palpitations Blurred vision Nausea Warmth Diaphoresis Lightheadedness	Shorter duration (<6 sec) Palpitations less common	Sudden onset or brief aura (déjà vu, olfactory, gustatory, visual)	Usually absent
Observations during the event	Pallor Diaphoresis Dilated pupils Slow pulse, low BP Incontinence may occur Brief clonic movements may occur	Blue, not pale Incontinence can occur Brief clonic movements can occur	Blue face, no pallor Frothing at the mouth Prolonged syncope (duration >5 min) Tongue biting Horizontal eye deviation Elevated pulse and BP Incontinence more likely* Tonic-clonic movements if grand mal	Normal color Not diaphoretic Eyes closed Normal pulse and BP No incontinence Prolonged duration (minutes) is common
Residual symptoms	Residual symptoms common Prolonged fatigue common (>90%) Oriented	Residual symptoms uncommon (unless prolonged unconsciousness) Oriented	Residual symptoms common Aching muscles Disoriented Fatigue Headache Slow recovery	Residual symptoms uncommon Oriented

*May be observed with any of these causes of syncope but more common with seizures.
From Mann DL, et al.: *Braunwald's heart disease*, ed 10, Philadelphia, 2015. Elsevier.

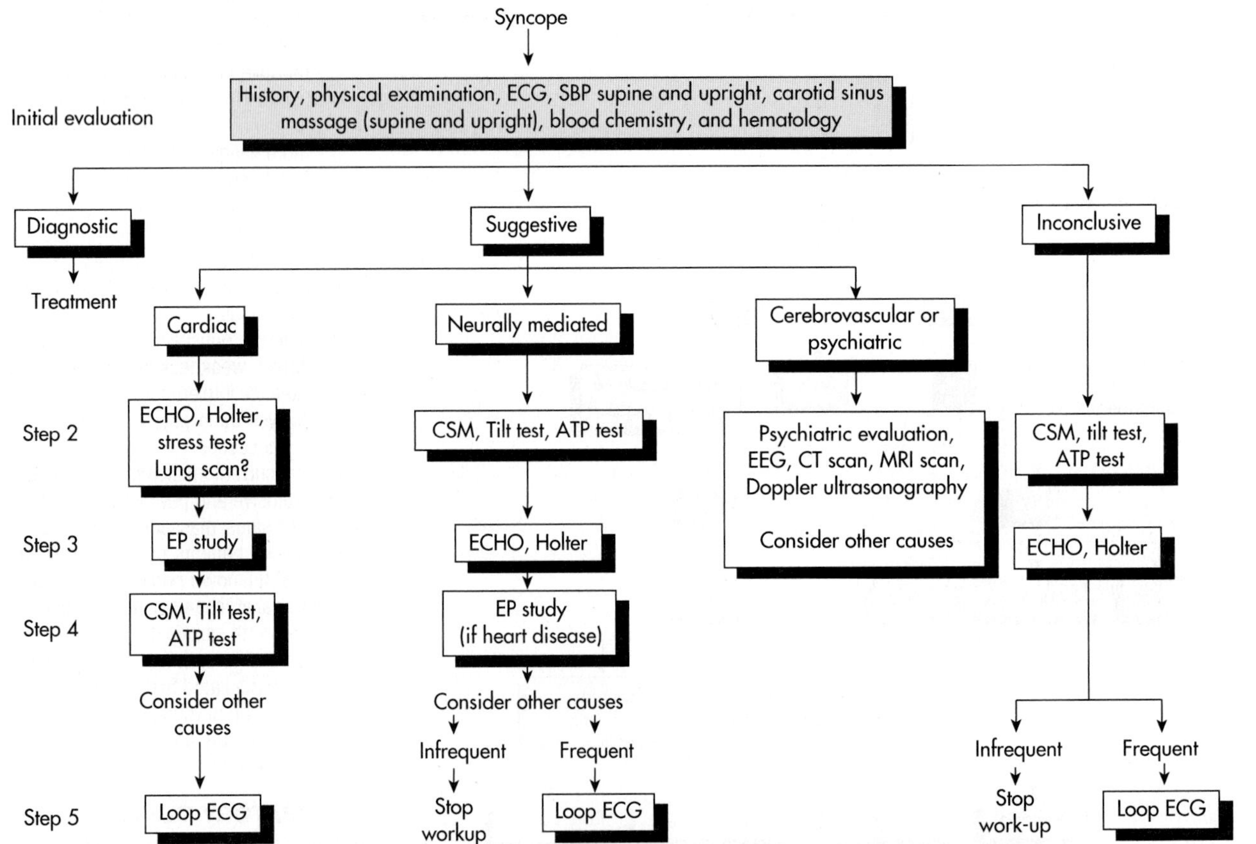

FIG. 2 An approach to the evaluation of syncope for all age groups. *ATP test,* Adenosine provocation test; *CSM,* carotid sinus massage; *ECG,* electrocardiogram; *ECHO,* echocardiogram; *EEG,* electroencephalography; *EP study,* electrophysiologic study; *SBP,* systolic blood pressure. (Fillit HM: *Brocklehurst's textbook of geriatric medicine and gerontology,* ed 8, Philadelphia, 2017, Elsevier.)

of the history and physical examination. The following are commonly ordered tests:

- Pregnancy test in women of childbearing age
- Complete blood count to look for anemia and signs of infection
- Electrolytes, blood urea nitrogen, creatinine, magnesium, and calcium to look for electrolyte abnormalities and evaluate fluid status
- Serum glucose level
- Cardiac troponins, especially if the patient gives a history of chest pain before the syncopal episode
- Drug and alcohol levels with suspected toxicity

IMAGING STUDIES

- ECG to rule out arrhythmias; may be diagnostic in 5% to 10% of patients.
- Echocardiography. Indicated in patients where initial evaluation suggests structural heart disease or have known heart disease.
- If seizure is suspected, MRI of the brain and electroencephalogram may be useful.
- If head trauma or neurologic signs on examination, CT or MRI may be helpful.
- If arrhythmias are suspected, a 24-hr Holter monitor or admission to a telemetry unit in high risk patients is appropriate. In general, Holter monitoring is rarely useful, revealing a cause for syncope in <3% of cases. Loop recorders that can be activated after syncopal episode to retrieve information about the cardiac rhythm during the preceding 4 min add considerable diagnostic yield in patients with unexplained syncope.
- Implantable cardiac monitors that function as permanent loop recorders or implantable cardioverter-defibrillators, which are placed subcutaneously in the pectoral region with the patient under local anesthesia, are useful in patients with cardiac syncope.
- Electrophysiologic studies may be indicated in patients with structural heart disease and/or recurrent syncope.

TILT-TABLE TESTING

- Useful to support a diagnosis of neurocardiogenic syncope. Patients age >50 yr should have stress testing before tilt-table testing. Positive results would preclude tilt-table testing.
- Indicated in patients with recurrent episodes of unexplained syncope as well as patients in high-risk occupations (e.g., pilots, bus drivers). The test is also useful for identifying patients with prominent bradycardic response who may benefit from implantation of a permanent pacemaker. The test is contraindicated in patients with recent stroke, MI, and severe coronary or carotid disease.
- It is performed by keeping the patient strapped in an upright posture on a tilt table with footboard support. The angle of the tilt table varies from 60 to 80 degrees. The duration of upright posture during tilt-table testing varies from 25 to 45 min.
- The hallmark of neurocardiogenic syncope is severe hypotension associated with a paradoxic bradycardia triggered by a specific stimulus. The diagnosis of neurocardiogenic syncope is likely if upright tilt testing reproduces these hemodynamic changes in <15 min and causes presyncope or syncope.
- Postural orthostatic tachycardia syndrome is diagnosed if there is a sustained heart rate increase of not less than 30 beats/minute or above 120 beats/min within 10 min of active standing or head-up tilt without associated orthostatic hypotension and with reproduction of symptoms.

PSYCHIATRIC EVALUATION

- May be indicated in young patients without heart disease who have frequently recurring transient loss of consciousness and other somatic symptoms.
- Generalized anxiety disorder, pain disorder, and major depression predispose patients to neurally mediated reactions and may result in syncope.

Rx TREATMENT

NONPHARMACOLOGIC THERAPY

- Ensure proper hydration; consider compression stockings and salt tablets in appropriate patients.
- Eliminate medications that may induce hypotension.

ACUTE GENERAL Rx

- Varies with the underlying etiology of syncope (e.g., pacemaker in patients with syncope resulting from complete heart block). Clinical variables for identification of high-risk syncope patients who may benefit from hospitalization or an accelerated outpatient evaluation are summarized in Table E3.
- Syncope caused by orthostatic hypotension is treated with volume replacement in patients with intravascular volume depletion. Also consider midodrine to promote venous return by adrenergic-mediated vasoconstriction and fludrocortisone for its mineralocorticoid effects to increase intravascular volume.

DISPOSITION

Prognosis varies with the age of the patient and the etiology of the syncope. In general:

- Benign prognosis (very low 1-yr morbidity rate) in patients:
  1. Age <30 yr and having noncardiac syncope
  2. Age <70 yr and having vasovagal or psychogenic syncope or syncope of unknown cause
- Poor prognosis (high mortality and morbidity rates) in patients with cardiac syncope, with presenting systolic BP <90 mm Hg.
- Patients with the following risk factors have a higher 1-yr mortality rate: Abnormal ECG, history of ventricular arrhythmia, history of congestive heart failure.

REFERRAL

Hospital admission in elderly patients without prior history of syncope or unknown etiology of their syncope and in any patients suspected of having cardiac syncope, with presenting systolic BP <90 mm Hg.

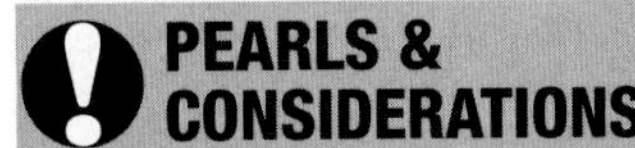

PEARLS & CONSIDERATIONS

COMMENTS

- The etiology of syncope is identified in <50% of cases during the initial evaluation.
- A thorough history and physical examination are the most productive means of establishing a diagnosis in patients with syncope.
- Driving restrictions vary based on state but consider restricting driving if syncope is frequent or unpredictable.

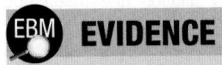

EVIDENCE

Available at ExpertConsult.com

SUGGESTED READINGS

Available at ExpertConsult.com

RELATED CONTENT

Syncope (Patient Information)
Orthostatic Hypotension (Related Key Topic)

AUTHORS: **COREY GOLDSMITH, M.D., JOSEPH S. KASS, M.D., J.D.,** and **W.U. TZU-CHING (TEDDY), M.D., M.P.H.**

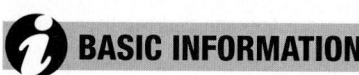

BASIC INFORMATION

DEFINITION

The syndrome of inappropriate antidiuresis (SIAD) is defined by the occurrence of "inappropriately" concentrated urine in patients with hypotonic hyponatremia and normal extracellular fluid (ECF) volume. The appropriate, osmotically driven, physiologic response to serum hypotonicity is inhibition of hypothalamic osmoreceptors, which results in suppression of antidiuretic hormone/arginine vasopressin (ADH) synthesis and release. The reduction in plasma ADH concentration decreases renal collecting duct arginine vasopressin receptor activation and lowers total body water (TBW) by increasing urine volume with urine osmolality that is lower than plasma osmolality. During this diuresis, there is relatively little loss of total body cations as the sum of total body exchangeable sodium and potassium $(Na + K)_e$. The urine is hypotonic with a relatively larger volume of electrolyte-free water (EFW), which represents the fractional volume of urine devoid of any electrolytes. The diuresis increases the serum sodium (S_{Na}, mEq/L) back toward normal. In the absence of elevated glucose or an exogenous osmole such as mannitol, the S_{Na} is primarily determined by the ratio of Na_e plus K_e (mEq) to TBW (L):

$$S_{Na} = \frac{(Na + K)_e}{TBW}$$

Hyponatremia results from a reduction of the numerator and/or increase of the denominator of this equation. In SIAD, TBW is expanded with a normal numerator. In hyponatremia from SIAD, EFW excretion is impaired. The severity of hyponatremia associated with SIAD reflects the severity of the defect in urinary dilution and magnitude of electrolyte-free fluid intake. Hemodynamic stimuli that stimulate ADH release preclude the diagnosis of SIAD and include decreased ECF volume (decreased Na_e), hypotension, and disorders characterized by decreased effective arterial blood volume. The latter group is manifested by increased ECF volume (edema from increased Na_e) and includes congestive heart failure, chronic pericardial disease, nephrotic syndrome, and cirrhosis.

The term *syndrome of inappropriate antidiuretic hormone* (SIADH) has been discarded by some because 10% to 15% of SIADH patients have suppressed or undetectable serum ADH concentrations. Others have nonosmotic stimulation of ADH. The group with suppressed ADH may have increased sensitivity of renal collecting duct cells to ADH, secretion of other ADH-like peptides, or altered renal hemodynamics that reduce sodium and water delivery to distal diluting sites, thereby preventing urinary dilution. Establishing a diagnosis of SIAD does not require the measurement of ADH levels or demonstration of high serum ADH concentrations. Patients with hypothyroidism and adrenal insufficiency are excluded from the definition of SIAD. SIAD is not diagnosed in acute or chronic kidney disease or when there has been recent loop diuretic administration. However, thiazide-induced hyponatremia is considered a drug-induced form of SIAD or SIAD-type physiology. Drugs that decrease electrolyte-free water excretion constitute another cause of SIAD, and represents a separate diagnostic entity.

SYNONYMS

SIADH
SIAD
Syndrome of inappropriate antidiuretic hormone secretion
Syndrome of inappropriate ADH release
Inappropriate secretion of antidiuretic hormone

ICD-10CM CODE

E22.2 Syndrome of inappropriate secretion of antidiuretic hormone

EPIDEMIOLOGY & DEMOGRAPHICS

INCIDENCE: Hyponatremia occurs in a significant proportion of hospitalized patients. SIAD is etiologic in nearly one half of these individuals. The adjusted odds ratio for in-hospital mortality in patients with hyponatremia at hospital admission is 1.47 (95% Confidence Interval, 1.33 to 1.62).

PHYSICAL FINDINGS & CLINICAL PRESENTATION

- Chronic hyponatremia is defined as an S_{Na} <130 mEq/L persisting for greater than 48 h with normal ECF volume. Patients are hemodynamically stable with no evidence of edema, ascites, pleural, or pericardial effusions.
- Manifestations of the precipitating cause: History of marathon running or other extreme endurance exercise, fever and delirium after 3,4-methylenedioxy-methamphetamine (ecstasy) administration, stigmata of alcoholism or malnutrition, fever and/or localizing symptoms related to pneumonia or other pulmonary disease, or headaches and visual field defects from an intracranial mass.
- If hyponatremia occurs rapidly, generally in less than 24 h, delirium, lethargy, or seizures may occur. Diminished reflexes and extensor plantar responses may occur with severe hyponatremia, generally considered as S_{Na} <120 mEq/L.
- Neurologic abnormalities, including ataxia, mood changes, and proximal muscle weakness, are frequent in chronic hyponatremia. Abnormalities may be subtle, despite severe hyponatremia.
- Drugs: Thiazide diuretics and selective serotonin reuptake inhibitor (SSRI) antidepressants are the two most common causes of drug-related hyponatremia. Narcotic analgesics, carbamazepine, phenothiazines, tricyclic antidepressants, MDMA (ecstasy), nicotine, clofibrate, haloperidol, NSAIDs, monoamine oxidase inhibitors, chlorpropamide, vasopressin, desmopressin, oxytocin, and chemotherapeutic agents (vincristine, vinblastine, cyclophosphamide) are additional causes.
- Neoplasms: Lung, oropharynx, stomach, duodenum, pancreas, brain, thymus, bladder, prostate, endometrium, mesothelioma, lymphoma, and Ewing sarcoma.
- Pulmonary disorders: Pneumonia, Aspergillosis, pulmonary abscess, tuberculosis, bronchiectasis, emphysema, cystic fibrosis, status asthmaticus, and respiratory failure associated with positive-pressure breathing.
- Intracranial pathology: Trauma, neoplasms, infections (meningitis, encephalitis, brain abscess), hemorrhage, hydrocephalus, multiple sclerosis, Guillain-Barré syndrome.
- Postoperative period: Surgical stress, positive pressure ventilation, anesthetic agents.
- Other: Acute intermittent porphyria, psychosis, delirium tremens, general anesthesia, endurance exercise.
- Table 1 summarizes common etiologies of SIAD.

DIFFERENTIAL DIAGNOSIS

- Hyponatremia associated with subclinical hypovolemia
- Solute-limited water excretion (e.g., "tea-and-toast" diet, beer-drinker's potomania)
- Primary polydipsia
- Endocrine disorders, including hypothyroidism and adrenal insufficiency
- Severe hypokalemia
- Hypertonic hyponatremia (hyperglycemia, iatrogenic administration of mannitol, sorbitol, glycine)
- Hyponatremia from subclinical heart or liver disease
- Pseudohyponatremia caused by extreme hyperglobulinemia or hyperlipidemia
- Reset osmostat: Regulation of ADH occurs at a lower-than-normal osmolal threshold, with intact urinary dilution and concentration

WORKUP

- Normal ECF volume by history and physical examination. No history of large-volume fluid losses. No generalized edema, ascites, or large pleural effusions.
- Laboratory evaluation (see "Laboratory Tests") is consistent with excessive ADH secretion or sensitivity in the absence of osmotic or hemodynamic stimuli for ADH secretion.
- Normal thyroid, adrenal, and cardiac function.
- No recent or concurrent use of loop diuretics.
- Failure to correct hyponatremia after ECF volume repletion by isotonic infusion of 0.9% saline solution.
- Correction of hyponatremia by solely fluid restriction is generally unsuccessful.
- Diagnostic criteria for SIADH are described in Table 2.

LABORATORY TESTS

- Normal or low BUN, creatinine
- Normal thyroid stimulating hormone
- S_{Na} less than the lower limit of normal

TABLE 1 Common Etiologies of the Syndrome of Inappropriate Antidiuretic Hormone Secretion (SIADH)

Tumors

Pulmonary/mediastinal (bronchogenic carcinoma, mesothelioma, thymoma)

Extrapulmonary (duodenal carcinoma, pancreatic carcinoma, ureteral/prostate carcinoma, uterine carcinoma, nasopharyngeal carcinoma, leukemia)

Central Nervous System Disorders

Mass lesions (tumors, brain abscesses, subdural hematoma)

Inflammatory diseases (encephalitis, meningitis, systemic lupus erythematosus, acute intermittent porphyria, multiple sclerosis)

Degenerative/demyelinating diseases (Guillain-Barré syndrome, spinal cord lesions)

Miscellaneous (subarachnoid hemorrhage, head trauma, acute psychosis, delirium tremens, pituitary stalk section, transsphenoidal adenomectomy, hydrocephalus)

Drug-Related

Stimulated release of AVP (nicotine, phenothiazines, tricyclics)

Direct renal effects and/or potentiation of AVP antidiuretic effects (desmopressin, oxytocin, prostaglandin synthesis inhibitors)

Mixed or uncertain actions (ACE inhibitors, carbamazepine and oxcarbazepine, chlorpropamide, clofibrate, clozapine, cyclophosphamide, 3,4-methylenedioxymethamphetamine (ecstasy), omeprazole; serotonin reuptake inhibitors (SSRIs), vincristine

Pulmonary

Infections (tuberculosis, acute bacterial and viral pneumonia, aspergillosis, empyema)

Mechanical/ventilatory causes (acute respiratory failure, COPD, positive-pressure ventilation)

Other Causes

Acquired immunodeficiency syndrome (AIDS) and AIDS-related complex

Prolonged strenuous exercise (marathon, triathlon, ultramarathon, hot-weather hiking)

Senile atrophy

Idiopathic

ACE, Angiotensin-converting enzyme; *AVP,* arginine vasopressin; *COPD,* chronic obstructive pulmonary disease.
From Melmed S: *Williams textbook of endocrinology,* ed 12, Philadelphia, 2011, Saunders.

TABLE 2 Diagnostic Criteria for the Syndrome of Inappropriate Antidiuretic Hormone Release

Essential Diagnostic Criteria

Decreased extracellular fluid effective osmolality (<270 mOsm/kg)

Inappropriate urinary concentration (>100 mOsm/kg)

Clinical normovolemia

Elevated urinary sodium concentration under conditions of normal salt and water intake

Absence of adrenal, thyroid, or pituitary insufficiency

Absence of chronic kidney disease

Absence of diuretic use

Supplemental Criteria

Abnormal water loading test (inability to excrete at least 90% of a 20 ml/kg water load in 4 h and/or failure to dilute urine osmolality to <100 mOsm/kg)

Plasma vasopressin level inappropriately elevated relative to the plasma osmolality

No significant correction of SNa with volume expansion, but improvement after fluid restriction

SNa, Serum sodium. From Floege J, et al.: *Comprehensive clinical nephrology,* ed 4, Philadelphia, 2010, Saunders.

- Decreased serum osmolality (<275 mOsm/kg) corrected for serum glucose and exogenous osmoles
- Decreased serum uric acid
- Urine osmolality >100 mOsm/kg with plasma hypotonicity
- Urine sodium usually >40 mEq/L with normal dietary salt intake

IMAGING STUDIES

Imaging is not routinely required for diagnosis. Imaging may be required to facilitate diagnosis of associated underlying pulmonary or CNS disease, or to rule-out intracranial pathology in cases of severe encephalopathy.

Rx TREATMENT

NONPHARMACOLOGIC THERAPY

With mild SIAD, reasonable degrees of fluid restriction (10–15 ml/kg/day) combined with increased solute loads (diets high in protein, sodium chloride, and potassium chloride) may increase EFW clearance sufficiently to normalize S_{Na}. Urea powder, commercially available as a "food supplement," can be ingested to enhance EFW excretion and increase S_{Na}. Nonpharmacologic therapy should not be used to increase S_{Na} rapidly when indicated for severe or symptomatic acute hyponatremia.

ACUTE GENERAL Rx

PHARMACOLOGIC THERAPY:

Rate of Correction: In chronic hyponatremia, avoid rapid S_{Na} correction rates to prevent neurologic injury from osmotic demyelination syndrome. All patients with moderate-to-severe hyponatremia should undergo serial monitoring of S_{Na} and S_K, urine volumes, and urine chemistries (osmolality, K, and Na) during the initial 48 h of admission and active therapy. Recommended rates of correction should not be exceeded. Most SIAD have chronic hyponatremia (developing over a period of greater than 24 h) associated with mild symptoms. Target rates of S_{Na} correction should not exceed 6–8 mEq/L/day in chronic hyponatremia. The S_{Na} should be actively lowered in patients who experience increases of >10 mEq/L during a 24-h period. The rate of S_{Na} change during conservative therapy or 0.9% infusion should be slow and relatively predictable during hypertonic saline administration, and urine volume will remain relatively low. If the patient has unrecognized ECF volume depletion, or the underlying etiology of SIAD resolves rapidly, a diuresis of a large volume of hypotonic urine may occur, with rapid rates of S_{Na} correction.

In the minority of patients with acute hyponatremia (duration <24 h), the goal of therapy is to increase S_{Na} sufficiently to prevent or reduce the severity of acute cerebral edema. The S_{Na} should be increased by only 4–6 mEq/L within the first 3 h if symptoms are mild-to-moderate and within the first hour if symptoms are severe (seizures, coma, obtundation).

Acute Hyponatremia: The rapid correction of S_{Na} required in acute hyponatremia requires administration of 3% saline with guidance by a specialist with expertise in this areas. Rates of S_{Na} correction may be greater if unrecognized ECF volume contraction is simultaneously repaired by the saline infusions. Concomitant intravenous furosemide therapy may increase urinary EFW loss as infused sodium is excreted and prevent undesirable increases in ECF volume.

Chronic Hyponatremia: The goal of therapy in chronic hyponatremia from SIAD is reduction of TBW to normal, while maintaining sodium and potassium stores at their normal levels. This is done as follows:

- Select a 24-hour target S_{Na} based on current S_{Na} and safe rate of correction (see "Rates of Correction").
- Estimate current TBW and total body cation content. Estimation of current TBW should consider the patient's baseline total body water, volume of additional retained water, and changes in Na_e or K_e.
- Calculate the target TBW that achieves the target S_{Na} of Step 1 (assume Na_e and K_e are constant).
- Calculate the 24-h net EFW loss required to attain the TBW determined in Step 3.
- Estimate and total other sources of EFW intake and loss (including insensible). Add/subtract this estimated volume to/from net target EFW (Step 4). Calculate total EFW volume loss required to attain target S_{Na}.
- Select an appropriate strategy to achieve the target EFW volume loss: Renal vasopressin receptor antagonist or combined loop diuretic administration with electrolyte replacement.

The following example demonstrates the method to determine the target TBW and EFW loss required to reach an appropriate S_{Na} target after 24 h of therapy for a patient with chronic hyponatremia:

- Example: The S_{Na} of a 75-kg minimally symptomatic elderly woman who chronically takes SSRI and hydrochlorothiazide is incidentally determined as 115 mEq/L.

1. *Step 1: Establish target S_{Na}*
   a. Target S_{Na} after 24 h = Current S_{Na} + 6 = 121 mEq/L
2. *Step 2: Estimate current TBW and total body cations*
   a. Current weight = 75 kg
   b. Normal adult TBW fraction = 0.5 (50%)
   c. Current TBW = 0.5 × 75 = 37.5 L
   d. Current number of total body cations = Current TBW × S_{Na} = 37.5 × 115 = 4313 mEq
3. *Step 3: Calculate target TBW*
   a. Target TBW = Current number of total body cations / Desired S_{Na} = 4313/121 = 35.6 L
4. *Step 4: Calculate net EFW loss*
   a. Target *net free water loss* at 24 h = Current TBW − Target TBW = 37.5 − 35.6 = 0.9 L
5. *Step 5: Calculate total urine EFW excretion*
   a. Target *total urine EFW excretion* (allowance for 1 L oral fluid intake and 0.5 L insensible loss) Urine EFW excretion = 0.9 + (1 − 0.5) = 1.4 L
6. *Step 6: Establish therapeutic strategy*

Loop Diuretic Plus Saline Strategy: The classical treatment strategy for SIAD is to increase urine volume and EFW loss via diuresis with a loop diuretic such as furosemide or bumetanide. These diuretics generate electrolyte-free water via urinary losses of Na and K, which are replaced at concentrations exceeding urine concentrations. NaCl and KCl tablets may be used to replace diuretic-induced losses of sodium and potassium, respectively. The table below considers only NaCl losses.

Periodic monitoring of S_{Na}, S_K, urine volume, and urine chemistries (osmolality, sodium, and potassium) is done to prevent excretion of urine volumes that will produce S_{Na} levels exceeding targets.

Use of DiZasopressin Receptor Antagonists: Selective type 2 vasopressin receptor (V_2) antagonists: Conivaptan (20 mg IV × 1 followed by continuous IV infusion of 20 to 40 mg/day for 2 to 4 days) and tolvaptan (15 to 60 mg/day orally, titrated daily from 15 mg as needed). Compared to furosemide and NaCl infusions, their use is relatively straightforward and convenient for patients and medical personnel. Urinary electrolyte losses are minimal, meaning that administration produces virtually electrolyte-free urine (Step 5). Therapeutic effects occur relatively quickly, facilitating rapid evaluation and dosing titration of inpatients. While the cost of the medications is considerable, the savings of just one hospital day offsets the cost of inpatient use.

Replacement Solutions	Cation (NaCl) mEq/L	Net Free Water Loss/L urine	Target Urine Output (L/24 hours)	Volume (L/ 24 hours) to Replace Electrolyte Loss
0.9% Saline	154	1 − (75/154) = 0.5	1.4/0.5 = 2.8	0.5 L/L UOP × (2.8 L) = 1.4 L
3% Saline	513	1 − (75/513) = 0.85	1.4/0.85 = 1.65	0.15 L/L UOP × 1.65 = 0.25 L

UOP, Urinary output.

CHRONIC Rx

- When SIAD is chronic, fluid restriction (<15 ml/kg) may be needed indefinitely in conjunction with high dietary electrolyte and protein content to enhance obligatory free water losses through osmotic diuresis.
- NaCl tablets, electrolyte or protein powders, and urea serve can be used to correct hyponatremia. Monthly monitoring of electrolytes is recommended in patients with chronic SIAD.
- Tolvaptan has been used chronically in phase 3 trials. Commercial labeling currently restricts use to 30 days because of concern about serious hepatotoxicity that occurred in trials of high-dose tolvaptan in patients with polycystic kidney disease.
- Demeclocycline 300 to 600 mg orally twice daily effectively increases electrolyte-free water. C^eH_2O in some patients. This is contraindicated in hepatic disease.

DISPOSITION

- Mortality exceeding 40% has been reported in patients with SNa <110 mEq/L.
- Hospital readmission rates are common in chronic SIAD when an underlying cause cannot be eliminated, especially if patients are unwilling or unable to restrict their fluid intake and follow dietary recommendations.
- Chronic, mild-to-moderate hyponatremia is associated with bone loss, falls, and increased fracture risk, particularly in elderly patients.

REFERRAL

Urgent emergency department evaluation and hospital admission are appropriate for moderate-to-severe hyponatremia due to SIAD, especially if acute or symptomatic, or for initiation of therapy. Because of the high risk of complications from overly aggressive or ineffective treatment, referral to a nephrologist, endocrinologist, or critical care physician is recommended.

SUGGESTED READINGS

Available at ExpertConsult.com

RELATED CONTENT

Syndrome of Inappropriate Secretion of Antidiuretic Hormone (Patient Information)

AUTHORS: **MARK D. FABER, M.D.,** and **JERRY YEE, M.D.**

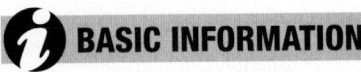

DEFINITION

Synthetic cannabinoids are manufactured variants of natural cannabinoids found in marijuana. Most are modeled after delta-9-tetrahydrocannabinol (THC), which is among the most psychoactive of the cannabinoids. The chemical structures of these substances are frequently altered in order to circumvent regulations and law enforcement. They are frequently sold as incense or herbal products, containing a variety of other herbal ingredients.

SYNONYMS

Chill out
Chill x
Crazy monkey
Herbs
Incense
K2
Spice
Spice diamond
Spice gold
There are over 700 commonly used synonyms for synthetic cannabinoids.

ICD-10CM CODES

F12.1	Cannabis abuse
F12.15	Cannabis abuse with psychotic disorder
F12. 98	Cannabis use, unspecified with other cannabis-induced disorder
F19.1	Other psychoactive substance abuse

EPIDEMIOLOGY & DEMOGRAPHICS

- Synthetic cannabinoids were developed in research laboratories in the 1980s and first emerged as a recreational drug in 2008.
- Prevalence and incidence have steadily increased, with over 7000 annual cases reported to regional poison control centers in the U.S.
- The majority of exposures occur in young men aged 20-30 yr as a result of intentional ingestion as a recreational drug. Adolescents 13-18 yr account for up to 25% of hospitalizations after ingestions.

PHYSICAL FINDINGS & CLINICAL PRESENTATION

- Synthetic cannabinoids are manufactured experimentally, with each variation carrying a new chemical signature. Frequently they are sold as a mixture with various herbs and other compounds. As such, physical symptoms may vary widely depending upon the route and type of substance ingested.
- The majority of symptoms are mild and self-limited; however, severe toxicities are common.
- Synthetic cannabinoids have much higher potency than natural marijuana, and thus greater potential for delirium, agitation, and psychosis.
- The most common symptoms across multiple studies are sinus tachycardia and neuropsychiatric symptoms (toxic psychosis, agitation, coma, CNS symptoms).
- Among the most commonly reported symptoms are:
  1. Tachycardia, palpitations, chest pain, hypotension, bradycardia, cardiac arrest
  2. Conjunctival injection, nystagmus, ataxia, sedation, seizures, syncope, respiratory depression, CNS depression, coma, emesis, hyperthermia, rhabdomyolysis, acute kidney injury
  3. Psychotic effects: Irritability, paranoia, anxiety, racing thoughts, hallucinations, delusions, psychosis, delirium
- There have been reports of myocardial infarction, subarachnoid hemorrhages, pneumothorax, and acute ischemic strokes after ingestion. Superwarfarin adulterants of synthetic cannabinoids can lead to clinically significant coagulopathy.[1]

ETIOLOGY

- The majority of synthetic compounds are cannabinoid receptor 1 and 2 (CB1 and CB2) agonists. Some versions have NDMA, serotonin, and other receptor affinity.
- Current compounds have higher cannabinoid receptor binding affinity, with resulting potency up to 800 times greater than THC.
- Metabolized by glucuronidation and oxidation by liver cytochrome oxidase enzymes and renally excreted.

Dx DIAGNOSIS

- Intoxication with synthetic cannabinoids is primarily a clinical diagnosis.
- Rapid urine drug screens designed to detect THC will not detect the presence of synthetic cannabinoids.
- Mass spectrometry and liquid chromatography can confirm the presence of synthetic compounds but have limited use in the timely treatment of the acutely toxic patient.

DIFFERENTIAL DIAGNOSIS

- Drug or alcohol intoxication
- Hypoglycemia
- Acute psychosis
- Status epilepticus or seizure disorder
- Toxidromes (tricyclic antidepressants, anticholinergic agents, organophosphates, sympathomimetics)

WORKUP

The diagnosis of synthetic cannabinoid intoxication is clinical. Workup is dictated by clinical symptoms and degree of toxicity.

[1] Kelkar AH, et al.: An outbreak of synthetic cannabinoid-associated coagulopathy in Illinois, *N Engl J Med* 379:1216–1223, 2018.

LABORATORY TESTS

- Mild intoxication usually does not require extensive laboratory studies.
- For severe toxicity:
  1. Serum electrolytes
  2. Blood urea nitrogen and creatinine, as there is increased risk for acute kidney injury
  3. Creatine kinase and urine myoglobin if concern for rhabdomyolysis
  4. Venous blood gas if concern for respiratory depression
  5. Serum lactate for increased risk of lactic acidosis
  6. Drug abuse screen for contaminants or coingestions
  7. Troponin or cardiac biomarkers, as there is increased risk for myocardial infarction in patients with chest pain

IMAGING STUDIES

Neuroimaging (CT or MRI of the brain) would be indicated if seizure is part of toxidrome.

OTHER TESTS

12-Lead electrocardiogram

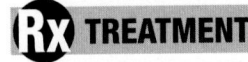

Treatment is supportive and directed at symptoms and complications of toxicity.

- Acute kidney injury is common. Fluid resuscitation should be started for the prevention and treatment of renal injury and rhabdomyolysis in most patients.
- Reassurance, decreased stimulation in a dimly lit room, and benzodiazepines for anxiety are useful in mild-to-moderate toxicity.
- Psychosis and agitation can usually be adequately controlled with benzodiazepines.
- Hyperthermia from seizures, myoclonus, and rhabdomyolysis should be treated aggressively. Evaporative cooling, benzodiazepines, and cooling blankets are usually sufficient.
  1. If intubation and paralysis are necessary, depolarizing agents such as succinylcholine should be avoided, as hyperkalemia from rhabdomyolysis is of concern.
  2. Antipyretics have no effect in temperature management.
- Seizures should be treated with benzodiazepines. Frequently, seizures are reported as a single nonsustained episode. Seizures unresponsive to benzodiazepines should be treated with pharmacologically induced coma and continuous EEG. Neuroimaging is recommended in patients with seizures.
- Dystonic symptoms are best treated with benzodiazepines rather than with anticholinergic agents such as diphenhydramine, which have the potential to worsen hyperthermia.
- Early administration of haloperidol in addition to antiemetics for the treatment of cannabinoid hyperemesis syndrome.

NONPHARMACOLOGIC THERAPY

Counseling addressing psychological and social issues

DISPOSITION

- Patients with mild-to-moderate symptoms can be observed for 6 hr in the emergency department and safely discharged after resolution of symptoms.
- Patients who remain symptomatic warrant admission to an appropriate level of care, based on the severity of their symptoms.

SUGGESTED READINGS

Available at ExpertConsult.com

AUTHORS: **CRAIG BLAKENEY, M.D.,** and **ALAN TAYLOR, M.D.**

BASIC INFORMATION

DEFINITION

Syphilis is a systemic sexually transmitted disease caused by the bacteria *Treponema pallidum*, with acute and chronic manifestations, characterized by primary skin lesions; secondary eruption involving skin and mucous membranes; long periods of latency; and late lesions of the skin, bone, viscera, central nervous system, and cardiovascular system.

SYNONYM

Lues

ICD-10CM CODES

A50	Congenital syphilis
A51.0	Primary genital syphilis
A51.1	Primary anal syphilis
A51.2	Primary syphilis of other sites
A51.3	Secondary syphilis of skin and mucous membranes
A51.4	Other secondary syphilis
A51.5	Early syphilis, latent
A51.9	Early syphilis, unspecified
A52	Late syphilis
A52.0	Cardiovascular and cerebrovascular syphilis
A52.1	Symptomatic neurosyphilis
A52.2	Asymptomatic neurosyphilis
A52.3	Neurosyphilis, unspecified
A52.8	Late syphilis, latent
A52.9	Late syphilis, unspecified
A53.9	Syphilis, unspecified

EPIDEMIOLOGY & DEMOGRAPHICS

- Most commonly diagnosed in people 20 to 30 yr old.
- Slightly more prevalent in men than women.
- Rates reached historic lows in the U.S. in 2000 but began increasing among males in 2001, and increase has continued. Rates are disproportionately higher among black and Hispanic men who have sex with men (MSM), compared with white MSM and among young MSM. Rates are also increasing in women, with highest rates in black women compared with Hispanic and white women.
- Usually more prevalent in urban areas and among people of lower socioeconomic status.
- Communicability is indefinite and variable. Communicable during primary, secondary, and latent mucocutaneous lesions in up to first 4 yr of latency. Most probable congenital transmission occurs in early maternal syphilis. Adequate penicillin treatment ends infectivity within 24 to 48 hr.

PHYSICAL FINDINGS & CLINICAL PRESENTATION

PRIMARY SYPHILIS:

- Characteristic lesion is a painless chancre on genitalia (Figs. E1 and E2), mouth, or anus; atypical primary lesions may occur.
- May appear 3 days to 12 wk (usually 3 wk) after exposure and may resolve without treatment within 6 wk.

SECONDARY SYPHILIS:

- Bacteremia associated with generalized lymphadenopathy and a characteristic maculopapular rash including palms, soles, trunk, and mucous membranes. Lesions may also be pustular, involve the mucosal surfaces. Constitutional, flulike symptoms may also occur, as well as mild disturbances of multiple organ systems.
- 60% to 80% have maculopapular lesions on palms and soles (Fig. E3).
- 21% to 58% have mucocutaneous or mucosal lesions (pharyngitis, tonsillitis, "mucous patch" lesion on oral and genital mucosa).
- Condylomata lata intertriginous papules (raised, gray-white lesions) form at areas of friction and moisture, such as the vulva (Fig. E4).
- Occurs 4 to 6 wk after appearance of chancre. Resolves within 1 wk to 12 mo. Can have relapsing episodes up to 5 yr after initial episode.

LATENT SYPHILIS—EARLY VS. LATE LATENT:

- Generally asymptomatic, can occur between 1 and 30 yr after a primary infection
- Seroreactivity without other evidence of primary or secondary disease
- Not sexually transmitted but may be transmitted from a pregnant woman to her fetus for up to 4 yr after acquiring the disease
- In early latent syphilis, disease can be transmitted even without the current presence of an active lesion. This is not the case in late latent syphilis
- Early latent: <12 mo from acquisition
- Late latent: >12 mo from acquisition, or time since infection is unknown

TERTIARY SYPHILIS:

- A form of late syphilis characterized by gummas (nodular, ulcerative lesions) that can involve the skin, mucous membranes, skeletal system, and viscera.
- Manifestations of cardiovascular syphilis include aortitis, aneurysm, or aortic regurgitation.
- Neurosyphilis may be asymptomatic or symptomatic. Tabes dorsalis, meningovascular syphilis, general paralysis, or insanity may occur. Iritis, choroidoretinitis, and leukoplakia may also occur.

ETIOLOGY

- *Treponema pallidum*, a spirochete
- Spread by sexual intercourse or by intrauterine transfer

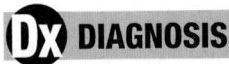

DIAGNOSIS

DIFFERENTIAL DIAGNOSIS

- Other genitoulcerative diseases such as herpes, chancroid (see Table 1)
- See Section III for a clinical algorithm for the evaluation of genital ulcer disease

WORKUP

Confirmation is primarily through laboratory diagnosis.

- Culture of lesions
- Serologic testing (see the following lab tests)
- Cerebrospinal fluid (CSF) testing

LABORATORY TESTS

- Dark-field microscopy of fluid from lesion to look for treponeme is the definitive method for diagnosis of early syphilis.
- Serologic testing:
  1. Nontreponemal tests: Venereal disease research laboratory (VDRL) or rapid plasma reagin (RPR).
  2. Treponemal tests: Fluorescent treponemal antibody absorbed (FTA-ABS) tests, the *T. pallidum* passive particle agglutination (TP-PA) assay, various enzyme immunoassays (EIAs), chemiluminescence immunoassays, immunoblots, or rapid treponemal assays.
  3. Antibody titers can assess for response to treatment and for reinfection in previously treated patients.
- Screening methods:
  1. Traditional: Screen with nontreponemal tests; confirmation with treponemal testing.
  2. Alternative: Screen with treponemal testing, confirm with nontreponemal testing. More false positives, less likely to miss early or latent syphilis.
- When the nontreponemal test is negative despite a positive screen, an additional treponemal screen may be helpful. Trials have shown that two positive treponemal screens help identify a population with likely prior

TABLE 1 Genital Ulcer Disease

Disease	Lesions	Lymphadenopathy	Systemic Symptoms
Primary syphilis	**Painless,** indurated, with a clean base, usually singular	Nontender, rubbery, nonsuppurative bilateral lymphadenopathy	None
Genital herpes	**Painful** vesicles, shallow, usually multiple	Tender, bilateral inguinal adenopathy	Present during primary infection
Chancroid	Tender papule, then **painful,** undermined purulent ulcer, single or multiple	Tender, regional, painful, suppurative nodes	None
Lymphogranuloma	Small, **painless** vesicle or papule progresses to an ulcer	Painful, matted, large nodes with fistulous tracts	Present after genital lesion heals

From Wein AJ et al: *Campbell-Walsh urology*, ed 11, Philadelphia, 2016, Elsevier.

or current syphilis, and treatment of these patients may be justifiable.
- In patients with neurosyphilis, serologic criteria for response to therapy is a fourfold or greater decrease in VDRL titer over 6 to 12 mo.
- Lumbar puncture (LP) for cerebrospinal fluid VDRL (CSF-VDRL) in patients with evidence of latent syphilis (good specificity, poor sensitivity). If negative with high suspicion, can also perform a CSF FTA-ABS (good sensitivity, less specificity). When reactive in the absence of substantial contamination of CSF with blood, it is considered diagnostic of neurosyphilis. The Centers for Disease Control and Prevention indications for LP are neurologic symptoms, treatment failure, any eye or ear involvement, or evidence of active syphilis (aortitis, gumma, iritis).
- HIV testing in all patients.

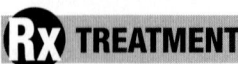

TREATMENT

ACUTE GENERAL Rx

- Primary, secondary, early latent:
  1. Penicillin G benzathine 2.4 million U IM once.
  2. Infants and children: Benzathine penicillin G 50,000 units/kg IM, up to the adult dose of 2.4 million units in a single dose.
  3. Nonpregnant penicillin-allergic patients: Doxycycline 100 mg bid × 14 days.
  4. Alternative regimens (contraindicated in MSM, persons with HIV, or pregnant women):
     a. Azithromycin 2 g PO × 1 dose
     b. Ceftriaxone 1-2 g IM or IV for 10-14 days
     c. Tetracycline 500 mg PO QID for 14 days
     d. Amoxicillin 3 g PO BID + probenecid 500 mg PO BID for 14 days
  5. Careful clinical and serologic follow-up of persons receiving any alternative therapy is essential.
  6. Persons with a penicillin allergy whose compliance with therapy or follow-up cannot be ensured should be desensitized and treated with benzathine penicillin.
- Late latent syphilis, tertiary syphilis (not neurosyphilis) in adults:
  1. Penicillin G benzathine 2.4 million U IM q wk × 3 wk.
  2. Nonpregnant penicillin-allergic patients: Doxycycline 100 mg PO BID × 4 wk.
- Neurosyphilis:
  1. Aqueous crystalline penicillin G 18 to 24 million U/day, administered as 3 to 4 million U IV q4h or continuous infusion for 10 to 14 days.
  2. Alternative regimen: Procaine penicillin 2.4 million U IM/day plus probenecid 500 mg PO qid, both for 10 to 14 days.
- Congenital syphilis:
  1. Aqueous crystalline penicillin G 50,000 U/kg/dose IV q12h × first 7 days of life and q8h after that for a total of 10 days OR procaine penicillin G 50,000 U/kg/dose IM/day × 10 days.
  2. An algorithm for evaluation and treatment of infants born to mothers with reactive serologic tests for syphilis is illustrated in Fig. E5.

DISPOSITION

- Repeat quantitative nontreponemal tests at 6 and 12 mo to ensure adequate treatment. For HIV-infected patients, repeat testing at 3, 6, 9, 12, and 24 mo. Pregnancy requires monthly tests until delivery.
- Findings indicating need for retreatment:
  1. If a fourfold increase in titer occurs and is sustained over testing performed >2 wk apart
  2. If initial high titer fails to drop by fourfold within a yr for early syphilis or 24 mo for late syphilis
  3. If signs persist, or patient develops new signs of infection
- Because treatment failure may be the result of unrecognized CNS infection, CSF examination can be considered in such situations. For retreatment, weekly infusions of benzathine penicillin G 2.4 million units IM for 3 wk is recommended, unless CSF examination indicates that neurosyphilis is present.
- Pregnant women without a fourfold drop in titer by 6 mo compared to pre-treatment titer need to be retreated.
- Cases should be reported to local or state health department for referral, follow-up, and partner notification.

REFERRAL

- Pregnant and possible congenital syphilis
- Pregnant and allergic to penicillin, who need to be desensitized for treatment
- Late latent syphilis with serious central nervous system, cardiovascular, or other organ system compromise

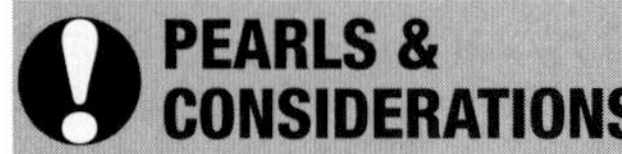

PEARLS & CONSIDERATIONS

- Jarisch-Herxheimer reaction (fever, myalgia, tachycardia, hypotension) may occur within 24 hr of treatment.
- Fig. E5 illustrates the course of untreated syphilis. One third of untreated patients develop CNS and/or cardiovascular sequelae.
- Up to 80% of those treated during late stages remain seropositive indefinitely.
- Treponemal tests remain positive even after adequate therapy.
- Male circumcision does not decrease the incidence of syphilis (unlike HIV, HSV-2, and HPV infection).
- Partner notification and treatment:
  1. Persons who are exposed within 90 days preceding the diagnosis of primary, secondary, or early latent syphilis in a sex partner might be infected even if seronegative; therefore, such persons should be treated presumptively.
  2. Persons who were exposed ≥90 days before the diagnosis of syphilis in a sex partner should be treated presumptively if serologic test results are not available immediately and the opportunity for follow-up is uncertain.

SUGGESTED READINGS

Available at ExpertConsult.com

RELATED CONTENT

Syphilis (Patient Information)
Tabes Dorsalis (Related Key Topic)

AUTHOR: **ASHWINI U. DHOKTE, M.D.**

BASIC INFORMATION

DEFINITION

Systemic lupus erythematosus (SLE) is a chronic inflammatory disorder characterized by autoantibody production responsible for antibody-mediated and immune complex deposition tissue damage. SLE involves multiple organs and systems and has heterogeneous disease patterns. Relapses and remissions are a common feature.

SYNONYMS

SLE
Lupus

ICD-10CM CODES

M32	Systemic lupus erythematosus
M32.0	Drug-induced systemic lupus erythematosus
M32.8	Other forms of systemic lupus erythematosus
M32.9	Systemic lupus erythematosus, unspecified
M32.10	Systemic lupus erythematosus, organ or system involvement unspecified
M32.11	Endocarditis in systemic lupus erythematosus
M32.12	Pericarditis in systemic lupus erythematosus
M32.13	Lung involvement in systemic lupus erythematosus
M32.14	Glomerular disease in systemic lupus erythematosus
M32.15	Tubulo-interstitial nephropathy in systemic lupus erythematosus
M32.19	Other organ or system involvement in systemic lupus erythematosus

EPIDEMIOLOGY & DEMOGRAPHICS

INCIDENCE: Varies across gender, race/ethnic groups, and geography from 20 to 70 cases per 100,000 persons. Prevalence higher among African Americans, Asian Americans, and Hispanics. There are an estimated 350,000 people with SLE in the U.S.

PREDOMINANT SEX: Female/male ratio is 9:1. The ratio is highest in reproductive age group, and about half of that in patients younger than 16 and older than 55.

PREDOMINANT AGE: Mean age at diagnosis is 31.

PHYSICAL FINDINGS & CLINICAL PRESENTATION

- Constitutional: Unexplained fever (rare in active SLE), fatigue (80% to 100% patients), malaise (see Table 1)
- Mucocutaneous lesions (more than 80% of patients): Acute (associated with + Ro antibody): malar rash (Fig. 1) sparing nasolabial folds (acute cutaneous lupus); annular or papulosquamous rash (subacute cutaneous lupus); Chronic: raised erythematous patches with subsequent edematous plaques and adherent scales (discoid cutaneous lupus), lupus profundus, lupus tumidus; alopecia, photosensitivity, nasal, or oropharyngeal ulcerations (classically painless, but discoid lesions [Fig. 2] may be painful); Raynaud's phenomenon; leukocytoclastic vasculitis, chilblains; livedo reticularis or livedo racemosa (secondary to antiphospholipid antibody syndrome); skin biopsy hallmark: interface dermatitis
- Musculoskeletal (about 90% of lupus patients): Arthralgias are more common than true arthritis, but nonerosive deforming arthritis is not rare; myositis
- Cardiac: Pericardial rub (pericarditis) is most common; valvular heart disease: valve nodules and thickening (Libman-Sacks endocarditis); congestive heart failure, myocarditis, premature atherosclerotic heart disease
- Pulmonary: Pleuritis (most common), acute or chronic pneumonitis, diffuse alveolar hemorrhage, pulmonary hypertension
- Gastrointestinal: Dysphagia, mesenteric vasculitis, peritonitis, pancreatitis, hepatitis
- Neuropsychiatric: Headache, psychosis, seizure, acute confusional states, peripheral or cranial neuropathy, transverse myelitis, stroke (may be associated with antiphospholipid syndrome), cognitive dysfunction
- Hematologic (about 50% of lupus patients): Anemia (hemolytic, anemia of chronic disease, aplastic anemia), thrombocytopenia, leukopenia, lymphadenopathy, secondary antiphospholipid antibody syndrome
- Renal: Acute renal failure, proteinuria, nephritic syndrome, nephrotic syndrome

ETIOLOGY

Lupus may develop in genetically susceptible individuals, triggered by endogenous and exogenous factors. SLE susceptibility involves MHC class II polymorphism with commonly observed association with HLA-DR-2, DR3, DR4, and DR8. SLE is also associated with inherited deficiencies of C1q, C2, C4a, others. There is predilection for familial clustering of SLE with risk in monozygotic twins—about 25% to 50%—and 5% in dizygotic twins. Environmental factors such as UV light, Epstein-Barr virus infection, and tobacco smoking may have a triggering role. Autoantibody production is the hallmark

TABLE 1 Potential Clinical Manifestations of Systemic Lupus Erythematosus

Target Organ	Potential Clinical Manifestations
Constitutional	Fatigue, anorexia, weight loss, fever, lymphadenopathy
Musculoskeletal	Arthritis, myositis, arthralgias, myalgias, avascular necrosis, osteoporosis
Skin	Malar rash, discoid rash, photosensitive rash, cutaneous vasculitis, livedo reticularis, periungual capillary abnormalities, Raynaud's phenomenon, alopecia, oral and nasal ulcers
Renal	Hypertension, proteinuria, hematuria, edema, nephrotic syndrome, renal failure
Cardiovascular	Pericarditis, myocarditis, conduction system abnormalities, Libman-Sacks endocarditis
Neurologic	Seizures, psychosis, cerebritis, stroke, transverse myelitis, depression, cognitive impairment, headaches, pseudotumor, peripheral neuropathy, chorea, optic neuritis, cranial nerve palsies
Pulmonary	Pleuritis, interstitial lung disease, pulmonary hemorrhage, pulmonary hypertension, pulmonary embolism
Hematologic	Immune-mediated cytopenias (hemolytic anemia, thrombocytopenia or leukopenia), anemia of chronic inflammation, hypercoagulability, thrombocytopenic thrombotic microangiopathy
Gastroenterology	Hepatosplenomegaly, pancreatitis, vasculitis affecting bowel, protein-losing enteropathy
Ocular	Retinal vasculitis, scleritis, episcleritis, papilledema

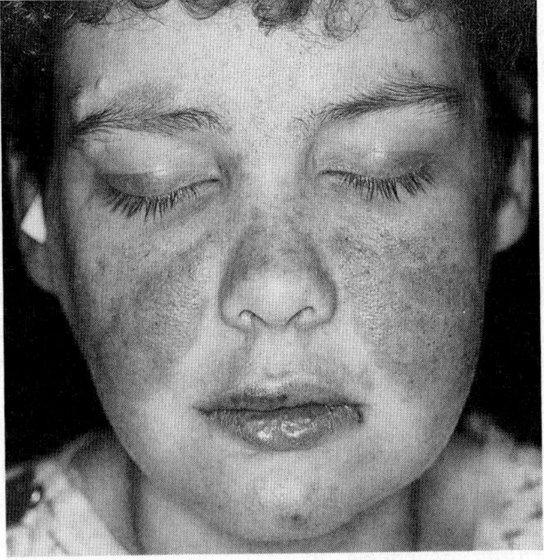

FIG. 1 Systemic lupus erythematosus. This young man has the typical malar rash of systemic lupus erythematosus. Note the prominent nasolabial sparing. (From Callen JP, et al.: *Dermatological signs of systemic disease*, ed 5, Philadelphia, 2017, Elsevier.)

 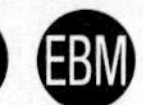

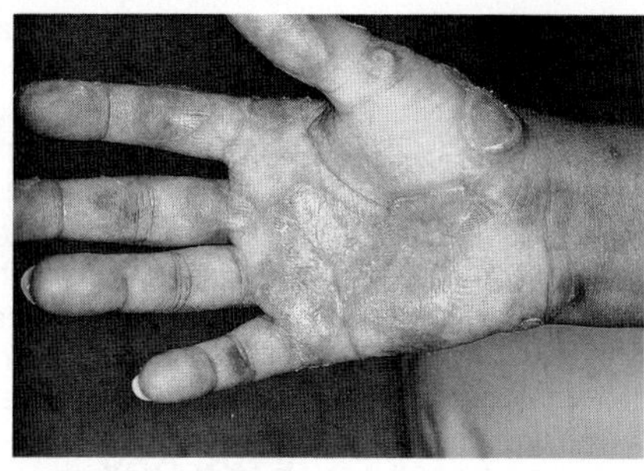

FIG. 2 Erosive lesions of discoid lupus erythematosus involving the palms. Typical lesions of discoid lupus erythematosus are present elsewhere. (From Callen JP, et al.: *Dermatological signs of systemic disease*, ed 5, Philadelphia, 2017, Elsevier.)

of disease development and diagnosis of SLE. Evidence supports the improper processing of nuclear proteins and nucleic acid from cell death. Impairments in neutrophil cell death via a process termed NET-osis (nuclear extracellular trap) contribute to the accumulation of nuclear debris. This, in turn, can lead to the presentation of self-nuclear material to plasmacytoid dendritic cells. Plasmacytoid dendritic cells propagate antibody and immune complex production via a type I interferon-dependent mechanism.

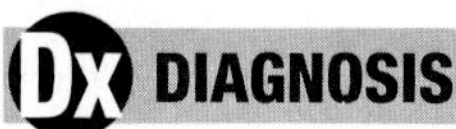

DIAGNOSIS

DIFFERENTIAL DIAGNOSIS

- Rheumatoid arthritis, mixed connective tissue disease, systemic vasculitis
- Neoplastic disorder
- Hematologic malignancy, paraneoplastic syndrome
- Systemic infection
- Other: Thrombotic thrombocytopenic purpura/hemolytic uremic syndrome, primary antiphospholipid antibody syndrome

EVALUATION

The diagnosis of SLE is suspected when any four or more of the following 1997 American College of Rheumatology (ACR) criteria (sensitivity 86%, specificity 93%) are present. These criteria were developed for research purposes, and diagnosis should be made on clinical grounds. The 2012 Systemic Lupus International Collaborating Clinics (SLICC) Classification Criteria (sensitivity 94%, specificity 92%) is also a validated tool for the diagnosis of SLE.

1997 ACR Criteria:

- Malar rash
- Discoid rash
- Photosensitivity (recurrence of unusual skin rash in sun-exposed areas)
- Oral or nasopharyngeal painless ulceration, observed by physician
- Arthritis (nonerosive)
- Serositis (pleuritis, pericarditis)
- Renal disorder (persistent proteinuria >0.5 g/day, or ≥3+ on dipstick if quantification not performed; cellular casts)
- Neurologic disorder (seizures, psychosis [in absence of offending drugs or metabolic derangement])
- Hematologic disorder:
  1. Hemolytic anemia with reticulocytosis
  2. Leukopenia (<4000/mm^3 total on two or more occasions)
  3. Lymphopenia (<1500/mm^3 on two or more occasions)
  4. Thrombocytopenia (<100,000/mm^3 in the absence of offending drugs)
- Immunologic disorder:
  1. Anti–double-stranded DNA antibody (anti-dsDNA)
  2. Anti-Smith antibody (anti-Sm)
  3. Antiphospholipid antibodies (anticardiolipin IgM or IgG, lupus anticoagulant, anti-beta-2 glycoprotein IgM or IgG, or false-positive fluorescent treponemal antibody absorption test or *Treponema pallidum* immobilization for 6 months)
- Antinuclear antibody (ANA): An abnormal titer of ANA by immunofluorescence or equivalent assay at any time in the absence of drugs known to be associated with drug-induced lupus syndrome

2012 SLICC Criteria:

SLE can be diagnosed if:

I. Biopsy-proven nephritis with either ANA or anti-dsDNA antibodies *or*
II. Patient satisfies four clinical criteria, requiring at least one clinical and at least one immunologic criterion
III. Clinical Criteria
   1. Acute cutaneous lupus (malar rash, bullous lupus, toxic epidermal necrolysis, photosensitive lupus rash, maculopapular lupus, subacute cutaneous lupus)
   2. Chronic cutaneous lupus (discoid, hypertrophic verrucous, panniculitis, mucosal lupus, lupus tumidus, chilblains lupus, lichen planus)
   3. Oral ulcers or nasal ulcers
   4. Nonscarring alopecia
   5. Synovitis (more than two joints or inflammatory arthralgias of more than two joints)
   6. Serositis (pleurisy for more than 1 day, pericardial pain for more than 1 day)
   7. Renal (>500 mg proteinuria/24 hr) or RBC casts)
   8. Neurologic (seizures, psychosis, mononeuritis multiplex, myelitis, peripheral or cranial neuropathy, acute confusional state)
   9. Hemolytic anemia
   10. Lymphopenia (<1000/mm^3 at least once)
   11. Thrombocytopenia (<100,000/mm^3 at least once)
IV. Immunologic Criteria
   1. ANA
   2. Anti-dsDNA (>2× laboratory reference range)
   3. Anti-Smith
   4. Antiphospholipid antibodies (lupus anticoagulant, RPR, anti-cardiolipin IgA, IgG, IgM, anti-β2 glycoprotein IgA, IgG, IgM)
   5. Low complement
   6. Direct Coombs test in the absence of hemolytic anemia

LABORATORY TESTS

Suggested initial laboratory evaluation of suspected SLE:

- ANA
  1. Complete blood count with differential, blood urea nitrogen and serum creatinine, urinalysis, ESR, PTT, complements (C3, C4)

Consider additional laboratory testing in a patient with strong suspicion for systemic lupus:

- Anti-dsDNA, anti-Smith, anti-SSA, anti-SSB, anti-RNP antibodies. Table 2 summarizes autoantibodies and clinical significance in SLE
- Lupus anticoagulant, RPR, anticardiolipin antibodies, anti-beta-2 glycoprotein antibodies especially in patients with thrombotic events or recurrent miscarriages
- Urinalysis for RBC, cellular casts
- Random spot urine protein: Urine creatinine ratio, 24-hr urine protein collection if proteinuria; >0.5 or >500 mg/24 hr is abnormal, respectively

  Direct Coombs test

IMAGING STUDIES

- Chest x-ray for evaluation of pulmonary involvement (pleural effusion, pulmonary infiltrates)
- Electrocardiogram for chest pain
- Echocardiogram if murmur, evidence of new or unexplained congestive heart failure, or suspected pericarditis
- Bedside and portable ultrasound use has been recently studied and is advocated for evaluation of inflamed joints in SLE patients

Rx TREATMENT

NONPHARMACOLOGIC THERAPY

- Avoidance of sunlight and use of high-SPF sunscreen (>35).
- Screening and counseling for modifiable cardiovascular risk factors such as cigarette smoking, diet, exercise, cholesterol, and uncontrolled HTN.
- Counseling for pregnancy planning for patients of childbearing age.
- Calcium and vitamin D supplementation for prevention of early osteoporosis (see "Clinical Pearls").

TABLE 2 Autoantibodies and Clinical Significance in Systemic Lupus Erythematosus (SLE)

Autoantibody	Prevalence in SLE	Clinical Significance
Antinuclear Antibody		
Anti-dsDNA	60%	95% specificity for SLE; fluctuates with disease activity; associated with glomerulonephritis
Anti-Smith	20%-30%	99% specificity for SLE; associated with anti-U1RNP antibodies
Anti-U1RNP	30%	Antibody associated with mixed connective tissue disease and lower frequency of glomerulonephritis
Anti-Ro/SSA	30%	Associated with Sjögren's syndrome, photosensitivity, SCLE, neonatal lupus, congenital heart block
Anti-La/SSB	20%	Associated with Sjögren's syndrome, SCLE, neonatal lupus, congenital heart block, anti-Ro/SSA
Antihistone	70%	Also associated with drug-induced lupus
Antiphospholipid	30%	Associated with arterial and venous thrombosis, pregnancy morbidity

Anti-dsDNA, Anti-double-stranded deoxyribonucleic acid; *SSA*, Anti-Sjögren's-syndrome-related antigen A; *SSB*, Anti-Sjögren's-syndrome-related antigen B; *SCLE*, subacute cutaneous lupus erythematosus.
From Firestein GS, et al.: *Kelley's textbook of rheumatology*, ed 9, Philadelphia, 2013, Saunders.

TABLE 3 Indications for Immunosuppressive Therapy in Systemic Lupus Erythematosus

General Indications

Involvement of major organs or extensive involvement of nonmajor organs (skin) refractory to other agents, or both

Failure to respond to or inability to taper corticosteroids to acceptable doses for long-term use

Specific Organ Involvement

Renal

Proliferative or membranous nephritis (nephritic or nephritic syndrome), or both

Hematologic

Severe thrombocytopenia (platelets <20,000/mm^3)

Thrombotic thrombocytopenic purpura–like syndrome

Severe hemolytic or aplastic anemia, or immune neutropenia not responding to glucocorticoids

Pulmonary

Lupus pneumonitis or alveolar hemorrhage, or both

Cardiac

Myocarditis with depressed left ventricular function, pericarditis with impending tamponade

Gastrointestinal

Abdominal vasculitis

Nervous system

Transverse myelitis, cerebritis, optic neuritis, psychosis refractory to corticosteroids, mononeuritis multiplex, severe peripheral neuropathy

From Firestein GS, et al.: *Kelly's textbook of rheumatology*, ed 9, Philadelphia, 2013, Saunders.

GENERAL Rx

- There are only four FDA-approved SLE medications: aspirin, steroids, hydroxychloroquine (1955), and belimumab (2011).
- Treatment should be targeted toward the involved organ(s).
- Limited and defined courses of corticosteroids are useful for a variety of SLE symptoms. Steroid therapy should be restricted to acute or subacute control of symptoms, due to the increased cardiovascular risk and increased organ damage associated with chronic steroid use.
- Consider checking G6PD in certain ethnic groups more predisposed to antimalarial-induced hemolytic anemia.
- Hydroxychloroquine has best evidence for reducing flares, organ damage, lipids, thrombosis; improving survival, augmenting action of mycophenolate mofetil (MMF) in lupus nephritis, and preventing seizures.
- Methotrexate or azathioprine is used as steroid-sparing drug. Indications for immunosuppressive therapy in SLE are described in Tables 3 and 4
- Joint pain and mild serositis are generally well controlled with nonsteroidal anti-inflammatory drugs or low-dose corticosteroids. Hydroxychloroquine and methotrexate are also effective for arthritis. Belimumab does well for joint manifestations. Leflunomide and rituximab may be considered for difficult arthritis.
- Cutaneous manifestations:
  1. Topical or intradermal corticosteroids are helpful for individual discoid lesions, especially in the scalp.
  2. Hydroxychloroquine alone or in combination with quinacrine and/or chloroquine could be considered for refractory skin disease.
  3. Refractory cases may be treated with belimumab, MMF, dapsone, or combination treatment.
- Hematologic manifestations:
  1. Corticosteroids are first-line therapy.
  2. Azathioprine can be used for thrombocytopenia or hemolytic anemia. Check for TPMT genetic mutation before the first use.
  3. Intravenous immunoglobulin (IVIG) or rituximab may be considered for severe leukopenia, autoimmune hemolytic anemia, or autoimmune thrombocytopenia.
- Central nervous system manifestations:
  1. Headaches are treated symptomatically. Most headaches will not be SLE-related and should be treated accordingly.
  2. Anticonvulsants and antipsychotics may be indicated.
  3. Standard therapy for other neuropsychiatric SLE symptoms is not established.
- Renal disease (Class III, IV or IV/V with cellular crescents lupus nephritis; see Table 5).

INDUCTION: 6-mo treatment

- The typical treatment induction period is 6 months. The use of intravenous cyclophosphamide (CYC) with corticosteroids given at monthly intervals is more effective in preserving renal function than is treatment with glucocorticoids alone. Low-dose "Euro-Lupus" protocol may be equally efficacious and less toxic for certain populations (e.g., Caucasians) than high-dose regimen. MMF is considered equivalent to CYC based on high-quality studies, with better tolerability and fertility profile. MMF may be preferred in African Americans and Hispanics. MMF or azathioprine is a good option for treatment maintenance.
- Severe nonrenal organ disease:
  1. Evidence from systematic randomized controlled trials for nonrenal lupus treatment is comparatively limited.
  2. High-dose intravenous CYC is used as induction treatment. Azathioprine or MMF may be used as maintenance.
  3. IVIG may be considered in severe disease especially when concomitant infection is present.
  4. Plasmapheresis or plasma exchange may be considered in critical situations: First-line therapy in Guillain-Barre syndrome, TTP, second line for SLE-related hemolytic anemia, cerebritis, and DAH. Infectious complications are common.
- Therapy targeting B cells:
  1. Rituximab: Anti-CD 20 monoclonal antibody. Randomized controlled trials for rituximab as an adjunct induction agent were negative in terms of both renal and nonrenal outcomes. An ongoing randomized controlled trial of rituximab

TABLE 4 Recommended Immunosuppressive Therapy for Major Organ Involvement in Systemic Lupus Erythematosus

Disease Severity	Induction Therapy	Maintenance Therapy
Mild	High-dose GC (0.5-1 mg/kg/day prednisone ×4-6 wk, tapered to 0.125 mg/kg every other day within 3 mo) alone or in combination with AZA (1-2 mg/kg/day)	Low-dose GC (prednisone ≤0.125 mg/kg on alternative days) alone or with AZA (1-2 mg/kg/day)
	If no remission within 3 mo, treat as moderately severe	Consider further gradual tapering at the end of each yr of remission
Moderate	MMF (2 g/day) (or AZA) with GC as above; if no remission after the first 6-12 mo, treat as severe	MMF tapered to 1.5 g/day for 6-12 mo and then to 1 g/day; consider further tapering at the end of each yr in remission Alternative: AZA (1-2 mg/kg/day)
Severe	Pulse IV-CYC alone or in combination with pulse IV-MP for the first 6 mo (background GC 0.5 mg/kg/day for 4 wk, then taper)	Quarterly pulses of IV-CYC for at least 1 yr beyond remission
	If no response, consider adding RTX or switch to MMF	Alternative: AZA (1-2 mg/kg/day), MMF (1-2 g/day)

AZA, Azathioprine; *CYC,* cyclophosphamide; *GC,* glucocorticoid; *IV,* intravenous; *MMF,* mycophenolate mofetil; *MP,* methylprednisolone; *RTX,* rituximab.
From Firestein GS, et al.: *Kelley's textbook of rheumatology,* ed 9, Philadelphia, 2013, Saunders.

TABLE 5 Severity of Lupus Nephritis*

Proliferative Disease	
Mild	Type III without severe histologic features (e.g., crescents, fibrinoid necrosis); low chronicity index (i.e., ≤3); normal renal function; nonnephrotic-range proteinuria
Moderately severe	Mild disease as defined above with partial or no response after the initial induction therapy or delayed remission (>12 months), or Focal proliferative nephritis with adverse histologic features or reproducible increase of at least 30% in serum creatinine levels, or Diffuse proliferative nephritis (class IV) without adverse histologic features
Severe	Moderately severe as defined above but not remitting after 6 to 12 mo of therapy, or Proliferative disease with impaired renal function and fibrinoid necrosis or crescents in >25% of glomeruli, or Mixed membranous and proliferative nephritis, or Proliferative nephritis with high chronicity alone or in combination with high activity (chronicity index >4 or chronicity index >3 and activity index >10), or Rapidly progressive glomerulonephritis (doubling of serum creatinine within 2 to 3 mo)
Membranous Nephropathy	
Mild	Nonnephrotic-range proteinuria with normal renal function
Moderate	Nephrotic-range proteinuria with normal renal function at presentation
Severe	Nephrotic-range proteinuria with impaired renal function at presentation (at least 30% increase in serum creatinine)

*Concomitant therapy with corticosteroids or other immunosuppressive drugs may modify urinary sediment and/or histologic findings and should be taken into consideration.
From Hochberg MC, et al.: *Rheumatology,* ed 5, St Louis, 2011, Mosby.

as add-on treatment to mycophenolate mofetil for lupus nephritis with no use of maintenance steroids was completed in December 2017 (Rituxilup trial). If preliminary data are positive, the study would provide the basis for a paradigm shift in treatment of lupus and lupus nephritis with little to no use of steroids.

2. Epratuzumab: An anti-CD 22 agent. Studies initially showed positive data, but in July 2015 both phase III trials for SLE failed to meet their primary endpoint and this medication is no longer studied.
3. Belimumab: Decreases activation of B cells. When used in addition to standard therapy, patients on belimumab showed improvement in cutaneous and musculoskeletal disease. Belimumab-treated patients had decreased SLE activity, a reduced time to disease flare, and lower glucocorticoid exposure. Safety data were good. Patients with central nervous system or serious kidney disease were excluded.
4. Abatacept: Downregulates T cell activation. Data is limited regarding improvement in arthritis, fatigue, sleep if added to routine therapy. Negative data as adjunct agent for lupus arthritis when added to MMF or CYC.
5. Interferon therapy: Interferon α (INFα) has been linked to increased disease activity in SLE. INFα blocking therapies are in phase II clinical trials. Sifalimumab, a monoclonal antibody against INFα, reduced moderate to severe mucocutaneous involvement in SLE and decreased active joint count and fatigue scores in preliminary data analysis. Development of sifalimumab has been terminated in favor of anifrolumab, a similar INFα blocking agent.

DISPOSITION

- Most patients with SLE experience remissions and exacerbations.
- Five-yr survival rate has improved to more than 90% in patients with newly diagnosed SLE since the advent of potent immunosuppressive therapy. The 15-yr survival rate is now 85%.
- Early death related to SLE activity and infections; late death due to CVD.
- Lupus nephritis progression rate to ESRD in 10% to 30% within 15 yr.
- African Americans, Asian Americans, and Hispanic Americans in general have a worse prognosis. The leading cause of death in SLE patients in developed countries is premature atherosclerosis. The quality of life for many SLE patients is poor due to fatigue, chronic pain, and cognitive impairment.

REFERRAL

- Rheumatology consultation for all patients with SLE
- Hematology consultation for patients with significant hematologic abnormalities (e.g., severe hemolytic anemia or thrombocytopenia)
- Nephrology consultation in patients with proteinuria and/or suspected renal involvement
- Dermatology consultation for patients with unexplained or unusual skin rash
- Cardiology consultation for patients with lupus carditis, arrhythmias

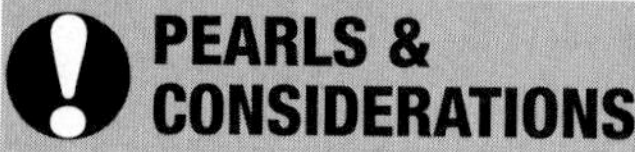

PEARLS & CONSIDERATIONS

- Arthritis in SLE often has no prolonged morning stiffness and is not erosive on x-rays; reversible joint deformities in lupus are termed Jaccoud's arthropathy.
- Myocardial infarction is 50 times more common in young female patients than in age-matched control group.
- Prevent adverse effects of medications: Consider prophylaxis for infections and appropriate vaccinations, ensure yearly Pap and other cancer screening as clinically indicated; for patients taking CYC, intervention to preserve bladder and fertility should be considered; manage bone health.
- Based on small clinical data a vitamin D level >40 may have modest reduction in disease activity; in addition vitamin D may reduce risk of thrombosis, based on oncology research.

SUGGESTED READINGS

Available at ExpertConsult.com

RELATED CONTENT

Systemic Lupus Erythematosus (Patient Information)
Discoid Lupus (Related Key Topic)

AUTHOR: **KATARZYNA GILEK-SEIBERT, M.D., RH.M.U.S.**

T

BASIC INFORMATION

DEFINITION

Takotsubo cardiomyopathy, also known as stress cardiomyopathy (SC), is a syndrome characterized by transient systolic and diastolic dysfunction with a characteristic ballooning of the apical and/or mid segments of the left ventricle (LV). It mimics acute myocardial infarction (MI); however, the difference lies in the absence of epicardial coronary occlusion. Typically, but not always, it is preceded by severe illness or intense emotional, physical, or psychological stress. Initially described in the 1990s in Japan, the systolic LV on left angiogram has a distinctive shape similar to a *tako-tsubo* pot with a narrow neck and round bottom, used by fishermen to trap octopi. The variants of SC include apical (81.7%), midventricular (14.6%), basal/reverse takotsubo (2.2%), and focal (1.5%).

SYNONYMS

Stress cardiomyopathy (SC)
Left ventricular apical ballooning syndrome (LVABS)
Ampulla cardiomyopathy
Broken heart syndrome
SC

ICD-10CM CODE

I51.81 Takotsubo syndrome

EPIDEMIOLOGY & DEMOGRAPHICS

INCIDENCE: Incidence is estimated to be ≈100 new cases per 1 million population per annum. The recurrence rate is 11.4% over 4 yr after initial presentation. Occurs mostly in summer; few cases in winter.

PREVALENCE: Studies suggest that 1% to 2% of patients presenting with troponin-positive acute coronary syndrome (ACS) have SC.

PREDOMINANT SEX AND AGE: On presentation, 90% are females, and 80% are females >50 yr of age. Mean age of presentation is 68.8 yr.

RISK FACTORS: SC can be triggered by severe medical illness, intense emotional psychosocial stress or physical stress (death of loved ones, domestic abuse, fierce arguments, financial hardships, severe pain, natural disasters, etc.), or chronic stress/distress. Sometimes there is no evident trigger; a positive life event (happy heart syndrome) can cause SC. Familial case series have raised the possibility of a genetic predisposition.

PHYSICAL FINDINGS & CLINICAL PRESENTATION

- Acute substernal chest pain, dyspnea, and syncope are the most common presenting complaints (International Takotsubo Registry study).
- Patients can present with clinical signs of heart failure (30%), serious ventricular arrhythmias, cardiogenic shock (10%), and sudden cardiac death are possible complications.

ETIOLOGY

The proposed mechanisms for an acute and reversible ventricular dysfunction include the following:

- Coronary spasm: In postmenopausal women, estrogen deficiency leads to endothelial vasomotor dysfunction. Lack of endothelial-dependent vasodilation causes excessive coronary vasoconstriction.
- Increased catecholamine from an acute event can be directly toxic to the myocardium.
- Microvascular dysfunction/aborted MI: Transient coronary occlusion by a fast-dissolving clot with spontaneous reperfusion.
- Abnormal myocardial architecture: The increased density of beta-adrenoreceptors in the apex makes it more sensitive to catecholamine and accounts for the apical ballooning.
- Fig. 1 depicts the interplay among triggers, pathogenic factors, and predisposing factors in SC.

DIAGNOSIS

Mayo Clinic proposed criteria (2008) for diagnosis of SC: All four criteria required to make diagnosis.

- Transient wall motion abnormalities of the left ventricular midsegments with or without apical segments in a noncoronary distribution (Fig. 2). A stressful trigger is often, but not always, present.
- Absence of obstructive coronary disease or angiographic evidence of acute plaque rupture.
- New ECG abnormalities (ST-segment elevation and/or T-wave inversion) or modest elevation in cardiac troponins.
- Absence of pheochromocytoma or myocarditis.

DIFFERENTIAL DIAGNOSIS

- Acute MI
- Cardiac syndrome X/microvascular angina
- Prinzmetal's angina
- Myocarditis
- Cocaine abuse
- Cerebrovascular disease with Takotsubo-like myocardial dysfunction
- Pheochromocytoma

WORKUP

- A high index of suspicion is required when a postmenopausal woman presents with ACS after intense stress.

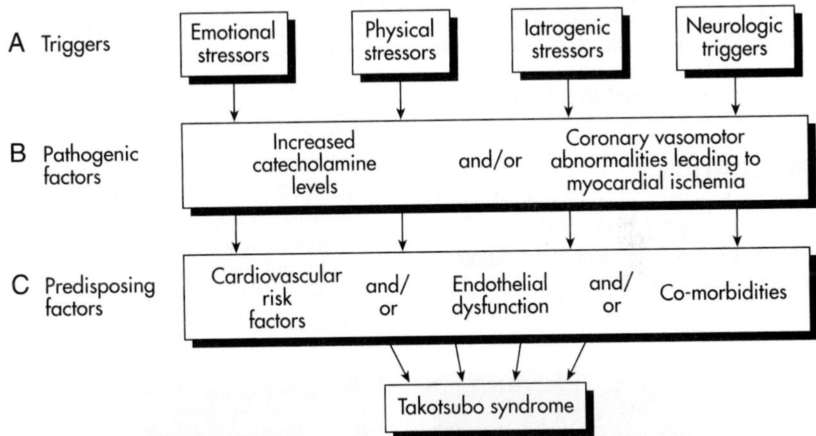

FIG. 1 The interplay among triggers, pathogenic factors, and predisposing factors in Takotsubo disease. (From Pelliccia F, et al.: Takotsubo syndrome [stress cardiomyopathy]: an intriguing clinical condition in search of its identity, *Am J Med* 127:699-704, 2014.)

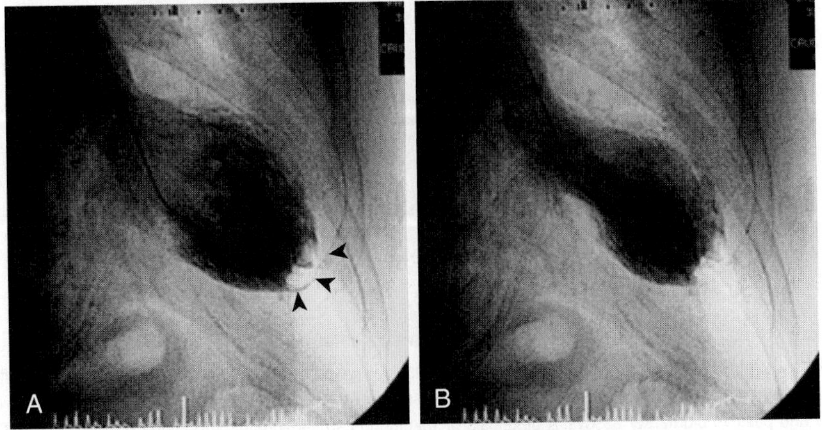

FIG. 2 A and B, Left ventriculogram showing apical ballooning characteristic of stress-induced cardiomyopathy. (From Mitsuma W, et al.: *JACC* 51[1]: cover, 2008.)

- Cardiology consult should be immediately obtained.
- Obstructive coronary artery disease needs to be ruled out.

LABORATORY TESTS

- Cardiac biomarkers (troponin, CK-MB) are often modestly elevated, but typically less than MI.
- Beta natriuretic peptide (BNP) levels are also commonly elevated.

IMAGING STUDIES

- Electrocardiographic (ECG): ST elevation in precordial leads (reciprocal changes typically absent), T-wave inversions (which may be dramatic) in the anterior or lateral leads, QT prolongation, and abnormal Q waves.
- Echocardiography (ECHO) typically shows the characteristic apical ballooning. Contrast ECHO is quite useful to exclude apical thrombus.
- SC is a diagnosis of exclusion. Left heart catheterization should be done to exclude obstructive coronary artery disease.
- Cardiac magnetic resonance imaging (Fig. 3) can show the absence of late gadolinium enhancement (seen in MI).
- Histopathologic findings: Interstitial infiltrates of mononuclear lymphocytes and macrophages with fibrosis and contraction band necrosis. Typically, atherosclerotic epicardial artery occlusion and MI is a coagulation necrosis.

COMPLICATIONS

- Approximately 20% have in-hospital complications including heart failure, cardiogenic shock (requiring mechanical support), life-threatening arrhythmias, acute mitral regurgitation, LV outflow tract (LVOT) obstruction, free wall rupture, and death.
- The presence of physical triggers, left ventricular ejection fraction <45%, acute neurologic or psychiatric disease, and first troponin >10× upper limit of normal predict high in-hospital complications.
- A reduced left ventricular ejection fraction is a common finding (86.5%) with recovery seen in days to weeks.
- The prognosis is worse for males.
- Even short-term LV dysfunction can lead to intraventricular thrombus formation (2.5%). This carries a great risk of cerebrovascular accident and distant embolization during the recovery phase.

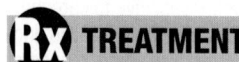

TREATMENT

Initially, patients should be treated for presumptive acute coronary syndrome until this is excluded.

NONPHARMACOLOGIC THERAPY

Supportive care such as the elimination of the physical or emotional trigger is important.

ACUTE GENERAL Rx

- Patients who are hemodynamically stable should be started on a beta-blocker, ACE inhibitor/angiotensin II receptor blockers, aldosterone antagonist, Sacubitril/valsartan, and diuretics if signs of volume overload.
- Patients in shock should get urgent ECHO to determine presence of LVOT obstruction.
- Cardiogenic shock without significant LVOT obstruction: Vasopressor and inotropic support may be required. May also benefit from an intraaortic balloon pump (IABP).
- Cardiogenic shock + LVOT obstruction: Fluid resuscitation if no significant pulmonary congestion. Increase preload by leg elevation or head tilt. Beta blockers will reduce contractility of basal segments and improve the obstruction. Phenylephrine should be used cautiously because it could increase the after-load and thus increase the gradient. IABP and inotropes will worsen the LVOT obstruction.

CHRONIC Rx

- Continued medical therapy and repeat ECHO (in 4-6 wk) to ensure normalization of systolic function (most patients normalize by this time).
- Duration of medical therapy is debatable. A period of 3 to 6 months has been suggested.
- Three months of anticoagulation is suggested if an intraventricular thrombus is detected.
- Recently published data could not find the protective effect of β-blockers in preventing the occurrence or recurrence of SC.
- Ace inhibition is associated with increased survival.

DISPOSITION

Carries a favorable prognosis compared to STEMI or NSTEMI; in-hospital mortality is approximately 2%. The recurrence rate is around 11%.

In a Medicare cohort, patients ≥85 yr of age had higher in-hospital, 30-day, 1-yr mortality, and 30-day readmission rates; hence, the need for good discharge planning is key.

REFERRAL

Follow-up with a cardiologist is suggested.

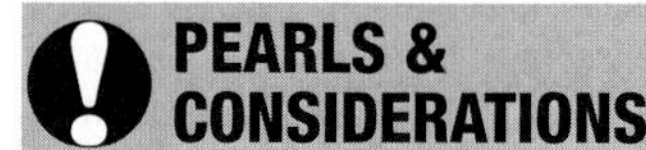

PEARLS & CONSIDERATIONS

COMMENTS

- The term *takotsubo* is the Japanese name for an octopus trap (*tako-tsubo*), which has a similar shape of the LV in systole during a left ventriculogram (see Fig. 2).
- Patients with takotsubo cardiomyopathy have a higher prevalence of neurologic or psychiatric disorders than those with an acute coronary syndrome.

PREVENTION

Minimizing stress may reduce incidence but no data to support this.

SUGGESTED READINGS

Available at ExpertConsult.com

AUTHORS: **MAXWELL EYRAM AFARI, M.D.,** and **MOSTAFA GHANIM, M.D.**

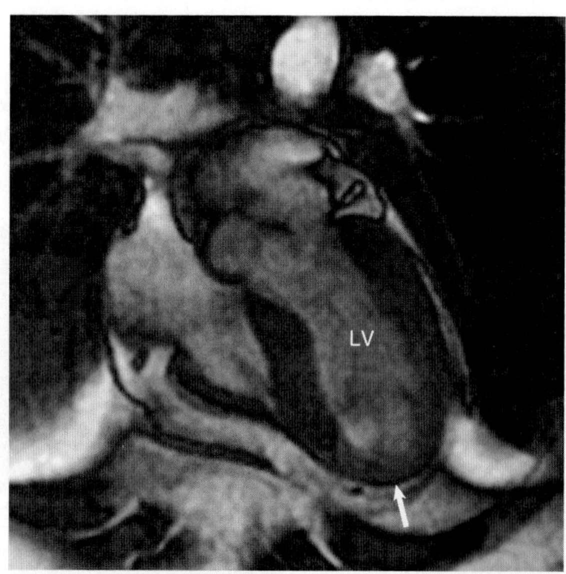

FIG. 3 Takotsubo cardiomyopathy. The patient was a 58-yr-old woman who was referred for CMR after a coronary angiogram revealed no obstructive disease despite the presence of ST-segment elevations on ECG and positive biomarker assays. A diagnosis of Takotsubo cardiomyopathy was made on the basis of the CMR image, which shows LV apical akinesis and ballooning (*arrow*). *LV,* Left ventricle. (From Mann DL, et al.: *Braunwald's heart disease*, ed 10, Philadelphia, 2015. Elsevier.)

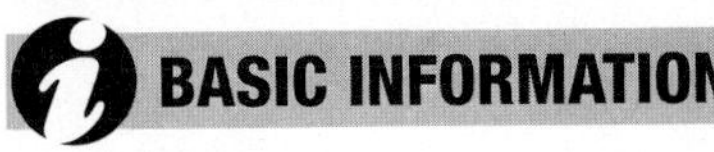

DEFINITION

Four species of adult tapeworm (cestodes) may infect humans as the definitive host: *Taenia saginata* (beef tapeworm), *Taenia solium* (pork tapeworm), *Diphyllobothrium latum* (fish tapeworm), and *Hymenolepis nana*. In addition, several tapeworms (*T. solium, T. crassiceps, T. multiceps*) can infect human tissue in their larval form, resulting in cysticercosis, and others infect in their intermediate forms, resulting in hydatid disease (see "Echinococcosis" in Section I). Table 1 describes common cestode parasites of humans, their typical vectors, and their usual symptoms.

SYNONYM

Cysticercosis (larval infection by *T. solium*)

ICD-10CM CODES
B68.0 *Taenia solium* taeniasis
B68.1 *Taenia saginata* taeniasis
B68.9 Taeniasis unspecified
B70.0 Diphyllobothriasis
B71.9 Cestode infection, unspecified

EPIDEMIOLOGY & DEMOGRAPHICS

INCIDENCE (IN U.S.):
- Diagnosed primarily in immigrants, particularly those from Latin America and Southeast Asia
- Varies widely by country of origin and dietary practices

PREVALENCE (IN U.S.):
- *T. saginata:* <0.1%
- *D. latum:* <0.05%
- *T. solium:* <0.1%
- *H. nana:* Sporadic, often in setting of outbreak

PREDOMINANT SEX: Equal sex distribution
PREDOMINANT AGE:
- *T. saginata, T. solium, D. latum:* 20 to 39 yr of age
- *H. nana* in setting of institution outbreaks: Children

PHYSICAL FINDINGS & CLINICAL PRESENTATION

Adult worms:
- Attach to bowel mucosa via suckers, hooks, or grooves depending on species
- Feed and grow, producing digestive/body/reproductive segments called proglottids
- Cause minimal or no symptoms or sequelae but occasionally can cause nausea, anorexia, or epigastric pain

Cysticercosis: Larval infection by *T. solium*:
- Mass lesions of brain (neurocysticercosis), soft tissue, viscera
- Neurocysticercosis may cause seizures, hydrocephalus (due to ventricle obstruction)

Prolonged infection with *D. latum*:
- Vitamin B_{12} deficiency
- Megaloblastic anemia

ETIOLOGY

TAPEWORM:
- Adult worms consist of a head (scolex), neck, and hundreds or thousands of proglottids. Each proglottid contains male and female reproductive organs, including eggs.
- Adult worm resides in small or large bowel; proglottids and eggs are passed in stool.
- *T. saginata* may produce up to 100,000 eggs/proglottid and *T. solium* up to 50,000 eggs/proglottid.
- Eggs are ingested by the animal intermediate host (Fig. 1).
- Eggs hatch into larvae.
- Larvae perforate the host intestinal wall and disseminate into skeletal muscle, brain, viscera.
- Develop into cysticerci (scolex inside a cyst) over several weeks.
- Humans eat infected beef (*T. saginata*), pork (*T. solium*), or fish (*D. latum*).
- Larval scolex attaches to intestinal wall and mature into adults within the GI lumen.
- *H. nana* infection is acquired by ingesting eggs in human or rodent feces.

CYSTICERCOSIS:
- Humans ingest eggs of *T. solium* in food contaminated with human feces that contain the eggs.
- Eggs hatch into larvae in gut and cross intestinal wall.
- Larvae disseminate widely through tissues (particularly soft tissue and CNS) forming cystic lesions containing either viable or nonviable larvae.

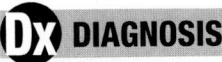

WORKUP

- Stool examination for eggs or proglottids (tapeworm):
  1. Eggs of *Taenia* spp. cannot be differentiated by microscopy, but the species can be identified through examination of the proglottids in stool
  2. Eggs of *Taenia* spp. are round and measure 30 to 40 micrometers
- Cerebral CT scan and MRI (neurocysticercosis)
- Serum antibody with ELISA confirmatory testing recommended for neurocysticercosis
- CBC may show eosinophilia

IMAGING STUDIES

- Tapeworm: Incidental finding on upper GI series
- Neurocysticercosis:
  1. Cerebral cysts are readily demonstrated by CT scan or MRI
  2. Calcified lesions are an incidental finding

TABLE 1 Common Cestode Parasites of Humans, Their Typical Vectors, and Their Usual Symptoms

Parasite Species	Developmental Stage Found in Humans	Common Name	Transmission Source	Symptoms Associated with Infection
Diphyllobothrium latum	Tapeworm	Fish tapeworm	Plerocercoid cysts in freshwater fish	Usually minimal; with prolonged or heavy infection, vitamin B_{12} deficiency
Hymenolepis nana	Tapeworm, cysticercoids	Dwarf tapeworm	Infected humans	Mild abdominal discomfort
Taenia saginata	Tapeworm	Beef tapeworm	Cysts in beef	Abdominal discomfort, proglottid migration
Taenia solium	Tapeworm	Pork tapeworm	Cysticerci in pork	Minimal
Taenia solium (Cysticercus cellulosae)	Cysticerci	Cysticercosis	Eggs from infected humans	Local inflammation, mass effect; if in central nervous system, seizures, hydrocephalus, arachnoiditis
Echinococcus granulosus	Larval cysts	Hydatid cyst disease	Eggs from infected dogs	Mass effect leading to pain, obstruction of adjacent organs; less commonly, secondary bacterial infection, distal spread of daughter cysts
Echinococcus multilocularis	Larval cysts	Alveolar cyst disease	Eggs from infected canines	Local invasion and mass effect leading to organ dysfunction; distal metastasis possible
Taenia multiceps	Larval cysts	Coenurosis, bladder worm	Eggs from infected dogs	Local inflammation and mass effect
Spirometra mansonoides	Larval cysts	Sparganosis	Cysts from infected copepods, frogs, snakes	Local inflammation and mass effect

Bennett JE et al: *Mandell, Douglas, and Bennett's principles and practice of infectious diseases*, ed 8, Philadelphia, 2015, WB Saunders.

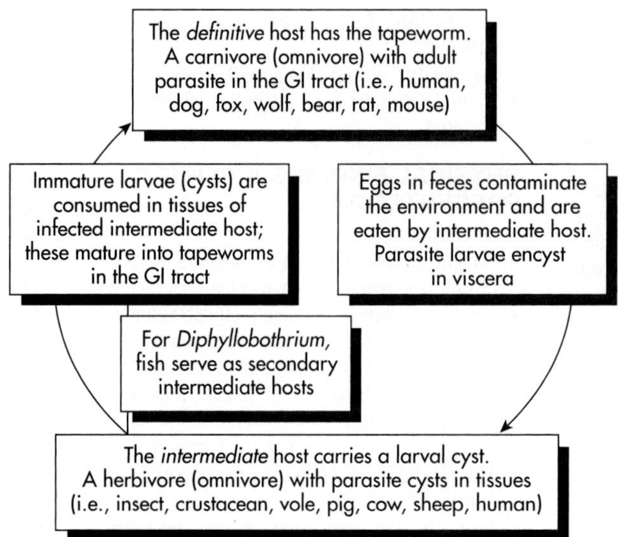

The *definitive* host has the tapeworm. A carnivore (omnivore) with adult parasite in the GI tract (i.e., human, dog, fox, wolf, bear, rat, mouse)
Eggs in feces contaminate the environment and are eaten by intermediate host. Parasite larvae encyst in viscera
The *intermediate* host carries a larval cyst. A herbivore (omnivore) with parasite cysts in tissues (i.e., insect, crustacean, vole, pig, cow, sheep, human)
For *Diphyllobothrium*, fish serve as secondary intermediate hosts
Immature larvae (cysts) are consumed in tissues of infected intermediate host; these mature into tapeworms in the GI tract

FIG. 1 Cestode parasites alternate larval and adult stages in two different hosts. *GI*, Gastrointestinal. (Bennett JE et al: *Mandell, Douglas, and Bennett's principles and practice of infectious diseases*, ed 8, Philadelphia, 2015, WB Saunders.)

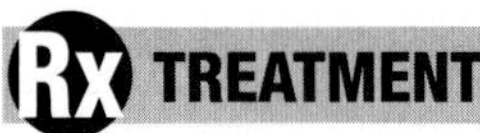

TREATMENT

ACUTE GENERAL Rx

- All adults and children with intestinal tapeworm infections should be treated with a single oral dose of praziquantel.
  1. *T. solium:* 5 to 10 mg/kg
  2. *T. saginata:* 5 to 10 mg/kg
  3. *D. latum:* 5 to 10 mg/kg
  4. *H. nana:* 25 mg/kg and a repeat dose 7 to 10 days later if heavy infection
- Praziquantel acts by causing changes in the teguments of the worms, allowing increased permeability to calcium ions, which then accumulate inside worm and cause paralysis.
- Repeat stool screening at 1 and 3 mo to confirm cure.
- Can use purgatives adjunctively to hasten clearance of deceased worms from intestine.
- An alternative therapy to praziquantel for fish, beef, or pork tapeworm infections is niclosamide, 2 g PO once for adults or 50 mg/kg orally once for children. For *H. nana* infections alternative is for adults: niclosamide 2 g PO × 7 days and for children: 11-34 kg: niclosamide 1 g PO on day 1 and then 500 mg/day for 6 days and 1.5 g for children over 34 kg PO on day 1 and then 1 g/day for 6 days.
- Therapy that may be considered for symptomatic cysticercosis:
  1. May regress spontaneously (i.e., no treatment, also okay for calcified parenchymal neurocysticercosis)
  2. Surgery, especially in cases of ventricular obstruction (neurocysticercosis)
  3. Albendazole 15 mg/kg/day (maximum: 1200 mg) PO for 10-14 days plus
  4. Praziquantel 50 mg/kg/day PO for 10-14 days plus
  5. Dexamethasone: 0.1 mg/kg/day often beginning 1-3 days before antiparasitic therapy × 10-14 days, plus/minus
  6. Antiseizure medication × 1 yr. Use of steroids in neurocysticercosis may reduce CNS inflammation and increase levels of albendazole in CNS.
- Medical therapy second line with:
  1. Ocular infections
  2. Cerebral infections in which local inflammation caused by destruction of the parasite may cause significant damage/inflammation (e.g. 4th ventricle infection)
- Adjunctive antiepileptics may be necessary for neurocysticercosis.

CHRONIC Rx

- Retreatment if required
- Avoidance of undercooked pork, meat, or fish
- Cysticercosis: Proper hand washing, proper disposal of human waste

DISPOSITION

- Neurologic follow-up for patients with neurocysticercosis
- Ophthalmologic follow-up for patients with ocular involvement

REFERRAL

Patients treated for neurocysticercosis should be evaluated by a physician experienced in managing this infection, if possible.

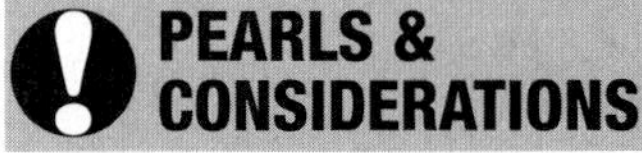

PEARLS & CONSIDERATIONS

COMMENTS

T. solium is the most dangerous of the tapeworms because of the potential for cysticercosis by means of autoinfection.

SUGGESTED READINGS

Available at ExpertConsult.com

RELATED CONTENT

Tapeworm Infection (Patient Information)
Cysticercosis (Related Key Topic)

AUTHOR: **RUSSELL J. MCCULLOH, M.D.**

BASIC INFORMATION

DEFINITION

Tardive dyskinesia (TD) is a neurological disorder of involuntary movements associated with the long-term use of antipsychotic medication, particularly first-generation antipsychotics. Patients exhibit rapid, repetitive, stereotypic movements that mostly involve the oral, lingual, trunk, and limb areas.

SYNONYMS

Orofacial dyskinesia
Tardive syndrome
TD

ICD-10CM CODE
G24.01 Drug induced subacute dyskinesia
DSM-5 CODE
335.85

EPIDEMIOLOGY & DEMOGRAPHICS

- The disorder is caused by dopamine-blocking antipsychotics (e.g., haloperidol) and antiemetics (e.g., metoclopramide, prochlorperazine, and promethazine).
- With first-generation antipsychotics, at least 20% of patients are affected with TD, and ~5% are expected to develop TD with each yr of antipsychotic treatment.
- The incidence of TD with second-generation antipsychotics is reduced only by about one third. With the increasing use of these medications, TD remains a serious problem.
- Risk increases with the duration of antipsychotic treatment, in female and in elderly patients, in patients with brain damage or dementia, with concurrent anticholinergic use, and in patients with nonschizophrenia diagnoses.

PHYSICAL FINDINGS & CLINICAL PRESENTATION

- TD is classically described as a chronic condition of insidious onset, but symptoms are variable over time and may even improve despite continued antipsychotic therapy.
- The condition typically appears with the reduction or withdrawal of the antipsychotic medications.
- TD classically involves stereotypic movements of the mouth and tongue, including lip smacking and puckering, tongue twisting and protrusion, and facial grimacing.
- TD may also involve slow, writhing movements of the trunk or choreoathetotic movements of the fingers and toes.
- The involuntary mouth movements associated with TD may be suppressed by voluntary actions (e.g., putting food in the mouth, talking).
- Variants of TD with similar treatment include tardive dystonia (e.g., torticollis, blepharospasm), tardive myoclonus, tardive akathisia, and tardive tics.

ETIOLOGY

TD is caused by chronic exposure to dopamine receptor antagonists that is thought to result in the upregulation of dopamine receptors in the basal ganglia as well as damage to striatal cholinergic neurons. Dysfunction of striatal GABAergic interneurons has also been implicated. It has been proposed that dopamine receptor hypersensitivity and neurodegenerative changes might cause altered synaptic plasticity of excitatory synapses onto striatal interneurons, resulting in an imbalance between the direct and indirect basal ganglia pathways.

Dx DIAGNOSIS

DIFFERENTIAL DIAGNOSIS

- Acute extrapyramidal symptoms (e.g., short-term withdrawal dyskinesias, Parkinsonism, akathisia)
- Basal ganglia movement disorders (e.g., Huntington chorea, Tourette's syndrome, levodopa-induced dyskinesia in Parkinson's disease, Wilson disease)
- Autoimmune diseases (Sydenham chorea, multiple sclerosis)
- Other causes of neurologic damage (e.g., lead or mercury toxicity, HIV, neurosyphilis, head injury, neurodegeneration from illicit substances)
- Mannerisms associated with disorganized type or catatonic type schizophrenia
- Hyperthyroidism-induced choreoathetosis
- Edentulous dyskinesias and improperly fitted dentures
- Rabbit syndrome (a rare variant of extrapyramidal symptoms with rapid vertical orofacial movements without tongue involvement); may respond to anticholinergic agents

WORKUP

TD is a diagnosis of exclusion, with emphasis on a complete neuropsychiatric and medication history and a thorough physical examination.

IMAGING STUDIES

Standard brain imaging is normal in patients with TD.

Rx TREATMENT

ACUTE GENERAL Rx

- Treatment is predicated on prevention: Limit the indications for antipsychotics; use the lowest effective dose; discontinue the drugs, when feasible; and monitor patients frequently. Anticholinergic medications may worsen symptoms.
- Switch to second-generation antipsychotics, if possible.

CHRONIC Rx

- If continued antipsychotic treatment is needed, switching to clozapine or quetiapine is the preferred initial treatment.
- Valbenazine and deutetrabenazine, inhibitors of the vesicular monoamine transporter 2 (VMAT2), are centrally acting synaptic dopamine depleters that are the first FDA-approved treatments for TD and are recommended as first-line treatment options when discontinuation of antipsychotic not indicated.
- Clonazepam and *Ginkgo biloba* probably improve TD. Amantadine and tetrabenazine may also improve TD and might be considered.
- For treatment-resistant, disabling TD, deep brain stimulation of internal globus pallidus seems to provide significant symptom reduction without exacerbation of psychiatric symptoms.
- TD is potentially irreversible in nearly two thirds of patients; thus, patients undergoing long-term treatment with dopamine receptor–blocking medications require frequent monitoring and aggressive management at the onset of TD symptoms.

REFERRAL

Movement disorder specialist consultation if symptoms are severe

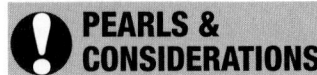

PEARLS & CONSIDERATIONS

- After removal of the causative medication, symptoms of tardive dyskinesia can take months to resolve or may become permanent (higher risk in elderly, female sex, prolonged use, and higher dose of causative medication).
- First-generation antipsychotics should be resumed to treat TD in the absence of active psychosis only as a last resort for persistent, disabling, and treatment-resistant TD.
- Avoid anticholinergic medications (e.g., benztropine), which may exacerbate TD symptoms.
- Recent evidence suggests increased overall mortality among patients with TD, which highlights the need for referral for more aggressive specialized interventions.

SUGGESTED READINGS

Available at ExpertConsult.com

RELATED CONTENT

Tardive Dyskinesia (Patient Information)

AUTHOR: **JOHN A. GRAY, M.D., PH.D.**

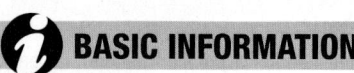

BASIC INFORMATION

DEFINITION

Temporomandibular joint (TMJ) syndrome refers to a group of disorders leading to symptoms of the TMJ. Temporomandibular joint disorders (TMD) can be classified as intraarticular (within the joint) or extraarticular (involving the surrounding musculature). The TMJ is a diarthrotic joint, meaning neither joint can move independently of the other because each is hinged at both ends. The joint is a true synovial joint capable of two actions of movement: translational and rotational. The articulating surfaces are the glenoid fossa of the temporal bone and the condylar process of the mandible, with the articular disk interposed between the two.

SYNONYMS

Temporomandibular dysfunction
Painful temporomandibular joint
TMJ
Temporomandibular disorders (TMD)

ICD-10CM CODE
N26.60 Temporomandibular joint disorder, unspecified

EPIDEMIOLOGY & DEMOGRAPHICS

- 15% to 25% of the population have symptoms of TMJ disorders at some point in their lives.
- Females are affected more often than males (up to 4:1 ratio).
- Occurs between the second and fourth decades of life.
- Usually unilateral, affecting either side with equal frequency.

PHYSICAL FINDINGS & CLINICAL PRESENTATION:

- Symptoms may appear or be worse during stressful life events.
  1. Often unilateral pain in the muscles of mastication, usually described as a "dull" ache
  2. Otalgia
  3. Odontalgia
  4. Headaches (frontal, temporal, retroorbital)
  5. Tinnitus
  6. Dizziness
  7. Clicking or popping sounds with movement of the TMJ
  8. Joint locking
- Physical exam findings:
  1. Tender to palpation over TMJ in external auditory meatus or preauricular region anterior to tragus
  2. Limited jaw opening or trismus
  3. Clicking or popping of TMJs with joint mobility
  4. Lateral deviation of mandible
  5. TMJ crepitus

ETIOLOGY

- Myofascial pain-dysfunction syndrome: The most common cause of TMJ syndrome and results from teeth grinding and clenching the jaw (bruxism)
- Internal TMJ derangement: Abnormal connection of the articular disk to the mandibular condyle as a result of disk displacement or chronic dislocations
- Degenerative joint disease
- Rheumatoid arthritis
- Gouty arthritis
- Pseudogout
- Ankylosing spondylitis
- Trauma (i.e., fractures)
- Congenital defects (i.e., aplasia, hypoplasia)
- Prior surgery (orthodontic, intraarticular steroid injection)
- Tumors

Dx DIAGNOSIS

Can be made based on history and physical examination in most cases.

DIFFERENTIAL DIAGNOSIS

Includes the list provided above. Myofascial pain-dysfunction syndrome, internal TMJ derangement, and degenerative joint disease represent >90% of all causes of TMJ syndrome. Others not mentioned include dental problems such as dental caries, loss of posterior teeth support, and Eagle's syndrome (stylohyoid syndrome, carotidynia, and trigeminal neuralgia). Alternative diagnoses such as otitis, mastoiditis, salivary gland disorders, migraine headache, sinusitis, postherpetic neuralgia, trigeminal neuralgia, glossopharyngeal neuralgia, and giant cell arteritis should always be excluded.

WORKUP

The diagnosis is based largely on history and physical examination findings. Radiographic imaging evaluation is used to exclude anatomic or systemic causes of disease when conservative management has failed.

LABORATORY TESTS

Laboratory examination is often not needed but may be helpful in ruling out certain conditions. CBC if infection is suspected. Rheumatoid factor if rheumatoid arthritis is suspected.

IMAGING STUDIES

- Plain radiographs: The most common views are the panoramic, transorbital, and transpharyngeal in both opened and closed positions.
- CT scan is highly accurate in diagnosing osseous derangements of the TMJ.
- MRI is the procedure of choice and has replaced arthrography in cases of disabling pain or if locking occurs. It is used to determine disk position and morphology along with degenerative bony changes.
- Arthrography is helpful in looking for meniscus involvement but is seldom performed anymore, as it is more invasive and less accurate than MRI for TMJ imaging.

Rx TREATMENT

NONPHARMACOLOGIC THERAPY

- Soft diet to rest the muscles of mastication
- Heat 15 to 20 min 4 to 6 times per day
- Massage of the masseter and temporalis muscles
- Formed splints or bite appliances to reduce compression of retrodiscal tissue (Fig. E1)
- Range-of-motion exercises
- Cognitive-behavioral therapy and biofeedback have been shown to reduce pain.
- Acupuncture

ACUTE GENERAL Rx

- NSAIDs: Ibuprofen 800 PO mg tid PRN or naproxen 500 mg PO bid prn, titrated to relieve symptoms
- Muscle relaxants or benzodiazepines at bedtime: Diazepam 2.5 to 5 mg PO tid PRN or amitriptyline 5 to 100 mg PO qd PRN
- In degenerative joint disease of the TMJ, intraarticular steroid injection can be tried
- Botulism toxin injections into the masticatory muscles
- Arthrocentesis with joint lavage and lysis of adhesions (Fig. E2)
- In patients with pain and clicking in the TMJ that is unresponsive to nonsurgical treatment, the disc should be repositioned arthroscopically or by open surgery (discoplasty) (see "Chronic Rx")

CHRONIC Rx

- Most of the above treatments are used for myofascial pain-dysfunction syndrome; however, they can be applied to other causes of TMJ syndrome. Surgery is usually a measure of last resort in patients who do not respond to nonpharmacologic and acute general treatment. Absolute indications for surgical therapy include neoplasms, growth abnormalities, and joint ankylosis.
- Surgical procedures include:
  1. Meniscoplasty
  2. Meniscectomy
  3. Subcondylar osteotomy
  4. TMJ reconstruction

DISPOSITION

The course depends on the underlying etiology; however, less than 5% of adults with temporomandibular symptoms develop chronic symptoms.

REFERRAL

All patients with TMJ syndrome refractory to conservative nonpharmacologic and acute therapy should be referred to a periodontist, oral maxillofacial surgeon, or ear-nose-throat surgeon.

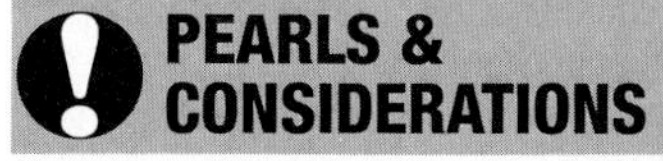

PEARLS & CONSIDERATIONS

Patients with rheumatoid arthritis involving the TMJ usually have bilateral involvement.

COMMENTS

Frequently, emotional stress initiates the myofascial pain-dysfunction, which accounts for 85% of all cases of TMJ syndrome.

SUGGESTED READING

Available at ExpertConsult.com

RELATED CONTENT

Temporomandibular Joint (TMJ) Syndrome (Patient Information)

AUTHOR: **LOUIS INSALACO, M.D.**

BASIC INFORMATION

Tension-type headache (TTH) is a highly prevalent primary headache disorder not associated with nausea or vomiting. Although previously thought to be caused by psychological factors and muscle contraction, current thinking implicates neurobiological mechanisms.

ICD-10CM CODES	
G44.209	Tension-type headache, unspecified, not intractable
G44.201	Tension-type headache, unspecified, intractable

EPIDEMIOLOGY & DEMOGRAPHICS

Most common type of headache, representing 70% of all headaches presenting to primary care physicians. Women are affected more often than men.

PHYSICAL FINDINGS & CLINICAL PRESENTATION

Headaches have an insidious progression, ranging from infrequent (<1 day per month) to chronic. Although considered a "featureless" headache disorder, either photophobia or phonophobia may still be present. Concurrent problems, such as anxiety, depression, and analgesic overuse, may aggravate the headaches. Patients may have pericranial tenderness to palpation on exam. The rest of the examination should be normal.

PATHOPHYSIOLOGY

- TTH is no longer thought to be due to either a psychological problem or abnormal muscle contraction. Similar to migraine, TTH is likely a heterogeneous disorder with several possible pathophysiologic mechanisms.
- In episodic TTH, peripheral mechanisms may predominate, whereas in chronic TTH, central mechanisms are involved.

Dx DIAGNOSIS

The International Headache Society criteria for tension-type headache are as follows:

- At least 10 headaches
- Lasting from 30 min to 7 days
- Having at least two of the following features:
  1. Bilateral
  2. Pressure or tightening (non-pulsating) quality
  3. Mild or moderate intensity
  4. Not aggravated by routine physical activity such as walking or climbing stairs
- Both of the following:
  1. No nausea or vomiting
  2. No more than one of either photophobia or phonophobia
- Not better accounted for by another diagnosis

DIFFERENTIAL DIAGNOSIS

- Migraine (would expect associated symptoms [i.e., nausea]; see topic "Headache, Migraine")
- Cervical spine disease
- Intracranial mass (may present with focal neurologic signs, seizures, or headache awakening patient from sleep)
- Idiopathic intracranial hypertension (found more often in obese women of childbearing age)
- Medication overuse headache
- Secondary headache (e.g., obstructive sleep apnea, temporomandibular joint syndrome, hypo- or hyperthyroidism, drug side effects)
- Section II describes the differential diagnosis of headaches

WORKUP

- Routine testing is not needed; the diagnosis may be established clinically.
- Thorough history to identify any red flag features (see topic "Headache, Migraine," SSNOOP5 mnemonic in differential diagnosis) and physical examination (looking for papilledema) for all patients being evaluated for headache.
- Neuroimaging, preferably with contrast-enhanced MRI, should be performed only when red flag features are identified by history or unexplained neurologic findings are present on examination.
- Erythrocyte sedimentation rate and C-reactive protein in patients 50 yr of age and older to screen for giant cell arteritis.

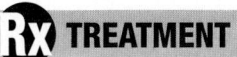

Rx TREATMENT

Current evidence supports synergistic benefits of combined nonpharmacologic and pharmacologic interventions. Nonpharmacologic therapy may include behavioral sleep modification, acupuncture, cognitive-behavioral therapy, relaxation training, and biofeedback.

ACUTE Rx

- Simple analgesics (i.e., NSAID, acetaminophen).
- Combination analgesics containing caffeine may be used as second-line treatment, although use on more than 10 days per month may lead to medication overuse headache.
- As with migraine headaches, narcotic- and barbiturate-containing analgesics should be avoided in tension-type headaches.

PREVENTIVE Rx

- Tricyclic antidepressants (e.g., amitriptyline 10 to 50 mg qhs) (first choice)
- Other options: Mirtazapine, venlafaxine, and tizanidine

DISPOSITION

The headache prognosis is generally favorable. Some patients will not respond to treatment.

REFERRAL

If red flags are present on history or exam or if the patient is not improving with treatment

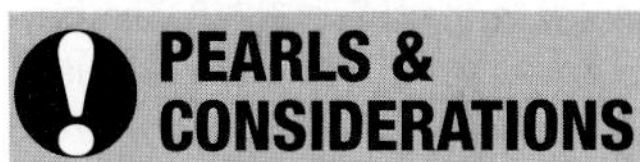

PEARLS & CONSIDERATIONS

It is imperative to avoid overuse of caffeine-, narcotic-, and barbiturate-containing medications because of the risk of rebound headaches.

SUGGESTED READINGS

Available at ExpertConsult.com

RELATED CONTENT

Tension Headache (Patient Information)

AUTHOR: **JONATHAN H. SMITH, M.D.**

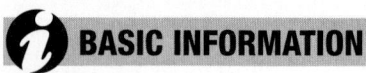

BASIC INFORMATION

DEFINITION

Testicular cancers are primary germ cell cancers originating in the testis.

SYNONYMS

Testis tumor
Testicular neoplasms

ICD-10CM CODES

C62.00	Malignant neoplasm of unspecified undescended testis
C62.01	Malignant neoplasm of undescended right testis
C62.02	Malignant neoplasm of undescended left testis
C62.10	Malignant neoplasm of unspecified descended testis
C62.11	Malignant neoplasm of descended right testis
C62.12	Malignant neoplasm of descended left testis
D40.10	Neoplasm of uncertain behavior of unspecified testis
D40.11	Neoplasm of uncertain behavior of right testis
D40.12	Neoplasm of uncertain behavior of left testis

EPIDEMIOLOGY & DEMOGRAPHICS

INCIDENCE: There will be an estimated 9310 new cases and 400 deaths associated with testicular cancer in the U.S. in 2018. The incidence is 5.4 cases per 100,000 men annually. White men have the highest incidence, whereas black men have the lowest incidence. Testicular cancer is the most common cancer diagnosis in men between 15 and 35 yr. The incidence has been gradually increasing since 1975.

PREVALENCE: It accounts for 1% to 2% of all cancers in males.

PHYSICAL FINDINGS & CLINICAL PRESENTATION

- Testicular cancer typically presents as a painless mass in the testis. Any mass within the testicle should be considered cancer until proven otherwise. It may be found by the patient, who brings it to the attention of a physician, or it may be found by a physician on a routine examination.
- Symptoms other than scrotal or testicular swelling are typically absent unless the cancer has metastasized (10% of patients at diagnosis). Occasionally a patient may report scrotal fullness or heaviness. About 10% of patients present with acute pain. Back pain secondary to enlarged retroperitoneal lymph nodes can occur. Gynecomastia from tumors that secrete beta-human chorionic gonadotropin (hCG) is found in 5% of men with testicular cancer.
- Testicular palpation should be performed with two hands. Transillumination may distinguish a solid mass (e.g., cancer) and a fluid-filled lesion (e.g., hydrocele or spermatocele). The mass is nontender; indeed, it is less sensitive than a normal testicle.

ETIOLOGY, CLASSIFICATION, & PATHOLOGY

- Cryptorchidism (undescended testes) is a major risk factor even if corrected by orchiopexy; however, treatment of undescended testis before puberty decreases the risk of testicular cancer from fivefold to twofold.
- Family history is an important risk factor (risk is 8-10 times as high in a brother of a person with testicular cancer and 4-6 times higher in sons of a father with testicular cancer)
- Other risk factors include genetic disorders (Down syndrome, testicular dysgenesis syndrome), Klinefelter syndrome, infertility, tobacco use, and white race (risk is highest among whites and lowest among blacks).
- Classification: Testicular cancers can be classified as pure seminomas or nonseminomatous germ cell tumors (embryonal carcinoma, choriocarcinoma, yolk sac carcinoma, teratoma, or mixed germ cell tumors).
- Germ-cell tumors appear to develop as a result of a tumorigenic event in utero that leads to a precursor lesion classified as intratubular germ-cell neoplasia. Approximately 90% of germ-cell tumors are associated with adjacent intratubular germ-cell neoplasia, which carries a 50% risk of testicular cancer within 5 yr.
- A genetic locus that confers a predisposition to testicular cancer is at 12q21, the location of the genes encoding the proteins involved in KITLG–KIT signaling. The development of intratubular germ-cell neoplasia may involve aberrantly activated KITLG–KIT in utero, which induces arrest of embryonic germ cells at the gonocyte stage; subsequently, overexpression of embryonic transcription factors leads to suppression of apoptosis, increased proliferation, and accumulation of mutations in gonocytes.
- The incidence of various subtypes of testicular cancers is as below:

Cell Type	Frequency (%)
Seminoma	42
Embryonal cell carcinoma	26
Teratocarcinoma	26
Teratoma	5
Choriocarcinoma	1

- Other rare types:
  1. Yolk sac carcinoma
  2. Mixed germ cell tumors
  3. Carcinoid tumor
  4. Sertoli cell tumors
  5. Leydig cell tumors
  6. Lymphoma
  7. Metastatic cancer to the testes

STAGING

- TNM staging system for testicular cancer is described on Table 2 and Table 3.
- The clinical stages consist of stage I, with tumor confined to the testis; stage II, with positive regional lymph nodes; and stage III, with metastases. Fig. 1 shows the clinical staging of testicular cancer.

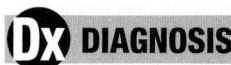

DIAGNOSIS

DIFFERENTIAL DIAGNOSIS

- Spermatocele
- Varicocele
- Hydrocele
- Epididymitis/orchitis
- Epidermoid cyst of the testicle
- Epididymis tumors
- Inguinal hernia
- Hematocele or testicular rupture
- Torsion of testicular appendage
- Skin cancer

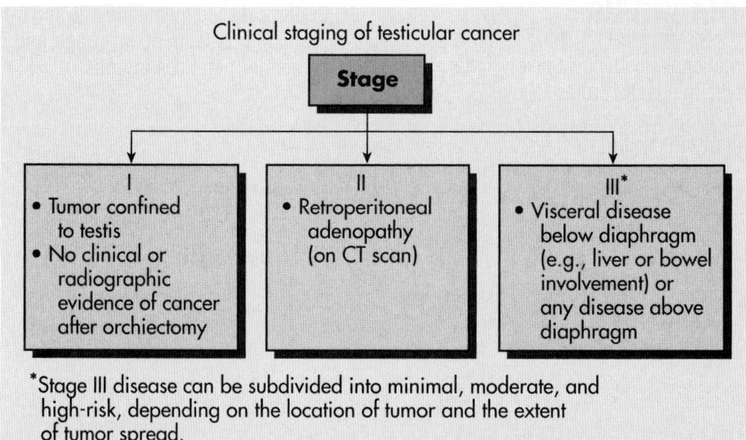

FIG. 1 Clinical staging of testicular cancer. The AJCC TNM staging system is less commonly used, because it is based upon histologic evaluation of the orchidectomy specimen and retroperitoneal periaortic lymph node dissection. Because the latter may not be performed in every patient, the clinical staging system is generally more practical. (From Skarin AT. *Atlas of diagnostic oncology,* ed 4, St Louis, 2010, Mosby.)

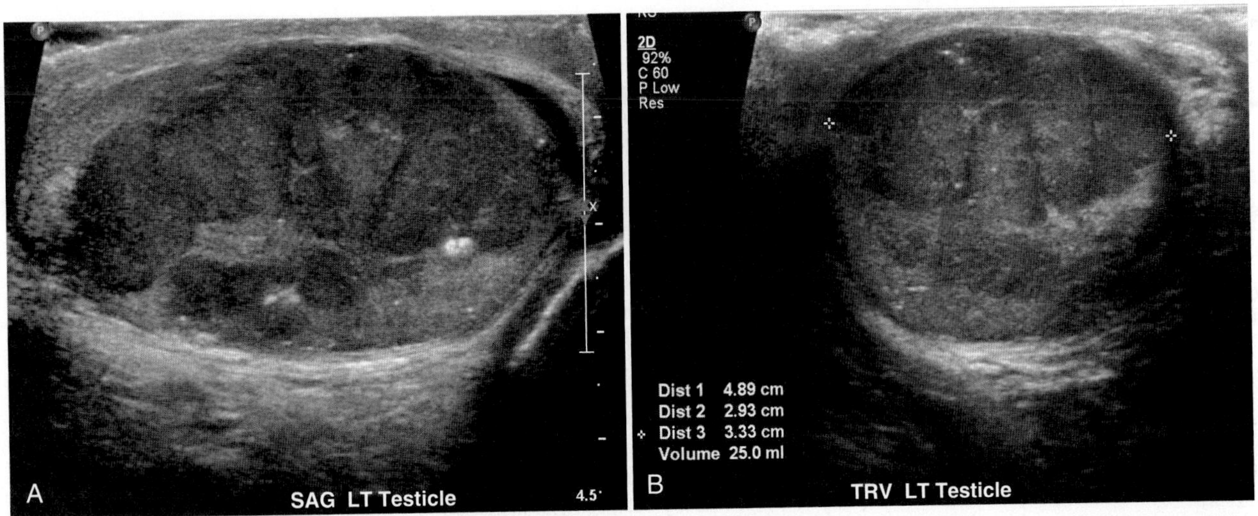

FIG. 2 Seminoma in an 18-year-old patient with painless left scrotal mass. A and **B,** Sagittal and transverse sonograms of the left testis demonstrate a testicular volume of 25 ml, with a lobulated, heterogeneous, relatively hypoechoic mass occupying most of the testis with a thin rim of normal testis and a few tiny clusters of calcification, as well as multiple, tiny, brightly echoic speckles both inside and outside the mass. The tiny speckles represent microlithiasis. (From Rumack CM et al: *Diagnostic ultrasound*, ed 4, Philadelphia, 2011, Elsevier.)

WORKUP

Physical examination, laboratory tests, and imaging studies (Fig. 2). A radical inguinal orchiectomy is diagnostic and therapeutic. Immunohistochemical analysis is used to determine the histologic composition of the tumor. Staging involves CT of chest, abdomen, and pelvis and measurement of beta subunit of human chorionic gonadotropins (β-hCG), alpha-fetoprotein (AFP), and lactate dehydrogenase (LDH).

LABORATORY TESTS

- Serum β-hCG is elevated in approximately 20% of patients with pure seminomas.
- Serum AFP is elevated in nonseminoma tumors, never elevated in patients with pure seminomas.

One or both of these tumor markers will be elevated in 70% of cases of testicular cancer.

- Serum lactate LDH level is elevated with rapid turnover of malignant cells.
- Testicular biopsy is contraindicated.

IMAGING STUDIES

- Testicular ultrasound
- CT scan of chest, pelvis, and abdomen
- MRI of the brain in patients with neurologic symptoms
- PET scan is not recommended (frequent false positives)

Rx TREATMENT

- Seminoma:
  1. Stage I: Most patients with clinical stage 1 are cured with orchiectomy. Radical inguinal orchiectomy plus one cycle of single-agent carboplatin chemotherapy or radiation therapy (RT) to the para-aortic lymph nodes was the standard of treatment for many yrs but has been eliminated in many instances and most patients are treated with active surveillance post-orchiectomy. More relapses are associated with surveillance (20% vs. 4% with radiotherapy or chemotherapy), but long-term survival approaches 100% irrespective of initial option chosen.[1]
  2. Stage II_A or II_B: RT or cisplatin-based chemotherapy (e.g., bleomycin, etoposide, and cisplatin [BEP]).
- Nonseminoma:
  1. Stage I_A: Radical orchiectomy plus nerve-sparing retroperitoneal lymph node dissection (RPLND).
  2. Stage I_B: Same as stage I_A plus two cycles of chemotherapy (bleomycin, etoposide, and cisplatin [BEP]).
  3. Stages II-III: Multiagent cisplatin-based chemotherapy regimens for three or four cycles depending on risk stratification (low/intermediate or high). RPLND is offered for residual lymph nodal disease after chemotherapy.
- Relapsed disease:
  1. Salvage chemotherapy using multiagent regimens is offered. Active drugs include ifosfamide, paclitaxel, cisplatin, vinblastine, and cisplatin.
  2. Chemotherapy-sensitive patients can be successfully treated with high-dose chemotherapy followed by autologous stem cell transplantation (ASCT).
- Posttreatment surveillance for testicular cancer survivors (annually):
  1. Fertility assessment
  2. Physical examination and skin examination (increased risk of dysplastic nevi)
  3. Testicular examination (3% to 4% risk of second testicular cancer)
  4. Serum tumor markers (hCG, AFP)
  5. Abdominal and pelvic CT every 3 to 4 months for 2 yr, every 6 to 12 months in third and fourth yr, and annually thereafter

[1] Hanna NH, Einhorn LH: Testicular cancer, discoveries and updates, *N Engl J Med* 371:2005–2016, 2014.

DISPOSITION

- The overall cure for testicular cancer is >95% (80% for metastatic disease). Patients with pure seminomas have a better prognosis. Prognosis can be determined by criteria established by the International Germ Cell Consensus Criteria (Table 1). Because treatment produces favorable outcomes even in advanced stages, the U.S. Preventive Services Task Force recommends against screening asymptomatic men for testicular cancer.
- There is an increased risk for metabolic syndrome (insulin resistance, hypertension, dyslipidemia, abdominal obesity) after radiation or chemotherapy. Additionally, effects on long-term reproductive health, lower fertility, hearing impairment, neuropathy, and Raynaud's phenomenon are long-term toxicities seen with chemotherapy use.
- Therapeutic radiation and chemotherapy are risk factors for cancers of thyroid, lymphoma, kidney, pancreas, stomach, and leukemia. There is also an increased risk for metabolic syndrome (insulin resistance, hypertension, dyslipidemia, abdominal obesity) after radiation or chemotherapy.

SUGGESTED READINGS

Available at ExpertConsult.com

RELATED CONTENT

Testicular Cancer (Patient Information)

AUTHOR: **BHARTI RATHORE, M.D.**

TABLE 1 International Germ Cell Consensus Criteria for Testicular Cancer

Nonseminoma	Seminoma
Good Prognosis	
Testis/retroperitoneal primary	Any primary site
And	*And*
No nonpulmonary visceral metastases	No nonpulmonary visceral metastases
And	*And*
Good markers—all of • AFP <1000 ng/ml and • hCG <5000 IU/L (1000 ng/ml) and • LDH <1.5 × upper limit of normal	Normal AFP, any hCG, any LDH
58% of nonseminomas	90% of seminomas
5-yr PFS 89%	5-yr PFS 82%
5-yr survival 92%	5-yr survival 86%
Intermediate Prognosis	
Testis/retroperitoneal primary	Any primary site
And	*And*
No nonpulmonary visceral metastases	Nonpulmonary visceral metastases
And	*And*
Intermediate markers—any of • AFP ≥1000 and ≤10,000 ng/ml or • hCG ≥5000 IU/L and ≤50,000 IU/L or • LDH ≥1.5 × normal and ≤10 × normal	Normal AFP, any hCG, any LDH
28% of nonseminomas	10% of seminomas
5-yr PFS 75%	5-yr PFS 67%
5-yr survival 80%	5-yr survival 72%
Poor Prognosis	
Mediastinal primary	No patients classified as
Or	poor prognosis
Nonpulmonary visceral metastases	
Or	
Poor markers—any of • AFP >10,000 ng/ml or • hCG >50,000 IU/L (10,000 ng/ml) or • LDH >10 × upper limit of normal	
16% of nonseminomas	
5-yr PFS 41%	
5-yr survival 48%	

AFP, α-fetoprotein; *hCG,* human chorionic gonadotrophin; *LDH,* lactate dehydrogenase; *PFS,* progression-free survival.
From Skarin AT: *Atlas of diagnostic oncology,* ed 4, St Louis, 2010, Mosby.

TABLE 2 TNM Staging for Testicular Cancer (*AJCC 8th Edition Staging Cancer Manual*)

pT Stage	Primary Tumor
pT_X	Primary tumor cannot be assessed
pT_0	No evidence of primary tumor
pT_{is}	Germ cell neoplasia *in situ*
pT_1	Tumor limited to testis (including rete testis invasion) without lymphovascular invasion pT_{1a}: Tumor smaller than 3 cm in size (seminoma only) pT_{1b}: Tumor 3 cm or larger in size (seminoma only)
pT_2	Tumor limited to testis (including rete testis invasion) with lymphovascular invasion OR tumor invading hilar soft tissue or epididymis or penetrating visceral mesothelial layer covering the external surface of tunica albuginea with or without lymphovascular invasion
pT_3	Tumor directly invades spermatic cord soft tissue with or without lymphovascular invasion
pT_4	Tumor invades scrotum with or without lymphovascular invasion
N Stage	**Regional Lymph Nodes**
N_x	Regional lymph nodes cannot be assessed
N_0	No regional lymph node metastasis
N_1	Metastasis with a lymph node mass 2 cm or smaller in greatest dimension OR multiple lymph nodes, none larger than 2 cm in greatest dimension
N_2	Metastasis with a lymph node mass larger than 2 cm but not larger than 5 cm in greatest dimension OR multiple lymph nodes, any one mass larger than 2 cm but not larger than 5 cm in greatest dimension
N_3	Metastasis with a lymph node mass larger than 5 cm in greatest dimension
M Stage	**Distant Metastasis**
M_0	No distant metastasis
M_1	Distant metastasis present M_{1a}: Nonretroperitoneal nodal or pulmonary metastases M_{1b}: Nonpulmonary visceral metastases
S	**Serum Tumor Markers**
S_x	Not available
S_0	Markers within normal levels
S_1	LDH <1.5 × N *and* hCG (mIU/ml) <5,000 *and* AFP (ng/ml) <1,000
S_2	LDH 1.5–10 × N *or* hCG (mIU/ml) 5,000–50,000 *or* AFP (ng/ml) 1,000–10,000
S_3	LDH >10 × N *or* hCG (mIU/ml) >50,000 *or* AFP (ng/ml) >10,000

AJCC, American Joint Committee on Cancer; *TNM,* tumor, necrosis, mestases.

TABLE 3 AJCC Prognostic Stage Groupings

Stage	T	N	M	S
0	pT_{is}	N_0	M_0	S_0
I	pT_{1-4}	N_0	M_0	S_X
I_A	pT_1	N_0	M_0	S_0
I_B	pT_{2-4}	N_0	M_0	S_0
I_S	Any T	N_0	M_0	S_{1-3}
II	Any T	N_{1-3}	M_0	S_X
II_A	Any T	N_1	M_0	S_0-S_1
II_B	Any T	N_2	M_0	S_0-S_1
II_C	Any T	N_3	M_0	S_0-S_1
III	Any T	Any N	M_1	S_X
III_A	Any T	Any N	M_{1a}	S_0-S_1
III_B	Any T	Any N	M_0-M_{1a}	S_2
III_C	Any T	Any N	M_0- M_{1a}	S_3
	Any T	Any N	M_{1b}	Any S

AJCC, American Joint Committee on Cancer.

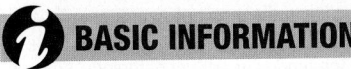

BASIC INFORMATION

DEFINITION

Testicular torsion is a twisting of the spermatic cord leading to cessation of testicular blood flow, ischemia, and infarction if left untreated.

SYNONYM

Spermatic cord torsion

ICD-10CM CODE
N44.03 Torsion of testis, unspecified

EPIDEMIOLOGY & DEMOGRAPHICS

INCIDENCE: Affects 1 in 4000 males <25 yr
PREDOMINANT AGE: Two thirds of all cases occur between the ages of 12 and 18 yr but may occur at any age, including antenatally.

PHYSICAL FINDINGS & CLINICAL PRESENTATION

- Typical sequence is sudden onset of hemiscrotal pain, then swelling, nausea, and vomiting without fever or urinary symptoms.
- Physical examination may reveal a tender firm testis, high-riding testis, horizontal lie of testis, absent cremasteric reflex, and no pain with elevation of testis. Absence of the cremasteric reflex (stroking or pinching the medial thigh causing contraction of cremaster muscle and elevation of testis) is the most sensitive physical finding.
- Painless testicular swelling occurs in 10%.
- One out of three patients reports previous episodes of spontaneously remitting scrotal pain.
- In the neonate, testicular torsion should be presumed in patients with a painless, discolored hemiscrotal swelling.
- In rare cases, torsion may involve an undescended testicle. In such situations an empty hemiscrotum is palpated with a tender lump in the inguinal area.

ETIOLOGY

- There are three types of testicular torsion: extravaginal, caused by nonadherence of the tunica vaginalis to the dartos layer; intravaginal torsion, caused by malrotation of the spermatic cord with the tunica vaginalis; and torsion of the testis below the epididymis. Intravaginal torsion accounts for 90% of cases.
- Torsion usually occurs in the absence of any precipitating events. Trauma accounts for <10% of cases.

Dx DIAGNOSIS

Diagnosis made mainly by clinical suspicion (Table E1). Color Doppler ultrasound evaluation or a nuclear testicular scan (Fig. E2) may help with diagnosis. Ultrasonography shows absent or decreased blood flow; scintigraphy reveals decreased perfusion on symptomatic side.

DIFFERENTIAL DIAGNOSIS

- Torsion of the testicular appendages (appendix testis)
- Testicular tumor
- Epididymitis
- Incarcerated inguinoscrotal hernia
- Orchitis
- Spermatocele
- Hydrocele, varicocele

WORKUP

The diagnosis is usually based on history and physical examination.

IMAGING STUDIES

- Doppler ultrasonic stethoscope (Doppler flowmetry) (Fig. E3)
- Radionuclide scrotal scanning (technetium-99m): Cold testicle (Fig. E2)

Rx TREATMENT

Surgical derotation of the spermatic cord followed by bilateral testicular fixation with nonabsorbable sutures. If affected testis is nonviable, orchiectomy of affected testis and orchiopexy of contralateral side are performed. Attempts at manual detorsion should not delay surgical consultation.

PROGNOSIS

- The degree of ischemia depends on the duration of torsion and the degree of rotation of the spermatic cord.
- There is an 80% testicular salvage rate if detorsion occurs within 12 hr of onset.
- After 24 hr, irreversible testicular infarction is expected.
- Because contralateral testes can be affected (immunologic process), if treatment delayed and blood flow does not return after detorsion, some recommend orchiectomy of the infarcted testicle.

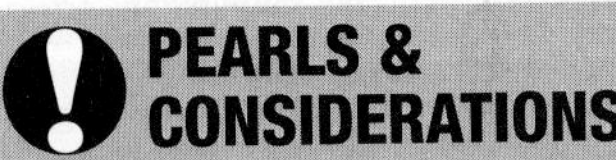

PEARLS & CONSIDERATIONS

- Manual detorsion by external rotation of the testis toward the thigh can be attempted for adolescent intravaginal torsion if an operating facility is not readily available.
- Extravaginal torsion is diagnosed in the newborn. Intravaginal torsion can occur at any age but is usually diagnosed in males ages 12 to 18 yr.

RELATED CONTENT

Testicular Torsion (Patient Information)

AUTHOR: **FRED F. FERRI, M.D.**

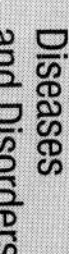

BASIC INFORMATION

DEFINITION

Thoracic outlet syndrome (TOS) describes a condition producing upper extremity symptoms believed to result from neurovascular compression at the thoracic outlet (Table 1). Three types are described on the basis of point of compression: (1) cervical rib and scalenus syndrome, in which abnormal scalene muscles or the presence of a cervical rib may cause compression; (2) costoclavicular syndrome, in which compression may occur under the clavicle; and (3) hyperabduction syndrome, in which compression may occur in the subcoracoid area. The compression occurs in three anatomical structures: arteries, veins, and nerves. TOS usually is caused by a combination of two factors: (1) having abnormal anatomy that creates compression in the thoracic outlet, (2) having some injury at the thoracic outlet.

- Neurogenic TOS: Caused by compression of brachial nerve plexus
- Arterial TOS: Caused by subclavian artery compression
- Venous TOS: Caused by compression of subclavian vein

SYNONYM

TOS

ICD-10CM CODE

G54.0 Brachial plexus disorders

EPIDEMIOLOGY & DEMOGRAPHICS

PREVALENCE: TOS is an uncommon disorder. Varies from source to source; presence of cervical ribs in 0.5% to 1% of population (50% bilateral), but most are asymptomatic. Approximately 90% of all TOS disorders are neurogenic, and the remaining 10% are arterial or venous.

PREDOMINANT SEX: Females affected more often than males (ratio of 3.5:1)

PREDOMINANT AGE: Rare in those aged <20 yr

PHYSICAL FINDINGS & CLINICAL PRESENTATION

- Symptoms and signs are related to the degree of involvement of each of the various structures at the level of the first rib.
- True venous or arterial involvement is not common.
- Diagnosis is most often used in the consideration of neural pain affecting the arm, which suggests involvement of the brachial plexus.
  1. Arterial compression: Pallor, paresthesias, diminished pulses, coolness, Raynaud's phenomenon, digital gangrene, supraclavicular bruit or mass, and stroke
  2. Venous compression: Edema and pain, thrombosis causing superficial venous dilation in the shoulder area
  3. Neurologic compression: Pain and/or paresthesia of neck, shoulder region, arm or hand, depending on the root involved with difficulty; intrinsic weakness and diminished sensation on examination
  4. Possible supraclavicular tenderness
  5. Provocative tests (Adson, Wright): May reproduce pain but are of disputed usefulness

ETIOLOGY

- Congenital cervical rib or fibrous extension of cervical rib
- Abnormal scalene muscle insertion
- Drooping of shoulder girdle from generalized hypotonia or trauma
- Narrowed costoclavicular interval as a result of downward and backward pressure on shoulder (sometimes seen in individuals who carry heavy backpacks), poor posturing, pregnancy
- Acute venous thrombosis with exercise (effort thrombosis)
- Bony abnormalities of first rib
- Abnormal fibromuscular bands
- Malunion of clavicle fracture

DIAGNOSIS

DIFFERENTIAL DIAGNOSIS

- Carpal tunnel syndrome
- Cervical radiculopathy
- Brachial neuritis
- Ulnar nerve compression (cubital tunnel syndrome)
- Complex regional pain syndrome
- Superior sulcus tumor

WORKUP

Fig. 1 describes a diagnostic algorithm for thoracic outlet syndrome. Preliminary criteria for the clinical diagnosis of neurogenic thoracic outlet syndrome are summarized in Table 2. Except for venous or arterial pathology, no ancillary diagnostic tests are reliable for diagnostic confirmation.

IMAGING STUDIES

- Electromyography, nerve conduction velocity studies to rule out carpal tunnel syndrome, cervical radiculopathy
- Ultrasound for initial evaluation for arterial or venous thoracic outlet syndrome
- Cervical spine radiographs to rule out cervical disk disease
- Chest radiograph to rule out lung tumor
- Computed tomography (CT) for detailed anatomical relationship of vascular structure to surrounding muscles and bones
- Contrast-enhanced magnetic angiography can be very useful in assessing vessel imaging while using provocative arm positions
- Arteriography or venography (Fig. E2) can be used for dynamic studies while performing upper extremity maneuvers and also performing thrombolysis, if needed

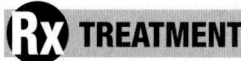

TREATMENT

ACUTE GENERAL Rx

- Sling for pain relief
- Physical therapy modalities plus shoulder girdle–strengthening exercises
- Postural reeducation
- Nonsteroidal antiinflammatory drugs
- Muscle relaxants

CHRONIC Rx

Surgical treatment is indicated:

- After failure of physical therapy
- With complications such as thrombosis, aneurysms
- With neurologic compressions
- With sympathetic cervical rib

Surgical options:

- Thoracic outlet decompression
- Cervical rib resection
- Thoracic sympathetectomy
- Vascular repair
- Catheter-directed thrombolysis

TABLE 1 Sites and Structures Compressed in Thoracic Outlet Syndrome

Site	Description	Abnormalities	Structures Compressed
Sternal-costovertebral circle	This aperture can be narrowed by bony variations	• Cervical first rib • First rib • Long transverse process	• Subclavian artery • Subclavian vein • Brachial plexus
Scalene muscle triangle	The scalenus anterior and middle muscle insert on the first rib, creating a tunnel	Scalenus anterior and middle	• Subclavian artery • Brachial plexus
First rib, clavicular space	The neurovascular structures lie above the rib and below the clavicle	• Costoclavicular ligament • Clavicle • First rib	• Subclavian vein • Subclavian artery • Brachial plexus
Behind the pectoralis minor muscle	The neurovascular structures travel to and from the arm behind this muscle	• Pectoralis minor • Costocoracoid ligament	• Subclavian vein • Subclavian artery • Brachial plexus

From Sellke FW et al: *Sabiston & Spencer surgery of the chest*, ed 9, Philadelphia, 2016, Elsevier.

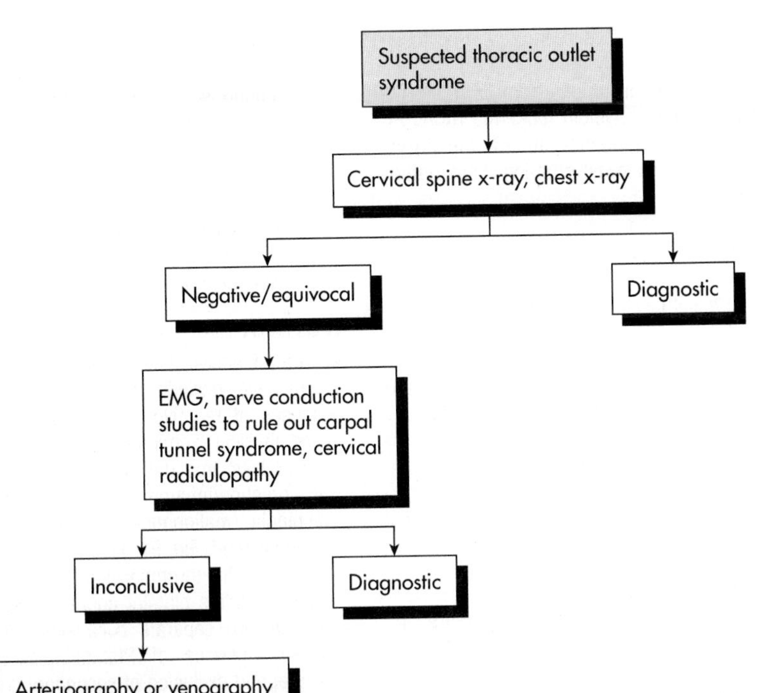

FIG. 1 Thoracic outlet syndrome. *EMG*, Electromyogram.

TABLE 2 Preliminary Criteria for the Clinical Diagnosis of Neurogenic Thoracic Outlet Syndrome

Unilateral or bilateral upper extremity symptoms that:
(1) Extend beyond the distribution of a single cervical nerve root or peripheral nerve
(2) Have been present for at least 12 wk
(3) Have not been explained satisfactorily by another condition
(4) Meet at least one criterion in at least four of the following five categories:

1. Principal symptoms	1A. Pain in the neck, upper back, shoulder, arm, or hand
	1B. Numbness; paresthesias; or weakness in the arm, hand, or digits
2. Symptom characteristics	2A. Pain, paresthesias, or weakness exacerbated with elevated arm positions
	2B. Pain, paresthesias, or weakness exacerbated by prolonged or repetitive arm or hand use or by prolonged work on a keyboard or other repetitive strain
	2C. Pain or paresthesias radiate down the arm from the supraclavicular or infraclavicular space
3. Clinical history	3A. Symptoms began after occupational, recreational, or accidental injury of the head, neck, or upper extremity, including repetitive upper extremity strain or overuse activity
	3B. Previous clavicle or first rib fracture or known cervical rib(s)
	3C. Previous cervical spine or peripheral nerve surgery without sustained improvement
	3D. Previous conservative or surgical treatment for thoracic outlet syndrome
4. Physical examination	4A. Local tenderness on palpation over scalene triangle or subcoracoid space
	4B. Arm, hand, or digit paresthesias on palpation over scalene triangle or subcoracoid space
	4C. Weak handgrip, intrinsic muscles, or digit 5 or thenar or hypothenar atrophy
5. Provocative maneuvers	5A. Positive upper limb tension test (ULTT)
	5B. Positive 1- or 3-min elevated arm stress test (EAST)

From Cameron JL, Cameron AM: *Current surgical therapy*, ed 12, Philadelphia, 2017, Elsevier.

DISPOSITION

- Nonsurgical treatment: Often successful for patients with pain as the primary symptom
- Complications of surgical treatment include transient dysesthesia, venous injury, arterial injuries, or brachial plexus injuries.

REFERRAL

For vascular surgery consultation when venous or arterial impairment is present

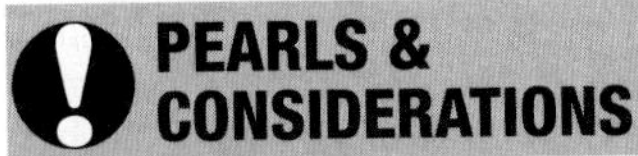

PEARLS & CONSIDERATIONS

COMMENTS

- True thoracic outlet syndrome is probably an uncommon condition.
- Diagnosis is often used to describe a wide variety of clinical symptoms.
- Considerable disagreement exists regarding the frequency of this disorder.

RELATED CONTENT

Thoracic Outlet Syndrome (Patient Information)

AUTHOR: **HISASHI TSUKADA, M.D., PH.D.**

BASIC INFORMATION

DEFINITION

Thrombocytosis is defined by an elevated platelet count (>450,000/ml) in peripheral blood. It is caused by overproduction of platelets (reactive thrombocytosis), or it may be caused by clonal expansion of megakaryocytes (clonal thrombocytosis). Reactive thrombocytosis is driven by excessive cytokines induced by various stimuli, such as trauma or inflammation. Clonal thrombocytosis is defined as chronic myeloproliferative neoplasms (MPNs), of which four subgroups are well characterized: chronic myelogenous leukemia (CML), polycythemia vera (PV), primary myelofibrosis (PMF), and essential thrombocythemia (ET). In addition, platelet count can be spuriously elevated in some conditions (see differential diagnosis). Extreme thrombocytosis is defined as platelet count >1 million/ml.

SYNONYMS

Thrombocythemia
Essential thrombocythemia
ET

ICD-10CM CODES

D47.3	Essential (hemorrhagic) thrombocythemia
D75.89	Other specified diseases of blood and blood-forming organs
D75.9	Disease of blood and blood-forming organs, unspecified
D77	Other disorders of blood and blood-forming organs in diseases classified elsewhere

EPIDEMIOLOGY & DEMOGRAPHICS

Reactive thrombocytosis is much more frequent than clonal thrombocytosis (70% vs. 22% in one series).

Epidemiology for essential thrombocytosis:

INCIDENCE: 2.5 cases/100,000 population/yr

PREVALENCE: Estimated as 24 cases/100,000 population

PREDOMINANT SEX AND AGE: The median age at diagnosis is 60 yr. Female:male ratio is 2:1.

PHYSICAL FINDINGS & CLINICAL PRESENTATION

- Regardless of the cause, a high platelet count may be associated with vasomotor symptoms such as headache, visual disturbances, dizziness, atypical chest pain, acral dysesthesia, and erythromelalgia.
- Thrombotic and bleeding complications can occur.
- Symptoms and complications are much more likely to occur in association with clonal thrombocytosis than reactive thrombocytosis.
- The degree of thrombocytosis does not predict the likelihood of clonal thrombocytosis and does not generally correlate to the risk of thrombosis.
- Splenomegaly is common with MPNs.
- Coexistent leukocytosis and erythrocytosis are common with CML and PV.
- Disease transformation from ET to PV, PMF, and acute myeloid leukemia (AML) is uncommon. In patients with ET, the 20-yr rate of leukemic transformation is estimated at 5%.

ETIOLOGY

- Essential thrombocytosis, a myeloproliferative neoplasm, is a clonal disorder of a multipotent hematopoietic progenitor cell.
- Abnormality in JAK2-STAT pathway (including *JAK2*, *CALR*, and *MPL* gene mutations) may play a role in pathogenesis of MPN.

DIAGNOSIS

DIFFERENTIAL DIAGNOSIS

- Spurious thrombocytosis:
  1. Mixed cryoglobulinemia
  2. Circulating cytoplasmic fragments in patients with leukemia, lymphoma, or severe hemolysis or burns can be counted as platelets
- Reactive thrombocytosis:
  1. Benign hematologic disorders
  2. Acute hemorrhage, iron deficiency anemia, hemolytic anemia
  3. Chronic infection, such as tuberculosis
  4. Acute and chronic inflammatory disorders
  5. Rheumatologic disorders
  6. Inflammatory bowel disease
  7. Celiac disease
  8. Functional and surgical asplenia
  9. Tissue damage
  10. Trauma, thermal burn
  11. Myocardial infarction
  12. Acute pancreatitis
  13. Recent surgery
  14. Renal failure, nephrotic syndrome
  15. Exercise
  16. Medications, such as vincristine, epinephrine
- Clonal thrombocytosis:
  1. CML
  2. PV
  3. PMF
  4. Myelodysplastic syndrome (5q-syndrome)
  5. AML with inv(3), t(3;3)
  6. Essential thrombocytosis (Box 1)

WORKUP

- Comprehensive history and physical examination to exclude many of the common causes of reactive thrombocytosis: History and physical examination suggestive of acute blood loss, iron deficiency, acute or chronic infection/inflammation, medication use, asplenia, malignancy, and trauma should be evaluated. Fig. E1 describes a diagnostic algorithm for thrombocytosis. The diagnosis of ET requires platelet counts $>450 \times 10^3$/ml on two separate occasions >4 weeks apart, absence of Philadelphia chromosome, and exclusion of secondary causes of thrombocytosis.
- Repeat CBC with peripheral blood smear and bone marrow biopsy (Figs. E2 and E3) to exclude spurious thrombocytosis.

LABORATORY TESTS

- CBC with peripheral blood smear: Howell-Jolly bodies and target cells are present in patients with asplenia; nucleated RBC, teardrop RBC and WBC precursors in patients with PMF
- Serum ferritin level: Low ferritin level suggests iron deficiency
- Serum C-reactive protein (CRP), ESR, and plasma fibrinogen: Nonspecific markers of infection or inflammation
- Philadelphia chromosome or BCR-ABL rearrangement: Positive in CML

BOX 1 World Health Organization Diagnostic Criteria for Essential Thrombocythemia

Diagnosis requires that all of the following criteria be met:

- Sustained platelet count $\geq 450 \times 10^9$/L[1]
- Bone marrow biopsy specimen showing proliferation mainly of the megakaryocytic lineage, with increased numbers of enlarged, mature megakaryocytes; no significant increase or left shift of neutrophil granulopoiesis or erythropoiesis
- Failure to meet the WHO criteria for polycythemia vera,[2] primary myelofibrosis,[3] BCR-ABL1–positive chronic myelogenous leukemia,[4] myelodysplastic syndrome,[5] or other myeloid neoplasms
- Demonstration of *JAK2 V617F* or other clonal marker; or, in the absence of *JAK2 V617F*, no evidence of reactive thrombocytosis[6]

[1]Sustained during the workup process.
[2]Requires the failure of iron replacement therapy to increase the hemoglobin level to the polycythemia vera range in the presence of decreased serum ferritin. Exclusion of polycythemia vera is based on hemoglobin and hematocrit levels; red cell mass measurement is not required.
[3]Requires the absence of relevant reticulin fibrosis, collagen fibrosis, peripheral blood leukoerythroblastosis, or markedly hypercellular marrow accompanied by megakaryocyte morphology typical for primary myelofibrosis—small to large megakaryocytes with an aberrant nuclear-to-cytoplasmic ratio and hyperchromatic, bulbous, or irregularly folded nuclei and dense clustering.
[4]Requires the absence of BCR-ABL1.
[5]Requires the absence of dyserythropoiesis and dysgranulopoiesis.
[6]Causes of reactive thrombocytosis include iron deficiency, splenectomy, surgery, infection, inflammation, connective tissue disease, metastatic cancer, and lymphoproliferative disorders.
WHO, World Health Organization.
From Swerdlow SH, et al. (eds): WHO classification of tumours of haematopoietic and lymphoid tissues, Lyon, France, 2008, IARC Press.

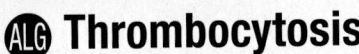

- Serum erythropoietin assay: Low to normal in PV and ET
- *JAK2* mutation analysis: PV and ET; *JAK2* mutation is found in 95% to 99% of patient with PV, in 40% to 60% of patients with PMF, and in about 50% to 55% of patients with ET
- MPL and CALR mutation analysis: Frequency is reported as 4% and 15% to 36%, respectively, in ET:
  1. These mutations are associated with differences in prognosis and risk of thrombosis.
  2. *JAK2, CALR,* and *MPL* mutations are mutually exclusive. They are not confined to a particular myeloproliferative neoplasm, and their absence does not exclude any of the MPNs.
  3. About 17% of patients with ET will be negative for *JAK2, CALR,* and *MPL* mutations.
- Bone marrow chromosome analysis: 5q-syndrome and other myelodysplastic syndrome, CML
- Bone marrow exam in ET may show clusters of abnormal megakaryocytes and increased reticulin fibrosis (see Fig. E3)

Rx TREATMENT

No therapies are known to alter survival or leukemic transformation in ET. Reactive thrombocytosis has been rarely associated with thrombosis or bleeding and generally does not require specific therapy.

ACUTE GENERAL Rx

- Vasomotor symptoms easily manageable with low-dose aspirin (<100 mg/day)
- Bleeding:
  1. Discontinue any platelet anti-aggregating agent, such as aspirin or nonsteroidal antiinflammatory agents.
  2. Evaluate for disseminated intravascular coagulopathy and coagulation factor deficiency. Acquired factor V deficiency is occasionally present in association with clonal thrombocytosis. In that case, treat with fresh frozen plasma infusion.
  3. In case of extreme thrombocytosis (platelet count generally >1,000,000/uL [1000×10^9/L]), acquired von Willebrand disease may occur. Immediate definitive therapy with a platelet-lowering agent is essential in this instance. Platelet pheresis should be reserved for cases of acute thrombosis or bleeding.
- Thrombosis:
  1. Arterial or venous thrombosis occurs in 20% to 30% of patients.
  2. If the platelet count is >800,000/ml, platelet apheresis coupled with a platelet-lowering agent should be considered with the goal of platelet count <400,000/mm^3.
  3. Anticoagulant therapy for 3 months to indefinite based on the presence or absence of additional thrombophilic defects.

CHRONIC Rx

Treatment strategies for ET are based on the presence or absence of risk factors for thrombosis. Smoking cessation and obesity management should be discussed with all patients with ET. In low-risk patients (age <60 yr, no history of thrombosis or hemorrhage, platelet count <1 million/ml), observation may be adequate. Treatment with low-dose aspirin is indicated in low-risk patients with vasomotor symptoms or with other indications for aspirin use. The cytoreductive therapy along with low-dose aspirin therapy is indicated in high-risk patients (age >60 yr and/or with previous history of thrombosis) regardless of vasomotor symptoms.

- Low-dose aspirin (81 mg/day) may be safe and effective in preventing vascular events. It is also effective in preventing recurrent vascular events in high-risk patients and in treating the vasomotor symptoms.
- Cytoreductive therapy (Table 1):
  1. Hydroxyurea (HU) versus anagrelide: HU plus aspirin is suggested to be safer and more effective than anagrelide plus aspirin in regard to thrombosis, bleeding, and transformation to PMF at 5 yr in a randomized trial. Monitor liver function tests and the degree of neutropenia or anemia with HU therapy.
  2. The incidence of leukemic conversion in patients with ET treated with HU alone is reported as <1%. Interferon alpha may be effective for controlling platelet count in patients failing treatment with HU.

TABLE 1 Choice of Drugs for Treatment of Patients with High-Risk Essential Thrombocythemia

Age (years)	Treatment of Choice	Second Line
<50	Interferon	Anagrelide Hydroxyurea
50-75	Hydroxyurea	Interferon Anagrelide
>75	Hydroxyurea	Anagrelide Busulfan

From Hoffman R, et al.: *Hematology, basic principles and practice*, ed 7, Philadelphia, 2018, Elsevier.

DISPOSITION

- Although long survival is expected in patients with ET, it is inferior to the sex- and age-matched U.S. population.
- An International Prognostic Score for Essential Thrombocythemia (IPSET) was proposed by International Working Group on Myelofibrosis Research and Treatment based on age, WBC count, and history of thromboembolism at diagnosis.

REFERRAL

Refer to hematologist/oncologist when platelet count is consistently elevated >450,000/mm^3 without causes for reactive thrombocytosis.

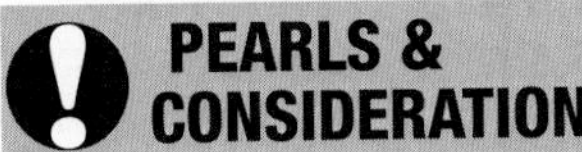

PEARLS & CONSIDERATION

COMMENTS

- Some patients with clinically apparent ET have Philadelphia chromosome or BCR-ABL rearrangement, even in the absence of other features of CML. It is suggested that it should be tested in all ET patients due to its potential therapeutic implications.
- The risk of bleeding with aspirin use in patients with ET is increased when the platelet count is >1 million/ml.

PATIENT & FAMILY EDUCATION

Smoking cessation is encouraged in both patients with ET and reactive thrombocytosis.

SUGGESTED READINGS

Available at ExpertConsult.com

AUTHOR: **JOHN L. REAGAN, M.D.**

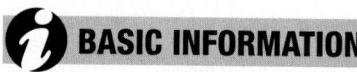

BASIC INFORMATION

DEFINITION

Superficial venous thrombophlebitis (SVT) is an inflammation of a vein with subsequent secondary thrombus formation. SVT most frequently involves superficial veins of the leg, but any superficial vein can be affected. SVT has been reported to occur in 125,000 people in the United States per year; however, the actual incidence is likely far greater. SVT is not always a benign condition. SVT should be regarded as the superficial venous manifestation of a systemic process known as venous thromboembolism (DVT, PE).

SYNONYMS

SVT
Superficial phlebitis
Superficial suppurative thrombophlebitis
Suppurative thrombophlebitis

ICD-10CM CODES

I80.00	Phlebitis and thrombophlebitis of superficial vessels of unspecified lower extremity
I80.8	Phlebitis and thrombophlebitis of other sites
I80.9	Phlebitis and thrombophlebitis of unspecified site

EPIDEMIOLOGY & DEMOGRAPHICS

- Approximately 30% to 45% of patients diagnosed with SVT are men with an average age of 54 yr.
- Approximately 55% to 70% of patients diagnosed with SVT are women with an average age of 58 yr.
- The overall recurrence of SVT is 18% over an average observation period of 15 mo, equally involving varicose and nonvaricose veins.
- The lifetime incidence of SVT in those with untreated varicose veins has been estimated at 25% to 50%.

PHYSICAL FINDINGS & CLINICAL PRESENTATION

- Subcutaneous vein is palpable as a tender cord or "wormlike" mass with increased warmth and erythema.
- Induration, redness, and tenderness are localized along the course of the vein. This linear appearance rather than circular appearance is useful to distinguish thrombophlebitis from other conditions (cellulitis, erythema nodosum).
- There is some swelling of the overlying skin and subcutaneous tissue but without generalized edema of the limb.
- Low-grade fever may be present.

ETIOLOGY

- In the lower extremity, 70% of SVT occurs in patients with varicose veins, with the great saphenous vein being most commonly involved (60% to 80%).
- Intravenous catheters and infusion of caustic drugs are the most common cause of upper-extremity SVT.
- Malignancy
- Pregnancy/puerperium
- Hypercoagulable states
- Previous
- DVT/SVT
- OCP (oral contraceptive pill)/HRT (hormone replacement therapy)

Dx DIAGNOSIS

DIFFERENTIAL DIAGNOSIS

Lymphangitis
Cellulitis
Erythema nodosum
Panniculitis
Acute lipodermatosclerosis

WORKUP

The clinical investigation includes not only the local findings but also the presence of varicose veins with or without the stigmata of chronic venous insufficiency. Today, duplex ultrasound is the most important additional diagnostic tool.

IMAGING STUDIES

- Duplex ultrasound offers the advantage of being inexpensive, noninvasive, and repeatable for follow-up examination.
- Ultrasonography confirms the diagnosis, shows the location of the thrombus and its location regarding the saphenofemoral and/or saphenopopliteal junctions.
- Ultrasound examination of patients with SVT has revealed that a concomitant DVT can exist in 15% to 20%.
- In up to 25% of these patients, the DVT may not be contiguous with the SVT and may be found in the contralateral leg.
- Therefore bilateral duplex exam is recommended in all cases of SVT that involve the main trunk of the great saphenous vein (GSV) or small saphenous vein (SSV).

Rx TREATMENT

NONPHARMACOLOGIC THERAPY

- Warm, moist compresses
- Do not restrict activity. Immediate mobilization with walking exercises

ACUTE GENERAL Rx

- Treatment guidelines for SVT are not well established because of the lack of controlled clinical trials. In general, the primary goal of management should be to prevent thrombus extension and the risk of venous thromboembolism. All other therapy is directed at patient comfort with analgesics and NSAIDs (in patients not receiving anticoagulants).
- In patients with migratory SVT, recurrent SVT, or SVT without varicose veins, the underlying condition should be investigated and treatment directed accordingly.
- The most common cause of upper-extremity SVT is an intravenous catheter. Treatment starts with removal of the cannula and application of warm compresses. The resultant lump may persist for months. No anticoagulant therapy is required.
- In patients with lower-extremity SVT in a varicose vein branch, control of pain with analgesics and the use of gradient compression stockings are usually sufficient. Patients are encouraged to continue their usual daily activities.
- Many investigators favor systemic anticoagulation when there is superficial thrombosis of 5 cm or more in length, the thrombus is within 1 cm of the saphenous junctions, or more than 5 cm of the saphenous trunk is involved, as shown by duplex ultrasonography. Anticoagulation is also reasonable for patients with SVT and cancer or previous DVT.
- The American College of Chest Physicians guidelines recommend anticoagulation for 45 days over no anticoagulation in patients with lower-extremity SVT within 1 cm of the saphenofemoral or saphenopopliteal junction.
- In the case of patients with varicose veins secondary to saphenous vein reflux, a catheter vein ablation procedure should be performed only after the acute SVT episode is over in order to avoid the thromboembolic complications induced by such procedures.

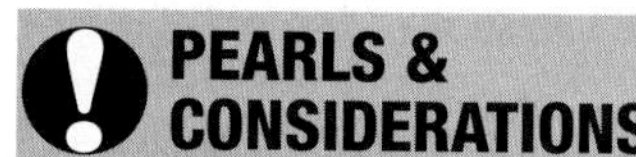

PEARLS & CONSIDERATIONS

SUPERFICIAL SUPPURATIVE THROMBOPHLEBITIS

- Superficial suppurative thrombophlebitis is associated with an intravenous catheter or multiple puncture sites secondary to IV drug abuse and is located primarily in the upper extremity.
- Clinical presentation is similar to that of nonsuppurative SVT but with associated fever, leukocytosis, and/or septicemia.
- Most cases of intravenous catheter sepsis are not complicated by suppurative thrombophlebitis; local IV catheter site infections occur in about 7% of cases and septicemia is found in only 1 of every 400 IV catheterizations.
- The incidence of peripheral vein suppurative thrombophlebitis is highest in patients with specific risk factors such as burns, steroids, and IV drug abuse.
- Treatment consists of antibiotics with adequate coverage of gram-negative rods and *Staphylococcus aureus,* including MRSA. Initial empirical treatment is with IV vancomycin 1 g q12h *plus* ceftriaxone 1 g IV q24h. Alternative regimen consists of daptomycin 6 mg/kg IV q 12h *plus* ceftriaxone 1 g IV q24h.

SUGGESTED READINGS

Available at ExpertConsult.com

RELATED CONTENT

Thrombophlebitis (Patient Information)
Deep Vein Thrombosis (Related Key Topic)

AUTHOR: **FRANK G. FORT, M.D., F.A.C.S., R.PH.S.**

BASIC INFORMATION

DEFINITION

Thrombotic thrombocytopenic purpura (TTP) is a rare disorder characterized by thrombocytopenia and microangiopathic hemolytic anemia; other hallmarks of the classic "pentad" such as neurologic impairment, renal dysfunction, and fever may also be present. The laboratory hallmark of TTP is a severe deficiency of the ADAMTS13 factor (activity <10%).

SYNONYM

TTP

ICD-10CM CODE
M31.1 Thrombotic microangiopathy

EPIDEMIOLOGY & DEMOGRAPHICS

- About 90% of new TTP cases are seen in adults (mostly females aged between 18 and 50 yr).
- The incidence of new TTP is 3-11 cases per million population per year. The prevalence is ~10 cases per million population.
- There is increased incidence in HIV/AIDS and during pregnancy.

PHYSICAL FINDINGS & CLINICAL PRESENTATION

- The disease often begins as a flulike illness ultimately followed by clinical and laboratory abnormalities.
- Most patients present with nonspecific constitutional symptoms (weakness, nausea, abdominal pain, vomiting).
- Purpura (secondary to thrombocytopenia).
- Jaundice, pallor (from hemolysis).
- Mucosal bleeding.
- Fever.
- Fluctuating levels of consciousness (caused by thrombotic occlusion of the cerebral vessels). However, one third of patients have no neurologic abnormalities.
- Renal failure and neurologic events are usually end-stage features.

ETIOLOGY

- Acquired TTP is an autoimmune disorder caused by autoantibody inhibition of ADAMTS13 activity. Hereditary TTP (also called Upshaw-Schulman syndrome) is caused by homozygous or compound heterozygous ADAMTS13 mutations (Table 1).
- Many drugs, including clopidogrel, ticlopidine, penicillin, antineoplastic agents (gemcitabine, mitomycin C), calcineurin inhibitors (cyclosporine), oral contraceptives, and quinine, have been associated with TTP.
- Other precipitating causes include infectious agents, pregnancy, malignancies, allogeneic stem cell transplantation, and neurologic disorders.

DIAGNOSIS

DIFFERENTIAL DIAGNOSIS

It is challenging to differentiate TTP from other thrombotic microangiopathies given the significant overlap in clinical presentation, but this distinction is critical in selecting an appropriate therapy for patients.

- Disseminated intravascular coagulation (DIC)
- Malignant hypertension
- Vasculitis
- Eclampsia or preeclampsia
- Hemolytic-uremic syndrome (HUS) and atypical HUS
- Gastroenteritis as a result of a serotoxin-producing serotype of *Escherichia coli*

WORKUP

- A comprehensive history, physical examination, and laboratory evaluation usually confirm the diagnosis (Fig. 1).

LABORATORY TESTS

- Severe anemia and thrombocytopenia (platelet count <50,000 or >50% reduction from previous counts).
- Peripheral blood smear (Fig. E2, Fig. E3) reveals numerous red cell fragments (schistocytes).
- Elevated blood urea nitrogen and creatinine.
- Evidence of hemolysis: Elevated reticulocyte count, indirect bilirubin, lactate dehydrogenase, decreased haptoglobin.
- Urinalysis: Hematuria (red blood cells [RBCs] and RBC casts in urine sediment) and proteinuria.
- Peripheral smear: Severely fragmented RBCs (schistocytes). More than 4% RBC fragments in the peripheral blood.
- No laboratory evidence of DIC (normal fibrin degradation product, fibrinogen).
- The diagnosis of hereditary TTP requires documentation of ADAMTS13 deficiency and an absence of ADAMTS13 autoantibody inhibitor, and confirmation requires documentation of ADAMTS13 mutations. Diagnostic criteria for acquired TTP are the presence of microangiopathic hemolytic anemia and thrombocytopenia without another apparent cause. An ADAMTS13 level indicating less than 10% of normal activity supports the clinical diagnosis of acquired TTP while moderately decreased levels of >20% suggest the presence of other diagnoses.

TREATMENT

ACUTE GENERAL Rx

- Discontinue potential offending agents. Initiate ADAMTS13 replacement by plasma infusion in patients with hereditary TTP.
- Daily therapeutic plasma exchange (TPE) with replacement of 1.0 to 1.5 times the predicted plasma volume of the patient is standard therapy for TTP. TPE should be continued for a minimum of 2 days after the platelet count returns to normal (>150,000 cells/m^3).
- High-dose plasma infusion (25 ml/kg/day) may be useful only if TPE cannot be promptly started and for patients with very severe or refractory disease between plasma exchange sessions. High-dose plasma infusions can cause volume overload in patients with renal insufficiency.
- Patients with hereditary TTP who experience severe plasma allergic reactions have been effectively treated with plasma-derived factor VIII concentrate that contains ADAMTS13.
- Corticosteroids (prednisone 1-2 mg/kg/day) are administered concomitantly with TPE, typically for a period of 3 to 4 weeks.
- The monoclonal anti-CD20 antibody rituximab has been traditionally used for treatment of suboptimally responsive TTP and results in remissions in the majority of patients. Frontline use of rituximab results in shorter hospitalization with fewer relapses but is likely resulting in overtreatment in many cases.

TABLE 1 Etiology, Epidemiology, and Pathogenesis of TTP, HUS, and ADAMTS13–Related Parameters

	Congenital TTP	Acquired TTP	HUS
Etiology	ADAMTS13 mutation	Antibody to ADAMTS13, endothelial cell activation	*Escherichia coli* or other microorganisms
Epidemiology	5-10 cases per year per million	≤1 case per year per million	1-5 cases per year per million, mainly in children
Pathogenesis	Defective cleavage of vWF multimers, massive secretion of ultra-large vWF multimers, increased platelet deposition under shear condition, occlusion of blood vessels in microcirculation		Intoxication with Shiga-like toxin, damage of endothelial cells, enterohemorrhagic colitis, renal disorder
ADAMTS13 antigen	Very low or absent	Low or variable	Normal or moderately decreased
ADAMTS13 activity	≤5%-10%	≤5%-10% or variable	30%-100%
Inhibitor against ADAMTS13	No	Mostly yes	No

ADAMTS13, A disintegrin and metalloproteinase with a thrombospondin type 1 motif, member 13; *HUS*, hemolytic uremic syndrome; *TTS*, thrombotic thrombocytopenic purpura; *vWF*, von Willebrand factor.
From McPherson RA, Pincus MR: *Henry's clinical diagnosis and management by laboratory methods*, ed 23, Philadelphia, 2017, Elsevier.

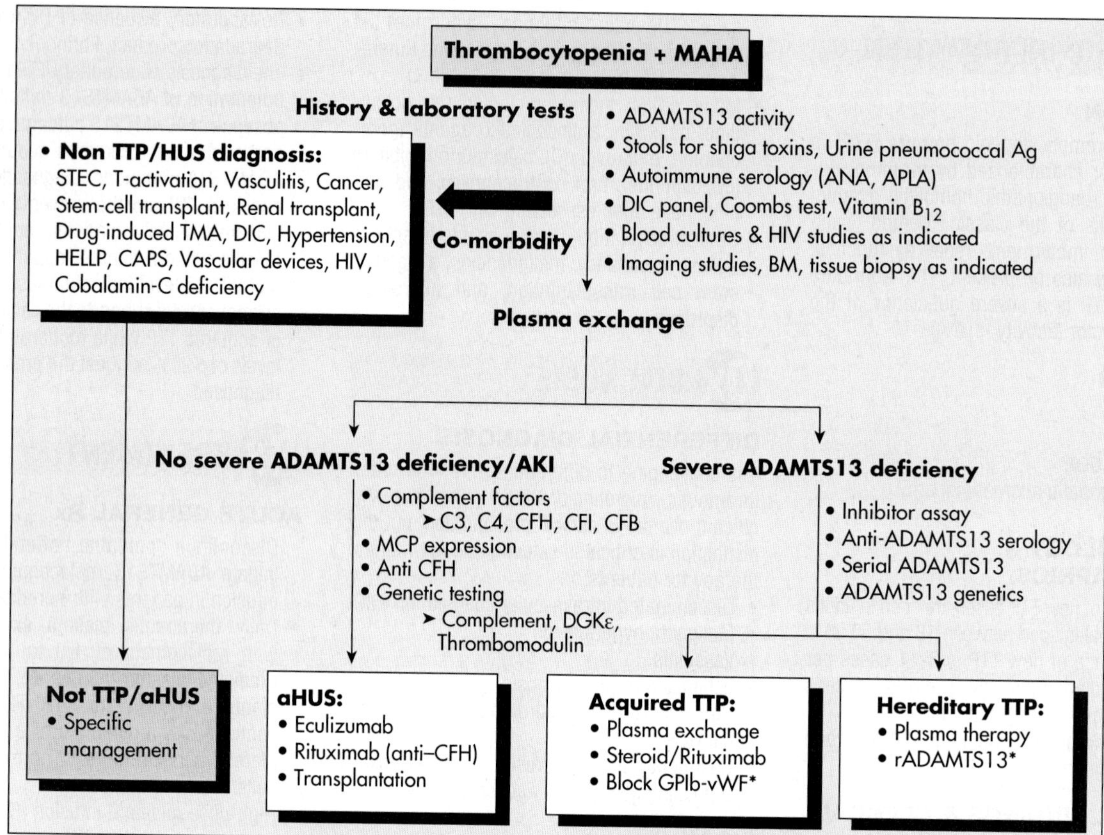

FIG. 1 An approach to diagnosis and management of thrombotic microangiopathies. *ADAMTS13*, A disintegrin and metalloproteinase with thrombospondin type 1 motifs, member 13; *Ag*, antigen; *aHUS*, atypical hemolytic uremic syndrome; *AKI*, acute kidney injury; *ANA*, antinuclear antibody; *APLA*, antiphospholipid antibodies; *BM*, bone marrow; *CAPS*, catastrophic antiphospholipid syndrome; *CFB*, complement factor B; *CFH*, complement factor H; *CFI*, complement factor I; *DGKE*, diacyl glycerol kinase ε; *DIC*, disseminated intravascular coagulation; *GP*, glycoprotein; *HELLP*, hemolysis, elevated liver enzymes, and low platelet count; *HIV*, human immunodeficiency virus; *HUS*, hemolytic uremic syndrome; *MAHA*, macroangiopathic hemolytic anemia; *MCP*, membrane cofactor protein; *rADAMTS13*, recombinant ADAMTS13; *STEC*, Shiga toxin-producing *E. coli*; *TMA*, thrombotic microangiopathy; *TTP*, thrombotic thrombocytopenic purpura; *vWF*, von Willebrand factor. *Bullet points* are diagnoses or therapies. *Indicates therapies under investigation. (From Hoffman R, et al.: *Hematology, basic principles and practice*, ed 7, Philadelphia, 2018, Elsevier.)

- Caplacizumab, an anti-von Willebrand factor, humanized, bivalent variable-domain-only immunoglobulin fragment. Inhibits the interaction between von Willebrand factor multimers and platelets. In a recent trial, treatment with caplacizumab was associated with faster normalization of the platelet count and a lower incidence of a composite of TTP-related death.[1]
- Platelet transfusions are contraindicated except in severely thrombocytopenic patients with documented bleeding or those who are facing surgery or other invasive procedures in the setting of severe thrombocytopenia.
- Use of antiplatelet agents (acetylsalicylic acid, dipyridamole) is controversial.
- Splenectomy is performed in refractory cases.
- Dialysis is rarely required.

CHRONIC Rx

- Relapsing TTP may be initially retreated with TPE.

[1] Scully M, et al.: Caplacizumab treatment for acquired thrombotic thrombocytopenic purpura, *N Engl J Med* 380(4):335–346, 2019.

- TTP unresponsive to conventional therapy is usually effectively treated with rituximab and occasionally with chemotherapy agents (vincristine, cyclophosphamide).
- Splenectomy done while patients are in remission has been used historically to decrease the frequency of relapses.

DISPOSITION

- Survival of patients with TTP currently exceeds 80% with TPE.
- Relapse occurs in 20% to 40% of patients who have achieved initial remission.

PEARLS & CONSIDERATIONS

COMMENTS

- The diagnosis of TTP should be considered in pregnant women with vague neurologic, gastrointestinal, or renal symptoms in either the obstetric triage or emergency department areas.
- TTP is fatal in 90% of patients without therapy.
- Phase 2 trials with caplacizumab, an anti–von Willebrand factor humanized single-variable-domain immunoglobulin used in patients with acquired TTP, have shown that it induces a faster resolution of the acute TTP episode than placebo, and the platelet-protective effect was maintained during the treatment period.
- Case reports have suggested a benefit of the proteasome inhibitor bortezomib, possibly due to elimination of the autoreactive plasma cells producing anti-ADAMTS13 antibodies in patients who are refractory to TPE and rituximab administration.

SUGGESTED READINGS

Available at ExpertConsult.com

RELATED CONTENT

Hemolytic Uremic Syndrome (Related Key Topic)

AUTHOR: **BHARTI RATHORE, M.D.**

BASIC INFORMATION

DEFINITION

Thyroid carcinoma is a primary neoplasm of the thyroid and consists of four major subtypes: papillary, follicular, anaplastic, and medullary.

SYNONYMS

Papillary carcinoma of thyroid
Follicular carcinoma of thyroid
Anaplastic carcinoma of thyroid
Medullary carcinoma of thyroid

ICD-10CM CODES

C73	Malignant neoplasm of thyroid gland
D09.3	Carcinoma in situ of thyroid and other endocrine glands
D34	Benign neoplasm of thyroid gland
D44.0	Neoplasm of uncertain behavior of thyroid gland

EPIDEMIOLOGY & DEMOGRAPHICS

- Thyroid cancer is the most common endocrine cancer, with an estimated 53,990 new cases and 2060 deaths occurring in 2018 in the U.S.
- Incidence is 13.9 per 100,000 people in the U.S. and increasing over last 4 decades.
- Female:male ratio is 3:1.
- Median age at diagnosis: 45 to 50 yr.
- Occult thyroid cancer is identified in 20% of autopsy specimens.

PHYSICAL FINDINGS & CLINICAL PRESENTATION

Thyroid cancer is often identified incidentally. Physical exam may reveal:

- Presence of thyroid nodule
- Hoarseness and cervical lymphadenopathy
- Painless swelling in the region of the thyroid

ETIOLOGY

- Risk factors: Prior neck irradiation.
- Multiple endocrine neoplasia II (medullary carcinoma).
- Inherited syndromes associated with thyroid cancer are described in Table 1.
- GLP-1 receptor agonists for the treatment of type 2 DM (e.g., exenatide, albiglutide) can increase the risk of medullary thyroid carcinoma (MTC).

TABLE 1 Inherited Syndromes Associated with Thyroid Cancer

Multiple endocrine neoplasia (MEN) 2A and 2B
Isolated familial medullary thyroid cancer
Gardner syndrome
Familial adenomatous polyposis
Carney complex
Cowden syndrome
Familial nonmedullary thyroid cancer

From Cameron JL, Cameron AM: *Current surgical therapy*, ed 10, Philadelphia, 2011, Saunders.

- Although formerly thought to be a single entity, papillary thyroid carcinoma encompasses several tumor types that have mutually exclusive mutations. BRAF V600E accounts for 60% of these mutations.
- Pathways to the development of thyroid cancer are depicted in Fig. E1.

Dx DIAGNOSIS

DIFFERENTIAL DIAGNOSIS

- Multinodular goiter
- Lymphocytic thyroiditis
- Ectopic thyroid

WORKUP

The workup of thyroid carcinoma includes laboratory evaluation and diagnostic imaging. Diagnosis is confirmed with fine-needle aspiration or surgical biopsy. At diagnosis, the vast majority of thyroid cancers are well differentiated, with excellent prognosis. The characteristics of thyroid carcinoma vary with the type:

- Papillary carcinoma (85%):
  1. Most frequently occurs in women during second or third decades
  2. Histologically, psammoma bodies (calcific bodies present in papillary projections) are pathognomonic; found in 35% to 45% of papillary thyroid carcinomas
  3. Majority are not papillary lesions but mixed papillary follicular carcinomas
  4. Spread is by lymphatics and by local invasion
- Follicular carcinoma (10%):
  1. More aggressive than papillary carcinoma
  2. Incidence increases with age
  3. Tends to metastasize hematogenously to bone, producing pathologic fractures
  4. Tends to concentrate iodine (useful for radiation therapy)
- Anaplastic carcinoma (1%):
  1. Very aggressive neoplasm
  2. Two major histologic types: Small cell (less aggressive, 5-yr survival approximately 20%) and giant cell (death usually within 6 mo of diagnosis)
- MTC (4%):
  1. Unifocal lesion: Found sporadically in elderly patients
  2. Bilateral lesions: Associated with pheochromocytoma and hyperparathyroidism; this combination is known as MEN-II and is inherited as an autosomal-dominant disorder

LABORATORY TESTS

- Thyroid function studies are generally normal. Thyroid-stimulating hormone (TSH), T4, and serum thyroglobulin levels should be obtained before thyroidectomy in patients with confirmed thyroid carcinoma. Serum thyroglobulin levels can be useful postoperatively to monitor recurrence of thyroid carcinoma (Fig. E2).
- Increased plasma calcitonin assay in patients with medullary carcinoma (tumors produce thyrocalcitonin). RET proto-oncogene sequencing and measurement of plasma free metanephrine and normetanephrine levels to rule out coexistent pheochromocytoma are recommended in all patients with medullary thyroid cancer.
- Fine-needle aspiration biopsy is the best method to assess a thyroid nodule (see "Thyroid Nodule" in Section I).

IMAGING STUDIES (FIG. E3)

- Thyroid ultrasound can detect solitary solid nodules that have a high risk of malignancy. However, a negative ultrasound does not exclude diagnosis of thyroid carcinoma.
- Thyroid scanning with iodine-123 or technetium-99m can identify hypofunctioning (cold) nodules, which are more likely to be malignant. However, warm nodules can also be malignant.

STAGING

- Stage I: Thyroid cancer of any size without distal spread in patient <45 yr. In patients >45 yr, tumor size ≤2 cm without local invasion or positive cervical lymph nodes
- Stage II: Distal spread in patient <45 yr. In patients >45 yr, tumors >2 cm but <4 cm without local invasion or positive cervical lymph nodes
- Stage III: Tumors >4 cm in patient >45 yr of age
- Stage IV: Distal spread in patient >45 yr of age

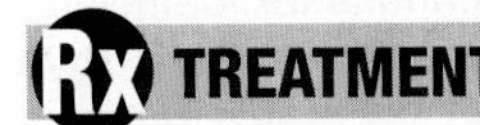

TREATMENT

ACUTE GENERAL Rx

- Papillary carcinoma:
  1. Total thyroidectomy is indicated if the patient has:
     a. Extrapyramidal extension of carcinoma
     b. Papillary carcinoma limited to thyroid but a positive history of irradiation to the neck
     c. Lesion >2 cm
  2. Lobectomy with isthmectomy may be considered in patients with intra-thyroid papillary carcinoma <2 cm and no history of neck or head irradiation; surgery should be followed with suppressive therapy with thyroid hormone because these tumors are TSH responsive. The accepted practice is to suppress serum TSH concentrations to <0.1 microunit/ml in patients with persistent disease, suppression to 0.1 to 0.5 microunit/ml in patients who are disease free but are at high risk of recurrence, and a goal TSH level of 0.3 to 2.0 microunits/ml in patients who are disease free and have a low risk of recurrence.
  3. Radioiodine ablation reduces rates of death and recurrence (Table 2). Radioiodine is administered for stages III and IV disease.
  4. In cases that have progressed after radioiodine therapy, oral targeted inhibitors (lenvantinib, sorafenib) have significant survival benefit.

- Follicular carcinoma:
  1. Total thyroidectomy followed by TSH suppression, as previously noted.
  2. Radiotherapy with iodine-131 followed by thyroid suppression therapy with triiodothyronine is useful in patients with metastasis (Table 2).
  3. In cases that have progressed after radioiodine therapy, oral targeted inhibitors (lenvantinib, sorafenib) have significant survival benefit.
- Anaplastic carcinoma:
  1. At diagnosis, this neoplasm is rarely operable; palliative surgery is indicated for extremely large tumor compressing the trachea.
  2. Management is usually restricted to radiation therapy or chemotherapy (combination of doxorubicin, cisplatin, and other antineoplastic agents) (Table 2); these measures rarely provide significant palliation.
- Medullary carcinoma:
  1. Thyroidectomy should be performed, followed by TSH suppression.
  2. Vandetanib and cabozantinib are oral tyrosine kinase inhibitors that are FDA-approved for treatment of symptomatic or progressive, unresectable, locally advanced or metastatic medullary thyroid cancer.
  3. Patients and their families should be screened for pheochromocytoma and hyperparathyroidism.

DISPOSITION

Overall 5 yr survival rate is 98.17, but prognosis varies with the type of thyroid carcinoma: 5-yr survival is over 80% for follicular carcinoma and is approximately 5% with anaplastic carcinoma (see Table 3).

PEARLS & CONSIDERATIONS

COMMENTS

- Follow-up surveillance involves neck ultrasound 6-12 mo after initial treatment and periodically and lab evaluation with TSH, serum thyroglobulin (T8), and thyroglobulin anitobdy (T8 Ab).
- Family members of patients with medullary carcinoma should be screened; DNA analysis for the detection of mutations in the *RET* gene structure permits the identification of *MEN IIA* gene carriers.
- While there is little controversy regarding the benefit of radioactive iodine in iodine-avid advanced-stage well-differentiated thyroid cancer, the indications for radioactive iodine following total thyroidectomy in patients with very low risk disease is controversial. Proponents argue that its use may destroy microscopic metastases, while opponents counter that the risk of secondary cancer due to radioactive iodine is not warranted in patients whose prognosis is typically excellent.
- Metastatic thyroid cancers that are refractory to radioiodine (iodine-131) are associated with a poor prognosis.
- Small-molecule tyrosine kinase inhibitors, including vandetanib, cabozantinib, sorafenib, and lenvatinib, are now FDA-approved and have shown clinical benefit with improved survival in advanced differentiated and medullary thyroid cancer.
- Targeted therapy with a combined regimen of BRAF inhibitors and MEK inhibitors (dabrafenib plus trametinib) is efficacious and approved in patients with metastatic BRAFV600E-mutated anaplastic thyroid cancer.

SUGGESTED READINGS

Available at ExpertConsult.com

RELATED CONTENT

Thyroid Cancer (Patient Information)
Thyroid Nodule (Related Key Topic)

AUTHOR: **BHARTI RATHORE, M.D.**

TABLE 2 Indications for Iodine-131 Treatment in Patients with Papillary, Follicular, or Hürthle Cell Thyroid Carcinoma after Initial Definitive Near-Total Thyroidectomy

No Indication
Adult patients at very low risk for cause-specific mortality or relapse: complete surgical resection, favorable histology, and limited extent of disease (e.g., PTC patients with MACIS scores <6; patients with tumor size <1 cm, N0, and M0).
Definite Indications
Distant metastasis at diagnosis
Incomplete tumor resection
Complete tumor resection but high risk for mortality or recurrence (e.g., PTC patients with MACIS scores ≥6 and pTNM stage II/III FTC or HCC)
Probable Indications
Incomplete surgery (less than near-total thyroidectomy, no lymph node dissection)
PTC or FTC in a child younger than 16 yr
If PTC, tall cell or columnar cell variant and diffuse sclerosing variant
If FTC, widely invasive or poorly differentiated tumor
Bulky nodal metastases

FTC, Follicular thyroid carcinoma; *HCC,* Hürthle cell carcinoma; *MACIS,* scoring system based on metastasis, age, completeness of resection, invasion, and size; *PTC,* papillary thyroid carcinoma; *pTNM,* pathologic tumor-node-metastasis classification.
From Melmed S, et al. (eds): *Williams textbook of endocrinology,* ed 12, Philadelphia, 2011, Saunders.

TABLE 3 Characteristics of Thyroid Cancers

Type of Cancer	Percentage of Thyroid Cancers	Age of Onset (Yr)	Treatment	Prognosis
Papillary	88	40-80	Thyroidectomy, followed by radioactive iodine ablation and TSH suppression	Good
Follicular	10	45-80	Thyroidectomy, followed by radioactive iodine ablation and TSH suppression	Fair to good
Medullary	3-4	20-50	Thyroidectomy and central compartment lymph node dissection and TSH suppression	Fair
Anaplastic	1	50-80	Isthmusectomy followed by palliative x-ray treatment	Poor
Lymphoma	<1	25-70	X-ray therapy and/or chemotherapy	Fair

From Andreoli TE, et al.: *Andreoli and Carpenter's Cecil essentials of medicine,* ed 8, Philadelphia, 2010, Saunders.

BASIC INFORMATION

DEFINITION

A thyroid nodule is an abnormality found on physical examination of the thyroid gland; nodules can be benign (70%) or malignant.

ICD-10CM CODES

E04.1	Nontoxic single thyroid nodule.
E05.2	Thyrotoxicosis with toxic single thyroid nodule.
E05.11	Thyrotoxicosis with toxic single thyroid nodule with thyrotoxic crisis or storm

EPIDEMIOLOGY & DEMOGRAPHICS

- Thyroid nodules are detected in 40% of the U.S. population.
- Thyroid nodules can be found in 50% of autopsies; however, only one in 10 is palpable.
- Malignancy is present in 5% to 15% of all thyroid nodules and in 7% to 9% of palpable nodules.
- Incidence of thyroid nodules increases after 45 yr. They are found more frequently in women (5% of women; 1% of men).
- History of prior head and neck irradiation increases the risk of thyroid cancer.
- Increased likelihood that nodule is malignant: Nodule increasing in size or >3 cm, regional lymphadenopathy, fixation to adjacent tissues, age <40 yr, symptoms of local invasion (dysphagia, hoarseness, neck pain, male sex, family history of thyroid cancer or polyposis [Gardner syndrome]), rapid growth during levothyroxine therapy, microcalcification within the nodule, and high intranodular vascular flow.

PHYSICAL FINDINGS & CLINICAL PRESENTATION

- Palpable, firm, and nontender nodule in the thyroid area should prompt suspicion of carcinoma. Signs of metastasis are regional lymphadenopathy and inspiratory stridor.
- Signs and symptoms of thyrotoxicosis can be found in functioning nodules.

ETIOLOGY

- History of prior head and neck irradiation
- Family history of pheochromocytoma, carcinoma of the thyroid, and hyperparathyroidism (medullary carcinoma of the thyroid is a component of MEN-II)

Dx DIAGNOSIS

DIFFERENTIAL DIAGNOSIS

- Thyroid carcinoma
- Multinodular goiter
- Thyroglossal duct cyst
- Epidermoid cyst
- Laryngocele
- Nonthyroid neck neoplasm
- Branchial cleft cyst

WORKUP

- Ultrasonography is an inexpensive and effective modality to stratify malignancy risk.
- Fine-needle aspiration (FNA) biopsy is the best diagnostic study; the accuracy can be >90%, but it is directly related to the level of experience of the physician and the cytopathologist interpreting the aspirate. FNA is not routinely recommended for thyroid nodules <1 cm in diameter unless there are significant risk factors (see above).
- FNA biopsy is less reliable with thyroid cystic lesions; surgical excision should be considered for most thyroid cysts not abolished by aspiration.
- A diagnostic approach to thyroid nodule is described in Fig. 1. Preoperative, ultrasonically guided FNA accurately classifies 62% to 85% of thyroid nodules as benign; however, 15% to 30% of aspirations yield indeterminate cytologic findings. Table 1 describes the probability of malignancy at histology based on FNA biopsy cytology.

LABORATORY TESTS

- Serum TSH should be obtained in all patients with thyroid nodules. If suppressed, obtain free T4 and free T3 and thyroid scan to rule out "hot nodule," indicative of hyperthyroid adenoma. Less than 1% of hyperfunctioning nodules are malignant. Typically FNA biopsy is not necessary in hot nodules.
- Thyroid-stimulating hormone (TSH), T4, and serum thyroglobulin levels should be obtained before thyroidectomy in patients with confirmed thyroid carcinoma on FNA biopsy.
- Serum calcitonin at random or after pentagastrin stimulation is useful when suspecting medullary carcinoma of the thyroid and in anyone with a family history of medullary thyroid carcinoma.
- Serum thyroid autoantibodies (see "Thyroiditis" in Section I) are useful in patients with multinodular goiter and when suspecting thyroiditis.
- Molecular analysis of thyroid tissue for the presence of *BRAF* and *RAS* mutations and for *RET/PTC* and *PAX8-PPAR* gamma 1 gene rearrangements can be used as a diagnostic tool, since 60% to 70% of thyroid cancers harbor at least one genetic mutation. The gene expression classifier profile can be used to identify a subpopulation of patients with a low likelihood of cancer, thereby avoiding unnecessary surgery in patients with indeterminate FNA. The gene expression classifier test has a high negative predictive value for cytologically indeterminate nodules (95% for an atypical or follicular lesion of undetermined significance, 94% for a follicular neoplasm, and 85% for a lesion suggestive of cancer).

IMAGING STUDIES

- Thyroid ultrasound (Fig. E2) is useful to evaluate the size of the thyroid and the number, composition (solid versus cystic), and dimensions of the thyroid nodule; solid thyroid nodules have a higher incidence of malignancy, but cystic nodules can also be malignant. The three characteristics on thyroid ultrasound most predictive of cancer are nodules >2 cm, microcalcifications, and entirely solid nodules.
- Thyroid scan can be performed with technetium-99m pertechnetate, iodine-123, or iodine-131. Iodine isotopes are preferred because up to 35% of nodules that appear functioning on pertechnetate scanning may appear nonfunctioning on radioiodine scanning. A thyroid scan:
  1. Classifies nodules as hyperfunctioning (hot), normally functioning (warm), or nonfunctioning (cold); cold nodules have a higher incidence of malignancy.
  2. Scan has difficulty evaluating nodules near the thyroid isthmus or at the periphery of the gland.
  3. Normal tissue over a nonfunctioning nodule might mask the nodule as "warm" or normally functioning.
- Both thyroid scan and ultrasound provide information about the risk of malignant neoplasia based on the characteristics of the thyroid nodule, but their value in the initial evaluation of a thyroid nodule is limited because neither provides a definite tissue diagnosis.

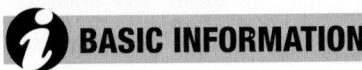

TREATMENT

GENERAL Rx

- Evaluation of results of FNA:
  1. Normal cells: May repeat biopsy during present evaluation or reevaluate patient after 3 to 6 mo of suppressive therapy (L-thyroxine, prescribed in doses to suppress the TSH level to 0.1-0.5).
     a. Failure to regress indicates increased likelihood of malignancy.
     b. Reliance on repeat FNA biopsy is preferable to routine surgery for nodules not responding to thyroxine.
- Indeterminate: Use of gene expression classifier profile. If suspicious, perform surgery; if benign, monitor with subsequent repeat FNA and gene expression classifier profile.
- Malignant cells: Surgery.

DISPOSITION

Variable with results of FNA biopsy

REFERRAL

Surgical referral for FNA biopsy

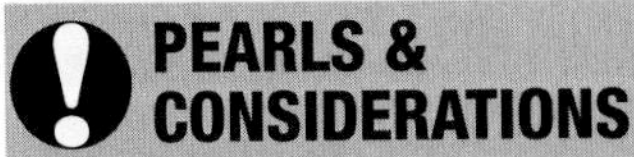

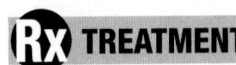

PEARLS & CONSIDERATIONS

COMMENTS

- Most solid, benign nodules grow; therefore, an increase in nodule volume alone is not a reliable predictor of malignancy.
- Thyroid nodules incidentally identified on fluorodeoxyglucose-PET (FDG-PET) scan done for other disorders has a much higher malignancy rate (30% to 50%).

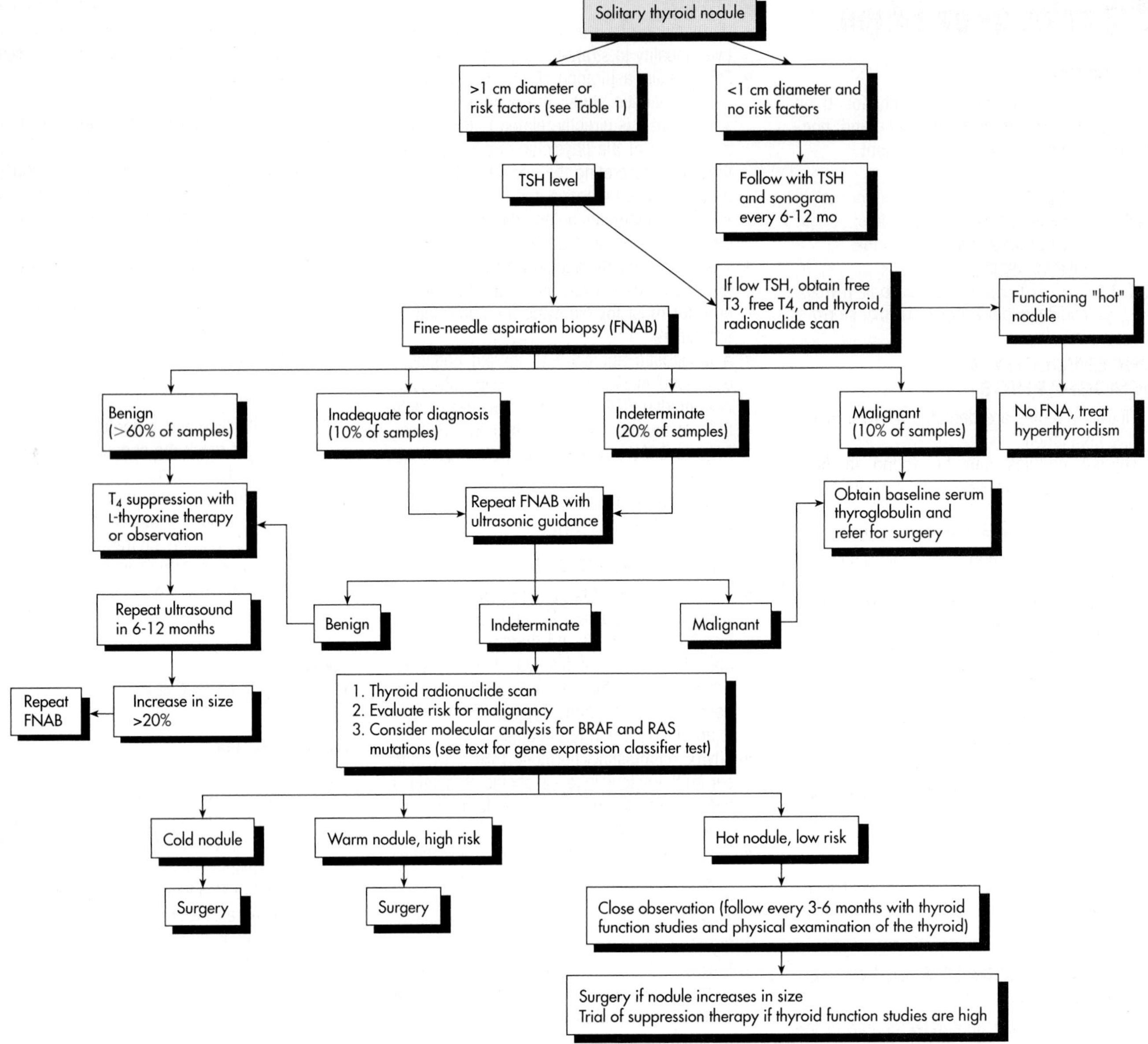

FIG. 1 Diagnostic algorithm for thyroid nodule. *FNA,* Fine needle aspiration; *T3,* triiodothyronine; *T4,* thyroxine; *TSH,* thyroid-stimulating hormone. (From Ferri F: *Ferri's best test,* ed 4, Philadelphia, Elsevier, 2017.)

TABLE 1 Clinical and Ultrasound Findings in Favor of Malignant Thyroid Nodules

Clinical Features	Ultrasound Findings
History	Higher suspicion
Young age (<20 yr) or older age (>60 yr)	Hypoechoic lesions
Male gender	Irregular margins
Neck irradiation during childhood or adolescence	Presence of microcalcifications
Rapid growth	Absence of halo
Recent changes in speaking, breathing, or swallowing	Internal or central blood flow
Family history of thyroid malignancy or MEN2	
Physical examination	Low suspicion
Firm and irregular consistency of nodule	Echo-free (cystic) lesion
Fixation to underlying or overlying tissues	Spongiform lesion
Vocal cord paralysis	
Regional lymphadenopathy	

MEN2, Multiple endocrine neoplasia II.
From Melmed S, Polonsky KS, Larsen PR et al: *Williams textbook of endocrinology,* ed 12, Philadelphia, 2011, Elsevier.

- Surgery is indicated in hard or fixed nodule, presence of dysphagia or hoarseness, and rapidly growing solid masses regardless of "benign" results on FNA.
- Suppressive therapy of malignant thyroid nodules postoperatively with thyroxine is indicated. The use of suppressive therapy for benign solitary nodules is controversial.

SUGGESTED READINGS

Available at ExpertConsult.com

RELATED CONTENT

Thyroid Nodule (Patient Information)
Thyroiditis (Related Key Topic)
Thyroid Cancer (Related Key Topic)

AUTHOR: **FRED F. FERRI, M.D.**

BASIC INFORMATION

DEFINITION

Thyroiditis is an inflammatory disease of the thyroid. It is a multifaceted disease with various etiologies, different clinical characteristics (depending on the stage), and distinct histopathology. Thyroiditis can be subdivided into three common types (Hashimoto, painful, and painless) and two rare forms (suppurative and Riedel). To add to the confusion, there are various synonyms for each form, and there is no internationally accepted classification of autoimmune thyroid disease.

SYNONYMS

Hashimoto's thyroiditis: Chronic lymphocytic thyroiditis, chronic autoimmune thyroiditis, lymphadenoid goiter

Painful subacute thyroiditis: Subacute thyroiditis, giant cell thyroiditis, de Quervain's thyroiditis, subacute granulomatous thyroiditis, pseudogranulomatous thyroiditis

Painless postpartum thyroiditis: Subacute lymphocytic thyroiditis, postpartum thyroiditis

Painless sporadic thyroiditis: Silent sporadic thyroiditis, subacute lymphocytic thyroiditis

Infectious thyroiditis: Acute suppurative thyroiditis, bacterial thyroiditis, microbial inflammatory thyroiditis, pyogenic thyroiditis

Riedel's thyroiditis: Fibrous thyroiditis

ICD-10CM CODES

E06.3 Autoimmune thyroiditis
E06.1 Subacute thyroiditis
E06.9 Thyroiditis, unspecified
E06.0 Acute thyroiditis
E06.5 Other chronic thyroiditis

PHYSICAL FINDINGS & CLINICAL PRESENTATION

- Thyroiditis typically has three phases: thyrotoxic hypothyroid (each lasting approximately 3 mo) and return to euthyroidism.
- Hashimoto: Patients may have signs of hyperthyroidism (tachycardia, diaphoresis, palpitations, weight loss) or hypothyroidism (fatigue, weight gain, delayed reflexes) depending on the stage of the disease. Usually there is diffuse, firm enlargement of the thyroid gland; the gland may also be of normal size (atrophic form with clinically manifested hypothyroidism).
- Painful subacute: Exquisitely tender, enlarged thyroid, fever; signs of hyperthyroidism are initially present; signs of hypothyroidism can subsequently develop.
- Painless thyroiditis: Clinical features are similar to subacute thyroiditis except for the absence of tenderness of the thyroid gland.
- Suppurative: Patient is febrile with severe neck pain, focal tenderness of the involved portion of the thyroid, erythema of the overlying skin.
- Riedel: Slowly enlarging hard mass in the anterior neck; often mistaken for thyroid cancer; signs of hypothyroidism occur in advanced stages.

ETIOLOGY

- Hashimoto: Autoimmune disorder that begins with the activation of CD4 (helper) T-lymphocytes specific for thyroid antigens. The etiologic factor for the activation of these cells is unknown
- Painful subacute: Possibly postviral; usually follows a respiratory illness not considered to be a form of autoimmune thyroiditis
- Painless thyroiditis: Frequently occurs postpartum
- Infectious (suppurative): Infectious etiology, generally bacterial, although fungi and parasites have also been implicated; often occurs in immunocompromised hosts or after a penetrating neck injury
- Riedel: Fibrous infiltration of the thyroid; etiology unknown
- Drug induced: Typically painless due to lithium, interferon-alfa, amiodarone, interleukin-2
- Radiation thyroiditis: Occurs 5 to 10 days after treatment with radioactive iodine; it is painful and may result in transient exacerbation of hyperthyroidism

DIAGNOSIS

DIFFERENTIAL DIAGNOSIS

- The hyperthyroid phase of Hashimoto's, subacute, and silent thyroiditis can be mistaken for Graves disease.
- Riedel thyroiditis can be mistaken for carcinoma of the thyroid.
- Painful subacute thyroiditis can be mistaken for infections of the oropharynx and trachea or for suppurative thyroiditis.
- Factitious hyperthyroidism can mimic silent thyroiditis.

WORKUP

- The diagnostic workup includes laboratory and radiologic evaluation to rule out other conditions that may mimic thyroiditis (see previously) and differentiate the various forms of thyroiditis.
- The patient's medical history may be helpful in differentiating the various types of thyroiditis (e.g., presentation after childbirth is suggestive of silent [postpartum, painless] thyroiditis; occurrence after a viral respiratory infection suggests subacute thyroiditis; history of penetrating injury to the neck indicates suppurative thyroiditis).

LABORATORY TESTS

- Thyroid-stimulating hormone, free T_4: May be normal or indicative of hypothyroidism or hyperthyroidism depending on the stage of the thyroiditis.
- White blood cell (WBC) with differential: Increased WBC with left shift occurs with subacute and suppurative thyroiditis.
- Antimicrosomal antibodies: Detected in >90% of patients with Hashimoto's thyroiditis and 50% to 80% of patients with silent thyroiditis.
- Serum thyroglobulin levels are elevated in patients with subacute and silent thyroiditis; this test is nonspecific but may be useful in monitoring the course of subacute thyroiditis and distinguishing silent thyroiditis from factitious hyperthyroidism (low or absent serum thyroglobulin level).

IMAGING STUDIES

Twenty-four–hour radioactive iodine uptake (RAIU) is useful to distinguish Graves disease (increased RAIU) from thyroiditis (normal or low RAIU). Table E1 summarizes factors that influence 24-hr thyroid iodide uptake.

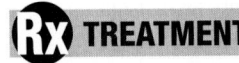

TREATMENT

ACUTE GENERAL Rx

- The duration of the thyrotoxic phase of thyroiditis is usually 10 to 12 wk. This phase is followed by a hypothyroid phase typically lasting up to 12 wk.
- Treat hypothyroid phase in symptomatic patients somatic with levothyroxine 25 to 50 mcg/day initially and monitor serum thyroid-stimulating hormone initially every 6 to 8 wk.
- Control symptoms of hyperthyroidism with beta-blockers (e.g., propranolol 20-40 mg PO q6h or atenolol).
- Control pain in patients with subacute thyroiditis with nonsteroidal antiinflammatory drugs. Prednisone 20 to 40 mg qd may be used if nonsteroidals are insufficient, but it should be gradually tapered off over several weeks.
- Use IV antibiotics and drain abscess (if present) in patients with suppurative thyroiditis.

DISPOSITION

- Hashimoto thyroiditis: Long-term prognosis is favorable; most patients recover their thyroid function.
- Painful subacute thyroiditis: Permanent hypothyroidism occurs in 10% of patients.
- Painless thyroiditis: 6% of patients have permanent hypothyroidism.
- Infectious thyroiditis: There is usually full recovery after treatment.
- Riedel thyroiditis: Hypothyroidism occurs when fibrous infiltration involves the entire thyroid.

REFERRAL

Surgical referral in patients with compression of adjacent neck structures and in some patients with infectious (suppurative) thyroiditis

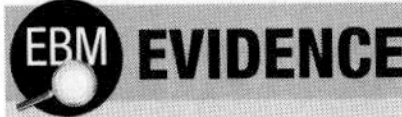

EVIDENCE

Available at ExpertConsult.com

Related Content

Thyroiditis (Patient Information)
Hyperthyroidism (Related Key Topic)
Hypothyroidism (Related Key Topic)

AUTHOR: **FRED F. FERRI, M.D.**

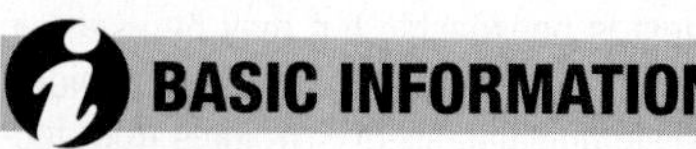

DEFINITION

Tinea capitis is a dermatophyte infection of hair shaft and follicles of the scalp, eyebrows, and eyelashes. It is a form of superficial mycosis. Etiologic agents are fungal species of the genera *Microsporum* and *Trichophyton.*

SYNONYMS

Ringworm of the scalp, ringworm of the head, gray patch tinea capitis, black dot tinea capitis, tinea tonsurans, herpes tonsurans, kerion, favus

ICD-10CM CODE
B35.0 Tinea barbae and tinea capitis

EPIDEMIOLOGY & DEMOGRAPHICS

Tinea capitis primarily affects prepubertal children with peak age between 3 and 7 yr old. Adult cases are rare, possibly because of the fungistatic effect of the sebum found in older persons. Urban living, large family size, low socioeconomic status, and crowded living conditions may contribute to an increased incidence of tinea capitis. The elderly and immunocompromised individuals have an increased risk of infection. The incidence of the disease varies worldwide; however, it is relatively low in the United States. It is reportedly widespread in parts of Central and South America, India, and Africa.

In the United States, peak incidence occurs in school-aged children of low socioeconomic status, with African American male children accounting for the greatest proportion of cases. About 3% to 8% of American children are affected, and 34% of household contacts are asymptomatic carriers.

PHYSICAL FINDINGS & CLINICAL PRESENTATION

- Classic triad of scalp scaling, alopecia, and cervical adenopathy. Table 1 summarizes clinical manifestations of tinea capitis in children.
- Most forms of tinea capitis begin with one or few round patches of scale (Fig. E1) or alopecia (Fig.E2).
- Primary lesions include plaques, papules, pustules, or nodules on the scalp (usually occipital region).
- Secondary lesions include scales, alopecia (usually reversible), erythema, exudates, and edema.
- Scalp pruritus may be present.
- Fever, pain, and lymphadenopathy (commonly postcervical) may occur with inflammatory lesions.
- Different clinical patterns of tinea capitis have been described:
  1. Gray patch: Lesions are scaly and well demarcated. The hairs within the patch break off a few millimeters above the scalp. One or several lesions may be present; sometimes the lesions join to form larger ones.
  2. Black dot: Early lesions with erythema and scaling patch are easily overlooked until areas of alopecia develop. Hairs within the patches break at the surface of the scalp, leaving behind a pattern of swollen black dots.
  3. Kerion (Fig. E3): Inflamed, exudative, pustular, boggy, tender nodules exhibiting marked edema, and hair loss seen in severe tinea capitis. Caused by immune response to the fungus. May lead to some scarring.
  4. Favus: Production of scutula (hair matted together with dermatophyte hyphae and keratin debris), characterized by yellow cup-shaped crusts around hair shafts. A fetid odor may be present.

TABLE 1 Clinical Manifestations of Tinea Capitis in Children

Clinical Feature	Comment
Scalp	
Alopecia	One or multiple patches; may simulate alopecia areata
Scaling	May be minimally inflammatory; may mimic seborrheic dermatitis
Erythema	Localized or widespread
Pustules	Differential diagnosis includes sterile folliculitis or bacterial folliculitis
"Black dots"	Alopecia with hair shafts broken off at surface of skin; may simulate trichotillomania
Kerion	Boggy, tender plaque with pustules and purulent discharge; represents a vigorous host immune response
Scarring	Rarely seen when untreated; usually follows kerion
Favus	Yellow, cup-shaped crusts around the hair
Other	
Lymphadenopathy	Common; cervical or occipital
Id reaction	Widespread, papular or papulovesicular eruption; extremity-predominant; usually seen after initiation of therapy; must be recognized as distinct from true drug reaction

From Paller AS, Mancini AJ: *Hurwitz clinical pediatric dermatology, a textbook of skin disorders of childhood and adolescence*, ed 5, 2016, Elsevier.

ETIOLOGY

Although fungi of the *Microsporum* or *Trichophyton* genera cause most cases of tinea capitis, causative species vary between geographical areas and across time. *T. tonsurans* is the predominant cause of tinea capitis, present in more than 90% of cases in North and Central America. *Microsporum canis, M. audouinii,* and *Trichophyton mentagrophytes* are less common. The most common causative species for black dot tinea capitis is *T. tonsurans*, while gray patch tinea capitis tends to be caused by *M. audouinii* and *M. canis.* Infection of the hair shaft is preceded by invasion of the stratum corneum of the scalp. Transmission of *T. tonsurans* occurs from person-to-person via infected persons or asymptomatic carriers, fallen infected hairs, animal vectors, and fomites. *M. audouinii* is commonly spread by dogs and cats. Infectious fungal particles may remain viable for many months. Even though the organism remains viable on combs, hairbrushes, and other fomites for long periods of time, the role of fomites in spreading the infection may vary in different geographic areas.

Dx DIAGNOSIS

DIFFERENTIAL DIAGNOSIS

Seborrheic dermatitis and psoriasis may be confused with tinea capitis. Other conditions that resemble tinea capitis include alopecia areata, impetigo, pediculosis, trichotillomania, traction alopecia, folliculitis, pseudopelade, seborrhea/atopic dermatitis, psoriasis, carbuncles, pyoderma, lichen ruber planus, and lupus erythematosus; these should also be considered in the differential. Table 2 highlights distinctive features of conditions that may be confused for tinea capitis.

WORKUP

- KOH testing of hair shaft extracted from the lesion, not the scale, because the *T. tonsurans* spores attach to or reside inside hair shafts and will rarely be found in the scales.
- Wood's ultraviolet light fluoresces blue-green on hair shafts for *Microsporum* infections but will fail to identify *T. tonsurans.*
- Fungal culture of hairs and scales on fungal medium such as Sabouraud agar may be used to confirm the diagnosis, especially if uncertain.
- Histology of biopsies with fungal staining in cases where mycology tests are negative because of treatment initiation.

Rx TREATMENT

- Griseofulvin is the gold standard FDA-approved treatment. Published studies show mean efficacy for griseofulvin treatment of about 68% for *Trichophyton* species and 88% for *Microsporum.* It is less costly than other drug options and has an excellent long-term safety profile. Micronized and ultramicronized preparations are absorbed better, and side effects are infrequent, especially when administered with fatty meals. Periodic monitoring of hematologic, liver, and renal function may be indicated, especially in prolonged treatment over 8 wk.
  1. **Children:** Griseofulvin is approved for children older than 2 yr of age: microsize griseofulvin 10 to 25 mg/kg PO per day in one single dose or two divided doses (maximum, 1 g/day; for tinea capitis, higher doses [20-25 mg/kg/day] have been recommended) or ultramicrosize griseofulvin,

TABLE 2 Differential Diagnosis of Tinea Capitis

Disorder	Differentiating Features
Psoriasis	Red skin with thick, uniform, silvery scale, sharply demarcated; often psoriasis at other body sites also
Dermatitis	Main possibility is seborrheic dermatitis: Usually more diffuse and has uniform fine scaling, rather than localized areas; doesn't typically cause alopecia or significant inflammation. May also be present on the face, especially the nasolabial fold, or as otitis externa. Atopic dermatitis is generally diffuse on scalp and almost inevitably present at other sites, but may coexist with tinea capitis, especially in children.
Pityriasis amiantacea	Thick sheets of asbestos-like scale, very adherent, generally a solitary patch. This may occur in various dermatoses.
Lichen simplex	Usually nape of neck; cobblestoned or lichenified skin thickening, with broken hairs that are not coated with scale
Alopecia areata	Usually not inflamed (may be mildly so), not scaly, usually sharply defined. "Exclamation mark" hairs occur but are not coated with fungus; "cadaverized" hairs especially cause difficulty, as they mimic black dot alopecia.
Scarring alopecias	Examples: Discoid lupus erythematosus, lichen planus of scalp; cause perifollicular inflammation around intact hairs; usually associated with lesions at other sites also. Dissecting cellulitis of scalp is also in this differential.
Bacterial infections	Impetigo causes crusting but little inflammation, and hairs are intact; carbuncle is deeper and very tender but may be in the differential of kerion
Trichotillomania	Broken hairs of unequal length, but hair shafts themselves and the scalp are normal
Damage from hairdressing processes	Usually clear from the timescale
Neoplasm	May be in the differential of kerion; usually slower-growing and mainly on elderly, balding scalp, whereas kerion is in children or young adults with previously intact hair

From White GM, Cox NH (eds): *Diseases of the skin, a color atlas and text,* ed 2, St Louis, 2006, Mosby.

5 to 15 mg/kg PO per day (maximum, 750 mg/day), in one single dose or two divided doses. Optimally, griseofulvin is given after a meal containing fat (e.g., peanut butter or ice cream). Recommended treatment length is 6 to 8 wk and should be continued 2 wk beyond clinical resolution (until hair regrowth occurs). Some children may require higher doses to achieve clinical cure.

2. **Adults and elderly persons:** Microsize griseofulvin 500 mg PO per day in one single dose or divided doses. The other option is ultramicrosize griseofulvin 375 mg PO per day in one single dose or divided doses. Recommended treatment length is 4 to 6 wk.

- Newer alternative treatments: Oral terbinafine, itraconazole, or fluconazole are comparable in efficacy and safety to griseofulvin, with possibly shorter treatment and better patient compliance. Preferred when resistant or when an allergy to griseofulvin is of concern. Monitoring of CBC, liver function tests, and renal function may be indicated.
  1. Terbinafine—4-wk course of therapy as effective as with griseofulvin. Dosages are 67.5 mg/day for patients weighing <20 kg; 125 mg/day for patients weighing 20 to 40 kg; and 250 mg for patients weighing >40 kg.
  2. Itraconazole—3.5 mg/kg daily for 4 to 6 wk or pulse therapy of 5 mg/kg daily for 1 wk each month for 2 to 3 mo (not approved for children)
  3. Fluconazole—the only oral antifungal agent approved for children <2 yr, 6 mg/kg/day for 6 wk in children (3-6 wk in adults) or 8 mg/kg weekly for 8 to 12 wk (cap at 150 mg weekly for adults)
- The adjuvant use of antifungal shampoos may be recommended for all patients and household contacts. Shampoo like selenium sulfide 2.5% used for 5 min or ketoconazole shampoo used 2 to 3 times/wk can help prevent infection or eradicate asymptomatic carrier state by inhibiting fungal growth.
- Severe inflammatory kerion can be managed with additional prednisone 40 mg daily (1 mg/kg/day in children) and tapering over 2 wk.
- Prompt treatment is indicated, as is examination of siblings and other household contacts for evidence of tinea capitis.
- Recommend follow-up visit every 2 to 4 wk with Wood light, microscopic study, and fungal culture. A mycologic documented cure is the goal of treatment.
- Pets that are infected or asymptomatic carriers should be treated.
- Children receiving treatment for tinea capitis may attend school once they start therapy with griseofulvin or other effective systemic agent.

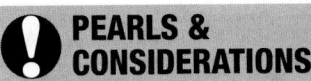

PEARLS & CONSIDERATIONS

- Systemic antifungal therapy is required for tinea capitis because topical antifungal medications are not effective.
- Shaving of the head, haircuts, or wearing a cap or scarf during treatment is unnecessary.
- Sharing of combs, hair ribbons, and hairbrushes should be discouraged.

COMMENTS

- Confirming the diagnosis of tinea capitis with a laboratory specimen is important because misdiagnosis will result in delay or improper treatment.
- Patients and their families should look for sources of infections and disinfect contaminated objects such as combs, brushes, towels, and headgear. Avoid sharing personal hygiene utensils.
- Culture of hairs and scalp dander facilitates carrier identification and prevention.

SUGGESTED READING

Available at ExpertConsult.com

RELATED CONTENT

Tinea Capitis (Patient Information)

AUTHORS: **PRIYA SARIN GUPTA, M.D., M.P.H., NADINE MBUYI, M.D.,** and **ALVARO M. RIVERA, M.D.**

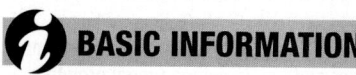

DEFINITION

Tinea corporis is a dermatophyte fungal infection caused by the genera *Trichophyton* or *Microsporum.* Tinea corporis includes all superficial dermatophyte infections of the skin other than those involving the scalp, beard, face, hands, feet, and groin.

SYNONYMS

Ringworm
Body ringworm
Tinea circinata

ICD-10CM CODE
B35.4 Tinea corporis

EPIDEMIOLOGY & DEMOGRAPHICS

- The disease is more common in warm climates.
- There is no predominant age or sex.

PHYSICAL FINDINGS & CLINICAL PRESENTATION

- Typically appears as single (Fig. E1) or multiple annular lesions with an advancing scaly border (Fig. E2); the margin is slightly raised, reddened (Fig. E3), and may be pustular.
- The central area becomes hypopigmented and less scaly as the active border progresses outward, thus the name "ringworm."
- The trunk and legs are primarily involved.
- Pruritus is variable.
- It is important to remember that recent topical corticosteroid use can significantly alter the appearance of the lesions.
- Tinea gladiatorum is a common problem for wrestlers.

ETIOLOGY

Trichophyton rubrum is the most common pathogen. Other common causes in the U.S. are *M. canis* and *T. mentagrophytes.* Table 1 summarizes common dermatophytes that cause tinea corporis.

Dx DIAGNOSIS

DIFFERENTIAL DIAGNOSIS

- Pityriasis rosea
- Erythema multiforme
- Psoriasis
- Cutaneous systemic lupus erythematosus
- Secondary syphilis
- Nummular eczema
- Eczema
- Granuloma annulare
- Lyme disease
- Tinea versicolor
- Contact dermatitis

WORKUP

Diagnosis is usually made on clinical grounds. It can be confirmed by direct visualization under the microscope of a small fragment of the scale using wet mount preparation and potassium hydroxide solution; dermatophytes appear as translucent branching filaments (hyphae) with lines of separation appearing at irregular intervals.

LABORATORY TESTS

- Microscopic examination of hyphae.
- Mycotic culture is usually not necessary.
- Biopsy is indicated only when the diagnosis is uncertain and the patient has not responded to treatment.
- HIV (widespread tinea corporis may be a presenting sign of AIDS).

Rx TREATMENT

NONPHARMACOLOGIC THERAPY

Affected areas should be kept clean and dry.

ACUTE GENERAL Rx

- Various creams are effective; the application area should include normal skin approximately 2 cm beyond the affected area:
  1. Butenafine cream applied qd for 14 days
  2. Terbinafine cream applied bid for 7-14 days
  3. Other effective topical agents are sulconazole, miconazole, clotrimazole, ketoconazole, naftifine, ciclopirox olamine, and efinaconazole
- Systemic therapy is reserved for severe cases and is usually given up to 4 wk; commonly used agents:
  1. Fluconazole, 150 mg once a week for 4 wk
  2. Terbinafine, 250 mg qd for 7-14 days
  3. Itraconazole, 200 mg/day for 1 wk

DISPOSITION

Majority of cases resolve without sequelae within 3 to 4 wk of therapy.

REFERRAL

Dermatology referral in patients with persistent or recurrent infections

RELATED CONTENT

Ringworm (Patient Information)
Tinea Capitis (Related Key Topic)
Tinea Cruris (Related Key Topic)

AUTHOR: **FRED F. FERRI, M.D.**

TABLE 1 Common Dermatophytes That Cause Tinea Corporis

Dermatophyte	Clinical features
Anthropophilic	
Trichophyton rubrum	Commonly harbored by hair follicles; may produce concentric rings; can recur; causative organism in nodular perifolliculitis (Majocchi granuloma) and most common cause of tinea corporis
T. tonsurans	Commonly seen in adults who care for children with tinea capitis caused by this organism
Epidermophyton floccosum	Generally restricted to groin or feet; responsible for eczema marginatum
T. concentricum	Responsible for tinea imbricata; infections typically chronic
T. interdigitale (previously *T. mentagrophytes* var. *interdigitale*)	Causes interdigital tinea pedis, tinea cruris, and onychomycosis
Zoophilic	
T. mentagrophytes (previously *T. mentagrophytes* var. *mentagrophytes*)	May be associated with dermatophytid reaction; causes inflammatory tinea pedis and tinea barbae; associated with exposure to small mammals
Microsporum canis	Associated with pet exposure (cat or dog)
T. verrucosum	May mimic bacterial furunculosis; associated with exposure to cattle
Geophilic	
M. gypseum	Frequently associated with outdoor/occupational exposure; lesions may be inflammatory or bullous

Bolognia J et al: *Dermatology,* ed 4, Philadelphia, 2018, Elsevier.

BASIC INFORMATION

DEFINITION

Tinea cruris is a dermatophyte infection of the groin.

SYNONYMS

Jock itch
Groin ringworm
Crotch itch

ICD-10CM CODE

B35.6 Tinea cruris

EPIDEMIOLOGY & DEMOGRAPHICS

- Most common during the summer in adolescent and young adult males.
- Males are affected more frequently than females; however, it has become more common in postpubertal females who are overweight or who often wear tight jeans or pantyhose.
- The infection often coexists with tinea pedis.

PHYSICAL FINDINGS & CLINICAL PRESENTATION

- It begins as a small erythematous, and scaling or crusted patch that spreads peripherally.
- Erythematous plaques have a half-moon shape and a scaling border.
- The acute inflammation tends to move down the inner thigh (Fig. E1) and usually spares the scrotum; in severe cases the fungus may spread onto the buttocks.
- Itching may be severe.
- Red papules, vesicles, and pustules may be present.
- An important diagnostic sign is the advancing well-defined border with a tendency toward central clearing.

ETIOLOGY

- Dermatophytes of the genera *Trichophyton, Epidermophyton,* and *Microsporum. T. rubrum and E. floccosum* are the most common infecting agents. Table 1 summarizes common causative agents of tinea cruris.
- Transmission from direct contact (e.g., infected persons, animals). The patient's feet should be evaluated as a source of infection because tinea cruris is often associated with tinea pedis.

DIAGNOSIS

DIFFERENTIAL DIAGNOSIS

- Candidal intertrigo
- Psoriasis
- Seborrheic dermatitis
- Erythrasma
- Contact dermatitis
- Tinea versicolor

WORKUP

Diagnosis is based on clinical presentation and demonstration of hyphae microscopically using potassium hydroxide.

LABORATORY TESTS

- Microscopic examination.
- Cultures are generally not necessary.

TREATMENT

NONPHARMACOLOGIC THERAPY

- Keep infected area clean and dry.
- Boxer shorts are preferred to briefs. The reduction of perspiration and enhancement of evaporation from the crural area are necessary prophylactic measures.

ACUTE GENERAL Rx

- Various topical antifungal agents are available:
  1. Butenafine cream, applied qd × 14 days
  2. Terbinafine cream, applied bid × 14 days
- Drying powders (e.g., miconazole nitrate) may be useful in patients with excessive perspiration.
- Oral antifungal therapy is generally reserved for cases unresponsive to topical agents or can be used along with topical agents in severe cases. Effective medications are fluconazole 200 mg qd × 7 days or 150 mg once a week for 4 wks, terbinafine 250 mg qd × 14 days, or itraconazole 200 mg/day for 7 days.

DISPOSITION

Most cases respond promptly to therapy with complete resolution within 2 to 3 wk.

RELATED CONTENT

Tinea Cruris (Patient Information)
Tinea Capitis (Related Key Topic)
Tinea Corporis (Related Key Topic)

AUTHOR: **FRED F. FERRI, M.D.**

TABLE 1 Tinea Cruris: Common Causative Pathogens

Dermatophyte	Clinical features
Trichophyton rubrum	• Most common cause of tinea cruris • Infection tends to be chronic • Fungus not viable in scale (e.g., on furniture, rugs, linens) for long periods of time • Frequent extension to buttocks, waist, and thighs
Epidermophyton floccosum	• Commonly associated with "epidemics" of tinea cruris in locker rooms or dormitories • Infection is acute (rarely chronic) • Arthroconidia are viable in scale (e.g., on furniture, rugs, linens) for long periods of time • Infection rarely extends beyond groin region • Causative agent of "eczema marginatum" (well demarcated borders with multiple small vesicles or, sometimes, vesiculopustules)
T. mentagrophytes (previously *T. mentagrophytes* var. *mentagrophytes*)	• Infection tends to be more severe and acute, with intense inflammation and pustule formation • May rapidly spread to the trunk and lower extremities, causing a severe inflammatory condition • Often acquired from animal dander

From Bolognia J et al: *Dermatology*, ed 4, Philadelphia, 2018, Elsevier.

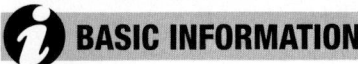

BASIC INFORMATION

DEFINITION

Tinea pedis is a dermatophyte infection of the feet.

SYNONYM

Athlete's foot

ICD-10CM CODE
B35.3 Tinea pedis

EPIDEMIOLOGY & DEMOGRAPHICS

- Most common dermatophyte infection
- Increased incidence in hot humid weather; occlusive footwear is a contributing factor
- Occurrence is rare before adolescence
- More common in adult males

PHYSICAL FINDINGS & CLINICAL PRESENTATION

- Typical presentation is variable and ranges from erythematous scaling plaques and isolated blisters to interdigital maceration (Fig.1). The four major types of tinea pedis are summarized in Fig. 2.
- The infection usually starts in the interdigital spaces of the foot. Most infections are found in the toe webs or on the soles.
- Fourth or fifth toes are most commonly involved.
- Pruritus is common and is most intense after removal of shoes and socks.
- Infection with *Trichophyton rubrum* often manifests with a "moccasin" distribution affecting the soles and lateral feet.

Tinea pedis caused by trichophyton mentagrophytes (interdigitale) can present with:

- Erythema and desquamation between the toes
- Multilocular bullae involving the thin skin of the plantar arch and along the sides of the feet and heel
- White superficial onychomycosis

ETIOLOGY

- Dermatophyte infection caused by *T. rubrum, Trichophyton mentagrophytes,* or less commonly *Epidermophyton floccosum*
- There may be an autosomal dominant predisposition to this form of infection.

Dx DIAGNOSIS

DIFFERENTIAL DIAGNOSIS

- Contact dermatitis
- Toe web infection (bacterial or candidal infection)
- Eczema
- Psoriasis
- Keratolysis exfoliativa
- Juvenile plantar dermatosis

WORKUP

- Diagnosis is usually made by clinical observation.
- Laboratory testing, when performed, generally consists of a simple potassium hydroxide preparation with mycologic examination under a light microscope to confirm the presence of dermatophytes.

LABORATORY TESTS

- Microscopic examination of a scale or the roof of a blister with 10% KOH under low or medium power will reveal hyphae.
- Mycologic culture is rarely indicated in the diagnosis of tinea pedis.
- Biopsy is reserved for when the diagnosis remains in question after testing or failure to respond to treatment.

Rx TREATMENT

NONPHARMACOLOGIC THERAPY

- Hyperhidrosis is a predisposing factor for tinea pedis. Keep infected area clean and dry. Aerate feet by using sandals when possible.
- Use 100% cotton socks rather than nylon socks to reduce moisture.
- Areas likely to become infected should be dried completely before being covered with clothes.

ACUTE GENERAL Rx

- Benzylamines: Butenafine HCl 1% cream applied bid for 1 wk or qd for 4 wk is effective in interdigital tinea pedis.
- Allylamines: Terbinafine cream applied bid × 14 days, or naftifine 1% cream applied qd or naftifine gel applied bid for 4 wk produces a significantly high cure rate.
- Imidazoles: Econazole, ketoconazole, miconazole, luliconazole, and clotrimazole cream are also effective agents. Clotrimazole 1% cream is an over-the-counter treatment. It should be applied to affected and surrounding area bid for up to 4 wk.
- Ciclopirox and tolnaftate are other antifungal agents available in cream, suspension, or gel. Tolnaftate is also available as a lotion, spray, or powder.
- When using topical preparations, the application area should include normal skin approximately 2 cm beyond the affected area.
- Areas of maceration can be treated with Burow solution soaks for 10 to 20 min bid followed by foot elevation.
- Oral agents (fluconazole 150 mg once per week for 4 wk, terbinafine 250 mg/day for 14 days, itraconazole 200 mg bid × 7 days, or griseofulvin 500-1000 mg/day for 14 days) can be used in combination with topical agents in resistant cases.

PEARLS & CONSIDERATIONS

- Use of tolnaftate powder (Tinactin) or Zeasorb medicated powder on the feet after bathing may be helpful in preventing recurrent tinea pedis in susceptible persons.
- Combination therapy of antifungal and corticosteroid (clotrimazole/betamethasone [Lotrisone]) should only be used when the diagnosis of fungal infection is confirmed and inflammation is a significant issue.
- Nystatin is not effective and should not be used.

RELATED CONTENT

Athlete's Foot (Patient Information)

AUTHOR: **FRED F. FERRI, M.D.**

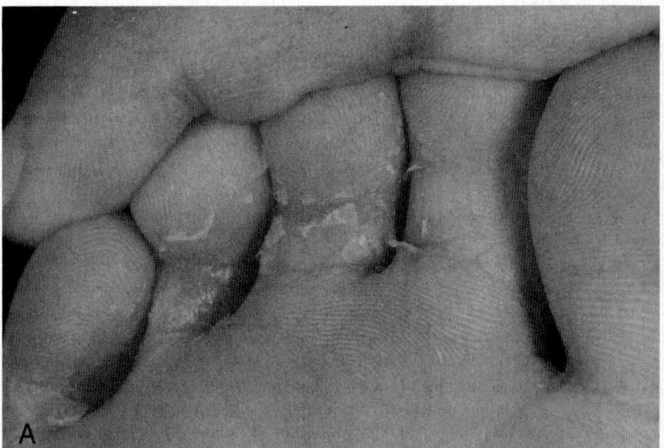

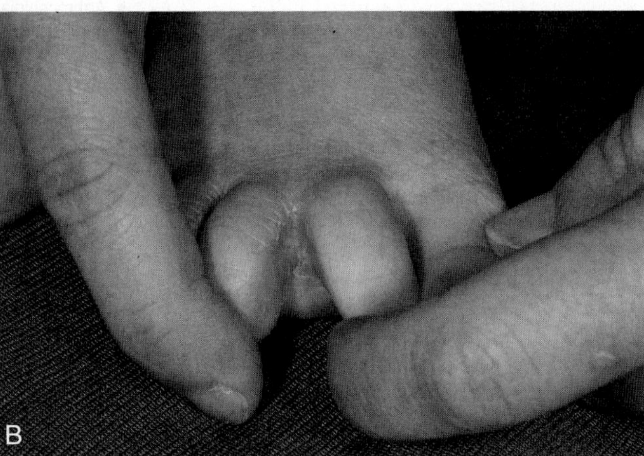

FIG. 1 Tinea pedis. This 6-year-old girl showed erythema and desquamation of the plantar foot and toes **(A)** and toe-web erythema and maceration **(B).** (From Paller AS, Mancini AJ: *Hurwitz clinical pediatric dermatology, a textbook of skin disorders of childhood and adolescence,* ed 5, 2016, Elsevier.)

THE FOUR MAJOR TYPES OF "TINEA PEDIS" CAUSED BY DERMATOPHYTES AND NON-DERMATOPHYTES			
Type	**Causative organism**	**Clinical features**	**Treatment considerations**
Moccasin	*Trichophyton rubrum* *Epidermophyton floccosum* *Neoscytalidium hyalinum* *N. dimidiatum*	Diffuse hyperkeratosis, erythema scaling and fissures on one or both plantar surfaces; frequently chronic and difficult to cure;* occasionally associated with immune deficiency	Topical antifungal plus product with urea or lactic acid; may require oral antifungal therapy
Interdigital	*T. interdigitale* (previously *mentagrophytes* var. *interdigitale*) *T. rubrum* *E. floccosum* *N. hyalinum* *N. dimidiatum* *Candida* spp. *Fusarium* spp.	Most common type; erythema, scaling, fissures and maceration in the web spaces; the two lateral web spaces are most commonly affected; "dermatophytosis complex" (fungal infection followed by bacterial invasion†) can develop; pruritus common; may extend to dorsum and sole of foot	Topical antifungal; may require topical or oral antibiotic if superimposed bacterial infection
Inflammatory (vesicular)	*T. mentagrophytes* (previously *T. mentagrophytes* var. *mentagrophytes*)	Vesicles and bullae on the medial foot; often associated with a dermatophytid reaction‡	Topical antifungal usually sufficient
Ulcerative	*T. rubrum* *T. interdigitale* (previously *T. mentagrophytes* var. *interdigitale*) *E. floccosum*	Typically an exacerbation of interdigital tinea pedis; ulcers and erosions in the web spaces; commonly secondarily infected with bacteria; seen in immunocompromised and diabetic patients	Topical antifungal; may require topical or oral antibiotics if secondary bacterial infection (common)

Dermatophytes   Non-dermatophytes

*Because of the thickness of stratum corneum on plantar surfaces and the inability of *T. rubrum* to elicit a sufficient immune response to eliminate the fungus.[21]

†Often *Pseudomonas, Proteus* spp., or *Staphylococcus aureus.*

‡Reaction to fungal elements presenting as a dyshidrotic-like eruption on the fingers and palms (culture negative for fungus).

FIG. 2 The four major types of tinea pedis caused by dermatophytes and nondermatophytes. (From Bolognia J et al: *Dermatology*, ed 4, Philadelphia, 2018, Elsevier.)

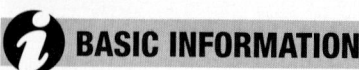

DEFINITION

Tinea unguium is defined as a persistent fungal infection affecting the toenails and fingernails.

SYNONYMS

Onychomycosis
Ringworm of the nails

ICD-10CM CODE
B35.1 Tinea unguium

EPIDEMIOLOGY & DEMOGRAPHICS

- Tinea unguium is most commonly found in people between the ages of 40 and 60 yr.
- Tinea unguium rarely occurs before puberty.
- Incidence: 20 to 100 cases/1000 population.
- Toenail infection is 4 to 6 times more common than fingernail infection.
- Tinea unguium affects men more often than women.
- Occurs more frequently in patients with diabetes, peripheral vascular disease, and any conditions resulting in the suppression of the immune system.
- Occlusive footwear, physical exercise followed by communal showering, and incompletely drying the feet predispose the individual to developing tinea unguium.

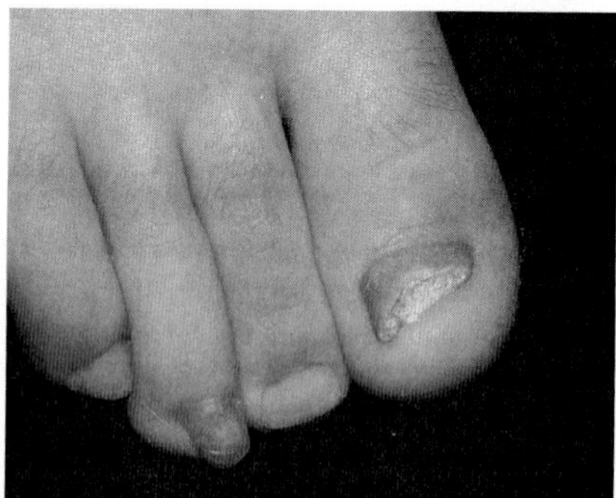

FIG. 1 Distal subungual onychomycosis in a 5-year-old. Note how heavily infected nails occur adjacent to totally normal nails. Cutting back the big toe's nail plate has revealed the friable subungual debris. This material is the most desirable for culture. (From White GM, Cox NH [eds]: *Diseases of the skin, a color atlas and text,* ed 2, St Louis, 2006, Mosby.)

PHYSICAL FINDINGS & CLINICAL PRESENTATION

- Tinea unguium causes nails to become thick, brittle, hard, distorted, and discolored (yellow to brown color) (Fig. 1). Eventually, the nail may loosen, separate from the nail bed, and fall off (Fig. 2).
- Tinea unguium is frequently associated with tinea pedis (athlete's foot).

ETIOLOGY

- The most common causes of tinea unguium are dermatophyte, yeast, and nondermatophyte molds.
- The dermatophyte *Trichophyton rubrum* accounts for 80% of all nail infections caused by fungus.
- *Trichophyton interdigitale* and *Trichophyton mentagrophytes* are other fungi causing tinea unguium.
- The yeast *Candida albicans* is responsible for 5% of the cases of tinea unguium and tends to involve fingernails more than toenails.
- Nondermatophyte molds *Scopulariopsis brevicaulis* and *Aspergillus niger,* although rare, can also cause tinea unguium.
- Tinea unguium is classified according to the clinical pattern of nail bed involvement. The main types are:
  1. Distal and lateral subungual tinea unguium (DLSO)
  2. Superficial tinea unguium
  3. Proximal subungual tinea unguium
  4. Endonyx tinea unguium
  5. Total dystrophic tinea unguium

Dx DIAGNOSIS

The diagnosis of tinea unguium is based on the clinical nail findings and confirmed by direct microscopy and culture.

DIFFERENTIAL DIAGNOSIS

- Psoriasis
- Contact dermatitis
- Lichen planus
- Subungual keratosis
- Paronychia
- Infection (e.g., *Pseudomonas*)
- Trauma
- Peripheral vascular disease
- Yellow nail syndrome

WORKUP

The workup of suspected tinea unguium is directed at confirming the diagnosis of tinea unguium by visualizing hyphae under the microscope by KOH prep or by culturing the organism. Although the standard for the diagnosis of fungal nail disease is a positive result on microscopic examination and culture of nail clippings with subungual debris or from surface debris in superficial white tinea unguium, treatment is often prescribed in the absence of confirmatory findings.

LABORATORY TESTS

- KOH prep: Specificity is high but sensitivity is variable
- Fungal cultures on Sabouraud medium: Culture may take 4 to 6 wk
- Dermatophyte test medium (DTM): An alternative to Sabouraud that takes only 3 to 7 days and can be done in office setting. A color change indicates dermatophyte growth.
- Nail plate biopsy with periodic acid–Schiff (PAS) stain
- Blood tests are not specific in the diagnosis of tinea unguium and therefore not useful

IMAGING STUDIES

- Imaging studies are not very specific in making the diagnosis of tinea unguium and not useful.
- If an infection is present and osteomyelitis is a consideration, an x-ray of the specific area and a bone scan may help establish the diagnosis.

CLASSIFICATION

- The Onychomycosis Severity Index (OSI) is a new classification system for grading the severity of tinea unguium.
- The OSI score is obtained by multiplying the score for the area of involvement (range, 0-5) by the score for the proximity of the disease to the matrix (range, 1-5). Ten points are added for the presence of a longitudinal streak or a patch (dermatophytoma) or for >2 mm of subungual hyperkeratosis.
- Mild tinea unguium corresponds to a score of 1 to 5; moderate to a score of 6 to 15; severe to a score of 16 to 35.
- Indicators of more severe onychomycosis are summarized in Table 1.

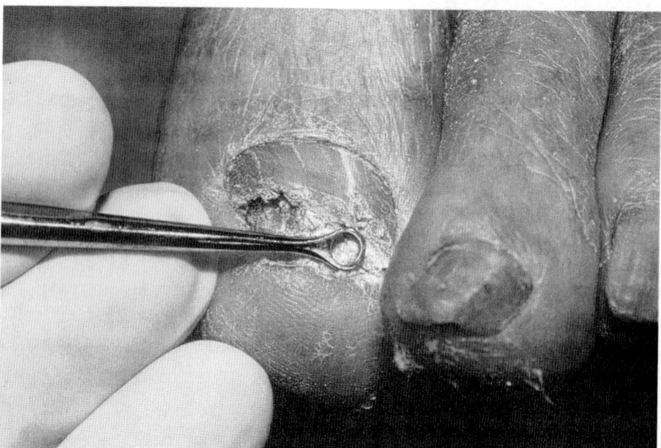

FIG. 2 Collection of nail for culture. The subungual debris is the most valuable material for culture. After the nail is cut back, a curette may be used. Clippings of the nail may be added to the culture. (From White GM, Cox NH [eds]: *Diseases of the skin, a color atlas and text,* ed 2, St Louis, 2006, Mosby.)

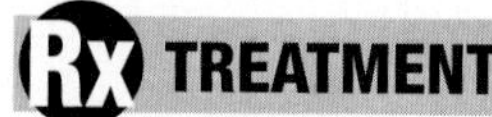

NONPHARMACOLOGIC THERAPY

- Surgical removal of the nail plate is a treatment option; however, the relapse rate is high.

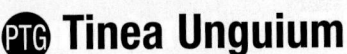

TABLE 1 Indicators of More Severe Onychomycosis with a Poor Response to Treatment

Nail factors	• Subungual hyperkeratosis >2 mm thick* • Significant lateral involvement • Dermatophytoma† • >50% involvement of nail bed • Slow nail growth rate • Total dystrophic onychomycosis • Matrix involvement
Patient factors	• Immunosuppression • Peripheral arterial disease • Poorly controlled diabetes mellitus

Adapted from Carney C, et al.: A new classification system for grading the severity of onychomycosis: Onychomycosis Severity Index. *Arch Dermatol* 2011; 147: pp. 1277-1282, From Bolognia J et al: *Dermatology*, ed 4, Philadelphia, 2018, Elsevier.

- Prevent reinfection by wearing properly fitted shoes, avoiding public showers, and keeping feet and nails clean and dry.
- Short-pulse laser therapy is fungicidal and is a newer treatment modality for tinea unguium. Most patients will require two to four treatments, each lasting 15 to 30 min. Laser therapy is useful in patients with contraindications to oral agents. It is, however, expensive ($250-$1000 per treatment) and not covered by most insurance plans.

ACUTE GENERAL Rx

- Topical antifungal creams are used for early superficial nail infections.
  1. Miconazole 2% cream applied over the nail plate bid.
  2. Clotrimazole 1% cream bid.
  3. Ciclopirox: Topical antifungal nail lacquer can be used for moderate tinea unguium that spares the lunula. Success rate <10%.
  4. Efinaconazole 10% topical solution (Jublia) is modestly effective in treating toenail tinea unguium due to *Trichophyton rubrum* and/or *Trichophyton mentagrophytes.* Dosage is 1 drop (2 drops for big toenail) once daily for 48 wk. Cost and formulary are limiting factors with this agent.
  5. Tavaborole 5% solution (Kerydin) is an oxaborole antifungal drug approved by the U.S. Food and Drug Administration (FDA) for topical treatment of toenail tinea unguium due to *T. rubrum* or *T. mentagrophytes.* It is applied to affected toenails once daily for 48 wk. It is modestly effective but much more expensive than topical ciclopirox 8% nail lacquer.
- Oral agents:
  1. Terbinafine:
     a. For toenails: 250 mg/day for 3 mo
     b. For fingernails: 250 mg/day for 6 wk
  2. Itraconazole:
     a. For toenails: 200 mg PO daily for 3 mo
     b. For fingernails: 200 mg PO daily for 6 wk
  3. Fluconazole: Not as effective as terbinafine or itraconazole:
     a. For toenails: 150 to 300 mg once weekly for 18 to 26 wk
     b. For fingernails: 150 to 300 mg once weekly for 12 to 16 wk
- All oral agents used for tinea unguium require periodic monitoring of liver function blood tests. Patients should be advised to watch for symptoms of drug-induced hepatitis (anorexia, fatigue, nausea, right upper quadrant pain) while taking these oral antifungal agents. They should stop their medication and contact their physician immediately if symptoms occur.
- Itraconazole is contraindicated in patients taking cisapride, astemizole, triazolam, midazolam, and terfenadine. Statins should be discontinued during itraconazole therapy. Itraconazole requires gastric acidity for absorption; patients should be advised not to take oral antacids, H_2 blockers, or proton pump inhibitors while taking itraconazole.
- Fluconazole is contraindicated in patients taking cisapride and terfenadine.
- Oral antifungal agents should not be initiated during pregnancy.

DISPOSITION

- Spontaneous remission of tinea unguium is rare.
- A disease-free toenail is reported to occur in approximately 25% to 50% of patients treated with the oral antifungal agents mentioned previously.

REFERRAL

- Podiatry consultation is indicated in diabetic patients for proper instruction in foot care, footwear, and nail debridement or surgical removal of the toenail.
- Dermatology consultation is indicated in patients refractory to treatment or if another diagnosis is considered (e.g., psoriasis).

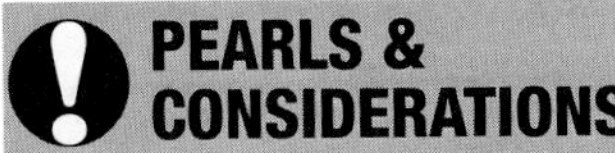

PEARLS & CONSIDERATIONS

COMMENTS

- The growth of fungus on an infected nail typically begins at the end of the nail and spreads under the nail plate to infect the nail bed as well.
- Carefully consider the informational insert regarding drug-drug interactions and contraindications before initiating oral antifungal agents.
- Meta-analysis showed cure rates with the oral agents as follows: terbinafine (about 75%), itraconazole (60% to 65%), and fluconazole (about 50%).

SUGGESTED READINGS

Available at ExpertConsult.com

RELATED CONTENT

Nail Fungus (Patient Information)
Ringworm (Patient Information)

AUTHOR: **GLENN G. FORT, M.D., M.P.H.**

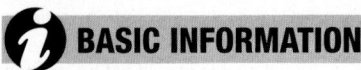

BASIC INFORMATION

DEFINITION

Tinea versicolor is a fungal infection of the skin caused by the yeast *Pityrosporum orbiculare (Malassezia furfur),* a commensal lipophilic fungus that lives in the hair follicles and stratum corneum.

SYNONYMS

Pityriasis versicolor

ICD-10CM CODES

B36.0 Pityriasis versicolor

EPIDEMIOLOGY & DEMOGRAPHICS

- Increased incidence in adolescence and young adulthood
- More common during the summer (hypopigmented lesions are more evident when the skin is tanned)

PHYSICAL FINDINGS & CLINICAL PRESENTATION

- Most lesions begin as multiple small, circular macules of various colors (Fig. E1) on the trunk and upper arms.
- The macules may be darker (Fig. E2) or lighter (Fig. E3) than the surrounding normal skin and will scale with scraping.
- Most frequent site of distribution is trunk.
- Facial lesions are more common in children (forehead is most common facial site).
- Eruption is generally of insidious onset and asymptomatic.
- Lesions may be hyperpigmented in blacks.
- Lesions may be inconspicuous in fair-complexioned individuals, especially during the winter.
- Most patients become aware of the eruption when the involved areas do not tan.
- Mild itching and inflammation around the patches may be present.
- Facial lesions may occur in infants and immunocompromised patients.

ETIOLOGY

The infection is caused by *Malassezia* species (*M. globosa, M. restricta, M. sympodialis, M. furfur, M. obtusa,* and *M. slooffiae*). Factors that favor proliferation are pregnancy, malnutrition, immunosuppression, oral contraceptives, and excess heat and humidity.

Dx DIAGNOSIS

DIFFERENTIAL DIAGNOSIS

- Vitiligo
- Pityriasis alba
- Secondary syphilis
- Pityriasis rosea
- Seborrheic dermatitis
- Postinflammatory hyperpigmentation or hypopigmentation
- Pityriasis rubra pilaris
- Syphilis
- Hansen disease

WORKUP

Diagnosis is based on clinical appearance. The *Malassezia* fungus is easily demonstrated in scraping of the profuse scales that cover the lesions. Identification of hyphae and budding spores ("spaghetti and meatballs" appearance) with microscopy confirms diagnosis.

LABORATORY TESTS

Microscopic examination with potassium hydroxide confirms diagnosis.

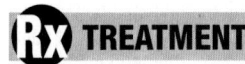

Rx TREATMENT

NONPHARMACOLOGIC THERAPY

Sunlight accelerates repigmentation of hypopigmented areas.

ACUTE GENERAL Rx

- Topical treatment: Selenium sulfide 2.5% suspension (Selsun or Exsel) applied daily for 30 min for 7 consecutive days results in a cure rate of 80% to 90%. The scalp can be shampooed monthly with selenium sulfide to reduce scalp colonization.
- Antifungal topical agents (e.g., miconazole, ciclopirox, clotrimazole) are also effective.
- Oral treatment can be given along with topical agents but is generally reserved for resistant cases. Effective agents are fluconazole and itraconazole. Table 1 summarizes treatment options for tinea versicolor.

DISPOSITION

The prognosis is good, with eradication of the fungus usually occurring within 3 to 4 wk of treatment; however, recurrence is common. After initial therapy, use of monthly application of selenium sulfide may lower risk of recurrence.

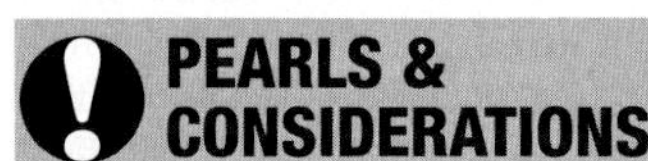

PEARLS & CONSIDERATIONS

COMMENTS

Patients should be informed that the hypopigmented areas will not disappear immediately after treatment and that several months may be necessary for the hypopigmented areas to regain their pigmentation.

RELATED CONTENT

Tinea Versicolor (Patient Information)

AUTHOR: **FRED F. FERRI, M.D.**

TABLE 1 Treatment of Tinea (Pityriasis) Versicolor

Initial therapy (often combination)	*Topical** • Antifungal shampoo applied as a body cleanser for 10-15 minutes before rinsing, twice weekly for 2-4 weeks 1. Selenium sulfide shampoo, 1% (OTC) or 2.5% 2. Ketoconazole shampoo, 1% (OTC) or 2% 3. Zinc pyrithione shampoo 4. Ciclopirox olamine shampoo, 1% • Antifungal cream applied several hand-widths beyond clinically visible lesions, daily to twice daily for 2 weeks 1. Imidazole, e.g., ketoconazole 2% cream 2. Ciclopirox olamine 0.77% cream, gel, or lotion *Oral*** • Fluconazole: 200 mg po daily × 5-7 days†; 200-300 mg weekly × 2-3 weeks; or 400 mg once • Itraconazole: 200 mg po daily × 5-7 days
Maintenance therapy to prevent recurrence	• Treat previously affected sites with topical imidazole daily for 2 weeks prior to anticipated sun exposure • Apply antifungal shampoo (see above) 1-2 times weekly

*Treatment of all the skin from the neck down to the knees may lead to higher success rates.

**Although there are few comparative studies of oral antifungal medications, cure rates of 98%-100% have been reported in several randomized controlled trials of itraconazole 200 mg daily × 5 days and an open-label study of fluconazole 300 mg weekly × 2 weeks.

†Based upon authors' personal experience.

From Bolognia J et al: *Dermatology*, ed 4, Philadelphia, 2018, Elsevier.

Oral ketoconazole is no longer indicated for treatment of superficial fungal infections due to risks of severe hepatotoxicity, QT prolongation, and serious drug interactions.

BASIC INFORMATION

DEFINITION

Tinnitus is a perceived sound in the absence of acoustic stimulus external to the head. It may be unilateral, bilateral, or lateral dominant. It is commonly described as a ringing, buzzing, roaring, hissing, whistling, humming, cricket-like, or pulsing sound. It is frequently a symptom associated with hearing loss, Ménière disease, acoustic neuroma, drug toxicity, depression, or an autoimmune inner ear disease. The sound may be internal and perceived only by the patient, called subjective or tonal tinnitus, or it may be heard by both the patient and the examiner, called objective or nontonal tinnitus.

ICD-10CM CODES

H93.1	Tinnitus
H93.2	Other abnormal auditory perceptions
H93.11	Tinnitus, right ear
H93.12	Tinnitus, left ear
H93.13	Tinnitus, bilateral
H93.19	Tinnitus, unspecified ear

EPIDEMIOLOGY & DEMOGRAPHICS

PREVALENCE:

- The American Tinnitus Association reports 50 to 60 million Americans have tinnitus for >6 mo.
- Prevalence increases steadily with age, peaking for persons aged 60 to 69 years.
- Prevalence in the U.S. based on National Health Interview Survey (NHIS) in 1996
  1. 2.98% all ages
  2. 0.26% for persons <18 yr old
  3. 1.6% for persons aged 18 to 44 yr
  4. 5.96% for persons aged 45 to 64 yr: 7.7% males, 4.3% females
  5. 9.6% for persons aged 65 to 74 yr: 12% males, 7.7% females
  6. 7.6% for persons >75 yr: 11.4% males, 5.3% females
  7. 2:1 South/Northeast regions
- Up to 18% of people in industrialized societies are mildly affected by chronic tinnitus, and 0.5% report tinnitus having a severe effect on their daily life.
- Only 20% of patients with persistent tinnitus ever seek medical evaluation.

PREDOMINANT SEX AND AGE: Persons most affected are male, Caucasian, elderly, persons with hearing impairment, persons living in southern U.S. For military veterans, tinnitus is the third most common service-related disability.

RISK FACTORS: Any condition causing hearing loss or damage to the auditory system can produce tinnitus. Cochlear damage from exposure to noise is the most common cause. Exposure to ototoxic drugs is also important.

PHYSICAL FINDINGS & CLINICAL PRESENTATION

- History should focus on exposure to loud noises, evidence of hearing loss, and ototoxic drugs.
- Patient should be screened for depression.
- Patient who complains of sound in ear may also complain of ear pain or fullness.
- Objective tinnitus is pulsatile and coincides with patient's pulse.
- Physical examination should focus on HEENT, neck, and neurologic exam.
- There may be no significant physical findings.

ETIOLOGY

- The mechanism behind tinnitus is poorly understood. It may originate at any point along the auditory pathway. Causes of tinnitus include injured cochlear hair cells, spontaneous activity in auditory nerve fibers, hyperactivity in the auditory nuclei in the brain stem, or a reduction in the suppressive activity of the central auditory cortex.
- Medications implicated in causing tinnitus include salicylates, NSAIDs, aminoglycosides, loop diuretics, valproate, quinine, chemotherapeutic agents, cisplatin, vincristine, and heavy metals such as lead.

Dx DIAGNOSIS

DIFFERENTIAL DIAGNOSIS

- Subjective/tonal tinnitus:
  1. Otologic: Tympanic membrane disorder, inner ear disorder (hair cells, organ of Corti), Ménière disease
  2. Ototoxic medications
  3. Neurologic: Multiple sclerosis, head trauma, cochlear nerve lesion, acoustic schwannoma, neurofibroma, meningioma
  4. Metabolic: Thyroid disorder, hyperlipidemia (leading to plaque formation), vitamin B_{12} deficiency
  5. Psychogenic: Depression, anxiety, fibromyalgia
  6. Infectious: Otitis media, Lyme disease, meningitis, syphilis
- Objective/nontonal tinnitus:
  1. Vascular: Arterial bruit, venous hum, arteriovenous malformation, vascular tumors
  2. Neurologic: Contraction of muscles of the eustachian tube, contraction of the stapedius muscle, contraction of the tensor tympani muscles, or a palatal myoclonus, glomus jugulare tumor
  3. Conductive: Patulous (wide-open) eustachian tube

WORKUP

- Audiometry.
- Tympanometry.
- Electronystagmography is used to evaluate for Ménière disease.
- An algorithm for tinnitus evaluation is described in Figs. E1 and E2.

LABORATORY TESTS

Evaluate for metabolic abnormalities: TSH, CBC, B_{12}, and lipid panel.

IMAGING STUDIES

- CT/MRI: To evaluate for subjective tinnitus
- MRI/MRA: To evaluate objective tinnitus
- Imaging should not be part of routine management. Clinicians must distinguish patients with bothersome tinnitus from patients with nonbothersome tinnitus. For patients without persistent and bothersome tinnitus, audiometric testing is optional.

Rx TREATMENT

NONPHARMACOLOGIC THERAPY

- It is best to avoid exposure to excessive noise, ototoxic agents, and to wear protective equipment in noisy environments, or mask the tinnitus through amplification of normal sounds with a hearing aid. Habituation techniques such as tinnitus retraining therapy may help. Cognitive behavioral therapy helps patients cope with tinnitus distress through biofeedback.
- Recent trials involving brain stimulation in the form of repetitive transcranial magnetic stimulation (rTMS have shown reduction in the perception or severity of tinnitus).[1]

ACUTE GENERAL Rx

- If the tinnitus is severe enough to cause suicidal symptoms, immediate referral to a psychiatrist and an otolaryngologist is recommended to minimize the time to diagnosis and optimize treatment.
- Patients with persistent symptoms or tinnitus accompanied by visual changes or headache should be evaluated for tumors such as acoustic neuroma.
- Clinicians should not routinely recommend anxiolytics, anticonvulsants, or intratympanic medications.

CHRONIC Rx

There is insufficient evidence to support the use of any medication, vitamin, or nutritional supplement to treat tinnitus. Empirical use of over-the-counter supplements or prescription medications should be discouraged.

DISPOSITION

Clinical course is variable. About 20% to 25% of patients with chronic tinnitus consider it a significant problem. Individualized tinnitus management programs can be beneficial in most patients.

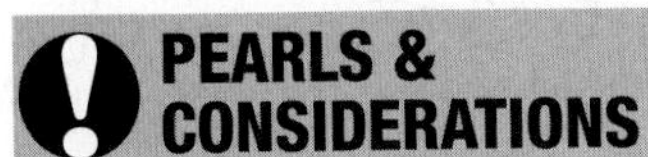

PEARLS & CONSIDERATIONS

PREVENTION

- Avoid loud, chronic noise and ototoxic drugs.
- Higher caffeine intake is associated with a lower risk of incidence of tinnitus in women.

RELATED CONTENT

Tinnitus (Patient Information)

AUTHORS: **VICKY H. BHAGAT, M.D., M.P.H.,** and **DAWN HOGAN, M.D.**

[1] Folmer RL et al: Repetitive transcranial magnetic stimulation treatment for chronic tinnitus: a randomized clinical trial, *JAMA Otolaryngol Head Neck Surg* 141(8):716-722, 2015.

BASIC INFORMATION

DEFINITION

The term *Torsade de Pointes* (TdP) refers to a polymorphic ventricular tachycardia (VT) associated with a prolonged QT interval and electrocardiographically characterized by QRS complexes of changing amplitude that appear to twist around the isoelectric line, hence the name *Torsade de Pointes*, or "twisting of the points" (Fig. 1).

Torsade is typically initiated by a short-long-short sequence of ventricular beats but can also be initiated by a short-coupled variant. Typically, TdP occurs in the setting of a markedly prolonged QT interval (>500 msec); the QTc prolongs even further during the long diastolic interval of a compensatory pause, leading to a polymorphic VT with a ventricular rate of 160 to 250 beats per minute, irregular RR intervals, and a cycling of the QRS axis through 180 degrees every 5 to 20 beats. It may be repetitive, nonsustained, or sustained and may degenerate into ventricular fibrillation. In some cases, the result is sudden cardiac death.

SYNONYMS

Torsades
TdP

ICD-10CM CODE

I47.2 Ventricular tachycardia

EPIDEMIOLOGY & DEMOGRAPHICS

INCIDENCE: The precise incidence of TdP is unclear but accounts for fewer than 5% of all sudden cardiac arrests. In congenital long QT syndromes (LQTS), TdP may occur in up to 6% of cases at rest and 9% of cases during an exercise test. Among drug-induced causes of TdP, the incidence may vary between <1% in cases of antibiotics and antipsychotics to 2% to 4% when caused by class III anti-arrhythmics such as sotalol, ibutilide, and dofetilide.

PREDOMINANT SEX AND AGE: Because testosterone shortens the QT interval, women have a longer baseline QT interval, which is believed to be the reason for a two- to threefold increased incidence of TdP in women.

GENETICS: Of the congenital LQTS channelopathies, long QT syndromes 1, 2, and 3 account for >70% of all cases. In general, the risk of TdP increases as the QT lengthens; however, there are also genotype-phenotype relationships that help define risk; for example, LQTS3 carries a higher risk of TdP than LQTS1. Similarly, the Jervell and Lange-Nielsen syndrome and Romano-Ward syndrome may lead to TdP.

It is also likely that genetic factors are at play in acquired LQT and in the development of TdP. For example, in large populations, the QT interval prolongs very little with the administration of QT-prolonging drugs such as fluoroquinolones; however, certain individuals will have markedly exaggerated QT prolongation that leads to TdP; this is likely due to some underlying genetic factor.

RISK FACTORS: TdP in patients with congenital LQTS is often initiated by an external trigger (Table 1). Triggers can include exercise, noise, emotion, sudden waking from sleep by an alarm clock, telephone ringing, thunder, swimming, or diving. TdP in LQT1 patients is classically triggered by vigorous exercise or swimming; in LQT2 by emotion, pregnancy, or noise; and in LQT3 when at rest or asleep. Risk factors for drug-induced TdP are outlined in Table 2.

The risk factors for developing TdP in patients with acquired long QT are extensive and are outlined in Table 3.

PATHOPHYSIOLOGY:

- Changes in the balance of transmembrane ionic currents lead to lengthening of the QT interval and to abnormal action potentials called early afterdepolarizations (EADs). An EAD, in the setting of electrical instability induced by the prolonged QT, initiates the torsades. Perpetuation may be caused by transmural entry, triggered activity, or abnormal automaticity. A distinct group of cells called the M cells, located in the mid-myocardium, has a less rapid delayed rectifier potassium current (IKr), and the cells are central to the genesis of TdP.
- Drugs with the potential to cause TdP most frequently inhibit the rapid potassium channels and result in prolongation of the action potential duration, producing a prolonged QT on ECG.

PHYSICAL FINDINGS & CLINICAL PRESENTATION

- Clinical features depend on whether the TdP is caused by acquired or congenital long QT syndrome. Congenital LQTS patients may have certain specific triggers, such as noise, exercise, and emotions (see "Risk Factors").
- Symptoms of the tachycardia itself include palpitations, pre-syncope, syncope (sometimes with jerking movements from myoclonus, often misinterpreted as seizures), and sudden cardiac death (SCD).
- Patients resuscitated from SCD have an especially ominous prognosis, with a relative risk of 12.9% of experiencing another cardiac arrest.

ETIOLOGY

The etiology or triggers of TdP may be congenital or acquired causes of QT prolongation (see Table 1). For a comprehensive list of drugs that can cause or have the potential to cause TdP, see "Patient/Family Education."

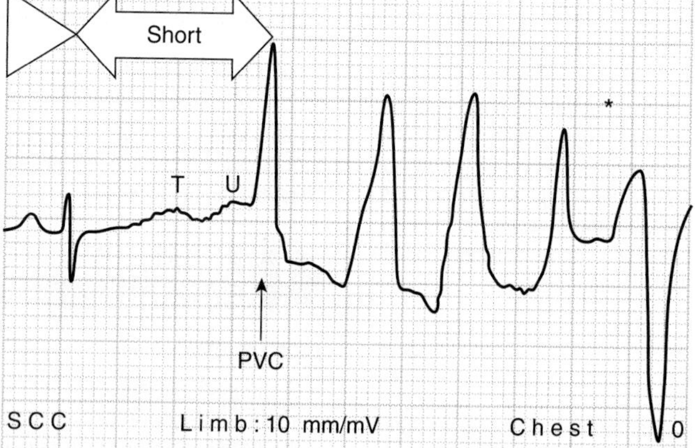

FIG. 1 Onset of Torsade de Pointes during the recording of a standard 12-lead ECG in a young male with a history of drug addiction treated with chronic methadone therapy who presented to a hospital emergency department after ingesting an overdose of prescription and over-the-counter drugs from his parent's drug cabinet. Classic ECG features evident in this rhythm strip include a prolonged QT interval with distorted T-U complex, initiation of the arrhythmia after a short-long-short cycle sequence by a PVC that falls near the peak of the distorted T-U complex, "warm-up" phenomenon with initial R-R cycles longer than subsequent cycles, and abrupt switching of QRS morphology from predominantly positive to predominantly negative complexes (asterisk). (From Drew BJ et al: Prevention of Torsade de Pointes in hospital settings: a scientific statement from the American Heart Association and the American College of Cardiology Foundation, *J Am Coll Cardiol* 55:934-947, 2010.)

DIAGNOSIS

DIFFERENTIAL DIAGNOSIS

Other causes of syncope

- Other causes of broad complex tachycardia such as:
  1. Polymorphic VT
  2. Wolff-Parkinson-White (WPW) syndrome with rapid atrial fibrillation
  3. ECG artifact

WORKUP

- ECG (Fig. 2) and telemetry are the mainstays of diagnosing TdP as they detect the arrhythmia, the preceding prolonged QT interval, and the long-short cycles that trigger it.
- Determination and treatment of the etiology of TdP (see Table 1) is key.

TABLE 1 Causes and Triggers of Torsade de Pointes

Congenital	• Romano-Ward syndrome (autosomal dominant) • Jervell and Lange-Nielsen syndrome (autosomal recessive) • LQTS channelopathies
Acquired	
Metabolic syndromes	• Hypokalemia • Hypocalcemia • Hypomagnesemia • Starvation • Anorexia nervosa • Liquid protein diets • Hypothyroidism
Bradyarrhythmias	• Sinus node dysfunction • Second- or third-degree AV block
Antiarrhythmic drugs	• Quinidine • Procainamide • Disopyramide • Amiodarone and dronedarone • Sotalol • Dofetilide, ibutilide, azimilide
Antimicrobial drugs	• Erythromycin, clarithromycin, azithromycin • Pentamidine • Azole antifungals like voriconazole • Fluoroquinolones such as levofloxacin and moxifloxacin • Chloroquine
Antihistaminics	• Terfenadine • Astemizole
Psychiatric drugs	• Phenothiazines • Thioridazine • Tricyclic antidepressants • Haloperidol • Risperidone • Selective serotonin reuptake inhibitors
Antineoplastic agents	• Tyrosine kinase inhibitors such as sunitinib, dasatinib • Vorinostat • Arsenic
Gastric motility agents	• Cisapride, domperidone
Opioid dependence drugs	• Methadone
Other factors	• Myocardial ischemia • Hypothermia • Intracranial disease • HIV infection • Connective tissue disease with anti-Ro/SSA antibodies • Periodic paralysis (Andersen syndrome) • Cocaine

TABLE 2 Risk Factors for Drug-Induced Torsade de Pointes

- Congenital long QT
- Female gender
- Electrolyte abnormalities (hypokalemia, hypomagnesemia, hypocalcemia)
- Diuretic use
- Bradycardia
- Cardiac hypertrophy
- Myocardial fibrosis
- Congestive heart failure
- Renal and liver insufficiency
- Coadministration of drugs blocking P450 isoenzyme CYP3A4
- High doses or rapid intravenous infusion of the drug
- Baseline electrocardiographic abnormalities (prolonged QT, T-wave lability)

From Gowda RM et al: Torsades de Pointes: the clinical considerations, *Int J Cardiol* 96(1):1-6, 2004.

TABLE 3 Risk Factors for Torsade de Pointes in Hospitalized Patients

- Clinically recognizable risk factors
- QTc >500 msec
- LQT2-type repolarization: Notched or "bifid" T-wave
- Use of QT-prolonging drugs
- Concurrent use of more than one QT-prolonging drug
- Rapid infusion by intravenous route
- Structural heart disease
- Congestive heart failure
- Myocardial infarction
- Advanced age
- Female sex
- Hypokalemia
- Hypomagnesemia
- Hypocalcemia
- Treatment with diuretics
- Impaired hepatic drug metabolism
- Bradycardia
- Sinus bradycardia, heart block, incomplete heart block with pauses
- Premature QRS complexes leading to short-long-short cycles
- Multiple clinically recognizable risk factors
- Occult (latent) congenital LQTS
- Genetic polymorphisms

From Drew BJ et al: Prevention of Torsade de Pointes in hospital settings: a scientific statement from the American Heart Association and the American College of Cardiology Foundation, *Circulation* 121(8):1047, 2010.

LABORATORY TESTS

- Electrolytes: Assess for hypokalemia, hypocalcemia, and hypomagnesemia
- Thyroid function tests
- Genetic studies if suspicion of congenital LQT syndrome

IMAGING STUDIES

- Echocardiography to rule out structural heart disease as a cause of VT.
- Stress test to rule out myocardial ischemia. Stress ECG with dynamic assessment of the QT interval during varying heart rates may be diagnostic of long QT syndromes and related TdP.
- CT scan of the head if intracranial disease is suspected.

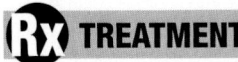

TREATMENT

The cornerstone of treatment comprises intravenous magnesium and acceleration of the heart rate, either by mechanical overdrive pacing or by infusion of isoproterenol. Withdrawal of causative drugs and correction of underlying causes such as electrolyte imbalances, hypothermia, and ischemia are also important.

NONPHARMACOLOGIC THERAPY

- Withdrawal of any offending drugs and correction of electrolyte abnormalities are recommended in patients presenting with TdP (Class I recommendation).
- Temporary atrial or ventricular overdrive pacing is a Class I recommendation for all causes of TdP if intravenous magnesium fails.
- Acute and long-term pacing is recommended for patients presenting with TdP due to heart block and symptomatic bradycardia (Class 1) or those with recurrent pause-dependent torsades (Class IIa).
- Active internal and external rewarming if hypothermia is the etiology.
- If TdP degenerates into ventricular fibrillation, defibrillation and advanced cardiac life support protocol should be followed.

ACUTE Rx

- Intravenous magnesium sulfate 1 to 2 g given over 1 to 2 min is first-line therapy for patients who present with LQTS and few episodes of TdP (Class IIa). Magnesium is not likely to be effective in patients with a normal QT interval
- Isoproterenol is reasonable as temporary treatment in patients with acute disease who present with recurrent pause-dependent TdP and who do not have congenital LQTS (Class IIa).
- Beta-blockade combined with pacing is reasonable acute therapy for patients who present with TdP and sinus bradycardia (Class IIa).

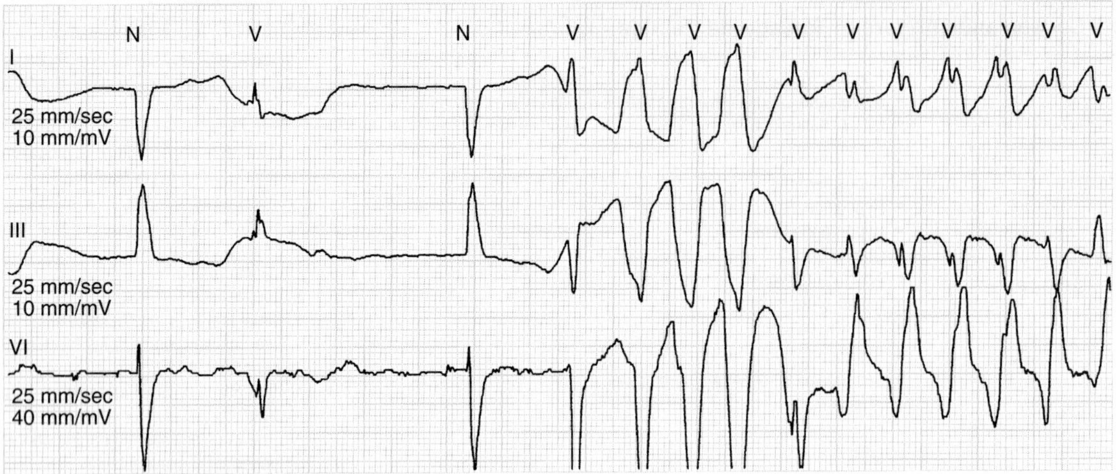

FIG. 2 Torsades de Pointes. This lead I, III, and V_1 rhythm strip shows sinus bradycardia with left bundle branch block and marked QT prolongation with premature ventricular contractions (R-on-T) that initiates a very rapid polymorphic ventricular tachycardia with the characteristic twisting of the QRS complex around the isoelectric baseline. Torsades des pointes literally means "twisting of the points." (From Olshansky B et al: *Arrhythmia essentials*, ed 2, Philadelphia, 2017, Elsevier.)

- Potassium repletion to 4.5 to 5 mmol/L may be considered for patients who present with TdP and hypokalemia (Class IIb).
- Intravenous lidocaine, oral mexiletine, or phenytoin may be considered in patients who present with LQT3 and TdP (Class IIb).
- TdP is usually self-limited, and cardioversion should be performed only as a last resort in the setting of pulseless VF because of the high likelihood of immediate recurrence of the TdP after cardioversion.

CHRONIC Rx

- TdP resulting from congenital LQTS is treated with beta-blockade, pacing, and implantable cardioverter-defibrillator (ICD) in high-risk cases. For patients who continue to have syncope despite maximal drug therapy, cervical-thoracic sympathectomy may be considered.
- Long-term pacing is recommended for patients presenting with TdP due to heart block and symptomatic bradycardia.
- Avoid use of QT-prolonging drugs.
- Lifestyle modification in case of congenital LQTS.
- In patients with eating disorders, nutritional rehabilitation will correct the QT prolongation over the long term (3-18 mo).
- Psychiatric evaluation of patients with drug overdose and eating disorders.

DISPOSITION

Patients with TdP should be monitored in an intensive care setting.

REFERRAL

Patients should have an urgent cardiology consultation.

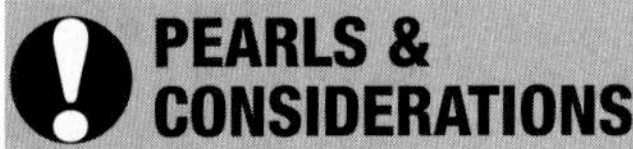

COMMENTS

- Identification of the etiology for TdP is key in diagnosis, management, and prognosis of this condition.
- Drugs associated with TdP vary greatly in their risk for arrhythmia; an updated list can be found at https://crediblemeds.org. The risk-benefit ratio should be assessed for each individual to determine whether the potential therapeutic benefit of a drug outweighs the risk for TdP.
- Risk factors for drug-induced TdP include older age, female sex, heart disease, electrolyte disorders (especially hypokalemia and hypomagnesemia), renal or hepatic dysfunction, bradycardia or rhythms with long pauses, treatment with more than one QT-prolonging drug, and genetic predisposition.
- After initiation of a drug associated with TdP, ECG signs indicative of risk for arrhythmia include an increase in QTc from predrug baseline of >60 msec, marked QTc interval prolongation >500 msec, T-U wave distortion that becomes more exaggerated in the beat after a pause, visible T-wave alternans, new-onset ventricular ectopy, and couplets and nonsustained polymorphic ventricular tachycardia initiated in the beat after a pause.

PREVENTION

The 2011 AHA/ACC scientific statement on prevention of TdP suggests a strategy of documenting the QTc interval before and at least every 8 to 12 hr after the initiation, increased dose, or overdose of QT-prolonging drugs. If QTc prolongation is observed, documentation of more frequent measurements is recommended. The duration of QTc monitoring depends upon the duration of treatment with the QT-prolonging drug and the drug half-life.

PATIENT/FAMILY EDUCATION

- Patients should be educated about avoiding use of QT-prolonging drugs. A complete list of these drugs can be found at https://crediblemeds.org.
- First-degree relatives of all patients with congenital LQTS should undergo genetic testing.
- Congenital LQTS patients should avoid certain specific triggers (e.g., swimming and exercise in LQTS 1 and LQTS 2 and acoustic stimuli in LQTS 2).
- It is recommended that all patients affected by LQTS avoid competitive sports activity.

RELATED TOPICS

Long QT Syndrome (Related Key Topic)

AUTHOR: **CHRISTOPHER PICKETT, M.D.**

BASIC INFORMATION

DEFINITION

Tourette syndrome (TS) is an inherited neuropsychiatric disorder characterized by motor, vocal, and phonic tics that change during the course of illness. Onset of symptoms is typically before the age of 18.

Tics are sudden, brief, intermittent, involuntary or semi-voluntary movements (motor tics), or sounds (phonic or vocal tics) that mimic fragments of normal behavior.

SYNONYMS

Gilles de la Tourette syndrome
TS
Tourette's disorder

ICD-10CM CODE
F95.2 Combined vocal and multiple motor tic disorder [de la Tourette]

EPIDEMIOLOGY & DEMOGRAPHICS

PREVALENCE (IN U.S.): Unknown; estimates range from 0.3% to 0.9% in children

PREDOMINANT SEX: Approximate male:female ratio of 4:1

PREDOMINANT AGE: Typical age of onset is between 2 and 15 yr (mean 5-7 yr).

PHYSICAL FINDINGS & CLINICAL PRESENTATION

- Neurologic examination is normal.
- Vocal and phonic tics are characterized as simple (e.g., clearing of throat, sniffing, grunting, sucking) or complex (e.g., repetition of short phrases, swearing [coprolalia]).
- Motor tics can be simple (e.g., blinking, grimacing, head jerking [Fig. 1]) or complex (e.g., gesturing [Fig. 2]). Tics wax, wane, change over time, and are often suppressed for short periods. Commonly, they are preceded by an urge to perform the tic.
- TS is often associated with a variety of behavioral symptoms, most commonly attention deficit hyperactivity disorder (ADHD) and obsessive-compulsive disorder (OCD).

TS can be diagnosed using the DSM-5 criteria as follows:

- Both multiple motor and one or more vocal tics must be present at some time during the illness, although not necessarily concurrently.
- The tics may wax and wane in frequency but have persisted for more than 1 yr since first tic onset.
- Age at onset is less than 18 yr.
- Disturbance is not attributable to the direct physiologic effects of a substance (e.g., stimulants) or another medical condition (e.g., Huntington disease or postviral encephalitis).

ETIOLOGY

The exact pathogenesis is unknown. Genetic predisposition is likely as there is a strong family history of OCD or TS in patients with tics, and twin studies provide evidence for the importance of genetic factors. Recent analysis of linkage in a two-generation pedigree has led to the identification of a mutation in the HDC gene encoding l-histidine decarboxylase, the rate-limiting enzyme in histamine biosynthesis, pointing to a role for histaminergic neurotransmission in the mechanism and modulation of TS and tics. Immunologic dysfunction is also being explored in the pathogenesis of this complex disorder.

Dx DIAGNOSIS

DIFFERENTIAL DIAGNOSIS

- Sydenham chorea: Occurs after infection with group A *Streptococcus.*
- Pediatric autoimmune neuropsychiatric disorder associated with group A streptococci (PANDAS).
- Sporadic tic disorders: Tics tend to be motor or vocal but not both.
- Head trauma.
- Drug intoxication: Many drugs are known to induce or exacerbate tic disorders, including methylphenidate, amphetamines, anticholinergics, and antihistamines.
- Postinfectious encephalitis.
- Inherited disorders: Huntington disease, neurodegeneration with brain iron accumulation, and neuroacanthocytosis. These conditions should have other observed abnormalities on neurologic examination.

WORKUP

Clinical observation and history to confirm diagnosis

LABORATORY TESTS

No definitive laboratory tests

IMAGING STUDIES

CT scan and MRI of brain are unremarkable in TS and unnecessary if the neurologic examination is within normal limits.

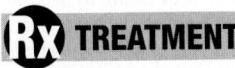

TREATMENT

NONPHARMACOLOGIC THERAPY

Multidisciplinary: Education of parents, teachers, psychologists, and school nurses is essential. Cognitive behavioral therapy, termed habit-reversal treatment, is efficacious in suppressing tics.

ACUTE GENERAL Rx

Dopamine-blocking agents may be used to acutely reduce the severity of tics. However, these agents carry a risk of side effects, such as acute dystonic reactions.

CHRONIC Rx

Tics only require long-term treatment when they interfere with an individual's psychosocial, educational, and occupational function.

TICS:

- Alpha-2 agonists, such as clonidine and guanfacine, are used for treatment of motor tics and are considered by some experts as first-line medications because of their favorable adverse effect profile. However, they are more beneficial for treatment of behavioral symptoms and are preferred for patients with predominant psychiatric disorders.
- Haloperidol and pimozide are the only U.S. Food and Drug Administration-approved neuroleptics for the treatment of tics in TS. Pimozide is started at a dose of 0.5 to 1.0 mg at night and increased every 5 to 7 days to a

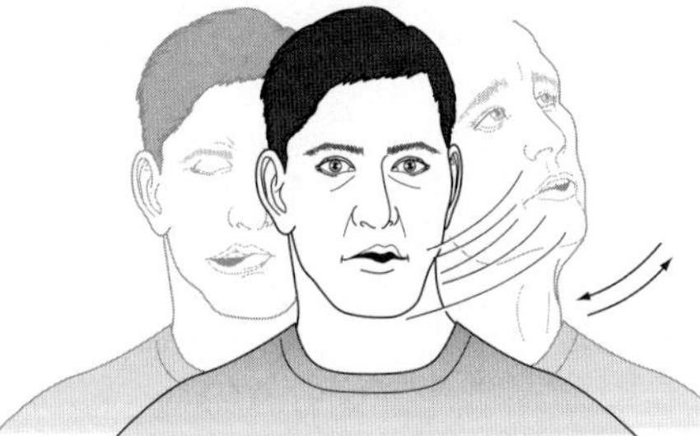

FIG. 1 This young man with Tourette disorder has multiple motor tics, including head jerking (head toss), grimacing of the right side of his mouth (half-smile), and depression of his forehead (frowning). Vocal tics of throat clearing and a short blowing sound accompany his motor tics. All of his tics continue throughout the day and briefly during sleep. Conversation, eating, and social situations have little influence, but with effort he can suppress his tics for several minutes. (From Kaufman DM, Geyer HL, Milstein MJ: *Kaufman's clinical neurology for psychiatrists*, ed 8, Philadelphia, 2017, Elsevier.)

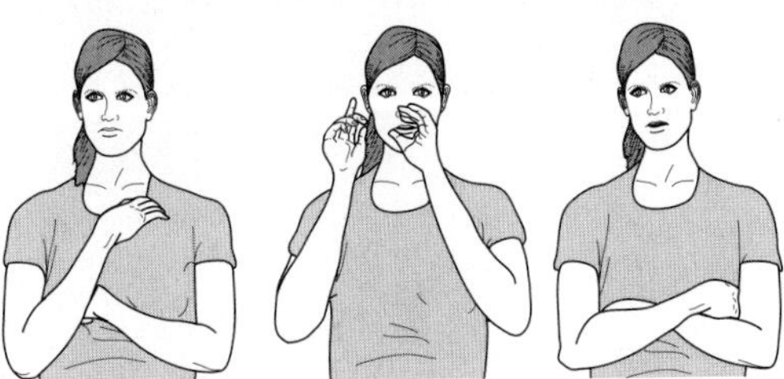

FIG. 2 This woman has compulsive obscene gestures—copropraxia. Similar to coprolalia, they have no affective or sexual content. (From Kaufman DM, Geyer HL, Milstein MJ: *Kaufman's clinical neurology for psychiatrists*, ed 8, Philadelphia, 2017, Elsevier.)

therapeutic dose of 2 to 8 mg. Haloperidol is started at a dose of 0.25 to 0.5 mg and can be increased to 1 to 4 mg depending on response and side effects. Use of neuroleptics carries a small but significant risk of tardive dyskinesia.

- Tetrabenazine is a dopamine-depleting agent that can be used effectively in TS patients to control tics. Tetrabenazine does not cause many of the typical side effects of neuroleptic medication. However, severe depression may occur with use of tetrabenazine. Newer deutetrabenazine and valbenazine (VMAT2 inhibitors) also can be considered and have randomized placebo-controlled trials in progress.
- Topiramate is an antiepileptic used off-label to treat tics.
- Botulinum toxin (local injection) is effective for focal tics like eye blinking and neck and shoulder tics. The benefits are temporary, lasting 3 to 6 months.
- Surgical treatment with deep brain stimulation is effective in some patients with disabling tics that are refractory to medications.

ADHD: Stimulants are useful for symptoms of ADHD but may exacerbate tics in 25% of patients. These medications should be used if troublesome behavioral symptoms persist.

OCD: Selective serotonin reuptake inhibitors, such as fluoxetine, are the most effective treatment for OCD.

DISPOSITION

- The intensity and frequency of tics typically diminishes during the later teenage years.
- One third of patients will achieve significant remission, although complete, lifelong remission is rare.
- One third will have mild, persistent, but "non-impairing" tics.

REFERRAL

Neurologist to confirm the initial diagnosis and for treatment in difficult cases

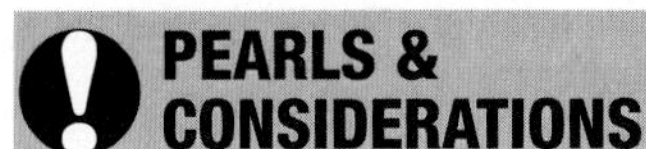

PEARLS & CONSIDERATIONS

- Tics do not need treatment unless they interfere with an individual's ability to function.
- Greater improvement in symptom severity among children with TS and chronic tic disorder has been reported with a comprehensive behavioral intervention compared with supportive therapy and education.
- An important part of treatment is appropriate evaluation and therapy of coexisting conditions (e.g., ADHD, OCD).
- Deep brain stimulation has shown promising results as an alternative therapy in patients with medically refractory disease.

COMMENTS

Patient education may be obtained from the Tourette Syndrome Association, 4240 Bell Blvd., Bayside, NY 11361-2864; 800-237-0717 or 718-224-2999; http://www.tsa-usa.org.

SUGGESTED READINGS

Available at ExpertConsult.com

RELATED CONTENT

Tourette Syndrome (Patient Information)

AUTHORS: **COREY GOLDSMITH, M.D., JOSEPH S. KASS, M.D., J.D.,** and **FARIHA ZAHEER, M.D.**

BASIC INFORMATION

DEFINITION

Toxic megacolon is a rare but severe complication of colonic inflammation, usually inflammatory bowel disease (IBD). It is characterized by total or segmental nonobstructive colonic distention (>6 cm) associated with systemic toxicity of inflammatory or infectious etiology.

SYNONYM

Toxic dilation of the colon

ICD ICD-10-CM CODES
K59.3 Megacolon, not elsewhere classified
A04.7 Megacolon due to *Clostridium difficile*

EPIDEMIOLOGY & DEMOGRAPHICS

INCIDENCE: Varies depending on etiology. Incidence in patients with ulcerative colitis (UC) is between 7% and 10% and approximately 1% and 5% in patients with Crohn. *Clostridium difficile* infections may be complicated by toxic megacolon in up to 3% of cases.
PEAK INCIDENCE: N/A
PREVALENCE: N/A
PREDOMINANT SEX AND AGE: With increasing rates of *Clostridium difficile (C. diff)* infections due to overuse of antibiotics and hypervirulent strains, patients ages 65 and older are at higher risk for developing toxic megacolon as a result of *C. diff* infection.
GENETICS: There are no known genetic factors that predispose patients to developing toxic megacolon associated with an inflammatory or infectious etiology.
RISK FACTORS: Major risk factors include inflammatory, infectious, and ischemic conditions of the colon, especially in individuals who are immunocompromised. Other risk factors include hypokalemia, use of narcotics or antidiarrheal agents, pregnancy, and recent instrumentation (such as colonoscopy).

PHYSICAL FINDINGS & CLINICAL PRESENTATION

- Patients with toxic megacolon usually appear severely ill. Clinical symptoms are similar to those of IBD and acute colitis and may include abdominal pain, diarrhea (usually bloody), and vomiting.
- Physical exam findings may include a distended, tender, and tympanic abdomen with reduced or absent bowel sounds. The patient may also present with signs of shock such as fever, tachycardia, mental status changes, and hypovolemia.
- Laboratory findings may include leukocytosis, anemia, and electrolyte abnormalities such as hypokalemia and hypoalbuminemia.

ETIOLOGY

- Most common etiologies are inflammatory conditions such as UC, Crohn, and Behçet's disease.
- Infections such as *C. diff, Salmonella, Shigella, E. coli,* cytomegalovirus, and *Entamoeba* can also be complicated by toxic megacolon.
- Other less common etiologies include ischemic colitis, malignancy such as lymphoma, and Kaposi sarcoma. In general, toxic megacolon is more likely to be associated with pancolitis than segmental colitis (Box 1).

DIAGNOSIS

DIFFERENTIAL DIAGNOSIS

Ischemic colitis, Crohn disease, ulcerative colitis

WORKUP

- General principles of workup include physical examination to evaluate for an acute abdomen, laboratory testing to detect electrolyte abnormalities, and plain radiography to evaluate for colonic dilation.
- Clinical criteria for toxic megacolon, proposed by Jalan et al in 1969, are still used. A diagnosis can be made if radiographic evidence of colonic distention >6 cm is present with at least three of the following: fever >38° C (100.4° F), heart rate >120, leukocytosis >10.5, or anemia. In addition, at least one of the following must also be present: dehydration, altered level of consciousness, electrolyte abnormalities, or hypotension.

LABORATORY TESTS

Initial testing should include a CBC, full chemistry panel, lactic acid, coagulation panel, liver function panel, and a type and screen.

IMAGING STUDIES

- All patients should initially receive a plain abdominal radiograph (Fig. 1) to assess for colonic dilation. Common findings include mucosal irregularity, loss of haustrations, "thumb printing" due to bowel wall edema, and thickening of the colonic wall with a continuous segment of air-filled colon >6 cm in diameter. The transverse or right colon is usually the most dilated segment seen.
- Computed tomography (CT) has been increasingly used to assess disease extent and for surgical planning (Fig. 2). It can also be helpful when differentiating between the various etiologies of toxic megacolon and to assess for complications such as intraabdominal hemorrhage or abscess.

BOX 1 Disorders Associated with Toxic Megacolon

- Inflammatory bowel disease
  1. Ulcerative colitis
  2. Crohn disease
- Infectious colitis
  1. *Salmonella, Shigella,* amoebic colitis
  2. *Clostridium difficile*
  3. Cytomegalovirus colitis
  4. HIV infection
- Cancer chemotherapy
- Ischemia

HIV, Human immunodeficiency virus.
From Vincent JL et al: *Textbook of critical care,* ed 6, Philadelphia, 2011, Saunders.

TREATMENT

Treatment includes both medical and surgical options. Principles of initial management include treating the underlying cause and managing symptoms of shock with early surgical and gastroenterology consultation.

NONPHARMACOLOGIC THERAPY

- Surgery may be required in up to 50% of patients with toxic megacolon who do not show clinical improvement within 24 to 48 hr. The preferred first-line surgical treatment is subtotal colectomy with an end ileostomy. Other options include total proctocolectomy or colon decompression via the Turnbull method.
- Timing of surgical treatment is still controversial, with many advocating for aggressive medical treatment and observation before surgical intervention. Definitive indications for early surgical treatment include perforation, persistent colonic hemorrhage, or rapid clinical deterioration.

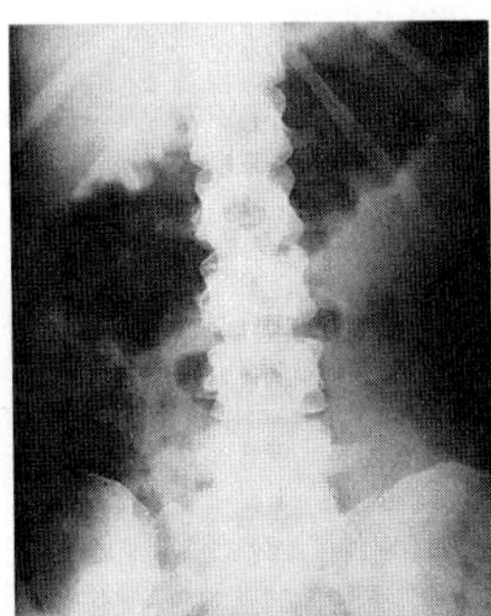

FIG. 1 Toxic megacolon secondary to ulcerative colitis. The smooth indentations seen along the margin of the colon represent pseudopolyps. (From Marx, JA et al [eds]: *Rosen's emergency medicine: concepts and clinical practice,* ed 7, Philadelphia, 2010, Elsevier.)

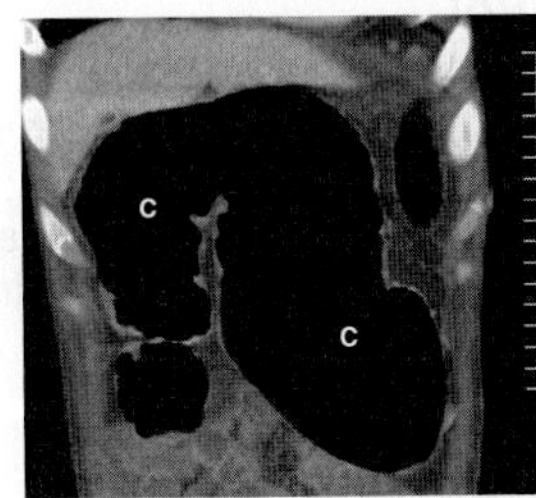

FIG. 2 Toxic megacolon. In a young patient with severe ulcerative colitis, coronal computed tomography demonstrates marked dilation of the colon (*c*) with thinning of its walls. The diameter of the lumen of the colon exceeds 7 cm. This finding places the patient at high risk of colon perforation. (From Webb WR et al: *Fundamentals of body CT,* ed 4, Philadelphia, 2015, WB Saunders.)

ACUTE GENERAL Rx

- Medications that impact colonic motility such as anticholinergics, opioids, and antidiarrheal agents should be discontinued and avoided.
- Electrolyte abnormalities, dehydration, and anemia are common clinical findings and should be addressed early. Fluid resuscitation with an isotonic solution (normal saline or lactated Ringer) and correction of electrolyte disturbances (especially hypokalemia) can help prevent worsening atony of the colonic wall. Patients with anemia from colonic hemorrhage should receive blood transfusion.
- Patients with systemic signs of infection or a suspected infectious etiology should receive broad-spectrum antibiotics. Infections due to *C. diff* should be treated with vancomycin (oral or rectal) or metronidazole (oral or IV). Toxic megacolon due to cytomegalovirus should be treated with ganciclovir IV.
- Patients with inflammatory etiologies such as UC or Crohn should receive high-dose IV steroids, either hydrocortisone 100 mg IV or methylprednisolone 60 mg IV. Steroids should not be used in patients with a confirmed infectious etiology.
- There are currently no data to support empiric treatment of toxic megacolon due to IBD with cyclosporine or infliximab. These treatment options should be reserved for patients who are not steroid responsive and should be limited to one attempt at clinical improvement so as not to delay surgical intervention.
- A management algorithm for toxic megacolon is outlined in Fig. 3.

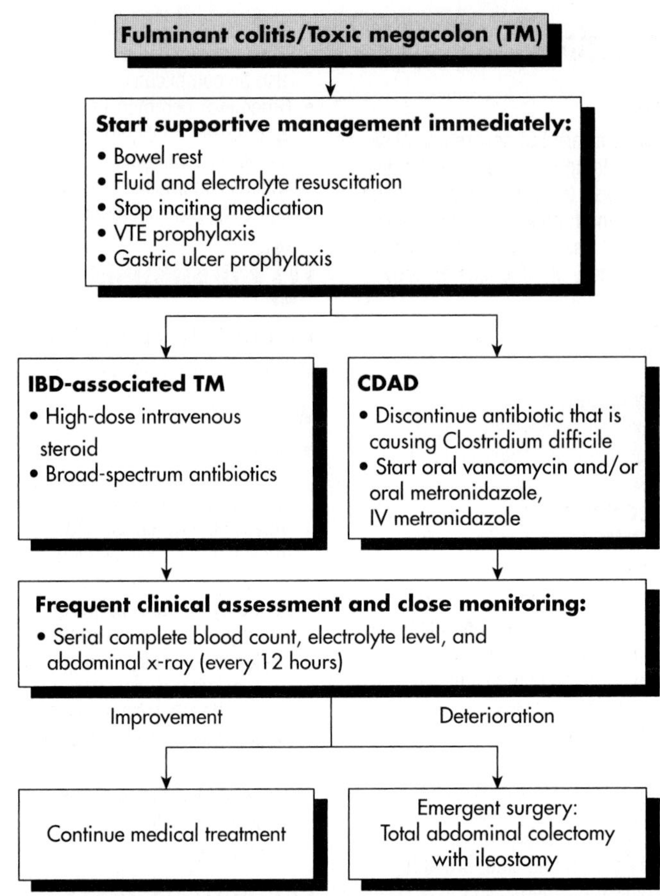

FIG. 3 Management algorithm for toxic megacolon. *CDAD, C. difficile*-associated disease; *IBD,* inflammatory bowel disease; *VTE,* venous thromboembolism. (From Cameron JL, Cameron AM: *Current surgical therapy*, ed 12, Philadelphia, 2017, Elsevier.)

CHRONIC Rx

Patients with IBD will need continued treatment for the underlying disease process once the acute processes associated with toxic megacolon have resolved.

COMPLEMENTARY AND ALTERNATIVE MEDICINE

N/A

DISPOSITION

All patients with toxic megacolon will require admission, possibly to the intensive care unit, depending on their clinical presentation.

REFERRAL

- Surgical consultation in all cases.
- All patients with toxic megacolon due to newly diagnosed IBD who are discharged from the hospital should be referred to a gastroenterologist for continued treatment.

PEARLS & CONSIDERATIONS

COMMENTS

- Early recognition and treatment of toxic megacolon is critical given the associated high morbidity and mortality.
- Anticholinergic medications, antidiarrheal agents, and opioids can precipitate or worsen toxic megacolon.
- Management includes medical and surgical treatment with inpatient hospitalization and treatment of the underlying cause.

PREVENTION

Prevention focuses on treatment of underlying causes of colitis to prevent complications such as toxic megacolon.

SUGGESTED READINGS

Available at ExpertConsult.com

RELATED CONTENT

Clostridium difficile Infection (Related Key Topic)
Crohn Disease (Related Key Topic)
Small Bowel Obstruction (Related Key Topic)
Ulcerative Colitis (Related Key Term)

AUTHOR: **STEVEN ROUGAS, M.D., M.S., F.A.C.E.P.**

BASIC INFORMATION

DEFINITION

Toxic shock syndrome (TSS) is an acute febrile illness resulting in multiple organ system dysfunction caused most commonly by a bacterial exotoxin. Disease characteristics also include hypotension, vomiting, myalgia, watery diarrhea, vascular collapse, and an erythematous sunburn-like cutaneous rash that desquamates during recovery. Box 1 summarizes the clinical case definition of toxic shock syndrome.

SYNONYM

TSS

ICD-10CM CODE

A48.3 Toxic shock syndrome

EPIDEMIOLOGY & DEMOGRAPHICS

- Case reported incidence peak: 14 cases per 100,000 menstruating women annually in 1980; has since fallen to 1 case per 100,000 persons
- Occurs most commonly between ages 10 and 30 yr in healthy, young, menstruating white females
- Case fatality ratio of 3%

PHYSICAL FINDINGS & CLINICAL PRESENTATION

- Fever (>38.0° C; 100.4° F)
- Diffuse macular erythrodermatous rash that involves both skin and mucous membranes, resembles sunburn, and also involves the palms and soles. The rash then desquamates 1 to 2 wk after disease onset in survivors
- Orthostatic hypotension
- Gastrointestinal symptoms: Vomiting, diarrhea, abdominal tenderness
- Constitutional symptoms: Myalgia, headache, photophobia, rigors, altered sensorium, conjunctivitis, arthralgia
- Respiratory symptoms: Dysphagia, pharyngeal hyperemia, strawberry tongue
- Genitourinary symptoms: Vaginal discharge, vaginal hyperemia, adnexal tenderness
- End-organ failure
- Severe hypotension and acute renal failure
- Hepatic failure
- Cardiovascular symptoms: Disseminated intravascular coagulation, pulmonary edema, acute respiratory distress syndrome (ARDS), endomyocarditis, heart block

ETIOLOGY

- Menstruation-associated TSS: 45% of cases associated with tampons, diaphragm, or vaginal sponge use. There has been a decline in these cases and in the case-fatality ratio.
- Non–menstruation-associated TSS: 55% of cases associated with puerperal sepsis, post-cesarean section endometritis, mastitis, sinusitis, wound or skin infection, septorhinoplasty (nasal packings), pelvic inflammatory disease, respiratory infections following influenza, enterocolitis, and burns. The number of cases is increasing and the case-fatality ratio has not declined.
- Causative agent: *Staphylococcus aureus* infection of a susceptible individual (10% of population lacking sufficient levels of antitoxin antibodies), which liberates the disease mediator TSST-1 (exotoxin). While most cases are caused by methicillin-susceptible *S. aureus* (MSSA), cases of TSS from methicillin-resistant *S. aureus* (MRSA) have occurred, particularly those due to the more virulent, community-associated MRSA strains.
- *S. aureus* exotoxins are superantigens that can activate large numbers of T cells (up to 20% at one time), resulting in a massive cytokine production: Interleukin (Il-1), Il-2, TNF, and interferon gamma that then mediate the signs and symptoms of the disease.
- Other causative agents: Coagulase-negative staphylococci producing enterotoxins B or C, and exotoxin A–producing group A beta-hemolytic streptococci.
- Risk factors for staphylococcal toxic shock syndrome are summarized in Box 2.

DIAGNOSIS

DIFFERENTIAL DIAGNOSIS

- Staphylococcal food poisoning
- Septic shock
- Mucocutaneous lymph node syndrome
- Scarlet fever
- Rocky Mountain spotted fever
- Meningococcemia
- Toxic epidermal necrolysis
- Kawasaki syndrome
- Leptospirosis
- Legionnaires' disease
- Hemolytic-uremic syndrome
- Stevens-Johnson syndrome
- Scalded skin syndrome
- Erythema multiforme
- Acute rheumatic fever

WORKUP

Broad-spectrum syndrome with multiorgan system involvement and variable but acute clinical presentation, including the following diagnostic criteria for staphylococcal toxic shock syndrome:

- Fever (>38° C; 100.4° F)
- Classic desquamating rash (1-2 wk)
- Hypotension/orthostatic systolic blood pressure ≤90 mm Hg
- Syncope
- Negative throat and cerebrospinal fluid cultures
- Negative serologic test for Rocky Mountain spotted fever, rubeola, and leptospirosis
- Clinical involvement of three or more of the following:
  1. Cardiopulmonary: ARDS, pulmonary edema, endomyocarditis, second- or third-degree atrioventricular block
  2. Central nervous system: Altered sensorium without focal neurologic findings
  3. Hematologic: Thrombocytopenia (platelets <100,000)

BOX 1 Clinical Case Definition of Toxic Shock Syndrome

Clinical Findings

- Fever: Temperature of ≥38.9°C (102°F)
- Rash: Diffuse macular erythroderma
- Desquamation: 1 to 2 weeks after onset of illness, particularly on palms, soles, fingers, and toes
- Hypotension: Systolic blood pressure ≤90 mm Hg for adults; <5th percentile by age for children <16 years; orthostatic drop in diastolic blood pressure of ≥15 mm Hg from lying to sitting; orthostatic syncope or orthostatic dizziness
- Involvement of three or more of the following organ systems:
  - Gastrointestinal: Vomiting or diarrhea at onset of illness
  - Muscular: Severe myalgia or creatinine phosphokinase level greater than twice the upper limit of normal for the laboratory
  - Mucous membrane: Vaginal, oropharyngeal, or conjunctival hyperemia
  - Renal: Blood urea nitrogen or serum creatinine greater than twice the upper limit of normal, or 5 or more white blood cells per high-power field in the absence of a urinary tract infection
  - Hepatic: Total bilirubin, aspartate transaminase, or alanine transaminase greater than twice the upper limit of normal for the laboratory
  - Hematologic: Platelets <100,000/mm^2
  - Central nervous system: Disorientation or alterations in consciousness without focal neurologic signs when fever and hypotension are absent
- Negative results on the following tests, if obtained:
  - Blood, throat, or cerebrospinal fluid cultures; blood culture may be positive for *Staphylococcus aureus*
  - Serologic tests for Rocky Mountain spotted fever, leptospirosis, or measles

Case Classification

- *Probable:* A case with 5 of the 6 clinical findings above
- *Confirmed:* A case with all 6 of the clinical findings above, including desquamation, unless the patient dies before desquamation can occur

From Wharton M, Chorba TL, Vogt RL et al: Case definitions for public health surveillance. *MMWR Recomm Rep.* 1990;39(RR-13):1–43, In Cherry JD et al: *Feigin and Cherry's pediatric infectious diseases*, ed 8, Philadelphia, 2019, Elsevier.

BOX 2 Risk Factors for Staphylococcal Toxic Shock Syndrome

I. Colonization of infection with toxin-producing *Staphylococcus aureus*
II. Absence of protective antitoxin antibody
III. Infected site
   A. Primary *S. aureus* infection
      - Carbuncle
      - Cellulitis
      - Dental abscess
      - Empyema
      - Endocarditis
      - Folliculitis
      - Mastitis
      - Osteomyelitis
      - Peritonitis
      - Peritonsillar abscess
      - Pneumonia
      - Pyarthrosis
      - Pyomyositis
      - Sinusitis
      - Tracheitis
   B. Postsurgical wound infection
      - Abdominal
      - Breast
      - Cesarean section
      - Dermatologic
      - Ear, nose, and throat
      - Genitourinary
      - Neurosurgery
      - Orthopedic
   C. Skin or mucous membrane disruption
      - Burns (chemical, scald, etc.)
      - Dermatitis
      - Influenza
      - Pharyngitis
      - Postpartum (vaginal delivery)
      - Superficial/penetrating trauma (insect bite, needle stick)
      - Viral infection
      - Varicella
   D. Foreign body placement
      - Augmentation mammoplasty
      - Catheters
      - Contraceptive sponge
      - Diaphragm
      - Surgical prostheses, stents, packing material, sutures
      - Tampons
   E. No obvious focus of infection (vaginal or pharyngeal colonization)

Cherry JD et al: *Feigin and Cherry's pediatric infectious diseases*, ed 8, Philadelphia, 2019, Elsevier.

TABLE 1 Staphylococcal Versus Streptococcal Toxic Shock Syndrome

Feature	Staphylococcal	Streptococcal
Age	Primarily 15-35 yr	Primarily 20-50 yr
Gender	Higher frequency in women	Men and women equally affected
Severe pain	Rare	Common
Hypotension	100%	100%
Erythroderma rash	Very common	Less common
Renal failure	Common	Common
Bacteremia	Low frequency	60%
Tissue necrosis	Rare	Common
Predisposing factors	Tampons, surgery	Cuts, burns, varicella
Thrombocytopenia	Common	Common
Mortality rate	<3%	30%-70%

From Mandell GL et al: *Principles and practice in infectious diseases*, ed 7, Philadelphia, 2008, Churchill Livingstone.

BOX 3 Therapeutic Principles for Management of Toxic Shock Syndrome

1. Identify the focus of infection; debride and irrigate extensively and remove any foreign material
2. Isolate the organism for antimicrobial susceptibility studies
3. Administer parenteral antimicrobial therapy to stop toxin production and eradicate the organism
4. Manage systemic multiorgan actions of toxins or mediators
5. Administer fluid therapy to maintain adequate venous return and cardiac filling pressure and prevent end-organ damage
6. Consider intravenous immunoglobulin for the following:
   - Disease refractory to initial fluid replacement and vasopressor support
   - A focus of infection that cannot be drained

Cherry JD et al: *Feigin and Cherry's pediatric infectious diseases*, ed 8, Philadelphia, 2019, Elsevier.

4. Liver: Elevated liver function test results
5. Renal: >5 cells/high-power field, negative urine cultures, azotemia, and increased creatinine (double normal)
6. Mucous membrane involvement: Vagina, oropharynx, conjunctiva
7. Musculoskeletal: Myalgia, creatine phosphokinase twice normal
8. Gastrointestinal: Vomiting, diarrhea

For streptococcal toxic shock syndrome the diagnostic criteria is as follows:

- Definite case: Isolation of group A β-hemolytic streptococci (GABHS) from a sterile site
- Probable case: Isolation of GABHS from a nonsterile site
- Hypotension: Presence of two of the following findings:
  1. Acute kidney injury or failure
  2. Elevated aminotransferase
  3. Erythematous macular rash, soft tissue necrosis
  4. Coagulopathy, including thrombocytopenia and disseminated intravascular coagulation
  5. Acute respiratory distress syndrome

LABORATORY TESTS

- Pan culture (cervix and vagina, throat, nasal passages, urine, blood, cerebrospinal fluid, wound) for *Staphylococcus, Streptococcus* (Table 1), and other pathogenic organisms
- Electrolytes to detect hypokalemia, hyponatremia
- Complete blood count with differential and clotting profile for anemia (normocytic or normochromic), thrombocytopenia, leukocytosis, coagulopathy, and bacteremia
- Chemistry profile to detect decreased protein, increased aspartate aminotransferase, increased alanine aminotransferase, hypocalcemia, elevated blood urea nitrogen and creatinine, hypophosphatemia, increased lactate dehydrogenase, increased creatine phosphokinase
- Urinalysis to detect white blood cells (>5 cells/high-power field), proteinemia, microhematuria
- Arterial blood gases to assess respiratory function and acid-base status
- Serologic tests considered for Rocky Mountain spotted fever, rubeola, and leptospirosis

IMAGING STUDIES

- Chest x-ray to evaluate pulmonary edema
- ECG to evaluate arrhythmia
- Sonography, CT scan, or MRI considered if pelvic abscess or tuboovarian abscess suspected

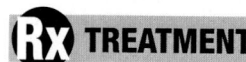

TREATMENT

NONPHARMACOLOGIC THERAPY

- Therapeutic principles for management of toxic shock syndrome are outlined in Box 3.
- For optimal outcome: High index of suspicion and early and aggressive supportive management in an ICU setting
- Aggressive fluid resuscitation (maintenance of circulating volume, cardiac output, systolic blood pressure)
- Thorough search for a localized infection or nidus: Incision and drainage, debridement, removal of tampon or vaginal sponge
- Central hemodynamic monitoring, Swan-Ganz catheter, and arterial line for surveillance of hemodynamic status and response to therapy
- Foley catheter to monitor hourly urine output
- Possible military antishock trousers as temporary measure
- Acute ventilator management if severe respiratory compromise
- Renal dialysis for severe renal impairment

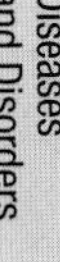

- Surgical intervention for indicated conditions (i.e., ruptured tubo-ovarian abscess, wound abscess, mastitis)
- Hyperbaric oxygen treatment can be used adjunctively

ACUTE GENERAL Rx

- Isotonic crystalloid (normal saline solution) for volume replacement following "7-3" rule (refers to the response in millimeters of mercury [mm Hg] of the pulmonary artery wedge pressure to volume replacement).
- Electrolyte replacement (K^+, C^+).
- Packed red blood cells, coagulation factor replacement, fresh frozen plasma to treat anemia or dilation and curettage.
- Vasopressor therapy for hypotension refractory to fluid volume replacement (e.g., dopamine beginning at 2-5 μg/kg/min).
- Steroids have been used but are not generally recommended due to lack of evidence of benefit.
- It is not clear whether antibiotics alter the course of acute TSS. Most authors recommend that patients receive 10 to 14 days of combination antibiotic therapy. In staphylococcal TSS, effective agents are clindamycin (900 mg IV every 8 hr in adults or 25-40 mg/kg per day in children) plus vancomycin (adults: 30 mg/kg per day IV in two divided doses; children: 40 mg/kg per day IV in four divided doses). Oxacillin or nafcillin sodium (2 g IV every 4 hr in adults; children: 100-150 mg/kg per 24 hr divided in four doses) can be used instead of vancomycin if TSS is due to MSSA. An alternative to vancomycin is linezolid.
- In streptococcal TSS, effective agents are penicillin G 24 million units/day in divided doses *plus* clindamycin 900 mg IV q8h. Alternative agents are ceftriaxone 2 g IV q24h *plus* clindamycin 900 mg IV q8h.
- Broad-spectrum antibiotic including gram-negative coverage added if concurrent sepsis suspected with TSS.
- Intravenous immune globulin (IVIG): While no controlled trials exist, most authors recommend IVIG (400 mg/kg in a single dose administered over several hours) in severe cases of TSS that are not responding to fluids or vasopressors. It may neutralize superantigen and decrease tissue damage.
- Tetracycline added if considering Rocky Mountain spotted fever.

CHRONIC Rx

- Severely ill patient: May require prolonged hospitalization and supportive management with gradual recovery and/or sequelae from severe end-organ involvement (ARDS or renal failure requiring dialysis)
- Majority of patients: Complete recovery
- Early-onset complications (within 2 wk):
  1. Skin desquamation
  2. Impaired digit sensation
  3. Denuded tongue
  4. Vocal cord paralysis
  5. Acute tubular necrosis
  6. ARDS
- Late-onset complications (after 8 wk):
  1. Nail splitting and loss
  2. Alopecia
  3. Central nervous system sequelae
  4. Renal impairment
  5. Cardiac dysfunction
- Recurrent TSS:
  1. More common in menstruation-related cases.
  2. Less common in patients treated with beta-lactamase–resistant antistaphylococcal antibiotics.
  3. Patients with history of TSS: If suspect signs and symptoms occur, have high index of suspicion and low threshold for evaluation and treatment.
  4. Screen for nasal carriage of *S. aureus* in patients with *S. aureus* TSS and treat with mupirocin in those with positive cultures.

PREVENTION

- Avoidance of tampons or use of low-absorbency tampons only (<4 hr in situ) and alternate with napkins
- Education for patients concerning signs and symptoms of TSS
- Avoidance of tampons for patients with history of TSS

DISPOSITION

- Complete recovery for most patients
- Long-term management of early- and late-onset complications for minority of patients

REFERRAL

- For multidisciplinary management, involving primary physician, gynecologist, internist, infectious disease specialist, and other supportive care specialists
- To tertiary-level hospital

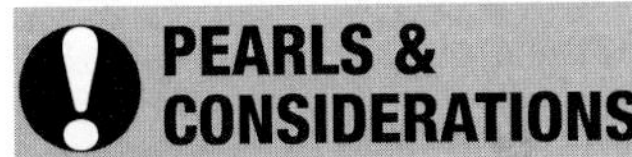

PEARLS & CONSIDERATIONS

COMMENTS

Antibiotic prophylaxis against invasive group A streptococcal infection with benzathine penicillin G plus rifampin, clindamycin, or azithromycin is recommended for immunocompromised household contacts of patients with streptococcal TSS-like syndrome.

SUGGESTED READINGS

Available at ExpertConsult.com

RELATED CONTENT

Toxic Shock Syndrome (Patient Information)

AUTHOR: **GLENN G. FORT, M.D., M.P.H.**

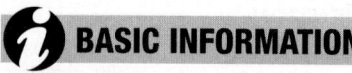

BASIC INFORMATION

DEFINITION

Toxoplasmosis is an infection caused by the protozoal parasite *Toxoplasma gondii* transmitted through ingestion of undercooked meat, undercooked shellfish, or cat feces.

ICD-10CM CODES	
B58.9	Toxoplasmosis, unspecified
B58.3	Pulmonary toxoplasmosis
B58.89	Toxoplasmosis with other organ involvement
P37.1	Congenital toxoplasmosis

EPIDEMIOLOGY & DEMOGRAPHICS

INCIDENCE (IN U.S.):

- Seroprevalence varies widely between different geographic locations, increasing with age, prevalence of cats in the area, and certain activities such as working in slaughterhouses or owning cats.
- Seroprevalence among women of childbearing age was 9.1% between 2009 and 2010.
- 0.23 cases of congenital toxoplasmosis per 10,000 live births between 2006 and 2014.
- Among patients with HIV, seroprevalence is approximately 11% in the U.S.

PREDOMINANT SEX: Equal gender distribution

PREDOMINANT AGE:

- Infancy (congenital infection)
- Prevalence increases with age

PEAK INCIDENCE: Temperate climates, with seroprevalence much higher in Latin America and Africa than in the U.S.

GENETICS: Congenital infection:

- Incidence and severity vary with the trimester of gestation during which the mother acquired infection.
  1. 10% to 25% (first trimester)
  2. 30% to 54% (second trimester)
  3. 60% to 65% (third trimester)
- Congenital infection occurring in the first trimester is the most severe.
- 89% to 100% of infections in the third trimester are asymptomatic.
- Risk to the fetus is not correlated with symptoms in the mother.

PHYSICAL FINDINGS & CLINICAL PRESENTATION

- Acquired (immunocompetent host): Usually subclinical, though may develop adenopathy, fatigue, and other constitutional symptoms that, while generally mild, can take weeks to resolve.
- Acquired (in patients with AIDS, CD4 count <100): Most common presentation is encephalitis with headache, confusion, and fever. May have motor weakness or other focal neurologic abnormalities and seizures. Can also present as pneumonitis, chorioretinitis, or other end-organ involvement.
- Acquired (immunocompromised patients):
  1. Encephalitis
  2. Myocarditis (especially in heart transplant patients)
  3. Pneumonitis
- Ocular infection in the immunocompetent host: If not congenital, then presents in second or third decade of life as a focal necrotizing retinitis with photophobia, blurred vision, pain, and potentially loss of central vision if the macula is involved.
- Congenital: Results from acute infection acquired by the mother within 6 to 8 weeks before conception or during gestation and is usually asymptomatic in the mother. In the infant, symptomatic disease is estimated at 40%. Ocular disease can include chorioretinitis and blindness, while CNS manifestations can include intracranial calcifications resulting in epilepsy, hydrocephalus, microcephaly, psychomotor or mental retardation, and encephalitis.

ETIOLOGY

- *Toxoplasma gondii:*
  1. Ubiquitous intracellular protozoan
  2. Present worldwide
  3. Cat is the definitive host (Fig. E1)
- Human infection:
  1. Ingestion of oocysts shed by cats in soil, litter boxes, vegetables
  2. Ingestion of inadequately cooked meat or shellfish containing tissue cysts
  3. Vertical transmission

Dx DIAGNOSIS

DIFFERENTIAL DIAGNOSIS

- Lymphadenopathy:
  1. Infectious mononucleosis
  2. Cytomegalovirus (CMV) mononucleosis
  3. Cat-scratch disease
  4. Sarcoidosis
  5. Tuberculosis
  6. Lymphoma
  7. Metastatic cancer
- Cerebral mass lesions in immunocompromised host:
  1. Lymphoma
  2. Tuberculosis
  3. Bacterial abscess
- Pneumonitis in immunocompromised host:
  1. *Pneumocystis jiroveci (carinii)* pneumonia
  2. Tuberculosis
  3. Fungal infection
- Chorioretinitis:
  1. Syphilis
  2. Tuberculosis
  3. Histoplasmosis (competent host)
  4. CMV
  5. Herpes simplex
  6. Fungal infection
  7. Tuberculosis
- Myocarditis:
  1. Organ rejection in heart transplant recipients
- Congenital infection:
  1. Rubella
  2. CMV
  3. Herpes simplex
  4. Syphilis
  5. Listeriosis
  6. Erythroblastosis fetalis
  7. Sepsis

WORKUP

- Acute infection, immunocompetent host:
  1. CBC
  2. *Toxoplasma* serology (IgG, IgM) in serial blood specimens 3 weeks apart
  3. Lymph node biopsy if diagnosis uncertain
- Immunocompromised host:
  1. CNS symptoms:
     a. Cerebral CT scan or MRI if CNS symptoms present
     b. Spinal tap, if safe
     c. Brain biopsy if no response to empiric therapy
  2. Ocular symptoms:
     a. Funduscopic examination
     b. Serologic studies
     c. Rarely, vitreous tap
  3. Pulmonary symptoms:
     a. Chest x-ray examination
     b. Bronchoalveolar lavage
     c. Transbronchial or open-lung biopsy
  4. Myocarditis:
     a. Cardiac enzymes
     b. Electrocardiogram
     c. Endomyocardial biopsy for definitive diagnosis
- Toxoplasmosis in pregnancy (Fig. 2):
  1. Initial maternal screening with IgM and IgG
     a. If negative, mother at risk of acute infection and should be retested monthly
     b. If both IgG and IgM positive, obtain IgA and IgE ELISA, AC/HS test
     c. IgA and IgE ELISA, AC/HS test elevated in acute infection
     d. Ig high for 1 yr or more
     e. IgG repeated 3 to 4 weeks later to determine if titer is stable
  2. Acute maternal infection not excluded or documented:
     a. Fetal blood sampling (for culture, Ig, IgA, IgE)
     b. Amniotic fluid polymerase chain reaction (PCR)
  3. Fetal ultrasound every other week if maternal infection documented:
- Congenital toxoplasmosis (Fig. 3):
  1. Placental histology
  2. Specific IgM or IgA in infant's blood

LABORATORY TESTS

- Antibody studies:
  1. More than one test necessary to establish diagnosis of acute toxoplasmosis
  2. IgM antibody:
     a. Appears 5 days into infection
     b. Peaks at 2 weeks
     c. Falls to low level or disappears within 2 months
     d. May persist at low levels for 1 yr or more
  3. Antibody not measurable:
     a. Ocular toxoplasmosis
     b. Reactivation
     c. Immunocompromised hosts
  4. IgG antibody:
     a. Appears 1 to 2 weeks after infection
     b. Peaks at 6 to 8 weeks
     c. Gradually declines over months to years

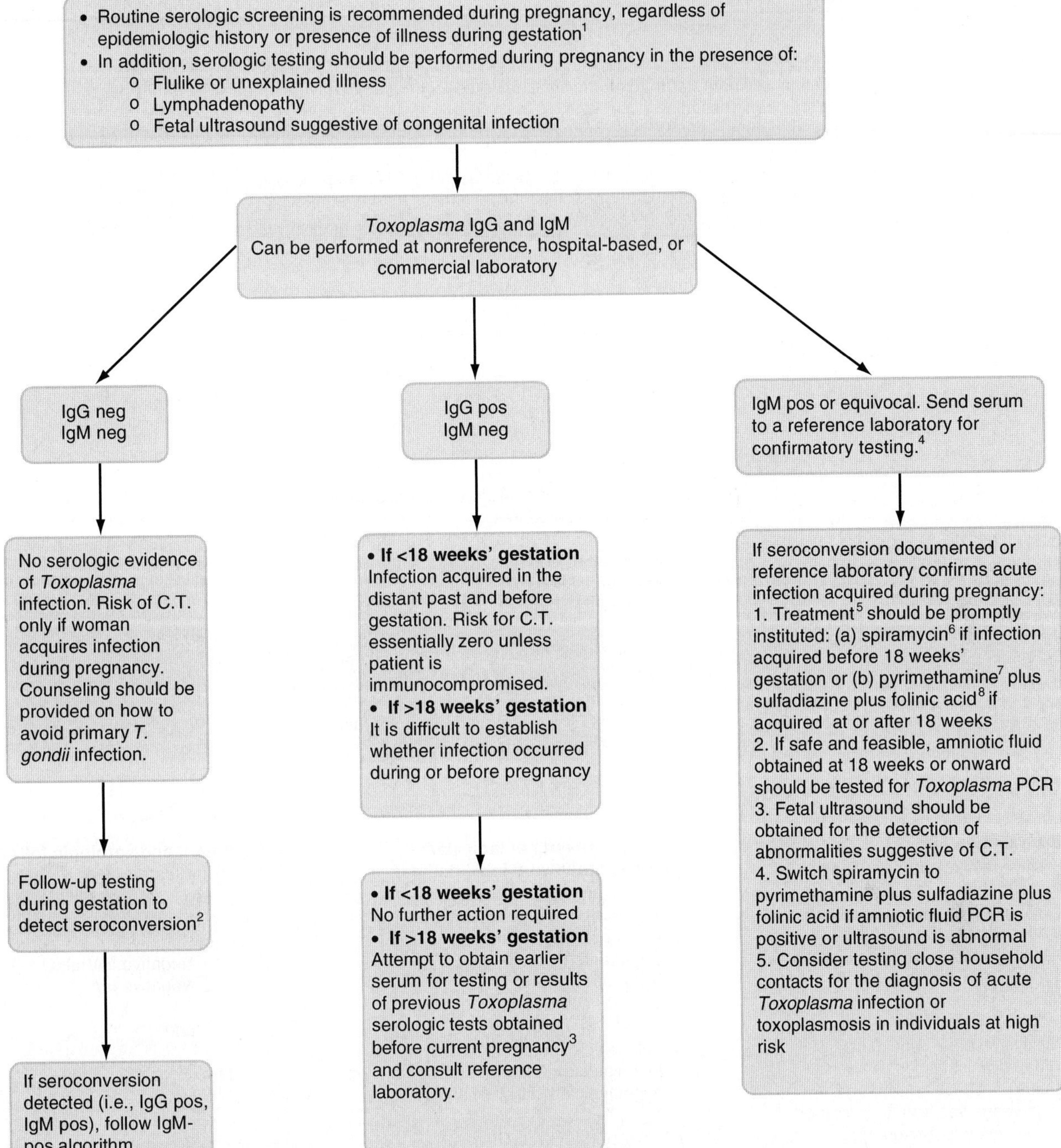

• Routine serologic screening is recommended during pregnancy, regardless of epidemiologic history or presence of illness during gestation1
• In addition, serologic testing should be performed during pregnancy in the presence of:
o Flulike or unexplained illness
o Lymphadenopathy
o Fetal ultrasound suggestive of congenital infection
Toxoplasma IgG and IgM
Can be performed at nonreference, hospital-based, or commercial laboratory
IgG neg
IgM neg
IgG pos
IgM neg
IgM pos or equivocal. Send serum to a reference laboratory for confirmatory testing.4
No serologic evidence of Toxoplasma infection. Risk of C.T. only if woman acquires infection during pregnancy. Counseling should be provided on how to avoid primary T. gondii infection.
• If <18 weeks' gestation
Infection acquired in the distant past and before gestation. Risk for C.T. essentially zero unless patient is immunocompromised.
• If >18 weeks' gestation
It is difficult to establish whether infection occurred during or before pregnancy
If seroconversion documented or reference laboratory confirms acute infection acquired during pregnancy:
1. Treatment5 should be promptly instituted: (a) spiramycin6 if infection acquired before 18 weeks' gestation or (b) pyrimethamine7 plus sulfadiazine plus folinic acid8 if acquired at or after 18 weeks
2. If safe and feasible, amniotic fluid obtained at 18 weeks or onward should be tested for Toxoplasma PCR
3. Fetal ultrasound should be obtained for the detection of abnormalities suggestive of C.T.
4. Switch spiramycin to pyrimethamine plus sulfadiazine plus folinic acid if amniotic fluid PCR is positive or ultrasound is abnormal
5. Consider testing close household contacts for the diagnosis of acute Toxoplasma infection or toxoplasmosis in individuals at high risk
Follow-up testing during gestation to detect seroconversion2
• If <18 weeks' gestation
No further action required
• If >18 weeks' gestation
Attempt to obtain earlier serum for testing or results of previous Toxoplasma serologic tests obtained before current pregnancy3 and consult reference laboratory.
If seroconversion detected (i.e., IgG pos, IgM pos), follow IgM-pos algorithm

FIG. 2 Diagnostic approach and management algorithm of toxoplasmosis during pregnancy. Most of the initial serologic screening can be accomplished by nonreference or commercial laboratories. Only positive immunoglobulin M results should be considered for additional testing and consultation with medical experts at a reference laboratory. *CT*, Congenital toxoplasmosis; *IgG*, immunoglobulin G; *IgM*, immunoglobulin M; *neg*, negative test result; *pos*, positive test result.[1] Up to 50% of women who acquire *Toxoplasma* infection during gestation do not have a known risk factor for acute infection or an illness suggestive of toxoplasmosis. Thus, to identify all women at risk, serologic screening should be performed in all pregnant women, along with other routine screening tests.[2] In a recent study from Lyon, France, monthly screening of seronegative pregnant women was reported to significantly decrease the risk of vertical transmission and of clinical signs at 3 years of age. Consider consultation with a physician expert in management of toxoplasmosis during pregnancy (e.g., in the U.S., Palo Alto Medical Foundation–*Toxoplasma* Serology Laboratory [PAMF-TSL], www.pamf.org/serology/; 650-853-4828; e-mail, toxolab@pamf.org; or U.S. [Chicago] National Collaborative Treatment Trial Study [NCCTS]; 773-834-4152).[4] Consider sending serum sample to a reference laboratory (e.g., PAMF-TSL).[5] Treatment regimens vary by country. The pyrimethamine-sulfadiazine-folinic acid regimen should not be offered to any pregnant woman before 12 weeks of gestation because of potential teratogenicity. In some centers in Europe, this regimen is offered at 14 weeks of gestation or later; in the U.S., it is recommended at 18 weeks or later.[6] Spiramycin is not commercially available in the U.S. It can be obtained at no cost and after consultation (with PAMF-TSL or the NCCTS through the U.S. Food and Drug Administration).[7] When using pyrimethamine, folic acid should be discontinued from the prenatal multivitamins. Folic acid can potentially counteract the antiparasitic effect of the drug.[8] Folic acid should not be erroneously used instead of folinic acid. (Bennett JE et al: *Mandell, Douglas, and Bennett's principles and practice of infectious diseases*, ed 8, Philadelphia, 2015, WB Saunders.)

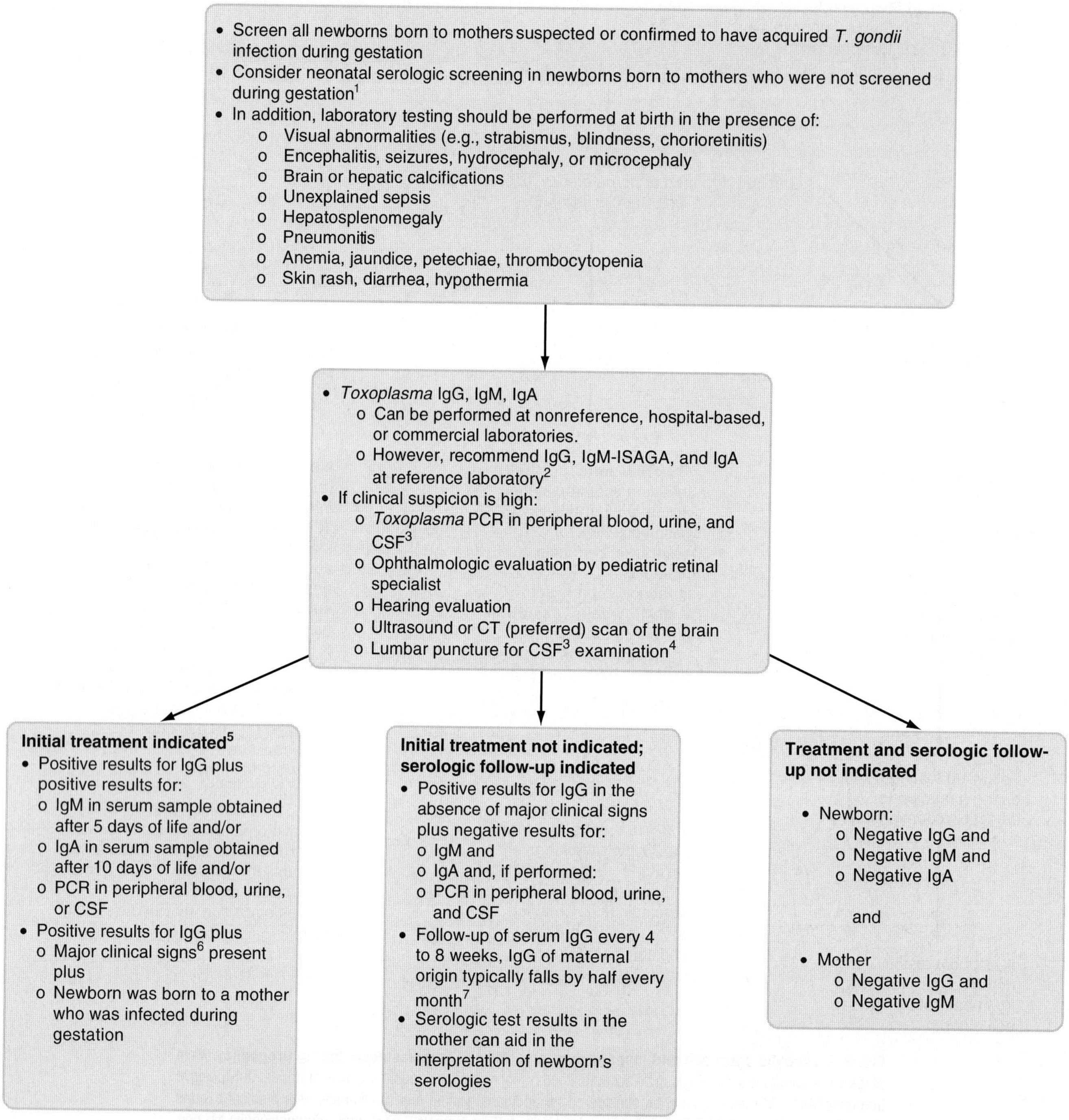

- Screen all newborns born to mothers suspected or confirmed to have acquired *T. gondii* infection during gestation
- Consider neonatal serologic screening in newborns born to mothers who were not screened during gestation[1]
- In addition, laboratory testing should be performed at birth in the presence of:
  - Visual abnormalities (e.g., strabismus, blindness, chorioretinitis)
  - Encephalitis, seizures, hydrocephaly, or microcephaly
  - Brain or hepatic calcifications
  - Unexplained sepsis
  - Hepatosplenomegaly
  - Pneumonitis
  - Anemia, jaundice, petechiae, thrombocytopenia
  - Skin rash, diarrhea, hypothermia

↓

- *Toxoplasma* IgG, IgM, IgA
  - Can be performed at nonreference, hospital-based, or commercial laboratories.
  - However, recommend IgG, IgM-ISAGA, and IgA at reference laboratory[2]
- If clinical suspicion is high:
  - *Toxoplasma* PCR in peripheral blood, urine, and CSF[3]
  - Ophthalmologic evaluation by pediatric retinal specialist
  - Hearing evaluation
  - Ultrasound or CT (preferred) scan of the brain
  - Lumbar puncture for CSF[3] examination[4]

↓

Initial treatment indicated[5]
- Positive results for IgG plus positive results for:
  - IgM in serum sample obtained after 5 days of life and/or
  - IgA in serum sample obtained after 10 days of life and/or
  - PCR in peripheral blood, urine, or CSF
- Positive results for IgG plus
  - Major clinical signs[6] present plus
  - Newborn was born to a mother who was infected during gestation

Initial treatment not indicated; serologic follow-up indicated
- Positive results for IgG in the absence of major clinical signs plus negative results for:
  - IgM and
  - IgA and, if performed:
  - PCR in peripheral blood, urine, and CSF
- Follow-up of serum IgG every 4 to 8 weeks, IgG of maternal origin typically falls by half every month[7]
- Serologic test results in the mother can aid in the interpretation of newborn's serologies

Treatment and serologic follow-up not indicated
- Newborn:
  - Negative IgG and
  - Negative IgM and
  - Negative IgA

and

- Mother
  - Negative IgG and
  - Negative IgM

FIG. 3 Diagnostic approach and management algorithm of the newborn whose mother has been suspected or confirmed to have acquired toxoplasmosis during gestation. *CSF*, Cerebrospinal fluid; *CT*, computed tomography; *IgG*, *IgM*, and *IgA*, immunoglobulins G, M, and A, respectively; *ISAGA*, immunosorbent agglutination assay; *PCR*, polymerase chain reaction.[1] Consider consultation with a physician expert in management of toxoplasmosis during pregnancy (e.g., in the U.S., Palo Alto Medical Foundation–*Toxoplasma* Serology Laboratory [PAMF-TSL], www.pamf.org/serology/; 650-853-4828; e-mail, toxolab@pamf.org; or U.S. [Chicago] National Collaborative Treatment Trial Study, 773-834-4152).[2] Consider sending serum sample to a reference laboratory (e.g., PAMF-TSL).[3] If lumbar puncture is clinically indicated, deemed safe, and feasible.[4] In an attempt to confirm the diagnosis of congenital toxoplasmosis, CSF should be sent for cell count and differential (congenital toxoplasmosis is one of the few causes of eosinophilic meningitis), protein (congenital toxoplasmosis is one of the few causes of extreme elevation of CSF protein), glucose, and *T. gondii* PCR.[5] The recommended regimen is pyrimethamine plus sulfadiazine plus folinic acid (see text).[6] Major clinical signs are referred here: chorioretinitis, brain calcifications, and hydrocephalus.[7] Maternally transferred IgG antibodies usually decline and disappear within 6 to 12 months of life. (Bennett JE et al: *Mandell, Douglas, and Bennett's principles and practice of infectious diseases*, ed 8, Philadelphia, 2015, WB Saunders.)

T

TABLE 1 Guidelines for Interpretation of Serologic Tests for Toxoplasmosis

IgG	IgM	IgG Avidity	Interpretation
Positive	Negative	—	Remote infection, immune. IgG avidity testing is best used when both IgG and IgM are positive and timing of infection is crucial, as in pregnancy (see below). False-negative IgM results occur in approximately 25% of cases when evaluating infection in the newborn. If infection is suspected in this setting, further testing (dye test, IgM EIA, IgA EIA, IgE EIA/ISAGA, PCRs, ideally with paired maternal serology tests—see text) is necessary in a reference laboratory (*Toxoplasma* Serology Laboratory, PAMF Research Institute, 795 El Camino Real, Ames Building Palo Alto, CA, 94301; 650-853-4828).
Positive	Positive or equivocal	High	Infection within the past 18 mo but likely >12 wk ago. If pregnant and beyond first trimester, consider sending specimen to reference laboratory for dye test, repeat IgG avidity and IgM EIA, IgA EIA, IgE EIA/ISAGA, and AC/HS testing (see above).
Positive	Positive or equivocal	Low	Infection within the past 12 wk. Consider sending specimen to a reference laboratory (see above) to time infection more accurately (dye test, repeat IgG avidity and IgM EIA, IgA EIA, IgE EIA/ISAGA, and AC/HS) in the setting of pregnancy.
Equivocal	Negative	—	Indeterminate. Test a new specimen or consider a different assay (IFA or ELISA).
Equivocal	Equivocal	—	Indeterminate. Test a new specimen or consider a different assay (IFA or ELISA).
Equivocal	Positive	—	Acute infection or false-positive IgM result. Test a second specimen; if IgG becomes positive or remains equivocal, consider sending specimen to a reference laboratory to time infection more accurately (dye test, IgG avidity, IgM EIA, IgA EIA, IgE EIA/ISAGA, AC/HS—see text) in the setting of pregnancy.
Negative	Negative	—	No evidence of *Toxoplasma* infection; not immune.
Negative	Equivocal	—	Either false-positive IgM result or possible recent infection. Obtain a new specimen and retest. If infection is recent, IgM and IgG should become positive, with low IgG avidity. If repeated testing is still IgG negative and IgM equivocal, patient is likely uninfected. Consider IgM ISAGA.
Negative	Positive	—	Acute infection or false-positive IgM result. Repeat testing on new specimen. If the result is the same, it is likely a false-positive IgM result. Consider IgM ISAGA.

AC/HS, Differential agglutination test; *EIA,* enzyme immunoassay; *ELISA,* enzyme-linked immunosorbent assay; *IFA,* immunofluorescence assay; *Ig,* immunoglobulin; *ISAGA,* immunosorbent agglutination assay; *PCR,* polymerase chain reaction.
From Cherry JD et al: *Feigin and Cherry's pediatric infectious diseases*, ed 8, Philadelphia, 2019, Elsevier.

Diseases and Disorders

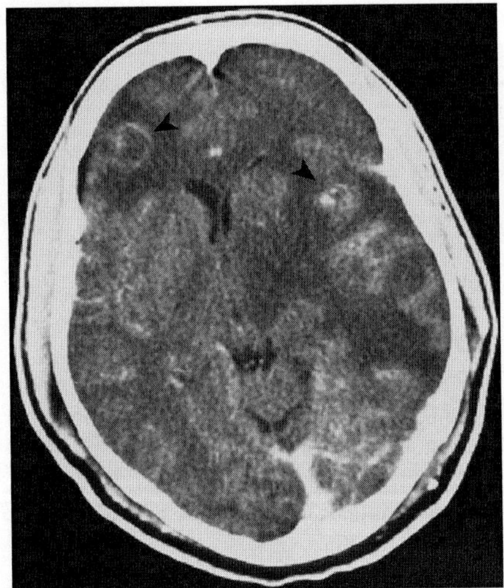

FIG. 4 Toxoplasmic encephalitis in person who has acquired immunodeficiency syndrome. A cranial computed tomography scan shows bilateral contrast-enhanced ring lesions with peripheral edema and mass effect. (From Cohen J, Powderly WG: *Infectious diseases,* ed 2, St Louis, 2004, Mosby.)

5. Guidelines for interpretation of serologic tests for toxoplasmosis are summarized in Table 1.

IMAGING STUDIES

- Chest x-ray if pulmonary involvement suspected
- Cerebral CT scan (Fig. 4) or MRI if encephalitis suspected

Rx TREATMENT

NONPHARMACOLOGIC THERAPY

- Selected cases of ocular infection:
  1. Photocoagulation
  2. Vitrectomy
  3. Lentectomy
- Selected cases of congenital cerebral infection:
  1. Ventricular shunting

ACUTE GENERAL Rx

- Acute infection, immunocompetent host:
  1. No treatment, unless severe and persistent symptoms or vital organ damage
- Acute infection, immunocompromised host, non-AIDS:
  1. Treat even if asymptomatic
  2. Duration:
     a. Until 4 to 6 weeks after resolution of all signs and symptoms
     b. Usually 6 months or longer
- Reactivated infection, immunocompromised host, non-AIDS:
  1. Treat if symptomatic
- Acute or reactivated infection, AIDS:
  1. Treat in all cases
  2. Induction course:
     a. 3 to 6 weeks
     b. Maintenance therapy continued for life; consider discontinuation of suppressive therapy if the patient has a good response to antiretroviral therapy and if the CD4 count remains >200 cells/mm^3 for more than 3 months
  3. Empiric therapy:
     a. AIDS with positive IgG
     b. Multiple ring-enhancing lesions on cerebral CT scan or MRI
     c. Response seen by day 7 in 71% and day 14 in 91%
- Ocular infection:
  1. Treat in all cases
  2. Therapy continued for 1 month or longer if needed
  3. Response seen in 70% within 10 days
  4. Retreat as needed
  5. Steroids may be indicated in patients with signs or symptoms of increased intracranial pressure
  6. Surgical treatment in selected cases
- Treatment regimens (Table 2):
  1. Pyrimethamine 200 mg loading dose once PO, then 50 mg (<60 kg) to 75 mg (>60 kg) q day; *plus*
  2. Leucovorin 10 to 20 mg PO qid, plus
  3. Sulfadiazine 1 (<60 kg) to 1.5 g (>60 kg) PO q6h

Other treatment options (if sulfa hypersensitivity or allergy is present): Pyrimethamine 50 to 75 mg/day PO with leucovorin 10 to 20 mg/day PO and either (1) clindamycin 600 mg q6h PO or IV (up to 1200 mg IV) q6h, or (2) clarithromycin 1 g PO bid, or (3) dapsone 100 mg/day PO, or (4) atovaquone 750 mg PO q6h.

- Acute infection in pregnancy:
  1. Treat immediately
  2. Risk of fetal infection reduced by 60% with treatment
     a. Seroconversion in the first trimester
        (1) Spiramycin 1 g every 8 hours

TABLE 2 Treatment of Toxoplasmosis

Disease	Medication	Dosage	Length of Therapy
Acute acquired—generally not treated unless severe or persistent symptoms, vital organ damage, or host immunosuppression[a]	Pyrimethamine *plus*	2 mg/kg/day for 2 days, then 1 mg/kg/day	4-6 wk or 2 wk after symptoms resolve for normal host; 4–6 wk beyond resolution for immunosuppressed hosts. In AIDS patients, treat until CD4+ count >200
	Sulfadiazine *plus*	75-100 mg/kg/day divided twice daily (maximum 4 g/day); consider the lower dose in children >20 kg (see text)	
	Folinic acid	5-20 mg 3 times weekly; use higher doses if marrow suppression	
Ocular, older child	Pyrimethamine *plus*	2 mg/kg/day for 2 days, then 1 mg/kg/day (maximum 50 mg/day)	4-6 wk or 2 wk after symptoms resolve
	Sulfadiazine *plus*	75-100 mg/kg/day divided twice daily (maximum 4 g/day); consider the lower dose in children >20 kg (see text)	Prednisone should be continued until resolution of sight-threatening active chorioretinitis
	Folinic acid *plus*	5-20 mg 3 times weekly	
	Prednisone	1 mg/kg/day divided twice daily	
Congenital	Pyrimethamine *plus*	2 mg/kg per day for 2 days, then 1 mg/kg/day for 6 mo, then 3 times weekly (M-W-F) for 6 mo	1 y
	Sulfadiazine *plus*	100 mg/kg per day divided twice daily	
	Folinic acid *plus*	5-10 mg 3 times weekly	
	Prednisone	1 mg/kg/day divided twice daily	Until resolution of elevated CSF protein level or sight-threatening active chorioretinitis
Pregnant women—acute infection first 21 wk of gestation	Spiramycin	3 g/day divided twice daily without food	Until fetal infection documented or excluded at 21 wk of gestation; if fetus infected, change to pyrimethamine plus sulfadiazine plus folinic acid until delivery
Pregnant women—fetal infection confirmed (amniotic fluid PCR positive)	Pyrimethamine *plus*	100 mg/day divided twice daily for 2 days, then 50 mg/day	Until delivery
	Sulfadiazine *plus*	3 g/day divided twice daily	
	Folinic acid	5-20 mg/day	

[a]For more detailed recommendations for patients with human immunodeficiency virus infection/AIDS, see http://aidsinfo.nih.gov/guidelines.
AIDS, Acquired immunodeficiency syndrome; *CSF,* cerebrospinal fluid; *PCR,* polymerase chain reaction.
From Cherry JD et al: *Feigin and Cherry's pediatric infectious diseases*, ed 8, Philadelphia, 2019, Elsevier.

b. Seroconversion beyond the first trimester or positive amniotic fluid PCR/ultrasound findings consistent with congenital toxoplasmosis:
   (1) Sulfadiazine 75 mg/kg/day in two divided doses ×2 days, then 50 mg/kg twice daily, *plus*
   (2) Pyrimethamine 50 mg bid ×2 days, then 50 mg PO daily, *plus*
   (3) Leucovorin 10 to 20 mg PO daily

- Postnatal treatment of congenital infection:
  1. Sulfadiazine 50 mg/kg PO bid, *plus*
  2. Pyrimethamine 2 mg/kg PO for 2 days, then 1 mg/kg PO daily for the first 2 to 6 months, then three times weekly, *plus*
  3. Leucovorin 5 to 20 mg PO three times weekly
  4. Minimum duration of treatment: 12 months

CHRONIC Rx

Maintenance therapy in AIDS patients because of the high risk (80%) of relapse:

- Pyrimethamine 25 mg PO qid
- Sulfadiazine 500 mg PO qid
- Leucovorin 10 to 20 mg PO qid

DISPOSITION

- Prognosis:
  1. Excellent in the immunocompetent host
  2. Good in ocular infection (although relapses are common)
- Treatment of acute infection in pregnancy:
  1. Reduces incidence and severity of congenital toxoplasmosis
- Treatment of congenital infection:
  1. Improvement in intellectual function
  2. Regression of retinal lesions
- AIDS:
  1. 70% to 95% response to therapy

REFERRAL

- To infectious disease expert:
  1. Immunocompromised hosts
  2. Pregnant women
  3. Difficulty in making a diagnosis or deciding on treatment
- To pediatric infectious disease expert:
  1. Congenital infection
- To obstetrician:
  1. Pregnant seronegative mother
  2. Acute seroconversion
- To ophthalmologist:
  1. Congenital infection
  2. Any case of ocular infection

PEARLS & CONSIDERATIONS

COMMENTS

- Prevention of toxoplasmosis is most important in seronegative pregnant women and immunocompromised hosts.
- Patient instructions:
  1. Cook meat to 66° C (150.8° F).
  2. Cook eggs.
  3. Do not drink unpasteurized milk.
  4. Wash hands thoroughly after handling raw meat.
  5. Wash kitchen surfaces that come in contact with raw meat.
  6. Wash fruits and vegetables.
  7. Avoid contact with materials potentially contaminated with cat feces.

SUGGESTED READINGS

Available at ExpertConsult.com

RELATED CONTENT

Toxoplasmosis (Patient Information)

AUTHORS: **PHILIP A. CHAN, M.D., M.S.,** and **GLENN G. FORT, M.D., M.P.H.**

BASIC INFORMATION

DEFINITION

Hemolytic transfusion reactions may be acute (occurring during or immediately after the transfusion) or delayed (occurring more than 24 hours after the transfusion). Acute hemolytic transfusion reaction (AHTR) is in vivo hemolysis most commonly caused by an alloantibody in a recipient's plasma to a cognate antigen on the donor red cells. The most commonly involved alloantibodies are to ABO antigens, but alloantibodies to minor blood group antigens have also been implicated. Typically the alloantibodies are of the IgM class, but complement fixing IgGs may also cause such a reaction. The clinical features vary, but usually there are high fever, chills, nausea, and backache. Red or brown urine may be passed due to hemoglobinuria. The plasma may show hemoglobinemia, and the direct Coombs test can be either positive or negative. Delayed hemolytic reactions are usually caused by an anamnestic alloantibody response upon re-exposure to cognate erythrocyte antigen. They are typically IgG and usually noncomplement fixing. They occur 1 to 10 days after transfusion. In delayed transfusion reactions, hemoglobinemia is unusual, and the only clinical manifestations may be fever, the serological finding of a newly positive indirect antiglobulin (indirect Coombs test), and/or the presence of a positive direct Coombs test. Delayed reactions can be clinically silent (called delayed serological hemolytic reactions) or manifest with fever, chills, nausea, vomiting, unexplained anemia, or jaundice. There is no specific treatment other than supportive care.

SYNONYMS

AHTR
DSTR
DHTR
Acute hemolytic transfusion reaction

ICD-10CM CODES

T80.9 Unspecified complication following infusion, transfusion and therapeutic injection
T80.3 ABO incompatibility reaction
T80.4 Rh incompatibility reaction
T80.8 Other complications following infusion, transfusion, and therapeutic injection

EPIDEMIOLOGY & DEMOGRAPHICS

- Acute intravascular hemolysis occurs in one to five per 50,000 transfusions.
- Delayed reactions occur about 1:1500 red cell transfusions.

PHYSICAL FINDINGS & CLINICAL PRESENTATION

- Fever, chills, nausea, tachycardia, chest pain, dyspnea, dizziness, bronchospasm.
- Lower back pain due to ischemic muscle pain or vasospasm hypotension.
- Severe reactions may occur in surgical patients under anesthesia who are unable to give any warning signs.
- Patients with delayed hemolytic transfusion reactions typically do not present as a clinical emergency. In most cases, presentation is with a low-grade fever from the generation of IL-1 or other proinflammatory cytokines. Hemoglobinuria and hemoglobinemia are rarely present. Unexplained anemia and jaundice are other possible presentations.
- Tables 1 and 2 summarize signs and symptoms of acute adverse reactions to blood transfusion. In the differential diagnosis of hemolysis.

ETIOLOGY

Most fatal hemolytic reactions are caused by clerical errors and mislabeled specimens.

DIAGNOSIS

DIFFERENTIAL DIAGNOSIS

- Septic reaction
- Transfusion-related acute lung injury

MANAGEMENT

The transfusion must be stopped immediately. The blood bank must be notified, and the donor transfusion bag must be returned to the blood bank along with a freshly drawn posttransfusion specimen. Table 3 summarizes immediate investigations in the case of an acute transfusion reaction.

LABORATORY TESTS

- The direct antiglobulin test (DAT) is usually positive in a delayed reaction, and preparation of an eluate will help identify the offending antibody.
- In some delayed reactions, the only finding is a positive indirect Coombs test, and the implicated alloantibody can be identified in an antibody panel.
- In acute reactions, the urine may show hemoglobinuria (wine-colored urine) and the plasma hemoglobinemia (pink plasma).
- Labs (Table 4): Decreased hematocrit and serum haptoglobin (haptoglobin low to 0 mg/dl). Elevated LDH, indirect bilirubin and creatinine, if acute.
- In acute cases, monitor coagulation status (PT, aPTT, fibrinogen) for disseminated intravascular coagulation.

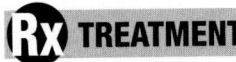

TREATMENT

NONPHARMACOLOGIC THERAPY

- Stop transfusion immediately. Test anticoagulated blood from the recipient for the presence of free hemoglobin in the plasma.
- Monitor vital signs closely and maintain IV access with a suitable crystalloid or colloid solution.
- Maintain an adequate airway.

ACUTE GENERAL Rx

- Treatment is supportive and consists of fluid resuscitation, vasopressor support, and mannitol.
- Vigorous IV hydration (0.9% NaCl or some other suitable crystalloid solution) to maintain urine flow at >100 ml/hr until hypotension is corrected and hemoglobinuria clears. IV furosemide may be necessary to maintain adequate renal flow.
- The addition of mannitol may prevent renal damage (controversial). Mannitol, if chosen, must be used with caution; if acute tubular necrosis occurs before mannitol infusion, pulmonary edema may occur as a result of the acute increase in intravascular volume secondary to fluid expansion.

TABLE 1 Signs and Symptoms of Acute Adverse Reactions to Blood Transfusion

Reaction	Fever	Chills/ Rigors	Nausea/ Vomiting	Chest Discomfort/Pain	Facial Flushing	Wheezing/ Dyspnea	Back/ Lumbar Pain	Discomfort at Infusion Site	Hypotension
Acute hemolytic	X	X	X	X	X	X	X	X	X
Febrile nonhemolytic	X	X		X	X				
Nonimmune hemolysis									
Acute lung injury	X			X		X			X
Allergic									
Massive transfusion complications									
Anaphylaxis	X	X	X	X	X	X	X	X	X
Passive cytokine infusion	X	X	X			X			
Hypervolemia						X			
Bacterial sepsis	X	X	X				X	X	X
Air embolus				X		X			

From Goldman L, Bennett JC [eds]: *Cecil's textbook of medicine,* ed 22, Philadelphia, 2004, Saunders.

TABLE 2 Types of Acute Transfusion Reactions

Reaction Type	Presenting Signs and Symptoms
Acute hemolytic	Fever, chills, dyspnea, vomiting, hypotension, tachycardia, infusion site pain, back pain, hemoglobinuria, hemoglobinemia, indirect hyperbilirubinemia, renal failure, DIC
Febrile reaction	Fever, chills, rigors
Allergic	Urticaria, pruritus, flushing, angioedema, dyspnea, bronchospasm stridor, hypotension, tachycardia, abdominal cramping
Hypervolemic	Dyspnea, tachycardia, hypertension, headache, jugular venous distention
Septic	Fever, chills, hypotension, tachycardia, vomiting
Transfusion-related acute lung injury	Dyspnea, hypoxemia, fever, hypotension

From Hoffman R et al: *Hematology, basic principles and practice*, ed 7, Philadelphia, 2018, Elsevier.

TABLE 3 Immediate Investigations in the Case of an Acute Transfusion Reaction

Check for hemolysis.
Perform visual examination of patient's plasma and urine (plasma and urine hemoglobin can be checked but this is not essential).
Blood film may show spherocytosis.
Bilirubin and lactate dehydrogenase (LDH) levels will be raised.
Check for incompatibility.
Check the documentation and the patient's identity.
Repeat ABO group of patient on pretransfusion and posttransfusion samples and of the donor unit(s).
Screen the patient for red cell antibodies pretransfusion and posttransfusion.
Repeat crossmatch with pretransfusion and posttransfusion samples.
Direct antiglobulin test (DAT) on pretransfusion and posttransfusion samples.
Eluate from patient's red cells.
Check for disseminated intravascular coagulation.
Perform blood count and film, coagulation screen, and fibrin degradation products (or D-dimers).
Check for renal dysfunction.
Check blood urea, creatinine, and electrolytes.
Check for bacterial infection.
Take blood cultures from the patient and donor unit including immediate Gram stain.

From Bain BJ, Bates I, Laffan MA: *Dacie and Lewis practical haematology*, ed 12, Philadelphia, 2017, Elsevier.

TABLE 4 Hemolytic Transfusion Reactions: Serologic Presentation

Type	Antibody Detectable Initially	Primary Antibody Type	Degree of Complement Binding	Example
Acute intravascular	Yes	IgM	Full (C1-9)	ABO system
Acute extravascular	Yes	IgG	None/partial	Rh system
Delayed intravascular	No	IgG	Full (C1-9)	Kidd system
Delayed extravascular	No	IgG	None/partial	Duffy system

From Hoffman R et al: *Hematology, basic principles and practice*, ed 7, Philadelphia, 2018, Elsevier.

- Monitor for the presence of disseminated intravascular coagulation. PT, aPTT, and fibrinogen levels should be closely monitored.
- If sepsis is suspected, culture as appropriate.

DISPOSITION

Mortality rate is 3% to 10% in severe transfusion reactions.

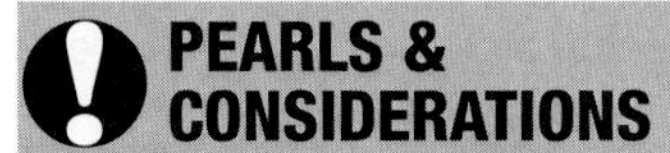

PEARLS & CONSIDERATIONS

COMMENTS

Hemolysis caused by minor antigen systems is generally less severe and may be delayed 1 to 10 days after transfusion.

SUGGESTED READINGS

Available at ExpertConsult.com

AUTHOR: **JOSEPH SWEENEY, M.D., F.A.C.P., F.R.C.PATH.**

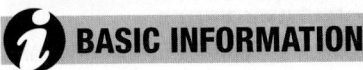

BASIC INFORMATION

DEFINITION
A clinical syndrome lasting up to 24 hours of sudden onset, severe anterograde and variable retrograde amnesia without loss of other neurologic function.

SYNONYM
TGA

ICD-10CM CODE
G45.4 Transient global amnesia

EPIDEMIOLOGY & DEMOGRAPHICS
INCIDENCE (IN U.S.): 3.4 to 10.4 per 100,000 people.
PEAK INCIDENCE: Most between ages 50 to 70 and equally common in men and women. In population older than 50 the incidence increases to 23.5 per 100,000 per year. TGA is also more common in individuals with migraine.[1]
RECURRENCE RATE: 2.9% to 23.8%

PHYSICAL FINDINGS & CLINICAL PRESENTATION[2]
- Cannot recall novel episodic information, repeatedly asking the same questions
- No impairment in consciousness or nonmemory cognitive domains, no focal neurologic deficit
- Complex procedural memory is often preserved (i.e., driving)
- Triggers include Valsalva maneuver, immersion in cold or hot, sexual intercourse, emotional stress
- Typically a single attack that is self-limited, with amnestic gap of the duration of episode

[1]Arena JE et al: Transient global amnesia, *Mayo Clin Proc* 90(2):264-272, 2015.
[2]Arena JE et al: Long-term outcome in patients with transient global amnesia: a population-based study, *Mayo Clin Proc* 92(3):399–405, 2017.

- Those with recent head injury or epilepsy diagnosis are excluded

ETIOLOGY
- Several proposed mechanisms of pathophysiology:
  1. Hypoperfusion or arterial ischemia of the hippocampi
  2. Internal jugular venous flow reversal causing venous hypertension to the medial temporal lobe
  3. Migraine phenomena with cortical spreading depression

Dx DIAGNOSIS

DIFFERENTIAL DIAGNOSIS
- Posterior cerebral artery transient ischemic attack: Can be associated with confusion or memory loss. Commonly with vascular risk factors and other focal neurologic signs (homonymous hemianopsia, aphasia, hemiparesis, hemisensory loss, hemi-body pain, oculomotor nerve palsy or vertical gaze palsy).
- Transient epileptic amnesia: Epilepsy syndrome, consisting of atypical TGA or recurrent attacks of amnesia, often less than one hour and upon waking, responsive to antiepileptic medications. Associated with olfactory hallucinations or oral automatisms. Interictal EEG may be abnormal. Hippocampal atrophy on MRI may be seen.
- Dissociative fugue, or transient dissociative amnesia: Extensive retrograde amnesia, loss of personal identity may occur, unlike in TGA where such is preserved.
- Hypoglycemia: Metabolic dysfunction can cause impairment in consciousness, focal signs, or prolonged cognitive impairment unlike TGA.

WORKUP
- Largely a clinical diagnosis, workup should focus on exclusion of vascular or epileptic source of symptoms.
- Collateral history of witnessed event and exclusion of prior event.
- Cognitive examination with evaluation of registration, delayed recall, and orientation.
- Careful cranial nerve examination to exclude posterior circulation stroke.

LABORATORY TESTS
- Complete blood count with erythrocyte sedimentation rate and C-reactive protein
- Serum chemistries, including lipid profile

DIAGNOSTIC STUDIES
- MRI of the brain may show reversible T2 hyperintensity or diffusion restriction exclusive to the hippocampi.
- EEG to exclude epileptiform activity.

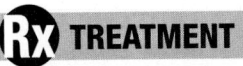

Rx TREATMENT

NONPHARMACOLOGIC THERAPY
Self-limited, not requiring specific pharmacologic or nonpharmacologic treatment

ACUTE GENERAL Rx
Investigate as an emergency.

CHRONIC Rx
- Does not lead to long-term sequela of memory loss. Complete recovery of cognitive function has been reported 5 days to 6 months after the episode.
- Low risk of subsequent ischemic cerebral stroke or seizures.

DISPOSITION
Due to the benign nature of transient global amnesia, rarely is continued followup necessary.

REFERRAL
Referral to a neurologist is necessary when the diagnosis is uncertain or with atypical features of the clinical presentation

AUTHOR: **RITUPARNA DAS, M.D.**

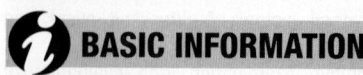

BASIC INFORMATION

DEFINITION

Transient ischemic attack (TIA) is a transient episode of neurologic dysfunction caused by focal brain, spinal cord, or retinal ischemia without acute infarction on MRI. TIA symptoms typically resolve within 60 min and by definition within 24 hours. Despite complete symptom resolution, 20% to 50% of patients clinically suspected to have suffered a TIA have evidence of acute tissue infarction on MRI.

SYNONYMS

TIA
Amaurosis fugax
Ophthalmologic TIA
"Mini-stroke"
Pre-stroke

ICD-10CM CODES

G45.9	Transient cerebral ischemic attack, unspecified
G45.8	Other transient cerebral ischemic attacks and related syndromes
Z86.73	Personal history of transient ischemic attack (TIA), and cerebral infarction without residual deficits

EPIDEMIOLOGY & DEMOGRAPHICS

INCIDENCE: 70 to 101 cases per 100,000 persons annually
PEAK INCIDENCE: After age 60 yr
PREVALENCE: 200,000 to 500,000 persons in the United States. The annual risk of stroke after either a TIA or minor stroke is approximately 3% to 4%.
PREDOMINANT SEX AND RACE: Males > females; African American > Caucasian
RISK FACTORS: Same as for ischemic stroke

PHYSICAL FINDINGS & CLINICAL PRESENTATION

- TIAs often present with transient neurologic symptoms including ipsilateral transient monocular blindness (amaurosis fugax), contralateral numbness or weakness, contralateral homonymous hemianopsia, and/or aphasia.
- Box 1 summarizes carotid artery TIAs.
- Vertebrobasilar artery TIAs are described in Box 2.

ETIOLOGY

Embolic (cardioembolism in 10% to 15%) large vessel atherothrombotic disease (20% to 25%) lacunar disease, hypoperfusion, hypercoagulable state, arteritis

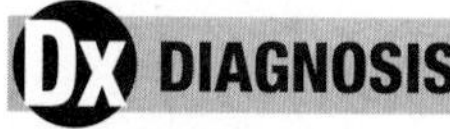

DIAGNOSIS

DIFFERENTIAL DIAGNOSIS

Seizures, hypoglycemia, hemiplegic migraine, intracranial hemorrhage, mass lesion, vestibular disease, Bell palsy, meningitis, multiple sclerosis, subdural hematoma, brain abscess, cervical or lumbar spine disease, conversion disorder

WORKUP

Given the high risk of stroke within the first 48 hours following TIA (up to 10%), hospital admission for workup is advised. Most of the immediate risk of stroke is secondary to carotid disease.

The American Heart Association recommends that the ABCD2 score be used in the evaluation of TIA. It consists of 1 point for age ≥60 yr, 1 point for BP ≥140 mm Hg systolic or ≥90 mm Hg diastolic, clinical features (2 points for unilateral weakness, 1 point for speech impairment), duration of TIA (2 points for duration ≥60 min, 1 point for duration 10-59 min), presence of diabetes mellitus (1 point). According to the guidelines, it is reasonable to hospitalize patients with TIA if they present within 72 hours and have an ABCD2 score ≥3. There is some debate about the usefulness of this scale since it fails to account for changes seen on echocardiogram, carotid Dopplers, or ECG that may place the patient at more imminent risk of stroke (carotid stenosis, Afib, cardiac thrombus, etc.). Alternatives to this scoring system are being investigated.

LABORATORY TESTS

Complete blood count, basic metabolic panel, prothrombin time, activated partial thromboplastin time, sedimentation rate, fasting lipid panel, serum glucose and hemoglobin A_{1c} (to detect latent diabetes mellitus), and TSH.

IMAGING STUDIES

- CT scan should be obtained to exclude hemorrhage; MRI with diffusion-weighted images if immediately available to determine whether infarction occurred.
- Imaging of the vessels should be obtained via magnetic resonance angiography (MRA) head and neck, computed tomography angiography (CTA) head and neck, or carotid Doppler/transcranial Doppler (CD/TCD). If symptoms are referrable to the posterior circulation, MRA or CTA should be obtained in lieu of CD/TCD.
- Transthoracic echocardiogram should be obtained.
- An echocardiogram with bubble should be obtained in all patients younger than 50 yr with TIA symptoms.

BOX 1 Carotid Artery Transient Ischemic Attacks

Symptoms
- Contralateral hemiparesis, hemianopia, hemisensory loss
- Aphasia, if dominant hemisphere
- Neglect and hemi-inattention, if nondominant hemisphere
- Ipsilateral amaurosis fugax

Associated findings
- Carotid bruit
- Retinal artery emboli

Tests
- Ultrasonography (carotid Doppler studies)
- Magnetic resonance imaging angiography (MRA)
- Cerebral arteriography

Therapy
- Medical: Platelet inhibitors (e.g., aspirin)
- Risk-reduction measures (e.g., control blood pressure, glucose levels, cholesterol)
- Surgical: Carotid endarterectomy, if stenosis >70% and symptomatic
- Endovascular: Placement of stent

From Kaufman DM, Geyer HL, Milstein MJ: *Kaufman's clinical neurology for psychiatrists*, ed 8, Philadelphia, 2017, Elsevier.

BOX 2 Vertebrobasilar Artery Transient Ischemic Attacks

Symptoms
- Vertigo, vomiting, tinnitus
- Circumoral paresthesias or numbness
- Dysarthria, dysphagia
- Drop attacks

Associated findings
- Nystagmus
- Ataxia
- Cranial nerve abnormalities

Tests
- Ultrasonography (transcranial Doppler studies)
- Magnetic resonance imaging angiography (MRA)
- Cerebral arteriography

Therapy
- Medical: Platelet inhibitors*
- Risk-reduction measures
- Surgical: None

*See Box 1.
From Kaufman DM, Geyer HL, Milstein MJ: *Kaufman's clinical neurology for psychiatrists*, ed 8, Philadelphia, 2017, Elsevier.

- Electrocardiogram should be obtained to exclude the presence of arrhythmias, namely atrial fibrillation.

At least 24 hours of heart rhythm monitoring should be accomplished to screen for arrhythmia. Many stroke centers now utilize prolonged ambulatory cardiac rhythm monitoring over several weeks to months to identify paroxysmal atrial fibrillation in select patients when there is a high index of clinical suspicion.

- Paroxysmal atrial fibrillation is common in patients with TIA. A recent study found that noninvasive ambulatory ECG monitoring for 30 days significantly improved the detection of atrial fibrillation by a factor of more than five and nearly doubled the rate of anticoagulant treatment as compared with the standard practice of short-duration ECG monitoring.

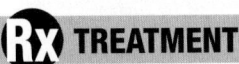

TREATMENT

NONPHARMACOLOGIC THERAPY

- Carotid endarterectomy or carotid stenting should be considered for patients found to have carotid stenosis of ≥50% as the cause for TIA. Please refer to the "Carotid Stenosis" chapter for more information.
- The practice of intracranial angioplasty and stenting has largely declined following the publication of negative results from clinical trials and is only used in select patients who fail maximal medical management with aggressive platelet inhibition, strict risk factor control such as hyperlipidemia, hypertension, diabetes mellitus, weight loss, treatment of sleep apnea, and smoking cessation among others.

ACUTE GENERAL Rx

- In the absence of contraindications, patients with atrial fibrillation should be considered for anticoagulation. Choices for anticoagulants include the direct oral anticoagulants (such as dabigatran, rivaroxaban, apixaban, edoxaban, betrixaban) and/or warfarin. In patients with TIA and atrial fibrillation or a cardiac thrombus, therapeutic anticoagulation should be achieved rapidly. Those who are not candidates for a direct oral anticoagulation and who will need chronic warfarin should first be started on either intravenous heparin or therapeutic anticoagulant doses of lovenox, along with warfarin, until target INR between 2.0 and 3.0 is achieved, at which point warfarin should be continued as monotherapy.
- Although no compelling evidence exists for the use of heparin in the acute treatment of TIAs without cardioembolic source, patients who develop recurrent symptoms within the same vascular territory that increase in duration, severity, and/or frequency (crescendo TIA/stuttering TIA) may benefit from its use pending cardiac and vascular imaging and identification of a possible source.

CHRONIC Rx

- Chronic therapy should be aimed at modifying the four major risk factors: hypertension, dyslipidemia, diabetes mellitus, and smoking cessation.
- Antiplatelet therapy should be used to reduce the risk of recurrent TIAs or subsequent stroke. Three antiplatelet agents are commonly used in stroke prevention: aspirin, aspirin/dipyridamole, and clopidogrel. All are reasonable choices but practitioners should consider their individual patient's comorbidities when selecting an antiplatelet agent.
- A direct oral anticoagulant of dose-adjusted warfarin (INR 2.0-3.0) or use of direct oral anticoagulants is indicated for prevention of future strokes in atrial fibrillation patients.

PEARLS & CONSIDERATIONS

- All cause mortality in 1 yr is 25% in patients diagnosed TIA.
- Dual antiplatelet therapy in acute TIA and minor stroke is being evaluated. A recent trial revealed that among patients with TIA or minor stroke who can be treated within 24 hours after the onset of symptoms, the combination of clopidogrel and aspirin is superior to aspirin alone for reducing the risk of stroke in the first 90 days but did increase the risk of hemorrhage. Most of the benefit was concentrated in the first seven to 30 days, so dual antiplatelet therapy may be reasonable in the first 30 days after TIA.
- Previous studies conducted between 1987 and 2003 estimated the risk of stroke or an acute coronary syndrome was 12% to 20% during the first 3 mo after a TIA. New data estimate the 1-yr risk to be 6.2%. Multiple infarctions on brain imaging, large-artery atherosclerosis, and an ABCD[1] score of 6 or 7 were each associated with more than a doubling of the risk of stroke.[2]

PREVENTION

- A healthy lifestyle and management of cardiovascular risk factors should be encouraged.
- The identification of insulin resistance as a risk factor for stroke and myocardial infarction raises the possibility that pioglitazone, which improves insulin sensitivity, might benefit patients with cerebrovascular disease. In a recent trial involving patients without a history of ischemic stroke or TIA, the risk of stroke or MI was lower among patients who received pioglitazone than among those who received placebo. Pioglitazone was also associated with a lower risk of diabetes but with a higher risk of weight gain, edema, and fracture.

PATIENT/FAMILY EDUCATION

Patients should be counseled on the early signs of stroke symptoms and instructed to promptly seek medical attention if they develop symptoms concerning for stroke. Patients should be encouraged to pursue a healthy lifestyle to include exercise and smoking cessation. In addition, patients should take an active role in controlling blood pressure and blood glucose. Further educational materials can be found online at http://www.strokecenter.org/.

SUGGESTED READINGS

Available at ExpertConsult.com

RELATED CONTENT

Transient Ischemic Attack (TIA) (Patient Information)
Carotid Stenosis (Related Key Topic)
Atrial Fibrillation (Related Key Topic)
Stroke, Acute Ischemic (Related Key Topic)
Stroke, Secondary Prevention (Related Key Topic)

AUTHORS: **COREY GOLDSMITH, M.D., JOSEPH S. KASS, M.D., J.D,** and **PRASHANTH KRISHNAMOHAN, M.D., M.B.B.S.**

[1] Amarenco P, et al.: One-year risk of stroke after transient ischemic attack or minor stroke, *N Engl J Med* 374:1533–1542, 2016.

[2] Kernan WN, et al.: Pioglitazone after ischemic stroke or transient ischemic attack, *N Engl J Med* 374:1321-1331, 2016.

BASIC INFORMATION

DEFINITION

Demyelination in a transverse region of the spinal cord due to an inflammatory process that leads to sensory and motor changes below the lesion as well as autonomic dysfunction. The term "transverse myelitis" of late refers to any cause of inflammatory myelopathy, irrespective of severity or degree of structural or functional interruption of pathways through a transverse spinal cord section. Patients usually experience bandlike symptoms, which is classically an area of altered sensation or pain in a horizontal (i.e., transverse) band usually at the dermatomal level corresponding to the lesion within the cord. Transverse myelitis that extends across three or more segments of the cord is referred to as longitudinally extensive transverse myelitis. The pathologic hallmark of transverse myelitis is the presence of focal collections of lymphocytes and monocytes with varying degrees of demyelination, axonal injury, and astroglial and microglial activation within the spinal cord.

SYNONYMS

Idiopathic transverse myelitis (ITM)
TM
ITM

ICD-10CM CODES

G37.3	Acute transverse myelitis in demyelinating disease of central nervous system
G04.89	Other myelitis

EPIDEMIOLOGY & DEMOGRAPHICS

INCIDENCE: Annual incidence ranges from 1.3 to 8 cases per million. The incidence increases to 24.6 cases per million annually if causes of acquired demyelination such as multiple sclerosis (MS) or neuromyelitis optic spectrum disorder are included.

PREVALENCE: Unknown

PREDOMINANT SEX: None, but female preponderance seen in cases associated with multiple sclerosis and neuromyelitis optica spectrum disorder.

GENETICS: No genetic predisposition has been shown.

PEAK INCIDENCE: Can occur at any age. Bimodal peak in the incidence between 10 to 19 yr and 30 to 39 yr. 20% of cases occur in children with a bimodal peak of incidence between 0 to 2 yr and 5 to 17 yr.

RISK FACTORS: Infection, vaccination

PHYSICAL FINDINGS & CLINICAL PRESENTATION

- The clinical signs are caused by an interruption in ascending and descending sensory, motor, and autonomic pathways in the transverse plane of the spinal cord, resulting in sensory-level weakness, and autonomic dysfunction at and below the level of the lesion.
- Rapid onset of symmetric or asymmetric paraparesis or paraplegia of the lower extremities over a few days, ascending paresthesia, sensory level at the trunk, back pain, sphincter dysfunction, and positive Babinski, which can be bilateral. The arms may also be involved if the cervical cord is involved, but cervical involvement is less common than thoracic involvement. In the acute phase the weakness is flaccid, with diminished deep tendon reflexes mimicking a peripheral neuropathy such as Guillain-Barré syndrome.
- One third to one half of patients present with localizing back pain.
- There is progression to nadir of clinical deficits between 4 hr and 21 days after symptom onset.
- Urinary incontinence or retention, GI disturbances (incontinence or constipation), and sexual dysfunction are common.
- Acute flaccid myelitis is a subtype of myelitis in which patients present with acute limb weakness and have primarily involvement of gray matter on spinal cord imaging.

ETIOLOGY

- Can be idiopathic demyelination (15% to 30%) that is a monophasic one-time event or demyelination secondary to neurologic or systemic conditions (Box 1).
- Secondary causes include postinfection, postvaccination, acute demyelinating encephalomyelitis (where transverse myelitis tends to be monophasic), and others such as multiple sclerosis, neuromyelitis optica spectrum disorder (NMOSD), connective tissue disorders such as systemic lupus, Sjögren syndrome, antiphospholipid antibody syndrome, sarcoidosis, and paraneoplastic conditions, which can be progressive or relapsing.
- Infectious causes of myelitis include HIV, syphilis, varicella zoster (associated with shingles), HTLV-1, Lyme disease, arboviruses such as West Nile virus (typically causing a poliomyelitis-type acute flaccid paralysis), or enteroviruses (typically causing acute flaccid paralysis mainly in children).
- About 50% of patients have had a recent upper respiratory infection.

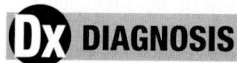

DIAGNOSIS

DIFFERENTIAL DIAGNOSIS

- MS (Table 1)
- Neuromyelitis optica spectrum disorder (NMOSD)
- Metastatic disease
- Spinal cord tumors
- Herniated or slipped discs
- Spinal stenosis
- Spinal epidural abscess
- Vascular malformation

BOX 1 Central Nervous System and Systemic Autoimmune Disorders Associated With Acute Transverse Myelitis

Central Nervous System Disorders
- Acute disseminated encephalomyelitis
- Multiple sclerosis
- Neuromyelitis optica

Systemic Autoimmune Disorders
- Antiphospholipid antibody syndrome
- Behçet disease
- Mixed connective tissue disorder
- Neurosarcoidosis
- Sjögren syndrome
- Systemic lupus erythematosus

From Cherry JD et al: *Feigin and Cherry's textbook of pediatric infectious diseases,* ed 8, Philadelphia, 2019, Elsevier.

TABLE 1 Distinguishing Acute Transverse Myelitis From Other Central Nervous System Demyelinating Disorders

Finding	ATM	ADEM	MS	NMO
Myelitis	+	+/–	+/– (partial)	+
Acute mental status changes	–	+	–	+/–
Optic neuritis	–	+/–	+/–	+/–
Abnormal brain MRI	–	+	+	+/–
CSF oligoclonal bands	–	+/–	+	+/–
Serum AQP4-IgG	–	–	–	+/–
Recurrences	+/–	+/–	+	+

+, Always present; +/–, variably present; –, usually absent.
ADEM, Acute disseminated encephalomyelitis; *AQP,* aquaporin 4; *ATM,* acute transverse myelitis; *CSF,* cerebrospinal fluid; *MRI,* magnetic resonance imaging; *MS,* multiple sclerosis; *NMO,* neuromyelitis optica.
From Cherry JD et al: *Feigin and Cherry's textbook of pediatric infectious diseases,* ed 8, Philadelphia, 2019, Elsevier.

TABLE 2 Suggested Diagnostic Workup for Recurrent Central Nervous System Demyelinating Disorders and Systemic Autoimmune Disorders Associated With Acute Transverse Myelitis

All Patients	Suggestive of Neuromyelitis Optica	Also Consider
Brain MRI with gadolinium	Ophthalmology consultation	Angiotensin-converting enzyme (serum, CSF)
CSF oligoclonal bands	Visual evoked potentials	Other autoantibodies
Antinuclear antibodies	Formal visual field testing	Anti-dsDNA
Antiphospholipid antibodies		Anti-La
Serum AQP4-IgG		Anti-Ro
		Anti-Smith

CSF, Cerebrospinal fluid; *MRI,* magnetic resonance imaging; *NMO,* neuromyelitis optica.
From Cherry JD et al: *Feigin and Cherry's textbook of pediatric infectious diseases,* ed 8, Philadelphia, 2019, Elsevier.

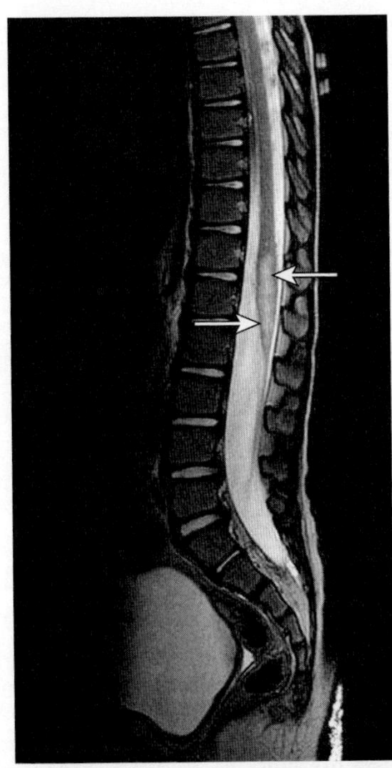

FIG. 1 Patient with clinical picture of transverse myelitis. Sagittal T2-weighted MRI of the distal cord shows central T2 hyperintensity within the conus medullaris *(arrows)* in this case of ADEM. An acute spinal cord infarct also could have this imaging appearance. (From Fuhrman BP et al: *Pediatric critical care,* ed 4, Philadelphia, 2011, Saunders.)

1. Spinal dural arteriovenous fistula (most common)
2. Arteriovenous malformation of the spinal cord

- Spinal cord infarction due to either anterior spinal artery or posterior spinal artery occlusion

WORKUP

Transverse myelitis (TM) should be suspected in patients with a history of rapid (hours to days) onset of motor weakness and sensory abnormalities with bladder or bowel dysfunction that is referable to the spinal cord. The dysfunction is bilateral (not necessarily symmetric) and there is a clearly defined sensory (dermatomal) level. It is important to distinguish idiopathic TM from TM due to MS or neuromyelitis optica spectrum disorder because idiopathic TM does not relapse and does not require long-term immunomodulatory therapy. A suggested diagnostic workup for recurrent CNS demyelinating disorders and systemic autoimmune disorders associated with acute transverse myelitis is summarized in Table 2.

IMAGING STUDIES

- Gadolinium-enhanced magnetic resonance imaging (MRI) of brain and MRI of the entire spine (Fig. 1, Fig. 2). This will show demyelinating lesion on T_2 with contrast enhancement. In MS there is usually a short segment lesion (less than three vertebral segments) that is dorsally located. Longitudinally extensive transverse myelitis that spans more than three or more segments of the cord is more typical of NMOSD.
- Computed tomography (CT) of the spine with and without contrast should be obtained if MRI is unavailable, but CT does not allow for visualization of the spinal cord itself.
- CT myelogram may also be obtained if MRI unavailable to evaluate for compression.
- Chest CT with and without contrast if sarcoidosis is suspected.

LABORATORY TESTS

- Lumbar puncture looking for CSF pleocytosis, oligoclonal bands for MS, or serology and PCR looking for infection (Table 3) such as varicella zoster virus and enterovirus PCR.
- ANA, hepatitis B serology, Lyme disease serology, VDRL, SSA, SSB, anticardiolipin antibody, lupus anticoagulant, copper, ceruloplasmin, vitamin B_{12}, RPR.
- Serum NMO-IgG and myelin oligodendrocyte glycoprotein (MOG) antibodies to evaluate for neuromyelitis optica spectrum disorder.
- If a paraneoplastic etiology is suspected, then appropriate antibodies should be ordered and appropriate cancer screening undertaken.

Rx TREATMENT

Corticosteroids (IV methylprednisolone 1 g/day for 3-7 days) are the first-line treatment for transverse myelitis.

NONPHARMACOLOGIC THERAPY

- Physical therapy
- Respiratory and oropharyngeal support

ACUTE GENERAL Rx

- High-dose IV corticosteroid (e.g., methylprednisolone 1000 mg/day for 3-7 days) to stop inflammatory damage to the spinal cord.
- Rescue therapy with plasma exchange may be helpful in patients who do not respond to corticosteroids.
- Combination therapy with plasmapheresis and corticosteroids or other immunosuppressive agents (e.g., rituximab or cyclophosphamide) may also be effective.
- Analgesia for pain.

CHRONIC Rx

- Baclofen or tizanidine for muscle spasms
- Gabapentin or pregabalin for neuropathic pain
- Low-molecular-weight heparin for DVT prophylaxis in patients with immobility

DISPOSITION

- One third of patients with transverse myelitis will have complete recovery, one third will have fair recovery, and one third have permanent disability and do not recover. Recurrence or relapse is possible, especially if the patient has MS, NMOSD, or sarcoidosis.
- Patients who need further care, including those with urinary retention, may need home nursing assistance. Some patients may benefit from rehabilitation, either inpatient or outpatient.

REFERRAL

- Consider physical therapy.
- Consider occupational therapy.
- Consider rehabilitation services.
- Consider psychiatric consultation (high incidence of long-term mood and anxiety disorders).

SUGGESTED READINGS

Available at ExpertConsult.com

AUTHORS: **PADMAJA SUDHAKAR, M.B.B.S.,** and **JOSEPH S. KASS, M.D., J.D.**

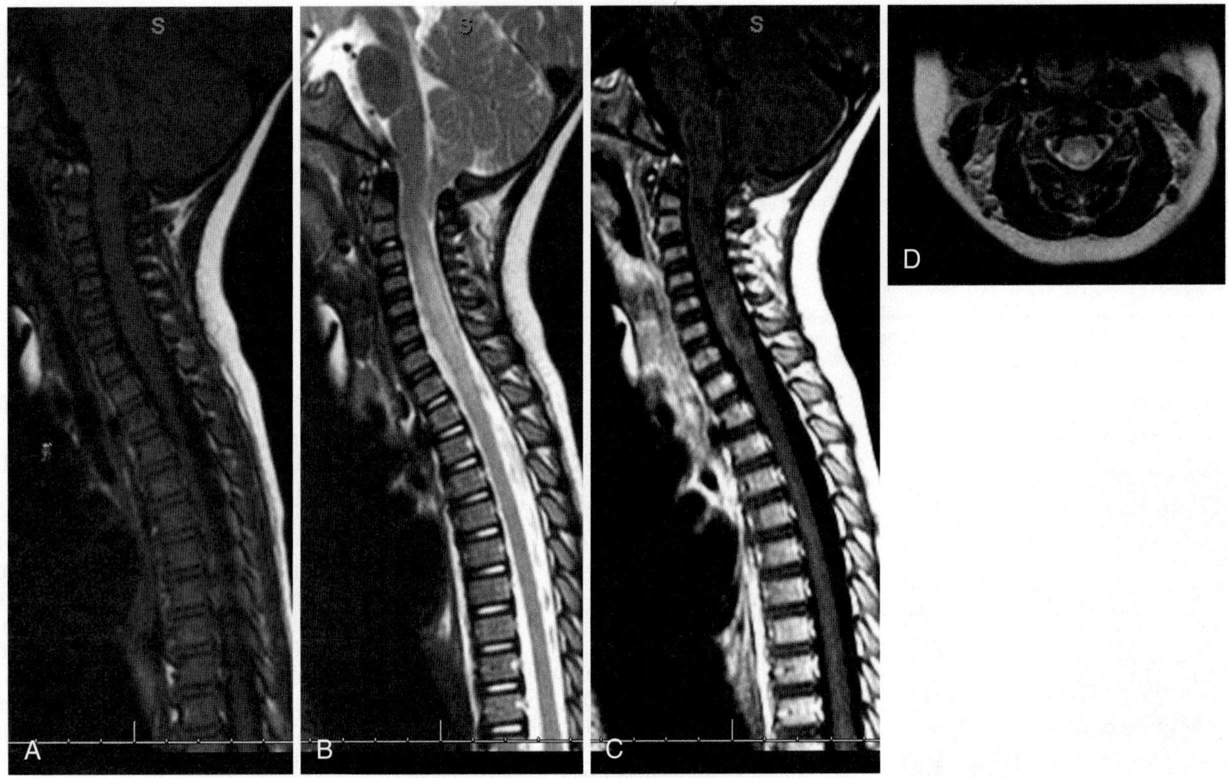

FIG. 2 Acute transverse myelitis of the cervical cord. (A) Sagittal T1-weighted magnetic resonance imaging (MRI) sequence through the cervical spinal cord demonstrating swelling of the cord. **(B)** T2-weighted MRI sequence of same patient revealing longitudinally extensive hyperintensity through the cervical cord. **(C)** T1-weighted MRI sequence with gadolinium revealing patchy enhancement of the cervical cord. **(D)** T2-weighted axial MRI sequence through the cervical cord revealing hyperintensity of both gray and white matter. (From Cherry JD et al: *Feigin and Cherry's textbook of pediatric infectious diseases,* ed 8, Philadelphia, 2019, Elsevier.)

TABLE 3 Suggested Diagnostic Workup for Infections Associated with Acute Transverse Myelitis

Blood	Cerebrospinal Fluid	Other
• Blood cultures • Acute and convalescent titers to *Borrelia burgdorferi,* EBV, *Mycoplasma pneumoniae*	• Bacterial culture • Viral culture • PCR testing for CMV, EBV, Enterovirus, HSV, *M. pneumoniae,* VZV	• Viral culture of stool and respiratory secretions • Consider stool ova and parasite testing and serum titers if parasitic infection is suspected

CMV, Cytomegalovirus; *EBV,* Epstein-Barr virus; *HSV,* herpes simplex virus; *PCR,* polymerase chain reaction; *VZV,* varicella zoster virus.
From Cherry JD et al: *Feigin and Cherry's textbook of pediatric infectious diseases,* ed 8, Philadelphia, 2019, Elsevier.

BASIC INFORMATION

DEFINITION

Impact to the head resulting in varying levels of cellular and macroscopic changes, detected with clinical examination supplemented by imaging studies. Maas et al have proposed this definition: "brain damage resulting from external forces, as a consequence of direct impact, rapid acceleration or deceleration, a penetrating object (e.g., gunshot) or blast waves from an explosion. The nature, intensity, direction, and duration of these forces determine the pattern and extent of damage."

SYNONYMS

TBI
Head injury
Concussion
Intracranial contusion

ICD-10CM CODES

S06.9 X0A	Intracranial injury
S06.1X7A	Traumatic cerebral edema with loss of consciousness of any duration with death due to brain injury prior to regaining consciousness, initial encounter
S06.2X9A	Diffuse traumatic brain injury with loss of consciousness of unspecified duration, initial encounter
S06.300A	Unspecified focal traumatic brain injury without loss of consciousness, initial encounter
S06.305A	Unspecified focal traumatic brain injury with loss of consciousness greater than 24 hours with return to pre-existing conscious level, initial encounter
S06.309A	Unspecified focal traumatic brain injury with loss of consciousness of unspecified duration, initial encounter

EPIDEMIOLOGY & DEMOGRAPHICS

Traumatic brain injury (TBI) is a worldwide leading cause of mortality in young individuals. Urbanization and increasing use of motor vehicles has led to an overall increase in TBI, especially in high-income and developing countries.

INCIDENCE: Globally, more than 10 million people suffer TBI resulting in mortality or requiring hospitalization each year. By the year 2020, it is projected that TBI will surpass many diseases as the major cause of death and disability worldwide. TBI likely accounts for 9% of global mortality and is a threat to health in every country in the world. The financial burden of TBI has been estimated to be greater than $60 billion per year in the United States alone. According to estimates from the CDC, about 2.5 million emergency department visits, including deaths and hospitalizations, were associated with TBI in 2010.

PREVALENCE: The prevalence of TBI in the United States has been estimated at approximately 5.3 million. In the European Union with 330 million inhabitants, approximately 7,775,000 new TBI cases occur each year. According to the CDC, combined rates of TBI-related hospitalizations, emergency department visits, and deaths have risen from 521/100,000 in 2000 to 823.7/100,000 in 2010.

PEAK INCIDENCE: Approximate incidence in the US per CDC data is 103/100,000 population. In the European Union, this is estimated to be at 235/100,000.

PREDOMINANT SEX AND AGE: TBI occurs more frequently in young adults, particularly males 15 to 25 yr of age, and has a high cost to society because of life years lost as a result of death and disability.

GENETICS: Work on the genetic basis and the susceptibility it affords in traumatic brain injury is being currently studied. The most recognized association between a genetic polymorphism and outcome involves the apolipoprotein E (*Apo E*) gene. The ε4 allele has been associated with poorer outcome after TBI. The same isoform is associated with Alzheimer's disease and increased deposition of amyloid beta lipoprotein after TBI. TBI and Apo E ε4 synergistically are also associated with a 10-fold increased risk for Alzheimer's disease as well as larger intracerebral hematomas and greater ischemia after TBI.

RISK FACTORS: N/A.

PHYSICAL FINDINGS & CLINICAL PRESENTATION

TBI patients can present with a spectrum of clinical symptoms including nausea, vomiting, headache, seizures, altered mental status, and/or coma. Stigmata of trauma, including bruises, scalp lacerations, and periorbital or mastoid ecchymosis suggesting skull base fractures, are telltale signs of possible underlying traumatic brain injury. Box 1 describes risk stratification in patients with minor head trauma. The spectrum of TBI is most commonly assessed using the Glasgow Coma Scale (GCS), which ranges from 3 to 15 and utilizes eye, motor, and verbal exams (Table 1).

ETIOLOGY

Etiology in most cases is impact related. Mechanical falls, motor vehicle accidents, and assaults resulting in direct or indirect trauma to the head from acceleration and rotational forces result in brain injury.

An estimated 283,000 children seek care in U.S. emergency departments each year for a sport- or recreation-related TBI. TBIs sustained in contact sports account for approximately 45% of these visits. Football, bicycling, basketball, playground activities, and soccer account for the highest number of emergency department visits.[1]

DIAGNOSIS

DIFFERENTIAL DIAGNOSIS

Differential diagnosis of TBI is quite limited; however, there are several considerations and diagnoses considered as a possibility within the realm of TBI. These are enumerated in the imaging section.

[1]Sarmiento K et al: Emergency Department Visits for Sports- and Recreation-Related Traumatic Brain Injuries Among Children — United States, 2010–2016, *MMWR* 68;241, 2019.

WORKUP

TBI workup is always a part of the advanced trauma life support (ATLS) protocol. Primary and secondary survey followed by imaging studies constitutes the standardized approach to TBI. Focused TBI workup includes:

- History: Including timing of injury, duration of loss of consciousness if applicable, seizures (if any), comorbidities, use of anticoagulants and antiplatelet agents (requires reversal in the event of intracranial blood on imaging).
- Neurological examination: Glasgow Coma Scale, cranial nerves, motor/sensory exam. Assess for scalp lacerations, specifically overlying a skull fracture as well as CSF otorrhea or rhinorrhea.
- CT imaging of the head if there is a significant history of impact to the head, polytrauma,

BOX 1 Risk Stratification in Patients with Minor Head Trauma

High Risk
- Focal neurologic findings
- Asymmetrical pupils
- Skull fracture on clinical examination
- Multiple trauma
- Serious, painful, distracting injuries
- External signs of trauma above the clavicles
- Initial Glasgow Coma Scale score of 14 or 15
- Loss of consciousness
- Posttraumatic confusion or amnesia
- Progressively worsening headache
- Vomiting
- Posttraumatic seizure
- History of bleeding disorder or anticoagulation
- Recent ingestion of intoxicants
- Unreliable or unknown history of injury
- Previous neurologic diagnosis
- Previous epilepsy
- Suspected child abuse
- Age above 60 years or below 2 years

Medium Risk
- Initial Glasgow Coma Scale score of 15
- Brief loss of consciousness
- Posttraumatic amnesia
- Vomiting
- Headache
- Intoxication

Low Risk
- Currently asymptomatic
- No other injuries
- No focality on examination
- Normal pupils
- No change in consciousness
- Intact orientation and memory
- Initial Glasgow Coma Scale score of 15
- Accurate history
- Trivial mechanism
- Injury less than 24 hours ago
- No or mild headache
- No vomiting
- No preexisting high-risk factors

TABLE 1 Glasgow Coma Scale (GCS)

Adult		Infant
Eye Opening	**E**	**Eye Opening**
Spontaneous	4	Spontaneous
To speech	3	To speech
To pain	2	To pain
No response	1	No response
Best Motor Response	**M**	**Best Motor Response**
Obeys verbal command	6	Normal movements
Localizes to pain	5	Localizes to pain
Withdraws to pain	4	Withdraws to pain
Flexion (decorticate)	3	Flexion (decorticate)
Extension (decerebrate)	2	Extension (decerebrate)
No response	1	No response
Best Verbal Response	**E**	**Best Verbal Response**
Oriented speech	5	Coos, babbles
Disoriented speech	4	Cries but consolable
Inappropriate words	3	Persistently irritable
Incomprehensible sounds	2	Grunts to pain/restless
No response	1	No response

Mild TBI: GCS 13-15, Moderate TBI: GCS 9-12, Severe TBI GCS 8 or less.

GCS can range from 3 to 15. If intubated, then verbal component is replaced by 'T'. Best possible score if intubated is 10T, and worst is 3T.

In obtunded patients, pain stimulus can be central or peripheral. In patients with suspected spinal cord injury and paralysis, central stimulus to elicit facial grimace can be used to assess motor and eye component.

BOX 2 American College of Emergency Physicians Clinical Policy Regarding Neuroimaging in Adults with Mild Traumatic Brain Injury

A noncontrast head CT is indicated (level-1 recommendation) in adults with LOC or posttraumatic amnesia only if one or more of the following is present:

- Headache
- Vomiting
- Age >60 years
- Drug or alcohol intoxication
- Deficits in short-term memory
- Physical evidence of trauma above the clavicle
- Posttraumatic seizure
- GCS score <15
- Focal neurologic deficit
- Coagulopathy

A noncontrast head CT should be considered (level-2 recommendation) in head trauma patients with no LOC or posttraumatic amnesia if there is:

- Focal neurologic deficit
- Vomiting
- Severe headache
- Age ≥ 65 years
- Physical signs of a basilar skull fracture
- GCS score <15
- Coagulopathy
- A dangerous mechanism (e.g., ejection from motor vehicle, pedestrian struck, fall of more than 3 feet or 5 stairs)

CT, Computed tomography; *GCS*, Glasgow Coma Scale; *LOC*, loss of consciousness.
From Marx JA et al: *Rosen's emergency medicine*, ed 8, Philadelphia, 2014, Elsevier.

positive loss of consciousness, or stigmata of trauma to the head. The American College of Emergency Physicians Clinical Policy Regarding Neuroimaging in adults with mild TBI is summarized in Box 2.

LABORATORY TESTS

Basic labs including CBC, basic metabolic panel, prothrombin time, activated partial thromboplastin time, urine drug screen, and ethanol blood level. Upcoming tests for platelet function analysis for unknown antiplatelet use are also being performed for early reversal with platelet replacement. These tests focus on an individual's responsiveness to antiplatelet agents and are available at most academic institutions. During the acute phase of severe TBI, protein biomarkers are thought to be released in the CSF and/or in the circulation by passing through the disrupted blood brain barrier. Currently no single protein biomarker can evaluate the extent of TBI pathology. Using a combination of complimentary biomarkers has been proposed as a means to assess potential damage from TBI (Figs. 1 and E2).

IMAGING STUDIES (TABLE 2)

CT imaging forms the current cornerstone of imaging modalities for head trauma. Usually, in addition to a plain CT of the head (Fig. 3), CTA head/neck and CT of the spine is helpful if arterial or C-spine injury is suspected, respectively. Other imaging modalities such as MRI can be helpful in certain situations but are typically adjuncts in the acute setting to CT-guided management. Canadian CT head rules are a useful guide in determining utility of obtaining a CT scan. These are based on risk factors:

HIGH-RISK:

- Failure to reach GCS of 15 within 2 hours
- Suspected open or any signs of basal skull fracture
- More than two episodes of vomiting
- Age older than 65

LOW RISK:

- Dangerous mechanism of injury or polytrauma
- Loss of consciousness lasting >30 minutes

Pathologies that can be identified with imaging are noted in the following:

- Primary extraaxial: Epidural, subdural, subarachnoid hemorrhage
- Primary intraaxial: Axonal injury, cortical contusion, intracerebral or intraventricular hemorrhage, encephalomalacia (from prior TBI or vascular insult)
- Skull fracture: Linear, depressed, open, involving frontal sinus or skull base
- Penetrating brain injury: Gunshot wounds, sharp objects resulting in parenchymal and vascular injury
- Vascular injury: Dissection, traumatic carotid-cavernous fistula (CCF), dural arteriovenous fistula (dAVF), pseudoaneurysm formation
- Secondary acute injury: Diffuse cerebral swelling/dysautoregulation (seen more commonly in children from posttraumatic hyperemia), infarction, infection from penetrating trauma, brain herniation from mass lesion or cerebral edema
- Secondary chronic injury: Hydrocephalus (posttraumatic due to disruption of normal CSF absorption pathways), encephalomalacia, CSF leak (from skull base fractures, manifests as otorrhea or rhinorrhea, leptomeningeal cyst (seen most commonly in infants, skull fracture resulting in underlying dural injury)

Rx TREATMENT

Prevention of secondary injury is the primary goal of prehospital and early in-hospital management. Most common mechanisms of secondary injury are either intracranial (ICP, hematoma) or systemic (hypoxia, hypovolemia, hypotension). Early categorization of head trauma patients according to the severity (based on GCS) and transport to facilities equipped with personnel and technology to deal with issues pertaining to head trauma has improved the overall management of head injury patients and prevention of secondary injury. Airway, breathing, and circulation, however, still remain the most important parameters to be stabilized and both directly and indirectly affect GCS and overall outcome. Trauma guidelines suggest

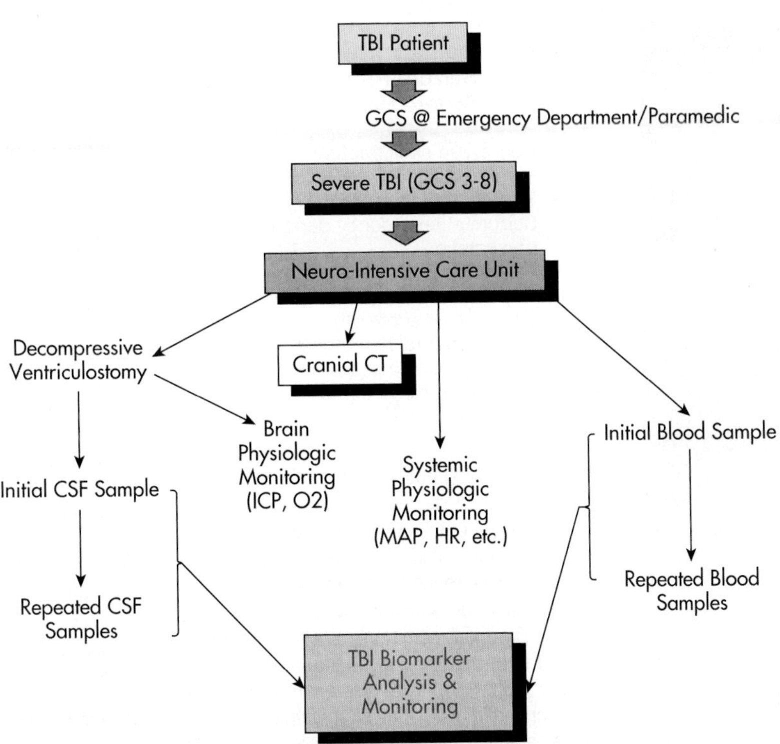

FIG. 1 Envisioned uses of brain biomarkers for severe traumatic brain injury *(TBI)* patient management. *CSF,* Cerebrospinal fluid; *CT,* computed tomography; *GCS,* Glasgow Coma Scale; *HR,* heart rate; *ICP,* intracranial pressure; *MAP,* mean arterial blood pressure. (From Vincent JL et al: *Textbook of critical care*, ed 7, Philadelphia, 2017, Elsevier.)

TABLE 2 Comparison of Head Imaging Modalities

	Computed Tomography Scans	Magnetic Resonance Imaging	Angiography	Skull Radiography
Advantages	Fast Patient accessible for monitoring Defines acute hemorrhages, mass effects, bone injuries, hydrocephalus, intraventricular blood, edema	Defines contusions and pericontusion edema, posttraumatic ischemic infarction, brainstem injuries	Helps localize acute traumatic lesions Defines vascular injuries, injuries to venous sinuses Detects mass effects	Readily available May help screen some patients for further imaging studies
Disadvantages	Artifacts arise from patient's movement, foreign bodies Streak artifacts may obscure brainstem or posterior fossa	Slow Patients not easily accessible for monitoring Does not define most acute hemorrhagic lesions Not useful for bone injuries	Does not define nature of acute lesion Does not detect infratentorial masses	Does not indicate presence or absence of intracranial injury
Indications	Acute severe head trauma Acute moderate head trauma Suspected depressed skull fracture High-risk minor head trauma Suspected child abuse in minor head trauma Deteriorating neurologic status	Persistent symptoms with postconcussive syndrome Suspected posttraumatic ischemic infarction Suspected contusions not seen on CT scan	Suspected vascular injury CT scan not available	CT scan may not be done Penetrating head trauma

CT, Computed tomography.
From Marx: *Rosen's emergency medicine: concepts and clinical practice,* J.A. Marx, R.S. Hockberger, R.M. Walls et al (eds.) 7 ed, 2010, Elsevier.

intubation should be performed in any patient with a GCS of 8 or less to prevent hypoxemia and hypercapnia. Intravenous fluid resuscitation should also be started early to prevent hypovolemia resulting in hypotension, shown to double mortality. Transfer to and care in a Level I trauma center are associated with better outcomes.

Details of in-hospital management including critical care and surgical intervention is beyond the scope of this text. Some important points are summarized below.

- ATLS protocol (airway, breathing, circulation, disability, exposure).
- Ventilatory support.
- Optimization of oxygenation, ventilation, and fluid status.
- CT head (Fig. E4) to evaluate for mass lesion (hematoma) or cerebral edema. These findings may necessitate either surgical intervention or ICP monitor placement. ATLS guidelines recommend maximum 30 minutes between initial assessment and CT head.
- In case of either a severe TBI (GCS 8 or less) or a moderate TBI (GCS 8 to 13) with an unreliable neurological exam, patients should be admitted to the intensive care unit for frequent neurological checks. TBI guidelines suggest ICP monitor placement for GCS 8 or less to monitor intracranial pressure closely. ICP monitors are of various kinds, and the most commonly used include external ventricular drain, intraparenchymal pressure monitor, and a bolt device with brain tissue oxygen pressure

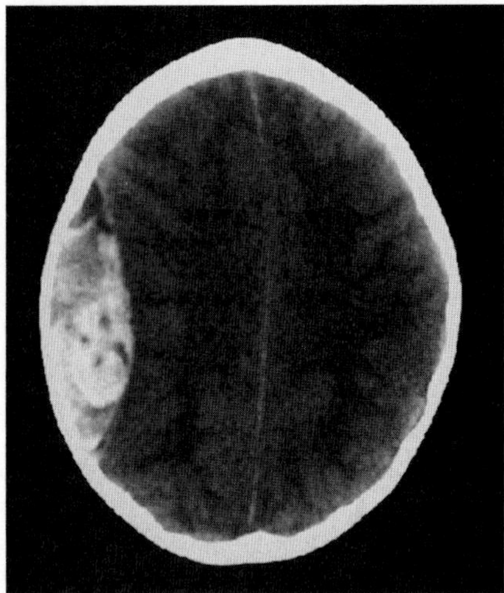

FIG. 3 Non–contrast-enhanced computed tomography scan of acute epidural hematoma at the level of right midconvexity. There is an associated mass effect and moderate midline shift. (From Marx: *Rosen's emergency medicine: concepts and clinical practice,* J.A. Marx, R.S. Hockberger, R.M. Walls et al [eds.] 7 ed, 2010, Elsevier.)

monitoring with fiberoptic pressure monitor. Recent research has also supported the use of brain tissue oxygen monitoring for severe TBI patients. Surgical decompression may involve evacuation of hematoma (epidural, subdural intraparenchymal contusion) through craniotomy alone (replacement of bone after completion of operation) versus decompressive craniectomy (complete removal of bone without replacement) in certain cases where cerebral edema is out of proportion to the presence of mass lesion. Skull fractures are treated depending on the morphology of the fracture. Open, depressed fractures require surgical debridement and elevation in most cases, in addition to broad-spectrum antibiotics.

- Avoid electrolyte imbalance, especially hyponatremia and hyperglycemia, which may contribute to cerebral edema and increase intracranial pressure.
- Elevation of head of bed to allow better venous drainage to reduce intracranial pressure.
- ICP management, which may include the following: drainage of cerebrospinal fluid via external ventricular drain, surgical hematoma evacuation, administration of hyperosmotic fluids to reduce edema, pharmacologic sedation and paralysis, pentobarbital-induced coma, and surgical decompression of the brain. In patients with traumatic brain injury, hypothermia can reduce intracranial hypertension, but recent trials in patients with an intracranial pressure of more than 20 mm Hg after TBI, therapeutic hypothermia, plus standard care to reduce intracranial pressure did not result in outcomes better than those with standard care alone. The new TBI guidelines do not recommend hypothermia.[2]
- Prevention of seizures in the acute setting. The most commonly used and studied drug is phenytoin. Indications for acute seizure prophylaxis in severe head trauma are described in Box 3. Levetiracetam (Keppra) is also a beneficial antiepileptic now commonly used in the TBI setting. Seizure prophylaxis, however, has not shown to prevent long-term development of traumatic epilepsy.
- DVT prophylaxis is recommended in almost all patients on hospital day 1 in addition to sequential compression devices (SCDs) for immobile or bedbound patients to prevent DVTs.
- Early initiation of parenteral nutrition.
- Early tracheostomy for ventilator-dependent patients is recommended to reduce mechanical ventilation days.

BOX 3 Indications for Acute Seizure Prophylaxis in Severe Head Trauma

- Depressed skull fracture
- Paralyzed and intubated patient
- Seizure at the time of injury
- Seizure at emergency department presentation
- Penetrating brain injury
- Severe head injury (Glasgow Coma Scale score ≤8)
- Acute subdural hematoma
- Acute epidural hematoma
- Acute intracranial hemorrhage
- Prior history of seizures

CHRONIC Rx

- TBI can lead to short- or long- term emotional, physiologic, and cognitive sequelae. Patients suffering from TBI are shown to benefit from neurocognitive, occupational, and physical therapy. The Glasgow Outcome Scale is a comprehensive measure of severity and eventual outcome of brain injury. Posttraumatic amnesia, age, length of coma, GCS score within the first 24 hours, and imaging study scales are some of the factors affecting outcome and dictating long-term prognosis.
- Chronic treatment addresses several sequelae of TBI, including, but not limited to, the following: dysautonomia, agitation, sleep disturbance, posttraumatic epilepsy, spasticity, dysphagia, syndrome of the trephined, posttraumatic hydrocephalus, apathy, fecal/urinary incontinence, headache, and neuropathic pain syndromes.

[2]Andrews PJD et al: Hypothermia for intracranial hypertension after traumatic brain injury, *N Engl J Med* 373:2103-2112, 2015.

COMPLEMENTARY AND ALTERNATIVE MEDICINE

Currently, there are no proven drugs that improve outcomes after TBI. Several pro-drugs are under study, with the hopes to have a single TBI cocktail that would enhance repair at the cellular and molecular pathway level. Neurostimulants such as amantadine, zolpidem, bromocriptine, amphetamine, and methylphenidate are used in the rehabilitation phase with anecdotal data, but good RCTs are lacking in this area.

DISPOSITION

Depending on severity of head injury, patients may require admission to a rehabilitation facility or discharge to home with outpatient neurocognitive therapy.

REFERRAL

Early transfer to a Level 1 Trauma Center with neurosurgical personnel if high-risk findings are noted on clinical exam or CT head, and is associated with better outcomes.

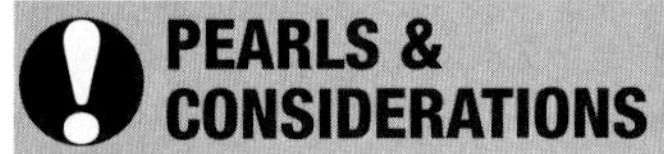

PEARLS & CONSIDERATIONS

TBI is major healthcare issue. Guidelines have been developed to address TBI in a timely and effective fashion. Clinical acumen and judgment, however, is irreplaceable and should be exercised for better patient care and outcomes. Early recognition of high-risk patients and early imaging and early evaluation at a Level 1 Trauma Center by a specialist are associated with improved outcomes. The goal of healthcare providers in the field or in the community is to identify patients who need this attention.

PATIENT/FAMILY EDUCATION

- Brain Injury Association of America http://www.biausa.org/
- Brain Injury Resource Center http://www.headinjury.com/linktbisup.htm

RELATED CONTENT

Concussion (Related Key Topic)
Postconcussive Syndrome (Related Key Topic)

AUTHORS: **FARHAN A. MIRZA, M.B.B.S.,** and **JUSTIN F. FRASER, M.D.**

BASIC INFORMATION

DEFINITION

Traveler's diarrhea (TD) is defined as 3 or more loose-to-watery stools, with or without associated fever, abdominal cramps, and vomiting, within a 24-hr period. It develops during or within 10 days of traveling to developing areas of the world.

SYNONYMS

TD
Enterotoxigenic *E. coli*
Enteroaggregative *E. coli*
Infectious diarrhea
Postinfectious irritable bowel syndrome

ICD-10CM CODE
A09 Infectious diarrhea

EPIDEMIOLOGY & DEMOGRAPHICS

Traveler's diarrhea is mostly caused by bacteria and other pathogens in food and water.

At least 1 episode of diarrhea occurs in 40% to 50% of travelers during their stay abroad. Table 1 describes pathogens and epidemiologic features associated with traveler's diarrhea.

INCIDENCE: High risk (>20%): South and Southeast Asia, Africa (except South Africa), South and Central America, and Mexico

Moderate risk (10% to 20%): Caribbean Islands, South Africa, Central and East Asia (including Russia and China), Eastern Europe, and the Middle East, including Israel

Low risk (<10%): Northern and Western Europe, Australia, New Zealand, United States, Canada, Singapore, Japan

PEAK INCIDENCE:
- Peak incidence occurs during the first week of travel and progressively declines after that
- Seasonal variation does exist for TD, with lower rates in the winter months

PREVALENCE: Acute and chronic diarrhea account for a third of medical visits by returned travelers as per the GeoSentinel database.

PREDOMINANT SEX AND AGE:
- Travelers in their 30s are at highest risk, possibly secondary to more adventurous travel.
- Gender does not seem to influence the risk for TD.
- Infants and toddlers are more likely to have a more severe form of TD and are more likely to need hospitalization.

GENETICS: Travelers with the O blood group are at higher risk for diarrhea caused by Norovirus and *Shigella*.

RISK FACTORS:
- Gastric acid protects against enteropathogens, so medications that reduce gastric acid secretion (i.e., PPI or H2-receptor blockers) are known to increase risk for TD by a factor of 12.
- Immunocompromised travelers such as those with HIV/AIDS are at higher risk for parasitic infections.
- Backpackers are at higher risk than those staying at a resort.
- Food bought from street vendors or prepared by persons not wearing gloves carries a higher risk.

PHYSICAL FINDINGS & CLINICAL PRESENTATION

- The clinical presentation does not allow determination of infectious cause.
- 90% of cases occur within 2 weeks of stay.
- Acute watery diarrhea predominates in 90% of patients.
- Signs of invasive infection, including fever and bloody/mucoid diarrhea, occur in 3% to 30%.
- Most patients report 3 to 5 bowel movements a day, but in 20% a higher frequency of up to 20 daily bowel movements occurs.
- Nausea (10% to 70%), vomiting (4% to 36%), abdominal cramps/tenesmus (80%), urgency (90%).
- Other: Myalgia, arthralgia, headache.
- Average episode resolves in 3 to 5 days.
- Prolonged symptoms lasting more than a week: 8% to 15%; chronic diarrhea >30 days: 1% to 3%.
- Severe episodes may result in electrolyte imbalance (K+ loss).
- 50% of all travelers are incapacitated for at least 24 hours, but up to 20% are ill in bed for 1 to 2 days.

ETIOLOGY

- *E. coli* (Table E2): Accounts for up to 60% of all cases of TD and is most prevalent in Central and South America, South Asia, and Africa. Table E3 summarizes etiology of traveler's diarrhea in Latin America, Africa, and Asia.
  1. Enterotoxigenic *E. coli* (ETEC): Produce heat labile and heat stable toxin and are the most common cause, accounting for 10% to 45% of cases. Frequently seen in Latin America, Africa, and South Asia.
  2. Enteroaggregative *E. coli* (EAEC): More commonly seen in Latin America.
  3. Other E. coli (enteropathogenic [EPEC], enteroinvasive [EIEC], enterohemorrhagic [EHEC]): Shiga toxin-producing or diffuse adhering *E. coli* are much less common.
- *Campylobacter*: 2% to 32% of cases. More common in Southeast Asia, where it is more frequent than ETEC.
- Shigella: 2% to 9%. More common in Africa.
- Salmonella: <5% of cases except in Asia, where it is seen in up to 10% of cases.
- Other bacteria: *Aeromonas, Arcobacter, Plesiomonas*, enterotoxigenic *Bacteroides fragilis, Vibrio cholera*, noncholera vibrios.
- Viral pathogens:
  1. Norovirus: Up to 17% of cases from Caribbean and Africa.
  2. Rotavirus: 4% to 7% of cases.
- Protozoans:
  1. *Entamoeba histolytica*: More common in South and Southeast Asia.
  2. *Giardia lamblia*: More common in South and Southeast Asia, especially Nepal.
  3. *Cryptosporidium, Cyclospora, Isospora.*

TABLE 1 Pathogens and Epidemiologic Features Associated with Traveler's Diarrhea

Organism	Approximate Percentage of Cases (%)	Epidemiologic Features
Enterotoxigenic *Escherichia coli*	15-50	Most important causative agent of traveler's diarrhea overall; not diagnosed by routine microbiologic methods
Enteroaggregative *E. coli*	20-35	Not diagnosed by routine microbiologic methods
Shigella spp. and enteroinvasive *E. coli*	10-25	Most important causes of dysentery. Enteroinvasive *E. coli* not diagnosed by routine microbiologic methods
Nontyphoidal *Salmonella* spp.	5-10	
Campylobacter jejuni	3-15	More common in Asia; antimicrobial resistance a concern
Aeromonas	5	
Plesiomonas	5	
Giardia lamblia	<2	Affects hikers and campers who drink from contaminated freshwater streams
Cryptosporidium hominis/parvum	<2	Occasional large-scale waterborne outbreaks
Cyclospora cayetanensis	<2	
Vibrio cholerae		Ongoing outbreaks in Haiti and Zimbabwe, and endemic in many countries in Asia; rare cause of disease in travelers
Norovirus		Outbreaks on cruise ships
Entamoeba histolytica		May cause liver abscess

From Bennett JE et al: *Mandell, Douglas, and Bennett's principles and practice of infectious diseases*, ed 8, Philadelphia, 2015, WB Saunders.

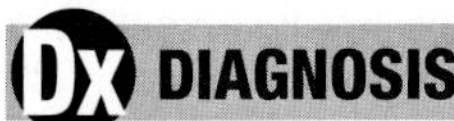

DIAGNOSIS

DIFFERENTIAL DIAGNOSIS

- Malaria
- Dengue fever
- Influenza
- Rocky Mountain spotted fever
- Irritable bowel syndrome
- Inflammatory bowel disease
- Shellfish poisoning
- Mushroom poisoning

WORKUP

- Most cases of TD are self-limiting, do not require workup, and are treated symptomatically without regard to etiologic agent.
- In patients with diarrhea, fever, and colitic symptoms (bloody stools, cramping), a stool culture should be obtained to look for specific bacterial pathogens.

LABORATORY TESTS

- Stool culture ×3 for bacterial pathogens.
- Stool for ova and parasites to help identify protozoans. Special stains such as modified acid fast or trichrome stain may be necessary for *Cryptosporidium, Cyclospora,* and *Isospora.*
- Blood cultures in patients with systemic illness to rule out *Salmonella* species.

Rx TREATMENT

NONPHARMACOLOGIC THERAPY

- Fluid replacement to treat volume depletion of diarrhea is important.
- Mild cases: Alternate fluids that contain salts and fluids that contain sugars, such as broths or fruit juices. Pedialyte is effective as an over-the-counter product.
- Severe cases: Oral rehydration solution (ORS) packets are available in most pharmacies. They should be mixed with clean water to replace lost electrolytes and are used until patient is urinating regularly. An alternative home-based solution can be made with: ½ teaspoon of salt, ½ teaspoon of baking soda, and 4 tablespoons of sugar in one liter of clean water.

ACUTE GENERAL Rx

- Antisecretory agents may reduce symptoms but do not treat underlying cause:
  1. Bismuth subsalicylate: 1 dose of 525 mg (2 tablets of Pepto-Bismol) PO every 30 min up to 8 doses a day. Can reduce number of bowel movements by 50%. Dosages are available for children based on weight, and the product is available in liquid or chewable tablet form.
  2. Loperamide: 4 mg PO, then 2 mg after each loose bowel movement, not to exceed 16 mg per day. Use for up to 48 hrs. Has antisecretory and antimotility effect. Antimotility drugs should not be used in cases of bloody diarrhea or dysentery (increased risk of colitis and colonic perforation). When used, they should be given only in conjunction with antimicrobial therapy.
- Antibiotics are warranted only for moderate to severe diarrhea (i.e., >4 bowel movements a day, fever, or blood, pus, or mucus in stool. Antibiotics can reduce duration of diarrhea by 1 to 2 days.
  1. Azithromycin: The preferred antibiotic for empiric treatment of moderate to severe TD. It is also the preferred agent for children and pregnant women. Dose of 1 gram PO is the single dose for women. Children: 10mg/kg/day single dose or for 3 days. Particularly effective against quinolone-resistant *Campylobacter* infections in Southeast Asia. Another option for children: Ceftriaxone 50 mg/kg/day IV once daily x 3 days.
     a. Ciprofloxacin: 500 mg twice a day for 1 to 3 days
     b. Levaquin: 500 mg a day for 1 to 3 days
  2. Fluoroquinolones are also effective agents for bacterial causes of TD, but resistance to fluoroquinolones is increasing. Cannot be used in children under 15 and in pregnant women:
  3. Rifaximin: 200 mg PO TID for 3 days for children age >12 and adults is effective for afebrile, noncolitic diarrhea such as ETEC. Does not treat *Salmonella, Shigella,* or *Campylobacter.*
  4. Rifamycin is now FDA approved for TD caused by non-invasive strains of *E. coli.* It is not recommended for TD complicated by fever and/or bloody stools. Dosage is 388 mg (2 tablets) bid x 3 days.
- Concerns of use of antibiotics:
  1. Widespread use of antibiotics has led to resistance. Tetracycline and sulfa agents such as Bactrim are no longer used due to widespread resistance.
  2. Antibiotic treatment may lead to prolonged colonization in infections with *Salmonella* and nontyphoid *Salmonella.*
  3. In cases of EHEC (Shiga toxin production) treatment with quinolones, but not rifaximin, may increase risk of complications such as hemolytic uremic syndrome.
  4. *Clostridia difficile* infection can occur with use of antibiotics.

PREVENTION BY ANTIBIOTICS AND NONANTIBIOTIC AGENTS

- Antibiotic prophylaxis can be considered for certain groups, such as persons with underlying illness, athletes, and politicians for up to 2 to 3 weeks. Ciprofloxacin 250 to 500 mg a day is effective in preventing 90% of TD. Rifaximin dosed daily has been shown to help prevent TD for U.S. travelers to Mexico, but not as effectively as Ciprofloxacin.
- Bismuth subsalicylate can be used. It must be given 4× daily and can cause black tongue and stools. As it contains salicylates, it can interact with anticoagulants and lead to toxicity in patients on long-term salicylate therapy.
- Probiotics are being studied for their potential use but evidence of their effectiveness is limited.

REFERRAL

Infectious diseases physician for more difficult cases lasting more than 72 hours

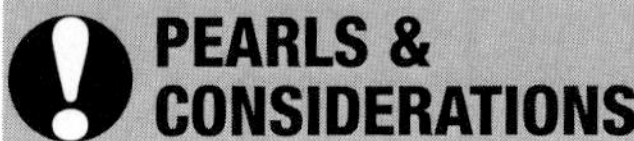

PEARLS & CONSIDERATIONS

- Travelers on cruises have lower incidence of TD than land-based trips, but cruise ship passengers and staff are at higher risk of large outbreaks of Norovirus that are difficult to contain. Norovirus infection needs only a low inoculum of virus to cause illness, and the virus is relatively resistant to cleaning.
- In up to 40% of cases of TD, no pathogen is identified.
- *Giardia* is the most frequent cause of long-lasting TD.

PREVENTION

- There are oral and injectable vaccines against *Salmonella typhi* available in the U.S.
- Dukoral oral vaccine is available in some countries such as Canada and Australia and in Europe to help prevent cholera and ETEC.

PATIENT/FAMILY EDUCATION

Food hygiene education: Wash hands often, especially after going to bathroom and before eating. Avoid raw fruits and vegetables (unless peeled and washed in clean water). Avoid undercooked meats, fish, and seafood. Avoid tap water and ice. Choose beverages in factory-sealed containers (such as bottled water and carbonated soft drinks). Try to avoid buffet-style foods.

SUGGESTED READINGS

Available at ExpertConsult.com

RELATED CONTENT

Traveler's Diarrhea (Patient Information)

AUTHOR: **GLENN G. FORT, M.D., M.P.H.**

BASIC INFORMATION

DEFINITION

Trigeminal neuralgia is an intense, usually unilateral, paroxysmal, stabbing pain in the sensory distribution of the trigeminal (cranial nerve V) nerve.

SYNONYM

Tic douloureux ("painful tics/spasms")

ICD-10CM CODE

G50.0 Trigeminal neuralgia

EPIDEMIOLOGY & DEMOGRAPHICS

INCIDENCE: 4 per 100,000
PEAK INCIDENCE: Incidence increases with age and peaks at 67 yr of age; onset in 90% of patients is after age 40.
PREVALENCE: 155 in 1 million
PREDOMINANT SEX AND AGE: Male:female ratio is 1:1.5.
RISK FACTORS: Most cases are idiopathic; age and multiple sclerosis are risk factors.

PHYSICAL FINDINGS & CLINICAL PRESENTATION

- Patients present with paroxysmal, unilateral facial pain that is usually described as shock-like, stabbing, or electric (Fig. 1).
- Pain can be spontaneous or triggered by touch, an air current, or activities such as shaving, eating, or brushing teeth.
- In severe cases, facial spasms can accompany the pain.
- Pain is usually described in distribution of the second (V2-maxillary) and third (V3-mandibular) divisions of the trigeminal nerve.
- The pain seldom lasts more than a few seconds to a minute.
- There is usually no sensory or motor loss.

ETIOLOGY

- Idiopathic or "classical": Cause usually unknown, likely an aberrant artery or vein compressing cranial nerve V at or near the pons. Neurovascular contact is also commonly found incidentally on imaging in asymptomatic individuals.
- Secondary: Accounts for up to 15% of cases; caused by nonvascular lesions such as a demyelinating plaque from multiple sclerosis or compression from a tumor near the pons.
- Box 1 summarizes causes of trigeminal neuralgia.

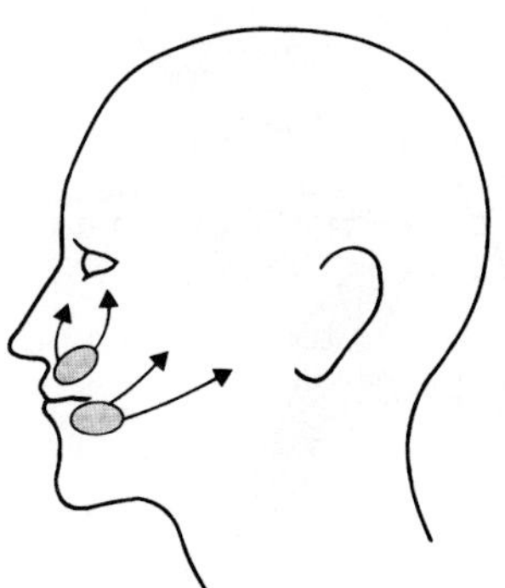

FIG. 1 Trigeminal neuralgia. The two most common sites of origin and radiation of pain are shown: mouth-ear and nose-orbit. Pain usually starts in the region of the encircled area and radiates in the directions shown.

DIAGNOSIS

DIFFERENTIAL DIAGNOSIS

- Trigeminal neuropathy
- Primary stabbing headache
- Short-lasting unilateral neuralgiform headache with conjunctival injection and tearing (SUNCT)
- Postherpetic neuralgia
- Glossopharyngeal neuralgia
- Dental pain

WORKUP

Trigeminal neuralgia is a clinical diagnosis (see previously).

IMAGING STUDIES

Neuroimaging (contrast-enhancing brain MRI) should be considered in young patients (<40 yr) with atypical symptoms (sensory loss, bilateral symptoms). MRI is useful to identify potential compressors or demyelinating causes. It detects nonvasular structure pathology in 15% of patients. Brain MRI is useful to identify neurovascular contrast between trigeminal nerve and superior cerebellar artery.

TREATMENT

PHARMACOLOGIC Rx

- Carbamazepine 400 to 800 mg, 2 to 3 times daily divided dosing is the recommended initial treatment. This can be titrated to pain relief by 100 to 200 mg every 3 days to a maximum of 1200 mg divided bid or tid.
- Oxcarbazepine can be used if carbamazepine is not tolerated due to side effects. Other medications include botulinum toxin type A, lidocaine, baclofen, phenytoin, gabapentin, clonazepam, lamotrigine, and levetiracetam.
- Drug combinations can be tried when one medication is partially effective before proceeding with secondary intervention.
- Spontaneous remissions may be seen in trigeminal neuralgia, and therefore periodic medication tapers should be considered if the patient is pain free.
- In the elderly population, caution should be used when initiating and titrating the above medications. Caution and extensive counseling should also be used in women of child-bearing age when initiating treatment with anti-seizure medications.

BOX 1 Causes of Trigeminal Neuralgia

Classical
Neurovascular compression by an artery or vein

Symptomatic
Saccular aneurysm
Arteriovenous malformation
Tumors/mass-lesions at cerebellopontine angle
- Vestibular schwannoma
- Meningioma
- Epidermoid

Primary demyelinating disorders
- Multiple sclerosis
- Charcot-Marie-Tooth disease (rare)

Infiltrative disorders
- Trigeminal amyloidoma

Nondemyelinating lesions
- Small infarct or angioma in the brainstem

Familial

Modified from Adams JG et al: *Emergency medicine, clinical essentials,* ed 2, Philadelphia, 2013, Elsevier.

NONPHARMACOLOGIC THERAPY

Patients with refractory pain eventually need secondary intervention such as microvascular decompression, selective nerve fiber destruction (rhizotomy), glycerol injection, thermal lesioning, chemical ablation, or gamma knife radiosurgery. Microvascular decompression is the only available nondestructive procedure and is effective in 75% of patients, and possesses observed long-term benefits.

DISPOSITION

- Most patients are responsive to initial pharmacologic treatment. Spontaneous remission is possible.
- Medical management is eventually ineffective in 30% to 50% of patients.

REFERRAL

Referral to a neurologist is appropriate if there is uncertainty about diagnosis or if symptoms are refractory to conservative management.

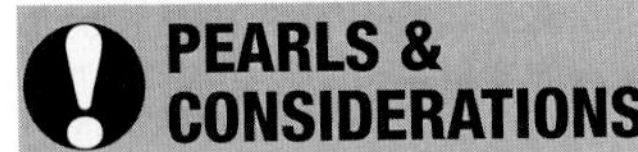

PEARLS & CONSIDERATIONS

In a young patient with trigeminal neuralgia, secondary causes such as multiple sclerosis should be considered, and an MRI of the head obtained. In secondary disease, initial therapy should address underlying secondary causes.

SUGGESTED READING

Available at ExpertConsult.com

RELATED CONTENT

Trigeminal Neuralgia (Patient Information)

AUTHOR: **JONATHAN H. SMITH, M.D.**

BASIC INFORMATION

DEFINITION

Pulmonary tuberculosis (TB) is an infection of the lung and, occasionally, surrounding structures, caused by the bacterium *Mycobacterium tuberculosis* (Mtb). Multidrug-resistant (MDR) TB is defined as disease caused by strains of Mtb that are at least resistant to treatment with isoniazid and rifampin; extensively drug-resistant (XDR) TB refers to disease caused by MDR strains that are also resistant to treatment with any fluoroquinolone and any of the injectable drugs used in the treatment of second-line anti-TB drugs.

SYNONYM

TB

ICD-10CM CODES
A15.0 Tuberculosis of lung
A15.7 Primary respiratory tuberculosis

EPIDEMIOLOGY & DEMOGRAPHICS

INCIDENCE (WORLDWIDE):
- One third of the world's population is infected with TB, and it is still one of the deadliest diseases known to humans.
- In 2015, there were 10.4 million new cases of active tuberculosis; 13% involved coinfection with HIV.
- 1.8 million deaths from TB, including 430,000 among HIV-infected patients; 310,000 incident cases of multidrug-resistant TB worldwide.
- Sub-Saharan Africa has the highest rates of active TB per capita.
- Absolute number of cases is highest in Asia, with India and China having the greatest burden of disease globally.

INCIDENCE (IN U.S.):
- In 2018, a total of 2029 new TB cases were reported in the U.S., representing a 0.7% decrease from 2017. The U.S. TB incidence in 2018 was 2.8 per 100,000 persons. The rate among non-U.S. born persons was >14 times that in the U.S. board persons.[3] Since 1993, TB case counts and rates have declined in the U.S (Fig. 1). As the number of cases decreases overall, an increasing percentage of cases occurs among non-U.S. born persons.
- >90% of new cases each year from reactivated prior infections.
- 9% newly infected.
- Only 10% of patients with purified protein derivative (PPD) conversions (higher [8%/yr] in HIV-positive patients) will develop TB, most within 1 to 2 yr.
- Two thirds of all new cases in racial and ethnic minorities.
- 80% of new cases in children in racial and ethnic minorities.
- Occurs most frequently in geographic areas and among populations with highest AIDS prevalence.
  1. Urban blacks and Hispanics between 25 and 45 yr old
  2. Poor, crowded urban communities
- Nearly 36% of new cases from new immigrants with top four countries being China, India, the Philippines, and Vietnam.
- In 2014 in the U.S., 1.3% of cases were MDR TB, which is a decline from 8.2% in 2008. There was one case of XDR TB in the U.S. in 2014 and one in 2015.

PREVALENCE (IN U.S.):
- Estimated 10 million people infected
- Varies widely among population groups

PREDOMINANT SEX:
- No specific predilection
- Male predominance in AIDS, shelters, and prisons reflected in disproportionate male incidence (Box 1)

PREDOMINANT AGE:
- Ages 24 to 45
- Childhood cases common among minorities
- Nursing home outbreaks among elderly

PEAK INCIDENCE:
- Infancy
- Teenage years
- Pregnancy
- Elderly
- HIV-positive patients at highest risk regardless of age

GENETICS:
- Populations with widespread low native resistance have been intensely infected when initially exposed to TB.
- Following elimination of those with least native resistance, incidence and prevalence of TB tends to decline.

PHYSICAL FINDINGS & CLINICAL PRESENTATION

- See "Etiology"
- Primary pulmonary TB infection generally asymptomatic
- Reactivation pulmonary TB:
  1. Fever
  2. Night sweats
  3. Cough
  4. Hemoptysis
  5. Scanty nonpurulent sputum
  6. Weight loss
- Progressive primary pulmonary TB disease: Same as reactivation pulmonary TB
- TB pleurisy:
  1. Pleuritic chest pain
  2. Fever
  3. Shortness of breath

BOX 1 High-Risk Groups for Tuberculosis Infection and Disease

Groups at High Risk for Exposure or Infection
- Close contacts of persons with tuberculosis
- Foreign-born persons from high-risk regions (Asia, Africa, Latin America, Russia, eastern Europe)
- Residents and employees of high-risk congregate settings (correctional institutions, nursing homes, homeless shelters, hospitals serving high-risk populations, drug treatment centers)
- Medically underserved, low-income populations
- High-risk racial or ethnic minority populations
- Injectable drug users
- Children exposed to adults in high-risk categories

Groups at Higher Risk for Disease Once Infected
- Immunosuppressed patients, including those with HIV
- Patients with recent tuberculosis infection (within past 2 years)
- Persons with certain medical conditions (diabetes mellitus, silicosis, cancer, end-stage renal disease, gastrectomy, body weight ≤90% of ideal)
- Injectable drug users
- History of inadequately treated tuberculosis
- Children age ≤4 years, especially infants

From Cherry JD et al: *Feigin and Cherry's textbook of pediatric infectious diseases*, ed 8, Philadelphia, 2019, Elsevier.

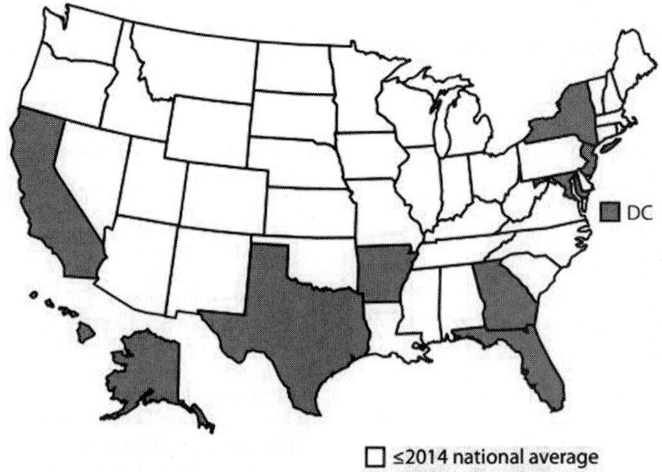

FIG. 1 Tuberculosis case rates (cases per 100,000) by state, 2014. (From Centers for Disease Control and Prevention. *Tuberculosis trends—United States*, 2014. *MMWR* 2015;64:265-9, in)

- Rare massive, suffocating, fatal hemoptysis secondary to erosion of pulmonary artery within a cavity (Rasmussen aneurysm)
- Chest examination:
  1. Not specific
  2. Usually underestimates extent of disease
  3. Rales accentuated following a cough (posttussive rales)

ETIOLOGY

- Mtb, a slow-growing, aerobic, non-spore-forming, nonmotile bacillus, with a lipid-rich cell wall:
  1. Lacks pigment
  2. Produces niacin
  3. Reduces nitrate
  4. Produces heat-labile catalase
  5. Mtb staining, acid-fast and acid-alcohol fast by Ziehl-Neelsen method, appearing as red, slightly bent, beaded rods 2 to 4 microns long (acid-fast bacilli [AFB]), against a blue background
  6. Polymerase chain reaction (PCR) to detect <10 organisms/ml in sputum (compared with the requisite 10,000 organisms/ml for AFB smear detection)
  7. Culture:
     a. Growth on solid media (Löwenstein-Jensen; Middlebrook 7H11) in 2 to 6 weeks
     b. Growth in liquid media (BACTEC, using a radioactive carbon source for early growth detection) often in 9 to 16 days
     c. Enhanced in a 5% to 10% carbon dioxide atmosphere
  8. DNA fingerprinting (based on restriction fragment length polymorphism [RFLP]):
     a. Facilitates immediate identification of MTB strains in early growing cultures
     b. False negatives possible if growth suboptimal
  9. Humans are the only reservoir for MTB
  10. Transmission:
     a. Facilitated by close exposure to high-velocity cough (unprotected by proper mask or respirators) from patient with AFB-positive sputum and cavitary lesions, producing aerosolized droplets containing AFB, which are inhaled directly into alveoli
     b. Occurs within prisons, nursing homes, and hospitals
- Pathogenesis:
  1. AFB (Mtb) ingested by macrophages in alveoli, then transported to regional lymph nodes, where spread is contained
  2. Some AFB may reach bloodstream and disseminate widely
  3. Primary TB (asymptomatic, minimal pneumonitis in lower or midlung fields, with hilar lymphadenopathy) essentially an intracellular infection, with multiplication of organisms continuing 2 to 12 weeks after primary exposure, until cell-mediated hypersensitivity (detected by positive skin test reaction to tuberculin PPD) matures, with subsequent containment of infection
  4. Local and disseminated AFB thus contained by T-cell–mediated immune responses:
     a. Recruitment of monocytes
     b. Transformation of lymphocytes with secretion of lymphokines
     c. Activation of macrophages and histiocytes
     d. Organization into granulomas, where organisms may survive within macrophages (Langhans giant cells), but within which multiplication essentially ceases (95%) and from which spread is prohibited
  5. Progressive primary pulmonary disease:
     a. May immediately follow the asymptomatic phase:
     b. Necrotizing pulmonary infiltrates
     c. Tuberculous bronchopneumonia
     d. Endobronchial TB
     e. Interstitial TB
     f. Widespread miliary lung lesions
  6. Postprimary TB pleurisy with pleural effusion:
     a. Develops after early primary infection, although often before conversion to positive PPD
     b. Results from pleural seeding from a peripheral lung lesion or rupture of lymph node into pleural space
     c. May produce a large (sometimes hemorrhagic) exudative effusion (with polymorphonuclear cells early, rapidly replaced by lymphocytes), frequently without pulmonary infiltrates
     d. Generally resolves without treatment
     e. Portends a high risk of subsequent clinical disease, and therefore must be diagnosed and treated early (pleural biopsy and culture) to prevent future catastrophic TB illness
     f. May result in disseminated extrapulmonary infection
  7. Reactivation pulmonary TB:
     a. Occurs months to years following primary TB
     b. Preferentially involves the apical posterior segments of the upper lobes and superior segments of the lower lobes
     c. Associated with necrosis and cavitation of involved lung, hemoptysis, chronic fever, night sweats, weight loss
     d. Spread within lung occurs via cough and inhalation
  8. Reinfection TB:
     a. May mimic reactivation TB
     b. Ruptured caseous foci and cavities, which may produce endobronchial spread
  9. Mtb in both progressive primary and reactivation pulmonary TB:
     a. Intracellular (macrophage) lesions (undergoing slow multiplication)
     b. Closed caseous lesions (undergoing slow multiplication)
     c. Extracellular, open cavities (undergoing rapid multiplication)
     d. INH and rifampin are bactericidal in all three sites
     e. Pyrazinamide (PZA) especially active within acidic macrophage environment
     f. Extrapulmonary reactivation disease also possible
  10. Rapid local progression and dissemination in infants with devastating illness before PPD conversion occurs
  11. Most symptoms (fever, weight loss, anorexia) and tissue destruction (caseous necrosis) from cytokines and cell-mediated immune responses
  12. Mtb has no important endotoxins or exotoxins
  13. Granuloma formation related to tumor necrosis factor (TNF) secreted by activated macrophages

Dx DIAGNOSIS

DIFFERENTIAL DIAGNOSIS

- Necrotizing pneumonia (anaerobic, gram-negative)
- Histoplasmosis
- Coccidioidomycosis
- Melioidosis
- Interstitial lung diseases (rarely)
- Cancer
- Sarcoidosis
- Silicosis
- Rare pneumonias:
  1. *Rhodococcus equi* (cavitation)
  2. *Bacillus cereus* (50% hemoptysis)
  3. *Eikenella corrodens* (cavitation)

WORKUP

- Sputum for AFB stains
- Chest x-ray (Fig. E2)
- PPD (tuberculin skin test [TST]):
  1. Recent conversion from negative to positive within 3 months of exposure is highly suggestive of recent infection.
  2. Single positive PPD is not helpful diagnostically.
  3. Negative PPD never rules out acute TB.
  4. Be certain that positive PPD does not reflect "booster phenomenon" (prior positive PPD may become negative after several yr and return to positive only after second repeated PPD; repeat second PPD within 1 wk), which thus may mimic skin test conversion.
  5. Positive PPD reaction is determined as follows:
     a. Induration after 72 hours of intradermal injection of 0.1 ml of 5 TU-PPD
     b. 5-mm induration if HIV-positive (or other severe immunosuppressed state affecting cellular immune function), close contact of active TB, fibrotic chest lesions
     c. 10-mm induration if in high–medical risk groups (immunosuppressive disease or therapy, renal failure, gastrectomy, silicosis, diabetes), foreign-born high-risk group (Southeast Asia, Latin

America, Africa, India), low socioeconomic groups, IV drug addict, prisoner, health care worker
   d. 15-mm induration if low risk
6. Anergy antigen testing (using mumps, *Candida,* tetanus toxoid) may identify patients who are truly anergic to PPD and these antigens, but results are often confusing. Not recommended.
7. Patients with TB may be selectively anergic only to PPD.
8. Positive PPD indicates prior infection but does not itself confirm active disease.

- Interferon gamma release assays (IGRAs): Diagnostic test for latent TB infection, known as the QuantiFERON TB Gold test (QFT-G) and T-SPOT.TB Assay. These blood tests measure interferon response to specific Mtb antigens. The test may assist in distinguishing true positive reactions from individuals with latent TB, from PPD reactions related to nontuberculous mycobacteria; prior BCG vaccination; or difficult-to-interpret skin-test results from people with dermatologic conditions or immediate allergic reactions to PPD. The diagnostic utility of the test as a replacement or supplement to the standard PPD is not yet fully determined. When IGRA is used for routine screening, positive results should be repeated routinely due to a high rate of false-positive results. IGRAs have a specificity >95% for diagnosis of latent TB. The sensitivity of the T-SPOT assay (90%) appears to be higher than the QFT-G test (80%). It should be noted that IGRA sensitivity is diminished by HIV infection.
- The Xpert MTB/RIF is an automated molecular test for *Mycobacterium tuberculosis* (MTB) and resistance to rifampin (RIF) that provides sensitive detection of TB and rifampin resistance directly from untreated sputum in less than 2 hours with minimal hands-on time.

LABORATORY TESTS

- Sputum for AFB stains and culture:
  1. Induced sputum if patient not coughing productively
- Sputum from bronchoscopy if high suspicion of TB with negative expectorated induced sputum for AFB:
  1. Positive AFB smear is essential before or shortly after treatment to ensure subsequent growth for definitive diagnosis and sensitivity testing
  2. Consider lung biopsy if sputum negative, especially if infiltrates are predominantly interstitial
- AFB stain-negative sputum may grow MTB subsequently
- Gastric aspirates reliable, especially in HIV-negative patients
- CBC:
  1. Variable values:
     a. WBCs: Low, normal, or elevated (including leukemoid reaction: >50,000)
     b. Normocytic, normochromic anemia often
  2. Rarely helpful diagnostically
- ESR usually elevated
- Thoracentesis:
  1. Exudative effusion:
     a. Elevated protein
     b. Decreased glucose
     c. Elevated WBCs (polymorphonuclear leukocytes early, replaced later by lymphocytes)
     d. May be hemorrhagic
  2. Pleural fluid usually AFB-negative
  3. Pleural biopsy often diagnostic—may need to be repeated for diagnosis
  4. Culture pleural biopsy tissue for AFB
- Bone marrow biopsy is often diagnostic in difficult-to-diagnose cases, especially miliary TB

IMAGING STUDIES

- Chest x-ray:
  1. Primary infection reflected by calcified peripheral lung nodule with calcified hilar lymph node
  2. Reactivation pulmonary TB:
     a. Necrosis
     b. Cavitation (especially on apical lordotic views)
     c. Fibrosis and hilar retraction
     d. Bronchopneumonia
     e. Interstitial infiltrates
     f. Miliary pattern
     g. Many of the previous findings may also accompany progressive primary TB
  3. TB pleurisy:
     a. Pleural effusion, often rapidly accumulating and massive
  4. TB activity not established by single chest x-ray examination
  5. Serial chest x-ray examinations are excellent indicators of progression or regression

Rx TREATMENT

NONPHARMACOLOGIC THERAPY

- Increased rest during acute phase of treatment
- High-calorie, high-protein diet to reverse malnutrition and enhance immune response to TB
- Isolation in negative-pressure rooms with high-volume air replacement and circulation, with health care provider wearing proper protective 0.5- to 1-micron filter respirators, until three consecutive sputum AFB smears are negative

ACUTE GENERAL Rx

- Compliance (rigid adherence to treatment regimen) chief determinant of success:
  1. Supervised directly observed therapy (DOT) recommended for all patients and mandatory for unreliable patients
- Preferred adult regimen: DOT
  1. Isoniazid (INH) 15 mg/kg (max 900 mg), rifampin 600 mg, ethambutol (EMB) 30 mg/kg (max 2500 mg), and pyrazinamide (PZA) (2 g [<50 kg]; 2.5 g [51 to 74 kg]; 3 g [>75 kg]) thrice weekly for 6 months
  2. Alternative, more complicated DOT regimens
- Rifapentine, a rifampin derivative with a much longer serum half-life, was shown to be as effective when administered weekly (with weekly isoniazid) as conventional regimens for drug-sensitive pulmonary TB in non–HIV-infected patients.
- Short-course daily therapy: Adult
  1. HIV-negative patient: 6 months total therapy (2 months INH 300 mg, rifampin 600 mg, and EMB 15 mg/kg [max 2500 mg]) and PZA (1.5 g [<50 kg]; 2 g [51-74 kg]; 2.5 g [>75 kg]) daily and until smear negative and sensitivity confirmed; then INH and rifampin daily for 4 months
  2. HIV-positive patient: 9 months total therapy (2 months INH, rifampin, EMB, and PZA daily until smear negative and sensitivity confirmed; then INH and rifampin qid for 7 months)
  3. Continue treatment at least 3 months following conversion to negative cultures.
- Drug resistance (often multiple drug resistance TB [MDRTB]) increased by:
  1 Prior treatment
  2. Acquisition of TB in developing countries
  3. Homelessness, incarceration
  4. AIDS, IVDA
  5. Known contact with MDRTB
- Never add single drug to failing regimen.
- Never treat TB with fewer than two to three drugs or two to three new additional drugs.
- Other medications used in MDR or XDRTB include moxifloxacin, cycloserine, aminoglycosides such as amikacin or kanamycin, clarithromycin, PAS, and ethionamide.
- Bedaquiline, a diarylquinoline antimycobacterial, is used for treatment of MDR-TB. Recommended dose is 400 mg once daily for 2 weeks, followed by 200 mg 3×/wk for weeks 3 to 24. Bedaquiline is administered in combination with ≥3 drugs to which it is susceptible.
- Monitor for clinical toxicity (especially hepatitis).
  1. Patient and physician awareness that anorexia, nausea, right upper quadrant pain, and unexplained malaise require immediate cessation of treatment.
  2. Evaluation of liver function testing:
     a. Minimal SGOT/SGPT elevations without symptoms generally transient and not clinically significant
- Preventive treatment for PPD conversion only (infection without disease):
  1. Must be certain that chest x-ray examination is negative and patient has no symptoms of TB
  2. Most important groups:
     a. HIV-positive and other severely immunocompromised patients
     b. Close contact with active TB
     c. Recent converter
     d. Old TB on chest x-ray examination
     e. IV drug addict
     f. Medical risk factor
     g. High-risk foreign country
     h. Homeless
     i. Box 2 summarizes persons in whom isoniazid (or other regimens) should be initiated to prevent progression to tuberculosis.

BOX 2 Persons in Whom Isoniazid (or Other Regimens) Should Be Initiated to Prevent Progression to Tuberculosis

Household members and other close associates of persons with potentially infectious tuberculosis
Contacts of any age with a Mantoux tuberculin skin test reading of 5 mm or greater and no documented history of reaction in the past, or with a positive interferon gamma release assay (IGRA), should be considered recently infected and receive therapy if they have not been treated previously.
Newly infected people, regardless of age, who have had a tuberculin skin test or IGRA conversion within the past 2 years
People with HIV infection who have a reaction of 5 mm or greater to a Mantoux test
People of any age with past tuberculosis infection who received inadequate treatment
People of any age with a positive tuberculin skin test or positive IGRA and an abnormal but stable chest radiograph
People with significant tuberculin reactions or positive IGRAs who have special clinical situations, including silicosis, diabetes mellitus, prolonged corticosteroid therapy, immunosuppressive therapy, hematologic malignant disease, or end-stage renal disease
All children and adolescents with a positive tuberculin skin test reaction or interferon release assay result

From Cherry JD et al: *Feigin and Cherry's textbook of pediatric infectious diseases*, ed 8, Philadelphia, 2019, Elsevier.

3. The traditional preventive therapy for persons with latent *M. tuberculosis* consists of INH 300 mg daily for 9-12 months (at least 12 months if HIV-positive patient). The CDC has issued recommendations for a new regimen consisting of isoniazid and rifapentine administered once a week for 12 weeks as directly observed therapy. Studies have demonstrated that this regimen is as effective as 9 months of isoniazid therapy for preventing tuberculosis. Patients who should not receive this regimen include children younger than 2 years, persons with HIV infection taking antiretroviral therapy, pregnant women or those who may become pregnant during the course of treatment, and patients who have latent *M. tuberculosis* infection that is presumed to be resistant to isoniazid or rifampin.
4. A recent open-label trial comparing a 9-month regimen of isoniazid with a 4-month regimin of rifampin revealed that the 4-month regimen of refampin was not inferior to the 9-month regimen of isoniazid for the prevention of active TB in persons with latent TB infection and was associated with a higher rate of treatment completion and better safety (Menzies D et al).

- Infants generally given prophylaxis immediately if recent contact with active TB (even if infant PPD negative), then retested with PPD in 3 months (continuing INH if PPD becomes positive and stopping INH if PPD remains negative).
- Chronic, stable PPD (several years) given INH prophylaxis generally only if patient is <35 years:
  1. INH toxicity may outweigh benefit
  2. Individualize decision
- Preventive therapy for suspected INH-resistant organisms is unclear.
- Pyridoxine (Vitamin B6) supplementation (25-50 mg daily) should be added to INH regimens in patients predisposed to neuropathy such as alcohol use, diabetes, uremia, malnutrition, and HIV.

CHRONIC Rx

- Generally not indicated beyond treatment described previously
- Prolonged treatment, supervised by infectious disease expert, in a few very complicated infections caused by resistant organisms

DISPOSITION

- Monthly follow-up by physician experienced in TB treatment
- Confirm sensitivity testing and alter treatment appropriately
- Frequent sputum samples until culture is negative
- Confirm chest x-ray regression at 2 to 3 months
- Approximately 5% of patients with drug-susceptible TB have a relapse after 6 months of first-line therapy, as do approximately 20% of patients after 4 months of short course therapy. Higher MIC values of isoniazid or rifampin in predominant isolates of *M. tuberculosis* are associated with a greater risk of relapse.[2]

REFERRAL

- To infectious disease expert for:
  1. HIV-positive patient
  2. Patient with suspected drug-resistant TB
  3. Patients previously treated for TB
  4. Patients whose fever has not decreased and sputum has not converted to negative in 2 to 4 weeks
  5. Patients with overwhelming pulmonary or extrapulmonary TB
- To pulmonologist for bronchoscopy or pleural biopsy

[2]Talwar A et al: Tuberculosis-United States, 2018, *MMWR* 68(11):257-262, 2019.
[3]Colangeli R et al: Bacterial factors that predict relapse after tuberculosis therapy, N Engl J Med 379:823-833, 2018.

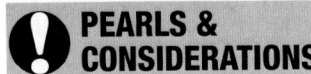

PEARLS & CONSIDERATIONS

COMMENTS

- All contacts (especially close household contacts and infants) should be properly tested for PPD conversions during 3 months following exposure.
- Those with positive PPD should be evaluated for active TB and properly treated or given prophylaxis.
- Previous treatment is a common risk factor for XDR and MDR TB.
- Evidence exists for the efficacy and safety of 6-month isoniazid monotherapy, rifampicin monotherapy, and combination therapies with 3 to 4 months of isoniazid and rifampicin.[1]

SUGGESTED READINGS

Available at ExpertConsult.com

AUTHOR: **GLENN G. FORT, M.D., M.P.H.**

[1]Zenner D et al: Treatment of latent tuberculosis infection, *Ann Intern Med* 167:248–255, 2017.

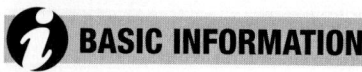

BASIC INFORMATION

DEFINITION

- Tumor lysis syndrome (TLS) is an oncologic emergency referring to the acute release of potentially injurious intracellular contents into the systemic circulation from tumor cell breakdown.
- TLS is a constellation of metabolic disturbances that occurs typically in the setting of rapid tumor cell lysis induced by cancer-targeted treatment (chemotherapy and/or other interventions such as embolization or radiation). However, spontaneous tumor cell turnover has induced TLS without precipitation by chemotherapy.
- TLS is characterized by hyperuricemia, hyperphosphatemia, hypocalcemia, hyperkalemia, and acute kidney injury (AKI), often with progressive oliguria.
- In the current 2004 Cairo and Bishop classification system, TLS may be defined by laboratory or clinical parameters. Grading of clinical tumor lysis syndrome is summarized in Table 1.
    1. **Laboratory TLS** is clinically silent and defined by the presence of at least two of the following biochemical variables within 3 days before or 7 days after initiation of chemotherapy despite adequate volume status and uric acid–lowering agents.
        a. Hyperuricemia:
            (1) Results from the rapid release and catabolism of intracellular nucleic acids.
            (2) Purine nucleic acids are metabolized to hypoxanthine, xanthine, and finally, uric acid.
            (3) In an acidic environment, uric acid can precipitate in the renal tubular lumen causing obstruction.
        b. Hyperkalemia
        c. Hyperphosphatemia:
            (1) Phosphate may precipitate with calcium to form calcium phosphate stones in renal tubules.
        d. Hypocalcemia:
            (1) Occurs secondary to precipitation with phosphorus.
    2. **Clinical TLS** occurs when laboratory TLS is complicated by at least one of the following clinical complications (severe renal impairment, cardiac arrhythmias, central nervous system toxicity, and/or death) that are not attributed to chemotherapy regimen.

SYNONYM

TLS

ICD-10CM CODE

E88.3 Tumor lysis syndrome

EPIDEMIOLOGY & DEMOGRAPHICS

INCIDENCE: The frequency of TLS is unknown, but it is the most common disease-related emergency encountered by physicians who treat children or adults with hematologic cancers. Incidence depends on cancer mass (greater mass correlates with greater cellular content release at cell death), patient characteristics (e.g., preexisting chronic kidney disease, volume depletion, hypotension), and supportive care. Tumor bulk, proliferation rate, and treatment sensitivity are associated with greater frequency of TLS.

PREVALENCE: Variable

PREDOMINANT SEX AND AGE:

- No sex predilection exists.
- Occurs in all age groups. Older adults are more susceptible to TLS due to a decline in glomerular filtration rate with age.

GENETICS: No racial predilection

RISK FACTORS:

- High tumor burden:
    1. Large-size tumor
    2. LDH >1500 IU/L
    3. WBC >25,000/mm^3
    4. Risk of TLS is further stratified by tumor type:
        a. High risk:
            (1) Burkitt lymphoma
            (2) High-grade non-Hodgkin's lymphoma
            (3) Lymphoblastic lymphoma
            (4) Acute T-cell leukemia
            (5) Other acute leukemias
        b. Moderate risk:
            (1) Low-grade lymphoma treated with chemotherapy/radiation/corticosteroids
            (2) Multiple myeloma
            (3) Breast carcinoma treated with chemotherapy/hormonal therapy
            (4) Small-cell lung carcinoma
            (5) Germ-cell tumors (e.g., seminoma, ovarian)
        c. Low risk
            (1) Low-grade lymphoma treated with interferon
            (2) Merkel cell carcinoma
            (3) Adenocarcinoma of the gastrointestinal tract
- Administration of certain agents, including:
    1. Paclitaxel
    2. Hydroxyurea
    3. Etoposide
    4. Fludarabine
    5. Sorafenib
- Extensive bone marrow involvement
- Elevated pretreatment uric acid, potassium, or phosphorus levels
- Tumor highly sensitive to treatment
- Volume depletion
- Chronic kidney disease
- Decreased urine output
- Acidic urine
- Tumor involvement of the kidney/renal vasculature
- Advanced age
- Post-transcatheter arterial chemoembolization (TACE), radiofrequency thermal ablation
- Chimeric Antigen Receptor T Cells therapy (CAR-T cell)

ETIOLOGY

Most commonly occurs in patients with acute leukemias; bulky, solid tumors; or high-grade lymphomas.

- Can occur spontaneously or after antitumor intervention (chemotherapy, radiation, etc.)
- Associated with administration of certain chemotherapeutic agents (whether intravenous, intrathecal, etc.):
    1. Paclitaxel
    2. Hydroxyurea
    3. Etoposide
    4. Fludarabine
- Spontaneous TLS:
    1. Rare
    2. Lysis of tumor cells without chemotherapy or in setting of minimal chemotherapy (e.g., steroid monotherapy in case of lymphomas)

TABLE 1 Grading of Clinical Tumor Lysis Syndrome

Stage I	Stage II	Stage III	Stage IV	Stage V
Renal failure	Serum creatinine = 1.5 UNL or creatinine clearance 30–45 ml/min	Serum creatinine = 1.5–3 UNL or creatinine clearance 20–30 ml/min	Serum creatinine = 3–6 UNL or creatinine clearance 10–20 ml/min	Serum creatinine >6 UNL or creatinine clearance <10 ml/min
Cardiac arrhythmia	Intervention not indicated	Nonurgent intervention indicated	Symptomatic and incompletely controlled or controlled with device (e.g., defibrillator)	Life-threatening (e.g., arrhythmia associated with heart failure, hypotension, syncope, shock)
Seizures	None	One brief, generalized seizure; seizure(s) well controlled by anti-convulsant, or infrequent focal motor seizures	Seizure in which consciousness is altered; poorly controlled seizure disorder, with generalized breakthrough seizures despite medical intervention	Seizure of any kind that is prolonged, repetitive, or difficult to control (e.g., status epilepticus, intractable epilepsy)

From Ronco C et al: *Critical care nephrology*, ed 3, Philadelphia, 2019, Elsevier.

3. Related to rapid cell turnover rate
4. Can be associated with pregnancy; fever; and rarely, generalized anesthesia in predisposed individuals
5. Hyperphosphatemia may not recur because of the reutilization of released phosphorus for resynthesis of newer tumor cells

PHYSICAL FINDINGS & CLINICAL PRESENTATION

CLINICAL PRESENTATION: Patients may present with a number of symptoms either before starting chemotherapy or commonly within 3 days after initiating cytotoxic treatment. Common symptoms include:

- Nausea
- Vomiting
- Edema
- Shortness of breath (from fluid overload or CHF)
- Lethargy or weakness
- Seizure
- Syncope
- Muscle cramp
- Tetany

PHYSICAL FINDINGS

- Associated with specific metabolic abnormalities, including hyperkalemia, hyperphosphatemia, hyperuricemia, and hypocalcemia
- Findings often overlap for these metabolic derangements

1. Hyperkalemia:
    a. Generalized weakness
    b. Paresthesias
    c. Paralysis
    d. ECG abnormalities:
        (1) Peaked T waves
        (2) Flattened P waves
        (3) Widened QRS complexes
        (4) Bradycardia
    a. Cardiac arrhythmias, including:
        (1) Ventricular tachycardia
        (2) Ventricular fibrillation
        (3) Asystole
        (4) Pulseless electrical activity
    b. Cardiac arrest
2. Hyperphosphatemia:
    a. Oliguric or anuric AKI
    b. Cardiac arrhythmias
3. Hypocalcemia:
    a. Paresthesias
    b. Tetany
    c. Neuromuscular irritability: Twitching, Chvostek's sign (nonspecific), and carpopedal spasm
    d. Bronchospasm
    e. ECG abnormalities, including:
        (1) Inverted T waves
        (2) Prolonged QT interval
        (3) Ventricular arrhythmias
        (4) Heart block
    f. Cardiac arrest

ETIOLOGY

- TLS is caused by massive release of intracellular contents into the bloodstream at the time of death of neoplastic cells. The pathophysiology of tumor lysis syndrome is illustrated in Fig. 1.
- Can occur spontaneously or after initiation of therapy in patients with:
    1. Acute leukemias
    2. Bulky solid tumors
    3. High-grade lymphomas
- Administration of certain agents:
    1. Paclitaxel
    2. Hydroxyurea
    3. Etoposide
    4. Fludarabine
- It has been reported in some cancer patients who received:
    1. Intrathecal administration of chemotherapy
    2. Rare causes: Pregnancy, fever, and rarely general anesthesia in predisposed individuals

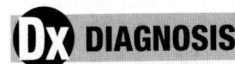

DIFFERENTIAL DIAGNOSIS

See "Acute Kidney Injury" topic in Section I.

LABORATORY TESTS

- Early identification of abnormal laboratory values may prevent or reduce complications of TLS.

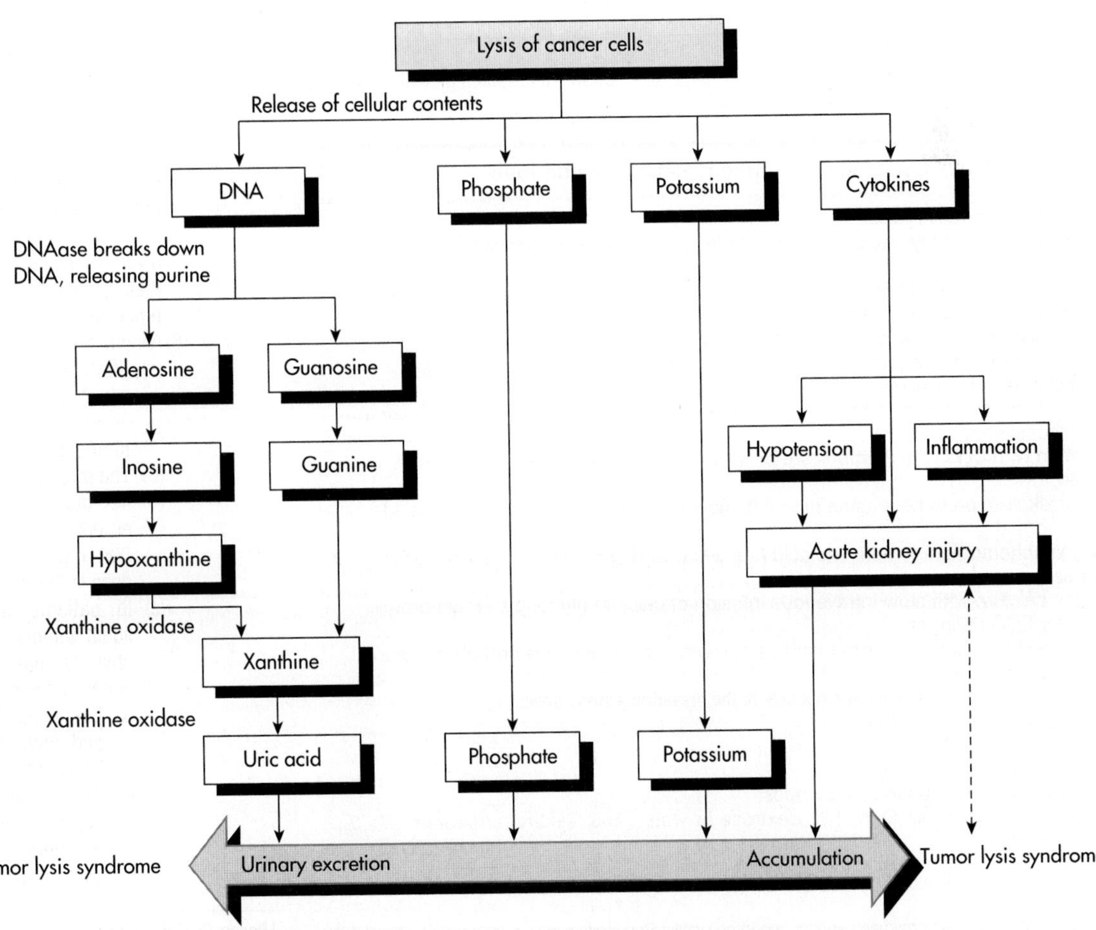

FIG. 1 Proposed pathophysiology of tumor lysis syndrome. (From Ronco C et al: *Critical care nephrology*, ed 3, Philadelphia, 2019, Elsevier.)

- Laboratory TLS is defined by the presence of at least two of the following biochemical criteria within 3 days before or 7 days after initiation of chemotherapy despite adequate volume repletion or use of uric acid-lowering agents:
  1. Uric acid:
     a. >8.0 mg/dl in adults or above the upper limit of the normal range for age in children
  2. Phosphorus:
     a. >4.5 mg/dl in adults or >6.5 mg/dl in children
  3. Potassium:
     a. >6.0 mEq/L
  4. Calcium:
     a. Corrected calcium <7.0 mg/dl or ionized calcium <1.12 mg/dl
- Patients should have careful and frequent laboratory and clinic monitoring:
  1. Perform frequent ECGs or continuous cardiac monitoring for arrhythmia detection
  2. Monitor renal status closely and follow daily weights and fluid intakes and outputs
  3. Monitor BUN, creatinine, phosphorus, potassium, calcium, uric acid, and LDH in high-risk patients before and up to 72 hours after initiating therapy:
     a. If evidence of TLS develops, laboratory parameters should be checked twice daily

IMAGING STUDIES

- Consider abdominal/renal ultrasound if kidney failure present
- Consider CT chest/abdominal/pelvis to evaluate for underlying malignancies

Rx TREATMENT

GENERAL PRINCIPLES

- Prevention is mainstay of therapy.
- Identify high-risk patients (evaluate extent of tumor burden, kidney function, and pathologic findings) to initiate prophylactic measures in a timely fashion. Delayed treatment may lead to life-threatening complications.
- Optimal treatment involves preservation of renal function and prevention of cardiac dysrhythmias and neuromuscular irritability.
- Any metabolic derangements should be corrected before starting cancer treatment.
- Prevention for high-risk patients without TLS:
  1. Prompt, vigorous volume repletion and administration of uricosuric agent are mainstays of therapy. Box 1 summarizes treatment recommendations for tumor lysis syndrome.
     a. Volume repletion:
        (1) Prevents volume depletion and corrects electrolyte derangement
        (2) Fluid intake (whether oral or intravenous) should be maintained at 2–3 L/m^2 per day
        (3) Begin 24 to 48 hours before initiating cancer treatment and continue for up to 72 hours after treatment
        (4) If intravenous fluids are required, isotonic solutions are appropriate (e.g., 0.9% saline or 1 L D_5W plus 3, 50-ml ampules of 1 M $NaHCO_3$)
        (5) Maintain urine output at 80–100 ml/m^2 per hour
        (6) Patients with underlying cardiac or kidney dysfunction should be monitored for volume overload and necessity for loop diuretics
        (7) Hypouricemic agents (e.g., allopurinol, rasburicase, and febuxostat). Uric acid is freely filtered at the glomerulus, and handling in the renal proximal tubule is a combination of reabsorption and secretion mediated by luminal urate/anion exchanger urate transporter 1 (URAT-1) and the basolateral organic anion transporter (OAT). When the capacity to transport luminal uric acid is overwhelmed, there is potential for uric acid to crystallize within the tubular lumen. An acidic urine pH favors this process. Uric acid crystals can cause direct tubular injury by obstruction. Furthermore, intratubular and parenchymatous uric acid precipitations causes renal injury by a granulomatous reaction and necrosis of the distal tubule epithelium through induction of chemokine-mediated inflammation from monocyte chemoattractant protein-1 (MCP-1) and macrophage migration inhibition factor (MIF). There are also crystal-independent mechanisms, which target hemodynamics: these include increased peritubular capillary pressures, increased vasoconstriction, and decreased blood flow. Uric acid also may prevent recovery from AKI in TLS, because it has been shown to inhibit proximal tubule cell proliferation. These diverse mechanisms are united in their propensity to cause AKI, as reported in Fig. 2.[1]
        (8) Allopurinol:
           (a) Xanthine oxidase inhibitor, which prevents the conversion of xanthine and hypoxanthine to uric acid.
           (b) The prophylactic dose is 200 to 400 mg/m^2 daily in 1 to 3 divided doses, up to a maximum of 800 mg daily. The treatment dose is 300 to 900 mg/day.
           (c) In patients with high-grade liquid tumors, Allopurinol prophylaxis may cause xanthine nephropathy/nephrolithiasis:
              - Low serum uric acid levels and high urinary xanthine levels aid in diagnosis
              - Consideration for reduction/cessation of allopurinol therapy should then be considered

BOX 1 Tumor Lysis Syndrome: Treatment Recommendations

When no metabolic aberration exists:
- Allopurinol 300 mg/day, reduce to 100 mg/day after 3 days of chemotherapy

OR
- Rasburicase 0.2 mg/kg IV daily × 5 days
- Hydration: 0.45% saline 3000 ml/day
- Initiate chemotherapy within 24-48 hours of admission
- Monitor serum chemistry values every 12-24 hours

When metabolic aberration exists:
- Allopurinol or rasburicase as above; reduce dose if hyperuricemia is controlled or for renal insufficiency
- Hydration with D_5W with 2 ampules/L of $NaCO_3$, add nonthiazide diuretics as needed
- Urinary alkalization to keep urine pH >7.0; may discontinue when serum uric acid level is normal
- Postpone chemotherapy until uric acid has decreased and electrolytes are stable
- Monitor serum chemistries every 6-8 hours
- Replace calcium with slow intravenous infusion of calcium gluconate (if symptomatic or for ECG changes)
- Treat hyperkalemia and hyperphosphatemia with exchange resins and phosphate binders, respectively

Criteria for hemodialysis in patients unresponsive to the measures listed above:
- Serum potassium >6.0 mEq/L
- Serum uric acid >20 mg/dl
- Serum phosphorus >10 mg/dl
- Fluid overload unresponsive to diuretics

Symptomatic hypercalcemia D_5W, 5% dextrose in water; *ECG*, electrocardiogram; *$NaCO_3$*, sodium carbonate.

From Parrillo JE, Dellinger RP: *Critical care medicine, principles of diagnosis and management in the adult*, ed 4, Philadelphia, 2014, Elsevier.
From Brudno JN et al: Toxicities of chimeric antigen receptor T cells: Recognition and management, *Blood*, May 20, 2016.

[1] Ronco C: *Critical care nephrology,* 3rd ed, Elsevier 2019.

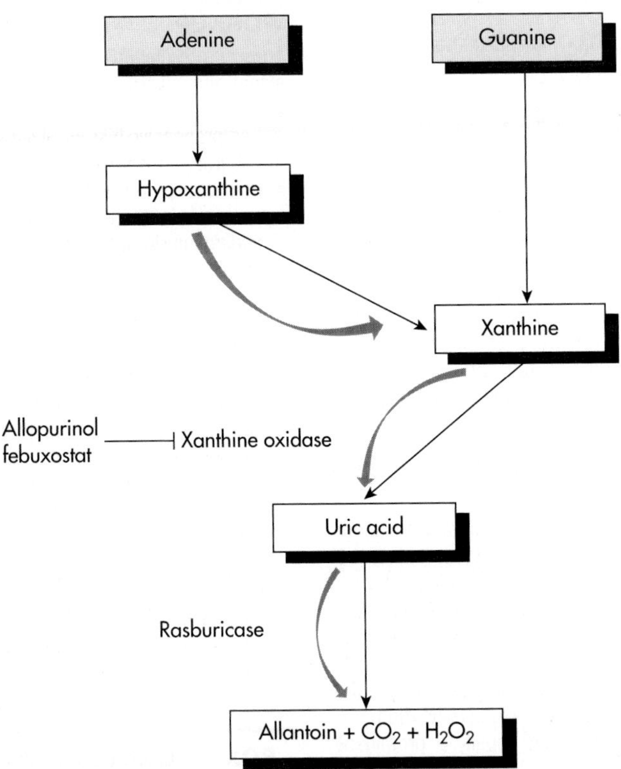

FIG. 2 Principles of therapy for the prevention and treatment of tumor lysis syndrome. (From Ronco C et al: *Critical care nephrology*, ed 3, Philadelphia, 2019, Elsevier.)

(9) Rasburicase:
   (a) Recombinant urate oxidase is used when uric acid levels cannot be lowered by standard measures
   (b) Given by intravenous or intramuscular route in dosages from 50 to 100 Units/kg per day for 1 to 5 days
   (c) Should not be administered at same time as allopurinol, because allopurinol reduces uric acid levels and may reduce rasburicase efficacy
   (d) Contraindicated in pregnancy and glucose-6-phosphate dehydrogenase deficiency due to hemolytic concerns
   (e) Cost is a limiting factor
(10) Febuxostat dose is 120 mg by mouth daily. It has fewer drug-drug interactions than allopurinol, and dose adjustment is not needed in patients with mild to moderate renal impairment. Cost is a limiting factor

a. Urinary alkalinization:
   (1) Uric acid more soluble at urinary alkaline pH
   (2) Remains controversial and has fallen out of favor
   (3) Contraindicated with hyperphosphatemia because of risk of calcium phosphate deposition leading to stones/nephrocalcinosis

TREATMENT OF PATIENTS WITH TUMOR LYSIS SYNDROME

- Principles:
  1. Early consultations for nephrology and critical care teams
  2. Preventive measures as indicated previously
  3. Aggressive treatment of electrolyte disturbances to prevent cardiac arrhythmias and neuromuscular irritability
     a. Arrhythmias tend to be resistant to conventional therapy
     b. Arrhythmias are a leading cause of death in patients with severe TLS
  4. Treatment of kidney failure
- Management of electrolyte disturbances:
  1. Multiple, coexisting electrolyte abnormalities may make conservative management strategies difficult.
     a. Systemic alkalinization may be required for concurrent hyperphosphatemia, hyperuricemia, and acidemia. Alkalinization may worsen hypocalcemia.
  2. Hyperuricemia:
     a. Uric acid–lowering agents including allopurinol or rasburicase
  3. Hyperkalemia:
     a. Low-potassium diet
     b. Intravenous calcium chloride/gluconate for ECG changes of hyperkalemia
     c. Intravenous infusions of glucose and insulin to shift potassium into intracellular compartments
     d. Oral potassium-exchange resins (not for acute management)
     e. Hemodialysis
  4. Hyperphosphatemia:
     a. Low phosphorus diet
     b. Intravenous infusion of glucose and insulin to shift phosphorus into cells
     c. Oral phosphate binders
  5. Hypocalcemia:
     a. Treat only if neuromuscular irritability is present
     b. Intravenous calcium chloride/gluconate
     c. Calcitriol can be used if the serum phosphorus level is normal, but is a relatively slow form of therapy
- Management of kidney failure:
  1. Perform standard workup for kidney failure, including urinalysis, urine microscopy, urinary electrolytes, kidney ultrasound, etc.
  2. Supportive care with intravenous fluids and diuretics (if required)
  3. Consider early dialysis if above methods fail (especially if cardiac abnormalities present)

REFERRAL

- Nephrology
- Critical care

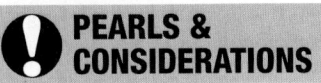

PEARLS & CONSIDERATIONS

COMMENTS

- TLS is an oncologic emergency, which can occur spontaneously, or, more commonly, during chemotherapy-related tumor cell lysis.
- TLS is associated with the release of several intracellular contents, including potassium, phosphorus, and uric acid. With concomitant renal failure, these products are retained to pathological levels, leading to cardiac and neurological abnormalities.
- Common risk factors for TLS include highly proliferative tumors and large tumor burdens (e.g., high-grade lymphomas and acute leukemias), and preexisting metabolic derangements and renal failure.
- High-risk patients should undergo prophylactic measures initiated 24 to 48 hours before initiation of cytotoxic agents.
- Prophylactic measures include aggressive intravenous volume repletion and administration of uric acid–lowering drugs.
- Frequent laboratory testing and monitoring of vital signs, intakes and outputs, and cardiac/neurological abnormalities are recommended.
- Complications may include continued electrolyte disturbances, renal failure, uremic complications, cardiac arrhythmias, and pulmonary edema from aggressive volume repletion.

SUGGESTED READINGS

Available at ExpertConsult.com

AUTHORS: **JESSE GOLDMAN, M.D., F.A.S.H.,** and **SANDEEP AGARWAL, M.D.**

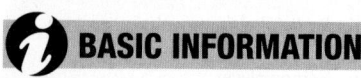

BASIC INFORMATION

DEFINITION

Ulcerative colitis (UC) is an idiopathic, remitting and relapsing, chronic inflammatory bowel disease that starts in the rectum and extends proximally.

SYNONYMS

UC
Inflammatory bowel disease (IBD)
Idiopathic proctocolitis
Pancolitis

ICD-10CM CODES

K51.0	Ulcerative pancolitis
K51.2	Ulcerative proctitis
K51.3	Ulcerative rectosigmoiditis
K51.5	Left-sided colitis
K51.90	Ulcerative colitis, unspecified, without complications
K51.80	Other ulcerative colitis without complications
K51.811	Other ulcerative colitis with rectal bleeding
K51.812	Other ulcerative colitis with intestinal obstruction
K51.813	Other ulcerative colitis with fistula
K51.814	Other ulcerative colitis with abscess
K51.818	Other ulcerative colitis with other complication
K51.819	Other ulcerative colitis with unspecified complications
K51.911	Ulcerative colitis, unspecified with rectal bleeding
K51.912	Ulcerative colitis, unspecified with intestinal obstruction
K51.913	Ulcerative colitis, unspecified with fistula
K51.914	Ulcerative colitis, unspecified with abscess
K51.918	Ulcerative colitis, unspecified with other complication
K51.919	Ulcerative colitis, unspecified with unspecified complications

EPIDEMIOLOGY & DEMOGRAPHICS

INCIDENCE: The incidence of UC is 9 to 12 cases per 100,000 persons per year in the U.S.; worldwide, the estimated incidence ranges from 1.2 to 20.3 cases per 100,000 person-years and its prevalence ranges from 7.6 to 246.0 per 100,000 persons. It is most common between ages 15 and 40 yr, with a second peak between 50 and 80 yr. The disease affects men and women at similar rates. Infection with nontyphoid salmonella or campylobacter is associated with an 8-10 time higher risk of developing ulcerative colitis in the following year. Worldwide UC is more common than Crohn disease.

PREVALENCE: The prevalence of UC is 7.6 to 246.0 cases per 100,000 per year. Higher prevalence in Ashkenazi Jewish descendants.

GEOGRAPHIC DISTRIBUTION: The highest incidence and prevalence of IBD are seen in northern Europe and North America, and the lowest in continental Asia.

GENETICS:
- Both specific and nonspecific gene variants are associated with UC.
- There are 47 loci associated with UC, of which 19 are specific for UC and 28 are shared with Crohn disease.
- Abnormalities in humoral and cellular adaptive immunity are also found in UC.

ETIOLOGY AND PATHOGENESIS

Accumulating evidence suggests that it may result from an inappropriate inflammatory response to environmental triggers and immune dysregulation involving CD4+ T-cell Th2 response in a genetically susceptible host.

PHYSICAL FINDINGS & CLINICAL PRESENTATION

- Patients with UC often present with acute onset of bloody diarrhea accompanied by tenesmus, fever, and dehydration. At presentation 40% of adults have proctitis, 40% have left-sided colitis, and 20% have pancolitis. Diarrhea is not always present in UC patients with proctosigmoiditis and proctitis, and patients may have constipation.
- Abdominal pain is not usually a prominent symptom. Abdominal distention and tenderness may indicate the presence of complications such as toxic megacolon.
- The onset of symptoms is typically acute and is generally followed by periods of spontaneous remission and frequent relapses.
- Fever, evidence of dehydration may be present during the acute flare-up.
- Evidence of extraintestinal manifestations may be present in nearly 25% of patients: Liver disease, sclerosing cholangitis, iritis, uveitis, episcleritis, arthritis, erythema nodosum, pyoderma gangrenosum, aphthous stomatitis. Box 1 summarizes common extraintestinal manifestations of UC.

Dx DIAGNOSIS

DIFFERENTIAL DIAGNOSIS (TABLE 1, BOX 2)

- Crohn disease
- Bacterial infections:
  1. Acute: *Campylobacter, Yersinia, Salmonella, Shigella, Chlamydia, Escherichia coli, Clostridium difficile*, gonococcal proctitis
  2. Chronic: Whipple disease, tuberculosis, enterocolitis
- Irritable bowel syndrome
- Protozoal and parasitic infections (amebiasis, giardiasis, cryptosporidiosis)
- Neoplasm (intestinal lymphoma, carcinoma of colon)
- Ischemic bowel disease
- Diverticulitis
- Celiac sprue, lymphocytic or collagenous colitis, radiation enteritis, endometriosis
- Solitary rectal ulcer
- Acute self-limited colitis
- Medication (NSAIDs, chemotherapy)

WORKUP

An accurate diagnosis of UC should define the extent and severity of inflammation. Diagnostic workup includes:
- Comprehensive history, physical examination.
- Laboratory tests (see "Laboratory Tests").
- Colonoscopy to establish the presence of mucosal inflammation; typical endoscopic findings in UC are areas of continuous friable mucosa; diffuse, uniform erythema replacing the usual mucosal vascular pattern (Table 2); and pseudopolyps. The transition from abnormal to normal tissue tends to be abrupt. Rectal involvement is invariably present if the disease is active. Pathologic findings suggestive of UC include crypt abscesses and atrophy, mucin depletion, basal plasmacytosis, basal lymphoid aggregates, increased lamina propria cellularity, and Paneth cell metaplasia.

LABORATORY TESTS

- Anemia and high erythrocyte sedimentation rate (in severe colitis) are common but normal levels do not rule out the disorder.

BOX 1 Common Extraintestinal Manifestations of Ulcerative Colitis

Cutaneous/Oral
Angular stomatitis
Aphthous stomatitis
Erythema nodosum
Oral ulcerations
Psoriasis
Pyoderma gangrenosum
Pyostomatitis vegetans
Sweet's syndrome (acute febrile neutrophilic dermatosis)

Ophthalmologic
Conjunctivitis
Episcleritis
Retinal vascular disease
Scleritis
Uveitis, iritis

Musculoskeletal
Ankylosing spondylitis
Osteomalacia
Osteonecrosis
Osteopenia
Osteoporosis
Peripheral arthropathy
Sacroiliitis

Hepatobiliary
Autoimmune hepatitis
Cholangiocarcinoma
Pericholangitis
PSC
Hepatic steatosis

Hematologic
Anemia of chronic disease
Autoimmune hemolytic anemia
Hypercoagulable state
Iron deficiency anemia
Leukocytosis or thrombocytosis
Leukopenia or thrombocytopenia

From Feldman M, Friedman LS, Brandt LJ: *Sleisenger and Fordtran's gastrointestinal and liver disease*, ed 10, Philadelphia, 2016, Elsevier.

TABLE 1 Features That Distinguish Ulcerative Colitis From Other Diagnoses

Diagnosis	Clinical Features	Radiologic and Colonoscopic Features	Histologic Features
UC	Bloody diarrhea	Extends proximally from rectum; fine mucosal ulceration	Distortion of crypts; acute and chronic diffuse inflammatory cell infiltrate; goblet cell depletion; crypt abscesses; lymphoid aggregates
Crohn colitis	Perianal lesions are common; may be associated with ileitis; frank bleeding is less common than in UC	Segmental disease; rectal sparing; strictures, fissures, ulcers, fistulas; small bowel involvement	Focal inflammation; submucosal involvement; granulomas; goblet cell preservation; transmural inflammation; fissuring
Ischemic colitis	Occurs in older adults; sudden onset, often painful; usually resolves spontaneously in several days	Segmental splenic flexure and sigmoid involvement are most common, with thumbprinting early and ulceration after 24-72 hr; rectal involvement is rare	Mucosal necrosis with ghost cells; congestion with red blood cells; hemosiderin-laden macrophages and fibrosis (when disease is chronic)
Microscopic colitis	Watery diarrhea; normal-appearing mucosa at colonoscopy	Usually normal	Chronic inflammatory infiltrate; increased intraepithelial lymphocytes (lymphocytic colitis) and/or subepithelial collagen band (collagenous colitis)
Infectious colitis	Sudden onset; identifiable source in some cases (e.g., *Salmonella* spp.); pain may predominate (e.g., *Campylobacter* spp.); pathogens are present in stool	Nonspecific findings	Crypt architecture is usually normal; edema, superficial neutrophilic infiltrate, crypt abscesses
Amebic colitis	History of travel to endemic area; amebae may be detected in a fresh stool specimen but ELISA for amebic lectin antigen is the preferable diagnostic test	Discrete ulcers; ameboma or strictures	Similar to UC; amebae present in lamina propria or in flask-shaped ulcers, identified by periodic acid–Schiff stain
Gonococcal proctitis	Rectal pain; pus	Granular changes in rectum	Intense polymorphonuclear neutrophil infiltration; purulent exudate; Gram-negative diplococci
Pseudomembranous colitis	Often a history of antibiotic use; characteristic pseudomembranes may be seen on sigmoidoscopy; *Clostridium difficile* toxin is detectable in stools	Edematous; shaggy outline of colon; pseudomembranes may be identified radiologically or seen at colonoscopy	May resemble acute ischemic colitis; summit lesions of fibrinopurulent exudate

ELISA, Enzyme-linked immunosorbent assay.
From Feldman M, Friedman LS, Brandt LJ: *Sleisenger and Fordtran's gastrointestinal and liver disease*, ed 10, Philadelphia, 2016, Elsevier.

- Potassium, magnesium, calcium, and albumin may be decreased.
- Antineutrophil cytoplasmic antibodies (ANCA) with a perinuclear staining pattern (pANCA) can be found in >45% of patients; there is an increased frequency in treatment-resistant left-sided colitis, suggesting a possible association between these antibodies and a relative resistance to medical therapy in patients with UC.
- Calprotectin is a protein that is measured in feces as a marker of intestinal mucosa leukocyte activity that may be useful for screening of patients with suspected IBD. Trials have shown that based on a pretest probability of IBD of 32% in adults, an abnormal fecal calprotectin test would increase the posttest probability to 91% and a normal result would reduce the probability to 3%.
- Fecal lactoferrin is also a sensitive marker of intestinal inflammation.
- Stool examinations for ova and parasites, stool culture, and testing for *Clostridium difficile* toxin and *E. coli* 0157:H7 may be useful to eliminate other causes of diarrhea in selected patients with risk factors.

IMAGING STUDIES

Image studies (plain radiography, CT scan [Fig. E1]) are generally reserved for suspected complications such as perforation of bowel or toxic megacolon.

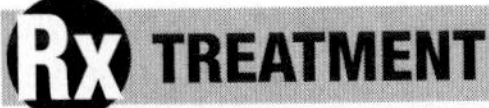

TREATMENT

NONPHARMACOLOGIC THERAPY

- Correct nutritional deficiencies; total parenteral nutrition with bowel rest may be necessary in severe cases. Folate supplementation may reduce the incidence of dysplasia and cancer in chronic UC.
- Avoid oral feedings during acute exacerbation to decrease colonic activity; a low-roughage diet may be helpful in early relapse.
- Psychotherapy is useful in most patients. Referral to self-help groups is also important because of the chronicity of the disease and the young age of the patients.

ACUTE GENERAL Rx

The therapeutic options vary with the degree of disease (mild, severe, fulminant) and areas of involvement (distal, extensive).

- Mild disease can be treated with 5-aminosalicylate agents (mesalamine, olsalazine, balsalazide, sulfasalazine). It can be administered as an enema (40 mg once daily at bedtime for 3-6 wk) or suppository (500 mg bid) for patients with distal colonic disease. Oral forms in which the 5-acetyl salicylic acid is in a slow-release or pH-dependent matrix (Pentasa 1 g qid, Asacol 800 mg PO tid) can deliver therapeutic concentrations to the more proximal small bowel or distal ileum. Olsalazine can be useful for maintenance of remission of UC in patients intolerant to sulfasalazine. Usual dose is 500 mg bid taken with food. Balsalazide is indicated for mild to moderately active UC. Usual dose is three 750-mg capsules tid. Probiotics may also be helpful in inducing remission in mild-to-moderate UC.
- Mild-to-moderate UC is often treated with a combination of rectal and oral 5-aminosalicylate. Refractory patients are candidates for oral glucocorticoids or immunosuppressive agents (e.g., cyclosporine). An algorithm for the management of mildly to moderately active UC is illustrated in Fig. 2.
- Severe disease usually responds to oral corticosteroids (e.g., prednisone 40-60 mg/day); the FDA has recently approved an extended-release formulation of the corticosteroid budesonide for induction of remission in mild to moderate ulcerative colitis. Corticosteroid suppositories or enemas are also useful for distal colitis. The immunosuppressant azathioprine or mercaptopurine also provides effective long-term treatment for Crohn disease. Fig. 3 describes an algorithm for the management of severely active UC.
- Biological agents are emerging treatment options for the management of ulcerative colitis. Infliximab, a chimeric monoclonal

BOX 2 Differential Diagnosis of Ulcerative Colitis

Infectious Causes
Aeromonas hydrophila
Campylobacter jejuni
Chlamydia spp.
Clostridium difficile
Cytomegalovirus
Entamoeba histolytica
Escherichia coli O157:H7, other EHEC
HSV
Listeria monocytogenes
Neisseria gonorrhoeae
Salmonella spp.
Schistosomiasis
Shigella spp.
Yersinia enterocolitica

Noninfectious Causes
Acute self-limited colitis
Behçet's disease
Crohn disease
Diversion colitis
Diverticulitis
Drugs and toxins
- Chemotherapy
- Gold
- Penicillamine

Eosinophilic colitis
Graft-versus-host disease
Ischemic colitis
Microscopic colitis
- Collagenous
- Lymphocytic

Neutropenic colitis (typhlitis)
NSAIDs
Radiation colitis
Segmental colitis associated with diverticulosis (SCAD)
Solitary rectal ulcer syndrome

EHEC, enterohemorrhagic *Escherichia coli*.
From Feldman M, Friedman LS, Brandt LJ: *Sleisenger and Fordtran's gastrointestinal and liver disease*, ed 10, Philadelphia, 2016, Elsevier.

antibody, has been shown to be effective in patients who have not responded to corticosteroid therapy. Newer TNF inhibitors include adalimumab (ADA), golimumab, and vedolizumab for treatment of moderate-to-severe ulcerative colitis. These agents can be used for induction and maintenance of remission in patients that have not responded to other therapies or are corticosteroid-dependent. Head-to-head trials of these biologic agents are necessary to establish the best therapeutic option.

- Fulminant disease generally requires hospital admission and parenteral corticosteroids (e.g., IV hydrocortisone 100 mg q6h). When bowel movements have returned to normal and the patient is able to eat normally, oral prednisone is resumed. IV cyclosporine can also be used in severe refractory cases; renal toxicity is a potential complication.
- Surgery is indicated in patients who do not respond to intensive medical therapy. Fig. 4 illustrates the surgical management of chronic UC.
- Proctocolectomy is usually curative in these patients and also eliminates the high risk of developing adenocarcinoma of the colon (10%-20% of patients develop it after 10 yr with the disease). Total proctocolectomy with ileal pouch-anal anastomosis (IPAA) is the procedure of choice for most patients who require elective surgery, since it preserves anal sphincter function. Continent ileostomy is an alternative procedure.

CHRONIC Rx

- Colonoscopic surveillance and multiple biopsies should be instituted approximately 10 yr after diagnosis because of the increased risk of colon carcinoma.
- Erythropoietin is useful in patients with anemia refractory to treatment with iron and vitamins.
- In patients on long-term steroid therapy, periodic bone density scans are recommended to screen for glucocorticoid-induced osteoporosis.

TABLE 2 Endoscopic Differentiation of Ulcerative Colitis and Crohn Disease

Feature	Ulcerative Colitis	Crohn Disease
Distribution	Diffuse inflammation that extends proximally from the anorectal junction	Rectal sparing, frequent skip lesions
Inflammation	Diffuse erythema, early loss of vascular markings with mucosal granularity or friability	Focal and asymmetrical, cobblestoning; granularity and friability less commonly seen
Ulceration	Small ulcers in a diffusely inflamed mucosa; deep, ragged ulcers in severe disease	Aphthoid ulcers, linear or serpiginous ulceration; intervening mucosa is often normal
Colonic lumen	Often narrowed in long-standing chronic disease; tubular colon; strictures are rare	Strictures are common

From Feldman M, Friedman LS, Brandt LJ: *Sleisenger and Fordtran's gastrointestinal and liver disease*, ed 10, Philadelphia, 2016, Elsevier.

DISPOSITION

- The natural history of the disease is one of remission and episodic flares.
- The clinical course is variable. ~66% of patients will achieve clinical remission with medical therapy, and nearly 80% of treatment-compliant patients maintain remission. 15% to 20% of patients eventually require colectomy. Pouchitis is the most common long-term complication of IPAA (up to 40% of patients). >75% of patients treated medically will experience relapse.

REFERRAL

- Gastrointestinal consultation for initial diagnostic sigmoidoscopy/colonoscopy in suspected cases
- Surgical referral for patients with severe disease unresponsive to medical therapy. Indications for surgery in patients with UC are summarized in Box 3.

SUGGESTED READINGS

Available at ExpertConsult.com

RELATED CONTENT

Ulcerative Colitis (Patient Information)

AUTHOR: **FRED F. FERRI, M.D.**

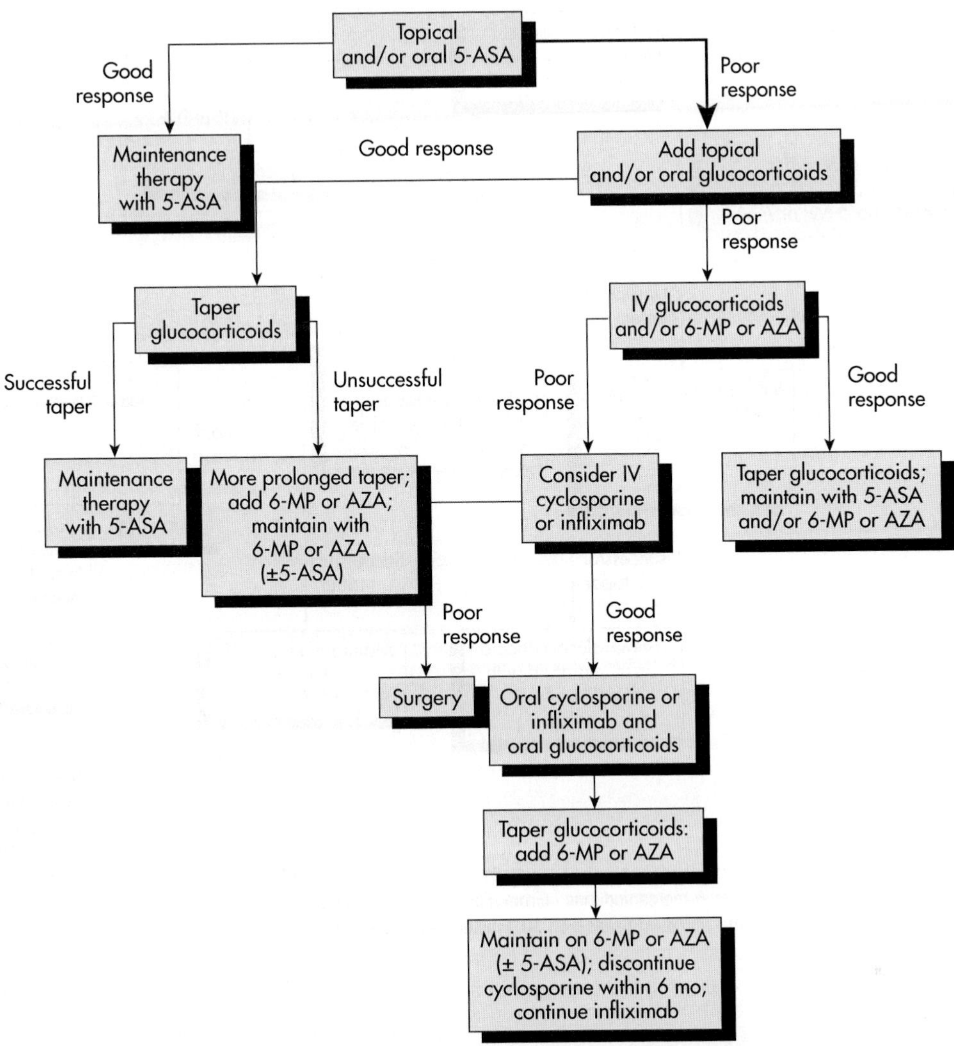

FIG. 2 Algorithm for the management of mildly to moderately active ulcerative colitis. *5-ASA*, 5-Aminosalicylate; *AZA*, azathioprine; *6-MP*, 6-mercaptopurine. (From Feldman M, Friedman LS, Brandt LJ: *Sleisenger and Fordtran's gastrointestinal and liver disease*, ed 10, Philadelphia, 2016, Elsevier.)

BOX 3 Indications for Surgery in Patients with Ulcerative Colitis

- Colonic dysplasia or carcinoma
- Colonic perforation
- Growth retardation
- Intolerable or unacceptable side effects of medical therapy
- Medically refractory disease
- Systemic complications that are recurrent or unmanageable
- Toxic megacolon
- Uncontrollable colonic hemorrhage

From Feldman M, Friedman LS, Brandt LJ: *Sleisenger and Fordtran's gastrointestinal and liver disease*, ed 10, Philadelphia, 2016, Elsevier.

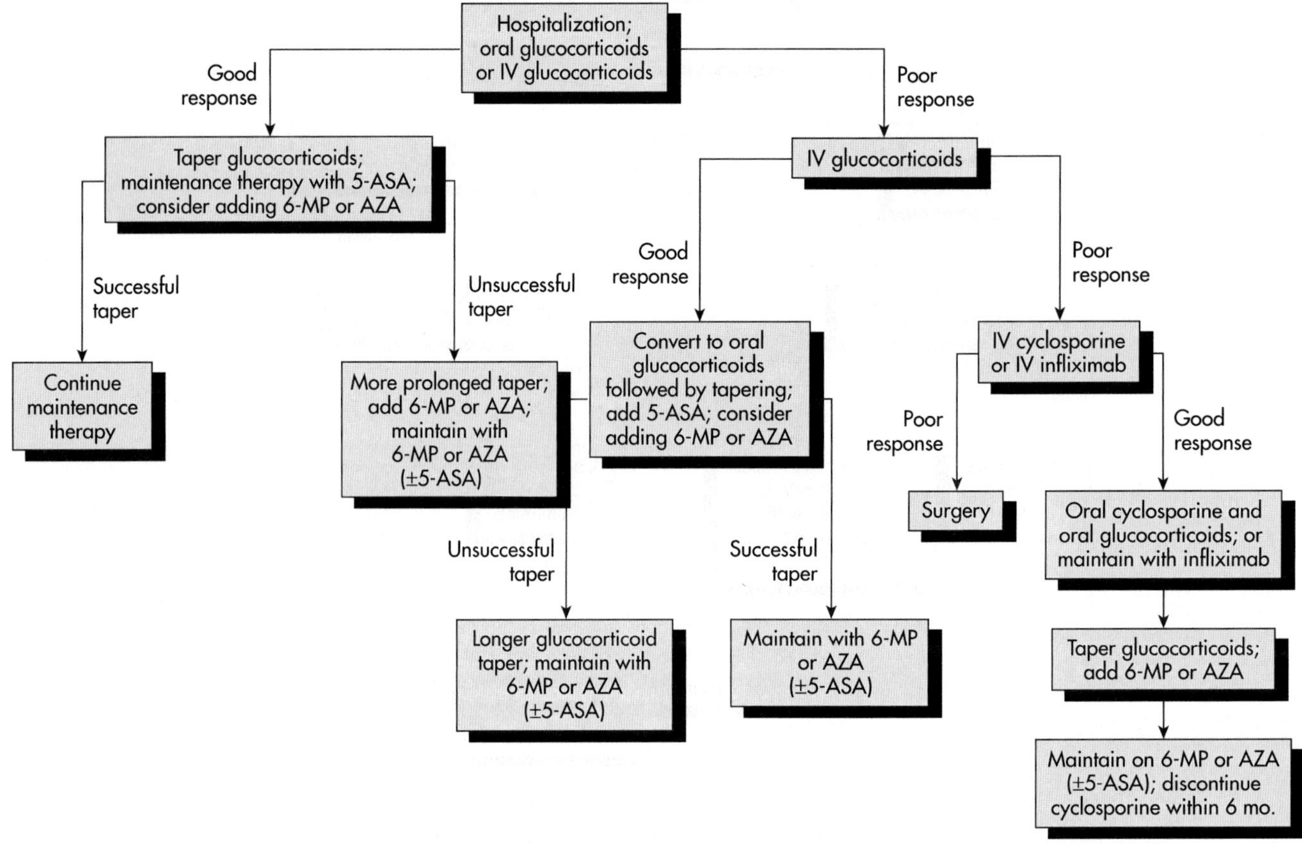

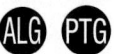

FIG. 3 Algorithm for the management of severely active ulcerative colitis. *5-ASA*, 5-Aminosalicylate; *AZA*, azathioprine; *6-MP*, 6-mercaptopurine. (From Feldman M, Friedman LS, Brandt LJ: *Sleisenger and Fordtran's gastrointestinal and liver disease*, ed 10, Philadelphia, 2016, Elsevier.)

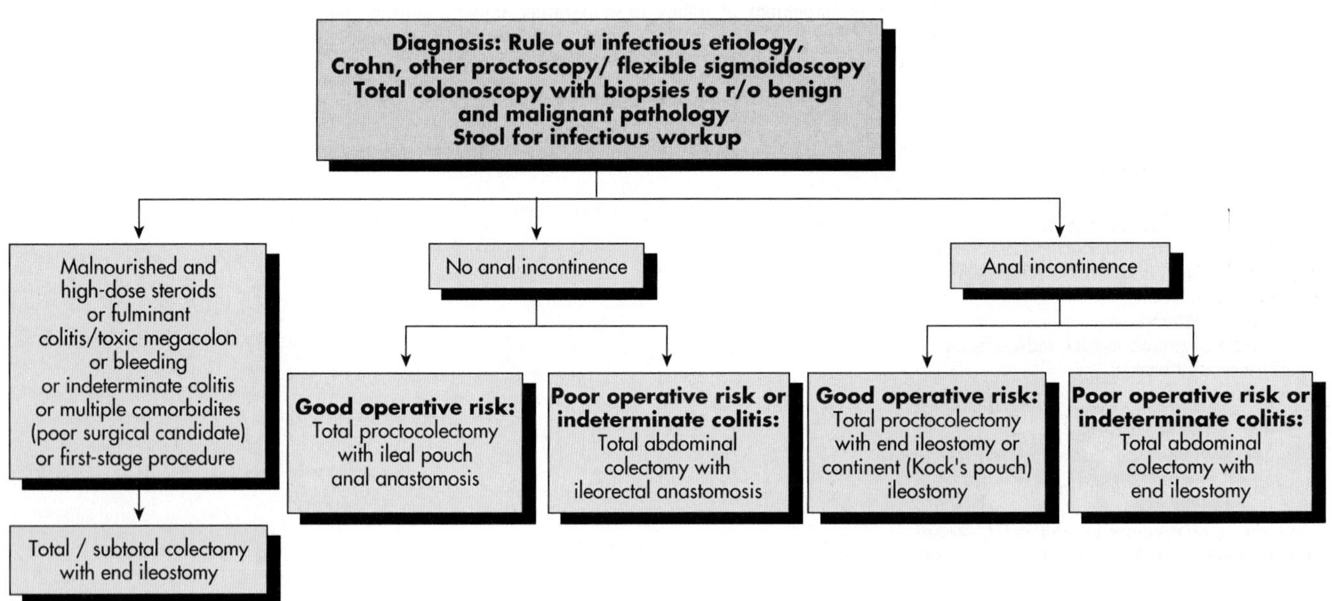

FIG. 4 Surgical management of chronic ulcerative colitis. (From Cameron JL, Cameron AM: *Current surgical therapy*, ed 12, Philadelphia, 2017, Elsevier.)

BASIC INFORMATION

DEFINITION

Unruptured intracranial aneurysms are acquired aneurysms found at bifurcations of major arteries. Most are found in the circle of Willis, with 85% being at the anterior circulation. Rupture of these aneurysms results in more than 80% of nontraumatic subarachnoid hemorrhages (SAH).

SYNONYMS

Berry aneurysms
Saccular aneurysms
UIAs

ICD-10CM CODE
I67.1 Cerebral aneurysm, nonruptured

EPIDEMIOLOGY & DEMOGRAPHICS

PEAK INCIDENCE: The incidence of UIAs is currently unknown.

PREVALENCE: The prevalence of UIAs is approximately 3% in a population without comorbidity and with a mean age of 50 yr.

PREDOMINANT SEX & AGE: UIAs are three times more common in women and are more likely to occur in those aged 60 and older. In the pediatric population, UIAs are twice as common in males.

GENETICS: No specific genetic mutations have been shown to cause UIAs. However, more than 19 single nucleotide polymorphisms (SNP) have been associated with sporadic aneurysms. SNPs on the EDNRA, CDKN2B, and SOX17 genes located on chromosomes 4, 8, and 9 have been found to have the strongest association with developing UIAs.

- Genetic disorders that increase the risk of UIAs include autosomal dominant polycystic kidney disease, Marfan's syndrome, Ehlers-Danlos syndrome type IV, multiple endocrine neoplasia type I, neurofibromatosis type 1, and hereditary hemorrhagic telangiectasia. Less commonly, aneurysms can occur with SLE, fibromuscular dysplasia, sickle-cell disease, and coarctation of the aorta.

RISK FACTORS: Risk factors include female gender, older age, family history, genetic factors, cigarette smoking, and hypertension.

- Risk factors that increase the risk of subarachnoid hemorrhage are also relevant to consider, as aneurysm rupture results in subarachnoid hemorrhages. These factors include heavy alcohol use, high dose estrogen, cocaine use in young populations, and low BMI.

PHYSICAL FINDINGS & CLINICAL PRESENTATION

UIAs often remain asymptomatic and undetected for long periods of time but also may present with nonspecific symptoms such as headaches or vertigo. A phase of aneurysm growth usually precedes any cases of rupture. Small aneurysms (<5mm) are likely to remain asymptomatic, while those that grow to a large size may compress surrounding structures and present with specific neurological deficits. Examples include third cranial nerve palsy due to an aneurysm of the posterior communicating or basilar arteries, hemiparesis due to middle cerebral artery aneurysms, and cavernous sinus syndrome due to aneurysms in the cavernous sinus. In rare cases, emboli may originate from aneurysms and cause transient ischemic attacks or infarctions in other regions.

ETIOLOGY

The development of aneurysms is a multifactorial process that involves hemodynamic stress, inflammation, and molecular changes that result in a weakened arterial wall. Saccular aneurysms form as protrusions that are often thin-walled and lack tunica media. Fusiform aneurysms are less common and form due to dilatation of the artery itself. It's currently thought that hemodynamic stress causes endothelial dysfunction and starts the process of arterial wall inflammation and remodeling, while other factors such as smoking and connective tissue disorders are contributory.

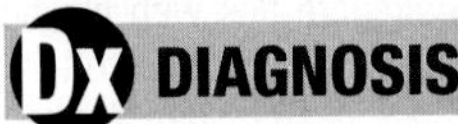

DIAGNOSIS

DIFFERENTIAL DIAGNOSIS

WORKUP

- The presence of UIAs should be investigated in those with a history of SAH.
- Patients with significant family history (>2 first degree relatives with UIA or SAH), ADPKD, coarctation of the aorta, or microcephalic osteodysplastic primordial dwarfism should be offered screening with MRA or CTA.

LABORATORY TEST

Lab tests are unrevealing when investigating UIAs.

IMAGING STUDIES

- Most UIAs are discovered incidentally on brain MRI or CT. However, MRA and CTA have been shown to detect smaller aneurysms and are the tests of choice in screening for UIAs. Patients with contraindications to contrast administration can be screened with MRA.
- Digital subtraction angiography is used when surgical treatment of UIA is considered.

TREATMENT

NONPHARMACOLOGIC THERAPY

- Reduction of risk factors such as smoking.
- Exercise is associated with a reduced risk of aneurysm formation and rupture.

ACUTE GENERAL Rx

- The main surgical treatments for UIAs are endovascular coiling and surgical clipping. However, there are few guidelines for surgical treatment of UIAs. Currently, it's believed that stable UIAs at <3mm should not undergo surgical treatment, while patients who present with headaches or nerve palsies likely should be treated surgically. Beyond this, a detailed discussion of the risks and benefits and an individualized treatment plan are necessary.
- Patients with known UIAs presenting with severe headaches or symptoms of nerve compression should raise high suspicion for development of SAH.

CHRONIC Rx

- Blood pressure management, with the goal of SBP <140.
- Aspirin use has been associated with lower risk of aneurysm rupture. A randomized, controlled trial is ongoing to investigate the use of aspirin in UIAs.

COMPLEMENTARY & ALTERNATIVE MEDICINE

None

DISPOSITION

The risk of rupture for patients managed conservatively is related to age, smoking status, blood pressure, size and location of the aneurysm, and history of previous SAH. This risk is estimated to be 1.4% in 1 yr and 3.4% in 5 yrs. Currently, it's recommended that those with family history, multiple UIAs, or a high number of risk factors should be monitored for aneurysm growth.

REFERRAL

Vascular neurology or neurosurgery

PREVENTION

Decreasing modifiable risk factors such as smoking

PATIENT/FAMILY EDUCATION

American Association of Neurological Surgeons
www.aans.org/Patients/Neurosurgical-Conditions-and-Treatments/Cerebral-Aneurysm

SUGGESTED READINGS

Available at ExpertConsult.com

RELATED CONTENT

Subarachnoid Hemorrhage (Related Key Topic)

AUTHORS: **SUDAD KAZZAZ, M.D.**, and **JOSEPH S. KASS, M.D., J.D.**

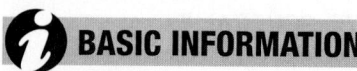

BASIC INFORMATION

DEFINITION

Urethritis is a well-defined clinical syndrome manifested by dysuria, a urethral discharge, or both.

SYNONYMS

Gonococcal urethritis
GCU

ICD-10CM CODE

A54.00 Gonococcal infection of lower genitourinary tract, unspecified

EPIDEMIOLOGY & DEMOGRAPHICS

- Urethritis commonly is divided into two major categories based on etiology: Gonococcal urethritis (GCU, *Neisseria gonorrhoeae* species) and nongonococcal urethritis (NGU, all other pathogens, most commonly *C. trachomatis.)*
- This differentiation is based historically on *N. gonorrhoeae*'s easy visualization on gram stain as gram-negative, kidney-shaped diplococci.
- NGU is twice as common as GCU in the U.S. NGU is the most common sexually transmitted disease (STD) syndrome occurring in men, accounting for 6 million office visits annually.
- In the United States, incidence varies greatly based on race and geography; the prevalence of GCU is disproportionately higher in the South and among black, non-Hispanic men. The urethra is the most common site of infection in all men. In heterosexual men, the pharynx is infected 7% of the time, and in homosexual men the pharynx is infected 40% of the time and the rectum 25% of the time. A single episode of intercourse with an infected partner carries a transmission risk of 20% for males; female partners of an infected male will contract the disease 80% of the time.

PHYSICAL FINDINGS & CLINICAL PRESENTATION

- Symptoms of GCU: Dysuria is the most common chief complaint in patients with GCU. Additional common complaints include discharge and pruritus. Purulent discharge, meatal edema, and urethral tenderness to palpation also may occur, and 5% to 10% of patients with GCU remain asymptomatic.
- GCU may spread to other parts of the GU system. Prostatic involvement can cause urinary frequency, urgency, and nocturia and may present with mucopurulent discharge. Epididymal involvement can result in unilateral testicular pain and edema.
- Time frame: The incubation period of GCU is variable but is commonly 4 to 7 days. Without treatment, urethritis will persist for 3 to 7 weeks, with 95% of men becoming asymptomatic after 3 months.
- Complications: Periurethritis leading to urethral stenosis can occur. Additionally, disseminated infection can lead to tenosynovitis and arthritis. Rarely, hepatitis, myocarditis, endocarditis, and meningitis can occur.

Dx DIAGNOSIS

DIFFERENTIAL DIAGNOSIS

- NGU
- Herpes simplex virus

LABORATORY TESTS

- Nucleic acid amplification tests (NAATs): These tests have largely replaced culture in many health care settings.. They are not more sensitive than culture for detecting *N. gonorrhoeae* in cervical or urethral specimen; however, they have specificities of >99% and retain sensitivity when used to test first catch urine or self-collected vaginal swabs. The performance of NAATs with respect to overall sensitivity, specificity, and ease of specimen transport is better than that of any of the other tests available for the diagnosis of chlamydial and gonococcal infections. NAATs should be used to detect chlamydia and gonorrhea except in cases of child sexual assault, rectal and oropharyngeal infections in prepubescent girls, and when evaluating a potential gonorrhea treatment failure in which case culture and susceptibility testing might be required.
- For culture and susceptibility testing: Rayon, Dacron, or calcium alginate tips with plastic or wire shafts should be used (not cotton-tipped swabs, which are bactericidal). A swab of the urethra should be performed within 2 to 4 hours after voiding to prevent bacterial washout with urination. Gram staining with modified Thayer-Martin media is indicated. Collect cultures of the pharynx and rectum when indicated for concomitant *Chlamydia* testing on all patients.
- Concomitant serologic testing for syphilis on all patients.
- Offer HIV counseling and testing to all patients.

Rx TREATMENT

NONPHARMACOLOGIC THERAPY

Behavioral management: Avoid intercourse until cure has been attained and sexual partners have been evaluated and treated.

ACUTE GENERAL Rx

- Ceftriaxone 250 mg IM ×1 dose *plus* azithromycin 1 g orally single dose
- Severe allergy to cephalosporins: High dose azithromycin with parenteral gentamicin or oral gemifloxacin

Alternative regimens:

- If ceftriaxone is not available: Cefotaxime 500 mg IM plus azithromycin.
- Oral therapy: Cefixime 400 mg PO ×1 dose *plus* azithromycin 1 g orally single dose. Cure rate with this regimen is lower than ceftriaxone plus azithromycin because cefixime does not provide as high, or as sustained, bactericidal blood levels as a 250 mg dose or ceftriaxone. Doxycycline 100 mg orally twice/day for 7 days can be substituted for azithromycin only in cases of allergy to azithromycin.
- Azithromycin as the second antimicrobial preferred over doxycycline due to the high prevalence of tetracycline resistance. There also is widespread resistance to penicillins, fluoroquinolones, macrolides, cephalosporins, and tetracyclines.
- The use of azithromycin as the second antimicrobial is preferred over doxycycline due to the high prevalence of tetracycline resistance.
- Fluoroquinolone antibiotics are no longer recommended to treat gonorrhea in the U.S.
- Dual treatment for gonococcal and chlamydial infections is based on antimicrobial resistance patterns and the lack of newly developed alternative treatments for gonorrhea.

CHRONIC Rx

Postgonococcal urethritis (PGU): Reinfection is the most common cause of recurrence. Repeat swab and culture of the urethra, pharynx, and rectum (where applicable) are mandatory. Persistence of polymorphonuclear cells (PMNs) with the absence of gram-negative intracellular diplococci suggests a diagnosis of PGU. This occurs when GCU is treated with a regimen that is ineffective against coincident chlamydial infection; it represents NGU after GCU. The syndrome should be treated as NGU. Persistence of *N. gonorrhoeae* by smear or culture requires treatment for *N. gonorrhoeae*.

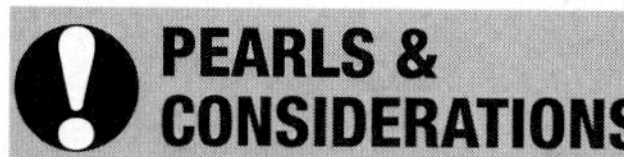

PEARLS & CONSIDERATIONS

COMMENTS

- Partner notification: The names and contact information of sexual partners should be gathered at the time of diagnosis and referred to the health department, or the patient can notify the contact directly. Expedited partner treatment is recommended by the Centers for Disease Control and Prevention (CDC) and is approved in several states. This consists of giving prescriptions to the infected patient for their partner(s) who has not been evaluated by a physician and is unlikely to seek medical care.
- On examination of the urethral smear, the presence of small numbers of PMNs provides objective evidence of urethritis. The complete absence of PMNs on a urethral smear argues against urethritis. If in addition to the PMNs there are gram-negative, intracellular diplococci, the diagnosis of gonorrhea is established.

SUGGESTED READINGS

Available at ExpertConsult.com

RELATED CONTENT

Evaluation of Patients with Dysuria and/or Urethral/Vaginal Discharge (Algorithm, Section III)
Gonococcal Urethritis (Patient Information)
Gonorrhea (Related Key Topic)

AUTHOR: **ROBIN METCALFE-KLAW, M.D.**

BASIC INFORMATION

DEFINITION

Nongonococcal urethritis (NGU) is urethral inflammation caused by any of several organisms (see "Etiology").

SYNONYMS

NGU
Nongonococcal urethritis

ICD-10CM CODES

A56.0 Chlamydial infection of lower genitourinary tract
N34.1 Nonspecific urethritis

EPIDEMIOLOGY & DEMOGRAPHICS

- Occurrence is 50% in sexually transmitted disease clinics. *Chlamydia trachomatis* is the most common notifiable disease in the U.S., with >1.3 million infections reported to the Centers for Disease Control and Prevention (CDC) in 2010.
- NGU most commonly affects men in a higher socioeconomic class, affecting heterosexual men more frequently than homosexual men.
- NGU carries a greater morbidity rate than gonococcal urethritis (GCU).

PHYSICAL FINDINGS & CLINICAL PRESENTATION

- Incubation period: 2 to 35 days.
- Symptoms: Dysuria, whitish-clear urethral discharge, and urethral itching. The onset of symptoms in NGU is less acute than GCU. The majority of persons with *C. trachomatis* infection are not aware of their infection because they do not have symptoms that would prompt them to seek medical care.
- Signs: Whitish-clear urethral discharge, meatal edema, and erythema. Infected women manifest pyuria, and the disease can present as acute urethral syndrome.

COMPLICATIONS

Epididymitis in heterosexual men may be linked to nonbacterial prostatitis, proctitis in homosexual men, or Reiter syndrome.

ETIOLOGY

- Most common agent is *Chlamydia* spp., an obligate intracellular parasite possessing both DNA and RNA, which replicates by binary fission. It causes 20% to 50% of NGU cases. Two species exist:
  1. *Chlamydia psittaci*
  2. *Chlamydia trachomatis* with its 15 serotypes:
     a. Serotypes A through C cause hyperendemic-blinding trachoma.
     b. Serotypes D through K cause genital tract infection.
     c. Serotypes L1 through L3 cause lymphogranuloma venereum.
- Other causes of NGU: *Mycoplasma genitalium* (found in 44% of treatment failures); *Ureaplasma urealyticum*, causing 15% to 30% of the cases of NGU; *Trichomonas vaginalis*; and herpes simplex virus. The cause of 20% of the cases of NGU has not been identified.
- Asymptomatic infection occurs in 28% of the contacts of women with chlamydial cervical infection.

DIAGNOSIS

DIFFERENTIAL DIAGNOSIS

- GCU
- Herpes simplex virus
- Trichomoniasis

LABORATORY TESTS

- Requires demonstration of urethritis and exclusion of infection with *N. gonorrhoeae.*
- Nucleic acid amplification tests (NAATs): These tests have replaced culture in many settings where persons are screened for asymptomatic genital infection. The performance of NAATs with respect to overall sensitivity, specificity, and ease of specimen transport is better than that of any of the other tests available for the diagnosis of chlamydial and gonococcal infections. NAATs should be used to detect chlamydia and gonorrhea except in cases of child sexual assault involving boys, rectal and oropharyngeal infections in prepubescent girls, and when evaluating a potential gonorrhea treatment failure, in which case culture and susceptibility testing might be required.
- *Chlamydia* culture: The appearance of PMNs on urethral smear confirms the diagnosis of urethritis. Because *Chlamydia* is an intracellular parasite of the columnar epithelium, the best specimen for culture is an endourethral swab taken from an area 2 to 4 cm inside the urethra. For culture, a Dacron-tipped swab is used; avoid calcium alginate or cotton swabs. The organism can only be grown in tissue culture, which is expensive.

TREATMENT

- Because it is impossible to differentiate among the common etiologies of NGU, the condition is treated syndromically, including in the initial treatment regimen those drugs effective against the common causative agents.
- In patients with isolated uncomplicated NGU, recommended regimens are azithromycin 1 g orally single dose or doxycycline 100 mg bid × 7 days. Recommended regimen in pregnancy is azithromycin, 1 g orally as a single dose.
- In patients with confirmed urethritis and unclear etiology, concurrent treatment for gonorrhea and *Chlamydia* is recommended. In these patients, uncomplicated infections of the urethra can be treated with combination of a single 1-g dose of oral azithromycin or 100 mg doxycycline bid × 7 days *plus* ceftriaxone 250 mg x 1 dose.
- In areas where *T. vaginitis* is prevalent, men who have sex with women and have persistent or recurrent urethritis should be presumably treated with metronidazole 2 g orally in a single dose of tinidazole 2 g orally in a single dose.

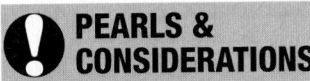

PEARLS & CONSIDERATIONS

COMMENTS

Partner notification: The names and contact information of all sexual partners within preceding 60 days should be gathered at the time of the visit and referred to the health department, or the patient notifies the contacts directly. Expedited partner treatment is recommended by the CDC and approved in several states. This consists of giving prescriptions to the infected patient for their partner(s) who have not been evaluated by a physician and are unlikely to seek medical care.

SUGGESTED READINGS

Available at ExpertConsult.com

RELATED CONTENT

Nongonococcal Urethritis (Patient Information)
Cervicitis (Related Key Topic)
Chlamydia Genital Infections (Related Key Topic)

AUTHOR: **ANTHONY SCISCIONE, D.O.**

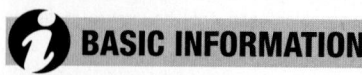

DEFINITION

Urinary tract infection (UTI) is a term that encompasses a broad range of clinical entities that have in common a positive urine culture. A conventional threshold is growth of >100,000 colony-forming units per milliliter from a midstream-catch urine sample. In symptomatic patients, a smaller number of bacteria (between 100 and 10,000 colony-forming units per milliliter of midstream urine) is recognized as an infection.

ICD-10CM CODES

N39.0	Urinary tract infection, site not specified
N99.521	Infection of other external stoma of urinary tract
N99.531	Infection of other stoma of urinary tract
N30.00	Acute cystitis without hematuria
N30.30	Trigonitis without hematuria
N30.20	Other chronic cystitis without hematuria

CLASSIFICATION

- Uncomplicated UTI: Occurs in a normal urinary tract and resolves rapidly with conventional antimicrobials. Patients have a low risk of upper UTI.
- Complicated UTI: Occurs in patients with coexisting pathology (strictures, stones, comorbidities [diabetes mellitus, multiple sclerosis, spinal cord injuries]). Patients are considered at high risk for upper UTI.
- First infection: The first documented UTI; tends to be uncomplicated and is easily treated.
- Unresolved bacteriuria: UTI in which the urinary tract is not sterilized during therapy. Main causes are bacterial resistance, patient noncompliance with medication, mixed bacterial infection, rapid reinfection, azotemia, infected stones, Munchausen syndrome, and papillary necrosis.
- Bacterial persistence: UTI in which the urine cultures become sterile during therapy, but a persistent source of infection gives rise to reinfection by the same organism. Causes include infected stone, chronic bacterial prostatitis, atrophic infected kidney, vesicovaginal or enterovesical fistulas, obstructive uropathy, infected pyelocaliceal diverticula, infected ureteral stump after nephrectomy, infected necrotic papillae from papillary necrosis, infected urachal cysts, infected medullary sponge kidney, urethral diverticula, and foreign bodies.
- Reinfection: UTI in which a new infection occurs with new pathogens at variable intervals after a previous infection has been eradicated.
- Relapse: The less common form of recurrent infection; occurs within 2 wk of treatment when the same organism reappears in the same site as the previous infection. Relapsing infections of the urinary tract most commonly occur in pyelonephritis, kidney obstruction from a stone, foreign body, and prostatitis.

EPIDEMIOLOGY & DEMOGRAPHICS

INCIDENCE:

- UTI is the most common bacterial infection encountered in the ambulatory care setting in the U.S. The self-reported annual incidence of UTI in women is 12%, and by age 32 half of all women report having had at least one UTI.
- In neonates: More common in boys as a result of anatomic abnormalities such as the posterior urethral valves.
- In preschool children: More common in girls (4.5% vs. 0.5% for boys).
- In adulthood: More common in women, with a 1% to 3% prevalence in nonpregnant women. Table 1 describes factors modulating risk for acute uncomplicated UTIs in women. In pregnancy at 12 wk, the incidence of asymptomatic bacteriuria is similar to nonpregnant women, at 2% to 10%. However, 25% to 30% of pregnant women with untreated asymptomatic bacteriuria develop acute pyelonephritis, especially in the second and third trimesters, and have a pyelonephritic recurrence rate of 10%. In adults aged ≥65 yr, at least 10% of men and 20% of women have bacteriuria.

PHYSICAL FINDINGS & CLINICAL PRESENTATION

- Typical symptoms of UTI include:
  1. Urinary frequency, urgency
  2. Dysuria
  3. Suprapubic pain
  4. Gross or microscopic hematuria
- The probability of cystitis is greater than 50% in women with any symptom of UTI and greater than 90% in women who have dysuria and frequency without vaginal symptoms.
- Clinical symptoms alone can be used to make the diagnosis of uncomplicated UTI in women without a urine culture.
- When negative cultures are associated with significant pyuria, vaginal discharge, or hematuria, infections with *Chlamydia trachomatis, Neisseria gonorrhoeae*, and *Trichomonas vaginalis* should be considered.
- Acute pyelonephritis presents with fever, flank or abdominal pain, chills, malaise, and vomiting. It is these systemic symptoms that distinguish pyelonephritis from cystitis. Complications of acute pyelonephritis are renal abscess, perinephric abscess, emphysematous pyelonephritis, and pyonephrosis.

ETIOLOGY & PATHOGENESIS

- Ascending infection via the urethra with bacterial flora from the genital and gastrointestinal tracts is the major pathway for UTI in women.
- Other risk factors: Incomplete bladder emptying due to neurologic disease, bladder outlet obstruction or urethral stricture, renal failure, diabetes, vesicoureteral reflux, fistula, urinary diversion, infected stones, age, pregnancy, instrumentation, and poor patient compliance.
- Catheters: All patients who require a long-term Foley catheter eventually develop significant levels of bacteriuria. Treatment is reserved for individuals who become symptomatic (leukocytosis, fever, chills, malaise, loss of appetite, etc.) Using prophylactic antibiotics to treat patients who have chronic catheters is not indicated because of the risk of acquiring bacteria resistant to antibiotic therapy.
- Once bacteria reach the urinary tract, three factors determine whether symptomatic infection occurs (Box E1). These factors also determine the anatomic level of the UTI:
  1. Virulence of the microorganism
  2. Inoculum size
  3. Adequacy of the host defense mechanisms
- Urinary pathogens: In 95% of UTIs the infecting organism is a member of the Enterobacteriaceae, enterococci, or, in young women, *Staphylococcus saprophyticus. Escherichia coli* is the most common pathogen (85% of UTI cases). In contrast, the organisms that commonly colonize the distal urethra and skin of both men and women and the vagina of women are *Staphylococcus epidermidis*, diphtheroids,

TABLE 1 Factors Modulating Risk for Acute Uncomplicated Urinary Tract Infections in Women

Host Determinants	Uropathogen Determinants
Behavioral: Sexual intercourse, use of spermicidal products, recent antimicrobial use, suboptimal voiding habits	*Escherichia coli* virulence determinants: P, S, Dr, and type I fimbriae; hemolysin; aerobactin; serum resistance
Genetic: Innate and adaptive immune response, enhanced epithelial cell adherence, antibacterial factors in urine and bladder mucosa, nonsecretor of ABO blood group antigens, P_1 blood group phenotype, reduced CXCR1 expression, previous history of recurrent cystitis	
Biologic: Estrogen deficiency in postmenopausal women, micturition	

From Floege J et al: *Comprehensive clinical nephrology,* ed 4, Philadelphia, 2010, Saunders.

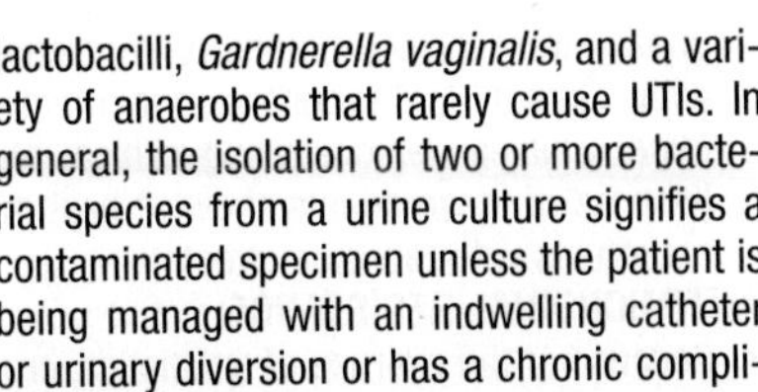

lactobacilli, *Gardnerella vaginalis*, and a variety of anaerobes that rarely cause UTIs. In general, the isolation of two or more bacterial species from a urine culture signifies a contaminated specimen unless the patient is being managed with an indwelling catheter or urinary diversion or has a chronic complicated infection.

- Defense mechanisms against cystitis: Low urine pH and high urine osmolarity, mucopolysaccharide glycosaminoglycan protective layer, normal bladder that empties completely, and low vaginal pH due to the presence of estrogen and resulting colonization of the genital tract by lactobacillus.
- In uncomplicated, nonpregnant patients, cystitis rarely progresses to pyelonephritis or other serious infections such as bacteremia.

Dx DIAGNOSIS (FIG. 1)

DIFFERENTIAL DIAGNOSIS

- Vaginitis
- Urethritis (gonococcal, nongonococcal, *Trichomonas*)
- Interstitial cystitis (painful bladder syndrome)
- Pelvic inflammatory disease
- Nephrolithiasis
- Structural urethral abnormalities such as diverticulum or stricture

LABORATORY TESTS

- Urinalysis with microscopic evaluation of clean-catch urine for bacteria and pyuria. The presence of ≥10 leukocytes/μl of unspun urine from a midstream catch indicates UTI.
- Dipstick urinalysis with the presence of nitrites or leukocyte esterase is indicative of UTI. However, dipstick urinalysis may not be useful in symptomatic patients with typical symptoms and a negative dipstick urinalysis does not exclude the diagnosis of UTI such cases.
- Urine culture and sensitivity are useful in complicated UTIs and to help guide therapy in women who fail initial therapy. They are generally not needed in uncomplicated UTIs.

IMAGING STUDIES

- Warranted only if renal infection or genitourinary abnormality is suspected
- CT urogram, voiding cystourethrogram, renal sonogram, and intravenous pyelogram
- Specialty examination: Cystoscopy and retrograde pyelography to rule out obstructive uropathy

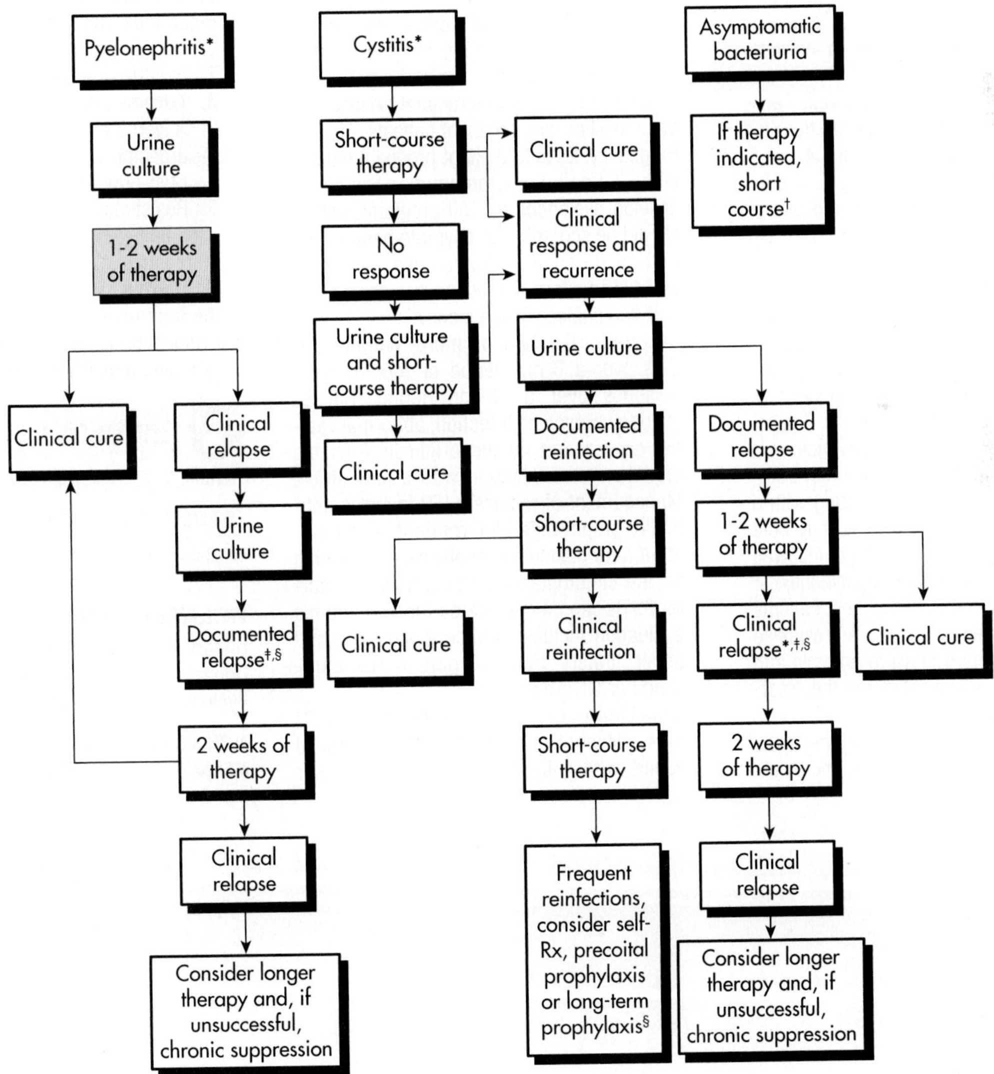

*Consider imaging studies in all men and in women with complicated urinary tract infection.
†No therapy except for renal transplant patients or prior to urologic procedures. Follow-up culture only in transplant patients.
‡Evaluate men for chronic bacterial prostatitis.
§Consider imaging studies in women.

FIG. 1 Approach to the management of urinary tract infection in nonpregnant adults. (From Bennett JE et al: *Mandell, Douglas, and Bennett's principles and practice of infectious diseases*, ed 8, Philadelphia, 2015, Saunders.)

 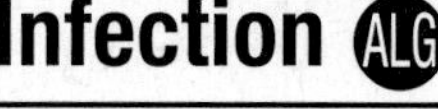

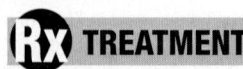

TREATMENT

NONPHARMACOLOGIC THERAPY

Urinary analgesics such as phenazopyridine and aggressive hydration

ACUTE GENERAL Rx

- First-line antimicrobials for uncomplicated UTI as recommended by the Infectious Disease Society of North America, the American Urologic Society, and ACOG include: nitrofurantoin, trimethoprim plus sulfamethoxazole (TMP-SMX), or fosfomycin.
- Antimicrobial stewardship and drug resistance needs to be considered when choosing antibiotic therapy. Empiric treatment with TMP-SMX is considered appropriate when resistance rates are below 20%. Nitrofurantoin continues to have the lowest rates of antimicrobial resistance. Beta lactam antibiotics may be appropriate in cases of known patient hypersensitivity to conventional first-line agents.
- Conventional therapy of 3 days with TMP-SMX or 5 for uncomplicated cystitis for nitrofurantoin, is generally appropriate.
- High rates of resistance and the potential for serious side effects should limit the use of fluoroquinolone antimicrobials. The U.S. FDA has warned against the use of fluoroquinolone antibiotics for routine infections when suitable alternatives are available.
- Pyelonephritis may be treated as an outpatient in stable, well-hydrated patients with close follow-up. Antimicrobial selection is ideally based on urine culture results. Empiric treatment with fluoroquinolone antimicrobials or TMP-SMX is acceptable. Initiation of treatment in the emergency room setting with a single parenteral dose of a long-acting beta lactam or aminoglycoside antibiotic followed by oral treatment with fluoroquinolones or TMP-SMX is an acceptable regimen. Patients should be assessed for a proper response to treatment within 48 hr. Nitrofurantoin and fosfomycin are not indicated for the treatment of pyelonephritis.
- Inpatient management of pyelonephritis should begin with parenteral antimicrobials followed by transition to oral agents based on clinical response and culture results.
- Pyelonephritis requires a total duration of 10 to 14 days of therapy, although evidence exists that 7 to 10 days may be equally effective in low-risk patients.

PEARLS & CONSIDERATIONS

COMMENTS

- Asymptomatic bacteriuria occurs commonly in postmenopausal women. Treatment of asymptomatic bacteriuria with antimicrobials is discouraged because it seldom resolves and can result in the development of drug-resistant organisms. Patients with cloudy or foul-smelling urine should be encouraged to aggressively hydrate to eliminate these symptoms. Postmenopausal women with vaginal atrophy can be treated with vaginal estrogen to reduce the incidence of bacteriuria. Exceptions include immunocompromised patients, patients with structural urinary tract abnormalities, and pregnant patients.
- Pregnancy: 25% to 30% of pregnant women with untreated asymptomatic bacteriuria develop pyelonephritis. All pregnant women should be screened for asymptomatic bacteriuria and treated. Nitrofurantoin, TMP-SMX, and beta lactam antibiotics are appropriate first-line choices in pregnancy.
- Recurrent UTI: Two or more symptomatic UTIs over a 6-mo period or four or more episodes over a 12-mo period. Causes include unresolved infection, abnormal vaginal colonization by the originally infecting organism, or reinfection with a new strain. Management of recurrent UTI includes antibiotic prophylaxis, intermittent self-treatment, and postcoital prophylaxis depending on the circumstances. Patients with recurrent UTIs can be considered for an anatomic evaluation including office cystoscopy and upper urinary tract imaging (renal ultrasound or CT urography).
- Nonantimicrobial strategies to prevent UTI have shown mixed results. Nonantimicrobial agents with antiseptic effects on the lower urinary tract include cranberry supplements with vitamin C, d-mannose, and methenamine. Studies demonstrating clinical effectiveness of these agents show at best modest effects with few side effects.

ANTIMICROBIAL RESISTANCE:

- Because of the overuse of antibiotics, organisms once sensitive to a number of antimicrobial agents are now increasingly resistant, making effective management of UTI and pyelonephritis more difficult and potentially more dangerous. Most important has been the increasing resistance to trimethoprim plus sulfamethoxazole (TMP-SMX), the current primary care provider drug of choice for acute uncomplicated UTI in women.
- Fluoroquinolone use for the treatment of acute cystitis in women should be avoided when suitable alternatives exist. The U.S. FDA has changed the labeling of quinolone antibiotics to reflect this recommendation.
- When choosing a treatment regimen, physicians should consider such factors as:
  1. In vitro susceptibility
  2. Adverse effects on individual patients
  3. Adverse effects on the population (stewardship)
  4. Cost-effectiveness
  5. Resistance rates in their respective communities
- Meropenem (1 g IV every 8 hr) or IV plazomicin (15 mg/kg BW once daily) are effective for the treatment of complicated UTIs and acute pyelonephritis caused by enterobacteriaceae, including multidrug-resistant strains.

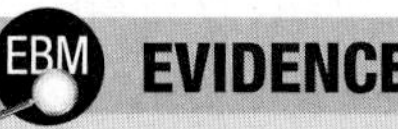

EVIDENCE

Available at ExpertConsult.com

SUGGESTED READINGS

Available at ExpertConsult.com

RELATED CONTENT

Urinary Tract Infection (Patient Information)
Urinary Tract Infection (Child) (Patient Information)
Pyelonephritis (Related Key Topic)

AUTHORS: **MATTHEW J. FAGAN, M.D., F.A.C.O.G.,** and **MEAGAN S. CRAMER, M.D.**

BASIC INFORMATION

DEFINITION

Urolithiasis is the presence of calculi within the urinary tract. The five major types of urinary stones are calcium oxalate (60% to 70%), calcium phosphate (20%), uric acid (7%), struvite (7%), and cystine (1%) (Table 1).

SYNONYMS

Kidney stones
Kidney calculi
Renal stones
Renal calculi
Ureteral stones
Ureteral calculi
Nephrolithiasis
Ureterolithiasis

ICD-10CM CODES

N20.9	Urinary calculus, unspecified
N20.0	Calculus of kidney
N20.1	Calculus of ureter
N20.2	Calculus of kidney with calculus of ureter
N21.0	Calculus in bladder
N21.1	Calculus in urethra
N21.8	Other lower urinary tract calculus
N21.9	Calculus of lower urinary tract, unspecified

EPIDEMIOLOGY & DEMOGRAPHICS

- Urinary stones affect approximately 1 in 11 people in the U.S., with a lifetime prevalence of approximately 10% in males and 7% in females.
- Peak incidence is in the fourth to sixth decade of life.
- Urolithiasis appears to be more common among whites than Hispanics, Asians, or African Americans.
- The incidence of urinary stone disease is increasing, likely due to increased use of cross-sectional imaging and changing dietary and lifestyle factors.
- The incidence of symptomatic urolithiasis is greatest during the summer as a result of increased temperature and resultant dehydration and urinary concentration.
- Annually, between 1 and 2 million emergency department visits are due to kidney stones and renal colic.
- Approximately 90% of all urinary stones are radiopaque. Uric acid stones and cystine stones are radiolucent.

TABLE 1 Stone Composition and Relative Occurrence

Stone Composition	Occurrence (%)
Calcium-containing stones	
Ca oxalate	60
Mixed Ca oxalate/ hydroxyapatite	20
Brushite	2
Noncalcium-containing stones	
Uric acid	7
Magnesium ammonium phosphate (struvite)	7
Cystine	1-3 (10% of stones in children)
Xanthine	<1
Medication-related stones	<1

From Lipshultz LI et al: *Urology and the primary care practitioner*, ed 3, Philadelphia, 2008, Elsevier.

PHYSICAL FINDINGS & CLINICAL PRESENTATION

Stones may be asymptomatic, or may cause the following signs and symptoms, often from urinary tract obstruction:

- Acute, often severe, flank pain (renal colic)
- Pain radiating from the flank downward and anteriorly with referred pain to the groin and genitalia (common as the stone progresses down the ureter)
- Low back and lower abdominal pain, often ipsilateral to the stone
- Nausea and vomiting
- Hematuria, gross or microscopic
- Inability to find a comfortable position
- Urinary urgency and frequency with distal ureteral stones mimicking a urinary tract infection
- Fever and chills accompanying acute colic with superimposed infection
- Elderly patients presenting with nonspecific and vague abdominal discomfort and pain

ETIOLOGY

- Urine composition: Supersaturation of various solutes and stone constituents is the driving force in kidney stone formation. Various metabolic abnormalities such as low or high urine pH, idiopathic hypercalciuria, hypocitraturia, hyperoxaluria and hyperuricosuria predispose patients to urinary stone formation.
- Low urine volume is the most common cause in many stone–formers.
- Dietary factors: Diets high in sodium and animal protein increase the risk of urinary stone formation. Very high dietary oxalate consumption and heavy intake of phosphoric acid-containing carbonated drinks likely increase the risk of stone formation. Foods with high potential renal acid load (PRAL) such as cheese and meats increase the risk of urinary stone formation, while fruits and vegetables with low PRAL may reduce the risk.
- Anatomic factors predisposing patients to urinary stasis: Malrotated, horseshoe, or ectopic kidney, vesicoureteral reflux in young children, bladder outlet obstruction, strictures.
- Disease states:
  1. Hyperparathyroidism with hypercalcemia and hypercalciuria
  2. Sarcoidosis with hypercalcemia
  3. Malabsorption (e.g., inflammatory bowel disease) with increased oxalate absorption
  4. Chronic diarrheal states
  5. Gastric bypass surgery with enteric hyperoxaluria
  6. Metabolic syndrome (e.g., diabetes, overweight) produces acidic urine predisposing patients to uric acid stones
  7. Gouty diathesis
  8. Primary hyperoxaluria: Genetic, rare, and usually presenting as a childhood disorder
  9. Medullary sponge kidney
  10. Hyperuricosuria (e.g., metabolic defects, dietary excess) (Box 1)
  11. Type I (distal tubule) renal tubular acidosis (>1% of calcium phosphate stones)
  12. Cystinuria: Autosomal recessive disorder produces 1% of stones
- Chronic infections: Urease-producing organisms (e.g., *Proteus* [most common], *Providencia, Pseudomonas, Klebsiella, Staphylococcus*) cause alkaline urine favoring struvite or magnesium ammonium phosphate crystal formation (Box 2).
- Medications: Protease inhibitors (e.g., indinavir, ritonavir), topiramate, and chronic laxative overuse.

BOX 1 Uric Acid Stones

Low urine pH (≤5.5)
High animal protein diet
Diarrhea
Insulin resistance (high body mass index, metabolic syndrome, type 2 diabetes)

Low Urine Volume
Inadequate fluid intake
Excessive extrarenal fluid losses
Diarrhea
Insensible losses (e.g., perspiration)

Hyperuricosuria
Excessive dietary purine intake
Hyperuricemia
- Gout
- Intracellular-to-extracellular uric acid shift
- Myeloproliferative disorders
- Tumor lysis syndrome

Inborn errors of metabolism
- Lesch–Nyhan syndrome
- Glucose-6-phosphatase deficiency

From Floege J, et al.: *Comprehensive clinical nephrology*, ed 4, Philadelphia, 2010, Saunders.

BOX 2 Factors Associated with Struvite Stone Formation

- Urease-producing bacteria:
  - *Proteus*
  - *Klebsiella*
  - *Providencia*
  - *Pseudomonas*
  - *Staphylococcus epidermidis*
  - *Haemophilus*
  - *Yersinia species*
  - *Serratia*
  - *Citrobacter*
  - *Ureaplasma*
- Elevated urinary pH

Modified from Floege J, et al.: *Comprehensive clinical nephrology*, ed 4, Philadelphia, 2010, Saunders.

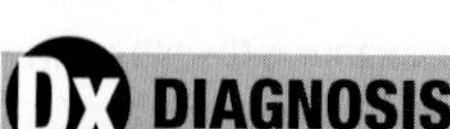

DIAGNOSIS

DIFFERENTIAL DIAGNOSIS

- Urinary tract infection (e.g., cystitis)
- Pyelonephritis
- Diverticulitis
- Appendicitis
- Pelvic inflammatory disease
- Ovarian pathology, including torsion
- Dysmenorrhea
- Ectopic pregnancy
- Small bowel obstruction
- Constipation
- Malignancy (primary urinary tract or retroperitoneal lymphadenopathy causing ureteral/kidney obstruction)
- Ureteropelvic junction obstruction
- Musculoskeletal back pain
- Factitious (illicit substance-seeking behavior), often with recurrent stone formers

The differential diagnosis of obstructive uropathy is described in Section II.

BOX 3 Indications for a Metabolic Stone Evaluation

Recurrent stone formers
Strong family history of stones
Intestinal disease (particularly chronic diarrhea)
Pathologic skeletal fractures
Osteoporosis
History of urinary tract infection with calculi
Personal history of gout
Infirm health (unable to tolerate repeat stone episodes)
Solitary kidney
Anatomic abnormalities
Renal insufficiency
Stones composed of cystine, uric acid, struvite

From Wein AJ, et al.: *Campbell-Walsh urology*, ed 11, Philadelphia, 2016, Elsevier.

WORKUP

- Stone composition of recovered stones should be determined by infrared spectroscopy or X-ray crystallography. Box 3 summarizes indications for a metabolic stone evaluation.
- Box 4 describes events in the medical history that may be significant with regard to urolithiasis.

LABORATORY TESTS

- Urinalysis: Hematuria is often present, but absence of hematuria does not exclude stones. Urine pH may help identify stone type: pH >7.5 is associated with struvite stones; pH <5.5 is generally associated with uric acid stones, and low serum bicarbonate concentration with urine pH ≥6 is consistent with a renal tubular acidosis.
- Urine culture and sensitivity results should be obtained selectively in patients who may have superimposed infections, based on clinical symptoms of dysuria, fever, chills, or urinalysis suggestive of infection, or when surgical intervention is planned.
- Serum chemistries include electrolytes, BUN, creatinine, calcium, phosphate, uric acid, and parathyroid hormone.
- Additional tests: 24-hr urine collection for volume, creatinine, calcium, uric acid, phosphate, oxalate, and citrate excretion is generally reserved for patients with recurrent stones, young patients, bilateral stones, and large stone burden. A 24-hr urine collection may be appropriate for motivated, first-time stone patients interested in preventing recurrent stones. An abbreviated evaluation of single-stone formers is described in Box 5. Table 2 summarizes diagnostic criteria for various disorders associated with urolithiasis.

BOX 4 Components of the Medical History That Are Significant for Urolithiasis

- Diseases associated with disturbances of calcium metabolism: Primary hyperparathyroidism, medullary sponge kidney, osteoporosis, immobilization, sarcoidosis, osteolytic metastases, plasmacytoma, neuroendocrine tumors, Paget disease
- Dietary history: Purine gluttony, calcium excess, milk alkali, oxalate excess, sodium excess, low citrus fruit intake
- Medications: Uricosurics, diuretics, analgesics, vitamins C and D, antacids (especially phosphorus-binding agents), acetazolamide, calcium channel blockers, triamterene, estrogens, theophylline, protease inhibitors (indinavir), sulfonamides
- Diseases associated with disturbances of oxalate metabolism: Primary hyperoxaluria types I and II, Crohn disease, ulcerative colitis, intestinal bypass surgery (especially jejunoileal bypass), ileal resection
- Diseases associated with disturbances of purine metabolism
- Intrinsic metabolic disorders: Anemia, neoplastic disorders (especially leukemias), intoxication, myocardial infarction, irradiation, cytotoxic chemotherapy
- Enzyme deficiency: Primary gout, Lesch–Nyhan syndrome
- Altered excretion: Renal insufficiency, metabolic acidosis
- Infectious history: Organisms (particularly *Proteus* and *Klebsiella*), febrile, upper tract involvement, and dates (if hospitalized)

Modified from Nseyo UO, et al. (eds): *Urology for primary care physicians*, Philadelphia, 1999, Saunders.

BOX 5 Abbreviated Evaluation of Single-Stone Formers

History
  Underlying predisposing conditions (as per Box 3 and Etiology section in text)
  Medications (calcium, vitamin C, vitamin D, acetazolamide, steroids)
  Dietary excesses, inadequate fluid intake, excessive fluid loss
Multichannel blood screen
  Basic metabolic panel (sodium, potassium, chloride, carbon dioxide, blood urea nitrogen, creatinine)
  Calcium
  Intact parathyroid hormone
  Uric acid
Urine
  Urinalysis
    pH >7.5: Infection lithiasis
    pH <5.5: Uric acid lithiasis
    Sediment for crystalluria
  Urine culture
    Urea-splitting organisms: Suggestive of infection lithiasis
  Qualitative cystine
Radiography
  Radiopaque stones: Calcium oxalate, calcium phosphate, magnesium ammonium phosphate (struvite), cystine.
  Radiolucent stones: Uric acid, xanthine, triamterene
  CT scan, renal ultrasound or intravenous pyelogram: Radiolucent stones, anatomic abnormalities
Stone analysis

Modified from Wein AJ, et al.: *Campbell–Walsh urology*, ed 11, Philadelphia, 2016, Elsevier.

IMAGING STUDIES

- Common diagnostic modalities for renal colic are summarized in Table 3.
- Noniodinated contrast CT scanning is rapid and accurate, has the greatest sensitivity (nearly 100%), and specificity (94% to 96%), and can identify almost all stone types in essentially all locations. CT scan is the best test upon which to base stone treatment recommendations, evaluate stone persistence or passage, and plan for surgery. Indinavir stones are a notable exception because they are poorly seen on noncontrast CT and usually require contrast-enhanced CT for visualization. A high index of suspicion is required for diagnosis.
- CT scans may be ordered by urologists planning surgical intervention because a CT yields information on adjacent organs and stone density that ultrasound and plain film radiography cannot reveal.
- Low-dose and ultra-low-dose CT protocols specific to kidney stone evaluation are becoming more common and readily available.
- Ultrasonography or ultrasound (Fig. E1) may be an adequate initial study to detect stones or stone presence (i.e., hydronephrosis), especially in patients known to have a history of stones and in patients where radiation should be avoided (e.g., pregnancy and children). Ultrasonography is 50% to 70% sensitive in detecting stones within the kidneys, and about 90% sensitive in detecting hydronephrosis.
- Point-of-care ultrasound use is increasing in emergency departments and some clinic settings.
- Initial ultrasonography may be associated with lower cumulative radiation exposure than initial CT, without significant differences in missing, serious, or alternative diagnoses; adverse events; pain scores; return emergency department visits; or hospitalizations. It is reasonable to use ultrasonography as the initial imaging modality in suspected nephrolithiasis and to monitor known stones.
- Accuracy of sonography in detecting distal ureteral stones is variable due to variable stone size, body habitus, and expertise of the technician and radiologist. The absence of an ipsilateral ureteral jet suggests renal blockage is possible and not pathognomonic.
- Abdominal radiography, or kidney-ureter-bladder x-ray (KUB), can identify radiopaque stones (e.g., calcium-containing but not pure radiolucent uric acid stones). However, 20% to 30% of stones will not be visible based on stone composition, poor film quality, or overlying structures (bowel gas or bone)

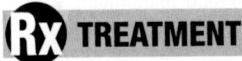

TREATMENT

ACUTE GENERAL Rx

- Diagnosis with labs, imaging, and patient history.
- Pain control: NSAIDs are excellent for managing renal colic (e.g., ketorolac, ibuprofen) and are preferred first-line agents. Opiates may be required for severe pain. Initial pain control with NSAIDs can reduce overall opiate dosing for

TABLE 2 Diagnostic Criteria

	SERUM			URINARY							
	Ca	P	PTH	Ca Fasting	Ca Load	Ca Restricted	UA	Ox	Cit	pH	Mg
Absorptive hypercalciuria type I	N	N	N	N	↑	↑	N	N	N	N	N
Absorptive hypercalciuria type II	N	N	N	↑	N	N	N	N	N	N	N
Renal hypercalciuria	N	N	↑	↑	↑	↑	N	N	N	N	N
Primary hyperparathyroidism	↑	↓	↑	↑	↑	↑	N	N	N	N	N
Unclassified hypercalciuria	N	N/↓	N	↑	↑	↑	N	N	N	N	N
Hyperuricosuria	N	N	N	N	N	N	↑	N	N	N	N
Enteric hyperoxaluria	N/↓	N/↓	N/↓	↓	↓	↓	↓	↑	↓	N	N
Hypocitraturia	N	N	N	N	N	N	N	N	↓	N	N
Renal tubular acidosis	N	N	N/↑	↑	N	N/↑	N	N	↓	N/↑	N
Hypomagnesuria	N	N	N	N	N	N	N/↓	N	↓	N	↓
Gouty diathesis	N	N	N	N	N	N	N/↑	N	N/↓	↓	N
Infection lithiasis	N	N	N	N	N	N	N	N	↓	↑	N

Fasting samples represent 2-hr collections obtained in morning after an overnight fast. Calcium load samples were obtained over a 4-hr period subsequent to oral ingestion of 1 g calcium. ↑, High; ↓, low; *Cit*, citrate; *Mg*, magnesium; *N*, normal; *Ox*, oxalate; *PTH*, immunoreactive parathyroid hormone; *UA*, uric acid.
From Wein AJ, et al.: *Campbell–Walsh urology*, ed 11, Philadelphia, 2016, Elsevier.

TABLE 3 Common Diagnostic Imaging Modalities for Renal Colic

Modality	Information Provided	Radiation Dose	Contrast	Approximate Cost	Time
CT	Renal and ureteral stones, stone size, location, number, evidence of obstruction Alternative diagnoses, such as AAA, appendicitis, and free air	4-10 mSv	No	$750-$1000	Less than 5 min to perform, 30 min for interpretation
CT with IV contrast	Same as noncontrast CT Delineation of renal masses Additional information about vascular dissections and mesenteric ischemia	4-10 mSv	Yes	$750-$1000	Less than 5 min, after delay to measure creatinine
CT with IV and oral contrast	Same as CT with IV contrast Potentially improved diagnosis of bowel abnormalities	4-10 mSv	Yes	$750-$1000	Less than 5 min, after delay of approximately 2 hr to ingest oral contrast
Intravenous urogram	Structural and functional information about obstruction Rarely, identification of other pathology, such as AAA	1.5 mSv	Yes	$350	Approximately 75 min
X-ray	Possible identification of stone, but cannot assess for hydronephrosis or most other pathology	0.5-1 mSv	No	$250	Less than 5 min
Ultrasound	Identification of hydronephrosis or hydroureter Possible identification of stone Used to assess for AAA or biliary disease	No	No	$150	Approximately 15-30 min—bedside ultrasound is quicker

AAA, Abdominal aortic aneurysm; *CT*, computed tomography; *IV*, intravenous.
From Lipshultz LI, et al.: *Urology and the primary care practitioner*, ed 3, Philadelphia, 2008, Elsevier.

 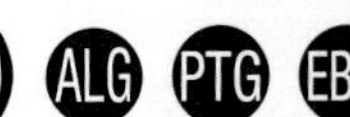

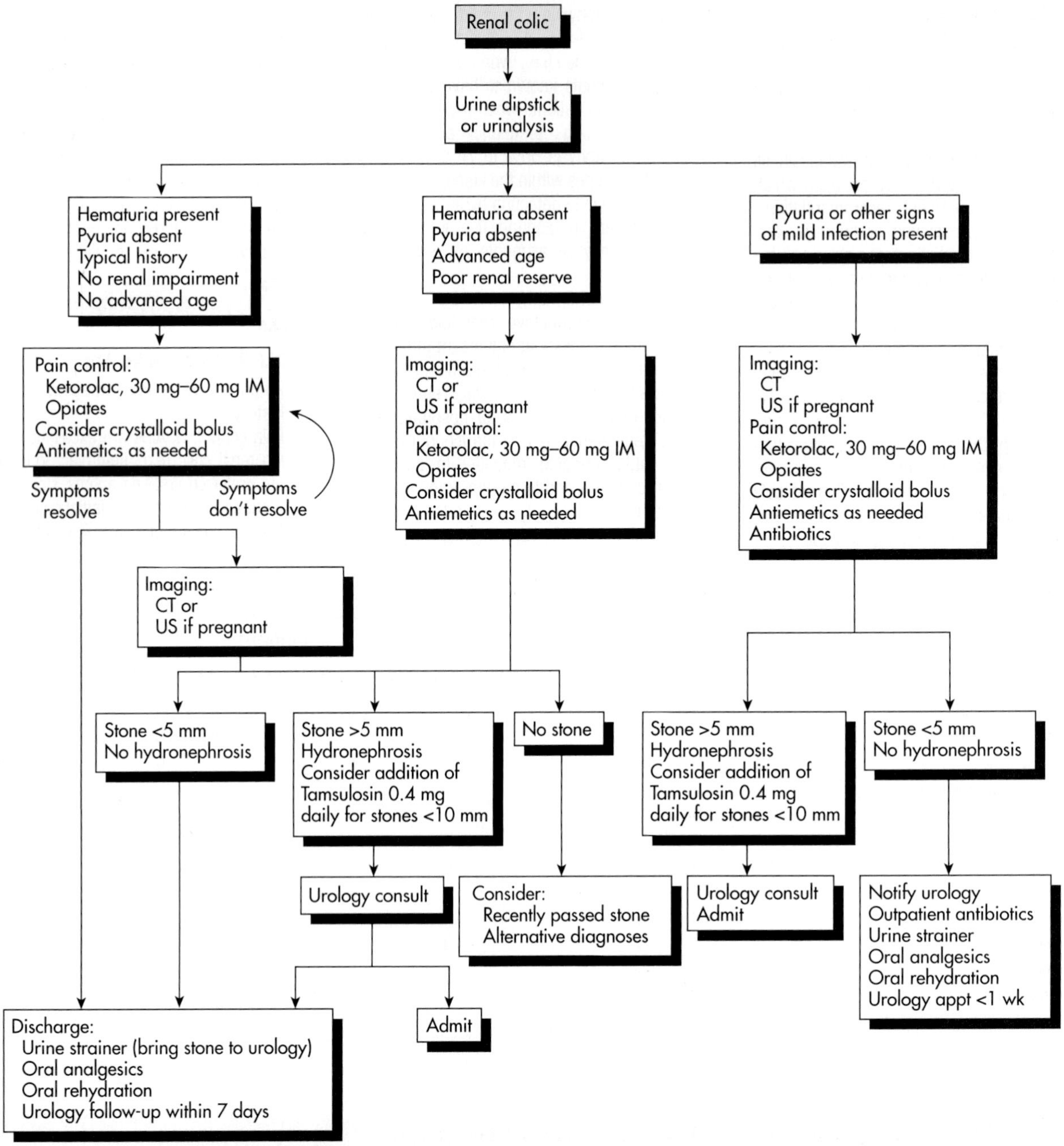

Renal colic

Urine dipstick or urinalysis

Hematuria present
Pyuria absent
Typical history
No renal impairment
No advanced age

Pain control:
Ketorolac, 30 mg–60 mg IM
Opiates
Consider crystalloid bolus
Antiemetics as needed

Symptoms resolve

Symptoms don't resolve

Imaging:
CT or
US if pregnant

Hematuria absent
Pyuria absent
Advanced age
Poor renal reserve

Imaging:
CT or
US if pregnant
Pain control:
Ketorolac, 30 mg–60 mg IM
Opiates
Consider crystalloid bolus
Antiemetics as needed

Pyuria or other signs of mild infection present

Imaging:
CT
US if pregnant
Pain control:
Ketorolac, 30 mg–60 mg IM
Opiates
Consider crystalloid bolus
Antiemetics as needed
Antibiotics

Stone <5 mm
No hydronephrosis

Stone >5 mm
Hydronephrosis
Consider addition of Tamsulosin 0.4 mg daily for stones <10 mm

No stone

Stone >5 mm
Hydronephrosis
Consider addition of Tamsulosin 0.4 mg daily for stones <10 mm

Stone <5 mm
No hydronephrosis

Urology consult

Consider:
Recently passed stone
Alternative diagnoses

Urology consult
Admit

Notify urology
Outpatient antibiotics
Urine strainer
Oral analgesics
Oral rehydration
Urology appt <1 wk

Discharge:
Urine strainer (bring stone to urology)
Oral analgesics
Oral rehydration
Urology follow-up within 7 days

Admit

FIG. 2 Guideline algorithm for the evaluation, treatment, and disposition of patients with presumed renal colic. *CT*, Computed tomography; *IV*, intravenously; *US*, ultrasonography. (Modified from Adams JG, et al.: *Emergency medicine, clinical essentials*, ed 2, Philadelphia, 2013, Elsevier.)

renal colic. Fig. 2 illustrates a guideline algorithm for the evaluation, treatment, and disposition of patients with presumed renal colic.

- IV fluids and antiemetics may be required.
- Patients with suspected urinary tract infections and obstructing stones require urgent kidney drainage (ureteral stent by a urologist or nephrostomy tube placement) and antibiotics. Patients with acute kidney injury or electrolyte derangements, or those whose pain cannot be controlled, also may require urgent kidney drainage.
- For patients who have a stone with a high probability of passage (i.e., small stone, especially distal ureter), medical expulsive therapy with α-blockers or calcium channel blockers (used less often due to side effects) may be helpful. New Level 1 evidence suggests that medical expulsive treatment may not be superior to placebo when considering all stone sizes; however, contemporary and numerous older studies have shown benefit to passage of distal stones ≥5 mm in size with the use of medical expulsive therapy.

PREVENTION

- Increase low-calorie fluid intake. Generally, patients at increased risk for stones should increase fluid intake to maintain a urine volume of 2 to 3 L/day.
- Recommended daily allowance of dietary calcium: 800 to 1200 mg/day. Lower calcium consumption results in less gut oxalate-binding and greater colonic oxalate absorption, which in turn increases urinary oxalate and risk for calcium-based stones.
- Limiting animal protein to one serving daily is often recommended.
- Greater fruit and vegetable intake increases urinary excretion of citrate (stone inhibitor).
- Dietary sodium restriction is recommended to <2 grams daily to decrease renal calcium excretion.
- Dietary oxalate restriction in patients with hyperoxaluria may be beneficial. However, low oxalate diets can be difficult to comply with and restrict many foods that promote and maintain cardiovascular health. Box 6 describes foods containing high levels of oxalate.
- Increased dietary citrate (e.g., lemons, limes, oranges).

- Stone specific therapy (Fig. 3):
  1. Uric acid calculi can be prevented or even dissolved at urine pH levels greater than 6 to 6.5. This often is accomplished with potassium citrate or sodium bicarbonate taken 2 or 3 times daily with food. Correction of metabolic syndrome, obesity and diabetes is also preventative for uric acid stones.
  2. Calcium stones:
     a. In general, cannot be dissolved and either persist, pass, or are removed.
     b. With hypercalciuria, thiazide diuretics and low-sodium diet are appropriate. Potassium citrate supplementation for patients with calcium stones and low 24-hr urine citrate excretion. Potassium citrate may also be effective with calcium stones even when urine citrate excretion is not low. Potassium citrate can treat the hypokalemia induced by thiazide diuretics.
     c. Urate-lowering treatment for patients with hyperuricosuria but not hypercalciuria.
  3. Struvite stones:
     a. Treating and preventing urinary tract infections reduces struvite stone formation and recurrence.
     b. Difficult to efficiently dissolve and rarely done due to treatment side effects and logistics.
     c. Urease inhibitor treatment by acetohydroxamic acid is considered for poor surgical candidates or those unable to fully clear stones. This agent is poorly tolerated and infrequently used in contemporary practice.
     d. Surgical interventions usually are required to remove struvite stones. Percutaneous nephrolithotomy (PCNL) and/or ureteroscopy are usually needed to adequately treat struvite stones as they facilitate active stone removal. Shock wave lithotripsy (SWL) can be used, but this does not actively remove the stones and may potentiate further UTIs.
  4. Cystine stones:
     a. High fluid intake of 3 to 4 L daily is the principal therapy, although it is hard to accomplish.
     b. Alkalinize urine to pH >6.5 to 7, often with potassium citrate.
     c. Thiol drugs such as penicillamine and tiopronin reduce the poorly soluble cystine to a soluble cysteine–drug complex. Tiopronin is better tolerated than penicillamine, but long-term compliance with both is infrequent.

BOX 6 Foods Containing High Levels of Oxalate

Tea (black)
Cocoa
Spinach
Mustard greens
Pokeweed
Swiss chard
Beets
Rhubarb
Okra
Berries (some)
Chocolate
Nuts
Wheat germ
Soy crackers
Pepper

From Wein AJ, et al.: *Campbell–Walsh urology*, ed 11, Philadelphia, 2016, Elsevier.

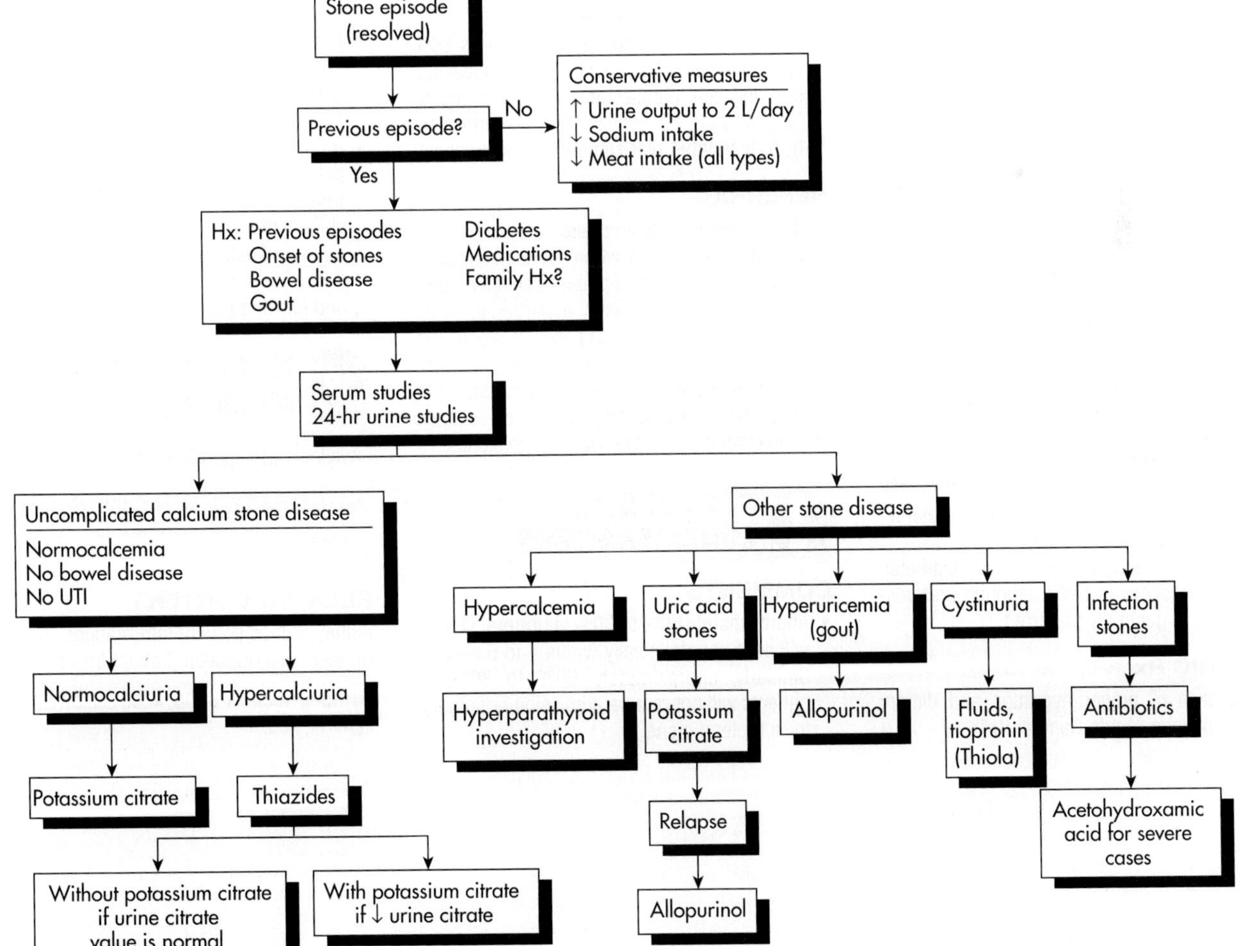

FIG. 3 Simplified treatment algorithm for the evaluation and medical management of urinary lithiasis. *Hx*, History; *UTI*, urinary tract infection. (Modified from C. Y. Pak.) (From Wein AJ, et al.: *Campbell–Walsh urology*, ed 11, Philadelphia, 2016, Elsevier.)

TABLE 4 Indications for Percutaneous Nephrolithotomy

Indicator	Description	Treatment
Stone size	≥1.5-2 cm or staghorn	
Composition*,**	Struvite stones	Complete removal necessary to reduce infection and minimize stone recurrence
	Calcium oxalate monohydrate and brushite stones	Difficult to pulverize by SWL
	Cystine stones	Difficult to pulverize by SWL
Stone position	Lower pole stones	Fragments less easily evacuated from dependent lower pole calyces; may not be accessible with ureteroscopy
Anatomic abnormalities	UPJ obstruction; calyceal diverticula; urinary diversion	Prevent passage of fragments after SWL; not always accessible with ureteroscopy
Patient characteristics	Morbid obesity; ureteral obstruction	Stone cannot be placed in focal point of SWL machine; not always accessible with ureteroscopy

SWL or ureteroscopy is the first choice for stone intervention, except in those circumstances that may favor PCNL. *SWL,* Extracorporeal shock wave lithotripsy; *PCNL,* percutaneous nephrolithotomy; *UPJ,* ureteropelvic junction.

*Stone composition can be defined with certainty only by direct stone analysis, but advances in imaging may ultimately provide a means to accurately assess stone composition in situ before treatment, thus allowing the urologist to select the treatment most likely to be successful.

**Ureteroscopy and laser lithotripsy also may be used to treat all stone types, including those listed in this table. Thus, stone size and location ultimately influence PCNL versus ureteroscopy decision.

Modified from Floege J, et al.: *Comprehensive clinical nephrology,* ed 4, Philadelphia, 2010, Saunders.

Surgical therapy:

1. Surgical treatment is needed for patients with severe pain unresponsive to medication, possible infection from an obstructing stone, acute kidney injury from ureteral obstruction, refractory nausea/vomiting, and prolonged kidney obstruction (i.e., risk of irreversible renal damage).
2. Ureteral stones can often be managed with ureteroscopy or SWL.
3. Stones in the kidney can be managed with ureteroscopy or SWL if <1 to 2 cm in diameter and in a favorable location. As a stone becomes larger and more complex, PCNL becomes the preferred means of management.
4. Indications for PCNL are described in Table 4.

- Guidelines for ureteral stone treatment:
  1. Proximal ureteral stones <1 cm diameter: SWL or ureteroscopy preferred.
  2. Proximal ureteral stones >1 cm diameter: SWL, ureteroscopy, or PCNL for complex and/or large stones.
  3. Distal ureteral stones <1 cm diameter: Ureteroscopy or SWL, although ureteroscopy is generally preferred.
  4. Distal ureteral stones >1 cm diameter: Ureteroscopy or SWL, although ureteroscopy is generally preferred.

CHRONIC Rx

Maintenance of proper hydration and dietary restrictions (see "Acute General Rx")

DISPOSITION

- >50% to 80% of patients will pass a ureteral stone within 4 to 6 weeks of presentation. Remember the "10 minus size of the stone in mm x 100% rule"; for example, a 3 mm stone has an approximately 70% chance of spontaneous passage while an 8 mm stone has only about a 20% chance.
- Lifetime stone recurrence is as high as 50% and depends on stone factors (composition, size, location, number of stones) and patient factors (anatomic, genetic, race, comorbidities, hydration status, diet, climate, and occupation).

REFERRAL

Urology referral is appropriate for any urinary stone patient, especially when spontaneous passage is unlikely; when a patient cannot be discharged from the emergency department; when a patient has an obstructing kidney stone and presumed or associated urinary tract infection; when there are large or recurrent stones; and when patients have solitary kidneys or complex anatomy that may predispose them to stones.

PEARLS & CONSIDERATIONS

COMMENTS

- Approximately 60% to 80% of ureteral stones will pass spontaneously within 4 to 6 weeks. Similarly, approximately 60% to 80% of patients will not require admission or surgery for a ureteral stone.
- Imaging is key to diagnosing urolithiases. Ultrasound or KUB is a suitable screening test, while CT scan is most accurate and often determines treatment recommendations.
- Consider NSAIDs as first-line therapy for pain control with kidney stones, unless there are contraindications (e.g., allergy or acute kidney injury).
- Patients should be referred to a urologist if they have large stones that are unlikely to pass spontaneously, multiple or bilateral stones at presentation, complex stones, or recurrent stones.
- An obstructing urinary stone in the setting of presumed urinary tract infection should be treated with prompt urinary tract drainage via insertion of a ureteral stent or percutaneous nephrostomy tube, and with antibiotics. Delays in renal drainage can lead to rapid and life-threatening sepsis.

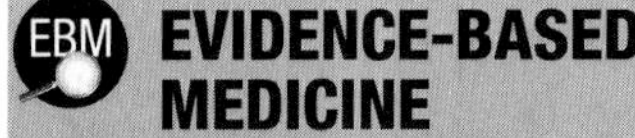

EVIDENCE-BASED MEDICINE

Available at ExpertConsult.com

SUGGESTED READINGS

Available at ExpertConsult.com

RELATED CONTENT

Kidney Stones (Patient Information)
Urinary Tract Infection (Patient Information)

AUTHORS: **AKSHAY SOOD, M.D.,** and **DAVID A. LEAVITT, M.D.**

BASIC INFORMATION

DEFINITION

Urticaria is a pruritic rash involving the epidermis and the upper portions of the dermis caused by localized capillary vasodilation and the release of histamine and other vasoactive mediators. It is followed by transudation of protein-rich fluid in the surrounding tissue and manifesting clinically with the presence of raised erythematous, circumscribed lesions with central pallor. Urticaria is classified according to its chronicity into acute (<6-wk duration) and chronic (>6-wk duration).

SYNONYMS

Hives
Wheals

ICD-10CM CODES
L50.0 Allergic urticaria
L50.1 Idiopathic urticaria
L50.2 Urticaria due to cold and heat
L50.8 Other urticaria
L50.9 Urticaria, unspecified
L50.6 Contact urticaria

EPIDEMIOLOGY & DEMOGRAPHICS

- Between 20% and 25% of the population will have at least one episode of urticaria during their lifetime.
- About 1% of the population is affected by chronic urticaria at a given time. It is more common in adults, with the average age of occurrence between the third and fifth decades of life. Females are twice as likely to be affected as males.
- Incidence is increased in atopic patients.

PHYSICAL FINDINGS & CLINICAL PRESENTATION

- Presence of elevated, erythematous, or white circumscribed lesions that change in size and shape over time (Fig. E1) in no specific distribution; they are characterized by extreme pruritus and evanescent in nature, with individual lesions generally lasting <24 hr in duration and disappear without scarring. If the patient has persistent symptoms, new lesions typically have a novel distribution.
- Stroking of the skin can lead to urticarial reaction (dermatographism) (Fig. 2).
- Angioedema occurs in approximately 40% of cases of urticaria and is caused by mast cell mediator release in the subcutaneous tissue and deep dermis.

ETIOLOGY

Acute urticaria (Table 1):

- Food allergies (e.g., shellfish [Fig. E3], eggs, strawberries, nuts, legumes, milk)
- Medication allergies (e.g., penicillin, aspirin, sulfonamides, hormone therapy)
- Insect sting allergies
- Systemic diseases (e.g., systemic lupus erythematosus, serum sickness, autoimmune thyroid disease, urticaria pigmentosa)
- Infections (viral infections such as hepatitis B and C, fungal infections, chronic bacterial infections, helminthic); viral upper respiratory infections are the predominant cause
- Contact (nonimmunologic) urticaria (e.g., caterpillars, plants)
- Other: Pregnancy, cryoglobulinemia, hair bleaches, chemicals, saliva, cosmetics, perfumes, pemphigoid, emotional stress, malignancy (lymphomas, endocrine tumors)
- Idiopathic urticaria is diagnosed in 50% of patients with chronic urticaria

Chronic urticaria

- Physical stimuli (e.g., pressure, exercise-induced, solar, cold, or cholinergic urticaria) are found in approximately 20% of patients.
- Between 30% and 40% of patients have anti-FcεRI antibodies, which could represent an autoimmune etiology, but their significance remains controversial at this time.
- Chronic idiopathic urticaria (CIU), also known as chronic spontaneous urticaria (CSU), is diagnosed in the remainder of cases.

DIAGNOSIS

DIFFERENTIAL DIAGNOSIS

- Erythema multiforme
- Erythema marginatum
- Erythema infectiosum
- Urticarial vasculitis
- Herpes gestationis
- Drug eruption
- Multiple insect bites
- Bullous pemphigoid
- Mastocytosis
- Mast cell activation syndrome
- Viral exanthema
- Pityriasis rosea
- Atopic dermatitis
- Contact dermatitis
- Henoch-Schönlein purpura

WORKUP

- It is useful to determine whether hives are acute or chronic; a medical history focused on various etiologic factors is necessary before embarking on extensive laboratory testing.
- Most cases of acute urticaria resolve spontaneously and diagnostic testing is not required. However, in patients with acute urticaria, it is crucial to consider anaphylaxis before further workup of urticaria because this may require urgent management.
- The etiology of chronic urticaria (CU) is often never determined, and no diagnostic testing may be necessary based on a detailed history and physical examination. Targeted laboratory testing based on clinical findings is appropriate.

LABORATORY TESTS

- If the history is consistent with allergen-induced contact urticaria, skin testing with allergen extracts and screening for dermatographism by attempting to elicit a wheal after application of linear skin pressure should be performed only after withholding antihistamines for 36 to 72 hr to prevent false-negative results.
- CBC with differential, ESR, TSH, and liver function tests should be considered only in patients with a remarkable history or physical exam for an underlying systemic condition. Routine testing is never indicated. Even with extensive testing, the cause of chronic urticaria is rarely established.
- Measurement of C4, C1 inhibitor antigenic level, and function and C1q may be helpful in patients who present with angioedema alone. In these patients, C1-inhibitor deficiency should be considered.
- Skin biopsy is helpful in patients with fever, arthralgias, and elevated erythrocyte sedimentation rate. Histologic evidence of leukocytoclasia (neutrophilic infiltration with fragmentation of nuclei) is indicative of urticarial vasculitis.
- When food or contact allergy is suspected in acute urticaria, testing can be performed using skin prick, immunoCAP, and radioallergosorbent testing.

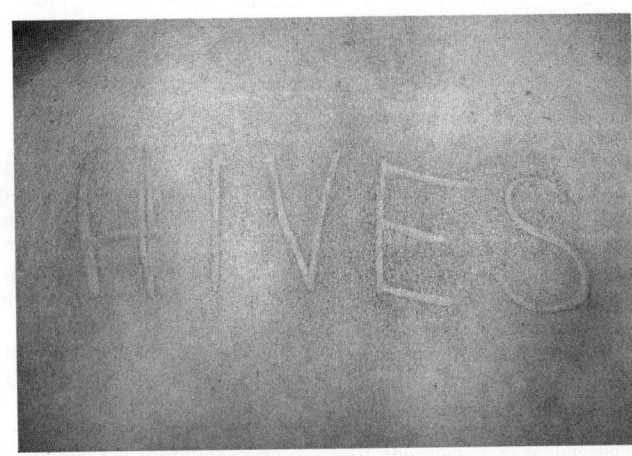

FIG. 2 Dermatographism. Stroking of the skin leads to the urticarial reaction. (From Callen JP et al: *Dermatological signs of systemic disease*, ed 5, Philadelphia, 2017, Elsevier.)

TABLE 1 Some Causes of Urticaria*

Some Causes of Urticaria*
Infections
Bacterial infections
Dental abscess
Sinusitis
Otitis
Pneumonitis
Gastritis
Hepatitis
Cholecystitis
Cystitis
Vaginitis
Fungal infections
Dermatophytes
Candida
Other infections/infestations
Scabies
Helminth
Protozoa
Trichomonas
Drugs and Chemicals
Salicylates
Indomethacin and other, newer nonsteroidal anti-inflammatory agents†
Opiates†
Radiocontrast material†
Penicillin (medication, milk, blue cheese)
Sulfonamides
Sodium benzoate
Douches
Ear drops or eye drops
Insulin
Menthol (cigarettes, toothpaste, iced tea, hand cream, lozenges, candy)
Tartrazine (vitamins, birth control pills, antibiotics, FDC yellow #5)
Foods
Nuts
Berries†
Fish
Seafood
Shellfish†
Bananas
Grapes
Tomatoes
Eggs†
Cheese
Inhalants
Animal danders
Pollen
Contactants
Wool
Silk
Occupational exposure
Potatoes
Antibiotics
Cosmetics
Dyes
Hairspray
Nail polish
Mouthwash
Toothpaste
Perfumes
Hand cream
Soap
Insect repellent
Physical Stimuli
Light
Pressure
Heat
Cold
Water
Vibration
Endocrinopathies
Thyroid disease
Diabetes mellitus
Pregnancy
Menstruation
Menopause
Systemic Diseases
Rheumatic fever
Connective tissue diseases (lupus erythematosus, Sjögren's syndrome, rheumatoid arthritis, Still disease, dermatomyositis, polymyositis, other)
Leukemia
Lymphoma
Acquired immunodeficiency disease
Ovarian tumors

*Partial list of most frequently described causes in each category.
†May be mediated by nonimmunologic mechanisms independent of IgE.
From Callen JP et al: *Dermatological signs of systemic disease*, ed 5, Philadelphia, 2017, Elsevier.

Rx TREATMENT

NONPHARMACOLOGIC THERAPY

Remove suspected etiologic agents (e.g., stop aspirin and all nonessential drugs) and avoid any foods that may have been observed to precipitate an attack.

ACUTE URTICARIA Rx

- Oral antihistamines: Use of second-generation H1 antihistamines (e.g., cetirizine 10 mg qd, levocetirizine 5 mg qd, loratadine 10 mg/day, fexofenadine 180 mg/day) as they are preferred over first-generation sedating antihistamines (e.g., hydroxyzine, diphenhydramine). Higher doses of second-generation antihistamines up to 4 times the FDA-approved dose may be required to achieve adequate control of symptoms.
- Leukotriene receptor antagonists (e.g., montelukast) can be added to H1 antagonists in refractory cases.
- Oral corticosteroids should be reserved for refractory cases and prescribed for a very limited course (e.g., prednisone 20 mg qd or 20 mg bid for 5 days).

CHRONIC URTICARIA Rx

Step-care approach for management of nonsedating chronic urticaria is described in Fig. E4.

- Step 1: Monotherapy with second-generation antihistamines. Avoidance of triggers (e.g., NSAIDs, alcohol, opiates, physical triggers).
- Step 2: One or more of the following:
  1. Dose advancement of second-generation antihistamine (up to 4 times the daily recommended dose).
  2. Add leukotriene receptor antagonist.
  3. Add first-generation antihistamine (hydroxyzine or doxepin) to be taken at bedtime.
- Step 3: Referral to allergy specialist for evaluation and management.
- Step 4: Add an alternate agent such as omalizumab (a monoclonal anti-IgE antibody that downregulates surface IgE receptors), cyclosporine, or other anti-inflammatory agents or immunosuppressants.
- Patient should be evaluated at each visit and if symptoms are well managed, should be considered for step down in treatment.

DISPOSITION

- Most cases of urticaria resolve within 6 wk.
- More than 50% of patients may not achieve satisfactory control of CIU with antihistamines alone and may require additional therapies. Median duration of CIU is between 3 to 5 yr, but it can often be present for much longer durations.

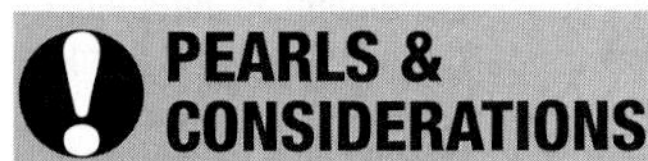

PEARLS & CONSIDERATIONS

COMMENTS

- Topical treatment (e.g., starch baths or oatmeal baths) may be temporarily soothing in selected patients; however, they are not recommended for long-term control of CIU.
- If individual urticarial lesions leave residual ecchymoses, pigmentation and/or lesions that typically last >24 hr at a single location, consider skin biopsy to evaluate for urticarial vasculitis.
- **Be judicious when prescribing NSAIDs in all CIU patients, as up to 30% of these patients will experience exacerbation of urticaria and angioedema.**

SUGGESTED READINGS

Available at ExpertConsult.com

RELATED CONTENT

Hives (Patient Information)
Urticaria, Chronic (Related Key Topic)

AUTHOR: **SHYAM JOSHI, M.D.**

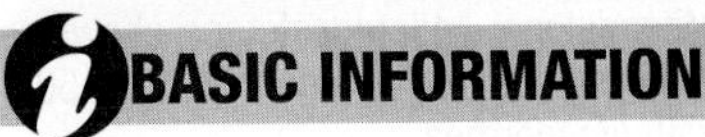

BASIC INFORMATION

DEFINITION

Uterine fibroids, also called leiomyomas or uterine myomas, are benign tumors of muscle cells of the myometrium and connective tissue. The incidence of malignancy is less than 1 in 1000. They are typically discrete nodular tumors that vary in size and number.

Fibroids are classified by location in the uterus relative to the myometrium.

- Subserosal: Located directly underneath the uterine serosa
- Intramural: Located in the myometrium proper
- Submucosal: Also known as intracavitary as they are located adjacent to the endometrium and protrude into the uterine cavity
- Pedunculated: Located on a pedicle or stalk, either from the serosa or in the cavity

Fibroids can also be located within the cervix, broad ligament, or diffusely in the body such as within the abdomen on peritoneum or within skin. Parasitic fibroids acquire a blood supply from a nonuterine source (Fig. 1).

SYNONYMS

Uterine leiomyomas
Uterine myomas
Fibroids

ICD-10CM CODES
D25.0 Submucous leiomyoma of uterus
D25.1 Intramural leiomyoma of uterus
D25.2 Subserosal leiomyoma of uterus
D25.9 Leiomyoma of uterus, unspecified

EPIDEMIOLOGY & DEMOGRAPHICS

- Estimated cumulative incidence of 70% to 80% in women by age 50.
- The most common benign solid pelvic tumor diagnosed in women and the most common reason for benign hysterectomy.
- More common in African American women than in Caucasian women.
- May occur singly but are often multiple.
- Approximately 50% of all fibroids are estimated to produce symptoms that impact women including restriction of social, physical, and work activities.
- Frequently diagnosed incidentally on pelvic examination.
- There is increased familial incidence.
- Potential to enlarge during pregnancy as well as regress after menopause.
- Approximately 200,000 hysterectomies, 30,000 myomectomies, and thousands of selective uterine-artery embolizations and high-intensity focused ultrasound procedures are performed annually in the U.S. to remove or destroy uterine fibroids.[1]

PHYSICAL FINDINGS & CLINICAL PRESENTATION

- Enlarged, irregular uterus on pelvic examination

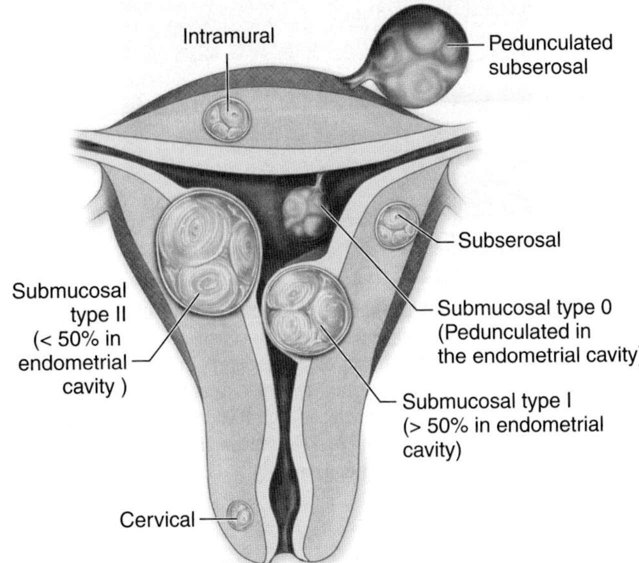

FIG. 1 Drawing of uterus in the coronal plane, illustrating possible location of uterine leiomyomas. (From Fielding JR, et al.: *Gynecologic imaging,* Philadelphia, 2011, Saunders.)

- Presenting symptoms:
  1. Abnormal uterine bleeding (most common)
  2. Chronic pelvic pain (dysmenorrhea, dyspareunia, pelvic pressure)
  3. Bulk symptoms (bloating, increase in abdominal girth)
  4. Anemia
  5. Acute pain (torsion of pedunculated fibroid, infarction, and degeneration)
  6. Urinary symptoms (frequency from bladder pressure, partial ureteral obstruction, complete ureteral obstruction, incontinence in setting of prolapse)
  7. GI symptoms (rectosigmoid compression with constipation or intestinal obstruction, pain with defecation)
  8. Prolapse through cervix of pedunculated submucosal fibroid
  9. Infertility
  10. Pregnancy complications including preterm birth, small fetus for gestational age, malpresentation, and potentially recurrent miscarriage

ETIOLOGY

Not well understood. It is suggested that fibroids arise from an original single smooth muscle cell in the myometrium. Each individual fibroid is monoclonal (all the cells are derived from one progenitor myocyte). Malignant degeneration of preexisting leiomyoma is extremely uncommon (<0.5%). There is a racial disparity in the prevalence, suggesting a genetic component, with most fibroids having a normal chromosomal makeup. A small group of women have an autosomal dominant disorder, hereditary leiomyomatosis and renal cell carcinoma syndrome, in which there is a genetic mutation in the fumarate hydratase gene, causing diminished suppressor function in fibroid formation.

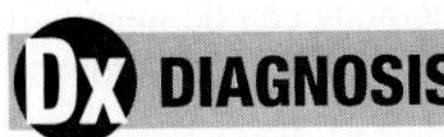

DIAGNOSIS

DIFFERENTIAL DIAGNOSIS

- Ovarian mass (neoplastic, nonneoplastic, endometrioma)
- Adenomyosis
- Endometriosis
- Endometrial polyp
- Endometrial carcinoma
- Leiomyosarcoma/uterine carcinosarcoma
- Inflammatory mass (reproductive organ or GI origin)
- Pregnancy

WORKUP

- Complete pelvic examination, including speculum exam as well as bimanual exam
- Estimation of size of uterus/mass and location of fibroids via imaging
- Endometrial sampling may be indicated (biopsy or dilation and curettage) when abnormal bleeding and pelvic mass are present
- If significant urinary symptoms are prominent, intravenous pyelogram to rule out impingement on urinary system

LABORATORY TESTS

- Pregnancy test
- Complete blood count
- BUN/creatinine
- TSH

IMAGING STUDIES

- Pelvic ultrasound (Fig. 2) is useful as a primary diagnostic modality. Transvaginal ultrasound commonly has higher diagnostic accuracy.
- MRI scan is helpful in planning treatment if malignancy is strongly suspected. Also important to localize fibroids, especially if myomectomy is contemplated. Size, number, and location of fibroids are also important if a minimally invasive myomectomy is considered.

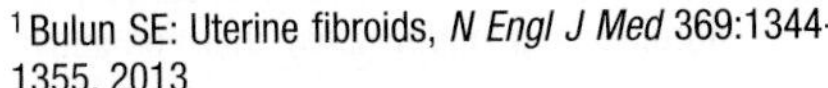

[1] Bulun SE: Uterine fibroids, *N Engl J Med* 369:1344-1355, 2013

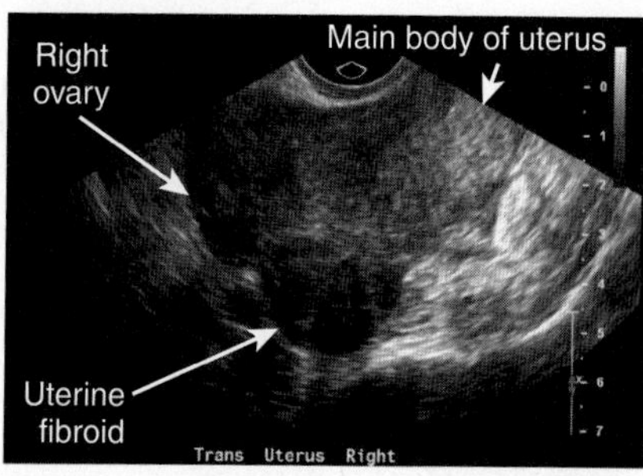

FIG. 2 Fibroid uterus: Endovaginal ultrasound. Ultrasound is the primary modality used for evaluation of uterine fibroids (leiomyomas). Typical features include a well-circumscribed appearance. Fibroids may be hypoechoic or hyperechoic relative to the uterus. They may be exophytic or intramural, or they may project into the uterine cavity. Whereas malignant uterine tumors may invade adjacent structures, a fibroid is contained within the uterine serosa. Uterine tumors, both benign and malignant, can show central necrosis, which usually appears hypoechoic with ultrasound. In this 38-year-old woman, the fibroid is exophytic. The right ovary lies adjacent and is difficult to distinguish in this case. (From Broder JS: *Diagnostic imaging for the emergency physician,* Philadelphia, 2011, Saunders.)

- Diagnostic hysteroscopy can be performed in the office and may provide direct evidence of intrauterine pathology or submucosal leiomyoma that distorts uterine cavity.
- Saline infusion sonography can be helpful in determining location and degree of intrusion into uterine cavity.

Rx TREATMENT

Management (Fig. 3) should be based on primary symptoms and may include observation with close follow-up, temporizing surgical therapies, embolization, medical management, or definitive surgical procedures. Treatment is generally indicated if bleeding is requiring blood transfusions, renal function is affected by size of the enlarged fibroid uterus, or when symptoms are present and are severe enough to be unacceptable to the patient.

NONSURGICAL Rx

- Patient observation and follow-up with periodic repeat pelvic examinations to ensure that tumors are not growing rapidly.
- Hormonal therapies can reduce bleeding symptoms and many have the added benefit of contraception. There is no evidence that exogenous estrogen or progestin increases risk of myomas.
  1. Combined hormonal methods with estrogen and progestin, including combined oral contraceptives, contraceptive patch, contraceptive vaginal ring.
  2. Progestin-only agents including oral progestins, intramuscular progestin injection, subcutaneous progestin implant, levonorgestrel IUD.
  3. Progesterone IUD can be used to treat menorrhagia, but intracavitary fibroids may be a relative contraindication.
  4. Ulipristal acetate, not yet available in the U.S. for treatment of fibroids, is a selective progesterone-receptor modulator that acts on progesterone receptors in myometrial and endometrial tissue and inhibits ovulation without significant effects on estradiol levels or antiglucocorticoid activity. Recent trials showed that treatment with ulipristal acetate for 13 wk effectively controlled excessive bleeding due to uterine fibroids and reduced the size of the fibroids.
- Gonadotropin-releasing hormone (GnRH) agonist use results in 40% to 60% reduction in uterine volume within 3 mo of initiating treatment. Hyperestrogenism, reversible bone loss, and hot flushes are associated with use. Consider low-dose progesterone replacement to minimize hypoestrogenic effects.
  1. Regrowth and return of bleeding symptoms occurs in approximately 50% of women treated within a few months after cessation.
  2. Indications for GnRH:
     a. Fertility preservation in women with large myomas before attempting conception or preoperative myectomy treatment
     b. Anemia treatment to normalize hemoglobin before surgery
     c. Women approaching menopause to avoid surgery
     d. Preoperative for large myomas to make vaginal hysterectomy, hysteroscopic resection/ablation, or laparoscopic destruction more feasible
     e. Women with medical contraindications for surgery
  3. Personal or medical indications for delaying surgery: Use of GnRH agonists may alter the consistency of the fibroid, making myomectomy more challenging.
- Nonhormonal medical therapies:
  1. Nonsteroidal anti-inflammatory drugs
  2. Tranexamic acid, an oral antifibrinolytic agent that prevents fibrinolysis of menstrual fluid, can decrease menorrhagia by 40% to 65%. Side effects include abdominal cramps, headaches, fatigue, and increase risk of venous thromboembolism.
- Other drugs used and under investigation:
  1. Danazol: Androgen and multienzyme inhibitor of steroidogenesis
  2. Mifepristone: Antiprogesterone shown to reduce the fibroid volume by 40% to 50% with amenorrhea
  3. Raloxifene: Selective estrogen receptor modulator, either alone or with a GnRH agonist, shown to reduce the fibroid volume 70% up to 1 yr but only in postmenopausal women
  4. Fadrozole: Aromatase inhibitor reported to have produced a 71% reduction in volume that is not yet available in the U.S.
  5. Vilaprisan: Selective progesterone receptor modulator (SPRM) currently in phase 3 trials showing decreasing amenorrhea rates and reduction in fibroid size

SURGICAL Rx

- Indications:
  1. Abnormal uterine bleeding with anemia refractory to hormonal therapy
  2. Chronic pain with severe dysmenorrhea, dyspareunia, or lower abdominal pressure/pain
  3. Acute pain, torsion, or prolapsing submucosal fibroid
  4. Urinary symptoms or signs such as hydronephrosis
  5. Rapid uterine enlargement premenopausal or any growth after menopause
  6. Infertility or recurrent pregnancy loss with submucous leiomyoma as only finding
  7. Enlarged uterus with compression symptoms or discomfort
- Procedures:
  1. Hysterectomy (definitive procedure): Vaginal, laparoscopic, robotic, or abdominal approach, dependent on surgical preference/expertise and uterine size.
  2. Myomectomy (to preserve fertility or due to patient preference): May be performed via abdominal, laparoscopic, or robotic approach.
  3. Vaginal myomectomy for prolapsed pedunculated submucous fibroid.
  4. Hysteroscopic resection: Typically at least 50% of the fibroid must be intracavitary for a hysteroscopic approach to be successful.
  5. Myolysis: Radio-frequency energy is used to ablate an individual fibroid and destroy the blood supply to that fibroid. Currently approved in the U.S. as a laparoscopic procedure performed under ultrasound guidance.
  6. Uterine artery embolization (UAE): Safe and effective short-term alternative to surgery, but its less invasive nature should be balanced against a higher rate for treatment failure or complications at 5 yr (32%) versus the surgery group (4%). Age 40 yr and under at embolization and history of previous myomectomy are significant predictors of embolization failure. If the patient wishes to preserve future fertility, UAE should not be performed.
  7. Endometrial ablation: Performed specifically to decrease menorrhagia
  8. MRI-guided focus ultrasound surgery for fibroids is a noninvasive thermoablative

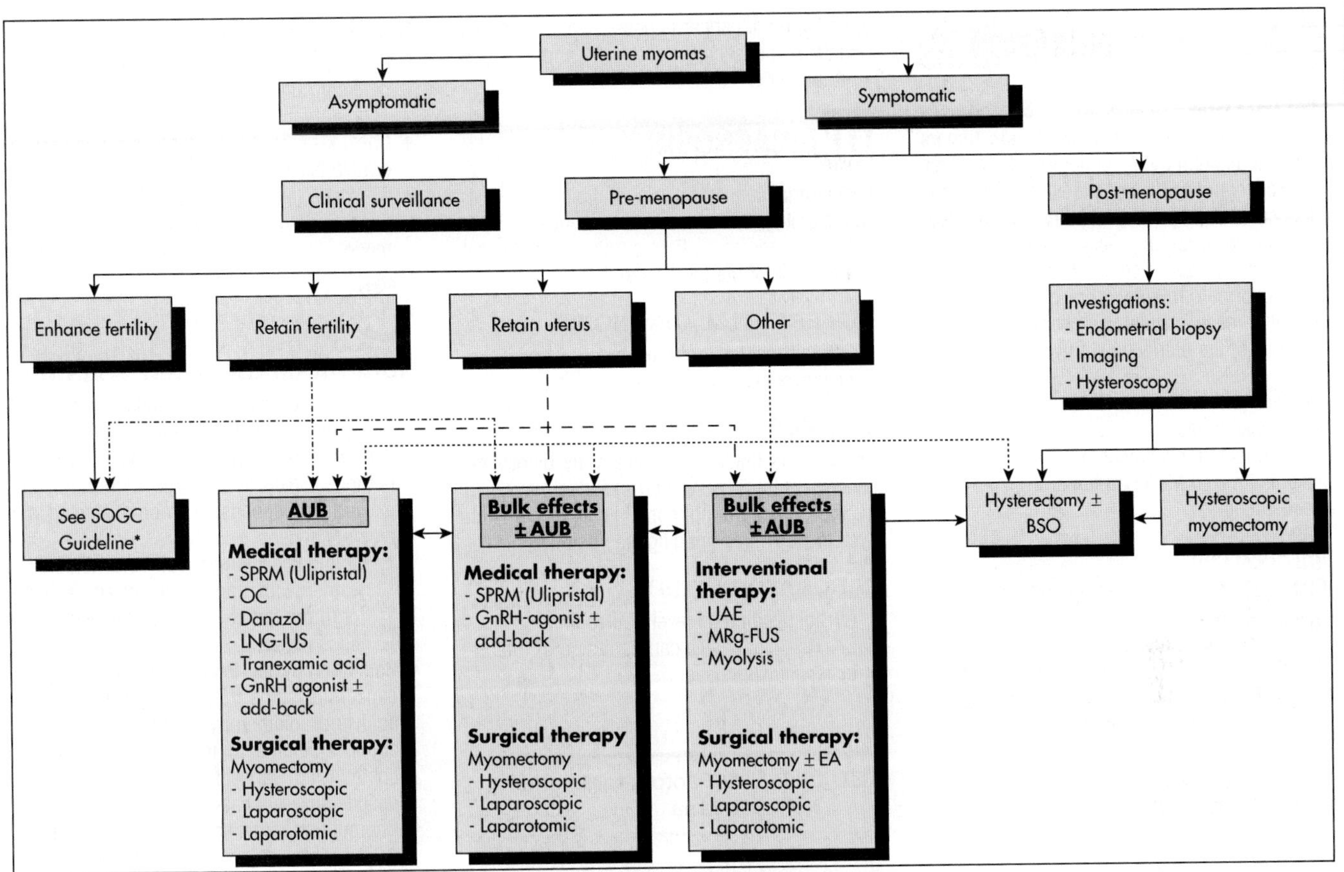

BSO: bilateral salpingo-oophorectomy; MRg-FUS: Magnetic resonance-guided focused ultrasound; OC: oral contraceptives

FIG. 3 Algorithm for the management of uterine fibroids. *GnRH*, Gonadotropin-releasing hormone; *UAE*, uterine artery embolization. (From Vilos GA, et al.: The management of uterine leiomyomas, *J Obstet Gynaecol Can* 37(2):163, 2015.)
*Carranza-Mamane B, Havelock J, Hemmings R; Society of Obstetrics and Gynaecology Canada Reproductive Endocrinology and Infertility Committee: The management of uterine fibroids in women with otherwise unexplained infertility. SOGC Clinical Practice Guidelines. *J Obstet Gynaecol Can*, 2015.

procedure that allows high-energy ultrasound waves to converge on a fibroid localized by MRI. Note, there is limited availability of this procedure.

COMPLICATIONS

- Red degeneration occurs when the fibroid outgrows its blood supply leading to hemorrhage in the center of the fibroid. This is typically seen in the second trimester of pregnancy but is a rare occurrence.
- Leiomyosarcoma (<0.1%). Recent concern has been voiced by the U.S. Food and Drug Administration (FDA) regarding the use of morcellation in minimally invasive surgery because of the possibility of spreading occult malignancy in the peritoneal cavity.

REFERRAL

Consultation with gynecologic oncologist if suspicious of malignancy

SUGGESTED READINGS

Available at ExpertConsult.com

RELATED CONTENT

Uterine Fibroids (Patient Information)
Dysfunctional Uterine Bleeding (Related Key Topic)

AUTHORS: **TERRI Q. HUYNH, M.D,** and **NIMA R. PATEL, M.D., M.S.**

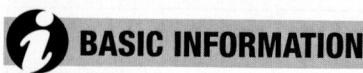

BASIC INFORMATION

DEFINITION

Cancers of the uterine corpus include tumors from the endometrium (endometrial cancers). The most common type of endometrial cancer is adenocarcinoma (includes endometrioid, clear cell, mucinous, and papillary serous subtypes). Uterine cancer also includes tumors that result from abnormal proliferation of cells originating from the mesenchymal, or connective tissue, elements of the uterine wall (myometrium).

SYNONYMS

Leiomyosarcomas
Endometrial stromal sarcoma
Malignant mixed Müllerian tumors
Adenosarcomas

ICD-10CM CODES

C54.1	Malignant neoplasm of endometrium
C54.2	Malignant neoplasm of the myometrium
C54.0	Malignant neoplasm of isthmus uteri
C54.8	Malignant neoplasm of overlapping sites of corpus uteri

EPIDEMIOLOGY & DEMOGRAPHICS

INCIDENCE: Incidence is 25.9 cases per 100,000 females per yr. Endometrial cancer remains the most common gynecologic malignancy in the U.S. Uterine cancer is one of the few cancers with increasing incidence and mortality in the U.S., reflecting in part increases in the prevalence of overweight and obesity since the 1980s. It is the fourth most common cancer diagnosed and the seventh most common cause of cancer death among U.S. women.[1]

PREVALENCE: Uterine sarcoma accounts for approximately 8% of all cancers of the uterine corpus and is associated with poor prognosis.

MEAN AGE AT DIAGNOSIS: 60 yr

RISK FACTORS: Box 1 describes risk factors for uterine sarcoma

PHYSICAL FINDINGS & CLINICAL PRESENTATION

- Abnormal vaginal bleeding is the most common symptom (90% of women with diagnosis).
- Vaginal discharge also may be a presenting symptom (10% of these patients have non-bloody discharge).
- May also present as pelvic pain or pressure and pelvic mass on examination (10% of women with uterine sarcoma)
- May appear as tumor protruding through the cervix as a fungating mass.
- Weight loss

ETIOLOGY

- The exact etiology is unknown.
- Endometrial cancer is possibly related to the balance between progesterone and estrogen in the body.

[1]Henley SJ et al: Uterine cancer incidence and mortality—United States, 1999-2016, *MMWR* 67(48):1333-1338, 2018.

DIAGNOSIS

Endometrial cancer: Endometrial biopsy or D&C with histologic evidence of malignancy.

Uterine sarcoma: Post-surgical histological examination of uterine tissue

DIFFERENTIAL DIAGNOSIS

- Endometrial hyperplasia
- Leiomyoma

WORKUP

Diagnosis is made histologically by biopsy for abnormal bleeding. Workup includes biopsy (in the office or operating room, in conjunction with hysteroscopy) and imaging (see below).

LABORATORY TESTS

- CBC depending on level of bleeding
- CA-125 (high levels can be a sign of metastasis, not diagnostic)

BOX 1 Risk Factors for Uterine Sarcoma

- Nulliparity
- Obesity
- History of pelvic radiation
- Exposure to tamoxifen

From Fielding JR et al: *Gynecologic imaging,* Philadelphia, 2011, Saunders.

BOX 2 Uterine Sarcoma Prognostic Factors

- Tumor stage
- Tumor grade
- Tumor size
- Patient age
- Vascular space involvement
- Mitotic count
- Residual disease at surgery
- Adjuvant chemotherapy

From Fielding JR et al: *Gynecologic imaging,* Philadelphia, 2011, Saunders.

BOX 3 Uterine Sarcoma: Key Points

- The disease mainly affects postmenopausal women.
- Most patients present early with postmenopausal bleeding.
- The primary treatment is hysterectomy.
- Adjuvant radiotherapy to the pelvis is used if poor prognosis features in stage 1 or if spread has occurred beyond the corpus.

From Greer IA et al: Mosby's *color atlas and text of obstetrics and gynecology,* London, 2001, Harcourt.

IMAGING STUDIES

- Pelvic ultrasound is a lower-cost method of detecting uterine corpus mass or thickened endometrial lining
- Chest x-ray is usually done as routine preoperative testing.
- CT scans (Fig. E1), MRI, and PET are useful for assessing tumor spread once diagnosis is made.

TREATMENT

NONPHARMACOLOGIC THERAPY

- Surgical excision is the mainstay of treatment, with or without lymph node mapping and with or without peritoneal lavage or peritoneal biopsies. Degree of removal and exploration depends on grading, staging, and type of cancer
  1. Hormonal treatment can be considered in women with stage 1 cancer and a desire for future fertility, although close monitoring is required.
- Radiotherapy is initiated in women with cancers at stage II or higher. The benefit of adjuvant radiotherapy in stage I endometrial adenocarcinoma to improve pelvic disease control and survival remains controversial despite several phase 3 trials.
- Chemotherapeutic agents have produced only partial and short-term responses.

DISPOSITION

- Survival varies with each type of sarcoma but is generally very poor. Box 2 describes uterine prognostic factors.
- 5-yr survival for localized (stage I) endometrial stromal sarcoma is 99% and drops to 69% for stage IV.
- 5-yr survival for leiomyosarcoma ranges from 63% for stage I to 14% for stage IV.
- 5-yr survival for undifferentiated sarcoma ranges from 70% for stage I to 23% for stage IV.

REFERRAL

Uterine sarcoma should be managed by a gynecologic oncologist and radiation oncologist. Key points in the management of uterine sarcoma are described in Box 3.

SUGGESTED READINGS

Available at ExpertConsult.com

RELATED CONTENT

Uterine Cancer (Patient Information)
Endometrial Cancer (Related Key Topic)

AUTHORS: **ASHWINI U. DHOKTE, M.D.**

BASIC INFORMATION

DEFINITION

Bleeding per vagina at any time during pregnancy must be regarded as abnormal and is associated with an increased likelihood of pregnancy complications.

SYNONYM

Hemorrhage

ICD-10CM CODES

O20.8	Other hemorrhage in early pregnancy
O20.9	Hemorrhage in early pregnancy, unspecified
O03.9	Complete or unspecified spontaneous abortion
O44.10	Placenta previa with hemorrhage, unspecified trimester
O45.8X9	Other premature separation of placenta, unspecified trimester

EPIDEMIOLOGY & DEMOGRAPHICS

- Common in U.S. and occurs in women of childbearing age.
- 20% to 25% of patients have vaginal spotting/bleeding in the first trimester.
- Early vaginal bleeding increases the risk of miscarriage (50%) and preterm birth.

PHYSICAL FINDINGS & CLINICAL PRESENTATION

- Bleeding: Ranges from scant to life-threatening with hemodynamic instability
- Color: Brown to bright red
- Can be painless or painful (cramps, back pain, severe abdominal pain)
- Fetal compromise: Ranges from none to fetal demise

DIAGNOSIS

DIFFERENTIAL DIAGNOSIS

- Any gestational age:
  1. Cervical lesions: Polyps, decidual reaction, neoplasia
  2. Vaginal trauma
  3. Cervicitis/vulvovaginitis
  4. Postcoital trauma
  5. Bleeding dyscrasias
- Gestation <20 wk:
  1. Implantation bleeding
  2. Spontaneous abortion
  3. Presence of intrauterine device
  4. Ectopic pregnancy (including cesarean scar and cervical pregnancy)
  5. Molar pregnancy
  6. Low-lying placenta/placenta previa
  7. hCG-secreting tumors, including gestational trophoblastic neoplasia or gestational choriocarcinoma (incidence is 1 in 1500-20,000 pregnancies)
- Gestation >20 wk:
  1. Molar pregnancy
  2. Placental disorders (low-lying placenta, placenta previa, placenta accreta)
  3. Placental abruption
  4. Vasa previa
  5. Marginal separation of the placenta
  6. Preterm labor
  7. Bloody show at term
  8. Uterine rupture
  9. Postpartum hemorrhage related to retroplacental myomas
  10. Rare etiologies such as uterine artery aneurysm or uterine arteriovenous malformations (AVM.) AVMs may be diagnosed following persistent vaginal bleeding after delivery or other uterine procedures
- Section II describes the differential diagnosis of vaginal bleeding in pregnancy.

WORKUP

- Gestation <20 wk
  1. Pelvic examination with vaginal/cervical cultures if appropriate
  2. Laparoscopy (if indicated)
  3. Laparotomy (rarely required)
  4. Ultrasound to verify viable intrauterine pregnancy when β-hCG levels achieve threshold values (≥1500 mIU/ml for transvaginal sonography). If viable intrauterine pregnancy, evaluate pregnancy and uterine cavity including placenta and placental location.
- Gestation >20 wk:
  1. Before pelvic examination, ultrasound for placental location, placental cord insertion, and placental evaluation
  2. If placenta previa or low-lying placenta, no bimanual examination
  3. If viable fetus, evaluation of fetal well-being as appropriate based on gestational age
  4. If suspected preterm labor, evaluate as clinically appropriate

LABORATORY TESTS

- Urine pregnancy test: If positive, get quantitative serum beta human chorionic gonadotropin (β-hCG). The following are typical although not entirely exclusive patterns:
  1. Early pregnancy: Follow serially every 48 hr
  2. Normal pregnancy: β-hCG doubles approximately every 48 hr
  3. Spontaneous abortion: β-hCG level will fall
  4. Ectopic pregnancy: β-hCG level will rise inappropriately (less than expected; threshold increase over 48 hr should be ≥66%)
  5. Molar pregnancy: β-hCG level is higher than expected for gestational age
- CBC
- Blood type and screen (Rh-negative patients need RhoGAM)
- Coagulation profile (particularly if moderate to heavy bleeding)
- Cervical/vaginal cultures, wet mount
- Pap smear for cervical malignancy; caution with biopsy as cervical biopsy sites in pregnancy can bleed extensively

IMAGING STUDIES

Ultrasound:

- 5 to 6 wk: Gestational sac (transvaginally); β-hCG >1500 mIU/ml is discriminatory level for visualization of a singleton gestation
- 6 to 7 wk: Fetal cardiac activity
- Molar pregnancy: Characteristic cluster of placental cysts
- Evaluate for evidence of subchorionic/submembranous hemorrhage
- Location of placenta and placental cord insertion (particularly if >20 wk)
- Degree of placental separation: Difficult to assess

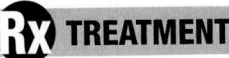

TREATMENT

NONPHARMACOLOGIC THERAPY

- Pelvic rest: No coitus, douching, or tampons
- Counseling: Genetic, bereavement (if indicated)
- For viable fetuses, ultrasound assessment of fetal growth and assessment of fetal well-being via external fetal monitoring as clinically appropriate
- Bed rest, if >20 wk (Recent studies show limited to no benefit of bed rest and possible increased medical and psychological risk to patients on activity restriction.)

ACUTE GENERAL Rx

- Hemodynamic stabilization with intravenous fluid administration and transfusion of blood products as clinically indicated
- Emergency D&C, laparoscopy, laparotomy, or cesarean delivery as necessary

REFERRAL

- If patient is unstable and needs emergency OB/GYN management and/or surgery
- If patient has suspected ectopic or molar pregnancy as immediate surgical treatment or medical intervention is indicated
- Perinatal consultation for high-risk pregnancies (placental disorders, placental abruption, vasa previa)
- Gynecologic oncology consultation if cervical carcinoma or hCG secreting tumor is suspected

SUGGESTED READINGS

Available at ExpertConsult.com

RELATED CONTENT

Abruptio Placentae (Related Key Topic)
Cervical Insufficiency (Related Key Topic)
Ectopic Pregnancy (Related Key Topic)
Molar Pregnancy (Related Key Topic)
Placenta Previa (Related Key Topic)
Sheehan's Syndrome (Related Key Topic)
Spontaneous Miscarriage (Related Key Topic)

AUTHOR: **JENNIFER B. MERRIMAN, M.D.**

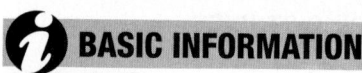

BASIC INFORMATION

DEFINITION

Vaginal malignancy is an abnormal proliferation of vaginal epithelium demonstrating malignant cells below the basement membrane.

SYNONYMS

Squamous cell carcinoma of the vagina
Adenocarcinoma of the vagina
Melanoma of the vagina
Sarcoma of the vagina
Endodermal sinus tumor

ICD-10CM CODE

C52 Malignant neoplasm of vagina

EPIDEMIOLOGY & DEMOGRAPHICS

INCIDENCE: There were an estimated 5170 new cases in 2018, and an estimated 910 deaths.

PREVALENCE: Vaginal cancer is the second rarest gynecologic cancer. It comprises 3% of malignancies of the female genital tract. It is more prevalent in women infected with HPV.

MEAN AGE AT DIAGNOSIS: Predominantly a disease of menopause. Mean age at diagnosis is 65.7 +/-14.3 yr.

PHYSICAL FINDINGS & CLINICAL PRESENTATION

- The signs and symptoms of invasive vaginal cancer (Fig. 1) are similar to those of cervical cancer. Majority of cases are asymptomatic.
- Postmenopausal vaginal bleeding and/or vaginal discharge are the most common symptoms.
- May also present as pelvic pain or pressure, dyspareunia, dysuria, malodor, or postcoital bleeding.
- May present as a vaginal lesion or abnormal Pap test.

ETIOLOGY

- The exact etiology is unknown.
- Approximately 80% to 90% of primary vaginal cancers are squamous cell carcinomas and 4% to 10% are adenocarcinomas.
- Most vaginal cancers are related to infection with HPV. It has been found in 65 percent of samples of invasive vaginal cancer and 93 percent of high-grade dysplastic vaginal lesions. Cervical cancers have similar risk factors.
- Vaginal intraepithelial neoplasia is believed to be a precursor for squamous cell carcinoma of the vagina.
- Prior pelvic radiation may be a risk factor.
- Clear-cell adenocarcinoma may be related to in utero diethylstilbestrol exposure (DES). Treatment of pregnant women with DES ended in the early 1970s, and it is anticipated that this spike in clear cell tumors will abate in the future.

Dx DIAGNOSIS

DIFFERENTIAL DIAGNOSIS

- Extension from another primary carcinoma is more common than primary vaginal cancer.
- Vaginitis.

WORKUP

- Diagnosis is made histologically by biopsy.
- Colposcopy and biopsy should follow suspicious Pap test.
- Cystoscopy, proctosigmoidoscopy, chest radiography, IV urography, and barium enema may be used for clinical staging.
- CT scan (Fig. 2), FDG, PET scan, and MRI are used to evaluate spread.
- Staging I to IV (Fig. 3).

IMAGING STUDIES

- Chest radiography, IV urography, and barium enema are used for staging.
- CT scan and MRI are good for assessing tumor spread.

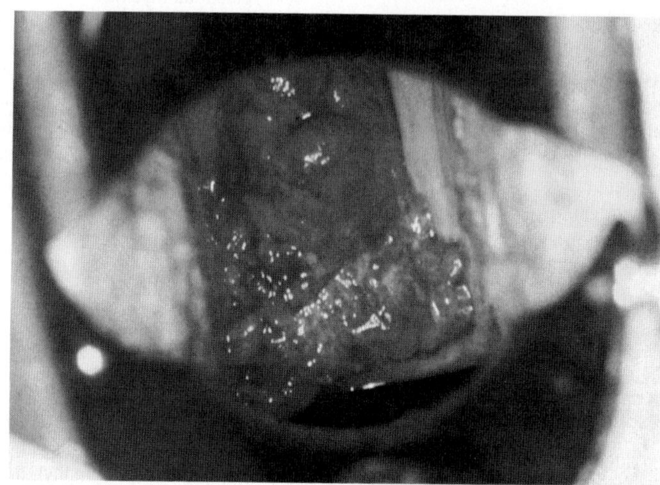

FIG 1 Lesion of the posterior fornix in squamous cell carcinoma. (From DiSaia, PJ et al: *Clinical Gynecologic Oncology*, ed 9, Philadelphia, 2018, Elsevier.)

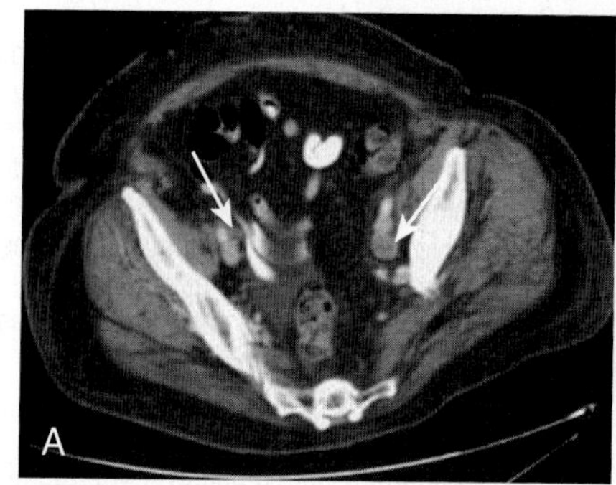
A

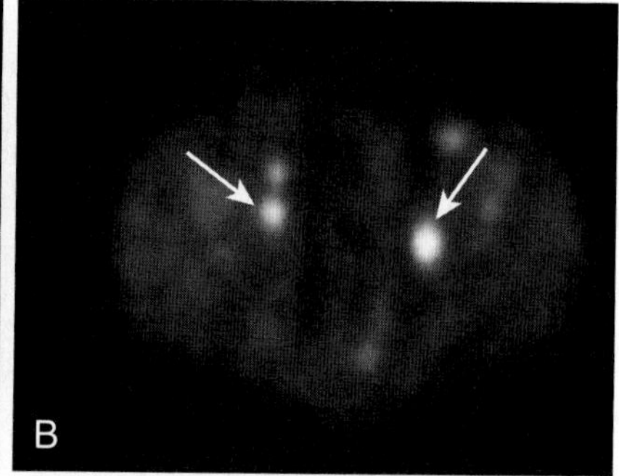
B

FIG. 2 Vaginal cancer with lymphadenopathy. A, computed tomography of pelvis showing mildly enlarged external iliac nodes suggestive of metastases *(arrows)*. **B,** Axial fluorodeoxyglucose-positron emission tomography scan showing hypermetabolic nodes as hyperintense spots confirming metastases. (From Abeloff MD: *Clinical oncology,* ed 3, Philadelphia, 2004, Churchill Livingstone.)

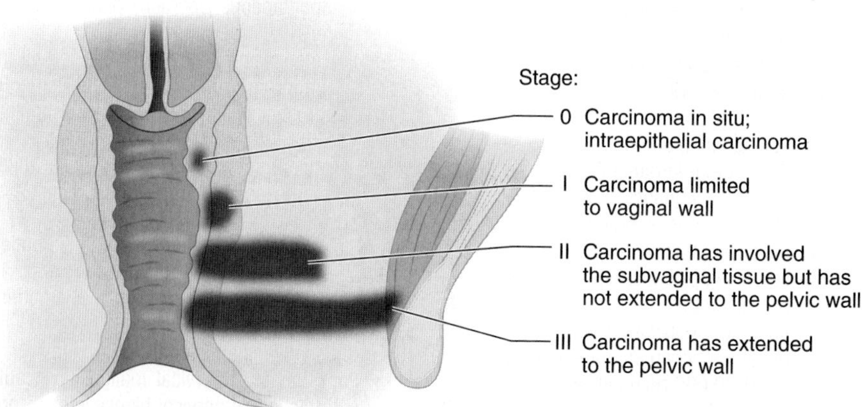
Stage:
0 Carcinoma in situ; intraepithelial carcinoma
I Carcinoma limited to vaginal wall
II Carcinoma has involved the subvaginal tissue but has not extended to the pelvic wall
III Carcinoma has extended to the pelvic wall

FIG. 3 Staging system for vaginal cancer. Metastatic disease that involves the bladder or rectum is stage IV_a. Metastatic disease beyond the pelvis is stage IV_b. (From Copeland LJ: *Textbook of gynecology,* ed 2, Philadelphia, 2000, Saunders.)

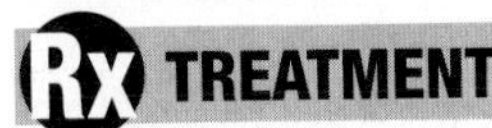

TREATMENT

- Radiation therapy is the mainstay of treatment.
- Stage I tumors that are small and confined to the posterior, upper third of the vagina may be treated with radical surgery.
- Other stages require a whole-pelvis, interstitial, and/or intracavitary radiation therapy.
- Chemotherapy is used in conjunction with radiotherapy in select select cases.
- Table 1 summarizes management of clear cell adenocarcinoma of the cervix and vagina.

DISPOSITION

Five-yr survival ranges from 85% for stage I to 13% for stage IV vaginal squamous cell carcinoma.

REFERRAL

Vaginal cancer should be managed by a gynecologic oncologist and radiation oncologist.

RELATED CONTENT

Vaginal Cancer (Patient Information)

SUGGESTED READING

Available at ExpertConsult.com

AUTHORS: **RUTH HENNEBERY, M.D.**, and **STEPHANIE JEAN, M.D.**

TABLE 1 Suggested Management of Clear Cell Adenocarcinoma of the Cervix and Vagina

Stage	Surgery	Radiation
Cervix		
I_b	Radical hysterectomy with clear vaginal margins and bilateral pelvic lymphadenectomy	5000 cGy of the whole pelvis in patients with positive pelvic nodes
II_a	Radical hysterectomy with bilateral pelvic lymphadenectomy and upper vaginectomy	5000 cGy of the whole pelvis in patients with positive pelvic nodes
II_b	Consider exenteration for radiation failures	5000 cGy of the whole pelvis, tandem, and ovoids
III_a and III_b	Consider exenteration for radiation failures	6000 cGy of the whole pelvis, tandem, and ovoids
IV	Individualize	
Vagina		
I (upper third of vagina)	Radical hysterectomy with bilateral pelvic lymphadenectomy and upper vaginectomy	5000 cGy of the whole pelvis in patients with positive nodes
I (lower two-thirds of vagina)	Radical hysterectomy with bilateral pelvic lymphadenectomy and total vaginectomy with vaginal reconstruction	5000 cGy of the whole pelvis, vaginal application, or interstitial implant
II	Consider exenteration for radiation failures	5000 cGy of the whole pelvis, interstitial implant
III	Consider exenteration for radiation failures	6000 cGy of the whole pelvis, interstitial implant
IV	Individualize	

From DiSaia PJ et al: *Clinical Gynecologic Oncology*, ed 9, Philadelphia, 2018, Elsevier.

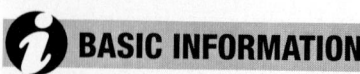

BASIC INFORMATION

DEFINITION

Prepubescent vulvovaginitis is an inflammatory condition of the vulva and vagina.

SYNONYM

Vulvovaginitis

ICD-10CM CODES
N76.0 Acute vaginitis
N76.1 Subacute and chronic vaginitis

EPIDEMIOLOGY & DEMOGRAPHICS

- Most common gynecologic problem of premenarchal girls.
- Prepubertal girls are susceptible to irritation and trauma because of the absence of protective hair and labial fat pads, as well as a lack of estrogenization leading to atrophic vaginal mucosa.
- Symptoms of vulvovaginitis and introital irritation and discharge account for 80% to 90% of gynecologic visits.
- Nonspecific etiology in approximately 75% of children with vulvovaginitis.
- Majority of vulvovaginitis in girls involves a primary irritation of the vulva with secondary involvement of the lower third of the vagina.

PHYSICAL FINDINGS & CLINICAL PRESENTATION

- Vulvar pain, dysuria, pruritus.
- Discharge is not a primary symptom but can occur.
- If present, vaginal discharge may be foul smelling or bloody.

ETIOLOGY

- Most commonly attributed to poor hygiene or nonspecific irritants. Etiologic factors in premenarcheal vulvovaginitis are summarized in Box 1.
- Hypoestrogenic state increases risk of infection or irritation due to:
  1. Higher vaginal pH (more hospitable to infectious agents)
  2. Underdeveloped labia minora and lack of significant adipose and hair of labia majora (less intrinsic protection of the vagina from trauma, irritants, infectious agents)
- Infections:
  1. Bacterial–often respiratory or enteric organisms
  2. Protozoal/parasitic
  3. Mycotic
  4. Viral
- Endocrine disorders
- Labial adhesions
- Skin disorders
- Sexual abuse
- Allergic substance
- Trauma
- Foreign body
- Masturbation
- Constipation

Section II describes the differential diagnosis of vaginal discharge in prepubertal girls.

Dx DIAGNOSIS

DIFFERENTIAL DIAGNOSIS

- Physiologic leukorrhea
- Foreign body
- Bacterial vaginosis
- Fungal vulvovaginitis
- Precocious puberty
- Sexual abuse and possibly an associated sexually transmitted infection such as gonorrhea, *Chlamydia*, or *Trichomonas*
- Pinworms

WORKUP

- Pelvic, genital examination; possibly speculum examination
- Rectal examination
- Vaginoscopy if considering a foreign body
- KOH and normal saline preparation of discharge
- Knee-chest position for examination may be easier for the child to tolerate. May need to consider exam under anesthesia for more thorough evaluation if necessary

Section III, "Vaginal Discharge," describes the evaluation of discharge.

LABORATORY TESTS

- Urinalysis to rule out urinary tract infection and diabetes
- Cultures including sexually transmitted diseases

Rx TREATMENT

NONPHARMACOLOGIC THERAPY

- Avoid tight clothing
- Appropriate hygiene education
- Avoid chemical irritants
- If foreign body, removal via irrigation or exam under anesthesia
- Reassurance

ACUTE GENERAL Rx

- *Streptococcal* and *staphylococcal* spp, *Haemophilus influenzae*: For children <20kg, ampicillin 25mg/kg q6h or amoxicillin 20mg/kg q12h for 5-10 days; for children >20kg, ampicillin 500mg q6h or amoxicillin 20mg/kg q12h for 5-10 days
- *Escherichia coli*: Azithromycin PO, 10mg/kg on day 1 and then 5mg/kg for 4 days
- *Proteus vulgaris*: TMP-SMX 5mg/kg q12h for 5-10 days
- *Chlamydia trachomatis*: For children <45kg, treat with erythromycin base or ethylsuccinate 50mg/kg/day PO QID x 14 days. For children ≥45kg but younger than 8 yr, treat with azithromycin 1g PO single dose. If older than 8 yr, also can consider doxycycline 100mg PO BID for 7 days.
- *Neisseria gonorrhoeae*: For children ≤45kg, treat with ceftriaxone 25-50mg/kg IV or IM in a single dose, not to exceed 125mg IM. Children >45kg should be treated with ceftriaxone 250mg IM plus azithromycin 1g PO once.
- *Trichomonas*: Metronidazole 125mg (or 15mg/kg/day) PO TID x 7 to 10 days
- Pinworms: Mebendazole 100mg chewable tablet, repeat in 2-3 weeks
- Labial agglutination: Spontaneous resolution or topical estrogen cream for 7 to 10 days. High degree of efficacy with topical estrogen

CHRONIC Rx

See "Referral."

DISPOSITION

Further education:
- Discuss appropriate hygiene.
- If sexually active, discuss pregnancy prevention and safe sexual practices. If there is suspicion of sexual abuse, report to child protective services.

REFERRAL

- To obstetrician/gynecologist, preferably a physician with specialized training in pediatric and adolescent gynecology if available
- To pediatrician

SUGGESTED READINGS

Available at ExpertConsult.com

RELATED CONTENT

Chlamydia Genital Infection (Related Key Topic)
Pruritus Vulvae (Related Key Topic)
Vaginitis, Fungal (Related Key Topic)
Vaginitis, *Trichomonas* (Related Key Topic)
Vaginosis, Bacterial (Related Key Topic)

AUTHOR: **MARGARET R. HINES, M.D.**

BOX 1 Etiologic Factors in Premenarcheal Vulvovaginitis

Bacterial Infections
Nonspecific mixed infections secondary to:
- Poor perineal hygiene
- Foreign body in vagina
- Respiratory tract infections
- Skin infections (impetigo)
- Urinary tract infection

Specific nonvenereal infection:
- Hemolytic streptococci (groups A, B, F)
- *Escherichia coli*
- *Shigella flexneri, Shigella sonnei*
- *Neisseria meningitidis, Neisseria sicca*
- *Haemophilus influenzae* type b, nontypeable strains
- *Streptococcus pneumoniae*
- *Corynebacterium diphtheriae*
- *Yersinia enterocolitica*
- *Mycobacterium tuberculosis*
- *Moraxella (Branhamella) catarrhalis*
- *Staphylococcus aureus*

Specific venereal infections:
- *Neisseria gonorrhoeae*
- *Treponema pallidum*
- *Chlamydia trachomatis*
- Chancroid *(Haemophilus ducreyi)*
- Granuloma inguinale

Bacterial vaginosis:
- *Gardnerella vaginalis*
- *Mobiluncus species*

Fungal infections:
- *Candida albicans*
- Other yeasts
- Dermatophytes

Protozoan and parasitic infections
- Trichomoniasis
- Amebiasis
- *Enterobius vermicularis*
- Hirudiniasis
- Schistosomiasis
- Other parasitic infections (ascariasis, trichuriasis)

Viral Infections
Venereal:
- Herpes simplex
- Condyloma acuminatum (papillomavirus)
- Molluscum contagiosum

Involvement as part of systemic infection:
- Measles
- Varicella
- Mononucleosis (Epstein-Barr virus)
- Coxsackievirus
- Smallpox

Infestations
- Pediculosis
- Scabies

Contact irritation or allergic reactions
- Bubble bath preparations
- Hair shampoos
- Vulvar deodorant sprays
- Soaps, laundry detergents
- Other medications

Vulvar or perineal skin diseases
Local:
- Seborrhea
- Lichen sclerosus et atrophicus
- Lichen planus
- Lichen simplex chronicus
- Premalignant leukoplakia
- Erythrasma (*Corynebacterium minutissimum*)
- Bartholinitis
- Skenitis

Involvement as part of a systemic disorder:
- Psoriasis
- Bullous pemphigoid
- Atopic dermatitis
- Drug eruption
- Generalized pruritus with excoriation
- Chronic liver disease
- Chronic renal disease
- Metabolic errors
- Psychosomatic
- Crohn disease
- Sjögren's syndrome
- Henoch-Schönlein purpura
- Histiocytosis
- Kawasaki disease
- Stevens-Johnson syndrome
- Typhoid
- Zinc deficiency

Physical factors
- Sand (sandbox)
- Chemical or thermal trauma
- Physical trauma (accidents, abuse, masturbation)
- Nylon, rayon underclothing
- Tight garments (maceration in warm climates)

Anatomic abnormalities:
- Neoplasms (sarcoma botryoides)
- Polyps
- Labial agglutination, adhesion
- Prolapsed urethra
- Ectopic ureter
- Rectal fistula
- Draining pelvic abscess via fistula

From Cherry JD et al: *Feigin and Cherry's textbook of pediatric infectious diseases*, ed 8, Philadelphia, 2019, Elsevier.

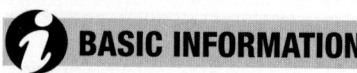

BASIC INFORMATION

DEFINITION

Trichomonas vulvovaginitis is the inflammation of vulva and vagina caused by *Trichomonas* spp.

SYNONYMS

Trichomonas vaginalis
Trichomoniasis
TV

ICD-10CM CODE

A59.01 Trichomonal vulvovaginitis

EPIDEMIOLOGY & DEMOGRAPHICS

- Acquired through sexual contact
- Diagnosed in
  1. 50% to 75% of prostitutes
  2. 5% to 15% of women visiting gynecology clinics
  3. 7% to 32% of women in sexually transmitted disease (STD) clinics
  4. 5% of women in family planning clinics
  5. 8% to 13% of black women, 0.8% to 1.8% of non-Hispanic white women
  6. >11% of women ≥40 yr old
- Most prevalent nonviral sexually transmitted infection in the U.S.

PHYSICAL FINDINGS & CLINICAL PRESENTATION

These symptoms and physical findings may or may not be present depending on the case:

- Yellow-green, malodorous vaginal discharge
- Vaginal and/or vulvar pruritus
- Dysuria
- Dyspareunia
- Intense erythema of the vaginal mucosa
- Cervical petechiae ("strawberry cervix")
- Infected men may have symptoms of urethritis, epididymitis, or prostatitis
- Asymptomatic in ~50% of women and 90% of men

ETIOLOGY

Single-cell protozoan *Trichomonas vaginalis*

RISK FACTORS

- Multiple sexual partners
- History of previous STDs
- HIV infection

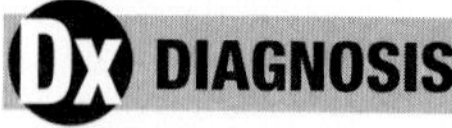

DIAGNOSIS

DIFFERENTIAL DIAGNOSIS (TABLE E1)

- Bacterial vaginosis
- Fungal vulvovaginitis
- Atrophic vulvovaginitis
- Vaginal or cervical infection with other sexually transmitted infections such as gonorrhea or chlamydia

WORKUP

- Pelvic examination
- Speculum examination
- Evaluation for mobile trichomonads seen on normal saline preparation (Fig. E1): 30% to 70% sensitivity; even lower sensitivity if there is a delay in evaluating slides
- Assessment of vaginal pH: Trichomonas is associated with elevated pH (>5) of vaginal discharge
- Laboratory testing (see below)

LABORATORY TESTS

- Nucleic acid amplification tests (NAATs) have been developed that combine excellent performance characteristics (sensitivity and specificity >95%) with a more rapid turnaround time compared with culture. Thus, they are now considered better laboratory tests than culture. There are two commercially available NAATs in the U.S.:
  1. APTIMA assays (Hologic Gen-Probe, San Diego, CA)
  2. BD Probe Tec TV Q^X Amplified DNA Assay (Becton Dickinson, Franklin Lakes, NJ)
- Rapid tests are also available:
  1. The OSOM Trichomonas Rapid test (Sekisui Diagnostics, Framingham, MA) is an antigen detection test on vaginal secretions. It provides results in 10 min and can be done as a point-of-care test. It has a sensitivity of 82% and a specificity of 97%-100%.
  2. The Affirm VP III (Becton Dickinson, Sparks, MD) is a DNA hybridization probe test; results are available within 45 min. Sensitivity is 63% and specificity is more than 99%.
- Culture, when available, is considered the traditional gold standard laboratory test for diagnosis of trichomonas, with sensitivity 75%-96% and specificity approaching 100%.

Rx TREATMENT

NONPHARMACOLOGIC THERAPY

Condom use: The best way to prevent trichomoniasis is through consistent and correct use of condoms during all penile-vaginal sexual encounters

ACUTE GENERAL Rx

- Preferred initial treatment: Metronidazole 2 g PO × 1 *or* tinidazole single 2-g oral dose in both sexes. Treatment of the sexual partner is essential to prevent reinfection.
- Alternative regimen: Metronidazole 500 mg PO BID × 7 days.
- Alcohol consumption should be avoided during treatment with metronidazole (at least 24 hr after completion of therapy) and tinidazole (at least 72 hr after completion of therapy) to reduce possibility of disulfiram-like reaction.
- CDC recommends retesting sexually active women within 3 mo of treatment to assess for possible reinfection.

CHRONIC Rx

- For persistent infections, the CDC recommends first trying metronidazole 500 mg PO BID × 7 days.
- If treatment is still unsuccessful, proceed with metronidazole or tinidazole 2 g PO daily × 7 days.
- Allergy, intolerance, or adverse reactions: Alternatives to metronidazole or tinidazole are not recommended. Patients who are allergic to nitroimidazoles can be managed by desensitization.
- Pregnancy:
  1. Associated with adverse outcomes (i.e., premature rupture of membranes, preterm delivery), although it is unclear whether treatment decreases the incidence of these outcomes.
  2. Treat with metronidazole 2 g PO × 1 day; avoid tinidazole as there is little known about tinidazole in pregnancy.

DISPOSITION

- *Trichomonas* infection is considered an STD; therefore, treatment of the sexual partner is necessary.
- *T. vaginalis* infection is associated with two- to threefold increased risk for HIV acquisition.
- *T. vaginalis* infection in pregnancy is associated with premature rupture of membranes, preterm birth, and delivery of low birthweight infants.

REFERRAL

To obstetrician/gynecologist for recurrence and pregnancy

SUGGESTED READINGS

Available at ExpertConsult.com

RELATED CONTENT

Trichomoniasis (Patient Information)
Pruritus Vulvae (Related Key Topic)

AUTHOR: **MARGARET R. HINES, M.D.**

BASIC INFORMATION

DEFINITION

Bacterial vaginosis (BV) is a polymicrobial infection in which anaerobic bacteria overgrow and replace the normal hydrogen peroxide-producing lactobacilli, resulting in thin, gray, and malodorous vaginal discharge.

SYNONYMS

Bacterial vaginosis
BV
Nonspecific vaginitis
Gardnerella vaginalis vaginitis

ICD-10CM CODES

N76.0 Acute vaginitis
N77.1 Vaginitis, vulvitis and vulvovaginitis in diseases classified elsewhere

EPIDEMIOLOGY & DEMOGRAPHICS

- Most common cause of vaginal discharge.
- Most common organisms include *Gardnerella vaginalis, Mycoplasma hominis, Bacteroides* species, *Peptostreptococcus* species, *Fusobacterium* species, *Prevotella* species, and *Atopobium vaginae* and other anaerobes.
- Women with BV are at increased risk for acquiring other sexually transmitted diseases (STDs) such as HIV, *N. gonorrhoeae*, *C. trachomatis,* and HSV-2. Also associated with pelvic inflammatory disease (PID) and complications after gynecologic surgery. Preoperative evaluation and treatment before planned hysterectomy or abortion decreases the infection complication rate.
- May be associated with low birthweight, premature rupture of membranes (PROM), and prematurity.
- BV may recur in 30% within the first 3 mo after treatment, which may be due to:
  1. Persistence of pathogenic bacteria
  2. Reinfection from exogenous sources including sexual partners
  3. Failure of the normal lactobacillus-dominant flora to reestablish
- Risk factors: Multiple female or male sexual partners, sexually transmitted infections, douching, tobacco use, lack of condom use, and lack of vaginal lactobacilli.

PHYSICAL FINDINGS & CLINICAL PRESENTATION

- 50% to 75% of patients are asymptomatic.
- A thin, dull, and gray homogeneous discharge (Fig. E1)
- Characterized by a "fishy" odor from the vagina
- Vaginal pH >4.5
- Clue cells on microscopic examination (Fig. E2)

ETIOLOGY

- *Gardnerella vaginalis* detected in 40% to 50% of vaginal secretions.
- Increase in vaginal pH secondary to decrease in hydrogen peroxide producing lactobacilli allows predominance of anaerobes that produce amines.
- It is unclear how the vaginal floral imbalance occurs and the role sexual activity plays in the pathogenesis of BV.
- *G. vaginalis* may be important in epithelial biofilm formation.
- Ethnicity and age may contribute to the vaginal microbial environment.

DIAGNOSIS

WORKUP

At least three of Amsel's clinical diagnostic criteria

- Sensitivity of 92% and specificity of 77%:
  1. Thin, gray, and homogeneous, malodorous discharge that adheres to the vaginal walls.
  2. Vaginal pH >4.5.
  3. Positive whiff-amine test:
     a. Conducted by placing wet mount specimen and adding 10% potassium hydroxide, which creates a fishy odor.
  4. More than 20% of the epithelial cells are clue cells on microscopy.
- Gram staining: Considered the gold-standard laboratory method to determine the concentration of lactobacilli and gram-negative and gram-positive bacteria.
- If microscopy is unavailable, other diagnostic tests include Affirm VPIII (Becton Dickinson, Sparks, M.D.), which is a DNA-hybridization probe test for high concentrations of *G. vaginalis*, and the OSOM BV Blue test (Sekisui Diagnostics, Framingham, MA), which detects vaginal fluid sialidase activity.
- Cultures are unnecessary.
- Pap smear is not a reliable test for BV.
- Rule out other causes such as vulvar diseases, STDs, and atrophic vaginitis.

TREATMENT

ACUTE GENERAL Rx

- Recommended regimens (similar efficacy):
  1. Metronidazole 500 mg PO BID for 7 days *or*
  2. Metronidazole 0.75% gel, one full applicator (5 gm) intravaginally daily for 5 days *or*
  3. Clindamycin 2% cream, one full applicator (5 gm) intravaginally at bedtime for 7 days
- Alternate regimens:
  1. Clindamycin 300 mg PO bid for 7 days or clindamycin 100 mg ovules intravaginally once at bedtime for 3 days. May be associated with antimicrobial resistance.
  2. Tinidazole 1g PO once daily for 5 days. Longer half life than metronidazole (~12-14 hr vs. ~6-7 hr)
  3. Secnidazole 2g PO once. Longer half life than metronidazole (~17 hr vs ~8 hr). Shown to be superior to placebo in plase 3 trial and at least as effective as metronidazole 500 mg PO BID in non-inferiority trial.
- Disulfiram-type reactions may occur while taking oral or topical metronidazole and patients should be advised to avoid alcohol while undergoing treatment.
- Sexual partners: It is not necessary to treat male partners of affected females; however, females who partner with females need to be aware of the signs and symptoms of BV, and treatment is indicated in this population if symptoms occur.
- Follow-up visits after treatment and resolution of symptoms are unnecessary, but patients are advised to return if symptoms recur.
- Not enough evidence for or against probiotic use for treatment and prevention.
- Clindamycin cream may weaken latex condoms if used together. Avoid treatment of asymptomatic patients.
- Treatment in pregnancy:
  1. Symptomatic pregnant patients with BV should be treated to relieve bothersome symptoms.
  2. Insufficient evidence to recommend routine screening for BV in asymptomatic pregnant women at high or low risk of preterm delivery.
  3. Can use oral or topical therapy for symptomatic pregnant women with same regimen as nonpregnant women.
  4. There is no evidence that metronidazole or clindamycin have any teratogenic effect during pregnancy. Tinidazole should be avoided in pregnancy.
- Recurrent BV:
  1. Condom use may help reduce the risk of recurrence.
  2. Chronic suppressive therapy has been proven to reduce the development or recurrence of BV.

PEARLS & CONSIDERATIONS

- BV is the most common cause of vaginitis in reproductive women.
- BV has been associated with PID, postprocedural gynecologic complications, and other STDs. It is reasonable to treat asymptomatic women who are to undergo gynecologic surgery and screen for other STDs.
- ACOG, USPSTF, and CDC all agree to not routinely screen and treat all pregnant women with asymptomatic BV to prevent preterm birth.

SUGGESTED READINGS

Available at ExpertConsult.com

RELATED CONTENT

Bacterial Vaginal Infections (Patient Information)

AUTHORS: **NEHA RANA, M.D.**, and **EMILY K. SAKS, M.D., M.S.C.E.**

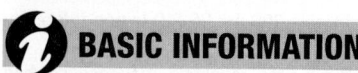

BASIC INFORMATION

DEFINITION

Enterococci are gram-positive, facultative anaerobic organisms usually oval in shape and can be seen as single cells, pairs, or chains. Vancomycin-resistant *Enterococcus* (VRE) are enterococci that have become resistant to vancomycin and several antibiotics normally used to treat enterococcal infections.

SYNONYM

VRE

ICD-10CM CODE

Z16.39 Resistance to other specified antimicrobial drug

EPIDEMIOLOGY & DEMOGRAPHICS

INCIDENCE: VRE may be associated with the use of specific classes of antibiotics.

PEAK INCIDENCE: VRE was first reported in Europe in 1986, and there has been a steady rise in the incidence of enterococcal strains resistant to vancomycin. In 2007, 80% of *E. faecium* isolates and 7% of *E. faecalis* isolates were resistant to vancomycin.

PREVALENCE: 80% of *E. faecium* are VRE; 69% of *E. faecalis* are VRE.

RISK FACTORS:

- Prior antimicrobial therapy, especially vancomycin
- Prolonged hospitalization
- Chronic medical conditions, renal failure
- Invasive devices
- ICU stay
- Colonization: VRE colonize the gastrointestinal tract; can be found on skin or perirectal swab culture or stool culture

PHYSICAL FINDINGS & CLINICAL PRESENTATION

Patients may be asymptomatic and have gastrointestinal colonization; it can be associated with diarrhea. In hospitalized patients, infection is associated with colonization and can cause wound infections, bacteremia, abscesses (intraabdominal), and, rarely, pneumonia, urinary tract infections, and endocarditis.

ETIOLOGY

- The Clinical and Laboratory Standards Institute uses the following MIC definitions for vancomycin susceptibility and resistance in enterococci:
    1. Vancomycin susceptible: ≤4 mcg/ml
    2. Vancomycin resistant: ≥32 mcg/ml
    3. Vancomycin intermediate: 8 to 16 mcg/ml (vancomycin not recommended)
- Enterococci are primarily found in the human digestive tract and female genital tract, where they make up a significant portion of the normal bacterial population in healthy people. Enterococci can cause urinary tract, wound, bloodstream, heart valve, and brain infections. In the great majority of cases, VRE infections occur in hospitalized patients who have compromised immune systems. Most cases of VRE are caused by the *E. faecium* strains that have acquired resistance when they came in contact with other bacteria and shared genetic information.
- VRE is most commonly transmitted from one patient to another by health care workers whose hands have become contaminated inadvertently with feces or fluids of a person carrying the organism. VRE are not airborne but can survive on surfaces for several weeks.

Dx DIAGNOSIS

DIFFERENTIAL DIAGNOSIS

- Other bacterial pathogens in blood, wounds, or urine.
- Once colonized, increased incidence to become infected

LABORATORY TESTS

- VRE rectal culture
- VRE stool culture
- Blood, urine, and wound cultures

Rx TREATMENT

- For rectal or stool colonization, therapy is not recommended.
- Therapy is complicated by the fact that strains exhibit inherent resistance to many commonly used antibiotics.
- More than 80% of vancomycin-resistant *E. faecium* strains are also resistant to ampicillin.
- In symptomatic patients, if VRE strains are known to be susceptible, potential therapeutic agents include:
    1. Linezolid: 600 mg IV or PO q12h
    2. Daptomycin: 4 mg/kg/day IV for nonbacteremia infections and 6 mg/kg/day IV for bacteremias
    3. Tigecycline: 100 mg IV load dose, then 50 mg IV q 12 hr. Although not specifically FDA approved for VRE strains, it offers an option for patients intolerant to other agents
    4. Quinupristin-dalfopristin (Synercid) only effective for *E. faecium* strains with no activity for *E. faecalis* strains: 7.5 mg/kg q8 to 12h. Can cause severe myalgias and arthralgias and venous irritation that often requires use of a central line, which has limited the use of this antibiotic
    5. Salvage regimens for severe VRE infections include:
        a. Daptomycin plus gentamicin and/or ampicillin or ceftaroline
        b. Daptomycin plus tigecycline
    6. The Healthcare Infection Control Practices Advisory Committee recommends that three negative stool/rectal cultures be obtained at weekly intervals to remove a patient from contact precautions.

REFERRAL

To infectious disease specialist

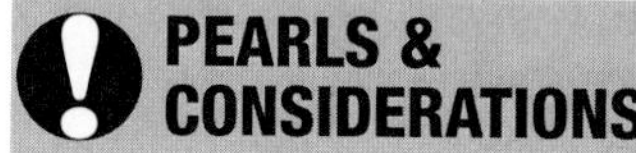

PEARLS & CONSIDERATIONS

COMMENTS

- Patients who are colonized with VRE have about an 8% rate of developing a true VRE infection in hospital or after discharge. The rate is higher in immunocompromised and severely ill patients.
- Incidence increases with comorbidity and hospitalization.
- The number of patients already colonized with VRE in a defined geographic area (colonization pressure) is the most significant factor for predicting new acquisition of VRE.
- An association between VRE colonization and *Clostridium difficile* infection has been reported in patients with hematologic malignancies.

PREVENTION

- Hand hygiene: Most important and practical method of preventing spread in hospital environment. Soap and water (used as a 30-sec wash) and alcohol-based hand rubs are effective, as is chlorhexidine.
- Cohorting and isolation techniques: Use of private rooms and use of gowns and gloves has been shown to decrease the risk of spread of multidrug-resistant bacteria.
- Cleaning contaminated objects or surfaces with standard hospital disinfectants, antibiotic management (prudent vancomycin use), and surveillance also help prevent spread.

SUGGESTED READINGS

Available at ExpertConsult.com

RELATED CONTENT

Health Care-Related Infections (Related Key Topic)

AUTHOR: **GLENN G. FORT, M.D., M.P.H.**

BASIC INFORMATION

DEFINITION

Vasculitis refers generically to inflammation occurring within the walls of blood vessels. Blood vessel inflammation can result in either perforation of affected vessels with hemorrhage into adjacent structures or thrombosis with subsequent ischemia and infarction of supplied tissues. Vasculitis can occur as a primary process or secondary to another connective tissue disease, infection, or drug exposure. The systemic vasculitides are a heterogeneous group of disorders (Table 1) characterized by blood vessel inflammation affecting vessels of varying size and location resulting in a wide range of clinical manifestations dictated largely by which vessels are affected (Fig. 1). Vasculitis is traditionally classified according to the size of the blood vessels predominantly affected (Table 2). Antineutrophilic cytoplasmic autoantibody (ANCA)-associated vasculitis (AAV) includes granulomatosis with polyangiitis (GPA); microscopic polyangiitis (MPA), including renal-limited vasculitis (RLV); and eosinophilic granulomatosis with polyangiitis (EGPA, Churg-Strauss). All are associated with ANCA and have similar features on renal histology (e.g., a focal necrotizing, and often crescentic, pauci-immune glomerulonephritis). Several of these are covered in individual topics, including topics on granulomatosis with polyangiitis (GPA), polyarteritis nodosa (PAN), giant cell arteritis (GCA), Takayasu arteritis, and Henoch-Schönlein purpura (HSP). Severity varies between and within specific vasculitides from a relatively benign, self-limited process to severe, life-threatening multisystem organ involvement with significant morbidity and mortality.

SYNONYM

None

ICD-10CM CODES

M30.0	Polyarteritis nodosa
M30.3	Mucocutaneous lymph node syndrome [Kawasaki]
M31.30 31	Wegener's granulomatosis without renal involvement
M31.5	Giant cell arteritis with polymyalgia rheumatica
M31.6	Other giant cell arteritis
M31.4	Aortic arch syndrome [Takayasu]
D 69.0	Allergic purpura
L95.9	Vasculitis limited to the skin, unspecified

EPIDEMIOLOGY & DEMOGRAPHICS

- The epidemiology and demographics of the various vasculitides vary by the individual disease and, where applicable, are covered under the relevant vasculitis disease chapters.
- The most common form of systemic vasculitis in the U.S. is giant cell arteritis, with an approximate incidence of 170 cases per 1 million per yr in individuals older than 50 yr.
- Antineutrophil cytoplasmic antibodies (ANCA)-associated vasculitis is significantly less common with aggregate incidence estimated at approximately 20 per million in the U.S.
- Age distribution can demonstrate significant variability between the vasculitides as shown by the fact that GCA generally does not occur before age 50, while 90% of cases of HSP occur in the pediatric population, and 80% of patients with Kawasaki disease are under age 5.

TABLE 1 Comparing the Vasculitides

Disease	Pathophysiology	Classic Features	Testing	Treatment
Giant cell arteritis	Mononuclear cell infiltration and giant cell formation	Headache, scalp tenderness, visual disturbance	ESR CRP biopsy	Prednisone and aspirin
Takayasu arteritis	Mononuclear cell infiltration and giant cell formation	Visual disturbance, chest pain, abdominal pain, differences in extremity blood pressure and pulses	Angiography	Prednisone Surgical or angiographic intervention
Polyarteritis nodosa	Polymorphonuclear infiltration	Fever, hypertension, myalgias, abdominal pain, hematuria, CHF, GI bleeding, orchitis	ESR, CRP biopsy Angiography	Prednisone (mild disease) plus cyclophosphamide (moderate-severe disease) Antiviral therapy if concurrent hepatitis B or C Azathioprine or methotrexate for maintenance of remission
Kawasaki disease	Polymorphonuclear infiltration	5-day fever, conjunctivitis, oral lesions, rash, red palms and soles, edema, cervical lymphadenopathy	ESR, CRP Leukocytosis Thrombocytosis Echocardiography	Aspirin plus IV gamma globulin
Granulomatosis with polyangiitis (Wegener granulomatosis)	Granuloma formation secondary to aggregating neutrophils	Upper and lower respiratory symptoms, renal insufficiency, skin lesions, visual disturbance	ESR CRP c-ANCA	Prednisone and methotrexate (mild disease) Cyclophosphamide or rituximab plus prednisone (moderate to severe disease)
Eosinophilic granulomatosis with polyangiitis (Churg-Strauss syndrome)	Eosinophilic infiltration Allergic granulomas	Allergic rhinitis, nasal polyps, asthma	Leukocytosis Eosinophilia ESR, CRP biopsy	Prednisone with or without cyclophosphamide
Henoch-Schönlein purpura	IgA complex deposition	Palpable purpura, arthralgias, GI disturbances, glomerulonephritis	Leukocytosis Eosinophilia Ig A elevation, skin biopsy	Usually self-limited NSAIDs Prednisone if necessary Rituximab (refractory cases)
Cryoglobulinemic vasculitis	Cold precipitable monoclonal or polyclonal immunoglobulins	Palpable purpura, glomerulonephritis, myalgias, weakness, peripheral neuropathy	Low complement levels, hepatitis C Renal biopsy	Rituximab with or without prednisone Peg interferon plus ribavirin (HCV infection)
Cutaneous leukocytoclastic vasculitis	Neutrophilic infiltration Mononuclear and eosinophilic infiltration	Palpable purpura, macules, vesicles, bullae, urticaria	Skin biopsy	Prednisone Colchicine Dapsone
Behçet syndrome	Polymorphonuclear infiltration	Recurrent oral aphthous ulcers, genital ulcers, skin lesions, visual disturbance	ESR, CRP leukocytosis Oral mucosa autoantibodies	Topical corticosteroids Prednisone with azathioprine (end-organ disease) Colchicine (aphthous ulcer and arthritis) Infliximab (refractory disease)

c-ANCA, Cytoplasmic antineutrophil cytoplasmic antibody; *CHF*, congestive heart failure; *CRP*, C-reactive protein; *ESR*, erythrocyte sedimentation rate; *GI*, gastrointestinal; *IgA*, immunoglobulin A; *IV*, intravenous.
From Adams JG, et al.: *Emergency medicine, clinical essentials*, ed 2, Philadelphia, 2013, Elsevier.

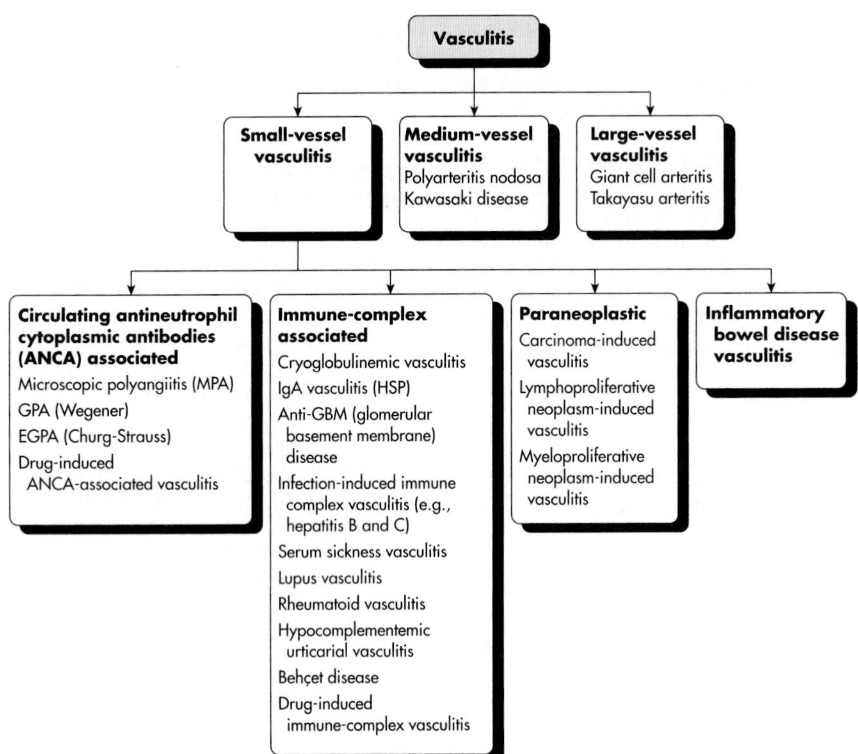

FIG. 1 Major categories of noninfectious vasculitis. Not included are vasculitides that are known to be caused by direct invasion of vessel walls by infectious pathogens, such as rickettsial vasculitis and neisserial vasculitis. *EGPA,* Eosinophilic granulomatous polyangiitis; *GPA,* granulomatous polyangiitis; *HSP,* Henoch-Schönlein purpura. (From Floege J, et al.: *Comprehensive clinical nephrology,* ed 6, Philadelphia, 2019, Saunders.)

- Although genetic factors clearly play a role in disease susceptibility, familial cases of vasculitis are rare.

PHYSICAL FINDINGS & CLINICAL PRESENTATION

- Clinical presentation often includes nonspecific constitutional symptoms including fever, malaise, headache, and weight loss.
- Signs and symptoms are generally dictated by the tropism of involved vessels.
- Skin manifestations of vasculitis include petechiae, palpable purpura (Fig. 2), subcutaneous nodules, livedo reticularis, ulcerations, and digital ischemia.
- Kidney involvement of medium-sized and large vessel vasculitis is often in the form of renovascular hypertension. Glomerulonephritis may be seen in small vessel vasculitis.
- Pulmonary small vessel involvement can cause alveolar hemorrhage, which can present with cough, dyspnea, and alveolar hemorrhage.
- Mononeuritis multiplex is the characteristic finding of vasculitis affecting the vasa nervorum of the peripheral nervous system.
- Gastrointestinal involvement of the mesenteric vasculature can cause postprandial pain, bleeding, and perforation.
- Arthritis, while nonspecific, can be present.
- Significant clinical variability exists between the various vasculitides, although overlapping symptoms may be seen.

ETIOLOGY

Most forms of systemic vasculitis are of unknown etiology. Cryoglobulinemia vasculitis is often secondary to hepatitis C infection, and cutaneous leukocytoclastic vasculitis is often related to a drug exposure.

Dx DIAGNOSIS

DIFFERENTIAL DIAGNOSIS

- Infective endocarditis
- Atrial myxoma
- Cholesterol emboli
- Malignancy
- Hypercoagulopathy
- Congenital collagen vascular disorder

WORKUP

- The diagnosis of most forms of systemic vasculitis relies on the history and physical examination as well as supportive laboratory testing. Table 3 describes differential diagnostic features of selected forms of small vessel vasculitis.
- Tissue biopsy is important in establishing an accurate diagnosis; biopsy sites should target affected tissues.
- Imaging such as mesenteric angiography can be supportive and may obviate the need for tissue biopsy.

LABORATORY TESTS

- Laboratory markers of systemic inflammation include an elevated erythrocyte sedimentation rate (ESR), C-reactive protein (CRP), and an anemia of chronic disease.
- ANCA targeting myeloperoxidase (MPO) and proteinase 3 (PR3) are frequently found in several small vessel vasculitides, including GPA (Wegener), microscopic polyangiitis (MPA), and Churg-Strauss syndrome (CSS).
- Hepatitis C antibodies and rheumatoid factor are often present in cryoglobulinemic vasculitis.
- Urinalysis in patients with glomerulonephritis due to small vessel ANCA-associated vasculitis will generally demonstrate hematuria with active urinary sediment with red blood cell casts and proteinuria.

IMAGING STUDIES

- Angiography can demonstrate vascular narrowing and aneurysm formation in suspected medium-size and large-vessel vasculitis.
- Pulmonary and sinus CT scans can demonstrate active pulmonary and upper airway disease in ANCA-associated vasculitis.

TABLE 2 Classification Scheme of Vasculitides According to Size of Predominant Blood Vessels Involved

- Primary vasculitides
- Predominantly large vessel vasculitides
- Takayasu arteritis
- Giant cell arteritis (temporal arteritis)
- Cogan syndrome
- Behçet's disease*
- Predominantly medium-sized vessel vasculitides
- Polyarteritis nodosa
- Cutaneous polyarteritis nodosa
- Buerger disease
- Kawasaki disease
- Primary angiitis of the central nervous system
- Predominantly small vessel vasculitides
- Immune complex mediated
- Goodpasture disease (anti-glomerular basement membrane disease)†
  1. Cutaneous leukocytoclastic angiitis ("hypersensitivity vasculitis")
  2. Henoch-Schönlein purpura
  3. Hypocomplementemic urticarial vasculitis
  4. Essential cryoglobulinemia‡
  5. Erythema elevatum diutinum
- ANCA-associated disorders§
  1. Granulomatosis with polyangiitis (GPA, Wegener granulomatosis)‡
  2. Microscopic polyangiitis (MPA)‡
  3. Eosinophilic granulomatosis with polyangiitis (EGPA, Churg-Strauss syndrome)‡
  4. Renal-limited vasculitis (RLV)
- Secondary forms of vasculitis
- Miscellaneous small vessel vasculitides
- Connective tissue disorders‡ (rheumatoid vasculitis, lupus erythematosus, Sjögren's syndrome, inflammatory myopathy)
- Inflammatory bowel disease
- Paraneoplastic
- Infection
- Drug-induced vasculitis: ANCA-associated, other

ANCA, Antineutrophil cytoplasmic antibody.
*May involve small, medium-sized, and large blood vessels.
†Immune complexes formed in situ, in contrast to other forms of immune complex–mediated vasculitis.
‡Frequent overlap of small and medium-sized blood vessel involvement.
§Not all forms of these disorders are always associated with ANCA.
From Firestein G, et al.: *Kelley's textbook of rheumatology,* ed 8, Philadelphia, 2008, Saunders.

Rx TREATMENT

Treatment of vasculitis depends on the specific type of vasculitis and is tailored to the severity of disease activity. Novel treatments are covered under the relevant vasculitis disease chapters.

ACUTE GENERAL Rx

- Systemic corticosteroids are generally required to gain initial control of active disease although mild cases of drug-induced cutaneous leukocytoclastic vasculitis can often be treated with NSAIDs and cessation of the offending medication.

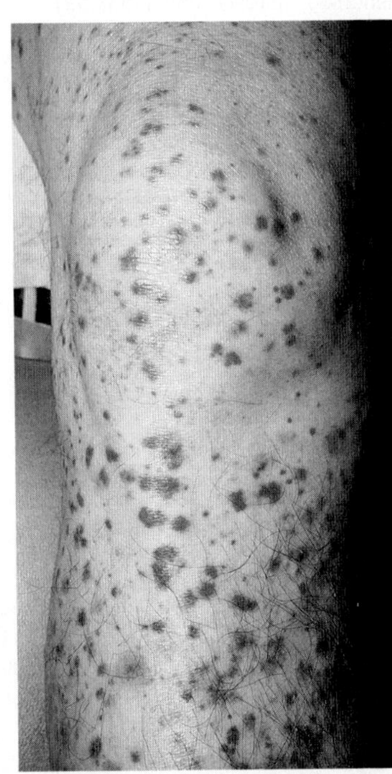

FIG. 2 Leukocytoclastic vasculitis, palpable purpura. (From James W, et al.: *Andrews' diseases of the skin, clinical dermatology,* ed 10, Philadelphia, 2005, Saunders.)

- GCA, HSP, and vasculitis limited to the skin, including cutaneous PAN, can often be managed without further immunosuppression.
- Major organ-threatening disease in systemic vasculitis has traditionally been treated with oral or intravenous cyclophosphamide for induction of remission.
- Studies have demonstrated noninferiority of rituximab compared to cyclophosphamide in ANCA-associated vasculitis with major organ involvement, and it is approved for this use.
- Rituximab with prednisone has also recently been shown to be effective in the treatment of relapsing flares of disease activity in ANCA-associated vasculitis.
- Similarly, rituximab has been used for maintenance of remission.
- Less severe disease such as granulomatosis with polyangiitis limited to the upper airways can be managed with methotrexate rather than cyclophosphamide.
- Trimethoprim/sulfamethoxazole should be used to prevent *Pneumocystis carinii* infection with concurrent immunosuppressive therapy.
- The goal of acute therapy is to induce remission of disease activity and is generally continued for 1 to 2 mo once this is achieved, at which point chronic therapy is used to prevent disease relapse.

CHRONIC Rx

- The goal of chronic therapy is to prevent disease relapse and minimize medication side effects.
- Steroids are gradually tapered as allowed by disease activity.
- Immunomodulatory agents such as methotrexate or azathioprine are commonly used for maintenance therapy in place of cyclophosphamide to reduce side effects.
- Cryoglobulinemic vasculitis due to chronic hepatitis C will often improve with treatment of the underlying viral infection.
- Rituximab may also be an appropriate remission maintenance agent in ANCA-associated vasculitis, although frequency of dosing and duration of therapy are not yet well characterized.

DISPOSITION

Varies widely among the various vasculitides

REFERRAL

Systemic vasculitis care is generally coordinated by a rheumatologist. Renal, pulmonary, neurologic, and gastrointestinal consultation is often needed when vasculitis involves these organ systems. Isolated cutaneous leukocytoclastic vasculitis is often managed by dermatology.

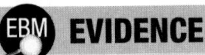

EVIDENCE

Available at ExpertConsult.com

SUGGESTED READINGS

Available at ExpertConsult.com

RELATED CONTENT

Cogan Syndrome (Related Key Topic)
Cryoglobulinemia (Related Key Topic)
Eosinophilic Granulomatosis with Polyangiitis (Related Key Topic)
Giant Cell Arteritis (Related Key Topic)
Granulomatosis with Polyangiitis (Related Key Topic)
Henoch-Schönlein Purpura (Related Key Topic)
Kawasaki Disease (Related Key Topic)
Microscopic Polyangiitis (Related Key Topic)
Polyarteritis Nodosa (Related Key Topic)
Takayasu Arteritis (Related Key Topic)

AUTHORS: **NICOLE B. YANG, M.D.,** and **ANTHONY M. REGINATO, PH.D. M.D.**

TABLE 3 Differential Diagnostic Features of Selected Forms of Small Vessel Vasculitis

Features	Microscopic Polyangiitis (MPA)	Granulomatosis with Polyangiitis (GPA)	Eosinophilic Granulomatosis with Polyangiitis	Henoch-Schönlein Purpura (HSP)	Cryoglobulinemic Vasculitis
Vasculitic signs and symptoms	+	+	+	+	+
IgA-dominant immune deposits	−	−	−	+	−
Cryoglobulins in blood and vessels	−	−	−	−	+
Antineutrophil cytoplasmic antibodies in blood	+	+	+	−	−
Necrotizing granulomas	−	+	+	−	−
Asthma and eosinophils	−	−	+	−	−

From Floege J, et al.: *Comprehensive clinical nephrology,* ed 4, Philadelphia, 2010, Saunders.

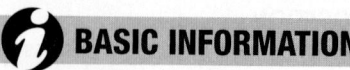

BASIC INFORMATION

DEFINITION

The spectrum of chronic venous disease (CVD) ranges from varicose veins to leg edema and skin manifestations consisting of hyperpigmentation, eczema, lipodermatosclerosis, and venous ulcer. These latter venous-specific skin changes constitute an advanced form of CVD known as chronic venous insufficiency (CVI).

SYNONYMS

Stasis dermatitis
Postthrombotic syndrome (PTS)
Chronic venous disease

ICD-10CM CODES

I87.2	Venous insufficiency (chronic) (peripheral)
I87.8	Other specified disorders of veins
I87.9	Disorder of vein, unspecified
I83.10	Varicose veins of unspecified lower extremity with inflammation

EPIDEMIOLOGY & DEMOGRAPHICS

- From 10% to 35% of adults in the United States have some form of CVI.
- Venous ulcers are the complication of CVI that results in the greatest morbidity and affects 4% of people over the age of 65.
- The population-based costs to the U.S. government for CVI treatment and venous ulcer care have been estimated at >$1 billion/yr.
- In addition, 4.6 million workdays/yr are lost to chronic venous-related diseases.

PHYSICAL FINDINGS & CLINICAL PRESENTATION

The manifestations of CVI can be viewed using the internationally accepted classification system, CEAP (clinical, etiology, anatomy, and pathophysiology) (Table 1). The spectrum of cutaneous changes of CVI in the affected leg include:

- Varicose eczema: The most common and earliest sign, this involves the skin above the medial ankle and consists of pruritic, red, and scaly eczematous patches and plaques.
- Hyperpigmentation: Caused by the breakdown of red blood cells and leads to hemosiderin deposition and dark staining of the skin (Fig. 1).
- Atrophie blanche: Usually presents as hypopigmented white patches with focal red punctate dots or telangiectasia surrounded by hyperpigmentation. Skin in this condition is avascular and prone to ulceration (Fig. 2).
- Lipodermatosclerosis: A chronic, brawny induration of the skin and underlying fat that usually involves the skin from medial malleolus up to the lower border of the calf. Progression of the disease leads to an "inverted champagne bottle" appearance. The induration and lack of perfusion of the skin in this area make it susceptible to ulcer formation.

TABLE 1 CEAP Classification

Clinical Classification	
C_0	No visible or palpable signs of venous disease
C_1	Telangiectasias or reticular veins
C_2	Varicose veins; diameter >3 mm
C_3	Edema
C_4	Changes in skin and subcutaneous tissue: Pigmentation, eczema, lipodermatosclerosis, or atrophie blanche
C_5	Healed venous ulcer
C_6	Active venous ulcer
	Each limb is further classified as asymptomatic (A) or symptomatic (S)
Etiologic Classification	
E_C	Congenital
E_P	Primary
E_S	Secondary (post-thrombotic)
E_N	No venous cause identified
Anatomic Classification	
A_S	Superficial veins
A_P	Perforator veins
A_O	Deep veins
A_N	No venous location identified
Pathophysiologic Classification	
P_R	Reflux
P_R	Obstruction
$P_{R,O}$	Reflux and obstruction
P_N	No venous pathophysiology identifiable

From Fillit HM: *Brocklehurst's textbook of geriatric medicine and gerontology*, ed 8, 2017, Elsevier.

FIG. 1 Stasis dermatitis, venous insufficiency. (From James WD, et al.: *Andrews' diseases of the skin*, ed 12, Philadelphia, 2016, Elsevier.)

ETIOLOGY

- CVI occurs as a result of sustained venous hypertension in the leg, which can be caused by the following:
  1. Primary: Vein valve failure with reflux in the superficial venous system or perforating veins (most common cause of CVI).
  2. Secondary: Post-thrombotic syndrome in which a deep vein thrombosis causes outflow obstruction *or*
  3. Combination of the two previous processes.
- This sustained elevation in venous pressure or venous hypertension results in pathologic effects in the skin and subcutaneous tissues such as edema, eczema, hyperpigmentation, fibrosis, and ultimately venous ulceration.

Dx DIAGNOSIS

The diagnosis and evaluation of CVI are directed primarily by a detailed history and physical examination.

DIFFERENTIAL DIAGNOSIS

- Contact dermatitis
- Atopic dermatitis
- Cellulitis
- Dermatophyte infection
- Pretibial myxedema
- Nummular eczema
- Xerosis
- Asteatotic eczema

WORKUP

The primary goal is to identify the cause of sustained venous hypertension. Fig. 3 describes the evaluation and management of chronic venous insufficiency.

LABORATORY TESTS

Generally not indicated

IMAGING STUDIES

- Evaluation of the patient is performed in the standing position with duplex ultrasonography to identify reflux in the superficial, deep, and perforating veins as well as obstruction of the deep veins.
- No exam of a leg with CVI is complete without palpation of pulses and/or determination of ankle-brachial index (ABI).

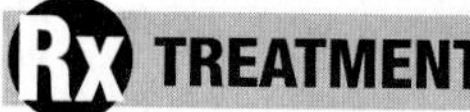

TREATMENT

NONPHARMACOLOGIC THERAPY

- Leg elevation above heart level for 30 min three to four times a day
- Weight reduction because obesity is a risk factor for DVT and CVI
- Walking exercises to improve calf function
- Physical therapy to improve ankle joint mobility
- For weeping skin lesions, wet-to-dry dressing changes

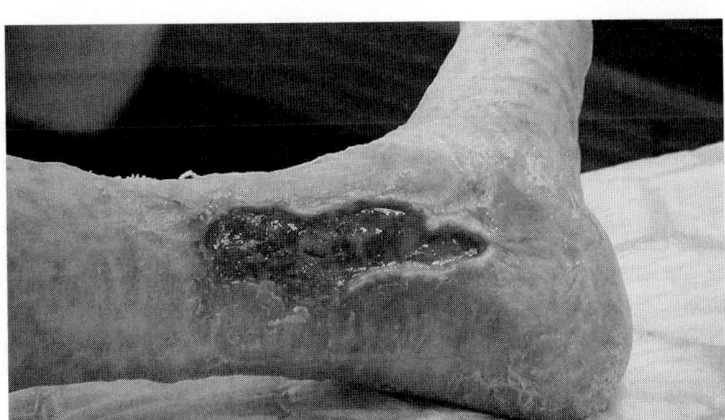

FIG. 2 Chronic venous ulcer likely to be resistant to treatment as it involves the space behind the medial malleolus, which is difficult to compress. (From Fillit HM: *Brocklehurst's textbook of geriatric medicine and gerontology*, ed 8, 2017, Elsevier.)

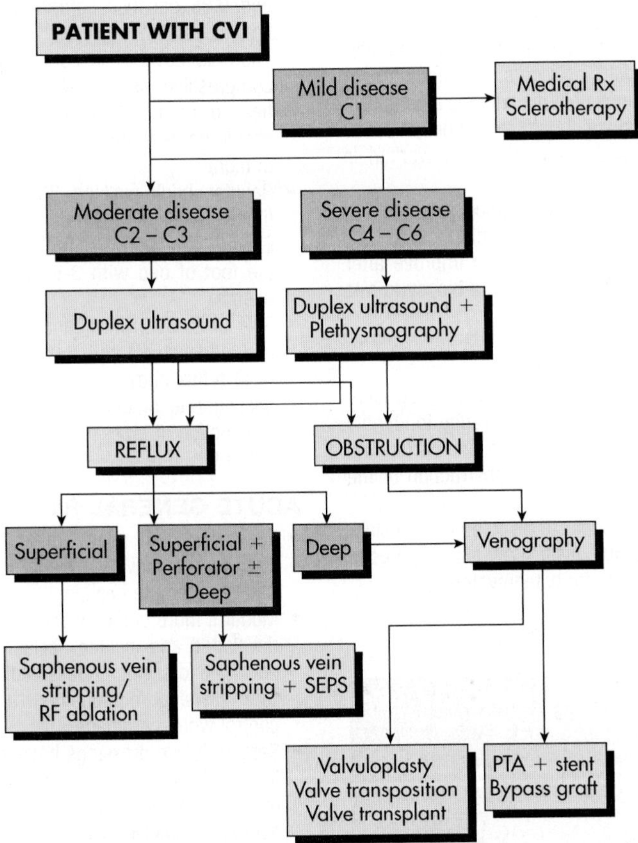

FIG. 3 Evaluation and management of chronic venous insufficiency. (From Cameron JA: *Current surgical therapy "varicose veins,"* Philadelphia, 2004, Saunders.)

ACUTE GENERAL Rx

- The fundamental role of compression in the treatment of CVI is well recognized and has been validated by randomized controlled trials (RCTs).
- The beneficial effects of gradient compression stockings (decrease in edema and control of discomfort) are due to their effect on microvascular hemodynamics and Starling forces.
- Below-knee compression stocking with a gradient of at least 20 to 30 mm Hg will control edema, alleviate pain, and improve the quality of life in CVI patients.
- Compression stockings are contraindicated in patients with an ABI of <0.6.
- Some patients (acute lipodermatosclerosis) may benefit from nonelastic compression with the Unna gel paste gauze boot to alleviate their symptoms and acute increase in their swelling. The Unna boot is changed once a week.
- Topical corticosteroid creams or ointments (e.g., triamcinolone 0.12% bid) may be used to help reduce inflammation and itching. Steroids should never be applied to ulcer.
- Antibiotics should only be used when treating a clinically apparent, culture-proved infection. Most secondary infections are the result of *Staphylococcus* or *Streptococcus* organisms.
- Diuretics have no role in the treatment of CVI-related edema.

CHRONIC Rx

- While conservative care is fundamental, patients with CVI should be considered for correction of their underlying venous hypertension.
- The majority of patients with CVI have superficial vein or perforator vein reflux as their underlying pathology and would benefit from the newer vein ablation procedures listed below.
  1. Endovenous ablation of superficial (saphenous) or perforator vein reflux.
  2. RF ablation with VNUS closure.
  3. Endovenous laser therapy (EVLT).
  4. Ultrasound-guided foam sclerotherapy.

COMPLEMENTARY & ALTERNATIVE MEDICINE

Several groups of drugs have been evaluated in the treatment of CVI, including coumarins, flavonoids, and saponosides (horse chestnut extracts). These drugs have venoactive properties and are widely used in Europe but are not approved for use in the U.S. The precise mechanism of action is not known. Horse chestnut seed extract has been found, in the short term, to be as effective as compression stockings in reducing pain and edema, but long-term efficacy has not been established.

REFERRAL

- Phlebology
- Vascular surgery
- Indications for referral:
  1. Skin and subcutaneous changes consistent with CVI
  2. Associated peripheral arterial insufficiency (PAD)
  3. Longstanding varicose vein disease
  4. Consideration for vein ablation procedure

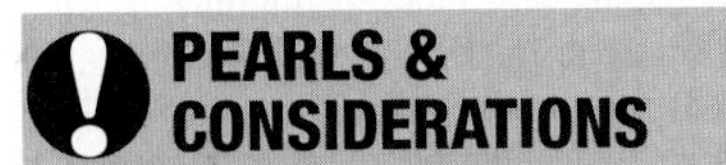

PEARLS & CONSIDERATIONS

COMMENTS

- Inflammatory skin changes from CVI are irreversible. The goal of therapy is to eliminate venous hypertension and prevent progression.
- Venous ulcers are often an end-stage manifestation of CVI. Refer to "Venous Ulcers" for more information.

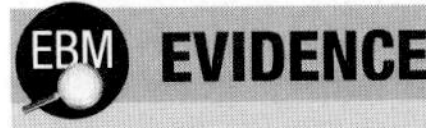

EVIDENCE

Available at ExpertConsult.com

SUGGESTED READINGS

Available at ExpertConsult.com

RELATED CONTENT

Stasis Dermatitis (Patient Information)
Varicose Veins (Related Key Topic)
Venous Ulcers (Related Key Topic)

AUTHOR: **FRANK G. FORT, M.D., F.A.C.S., R.PH.S.**

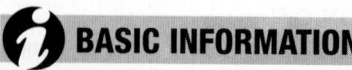

BASIC INFORMATION

DEFINITION

Venous ulcers are defined as chronic defects of the skin that fail to heal spontaneously and persist for longer than 4 wk. Venous ulcers account for about 70% of all lower-extremity ulcerations. They are usually located in the "gaiter" region and can be accompanied by varicose veins, edema, hyperpigmentation, and lipodermatosclerosis. Venous ulceration develops in patients as a result of sustained venous hypertension.

SYNONYM

Stasis ulcers

ICD-10CM CODES

I87.2	Venous insufficiency (chronic) (peripheral)
L97.909	Non-pressure chronic ulcer of unspecified part of unspecified lower leg with unspecified severity

EPIDEMIOLOGY & DEMOGRAPHICS

In industrialized nations, up to 1.5% of the population will suffer from venous ulcers. In patients ≥65 yr, the incidence increases to 4%. In the U.S., >500,000 people suffer from stasis ulcers.

RISK FACTORS

- Obesity
- Increasing age
- Family history of chronic venous insufficiency
- History of deep venous thromboembolism

PHYSICAL FINDINGS & CLINICAL PRESENTATION

Venous ulcers are most commonly located in the lower leg just above the ankle (gaiter region). They are a partial-thickness, irregularly shaped wound with well-defined borders with granulation tissue and fibrin present in the ulcer base (Fig. 1). Venous ulcers are relatively painless and are surrounded by brown-stained skin and/or dry, itchy, and reddened skin. In about 50% of patients, there are visible varicose veins in an aching, swollen leg.

ETIOLOGY

The exact mechanism of the role of venous hypertension in the etiology of venous ulcers is not certain. Hemodynamic forces such as venous hypertension, circulatory stasis, and modified conditions of shear stress appear to play an important role in an inflammatory reaction accompanied by leukocyte activation that clinically leads to fibrosclerotic remodeling of the skin and then to ulceration.

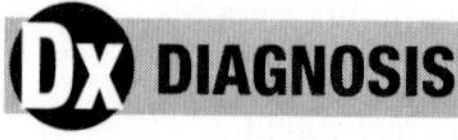

DIAGNOSIS

DIFFERENTIAL DIAGNOSIS

- Arterial ulcer
- Neurotrophic ulcers (located predominantly in the foot)
- Vasculitis
- Pyoderma gangrenosum
- Ulcerated skin tumors like basal cell or squamous cell carcinoma (Marjolin ulcer)
- Rheumatoid arthritis

WORKUP

- The history and clinical signs and symptoms of leg ulcers are often misleading and may not differentiate venous ulcers from other leg ulcers; about 30% of leg ulcers are not of venous origin.
- Measurement of the ankle-brachial index (ABI) is essential in excluding peripheral arterial disease (PAD), which can be present in 20% of patients and is required before starting compression therapy. Arterial insufficiency is suggested by an ABI <0.9.
- Patients with lower-extremity ulcers should also be evaluated for diabetes.
- Coagulation defects have been found in 40% of patients with leg ulcers. This finding suggests that many patients with leg ulcers have a known or suspected history of deep venous thrombosis and a thrombophilia workup is indicated.
- If vasculitis is suspected, a biopsy of the edge of the ulcer can confirm the diagnosis.
- Any wound that has failed to improve after therapy of 4 wk should have a biopsy to rule out malignancy.

IMAGING STUDIES

- Evaluation of patients with venous leg ulcer should include duplex sonography to identify reflux in the superficial, deep, and perforating veins as well as possible obstruction of the deep veins.
- If the ulcer appears to be infected, consider tissue for culture, plain x-ray films, and bone scan to evaluate for osteomyelitis.

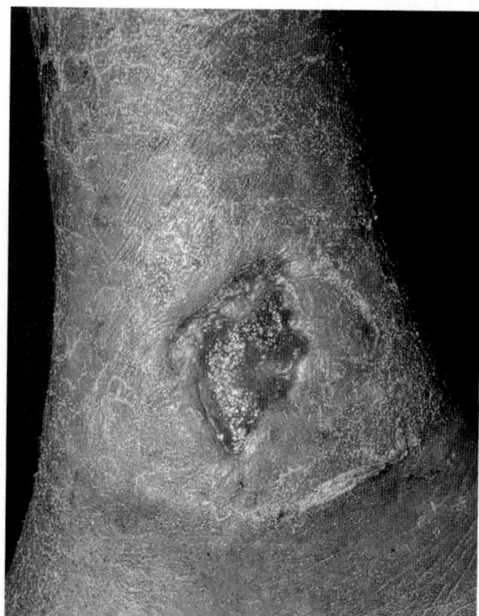

FIG. 1 Stasis ulcer. Any ulcer in this location with surrounding edema, redness, and scale is typical of a stasis ulcer. (From White GM, Cox NH [eds]: *Diseases of the skin, a color atlas and text,* ed 2, St Louis, 2006, Mosby.)

TREATMENT

NONPHARMACOLOGIC THERAPY

- Fig. 2 describes an algorithm for the treatment of venous ulcers.
- Surgical debridement to remove all nonviable material can be accomplished in the office setting with the use of a topical Xylocaine gel. Debridement produces the release of growth factors that allow the development of healthy granulation tissue and the initiation of the healing process.
- The first-line treatment of ulcers includes below-knee compression stockings to improve venous return to the heart, thereby decreasing edema, inflammation, and tissue ischemia (used only if the ABI is between 0.6 and 0.85 because compression can cause limb ischemia).
- There is Level A evidence that graduated compression stockings alone can lead to healing of a venous ulcer. The stockings should be worn during the day and removed at night.
- Regular, brisk walking 30 min a day, five times a week is recommended.
- Elevate leg above heart level and raise the foot of bed with 3-in blocks to reduce edema.
- Role of surgery: In a randomized controlled trial, endovenous catheter ablation of superficial reflux showed no improvement in the healing rate of ulcers but did demonstrate a reduction of ulcer recurrence from 28% to 12% at 12 mo.

ACUTE GENERAL Rx

- Dressings are used under compression stockings to provide a clean, moist environment to promote healing.
- Modern, more complex dressings have been developed and include occlusive and semiocclusive dressings, classified according to their physical composition and ability to control wound drainage.
- Semiocclusive dressings have varying ability to absorb wound drainage. Some examples of this type are hydrocolloids (DuoDerm), hydrogels (DuoDerm hydrogel), foam dressings (Allevyn), and alginates.
- Biologic wound dressings (Apligraf) and tissue-engineered products (Oasis) have been developed, and these products can either directly provide growth factors or indirectly stimulate growth factors in the ulcer bed.
- Pentoxifylline (800 mg tid) has been shown to be an effective adjuvant to compression therapy as reported in a meta-analysis of nine clinical trials.
- Skin grafting should be considered for large or refractory ulcers as long as the wound is clean and there is healthy granulation tissue.
- Published randomized clinical trials on the value of the different types of dressings in the management of leg ulcers have not shown effects on ulcer healing. Despite the lack of evidence to support their use, modern dressings remain a part of the standard of

care. Decisions regarding their use should be based on local cost of the dressings and the physician's clinical experience.
- Trials involving the use of weekly, low-dose, high-frequency ultrasound for hard-to-heal venous leg ulcers do not support adding therapeutic ultrasound to standard care for venous leg ulcers.

DISPOSITION

The overall prognosis for this condition is poor; the healing rate depends on the initial size of the ulcer. Although 65% to 70% of venous ulcers are healed within 6 mo, the 5-yr recurrence rate of healed venous ulcers can be as high as 40%. Maintenance of lifelong compression therapy is recommended.

REFERRAL

All patients should be evaluated weekly during the first month of therapy. Nonhealing ulcers with little to no improvement should also be referred to a wound care clinic.

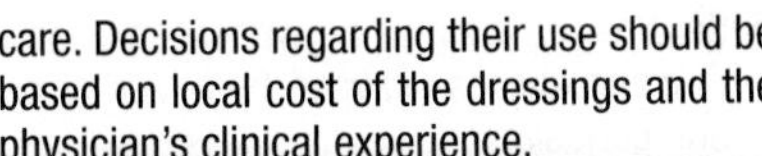

EVIDENCE

Available at ExpertConsult.com

SUGGESTED READINGS

Available at ExpertConsult.com

AUTHOR: **FRANK G. FORT, M.D., F.A.C.S., R.PH.S.**

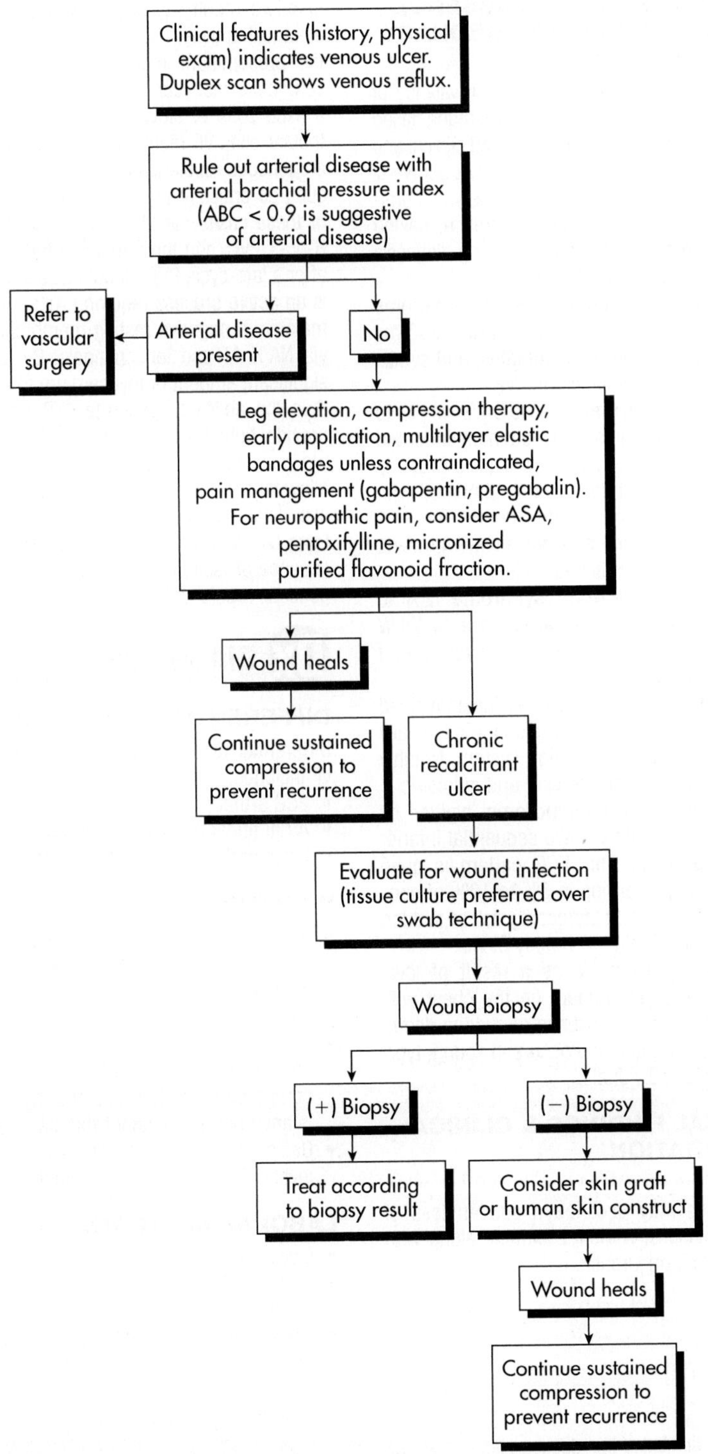

FIG. 2 Algorithm for the care of a patient with a venous leg ulcer.

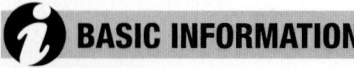

BASIC INFORMATION

DEFINITION

Ventricular fibrillation (VF) is a rapid, disorganized ventricular arrhythmia (Fig. 1) that renders the ventricle unable to contract in a synchronized manner resulting in no meaningful cardiac output or blood pressure and, if not rapidly interrupted, death. The ECG appearance of VF can evolve rapidly over the course of minutes as the heart becomes more ischemic. Upon initiation, QRST complexes in VF often appear coarse with grossly irregular oscillating complexes of variable rate, axis, and morphology. As VF continues, the QRST complexes become finer, lower amplitude, and slower, eventually resulting in asystole. VF is the leading mechanism of sudden cardiac death.

ICD-10CM CODE
I49.01 Ventricular fibrillation

EPIDEMIOLOGY & DEMOGRAPHICS

INCIDENCE: A peak incidence of VF occurs in the first 48 hr after an acute myocardial infarction (MI). The true incidence of VF is impossible to know because the majority of these episodes are in unmonitored patients and result in sudden cardiac death. Sudden cardiac death, as determined by death certificate analysis, is estimated to account for 400,000 to 450,000 deaths per year in the U.S. In small studies in which patients were wearing monitoring at the time of death, the majority of sudden cardiac deaths were caused by VF (60%-70%). The true proportion of sudden cardiac deaths caused by VF is highly dependent on the population studied.

MAJOR RISK FACTORS:
- Between 80% and 90% of sudden cardiac death and VF cases occur in patients with coronary artery disease (CAD) or systolic dysfunction, with only about 15% of VF cases occurring in a "normal" heart at autopsy.
- Between 60% and 70% of patients with VF have CAD.
- Between 5% and 15% of events are secondary to structural heart disease (congenital coronary anatomy, myocarditis, hypertrophic cardiomyopathy, arrhythmogenic right ventricular cardiomyopathy). This frequency increases when under the age of 35 yr.
- Between 5% and 10% of events occur in the absence of ischemic or structural heart disease. These events are more common before the age of 35 and include inherited channelopathies and trauma-induced (commotio cordis) etiologies.

RISK FACTORS FOR VF IN PATIENTS PRESENTING WITH ISCHEMIC CORONARY HEART DISEASE

- STEMI as opposed to NSTEMI
- Larger infarcts
- Inferior infarcts
- Baseline repolarization abnormalities
- Hypokalemia
- Male sex
- History of tobacco abuse
- Absence of pre-infarct angina

ETIOLOGIES OF VF IN ABSENCE OF STRUCTURAL OR CORONARY HEART DISEASE

- **Long QT syndrome**: Estimated prevalence of 1:2000 to 1:5000; the diagnosis is made based on combination of ECG findings and clinical and family history collectively compiled as Schwartz criteria. Typically inherited as autosomal dominant mutation with variable penetrance, making genetic testing helpful for confirming diagnosis or screening family members.
- **Short QT syndrome**: Inherited syndrome characterized by both a short QTc (<350 ms in males and 360 ms in females) and symptomatic atrial fibrillation and VF.
- **Brugada syndrome**: Prevalence is 5 to 50:10,000 of autosomal dominant inherited mutation characterized by a classic Brugada pattern on ECG in leads V1-2 combined with syncope or clinical sudden death. The ECG pattern is mutable and not always present. Genetic testing is limited.
- **Wolff-Parkinson-White syndrome**: 2% to 3% of sudden cardiac arrest due to WPW caused by AF conducting down bypass tract degenerating into VF.
- **Idiopathic VF**: Diagnosis of exclusion typified by VF induced by early coupled PVCs typically emanating from conduction system. Notably suppressed by isoproterenol and quinidine.
- **Early repolarization syndrome**: typified by 1-mm ST elevation in two sequential inferior or lateral leads. This ECG pattern is quite nonspecific, occurring in 5% to 10% of general population and increasing risk of sudden death by threefold, or roughly 0.3%.
- **Commotio cordis**: VF as a result of low-velocity projectile impact on the chest wall inducing VF in the absence of sudden death. This is uncommon and occurs in young, typically male, individuals.

PHYSICAL FINDINGS & CLINICAL PRESENTATION

- Patients are unconscious, without BP or pulse.
- Witnesses may describe a sudden loss of consciousness, without breathing along with a cyanotic appearance.
- Seizure activity may be witnessed after loss of consciousness caused by a lack of cerebral perfusion.

ETIOLOGY

In roughly 80% of patients with VT/VF there is increased ventricular ectopy prior to sustained ventricular arrhythmia. VF is thought to develop in one of three ways: (1) degeneration of sustained monomorphic VT, (2) degeneration of sustained polymorphic VT, or (3) development of VF as a primary event. The mechanism of VF is thought to involve multiple rotating spiral waves of micro reentry without any overall organized electrical activity. This is distinctly different from the predominant mechanism of monomorphic ventricular tachycardia, which is reentry around a fixed zone of slow conduction, typically ventricular scar. VF results from a substrate of heterogeneous repolarization and a triggering event such as critically timed PVC. In about one third of these cases the PVC initiates VT by an early R-on-T PVC, and the remaining two thirds occur after a late-cycle PVC. Repolarization of the heart is an active process requiring ATP to obtain and maintain a negative resting membrane potential via NA/K ATPase ion channels. By depriving a significant amount of myocardium to oxygen and thus the ability to generate ATP, ischemia can provide both the substrate of VF by impairing the ischemic area's ability to fully repolarize and allow for a triggering event by allowing spontaneous depolarization. Genetic conditions such as Long QT syndrome can also predispose to VF in absence of ischemia by providing more heterogeneous repolarization within the myocardium.

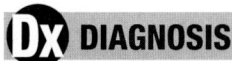

DIAGNOSIS

DIFFERENTIAL DIAGNOSIS

Differential diagnosis of an ECG suspicious of VF includes:
- ECG artifact
- Atrial fibrillation with aberration
- Polymorphic ventricular tachycardia

WORKUP

- Ischemia evaluation is paramount. Cardiac biomarkers should be checked and cardiac catheterization should be performed in most cases.
- A 12-lead ECG of the tachycardia should always be obtained and, whenever possible, compared to the ECG in sinus rhythm if there is any uncertainty about the diagnosis.
- Basic lab testing with focus on electrolytes levels (K and Mg) and hemoglobin.

LABORATORY TESTS

- Electrolyte levels potassium, magnesium
- Hemoglobin level
- Cardiac biomarkers
- Genetic testing should be reserved for specific situations such as when there is a concern for genetically mediated conditions such as hypertrophic cardiomyopathy, catecholaminergic polymorphic ventricular tachycardia or Brugada syndrome

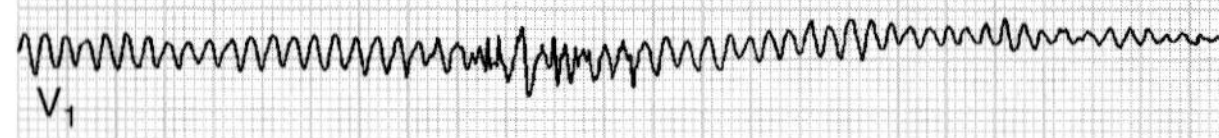

FIG. 1 Ventricular fibrillation. This rhythm strip shows ventricular fibrillation that degenerates further into fine ventricular fibrillation. (From Olshansky B et al: *Arrhythmia essentials*, ed 2, Philadelphia, 2017, Elsevier.)

IMAGING STUDIES

- Echocardiogram (rule out structural heart disease).
- Diagnostic coronary angiography (rule out ischemic etiology).
- Cardiac MRI is indicated if the previous tests are unable to establish the cause of the arrhythmia and to rule out cardiomyopathies such as cardiac sarcoidosis, amyloid, LV noncompaction, arrhythmogenic right ventricular dysplasia.

Rx TREATMENT

ACUTE GENERAL Rx

- Patients with VF are hemodynamically unstable and require emergent unsynchronized defibrillation along with appropriate high-quality CPR as per ACLS protocols.
- Antiarrhythmic therapy with IV amiodarone and/or IV lidocaine is appropriate, particularly if patients have more than one event. IV lidocaine is particularly effective if VF is mediated by cardiac ischemia. Cardiac catheterization is recommended provided no contraindications exist. IV beta blockers are also recommended provided the patient is not in shock and blood pressure is permissive. If the patient is unresponsive after appropriate CPR a hypothermia protocol should be considered to aid in neurologic recovery. If the patient is having multiple episodes of VF despite these measures and is still awake between episodes, sedation and intubation are appropriate to reduce adrenergic drive. Cardiac electrophysiology consultation is appropriate for management of VF.
- Electrolyte supplementation is essential if hypokalemia or hypomagnesemia is detected.

CHRONIC Rx

After acute stabilization has occurred, chronic treatment is dependent on circumstances surrounding VF. If VF occurred within 48 hr of a large MI, then relief of ischemia via PCI, CABG, or lytic therapy is the primary treatment. A patient who has a well-defined ischemic trigger that has been satisfactorily treated likely will not require an implantable cardiac defibrillator, but a wearable external defibrillator could be considered under certain circumstances. Patients with VF in the periinfarction period who survive to hospital discharge have a prognosis similar to patients without arrhythmias in the peri-infarction period. ICD implantation is recommended in patients when there is no clearly reversible trigger, such as acute MI, commotio cordis, or drug overdose. If an inherited ion channelopathy is suspected, such as long QT, Brugada syndrome, or CPVT, genetic testing should be performed, but an ICD is appropriate even before definitive diagnosis is made for secondary prevention of sudden death from VF. If the etiology of VF is unknown after standard workup, cardiac MRI is suggested to work up cardiac sarcoid, hypertrophic cardiomyopathy, arrhythmogenic right ventricular cardiomyopathy. If indicated, then cardiac MRI should be done before ICD implantation. If a patient is subsequently diagnosed with inherited arrhythmia syndrome, familial screening should be discussed with the patient.

Cardiac echocardiography plays an important role in long-term risk stratification as well. If a patient's EF remains <35% 3 mo after appropriate revascularization and institution of appropriate heart failure therapy (ACE, beta-blocker therapy), then consideration of ICD is appropriate at that time.

Chronic therapy with antiarrhythmic medications such as amiodarone, mexiletine, or sotalol may be needed even after ICD implantation if the patient presents with multiple appropriate shocks. Continued focus on the trigger of VF such as ischemia or electrolyte disturbance is also critical. Cardiac ablation has been described in rare cases if a distinct triggering PVC is isolated, but this is not as commonly employed as ablation for VT.

DISPOSITION

Patients with sustained VF should be managed in an ICU because of the risk of degeneration to a hemodynamically unstable rhythm. A cardiologist or cardiac electrophysiologist should be consulted.

REFERRAL

All patients with VF should be referred to a cardiologist or a cardiac electrophysiologist.

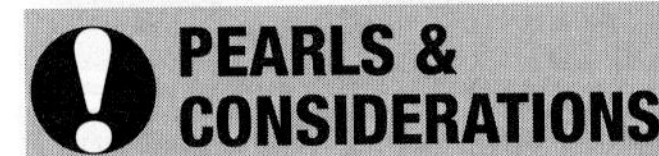

PEARLS & CONSIDERATIONS

COMMENTS

- Effective VF treatment is strongly dependent on identifying and treating the inciting trigger (i.e., ischemia, cardiogenic shock) while using antiarrhythmic therapy IV amiodarone +/- IV lidocaine for stabilization.
- Hypothermia protocol should be considered in patients who have return of spontaneous circulation after VF arrest who remain comatose upon presentation.
- ICDs are indicated for secondary prevention of VF independent of the substrate in the absence of a clearly reversible trigger.
- In the peri-infarction period, VT, particularly VT occurring more than 48 hr after MI, is far more predictive of subsequent out-of-hospital sudden death than VF and as such often warrants earlier ICD therapy consideration.
- In managing patients with multiple VF events (VF storm), therapies to reduce adrenergic drive are important, such as IV beta blockers as BP tolerates, aggressive IV sedation with propofol or Versed, or fentanyl along with intubation and electrolyte repletion.
- In patients with suspected long QT or Brugada syndrome, VF storm may be managed differently than VF in an ischemic setting or with structural cardiomyopathy. Long QT syndrome VF storm may prompt use of isoproterenol, magnesium repletion, and consideration of atrial pacing to prevent bradycardia. In treating Brugada syndrome VF storm, use of isoproterenol, quinidine, and treatment of fever if it exists can be helpful.

PATIENT/FAMILY EDUCATION

Patients with familial or genetic causes of ventricular arrhythmias should have family screening of first-degree relatives.

SUGGESTED READING

Available at ExpertConsult.com

RELATED CONTENT

Arrhythmogenic Right Ventricular Dysplasia (Related Key Topic)
Brugada Syndrome (Related Key Topic)
Hypertrophic Cardiomyopathy (Related Key Topic)
Long QT Syndrome (Related Key Topic)
Torsade de Pointes (Related Key Topic)

AUTHORS: **GERARD H. DALY, M.D., M.S.,** and **SHAW NATAN, M.D.**

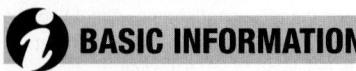

BASIC INFORMATION

DEFINITION

- *Ventricular septal defect* (VSD) refers to an abnormal communication through the septum that separates the right and left ventricles of the heart.
- VSDs may be large or small, single or multiple.
- VSDs can be classified according to their location, either within the muscular septum (muscular defects) or at its margins:
  1. Membranous (75% to 80%): This is the most common type of defect. The septal leaflet of the tricuspid valve may become adherent and form a "pouch" of the septum that can limit the left-to-right shunting and lead to self-closure.
  2. Muscular or trabecular (5% to 20%): This defect is entirely surrounded by muscular tissue. Often has less hemodynamic impact, and spontaneous closure is common.
  3. Canal or inlet (8%): This defect commonly lies beneath the septal leaflet of the tricuspid valve; associated with Down syndrome.
  4. Subarterial, outlet, infundibular, or supracristal (5%): This is the least common type of defect. It is usually found beneath the aortic valve, and it may lead to aortic regurgitation. High prevalence in Asian population.

SYNONYM

VSD

ICD-10CM CODES

Q21.0	Ventricular septal defect
I23.2	Ventricular septal defect as current complication following acute myocardial infarction

EPIDEMIOLOGY & DEMOGRAPHICS

- VSDs are one of the most common congenital heart abnormalities.
- VSD accounts for ~25% of all congenital heart defects in children and for approximately 10% of defects in adults (the decrease is a result of spontaneous closure that occurs by adulthood, with the majority occurring prior to 3 yr of age).
- The prevalence of VSD is 3 to 4 infants per 1000 live births and 0.5/1000 adults.
- VSD is found with equal frequency among both males and females.
- VSD may be associated with the following conditions:
  1. Atrial septal defect (35%)
  2. Patent ductus arteriosus (22%)
  3. Coarctation of the aorta (17%)
  4. Subvalvular aortic stenosis (4%)
  5. Subpulmonic stenosis, usually associated with progressive aortic regurgitation caused by prolapse of the aortic cusp through the defect
- Multiple VSDs are more prevalent among patients with tetralogy of Fallot and double-outlet right ventricular defects.

PHYSICAL FINDINGS & CLINICAL PRESENTATION

- Clinical presentation depends on the direction and volume of the VSD shunt, which is dictated by the size of the defect as well as by the relative resistances of pulmonary and systemic vascular beds. Fig. 1 illustrates the physiology of VSD.
  1. Defects of ≤25% of the aortic annulus diameter are small or restrictive defects (Q_p:Q_s <1.5:1). These typically involve small left-to-right shunts, no left ventricular volume overload, and no pulmonary artery hypertension (PAH).
  2. Defects that are 25% to 75% of aortic annulus diameter are considered to be moderate in size. Small to moderate left-to-right shunting (Q_p:Q_s 1.5-2:1)., mild to moderate left ventricular volume overload, and mild or no PAH are seen. Patients may have symptoms of congestive heart failure that may improve with medical therapy or with age as the defect decreases in size relative to increasing body size.

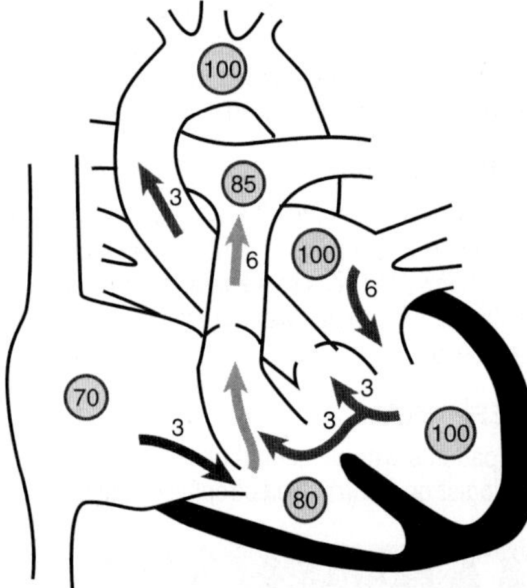

FIG. 1 Physiology of a large ventricular septal defect (VSD). Circled numbers represent oxygen saturation values. The numbers next to the *arrows* represent volumes of blood flow (in L/min/m^2). This illustration shows a hypothetical patient with a pulmonary-to-systemic blood flow ratio (Qp:Qs) of 2:1. Desaturated blood enters the right atrium from the vena cava at a volume of 3 L/min/m^2 and flows across the tricuspid valve. An additional 3 L of blood shunts left to right across the VSD, the result being an increase in oxygen saturation in the right ventricle. Six liters of blood is ejected into the lungs. Pulmonary arterial saturation may be further increased because of incomplete mixing at right ventricular level. Six liters returns to the left atrium, crosses the mitral valve, and causes a mid-diastolic flow rumble. Three liters of this volume shunts left to right across the VSD, and 3 L is ejected into the ascending aorta (normal cardiac output). (From Kliegman RM, et al.: *Nelson textbook of pediatrics,* ed 19, Philadelphia, 2011, Saunders.)

  3. Defects of ≥75% of the aortic annulus diameter usually have moderate to large left-to-right shunting (Q_p:Q_s >2:1)., left ventricular volume overload, and PAH. These patients usually have a history of congestive heart failure, or they may possibly develop right-to-left shunting (Q_p:Q_s <1:1). in the setting of Eisenmenger's syndrome during late childhood, adolescence, or young adulthood. Eisenmenger's syndrome—resulting from chronic elevations of pressure and flow—is associated with functional and structural alterations within the pulmonary vasculature.
- Infants may be asymptomatic at birth because of elevated pulmonary artery resistance. During the first few weeks of life, pulmonary arterial resistance decreases, thereby allowing for more left-to-right shunting through the VSD. This results in a subsequent increase in flow into the lungs, the left atrium, and the left ventricle, which can potentially cause left ventricular volume overload. Tachypnea, failure to thrive, and congestive heart failure may then ensue.
- In adults with VSD, the shunt is left to right in the absence of pulmonary stenosis and pulmonary hypertension. Patients typically manifest symptoms of left-sided heart failure from left ventricular volume overload and associated eccentric hypertrophy (e.g., shortness of breath, orthopnea, dyspnea on exertion). Presence of relevant longstanding PAH could ultimately lead to right-ventricular hypertrophy and dilation.
- A spectrum of physical findings may be seen, including the following:
  1. Machine-like holosystolic murmur that is heard best along the left sternal border
  2. Murmur becomes shorter as right heart pressures increase
  3. Systolic thrill
  4. Mid-diastolic rumble heard at the apex (increased mitral flow)
  5. S_3 heart sound
  6. Rales
- With the development of pulmonary hypertension, the following occur:
  1. An augmented pulmonic component of the S_2 heart sound and decrescendo diastolic murmur indicating pulmonary regurgitation
  2. Cyanosis, clubbing, right ventricular heave, and signs of right heart failure (i.e., as seen with Eisenmenger's complex, with a reversal of the shunt in a right-to-left direction)

ETIOLOGY

- VSD is usually congenital but can be acquired.
- Acquired VSD may result from postsurgical residual leak, trauma, or myocardial infarction.
- Postinfarct ventricular septal defect (PIVSD) typically occurs 1 to 5 days after the event in 0.2% of patients in the current fibrinolytic or primary angioplasty era.

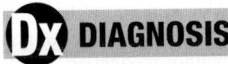

DIAGNOSIS

The diagnosis of VSD can be suspected during a physical examination. Imaging studies—particularly transthoracic echocardiography with color Doppler—establish the diagnosis.

DIFFERENTIAL DIAGNOSIS

On the basis of the physical examination alone, the diagnosis of VSD may be confused with other causes of systolic murmurs, such as mitral regurgitation, tricuspid regurgitation, aortic stenosis, pulmonary stenosis, and hypertrophic cardiomyopathy.

WORKUP

Any person who is suspected of having a VSD should undergo an ECG, a chest radiograph, and an echocardiogram.

LABORATORY TESTS

- Laboratory tests are not specific.
- The CBC may show polycythemia, especially in patients with Eisenmenger's complex.
- Arterial blood gas results may demonstrate hypoxemia, which does not correct with supplemental oxygen.

IMAGING STUDIES

- ECG findings vary in accordance with the size of the VSD and depending on whether pulmonary hypertension is present. Volume loading of the left ventricle might result in left-ventricular hypertrophy and left atrial enlargement, whereas raised right-ventricular pressure due to either pulmonary hypertension or obstruction to the pulmonary outflow tract could lead to right-ventricular hypertrophy findings.
- Chest x-ray findings in patients with VSD include the following:
  1. Cardiomegaly that results from left ventricular volume overload that directly relates to the magnitude of the shunt
  2. The enlargement of the proximal pulmonary arteries along with the redistribution and pruning of the distal pulmonary vessels as a result of sustained pulmonary hypertension (Fig. 2, *A*)
- Echocardiography is the imaging modality of choice for the diagnosis of VSD:
  1. Two-dimensional echocardiography and color Doppler display the size and location of the VSD (Fig. 2, *B*), the chamber sizes, ventricular function, the presence of aortic valve prolapse or regurgitation, outflow tract obstruction, and the presence of tricuspid regurgitation.
  2. Continuous-wave Doppler approximates the gradient between the left and right ventricles and estimates the pulmonary artery pressure.
  3. The magnitude of the shunt can be determined by the calculation of the pulmonary-to-systemic flow ratio with the use of echocardiography.
- Heart catheterization is primarily indicated to assess operability of VSD patients with PAH based on their pulmonary vascular resistance (PVR) and in patients in whom the noninvasive testing was inconclusive, and further information, such as quantification of shunting and assessment of pulmonary pressures, is required.
- MRI, computed tomography or (3D) transesophageal echocardiography can be useful to assess the pulmonary artery, the pulmonary vein, and the aortic anatomy and to confirm the anatomy of unusual VSDs (e.g., inlet or apical defects) that are inadequately visualized with conventional surface echocardiography.

Rx TREATMENT

The decision to close a VSD depends on the type, size, and shunt severity as well as the patient's pulmonary vascular resistance, functional capacity, and associated valvular abnormalities.

NONPHARMACOLOGIC THERAPY

- Young children and adults with a small, asymptomatic VSD with a large left-to-right ventricular pressure gradient, a pulmonary-to-systemic blood flow ratio (Qp/Qs) of less than 1.5:1, and no evidence of pulmonary hypertension can be observed (i.e., restrictive defect).
- Oxygen for hypoxemia and a low-salt diet are recommended for patients with congestive heart failure.

ACUTE GENERAL & CHRONIC Rx

Closure of the VSD is indicated for the following patients:

- Infants with congestive heart failure and failure to thrive. Unrestrictive VSDs require surgical intervention within the first 2 yr of life to prevent PAH.
- Children between the ages of 1 and 6 yr with persistent VSD and a Qp/Qs of ≥2.
- Adults with a Qp/Qs of ≥2 and clinical evidence of left-ventricular volume overload (class I, level of evidence B), positive history of infective endocarditis (IE) (class I, level of evidence C), adults with a Qp/Qs of >1.5 with pulmonary artery pressure that is less than two thirds of the systemic pressure and pulmonary vascular resistance that is less than two thirds of the systemic vascular resistance (class IIa, level of evidence B), and adults with a Qp/Qs of >1.5 in the presence of left ventricular systolic or diastolic failure (class IIa, level of evidence B).
- Surgical closure is not indicated for VSD with severe irreversible PAH with high PVR (class III, level of evidence B). Although the exact PVR at which a child with VSD and pulmonary arterial hypertension is considered inoperable has not been determined, the consensus is that a PVR of <4 Wood units/m^2 is considered optimal. PVR of between 4 and 8 wood units/m^2 is considered on a case-by-case basis. There are no definitive guidelines on the use of vasoreactivity as a preoperative predictor, but a >20% decrease in PVR during vasodilator testing is considered a positive response. Some progress has been made in attempts to use pharmacotherapy to decrease PVR to allow for surgical correction.

Surgical closure with Dacron or Gore-Tex patches or primary surgical closure has long

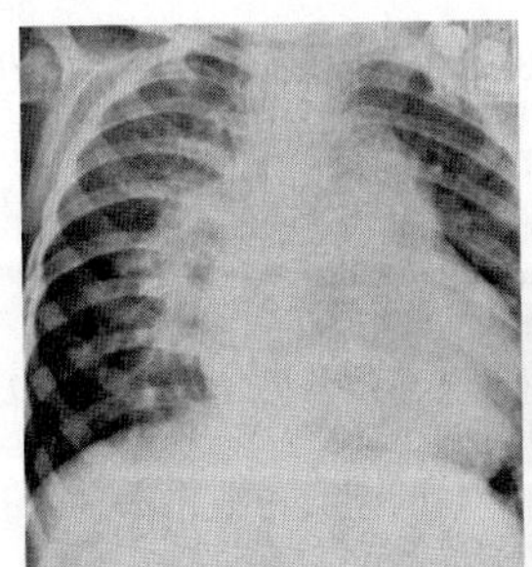

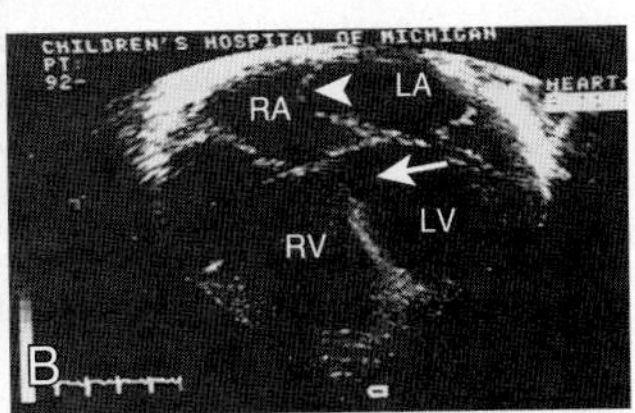

FIG. 2 A, Chest roentgenogram of a child with a large ventricular septal defect, large pulmonary blood flow, and pulmonary hypertension but only mild elevation of peripheral vascular resistance. This is reflected in the evidence of left and right ventricular enlargement, the enlargement of the main pulmonary artery, and a marked increase in pulmonary blood flow. **B,** Apical four-chamber echocardiographic view of ventricular septal defect *(large arrow)*. The small arrow points to the interatrial septum. *LA,* Left atrium; *LV,* left ventricle; *RA,* right atrium; *RV,* right ventricle. (**A** From Pacifico AD et al: Surgical treatment of ventricular septal defect. In Sabiston DC Jr, Spencer FC [eds]: *Surgery of the chest,* ed 5, Philadelphia, 1990, Saunders. **B** courtesy of Richard Humes, M.D., Children's Hospital of Michigan, Detroit.)

been the gold standard of therapy. It has low operative mortality (<2%) at experienced centers. However, surgery still carries a small risk of complete heart block, postpericardiotomy syndrome, wound infection, and neurologic sequelae related to cardiopulmonary bypass. The transcatheter approach to VSD closure is becoming an increasingly accepted modality of treatment for appropriately selected patients. Some studies have shown similar success rates for both surgical and percutaneous closures, and there are significantly fewer complications, days in the hospital, and blood transfusions after percutaneous closures. For patients with difficult vascular access, a periventricular approach using a partial median sternotomy allows for a less invasive repair, often without cardiopulmonary bypass.

Catheter-based closure in muscular VSD may be considered, especially if the VSD is remote from the tricuspid valve and the aorta, if the VSD is associated with severe left-sided heart chamber enlargement, or if there is PAH (class IIb, level of evidence C). Device closure is indicated in residual defects after prior attempts at surgical closure, restrictive VSDs with either a significant left-to-right shunt (Qp/Qs >1.5:1) or history of IE, trauma, or iatrogenic artifacts after surgical replacement of the aortic valve.

Surgery still remains the treatment of choice in patients with large defects, coexistent congenital anomalies requiring surgical correction, and defects with close proximity to the aortic valve. Subpulmonic VSDs may require surgery due to the increased risk of aortic valve prolapse. Perimembranous VSD with more than trivial aortic regurgitation should be referred to surgery. Availability of early reperfusion therapy has led to a decline in incidence of PIVSDs. Surgical closure remains the gold standard in the acute setting or for large (>15 mm) septal ruptures. In the subacute or chronic setting, small or medium PIVSD (<15 mm) can be treated with percutaneous closure with comparable mortality to surgery. Percutaneous closure may also be considered as a temporizing measure to clinically stabilize patients prior to surgical correction. PIVSDs generally arise within 3 to 5 days of the acute event, and even earlier following reperfusion therapy. PIVSDs usually carry a high mortality rate of ~95% of those treated medically and ~50% with surgical repair. Surgical management within 10 days has better outcomes than waiting for cardiac stabilization.

DISPOSITION

- The natural history of an isolated VSD depends on the type of defect, its size, and any associated abnormalities.
- ~75% to 80% of small VSDs close spontaneously by the time the patient reaches the age of 10 yr.
- Only 10% to 15% of large VSDs will close spontaneously.
- Large VSDs that are left untreated may lead to arrhythmias, congestive heart failure, PAH, and Eisenmenger's complex.
- Eisenmenger's complex carries a poor prognosis, with most patients dying before the age of 40 yr.
- Issues to monitor in adults with unrepaired or repaired and catheter-closed VSDs include the following:
  1. Development of aortic regurgitation
  2. Assessment of associated coronary artery disease
  3. Development of tricuspid regurgitation
  4. Assessment of the degree of left-to-right shunting (in unrepaired or residual VSD after repair)
  5. Ventricular dysfunction
  6. Assessment of pulmonary pressure
  7. Development of subpulmonary stenosis (usually as a result of midcavity obstruction of the right ventricle due to hypertrophy of muscle bands, also referred to as a double-chambered right ventricle)
  8. Development of discrete subaortic stenosis
  9. Development of arrhythmia or heart block
  10. Thromboembolic complications
  11. Infective endocarditis
- After closure, late survival is excellent when ventricular function is normal. PAH may improve, progress, or remain the same. Late operations may be required for tricuspid or aortic regurgitation.

REFERRAL

All infants and children diagnosed with VSD should be referred to a pediatric cardiologist. Adults with VSD should be referred to an adult cardiologist. Cardiothoracic surgeons who have experience with congenital heart disease surgery should be consulted if surgery is indicated.

FOLLOW-UP

- Adults with no residual VSD, no associated lesions, and normal pulmonary artery pressure do not require continued follow-up at a regional adult congenital heart disease (ACHD) center.
- Adults with VSD with residual heart failure, shunts, PAH, AR, or RV outflow tract (RVOT) or LV outflow tract (LVOT) obstruction should be seen at least annually at an ACHD regional center (class I, level of evidence C).
- Adults with a small residual VSD and no other lesions should be seen every 3 to 5 yr at an ACHD regional center (class I, level of evidence C).
- Adults with device closure of a VSD should be followed up every 1 to 2 yr at an ACHD center depending on the location of the VSD and other factors (class I, level of evidence C).
- Patients who develop bifascicular block or transient trifascicular block after VSD closure are at risk in later years for the development of complete heart block and should be followed up yearly by history and ECG and have periodic ambulatory monitoring and/or exercise testing.

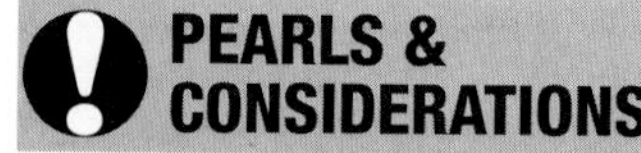

PEARLS & CONSIDERATIONS

COMMENTS

- A loud murmur does not imply a large VSD. Small, hemodynamically insignificant VSDs can cause loud murmurs.
- In patients with Eisenmenger's complex, the right-to-left shunting across the VSD is usually not associated with an audible murmur.
- Air-eliminating filters should be used on intravenous lines to prevent air embolism in patients with cyanosis indicating right-to-left shunting.
- The risk of patients with unrepaired VSD developing infective endocarditis is 4%. The risk is higher if aortic insufficiency is present.
- For patients with endocarditis, routine antibiotic prophylaxis for dental or surgical procedures is not indicated for isolated VSDs, except in the following circumstances:
  1. In the presence of complex congenital heart disease with cyanosis
  2. In the presence of a residual VSD after surgical closure
  3. During the first 6 months after surgical patch or percutaneous transcatheter closure
- Any patient with a newly diagnosed murmur or hemodynamic compromise after a myocardial infarction should undergo evaluation for possible VSD.
- Pregnancy with a VSD is generally well tolerated in women with small VSDs, no pulmonary artery hypertension, and no associated lesions. Women with large shunts may experience arrhythmias, ventricular dysfunction, and the progression of pulmonary hypertension.
- Women with VSDs and severe pulmonary artery hypertension or Eisenmenger's physiology should be counseled against pregnancy because of associated excessive maternal and fetal mortality.

SUGGESTED READINGS

Available at ExpertConsult.com

RELATED CONTENT

Ventricular Septal Defect (VSD) (Patient Information)

AUTHORS: **JOHANNES STEINER, M.D.,** and **TRACE BARRETT, M.D.**

BASIC INFORMATION

DEFINITION

- Ventricular tachycardia (VT) can be classified based on time (duration) or morphology.
- Nonsustained ventricular tachycardia (NSVT) is defined as beats originating from the ventricle, lasting from 3 to 30 seconds or for <30 seconds, at a rate >100/min.
- Sustained ventricular tachycardia is defined as above but lasts >30 seconds or produces symptoms in the patient and/or requires early intervention due to hemodynamic embarrassment.
- Ventricular tachycardia can be monomorphic or polymorphic, and the etiology, significance, and treatment of these two types of VT are different.

SYNONYMS

VT
Nonsustained paroxysmal ventricular tachycardia (NSVT) (Fig. 1)
Sustained ventricular tachycardia
Ventricular tachycardia, monomorphic
Ventricular tachycardia, nonsustained
Ventricular tachycardia, paroxysmal
Ventricular tachycardia, polymorphic
Ventricular tachycardia, sustained

ICD-10CM CODE

I47.2 Ventricular tachycardia

EPIDEMIOLOGY & DEMOGRAPHICS

INCIDENCE: The actual incidence and prevalence of VT in the general population is unknown. VT, especially NSVT, can be seen in both structurally normal and abnormal hearts, although it is far more common in the latter. In apparently healthy, asymptomatic individuals, the incidence is estimated at 0% to 3% (1).

For details on incidence of NSVT in various cardiac conditions, please refer to Table 1.

RISK FACTORS: The presence of structural heart disease is a strong risk factor for VT, but there are multiple, specific types of VT seen in patients without any structural heart disease.

PHYSICAL FINDINGS & CLINICAL PRESENTATION

- Patients may be asymptomatic, or they may present with any combination of palpitations, dizziness, syncope, chest pain, shortness of breath, seizures, or even cardiac arrest.
- History of structural heart disease, especially coronary artery disease and a prior myocardial infarction, is a strong predictor of VT. Patients may also have a history of pacemaker or defibrillator implantation. A family history of sudden death must also be sought.
- Physical findings of AV dissociation may be seen by the astute observer. These include cannon A waves in the neck and variability in intensity of heart sounds. The patient may also present physical findings of congestive heart failure including an S3 gallop, pedal edema, or crackles at the lung bases.

Fig. 2 shows initiation and termination of VT by means of programmed ventricular stimulation.

ETIOLOGY

Sustained monomorphic VT (Fig. 3) is mostly caused by reentry around a scar in the ventricular wall. The scar is most commonly the result of an old myocardial infarction, but arrhythmogenic RV cardiomyopathy (ARVC), nonischemic dilated cardiomyopathy, sarcoidosis, Chagas disease, tuberculosis, surgical incisions for repair of congenital heart disease, and ventricular volume reduction surgery can all cause scars in the myocardium. Fibrosis in the scar creates areas of anatomical conduction block, and fibrosis between surviving myocytes reduces cell-to-cell coupling, thereby distorting the path of propagation and causing areas of slow conduction, which promotes reentry.

Monomorphic VT can also be seen in patients without any evidence of structural heart disease (idiopathic VT). This subgroup represents 10% of all patients with VT and includes RVOT VT and fascicular VT. Common sites of origin of idiopathic VT include the right ventricular outflow tract (most common), the left ventricular outflow tract, the regions near the anterior and posterior left fascicles, and the papillary muscles.

Polymorphic VT is usually the result of active myocardial ischemia, electrolyte abnormalities (hypokalemia, hypomagnesemia), or genetic conditions such as LQTS, BRS, and CPVT. It may also be seen in HCM, various types of nonischemic cardiomyopathy, and idiopathic VF. The mechanisms are poorly understood but likely involve an initiating trigger that interacts with multiple rotors in the substrate to maintain the arrhythmia.

DIAGNOSIS

DIFFERENTIAL DIAGNOSIS

Differential diagnosis of an ECG suspicious of VT includes:

- SVT with aberrancy, either with a preexisting bundle branch block or a rate-related bundle branch block
- SVT in a patient taking anti-arrhythmic drugs, e.g., IA or IC agents
- Antidromic tachycardia from ventricular preexcitation
- Ventricular paced rhythms
- ECG artifact

TABLE 1 Reported Prevalence of Nonsustained Ventricular Tachycardia in Different Cardiac Conditions

Condition	Prevalence
Apparently healthy individuals	0%-3%
Non-ST ACS (2 to 9 days after admission)	18%-25%
Acute MI (early phase)	45%-75%
Reperfused acute MI (later than 1 week)	7%-13%
Heart failure (LVEF <30-40%)	30%-80%
DCM	40%-50%
HCM	25%-80%
Significant valve disease	≤25%
Hypertension	8%
Hypertension and left ventricular hypertrophy	12%-28%

DCM, Dilated cardiomyopathy; *HCM*, hypertrophic cardiomyopathy; *LVEF*, left ventricular ejection fraction; *MI*, myocardial infarction; *Non-ST ACS*, non–ST-segment elevation acute coronary syndrome.

From Saksena S et al: *Electrophysiological disorders of the heart*, ed 2, Philadelphia, 2011, Saunders.

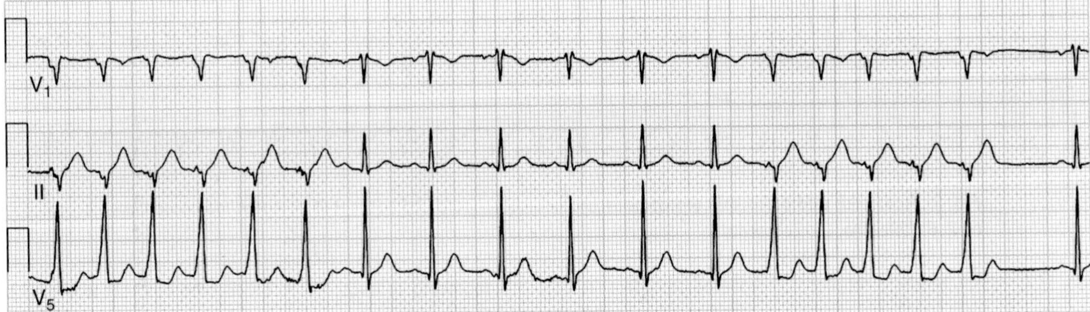

FIG. 1 Nonsustained ventricular tachycardia. This lead V_1, *II*, and V_5 rhythm strip shows repetitive runs of nonsustained wide QRS complex tachycardias (five to six beats long, rate ~125-135 bpm) that represent nonsustained ventricular tachycardia. The second run is followed by a compensatory pause. There is AV dissociation evident in the first run on lead V_1. (From Olshansky B et al: *Arrhythmia essentials*, ed 2, Philadelphia, 2017, Elsevier.)

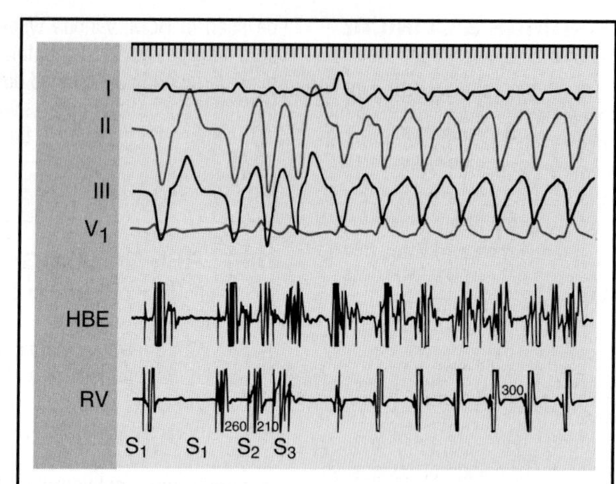

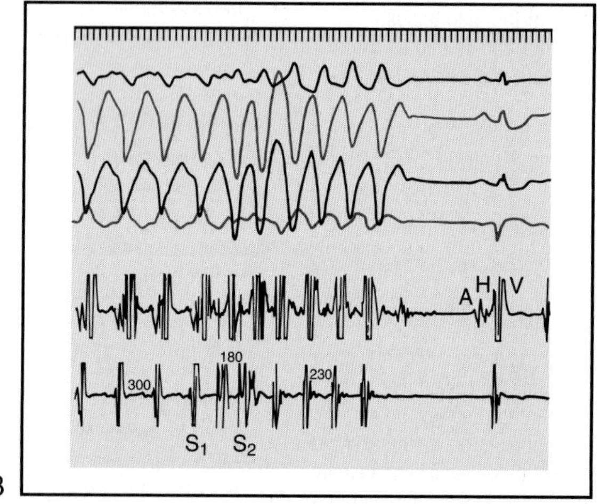

FIG. 2 Initiation and termination of ventricular tachycardia (VT) by means of programmed ventricular stimulation. The last two ventricular paced beats at a cycle length of 600 milliseconds are shown in **(A)**. A premature stimulus *(S_2)* at an *S_1–S_2* interval of 260 milliseconds and another premature stimulus *(S_3)* at a cycle length of 210 milliseconds initiate a sustained monomorphic VT at a cycle length of 300 milliseconds. **B,** Two premature ventricular stimuli *(S_1–S_2)* create an unstable VT that persists for several beats at a shorter cycle length (230 milliseconds) and then terminates, followed by sinus rhythm. *HBE,* His bundle electrogram; *RV,* right ventricle. (From Bonow RO et al: *Heart disease,* ed 9. Philadelphia, 2012, Saunders.)

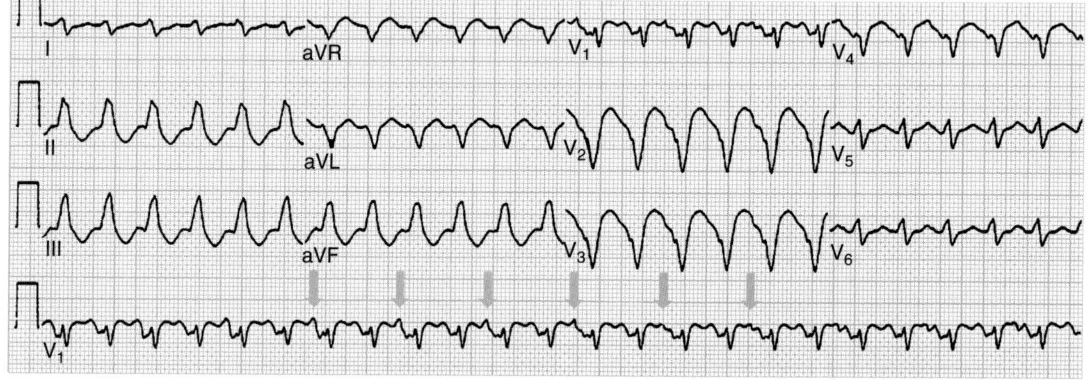

FIG. 3 Sustained monomorphic ventricular tachycardia. (From Olshansky B et al: *Arrhythmia essentials,* ed 2, Philadelphia, 2017, Elsevier.)

The following ECG characteristics strongly favor VT as opposed to SVT: Northwest (right superior) axis, QRS width >160 ms, AV dissociation, fusion beats, and capture beats. The last three are highly specific for VT.

Additional assessment is based upon QRS morphology. Most VT can be classified as either RBBB-type (overall positive in V1) or LBBB-type (overall negative in V1). The following criteria favoring VT can be applied for the respective types:

- RBBB type: Monophasic R; notched waveform with a taller left peak Rr'; biphasic RS or QR pattern.
- LBBB type in V1: R-wave >30 ms, slurred or notched S wave downstroke, delayed S nadir (QRS onset to S nadir >60 ms).
- LBBB type in V6: VT is favored in presence of a QS pattern, rS pattern (R-to-S <1) in RBBB-type tachycardias; QRS onset to predominant peak or nadir in lead V6 of 70 ms.

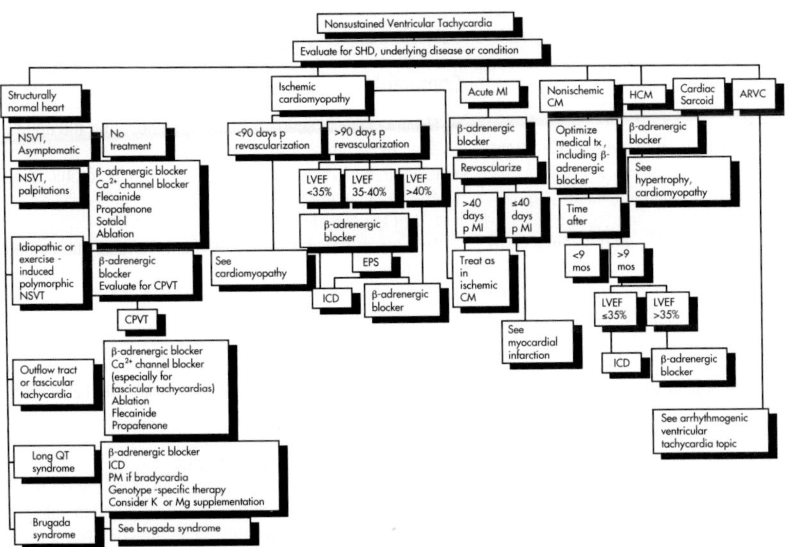

FIG. 4 Nonsustained ventricular tachycardia. *ARVC,* Arrhythmogenic right ventricular cardiomyopathy; *CM,* cardiomyopathy; *CPVT,* catecholaminergic polymorphic ventricular tachycardia; *EP,* electrophysiologic study; *HCM,* hypertrophic cardiomyopathy; *ICD,* implantable cardioverter defibrillator; *LVEF,* left ventricular ejection fraction; *MI,* myocardial infarction; *NSVT,* nonsustained ventricular tachycardia; *PM,* pacemaker. (Modified from Olshansky B et al: *Arrhythmia essentials,* ed 2, Philadelphia, 2017, Elsevier.)

- aVR: Presence of an initial R-wave in AVR and width of an initial r or q wave >40 ms.

WORKUP

- Lab testing should especially focus on checking K and Mg levels.
- A full 12-lead ECG of the tachycardia should always be obtained, whenever possible, and compared to the ECG in sinus rhythm if there is any uncertainty about the diagnosis.
- This should be followed by an echocardiogram and ischemia evaluation with diagnostic coronary angiography and/or nuclear stress testing. Exercise testing should be performed because it may aid in provoking as well as establishing patient response to exercise-induced arrhythmias, including catecholaminergic *polymorphic* VT.
- An MRI of the heart is indicated if these tests are unable to establish the cause of the arrhythmia.
- Ambulatory ECG, event monitors, and implantable recorders are appropriate to evaluate for QT interval changes and T-wave alternans, judge therapy, evaluate risk, and to allow for symptom-rhythm correlation.
- Electrophysiologic testing is useful for the inducibility of VT, to guide ablation, the evaluation of drug effects, the assessment of the risk of recurrent VT, the loss of consciousness with arrhythmia as a suspected cause, and the assessment of indications for ICD therapy.

LABORATORY TESTS

- Potassium, magnesium
- Genetic testing should be reserved for specific situations, i.e., when there is a concern for genetically mediated conditions such as LQTS, HCM, CPVT, or BRS

IMAGING STUDIES

An echocardiogram and ischemia evaluation with diagnostic coronary angiography and/or nuclear stress testing is recommended to rule out structural heart disease and ischemia. An MRI of the heart is indicated if these tests are unable to establish the cause of the arrhythmia, to rule out cardiomyopathies such as cardiac sarcoidosis, amyloid, LV noncompaction, arrhythmogenic right ventricular dysplasia, etc.

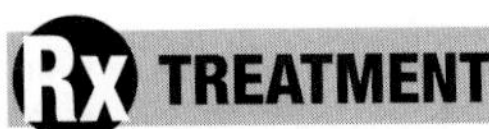

TREATMENT

ACUTE GENERAL Rx

Patients with VT may become hemodynamically unstable very quickly. In such situations emergency synchronized cardioversion (or defibrillation for polymorphic rhythms) is needed. Those who subsequently become pulseless or unresponsive should be managed as per standard ACLS resuscitation protocols. An approach to nonsustained tachycardia is described in Fig. 4 and Table 2. Table 3 and Fig. 5 illustrate the management of sustained ventricular tachycardia.

If the patient is hemodynamically stable, either IV amiodarone, lidocaine (especially if there is a suspicion of ongoing ischemia), or procainamide may be used. In the case of a patient with sustained monomorphic VT and a known structurally normal heart, IV beta blockers or calcium blockers may be used. It must be remembered that use of all these agents may be associated with hemodynamic deterioration and an external defibrillator must be made available at all times.

Electrolyte supplementation is essential if hypokalemia or hypomagnesemia is detected.

CHRONIC Rx

An implantable cardioverter-defibrillator (ICD) is indicated for all cases of hemodynamically untolerated monomorphic VT in patients with structural heart disease or prior MI (in the absence of a successful catheter ablation that eliminates all VT, which is usually possible only in patients with normal LVEF and stable VT), since it indicates the presence of a scar and risk of subsequent arrhythmias. Patients with idiopathic VT and structurally normal hearts generally do not require an ICD, but in cases of syncope associated with VT that cannot be successfully treated with ablation, it may be considered. For polymorphic VT, a reversible cause such as ischemia or electrolyte disturbances can sometimes be found, and an ICD may not be appropriate under these circumstances.

Chronic therapy with antiarrhythmic medications such as amiodarone, mexiletine, or sotalol may be needed even after ICD implantation if the patient presents with multiple appropriate shocks. Cather ablation of VT, particularly if performed early after first appropriate ICD discharge, is also very effective in preventing further ICD discharges and is associated with improved acute and long-term outcomes. For patients with refractory VT, surgical cardiac sympathetic denervation may be beneficial.

DISPOSITION

Patients with sustained VT, either monomorphic or polymorphic, should always be managed in an intensive care unit due to the risk of degeneration to a hemodynamically unstable rhythm. An electrophysiologist should be consulted.

REFERRAL

All patients with VT or NSVT should be referred to a cardiologist or a cardiac electrophysiologist.

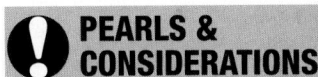

PEARLS & CONSIDERATIONS

COMMENTS

- Use of antiarrhythmic drugs, especially IC agents, to treat NSVT is associated with increased mortality (CAST trial), while beta blockers have been shown to be helpful.
- In patients with coronary disease, NSVT has not been shown to have an adverse significance if LVEF is >40%. If the EF is below 40%, the MUSTT trial showed a benefit of EP-guided ICD therapy over antiarrhythmic agents such as mexiletine, propafenone, sotalol, or amiodarone. Patients with LVEF <35% are candidates for prophylactic ICD implantation based on the MADIT II and SCDHeFt trials.
- In hypertrophic cardiomyopathy, NSVT does seem to confer an increased risk of sudden death, especially if symptomatic, prolonged, or repetitive.
- There are certain conditions in which NSVT does not seem to have an adverse significance and does not predict sudden cardiac death. These include nonischemic dilated cardiomyopathy, mitral valve prolapse, mitral regurgitation, and absence of structural heart disease.

PATIENT/FAMILY EDUCATION

Patients with familial or genetic causes of ventricular tachycardia should have family screening of first-degree relatives.

TABLE 2 Management of Nonsustained Monomorphic and Polymorphic Ventricular Tachycardia

Setting	Therapy	Comments
Normal LV function	• No symptoms, no heart disease: No therapy • Young patient with bidirectional (or polymorphic) VT that may be life-threatening (CPVT): β-adrenergic blocker • Symptoms of palpitations, no heart disease: β-adrenergic blocker (e.g., acebutolol, 200-800 per day) • Idiopathic LV fascicular tachycardia (RBBB left axis QRS morphology): Verapamil • If LBBB (inferior axis morphology), β-adrenergic blocker is first line. Other drugs: Sotalol (started in hospital), propafenone, flecainide, amiodarone. • RF ablation is curative for this type of VT in more than 95% if it can be initiated and mapped in the EP laboratory. • CAD, no symptoms: β-adrenergic blocker, no additional antiarrhythmic therapy • CAD with symptoms, β-adrenergic blocker, sotalol, amiodarone (started in the hospital) • Polymorphic NSVT 1. In the setting of the long QT with syncope, treatment is required. 2. Genotyping is available. 3. β-Adrenergic blockers are the first choice for long QT type I. 4. With syncope or family history of sudden death, LQT2 or LQT3: ICD.	• Multiple clinical scenarios exist depending on the age of patient, heart disease, and symptoms. • Idiopathic VT may occur in repetitive monomorphic variety and be symptomatic. 1. Not life-threatening. 2. Is exacerbated by exercise, mental stress, and catecholamines. • Idiopathic polymorphic VT in the young can be potentially life-threatening. 1. Treat with β-adrenergic blocker. 2. Consider genotyping for CPVT. • Consider RV cardiomyopathy (dysplasia) with LBBB/noninferior axis morphology. • Consider ischemia. • The 12-lead morphology is helpful. 1. If LBBB with inferior axis, it is likely from the RV or LV/aortic cusp outflow tract in normal hearts and is ablatable. 2. If QRS is negative in I and aVL, it may be arising from the septum. 3. If it is positive in these leads, it may be arising from the free wall and may be adenosine sensitive. 4. VTs may respond to β-adrenergic blockers, verapamil, and most antiarrhythmic drugs. • If it is a RBBB left axis QRS pattern, it may be a reentrant idiopathic VT from the LV apical septum. 1. Thought to be due to fascicular reentry. 2. Can be cured with RF ablation. 3. Is sensitive to verapamil (only use if known to be this type of VT). • Even patients with normal hearts may be at slightly higher risk for CA compared with the general population, but further evaluation and therapy is not beneficial. • Polymorphic tachycardia may be due to ischemia or infarction and may be transient.
Ischemic cardiomyopathy	• For LVEF ≤30%, more than 1 mo after MI, 3 mo after revascularization, ICD implantation. • For LVEF ≤35%, NYHA FC II-III, ICD implantation is recommended. • For LVEF ≤40%, EP study is recommended, and if sustained VT is induced, ICD should be implanted. • For NYHA FC III-IV heart failure, LVEF ≤35%, and QRS duration >120 ms, cardiac resynchronization therapy is recommended.	• Increased risk of sudden death. • Increased risk is not related to length of episodes. • EP testing may risk stratify.
Nonischemic cardiomyopathy	• β-adrenergic blockers, ACE inhibitors, and other optimal therapies for heart failure • For LVEF ≤35%, NYHA FC II-III, ICD is recommended. • For NYHA FC III-IV heart failure, LVEF ≤35%, and QRS duration >120 ms, cardiac resynchronization therapy is recommended.	
HCM	• β-adrenergic blocker, especially if symptomatic • Memory loop event recorders may be beneficial in correlating symptoms with arrhythmias. • No indication for amiodarone or other antiarrhythmic drugs if asymptomatic • Start amiodarone, if symptomatic, in the hospital. • ICD if 1. Septum >30 mm 2. Syncope 3. NSVT 4. Family history of sudden death 5. High-risk genotype 6. If prior CA 7. Sustained VT/VF	• Potentially indicative of a malignant, life-threatening ventricular arrhythmia. • EP testing of no proven benefit in this setting.
MI	• No specific therapy • Assess LV function. • β-Adrenergic blocker as part of the post-MI regimen • If continued NSVT and impaired LV function (LVEF <0.40) after 4-6 wk, consider ICD and suppressive antiarrhythmic therapy to slow VT rate and prevent shocks.	• Little prognostic meaning early after MI. Predictive value increases with increasing time from MI. • If polymorphic, consider ischemia (or electrolyte disturbance if the QT interval is prolonged). • May represent a coronary reperfusion injury rhythm.
Preoperative	• If noncardiac surgery planned, assess symptoms, longevity of the problem, drugs • If recent onset: Assess LV function • If LVEF ≤0.40, and if CAD, consider EP test • If no CHF LVEF ≤0.30, ICD. If CHF and LVEF ≤0.35, ICD	

TABLE 2 Management of Nonsustained Monomorphic and Polymorphic Ventricular Tachycardia—cont'd

Setting	Therapy	Comments
Postoperative	• No therapy • Has little prognostic meaning early after surgery • Resolves spontaneously in the great majority • Evaluate for underlying heart disease if risk factors are present. • Plan follow-up Holter monitor. If episodes continue, consider EP test. If induced VT, consider ICD if LVEF ≤0.40 or other criteria met (ischemic, nonischemic cardiomyopathy; discussed previously). • If asymptomatic, treat based on monitor results or based on EP test results.	

ACE, Angiotensin-converting enzyme; *CA*, cardiac arrest; *CABG*, coronary artery bypass graft; *CAD*, coronary artery disease; *CPVT*, catecholaminergic polymorphic ventricular tachycardia; *EP*, electrophysiologic; *FC*, functional class; *HCM*, hypertrophic cardiomyopathy; *ICD*, implantable cardioverter defibrillator; *LBBB*, left bundle branch block; *LV*, left ventricular; *LVEF*, left ventricular ejection fraction; *MI*, myocardial infarction; *NSVT*, nonsustained ventricular tachycardia; *NYHA*, New York Heart Association; *RBBB*, right bundle branch block; *RF*, radiofrequency; *RV*, right ventricular; *VT*, ventricular tachycardia.

From Olshansky B et al: *Arrhythmia essentials*, ed 2, Philadelphia, 2017, Elsevier.

TABLE 3 Management of Sustained Ventricular Tachycardia

Setting	Therapy	Comments
Acute therapy • Monomorphic VT well tolerated (patient awake and alert, no angina, no CHF, stable BP)	• First line: Amiodarone 150 mg over 10 min followed by 1mg/min for 6 h followed by 0.5 mg/min 1. May combine amiodarone IV with oral drug and with IV lidocaine if needed 2. Lidocaine 1.5-2 mg/kg (but only effective in <15%) • Second line: Procainamide 10-15 mg/kg at 25 mg/min (or less), assessing the BP carefully 1. Procainamide can slow VT and may be effective in an additional 20% to 30% 2. Amiodarone is probably more effective than procainamide, safer, and better tolerated • Third line: Cardioversion after adequate anesthesia • Do not cardiovert while awake • Fourth line: Antitachycardia pacing via a temporary transvenous pacing lead	• Assess cause and hemodynamic tolerance. 1. Guidance of therapy is dependent on the clinical status of the patient. 2. VT can always degenerate to VF even if it is at first stable. • IV amiodarone is emerging as first-line therapy for sustained monomorphic VT due to lack of efficacy of other drugs. • Procainamide has a negative inotropic effect. • Temporary transvenous pacing requires time and experienced personnel to accomplish.
Acute therapy, MI	• Same as above but degree of urgency in treatment is greater. • The length of time in VT, even if apparently tolerated, should be minimized. • Lidocaine is associated with no improvement in mortality.	• Monomorphic VT 1. May not increase long-term mortality. 2. Can be ischemia induced but this is rare (<3% of all MIs). 3. Tends to indicate "an electrical reentry circuit" of damaged myocardium.
Acute therapy, polymorphic VT • Normal QT interval • Patient stable	• If stable and the patient is awake (very rare): 1. If ineffective, DC shock (200 J >300-360 J) after anesthetized • IV β-adrenergic blockade as tolerated	• Assess cause and hemodynamic tolerance. • Rule out ischemia, infarction, electrolyte abnormality (low K^+ or Mg^{2+}), or adverse drug effect. • Assess age, underlying disease process and LV function, potential causative factors (e.g., exercise). • Therapy depends on the clinical status, which can always degenerate to VF even if it appears to be stable. • IV amiodarone may be effective, but there are no data on well-tolerated polymorphic VT.
Chronic prevention • No structural heart disease • Idiopathic VT, usually in young patient • Often exercise- or stress-induced • Rule out RV cardiomyopathy (dysplasia) with MRI	• First line: β-adrenergic blocker titrated to the highest tolerated dose • If recurrent episodes (with moderate or severe symptoms) occur: RF catheter ablation • The success for LBBB inferior axis and for RBBB superior axis VT ablation is 90% to 95% • RF ablation is first line if patient has syncope, hemodynamic intolerance, or patient preference	• Monomorphic VT can be highly symptomatic but is almost never "malignant" and life-threatening. • LBBB/inferior axis VT is usually from the outflow tract. 1. If the QRS is negative in I and aVL, suspect a septal or LV origin. 2. If it is positive in these leads, suspect a free wall origin. 3. The mechanism may be due to triggered automaticity. Highly amenable to RF ablation. • RBBB/superior axis VTs are likely due to reentry in the Purkinje system. 1. Are verapamil sensitive. 2. Can be successfully ablated. • For LBBB, noninferior axis morphology VTs, r/o ARVC.

Continued

TABLE 3 Management of Sustained Ventricular Tachycardia—cont'd

Setting	Therapy	Comments
Prior MI, ischemia can be provoked	• If monomorphic, suspect a substrate that is due to scar, not ischemia. • If polymorphic, suspect ischemia or infarction. • Consider a functional stress test or coronary angiogram and revascularization if ischemic. • ICD implantation if hemodynamically significant sustained VT/VF • Ablation can be successful in >50% but with a high rate of long-term recurrence 1. Used as adjunctive therapy to ICD implantation 2. May be used to reduce recurrent ICD shocks • Adjunctive antiarrhythmic drugs include amiodarone or sotalol	• May also be associated with VF. • Rarely, monomorphic VT is due to ischemia alone, but always suspect substrate even if episodes occur relatively soon after infarction. 1. If an antiarrhythmic drug is being used, consider the possibility of a proarrhythmic effect. • Most patients (>95%) with chronic VT due to CAD will be inducible in the EP laboratory, but this does not change treatment strategy.

ARVC, arrhythmogenic right ventricular cardiomyopathy; *BP,* blood pressure; *EP,* electrophysiologic; *ICD,* implantable cardioverter defibrillator; *IV,* intravenous; *LBBB,* left bundle branch block; *LV,* left ventricular; *MI,* myocardial infarction; *MRI,* magnetic resonance imaging; *RBBB,* right bundle branch block; *RF,* radiofrequency; *RV,* right ventricular; *VF,* ventricular fibrillation; *VT,* ventricular tachycardia.

From Olshansky B et al: *Arrhythmia essentials*, ed 2, Philadelphia, 2017, Elsevier.

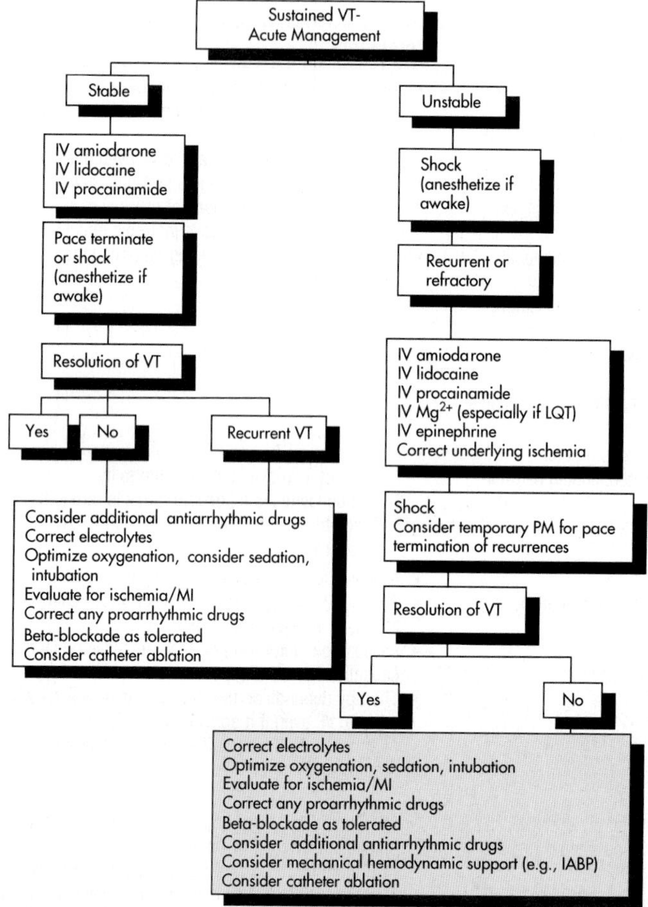

FIG. 5 Sustained ventricular tachycardia—acute management. *IABP,* Intra-aortic balloon pump; *IV,* intravenous; *LQT,* long QT interval; *MI,* myocardial infarction; *PM,* pacemaker; *VT,* ventricular tachycardia. (From Olshansky B et al: *Arrhythmia essentials*, ed 2, Philadelphia, 2017, Elsevier.)

SUGGESTED READINGS

Available at ExpertConsult.com

RELATED TOPICS

Arrhythmogenic Right Ventricular Dysplasia (Related Key Topic)
Brugada Syndrome (Related Key Topic)
Long QT Syndrome (Related Key Topic)
Torsade de Pointes (Related Key Topic)

AUTHOR: **SIMON GRINGUT, M.D.**

BASIC INFORMATION

DEFINITION

Vertebral compression fractures (VCFs) are defined as fractures of spinal vertebrae in which a bony surface is driven toward another bony surface. These fractures are classified as radiographic reductions in vertebral body height of more than 15%.

SYNONYMS

Thoracolumbar vertebral compression fractures
Osteoporotic fractures
VCF

ICD-10CM CODES

M80.0	Post-menopausal osteoporosis with pathologic fracture
M80.4	Drug-induced osteoporosis with pathological fracture
M80.5	Idiopathic osteoporosis with pathological fracture
M80.8	Other osteoporosis with pathological fracture
M80.9	Unspecified osteoporosis with pathological fracture
S32.009A	Unspecified fracture of unspecified lumbar vertebra, initial encounter for closed fracture
S22.009A	Unspecified fracture of unspecified thoracic vertebra, initial encounter for closed fracture

EPIDEMIOLOGY & DEMOGRAPHICS

~700,000 VCFs occur in the United States each year, and they affect up to 25% of postmenopausal women. They are the most common complication of osteoporosis. The prevalence increases with age, reaching a peak of 40% to 50% among women aged >80 yr. Compression fractures are also a major concern among men, although their rates of VCF are lower.

RISK FACTORS:

- Modifiable: Tobacco or alcohol use, osteoporosis, estrogen deficiency (i.e., early menopause, bilateral oophorectomy, premenopausal amenorrhea for >1 yr), frailty, impaired vision, abusive situations, inadequate physical activity, low body mass index, and deficiency of vitamin D or calcium.
- Nonmodifiable: Advanced age, female gender, dementia, Caucasian descent, history of fractures in adulthood and among first-degree relatives, and falls.

PHYSICAL FINDINGS & CLINICAL PRESENTATION

- Asymptomatic: Most VCFs are asymptomatic, except for height loss or kyphosis (i.e., dowager's hump [Fig. 1]), which is often a sign of multiple VCFs and height loss of >6 cm has a sensitivity/specificity of 94% and 30%, respectively, for VCF.
- Symptomatic: When symptomatic, VCFs usually present as acute back pain after activity (e.g., bending, lifting) or coughing; neck strain and radicular rib pain may also be present.

ETIOLOGY

- VCFs take place when the combination of bending and the axial load on the spine exceed the strength of the vertebral body.
- The primary etiology of VCF is osteoporosis, though a pathologic fracture from an underlying malignancy, typically metastatic disease, must be ruled out.

Dx DIAGNOSIS

DIFFERENTIAL DIAGNOSIS

- Osteoporosis
- Malignancy, most often metastases
- Hyperparathyroidism
- Osteomalacia
- Granulomatous diseases (e.g., tuberculosis)
- Hematologic/oncologic diseases (e.g., multiple myeloma, primary bone malignancy)

WORKUP

- Only one third of VCFs are diagnosed. Guidelines for patient selection for vertebral fractural assessment are described in Box 1.
- VCFs can be clinically suspected from the history and physical alone, though they are often diagnosed incidentally by imaging performed for another indication.
- There may or may not be a specific injury or a remembered event that led to the VCF.

LABORATORY TESTS

Tests to rule out infection or cancer may be helpful, such as a CBC, an erythrocyte sedimentation rate, an alkaline phosphatase level, and a C-reactive protein level; these tests can be reserved for individuals for whom there is clinical suspicion.

IMAGING STUDIES

- Plain frontal and lateral radiographs (x-rays) are the initial imaging method (Fig. 1) and may be sufficient, particularly when no neurologic abnormalities are present. MRI and computed tomography (CT) scans may be uncomfortable or painful for the patient, especially during the acute phase.
- Although CT scans are not routinely necessary for the diagnosis, they can be helpful for visualizing fractures that are not seen on plain films, for evaluating the integrity of the posterior vertebral wall, for ruling out other causes of back pain, for detecting spinal canal narrowing, and for assessing instability.
- MRI may be useful when spinal cord compression is suspected, if neurologic symptoms are present, or to distinguish malignancy from osteoporosis (e.g., in patients <55 yr with VCF after minimal or no trauma).
- Bone density studies may be helpful to determine the severity of osteoporosis, which is a key risk factor for future fractures.

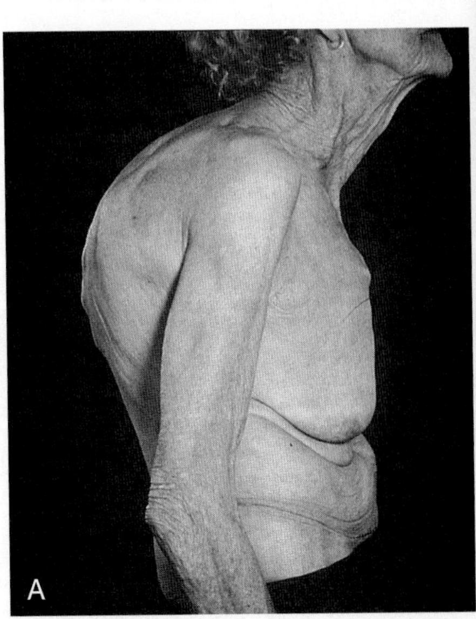

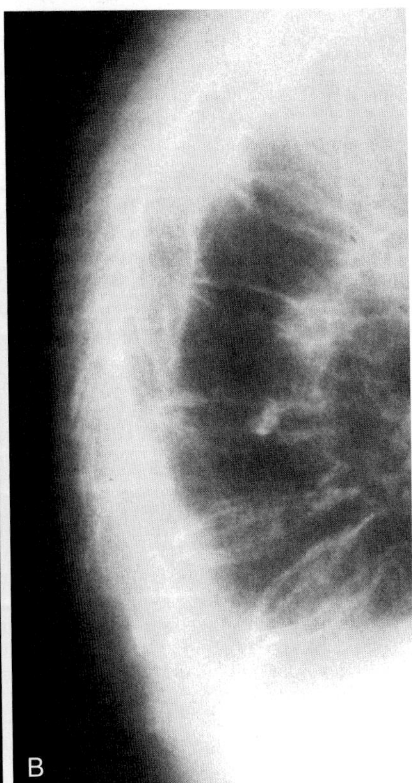

FIG. 1 Dowager's hump. A, Marked thoracic kyphosis due to multiple osteoporotic fractures in an elderly woman with corresponding radiograph **(B)**. (From Hochberg MC, et al. [eds]: *Rheumatology,* ed 3, St Louis, 2003, Mosby.)

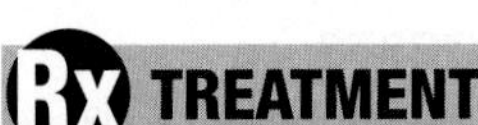

TREATMENT

NONPHARMACOLOGIC THERAPY

- Physical therapy.
- External back braces: Frequently recommended to relieve pain and improve mobility, however, controlled trials have not shown any effect in patients with vertebral compression fractures.
- Exercise programs: Getting active as soon as possible is extremely important for both short-and long-term recovery.

ACUTE GENERAL Rx

- Analgesics are first line for pain control, including acetaminophen and opioids (oral or parenteral), and pain can be expected to diminish over 4 to 6 wk.
- Nonsteroidal antiinflammatory drugs are helpful but must be used with caution among elderly patients or when contraindicated.
- Muscle relaxants should be used judiciously because they have significant side effects, particularly in the elderly.
- Intranasal calcitonin (200 units once daily, alternating nostrils) has been shown in some small trials to hasten relief from pain when used as an adjunct to oral analgesics, and a 2- to 4-wk course may be useful for patients who do not achieve adequate control with oral analgesics alone.
- Early mobilization with physical therapy is important for recovery and prevention of subsequent fractures.
- The efficacy of vertebroplasty versus kyphoplasty versus conservative treatment remains controversial.
- Percutaneous vertebroplasty involves the injection of acrylic bone cement into the affected vertebral body in an effort to stabilize the fracture and reduce pain, whereas in kyphoplasty, a high-pressure inflatable bone tamp or balloon is expanded within the body of the affected vertebra to restore prefracture vertebral height before the injection of bone cement. These two procedures were thought to be helpful in patients who did not respond to conservative therapy; however, further studies showed them to be no more effective than sham procedures (Buchbinder et al, 2009; Kallmes et al, 2009). Nonetheless, Klazen et al (2010) demonstrated in an open-label prospective randomized trial that for the subgroup of patients with acute osteoporotic VCFs and persistent pain, percutaneous vertebroplasty may provide immediate pain relief, sustained for at least a year, which may be significantly greater than that achieved with conservative treatment. Zampini (2010) showed in a nonrandomized cohort study that elderly patients who underwent kyphoplasty were more likely to be discharged home. McCullough et al (2013) analyzed Medicare claims of patients with VCF treated with kyphoplasty or vertebroplasty compared with medical management and found no difference in mortality or major medical outcomes but decreased health care utilization in the conservatively managed group. These procedures are still in their infancy, and more answers should be forthcoming as to their efficacy, as well as questions regarding the amount of time that conservative therapy alone should be pursued and which procedure, if any, should be advised. Most current guidelines recommend 4 to 6 wk of medical therapy before pursuing surgical intervention in neurologically intact VCF.

CHRONIC Rx

Osteoporosis should be treated with the reduction of risk factors (e.g., smoking, alcohol), diet, exercise, calcium and vitamin D supplements, and with medications used to treat osteoporosis (e.g., bisphosphonates).

REFERRAL

Referral is indicated for neurologic abnormalities, unremitting pain, instability, continued disability, or when the investigation of the cause of the fracture reveals serious underlying pathology.

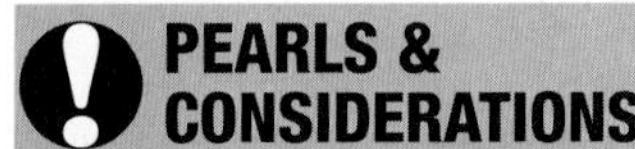

PEARLS & CONSIDERATIONS

Prevention of osteoporosis and conservative therapy remain the mainstay of treatment.

COMMENTS

- VCFs should be suspected in anyone aged >50 yr with the acute onset of low back pain. There are many opportunities for diagnosis and treatment that are easy to miss, especially for males.
- Solitary vertebral fractures higher than T7 are unusual and should raise suspicion for other pathologic causes.
- Diagnosing and treating osteoporosis reduce the incidence of VCFs.
- Getting people with VCF physically active as soon as possible will be efficacious both acutely and in the long term.
- In general, VCF will be best managed through a partnership of the patient, the primary care physician, an orthopedist, a physical therapist, a dietitian, and a social worker.

PREVENTION

Reducing the effects of modifiable risk factors is key.

SUGGESTED READINGS

Available at ExpertConsult.com

AUTHOR: **FRED F. FERRI, M.D.**

BOX 1 2007 ISCD Guidelines for Patient Selection for Vertebral Fractural Assessment

- Postmenopausal women with low bone mass (osteopenia) by BMD criteria, *plus* any one of the following: age >70 yr, historical height loss >4 cm (1.6 in), or prospective height loss >2 cm (0.8 in), self-reported vertebral fracture (not previously documented)
- Two or more of the following: age 60 to 69 yr, self-reported prior non-vertebral fracture, historical height loss of 2 to 4 cm, or chronic systemic diseases associated with increased risk of vertebral fractures (e.g., moderate to severe COPD or COAD, seropositive rheumatoid arthritis, Crohn's disease)
- Men with low bone mass (osteopenia) by BMD criteria, *plus* any one of the following: age >80 yr, historical height loss >6 cm (2.4 in), prospective height loss >3 cm (1.2 in), self-reported vertebral fracture (not previously documented)
- Two or more of the following: age 70 to 79 yr, self-reported prior non-vertebral fracture, historical height loss of 3 to 6 cm, on pharmacologic androgen deprivation therapy or following orchiectomy, chronic systemic diseases associated with increased risk of vertebral fractures (e.g., moderate to severe COPD or COAD, seropositive rheumatoid arthritis, Crohn's disease)
- Women or men on chronic glucocorticoid therapy (equivalent to 5 mg or more of prednisone daily for 3 mo or longer)
- Postmenopausal women or men with osteoporosis by BMD criteria, if documentation of one or more vertebral fractures will alter clinical management

BMD, Bone mineral density; *COAD,* chronic obstructive airways disease; *COPD,* chronic obstructive pulmonary disease; *ISCD,* International Society for Clinical Densitometry.

Reproduced with permission from the International Society for Clinical Densitometry.
From Hochberg MC, et al.: *Rheumatology,* ed 5, St Louis, 2011, Mosby.

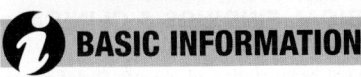

BASIC INFORMATION

DEFINITION

Vestibular neuronitis is a syndrome of sudden-onset dysfunction of the peripheral vestibular system, often severe, with prolonged vertigo, nausea, and vomiting.

SYNONYMS

Vestibular neuritis
Acute neuritis
Neurolabyrinthitis
Vestibular neuropathy

ICD-10CM CODES

H81.2	Vestibular neuronitis
H81.23	Vestibular neuronitis, bilateral
H81.20	Vestibular neuronitis, unspecified ear
H81.21	Vestibular neuronitis, right ear
H81.22	Vestibular neuronitis, left ear

EPIDEMIOLOGY & DEMOGRAPHICS

Vestibular neuritis is the second most common cause of peripheral vestibular vertigo with an incidence of about 3.5:100,000 population. Although etiology remains uncertain, it is thought to result from viral infection causing selective inflammation of the vestibular nerve. Infectious origin is supported by the fact that it occurs in epidemics, may affect several family members, and occurs more commonly in spring and early summer. The male:female ratio is nearly 1:1. There is selective damage to the superior part of the vestibular labyrinth, supplied by the superior vestibular portion of the eighth cranial nerve.

PHYSICAL FINDINGS & CLINICAL PRESENTATION

COURSE: Develops acutely over a period of hours and resolves over periods of days or weeks, although long-term sequelae may occur, such as residual imbalance and nonspecific dizziness persisting for months. Symptoms include vertigo, spontaneous peripheral nystagmus (predominantly horizontal), positive head-thrust test, and imbalance. Patients report intense sensation of rotation and difficulty standing and walking and tend to veer toward the affected side; autonomic symptoms occur with pallor, sweating, nausea, and vomiting.

ETIOLOGY

Etiology remains uncertain but viral and post-viral inflammatory disorders are suspected. Herpes zoster, reactivation of herpes simplex type I, and other viruses have been implicated, but evidence is circumstantial.

Dx DIAGNOSIS

DIFFERENTIAL DIAGNOSIS

- Labyrinthitis: Similar symptoms of vertigo, with the addition of unilateral hearing loss
- Labyrinthine infarction
- Acoustic neuroma
- Perilymph fistula
- Brain stem and cerebellar infarction
- Migraine-associated vertigo
- Meniere disease
- Multiple sclerosis

WORKUP

- Patient may fall toward affected side when attempting ambulation or during Romberg tests.
- Hallpike maneuver: Checking for nystagmus and asking about re-creation of vertigo symptoms
- Head-thrust test: Grasp patient's head, apply brief small-amplitude rapid head turn, first to one side and then the other; patient fixates on examiner's nose: positive test is lack of or slowing of corrective eye movements ("saccades") on affected side. A positive test supports the diagnosis of vestibular neuronitis.
- Laboratory testing and imaging are generally not indicated but may help rule out other etiologies.

LABORATORY TESTS

- Electronystagmography (ENG): A battery of eye movement tests that may provide an objective assessment of the vestibular and oculomotor systems and may help localize the lesion's site
- Audiogram: Normal

IMAGING STUDIES

Brain imaging: CT or MRI—normal

Rx TREATMENT

NONPHARMACOLOGIC THERAPY

Vestibular exercises, when tolerated, will accelerate recovery.

ACUTE GENERAL Rx

Most treatments are empirical and related to symptoms. Further studies are needed.

- Corticosteroids: Corticosteroids are often prescribed, although a Cochrane Review finds that there is insufficient evidence for administration. Some studies have shown that glucocorticoids administered within 3 days after onset of vestibular neuronitis may improve long-time recovery of vestibular function and reduce the length of hospital stay and may improve the caloric extent and recovery of canal paresis while others show no significant difference.
- Antihistamines: e.g., meclizine, dimenhydrinate, promethazine
- Anticholinergics: Scopolamine
- Antiemetics: Droperidol, prochlorperazine
- Benzodiazepines: e.g., diazepam, valium, lorazepam
- Valacyclovir, either alone or in combination, is likely ineffective in treating vestibular neuronitis

CHRONIC Rx

- Vestibular rehabilitation exercises
- Anti-GABA agents
- Antihistamines

DISPOSITION

Most patients can be treated as outpatients, but inpatient care may be required in cases where vomiting is uncontrollable. If dehydrated because of severe vomiting, sufferers may require brief parenteral therapy.

REFERRAL

- ENT: If diagnosis uncertain, and if these patients are at risk for benign paroxysmal positional vertigo (BPPV) subsequently; also if symptoms linger
- Neurology: If question of central origin or migraine

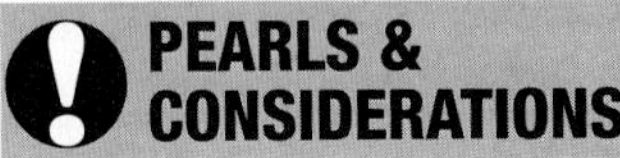

PEARLS & CONSIDERATIONS

COMMENTS

- Diagnosis unlikely to be vestibular neuronitis if hearing is impaired or other neurologic signs and symptoms are present.
- Although patients may recover from dramatic acute symptoms, subtle vestibular deficits may linger for prolonged period, if not indefinitely (i.e., residual imbalance and nonspecific dizziness).
- Program of vestibular habituation head movement exercises can reduce imbalance symptoms.

PATIENT & FAMILY EDUCATION

Vestibular Disorders Association: http://www.vestibular.org

SUGGESTED READINGS

Available at ExpertConsult.com

RELATED CONTENT

Benign Paroxysmal Positional Vertigo (Related Key Topic)
Meniere's Disease (Related Key Topic)
Labyrinthitis (Related Key Topic)

AUTHOR: **ROCCO J. RICHARDS, M.D.**

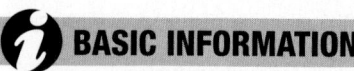

BASIC INFORMATION

- Vitamin D is a hormone and a steroid and, by definition, not a vitamin. There are two forms of vitamin D: vitamin D_2 and vitamin D_3.
- Vitamin D_2 (ergocalciferol) is mainly found in some plant foods.
- Vitamin D_3 (cholecalciferol) is produced in skin exposed to ultraviolet (UV) B radiation from sunlight (Fig. 1). Gloson, Whistler, and DeBoot independently described rickets in the mid-seventeenth century. Sniadecki first reported the association of rickets with inadequate exposure to sunlight in 1822.
- The major functions of vitamin D include:
  1. Increasing calcium and phosphorus absorption from the small intestines.
  2. Promoting the maturation of osteoclast to resorb calcium from bones.

DEFINITION

Vitamin D deficiency is characterized by hypocalcemia and/or hypophosphatemia leading to impaired bone mineralization. It is classified as a serum 25-hydroxyvitamin D (25[OH]D) level of <20 ng/ml (50 nmol/L). This standard definition of vitamin D deficiency has been recently challenged, and some endocrinologists recommend a cutoff of 12 mg/ml for vitamin D deficiency.[1]

The consequences of vitamin D deficiency include:

- Bone disease (rickets, osteoporosis, low bone mass)
- May impair reproductive success
- Decrease the ability to combat infection (especially TB, influenza, viral infection)
- May induce or worsen autoimmune disorders
- May increase the incidence of death due to heart disease, IBD, fracture, and cancer of the breast, colon, and prostate
- Subclinical vitamin D deficiency may occur in developed countries and be associated with increased fall risk, possible fractures, and osteoporosis.

SYNONYMS

The sunshine vitamin
The antirachitic factor
Cholecalciferol

ICD-10CM CODE

E55.9 Vitamin D deficiency, unspecified

EPIDEMIOLOGY & DEMOGRAPHICS

INCIDENCE:

- Vitamin D insufficiency is very high among older adults and hospitalized and institutionalized people.
- Worldwide deficiency and insufficiency affect about 1 billion people.
- Children and young adults: 40% to 50% of preadolescent Caucasian girls, and Hispanic and African American adolescents, are vitamin D deficient.

[1]Shah S et al: Serum 25-hydroxyvitamin D insufficiency in search of a bone disease, *J Clin Endocrinol Metab*, 102:2321-2328, 2017.

PEAK INCIDENCE: In the U.S., 40% to 100% of the elderly are vitamin D deficient.

60% of nursing home residents may be vitamin D deficient.

PREVALENCE: 42% of African American girls and women 15 to 49 yr old have 25(OH)D levels <20 ng/dl.

PREDOMINANT SEX AND AGE:

- Decreased skin production of vitamin D with age
- Increased prevalence among darker-skinned individuals

RISK FACTORS:

- Age (due to decreased ability to produce D_3)
- Sunshine-deficient areas (geographic location, living in higher latitudes)
- Dark-skinned individuals (melanin competes with vitamin D_3 precursors for UV photons and thus decreases pre-D_3 formation)
- Obese individuals
- Institutionalized individuals
- Pregnant and lactating women
- Use of sunscreen (sun radiation that causes skin cancer also produces pre-vitamin D_3 in skin)
- Patients on certain medications that antagonize vitamin D action (phenobarbital, phenytoin)
- Intestinal resection
- Severe chronic liver diseases (such as cirrhosis)
- Kidney disease (e.g., nephritic syndrome)
- Sarcoidosis and lymphomas (increased catabolism of 25[OH]D to 1,25[OH]2D)
- Intestinal malabsorption disease (caused by celiac sprue, cystic fibrosis, Whipple's disease)

PHYSICAL FINDINGS & CLINICAL PRESENTATION

- Clinical presentation of vitamin D deficiency is dependent on the duration and severity of deficiency.
- Most patients with mild to moderate vitamin D deficiency are asymptomatic.
- Severe deficiency may lead to rickets (in children), osteomalacia (in adults), bone demineralization, hypokalemia, and phosphaturia.
- Rickets—seen in children; caused by defective mineralization in the skeleton (Fig. E2).
  1. Bowing of the legs
  2. Leg bone pain
  3. Delayed growth
  4. Seizure due to hypocalcemia
- Osteomalacia—seen in adults
  1. Periosteal bone pain (best detected by putting firm pressure on tibia or sternal bones)
  2. Proximal muscle weakness
  3. Chronic muscle aches/pain
- Fracture with very minimal trauma (brittle and easily broken bones)
- Severe hypocalcemia—especially in late vitamin D deficiency leading to seizure tetany
- Hypophosphatemia
- Paresthesia
- Tetany
- Muscle cramps

ETIOLOGY

- Inadequate exposure to sunlight, such as:
  1. During winter
  2. In nursing home and health care institution residents
  3. With excessive use of sunscreen

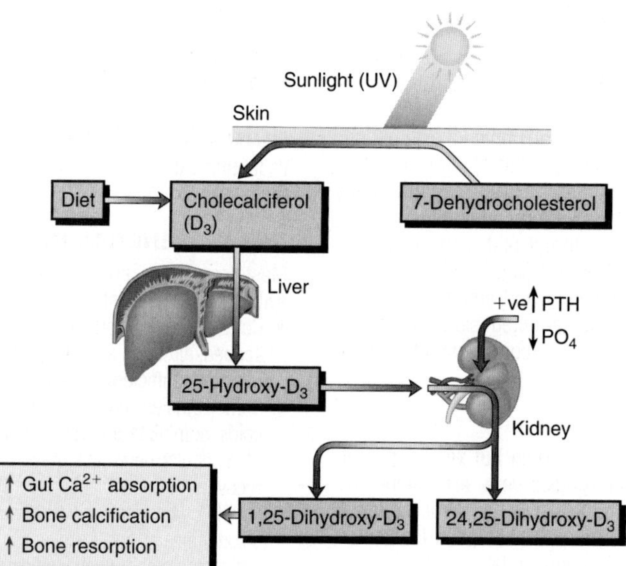

FIG. 1 The metabolism and actions of vitamin D. The primary source of vitamin D in humans is photoactivation in the skin of 7-dehydrocholesterol to cholecalciferol, which is then converted first in the liver to 25-hydroxyvitamin D and subsequently in the kidney to the much more active form, 1,25-dihydroxycholecalciferol (1,25[OH]$_2$,D$_3$). Regulation of the latter step is by PTH, phosphate, and feedback inhibition by 1,25(OH)$_2$,D$_3$. This step can also occur in lymphomatous and sarcoid tissue, resulting in the hypercalcemia that may complicate these diseases. (From Ballinger A: *Kumar & Clark's essentials of clinical medicine,* ed 6, Edinburgh, 2012, Saunders.)

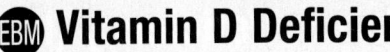

- Medications:
  1. Individuals on certain medications, such as phenobarbital, phenytoin, and rifampin (antagonize vitamin D action/increase vitamin D catabolism)
- Diseases and disease states:
  1. Diseases causing vitamin D malabsorption:
     a. Cystic fibrosis
     b. Whipple disease
     c. Celiac sprue
  2. Diseases increasing vitamin D catabolism:
     a. Lymphoma
     b. Sarcoidosis
  3. Intestinal resection
  4. Decreased 25(OH)D production:
     a. Kidney disease
     b. Liver cirrhosis

DIAGNOSIS

DIFFERENTIAL DIAGNOSIS

- Arthritis
- Fibromyalgia

WORKUP

- Population-wide screening for vitamin D deficiency is not recommended because evidence to support this practice is lacking.
- Screening is needed for individuals at risk (osteoporosis, history of falls, obese persons, pregnant and lactating women, diseases causing vitamin D malabsorption, African Americans). Workup involves blood and urine tests as well as radiography, as outlined in the next section.

LABORATORY TESTS

- Serum 25(OH)D: This is the best test to determine vitamin D status.
- Parathyroid hormone (PTH): Increased levels in vitamin D insufficiency. It is a marker of vitamin D insufficiency.
- Increased (serum or bone) alkaline phosphatase.
- Decreased 24-hour urine calcium (patient should not be on a thiazide).
- In patients at risk for osteomalacia [s-25(OH) D is less than 10 ng/ml], check Ca, Ph, alkaline phosphatase, PTH, BMP, and tissue transglutaminase antibodies.

IMAGING STUDIES

- Radiographs may show:
  1. Pseudofractures of the pelvis, femur, metatarsals
  2. Nontraumatic fractures
- Bone density:
  1. Decreased bone mineral density (osteopenia or osteoporosis). Note that bone mineral density is not routinely performed in patients whose only risk factor is decreased Vitamin D levels.

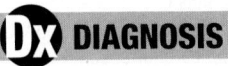

TREATMENT

NONPHARMACOLOGIC THERAPY

- Natural sources of vitamin D. These include:
  1. Exposure to sunlight. A mild sunburn is equivalent to consuming 10,000 to 25,000 IU of dietary vitamin D.
  2. Dietary sources are not enough to meet daily requirements. Oily fish such as salmon, cod, and mackerel are rich sources of vitamin D_3.
- Foods fortified with vitamin D.
  1. Mainly fortified dairy products.
  2. Fortified orange juice.

ACUTE GENERAL Rx

- Treating deficiency (general population):
  1. Cholecalciferol (Vitamin D_3), when available, is preferred for Vitamin D supplementation.
     a. 50,000 IU of vitamin D every week for 8 weeks, *or*
     b. 6000 IU daily to achieve a serum level of 25(OH)D of at least 30 ng/ml.
- Maintenance measures after treatment (general population): 1500 to 2000 IU daily.
- Treating deficiency (obese patients, patients with malabsorption syndromes, or those taking certain medications, as indicated earlier).
  1. 6000 to 10,000 IU daily.
- Maintenance measures after treatment (obese patients, patients with malabsorption syndromes, or those taking certain medications, as indicated earlier):
  1. 3000 to 6000 IU daily.
- After treating deficiency, recheck 25(OH)D in 12 to 16 weeks.

If deficiency persists after several attempts at treatment, try UV B light therapy

REFERRAL

Referral to an endocrinologist is recommended if there is no response to treatment.

PREVENTION

- Food fortification with vitamin D_2 or vitamin D_3.
- Adequate sun exposure, for example, exposure in the middle of the day (between 10:00 AM and 3:00 PM).
- Use vitamin D_3 for supplementation when available.
- Vitamin D supplementation (per the Endocrine Society):
  1. Infants (age range 1-12 mo) require at least 400 IU/day of vitamin D
  2. Children (age range 1-18 yr) require 600 IU/day of vitamin D
  3. Adult supplementation (adults 19-70 yr): 600 IU of vitamin D daily
  4. Adult supplementation (persons ≥70 yr): 800 IU of vitamin D daily
  5. Exceptions: Pregnant or lactating women, obese persons, and patients on antiseizure medications, steroids, antifungals, and AIDS medications should be given 2× to 3× more vitamin D
- Screening: Routine screening for low-risk adults is not recommended. Screening is recommended only for individuals at high risk for vitamin D deficiency such as blacks and Hispanics, obese individuals (BMI >30 kg/m^2), patients with osteoporosis, the elderly, and patients with certain chronic diseases (see "Risk Factors"). According to the U.S. Preventive Services Task Force (USPSTF), current evidence is insufficient to assess the balance of benefits and harms of screening for vitamin D deficiency in asymptomatic adults.

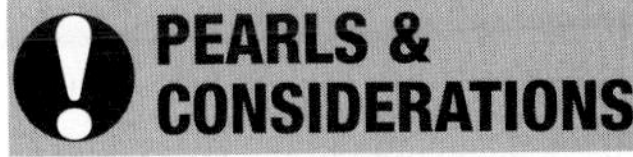

PEARLS & CONSIDERATIONS

- In the U.S., vitamin D supplements are available by prescription as vitamin D_2 (ergocalciferol) or over the counter as vitamin D_3 (cholecalciferol, usually in 400-1000-IU doses). Both vitamin D_2 and vitamin D_3 are acceptable as supplements. On average, oral vitamin D_3 raises blood levels more than does vitamin D_2.
- Upper limit of maintenance tolerability in healthy adults is 4000 IU a day. More than 4000 IU of vitamin D daily in nondeficient individuals increases the risk of harm. High-level supplements (>10,000 IU daily) are associated with kidney and tissue damage.
- Vitamin D supplementation is recommended for fall prevention. High-dose vitamin D supplementation (≥800 IU daily) has been shown to be favorable in the prevention of hip fracture and any nonvertebral fracture in persons 65 years of age or older.
- Prescribing more than the recommended daily amount to improve quality of life or prevent cardiovascular disease or death is not advised.
- Trials have shown that low vitamin D levels are associated with depressive symptoms, especially in persons with a history of depression. These findings suggest that measuring vitamin D levels may be useful in patients with a history of depression.
- Vitamin D supplementation, administered with calcium, has been shown to lower the risk for falling and improve muscle strength in the elderly, especially in older vitamin D–deficient women who are at high baseline risk for falling.
- The treatment of vitamin D insufficiency in asymptomatic persons might reduce mortality risk in institutionalized elderly persons and risks for falls but not fractures.
- Recent data suggest that vitamin D deficiency is associated with the risk of developing certain cancers (including breast, colon, and prostate).
- Vitamin D deficiency is associated with some autoimmune diseases (types 1 and 2 diabetes, metabolic syndrome, multiple sclerosis).

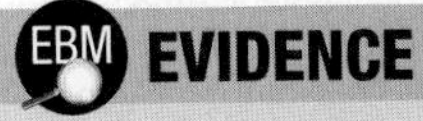

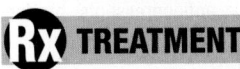

EVIDENCE

Available at ExpertConsult.com

SUGGESTED READINGS

Available at ExpertConsult.com

RELATED CONTENT

Vitamin D Deficiency (Patient Information)
Rickets (Related Key Topic)
Vitamin Deficiency (Related Key Topic)

AUTHOR: **DANIEL K. ASIEDU, M.D., PH.D., F.A.C.P.**

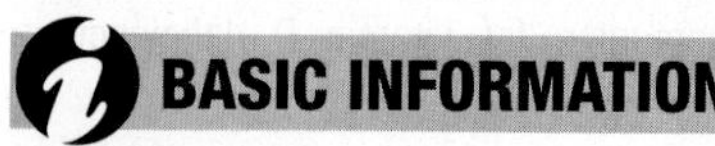

BASIC INFORMATION

DEFINITION

Vitamins are organic compounds that cannot be synthesized by humans but are required as nutrients in minute amounts for normal metabolism. Vitamins have several different functions: They may regulate cell growth and differentiation, as catalysts, as antioxidants, and as co-enzymes. Vitamins are classified as either fat soluble (vitamins A, D, E, K) or water soluble (B group of vitamins and C). Deficiency of most vitamins is rare in Western countries. Certain groups may be prone to vitamin deficiency, and these are discussed here. Vitamin D deficiency is discussed in a separate topic.

SYNONYMS

Hypovitaminosis
Vitamin A: Retinol
Vitamin E: Alpha tocopherol
Vitamin K: Phytonadione or menadiol
Vitamin B_1: Thiamine
Vitamin B_2: Riboflavin
Niacin: Vitamin B_3; nicotinic acid
Vitamin B_5: Pantothenic acid
Vitamin B_6: Pyridoxine; pyridoxal phosphate
Folic acid: Vitamin B_9; folate
Vitamin B_{12}: Cyanocobalamin
Vitamin C: Ascorbic acid

ICD-10CM CODES

E50	Vitamin A deficiency
E51	Thiamine deficiency
E53	Deficiency of other B group vitamins
E55	Vitamin D deficiency
E56	Other vitamin deficiencies
E56.0	Deficiency of vitamin E
E56.1	Deficiency of vitamin K
E53.0	Riboflavin deficiency
E52	Niacin deficiency [pellagra]
E53.1	Pyridoxine deficiency
E53.8	Deficiency of other specified B group vitamins
E54	Ascorbic acid deficiency

EPIDEMIOLOGY & DEMOGRAPHICS

Deficiency can occur in all age groups but is most common in the elderly.

- Vitamin A deficiency: Affects 250 million preschool children worldwide.
- Vitamin K deficiency: Varies by geographic regions; no race predilection; affects both sexes equally. Encountered often in infants.
- Vitamin B_1 (thiamine) deficiency: Incidence is unknown; no sex, race, or age predilection.
- Vitamin B_2 (riboflavin): More common than previously appreciated. Deficiency is referred to as ariboflavinosis.
- Vitamin B_5 (pantothenic acid) deficiency: Rare, as it is present in all foods.
- Vitamin B_{12} (cobalamin) deficiency: Relatively common. Occurs in all age groups but more common in the elderly.
- Vitamin B_9 (folic acid) deficiency: Mandatory fortification started in 1998. Prevalence before fortification 16% and after 0.5%. Neural tube defect associated with low maternal folate status during pregnancy. Pregnant women and the elderly are at greatest risk of folic acid deficiency.
- Vitamin C (ascorbic acid) deficiency: Smokers and low-income persons are at increased risk.

Fig. 1 shows environmental and nutritional factors in disease.

PHYSICAL FINDINGS & CLINICAL PRESENTATION

- Vitamin A: Xerophthalmia, xerosis of the cornea, keratomalacia, Bitot spots (abnormal squamous cell proliferation and keratinization of the conjunctiva), nyctalopia (poor adaptation to darkness)/night blindness, poor bone growth, dry skin and hair, follicular hyperkeratosis (caused by blockage of hair follicles by keratin), pruritus, broken fingernails
- Vitamin K: Clinical manifestation usually occurs if hypoprothrombinemia is present. Major symptom is bleeding to minor trauma. Also can show easy bruisability, epistaxis, hematoma, or gum bleeding
- Vitamin E: Nerve dysfunction (ataxia; hyporeflexia, peripheral neuropathy); bone weakness
- Vitamin B_1 (thiamine):
  - * Beriberi, which has two subtypes (infantile and adult). Adult type is described below:
    1. Dry beriberi (affecting the nervous system): Symmetrical peripheral neuropathy (with sensory and motor impairments), Wernicke encephalopathy (nystagmus, ataxia, ophthalmoplegia, and confusion), Korsakoff syndrome (impaired short-term memory loss and confabulation but normal cognition)
    2. Wet beriberi (affecting the cardiovascular system): Cardiomegaly, cardiomyopathy, heart failure, tachycardia, hypotension, chest pain, peripheral edema
    3. Gastrointestinal (GI): Anorexia; constipation
- Vitamin B_2 (riboflavin):
  1. Cheilosis (chapping and fissure of the lip)
  2. Glossitis (sore red tongue)
  3. Oily, scaly rashes on nasolabial folds, eyelids, scrotum, labia majora
  4. Red itchy eyes
  5. Normocytic or normochromic anemia
  6. Peripheral neuropathy
- Vitamin B_3 (niacin):
  1. Pellagra (4 *Ds*—diarrhea, dermatitis, dementia, and ultimately death)
  2. Hyperpigmentation of sun-exposed skin
  3. "Raw beef" swollen and painful tongue
  4. Deficiency can be seen in prolonged use of Isoniazid, in carcinoid syndrome, and in Hartnup syndrome
- Vitamin B_5 (pantothenic acid):
  1. Deficiency is rare
  2. Deficiency leads to "burning feet syndrome" (distal paresthesia and dysesthesia)
  3. Anemia
  4. GI symptoms
- Vitamin B_6 (Pyridoxine): Rare to see overt deficiency.
  1. Mild deficiency—glossitis, cheilosis, impaired proprioception; sensory ataxia, confusion, depression
  2. Severe deficiency—seborrheic dermatitis, seizure, microcytic
- Vitamin B_{12} (cyanocobalamin):
  1. Megaloblastic anemia (pernicious anemia)
  2. Neurologic symptoms including peripheral neuropathy, ataxia (shuffling gait), paresthesia; subacute degeneration of the spinal cord (demyelination of the dorsal column), visual disturbances due to optic atrophy
  3. Glossitis and GI symptoms such as nausea, vomiting, and anorexia are also common
  4. Patients may also have dementia/mental sluggishness, depression, and weakness
- Vitamin B_9 (folic acid):
  1. Patchy hyperpigmentation of skin (especially between fingers and toes) and mucous membranes
  2. Moderate fever (temp <102° F; 38.9° C) despite the absence of infection
  3. Neural tube defect
  4. Angular stomatitis
  5. Red, beefy, smooth, and shiny tongue
  6. Megaloblastic anemia
- Vitamin C: Scurvy (bruising, petechiae, follicular hyperkeratosis, perifollicular hemorrhage), poor wound healing, fatigue, gingivitis/bleeding gums, weight loss, bone abnormalities (Fig. E2)

ETIOLOGY

- Fat-soluble vitamins (vitamins A, D, E, K):
  1. Decreased ingestion, malnutrition, eating disorders
  2. Diseases that affect fat absorption decrease the absorption of fat-soluble vitamins—for example, cystic fibrosis, celiac sprue, inflammatory bowel disease, cholestasis, hepatobiliary disease, small bowel surgery
  3. Change in vitamin metabolism:
     a. Alcoholism
     b. Drugs such as cholestyramine, warfarin, anticonvulsants, antibiotics (e.g., cephalosporins)
     c. Chronic kidney disease
- Increased risk in:
  1. Vegans
  2. Recent immigrants
  3. Refugees
  4. Toddlers/preschoolers living below the poverty line
- Water-soluble vitamins (the B group of vitamins and vitamin C)—there are several etiologic factors, including:
  1. Inadequate intake
  2. Decreased absorption
  3. Alcoholism
  4. Pregnancy/lactation
  5. Peritoneal dialysis
  6. Medications (e.g., isoniazid, phenothiazines, tricyclic antidepressants, metformin [Vit B_{12}])
  7. Malabsorption
  8. Low income
  9. Advanced age
- Vitamin B_{12} deficiency—caused by:
  1. Insufficient dietary intake, as in strict vegans
  2. Decreased absorption secondary to intrinsic factor deficiency, decreased

Vitamin	Function	Consequences of deficiency
A	Retinal function, epithelial growth control	Night blindness, keratomalacia, xerophthalmia
B_1 (thiamine)	Co-enzyme	Beri beri, Wernicke's encephalopathy
B_2 (riboflavin)	Co-enzyme	Dermatitis, glossitis, keratitis, neuropathy, confusion
B_6 (pyridoxine)	Co-enzyme	Neuropathy
B_{12} (cobalamin)	Nucleic acid synthesis	Megaloblastic anemia Subacute combined degeneration of spinal cord
Niacin	Co-enzyme NAD, NADP	Pellagra (diarrhea, dermatitis, and dementia)
Folate	Co-enzyme in nucleic acid synthesis	Megaloblastic anemia, villous atrophy of gut
Vitamin C	Co-factor in hydroxylation	Scurvy
Vitamin D	Calcium and phosphate absorption	Rickets (childhood) Osteomalacia (adults)
Vitamin E	Antioxidant	Spinocerebellar degeneration
Vitamin K	Co-factor for coagulation factor synthesis	Bleeding due to coagulation defects

FIG. 1 Environmental and nutritional factors in disease. (From Stevens A: *Core pathology,* St Louis, 2009, Elsevier.)

intrinsic factor secretion, gastric atrophy, gastrectomy/gastric bypass
3. Terminal ileum disease such as celiac disease, enteritis, tropical sprue
- Folic acid deficiency:
  1. Increased needs can lead to deficiency (e.g., pregnancy, lactation, malignancy)
  2. Derangement of folate metabolism by:
     1. Medication (e.g., methotrexate)
     2. Disease (e.g., hypothyroidism)
     3. Increased excretion: As seen in alcoholics

Dx DIAGNOSIS

WORKUP/LABORATORY TESTS

General initial laboratory tests include:
- Complete blood cell count (CBC)
- Liver function tests (LFTs)
- Basic metabolic panel (BMP)
- Albumin
- Measurement of serum levels of the specific vitamin in question

Specific tests may be considered in the following cases:
- Vitamin A:
  1. Serum retinol level (best test, a direct measure, expensive)
  2. Retinol binding protein (easier to perform, less expensive)
  3. Dark-adaptation threshold test
- Vitamin K:
  1. Prothrombin time/partial thromboplastin time (PT/PTT)
  2. Prothrombin
  3. Des-gamma-carboxyprothrombin (most sensitive test).
  4. Niacin: Urine-*N*-methylnicotinamide (level <0.8 mg/day indicates niacin deficiency)
- Vitamin B_1 (thiamine):
  1. Blood thiamine levels
  2. Thiamine pyrophosphate levels in blood
  3. Erythrocyte thiamine transketolase activity (ETKA)
  4. Urinary thiamine excretion
- Vitamin B_3 (niacin):
  1. Check urinary N-methylnicotinamide or erythrocyte NAD/NADP ratio (tests are not readily available)
- Vitamin B_2:
  1. Check plasma riboflavin concentration
- Vitamin B_{12}
  1. Serum vitamin B_{12} <190 pg/ml is diagnostic of vitamin B_{12} deficiency
  2. Serum methylmalonic acid, which is elevated in B_{12} deficiency
  3. Antiparietal antibody
  4. Intrinsic factor antibody is decreased
  5. Blood smear shows macrocytosis and hypersegmentation of megaloblasts
  6. CBC shows increased mean corpuscle volume (MCV)
  7. Megaloblastic anemia
- Folic acid:
  1. Check serum folate level
  2. Additional testing includes checking for serum homocysteine level, which will be elevated
  3. Red cell folate level shows chronic folate status

Rx TREATMENT

Most of the vitamins are available over the counter individually or in different multivitamin formulations.
- Specific vitamins:
- Vitamin A deficiency: Treat with oral supplementation 10,000 IU daily.
  1. Consume vitamin A–rich foods such as liver, beef, carrots, oranges, mangoes.
  2. Five servings of fruit and vegetables give enough carotenoids for a day.
- Vitamin K deficiency: Treatment depends on the severity of bleeding, administered subcutaneously (SQ) or intramuscularly (IM).
- Vitamin B_1 (thiamine) deficiency: Give intramuscular thiamine 50 mg for several days.
  1. If B_1 deficiency is suspected and patient needs intravenous glucose, give thiamine first before intravenous glucose. This prevents the development of Korsakoff psychosis.
- Vitamin B_{12} deficiency: Give 1000 mcg IM daily for 7 days, then once a week for 1 mo, then once a month indefinitely.
  1. A potential option is oral supplementation.
- Folic acid deficiency: Daily requirement is 400 to 1000 mcg (1 mg) daily.
  1. Centers for Disease Control and Prevention (CDC) recommend that women of childbearing age take 400 mcg of folic acid daily.

SUGGESTED READINGS

Available at ExpertConsult.com

RELATED CONTENT

Anemia, Pernicious (Related Key Topic)
Rickets (Related Key Topic)
Vitamin D Deficiency (Related Key Topic)
Wernicke Syndrome (Related Key Topic)
Vitamins and Their Functions (Appendix IIb)

AUTHOR: **DANIEL K. ASIEDU, M.D., PH.D., F.A.C.P.**

BASIC INFORMATION

DEFINITION

von Willebrand's disease is an inherited disorder of hemostasis characterized by a quantitative or qualitative deficiency in von Willebrand factor (vWF), a protein product of a gene located on the short arm of chromosome 12. The vWF factor is mostly synthesized in endothelial cells. von Willebrand's disease results from a failure to synthesize or secrete vWF or an accelerated clearance of vWF. vWF is the carrier protein for clotting factor VIII (FVIII:C). vWF binds to denuded subendothelial collagen or glycosaminoglycans and causes platelets to adhere by acting as a ligand for glycoprotein IB on the platelet surface. This latter activity is measured in the laboratory by a test called the ristocetin cofactor (RCF). vWF circulates in plasma as a multimeric protein consisting of protomers attached by disulfide bonds. By definition, vWD is present if the level RCF is <30% of normal. A clinical entity known as low vWF exists when the level is between 30% and 60%. Such patients may exhibit a bleeding phenotype. Previously, this was considered mild vWD. There are several subtypes of von Willebrand's disease. The most common type (80% of cases) is type I, where levels of vWF, FVIII:C, and RCF are reduced but concordant. Within type 1, there is type 1 mild, which is common; type 1 severe (T1S), which is rare; and type 1 C, in which the low vWF is due to accelerated clearance. There are four type 2 subtypes: type 2A, type 2B, type 2N, and type 2M. All the type 2 variants are due to a qualitative defect in vWF and show a discordancy between levels of RCF and FVIII:C. The type 2 vWD variants are characterized by low levels of RCF. Type 3 is rare and either an autosomal recessive disorder or double heterozygote and characterized by a near-complete quantitative deficiency of vWF and very low FVIII:C. Acquired vWD disease is a rare disorder that presents with mucocutaneous bleeding abnormalities and no clinical family history. It is seen often in association with hematoproliferative or autoimmune disorder or may occur in hypothyroidism. Successful treatment of the associated illness can reverse the clinical and laboratory manifestations.

SYNONYMS

Pseudohemophilia
vWD

ICD-10CM CODE

D68.0 von Willebrand's disease

EPIDEMIOLOGY & DEMOGRAPHICS

- Autosomal-dominant disorder predominantly; rarely recessive or double-heterozygotic.
- Most common inherited bleeding disorder.
- Prevalence is 0.6% to 1.3% in general population, according to screening studies; estimates based on referral for symptoms of bleeding suggest a prevalence of 1 case per 10,000 persons.

PHYSICAL FINDINGS & CLINICAL PRESENTATION

- Generally normal physical examination
- Mucosal bleeding (gingival bleeding, epistaxis) and gastrointestinal bleeding may occur.
- Easy bruising
- Bleeding after surgery or dental extraction, menorrhagia
- Rarely, muscle or joint bleeding in type 3

ETIOLOGY

Quantitative or qualitative deficiency of vWF (see "Definition").

DIAGNOSIS

The diagnosis of von Willebrand's disease generally requires two criteria: (1) a personal history, family history, or physical evidence of mucocutaneous bleeding and (2) a qualitative or quantitative decrease in functional activity of von Willebrand's disease. The American Society of Hematology states that a definitive diagnosis of vWD may be made if RCF levels are <30 IU/dl.

DIFFERENTIAL DIAGNOSIS

Platelet function disorders, clotting factor deficiencies

WORKUP (FIG. 1)

SCREENING LABORATORY TESTS:

- Laboratory evaluation (Table 1).

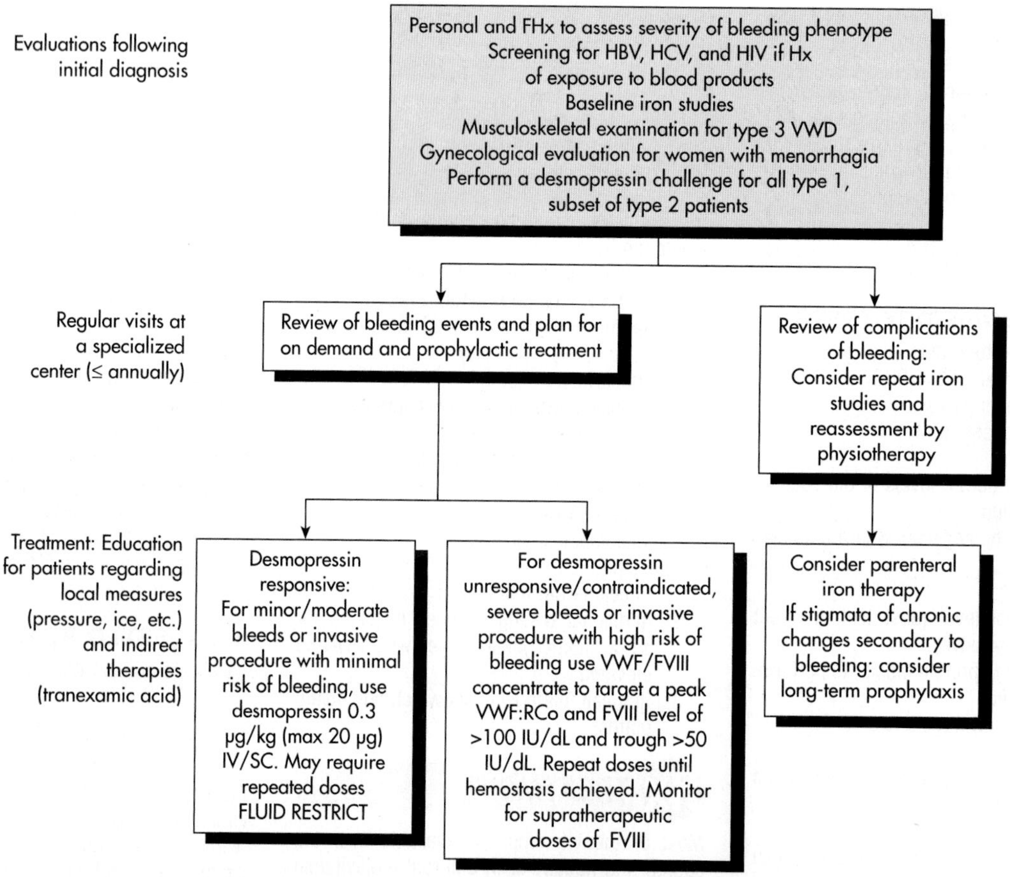

Evaluations following initial diagnosis

Personal and FHx to assess severity of bleeding phenotype
Screening for HBV, HCV, and HIV if Hx of exposure to blood products
Baseline iron studies
Musculoskeletal examination for type 3 VWD
Gynecological evaluation for women with menorrhagia
Perform a desmopressin challenge for all type 1, subset of type 2 patients

Regular visits at a specialized center (≤ annually)

Review of bleeding events and plan for on demand and prophylactic treatment

Review of complications of bleeding: Consider repeat iron studies and reassessment by physiotherapy

Treatment: Education for patients regarding local measures (pressure, ice, etc.) and indirect therapies (tranexamic acid)

Desmopressin responsive: For minor/moderate bleeds or invasive procedure with minimal risk of bleeding, use desmopressin 0.3 μg/kg (max 20 μg) IV/SC. May require repeated doses FLUID RESTRICT

For desmopressin unresponsive/contraindicated, severe bleeds or invasive procedure with high risk of bleeding use VWF/FVIII concentrate to target a peak VWF:RCo and FVIII level of >100 IU/dL and trough >50 IU/dL. Repeat doses until hemostasis achieved. Monitor for supratherapeutic doses of FVIII

Consider parenteral iron therapy
If stigmata of chronic changes secondary to bleeding: consider long-term prophylaxis

FIG. 1 Approach to the Management of von Willebrand Disease. *FHx,* Family history; *FVIII,* factor VIII; *HBV,* hepatitis B virus; *HCV,* hepatitis C virus; *HIV,* human immunodeficiency virus; *Hx,* history; *IV,* intravenous; *RCo,* ristocetin cofactor; *SC,* subcutaneous; *VWD,* von Willebrand disease; *VWF,* von Willebrand factor. (From Hoffman R: *Hematology, basic principles and practice*, ed 7, Philadelphia, 2018, Elsevier.)

TABLE 1 Table of Investigations

vWD Type	vWF:RCo IU/dl[a]	vWF:Ag IU/dl[a]	RCo/Ag IU/dl[a]	FVIII:C IU/dl[a]	Multimer Pattern[b]	Other
1	Low	Low	Equivalent	~1.5× vWF:Ag	Normal	
2A	Low	Low	vWF:RCo < vWF:Ag	Low or normal	Abnormal ↓ HMWM	
2B	Low	Low	vWF:RCo < vWF:Ag	Low or normal	Abnormal ↓ HMWM	↑ RIPA[c](↓ platelet count)
2M	Low	Low	vWF:RCo < vWF:Ag	Low or normal	Normal	
2N	Normal/low	Normal/low	Equivalent	<30	Normal	↓ vWF:FVIIIB[d]
3	Absent	Absent	NA	<10	Absent	

Ag, Antigen; *FVIII:C,* FVIII level; *NA,* not applicable; *RCo,* ristocetin cofactor; *RIPA,* ristocetin-induced platelet aggregation; *vWD,* von Willebrand's disease; *vWF:FVIIIB,* FVIII-binding assay.
[a]Relative to the reference range (approximate values); vWF:RCo (50–200 IU/dl); vWF:Ag (50–200 IU/dl); FVIII:C (50–150 IU/dl).
[b]HMWM, High-molecular-weight multimers.
[c]Increased agglutination at low concentrations of ristocetin.
[d]The ability of vWF to bind and protect FVIII is reduced. vWF and FVIII levels can look exactly like those in males with mild hemophilia A or in symptomatic hemophilia A carrier females.
From Hoffman R: *Hematology, basic principles and practice,* ed 7, Philadelphia, 2018, Elsevier.

TABLE 2 Desmopressin Responsiveness in the Various Subtypes of von Willebrand's Disease

vWD Type	vWF:RCo	vWF:Ag	RCo/Ag	FVIII:C IU/dl	vWF:CB	vWF:CB/vWF:Ag
1	Increase	Increase	Remains >0.7	Increase	Increase	Remains >0.7
2A	No/little change	Increase	Remains <0.7	Increase	No/little change	Remains <0.7
2M (GP1B-binding dysfunction)	No/little change	Increase	Remains <0.7	Increase	Increase	Remains >0.7
3	No/little change	No/little change		No/little change	No/little change	

*Ag,*Antigen; *FVIII:C,*factor VIII level; *GP1B,*glycoprotein 1B; *RCo,*ristocetin cofactor; *vWD,* von Willebrand's disease; *vWF,*von Willebrand factor; *vWF:CB,* collagen assays-binding.
Modified from Favaloro EJ: Rethinking the diagnosis of von Willebrand disease. *Thromb Res* 127;Suppl 2:17, 2011; In Hoffman R: *Hematology, basic principles and practice,* ed 7, Philadelphia, 2018, Elsevier.

- Initial testing includes prothrombin time (normal), partial thromboplastin time (normal or slightly increased), platelet count (normal), and PFA-100 (abnormal or may show high normal values in type 1 vWD).

SPECIFIC LABORATORY TESTS

- Factor VIII coagulant activity (FVIII:C, typically decreased, may be normal in some Type 2 variants).
- vWF antigen, ristocetin cofactor (RCF), and collagen binding assay (these typically are decreased and may be concordant as in type 1 and type 3, or discordant as in type 2 variants).
- Normal platelet number and morphology.
- Prolonged bleeding time, or more commonly, prolonged PFA-100 closure times.
- von Willebrand propeptide. This measures the N-terminal propeptide of vWF. This vWFpp is secreted in equimolar amounts to the mature vWF. The ratio of vWFpp to vWF can assist in identifying vWD due to rapid clearance, as in type1C.
- Multimeric analysis: Type 2A von Willebrand's disease can be distinguished from type I by absence of medium- and high-molecular-weight multimers.
- Type 2B von Willebrand's disease is distinguished from Type I by the absence of high-molecular-weight multimers.
- Type 2N is a defect in the factor VIII:C binding and has normal vWF levels but very low factor VIII:C with normal multimer pattern
- Type 2M is a defect in binding to platelets (low RCF, low CBA) but normal multimers.

Rx TREATMENT

NONPHARMACOLOGIC THERAPY

- Avoidance of aspirin and other nonsteroidal antiinflammatory drugs
- Use of antifibrinolytics such as tranexamic acid, especially for menorrhagia or oral bleeding

GENERAL Rx

- Treatment of von Willebrand's disease is based on normalizing factor VIII levels and von Willebrand factor at the time of spontaneous bleeding or before an intervention.
- Use of DDAVP (Table 2): DDAVP binds to V2 receptors in certain endothelial cells and causes the release of vWF. This is suitable for the management of the milder forms of vWD. Dose is 0.3 mcg/kg in 50 to 100 ml of normal saline solution IV infused over 20 min. DDAVP is also available as a nasal spray (dose of 150 mcg spray administered to each nostril) as a preparation for minor surgery and management of minor bleeding episodes.
- When a patient undergoes surgery or receives repeated therapeutic doses of concentrates, use of a plasma-derived vWF concentrate such as Humate-P or a new recombinant vWF (Vonvendi) may need to be administered.

SUGGESTED READINGS

Available at ExpertConsult.com

AUTHOR: **JOSEPH SWEENEY, M.D., F.A.C.P., F.R.C.PATH.**

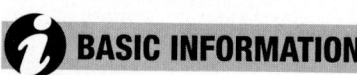

DEFINITION

Waldenström's macroglobulinemia (WM) is an indolent B-cell lymphoplasmacytic lymphoma (LPL) characterized by lymphoplasmacytic infiltration in the bone marrow (BM) and other organs, and a monoclonal immunoglobulin M (IgM) paraprotein in the serum. Less than 5% of LPL secrete IgG, IgA, or light chains. Rare nonsecretory cases exist.

SYNONYMS

WM
Monoclonal macroglobulinemia
Lymphoplasmacytic lymphoma

ICD-10CM CODE
C88.0 Waldenström's macroglobulinemia

EPIDEMIOLOGY & DEMOGRAPHICS

- Accounts for 2% of all hematologic cancers
- 1500 new cases diagnosed every yr in the U.S.
- Overall incidence: 3.4 per million person-yr in men, 1.7 per million person-yr in women
- Median age at diagnosis: 72 yr
- More common among men than women and among whites than blacks

PHYSICAL FINDINGS & CLINICAL PRESENTATION

- 30% to 50% of patients can be asymptomatic at presentation
- Weakness, fatigue, and pallor, usually associated with anemia (50%)
- Fever, night sweats, and weight loss (30%)
- Peripheral sensory neuropathy associated with IgM demyelinating antibodies, usually affecting the feet symmetrically (20%)
- Lymphadenopathy (15%)
- Hepatosplenomegaly (15%)
- Hyperviscosity syndrome (10%), characterized by headaches, recurrent nosebleeds, blurry vision due to retinal hemorrhages; retinal vein link: sausage shaped
- Acrocyanosis, livedo reticularis, and purpura, usually associated with symptomatic cryoglobulinemia (5% to 10%)
- Peripheral ulcerations associated with severe cryoglobulinemia
- Hemolytic anemia caused by cold agglutinin disease (5%)
- Amyloidosis causing renal dysfunction, neuropathy, and/or cardiac dysfunction (<5%)
- Meningeal signs caused by CNS involvement by WM (Bing Neel syndrome; 1%)

ETIOLOGY

- The main risk factor for development of WM is having IgM monoclonal gammopathy of unknown significance (MGUS).
- Other risk factors are older age and male sex.
- Multiple reports suggest familial clustering in about 20% of the patients, which may indicate a genetic predisposition to WM and other blood cancers.
- Approximately 20% of the patients have an Ashkenazi Jewish ancestry.
- Radiation exposure, occupational chemicals, viral infection (hepatitis C) and chronic inflammatory stimulation have been suggested, but there is insufficient evidence to substantiate these hypotheses.
- There is an increased risk of WM in people with a personal history of autoimmune diseases.

Dx DIAGNOSIS

The diagnosis of WM is usually established by laboratory blood tests and by bone marrow (BM) biopsy. Diagnosis requires demonstration of LPL involving the BM space and the presence of an IgM monoclonal paraprotein. MYD88 L265P is a commonly recurring mutation in WM seen in >90% of the patients with WM and 50% to 60% of patients with IgM MGUS and can be useful in differentiating WM from other IgM-secreting B-cell disorders such as marginal zone lymphoma, IgM multiple myeloma, and atypical forms of chronic lymphocytic. Non-L265P MYD88 mutations rarely have been described (<5%) and should be excluded in patients who test negative for MYD88 L265P by PCR-based assays. Mutations in the *CXCR4* gene have been described in 40% of patients, and may impact clinical presentation and response to ibrutinib treatment.

DIFFERENTIAL DIAGNOSIS

- IgM MGUS
- IgM multiple myeloma
- Marginal zone lymphoma
- Atypical chronic lymphocytic leukemia

WORKUP

In any patient suspected of having WM, specific blood tests (CBC, serum or urine protein electrophoresis [SPEP or UPEP, respectively], serum IgM level, beta 2-microglobulin, serum viscosity) should be ordered. BM biopsy confirms the diagnosis. *MYD88* mutation testing can be helpful in supporting the diagnosis of WM.

LABORATORY TESTS

- CBC with differential:
  1. Anemia is a common finding, with a median hemoglobin value of approximately 10 g/dl. WBC count is usually normal; thrombocytopenia can occur.
  2. Peripheral smear may reveal "stacked coin" rouleaux formations and malignant lymphoid cells in some patients.
- SPEP: Homogeneous M spike (monoclonal gammopathy).
- Immunoelectrophoresis: Confirms IgM responsible for the M spike. Table 1 describes physicochemical and immunologic properties of the monoclonal IgM protein in WM.
- Serum IgM levels are high, generally >3000 mg/dl.
- High serum beta 2-microglobulin levels are associated with poor prognosis.
- Serum viscosity. Hyperviscosity usually occurs when the serum viscosity is four times the viscosity of normal serum; classic feature although presents in only 10% of cases.
- Cryoglobulins or cold agglutinins may be present.
- BM biopsy: BM reveals infiltration by a lymphoplasmacytic cell population constituted by small lymphocytes with

TABLE 1 Physicochemical and Immunologic Properties of the Monoclonal Immunoglobulin M Protein in Waldenström's Macroglobulinemia

Properties of IgM Monoclonal Protein	Diagnostic Condition	Clinical Manifestations
Pentameric structure	Hyperviscosity	Headaches, blurred vision, epistaxis, retinal hemorrhages, leg cramps, impaired mentation, intracranial hemorrhage
Precipitation on cooling	Cryoglobulinemia (type I)	Raynaud's phenomenon, acrocyanosis, ulcers, purpura, cold urticaria
Autoantibody activity to myelin-associated glycoprotein, ganglioside M_1, sulfatide moieties on peripheral nerve sheaths	Peripheral neuropathies	Sensorimotor neuropathies, painful neuropathies, ataxic gait, bilateral foot drop
Autoantibody activity to IgG	Cryoglobulinemia (type II)	Purpura, arthralgia, renal failure, sensorimotor neuropathies
Autoantibody activity to red blood cell antigens	Cold agglutinins	Hemolytic anemia, Raynaud's phenomenon, acrocyanosis, livedo reticularis
Tissue deposition as amorphous aggregates	Organ dysfunction	Skin: Bullous skin disease, papules, Schnitzler syndrome Gastrointestinal: Diarrhea, malabsorption, bleeding Kidney: Proteinuria, renal failure (light-chain component)
Tissue deposition as amyloid fibrils (light-chain component most common)	Organ dysfunction	Fatigue, weight loss, edema, hepatomegaly, macroglossia, organ dysfunction of involved organs (heart, kidney, liver, peripheral sensory and autonomic nerves)

IgM, Immunoglobulin M.
From Hoffman R et al: *Hematology, basic principles and practice*, ed 7, Philadelphia, 2018, Elsevier.

evidence of plasmacytoid and plasma cell differentiation. The BM infiltration should be confirmed by immunophenotypic studies (flow cytometry and immunohistochemistry) showing the following profile: sIgM+CD19+CD20+CD22+CD79+.

IMAGING STUDIES

CT of the chest, abdomen, and pelvis may show lymphadenopathy, hepatosplenomegaly, and rarely, extralymphatic/extramedullary areas of disease.

TABLE 2 Summary of Consensus Response Criteria for Waldenström's Macroglobulinemia

Response Type	Abbreviation	Criteria
Complete response	CR	Absence of serum monoclonal IgM protein by immunofixation Normal serum IgM level Complete resolution of extramedullary disease (i.e., lymphadenopathy/splenomegaly if present at baseline) Morphologically normal bone marrow aspirate and trephine biopsy
Very good partial response	VGPR	Monoclonal IgM protein is detectable 90% reduction in serum IgM level from baseline or normalization of serum IgM level Complete resolution of extramedullary disease (i.e., lymphadenopathy/splenomegaly if present at baseline) No new signs or symptoms of active disease
Partial response	PR	Monoclonal IgM protein is detectable ≥50% but <90% reduction in serum IgM level from baseline Reduction in extramedullary disease (i.e., lymphadenopathy/splenomegaly if present at baseline) No new signs or symptoms of active disease
Minor response	MR	Monoclonal IgM protein is detectable ≥25% but <50% reduction in serum IgM level from baseline No new signs or symptoms of active disease
Stable disease	SD	Monoclonal IgM protein is detectable <25% reduction and <25% increase in serum IgM level from baseline No progression in extramedullary disease (i.e., lymphadenopathy/splenomegaly) No new signs or symptoms of active disease
Progressive disease	PD	>25% increase in serum IgM level from lowest nadir (requires confirmation) and/or progression in clinical features attributable to the disease

IgM, Immunoglobulin M.
Owen RG, Kyle RA, Stone MJ et al: Response assessment in Waldenström macroglobulinemia. *Br J Haematol* 160:171, 2013. In Hoffman R et al: *Hematology, basic principles and practice*, ed 7, Philadelphia, 2018, Elsevier.

Rx TREATMENT

- Because of the incurable nature of WM, the aim of treatment is to relieve symptoms and reduce the risk of organ damage. Initiation of therapy should not be based on the IgM levels alone because this may not correlate with either disease burden or symptomatic status. Patients with smoldering or asymptomatic WM and preserved hematologic function should be observed without therapy.
- Initiation of therapy is appropriate for patients with constitutional symptoms. Considerations for the initiation of treatment include the following: significant adenopathy or organomegaly, symptomatic hyperviscosity, moderate to severe neuropathy, amyloidosis, symptomatic cryoglobulinemia or cold agglutinin disease, hemoglobin concentration <10 g/dl, or evidence of disease transformation.
- Treatment is directed at both hyperviscosity and the lymphoproliferative disorder itself.

NONPHARMACOLOGIC THERAPY

Asymptomatic patients do not require treatment, and these patients should be monitored periodically for the onset of symptoms or changes in blood tests (e.g., worsening anemia, thrombocytopenia, rising IgM levels, and serum viscosity). Plasmapheresis should be the initial treatment in patients with symptoms of hyperviscosity or cryoglobulinemia followed immediately by more definitive therapy.

INITIAL Rx

- Treatment of the lymphoproliferative disorder includes single or combination therapy. There is no universally agreed upon standard of care:
  1. Combination regimens include BDR (bortezomib, dexamethasone, rituximab) and bendamustine/rituximab. These should be used in patients with severe constitutional symptoms, symptomatic bulky disease, hyperviscosity, or profound hematologic compromise. Response rates are ~90% with any of these regimens.
  2. Rituximab, a monoclonal anti-CD20 antibody, can be used in symptomatic patients with modest hematologic compromise, IgM-related neuropathy, or hemolytic anemia unresponsive to corticosteroids. Response rates are 40% to 50%.
  3. In April 2015, the FDA granted approval for the oral Bruton tyrosine kinase inhibitor ibrutinib to be used in patients with symptomatic WM. The response rate to ibrutinib is 90%, with a median time to response of 4 weeks. Major responses were absent in patients who do not carry the MYD88 mutation. The response was delayed in patients who carry any *CXCR4* mutation.
  4. In August 2018, the FDA approved the combination of ibrutinib and rituximab for the treatment of symptomatic WM patients. The combination was associated with higher response rate and longer median progression-free survival than rituximab and placebo.

RX ON RELAPSED/REFRACTORY DISEASE

- Rituximab can be used as maintenance therapy.
- Refractory patients can be retried on original therapy if length of response from initial therapy is >3 yr. If the response from the initial therapy was <3 yr, alternative first-line agents can be used.
- Other treatment options: Carfilzomib, cyclophosphamide, fludarabine, ofatumumab, thalidomide, everolimus, and clinical trials.

Autologous stem cell transplantation should be considered in patients with highly refractory disease.

DISPOSITION

- The progression of WM is slow and insidious, with median survival from time of diagnosis of about 10 yr. Table 2 summarizes consensus response criteria for Waldenström's macroglobulinemia.
- Younger patients tend to have more prolonged survival.
- About 10% to 20% of patients die from progression of the disease.
- Some patients develop acute myelogenous leukemia, usually secondary to exposure to chemotherapy, and some patients can develop more aggressive lymphomas.
- The risk of thyroid cancer, kidney cancer, and melanoma is increased in patients with WM.
- A staging system using age, serum beta 2-microglobulin level, hemoglobin level, platelet count and serum IgM concentration before treatment provide insight into prognosis and survival. Prognostic scoring systems in Waldenström's macroglobulinemia are summarized in Table 3.

TABLE 3 Prognostic Scoring Systems in Waldenström's Macroglobulinemia

Study	Adverse Prognostic Factors	Number of Groups	Survival
Gobbi et al[1]	Hgb <9 g/dl	0–1 prognostic factors	Median: 48 months
	Age >70 years	2–4 prognostic factors	Median: 80 months
	Weight loss		
	Cryoglobulinemia		
Morel et al[2]	Age ≥65 years	0–1 prognostic factors	5-year: 87% of patients
	Albumin <4 g/dl	2 prognostic factors	5-year: 62%
	Number of cytopenias:	3–4 prognostic factors	5-year: 25%
	Hgb <12 g/dl		
	Platelets $<150 \times 10^9$/L		
	WBC $<4 \times 10^9$/L		
Dhodapkar et al[3]	β_2M ≥3 g/dl	β_2M <3 mg/dl + Hgb ≥12 g/dl	5-year: 87% of patients
	Hgb <12 g/dl	β_2M <3 mg/dl + Hgb <12 g/dl	5-year: 63%
	IgM <4 g/dl	β_2M ≥3 mg/dl + IgM ≥4 g/dl	5-year: 53%
		β_2M ≥3 mg/dl + IgM <4 g/dl	5-year: 21%
Dimopoulos et al[4]	Albumin ≤3.5 g/dl	Albumin ≥3.5 g/dl + β_2M <3.5 mg/dl	Median: NR
	β_2M ≥3.5 mg/L	Albumin ≤3.5 g/dl + β_2M <3.5 or	Median: 116 months
		β_2M 3.5–5.5 mg/dl	Median: 54 months
		β_2M >5.5 mg/dl	
Morel et al[5]	Age >65 years	0–1 prognostic factors (excluding age)	5 year: 87% of patients
	Hgb <11.5 g/dl	2 prognostic factors (or age >65 years)	5 year: 68%
	Platelets $<100 \times 10^9$/L	3–5 prognostic factors	5 year: 36%
	β_2M >3 mg/L		
	IgM >7 g/dl		

β_2M, β_2-microbloulin; *Hgb*, hemoglobulin; *IgM*, immunoglobulin M; *NR*, not reported; *WBC*, white blood cell count.

[1] Gobbi PG, Bettini R, Montecucco C et al: Study of prognosis in Waldenström's macroglobulinemia: A proposal for a simple binary classification with clinical and investigational utility. *Blood* 83:2939, 1994. [2] Morel P, Monconduit M, Jacomy D et al: Prognostic factors in Waldenström macroglobulinemia: A report on 232 patients with the description of a new scoring system and its validation on 253 other patients. *Blood* 96:852, 2000. [3] Dhodapkar MV, Jacobson JL, Gertz MA et al: Prognostic factors and response to fludarabine therapy in patients with Waldenström macroglobulinemia: Results of United States intergroup trial (Southwest Oncology Group S9003). *Blood* 98:41, 2001. [4] Dimopoulos M, Gika D, Zervas K et al: The international staging system for multiple myeloma is applicable in symptomatic Waldenström's macroglobulinemia. *Leuk Lymphoma* 45:1809, 2004. [5] Morel P, Duhamel A, Gobbi P et al: International prognostic scoring system for Waldenström macroglobulinemia. *Blood* 113:4163, 2009.

From Hoffman R et al: *Hematology, basic principles and practice*, ed 7, Philadelphia, 2018, Elsevier.

REFERRAL

A hematology consultation is helpful in guiding future workup, treatment, and monitoring. Participation in clinical trials is highly encouraged in patients with WM.

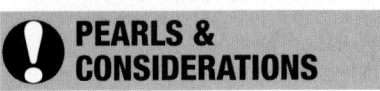

PEARLS & CONSIDERATIONS

COMMENTS

WM was first described in 1944 by the Swedish physician Jan Gösta Waldenström, who also described the X-linked Bruton agammaglobulinemia.

SUGGESTED READINGS

Available at ExpertConsult.com

AUTHORS: **JORGE J. CASTILLO, M.D.,** and **STEVEN P. TREON, M.D.**

BASIC INFORMATION

DEFINITION

Warts are benign epidermal lesions caused by human papillomavirus (HPV).

SYNONYMS

Verruca vulgaris (common warts)
Verruca plana (flat warts)
Condyloma acuminatum (venereal warts)
Verruca plantaris (plantar warts)
Mosaic warts (cluster of many warts)
HPV infection

ICD-10CM CODES	
B07.9	Viral wart, unspecified
B07.8	Other viral warts
A63.0	Anogenital (venereal) warts
B07.0	Plantar wart

EPIDEMIOLOGY & DEMOGRAPHICS

- Risk factors include use of communal showers, occupational handling of meat, and immunosuppression. Common warts occur most frequently in children and young adults.
- Anogenital warts are most common in young, sexually active patients. Genital warts are the most common viral sexually transmitted disease in the United States, with up to 79 million Americans carrying the causative virus, and 14 million persons are newly infected each year in the U.S.
- Persistent infection with oncogenic HPV types can cause cervical cancer in women as well as other anogenital and oropharyngeal cancers in women and men. 66% of cervical cancers, 55% of vaginal cancers, 79% of anal cancers, and 62% of oropharyngeal cancers are attributable to HPV types 16 or 18.
- Common warts are longer lasting and more frequent in immunocompromised patients (e.g., lymphoma, AIDS, immunosuppressive drugs).
- Plantar warts occur most frequently at points of maximal pressure (over the heads of the metatarsal bones or on the heels).

PHYSICAL FINDINGS & CLINICAL PRESENTATION

- Common warts (Fig. 1) have an initial appearance of a flesh-colored papule with a rough surface; they subsequently develop a hyperkeratotic appearance with black dots on the surface (thrombosed capillaries). They may be single or multiple and are most common on the hands.
- Warts obscure normal skin lines (important diagnostic feature). Cylindrical projections from the wart may become fused, forming a mosaic pattern.
- Flat warts (Fig. 2) generally are pink or light yellow, slightly elevated, and often found on the forehead, back of hands, mouth, and beard area. They often occur in lines corresponding to trauma (e.g., a scratch), are often misdiagnosed (particularly when present on the face), and are inappropriately treated with topical corticosteroids.
- Filiform warts have a fingerlike appearance with various projections; they are generally found near the mouth, beard, or periorbital and paranasal regions.
- Plantar warts (Fig. 3) are slightly raised and have a roughened surface; they may cause pain when walking; as they involute, small hemorrhages (caused by thrombosed capillaries) may be noted.
- Genital warts (Fig. 4) are generally pale pink with several projections and a broad base. They may coalesce in the perineal area to form masses with a cauliflower-like appearance. Intraanal warts occur predominantly in patients who have had receptive anal intercourse, in contrast with perianal warts, which may occur in men and women without a history of anal sex.
- Genital warts on the cervical epithelium can produce subclinical changes that may be noted on Pap smear or colposcopy.

ETIOLOGY

- HPV infection; >150 types of viral DNA have been identified. Transmission of warts is by direct contact. Approximately 40 different types of HPV are transmitted through sexual contact.
- Genital warts: 90% are caused by HPV types 6 or 11. HPV types 16, 18, 31, 33, and 35 are found occasionally in visible genital warts (usually as coinfections with HPV 6 or 11) and can be associated with foci of high-grade, intraepithelial neoplasia, particularly in persons who are infected with HIV infection. In addition to warts on genital areas, HPV types 6 and 11 have been associated with conjunctival, nasal, oral, and laryngeal warts.

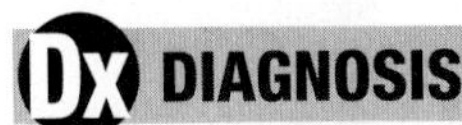

DIAGNOSIS

DIFFERENTIAL DIAGNOSIS

- Molluscum contagiosum
- Condyloma latum
- Acrochordon (skin tags) or seborrheic keratosis
- Epidermal nevi
- Hypertrophic actinic keratosis
- Squamous cell carcinomas
- Acquired digital fibrokeratoma
- Varicella-zoster virus in patients with AIDS

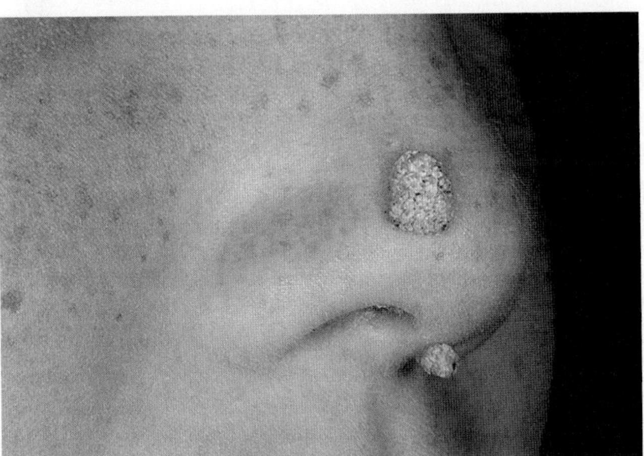

FIG. 1 Common warts. A dome-shaped lesion of the lateral nose and a filiform lesion of the columella. (From Paller AS, Mancini AJ: *Hurwitz clinical pediatric dermatology, a textbook of skin disorders of childhood and adolescence,* ed 5, 2016, Elsevier.)

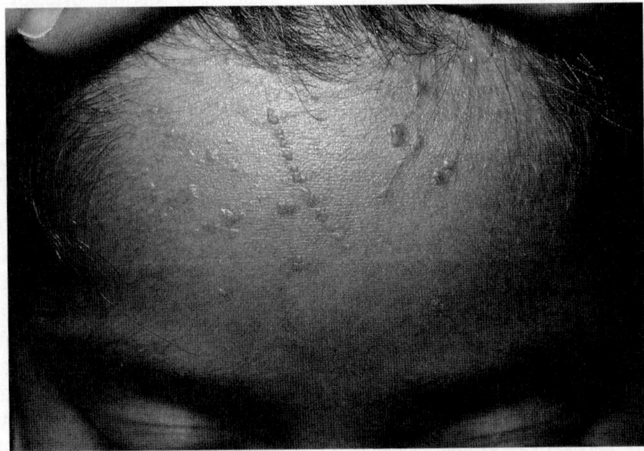

FIG. 2 Flat warts with koebnerization. Flat papules on the forehead, with a linear configuration (Koebner phenomenon) at sites of autoinoculation. (From Paller AS, Mancini AJ: *Hurwitz clinical pediatric dermatology, a textbook of skin disorders of childhood and adolescence,* ed 5, 2016, Elsevier.)

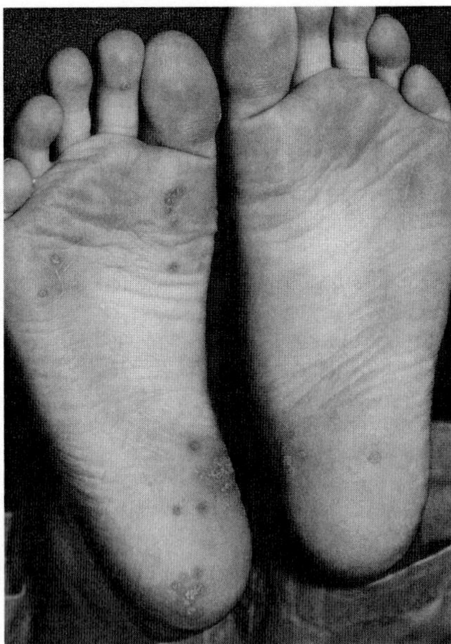

FIG. 3 Plantar warts. Verrucous papules on the plantar surfaces. (From Paller AS, Mancini AJ: *Hurwitz clinical pediatric dermatology, a textbook of skin disorders of childhood and adolescence,* ed 5, 2016, Elsevier.)

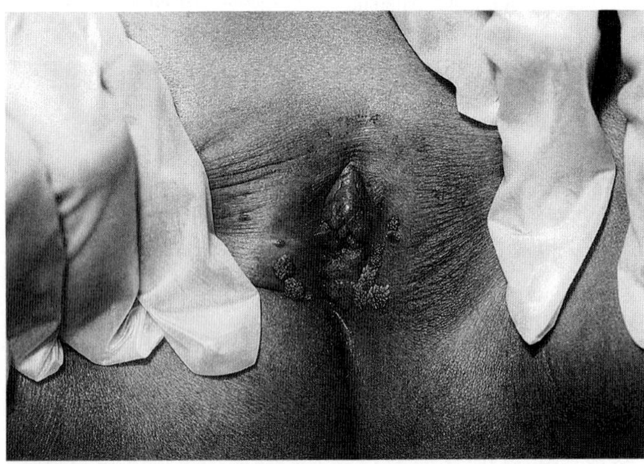

FIG. 4 Condylomata acuminata. Verrucous papules of the labial surfaces, with a large, vegetative lesion protruding from the vagina. This toddler had been sexually abused. (From Paller AS, Mancini AJ: Hurwitz clinical pediatric dermatology, a textbook of skin disorders of childhood and adolescence, ed 5, 2016, Elsevier.)

- Recurrent infantile digital fibroma
- Plantar corns (may be mistaken for plantar warts)

WORKUP

- Diagnosis is generally based on clinical findings.
- Suspect lesions should be biopsied.
- The application of 3% to 5% acetic acid, which causes skin color to turn white, has been used by some providers to detect HPV-infected genital mucosa. However, acetic acid application is not a specific test for HPV infection. Therefore, the routine use of this procedure for screening to detect mucosal changes attributed to HPV infection is not recommended.

LABORATORY TESTS

- Screening for cervical cancer with cytology, which is performed by either Pap smear or liquid-based cytology. Screening guidelines recommend starting screening at age 21. Annual cytology is recommended until at least three normal cytology results are obtained.
- Colposcopy with biopsy is recommended in patients with cervical squamous cell changes.

Rx TREATMENT

NONPHARMACOLOGIC THERAPY

- Importance of use of condoms to reduce transmission of genital warts should be emphasized.
- Watchful waiting is an acceptable option in the treatment of nongenital cutaneous warts because many warts will disappear without intervention over time. However, many patients often request treatment because of social stigma or discomfort.
- Plantar warts that are not painful do not need treatment.
- Factors that influence selection of treatment include wart size, wart number, anatomic site of the wart, wart morphology, patient preference, cost of treatment, convenience, adverse effects, and provider experience. Factors that might affect response to therapy include the presence of immunosuppression and compliance with therapy.

GENERAL Rx

- Common warts:
  1. Application of topical salicylic acid 17%. Soak area for 5 min in warm water and dry. Apply thin layer once or twice daily for up to 12 wk, avoiding normal skin. Bandage.
  2. Liquid nitrogen and electrocautery are also common methods of removal. Cure rates for cryotherapy are 50% to 70% after three to four treatments.
  3. Blunt dissection can be used in large lesions or resistant lesions.
  4. Duct tape occlusion is also effective for treating common warts. It is cut to cover warts and left in place for 6 days. It is removed after 6 days and the warts are soaked in water and then filed with pumice stones. New tape is applied 12 hr later. This treatment can be repeated until warts resolve.
  5. Recalcitrant warts can be treated with injection of *Candida* or mumps skin antigen into the wart every 3 to 4 wk for up to three treatments, photodynamic therapy with aminolevulinic acid, pulsed dye laser, and intralesional bleomycin.
- Filiform warts: Surgical removal is necessary.
- Flat warts: Generally more difficult to treat.
  1. Tretinoin cream applied at bedtime over the involved area for several weeks may be effective.
  2. Application of liquid nitrogen.
  3. Electrocautery.
  4. 5-Fluorouracil cream applied once or twice a day for 3 to 5 wk is also effective. Persistent hyperpigmentation may occur after Efudex use.
- Plantar warts:
  1. Salicylic acid therapy (e.g., Occlusal-HP). Soak wart in warm water for 5 min, remove loose tissue, dry. Apply to area, allow to dry, reapply. Use once or twice daily; maximum 12 wk. Use of 40% salicylic acid plasters (Mediplast) is also a safe, nonscarring treatment; it is particularly useful in treating mosaic warts covering a large area.
  2. Blunt dissection is also a fast and effective treatment modality.
  3. Laser therapy can be used for plantar warts and recurrent warts; however, it leaves open wounds that require 4 to 6 wk to fill with granulation tissue.
  4. Interlesional bleomycin is also effective but generally used when all other treatments fail.
- Genital warts:
  1. Can be effectively treated with 20% podophyllin resin in compound tincture of

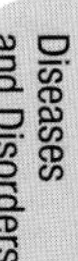

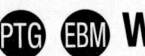

benzoin applied with a cotton tip applicator by the treating physician and allowed to air dry. The treatment can be repeated weekly if necessary.

2. Podofilox (Condylox 0.5% gel) is available for application by the patient. Local adverse effects include pain, burning, and inflammation at the site.
3. Cryosurgery with liquid nitrogen delivered with a probe or as a spray is effective for treating smaller genital warts.
4. Carbon dioxide laser can also be used for treating primary or recurrent genital warts (cure rate >90%).
5. Imiquimod cream, 5%, is a patient-applied immune response modifier effective in the treatment of external genital and perianal warts (complete clearing of genital warts in >70% of females and >30% of males in 4-16 wk). Sexual contact should be avoided while the cream is on the skin. It is applied 3 times per wk before normal sleeping hours and is left on the skin for 6 to 10 hr.
6. Sinecatechins (Veregen), a botanical drug product, is also effective for treatment of external genital and perianal warts. Formulation is a 15% ointment applied to affected area tid for up to 16 wk.

- Application of trichloroacetic acid or bichloracetic acid 80% to 90% is also effective for external genital warts. A small amount should be applied only to warts and allowed to dry, at which time a white "frosting" develops. This treatment can be repeated weekly if necessary.

DISPOSITION

- Warts can be effectively treated with the previous modalities with complete resolution in the majority of patients; however, the recurrence rate is high.
- Cervical carcinomas and precancerous lesions in women are associated with genital papillomavirus infection.
- Squamous cell anal cancer is also associated with a history of genital warts.

REFERRAL

- Dermatology referral for warts resistant to conservative therapy
- Surgical referral in selected cases
- Sexually transmitted disease counseling for patients with anogenital warts

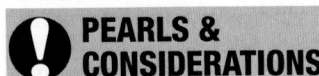

PEARLS & CONSIDERATIONS

COMMENTS

- Subungual and periungual warts are generally more resistant to treatment. Dermatology referral for cryosurgery is recommended in resistant cases.
- Examination of sex partners is not necessary for the management of genital warts because no data indicate that reinfection plays a role.

PREVENTION

- Two HPV vaccines (Gardasil, Gardasil-9, Cervarix) have been licensed in the United States. ACIP recommends routine vaccination with HPV4 or HPV2 for females aged 11 to 12 yr and HPV4 for males aged 11 to 12 yr. Vaccination is also recommended for females aged 13 to 26 yr and for males aged 13 through 21 yr who were not vaccinated previously. Males aged 22 through 26 may be vaccinated. ACIP recommends vaccination of men who have sex with men and immunocompromised persons (including those with infection) through age 26 yr if not previously vaccinated. The 9-valent HPV vaccine (Gardasil-9) is approved for use in girls and women 9 to 26 yr old and boys 9 to 15 yr old. It is indicated to prevent diseases associated with HPV infection with types 6, 11, 16, 18, 31, 33, 45, 52, and 58. It appears to be more effective than the other 2 currently available vaccines. It consists of two doses. The first dose is administered at 11 to 12 yr of age, and the second dose 6 to 12 mo later. However, if the second dose is given less than 5 mo apart, a third dose will be needed at age 9 to 14. Patients with a weak immune system and in those starting vaccination at age 15 to 26 yr will need three doses.
- Male circumcision decreases heterosexual transmission of HPV.

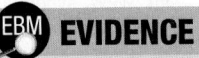

EVIDENCE

Available at ExpertConsult.com

SUGGESTED READINGS

Available at ExpertConsult.com

RELATED CONTENT

Human Papillomavirus Infection (Patient Information)
Warts (Patient Information)
Condyloma Acuminatum (Related Key Topic)

AUTHOR: **FRED F. FERRI, M.D.**

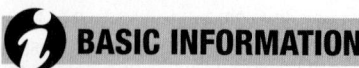

BASIC INFORMATION

DEFINITION

Wolff-Parkinson-White (WPW) syndrome is a congenital heart condition in which, in addition to the normal electrical conduction through the atrioventricular (AV) node, there is an accessory pathway (AP) that connects the atria to the ventricles. Consequently, a portion of the ventricular myocardium is depolarized via the AP earlier than the normal AV nodal conduction, resulting in ventricular preexcitation. The terms "WPW syndrome" and "WPW pattern" often are used in describing patients with ventricular preexcitation. Patients with WPW syndrome have ECG findings of preexcitation, including short PR and slurring of the initial segment of the QRS complex known as the delta wave together with symptoms suggestive of arrhythmia or documented arrhythmia, which may be atrioventricular (AV) reentrant tachycardia, atrial fibrillation (AF), or both. Patients with the WPW pattern have characteristic ECG findings of preexcitation without evidence of arrhythmia.

SYNONYMS

Preexcitation syndrome
WPW

ICD-10CM CODE

I45.6 Pre-excitation syndrome

EPIDEMIOLOGY & DEMOGRAPHICS

- The prevalence of a WPW pattern on the surface ECG is 0.1% to 0.3% in the general population. The prevalence is increased to 0.55% in first-degree relatives of affected patients. It is estimated that approximately 65% of adolescents and 40% of individuals older than 30 yr with WPW pattern on a resting ECG are asymptomatic.
- The prevalence of WPW is higher among males and decreases with age.
- Most patients with WPW have structurally normal hearts, but it may also occur in patients with congenital heart disease, most notably in patients with Ebstein's anomaly, which is associated with right-side AP and often multiple and slowly conducting APs.

PHYSICAL FINDINGS & CLINICAL PRESENTATION

- The physical examination is usually unremarkable.
- Symptoms are typically related to tachyarrhythmias, including the following:
  1. Palpitations, lightheadedness, anxiety, dyspnea, or chest pain
  2. Syncope or near syncope
  3. Sudden cardiac death
- The common arrhythmias in WPW syndrome are:
  1. Supraventricular tachycardia: AV reciprocating tachycardia (AVRT). This is the most common arrhythmia, further classified as orthodromic AVRT (narrow complex tachycardia, with antegrade conduction through the AV node and retrograde conduction via the AP that occurs in 70% of symptomatic patients) or antidromic AVRT (wide complex tachycardia with antegrade conduction via the AP and retrogradely through the AV node, which occurs in 4% to 5% of patients).
  2. AF (~10% to 38%), the second most common tachycardia, can be complicated by a very rapid ventricular response due to conduction over the AP, which can lead to ventricular fibrillation (VF) and sudden death. This risk is dependent on the antegrade refractory period of AP during AF.
  3. The risk of sudden death in symptomatic patients with WPW syndrome is estimated to be approximately 0.25% per year or 3% to 4% over a lifetime.
- In a meta-analysis including approximately 2000 subjects with asymptomatic WPW, children had a sudden death rate of 1.9 compared with 0.9 in adults per 1000 patient years of follow-up. This incidence is comparable with the estimated 0.1% per year risk of death in the general population in Europe, Japan, and the United States.

ETIOLOGY & PATHOGENESIS

- APs are thought to be an embryologic remnant, as substantiated by reports of SVT in uterus and by a greater prevalence of WPW in newborns and infants.
- Left free wall APs are most common followed by posteroseptal, right free wall, and anteroseptal locations.
- Some patients with WPW syndrome (~5% to 10%) have multiple APs.
- In subjects with WPW, two parallel routes of AV conduction are present: One is subject to delay through the AV node, and the other occurs without delay through the AP and results in preexcitation of the ventricles. The resulting QRS complex is a fusion beat, as a portion of the ventricle is preexcited and activated via the AP giving rise to the delta wave, and the remainder of the ventricle is activated by the normal activation pathway (Fig. 1).

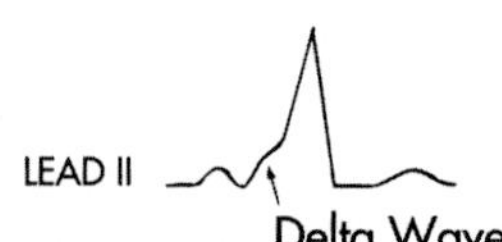

FIG. 1 With Wolff-Parkinson-White (WPW) syndrome, an abnormal accessory pathway called a bypass tract connects the atria and the ventricles. (From Goldberger AL [ed]: *Clinical electrocardiography: a simplified approach,* ed 6, St, Louis, 1999, Mosby.)

- Reciprocating tachycardias occur when conduction is anterograde in one pathway (usually the AV node, i.e., orthodromic AVRT) and retrograde in the other (usually the AP) as a result of different refractory periods. This is usually initiated by a premature atrial or ventricular depolarization.

Dx DIAGNOSIS

- Three basic features characterize the ECG abnormalities associated with WPW pattern:
  1. PR interval <120 ms.
  2. QRS complex can be >120 ms with a slurred, slowly rising onset of QRS in some leads (delta wave) and a normal terminal QRS portion. The width of the QRS complex depends on the amount of preexcitation ventricular tissue.
  3. Secondary ST-T wave changes directed in an opposite direction to the major delta and QRS vectors may be present.
- ECG patterns with abnormal QRS complexes and ST and T changes can mask or mimic myocardial infarction (in particular posteroseptal AP with negative delta waves in the inferior wall, which mimics old inferior wall myocardial infarction), bundle branch block (Fig. 2), or ventricular hypertrophy.
- Most commonly seen tachycardia (orthodromic AVRT) is characterized by a normal QRS with a regular rate of 150 to 250 bpm. Onset and termination are abrupt.
- Variants of preexcitation:
  1. Lown-Ganong-Levine syndrome is characterized by a short PR interval, a narrow QRS complex without a delta wave, and a clinical syndrome of paroxysmal SVTs. Postulated mechanisms to the short PR interval include a variant of the normal, enhanced sympathetic tone or specialized intra-nodal fibers with enhanced AV nodal conduction.
  2. Atriofascicular accessory pathway (Mahaim fiber): A slowly conducting AP with AV-nodal like properties, which connects the right atrium with the right bundle branch or the apical myocardium. In the baseline state, minimal or no preexcitation may be present. During preexcitation the QRS appears like a typical LBBB pattern.
  3. Nodoventricular or nodofascicular APs: Rare variants that connect the AV node and the ventricle or the bundle branch appropriately.
- An electrophysiology study is the gold standard to confirm the diagnosis, determine the location, and assess the conduction properties of the AP.

RISK STRATIFICATION

- Intermittent and abrupt loss of preexcitation on a beat-to-beat basis is indicative of lower risk, assessed with Holter monitoring or with an exercise stress test. The loss of preexcitation after administration of the antiarrhythmic drug procainamide has also been used to indicate a low-risk subgroup.

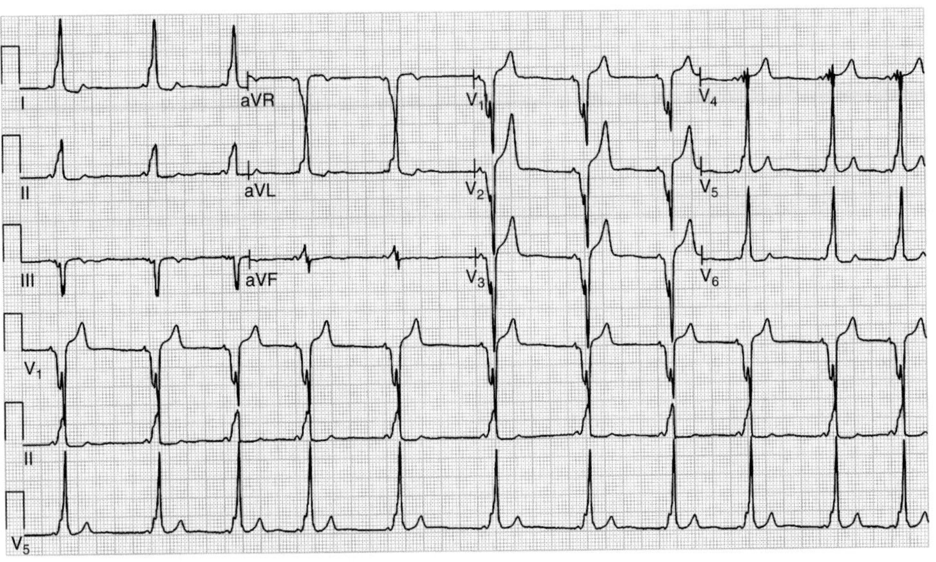

FIG. 2 Wolff-Parkinson-White syndrome. This 12-lead ECG with rhythm strips shows preexcitation with an accessory pathway connecting the right atrium to the right ventricle. This gives rise to a pattern like LBBB because the ventricles are activated over the right-sided accessory pathway. The tracing shows the typical characteristics of WPW syndrome, including a short PR interval, a wide QRS complex, and a delta wave. (From Olshansky B, et al.: *Arrhythmia essentials*, ed 2, Philadelphia, 2017, Elsevier.)

BOX 1 Goals of Electrophysiologic Evaluation in Patients with Wolff-Parkinson-White Syndrome

- Confirmation of the presence of an accessory pathway (AP)
- Evaluation for the presence of multiple APs
- Localization of the AP(s)
- Evaluation of the refractory period of the AP and its implications for life-threatening arrhythmias
- Induction and evaluation of tachycardias
- Demonstration of the AP role in the tachycardia
- Evaluation of other tachycardias not dependent on the presence of the AP
- Ablation of the AP, when indicated.

From Issa Z, et al.: *Clinical arrhythmology and electrophysiology*, ed 2, Philadelphia, 2012, Saunders.

- In patients with a persistent preexcitation pattern, electrophysiology study is the procedure of choice for risk stratification.

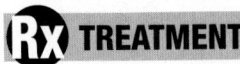

TREATMENT

Goals of electrophysiologic evaluation in patients with WPW syndrome are described in Box 1.

ACUTE MANAGEMENT

- Urgent cardioversion, for an acute tachycardia episode with hemodynamic instability.
- Narrow QRS tachycardia (c/w orthodromic AVRT):
  1. Vagal maneuvers and/or IV adenosine.
  2. IV beta blockers, diltiazem, or verapamil can be administered for regular and **narrow** QRS tachycardia, implying antegrade conduction via the AV node, when the patient is hemodynamically stable and IV adenosine is ineffective.
- Wide QRS complex tachycardias (WCTs):
  1. Most commonly caused by atrial fibrillation with antegrade conduction via the AP and the AV node. AV nodal blocking therapies (i.e., beta blockers, calcium channel blockers, digoxin, and adenosine) are potentially dangerous and should be avoided in these cases because of the risk of causing VF by enhancement of the ventricular response through the accessory pathway when the AV node is blocked and the blood pressure is lowered.
  2. Stable patients with preexcited AF can be managed with IV procainamide. Electrical cardioversion should be performed if the patient is hemodynamically unstable.
  3. In a patient with WCT due to antidromic tachycardia, drug treatment may be directed at the AP or at the AV node because both are critical components of the tachycardia circuit.

Long-term management:

- Asymptomatic:
  1. In low-risk patients with intermittent loss of preexcitation, AP effective refractory period (APERP) ≤250, or shortest preexcited RR interval (SPERRI) ≤250 ms, no therapy is required.
  2. In high-risk patients with APERP ≥250 ms or SPERRI≥ 250 ms, competitive athletes, or high-risk occupation (i.e., pilots), ablation should be considered.
- Symptomatic:
  1. Patients who presented with aborted sudden cardiac death, preexcited tachycardia (i.e., atrial fibrillation, flutter, atrial tachycardia), or syncope suggestive of cardiac origin should undergo an electrophysiology study for further characterization and ablation of the AP accordingly.
  2. Patients with symptomatic palpitations or documented AVRT should be offered an electrophysiology study and ablation of the AP to prevent recurrence and to allow the patient to avoid long-term medical therapy. Ongoing management for stable patients with history of orthodromic AVRT who are not candidates for, or prefer not to undergo, catheter ablation:
     - Class IC antiarrhythmics (flecainide, propafenone), in the absence of structural heart disease.
     - Class III antiarrhythmics (amiodarone, sotalol).
     - Oral beta blockers, diltiazem, or verapamil.

SUGGESTED READINGS

Available at ExpertConsult.com

RELATED CONTENT

Wolff-Parkinson-White Syndrome (Patient Information)

AUTHORS: **YUVAL KONSTANTINO, M.D.,** and **MOTI HAIM, M.D.**

Differential Diagnosis

ABDOMINAL DISTENTION

ICD-10CM # R14.0 Abdominal distension (gaseous)

NONMECHANICAL OBSTRUCTION

Excessive intraluminal gas.
Intraabdominal infection.
Trauma.
Retroperitoneal irritation (renal colic, neoplasms, infections, hemorrhage).
Vascular insufficiency (thrombosis, embolism).
Mechanical ventilation.
Extraabdominal infection (sepsis, pneumonia, empyema, osteomyelitis of spine).
Metabolic/toxic abnormalities (hypokalemia, uremia, lead poisoning).
Chemical irritation (perforated ulcer, bile, pancreatitis).
Peritoneal inflammation.
Severe pain, pain medications.

MECHANICAL OBSTRUCTION

Neoplasm (intraluminal, extraluminal).
Adhesions, endometriosis.
Infection (intraabdominal abscess, diverticulitis).
Gallstones.
Foreign body, bezoars.
Pregnancy.
Hernias.
Volvulus.
Stenosis at surgical anastomosis, radiation stenosis.
Fecaliths.
Inflammatory bowel disease.
Gastric outlet obstruction.
Hematoma.
Other: parasites, superior mesenteric artery (SMA) syndrome, pneumatosis intestinalis, annular pancreas, Hirschsprung disease, intussusception, meconium.

ABDOMINAL PAIN, ADOLESCENCE[55]

ICD-10CM # R10.817 Generalized abdominal tenderness
R10.827 Generalized rebound abdominal tenderness

Acute gastroenteritis.
Irritable bowel syndrome (IBS).
Anxiety.
Mittelschmerz.
Appendicitis.
Inflammatory bowel disease.
Peptic ulcer disease (PUD).
Cholecystitis.
Neoplasm.
Diabetic ketoacidosis.
Functional abdominal pain.
Pelvic inflammatory disease (PID).
Pregnancy.
Pyelonephritis.
Renal stone.
Trauma.

ABDOMINAL PAIN, CHILDHOOD[55]

ICD-10CM # R10.817 Generalized abdominal tenderness
R10.827 Generalized rebound abdominal tenderness

Acute gastroenteritis.
Appendicitis.
Constipation.
Cholecystitis, acute.
Intestinal obstruction.
Pancreatitis.
Neoplasm.
Inflammatory bowel disease.
Other:
  Functional abdominal pain.
  Pyelonephritis.
  Pneumonia.
  Diabetic ketoacidosis.
  Heavy metal poisoning.
  Sickle cell crisis.
  Trauma.
  Anxiety.
  Sexual abuse.

ABDOMINAL PAIN, CHRONIC LOWER[81]

ICD-10CM # R10.814 Left lower quadrant abdominal tenderness
R10.824 Left lower quadrant rebound abdominal tenderness
R10.813 Right lower quadrant abdominal tenderness
R10.823 Right lower quadrant rebound abdominal tenderness
R10.30 Lower abdominal pain, unspecified

ORGANIC DISORDERS

Common

Gynecologic disease.
Lactase deficiency.
Diverticulitis/diverticulosis.
Crohn's disease.
Intestinal obstruction.

Uncommon

Chronic intestinal pseudoobstruction.
Mesenteric ischemia.
Malignancy (e.g., ovarian carcinoma).
Abdominal wall pain.
Spinal disease.
Testicular disease.
Metabolic diseases (e.g., diabetes mellitus, familial Mediterranean fever, C1 esterase deficiency [angioneurotic edema], porphyria, lead poisoning, tabes dorsalis, renal failure).

FUNCTIONAL DISORDERS

Common

Irritable bowel syndrome.
Functional abdominal bloating.

Uncommon

Functional abdominal pain.

ABDOMINAL PAIN, DIFFUSE

ICD-10CM # R10.817 Generalized abdominal tenderness
R10.827 Generalized rebound abdominal tenderness

Early appendicitis.
Aortic aneurysm.
Gastroenteritis.
Intestinal obstruction.
Diverticulitis.
Peritonitis.
Mesenteric insufficiency or infarction.
Pancreatitis.
Inflammatory bowel disease.
Irritable bowel.
Mesenteric adenitis.
Metabolic: toxins, lead poisoning, uremia, drug overdose, diabetic ketoacidosis (DKA), heavy metal poisoning.
Sickle cell crisis.
Pneumonia (rare).
Trauma.
Urinary tract infection, PID.
Other: anxiety, acute intermittent porphyria, tabes dorsalis, periarteritis nodosa, Henoch-Schönlein purpura, adrenal insufficiency.

ABDOMINAL PAIN, EPIGASTRIC

ICD-10CM # R10.816 Epigastric abdominal tenderness
R10.826 Epigastric rebound abdominal tenderness

Gastric: PUD, gastric outlet obstruction, gastric ulcer.
Duodenal: PUD, duodenitis.
Biliary: cholecystitis, cholangitis, biliary dyskinesia.
Hepatic: hepatitis.
Pancreatic: pancreatitis.
Intestinal: high small bowel obstruction, early appendicitis.
Cardiac: angina, MI, pericarditis.
Pulmonary: pneumonia, pleurisy, pneumothorax.
Subphrenic abscess.
Vascular: dissecting aneurysm, mesenteric ischemia.
Psychiatric: anxiety.

ABDOMINAL PAIN, EXTRAABDOMINAL AND SYSTEMIC CAUSES[26]

ICD-10CM # R10.817 Generalized abdominal tenderness

EXTRAABDOMINAL AND SYSTEMIC CAUSES OF ACUTE ABDOMINAL PAIN

Cardiac

Endocarditis.
Heart failure.
Myocardial ischemia and infarction.
Myocarditis.

Thoracic

Empyema.
Esophageal rupture (Boerhaave's syndrome).
Esophageal spasm.
Esophagitis.
Pleurodynia (Bornholm's disease).
Pneumonitis.
Pneumothorax.
Pulmonary embolism and infarction.

Hematologic

Acute leukemia.
Hemolytic anemia.
Henoch-Schönlein purpura.
Sickle cell disease.

Metabolic

Acute adrenal insufficiency (Addison's disease).
Diabetes mellitus (especially with ketoacidosis).
Hyperlipidemia.
Hyperparathyroidism.
Hypersensitivity reactions (e.g., to insect bites, reptile venoms).
Lead poisoning.
Porphyria.
Toxins.
Uremia.

Infections

Herpes zoster.
Osteomyelitis.
Typhoid fever.

Neurologic

Abdominal epilepsy.
Radiculopathy, spinal cord or peripheral nerve tumors, degenerative arthritis of spine, herniated vertebral disk.
Tabes dorsalis.

Miscellaneous

Angioedema.
Familial Mediterranean fever.
Heat stroke.
Muscle contusion, hematoma, tumor.
Narcotic withdrawal.
Psychiatric disorders.

ABDOMINAL PAIN, INFANCY[55]

ICD-10CM #		
	R10.817	Generalized abdominal tenderness
	R10.827	Generalized rebound abdominal tenderness

Acute gastroenteritis.
Appendicitis.
Intussusception.
Volvulus.
Meckel diverticulum.
Other: colic, trauma.

ABDOMINAL PAIN, LEFT LOWER QUADRANT

ICD-10CM #		
	R10.814	Left lower quadrant abdominal tenderness
	R10.824	Left lower quadrant rebound abdominal tenderness

Intestinal: diverticulitis, diverticulosis, intestinal obstruction, perforated ulcer, inflammatory bowel disease, perforated descending colon, inguinal hernia, neoplasm, appendicitis.
Reproductive: ectopic pregnancy, ovarian cyst, torsion of ovarian cyst, tuboovarian abscess, mittelschmerz, endometriosis, seminal vesiculitis.
Renal: renal or ureteral calculi, pyelonephritis, neoplasm.
Vascular: leaking aortic aneurysm.
Psoas abscess.
Trauma.

ABDOMINAL PAIN, LEFT UPPER QUADRANT

ICD-10CM #		
	R19.02	Left upper quadrant abdominal swelling, mass, and lump

Gastric: PUD, gastritis, pyloric stenosis, hiatal hernia.
Pancreatic: pancreatitis, neoplasm, stone in pancreatic duct or ampulla.
Cardiac: MI, angina pectoris.
Splenic: splenomegaly, ruptured spleen, splenic abscess, splenic infarction.
Renal: calculi, pyelonephritis, neoplasm.
Pulmonary: pneumonia, empyema, pulmonary infarction.
Vascular: ruptured aortic aneurysm.
Cutaneous: herpes zoster.
Trauma.
Intestinal: high fecal impaction, perforated colon, diverticulitis.

ABDOMINAL PAIN, NONSURGICAL CAUSES

ICD-10CM #		
	R19.8	Other specified symptoms and signs involving the digestive system and abdomen
	R10.817	Generalized abdominal tenderness

Irritable bowel syndrome.
Urinary tract infection, pyelonephritis, salpingitis, PID.
Gastroenteritis, gastritis, peptic ulcer.
Diverticular spasm.
Hepatitis, mononucleosis.
Pancreatitis.
Inferior wall myocardial infarction.
Basilar pneumonia, pulmonary embolism.
Diabetic ketoacidosis.
Strain or hematoma of rectus muscle.
Ruptured Graafian follicle.
Herpes zoster.
Nerve root compression.
Sickle cell crisis.
Acute adrenal insufficiency.
Other: acute porphyria, familial Mediterranean fever, tabes dorsalis, anxiety, sexual abuse.

ABDOMINAL PAIN, PERIUMBILICAL

ICD-10CM #		
	R10.815	Periumbilic abdominal tenderness
	R10.825	Periumbilic rebound abdominal tenderness

Intestinal: small bowel obstruction or gangrene, early appendicitis.
Vascular: mesenteric thrombosis, dissecting aortic aneurysm.
Pancreatic: pancreatitis.
Metabolic: uremia, DKA.
Trauma.

ABDOMINAL PAIN, POORLY LOCALIZED[55]

ICD-10CM #		
	R10.819	Abdominal tenderness, unspecified site

EXTRAABDOMINAL

Metabolic

DKA, acute intermittent porphyria, hyperthyroidism, hypothyroidism, hypercalcemia, hypokalemia, uremia, hyperlipidemia, hyperparathyroidism.

Hematologic

Sickle cell crisis, leukemia or lymphoma, Henoch-Schönlein purpura.

Infectious

Infectious mononucleosis, Rocky Mountain spotted fever, acquired immunodeficiency syndrome (AIDS), streptococcal pharyngitis (in children), herpes zoster.

Drugs and Toxins

Heavy metal poisoning, black widow spider bites, withdrawal syndromes, mushroom ingestion.

Referred Pain

Pulmonary: pneumonia, pulmonary embolism, pneumothorax.
Cardiac: angina, MI, pericarditis, myocarditis.
Genitourinary: prostatitis, epididymitis, orchitis, testicular torsion.
Musculoskeletal: rectus sheath hematoma.

Functional

Somatization disorder, malingering, hypochondriasis, Munchausen syndrome.

INTRAABDOMINAL

Early appendicitis, gastroenteritis, peritonitis, pancreatitis, abdominal aortic aneurysm, mesenteric insufficiency or infarction, intestinal obstruction, volvulus, ulcerative colitis.

ABDOMINAL PAIN, POST-CHOLECYSTECTOMY[26]

ICD-10CM # R10.817 Generalized abdominal tenderness

CAUSES OF ABDOMINAL PAIN AFTER CHOLECYSTECTOMY

Biliary Causes
Biliary stricture.
Biliary tract malignancy.
Choledocholithiasis.
Choledochocele.
Cystic duct remnant.
SOD.

Pancreatic Causes
Pancreatitis.
Pseudocyst.
Malignancy.

Other GI Disorders
Esophageal motor disorders.
GERD.
Intestinal malignancy.
Intraabdominal adhesions.
IBS.
Mesenteric ischemia.
PUD.

Extraintestinal Disorders
Coronary artery disease.
Intercostal neuritis.
Neurologic disorders.
Psychiatric disorders.
Wound neuroma.

ABDOMINAL PAIN, PREGNANCY

ICD-10CM # R10.817 Generalized abdominal tenderness
R10.827 Generalized rebound abdominal tenderness

GYNECOLOGIC (GESTATIONAL AGE IN PARENTHESES)

Miscarriage	(<20 wk; 80% <12 wk)
Septic abortion	(<20 wk)
Ectopic pregnancy	(<14 wk)
Corpus luteum cyst rupture	(<12 wk)
Ovarian torsion	(especially <24 wk)
Pelvic inflammatory disease	(<12 wk)
Chorioamnionitis	(>16 wk)
Abruptio placentae	(>16 wk)

NONGYNECOLOGIC

Appendicitis	(Throughout)
Cholecystitis	(Throughout)
Hepatitis	(Throughout)
Pyelonephritis	(Throughout)
Preeclampsia	(>20 wk)

ABDOMINAL PAIN, RIGHT LOWER QUADRANT

ICD-10CM # R10.813 Right lower quadrant abdominal tenderness
R10.823 Right lower quadrant rebound abdominal tenderness

Intestinal: acute appendicitis, regional enteritis, incarcerated hernia, cecal diverticulitis, intestinal obstruction, perforated ulcer, perforated cecum, Meckel diverticulitis.
Reproductive: ectopic pregnancy, ovarian cyst, torsion of ovarian cyst, salpingitis, tuboovarian abscess, mittelschmerz, endometriosis, seminal vesiculitis.
Renal: renal and ureteral calculi, neoplasms, pyelonephritis.
Vascular: leaking aortic aneurysm.
Cutaneous: herpes zoster.
Psoas abscess.
Trauma.
Cholecystitis.

ABDOMINAL PAIN, RIGHT UPPER QUADRANT

ICD-10CM # R10.811 Right upper quadrant abdominal tenderness
R10.821 Right upper quadrant rebound abdominal tenderness

Biliary: calculi, infection, inflammation, neoplasm.
Hepatic: hepatitis, abscess, hepatic congestion, neoplasm, trauma.
Gastric: PUD, pyloric stenosis, neoplasm, alcoholic gastritis, hiatal hernia.
Pancreatic: pancreatitis, neoplasm, stone in pancreatic duct or ampulla.
Renal: calculi, infection, inflammation, neoplasm, rupture of kidney.
Pulmonary: pneumonia, pulmonary infarction, right-sided pleurisy.
Intestinal: retrocecal appendicitis, intestinal obstruction, high fecal impaction, diverticulitis.
Cardiac: myocardial ischemia (particularly involving the inferior wall), pericarditis.
Cutaneous: herpes zoster.
Trauma.
Fitz-Hugh-Curtis syndrome (perihepatitis).

ABDOMINAL PAIN, RIGHT UPPER QUADRANT, DIFFERENTIAL DIAGNOSIS IN PREGNANCY[30]

ICD-10CM # R10.811 Right upper quadrant abdominal tenderness
R10.821 Right upper quadrant rebound abdominal tenderness

DIFFERENTIAL DIAGNOSIS OF RIGHT UPPER QUADRANT ABDOMINAL PAIN DURING PREGNANCY

Hepatic Disorders:
- Hepatitis.
- Hepatic vascular engorgement.
- Hepatic hematoma.
- Hepatic malignancy.

Biliary Tract Disease:
- Biliary colic.
- Choledocholithiasis.
- Cholangitis.
- Cholecystitis.

Diseases Related to Pregnancy:
- Preeclampsia or eclampsia.
- Hemolysis, elevated liver enzymes, and low platelet count (HELLP) syndrome.
- Acute fatty liver of pregnancy.
- Hepatic hemorrhage or rupture.

Renal Disorders:
- Pyelonephritis.
- Nephrolithiasis.

Gastrointestinal Disorders:
- Peptic ulcer disease.
- Perforated duodenal ulcer.

Other Conditions in RUQ:
- Rib fracture.
- Shingles.

Referred Pain from Other Organ Disease:
- Pneumonia.
- Pulmonary embolus or infarct.
- Pleural effusion.
- Radiculopathy.
- Inferior wall myocardial infarction.
- Colon cancer.

ABDOMINAL PAIN, SUPRAPUBIC

ICD-10CM # R10.30 Lower abdominal pain, unspecified

Intestinal: colon obstruction or gangrene, diverticulitis, appendicitis.
Reproductive system: ectopic pregnancy, mittelschmerz, torsion of ovarian cyst, PID, salpingitis, endometriosis, rupture of endometrioma.
Cystitis, rupture of urinary bladder.

ABDOMINAL WALL MASSES[81]

ICD-10CM # R19.00 Intraabdominal and pelvic swelling, mass and lump, unspecified site

LUMPS ARISING IN THE SKIN AND SUBCUTANEOUS FAT (THAT COULD OCCUR ANYWHERE ON THE BODY)

Lipoma.
Sebaceous cyst.

LUMPS ARISING IN THE SKIN AND SUBCUTANEOUS FAT (SPECIFIC TO THE ANTERIOR ABDOMINAL WALL)

Tumor nodule of the umbilicus (secondary to the intraperitoneal malignancy, also called *Sister Mary Joseph nodule*).

LUMPS ARISING IN THE FASCIA AND MUSCLE

Rectus sheath hematoma (usually painful).
Desmoid tumor (associated with Gardner's syndrome).

HERNIA

Incisional:	It has an overlying scar. The sac may be very much larger than the neck of the hernia.
Umbilical:	The hernia is through the umbilical scar. Those presenting at birth commonly resolve in the first years of life.
Paraumbilical:	The neck is just lateral to the umbilical scar. Patients usually present later in life.
Epigastric:	It occurs in the midline between the xiphoid process and the umbilicus. They are usually small (<2 cm). They result when a knuckle of extraperitoneal fat extrudes through a small defect in the linea alba. Commonly irreducible and without an expansile cough impulse.
Spigelian:	A rare hernia found along the linea semilunaris at the lateral edge of the rectus sheath, most commonly a third of the way between the umbilicus and the pubis.

DIVARICATION OF THE RECTI

Supraumbilical elliptical swelling of the attenuated linea alba (no cough impulse).

ABORTION, RECURRENT

ICD-10CM # P01.8 Newborn (suspected to be) affected by other maternal complications of pregnancy

Congenital anatomic abnormalities.
Adhesions (uterine synechiae).
Uterine fibroids.
Endometriosis.
Endocrine abnormalities (luteal phase insufficiency, hypothyroidism, uncontrolled diabetes mellitus [DM]).
Parenteral chromosome abnormalities.
Maternal infections (cervical mycoplasma, ureaplasma, chlamydia).
DES exposure, heavy metal exposure.
Thrombocytosis.
Allogenic immunity, autoimmunity, lupus anticoagulant.

ACALCULOUS GALLBLADDER DISEASE[19]

ICD-10CM # K82.9 Other diseases of gallbladder

Biliary tract anomaly (e.g., choledochal cyst).
Bone marrow transplant.
Burns.
Chemotherapy in oncology patients.
Critical illness in intensive care unit patients.
Crohn's disease, Henoch-Schönlein purpura, Kawasaki disease, systemic lupus erythematosus.
Infectious agents (atypical microbes).
Microlithiasis.
Postoperative state (e.g., cardiac surgery).
Sepsis.
Sludge.
Systemic inflammatory states.
Total parenteral nutrition.
Traumatic spinal cord injury.

ACHES AND PAINS, DIFFUSE[48]

ICD-10CM # M25.50 Pain in unspecified joint

Postviral arthralgias/myalgias.
Bilateral soft tissue rheumatism.
Overuse syndromes.
Fibrositis.
Hypothyroidism.
Metabolic bone disease.
Paraneoplastic syndrome.
Myopathy (polymyositis, dermatomyositis).
Rheumatoid arthritis (RA).
Sjögren's syndrome.
Polymyalgia rheumatica.
Hypermobility.
Benign arthralgias/myalgias.
Chronic fatigue syndrome.
Hypophosphatemia.

ACIDOSIS, HYPERCHLOREMIC METABOLIC[83]

ICD-10CM # E87.2 Acidosis

GASTROINTESTINAL BICARBONATE LOSS

Diarrhea.
External pancreatic or small bowel drainage.
Ureterosigmoidostomy, jejunal loop.
Drugs:
- Calcium chloride (acidifying agent).
- Magnesium sulfate (diarrhea).
- Cholestyramine (bile acid diarrhea).

RENAL ACIDOSIS

Hypokalemic:
- Proximal RTA (type 2).
- Distal (classic) RTA (type 1).
- Drug-induced hypokalemia:
  - Acetazolamide (proximal RTA).
  - Amphotericin B (distal RTA).

Hyperkalemic:
- Generalized distal nephron dysfunction (type 4 RTA).
- Mineralocorticoid deficiency or resistance (pseudohypoaldosteronism type 1) PHA-I, PHA-II.
- ↓ Na^+ delivery to distal nephron.
- Tubulointerstitial disease.
- Ammonium excretion defect.
- Drug-induced hyperkalemia:
  - Potassium-sparing diuretics (amiloride, triamterene, spironolactone).
  - Trimethoprim.
  - Pentamidine.
  - Angiotensin-converting enzyme inhibitors and angiotensin II receptor blockers.
  - Nonsteroidal antiinflammatory drugs.
  - Cyclosporine, tacrolimus.

Normokalemic:
- Early renal insufficiency.

OTHER

Acid loads (ammonium chloride, hyperalimentation).
Loss of potential bicarbonate: ketosis with ketone excretion.
Dilution acidosis (rapid saline administration).
Hippurate.
Cation-exchange resins.

ACIDOSIS, LACTIC[83]

ICD-10CM # E87.2 Acidosis

CAUSES OF LACTIC ACIDOSIS

L-Lactic Acidosis

Conditions associated with type A lactic acidosis:
- Poor tissue perfusion.
- Shock:
  - Cardiogenic.
  - Hemorrhagic.
  - Septic.
- Profound hypoxemia:
  - Severe asthma.
  - Carbon monoxide poisoning.

Conditions associated with type B lactic acidosis:
- Liver disease.
- Metformin.
- Inborn errors of metabolism.
- Pyroglutamic acidosis.
- Kombucha tea.

d-Lactic Acidosis

Short bowel syndrome.
Ischemic bowel.
Small bowel obstruction.

ACIDOSIS, METABOLIC

ICD-10CM # E87.2 Acidosis

METABOLIC ACIDOSIS WITH INCREASED ANION GAP (AG ACIDOSIS)

Lactic acidosis.
Ketoacidosis (DM, alcoholic ketoacidosis).
Uremia (chronic renal failure).
Ingestion of toxins (paraldehyde, methanol, salicylate, ethylene glycol).
High-fat diet (mild acidosis).

METABOLIC ACIDOSIS WITH NORMAL AG (HYPERCHLOREMIC ACIDOSIS)

Renal tubular acidosis (including acidosis of aldosterone deficiency).
Intestinal loss of HCO_3^- (diarrhea, pancreatic fistula).
Carbonic anhydrase inhibitors (e.g., acetazolamide).
Dilutional acidosis (as a result of rapid infusion of bicarbonate-free isotonic saline).
Ingestion of exogenous acids (ammonium chloride, methionine, cystine, calcium chloride).
Ileostomy.
Ureterosigmoidostomy.
Drugs: amiloride, triamterene, spironolactone, β-blockers.

ACIDOSIS, RESPIRATORY

ICD-10CM # E87.2 Acidosis

Pulmonary disease (COPD, severe pneumonia, pulmonary edema, interstitial fibrosis).
Airway obstruction (foreign body, severe bronchospasm, laryngospasm).
Thoracic cage disorders (pneumothorax, flail chest, kyphoscoliosis).
Defects in muscles of respiration (myasthenia gravis, hypokalemia, muscular dystrophy).
Defects in peripheral nervous system (amyotrophic lateral sclerosis, poliomyelitis, Guillain-Barré syndrome, botulism, tetanus, organophosphate poisoning, spinal cord injury).
Depression of respiratory center (anesthesia, narcotics, sedatives, vertebral artery embolism or thrombosis, increased intracranial pressure).
Failure of mechanical ventilator.

ACUTE KIDNEY INJURY AND LIVER DISEASE, CAUSES[27,28]

ICD-10CM #		
	S37.009A	Unspecified injury of unspecified kidney, initial encounter
	K76.89	Other specified diseases of liver

Prerenal uremia:	Diuretic use, GI loss, peritoneal aspiration, hypoalbuminemia.
Hepatorenal syndrome	
Acute tubular necrosis:	Hyperbilirubinemia, sepsis, toxic shock syndrome.
Drugs:	Acetaminophen (paracetamol), NSAIDs, tetracycline, rifampicin, isoniazid, anesthetic agents, sulfonamides, allopurinol, methotrexate.
Infections:	Hepatitis C and cryoglobulinemia, hepatitis B and polyarteritis nodosa, leptospirosis, hantavirus, Epstein-Barr virus, gram-negative sepsis, spontaneous bacterial peritonitis.
Other:	Papillary necrosis and obstruction, inhalation of chlorinated hydrocarbons, mushroom poisoning (*Amanita phalloides*).

ACUTE KIDNEY INJURY DUE TO INTRINSIC RENAL DISEASES[57]

ICD-10CM # Varies with specific diagnosis

INTRINSIC RENAL DISEASES THAT CAUSE ACUTE KIDNEY INJURY

Vascular Diseases
Large-Vessel Diseases
Renal artery thrombosis or stenosis.
Renal vein thrombosis.
Atheroembolic disease.
Small- and Medium-Vessel Diseases
Scleroderma.
Malignant hypertension.
Hemolytic uremic syndrome.
Thrombotic thrombocytopenic purpura.
HIV-associated microangiopathy.
Glomerular Diseases
Systemic Diseases
Systemic lupus erythematosus.
Infective endocarditis.
Systemic vasculitis (e.g., periarteritis nodosa, granulomatosis with polyangiitis).
Henoch-Schönlein purpura.
HIV-associated nephropathy.
Essential mixed cryoglobulinemia.
Goodpasture's syndrome.
Primary Renal Diseases
Poststreptococcal glomerulonephritis.
Other postinfectious glomerulonephritis.
Rapidly progressive glomerulonephritis.
Tubulointerstitial Diseases and Conditions
Drugs (many).
Toxins (e.g., heavy metals, ethylene glycol).
Infections.
Multiple myeloma.
Acute Tubular Necrosis
Ischemia
Shock.
Sepsis.
Severe prerenal azotemia.
Nephrotoxins
Antibiotics.
Radiographic contrast agents.
Myoglobinuria.
Hemoglobinuria.
Other Diseases and Conditions
Severe liver disease.
Allergic reactions.
NSAIDs.

ACUTE KIDNEY INJURY, HIV PATIENT, CAUSES[27,28]

ICD-10CM # S37.009A Unspecified injury of unspecified kidney, initial encounter with B20 human immunodeficiency virus (HIV) disease

Prerenal:	Diarrhea, nausea and vomiting, cirrhosis and hepatorenal syndrome, sepsis.
Vascular:	Thrombotic microangiopathy
Glomerular:	Immune complex glomerulonephritis (MPGN secondary to hepatitis C virus, postinfectious glomerulonephritis), HIVAN.
Acute tubular necrosis:	Sepsis, hypotension, nephrotoxins (aminoglycosides, amphotericin, acyclovir, cidofovir, tenofovir, pentamidine).
Acute interstitial nephritis:	Drug-induced (co-trimoxazole), rifampicin, foscarnet, nevirapine), CMV infection, DILS.
Drug-induced intratubular obstruction:	Sulfadiazine, indinavir, foscarnet, acyclovir.
Postrenal obstruction:	Stones, tuberculosis, fungal ball, tumor.
Associated with IV drug use:	Sepsis, endocarditis, heroin-associated nephropathy (FSGS), rhabdomyolysis.

CMV, Cytomegalovirus; *DILS,* diffusive infiltrative lymphocytosis syndrome; *FSGS,* focal segmental glomerulosclerosis; *HIVAN,* HIV-associated nephropathy; *MPGN,* membranoproliferative glomerulonephritis.

ACUTE KIDNEY INJURY IN SPECIFIC CLINICAL SETTINGS[74]

ICD-10CM # N17.9 Acute kidney failure, unspecified

MAJOR CAUSES OF ACUTE KIDNEY INJURY IN SPECIFIC CLINICAL SETTINGS

AKI in the Cancer Patient
Prerenal azotemia.
- Hypovolemia (e.g., poor intake, vomiting, diarrhea).

Intrinsic AKI.
- Exogenous nephrotoxins: chemotherapy, antibiotics, contrast media.
- Endogenous toxins: hyperuricemia, hypercalcemia, tumor lysis, paraproteins.
- Other: radiation, HUS/TTP, glomerulonephritis, amyloid, malignant infiltration.

Postrenal AKI.
- Ureteric or bladder neck obstruction.

AKI after Cardiac Surgery
Prerenal azotemia.
- Hypovolemia (surgical losses, diuretics), cardiac failure, vasodilators.

Intrinsic AKI.
- Ischemic ATN (even in absence of hypotension).
- Atheroembolic disease after aortic manipulation/intraaortic balloon pump.
- Preoperative or perioperative administration of contrast medium.
- Allergic interstitial nephritis induced by perioperative antibiotics.

Postrenal AKI.
Obstructed urinary catheter, exacerbation of voiding dysfunction.

AKI in Pregnancy

Prerenal azotemia.
Acute fatty liver of pregnancy with fulminant hepatic failure.
Intrinsic AKI.
Preeclampsia or eclampsia.
Postpartum HUS/TTP.
HELLP syndrome.
Ischemia: postpartum hemorrhage, abruptio placentae, amniotic fluid embolus.
Direct toxicity of illegal abortifacients.
Postrenal AKI.
Obstruction with pyelonephritis.

AKI after Solid Organ or Bone Marrow Transplantation

Prerenal azotemia.
Intravascular volume depletion (e.g., diuretic therapy).
Vasoactive drugs (e.g., calcineurin inhibitors, amphotericin B).
Hepatorenal syndrome, venoocclusive disease of liver (BMT).
Intrinsic AKI.
Postoperative ischemic ATN (even in absence of hypotension).
Sepsis.
Exogenous nephrotoxins: aminoglycosides, amphotericin B, radiocontrast media.
HUS/TTP (e.g., cyclosporine or myeloablative radiotherapy related).
Allergic tubulointerstitial nephritis.
Postrenal AKI.
Obstructed urinary catheter.

AKI and Pulmonary Disease (Pulmonary Renal Syndrome)

Prerenal azotemia.
Diminished cardiac output complicating pulmonary embolism, severe pulmonary hypertension, or positive-pressure mechanical ventilation.
Intrinsic AKI.
Vasculitis.
Goodpasture's syndrome, ANCA-associated vasculitis, SLE, eosinophilic granulomatosis with polyangiitis, polyarteritis nodosa, cryoglobulinemia, right-sided endocarditis, lymphomatoid granulomatosis, sarcoidosis, scleroderma.
Toxins.
Ingestion of paraquat or diquat.
Infections.
Legionnaires' disease, *Mycoplasma* infection, tuberculosis, disseminated viral or fungal infection.
AKI from any cause with hypervolemia and pulmonary edema.
Lung cancer with hypercalcemia, tumor lysis, or glomerulonephritis.

AKI and Liver Disease

Prerenal azotemia.
Reduced true (GI hemorrhage, GI losses from lactulose, diuretics, large-volume paracentesis) circulatory volume or effective (hypoalbuminemia, splanchnic vasodilation).
Hepatorenal syndrome type 1 or 2.
Tense ascites with abdominal compartment syndrome.
Intrinsic AKI.
Ischemic (severe hypoperfusion—see earlier) or direct nephrotoxicity and hepatotoxicity of drugs or toxins (e.g., carbon tetrachloride, acetaminophen, tetracyclines, methoxyflurane).
Tubulointerstitial nephritis plus hepatitis caused by drugs (e.g., sulfonamides, rifampin, phenytoin, allopurinol, phenindione), infections (leptospirosis, brucellosis, Epstein-Barr virus infection, cytomegalovirus infection), malignant infiltration (leukemia, lymphoma), or sarcoidosis.
Glomerulonephritis or vasculitis (e.g., polyarteritis nodosa, ANCA-associated glomerulonephritis, cryoglobulinemia, SLE, postinfectious hepatitis or liver abscess.

AKI and Nephrotic Syndrome

Prerenal azotemia.
Intravascular volume depletion (diuretic therapy, hypoalbuminemia).
Intrinsic AKI.
Manifestation of primary glomerular disease.
Collapsing glomerulopathy (e.g., HIV, pamidronate).
Associated ATN (older hypertensive males).
Associated interstitial nephritis (NSAIDs, rifampin, interferon alfa).
Other—amyloid or light-chain deposition disease, renal vein thrombosis, severe interstitial edema.

AKI, Acute kidney injury; *ANCA,* antineutrophil cytoplasmic antibody; *ATN,* acute tubular necrosis; *BMT,* bone marrow transplantation; *GI,* gastrointestinal; *HELLP,* *h*emolysis, *e*levated *l*iver enzymes, *l*ow *p*latelets; *HIV,* human immunodeficiency virus; *HUS,* hemolytic uremic syndrome; *NSAID,* nonsteroidal antiinflammatory drug; *SLE,* systemic lupus erythematosus; *TTP,* thrombotic thrombocytopenic purpura.

ACUTE KIDNEY INJURY, PIGMENT INDUCED[57]

ICD-10CM #	Varies with specific diagnosis

CAUSES OF PIGMENT-INDUCED ACUTE KIDNEY INJURY

Rhabdomyolysis and myoglobinuria.
Vigorous exercise.
Arterial embolization.
Status epilepticus.
Status asthmaticus.
Coma-induced and pressure-induced myonecrosis.
Heat stress.
Diabetic ketoacidosis.
Myopathy.
Alcoholism.
Hypokalemia.
Hypophosphatemia.
Hemoglobinuria.
Transfusion reactions.
Snake envenomation.
Malaria.
Mechanical destruction of RBCs by prosthetic valves.
G6PD deficiency.

G6PD, glucose-6-phosphate dehydrogenase.

ACUTE LUNG INJURY, DISEASE AND DISORDERS ASSOCIATIONS[58]

ICD-10CM #	S27.3 Injury, lung

CLINICAL DISORDERS ASSOCIATED WITH ACUTE LUNG INJURY

Infectious Causes

Gram-negative or gram-positive sepsis.
Bacterial pneumonia.
Viral pneumonia.
Fungal pneumonia
Parasitic infections.
Mycobacterial disease.

Aspiration

Gastric acid.
Food and other particulate matter.
Fresh or sea water (near drowning).
Hydrocarbon fluids.

Trauma

Lung contusion.
Fat emboli.
Nonthoracic trauma.
Thermal injury (burns).
Blast injury (explosion, lightning).
Overdistention (mechanical ventilation).
Inhaled gases (phosgene, ammonia).

Hemodynamic Disturbances

Shock of any etiology.
Anaphylaxis.
High-altitude pulmonary edema.
Reperfusion.
Air embolism.
Amniotic fluid embolism.

Drugs

Heroin.
Methadone.
Propoxyphene.
Naloxone.
Cocaine.
Barbiturates.
Colchicine.
Salicylates.
Ethchlorvynol.
Interleukin-2.
Protamine.
Hydrochlorothiazide.

Hematologic Disorders

Disseminated intravascular coagulation.
Incompatible blood transfusion.
Rh incompatibility.
Antileukocyte antibodies.
Leukoagglutinin reactions.
Post–cardiopulmonary bypass, pump oxygenator.

Metabolic Disorders

Pancreatitis.
Diabetic ketoacidosis.

Neurologic Disorders
Head trauma.
Grand mal seizures.
Increased intracranial pressure (any cause).
Subarachnoid or intracerebral hemorrhage.
Miscellaneous Disorders
Lung reexpansion.
Upper airway obstruction.

ACUTE SCROTUM

ICD-10CM # R10.2 Pelvic and perineal pain

Testicular torsion.
Epididymitis.
Testicular neoplasm.
Orchitis.
Trauma.

ADNEXAL MASS[55]

ICD-10CM # R19.00 Intraabdominal and pelvic swelling, mass and lump, unspecified site

Ovary (neoplasm, endometriosis, functional cyst).
Fallopian tube (ectopic pregnancy, neoplasm, tuboovarian abscess, hydrosalpinx, paratubal cyst).
Uterus (fibroid, neoplasm).
Retroperitoneum (neoplasm, abdominal wall hematoma or abscess).
Urinary tract (pelvic kidney, distended bladder, urachal cyst).
Inflammatory bowel disease.
GI tract neoplasm.
Diverticular disease.
Appendicitis.
Bowel loop with feces.

ADRENAL CALCIFICATIONS[69]

ICD-10CM # E27.8 Other specified disorder of adrenal gland

CAUSES OF ADRENAL CALCIFICATION

Infection:
- Tuberculosis.
- Histoplasmosis.
- *Echinococcus.*

Prior hemorrhage.
Neoplasm:
- Adrenocortical carcinoma.
- Myelolipoma.
- Pheochromocytoma.

Hemangioma (rare).

ADRENAL CYSTIC LESIONS[69]

ICD-10CM # E27.8 Other specified disorder of adrenal gland

CYSTIC ADRENAL LESIONS

Pseudocyst.
Endothelial cyst.
Epithelial cyst.
Infection (*Echinococcus,* abscess).
Necrotic neoplasm.
Cystic pheochromocytoma.
Lymphangioma.

ADRENAL INSUFFICIENCY, CRITICALLY ILL PATIENT[68]

ICD-10CM # E27.40 Unspecified adrenocortical insufficiency

CAUSES OF ADRENAL INSUFFICIENCY IN CRITICALLY ILL PATIENTS

Reversible Dysfunction of the HPA Axis
Sepsis/septic shock.
Acute lung injury.
Burns.
Pancreatitis.
Liver failure.
Hypothermia.
Drugs:
- Etomidate (primary AI).
- Corticosteroids (secondary AI).
- Ketoconazole (primary AI).
- Megestrol acetate (secondary AI).
- Rifampin (increased cortisol metabolism).
- Phenytoin (increased cortisol metabolism).
- Metyrapone (primary AI).
- Mitotane (primary AI).

Primary Adrenal Insufficiency (Adrenal Failure)
Autoimmune adrenalitis.
HIV infection:
- HART therapy.
- HIV virus.
- CMV.

Metastatic carcinoma:
- Lung.
- Breast.
- Kidney.

Systemic fungal infection:
- Histoplasmosis.
- Cryptococcus.
- Blastomycosis.

Tuberculosis.
Adrenal hemorrhage/infarction:
- DIC.
- Meningococcemia.
- Anticoagulation.
- Antiphospholipid syndrome.
- HIT.
- Trauma.

AI, Adrenal insufficiency; *CMV,* cytomegalovirus; *DIC,* disseminated intravascular coagulation; *HIT,* heparin-induced thrombocytopenia; *HPA,* hypothalamic-pituitary axis.

ADRENAL MASSES[77]

ICD-10CM # C74.90 Malignant neoplasm of unspecified part of unspecified adrenal gland
E27.8 Other specified disorders of adrenal gland

UNILATERAL ADRENAL MASSES

Functional Lesions
Adrenal adenoma.
Adrenal carcinoma.
Pheochromocytoma.
Primary aldosteronism, adenomatous type.
Nonfunctional Lesions
Incidentaloma of adrenal.
Ganglioneuroma.
Myelolipoma.
Hematoma.
Adenolipoma.
Metastasis.

BILATERAL ADRENAL MASSES

Functional Lesions
ACTH-dependent Cushing's syndrome.
Congenital adrenal hyperplasia.
Pheochromocytoma.
Conn's syndrome, hyperplastic variety.
Micronodular adrenal disease.
Idiopathic bilateral adrenal hypertrophy.
Nonfunctional Lesions
Infection (tuberculosis, fungi).
Infiltration (leukemia, lymphoma).
Replacement (amyloidosis).
Hemorrhage.
Bilateral metastases.

ADRENAL PSEUDOMASSES[69]

ICD-10CM # E27.8 Other specified disorder of adrenal gland

Thickened diaphragmatic crus.
Accessory spleen.
Gastric fundus.
Gastric diverticulum.
Renal vein.
Retrocrural and retroperitoneal adenopathy.
Upper-pole renal cysts and tumors.
Pancreatic tumors.
Hypertrophied caudate lobe of liver.
Fluid-filled colon interposed between stomach and kidney.

ADRENERGIC TOXIDROME[68]

ICD-10CM # T44.8X1S Poisoning by centrally acting and adrenergic-neuron-blocking agents, accidental (unintentional), sequela

COMMON CAUSES OF THE ADRENERGIC TOXIDROME

Recreational drugs:
Cocaine.
Amphetamines and other "designer drugs"[a]—"ecstasy" (3,4-methylenedioxymethamphetamine [MDMA]); 3,4-methylenedioxyamphetamine (MDA); 3,4-methylenedioxyethylamphetamine (MDEA); paramethoxyamphetamine (PMA); methamphetamine.

[a]Up to 80% of ecstasy tablets sold in Australia are actually methamphetamine.

Differential Diagnosis II

β_1-Adrenergic agents:
- Salbutamol.
- Theophylline.

Inotropic agents:
- Norepinephrine.
- Epinephrine.
- Isoproterenol.

Over-the-counter cough and cold preparations and nasal decongestants:
- Phenylpropanolamine.
- Pseudoephedrine.

Amphetamine-like agents prescribed for ADD or weight loss:
- Methylphenidate.
- Dextroamphetamine.

Psychostimulants.

ADD, Attention deficit disorder.

ADRENOCORTICAL HYPERFUNCTION[3]

ICD-10CM # E26.9 Hyperaldosteronism, unspecified

SYNDROMES OF ADRENOCORTICAL HYPERFUNCTION

States of Glucocorticoid Excess

Physiologic states

Stress.
Strenuous exercise.
Last trimester of pregnancy.

Pathologic States

Psychiatric conditions (pseudo-Cushing's disorders):
- Depression.
- Alcoholism.
- Anorexia nervosa.
- Panic disorders.
- Alcohol and drug withdrawal.

ACTH-dependent states:
- Pituitary adenoma (Cushing's disease).
- Ectopic ACTH syndrome.
- Bronchial carcinoid.
- Thymic carcinoid.
- Islet cell tumor.
- Small cell lung carcinoma.
- Ectopic CRH secretion.

ACTH-independent states:
- Adrenal adenoma.
- Adrenal carcinoma.
- Micronodular adrenal disease.

Exogenous Sources

Glucocorticoid intake.
ACTH intake.

States of Mineralocorticoid Excess

Primary Aldosteronism

Aldosterone-secreting adenoma.
Bilateral adrenal hyperplasia.
Aldosterone-secreting carcinoma.
Glucocorticoid-suppressible hyperaldosteronism.

Adrenal Enzyme Deficiencies

11b-Hydroxylase deficiency.
17a-Hydroxylase deficiency.
11b-Hydroxysteroid dehydrogenase, type II.

Exogenous Mineralocorticoids

Licorice.
Carbenoxolone.
Fludrocortisone.

Secondary Hyperaldosteronism

Associated with hypertension:
- Accelerated hypertension.
- Renovascular hypertension.
- Estrogen administration.
- Renin-secreting tumors.

Without hypertension:
- Bartter syndrome.
- Sodium-wasting nephropathy.
- Renal tubular acidosis.
- Diuretic and laxative abuse.
- Edematous states (cirrhosis, nephrosis, congestive heart failure).

ACTH, Adrenocorticotropin hormone; *CRH,* corticotropin-releasing hormone.

ADRENOCORTICAL HYPOFUNCTION

ICD-10CM # E27.49 Other adrenocortical insufficiency

SYNDROMES OF ADRENOCORTICAL HYPOFUNCTION

Primary Adrenal Disorders

Combined Glucocorticoid and Mineralocorticoid Deficiency

Autoimmune:
- Isolated autoimmune disease (Addison disease).
- Polyglandular autoimmune syndrome, type I.
- Polyglandular autoimmune syndrome, type II.

Infectious:
- Tuberculosis.
- Fungal.
- Cytomegalovirus.
- Human immunodeficiency virus.

Vascular:
- Bilateral adrenal hemorrhage.
- Sepsis.
- Coagulopathy.
- Thrombosis; embolism.
- Adrenal infarction.

Infiltration:
- Metastatic carcinoma and lymphoma.
- Sarcoidosis.
- Amyloidosis.
- Hemochromatosis.

Congenital:
- Congenital adrenal hyperplasia.
  - 21-Hydroxylase deficiency.
  - 3b-ol Dehydrogenase deficiency.
  - 20,22-Desmolase deficiency.

Adrenal unresponsiveness to ACTH.
Congenital adrenal hypoplasia.
Adrenoleukodystrophy.
Adrenomyeloneuropathy.

Iatrogenic

Bilateral adrenalectomy.
Drugs:
- Metyrapone, aminoglutethimide, trilostane, ketoconazole, o,p¢-DDD, mifepristone.

Mineralocorticoid deficiency without glucocorticoid deficiency

Corticosterone methyl oxidase deficiency.
Isolated zona glomerulosa defect.
Heparin therapy.
Critical illness.
Converting-enzyme inhibitors.

Secondary Adrenal Disorders

Secondary Adrenal Insufficiency

Hypothalamic-pituitary dysfunction.
Exogenous glucocorticoids.
After removal of an ACTH-secreting tumor.

Hyporeninemic Hypoaldosteronism

Diabetic nephropathy.
Tubulointerstitial diseases.
Obstructive uropathy.
Autonomic neuropathy.
Nonsteroidal antiinflammatory drugs.
β-Adrenergic drugs.

ACTH, Adrenocorticotropic hormone.

ADVERSE FOOD REACTIONS, DIFFERENTIAL DIAGNOSIS[51]

ICD-10CM # T78.1XXA Other adverse food reactions, not elsewhere classified, initial encounter

GASTROINTESTINAL DISORDERS (WITH VOMITING AND/OR DIARRHEA)

Structural abnormalities (pyloric stenosis, Hirschsprung's disease).

Enzyme deficiencies (primary or secondary):
- Disaccharidase deficiency—lactase, fructase, sucrase-isomaltase.
- Galactosemia.

Other: pancreatic insufficiency (cystic fibrosis), peptic disease.

CONTAMINANTS AND ADDITIVES

Flavorings and preservatives—rarely cause symptoms: Sodium metabisulfite, monosodium glutamate, nitrites.

Dyes and colorings—very rarely cause symptoms (urticaria, eczema): Tartrazine.

Toxins: Bacterial, fungal (aflatoxin), fish-related (scombroid, ciguatera).

Infectious organisms:
- Bacteria *(Salmonella, Escherichia coli, Shigella).*
- Virus (rotavirus, enterovirus).
- Parasites (*Giardia, Akis simplex* [in fish]).

Accidental contaminants: Heavy metals, pesticides.

Pharmacologic agents: Caffeine, glycosidal alkaloid solanine (potato spuds), histamine (fish), serotonin (banana, tomato), tryptamine (tomato), tyramine (cheese).

PSYCHOLOGIC REACTIONS

Food phobias.

ADYNAMIC ILEUS[55]

ICD-10CM # K56.0 Paralytic ileus
K56.7 Ileus, unspecified

Abdominal trauma.
Infection (retroperitoneal, pelvic, intrathoracic).
Laparotomy.
Metabolic disease (hypokalemia).
Renal colic.
Skeletal injury (rib fracture, vertebral fracture).
Medications (e.g., narcotics).

AEROPHAGIA (BELCHING, ERUCTATION)

ICD-10CM #		
	R14.0	Abdominal distention (gaseous)
	R14.1	Gas pain
	R14.2	Eructation
	R14.3	Flatulence

Anxiety disorders.
Rapid food ingestion.
Carbonated beverages.
Nursing infants (especially when nursing in horizontal position).
Eating or drinking in supine position.
Gum chewing.
Poorly fitting dentures, orthodontic appliances.
Hiatal hernia, gastritis, nonulcer dyspepsia.
Cholelithiasis, cholecystitis.
Ingestion of legumes, onions, peppers.

AIR-SPACE OPACIFICATION ON X-RAY[36]

ICD-10CM #		
	R91.8	Other nonspecific abnormal finding of lung field

CAUSES OF AIR-SPACE OPACIFICATION

Edema
Cardiogenic.
Non-cardiogenic.
Inflammation/Infection
Granulomatosis with polyangiitis.
Cryptogenic organizing pneumonia.
Blood
Idiopathic pulmonary hemosiderosis.
Antibasement membrane antibody disease.
Systemic lupus erythematosus.
Miscellaneous Causes
Eosinophilic pneumonia.
Alveolar proteinosis.
Alveolar cell carcinoma.
Alveolar microlithiasis.
Lymphoma (MALToma).
Sarcoidosis.

AIRWAY OBSTRUCTION, PEDIATRIC AGE[41]

ICD-10CM #		
	J44.9	Chronic obstructive pulmonary disease, unspecified
	T17.900A	Unspecified foreign body in respiratory tract, part unspecified causing asphyxiation, initial encounter
	T17.908A	Unspecified foreign body in respiratory tract, part unspecified causing other injury, initial encounter
	T17.910A	Gastric contents in respiratory tract, part unspecified causing asphyxiation, initial encounter
	T17.918A	Gastric contents in respiratory tract, part unspecified causing other injury, initial encounter
	T17.920A	Food in respiratory tract, part unspecified causing asphyxiation, initial encounter
	T17.928A	Food in respiratory tract, part unspecified causing other injury, initial encounter
	T17.990A	Other foreign object in respiratory tract, part unspecified in causing asphyxiation, initial encounter
	T17.998A	Other foreign object in respiratory tract, part unspecified causing other injury, initial encounter
	J38.5	Laryngeal spasm
	J68.9	Unspecified respiratory condition due to chemicals, gases, fumes, and vapors

CONGENITAL CAUSES

Craniofacial dysmorphism.
Hemangioma.
Laryngeal cleft/web.
Laryngoceles, cysts.
Laryngomalacia.
Macroglossia.
Tracheal stenosis.
Vascular ring.
Vocal cord paralysis.

ACQUIRED INFECTIOUS CAUSES

Acute laryngotracheobronchitis.
Epiglottitis.
Laryngeal papillomatosis.
Membranous croup (bacterial tracheitis).
Mononucleosis.
Retropharyngeal abscess.
Spasmodic croup.
Diphtheria.

ACQUIRED NONINFECTIOUS CAUSES

Anaphylaxis.
Foreign body aspiration.
Supraglottic hypotonia.
Thermal/chemical burn.
Trauma.
Vocal cord paralysis.
Angioneurotic edema.

AKINETIC/RIGID SYNDROME[3]

ICD-10CM #		
	R29.8	Akinesis

Parkinsonism (idiopathic, drug-induced).
Catatonia (psychosis).
Progressive supranuclear palsy.
Multisystem atrophy (Shy-Drager syndrome, olivopontocerebellar atrophy).
Diffuse Lewy-body disease.
Toxins (MPTP, manganese, carbon monoxide).
Huntington's disease and other hereditary neurodegenerative disorders.

ALCOHOL-RELATED SEIZURES[57]

ICD-10CM #		
	F10.232	Alcohol dependence with withdrawal with perceptual disturbance

DIFFERENTIAL DIAGNOSIS OF ALCOHOL-RELATED SEIZURES

Withdrawal (alcohol or drugs).
Exacerbation of idiopathic or posttraumatic seizures.
Acute intoxication (amphetamines, anticholinergics, cocaine, isoniazid, organophosphates, phenothiazines, tricyclic antidepressants, salicylates, lithium).
Metabolic (hypoglycemia, hyponatremia, hypernatremia, hypocalcemia, hepatic failure).
Infectious (meningitis, encephalitis, brain abscess).
Trauma (intracranial hemorrhage).
Cerebrovascular accident.
Sleep deprivation.
Noncompliance with anticonvulsants.

ALKALOSIS, METABOLIC

ICD-10CM #		
	E87.3	Alkalosis

CAUSES OF METABOLIC ALKALOSIS

Exogenous HCO_3^- loads
Acute alkali administration.
Milk-alkali syndrome.
Effective Extracellular Volume Contraction, Normotension, Hypokalemia, and Secondary Hyperreninemic Hyperaldosteronism
GI origin:
- Vomiting.
- Gastric aspiration.
- Congenital chloridorrhea.
- Villous adenoma.
- Combined administration of sodium polystyrene sulfonate (Kayexalate and aluminum hydroxide).

Renal origin:
- Diuretics (especially thiazides and loop diuretics).
- Acute.
- Chronic.
- Edematous states.
- Posthypercapnic state.
- Hypercalcemia-hypoparathyroidism.

Recovery from lactic acidosis or ketoacidosis.
Nonreabsorbable anions such as penicillin, carbenicillin.
Mg++ deficiency.
K+ depletion.
Bartter syndrome (loss-of-function mutation of Cl– transport in thick ascending limb of Henle loop).
Gitelman syndrome (loss-of-function mutation in Na+/Cl– cotransporter).
Carbohydrate refeeding after starvation.

Extracellular Volume Expansion, Hypertension, K+ Deficiency, and Hypermineralocorticoidism

Associated with high renin:
- Renal artery stenosis.
- Accelerated hypertension.
- Renin-secreting tumor.
- Estrogen therapy.

Associated with low renin:
- Primary aldosteronism.
- Adenoma.
- Hyperplasia.
- Carcinoma.
- Glucocorticoid suppressible.

Adrenal enzymatic defects:
- 11β-Hydroxylase deficiency.
- 17α-Hydroxylase deficiency.

Cushing syndrome or disease:
- Ectopic corticotropin.
- Adrenal carcinoma.
- Adrenal adenoma.
- Primary pituitary.

Other:
- Licorice.
- Carbenoxolone.
- Chewer's tobacco.
- Lydia Pinkham tablets.

Gain-of-Function Mutation of ENaC with Extracellular Fluid Volume Expansion, Hypertension, K+ Deficiency, and Hyporeninemic Hypoaldosteronism

Liddle syndrome.

ALKALOSIS, RESPIRATORY

ICD-10CM #		
	E87.3	Alkalosis

Hypoxemia (pneumonia, pulmonary embolism, atelectasis, high-altitude living).
Drugs (salicylates, xanthenes, progesterone, epinephrine, thyroxine, nicotine).
Central nervous system (CNS) disorders (tumor, cerebrovascular accident [CVA], trauma, infections).
Psychogenic hyperventilation (anxiety, hysteria).
Hepatic encephalopathy.
Gram-negative sepsis.
Hyponatremia.
Sudden recovery from metabolic acidosis.
Assisted ventilation.

ALOPECIA[32,61]

ICD-10CM #		
	L65.9	Nonscarring hair loss, unspecified
	L63.2	Ophiasis
	L63.8	Other alopecia areata
	Q84.0	Congenital alopecia
	Q84.1	Congenital morphological disturbances of hair, not elsewhere classified
	Q84.2	Other congenital malformations of hair
	F54	Psychological and behavioral factors associated with disorders or diseases classified elsewhere

SCARRING ALOPECIA

Congenital (aplasia cutis).
Tinea capitis with inflammation (kerion).
Bacterial folliculitis.
Discoid lupus erythematosus.
Lichen planopilaris.
Folliculitis decalvans.
Neoplasm.
Trauma.

NONSCARRING ALOPECIA

Cosmetic treatment.
Tinea capitis.
Structural hair shaft disease.
Trichotillomania (hair pulling).
Anagen arrest.
Telogen arrest.
Alopecia areata.
Androgenetic alopecia.

ALOPECIA AND HYPOTRICHOSIS, IN CHILDREN AND ADOLESCENTS

ICD-10CM #		
	L65.9	Nonscarring hair loss, unspecified
	L63.2	Ophiasis
	L63.8	Other alopecia areata
	Q84.0	Congenital alopecia
	Q84.1	Congenital morphological disturbances of hair, not elsewhere classified
	Q84.2	Other congenital malformations Of hair

Congenital total alopecia: atrichia with papules, Moynahan alopecia syndrome.
Congenital localized alopecia: aplasia cutis, triangular alopecia, sebaceous nevus.
Hereditary hypotrichosis: Marie-Unna syndrome, hypotrichosis with juvenile macular dystrophy, hypotrichosis–Mari type, ichthyosis with hypotrichosis, cartilage-hair hypoplasia, Hallermann-Streiff syndrome, trichorhinophalangeal syndrome, ectodermal dysplasia ("pure" hair and nail and other ectodermal dysplasias).
Diffuse alopecia of endocrine origin: hypopituitarism, hypothyroidism, hypoparathyroidism, hyperthyroidism.
Alopecia of nutritional origin: marasmus, kwashiorkor, iron deficiency, zinc deficiency (acrodermatitis enteropathica), gluten-sensitive enteropathy, essential fatty acid deficiency, biotinidase deficiency.
Disturbances of the hair cycle: telogen effluvium.
Toxic alopecia: anagen effluvium.
Autoimmune alopecia: alopecia areata.
Traumatic alopecia: traction alopecia, trichotillomania.
Cicatricial alopecia: lupus erythematosus, lichen planopilaris, pseudopelade, morphea (en coup de saber), dermatomyositis, infection (kerion, favus, tuberculosis, syphilis, folliculitis, leishmaniasis, herpes zoster, varicella), acne keloidalis, follicular mucinosis, sarcoidosis.
Hair shaft abnormalities: monilethrix, pili annulati, pili torti, trichorrhexis invaginata, trichorrhexis nodosa, woolly hair syndrome, Menkes disease, trichothiodystrophy, tricho-dento-osseous syndrome, uncombable hair syndrome (spun-glass hair, pili trianguli et canaliculi).

ALOPECIA, DRUG-INDUCED

ICD-10CM #		
	L65.9	Nonscarring hair loss, unspecified
	L63.8	Alopecia areata

DRUGS REPORTED TO INDUCE HAIR LOSS

ACE inhibitors (captopril, enalapril, moexipril, ramipril).
Allopurinol.
Amiodarone.
Amphetamines.[1,2]
Analgesics, antiinflammatories (ibuprofen, indomethacin, naproxen).
Androgens.[3]
Anticoagulants (coumarin, dextran, heparin/heparinoids).
Antiepileptics (carbamazepine, hydantoins, lamotrigine, troxidone, valproic acid, vigabatrin).
Antipsychotics (flupenthixol decanoate, fluphenazine decanoate).
Antithyroid drugs (carbimazole, iodine, thiouracil).
Appetite suppressants.
Aromatase inhibitors (fadrozole, 4-OHA, vorozole).
Benzimidazoles (albendazole, mebendazole)
β-Blockers (levobunolol, metoprolol, nadolol, propranolol, timolol).
Bromocriptine.
Buspirone.
Butyrophenones.
Cantharidin.
Chloramphenicol.
Cholestyramine.
Cidofovir.
Cimetidine.
Clonazepam.
Clotrimazole.

[1] Established by multiple reports or proved by rechallenge.
[2] Involvement principally of cancellous bone.
[3] May produce androgenetic alopecia.

Colchicine.
Contraceptives (oral).[4]
Danazol.
Diazoxide.
Diclofenac.
Dixyrazine.
Ethambutol.
Ethionamide.
Fibrates (clofibrate, fenofibrate).
G-CSF (granulocyte-colony stimulating factor).
Gefitinib.[5]
Gentamicin.
Glatiramer acetate.
Glibenclamide.
Gold salts.
Haloperidol.
Immunoglobulins.
Indanediones.
Indinavir.
Interferons.
Isonicotinic acid hydrazide.[6]
Leflunomide.
Levodopa.
Lithium.
Maprotiline.
Mesalazine.
Methyldopa.
Methysergide.
Metyrapone.
Minoxidil.
Nicotinic acid.
Nitrofurantoin.
Octreotide.
Olanzapine.
Pentosan polysulfate.
Phenindione.
Potassium thiocyanate.
Pyridostigmine.
Radiation (<700 Gy).
Retinoids (acitretin, etretinate, isotretinoin).
Retinol (vitamin A).
Risperidone.
Salicylates.
Serotonin reuptake inhibitors (fluoxetine, fluvoxamine, paroxetine, sertraline).
Sorafenib.
Spironolactone.
Strontium ranelate.
Sulfasalazine.
Tamoxifen.
Terbinafine.
Terfenadine.
Thiamphenicol.
Thyroxine.
Tocopherol (vitamin E).
Trazodone.
Triazoles (fluconazole, itraconazole).
Tricyclic antidepressants (amitriptyline, desipramine, doxepin, imipramine, maprotiline).
Trimethadione.
Triparanol.
Vasopressin.

†Hair loss usually severe.
[4]May produce telogen effluvium 3 months after discontinuation.
[5]Involvement of cancellous and cortical bone.
[6]May produce anagen effluvium.

ALVEOLAR CONSOLIDATION

ICD-10CM #		
	J18.2	Hypostatic pneumonia, unspecified organism
	J81.1	Hypostatic pneumonia, unspecified organism

Infection.
Neoplasm (bronchoalveolar carcinoma, lymphoma).
Aspiration.
Trauma.
Hemorrhage (granulomatosis with polyangiitis, Goodpasture's, bleeding diathesis).
ARDS.
CHF.
Renal failure.
Eosinophilic pneumonia.
Bronchiolitis obliterans.
Pulmonary alveolar proteinosis.

ALVEOLAR HEMORRHAGE[61]

ICD-10CM #		
	P26.1	Massive pulmonary hemorrhage originating in the perinatal period
	K08.8	Alveolar hemorrhage
	P26.8	Other pulmonary hemorrhages originating in the perinatal period

Hematologic disorders (coagulopathies, thrombocytopenia).
Goodpasture's syndrome (anti-basement membrane antibody disease).
Granulomatosis with polyangiitis.
Immune complex-mediated vasculitis.
Idiopathic pulmonary hemosiderosis.
Drugs (penicillamine).
Lymphangiogram contrast.
Mitral stenosis.

AMENORRHEA

ICD-10CM #		
	N91.2	Amenorrhea, unspecified

PREGNANCY

Early Menopause

Hypothalamic Dysfunction

Defective synthesis or release of LHRH, anorexia nervosa, stress, exercise.

Pituitary Dysfunction

Neoplasm, postpartum hemorrhage, surgery, radiotherapy.

Ovarian Dysfunction

Gonadal dysgenesis, 17a-hydroxylase deficiency, premature ovarian failure, polycystic ovarian disease, gonadal stromal tumors.

UTEROVAGINAL ABNORMALITIES

Congenital: imperforate hymen, imperforate cervix, imperforate or absent vagina, Müllerian agenesis.
Acquired: destruction of endometrium with curettage (Asherman's syndrome), closure of cervix or vagina caused by traumatic injury, hysterectomy.

OTHER

Metabolic diseases (liver, kidney), malnutrition, rapid weight loss, exogenous obesity, endocrine abnormalities (Cushing's syndrome, Graves disease, hypothyroidism).

AMNESIA

ICD-10CM #		
	F19.96	Other psychoactive substance use, unspecified with psychoactive substance-induced persisting amnestic disorder
	F44.0	Dissociative amnesia
	R41.2	Retrograde amnesia
	G45.4	Transient global amnesia

Degenerative diseases (e.g., Alzheimer's, Huntington's disease).
CVA (especially when involving thalamus, basal forebrain, and hippocampus).
Head trauma.
Postsurgical (e.g., mammillary body surgery, bilateral temporal lobectomy).
Infections (herpes simplex encephalitis, meningitis).
Wernicke-Korsakoff syndrome.
Cerebral hypoxia.
Hypoglycemia.
CNS neoplasms.
Creutzfeldt-Jakob disease.
Medications (e.g., midazolam and other benzodiazepines).
Psychosis.
Malingering.

AMNIOTIC FLUID α-FETOPROTEIN ELEVATION[36]

ICD-10CM #		
	Z36	Encounter for antenatal screening of mother

CAUSES OF ELEVATED AMNIOTIC FLUID α-FETOPROTEIN

Craniospinal defect (open neural tube defect).
Omphalocele.
Gastroschisis.
Duodenal atresia.
Congenital nephrosis.
Cystic hygroma.
Unbalanced D/G dislocation.
Down, Tay-Sachs, Klinefelter, Turner syndromes.
Fetal tumors.
Epidermolysis bullosa.
Pilonidal sinus.
Rhesus disease.
Fetal demise.
Incorrect dates.
Multiple pregnancies.

ANAL ABSCESS AND FISTULA[81]

ICD-10CM #		
	K61.0	Anal abscess
	K61.1	Rectal abscess
	K61.3	Ischiorectal abscess
	K60.3	Anal fistula

Primary anal gland infection.
Secondary abscess:
- Inflammatory bowel disease:
  - Crohn disease.
  - Ulcerative colitis.
- Infection:
  - Tuberculosis.
  - Actinomycosis.
  - Threadworm.
- Trauma.
- Leukopenia.
- Immunosuppression:
  - HIV.
  - Drugs.
- Rectal cancer.
- Diabetes mellitus.

ANAL INCONTINENCE[55]

ICD-10CM #	R15.9	Full incontinence of feces

TRAUMATIC

Nerve injured in surgery.
Spinal cord injury.
Obstetric trauma.
Sphincter injury.

NEUROLOGIC

Spinal cord lesions.
Dementia.
Autonomic neuropathy (e.g., DM).
Obstetrics: pudendal nerve stretched during surgery.
Hirschsprung disease.

MASS EFFECT

Carcinoma of anal canal.
Carcinoma of rectum.
Foreign body.
Fecal impaction.
Hemorrhoids.

MEDICAL

Procidentia.
Inflammatory disease.
Diarrhea.
Laxative abuse.

PEDIATRIC

Congenital.
Meningocele.
Myelomeningocele.
Spina bifida.
After corrective surgery for imperforate anus.
Sexual abuse.
Encopresis.

ANAPHYLAXIS[47]

ICD-10CM #	T78.2	Anaphylactic shock, unspecified, initial encounter

PULMONARY

Laryngeal edema.
Epiglottitis.
Foreign body aspiration.
Pulmonary embolus.
Asphyxiation.
Hyperventilation.

CARDIOVASCULAR

Myocardial infarction.
Arrhythmia.
Hypovolemic shock.
Cardiac arrest.

CNS

Vasovagal reaction.
CVA.
Seizure disorder.
Drug overdose.

ENDOCRINE

Hypoglycemia.
Pheochromocytoma.
Carcinoid syndrome.
Catamenial (progesterone-induced anaphylaxis).

PSYCHIATRIC

Vocal cord dysfunction syndrome.
Munchausen syndrome.
Panic attack/globus hystericus.

OTHER

Hereditary angioedema.
Cord urticaria.
Idiopathic urticaria.
Mastocytosis.
Serum sickness.
Idiopathic capillary leak syndrome.
Sulfite exposure.
Scombroid poisoning (tuna, blue fish, mackerel).

ANAPHYLAXIS MIMICS[65]

ICD-10CM #	Varies with specific diagnosis

CONDITIONS THAT MIMIC ANAPHYLAXIS

Vasovagal episodes.
Acute pulmonary events:
- Acute asthmatic attacks.
- Acute pulmonary edema.
- Pulmonary embolus.
- Spontaneous pneumothorax.
- Foreign body aspiration.

Acute cardiac events:
- Supraventricular tachycardias.
- Acute myocardial infarction/ischemia.

Drug overdoses.
Insulin shock.
Carcinoid attacks.

ANAPHYLAXIS, PATHOPHYSIOLOGIC CLASSIFICATION[2]

ICD-10CM #	T78.2	Anaphylactic shock, unspecified, initial encounter

PATHOPHYSIOLOGIC CLASSIFICATION OF ANAPHYLAXIS

IgE Dependent, Immunologic

Foods.
Drugs.
Insect stings and bites.
Exercise (food dependent).
Other causes.

IgE Independent, Immunologic

Immune aggregates.
IgG anti-IgA.
Cytotoxic.
Disturbance of arachidonic acid metabolism:
- Aspirin.
- Other nonsteroidal antiinflammatory drugs.

Activation of kallikrein-kinin contact system:
- Dialysis membranes.
- Radiocontrast media.

Multimediator recruitment:
- Complement.
- Clotting.
- Clot lysis.
- Kallikrein-kinin contact system.

Other causes

Nonimmunologic

Direct mediator release from mast cells and basophils:
- Drugs, e.g., opiates.
- Physical factors, e.g., cold and sunlight.

Exercise
c-kit Mutation (D816V)
Other causes

Idiopathic

ANAPHYLACTOID SYNDROME OF PREGNANCY[1]

ICD-10CM #	O88.113	Amniotic fluid embolism in pregnancy, third semester

CARDIOVASCULAR COLLAPSE, HYPOTENSION

Acute coronary syndromes, myocardial infarction.
Cardiomyopathy.
Pulmonary embolism.
Anesthesia complications, transfusion reaction.
Sepsis, systemic inflammatory response syndrome.

RESPIRATORY ARREST

Pulmonary embolism, air embolism.
Anesthesia complications, transfusion reaction.
Aspiration.

ALTERED MENTAL STATUS, SEIZURE

Eclampsia.
Cerebrovascular accident.
Hypoglycemia.

COAGULOPATHY

Disseminated intravascular coagulation.
Consumptive coagulopathy from hemorrhage.

ANDROGEN EXCESS, REPRODUCTIVE-AGE WOMAN

ICD-10CM # E28.1 Androgen excess

Polycystic ovary syndrome.
Idiopathic.
Medications (e.g., anabolizing agents, testosterone, danazol).
Pregnancy (luteoma, hyperreaction luteinalis).
Sertoli-Leydig ovarian neoplasm.
Adrenal adenoma or hyperplasia.
Cushing's syndrome.
Glucocorticoid resistance.
Hypothyroidism.
Hyperprolactinemia.

ANDROGEN RESISTANCE[59]

ICD-10CM # E34.5 Androgen resistance syndrome

CONGENITAL OR DEVELOPMENTAL DISORDERS

Uncommon causes:
- Kennedy disease (spinal and bulbar muscular atrophy).
- Partial androgen insensitivity syndrome (AR mutations).
- 5α-reductase type 2 deficiency.
- Complete androgen insensitivity syndrome (female phenotype).

ACQUIRED DISORDERS

Common causes:
- AR antagonists (bicalutamide, nilutamide).
- Drugs (spironolactone, cyproterone acetate, marijuana, histamine 2 receptor antagonists).

Uncommon causes:
- Celiac disease.

ANEMIA, APLASTIC[43]

ICD-10CM # D61.09 Other constitutional aplastic anemia

ACQUIRED APLASTIC ANEMIA

Secondary aplastic anemia.
Irradiation.
Drugs and chemicals.
Regular effects.
Cytotoxic agents.
Benzene.
Idiosyncratic reactions.
Chloramphenicol.
Nonsteroidal antiinflammatory drugs.
Antiepileptics.
Gold.
Other drugs and chemicals.
Viruses.
Epstein-Barr virus (infectious mononucleosis).
Hepatitis virus (non-A, non-B, non-C, non-G hepatitis).
Parvovirus (transient aplastic crisis, some pure red cell aplasia).
Human immunodeficiency virus (acquired immunodeficiency syndrome).
Immune diseases.
Eosinophilic fasciitis.
Hyperimmunoglobulinemia.
Thymoma and thymic carcinoma.
Graft-versus-host disease in immunodeficiency.
Paroxysmal nocturnal hemoglobinuria.
Pregnancy.
Idiopathic aplastic anemia.

INHERITED APLASTIC ANEMIA

Fanconi anemia.
Dyskeratosis congenita.
Shwachman-Diamond syndrome.
Reticular dysgenesis.
Amegakaryocytic thrombocytopenia.
Familial aplastic anemias.
Preleukemia (e.g., monosomy 7).
Nonhematologic syndromes (e.g., Down, Dubowitz, Seckel).

ANEMIA, APLASTIC, DUE TO DRUGS AND CHEMICALS[1]

ICD-10CM #		
	D61.1	Drug-induced aplastic anemia
	D61.2	Aplastic anemia due to other external agents
	D61.89	Other specified aplastic anemias and other bone marrow failure syndromes

Agents that regularly produce marrow depression as a major toxic effect when used in commonly employed doses or normal exposures:
- Cytotoxic drugs used in cancer chemotherapy.
- Alkylating agents (busulfan, melphalan, cyclophosphamide).
- Antimetabolites (antifolic compounds, nucleotide analogs), antimitotics (vincristine, vinblastine, colchicine).
- Some antibiotics (daunorubicin, doxorubicin [Adriamycin]).
- Benzene (and less often benzene-containing chemicals; kerosene, carbon tetrachloride, Stoddard's solvent, chlorophenols).

Agents probably associated with aplastic anemia but with a relatively low probability relative to their use:
- Chloramphenicol.
- Insecticides.
- Antiprotozoals (quinacrine and chloroquine).
- Nonsteroidal antiinflammatory drugs (including phenylbutazone, indomethacin, ibuprofen, sulindac, diclofenac, naproxen, piroxicam, fenoprofen, fenbufen, aspirin).
- Anticonvulsants (hydantoins, carbamazepine, phenacemide, ethosuximide).
- Gold, arsenic, and other heavy metals such as bismuth and mercury.
- Sulfonamides as a class.
- Antithyroid medications (methimazole, methylthiouracil, propylthiouracil).
- Antidiabetes drugs (tolbutamide, carbutamide, chlorpropamide).
- Carbonic anhydrase inhibitors (acetazolamide, methazolamide, mesalazine).
- D-Penicillamine.
- 2-Chlorodeoxyadenosine.

Agents more rarely associated with aplastic anemia:
- Antibiotics (streptomycin, tetracycline, methicillin, ampicillin, mebendazole and albendazole, sulfonamides, flucytosine, mefloquine, dapsone).
- Antihistamines (cimetidine, ranitidine, chlorpheniramine).
- Sedatives and tranquilizers (chlorpromazine, prochlorperazine, piperacetazine, chlordiazepoxide, meprobamate, methyprylon, remoxipride).
- Antiarrhythmics (tocainide, amiodarone).
- Allopurinol (can potentiate marrow suppression by cytotoxic drugs).
- Ticlopidine.
- Methyldopa.
- Quinidine.
- Lithium.
- Guanidine.
- Canthaxanthin.
- Thiocyanate.
- Carbimazole.
- Cyanamide.
- Deferoxamine.
- Amphetamines.

ANEMIA, CAUSES IN PREGNANCY[30]

ICD-10CM #		
	D50.8	Other iron deficiency anemias
	D50.9	Iron deficiency anemia, unspecified
	D51.0	Vitamin B_{12} deficiency anemia due to intrinsic factor deficiency
	D51.1	Vitamin B_{12} deficiency anemia due to selective vitamin B_{12} malabsorption with proteinuria
	D51.3	Other dietary vitamin B_{12} deficiency anemia
	D51.8	Other vitamin B_{12} deficiency anemias
	D52.0	Dietary folate deficiency anemia
	D52.1	Drug-induced folate deficiency anemia
	D52.8	Other folate deficiency anemias
	D52.9	Folate deficiency anemia, unspecified
	D53.1	Other megaloblastic anemias, not elsewhere classified
	D53.0	Protein deficiency anemia
	D53.2	Scorbutic anemia
	D53.8	Other specified nutritional anemias
	D53.9	Nutritional anemia, unspecified
	D64.0	Hereditary sideroblastic anemia

D64.1	Secondary sideroblastic anemia due to disease
D64.2	Secondary sideroblastic anemia due to drugs and toxins
D64.3	Other sideroblastic anemias

CAUSES OF ANEMIA DURING PREGNANCY

Common Causes—85% of Anemia:
- Physiologic anemia.
- Iron deficiency.

Uncommon Causes:
- Folic acid deficiency.
- Vitamin B_{12} deficiency (due to the rapid increase in bariatric surgery).
- Hemoglobinopathies:
  - Sickle cell disease.
  - Hemoglobin SC.
  - β-Thalassemia minor.
- Bariatric surgery.
- GI bleeding.

Rare Causes:
- Hemoglobinopathies.
  - β-Thalassemia major.
  - α-Thalassemia.
- Syndromes of chronic hemolysis:
  - Hereditary spherocytosis.
  - Paroxysmal nocturnal hemoglobinuria.

Hematologic malignancy.

ANEMIA, DRUG-INDUCED[38]

ICD-10CM #		
	D61.1	Drug-induced aplastic anemia

DRUGS THAT MAY INTERFERE WITH RED CELL PRODUCTION BY INDUCING MARROW SUPPRESSION OR APLASIA

Alcohol.
Antineoplastic drugs.
Antithyroid drugs.
Antibiotics.
Oral hypoglycemic agents.
Phenylbutazone.
Azidothymidine (AZT).

DRUGS THAT INTERFERE WITH VITAMIN B_{12}, FOLATE, OR IRON ABSORPTION OR UTILIZATION

Nitrous oxide.
Anticonvulsant drugs.
Antineoplastic drugs.
Isoniazid.
Cycloserine A.

DRUGS CAPABLE OF PROMOTING HEMOLYSIS

Immune Mediated

Penicillins.
Quinine.
α-methyldopa.
Procainamide.
Mitomycin C.

Oxidative Stress

Antimalarials.
Sulfonamide drugs.
Nalidixic acid.

DRUGS THAT MAY PRODUCE OR PROMOTE BLOOD LOSS

Aspirin.
Alcohol.
Nonsteroidal antiinflammatory agents.
Corticosteroids.
Anticoagulants.

ANEMIA, HYPOCHROMIC[43]

ICD-10CM #		
	D50.8	Other iron deficiency anemias
	D50.9	Iron deficiency anemia, unspecified
	D64.0	Hereditary sideroblastic anemia
	D64.1	Secondary sideroblastic anemia due to disease
	D64.2	Secondary sideroblastic anemia due to drugs and toxins
	D64.3	Other sideroblastic anemias

DECREASED BODY IRON STORES

Iron-deficiency anemia.

NORMAL OR INCREASED BODY IRON STORES

Impaired iron metabolism.
Anemia of chronic disease.
Defective absorption, transport, or use of iron.
Disorders of globin synthesis:
- Thalassemia.
- Other microcytic hemoglobinopathies.

Disorders of heme synthesis: sideroblastic anemias:
- Hereditary.
- Acquired.

ANEMIA, LOW RETICULOCYTE COUNT[3]

ICD-10CM #		
	D64.9	Anemia, unspecified

MICROCYTIC ANEMIA (MCV <80)

Iron deficiency.
Thalassemia minor.
Sideroblastic anemia.
Lead poisoning.

MACROCYTIC ANEMIA (MCV >100)

Megaloblastic anemias.
Folate deficiency.
Vitamin B_{12} deficiency.
Drug-induced megaloblastic anemia.
Nonmegaloblastic macrocytosis.
Liver disease.
Hypothyroidism.

NORMOCYTIC ANEMIA (MCV 80-100)

Early iron deficiency.
Aplastic anemia.
Myelophthisic disorders.
Endocrinopathies.
Anemia of chronic disease.
Uremia.
Mixed nutritional deficiency.

ANEMIA, MEGALOBLASTIC[77]

ICD-10CM #		
	D51.0	Vitamin B_{12} deficiency anemia due to intrinsic factor deficiency
	D51.1	Vitamin B_{12} deficiency anemia due to selective vitamin B_{12} malabsorption with proteinuria
	D51.3	Other dietary vitamin B_{12} deficiency anemia
	D51.8	Other vitamin B_{12} deficiency anemias
	D52.0	Dietary folate deficiency anemia
	D52.1	Drug-induced folate deficiency anemia
	D52.8	Other folate deficiency anemias
	D52.9	Folate deficiency anemia, unspecified
	D53.1	Other megaloblastic anemias, not elsewhere classified
	D53.0	Protein deficiency anemia
	D53.2	Scorbutic anemia
	D53.8	Other specified nutritional anemias
	D53.9	Nutritional anemia, unspecified

COBALAMIN (CBL) DEFICIENCY

Nutritional CBL Deficiency (Insufficient CBL Intake)

Vegetarians, vegans, breastfed infants of mothers with pernicious anemia.

Abnormal Intragastric Events (Inadequate Proteolysis of Food CBL)

Atrophic gastritis, partial gastrectomy with hypochlorhydria.

Loss/Atrophy of Gastric Oxyntic Mucosa (Deficient Intrinsic Factor [If] Molecules)

Total or partial gastrectomy, pernicious anemia (PA), caustic destruction (lye).

Abnormal Events in Small Bowel Lumen

Inadequate pancreatic protease (R-CBL not degraded, CBL not transferred to IF).
- Insufficiency of pancreatic protease—pancreatic insufficiency.
- Inactivation of pancreatic protease—Zollinger-Ellison syndrome.

Usurping of luminal CBL (inadequate CBL binding to IF).
- By bacteria—stasis syndromes (blind loops, pouches of diverticulosis, strictures, fistulas, anastomoses); impaired bowel motility

(scleroderma, pseudoobstruction), hypogammaglobulinemia.
By *Diphyllobothrium latum.*

Disorders of Ileal Mucosa/IF Receptors (IF-CBL not Bound to IF Receptors)

Diminished or absent IF receptors—ileal bypass/resection/fistula.
Abnormal mucosal architecture/function—tropical/nontropical sprue, Crohn's disease, TB ileitis, infiltration by lymphomas, amyloidosis.
IF-/post IF-receptor defects—Imerslund-Gräsbeck syndrome, TC II deficiency.
Drug-induced effects (slow K, biguanides, cholestyramine, colchicine, neomycin, PAS).

DISORDERS OF PLASMA CBL TRANSPORT (TC II-CBL NOT DELIVERED TO TC II RECEPTORS)

Congenital TC II deficiency, defective binding of TC II-CBL to TC II receptors (rare).

METABOLIC DISORDERS (CBL NOT UTILIZED BY CELL)

Inborn enzyme errors (rare).
Acquired disorders: (CBL oxidized to cob[III] alamin)—N_2O inhalation.

FOLATE DEFICIENCY

Nutritional Causes

Decreased dietary intake—poverty and famine (associated with kwashiorkor, marasmus), institutionalized individuals (psychiatric/nursing homes), chronic debilitating disease/goats' milk (low in folate), special diets (slimming), cultural/ethnic cooking techniques (food folate destroyed) or habits (folate-rich foods not consumed).
Decreased diet and increased requirements:
Physiologic: pregnancy and lactation, prematurity, infancy.
Pathologic: intrinsic hematologic disease (autoimmune hemolytic disease), drugs, malaria; hemoglobinopathies (SS, thalassemia), RBC membrane defects (hereditary spherocytosis, paroxysmal nocturnal hemoglobinopathy); abnormal hematopoiesis (leukemia/lymphoma, myelodysplastic syndrome, agnogenic myeloid metaplasia with myelofibrosis); infiltration with malignant disease; dermatologic (psoriasis).

Folate Malabsorption

With normal intestinal mucosa:
Some drugs (controversial).
Congenital folate malabsorption (rare).
With mucosal abnormalities—tropical and nontropical sprue, regional enteritis.

Defective Cellular Folate Uptake—Familial Aplastic Anemia (Rare), Inadequate Cellular Utilization

Folate antagonists (methotrexate).
Hereditary enzyme deficiencies involving folate.

Drugs (Multiple Effects on Folate Metabolism)

Alcohol, sulfasalazine, triamterene, pyrimethamine, trimethoprim-sulfamethoxazole, diphenylhydantoin, barbiturates.

MISCELLANEOUS MEGALOBLASTIC ANEMIAS (NOT CAUSED BY CBL OR FOLATE DEFICIENCY)

Congenital Disorders of DNA Synthesis (Rare)

Orotic aciduria, Lesch-Nyhan syndrome, congenital dyserythropoietic anemia.

Acquired Disorders of DNA Synthesis

Thiamine-responsive megaloblastosis (rare).
Malignancy—erythroleukemia—refractory sideroblastic anemias—all antineoplastic drugs that inhibit DNA synthesis.
Toxins—alcohol.

ANEMIA, MICROCYTIC, HYPOCHROMIC, DIFFERENTIAL DIAGNOSIS[42]

ICD-10CM #		
	D50.8	Other iron deficiency anemias
	D50.9	Iron deficiency anemia, unspecified
	D64.0	Hereditary sideroblastic anemia
	D64.1	Secondary sideroblastic anemia due to disease
	D64.2	Secondary sideroblastic anemia due to drugs and toxins
	D64.3	Other sideroblastic anemias

DIFFERENTIAL DIAGNOSIS OF MICROCYTIC HYPOCHROMIC ANEMIA

Decreased Body Iron Stores

Iron-deficiency anemia.

Normal or Increased Body Iron Stores

Anemia of chronic disease.
Defective absorption, transport, or use of iron.
Iron-refractory, iron-deficiency anemia after parenteral iron.
Atransferrinemia.
Aceruloplasminemia.
Divalent metal transporter 1 (DMT1 or SLC11A2) deficiency.
Ferroportin-associated hemochromatosis with impaired iron export (type 4A).
Heme oxygenase 1 deficiency.
Disorders of globin synthesis.

Decreased Body Iron Stores

Thalassemia.
Other microcytic hemoglobinopathies.
Disorders of heme synthesis:
Sideroblastic anemias.
Hereditary.
Acquired.

ANERGY, CUTANEOUS[77]

ICD-10CM #		
	D89.9	Disorder involving the immune mechanism, unspecified

IMMUNOLOGIC

Acquired (AIDS, acute leukemia, carcinoma, CLL, Hodgkin's lymphoma, NHL).
Congenital (ataxia-telangiectasia, Di George's syndrome, severe combined immunodeficiency, Wiskott-Aldrich syndrome).

INFECTIONS

Bacterial (bacterial pneumonia, brucellosis).
Disseminated mycotic infections.
Mycobacterial (lepromatous leprosy, TB).
Viral (varicella, hepatitis, influenza, mononucleosis, measles, mumps).

IMMUNOSUPPRESSIVE MEDICATIONS

Systemic corticosteroids.
Methotrexate, cyclophosphamide.
Rifampin.

OTHER

Alcoholic cirrhosis, biliary cirrhosis, sarcoidosis, rheumatic disease.
Diabetes, Crohn's disease, uremia.
Anemia, pyridoxine deficiency, sickle cell anemia.
Burns, malnutrition, pregnancy, old age, surgery.

ANEURYSMS, THORACIC AORTA

ICD-10CM #		
	I71.2	Thoracic aortic aneurysm, without rupture

Trauma.
Infection.
Inflammatory (syphilis, Takayasu's disease).
Collagen vascular disease (RA, ankylosing spondylitis).
Annuloaortic ectasia (Marfan's syndrome, Ehlers-Danlos syndrome).
Congenital.
Coarctation.
Cystic medial necrosis.

ANHIDROSIS

ICD-10CM #		
	L74.0	Miliaria rubra
	L74.1	Miliaria crystallina
	L74.2	Miliaria profunda

Drugs (anticholinergics).
Dehydration.
Hysteria.
Obstruction of sweat ducts (e.g., inflammation, miliaria).
Local radiant heat or pressure.
CNS lesions (medulla, hypothalamus, pons).
Spinal cord lesions.
Lesions of sympathetic nerves.
Congenital sweat gland disturbances.

ANION GAP ACIDOSIS[83]

ICD-10CM #		
	E87.2	Acidosis

CLINICAL CAUSES OF HIGH ANION GAP AND NORMAL ANION GAP ACIDOSIS

High Anion Gap

Ketoacidosis:
- Diabetic ketoacidosis (acetoacetate).
- Alcoholic (β-hydroxybutyrate).
- Starvation.

Lactic acid acidosis:
- L-Lactic acid acidosis (types A and B).
- D-Lactic acid acidosis.
- Renal failure: sulfate, phosphate, urate, hippurate.

Ingestions (toxins and their metabolites):
- Ethylene glycol → glycolate, oxalate.
- Methyl alcohol → formate.
- Salicylate → ketones, lactate, salicylate.
- Paraldehyde → organic anions.
- Toluene → hippurate (commonly presents with normal anion gap).
- Propylene glycol → lactate.
- Pyroglutamic acidosis (acetaminophen use) → 5-oxoproline.

Normal Anion Gap

GI loss of HCO_3^- (negative urine anion gap):
- Diarrhea.
- Fistula, external.

Renal loss of HCO_3^- or failure to excrete NH_4^+ (positive urine anion gap):
- Proximal renal tubular acidosis (RTA type 2).
- Acetazolamide.
- Classic distal renal tubular acidosis (low serum K^+) RTA type 1.
- Generalized distal renal tubular defect (high serum K^+) RTA type 4.

Miscellaneous:
- NH_4Cl ingestion.
- Sulfur ingestion.
- Dilutional acidosis.
- Late stages in treatment of diabetic ketoacidosis.

ANION GAP INCREASE

ICD-10CM # E87.8 Other disorders of electrolyte and fluid balance, not elsewhere classified

Uremia.
Ketoacidosis (diabetic, starvation, alcoholic).
Lactic acidosis.
Ethylene glycol poisoning.
Salicylate overdose.
Methanol poisoning.

ANISOCORIA

ICD-10CM # H57.02 Anisocoria

Mydriatic or miotic drugs.
Prosthetic eye.
Inflammation (keratitis, iridocyclitis).
Infections (herpes zoster, syphilis, meningitis, encephalitis, TB, diphtheria, botulism).
Subdural hemorrhage.
Cavernous sinus thrombosis.
Intracranial neoplasm.
Cerebral aneurysm.
Glaucoma.
CNS degenerative diseases.
Internal carotid ischemia.
Toxic polyneuritis (alcohol, lead).
Adie syndrome.
Horner syndrome.
DM.
Trauma.
Congenital.

ANORECTAL DISEASE, AIDS PATIENT[26]

ICD-10CM # Varies with specific diagnosis

DIFFERENTIAL DIAGNOSIS OF ANORECTAL DISEASE IN PATIENTS WITH AIDS

Infections

Bacteria

*Chlamydia trachomatis.**
Lymphogranuloma venereum.
*Neisseria gonorrhoeae.**
Shigella flexneri.
Mycobacterium tuberculosis.

Protozoa

Entamoeba histolytica.
- *Leishmania donovani.*

Viruses

HSV.*
Cytomegalovirus.*

Fungi

Candida albicans.
- *Histoplasma capsulatum.*

Neoplasms

Lymphoma.*
- Kaposi's sarcoma.
- Squamous cell carcinoma.
- Cloacogenic carcinoma.
- Condyloma acuminatum.

Other

Idiopathic ulcers.*
- Perirectal abscess, fistula.*

---

*More frequent diagnosis.

ANOREXIA[81]

ICD-10CM # R63.0 Anorexia

SELECTED CAUSES OF ANOREXIA

Gastrointestinal Tract/Liver

Gastric outlet obstruction or small bowel obstruction.
Gastric cancer.
Hepatic metastases.
Acute viral hepatitis.

Metabolic

Addison's disease.
Hypopituitarism.
Hyperparathyroidism.

Functional

Extremely unpleasant sight/smell.

Systemic

Chronic pain.
Renal failure.
Severe congestive heart failure.
Respiratory failure.

Psychiatric

Depression.
Anorexia nervosa.

Medications

Digoxin.
Narcotic analgesics.
Diuretics.
Antihypertensives.
Chemotherapeutic agents.
Amphetamines.

Miscellaneous

Excessive smoking.
Excessive alcohol intake.
Oral cavity disease.
Thiamine deficiency.
Early pregnancy.
Hypogeusia or dysgeusia.

ANOVULATION

ICD-10CM # N97.0 Female infertility associated with anovulation

Anorexia and bulimia.
Strenuous exercise.
Weight loss/malnutrition.
Empty sella syndrome.
Pituitary disorders (infarction, infection, trauma, irradiation, surgery, microadenomas, macroadenomas).
Idiopathic hypopituitarism.
Drug induced.
Thyroid dysfunction (hypothyroidism, hyperthyroidism).
Systemic diseases (e.g., liver disease).
Adrenal hyperfunction (Cushing's syndrome, congenital adrenal hyperplasia).
Polycystic ovarian syndrome.
Isolated gonadotropin deficiency.

APPENDICITIS, DIFFERENTIAL DIAGNOSIS IN PREGNANCY[30]

ICD-10CM # Varies with specific diagnosis

DIFFERENTIAL DIAGNOSIS OF APPENDICITIS DURING PREGNANCY

Gynecologic Conditions

Ruptured ovarian cyst.
Adnexal torsion.
Pelvic inflammatory disease or salpingitis.
Endometriosis.
Ovarian cancer.

Obstetrical Causes

Abruptio placentae.
Chorioamnionitis.
Endometritis.
Uterine fibroid degeneration.
Labor (preterm or term).
Viscus perforation after abortion.
Ruptured ectopic pregnancy.

Gastrointestinal Causes
Crohn's disease.
Colonic diverticulitis (right side).
Cholecystitis.
Pancreatitis.
Mesenteric lymphadenitis.
Gastroenteritis.
Colon cancer.
Intestinal obstruction.
Hernia (incarcerated inguinal or internal).
Colonic intussusception.
Ruptured Meckel's diverticulum.
Colonic perforation.
Acute mesenteric ischemia.
Other Causes
Pyelonephritis.
Urolithiasis.

APPETITE LOSS IN INFANTS AND CHILDREN[41]

ICD-10CM #	R63.0	Anorexia
	F50.8	Other eating disorders
	F98.29	Other feeding disorders of infancy and early childhood

ORGANIC DISEASE

Infection (Acute or Chronic) Neurologic
Congenital degenerative disease.
Hypothalamic lesion.
Increased intracranial pressure (including a brain tumor).
Swallowing disorders (neuromuscular).
Gastrointestinal
Oral lesions (e.g., thrush or herpes simplex).
Gastroesophageal reflux.
Obstruction (especially with gastric or intestinal distention).
Inflammatory bowel disease.
Celiac disease.
Constipation.
Cardiac
Congestive heart failure (especially associated with cyanotic lesions).
Metabolic
Renal failure and/or renal tubule acidosis.
Liver failure.
Congenital metabolic disease.
Lead poisoning.
Nutritional
Marasmus.
Iron deficiency.
Zinc deficiency.
Fever
RA.
Rheumatic fever.
Drugs
Morphine.
Digitalis.
Antimetabolites.
Methylphenidate.
Amphetamines.
Miscellaneous
Prolonged restriction of oral feedings, beginning in the neonatal period.
Systemic lupus erythematosus (SLE).
Tumor.

PSYCHOLOGIC FACTORS

Anxiety, fear, depression, mania (limbic influence on the hypothalamus).
Avoidance of symptoms associated with meals (abdominal pain, diarrhea, bloating, urgency, dumping syndrome).
Anorexia nervosa.
Excessive weight loss and food aversion in athletes, simulating anorexia nervosa.

ARTERIAL OCCLUSION[33]

ICD-10CM #	I74.3	Embolism and thrombosis of arteries of the lower extremities
	I74.2	Embolism and thrombosis of arteries of the upper extremities

Thromboembolism (post-MI, mitral stenosis, rheumatic valve disease, atrial fibrillation, atrial myxoma, marantic endocarditis, bacterial endocarditis, Libman-Sacks endocarditis).
Atheroembolism (microemboli composed of cholesterol, calcium, and platelets from proximal atherosclerotic plaques).
Arterial thrombosis (endothelial injury, altered arterial blood flow, trauma, severe atherosclerosis, acute vasculitis).
Vasospasm.
Trauma.
Hypercoagulable states.
Miscellaneous (irradiation, drugs, infections, necrotizing).

ARTHRITIS AND ABDOMINAL PAIN

ICD-10CM #	M00.9	Pyogenic arthritis, unspecified
	R10.817	Generalized abdominal tenderness
	M02.9	Reactive arthropathy

Viral syndrome.
Inflammatory bowel disease.
Celiac disease.
Vasculitis.
SLE.
RA.
Scleroderma.
Amyloidosis.
Chronic hepatitis C.
Whipple's disease.
Polyarteritis nodosa.
Behçet's disease.
Familial Mediterranean fever.
Blind loop syndrome.
Babesiosis.
Lyme disease.
Ehrlichiosis.

ARTHRITIS AND DIARRHEA

ICD-10CM #	M00.9	Pyogenic arthritis, unspecified
	R19.7	Diarrhea, unspecified

Viral syndrome.
Inflammatory bowel disease.
Celiac disease.
Whipple's disease.
Enterogenic (bacterial) reactive arthritis.
Collagenous colitis.
Behçet's disease.
Hyperthyroidism.
Spondyloarthropathy.
Blind loop syndrome.

ARTHRITIS AND EYE LESIONS[16]

ICD-10CM #	M00.9	Pyogenic arthritis, unspecified
	M02.3	Reiter disease
	M02.9	Reactive arthropathy

SLE.
Sjögren syndrome.
Behçet's syndrome.
Sarcoidosis.
Subacute bacterial endocarditis (SBE).
Lyme disease.
Granulomatosis with polyangiitis.
Giant cell arteritis.
Takayasu's arteritis.
RA, JRA.
Scleroderma.
Inflammatory bowel disease.
Whipple's disease.
Ankylosing spondylitis.
Reactive arthritis.
Psoriatic arthritis.

ARTHRITIS AND HEART MURMUR[16]

ICD-10CM #	M00.9	Pyogenic arthritis, unspecified
	I01.8	Other acute rheumatic heart disease
	M02.9	Reactive arthropathy

SBE.
Cardiac myxoma.
Ankylosing spondylitis.
Reactive arthritis.
Acute rheumatic fever.
RA.
SLE with Libman-Sacks endocarditis.
Relapsing polychondritis.

ARTHRITIS AND MUSCLE WEAKNESS[18]

ICD-10CM #	M00.9	Pyogenic arthritis, unspecified
	M62.9	Disorder of muscle, unspecified
	M02.9	Reactive arthropathy

RA.
Ankylosing spondylitis.
Polymyositis.
Dermatomyositis.
SLE, scleroderma, mixed connective tissue disease.
Sarcoidosis.
HIV-associated arthritis.
Whipple's disease.

ARTHRITIS AND RASH[16]

ICD-10CM #		
	M00.9	Pyogenic arthritis, unspecified
	R21	Rash and other nonspecific skin eruption
	M02.9	Reactive arthropathy

Chronic urticaria.
Vasculitic urticaria.
SLE.
Dermatomyositis.
Polymyositis.
Psoriatic arthritis.
Reactive arthritis.
Chronic sarcoidosis.
Serum sickness.
Sweet's syndrome.
Leprosy.

ARTHRITIS AND SUBCUTANEOUS NODULES[16]

ICD-10CM #		
	M00.9	Pyogenic arthritis, unspecified
	A18.4	Tuberculosis of skin and subcutaneous tissue
	M02.9	Reactive arthropathy

RA.
Gout.
Pseudogout (rare).
Sarcoidosis.
Light chain (LA) amyloidosis (primary, multiple myeloma).
Acute rheumatic fever (ARF).
Hemochromatosis.
Whipple's disease.
Multicentric reticulohistiocytosis.

ARTHRITIS AND WEIGHT LOSS[16]

ICD-10CM #		
	M00.9	Pyogenic arthritis, unspecified
	R63.4	Abnormal weight loss
	M02.9	Reactive arthropathy

Severe RA.
RA with vasculitis.
Reactive arthritis.
RA or psoriatic arthritis or ankylosing spondylitis with amyloidosis.
Cancer.
Enteropathic arthritis (Crohn's, ulcerative colitis).
HIV infection.
Whipple's disease.
Blind loop syndrome.
Scleroderma with intestinal bacterial overgrowth.

ARTHRITIS OR EXTREMITY PAIN, IN CHILDREN AND ADOLESCENTS[51]

ICD-10CM #		
	M02.9	Reactive arthropathy

CAUSES OF ARTHRITIS OR EXTREMITY PAIN IN CHILDREN AND ADOLESCENTS

Rheumatic and Inflammatory Diseases
Juvenile idiopathic arthritis.
Systemic lupus erythematosus.
Juvenile dermatomyositis.
Polyarteritis.
Vasculitis.
Scleroderma.
Sjögren syndrome.
Behçet's disease.
Overlap syndromes.
Granulomatosis with polyangiitis (Wegener granulomatosis).
Sarcoidosis.
Kawasaki syndrome.
Henoch-Schönlein purpura.
Chronic recurrent multifocal osteomyelitis.
Seronegative Spondyloarthropathies
Juvenile ankylosing spondylitis.
Inflammatory bowel disease.
Psoriatic arthritis.
Reactive arthritis associated with urethritis, iridocyclitis, and mucocutaneous lesions.
Infectious Illnesses
Bacterial arthritis (septic arthritis, *Staphylococcus aureus,* pneumococcus, gonococcus, *Haemophilus influenzae*).
Lyme disease.
Viral illness (parvovirus, rubella, mumps, Epstein-Barr virus, hepatitis B).
Fungal arthritis.
Mycobacterial infection.
Spirochetal infection.
Endocarditis.
Reactive Arthritis
Acute rheumatic fever.
Reactive arthritis (postinfectious due to *Shigella, Salmonella, Yersinia, Chlamydia,* or meningococcus).
Serum sickness.
Toxic synovitis of the hip.
Postimmunization.
Immunodeficiencies
Hypogammaglobulinemia.
Immunoglobulin A deficiency.
Human immunodeficiency virus.
Congenital and Metabolic Disorders
Gout.
Pseudogout.
Mucopolysaccharidoses.
Thyroid disease (hypothyroidism, hyperthyroidism).
Hyperparathyroidism.
Vitamin C deficiency (scurvy).
Hereditary connective tissue disease (Marfan syndrome, Ehlers-Danlos syndrome).
Fabry disease.
Farber disease.
Amyloidosis (familial Mediterranean fever).
Bone and Cartilage Disorders
Trauma.
Patellofemoral syndrome.
Hypermobility syndrome.
Osteochondritis dissecans.
Avascular necrosis (including Legg-Calvé-Perthes disease).
Hypertrophic osteoarthropathy.
Slipped capital femoral epiphysis.
Osteolysis.
Benign bone tumors (including osteoid osteoma).
Histiocytosis.
Rickets.
Neuropathic Disorders
Peripheral neuropathies.
Carpal tunnel syndrome.
Charcot joints.
Neoplastic Disorders
Leukemia.
Neuroblastoma.
Lymphoma.
Bone tumors (osteosarcoma, Ewing sarcoma).
Histiocytic syndromes.
Synovial tumors.
Hematologic Disorders
Hemophilia.
Hemoglobinopathies (including sickle cell disease).
Miscellaneous Disorders
Pigmented villonodular synovitis.
Plant-thorn synovitis (foreign body arthritis).
Myositis ossificans.
Eosinophilic fasciitis.
Tendinitis (overuse injury).
Raynaud phenomenon.
Pain Syndromes
Fibromyalgia.
Growing pains.
Depression (with somatization).
Reflex sympathetic dystrophy.
Regional myofascial pain syndromes.

ARTHRITIS, AXIAL SKELETON

ICD-10CM #		
	M45.9	Ankylosing spondylitis of unspecified sites in spine
	L40.54	Psoriatic juvenile arthropathy
	L40.59	Other psoriatic arthropathy
	M15.9	Polyosteoarthritis, unspecified
	M45.9	Ankylosing spondylitis of unspecified sites in spine

RA.
Psoriatic arthritis.
Reiter's syndrome (reactive arthritis).
Ankylosing spondylitis.
Juvenile RA.
Degenerative disease of the nucleus pulposus.
Spondylosis deformans.
Diffuse idiopathic skeletal hyperostosis (DISH).
Alkaptonuria.
Infection.

ARTHRITIS, CHRONIC, MONOARTICULAR OR OLIGOARTICULAR, INFECTIOUS CAUSES[10]

ICD-10CM #	Varies with specific diagnosis

INFECTIOUS CAUSES OF CHRONIC MONARTICULAR OR OLIGOARTICULAR ARTHRITIS

Bacterial
Borrelia burgdorferi.
Tropheryma whipplei.
Treponema pallidum.
Nocardia spp.
Fungi
Candida spp.
Cryptococcus neoformans.
Blastomyces dermatitidis.
Coccidioides spp.
Paracoccidioides brasiliensis.
Sporothrix schenckii.
Aspergillus spp. and other molds, including *Rhizopus, Scedosporium,* and *Fusarium.*
Mycobacteria
Mycobacterium tuberculosis.
M. kansasii.
M. marinum.
M. avium-intracellulare complex.
M. terrae.
M. fortuitum, M. chelonae, M. abscessus.
M. haemophilum.
M. leprae.
Parasites
Helminths.
Filariae.

ARTHRITIS, FEVER, AND RASH[16]

ICD-10CM #	M00.9	Pyogenic arthritis, unspecified
	M02.9	Reactive arthropathy
	R21	Rash and other nonspecific skin eruption
	R50.9	Fever, unspecified

Rubella, parvovirus B19.
Gonococcemia, meningococcemia.
Secondary syphilis, Lyme borreliosis.
Adult acute rheumatic fever, adult Still's disease, adult Kawasaki disease.
Vasculitic urticaria.
Acute sarcoidosis.
Familial Mediterranean fever.
Hyperimmunoglobulinemia D and periodic fever syndrome.

ARTHRITIS, MONOARTICULAR AND OLIGOARTICULAR[7]

ICD-10CM #	M19.90	Unspecified osteoarthritis, unspecified site
	M01.X0	Direct infection of unspecified joint in infectious and parasitic diseases classified elsewhere
	M13.10	Monoarthritis, not elsewhere classified, unspecified site

Septic arthritis (*S. aureus, Neisseria gonorrhoeae,* meningococci, streptococci, *Streptococcus pneumoniae,* enteric gram-negative bacilli).
Crystalline-induced arthritis (gout, pseudogout, calcium oxalate, hydroxyapatite and other basic calcium/phosphate crystals).
Traumatic joint injury.
Hemarthrosis.
Monoarticular or oligoarticular flare of an inflammatory polyarticular rheumatic disease (RA, psoriatic arthritis, Reiter syndrome [reactive arthritis], SLE).

ARTHRITIS, PEDIATRIC AGE[41]

ICD-10CM #	M01.X0	Direct infection of unspecified joint in infectious and parasitic diseases classified elsewhere
	M08.00	Unspecified juvenile rheumatoid arthritis of unspecified site
	M08.3	Juvenile rheumatoid polyarthritis (seronegative)
	M08.40	Pauciarticular juvenile rheumatoid arthritis, unspecified site

RHEUMATIC DISEASES OF CHILDHOOD

Acute rheumatic fever.
SLE.
Juvenile ankylosing spondylitis.
Polymyositis and dermatomyositis.
Vasculitis.
Scleroderma.
Psoriatic arthritis.
Mixed connective tissue disease and overlap syndromes.
Kawasaki disease.
Behçet's syndrome.
Familial Mediterranean fever.
Reiter's syndrome (reactive arthritis).
Reflex sympathetic dystrophy.
Fibromyalgia (fibrositis).

INFECTIOUS DISEASES

Bacterial arthritis.
Viral or postviral arthritis.
Fungal arthritis.
Osteomyelitis.
Reactive arthritis.

NEOPLASTIC DISEASES

Leukemia.
Lymphoma.
Neuroblastoma.
Primary bone tumors.

NONINFLAMMATORY DISORDERS

Trauma.
Avascular necrosis syndromes.
Osteochondroses.
Slipped capital femoral epiphysis.
Diskitis.
Patellofemoral dysfunction (chondromalacia patellae).
Toxic synovitis of the hip.
Overuse syndromes.

GENETIC OR CONGENITAL SYNDROMES

Hematologic Disorders
Sickle cell disease.
Hemophilia.

INFLAMMATORY BOWEL DISEASE

Miscellaneous
Growing pains.
Psychogenic arthralgias (conversion reactions).
Hypermobility syndrome.
Villonodular synovitis.
Foreign body arthritis.

ARTHRITIS, POLYARTICULAR

ICD-10CM #	M15.0	Primary generalized (osteo)arthritis
	M12.89	Other specific arthropathies, not elsewhere classified, multiple sites
	M08.3	Juvenile rheumatoid polyarthritis (seronegative)

RA, juvenile (rheumatoid) polyarthritis.
SLE, other connective tissue diseases, erythema nodosum, palindromic rheumatism, relapsing polychondritis.
Psoriatic arthritis, ankylosing spondylitis.
Sarcoidosis.
Lyme arthritis, bacterial endocarditis, *Neisseria gonorrhoeae* infection, rheumatic fever, Reiter's disease (reactive arthritis).
Crystal deposition disease.
Hypersensitivity to serum or drugs.
Hepatitis B, HIV, rubella, mumps.
Other: serum sickness, leukemias, lymphomas, enteropathic arthropathy, Whipple disease, Behçet's syndrome, Henoch-Schönlein purpura, familial Mediterranean fever, hypertrophic pulmonary osteoarthropathy.

ASCITES

ICD-10CM #	R18.0	Malignant ascites
	C78.6	Secondary malignant neoplasm of retroperitoneum and peritoneum
	I89.8	Other specified noninfective disorders of lymphatic vessels and lymph nodes

Hypoalbuminemia: nephrotic syndrome, protein-losing gastroenteropathy, starvation.
Cirrhosis.
Hepatic congestion: CHF, constrictive pericarditis, tricuspid insufficiency, hepatic vein obstruction (Budd-Chiari syndrome), inferior vena cava or portal vein obstruction.
Peritoneal infections: TB and other bacterial infections, fungal diseases, parasites.
Neoplasms: primary hepatic neoplasms, metastases to liver or peritoneum, lymphomas, leukemias, myeloid metaplasia.
Lymphatic obstruction: mediastinal tumors, trauma to the thoracic duct, filariasis.
Ovarian disease: Meigs syndrome, struma ovarii.
Chronic pancreatitis or pseudocyst: pancreatic ascites.
Leakage of bile: bile ascites.
Urinary obstruction or trauma: urine ascites.
Myxedema.
Chylous ascites.

ASPIRATION LUNG INJURY, CHILDREN[51]

ICD-10CM #		
	P24.8	Neonatal aspiration syndromes

CONDITIONS PREDISPOSING TO ASPIRATION LUNG INJURY IN CHILDREN

Anatomic and Mechanical

Tracheoesophageal fistula.
Laryngeal cleft.
Vascular ring.
Cleft palate.
Micrognathia.
Macroglossia.
Achalasia.
Esophageal foreign body.
Tracheostomy.
Endotracheal tube.
Nasoenteric tube.
Collagen vascular disease (scleroderma, dermatomyositis).
Gastroesophageal reflux disease.
Obesity.

Neuromuscular

Altered consciousness.
Immaturity of swallowing/prematurity.
Dysautonomia.
Increased intracranial pressure.
Hydrocephalus.
Vocal cord paralysis.
Cerebral palsy.
Muscular dystrophy.
Myasthenia gravis.
Guillain-Barré syndrome.
Werdnig-Hoffmann disease.
Ataxia-telangiectasia.
Cerebral vascular accident.

Miscellaneous

Poor oral hygiene.
Gingivitis.
Prolonged hospitalization.
Gastric outlet or intestinal obstruction.
Poor feeding techniques (bottle propping, overfeeding, inappropriate foods for toddlers).
Bronchopulmonary dysplasia.
Viral infection.

ASTHENIA

ICD-10CM #		
	G93.3	Postviral fatigue syndrome
	R53.1	Weakness
	R53.81	Other malaise
	R53.83	Other fatigue

Depression.
Chronic fatigue syndrome.
Sleep disorders.
Anemia.
Hypothyroidism.
Sedentary lifestyle.
Medications (e.g., narcotics, sedatives).
Infections.
Dehydration/electrolyte disorders.
COPD and other pulmonary disorders.
Renal failure.
CHF.
Diabetes.
Addison disease.
Paraneoplastic syndrome.

ASTHMA, CHILDHOOD[9]

ICD-10CM #		
	J45.20	Mild intermittent asthma, uncomplicated
	J45.22	Mild intermittent asthma with status asthmaticus

INFECTIONS

Bronchiolitis (RSV).
Pneumonia.
Croup.
Tuberculosis, histoplasmosis.
Bronchiectasis.
Bronchiolitis obliterans.
Bronchitis.
Sinusitis.

ANATOMIC, CONGENITAL

Cystic fibrosis.
Vascular rings.
Ciliary dyskinesia.
B-lymphocyte immune defect.
Congestive heart failure.
Laryngotracheomalacia.
Tumor, lymphoma.
H-type tracheoesophageal fistula.
Repaired tracheoesophageal fistula.
Gastroesophageal reflux.

VASCULITIS, HYPERSENSITIVITY

Allergic bronchopulmonary aspergillosis.
Allergic alveolitis, hypersensitivity pneumonitis.
Churg-Strauss syndrome.
Periarteritis nodosa.

OTHER

Foreign body aspiration.
Pulmonary thromboembolism.
Psychogenic cough.
Sarcoidosis.
Bronchopulmonary dysplasia.
Vocal cord dysfunction.

ATAXIA

ICD-10CM #		
	R27.0	Ataxia, unspecified
	R27.8	Other lack of coordination
	R27.9	Unspecified lack of coordination
	F10.229	Alcohol dependence with intoxication, unspecified
	F10.20	Alcohol dependence, uncomplicated
	G11.1	Early-onset cerebellar ataxia
	G31.89	Other specified degenerative diseases of nervous system
	F44.4	Conversion sisorder with motor symptom or deficit
	F44.6	Conversion disorder with sensory symptom or deficit

Vertebral-basilar artery ischemia.
Diabetic neuropathy.
Tabes dorsalis.
Vitamin B_{12} deficiency.
Multiple sclerosis and other demyelinating diseases.
Meningomyelopathy.
Cerebellar neoplasms, hemorrhage, abscess, infarct.
Nutritional (Wernicke encephalopathy).
Paraneoplastic syndromes.
Parainfectious: Guillain-Barré syndrome, acute ataxia of childhood and young adults.
Toxins: phenytoin, alcohol, sedatives, organophosphates.
Wilson's disease (hepatolenticular degeneration).
Hypothyroidism.
Myopathy.
Cerebellar and spinocerebellar degeneration: ataxia/telangiectasia, Friedreich ataxia.
Frontal lobe lesions: tumors, thrombosis of anterior cerebral artery, hydrocephalus.
Labyrinthine destruction: neoplasm, injury, inflammation, compression.
Hysteria.
AIDS.

ATAXIA, ACUTE OR RECURRENT[23]

ICD-10CM #		
	R27.0	Ataxia, unspecified
	R27.8	Other lack of coordination
	R27.9	Unspecified lack of coordination
	F10.229	Alcohol dependence with intoxication, unspecified
	F10.20	Alcohol dependence, uncomplicated
	G11.1	Early-onset cerebellar ataxia
	G31.89	Other specified degenerative diseases of nervous system

	F44.4	Conversion disorder with motor symptom or deficit
	F44.6	Conversion disorder with sensory symptom or deficit

Drug ingestion (e.g., phenytoin, carbamazepine, sedatives, hypnotics, and phencyclidine) or intoxication (e.g., alcohol, ethylene glycol, hydrocarbon fumes, lead, mercury, or thallium).
Postinfectious (cerebellitis [e.g., varicella], acute disseminated encephalomyelitis).
Head trauma.
Basilar migraine.
Benign paroxysmal vertigo (migraine equivalent).
Brain tumor or neuroblastoma (if accompanied by opsoclonus or myoclonus [i.e., "dancing eyes, dancing feet"]).
Hydrocephalus.
Infection (e.g., labyrinthitis, abscess).
Seizure (ictal or postictal).
Vascular events (e.g., cerebellar hemorrhage or stroke).
Miller-Fisher variant of Guillain-Barré syndrome (ataxia, ophthalmoplegia, and areflexia). Warning: If bulbar signs present, disease is likely progressive; patient may lose ability to protect airway and/or ability to breathe.
Inherited ataxias.
Inborn errors of metabolism (e.g., mitochondrial disorders, amino-acidopathies, urea cycle defects).
Conversion reaction.
Multiple sclerosis.

ATAXIA, CEREBELLAR, ADULT ONSET[75]

ICD-10CM #	G11.0	Congenital nonprogressive ataxia
	G11.2	Late-onset cerebellar ataxia

CAUSES OF ADULT ONSET CEREBELLAR ATAXIA

Inherited
Later onset SCA syndromes.
Rarely Friedreich ataxia.
Congenital
Arnold–Chiari malformation (cerebellar ectopia).
Inflammatory
Multiple sclerosis.
Sarcoidosis.
Infections (TB, viral).
Neoplastic
Often metastatic in adults.
Meningioma, neurofibroma.
Hemangioblastoma.
Paraneoplastic
Usually with small cell bronchial carcinoma.
Vascular
Infarction, hemorrhage.
Arteriovenous malformations.
Trauma
Head injury.
Postsurgical.
Toxic
Alcohol, phenytoin, solvent abuse.
Endocrine
Hypothyroidism (very rare).
Degenerative
Multiple system atrophy (MSA).

ATAXIA, CEREBELLAR, CHILDREN[75]

ICD-10CM #	G11.0	Congenital nonprogressive ataxia
	G11.2	Late-onset cerebellar ataxia

CAUSES OF CEREBELLAR ATAXIA IN CHILDREN

Congenital Malformations
Cerebellar agenesis/hypoplasia.
Dandy–Walker syndrome.
Arnold–Chiari malformation.
Hereditary Ataxias
Friedreich ataxia.
Trauma
Birth trauma.
Head injury in childhood.
Infectious
Secondary to bacterial meningitis.
Secondary to encephalitis.
Hydrocephalus
Tumors
Medulloblastoma.
Astrocytoma.
Hemangioblastoma.

ATAXIA, CHRONIC OR PROGRESSIVE[23]

ICD-10CM #	R27.0	Ataxia, unspecified
	R27.8	Other lack of coordination
	R27.9	Unspecified lack of coordination
	G11.1	Early-onset cerebellar ataxia
	G11.0	Congenital nonprogressive ataxia
	G11.2	Late-onset cerebellar ataxia
	G11.3	Cerebellar ataxia with defective DNA repair
	G11.8	Other hereditary ataxia

Hydrocephalus.
Hypothyroidism.
Tumor or paraneoplastic syndrome.
Low vitamin E levels (e.g., cystic fibrosis).
Wilson disease.
Inborn errors of metabolism.
Inherited ataxias (e.g., ataxia-telangiectasia, Friedreich ataxia).

ATAXIA IN CHILDHOOD[79]

ICD-10CM #	G11.1	Early-onset cerebellar ataxia

SELECTED CAUSES OF ATAXIA IN CHILDHOOD

Congenital:
- Agenesis of vermis of the cerebellum.
- Aplasia or dysplasia of the cerebellum.
- Basilar impression.
- Cerebellar dysplasia with microgyria, macrogyria, or agyria.
- Cervical spinal bifida with herniation of the cerebellum (Chiari malformation, type 3).
- Chiari malformation.
- Dandy-Walker syndrome.
- Encephalocele.
- Hydrocephalus (progressive).
- Hypoplasia of the cerebellum.

Degenerative and/or genetic:
- Acute intermittent cerebellar ataxia.
- Ataxia, retinitis pigmentosa, deafness, vestibular abnormality, and intellectual deterioration.
- Ataxia-telangiectasia.
- Biemond posterior column ataxia.
- Cerebellar ataxia with deafness, anosmia, absent caloric responses, nonreactive pupils, and hyporeflexia.
- Cockayne syndrome.
- Dentate cerebellar ataxia (dyssynergia cerebellaris progressiva).
- Familial ataxia with macular degeneration.
- Friedreich ataxia.
- Hereditary cerebellar ataxia, intellectual retardation, choreoathetosis, and eunuchoidism.
- Hereditary cerebellar ataxia with myotonia and cataracts.
- Hypertrophic interstitial neuritis.
- Marie ataxia.
- Marinesco-Sjögren syndrome.
- Pelizaeus-Merzbacher disease.
- Periodic attacks of vertigo, diplopia, and ataxia—autosomal dominant inheritance.
- Posterior and lateral column difficulties, nystagmus, and muscle atrophy.
- Progressive cerebellar ataxia and epilepsy.
- Ramsay Hunt syndrome (myoclonic seizures and ataxia).
- Roussy-Lévy syndrome.
- Spinocerebellar ataxia (SCAs); olivopontocerebellar ataxias.

Endocrinologic:
- Cretinism.
- Hypothyroidism.

Infectious or postinfectious:
- Acute cerebellar ataxia.
- Acute disseminated encephalomyelitis.
- Cerebellar abscess.
- Coxsackievirus.
- Diphtheria.
- Echovirus.
- Fisher syndrome.
- Infectious mononucleosis (Epstein-Barr virus infection).
- Infectious polyneuropathy.
- Japanese B encephalitis.
- Mumps encephalitis.
- *Mycoplasma pneumoniae.*
- Pertussis.
- Polio.

Postbacterial meningitis.
Rubeola.
Tuberculosis.
Typhoid.
Varicella.
Metabolic:
Abetalipoproteinemia.
Argininosuccinic aciduria.
Ataxia with vitamin E deficiency (AVED).
GM2 gangliosidosis (late).
Hartnup disease.
Hyperalaninemia.
Hyperammonemia I and II.
Hypoglycemia.
Kearns-Sayre syndrome.
Leigh disease.
Maple syrup urine disease (intermittent).
MERRF (Myoclonic epilepsy with ragged red fibers).
Metachromatic leukodystrophy.
Mitochondrial complex defects (I, III, IV).
Multiple carboxylase deficiency (biotinidase deficiency).
Neuronal ceroid-lipofuscinosis.
Neuropathy, ataxia, retinitis pigmentosa (NARP).
Niemann-Pick disease (late infantile).
5-Oxoprolinuria.
Pyruvate decarboxylase deficiency.
Refsum disease.
Sialidosis.
Triose-phosphate isomerase deficiency.
Tryptophanuria.
Wernicke encephalopathy (thiamine or B1 deficiency).
Neoplastic:
Frontal lobe tumors.
Hemispheric cerebellar tumors.
Midline cerebellar tumors.
Neuroblastoma.
Pontine tumors (primarily gliomas).
Spinal cord tumors.
Primary psychogenic:
Conversion reaction.
Toxic:
Alcohol.
Benzodiazepines.
Carbamazepine.
Clonazepam.
Lead encephalopathy.
Phenobarbital.
Phenytoin.
Primidone.
Tick paralysis poisoning.
Traumatic:
Acute cerebellar edema.
Acute frontal lobe edema.
Vascular:
Angioblastoma of cerebellum.
Basilar migraine.
Cerebellar embolism.
Cerebellar hemorrhage.
Cerebellar thrombosis.
Posterior cerebellar artery disease.
Vasculitis.
von Hippel-Lindau disease.

ATAXIA, TOXIC CAUSES[79]

ICD-10CM # R27.0 Early-onset cerebellar ataxia

SELECTED TOXIC CAUSES OF ATAXIA

Medications:
Acetohexamide.
Amiodarone.
Anticholinergic agents.
Antidepressants, including selective serotonin reuptake inhibitors.
Antiepileptic drugs.
Antihistamines.
Antimicrobials, antifungals.
Antineoplastics.
Antiparasitics.
Baclofen.
Buspirone.
Dextromethorphan.
Disulfiram.
Ethanol.
Fenfluramine.
Lithium.
Lysergic acid diethylamide (LSD), phencyclidine palmitate (PCP).
Mexiletine.
Sedatives, narcotics.
Industrial toxins:
Aluminum compounds.
Butyl alcohol.
Carbon monoxide.
Carbon tetrachloride.
Ethylene glycol.
Formaldehyde.
Gasoline.
Manganese.
Metaldehyde (snail bait, fire starters).
Paradichlorobenzene (moth repellent, diaper pail deodorant).
Rodenticides: aluminum phosphide, sodium monofluoroacetate.
Solvents.
Biologic toxins:
Belladonna, hyoscyamine.
Buckeye (*Aesculus* spp.).
Mayapple (*Podophyllum peltatum*).
Mescaline, peyote.
Podophyllum (ingested).
Poison hemlock (*Conium maculatum*).

ATELECTASIS

ICD-10CM # J98.11 Atelectasis

Lung neoplasm (primary or metastatic).
Infection (pneumonia, TB, fungal, histoplasmosis).
Postoperative (lower lobes).
Sarcoidosis.
Mucoid impaction.
Foreign body.
Postinflammatory (middle lobe syndrome).
Pneumothorax.
Pleural effusion.
Pneumoconiosis.
Interstitial fibrosis.
Bulla.
Mediastinal or adjacent mass.

ATRIAL ENLARGEMENT, LEFT ATRIUM[36]

ICD-10CM # I51.7 Cardiomegaly

CAUSES OF LARGE LEFT ATRIUM

Causes Due to Volume Overload
Mitral regurgitation (often with left ventricular failure).
Ventricular septal defect.
Patent ductus arteriosus.
Atrial septal defect with shunt reversal (i.e., pulmonary hypertension).
ASD with tricuspid atresia (obligatory shunt reversal).
Aortopulmonary window.
Causes Due to Pressure Overload
Mitral stenosis.
Noncompliant left ventricle: hypertension, hypertrophic cardiomyopathy, aortic stenosis.
Left ventricular failure (often with secondary mitral regurgitation).
Left atrial myxoma.
Other Causes (Both Rare)
Atrial fibrillation.
Isolated/idiopathic.

ATRIAL ENLARGEMENT, RIGHT ATRIUM

ICD-10CM # I51.7 Cardiomegaly

Right ventricular failure.
Atrial septal defect.
Tricuspid regurgitation.
Tricuspid stenosis.
Pulmonary hypertension.
Restrictive cardiomyopathy.
Right atrial myxoma.
Ebstein anomaly.
Anomalous pulmonary venous drainage to the right atrium.
Endomyocardial fibrosis.
Sinus of Valsalva fistula.
Arrhythmogenic right ventricular dysplasia.

ATYPICAL LYMPHOCYTOSIS, HETEROPHIL NEGATIVE, INFECTIOUS CAUSES[3]

ICD-10CM # D72.820 Lymphocytosis (symptomatic)

MOST COMMON INFECTIOUS CAUSES OF HETEROPHIL-NEGATIVE ATYPICAL LYMPHOCYTOSIS

Babesiosis.
Cytomegalovirus.
Epstein-Barr virus (particularly in children).
Human herpesvirus 6.
Human immunodeficiency virus (especially during acute seroconversion).
Infectious mononucleosis.
Malaria.
Measles.
Toxoplasmosis.
Varicella.
Infectious hepatitis.

AV NODAL BLOCK[33]

ICD-10CM # I44.30 Unspecified atrioventricular block
I44.2 Atrioventricular block, complete

Idiopathic fibrosis (Lenègre disease).
Sclerodegenerative processes (e.g., Lev disease with calcification of the mitral and aortic annuli).
AV node radiofrequency ablation procedure.
Medications (e.g., digoxin, beta-blockers, calcium channel blockers, class III antiarrhythmics).
Acute inferior wall MI.
Myocarditis.
Infections (endocarditis, Lyme disease).
Infiltrative diseases (e.g., hemochromatosis, sarcoidosis, amyloidosis).
Trauma (including cardiac surgical procedures).
Collagen vascular diseases.
Aortic root diseases (e.g., spondylitis).
Electrolyte abnormalities (e.g., hyperkalemia).

BACK PAIN

ICD-10CM # M54.89 Other dorsalgia
M54.9 Dorsalgia, unspecified
M54.5 Low back pain
F45.42 Pain disorder with related psychological factors
M54.08 Panniculitis affecting regions of neck and back, sacral and sacrococcygeal region
S23.9XXA Sprain of unspecified parts of thorax, initial encounter
M43.27 Fusion of spine, lumbosacral region
M43.28 Fusion of spine, sacral and sacrococcygeal region
M53.2X7 Spinal instabilities, lumbosacral region
M53.3 Sacrococcygeal disorders, not elsewhere classified

Trauma: injury to bone, joint, or ligament.
Mechanical: pregnancy, obesity, fatigue, scoliosis.
Degenerative: osteoarthritis.
Infections: osteomyelitis, subarachnoid or spinal abscess, TB, meningitis, basilar pneumonia.
Metabolic: osteoporosis, osteomalacia.
Vascular: leaking aortic aneurysm, subarachnoid or spinal hemorrhage/infarction.
Neoplastic: myeloma, Hodgkin's disease, carcinoma of pancreas, metastatic neoplasm from breast, prostate, lung.
GI: penetrating ulcer, pancreatitis, cholelithiasis, inflammatory bowel disease.
Renal: hydronephrosis, calculus, neoplasm, renal infarction, pyelonephritis.
Hematologic: sickle cell crisis, acute hemolysis.
Gynecologic: neoplasm of uterus or ovary, dysmenorrhea, salpingitis, uterine prolapse.
Inflammatory: ankylosing spondylitis, psoriatic arthritis, Reiter syndrome (reactive arthritis).
Lumbosacral strain.
Psychogenic: malingering, hysteria, anxiety.
Endocrine: adrenal hemorrhage or infarction.

BACK PAIN, CHILDREN AND ADOLESCENTS[51]

ICD-10CM # M54.5 Low back pain
M54.9 Dorsalgia

INFLAMMATORY OR INFECTIOUS

Diskitis.
Vertebral osteomyelitis (pyogenic, tuberculous).
Spinal epidural abscess.
Pyelonephritis.
Pancreatitis.

RHEUMATOLOGIC

Pauciarticular juvenile rheumatoid arthritis.
Reiter syndrome (reactive arthritis).
Ankylosing spondylitis.
Psoriatic arthritis.

DEVELOPMENTAL

Spondylolysis.
Spondylolisthesis.
Scheuermann disease.
Scoliosis.

TRAUMATIC (ACUTE VERSUS REPETITIVE)

Hip-pelvis anomalies.
Herniated disk.
Overuse syndromes.
Vertebral stress fractures.
Upper cervical spine instability.

NEOPLASTIC

Vertebral Tumors

Benign

Eosinophilic granuloma.
Aneurysmal bone cyst.
Osteoid osteoma.
Osteoblastoma.

Malignant

Osteogenic sarcoma.
Leukemia.
Lymphoma.
Metastatic tumors.

Spinal Cord, Ganglia, and Nerve Roots

Intramedullary spinal cord tumor.
Sympathetic chain.
Ganglioneuroma.
Ganglioneuroblastoma.
Neuroblastoma.

OTHER

Intraabdominal or pelvic pathology.
Following lumbar puncture.
Conversion reaction.
Juvenile osteoporosis.

BACK PAIN, LOW, ACUTE[7]

ICD-10CM # M54.5 Low back pain

DIFFERENTIAL CONSIDERATIONS IN ACUTE LOW BACK PAIN

Emergent

Aortic dissection.
Cauda equina syndrome.
Epidural abscess or hematoma.
Meningitis.
Ruptured/expanding aortic aneurysm.
Spinal fracture or subluxation with cord or root impingement.

Urgent

Back pain with neurologic deficits.
Disk herniation causing neurologic compromise.
Malignancy.
Sciatica with motor nerve root compression.
Spinal fractures without cord impingement.
Spinal stenosis.
Transverse myelitis.
Vertebral osteomyelitis.

Common or Stable

Acute ligamentous injury.
Acute muscle strain.
Ankylosing spondylitis.
Degenerative joint disease.
Intervertebral disk disease without impingement.
Pathologic fracture without impingement.
Seropositive arthritis.
Spondylolisthesis.

Referred or Visceral

Cholecystitis.
Esophageal disease.
Nephrolithiasis.
Ovarian torsion, mass, or tumor.
Pancreatitis.
Peptic ulcer disease.
Pleural effusion.
Pneumonia.
Pulmonary embolism.
Pyelonephritis.
Retroperitoneal hemorrhage or mass.

BACK PAIN, VISCEROGENIC ORIGIN

ICD-10CM # F45.41 Pain disorder exclusively related to psychological factors
M54 Dorsalgia
M54.5 Low back pain

Urolithiasis.
Aortic aneurysm.
Colorectal carcinoma.
Endometriosis.
Tubal pregnancy.
Prostatitis.
Peptic ulcer.
Pancreatitis.
Diverticular spasm.
Metastatic neoplasm (e.g., bladder, uterus, ovary, kidney).

BACTERIAL OVERGROWTH, SMALL INTESTINE[81]

ICD-10CM # A04.9 Bacterial intestinal infection, unspecified

Gastric surgery—Billroth II.
Small bowel diverticula.
Small bowel stricture:
Crohn disease.
Radiation enteritis.
Impaired small intestinal motility:
Scleroderma.
Diabetes mellitus.
Chronic intestinal pseudoobstruction.
Miscellaneous/multifactorial:
Elderly.
Immune deficiency syndromes.
Chronic pancreatitis.
Cirrhosis.

BALLISM[7]

ICD-10CM # G25.4 Drug-induced chorea
G25.5 Other chorea

Cerebral infarction or hemorrhage.
Medications (e.g., dopamine agonists, phenytoin).
CNS neoplasm (primary or metastatic).
Nonketotic hyperosmolar state.

[7]Violent, flinging, nonpatterned rapid movements

BILE DUCT, DILATED[81]

ICD-10CM # K83.1 Obstruction of bile duct

Normal variant.
Post-cholecystectomy.
Unsuspected bile duct stone.
Sphincter of Oddi stenosis.
Occult bile duct stricture.
Previous bile duct injury.
Early carcinoma of the pancreas, carcinoma of the bile duct, or carcinoma of the ampulla.
Extrinsic compression of the bile duct by a primary or secondary neoplasm.

BILIARY OBSTRUCTION[69]

ICD-10CM # Varies with specific diagnosis

CAUSES OF BILIARY OBSTRUCTION

Benign Miscellaneous
Choledocholithiasis.*
Hemobilia.*
Congenital biliary diseases.*
Caroli disease.*
Choledochal cysts.
Cholangitis.
Infectious.
Acute pyogenic cholangitis.*
Biliary parasites.*
Recurrent pyogenic cholangitis.*
HIV cholangiopathy.
Sclerosing cholangitis.
Neoplasms
Cholangiocarcinoma.
Gallbladder carcinoma.
Locally invasive tumors (esp. pancreatic adenocarcinoma).
Ampullary tumors.
Metastases.
Extrinsic compression
Mirizzi syndrome.
Pancreatitis.
Adenopathy.

*Denotes causes of painful jaundice.

BILIARY TREE, REFLUX OF GAS OR BOWEL[84]

ICD-10CM # Varies with specific diagnosis

CAUSES OF REFLUX OF GAS OR BOWEL CONTRAST INTO THE BILIARY TREE

Iatrogenic.
Sphincterotomy.
Choledochojejunostomy.
Gallstone fistula.
Cholecystoduodenal fistula.
Perforated ulcer.
Choledochoduodenal fistula.
Carcinoma.
Choledochoenteric fistula.

BLADDER (URINARY) WALL THICKENING[69]

ICD-10CM # Varies with specific diagnosis

CAUSES OF BLADDER WALL THICKENING

Focal
Neoplasm
Transitional cell carcinoma.
Squamous cell carcinoma.
Adenocarcinoma.
Lymphoma.
Metastases.
Infectious/Inflammatory.
Tuberculosis (acute).
Schistosomiasis (acute).
Cystitis.
Malakoplakia.
Cystitis cystica.
Cystitis glandularis.
Fistula.
Medical Diseases
Endometriosis.
Amyloidosis.
Trauma
Hematoma.
Diffuse
Neoplasm
Transitional cell carcinoma.
Squamous cell carcinoma.
Adenocarcinoma.
Infectious/Inflammatory
Cystitis.
Tuberculosis (chronic).
Schistosomiasis (chronic).
Medical Diseases
Interstitial cystitis.
Amyloidosis.
Neurogenic Bladder
Detrusor hyperreflexia.
Bladder Outlet Obstruction
With muscular hypertrophy.

BLEEDING, GI IN PATIENTS WITH AIDS[26]

ICD-10CM # K92.2 Gastrointestinal bleeding, unspecified

(EXCLUDING NON-AIDS-SPECIFIC DIAGNOSES)

Esophagus
Candida spp.*
Cytomegalovirus.*
HSV.
Idiopathic ulcer.
Stomach
Cytomegalovirus.*
Kaposi sarcoma.*
Cryptosporidiosis.
Lymphoma.
Small Intestine
Kaposi sarcoma.
Lymphoma.
Cytomegalovirus.
Salmonella spp.
Cryptosporidium.
Colon
Cytomegalovirus.*
Kaposi sarcoma.*
Entamoeba histolytica.
Campylobacter jejuni.
Clostridium difficile.
Shigella spp.
Idiopathic ulcerations.
Lymphoma.

*More frequent diagnosis.

BLEEDING, LOWER GI

ICD-10CM # K92.2 Gastrointestinal hemorrhage, unspecified

(ORIGINATING BELOW THE LIGAMENT OF TREITZ)

Small Intestine
Ischemic bowel disease (mesenteric thrombosis, embolism, vasculitis, trauma).
Small bowel neoplasm: leiomyomas, carcinoids.
Hereditary hemorrhagic telangiectasia (Rendu-Osler-Weber syndrome).
Meckel diverticulum and other small intestine diverticula.
Aortoenteric fistula.
Intestinal hemangiomas: blue rubber-bleb nevi, intestinal hemangiomas, cutaneous vascular nevi.
Hamartomatous polyps: Peutz-Jeghers syndrome (intestinal polyps, mucocutaneous pigmentation).
Infections of small bowel: tuberculous enteritis, enteritis necroticans.
Volvulus.

Intussusception.
Lymphoma of small bowel, sarcoma, Kaposi sarcoma.
Irradiation ileitis.
AV malformation of small intestine.
Inflammatory bowel disease.
Polyarteritis nodosa.
Other: pancreatoenteric fistulas, Henoch-Schönlein purpura, Ehlers-Danlos syndrome, SLE, amyloidosis, metastatic melanoma.

Colon

Carcinoma (particularly left colon).
Diverticular disease.
Inflammatory bowel disease.
Ischemic colitis.
Colonic polyps.
Vascular abnormalities: angiodysplasia, vascular ectasia.
Radiation colitis.
Infectious colitis.
Uremic colitis.
Aortoenteric fistula.
Lymphoma of large bowel.
Hemorrhoids.
Anal fissure.
Trauma, foreign body.
Solitary rectal/cecal ulcers.
Long-distance running.

BLEEDING, LOWER GI, PEDIATRIC[7]

ICD-10CM # K92.2 Gastrointestinal hemorrhage, unspecified

<3 MO

Swallowed maternal blood.
Infectious colitis.
Milk allergy.
Bleeding diathesis.
Intussusception.
Midgut volvulus.
Meckel diverticulum.
Necrotizing enterocolitis.

<2 YR

Anal fissure.
Infectious colitis.
Milk allergy.
Colitis.
Intussusception.
Meckel diverticulum.
Polyp.
Duplication.
Hemolytic-uremic syndrome.
Inflammatory bowel disease.
Pseudomembranous enterocolitis.

<5 YR

Infectious colitis.
Anal fissure.
Polyp.
Intussusception.
Meckel diverticulum.
Henoch-Schönlein purpura.
Hemolytic-uremic syndrome.
Inflammatory bowel disease.
Pseudomembranous enterocolitis.

5 TO 18 YR

Infectious colitis.
Inflammatory bowel disease.
Pseudomembranous enterocolitis.
Polyp.
Hemolytic-uremic syndrome.
Hemorrhoids.

BLEEDING, RECTAL[81]

ICD-10CM # K92.2 Gastrointestinal hemorrhage, unspecified

IN PATIENTS <40 YR

Very Common

Hemorrhoids.
Anal fissure.
Inflammatory bowel disease (mainly proctitis).

Less Common

Polyps (hamartomatous or adenomatous).
Infective colitis.
Meckel diverticulum.
Intussusception.

Rare

Colorectal cancer.

IN PATIENTS >40 YR

Hemorrhoids.
Anal fissure.
Colorectal cancer.
Colorectal polyps (mostly adenomas).
Angiodysplasia.
Diverticular disease.
Inflammatory bowel disease.
Ischemic colitis.
Infective colitis.

BLEEDING, THIRD TRIMESTER[1]

ICD-10CM # N93.9 Abnormal uterine and vaginal bleeding, unspecified

Placental abruption.
Placenta previa.
Bloody show (extrusion of cervical mucus).
Vasa previa.
Disseminated intravascular coagulopathy.
Uterine rupture.
Cervicitis, cervical cancer, or other cervical abnormality.
Vaginal laceration.

BLEEDING, UPPER GI

ICD-10CM # K92.2 Gastrointestinal hemorrhage, unspecified

(ORIGINATING ABOVE THE LIGAMENT OF TREITZ)

Swallowed Hemoptysis

Oral or pharyngeal lesions: swallowed blood from nose or oropharynx.
Esophageal: varices, ulceration, esophagitis, Mallory-Weiss tear, carcinoma, trauma.
Gastric: peptic ulcer (including Cushing and Curling ulcers), gastritis, angiodysplasia, gastric neoplasms, hiatal hernia, gastric diverticulum, pseudoxanthoma elasticum, Rendu-Osler-Weber syndrome.
Duodenal: peptic ulcer, duodenitis, angiodysplasia, aortoduodenal fistula, duodenal diverticulum, duodenal tumors, carcinoma of ampulla of Vater, parasites (e.g., hookworm), Crohn's disease.
Biliary: hematobilia (e.g., penetrating injury to liver, hepatobiliary malignancy, endoscopic papillotomy).

BLEEDING, UPPER GI, PEDIATRIC[7]

ICD-10CM # K92.2 Gastrointestinal hemorrhage, unspecified

<3 MO

Swallowed maternal blood.
Gastritis.
Ulcer, stress.
Bleeding diathesis.
Foreign body (NG tube).
Vascular malformation.
Duplication.

<2 YR

Esophagitis.
Gastritis.
Ulcer.
Pyloric stenosis.
Mallory-Weiss syndrome.
Vascular malformation.
Duplication.

<5 YR

Esophagitis.
Gastritis.
Ulcer.
Esophageal varices.
Foreign body.
Mallory-Weiss syndrome.
Hemophilia.
Vascular malformations.

5 TO 18 YR

Esophagitis.
Gastritis.
Ulcer.
Esophageal varices.
Mallory-Weiss syndrome.
Inflammatory bowel disease.
Hemophilia.
Vascular malformation.

BLEEDING, VAGINAL, NON-PREGNANT FEMALE[1]

ICD-10CM # N93.9 Abnormal uterine and vaginal bleeding, unspecified

TRAUMA

Blunt force.
Penetrating force.
Foreign bodies.

INFECTIOUS

Vaginitis.
Cervicitis.
Endometritis.

DYSFUNCTIONAL UTERINE BLEEDING

Ovulatory.
Anovulatory.
Adenomyosis.

BENIGN GROWTHS

Uterine leiomyomas.
Cervical polyps.

MALIGNANCY

Vulvar.
Cervical.
Uterine.
Ovarian.

SYSTEMIC DISEASE

Medications

Anticoagulation (warfarin [Coumadin], low-molecular-weight heparin, clopidogrel [Plavix]).
Antipsychotics.
Corticosteroids.
Tamoxifen.
Selective serotonin reuptake inhibitors.
Contraceptives (oral, intrauterine devices, intramuscular).

BLINDNESS, GERIATRIC AGE

ICD-10CM # H54.8 Legal blindness, as defined in USA

Cataracts.
Glaucoma.
Diabetic retinopathy.
Macular degeneration.
Trauma.
CVA.
Corneal scarring.
Giant cell arteritis.
Ocular herpes zoster.

BLINDNESS, MONOCULAR, TRANSIENT

ICD-10CM # H54.41 Blindness, right eye, normal vision left eye
H54.42 Blindness, left eye, normal vision right eye

Migraine (vasospasm).
Embolic cerebrovascular disease.
Intermittent angle-closure glaucoma.
Partial retinal vein occlusion.
Hyphema.
Optic disc edema.
Giant cell arteritis.
Psychogenic.
Hypotension.
Hypercoagulopathy disorders.
Multiple sclerosis.

BLINDNESS, PEDIATRIC AGE[52]

ICD-10CM # H54.41 Blindness, right eye, normal vision left eye
H54.42 Blindness, left eye, normal vision right eye

CONGENITAL

Optic nerve hypoplasia or aplasia.
Optic coloboma.
Congenital hydrocephalus.
Hydranencephaly.
Porencephaly.
Microencephaly.
Encephalocele, particularly occipital type.
Morning glory disc.
Aniridia.
Anterior microphthalmia.
Peter anomaly.
Persistent pupillary membrane.
Glaucoma.
Cataracts.
Persistent hyperplastic primary vitreous.

PHAKOMATOSES

Tuberous sclerosis.
Neurofibromatosis (special association with optic glioma).
Sturge-Weber syndrome.
von Hippel–Lindau disease.

TUMORS

Retinoblastoma.
Optic glioma.
Perioptic meningioma.
Craniopharyngioma.
Cerebral glioma.
Posterior and intraventricular tumors when complicated by hydrocephalus.
Pseudotumor cerebri.

NEURODEGENERATIVE DISEASES

Cerebral storage disease.
Gangliosidoses, particularly Tay-Sachs disease (infantile amaurotic familial idiocy), Sandhoff variant, generalized gangliosidosis.
Other lipidoses and ceroid lipofuscinoses, particularly the late-onset amaurotic familial idiocies such as those of Jansky-Bielschowsky and of Batten-Mayou-Spielmeyer-Vogt.
Mucopolysaccharidoses, particularly Hurler syndrome and Hunter syndrome.
Leukodystrophies (dysmyelination disorders), particularly metachromatic leukodystrophy and Canavan disease.
Demyelinating sclerosis (myelinoclastic diseases), especially Schilder disease and Devic neuromyelitis optica.
Special types: Dawson disease, Leigh disease, Bassen-Kornzweig syndrome, Refsum disease.
Retinal degenerations: retinitis pigmentosa and its variants, Leber congenital type.
Optic atrophies: congenital autosomal recessive type, infantile and congenital autosomal dominant types, Leber disease, and atrophies associated with hereditary ataxias—the types of Behr, of Marie, and of Sanger-Brown.

INFECTIOUS PROCESSES

Encephalitis, especially in the prenatal infection syndromes caused by *Toxoplasma gondii*, cytomegalovirus, rubella virus, *Treponema pallidum*, herpes simplex.
Meningitis, arachnoiditis.
Chorioretinitis.
Endophthalmitis.
Keratitis.

HEMATOLOGIC DISORDERS

Leukemia with CNS involvement.

VASCULAR AND CIRCULATORY DISORDERS

Collagen vascular diseases.
Arteriovenous malformations—intracerebral hemorrhage, subarachnoid hemorrhage.
Central retinal occlusion.

TRAUMA

Contusion or avulsion of optic nerves, chiasm, globe, cornea.
Cerebral contusion or laceration.
Intracerebral, subarachnoid, or subdural hemorrhage.

DRUGS AND TOXINS OTHER

Retinopathy of prematurity.
Sclerocornea.
Conversion reaction.
Optic neuritis.
Osteopetrosis.

BLISTERS, SUBEPIDERMAL

ICD-10CM # T07 Unspecified multiple injuries

Burns.
Porphyria cutanea tarda.
Bullous pemphigoid.
Bullous drug reaction.
Arthropod bite reaction.
Toxic epidermal necrosis.
Dermatitis herpetiformis.
Polymorphous light eruption.
Variegate porphyria.
SLE.
Epidermolysis bullosa.
Pseudoporphyria.
Acute graft-versus-host reaction.
Linear IgA disease.
Leukocytoclastic vasculitis.
Pressure necrosis.
Urticaria pigmentosa.
Amyloidosis.

BONE AND/OR SOFT TISSUE HYPERTROPHY[66]

ICD-10CM # M85.80 Other specified disorders of bone density and structure, unspecified site

DISORDERS ASSOCIATED WITH BONE AND/OR SOFT TISSUE HYPERTROPHY

Conditions Associated with Generalized Overgrowth

Pituitary gigantism and acromegaly.
Other endocrine disorders.
Cerebral gigantism (Sotos).

Conditions Associated with Limb Hemihypertrophy

Lipomatosis.
Idiopathic congenital hemihypertrophy (associated with tumors, e.g., Wilms tumor, adrenocortical tumors, hepatoblastoma).
Proteus syndrome (capillary port-wine hemangiomas, lymphangiomas, lipomas, epidermal nevi, hypertrophy hands and feet, macrocephaly).
Maffucci syndrome (enchondromas, exostosis, lymphangiomas, venous angiomas).
Klippel-Trenaunay syndrome (capillary port-wine hemangiomas, varicosities, lymphangiomas).
Parkes Weber syndrome (capillary port-wine hemangiomas, varicosities, arteriovenous fistula).
Blue rubber bleb nevus syndrome (cavernous hemangiomas of skin, GI tract).
Other angiodysplasias (e.g., Servelle-Martorell syndrome; venous arterial malformations with limb hypertrophy and bony hypoplasia).
Beckwith-Wiedemann syndrome (macroglossia, visceromegaly, omphaloceles, hemihypertrophy, etc.).

Conditions Associated with Macrodactyly

Neurofibromatosis.
Macrodystrophia lipomatosa.
Proteus syndrome.
Bannayan-Zonana syndrome (lipomatosis, angiomatosis, macrocephaly).
Hemangiomatosis and other vascular malformations (Klippel-Trenaunay and Parkes Weber).
Lymphangiomatosis.
Arteriovenous malformation.
Maffucci syndrome, Ollier disease.
Epidermal nevus syndrome.

BONE DENSITY, DECREASED, GENERALIZED[36]

ICD-10CM #		
	M85.80	Other specified disorders of bone density and structure, unspecified site

DISORDERS ASSOCIATED WITH GENERALIZED LOSS OF BONE DENSITY

Disorders of Multiple or Uncertain Cause

Senile osteoporosis.[8]
Juvenile osteoporosis.
Osteogenesis imperfecta.[9]

Secondary Bone Disorders

Endocrine

Adrenal cortex.
 Cushing's disease.
 Addison disease.
Gonadal disorders.
 Postmenopausal osteoporosis.
 Hypogonadism.
Pituitary.
 Acromegaly.
 Hypopituitarism.
Pancreas.
 Diabetes mellitus.
Thyroid.
 Hyperthyroidism.
 Hypothyroidism.
Parathyroid.
 Hyperparathyroidism.

Marrow Replacement and Expansion

Myeloma.
Leukemia.
Lymphoma.
Metastatic disease.
Gaucher disease.
Anemias (sickle cell, thalassaemia, hemophilia).

Drugs and Other Substances

Steroids.
Heparin (osteoporosis).
Anticonvulsants (osteomalacia).
Immunosuppressants.
Alcohol.

Chronic Disease

Chronic renal disease.
Hepatic insufficiency.
GI malabsorption syndromes.
Chronic inflammatory polyarthropathies.
Chronic debility or immobilization.

[8] Patients who cannot synthesize Lewis blood group antigens (~5% of the population) do not produce CA–19–9 antigen.
[9] Common cause of decrease in bone density in children.
*Common cause of decrease in bone density in adults.

BONE DENSITY, DECREASED, LOCALIZED[36]

ICD-10CM #		
	Z82.62	Family history of osteoporosis
	M85.80	Other specified disorders of bone density and structure, unspecified site

DISORDERS ASSOCIATED WITH LOCALIZED LOSS OF BONE DENSITY

Disuse osteoporosis.[10]
Reflex sympathetic dystrophy (Sudeck).
Osteolytic syndromes.
 Acro-osteolysis, primary and secondary.
 Massive osteolysis of Gorham.
 Carpotarsal osteolysis.
Transient regional osteoporosis.
Neuromuscular disorders.
Infection.
Arthropathies.
Tumors, primary and secondary, myelomatosis.

[10] Common causes.

BONE LESIONS, PREFERENTIAL SITE OF ORIGIN[76]

ICD-10CM #		
	C41.0	Malignant neoplasm of bones of skull and face
	C41.1	Malignant neoplasm of mandible
	C41.2	Malignant neoplasm of vertebral column
	C41.3	Malignant neoplasm of ribs, sternum and clavicle
	C40.00	Malignant neoplasm of scapula and long bones of unspecified upper limb
	C40.10	Malignant neoplasm of short bones of unspecified upper limb
	C41.4	Malignant neoplasm of pelvic bones, sacrum, and coccyx
	C40.20	Malignant neoplasm of long bones of unspecified lower limb
	C40.30	Malignant neoplasm of short bones of unspecified lower limb
	C41.9	Malignant neoplasm of bone and articular cartilage, unspecified
	C79.51	Secondary malignant neoplasm of bone
	C79.52	Secondary malignant neoplasm of bone marrow

EPIPHYSIS

Chondroblastoma.
Giant cell tumor—after fusion of growth plate.
Langerhans cell histiocytosis.
Clear cell chondrosarcoma.
Osteosarcoma.

METAPHYSIS

Parosteal sarcoma.
Chondrosarcoma.
Fibrosarcoma.
Nonossifying fibroma.
Giant cell tumor—before fusion of growth plate.
Unicameral bone cyst.
Aneurysmal bone cyst.

DIAPHYSIS

Myeloma.
Ewing tumor.
Reticulum cell sarcoma.

METADIAPHYSEAL

Fibrosarcoma.
Fibrous dysplasia.
Enchondroma.
Osteoid osteoma.
Chondromyofibroma.

BONE MARROW FAILURE SYNDROMES, INHERITED[43]

ICD-10CM # D61.89 Other specified aplastic anemias and other bone marrow failure syndromes

BI-LINEAGE AND TRI-LINEAGE CYTOPENIAS

Fanconi anemia.
Shwachman-Diamond syndrome.
Dyskeratosis congenita.
Amegakaryocytic thrombocytopenia:
 Other inherited thrombocytopenia disorders.
Other genetic syndromes:
 Down syndrome.
 Dubowitz syndrome.
 Seckel syndrome.
 Reticular dysgenesis.
 Schimke immunoosseous dysplasia.
 Noonan syndrome.
 Cartilage-hair hypoplasia.
 Familial marrow failure (non-Fanconi).

UNI-LINEAGE CYTOPENIA

Diamond-Blackfan anemia.
Kostmann syndrome/Congenital neutropenia:
 ELA2 mutations.
 HAX1 mutations.
 GFI1 mutations.
 WASP mutations.
 Constitutive cell surface G-CSF-R mutations.
Other inherited neutropenia syndromes:
 Barth syndrome.
 Glycogen storage disease 1b.
 Miscellaneous.
Thrombocytopenia with absent radii.
Congenital dyserythropoietic anemias (CDAs):
 Types I, II, III, IV.
 Variants.
 Nonclassifiable CDAs.
 Groups IV, V, VI, VII.

BONE MARROW FIBROSIS[32]

ICD-10CM # D75.9 Disease of blood and blood-forming organs, unspecified

MYELOID DISORDERS

Myelofibrosis with myeloid metaplasia.
Metastatic cancer.
Chronic myeloid leukemia.
Myelodysplastic syndrome.
Atypical myeloid disorder.
Acute megakaryocytic leukemia.
Other acute myeloid leukemias.
Gray platelet syndrome.

LYMPHOID DISORDERS

Hairy cell leukemia.
Multiple myeloma.
Lymphoma.

NONHEMATOLOGIC DISORDERS

Connective tissue disorder.
Infections (tuberculosis, kala-azar).
Vitamin D deficiency (rickets).
Renal osteodystrophy.

BONE MASS, LOW[3]

ICD-10CM # M85.80 Other specified disorders of bone density and structure, unspecified site

SECONDARY CAUSES OF LOW BONE MASS

Endocrine Diseases
Female hypogonadism.
Hyperprolactinemia.
Hypothalamic amenorrhea.
Anorexia nervosa.
Premature and primary ovarian failure.
Female athlete triad.
Male hypogonadism.
Primary gonadal failure (e.g., Klinefelter syndrome).
Secondary gonadal failure (e.g., idiopathic hypogonadotropic hypogonadism, androgen deprivation therapy for prostate cancer).
Hyperthyroidism.
Hyperparathyroidism.
Hypercortisolism.
Vitamin D insufficiency or deficiency.
Gastrointestinal Diseases
Subtotal gastrectomy.
Gastric bypass surgery.
Malabsorption syndromes.
Chronic obstructive jaundice.
Primary biliary cirrhosis and other cirrhoses.
Bone Marrow Disorders
Multiple myeloma.
Monoclonal gammopathy of unknown significance (MGUS).
Lymphoma.
Leukemia.
Hemolytic anemias.
Systemic mastocytosis.
Disseminated carcinoma.
Connective Tissue Diseases
Osteogenesis imperfecta.
Ehlers-Danlos syndrome.
Marfan syndrome.
Homocystinuria.
Drugs
Alcohol.
Antiseizure medications.
Aromatase inhibitors.
Chemotherapy.
Cyclosporine.
Depo-medroxyprogesterone.
Excess thyroid hormone.
Glucocorticoids.
Gonadotropin-releasing hormone agonists.
Heparin.
Miscellaneous Causes
Immobilization.
Rheumatoid arthritis.
Chronic obstructive pulmonary disease.
Weight loss.

BONE MINERAL DENSITY, INCREASED

ICD-10CM # M89.30 Hypertrophy of bone, unspecified site
M89.8X9 Other specified disorders of bone, unspecified site
M94.8X9 Other specified disorders of cartilage, unspecified sites

Paget disease of bone.
Skeletal metastases.
DISH.
Osteonecrosis.
Sarcoidosis.
Hypoparathyroidism, pseudohypoparathyroidism.
Milk-alkali syndrome.
Osteopetrosis.
Hypervitaminosis A or D.
Dysplasias (craniodiaphyseal, craniometaphyseal, frontometaphyseal).
Endosteal hyperostosis.
Fluorosis.
Heavy metal poisoning.
Ionizing radiation.
Other: lymphoma, leukemia, mastocytosis, multiple myeloma, polycythemia vera.

BONE PAIN

ICD-10CM # M89.8 Pain, bone

Trauma.
Neoplasm (primary or metastatic).
Osteoporosis with compression fracture.
Paget disease of bone.
Infection (osteomyelitis, septic arthritis).
Osteomalacia.
Viral syndrome.
Sickle cell disease.
Anxiety.

BONE RESORPTION[76]

ICD-10CM # M89.9 Disorder of bone, unspecified
M94.9 Disorder of cartilage, unspecified

DISTAL CLAVICLE

Hyperparathyroidism.
RA.
Scleroderma.
Posttraumatic osteolysis.
Progeria.
Pycnodysostosis.
Cleidocranial dysplasia.

INFERIOR ASPECT OF RIBS

Vascular impression, associated with but not limited to coarctation of the aorta.
Hyperparathyroidism.
Neurofibromatosis.

TERMINAL PHALANGEAL TUFTS

Scleroderma.
Raynaud's phenomenon.

Vascular disease.
Frostbite, electrical burns.
Psoriasis.
Tabes dorsalis.
Hyperparathyroidism.

GENERALIZED RESORPTION

Paraplegia.
Myositis ossificans.
Osteoporosis.

BOWEL WALL THICKENING[84]

ICD-10CM #	Varies with specific diagnosis

BENIGN VERSUS MALIGNANT BOWEL WALL THICKENING

Benign

Homogeneous attenuation.
Symmetrical.
Circumferential.
Thickening <1 cm.
Segmental or diffuse involvement.
Double halo sign.
Dark inner ring.
Bright outer ring.
Target sign.
Bright inner ring.
Dark middle ring.
Bright outer ring.

Malignant

Heterogeneous attenuation.
Asymmetrical.
Eccentric.
Thickening >1 to 2 cm.
Focal mass.
Abrupt transition.
Lobulated contour.
Spiculated contour.
Narrowed bowel lumen.
Enlarged lymph nodes.
Liver metastases.

BOW LEGS (GENU VARUM), CLASSIFICATION[51]

ICD-10CM #	E64.3	Genu varum, acquired
	Q74.1	Congenital malformation of knee

PHYSIOLOGIC

Asymmetric Growth

Tibia vara (Blount disease).
  Infantile.
  Juvenile.
  Adolescent.
Focal fibrocartilaginous dysplasia.
Physeal injury.
Trauma.
Infection.
Tumor.

METABOLIC DISORDERS

Vitamin D deficiency (nutritional rickets).
Vitamin D–resistant rickets.
Hypophosphatasia.

SKELETAL DYSPLASIA

Metaphyseal dysplasia.
Achondroplasia.
Enchondromatosis.

BRACHYCARDIA, ICU PATIENT[83]

ICD-10CM #	R00.1	Bradycardia, unspecified

COMMON CAUSES OF BRADYCARDIA IN THE ICU

Medications: antiarrhythmics, β-blockers, calcium channel blockers, clonidine, dexmedetomidine, digoxin, lithium, opioids, phenytoin, and propofol.
Age-related degeneration.
Cardiac ischemia.
Electrolyte abnormalities.
Elevated intracranial pressure.
Elevated vagal tone.
Endotracheal intubation.
Hypertension.
Hypothermia.
Hypothyroidism.
Hypoxia.
Inflammatory disease.
Obstructive sleep apnea.
Post-cardiac surgery

BRADYCARDIA, SINUS[33]

ICD-10CM #	I49.8	Other specified cardiac arrhythmias
	R00.1	Bradycardia, unspecified

Idiopathic.
Degenerative processes (e.g., Lev disease, Lenègre disease).

Medications

  β-Blockers.
  Some calcium channel blockers (diltiazem, verapamil).
  Digoxin (when vagal tone is high).
  Class I antiarrhythmic agents (e.g., procainamide).
  Class III antiarrhythmic agents (amiodarone, sotalol).
  Clonidine.
  Lithium carbonate.

ACUTE MYOCARDIAL ISCHEMIA AND INFARCTION

Right or left circumflex coronary artery occlusion or spasm.
High vagal tone (e.g., athletes).

BRAIN MASS[1]

ICD-10CM #	C71	Malignant neoplasm of brain
	D33	Benign neoplasm of brain
	I61.9	Intracranial hemorrhage, unspecified

METASTATIC BRAIN TUMOR

Primary Brain Tumor

Meningioma.
Glioma.
Pituitary adenoma.
Vestibular schwannoma.
Primary or secondary CNS lymphoma.

Infections

Abscess.
Toxoplasmosis.
Neurocysticercosis.
Tuberculoma.
Progressive multifocal leukoencephalopathy.

VASCULAR DISEASE

Hemorrhage

Anomalies (arteriovenous malformation).
Intratumoral.
Hypertensive.

Infarct

Embolism.
Thrombosis (sinus venous).

Inflammatory

Multiple sclerosis.
Encephalomyelitis.

BREAST INFLAMMATORY LESION[24]

ICD-10CM #	N61	Inflammatory disorders of breast
	N60.19	Diffuse cystic mastopathy of unspecified breast
	P39.0	Neonatal infective mastitis
	P83.4	Breast engorgement of newborn

Mastitis (*S. aureus*, β-hemolytic *Streptococcus*).
Trauma.
Foreign body (sutures, breast implants).
Granuloma (TB, fungal).
Fat necrosis post biopsy.
Necrosis or infarction (anticoagulant therapy, pregnancy).
Breast malignancy.

BREAST MASS

ICD-10CM #	N63	Unspecified lump in breast

Fibrocystic breasts.
Benign tumors (fibroadenoma, papilloma).
Mastitis (acute bacterial mastitis, chronic mastitis).
Malignant neoplasm.
Fat necrosis.
Hematoma.
Duct ectasia.
Mammary adenosis.

BREATH ODOR[73]

ICD-10CM #	R19.6	Halitosis

Sweet, fruity: DKA, starvation ketosis.
Fishy, stale: uremia (trimethylamines).

Ammonia-like: uremia (ammonia).
Musty fish, clover: fetor hepaticus (hepatic failure).
Foul, feculent: intestinal obstruction/diverticulum.
Foul, putrid: nasal/sinus pathology (infection, foreign body, cancer), respiratory infections (empyema, lung abscess, bronchiectasis).
Halitosis: tonsillitis, gingivitis, respiratory infections, Vincent angina, gastroesophageal reflux, achalasia, certain foods (garlic, onions, protein drinks, etc.)
Cinnamon: pulmonary TB.

BREATHING, NOISY[73]

ICD-10CM #	Code	Description
	R06.00	Dyspnea, unspecified
	R06.09	Other forms of dyspnea
	R06.3	Periodic breathing
	R06.83	Snoring
	R06.89	Other abnormalities of breathing
	R06.1	Stridor

Infection: upper respiratory infection, peritonsillar abscess, retropharyngeal abscess, epiglottitis, laryngitis, tracheitis, bronchitis, bronchiolitis.
Irritants and allergens: hyperactive airway, asthma (reactive airway disease), rhinitis, angioneurotic edema.
Compression from outside of the airway: esophageal cysts or foreign body, neoplasms, lymphadenopathy.
Congenital malformation and abnormality: vascular rings, laryngeal webs, laryngomalacia, tracheomalacia, hemangiomas within the upper airway, stenoses within the upper airway, cystic fibrosis.
Acquired abnormality (at every level of the airway): nasal polyps, hypertrophied adenoids and/or tonsils, foreign body, intraluminal tumors, bronchiectasis.
Neurogenic disorder: vocal cord paralysis.

BRONCHIAL OBSTRUCTION[36]

ICD-10CM # J98.0 Tracheobronchial collapse

CAUSES OF BRONCHIAL OBSTRUCTION

Outside the Bronchus
Lymph nodes and other masses.
In the Wall of the Bronchus
Tumors
Lung carcinoma (commonly squamous cell).
Bronchial carcinoid.
Metastasis.
Hamartoma.
Inflammation
Tuberculosis.
Sarcoidosis.
Granulomatosis with polyangiitis.
Inflammatory bowel disease.
Bronchomalacia
Broncholith.
Inside the Bronchus
Mucus plug.
Inhaled foreign body.

BRONCHOPLEURAL FISTULA[36]

ICD-10CM # J86.0 Bronchopleural fistula

CAUSES OF BRONCHOPLEURAL FISTULA

Trauma
Penetrating.
Iatrogenic (especially postpneumonectomy, postlobectomy, postbiopsy).
Infection
Necrotizing pneumonia.
Empyema.
Tuberculosis.
Septic embolus.
Infected pulmonary infarct.

BROWN URINE

ICD-10CM # R82 Other abnormal findings in urine

Bile pigments.
Myoglobin.
Concentrated urine.
Use of multivitamin supplements.
Medications (antimalarials, metronidazole, nitrofurantoin, levodopa, methyldopa, phenazopyridine).
Diet rich in fava beans.
Urinary tract infection.

BRUISING

ICD-10CM # I99.8 Other disorder of circulatory system

Medication-induced (warfarin, aspirin, NSAIDs, prednisone).
Alcohol abuse.
Senile purpura.
Purpura simplex.
Physical abuse.
Vasculitis.
Platelet disorders.
Coagulation factor deficiencies.
Cushing's disease.
Vitamin C deficiency.
Marfan syndrome.
Ehlers-Danlos syndrome.
Disseminated intravascular coagulation.
Leukemia.
Hereditary hemorrhagic telangiectasia.

BULLOUS DISEASES

ICD-10CM #	Code	Description
	L13.9	Bullous disorder, unspecified
	L12.0	Bullous pemphigoid
	L12.8	Other pemphigoid
	L10.0	Pemphigus vulgaris
	L10.1	Pemphigus vegetans
	L10.2	Pemphigus foliaceous
	L10.4	Pemphigus erythematosus
	L10.9	Pemphigus, unspecified

Bullous pemphigoid.
Pemphigus vulgaris.
Pemphigus foliaceus.
Paraneoplastic pemphigus.
Cicatricial pemphigoid.
Erythema multiforme.
Dermatitis herpetiformis.
Herpes gestationis.
Impetigo.
Erosive lichen planus.
Linear IgA bullous dermatosis.
Epidermolysis bullosa acquisita

CAFÉ-AU-LAIT SPOTS[51]

ICD-10CM # L81.3 Cafe au lait apots

Neurofibromatosis types 1 and 2.
McCune-Albright syndrome.
Russell-Silver syndrome.
Ataxia-telangiectasia.
Fanconi anemia.
Tuberous sclerosis.
Bloom syndrome.
Basal cell nevus syndrome.
Gaucher disease.
Chédiak-Higashi syndrome.
Hunter syndrome.
Maffucci syndrome.
Multiple mucosal neuroma syndrome.
Watson syndrome.
Proteus syndrome.
Turner syndrome.
Ring chromosome syndrome.
Jaffe-Campanacci syndrome.

CALCIFICATION ON CHEST X-RAY

ICD-10CM #	Code	Description
	J98.4	Calcification of lung
	M51.84	Other intervertebral disc disorders, thoracic region
	M51.85	Other intervertebral disc disorders, thoracolumbar region

Lung neoplasm (primary or metastatic).
Silicosis.
Idiopathic pulmonary fibrosis.
Tuberculosis.
Histoplasmosis.
Disseminated varicella infection.
Mitral stenosis (end-stage).
Secondary hyperparathyroidism.

CALCIFICATIONS, ABDOMINAL, NONVISCERAL ON X-RAY[36]

ICD-10CM # M61.9 Calcification and ossification of muscle, unspecified

NONVISCERAL ABDOMINAL CALCIFICATION

Common
Atherosclerosis.
Mesenteric lymph nodes.

Phleboliths.
Aneurysm.
Dermoid cyst.
Differentiate
Rib cartilage.
Injections in the buttocks.
Uncommon
Infestations.
Armillifer armillatus.
Cysticercosis.
Guinea worm.
Hydatid.
Tumors.
Lipoma.
Hemangioma.
Neuroblastoma.
Osteo/chondrosarcoma of soft tissues.
Retroperitoneal sarcoma of soft tissues.
Peritoneal metastases.
Pheochromocytoma.
Tuberculosis.
Peritonitis.
Psoas abscess.
Meconium peritonitis.
Pseudomyxoma Peritonei
Mesenteric cyst.
Pancreatitis with saponification.
Lithopedion.
Appendices Epiploicae
Ligaments.
Foreign bodies.
Posttraumatic buttock cysts.

CALCIFICATIONS, ADRENAL GLAND ON X-RAY[36]

ICD-10CM #	E27.4	Calcification, adrenal gland

ADRENAL GLAND CALCIFICATION

Common
Idiopathic.
Hemorrhage.
Tuberculosis.
Neuroblastoma/ganglioneuroma.
Pheochromocytoma.
Uncommon
Other tumors:
Adenoma.
Carcinoma.
Dermoid.
Addison disease.
Cyst.
Histoplasmosis.

CALCIFICATIONS, CARDIAC ON X-RAY[36]

ICD-10CM #	I51.5	Calcification, myocardium
	I25.1	Calcification, arteriosclerotic

CAUSES OF VISIBLE CALCIFICATION WITHIN THE HEART

Coronary Artery
Atherosclerosis.
Aortic Root
Atherosclerotic aorta.
Thrombus.
Syphilis.
Ankylosing spondylitis.
Homograft calcification.
Pericardium
Chronic pericarditis, tuberculosis, hemopericardium, pyogenic or viral pericarditis.
Posttraumatic.
Postoperative.
Uremic pericarditis.
Asbestosis (may be pleural calcification applied to pericardium).
Myocardium
Ventricular aneurysm (may mimic pericardial calcification).
Calcified myocardial infarction.
Postmyocarditis.
Endocardium
Endomyocardial fibrosis.
Thrombus.
Valve Cusps
Calcified valves (particularly mitral and aortic valves).
Mitral annulus calcification.
Homograft calcification.
Old vegetation.
Valve Annulus
Submitral.
Mitral.
Aortic.
Left Atrium
Wall.
Thrombus.
Atrial myxoma.
Pulmonary Artery
Pulmonary hypertension.
Postoperative.
Postoperative serumoma calcified hydatid cyst.

CALCIFICATIONS, CUTANEOUS

ICD-10CM #	L94.2	Calcinosis cutis
	L98.8	Other specified disorders of the skin and subcutaneous tissue

Calcification, Raynaud's phenomenon, esophageal dysmotility, sclerodactyly, and telangiectasia (CREST) syndrome.
Trauma.
Pancreatitis or pancreatic cancer.
Chronic renal failure.
Sarcoidosis.
Hyperparathyroidism.
Milk-alkali syndrome.
Hypervitaminosis D.
Panniculitis.
Idiopathic.
Iatrogenic (e.g., application of calcium alginate dressing to skin).
Multiple myeloma.
Dermatomyositis.
Parasitic infections.
Leukemia.
Lymphoma.

CALCIFICATIONS, GENITAL TRACT, FEMALE ON X-RAY[36]

ICD-10CM #	E83.59	Other disorders of calcium metabolism

FEMALE GENITAL TRACT CALCIFICATION

Uterus
Leiomyomas.
Squamous cell carcinoma.
Adenocarcinoma of endometrium.
Leiomyosarcoma.
Lithopedion.
Fallopian Tubes
Ovary.
Dermoid cyst.
Serous cystadenoma/carcinoma.
Tuberculosis.
Cysts.
Autoamputation.

CALCIFICATIONS, LIVER ON X-RAY[36]

ICD-10CM #	K76.89	Other specified diseases of liver
	NEC K75.3	Granuloma, hepatic

LIVER CALCIFICATION

Common
Granuloma (tuberculosis, histoplasmosis, brucellosis).
Multiple scattered round densities.
Hydatid cyst.
Fine curvilinear in wall, or dense and irregular if contracted.
Primary liver tumor (hemangioma, hepatoblastoma, hepatoma, cholangiocarcinoma).
Irregular patterns or multiple nodules.
Metastases (mucinous primary of colon or breast, cystadenocarcinoma of ovary).
Finely stippled, may be extensive.
Uncommon
Hepatic artery aneurysm.
Armillifer armillatus infestation.
Chronic granulomatous disease of childhood.
Cyst (congenital or acquired).
Hematoma.
Intrahepatic gallstones.
Old liver abscess.
Portal vein thrombosis.
Differentiate
Hemochromatosis.
Thorotrast, thallium, iron.

CALCIFICATIONS, PANCREAS ON X-RAY[36]

ICD-10CM #	K86.8	Calcification, pancreas

PANCREATIC CALCIFICATION

Common
Chronic pancreatitis.
Uncommon
Acute pancreatitis (saponification).
Tumors.

Cystadenoma.
Cystadenocarcinoma.
Islet cell tumor.
Metastases.
Hereditary pancreatitis (large clumps).
Hemorrhage.
Hyperparathyroidism.
Pseudocyst.
Cavernous lymphangioma.
Mucoviscidosis.
Kwashiorkor.

CALCIFICATIONS, SPLEEN ON X-RAY[36]

ICD-10CM # D73.8 Calcification, spleen

SPLENIC CALCIFICATION

Larger than 10 mm
Splenic artery aneurysm.
Splenic artery atheroma.
Cyst:
Posttraumatic.
Dermoid.
Epidermoid.
Hydatid.
Hematoma.
Infarct.
Abscess.
Tuberculosis.

Smaller than 10 mm
Histoplasmosis.
Tuberculosis.
Phleboliths.
Armillifer armillatus infestation.
Brucellosis.
Infarcts.

CALCIFICATIONS, VALVULAR ON X-RAY[36]

ICD-10CM # I51.5 Calcification, heart

CAUSES OF RADIOGRAPHICALLY VISIBLE VALVE CALCIFICATION

Aortic Valve
Rheumatic aortic valve disease.
Bicuspid aortic valve.
Age/degenerate aortic valve.
Syphilis.
Ankylosing spondylitis.
Homograft calcification.

Mitral Valve
Rheumatic mitral valve disease.
Mitral annulus calcification.
Old vegetation (may only be visible on CT).
Homograft calcification.

Pulmonary Valve
Congenital pulmonary valve stenosis.
Rheumatic pulmonary valve disease (rare).
Fallot tetralogy (usually after repair).
Pulmonary hypertension.
Homograft calcification.

Tricuspid Valve
Rheumatic tricuspid valve disease.
Old vegetation (may only be visible on ultrafast CT).

CALCIUM STONES

ICD-10CM # N20.9 Urinary calculus, unspecified

Medications (e.g., antacids, loop diuretics, vitamin D, acetazolamide, glucocorticoids).
Primary hyperparathyroidism.
Hypercalcemia from malignancy.
Sarcoidosis.
Prolonged immobilization.
Hyperoxaluria (e.g., Crohn's disease, celiac disease, chronic pancreatitis).
Hyperuricosuria (e.g., hyperuricemia, excessive dietary purine, allopurinol, probenecid).
Renal tubular acidosis.
Milk-alkali syndrome.
Thyrotoxicosis.
Hypocitraturia (e.g., metabolic acidosis, hypomagnesemia, hypokalemia).

CARDIAC ARREST, NONTRAUMATIC[55]

ICD-10CM # I46.9 Cardiac arrest, cause unspecified

Cardiac (coronary artery disease, cardiomyopathies, structural abnormalities, valve dysfunction, arrhythmias).
Respiratory (upper airway obstruction, hypoventilation, pulmonary embolism, asthma, COPD exacerbation, pulmonary edema).
Circulatory (tension pneumothorax, pericardial tamponade, PE, hemorrhage, sepsis).
Electrolyte abnormalities (hypokalemia or hyperkalemia, hypomagnesemia or hypermagnesemia, hypocalcemia).
Medications (tricyclic antidepressants, digoxin, theophylline, calcium channel blockers).
Drug abuse (cocaine, heroin, amphetamines).
Toxins (carbon monoxide, cyanide).
Environmental (drowning/near-drowning, electrocution, lightning, hypothermia or hyperthermia, venomous snakes).

CARDIAC DEATH, SUDDEN[3]

ICD-10CM # Z86.74 Personal history of sudden cardiac arrest

Ventricular tachycardia.
Bradyarrhythmia, sick sinus syndrome.
Aortic stenosis.
Tetralogy of Fallot.
Pericardial tamponade.
Cardiac tumors.
Complications of infective endocarditis.
Hypertrophic cardiomyopathy (arrhythmia or obstruction).
Myocardial ischemia.
Atherosclerosis.
Prinzmetal angina.
Kawasaki arteritis.

CARDIAC ENLARGEMENT[33]

ICD-10CM # I51.7 Cardiomegaly
Q23.8 Other congenital malformations of aortic and mitral valves
Q24.8 Other specified congenital malformations of heart
I11.9 Hypertensive heart disease without heart failure

CHAMBER ENLARGEMENT

Chronic Volume Overload
Mitral or aortic regurgitation.
Left-to-right shunt (PDA, VSD, AV fistula).

Cardiomyopathy
Ischemic.
Nonischemic.

Decompensated Pressure Overload
Aortic stenosis.
Hypertension.

High-Output States
Severe anemia.
Thyrotoxicosis.

Bradycardia
Severe sinus bradycardia.
Complete heart block.

LEFT ATRIUM

LV failure of any cause.
Mitral valve disease.
Myxoma.

RIGHT VENTRICLE

Chronic volume overload.
Tricuspid or pulmonic regurgitation.
Left-to-right shunt (ASD).
Decompensated pressure overload:
Pulmonic stenosis.
Pulmonary artery hypertension:
Primary.
Secondary (PE, COPD).
Pulmonary venoocclusive disease.

RIGHT ATRIUM

RV failure of any cause.
Tricuspid valve disease.
Myxoma.
Ebstein anomaly.

MULTICHAMBER ENLARGEMENT

Hypertrophic cardiomyopathy.
Acromegaly.
Severe obesity.

PERICARDIAL DISEASE

Pericardial effusion with or without tamponade.
Effusive constrictive disease.
Pericardial cyst, loculated effusion.

PSEUDOCARDIOMEGALY

Epicardial fat.
Chest wall deformity (pectus excavatum, straight back syndrome).
Low lung volumes.
AP chest x-ray.
Mediastinal tumor, cyst.

CARDIAC MURMURS

ICD-10CM # R01.0 Benign and innocent cardiac murmurs
R01.1 Cardiac murmur, unspecified

SYSTOLIC

Mitral regurgitation (MR).
Tricuspid regurgitation (TR).
Ventricular septal defect (VSD).
Aortic stenosis (AS).
Idiopathic hypertrophic subaortic stenosis (IHSS).
Pulmonic stenosis (PS).
Innocent murmur of childhood.
Coarctation of aorta.
Mitral valve prolapse (MVP).

DIASTOLIC

Aortic regurgitation (AR).
Atrial myxoma.
Mitral stenosis (MS).
Pulmonary artery branch stenosis.
Tricuspid stenosis (TS).
Graham Steell murmur (diastolic decrescendo murmur heard in severe pulmonary hypertension).
Pulmonic regurgitation (PR).
Severe mitral regurgitation (MR).
Austin Flint murmur (diastolic rumble heard in severe AR).
Severe VSD and patent ductus arteriosus.

CONTINUOUS

Patent ductus arteriosus.
Pulmonary AV fistula.

CARDIAC TUMORS[34]

ICD-10CM #		
	C38.0	Malignant neoplasm of heart
	D15.1	Benign neoplasm of heart

PRIMARY

Benign.
- Myxoma.
- Lipoma.
- Fibroma.
- Rhabdomyoma.
- Fibroelastoma.

Malignant.
- Sarcoma.
- Mesothelioma.
- Lymphoma.

SECONDARY

Direct Extension

Lung cancer.
Breast cancer.
Mediastinal tumors.

Metastatic Tumors

Malignant melanoma.
Leukemia.
Lymphoma.

Venous Extension

Renal cell cancer.
Adrenal cancer.
Liver cancer.

CARDIOEMBOLISM

ICD-10CM #		
	I21.3 ST	Elevation (STEMI) myocardial infarction of unspecified site
	I21.9	Acute myocardial infarction, unspecified

Acute MI.
Atrial fibrillation.
Left ventricular aneurysm.
Valvular heart disease (e.g., rheumatic mitral valve disease, mitral valve prolapse).
Dilated cardiomyopathy.
Atrial septal defect.
Patent foramen ovale.
Cardioversion for atrial fibrillation.
Infective endocarditis.
Atrial septal aneurysm.
Sick sinus syndrome and cardiac arrhythmias.
Nonbacterial thrombotic endocarditis.
Prosthetic heart valves.
Atrial myxoma and other intracardiac tumors.
Cyanotic heart disease.
Balloon angioplasty.
Coronary artery bypass grafting.
Aneurysms of sinus of Valsalva.
Other: VVI pacing, ventricular support devices, heart transplantation, intracardiac defects with paradoxical embolism.

CARDIOGENIC SHOCK

ICD-10CM #		
	R57.0	Cardiogenic shock

Myocardial infarction.
Arrhythmias.
Pericardial effusion/tamponade.
Chest trauma.
Valvular heart disease.
Myocarditis.
Cardiomyopathy.
CHF, end-stage.

CATARACTS, PEDIATRIC AGE

ICD-10CM #		
	H26.0	Infantile, juvenile and presenile cataracts

DEVELOPMENTAL VARIANTS

Prematurity (Y-suture vacuoles) with or without retinopathy of prematurity.

GENETIC DISORDERS

Simple Mendelian Inheritance

Autosomal dominant (most common).
Autosomal recessive.
X-linked.

Major Chromosomal Defects

Trisomy disorders (13, 18, 21).
Turner syndrome (45X).
Deletion syndromes (11p13, 18p, 18q).
Duplication syndromes (3q, 20p, 10q).

Multisystem Genetic Disorders

Alport syndrome (hearing loss, renal disease).
Alström syndrome (nerve deafness, diabetes mellitus).
Apert disease (craniosynostosis, syndactyly).
Cockayne syndrome (premature senility, skin photosensitivity).
Conradi disease (chondrodysplasia punctata).
Crouzon disease (dysostosis craniofacialis).
Hallermann-Streiff syndrome (microphthalmia, small pinched nose, skin atrophy, hypotrichosis).
Hypohidrotic ectodermal dysplasia (anomalous dentition, hypohidrosis, hypotrichosis).
Ichthyosis (keratinizing disorder with thick, scaly skin).
Incontinentia pigmenti (dental anomalies, mental retardation, cutaneous lesions).
Lowe syndrome (oculocerebrorenal syndrome: hypotonia, renal disease).
Marfan syndrome.
Marinesco-Sjögren syndrome (cerebellar ataxia, hypotonia).
Meckel-Gruber syndrome (renal dysplasia, encephalocele).
Myotonic dystrophy.
Nail-patella syndrome (renal dysfunction, dysplastic nails, hypoplastic patella).
Nevoid basal cell carcinoma syndrome (autosomal dominant, basal cell carcinoma erupts in childhood).
Peters anomaly (corneal opacifications with iris-corneal dysgenesis).
Reiger syndrome (iris dysplasia, myotonic dystrophy).
Rothmund-Thomson syndrome (poikiloderma: skin atrophy).
Rubinstein-Taybi syndrome (broad great toe, mental retardation).
Smith-Lemli-Opitz syndrome (toe syndactyly, hypospadias, mental retardation).
Sotos syndrome (cerebral gigantism).
Spondyloepiphyseal dysplasia (dwarfism, short trunk).
Werner syndrome (premature aging in 2nd decade of life).

Inborn Errors of Metabolism

Abetalipoproteinemia (absent chylomicrons, retinal degeneration).
Fabry disease (α-galactosidase A deficiency).
Galactokinase deficiency.
Galactosemia (galactose-1-phosphate uridyl transferase deficiency).
Homocystinemia (subluxation of lens, mental retardation).
Mannosidosis (acid α-mannosidase deficiency).
Niemann-Pick disease (sphingomyelinase deficiency).
Refsum disease (phytanic acid α-hydrolase deficiency).
Wilson disease (accumulation of copper leads to cirrhosis and neurologic symptoms).

ENDOCRINOPATHIES

Hypocalcemia (hypoparathyroidism).
Hypoglycemia.
Diabetes mellitus.

CONGENITAL INFECTIONS

Toxoplasmosis.
Cytomegalovirus infection.
Syphilis.
Rubella.
Perinatal herpes simplex infection.
Measles (rubeola).
Poliomyelitis.
Influenza.
Varicella-zoster.

OCULAR ANOMALIES

Microphthalmia.
Coloboma.
Aniridia.

Mesodermal dysgenesis.
Persistent papillary membrane.
Posterior lenticonus.
Persistent hyperplastic primary vitreous.
Primitive hyaloid vascular system.

MISCELLANEOUS DISORDERS

Atopic dermatitis.
Drugs (corticosteroids).
Radiation.
Trauma.
Idiopathic.

CAVITARY LESION ON CHEST X-RAY[35]

ICD-10CM # R91.8 Other nonspecific abnormal finding of lung field

NECROTIZING INFECTIONS

Bacteria: anaerobes, *Staphylococcus aureus*, enteric gram-negative bacteria, *Pseudomonas aeruginosa*, Legionella species, *Haemophilus influenzae*, *Streptococcus pyogenes*, *Streptococcus pneumoniae*, *Rhodococcus*, *Actinomyces*.
Mycobacteria: *Mycobacterium tuberculosis*, *Mycobacterium kansasii*, MAI.
Bacteria-like: *Nocardia species*.
Fungi: *Coccidioides immitis*, *Histoplasma capsulatum*, *Blastomyces hominis*, *Aspergillus* species, *Mucor* species.
Parasitic: *Entamoeba histolytica*, *Echinococcus*, *Paragonimus westermani*.

CAVITARY INFARCTION

Bland infarction (with or without superimposed infection).
Lung contusion.

SEPTIC EMBOLISM

S. aureus, anaerobes, others.

VASCULITIS

Granulomatosis with polyangiitis, periarteritis.

NEOPLASMS

Bronchogenic carcinoma, metastatic carcinoma, lymphoma.

MISCELLANEOUS LESIONS

Cysts, blebs, bullae, or pneumatocele with or without fluid collections.
Sequestration.
Empyema with air-fluid level.
Bronchiectasis.

CEREBRAL INFARCTION SECONDARY TO INHERITED DISORDERS

ICD-10CM # I63.50 Cerebral infarction due to unspecified occlusion or stenosis of unspecified cerebral artery

Homocystinuria.
Marfan syndrome.
Ehlers-Danlos syndrome.
Rendu-Osler-Weber syndrome.
Pseudoxanthoma elasticum.
Fabry disease.

CEREBRAL VASCULITIS, CAUSES[29]

ICD-10CM # Varies with specific diagnosis

PRIMARY CEREBRAL VASCULITIDES

Takayasu arteritis.
Primary cerebral vasculitis.
Polyarteritis nodosa.

SECONDARY VASCULITIDES

Immune Disorders

Systemic lupus erythematosus.
Wegener granulomatosis.
Kawasaki syndrome.
Sarcoidosis.
Henoch-Schönlein purpura.

Primary Intracranial Infections

Bacterial meningitis (especially *Diplococcus pneumoniae*).
Tuberculous meningitis.
Mycotic infections.
Cat-scratch disease.
Human immunodeficiency virus/acquired immunodeficiency syndrome.
Malaria.
Lyme disease.
Rickettsial infections.
Brucellosis.

CEREBROVASCULAR DISEASE, ISCHEMIC[87]

ICD-10CM # I67.9 Cerebrovascular disease, unspecified

VASCULAR DISORDERS

Large-vessel atherothrombotic disease.
Lacunar disease.
Arterial-to-arterial embolization.
Carotid or vertebral artery dissection.
Fibromuscular dysplasia.
Migraine.
Venous thrombosis.
Radiation.
Complications of arteriography.
Multiple, progressive intracranial arterial occlusions.

INFLAMMATORY DISORDERS

Giant cell arteritis.
Polyarteritis nodosa.
SLE.
Granulomatous angiitis.
Takayasu disease.
Arteritis associated with amphetamine, cocaine, or phenylpropanolamine.
Syphilis, mucormycosis.
Sjögren syndrome.
Behçet's syndrome.

CARDIAC DISORDERS

Rheumatic heart disease.
Mural thrombus.
Arrhythmias.
Mitral valve prolapse.
Prosthetic heart valve.
Endocarditis.
Myxoma.
Paradoxical embolus.

HEMATOLOGIC DISORDERS

Thrombotic thrombocytopenic purpura.
Sickle cell disease.
Hypercoagulable states.
Polycythemia.
Thrombocytosis.
Leukocytosis.
Lupus anticoagulant.

CERVICAL INSTABILITY, PEDIATRIC

ICD-10CM # M50 Cervical disc disorders

CONGENITAL

Vertebral (Bony Anomalies)

Cranioocipital defects (occipital vertebrae, basilar impression, occipital dysplasias, condylar hypoplasia, occipitalized atlas).
Atlantoaxial defects (aplasia of atlas arch, aplasia of odontoid process).
Subaxial anomalies (failure of segmentation and/or fusion, spina bifida, spondylolisthesis).

Ligamentous or Combined Anomalies

Found at birth as an element of somatogenic aberration.

Syndromic Disorders

Down syndrome.
Klippel-Feil syndrome.
22q11.2 deletion syndrome.
Larsen syndrome.
Marfan syndrome.
Ehlers-Danlos syndrome.

ACQUIRED

Trauma.
Infection (pyogenic, granulomatous).
Tumor (including neurofibromatosis).
Inflammatory conditions (e.g., juvenile rheumatoid arthritis).
Osteochondrodysplasias (e.g., achondroplasia, diastrophic dysplasia, metatropic dysplasia, spondyloepiphyseal dysplasia).
Storage disorders (e.g., mucopolysaccharidoses).
Metabolic disorders (rickets).
Miscellaneous (including osteogenesis imperfecta, sequela of surgery).

CHEST PAIN, CHILDREN[9]

ICD-10CM # R07.9 Chest pain, unspecified
R07.82 Intercostal pain
R07.89 Other chest pain
R07.1 Chest pain on breathing
R07.81 Pleurodynia

MUSCULOSKELETAL (COMMON)

Trauma (accidental, abuse).
Exercise, overuse injury (strain, bursitis).
Costochondritis (Tietze syndrome).
Herpes zoster (cutaneous).
Pleurodynia.
Fibrositis.
Slipping rib.
Sickle cell anemia vasoocclusive crisis.
Osteomyelitis (rare).
Primary or metastatic tumor (rare).

PULMONARY (COMMON)

Pneumonia.
Pleurisy.
Asthma.
Chronic cough.
Pneumothorax.
Infarction (sickle cell anemia).
Foreign body.
Embolism (rare).
Pulmonary hypertension (rare).
Tumor (rare).

GASTROINTESTINAL (LESS COMMON)

Esophagitis (gastroesophageal reflux).
Esophageal foreign body.
Esophageal spasm.
Cholecystitis.
Subdiaphragmatic abscess.
Perihepatitis (Fitz-Hugh-Curtis syndrome).
Peptic ulcer disease.

CARDIAC (LESS COMMON)

Pericarditis.
Postpericardiotomy syndrome.
Endocarditis.
Mitral valve prolapse.
Aortic or subaortic stenosis.
Arrhythmias.
Marfan syndrome (dissecting aortic aneurysm).
Anomalous coronary artery.
Kawasaki disease.
Cocaine, sympathomimetic ingestion.
Angina (familial hypercholesterolemia).

IDIOPATHIC (COMMON)

Anxiety, hyperventilation.
Panic disorder.

OTHER (LESS COMMON)

Spinal cord or nerve root compression.
Breast-related pathologic condition.
Castleman disease (lymph node neoplasm).

CHEST PAIN, NONPLEURITIC[20]

ICD-10CM #		
	R07.9	Chest pain, unspecified
	R07.82	Intercostal pain
	R07.89	Other chest pain

Cardiac: myocardial ischemia/infarction, myocarditis.
Esophageal: spasm, esophagitis, ulceration, neoplasm, achalasia, diverticula, foreign body.
Referred pain from subdiaphragmatic GI structures.
Gastric and duodenal: hiatal hernia, neoplasm, PUD.
Gallbladder and biliary: cholecystitis, cholelithiasis, impacted stone, neoplasm.
Pancreatic: pancreatitis, neoplasm.
Dissecting aortic aneurysm.
Pain originating from skin, breasts, and musculoskeletal structures: herpes zoster, mastitis, cervical spondylosis.
Mediastinal tumors: lymphoma, thymoma.
Pulmonary: neoplasm, pneumonia, pulmonary embolism/infarction.
Psychoneurosis.
Chest pain associated with mitral valve prolapse.

CHEST PAIN, PLEURITIC

ICD-10CM #		
	R07.1	Chest pain on breathing
	R07.81	Pleurodynia

Cardiac: pericarditis, postpericardiotomy/Dressler syndrome.
Pulmonary: pneumothorax, hemothorax, embolism/infarction, pneumonia, empyema, neoplasm, bronchiectasis, pneumomediastinum, TB, carcinomatous effusion.
GI: liver abscess, pancreatitis, esophageal rupture, Whipple disease with associated pericarditis or pleuritis.
Subdiaphragmatic abscess.
Pain originating from skin and musculoskeletal tissues: costochondritis, chest wall trauma, fractured rib, interstitial fibrositis, myositis, strain of pectoralis muscle, herpes zoster, soft tissue and bone tumors.
Collagen vascular diseases with pleuritis.
Psychoneurosis.
Familial Mediterranean fever.

CHEST WALL TUMORS, PRIMARY[15]

ICD-10CM # Varies with specific diagnosis

SOFT TISSUE

Benign
Lipoma.
Hemangioma.
Lymphangioma.
Fibroma.
Rhabdomyoma.
Neurofibroma.
Desmoid tumor.
Malignant
Malignant fibrous histiocytoma.
Rhabdosarcoma.
Liposarcoma.
Neurofibrosarcoma.
Leiomyosarcoma.

BONY AND CARTILAGINOUS

Benign
Fibrous dysplasia.
Osteochondroma.
Chondroma.
Askin tumor.
Plasmacytoma.
Malignant
Chondrosarcoma.
Osteogenic sarcoma.
Ewing sarcoma.

CHIASMAL DISEASE[12]

ICD-10CM # Varies with specific diagnosis

CAUSES OF CHIASMAL DISEASE

Tumors
Pituitary adenomas.
Craniopharyngioma.
Meningioma.
Glioma.
Chordoma.
Dysgerminoma.
Nasopharyngeal tumors.
Metastases.
Non-neoplastic masses
Aneurysm.
Rathke pouch cysts.
Fibrous dysplasia.
Sphenoidal sinus mucocele.
Arachnoid cysts.
Miscellaneous
Demyelination.
Inflammation (e.g., sarcoidosis).
Trauma.
Radiation-induced necrosis.
Toxicity (e.g., ethambutol).
Vasculitis.

CHILDHOOD EOSINOPHILIA

ICD-10CM # D72.1 Eosinophilia

PHYSIOLOGIC

Prematurity.
Infants receiving hyperalimentation.
Familial.

INFECTIOUS

Parasitic (with tissue-invasive helminths, e.g., trichinosis, strongyloidiasis, pneumocystosis, filariasis, cysticercosis, cutaneous and visceral larva migrans, echinococcosis).
Bacterial (brucellosis, tularemia, cat-scratch disease, *Chlamydia*).
Fungal (histoplasmosis, blastomycosis, coccidioidomycosis, allergic bronchopulmonary aspergillosis).
Mycobacterial (tuberculosis, leprosy).
Viral (hepatitis A, hepatitis B, hepatitis C, Epstein-Barr virus).

PULMONARY

Allergic (rhinitis, asthma).
Loeffler syndrome.
Hypersensitivity pneumonitis.
Eosinophilic pneumonia.
Pulmonary interstitial eosinophilia.

DERMATOLOGIC

Atopic dermatitis.
Pemphigus.
Dermatitis herpetiformis.
Infantile eosinophilic pustular folliculitis.
Episodic angioedema and urticaria.
Eosinophilic fasciitis (Schulman syndrome).
Eosinophilic cellulitis (Wells syndrome).
Kimura disease.

ONCOLOGIC

Neoplasm (lung, GI, uterine).
Hodgkin's disease.
Leukemia.
Myelofibrosis.

IMMUNOLOGIC

T-cell immunodeficiencies.
Hyperimmunoglobulin E (Job) syndrome.
Wiskott-Aldrich syndrome.
Graft-versus-host disease.
Drug hypersensitivity.
Postirradiation.
Postsplenectomy.

ENDOCRINE

Postadrenalectomy.
Addison disease.
Panhypopituitarism.

CARDIOVASCULAR

Loeffler disease (fibroplastic endocarditis).
Congenital heart disease.
Hypersensitivity vasculitis.

GASTROINTESTINAL

Milk protein allergy.
Inflammatory bowel disease.
Eosinophilic esophagitis.
Eosinophilic gastroenteritis.

CHOLANGITIS, ACUTE[15]

ICD-10CM # K83.0 Cholangitis

NONIATROGENIC

Benign Conditions

Choledocholithiasis.
- Primary.
- Secondary.

Pancreatitis (chronic/acute), including pancreatic pseudocyst.
Papillary stenosis.
Mirizzi syndrome.
Choledochal cysts (type V, Caroli disease).
Primary sclerosing cholangitis.

Malignancies

Pancreatic cancer.
Cholangiocarcinoma.
Porta hepatis tumor/metastasis.

IATROGENIC

Obstructed biliary endoprosthesis.
Iatrogenic biliary stricture.
Direct surgical trauma.
Ischemia-induced stricture.
Anastomotic stricture (biliobiliary/bilioenteric anastomosis).

CHOLESTASIS[32]

ICD-10CM # K80.65 Calculus of gallbladder and bile duct with chronic cholecystitis with obstruction

EXTRAHEPATIC

Choledocholithiasis.
Bile duct stricture.
Cholangiocarcinoma.
Pancreatic carcinoma.
Chronic pancreatitis.
Papillary stenosis.
Ampullary cancer.
Primary sclerosing cholangitis.
Choledochal cysts.
Parasites (e.g., ascaris, clonorchis).
AIDS.
Cholangiography.
Biliary atresia.
Portal lymphadenopathy.
Mirizzi syndrome.

INTRAHEPATIC

Viral hepatitis.
Alcoholic hepatitis.
Drug induced.
Ductopenia syndromes.
Primary biliary cirrhosis.
Benign recurrent intrahepatic cholestasis.
Byler disease.
Primary sclerosing cholangitis.
Alagille syndrome.
Sarcoid.
Lymphoma.
Postoperative.
Total parenteral nutrition.
α-1-antitrypsin deficiency.

CHOLESTASIS, NEONATAL AND INFANTILE, DIFFERENTIAL DIAGNOSIS[51]

ICD-10CM # O26.6 Liver disorders in pregnancy, childbirth and the puerperium

INFECTIOUS

Generalized bacterial sepsis.
Viral hepatitis.
- Hepatitis A, B, C, D.
- Cytomegalovirus.
- Rubella virus.
- Herpesvirus: herpes simplex, human herpesvirus 6 and 7.
- Varicella virus.
- Coxsackievirus.
- Echovirus.
- Reovirus type 3.
- Parvovirus B19.
- HIV.
- Adenovirus.

Others.
- Toxoplasmosis.
- Syphilis.
- Tuberculosis.
- Listeriosis.
- Urinary tract infection.

TOXIC

Sepsis.
Parenteral nutrition related.
Drug related.

METABOLIC

Disorders of amino acid metabolism.
- Tyrosinemia.

Disorders of lipid metabolism.
- Wolman disease.
- Niemann-Pick disease (type C).
- Gaucher disease.

Cholesterol ester storage disease.
Disorders of carbohydrate metabolism.
- Galactosemia.
- Fructosemia.
- Glycogenosis IV.

Disorders of bile acid biosynthesis.
Other metabolic defects.
- α1-Antitrypsin deficiency.
- Cystic fibrosis.
- Hypopituitarism.
- Hypothyroidism.
- Zellweger (cerebrohepatorenal) syndrome.
- Neonatal iron storage disease.
- Indian childhood cirrhosis/infantile copper overload.
- Congenital disorders of glycosylation.
- Mitochondrial hepatopathies.
- Citrin deficiency.

GENETIC OR CHROMOSOMAL

Trisomy 17, 18, 21.
Donahue syndrome.

INTRAHEPATIC CHOLESTASIS SYNDROMES

"Idiopathic" neonatal hepatitis.
Alagille syndrome (arteriohepatic dysplasia).
Nonsyndromic bile duct paucity syndrome.
Intrahepatic cholestasis (PFIC):
- FIC-1 deficiency.
- BSEP deficiency.
- MDR3 deficiency.

Familial benign recurrent cholestasis associated with lymphedema (Aagenaes).
Congenital hepatic fibrosis.
Caroli disease (cystic dilatation of intrahepatic ducts).

EXTRAHEPATIC DISEASES

Biliary atresia.
Sclerosing cholangitis.
Bile duct stricture/stenosis.
Choledochal-pancreaticoductal junction anomaly.
Spontaneous perforation of the bile duct.
Choledochal cyst.
Mass (neoplasia, stone).
Bile/mucous plug ("inspissated bile").

MISCELLANEOUS

Shock and hypoperfusion.
Associated with enteritis.
Associated with intestinal obstruction.
Neonatal lupus erythematosus.

Myeloproliferative disease (trisomy 21).
Hemophagocytic lymphohistiocytosis.
Arthrogryposis cholestatic pigmentary syndrome.

CHOLESTATIC LIVER ENZYME ELEVATION, EXTRAHEPATIC CAUSES[26]

ICD-10CM # Varies with Specific Diagnosis

EXTRAHEPATIC CAUSES OF CHOLESTATIC LIVER ENZYMES IN ADULTS

Intrinsic

Choledocholithiasis.
Immune-mediated duct injury.
  Autoimmune pancreatitis.
  PSC.
Malignancy.
  Ampullary cancer.
  Cholangiocarcinoma.
Infections.
  AIDS cholangiopathy.
    Cytomegalovirus.
    Cryptosporidiosis.
    Microsporidiosis.
  Parasitic infections.
    Ascariasis.

Extrinsic

Malignancy.
  Gallbladder cancer.
  Metastases, including portal adenopathy from metastases.
  Pancreatic cancer.
Mirizzi syndrome.
Pancreatitis.
Pancreatic pseudocyst.

CHOLESTATIC LIVER ENZYME ELEVATION, INTRAHEPATIC CAUSES[26]

ICD-10CM # Varies with specific causes

INTRAHEPATIC CAUSES OF CHOLESTATIC LIVER ENZYME ELEVATIONS IN ADULTS

Drugs[11]

Bland cholestasis.
  Anabolic steroids.
  Estrogens.
Cholestatic hepatitis.
  Angiotensin-converting enzyme inhibitors: captopril, enalapril.
  Antimicrobials: amoxicillin-clavulanic acid, ketoconazole.
  Azathioprine.
  Chlorpromazine.
  NSAIDs: sulindac, piroxicam.
Granulomatous hepatitis.
  Allopurinol.
  Antibiotics: sulfonamides.
  Antiepileptics: carbamazepine, phenytoin.
  Cardiovascular agents: hydralazine, procainamide, quinidine.
  Phenylbutazone.
Vanishing bile duct syndrome.
  Amoxicillin-clavulanic acid.
  Chlorpromazine.
  Dicloxacillin.
  Flucloxacillin.
  Macrolides.

PBC

PSC

Granulomatous Liver Disease

Infections:
  Brucellosis.
  Fungal: histoplasmosis, coccidioidomycosis.
  Leprosy.
  Q fever.
  Schistosomiasis.
  TB, *Mycobacterium avium* complex, bacillus Calmette-Guérin.
Sarcoidosis.
Idiopathic granulomatous hepatitis.
Other:
  Crohn's disease.
  Heavy metal exposure: beryllium, copper.
  Hodgkin's disease.

Viral Hepatitis

HAV and HEV.
HBV and HCV, including fibrosing cholestatic hepatitis.
EBV.
Cytomegalovirus.

Idiopathic Adulthood Ductopenia

Genetic Conditions

Progressive familial intrahepatic cholestasis:
  Type 1 (formerly Byler disease).
  Type 2.
  Type 3.
Benign recurrent intrahepatic cholestasis:
  Type 1.
  Type 2.
CF.

Malignancy

Hepatocellular carcinoma.
Metastatic disease.
Paraneoplastic syndrome:
  Non-Hodgkin's lymphoma.
  Prostate cancer.
  Renal cell cancer.

Infiltrative Liver Disease

Amyloidosis.
Lymphoma.

Intrahepatic Cholestasis of Pregnancy

TPN
  Graft-versus-Host Disease
  Sepsis

[11] Categorized by histologic pattern. Drug lists are not meant to be comprehensive.

CHOREA

ICD-10CM # G25.4 Drug-induced chorea
G25.5 Other chorea

Medications (e.g., neuroleptics, tricyclics, antiparkinsonian drugs).
Cerebral palsy.
Huntington disease.
Benign hereditary chorea.
Thyroid disorder (hyperthyroidism, hypothyroidism).
Friedreich ataxia.
Ataxia-telangiectasia.
Hypoglycemia, hyperglycemia.
Electrolyte abnormalities (hyponatremia, hypocalcemia, hypomagnesemia, hypernatremia).
Vitamin B_{12} deficiency.
SLE.
Wilson's disease.
Alcohol.
Cocaine.
Carbon monoxide poisoning.
Mercury poisoning.

CHOREA, PEDIATRIC PATIENT[79]

ICD-10CM # G25.5 Other chorea

CAUSES OF CHOREA IN CHILDHOOD

Static Injury/Structural Disorders

Cerebral palsy.
Stroke.
Trauma.
Moyamoya disease.
Vasculitis.
Tumors.
Congenital malformations.
Joubert syndrome.

Hereditary/Degenerative Disorders

Ataxia-telangiectasia (A-T), and Ataxia-Telangiectasia-Like Disorder (ATLD).
Ataxia oculomotor apraxia (AOA) (includes AOA-1, AOA-2, and early onset cerebellar ataxia and hypoalbuminemia [EOCA-HA]).
Fahr disease.
Pantothenate kinase-associated neurodegeneration (PKAN, associated with mutations in the pantothenate kinase-2 (*PANK-2*) gene), and other causes of neuronal brain iron accumulation (NBIA).

Metabolic Disorders

Acyl-coA dehydrogenase deficiencies.
Mitochondrial disorders, including Leigh syndrome.
GM_1 gangliosidosis.
Lesch-Nyhan disease.
Niemann-Pick type C.
Methylmalonic aciduria.
Nonketotic hyperglycemia.
Kernicterus.
Hypoparathyroidism.
Propionic acidemia.
Hypernatremia.
Hypomagnesemia.
Hypocalcemia.
Hypo- or hyperglycemia.
Vitamin E deficiency or malabsorption.
Bassen-Kornzweig syndrome.
Complications of cardiac bypass.

Infectious/Parainfectious Disease

Encephalitis/postencephalitis.

Immune-Mediated/Demyelinating Disorders

Sydenham chorea.
Lupus erythematosus.
Henoch-Schönlein purpura.
Anticardiolipin or antiphospholipid antibody syndrome.

Anti-NMDA antibody syndrome.

Drugs/Toxins

Neuroleptic medications, and neuroleptic-like antiemetics (haloperidol, chlorpromazine, pimozide, prochlorperazine, metoclopramide).
Calcium channel blockers (flunarizine, cinnarizine).
Antiseizure medications (phenytoin, carbamazepine, valproate, phenobarbital).
Anticholinergic medications (trihexyphenidyl, benztropine).
Antihistamines.
Tricyclic antidepressants.
Clomipramine.
Stimulants (including methylphenidate, dexamphetamine, pemoline, and bronchodilators).
Clonidine.
L-dopa.
Cocaine.
Bismuth.
Lithium.
Manganese.
Ethanol.
Carbon monoxide.
Oral contraceptives.
General anesthesia (including propofol)—during induction or emergence.

Paroxysmal Disorders

Complex migraine.
Alternating hemiplegia of childhood.
Paroxysmal kinesigenic dyskinesia (PKD).
Paroxysmal nonkinesigenic dyskinesia (PNKD).
Paroxysmal exercise-induced dyskinesia (PED).

Endocrine Disorders

Hyperthyroidism.
Pheochromocytoma.

CHOREOATHETOSIS[61]

ICD-10CM # G25.5 Choreoathetosis

SYSTEMIC DISEASES

SLE.
Polycythemia.
Thyrotoxicosis.
Rheumatic fever.
Cirrhosis of the liver (acquired hepatocerebral degeneration).
DM.
Wilson disease.

PRIMARY DEGENERATIVE BRAIN DISEASES

Huntington chorea.
Olivopontocerebellar atrophies.
Neuroacanthocytosis.

FOCAL BRAIN DISEASES

Hemichorea.
Stroke.
Tumor.
Arteriovenous malformation.

DRUG-INDUCED CHOREOATHETOSIS

Parkinson's Disease Drugs

Levodopa.

EPILEPSY DRUGS

Phenytoin.
Carbamazepine.
Phenobarbital.
Gabapentin.
Valproate.

Psychostimulant Drugs

Cocaine.
Amphetamine.
Methamphetamine.
Dextroamphetamine.
Methylphenidate.
Pemoline.

Psychotropic Drugs

Lithium.
Tricyclic antidepressant drugs.

Oral Contraceptive Drugs

Cimetidine

CHYLOTHORAX

ICD-10CM # I89.8 Other specified noninfective disorders of lymphatic vessels and lymph nodes

Post-lymph node dissection of neck or chest.
Subclavian venous catheterization.
Thoracic aneurysm repair.
Trauma to chest and neck.
Mediastinal tumor resection.
Esophagectomy, pneumonectomy.
Lymphangitis, mediastinitis.
Neoplasms (lymphoma, carcinoma of esophagus, lung, mediastinal malignancies).
Sympathectomy.
Venous thrombosis.
Congenital.

CLOUDY URINE

ICD-10CM # R82 Other abnormal findings in urine

Concentrated urine.
Use of multivitamin supplements.
Diet high in purine-rich foods.
Pyuria.
Phosphaturia.
Urinary tract infection.
Lipiduria.
Chyluria.
Hyperoxaluria.

CLUBBING

ICD-10CM # R68.3 Clubbing of fingers

Pulmonary neoplasm (lung, pleura).
Other neoplasm (GI, liver, Hodgkin's, thymus, osteogenic sarcoma).
Pulmonary infectious process (empyema, abscess, bronchiectasis, TB, chronic pneumonitis).
Extrapulmonary infectious process (subacute bacterial endocarditis, intestinal TB, bacterial or amebic dysentery, arterial graft sepsis).
Pneumoconiosis.
Cystic fibrosis.
Sarcoidosis.
Cyanotic congenital heart disease.
Endocrine (Graves disease, hyperparathyroidism).
Inflammatory bowel disease.
Celiac disease.
Chronic liver disease, cirrhosis (particularly biliary and juvenile).
Pulmonary AV malformations.
Idiopathic.
Thyroid acropachy.
Hereditary (pachydermoperiostosis).
Chronic trauma (jackhammer operators, machine workers).

COBALAMIN DEFICIENCY[43]

ICD-10CM # E53.8 Deficiency of other specified B group vitamins

ETIOPATHOPHYSIOLOGIC CLASSIFICATION OF COBALAMIN DEFICIENCY

Nutritional cobalamin deficiency (i.e., insufficient cobalamin intake):
- Vegetarians, poverty-imposed near-vegetarians, breastfed infants of mothers with pernicious anemia.

Abnormal intragastric events (i.e., inadequate proteolysis of food cobalamin):
- Atrophic gastritis, partial gastritis with hypochlorhydria, proton-pump inhibitors, H_2 blockers.

Loss or atrophy of gastric oxyntic mucosa (i.e., deficient intrinsic factor [IF] molecules):
- Total or partial gastrectomy, pernicious anemia, caustic destruction (lye).

Abnormal events in small bowel lumen:
- Inadequate pancreatic protease (e.g., R-cobalamin not degraded, cobalamin not transferred to IF):
  - Insufficient pancreatic protease (i.e., pancreatic insufficiency).
  - Inactivation of pancreatic protease (i.e., Zollinger–Ellison syndrome).
- Usurping of luminal cobalamin (i.e., inadequate cobalamin binding to IF):
  - By bacteria, during stasis syndromes (e.g., blind loops, pouches of diverticulosis, strictures, fistulas, anastomosis), impaired bowel motility (e.g., scleroderma), hypogammaglobulinemia.
- By *Diphyllobothrium latum* (fish tapeworm).

Disorders of ileal mucosa/IF–cobalamin receptors (i.e., IF–cobalamin not bound to IF–cobalamin receptors):
- Diminished or absent IF–cobalamin receptors (e.g., ileal bypass, resection, fistula).
- Abnormal mucosal architecture/function (e.g., tropical or nontropical sprue, Crohn's disease, tuberculosis ileitis, infiltration by lymphomas, amyloidosis).
- IF-/post-IF–cobalamin receptor defects (e.g., Imerslund–Gräsbeck syndrome, transcobalamin II [TC II] deficiency).
- Drug effects (e.g., slow K, metformin, cholestyramine, colchicine, neomycin).

Disorders of plasma cobalamin transport (i.e., TC II–cobalamin not delivered to TC II receptors):
- Congenital TC II deficiency, defective binding of TC II–cobalamin to TC II receptors (rare).

Metabolic disorders (i.e., cobalamin not used by cells):
- Inborn enzyme errors (rare).
- Acquired disorders (e.g., cobalamin functionally inactivated by irreversible oxidation, N_2O inhalation).

COGNITIVE IMPAIRMENT[78]

ICD-10CM # G31.84 Mild cognitive impairment, so stated

CAUSES OF COGNITIVE IMPAIRMENT: DIAGNOSES BY CATEGORIES WITH REPRESENTATIVE EXAMPLES

Degenerative:
Alzheimer's disease.
Frontotemporal dementias.
Dementia with Lewy bodies.
Corticobasal degeneration.
Huntington disease.
Wilson's disease.
Parkinson's disease.
Multiple system atrophy.
Progressive supranuclear palsy.

Psychiatric:
Depression.
Schizophrenia.

Vascular:
Vascular dementia.
Binswanger encephalopathy.
Amyloid dementia.
Diffuse hypoxic/ischemic injury.

Obstructive:
Normal-pressure hydrocephalus.
Obstructive hydrocephalus.

Traumatic:
Chronic subdural hematoma.
Chronic traumatic encephalopathy.
Post-concussion syndrome.

Neoplastic:
Tumor: malignant, primary and secondary.
Tumor: benign (e.g., frontal meningioma).
Paraneoplastic limbic encephalitis.

Infections:
Chronic meningitis.
Post-herpes encephalitis.
Focal cerebritis/abscesses.
HIV dementia.
HIV-associated infection.
Syphilis.
Lyme encephalopathy.
Subacute sclerosing panencephalitis.
Creutzfeldt–Jakob disease.
Progressive multifocal leukoencephalopathy.
Parenchymal sarcoidosis.
Chronic systemic infection.

Demyelinating:
Multiple sclerosis.
Adrenoleukodystrophy.
Metachromatic leukodystrophy.

Autoimmune:
Systemic lupus erythematosus.
Polyarteritis nodosa.

Drugs/Toxins
Medications:
- Anticholinergics.
- Antihistamines.
- Anticonvulsants.
- β-blockers.
- Sedative–hypnotics.

Substance abuse:
Alcohol.
Inhalants.
Phencyclidine (PCP).

Toxins
Arsenic.
Bromide.
Carbon monoxide.
Lead.
Mercury.
Organophosphates.

COLIC, ACUTE ABDOMINAL[81]

ICD-10CM # R10.0 Acute abdomen

Acute gastroenteritis.
Food poisoning.
Nonspecific causes.
Constipation.
Gastric outlet obstruction:
- Chronic peptic ulceration.
- Gastric cancer.

Small bowel obstruction:
- Adhesions:
  - Postsurgical.
  - Inflammatory (e.g., diverticular).
  - Radiation.
  - Meckel diverticulum.
  - Metastatic.
- Stricture:
  - Ischemic.
  - Radiation.
  - Inflammatory (e.g., Crohn disease).
- Volvulus intussusception:
  - Tumor (e.g., Peutz-Jeghers syndrome).
  - Superior mesenteric artery syndrome.
- Intraluminal bolus:
  - Gallstone.
  - Bezoar.
- Hernia:
  - Abdominal wall.
  - Internal.
- Neoplasm:
  - Benign (e.g., leiomyoma).
  - Malignant (e.g., carcinoid tumor, adenocarcinoma).

Large bowel obstruction:
- Colon cancer.
- Diverticular disease.
- Volvulus.

Uterine:
- Missed abortion.
- Parturition.
- Period pain.

COLON ISCHEMIA[26]

ICD-10CM # Varies with specific diagnosis

CAUSES OF COLON ISCHEMIA

Acute pancreatitis.
Allergy.
Amyloidosis.
Heart failure or cardiac arrhythmias.
Hematologic disorders and coagulopathies:
- Activated protein C resistance.
- Antithrombin deficiency.
- Factor V Leiden mutation.
- Paroxysmal nocturnal hemoglobinuria.
- Polycythemia vera.
- Protein C and S deficiencies.
- Prothrombin G20210A mutation.
- Sickle cell disease.

Infection:
- Bacteria (*Escherichia coli* O157:H7).
- Parasites (*Angiostrongylus costaricensis*).
- Viruses (HBV, HCV, cytomegalovirus).

Inferior mesenteric artery thrombosis.
Long-distance running.
Medications and toxins:
- Alosetron.
- Cocaine.
- Danazol.
- Digitalis compounds.
- Ergots.
- Estrogens.
- Flutamide.
- Glycerin enema.
- Gold salts.
- Immunosuppressive agents.
- Interferon-α.
- Methamphetamine.
- NSAIDs.
- Penicillin.
- Phenylephrine.
- Polyethylene glycol 3350 colon lavage solutions.
- Pit viper toxin.
- Progestins.
- Pseudoephedrine.
- Psychotropic drugs.
- Saline laxatives.
- Sumatriptan.
- Tegaserod.
- Vasopressin.

Pheochromocytoma.
Ruptured ectopic pregnancy.
Shock.
Strangulated hernia.
Surgery/procedures:
- Aortic aneurysmectomy.
- Aortoiliac reconstruction.
- Barium enema.
- Colectomy with inferior mesenteric artery ligation.
- Colon bypass.
- Colonoscopy.
- Exchange transfusions.
- Gynecologic operations.
- Lumbar aortography.

Thromboembolism:
- Cholesterol (atheroembolism).
- Myxoma (left atrial).

Trauma (blunt or penetrating).
Vasculitis and vasculopathy:
- Buerger disease.
- Eosinophilic granulomatosis with angiitis.
- Fibromuscular dysplasia.

Kawasaki disease.
Polyarteritis nodosa.
Rheumatoid vasculitis.
SLE.
Takayasu arteritis.
Volvulus.

COLOR CHANGES, CUTANEOUS[73]

ICD-10CM # L81.9 Disorder of pigmentation, unspecified

BROWN

Generalized: pituitary, adrenal, liver disease, ACTH-producing tumor (e.g., oat cell lung carcinoma).
Localized: nevi, neurofibromatosis.

WHITE

Generalized: albinism.
Localized: vitiligo, Raynaud's syndrome.

RED (ERYTHEMA)

Generalized: fever, polycythemia, urticaria, viral exanthems.
Localized: inflammation, infection, Raynaud's syndrome.

YELLOW

Generalized: liver disease, chronic renal disease, anemia.
Generalized (except sclera): hypothyroidism, increased intake of vegetables containing carotene.
Localized: resolving hematoma, infection, peripheral vascular insufficiency.

BLUE

Lips, mouth, nail beds: cardiovascular and pulmonary diseases, Raynaud's.

COMA

ICD-10CM # R40.20 Unspecified coma

Vascular: hemorrhage, thrombosis, embolism.
CNS infections: meningitis, encephalitis, cerebral abscess.
Cerebral neoplasms with herniation.
Head injury: subdural hematoma, cerebral concussion, cerebral contusion.
Drugs: narcotics, sedatives, hypnotics.
Ingestion or inhalation of toxins: CO, alcohol, lead.
Metabolic disturbances.
Hypoxia.
Acid-base disorders.
Hypoglycemia, hyperglycemia.
Hepatic failure.
Electrolyte disorders.
Uremia.
Hypothyroidism.
Hypothermia, hyperthermia.
Hypotension, malignant hypertension.
Postictal.

COMA, NORMAL COMPUTED TOMOGRAPHY[3]

ICD-10CM # R40.20 Unspecified coma

MENINGEAL DISORDERS

Subarachnoid hemorrhage (uncommon).
Bacterial meningitis.
Encephalitis.
Subdural empyema.

EXOGENOUS TOXINS

Sedative drugs and barbiturates.
Anesthetics and γ-hydroxybutyrate.[12]
Alcohols.
Stimulants:
- Phencyclidines.[13]
- Cocaine and amphetamines.[14]

Psychotropic drugs:
- Cyclic antidepressants.
- Phenothiazines.
- Lithium.

Anticonvulsants.
Opioids.
Clonidine.[15]
Penicillins.
Salicylates.
Anticholinergics.
Carbon monoxide, cyanide, and methemoglobinemia.

ENDOGENOUS TOXINS/DEFICIENCIES/DERANGEMENTS

Hypoxia and ischemia.
Hypoglycemia.
Hypercalcemia.
Osmolar:
- Hyperglycemia.
- Hyponatremia.
- Hypernatremia.

Organ system failure:
- Hepatic encephalopathy.
- Uremic encephalopathy.
- Pulmonary insufficiency (carbon dioxide narcosis).

SEIZURES

Prolonged postictal state.
Spike-wave stupor.

HYPOTHERMIA OR HYPERTHERMIA

Brain stem ischemia.
Basilar artery stroke.
Brain stem or cerebellar hemorrhage.
Conversion or malingering.

[12] General anesthetic, similar to g-aminobutyric acid; recreational drug and body building aid. Rapid onset, rapid recovery often with myoclonic jerking and confusion. Deep coma (2–3 hr; Glasgow Coma Scale = 3) with maintenance of vital signs.
[13] Coma associated with cholinergic signs: lacrimation, salivation, bronchorrhea, and hyperthermia.
[14] Coma after seizures or status (i.e., a prolonged postictal state).
[15] An antihypertensive agent active through the opiate receptor system; frequent overdose when used to treat narcotic withdrawal..

COMA, PEDIATRIC POPULATION[67]

ICD-10CM # R40.20 Unspecified coma

ANOXIA

Birth asphyxia.
Carbon monoxide poisoning.
Croup/epiglottitis.
Meconium aspiration.

INFECTION

Hemolysis.
Blood loss.
Hydrops fetalis.
Infection.
Meningoencephalitis.
Sepsis.
Postimmunization encephalitis.

INCREASED INTRACRANIAL PRESSURE

Anoxia.
Inborn metabolic errors.
Toxic encephalopathy.
Reye syndrome.
Head trauma/intracranial bleed.
Hydrocephalus.
Posterior fossa tumors.

HYPERTENSIVE ENCEPHALOPATHY

Coarctation of aorta.
Nephritis.
Vasculitis.
Pheochromocytoma.

ISCHEMIA

Hypoplastic left heart.
Shunting lesions.
Aortic stenosis.
Cardiovascular collapse (any cause).

PURPURIC CAUSES

Disseminated intravascular coagulation.
Hemolytic-uremic syndrome.
Leukemia.
Thrombotic purpura.

HYPERCAPNIA

Cystic fibrosis.
Bronchopulmonary dysplasia.
Congenital lung anomalies.

NEOPLASM

Medulloblastoma.
Glioma of brain stem.
Posterior fossa tumors.

DRUGS/TOXINS

Maternal sedation.
Alcohol.
Any drug.
Lead.
Salicylism.
Arsenic.
Pesticides.

ELECTROLYTE ABNORMALITIES

Hypernatremia (diarrhea, dehydration, salt poisoning).
Hyponatremia (SIADH, androgenital syndrome, gastroenteritis).
Hyperkalemia (renal failure, salicylism, androgenitalism).
Hypokalemia (diarrhea, hyperaldosteronism, salicylism, DKA).
Hypocalcemia (vitamin D deficiency, hyperparathyroidism).
Severe acidosis (sepsis, cold injury, salicylism, DKA).

HYPOGLYCEMIA

Birth injury or stress.
Diabetes.
Alcohol.
Salicylism.
Hyperinsulinemia.
Iatrogenic.

POSTSEIZURE

Renal Causes
Nephritis.
Hypoplastic kidneys.
Hepatic Causes
Acute hepatitis.
Fulminant hepatic failure.
Inborn metabolic errors.
Bile duct atresia.

COMPRESSION SYNDROMES, NEUROVASCULAR CAUSES[65]

ICD-10CM #		
	M47.016	Anterior spinal artery compression syndromes, lumbar region
	M47.019	Anterior spinal artery compression syndromes, site unspecified
	M47.013	Anterior spinal artery compression syndromes, cervicothoracic region
	M47.021	Vertebral artery compression syndromes, occipito-atlanto-axial region
	M47.022	Vertebral artery compression syndromes, cervical region

Anatomic
Potential sites of neurovascular compression:
- Interscalene triangle.
- Costoclavicular space.
- Subcoracoid area.

Congenital
Cervical rib and its fascial remnants.
Rudimentary first thoracic rib.
Scalene muscles:
- Anterior.
- Middle.
- Minimus.

Adventitious fibrous bands.
Bifid clavicle or first rib.
Exostosis of first thoracic rib.
Enlarged transverse process of C7.
Omohyoid muscle.
Anomalous course of transverse cervical artery.
Abnormal lateral insertion of costoclavicular ligament.
Flat clavicle.
Traumatic
Fracture of clavicle.
Dislocation of head of humerus.
Crushing injury to upper thorax.
Sudden, unaccustomed muscular efforts involving shoulder girdle muscles.
Cervical spondylosis and injuries to cervical spine.

CONGESTIVE HEART FAILURE AND CARDIOMYOPATHY[3]

ICD-10CM #		
	I50.9	Heart failure, unspecified
	I42.7	Cardiomyopathy due to drug and external agent

CAUSES OF CONGESTIVE HEART FAILURE AND CARDIOMYOPATHY

Coronary Artery Disease
Acute ischemia.
Myocardial infarction.
Ischemic cardiomyopathy with hibernating myocardium.
Idiopathic
Idiopathic dilated cardiomyopathy.
Idiopathic restrictive cardiomyopathy.
Peripartum.
Pressure Overload
Hypertension.
Aortic stenosis.
Volume Overload
Mitral regurgitation.
Aortic insufficiency.
Anemia.
Atrioventricular fistula.
Toxins
Ethanol.
Cocaine.
Doxorubicin (Adriamycin).
Methamphetamine.
Metabolic-Endocrine
Thiamine deficiency.
Diabetes.
Hemochromatosis.
Thyrotoxicosis.
Obesity.
Infiltrative
Amyloidosis.
Inflammatory
Viral myocarditis.
Hereditary
Hypertrophic.
Dilated.

Genetic bases for these cardiomyopathies have been identified in a large number of individual patients and families. Most of the mutations have been found in cardiac contractile or structural proteins.

CONGESTIVE HEART FAILURE, INFANT[1]

ICD-10CM # I05.9 Heart failure, unspecified

Critical coarctation of the aorta.
Interrupted aortic arch.
Congenital aortic stenosis.
Hypoplastic left heart syndrome.
Large ventricular septal defect.
Truncus arteriosus.
Unrecognized supraventricular tachycardia.
Cardiac tamponade.
Myocarditis.

CONJUNCTIVAL NEOPLASM

ICD-10CM # Varies with specific diagnosis

MALIGNANT

Squamous cell carcinoma.
Melanoma.
Sebaceous carcinoma.
Kaposi sarcoma.
Metastatic neoplasms.

BENIGN

Melanocytic nevus.
Squamous papilloma.
Hemangioma.
Lymphangioma.
Myxoma.

CONSCIOUSNESS IMPAIRMENT, ACUTE, IN CRITICALLY ILL PATIENT

ICD-10CM # F05.9 Delirium, unspecified

GENERAL CAUSES OF ACUTELY IMPAIRED CONSCIOUSNESS IN THE CRITICALLY ILL

Infection
Sepsis encephalopathy.
CNS infection.
Drugs
Narcotics.
Benzodiazepines.
Anticholinergics.
Anticonvulsants.
Tricyclic antidepressants.
Selective serotonin uptake inhibitors.
Phenothiazines.
Steroids.
Immunosuppressants (cyclosporine, FK-506, OKT3).
Anesthetics.
Electrolyte and Acid-Base Disturbances
Hyponatremia.
Hypernatremia.
Hypercalcemia.
Hypermagnesemia.
Severe acidemia and alkalemia.
Organ System Failure
Shock.
Renal failure.
Hepatic failure.
Pancreatitis.
Respiratory failure (hypoxia, hypercapnia).

Endocrine Disorders
Hypoglycemia.
Hyperglycemia.
Hypothyroidism.
Hyperthyroidism.
Pituitary apoplexy.
Drug Withdrawal
Alcohol.
Opiates.
Barbiturates.
Benzodiazepines.
Vascular Causes
Shock.
Hypotension.
Hypertensive encephalopathy.
CNS vasculitis.
Cerebral venous sinus thrombosis.
Central Nervous System Disorders
Hemorrhage.
Stroke.
Brain edema.
Hydrocephalus.
Increased intracranial pressure.
Meningitis.
Ventriculitis.
Brain abscess.
Subdural empyema.
Seizures.
Vasculitis.
Seizures
Convulsive and nonconvulsive status epilepticus.
Miscellaneous
Fat embolism syndrome.
Neuroleptic malignant syndrome.
Thiamine deficiency (Wernicke encephalopathy).
Psychogenic unresponsiveness.

CONSTIPATION

ICD-10CM # K59.00 Constipation, unspecified

Intestinal obstruction.
Fecal impaction.
Diverticular disease.
GI neoplasm.
Strangulated femoral hernia.
Gallstone ileus.
Tuberculous stricture.
Adhesions.
Ameboma.
Volvulus.
Intussusception.
Inflammatory bowel disease.
Hematoma of bowel wall, secondary to trauma or anticoagulants.
Poor dietary habits: insufficient bulk in diet, inadequate fluid intake.
Change from daily routine: travel, hospital admission, physical inactivity.
Acute abdominal conditions: renal colic, salpingitis, biliary colic, appendicitis, ischemia.
Hypercalcemia or hypokalemia, uremia.
Irritable bowel syndrome, pregnancy, anorexia nervosa, depression.
Painful anal conditions: hemorrhoids, fissure, stricture.
Decreased intestinal peristalsis: old age, spinal cord injuries, myxedema, diabetes, multiple sclerosis, Parkinsonism and other neurologic diseases.
Drugs: codeine, morphine, antacids with aluminum, verapamil, anticonvulsants, anticholinergics, disopyramide, cholestyramine, alosetron, iron supplements.
Hirschsprung disease, meconium ileus, congenital atresia in infants.

CONSTIPATION, ADULT PATIENT[81]

ICD-10CM # K59.00 Constipation, unspecified

NO GROSS STRUCTURAL ABNORMALITY

Inadequate fiber intake.
Irritable bowel syndrome (associated with abdominal pain) or functional constipation.
Idiopathic slow-transit constipation.
"Obstructed defecation" pelvic floor dysfunction (or dyssynergia).

STRUCTURAL DISORDERS

Anal fissure, infection, or stenosis.
Colon cancer or stricture.
Aganglionosis and/or abnormal myenteric plexus:
Hirschsprung disease.
Chagas disease.
Neuropathic pseudoobstruction.
Abnormal colonic muscle:
Myopathy.
Dystrophia myotonica.
Systemic sclerosis.
Idiopathic megarectum and/or megacolon.
Proximal megacolon.

NEUROLOGIC CAUSES

Diabetic autonomic neuropathy.
Damage to the sacral parasympathetic outflow.
Spinal cord damage or disease (e.g., multiple sclerosis).
Parkinson's disease.
Blunting of consciousness, mental retardation, psychosis.
Pain induced by straining (e.g., sciatic nerve compression).

ENDOCRINE OR METABOLIC CAUSES

Hypothyroidism.
Hypercalcemia.
Porphyria.
Pregnancy.

PSYCHOLOGIC DISORDERS

Depression.
Anorexia nervosa.
Denied bowel habit.
Drug Side Effects

COPD DECOMPENSATION[57]

ICD-10CM # J44.1 Chronic obstructive pulmonary distress with acute exacerbation

CAUSES OF ACUTE DECOMPENSATION IN THE PATIENT WITH CHRONIC OBSTRUCTIVE PULMONARY DISEASE

Acute Exacerbations
Infectious
Viral.
Rhinovirus, respiratory syncytial virus, coronavirus, influenza virus.
Bacterial.
Haemophilus influenzae, Streptococcus pneumoniae, Moraxella (Branhamella) catarrhalis, Pseudomonas aeruginosa.
Atypical bacteria.
Chlamydia pneumoniae, Legionella.
Air Pollution
Nitrogen dioxide.
Ozone.
Particulates, dust.
Other Critical Events
Pneumothorax.
Pulmonary embolism.
Lobar atelectasis.
Congestive heart failure.
Pneumonia.
Pulmonary compression (e.g., obesity, ascites, gastric distention, pleural effusion).
Trauma (e.g., rib fractures, pulmonary contusion).
Neuromuscular and metabolic disorders.
Unrelated treatable chronic pulmonary disease (bronchiectasis, tuberculosis, sarcoidosis).
Noncompliance with prescribed treatment regimens.
Iatrogenic.
Inadequate therapy.
Inappropriate therapy (e.g., deleterious drugs).

CORNEAL SENSATION, DECREASED

ICD-10CM # H18.899 Other specified disorders of cornea, unspecified eye

Herpes (simplex, zoster).
Contact lens wear.
Topical agents (NSAIDs, anesthetics, beta-blockers).
Diabetes.
Eye trauma.
Postsurgery.

COUGH

ICD-10CM # R05 Cough

Infectious process (viral, bacterial).
Postinfectious.
"Smoker's cough."
Rhinitis (allergic, vasomotor, postinfectious).
Asthma.
Exposure to irritants (noxious fumes, smoke, cold air).
Drug-induced (especially ACE inhibitors, beta-blockers).
GERD.
Interstitial lung disease.
Lung neoplasms.

Lymphomas, mediastinal neoplasms.
Bronchiectasis.
Cardiac (CHF, pulmonary edema, mitral stenosis, pericardial inflammation).
Recurrent aspiration.
Inflammation of larynx, pleura, diaphragm, mediastinum.
Cystic fibrosis.
Anxiety.
Other: pulmonary embolism, foreign body inhalation, aortic aneurysm, Zenker diverticulum, osteophytes, substernal thyroid, thyroiditis, PMR.

COUGH, CHRONIC, ADULT PATIENT[2]

ICD-10CM # R05 Cough

CAUSES OF CHRONIC COUGH IN ADULTS

Intrathoracic Causes

Lungs and Airways

Asthma.
Nonasthmatic eosinophilic bronchitis.
Chronic bronchitis.
Bronchiectasis.
ACEIs.
Inhaled medications.
Chronic exposure to environmental and occupational irritants.
Bronchogenic and metastatic carcinoma.
Bronchial carcinoid.
Foreign body or endobronchial suture.
Broncholith.
Infectious and noninfectious bronchiolitis.
Chronic infectious pneumonias (e.g., bacterial, tuberculous, fungal, parasitic).
Chronic infectious tracheobronchitis (as in tuberculosis or aspergillosis).
Chronic interstitial lung disease (e.g., sarcoidosis, HSP, IPF, asbestosis).
Pulmonary vasculitis (as in granulomatosis with polyangiitis).
Sjögren syndrome with xerotrachea.
Relapsing polychondritis.

Pleura

Chronic effusion.

Diaphragm

Transvenous pacemaker stimulation.

Mediastinum

Neural tumors.
Thymoma.
Teratoma.
Lymphoma.
Metastatic lymphadenopathy.
Intrathoracic goiter.
Bronchogenic cyst.

Cardiovascular

Mitral stenosis.
Left ventricular failure.
Pulmonary thromboembolism.
Enlarged left atrium.
Vascular ring.
Aberrant innominate artery.
Aortic aneurysm.
Pericardial stimulation by transvenous pacemaker.

Extrathoracic Causes

Head and Neck

Rhinitis and sinusitis.
Nasal polyps.
Rhinolith.
Oropharyngeal dysphagia.
Laryngeal disorders (e.g., vocal fold dysfunction, laryngomalacia).
Postviral vagal neuropathy.
Recurrent aspiration.
Elongated uvula.
Chronically infected tonsils.
Neurilemmoma of vagus nerve.
Neuroma of internal laryngeal nerve.
Ascending palatine artery aneurysm.
Osteophytes of cervical spine.
Mammomanogamus (Syngamus) laryngeus infection.
Thyroiditis.

Upper Gastrointestinal

Gastroesophageal reflux disease.
Esophageal cyst or diverticulum.
Tracheoesophageal fistula.

Central Nervous System

Psychogenic or habit cough.
Tic disorders.
Gilles de la Tourette syndrome.

ACEI, Angiotensin-converting enzyme inhibitor; *HSP,* hypersensitivity pneumonitis; *IPF,* idiopathic pulmonary fibrosis.

CUTANEOUS INFECTIONS, ATHLETES

ICD-10CM # L08.9 Local infection of the skin and subcutaneous tissue, unspecified

Tinea pedis.
Tinea cruris.
Molluscum contagiosum.
Herpes simplex.
Verruca vulgaris.
Folliculitis.
Impetigo.
Furuncles.
Otitis externa.
Erythrasma.

CYANOSIS[7]

ICD-10CM # R23.0 Cyanosis

DIFFERENTIAL DIAGNOSIS OF CYANOSIS

Peripheral Cyanosis

Low cardiac output states

Shock.
Left ventricular failure.
Hypovolemia.

Environmental exposure (cold)

Air or water.

Arterial occlusion

Thrombosis.
Embolism.
Vasospasm (Raynaud's phenomenon).
Peripheral vascular disease.
Venous obstruction

Redistribution of blood flow from extremities

Central Cyanosis

Decreased arterial oxygen saturation

High altitude (>8000 ft).
Impaired pulmonary function.
- Hypoventilation.
- Impaired oxygen diffusion.
- Ventilation-perfusion mismatching.
  - Pulmonary embolism.
  - Acute respiratory distress syndrome.
  - Pulmonary hypertension.
- Respiratory compromise.
  - Upper airway obstruction.
  - Pneumonia.
  - Diaphragmatic hernia.
  - Tension pneumothorax.
  - Polycythemia.

Anatomic Shunts

Pulmonary arteriovenous fistulae and intrapulmonary shunts.
Cerebral, hepatic, peripheral arteriovenous fistulae.
Cyanotic congenital heart disease.
- Endocardial cushion defects.
- Ventricular septal defects.
- Coarctation of aorta.
- Tetralogy of Fallot.
- Total anomalous pulmonary venous drainage.
- Hypoplastic left ventricle.
- Pulmonary vein stenosis.
- Tricuspid atresia and anomalies.
- Premature closure of foramen ovale.
- Dextrocardia.
- Pulmonary stenosis of atrial septal defect.
- Patent ductus arteriosus with reversed shunt.

Abnormal Hemoglobin

Methemoglobinemia.
- Hereditary.
- Acquired.

Sulfhemoglobinemia.
Mutant hemoglobin with low oxygen affinity (e.g., hemoglobin Kansas).

CYANOSIS, NEONATAL[1]

ICD-10CM # R23.0 Cyanosis

RESPIRATORY

Upper Airway

Choanal atresia.
Macroglossia.
Glossoptosis (secondary to micrognathia).
Laryngomalacia.
Laryngeal web or cyst.
Vascular anomalies (e.g., cystic hygromas, rings).
Subglottic stenosis (commonly secondary to intubation).
Foreign body.

Lower Airway

Pneumonia.
Bronchiolitis.
Pulmonary edema.
Atelectasis.
Bronchopulmonary dysplasia.

SYSTEMIC

Sepsis.
Trauma.
Poisons.

CARDIAC

Cyanotic congenital heart diseases.
Transposition of the great vessels (most common neonatal).
Tetralogy of Fallot.
Truncus arteriosus.
Tricuspid atresia.
Total anomalous pulmonary venous return.
Ebstein anomaly.
GI.
Gastroesophageal reflux.

NEUROLOGIC

Seizures.
Central hypoventilation syndrome (Ondine curse).
Spinal muscular atrophy type I (Werdnig-Hoffmann).
Botulism.
Congenital myopathies.

HEMATOLOGIC

Methemoglobinemia.

CYTOPENIAS, OLDER ADULTS[44]

ICD-10CM #	D46.A	Refractory cytopenia with multilineage dysplasia

Differential diagnosis for common causes of cytopenias in older adults:
Cytopenia of one or more lineages.
Hematologic neoplasm.
Vitamin B_{12} deficiency.
Autoimmune disorder.
Consumptive coagulopathy.
Systemic inflammation.
Alcohol.
Splenomegaly.
Thyroid dysfunction.
Human immunodeficiency virus

DAYTIME SLEEPINESS

ICD-10CM #	R53.82	Chronic fatigue, unspecified

Sleep deprivation.
Medication induced (e.g., benzodiazepines, beta-blockers, narcotics, sedative antidepressants, gabapentin).
Depression.
Obstructive sleep apnea.
Medical illness (e.g., severe anemia, hypothyroidism, COPD, hepatic failure, renal insufficiency, CHF, electrolyte disturbances).
Circadian rhythm abnormalities (e.g., jet lag, shift work sleep disorder).
Restless legs syndrome.
Posttrauma.
Narcolepsy.
Neurologic disorders (e.g., neurodegenerative disorders; parkinsonism; multiple sclerosis; lesions affecting thalamus, hypothalamus, or brain stem).

DELAYED PASSAGE OF MECONIUM[36]

ICD-10CM #	P76.0	Meconium plug syndrome

Ileal atresia.
Meconium ileus.
Functional immaturity of the colon.
Colon atresia.
Anorectal malformations.
Hirschsprung disease.
Megacystis-microcolon-intestinal hypoperistalsis syndrome.
Extrinsic compression of the distal bowel by a mass lesion.
 Mesenteric cyst.
 Enteric duplication cyst.
Paralytic ileus, sepsis, drugs, and metabolic upset.

DELIRIUM[55]

ICD-10CM #	R40.0	Somnolence
	R40.1	Stupor
	F05	Delirium due to known physiological condition

PHARMACOLOGIC AGENTS

Anxiolytics (benzodiazepines).
Antidepressants (e.g., amitriptyline, doxepin, imipramine).
Cardiovascular agents (e.g., methyldopa, digitalis, reserpine, propranolol, procainamide, captopril, disopyramide).
Antihistamine.
Cimetidine.
Corticosteroids.
Antineoplastics.
Drugs of abuse (alcohol, cannabis, amphetamines, cocaine, hallucinogens, opioids, sedative-hypnotics, phencyclidine).

METABOLIC DISORDERS

Hypercalcemia.
Hypercarbia.
Hypoglycemia.
Hyponatremia.
Hypoxia.

INFLAMMATORY DISORDERS

Sarcoidosis.
SLE.
Giant cell arteritis.

ORGAN FAILURE

Hepatic encephalopathy.
Uremia.

NEUROLOGIC DISORDERS

Alzheimer's disease.
CVA.
Encephalitis (including HIV).
Encephalopathies.
Epilepsy.
Huntington disease.
Multiple sclerosis.
Neoplasms.
Normal-pressure hydrocephalus.
Parkinson's disease.
Pick disease.
Wilson disease.

ENDOCRINE DISORDERS

Addison disease.
Cushing disease.
Panhypopituitarism.
Parathyroid disease.
Postpartum psychosis.
Recurrent menstrual psychosis.
Sydenham chorea.
Thyroid disease.

DEFICIENCY STATES

Niacin.
Thiamine, vitamin B_{12}, and folate.

DELIRIUM AND AGITATION, DRUG-INDUCED

ICD-10CM #	F05.9	Delirium, unspecified

COMMONLY USED DRUGS ASSOCIATED WITH DELIRIUM AND AGITATION

Benzodiazepines.
Opiates (especially meperidine).
Anticholinergics.
Antihistamines.
H_2 blockers.
Antibiotics.
Corticosteroids.
Metoclopramide.

DELIRIUM, AGITATED[7]

ICD-10CM #	F05	Delirium due to known physiological condition

Metabolic causes:
 Electrolyte abnormalities.
 Hypoglycemia.
 Hypoxia.
 Uremia/hyperammonemia.
Structural lesions of the CNS:
 Trauma.
 Stroke.
 Hemorrhage.
 Mass.
Endocrine disease:
 Thyrotoxicosis.
Infections:
 Bacterial/viral meningitis/encephalitis.
Toxicologic causes:
 Sympathomimetic/stimulants.
 Cocaine.
 Amphetamines and derivatives.
 Caffeine.
 Phencyclidine/ketamine.
 Anticholinergics.
 Serotonin syndrome.
 Sedative-hypnotic withdrawal.
Heatstroke.
Postictal state.

CNS, Central nervous system.

DELIRIUM, DIALYSIS PATIENT[55]

ICD-10CM #		
	F05	Delirium due to known physiological condition
	F06.8	Other specified mental disorders due to known physiological condition

STRUCTURAL

Cerebrovascular accident (particularly hemorrhage).
Subdural hematoma.
Intracerebral abscess.
Brain tumor.

METABOLIC

Disequilibrium syndrome.
Uremia.
Drug effects.
Meningitis.
Hypertensive encephalopathy.
Hypotension.
Postictal state.
Hypernatremia or hyponatremia.
Hypercalcemia.
Hypermagnesemia.
Hypoglycemia.
Severe hyperglycemia.
Hypoxemia.
Dialysis dementia.

DEMENTIA, ADOLESCENT PATIENT[49]

ICD-10CM #		
	F03	Unspecified dementia
	F03.90	Unspecified dementia without behavioral disturbance

CAUSES OF DEMENTIA IN ADOLESCENTS

Autoimmune or inflammatory diseases:
- Paraneoplastic syndromes, including NMDA antibody encephalitis.
- Vasculitis.

Cerebral and noncerebral neoplasms:
- Chemotherapy (intrathecal).
- Radiotherapy treatment.

Drug, inhalant, and alcohol abuse, including overdose.
Head trauma, including child abuse.
Infections:
- HIV-associated dementia.
- Variant Creutzfeldt–Jakob disease (vCJD).
- Subacute sclerosing panencephalitis (SSPE).

Metabolic abnormalities:
- Adrenoleukodystrophy.
- Wilson disease.

Neurodegenerative illnesses:
- Huntington disease.
- Metachromatic leukodystrophy.
- Other rare, usually genetically transmitted, illnesses.

DEMYELINATING DISEASES[87]

ICD-10CM #		
	G37.9	Demyelinating disease of central nervous system, unspecified

MULTIPLE SCLEROSIS

Relapsing and chronic progressive forms.
Acute multiple sclerosis.
Neuromyelitis optica (Devic disease).

DIFFUSE CEREBRAL SCLEROSIS

Schilder encephalitis periaxialis diffusa.
Baló concentric sclerosis.

ACUTE DISSEMINATED ENCEPHALOMYELITIS

After measles, chickenpox, rubella, influenza, mumps.
After rabies or smallpox vaccination.

NECROTIZING HEMORRHAGIC ENCEPHALITIS

Hemorrhagic leukoencephalitis.

LEUKODYSTROPHIES

Krabbe globoid leukodystrophy.
Metachromatic leukodystrophy.
Adrenoleukodystrophy.
Adrenomyeloneuropathy.
Pelizaeus-Merzbacher leukodystrophy.
Canavan disease.
Alexander disease.

DIAPHRAGM ELEVATION, BILATERAL, SYMMETRICAL[36]

ICD-10CM #		
	J98.6	Disorders of diaphragm

CAUSES OF BILATERAL SYMMETRICAL ELEVATION OF THE DIAPHRAGM

Supine position.
Poor inspiration.
Obesity.
Pregnancy.
Abdominal distention (ascites, intestinal obstruction, abdominal mass).
Diffuse pulmonary fibrosis.
Lymphangitis carcinomatosa.
Disseminated lupus erythematosus.
Bilateral basal pulmonary emboli.
Painful conditions (after abdominal surgery).
Bilateral diaphragmatic paralysis.

DIAPHRAGM ELEVATION, UNILATERAL[36]

ICD-10CM #		
	J98.6	Disorders of diaphragm

CAUSES OF UNILATERAL ELEVATION OF THE DIAPHRAGM

Posture—lateral decubitus position (dependent side).
Gaseous distention of stomach or colon.
Dorsal scoliosis.
Pulmonary hypoplasia.
Pulmonary collapse.
Phrenic nerve palsy.
Eventration.
Pneumonia or pleurisy.
Pulmonary thromboembolism.
Rib fracture and other painful conditions.
Subphrenic infection.
Subphrenic mass.

DIARRHEA, ACUTE WATERY AND BLOODY[81]

ICD-10CM #		
	K52.2	Allergic and dietetic gastroenteritis and colitis
	K52.89	Other specified noninfective gastroenteritis and colitis
	R19.7	Diarrhea, unspecified

ACUTE WATERY DIARRHEA

GI infections:
- Protozoal (e.g., *Giardia*).
- Bacterial (e.g., enterotoxigenic *Escherichia coli*, cholera).
- Viral (e.g., rotavirus, Norwalk virus).

Drugs.
Toxins.
Dietary constituents (e.g., lactose intolerance).
Onset of chronic diarrheal illness.

ACUTE BLOODY DIARRHEA

Infectious colitis:
- Confluent proctocolitis (e.g., *Shigella, Campylobacter, Salmonella, Entamoeba histolytica*).
- Segmental colitis (e.g., *Campylobacter, Salmonella,* enteroinvasive *E. coli, Aeromonas, E. histolytica*).
- Drug-induced colitis (e.g., nonsteroidal anti-inflammatory drugs [NSAIDs]).
- Inflammatory bowel disease.
- Ischemic colitis (usually elderly patient with underlying heart disease or arrhythmias).
- Antibiotic-associated colitis.

DIARRHEA, CRITICALLY ILL PATIENT[74]

ICD-10CM #		
	R19.7	Diarrhea, unspecified

COMMON CAUSES OF DIARRHEA IN CRITICALLY ILL PATIENTS

Medication

Antibiotics.
H2-recepter antagonists, antacids.
Drugs: significant amounts of sorbitol, magnesium, or hypertonic medications.
Laxative use (unintended).

Gastrointestinal Dysfunction

Gastric or small bowel resection.
Inflammatory bowel disease.
Pancreatic insufficiency.
Radiation enteritis.
Sprue.
Protein-losing gastroenteropathies.
Bowel impaction (paradoxic).

Malnutrition
Hypoproteinemia.
Micronutrient deficiencies.
Enteral Nutrition–Associated
Excessive feeding rate, concentration, volume, or osmolality.
Adaptation in malnourished patients or those whose GI tract has not been used recently.
Intolerance or allergy to feeding formula.
Infection
Clostridium difficile enterocolitis.
Opportunistic GI infection.
Significant amounts of contaminated feeding formula.
Altered GI flora.
Endocrine Dysfunction
Diabetes mellitus.
Hyperthyroidism.
Hypocortisolism.

DIARRHEA, INFECTIOUS[7]

ICD-10CM # A09 Infectious gastroenteritis and colitis, unspecified

ETIOLOGIC AGENTS OF INFECTIOUS DIARRHEA

Viral (60% of Cases)
Astrovirus.
Calicivirus.
Coronavirus.
Cytomegalovirus.[16]
Enteric adenovirus.
Hepatitis A through G.
Herpes simplex virus.
HIV enteropathy.
Norwalk like agents.
Pararotavirus.
Norwalk virus.
Picornavirus.
Rotavirus.
Small round viruses.
Bacterial (20% of Cases)
Invasive
Aeromonas spp.
Campylobacter spp.
Clostridium difficile.
Enteroinvasive *E. coli.*
Mycobacterium spp.
Plesiomonas shigelloides.
Salmonella spp.
Shigella spp.
Vibrio fluvialis.
Vibrio parahaemolyticus.
Vibrio vulnificus.
Yersinia enterocolitica.
Yersinia pseudotuberculosis.
Toxigenic
Food poisoning with preformed toxins.
Bacillus cereus.
Clostridium botulinum.
Staphylococcus aureus.
Toxin formation after colonization.
Aeromonas hydrophila.
Clostridium perfringens.
Enterohemorrhagic *E. coli* 0157:H7.
Enterotoxigenic *E. coli.*
Klebsiella pneumoniae.
Shigella spp.
Vibrio cholerae.
Other bacteria
Parasitic (5% of Cases)
Protozoa
Balantidium coli.
Blastocystis hominis.
Cryptosporidium.
Cyclospora.
Dientamoeba fragilis.
Entamoeba histolytica.
Entamoeba polecki.
Enteromonas hominis.
Giardia lamblia.
Isospora belli.
Microsporidia.
Sarcocystis hominis.
Helminths
Angiostrongylus costaricense.
Anisakiasis.
Ascaris lumbricoides.
Diphyllobothrium latum.
Enterobius vermicularis.
Hookworms.
Schistosoma spp.
Strongyloides stercoralis.
Taenia spp.
Trichinella spiralis.
Trichuris trichiura.

[16]Associated with fever, abdominal pain, and fecal red blood cells or white blood cells. % indicates the estimated contribution to total cases.

DIARRHEA, NONINFECTIOUS[7]

ICD-10CM # K59.1 Functional diarrhea

CAUSES OF NONINFECTIOUS DIARRHEA

Toxins
Drugs
ACE inhibitors.
Alprazolam.
Antacids (Mg).
Antibiotics.
Antidepressants.
Antiepileptic drugs.
Antihypertensives.
Antiparkinson drugs.
Beta-blockers.
Caffeine.
Cardiac antiarrhythmics.
Chemotherapy agents.
Cholesterol-lowering drugs.
Cholinergic agents.
Cholinesterase inhibitors.
Colchicine.
Digitalis.
Diuretics.
Flurouracil.
Fluoxetine.
Histamine H_2-receptor antagonists.
Hydralazine.
Lactulose.
Laxatives/cathartics.
Levodopa.
Lithium.
NSAIDs.
Neomycin.
Podophyllin.
Procainamide.
Prostaglandins.
Quinidine.
Ricinoleic acid.
Theophylline.
Thyroid hormone.
Valproic acid.
Dietetic foods
Mannitol.
Sorbitol.
Xylitol.
Fish-associated toxins
Amnestic shellfish poisoning.
Ciguatera.
Echinoderms.
Neurotoxic shellfish poisoning.
Paralytic shellfish poisoning.
Scombroid.
Tetroton.
Plant-associated toxins
Herbal preparations.
Horse chestnut.
Mushrooms—*Amanita* spp.
Nicotine.
Other plant toxins:
Pesticides—organophosphates.
Pokeweed.
Rhubarb.
Miscellaneous:
Allergic reactions.
Carbon monoxide poisoning.
Ethanol.
Heavy metals.
Monosodium glutamate (MSG).
Opiate withdrawal.
Gastrointestinal Pathology
Appendicitis.
Autonomic dysfunction.
Bile acid malabsorption.
Blind loop.
Bowel obstruction.
Celiac disease.
Cirrhosis.
Defects in amino acid transport.
Diverticular disease.
Familial dysautonomia.
Fecal impaction.
Fecal incontinence.
GI bleed.
GI cancer.
Hirschsprung disease.
Inflammatory bowel disease (ulcerative colitis, Crohn's disease).
Intussusception.
Irritable bowel syndrome.
Ischemic bowel.
Lactose/fructose intolerance.
Malabsorption syndromes.
Malrotation.
Postsurgical.
Postvagotomy.
Radiation therapy.
Short gut syndrome.
Small bowel resection.

Strictures.
Toxic megacolon.
Tropical sprue.
Volvulus.
Whipple disease.

Endocrine Related

Carcinoid syndrome (serotonin).
Hormonal hypersecretion.
Hyperthyroidism (thyroid hormone).
Medullary carcinoma of the thyroid (calcitonin).
Pancreatic cholera (VIP).
Somatostatinoma (somatostatin).
Systemic mastocytosis (histamine).
Zollinger-Ellison syndrome (gastrin).

Endocrine pathology

Adrenal insufficiency.
Diabetes enteropathy.
Hypoparathyroidism.
Pancreatic insufficiency.

Systemic Illness/Other

Alcoholism.
Amyloidosis.
Connective tissue disease.
Cystic fibrosis.
Ectopic pregnancy.
Hemolytic-uremic syndrome.
Henoch-Schönlein purpura.
Lymphoma.
Otitis media—infants.
Pelvic inflammatory disease.
Pneumonia/sepsis.
Pyelonephritis.
Scleroderma/SLE.
Severe malnutrition.
Stevens-Johnson syndrome.
Toxic shock syndrome.
Wilson's disease.
Miscellaneous:
- Factitious diarrhea.
- Runner's diarrhea.

ACE, Angiotensin-converting enzyme; *GI*, gastrointestinal; *NSAIDs*, nonsteroidal antiinflammatory drugs; *SLE*, systemic lupus erythematosus; *VIP*, vasoactive intestinal polypeptide.

DIARRHEA IN PATIENTS WITH AIDS[26]

ICD-10CM # R19.7 Diarrhea, unspecified

PROTOZOA

*Microsporidium.**
Cryptosporidium spp.*
Isospora belli.
Toxoplasma spp.
Giardia lamblia.
Entamoeba histolytica.
Leishmania donovani.
Blastocystis hominis.
Cyclospora spp.
Pneumocystis jiroveci.

BACTERIA

Clostridium difficile.
Salmonella spp.
Shigella spp.*
*Campylobacter jejuni.**
Mycobacterium avium complex.
Mycobacterium tuberculosis.
SIBO.
Vibrio spp.

VIRUSES

CMV.*
HSV.
Adenoviruses.
Rotavirus spp.
Norovirus.
HIV.

FUNGI

Histoplasmosis.
Coccidioidomycosis.
Cryptococcosis.
Candidiasis.
Penicillium marneffei.

NEOPLASMS

Lymphoma.
Kaposi sarcoma.

IDIOPATHIC

"AIDS enteropathy."

DRUG INDUCED

HIV protease inhibitors.

PANCREATIC DISEASE

Pancreatic insufficiency.
Chronic pancreatitis.
Infectious pancreatitis (CMV, MAC).
Drug-induced pancreatitis (e.g., pentamidine).

CMV, cytomegalovirus.
*More frequent cause.

DIARRHEA, TUBE-FED PATIENT[32]

ICD-10CM # K91.89 Other postprocedural complications and disorders of digestive system

COMMON CAUSES UNRELATED TO TUBE FEEDING

Elixir medications containing sorbitol.
Magnesium-containing antacids.
Antibiotic-induced sterile gut.
Pseudomembranous colitis.

POSSIBLE CAUSES RELATED TO TUBE FEEDING

Inadequate fiber to form stool bulk.
High fat content of formula (in the presence of fat malabsorption syndrome).
Bacterial contamination of enteral products and delivery systems (causal association with diarrhea not documented).
Rapid advancement in rate (after the GI tract is unused for prolonged periods).

UNLIKELY CAUSES RELATED TO TUBE FEEDING

Formula hyperosmolality (proven not to be the cause of diarrhea).
Lactose (absent from nearly all enteral feeding formulas).

DIPLOPIA, BINOCULAR

ICD-10CM # H53.2 Diplopia

Cranial nerve palsy (3rd, 4th, 6th).
Thyroid eye disease.
Myasthenia gravis.
Decompensated strabismus.
Orbital trauma with blowout fracture.
Orbital pseudotumor.
Cavernous sinus thrombosis.

DIPLOPIA, MONOCULAR

ICD-10CM # H53.2 Diplopia

Postoperative corrected long-standing tropia.
Defective contact lenses.
Poorly fitting bifocals.
Trauma to iris.
Corneal disorder (e.g., dry eye, astigmatism).
Cataracts.
Lens subluxation.
Nystagmus.
Eyelid twitching.
Foreign body in aqueous or vitreous media.
Migraine.
Lesions of occipital cortex.
Psychogenic.

DIPLOPIA, VERTICAL

ICD-10CM # H53.2 Diplopia

- Myasthenia.
- Superior oblique palsy.
- Myositis or pseudotumor with orbital involvement.
- Lymphoma or metastases affecting the orbits.
- Brain stem or cerebellar lesions.
- Hydrocephalus.
- Third nerve palsy.
- Botulism.
- Wernicke encephalopathy.
- Dysthyroid orbitopathy (muscle infiltration).

DYSENTERY AND INFLAMMATORY ENTEROCOLITIS[10]

ICD-10CM # Varies with specific diagnosis

DIFFERENTIAL DIAGNOSIS OF ACUTE BACTERIAL DYSENTERY AND INFLAMMATORY ENTEROCOLITIS

Specific Infectious Processes

Bacillary dysentery (*Shigella dysenteriae, Shigella flexneri, Shigella sonnei, Shigella boydii; invasive Escherichia coli*).
Campylobacteriosis (*Campylobacter jejuni*).

Amebic dysentery (*Entamoeba histolytica*).
Ciliary dysentery (*Balantidium coli*).
Vibriosis (*Vibrio parahaemolyticus*).
Salmonellosis (*Salmonella typhimurium*).
Typhoid fever (*Salmonella typhi*).
Enteric fever (*Salmonella choleraesuis, Salmonella paratyphi*).
Yersiniosis (*Yersinia enterocolitica*).

Proctitis

Gonococcal (*Neisseria gonorrhoeae*).
Herpetic (*herpes simplex virus*).
Chlamydial (*Chlamydia trachomatis*).
Syphilitic (*Treponema pallidum*).

Other Syndromes

Necrotizing enterocolitis of the newborn.
Enteritis necroticans.
Pseudomembranous enterocolitis or *Clostridium difficile* colitis without overt pseudomembranes (*C. difficile*).
Diverticulitis.
Typhlitis.

Chronic Inflammatory Processes

Enteropathogenic and enteroaggregative *E. coli.*
Syphilis.
GI tuberculosis.
GI mycosis (including *Basidiobolus ranarum*).
Parasitic enteritis.

Syndromes without Known Infectious Cause

Idiopathic ulcerative colitis.
Crohn's disease.
Radiation enteritis.
Ischemic colitis.
Allergic enteritis.
Brainerd diarrhea.

DIZZINESS

ICD-10CM # R42 Dizziness and giddiness

- Viral syndrome.
- Anxiety, hyperventilation.
- Benign positional paroxysmal vertigo.
- Medications (e.g., sedatives, antihypertensives, analgesics).
- Withdrawal from medications (e.g., benzodiazepines, SSRIs).
- Alcohol or drug abuse.
- Postural hypotension.
- Hypoglycemia, hyperglycemia.
- Hematologic disorders (e.g., anemia, polycythemia, leukemia).
- Head trauma.
- Ménière's disease.
- Vertebrobasilar ischemia.
- Cervical osteoarthritis.
- Cardiac abnormalities (arrhythmias, cardiomyopathy, CHF, pericarditis).
- Multiple sclerosis.
- Peripheral vestibulopathy.
- Air or sea travel.
- Electrolyte abnormalities.
- Eye problems (cornea, lens, retina).
- Migraine.
- Brain stem infarct.
- Autonomic neuropathy.
- Chronic otomastoiditis.
- Complex partial seizures.
- Ramsey Hunt syndrome.
- Arteritis.
- Syncope and presyncope.
- Perilymph fistula.
- Cerebellopontine tumor.
- Hepatic or renal disease.

DRY EYE

ICD-10CM # H04.129 Dry eye syndrome of unspecified lacrimal gland

Contacts.
Medications (antihistamines, clonidine, beta-blockers, ibuprofen, scopolamine).
Keratoconjunctivitis sicca.
Trauma.
Environmental causes (air conditioning in patient with contacts).

DYSLIPOPROTEINEMIAS, SECONDARY CAUSES[11]

ICD-10CM # E78.4 Other hyperlipidemia

Cause	Disorder
Metabolic	Diabetes. Lipodystrophy. Glycogen storage disorders.
Renal	Chronic renal failure. Glomerulonephritis with nephritic syndrome.
Hepatic	Cirrhosis. Biliary obstruction. Porphyria.
Hormonal	Estrogens. Progesterones. Growth hormone. Thyroid disorders (hypothyroidism) Corticosteroids.
Lifestyle	Physical inactivity. Obesity. Diet rich in fats, saturated fats. Alcohol intake. Smoking.
Medications	Retinoic acid derivatives. Glucocorticoids. Exogenous estrogens. Thiazide diuretics. Beta-adrenergic blockers (non-selective). Testosterone and other anabolic steroids. Immunosuppressive medications (cyclosporine). Antiviral medications (human immunodeficiency virus protease inhibitors) Antischizophrenic agents.

DYSPAREUNIA[24]

ICD-10CM #

N94.1	Dyspareunia
N44.8	Other noninflammatory disorders of the testis
N50.8	Other specified disorders of male genital organs
N53.12	Painful ejaculation
F52.6	Dyspareunia not due to a substance or known physiological condition

INTROITAL

Vaginismus.
Intact or rigid hymen.
Clitoral problems.
Vulvovaginitis.
Vaginal atrophy: hypoestrogen.
Vulvar dystrophy.
Bartholin or Skene gland infection.
Inadequate lubrication.
Operative scarring.

MIDVAGINAL

Urethritis.
Trigonitis.
Cystitis.
Short vagina.
Operative scarring.
Inadequate lubrication.

DEEP

Endometriosis.
Pelvic infection.
Uterine retroversion.
Ovarian pathology.
GI.
Orthopedic.
Abnormal penile size or shape.

DYSPEPSIA AND PYROSIS, DIFFERENTIAL DIAGNOSIS DURING PREGNANCY[30]

ICD-10CM #

K30	Dyspepsia, atonic
F45.3	Dyspepsia, psychogenic

DIFFERENTIAL DIAGNOSIS OF DYSPEPSIA OR PYROSIS DURING PREGNANCY

Gastroesophageal reflux disease.
Peptic ulcer disease.
Nausea and vomiting of pregnancy.
Hyperemesis gravidarum.
Pancreatitis.
Biliary colic.
Acute cholecystitis.
Viral hepatitis.
Appendicitis.
Acute fatty liver of pregnancy (in late pregnancy).
Irritable bowel syndrome/nonulcer dyspepsia.

DYSPHAGIA

ICD-10CM # R13.10 Dysphagia, unspecified

Esophageal obstruction: neoplasm, foreign body, achalasia, stricture, spasm, esophageal web, diverticulum, Schatzki ring.
Peptic esophagitis with stricture, Barrett stricture.
External esophageal compression: neoplasms (thyroid neoplasm, lymphoma, mediastinal tumors), thyroid enlargement, aortic aneurysm, vertebral spurs, aberrant right subclavian artery (dysphagia lusoria).
Hiatal hernia, GERD.
Oropharyngeal lesions: pharyngitis, glossitis, stomatitis, neoplasms.
Hysteria: globus hystericus.
Neurologic and/or neuromuscular disturbances: bulbar paralysis, myasthenia gravis, ALS, multiple sclerosis, Parkinsonism, CVA, diabetic neuropathy.
Toxins: poisoning, botulism, tetanus, postdiphtheritic dysphagia.
Systemic diseases: scleroderma, amyloidosis, dermatomyositis.
Candida and herpes esophagitis.
Presbyesophagus.

DYSPHAGIA, ESOPHAGEAL[26]

ICD-10CM # R13-14 Dysphagia, pharyngoesophageal phase

COMMON CAUSES OF ESOPHAGEAL DYSPHAGIA

Motility (Neuromuscular) Disorders

Primary

Achalasia.
Distal esophageal spasm.
Hypercontractile (jackhammer) esophagus.
Hypertensive LES.
Nutcracker (high-pressure) esophagus.
Other peristaltic abnormalities.[17]

Secondary

Chagas disease.
Reflux-related dysmotility.
Scleroderma and other rheumatologic disorders.

Structural (Mechanical) Disorders

Intrinsic

Carcinoma and benign tumors.
Diverticula.
Eosinophilic esophagitis.
Esophageal rings and webs (other than Schatzki ring).
Foreign body.
Lower esophageal (Schatzki) ring.
Medication-induced stricture.
Peptic stricture.

Extrinsic

Mediastinal mass.
Spinal osteophytes.
Vascular compression.

LES, lower esophageal sphincter.

[17] Peristaltic abnormalities include absent peristalsis and weak peristalsis, as well as hypertensive peristalsis (nutcracker esophagus).

DYSPHAGIA, OROPHARYNGEAL[81]

ICD-10CM # R13.12 Dysphagia, oropharyngeal phase

FUNCTIONAL DISORDERS

Central Nervous System

Stroke.
Head injury.
Parkinson's disease.
Motor neuron disease.
Multiple sclerosis.
Tumor.
Drugs (e.g., phenothiazines).
Malformations (e.g., syrinx, Arnold–Chiari).

Neural

Motor neuron disease.
Myasthenia gravis.
Radiotherapy.
Poliomyelitis.
Familial dysautonomia.

Muscle

Autoimmune myopathy (polymyositis, dermatomyositis, systemic lupus erythematosus).
Thyrotoxic myopathy.
Guillain-Barré motor neuropathy.
Muscular dystrophies.

STRUCTURAL DISORDERS

Head/neck surgery.
Stricture.
Radiotherapy.
Tumor.
Pharyngeal pouch.
Web.
Extrinsic (e.g., osteophytes).

MISCELLANEOUS

Xerostomia.

DYSPNEA

ICD-10CM # R06.9 Unspecified abnormalities of breathing

Upper airway obstruction: trauma, neoplasm, epiglottitis, laryngeal edema, tongue retraction, laryngospasm, abductor paralysis of vocal cords, aspiration of foreign body.
Lower airway obstruction: neoplasm, COPD, asthma, aspiration of foreign body.
Pulmonary infection: pneumonia, abscess, empyema, TB, bronchiectasis.
Pulmonary hypertension.
Pulmonary embolism/infarction.
Parenchymal lung disease.
Pulmonary vascular congestion.
Cardiac disease: ASHD, valvular lesions, cardiac dysrhythmias, cardiomyopathy, pericardial effusion, cardiac shunts.
Space-occupying lesions: neoplasm, large hiatal hernia, pleural effusions.
Disease of chest wall: severe kyphoscoliosis, fractured ribs, sternal compression, morbid obesity.
Neurologic dysfunction: Guillain-Barré syndrome, botulism, polio, spinal cord injury.
Interstitial pulmonary disease: sarcoidosis, collagen vascular diseases, DIP, Hamman-Rich pneumonitis, etc.
Pneumoconioses: silicosis, berylliosis, etc.
Mesothelioma.
Pneumothorax, hemothorax, pleural effusion.
Inhalation of toxins.
Cholinergic drug intoxication.
Carcinoid syndrome.
Hematologic: anemia, polycythemia, hemoglobinopathies.
Thyrotoxicosis, myxedema.
Diaphragmatic compression caused by abdominal distention, subphrenic abscess, ascites.
Lung resection.
Metabolic abnormalities: uremia, hepatic coma, DKA.
Sepsis.
Atelectasis.
Psychoneurosis.
Diaphragmatic paralysis.
Pregnancy.

DYSTONIA, PEDIATRIC PATIENT[79]

ICD-10CM #		
	G24.9	Dystonia, unspecified
	G24.2	Idiopathic nonfamilial dystonia
	G24.1	Genetic torsion dystonia

CAUSES OF DYSTONIA IN CHILDHOOD

Static Injury/Structural Disorders

Cerebral palsy.
Hypoxic-ischemic injury.
Kernicterus.
Head trauma.
Encephalitis.
Tumors.
Stroke in the basal ganglia (which may be due to vascular abnormalities or varicella).
Congenital malformations affecting basal ganglia.

Hereditary/Degenerative Disorders

DYT1 (autosomal dominant, TorsinA).
DYT2 (autosomal-recessive, Hippocalcin).
DYT4 (autosomal dominant, β-tubulin 4a).
DYT5 (autosomal dominant, GTP cyclohydrolase 1).
DYT6 (autosomal dominant, THAP1).
DYT8 (autosomal dominant, Myofibrillogenesis regulator 1).
DYT9 (autosomal dominant, GLUT1).
DYT10 (autosomal dominant, PRRT2).
DYT11 (autosomal dominant [maternal imprinting], ε-Sarcoglycan).
DYT12 (autosomal dominant, Na^+/K^+ATPase $\alpha 3$ subunit).
DYT15 (autosomal dominant, unknown).
DYT16 (autosomal recessive, Protein kinase activator PRKRA).
Pantothenate kinase-associated neurodegeneration (PKAN; neuronal brain iron accumulation type 1, due to mutations in *PANK2*).
PLA2G6-associated neurodegeneration (PLAN).

Huntington disease (Westphal variant, IT15–4p16.3).
Spinocerebellar ataxias (SCAs, particularly SCA3/Machado-Joseph disease).
Striatal necrosis.
Leigh syndrome.
Neuroacanthocytosis.
HARP syndrome (hypoprebetalipoproteinemia, acanthocytosis, retinitis pigmentosa, and pallidal degeneration).
Tay-Sachs disease.
Sandhoff disease.
Niemann-Pick type C.

Metabolic Disease

Glutaric aciduria types 1 and 2.
Acyl-CoA dehydrogenase deficiencies.
Neurotransmitter disorders.
Mitochondrial disorders.
GM $_1$ gangliosidosis.
Lesch-Nyhan disease.
Wilson disease.
Vitamin E deficiency.
Methylmalonic aciduria.
Tyrosinemia.

Drugs/Toxins

Neuroleptic and neuroleptic-like antiemetic medications (haloperidol, chlorpromazine, olanzapine, risperidone, prochlorperazine).
Calcium channel blockers.
Stimulants (amphetamine, cocaine, ergot alkaloids).
Anticonvulsants (carbamazepine, phenytoin).
Thallium.
Manganese.
Carbon monoxide.
Ethylene glycol.
Cyanide.
Methanol.

Paroxysmal Disorders

Paroxysmal kinesigenic dyskinesia (PKD).
Paroxysmal nonkinesigenic dyskinesia (PNKD).
Exercise-induced dyskinesia (PED).

DYSURIA

ICD-10CM # R30.0 Dysuria
R30.9 Painful micturition, unspecified

Urinary tract infection.
Estrogen deficiency (in postmenopausal female).
Vaginitis.
Genital infection (e.g., herpes, condyloma).
Interstitial cystitis.
Chemical irritation (e.g., deodorant aerosols, douches).
Meatal stenosis or stricture.
Reiter syndrome.
Bladder neoplasm.
GI etiology (diverticulitis, Crohn’s disease).
Impaired bladder or sphincter action.
Urethral carbuncle.
Chronic fibrosis posttrauma.
Radiation therapy.
Prostatitis.
Urethritis (gonococcal, *Chlamydia*).
Behçet syndrome.
Stevens-Johnson syndrome.

EARACHE[71]

ICD-10CM # H92.09 Otalgia, unspecified ear

Otitis media.
Serous otitis media.
Eustachitis.
Otitis externa.
Otitic barotrauma.
Mastoiditis.
Foreign body.
Impacted cerumen.
Referred otalgia, as with TMJ dysfunction, dental problems, and tumors.

ECTOPIC ACTH SECRETION[32]

ICD-10CM # E34.2 Ectopic hormone secretion, not elsewhere classified

Small cell carcinoma of lung.
Endocrine tumors of foregut origin:
- Thymic carcinoid.
- Islet cell tumor.
- Medullary carcinoid, thyroid.
- Bronchial carcinoid.

Pheochromocytoma.
Ovarian tumors.

EDEMA, CHILDREN[41]

ICD-10CM # R60.0 Localized edema
R60.1 Generalized edema
R60.9 Edema, unspecified

CARDIOVASCULAR

Congestive heart failure.
Acute thrombi or emboli.
Vasculitis of many types.

RENAL

Nephrotic syndrome.
Glomerulonephritis of many types.
End-stage renal failure.

ENDOCRINE OR METABOLIC

Thyroid disease.
Starvation.
Hereditary angioedema.

IATROGENIC

Drugs (diuretics and steroids).
Water or salt overload.

HEMATOLOGIC

Hemolytic disease of the newborn.

GASTROINTESTINAL

Hepatic cirrhosis.
Protein-losing enteritis.
Lymphangiectasis.
Cystic fibrosis.
Celiac disease.
Enteritis of many types.

LYMPHATIC ABNORMALITIES

Congenital (gonadal dysgenesis).
Acquired.

EDEMA, GENERALIZED

ICD-10CM # R60.0 Localized edema
R60.1 Generalized edema
R60.9 Edema, unspecified

Congestive heart failure (CHF).
Cirrhosis.
Nephrotic syndrome.
Pregnancy.
Idiopathic.
Acute nephritic syndrome.
Myxedema.
Medications (NSAIDs, estrogens, vasodilators).

EDEMA, LEG, UNILATERAL[55]

ICD-10CM # R60.0 Localized edema
R60.9 Edema, unspecified

WITH PAIN

DVT.
Postphlebitic syndrome.
Popliteal cyst rupture.
Gastrocnemius rupture.
Cellulitis.
Psoas or other abscess.

WITHOUT PAIN

DVT.
Postphlebitic syndrome.
Other venous insufficiency (after saphenous vein harvest, varicosities).
Lymphatic obstruction/lymphedema (carcinoma, lymphoma, sarcoidosis, filariasis, retroperitoneal fibrosis).

EDEMA OF LOWER EXTREMITIES

ICD-10CM # R60.0 Localized edema
R60.9 Edema, unspecified

CHF (right-sided).
Hepatic cirrhosis.
Nephrosis.
Myxedema.
Lymphedema.
Pregnancy.
Abdominal mass: neoplasm, cyst.
Venous compression from abdominal aneurysm.
Varicose veins.
Bilateral cellulitis.
Bilateral thrombophlebitis.
Vena cava thrombosis, venous thrombosis.
Retroperitoneal fibrosis.

EJECTION SOUND OR CLICK

ICD-10CM # R01.2 Other cardiac sounds

Aortic regurgitation.
Aortic root dilatation.
Systemic hypertension.
Chronic pulmonary hypertension.
Tetralogy of Fallot.
Atrial septal defect.
Pulmonary valve stenosis.
Aortic aneurysm.

ELBOW PAIN

ICD-10CM # M25.529 Pain in unspecified elbow

Trauma.
Infection.
Inflammatory arthritis.
Lateral or medial epicondylitis.
Entrapment neuropathy.
Olecranon bursitis.
Osteoarthritis.
Gout.
Cervical disease (referred pain).
Shoulder disease (referred pain).
Partial subluxation.
Synovial osteochondromatosis.
Loose body.

ELEVATED HEMIDIAPHRAGM

ICD-10CM # J98.6 Disorders of diaphragm
Q79.0 Congenital diaphragmatic hernia
Q79.1 Other congenital malformations of diaphragm

Neoplasm (bronchogenic carcinoma, mediastinal neoplasm, intrahepatic lesion).
Substernal thyroid.
Infectious process (pneumonia, empyema, TB, subphrenic abscess, hepatic abscess).
Atelectasis.
Idiopathic.
Eventration.
Phrenic nerve dysfunction (myelitis, myotonia, herpes zoster).
Trauma to phrenic nerve or diaphragm (e.g., surgery).
Aortic aneurysm.
Intraabdominal mass.
Pulmonary infarction.
Pleurisy.
Radiation therapy.
Rib fracture.

EMBOLI, ARTERIAL[55]

ICD-10CM # I74.3 Embolism and thrombosis of arteries of the lower extremities
I74.2 Embolism and thrombosis of arteries of the upper extremities

Myocardial infarction with mural thrombi.
Atrial fibrillation.
Cardiomyopathies.
Prosthetic heart valves.
CHF.
Endocarditis.
Left ventricular aneurysm.
Left atrial myxoma.
Sick sinus syndrome.
Paradoxical embolus from venous thrombosis.
Aneurysms of large blood vessels.
Atheromatous ulcers of large blood vessels.

EMESIS, PEDIATRIC AGE[41]

ICD-10CM # R11.10 Vomiting, unspecified
R11.11 Vomiting without nausea
R11.12 Projectile vomiting

INFANCY

Gastrointestinal Tract

Congenital

Regurgitation—chalasia, gastroesophageal reflux.
Atresia—stenosis (tracheoesophageal fistula, prepyloric diaphragm, intestinal atresia).
Duplication.
Volvulus (errors in rotation and fixation, Meckel diverticulum).
Congenital bands.
Hirschsprung disease.
Meconium ileus (cystic fibrosis), meconium plug.

Acquired

Acute infectious gastroenteritis, food poisoning (staphylococcal, clostridial).
Pyloric stenosis.
Gastritis, duodenitis.
Intussusception.
Incarcerated hernia—inguinal, internal secondary to old adhesions.
Cow's milk protein intolerance, food allergy, eosinophilic gastroenteritis.
Disaccharidase deficiency.
Celiac disease—presents after introduction of gluten in diet; inherited risk.
Adynamic ileus—the mediator for many nongastrointestinal causes.
Neonatal necrotizing enterocolitis.
Chronic granulomatous disease with gastric outlet obstruction.

Nongastrointestinal Tract

Infectious—otitis, urinary tract infection, pneumonia, upper respiratory tract infection, sepsis, meningitis.
Metabolic—aminoaciduria and organic aciduria, galactosemia, fructosemia, adrenogenital syndrome, renal tubular acidosis, diabetic ketoacidosis, Reye syndrome.
CNS—trauma, tumor, infection, diencephalic syndrome, rumination, autonomic responses (pain, shock).
Medications—anticholinergics, aspirin, alcohol, idiosyncratic reaction (e.g., codeine).

CHILDHOOD

Gastrointestinal Tract

Peptic ulcer—vomiting is a common presentation in children younger than 6 yr old.
Trauma—duodenal hematoma, traumatic pancreatitis, perforated bowel.
Pancreatitis—mumps, trauma, cystic fibrosis, hyperparathyroidism, hyperlipidemia, organic acidemias.
Crohn's disease.
Idiopathic intestinal pseudoobstruction.
Superior mesenteric artery syndrome.

Nongastrointestinal Tract

CNS—cyclic vomiting, migraine, anorexia nervosa, bulimia.

ENCEPHALOMYELITIS, NONVIRAL CAUSES[55]

ICD-10CM # G04.81 Other encephalitis and encephalomyelitis

Subacute bacterial endocarditis.
Rocky Mountain spotted fever.
Typhus.
Ehrlichia.
Q fever.
Chlamydia.
Mycoplasma.
Legionella.
Brucellosis.
Listeria.
Whipple disease.
Cat-scratch disease.
Syphilis (meningovascular).
Relapsing fever.
Lyme disease.
Leptospirosis.
Nocardia.
Actinomycosis.
Tuberculosis.
Cryptococcus.
Histoplasma.
Toxoplasma.
Plasmodium falciparum.
Trypanosomiasis.
Behçet's disease.
Vasculitis.
Carcinoma.
Drug reactions.

ENCEPHALOPATHY, HYPERTENSIVE[83]

ICD-10CM # Varies with specific diagnosis

Cerebral infarction.
Subarachnoid hemorrhage.
Intracerebral hemorrhage.
Subdural or epidural hematoma.
Brain tumor or other mass lesion.
Seizure disorder.
CNS vasculitis.
Encephalitis/meningitis.
Drug ingestion.
Drug withdrawal.

ENCEPHALOPATHY, METABOLIC[77]

ICD-10CM # F10.27 Alcohol dependence with alcohol-induced persisting dementia
K72.90 Hepatic failure, unspecified without coma
K72.91 Hepatic failure, unspecified with coma

	G92	Toxic encephalopathy
	T56.0X1A	Toxic effect of lead and its compounds, accidental (unintentional), initial encounter
	T56.0X2A	Toxic effect of lead and its compounds, intentional self-harm, initial encounter

Substrate deficiency: hypoxia/ischemia, carbon monoxide poisoning, hypoglycemia.
Cofactor deficiency: thiamine, vitamin B_{12}, pyridoxine (INH administration).
Electrolyte disorders: hyponatremia, hypercalcemia, carbon dioxide narcosis, dialysis, hypermagnesemia, disequilibrium syndrome.
Endocrinopathies: DKA, hyperosmolar coma, hypothyroidism, hyperadrenocorticism, hyperparathyroidism.
Endogenous toxins: liver disease, uremia, porphyria.
Exogenous toxins: drug overdose (sedative/hypnotics, ethanol, narcotics, salicylates, tricyclic antidepressants), drug withdrawal, toxicity of therapeutic medications, industrial toxins (e.g., organophosphates, heavy metals), sepsis.
Heat stroke.
Epilepsy (postictal).

ENDOMETRIAL THICKENING[69]

ICD-10CM # Varies with specific diagnosis

CAUSES OF ENDOMETRIAL THICKENING

Early intrauterine pregnancy.
Incomplete abortion.
Ectopic pregnancy.
Retained products of conception.
Trophoblastic disease.
Endometritis.
Adhesions.
Hyperplasia.
Polyps.
Carcinoma.

ENTERIC FEVER[19]

ICD-10CM #	A01.00	Typhoid fever, unspecified
	A01.3	Paratyphoid fever
	R50.9	Fever, unspecified

Epstein-Barr infection.
Dengue.
Tuberculosis.
Brucellosis.
Bartonella henselae.
Leptospirosis.
Tularemia.
Ehrlichiosis.
Plague.
Typhus.
Malaria.
Disseminated histoplasmosis.

ENTHESOPATHY

ICD-10CM # M46.00 Spinal enthesopathy, site unspecified

Viremia or bacteremia.
Ankylosing spondylitis.
Psoriatic arthritis.
Drug-induced (quinolones, etretinate).
Reactive arthritis.
DISH.
Reiter syndrome.

EOSINOPHILIA, DISEASE ASSOCIATIONS[54]

ICD-10CM #	D72.1	Eosinophilia
	NEC J82	Eosinophilia, pulmonary

DISEASES, SYNDROMES, AND CONDITIONS COMMONLY ASSOCIATED WITH PERIPHERAL BLOOD EOSINOPHILIA AND/OR TISSUE EOSINOPHILIA

Infectious Agents

Parasitic Infections

Tropical eosinophilia.
Visceral larval migrans (VLM, toxocariasis).
Helminth infections.
Filariasis (*Wuchereria bancrofti, Brugia malay*).
Onchocerciasis.
Schistosomiasis.
Fascioliasis.
Paragonimiasis.
Strongyloidiasis.
Trichinosis.
Hookworm.
Ascariasis.
Echinococcosis/hydatid disease.

Fungal Infections

Coccidioidomycosis.
Cryptococcosis (CSF eosinophilia) in HIV.

Allergic Diseases

Asthma (atopic and intrinsic, nasal polyps, aspirin intolerance syndromes).
Bronchopulmonary aspergillosis.
Allergic rhinitis.
Urticarias (acute allergic and chronic idiopathic).
Atopic dermatitis.
Acute drug (hypersensitivity) reactions (interstitial nephritis, cholestatic hepatitis, exfoliative dermatitis).

Respiratory Tract Disorders

Hypersensitivity pneumonitis (rare).
Allergic bronchopulmonary aspergillosis.
Eosinophilic pneumonia.
Transient pulmonary infiltrates (Löeffler syndrome).
Prolonged pulmonary infiltrates with eosinophilia (PIE syndrome).
Tropical pulmonary eosinophilia (TPE).
Bronchiectasis.
Cystic fibrosis.

Endocrinologic Disorders

Addison disease.

Gastrointestinal Diseases

Inflammatory bowel disease (IBD).
Eosinophilic gastroenteritis, eosinophilic esophagitis (EE).
Allergic gastroenteritis (young children).
Celiac disease (when associated with EE).

Toxic Reactions to Ingested Agents

Eosinophil myalgia syndrome (L-tryptophan).
Toxic oil syndrome.

Reactions to Cytokine Therapies

IL-2 and IL-2 plus lymphokine activated killer (LAK) cells.
GM-CSF therapy.

Cutaneous Disorders

Atopic dermatitis.
Immunologic skin diseases.
Scabies.
Myiasis.
Chlamydial pneumonia of infancy.
Scarlet fever and pneumococcal pneumonia (convalescent phase).
Cat scratch disease.
Eosinophilic cellulitis (Wells syndrome).
Episodic angioedema with eosinophilia.
Chronic idiopathic urticaria.
Bullous pemphigoid.
Herpes gestationis.
Angioblastic lymphoid hyperplasia (Kimura disease).

Immunodeficiency Syndromes

Wiskott-Aldrich syndrome.
Selective IgA deficiency with atopy.
Hyper-IgE recurrent infection syndrome (Job syndrome).
Swiss-type and sex-linked combined immunodeficiency.
Nezelof syndrome.
Graft-versus-host-disease (GVHD).

Connective Tissue Diseases

Vasculitis/Collagen Vascular Disorders

Hypersensitivity vasculitis.
Allergic granulomatosis with angiitis (Churg-Strauss syndrome).
Serum sickness.
Eosinophilic fasciitis.
Sjögren syndrome.
Rheumatoid arthritis (severe).

Neoplastic, Myeloproliferative, and Ly Neoplasms and Syndromes

Neoplastic

Ovarian carcinoma.
Solid tumors (mucin-secreting, epithelial cell origin).
Chronic eosinophil leukemia.
Idiopathic hypereosinophilic syndromes (HES).
Systemic mastocytosis.

Myeloproliferative

Chronic myelogenous leukemia (CML) acute myelogenous leukemia (AML) and myelodysplastic syndrome (MDS).
Myelomonocytic leukemia with bone marrow eosinophilia (M4Eo, inversion 16).

Lymphoproliferative

T-cell lymphocytic leukemia.
Lymphomas (T cell, Hodgkin disease).
Angioimmunoblastic lymphadenopathy.

Rare Causes

- Chronic active hepatitis.
- Chronic dialysis.
- Acute pancreatitis.
- Postirradiation.
- Hypopituitarism.

EOSINOPHILIA, GI[26]

ICD-10CM #	D72.1	Eosinophilia

CAUSES OF GI EOSINOPHILIA

GERD.
Eosinophilic GI disorders.
- Eosinophilic esophagitis.
  - Connective tissue disease-associated eosinophilic esophagitis.
  - Familial eosinophilic esophagitis.
- Eosinophilic gastritis.
- Eosinophilic enteritis.
- Eosinophilic gastroenteritis.

Infections.
- Schistosomiasis.
- Anisakiasis.
- GI basidiobolomycosis.
- Toxocariasis.

Celiac disease.
Hypereosinophilic syndrome.
Drug hypersensitivity response.
IBD.
Transplant-associated eosinophilic enteritis.
Eosinophilic granulomatosis with polyangiitis.
Toxic injury.
Graft-versus-host disease.

EOSINOPHILIC LUNG DISEASE[36]

ICD-10CM #	NEC J82	Eosinophilia, pulmonary

IDIOPATHIC

Simple pulmonary eosinophilia (Löffler's syndrome).
Acute eosinophilic pneumonia.
Chronic eosinophilic pneumonia.
Hypereosinophilic syndrome.

DRUG-INDUCED

Aminosalicylic acid.
Para-aminosalicylic acid.
NSAIDs.
Captopril.
Cocaine.
Minocycline.
Nitrofurantoin.
Phenytoin.

INFECTION

Parasitic (ascariasis, paragonimiasis. tropical eosinophilia).
Fungal (aspergillus).
Bacterial (TB, atypical mycobacterial infection, brucella).
Viral (respiratory syncytial virus).

IMMUNOLOGIC DISEASES

Granulomatosis with polyangiitis.
Churg–Strauss syndrome.
Rheumatoid disease.
Sarcoidosis.

NEOPLASMS

Bronchogenic carcinoma.
Bronchial carcinoid.
Lymphoma (Hodgkin's, non-Hodgkin's).

EOSINOPHILIA, PARASITIC CAUSES[10]

ICD-10CM #	Varies with specific diagnosis

PARASITIC CAUSES OF EOSINOPHILIA

Widespread Geographic Distribution

Ascariasis (migratory phase).
Hookworm.†
Strongyloidiasis.*‡
Tropical pulmonary eosinophilia.
Lymphatic filariasis.
Schistosomiasis.
Toxocariasis.
Cysticercosis (*Taenia solium*).
Echinococcosis (cyst rupture).
Trichinosis.
Trichuriasis.
Aberrant helminthiasis from animals.

Limited Geographic Distribution

Clonorchiasis.
Paragonimiasis.
Fascioliasis.
Angiostrongyliasis.
Opisthorchiasis.
Onchocerciasis, loiasis, and other nonlymphatic filariases.
Gnathostomiasis.
Capillariasis.
Trichostrongyliasis.

EPIGASTRIC PAIN[81]

ICD-10CM #	R10.816	Epigastric abdominal tenderness
	R10.826	Epigastric rebound abdominal tenderness

Peptic ulceration (uncomplicated).[18]
Peptic ulceration (perforated).
Biliary colic.
Acute pancreatitis.
Abdominal aortic aneurysm.
Anxiety.
Inferior wall MI.

EPILEPSY

ICD-10CM #	G40.909	Epilepsy, unspecified, not intractable, without status epilepticus

Psychogenic spells.
Transient ischemic attack.
Hypoglycemia.
Syncope.
Narcolepsy.
Migraine.
Paroxysmal vertigo.
Arrhythmias.
Drug reaction.

† Moderate to marked during larval migration in early infection; most often absent or very mild during chronic infection.
* Most frequent parasitic causes of massive eosinophilia (>5000/mm^3).
‡ Absent in disseminated infection in compromised hosts.
[18] Conditions that also cause right upper quadrant pain

EPILEPSY MIMICS, PEDIATRIC PATIENT[79]

ICD-10CM #	Varies with specific diagnosis

DISORDERS THAT MAY MIMIC CHILDHOOD EPILEPSY

Confused with Generalized Tonic–Clonic Seizures

Pallid syncope (reflex anoxic seizure).
Vasodepressor syncope (reflex anoxic seizure).
Cyanotic breath-holding attacks.
Collapsing attacks with cardiac dysrhythmias.
Cataplexy.

Confused with Generalized Absence Seizures

Behavioral staring attacks.
Complex partial (dyscognitive) seizures.
Tic disorder.

Confused with Complex Partial (Dyscognitive) Seizures

Self-stimulatory behavior, especially in children with autistic spectrum disorders.
Sleep walking.
Night terrors.
Temper tantrums with amnesia for the rage event.
Benign paroxysmal vertigo.
Migraine-related disorders.

Confused with Epileptic Myoclonus

Physiologic hypnagogic myoclonus.
Benign infantile sleep myoclonus.
Startle disease.

EPILEPSY SYNDROMES, AGE SPECIFIC[19]

ICD-10CM #	G40.90	Epilepsy, unspecified, not intractable
	G40.301	Generalized idiopathic epilepsy and epileptic syndromes, not intractable, with status epilepticus
	G40.40	Other generalized epilepsy and epileptic syndromes, not intractable

EPILEPSY SYNDROMES BY AGE OF ONSET

Neonatal

Benign familial neonatal epilepsy.
Early myoclonic encephalopathy.
Ohtahara syndrome.

Infancy

Epilepsy of infancy with migrating focal seizures.
West syndrome (infantile spasms, hypsarrhythmia; to be distinguished from benign myoclonus of early infancy, a nonepilepsy).

Differential Diagnosis II

Myoclonic epilepsy in infancy (benign Dravet variant).
Benign infantile epilepsy.
Benign familial infantile epilepsy.
Severe myoclonic epilepsy of infancy (classic Dravet syndrome).
Myoclonic encephalopathy in nonprogressive disorders.

Childhood

Genetic epilepsy with febrile seizures plus (GEFS +; can begin in infancy).
Panayiotopoulos syndrome.
Epilepsy with myoclonic atonic (previously astatic) seizures (Doose syndrome).
Benign epilepsy with centrotemporal spikes (BECTS, or benign rolandic epilepsy).
Autosomal-dominant nocturnal frontal lobe epilepsy (ADNFLE).
Late-onset childhood occipital epilepsy (Gastaut syndrome).
Epilepsy with myoclonic absences (Tassinari syndrome).
Lennox–Gastaut syndrome.
Epileptic encephalopathy with continuous spike-and-wave during sleep (CSWS).
Landau–Kleffner syndrome (LKS).
Childhood absence epilepsy (pyknolepsy).
Generalized epilepsy with eyelid myoclonia (Jeavons syndrome).*

Adolescence–Adult

Juvenile absence epilepsy (JAE).
Juvenile myoclonic epilepsy (JME).
Epilepsy with generalized tonic-clonic seizures alone.
Progressive myoclonus epilepsies (PME).
Autosomal-dominant epilepsy with auditory features.
Other familial temporal lobe epilepsies.

Less Specific Age Relationship

Familial focal epilepsy with variable foci (childhood to adult).
Reflex epilepsies (e.g., photosensitive, audiogenic, or reading-induced seizures; may or may not coexist with spontaneous seizures).

*Not listed as a syndrome by ILAE but instead recognized under absence seizures with special features.
(Adapted from Berg AT, Berkovic SF, Brodie MJ, et al: *Epilepsia* 51:676–685, 2010.)

EPISTAXIS

ICD-10CM # R04.0 Epistaxis

Trauma.
Medications (nasal sprays, NSAIDs, anticoagulants, antiplatelets).
Nasal polyps.
Cocaine use.
Coagulopathy (hemophilia, liver disease, DIC, thrombocytopenia).
Systemic disorders (hypertension, uremia).
Infections.
Anatomic malformations.
Rhinitis.
Nasal polyps.
Local neoplasms (benign and malignant).
Desiccation.
Foreign body.

ERECTILE DYSFUNCTION, ORGANIC[67]

ICD-10CM # N52.9 Male erectile dysfunction, unspecified

Neurogenic abnormalities: somatic nerve neuropathy, CNS abnormalities.
Psychogenic causes: depression, performance anxiety, marital conflict.
Endocrine causes: hyperprolactinemia, hypogonadotropic hypogonadism, testicular failure, estrogen excess.
Trauma: pelvic fracture, prostate surgery, penile fracture.
Systemic disease: DM, renal failure, hepatic cirrhosis.
Medications: diuretics, antidepressants, H_2 blockers, exogenous hormones, alcohol, antihypertensives, nicotine abuse, finasteride, etc.
Structural abnormalities: Peyronie's disease.

EROSIONS, GENITALIA

ICD-10CM # N36.8 Other specified disorders of urethra

Candidiasis.
Intraepithelial neoplasia.
Squamous cell carcinoma.
Lichen planus.
Pemphigus vulgaris.
Erythema multiforme.
Lichen sclerosus.
Bullous pemphigoid.
Extramammary Paget disease.
Impetigo.

ERYTHEMATOUS ANNULAR SKIN LESIONS

ICD-10CM # L53.8 Other specified erythematous conditions

Tinea corporis.
Warfarin plaques.
Erythema multiforme.
Erythema annulare.
Cutaneous lupus.
Cutaneous sarcoidosis.
Trauma.
Acute febrile neutrophilic dermatosis (Sweet syndrome).

ERYTHROCYTOSIS[43]

ICD-10CM # D75.0 Familial erythrocytosis

CAUSES OF ERYTHROCYTOSIS

Relative or Spurious Erythrocytosis (Normal Red Cell Mass)

Hemoconcentration secondary to dehydration (diarrhea, diaphoresis, diuretics, water deprivation, emesis, ethanol, hypertension, preeclampsia, pheochromocytoma, carbon monoxide intoxication).

True or Absolute Erythrocytosis

Polycythemia vera.
Primary congenital polycythemia.
Secondary erythrocytosis caused by:
- Congenital causes (e.g., activating mutation of erythropoietin receptor).
- Hypoxia caused by carbon monoxide poisoning, high oxygen affinity hemoglobin, high-altitude residence, chronic pulmonary disease, hypoventilation syndromes such as sleep apnea, right to left cardiac shunt, neurologic defects involving the respiratory center.
- Nonhypoxic causes with pathologic erythropoietin production.
- Renal disease (cysts, hydronephrosis, renal artery stenosis, focal glomerulonephritis, renal transplantation).
- Tumors (renal cell cancer, hepatocellular carcinoma, cerebellar hemangioblastoma, uterine fibromyoma, adrenal tumors, meningioma, pheochromocytoma).
- Drug-associated causes:
  - Androgen therapy.
  - Exogenous erythropoietin growth factor therapy.

ERYTHRODERMA

ICD-10CM # L53.9 Erythematous condition, unspecified

Drug reaction (e.g., allopurinol, ampicillin, phenytoin, vancomycin, dapsone, omeprazole, carbamazepine).
Atopic dermatitis.
Psoriasis.
Contact dermatitis.
Idiopathic.
Pityriasis rubra.
Chronic actinic dermatitis.
Bullous pemphigoid.
Paraneoplastic.
Cutaneous T-cell lymphoma.
Connective tissue disease.
Hypereosinophilia syndrome.

ESOPHAGEAL PERFORATION[55]

ICD-10CM # K22.3 Perforation of esophagus
S27.819A Unspecified injury of esophagus (thoracic part), initial encounter

Trauma.
Caustic burns.
Iatrogenic.
Foreign bodies.
Spontaneous rupture (Boerhaave syndrome).
Postoperative breakdown of anastomosis.

ESOPHAGEAL STRICTURES[72]

ICD-10CM # Varies with specific diagnosis

BENIGN

Congenital

Esophageal atresia.
Tracheoesophageal fistula.
Web.

ACQUIRED

Peptic:
- Gastroesophageal reflux.
- Scleroderma.

Schatzki ring.
Caustic ingestion.
Drug-induced:
- Anticholinergic medications.
- Aspirin.
- Ferrous sulfate.
- Fosamax.
- Nonsteroidal antiinflammatory.
- Quinidine.
- Potassium supplements.
- Tetracycline.
- Vitamin C.

Eosinophilic esophagitis.
Iatrogenic:
- Variceal ligation/injection.
- Endoscopic mucosal resection.
- Ablation therapy (cryotherapy/radiofrequency).
- Postoperative (anastomotic).
- Radiation.
- Instrumentation.
- Nasogastric tube.

Infections:
- Fungal: moniliasis.
- Bacterial: syphilis.
- Mycobacterial: tuberculosis.

Granulomatous:
- Crohn's disease.

Dermatosis:
- Epidermolysis bullosa dystrophica.
- Pemphigoid.
- Behçet disease.

MALIGNANT

Primary.
Secondary.

ESOPHAGEAL TUMORS, BENIGN[72]

ICD-10CM # Varies with specific diagnosis

CLASSIFICATION OF BENIGN ESOPHAGEAL TUMORS

Mucosa (First and Second Esophageal Ultrasound [EUS] Layers)

Squamous papilloma.
Fibrovascular polyp.
Retention cyst.

Submucosa (Third EUS Layer)

Lipoma.
Fibroma.
Neurofibroma.
Granular cell tumor.
Hemangiomas.
Salivary gland–type tumor.

Muscularis Propria (Fourth EUS Layer)

Leiomyoma.
Duplication cyst.

Periesophageal Tissue (Fifth EUS Layer)

Foregut cyst.

ESOPHAGITIS[55]

ICD-10CM # K20.9 Esophagitis, unspecified

INFECTIOUS

Candidiasis.
Cytomegalovirus.
Herpes simplex virus.
HIV infection, acute.

NONINFECTIOUS

Gastroesophageal reflux.
Mucositis from cancer chemotherapy.
Mucositis from radiation therapy.
Aphthous ulcers.

ESOPHAGUS, SYSTEMIC DISEASES[72]

ICD-10CM # Varies with specific diagnosis

SYSTEMIC DISEASES OF THE ESOPHAGUS

Connective Tissue Disorders

Scleroderma.
Systemic lupus erythematosus.
Polymyositis.
Dermatomyositis.
Mixed connective tissue disorder.
Raynaud syndrome.

Allergic Disease

Eosinophilic esophagitis.

Metabolic Diseases

Amyloidosis.
Diabetes mellitus.
Hypothyroidism.
Hyperthyroidism.

Dermatologic Diseases

Epidermolysis bullosa.
Pemphigus vulgaris.
Pemphigoid.
Erythema multiforme.
Lichen planus.
Behçet disease.

Infectious Diseases

Histoplasmosis.
Tuberculosis.
Actinomycosis.
Immunocompromised host:
- Fungal: *Candida* species.
- Viral: herpes simplex, cytomegalovirus.
- Mycobacterial.
- Bacterial: *Streptococcus viridans*, *Staphylococcus*, bacilli, *Treponema pallidum*.
- Protozoal.

Miscellaneous Disorders

Sarcoidosis.
Crohn's disease.

ESOTROPIA

ICD-10CM # H50.00 Unspecified esotropia
H50.43 Accommodative component in esotropia
H50.05 Alternating esotropia

Congenital.
Accommodative esotropia.
Myasthenia gravis.
Abducens palsy.
Pseudo-sixth nerve palsy.
Medial rectus entrapment (e.g., blowout fracture).
Posterior internuclear ophthalmoplegia.
Wernicke encephalopathy.
Thyroid myopathy.
Chiari malformation.

EXANTHEMS

ICD-10CM # R21 Rash and other nonspecific skin eruption

Measles.
Rubella.
Erythema infectiosum (fifth disease).
Roseola exanthema.
Varicella.
Enterovirus.
Adenovirus.
Epstein-Barr virus.
Kawasaki disease.
Staphylococcal scalded skin.
Scarlet fever.
Meningococcemia.
Rocky Mountain spotted fever.

EYELID NEOPLASM

ICD-10CM # C44.101 Unspecified malignant neoplasm of skin of unspecified eyelid, including canthus

MALIGNANT

Melanoma.
Basal cell carcinoma.
Squamous cell carcinoma.
Bowen disease.
Sebaceous cell carcinoma.
Metastatic lymphoma/leukemia.

BENIGN

Melanocytic nevus.
Pilar, eccrine, or apocrine tumor.
Neurofibroma.
Keratosis.
Squamous papilloma.
Keratoacanthoma.

EYELID RETRACTION

ICD-10CM # H02.89 Other specified disorders of eyelid

Congenital.
Graves ophthalmopathy.
Myasthenia gravis.
Postsurgical.
Guillain-Barré syndrome.

Cerebellar disease.
Horizontal gaze palsy.
Partial palsy of superior rectus muscle.
Encephalitis.
Closed head injury.
Disseminated sclerosis.
Eye trauma.
Contact lens wear.
Proptosis.
Eyelid neoplasm.
Atopic dermatitis.
Herpes zoster ophthalmicus.
Botulinum toxin injection.
Cyclic oculomotor paralysis.
Spheroid wing meningioma.
Hepatic cirrhosis.
Down syndrome.
Essential hypertension.
Meningitis.
Paget disease of bone.

EYE PAIN

ICD-10CM # H57.13 Ocular pain, bilateral

Foreign body.
Herpes zoster.
Trauma.
Conjunctivitis.
Iritis.
Iridocyclitis.
Uveitis.
Blepharitis.
Ingrown lashes.
Orbital or periorbital cellulitis/abscess.
Sinusitis.
Headache.
Glaucoma.
Inflammation of lacrimal gland.
Tic douloureux.
Cerebral aneurysm.
Cerebral neoplasm.
Entropion.
Retrobulbar neuritis.
UV light.
Dry eyes.
Irritation or inflammation from eye drops, dust, cosmetics, etc.

FACIAL PAIN

ICD-10CM # G50.1 Atypical facial pain

Infection, abscess.
Postherpetic neuralgia.
Trauma, posttraumatic neuralgia.
Tic douloureux.
Cluster headache, "lower-half headache."
Geniculate neuralgia.
Anxiety, somatization syndrome.
Glossopharyngeal neuralgia.
Carotidynia.

FACIAL PARALYSIS[61]

ICD-10CM # G51.0 Bell palsy

INFECTION

Bacterial: otitis media, mastoiditis, meningitis, Lyme disease.
Viral: herpes zoster, mononucleosis, varicella, rubella, mumps, Bell palsy.
Mycobacterial: TB, meningitis, leprosy.
Miscellaneous: syphilis, malaria.

TRAUMA

Temporal bone fracture, facial laceration.
Surgery.

NEOPLASM

Malignant: squamous cell carcinoma, basal cell and adenocystic tumors, leukemia, parotid neoplasms, metastatic tumors.
Benign: facial nerve neuroma, vestibular schwannoma, congenital cholesteatoma.

IMMUNOLOGIC

Guillain-Barré syndrome, periarteritis nodosa.
Reaction to tetanus antiserum.

METABOLIC

Pregnancy.
Hypothyroidism.
DM.

FAILURE TO THRIVE

ICD-10CM # R62.50 Unspecified lack of expected normal physiological development in childhood

PSYCHOSOCIAL/BEHAVIORAL

Inadequate diet because of poverty/food insufficiency, errors in food preparation.
Poor parenting skills (lack of knowledge of sufficient diet).
Child/parent interaction problems (autonomy struggles, coercive feeding, maternal depression).
Food refusal.
Rumination.
Parental cognitive or mental health problems.
Child abuse or neglect; emotional deprivation.

NEUROLOGIC

Cerebral palsy.
Hypothalamic and other CNS tumors (diencephalic syndrome).
Neuromuscular disorders.
Neurodegenerative disorders.

RENAL

Recurrent urinary tract infection.
Renal tubular acidosis.
Renal failure.

ENDOCRINE

Diabetes mellitus.
Diabetes insipidus.
Hypothyroidism/hyperthyroidism.
Growth hormone deficiency.
Adrenal insufficiency.

GENETIC/METABOLIC/CONGENITAL

Sickle cell disease.
Inborn errors of metabolism (organic acidosis, hyperammonemia, storage disease).
Fetal alcohol syndrome.
Skeletal dysplasias.
Chromosomal disorders.
Multiple congenital anomaly syndromes (VATER [vertebral defects, imperforate anus, tracheoesophageal fistula, radial and renal dysplasia], CHARGE [coloboma, heart disease, atresia choanae, retarded growth and retarded development and/or CNS anomalies, genital hypoplasia, ear anomalies and/or deafness]).

GASTROINTESTINAL

Pyloric stenosis.
Gastroesophageal reflux.
Repair of tracheoesophageal fistula.
Malrotation.
Malabsorption syndromes.
Celiac disease.
Milk intolerance: lactose, protein.
Pancreatic insufficiency syndromes (cystic fibrosis).
Chronic cholestasis.
Inflammatory bowel disease.
Chronic congenital diarrhea states.
Short bowel syndrome.
Pseudoobstruction.
Hirschsprung disease.
Food allergy.

CARDIAC

Cyanotic heart lesions.
Congestive heart failure.
Vascular rings.

PULMONARY/RESPIRATORY

Severe asthma.
Cystic fibrosis; bronchiectasis.
Chronic respiratory failure.
Bronchopulmonary dysplasia.
Adenoid/tonsillar hypertrophy.
Obstructive sleep apnea.

MISCELLANEOUS

Collagen vascular disease.
Malignancy.
Primary immunodeficiency.
Transplantation.

INFECTIONS

Perinatal infection (TORCHES [toxoplasma, other, rubella, cytomegalovirus, herpes simplex]).
Occult/chronic infections.
Parasitic infestation.
Tuberculosis.
HIV.

FATIGUE

ICD-10CM # R53.83 Other fatigue
F48.0 Neurasthenia

Depression.
Anxiety, emotional stress.
Inadequate sleep.
Chronic fatigue syndrome.
Prolonged physical activity.
Pregnancy and postpartum period.
Anemia.

Hypothyroidism.
Medications (β-blockers, anxiolytics, antidepressants, sedating antihistamines, clonidine, methyldopa).
Viral or bacterial infections.
Sleep apnea syndrome.
Dieting.
Renal failure, CHF, COPD, liver disease.

FATIGUE, CHRONIC

ICD-10CM #	R53.83	Other fatigue
	F48.0	Neurasthenia

CHRONIC INFECTIONS

Hepatitis C.
Lyme disease.
Parasitic and fungal infections.
Tuberculosis.
Human immunodeficiency virus.
Xenotropic murine leukemia retrovirus.

SLEEP DISORDERS

Obstructive sleep apnea.
Restless leg syndrome.
Circadian rhythm disorder.
Upper airway resistance syndrome.
Narcolepsy/parasomnias.
Alpha-delta sleep disorder.

ENDOCRINE/METABOLIC DISORDERS

Addison disease.
Cushing's syndrome.
Poorly controlled diabetes.
Thyroid disorders.
Hemochromatosis.
Hypopituitarism.
Diabetes insipidus.

GENERAL MEDICAL DISORDERS

Anemia (any cause).
Chronic renal/hepatic failure.
Malnutrition.
Medication side effects.
Chronic pain disorders.

PSYCHOLOGICAL

Mood disorders (depression, anxiety, bipolar).
Schizophrenia.
Posttraumatic stress disorder.
Anorexia nervosa/bulimia.
Childhood abuse and/or neglect.

CHRONIC INFLAMMATION

Rheumatoid arthritis.
Systemic lupus erythematosus.
Sjögren syndrome.
Polymyositis/dermatomyositis.
Vasculitis.
Sarcoidosis.

CARDIOPULMONARY

Congestive heart failure.
Neurally mediated hypotension.
Postural orthostatic tachycardia syndrome.
Pulmonary hypertension.
Chronic obstructive pulmonary disease.
Mitral valve prolapse.

GASTROINTESTINAL

Celiac disease.
Inflammatory bowel disease.
Autoimmune hepatitis.
Hepatic cirrhosis.

MALIGNANCY

Lymphoma and occult malignancies.
Postchemotherapy syndrome.

NEUROLOGIC DISORDERS

Multiple sclerosis.
Myasthenia gravis.
Muscular dystrophies.
Parkinson's disease.
Early dementia.

LIFESTYLE FACTORS

Chronic overwork.
Persistent unresolved stress.
Inadequate exercise.
Morbid obesity (body mass index >40).
Alcoholism/drug abuse.

FATTY LIVER

ICD-10CM #	K76.0	Fatty (change of) liver, not elsewhere classified
	K76.89	Other specified diseases of liver

Obesity.
Alcohol abuse.
DM.
Acute fatty liver of pregnancy.
Medications (tetracycline, valproic acid, glucocorticoids, amiodarone, estrogen, methotrexate).
Reye syndrome.
Wilson's disease.
Nonalcoholic steatosis.

FEVER, ABDOMINAL PAIN, JAUNDICE IN PEDIATRIC PATIENT[19]

ICD-10CM #	R50.9	Fever, unspecified

Cholangitis.
Cholecystitis.
Cholelithiasis.
Sepsis.
Hepatitis.
Choledochal cyst.
Pancreatitis.
Urinary tract infection.
Leptospirosis and other systemic infections with hepatic involvement.
Spontaneous perforation of common bile duct.
Biliary cyst.
Appendicitis.

FEVER AND CARDIOPULMONARY FAILURE[25]

ICD-10CM #	R50.9	Fever, unspecified

DIFFERENTIAL DIAGNOSIS OF FEVER AND RAPIDLY PROGRESSIVE CARDIOPULMONARY FAILURE

Bacterial Infection

Severe community-acquired pneumonia.
Meningitis, endocarditis.
Rickettsial disease (babesiois, ehrlichiosis, Rocky Mountain spotted fever, scrub typhus, Mediterranean spotted fever).
Q-Fever (*Coxiella burnetii*).
Brucellosis.
Plague (*Yersinia pestis*).
Tularemia (*Francisella tularensis*).
Typhoid fever/salmonellosis.
Leptospirosis (*Leptospira interrogans*).
Anthrax.
Mycobacterial infections.

Viral Infections

Viral pneumonia (influenza, CMV, EBV, VZV, SARS).
Hantavirus.
Dengue fever and yellow fever.
Hemorrhagic fever (Lassa, Marburg, or Ebola viruses).

Fungal Infections

Coccidiomycosis.
Cryptococcus.
Histoplasmosis.
Blastomycosis.

Parasitic Infections

Malaria.
Leishmaniasis.
Schistosomiasis.
Strongyloides.

Noninfectious Causes

Inflammatory:
- Rapid-onset interstitial pneumonia (acute interstitial pneumonia, acute hypersensitivity pneumonitis).
- Acute eosinophilic pneumonia.
- ARDS due to other causes (inhalation injury, drug overdose, trauma).

Rheumatologic disorders:
- Wegener granulomatosis, Churg-Strauss disease, Goodpasture syndrome.
- Systemic lupus erythematosus, antiphospholipid syndrome.

Other:
- Malignancy, lymphoma, lymphoproliferative disease, leukemia.
- Pulmonary embolism, aortic dissection, acute myocardial infarction.
- Adrenal insufficiency, thyroid storm.

ARDS, acute respiratory distress syndrome; *CMV*, Cytomegalovirus; *EBV*, Epstein-Barr virus; *SARS*, severe acute respiratory syndrome; *VZV*, varicella zoster virus.

FEVER AND JAUNDICE

ICD-10CM #	R50.9	Fever, unspecified
	R17	Unspecified jaundice

Bacterial sepsis.
Cholangitis.
Hepatic abscess.
Leptospirosis.
Malaria.
Viral hepatitis.
Yellow fever.

FEVER AND LYMPHADENOPATHY

ICD-10CM #	R59.9	Enlarged lymph nodes, unspecified
	R50.9	Fever, unspecified

REGIONAL

Cervical

Streptococci.
Tuberculosis.
Viral upper respiratory infection.

Peripheral

Bartonella henselae.
Herpesviruses.
Lymphoma.
Metastatic cancer.
Sporotrichosis.
Streptococci.

Inguinal

Chancroid.
Herpes.
Lymphogranuloma venereum.
Syphilis (primary).

GENERALIZED

Cytomegalovirus.
Epstein-Barr virus.
HIV.
Lymphoma.
Sarcoidosis.
Syphilis (secondary).
Toxoplasmosis.
Viral hepatitis.

FEVER AND RASH

ICD-10CM #	R21	Rash and other nonspecific skin eruption
	R21	Rash and other nonspecific skin eruption
	R50.9	Fever, unspecified

Drug hypersensitivity: penicillin, sulfonamides, thiazides, anticonvulsants, allopurinol.
Viral infection: measles, rubella, varicella, erythema infectiosum, roseola, enterovirus infection, viral hepatitis, infectious mononucleosis, acute HIV.
Other infections: meningococcemia, staphylococcemia, scarlet fever, typhoid fever, *Pseudomonas* bacteremia, Rocky Mountain spotted fever, Lyme disease, secondary syphilis, bacterial endocarditis, babesiosis, brucellosis, listeriosis.
Serum sickness.
Erythema multiforme.
Erythema marginatum.
Erythema nodosum.
SLE.
Dermatomyositis.
Allergic vasculitis.
Pityriasis rosea.
Herpes zoster.

FEVER AND RASH IN ICU[81]

ICD-10CM #	R21	Rash and other nonspecific skin eruption
	R50.9	Fever, unspecified

DIFFERENTIAL DIAGNOSTIC CLINICAL FEATURES OF FEVER AND RASH IN THE ICU

Rash with Shock

Infectious causes: toxic shock syndrome, meningococcemia, postsplenectomy sepsis, overwhelming *Staphylococcus aureus* bacteremia/acute bacterial endocarditis, arboviral hemorrhagic fevers, hemorrhagic smallpox, *Vibrio vulnificus*, gas gangrene, dengue fever.
Noninfectious cause: systemic lupus erythematosus (on steroids).

RASH WITH MENTAL CHANGES

Infectious causes: Rocky Mountain spotted fever, meningococcemia (with meningitis), *S. aureus* acute bacterial endocarditis, Chikungunya fever, typhus.
Noninfectious cause: systemic lupus erythematosus.

RASH WITH CONJUNCTIVAL SUFFUSION

Infectious causes: Rocky Mountain spotted fever, dengue fever, arboviral hemorrhagic fevers, toxic shock syndrome.
Noninfectious cause: adult Kawasaki disease.

RASH WITH RELATIVE BRADYCARDIA

Infectious causes: Rocky Mountain spotted fever, typhus, dengue fever, typhoid, arboviral hemorrhagic fevers.
Noninfectious cause: drug rash.

RASH WITH ABDOMINAL PAIN

Infectious causes: *V. vulnificus,* gas gangrene, *Clostridium sordelli,* scarlet fever.
Noninfectious causes: cholesterol emboli syndrome, systemic lupus erythematosus.

RASH ON PALMS AND SOLES

Infectious causes: Rocky Mountain spotted fever, toxic shock syndrome, chickenpox, smallpox, monkeypox, scarlet fever.
Noninfectious cause: drug rash.

RASH WITH DIARRHEA

Infectious causes: *V. vulnificus,* gas gangrene, toxic shock syndrome, dengue fever, arboviral hemorrhagic fevers.
Noninfectious cause: none.

RASH WITH EDEMA OF DORSUM OF HANDS/FEET

Infectious causes: Rocky Mountain spotted fever, toxic shock syndrome.
Noninfectious cause: adult Kawasaki disease.

RASH WITH BULLAE

Infectious causes: *V. vulnificus, S. aureus* complicated skin/skin structure infection, gas gangrene.
Noninfectious cause: none.

RASH WITH HEART MURMUR

Infectious cause: acute bacterial endocarditis.
Noninfectious cause: systemic lupus erythematosus.

Rash with gangrene of nose tip
Infectious cause: *S. aureus* acute bacterial endocarditis.
Noninfectious causes: systemic lupus erythematosus, vasculitis.

RASH WITH CEREBROVASCULAR ACCIDENT

Infectious causes: cholesterol emboli syndrome, *S. aureus* acute bacterial endocarditis.
Noninfectious cause: none.

RASH WITH SPLENOMEGALY

Infectious causes: Rocky Mountain spotted fever, typhus.
Noninfectious causes: systemic lupus erythematosus, adult Kawasaki disease.

RASH WITH DEAFNESS

Infectious causes: Rocky Mountain spotted fever, typhus, meningococcal meningitis.
Noninfectious cause: none.

RASH WITH HEPATOSPLENOMEGALY

Infectious causes: Rocky Mountain spotted fever, typhus.
Noninfectious cause: atypical measles.

RASH WITH HEPATOMEGALY

Infectious cause: typhus.
Noninfectious cause: none.

FEVER, AFTER TRAVEL TO THE TROPICS[3]

ICD-10CM #	R50.81	Fever presenting with conditions classified elsewhere

CAUSES OF FEVER AFTER TRAVEL TO THE TROPICS

80% of Specific Infections Causing Fever (Includes Respiratory and Urinary Tract Infection)

Malaria.
Viral hepatitis.
Febrile illness unrelated to foreign travel.
Dengue fever.
Enteric fever (typhoid and paratyphoid fevers).

Other Causes

- Gastroenteritis.
- Rickettsia.
- Leptospirosis.
- Schistosomiasis.
- Amebic liver abscess.
- Tuberculosis.
- Acute HIV infection.
- Others.

FEVER, COMMON INFECTIOUS CAUSES[83]

ICD-10CM #	R50.9	Fever, unspecified

CENTRAL NERVOUS SYSTEM

Meningitis:
- Encephalitis.
- Brain abscess.
- Epidural abscess.

HEAD AND NECK

Acute suppurative parotitis:
- Acute sinusitis.
- Parapharyngeal and retropharyngeal space infections.
- Acute suppurative otitis media.

CARDIOVASCULAR

Catheter-related infection:
- Endocarditis.

PULMONARY AND MEDIASTINAL

Pneumonia:
- Empyema.
- Mediastinitis.

HEPATOBILIARY AND GASTROINTESTINAL

Diverticulitis:
- Appendicitis.
- Peritonitis (spontaneous or secondary).
- Intraperitoneal abscess.
- Perirectal abscess.
- Infected pancreatitis.
- Acute cholecystitis.
- Cholangitis.
- Hepatic abscess.
- Acute viral hepatitis.

GENITOURINARY

Bacterial or fungal cystitis:
- Pyelonephritis.
- Perinephric abscess.
- Tubo-ovarian abscess.
- Endometritis.
- Prostatitis.

BREAST

Mastitis:
- Breast abscess.

CUTANEOUS AND MUSCULAR

Cellulitis:
- Suppurative wound infection.
- Necrotizing fasciitis.
- Bacterial myositis or myonecrosis.
- Herpes zoster.

OSSEOUS

Osteomyelitis.

FEVER, DRUG-INDUCED[34]

ICD-10CM # R50.2 Drug induced fever

SELECTED AGENTS ASSOCIATED WITH DRUG-INDUCED FEVER

Common

Antimicrobial:
- Amphotericin B.
- β-Lactams.
- Sulfonamides.

Cardiovascular:
- Procainamide.
- Quinidine.

CNS:
- Carbamazepine.
- Phenytoin.

Miscellaneous:
- Bleomycin.
- Interferon-α.
- Interleukin-2.

Less Common

Antimicrobial:
- Clindamycin.
- Fluoroquinolones.
- Rifampin.

Cardiovascular:
- Diltiazem.
- Hydralazine.

CNS:
- Haloperidol.
- Serotonin reuptake inhibitors.

Miscellaneous:
- Allopurinol.
- Cimetidine.
- Tacrolimus.

FEVER, HOSPITAL ASSOCIATED[34]

ICD-10CM # R50.2 Drug induced fever
R50.9 Fever, unspecified

SELECTED CAUSES OF HOSPITAL-ASSOCIATED FEVER

Common

Infectious:
- *Clostridium difficile* enterocolitis.
- Pneumonia.
- Surgical wound.
- Urinary tract.
- Vascular catheter.

Noninfectious:
- Drug-induced fever.
- Hematoma.
- Immediate postoperative state.
- Transfusion reaction.
- Venous thromboembolism.

Less Common

Infectious:
- Biliary tract disease.
- Endometritis.
- Intraabdominal abscess.
- Mediastinitis.
- Sinusitis.

Noninfectious:
- Adrenal insufficiency.
- Gout.
- Myocardial infarction.
- Organ infarction.
- Pancreatitis.

FEVER IN RETURNING TRAVELERS AND IMMIGRANTS[61]

ICD-10CM # R50.81 Fever presenting with conditions classified elsewhere

COMMON*

Acute respiratory tract infection (worldwide).
Gastroenteritis (worldwide) [foodborne, waterborne, fecal-oral].
Enteric fever, including typhoid (worldwide) [food, water].
Urinary tract infection (worldwide) [sexual contact].
Drug reactions [antibiotics, prophylactic agents, other] {rash frequent}.
Malaria (tropics, limited areas of temperate zones) [mosquitoes].
Arboviruses (Africa; tropics) [mosquitoes, ticks, mites].
Dengue (Asia, Caribbean, Africa) [mosquitoes].
Viral hepatitis (worldwide).
Hepatitis A (worldwide) [food, fecal-oral].
Hepatitis B (worldwide, especially Asia, sub-Saharan Africa) [sexual contact] {long incubation period}.
Hepatitis C (worldwide) [blood or sexual contact].
Hepatitis E (Asia, North Africa, Mexico, others) [food, water].
Tuberculosis (worldwide) [airborne, milk] {long period to symptomatic infection}.
Sexually transmitted diseases (worldwide) [sexual contact].

LESS COMMON*

Filariasis (Asia, Africa, South America) [biting insects] {long incubation period, eosinophilia}.
Measles (developing world) [airborne] {in susceptible individual}.
Amebic abscess (worldwide) [food].
Brucellosis (worldwide) [milk, cheese, food, animal contact].
Listeriosis (worldwide) [foodborne] {meningitis}.
Leptospirosis (worldwide) [animal contact, open fresh water] {jaundice, meningitis}.
Strongyloidiasis (warm and tropical areas) [soil contact] {eosinophilia}.
Toxoplasmosis (worldwide) [undercooked meat].

RARE

Relapsing fever (western Americas, Asia, northern Africa) [ticks, lice].
Hemorrhagic fevers (worldwide) [arthropod and nonarthropod transmitted].
Yellow fever (tropics) [mosquitoes] {hepatitis}.
Hemorrhagic fever with renal syndrome (Europe, Asia, North America) [rodent urine] {renal impairment}.
Hantavirus pulmonary syndrome (western North America, other) [rodent urine] {respiratory distress syndrome}.

*Diagnoses for which particular symptoms are indicative are in *italics.* Exposure to regions of the world that are most likely to be significant to the diagnosis are presented in (parentheses). Vectors, risk behaviors, and sources associated with acquisition are presented in [brackets]. Special clinical characteristics are listed within {braces}.

*Diagnoses for which particular symptoms are indicative are in *italics.* Exposure to regions of the world that are most likely to be significant to the diagnosis are presented in (parentheses). Vectors, risk behaviors, and sources associated with acquisition are presented in [brackets]. Special clinical characteristics are listed within {braces}.

Lassa fever (Africa) [rodent excreta, person to person] {high mortality rate}
Other—chikungunya, Rift Valley, Ebola-Marburg, etc. (various) [insect bites, rodent excreta, aerosols, person to person] {often severe}.
Rickettsial infections {rashes and eschars}.
Leishmaniasis, visceral (Middle East, Mediterranean, Africa, Asia, South America) [biting flies] {long incubation period}.
Acute schistosomiasis (Africa, Asia, South America, Caribbean) [fresh water].
Chagas' disease (South and Central America) [reduviid bug bites] {often asymptomatic}.
African trypanosomiasis (Africa) [tsetse fly bite] {neurologic syndromes, sleeping sickness}.
Bartonellosis (South America) [sandfly bite] {skin nodules}.
HIV infection/AIDS (worldwide) [sexual and blood contact].
Trichinosis (worldwide) [undercooked meat] {eosinophilia}.
Plague (temperate and tropical plains) [animal exposures and fleas].
Tularemia (worldwide) [animal contact, fleas, aerosols] {ulcers, lymph nodes}.
Anthrax (worldwide) [animal, animal product contact] {ulcers}.
Lyme disease (North America, Europe) [tick bites] {arthritis, meningitis, cardiac abnormalities}.

FEVER, NONINFECTIOUS CAUSES[7]

ICD-10CM # R50.9 Fever, unspecified

DIFFERENTIAL DIAGNOSIS—NONINFECTIOUS CAUSES OF FEVER

Critical Diagnoses
Acute myocardial infarction.
Pulmonary embolism/infarction.
Intracranial hemorrhage.
Cerebrovascular accident.
Neuroleptic-malignant syndrome.
Thyroid storm.
Acute adrenal insufficiency.
Transfusion reaction.
Pulmonary edema.

Emergent Diagnoses
Congestive heart failure.
Dehydration.
Recent seizure.
Sickle cell disease.
Transplant rejection.
Pancreatitis.
Deep vein thrombosis.

Nonemergent Diagnoses
Drug fever.
Malignancy.
Gout.
Sarcoidosis.
Crohn's disease.
Postmyocardiotomy syndrome.

FEVER OF UNKNOWN ORIGIN, PEDIATRIC PATIENT[19]

ICD-10CM # R50.9 Fever, Unspecified

INFECTIOUS DISEASES

Bacterial
Bacterial endocarditis.
Brucellosis.
Cat-scratch disease.
Leptospirosis.
Liver abscess.
Mastoiditis (chronic).
Osteomyelitis.
Pelvic abscess.
Perinephric abscess.
Pyelonephritis.
Salmonellosis.
Sinusitis.
Subdiaphragmatic abscess.
Tuberculosis.
Tularemia.

Viral
Adenovirus.
Arboviruses.
Cytomegalovirus.
Epstein-Barr virus (infectious mononucleosis).
Hepatitis viruses.

Chlamydial
Lymphogranuloma venereum.
Psittacosis.

Rickettsial
Q fever.
Rocky Mountain spotted fever.

Fungal
Blastomycosis (nonpulmonary).
Histoplasmosis (disseminated).

Parasitic
Malaria.
Toxoplasmosis.
Visceral larva migrans.

Unclassified
Sarcoidosis.

Collagen Vascular Diseases
Juvenile rheumatoid arthritis.
Polyarteritis nodosa.
Systemic lupus erythematosus.

Malignancies
Hodgkin's disease.
Leukemia and lymphoma.
Neuroblastoma.

Miscellaneous
Central diabetes insipidus.
Drug fever.
Ectodermal dysplasia.
Factitious fever.
Familial dysautonomia.
Granulomatous colitis.
Hemophagocytic lymphohistiocytosis.
Infantile cortical hyperostosis.
Kikuchi-Fujimoto disease.
Nephrogenic diabetes insipidus.
Pancreatitis.
Periodic fever.
Serum sickness.
Thyrotoxicosis.
Ulcerative colitis.

FEVER, POSTPARTUM[1]

ICD-10CM # R50.9 Fever, unspecified

MOST COMMON

Metritis.
Urinary tract infection.
Pneumonia.
Wound infection.
Mastitis.
Superficial or deep vein thrombosis.

MOST THREATENING

Toxic shock syndrome.
Necrotizing fasciitis.
Pelvic phlegmon.
Pelvic abscess.
Peritonitis.
Septic pelvic thrombosis.
Breast abscess.

FEVER, PERIODIC[29]

ICD-10CM # R50.9 Fever, unspecified

HEREDITARY

Nonhereditary
Infectious
Hidden infectious focus (e.g., aortoenteric fistula, Caroli disease).
Recurrent reinfection (e.g., chronic meningococcemia, host defense defect).
Specific infection (e.g., Whipple disease, malaria).
Noninfectious inflammatory disorder, e.g.:
- Adult-onset Still disease.
- Juvenile chronic rheumatoid arthritis.
- Periodic fever, aphthous stomatitis, pharyngitis, and adenitis.
- Schnitzler syndrome.
- Behçet's syndrome.
- Crohn's disease.
- Sarcoidosis.
- Extrinsic alveolitis.
- Humidifier lung, polymer fume fever.
- Neoplastic.

Lymphoma (e.g., Hodgkin's disease, angioimmunoblastic lymphoma).
Solid tumor (e.g., pheochromocytoma, myxoma, colon carcinoma).
Vascular (e.g., recurrent pulmonary embolism)
Hypothalamic
Psychogenic periodic fever.
Factitious or fraudulent.

FEVER, PEDIATRIC, ACUTE[1]

ICD-10CM # R50.9 Fever, unspecified

COMMON VIRAL INFECTIONS

Central Nervous System
Meningitis.
Encephalitis.
Tumor.
Brain abscess.

Head, Ears, Eyes, Nose, and Throat
Otitis media.
Pharyngitis.
Retropharyngeal abscess.
Peritonsillar abscess.
Lateral pharyngeal wall abscess.
Stomatitis.
Influenza.
Sinusitis.
Parotitis.
Cervical adenitis.
Periorbital cellulitis.

Orbital cellulitis or abscess.

Respiratory System

Bronchiolitis.
Croup.
Epiglottitis.
Pneumonia.
Upper respiratory infection.

Cardiovascular System

Myocarditis.
Pericarditis.
Endocarditis.

Genitourinary System

Urinary tract infection.
Tuboovarian abscess.

Gastrointestinal Tract

Acute viral gastroenteritis.
Bacterial enteritis.
Appendicitis.

Focal Soft Tissue Infections

Cellulitis.

Musculoskeletal System

Osteomyelitis.
Septic arthritis.

Rheumatologic Disorders

Acute rheumatic fever.
Juvenile rheumatoid arthritis.
Henoch-Schönlein purpura.

Vasculitis

Behçet syndrome.

Malignancy

Leukemia.
Lymphoma.
Sarcoma.

Systemic Illness

Bacteremia.
Viremia.
Sepsis.
Kawasaki disease.
Toxic shock syndrome.
Rocky Mountain spotted fever.
Meningococcemia.

MISCELLANEOUS DISORDERS

Toxicologic

Anticholinergic toxidromes.
Salicylate overdose.
Amphetamine.
Cocaine.

Endocrine

Thyrotoxicosis.

FEVER, RECURRENT OR PERIODIC, IN CHILDREN[51]

ICD-10CM #		
	R50.2	Drug induced fever
	R50.9	Fever, unspecified

INFECTIOUS DISEASES

Brucellosis.
Rat-bite fever.
Relapsing fever.

RHEUMATIC DISEASES

Juvenile idiopathic arthritis (systemic onset).
Behçet disease.
Systemic lupus erythematosus.
Relapsing polychondritis.
Crohn's disease.

HEREDITARY AUTOINFLAMMATORY SYNDROMES

Familial Mediterranean fever (FMF).
Cryopyrinopathies:
- Familial cold autoinflammatory syndrome (FCAS).
- Muckle-Wells syndrome (MWS).
- Chronic infantile neurologic cutaneous and articular (CINCA) syndrome, also called neonatal-onset multisystem inflammatory disease (NOMID).

Tumor necrosis factor receptor–associated periodic syndrome (TRAPS).
Hyperimmunoglobulinemia D with periodic fever syndrome (HIDS).

CYCLIC HEMATOPOIESIS

Hereditary form.
Acquired form.

IDIOPATHIC CONDITIONS

Periodic fever with aphthous stomatitis, pharyngitis, and adenitis (PFAPA).

FEVER WITH MACULOPAPULAR OR PETECHIAL RASH[65]

ICD-10CM #		
ICD-10CM #	R21	Rash and nonspecific skin eruption
ICD-10CM #	R50.9	Fever, unspecified

DIFFERENTIAL DIAGNOSIS OF FEVER WITH MACULOPAPULAR OR PETECHIAL RASH

Rocky Mountain spotted fever.
Meningococcal disease.
Enteroviral infection (echovirus and coxsackievirus).
Human herpesvirus 6 infection (roseola).
Human parvovirus B19 infection (fifth disease).
Epstein-Barr virus infection.
Disseminated gonococcal infection.
Murine typhus.
Ehrlichiosis.
Group A streptococcal pharyngitis.
Mycoplasma pneumoniae Infection.
Leptospirosis.
Secondary syphilis.
Kawasaki disease.
Thrombotic thrombocytopenic purpura (TTP).
Drug reactions.
Immune complex–mediated illness.
Toxic shock syndrome.
Erythema multiforme.
Stevens-Johnson syndrome.

FINGER LESIONS, INFLAMMATORY

ICD-10CM #		
	B08.8	Other specified viral infections characterized by skin and mucous membrane lesions
	L03.0	Cellulitis of finger and toe

Paronychia.
Herpes simplex type 1 (herpetic whitlow).
Dyshidrotic eczema (pompholyx).
Herpes zoster.
Bacterial endocarditis (Osler's nodes).
Psoriatic arthritis.

FLACCID PARALYSIS, ACUTE, DIFFERENTIAL DIAGNOSIS[51]

ICD-10CM #		
	G83.9	Paralytic syndrome, unspecified

Brain stem stroke.
Brain stem encephalitis.
Acute anterior poliomyelitis.
- Caused by poliovirus.
- Caused by other neurotropic viruses.

Acute myelopathy.
- Space-occupying lesions.
- Acute transverse myelitis.

Peripheral neuropathy.
- Guillain-Barré syndrome.
- Post-rabies vaccine neuropathy.
- Diphtheritic neuropathy.
- Heavy metals, biologic toxins, or drug intoxication.
- Acute intermittent porphyria.
- Vasculitic neuropathy.
- Critical illness neuropathy.
- Lymphomatous neuropathy.

Disorders of neuromuscular transmission.
- Myasthenia gravis.
- Biologic or industrial toxins.
- Tic paralysis.

Disorders of muscle.
- Hypokalemia.
- Hypophosphatemia.
- Inflammatory myopathy.
- Acute rhabdomyolysis.
- Trichinosis.
- Periodic paralyses.

FLATULENCE AND BLOATING[71]

ICD-10CM #		
	R14.0	Abdominal distension (gaseous)
	R14.1	Gas pain
	R14.2	Eructation
	R14.3	Flatulence

Ingestion of nonabsorbable carbohydrates.
Ingestion of carbonated beverages.
Malabsorption: pancreatic insufficiency, biliary disease, celiac disease, bacterial overgrowth in small intestine.
Lactase deficiency.
Irritable bowel syndrome.
Anxiety disorders.
Food poisoning, giardiasis.

FLUSHING[60]

ICD-10CM #		
	R23.2	Flushing

Physiologic flushing: menopause, ingestion of monosodium glutamate (Chinese restaurant syndrome), ingestion of hot drinks.
Drugs: alcohol (with or without disulfiram, metronidazole, or chlorpropamide), nicotinic acid,

diltiazem, nifedipine, levodopa, bromocriptine, vancomycin, amyl nitrate.
Neoplastic disorders: carcinoid syndrome, VIPoma syndrome, medullary carcinoma of thyroid, systemic mastocytosis, basophilic chronic myelocytic leukemia, renal cell carcinoma.
Anxiety.
Agnogenic flushing.

FOLATE DEFICIENCY[43]

ICD-10CM #		
	D52.0	Dietary folate deficiency anemia
	D52.1	Drug-induced folate deficiency anemia
	D52.8	Other folate deficiency anemias
	D52.9	Folate deficiency anemia, unspecified

ETIOPATHOPHYSIOLOGIC CLASSIFICATION OF FOLATE DEFICIENCY

Nutritional causes:
- Decreased dietary intake:
  - Poverty and famine.
  - Institutionalized individuals (e.g., psychiatric, nursing homes), chronic debilitating disease.
  - Prolonged feeding of infants with goat's milk, special slimming diets or food fads (i.e., folate-rich foods not consumed), cultural or ethnic cooking techniques (i.e., food folate destroyed).
- Decreased diet and increased requirements:
  - Physiologic (e.g., pregnancy and lactation, prematurity, hyperemesis gravidarum, infancy).
  - Pathologic (e.g., intrinsic hematologic diseases involving hemolysis with compensatory erythropoiesis, abnormal hematopoiesis, or bone marrow infiltration with malignant disease and dermatologic disease such as psoriasis).

Folate malabsorption:
- With normal intestinal mucosa:
  - Some drugs (controversial).
  - Congenital folate malabsorption (rare).
  - With mucosal abnormalities (e.g., tropical and nontropical sprue, regional enteritis).

Defective cellular folate uptake:
- Familial aplastic anemia (rare).
- Acute cerebral folate deficiency.

Inadequate cellular use:
- Folate antagonists (e.g., methotrexate).
- Hereditary enzyme deficiencies involving folate.

Drugs:
- Multiple effects on folate metabolism (e.g., alcohol, sulfasalazine, triamterene, pyrimethamine, trimethoprim-sulfamethoxazole, diphenylhydantoin, barbiturates).

Acute folate deficiency:
- Intensive care unit setting.
- Uncertain origin.

FOOT AND ANKLE PAIN[27]

ICD-10CM #		
	M25.5	Pain in joint
	M25.9	Joint disorder, unspecified

TENDON, LIGAMENT, AND MUSCLE

Gastrocnemius-soleus strain.
Plantaris rupture.
Anterior talofibular ligament tear.
Calcaneofibular ligament tear.
Deltoid ligament tear.
Anterolateral impingement due to complete tear of anterior talofibular ligament and anterior inferior tibiofibular ligament.
Syndesmotic impingement due to tear of syndesmosis.
Sinus tarsi syndrome (lateral hindfoot pain and instability due to injury of contents of the sinus and tarsal tunnel).
Achilles tendinitis.
Achilles rupture.
Plantar fasciitis.
Posterior tibial tendon dysfunction.
Flexor hallucis longus dysfunction.
Tibialis anterior tendon tear.
Peroneus brevis tendon tear.

BONE

Fracture of talus.
Calcaneal fracture.
Navicular fractures.
Lisfranc fracture-dislocation (fracture of the first metatarsal base with dislocation of medial cuneiform).
Metatarsal stress fracture.
Freiberg infraction (sclerosis and flattening of the second metatarsal head due to trauma or microtrauma).
Avascular necrosis of the talus.
Fracture of the phalanges.
Fracture of the sesamoids.
Sesamoiditis.
Metatarsalgia.

JOINT

Osteoarthritis.
Gout.
Rheumatoid arthritis.
Other inflammatory arthritides.
Charcot joint.
Osteochondral lesion of the talus.

PERIARTICULAR STRUCTURES

Shin splint (periosteal avulsion and periostitis at the insertion of the medial soleus due to repetitive overuse, such as in running and hiking).
Hallux rigidus.
Hallux valgus.
Ingrown toenail.
Toe deformities.
Turf toe (sprain of the first metatarsophalangeal joint due to hyperextension forces).
Plantar fasciitis.
Plantar fibromatosis.

NERVES

Anterior tarsal tunnel syndrome (involvement of deep peroneal nerve under the superficial fascia of the ankle).
Morton neuroma.

VESSELS

Atherosclerosis.
Compartment syndrome.

REFERRED PAIN

Complex regional pain syndrome.

FOOT AND ANKLE PAIN, IN DIFFERENT AGE GROUPS[18]

ICD-10CM #		
	M25.579	Pain in unspecified ankle and joints of unspecified foot

COMMON CAUSES OF FOOT AND ANKLE PAIN IN DIFFERENT AGE GROUPS

Childhood (2-10 yr)

Intraarticular
Club foot.
Congenital midfoot and forefoot deformities.
Septic arthritis.

Periarticular
Osteomyelitis.

Adolescence (10-18 yr)

Intraarticular
Arch disorders (pes cavus, pes planus).

Periarticular
Osteomyelitis.
Tumors.

Early Adulthood (18-30 yr)

Intraarticular
Metatarsalgia.
Hallux valgus.
Hallux rigidus.
Osteochondritis.
Accessory ossicles.

Periarticular
Achilles tendonitis.
Achilles tendon rupture.
Fasciitis.

Referred
Lumbar spine.
Knee.

Adulthood (30-50 yr)

Intraarticular
Osteoarthritis.
Inflammatory arthritis.
Gout.
Metatarsalgia.
Hallux valgus.
Hallux rigidus.
Osteochondritis.
Accessory ossicles.

Periarticular
Ischemic foot pain.
Diabetes.
Bursitis.
Tendonitis.
Plantar fasciitis.
Corns.

Referred
Lumbar spine.
Knee.
Old Age (>50 yr)
Intraarticular
Osteoarthritis.
Inflammatory arthritis.
Gout.
Metatarsalgia.
Hallux valgus.
Hallux rigidus.
Periarticular
Ischemic foot pain.
Diabetes.
Bursitis.
Tendonitis.
Plantar fasciitis.
Corns.
Referred
Lumbar spine.
Knee.

FOOT DERMATITIS

ICD-10CM #	B35.3	Tinea pedis
	K25	Unspecified contact dermatitis

Tinea pedis.
Dyshidrotic eczema.
Tylosis (mechanically induced hyperkeratosis, fissuring, and dryness).
Allergic contact dermatitis.
Psoriasis.
Peripheral vascular insufficiency.
Neuropathic foot ulcers (DM, poorly fitting shoes).
Acquired plantar keratoderma.
Sézary syndrome.

FOOTDROP

ICD-10CM #	M21.379	Foot drop, unspecified foot

Peripheral neuropathy.
L5 radiculopathy.
Peroneal nerve compression.
Sciatic nerve palsy.
Scapuloperoneal syndromes.
Spasticity.
Peroneal nerve compression.
Myopathy.
Dystonia.

FOOT LESION, ULCERATING

ICD-10CM #	S90.929A	Unspecified superficial injury of unspecified foot, initial encounter
	S90.933A	Unspecified superficial injury of unspecified great toe, initial encounter
	S90.936A	Unspecified superficial injury of unspecified lesser toe(s), initial encounter
	L08.89	Other specified local infections of the skin and subcutaneous tissue

Cellulitis.
Plantar wart.
Squamous cell carcinoma.
Actinomycosis (Madura foot).
Plantar fibromatosis.
Pseudoepitheliomatous hyperplasia.

FOOT PAIN

ICD-10CM #	M25.579	Pain in unspecified ankle and joints of unspecified foot

Trauma (fractures, musculoskeletal and ligamentous strain).
Inflammation (plantar fasciitis, Achilles tendonitis or bursitis, calcaneal apophysitis).
Arterial insufficiency, Raynaud's phenomenon, thromboangiitis obliterans.
Gout, pseudogout.
Calcaneal spur.
Infection (cellulitis, abscess, lymphangitis, gangrene).
Decubitus ulcer.
Paronychia, ingrown toenail.
Thrombophlebitis, postphlebitic syndrome.

FOOT PAIN BY AGE[51]

ICD-10CM #	M25.579	Pain in unspecified ankle and joints of unspecified foot

0-6 YEARS

Poorly fitting shoes.
Foreign body.
Fracture.
Osteomyelitis.
Leukemia.
Puncture wound.
Drawing of blood.
Dactylitis.
Juvenile rheumatoid arthritis (JRA).

6-12 YEARS

Poorly fitting shoes.
Sever disease.
Enthesopathy (JRA).
Foreign body.
Accessory navicular.
Tarsal coalition.
Ewing sarcoma.
Hypermobile flatfoot.
Trauma (sprains, fractures).
Puncture wound.

12-20 YEARS

Poorly fitting shoes.
Stress fracture.
Foreign body.
Ingrown toenail.
Metatarsalgia.
Plantar fasciitis.
Osteochondroses (avascular necrosis).
Freiberg infarction.
Köhler disease.
Achilles tendinitis.
Trauma (sprains).
Plantar warts.
Tarsal coalition.

FOREARM AND HAND PAIN

ICD-10CM #	S59.809A	Other specified injuries of unspecified elbow, initial encounter
	S59.919A	Unspecified injury of unspecified forearm, initial encounter
	S69.80XA	Other specified injuries of unspecified wrist, hand, and finger(s), initial encounter
	S69.90XA	Unspecified injury of unspecified wrist, hand, and finger(s), initial encounter

Epicondylitis.
Tenosynovitis.
Osteoarthritis.
Cubital tunnel syndrome.
Carpal tunnel syndrome.
Trauma.
Herpes zoster.
Peripheral vascular insufficiency.
Infection (cellulitis, abscess).

FOREARM FRACTURES[3]

ICD-10CM #	S52	Fracture of forearm

TRAUMATIC

Wrist sprain, elbow sprain.
Ligamentous injuries, forearm contusions, hematomas.
Dislocations of the elbow or wrist (including nursemaid's elbow).

INFECTIOUS

Cellulitis of the forearm, abscesses.
Necrotizing fasciitis.

VASCULAR

Acute arterial occlusion.
Venous thrombosis.

NEUROLOGIC

Neurapraxias, carpal tunnel syndrome.
Systemic neurologic syndromes involving the nerves of the upper extremities.

ARTHRITIS

Septic joint, gonococcal arthritis, rheumatoid arthritis, osteoarthritis.
Pseudogout, gout.
Systemic lupus erythematosus, rheumatic fever, viral syndrome.
Reiter syndrome, Lyme disease, serum sickness.

OTHER

Olecranon bursitis, soft tissue masses.
Normal growth plates, nutrient vessels.

GAIT ABNORMALITY

ICD-10CM #		
	R26.0	Ataxic gait
	R26.1	Paralytic gait
	R26.89	Other abnormalities of gait and mobility
	R26.9	Unspecified abnormalities of gait and mobility

Parkinsonism.
Degenerative joint disease (hips, back, knees).
Multiple sclerosis.
Trauma, foot pain.
CVA.
Cerebellar lesions.
Infections (tabes, encephalitis, meningitis).
Sensory ataxia.
Dystonia, cerebral palsy, neuromuscular disorders.
Metabolic abnormalities.

GALACTORRHEA[61]

ICD-10CM #		
	N64.3	Galactorrhea not associated with childbirth

Prolonged suckling.
Drugs (INH, phenothiazines, reserpine derivatives, amphetamines, spironolactone and tricyclic antidepressants).
Major stressors (surgery, trauma).
Hypothyroidism.
Pituitary tumors.

GALLBLADDER SONOGRAPHIC NON-VISUALIZATION[69]

ICD-10CM # Varies with specific diagnosis

CAUSES OF SONOGRAPHIC NONVISUALIZATION OF GALLBLADDER

Previous cholecystectomy.
Physiologic contraction.
Fibrosed gallbladder duct—chronic cholecystitis.
Air-filled gallbladder or emphysematous cholecystitis.
Tumefactive sludge.
Agenesis of gallbladder.
Ectopic location.

GALLBLADDER WALL THICKENING[69]

ICD-10CM # Varies with specific diagnosis

CAUSES OF GALLBLADDER WALL THICKENING

Generalized Edematous States
Congestive heart failure.
Renal failure.
End-stage cirrhosis.
Hypoalbuminemia.
Inflammatory Conditions
Primary:
Acute cholecystitis.
Cholangitis.
Chronic cholecystitis.
Secondary:
Acute hepatitis.
Perforated duodenal ulcer.
Pancreatitis.
Diverticulitis/colitis.
Neoplastic Conditions
Gallbladder adenocarcinoma.
Metastases.
Miscellaneous
Adenomyomatosis.
Mural varicosities.

GALLSTONE DISEASE, PEDIATRIC PATIENT[19]

ICD-10CM #		
	K80.20	Calculus of gallbladder without cholecystitis without obstruction

Biliary tract anomaly (e.g., choledochal cyst).
Cephalosporin use.
Crohn's disease.
Cystic fibrosis.
Genetic predisposition (e.g., ABCB4, UGT1A1 mutations).
Hemolytic disorders (e.g., sickle-cell anemia, hereditary spherocytosis).
Hispanic or Latino ancestry.
Malabsorption.
Metabolic syndrome.
Obesity.
Parasitic disease (*Ascaris lumbricoides*).
Pregnancy.
Rapid weight loss.
Solid organ and hematologic transplant (e.g., liver, kidney, heart, bone marrow).
Total parenteral nutrition.

GASTRIC DILATATION[36]

ICD-10CM #		
	K31.0	Acute dilatation of stomach

CAUSES OF A MASSIVELY DILATED STOMACH

Mechanical Gastric Outlet Obstruction
Duodenal or pyloric canal ulceration.
Carcinoma of pyloric antrum.
Extrinsic compression.
Paralytic Ileus
Surgery.
Trauma.
Peritonitis.
Pancreatitis.
Cholecystitis.
Diabetes mellitus.
Hepatic coma.
Drugs.
Gastric Volvulus
Intubation.
Air swallowing.

GASTRIC EMPTYING, DELAYED[3]

ICD-10CM #		
	K30	Functional dyspepsia

CAUSES OF DELAYED GASTRIC EMPTYING

Mechanical Causes
Peptic ulcer disease, scarred pylorus.
Malignancy: gastric cancer, gastric lymphoma, pancreatic cancer.
Gastric surgery: vagotomy, gastric resection, Roux-en-Y anastomosis.
Crohn's disease.
Endocrine and Metabolic Causes
Diabetes mellitus.
Hypothyroidism.
Hypoadrenal states.
Electrolyte abnormalities.
Chronic renal failure.
Medications.
Anticholinergics.
Opiates.
Dopamine agonists.
Tricyclic antidepressants.
Abnormalities of Gastric Smooth Muscle
Scleroderma.
Polymyositis, dermatomyositis.
Amyloidosis.
Pseudoobstruction.
Myotonic dystrophy.
Neuropathy.
Scleroderma.
Amyloidosis.
Autonomic neuropathy.
Central Nervous System or Psychiatric Disorders
Brain stem tumors.
Spinal cord injury.
Anorexia nervosa.
Stress.
Miscellaneous
Idiopathic gastroparesis.
Gastroesophageal reflux disease.
Nonulcer (functional) dyspepsia.
Cancer cachexia or anorexia.

GASTRIC EMPTYING, RAPID

ICD-10CM #		
	K30	Functional dyspepsia

Pancreatic insufficiency.
Dumping syndrome.
Peptic ulcer.
Celiac disease.
Promotility agents.
Zollinger-Ellison disease.

GENITAL DISCHARGE, FEMALE[24]

ICD-10CM #		
	N94.9	Unspecified condition associated with female genital organs and menstrual cycle

Physiologic discharge: cervical mucus, vaginal transudation, bacteria, squamous epithelial cells.
Individual variation.
Pregnancy.
Sexual response.
Menstrual cycle variation.
Infection.
Foreign body: tampon, cervical cap, other.
Neoplasm.

Fistula.
IUD.
Cervical ectropion.
Spermicide.
Nongenital causes: urinary incontinence, urinary tract fistula, Crohn's disease, rectovaginal fistula.

GENITAL LESIONS, INFECTIOUS CAUSES[10]

ICD-10CM # Varies with specific diagnosis

INFECTIOUS CAUSES OF GENITAL LESIONS

Sexually Transmitted Infections

Syphilis:
  Primary (chancre).
  Secondary (condyloma latum).
Herpes simplex virus types 1 and 2.
Chancroid *(Haemophilus ducreyi).*
Lymphogranuloma venereum.
Granuloma inguinale (donovanosis).
Human papillomavirus.
Sarcoptes scabiei.
Molluscum contagiosum.

Nonsexually Transmitted Infections

Folliculitis.
Tuberculosis.
Tularemia.
Histoplasmosis.
Candida (balanitis or vaginitis).
Amebiasis.

GENITAL LESIONS, NONINFECTIOUS CAUSES[10]

ICD-10CM # Varies with specific diagnosis

NONVENEREAL CAUSES OF GENITAL LESIONS

Trauma.
Malignancies (e.g., squamous cell carcinoma).
Behçet's syndrome.
Lipschütz vulvar ulcers.
Peyronie disease.
Fixed-drug eruption.
Eczema.
Psoriasis.
Inflammatory bowel disease.
Contact dermatitis.
Lichen planus.
Hidradenitis suppurativa.
Postinflammatory hypopigmentation.
Aphthous ulcers (associated with human immunodeficiency virus).

GENITAL SORES[3]

ICD-10CM #		
	A60.9	Anogenital herpesviral infection, unspecified
	A51.0	Primary genital syphilis
	A63.0	Anogenital (venereal) warts
	A57	Chancroid
	A58	Granuloma inguinale
	A55	Chlamydial lymphogranuloma (venereum)
	N94.89	Other specified conditions associated with female genital organs and menstrual cycle
	N50.8	Other specified disorders of male genital organs

Herpes genitalis.
Syphilis.
Chancroid.
Lymphogranuloma venereum.
Granuloma inguinale.
Condyloma acuminatum.
Neoplastic lesion.
Trauma.

GLOMERULONEPHRITIS ASSOCIATED WITH MALIGNANCY[74]

ICD-10CM # N00.9 Acute nephritic syndrome with unspecified morphologic changes

Membranous glomerulonephritis.
Breast cancer.
Lung cancer.
Colon cancer.
Prostate cancer.
Graft-versus-host disease.
Minimal change disease.
Hodgkin's lymphoma.
Non-Hodgkin's lymphoma.
Graft-versus-host disease.
Case reports.
Immunoglobulin A nephritis.
Antineutrophil cytoplasmic antibody vasculitis.
Focal segmental glomerulosclerosis.

GLOMERULONEPHRITIS, RAPIDLY PROGRESSIVE[3]

ICD-10CM # N05.9 Unspecified nephritic syndrome with unspecified morphologic changes

DIFFERENTIAL DIAGNOSIS OF RAPIDLY PROGRESSIVE GLOMERULONEPHRITIS

Linear Immune Staining

Anti-GBM disease.
Goodpasture syndrome.
Rarely membranous glomerulonephritis.

Granular Immune Staining

Subacute bacterial endocarditis (past infectious).
Lupus nephritis.
Cryoglobulinemia.
Membranoproliferative glomerulonephritis (type II more than type I).
Immunoglobulin A nephropathy, Henoch-Schönlein purpura.
Idiopathic.

No Immune Staining (Pauci-immune)

Antineutrophil cytoplasmic antibody-associated vasculitis (Wegener granulomatosis, microscopic polyangiitis, Churg-Strauss syndrome).
Idiopathic.

GLOMERULOPATHIES, THROMBOTIC, MICROANGIOPATHIC[3]

ICD-10CM # M31.1 Thrombotic microangiopathy

THROMBOTIC MICROANGIOPATHIC GLOMERULOPATHIES

Thrombotic thrombocytopenic purpura.
Hemolytic-uremic syndrome.
Malignant hypertension.
Scleroderma renal crisis.
Preeclampsia, eclampsia.
HELLP syndrome (hemolysis, elevated liver enzymes, low platelets).
Antiphospholipid antibody syndrome.
Drugs: oral contraceptives, quinine, cyclosporine, tacrolimus, ticlopidine, clopidogrel.

GLOMERULOSCLEROSIS, FOCAL SEGMENTAL[3]

ICD-10CM # N03.3 Chronic nephritic syndrome with diffuse mesangial proliferative glomerulonephritis

ETIOLOGY OF FOCAL SEGMENTAL GLOMERULOSCLEROSIS (FSGS)

Primary idiopathic FSGS.
Secondary FSGS.
HIV (usually collapsing variant).
Reflux nephropathy.
Heroin abuse.
Sickle cell disease.
Oligomeganephronia.
Renal dysgenesis or agenesis (low nephron mass).
Radiation nephritis.
Familial podocytopathies.
NPHS1 (nephrin) mutation.
NPHS2 (podocin) mutation.
TRPC6 (cation channel) mutation.
ACTN4 (a-actinin 4 mutation).

GLOSSODYNIA[81]

ICD-10CM # K14.6 Glossodynia

DENTURE-RELATED

Dentures (ill-fitting, monomer from denture base).
Dental plaque.
Oral parafunction.

INFECTIVE/DERMATOLOGIC

Candidiasis.
Lichen planus.

DEFICIENCY STATES

Iron, B12, folate, B2 (riboflavin), B6 (pyridoxine), zinc.

ENDOCRINE

Diabetes.
Myxedema.
Hormonal changes occurring during menopause.

NEUROLOGICALLY MEDIATED

Referred from tonsils, teeth.
Lingual nerve neuropathy.
Glossopharyngeal neuralgia.
Esophageal reflux.

IATROGENIC

Mouthwash.

XEROSTOMIA

PSYCHOGENIC

IDIOPATHIC

GLUCOCORTICOID DEFICIENCY[32]

ICD-10CM #		
	E27.1	Primary adrenocortical insufficiency
	E27.3	Drug-induced adrenocortical insufficiency

ACTH-independent causes.
TB.
Autoimmune (idiopathic).
Other rare causes:
- Fungal infection.
- Adrenal hemorrhage.
- Metastases.
- Sarcoidosis.
- Amyloidosis.
- Adrenoleukodystrophy.
- Adrenomyeloneuropathy.
- HIV infection.
- Congenital adrenal hyperplasia.
- Medications (e.g., ketoconazole).

ACTH-dependent causes:
- Hypothalamic-pituitary-adrenal suppression.
- Exogenous.
- Glucocorticoid.
- ACTH.
- Endogenous—cure of Cushing's syndrome.

Hypothalamic-pituitary lesions.
- Neoplasm:
  - Primary pituitary tumor.
  - Metastatic tumor.
  - Craniopharyngioma.
- Infection:
  - Tuberculosis.
  - Actinomycosis.
  - Nocardiosis.

Sarcoid.
Head trauma.
Isolated ACTH deficiency.

GOITER

ICD-10CM #		
	E01.2	Iodine-deficiency related (endemic) goiter, unspecified
	E04.9	Nontoxic goiter, unspecified
	E07.1	Dyshormogenetic goiter
	E01.2	Iodine-deficiency related (endemic) goiter, unspecified
	E04.2	Nontoxic multinodular goiter
	E04.0	Nontoxic diffuse goiter
	E05.10	Thyrotoxicosis with toxic single thyroid nodule without thyrotoxic crisis or storm

Thyroiditis.
Toxic multinodular goiter.
Graves disease.
Medications (PTU, methimazole, sulfonamides, sulfonylureas, ethionamide, amiodarone, lithium, etc.).
Iodine deficiency.
Sarcoidosis, amyloidosis.
Defective thyroid hormone synthesis.
Resistance to thyroid hormone.

GRANULOMATOUS DERMATITIDES

ICD-10CM #		
	L92.9	Granulomatous disorder of the skin and subcutaneous tissue, unspecified

Granuloma annulare.
Sarcoidosis.
Necrobiosis lipoidica diabeticorum.
Cutaneous Crohn's disease.
Rheumatoid nodules.
Annular elastolytic giant cell granuloma (actinic granuloma).
Foreign body granuloma.

GRANULOMATOUS DISORDERS[70]

ICD-10CM #		
	M31.30	Granulomatosis with polyangiitis without renal involvement
	K75.3	Granulomatous hepatitis
	L92.9	Granulomatous disorder of skin and subcutaneous tissue, unspecified

INFECTIONS

Fungi
Histoplasma.
Coccidioides.
Blastomyces.
Sporothrix.
Aspergillus.
Cryptococcus.

Protozoa
Toxoplasma.
Leishmania.

Metazoa
Toxocara.
Schistosoma.

Spirochetes
Treponema pallidum.
T. pertenue.
T. carateum.

Mycobacteria
M. tuberculosis.
M. leprae.
M. kansasii.
M. marinum.
M. avian.
Bacille Calmette-Guérin (BCG) vaccine.

Bacteria
Brucella.
Yersinia.

Other Infections
Cat-scratch disease.
Lymphogranuloma.

NEOPLASIA

Carcinoma.
Reticulosis.
Pinealoma.
Dysgerminoma.
Seminoma.
Reticulum cell sarcoma.
Malignant nasal granuloma.

CHEMICALS

Beryllium.
Zirconium.
Silica.
Starch.

IMMUNOLOGIC ABERRATIONS

Sarcoidosis.
Crohn's disease.
Primary biliary cirrhosis.
Granulomatosis with polyangiitis.
Giant cell arteritis.
Peyronie's disease.
Hypogammaglobulinemia.
SLE.
Lymphomatoid granulomatosis.
Histiocytosis X.
Hepatic granulomatous disease.
Immune complex disease.
Rosenthal-Melkersson syndrome.
Churg-Strauss allergic granulomatosis.

LEUKOCYTE OXIDASE DEFECT

Chronic granulomatous disease of childhood.

EXTRINSIC ALLERGIC ALVEOLITIS

Farmer's lung.
Bird fancier's.
Mushroom worker's.
Suberosis (cork dust).
Bagassosis.
Maple bark stripper's.
Paprika splitter's.
Coffee bean.
Spatlese lung.

OTHER DISORDERS

Whipple disease.
Pyrexia of unknown origin.
Radiotherapy.
Cancer chemotherapy.

Panniculitis.
Chalazion.
Sebaceous cyst.
Dermoid.
Sea urchin spine injury.

GRANULOMATOUS LIVER DISEASE

ICD-10CM #	K75.3	Granulomatous hepatitis

Sarcoidosis.
Granulomatosis with polyangiitis.
Vasculitis.
Inflammatory bowel disease.
Allergic granulomatosis.
Erythema nodosum.
Infections (fungal, viral, parasitic).
Primary biliary cirrhosis.
Lymphoma.
Hodgkin's disease.
Drugs (e.g., allopurinol, hydralazine, sulfonamides, penicillins).
Toxins (copper sulfate, beryllium).

GREEN OR BLUE URINE

ICD-10CM #	R82	Other abnormal findings in urine

Pseudomonal urinary tract infection
Medications: triamterene, amitriptyline, IV cimetidine, IV promethazine.
Biliverdin.
Dyes (methylene blue, indigo carmine).

GROIN LUMP[81]

ICD-10CM #	R19.09	Other intraabdominal and pelvic swelling, mass and lump
	R22.9	Localized swelling, mass and lump, unspecified

COMMON CAUSES

Inguinal hernia.
Femoral hernia.
Lymph node.

OTHER CAUSES

Saphena varix.
Femoral artery aneurysm/pseudoaneurysm.
Psoas abscess.
Lipoma of the cord.
Encysted hydrocele of the cord (male).
Testicular maldescent (male).
Hydrocele of canal of Nuck (female).

GROIN MASSES

ICD-10CM #	R22.9	Localized swelling, mass and lump, unspecified
	S39.848A	Other specified injuries of external genitals, initial encounter

Hernia (inguinal, femoral).
Hydrocele.
Varicocele.
Sebaceous cyst.
Hidradenitis of inguinal apocrine glands.
Neoplasm: lymphoma, metastases.
Lipoma.
Hematoma.
Reactive inguinal adenopathy, femoral adenitis.
Folliculitis, psoas abscess.
Epididymitis, testicular torsion, ectopic testes.
Aneurysm or pseudoaneurysm of femoral artery.

GROIN PAIN[15]

ICD-10CM #	R52	Pain, unspecified

DIFFERENTIAL DIAGNOSIS OF GROIN PAIN

Surgery
Workers' Compensation.
Hernia.
Recurrent hernia.
Posthernia.
Orthopedic
Hip disorders.
- Acetabular labral tears.
- Avascular necrosis.
- Chondritis dissecans.
- Legg-Calvé-Perthes disease.
- Osteoarthritis.
- Pelvic stress fractures.
- Slipped femoral capital epiphysis.
- Synovitis.

Urology
Cystitis.
Epididymitis.
Nephrolithiasis.
Prostate cancer.
Prostatitis.
Torsion of testes.
Urethral extravasation.
Urinary tract infection.
Vas granuloma/fibrosis.
Dermatology
Lymphadenitis.
Psoriasis/burn.
Sebaceous cyst/hidradenitis.
Thrombophlebitis/cellulitis.
Neurosurgery
Disk disease.
Spinal injuries, inflammation, tumors.
Spondylolisthesis.
Spondylolysis.
Rheumatology
Connective tissue disorders.
Iliopsoas bursitis.
Osteitis pubis.
Systemic lupus erythematosus.
Neurology
Lumbosacral disorders.
Neurofibromatosis.
Infectious Disease
Herpes zoster.
HIV/tuberculosis.
Lyme disease.
Psoas abscess.
Sports Medicine
"Sports hernia" (adductor strains).
Gilmore groin.
Vascular
Abscess hematoma.
Post-vein stripping.
Pseudoaneurysm.
Vascular graft.
Gastroenterology
Appendicitis/adhesions.
Diverticulitis.
Inflammatory retroperitoneal phlegmon (pancreatitis).
Meckel diverticulum.
Granulomatous colitis.
Gynecology
Cesarean section.
Cervical cancer.
Endometriosis.
Tubal/ovarian disorders.

GROIN PAIN, ACTIVE PATIENT[80]

ICD-10CM #	S39.848A	Other specified injuries of external genitals, initial encounter
	R52	Pain, unspecified

MUSCULOSKELETAL

Avascular necrosis of the femoral head.
Avulsion fracture (lesser trochanter, anterior superior iliac spine, anterior inferior iliac spine).
Bursitis (iliopectineal, trochanteric).
Entrapment of the ilioinguinal or iliofemoral nerve.
Gracilis syndrome.
Muscle tear (adductors, iliopsoas, rectus abdominis, gracilis, sartorius, rectus femoris).
Myositis ossificans of the hip muscles.
Osteitis pubis.
Osteoarthritis of the femoral head.
Slipped capital femoral epiphysis.
Stress fracture of the femoral head or neck and pubis.
Synovitis.

HERNIA-RELATED

Avulsion of the internal oblique muscle in the conjoined tendon.
Defect at the insertion of the rectus abdominis muscle.
Direct inguinal hernia.
Femoral ring hernia.
Indirect inguinal hernia.
Inguinal canal weakness.

UROLOGIC

Epididymitis.
Fracture of the testis.
Hydrocele.
Kidney stone.
Posterior urethritis.
Prostatitis.
Testicular cancer.
Torsion of the testis.

Urinary tract infection.
Varicocele.

GYNECOLOGIC

Ectopic pregnancy.
Ovarian cyst.
Pelvic inflammatory disease.
Torsion of the ovary.
Vaginitis.

LYMPHATIC ENLARGEMENT IN GROIN

GYNECOMASTIA

ICD-10CM #	N62	Hypertrophy of breast

Physiologic (puberty, newborns, aging).
Drugs (estrogen and estrogen precursors, 5-a reductase inhibitors, digitalis, testosterone and exogenous androgens, clomiphene, cimetidine, spironolactone, ketoconazole, amiodarone, ACE inhibitors, isoniazid, phenytoin, methyldopa, metoclopramide, phenothiazine).
Increased prolactin level (prolactinoma).
Liver disease.
Adrenal disease.
Thyrotoxicosis.
Increased estrogen production (hCG-producing tumor, testicular tumor, bronchogenic carcinoma).
Secondary hypogonadism.
Primary gonadal failure (trauma, castration, viral orchitis, granulomatous disease).
Defects in androgen synthesis.
Testosterone deficiency.
Klinefelter syndrome.

HAIR LOSS[37]

ICD-10CM #	L63.8	Other alopecia areata
	L63.9	Alopecia areata, unspecified
	L64.0	Drug-induced androgenic alopecia
	L64.8	Other androgenic alopecia

GENERALIZED

Acute blood loss.*
Childbirth.
Crash diets (inadequate protein).
Drugs:
Coumarin.
Heparin.
Propranolol.
Vitamin A.
High fever.
Hypothyroidism and hyperthyroidisms.
Physical stress (e.g., surgery).
Physiologic stress (e.g., neonate).
Psychologic stress.
Severe illness (e.g., systemic lupus erythematosus).
Cancer chemotherapeutic agents.

*Diffuse, uniform loss, but many hairs left randomly distributed in area of loss.

Poisoning:
Thallium (rat poison).
Arsenic.
Radiation therapy.
Secondary syphilis: "moth eaten" alopecia.

LOCALIZED

Androgenetic alopecia:†
Male pattern.
Female pattern.
Hirsutism.
Alopecia areata.
Trichotillomania.
Traction alopecia.
Scarring alopecia:
Developmental defects: aplasia cutis.
Physical injury: burns, pressure.
Infection:
Fungal: kerion.
Bacterial: folliculitis, furuncle.
Viral: herpes zoster.
Neoplasms:
Metastatic carcinoma.
Sclerosing basal cell carcinoma.
Lupus erythematosus.
Lichen planus.
Cicatricial pemphigoid.
Scleroderma.

†Most or all hair missing from involved area.

HALITOSIS

ICD-10CM #	R19.6	Halitosis

Tobacco use.
Alcohol use.
Dry mouth (mouth breathing, inadequate fluid intake).
Foods (onion, garlic, meats, nuts, protein drinks).
Disease of mouth or nose (infections, cancer, inflammation).
Medications (antihistamines, antidepressants).
Systemic disorders (diabetes, uremia).
GI disorders (esophageal diverticula, hiatal hernia, GERD, achalasia).
Sinusitis.
Pulmonary disorders (bronchiectasis, pneumonia, neoplasms, TB).

HALLUCINATIONS, VISUAL, NEUROLOGIC CAUSES[49]

ICD-10CM #	R44.1	Visual hallucinations

Blindness/sensory deprivation—Charles Bonnet syndrome.
Palinopsia.
Dementia-producing diseases:
Alzheimer.
Dementia with Lewy bodies.*
Parkinson.†
Intoxications:
Alcoholic hallucinosis.
Delirium tremens (DTs).
Hallucinogens:
Amphetamines.
Cocaine.
Lysergic acid diethylamide (LSD).
Phencyclidine (PCP).
Medicines:
Atropine, scopolamine.
Levodopa and dopamine agonists.
Steroids.
Migraine with aura (classic migraine).
Narcolepsy: hypnopompic (awakening) and hypnagogic (falling asleep) hallucinations.
Seizures.
Peduncular hallucinations.

*Although visual hallucinations are likely to complicate almost any form of dementia, they are characteristic of dementia with Lewy bodies disease.
†Dopaminergic medications such as levodopa-carbidopa (Sinemet) are more likely than Parkinson disease itself to produce hallucinations.

HAND PAIN AND SWELLING[16]

ICD-10CM #	729.5	Pain in limb

Trauma.
Gout.
Pseudogout.
Cellulitis.
Lymphangitis.
DVT of upper extremity.
Thrombophlebitis.
RA.
Remitting seronegative symmetrical synovitis with pitting edema (RS3PE).
Polymyalgia rheumatica.
Mixed connective tissue disease.
Scleroderma.
Rupture of the olecranon bursa.
Metzger syndrome (neoplasia).
The puffy hand of drug addiction.
Reflex sympathetic dystrophy.
Eosinophilic fasciitis.
Sickle cell (hand-foot syndrome).
Leprosy.
Factitial (the rubber band syndrome).

HEADACHE[31]

ICD-10CM #	G44.1	Vascular headache, not elsewhere classified
	R51	Headache
	G44.209	Tension-type headache, unspecified, not intractable
	G44.009	Cluster headache syndrome, unspecified, not intractable
	G43.909	Migraine, unspecified, not intractable, without status migrainosus
	G44.1	Vascular headache, not elsewhere classified

Vascular: migraine, cluster headaches, temporal arteritis, hypertension, cavernous sinus thrombosis.
Musculoskeletal: neck and shoulder muscle contraction, strain of extraocular and/or intraocular muscles, cervical spondylosis, temporomandibular arthritis.

Infections: meningitis, encephalitis, brain abscess, sepsis, sinusitis, osteomyelitis, parotitis, mastoiditis.
Cerebral neoplasm.
Subdural hematoma.
Cerebral hemorrhage/infarct.
Pseudotumor cerebri.
Normal-pressure hydrocephalus (NPH).
Postlumbar puncture.
Cerebral aneurysm, arteriovenous malformations.
Posttrauma.
Dental problems: abscess, periodontitis, poorly fitting dentures.
Trigeminal neuralgia, glossopharyngeal neuralgia.
Otitis and other ear diseases.
Glaucoma and other eye diseases.
Metabolic: uremia, carbon monoxide inhalation, hypoxia.
Pheochromocytoma, hypoglycemia, hypothyroidism.
Effort induced: benign exertional headache, cough, headache, coital cephalalgia.
Drugs: alcohol, nitrates, histamine antagonists.
Paget disease of the skull.
Emotional, psychiatric.

HEADACHE, ACUTE[23]

ICD-10CM #	R51	Headache

DIFFERENTIAL DIAGNOSIS OF ACUTE HEADACHE

Evaluation of the first acute headache should exclude pathologic causes listed here before consideration of more common etiologies.
Increased intracranial pressure (ICP): trauma, hemorrhage, tumor, hydrocephalus, pseudotumor cerebri, abscess, arachnoid cyst, cerebral edema.
Decreased ICP: after ventriculoperitoneal shunt, lumbar puncture, cerebrospinal fluid leak from basilar skull fracture.
Meningeal inflammation: meningitis, leukemia, subarachnoid or subdural hemorrhage.
Vascular: Vasculitis, arteriovenous malformation, hypertension, cerebrovascular accident.
Bone, soft tissue: referred pain from scalp, eyes, ears, sinuses, nose, teeth, pharynx, cervical spine, temporomandibular joint.
Infection: systemic infection, encephalitis, sinusitis, etc.
First migraine.

HEADACHE AND FACIAL PAIN[77]

ICD-10CM #	R51	Headache
	G44.1	Vascular headache, not elsewhere classified

VASCULAR HEADACHES

Migraine

Migraine with headaches and inconspicuous neurologic features:
- Migraine without aura ("common migraine").

Migraine with headaches and conspicuous neurologic features:
- With transient neurologic symptoms:
  - Migraine with typical aura ("classic migraine").
  - Sensory, basilar, and hemiplegic migraine.
- With prolonged or permanent neurologic features ("complicated migraine"):
  - Ophthalmoplegic migraine.
  - Migrainous infarction.

Migraine without headaches but with conspicuous neurologic features ("migraine equivalents"):
- Abdominal migraine.
- Benign paroxysmal vertigo of childhood.
- Migraine aura without headache ("isolated auras," transient migrainous accompaniments).

Cluster Headaches

Episodic cluster headache ("cyclic cluster headaches").
Chronic cluster headaches.
Chronic paroxysmal hemicrania.

Other Vascular Headaches

Headaches of reactive vasodilation (fever, drug-induced, postictal, hypoglycemia, hypoxia, hypercarbia, hyperthyroidism).
Headaches associated with arterial hypertension:
- Chronic severe hypertension (diastolic 120 mm Hg).
- Paroxysmal severe hypertension (pheochromocytoma, some coital headaches).

Headaches caused by cranial arteritis:
- Giant cell arteritis ("temporal arteritis").
- Other vasculitides.

HEADACHES ASSOCIATED WITH DEMONSTRABLE MUSCLE SPASM

Headache caused by posturally induced or perilesional muscle spasm:
- Headaches of sustained or impaired posture (e.g., prolonged close work, driving).
- Headaches associated with cervical spondylosis and other diseases of cervical spine.
- Myofascial pain dysfunction syndrome (headache or facial pain associated with disorders of teeth, jaws, and related structures, or "TMJ syndrome").

Headaches caused by psychophysiologic muscular contraction ("muscle contraction headaches," or tension-type headache associated with disorder of pericranial muscles).

HEADACHES AND FACIAL PAIN WITHOUT DEMONSTRABLE PHYSICAL SUBSTRATE

Headaches of uncertain etiology:
- "Tension headaches" (tension-type headache unassociated with disorder of pericranial muscles).
- Some forms of posttraumatic headache.

Psychogenic headaches (e.g., hypochondriacal, conversional, delusional, malingered).
Facial pain of uncertain etiology ("atypical facial pain").

COMBINED TENSION-MIGRAINE HEADACHES

Episodic migraine superimposed on chronic tension headaches.
Chronic daily headaches:
- Associated with analgesic and/or ergotamine overuse ("rebound headaches").
- Not associated with drug overuse.

HEADACHES AND HEAD PAINS CAUSED BY DISEASES OF EYES, EARS, NOSE, SINUSES, TEETH, OR SKULL

Headaches Caused by Meningeal Inflammation

Subarachnoid hemorrhage.
Meningitis and meningoencephalitis.
Others (e.g., meningeal carcinomatosis).

HEADACHES ASSOCIATED WITH ALTERED INTRACRANIAL PRESSURE ("TRACTION HEADACHES")

Increased Intracranial Pressure

Intracranial mass lesions (neoplasm, hematoma, abscess, etc.).
Hydrocephalus.
Benign intracranial hypertension.
Venous sinus thrombosis.

Decreased Intracranial Pressure

Post–lumbar puncture headaches.
Spontaneous hypoliquorrheic headaches.

HEADACHES AND HEAD PAINS CAUSED BY CRANIAL NEURALGIAS

Presumed Irritation of Superficial Nerves

Occipital neuralgia.
Supraorbital neuralgia.

Presumed Irritation of Intracranial Nerves

Trigeminal neuralgia ("tic douloureux").
Glossopharyngeal neuralgia.

HEADACHE, CHRONIC[23]

ICD-10CM #	R51	Headache

DIFFERENTIAL DIAGNOSIS OF RECURRENT OR CHRONIC HEADACHES

Migraine (with or without aura).
Tension.
Analgesic rebound.
Caffeine withdrawal.
Sleep deprivation (e.g., in children with sleep apnea) or chronic hypoxia.
Tumor.
Psychogenic: Conversion disorder, malingering.
Cluster headache.

HEAD AND NECK, SOFT TISSUE MASSES

ICD-10CM #	R22.0	Localized swelling, mass and lump, head
	R22.1	Localized swelling, mass and lump, neck

Lipoma.
Pilar cyst.
Epidermal inclusion cyst.
Dermoid cyst.
Bone cyst.

Hemangioma.
Eosinophilic granuloma.
Other: facial nerve neuroma, teratoma, rhabdomyoma, rhabdomyosarcoma, branchial cleft cyst.

HEARING LOSS, ACUTE[55]

ICD-10CM # H91.23 Sudden idiopathic hearing loss, bilateral

Infectious: mumps, measles, influenza, herpes simplex, herpes zoster, CMV, mononucleosis, syphilis.
Vascular: macroglobulinemia, sickle cell disease, Berger disease, leukemia, polycythemia, fat emboli, hypercoagulable states.
Metabolic: diabetes, pregnancy, hyperlipoproteinemia.
Conductive: cerumen impaction, foreign bodies, otitis media, otitis externa, barotrauma, trauma.
Medications: aminoglycosides, loop diuretics, antineoplastics, salicylates, vancomycin.
Neoplasm: acoustic neuroma, metastatic neoplasm.

HEARTBURN AND INDIGESTION[71]

ICD-10CM # R12 Heartburn
K30 Functional dyspepsia

Reflux esophagitis.
Gastritis.
Nonulcer dyspepsia.
Functional GI disorder (anxiety disorder, social/environmental stresses).
Excessive intestinal gas (ingestion of flatulogenic foods, GI stasis, constipation).
Gas entrapment (hepatitis or splenic flexure syndrome).
Neoplasm (adenocarcinoma of stomach or esophagus, lymphoma).
Gallbladder disease.

HEART DISEASE, TRAUMATIC CAUSES[56]

ICD-10CM # S26.020 Mild laceration of heart with hemopericardium
S26.021 Moderate laceration of heart with hemopericardium
S26.022 Major laceration of heart with hemopericardium

Penetrating:
- Stab wounds: knives, swords, ice picks, fence posts, wire, sports.
- Projectile wounds: handguns, rifles, nail guns, lawnmower projectiles.
- Shotgun wounds: pellets, close-range versus distant.

Nonpenetrating (blunt):
- Motor vehicle accident:
  - Seat belt.
  - Air bag.
  - Dashboard/steering wheel.
- Vehicular-pedestrian accident.
- Falls from a height.
- Crushing: industrial accident.
- Blasts: improvised explosive devices, grenades, fragments (combined blunt/penetrating).
- Assault.
- Sternal or rib fractures.
- Recreational: sporting events (e.g., rodeo, baseball).

Iatrogenic:
- Catheter induced.
- Pericardiocentesis induced.
- Percutaneous.

Metabolic:
- Traumatic response to injury.
- "Stunning."
- Systemic inflammatory response syndrome.

Others:
- Burn.
- Electrical.
- Factitious (needles, foreign bodies).
- Embolic.

HEART FAILURE WITH PRESERVED LEFT VENTRICULAR EJECTION FRACTION[34]

ICD-10CM # I50.9 Heart failure, unspecified

CAUSES OF (AND ALTERNATIVE EXPLANATIONS FOR) HEART FAILURE WITH PRESERVED LEFT VENTRICULAR EJECTION FRACTION (>45%–50%)

Inaccurate diagnosis of heart failure (e.g., pulmonary disease, obesity).
Inaccurate measurements of ejection fraction.
Systolic function overestimated by ejection fraction (e.g., mitral regurgitation).
Episodic, unrecognized systolic dysfunction.
Intermittent ischemia.
Arrhythmia.
Severe hypertension.
Alcohol abuse.
Diastolic dysfunction.
Abnormalities of myocardial relaxation:
- Ischemia.
- Hypertrophy.

Abnormalities of myocardial compliance:
- Hypertrophy.
- Aging.
- Fibrosis.
- Diabetes mellitus.
- Infiltrative disease (amyloidosis, sarcoidosis).
- Storage disease (hemochromatosis).
- Endomyocardial disease (endomyocardial fibrosis, radiation, anthracyclines).

Pericardial disease (constriction, tamponade).

HEART FAILURE, ACUTE[7]

ICD-10CM # I50.9 Heart failure, unspecified

COMMON PRECIPITATING CAUSES OF ACUTE HF

Systemic hypertension.
Myocardial infarction or ischemia.
Dysrhythmia.
Systemic infection.
Anemia.
Dietary, physical, environmental, and emotional excesses.
Pregnancy.
Thyrotoxicosis or hypothyroidism.
Acute myocarditis.
Acute valvular dysfunction.
Pulmonary embolus.
Pharmacologic complications.

HEART FAILURE, CHRONIC[11]

ICD-10CM # I50.9 Heart failure, unspecified

Myocardial disease.
Coronary artery disease.
- Myocardial infarction.[19]
- Myocardial ischemia.

Chronic pressure overload.
- Hypertension.
- Obstructive valvular disease.

Chronic volume overload.
- Regurgitant valvular disease.
- Intracardiac (left-to-right) shunting.
- Extracardiac shunting.

Nonischemic dilated cardiomyopathy.
- Familial or genetic disorders.
- Infiltrative disorders.
- Toxic or drug-induced damage.
- Metabolic disorder.
- Viral or other infectious agents.

Disorders of rate and rhythm.
- Chronic bradyarrhythmias.
- Chronic tachyarrhythmias.

Pulmonary heart disease.
- Cor pulmonale.
- Pulmonary vascular disorders.

High-output states.
Metabolic disorders.
- Thyrotoxicosis.
- Nutritional disorders (beriberi).

Excessive blood flow requirements.
- Systemic arteriovenous shunting.
- Chronic anemia.

HEART FAILURE, CONGENITAL HEART DISEASE CAUSES[64]

ICD-10CM # I50.9 Heart failure, unspecified

[19] Indicates conditions that can also lead to HF with a preserved EF.

CAUSES OF CONGESTIVE HEART FAILURE RESULTING FROM CONGENITAL HEART DISEASE

Age of Onset	Cause
At birth:	HLHS. Volume overload lesions: Severe tricuspid or pulmonary insufficiency. Large systemic arteriovenous fistula.
First week	TGA. PDA in small premature infants. HLHS (with more favorable anatomy). TAPVR, particularly those with pulmonary venous obstruction. Others. Systemic arteriovenous fistula. Critical AS or PS.
1–4 wk	COA with associated anomalies. Critical AS. Large left-to-right shunt lesions (VSD, PDA) in premature infants. All other lesions previously listed.
4–6 wk	Some left-to-right shunt lesions such as ECD.
6 wk–4 mo	Large VSD. Large PDA. Others, such as anomalous left coronary artery from the PA.

AS, Aortic stenosis; *COA*, coarctation of the aorta; *ECD*, endocardial cushion defect; *HLHS*, hypoplastic left heart syndrome; *PA*, pulmonary artery; *PDA*, patent ductus arteriosus; *PS*, pulmonary stenosis; *TAPVR*, total anomalous pulmonary venous return; *TGA*, transposition of the great arteries; *VSD*, ventricular septal defect.

HEART FAILURE, PATHOGENIC CAUSES[34]

ICD-10CM # I50.9 Heart failure, unspecified

IMPAIRED SYSTOLIC (CONTRACTILE) FUNCTION

Ischemic damage or dysfunction:
- Myocardial infarction.
- Persistent or intermittent myocardial ischemia.
- Hypoperfusion (shock).

Chronic pressure overloading:
- Hypertension.
- Obstructive valvular disease.

Chronic volume overload:
- Regurgitant valvular disease.
- Intracardiac left-to-right shunting.
- Extracardiac shunting.

Nonischemic dilated cardiomyopathy:
- Familial/genetic disorders.
- Toxic/drug-induced damage
- Immunologically mediated necrosis.
- Infectious agents.
- Metabolic disorders.
- Infiltrative processes.
- Idiopathic conditions.

IMPAIRED DIASTOLIC FUNCTION (RESTRICTED FILLING, INCREASED STIFFNESS)

Pathologic myocardial hypertrophy:
- Primary (hypertrophic cardiomyopathies).
- Secondary (hypertension).
- Aging.
- Ischemic fibrosis.
- Restrictive cardiomyopathy:
  - Infiltrative disorders (amyloidosis, sarcoidosis).
  - Storage diseases (hemochromatosis, genetic abnormalities).

Endomyocardial disorders.

MECHANICAL ABNORMALITIES

Intracardiac:
- Obstructive valvular disease.
- Regurgitant valvular disease.
- Intracardiac shunts.
- Other congenital abnormalities.

Extracardiac:
- Obstructive (coarctation, supravalvular aortic stenosis).
- Left-to-right shunting (patent ductus arteriosus).

DISORDERS OF RATE AND RHYTHM

- Bradyarrhythmias (sinus node dysfunction, conduction abnormalities).
- Tachyarrhythmias (ineffective rhythms, chronic tachycardia).

PULMONARY HEART DISEASE

- Cor pulmonale.
- Pulmonary vascular disorders.

HIGH-OUTPUT STATES

Metabolic disorders:
- Thyrotoxicosis.
- Nutritional disorders (beriberi).
- Excessive blood flow requirements:
  - Chronic anemia.
  - Systemic arteriovenous shunting.

HEART FAILURE, PREGNANCY

ICD-10CM # I50.9 Heart failure, unspecified

Congenital valvular heart disease exacerbated by pregnancy.
Peripartum cardiomyopathy.
Untreated thyrotoxicosis.
Hypothyroidism.
Pulmonary hypertension.
Myocardial infarction.

HEAT STROKE[1]

ICD-10CM # T67.0 Heatstroke and sunstroke

Sepsis.
Encephalitis.
Meningitis.
Brain abscess.
Malaria (cerebral falciparum).
Typhoid fever.
Tetanus.
Alcohol withdrawal syndrome.
Neuroleptic malignant syndrome (see Tips and Tricks box).
Anticholinergic toxicity.
Salicylate toxicity.
Phencyclidine hydrochloride (PCP), cocaine, or amphetamine toxicity.
Status epilepticus.
Cerebral hemorrhage.
Diabetic ketoacidosis.
Thyroid storm.

HEEL PAIN

ICD-10CM # M25.50 Pain in unspecified joint

Achilles tendonitis/tendinopathy (insertional, noninsertional).
Retrocalcaneal bursitis (superficial, deep).
Plantar fasciopathy.
Neuropathy (tarsal tunnel, posterior tibial nerve [medial calcaneal branch], abductor digiti quinti).
Calcaneal stress fracture.
Puncture wound, foreign body.
Cellulitis.
Spondyloarthropathy.
Fat pad atrophy.
Soft tissue tumor.
S1 radiculopathy.
Paget disease of bone.
Haglund deformity.
Primary or metastatic bone tumor.

HEEL PAIN, PLANTAR[48]

ICD-10CM # M79.609 Pain in unspecified limb

SKIN

Keratoses.
Verruca.
Ulcer.
Fissure.

CONNECTIVE TISSUE

Fat
Atrophy.
Panniculitis.

Dense Connective Tissue
Inflammatory fasciitis.
Fibromatosis.
Enthesopathy.
Bursitis.

Bone (Calcaneus)
Stress fracture.
Paget disease.
Benign bone cyst/tumor.
Malignant bone tumor.
Metabolic bone disease (osteopenia).

Nerve
Tarsal tunnel.
Plantar nerve entrapment.
S1 nerve root radiculopathy.
Painful peripheral neuropathy.

INFECTION

Dermatomycoses.
Acute osteomyelitis.
Plantar abscess.

MISCELLANEOUS

Foreign body.
Nonunion calcaneus fracture.
Psychogenic.
Idiopathic.

HEMARTHROSIS

ICD-10CM # T14.90 Injury, unspecified

Trauma.
Anticoagulant therapy.
Thrombocytopenia, thrombocytosis.
Bleeding disorders (e.g., von Willebrand's disease).
Charcot joint.
Idiopathic.
Other: pigmented villonodular synovitis, hemangioma, synovioma, AV fistula, ruptured aneurysm.

HEMATEMESIS[81]

ICD-10CM # K92.0 Hematemesis

CAUSES OF HEMATEMESIS

Very Common
Gastric or duodenal ulcer or erosions.
Common
Mallory-Weiss tear (a laceration at the gastroesophageal junction).
Ulcerative esophagitis.
Esophageal varices.
Uncommon
Vascular malformations.
Ulcerated GI stromal tumor.
Carcinoma of esophagus or stomach.
Aortoenteric fistula.

HEMATURIA

ICD-10CM # R31.9 Hematuria, unspecified

Use the mnemonic TICS:

T (Trauma): blow to kidney, insertion of Foley catheter or foreign body in urethra, prolonged and severe exercise, very rapid emptying of overdistended bladder.
(Tumor): hypernephroma, Wilms tumor, papillary carcinoma of the bladder, prostatic and urethral neoplasms.
(Toxins): turpentine, phenols, sulfonamides and other antibiotics, cyclophosphamide, NSAIDs.
I (Infections): glomerulonephritis, TB, cystitis, prostatitis, urethritis, *Schistosoma haematobium,* yellow fever, blackwater fever.
(Inflammatory processes): Goodpasture syndrome, periarteritis, postirradiation.
C (Calculi): renal, ureteral, bladder, urethra.
(Cysts): simple cysts, polycystic disease.
(Congenital anomalies): hemangiomas, aneurysms, AVM.
S (Surgery): invasive procedures, prostatic resection, cystoscopy.
(Sickle cell disease and other hematologic disturbances): hemophilia, thrombocytopenia, anticoagulants.
(Somewhere else): bleeding genitals, factitious (drug addicts).

HEMATURIA, DIFFERENTIAL BASED ON AGE AND SEX

ICD-10CM # R31.9 Hematuria, unspecified

0 TO 20 YR

Acute urinary tract infections.
Acute glomerulonephritis.
Congenital urinary tract anomalies with obstruction.
Trauma to genitals.

20 TO 40 YR

Acute urinary tract infection.
Trauma to genitals.
Urolithiasis.
Bladder cancer.

40 TO 60 YR (WOMEN)

Acute urinary tract infection.
Bladder cancer.
Urolithiasis.

40 TO 60 YR (MEN)

Acute urinary tract infection.
Bladder cancer.
Urolithiasis.

60 YR AND OLDER (WOMEN)

Acute urinary tract infection.
Bladder cancer.
Vaginal trauma or irritation.
Urolithiasis.

60 YR AND OLDER (MEN)

Acute urinary tract infection.
Benign prostatic hyperplasia.
Bladder cancer.
Urolithiasis.
Trauma.

HEMATURIA, IN CHILDREN[7]

ICD-10CM # R31.9 Hematuria, unspecified

EXTRARENAL

Trauma.
Meatal stenosis or posterior urethral valves.
Exercise.
Menstruation or rectal bleeding.
Foreign bodies.
Cystitis, urethritis, or epididymitis.

INTRARENAL

Pyelonephritis.
Renal or bladder stones or tumors.
Poststrepotococcal or idiopathic glomerulonephritis.
Acute interstitial nephritis.
Acute tubular necrosis.
Basement membrane glomerular disease.
Renal vein or arterial thrombosis.
Recurrent familial hematuria.
Polycystic kidney disease.

SYSTEMIC

Henoch-Schönlein purpura.
Systemic lupus erythematosus.
Hemolytic-uremic syndrome.
Infectious mononucleosis.
Sickle cell disease or other hemoglobinopathies.
Bacterial endocarditis or artificial cardiac valves.
Bleeding disorders, warfarin, or aspirin.
Medications such as amitriptyline or chlorpromazine, radiocontrast dyes.
Munchausen syndrome or factitious.

HEMIPARESIS/HEMIPLEGIA

ICD-10CM #		
	G81.00	Flaccid hemiplegia affecting unspecified side
	G81.10	Spastic hemiplegia affecting unspecified side

CVA.
Transient ischemic attack.
Cerebral neoplasm.
Multiple sclerosis or other demyelinating disorder.
CNS infection.
Migraine.
Hypoglycemia
Subdural hematoma.
Vasculitis.
Todd paralysis.
Epidural hematoma.
Metabolic (hyperosmolar state, electrolyte imbalance).
Psychiatric disorders.
Congenital disorders.
Leukodystrophies.

HEMOLYSIS AND HEMOGLOBINURIA

ICD-10CM #		
	P55.8	Other hemolytic diseases of newborn
	P55.9	Hemolytic disease of newborn, unspecified
	R82.3	Hemoglobinuria

Erythrocyte trauma (prosthetic cardiac valves, marching and severe trauma, extensive burns).
Infections (malaria, *Bartonella, Clostridium welchii*).
Brown recluse spider bite.
Incompatible blood transfusions.
Hemolytic-uremic syndrome.
Thrombotic thrombocytopenic purpura (TTP).
Paroxysmal nocturnal hemoglobinuria (PNH).
Drugs (penicillins, quinidine, methyldopa, sulfonamides, nitrofurantoin).
Erythrocyte enzyme deficiencies (e.g., exposure to fava beans in patients with glucose- 6-phosphate dehydrogenase deficiency).

HEMOLYSIS, INTRAVASCULAR

ICD-10CM #		
	D59.6	Hemoglobinuria due to hemolysis from other external causes
	D59.8	Other acquired hemolytic anemias

- Infections.
- Exertional hemolysis (e.g., prolonged march).
- Valve hemolysis.
- Microangiopathic hemolytic anemia.
- Osmotic and chemical agents.
- Thermal injury.
- Cold agglutinins.
- Venoms (snakes, spiders).
- Paroxysmal nocturnal hemoglobinuria (PNH).

HEMOLYSIS, MECHANICAL

ICD-10CM #		
	D59.4	Other nonautoimmune hemolytic anemias

Prosthetic heart valves.
Aortic stenosis.
Malignant hypertension.
Metastatic adenocarcinoma.
Traumatic exercise.
Renal transplants.
Renal cortical necrosis.
Glomerulonephritis.
Thrombotic thrombocytopenic purpura (TTP), hemolytic-uremic syndrome (HUS).
Renal vasculitis.
Scleroderma.
Diabetes mellitus.

HEMOLYSIS, OXIDATIVE, DRUG-INDUCED[44]

ICD-10CM #		
	D59	Acquired hemolytic anemia
	D59.1	Other autoimmune hemolytic anemias

AGENTS THAT CUASE OXIDATIVE HEMOLYSIS

Therapeutic Agents
Nitrofurantoin (Furadantin).
Sulfasalazine (Azulfidine).
p-Aminosalicylic acid.
Phenazopyridine (Pyridium).
Clotrimoxazole.
Quinolones.
Phenacetin.
Rasburicase.
Dapsone and other sulfones.
Primaquine.
Recreational Drugs
Isobutyl nitrate.
Amyl nitrite.
Miscellaneous Agents
Naphthalene mothballs.
Methylene blue.
Paraquat.
Hydrogen peroxide.

HEMOPERITONEUM

ICD-10CM #		
	K66.1	Hemoperitoneum

Ruptured Graafian follicle.
Ruptured spleen.
Ectopic pregnancy.
Traumatic laceration of liver.
Ruptured aneurysm.
Ruptured bladder.
Traumatic laceration of bowel, pancreas, uterus.

HEMOPTYSIS

ICD-10CM #		
	R04.2	Hemoptysis

CARDIOVASCULAR

Pulmonary embolism/infarction.
Left ventricular failure.
Mitral stenosis.
AV fistula.
Severe hypertension.
Erosion of aortic aneurysm.

PULMONARY

Neoplasm (primary or metastatic).
Infection.
Pneumonia: *Streptococcus pneumoniae, Klebsiella pneumoniae, Staphylococcus aureus, Legionella pneumophila.*
Bronchiectasis.
Abscess.
TB.
Bronchitis.
Fungal infections (aspergillosis, coccidioidomycosis).
Parasitic infections (amebiasis, ascariasis, paragonimiasis).
Vasculitis: granulomatosis with polyangiitis, Churg-Strauss syndrome, Henoch-Schönlein purpura.
Goodpasture syndrome.
Trauma (needle biopsy, foreign body, right-sided heart catheterization, prolonged and severe cough).
Cystic fibrosis, bullous emphysema.
Pulmonary sequestration.
Pulmonary AV fistula.
SLE.
Idiopathic pulmonary hemosiderosis.
Drugs: aspirin, anticoagulants, penicillamine.
Pulmonary hypertension.
Mediastinal fibrosis.

OTHER

Epistaxis, trauma.
Laryngeal bleeding (laryngitis, laryngeal neoplasm).
Hematologic disorders (clotting abnormalities, DIC, thrombocytopenia).

HEMORRHAGIC CYSTITIS[85]

ICD-10CM #		
	N39.0	Urinary tract infection

DIFFERENTIAL DIAGNOSIS FOR HEMORRHAGIC CYSTITIS[20]

Infectious:
 Bacterial.
 Viral (especially BK virus, adenovirus).
 Fungal.
 Parasitic.
Trauma:
 External.
 Postsurgical (e.g., transurethral resection of the bladder).
Malignancy:
 Bladder primary.
 Bladder invasion from local/distant primary.
Vascular malformation.
Chemical exposure:
 Cyclophosphamide.
 Ifosfamide.
 Busulfan.
 Thiotepa.
 Temozolomide.
 Aniline dye.
 Ether.
 Nonoxynol-9 (accidental urethral insertion of vaginal contraceptive).
Radiation therapy history (e.g., prostate cancer, cervical cancer).
Medication induced:
 Penicillin and derivatives (via immune reaction).
 Bleomycin.
 Danazol.
 Tiaprofenic.
 Allopurinol.
 Phensuximide.
 Methenamine mandelate.
 Acetic acid.
Manifestation of systemic disease:
 Amyloidosis.
 Rheumatoid arthritis.
 Crohn's disease.

[20] Bleeding localized to bladder after diagnostic workup for gross hematuria with cystoscopy, urine cytology, and upper tract imaging is without clear cause of alternative bleeding source.

HEPATIC CYSTS[77]

ICD-10CM #		
	Q44.6	Cystic disease of liver
	B67.8	Echinococcosis, unspecified, of liver

CONGENITAL HEPATIC CYSTS

Parenchymal: solitary cyst, polycystic disease.
Ductal: localized dilatation, multiple cystic dilatations of intrahepatic ducts (Caroli disease).

ACQUIRED HEPATIC CYSTS

Inflammatory cysts: retention cysts, echinococcal cyst, amebic cyst.
Neoplastic cyst.
Peliosis hepatis.

HEPATIC DYSFUNCTION, POSTOPERATIVE[26]

ICD-10CM #		
	K91.82	Postprocedural hepatic failure

CAUSES OF POSTOPERATIVE HEPATIC DYSFUNCTION

Hepatocellular Injury (predominant serum ALT elevation, with or without hyperbilirubinemia)
Acute transfusion-associated viral hepatitis.
Hepatic allograft rejection.
Hepatic artery thrombosis.
Inhalational anesthetics: halothane, others.
Ischemic hepatitis (shock liver).
Other drugs—antihypertensives (e.g., labetalol), heparin.

Unrecognized chronic liver disease: NASH, hepatitis C, other disorders.
Cholestatic Jaundice (elevated serum alkaline phosphatase ± ALT; direct hyperbilirubinemia)
Acalculous cholecystitis.
Benign postoperative cholestasis.
Bile duct injury: after cholecystectomy or liver transplantation.
Bile duct obstruction: gallstones, pancreatitis.
Cardiac bypass of prolonged duration.
Cholangitis.
Drugs: amoxicillin-clavulanic acid, chlorpromazine, erythromycin, telithromycin, trimethoprim/sulfamethoxazole, warfarin, others.
Hemobilia.
Microlithiasis (biliary sludge).
Prolonged TPN.
Sepsis.
Indirect Hyperbilirubinemia (serum alkaline phosphatase and ALT often normal)
Gilbert syndrome.
Hemolytic anemia (G6PD deficiency, other causes).
Multiple transfusions.
Resorbing hematoma.

G6PD, Glucose-6-phosphate dehydrogenase; *NASH*, nonalcoholic steatohepatitis.

HEPATIC GRANULOMAS[3]

ICD-10CM # K75.3 Granulomatous hepatitis

INFECTIONS

Bacterial, spirochetal: TB and atypical mycobacterial infections, tularemia, brucellosis, leprosy, syphilis, Whipple disease, listeriosis.
Viral: mononucleosis, CMV.
Rickettsial: Q fever.
Fungal: coccidioidomycosis, histoplasmosis, cryptococcal infections, actinomycosis, aspergillosis, nocardiosis.
Parasitic: schistosomiasis, clonorchiasis, toxocariasis, ascariasis, toxoplasmosis, amebiasis.

HEPATOBILIARY DISORDERS

Primary biliary cirrhosis, granulomatous hepatitis, jejunoileal bypass.

SYSTEMIC DISORDERS

Sarcoidosis, granulomatosis with polyangiitis, inflammatory bowel disease, Hodgkin's disease, lymphoma.

DRUGS/TOXINS

Beryllium, parenteral foreign material (starch, talc, silicone, etc.), phenylbutazone, α-methyldopa, procainamide, allopurinol, phenytoin, nitrofurantoin, hydralazine.

HEPATITIS, ACUTE[55]

ICD-10CM #		
	B17.8	Acute viral hepatitis, unspecified
	B15	Acute hepatitis A
	B16	Acute hepatitis B
	B17.1	Acute hepatitis C
	B17.2	Acute hepatitis E

Infectious:
Hepatitis A, B, C, D, E.
Epstein-Barr virus.
Cytomegalovirus.
Herpes simplex virus.
Yellow fever.
Leptospirosis.
Q fever.
HIV.
Brucellosis.
Lyme disease.
Syphilis.
Noninfectious:
Drug induced.
Autoimmune.
Ischemic.
Acute fatty liver of pregnancy.
Acute Budd-Chiari syndrome.
Wilson's disease.

HEPATITIS, CHRONIC[55]

ICD-10CM #		
	K73.9	Chronic hepatitis, unspecified
	B18.0	Chronic viral hepatitis B with δ-agent
	B18.2	Chronic viral hepatitis C

Chronic viral hepatitis:
Hepatitis B.
Hepatitis C.
Hepatitis D.
Autoimmune hepatitis and variant syndromes.
Hereditary hemochromatosis.
Wilson's disease.
α_1-Antitrypsin deficiency.
Fatty liver and nonalcoholic steatohepatitis.
Alcoholic liver disease.
Drug-induced liver disease.
Hepatic granulomas:
Infectious.
Drug induced.
Neoplastic.
Idiopathic.

HEPATITIS, IN CHILDREN[51]

ICD-10CM #		
	B17.9	Acute viral hepatitis, unspecified
	K73.9	Chronic hepatitis, unspecified

CAUSES AND DIFFERENTIAL DIAGNOSIS OF HEPATITIS IN CHILDREN

Infectious
Hepatotropic viruses:
HAV.
HBV.
HCV.
HDV.
HEV.
Hepatitis non–A-E viruses.
Systemic infection that can include hepatitis:
Adenovirus.
Arbovirus.
Coxsackievirus.
Cytomegalovirus.
Enterovirus.
Epstein-Barr virus.
"Exotic" viruses (e.g., yellow fever).
Herpes simplex virus.
Human immunodeficiency virus.
Paramyxovirus.
Rubella.
Varicella zoster.
Other.
Nonviral liver infections
Abscess.
Amebiasis.
Bacterial sepsis.
Brucellosis.
Fitz-Hugh-Curtis syndrome.
Histoplasmosis.
Leptospirosis.
Tuberculosis.
Other.
Autoimmune
Autoimmune hepatitis.
Sclerosing cholangitis.
Other (e.g., systemic lupus erythematosus, juvenile rheumatoid arthritis).
Metabolic
α1-Antitrypsin deficiency.
Tyrosinemia.
Wilson disease.
Other.
Toxic
Iatrogenic or drug induced (e.g., acetaminophen).
Environmental (e.g., pesticides).
Anatomic
Choledochal cyst.
Biliary atresia.
Other.
Hemodynamic
Shock.
Congestive heart failure.
Budd-Chiari syndrome.
Other.
Nonalcoholic Fatty Liver Disease
Idiopathic.
Reye's syndrome.
Other.

HEPATOMEGALY

ICD-10CM #		
	R16.0	Hepatomegaly, not elsewhere classified

FREQUENT JAUNDICE

Infectious hepatitis.
Toxic hepatitis.
Carcinoma: liver, pancreas, bile ducts, metastatic neoplasm to liver.
Cirrhosis.
Obstruction of common bile duct.
Alcoholic hepatitis.
Biliary cirrhosis.
Cholangitis.
Hemochromatosis with cirrhosis.

INFREQUENT JAUNDICE

CHF.
Amyloidosis.
Liver abscess.
Sarcoidosis.

Infectious mononucleosis.
Alcoholic fatty infiltration.
Nonalcoholic steatohepatitis.
Lymphoma.
Leukemia.
Budd-Chiari syndrome.
Myelofibrosis with myeloid metaplasia.
Familial hyperlipoproteinemia type 1.
Other: amebiasis, hydatid disease of liver, schistosomiasis, kala-azar *(Leishmania donovani),* Hurler syndrome, Gaucher disease, kwashiorkor.

HEPATOMEGALY, BY SHAPE OF LIVER[81]

ICD-10CM # R16.0 Hepatomegaly, not elsewhere classified

DIFFUSELY ENLARGED AND SMOOTH

Massive

Metastatic disease.
Alcoholic liver disease with fatty infiltration.
Myeloproliferative diseases (e.g., polycythemia rubra vera, myelofibrosis).

Moderate

The above causes.
Hemochromatosis.
Hematologic disease (e.g., chronic myeloid leukemia, lymphoma).
Fatty liver (e.g., diabetes mellitus, obesity).
Infiltrative disorders (e.g., amyloid).

Mild

The above causes.
Hepatitis (viral, drugs).
Cirrhosis.
Biliary obstruction.
Granulomatous disorders (e.g., sarcoid).
HIV infection.

DIFFUSELY ENLARGED AND IRREGULAR

Metastatic disease.
Cirrhosis.
Hydatid disease.
Polycystic liver disease.

LOCALIZED SWELLINGS

Riedel lobe (a normal variant—the lobe may be palpable in the right lumbar region).
Metastasis.
Large simple hepatic cyst.
Hydatid cyst.
Hepatoma.
Liver abscess (e.g., amebic abscess).

HERMAPHRODITISM[9]

ICD-10CM # Q56.3 Pseudohermaphroditism, unspecified
Q56.4 Indeterminate sex, unspecified

Female Pseudohermaphroditism
- Androgen exposure:
  - Fetal source:
    - 21-Hydroxylase (P450 c21) deficiency.
    - 11β-Hydroxylase (P450 c11) deficiency.
    - 3β-Hydroxysteroid dehydrogenase II (3β-HSD II) deficiency.
    - Aromatase (P450arom) deficiency.
  - Maternal source.
  - Virilizing ovarian tumor.
  - Virilizing adrenal tumor.
  - Androgenic drugs.
- Undetermined origin:
  - Associated with genitourinary and GI tract defects.

MALE PSEUDOHERMAPHRODITISM

- Defects in testicular differentiation:
  - Denys-Drash syndrome (mutation in WT1 gene).
  - WAGR syndrome (*W*ilms tumor, *a*niridia, *g*enitourinary malformation, *r*etardation).
  - Deletion of 11p13.
  - Camptomelic syndrome (autosomal gene at 17q24.3-q25.1) and SOX 9 mutation.
  - XY pure gonadal dysgenesis (Swyer syndrome).
  - Mutation in SRY gene.
  - Unknown cause.
  - XY gonadal agenesis.
- Deficiency of testicular hormones:
  - Leydig cell aplasia.
  - Mutation in LH receptor.
  - Lipoid adrenal hyperplasia (P450 scc) deficiency; mutation in StAR (steroidogenic acute regulatory protein).
  - 3α-HSD II deficiency.
  - 17-Hydroxylase/17, 20-lyase (P450 c17) deficiency.
  - Persistent müllerian duct syndrome.
  - Gene mutations, müllerian-inhibiting substance (MIS).
  - Receptor defects for MIS.
- Defect in androgen action:
  - 5α-Reductase II mutations.
  - Androgen receptor defects:
    - Complete androgen insensitivity syndrome.
    - Partial androgen insensitivity syndrome.
    - Reifenstein and other syndromes.
    - Smith-Lemli-Opitz syndrome.
- Defect in conversion of 7-dehydrocholesterol to cholesterol.

TRUE HERMAPHRODITISM

XX.
XY.
XX/XY chimeras.

HICCUPS[47]

ICD-10CM # R06.6 Hiccough

TRANSIENT HICCUPS

Sudden excitement, emotion.
Gastric distention.
Esophageal obstruction.
Alcohol ingestion.
Sudden change in temperature.

PERSISTENT OR CHRONIC HICCUPS

Toxic/metabolic: uremia, DM, hyperventilation, hypocalcemia, hypokalemia, hyponatremia, gout, fever.
Drugs: benzodiazepines, steroids, α-methyldopa, barbiturates.
Surgery/general anesthesia.
Thoracic/diaphragmatic disorders: pneumonia, lung cancer, asthma, pleuritis, pericarditis, myocardial infarction, aortic aneurysm, esophagitis, esophageal obstruction, diaphragmatic hernia or irritation.
Abdominal disorders: gastric ulcer or cancer, hepatobiliary or pancreatic disease, IBD, bowel obstruction, intraabdominal or subphrenic abscess, prostatic infection or cancer.
CNS disorders: traumatic, infectious, vascular, structural.
Ear, nose, and throat disorders: pharyngitis, laryngitis, tumor, irritation of auditory canal.
Psychogenic disorders.
Idiopathic disorders.

HILAR AND MEDIASTINAL LYMPH NODE ENLARGEMENT[34]

ICD-10CM # R59.0 Mediastinal adenopathy

DISORDERS ASSOCIATED WITH HILAR AND MEDIASTINAL LYMPH NODE ENLARGEMENT

Sarcoidosis.
Lymphoma.
Fungal disease.
Tuberculosis.
Metastatic cancer.
Silicosis, coal worker's pneumoconiosis, beryllium lung.

HIP PAIN, CHILDREN[55]

ICD-10CM # S79.819A Other specified injuries of unspecified hip, initial encounter
S79.829A Other specified injuries of unspecified thigh, initial encounter
S79.919A Unspecified injury of unspecified hip, initial encounter

TRAUMA

Hip or pelvis fractures.
Overuse injuries.

INFECTION

Septic arthritis.
Osteomyelitis.

INFLAMMATION

Transient synovitis.
Juvenile RA.
Rheumatic fever.

NEOPLASM

Leukemia.
Osteogenic or Ewing sarcoma.
Metastatic disease.

HEMATOLOGIC DISORDERS

Hemophilia.
Sickle cell anemia.

MISCELLANEOUS

Legg-Calvé-Perthes disease.
Slipped capital femoral epiphysis.

HIP PAIN, DIFFERENTIAL DIAGNOSIS[40]

ICD-10CM # M25.559 Pain in unspecified hip

ARTICULAR

Inflammatory joint disease
Rheumatoid arthritis.
Spondyloarthropathies.
Polymyalgia rheumatica.
Degenerative joint disease
Primary osteoarthritis.
Secondary osteoarthritis.
Metabolic joint diseases
Gout.
Pseudogout.
Ochronosis.
Hemochromatosis.
Wilson's disease.
Acromegaly.
Femoroacetabular impingement
Acetabular labral tear
Infections
Tumors
- Benign.
  - Pigmented villonodular sclerosis.
  - Osteochondromatosis.
- Malignant.
  - Synovial sarcoma.
  - Synovial metastasis.

Hemarthrosis
In children:
- Toxic synovitis.
- Juvenile chronic arthritis.

REFERRED PAIN

Thoracolumbar spine.
- Intraabdominal structures.
- Retroperitoneal structures.

PERIARTICULAR

Bursitis.
- Trochanteric.
- Iliopsoas.
- Ischiogluteal.

Tendinitis.
- Trochanteric.
- Adductor.

Acute calcific periarthritis.
Heterotropic ossification.

OSSEOUS

Bone lesions.
Fractures.
Neoplasms.
Infection.
Osteonecrosis of the femoral head.
Paget disease.
Metabolic bone disease.
Stress fracture.
Transient osteoporosis.
In children:
- Congenital dislocation of the hip.
- Acetabular dysplasia.
- Coxa vara.
- Slipped capital femoral epiphysis.
- Legg-Calvé-Perthes disease.
- Rickets.

NEUROLOGIC

Entrapment neuropathies.
Lateral femoral cutaneous nerve (meralgia paresthetica).
Lumbar nerve root compression.
L2, L3, and L4.

VASCULAR

Atherosclerosis of aorta, iliac vessels.

HIP PAIN, IN DIFFERENT AGE GROUPS[18]

ICD-10CM # M25.559 Pain in unspecified hip

COMMON CAUSES OF HIP PAIN IN DIFFERENT AGE GROUPS

Childhood (2-10 yr)
Intraarticular
Developmental dislocation of the hip.
Perthes disease.
Irritable hip.
Rickets.
Periarticular
Osteomyelitis.
Referred
Abdominal.

Adolescence (10-18 yr)
Intraarticular
Slipped upper femoral epiphysis.
Torn labrum.
Periarticular
Trochanteric bursitis.
Snapping hip.
Osteomyelitis.
Tumors.
Referred
Abdominal.
Lumbar spine.

Early Adulthood (18-30 yr)
Intraarticular
Inflammatory arthritis.
Torn labrum.
Periarticular
Bursitis.
Referred
Abdominal.
Lumbar spine.

Adulthood (30-50 yr)
Intraarticular
Osteoarthritis.
Inflammatory arthritis.
Osteonecrosis.
Transient osteoporosis.
Periarticular
Bursitis.
Referred
Abdominal.
Lumbar spine.

Old Age (>50 yr)
Intraarticular
Osteoarthritis.
Inflammatory arthritis.
Referred
Abdominal.
Lumbar spine.

HIP PAIN WITHOUT OBVIOUS FRACTURE[7]

ICD-10CM # R52 Pain, unspecified
M25.559 Pain in unspecified hip

DIFFERENTIAL DIAGNOSIS OF A PAINFUL HIP WITHOUT OBVIOUS FRACTURE

Referred pain (lumbar spine, hip, or knee).
Avascular necrosis of the femoral head.
Degenerative joint disease or osteoarthritis.
Herniation of a lumbar disk.
Diskitis.
Toxic synovitis of the hip.
Septic arthritis.
Bursitis.
Tendonitis.
Ligamentous injuries of the knee or hip.
Occult fracture.
Slipped capital femoral epiphysis.
Perthes disease.
Tumor (lymphoma).
Deep venous thrombosis.
Arterial insufficiency.
Osteomyelitis.
Iliopsoas abscess.
Retroperitoneal hematoma.
Inguinal hernia.
Inguinal lymphadenopathy.
Genitourinary complaints.
Sports-related hernia.

HIRSUTISM

ICD-10CM # L68.0 Hirsutism

- Idiopathic: familial, possibly increased sensitivity to androgens.
- Menopause.
- Polycystic ovarian syndrome.
- Drugs: androgens, anabolic steroids, methyltestosterone, minoxidil, diazoxide, phenytoin, glucocorticoids, cyclosporine.
- Congenital adrenal hyperplasia.
- Adrenal virilizing tumor.
- Ovarian virilizing tumor: arrhenoblastoma, hilus cell tumor.
- Pituitary adenoma.
- Cushing's syndrome.
- Hypothyroidism (congenital and juvenile).
- Acromegaly.
- Testicular feminization.

HIV INFECTION, ANORECTAL LESIONS[55]

ICD-10CM # B20 Human immunodeficiency virus [HIV] disease
Z21 Asymptomatic human immunodeficiency virus [HIV] infection status

COMMON CONDITIONS

Anal fissure.
Abscess and fistula.
Hemorrhoids.
Pruritus ani.
Pilonidal disease.

COMMON STDS

Gonorrhea.
Chlamydia.
Herpes.
Chancroid.
Syphilis.
Condylomata acuminata.

ATYPICAL CONDITIONS

Infectious: TB, CMV, actinomycosis, cryptococcus.
Neoplastic: lymphoma, Kaposi sarcoma, squamous cell carcinoma.
Other: idiopathic and ulcer.

HIV INFECTION, CHEST RADIOGRAPHIC ABNORMALITIES[55]

ICD-10CM #		
	B20	Human immunodeficiency virus [HIV] disease
	Z21	Asymptomatic human immunodeficiency virus [HIV] infection status

DIFFUSE INTERSTITIAL INFILTRATION

Pneumocystis jiroveci.
Cytomegalovirus.
Mycobacterium tuberculosis.
Mycobacterium avium complex.
Histoplasmosis.
Coccidioidomycosis.
Lymphoid interstitial pneumonitis.

FOCAL CONSOLIDATION

Bacterial pneumonia.
Mycoplasma pneumoniae.
Pneumocystis jiroveci.
Mycobacterium tuberculosis.
Mycobacterium avium complex.

NODULAR LESIONS

- Kaposi sarcoma.
- *Mycobacterium tuberculosis.*
- *Mycobacterium avium complex.*
- Fungal lesions.
- Toxoplasmosis.

CAVITARY LESIONS

- *Pneumocystis jiroveci.*
- *Mycobacterium tuberculosis.*
- Bacterial infection.

PLEURAL EFFUSION

Kaposi sarcoma.
(Small effusion may be associated with any infection).

ADENOPATHY

Kaposi sarcoma.
Lymphoma.
Mycobacterium tuberculosis.
Cryptococcus.

PNEUMOTHORAX

Kaposi sarcoma.

HIV INFECTION, COGNITIVE IMPAIRMENT[55]

ICD-10CM #		
	B20	Human immunodeficiency virus [HIV] disease

EARLY TO MID-STAGE HIV DISEASE

Depression.
Alcohol and substance abuse.
Medication-induced cognitive impairment.
Metabolic encephalopathies.
HIV-related cognitive impairment.

ADVANCED HIV DISEASE (CD4+ <100/MM^3)

- Opportunistic infection of CNS.
- Neurosyphilis.
- CNS lymphoma.
- Progressive multifocal leukoencephalopathy.
- Depression.
- Metabolic encephalopathies.
- Medication-induced cognitive impairment.
- Stroke.
- HIV dementia.

HIV INFECTION, CUTANEOUS MANIFESTATIONS[47]

ICD-10CM #		
	B20	Human immunodeficiency virus [HIV] disease
	Z21	Asymptomatic human immunodeficiency virus [HIV] infection status

BACTERIAL INFECTION

Bacillary angiomatosis: numerous angiomatous nodules associated with fever, chills, weight loss.
Staphylococcus aureus: folliculitis, ecthyma, impetigo, bullous impetigo, furuncles, carbuncles.
Syphilis: may occur in different forms (primary, secondary, tertiary); chancre may become painful because of secondary infection.

FUNGAL INFECTION

Candidiasis: mucous membranes (oral, vulvovaginal), less commonly candida intertrigo or paronychia.
Cryptococcoses: papules or nodules that strongly resemble molluscum contagiosum; other forms include pustules, purpuric papules, and vegetating plaques.
Seborrheic dermatitis: scaling and erythema in the hair-bearing areas (eyebrows, scalp, chest, and pubic area).

ARTHROPOD INFESTATIONS

Scabies: pruritus with or without rash, usually generalized but can be limited to a single digit.

VIRAL INFECTION

Herpes simplex: vesicular lesion in clusters; perianal, genital, orofacial, or digital; can be disseminated.
Herpes zoster: painful dermatomal vesicles that may ulcerate or disseminate.
HIV: discrete erythematous macules and papules on the upper trunk, palms, and soles are the most characteristic cutaneous finding of acute HIV infection.
Human papillomavirus: genital warts (may become unusually extensive).
Kaposi sarcoma (herpesvirus): erythematous macules or papules; enlarge at varying rates; violaceous nodules or plaques; occasionally painful.
Molluscum contagiosum: discrete umbilicated papules commonly on the face, neck, and intertriginous sites (axilla, groin, or buttocks).

NONINFECTIOUS

Drug reactions: more frequent and severe in HIV patients.
Nutritional deficiencies: mainly seen in children and patients with chronic diarrhea; diffuse skin manifestations, depending upon the deficiency.
Psoriasis: scaly lesions; diffuse or localized; can be associated with arthritis.
Vasculitis: palpable purpuric eruption (can resemble septic emboli).

HIV INFECTION, ESOPHAGEAL DISEASE

ICD-10CM #		
	B20	Human immunodeficiency virus [HIV] disease
	K21.9	Gastro-esophageal reflux disease without esophagitis

Candida infection.
Cytomegalovirus infection.
Aphthous ulcer.
Herpes simplex.

HIV INFECTION, HEPATIC DISEASE[55]

ICD-10CM #		
	B20	Human immunodeficiency virus [HIV] disease

VIRUSES

Hepatitis A.
Hepatitis B.
Hepatitis C.
Hepatitis D (with HBV).
Epstein-Barr virus.
Cytomegalovirus.
Herpes simplex virus.
Adenovirus.
Varicella-zoster virus.

MYCOBACTERIA

Mycobacterium avium complex.
Mycobacterium tuberculosis.

FUNGI

Histoplasma capsulatum.
Cryptococcus neoformans.

Coccidioides immitis.
Candida albicans.
Pneumocystis jiroveci.
Penicillium marneffei.

PROTOZOA

Toxoplasma gondii.
Cryptosporidium parvum.
Microsporida.
Schistosoma.

BACTERIA

Bartonella henselae (peliosis hepatis).

MALIGNANCY

- Kaposi sarcoma (HHV-8).
- Non-Hodgkin's lymphoma.
- Hepatocellular carcinoma.

MEDICATIONS

Zidovudine.
Didanosine.
Ritonavir.
Other HIV-1 protease inhibitors.
Fluconazole.
Macrolide antibiotics.
Isoniazid.
Rifampin.
Trimethoprim-sulfamethoxazole.

HIV INFECTION, LOWER GI TRACT DISEASE[55]

ICD-10CM # B20 Human immunodeficiency virus [HIV] disease

CAUSES OF ENTEROCOLITIS

Bacteria
Campylobacter jejuni and other spp.
Salmonella spp.
Shigella flexneri.
Aeromonas hydrophila.
Plesiomonas shigelloides.
Yersinia enterocolitica.
Vibrio spp.
Mycobacterium avium complex.
Mycobacterium tuberculosis.
Escherichia coli (enterotoxigenic, enteroadherent).
Bacterial overgrowth.
Clostridium difficile (toxin).
Parasites
Cryptosporidium parvum.
Microsporida (*Enterocytozoon bieneusi, Septata intestinalis*).
Isospora belli.
Entamoeba histolytica.
Giardia lamblia.
Cyclospora cayetanensis.
Viruses
Cytomegalovirus.
Adenovirus.
Calicivirus.
Astrovirus.
Picobirnavirus.
Human immunodeficiency virus.
Fungi
Histoplasma capsulatum.

CAUSES OF PROCTITIS

Bacteria
Chlamydia trachomatis.
Neisseria gonorrhoeae.
Treponema pallidum.
Viruses
Herpes simplex.
Cytomegalovirus.

HIV INFECTION, MUSCULOSKELETAL DISORDERS[66]

ICD-10CM # B20 Human immunodeficiency virus [HIV] disease

MUSCULOSKELETAL DISORDERS ASSOCIATED WITH HIV INFECTION

Joints, Ligaments, and Soft Tissues
Painful articular syndrome.
HIV-associated arthritis.
Reactive arthritis.
Septic arthritis.
Psoriatic arthritis.
Diffuse infiltrative lymphocytosis syndrome.
Systemic lupus erythematosus.
Rheumatoid arthritis.
Vasculitis (polyarteritis nodosa, drug induced).
Immune reconstitution inflammatory syndrome.
Cellulitis and soft tissue abscesses.
Fasciitis (including necrotizing fasciitis).
Bursitis and tenosynovitis.
Muscles
HIV myopathy.
Nucleoside reverse transcriptase inhibitor (NRTI) myopathy.
Muscle infections (pyomyositis, toxoplasmosis).
Other (rhabdomyolysis, non-Hodgkin's lymphoma, myasthenia gravis, nemaline [rod] myopathy, and inclusion body myositis).
Bones
Osteomyelitis.
Osteopenia and osteoporosis.
Osteonecrosis.
Hypertrophic osteoarthropathy.
Opportunistic Infections, HIV/AIDS-Defining Neoplastic Disorders, and Other Disorders Affecting Any Part of the Musculoskeletal System in HIV Infection
Neoplasia:
  Kaposi sarcoma.
  Non-Hodgkin's lymphoma.
  Hodgkin's lymphoma.
  Leiomyosarcoma.
  Ewing sarcoma.
Infection:
  Tuberculosis.
  Disseminated *Mycobacterium avium* complex infection.
  Coccidioidomycosis.
  Toxoplasmosis.
  Bacillary angiomatosis.
Other:
  HIV-related lipodystrophy.
  HIV wasting syndrome.

HIV INFECTION, OCULAR MANIFESTATIONS[77]

ICD-10CM # B20 Human immunodeficiency virus [HIV] disease
Z21 Asymptomatic human immunodeficiency virus [HIV] infection status

EYELIDS

Molluscum contagiosum.
Kaposi sarcoma.

CORNEA/CONJUNCTIVA

Keratoconjunctivitis sicca.
Bacterial/fungal ulcerative keratitis.
Herpes simplex.
Herpes zoster ophthalmicus.
Conjunctival microvasculopathy.
Kaposi sarcoma.

RETINA, CHOROID, AND VITREOUS

Microvasculopathy.
Endophthalmitis.
Cytomegalovirus retinitis.
Acute retinal necrosis.
Syphilis.
Toxoplasmosis.
Pneumocystis choroidopathy.
Cryptococcosis.
Mycobacterial infection.
Intraocular lymphoma.
Candidiasis.
Histoplasmosis.

DRUGS ASSOCIATED WITH OCULAR TOXICITY

Rifabutin.
Didanosine.

NEUROOPHTHALMIC

Disc edema.
Primary or secondary optic neuropathy.
Cranial nerve palsies.

ORBITAL

Lymphoma.
Infection.
Pseudotumor.

HIV INFECTION, PULMONARY DISEASE[10,55]

ICD-10CM # B20 Human immunodeficiency virus [HIV] disease
I28.8 Other diseases of pulmonary vessels

RADIOGRAPHIC APPEARANCE

Diffuse Interstitial Infiltrates
Pneumocystis jiroveci.
Mycobacterium tuberculosis, especially with advanced human immunodeficiency virus disease.
Histoplasma capsulatum.
Coccidioides spp.

Cryptococcus neoformans.
Toxoplasma gondii.
Cytomegalovirus.
Influenza.
Lymphocytic interstitial pneumonitis.
Abacavir hypersensitivity.

Focal Consolidation

Pyogenic bacterial pneumonia from *Streptococcus pneumoniae, Haemophilus influenzae.*
M. tuberculosis.
Legionella spp.
Rhodococcus equi.

Hilar Adenopathy

M. tuberculosis.
H. capsulatum.
Coccidioides spp.
Non-Hodgkin's or Hodgkin's lymphoma.
Mycobacterium avium complex.

Cavitary Disease

Pyogenic bacterial pneumonia from *Pseudomonas aeruginosa, Staphylococcus aureus*, Enterobacteriaceae.
M. tuberculosis.
C. neoformans.
R. equi.
Aspergillus spp.
Nocardia spp.
Mycobacterium avium complex.
P. jiroveci.

Nodules or Masses

M. tuberculosis.
C. neoformans.
Aspergillus spp.
H. capsulatum.
Nocardia spp.
Non-Hodgkin's lymphoma.
Kaposi sarcoma.
Lung cancer.

Normal Radiograph

P. jiroveci.
M. tuberculosis.

CAUSES

Mycobacterial

M. tuberculosis.
M. kansasii.
M. avium complex.
Other nontuberculous mycobacteria.

Other Bacterial

Streptococcus pneumoniae.
Staphylococcus aureus.
Haemophilus influenzae.
Enterobacteriaceae.
Pseudomonas aeruginosa.
Moraxella catarrhalis.
Group A *Streptococcus.*
Nocardia spp.
Rhodococcus equi.
Chlamydia pneumoniae.

Fungal

Pneumocystis carinii.
Cryptococcus neoformans.
Histoplasma capsulatum.
Coccidioides immitis.
Aspergillus spp.
Blastomyces dermatitidis.
Penicillium marneffei.

Viral

Cytomegalovirus.
Herpes simplex virus.
Adenovirus.
Respiratory syncytial virus.
Influenza viruses.
Parainfluenza virus.

Other

Toxoplasma gondii.
Strongyloides stercoralis.
Kaposi sarcoma.
Lymphoma.
Lung cancer.
Lymphocytic interstitial pneumonitis.
Nonspecific interstitial pneumonitis.
Bronchiolitis obliterans with organizing pneumonia.
Pulmonary hypertension.
Emphysema-like or bullous disease.
Pneumothorax.
Congestive heart failure.
Diffuse alveolar damage.
Pulmonary embolus.

HOARSENESS

ICD-10CM # R49.8 Other voice and resonance disorders

Allergic rhinitis.
Infections (laryngitis, epiglottitis, tracheitis, croup).
Vocal cord polyps.
Voice strain.
Irritants (tobacco smoke).
Vocal cord trauma (intubation, surgery).
Neoplastic involvement of vocal cord (primary or metastatic).
Neurologic abnormalities (multiple sclerosis, ALS, parkinsonism).
Endocrine abnormalities (puberty, menopause, hypothyroidism).
Other (laryngeal webs or cysts, psychogenic, muscle tension abnormalities).

HYDROCEPHALUS

ICD-10CM # G91.1 Obstructive hydrocephalus

Head trauma.
Brain neoplasm (primary or metastatic).
Spinal cord tumor.
Cerebellar infarction.
Exudative or granulomatous meningitis.
Cerebellar hemorrhage.
Subarachnoid hemorrhage.
Aqueductal stenosis.
Third ventricle colloid cyst.
Hindbrain malformation.
Viral encephalitis.
Metastases to leptomeninges.

HYPERCALCEMIA

ICD-10CM # E83.52 Hypercalcemia

Malignancy: increased bone resorption via osteoclast-activating factors, secretion of PTH-like substances, prostaglandin E_2, direct erosion by tumor cells, transforming growth factors, colony-stimulating activity.

Hypercalcemia is common in the following neoplasms:

Solid tumors: breast, lung, pancreas, kidneys, ovary.

Hematologic cancers: myeloma, lymphosarcoma, adult T-cell lymphoma, Burkitt lymphoma.

Hyperparathyroidism: increased bone resorption, GI absorption, and renal absorption; etiology:

Parathyroid hyperplasia, adenoma.

Hyperparathyroidism or renal failure with secondary hyperparathyroidism.

Granulomatous disorders: increased GI absorption (e.g., sarcoidosis).
Paget disease: increased bone resorption, seen only during periods of immobilization.
Vitamin D intoxication, milk-alkali syndrome; increased GI absorption.
Thiazides: increased renal absorption.
Other causes: familial hypocalciuric hypercalcemia, thyrotoxicosis, adrenal insufficiency, prolonged immobilization, vitamin A intoxication, recovery from acute renal failure, lithium administration, pheochromocytoma, disseminated SLE.

HYPERCALCEMIA, MALIGNANCY-INDUCED

ICD-10CM # E83.52 Hypercalcemia

Lung carcinoma	(6% frequency, 35% of hypercalcemic cases)
Breast carcinoma	(10% frequency, 25% of hypercalcemic cases)
Multiple myeloma	(33% frequency, 10% of hypercalcemic cases)
Lymphoma	(4% of hypercalcemic cases)
Genitourinary cancer	(6% of hypercalcemic cases)

HYPERCAPNIA, PERSISTENT[77]

ICD-10CM # R06.00 Dyspnea, unspecified
R06.09 Other forms of dyspnea
R06.89 Other abnormalities of breathing

Hypercapnia with normal lungs: CNS disturbances (CVA, parkinsonism, encephalitis), metabolic alkalosis, myxedema, primary alveolar hypoventilation, spinal cord lesions.
Diseases of the chest wall (e.g., kyphoscoliosis, ankylosing spondylitis).
Neuromuscular disorders (e.g., myasthenia gravis, Guillain-Barré syndrome, amyotrophic lateral sclerosis, muscular dystrophy, poliomyelitis).
COPD.

HYPERCOAGULABLE STATE, ASSOCIATED DISORDERS[43]

ICD-10CM # D68.69 Other thrombophilia

Systemic lupus erythematosus in association with the presence of a lupus anticoagulant or antiphospholipid antibodies.

MALIGNANCY

Disease-related: includes migratory superficial thrombophlebitis (Trousseau syndrome), nonbacterial thrombotic endocarditis, thrombosis associated with chronic DIC, thrombotic microangiopathy.
Treatment-related: associated with the administration of various chemotherapeutic agents (L-asparaginase, mitomycin, some adjuvant chemotherapeutic agents for treatment of breast cancer, thalidomide or lenalidomide in conjunction with high doses of dexamethasone).
Infusion of prothrombin complex concentrates.
Nephrotic syndrome.
Heparin-induced thrombocytopenia.
Myeloproliferative disorders.
Paroxysmal nocturnal hemoglobinuria.

DIC, Disseminated intravascular coagulopathy.

HYPERGASTRINEMIA

ICD-10CM # E16.4 Abnormal secretion of gastrin

Decreased gastrin release inhibition from medications (proton pump inhibitors [PPIs], H_2 receptor antagonists), vagotomy.
Chronic renal failure.
Hypochlorhydria due to atrophic gastritis, gastric carcinoma, pernicious anemia.
Gastrinoma (Zollinger-Ellison syndrome).
Pyloric obstruction.
Hyperplasia of antral G cells.
RA.

HYPERHIDROSIS[9]

ICD-10CM # R61 Generalized hyperhidrosis

CORTICAL

Emotional.
Familial dysautonomia.
Congenital ichthyosiform erythroderma.
Epidermolysis bullosa.
Nail-patella syndrome.
Jadassohn-Lewandowsky syndrome.
Pachyonychia congenita.
Palmoplantar keratoderma.

HYPOTHALAMIC

Drugs
Antipyretics.
Emetics.
Insulin.
Meperidine.
Exercise Infection
Defervescence.
Chronic illness.
Metabolic
Debility.
DM.
Hyperpituitarism.
Hyperthyroidism.
Hypoglycemia.
Obesity.
Porphyria.
Pregnancy.
Rickets.
Infantile scurvy.
Cardiovascular
Heart failure.
Shock.
Vasomotor
Cold injury.
Raynaud's phenomenon.
RA.
Neurologic
Abscess.
Familial dysautonomia.
Postencephalitic.
Tumor.
Miscellaneous
Chédiak-Higashi syndrome.
Compensatory.
Phenylketonuria.
Pheochromocytoma.
Vitiligo.
Medullary
Physiologic gustatory sweating.
Encephalitis.
Granulosis rubra nasi.
Syringomyelia.
Thoracic sympathetic trunk injury.
Spinal
Cord transection.
Syringomyelia.
Changes in Blood Flow
Mallucci syndrome.
Arteriovenous fistula.
Klippel-Trenaunay syndrome.
Glomus tumor.
Blue rubber bleb nevus syndrome.

HYPERKALEMIA

ICD-10CM # E87.5 Hyperkalemia

Pseudohyperkalemia.
- Hemolyzed specimen.
- Severe thrombocytosis (platelet count 0.106 ml).
- Severe leukocytosis (white blood cell count 0.105 ml).
- Fist clenching during phlebotomy.

Excessive potassium intake (often in setting of impaired excretion).
- Potassium replacement therapy.
- High-potassium diet.
- Salt substitutes with potassium.
- Potassium salts of antibiotics.

Decreased renal excretion.
- Potassium-sparing diuretics (e.g., spironolactone, triamterene, amiloride).
- Renal insufficiency.
- Mineralocorticoid deficiency.
- Hyporeninemic hypoaldosteronism.
- Tubular unresponsiveness to aldosterone (e.g., SLE, multiple myeloma, sickle cell disease).
- Type 4 RTA.
- ACE inhibitors.
- Heparin administration.
- NSAIDs.
- Trimethoprim-sulfamethoxazole.
- Beta-blockers.
- Pentamidine.

Redistribution (excessive cellular release).
- Acidemia (each 0.1 decrease in pH increases the serum potassium by 0.4 to 0.6 mEq/L). Lactic acidosis and ketoacidosis cause minimal redistribution.
- Insulin deficiency.
- Drugs (e.g., succinylcholine, markedly increased digitalis level, arginine, beta-adrenergic blockers).
- Hypertonicity.
- Hemolysis.
- Tissue necrosis, rhabdomyolysis, burns.
- Hyperkalemic periodic paralysis.

HYPERKALEMIA, DRUG-INDUCED[83]

ICD-10CM # E87.5 Hyperkalemia

IMPAIRED RENIN-ALDOSTERONE ELABORATION/FUNCTION

Cyclooxygenase inhibitors (NSAIDs).
β-Adrenergic antagonists.
Spironolactone.
Angiotensin-converting enzyme inhibitors and angiotensin II receptor blockers.
Heparin.

INHIBITORS OF RENAL POTASSIUM SECRETION

Potassium-sparing diuretics (amiloride, triamterene).
Trimethoprim.
Pentamidine.
Cyclosporine.
Digitalis overdose.
Lithium.

ALTERED POTASSIUM DISTRIBUTION

Insulin antagonists (somatostatin, diazoxide).
β-Adrenergic antagonists.
α-Adrenergic agonists.
Hypertonic solutions.
Digitalis.
Succinylcholine.
Arginine hydrochloride, lysine hydrochloride.

HYPERKALEMIA IN CHILDREN[74]

ICD-10CM # E87.5 Hyperkalemia

MOST RELEVANT CAUSES OF HYPERKALEMIA IN PEDIATRIC PATIENTS

Pseudohyperkalemia
Improper collection of blood.
Hematologic disorders: leukocytosis, thrombocytosis, spherocytosis.
Transcellular Shift of Potassium
Acidosis.
Insulin deficiency.
Hyperosmolality.
Exercise with nonselective β-blockers.
Familial hyperkalemic periodic paralysis.

Increased Potassium Load
From exogenous origin: pharmacologic supplements.
From endogenous origin (cellular lysis): burns, trauma, intravascular hemolysis, rhabdomyolysis, tumor mass destruction.
Decreased Urinary Excretion
Renal failure.
Mineralocorticoid deficiency.
Addison disease.
Hypoaldosteronism.
Mineralocorticoid resistance.
Type 1 and type 2 pseudohypoaldosteronism.
Renal tubular acidosis: type 4 and hyperkalemic form of type 1.
"Hyperkalemic" drugs: potassium-sparing diuretics, trimethoprim, calcineurin inhibitors, blockers of the renin angiotensin aldosterone system.

HYPERKINETIC MOVEMENT DISORDERS[63]

ICD-10CM #		
	F90.8	Attention-deficit hyperactivity disorder, other type
	E83.00	Disorder of copper metabolism, unspecified
	E83.01	Wilson's disease
	E83.09	Other disorders of copper metabolism
	G24.02	Drug induced acute dystonia
	G24.1	Genetic torsion dystonia

Chorea, choreoathetosis: drug-induced, Huntington chorea, Sydenham chorea.
Tardive dyskinesia (e.g., phenothiazines).
Hemiballismus (lacunar CVA near subthalamic nuclei in basal ganglia, metastatic lesions, toxoplasmosis [in AIDS]).
Dystonia (idiopathic, familial, drug-induced [prochlorperazine, metoclopramide]), Wilson's disease.
Liver failure.
Thyrotoxicosis.
SLE, polycythemia.

HYPERMAGNESEMIA

ICD-10CM #		
	E83.40	Disorders of magnesium metabolism, unspecified
	E83.41	Hypermagnesemia

Renal failure (decreased GFR).
Decreased renal excretion secondary to salt depletion.
Abuse of antacids and laxatives containing magnesium in patients with renal insufficiency.
Endocrinopathies (deficiency of mineralocorticoid or thyroid hormone).
Increased tissue breakdown (rhabdomyolysis).
Redistribution: acute DKA, pheochromocytoma.
Other: lithium, volume depletion, familial hypocalciuric hypercalcemia.

HYPEROSTOSIS, CORTICAL BONE[36]

ICD-10CM #		
	M48.19	Ankylosing hyperostosis [Forestier], multiple sites in spine

DISORDERS ASSOCIATED WITH HYPEROSTOSIS OF CORTICAL BONE

Progressive diaphyseal dysplasia.
Endosteal hyperostosis.
Pachydermoperiostosis.
Hypertrophic oseoarthropathy.
Thyroid acropachy.
Hypervitaminosis A.
Paget disease.
Infantile cortical hyperostosis.

HYPERPHOSPHATEMIA

ICD-10CM #		
	E83.30	Disorder of phosphorus metabolism, unspecified

Excessive phosphate administration.
Excessive oral intake or IV administration.
Laxatives containing phosphate (phosphate tablets, phosphate enemas).
Decreased renal phosphate excretion.
Acute or chronic renal failure.
Hypoparathyroidism or pseudohypoparathyroidism.
Acromegaly, thyrotoxicosis.
Bisphosphonate therapy.
Tumor calcinosis.
Sickle cell anemia.
Transcellular shift out of cells.
Chemotherapy of lymphoma or leukemia, tumor lysis syndrome, hemolysis.
Acidosis.
Rhabdomyolysis, malignant hyperthermia.
Artifact: in vitro hemolysis.
Pseudohyperphosphatemia: hyperlipidemia, paraproteinemia, hyperbilirubinemia.

HYPERPHOSPHATEMIA IN CHILDREN[74]

ICD-10CM #		
	E83.30	Disorder of phosphorus metabolism, unspecified

CAUSES OF HYPERPHOSPHATEMIA

Impaired Renal Excretion of Phosphate
Renal insufficiency.
Hypoparathyroidism, pseudohypoparathyroidism.
Transient parathyroid resistance of infancy.
Acromegaly.
Tumoral calcinosis.
Hyperthyroidism.
Juvenile hypogonadism.
High ambient temperature.
Heparin.
Bisphosphonate etidronate.
Increased Phosphate Intake
Exogenous Loads
Phosphate salts: laxatives and enemas.
Vitamin D intoxication.
Blood transfusion.
White phosphorus burns.
Liposomal amphotericin B.
Fosphenytoin.
Parenteral phosphate.
Endogenous Loads
Crush injury.
Rhabdomyolysis.
Cytotoxic therapy of neoplasms: tumor lysis.
Hemolysis.
Malignant hyperthermia.
Catabolic states.
Lactic acidosis.
Fulminant hepatitis.
Transcellular Shift of Phosphate
Cellular shift in diabetes ketoacidosis.
Metabolic acidosis.
Respiratory acidosis.
Miscellaneous
Hyperostosis.

HYPERPIGMENTATION[14]

ICD-10CM #		
	L81.4	Other melanin hyperpigmentation

Addison disease.[21]
Arsenic ingestion.
ACTH- or MSH-producing tumors (e.g., oat cell carcinoma of the lung).
Drug induced (e.g., antimalarials, some cytotoxic agents).
Hemochromatosis ("bronze" diabetes).
Malabsorption syndrome (Whipple disease and celiac sprue).
Melanoma.
Melanotropic hormone injection.
Pheochromocytoma.
Porphyrias (porphyria cutanea tarda and variegate porphyria).
Pregnancy.
Progressive systemic sclerosis and related conditions.
PUVA therapy (psoralen administration) for psoriasis and vitiligo.

ACTH, Adrenocorticotropic hormone; *MSH,* melanocyte-stimulating hormone; *PUVA,* psoralen plus ultraviolet A.
[21] Accentuation on sun-exposed surfaces.

HYPERPROLACTINEMIA[59]

ICD-10CM #		
	E22.1	Hyperprolactinemia

PHYSIOLOGIC

Pregnancy.
Lactation.
Stress.
Sleep.
Coitus.
Exercise.

PATHOLOGIC

Hypothalamic-Pituitary Stalk Damage

Tumors: craniopharyngioma, suprasellar pituitary mass extension, meningioma, dysgerminoma, hypothalamic metastases.
Granulomas.
Infiltrations.
Rathke cyst.
Irradiation.
Trauma: pituitary stalk section, sellar surgery, head trauma.

Pituitary

Prolactinoma.
Acromegaly.
Macroadenoma (compressive).
Idiopathic.
Plurihormonal adenoma.
Lymphocytic hypophysitis or parasellar mass.
Macroprolactinemia.

Systemic Disorders

Chronic renal failure.
Polycystic ovary syndrome.
Cirrhosis.
Pseudocyesis.
Epileptic seizures.
Cranial irradiation.
Chest: neurogenic chest wall trauma, surgery, herpes zoster.

PHARMACOLOGIC

Neuropeptide

Thyrotropin-releasing hormone.

Drug-Induced Hypersecretion

Dopamine receptor blockers:
Phenothiazines: chlorpromazine, perphenazine.
Butyrophenones: haloperidol.
Thioxanthenes.
Metoclopramide.
Dopamine synthesis inhibitors:
α-Methyldopa.
Catecholamine depleters:
Reserpine.

Cholinergic Agonist

Physostigmine.

Antihypertensives

Labetalol.
Reserpine.
Verapamil.

H_2 Antihistamines

Cimetidine.
Ranitidine.

Estrogens

Oral contraceptives.
Oral contraceptive withdrawal.

Anticonvulsant

Phenytoin.

Anesthetics

Neuroleptics

Chlorpromazine.
Risperidone.
Promazine.
Promethazine.
Trifluoperazine.
Fluphenazine.
Butaperazine.
Perphenazine.
Thiethylperazine.
Thioridazine.
Haloperidol.
Pimozide.
Thiothixene.
Molindone.

Opiates and Opiate Antagonists

Heroin.
Methadone.
Apomorphine.
Morphine.

Antidepressants

Tricyclic antidepressants: chlorimipramine, amitriptyline.
Selective serotonin reuptake inhibitors: fluoxetine.

HYPERSPLENISM, ASSOCIATED CONDITIONS

ICD-10CM # D73.1 Hypersplenism

Cirrhosis.
Portal vein thrombosis.
Myeloproliferative diseases.
Lymphomas.
Leukemias.
Splenic vein thrombosis.
Autoimmune disease.
Sickle cell disease.
Thalassemias.
Gaucher disease.
Niemann-Pick disease.

HYPERTENSION, ADRENOCORTICAL CAUSES[59]

ICD-10CM # I15.8 Other secondary hypertension

LOW RENIN AND HIGH ALDOSTERONE

Primary Aldosteronism

Aldosterone-producing adenoma (APA)	35% of cases
Bilateral idiopathic hyperplasia (IHA)	60% of cases
Primary (unilateral) adrenal hyperplasia	2% of cases
Aldosterone-producing adrenocortical carcinoma	<1% of cases
Familial hyperaldosteronism (FH)	
Glucocorticoid-remediable aldosteronism (FH type I)	<1% of cases
FH type II (APA or IHA)—<2% of cases	
Ectopic aldosterone-producing adenoma or carcinoma	<0.1% of cases

LOW RENIN AND LOW ALDOSTERONE

Hyperdeoxycorticosteronism

Congenital adrenal hyperplasia.
11β-Hydroxylase deficiency.
17α-Hydroxylase deficiency.
Deoxycorticosterone-producing tumor.
Primary cortisol resistance.
Apparent mineralocorticoid excess (AME)/11β-HSD[22] deficiency.
Genetic: Type 1 AME.
Acquired: Licorice or carbenoxolone ingestion (type 1 AME), Cushing's syndrome (type 2 AME).

Cushing's Syndrome

Exogenous glucocorticoid administration—most common cause.
Endogenous.
ACTH[23]-dependent—85% of cases: Pituitary, ectopic.
ACTH-independent—15% of cases: Unilateral adrenal disease (adenoma or carcinoma), bilateral adrenal disease (massive macronodular hyperplasia [rare], primary pigmented nodular adrenal disease [rare]).

[22] *HSD,* hydroxysteroid dehydrogenase
[23] ACTH, corticotropina

HYPERTENSION, ENDOCRINE CAUSES[59]

ICD-10CM # I15.8 Other secondary hypertension

ADRENAL-DEPENDENT CAUSES

Pheochromocytoma.
Primary aldosteronism.
Hyperdeoxycorticosteronism:
Congenital adrenal hyperplasia: 11β-Hydroxylase deficiency, 17α-hydroxylase deficiency.
Deoxycorticosterone-producing tumor.
Primary cortisol resistance.
Cushing's syndrome.

AME/11β-HSD (HYDROXYSTEROID DEHYDROGENASE) DEFICIENCY

Genetic:
Type 1 apparent mineralocorticoid excess (AME).
Acquired:
Licorice or carbenoxolone ingestion (type 1 AME).
Cushing's syndrome (type 2 AME).

THYROID-DEPENDENT CAUSES

Hypothyroidism.
Hyperthyroidism.

PARATHYROID-DEPENDENT CAUSES

Hyperparathyroidism.

PITUITARY-DEPENDENT CAUSES

Acromegaly.
Cushing's syndrome.

HYPERTENSION, IN CHILDREN[7]

ICD-10CM # I10 Essential (primary) hypertension

PRIMARY

Essential hypertension.

SECONDARY

Renal

Glomerulonephritis.
Henoch-Schönlein purpura.
Pyelonephritis.
Obstruction of reflux.
Polycystic kidney disease.
Diabetic nephropathy.
Trauma.
Renal transplant or hemodialysis.
Tuberous sclerosis.
Systemic lupus nephritis.

Endocrine

Pheochromocytoma.
Cushing's syndrome.
Congenital adrenal hyperplasia.
Corticosteroid treatment.
Hyperthyroidism.
Neuroblastoma.
Ovarian tumor.

Cardiac

Congestive heart failure.
Coarctation of the aorta.

Vascular

Hemolytic-uremic syndrome.
Kawasaki syndrome.
Renal artery thrombosis or stenosis.

Neurologic

CNS tumor or infection.
CNS trauma or abuse.
Increased intracranial pressure.
Guillain-Barré syndrome.

Neoplastic

Neuroblastoma.
Wilms tumor.
Pheochromocytoma.
Adrenal carcinoma.

Drugs

Corticosteroids.
Cocaine.
Sympathomimetics.
Oral contraceptives.
Phencyclidine.
Beta-blocker or clonidine withdrawal.
Lead, mercury.

Others

Iatrogenic fluid overload.
Volume overload from end-stage renal disease.

HYPERTENSION, RESISTANT[74]

ICD-10CM # I10 Essential (primary) hypertension
ICD-10CM # I15 Secondary hypertension

CAUSES OF RESISTANT HYPERTENSION

Pseudoresistance.
- White coat hypertension or office elevations.
- Pseudohypertension in older patients.
- Use of small cuff on very obese arm.

Nonadherence to therapeutic regimen.
Volume overload.
Drug-related causes.
- Antihypertensive drug dosage too low.
- Wrong type of diuretic.
- Inappropriate combinations of antihypertensive drugs.

Drug actions and interactions.
- Sympathomimetics.
- Nasal decongestants.
- Appetite suppressants.
- Cocaine.
- Caffeine.
- Oral contraceptives.
- Adrenal steroids.
- Licorice (may be found in chewing tobacco).
- Cyclosporine, tacrolimus.
- Erythropoiesis-stimulating agents (ESAs) and Erythropoietin.
- Antidepressants.
- Nonsteroidal antiinflammatory drugs.

Concomitant conditions.
- Obesity.
- Sleep apnea.
- Ethanol intake >1 oz (30 ml)/day.
- Anxiety, hyperventilation.

Secondary causes of hypertension.
- Renovascular hypertension.
- Primary aldosteronism.
- Pheochromocytoma.
- Hypothyroidism.
- Hyperthyroidism.
- Hyperparathyroidism.
- Aortic coarctation.
- Renal disease.

HYPERTENSIVE CRISIS SYNDROMES[83]

ICD-10CM # I13 Hypertensive heart and renal disease
I15 Secondary hypertension

Malignant hypertension.
Nonmalignant hypertension with target organ disorders:
- Patient requiring emergency surgery with poorly controlled hypertension.
- Hyperviscosity syndrome.
- Postoperative patient.
- Renal transplant patient: acute rejection, transplant renal artery stenosis.
- Quadriplegic patient with autonomic hyperreflexia.
- Severe burns.
- Acute aortic dissection.
- Intracranial hemorrhage, ischemic stroke, or subarachnoid hemorrhage.
- Hypertensive encephalopathy.
- Myocardial ischemia/acute left ventricular failure.
- Preeclampsia/eclampsia.
- Antiphospholipid antibody syndrome.
- Acute renal failure:
  - Scleroderma renal crisis.
  - Chronic glomerulonephritis.
  - Reflux nephropathy.
  - Analgesic nephropathy.
  - Acute glomerulonephritis.
  - Radiation nephritis.
  - Ask-Upmark kidney.
  - Chronic lead intoxication.
- Renovascular hypertension:
  - Fibromuscular dysplasia.
  - Atherosclerosis.
- Endocrine hypertension:
  - Congenital adrenal hyperplasia.
  - Pheochromocytoma.
  - Oral contraceptives.
  - Aldosteronism.
  - Cushing's disease.
  - Systemic vasculitis.
  - Atheroembolic renal crisis.
- Drugs:
  - Oral contraceptives.
  - Nonsteroidal antiinflammatory agents.
  - Atropine.
  - Corticosteroids.
  - Sympathomimetics.
  - Cyclosporine.
  - Erythropoietin.
- Lead intoxication.
- Catecholamine excess states:
  - Pheochromocytoma.
  - MAO/tyramine interaction.
  - Antihypertensive withdrawal.
  - Cocaine intoxication, sympathomimetic overdose.

HYPERTRICHOSIS[17]

ICD-10CM #		
	L68.0	Hirsutism
	L68.1	Acquired hypertrichosis lanuginosa
	L68.3	Polytrichia
	L68.9	Hypertrichosis, unspecified
	Q84.1	Congenital morphological disturbances of hair, not elsewhere classified

DRUGS

Dilantin.
Streptomycin.
Hexachlorobenzene.
Penicillamine.
Diazoxide.
Minoxidil.
Cyclosporine.

SYSTEMIC ILLNESS

Hypothyroidism.
Anorexia nervosa.
Malnutrition.
Porphyria.
Dermatomyositis.

IDIOPATHIC

HYPERTROPHIC OSTEOARTHROPATHY

ICD-10CM # M89.40 Other hypertrophic osteoarthropathy, unspecified site

Idiopathic.
Pulmonary disease (e.g., pulmonary fibrosis, cystic fibrosis, sarcoidosis).
Bronchogenic carcinoma.
AIDS.
GI neoplasm (e.g., esophagus, colon).
Hepatic neoplasm, cirrhosis.
Cardiovascular diseases, aortic aneurysm, aortic prosthesis.
Congenital cyanotic heart disease, patent ductus arteriosus.

Pulmonary infections, bacterial endocarditis, amebic dysentery.
Inflammatory bowel disease.
Connective tissue diseases.
Lymphomas.
Thyroid acropachy.

HYPERVENTILATION, PERSISTENT[77]

ICD-10CM # R06.4 Hyperventilation

Fibrotic lung disease.
Metabolic acidosis (e.g., diabetes, uremia).
CNS disorders (midbrain and pontine lesions).
Hepatic coma.
Salicylate intoxication.
Fever.
Sepsis.
Psychogenic (e.g., anxiety).

HYPOCALCEMIA

ICD-10CM # E83.51 Hypocalcemia

Renal insufficiency: hypocalcemia caused by:
- Increased calcium deposits in bone and soft tissue secondary to increased serum phosphate level.
- Decreased production of 1,25-dihydroxyvitamin D.
- Excessive loss of 25-OHD (nephrotic syndrome).

Hypoalbuminemia: each decrease in serum albumin (g/L) will decrease serum calcium by 0.8 mg/dl but will not change free (ionized) calcium.
Vitamin D deficiency:
- Malabsorption (most common cause).
- Inadequate intake.
- Decreased production of 1,25-dihydroxyvitamin D (vitamin D–dependent rickets, renal failure).
- Decreased production of 25-OHD (parenchymal liver disease).
- Accelerated 25-OHD catabolism (phenytoin, phenobarbital).
- End-organ resistance to 1,25-dihydroxyvitamin D.

Hypomagnesemia: hypocalcemia caused by:
- Decreased PTH secretion.
- Inhibition of PTH effect on bone.

Pancreatitis, hyperphosphatemia, osteoblastic metastases: hypocalcemia is secondary to increased calcium deposits (bone, abdomen).
Pseudohypoparathyroidism (PHP): autosomal recessive disorder characterized by short stature, shortening of metacarpal bones, obesity, and mental retardation; the hypocalcemia is secondary to congenital end-organ resistance to PTH.
Idiopathic hypoparathyroidism, surgical removal of parathyroids (e.g., neck surgery).
"Hungry bones syndrome": rapid transfer of calcium from plasma into bones after removal of a parathyroid tumor.
Sepsis.
Massive blood transfusion (as a result of EDTA in blood).

HYPOCALCEMIA IN PEDIATRIC PATIENTS[74]

ICD-10CM # E83.51 Hypocalcemia

CAUSES OF HYPOCALCEMIA

Neonatal Hypocalcemia

Early neonatal hypocalcemia (first few days of life)
Maternal hyperparathyroidism.
Maternal diabetes mellitus.
Toxemia of pregnancy.
Sepsis.
SGA, IUGR, prematurity.
Asphyxia.
Transfusion (citrated blood products).
Congenital rubella.
Hypomagnesemia.
Respiratory or metabolic alkalosis.

Late neonatal hypocalcemia (fourth to tenth day of life)
Vitamin D deficiency: nutritional deficiency; VDR loss-of-function mutation; deficient 1α-hydroxylase activity.
Phosphate overload: excessive intake of evaporated/whole milk.
Nutritional calcium deficiency.
Hypomagnesemia.
Hypoalbuminemia (nephrotic syndrome).
Transfusion (citrated blood products).
Acute/chronic kidney insufficiency.
Diuretics (furosemide).
Organic acidemia.
Primary hypoparathyroidism: DiGeorge syndrome; familial hypoparathyroidism; pseudohypoparathyroidism; Kenny-Caffey syndrome; partial deletion of GCMB; retardation dysmorphism syndrome; Pearson mitochondriopathy; Kerns-Sayre mitochondriopathy; PTH gene defects; CaSR-activating gene mutation.

Hypocalcemia in Childhood

Parathyroid-related hypocalcemia
Primary hypoparathyroidism: DiGeorge syndrome; familial hypoparathyroidism; pseudohypoparathyroidism; Kenny-Caffey syndrome; Sanjad-Sakati syndrome; partial deletion of GCMB; retardation dysmorphism syndrome; Pearson mitochondropathy; Kerns-Sayre mitochondropathy; PTH gene defects; CaSR-activating gene mutation; Bartter syndrome type 5.
Secondary hypoparathyroidism: radiation; surgery; infiltration (hemochromatosis, thalassemia, Wilson's disease).
Autoimmune polyglandular syndrome type 1.

Vitamin D–related hypocalcemia
Nutritional vitamin D deficiency.
Defective 1α-hydroxylase activity.
VDR loss-of-function mutation.

Nutritional calcium deficiency

Hypomagnesemia

Hyperphosphatemia: kidney failure; rhabdomyolysis; tumor lysis

Hypoalbuminemia (nephrotic syndrome)

Medications: diuretics; chemotherapy; transfusion (citrated blood)

Organic acidemia (IVA, MMA, PPA)

CaSR, Calcium-sensing receptor; *GCMB,* glial cell missing homolog B (a parathyroid-specific transcription factor); *IUGR,* intrauterine growth retardation; *IVA,* isovaleric acidemia; *MMA,* methylmalonic acidemia; *PPA,* propionic acidemia; *PTH,* parathyroid hormone; *SGA,* small for gestational age; *VDR,* vitamin D receptor.

HYPOCAPNIA

ICD-10CM # R06.8 Hypoventilation

Hyperventilation.
Pneumonia, pneumonitis.
Fever, sepsis.
Medications (salicylates, beta-adrenergic agonists, progesterone, methylxanthines).
Pulmonary disease (asthma, interstitial fibrosis).
Pulmonary embolism.
Hepatic failure.
Metabolic acidosis.
High altitude.
CHF.
Pregnancy.
Pain.
CNS lesions.

HYPOGLYCEMIA

ICD-10CM #		
	E16.2	Hypoglycemia, unspecified
	E10.65	Type 1 diabetes mellitus with hyperglycemia
	E15	Nondiabetic hypoglycemic coma
	K91.2	Postsurgical malabsorption, not elsewhere classified
	E16.2	Hypoglycemia, unspecified

Oral hypoglycemics (therapeutic, factitious).
Exogenous insulin (therapeutic, factitious).
Postoperative gastric emptying (alimentary hyperinsulinism).
Severe malnutrition.
Liver disease.
Hypermetabolic state (sepsis).
Ketotic hypoglycemia.
Insulinoma.
Antibodies to endogenous insulin.
Hormone deficiencies (glucagon, growth hormone, hypoadrenalism).
Enzyme disorders in metabolism of glycogen, hexose, glycolysis, and Krebs cycle.
Idiopathic.

HYPOGLYCEMIA, IN INFANTS AND CHILDREN[51]

ICD-10CM # E16.2 Hypoglycemia, unspecified

CLASSIFICATION OF HYPOGLYCEMIA IN INFANTS AND CHILDREN

Neonatal Transient Hypoglycemia

Associated with Inadequate Substrate or Immature Enzyme Function in Otherwise Normal Neonates
Prematurity.

Small for gestational age.
Normal newborn.
Transient Neonatal Hyperinsulinism Also Present in
Infant of diabetic mother.
Discordant twin.
Birth asphyxia.
Infant of toxemic mother.

NEONATAL, INFANTILE, OR CHILDHOOD PERSISTENT HYPOGLYCEMIAS

Hormonal Disorders
Hyperinsulinism.
Recessive K_{ATP} channel HI.
Recessive HADH (hydroxyl acyl CoA dehydrogenase) mutation HI.
Recessive UCP2 (mitochondrial uncoupling protein 2) mutation HI.
Focal K_{ATP} channel HI.
Dominant K_{ATP} channel HI.
Dominant glucokinase HI.
Dominant glutamate dehydrogenase HI (hyperinsulinism/hyperammonemia syndrome).
Dominant mutation in HNF4A (hepatic nuclear factor 4 alpha) HI with MODY later in life.
Dominant mutation in SLC16A1 (the pyruvate transporter)-exercise-induced hypoglycemia.
Acquired islet adenoma.
Beckwith-Wiedemann syndrome.
Insulin administration (Munchausen syndrome by proxy).
Oral sulfonylurea drugs.
Congenital disorders of glycosylation.
Counter-Regulatory Hormone Deficiency
Panhypopituitarism.
Isolated growth hormone deficiency.
Addison disease.
Epinephrine deficiency.
Glycogenolysis and Gluconeogenesis Disorders
Glucose-6-phosphatase deficiency (GSD 1a).
Glucose-6-phosphate translocase deficiency (GSD 1b).
Amylo-1,6-glucosidase (debranching enzyme) deficiency (GSD 3).
Liver phosphorylase deficiency (GSD 6).
Phosphorylase kinase deficiency (GSD 9).
Glycogen synthetase deficiency (GSD 0).
Fructose-1,6-diphosphatase deficiency.
Pyruvate carboxylase deficiency.
Galactosemia.
Hereditary fructose intolerance.
Lipolysis Disorders
Fatty Acid Oxidation Disorders
Carnitine transporter deficiency (primary carnitine deficiency).
Carnitine palmitoyltransferase-1 deficiency.
Carnitine translocase deficiency.
Carnitine palmitoyltransferase-2 deficiency.
Secondary carnitine deficiencies.
Very long-, long-, medium-, short-chain acyl-CoA dehydrogenase deficiency.

OTHER ETIOLOGIES

Substrate-Limited
Ketotic hypoglycemia.
Poisoning: drugs.
Salicylates.
Alcohol.
Oral hypoglycemic agents.
Insulin.
Propranolol.
Pentamidine.
Quinine.
Disopyramide.
Ackee fruit (unripe): hypoglycin.
Vacor (rat poison).
Trimethoprim-sulfamethoxazole (with renal failure).
Liver Disease
Reye syndrome.
Hepatitis.
Cirrhosis.
Hepatoma.
Amino Acid and Organic Acid Disorders
Maple syrup urine disease.
Propionic acidemia.
Methylmalonic acidemia.
Tyrosinosis.
Glutaric aciduria.
3-Hydroxy-3-methylglutaric aciduria.
Systemic Disorders
Sepsis.
Carcinoma/sarcoma (secreting—insulin-like growth factor II).
Heart failure.
Malnutrition.
Malabsorption.
Anti-insulin receptor antibodies.
Anti-insulin antibodies.
Neonatal hyperviscosity.
Renal failure.
Diarrhea.
Burns.
Shock.
Postsurgical.
Pseudohypoglycemia (leukocytosis, polycythemia).
Excessive insulin therapy of insulin-dependent diabetes mellitus.
Factitious.
Nissen fundoplication (dumping syndrome).
Falciparum malaria.

GSD, Glycogen storage disease; *HI,* hyperinsulinemia; K_{ATP}, regulated potassium channel.

HYPOGONADISM

ICD-10CM #		
	E28.310	Symptomatic premature menopause
	E29.1	Testicular hypofunction
	E28.39	Other primary ovarian failure
	E23.6	Other disorders of pituitary gland

HYPERGONADOTROPIC HYPOGONADISM

Hormone resistance (androgen, LH insensitivity).
Gonadal defects (e.g., Klinefelter syndrome, myotonic dystrophy).
Drug-induced (e.g., spironolactone, cytotoxins).
Alcoholism, radiation-induced.
Mumps orchitis.
Anatomic defects, castration.

HYPOGONADOTROPIC HYPOGONADISM

Pituitary lesions (neoplasms, granulomas, infarction, hemochromatosis, vasculitis).
Drug-induced (e.g., glucocorticoids).
Hyperprolactinemia.
Genetic disorders (Laurence-Moon-Biedl syndrome, Prader-Willi).
Delayed puberty.
Other: chronic disease, nutritional deficiency, Kallmann syndrome, idiopathic isolated LH or FSH deficiency.

HYPOKALEMIA

ICD-10CM #	E87.6	Hypokalemia

Cellular shift (redistribution) and undetermined mechanisms.
Alkalosis (each 0.1 increase in pH decreases serum potassium by 0.4 to 0.6 mEq/L).
Insulin administration.
Vitamin B_{12} therapy for megaloblastic anemias, acute leukemias.
Hypokalemic periodic paralysis: rare familial disorder manifested by recurrent attacks of flaccid paralysis and hypokalemia.
Beta-adrenergic agonists (e.g., terbutaline), decongestants, bronchodilators, theophylline, caffeine.
Barium poisoning, toluene intoxication, verapamil intoxication, chloroquine intoxication.
Correction of digoxin intoxication with digoxin antibody fragments (Digibind).
Increased renal excretion.
Drugs:
- Diuretics, including carbonic anhydrase inhibitors (e.g., acetazolamide).
- Amphotericin B.
- High-dose sodium penicillin, nafcillin, ampicillin, or carbenicillin.
- Cisplatin.
- Aminoglycosides.
- Corticosteroids, mineralocorticoids.
- Foscarnet sodium.

RTA: distal (type 1) or proximal (type 2).
Diabetic ketoacidosis (DKA), ureteroenterostomy.
Magnesium deficiency.
Postobstruction diuresis, diuretic phase of ATN.
Osmotic diuresis (e.g., mannitol).
Bartter syndrome: hyperplasia of juxtaglomerular cells leading to increased renin and aldosterone, metabolic alkalosis, hypokalemia, muscle weakness, and tetany (seen in young adults).
Increased mineralocorticoid activity (primary or secondary aldosteronism), Cushing's syndrome.
Chronic metabolic alkalosis from loss of gastric fluid (increased renal potassium secretion).
GI loss:
- Vomiting, nasogastric suction.
- Diarrhea.
- Laxative abuse.
- Villous adenoma.
- Fistulas.
- Inadequate dietary intake (e.g., anorexia nervosa).

Cutaneous loss (excessive sweating).
High dietary sodium intake, excessive use of licorice.

HYPOKALEMIA IN PEDIATRIC PATIENTS[74]

ICD-10CM # E87.6 Hypokalemia

MOST RELEVANT CAUSES OF HYPOKALEMIA IN PEDIATRIC PATIENTS

Acute Redistribution of Potassium to the Intracellular Compartment

Metabolic alkalosis.
Insulin administration.
Hypokalemic periodic paralysis.

Prolonged Lack of Intake

Increased Renal Loss

Drugs: diuretics, antibiotics, aminoglycosides, penicillin, amphotericin B, capreomycin.
Metabolic acidosis and diabetic ketoacidosis.
Increased mineralocorticoid activity.
Cushing's syndrome.
Congenital adrenal hyperplasia.
Primary or secondary hyperaldosteronism.
Primary tubulopathies.
Bartter syndrome.
Gitelman syndrome.
Liddle syndrome.
Types 1 and 2 renal tubular acidosis.
Epilepsy, ataxia, sensorineural deafness, and tubulopathy (EAST) syndrome.
Fanconi syndrome.

Increased Gastrointestinal Loss

Vomiting (hypertrophic pyloric stenosis).
Diarrhea.

HYPOMAGNESEMIA

ICD-10CM # E83.40 Disorders of magnesium metabolism, unspecified
E83.42 Hypomagnesemia

GASTROINTESTINAL AND NUTRITIONAL

Defective GI absorption (malabsorption).
Inadequate dietary intake (e.g., alcoholics).
Parenteral therapy without magnesium.
Chronic diarrhea, villous adenoma, prolonged nasogastric suction, fistulas (small bowel, biliary).

EXCESSIVE RENAL LOSSES

Diuretics.
RTA.
Diuretic phase of ATN.
Endocrine disturbances (DKA, hyperaldosteronism, hyperthyroidism, hyperparathyroidism), SIADH, Bartter syndrome, hypercalciuria, hypokalemia.
Cisplatin, alcohol, cyclosporine, digoxin, pentamidine, mannitol, amphotericin B, foscarnet, methotrexate.
Antibiotics (gentamicin, ticarcillin, carbenicillin).
Redistribution: hypoalbuminemia, cirrhosis, administration of insulin and glucose, theophylline, epinephrine, acute pancreatitis, cardiopulmonary bypass.
Miscellaneous: sweating, burns, prolonged exercise, lactation, "hungry-bones" syndrome.

HYPOMAGNESEMIA IN PEDIATRIC PATIENTS[74]

ICD-10CM # E83.42 Hypomagnesemia

MAIN CAUSES OF HYPOMAGNESEMIA IN CHILDREN

Primary Inherited Disorders

Familial hypomagnesemia with hypercalciuria and nephrocalcinosis.
Hypomagnesemia with secondary hypocalcemia.
Autosomal dominant hypomagnesemia.
Isolated autosomal recessive hypomagnesemia with normocalciuria.
Activating mutations of calcium-sensing receptor.
Gitelman syndrome.
Bartter syndrome.

Secondary Disorders

Decreased GI absorption:
- Malabsorptive syndromes.
- Vomiting and diarrhea.

Increased urinary excretion:
- Extracellular volume expansion.
- Polyuric states: obstructive uropathy, kidney transplant.

Drugs:
- Diuretics.
- Calcineurin antagonists.
- Others: cisplatinum, aminoglycosides, amphotericin B.
- Metabolic acidosis.

Miscellaneous: "hungry bone," low-birth-weight newborn, infant of diabetic mother.

HYPONATREMIA

ICD-10CM # E87.1 Hypo-osmolality and hyponatremia

Renal loss from renal disease, diuretics.
GI loss (diarrhea, vomiting, suction).
Hypertonic hyponatremia (e.g., increased serum osmolality from hyperglycemia).
Transcutaneous loss (extensive burns, excessive sweating).
Fluid sequestration (e.g., ascites).
Osmotic diuresis (e.g., mannitol, glucose).
Dilutional (psychogenic polydipsia, iatrogenic).
Syndrome of inappropriate antidiuretic hormone secretion.
Edema with water and sodium retention.
Artifact (e.g., severe hyperlipidemia).
Laboratory error.
Adrenal insufficiency.

HYPOPHOSPHATEMIA

ICD-10CM # E83.30 Disorder of phosphorus metabolism, unspecified
E83.31 Familial hypophosphatemia

Decreased intake (prolonged starvation [alcoholics], hyperalimentation, or IV infusion without phosphate).
Malabsorption.
Phosphate-binding antacids.
Renal loss:
- RTA.
- Fanconi syndrome, vitamin D–resistant rickets.
- ATN (diuretic phase).
- Hyperparathyroidism (primary or secondary).
- Familial hypophosphatemia.
- Hypokalemia, hypomagnesemia.
- Acute volume expansion.
- Glycosuria, idiopathic hypercalciuria.
- Acetazolamide.

Transcellular shift into cells:
- Alcohol withdrawal.
- DKA (recovery phase).
- Glucose-insulin or catecholamine infusion.
- Anabolic steroids.
- Total parenteral nutrition.
- Theophylline overdose.
- Severe hyperthermia; recovery from hypothermia.
- "Hungry bones" syndrome.

HYPOPHOSPHATEMIA IN PEDIATRIC PATIENTS[74]

ICD-10CM # E83.30 Disorder of phosphorus metabolism, unspecified

CAUSES OF HYPOPHOSPHATEMIA

Decreased Phosphate Intake

Starvation, inadequate phosphate intake, chronic diarrhea, chronic alcoholism.
Total parenteral nutrition with insufficient phosphate content.

Increased Loss of Phosphate

Increased renal phosphate excretion:
- Primary hyperparathyroidism.
- Secondary hyperparathyroidism: vitamin D deficiency or resistance (including 1α-hydroxylase deficiency, VDR mutations, VDDR); imatinib.
- Excess FGF-23 or phosphatonins: X-linked hypophosphatemia, AD hypophosphatemic rickets, tumor-induced osteomalacia, epidermal nevus, McCune-Albright syndrome.
- Fanconi syndrome, cystinosis, Wilson's disease, Dent disease, Lowe syndrome, multiple myeloma, amyloidosis, heavy-metal toxicity, rewarming of hyperthermia, Na/Pi-IIa and Na/Pi-IIc mutation (HHRH).
- PTHrP-dependent hypercalcemia of malignancy.
- Hypomagnesemia.

Decreased intestinal absorption:
- Vitamin D deficiency or resistance (VDDR I and II).
- Malabsorption.

Increased intestinal loss:
- Phosphate binding antacids used in treating peptic ulcers.

Increased loss from other routes:
- Skin: severe burns.
- Vomiting.

Phosphate Shifting from Extracellular Compartment to Cells and Bones

Diabetic ketoacidosis.
Alcohol intoxication.
Acute respiratory alkalosis, salicylate intoxication, gram-negative sepsis, toxic shock syndrome, acute gout.
Refeeding syndromes from starvation, anorexia nervosa, hepatic failure: acute intravenous glucose, fructose, glycerol.
Rapid cellular proliferation: intensive erythropoietin therapy, GM-CSF therapy, leukemic blast crisis.
Recovery from hypothermia.
Heat stroke.
Post parathyroidectomy; "hungry bone" disease: osteoblastic metastases, antiresorptive treatment of severe Paget disease.
Catecholamine (albuterol, dopamine, terbutaline, epinephrine).
Thyrotoxic periodic paralysis.
Hypocalcemic periodic paralysis.

Miscellaneous

Hyperaldosteronism.
Oncogenic hypophosphatemia.
Post kidney transplantation.
Post partial hepatectomy.
High-dose corticosteroids, estrogens.
Medications: ifosfamide; toluene; calcitonin; bisphosphonate; tenofovir; paraquat, cisplatin; acetazolamide and other diuretics.
Post obstructive diuresis.

AD, Autosomal dominant; *FGF-23,* fibroblast growth factor 23; *GM-CSF,* granulocyte-macrophage colony-stimulating factor; *HHRH,* hereditary hypophosphatemic rickets with hypercalciuria; *Na/Pi-II,* type II sodium-dependent phosphate cotransporter; *PTHrP,* parathyroid hormone–related peptide; *VDR,* vitamin D receptor; *VDDR,* vitamin D–dependent rickets.

HYPOPIGMENTATION

ICD-10CM # L81.9 Disorder of pigmentation, unspecified

Vitiligo.
Tinea versicolor.
Atopic dermatitis.
Chemical leukoderma.
Idiopathic hypomelanosis.
Sarcoidosis.
SLE.
Scleroderma.
Oculocutaneous albinism.
Phenylketonuria.
Nevoid hypopigmentation.

HYPOTENSION, POSTURAL

ICD-10CM # I95.89 Other hypotension

Antihypertensive medications (especially a-blockers, diuretics, ACE inhibitors).
Volume depletion (hemorrhage, dehydration).
Impaired cardiac output (constrictive pericarditis, aortic stenosis).
Peripheral autonomic dysfunction (DM, Guillain-Barré).
Idiopathic orthostatic hypotension.
Central autonomic dysfunction (Shy-Drager syndrome).
Peripheral venous disease.
Adrenal insufficiency.

HYPOTHYROIDISM, CONGENITAL[51]

ICD-10CM # E03.0 Congenital hypothyroidism with diffuse goiter
E03.1 Congenital hypothyroidism without goiter

ETIOLOGIC CLASSIFICATION OF CONGENITAL HYPOTHYROIDISM

Primary Hypothyroidism

Defect of fetal thyroid development (dysgenesis):
- Aplasia.
- Hypoplasia.
- Ectopia.

Defect in thyroid hormone synthesis (dyshormonogenesis):
- Iodide transport defect: mutation in thyroglobulin gene.
- Thyroid organification, or coupling defect: mutation in thyroid peroxidase gene.
- Defects in H_2O_2 generation: mutations in DUOXA2 maturation factor or *DUOX2* gene.
- Thyroglobulin synthesis defect: mutation in thyroglobulin gene.
- Deiodination defect: mutation in *DEHAL1* gene.

TSH unresponsiveness:
- $G_s\alpha$ mutation (e.g., type 1A pseudohypothyroidism).
- Mutation in TSH receptor.

Defect in thyroid hormone transport: mutation in monocarboxylate transporter 8 *(MCT8)* gene.
Iodine deficiency (endemic goiter).
Maternal antibodies: thyrotropin receptor–blocking antibody (TRBAb, also termed *thyrotropin-binding inhibitor immunoglobulin*).
Maternal medications:
- Iodides, amiodarone.
- Propylthiouracil, methimazole.
- Radioiodine.

CENTRAL (HYPOPITUITARY) HYPOTHYROIDISM

PIT-1 mutations:
- Deficiency of thyroid-stimulating hormone (TSH).
- Deficiency of growth hormone.
- Deficiency of prolactin.

PROP-1 mutations:
- Deficiency of TSH.
- Deficiency of growth hormone.
- Deficiency of prolactin.
- Deficiency of luteinizing hormone.
- Deficiency of follicle-stimulating hormone.
- ±Deficiency of adrenocorticotropic hormone.

TSH deficiency: mutation in TSH β subunit gene (manifests as primary hypothyroidism with elevated TSH level).
Multiple pituitary deficiencies (e.g., craniopharyngioma).
Thyroid-releasing hormone (TRH) deficiency:
- Isolated.
- Multiple hypothalamic deficiencies (e.g., septooptic dysplasia).

TRH unresponsiveness.
Mutations in TRH receptor.

HYPOTONIA, INFANTILE, DIFFERENTIAL DIAGNOSIS[51]

ICD-10CM # H44.40 Unspecified hypotony of eye

Cerebral hypotonia.
- Benign congenital hypotonia.
- Chromosome disorders.
- Prader-Willi syndrome.
- Trisomy.
- Chronic nonprogressive encephalopathy.
- Cerebral malformation.
- Perinatal distress.
- Postnatal disorders.
- Peroxisomal disorders.
- Cerebrohepatorenal syndrome (Zellweger syndrome).
- Neonatal adrenoleukodystrophy.
- Other genetic defects.
- Familial dysautonomia.
- Oculocerebrorenal syndrome (Lowe syndrome).
- Other metabolic defects.
- Acid maltase deficiency (see "Metabolic Myopathies").
- Infantile G_{M_1} gangliosidosis.

Spinal cord disorders.
Spinal muscular atrophies.
- Acute infantile.
- Autosomal dominant.
- Autosomal recessive.
- Cytochrome-*c* oxidase deficiency.
- X-linked.

Chronic infantile.
- Autosomal dominant.
- Autosomal recessive.
- Congenital cervical spinal muscular atrophy.
- Infantile neuronal degeneration.
- Neurogenic arthrogryposis.

Polyneuropathies.
- Congenital hypomyelinating neuropathy.
- Giant axonal neuropathy.
- Hereditary motor-sensory neuropathies.

Disorders of neuromuscular transmission.
- Familial infantile myasthenia.
- Infantile botulism.
- Transitory myasthenia gravis.
- Fiber-type disproportion myopathies.
- Central core disease.
- Congenital fiber-type disproportion myopathy.
- Myotubular (centronuclear) myopathy.
- Acute.
- Chronic.
- Nemaline (rod) myopathy.
- Autosomal dominant.
- Autosomal recessive.

Metabolic myopathies.
- Acid maltase deficiency.
- Cytochrome-*c* oxidase deficiency.

Muscular dystrophies.
- Bethlem myopathy.
- Congenital dystrophinopathy.

Congenital muscular dystrophy.
Merosin deficiency, primary.
Merosin deficiency, secondary.
Merosin positive.
Congenital myotonic dystrophy.

HYPOTONIC POLYURIA[74]

ICD-10CM # Varies with specific diagnosis

CAUSES OF HYPOTONIC POLYURIA

Central (Neurogenic) Diabetes Insipidus

Congenital (congenital malformations, autosomal dominant, arginine vasopressin [AVP] neurophysin gene mutations).
Drug- or toxin-induced (ethanol, diphenylhydantoin, snake venom).
Granulomatous (histiocytosis, sarcoidosis).
Neoplastic (craniopharyngioma, germinoma, lymphoma, leukemia, meningioma, pituitary tumor; metastases).
Infectious (meningitis, tuberculosis, encephalitis).
Inflammatory, autoimmune (lymphocytic infundibuloneurohypophysitis).
Trauma (neurosurgery, deceleration injury).
Vascular (cerebral hemorrhage or infarction, brain death).
Idiopathic.

Osmoreceptor Dysfunction

Granulomatous (histiocytosis, sarcoidosis).
Neoplastic (craniopharyngioma, pinealoma, meningioma, metastases).
Vascular (anterior communicating artery aneurysm or ligation, intrahypothalamic hemorrhage).
Other (hydrocephalus, ventricular or suprasellar cyst, trauma, degenerative diseases).
Idiopathic.

Increased AVP Metabolism

Pregnancy

Nephrogenic Diabetes Insipidus

Congenital (X-linked recessive, AVP V2 receptor gene mutations, autosomal recessive or dominant, aquaporin-2 water channel gene mutations).
Drug-induced (demeclocycline, lithium, cisplatin, methoxyflurane).
Hypercalcemia.
Hypokalemia.
Infiltrating lesions (sarcoidosis, amyloidosis).
Vascular (sickle cell anemia).
Mechanical (polycystic kidney disease, bilateral ureteral obstruction).
Solute diuresis (glucose, mannitol, sodium, radiocontrast dyes).
Idiopathic.

Primary Polydipsia

Psychogenic (schizophrenia, obsessive-compulsive behaviors).
Dipsogenic (downward resetting of thirst threshold, idiopathic or similar lesions, as with central DI).

HYPOVOLEMIA[74]

ICD-10CM # Varies with specific diagnosis

CAUSES OF ABSOLUTE AND RELATIVE HYPOVOLEMIA

Absolute

Extrarenal

GI fluid loss.
Bleeding.
Skin fluid loss.
Respiratory fluid loss.
Extracorporeal ultrafiltration.

Renal

Diuretics.
Obstructive uropathy/postobstructive diuresis.
Hormone deficiency.
Hypoaldosteronism.
Adrenal insufficiency.
Na+ wasting tubulopathies.
Genetic.
Acquired tubulointerstitial disease.

Relative

Extrarenal

Edematous states.
Heart failure.
Cirrhosis.
Generalized vasodilation.
Sepsis.
Drugs.
Pregnancy.
Third-space loss.

Renal

Severe nephrotic syndrome.

HYPOVOLEMIC SHOCK, PEDIATRIC POPULATION[29]

ICD-10CM # R57.1 Hypovolemic shock
R57.8 Other shock

ETIOLOGIES OF HYPOVOLEMIC SHOCK

Whole blood loss.
Absolute loss: hemorrhage.
External bleeding.
Internal bleeding.
  GI.
  Intraabdominal (spleen, liver).
  Major vessel injury.
  Intracranial (in infants).
  Fractures.
Relative loss.
  Pharmacologic (barbiturates, vasodilators).
  Positive pressure ventilation.
  Spinal cord injury.
  Sepsis.
  Anaphylaxis.
Plasma loss.
Burns.
Capillary leak syndromes.
  Inflammation, sepsis.
  Anaphylaxis.
Protein-losing syndromes.
Fluid and electrolyte loss.
Vomiting and diarrhea.
Excessive diuretic use.
Endocrine:
  Adrenal insufficiency.
  Diabetes insipidus.
  Diabetes mellitus.

HYPOXEMIA AND HYPERCAPNIC RESPIRATORY FAILURE[65]

ICD-10CM # Varies with specific diagnosis

COMMON CAUSES OF HYPOXEMIC AND HYPERCAPNIC RESPIRATORY FAILURE

Brain

Bulbar poliomyelitis.
Central alveolar hypoventilation.
Cerebrovascular accident.
Cerebral malignancy.
Drug overdose (e.g., narcotic, sedative/hypnotic).
Elevated intracranial pressure.
Encephalitis and meningitis.
Pontine herniation.
Postoperative anesthetic depression.

Spinal Cord

Amyotrophic lateral sclerosis.
Cervical cordotomy.
Guillain-Barré syndrome.
Poliomyelitis.
Spinal cord trauma.

Neuromuscular System

Acute intermittent porphyria.
Botulism.
Cholinergic crisis.
Curariform drugs.
Electrolyte disorders (e.g., hypophosphatemia, hypomagnesemia).
Hypokalemic periodic paralysis.
Multiple sclerosis.
Myasthenia gravis.
Myxedema.
Neuromuscular blocking antibiotics (e.g., polymyxin, streptomycin).
Organophosphate insecticides.
Peripheral neuritis.
Polymyositis.
Respiratory muscle fatigue—critical illness polyneuropathy/polymyopathy.
Tetanus.

Upper Airway

Epiglottitis and laryngotracheitis.
Large tonsils and adenoids.
Obstructive sleep apnea.
Postintubation laryngeal edema.
Tracheal obstruction.
Vocal cord paralysis.

Thorax and Pleura

Chest wall burn with eschar formation.
Chest wall trauma—flail chest.
Kyphoscoliosis.
Massive abdominal distention.
Massive obesity.
Muscular dystrophy.
Large pleural effusion/pleural fibrosis.
Pneumothorax.
Rheumatoid spondylitis.
Thoracoplasty.

Cardiovascular System

Cardiogenic pulmonary edema.
Left ventricular failure.
Mitral stenosis.

Biventricular failure.
Fat embolism.
Snake bite.
Uremia.
Volume overload.
Pulmonary veno-occlusive disease.

Lower Airway and Alveoli

Acute respiratory distress syndrome (ARDS).
Aspiration.
Asthma.
Atelectasis.
Bronchiectasis.
Bronchiolitis.
Chronic obstructive pulmonary disease.
Cystic fibrosis.
Interstitial lung disease.
Massive bilateral pneumonia.
Near-drowning.
Pancreatitis.
Pulmonary contusion.
Radiation lung injury.
Sepsis.
Smoke inhalation.
Surgical resection of lung parenchym.

ILIAC FOSSA PAIN, LEFT SIDED[81]

ICD-10CM #	M25.5	Pain in joint

GASTROINTESTINAL CAUSES OF ACUTE LEFT ILIAC FOSSA PAIN

Nonspecific left iliac fossa pain including constipation.
Acute gastroenteritis.
Acute diverticulitis.
Colonic carcinoma.
Colonic ischemia.
Localized small bowel perforation.

ILIAC FOSSA PAIN, RIGHT SIDED[81]

ICD-10CM #	M25.5	Pain in joint

DIFFERENTIAL DIAGNOSIS OF RIGHT ILIAC FOSSA PAIN

Gastrointestinal Causes

Nonspecific right iliac fossa pain.
Acute appendicitis.
Mesenteric adenitis.
Terminal ileitis.
Acute inflammation of Meckel diverticulum.
Crohn's disease of the terminal ileum.
Cecal carcinoma.
Inflammatory cecal lesion (e.g., diverticulitis in a solitary cecal diverticulum).
Inflammatory lesion of the terminal ileum (e.g., foreign body perforation).

Non-Gastrointestinal Causes

Ruptured ovarian follicle (mittelschmerz).
Acute salpingitis (pelvic inflammatory disease).
Rupture/torsion or hemorrhage of an ovarian cyst.
Endometriosis.
Ectopic pregnancy.
Urinary tract infection.

IMMUNODEFICIENCY, CONGENITAL (PRIMARY)

ICD-10CM #	D80.0	Hereditary hyopgammaglobulinemia
	D80.1	Nonfamilial hypogammaglobulinemia
	D80.2	Selective deficiency of IgA
	D80.3	Selective deficiency of IgG
	D80.4	Selective deficiency of IgM

CONGENITAL (PRIMARY) CAUSES OF IMMUNODEFICIENCY

T-lymphocyte Deficiencies

DiGeorge syndrome (thymic aplasia with reduced CD4 and CD3 cells).
Purine nucleoside phosphorylase deficiency (marked T-cell depletion).

B-lymphocyte Deficiencies

Bruton X-linked agammaglobulinemia (absence of B cells, plasma cells, and antibody).
Selective immunoglobulin G (IgG) subclass deficiencies.
Selective IgA deficiency.
Hyper-IgM immunodeficiency (elevated IgM but reduced IgG and IgA).

Mixed T- and B-lymphocyte Deficiencies

Common variable immunodeficiency (leads to various B-cell activation or differentiation defects and gradual deterioration of T-cell number and function).
Severe combined immunodeficiency (severe reduction in IgG and absence of T cells).
Wiskott-Aldrich syndrome (decreased T-cell number and function, low IgM, occasionally low IgG).
Ataxia-telangiectasia (decreased T-cell number and function; IgA, IgE, IgG_2, and IgG_4 deficiency).

Disorders of Complement

C3 deficiency (congenital absence of C3 or consumption of C3 due to deficiency of C3b inactivator).

Phagocyte Defects

Chronic granulomatous disease (defect in nicotinamide adenine dinucleotide phosphate oxidase in phagocytic cells).
Chédiak-Higashi syndrome (impaired microbicidal activity of phagocytes).
Kostmann syndrome, Shwachman-Diamond syndrome, cyclic neutropenia (low neutrophil count).

IMPOTENCE[60]

ICD-10CM #	F52.21	Male erectile disorder
	F52.8	Other sexual dysfunction not due to a substance or known physiological condition
	N52.9	Male erectile dysfunction, unspecified

Psychogenic.
Endocrine: hyperprolactinemia, DM, Cushing's syndrome, hypothyroidism or hyperthyroidism, abnormality of hypothalamic-pituitary-testicular axis.
Vascular: arterial insufficiency, venous leakage, AV malformation, local trauma.
Medications.
Neurogenic: autonomic or sensory neuropathy, spinal cord trauma or tumor, CVA, multiple sclerosis, temporal lobe epilepsy.
Systemic illness: renal failure, COPD, cirrhosis of liver, myotonic dystrophy.
Peyronie's disease.
Prostatectomy.

INCONTINENCE, FECAL[81]

ICD-10CM #	R15.9	Full incontinence of feces

NORMAL SPHINCTER

Diarrhea.
Anorectal conditions:
- Rectal carcinoma.
- Inflammatory bowel disease.
- Hemorrhoids.
- Mucosal prolapse.
- Fissure-in-ano.
- Abnormal rectal sensation.

ABNORMAL SPHINCTER

Congenital abnormalities.
Anal sepsis.
Neurologic conditions.
Rectal prolapse.
Sphincter trauma.
Neurogenic (idiopathic) incontinence.

INFECTIOUS DIARRHEA IN TROPICS[26]

ICD-10CM #	R19.7	Diarrhea, unspecified

CAUSES OF INFECTIOUS DIARRHEA IN THE TROPICS

Bacteria

- *Aeromonas hydrophila.*
- *Arcobacter butzleri.*
- *Bacteroides fragilis,* enterotoxigenic.
- *Campylobacter jejuni.*
- *Escherichia coli:* enterotoxigenic, enteroaggregative, enteroinvasive, enterohemorrhagic.
- *Laribacter hongkongensis.*
- *Plesiomonas shigelloides.*
- *Salmonella,* non-typhoidal.
- *Shigella species: S. dysenteriae, S. flexneri, S. sonnei, S. boydii.*
- *Vibrio cholerae* 01, 0139, non-01 non-0139.
- *Vibrio parahaemolyticus.*
- *Yersinia enterocolitica.*

Helminths

- *Paracapillaria philippinensis.*
- *Fasciolopsis buski.*
- Heterophyiasis *(Metagonimus yokogawai, Haplorchis taichui).*
- *Schistosoma mansoni.*
- *Strongyloides stercoralis.*

Protozoa

- *Blastocystis hominis.*
- *Cryptosporidium parvum.*
- *Cyclospora cayetanensis.*
- *Encephalitozoon intestinalis.*
- *Enterocytozoon bieneusi.*

Giardia lamblia.
Isospora belli.
Leishmania donovani.

Viruses

Astroviruses.
Caliciviruses: norovirus and sapovirus.
Enteric adenoviruses.
HIV.
Picornaviruses.
Rotavirus.

INFERTILITY, FEMALE[32]

ICD-10CM #	N97.9	Female infertility, unspecified

FALLOPIAN TUBE PATHOLOGY

PID or puerperal infection.
Congenital anomalies.
Endometriosis.
Secondary to past peritonitis of nongenital origin.
Amenorrhea and anovulation.
Minor anovulatory disturbances.

CERVICAL AND UTERINE FACTORS

Leiomyomas and polyps.
Uterine anomalies.
Intrauterine synechiae (Asherman syndrome).
Destroyed endocervical glands (postsurgery or postinfection).

VAGINAL FACTORS

Congenital absence of vagina.
Imperforate hymen.
Vaginismus.
Vaginitis.

IMMUNOLOGIC FACTORS

Sperm-immobilizing antibodies.
Sperm-agglutinating antibodies.

NUTRITIONAL AND METABOLIC FACTORS

Thyroid disorders.
DM.
Severe nutritional disturbances.

INFERTILITY, MALE[32]

ICD-10CM #	N46.9	Male infertility, unspecified

DECREASED PRODUCTION OF SPERMATOZOA

Varicocele.
Testicular failure.
Endocrine disorders.
Cryptorchidism.
Stress, smoking, caffeine, nicotine, recreational drugs.

DUCTAL OBSTRUCTION

Epididymal (postinfection).
Congenital absence of vas deferens.
Ejaculatory duct (postinfection).
Postvasectomy.

INABILITY TO DELIVER SPERM INTO VAGINA

Ejaculatory disturbances.
Hypospadias.
Sexual problems (i.e., impotence), medical or psychological.

ABNORMAL SEMEN

Infection.
Abnormal volume.
Abnormal viscosity.
Abnormal sperm motion.

IMMUNOLOGIC FACTORS

Sperm-immobilizing antibodies.
Sperm-agglutinating antibodies.

INSOMNIA[71]

ICD-10CM #	780.51	Insomnia with sleep apnea
	G47.00	Insomnia, unspecified
	F51.01	Primary insomnia
	F51.03	Paradoxical insomnia
	F51.09	Other insomnia not due to a substance or known physiological condition

Anxiety disorder, psychophysiologic insomnia.
Depression.
Drugs (e.g., caffeine, amphetamines, cocaine), hypnotic-dependent sleep disorder.
Pain, fibromyalgia.
Inadequate sleep hygiene.
Restless leg syndrome.
Obstructive sleep apnea.
Sleep bruxism.
Medical illness (e.g., GERD, sleep-related asthma, parkinsonism and movement disorders).
Narcolepsy.
Other: periodic leg movement of sleep, central sleep apnea, REM behavioral disorder.

INTESTINAL PSEUDOOBSTRUCTION[77]

ICD-10CM #	K56.0	Paralytic ileus
	K56.7	Ileus, unspecified
	K59.9	Functional intestinal disorder, unspecified

"PRIMARY" (IDIOPATHIC INTESTINAL PSEUDOOBSTRUCTION)

Hollow visceral myopathy:
Familial.
Sporadic.
Neuropathic:
Abnormal myenteric plexus.
Normal myenteric plexus.

SECONDARY

Scleroderma.
Myxedema.
Amyloidosis.
Muscular dystrophy.
Hypokalemia.
Chronic renal failure.
DM.
Drug toxicity caused by:
Anticholinergics.
Opiate narcotics.
Ogilvie syndrome.

INTRAABDOMINAL MASS LESION, NEONATAL[36]

ICD-10CM #	R19.00	Intraabdominal and pelvic swelling, mass and lump, unspecified site

CAUSES OF A NEONATAL INTRA-ABDOMINAL MASS LESION

Complicated meconium ileus.
Dilated bowel proximal to an obstruction.
Mesenteric or duplication cyst.
Abscess.
GU causes:
Hydronephrosis.
Renal cystic disease.
Mesoblastic nephroma.
Wilms tumor.
Adrenal hemorrhage.
Neuroblastoma.
Retroperitoneal teratoma.
Ovarian cyst.
Hydrometrocolpos.
Hemangioendothelioma.
Hepatoblastoma.
Choledochal, hepatic, or splenic cysts.

INTRACEREBRAL HEMORRHAGE, NONHYPERTENSIVE CAUSES

ICD-10CM #	I61.9	Nontraumatic intracerebral hemorrhage, unspecified

Trauma.
Anticoagulation.
Intracranial tumors.
Vascular malformations.
Bleeding disorders.
Vasculitides (e.g., polyarteritis nodosa, granulomatous angiitis).
Cocaine and other sympathomimetic agents.
Cerebral amyloid angiopathy.

INTRACRANIAL LESION

ICD-10CM #	G93.89	Other specified disorders of brain

Tumor (primary or metastatic).
Abscess.
Stroke.
Intracranial hemorrhage.
Angioma.
Multiple sclerosis (initial single lesion).
Granuloma.
Herpes encephalitis.
Artifact.

INTRAOCULAR NEOPLASM

ICD-10CM #	C69.9	Malignant disorder of eye, unspecified

MALIGNANT
Retinoblastoma.
Melanoma.
Reticulum cell sarcoma.
Metastatic tumor.

BENIGN
Melanocytic nevus.
Hemangioma.
Reactive lymphoid hyperplasia.

IRON METABOLISM DISORDERS[5]

ICD-10CM # E83.10 Disorder of iron metabolism, unspecified

IRON DEFICIENCY
Deficient Iron Intake
Diet of low bioavailability.
Increased physiological requirements due to rapid growth in early childhood and in adolescence.
Blood loss.
Physiological (e.g., menstruation).
Pathological (e.g., GI).
Malabsorption of Iron
Reduced or absent gastric acid secretion (e.g., after partial or total gastrectomy or with atrophic gastritis).
Reduced duodenal absorption (e.g., in coeliac disease).
Bypass of stomach and duodenum (bariatric surgery).
Rare, inherited iron-refractory iron-deficiency anemia (e.g., deficiency of TMPRSS6 [transmembrane protease, serine 6], also known as matriptase-2).
Redistribution of Iron
Macrophage iron accumulation in reticuloendothelial system in inflammatory, infectious, or malignant diseases (anemia of chronic disease, also known as anemia of inflammation).
Macrophage iron accumulation within the lungs in idiopathic pulmonary hemosiderosis.
Iron Overload
Due to Increased Iron Absorption
Hereditary hemochromatosis—commonly (among Northern Europeans) homozygosity for *HFE* C282Y but sometimes involving non-C282Y *HFE* or other genes (*HAMP, HFE2* [encoding hemojuvelin], *TFR2, SLC40A1*).
Substantial ineffective erythropoiesis (e.g., β thalassemia intermedia and major, some types of sideroblastic anemia, congenital dyserythropoietic anemia).
Sub-Saharan iron overload ("Bantu siderosis")—only in combination with increased dietary iron.
Other rare inherited disorders (e.g., congenital atransferrinemia, DMT1 deficiency, aceruloplasminemia).
Inappropriate iron therapy (rare).

DUE TO MULTIPLE BLOOD TRANSFUSIONS FOR REFRACTORY ANEMIAS OR FOR OTHER REASONS
Thalassemia major.
Aplastic anemia.
Myelodysplastic syndromes.
Sickle cell disease (when regularly transfused).

IRON OVERLOAD[43]

ICD-10CM # E83.10 Disorder of iron metabolism, unspecified

HEREDITARY IRON OVERLOAD
Hereditary hemochromatosis:
HFE-associated (type 1).
Non–HFE-associated:
Transferrin receptor 2–associated (type 3).
Juvenile hemochromatosis (type 2):
Hemojuvelin-associated (type 2A).
Hepcidin-associated (type 2B).
Autosomal dominant hemochromatosis:
Ferroportin-associated (type 4).
DMT1-associated hemochromatosis.
Atransferrinemia.
Aceruloplasminemia.

ACQUIRED IRON OVERLOAD
Iron-loading anemias (refractory anemias with hypercellular erythroid marrow).
Chronic liver disease.
Porphyria cutanea tarda.
Insulin resistance–associated hepatic iron overload.
African dietary iron overload.[24]
Medical iron ingestion.
Parenteral iron overload:
Transfusional iron overload.
Inadvertent iron overload from therapeutic injections.

PERINATAL IRON OVERLOAD
Neonatal hemochromatosis.
Trichohepatoenteric syndrome.
Cerebrohepatorenal syndrome.
GRACILE[25] (Fellman) syndrome.

FOCAL SEQUESTRATION OF IRON
Idiopathic pulmonary hemosiderosis.
Renal hemosiderosis.
Associated with neurologic abnormalities:
Pantothenate kinase–associated neurodegeneration (formerly called Hallervorden-Spatz syndrome).
Neuroferritinopathy.
Friedreich ataxia.

[24] May have a genetic component.
[25] *GRACILE,* Growth retardation, aminoaciduria, cholestasis, iron overload, lactic acidosis, and early death.

ISCHEMIA, UPPER EXTREMITY, CAUSES[15]

ICD-10CM # S45.809A Unspecified injury of other specified blood vessels at shoulder and upper arm level, unspecified arm, initial encounter

VASOSPASM
Raynaud's disease.
Medication induced: vasopressors, b-blockers.
Ergot poisoning.

INTRINSIC ARTERIAL DISEASE
Atherosclerosis.
Radiation arteritis.
Azotemic arteriopathy.
Spontaneous dissection.
Fibromuscular dysplasia.

INFLAMMATORY DISEASES
Connective tissue disorders.
Buerger disease.
Takayasu arteritis.
Temporal (giant cell) arteritis.
Hypersensitivity angiitis.

NONINFLAMMATORY MEDICAL DISEASE
Thrombophilic states.
Myeloproliferative disorders.
Cold injury.
Hepatitis-associated vasculitis.
Cryoglobulinemia.
Vinyl chloride exposure.

EMBOLISM
Cardiac (most common).
Proximal aneurysm.
Arterial thoracic outlet syndrome.
Atheroembolism.
Paradoxic embolus (with accompanying septal defect).

TRAUMA
Iatrogenic.
Blunt arterial injury.
Penetrating arterial injury.
Hypothenar hammer syndrome.
Vibration.

ISCHEMIC BOWEL DISEASE[1]

ICD-10CM # K55.1 Vascular disorder of intestine
I99 Other and unspecified disorders of circulatory system

Abdominal aortic aneurysm: rupture or expansion.
Perforated ulcer or viscus.
Ruptured ectopic pregnancy (woman of childbearing age).
Incarcerated or strangulated hernia.
Septic shock.
Intussusception.
Volvulus.
Salpingitis or tuboovarian abscess.
Torsion of the ovary or testicle.
Appendicitis.
Pelvic mass or torsion.
Pancreatitis.
Diverticulitis.
Ruptured ovarian cyst.
Renal colic.
Biliary colic.
Also consider atypical manifestations of:
Inferior wall myocardial infarction.
Pulmonary embolism.

Pneumonia.
Diabetic ketoacidosis.
Acute glaucoma.
Differential diagnoses are listed in order of urgency.

ISCHEMIC COLITIS, NONOCCLUSIVE[47]

ICD-10CM #		
	K55.1	Chronic vascular disorders of intestine

ACUTE DIMINUTION OF COLONIC INTRAMURAL BLOOD FLOW

Small Vessel Obstruction

Collagen-vascular disease.
Vasculitis, diabetes.
Oral contraceptives.

Nonocclusive Hypoperfusion

Hemorrhage.
CHF, MI, arrhythmias.
Sepsis.
Vasoconstricting agents: vasopressin, ergot.
Increased viscosity: polycythemia, sickle cell disease, thrombocytosis.

INCREASED DEMAND ON MARGINAL BLOOD FLOW

Increased Motility

Mass lesion, stricture.
Constipation.

Increased Intraluminal Pressure

Bowel obstruction.
Colonoscopy.
Barium enema.

ISCHEMIC NECROSIS OF CARTILAGE AND BONE[32]

ICD-10CM #		
	M89.9	Disorder of bone, unspecified
	M94.9	Disorder of cartilage, unspecified

ENDOCRINE/METABOLIC

Ethanol abuse.
Glucocorticoid therapy.
Cushing's disease.
DM.
Hyperuricemia.
Osteomalacia.
Hyperlipidemia.

STORAGE DISEASES (E.G., GAUCHER DISEASE)

Hemoglobinopathies (e.g., sickle cell disease).
Trauma (e.g., dislocation, fracture).
HIV infection.
Dysbaric conditions (e.g., caisson disease).
Collagen-vascular disorders.
Irradiation.
Pancreatitis.
Organ transplantation.
Hemodialysis.
Burns.
Intravascular coagulation.
Idiopathic, familial.

JAUNDICE

ICD-10CM #		
	R17	Unspecified jaundice
	K83.8	Other specified diseases of biliary tract
	E80.7	Disorder of bilirubin metabolism, unspecified

PREDOMINANCE OF DIRECT (CONJUGATED) BILIRUBIN

Extrahepatic obstruction.
Common duct abnormalities: calculi, neoplasm, stricture, cyst, sclerosing cholangitis.
Metastatic carcinoma.
Pancreatic carcinoma, pseudocyst.
Ampullary carcinoma.
Hepatocellular disease: hepatitis, cirrhosis.
Drugs: estrogens, phenothiazines, captopril, methyltestosterone, labetalol.
Cholestatic jaundice of pregnancy.
Hereditary disorders: Dubin-Johnson syndrome, Rotor syndrome.
Recurrent benign intrahepatic cholestasis.

PREDOMINANCE OF INDIRECT (UNCONJUGATED) BILIRUBIN

Hemolysis: hereditary and acquired hemolytic anemias.
Inefficient marrow production.
Impaired hepatic conjugation: chloramphenicol.
Neonatal jaundice.
Hereditary disorders: Gilbert syndrome, Crigler-Najjar syndrome.

JAUNDICE, CLASSIFICATION[3]

ICD-10CM #		
	R17	Unspecified jaundice

PREHEPATIC (PREDOMINANTLY UNCONJUGATED HYPERBILIRUBINEMIA)

Overproduction

Hemolysis (e.g., spherocytosis, sickle cell disease, hemolysis of the newborn, autoimmune disorders).
Ineffective erythropoiesis (e.g., megaloblastic anemias).
Hematomas.
Pulmonary emboli.

HEPATIC (UNCONJUGATED HYPERBILIRUBINEMIA)

Decreased Hepatic Uptake

Gilbert syndrome.
Drugs (e.g., rifampin, radiographic contrast agents).
Neonatal jaundice.
Posthepatitis.
Decreased cystolic binding proteins (e.g., newborn or premature infants).
Portacaval shunt.
Prolonged fasting.

Decreased Conjugation Due to Limited Glucuronyl Transferase Activity

Gilbert disease.
Crigler-Najjar syndrome, types I and II.
Neonatal jaundice.
Breast-milk jaundice.
Chronic persistent hepatitis.
Wilson's disease.
Noncirrhotic portal fibrosis.
Drug inhibition (e.g., chloramphenicol).

PREDOMINANTLY CONJUGATED HYPERBILIRUBINEMIA

Impaired Hepatic Excretion

Familial disorders (Dubin-Johnson syndrome, Rotor syndrome, benign recurrent cholestasis, cholestasis of pregnancy).
Hepatocellular infiltrative disorders.
Liver metastasis.
Liver cirrhosis.
Hepatitis (viral, bacterial, parasitic, autoimmune, ethanol, and drug-induced).
Drug-induced cholestasis (especially chlorpromazine, erythromycin estolate, isoniazid, halothane).
Primary biliary cirrhosis.
Primary sclerosing cholangitis.
Pericholangitis.
Congestive heart failure.
Shock.
Toxemia of pregnancy.
Sarcoidosis.
Hepatic trauma.
Amyloidosis.
Autoimmune cholangiopathy.
Vanishing bile duct syndrome.
Sepsis.
Postoperative complications.

EXTRAHEPATIC

Extrahepatic Biliary Obstruction

Gallstones, choledocholithiasis.
Cholecystitis.
Tumors of the head of the pancreas (adenocarcinoma, mucinous duct ectasia, neuroendocrine tumors, metastasis).
Tumors of bile ducts (cholangiocarcinoma, Klatskin tumor: cholangiocarcinoma at the bifurcation).
Gallbladder cancer.
Tumors of the ampulla of Vater (adenoma, adenocarcinoma).
Tumors of the duodenum (adenocarcinoma, lymphoma).
Hemobilia (blood in the biliary tree).
Biliary strictures (postcholecystectomy, post-liver transplantation, primary sclerosing cholangitis).
Congential disorders (biliary atresia, idiopathic dilation of common bile duct, cystic fibrosis).
Metastasis to the hepatic hilum.
Primary bile duct lymphoma.
Cholangiopathy of acquired immunodeficiency syndrome.
Choledochal cysts.
Infectious cholangiopathy *(Clonorchis sinensis, Ascaris lumbricoides, Fasciola hepatica).*
Chronic pancreatitis (fibrosis of the head of the pancreas).

JAUNDICE, NEONATAL[3]

ICD-10CM #		
	P59.9	Neonatal jaundice, unspecified

PREHEPATIC

Hereditary spherocytosis.
Nonspherocytic hemolytic anemia (glucose-6-phosphate dehydrogenase deficiency, α-thalassemia, vitamin K_3–induced hemolysis, pyruvate kinase deficiency).

HEPATIC

Crigler-Najjar syndrome, types I and II.
α_1-Antitrypsin deficiency.
Sepsis.
Drug-induced.
Hypothyroidism.
Breast-milk jaundice.
Fetomaternal blood group incompatibility (Rhesus, Landsteiner groups ABO).

POSTHEPATIC

Extrahepatic biliary obstruction.
Biliary atresia.
Bile duct paucity.
Alagille syndrome.

JOINT AND PERIARTICULAR PAIN, ACUTE[27]

ICD-10CM #	M25.50	Joint pain

COMMON ACUTE MONOARTHRITIS

Septic arthritis (nongonococcal, gonococcal).
Crystal arthritis (gout, pseudogout).
Reactive arthritides.
Lyme disease.
Plant thorn synovitis.
Other infections (mycobacterial, viral, soft tissue).

TRAUMA OR INTERNAL DERANGEMENT

Loose bodies.
Stress fractures.
Ischemic necrosis.
Hemarthrosis.

ACUTE MONOARTHRITIS OR POLYARTHRITIS

Psoriatic arthritis.
Enteropathic arthritis.
Rheumatoid arthritis/palindromic rheumatism.
Juvenile inflammatory arthritides.

MONOARTHROPATHIES FROM NONINFLAMMATORY DISEASE

Osteoarthritis.
Charcot joints.
Storage diseases (hemochromatosis, ochronosis).

SYNOVIAL DISEASES

Pigmented villonodular synovitis.
Lipoma arborescens.
Synovial osteochondromatosis.
Reflex sympathetic dystrophy.
Sarcoidosis.
Amyloid.

ACUTE MONOARTHRITIS OF SYSTEMIC DISEASE

Systemic lupus erythematosus.
Vasculitides (antineutrophil cytoplasmic antibody positive and negative).
Henoch-Schönlein purpura.
Behçet's disease.
Bacterial endocarditis.
Familial Mediterranean fever.
Relapsing polychondritis.

SOFT TISSUE LESIONS

Bone Diseases

Paget disease.
Osteomyelitis (Brodie abscess).
Osteogenic/osteoid tumors.
Metastatic disease.
Pulmonary hypertrophic osteoarthropathy.

This table shows the causes of inflammation in any one joint (monoarthritis) and pain around the joint that presents without inflammation (monoarthropathy).

JOINT PAIN, ANTERIOR HIP, MEDIAL THIGH, KNEE[61]

ICD-10CM #	M25.50	Pain in unspecified joint
	M25.559	Pain in unspecified hip
	M25.569	Pain in unspecified knee

ACUTE

Acute rheumatic fever.
Adductor muscle strain.
Avascular necrosis.
Crystal arthritis.
Femoral artery (pseudo) aneurysm.
Fracture (femoral neck or intertrochanteric).
Hemarthrosis.
Hernia.
Herpes zoster.
Iliopectineal bursitis.
Iliopsoas tendinitis.
Inguinal lymphadenitis.
Osteomalacia.
Painful transient osteoporosis of hip.
Septic arthritis.

SUBACUTE AND CHRONIC

Adductory muscle strain.
Amyloidosis.
Acute rheumatic fever.
Femoral artery aneurysm.
Hernia (inguinal or femoral).
Iliopectineal bursitis.
Iliopsoas tendinitis.
Inguinal lymphadenopathy.
Osteochondromatosis.
Osteomyelitis.
Osteitis deformans (Paget disease).
Osteomalacia (pseudofracture).
Postherpetic neuralgia.
Sterile synovitis (e.g., RA, psoriatic, SLE).

JOINT PAIN, HIP, LATERAL THIGH[61]

ICD-10CM #	S79.919A	Unspecified injury of unspecified hip, initial encounter
	S79.929A	Unspecified injury of unspecified thigh, initial encounter
	M25.9	Joint disorder, unspecified

ACUTE

Herpes zoster.
Iliotibial tendinitis.
Impacted fracture of femoral neck.
Lateral femoral cutaneous neuropathy (meralgia paresthetica).
Radiculopathy: L4-5.
Trochanteric avulsion fracture (greater trochanter).
Trochanteric bursitis.
Trochanteric fracture.

SUBACUTE AND CHRONIC

Lateral femoral cutaneous neuropathy (meralgia paresthetica).
Osteomyelitis.
Postherpetic neuralgia.
Radiculopathy: L4-5.
Tumors.

JOINT PAIN, POLYARTICULAR

ICD-10CM #	M25.50	Pain in unspecified joint

Osteoarthritis.
RA.
Fibromyalgia.
Viral syndrome (e.g., human parvovirus B19 infection).
SLE.
Psoriatic arthritis.
Ankylosing spondylitis.

JOINT PAIN, POSTERIOR HIPS, THIGH, BUTTOCKS[61]

ICD-10CM #	M25.50	Pain in unspecified joint
	M25.559	Pain in unspecified hip
	M25.569	Pain in unspecified knee

ACUTE

Gluteal muscle strain.
Herpes zoster.
Ischial bursitis.
Ischial or sacral fracture.
Osteomalacia (pseudofracture).
Sciatic neuropathy.
Radiculopathy: L5-S1.

SUBACUTE AND CHRONIC

Gluteal muscle strain.
Ischial bursitis.
Lumbar spinal stenosis.
Osteoarthritis of hip.
Osteitis deformans (Paget disease).
Osteomyelitis.
Osteochondromatosis.
Osteomalacia (pseudofracture).
Postherpetic neuralgia.
Radiculopathy: L5-S1.
Tumors.

JOINT SWELLING

ICD-10CM #	M25.40	Effusion, unspecified joint

Trauma.
Osteoarthritis.
Gout.
Pyogenic arthritis.
Pseudogout.
RA.
Viral syndrome.

JUGULAR VENOUS DISTENTION

ICD-10CM # I99.8 Other disorder of circulatory system

Right-sided heart failure.
Cardiac tamponade.
Constrictive pericarditis.
Goiter.
Tension pneumothorax.
Pulmonary hypertension.
Cardiomyopathy (restrictive).
Superior vena cava syndrome.
Valsalva maneuver.
Right atrial myxoma.
COPD.

KERATITIS, NONINFECTIOUS

ICD-10CM # H16.9 Unspecified keratitis

Collagen vascular disease.
Atopic keratoconjunctivitis.
Chemical injury.
Thermal injury.
Ectropion/entropion.
Lid defects.
Exophthalmos.
Keratoconjunctivitis sicca.
Erythema multiforme.
Mucous membrane pemphigoid.
DM (delayed epithelial healing).
Neuroparalytic (cranial nerve VII).
Neurotrophic (diabetes, cranial nerve V).

KIDNEY CYSTIC DISEASE[85]

ICD-10CM # Varies with specific diagnosis

CYSTIC DISEASES OF THE KIDNEY

Inheritable

Autosomal recessive (infantile) polycystic kidney disease.
Autosomal dominant (adult) polycystic kidney disease.
Juvenile nephronophthisis and medullary cystic disease complex.
Juvenile nephronophthisis (autosomal recessive).
Medullary cystic disease (autosomal dominant).
Congenital nephrosis (familial nephrotic syndrome) (autosomal recessive).
Familial hypoplastic glomerulocystic disease (autosomal dominant).
Multiple malformation syndromes with renal cysts (e.g., tuberous sclerosis, von Hippel-Lindau disease).

Nonheritable

Multicystic kidney (multicystic dysplastic kidney).
Benign multilocular cyst (cystic nephroma).
Simple cysts.
Medullary sponge kidney.
Sporadic glomerulocystic kidney disease.
Acquired renal cystic disease.
Calyceal diverticulum (pyelogenic cyst).

KIDNEY ENLARGEMENT, UNILATERAL[81]

ICD-10CM # N13.30 Unspecified hydronephrosis

Hydronephrosis (may be bilateral).
Polycystic kidney (may be bilateral).
Simple cyst of kidney.
Renal cell carcinoma.
Pyonephrosis (may be bilateral).
Acute renal vein thrombosis.

KIDNEY INJURY, CANCER PATIENTS[74]

ICD-10CM # Varies with specific diagnosis

CAUSES OF ACUTE KIDNEY INJURY IN CANCER PATIENTS

Prerenal

Sepsis

Volume depletion (vomiting, diarrhea, mucositis).
Hepatorenal syndrome (venoocclusive disease of the liver).
Capillary leak syndrome (interleukin-2 administration).
Hypercalcemia.

Intrinsic

Acute tubular necrosis

Ischemia (sepsis/shock).
Nephrotoxic (aminoglycosides, amphotericin B, chemotherapy).

Tubulointerstitial nephritis

Tumor lysis syndrome (urate and phosphate nephropathy).
Allergic reaction.
Pyelonephritis.
Opportunistic infections.
Infiltration (lymphoma/leukemia).

Vascular

Thrombotic microangiopathy.
Cancer treated.
Drug induced.
Bone marrow transplantation.
Radiation injury.

Amyloidosis

Light-chain deposition disease

Paraneoplastic syndromes (membranous, antineutrophil cytoplasmic antibody associated, focal segmental glomerulosclerosis)

Postrenal

Intrarenal (urate, acyclovir, methotrexate)

Extrarenal (retroperitoneal fibrosis, lymphadenopathy, direct invasion)

KNEE PAIN[61]

ICD-10CM #	Code	Description
	S83.419A	Sprain of medial collateral ligament of unspecified knee, initial encounter
	S83.509A	Sprain of unspecified cruciate ligament of unspecified knee, initial encounter
	M23.50	Chronic instability of knee, unspecified knee
	M23.8X9	Other internal derangements of unspecified knee
	S83.289A	Other tear of lateral meniscus, current injury, unspecified knee, initial encounter
	S83.249A	Other tear of medial meniscus, current injury, unspecified knee, initial encounter
	M25.669	Stiffness of unspecified knee, not elsewhere classified

DIFFUSE

Articular.
Anterior.
Prepatellar bursitis.
Patellar tendon enthesopathy.
Chondromalacia patellae.
Patellofemoral osteoarthritis.
Cruciate ligament injury.
Medial plica syndrome.

MEDIAL

Anserine bursitis.
Spontaneous osteonecrosis.
Osteoarthritis.
Medial meniscal tear.
Medial collateral ligament bursitis.
Referred pain from hip and L3.
Fibromyalgia.

LATERAL

Iliotibial band syndrome.
Meniscal cyst.
Lateral meniscal tear.
Collateral ligament.
Peroneal tenosynovitis.

POSTERIOR

Popliteal cyst (Baker's cyst).
Tendinitis.
Aneurysms, ganglions, sarcoma.

KNEE PAIN, IN DIFFERENT AGE GROUPS[18]

ICD-10CM # M25.569 Pain in unspecified knee

COMMON CAUSES OF KNEE PAIN IN DIFFERENT AGE GROUPS

Childhood (2-10 yr)
Intraarticular
Juvenile arthritis.
Osteochondritis dissecans.
Infection.
Torn discoid meniscus.
Periarticular
Osteomyelitis.
Referred
Perthes disease.
Irritable hip.
Adolescence (10-18 yr)
Intraarticular
Osteochondritis dissecans.
Torn meniscus.
Anterior knee pain syndrome.
Patellar instability.
Periarticular
Osgood–Schlatter disease.
Sinding–Larsen–Johansson syndrome.
Osteomyelitis.
Bone tumors.
Referred
Slipped upper femoral epiphysis.
Early Adulthood (18-30 yr)
Intraarticular
Torn meniscus.
Patellar instability.
Anterior knee pain syndrome.
Inflammatory arthritis.
Periarticular
Ligament injuries.
Bursitis.
Adulthood (30-50 yr)
Intraarticular
Degenerate meniscal tears.
Osteoarthritis.
Inflammatory arthritis.
Periarticular
Bursitis.
Referred
Osteoarthritis of hip.
Spinal disorders.
Old Age (>50 yr)
Intraarticular
Osteoarthritis.
Inflammatory arthritis.
Periarticular
Bursitis.
Referred
Osteoarthritis of hip.
Spinal disorders.

LARGE BOWEL STRICTURE[36]

ICD-10CM #	S36.5	Injury of colon

CAUSES OF LARGE BOWEL STRICTURES

Physiologic:
- Spasm.
- Distended bladder.

Maligant:
- Annular carcinoma.
- Scirrhous carcinoma.
- Lymphoma.

Diverticular disease:
- Muscle thickening.
- Pericolic abscess.
- Superimposed malignancy.

Ischemia.
Radiation colitis.
Inflammatory bowel disease:
- Ulcerative colitis.
- Crohn's disease.
- Tuberculosis.
- Lymphogranuloma venereum.
- Amebiasis.

Extrinsic disease:
- Intraabdominal masses.
- Metastatic carcinoma.
- Endometriosis.
- Pelvic lipomatosis.
- Cholecystitis.
- Pancreatitis.

Miscellaneous:
- Postoperative anastomosis.
- Trauma.
- Hirschsprung disease.

LEFT AXIS DEVIATION[50]

ICD-10CM #	I44.7	Left bundle-branch block, unspecified
	I44.4	Left anterior fascicular block
	I44.5	Left posterior fascicular block
	I44.60	Unspecified fascicular block
	I44.69	Other fascicular block

Normal variation.
Left anterior fascicular block (hemiblock).
Left bundle branch block.
Left ventricular hypertrophy.
Mechanical shifts causing a horizontal heart, high diaphragm, pregnancy, ascites.
Some forms of ventricular tachycardia.
Endocardial cushion defects and other congenital heart disease.

LEFT BUNDLE BRANCH BLOCK

ICD-10CM #	I44.7	Left bundle-branch block, unspecified

Ischemic heart disease.
Electrolyte abnormalities (e.g., hyperkalemia).
Cardiomyopathy.
Idiopathic.
LVH.
Pulmonary embolism.
Cardiac trauma.
Bacterial endocarditis.

LEG CRAMPS, NOCTURNAL

ICD-10CM #	R25.2	Cramp and spasm

Diabetic neuropathy.
Medications.
Electrolyte abnormalities (hypokalemia, hyponatremia, hypocalcemia, hyperkalemia, hypophosphatemia).
Respiratory alkalosis.
Uremia.
Hemodialysis.
Peripheral nerve injury.
ALS.
Alcohol use.
Heat cramps.
Vitamin B_{12} deficiency.
Hyperthyroidism.
Contractures.
DVT.
Hypoglycemia.
Peripheral vascular insufficiency.
Baker's cyst.

LEG LENGTH DISCREPANCIES[52]

ICD-10CM #	M21.759	Unequal limb length (acquired), unspecified femur
	M21.769	Unequal limb length (acquired), unspecified tibia and fibula
	Q72.899	Other reduction defects of unspecified lower limb

CONGENITAL

Proximal femoral local deficiency.
Coxa vara.
Hemiatrophy-hemihypertrophy (anisomelia).
Developmental dysplasia of the hip.

DEVELOPMENTAL

Legg-Calvé-Perthes disease.

NEUROMUSCULAR

Polio.
Cerebral palsy (hemiplegia).

INFECTIOUS

Pyogenic osteomyelitis with physeal damage.

TRAUMA

Physeal injury with premature closure.
Overgrowth.
Malunion (shortening).

TUMOR

Physeal destruction.
Radiation-induced physeal injury.
Overgrowth.

LEG MOVEMENT WHEN STANDING, INVOLUNTARY

ICD-10CM #	R25.8	Other abnormal involuntary movements

Benign essential tremor.
Orthostatic tremor.
Spastic ataxia.
Cerebellar truncal tremor.
Postanoxic myoclonus.

LEG PAIN WITH EXERCISE

ICD-10CM #	R25.2	Cramp and spasm

Shin splints.
Arteriosclerosis obliterans.
Neurogenic (spinal cord compression or ischemia).
Venous claudication.
Popliteal cyst.
DVT.
Thromboangiitis obliterans.
Adventitial cysts.
Popliteal artery entrapment syndrome.
McArdle syndrome.

LEG SWELLING[1]

ICD-10CM # R60.0 Localized edema

Deep vein thrombosis.
Cellulitis.
Baker cyst rupture or inflammation.
Congestive heart failure.
Renal failure.
Liver failure.
Inferior vena cava compression.
Musculoskeletal trauma.
Polyarteritis nodosa.
Erythema nodosum.
Myositis.
Tendinitis.
Lymphedema.
Superficial thrombophlebitis.
Compartment syndrome.

LEG ULCERS[61]

ICD-10CM # I70.25 Atherosclerosis of native arteries of other extremities with ulceration
L97.909 Non-pressure chronic ulcer of unspecified part of unspecified lower leg with unspecified severity

VASCULAR

Arterial: arteriosclerosis, thromboangiitis obliterans, AV malformation, cholesterol emboli.
Venous: superficial varicosities, incompetent perforators, DVT, lymphatic abnormalities.

VASCULITIS HEMATOLOGIC

Sickle cell anemia, thalassemia, polycythemia vera, leukemia, cold agglutinin disease.
Macroglobulinemia, protein C and protein S deficiency, cryoglobulinemia, lupus anticoagulant, antiphospholipid syndrome.

INFECTIOUS

Fungal: Blastomycosis, coccidioidomycosis, histoplasmosis, sporotrichosis.
Bacterial: Furuncle, ecthyma, septic emboli.
Protozoal: leishmaniasis.

METABOLIC

Necrobiosis lipoidica diabeticorum.
Localized bullous pemphigoid.
Gout, calcinosis cutis, Gaucher disease.

TUMORS

Basal cell carcinoma, squamous cell carcinoma, melanoma.
Mycosis fungoides, Kaposi sarcoma, metastatic neoplasms.

TRAUMA

Burns, cold injury, radiation dermatitis.
Insect bites.
Factitial, excessive pressure.

NEUROPATHIC

Diabetic trophic ulcers.
Tabes dorsalis, syringomyelia.

DRUGS

Warfarin, IV colchicine extravasation, methotrexate, halogens, ergotism, hydroxyurea.

PANNICULITIS

Weber-Christian disease.
Pancreatic fat necrosis, alpha-antitrypsinase deficiency.

LEPTOMENINGEAL LESIONS

ICD-10CM # G03.9 Leptomeningitis

Metastases.
Multiple sclerosis.
Bacterial or viral meningitis.
Vasculitis.
Lyme disease.
Tuberculosis.
Fungal infections (e.g., *Cryptococcus*).
Sarcoidosis.
Granulomatosis with polyangiitis.
Neurocysticercosis.
Rheumatoid nodules.
Histiocytosis.

LEUKOCORIA

ICD-10CM # H57.9 Unspecified disorder of eye and adnexa

Cataract.
Retinal detachment.
Retinoblastoma.
Retinal telangiectasia.
Retrolenticular vascularized membrane.
Familial exudative vitreoretinopathy.

LID RETRACTION, CAUSES[46]

ICD-10CM # H02.539 Eyelid retraction unspecified eye, unspecified lid

Thyroid eye disease.
Neurogenic:
- Contralateral unilateral ptosis.
- Unopposed levator action due to facial palsy.
- 3rd nerve misdirection.
- Marcus Gunn jaw-winking syndrome.
- Collier sign of the dorsal midbrain (Parinaud syndrome).
- Infantile hydrocephalus (setting sun sign).
- Parkinsonism.
- Sympathomimetic drops.

Mechanical:
- Surgical over-correction of ptosis.
- Scarring of upper lid skin.

Congenital:
- Isolated.
- Duane retraction syndrome.
- Down syndrome.
- Transient "eye popping" reflex in normal infants.

Miscellaneous:
- Prominent globe (pseudo-lid retraction).
- Uremia (Summerskill sign).
- Idiopathic.

LIGHT-NEAR DISSOCIATION[12]

ICD-10CM # Varies with specific diagnosis

CAUSES OF LIGHT-NEAR DISSOCIATION

Unilateral

Afferent conduction defect.
Adie pupil.
Herpes zoster ophthalmicus.
Aberrant regeneration of the third cranial nerve.

Bilateral

Neurosyphilis.
Type 1 diabetes mellitus.
Myotonic dystrophy.
Parinaud (dorsal midbrain) syndrome.
Familial amyloidosis.
Encephalitis.
Chronic alcoholism.

LIMB ISCHEMIA, ACUTE, NONTRAUMATIC[15]

ICD-10CM # Atherosclerosis of arteries of extremities

CAUSES OF NONTRAUMATIC ACUTE LIMB ISCHEMIA

Atherosclerotic

In situ thrombosis.
Atheroembolism from thoracic aortic aneurysm/abdominal aortic aneurysm.
Femoral/popliteal aneurysm with or without compression.
Dissection.

Nonatherosclerotic

Embolism from cardiac thrombosis (atrial fibrillation, post–myocardial infarction akinesis).
Graft thrombosis, graft aneurysm.
Mycotic emboli.
Raynaud's syndrome.
Arteritis with thrombosis.
Inherited and acquired hypercoagulable states.
Drug-induced vasospasm.
External compression (Baker's cyst, popliteal entrapment).

Mimics

Phlegmasia cerulea dolens.
Acute neuropathy.
Hypovolemia.
Systemic shock.

LIMP

ICD-10CM #		
	R26.0	Ataxic gait
	R26.1	Paralytic gait
	R26.89	Other abnormalities of gait and mobility
	R26.9	Unspecified abnormalities of gait and mobility
	M25.80	Other specified joint disorders, unspecified joint
	F44.4	Conversion disorder with motor symptom or deficit
	F44.6	Conversion disorder with sensory symptom or deficit

Degenerative joint disease, osteochondritis dissecans, chondromalacia patellae.
Trauma to extremities, vertebral disk, hips.
Poorly fitting shoes, foreign body in shoe, unequal leg length.
Splinter in foot.
Joint infection (septic arthritis, osteomyelitis), viral arthritis.
Abdominal pain (e.g., appendicitis, incarcerated hernia), testicular torsion.
Polio, neuromuscular disorders, Guillain-Barré syndrome, multiple sclerosis.
Osgood-Schlatter disease.
Legg-Calvé-Perthes disease.
Factitious, somatization syndrome.
Neoplasm (local or metastatic).
Other: diskitis, periostitis, sickle cell disease, hemophilia.

LIMPING, PEDIATRIC AGE[52]

ICD-10CM #		
	R26.0	Ataxic gait
	R26.1	Paralytic gait
	R26.89	Other abnormalities of gait and mobility
	R26.9	Unspecified abnormalities of gait and mobility

TODDLER (1-3 YR)

Infection:
- Septic arthritis:
  - Hip.
  - Knee.
- Osteomyelitis.
- Diskitis.

Occult trauma:
- Toddler's fracture.

Neoplasia.

CHILDHOOD (4-10 YR)

Infection:
- Septic arthritis:
  - Hip.
  - Knee.
- Osteomyelitis.
- Diskitis.
- Transient synovitis, hip.

LCPD.
Tarsal coalition.
Rheumatologic disorder:
- JRA.

Trauma.
Neoplasia.

ADOLESCENCE (11+ YR)

SCFE.
Rheumatologic disorder:
- JRA.
- Trauma.
- Tarsal coalition.
- Hip dislocation (DDH).
- Neoplasia.

DDH, Developmental dysplasia of the hip; *JRA,* juvenile RA; *LCPD,* Legg-Calvé-Perthes disease; *SCFE,* slipped capital femoral epiphysis.

LIVEDO RETICULARIS

ICD-10CM #		
	L95.0	Livedoid vasculitis

Emboli (SBE, left atrial myxoma, cholesterol emboli).
Thrombocythemia or polycythemia.
Antiphospholipid antibody syndrome.
Cryoglobulinemia, cryofibrinogenemia.
Leukocytoclastic vasculitis.
SLE, RA, dermatomyositis.
Pancreatitis.
Drugs (quinine, quinidine, amantadine, catecholamines).
Physiologic (cutis marmorata).
Congenital.

LIVER DISEASE, PREGNANCY[81]

ICD-10CM #		
	K75.89	Other specified inflammatory liver diseases

INCIDENTAL TO PREGNANCY

Viral hepatitis.
Alcohol related.
Autoimmune chronic active hepatitis.

RELATED TO PREGNANCY (POSSIBLY INFLUENCED BY HORMONES PRESENT IN PREGNANCY)

Complicated gallstone disease.
Hepatic adenoma.
Focal nodular hyperplasia.
Budd-Chiari syndrome.

SPECIFIC TO PREGNANCY

Severe hyperemesis gravidarum.
Benign intrahepatic cholestasis.
Acute fatty liver of pregnancy.
Preeclampsia (HELLP).

LIVER LESIONS, BENIGN, OFTEN CONFUSED WITH MALIGNANCY

ICD-10CM #		
	K76.1	Chronic passive congestion of liver
	K76.89	Other specified diseases of liver

Fatty infiltration.
Adenoma.
Hemangioma.
Cysts.
Flow artifacts.
Focal nodular hyperplasia.
Nonenhanced vessels.

LOWER GI ULCERATIVE LESIONS[22]

ICD-10CM #	
	Code varies with specific diagnosis

INFECTIOUS

Epstein-Barr virus.
Human immunodeficiency virus.
Cytomegalovirus.
Herpes simplex.
Herpes zoster.
Syphilis.
Erosive candidiasis.
Mycobacterial infection.
Chancroid.
Lymphogranuloma venereum.

NOT INFECTIOUS

Behçet's syndrome.
Excoriation.
Aphthous (idiopathic) ulcer.
Erythema multiforme.
Carcinoma.

LOW-VOLTAGE ECG

ICD-10CM #		
	R94.31	Abnormal electrocardiogram [ECG] [EKG]

Hypothyroidism.
Obesity.
Pericardial effusion.
Anasarca.
Pleural effusion.
Pneumothorax.
Amyloidosis.
Aortic stenosis.

LUNG CANCER, OCCUPATIONAL CAUSES[36]

ICD-10CM #		
	C34.90	Malignant neoplasm of unspecified part of unspecified bronchus or lung

CAUSES OF OCCUPATIONAL LUNG CANCER

Asbestos	Lagging, insulation
Arsenic	Metal smelting, pesticide manufacture
Beryllium	Electronics, dental prosthetic manufacture
Chromium	Coloring pigment production, electroplating
Nickel	Electroplating
Silica	Grinding, quarrying, sandblasting
Radon	Mining
Uranium	Mining

LUNG DISEASE AND GASTROINTESTINAL AND LIVER INVOLVEMENT[58]

ICD-10CM # Varies with specific diagnosis

ESOPHAGEAL REFLUX

Aspiration pneumonia.
Asthma.
Scleroderma.
Bronchitis.
Bronchiectasis.
Cough.
Pulmonary fibrosis.
Mycobacterial disease.

INFLAMMATORY BOWEL DISEASE

Bronchitis.
Bronchiectasis.
Bronchiolitis.
Colobronchial fistula.
Desquamative interstitial lung disease.
Drug reactions for agents that treat inflammatory bowel disease.
Eosinophilic lung disease.
Interstitial lung disease.
Necrobiotic nodules.
Obstructive lung disease.
Organizing pneumonia.
Reduced diffusing capacity.
Sarcoidosis.
Serositis affecting pleura or pericarditis.
Tracheal stenosis.

LIVER

Alpha1-antitrypsin deficiency.
Chronic active hepatitis.
Hepatopulmonary syndrome.
Portapulmonary hypertension.
Primary biliary cirrhosis.
Hepatosplenomegaly:
- Amyloidosis.
- Collagen vascular disease.
- Eosinophilic granulomatosis.
- Lymphatic interstitial pneumonia.
- Sarcoidosis.

LUNG DISEASE AND RENAL INVOLVEMENT[58]

ICD-10CM # Varies with specific diagnosis

LUNG DISEASE WITH RENAL INVOLVEMENT

Glomerulonephritis

Systemic vasculitis.
Collagen vascular disease.
Antibasement membrane.
Sarcoidosis.

Nephrotic Syndrome

Amyloidosis.
Disseminated Langerhans cell histiocytosis.
Drug-induced lung disease.
Paraneoplastic syndrome.
Post transplantation.
Pulmonary hydatid disease.
Systemic lupus erythematosus.
Vasculitis.
Venous thrombosis.

Renal Mass

Lymphangioleiomyomatosis.
Metastasis neoplasm.
Renal carcinoid.
Tuberous sclerosis.
Granulomatosis with polyangiitis.

Nephrolithiasis

Alveolar proteinosis.
Cystic fibrosis.
Hypercalcemic syndromes.
Osteolysis from mycobacteria or fungi.
Sarcoidosis.

Systemic Hypertension

Collagen vascular disease.
Diffuse alveolar hemorrhage.
Pulmonary renal syndromes.
Neurofibromatosis.
Sleep apnea.

LUNG DISEASE AND SKIN AND SUBCUTANEOUS LESIONS[58]

ICD-10CM # Varies with specific diagnosis

SKIN AND SUBCUTANEOUS LESIONS ASSOCIATED WITH LUNG DISEASE

Skin Lesions

Diffuse pigment change.
- Acanthosis nigricans—lung neoplasm.
- Albinism—Hermansky-Pudlak syndrome.
- Bronze pigmentation—hemosiderosis.
- Gray-brown—Whipple disease.

Cutaneous draining sinus.
- Fungal infections (especially histoplasmosis).
- Mycobacterial infections (especially tuberculosis).
- Neoplasms (especially mesothelial tumors).
- Necrotizing vasculitis.
- Other bacterial infections (especially actinomycosis).

Cutaneous ulcers.
- Beryllium disease.
- Chronic venous insufficiency.
- Fungal infections (especially histoplasmosis).
- Mycobacterial disease.
- Necrotizing vasculitis.
- Parasitic disease.
- Polycythemia.
- Sickle cell disease.
- Tularemia.

Cutaneous vasculitis.
- Behçet's syndrome.
- Churg-Strauss syndrome.
- Collagen vascular disease.
- Sarcoidosis.
- Granulomatosis with polyangiitis.

Erythema multiforme.
- Drug reactions.
- Fungi (especially coccidiomycosis).
- Mycoplasma and other infectious agents.
- Neoplasms.
- Exfoliative dermatitis.
- Adverse drug reactions.
- Chemotherapy.
- Disseminated malignancy.
- Graft-versus-host disease.
- Radiation therapy.

Flushing.
- Bronchial carcinoid, pheochromocytoma, other neoplasms.
- Carbon dioxide, cyanide, and other toxins.
- Drugs.
- Foods and vasodilatory substances.
- Hormones.
- Mastocytosis.
- Metabolic states (e.g., hyperthyroidism, fever).

Macular rash.
- Anti-basement membrane disease.
- Café-au-lait spots (neurofibromatosis).
- Coal miner's scars.
- Collagen vascular disease.
- Idiopathic pulmonary fibrosis.
- Rose spots (psittacosis).
- Sarcoidosis.
- Syphilis.
- Viral pneumonia.

Maculopapular rash.
- Amyloidosis.
- Drug-induced lung disease.
- Collagen vascular disease.
- Gaucher disease.
- Kaposi sarcoma.
- Lung neoplasm.
- Lymphomatoid granulomatosis.
- Lymphoma.
- Parasites.
- Sarcoidosis.
- Syphilis.
- Vasculitis.
- Viral pneumonia

Telangiectasia
- Arteriovenous malformation.
- Ataxia-telangiectasia.
- Carcinoid syndrome.
- Cushing's disease.
- Hepatopulmonary syndrome and other chronic liver diseases.
- Hereditary hemorrhagic telangiectasia (Osler-Weber-Rendu).
- Mastocytosis.
- Systemic sclerosis and other collagen vascular diseases.

Urticaria
- Asthma.
- Drug reactions.
- Cystic fibrosis.
- Exercise-induced urticaria.
- Food allergy.
- Hereditary angioneurotic edema.
- Inhaled antigens.
- Insect bites and stings.
- Infectious agents, such as mycoplasma and helicobacter.
- Mastocytosis.
- Occupational sensitization.
- Parasites.
- Vasculitis.

Nail Changes with Lung Disease

Color changes:
- Cigarette smoking discoloration.
- Splinter hemorrhages.

Yellow nail syndrome.
Beau lines (any severe illness):
Dermatomyositis.
Sarcoidosis.
Seronegative arthropathies.
Systemic sclerosis.

Lung Disease with Subcutaneous Involvement

Adenopathy:
Environmental mycobacteria.
Fungal infections.
Human immunodeficiency visurs infections.
Metastatic neoplasm.
Leukemia.
Lymphoma.
Sarcoidosis.
Tuberculosis.

Calcinosis:
Dermatomyositis.
Metastatic osteosarcoma.
Mixed connective tissue disease.
Scleroderma.
Tuberculosis.
Uremic metastatic calcification.

Erythema induratum (Bazin disease):
Aortic stenosis.
Cryoglobulinemia.
Nodular vasculitis.
Panniculitis.
Peripheral neuropathy.
Takayasu disease.
Streptococcus infection.
Tuberculosis and other mycobacterial disease.
Weber-Christian disease.

Erythema nodosa:
Neoplasm.
Other infectious and inflammatory diseases.
Primary coccidiomycosis, histoplasmosis.
Primary tuberculosis.
Psittacosis.
Sarcoidosis.

Subcutaneous nodules:
Amyloidosis.
Neoplasm.
Neurofibromatosis.
Rheumatoid arthritis.
Tuberous sclerosis (angiofibromas).
von Recklinghausen.
Weber-Christian disease.

Lung Disease with Salivary Gland Enlargement

Bulimia and aspiration.
Gaucher disease.
Lymphoid interstitial pneumonitis.
Lymphatic carcinoma.
Lymphoma.
Other causes of lymphadenopathy.
Sarcoidosis.
Sjögren syndrome.

LUNG DISEASE WITH BONE, JOINT, NERVE, AND MUSCLE INVOLVEMENT[58]

ICD-10CM # Varies with specific diagnosis

ARTHRITIS

Ankylosing spondylitis.
Collagen vascular diseases.
Reactive arthritis.
Sarcoidosis.
Systemic vasculitis.
Tuberculosis.

BONE LESIONS

Ankylosing spondylitis.
Blastomycosis and other fungal disease.
Collagen vascular diseases.
Eosinophilic granulomatosis.
Fibrous histiocytoma.
Gaucher disease.
Neoplasm.
Sarcoidosis.
Tuberculosis.

MUSCLE DISEASE

Collagen vascular disease.
L-Tryptophan.
Diabetes insipidus.
Eosinophilic granulomatosis.
Polymyositis.
Sarcoidosis.

NEUROLOGIC DISEASE

Acute inflammatory polyneuropathy.
Amyotrophic lateral sclerosis.
Aspiration.
Botulism.
Lambert-Eaton syndrome.
Myasthenia gravis.
Organophosphate poisoning.
Polio and postpolio syndrome.
Sarcoidosis.
Churg-Strauss syndrome.
Granulomatosis with polyangiitis.

LUNG TUMORS, BENIGN[72]

ICD-10CM # Varies with specific disorder

COMMON BENIGN TUMORS OF THE LUNG BASED ON CELLS OF ORIGIN

Tumors of Epithelial Origin

Mucous gland adenoma.
Clara cell adenoma.
Mucous cystadenoma.
Pleomorphic adenoma.

Tumors of Mesenchymal Origin

Hamartoma.
Inflammatory pseudotumor.
Chondroma.
Fibroma.
Benign endobronchial fibrous histiocytoma.
Leiomyoma.
Lipoma.
Lymphatic lesions.

Tumors of Miscellaneous Origin

Nodular pulmonary amyloidosis.
Clear cell tumor (sugar tumor).
Thymoma.
Granular cell tumor.
Teratoma.
Pulmonary paraganglioma.

LUNG VOLUMES IN DIFFUSE LUNG DISEASE[34]

ICD-10CM # Varies with specific disorder

LARGE LUNG VOLUMES

Emphysema.
Chonic asthma.
Diffuse bronchiolitis obliterans.
Highly trained athletes.
Lymphangioleiomyomatosis.

SMALL LUNG VOLUMES

End-stage lung fibrosis.
Bilateral diaphragmatic paralysis.
Massive ascites.

NORMAL LUNG VOLUMES

Sarcoidosis.
Langerhans cell histiocytosis.
Neurofibromatosis.
Emphysema with pulmonary fibrosis.

LYMPHADENOPATHY[32]

ICD-10CM # R59.9 Enlarged lymph nodes, unspecified

GENERALIZED

AIDS.
Lymphoma: Hodgkin's disease, non-Hodgkin's lymphoma.
Leukemias, reticuloendotheliosis.
Infectious mononucleosis, CMV, and other viral infections.
Diffuse skin infection: generalized furunculosis, multiple tick bites.
Parasitic infections: toxoplasmosis, filariasis, leishmaniasis, Chagas' disease.
Serum sickness.
Collagen vascular diseases (RA, SLE).
Dengue (arbovirus infection).
Sarcoidosis and other granulomatous diseases.
Drugs: INH, hydantoin derivatives, antithyroid and antileprosy drugs.
Secondary syphilis.
Hyperthyroidism, lipid-storage diseases.

LOCALIZED

Cervical Nodes

Infections of the head, neck, ears, sinuses, scalp, pharynx.
Mononucleosis.
Lymphoma.
TB.
Malignancy of head and neck.
Rubella.

Scalene/Supraclavicular Nodes

Lymphoma.
Lung neoplasm.
Bacterial or fungal infection of thorax or retroperitoneum.
GI malignancy.

Axillary Nodes

Infections of hands and arms.
Cat-scratch disease.
Neoplasm (lymphoma, melanoma, breast carcinoma).

Brucellosis.
Epitrochlear Nodes
Infections of the hand.
Lymphoma.
Tularemia.
Sarcoidosis, secondary syphilis (usually bilateral).
Inguinal Nodes
Infections of leg or foot, folliculitis (pubic hair).
LGV, syphilis.
Lymphoma.
Pelvic malignancy.
Pasteurella pestis.
Hilar Nodes
Sarcoidosis.
TB.
Lung carcinoma.
Fungal infections, systemic.
Mediastinal Nodes
Sarcoidosis.
Lymphoma.
Lung neoplasm.
TB.
Mononucleosis.
Histoplasmosis.
Abdominal/Retroperitoneal Nodes
Lymphoma.
TB.
Neoplasm (ovary, testes, prostate, and other malignancies).

LYMPHANGITIS[55]

ICD-10CM # I89.1 Lymphangitis

Acute:
- Group A streptococci.
- *Staphylococcus aureus.*
- *Pasteurella multocida.*

Chronic:
- *Sporothrix schenckii* (sporotrichosis).
- *Mycobacterium marinum* (swimming pool granuloma).
- *Mycobacterium kansasii.*
- *Nocardia brasiliensis.*
- *W. bancrofti.*

LYMPHEDEMA[45]

ICD-10CM #		
	I89.0	Lymphedema, not elsewhere classified
	I97.2	Postmastectomy lymphedema syndrome
	Q82.0	Hereditary lymphedema

CLASSIFICATION OF LYMPHEDEMA

Primary lymphedema
Congenital lymphedema (Milroy disease).
Lymphedema praecox.
Lymphedema tarda.
Syndromes associated with primary lymphedema
Yellow nail syndrome.
Turner syndrome.
Noonan syndrome.
Pes cavus.
Phakomatosis pigmentovascularis.
Distichiasis-lymphedema.
Emberger syndrome.
WILD syndrome.
Hypotrichosis-telangiectasia-lymphedema syndrome.
Cutaneous disorders sometimes associated with primary lymphedema
Yellow nails.
Hemangiomas.
Xanthomatosis and chylous lymphedema.
Congenital absence of nails.
Secondary lymphedema
Postmastectomy lymphedema.
Melphalan isolated limb perfusion.
Malignant occlusion with obstruction.
Extrinsic pressure.
Factitial lymphedema.
Postradiation therapy.
Following recurrent lymphangitis/cellulitis.
Lymphedema of upper limb in recurrent eczema.
Granulomatous disease.
Rosaceous lymphedema.
Primary amyloidosis.
Complications of lymphedema
Cellulitis of lymphedema.
Elephantiasis nostra verrucosa.
Ulceration.
Lymphangiosarcoma.

LYMPHOCYTOSIS, ATYPICAL[55]

ICD-10CM # D72.89 Other specified disorders of white blood cells

Epstein-Barr virus primary infection (infectious mononucleosis).
Cytomegalovirus primary infection (heterophile-negative mono).
Human herpesvirus 6 primary infection (roseola).
Primary HIV infection.
Toxoplasmosis.
Acute viral hepatitis.
Rubella, mumps.
Drug reactions (e.g., phenytoin, sulfa).

MACROTHROMBOCYTOPENIA, INHERITED[43]

ICD-10CM # Varies with specific disorder

Bernard-Soulier syndrome.
MHY9-related disorders:
- May-Hegglin anomaly.
- Sebastian syndrome.
- Fechtner syndrome.
- Epstein syndrome.

Gray platelet syndrome.
Montreal platelet syndrome.
Mediterranean macrothrombocytopenia.
Mediterranean stomatocytosis/macrothrombocytemia.
GATA1 mutations.
Sialyl-Lewis-S antigen deficiency.
Paris-Trousseau syndrome.
Platelet-type von Willebrand's disease.

MACULAR CRYSTALS[12]

ICD-10CM # Varies with specific diagnosis

OTHER CAUSES OF MACULAR CRYSTALS

Primary hyperoxaluria.
Bietti corneoretinal crystalline dystrophy.
Cystinosis.
Sjögren–Larsson syndrome.
Gyrate atrophy.
Acquired parafoveal telangiectasis.
Talc-corn starch emboli.
West African crystalline maculopathy.

MADAROSIS[12]

ICD-10CM # H02.729 Madarosis of unspecified eye, unspecified eyelid and periocular area

CAUSES OF MADAROSIS

Local
Chronic anterior lid margin disease.
Infiltrating lid tumors.
Burns.
Radiotherapy or cryotherapy of lid tumors.
Skin disorders
Generalized alopecia.
Psoriasis.
Systemic diseases.
Myxoedema.
Systemic lupus erythematosus.
Acquired syphilis.
Lepromatous leprosy.
Following removal
Procedures for trichiasis.
Trichotillomania (psychiatric disorder of hair removal).

MALABSORPTION[81]

ICD-10CM # K90.89 Other intestinal malabsorption

CAUSES OF MALABSORPTION

More Common
Celiac disease.
Chronic pancreatitis.
Post gastrectomy.
Crohn's disease.
Small bowel resection.
Small intestinal bacterial overgrowth.
Lactase deficiency.
Less Common
AIDS (*Myobacterium avium* intracellulare, AIDS enteropathy).
Whipple disease.
Intestinal lymphoma.
Immunoproliferative small intestinal disease (alpha heavy chain disease).
Radiation enteritis.
Collagenous sprue.
Tropical sprue.
Non-granulomatous ulcerative jejunoileitis.
Eosinophilic gastroenteritis.
Amyloidosis.

Zollinger-Ellison syndrome.
Intestinal lymphangiectasia.
Systemic mastocytosis.
Chronic mesenteric ischemia.
Abetalipoproteinemia (autosomal recessive).

MALABSORPTION SYNDROME IN TROPICS[26]

ICD-10CM # K90.89 Other intestinal malabsorption

CAUSES OF MALABSORPTION SYNDROME IN THE TROPICS

SIBO
- Following ulcer surgery.
- Secondary to intestinal TB and Crohn's disease.

Infections

Bacteria
- *Mycobac*terium avium intracellulare complex.
- Mycobact*erium tuberculosis.*

Helminths
- *Paracapill*aria philippinensis.
- Strongyloides *stercoralis.*

Protozoa
- *Cryptospori*dium parvum.
- Cyclospora cayetanensis.
- Encephalitozoon intestinalis.
- Enterocytozoon bieneusi.
- Giardia lamblia.
- Isospora belli.
- Leishmania *donovani.*

Lymphatic Obstruction
- Intestinal lymphangiectasia.

Mucosal Diseases
- Autoimmune enteropathy.
- Celiac disease.
- Eosinophilic gastroenteritis.
- HIV enteropathy.
- Immunoproliferative small intestinal disease.
- Intestinal lymphoma.
- Primary immunodeficiencies.
- Tropical sprue.

Neonatal Diseases
- Microvillus inclusion disease.
- Tufting enteropathy.

Pancreatic Insufficiency
- Alcoholic pancreatitis.
- CF.
- Tropical pancreatitis.

Specific Transport Disorders
- Abetalipoproteinemia.
- Fructose malabsorption.
- Glucose-galactose malabsorption.
- Hypolactasia.
- Sucrose intolerance.

MALNUTRITION, CAUSES IN EARLY LIFE[51]

ICD-10CM # E46 Unspecified protein-energy malnutrition

0-6 MO

Breastfeeding difficulties.
Improper formula preparation.
Impaired parent/child interaction.
Congenital syndromes.
Prenatal infections or teratogenic exposures.
Poor feeding (sucking, swallowing) or feeding refusal (aversion).
Maternal psychological disorder (depression or attachment disorder).
Congenital heart disease.
Cystic fibrosis.
Neurologic abnormalities.
Child neglect.
Recurrent infections.

6-12 MO

Celiac disease.
Food intolerance.
Child neglect.
Delayed introduction of age-appropriate foods or poor transition to food.
Recurrent infections.
Food allergy.

AFTER INFANCY

Acquired chronic diseases.
Highly distractible child.
Inappropriate mealtime environment.
Inappropriate diet (e.g., excessive juice consumption, avoidance of high-calorie foods).
Recurrent infections.

MEDIASTINAL COMPARTMENTS, ANATOMY AND PATHOLOGY[86]

ICD-10CM # Varies with specific disorder

ANTERIOR

Normal Structures

Lymph nodes.
Connective tissue.
Thymus (remnant in adults).

Masses

Thymoma.
Germ cell neoplasm.
Lymphoma.
Thyroid enlargement (intrathoracic goiter).
Other tumors.

MIDDLE

Normal Structures

Pericardium.
Heart.
Vessels: ascending aorta, venae cavae, main pulmonary arteries.
Trachea.
Lymph nodes.
Nerves: phrenic, upper vagus.

Masses

Carcinoma.
Lymphoma.
Pericardial cyst.
Bronchogenic cyst.
Benign lymph node enlargement (granulomatous disease).

POSTERIOR

Normal Structures

Vessels: descending aorta.
Esophagus.
Vertebral column.
Nerves: sympathetic chain, lower vagus.
Lymph nodes.
Connective tissue.

Masses

Neurogenic tumor.
Diaphragmatic hernia.

MEDIASTINAL MASSES OR WIDENING ON CHEST X-RAY

ICD-10CM # R59.9 Enlarged lymph nodes, unspecified
J98.5 Diseases of mediastinum, not elsewhere classified

Lymphoma: Hodgkin's disease and non-Hodgkin's lymphoma.
Sarcoidosis.
Vascular: aortic aneurysm, ectasia, or tortuosity of aorta or bronchocephalic vessels.
Carcinoma: lungs, esophagus.
Esophageal diverticula.
Hiatal hernia.
Achalasia.
Prominent pulmonary outflow tract: pulmonary hypertension, pulmonary embolism, right-to-left shunts.
Trauma: mediastinal hemorrhage.
Pneumomediastinum.
Lymphadenopathy caused by silicosis and other pneumoconioses.
Leukemias.
Infections: TB, viral (rare), *Mycoplasma* (rare), fungal, tularemia.
Substernal thyroid.
Thymoma.
Teratoma.
Bronchogenic cyst.
Pericardial cyst.
Neurofibroma, neurosarcoma, ganglioneuroma.

MEDIASTINAL MASSES, SITES OF ORIGIN[84]

ICD-10CM # Varies with specific diagnosis

DIFFERENTIAL DIAGNOSIS OF MEDIASTINAL MASSES BASED ON COMMON SITES OF ORIGIN

Prevascular space (anterior mediastinum)

Thymic masses.
Thymoma.
Thymic carcinoma.
Thymic neuroendocrine tumor.
Thymolipoma.
Thymic cyst.
Thymic hyperplasia.
Thymic lymphoma.
Germ cell tumors.
Teratoma and dermoid cyst.
Seminoma.
Nonseminomatous germ cell tumors.
Thyroid abnormalities (goiter and neoplasm).
Parathyroid tumor or hyperplasia.
Lymph node masses (particularly Hodgkin's lymphoma).
Vascular abnormalities (aorta and great vessels).
Mesenchymal abnormalities (e.g., lipomatosis, lipoma).

Foregut cyst.
Lymphangioma.
Hemangioma.
Retrosternal space (anterior mediastinum)
Lymph node masses.
Pretracheal space (middle mediastinum)
Lymph node masses.
Lung carcinoma.
Sarcoidosis.
Lymphoma (particularly Hodgkin's disease).
Metastases.
Infections (e.g., tuberculosis).
Foregut cyst.
Tracheal tumor.
Mesenchymal masses (e.g., lipomatosis, lipoma).
Thyroid abnormalities.
Vascular abnormalities (aorta and great vessels).
Lymphangioma and hemangioma.
Aortopulmonary window (middle mediastinum)
Lymph node masses.
Lung carcinoma.
Sarcoidosis.
Lymphoma.
Metastases.
Infections (e.g., tuberculosis).
Mesenchymal masses (e.g., lipomatosis, lipoma).
Vascular abnormalities (aorta or pulmonary artery).
Chemodectoma.
Foregut cyst.
Subcarinal space and azygoesophageal recess (middle mediastinum)
Lymph node masses.
Lung carcinoma.
Sarcoidosis.
Lymphoma.
Metastases.
Infections (e.g., tuberculosis).
Foregut cyst.
Dilated azygos vein.
Esophageal masses.
Varices.
Hernia.
Paravertebral masses (posterior mediastinum)
Neurogenic tumor.
Nerve sheath tumors.
Sympathetic ganglia tumors.
Paraganglioma.
Meningocele.
Foregut cyst.
Neurenteric cyst.
Thoracic spine abnormalities.
Extramedullary hematopoiesis.
Fluid collections and pseudocyst.
Vascular abnormalities.
Hernias.
Esophageal masses.
Varices.
Mesenchymal masses (e.g., lipomatosis, lipoma).
Lymph node masses.
Lymphoma (particularly non-Hodgkin's).
Metastases.
Dilated azygos or hemiazygos vein.
Hernia.
Lymphangioma and hemangioma.
Thymic mass or germ cell tumor.
Anterior cardiophrenic angle masses.
Lymph node masses (particularly lymphoma and metastases).
Pericardial cyst.
Fat pad.
Morgagni hernia.
Thymic masses.
Germ cell tumors.

MEDIASTINITIS, ACUTE[55]

ICD-10CM # J98.5 Diseases of mediastinum, not elsewhere classified

Esophageal perforation.
Iatrogenic.
EGD, esophageal dilation, esophageal variceal sclerotherapy, nasogastric tube, Sengstaken-Blackmore tube, endotracheal intubation, esophageal surgery, paraesophageal surgery, transesophageal echocardiography, anterior stabilization of cervical vertebral bodies.
Swallowed foreign bodies.
Trauma.
Spontaneous perforation (e.g., emesis, carcinoma).
Head and neck infections (e.g., tonsillitis, pharyngitis, parotitis, epiglottitis, odontogenic).
Infections originating at another site (e.g., TB, pneumonia, pancreatitis, osteomyelitis of sternum, clavicle, ribs).
Cardiothoracic surgery (median sternotomy) (e.g., CABG, valve replacement, other types of cardiothoracic surgery).

MELANONYCHIA

ICD-10CM # NEC L81.4 Melanin hyperpigmentation

Pregnancy.
Trauma.
Medications (e.g., AZT, 5-fluorouracil, doxorubicin, psoralens).
Nail matrix nevus.
HIV infection.
Onychomycosis.
Melanocyte hyperplasia.
Verrucae.
Pustular psoriasis.
Lichen planus.
Basal cell carcinoma.
Nail matrix melanoma.
Subungual keratosis.
Addison disease.
Bowen disease.

MEMORY LOSS SYMPTOMS, ELDERLY PATIENTS

ICD-10CM # R41.2 Retrograde amnesia

Age-related mild cognitive impairment.
Depression (pseudodementia).
Medications (e.g., anticholinergics, sedatives).
Hypothyroidism.
Chronic hypoxia.
Cerebrovascular infarcts.
Alzheimer disease.
Hepatic disease.
Chronic renal failure.
Hyperthyroidism.
Frontotemporal dementia.
Lewy body dementia.

MENINGITIS, CHRONIC[55]

ICD-10CM # G03.1 Chronic meningitis

TB.
Fungal CNS infection.
Tertiary syphilis.
CNS neoplasm.
Metabolic encephalopathies.
Multiple sclerosis.
Chronic subdural hematoma.
SLE cerebritis.
Encephalitides.
Sarcoidosis.
NSAIDs.
Behçet's syndrome.
Anatomic defects (traumatic, congenital, postoperative).
Granulomatous angiitis.

MENINGITIS, RECURRENT[55]

ICD-10CM # G03.2 Benign recurrent meningitis [Mollaret]

Drug induced (with rechallenge).
Parameningeal focus:
Infection (sinusitis, mastoiditis, osteomyelitis, brain abscess).
Tumor (epidermoid cyst, craniopharyngioma).
Posttraumatic (bacterial).
Mollaret meningitis.
SLE.
Herpes simplex virus.

MENTAL STATUS CHANGES AND COMA[7]

ICD-10CM # R41.82 Altered mental status, unspecified

METABOLIC/SYSTEMIC ETIOLOGY OF ALTERED MENTAL STATUS AND COMA

Hypoxia
Severe pulmonary disease (hypoventilation).
Severe anemia.
Environmental/toxin:
Methemoglobinemia.
Cyanide.
Carbon monoxide.
Decreased atmospheric oxygen (high altitude).
Near-drowning.
Disorders of Glucose
Hypoglycemia:
Chronic alcohol abuse and liver disease.
Excessive use of insulin or other hypoglycemic agents.
Insulinoma.
Hyperglycemia:
Diabetic ketoacidosis.
Nonketotic hyperosmolar coma.

Decreased Cerebral Blood Flow

Hypovolemic shock.
Cardiac:
- Vasovagal syncope.
- Arrhythmias.
- Myocardial infarction.
- Valvular disorders.
- Congestive heart failure.
- Pericardial effusion/tamponade.
- Myocarditis.

Infectious:
- Septic shock.
- Bacterial meningitis.

Vascular/hematologic:
- Hypertensive encephalopathy.
- Pseudotumor cerebri.
- Hyperviscosity (sickle cell, polycythemia).
- Hyperventilation.
- Cerebral lupus vasculitis.
- Thrombotic thrombocytopenic purpura.
- Disseminated intravascular coagulation.

Metabolic Cofactor Deficiency

Thiamine (Wernicke-Korsakoff syndrome).
Pyridoxine (isoniazid overdose).
Folic acid (chronic alcohol abuse).
Cyanocobalamin.
Niacin.

Electrolyte/pH Disturbances

Acidosis/alkalosis.
Hypernatremia/hyponatremia.[26]
Hypercalcemia/hypocalcemia.
Hypophosphatemia.
Hypermagnesemia/hypomagnesemia.

Endocrine Disorders

Myxedema coma, thyrotoxicosis.
Hypopituitarism.
Addison disease (primary or secondary).
Cushing's disease.
Pheochromocytoma.
Hyperparathyroidism/hypoparathyroidism.

Endogenous Toxins

Hyperammonemia (liver failure).
Uremia (renal disease).
Carbon dioxide narcosis (pulmonary disease).
Porphyria.

Exogenous Toxins

Alcohols:
- Ethanol, isopropyl alcohol, methanol, ethylene glycol.

Acid poisons:
- Salicylates.
- Paraldehyde.
- Ammonium chloride.

Antidepressant medications:
- Lithium.
- Tricyclic antidepressants (TCAs).
- Selective serotonin reuptake inhibitors (SSRIs).
- Monamine oxidase inhibitors (MAOIs).

Stimulants:
- Amphetamines/methamphetamines.
- Cocaine.
- Over-the-counter sympathomimetics.

Narcotics/opiates:
- Morphine.
- Heroin.
- Codeine, oxycodone, meperidine, hydrocodone.
- Methadone.
- Fentanyl.
- Propoxyphene.

Sedative-hypnotics:
- Benzodiazepines.
- Barbiturates.
- Rohypnol.
- Bromide.

Hallucinogens:
- Lysergic acid diethylamide (LSD).
- Marijuana.
- Mescaline, peyote.
- Mushrooms.
- Phencyclidine (PCP).

Herbs/plants:
- Aconite.
- Jimson weed.
- Morning glory.

Volatile substances:
- Hydrocarbons (gasoline, butane, toluene, benzene, chloroform).
- Nitrites.
- Anesthetic agents (nitrous oxide, ether).

Other:
- γ-Hydroxybutyrate (GHB).
- Ketamine.
- Penicillin.
- Cardiac glycosides.
- Anticonvulsants.
- Steroids.
- Heavy metals.
- Cimetidine.
- Organophosphates.

Disorders of Temperature Regulation/ Environmental

Hypothermia.
Heat stroke.
Malignant hyperthermia.
Neuroleptic malignant syndrome.
High-altitude cerebral edema (HACE).
Dysbarism.

Primary Glial or Neuronal Disorders

Adrenoleukodystrophy.
Creutzfeldt-Jakob disease.
Progressive multifocal leukoencephalopathy.
Marchiafava-Bignami disease.
Gliomatosis cerebri.
Central pontine myelinolysis.

Other Disorders of Unknown Etiology

Seizures.
Postictal states.
Reye syndrome.[27]
Intussusception.

---

[26] Can be associated with dilution of formula in infant feeding.
[27] Prominent in the pediatric population.

MENTAL STATUS CHANGES AND COMA, STRUCTURAL CAUSES[1]

ICD-10CM # R40.1 Stupor

COMMON AGE-RELATED CAUSES OF ALTERED MENTAL STATUS AND COMA

Infant

Infection.
Trauma, abuse.
Metabolic.

Child

Toxic ingestion.

Adolescent, Young Adult

Toxic ingestion.
Recreational drug use.
Trauma.

Elderly

- Medication changes.
- Over-the-counter medications.
- Infection.
- Alterations in living environment.
- Stroke.
- Trauma.

MENTAL STATUS CHANGES AND COMA, METABOLIC AND SYSTEMIC CAUSES

ICD-10CM # CM40.1

METABOLIC AND SYSTEMIC CAUSES OF ALTERED MENTAL STATUS AND COMA

Hypoxia, Hypercapnia

Severe pulmonary disease (hypoventilation).
Severe anemia.
Environmental, toxic.
Methemoglobinemia.
Cyanide.
Carbon monoxide.
Decreased atmospheric oxygen (high altitude).
Near-drowning.

Glucose Disorders

Hypoglycemia:
- Chronic alcohol abuse and liver disease.
- Excessive dosage of insulin or other hypoglycemic agents.
- Insulinoma.

Hyperglycemia:
- Diabetic ketoacidosis.
- Nonketotic hyperosmolar coma.

Decreased Cerebral Blood Flow

Hypovolemic shock.
Cardiac:
- Vasovagal syncope.
- Arrhythmias.
- Myocardial infarction.
- Valvular disorders.
- Congestive heart failure.
- Pericardial effusion, tamponade.
- Myocarditis.

Infectious
- Septic shock.
- Bacterial meningitis.

Vascular, hematologic
- Hypertensive encephalopathy.
- Pseudotumor cerebri.
- Hyperviscosity (sickle cell, polycythemia).
- Hyperventilation.
- Cerebral vasculitis as a manifestation of systemic lupus erythematosus.
- Thrombotic thrombocytopenic purpura.
- Disseminated intravascular coagulation.

Metabolic Cofactor Deficiency

Thiamine (Wernicke-Korsakoff syndrome).
Pyridoxine (isoniazid overdose).
Folic acid (chronic alcohol abuse).
Cyanocobalamin.
Niacin.

Electrolyte, pH Disturbances
Acidosis, alkalosis.
Hypernatremia, hyponatremia.[28]
Hypercalcemia, hypocalcemia.
Hypophosphatemia.
Hypermagnesemia, hypomagnesemia.
Endocrine Disorders
Myxedema coma, thyrotoxicosis.
Hypopituitarism.
Addison disease (primary or secondary).
Cushing's disease.
Pheochromocytoma.
Hyperparathyroidism, hypoparathyroidism.
Endogenous Toxins
Hyperammonemia (liver failure).
Uremia (renal disease).
Carbon dioxide narcosis (pulmonary disease).
Porphyria.
Exogenous Toxins
Alcohols:
- Ethanol, isopropyl alcohol, methanol, ethylene glycol.

Acid poisons:
- Salicylates.
- Paraldehyde.
- Ammonium chloride.

Antidepressant medications:
- Lithium.
- Tricyclic antidepressants.
- Selective serotonin reuptake inhibitors.
- Monoamine oxidase inhibitors.

Stimulants:
- Amphetamines, methamphetamines.
- Cocaine.
- Over-the-counter sympathomimetics.

Narcotics, opiates:
- Morphine.
- Heroin.
- Codeine, oxycodone, meperidine, hydrocodone.
- Methadone.
- Fentanyl.
- Propoxyphene.

Sedative-hypnotics:
- Benzodiazepines.
- Barbiturates.
- Rohypnol.
- Bromide.

Hallucinogens:
- Lysergic acid diethylamide.
- Marijuana.
- Mescaline, peyote.
- Mushrooms.
- Phencyclidine.

Herbs, plants:
- Aconite.
- Jimsonweed.
- Morning glory.

Volatile substances:
- Hydrocarbons (gasoline, butane, toluene, benzene, chloroform).
- Nitrites.
- Anesthetic agents (nitrous oxide, ether).

Other:
- γ-Hydroxybutyrate.
- Ketamine.
- Penicillin.
- Cardiac glycosides.
- Anticonvulsants.
- Steroids.
- Heavy metals.
- Cimetidine.
- Organophosphates.

Disorders of Temperature Regulation, Environmental
Hypothermia.
Heat stroke.
Malignant hyperthermia.
Neuroleptic malignant syndrome.
High-altitude cerebral edema.
Dysbarism.
Primary Glial or Neuronal Disorders
Adrenoleukodystrophy.
Creutzfeldt-Jakob disease.
Progressive multifocal leukoencephalopathy.
Marchiafava-Bignami disease.
Gliomatosis cerebri.
Central pontine myelinolysis.
Other Disorders with Unknown Etiology
Seizures.
Postictal states.
Reye's syndrome.
Intussusception.

[28] Can be associated with dilution of formula in infant feeding.

MESENTERIC ARTERIAL EMBOLISM, ASSOCIATED FACTORS[7]

ICD-10CM # I74.09 Other arterial embolism and thrombosis of abdominal aorta

FACTORS ASSOCIATED WITH MESENTERIC ARTERIAL EMBOLISM

Coronary artery disease:
- Post-myocardial infarction mural thrombi.
- Congestive heart failure.

Valvular heart disease:
- Rheumatic mitral valve disease.
- Nonbacterial endocarditis.

Arrhythmias:
- Chronic atrial fibrillation.

Aortic aneurysms or dissections.
Coronary angiography.

MESENTERIC ISCHEMIA, NONOCCLUSIVE[55]

ICD-10CM # K55.0 Acute vascular disorders of intestine
K55.1 Chronic vascular disorders of intestine
S35.8X9A Unspecified injury of other blood vessels at abdomen, lower back and pelvis level, initial encounter

- Cardiovascular disease resulting in low-flow states (CHF, cardiogenic shock, post cardiopulmonary bypass, dysrhythmias).
- Septic shock.
- Drug induced (cocaine, vasopressors, ergot alkaloid poisoning).

MESENTERIC VENOUS THROMBOSIS[55]

ICD-10CM # I82.91 Chronic embolism and thrombosis of unspecified vein

Hypercoagulable states (protein C or S deficiency, antithrombin III deficiency, Factor V Leyden, malignancy, polycythemia vera, sickle cell disease, homocystinemia, lupus anticoagulant, cardiolipin antibody).
Trauma (operative venous injury, abdominal trauma, postsplenectomy).
Inflammatory conditions (pancreatitis, diverticulitis, appendicitis, cholangitis).
Other: CHF, renal failure, portal hypertension, decompression sickness.

METASTATIC NEOPLASMS

ICD-10CM # C79.51 Secondary malignant neoplasm of bone
C79.52 Secondary malignant neoplasm of bone marrow
C79.31 Secondary malignant neoplasm of brain
C78.7 Secondary malignant neoplasm of liver and intrahepatic bile duct
C78.00 Secondary malignant neoplasm of unspecified lung

To: Bone
Breast.
Lung.
Prostate.
Thyroid.
Kidney.
Bladder.
Endometrium.
Cervix.
Melanoma.

To: Brain
Lung.
Breast.
Melanoma.
GU tract.
Colon.
Sinuses.
Sarcoma.
Skin.
Thyroid.

To: Liver
Colon.
Stomach.
Pancreas.
Breast.
Lymphomas.
Bronchus.
Lung.
Sarcoma.
Choriocarcinoma.
Kidney.

To: Lung
Breast.
Colon.
Kidney.
Testis.
Stomach.
Thyroid.
Melanoma.

METHEMOGLOBINEMIA, DRUG-INDUCED[42]

ICD-10CM # D74 Methaemoglobinaemia

SUBSTANCES ASSOCIATED WITH METHAEMOGLOBINAEMIA

Acetaminophen (nitrobenzene derivative).
Acetanilide.
Local anesthetics:
- Benzocaine.
- Lidocaine.
- Prilocaine.

Aniline dyes.
Celecoxib.
Dapsone.
Flutamide.
Ifosfamide.
Metoclopramide.
Nitric oxide.
Nitrites:
  Amyl nitrite.
  Isobutyl nitrite.
  Sodium nitrite.
  Nitrates (bacterial conversion to nitrites).
Nitrobenzenes/nitrobenzoates.
Nitroethane (nail polish remover).
Nitrofurans.
Nitroglycerin.
Paraquat/monolinuron.
Phenacetin.
Phenazopyridine (pyridium).
Primaquine.
Rasburicase.
Sulfamethoxazole.

MICROCEPHALY[9]

ICD-10CM # Q02 Microcephaly

PRIMARY (GENETIC)

Familial (autosomal recessive).
Autosomal dominant.
Syndromes:
  Down (21-trisomy).
  Edward (18-trisomy).
  Cri-du-chat (5 p-).
  Cornelia de Lange.
  Rubinstein-Taybi.
  Smith-Lemli-Opitz.

SECONDARY (NONGENETIC)

Radiation.
Congenital infections:
  Cytomegalovirus.
  Rubella.
  Toxoplasmosis.
Drugs:
  Fetal alcohol.
  Fetal hydantoin.
Meningitis/encephalitis.
Malnutrition.
Metabolic.
Hyperthermia.
Hypoxic-ischemic encephalopathy.

MICROPENIS[60]

ICD-10CM # N48.89 Other specified disorders of penis
Q55.62 Hypoplasia of penis

HYPOGONADOTROPIC HYPOGONADISM (HYPOTHALAMIC OR PITUITARY DEFICIENCIES)

Kallmann syndrome: autosomal dominant; associated with hyposmia.
Prader-Willi syndrome: hypotonia, mental retardation, obesity, small hands and feet.
Rud syndrome: hyposomia, ichthyosis, mental retardation.
De Morsier syndrome (septooptic dysplasia): hypopituitarism, hypoplastic optic discs, absent septum pellucidum.

HYPERGONADOTROPIC HYPOGONADISM

Primary testicular defect: disorders of testicular differentiation or inborn errors of testosterone synthesis.
Klinefelter syndrome.
Other X polysomies (i.e., XXXXY, XXXY).
Robinow syndrome: brachymesomelic dwarfism, dysmorphic facies.

PARTIAL ANDROGEN INSENSITIVITY

Idiopathic
Defective morphogenesis of the penis.

MIOSIS

ICD-10CM # H57.03 Miosis

Medications (e.g., morphine, pilocarpine).
Neurosyphilis.
Congenital.
Iritis.
CNS pontine lesion.
CNS infections.
Cavernous sinus thrombosis.
Inflammation/irritation of cornea or conjunctiva.

MONOARTHRITIS, ACUTE

ICD-10CM # M13.10 Monoarthritis, not elsewhere classified, unspecified site

Overuse.
Trauma.
Gout.
Pseudogout.
Osteoarthritis.
Infectious arthritis (e.g., gonococcal, Lyme disease, viral, mycobacteria, fungi).
Osteomyelitis.
Avascular necrosis of bone.
Hemarthrosis.
Bowel disease–associated arthritis.
Bone malignancy.
Psoriatic arthritis.
Juvenile RA.
Sarcoidosis.
Hemoglobinopathies.
Vasculitic syndromes.
Behçet's syndrome.
Foreign body synovitis.
Hypertrophic pulmonary osteoarthropathy.
Amyloidosis, familial Mediterranean fever.

MONOCYTOSIS[43]

ICD-10CM # D72.821 Monocytosis (symptomatic)

Inflammatory diseases:
  Autoimmune/granulomatous.
  Systemic lupus erythematosus.
  Rheumatoid arthritis.
  Giant cell arteritis.
  Myositis.
  Polyarteritis.
  Ulcerative colitis.
  Regional enteritis.
  Sarcoidosis.
Infectious diseases:
  Tuberculosis.
  Syphilis.
  Subacute bacterial endocarditis.
Malignant disorders:
  Preleukemia.
  Nonlymphocytic leukemia.
  Histiocytoses.
  Hodgkin's disease.
  Non-Hodgkin's lymphoma.
  Carcinomas.
Miscellaneous:
  Chronic neutropenia.
  Post splenectomy.

MONONEUROPATHY

ICD-10CM # G58.9 Mononeuropathy, unspecified

Herpes zoster.
Herpes simplex.
Vasculitis.
Trauma, compression.
Diabetes.
Postinfectious or inflammatory.

MONONEUROPATHY, ISOLATED[7]

ICD-10CM # G56.90 Unspecified mononeuropathy of unspecified upper limb

UPPER EXTREMITY

Radial nerve:
  Axilla.
  Humerus.
  Elbow (posterior interosseous neuropathy).
  Wrist (superficial cutaneous radial neuropathy).
Ulnar nerve:
  Axilla.
  Humerus.
  Elbow.
  Condylar groove.
  Cubital tunnel.
Wrist (Guyon canal).
Hand:
  Superficial terminal ulnar neuropathy.
  Deep terminal ulnar neuropathy.
    Proximal hypothenar.
    Distal hypothenar.
Median nerve.
Axilla.
Humerus (musculocutaneous mononeuropathy).
Forearm:
  Anterior interosseus.
  Pronator syndrome.
Wrist (carpal tunnel).
Hand (recurrent motor branch).
Suprascapular mononeuropathy:
  Axillary mononeuropathy.

LOWER EXTREMITY

Sciatic nerve.
Femoral nerve:

Iliacus compartment (proximal).
Saphenous mononeuropathy (distal).
Lateral femoral cutaneous (meralgia paresthetica).
Peroneal nerve:
Common peroneal mononeuropathy (fibular head, popliteal fossa).
Deep peroneal mononeuropathy (anterior compartment).
Tibial nerve:
Popliteal fossa (proximal).
Tarsal tunnel (distal).
Sural nerve:
Popliteal fossa, calf (proximal).
Fifth metatarsal base (distal).
Plantar nerve:
Distal to tarsal tunnel.
Interdigital neuropathies (Morton neuroma).
Obturator mononeuropathy.

MONONEUROPATHY MULTIPLEX[57]

ICD-10CM # G58.9 Mononeuropathy, unspecified

MONONEUROPATHY MULTIPLEX

Vasculitis
Systemic vasculitis:
Polyarteritis nodosa.
Rheumatoid arthritis.
Systemic lupus erythematosus.
Sjögren syndrome (keratoconjunctivitis sicca).
Nonsystemic vasculitis
Diabetes mellitus
Neoplastic
Paraneoplastic.
Direct infiltration.
Infectious
Lyme disease.
HIV infection.
Sarcoid
Toxic (lead)
Transient (polycythemia vera)
Cryoglobulinemia (hepatitis C)

MONONUCLEOSIS, MONOSPOT NEGATIVE[3]

ICD-10CM # B27.90 Infectious mononucleosis, unspecified without complication

DIFFERENTIAL DIAGNOSIS OF MONOSPOT-NEGATIVE MONONUCLEOSIS

Acute HIV infection.
EBV mononucleosis (particularly in children).
Cytomegalovirus.
Acute toxoplasmosis.
Streptococcal pharyngitis.
Acute hepatitis B infection.

EBV, Epstein-Barr virus; *HIV,* human immunodeficiency virus.

MOVEMENT DISORDER, PEDIATRIC PATIENT[49]

ICD-10CM # G25.9 Extrapyramidal and movement disorder, unspecified

COMMONLY CITED MOVEMENT DISORDERS THAT MAY BEGIN IN CHILDHOOD OR ADOLESCENCE

Early Childhood
Athetosis or choreoathetosis.
Lesch–Nyhan syndrome.*
Childhood
Dopa-responsive dystonia.*
Dystonia associated with *DYT1* gene.*
Myoclonus from subacute sclerosing panencephalitis (SSPE).
Parkinson's disease.
Sydenham chorea.
Tourette's syndrome.*
Withdrawal-emergent dyskinesia.
Adolescence
Essential tremor.*
Huntington disease (juvenile Huntington disease).*
Medication- and drug-induced movements.
Tardive dyskinesias.
Wilson's disease.*

MOVEMENT DISORDERS AND COGNITIVE IMPAIRMENT[49]

ICD-10CM # G25.9 Extrapyramidal and movement disorder, unspecified

MOVEMENT DISORDERS ASSOCIATED WITH COGNITIVE IMPAIRMENT

Young Children
Athetosis or choreoathetosis.*
Lesch–Nyhan syndrome.
Rett syndrome.
Older Children and Adolescents
Huntington disease.
Subacute sclerosing panencephalitis.
Wilson disease.
Adults
Creutzfeldt-Jakob disease.†
Huntington disease.
Parkinson's disease.

*Genetic transmission.
*Despite incapacitating movements, many choreoathetosis patients have no mental retardation.
†Myoclonus.

MOVEMENT DISORDERS, NEUROLEPTIC-INDUCED[49]

ICD-10CM # G25.70 Drug-induced movement disorder, unspecified

Acute dyskinesias:
Akathisia.
Neuroleptic-malignant syndrome.
Oculogyric crisis and other dystonias.
Tardive dyskinesias:
Akathisia.
Dystonia.
Oral-buccal-lingual dyskinesia.*
Tics.
Tremor.
Stereotypies.
Dose-dependent dyskinesia:
Parkinsonism.
Withdrawal-emergent dyskinesias.

*Commonly referred to as "tardive dyskinesia"

MUSCLE DISEASE[75]

ICD-10CM # M60.009 Infective myositis, unspecified site

CLASSIFICATION OF MUSCLE DISEASE

Muscular Dystrophies
Duchenne.
Becker.
Limb girdle.
Childhood.
Facioscapulohumeral.
Myotonic Disorders
Dystrophia myotonica.
Myotonica congenita.
Inflammatory
Infective: bacterial, viral, parasitic.
Unknown cause: polymyositis, dermatomyositis, sarcoidosis.
Endocrine
Thyroid disease—hyper- and hypothyroidism.
Cushing's disease.
Addison disease.
Hyperparathyroidism.
Metabolic
- Glycogen storage diseases.
- Periodic paralyses.
- Mitochondrial diseases.

Drug-induced
- Corticosteroids.
- Chloroquine.
- Amiodarone.
- Penicillamine.
- Alcohol.
- Zidovudine.
- Clofibrate.

Other
- Inclusion body myositis.

MUSCLE WEAKNESS

ICD-10CM # M62.9 Disorder of muscle, unspecified

Physical deconditioning.
Impaired cardiac output (e.g., mitral stenosis, mitral regurgitation).
Uremia, liver failure.
Electrolyte abnormalities (hypokalemia, hyperkalemia, hypophosphatemia, hypercalcemia), hypoglycemia.
Drug induced (e.g., statin myopathy).
Muscular dystrophies.
Steroid myopathy.
Alcoholic myopathy.
Myasthenia gravis, Lambert-Eaton syndrome.

Infections (polio, botulism, HIV, hepatitis, diphtheria, tick paralysis, neurosyphilis, brucellosis, TB, trichinosis).
Pernicious anemia, other anemias, beriberi.
Psychiatric illness (depression, somatization syndrome).
Organophosphate or arsenic poisoning.
Inflammatory myopathies (e.g., collagen vascular disease, RA, sarcoidosis).
Endocrinopathies (e.g., adrenal insufficiency, hypothyroidism), diabetic neuropathy.
Other: motor neuron disease, mitochondrial myopathy, l-tryptophan (eosinophilia-myalgia), rhabdomyolysis, glycogen storage disease, lipid storage disease.

MUSCLE WEAKNESS, LOWER MOTOR NEURON VERSUS UPPER MOTOR NEURON

ICD-10CM # M62.9 Disorder of muscle, unspecified

LOWER MOTOR NEURON

Weakness, usually severe.
Marked muscle atrophy.
Fasciculations.
Decreased muscle stretch reflexes.
Clonus not present.
Flaccidity.
No Babinski sign.
Asymmetric and may involve one limb only in the beginning to become generalized as the disease progresses.

UPPER MOTOR NEURON

Weakness, usually less severe.
Minimal disuse muscle atrophy.
No fasciculations.
Increased muscle stretch reflexes.
Clonus may be present.
Spasticity.
Babinski sign.
Often initial impairment of only skilled movements.
In the limbs the following muscles may be the only ones weak or weaker than the others: triceps; wrist and finger extensors; interossei; iliopsoas; hamstrings; and foot dorsiflexors, inverters, and extroverters.

MUSCULOSKELETAL BENIGN TUMORS AND TUMORLIKE LESIONS[66]

ICD-10CM # Varies with specific diagnosis

Fibrous dysplasia.
Enchondromatosis.
Osteochondromatosis.
Synovial cysts.
Brown tumors in hyperparathyroidism.
Langerhans cell histiocytosis (eosinophilic granuloma).
Hemangiomatosis.
Bone islands, osteoma (Gardner syndrome).
Fibrous cortical defect, nonossifying fibroma.
Giant cell tumor.
Neurofibromatosis.
Amyloidosis.
Mastocytosis.
SAPHO, chronic multifocal osteomyelitis.

SAPHO, Synovitis, acne, pustulosis, hyperostosis, osteitis.

MUSCULOSKELETAL MALIGNANT TUMORS AND TUMORLIKE LESIONS[66]

ICD-10CM # Varies with specific diagnosis

Metastases.
Myeloma.
Angiosarcoma.
Leukemia.
Neuroblastoma.
Ewing sarcoma.
Osteosarcomatosis.
Lymphoma.

MYDRIASIS

ICD-10CM # H57.04 Mydriasis

Coma.
Medications (cocaine, atropine, epinephrine, etc.).
Glaucoma.
Cerebral aneurysm.
Ocular trauma.
Head trauma.
Optic atrophy.
Cerebral neoplasm.
Iridocyclitis.

MYELIN DISORDERS

ICD-10CM # Varies with specific diagnosis

Multiple sclerosis.
Vitamin B_{12} deficiency.
Radiation.
Hypoxia.
Toxicity from carbon monoxide, alcohol, mercury.
Progressive multifocal encephalopathy.
Acute disseminated encephalomyelitis.
Acute hemorrhagic leukoencephalopathy.
Phenylketonuria.
Adrenoleukodystrophy.
Krabbe disease.

MYELITIS[83]

ICD-10CM # G04.91 Myelitis, unspecified
G04.89 Other myelitis

Viral
HIV.
HSV-1 and HSV-2.
VZV.
CMV.
EBV.
WNV.
HTLV.
Bacterial
Mycoplasma pneumoniae.
Borrelia burgdorferi.
Treponema pallidum.
Pyogenic bacteria.
Mycobacterium tuberculosis.
Fungal
Coccidioides immitis.
Actinomyces.
Aspergillus.
Blastomyces dermatitidis.
Histoplasmosis.
Immune-Mediated
Multiple sclerosis.
Neuromyelitis optica.
Connective tissue disorders (neuro-lupus, neuro-Sjögren).
Neurosarcoidosis.
Paraneoplastic.
Noninflammatory Myelopathies
Vitamin B_{12} deficiency.
Folic acid deficiency.
Copper deficiency.
Vitamin E deficiency.
Nitrous oxide toxicity.
Heroin.
Radiation myelopathy.
Traumatic/compressive myelopathy.
Vascular myelopathy.

MYELOPATHY AND MYELITIS[77]

ICD-10CM # M51.9 Unspecified thoracic, thoracolumbar and lumbosacral intervertebral disc disorder
G95.9 Disease of spinal cord, unspecified

INFLAMMATORY

Infectious: spirochetal TB, zoster, rabies, HIV, polio, rickettsial, fungal, parasitic.
Noninfectious: idiopathic transverse myelitis, multiple sclerosis.

TOXIC/METABOLIC

DM, pernicious anemia, chronic liver disease, pellagra, arsenic.

TRAUMA COMPRESSION

Spinal neoplasm, cervical spondylosis, epidural abscess, epidural hematoma.

VASCULAR

AV malformation, SLE, periarteritis nodosa, dissecting aortic aneurysm.

PHYSICAL AGENTS

Electrical injury, irradiation.

NEOPLASTIC

Spinal cord tumors, paraneoplastic myelopathy.

MYOCARDIAL ISCHEMIA[77]

ICD-10CM # I25.5 Ischemic cardiomyopathy
I25.89 Other forms of chronic ischemic heart disease
I25.9 Chronic ischemic heart disease, unspecified
I24.8 Other forms of acute ischemic heart disease

Atherosclerotic obstructive coronary artery disease.

Nonatherosclerotic coronary artery disease:
- Coronary artery spasm.
- Congenital coronary artery anomalies:
  - Anomalous origin of coronary artery from pulmonary artery.
  - Aberrant origin of coronary artery from aorta or another coronary artery.
  - Coronary arteriovenous fistula.
  - Coronary artery aneurysm.

Acquired disorders of coronary arteries:
- Coronary artery embolism.
- Dissection:
  - Surgical.
  - During percutaneous coronary angioplasty.
  - Aortic dissection.
  - Spontaneous (e.g., during pregnancy).
- Extrinsic compression:
  - Tumors.
  - Granulomas.
  - Amyloidosis.
- Collagen-vascular disease:
  - Polyarteritis nodosa.
  - Temporal arteritis.
  - RA.
  - SLE.
  - Scleroderma.
- Miscellaneous disorders:
  - Irradiation.
  - Trauma.
  - Kawasaki disease.

Syphilis.

Hereditary disorders:
- Pseudoxanthoma elasticum.
- Gargoylism.
- Progeria.
- Homocystinuria.
- Primary oxaluria.

"Functional" causes of myocardial ischemia in absence of anatomic coronary artery disease:
- Syndrome X.
- Hypertrophic cardiomyopathy.
- Dilated cardiomyopathy.
- Muscle bridge.
- Hypertensive heart disease.
- Pulmonary hypertension.
- Valvular heart disease; aortic stenosis, aortic regurgitation.

MYOCLONUS

ICD-10CM # G25.3 Myoclonus

Physiologic (e.g., exercise or anxiety induced).
Renal failure.
Hepatic failure.
Hyponatremia.
Hypoglycemia or severe hyperglycemia.
Postdialysis.
Epileptic myoclonus.
Postencephalitis.
CNS lesion (stroke, neoplasm).
CNS trauma.
Parkinson's disease.
Medications (e.g., tricyclics, L-dopa).
Friedreich ataxia.
Ataxia-telangiectasia.
Wilson's disease.
Huntington disease.
Progressive supranuclear palsy.
Heavy metal poisoning.
Benign familial.

MYOCLONUS, DRUG-INDUCED[79]

ICD-10CM # G25.79 Other drug-induced movement disorders

SELECTED AGENTS ASSOCIATED WITH MYOCLONUS

Medications

Antibiotics (β-lactams).
Antidepressants.
Antineoplastics: busulfan, chlorambucil.
Carbamazepine, vigabatrin.
Clozapine.
l-DOPA.
Lidocaine.
Lithium.
Lorazepam (preterm infants).
Methaqualone.
Morphine.
Nitroprusside.
Piperazine.

Industrial Toxins

Camphor.
Chlorophenoxy herbicides.
Gasoline.

Biological Toxins

Buckeye (*Aesculus* spp.).
Lupine.
Shellfish (domoic acid poisoning).

MYOPATHIC SYNDROMES, DRUG-INDUCED[40]

ICD-10CM # G72.9 Myopathy, unspecified

TYPE OF MYOPATHY

Necrotizing myopathy.
Inflammatory myopathy.
Mitochondrial myopathy.
Hypokalemic myopathy.
Antimicrotubular myopathy.
Lysosomal storage myopathy.
Corticosteroid myopathy.
Others.

DRUGS

HMG-CoA reductase inhibitors (statins), fibrates, alcohol.
Penicillamine, interferon-a, procainamide.
Zidovudine.
Diuretics, laxatives, licorice, amphotericin B, alcohol.
Colchicine, vincristine.
Chloroquine, hydroxychloroquine, quinacrine, amiodarone, perhexiline.
Corticosteroids, especially fluorinated.
Ipecac syrup, emetine.

MYOPATHIES ASSOCIATED WITH REST PAIN[40]

ICD-10CM # G72.9 Myopathy, unspecified

Childhood dermatomyositis.
Hypothyroid myopathy.
Acute alcoholic myopathy.
Drug-induced myopathies.
Infectious myopathies.
Myopathies associated with metabolic bone disease.
Carnitine palmitoyl transferase deficiency.
Rhabdomyolysis from any cause.

MYOPATHIES, HIV ASSOCIATED[27]

ICD-10CM # R25.2

HIV-Associated Myopathies	Myopathies Secondary to Antiretrovirals	Others
HIV polymyositis.	Zidovudine myopathy.	Opportunistic infections involving muscle (toxoplasmosis).
Inclusion body myositis.	Toxic mitochondrial myopathies related to other NRTIs.	Tumor infiltrations of skeletal muscle.
Nemaline myopathy.		Rhabdomyolysis.
Diffuse infiltrative lymphocytosis syndrome.	HIV-associated lipodystrophy syndrome.	
HIV wasting syndrome.	Immune reconstitution syndrome related to ART.	
Vasculitic processes.		
Myasthenia gravis and other myasthenic syndromes.		
Chronic fatigue and fibromyalgia.		

NRTIs, nucleoside reverse transcriptase inhibitors; *ART,* antiretroviral therapy.

MYOPATHIES, INFECTIOUS

ICD-10CM # G72.9 Myopathy, unspecified

HIV.
Viral myositis.
Trichinosis.
Toxoplasmosis.
Cysticercosis.

MYOPATHIES, INFLAMMATORY

ICD-10CM # G72.9 Myopathy, unspecified

SLE, RA.
Sarcoidosis.
Paraneoplastic syndrome.
Polymyositis, dermatomyositis.
Polyarteritis nodosa.
Mixed connective tissue disease.
Scleroderma.
Inclusion body myositis.
Sjögren syndrome.
Cimetidine, D-penicillamine.

MYOPATHIES, METABOLIC[40]

ICD-10CM # G72.9 Myopathy, unspecified

DISORDERED GLYCOGEN METABOLISM

Myophosphorylase deficiency (McArdle disease).
Phosphorylase b kinase deficiency.
Phosphofructokinase deficiency.
Debrancher enzyme deficiency.
Brancher enzyme deficiency.
Phosphoglycerate kinase deficiency.
Phosphoglycerate mutase deficiency.
Lactate dehydrogenase deficiency.
Acid maltase deficiency.
Aldolase deficiency.
b-Enolase deficiency.

DISORDERED LIPID METABOLISM

Carnitine deficiencies.
Carnitine palmitoyltransferase deficiency.
Fatty acid acyl-CoA dehydrogenase deficiencies.

MITOCHONDRIAL MYOPATHIES

Coenzyme Q10 deficiency.
Respiratory chain complex deficiencies.

ENDOCRINE

Acromegaly.
Hypothyroidism.
Hyperthyroidism.
Hyperparathyroidism.
Cushing's disease.
Addison disease.
Hyperaldosteronism.

METABOLIC-NUTRITIONAL

Uremia.
Hepatic failure.
Malabsorption.
Periodic paralysis.
Vitamin D deficiency.
Vitamin E deficiency.

ELECTROLYTE DISORDERS

Sodium: hypernatremia and hyponatremia.
Potassium: hyperkalemia and hypokalemia.
Calcium: hypercalcemia and hypocalcemia.
Phosphate: hypophosphatemia.
Magnesium: hypomagnesemia.

MYOPATHIES, TOXIC[3]

ICD-10CM # G72.2 Myopathy due to other toxic agents

Inflammatory: cimetidine, D-penicillamine.
Noninflammatory necrotizing or vacuolar: cholesterol-lowering agents, chloroquine, colchicine.
Acute muscle necrosis and myoglobinuria: cholesterol-lowering drugs, alcohol, cocaine.
Malignant hyperthermia: halothane, ethylene, others; succinylcholine.
Mitochondrial: zidovudine.
Myosin loss: nondepolarizing neuromuscular blocking agents; glucocorticoids.

MYOSITIS, INFECTIOUS CAUSES[40]

ICD-10CM # M60.009 Infective myositis, unspecified site

VIRAL

Influenza A and B viruses.
Enteroviruses (coxsackieviruses, echoviruses).
Human immunodeficiency virus.
Human T-cell lymphotrophic virus type 1.
Hepatitis B and C viruses.
Cytomegalovirus.
Epstein-Barr virus.
Adenovirus.
Varicella-zoster virus.
Parainfluenza.

PARASITIC

Trichinella species.
Echinococcus species.
Schistosoma species.
Toxoplasma gondii.
Trypanosoma cruzi.
Sarcocystis species.

BACTERIAL

Staphylococcus aureus.
Streptococcus, groups A and B.
Aeromonas hydrophila.
Borrelia burgdorferi.
Clostridium perfringens.
Anaerobic streptococci.
Mycobacterium species.
Rickettsia species.

FUNGAL

Candida species.
Cryptococcus neoformans.
Microsporida.

MYOSITIS, INFLAMMATORY[3]

ICD-10CM # M60.009 Infective myositis, unspecified site
M60.9 Myositis, unspecified
M60.10 Interstitial myositis of unspecified site

INFECTIOUS

Viral myositis:
- Retroviruses (HIV, HTLV-I).
- Enteroviruses (echovirus, Coxsackievirus).
- Other viruses (influenza, hepatitis A and B, Epstein-Barr virus).

Bacterial: pyomyositis.
Parasites: trichinosis, cysticercosis.
Fungi: candidiasis.

IDIOPATHIC

Granulomatous myositis (sarcoid, giant cell).
Eosinophilic myositis.
Eosinophilia-myalgia syndrome.

ENDOCRINE/METABOLIC DISORDERS

Hypothyroidism.
Hyperthyroidism.
Hypercortisolism.
Hyperparathyroidism.
Hypoparathyroidism.
Hypocalcemia.
Hypokalemia.

METABOLIC MYOPATHIES

Myophosphorylase deficiency (McArdle disease).
Phosphofructokinase deficiency.
Myoadenylate deaminase deficiency.
Acid maltase deficiency.
Lipid storage diseases.
Acute rhabdomyolysis.

DRUG-INDUCED MYOPATHIES

Alcohol.
d-Penicillamine.
Zidovudine.
Colchicine.
Chloroquine, hydroxychloroquine.
Lipid-lowering agents.
Cyclosporine.
Cocaine, heroin, barbiturates.
Corticosteroids.

NEUROLOGIC DISORDERS

Muscular dystrophies.
Congenital myopathies.
Motor neuron disease.
Guillain-Barré syndrome.
Myasthenia gravis.

NAIL CLUBBING

ICD-10CM # R68.3 Clubbing of nails

COPD.
Pulmonary malignancy.
Cirrhosis.
Inflammatory bowel disease.
Chronic bronchitis.
Congenital heart disease.
Endocarditis.
AV malformations.
Asbestosis.
Trauma.
Idiopathic.

NAIL, HORIZONTAL WHITE LINES (BEAU LINES)

ICD-10CM # L60.4 Beau lines

Malnutrition.
Idiopathic.
Trauma.
Prolonged systemic illnesses.
Pemphigus.
Raynaud's disease.

NAIL KOILONYCHIA

ICD-10CM # L60.8 Other nail disorders

Trauma.
Iron deficiency.
SLE.
Hemochromatosis.
Raynaud's disease.
Nail-patella syndrome.
Idiopathic.

NAIL ONYCHOLYSIS

ICD-10CM # L60.1 Onycholysis

Infection.
Trauma.
Psoriasis.
Connective tissue disorders.
Sarcoidosis.
Hyperthyroidism.
Amyloidosis.
Nutritional deficiencies.

NAIL PITTING

ICD-10CM # L60.8 Other nail disorders

Psoriasis.
Alopecia areata.
Reiter syndrome.
Trauma.
Idiopathic.

NAIL SPLINTER HEMORRHAGE

ICD-10CM # L60.8 Other nail disorders

SBE.
Trauma.
Malignancies.
Oral contraceptives.
Pregnancy.
SLE.
Antiphospholipid syndrome.
Psoriasis.
RA.
Peptic ulcer disease.

NAIL STRIATIONS

ICD-10CM # L60.8 Other nail disorders

Psoriasis.
Alopecia areata.
Trauma.
Atopic dermatitis.
Vitiligo.

NAIL TELANGIECTASIA

ICD-10CM # L60.8 Other nail disorders

RA.
Scleroderma.
Trauma.
SLE.
Dermatomyositis.

NAIL WHITENING (TERRY NAILS)

ICD-10CM # L60.8 Other nail disorders

Malnutrition.
Trauma.
Liver disease (cirrhosis, hepatic failure).
DM.
Hyperthyroidism.
Idiopathic.

NAIL YELLOWING

ICD-10CM # L60.8 Other nail disorders

Tobacco abuse.
Nephrotic syndrome.
Chronic infections (TB, sinusitis).
Bronchiectasis.
Lymphedema.
Raynaud's disease.
RA.
Pleural effusions.
Thyroiditis.
Immunodeficiency.

NASAL AND PARANASAL SINUS TUMORS[36]

ICD-10CM # C30.0 Malignant neoplasm of nasal cavity

BENIGN AND MALIGNANT NASAL AND PARANASAL SINUS TUMORS

Epithelial Tumors

BENIGN

Papilloma.
Adenoma.
Inverting papilloma.

MALIGNANT

Squamous carcinoma.
Adenocarcinoma.
Melanoma.
Adenoid cystic carcinoma.
Malignant salivary tumors.

MESENCHYMAL TUMORS

Benign

Osteoma.
Ossifying fibroma complex.
Angiofibroma.
Chondroma.

Malignant

Osteogenic sarcoma.
Fibrosarcoma.
Angiosarcoma.
Chondrosarcoma.
Lymphoma.
Rhabdomyosarcoma.

NASAL MASSES, CONGENITAL[36]

ICD-10CM # J34.1 Cyst and mucocele of nose and nasal sinus
J34.89 Other specified disorders of nose and nasal sinuses

Dermoid.
Nasal cerebral heterotopia (glioma).
Frontal meningoencephalocele.
Nasolacrimal duct mucocele.
Nasal hamartoma.
Nasal hemangioma.

NAUSEA AND VOMITING

ICD-10CM # R11.2 Nausea with vomiting, unspecified

Infections (viral, bacterial).
Intestinal obstruction.
Metabolic (uremia, electrolyte abnormalities, DKA, acidosis, etc.).
Severe pain.
Anxiety, fear.
Psychiatric disorders (bulimia, anorexia nervosa).
Pregnancy.
Medications (NSAIDs, erythromycin, morphine, codeine, aminophylline, chemotherapeutic agents, etc.).
Withdrawal from substance abuse (drugs, alcohol).
Head trauma.
Vestibular or middle ear disease.
Migraine headache.
CNS neoplasms.
Radiation sickness.
PUD.
Carcinoma of GI tract.
Reye syndrome.
Eye disorders.
Abdominal trauma.

NAUSEA AND VOMITING, CAUSES DURING PREGNANCY[30]

ICD-10CM # R11.2 Nausea with vomiting, unspecified

DIFFERENTIAL DIAGNOSIS OF NAUSEA AND VOMITING DURING PREGNANCY

Nausea and vomiting of pregnancy.
Hyperemesis gravidarum.
Pancreatitis.
Symptomatic cholelithiasis.
Viral hepatitis.
Peptic ulcer disease.
Gastric cancer.
Intestinal obstruction.
Intestinal pseudoobstruction.
Gastroparesis diabeticorum.
Gastritis.
Gastroesophageal reflux disease.
Acute pyelonephritis.
Drug toxicity.
Vagotomy.
Preeclampsia/eclampsia.
Acute fatty liver of pregnancy.
Hemolysis, elevated liver enzymes, and low platelets (HELLP) syndrome.
Anorexia nervosa/bulimia.
Other neuropsychiatric disorders.

NAUSEA AND VOMITING, CHRONIC[26]

ICD-10CM # R11.2 Nausea with vomiting, unspecified

DIFFERENTIAL DIAGNOSIS OF CHRONIC NAUSEA AND VOMITING

Mechanical GI tract obstruction (pylorus, bile duct, small intestine, colon)
Mucosal inflammation
Peritoneal irritation
Carcinomas (e.g., gastric, ovarian, renal, bronchogenic)

Metabolic/endocrine disorders (diabetic mellitus, hypothyroidism, hyperthyroidism, adrenal insufficiency, uremia)
Medications (anticholinergics, narcotics, L-dopa, progesterone, calcium channel blockers, digitalis, NSAIDs, antidysrhythmic agents, lubiprostone, cannabis, metformin, amylin analogs)
Gastroparesis
Gastric dysrhythmias (tachygastria, bradygastria, mixed)
CNS disorders (tumors, migraine, seizures, stroke, orthostatic intolerance)
Psychogenic disorders (anorexia nervosa, bulimia nervosa)

NECK AND ARM PAIN

ICD-10CM #		
	M54.2	Cervicalgia
	S46.919A	Strain of unspecified muscle, fascia and tendon at shoulder and upper arm level, unspecified arm, initial encounter

Cervical disk syndrome.
Trauma, musculoskeletal strain.
Rotator cuff syndrome.
Bicipital tendonitis.
Glenohumeral arthritis.
Acromioclavicular arthritis.
Thoracic outlet syndrome.
Pancoast tumor.
Infection (cellulitis, abscess).
Angina pectoris.

NECK MASS[61]

ICD-10CM # R22.1 Localized swelling, mass and lump, neck

CONGENITAL ANOMALIES

Thyroglossal duct cyst.
Bronchial apparatus anomalies.
Teratomas.
Ranula.
Dermoid cysts.
Hemangioma.
Laryngoceles.
Cystic hygroma.

NONNEOPLASTIC INFLAMMATORY ETIOLOGIES

Folliculitis.
Adenopathy secondary to peritonsillar abscess.
Retropharyngeal or parapharyngeal abscess.
Salivary gland infections.
Viral infections (mononucleosis, HIV, CMV).
TB.
Cat-scratch disease.
Toxoplasmosis.
Actinomyces.
Atypical mycobacterium.
Jugular vein thrombus.

NEOPLASM (PRIMARY OR METASTATIC)

LIPOMA

NECK PAIN[61]

ICD-10CM # M54.2 Cervicalgia

INFLAMMATORY DISEASES

RA.
Spondyloarthropathies.
Juvenile RA.

NONINFLAMMATORY DISEASE

Cervical osteoarthritis.
Diskogenic neck pain.
Diffuse idiopathic skeletal hyperostosis.
Fibromyalgia or myofascial pain.

INFECTIOUS CAUSES

Meningitis.
Osteomyelitis.
Infectious diskitis.

NEOPLASMS

Primary.
Metastatic.

REFERRED PAIN

Temporomandibular joint pain.
Cardiac pain.
Diaphragmatic irritation.
GI sources (gastric ulcer, gallbladder, pancreas).

NECK PAIN FROM RHEUMATOLOGIC DISORDERS[27]

ICD-10CM # M54.2 Cervicalgia

Rheumatoid arthritis:
- Without disease of the C1-C2 joint.
- With structural cervical abnormalities: C1-C2 subluxation, C1-C2 facet involvement.

Spondyloarthropathies.
Reactive arthritis.
Psoriatic arthritis.
Enteropathic arthritis.
Polymyalgia rheumatica.
Osteoarthritis.
Fibromyalgia.
Nonspecific musculoskeletal pain.
Miscellaneous spondyloarthropathies:
- Whipple disease.
- Behçet's disease.
- Paget disease.
- Acromegaly.
- Ossification of the posterior longitudinal ligament.
- Diffuse idiopathic skeletal hyperostosis.

NECROTIZING PNEUMONIAS[3]

ICD-10CM # J15.8 Pneumonia due to other specified bacteria

COMMON

Tuberculosis.
Staphylococcus.
Gram-negative bacilli.
Anaerobes.
Fungi.
Pneumocystis jirovecii.

RARE

Streptococcus pneumoniae.
Legionella.
Viruses.
Mycoplasma pneumoniae.

NEPHRITIC SYNDROME, ACUTE[3]

ICD-10CM # N00.8 Acute nephritic syndrome with other morphologic changes

LOW SERUM COMPLEMENT LEVEL

Acute postinfectious glomerulonephritis.
Membranoproliferative glomerulonephritis.
SLE.
Subacute bacterial endocarditis.
Visceral abscess "shunt" nephritis.
Cryoglobulinemia.

NORMAL SERUM COMPLEMENT LEVEL

IgA nephropathy.
Antiglomerular basement membrane disease.
Polyarteritis nodosa.
Granulomatosis with polyangiitis.
Henoch-Schönlein purpura.
Goodpasture syndrome.

NEPHROCALCINOSIS

ICD-10CM # E83.59 Other disorders of calcium metabolism

Sarcoidosis.
Hyperparathyroidism.
Chronic glomerulonephritis.
Milk-alkali syndrome.
Distal renal tubular acidosis.
Medullary sponge kidney.
Bartter syndrome.
Hypervitaminosis D.
Idiopathic hypercalciuria.
Hyperoxaluria.
Cortical necrosis.
Tuberculosis.
Idiopathic hypercalciuria.
Rapidly progressive osteoporosis.

NEPHROPATHY, OBSTRUCTIVE[85]

ICD-10CM # Varies with specific diagnosis

POSSIBLE CAUSES OF OBSTRUCTIVE NEPHROPATHY

Renal

Congenital

Polycystic kidney.
Renal cyst.
Peripelvic cyst.
Ureteropelvic junction obstruction.

Neoplastic
Wilms tumor.
Renal cell carcinoma.
Transitional cell carcinoma of the collecting system.
Multiple myeloma.
Inflammatory
Tuberculosis.
Echinococcus infection.
Metabolic
Calculi.
Miscellaneous
Sloughed papillae.
Trauma.
Renal artery aneurysm.
URETER
Congenital
Stricture.
Ureterocele.
Obstructing megaureter.
Retrocaval ureter.
Prune belly syndrome.
Neoplastic
Primary carcinoma of ureter.
Metastatic carcinoma.
Inflammatory
Tuberculosis.
Amyloidosis.
Schistosomiasis.
Abscess.
Ureteritis cystica.
Endometriosis.
Miscellaneous
Retroperitoneal fibrosis.
Pelvic lipomatosis.
Aortic aneurysm.
Radiation therapy.
Lymphocele.
Trauma.
Urinoma.
Pregnancy.
Radiofrequency ablation.
BLADDER AND URETHRA
Congenital
Posterior urethral valve.
Phimosis.
Hydrocolpos.
Neoplastic
Bladder carcinoma.
Prostate carcinoma.
Carcinoma of urethra.
Carcinoma of penis.
Inflammatory
Prostatitis.
Paraurethral abscess.
Miscellaneous
Benign prostatic hypertrophy.
Neurogenic bladder.
Urethral stricture.

NEUROGENIC BLADDER[62]

ICD-10CM #	N31.9	Neuromuscular dysfunction of bladder, unspecified

SUPRATENTORIAL

CVA.
Parkinson's disease.
Alzheimer's disease.
Cerebral palsy.

SPINAL CORD

Spinal cord injury.
Spinal stenosis.
Central cord syndrome.
ALS.
Multiple sclerosis.
Myelodysplasia.

PERIPHERAL NEUROPATHY

Diabetes.
Alcohol.
Shingles.
Syphilis.

NEUROLOGIC DEFICIT, FOCAL[55]

ICD-10CM #	G45.9	Transient cerebral ischemic attack, unspecified
	I67.848	Other cerebrovascular vasospasm and vasoconstriction

TRAUMATIC: INTRACRANIAL, INTRASPINAL

Subdural hematoma.
Intraparenchymal hemorrhage.
Epidural hematoma.
Traumatic hemorrhagic necrosis.

INFECTIOUS

Brain abscess.
Epidural and subdural abscesses.
Meningitis.

NEOPLASTIC

Primary CNS tumors.
Metastatic tumors.
Syringomyelia.
Vascular.
Thrombosis.
Embolism.
Spontaneous hemorrhage: arteriovenous malformation, aneurysm, hypertensive.

METABOLIC

Hypoglycemia.
B_{12} deficiency.
Postseizure.
Hyperosmolar nonketotic.

OTHER

Migraine.
Bell palsy.
Psychogenic.

NEUROLOGIC DEFICIT, MULTIFOCAL[55]

ICD-10CM #	I67.89	Other cerebrovascular disease
	G45.9	Transient cerebral ischemic attack, unspecified
	I67.848	Other cerebrovascular vasospasm and vasoconstriction

Acute disseminated encephalomyelitis: postviral or postimmunization.
Infectious encephalomyelitis: poliovirus, enteroviruses, arbovirus, herpes zoster, Epstein-Barr virus.
Granulomatous encephalomyelitis: sarcoid.
Autoimmune: SLE.
Other: familial spinocerebellar degenerations.

NEUROMUSCULAR JUNCTION DYSFUNCTION[3]

ICD-10CM #	N31.9	Neuromuscular dysfunction of bladder, unspecified

DISORDERS OF THE NEUROMUSCULAR JUNCTION

Autoimmune
Myasthenia gravis.
Lambert-Eaton myasthenic syndrome.
Congenital
Presynaptic defects in ACh resynthesis, packaging, or release.
Synaptic defect: congenital end plate AChE deficiency.
Postsynaptic defects: slow-channel syndromes.
Postsynaptic defects: decreased response to ACh:
Fast-channel syndromes.
AChR deficiency without kinetic abnormality.
Familial limb-girdle myasthenia.
Toxic
Botulism.
Drug-induced disorders.
Organophosphate intoxication.

Ach, Acetylcholine; *AChE,* acetylcholinesterase; *AChR,* acetylcholine receptor.

NEURONOPATHIES, SENSORY (GANGLIONOPATHIES)[7]

ICD-10CM #	G60.0	Hereditary motor and sensory neuropathy

Herpes:
Herpes simplex I and II.
Varicella zoster (shingles).
Inflammatory sensory polyganglionopathy (ISP).
Paraneoplastic.
Primary biliary cirrhosis.
Sjögren syndrome (keratoconjunctivitis sicca).
Toxin-induced:
Pyridoxine (vitamin B_6) overdose.
Metals:
Platinum (cisplatin).
Methyl mercury.
Vitamin E deficiency.

NEUROPATHIC BLADDER

ICD-10CM #	N31.9	Neuromuscular dysfunction of bladder, unspecified

Diabetes.
Stroke.

Multiple sclerosis.
Parkinson's disease.
Dementia.
Encephalopathy.
Brain trauma.
Spinal cord trauma.
Pelvic surgery.
Spina bifida.

NEUROPATHIES WITH FACIAL NERVE INVOLVEMENT

ICD-10CM #	G51.8	Other disorders of facial nerve

Sarcoidosis.
HIV.
Lyme disease.
Guillain-Barré.
Others: chronic inflammatory polyneuropathy, Tangier disease, amyloidosis.

NEUROPATHIES, AUTONOMIC[51]

ICD-10CM #	G63	Polyneuropathy in diseases classified elsewhere

GUILLAIN-BARRÉ SYNDROME

Non–Gulllain-Barré syndrome autoimmunity.
Paraneoplastic (type I antineuronal nuclear antibody).
Lambert-Eaton syndrome.
Antibodies to neuronal nicotinc acetylcholine receptors.
Antibodies to P/Q type calcium channels.
Other autoantibodies.
Systemic lupus erythematosus.

HEREDITARY

Type I autosomal dominant.
Type II autosomal recessive (Morvan disease).
Type III autosomal recessive (Riley-Day).
Type IV autosomal recessive (congenital insensitivity to pain with anhidrosis).
Type V absence of pain.

METABOLIC

Fabry disease.
Diabetes mellitus.
Tangier disease.
Porphyria.

INFECTIOUS

HIV.
Chagas' disease.
Botulism.
Leprosy.
Diphtheria.

OTHER

Triple A (Allgrove) syndrome.
Navajo Indian neuropathy.
Multiple endocrine neoplasia type 2b.
TOXINS

NEUROPATHIES, AUTONOMIC, PERIPHERAL, CAUSES[34]

ICD-10CM #	G90.09	Other idiopathic peripheral autonomic neuropathy

METABOLIC

Diabetes mellitus.
Alcohol.
Acute intermittent porphyria.
Uremia.

AUTOIMMUNE

Autoimmune autonomic ganglionopathy.
Guillain-Barré syndrome.
Morvan syndrome.
Lambert-Eaton myasthenic syndrome.
Chronic inflammatory demyelinating polyradiculoneuropathy.
Sjögren syndrome.
Systemic lupus erythematosus.
Mixed connective tissue diseases.

PARAPROTEINEMIC

Amyloidosis.

NUTRITIONAL

Cyanocobalamin deficiency.
Thiamine deficiency.
Gluten-sensitive neuropathy.

TOXIC

Heavy metals.
Organic solvents.
Organophosphates.
Vacor.
Acrylamide.

DRUG INDUCED

Cisplatin.
Vincristine.
Amiodarone.
Metronidazole.
Perhexiline.
Paclitaxel.

INFECTIOUS

HIV.
Leprosy.
Chagas' disease.
Botulism.
Diphtheria.
Lyme disease.

GENETIC

Hereditary sensory and autonomic neuropathies:
- Types I and II.
- Type III (familial dysautonomia).
- Type IV (congenital insensitivity to pain).
- Type V.

Fabry disease.

IDIOPATHIC

Adie syndrome.
Ross syndrome.
Acute cholinergic neuropathy.
Chronic idiopathic anhidrosis.
Amyotrophic lateral sclerosis.

NEUROPATHIES, PAINFUL[87]

ICD-10CM #	G58.9	Mononeuropathy, unspecified
	G62.1	Alcoholic polyneuropathy
	G61.89	Other inflammatory polyneuropathies
	G60.0	Hereditary motor and sensory neuropathy
	E11.42	Type 2 diabetes mellitus with diabetic polyneuropathy
	E10.42	Type 1 diabetes mellitus with diabetic polyneuropathy

MONONEUROPATHIES

Compressive neuropathy (carpal tunnel, meralgia paresthetica).
Trigeminal neuralgia.
Ischemic neuropathy.
Polyarteritis nodosa.
Diabetic mononeuropathy.
Herpes zoster.
Idiopathic and familial brachial plexopathy.

POLYNEUROPATHIES

DM.
Paraneoplastic sensory neuropathy.
Nutritional neuropathy.
Multiple myeloma.
Amyloid.
Dominantly inherited sensory neuropathy.
Toxic (arsenic, thallium, metronidazole).
AIDS-associated neuropathy.
Tangier disease.
Fabry disease.

NEUROPATHIES, PERIPHERAL, ASYMMETRICAL PROXIMAL/DISTAL[7]

ICD-10CM #	G99.0	Autonomic neuropathy in diseases classified elsewhere

BRACHIAL PLEXOPATHY

Open

Direct plexus injury (knife or gunshot wound).
Neurovascular (plexus ischemia).
Iatrogenic (central line insertion).

Closed

Traction injuries:
- "Stingers."
- Traction neurapraxia.
- Partial or complete nerve root avulsion.

Radiation.
Neoplastic.
Idiopathic brachial plexitis.
Thoracic outlet.

LUMBOSACRAL PLEXOPATHIES

Open

Closed

Traction injuries:
- Pelvic double vertical shearing fracture.
- Posterior hip dislocation.
- Retroperitoneal hemorrhage.

Vasospastic (deep buttock injection).
Neoplastic.
Radiation.
Idiopathic lumbosacral plexitis.
Infectious:
- Herpesvirus (sacrococcygeal).
- Herpes simplex II.
- Herpes zoster.

Cytomegalovirus (CMV) polyradiculopathy (HIV).

NEUROPATHIES, TOXIC AND METABOLIC[51]

ICD-10CM # NEC G62.2 Toxic neuropathy

METALS

Arsenic (insecticide, herbicide).
Lead (paint, batteries, pottery).
Mercury (metallic, vapor).
Thallium (rodenticides).
Gold.

OCCUPATIONAL OR INDUSTRIAL CHEMICALS

Acrylamide (grouting, flocculation).
Carbon disulfide (solvent).
Cyanide.
Dichlorophenoxyacetate.
Dimethylaminopropionitrite.
Ethylene oxide (gas sterilization).
Hexacarbons (glue, solvents).
Organophosphates (insecticides, petroleum additive).
Polychlorinated biphenyls.
Tetrachlorbiphenyl.
Trichloroethylene.

DRUGS

Amiodarone.
Chloramphenicol.
Chloroquine.
Cisplatin.
Colchicine.
Dapsone.
Ethambutol.
Ethanol.
Gold.
Hydralazine.
Isoniazid.
Metronidazole.
Nitrofurantoin.
Nitrous oxide.
Nucleosides (antiretroviral agents ddC, ddl, d4T, others).
Penicillamine.
Pentamidine.
Phenytoin.
Pyridoxine (excessive).
Statins.
Stilbamidine.
Suramin.
Taxanes (paclitaxel, docetaxel).
Thalidomide.
Tryptophan (eosinophilia-myalgia syndrome).
Vincristine.

METABOLIC DISORDER

Fabry disease.
Krabbe disease.
Leukodystrophies.
Porphyria.
Tangier disease.
Tyrosinemia.
Uremia.

NEUTROPENIA, DRUG-INDUCED[42]

ICD-10CM # D70

DRUGS COMMONLY ASSOCIATED WITH NEUTROPENIA

Antibiotics:
- Vancomycin.
- Semisynthetic penicillins.
- Chloramphenicol.
- Sulfa.
- Linezolid.

Antithyroid drugs:
- Methimazole.
- Propylthiouracil.

Cardiovascular:
- Ticlopidine.
- Procainamide.

Antipsychotics:
- Clozapine.
- Olanzapine.
- Chlorpromazine.

Anticonvulsants:
- Phenytoin.
- Carbamazepine
- Valproic acid.

Antiinflammatory agents:
- Indomethacin.
- Sulfasalazine.
- Phenylbutazone.

H2 blockers:
- Cimetidine.
- Ranitidine.

Analgesics:
- Dipyrone.

Antineoplastic:
- Rituximab.

Anthelminthic:
- Levamisole.

NEUTROPENIA WITH DECREASED MARROW RESERVE[43]

ICD-10CM # D70.8 Other neutropenia

PRIMARY

Severe congenital neutropenia.
Shwachman–Diamond syndrome.
Cyclic neutropenia.

SECONDARY

Lymphoproliferative disorder of granular lymphocytes.
Chemotherapy.
Drug induced (nonimmune).
Nutritional.
Viral infection (varicella, EBV, measles, CMV, hepatitis, HIV).

NEUTROPENIA WITH NORMAL MARROW RESERVE[43]

ICD-10CM # D70.9 Neutropenia, unspecified

Chronic benign neutropenia of infancy and childhood.
Ethnic or benign familial neutropenia.
Autoimmune neutropenia.
Alloimmune neutropenia.
Drug-induced neutropenia.
Infection-related neutropenia.
Hypersplenism.

NEUTROPENIA, IN CHILDHOOD[82]

ICD-10CM # D70.8 Other neutropenia
D70.9 Neutropenia unspecified

ACQUIRED

Infection.
Immune mediated.
Hypersplenism.
Vitamin B_{12}, folate, copper deficiency.
Drugs or toxic substances.
Aplastic anemia.
Malignancies or preleukemic disorders.
Ionizing radiation.

CONGENITAL

Cyclic neutropenia.
Severe congenital neutropenia (Kostmann syndrome).
Chronic benign neutropenia of childhood.
Shwachman-Diamond syndrome.
Fanconi anemia.
Metabolic disorders (amino acidopathies, Barth syndrome, glycogen storage disorders).
Osteopetrosis.
Neutropenia with pigmentation abnormalities, e.g., Chédiak-Higashi.

NEUTROPHILIA[43]

ICD-10CM # D72.0 Neutrophilia, hereditary giant
D71 Functional disorders of polymorphonuclear neutrophils

CLASSIFICATION OF NEUTROPHILIA

Primary (No Other Evident Associated Disease)

Hereditary neutrophilia.
Chronic idiopathic neutrophilia.
Chronic myelogenous leukemia (CML) and other myeloproliferative diseases.
Familial myeloproliferative disease.

Congenital anomalies and leukemoid reaction.
Leukocyte adhesion factor deficiency (LAD).
Familial cold urticaria and leukocytosis.
Secondary
Infection.
Stress neutrophilia.
Chronic inflammation.
Drug induced.
Nonhematologic malignancy.
Generalized marrow stimulation as in hemolysis.
Asplenia and hyposplenism.

NIPPLE LESIONS

ICD-10CM # Varies with specific diagnosis

Contact dermatitis.
Trauma.
Paget disease.
Sebaceous hyperplasia.
Neurofibroma.
Accessory nipple.
Papillary adenoma.
Nevoid hyperkeratosis.
Cellulitis.

NODULAR LESIONS, SKIN

ICD-10CM #	R22.9	Localized swelling, mass and lump, unspecified

Lipoma.
Cherry angioma.
Angiokeratoma.
Hemangioma.
Classic Kaposi sarcoma.
Nodular melanoma.
Pyogenic granuloma.
Angiosarcoma.
Eccrine poroma.

NODULES, PAINFUL

ICD-10CM #	R22.9	Localized swelling, mass and lump, unspecified

Arthropod bite or sting.
Erythema nodosum.
Glomus tumor.
Neuroma.
Leiomyoma.
Angiolipoma.
Dermatofibroma.
Osler node.
Blue rubber bleb nevus.
Vasculitis.
Sweet syndrome.

NYSTAGMUS

ICD-10CM #	H55.00	Unspecified nystagmus
	H55.89	Other irregular eye movements

Medications (meperidine, barbiturates, phenytoin, phenothiazines, etc.).
Multiple sclerosis.
Congenital.
Neoplasm (cerebellar, brain stem, cerebral).
Labyrinthine or vestibular lesions.
CNS infections.
Optic atrophy.
Other: Arnold–Chiari malformation, syringobulbia, chorioretinitis, meningeal cysts.

NYSTAGMUS, MONOCULAR

ICD-10CM #	H55.09	Other forms of nystagmus
	H55.00	Unspecified nystagmus

Amblyopia.
Strabismus.
Multiple sclerosis.
Monocular blindness.
Internuclear ophthalmoplegia.
Lid fasciculations.
Brain stem infarct.

ODYNOPHAGIA[81]

ICD-10CM # Varies with specific diagnosis

CAUSES OF ODYNOPHAGIA

Infections
Herpes simplex virus.
Cytomegalovirus.
Candidiasis.
Chemical, Inflammatory
Gastroesophageal reflux.
Drug induced (Slow-K, tetracyclines, quinidine).
Radiation.
Graft-versus-host disease.
Crohn's disease.
Dermatologic diseases (pemphigus and pemphigoid).

OPACIFICATION OF HEMIDIAPHRAGM ON X-RAY[36]

ICD-10CM # Varies with specific diagnosis

CAUSES OF OPACIFICATION OF A HEMITHORAX

Pleural effusion.
Consolidation.
Collapse.
Massive tumor.
Fibrothorax.
Combination of above lesions.
Pneumonectomy.
Lung agenesis.

OPHTHALMOPLEGIA[3]

ICD-10CM #	H51.9	Unspecified disorder of binocular movement
	H49.00	Third [oculomotor] nerve palsy, unspecified eye

BILATERAL

Botulism.
Myasthenia gravis.
Wernicke encephalopathy.
Acute cranial polyneuropathy.
Brain stem stroke.

UNILATERAL

Carotid-posterior (3rd cranial nerve, pupil involved communicating aneurysm).
Diabetic-idiopathic (3rd or 6th cranial nerve, pupil spared).
Myasthenia gravis.
Brain stem stroke.

OPSOCLONUS[29]

ICD-10CM #	H55.89	Other irregular eye movements

Multiple sclerosis.
Encephalitis.
CNS lymphoma.
Hydrocephalus.
Pontine hemorrhage.
Thalamic disorder (glioma, hemorrhage).
Hyperosmolar coma.
Carcinoma, paraneoplastic.
Cocaine.
Medications (e.g., phenytoin, haloperidol, amitriptyline, diazepam, vidarabine).

[29] Spontaneous, multivector, chaotic eye movement

OPTIC ATROPHY[75]

ICD-10CM #	H47.20	Unspecified optic atrophy

CAUSES OF OPTIC ATROPHY

Optic Nerve Compression
Pituitary tumor.
Carotid aneurysm.
Glaucoma.
Optic nerve tumor.
Sphenoid meningioma.
Olfactory groove meningioma.
Optic Neuritis Following Long-standing Papilledema Central Retinal Artery Occlusion Toxic/Metabolic
Diabetes.
Methyl alcohol.
Tobacco.
Quinine.
Ethambutol.
Lead and arsenic.
Anemia.
Secondary to Retinal Disease
Senile macular degeneration.
Retinitis pigmentosa.
Severe chorioretinitis.
Secondary to Trauma
Orbital fracture.
Hereditary
Leber optic atrophy.
Hereditary ataxias.
Spinocerebellar degeneration.

OPTIC DISC ELEVATION[12]

ICD-10CM # Varies with specific diagnosis

CAUSES OF OPTIC DISC ELEVATION

Papilloedema.
Accelerated hypertension.
Anterior optic neuropathy.
Ischemic.
Inflammatory.
Infiltrative.
Compressive, including orbital disease.
Pseudopapilloedema.
Disc drusen.
Tilted optic disc.
Peripapillary myelinated nerve fibers.
Crowded disc in hypermetropia.
Mitochondrial optic neuropathies.
Leber hereditary optic neuropathy.
Methanol poisoning.
Intraocular disease.
Central retinal vein occlusion.
Uveitis.
Posterior scleritis.
Hypotony.

ORAL MUCOSA, ERYTHEMATOUS LESIONS[20]

ICD-10CM #		
	K12.2	Cellulitis and abscess of mouth
	K13.70	Unspecified lesions of oral mucosa
	K13.79	Other lesions of oral mucosa

Allergy.
Erythroplakia.
Candidiasis.
Geographic tongue.
Stomatitis areata migrans.
Plasma cell gingivitis.
Pemphigus vulgaris.

ORAL MUCOSA, PIGMENTED LESIONS[20]

ICD-10CM #		
	K12.2	Cellulitis and abscess of mouth
	K13.70	Unspecified lesions of oral mucosa
	K13.79	Other lesions of oral mucosa
	K13.5	Oral submucous fibrosis

Racial pigmentation.
Oral melanotic macule.
Peutz-Jeghers syndrome.
Neurofibromatosis.
Albright syndrome.
Addison disease.
Chloasma.
Drug reaction: quinacrine, Minocin, chlorpromazine, Myleran.
Amalgam tattoo.
Lead line.
Smoker's melanosis.
Nevi.
Melanoma.

ORAL MUCOSA, PUNCTATE EROSIVE LESIONS[20]

ICD-10CM #		
	K12.2	Cellulitis and abscess of mouth
	K13.70	Unspecified lesions of oral mucosa
	K13.79	Other lesions of oral mucosa

Viral lesion: herpes simplex, coxsackievirus (A, B, A16), herpes zoster.
Aphthous stomatitis.
Sutton disease (giant aphthae).
Behçet's syndrome.
Reiter syndrome.
Neutropenia.
Acute necrotizing ulcerative gingivostomatitis (ANUG).
Drug reaction.
Inflammatory bowel disease.
Contact allergy.

ORAL MUCOSA, WHITE LESIONS[20]

ICD-10CM #		
	K12.2	Cellulitis and abscess of mouth
	K13.70	Unspecified lesions of oral mucosa
	K13.79	Other lesions of oral mucosa
	K13.5	Oral submucous fibrosis

Leukoplakia.
White, hairy leukoplakia.
Squamous cell carcinoma.
Lichen planus.
Stomatitis nicotinica.
Benign intraepithelial dyskeratosis.
White spongy nevus.
Leukoedema.
Darier-White disease.
Pachyonychia congenital.
Candidiasis.
Allergy.
SLE.

ORAL ULCERS, ACUTE

ICD-10CM #		
	K13.70	Unspecified lesions of oral mucosa
	K13.79	Other lesions of oral mucosa

Trauma (including thermal trauma).
Aphthous stomatitis.
Syphilis.
Herpes simplex infection.
Herpes zoster.

ORAL VESICLES AND ULCERS[3]

ICD-10CM #		
	K13.70	Unspecified lesions of oral mucosa
	K13.79	Other lesions of oral mucosa

Aphthous stomatitis.
Primary herpes simplex infection.
Vincent stomatitis.
Syphilis.
Coxsackievirus A (herpangina).
Fungi (histoplasmosis).
Behçet's syndrome.
SLE.
Reiter syndrome.
Crohn's disease.
Erythema multiforme.
Pemphigus.
Pemphigoid.

ORBITAL INFLAMMATION[12]

ICD-10CM #		
	H05.019	Cellulitis of unspecified orbit
	C69.10	Malignant neoplasm of unspecified orbit
	D31.60	Benign neoplasm of unspecified orbit
	H05.029	Osteomyelitis of unspecified orbit
	H05.049	Tenonitis of unspecified orbit
	H05.229	Edema of unspecified orbit
	H05.239	Hemorrhage of unspecified orbit

DIFFERENTIAL DIAGNOSIS OF AN ACUTELY INFLAMED ORBIT

Infection
Bacterial orbital cellulitis.
Fungal orbital infection.
Dacryocystitis.
Infective dacryoadenitis.
Vascular lesions
Acute orbital hemorrhage,
Cavernous sinus thrombosis.
Carotid–cavernous fistula.
Neoplasia
Rapidly progressive retinoblastoma.
Lacrimal gland tumor.
Other neoplasms (e.g., metastatic lesion with inflammation, lymphoma, Waldenström macroglobulinemia).
Rhabdomyosarcoma, leukemia, lymphangioma, or neuroblastoma in children
Endocrine
Thyroid eye disease of rapid onset.
Non-neoplastic inflammation
Idiopathic orbital inflammatory disease.
Tolosa–Hunt syndrome.
Orbital myositis.
Acute allergic conjunctivitis with lid swelling.
Herpes zoster ophthalmicus.
Herpes simplex skin rash.
Sarcoidosis.
Vasculitides: Wegener granulomatosis, polyarteritis nodosa.
Scleritis, including posterior scleritis.
Ruptured dermoid cyst.

ORBITAL LESIONS, CALCIFIED

ICD-10CM #		
	H05.89	Other disorders of orbit

Chronic inflammation.
Phlebolith.

Dermoid cyst.
Mucocele walls.
Tumors (lacrimal gland, fibro-osseous).
Meningioma (optic sheath).
Lymphangioma.
Orbital varix.

ORBITAL LESIONS, CYSTIC

ICD-10CM # H05.9 Unspecified disorder of orbit

Sweat gland cyst.
Dermoid cyst.
Lacrimal gland cyst.
Abscess.
Conjunctival cyst.
Lymphangioma.
Schwannoma.

ORGASM DYSFUNCTION[24]

ICD-10CM # F52.31 Female orgasmic disorder
F52.32 Male orgasmic disorder

Anorgasmia: inadequate stimulation or learning.
Spinal cord lesion or injury.
Multiple sclerosis.
Alcoholic neuropathy.
Amyotrophic lateral sclerosis.
Spinal cord accident.
Spinal cord trauma.
Peripheral nerve damage.
Radical pelvic surgery.
Herniated lumbar disk.
Hypothyroidism.
Addison disease.
Cushing's disease.
Acromegaly.
Hypopituitarism.
Pharmacologic agents (e.g., SSRIs, beta-blockers).
Psychogenic.

OROFACIAL PAIN

ICD-10CM # R51 Facial pain

Dental abscess.
Sinusitis.
Otitis media.
Otitis externa.
Wisdom tooth eruption.
Sialoadenitis.
Herpes zoster.
Trigeminal neuralgia.
Parotitis.
Anxiety disorder.
Malingering.

OSTEOLYTIC BENIGN BONE LESIONS, MULTIPLE[66]

ICD-10CM # Varies with specific diagnosis

COMMON MULTIPLE OSTEOLYTIC BENIGN LESIONS

Cystic lesions in joint disease.
Amyloidosis.
Brown tumors in hyperparathyroidism.
Enchondromatosis.
Fibrous dysplasia.
Osteomyelitis (including tuberculosis, hydatid, sarcoid, etc.).
Massive osteolysis (Gorham disease).
Mastocytosis.
Neurofibromatosis.
Langerhans cell histiocytosis (histiocytosis X).

OSTEOMYELITIS, PEDIATRIC PATIENT[19]

ICD-10CM # M86 Osteomyelitis

Fractures.
Thrombophlebitis.
Scurvy.
Septicemia.
Cellulitis.
Septic bursitis.
Myositis.
Pyomyositis.
Rheumatic fever.
Toxic synovitis.
Reactive arthritis.
Complex regional pain syndrome.
Chronic recurrent multifocal osteomyelitis.
Osteoid osteoma.
Langerhans cell histiocytosis.
Leukemia.
Ewing sarcoma.
Malignant primary bone tumors.
Bone infarction (sickle-cell or Gaucher disease).

OSTEOPOROSIS IN CHILDREN[66]

ICD-10CM # M81.8 Other osteoporosis without current pathological fracture

CAUSES OF OSTEOPOROSIS IN CHILDREN

Systemic long-term oral glucocorticoid therapy.
Chronic inflammatory disease (e.g., juvenile inflammatory arthritis).
Hypogonadism—primary or secondary.
Prolonged immobilization.
Osteogenesis imperfecta.
Idiopathic juvenile osteoporosis.

OSTEOPOROSIS, SECONDARY CAUSES

ICD-10CM # M81.0 Age-related osteoporosis without current pathological fracture

Medication induced (e.g., glucocorticoids, anticonvulsants, heparin, LHRH agonists or antagonists).
Hyperparathyroidism.
Hyperthyroidism.
Prolonged immobilization.
Chronic renal failure.
Sickle cell disease.
Multiple myeloma.
Myeloproliferative diseases.
Leukemias and lymphomas.
Acromegaly.
Prolactinoma.
DM.
Total parenteral nutrition.
Malabsorption.
Chronic hypophosphatemia.
Connective tissue disorders (e.g., osteogenesis imperfecta, Marfan syndrome, Ehlers-Danlos).
Hepatobiliary disease.
Postgastrectomy.
Aluminum-containing antacids.
Systemic mastocytosis.
Homocystinuria.

OSTEOSCLEROSIS, DIFFUSE[36]

ICD-10CM # Q77.4 Congenital osteosclerosis

DISORDERS ASSOCIATED WITH DIFFUSE OSTEOSCLEROSIS

Neoplastic Causes[30]

Prostate carcinoma, breast carcinoma, GI adenocarcinoma, carcinoid tumors, transitional cell carcinoma of the bladder, myeloma, lymphoma, leukemia.

Hematologic Causes

Sickle cell disorders, mastocytosis, myelofibrosis, polycythemia vera.

Metabolic Causes

Renal osteodystrophy, primary hyperparathyoidism, familial hypophosphatemic osteomalacia, hypervitaminosis D, fluorosis, hypoparathyroidism, pseudohypoparathyroidism.

Primary Osseous Disorders[31]

Osteoporosis.
Pyknodysostosis.
Paget disease.

---

[30] Involvement principally of cancellous bone
[31] Involvement of cancellous and cortical bone

OSTEOSCLEROTIC BENIGN BONE LESIONS, MULTIPLE[66]

ICD-10CM #

COMMON MULTIPLE OSTEOSCLEROTIC BENIGN LESIONS

Bone infarcts.
Bone islands.
Callus.
Osteomyelitis (chronic, multifocal).
Paget disease.
Fibrous dysplasia.
Enchondromatosis.
Mastocytosis.
Matured benign lesions (e.g., nonossifying fibromas).
Osteomas (Gardner syndrome).
Osteopathia striata.
Osteopoikilosis.

OVARIAN ENLARGEMENT, NONNEOPLASTIC[22]

ICD-10CM #		
	N83.209	Unspecified ovarian cyst, unspecified side
	N83.29	Other ovarian cysts
	N80.1	Endometriosis of ovary
	000.209	Unspecified ovarian pregnancy without intrauterine pregnancy

NON-NEOPLASTIC CAUSES OF OVARIAN ENLARGEMENT IN THE NONPREGNANT PATIENT

Functional

Hemorrhagic corpus luteum.
Follicle cyst.
Cortical stromal hyperplasia (hyperthecosis).
Polycystic ovarian syndrome (PCOS).
Mesothelial/müllerian.
Endometriotic cyst.
Xanthomatous pseudotumor.
Cystic adhesions/cystic mesothelioma.
Simple cyst.

Vascular

Ovarian torsion/infarction.
Massive ovarian edema.

OVULATORY DYSFUNCTION[47]

ICD-10CM #		
	N97.0	Female infertility associated with anovulation
	N92.3	Ovulation bleeding

HYPERANDROGENIC ANOVULATION

Polycystic ovarian syndrome.
Late-onset congenital adrenal hyperplasias.
Ovarian hyperthecosis.
Androgen-producing ovarian tumors.
Androgen-producing adrenal tumors.
Cushing's syndrome.

HYPOESTROGENIC ANOVULATION (HYPOTHALAMIC OR PITUITARY ETIOLOGY)

Hypogonadotropic Hypoestrogenic States

Reversible:
- Functional hypothalamic amenorrheas:
  - Eating disorders (anorexia nervosa, excessive weight loss).
  - Excessive athletic training.

Neoplastic:
- Craniopharyngioma.
- Pituitary stalk compression.

Infiltrative diseases:
- Histiocytosis-X.
- Sarcoidosis.

Hypophysitis.

Pituitary adenomas:
- Hyperprolactinemia.
- Euprolactinemic galactorrhea.

Endocrinopathies:
- Hypothyroidism/hyperthyroidism.
- Cushing's disease.

Irreversible:
- Kallmann syndrome.
- Isolated gonadotropin deficiency (hypothalamic or pituitary origin).
- Panhypopituitarism/pituitary insufficiency:
  - Sheehan syndrome, pituitary apoplexy.
  - Pituitary irradiation or ablation.

Hypergonadotropic Hypoestrogenic States

Physiologic states:
- Menopause.
- Perimenopause.

Premature ovarian failure.

Immune-related:
- Radiation/chemotherapy-induced.

Ovarian dysgenesis.
Turner syndrome.
46XX with mutations of X.
Androgen insensitivity syndrome.

MISCELLANEOUS

Endometriosis.
Luteal phase defect.

PAIN, MIDFOOT

ICD-10CM #		
	M25.579	Pain in unspecified ankle and joints of unspecified foot

MEDIAL ASPECT

Tendonitis of posterior tibialis.
Tendonitis of flexor digitorum longus.
Tendonitis of flexor hallucis longus.
Infection (osteomyelitis, septic arthritis, cellulitis) of foot.
Peripheral vascular insufficiency.
Fracture.
Osteoarthritis.
Gout, pseudogout.
Neuropathy.
Tumor.

LATERAL ASPECT

Peroneus longus tendonitis.
Peroneus brevis tendonitis.
Infection (osteomyelitis, septic arthritis, cellulitis) of foot.
Peripheral vascular insufficiency.
Fracture.
Osteoarthritis.
Gout, pseudogout.
Neuropathy.
Tumor.

PAIN, PLANTAR ASPECT, HEEL

ICD-10CM #		
	M25.579	Pain in unspecified ankle and joints of unspecified foot

Plantar fasciitis.
Tarsal tunnel syndrome.
Neuroma.
Infection (osteomyelitis, septic arthritis, cellulitis) of foot.
Peripheral vascular insufficiency.
Fracture.
Bone cyst.
Osteoarthritis.
Gout, pseudogout.
Neuropathy.
Tumor.
Heel pad atrophy.
Plantar fascia rupture.

PAIN, POSTERIOR HEEL

ICD-10CM #		
	M79.609	Pain in unspecified limb

Achilles tendonitis.
Retrocalcaneal bursitis.
Retroachilles bursitis.
Infection (osteomyelitis, septic arthritis, cellulitis) of foot.
Peripheral vascular insufficiency.
Fracture.
Osteoarthritis.
Gout, pseudogout.
Neuropathy.
Tumor.

PALINDROMIC RHEUMATISM[16]

ICD-10CM #		
	M12.30	Palindromic rheumatism, unspecified site
	M12.319	Palindromic rheumatism, unspecified shoulder
	M12.329	Palindromic rheumatism, unspecified elbow
	M12.339	Palindromic rheumatism, unspecified wrist
	M12.349	Palindromic rheumatism, unspecified hand
	M12.359	Palindromic rheumatism, unspecified hip
	M12.369	Palindromic rheumatism, unspecified knee
	M12.379	Palindromic rheumatism, unspecified ankle and foot
	M12.38	Palindromic rheumatism, vertebrae
	M12.39	Palindromic rheumatism, multiple sites

Palindromic RA.
Essential palindromic rheumatism.
Crystal synovitis (gout, CPPD, pseudogout, calcific periarthritis).
Lyme borreliosis, stages 2 and 3.
Sarcoidosis.
Whipple disease.
Acute rheumatic fever.
Reactive arthritis (rare).

PALMOPLANTAR HYPERKERATOSIS

ICD-10CM #		
	L85.1	Acquired keratosis [keratoderma] palmaris et plantaris
	L85.2	Keratosis punctata (palmaris et plantaris)
	L87.0	Keratosis follicularis et parafollicularis in cutem penetrans

Superficial skin infection.
Chronic eczema.
Repeated trauma.
Psoriasis.
Reiter syndrome.
Paraneoplastic acrokeratosis.

PALPITATIONS[71]

ICD-10CM #		
	R00.2	Palpitations

Anxiety.
Electrolyte abnormalities (hypokalemia, hypomagnesemia).
Exercise.
Hyperthyroidism.
Ischemic heart disease.
Ingestion of stimulant drugs (cocaine, amphetamines, caffeine).
Medications (digoxin, beta-blockers, calcium channel antagonists, hydralazines, diuretics, minoxidil).
Hypoglycemia in type 1 DM.
Mitral valve prolapse.
Wolff-Parkinson-White (WPW) syndrome.
Sick sinus syndrome.

PANCREATIC CALCIFICATIONS

ICD-10CM #		
	K86.1	Other chronic pancreatitis
	K86.8	Other specified diseases of pancreas

Chronic pancreatitis.
Hyperparathyroidism.
Metastatic neoplasm.
Pseudocyst.
Hereditary pancreatitis.
Cystoadenoma.
Cystoadenocarcinoma.
Cavernous lymphangioma.
Hemorrhage.
Acute pancreatitis (saponification).

PANCREATIC CYSTIC LESIONS[84]

ICD-10CM #		
	K86.2	Cyst of pancreas
	K86.3	Pseudocyst of pancreas

Pseudocyst.
Serous cystadenoma.
Mucinous cystic neoplasm.
Intraductal papillary mucinous neoplasm.
Solid and papillary epithelial neoplasm.
True epithelial cyst.
Duodenal diverticulum.
Cystic neuroendocrine tumors.
Ductal adenocarcinoma with cystic degeneration.
Cystic metastases.
Cystic degeneration in sarcoma, hemangioma, and paraganglioma.

PANCREATIC SOLID LESIONS[84]

ICD-10CM #		
	C25.9	Malignant neoplasm of pancreas, unspecified
	D13.6	Benign neoplasm of pancreas

Neoplastic solid tumors.
Ductal adenocarcinoma.
Pancreatic neuroendocrine tumor.
Pancreatic lymphoma.
Metastases to the pancreas.
Solid pseudopapillary tumor.
Pancreaticoblastoma.
Acinar cell carcinoma.
Mesenchymal tumors (sarcoma, fibrous histiocytoma, etc.).
Nonneoplastic solid lesions.
Focal chronic pancreatitis.
Autoimmune pancreatitis.
Groove pancreatitis.
Focal sparing of diffuse pancreatic fatty infiltration.
Intrapancreatic accessory spleen.
Developmental pancreas lobulation.
Sarcoidosis of the pancreas.

PANCREATITIS, ACUTE, IN CHILDREN[51]

ICD-10CM #		
	K85	Acute pancreatitis

CAUSES OF ACUTE PANCREATITIS IN CHILDREN

Drugs and Toxins

Acetaminophen overdose.
Alcohol.
L-Asparaginase.
Azathioprine.
Carbamazepine.
Cimetidine.
Corticosteroids.
Enalapril.
Erythromycin.
Estrogen.
Furosemide.
Isoniazid.
Lisinopril.
6-Mercaptopurine.
Methyldopa.
Metronidazole.
Organophosphate poisoning.
Pentamidine.
Retrovirals: DDC, DDI, tenofovir.
Sulfonamides: mesalamine, 5-aminosalicylates, sulfasalazine, trimethoprim/sulfamethoxazole.
Sulindac.
Tetracycline.
Thiazides.
Valproic acid.
Venom (spider, scorpion, Gila monster lizard).
Vincristine.

Genetic

Cationic trypsinogen gene *(PRSS1).*
Chymotrypsin C gene *(CTRC).*
Cystic fibrosis gene *(CFTR).*
Trypsin inhibitor gene *(SPINK1).*

Infectious

Ascariasis.
Coxsackie B virus.
Epstein-Barr virus.
Hepatitis A, B.
Influenza A, B.
Leptospirosis.
Malaria.
Measles.
Mumps.
Mycoplasma.
Reye's syndrome: varicella, influenza B.
Rubella.
Rubeola.
Septic shock.

Obstructive

Ampullary disease.
Ascariasis.
Biliary tract malformations.
Choledochal cyst.
Choledochocele.
Cholelithiasis, microlithiasis, and choledocholithiasis (stones or sludge).
Duplication cyst.
Endoscopic retrograde cholangiopancreatography (ERCP) complication.
Pancreas divisum.
Pancreatic ductal abnormalities.
Postoperative.
Sphincter of Oddi dysfunction.
Tumor.

Systemic Disease

Autoimmune pancreatitis.
Brain tumor.
Collagen vascular diseases.
Crohn's disease.
Diabetes mellitus.
Head trauma.
Hemochromatosis.
Hemolytic-uremic syndrome.
Hyperlipidemia: type I, IV, V.
Hyperparathyroidism/Hypercalcemia.
Kawasaki disease.
Malnutrition.
Organic acidemia.
Peptic ulcer.
Periarteritis nodosa.
Renal failure.
Systemic lupus erythematosus.
Transplantation: bone marrow, heart, liver, kidney, pancreas.
Vasculitis.

Traumatic

Blunt injury.
Burns.
Child abuse.
Hypothermia.
Surgical trauma.
Total body cast.

PANCREATITIS, DRUG-INDUCED[7]

ICD-10CM # K85.3 Drug induced acute pancreatitis

DEFINITE

Acetaminophen.
Azathioprine.
Cimetidine.
Cisplatin.
Corticosteroids.
Didanosine.
Erythromycin.
Estrogens.
Ethyl alcohol.
Furosemide.
L-Asparaginase.
Mercaptopurine.
Metronidazole.
Methyldopa.
Nitrofurantoin.
Octreotide.
Organophosphates.
Pentamidine.
Ranitidine.
Tetracycline.
Salicylates.
Sulfonamides, trimethoprim-sulfamethoxazole, sulfasalazine.
Sulindac.
Valproic acid.

POSSIBLE

Bumetanide.
Carbamazepine.
Chlorthalidone.
Clonidine.
Colchicine.
Cyclosporine.
Cytarabine.
Diazoxide.
Enalapril.
Ergotamine.
Ethacrynic acid.
Indomethacin.
Isoniazid.
Isotretinoin.
Mefenamic acid.
Opiates.
Phenformin.
Piroxicam.
Procainamide.
Rifampin.
Thiazides.

PANCYTOPENIA[43]

ICD-10CM # D61.818 Other pancytopenia

PANCYTOPENIA WITH HYPOCELLULAR BONE MARROW

Acquired aplastic anemia.
Inherited aplastic anemia (Fanconi anemia and others).
Some myelodysplasia syndromes.
Rare aleukemic leukemia (acute myelogenous leukemia).
Some acute lymphoblastic leukemias.
Some lymphomas of bone marrow.

PANCYTOPENIA WITH CELLULAR BONE MARROW

Primary bone marrow diseases.
Myelodysplasia syndromes.
Paroxysmal nocturnal hemoglobinuria.
Myelofibrosis.
Some aleukemic leukemias.
Myelophthisis.
Bone marrow lymphoma.
Hairy cell leukemia.
Secondary to systemic diseases.
Systemic lupus erythematosus, Sjögren syndrome.
Hypersplenism.
Vitamin B_{12}, folate deficiency (familial defect).
Overwhelming infection.
Alcohol.
Brucellosis.
Ehrlichiosis.
Sarcoidosis.
Tuberculosis and atypical mycobacteria.

HYPOCELLULAR BONE MARROW ± CYTOPENIA

Q fever.
Legionnaires' disease.
Mycobacteria.
Tuberculosis.[32]
Anorexia nervosa, starvation.
Hypothyroidism.

[32] Pancytopenia in tuberculosis only rarely is associated with a hypocellular bone marrow at biopsy or autopsy. Marrow failure in the setting of tuberculosis is almost always fatal; exceptional patients probably had underlying myelodysplasia or acute leukemia.

PANCYTOPENIA SYNDROME, INHERITED[51]

ICD-10CM # D61.818 Other pancytopenia

Fanconi anemia.
Shwachman-Diamond syndrome.
Dyskeratosis congenita.
Congenital amegakaryocytic thrombocytopenia.
Unclassified inherited bone marrow failure syndromes.
Other genetic syndromes:
- Down syndrome.
- Dubowitz syndrome.
- Seckel syndrome.
- Reticular dysgenesis.
- Schimke immunoosseous dysplasia.
- Familial aplastic anemia (non-Fanconi).
- Cartilage-hair hypoplasia.
- Noonan syndrome.

PAPILLEDEMA

ICD-10CM # H47.10 Unspecified papilledema

CNS infections (viral, bacterial, fungal).
Medications (lithium, cisplatin, corticosteroids, tetracycline, etc.).
Head trauma.
CNS neoplasm (primary or metastatic).
Pseudotumor cerebri.
Cavernous sinus thrombosis.
SLE.
Sarcoidosis.
Subarachnoid hemorrhage.
Carbon dioxide retention.
Arnold–Chiari malformation and other developmental or congenital malformations.
Orbital lesions.
Central retinal vein occlusion.
Hypertensive encephalopathy.
Metabolic abnormalities.

PAPULOSQUAMOUS DISEASES[32]

ICD-10CM # L98.8 Other specified disorders of the skin and subcutaneous tissue

Psoriasis.
Pityriasis rubra pilaris.
Pityriasis rosea.
Lichen planus.
Lichen nitidus.
Secondary syphilis.
Pityriasis lichenoides.
Parapsoriasis.
Mycosis fungoides.
Dermatophytosis.
Tinea versicolor.

PARALYSIS AND MUSCULAR RIGIDITY, DRUG-INDUCED[79]

ICD-10CM # G83 Other paralytic syndromes
R29.818 Other symptoms and signs involving the nervous system

SELECTED AGENTS ASSOCIATED WITH PARALYSIS AND MUSCULAR RIGIDITY

Paralysis

Medications and Industrial Toxins

Aminoglycoside antibiotics.
Beta blockers.
Chloroquine (with color vision shift).
Cholinesterase inhibitors: neostigmine, pyridostigmine.
D-Penicillamine.
Pesticides: organophosphates, carbamates.
Pyrithioxine.
Trimethadione.

Biologic Toxins

Cobra venom.
Poison hemlock (Conium maculatum).
Scorpion fish (Scorpaenidae).
Snake venom, ticks, botulinum toxin.
Star of Bethlehem (Hippobroma longiflora).
Sweet pea (Lathyrus odoratus).
Tetrodotoxin (puffer fish, blue-ringed octopus, others).

Muscular Rigidity

Black widow spider venom (Latrodectus mactans).
Strychnine (Strychnos nux vomica, "slang nut").
Tetanus toxin.

PARANEOPLASTIC NEUROLOGIC SYNDROMES

ICD-10CM # G13.0 Paraneoplastic neuromyopathy and neuropathy

Lambert-Eaton myasthenic syndrome.
Myasthenia gravis.
Guillain-Barré syndrome.
Amyotrophic lateral sclerosis.
Dermatomyositis.
Carcinoid myopathy.
Cerebellar degeneration.
Encephalomyelitis.
Optic neuritis, uveitis, retinopathy.
Stiff-man syndrome.
Autonomic neuropathy.
Brachial neuritis.
Sensory neuropathy.
Progressive multifocal leukoencephalopathy.

PARANEOPLASTIC SYNDROMES, ENDOCRINE[77]

ICD-10CM # G13.0 Paraneoplastic neuromyopathy and neuropathy

Hypercalcemia.
Syndrome of inappropriate secretion of antidiuretic hormone.
Hypoglycemia.
Zollinger-Ellison syndrome.
Ectopic secretion of human chorionic gonadotropin.
Cushing's syndrome.

PARANEOPLASTIC SYNDROMES, NONENDOCRINE[77]

ICD-10CM # G13.0 Paraneoplastic neuromyopathy and neuropathy

CUTANEOUS

Dermatomyositis.
Acanthosis nigricans.
Sweet syndrome.
Erythema gyratum repens.
Systemic nodular panniculitis (Weber-Christian disease).

RENAL

Nephrotic syndrome.
Nephrogenic diabetes insipidus.

NEUROLOGIC

Subacute cerebellar degeneration.
Progressive multifocal leukoencephalopathy.
Subacute motor neuropathy.
Sensory neuropathy.
Ascending acute polyneuropathy (Guillain-Barré syndrome).
Myasthenic syndrome (Eaton-Lambert syndrome).

HEMATOLOGIC

Microangiopathic hemolytic anemia.
Migratory thrombophlebitis (Trousseau syndrome).
Anemia of chronic disease.

RHEUMATOLOGIC

Polymyalgia rheumatica.
Hypertrophic pulmonary osteoarthropathy.

PARAPARESIS, ACUTE OR SUBACUTE[75]

ICD-10CM # G82.2 Paraparesis

CAUSES OF ACUTE OR SUBACUTE PARAPARESIS

Trauma to a Previously Normal Spine

Vertebral Disease

Metastatic carcinoma.
Cervical spondylosis.
Dorsal disk prolapse.
Paget disease.
Rheumatoid arthritis.
Pott disease of spine.

Tumors

Extradural or intradural carcinoma, lymphoma, myeloma, leukemia.
Dorsal meningioma.
Neurofibroma.

Hematologic Disease

Any cause of thrombocytopenia.
Other clotting disorders.
Leukemia.
Anticoagulant treatment.
Epidural or intramedullary hemorrhage.

Infection

Epidural abscess.
TB abscess.
Syphilitic myelitis.
HIV infection.
Vascular myelopathy.

Vascular

Anterior spinal artery occlusion.
Infarction secondary to hypotension.
Embolic infarction.
Infarction secondary to aortic dissection.
Arteriovenous malformation: infarction or hemorrhage.
Primary intramedullary hemorrhage.
Vasculitis—polyarteritis nodosa (PAN).

Inflammatory

Myelitis of unknown cause.
Multiple sclerosis.
Systemic lupus erythematosus.
Sarcoidosis.

Metabolic

Subacute degeneration of the cord.

PARAPARESIS, CHRONIC PROGRESSIVE[75]

ICD-10CM # G82.2 Paraparesis

CAUSES OF CHRONIC PROGRESSIVE PARAPARESIS

Vertebral Disease

Cervical spondylosis.
Dorsal disk prolapse.
Rheumatoid arthritis.
Pott disease of spine.
Ankylosing spondylitis.

Tumors

Meningioma.
Neurofibroma.
Glioma.
Ependymoma.
Chordoma.
Lipoma.

Syringomyelia

With Arnold–Chiari malformation.
With tumor.
Posttraumatic.

Infection

Tropical spastic paraparesis (HTLV 1 infection).
Syphilitic myelitis.

Vascular

Arteriovenous malformation.

Inflammatory

Multiple sclerosis.
Sarcoidosis.
Radiation myelopathy.
Arachnoiditis.

Metabolic

Subacute combined degeneration of the cord.
Paget disease.

Degenerative

Motor neuron disease.

Hereditary

Hereditary spastic paraplegia.

PARAPARESIS, PAINLESS[49]

ICD-10CM # G82 Paraplegia (paraparesis) and quadriplegia (quadriparesis)

FREQUENTLY OCCURRING CAUSES OF PAINLESS PARAPARESIS

Inflammatory CNS diseases:
- Multiple sclerosis (MS).
- Neuromyelitis optica (NMO).

Genetic disorders:
- Spinal cerebellar ataxias (SCAs).
- Hereditary spastic paraparesis (HSP).

Infectious illnesses:
- Human T-lymphotropic virus type 1 (HTLV-1) myelopathy.

Compressive lesions*:
- Cervical spondylosis.
- Spinal meningiomas.
- Metastatic tumors.

Neurodegenerative illnesses:
- ALS.

Nutritional deficiencies:
- Copper deficiency.
- Vitamin B12 deficiency (combined system disease).

*May be associated with spine pain.

PARAPLEGIA

ICD-10CM #		
	G82.20	Paraplegia, unspecified
	G80.1	Spastic diplegic cerebral palsy
	I69.969	Other paralytic syndrome following unspecified cerebrovascular disease affecting unspecified side

Trauma: penetrating wounds to motor cortex, fracture-dislocation of vertebral column with compression of spinal cord or cauda equina, prolapsed disk, electrical injuries.
Neoplasm: parasagittal region, vertebrae, meninges, spinal cord, cauda equina, Hodgkin's disease, NHL, leukemic deposits, pelvic neoplasms.
Multiple sclerosis and other demyelinating disorders.
Mechanical compression of spinal cord, cauda equina, or lumbosacral plexus: Paget disease, kyphoscoliosis, herniation of intervertebral disk, spondylosis, ankylosing spondylitis, RA, aortic aneurysm.
Infections: spinal abscess, syphilis, TB, poliomyelitis, leprosy.
Thrombosis of superior sagittal sinus.
Polyneuritis: Guillain-Barré syndrome, diabetes, alcohol, beriberi, heavy metals.
Heredofamilial muscular dystrophies.
ALS.
Congenital and familial conditions: syringomyelia, myelomeningocele, myelodysplasia.
Hysteria.

PARASELLAR MASSES[59]

ICD-10CM # Varies with specific diagnosis

GENETIC

Transcription factor mutations (e.g., PROP1[33]).

CYSTS

Rathke.
Arachnoid.
Epidermoid.
Dermoid.

TUMORS

Hormone-secreting or nonfunctional pituitary adenoma.
Granular cell tumor.
Craniopharyngioma (cystic components).
Chordoma.
Meningioma.
Sarcoma.
Glioma.
Schwannoma.
Germ cell tumor.
Vascular tumor.
Solid or hematological metastasis.

MALFORMATION AND HAMARTOMAS

Ectopic pituitary, neurohypophyseal, or salivary tissue.
Hypothalamic hamartoma.
Gangliocytoma.

MISCELLANEOUS LESIONS

Aneurysms.
Hypophysitis.
Infections.
Sarcoidosis.
Giant cell granuloma.
Histiocytosis X.

PARESTHESIAS

ICD-10CM #		
	R20.2	Paresthesia of skin
	G54.8	Other nerve root and plexus disorders

Multiple sclerosis.
Nutritional deficiencies (thiamin, vitamin B_{12}, folic acid).
Compression of spinal cord or peripheral nerves.
Medications (e.g., INH, lithium, nitrofurantoin, gold, cisplatin, hydralazine, amitriptyline, sulfonamides, amiodarone, metronidazole, dapsone, disulfiram, chloramphenicol).
Toxic chemicals (e.g., lead, arsenic, cyanide, mercury, organophosphates).
DM.
Myxedema.
Alcohol.
Sarcoidosis.
Neoplasms.
Infections (HIV, Lyme disease, herpes zoster, leprosy, diphtheria).
Charcot-Marie-Tooth syndrome and other hereditary neuropathies.
Guillain-Barré neuropathy.

PARKINSONISM[79]

ICD-10CM #		
	G20	Parkinson disease
	G21	Secondary parkinsonism
	G21.9	Secondary parkinsonism, unspecified
	G21.19	Other drug-induced Secondary parkinsonism
	G21.4	Vascular parkinsonism
	G21.2	Secondary parkinsonism due to other external agents

CAUSES OF PARKINSONISM

Static Injury/Structural Disorders
Basal ganglia infarcts.
Brain tumor.
Hydrocephalus.
Hereditary/Degenerative Disorders
Juvenile Parkinson's disease.
Spinocerebellar ataxia.
Huntington disease (Westphal variant).
Pallidal-pyramidal disorder.
Neurdegeneration with brain iron accumulation (NBIA).
Pantothenate kinase-associated neurodegeneration (PKAN).
Rett syndrome.
Pelizaeus-Merzbacher disease.
Machado-Joseph disease (spinocerebellar ataxia type 3).
Neuronal ceroid lipofuscinoses.
Neuronal intranuclear inclusion body disease.
Metabolic Disorders
Dopa-responsive dystonia.
Tyrosine hydroxylase deficiency and other abnormalities of bioamine metabolism.
Abnormalities of folate metabolism.
Wilson disease.
Basal ganglia calcification (Fahr syndrome, hypoparathyroidism).
Infectious/Para-Infectious Disorders
Encephalitis lethargica (Von Economo disease).
Autoimmune encephalitides, including anti-NMDA receptor associated encephalitis.
Viral encephalitis.
Acute demyelinating encephalomyelitis.
Drugs/Toxins
1-methyl-4-phenyl-1,2,3,6-tetrahydropyridine (MPTP) poisoning.
Rotenone.
Tetrabenazine.
Reserpine.
Methyldopa.
Sedatives.
Neuroleptics.
Antiemetics.
Calcium channel blockers.
Isoniazid.
Serotonin reuptake inhibitors (sertraline, fluoxetine).
Meperidine.
Disorders That Mimic Parkinsonism
Catatonia.
Spasticity.
Hypothyroidism.
Depression (with psychomotor retardation).

PARKINSONISM AND OTHER ACUTE EXTRAPYRAMIDAL REACTIONS, DRUG-INDUCED[79]

ICD-10CM #		
	G21.19	Other drug-induced secondary parkinsonism

SELECTED AGENTS ASSOCIATED WITH PARKINSONISM AND OTHER ACUTE EXTRAPYRAMIDAL REACTIONS

Medications
Amiodarone.
Anticholinergic agents: benztropine.
Antidepressants (including selective serotonin reuptake inhibitors).
Antiepileptic drugs.
Antifungal agents.
Antihistamines.
Antipsychotics and related drugs (including "novel" agents).
Bethanechol.
Bupropion (acute).

[33] PROP1, prophet of Pit1 (paired-like homeodomain transcription factor).

Buspirone.
Captopril (acute).
Clonazepam.
Diazoxide.
Digoxin (chorea).
Estrogen (chorea).
Heroin.
Ketamine.
l-DOPA.
Lithium (chorea).
l-Methyl-4-phenyl-1,2,3,6,-tetrahydropyridine (MPTP).
Metronidazole (oculogyric crisis).
Ofloxacin (Tourettelike syndrome).
Opiates/opiods.
Reserpine.
Stimulants.
Sulfasalazine (chorea).
Vinblastine.

Industrial Toxins

Carbon monoxide.
Metals: manganese, thallium, aluminum.
Methanol.
Trichloroethylene.

Biologic Toxins

Arthrinium mycotoxin.

PARKINSONISM-PLUS SYNDROMES

ICD-10CM #	G21.8	Other secondary parkinsonism

Parkinson's disease.
Shy-Drager syndrome.
Corticobasal degeneration.
Olivo-ponto-cerebellar atrophy.
Dementia with Lewy bodies.
Progressive supranuclear palsy.
Striatonigral degeneration.

PAROTID SWELLING[8]

ICD-10CM #	K11.20	Sialoadenitis, unspecified
	B26.9	Mumps without complication
	K11.8	Other diseases of salivary glands
	K11.5	Sialolithiasis
	K11.3	Abscess of salivary gland

INFECTIOUS

Mumps.
Parainfluenza.
Influenza.
Cytomegalovirus infection.
Coxsackievirus infection.
Lymphocytic choriomeningitis.
Echovirus infection.
Suppuration (bacterial).
Actinomyces infection.
Mycobacterial infection.
Cat-scratch disease.

NONINFECTIOUS

Drug hypersensitivity (thiouracil, phenothiazines, thiocyanate, iodides, copper, isoprenaline, lead, mercury, phenylbutazone).
Sarcoidosis.
Tumors, mixed.
Hemangioma, lymphangioma.
Sialectasis.
Sjögren syndrome.
Mikulicz syndrome (scleroderma, mixed connective tissue disease, SLE).
Recurrent idiopathic parotitis.
Pneumoparotitis.
Trauma.
Sialolithiasis.
Foreign body.
Cystic fibrosis.
Malnutrition (marasmus, alcohol cirrhosis).
Dehydration.
DM.
Waldenström macroglobulinemia.
Reiter syndrome (reactive arthritis).
Amyloidosis.

NONPAROTID SWELLING

Hypertrophy of masseter muscle.
Lymphadenopathy.
Rheumatoid mandibular joint swelling.
Tumors of jaw.
Infantile cortical hyperostosis.

PELVIC AVULSION FRACTURES[66]

ICD-10CM #	M84.350A	Stress fracture pelvis, initial encounter
	M84.454A	Pathological fracture pelvis, initial encounter

ACUTE AVULSION FRACTURE

Nontraumatic avulsion fracture	Bone metastasis, prior graft harvesting.
Soft tissue injury	Tendon tear, muscle strain.
Aggressive-looking appearance	Osteomyelitis, tumor.
Incidental normal variant	Accessory bone.

CHRONIC AVULSION FRACTURE

Apophyseal avulsion injury	Apophysitis, traction periostitis.
Soft tissue injury	Bursitis, degenerative tendinopathy, calcific tendinitis.

PELVIC MASS

ICD-10CM #	R19.09	Other intraabdominal and pelvic swelling, mass and lump

Hemorrhagic ovarian cyst.
Simple ovarian cyst (follicle or corpus luteum).
Ovarian carcinoma, carcinoma of fallopian tube, colorectal carcinoma, metastatic carcinoma, prostate carcinoma, bladder carcinoma, lymphoma, Hodgkin's disease.
Cystadenoma, teratoma, endometrioma.
Leiomyoma.
Leiomyosarcoma.
Diverticulitis, diverticular abscess.
Appendiceal abscess, tuboovarian abscess.
Ectopic pregnancy, intrauterine pregnancy.
Paraovarian cyst.
Hydrosalpinx.

PELVIC PAIN, CAUSES IN WOMEN[7]

ICD-10CM #	N94	Pain and other conditions associated with female genital organs and menstrual cycle
	G10.2	Pelvic and perineal pain
	G89.4	Chronic pain syndrome

POTENTIAL CAUSES OF PELVIC PAIN IN WOMEN

Reproductive Tract

Ovarian torsion.
Ovarian cyst.
Salpingitis/tubo-ovarian abscess.
Septic pelvic thrombophlebitis.
Endometritis.
Endometriosis.
Uterine perforation.
Uterine fibroids.
Dysmenorrhea.

Pregnancy-related

First Trimester

Ectopic pregnancy.
Threatened abortion.
Nonviable pregnancy.
Ovarian hyperstimulation syndrome.

Second and Third Trimesters

Placenta previa.
Placental abruption.
Round ligament pain.

Intestinal Tract

Appendicitis.
Diverticulitis.
Ischemic bowel.
Perforated viscus.
Bowel obstruction.
Incarcerated/strangulated hernia.
Inflammatory bowel disease.
Gastroenteritis.

Urinary Tract

Pyelonephritis.
Cystitis.
Ureteral stone.

PELVIC PAIN, CHRONIC[17]

ICD-10CM #	N94.89	Other specified conditions associated with female genital organs and menstrual cycle

	R10.10	Upper abdominal pain, unspecified
	R10.2	Pelvic and perineal pain
	R10.30	Lower abdominal pain, unspecified

GYNECOLOGIC DISORDERS

Primary dysmenorrhea.
Endometriosis.
Adenomyosis.
Adhesions.
Fibroids.
Retained ovary syndrome after hysterectomy.
Previous tubal ligation.
Chronic pelvic infection.

MUSCULOSKELETAL DISORDERS

Myofascial pain syndrome.

GASTROINTESTINAL DISORDERS

Irritable bowel syndrome.
Inflammatory bowel disease.

URINARY TRACT DISORDERS

Interstitial cystitis.
Nonbacterial urethritis.

PELVIC PAIN, GENITAL ORIGIN[55]

ICD-10CM #		
	N94.89	Other specified conditions associated with female genital organs and menstrual cycle
	R10.10	Upper abdominal pain, unspecified
	R10.2	Pelvic and perineal pain
	R10.30	Lower abdominal pain, unspecified

PERITONEAL IRRITATION

Ruptured ectopic pregnancy.
Ovarian cyst rupture.
Ruptured tuboovarian abscess.
Uterine perforation.

TORSION

Ovarian cyst or tumor.
Pedunculated fibroid.

INTRATUMOR HEMORRHAGE OR INFARCTION

Ovarian cyst.
Solid ovarian tumor.
Uterine leiomyoma.

INFECTION

Endometritis.
Pelvic inflammatory disease.
Trichomonas cervicitis or vaginitis.
Tuboovarian abscess.

PREGNANCY-RELATED

First Trimester

Ectopic pregnancy.
Abortion.
Corpus luteum hematoma.

Late Pregnancy

Placental problems.
Preeclampsia.
Premature labor.

MISCELLANEOUS

Endometriosis.
Foreign objects.
Pelvic adhesions.
Pelvic neoplasm.
Primary dysmenorrhea.

PELVIC PAIN, NON-PREGNANT FEMALE[1]

ICD-10CM #		
	N94.89	Other specified conditions associated with female genital organs and menstrual cycle
	R10.2	Pelvic and perineal pain
	R10.10	Upper abdominal pain, unspecified
	R10.30	Lower abdominal pain, unspecified

DIFFERENTIAL DIAGNOSIS OF PELVIC PAIN IN NONPREGNANT FEMALES

Gynecologic Diagnoses

Infectious:
- Vaginitis.
- Cervicitis.
- Endometritis.
- Tuboovarian abscess.
- Pelvic inflammatory disease.

Ovarian:
- Ovarian torsion.
- Ruptured ovarian cyst.
- Ovarian tumor.
- Degenerating ovarian tumor.
- Mittelschmerz.

Cervical:
- Cervical polyps.
- Cervical stenosis.
- Cervical cancer.

Uterine:
- Uterine fibroids.
- Degenerating uterine fibroids.
- Adenomyosis.
- Endometrial carcinoma.

Extrauterine:
- Endometriosis.
- Adhesions.
- Residual accessory ovary.

Nongynecologic Diagnoses

GI:
- Acute appendicitis.
- Mesenteric lymphadenitis.
- Diverticulitis.
- Inflammatory bowel disease.
- Irritable bowel syndrome.
- Bowel obstruction.
- Intraabdominal abscess.
- Colorectal carcinoma.

Urinary:
- Cystitis.
- Renal colic.
- Bladder cancer.

Musculoskeletal:
- Abdominal wall pain.
- Lumbar back pain.
- Fibromyalgia.
- Muscular strain.
- Piriformis syndrome.

Neurologic:
- Lumbar radiculopathy.
- Shingles.
- Spondylosis.

Psychologic:
- Personality disorders.
- Major depressive disorder.

PENILE RASH

ICD-10CM #		
	R21	Rash and other nonspecific skin eruption

Herpes simplex 2.
Balanitis (Candida).
Condyloma acuminatum.
Molluscum contagiosum.
Scabies.
Pediculosis pubis.
Pearly penile papules.
Lichen nitidus.
Fox-Fordyce disease (follicular papules).
Trauma.

PERIANAL PAIN[81]

ICD-10CM #		
	K62.89	Other specified diseases of anus and rectum

Fissure-in-ano

Anal sepsis:
- Anal abscess
- Anal fistula

Hemorrhoids:
- Internal hemorrhoids
- External hemorrhoids

Pruritus ani

Proctalgia fugax

Chronic perianal pain syndromes:
- Coccygodynia
- Descending perineum syndrome
- Levator ani syndrome
- Idiopathic perineal pain

PERICARDIAL EFFUSION

ICD-10CM #		
	I30.9	Acute pericarditis, unspecified
	I31.3	Pericardial effusion

Pericarditis.
Uremia.
Myxedema.
Neoplasm (leukemia, lymphoma, metastatic).
Hemorrhage (trauma, leakage of thoracic aneurysm).
SLE, rheumatoid disease.
Myocardial infarction.

PERIPHERAL ARTERIAL DISEASE, NONATHEROSCLEROTIC CAUSES[44]

ICD-10CM #		
	I73.9	Peripheral vascular disease, unspecified
	I73.8	Other specified peripheral vascular diseases
	I79.8	Other disorders of arteries, arterioles, and capillaries in diseases classified elsewhere

NONATHEROSCLEROTIC CAUSES OF PERIPHERAL ARTERY DISEASE

Thromboembolism.
Atheroembolism.
Vasculitides:
- Large vessel vasculitides, such as giant cell arteritis and Takayasu arteritis.
- Small vessel vasculitides, such as thromboangiitis obliterans (Buerger disease).

Trauma.
Popliteal artery entrapment.
Cystic adventitial disease.
Fibromuscular dysplasia.
Iliac artery endofibrosis.

PERIODIC PARALYSIS, HYPERKALEMIC

ICD-10CM #		
	G83.9	Paralytic syndrome, unspecified

Chronic renal failure.
Renal insufficiency with excessive potassium supplementation.
Potassium-sparing diuretics.
Endocrinopathies (hypoaldosteronism, adrenal insufficiency).

PERIODIC PARALYSIS, HYPOKALEMIC

ICD-10CM #		
	G83.9	Paralytic syndrome, unspecified

Chronic diarrhea (laxative abuse, sprue, villous adenoma).
Potassium-depleting diuretics.
Medications (amphotericin B, corticosteroids).
Chronic licorice ingestion.
Thyrotoxicosis.
Renal tubular acidosis.
Conn syndrome.
Bartter syndrome.
Barium intoxication.

PERITONEAL CARCINOMATOSIS[32]

ICD-10CM #		
	C78.6	Secondary malignant neoplasm of retroperitoneum and peritoneum

PRIMARY DISORDERS OF THE PERITONEUM: MESOTHELIOMA

Metastatic spread from:
- Stomach.
- Colon.
- Pancreas.
- Carcinoid.

Other Intraabdominal Organs
Ovary.
Pseudomyxoma peritonei.
Extraabdominal Primary Tumors
Breast.
Lung.
Hematologic Malignancy
Lymphoma.

PERITONEAL EFFUSION[39]

ICD-10CM #		
	R18	Ascites
	R85.9	Unspecified abnormal finding in specimens from digestive organs and abdominal cavity
	R88.8	Abnormal findings in other body fluids and substances

TRANSUDATES

Increased hydrostatic pressure or decreased plasma oncotic pressure.
Congestive heart failure.
Hepatic cirrhosis.
Hypoproteinemia.

EXUDATES

Increased capillary permeability or decreased lymphatic resorption.
Infections (TB, spontaneous bacterial peritonitis, secondary bacterial peritonitis).
Neoplasms (hepatoma, metastatic carcinoma, lymphoma, mesothelioma).
Trauma.
Pancreatitis.
Bile peritonitis (e.g., ruptured gallbladder).

CHYLOUS EFFUSION

Damage or obstruction to thoracic duct.
Trauma.
Lymphoma.
Carcinoma.
Tuberculosis.
Parasitic infection.

PERIUMBILICAL SWELLING

ICD-10CM #		
	R19.00	Intraabdominal and pelvic swelling, mass and lump, unspecified site

Umbilical hernia.
Lipoma.
Epigastric hernia.
Umbilical granuloma.
Omphalocele.
Gastroschisis.
Caput medusae.

PHARYNGEAL OBSTRUCTION, CAUSES[58]

ICD-10CM #	
	Varies with specific diagnosis

CAUSES OF PHARYNGEAL OBSTRUCTION

Malignant or benign tumors (e.g., papillomas, polyps).
Infection (e.g., croup, epiglottitis, tonsillar abscess).
Edema or hypertrophy (e.g., angioneurotic edema, anaphylactic reactions, postradiation therapy, obstructive sleep apnea).
Trauma (e.g., cricoid fracture, cervical subluxation, precervical hematoma).
Burn injury.
Extrinsic compression (e.g., goiter or pregnancy-related thyroid enlargement).
Foreign body.
Congenital web (infants).
Sarcoidosis and other granulomatous diseases.
Amyloid.

PHEOCHROMOCYTOMA-TYPE SPELLS[59]

ICD-10CM #		
	I15.2	Hypertension due to pheochromocytoma

DIFFERENTIAL DIAGNOSIS OF PHEOCHROMOCYTOMA-TYPE SPELLS

Endocrine Causes
Carbohydrate intolerance.
Hyperadrenergic spells.
Hypoglycemia.
Pancreatic tumors (e.g., insulinoma).
Pheochromocytoma.
Primary hypogonadism (menopausal syndrome).
Thyrotoxicosis.
Cardiovascular Causes
Angina.
Cardiovascular deconditioning.
Labile essential hypertension.
Orthostatic hypotension.
Paroxysmal cardiac arrhythmia.
Pulmonary edema.
Renovascular disease.
Syncope (e.g., vasovagal reaction).
Psychologic Causes
Factitious (e.g., drugs, Valsalva).
Hyperventilation.
Severe anxiety and panic disorders.
Somatization disorder.
Pharmacologic Causes
Chlorpropamide-alcohol flush.
Combination of a monoamine oxidase inhibitor and a decongestant.
Illegal drug ingestion (cocaine, phencyclidine, lysergic acid diethylamide).
Sympathomimetic drug ingestion.
Vancomycin ("red man syndrome").
Withdrawal of adrenergic-inhibitor.
Neurologic Causes
Autonomic neuropathy.
Cerebrovascular insufficiency.
Diencephalic epilepsy (autonomic seizures).

Migraine headache.
Postural orthostatic tachycardia syndrome.
Stroke.

Other Causes

Carcinoid syndrome.
Mast cell disease.
Recurrent idiopathic anaphylaxis.
Unexplained flushing spells.

PHOTODERMATOSES[32]

ICD-10CM #	L56.0	Drug phototoxic response
	L56.1	Drug photoallergic response
	L56.2	Photocontact dermatitis [berloque dermatitis]

Polymorphous light eruption.
Chronic actinic dermatitis.
Solar urticaria.
Phototoxicity and photoallergy.
Porphyrias.

PHOTOSENSITIVITY

ICD-10CM #	L56.0	Drug phototoxic response
	L56.1	Drug photoallergic response
	L56.2	Photocontact dermatitis [berloque dermatitis]

Solar urticaria.
Photoallergic reaction.
Phototoxic reaction.
Polymorphous light eruption.
Porphyria cutanea tarda.
SLE.
Drug induced (e.g., tetracyclines).

PIGMENTURIA[7]

ICD-10CM #	R82	Other abnormal findings in urine

HEMOGLOBINURIA

Hemolysis.

HEMATURIA

Renal causes.
Trauma.

ACUTE INTERMITTENT PORPHYRIA

Bilirubinuria

Food

Beets.

Drugs

Vitamin B_{12}.
Rifampin.
Phenytoin.
Laxatives.

PITUITARY REGION TUMORS[36]

ICD-10CM # Varies with specific diagnosis

PRIMARY TUMORS IN THE SELLAR AND PARASELLAR REGION

Pituitary macroadenoma.
Meningioma.
Schwannoma (e.g., of fifth nerve).
Chordoma.
Chondrosarcoma.
Crangiopharyngioma.
Rathke cleft cyst.
Dermoid.
Epidermoid.
Tuber cinereum hamartoma.
Optic glioma.
Germ cell tumors.

PLATELET DYSFUNCTION, DRUG-INDUCED[44]

ICD-10CM #	D69.1	Qualitative platelet defects

ANTI-PLATELET DRUGS

COX inhibitors: aspirin.
ADP receptor antagonists:
Thienopyridines: clopidogrel, ticlopidine, prasugrel.
Nonthienopyridines: ticagrelor, cangrelor.
$\alpha_{IIb}\beta_3$ inhibitors: abciximab, eptifibatide, tirofiban.
PDE inhibitors:
Nonselective PDE inhibitors: pentoxifylline, caffeine, theophylline.
PDE3 inhibitors: cilostazol, milrinone, anagrelide.
PDE5 inhibitors: dipyridamole, sildenafil.
Adenyl cyclase stimulators: epoprostenol, iloprost, beraprost.
Drugs that adversely affect platelet function.
NSAIDs: ibuprofen, naproxen, indomethacin.
Cardiovascular agents:
Calcium channel blockers: nifedipine, diltiazem, verapamil.
β-Blockers: propranolol.
Vasodilators: nitrates, nitroprusside.
Diuretics: furosemide.
Angiotensin II receptor antagonist: losartan, valsartan, and olmesartan.
Antibiotics: β-lactams, amphotericin, hydroxychloroquine, nitrofurantoin.
Antifungal drugs: Miconazole, amphotericin B;
Psychiatric drugs: TCAs, fluoxetine, chlorpromazine, promethazine, trifluoperazine.
Oncologic drugs: mithramycin, daunorubicin, BCNU, asparaginase, vincristine, dasatinib, ibritunib.
Anesthetics: dibucaine, procaine, halothane, sevoflurane, propofol.
Plasma expanders: dextran, hydroxyl ethyl starch.
Heparins and thrombolytic agents.
Miscellaneous: clofibrate, statins, cocaine, ketanserin, radiographic contrast agents, antihistamines, immunosuppressive drugs.

ADP, Adenosine diphosphate; *BCNU,* carmustine; *COX,* cyclooxygenase; *NSAID,* nonsteroidal antiinflammatory drug; *PDE,* phosphodiesterase; *TCA,* tricyclic antidepressant.

PLEURAL EFFUSIONS

ICD-10CM #	J91.8	Pleural effusion in other conditions classified elsewhere

EXUDATIVE

Neoplasm: bronchogenic carcinoma, breast carcinoma, mesothelioma, lymphoma, ovarian carcinoma, multiple myeloma, leukemia, Meigs syndrome.
Infections: viral pneumonia, bacterial pneumonia, *Mycoplasma,* TB, fungal and parasitic diseases, extension from subphrenic abscess.
Trauma.
Collagen vascular diseases: SLE, RA, scleroderma, polyarteritis, granulomatosis with polyangiitis.
Pulmonary infarction.
Pancreatitis.
Postcardiotomy/Dressler syndrome.
Drug-induced SLE (hydralazine, procainamide).
Postabdominal surgery.
Ruptured esophagus.
Chronic effusion secondary to congestive failure.

TRANSUDATIVE

CHF.
Hepatic cirrhosis.
Nephrotic syndrome.
Hypoproteinemia from any cause.
Meig syndrome.

PLEURAL EFFUSIONS, MALIGNANCY-ASSOCIATED

ICD-10CM #	C78.2	Secondary malignant neoplasm of pleura

Lung cancer	(30% to 40%)
Breast cancer	(20% to 25%)
Lymphoma	(10% to 15%)
Leukemia	(5% to 10%)
GI tract	(5%)
GU tract	(5%)
Reproductive	(3%)

PLEURAL HYPERPLASIA[72]

ICD-10CM # Varies with specific diagnosis

BENIGN CAUSES OF PLEURAL HYPERPLASIA

Pleural infections.
Radiation.
Surgery.
Trauma.
Intracavitary treatments (chemotherapy or sclerosing agents).
Collagen vascular diseases.
Systemic immune diseases (systemic lupus erythematosus, rheumatoid arthritis, Sjögren syndrome, Wegener granulomatosis).
Subpleural pulmonary abnormalities (infarction, infection, neoplasia).
Pneumothorax.
Drug reactions (nitrofurantoin, bromocriptine, methysergide, procarbazine).
Pancreatitis, uremia.
Pneumoconiosis (asbestosis).

PLEURAL MASSES[72]

ICD-10CM # Varies with specific diagnosis

CAUSES OF PLEURAL MASSES

- Inflammatory pleural reactions:
  - Reactive mesothelial hyperplasia or organizing pleuritis versus atypical mesothelial hyperplasia.
  - Nodular pleural plaques.
- Pulmonary tumors that may resemble pleural tumors:
  - Inflammatory pseudotumor of the lung.
- Benign pleural tumors:
  - Solitary fibrous tumor.
  - Lipomas and lipoblastomas.
  - Adenomatous tumors.
  - Calcifying fibrous tumors.
  - Mesothelial cysts.
  - Multicystic mesothelioma.
  - Schwannoma.
- Pleural tumors with low malignant potential:
  - Desmoid tumors.
  - Well-differentiated papillary mesothelioma.
  - Pleural thymoma.
- Primary malignant pleural tumors that may look like benign tumors:
  - Malignant solitary fibrous tumor.
  - Pleuropulmonary blastoma.
  - Localized malignant mesothelioma.
  - Vascular sarcoma.
  - Liposarcoma.
  - Pleuropulmonary synovial sarcoma.
  - Askin tumor or primitive neuroectodermal tumor (PNET).
  - Desmoplastic small round cell tumor.
- Malignant pleural tumors:
  - Metastatic malignancies to the pleura.
  - Malignant mesothelioma.

PNEUMATOSIS INTESTINALIS IN NEONATE AND OLDER CHILD[36]

ICD-10CM #	Varies with specific diagnosis

CAUSES OF PNEUMATOSIS INTESTINALIS IN THE NEONATE AND THE OLDER CHILD

- Necrotizing enterocolitis.
- Bowel ischemia, inflammation, and obstruction.
- Cyanotic congenital heart disease.
- Hirschsprung disease.
- Gastroschisis.
- Anorectal atresia.
- Inflammatory bowel disease.
- Lymphoma.
- Leukemia.
- CMV and rotavirus gastroenteritis.
- Colonoscopy.
- Caustic ingestion.
- Short bowel syndrome.
- Congenital immune deficiency states.
- *Clostridium* infection.
- Chronic steroid use.
- Posthepatic, renal, or bone marrow transplant.
- Collagen vascular disease.
- Graft-versus-host disease.
- AIDS.

PNEUMONIA, CHRONIC[10]

ICD-10CM #		
	J15.9	Unspecified bacterial pneumonia
	J12.9	Viral pneumonia, unspecified
	B25.0	Cytomegaloviral pneumonitis
	J18.0	Bronchopneumonia, unspecified organism

INFECTIOUS AGENTS THAT TYPICALLY CAUSE CHRONIC PNEUMONIA

Bacteria

Mixed aerobic and anaerobic bacteria.
Actinomyces spp.
Nocardia spp.
Rhodococcus equi.
Burkholderia pseudomallei.

Mycobacteria

Mycobacterium tuberculosis.
Mycobacterium kansasii.
Mycobacterium avium complex.
Mycobacterium abscessus.
Mycobacterium terrae.

Fungi

Aspergillus spp.
Blastomyces dermatitidis.
Coccidioides spp.
Cryptococcus neoformans.
Cryptococcus gattii.
Dark-walled molds.
Emmonsia parvum var. crescens.
Histoplasma capsulatum.
Sporothrix schenckii complex.
Paracoccidioides brasiliensis.
Penicillium marneffei.
Scedosporium apiospermum.

Parasites

Dirofilaria.
Echinococcus granulosus.
Filaria (tropical pulmonary eosinophilia).
Paragonimus westermani.

NONINFECTIOUS CAUSES OF CHRONIC PNEUMONIA

Neoplasia

Carcinoma (primary or metastatic).
Hodgkin's disease and non-Hodgkin's lymphoma.
Other lymphoproliferative disorders.

Cystic Fibrosis

Sarcoidosis

Amyloidosis
Vasculitis (Autoimmune Diseases)
Systemic lupus erythematosus.
Polyarteritis nodosa.
Granulomatosis with polyangiitis.
Allergic angiitis and granulomatosis (Churg-Strauss syndrome).
Goodpasture syndrome.
Microscopic polyangiitis.
Lymphomatoid granulomatosis.
Progressive systemic sclerosis.
Rheumatoid arthritis.
Mixed connective tissue syndrome (overlap syndrome).

Chemicals, Drugs

Radiation

Recurrent Pulmonary Emboli

Bronchial Obstruction with Atelectasis (e.g., Tumor, Foreign Body)

Pulmonary Sequestration
Pulmonary Infiltration with Eosinophilia Syndrome
Löffler syndrome—usually transient.
Pneumonia plus asthma (e.g., allergic bronchopulmonary aspergillosis).
Bronchocentric granulomatosis.
Chronic eosinophilic pneumonia.

Pneumoconiosis

Asbestosis.
Berylliosis.
Silicosis.
Anthracosilicosis.

Chronic Form of Extrinsic Allergic Alveolitis (Hypersensitivity Pneumonitis)

OTHER LUNG DISEASES: CAUSE UNKNOWN

Chronic Organizing Pneumonia

Chronic Interstitial Pneumonia (Fibrosing Alveolitis, Idiopathic Pulmonary Fibrosis)

Usual interstitial pneumonia (UIP).
Desquamative interstitial pneumonia (DIP).
Lymphocytic interstitial pneumonia (LIP).
Giant cell interstitial pneumonia (GIP).
Eosinophilic granuloma (histiocytosis X).
Lymphangioleiomyomatosis.
Pulmonary alveolar proteinosis.
Pulmonary alveolar microlithiasis.
Idiopathic pulmonary hemosiderosis.
Angiocentric immunoproliferative lesions.

PNEUMONIA MIMICS[13]

ICD-10CM #	Varies with specific diagnosis

NONINFECTIOUS CAUSES THAT MAY PRESENT AS PNEUMONIA

Radiologic Technique

Inadequate inspiration.
Breast shadow.
Thymus.
Uneven grid on film.
Underpenetrated film.

Primary Pulmonary

Asthma.
Bronchiectasis.
Atelectasis.
Bronchopulmonary dysplasia.
Cystic fibrosis.
Pulmonary sequestration.
Congenital cystic adenomatoid malformation.
α_1-Antitrypsin deficiency.

Aspiration

Foreign body.
Chemical.
Recurrent caused by anatomic or physiologic disorders.

Primary Cardiac

Congenital heart disease.
CHF.

Pulmonary Infarction
Sickle cell vasoocclusive crisis.
Pulmonary embolism.
Collagen Vascular Disorders
Acute Respiratory Distress Syndrome
Pleural Effusion.
Neoplasm.
From Boyer KM: Nonbacterial pneumonia. In Feigin RD, Cherry JD (eds): *Textbook of pediatric infectious diseases,* ed 4, Philadelphia, WB Saunders, 1998, pp 260-273.

PNEUMONIA, NONRESPONDING, CAUSES[58]

ICD-10CM #		
	J15.9	Unspecified bacterial pneumonia
	J12.9	Viral pneumonia, unspecified
	B25.0	Cytomegaloviral pneumonitis
	J18.0	Bronchopneumonia, unspecified organism

CAUSES OF NONRESPONDING PNEUMONIA

Infectious Pneumonia
Resistant microorganisms:
- Community-acquired pneumonia (e.g., *Streptococcus pneumoniae, Staphylococcus aureus*).
- *Nosocomial pneumonia* (e.g., *Acinetobacter*, methicillin-resistant *Staphylococcus aureus* (MRSA), *Pseudomonas aeruginosa*).

Uncommon microorganisms (e.g., *Mycobacterium tuberculosis, Nocardia* spp., fungi, *Pneumocystis jirovecii*).
Complications of pneumonia:
- Empyema.
- Abscess or necrotizing pneumonia.
- Metastatic infection.

Noninfectious Pneumonia
Neoplasms.
Pulmonary hemorrhage.
Pulmonary embolism.
Sarcoidosis.
Eosinophilic pneumonia.
Pulmonary edema.
Acute respiratory distress syndrome.
Bronchiolitis obliterans with organizing pneumonia.
Drug-induced pulmonary disease.
Pulmonary vasculitis.

PNEUMONIA, RECURRENT

ICD-10CM #		
	J15.9	Unspecified bacterial pneumonia
	J12.9	Viral pneumonia, unspecified
	B25.0	Cytomegaloviral pneumonitis
	J18.0	Bronchopneumonia, unspecified organism

Mechanical obstruction from neoplasm.
Chronic aspiration (tube feeding, alcoholism, CVA, neuromuscular disorders, seizure disorder, inability to cough).
Bronchiectasis.
Kyphoscoliosis.
COPD, CHF, asthma, silicosis, pulmonary fibrosis, cystic fibrosis.
Pulmonary TB, chronic sinusitis.
Immunosuppression (HIV, corticosteroids, leukemia, chemotherapy, splenectomy).

PNEUMOPERITONEUM, NEONATAL[36]

ICD-10CM #	Varies with specific diagnosis

CAUSES OF NEONATAL PNEUMOPERITONEUM

Necrotizing enterocolitis.
Spontaneous perforation of a hollow viscus.
- Stomach.
- Duodenum.
- Ileum.
- Colon.

Malrotation and volvulus.
Distal obstruction.
Perforation of Meckel diverticulum.
Anterior abdominal wall defects.
- Pentalogy of Cantrell.
- Omphalocele.
- Gastroschisis.
- Cloacal exstrophy.

Stress and peptic ulcers.
Mechanical ventilation (air leak) or resuscitation ("bagging").
Post-laparotomy.
Iatrogenic gastric perforation with an orogastric tube.
Iatrogenic colon perforation.
- Thermometer.
- During an enema.

Indomethacin.
Dexamethasone treatment.

PNEUMOTHORAX, IN CHILDREN[51]

ICD-10CM #		
	J93.0	Spontaneous tension pneumothorax
	J93	Pneumothorax
	J93.9	Pneumothorax unspecified

SPONTANEOUS

Primary idiopathic—usually resulting from ruptured subpleural blebs.
Secondary blebs.
Congenital lung disease:
- Congenital cystic adenomatoid malformation.
- Bronchogenic cysts.
- Pulmonary hypoplasia.

Conditions associated with increased intrathoracic pressure:
- Asthma.
- Bronchiolitis.
- Air-block syndrome in neonates.
- Cystic fibrosis.
- Airway foreign body.

Infection:
- Pneumatocele.
- Lung abscess.
- Bronchopleural fistula.

Diffuse lung disease:
- Langerhans cell histiocytosis.
- Tuberous sclerosis.
- Marfan syndrome.
- Ehlers-Danlos syndrome.

Metastatic neoplasm—usually osteosarcoma (rare).

TRAUMATIC

Noniatrogenic:
- Penetrating trauma.
- Blunt trauma.
- Loud music (air pressure).

Iatrogenic:
- Thoracotomy.
- Thoracoscopy, thoracentesis.
- Tracheostomy.
- Tube or needle puncture.

Mechanical ventilation.

POLIOSIS[12]

ICD-10CM #	Varies with specific diagnosis

CAUSES OF POLIOSIS

Ocular
Chronic anterior blepharitis.
Sympathetic ophthalmitis.
Idiopathic uveitis.
Systemic
Vogt–Koyanagi–Harada syndrome.
Waardenburg syndrome.
Vitiligo.
Marfan syndrome.
Tuberous sclerosis.

POLYCYTHEMIA

ICD-10CM #		
	D45	Polycythemia primary
	D75.1	Polycythemia secondary

Tobacco abuse.
Chronic lung disease.
High altitude.
Sleep apnea.
Right-to-left cardiac shunts.
Erythropoietin administration.
Androgens/anabolic steroids.
Polycystic kidney disease.
Renal cell carcinoma.
Hepatocellular carcinoma.
Polycythemia vera.
Carbon monoxide exposure.
Primary familial and congenital polycythemia.
High-oxygen–affinity hemoglobins.
Uterine leiomyoma, meningioma, pheochromocytoma, parathyroid carcinoma.
Cobalt exposure.

POLYCYTHEMIAS, DIFFERENTIAL DIAGNOSIS[42]

ICD-10CM #		
	D45	Polycythemia primary
	D75.1	Polycythemia secondary

DIFFERENTIAL DIAGNOSIS OF THE POLYCYTHEMIAS

Relative or Spurious Polycythemia

Decreased plasma volume—reduced fluid intake, marked loss of body fluids (diaphoresis, vomiting, diarrhea, "third spacing").
Gaisböck syndrome.
Overfilling of blood in collection vacuum tubes.
Absolute polycythemia
Secondary polycythemia.
Acquired.
Hypoxia.
- Pulmonary disease.
- Cyanotic congenital heart disease.
- Hypoventilation syndromes:
  - Sleep apnea.
  - Pickwickian syndrome.
  - High altitude.
  - Smokers' polycythemia, hookah polycythemia, carbon monoxide intoxication caused by industrial exposure.

Postrenal transplantation erythrocytosis.
Aberrant erythropoietin production.
Tumors:
- Renal cell carcinoma.
- Wilms tumor.
- Hepatic carcinoma.
- Uterine leiomyomata.

Virilizing ovarian tumors.
Vascular cerebellar tumors.
Miscellaneous renal and hepatic disorders:
- Solitary renal cysts.
- Polycystic kidney disease.
- Renal artery stenosis hydronephrosis.
- Viral hepatitis.

Endocrine disorders:
- Cushing's syndrome.
- Primary aldosteronism.
- Androgen use.
- Erythropoietin use.
- Congenital Polycythemias:
  - Abnormal high-affinity hemoglobin variants.
  - Bisphosphoglycerate deficiency.
  - Congenital methemoglobinemia.
  - Chuvash polycythemia (von Hippel Lindau mutations).
  - Prolyl hydroxylase mutations.

Hypoxia-inducible factor gene mutations.
Primary polycythemias:
- Primary congenital and familial polycythemia.
- Polycythemia vera.

POLYCYTHEMIA, RELATIVE VERSUS ABSOLUTE[43]

ICD-10CM #	D75.1	Secondary polycythemia

RELATIVE OR SPURIOUS POLYCYTHEMIA

Decreased plasma volume—reduced fluid intake, marked loss of body fluids (diaphoresis, vomiting, diarrhea, "third-spacing").
Gaisböck syndrome.
Overfilling of blood in collection vacuum tubes.

ABSOLUTE POLYCYTHEMIA

Primary Congenital and Familial Polycythemia

Secondary Polycythemia Acquired

Hypoxia:
- Pulmonary disease.
- Cyanotic congenital heart disease.
- Hypoventilation syndromes—sleep apnea, Pickwickian syndrome.

High altitude.
Smokers' polycythemia, carbon monoxide intoxication due to industrial exposure.
Postrenal transplantation erythrocytosis.
Aberrant erythropoietin production
Tumors—renal cell carcinoma, Wilms tumor, hepatic carcinoma, uterine leiomyomata, virilizing ovarian tumors, vascular cerebellar tumors.
Miscellaneous renal and hepatic disorders—solitary renal cysts, polycystic kidney disease, renal artery stenosis, hydronephrosis, viral hepatitis.
Endocrine disorders—Cushing's syndrome, primary aldosteronism.
Androgen use.
Erythropoietin use.
Congenital:
- Abnormal high-affinity hemoglobin variants.
- Bisphosphoglycerate deficiency.
- Congenital methemoglobinemia.
- Chuvash polycythemia (von Hippel–Lindau mutations).
- Prolyl hydroxylase mutations.

POLYCYTHEMIA VERA

POLYMYALGIAS[40]

ICD-10CM #	M35.3	Polymyalgia rheumatica

DISEASE ENTITIES WITH POLYMYALGIAS

Rheumatoid arthritis.
Rotator cuff syndrome.
Osteoarthritis of shoulder and hip joints.
Fibromyalgia.
Polymyositis/dermatomyositis.
Spondyloarthritis.
Systemic lupus erythematosus.
Vasculitides.
Paraneoplastic myalgias.
Infection-associated myalgias.
Statin therapy.
RS3PE (remitting seronegative symmetric synovitis and pitting edema).
Parkinson's disease.
Hypothyroidism.

POLYNEUROPATHY[87]

ICD-10CM #	G61.9	Inflammatory polyneuropathy, unspecified

PREDOMINANTLY MOTOR

Guillain-Barré syndrome.
Porphyria.
Diphtheria.
Lead.
Hereditary sensorimotor neuropathy, types I and II.
Paraneoplastic neuropathy.

PREDOMINANTLY SENSORY

Diabetes.
Amyloidosis.
Leprosy.
Lyme disease.
Paraneoplastic neuropathy.
Vitamin B_{12} deficiency.
Hereditary sensory neuropathy, types I-IV.

PREDOMINANTLY AUTONOMIC

Diabetes.
Amyloidosis.
Alcoholic neuropathy.
Familial dysautonomias.

MIXED SENSORIMOTOR

Systemic diseases: renal failure, hypothyroidism, acromegaly, RA, periarteritis nodosa, SLE, multiple myeloma, macroglobulinemia, remote effect of malignancy.
Medications: isoniazid, nitrofurantoin, ethambutol, chloramphenicol, chloroquine, vincristine, vinblastine, dapsone, disulfiram, diphenylhydantoin, cisplatin, 1-tryptophan.
Environmental toxins: *N*-hexane, methyl *N*-butyl ketone, acrylamide, carbon disulfide, carbon monoxide, hexachlorophene, organophosphates.
Deficiency disorders: malabsorption, alcoholism, vitamin B_1 deficiency, Refsum disease, metachromatic leukodystrophy.

POLYNEUROPATHY, DEMYELINATING[7]

ICD-10CM #	G37.9	Demyelinating disease of central nervous system, unspecified

Guillain-Barré syndrome.
- Acute inflammatory demyelinating polyradiculoneuropathy (AIDP).
- Acute motor axonal neuropathy (AMAN).
- Acute motor and sensory axonal neuropathy (AMSAN).
- Miller Fisher syndrome.

Chronic inflammatory demyelinating polyradiculoplexo-neuropathy.
Malignancy.
HIV.
Hepatitis B.
Buckthorn.
Diphtheria.

POLYNEUROPATHY, DISTAL SENSORIMOTOR[7]

ICD-10CM #	G63	Polyneuropathy in diseases classified elsewhere

Diabetes mellitus.
Alcoholism.
Neoplastic or paraneoplastic.

Hereditary motor and sensory neuropathies (Charcot-Marie-Tooth).
Cryptogenic sensorimotor polyneuropathies (CSPN).
HIV.
Toxins:
Organic or industrial agents:
Acrylamide.
Allyl chloride.
Carbon disulfide.
Ethylene oxide.
Hexacarbons.
Methyl bromide.
Organophosphate-induced delayed polyneuropathy (OPIDP).
Polychlorinated biphenyls (PCBs).
Trichloroethylene.
Vacor.
Metals:
Arsenic.
Gold.
Mercury (inorganic).
Thallium.
Therapeutic agents:
Amiodarone.
Antiretrovirals.
Dapsone.
Disulfiram.
Isoniazid.
Metronidazole.
Nitrofurantoin.
Paclitaxel (Taxol).
Phenytoin.
Statins (HMG-CoA reductase inhibitors).
Thalidomide.
Vinca alkaloids (vincristine, vinblastine).
Nutritional:
Beriberi (thiamine or vitamin B1).
Pellagra (niacin, B vitamins).
Pernicious anemia (vitamin B12).
Pyridoxine deficiency (vitamin B_6).
End-organ dysfunction:
Acromegaly.
Chronic pulmonary disease.
Hypothyroidism.
Renal failure (uremic neuropathy).
Paraproteinemias:
Amyloidosis.
Monoclonal gammopathy of unknown significance (MGUS).
Multiple myeloma.
Waldenström macroglobulinemia.
Porphyria.

HMG-CoA, Hydroxymethylglutaryl coenzyme A.

POLYNEUROPATHY, DRUG-INDUCED[87]

ICD-10CM # G62.0 Drug-induced polyneuropathy

DRUGS IN ONCOLOGY

Vincristine.
Procarbazine.
Cisplatin.
Misonidazole.
Metronidazole
Taxol.

DRUGS IN INFECTIOUS DISEASES

Isoniazid.
Nitrofurantoin.
Dapsone.
ddC (dideoxycytidine).
ddI (dideoxyinosine).

DRUGS IN CARDIOLOGY

Hydralazine.
Perhexiline maleate.
Procainamide.
Disopyramide.

DRUGS IN RHEUMATOLOGY

Gold salts.
Chloroquine.

DRUGS IN NEUROLOGY AND PSYCHIATRY

Diphenylhydantoin.
Glutethimide.
Methaqualone.

MISCELLANEOUS

Disulfiram (Antabuse).
Vitamin: (pyridoxine in megadoses).

POLYNEUROPATHY, SYMMETRIC[87]

ICD-10CM # G61.9 Inflammatory polyneuropathy, unspecified

ACQUIRED NEUROPATHIES

Toxic:
Drugs.
Industrial toxins.
Heavy metals.
Abused substances.
Metabolic/endocrine:
Diabetes.
Chronic renal failure.
Hypothyroidism.
Polyneuropathy of critical illness.
Nutritional deficiency:
Vitamin B_12 deficiency.
Alcoholism.
Vitamin E deficiency.
Paraneoplastic:
Carcinoma.
Lymphoma.
Plasma cell dyscrasia:
Myeloma, typical, atypical, and solitary forms.
Primary systemic amyloidosis.
Idiopathic chronic inflammatory demyelinating polyneuropathies.
Polyneuropathies associated with peripheral nerve autoantibodies.
AIDS.

INHERITED NEUROPATHIES

Neuropathies with Biochemical Markers

- Refsum disease.
- Bassen-Kornzweig disease.
- Tangier disease.
- Metachromatic leukodystrophy.
- Krabbe disease.
- Adrenomyeloneuropathy.
- Fabry disease.

Neuropathies without Biochemical Markers or Systemic Involvement

Hereditary motor neuropathy.
Hereditary sensory neuropathy.
Hereditary sensorimotor neuropathy.

POLYURIA

ICD-10CM # R35.8 Other polyuria

DM.
Diabetes insipidus.
Primary polydipsia (compulsive water drinking).
Hypercalcemia.
Hypokalemia.
Postobstructive uropathy.
Diuretic phase of renal failure.
Drugs: diuretics, caffeine, alcohol, lithium.
Sickle cell trait or disease, chronic pyelonephritis (failure to concentrate urine).
Anxiety, cold weather.

POPLITEAL SWELLING

ICD-10CM#		
	I87.1	Compression of vein
	I72.4	Aneurysm of artery of lower extremity
	S85.009A	Unspecified injury of popliteal artery, unspecified leg, initial encounter
	I77.3	Arterial fibromuscular dysplasia
	M71.20	Synovial cyst of popliteal space [Baker], unspecified knee
	I80.3	Phlebitis and thrombophlebitis of lower extremities, unspecified
	M66.369	Spontaneous rupture of flexor tendons, unspecified lower leg

Phlebitis (superficial).
Lymphadenitis.
Trauma: fractured tibia or fibula, contusion, traumatic neuroma.
DVT.
Ruptured varicose vein.
Baker's cyst.
Popliteal abscess.
Osteomyelitis.
Ruptured tendon.
Aneurysm of popliteal artery.
Neoplasm: lipoma, osteogenic sarcoma, neurofibroma, fibrosarcoma.

PORTAL HYPERTENSION[3]

ICD-10CM # K76.6 Portal hypertension

INCREASED RESISTANCE TO FLOW

Presinusoidal

Portal or splenic vein occlusion (thrombosis, tumor).
Schistosomiasis.
Congenital hepatic fibrosis.

Sarcoidosis.
Sinusoidal
Cirrhosis (all causes).
Alcoholic hepatitis.
Postsinusoidal
Venoocclusive disease.
Budd-Chiari syndrome.
Constrictive pericarditis.

INCREASED PORTAL BLOOD FLOW

Splenomegaly not caused by liver disease.
Arterioportal fistula.

POSTMENOPAUSAL BLEEDING

ICD-10CM #	N95.0	Postmenopausal bleeding

Hormone replacement therapy.
Neoplasm (uterine, ovarian, cervical, vaginal, vulvar).
Atrophic vaginitis.
Vaginal infection.
Polyp.
Extragenital (GI, urinary).
Tamoxifen.
Trauma.

POSTURAL HYPOTENSION, NONNEUROLOGIC CAUSES

ICD-10CM #	I95.1	Orthostatic hypotension

Diuretics and hypertensive agents.
GI hemorrhage.
Alcohol.
Excessive heat.
Rapid volume loss from diarrhea, vomiting.
Hemodialysis.
Extensive burns.
Pyrexia.
Aortic stenosis (impaired output).
Constrictive pericarditis, atrial myxoma (impaired cardiac filling).
Adrenal insufficiency.
Diabetes insipidus.
Vasodilatory agents (e.g., nitrates).

PREMATURE GRAYING, SCALP HAIR

ICD-10CM #	Varies with specific diagnosis

Chemical exposure (e.g., phenol/catechol derivatives, sulfhydryls, arsenic).
Physical agents (e.g., ionizing radiation, lasers).
Hyperthyroidism.
Vitamin B_{12} deficiency.
Down syndrome.
Chronic and severe protein deficiency.
Vitiligo.
Idiopathic.
Myotonic dystrophy.
Ataxia-telangiectasia.
Progeria.
Werner syndrome.

PREMATURE VENTRICULAR CONTRACTIONS AND VENTRICULAR TACHYCARDIA[7]

ICD-10CM #	I49.40	Unspecified premature depolarization
	I47.2	Ventricular tachycardia

CAUSES OF PREMATURE VENTRICULAR CONTRACTIONS AND VENTRICULAR TACHYCARDIA

Acute or previous myocardial infarction/ischemia.
Hypokalemia.
Hypoxemia.
Ischemic heart disease.
Valvular disease.
Catecholamine excess.[34]
Other drug intoxications (especially cyclic antidepressants).
Idiopathic causes.[35]
Digitalis toxicity.
Hypomagnesemia.
Hypercapnia.
Class I antidysrhythymic agents.
Ethanol.
Myocardial contusion.
Cardiomyopathy.
Acidosis.
Alkalosis.
Methylxanthine toxicity.

---

[34] Relative increase in sympathetic tone from drugs (direct or indirect) or conditions that augment catecholamine release or decrease parasympathetic tone.

[35] Isolated premature ventricular contractions (PVCs) can occur in up to 50% of young subjects without obvious cardiac or noncardiac disease; however, multiform and repetitive PVCs and ventricular tachycardia are rarely seen in this population.

PRESACRAL MASSES IN CHILDREN[69]

ICD-10CM #	Varies with specific diagnosis

PRESACRAL MASSES IN CHILDREN

Solid
Sacrococcygeal teratoma.
Neuroblastoma.
Rhabdomyosarcoma.
Fibroma.
Lipoma.
Leiomyoma.
Lymphoma.
Hemangioendothelioma.
Sacral bone tumors.
Cystic
Abscess.
Rectal duplication.
Hematoma.
Lymphocele.
Neurenteric cyst.
Sacral osteomyelitis.
Ulcerative colitis.
Anterior meningocele.

PROLONGED QT SYNDROMES[57]

ICD-10CM #	I45.81	Long QT syndrome

CLASSIFICATION AND CAUSES OF PROLONGED QT SYNDROMES THAT PRODUCE TORSADES DE POINTES

Pause Dependent (Acquired)
Drug induced: Class IA and IC antidysrhythmics; many phenothiazines and butyrophenones (notably haloperidol and droperidol), cyclic antidepressants, antibiotics (especially macrolides), organophosphates, antihistamines, antifungals, antiseizure and antiemetic agents.
Electrolyte abnormalities: hypokalemia, hypomagnesemia, hypocalcemia (rarely).
Diet related: starvation, low protein.
Severe bradycardia or atrioventricular block.
Hypothyroidism.
Contrast injection.
Cerebrovascular accident (especially intraparenchymal).
Myocardial ischemia.
Adrenergic Dependent (Tachycardia Prompted)
Congenital:
- Jervell and Lange-Nielsen syndrome (deafness, autosomal recessive).
- Romano-Ward syndrome (normal hearing, autosomal dominant).
- Sporadic (normal hearing, no familial tendency).
- Mitral valve prolapse.

Acquired (Rare):
- Cerebrovascular disease (especially subarachnoid hemorrhage).
- Autonomic surgery: radical neck dissection, carotid endarterectomy, truncal vagotomy.

PROPTOSIS[63]

ICD-10CM #	H05.20	Unspecified exophthalmos
	H05.2	Ocular proptosis

Thyrotoxicosis.
Orbital pseudotumor.
Optic nerve tumor.
Cavernous sinus AV fistula, cavernous sinus thrombosis.
Cellulitis.
Metastatic tumor to orbit.

PROPTOSIS AND PALATAL NECROTIC ULCERS

ICD-10CM #	K13.70	Unspecified lesions of oral mucosa
	K13.79	Other lesions of oral mucosa
	H05.20	Unspecified exophthalmos

Cavernous sinus thrombosis.
Bacterial orbital cellulitis.
Metastatic neoplasm.
Rhinocerebral mucormycosis.
Ecthyma gangrenosum.
CNS aspergillosis.

PROTEIN-LOSING ENTEROPATHY, PEDIATRIC AGE[51]

ICD-10CM #	E44.0	Moderate protein-energy malnutrition

CAUSES OF PROTEIN-LOSING ENTEROPATHY

Mucosal inflammation:
Infection:
- Cytomegalovirus.
- Bacterial overgrowth.
- Invasive bacterial infection.

Gastric inflammation:
- Ménétrier disease.
- Eosinophilic gastroenteropathy.

Intestinal inflammation:
- Celiac disease.
- Crohn's disease.

Eosinophilic gastroenteropathy:
- Tropical sprue.
- Radiation enteritis.

Primary intestinal lymphangiectasia.
Secondary intestinal lymphangiectasia:
- Constrictive pericarditis.
- Congestive heart failure.
- Post–Fontan procedure.
- Malrotation.
- Lymphoma.
- Sarcoidosis.
- Radiation therapy.
- Colonic inflammation:
  - Inflammatory bowel diseases.
  - Necrotizing enterocolitis.
- Congenital disorders of glycosylation.

PROTEINURIA

ICD-10CM #	R80.9	Proteinuria, unspecified

Nephrotic syndrome as a result of primary renal diseases.
Malignant hypertension.
Malignancies: multiple myeloma, leukemias, Hodgkin's disease.
CHF.
DM.
SLE, RA.
Sickle cell disease.
Goodpasture syndrome.
Malaria.
Amyloidosis, sarcoidosis.
Tubular lesions: cystinosis.
Functional (after heavy exercise).
Pyelonephritis.
Pregnancy.
Constrictive pericarditis.
Renal vein thrombosis.
Toxic nephropathies: heavy metals, drugs.
Radiation nephritis.
Orthostatic (postural) proteinuria.
Benign proteinuria: fever, heat, or cold exposure.

PRURITUS

ICD-10CM #	L29.9	Pruritus, unspecified
	L29.3	Anogenital pruritus, unspecified

Dry skin.
Drug-induced eruption, fiberglass exposure.
Scabies.
Skin diseases.
Myeloproliferative disorders: mycosis fungoides, Hodgkin's lymphoma, multiple myeloma, polycythemia vera.
Cholestatic liver disease.
Endocrine disorders: DM, thyroid disease, carcinoid, pregnancy.
Carcinoma: breast, lung, gastric.
Chronic renal failure.
Iron deficiency.
AIDS.
Neurosis.
Sjögren syndrome.

PRURITUS ANI[57]

ICD-10CM #	L29.0	Pruritus ani

FECAL IRRITATION

Poor hygiene.
Anorectal conditions (fissure, fistula, hemorrhoids, skin tags, perianal clefts).
Spicy foods, citrus foods, caffeine, colchicine, quinidine.

CONTACT DERMATITIS

Anesthetic agents, topical corticosteroids, perfumed soap.

DERMATOLOGIC DISORDERS

Psoriasis, seborrhea, lichen simplex or sclerosus.

SYSTEMIC DISORDERS

Chronic renal failure, myxedema, DM, thyrotoxicosis, polycythemia vera, Hodgkin's disease.

SEXUALLY TRANSMITTED DISEASES

Syphilis, herpes simplex virus, human papillomavirus.

OTHER INFECTIOUS AGENTS

Pinworms.
Scabies.
Bacterial infection, viral infection.

PRURITUS VULVAE[75]

ICD-10CM #	L29.3	Anogenital pruritus, unspecified

CAUSES OF PRURITUS VULVAE

Diseases Special to Vulval Skin
Lichen sclerosus et atrophicus.
Leukoplakia.
Carcinoma.

Skin Disease
Psoriasis.
Atopic dermatitis.
Irritant and allergic contact dermatitis (especially medicaments).

Infection
Candidiasis.
Trichomonas.

Infestation
Pediculosis.

Psychogenic
Anxiety.
Depression.

Unknown

PSEUDOCYANOSIS, ETIOLOGY

ICD-10CM #	Varies with etiology

Medications: amiodarone, minocycline, chlorpromazine.
Heavy metals:
- Gold (systemic absorption).
- Silver (systemic absorption).

Local contact with color dyes, gold, silver.

PSEUDOHERMAPHRODITISM, FEMALE

ICD-10CM #	E25.0	Congenital adrenogenital disorders associated with enzyme deficiency
	E25.8	Other adrenogenital disorders
	E25.9	Adrenogenital disorder, unspecified
	Q56.3	Pseudohermaphroditism, unspecified
	Q56.4	Indeterminate sex, unspecified

Congenital adrenal hyperplasia.
Maternal use of testosterone or related steroids.
Virilizing ovarian or adrenal tumor.
Virilizing luteoma of pregnancy.
Disturbances in differentiation of urogenital structures, non-androgen related.
Maternal virilizing adrenal hyperplasia.
Fetal P450 aromatase deficiency.

PSEUDOHERMAPHRODITISM, MALE

ICD-10CM#	E25.0	Congenital adrenogenital disorders associated with enzyme deficiency
	E25.8	Other adrenogenital disorders
	E25.9	Adrenogenital disorder, unspecified
	Q56.3	Pseudohermaphroditism, unspecified
	Q56.4	Indeterminate sex, unspecified

Maternal ingestion of progestogens.
End-organ resistance to androgenic hormones.

5-α-reductase-2 deficiency.
XY gonadal dysgenesis.
Testicular regression syndrome.
Defects in testosterone metabolism by peripheral tissues.
Testosterone biosynthesis defects.

PSEUDOINFARCTION[50]

ICD-10CM #	Varies with specific diagnosis

Cardiac tumors, primary and secondary.
Cardiomyopathy (particularly hypertrophic and dilated).
Chagas' disease.
Chest deformity.
COPD (particularly emphysema).
HIV infection.
Hyperkalemia.
Left anterior fascicular block.
Left bundle branch block.
Left ventricular hypertrophy.
Myocarditis and pericarditis.
Normal variant.
Pneumothorax.
Poor R wave progression, rotational changes, and lead placement.
Pulmonary embolism.
Trauma to chest (nonpenetrating).
Wolff-Parkinson-White syndrome.
Rare causes: pancreatitis, amyloidosis, sarcoidosis, scleroderma.

PSYCHOSIS[61]

ICD-10CM #	# F29	Unspecified psychosis not due to a substance or known physiological condition
	F29	Unspecified psychosis not due to a substance or known physiological condition
	F10.231	Alcohol dependence with withdrawal delirium
	F01.51	Vascular dementia with behavioral disturbance

PRIMARY

Schizophrenia related.[36]
Major depression.
Dementia.
Bipolar disorder.

SECONDARY

Drug use.[37]
Drug withdrawal. [38]
Drug toxicity.[39]
Charles Bonnet syndrome.
Infections (pneumonia).
Electrolyte imbalance.
Syphilis.
Congestive heart failure.
Parkinson's disease.
Trauma to temporal lobe.
Postpartum psychosis.
Hypothyroidism/hyperthyroidism.
Hypomagnesemia.
Epilepsy.
Meningitis.
Encephalitis.
Brain abscess.
Herpes encephalopathy.
Hypoxia.
Hypercarbia.
Hypoglycemia.
Thiamine deficiency.
Postoperative states.

[36] Includes schizophrenia, schizophreniform disorder, brief reactive psychosis.
[37] Includes hypnotics, glucocorticoids, marijuana, phencyclidine, atropine, dopaminergic agents (e.g., amantadine, bromocriptine, l-dopa), immunosuppressants.
[38] Includes alcohol, barbiturates, benzodiazepines.
[39] Includes digitalis, theophylline, cimetidine, anticholinergics, glucocorticoids, catecholaminergic agents.

PSYCHOSIS, MEDICAL DISORDERS-INDUCED[57]

ICD-10CM #	F29	Unspecified psychosis not due to a substance or known physiological condition
	F53	Puerperal psychosis

MEDICAL DISORDERS THAT MAY CAUSE ACUTE PSYCHOSIS

Metabolic Disorders
Hypercalcemia.
Hypercarbia.
Hypoglycemia.
Hyponatremia.
Hypoxia.
Inflammatory Disorders
Sarcoidosis.
Systemic lupus erythematosus.
Temporal (giant cell) arteritis.
Organ Failure
Hepatic encephalopathy.
Uremia.
Neurologic Disorders
Alzheimer's disease.
Cerebrovascular disease.
Encephalitis (including HIV infection).
Encephalopathies.
Epilepsy.
Huntington disease.
Multiple sclerosis.
Neoplasms.
Normal-pressure hydrocephalus.
Parkinson's disease.
Pick disease.
Wilson's disease.
Endocrine disorders
Addison disease.
Cushing's disease.
Panhypopituitarism.
Parathyroid disease.
Postpartum psychosis.
Recurrent menstrual psychosis.
Sydenham chorea.
Thyroid disease.
Deficiency States
Niacin.
Thiamine.
Vitamin B_{12} and folate.

PSYCHOSIS, MEDICATION-INDUCED[57]

ICD-10CM #	F10.5	Psychotic disorder due to psychoactive substance use

PHARMACOLOGIC AGENTS THAT MAY CAUSE ACUTE PSYCHOSIS

Antianxiety Agents
Alprazolam.
Chlordiazepoxide.
Clonazepam.
Clorazepate.
Diazepam.
Ethchlorvynol.
Antibiotics
Isoniazid.
Rifampin.
Anticonvulsants
Ethosuximide.
Phenobarbital.
Phenytoin.
Primidone.
Antidepressants
Amitriptyline.
Doxepin.
Imipramine.
Protriptyline.
Trimipramine.
Cardiovascular Drugs
Captopril.
Digitalis.
Disopyramide.
Methyldopa.
Procainamide.
Propranolol.
Reserpine.
Drugs of Abuse
Alcohol.
Amphetamines.
Cannabis.
Cocaine.
Hallucinogens.
Opioids.
Phencyclidine.
Sedative-hypnotics.
Miscellaneous Drugs
Antihistamines.
Antineoplastics.
Bromides.
Cimetidine.
Corticosteroids.
Disulfiram.
Heavy metals.

PTOSIS

ICD-10CM #	H02.409	Unspecified ptosis of unspecified eyelid
	Q10.0	Congenital ptosis

H02.419	Mechanical ptosis of unspecified eyelid
H02.429	Myogenic ptosis of unspecified eyelid
H02.439	Paralytic ptosis unspecified eyelid

Third nerve palsy.
Myasthenia gravis.
Horner syndrome.
Senile ptosis.

PUBERTY, DELAYED[60]

ICD-10CM # E30.0 Delayed puberty

NORMAL OR LOW SERUM GONADOTROPIN LEVELS

Constitutional delay in growth and development.
Hypothalamic and/or pituitary disorders:
- Isolated deficiency of growth hormone.
- Isolated deficiency of Gn-RH.
- Isolated deficiency of LH and/or FSH.
- Multiple anterior pituitary hormone deficiencies.
- Associated with congenital anomalies: Kallmann syndrome; Prader-Willi syndrome; Laurence-Moon-Biedl syndrome; Friedreich ataxia.
- Trauma.
- Postinfection.
- Hyperprolactinemia.
- Postirradiation.
- Infiltrative disease (histiocytosis).
- Tumor.
- Autoimmune hypophysitis.
- Idiopathic.

Functional:
- Chronic endocrinologic or systemic disorders.
- Emotional disorders.
- Drugs: cannabis.

INCREASED SERUM GONADOTROPIN LEVELS

Gonadal abnormalities:
- Congenital:
  - Gonadal dysgenesis.
  - Klinefelter syndrome.
  - Bilateral anorchism.
  - Resistant ovary syndrome.
  - Myotonic dystrophy in males.
  - 17-Hydroxylase deficiency in females.
  - Galactosemia.
- Acquired:
  - Bilateral gonadal failure resulting from trauma or infection or after surgery, irradiation, or chemotherapy.
  - Oophoritis: isolated or with other autoimmune disorders.
- Uterine or vaginal disorders:
  - Absence of uterus and/or vagina.
  - Testicular feminization: complete or incomplete androgen insensitivity.

PUBERTY, PRECOCIOUS

ICD-10CM #		
	E25.0	Congenital adrenogenital disorders associated with enzyme deficiency
	E25.8	Other adrenogenital disorders
	E25.9	Adrenogenital disorder, unspecified

Idiopathic.
Congenital virilizing adrenal hyperplasia.
Hypothalamic tumors.
Head trauma.
Hydrocephalus.
Degenerative CNS disease.
Arachnoid cyst.
Sex chromosome abnormalities (e.g., 47, XXY, 48, XXXY).
Perinatal asphyxia.
CNS infection (e.g., meningitis, encephalitis).

PULMONARY CRACKLES

ICD-10CM # R09.8 Friction sounds, chest

Pneumonia.
Left ventricular failure.
Asbestosis, silicosis, interstitial lung disease.
Chronic bronchitis.
Alveolitis (allergic, fibrosing).
Neoplasm.

PULMONARY CYSTS ON X-RAY[36]

ICD-10CM #		
	Q33.0	Polycystic lungs, congenital
	J98.4	Pulmonary manifestations

CAUSES OF CYSTS IN THE LUNG ON CHEST RADIOGRAPH

Cystic fibrosis.
Cystic bronchiectasis.
Bronchopulmonary dysplasia (neonate and older).
Tuberculosis (apical thick walled).
Pulmonary abscess (thick wall, fluid level).
Empyema.
Streptococcal pneumatocele (thin wall, postinfective).
Cavitating pneumonia.
Mycetoma (apical cyst with contents).
Cystic congenital adenomatoid malformation (basal cysts of varying size).
Diaphragmatic hernia (cysts of similar size).
Hiatal hernia (posterior).
Morgagni hernia (midline anterior).
Bronchopulmonary sequestration (basal).
Congenital lobar emphysema.
Hydatid disease (in endemic areas).
Kerosene inhalation (pneumatocele).
Histiocytosis and other causes of interstitial disease.

PULMONARY EDEMA, NONCARDIOGENIC[36]

ICD-10CM # J81.0 Acute pulmonary edema

CAUSES OF NONCARDIOGENIC PULMONARY EDEMA

Adult respiratory distress syndrome.
Drowning.
Asphyxia.
Upper airway obstruction (usually with cardiomegaly).
High altitude.
Increased intracranial pressure.
Postictal.
Noxious gases:
- Smoke.
- Nitrous dioxide (silo filler's disease).
- Sulfur dioxide.
- Nitrogen mustard.

Drugs:
- Aspirin.
- Diazepam, chlordiazepoxide, barbiturates.
- Narcotics (heroin, methadone, morphine).
- β-adrenergic drugs (terbutaline).
- Contrast media.
- Colchicine.
- Fluorescein.
- Hydrochlorothiazide.
- Nitrofurantoin.
- Propoxyphene.

Poisons:
- Parathion.

Transfusion reactions.
Renal failure: transplantation.
Bone marrow transplantation.
Fat embolism.
Pancreatitis.

PULMONARY EOSINOPHILIA[2]

ICD-10CM # NEC J82 Eosinophilia, pulmonary

TYPES AND CAUSES OF PULMONARY EOSINOPHILIA

Drug- and toxin-induced eosinophilic lung diseases.
Helminth and fungal infection-related eosinophilic lung diseases:
- Transpulmonary passage of larvae (i.e., Löffler syndrome): *Ascaris,* hookworm, *Strongyloides.*
- Pulmonary parenchymal invasion: mostly helminths, paragonimiasis.
- Heavy hematogenous seeding with helminths: trichinellosis, disseminated strongyloidiasis, cutaneous and visceral larva migrans, schistosomiasis.
- Tropical pulmonary eosinophilia: filaria.
- Allergic bronchopulmonary aspergillosis.

Chronic eosinophilic pneumonia.
Acute eosinophilic pneumonia.
Churg-Strauss syndrome (vasculitis).
Other: neoplasia, idiopathic hypereosinophilic syndrome, bronchocentric granulomatosis.

PULMONARY HEMORRHAGE, FOCAL[65]

ICD-10CM # R04.8 Pulmonary hemorrhage

CAUSES OF FOCAL PULMONARY HEMORRHAGE

Iatrogenic Disorders

Bronchoscopy.
Lung biopsy.
Pulmonary artery catheterization.

Transtracheal aspiration.
Radiofrequency ablation.
Brachytherapy.

Infectious Disorders

Lung abscess.
Mycetoma.
Necrotizing pneumonia (*Staphylococcus aureus,* gram-negative aerobes, *Legionella,* Actinomyces species, *Stenotrophomonas, Kytococcus sedentarius,* Leptospira species, Yersinia pestis, Francisella tularensis).
Parasitic infection (paragonimiasis, amebiasis, ascariasis, clonorchiasis, echinococcosis, hookworm infestation, strongyloidiasis, trichinosis, schistosomiasis).
Parenchymal fungal infection (aspergillosis, mucormycosis, coccidioidomycosis, histoplasmosis, maduromycosis, botryomycosis).
Tuberculosis (active or inactive).
Viral tracheitis.
Herpetic tracheobronchitis.

Interstitial Lung Diseases

Lymphangioleiomyomatosis.
Sarcoidosis.
Tuberous sclerosis.
Pneumoconiosis.
Langerhans cell granulomatosis.

Miscellaneous Disorders

Amyloidosis.
Bronchogenic cyst.
Broncholithiasis.
Bronchopleural fistula.
Thoracic endometriosis.
Foreign body.
Tracheopathia osteoplastica.
Lipoid pneumonia.
Organophosphate aspiration.
Chronic pancreatitis.

Neoplastic Disorders

Bronchial adenoma.
Lung cancer.
Tracheal tumors (mucoepidermoid, squamous cell, adenoid cystic, glomus).
Pulmonary blastoma.
Pleuropulmonary angiosarcoma.
Sarcoma (synovial, myofibroblastic).
Clear cell tumor.
Metastatic disease (prostate, renal, breast, ovarian).
Tracheobronchial schwannoma.

Pulmonary Airway Diseases

Bronchiectasis.
Bronchitis.
Granulomatous tracheobronchitis (ulcerative colitis, Crohn's disease, granulomatosis with polyangiitis).
Cystic fibrosis.
Bullous emphysema.

Traumatic Injury

Blunt chest trauma.
Penetrating injury.
Ruptured bronchus.
Lightning injury.
Thoracic splenosis.

Vascular Disorders

Pulmonary embolism, infarction.
Systemic cholesterol emboli.
Intralobar sequestration.
Pulmonary artery aneurysms.
Behçet's disease, Hughes-Stovin syndrome, traumatic pseudoaneurysms.
Acquired arteriovenous malformations.
Osler-Weber-Rendu syndrome (hereditary hemorrhagic telangiectasia).
Takayasu arteritis.
Aortic aneurysms.
Trachea–innominate artery fistulas.
Scimitar syndrome.
Vena cava-bronchial.
Dieulafoy disease of bronchus.
Ventriculopulmonary fistulas.
Hemangioma (sclerosing, cavernous, tracheal).

PULMONARY HEMORRHAGE, PEDIATRIC AGE

ICD-10CM #	P26.9	Pulmonary hemorrhage newborn

CAUSES OF PULMONARY HEMORRHAGE (HEMOPTYSIS)

Focal Hemorrhage

Bronchitis and bronchiectasis (especially cystic fibrosis related).
Infection (acute or chronic), pneumonia, abscess.
Tuberculosis.
Trauma.
Pulmonary arteriovenous malformation.
Foreign body (chronic).
Neoplasm including hemangioma.
Pulmonary embolus with or without infarction.
Bronchogenic cysts.
Diffuse hemorrhage
Idiopathic of infancy.
Congenital heart disease (including pulmonary hypertension, venoocclusive disease, congestive heart failure).
Prematurity.
Cow's milk hyperreactivity (Heiner syndrome).
Goodpasture syndrome.
Collagen vascular diseases (systemic lupus erythematosus, rheumatoid arthritis).
Henoch-Schönlein purpura and vasculitic disorders.
Granulomatous disease (Wegener granulomatosis).
Celiac disease.
Coagulopathy (congenital or acquired).
Malignancy.
Immunodeficiency.
Exogenous toxins.
Hyperammonemia.
Pulmonary hypertension.
Pulmonary alveolar hemosiderosis.
Tuberous sclerosis.
Lymphangiomyomatosis or lymphangioleiomyomatosis.
Physical injury or abuse.

PULMONARY HEMORRHAGIC SYNDROMES, DIFFUSE[36]

ICD-10CM #	P26.1	Massive pulmonary hemorrhage originating in the perinatal period
	R04.8	Pulmonary hemorrhage

CLASSIFICATION OF DIFFUSE PULMONARY HEMORRHAGE SYNDROMES

Non-immunocompromised patients

Antibasement membrane antibody disease/Goodpasture syndrome.
Diseases of presumed immune etiology, with or without nephropathy:
- Systemic lupus erythematosus.
- Rheumatoid arthritis.
- Systemic sclerosis.
- Systemic necrotizing vasculitis.
- Granulomatosis with polyangiitis.
- Microscopic polyarteritis.

Diseases with no known immune etiology:
- Idiopathic pulmonary hemosiderosis.
- Rapidly progressive glomerulonephritis without immune complexes.
- Fibrillary glomerulonephritis.
- Drug-induced (anticoagulants, trimellitic anhydride, cocaine, lymphangiography).
- Valvular heart disease.
- Disseminated intravascular coagulation.
- Acute lung injury.
- Tumors.

Immunocompromised Patients

Blood dyscrasias.
Infection.
Tumors.

PULMONARY INFILTRATES, IMMUNOCOMPROMISED HOST[86]

ICD-10CM #	J82	Pulmonary eosinophilia, not elsewhere classified
	J98.4	Other disorders of lung

CAUSES OF PULMONARY INFILTRATES IN THE IMMUNOCOMPROMISED HOST

Infections:
- Bacteria:
  - Gram-positive cocci, especially *Staphylococcus.*
  - Gram-negative bacilli.
  - *Mycobacterium tuberculosis.*
  - Nontuberculous mycobacteria.
  - Nocardia.
- Viruses:
  - Cytomegalovirus.
  - Herpesvirus.
- Fungi:
  - *Aspergillus.*
  - *Cryptococcus.*
  - *Candida.*
  - *Mucor.*
  - *Pneumocystis jiroveci.*
- Protozoa:
  - Toxoplasma gondii (rare).
- Pulmonary effects of therapy:
  1. Chemotherapeutic agents.
  2. Radiation therapy.
  3. Pulmonary hemorrhage.
  4. Congestive heart failure.
  5. Disseminated malignancy.
  6. Nonspecified interstitial pneumonitis (no defined etiology).

PULMONARY LESIONS

ICD-10CM#		
	J98.4	Other disorders of lung
	J70.9	Respiratory conditions due to unspecified external agent
	S27.309A	Unspecified injury of lung, unspecified, initial encounter

TB.
Legionella pneumonia.
Mycoplasma pneumonia.
Viral pneumonia.
Pneumocystis carinii.
Hypersensitivity pneumonitis.
Aspiration pneumonia.
Fungal disease (aspergillosis, histoplasmosis).
ARDS associated with pneumonia.
Psittacosis.
Sarcoidosis.
Septic emboli.
Metastatic cancer.
Multiple pulmonary emboli.
Rheumatoid nodules.

PULMONARY MASS, SOLITARY, CAUSES[36]

ICD-10CM #	R91.1	Solitary pulmonary nodule

CAUSES OF A SOLITARY PULMONARY MASS

Bronchial carcinoma.
Bronchial carcinoid.
Granuloma.
Hamartoma.
Metastasis.
Chronic pneumonia or abscess.
Hydatid cyst.
Pulmonary hematoma.
Bronchocele.
Fungus ball.
Massive fibrosis in coal workers.
Bronchogenic cyst.
Sequestration.
Arteriovenous malformation.
Pulmonary infarct.
Round atelectasis.

PULMONARY MASS, SOLITARY, MIMICS[36]

ICD-10CM #	Varies with specific diagnosis

SIMULANTS OF A SOLITARY PULMONARY MASS

Extrathoracic artifacts.
Cutaneous masses.
Bony lesions.
Pleural tumors or plaques.
Encysted pleural fluid.
Pulmonary vessels.

PULMONARY NODULE, SOLITARY

ICD-10CM #	J98.4	Other disorders of lung

Bronchogenic carcinoma.
Granuloma from histoplasmosis.
TB granuloma.
Granuloma from coccidioidomycosis.
Metastatic carcinoma.
Bronchial adenoma.
Bronchogenic cyst.
Hamartoma.
AV malformation.
Other: fibroma, intrapulmonary lymph node, sclerosing hemangioma, bronchopulmonary sequestration.

PULMONARY–RENAL SYNDROMES, CAUSES[28]

ICD-10CM #	Varies with specific diagnosis

Systemic vasculitis	Anti-GBM disease (Goodpasture). ANCA associated: Granulomatosis with polyangiitis. Microscopic polyarteritis. Churg-Strauss syndrome. Drugs (penicillamine, hydralazine, propylthiouracil). Immune complex disease. Lupus erythematosus. Henoch-Schönlein purpura. Mixed cryoglobulinemia. Rheumatoid vasculitis.
Infection	Severe bacterial pneumonia; postinfectious glomerulonephritis; *Legionella;* hantavirus; opportunistic infection in immunocompromised patients; infective endocarditis.
Pulmonary edema and AKI	Volume overload; severe left ventricular failure.
Multiorgan failure	Acute respiratory distress syndrome and AKI.
Other	Paraquat poisoning; renal vein or IVC thrombosis with pulmonary emboli.

AKI, Acute kidney injury; *ANCA,* anti-neutrophil cytoplasmic antibody; *GBM,* glomerular basement membrane; *IVC,* inferior vena cava.

PULSELESS ELECTRICAL ACTIVITY

ICD-10CM #	I46.9	Cardiac arrest, cause unspecified

Hypovolemia.
Hypoxia.
Hyperkalemia.
Acidosis.
Cardiac tamponade.
Tension pneumothorax.
Pulmonary embolus.
Drug overdose.
Hypothermia.

PUPILLARY DILATATION, POOR RESPONSE TO DARKNESS

ICD-10CM #	H21.569	Pupillary abnormality, unspecified eye

Drugs (narcotics, general anesthetics, cholinergics).
Acute trauma (spasm from prostaglandin release).
Inflammation, infection (interruption of inhibitory fibers to the Edinger-Westphal nucleus).
Old age (loss of inhibition at midbrain from reticular activating formation).
Horner syndrome (sympathetic neuron interruption).
Adie syndrome tonic pupil.
Lymphoma.
Congenital miosis.

PURPURA

ICD-10CM #		
	D69.2	Other nonthrombocytopenic purpura
	D69.0	Allergic purpura
	D69.49	Other primary thrombocytopenia
	M31.1	Thrombotic microangiopathy

THROMBOTIC

Trauma.
Septic emboli, atheromatous emboli.
DIC.
Thrombocytopenia.
Meningococcemia.
Rocky Mountain spotted fever.
Hemolytic-uremic syndrome.
Viral infection: echo, coxsackie.
Scurvy.
Other: left atrial myxoma, cryoglobulinemia, vasculitis, hyperglobulinemic purpura.

PURPURA, NONPALPABLE[43]

ICD-10CM #	D69.2	Other nonthrombocytopenic purpura

INCREASED TRANSMURAL PRESSURE GRADIENT

Acute (Valsalva, coughing, vomiting, high altitude, weight lifting).
Chronic—Venous stasis.

DECREASED MECHANICAL INTEGRITY OF MICROCIRCULATION AND SUPPORTING TISSUES

Age related (infancy and actinic purpura).
Glucocorticoid excess—Cushing's syndrome and glucocorticoid therapy.
Vitamin C deficiency (scurvy).
Abnormal connective tissue—Ehlers-Danlos syndrome.

Amyloid infiltration of blood vessels.
Colloid milium.
Hormonal—Female easy bruising syndrome (purpura simplex).
Lorenzo's oil.
MELAS syndrome.

TRAUMA TO BLOOD VESSELS

Physical:
- Injuries.
- Child abuse.
- Factitial purpura.

Ultraviolet purpura:
- Purpuric sunburn.
- Solar purpura.

Infectious:
- Bacterial.
- Rickettsial.
- Fungal.
- Viral.
- Parasitic.

Embolic:
- Infectious organisms.
- Atheroemboli (cholesterol crystal emboli).
- Fat emboli.

Allergic and/or inflammatory:
- Serum sickness.
- Pigmented purpuric eruptions.
- Pyoderma gangrenosum.
- Contact dermatitis.
- Familial Mediterranean fever.

Neoplastic.
Metabolic:
- Erythropoietic porphyria.
- Calciphylaxis.

Immunoglobulin related (hyperglobulinemic purpura of Waldenström and light-chain vasculitis).
Drug related.
Thrombotic:
- Disseminated intravascular coagulation.
- Warfarin (Coumadin)-induced skin necrosis.
- Protein C or protein S deficiency, factor V Leiden, prothrombin G20201A.
- Purpura fulminans.
- Paroxysmal nocturnal hemoglobinuria.
- Antiphospholipid antibody syndrome.
- Hemangioma with thrombocytopenia and consumptive coagulopathy (Kasabach-Merritt syndrome).

UNKNOWN CAUSE—PSYCHOGENIC PURPURA

PURPURA, NONPURPURIC DISORDERS SIMULATING PURPURA[3]

ICD-10CM #	Varies with specific diagnosis

Disorders with telangiectasias:
- Cherry angiomas.
- Hereditary hemorrhagic telangiectasia.
- Chronic actinic telangiectasia.
- Scleroderma.
- CREST syndrome.
- Ataxia-telangiectasia.
- Chronic liver disease.
- Pregnancy-related telangiectasia.

Kaposi sarcoma and other vascular sarcomas.
Fabry disease.
Neonatal extramedullary hematopoiesis.
Angioma serpiginosum.

PURPURA, PALPABLE[43]

ICD-10CM #	D69.2	Other nonthrombocytopenic purpura

Cutaneous vasculitis:
- Systemic vasculitides.
- Paraneoplastic vasculitis.
- Henoch-Schönlein purpura.
- Acute hemorrhagic edema of infancy.
- Livedoid vasculitis.
- Idiopathic.
- Urticarial.

Cryoglobulinemia.
Cryofibrinogenemia.
Primary cutaneous diseases.

QT INTERVAL PROLONGATION[50]

ICD-10CM #	R94.31	Abnormal electrocardiogram [ECG] [EKG]
	I45.81	Long QT syndrome

Drugs:
- Class I antiarrhythmics (e.g., disopyramide, procainamide, quinidine).
- Class III antiarrhythmics.
- Tricyclic antidepressants.
- Phenothiazines.
- Astemizole.
- Terfenadine.
- Adenosine.
- Antibiotics (e.g., erythromycin and other macrolides):
  - Antifungal agents.
  - Pentamidine, chloroquine.

Ischemic heart disease.
Cerebrovascular disease.
Rheumatic fever.
Myocarditis.
Mitral valve prolapse.
Electrolyte abnormalities.
Hypocalcemia.
Hypothyroidism.
Liquid protein diets.
Organophosphate insecticides.
Congenital prolonged QT syndrome.

RADIATION-INDUCED NEOPLASMS[76]

ICD-10CM #	Varies with specific diagnosis

RADIATION-INDUCED NEOPLASMS

Osteochondroma

Benign.
Exclusively with childhood irradiation.
Histologically identical to spontaneous osteochondroma.

Sarcoma

Malignant.
Latent period of 4 years or more.
Histologically identical to spontaneous sarcoma.
Commonly malignant fibrous histiocytoma or osteosarcoma.
Occurs in either bone or soft tissue.

Tumors in Other Organ Systems

Squamous cell cancer of the skin.
Breast cancer.
Leukemia, with shorter latent period than sarcoma.

RECTAL MASS, PALPABLE[81]

ICD-10CM #	R22.9	Localized swelling, mass and lump, unspecified

Rectal carcinoma.
Rectal polyp.
Hypertrophied anal papilla.
Diverticular phlegmon (prolapsing into the pouch of Douglas).
Sigmoid colon carcinoma (prolapsing into the pouch of Douglas).
Metastatic deposits at the pelvic reflection (Blumer shelf).
Primary pelvic malignancy (uterine, ovarian, prostatic, or cervical).
Mesorectal lymph nodes.
Endometriosis.
Solitary rectal ulcer syndrome.
Foreign body.
Feces.
Presacral cyst.
Amebic granuloma.
Vaginal tampon and even the pubic bone may be mistaken for a rectal mass.

RECTAL PAIN

ICD-10CM #	K62.89	Other specified diseases of anus and rectum

Anal fissure.
Thrombosed hemorrhoid.
Anorectal abscess.
Foreign bodies.
Fecal impaction.
Endometriosis.
Neoplasms (primary or metastatic).
Pelvic inflammatory disease.
Inflammation of sacral nerves.
Compression of sacral nerves.
Prostatitis.
Other: proctalgia fugax, uterine abnormalities, myopathies, coccygodynia.

RED BLOOD CELL APLASIA, ACQUIRED, ETIOLOGY

ICD-10CM #	D61.01	Constitutional (pure) red blood cell aplasia

Idiopathic (>50% of cases).
Medications (most frequent with phenytoin).
Non-Hodgkin's lymphoma.
Viral infections (parvovirus B19, EB virus, mumps, hepatitis).
Myelodysplastic syndromes.
Thymoma.
Autoimmune diseases.

Allogenic bone marrow transplant from ABO incompatible donor.
Pregnancy.

RED BLOOD CELL FRAGMENTATION HEMOLYSIS, CAUSES[42]

ICD-10CM #	Varies with specific disorder

CAUSES OF RED BLOOD CELL FRAGMENTATION HEMOLYSIS

Damaged microvasculature.
Thrombotic thrombocytopenic purpura–hemolytic uremic syndrome (TTP–HUS).
Associated with pregnancy: preeclampsia or eclampsia; hemolysis plus elevated liver enzymes plus low platelets (HELLP syndrome).
Associated with malignancy, with or without mitomycin C treatment.
Vasculitis: polyarteritis, Wegener granulomatosis, acute glomerulonephritis, or *Rickettsia*-like infections.
Systemic lupus erythematosus.
Abnormalities of renal vasculature: malignant hypertension, acute glomerulonephritis, scleroderma, or allograft rejection with or without cyclosporine treatment.
Disseminated intravascular coagulation.
Malignant hypertension.
Catastrophic antiphospholipid antibody syndrome.
Atrioventricular malformations.
Kasabach-Merritt syndrome.
Hemangioendotheliomas.
Atrioventricular shunts for congenital and acquired conditions (e.g., stents, coils, transjugular intrahepatic portosystemic shunt, Levine shunts).
Cardiac abnormalities:
- Replaced valve, prosthesis, graft, or patch.
- Aortic stenosis or regurgitant jets (e.g., in ruptured sinus of Valsalva).

Drugs:
- Cyclosporine.
- Mitomycin.
- Ticlopidine.
- Clopidogrel.
- Tacrolimus.
- Cocaine.

Systemic infection:
- Bacterial endocarditis.
- Brucellosis.
- Cytomegalovirus.
- Human immunodeficiency virus.
- Ehrlichiosis.
- Rocky Mountain spotted fever.

RED EYE

ICD-10CM #	H57.8	Other specified disorders of eye and adnexa

Infectious conjunctivitis (bacterial, viral).
Allergic conjunctivitis.
Acute glaucoma.
Keratitis (bacterial, viral).
Iritis.
Trauma.

RED EYE, ACUTE[4]

ICD-10CM #	H57.8

Obvious open globe.
Corneal abrasion.
Corneal ulcer.
Subconjunctival hemorrhage.
Hyphema.
Occult open globe.
Herpes simplex virus glaucoma.
Iritis, traumatic iritis.
Scleritis.
Conjunctivitis.
Blepharitis.
Ultraviolet keratitis.
Episcleritis.
Conjunctival foreign body.
Dry eye.
Contact lens overwear syndrome.

RED HOT JOINT

ICD-10CM #	Varies with specific diagnosis

Trauma.
Gout.
Infection (septic joint).
Pseudogout (calcium pyrophosphate dehydrate crystal deposition).
Psoriatic arthropathy.
Reactive arthritis.
Palindromic rheumatism.

RED URINE

ICD-10CM #	R39.19	Other difficulties with micturition

Hematuria.
Porphyrins.
Hemoglobinuria.
Myoglobinuria.
Medications (phenazopyridine, aminosalicylic acid, deferoxamine, phenazopyridine, phenolphthalein, NSAIDs, rifampin, phenytoin, methyldopa, doxorubicin, phenacetin).
Foods (beets, berries, maize).
Urate crystalluria.

RENAL ALLOGRAFT DYSFUNCTION[34]

ICD-10CM #	T86.1	Complications of renal allograft

IMMEDIATE/DELAYED GRAFT FUNCTION (1-3 DAYS)

Acute tubular necrosis.
Hyperacute humoral rejection.
Urinary leak or obstruction.
Renal artery or vein thrombosis.
Recurrence of disease (e.g., focal segmental glomerulosclerosis).

EARLY POSTTRANSPLANTATION PERIOD (FIRST MONTH)

Acute cellular rejection.
Acute humoral rejection.
Calcineurin inhibitor toxicity.
Urinary tract obstruction.
Volume depletion.
Recurrence of disease.

Late Acute Dysfunction

Acute rejection.
Cyclosporine or tacrolimus toxicity.
Recurrence of primary disease.
Tubulointerstitial nephritis, drug-induced.
Renal artery stenosis.
Infection (bacterial urinary tract infection [UTI], cytomegalovirus, BK virus).
Hemodynamic (volume; use of angiotensin-converting enzyme inhibitor, angiotensin II receptor blocker).

Chronic Dysfunction

Chronic rejection.
Cyclosporine or tacrolimus toxicity.
Recurrent renal disease.
De novo renal disease.
Urinary tract obstruction.
Bacterial UTI.
Hypertensive nephrosclerosis.

RENAL ARTERY OCCLUSION, CAUSES

ICD-10CM #	N28.0	Ischemia and infarction of kidney

Atrial fibrillation.
Angiography or stent placement.
Abdominal aortic surgery.
Trauma.
Renal artery aneurysm/dissection.
Vasculitis.
Thrombosis in patient with fibromuscular dysplasia.
Atherosclerosis.
Septic embolism.
Mural thrombus thromboembolism.
Atrial myxoma thromboembolism.
Mitral stenosis thromboembolism.
Prosthetic valve thromboembolism.
Renal cell carcinoma.

RENAL COLIC[4]

ICD-10CM #	N23	Unspecified renal colic

Vascular:
- Abdominal aortic aneurysm.
- Aortic dissection.
- Renal artery dissection.
- Renal artery stenosis.
- Renal vein thrombosis.
- Renal infarct.
- Mesenteric ischemia.
- Retroperitoneal hemorrhage.

GI:
- Incarcerated hernia.
- Appendicitis.
- Cholecystitis.
- Biliary colic.
- Pancreatitis.

Bowel obstruction.
Diverticulitis.
Gynecologic:
Ectopic pregnancy.
Ovarian torsion.
Tuboovarian abscess.
Pelvic inflammatory disease.
Endometriosis.
Genitourinary:
Testicular torsion.
Pyelonephritis.
Perinephric abscess.
Urinary tract tumor.
Renal papillary necrosis.
Upper urinary tract hemorrhage.
Musculoskeletal:
Lumbar strain.
Radiculopathy.
Disk herniation.
Vertebral compression fracture.
Dermatologic:
Herpes zoster.
Miscellaneous:
Factitious.

RENAL CYSTIC DISORDERS

ICD-10CM #	Q61.01	Congenital single renal cyst

Simple cysts.
Acquired cystic kidney disease.
Autosomal dominant polycystic kidney disease.
Autosomal recessive polycystic kidney disease.
Medullary cystic disease.
Medullary sponge kidney.

RENAL DISEASE, SKIN MANIFESTATIONS[74]

ICD-10CM #	Varies with specific diagnosis

SKIN MANIFESTATIONS SECONDARY TO RENAL DISEASE

Nonspecific
Pruritus.
Xerosis.
Acquired ichthyosis.
Pigmentary alteration.
Pallor (secondary to anemia).
Hyperpigmentation.
Dyspigmentation (yellow tint).
Infections (fungal, bacterial, viral).
Purpura.

Somewhat Specific
Acquired perforating dermatosis.
Calciphylaxis.
Metastatic calcification.
Blistering disorders.
Porphyria cutanea tarda.
Pseudoporphyria.
Eruptive xanthomas.
Pseudo–Kaposi sarcoma.

Specific
Nephrogenic systemic fibrosis.
Dialysis-associated steal syndrome.
Metastatic renal cell carcinoma.
Dialysis-related amyloidosis.
Arteriovenous shunt dermatitis.
Uremic frost.

RENAL FAILURE, ACUTE, PIGMENT-INDUCED[7]

ICD-10CM #	N19	Unspecified kidney failure

CAUSES OF PIGMENT-INDUCED ACUTE RENAL FAILURE

Rhabdomyolysis and myoglobinuria.
Vigorous exercise.
Arterial embolization.
Status epilepticus.
Status asthmaticus.
Coma-induced and pressure-induced myonecrosis.
Heat stress.
Diabetic ketoacidosis.
Myopathy.
Alcoholism.
Hypokalemia.
Hypophosphatemia.
Hemoglobinuria.
Transfusion reactions.
Snake envenomation.
Malaria.
Mechanical destruction of RBCs by prosthetic valves.
G6PD deficiency.

G6PD, Glucose-6-phosphate dehydrogenase; *RBCs,* red blood cells.

RENAL FAILURE, CHRONIC[34]

ICD-10CM #	N18.9	Chronic kidney disease, unspecified

CAUSES OF CHRONIC RENAL FAILURE

Diabetic glomerulosclerosis (systemic disease involving the kidney).
Hypertensive nephrosclerosis.
Glomerular disease:
Glomerulonephritis.
Amyloidosis, light chain disease (systemic disease involving the kidney).
Systemic lupus erythematosus, Wegener granulomatosis (systemic disease involving the kidney).
Tubulointerstitial disease:
Reflux nephropathy (chronic pyelonephritis).
Analgesic nephropathy.
Obstructive nephropathy (stones, benign prostatic hypertrophy).
Myeloma kidney (systemic disease involving the kidney).
Vascular disease:
Scleroderma (systemic disease involving the kidney).
Vasculitis (systemic disease involving the kidney).
Renovascular renal failure (ischemic nephropathy).
Atheroembolic renal disease (systemic disease involving the kidney).
Cystic disease:
Autosomal dominant polycystic kidney disease.
Medullary cystic kidney disease.

RENAL FAILURE, INTRINSIC OR PARENCHYMAL CAUSES[77]

ICD-10CM #	N17.0	Acute kidney failure with tubular necrosis
	N17.1	Acute kidney failure with acute cortical necrosis
	N17.2	Acute kidney failure with medullary necrosis
	N17.8	Other acute kidney failure
	N17.9	Acute kidney failure, unspecified
	N18.9	Chronic kidney disease, unspecified

ABNORMALITIES OF THE VASCULATURE

Renal arteries: atherosclerosis, thromboembolism, arteritis.
Renal veins: thrombosis.
Microvasculature: vasculitis, thrombotic microangiopathy.

ABNORMALITIES OF GLOMERULI (ACUTE GLOMERULONEPHRITIS)

Antiglomerular membrane disease (Goodpasture syndrome).
Immune complex glomerulonephritis: SLE, postinfectious, idiopathic, membranoproliferative.

ABNORMALITIES OF INTERSTITIUM (ACUTE INTERSTITIAL NEPHRITIS)

Drugs (e.g., antibiotics, NSAIDs, diuretics, anticonvulsants, allopurinol).
Infectious pyelonephritis.
Infiltrative: lymphoma, leukemia, sarcoidosis.

ABNORMALITIES OF TUBULES

Physical obstruction (uric acid, oxalate, light chains).
Acute tubular necrosis:
Ischemic.
Toxic (antibiotics, chemotherapy, immunosuppressives, radiocontrast dyes, heavy metals, myoglobin, hemolyzed RBCs).

RENAL FAILURE, POSTRENAL CAUSES[77]

ICD-10CM #	N17.0	Acute kidney failure with tubular necrosis
	N17.1	Acute kidney failure with acute cortical necrosis
	N17.2	Acute kidney failure with medullary necrosis

	N17.8	Other acute kidney failure
	N17.9	Acute kidney failure, unspecified
	N18.9	Chronic kidney disease, unspecified

URETER AND RENAL PELVIS

Intrinsic obstruction:
- Blood clots.
- Stones.
- Sloughed papillae: diabetes, sickle cell disease, analgesic nephropathy.
- Inflammatory: fungus ball.

Extrinsic obstruction:
- Malignancy.
- Retroperitoneal fibrosis.
- Iatrogenic: inadvertent ligation of ureters.

BLADDER

Prostatic hypertrophy or malignancy.
Neuropathic bladder.
Blood clots.
Bladder cancer.
Stones.

URETHRAL

Strictures.
Congenital valves.

RENAL FAILURE, PRERENAL CAUSES[77]

ICD-10CM #	N17.0	Acute kidney failure with tubular necrosis
	N17.1	Acute kidney failure with acute cortical necrosis
	N17.2	Acute kidney failure with medullary necrosis
	N17.8	Other acute kidney failure
	N17.9	Acute kidney failure, unspecified
	N18.9	Chronic kidney disease, unspecified

DECREASED CARDIAC OUTPUT

CHF.
Arrhythmias.
Pericardial constriction or tamponade.
Pulmonary embolism.

HYPOVOLEMIA

GI tract loss (vomiting, diarrhea, nasogastric suction).
Blood losses (trauma, GI tract surgery).
Renal losses (diuretics, mineralocorticoid deficiency, postobstructive diuresis).
Skin losses (burns).

VOLUME REDISTRIBUTION (DECREASE IN EFFECTIVE BLOOD VOLUME)

Hypoalbuminemic states (cirrhosis, nephrosis).
Sequestration of fluid in "third" space (ischemic bowel, peritonitis, pancreatitis).
Peripheral vasodilation (sepsis, vasodilators, anaphylaxis).

ALTERED RENAL VASCULAR RESISTANCE

Increase in afferent vascular resistance (NSAIDs, liver disease, sepsis, hypercalcemia, cyclosporine).
Decrease in efferent arteriolar tone (ACE inhibitors).

RENAL INFARCTION[28]

ICD-10CM #	N28.0	Ischemia and infarction of kidney

CAUSES OF RENAL INFARCTION

Thrombosis: Spontaneous

Atherosclerotic disease of aorta and renal artery.
Fibromuscular dysplasia of renal artery.
Aneurysms of aorta or renal artery.
Dissection of aorta or renal artery.
- Marfan syndrome.
- Ehlers-Danlos syndrome.

Vasculitis involving renal artery.
- Polyarteritis nodosa.
- Takayasu arteritis.
- Kawasaki disease.
- Thromboangiitis obliterans.
- Other necrotizing vasculitides.

Inflammatory disease of the aorta or renal artery.
- Syphilis.
- Tuberculosis.
- Mycoses.

Hypercoagulable states.
- Nephrotic syndrome.
- Antiphospholipid syndrome.
- Antithrombin III deficiency.
- Homocystinuria.

Thrombotic microangiopathies.
- Hemolytic-uremic syndrome.
- Thrombotic thrombocytopenic purpura.
- Antiphospholipid syndrome.
- Malignant hypertension.
- Scleroderma.
- Sickle cell nephropathy.
- Polycythemia vera.
- Postpartum hemolytic-uremic syndrome.
- Hyperacute vascular allograft rejection.

Thrombosis: Induced

Traumatic.
Following endovascular intervention.
Post renal transplantation.

Embolism

Cardiac source.
- Atrial fibrillation or other arrhythmias.
- Native and prosthetic valvular heart disease.
- Infective endocarditis.
- Marantic endocarditis.

Myocardial infarction with mural thrombi.
- Left atrial myxoma or other tumor.

Noncardiac sources.
- Atheromatous embolic disease.
- Paradoxical emboli.
- Fat emboli.
- Tumor emboli.

Therapeutic renal embolization.
Segmental renal infarction of childhood.
Cisplatinum and gemcitabine.
Sickle cell disease or sickle cell trait.

RENAL PARENCHYMAL DISEASE, CHRONIC[36]

ICD-10CM #	N28.9	Disorder of kidney and ureter, unspecified

DIFFERENTIAL DIAGNOSIS OF CHRONIC RENAL PARENCHYMAL DISEASE

No Papillary/Caliceal Abnormality

Diffuse Parenchymal Loss

Bilateral:
- Chronic glomerulonephritis.
- Diffuse small-vessel disease.
- Hereditary nephropathies.

Unilateral:
- Renal artery stenosis.
- Postirradiation.
- Rare:
  - Hypoplastic kidney.
  - Postobstructive atrophy.

FOCAL PARENCHYMAL LOSS

Infarct.
Previous trauma.

Papillary/Caliceal Abnormality

Diffuse Parenchymal Loss

Obstructive nephropathy.
Generalized reflux nephropathy.

No Parenchymal Loss

Papillary necrosis.
TB.
Medullary sponge kidney.
Megacalices.
Pelvicaliceal cyst.

Focal Parenchymal Loss

Focal reflux nephropathy (chronic atrophic pyelonephritis).
TB.
Calculus disease.

RENAL VEIN THROMBOSIS, CAUSES

ICD-10CM #	I82.3	Embolism and thrombosis of renal vein

Nephrotic syndrome.
Renal cell carcinoma.
Aortic aneurysm causing compression.
Lymphadenopathy.
Retroperitoneal fibrosis.
Estrogen therapy.
Pregnancy.
Renal cell carcinoma with vein invasion.
Severe dehydration.

RESPIRATORY DISTRESS IN THE NEWBORN, CAUSES[30]

ICD-10CM #	J96.00	Acute respiratory failure

Respiratory Distress in the Newborn

Noncardiopulmonary

Hypothermia or hyperthermia.
Hypoglycemia.
Metabolic acidosis.

Drug intoxications; withdrawal.
Polycythemia.
CNS insult.
Asphyxia.
Hemorrhage.
Neuromuscular disease.
Werdnig-Hoffman disease.
Myopathies.
Phrenic nerve injury.
Skeletal abnormalities.
Asphyxiating thoracic dystrophy.

Cardiovascular

Left-sided outflow obstruction.
Hypoplastic left heart.
Aortic stenosis.
Coarctation of the aorta.
Cyanotic lesions.
Transposition of the great vessels.
Total anomalous pulmonary venous return
Tricuspid atresia.
Right-sided outflow obstruction.

Pulmonary

Upper airway obstruction.
Choanal atresia.
Vocal cord paralysis.
Meconium aspiration.
Clear fluid aspiration.
Transient tachypnea.
Pneumonia.
Pulmonary hypoplasia.
Primary.
Secondary.
Hyaline membrane disease.
Pneumothorax.
Pleural effusions.
Mass lesions.
Lobar emphysema.
Cystic adenomatoid malformation.

RESPIRATORY FAILURE, HYPOVENTILATORY[61]

ICD-10CM #		
	J96.00	Acute respiratory failure, unspecified whether with hypoxia or hypercapnia
	J96.90	Respiratory failure, unspecified, unspecified whether with hypoxia or hypercapnia

ABNORMAL RESPIRATORY CAPACITY (NORMAL RESPIRATORY WORKLOADS)

Acute depression of CNS:
  Various causes.
Chronic central hypoventilation syndromes:
  Obesity-hypoventilation syndrome.
  Sleep apnea syndrome.
  Hypothyroidism.
  Shy-Drager syndrome (multisystem atrophy syndrome).
Acute toxic paralysis syndromes:
  Botulism.
  Tetanus.
  Toxic ingestion or bites.
  Organophosphate poisoning.
Neuromuscular disorders (acute and chronic):
  Myasthenia gravis.
  Guillain-Barré syndrome.
  Drugs.
  Amyotrophic lateral sclerosis.
  Muscular dystrophies.
  Polymyositis.
  Spinal cord injury.
  Traumatic phrenic nerve paralysis.

ABNORMAL PULMONARY WORKLOADS

Chronic obstructive pulmonary disease:
  Chronic bronchitis.
  Asthmatic bronchitis.
  Emphysema.
Asthma and acute bronchial hyperreactivity syndromes.
Upper airway obstruction.
Interstitial lung diseases.

ABNORMAL EXTRAPULMONARY WORKLOADS

Chronic thoracic cage disorders:
  Severe kyphoscoliosis.
  After thoracoplasty.
  After thoracic cage injury.
Acute thoracic cage trauma and burns.
Pneumothorax.
Pleural fibrosis and effusions.
Abdominal processes.

RESPIRATORY MUSCLE WEAKNESS[65]

ICD-10CM #	Varies with specific diagnosis

CAUSES OF DECREASED RESPIRATORY MUSCLE STRENGTH OR ENDURANCE

Disorders of the phrenic nerve:
  Guillain-Barré syndrome.
  Poliomyelitis.
Respiratory muscle atrophy.
Disorders of neuromuscular transmission:
  Myasthenia gravis.
  Ventilator dependence.
  Malnutrition.
  Myopathy.
  Critical illness polyneuropathy/myopathy.
Altered diaphragmatic force-length relationship:
  Dynamic hyperinflation and diaphragmatic flattening.

RETINOPATHY, HYPERTENSIVE

ICD-10CM #	H35.039	Hypertensive retinopathy, unspecified eye

Retinal venous obstruction.
Diabetic retinopathy.
Ocular ischemic syndrome.
Hyperviscosity.
Tortuosity of retinal artery.

RHINITIS

ICD-10CM #		
	J31.0	Chronic rhinitis
	J30.0	Vasomotor rhinitis
	J30.1	Allergic rhinitis due to pollen
	J30.2	Other seasonal allergic rhinitis
	J30.5	Allergic rhinitis due to food
	J30.89	Other allergic rhinitis
	J30.9	Allergic rhinitis, unspecified

Allergic rhinitis.
Infectious rhinitis.
Vasomotor rhinitis.
Exercise-induced rhinitis.
Emotional rhinitis.
Rhinitis medicamentosa.
Hormone-mediated rhinitis (menses, pregnancy, oral contraceptives, hypothyroidism).
GERD.
Chemical- or irritant-induced rhinitis.
Rhinitis mimics:
  Deviated septum.
  Enlarged adenoids.
  Nasal polyps/tumors.
  Foreign bodies.
  CSF rhinorrhea.
  Sarcoidosis.
  Midline granuloma.
  Granulomatosis with polyangiitis.
  SLE.
  Sjögren syndrome.

RHINITIS, CHRONIC[2]

ICD-10CM #	J31.0	Chronic rhinitis

CLASSIFICATION OF CHRONIC RHINITIS

Allergic

Systemic.
Local (entopy).

Work-Related

Irritant.
Corrosive.
Immunologic.

Infectious (Rhinosinusitis)

Allergic.
Nonallergic.

Nonallergic

Idiopathic.
Nonallergic with eosinophilia.
Atrophic.
Primary.
Secondary.
Medication-related.
Topical vasoconstrictors (rhinitis medicamentosa).
Oral medications.
Exercise-induced.
Cold air–induced.
Gustatory.
Hormonal.
Aging.
Systemic diseases.

RHINOSINUSITIS, DIFFERENTIAL DIAGNOSIS[58]

ICD-10CM #	Varies with specific diagnosis

DIFFERENTIAL DIAGNOSIS OF RHINOSINUSITIS

Allergic Rhinitis

Seasonal.
Perennial.
Combined seasonal and perennial.
Allergic fungal rhinosinusitis.

Nonallergic Rhinitis

Nonallergic, noninflammatory idiopathic rhinopathy (vasomotor rhinitis).
Nonallergic rhinitis with eosinophilia syndrome (NARES).
Cold dry air–induced rhinitis.
Gustatory rhinitis.

Infectious Rhinosinusitis

Bacterial.
Viral.
Fungal.
Granulomatous.

Drug-Induced Rhinitis

Oral contraceptives.
Various antihypertensives and ocular β-blockers.
Topical decongestants (rhinitis medicamentosa).
Phosphodiesterase-5 antagonists.

Mechanical Causes of Rhinosinusitis

Septal deviation.
Nasal foreign body.
Choanal atresia or stenosis.
Adenoid hypertrophy.
Encephalocele.
Glioma.
Dermoid.

Innate and Acquired Immunity Disorders

Congenital or acquired immunodeficiencies.
Cystic fibrosis.
Immotile cilia syndrome.

Systemic Inflammatory Disorders

Sarcoidosis.
Granulomatosis with polyangiitis.
Vasculitis.

Neoplastic Causes

Benign:
- Polyps.
- Nasopharyngeal angiofibroma.
- Inverting papilloma.

Malignant:
- Adenocarcinoma.
- Squamous cell carcinoma.
- Aesthesioneuroblastoma.
- Lymphoma.
- Rhabdomyosarcoma.

RIB DEFECTS ON X-RAY[36]

ICD-10CM #	Varies with specific diagnosis

CAUSES OF SUPERIOR MARGINAL RIB DEFECTS

Normal

Isolated defects.
Projectional artifacts (due to lordosis).

Neurologic

Paralytic poliomyelitis.
Quadriparesis.

Collagen Vascular Disease

Rheumatoid arthritis.
SLE.
Systemic sclerosis.

Local Pressure

Chest drainage tube.
Osteochondroma.
Neural tumor.
Coarctation of aorta.

Hyperparathyroidism Miscellaneous

Osteogenesis imperfecta.
Marfan syndrome.

RIB NOTCHING ON X-RAY[36]

ICD-10CM #	Varies with specific diagnosis

CAUSES OF INFERIOR RIB NOTCHING

Arterial

AORTIC OBSTRUCTION

Aortic coarctation.
Aortic thrombosis.
Aortitis.

SUBCLAVIAN ARTERY OBSTRUCTION

Blalock-Taussig operation.
Arteritis.
Atherosclerotic occlusion.

PULMONARY OLIGEMIA

Pulmonary atresia.
Tetralogy of Fallot.
Multiple pulmonary arterial stenoses.
Venous

CHRONIC SUPERIOR VENA CAVAL OBSTRUCTION

Arteriovenous

Arteriovenous Malformation

Pulmonary.
Chest wall.
Neural
Neurofibromas

RIGHT AXIS DEVIATION[50]

ICD-10CM #	Varies with specific diagnosis

Normal variation.
Right ventricular hypertrophy.
Left posterior fascicular block.
Lateral myocardial infarction.
Pulmonary embolism.
Dextrocardia.
Mechanical shifts or emphysema causing a vertical heart.

SALIVARY GLAND ENLARGEMENT

ICD-10CM #	K11.1	Hypertrophy of salivary gland

Neoplasm.
Sialolithiasis.
Infection (mumps, bacterial infection, HIV, TB).
Sarcoidosis.
Idiopathic.
Acromegaly.
Anorexia/bulimia.
Chronic pancreatitis.
Medications (e.g., phenylbutazone).
Cirrhosis.
DM.

SALIVARY GLAND SECRETION, DECREASED

ICD-10CM #	K11.7	Disturbances of salivary secretion
	R68.2	Dry mouth, unspecified

Medications (antihistamines, antidepressants, neuroleptics, antihypertensives).
Dehydration.
Anxiety.
Sjögren syndrome.
Sarcoidosis.
Mumps.
Amyloidosis.
CNS disorders.
Head and neck radiation.

SCLERODERMA-LIKE SYNDROMES[3]

ICD-10CM #	Varies with specific diagnosis

OTHER DISEASES

Morphea.
Eosinophilic fasciitis.
Scleredema (of Buschke).
Scleromyxedema.
Graft-versus-host disease.
Nephrogenic-fibrosing dermopathy.

ENVIRONMENTAL AGENTS AND DRUGS

Bleomycin.
l-Tryptophan.
Organic solvents.
Pentazocine.
Toxic oil syndrome.
Vinyl chloride disease.
Gadolinium.

SCROTAL CALCIFICATIONS[69]

ICD-10CM #	Varies with specific diagnosis

SCROTAL CALCIFICATIONS

Testicular

Solitary, postinflammatory granulomatous, vascular.
Microlithiasis.
"Burned-out" germ cell tumor.
Large-cell calcifying Sertoli cell tumor.
Teratoma.
Mixed germ cell tumor.
Sarcoid.
TB.
Chronic infarct.

Extratesticular

Tunica vaginalis "scrotal pearls."
Chronic epididymitis.
Schistosomiasis.

SCROTAL MASSES, BOYS AND ADOLESCENTS[51]

ICD-10CM #	R22.9	Localized swelling, mass and lump, unspecified

PAINFUL

Testicular torsion.
Torsion of appendix testis.
Epididymitis.
Trauma: ruptured testis, hematocele.
Inguinal hernia (incarcerated).
Mumps orchitis.

PAINLESS

Hydrocele.
Inguinal hernia.[40]
Varicocele.
Spermatocele.
Testicular tumor.
Henoch-Schönlein purpura.
Idiopathic scrotal edema.

[40] May be associated with discomfort.

SCROTAL PAIN[61]

ICD-10CM#	S31.30XA	Unspecified open wound of scrotum and testes, initial encounter
	N50.9	Disorder of male genital organs, unspecified
	R10.2	Pelvic and perineal pain
	N49.9	Inflammatory disorder of unspecified male genital organ
	N50.1	Vascular disorders of male genital organs
	N49.9	Inflammatory disorder of unspecified male genital organ

Torsion:
- Appendages.
- Spermatic cord.

Infection:
- Orchitis.
- Abscess.
- Epididymitis.

Neoplasia:
- Benign.
- Malignant.

Incarcerated hernia.
Trauma.
Hydrocele.
Spermatocele.
Varicocele.

SCROTAL PAIN, ADOLESCENT OR PEDIATRIC PATIENT[85]

ICD-10CM #	Varies with specific diagnosis

DIFFERENTIAL DIAGNOSIS OF PEDIATRIC ADOLESCENT ACUTE SCROTAL PAIN

Appendage torsion:
- Appendix testis.
- Other appendage (epididymis, paradidymis, vas aberrans).

Spermatic cord torsion:
- Intravaginal, acute or intermittent.
- Extravaginal.

Epididymitis:
- Infectious.
  - Urinary tract infection.
  - Sexually transmitted disease.
  - Viral
- Sterile or traumatic.

Scrotal edema or erythema:
- Diaper dermatitis, insect bite, or other skin lesions.
- Idiopathic scrotal edema.

Orchitis:
- Associated with epididymitis with or without abscess.
- Vasculitis (e.g., Henoch-Schönlein purpura).
- Viral illness (mumps).

Trauma:
- Hematocele or scrotal contusion or testis rupture.

Hernia or hydrocele:
- Inguinal hernia with or without incarceration.
- Communicating hydrocele.
- Encysted hydrocele with or without torsion.
- Associated with acute abdominal pathology (e.g., appendicitis, peritonitis).

Varicocele.

Intrascrotal mass:
- Cystic dysplasia or tumor of testis.
- Epididymal cyst, spermatocele or tumor.
- Other paratesticular tumors.

Musculoskeletal pain from inguinal tendonitis or muscle strain.

Referred pain (e.g., ureteral calculus or anomaly).

SCROTAL SWELLING

ICD-10CM #	N50.8	Other specified disorders of male genital organs

Hydrocele.
Varicocele.
Neoplasm.
Acute epididymitis.
Orchitis.
Trauma.
Hernia.
Torsion of spermatic cord.
Torsion of epididymis.
Torsion of testis.
Insect bite.
Folliculitis.
Sebaceous cyst.
Thrombosis of spermatic vein.
Other: lymphedema, dermatitis, fat necrosis, Henoch-Schönlein purpura, idiopathic scrotal edema.

SEIZURE

ICD-10CM #	R56.9	Unspecified convulsions

Syncope.
Alcohol abuse/withdrawal.
TIA.
Hemiparetic migraine.
Psychiatric disorders.
Carotid sinus hypersensitivity.
Hyperventilation, prolonged breath holding.
Hypoglycemia.
Narcolepsy.
Movement disorders (tics, hemiballismus).
Hyponatremia.
Brain tumor (primary or metastatic).
Tetanus.
Strychnine, phencyclidine poisoning.

SEIZURE, PEDIATRIC[7]

ICD-10CM #	R56.9	Unspecified convulsions
	P90	Convulsions of newborn

First Month of Life

First Day

Hypoxia.
Drugs.
Trauma.
Infection.
Hyperglycemia.
Hypoglycemia.
Pyridoxine deficiency.

Day 2-3

Infection.
Drug withdrawal.
Hypoglycemia.
Hypocalcemia.
Developmental malformation.
Intracranial hemorrhage.
Inborn error of metabolism.
Hyponatremia or hypernatremia.

Day >4

Infection.
Hypocalcemia.
Hyperphosphatemia.
Hyponatremia.
Developmental malformation.
Drug withdrawal.
Inborn error of metabolism.

1 TO 6 MO

As above.

6 MO TO 3 YR

Febrile seizures.
Birth injury.
Infection.
Toxin.
Trauma.
Metabolic disorder.
Cerebral degenerative disease.

>3 YR

Idiopathic.
Infection.
Trauma.
Cerebral degenerative disease.

SEIZURE MIMICS[3]

ICD-10CM # Varies with specific diagnosis

NON-EPILEPTIC EPISODIC DISORDERS THAT MAY RESEMBLE SEIZURES

Movement disorders: myoclonus, paroxysmal choreoathetosis, episodic ataxias, hyperexplexia (startle disease).
Migraine: confusional, vertebrobasilar, visual auras.
Syncope.
Behavioral and psychiatric: psychogenic nonepileptic attacks (pseudoseizures), hyperventilation syndrome, panic or anxiety disorder, dissociative states.
Cataplexy (usually associated with narcolepsy).
Transient ischemic attack.
Alcoholic blackouts.
Hypoglycemia.

SEXUAL DIFFERENTIATION ABNORMALITIES[85]

ICD-10CM # Varies with specific diagnosis

ABNORMAL SEXUAL DIFFERENTIATION

1. Disorders of gonadal differentiation.
   Seminiferous tubule dysgenesis.
   Klinefelter syndrome.
   46,XX male.
   Syndromes of gonadal dysgenesis:
      Turner syndrome.
      Pure gonadal dysgenesis.
      Mixed gonadal dysgenesis.
      Partial gonadal dysgenesis (dysgenetic male pseudohermaphroditism).
      Bilateral vanishing testis, testicular regression syndromes.
2. Ovotesticular DSD (true hermaphroditism).
3. 46,XX DSD (masculinized female).
   Congenital adrenal hyperplasia (21-hydroxylase, 11β-hydroxylase, 3β-hydroxysteroid dehydrogenase deficiencies).
   Maternal androgens.
4. 46,XY DSD (undermasculinized male).
   Leydig cell agenesis, unresponsiveness.
   Disorders of testosterone biosynthesis.
   Variants of congenital adrenal hyperplasia affecting corticosteroid and testosterone synthesis:
      StAR deficiency (congenital lipoid adrenal hyperplasia).
      Cytochrome P450 oxidoreductase (POR) deficiency.
      3β-Hydroxysteroid dehydrogenase deficiency.
      17β-Hydroxylase deficiency.
   Disorders of testosterone biosynthesis:
      17,20-Lyase deficiency.
      17β-Hydroxysteroid oxidoreductase deficiency.
   Disorders of androgen-dependent target tissue:
      Androgen receptor and postreceptor defects.
      Syndrome of complete (severe) androgen insensitivity.
      Syndrome of partial androgen insensitivity.
      Mild androgen insensitivity syndrome (MAIS).
   Disorders of testosterone metabolism by peripheral tissues:
      5α-Reductase deficiency.
      Disorders of synthesis, secretion, or response to müllerian-inhibiting substance.
   Persistent müllerian duct syndrome.
5. Unclassified forms.
   In females: Mayer-Rokitansky-Küster-Hauser syndrome.
   DSD, disorder of sex development.

SEXUAL DYSFUNCTION, FEMALE[3]

ICD-10CM # R37 Sexual dysfunction, unspecified

FACTORS THAT MAY INFLUENCE SEXUAL FUNCTIONING IN WOMEN

Biological

Medications (e.g., antidepressants, antihypertensives).
Vaginal atrophy, pain with intercourse.
Low testosterone levels (e.g., bilateral oophorectomy).
Illness (e.g., diabetes, hypothyroidism, cerebrovascular accident).
Sleep disturbances, fatigue.
Disability or pain from illness (e.g., arthritis).
Incontinence.

Psychological

Depression.
Body image.

Interpersonal

Marital issues.
Poor communication.
Partner's sexual problems (e.g., erectile dysfunction).
Partner's health problems (e.g., myocardial infarction).

Sociocultural

Ageism ("too old" to want sex).
Multiple other obligations and commitments.
Lack of partner.

SEXUALLY TRANSMITTED DISEASES, ANORECTAL REGION[57]

ICD-10CM # K62.89 Other specified diseases of anus and rectum

ULCERATIVE

Lymphogranuloma venereum.
Herpes simplex virus.
Early (primary) syphilis.
Chancroid *(Haemophilus ducreyi).*
Cytomegalovirus.
Idiopathic (usually HIV positive).

NONULCERATIVE

Condyloma acuminatum.
Gonorrhea.
Chlamydia *(Chlamydia trachomatis).*
Syphilis.

SEXUAL PRECOCITY[88]

ICD-10CM #		
	E30.1	Precocious puberty
	E30.8	Other disorders of puberty

TRUE PRECOCIOUS PUBERTY

Premature reactivation of LHRH pulse generator.

INCOMPLETE SEXUAL PRECOCITY

(Pituitary gonadotropin independent).

Males

Chorionic gonadotropin-secreting tumor.
Leydig cell tumor.
Familial testotoxicosis.
Virilizing congenital adrenal hyperplasia.
Virilizing adrenal tumor.
Premature adrenarche.

Females

Granulosa cell tumor (follicular cysts may be manifested similarly).
Follicular cyst.
Feminizing adrenal tumor.
Premature thelarche.
Premature adrenarche.
Late-onset virilizing congenital adrenal hyperplasia.

In Both Sexes

McCune-Albright syndrome.
Primary hypothyroidism.

SHOULDER PAIN

ICD-10CM #		
	M24.819	Other specific joint derangements of unspecified shoulder, not elsewhere classified
	M75.80	Other shoulder lesions, unspecified shoulder
	S43.409A	Unspecified sprain of unspecified shoulder joint, initial encounter
	S46.919A	Strain of unspecified muscle, fascia and tendon at shoulder and upper arm level, unspecified arm, initial encounter

WITH LOCAL FINDINGS IN SHOULDER

Trauma: contusion, fracture, muscle strain, trauma to spinal cord.
Arthrosis, arthritis, RA, ankylosing spondylitis.
Bursitis, synovitis, tendinitis, tenosynovitis.
Aseptic (avascular) necrosis.
Local infection: septic arthritis, osteomyelitis, abscess, herpes zoster, TB.

WITHOUT LOCAL FINDINGS IN SHOULDER

Cardiovascular disorders: ischemic heart disease, pericarditis, aortic aneurysm.
Subdiaphragmatic abscess, liver abscess.
Cholelithiasis, cholecystitis.
Pulmonary lesions: apical bronchial carcinoma, pleurisy, pneumothorax, pneumonia.
GI lesions: PUD, gastric neoplasm, peptic esophagitis.
Pancreatic lesions: carcinoma, calculi, pancreatitis.
CNS abnormalities: neoplasm, vascular abnormalities.
Multiple sclerosis.
Syringomyelia.
Polymyositis/dermatomyositis.
Psychogenic.
Polymyalgia rheumatica.
Ectopic pregnancy.

SHOULDER PAIN BY LOCATION

ICD-10CM #		
	M75.80	Other shoulder lesions, unspecified shoulder
	S43.499A	Other sprain of unspecified shoulder joint, initial encounter
	S46.019A	Strain of muscle(s) and tendon(s) of the rotator cuff of unspecified shoulder, initial encounter
	S46.819A	Strain of other muscles, fascia and tendons at shoulder and upper arm level, unspecified arm, initial encounter

TOP OF SHOULDER (C4)

Cervical source.
Acromioclavicular.
Sternoclavicular.
Diaphragmatic.

SUPEROLATERAL (C5)

Rotator cuff tendinitis.
Impingement.
Adhesive capsulitis.
Glenohumeral arthritis.

ANTERIOR

Bicipital tendinitis and rupture.
Glenoid labral tear.
Adhesive capsulitis.
Glenohumeral arthritis.
Osteonecrosis.

AXILLARY

Neoplasm (Pancoast, mediastinal).
Herpes zoster.

SHOULDER PAIN, IN DIFFERENT AGE GROUPS[18]

ICD-10CM # M25.519 Pain in unspecified shoulder

COMMON CAUSES OF SHOULDER PAIN IN DIFFERENT AGE GROUPS

Childhood (2-10 yr)

Intraarticular

Instability.

Periarticular

Osteochondromas.

Adolescence (10-18 yr)

Intraarticular

Instability.

Early Adulthood (18-30 yr)

Intraarticular

Instability.
Acromioclavicular joint sprain.

Periarticular

Calcific tendonitis.
Impingement.

Referred

Cervical.

Adulthood (30-60 yr)

Intraarticular

Osteochondritis.
Osteoarthritis.
Frozen shoulder.
Inflammatory arthritis.

Periarticular

Calcific tendonitis.
Impingement.
Rotator cuff tear.
Bicipital tendonitis.

Referred

Cervical.

Old Age (>60 yr)

Intraarticular

Osteochondritis.
Osteoarthritis.
Frozen shoulder.
Inflammatory arthritis.

Periarticular

Impingement.
Rotator cuff tear.

Referred

Cervical.

SINUS NODE DYSFUNCTION[34]

ICD-10CM # Varies with specific diagnosis

CAUSES OF SINUS NODE DYSFUNCTION

Intrinsic

Hypothyroidism.
Fibrocalcific degeneration.
Increased vagal tone, especially in sleep apnea.
Congenital mutations.
Scleroderma.
Amyloidosis.
Chagas' disease.

Extrinsic

Trauma, including cardiac surgery.
Drugs:
  Calcium-channel blockers.
  β-Blockers.
  Digoxin.
  Antiarrhythmic medications (amiodarone, dronedarone, sotalol, flecainide, propafenone).
  Lithium.

SINUS OSTIAL OBSTRUCTION[10]

ICD-10CM # Varies with specific diagnosis

FACTORS THAT PREDISPOSE TO SINUS OSTIAL OBSTRUCTION

Mucosal Swelling

Systemic factors:
  Viral upper respiratory infection.
  Allergic inflammation.
  Cystic fibrosis.
  Immune disorders.
  Ciliary dyskinesia.
  Tobacco smoke.
Local insult:
  Facial trauma.
  Swimming, diving.
  Rhinitis medicamentosa.
  Nasal intubation.

Mechanical Obstruction

Choanal atresia.
Deviated septum.
Nasal polyps.
Foreign body.
Tumor.
Ethmoid bullae.

SINUS TACHYCARDIA[65]

ICD-10CM # R00.0 Tachycardia, unspecified

DIFFERENTIAL DIAGNOSIS OF SINUS TACHYCARDIA

Etiologic Category

Specific Disorders

Hemodynamic:
  Heart failure—systolic and diastolic heart failure caused by ischemic, valvular, or nonischemic myopathy.
  Loss of circulating blood volume—GI bleeding, anemia, shifts of intravascular fluid due to changes in colloidal osmotic pressure or inflammation.
  Septic shock—dehydration.
  Vascular shunts—intracardiac as well as aortovenous malformations, fistulas.
  Pulmonary embolism.
Metabolic and neurohumoral:
  Sepsis—infections and inflammatory conditions.
  Hyperthyroidism.
  Paget disease of the bone.
  Pheochromocytoma.
  Carcinoid syndrome.
  Beriberi heart disease.
  Carcinoma.

Hyperpyrexia.
Acidosis.
Exercise.
Pharmacologic:
Sympathomimetic agents—isoproterenol, epinephrine, or dopamine.
Vagolytic agents, atropine, scopolamine.
Vasodilators—nitrates, angiotensin-converting enzyme inhibitors, angiotensin receptor blockers, hydrazine, as well as centrally acting vasodilators.
Thyroid preparations, caffeine and nicotine.
Bronchodilators, including theophylline and terbutaline.
Anesthetic agents, including spinal anesthetics, causing peripheral vasodilation.
Drugs of abuse—amphetamines, cocaine, "ecstasy," cannabis.
Neurologic/psychological:
Pain.
Fear, anxiety, and hysteria.
Hyper-beta adrenergic phase of neurocardiogenic syncope.
Autonomic dysfunction such as with diabetes.

SKIN AND RENAL[74]

ICD-10CM # Varies with specific diagnosis

SELECTED CONDITIONS WITH CONCURRENT SKIN AND RENAL INVOLVEMENT

More Common
Lupus erythematosus.
Leukocytoclastic vasculitis.
Henoch-Schönlein purpura.
Mixed cryoglobulinemia.
Diabetes mellitus.
Systemic vasculitis.
Less Common
Nail-patella syndrome.
Hemolytic-uremic syndrome.
Toxic shock syndrome.
Mixed connective tissue disease.
Dermatomyositis.
Rheumatoid arthritis.
Sjögren syndrome.
Dermatitis herpetiformis.
Sarcoidosis.
Systemic sclerosis.
Ulcerative colitis.
Amyloidosis.
Toxic epidermolysis.
Hypothyroidism.
Graves disease.
Fabry disease.
Neurofibromatosis.
Hurler syndrome.
Castleman disease.
Infectious endocarditis.
Staphylococcal scalded skin syndrome (in adults).

SKIN INDURATION, CHRONIC[40]

ICD-10CM # Varies with specific diagnosis

CONDITIONS ASSOCIATED WITH CHRONIC SKIN INDURATION

Systemic sclerosis.
Localized scleroderma.
Scleroderma variants.
Scleredema.
Scleredema adultorum of Buschke.
Scleredema diabeticorum.
Scleredema neonatorum.
Scleromyxedema.
Nephrogenic fibrosing dermopathy.
Eosinophilic syndromes.
Eosinophilic fasciitis (diffuse fasciitis with eosinophilia, Schulman disease).
Eosinophilia-myalgia syndrome.
Toxic oil syndrome.
Chronic graft-versus-host disease.
Pseudoscleroderma (local injection of vitamin K, bleomycin, pentazocine).
Metabolic diseases.
Porphyria cutanea tarda.
Phenylketonuria.
Werner syndrome.
Acromegaly.
Pachydermoperiostitis.
Polyneuropathy, organomegaly, endocrinopathy, monoclonal gammopathy (POEMS).
Stiff skin syndrome.
Reflex sympathetic dystrophy.
Hemiplegia.

SMALL BOWEL MASSES[81]

ICD-10CM # Varies with specific diagnosis

Cyst:
Mesenteric cyst.
Tumor:
Benign.
Malignant.
Intussusception.
Inflammation:
Crohn's disease.

SMALL BOWEL OBSTRUCTION[57]

ICD-10CM #		
	K56.5	Intestinal adhesions [bands] with obstruction (postprocedural) (postinfection)
	Q41.9	Congenital absence, atresia and stenosis of small intestine, part unspecified

INTRINSIC

Congenital (atresia, stenosis).
Inflammatory (Crohn's, radiation enteritis).
Neoplasms (metastatic or primary).
Intussusception.
Traumatic (hematoma).

EXTRINSIC

Hernias (internal and external).
Adhesions.
Volvulus.
Compressing masses (tumors, abscesses, hematomas).

INTRALUMINAL

Foreign body.
Gallstones.
Bezoars.
Barium.
Ascaris infestation.

SMALL INTESTINE ULCERATION

ICD-10CM # K63.3 Ulcer of intestine

Inflammatory bowel disease.
Celiac disease.
Vasculitis, SLE, Behçet's syndrome.
Uremia.
Infections (*Campylobacter,* TB, *Yersinia,* parasites, typhoid, cytomegalovirus [CMV], *Clostridium).*
Mesenteric insufficiency.
Neoplasms.
Radiation.
Drugs (salicylates, potassium, indomethacin, antimetabolites).
Meckel diverticulum.
Zollinger-Ellison syndrome.
Lymphocytic enterocolitis.
Stomal ulceration.

SMELL DISTURBANCE

ICD-10CM # R43.8 Other disturbances of smell and taste

Upper respiratory tract infection.
Nasal or paranasal sinus disease.
Exposure to noxious vapors.
Head trauma.
Idiopathic.
Dental caries, periodontal disease.
Medications.

SODIUM RETENTION, RENAL CAUSES[74]

ICD-10CM # Varies with specific diagnosis

CAUSES OF RENAL SODIUM RETENTION

Primary
Oliguric acute kidney injury.
Chronic kidney disease.
Glomerular disease.
Severe bilateral renal artery stenosis.
Na^+-retaining tubulopathies (genetic).
Mineralocorticoid excess.
Secondary
Heart failure.
Cirrhosis.
Idiopathic edema.

SOFT TISSUE MASS MIMICKING MALIGNANCY[66]

ICD-10CM # Varies with specific diagnosis

OVERVIEW OF DISEASES THAT CAN PRESENT AS A SOFT TISSUE MASS MIMICKING MALIGNANCY

Etiology	Disease Entity
Trauma:	Muscle contusion. Hematoma. Muscle herniation. Calcific myonecrosis. Hypothenar hammer syndrome. Myositis ossificans.
Metabolic:	Diabetic myopathy. Gout. Pseudogout. Calcific tendinosis.
Congenital:	Accessory muscle.
Infectious:	Necrotizing fasciitis. Abscess. Pyomyositis. Hydatid cystic disease. Cat-scratch disease. Actinomycosis.
Inflammation:	Bursitis. Sarcoidosis. Foreign body reaction. Injection granuloma. Granuloma annulare. Epidermal inclusion cyst.
Vascular:	Adventitial cystic disease. Pseudoaneurysm. Thrombosed vein. Arteriovenous vascular malformation.
Miscellaneous:	Focal myositis. Amyloid tumor of soft tissue.

SOFT TISSUE TUMORS, PEDIATRIC PATIENTS[66]

ICD-10CM # Varies with specific diagnosis

PEDIATRIC SOFT TISSUE TUMORS

Vascular lesions:
- Hemangioma of infancy.*
- Congenital hemangioma.
- Hemangioendothelioma (Kasabach-Merritt syndrome).
- Arteriovenous malformation.
- Venous malformations.
- Lymphatic malformation (lymphangioma, cystic hygroma).
- Capillary malformation.

Adipocytic tumors:
- Lipoma.
- Lipoblastoma.
- Liposarcoma.

Fibrohistiocytic tumors:
- Pigmented villonodular synovitis.
- Giant cell tumor of tendon sheath.

Fibroblastic and myofibroblastic tumors:
- Nodular fasciitis.
- Fibrous hamartoma of infancy.
- Myofibroma, myofibromatosis.
- Infantile fibrosarcoma.
- Fibromatosis colli.

Neurogenic tumors:
- Schwannoma.
- Neurofibroma.
- Malignant nerve sheath tumor.

Leiomyoma.
Rhabdomyosarcoma.
Tumors of uncertain differentiation:
- Synovial cell sarcoma.
- Primitive neuroectodermal tumor (Ewing sarcoma).

Pilomatricoma.

*Lesions with MR-specific features.

SORE THROAT[7]

ICD-10CM # J02 Acute pharyngitis

DIFFERENTIAL DIAGNOSIS FOR SORE THROAT

Infectious Causes

Aerobes

Common:
- *Streptococcus pyogenes* (GABHS).
- GABHS.
- *Peptostreptococcus* spp.
- Non–group A streptococcus.
- *Neisseria gonorrhoeae.*
- *Neisseria meningitides.*
- *Mycoplasma pneumoniae.*
- *Arcanobacterium hemolyticum.*
- *Chlamydia trachomatis.*
- *Staphylococcus aureus.*

Uncommon:
- *Haemophilus influenzae.*
- *Haemophilus parainfluenzae.*
- *Coccidioides* spp.
- *Corynebacterium diphtheriae.*
- *Streptococcus pneumoniae.*
- *Yersinia enterocolitica.*
- *Treponema pallidum.*
- *Francisella tularensis.*
- *Legionella pneumophila.*
- *Mycobacterium spp.*

ANAEROBES

Bacteroides spp.
Peptococcus spp.
Clostridium spp.
Fusobacterium spp.
Prevotella spp.

OTHER

Candida spp.

VIRAL

Rhinovirus.
Adenovirus.
Coronavirus.
Herpes simplex 1, 2.
Influenza A, B.
Parainfluenza.
Cytomegalovirus.
Epstein-Barr.
Varicella-zoster.
Hepatitis virus.

Noninfectious Causes

SYSTEMIC

Kawasaki disease.
Stevens-Johnson syndrome.
Cyclic neutropenia.
Thyroiditis.
Connective tissue disease.

TRAUMA, MISCELLANEOUS

Penetrating injury.
Angioneurotic edema.
Retained foreign body.
Anomalous aortic arch.
Laryngeal fracture.
Calcific retropharyngeal tendinitis.
Retropharyngeal hematoma.
Caustic exposure.

TUMOR

Tongue.
Larynx.
Thyroid.
Leukemia.

SPASTIC PARAPLEGIAS

ICD-10CM # G82.20 Paraplegia, unspecified

Cervical spondylosis.
Friedreich ataxia.
Multiple sclerosis.
Spinal cord tumor.
HIV.
Tertiary syphilis.
Vitamin B_{12} deficiency.
Spinocerebellar ataxias.
Syringomyelia.
Spinal cord AV malformations.
Adrenoleukodystrophy.

SPINAL CORD COMPRESSION, EPIDURAL

ICD-10CM # Varies with specific diagnosis

Osteoarthritis.
Meningioma.
Spinal epidural abscess.
Spinal epidural hematoma.
Spinal epidural vascular malformations.
RA.
Metastatic cancer (vertebral, intramedullary, leptomeninges).
Radiation myelopathy.
Neurofibroma.
Sarcoidosis.
Paraneoplastic myelopathy.
Histiocytosis.

SPINAL CORD DYSFUNCTION

ICD-10CM # G95.9 Disease of spinal cord, unspecified
Q07.9 Congenital malformation of nervous system, unspecified
D51.1 Vitamin B_{12} deficiency anemia due to selective vitamin B_{12} malabsorption with proteinuria

D51.3	Other dietary vitamin B_{12} deficiency anemia
D51.8	Other vitamin B_{12} deficiency anemias
G95.89	Other specified diseases of spinal cord
G95.19	Other vascular myelopathies

Trauma.
Multiple sclerosis.
Transverse myelitis.
Neoplasm (primary, metastatic).
Syringomyelia.
Spinal epidural abscess.
HIV myelopathy.
Diskitis.
Spinal epidural hematoma.
Spinal cord infarction.
Spinal AV malformation.
Subarachnoid hemorrhage.

SPINAL CORD DYSFUNCTION, NONTRAUMATIC[7]

ICD-10CM # Q07.9 Congenital malformation of nervous system, unspecified

NONTRAUMATIC ETIOLOGIES OF SPINAL CORD DYSFUNCTION

Processes Affecting the Spinal Cord or Blood Supply Directly
Multiple sclerosis.
Transverse myelitis.
Spinal arteriovenous malformation/subarachnoid hemorrhage.
Syringomyelia.
HIV myelopathy.
Other myelopathies.
Spinal cord infarction.
Compressive Lesions Affecting the Spinal Cord
Spinal epidural abscess.
Spinal epidural hematoma.
Diskitis.
Neoplasm.
Metastatic.
Primary CNS.

HIV, Human immunodeficiency virus; *CNS,* central nervous system.

SPINAL CORD ISCHEMIC SYNDROMES

ICD-10CM # Varies with specific diagnosis

Systemic hypotension.
Venous or arterial occlusion.
Arterial dissection.
Thromboembolism.
Endovascular procedures.
Vasculitis.
Fibrocartilaginous embolism.
Regional hemodynamic compromise.

SPINAL TUMORS[32]

ICD-10CM # Varies with specific diagnosis

EXTRADURAL

Metastases.
Primary bone tumors arising in spine.

INTRADURAL EXTRAMEDULLARY

Meningiomas.
Neurofibromas.
Schwannomas.
Lipomas.
Arachnoid cysts.
Epidermoid cysts.
Metastasis.

INTRAMEDULLARY

Ependymoma.
Glioma.
Hemangioblastoma.
Lipoma.
Metastases.

SPLENIC CYSTS, CLASSIFICATION[15]

ICD-10CM # D73.4 Cyst of spleen

- Primary (true).
- Parasitic.
- Nonparasitic.
- Congenital.
- Epidermoid.
- Dermoid.
- Mesothelial (serous).
- Transitional.
- Neoplastic.
- Secondary (false): pseudocysts.
- Traumatic.
- Degenerative.
- Inflammatory.
- Hemorrhagic.

SPLENIC MASSES, FOCAL SOLID[69]

ICD-10CM # Varies with specific diagnosis

FOCAL SOLID SPLENIC MASSES

Benign
Hemangioma.
Hamartoma.
Littoral cell angioma.
Lymphangioma.
Sclerosing angiomatoid nodular transformation (SANT).
Inflammatory pseudotumor.
Malignant
Lymphoma.
Metastases.
Angiosarcoma.
Hemangiopericytoma.
Other
Infarct.

SPLENIC NODULES[69]

ICD-10CM # Varies with specific diagnosis

CAUSES OF SPLENIC NODULES

Infectious
Tuberculosis/Mycobacterium avium-intracellulare complex.
Pyogenic abscesses.
Histoplasmosis.
Candida abscesses.
Cat-scratch disease.
Pneumocystis jiroveci (formerly P. carinii pneumonia).
Inflammatory
Sarcoidosis.
Malignant
Lymphoma.
Metastases.
Other
Gamna-Gandy bodies.
Gaucher disease.

SPLENIC TUMORS, CLASSIFICATION[15]

ICD-10CM # C26.1 Malignant neoplasm of spleen

- Malignant.
- Lymphoproliferative disease.
- Non-Hodgkin's lymphoma.
- Hodgkin's disease.
- Hairy cell leukemia.
- Chronic lymphocytic leukemia.
- Myeloproliferative disease.
- Chronic myelogenous leukemia.
- Myelofibrosis.
- Primary tumors.
- Angiosarcoma.
- Metastatic tumors.
- Benign.
- Hemangiomas.
- Hamartomas.
- Lymphangiomas.
- Sclerosing angiomatoid nodular transformation (SANT).

SPLENOMEGALY

ICD-10CM #		
	R16.1	Splenomegaly, not elsewhere classified
	D73.2	Chronic congestive splenomegaly
	R16.1	Splenomegaly, not elsewhere classified

Hepatic cirrhosis.
Neoplastic involvement: CML, CLL, lymphoma, multiple myeloma.
Bacterial infections: TB, infectious endocarditis, typhoid fever, splenic abscess.
Viral infections: infectious mononucleosis, viral hepatitis, HIV.
Gaucher disease and other lipid storage diseases.
Sarcoidosis.
Parasitic infections (malaria, kala-azar, histoplasmosis).

Hereditary and acquired hemolytic anemias.
Idiopathic thrombocytopenic purpura (ITP).
Collagen vascular disorders: SLE, RA (Felty syndrome), polyarteritis nodosa.
Serum sickness, drug hypersensitivity reaction.
Splenic cysts and benign tumors: hemangioma, lymphangioma.
Thrombosis of splenic or portal vein.
Polycythemia vera, myeloid metaplasia.

SPLENOMEGALY AND HEPATOMEGALY[81]

ICD-10CM #		
	R16.1	Splenomegaly, not elsewhere classified
	R16.0	Hepatomegaly, not elsewhere classified

CAUSES OF SPLENOMEGALY AND HEPATOSPLENOMEGALY

Massive Splenomegaly

Hematologic disease (e.g., chronic myeloid leukemia, myelofibrosis).

Moderate Splenomegaly

The above causes.
Portal hypertension.
Hematologic disease (e.g., lymphoma, leukemia, thalassemia).
Storage disease (e.g., Gaucher disease).

Small Splenomegaly

The above causes.
Infective (hepatitis, leptospirosis, malaria, bacterial endocarditis).
Hematologic disease (e.g., hemolytic anemias, essential thrombocythemia, polycythemia rubra vera).
Connective tissue diseases or vasculitis (e.g., rheumatoid arthritis, systemic lupus erythematosus, polyarteritis nodosa).
Solitary cyst, polycystic syndrome, hydatid cyst.
Infiltration (amyloid, sarcoid).

Hepatosplenomegaly

Chronic liver disease with portal hypertension.
Hematologic disease (e.g., myeloproliferative disease, lymphoma).
Infection (e.g., amyloid, sarcoid).
Connective tissue disease (e.g., systemic lupus erythematosus).

SPLENOMEGALY AND HYPERSPLENISM[44]

ICD-10CM #		
	R16.1	Splenomegaly, not elsewhere classified
	D73.1	Hypersplenism
	D73.81	Neutropenic splenomegaly

DIFFERENTIAL DIAGNOSIS OF SPLENOMEGALY AND HYPERSPLENISM

Infections

Acute

Viral (viral hepatitis, infectious mononucleosis, CMV infection).
Bacterial (septicemia, salmonellosis, brucellosis, splenic abscess).
Parasite (toxoplasmosis).

Subacute and Chronic

Subacute bacterial endocarditis.
Tuberculosis.
Malaria.
Kala-azar.
Fungal disease.

Inflammation

Felty syndrome.
SLE.
Serum sickness.
Rheumatic fever.
Sarcoidosis.
ALPS.

Congestive Splenomegaly

Intrahepatic

Cirrhosis.

Extrahepatic

Portal vein obstruction.
Splenic vein obstruction.
Hepatic vein occlusion (Budd-Chiari syndrome).

Chronic Passive Congestion

Heart failure.

Hematologic Disorders

RBC disorders: hemolytic anemias, thalassemia, sickle cell disorders.

Neoplasia

Malignant

MPDs.
Myeloid metaplasia.
Polycythemia rubra vera.
Essential thrombocythemia.
Chronic leukemia.
Chronic myeloid leukemia.
Chronic lymphocytic leukemia.
Hairy cell leukemia.
Lymphoma.
Acute leukemia.
Malignant histiocytosis.

Benign

Hamartoma.
Hemangioma.
Lymphangioma.
Fibroma.

Storage Diseases

Gaucher disease.
Niemann-Pick disease.

Miscellaneous

Amyloidosis.
Cysts.

ALPS, Autoimmune lymphoproliferative syndrome; *CMV,* cytomegalovirus; *MPD,* myeloproliferative disorder; *RBC,* red blood cell; *SLE,* systemic lupus erythematosus.

SPLENOMEGALY, CHILDREN[43]

ICD-10CM #		
	R16.1	Splenomegaly, not elsewhere classified

DISORDERS OF THE BLOOD

Hemolytic anemia: congenital/acquired.
Thalassemia.
Sickle cell disease.
Leukemia.
Osteopetrosis.
Myelofibrosis/myeloid metaplasia/thrombocythemia.

INFECTIONS: ACUTE AND CHRONIC

Viral:
- Congenital (e.g., TORCH association).
- Mononucleosis (e.g., EBV, CMV infection).
- Virus-associated hemophagocytic syndrome.
- Human immunodeficiency virus.

Bacterial:
- Sepsis/abscess.
- Brucellosis.
- Salmonellosis.
- Tularemia.
- Tuberculosis.
- Subacute bacterial endocarditis.
- Syphilis.
- Lyme disease.

Fungal:
- Histoplasmosis (disseminated).

Rickettsial:
- Rocky Mountain spotted fever.
- Cat scratch disease.

Parasitic:
- Toxoplasmosis.
- Malaria.
- Leishmaniasis (kala-azar).
- Schistosomiasis.
- Echinococcosis.

HEPATIC/PORTAL SYSTEM DISORDERS

Acute/chronic active hepatitis.
Cirrhosis/hepatic fibrosis/biliary atresia.
Portal or splenic venous obstruction (Banti syndrome).

AUTOIMMUNE DISEASE

Juvenile rheumatoid arthritis.
Systemic lupus erythematosus.
Autoimmune lymphoproliferative syndrome (Canale–Smith syndrome).

NEOPLASMS/CYSTS

Lymphomas (Hodgkin and non-Hodgkin).
Hemangiomas/lymphangiomas.
Hamartomas.
Congenital or acquired (posttraumatic) cysts.

STORAGE DISEASES/INBORN ERRORS OF METABOLISM

Lipidoses: Gaucher disease, Niemann–Pick disease, others.
Mucopolysaccharidoses.
Defects in carbohydrate metabolism: galactosemia, fructose intolerance.
Sea-blue histiocyte syndrome.

MISCELLANEOUS DISORDERS

Histiocytoses:
- Reactive.
- Langerhans cell.
- Malignant.

Sarcoidosis.
Congestive heart failure.
Familial Mediterranean fever.

CMV, Cytomegalovirus; *EBV,* Epstein-Barr virus; *TORCH,* toxoplasmosis, other infections, rubella, cytomegalovirus infection, herpes simplex.

SPONTANEOUS PNEUMOTHORAX[57]

ICD-10CM #		
	J93.0	Spontaneous tension pneumothorax
	J93.11	Primary spontaneous pneumothorax
	J93.12	Secondary spontaneous pneumothorax

CAUSES OF SECONDARY SPONTANEOUS PNEUMOTHORAX

Airway Disease

Chronic obstructive pulmonary disease.
Asthma.
Cystic fibrosis.

Infections

Necrotizing bacterial pneumonia, lung abscess.
Pneumocystis jiroveci pneumonia.
Tuberculosis.

Interstitial Lung Disease

Sarcoidosis.
Idiopathic pulmonary fibrosis.
Lymphangiomyomatosis.
Tuberous sclerosis.
Pneumoconioses.

Neoplasms

Primary lung cancers.
Pulmonary or pleural metastases.

Miscellaneous

Connective tissue diseases.
Pulmonary infarction.
Endometriosis, catamenial pneumothorax.

STATURAL OVERGROWTH[59]

ICD-10CM #		
	E34.4	Constitutional tall stature

FETAL OVERGROWTH

Maternal diabetes mellitus.
Cerebral gigantism (Sotos syndrome).
Weaver syndrome.
Beckwith-Wiedemann syndrome.
Other insulin-like growth factor 2 (IGF2) excess syndromes.

POSTNATAL OVERGROWTH LEADING TO CHILDHOOD TALL STATURE

Familial (constitutional) tall stature.
Cerebral gigantism.
Beckwith-Wiedemann syndrome.
Exogenous obesity.
Excess growth hormone (GH) secretion (pituitary gigantism).
McCune-Albright syndrome or multiple endocrine neoplasia (MEN) associated with excess GH secretion.
Precocious puberty.
Marfan syndrome.
Klinefelter syndrome (XXY).
Weaver syndrome.
Fragile X syndrome.
Homocystinuria.
XYY.
Hyperthyroidism.

POSTNATAL OVERGROWTH LEADING TO ADULT TALL STATURE

Familial (constitutional) tall stature.
Androgen or estrogen deficiency/estrogen resistance (in males).
Testicular feminization.
Excess GH secretion.
Marfan syndrome.
Klinefelter syndrome (XXY).
XYY.

STEATOHEPATITIS

ICD-10CM #		
	K76.0	Fatty (change of) liver, not elsewhere classified
	K76.89	Other specified diseases of liver

Alcohol abuse.
Obesity.
DM.
Parenteral nutrition.
Medications (high-dose estrogen, amiodarone, corticosteroids, methotrexate, nifedipine).
Jejunoileal bypass.
Abetalipoproteinemia.
Wilson's disease, Weber-Christian disease.

STOMATITIS, BULLOUS

ICD-10CM #		
	K12.30	Oral mucositis (ulcerative), unspecified

Erythema multiforme.
Erosive lichen planus.
Bullous pemphigoid.
SLE.
Pemphigus vulgaris.
Mucous membrane pemphigoid.

STRIDOR IN NEONATES[1]

ICD-10CM #		
	R06.1	Stridor

INTRINSIC LESIONS

Larynx

Laryngomalacia.
Infection (laryngitis).
Vocal cord paralysis.
Laryngeal web.
Laryngocele or laryngeal cyst.
Laryngotracheal esophageal cleft.
Foreign body.

Trachea

Tracheomalacia.
Tracheal stenosis.
Tracheoesophageal fistula.
Subglottic hemangioma.
Tracheal web.

Extrinsic Compression

Vascular ring.
Anomalous innominate artery.
Mediastinal mass.
Esophageal foreign body.

Other

Macroglossia.
Gastroesophageal reflux.

STRIDOR, PEDIATRIC AGE[9]

ICD-10CM #		
	R06.1	Stridor

RECURRENT

Allergic (spasmodic) croup.
Respiratory infections in a child with otherwise asymptomatic anatomic narrowing of the large airways.
Laryngomalacia.

PERSISTENT

Laryngeal obstruction:
- Laryngomalacia.
- Papillomas, other tumors.
- Cysts and laryngoceles.
- Laryngeal webs.
- Bilateral abductor paralysis of the cords.
- Foreign body.

Tracheobronchial disease:
- Tracheomalacia.
- Subglottic tracheal webs.

Endotracheal, endobronchial tumors.
Subglottic tracheal stenosis.
Congenital.
Acquired.
Extrinsic masses.
Mediastinal masses.
Vascular ring.
Lobar emphysema.
Bronchogenic cysts.
Thyroid enlargement.
Esophageal foreign body.
Tracheoesophageal fistulas.
Other.
Gastroesophageal reflux.
Macroglossia, Pierre Robin syndrome.
Cri-du-chat syndrome.
Hysterical stridor.
Hypocalcemia.

STROKE[77]

ICD-10CM #	
	Varies with specific diagnosis

STROKE "MIMICS"

Hypoglycemia.
Drug overdose or intoxication.
Hysterical conversion reaction.
Hyperventilation.
Metabolic encephalopathy.
Migraine.
Syncope.
Transient global amnesia.
Seizures.
Vestibular vertigo.

STROKE, PEDIATRIC AGE[52]

ICD-10CM #		
	I67.89	Other cerebrovascular disease

CARDIAC DISEASE

Congenital:
- Aortic stenosis.
- Mitral stenosis; mitral prolapse.

Ventricular septal defects.
Patent ductus arteriosus.
Cyanotic congenital heart disease involving right-to-left shunt.

Acquired:
- Endocarditis (bacterial, SLE).
- Kawasaki disease.
- Cardiomyopathy.
- Atrial myxoma.
- Arrhythmia.
- Paradoxical emboli through patent foramen ovale.
- Rheumatic fever.
- Prosthetic heart valve.

HEMATOLOGIC ABNORMALITIES

Hemoglobinopathies:
- Sickle cell (SS) disease.
- Sickle (SC) disease.

Polycythemia.
Leukemia/lymphoma.
Thrombocytopenia.
Thrombocytosis.
Disorders of coagulation:
- Protein C deficiency.
- Protein S deficiency.
- Factor V Leiden.
- Antithrombin III deficiency.
- Lupus anticoagulant.

Oral contraceptive pill use.
Pregnancy and the postpartum state.
Disseminated intravascular coagulation.
Paroxysmal nocturnal hemoglobinuria.
Inflammatory bowel disease (thrombosis).

INFLAMMATORY DISORDERS

Meningitis:
- Viral.
- Bacterial.
- Tuberculosis.

Systemic infection:
- Viremia.
- Bacteremia.
- Local head and neck infections.

Drug-induced inflammation:
- Amphetamine.
- Cocaine.

Autoimmune disease:
- SLE.
- Juvenile RA.
- Takayasu arteritis.
- Mixed connective tissue disease.
- Polyarteritis nodosum.
- Primary CNS vasculitis.
- Sarcoidosis.
- Behçet's syndrome.
- Granulomatosis with polyangiitis.

METABOLIC DISEASE ASSOCIATED WITH STROKE

Homocystinuria.
Pseudoxanthoma elasticum.
Fabry disease.
Sulfite oxidase deficiency.
Mitochondrial disorders:
- MELAS.
- Leigh syndrome.

Ornithine transcarbamylase deficiency.

INTRACEREBRAL VASCULAR PROCESSES

Ruptured aneurysm.
Arteriovenous malformation.
Fibromuscular dysplasia.
Moyamoya disease.
Migraine headache.
Postsubarachnoid hemorrhage vasospasm.
Hereditary hemorrhagic telangiectasia.
Sturge-Weber syndrome.
Carotid artery dissection.
Postvaricella.

TRAUMA AND OTHER EXTERNAL CAUSES

Child abuse.
Head trauma/neck trauma.
Oral trauma.
Placental embolism.
ECMO therapy.

CNS, Central nervous system; *ECMO,* extracorporeal membrane oxygenation; *MELAS,* mitochondrial encephalomyopathy, lactic acidosis, and stroke.

STROKE, YOUNG ADULT, CAUSES[3]

ICD-10CM #		
	I64	Stroke
	I67.89	Other cerebrovascular disease

Cardiac factors (ASD, MVP, patent foramen ovale).
Inflammatory factors (SLE, polyarteritis nodosa).
Infections (endocarditis, neurosyphilis).
Drugs (cocaine, heroin, oral contraceptives, decongestants).
Arterial dissection.
Hematolic factors (DIC, TTP, deficiency of protein S, protein C, antithrombin III).
Migraine.
Postpartum angiopathy.
Other: premature atherosclerosis, fibromuscular dysplasia.

ST-SEGMENT DEPRESSION, NONCORONARY CAUSES[11]

ICD-10CM #		
	R94.31	Abnormal electrocardiogram

NONCORONARY CAUSES OF ST-SEGMENT DEPRESSION

Anemia.
Cardiomyopathy.
Digitalis use.
Glucose load.
Hyperventilation.
Hypokalemia.
Intraventricular conduction disturbance.
Left ventricular hypertrophy.
Mitral valve prolapse.
Preexcitation syndrome.
Severe aortic stenosis.
Severe hypertension.
Severe hypoxia.
Severe volume overload (aortic, mitral regurgitation).
Sudden excessive exercise.
Supraventricular tachyarrhythmias.

ST-SEGMENT ELEVATION[1]

ICD-10CM #		
	R94.31	Abnormal electrocardiogram [ECG] [EKG]

DIFFERENTIAL DIAGNOSIS OF ST-SEGMENT ELEVATION ON ELECTROCARDIOGRAPHY

ST-segment elevation myocardial infarction.
Pericarditis.
Benign early repolarization.
Left bundle branch block.
Left ventricular hypertrophy.
Left ventricular aneurysm.
Paced ventricular rhythms.
Prinzmetal angina.
Hyperkalemia.
Hypothermia with Osborne waves.
Intracranial hemorrhage.
Brugada syndrome.
Normal variant.

ST SEGMENT ELEVATIONS, NONISCHEMIC

ICD-10CM #		
	R94.31	Abnormal electrocardiogram [ECG] [EKG]

Early repolarization.
Acute pericarditis.
LVH.
Normal pattern variant.
LBBB.
Pulmonary embolism.
Hyperkalemia.
Postcardioversion.

SUDDEN CARDIAC DEATH[56]

ICD-10CM #		
	Z86.74	Personal history of sudden cardiac arrest
	Z82.41	Family history of sudden cardiac death

CAUSES OF AND CONTRIBUTING FACTORS IN SUDDEN CARDIAC DEATH

Coronary Artery Abnormalities

Coronary atherosclerosis:
- Chronic coronary atherosclerosis with acute or transient myocardial ischemia—thrombosis, spasm, physical stress.
- Acute myocardial infarction, onset and early phase.
- Chronic atherosclerosis with a change in myocardial substrate, including previous myocardial infarction.

Congenital abnormalities of coronary arteries:
- Anomalous origin from the pulmonary artery.
- Other coronary arteriovenous fistula.
- Origin of a left coronary branch from the right or noncoronary sinus of Valsalva.
- Origin of the right coronary artery from the left sinus of Valsalva.
- Hypoplastic or aplastic coronary arteries.
- Coronary-intracardiac shunt.

Coronary artery embolism:
- Aortic or mitral endocarditis.
- Prosthetic aortic or mitral valves.
- Abnormal native valves or left ventricular mural thrombus.
- Platelet embolism.

Coronary arteritis:
- Polyarteritis nodosa, progressive systemic sclerosis, giant cell arteritis.
- Mucocutaneous lymph node syndrome (Kawasaki disease).
- Syphilitic coronary ostial stenosis.

Miscellaneous mechanical obstruction of the coronary arteries:
- Coronary artery dissection in Marfan syndrome.
- Coronary artery dissection in pregnancy.
- Prolapse of aortic valve myxomatous polyps into the coronary ostia.
- Dissection or rupture of the sinus of Valsalva.

Functional obstruction of the coronary arteries:
- Coronary artery spasm with or without atherosclerosis.
- Myocardial bridges.

Hypertrophy of the Ventricular Myocardium

Left ventricular hypertrophy associated with coronary heart disease.

Hypertensive heart disease without significant coronary atherosclerosis.

Hypertrophic myocardium secondary to valvular heart disease.

Hypertrophic cardiomyopathy:
- Obstructive.
- Nonobstructive.

Primary or secondary pulmonary hypertension:
- Advanced chronic right ventricular overload.
- Pulmonary hypertension in pregnancy (highest risk peripartum).

Myocardial Diseases and Dysfunction, with or without Heart Failure

Chronic congestive heart failure:
- Ischemic cardiomyopathy.
- Idiopathic dilated cardiomyopathy, acquired.
- Hereditary dilated cardiomyopathy.
- Alcoholic cardiomyopathy.
- Hypertensive cardiomyopathy.
- Postmyocarditis cardiomyopathy.
- Peripartum cardiomyopathy.
- Idiopathic fibrosis.

Acute and subacute cardiac failure:
- Massive acute myocardial infarction.
- Myocarditis, acute or fulminant.
- Acute alcoholic cardiac dysfunction.
- Takotsubo syndrome (uncertain risk for sudden death).
- Ball valve embolism in aortic stenosis or prosthesis.
- Mechanical disruptions of cardiac structures:
  - Rupture of the ventricular free wall.
  - Disruption of the mitral apparatus:
    - Papillary muscle.
    - Chordae tendineae.
    - Leaflet.
  - Rupture of the interventricular septum.
- Acute pulmonary edema in noncompliant ventricles.

Inflammatory, Infiltrative, Neoplastic, and Degenerative Processes

Viral myocarditis, with or without ventricular dysfunction:
- Acute phase.
- Postmyocarditis interstitial fibrosis.

Myocarditis associated with the vasculitides.

Sarcoidosis.

Progressive systemic sclerosis.

Amyloidosis.

Hemochromatosis.

Idiopathic giant cell myocarditis.

Chagas' disease.

Cardiac ganglionitis.

Arrhythmogenic right ventricular dysplasia, right ventricular cardiomyopathy.

Neuromuscular diseases (e.g., muscular dystrophy, Friedreich ataxia, myotonic dystrophy).

Intramural tumors:
- Primary.
- Metastatic.

Obstructive intracavitary tumors:
- Neoplastic.
- Thrombotic.

Diseases of the Cardiac Valves

Valvular aortic stenosis/insufficiency.

Mitral valve disruption.

Mitral valve prolapse.

Endocarditis.

Prosthetic valve dysfunction.

Congenital Heart Disease

Congenital aortic (potentially high risk) or pulmonic (low risk) valve stenosis:

Congenital septal defects with Eisenmenger physiology:
- Advanced disease.
- During labor and delivery.

Late after surgical repair of congenital lesions (e.g., tetralogy of Fallot).

Electrophysiologic Abnormalities

Abnormalities of the conducting system:
- Fibrosis of the His-Purkinje system.
  - Primary degeneration (Lenègre disease).
  - Secondary to fibrosis and calcification of the "cardiac skeleton" (Lev disease).
  - Postviral conducting system fibrosis.
  - Hereditary conducting system disease.
- Anomalous pathways of conduction (Wolff-Parkinson-White syndrome, short refractory period bypass).

Abnormalities of repolarization:
- Congenital abnormalities in duration of the QT interval:
  - Congenital long–QT interval syndromes.
    - Romano-Ward syndrome (without deafness).
    - Jervell and Lange-Nielsen syndrome (with deafness).
  - Congenital short–QT interval syndrome.
- Acquired (or provoked) long–QT interval syndromes:
  - Drug effect (with genetic predisposition?):
    - Cardiac, antiarrhythmic.
    - Noncardiac.
    - Drug interactions.
  - Electrolyte abnormality (response modified by genetic predisposition?):
  - Toxic substances.
  - Hypothermia.
  - CNS injury, subarachnoid hemorrhage.
- Brugada syndrome—right bundle branch block and ST-segment elevations in the absence of ischemia:
  - Early repolarization syndrome.

Ventricular fibrillation of unknown or uncertain cause:
- Absence of identifiable structural or functional causes:
  - "Idiopathic" ventricular fibrillation.
  - Short-coupled torsades de pointes, polymorphic ventricular tachycardia.
  - Nonspecific fibrofatty infiltration in a previously healthy victim (variation of right ventricular dysplasia?).
- Sleep-death in Southeast Asians (see VIIB3, Brugada syndrome):
  - Bangungut.
  - Pokkuri.
  - Lai-tai.

Electrical Instability Related to Neurohumoral and Central Nervous System Influences

Catecholaminergic polymorphic ventricular tachycardia.

Other catecholamine-dependent arrhythmias.

CNS related:
- Psychic stress, emotional extremes (Takotsubo syndrome).
- Auditory related.
- "Voodoo death" in primitive cultures.
- Diseases of the cardiac nerves.
- Arrhythmia expression in congenital long–QT interval syndrome.

Sudden Infant Death Syndrome and Sudden Death in Children

Sudden infant death syndrome:
- Immature respiratory control function.
- Long–QT interval syndrome.
- Congenital heart disease.
- Myocarditis.

Sudden death in children:
- Eisenmenger syndrome, aortic stenosis, hypertrophic cardiomyopathy, pulmonary atresia.
- After corrective surgery for congenital heart disease.
- Myocarditis.
- Genetic disorders of electrical function (e.g., long–QT interval syndrome).
- No identified structural or functional cause.

Miscellaneous

Sudden death during extreme physical activity (seek predisposing causes).

Commotio cordis—blunt chest trauma.

Mechanical interference with venous return:
- Acute cardiac tamponade.
- Massive pulmonary embolism.
- Acute intracardiac thrombosis.

Dissecting aneurysm of the aorta.

Toxic and metabolic disturbances (other than the QT interval effects listed above):
- Electrolyte disturbances.
- Metabolic disturbances.
- Proarrhythmic effects of antiarrhythmic drugs.
- Proarrhythmic effects of noncardiac drugs.

Mimics sudden cardiac death:
- "Café coronary."
- Acute alcoholic states ("holiday heart").
- Acute asthmatic attacks.
- Air or amniotic fluid embolism.

SUDDEN DEATH, PEDIATRIC AGE[9]

ICD-10CM # R99 Ill-defined and unknown cause of mortality

SIDS AND SIDS "MIMICS"

SIDS.
Long QT syndromes.
Inborn errors of metabolism.
Child abuse.
Myocarditis.
Duct-dependent congenital heart disease.

CORRECTED OR UNOPERATED CONGENITAL HEART DISEASE

Aortic stenosis.
Tetralogy of Fallot.
Transposition of great vessels (postoperative atrial switch).
Mitral valve prolapse.
Hematologic left heart syndrome.
Eisenmenger syndrome.

CORONARY ARTERIAL DISEASE

Anomalous origin.
Anomalous tract.
Kawasaki disease.
Periarteritis.
Arterial dissection.
Marfan syndrome.
Myocardial infarction.

MYOCARDIAL DISEASE

Myocarditis.
Hypertrophic cardiomyopathy.
Dilated cardiomyopathy.
Arrhythmogenic right ventricular dysplasia.

CONDUCTION SYSTEM ABNORMALITY/ARRHYTHMIA

Long Q-T syndromes.
Proarrhythmic drugs.
Preexcitation syndromes.
Heart block.
Commotio cordis.
Idiopathic ventricular fibrillation.
Heart tumor.

MISCELLANEOUS

Pulmonary hypertension.
Pulmonary embolism.
Heat stroke.
Cocaine.
Anorexia nervosa.
Electrolyte disturbances.

SIDS, Sudden infant death syndrome.

SUDDEN DEATH, YOUNG ATHLETE

ICD-10CM # R99 Ill-defined and unknown cause of mortality

Hypertrophic cardiomyopathy.
Coronary artery anomalies.
Myocarditis.
Ruptured aortic aneurysm (Marfan syndrome).
Arrhythmias.
Aortic valve stenosis.
Asthma.
Trauma (cerebral, cardiac).
Drug and alcohol abuse.
Heat stroke.
Cardiac sarcoidosis.
Atherosclerotic coronary artery disease.
Dilated cardiomyopathy.

SWOLLEN LIMB

ICD-10CM # M79.89 Other specified soft tissue disorders

Trauma.
Insect bite.
Abscess.
Lymphedema.
Thrombophlebitis.
Lipoma.
Neurofibroma.
Postphlebitic syndrome.
Myositis ossificans.
Nephrosis, cirrhosis, CHF.
Hypoalbuminemia.
Varicose veins.

TALL STATURE[60]

ICD-10CM # E22.0 Acromegaly and pituitary gigantism

CONSTITUTIONAL (FAMILIAL OR GENETIC)—MOST COMMON CAUSE

Endocrine Causes

Growth hormone excess—gigantism.
Sexual precocity (tall as children, short as adults):
  True sexual precocity.
  Pseudosexual precocity.
Androgen deficiency:
  Klinefelter syndrome.
  Bilateral anorchism.

GENETIC CAUSES

Klinefelter syndrome.
Syndromes of XYY, XXYY.

MISCELLANEOUS SYNDROMES AND DISORDERS

Cerebral gigantism or Sotos syndrome: prominent forehead, hypertelorism, high arched palate, dolichocephaly, mental retardation, large hands and feet, and premature eruption of teeth. Large at birth, with most rapid growth in first 4 yr of life.
Marfan syndrome: disorder of mesodermal tissues, subluxation of the lenses, arachnodactyly, and aortic aneurysm.
Homocystinuria: same phenotype as Marfan syndrome.
Obesity: tall as infants, children, and adolescents.
Total lipodystrophy: large hands and feet, generalized loss of subcutaneous fat, insulin-resistant DM, and hepatomegaly.
Beckwith-Wiedemann syndrome: neonatal tallness, omphalocele, macroglossia, and neonatal hypoglycemia.
Weaver-Smith syndrome: excessive intrauterine growth, mental retardation, megalocephaly, widened bifrontal diameter, hypertelorism, large ears, micrognathia, camptodactyly, broad thumbs, and limited extension of elbows and knees.
Marshall-Smith syndrome: excessive intrauterine growth, mental retardation, blue sclerae, failure to thrive, and early death.

TARDIVE DYSKINESIA[31]

ICD-10CM #	R27.9	Unspecified lack of coordination
	F44.4	Conversion disorder with motor symptom or deficit
	F44.6	Conversion disorder with sensory symptom or deficit
	G24.4	Idiopathic orofacial dystonia

DIFFERENTIAL DIAGNOSIS

Medications (antidepressants, anticholinergics, amphetamines, lithium, l-dopa, phenytoin).
Brain neoplasms.
Ill-fitting dentures.
Huntington disease.
Idiopathic dystonias (tics, blepharospasm, aging).
Wilson's disease.
Extrapyramidal syndrome (postanoxic or postencephalitic).
Torsion dystonia.

TASTE AND SMELL LOSS[3]

ICD-10CM #	R43.0	Anosmia
	R43.1	Parosmia
	R43.2	Parageusia

TASTE

Local: radiation therapy.
Systemic: cancer, renal failure, hepatic failure, nutritional deficiency (vitamin B_{12}, zinc), Cushing's syndrome, hypothyroidism, DM, infection (influenza), drugs (antirheumatic and antiproliferative).
Neurologic: Bell palsy, familial dysautonomia, multiple sclerosis.

SMELL

Local: allergic rhinitis, sinusitis, nasal polyposis, bronchial asthma.
Systemic: renal failure, hepatic failure, nutritional deficiency (vitamin B_{12}), Cushing's syndrome, hypothyroidism, DM, infection (viral hepatitis, influenza), drugs (nasal sprays, antibiotics).
Neurologic: head trauma, multiple sclerosis, Parkinson's disease, frontal brain tumor.

TELANGIECTASIA

ICD-10CM #		
	I78.8	Other diseases of capillaries
	I78.9	Disease of capillaries, unspecified

Oral contraceptive agents.
Pregnancy.
Rosacea.
Varicose veins.
Trauma.
Drug induced (corticosteroids, systemic or topical).
Spider telangiectases.
Hepatic cirrhosis.
Mastocytosis.
SLE, dermatomyositis, systemic sclerosis.

TENDINOPATHY[57]

ICD-10CM #		
	M67.90	Unspecified disorder of synovium and tendon, unspecified site
	M71.9	Bursopathy, unspecified

INTRINSIC FACTORS

Anatomic Factors
Malalignment.
Muscle weakness or imbalance.
Muscle inflexibility.
Decreased vascularity.
Systemic Factors
Inflammatory conditions (e.g., SLE).
Pregnancy.
Quinolone-induced tendinopathy.
Age-Related Factors
Tendon degeneration.
Increased tendon stiffness.
Tendon calcification.
Decreased vascularity.

EXTRINSIC FACTORS

Repetitive Mechanical Load
Excessive duration.
Excessive frequency.
Excessive intensity.
Poor technique.
Workplace factors.
Equipment Problems
Footwear.
Athletic field surface.
Equipment factors (e.g., racquet size).
Protective gear.

TESTICULAR CYSTIC LESIONS[69]

ICD-10CM #	
	Varies with specific diagnosis

Benign
Tunica albuginea cysts.
Tunica vaginalis cysts.
Intratesticular cysts.
Tubular ectasia of rete testis.
Cystic dysplasia.
Epidermoid cysts.
Abscess.
Malignant
Nonseminomatous germ cell tumor.
Necrosis or hemorrhage in tumor.
Tubular obstruction by tumor.
Lymphoma.

TESTICULAR FAILURE[21]

ICD-10CM #		
	E29	Testicular dysfunction

PRIMARY

Klinefelter syndrome (XXY).
XYY.
Vanishing testes syndrome (in utero or early postnatal torsion).
Noonan syndrome.
Varicocele.
Myotonic dystrophy.
Orchitis (mumps, gonorrhea).
Cryptorchidism.
Chemical exposure.
Irradiation to testes.
Spinal cord injury.
Polyglandular failure.
Idiopathic oligospermia or azoospermia.
Germinal cell aplasia (Sertoli cell–only syndrome).
Idiopathic testicular failure.
Testicular torsion.
Testicular trauma.
Diethylstilbestrol (maternal use during pregnancy leading to in utero estrogen exposure).
Testicular tumor with subsequent irradiation therapy, chemotherapy, or surgery (retroperitoneal lymph node dissection or orchiectomy).

SECONDARY

Delayed puberty.
Kallmann syndrome.
Isolated gonadotropin deficiency.
Prader-Labhart-Willi syndrome.
Lawrence-Moon-Biedl syndrome.
CNS irradiation.
Prepubertal panhypopituitarism.
Postpubertal panhypopituitarism.
Hypogonadism secondary to hyperprolactinemia.
Adrenogenital syndrome.
Chronic liver disease.
Chronic renal failure/uremia.
Hemochromatosis.
Cushing's syndrome.
Malnutrition.
Massive obesity.
Sickle cell anemia.
Hyper/hypothyroidism.
Anabolic steroid use.

TESTICULAR PAIN

ICD-10CM #		
	N50.9	Disorder of male genital organs, unspecified
	R10.2	Pelvic and perineal pain

Testicular torsion.
Trauma.
Epididymitis.
Orchitis.
Neoplasm.
Urolithiasis.
Inguinal hernia.
Infection (cellulitis, abscess, folliculitis).
Anxiety.

TESTICULAR SIZE VARIATIONS[21]

ICD-10CM #		
	N50.0	Atrophy of testis
	N44.2	Benign cyst of testis
	N44.8	Other noninflammatory disorders of the testis
	N50.3	Cyst of epididymis
	N50.8	Other specified disorders of male genital organs
	N53.12	Painful ejaculation
	E29.1	Testicular hypofunction

SMALL TESTES

Hypothalamic-pituitary dysfunction.
Gonadotropin deficiency.
Growth hormone deficiency.
Normal variant.
Primary hypogonadism.
Autoimmune destruction.
Chemotherapy.
Cryptorchidism.
Irradiation.
Klinefelter syndrome.
Orchiditis.
Testicular regression syndrome.
Torsion.
Trauma.

LARGE TESTES

Adrenal rest tissue.
Compensatory.
Fragile X syndrome.
Idiopathic.
Tumor.

TETANUS[57]

ICD-10CM #		
	A35	Other tetanus

TETANUS "MIMICS"

Acute abdomen.
Black widow spider bite.
Dental abscess.
Dislocated mandible.
Dystonic reaction.
Encephalitis.
Head trauma.
Hyperventilation syndrome.
Hypocalcemia.
Meningitis.
Peritonsillar abscess.
Progressive fluctuating muscular rigidity (stiff-man syndrome).
Psychogenic.
Rabies.
Sepsis.
Subarachnoid hemorrhage.

Status epilepticus.
Strychnine poisoning.
Temporomandibular joint syndrome.

THROMBOCYTOPENIA

ICD-10CM #		
	D47.3	Essential (hemorrhagic) thrombocythemia
	D69.59	Other secondary thrombocytopenia
	D69.6	Thrombocytopenia, unspecified

INCREASED DESTRUCTION

Immunologic

Drugs: quinine, quinidine, digitalis, procainamide, thiazide diuretics, sulfonamides, phenytoin, aspirin, penicillin, heparin, gold, meprobamate, sulfa drugs, phenylbutazone, NSAIDs, methyldopa, cimetidine, furosemide, INH, cephalosporins, chlorpropamide, organic arsenicals, chloroquine, platelet glycoprotein IIb/IIIa receptor inhibitors, ranitidine, indomethacin, carboplatin, ticlopidine, clopidogrel.
Idiopathic thrombocytopenic purpura (ITP).
Transfusion reaction: transfusion of platelets with plasminogen activator (PLA) in recipients without PLA-1.
Fetal/maternal incompatibility.
Collagen vascular diseases (e.g., SLE).
Autoimmune hemolytic anemia.
Lymphoreticular disorders (e.g., CLL).

Nonimmunologic

Prosthetic heart valves.
Thrombotic thrombocytopenic purpura (TTP).
Sepsis.
DIC.
Hemolytic-uremic syndrome (HUS).
Giant cavernous hemangioma.

DECREASED PRODUCTION

Abnormal marrow.
Marrow infiltration (e.g., leukemia, lymphoma, fibrosis).
Marrow suppression (e.g., chemotherapy, alcohol, radiation).
Hereditary disorders.
Wiskott-Aldrich syndrome: X-linked disorder characterized by thrombocytopenia, eczema, and repeated infections.
May-Hegglin anomaly: increased megakaryocytes but ineffective thrombopoiesis.
Vitamin deficiencies (e.g., vitamin B_{12}, folic acid).

SPLENIC SEQUESTRATION, HYPERSPLENISM

DILUTIONAL, AS A RESULT OF MASSIVE TRANSFUSION

THROMBOCYTOPENIA, IN PREGNANCY[43]

ICD-10CM #		
	D69.59	Other secondary thrombocytopenia

Incidental thrombocytopenia of pregnancy (gestational thrombocytopenia).
Preeclampsia/eclampsia.[41]
Peripartum/postpartum thrombotic microangiopathy.
Disseminated intravascular coagulation (DIC) secondary to:
Abruptio placentae.
Endometritis.
Amniotic fluid embolism.
Retained fetus.
Thrombotic thrombocytopenic purpura.
Hemolytic-uremic syndrome.

[41] Preeclampsia/eclampsia usually is not associated with overt DIC.

THROMBOCYTOPENIA, INHERITED DISORDERS[3]

ICD-10CM #		
	D47.3	Essential (hemorrhagic) thrombocythemia

Amegakaryocytic thrombocytopenia.
Thrombocytopenia–absent radii.
MYH9-related thrombocytopenia:
May-Hegglin anomaly.
Fechtner syndrome.
Epstein syndrome.
Sebastian syndrome.
X-linked macrothrombocytopenia.
Wiskott-Aldrich syndrome.
X-linked thrombocytopenia.
Thrombocytopenia and radioulnar synostosis.
Familial platelet disorder—AML.
Familial dominant thrombocytopenia.
Paris-Trousseau thrombocytopenia.
Bernard-Soulier syndrome.
Bernard-Soulier carrier/Mediterranean macrothrombocytopenia.

THROMBOCYTOPENIA IN NEWBORNS, DIFFERENTIAL DIAGNOSIS[42]

ICD-10CM #		
	D47.3	Essential (hemorrhagic) thrombocythemia
	D69.59	Other secondary thrombocytopenia
	D69.6	Thrombocytopenia, unspecified

DIFFERENTIAL DIAGNOSIS OF THROMBOCYTOPENIA IN NEWBORNS

Perinatal hypoxemia
Placental insufficiency
Congenital infection
Sepsis.
Toxoplasmosis.
Rubella.
Cytomegalovirus.
Autoimmune
Maternal immune thrombocytopenia.
Maternal systemic lupus erythematosus.
Disseminated intravascular coagulation
Maternal drug exposure
Congenital heart disease
Hereditary thrombocytopenia
MYH9 macrothrombocytopenia (including May-Hegglin anomaly).
Thrombocytopenia absent radii syndrome.
Amegakaryocytic thrombocytopenia.
Wiskott-Aldrich syndrome.
Fanconi anemia.
Hemangioma with thrombocytopenia
Kasabach-Merritt syndrome.
Bone marrow infiltration
Congenital leukemia.

THROMBOCYTOSIS

ICD-10CM #		
	D75.9	Disease of blood and blood-forming organs, unspecified

Iron deficiency.
Posthemorrhage.
Neoplasms (GI tract).
CML.
Polycythemia vera.
Myelofibrosis with myeloid metaplasia.
Infections.
After splenectomy.
Postpartum.
Hemophilia.
Pancreatitis.
Cirrhosis.
Idiopathic.

THROMBOSIS OR THROMBOTIC DIATHESIS[3]

ICD-10CM #		
	I74.09	Other arterial embolism and thrombosis of abdominal aorta

DIFFERENTIAL DIAGNOSIS OF THE PATIENT PRESENTING WITH THROMBOSIS OR THROMBOTIC DIATHESIS

Inherited (Primary) Hypercoagulable States

Activated protein C resistance caused by factor V Leiden mutation.
Prothrombin gene mutation (G to A transition at position 20210 in the 3-untranslated region).
Antithrombin III deficiency.
Protein C deficiency.
Protein S deficiency.
Dysfibrinogenemias (rare).

Acquired (Secondary) Hypercoagulable States

In association with physiologic or thrombogenic stimuli:
Pregnancy (especially the postpartum period).
Estrogen use (oral contraceptives, hormone replacement therapy).
Immobilization.
Trauma.
Postoperative state.
Advancing age.
Obesity.
Prolonged air travel.
Lupus anticoagulant or antiphospholipid antibody syndrome.
In association with other clinical disorders.

Mixed/Unknown

Activated protein C resistance in the absence of factor V Leiden.
Elevated factor VIII level.
Elevated factor XI level.

Elevated factor IX level.
Elevated thrombin activatable fibrinolysis inhibitor (TAFI) level.
Decreased free tissue factor pathway inhibitor (TFPI) level.
Decreased plasma fibrinolytic activity.

THYMIC MASSES[72]

ICD-10CM # Varies with specific diagnosis

THYMIC MASSES

Thymic hyperplasia.
Thymoma.
Thymic carcinoma.
Thymic neuroendocrine tumors:
- Carcinoid.
- Small-cell carcinoma.

Thymic cysts (not rhizomatous).
Thymolipoma.
Metastases to the thymus.

THYMOMA, DISEASES ASSOCIATIONS[72]

ICD-10CM # Varies with specific diagnosis

SYSTEMIC DISEASES MOST COMMONLY ASSOCIATED WITH THYMOMA

Myasthenia gravis.
Cytopenias (most commonly red cell hypoplasia).
Nonthymic malignancies.
Hypogammaglobulinemia.
Systemic lupus erythematosus.
Polymyositis.
Rheumatoid arthritis.
Thyroiditis.
Sjögren syndrome.
Ulcerative colitis.

THYROMEGALY

ICD-10CM # Varies with specific diagnosis

Goiter.
Graves disease.
Thyroiditis (lymphocytic, granulomatous, suppurative).
Toxic adenoma.
Neoplasm (primary, metastatic).

THYROTOXICOSIS[59]

ICD-10CM # E05.80 Other thyrotoxicosis without thyrotoxic crisis or storm

CAUSES OF THYROTOXICOSIS

Sustained Hormone Overproduction (Hyperthyroidism)

Low TSH, High RAIU:
- Graves disease (von Basedow disease).
- Toxic multinodular goiter.
- Toxic adenoma.
- Chorionic gonadotropin-induced.
  - Gestational hyperthyroidism: physiologic hyperthyroidism of pregnancy, familial gestational hyperthyroidism due to TSH receptor mutations.
  - Trophoblastic tumors.

Inherited nonimmune hyperthyroidism associated with TSH receptor or G protein mutations.
Low TSH, Low RAIU:
- Iodide-induced hyperthyroidism (Jod-Basedow effect).
- Amiodarone-associated hyperthyroidism due to iodide release.

Struma Ovarii:
- Metastatic functioning thyroid carcinoma.

Normal or Elevated TSH:
- TSH-secreting pituitary tumors.
- Thyroid hormone resistance with pituitary predominance.

Transient Hormone Excess (Thyrotoxicosis)

Low TSH, Low RAIU
- Thyroiditis.
- Autoimmune: lymphocytic thyroiditis (silent thyroiditis, painless thyroiditis, postpartum thyroiditis), acute exacerbation of Hashimoto disease.

Viral or postviral.
Subacute (granulomatous, painful, postviral) thyroiditis.
Drug-induced or associated thyroiditis.
- Amiodarone.
- Lithium, interferon-α, interleukin-2, GM-CSF.

Infectious thyroiditis.
Exogenous Thyroid Hormone:
- Iatrogenic overreplacement.
- Thyrotoxicosis factitia.
- Ingestion of natural products containing thyroid hormone.
  - "Hamburger" thyrotoxicosis.
  - Natural foodstuffs.
  - Thyromimetic compounds (e.g., tiratricol PLB).
  - Occupational exposure to thyroid hormone (e.g., pill manufacturing, veterinary occupations).

GM-CSF, granulocyte-macrophage colony-stimulating factor; *RAIU*, radioactive iodine uptake; *TSH*, thyroid-stimulating hormone.

TICK-RELATED INFECTIONS

ICD-10CM #		
	A77.0	Spotted fever due to Rickettsia rickettsii
	A93.2	Colorado tick fever
	B60.0	Babesiosis
	A77.8	Other spotted fevers
	A69.20	Lyme disease, unspecified

Lyme disease.
Rocky Mountain spotted fever.
Babesiosis.
Tularemia.
Q fever.
Colorado tick fever.
Ehrlichiosis.
Relapsing fever.

TICS

ICD-10CM # F95.9 Tic disorder, unspecified

Tourette's syndrome.
Physiologic tic.
Anxiety disorder.
Huntington disease.
Medications (e.g., antipsychotics, carbamazepine, phenytoin, phenobarbital).
Encephalitis.
Head trauma.
Schizophrenia.
Carbon monoxide poisoning.
Stroke.
Sydenham chorea.
Creutzfeldt-Jakob disease.

TORSADES DE POINTES[50]

ICD-10CM # I47.2 Ventricular tachycardia

Antiarrhythmics known to increase the QT interval (e.g., quinidine, procainamide, amiodarone, disopyramide, sotalol).
Tricyclic antidepressants and phenothiazines.
Histamine (H_1) antagonists (e.g., astemizole, terfenadine).
Antiviral and antifungal agents and antibiotics.
Hypokinemia.
Hypomagnesemia.
Insecticide poisoning.
Bradyarrhythmias.
Congenital long QT syndrome.
Subarachnoid hemorrhage.
Chloroquinine, pentamidine.
Cocaine abuse.

TOXIC MEGACOLON, CAUSES[15]

ICD-10CM # K59.3 Megacolon, not elsewhere classified

INFLAMMATORY

Ulcerative colitis.
Crohn's disease.

INFECTIOUS

Bacterial.
- *Clostridium difficile* pseudomembranous colitis.
- *Salmonella* (typhoid and nontyphoid).
- *Shigella.*
- *Campylobacter.*
- *Yersinia.*

Parasitic.
- *Entamoeba histolytica.*
- *Cryptosporidium.*

Viral.
- Cytomegalovirus colitis.

OTHER

Ischemia.
Kaposi sarcoma.

TRACHEOBRONCHIAL NARROWING ON X-RAY[36]

ICD-10CM # Varies with specific diagnosis

CAUSES OF TRACHEOBRONCHIAL NARROWING

Long-Segment/Diffuse Narrowing

Sarcoidosis.
Amyloidosis.
Granulomatosis with polyangiitis.
Relapsing polychondritis.
Tracheobronchopathia osteochondroplastica.
Pemphigoid.

Short-Segment Narrowing

Previous intubation or tracheostomy.
Congenital stenosis or web.
Extrinsic compression (from thyroid).
Adenoid cystic carcinoma.
Squamous carcinoma.

TREMOR

ICD-10CM #		
	R25.0	Abnormal head movements
	R25.1	Tremor, unspecified
	R25.2	Cramp and spasm
	R25.3	Fasciculation
	R25.9	Unspecified abnormal involuntary movements
	G25.0	Essential tremor
	G25.1	Drug-induced tremor
	G25.2	Other specified forms of tremor

REST TREMORS

Parkinson's disease.
Other parkinsonian syndromes (less commonly).
Midbrain (rubral) tremor: rest <postural <kinetic.
Wilson's disease (also acquired hepatocerebral degeneration).
Essential tremor—only if severe: rest <postural and action.

POSTURAL AND ACTION (TERMINAL) TREMORS

Physiologic tremor.
Exaggerated physiologic tremor (these factors can also aggravate other forms of tremor).
- Stress, fatigue, anxiety, emotion.
- Endocrine: hypoglycemia, thyrotoxicosis, pheochromocytoma, adrenocorticosteroids.
- Drugs and toxins: b-agonists, dopamine agonists, amphetamines, lithium, tricyclic antidepressants, neuroleptics, theophylline, caffeine, valproic acid, alcohol withdrawal, mercury (Hatter shakes), lead, arsenic, others.

Essential tremor (familial or sporadic).
Primary writing tremor.
With other CNS disorders:
- Parkinson's disease.
- Other akinetic-rigid syndromes.
- Idiopathic dystonia, including focal dystonias.

With peripheral neuropathy:
- Charcot-Marie-Tooth syndrome (controversial whether to call this the Roussy-Levy syndrome).
- Variety of other peripheral neuropathies (especially dysgammaglobulinemia).

Cerebellar tremor.

KINETIC (INTENTION) TREMOR

Disease of cerebellar outflow (dentate nucleus and superior cerebellar peduncle): multiple sclerosis, trauma, tumor, vascular disease, Wilson's acquired hepatocerebral degeneration, drugs, toxins (e.g., mercury), others.

MISCELLANEOUS RHYTHMICAL MOVEMENT DISORDERS

Psychogenic tremor.
Orthostatic tremor.
Rhythmical movements in dystonia (dystonic tremor).
Rhythmical myoclonus (segmental myoclonus—e.g., palatal or branchial myoclonus, spinal myoclonus, limb myorhythmia).
Oscillatory myoclonus.
Asterixis.
Clonus.
Epilepsia partialis continua.
Hereditary chin quivering.
Spasmus nutans.
Head bobbing with third ventricular cysts.
Nystagmus.

TREMOR, IN CHILDREN, CAUSES[51]

ICD-10CM #		
	R25.0	Abnormal head movements
	R25.1	Tremor, unspecified
	R25.2	Cramp and spasm
	R25.3	Fasciculation
	R25.9	Unspecified abnormal involuntary movements

BENIGN

Enhanced physiologic tremor.
Shuddering attacks.
Jitteriness.
Spasmus nutans.

STATIC INJURY/STRUCTURAL

Cerebellar malformation.
Stroke (particularly in the midbrain or cerebellum).
Multiple sclerosis.

HEREDITARY/DEGENERATIVE

Familial essential tremor.
Fragile X premutation.
Wilson's disease.
Huntington disease.
Juvenile parkinsonism (tremor is rare).
Pallidonigral degeneration.

METABOLIC

Hyperthyroidism.
Hyperadrenergic state (including pheochromocytoma and neuroblastoma).
Hypomagnesemia.
Hypocalcemia.
Hypoglycemia.
Hepatic encephalopathy.
Vitamin B_{12} deficiency.
Inborn errors of metabolism.
Mitochondrial disorders.

DRUGS/TOXINS

Valproate, phenytoin, carbamazepine, lamotrigine, gabapentin, lithium, tricyclic antidepressants, stimulants (cocaine, amphetamine, caffeine, thyroxine, bronchodilators), neuroleptics, cyclosporin, toluene, mercury, thallium, amiodarone, nicotine, lead, manganese, arsenic, cyanide, naphthalene, ethanol, lindane, serotonin reuptake inhibitors.

PERIPHERAL NEUROPATHIES

PSYCHOGENIC

TRICHOMEGALY[12]

ICD-10CM # Not available

CAUSES OF TRICHOMEGALY

Drug-induced: topical prostaglandin analogues, phenytoin and cyclosporine.
Malnutrition.
AIDS.
Porphyria.
Hypothyroidism.
Familial.
Congenital: Oliver–McFarlane, Cornelia de Lange, Goldstein-Hutt, Hermansky–Pudlak syndromes.

TUBULOINTERSTITIAL DISEASE, ACUTE[32]

ICD-10CM #		
	N17.0	Acute kidney failure with tubular necrosis

DRUGS

Antibiotics, penicillins, cephalosporins, rifampin.
Sulfonamides: cotrimoxazole, sulfamethoxazole.
NSAIDs: propionic acid derivatives.
Miscellaneous: phenytoin, thiazides, allopurinol, cimetidine, ifosfamide.

INFECTIONS

Invasion of renal parenchyma.
Reaction to systemic infections: streptococcal, diphtheria, hantavirus.

SYSTEMIC DISEASES

Immune mediated: SLE, transplanted kidney, cryoglobulinemias.
Metabolic: urate, oxalate.
Neoplastic: lymphoproliferative diseases.

IDIOPATHIC

TUBULOINTERSTITIAL KIDNEY DISEASE[32]

ICD-10CM #		
	N17.0	Acute kidney failure with tubular necrosis

Ischemic and toxic acute tubular necrosis.
Allergic interstitial nephritis.
Interstitial nephritis secondary to immune complex-related collagen vascular disease (e.g., SLE, Sjögren).
Granulomatous diseases (sarcoidosis, uveitis).
Pigment-related tubular injury (myoglobinuria, hemoglobinuria).

Hypercalcemia with nephrocalcinosis.
Tubular obstruction (drugs such as indinavir, uric acid in tumor lysis syndrome).
Myeloma kidney or cast nephropathy.
Infection-related interstitial nephritis: *Legionella, Leptospira.*
Infiltrative diseases (e.g., lymphoma).

TUMOR MARKERS ELEVATION[81]

ICD-10CM #	R97.8	Other abnormal tumor markers

CAUSES OF ELEVATED LEVELS OF TUMOR MARKERS

Carcinoembryonic Antigen (CEA)

Colonic cancer (higher levels if the tumor is more differentiated or is extensive or has spread to the liver).
Lung or breast cancer; seminoma.
Cigarette smokers.
Cirrhosis, inflammatory bowel disease, rectal polyps, pancreatitis.
Advanced age.

Alpha-Fetoprotein

Hepatocellular cancer: very high titers or a rising titer is strongly suggestive, but >10% of patients do not have an elevated level.
Hepatic regeneration (e.g., cirrhosis, alcoholic or viral hepatitis).
Cancer of the stomach, colon, pancreas, or lung.
Teratocarcinoma or embryonal cell carcinoma (testis, ovary, extragonadal).
Pregnancy.
Ataxia-telangiectasia.
Normal variant.

Prostate-Specific Antigen

Prostate carcinoma (localized disease).
Prostatic hyperplasia.
Prostatitis.
Prostatic infarction.

Cancer-Associated Antigen (CA-19-9)[42]

Pancreatic carcinoma (80% with advanced, well-differentiated cancer have an elevated level).
Other GI cancers: colon, stomach, bile duct.
Acute or chronic pancreatitis.
Chronic liver disease.
Biliary tract disease.

[42] Patients who cannot synthesize Lewis blood group antigens (~5% of the population) do not produce CA-19–9 antigen.

UREMIC ENCEPHALOPATHY, DIFFERENTIAL DIAGNOSIS[28]

ICD-10CM #	G93.40	Encephalopathy, unspecified

Differential Diagnosis	Comment
Hypertensive encephalopathy	
Systemic inflammatory response syndrome (SIRS):	Observed in septic patients.
Systemic vasculitis:	Vasculitis or lupus with cerebral involvement.
Drug-induced neurotoxicity	
Analgesics:	Meperidine, codeine, morphine, gabapentin.
Antibiotics:	High-dose penicillins (may cause seizures), acyclovir, ethambutol (optic nerve damage), erythromycin and aminoglycosides (may cause ototoxicity), nitrofurantoin and isoniazid (peripheral neuropathy).
Psychotropics:	Lithium, haloperidol, clonazepam, diazepam, chlorpromazine.
Immunosuppressants:	Cyclosporine, tacrolimus.
Chemotherapeutics:	Cisplatinum, ifosfamide.
Others:	High doses of loop diuretics (ototoxic), ephedrine, methyldopa, aluminum.
Cerebral atheroembolic disease:	Follows recent aortic or cardiac angiography; associated with peripheral manifestations, including lower extremity cyanosis, livedo reticularis, and eosinophilia.
Subdural hematoma	
Posterior leukoencephalopathy:	Observed particularly following renal transplantation due to reversible, abnormal permeability of the blood-brain barrier Often manifests as headache followed by mental depression, visual loss, and seizures in the context of volume expansion, acute hypertension, and often treatment with corticosteroids or calcineurin inhibitors Lesions in the parietal, temporal, and occipital lobes may be seen on imaging studies.

URETERAL COLIC[53]

ICD-10CM #	R33.8	Other retention of urine
	N13.8	Other obstructive and reflux uropathy

DIAGNOSTIC DIFFERENTIALS OF RENAL OR URETERAL COLIC

Acute cholecystitis, acute cholelithiasis.
Acute appendicitis.
Pelvic inflammatory disease.
Diverticulosis and/or diverticulitis.
Intestinal obstruction.
Leaking abdominal aortic aneurysm.
Musculoskeletal sprains.
Herniated disk.
Hepes zoster (shingles).
GI dysfunction with ileus and/or toxic colonic dilatation.

URETERAL STRICTURE[85]

ICD-10CM #	Varies with specific diagnosis

ETIOLOGY OF URETERAL STRICTURE

Malignancy (e.g., transitional cell carcinoma, cervical cancer).
Ureteral calculus.
Radiation.
Ischemia or trauma caused by surgical dissection.
Periureteral fibrosis caused by abdominal aortic aneurysm or endometriosis.
Endoscopic instrumentation.
Renal ablation injury.
Infection (tuberculosis).
Idiopathic condition.

URETERIC OBSTRUCTION, CONGENITAL[36]

ICD-10CM #	N13.8	Other obstructive and reflux uropathy
	N20.9	Urolithiasis

CONGENITAL CAUSES OF URETERIC OBSTRUCTION

Primary megaureter.
Ureterocele (ectopic and orthotopic).
Ureteric valve.
Distal ureteric stenosis.
Ureteric atresia.
Circumcaval ureter and variants.
Bladder diverticulum.

URETHRAL BLEEDING[85]

ICD-10CM #	Varies with specific diagnosis

DIFFERENTIAL DIAGNOSIS FOR URETHRAL BLEEDING

Male

Trauma:
Blunt (straddle injury, kick to perineum).

Penetrating (foreign body insertion, failed urethral catheterization).
Intercourse related (penile fracture, masturbation).
Urethritis:
Bacterial (gonococcal, nongonococcal).
Viral.
Chemical.
Autoimmune (Reiter syndrome).
Malignancy:
Urothelial carcinoma.
Squamous cell carcinoma (meatus/glans).
Condyloma.
Calculus disease.

Female

Trauma:
Blunt (pelvic fracture).
Penetrating (foreign body).
Urethral diverticulum.
Urethral caruncle.
Urethritis.
Malignancy.
Calculus disease.

URETHRAL DISCHARGE AND DYSURIA

ICD-10CM #	Code	Description
	R36.0	Urethral discharge without blood
	R36.9	Urethral discharge, unspecified
	N36.9	Urethral disorder, unspecified
	N39.9	Disorder of urinary system, unspecified
	R30.0	Dysuria
	R30.9	Painful micturition, unspecified

Urethritis (gonococcal, chlamydial, trichomonal).
Cystitis.
Prostatitis.
Vaginitis (candidiasis, chemical).
Meatal stenosis.
Interstitial cystitis.
Trauma (foreign body, masturbation, horseback or bike riding).

URETHRAL OBSTRUCTION, CHILDREN[36]

ICD-10CM #	Code	Description
	N13.8	Other obstructive and reflux uropathy

CAUSES OF URETHRAL OBSTRUCTION IN CHILDREN

Intrinsic Lesions

Valve (posterior, anterior, saccular diverticulum).
Stenosis, atresia.
Inflammatory stricture.
Traumatic stricture:
External trauma (saddle injury, and so on).
Iatrogenic trauma (catheter, cystoscopy, surgery).
Urethral "tumors":
Girls: leiomyoma.
Boys: polyp, rhabdomyosarcoma.
Miscellaneous (epidermolysis bullosa).

Extrinsic Lesions

Presacral mass dissecting inferiorly (tumor, cyst).
Fecal impaction (Hirschsprung, postrepair anal atresia, habitual constipation, neuropathy).
Mass originating in genital organs:
Boys: utricle cyst, prostate rhabdomyosarcoma, seminal vesicle cyst, Cowper duct cyst.
Girls: hydrometrocolpos, hydrocolpos, fused labia.

URETHRITIS, PEDIATRIC PATIENT[19]

ICD-10CM #	Code	Description
	N34.1	Nonspecific urethritis
	N34.2	Other urethritis

ETIOLOGY OF URETHRITIS

Infectious	Noninfectious
Sexually Transmitted Infections	**Vasculitides**
Neisseria gonorrhoeae.	Reiter syndrome.
Chlamydia trachomatis.	Erythema multiforme.
Trichomonas vaginalis.	Kawasaki disease.
Herpes simplex virus type 2.	**Mechanical**
Mycoplasma spp.	Masturbation.
Non–Sexually Transmitted Infections	Foreign body.
Staphylococcus saprophyticus.	Trauma.
Enterobacteriaceae.	Dysfunctional elimination.
Gardnerella vaginalis.	**Chemical**
Streptococcus spp.	Soaps.
Enterobius vermicularis.	Detergents.
	Drugs.

URIC ACID STONES

ICD-10CM #	Code	Description
	N20.9	Urolithiasis

Hyperuricemia.
Excessive dietary purine.
Medications (salicylates, allopurinol, probenecid).
Urine pH <5.5 (e.g., diarrhea, high animal protein diet).
Decreased urine output (dehydration, malabsorption, diarrhea, inadequate fluid intake).
Tumor lysis.
Hemolytic anemia.
Myeloproliferative disorders.

URINARY INCONTINENCE, CHILDREN[51]

ICD-10CM #	Code	Description
	R32	Unspecified urinary incontinence

CAUSES OF URINARY INCONTINENCE IN CHILDHOOD

Overactive bladder.
Infrequent voiding.
Detrusor-sphincter dyssynergia.
Non-neurogenic neurogenic bladder (Hinman syndrome).
Vaginal voiding.
Giggle incontinence.
Cystitis.
Bladder outlet obstruction (posterior urethral valves).
Ectopic ureter and fistula.
Sphincter abnormality (epispadias, exstrophy; urogenital sinus abnormality).
Neuropathic.
Overflow incontinence.
Traumatic.
Iatrogenic.
Behavioral.
Combination.

URINARY RETENTION[53]

ICD-10CM #	Code	Description
	R33.9	Retention of urine, unspecified

COMMON CAUSES OF URINARY RETENTION

Obstructive Cause

Urethral stricture.
Enlarged prostate.
Lower genitourinary tract malignancy.
Pelvic malignancy.
Bladder stones.
Foreign body.
Blood clot.
Posterior urethral valves.
Ureterocele.

Primary Detrusor Insufficiency

Detrusor areflexia.
Multiple sclerosis.
Iatrogenic injury during abdominal or back surgery.
Spinal cord injury.
Myelomeningocele.

URINARY RETENTION, ACUTE

ICD-10CM #	Code	Description
	R33.9	Retention of urine, unspecified

Mechanical obstruction: urethral stone, foreign body, urethral stricture, BPH, prostate carcinoma, prostatitis, trauma with hematoma formation.
Neurogenic bladder.
Neurologic disease (MS, parkinsonism, tabes dorsalis, CVA).
Spinal cord injury.
CNS neoplasm (primary or metastatic).
Spinal anesthesia.
Lower urinary tract instrumentation.
Medications (antihistamines, antidepressants, narcotics, anticholinergics).
Abdominal or pelvic surgery.
Alcohol toxicity.
Pregnancy.
Anxiety.
Encephalitis.
Postoperative pain.
Spina bifida occulta.

URINARY TRACT BLEEDING, UPPER[85]

ICD-10CM # Varies with specific diagnosis

DIFFERENTIAL DIAGNOSIS FOR UPPER URINARY TRACT BLEEDING

Renal glomerular diseases:
- IgA nephropathy (Berger disease).
- Thin basement membrane disease.
- Acute glomerulonephritis (e.g., poststreptococcal).
- Lupus nephritis.
- Hereditary nephritis (e.g., Alport syndrome).

Renal tubulointerstitial diseases:
- Papillary necrosis.
- Sickle cell nephropathy.
- Analgesic nephropathy.
- Polycystic kidney disease.
- Medullary sponge kidney.

Vasculitis:
- Henoch-Schönlein purpura.
- Wegener granulomatosis.

Infection:
- Pyelonephritis.
- Xanthogranulomatous pyelonephritis.
- Renal tuberculosis.
- Fungal infection.

Obstruction:
- Ureteropelvic junction obstruction.
- Ureteral stricture.

Nephrolithiasis.

Malignancy:
- Renal cortical tumors (renal cell carcinoma, benign tumors).
- Upper tract urothelial carcinoma.

Fibroepithelial polyp.

Vascular diseases:
- Renal arteriovenous malformations (congenital, acquired).
- Iliac arterio-ureteral fistula.
- Renal artery aneurysm (especially ruptured).
- Renal artery pseudoaneurysm.
- Renal artery and/or vein thrombosis.
- Hemangioma.
- Atheroembolic disease.
- Nutcracker syndrome.
- Loin-pain hematuria syndrome.

Trauma:
- Blunt.
- Penetrating.

Lateralizing essential hematuria.

URINARY TRACT OBSTRUCTION[34]

ICD-10CM #		
	N21.8	Other lower urinary tract calculus
	N20.9	Urolithiasis

INTRARENAL

Uric acid nephropathy.
Sulfonamide precipitates.
Acyclovir, indinavir precipitates.
Multiple myeloma.

URETERAL

Intrinsic

Intraluminal:
- Nephrolithiasis.
- Papillary necrosis.
- Blood clots.
- Fungus balls.

Intramural:
- Ureteropelvic junction dysfunction.
- Ureterovesical junction dysfunction.
- Ureteral valve, polyp, or tumor.
- Ureteral stricture:
  - Schistosomiasis.
  - Tuberculosis.
  - Scarring from instrumentation.
  - Drugs (e.g., NSAIDs).

Extrinsic

Vascular system:
- Aneurysm: abdominal aorta or iliac vessels.
- Aberrant vessels: ureteropelvic junction.
- Venous: retrocaval ureter.

GI tract:
- Crohn's disease.
- Diverticulitis.
- Appendiceal abscess.
- Colon cancer.
- Pancreatic tumor, abscess, or cyst.

Reproductive system:
- Uterus: pregnancy, prolapse, tumor, endometriosis.
- Ovary: abscess, tumor, ovarian remnants.
- Gartner duct cyst, tuboovarian abscess.

Retroperitoneal disease:
- Retroperitoneal fibrosis: radiation, drugs, idiopathic.
- Inflammatory: tuberculosis, sarcoidosis.
- Hematoma.
- Primary tumor (e.g., lymphoma, sarcoma).
- Metastatic tumor (e.g., cervix, ovarian, bladder, colon).
- Lymphocele.
- Pelvic lipomatosis.

BLADDER

Neurogenic bladder:
- Diabetes mellitus.
- Spinal cord defect.
- Trauma.
- Multiple sclerosis.
- Stroke.
- Parkinson's disease.
- Spinal anesthesia.
- Anticholinergics.

Bladder neck dysfunction.
Bladder calculus.
Bladder cancer.

URETHRA

Urethral stricture.
Prostate hypertrophy or cancer.
Obstruction from instrumentation.

URINARY TRACT OBSTRUCTION, CONGENITAL CAUSES[74]

ICD-10CM # Varies with specific diagnosis

CONGENITAL CAUSES OF URINARY TRACT OBSTRUCTION

Ureteropelvic Junction

Ureteropelvic junction obstruction.

Proximal and Middle Ureter

Ureteral folds.
Ureteral valves.
Strictures.
Benign fibroepithelial polyps.
Retrocaval ureter.

Distal Ureter

Ureterovesical junction obstruction.
Vesicoureteral reflux.
Prune-belly syndrome.
Ureteroceles.

Bladder

Bladder diverticula.
Neurologic conditions (e.g., spina bifida).

Urethra

Posterior urethral valves.
Urethral diverticula.
Anterior urethral valves.
Urethral atresia.
Labial fusion.

URINE CASTS

ICD-10CM #	R82.99	Other abnormal findings in urine

Normal finding.
Pyelonephritis.
Chronic renal disease.
Nephrotic syndrome.
Acute tubular necrosis.
Interstitial nephritis.
Nephritic syndrome.
Glomerulonephritis.
Eclampsia.
Heavy metal ingestion.
Allograft rejection.
Hypothyroidism.

URINE COLOR ABNORMALITIES[53]

ICD-10CM #		
	R82.5	Elevated urine levels of drugs, medicaments and biological substances
	R82.99	Other abnormal findings in urine

COMMON CAUSES OF ABNORMAL URINE COLOR

Colorless

DISEASE

Diabetes mellitus.
Diabetes insipidus.

DRUG

Ethyl alcohol.
Diuretics.

MISCELLANEOUS

Overhydration.

Yellow-orange

DRUG
Tetracycline.
Flutamide.
Pyridium.
Azo Gantrisin (Roche Labs, Nutley, NJ).
Sulfasalazine.
Vitamin B.

MISCELLANEOUS
Dehydration.

Milky White

DISEASE
Urinary tract infection/pyuria.

Blue-green

DISEASE
Pseudomonas urinary tract infection.

DRUG
Methylene blue.
Urised (Polymedica Pharmaceuticals, Woburn, MA).
Indigo carmine.
Doan pills (Novartis Consumer Health, Parsippany, NJ).
Clorets (Cadbury Adams, Parsippany, NJ).
Amitriptyline.

Red-brown

DISEASE
Hematuria.
Hemolytic anemia.
Hemoglobinuria.
Lead poisoning.
Mercury poisoning.
Porphyria.

DRUG
Rifampin.
Ex-Lax (Novartis Consumer Health, Parsippany, NJ).
Phenolphthalein.
Phenothiazines.
Nitrofurantoin.
Doxorubicin.

MISCELLANEOUS
Beets.
Blackberries.
Rhubarb.

Brown-black

DISEASE
Fecaluria.
Methemoglobinuria.
Melaninuria.

DRUG
Metronidazole.
Methyldopa.
Methocarbamol.

MISCELLANEOUS
Fava beans.
Aloe.

URINE, RED[62]

ICD-10CM # Varies with specific diagnosis

WITH A POSITIVE DIPSTICK
Hematuria.
Hemoglobinuria: negative urinalysis.
Myoglobinuria: negative urinalysis.

WITH A NEGATIVE DIPSTICK
Drugs
Aminosalicylic acid.
Deferoxamine mesylate.
Ibuprofen.
Phenacetin.
Phenolphthalein.
Phensuximide.
Rifampin.
Anthraquinone laxatives.
Doxorubicin.
Methyldopa.
Phenazopyridine.
Phenothiazine.
Phenytoin.

Dyes
Azo dyes.
Eosin.

Foods
Beets, berries, maize.
Rhodamine B.

Metabolic
Porphyrins.
Serratia marcescens (red diaper syndrome).
Urate crystalluria.

UROLITHIASIS-LIKE PAIN[74]

ICD-10CM # Varies with specific diagnosis

DIFFERENTIAL DIAGNOSIS OF UROLITHIASIS-LIKE PAIN
Category
Disorders

Renal:
- Pyelonephritis.
- Blood clot.
- Renal infarction.
- Tumor (kidney or pelvis).
- Papillary necrosis.

Ureteral:
- Tumor.
- Blood clot.
- Stricture.

Bladder:
- Tumor.
- Blood clot.
- Urinary retention.

Intraabdominal:
- Peritonitis.
- Appendicitis.
- Biliary disease.
- Bowel obstruction.
- Vascular disorder.
- Aortic aneurysm.
- Mesenteric insufficiency.

Retroperitoneal:
- Lymphadenopathy.
- Fibrosis.
- Tumor.

Gynecologic:
- Ectopic or tubal pregnancy.
- Ovarian torsion, cyst rupture.
- Pelvic inflammatory disease.
- Cervical cancer.
- Endometriosis.
- Ovarian vein syndrome.

Neuromuscular:
- Muscle pain.
- Rib fracture.
- Radiculitis.

Infectious:
- Herpes zoster.
- Pleuritis, pneumonia.
- Fungal bezoar.

UROPATHY, OBSTRUCTIVE[77]

ICD-10CM #	N13.9	Obstructive and reflux uropathy, unspecified
	N20.9	Urolithiasis

INTRINSIC CAUSES
Intraluminal
Intratubular deposition of crystals (uric acid, sulfas).
Stones.
Papillary tissue.
Blood clots.

Intramural
Functional.
Ureter (ureteropelvic or ureterovesical dysfunction).
Bladder (neurogenic): spinal cord defect or trauma, diabetes, multiple sclerosis, Parkinson's disease, cerebrovascular accidents.
Bladder neck dysfunction.

Anatomic
Tumors.
Infection, granuloma.
Strictures.

EXTRINSIC CAUSES
Originating in the Reproductive System
Prostate: benign hypertrophy or cancer.
Uterus: pregnancy, tumors, prolapse, endometriosis.
Ovary: abscess, tumor, cysts.

Originating in the Vascular System
Aneurysms (aorta, iliac vessels).
Aberrant arteries (ureteropelvic junction).
Venous (ovarian veins, retrocaval ureter).

Originating in the Gastrointestinal Tract
- Crohn's disease.
- Pancreatitis.
- Appendicitis.
- Tumors.

Originating in the Retroperitoneal Space
- Inflammations.
- Fibrosis.
- Tumor, hematomas.

UROSEPSIS[53]

ICD-10CM # A41.9 Sepsis, unspecified organism

COMMON CAUSES OF UROSEPSIS
Obstructing ureteral stone with pyonephrosis.
Staghorn calculus with urinary tract infection.

Ureteral obstruction with proximal urinary tract infection.
Urinary retention with urinary tract infection.
Acute prostatitis with prostatic abscess.
Perinephric abscess or renal carbuncle.
Urethral stricture with periurethral abscess.
Fournier gangrene.
Foreign body within urinary tract (e.g., Foley catheter).

UTERINE BLEEDING, ABNORMAL[24]

ICD-10CM #	N92.6	Irregular menstruation, unspecified
	N93.9	Abnormal uterine and vaginal bleeding, unspecified

PREGNANCY

Threatened abortion.
Incomplete abortion.
Complete abortion.
Molar pregnancy.
Ectopic pregnancy.
Retained products of conception.

OVULATORY

Vulva: infection, laceration, tumor.
Vagina: infection, laceration, tumor, foreign body.
Cervix: polyps, cervical erosion, cervicitis, carcinoma.
Uterus: fibroids (submucous fibroids most likely to cause abnormal bleeding), polyps, adenomyosis, endometritis, intrauterine device, atrophic endometrium.
Pregnancy complications: ectopic pregnancy; threatened, incomplete, complete abortion; retained products of conception.
Abnormality of clotting system.
Midcycle bleeding.
Halban disease (persistent corpus luteum).
Menorrhagia.
Pelvic inflammatory disease.

ANOVULATORY

Physiologic causes:
Puberty.
Perimenopausal.
Pathologic causes:
- Ovarian failure (FSH over 40 IU/ml).
- Hyperandrogenism.
- Hyperprolactinemia.
- Obesity.
- Hypothalamic dysfunction (polycystic ovaries); LH/FSH ratio greater than 2:1.
- Hyperplasia.
- Endometrial carcinoma.
- Estrogen-producing tumors.
- Hypothyroidism.

UVEITIS, PEDIATRIC AGE

ICD-10CM #	H20.9	Anterior uveitis

ANTERIOR UVEITIS

Juvenile rheumatoid arthritis (pauciarticular).
Sarcoidosis.
Trauma.
Tuberculosis.
Kawasaki disease.
Ulcerative colitis.
Postinfectious (enteric or genital) with arthritis and rash.
Spirochetal (syphilis, leptospiral).
Heterochromic iridocyclitis (Fuchs).
Viral (herpes simplex, herpes zoster).
Ankylosing spondylitis.
Stevens-Johnson syndrome.
Idiopathic.
Drugs.

POSTERIOR UVEITIS (CHOROIDITIS—MAY INVOLVE RETINA)

Toxoplasmosis.
Parasites (toxocariasis).
Sarcoidosis.
Tuberculosis.
Viral (rubella, herpes simplex, HIV, cytomegalovirus).
Subacute sclerosing panencephalitis.
Idiopathic.

ANTERIOR AND/OR POSTERIOR UVEITIS

Sympathetic ophthalmia (trauma to other eye).
Vogt-Koyanagi-Harada syndrome (uveo-otocutaneous syndrome: poliosis, vitiligo, deafness, tinnitus, uveitis, aseptic meningitis, retinitis).
Behçet's syndrome.
Lyme disease.

VAGINAL BLEEDING, PREGNANCY[17]

ICD-10CM #	N93.9	Abnormal uterine and vaginal bleeding, unspecified

FIRST TRIMESTER

Implantation bleeding.
Abortion.
- Threatened.
- Complete.
- Incomplete.
- Missed.

Ectopic pregnancy.
Neoplasia.
Hydatidiform mole.
Cervix.

THIRD TRIMESTER

Placenta previa.
Placental abruption.
Premature labor.
Choriocarcinoma.

VAGINAL DISCHARGE, PREPUBERTAL GIRLS[41]

ICD-10CM #	N89.8	Other specified noninflammatory disorders of vagina

Irritative (bubble baths, sand).
Poor perineal hygiene.
Foreign body.
Associated systemic illness (group A streptococci, chickenpox).
Infections.
Escherichia coli with foreign body.
Shigella organisms.
Yersinia organisms.
Infections (consider sexual abuse):
- *Chlamydia trachomatis.*
- *Neisseria gonorrhoeae.*
- *Trichomonas vaginalis.*

Tumor (rare).

VALVULAR HEART DISEASE[3]

ICD-10CM #	Varies with specific diagnosis

MAJOR CAUSES OF VALVULAR HEART DISEASE IN ADULTS

Aortic Stenosis

Bicuspid aortic valve.
Rheumatic fever.
Degenerative stenosis.

Aortic Regurgitation

Bicuspid aortic valve.
Aortic dissection.
Endocarditis.
Rheumatic fever.
Aortic root dilation.

Mitral Stenosis

Rheumatic fever.

Mitral Regurgitation

CHRONIC

Mitral valve prolapse.
Left ventricular dilation.
Posterior wall myocardial infarction.
Rheumatic fever.
Endocarditis.

ACUTE

Posterior wall or papillary muscle ischemia.
Papillary muscle or chordal rupture.
Endocarditis.
Prosthetic valve dysfunction.
Systolic anterior motion of mitral valve.

TRICUSPID REGURGITATION

Functional (annular) dilation.
Tricuspid valve prolapse.
Endocarditis.
Carcinoid heart disease.

VASCULAR LESIONS OF GI TRACT[26]

ICD-10CM #	Varies with specific diagnosis

Primary Vascular Lesions

Aneurysms of the aorta and its branches.
Angioectasia (angiodysplasia, vascular ectasia).
Arteriovenous malformation.
Blue rubber bleb nevus.
Capillary phlebectasia.
Dieulafoy lesion.
Glomus tumor.
Hemangioma.
Hemangiomatosis.
Hemangioendothelioma.
Hemangiopericytoma.

Hemangiosarcoma.
Hemorrhoids.
Kaposi sarcoma.

Diseases and Syndromes with Vascular Lesions

Blue rubber bleb nevus syndrome.
Ehlers-Danlos syndrome.
Hereditary hemorrhagic telangiectasia (Osler-Weber-Rendu disease).
Klippel-Trenaunay or Parkes Weber syndrome.
Kohlmeier-Degos syndrome.
Marfan syndrome.
Pseudoxanthoma elasticum.
PSS (scleroderma, CREST).
Scurvy.
Turner syndrome.
von Willebrand's disease.

Systemic Disorders Associated with Vascular Lesions

Portal hypertension:
- Congestive gastropathy and colopathy.
- GAVE (watermelon stomach).
- Spider telangiectasias.
- Varices.

Renal failure:
- GI telangiectasias.
- GAVE (watermelon stomach).

Vasculitis (e.g., polyarteritis nodosa).
Iatrogenic lesions:
- Radiation telangiectasia.

CREST, Calcinosis, Raynaud's phenomenon, esophageal dysmotility, sclerodactyly, telangiectasia; *GAVE,* gastric antral vascular ectasia

VASCULITIS, CLASSIFICATION[57]

ICD-10CM # I77.6 Arteritis, unspecified

LARGE VESSEL DISEASE

Arteritis

Giant cell arteritis.
Takayasu arteritis.
Arteritis associated with Reiter syndrome (reactive arthritis), ankylosing spondylitis.

MEDIUM AND SMALL VESSEL DISEASE

Polyarteritis Nodosa

Primary (idiopathic).
Associated with viruses (hepatitis B or C, CMV, HIV, herpes zoster).
Associated with malignancy (hairy cell leukemia).
Familial Mediterranean fever.

Granulomatous Vasculitis

Granulomatosis with polyangiitis.
Lymphomatoid granulomatosis.

Behçet's Disease

Kawasaki Disease (Mucocutaneous Lymph Node Syndrome)

PREDOMINANTLY SMALL VESSEL DISEASE

Hypersensitivity Vasculitis (Leukocytoclastic Vasculitis)

Henoch-Schönlein purpura.
Mixed cryoglobulinemia.
Serum sickness.
Vasculitis associated with connective tissue diseases (SLE, Sjögren syndrome).
Vasculitis associated with specific syndromes:
- Primary biliary cirrhosis.
- Lyme disease.
- Chronic active hepatitis.
- Drug-induced vasculitis.

Churg-Strauss Syndrome

Goodpasture Syndrome

Erythema Nodosum

Panniculitis

Buerger Disease (Thrombophlebitis Obliterans)

VASCULITIS (DISEASES THAT MIMIC VASCULITIS)[61]

ICD-10CM # Varies with specific diagnosis

EMBOLIC DISEASE

Infectious or marantic endocarditis.
Cardiac mural thrombus.
Atrial myxoma.
Cholesterol embolization syndrome.

NONINFLAMMATORY VESSEL WALL DISRUPTION

Atherosclerosis.
Arterial fibromuscular dysplasia.
Drug effects (vasoconstrictors, anticoagulants).
Radiation.
Genetic disease (neurofibromatosis, Ehlers-Danlos syndrome).
Amyloidosis.
Intravascular malignant lymphoma.

DIFFUSE COAGULATION

Disseminated intravascular coagulation.
Thrombotic thrombocytopenic purpura.
Hemolytic-uremic syndrome.
Protein C and S deficiencies, factor V/Leiden mutation.
Antiphospholipid syndrome.

VEGETATIVE STATE, PERSISTENT[3]

ICD-10CM # R40.3 Persistent vegetative state

PERSISTENT VEGETATIVE STATE: COMMON CAUSES[43]

Trauma (diffuse axonal injury).
Cardiac arrest and hypoperfusion (laminar necrosis of cortical mantle and/or thalamic necrosis).
Bihemispheric infarctions.
Purulent meningitis or encephalitis (cortical injury).
Carbon monoxide.
Prolonged hypoglycemic coma.

---

[43] A vegetative state may not necessarily begin with coma but can also develop as the end stage of neurodegenerative diseases (e.g., Alzheimer's disease) of adults or children and can accompany severe congenital developmental abnormalities of the brain such as anencephaly.

VENTILATION–PERFUSION MISMATCH ON LUNG SCAN

ICD-10CM # Varies with specific diagnosis

Pulmonary embolism.
Emphysema.
Irradiation.
Pulmonary hypertension.
AV malformations.
Pulmonary thrombosis.
External compression of pulmonary artery (neoplasm, cysts, fibrosing mediastinitis).
Vasculitis.
Tuberculosis.
Pulmonary thrombosis.
Congenital (pulmonary artery hypoplasia, congenital heart disease with upper lobe diversion).
Sequestered segment.
Parasitic lung disease.
Intraluminal obstruction from catheter fragments.

VENTRICULAR FAILURE

ICD-10CM # I51.9 Heart disease, unspecified

LEFT VENTRICULAR FAILURE

Systemic hypertension.
Valvular heart disease (AS, AR, MR).
Cardiomyopathy, myocarditis.
Bacterial endocarditis.
Myocardial infarction.
Idiopathic hypertrophic subaortic stenosis.

RIGHT VENTRICULAR FAILURE

Valvular heart disease (mitral stenosis).
Pulmonary hypertension.
Bacterial endocarditis (right-sided).
Right ventricular infarction.

BIVENTRICULAR FAILURE

Left ventricular failure.
Cardiomyopathy.
Myocarditis
Arrhythmias.
Anemia.
Thyrotoxicosis.
Arteriovenous fistula.
Paget disease.
Beriberi.

VERRUCOUS LESIONS

ICD-10CM # Varies with specific diagnosis

Warts.
Seborrheic keratosis.
Lichen simplex.
Acanthosis nigricans.
Scabies (Norwegian, crusted).
Verrucous carcinoma.
Nevus sebaceous.
Deep fungal infection.

VERTIGO

ICD-10CM #		
	R42	Dizziness and giddiness
	H81.13	Benign paroxysmal vertigo, bilateral
	H81.49	Vertigo of central origin, unspecified ear
	H81.399	Other peripheral vertigo, unspecified ear
	H81.23	Vestibular neuronitis, bilateral

PERIPHERAL

Otitis media.
Acute labyrinthitis.
Vestibular neuronitis.
Benign positional vertigo.
Ménière's disease.
Ototoxic drugs: streptomycin, gentamicin.
Lesions of the eighth nerve: acoustic neuroma, meningioma, mononeuropathy, metastatic carcinoma.
Mastoiditis.

CNS OR SYSTEMIC

Vertebrobasilar artery insufficiency.
Posterior fossa tumor or other brain tumors.
Infarction/hemorrhage of cerebral cortex, cerebellum, or brain stem.
Basilar migraine.
Metabolic: drugs, hypoxia, anemia, fever.
Hypotension/severe hypertension.
Multiple sclerosis.
CNS infections: viral, bacterial.
Temporal lobe epilepsy.
Arnold–Chiari malformation, syringobulbia.
Psychogenic: ventilation, hysteria.

VERTIGO, CENTRAL[1]

ICD-10CM #		
	R42	Vertigo NOS

MAJOR CAUSES OF CENTRAL VERTIGO

Demyelination:
- Acquired.
- Leukodystrophies.
- Multiple sclerosis.

Familial disorders:
- Friedreich ataxia.
- Spinocerebellar ataxia.
- Familial episodic ataxia (type 1 and type 2).
- Olivopontocerebellar atrophy.

CNS infections:
- Lyme neuroborreliosis.
- Meningitis.
- Tuberculosis.

Intrinsic brainstem lesion:
- Tumor.
- Arteriovenous malformation.
- Trauma.

Migraine:
- Basilar.
- Benign paroxysmal positional vertigo of childhood.

Toxins:
- Drugs, alcohol.
- Analgesics.
- Anticonvulsants.
- Antihypertensives.
- Hypnotics.
- Tranquilizers.

Metabolic and endocrine disorders:
- Hyperinsulinism.
- Impaired glucose tolerance.
- Diabetes mellitus.
- Hypertriglyceridemia.
- Hypothyroidism.

Systemic conditions:
- Paget disease.

Stroke/ischemia:
- Vertebrobasilar.
- Cerebellar.
- Posterior inferior cerebellar artery syndrome.
- Lateral medullary syndrome.
- Medial medullary infarct.
- Basilar artery syndrome.
- Anterior inferior cerebellar artery.

Other causes of posterior ischemia:
- Subclavian steal syndrome.
- Rotational vertebral artery occlusion syndrome.
- Vertebral artery dissection.
- Vertebral or basilar artery dolichoectasia.
- Neoplasm of the fourth ventricle.
- Chiari malformation.
- Superficial siderosis of the CNS.
- Vestibular epilepsy.

VESICULOBULLOUS DISEASES[32]

ICD-10CM #		
	L94.2	Calcinosis cutis
	L98.8	Other specified disorders of the skin and subcutaneous tissue

IMMUNOLOGICALLY MEDIATED DISEASES

Bullous pemphigoid.
Herpes gestationis.
Mucous membrane pemphigoid.
Epidermolysis bullosa acquisita.
Dermatitis herpetiformis.
Pemphigus (vulgaris, foliaceus, paraneoplastic).

HYPERSENSITIVITY DISEASES

Erythema multiforme minor.
Erythema multiforme major (Stevens-Johnson syndrome).
Toxic epidermal necrolysis.

METABOLIC DISEASES

Porphyria cutanea tarda.
Pseudoporphyria.
Diabetic blisters.

INHERITED GENETIC DISORDERS

Epidermolysis bullosa:
- Simplex.
- Junctional.
- Dystrophic.

INFECTIOUS DISEASES

Impetigo.
Staphylococcal scalded skin syndrome.
Herpes simplex.
Varicella.
Herpes zoster.

VISION LOSS, ACUTE, PAINFUL

ICD-10CM #		
	H53.139	Sudden visual loss, unspecified eye

Acute angle-closure glaucoma.
Corneal ulcer.
Uveitis.
Endophthalmitis.
Factitious.
Somatization syndrome.
Trauma.

VISION LOSS, ACUTE, PAINLESS

ICD-10CM #		
	H53.139	Sudden visual loss, unspecified eye

Retinal artery occlusion.
Optic neuritis.
Retinal vein occlusion.
Vitreous hemorrhage.
Retinal detachment.
Exudative macular degeneration.
CVA.
Ischemic optic neuropathy.
Factitious.
Somatization syndrome, anxiety reaction.

VISION LOSS AFTER DIVING[4]

ICD-10CM #	
	H53.139

DIFFERENTIAL DIAGNOSIS OF DECREASED VISION AFTER DIVING

Decompression sickness.
Arterial gas embolism.
Bubbles under contact lenses.
Displaced contact lens.
Antifog agent keratopathy.
Contact lens adherence syndrome.
Transdermal scopolamine
Hyperoxic myopia.
Oxymetazoline optic neuropathy.
Diving-induced migraine phenomena.
Eye disorders not related to diving.

VISION LOSS, CHILDREN

ICD-10CM #		
	H53.9	Unspecified visual disturbance

Craniopharyngioma.
Hereditary optic atrophy.
Optic nerve glioma.
Glioma of chiasm.
Albinism.
Optic nerve hypoplasia.

VISION LOSS, CHRONIC, PROGRESSIVE

ICD-10CM #	H54.7	Unspecified visual loss

Cataract.
Macular degeneration.
Cerebral neoplasm.
Refractive error.
Open-angle glaucoma.

VISION LOSS, MONOCULAR, TRANSIENT

ICD-10CM #	H54.7	Unspecified visual loss

Thromboembolism.
Vasculitis.
Migraine (vasospasm).
Anxiety reaction.
CNS tumor.
Temporal arteritis.
Multiple sclerosis.

VITREOUS HEMORRHAGE[46]

ICD-10CM #	H43.13	Vitreous hemorrhage, bilateral

CAUSES OF VITREOUS HEMORRHAGE

Acute posterior vitreous detachment associated either with a retinal tear or avulsion of a peripheral vessel.
Proliferative retinopathies:
- Diabetic.
- Following retinal vein occlusion.
- Sickle cell disease.
- Eales disease.
- Vasculitis.

Miscellaneous retinal disorders:
- Macroaneurysm.
- Telangiectasis.
- Capillary hemangioma.

Trauma:
- Blunt.
- Penetrating.
- Iatrogenic.

Systemic:
- Bleeding disorders.
- Terson syndrome.

VOCAL CORD PARALYSIS

ICD-10CM #	J38.00	Paralysis of vocal cords and larynx, unspecified
	J38.01	Paralysis of vocal cords and larynx, unilateral
	J38.02	Paralysis of vocal cords and larynx, bilateral

Neoplasm: primary or metastatic (e.g., lung, thyroid, parathyroid, mediastinum).
Neck surgery (parathyroid, thyroid, carotid endarterectomy, cervical spine).
Idiopathic.
Viral, bacterial, or fungal infection.
Trauma (intubation, penetrating neck injury).
Cardiac surgery.
RA.
Multiple sclerosis.
Parkinsonism.
Toxic neuropathy.
CVA.
CNS abnormalities: hydrocephalus, Arnold–Chiari malformation, meningomyelocele.

VOLUME DEPLETION[3]

ICD-10CM #	E86.9	Volume depletion, unspecified

GI losses:
- Upper: bleeding, nasogastric suction, vomiting.
- Lower: bleeding, diarrhea, enteric or pancreatic fistula, tube drainage.

Renal losses:
- Salt and water: diuretics, osmotic diuresis, postobstructive diuresis, acute tubular necrosis (recovery phase), salt-losing nephropathy, adrenal insufficiency, renal tubular acidosis.

Water loss: diabetes insipidus.
Skin and respiratory losses:
- Sweat, burns, insensible losses.

Sequestration without external fluid loss:
- Intestinal obstruction, peritonitis, pancreatitis, rhabdomyolysis, internal bleeding.

VOLUME EXCESS[3]

ICD-10CM #	Varies with specific diagnosis

Primary Renal Sodium Retention (Increased Effective Circulating Volume)

Renal failure, nephritic syndrome, acute glomerulonephritis.
Primary hyperaldosteronism.
Cushing's syndrome.
Liver disease.

Secondary Renal Sodium Retention (Decreased Effective Circulating Volume)

Heart failure.
Liver disease.
Nephrotic syndrome (minimal change disease).
Pregnancy.

VOMITING

ICD-10CM #	R11.10	Vomiting, unspecified
	R11.11	Vomiting without nausea
	R11.12	Projectile vomiting

GI disturbances:
- Obstruction: esophageal, pyloric, intestinal.
- Infections: viral or bacterial enteritis, viral hepatitis, food poisoning, gastroenteritis.
- Pancreatitis.
- Appendicitis.
- Biliary colic.
- Peritonitis.
- Perforated bowel.
- Diabetic gastroparesis.

Other: gastritis, PUD, IBD, GI tract neoplasms.
Drugs: morphine, digitalis, cytotoxic agents, bromocriptine.
Severe pain: MI, renal colic.
Metabolic disorders: uremia, acidosis/alkalosis, hyperglycemia, DKA, thyrotoxicosis.
Trauma: blows to the testicles, epigastrium.
Vertigo.
Reye syndrome.
Increased intracranial pressure.
CNS disturbances: trauma, hemorrhage, infarction, neoplasm, infection, hypertensive encephalopathy, migraine.
Radiation sickness.
Nausea and vomiting of pregnancy, hyperemesis gravidarum.
Motion sickness.
Bulimia, anorexia nervosa.
Psychogenic: emotional disturbances, offensive sights or smells.
Severe coughing.
Pyelonephritis.
Boerhaave syndrome.
Carbon monoxide poisoning.

VOMITING, NEONATAL[1]

ICD-10CM #	R11.10	Vomiting, unspecified

CAUSES OF NEONATAL VOMITING

Anatomic Causes

Esophagus, trachea, great vessels:
- Stricture.
- Web.
- Tracheoesophageal fistula.
- Laryngeal cleft.
- Double aortic arch.

Stomach and duodenum:
- Pyloric stenosis.
- Duodenal atresia (usually noted on the first day of life).

Small and large intestine:
- Volvulus secondary to malrotation.
- Incarcerated hernia.
- Hirschsprung disease (secondary to obstipation).
- Necrotizing enterocolitis.

Genitourinary:
- Testicular torsion.

Nonanatomic Causes

Infection:
- Septicemia.
- Meningitis.
- Urinary tract infection.
- Gastroenteritis.
- Otitis media

Increased intracranial pressure:
- Cerebral edema.
- Subdural hematoma.
- Hydrocephalus.
- Brain tumor.

Congenital adrenal hyperplasia (salt-losing variety).
Inborn errors of metabolism.
Renal disease.

VULVAR LESIONS[24]

ICD-10CM #		
	N77.0	Ulceration of vulva in diseases classified elsewhere
	N90.7	Vulvar cyst
	N90.89	Other specified noninflammatory disorders of vulva and perineum
	D07.1	Carcinoma in situ of vulva
	N90.5	Atrophy of vulva

RED LESION

Infection/Infestation

Fungal infection:
- *Candida.*
- *Tinea cruris.*
- Intertrigo.
- *Pityriasis versicolor.*

Sarcoptes scabiei.
Erythrasma: *Corynebacterium minutissimum.*
Granuloma inguinale: Calymmatobacterium granulomatis.
Folliculitis: *Staphylococcus aureus.*
Hidradenitis suppurativa.
Behçet's syndrome.

Inflammation

Reactive vulvitis.
Chemical irritation:
- Detergent.
- Dyes.
- Perfume.
- Spermicide.
- Lubricants.
- Hygiene sprays.
- *Podophyllum.*
- Topical 5-FU.
- Saliva.
- Gentian violet.
- Semen.

Mechanical trauma: scratching.
Vestibular adenitis.
Essential vulvodynia.
Psoriasis.
Seborrheic dermatitis.

Neoplasm

Vulvar intraepithelial neoplasia (VIN):
- Mild dysplasia.
- Moderate dysplasia.
- Severe dysplasia.
- Carcinoma-in-situ.

Vulvar dystrophy.
Bowen disease.
Invasive cancer:
- Squamous cell carcinoma.
- Malignant melanoma.
- Sarcoma.
- Basal cell carcinoma.
- Adenocarcinoma.
- Paget disease.
- Undifferentiated.

WHITE LESION

Vulvar dystrophy:
- Lichen sclerosus.
- Vulvar dystrophy.
- Vulvar hyperplasia.
- Mixed dystrophy.

VIN.
Vitiligo.
Partial albinism.
Intertrigo.
Radiation treatment.

DARK LESION

Lentigo.
Nevi (mole).
Neoplasm (see "Neoplasm, Vulvar," below).
Reactive hyperpigmentation.
Seborrheic keratosis.
Pubic lice.

ULCERATIVE LESION

Infection

Herpes simplex.
Vaccinia.
Treponema pallidum.
Granuloma inguinale.
Pyoderma.
Tuberculosis.

Noninfectious

Behçet's disease.
Crohn's disease.
Pemphigus.
Pemphigoid.
Hidradenitis suppurativa (see "Neoplasm, Vulvar," below).

Neoplasm

Basal cell carcinoma.
Squamous cell carcinoma.
Vulvar tumor <1 cm:
- Condyloma acuminatum.
- Molluscum contagiosum.
- Epidermal inclusion.
- Vestibular cyst.
- Mesonephric duct.
- VIN.
- Hemangioma.
- Hidradenoma.
- Neurofibroma.
- Syringoma.
- Accessory breast tissue.
- Acrochordon.
- Endometriosis.
- Fox-Fordyce disease.
- Pilonidal sinus.

Vulvar tumor >1 cm:
- Bartholin cyst or abscess.
- Lymphogranuloma venereum.
- Fibroma.
- Lipoma.
- Verrucous carcinoma.
- Squamous cell carcinoma.
- Hernia.
- Edema.
- Hematoma.
- Acrochordon.
- Epidermal cysts.
- Neurofibromatosis.
- Accessory breast tissue.

VULVAR PAIN[22]

ICD-10CM #		
	R10.2	Pelvic and perineal pain

DISEASES ASSOCIATED WITH VULVAR PAIN, NOT QUALIFYING FOR THE DIAGNOSIS OF VULVODYNIA

Podophyllin overdose.
Condylox (podofilox) overdose.
Behçet disease.
Aphthous ulcers.
Herpes (simplex and zoster).
Candidiasis.
Trichomonas.
Chancroid.
Sjögren syndrome.
Contact dermatitis.
Endometriosis.
Pemphigus.
Pemphigoid.
Atrophy.
Lichen sclerosus.
Lichen planus.
Crohn's disease.
Bartholin abscess.
Trauma.
Imperforate hymen.
Prolapsed urethra.
Vulvar intraepithelial neoplasia.
Carcinoma.

VULVITIS, GRANULOMATOUS

ICD-10CM #		
	N76.2	Acute vulvitis
	N76.3	Subacute and chronic vulvitis

Differential diagnosis of granulomatous vulvitis.
Syphilis.
Lymphogranuloma venereum.
Mycobacteria.
Fungus.
Bacillary angiomatosis.
Folliculitis.
Ruptured pilosebaceous unit.
Ruptured cyst.
Crohn's disease.
Vulvitis granulomatosa.
Hydradenitis suppurativa.

WEAKNESS, ACUTE, EMERGENT[57]

ICD-10CM #		
	M62.81	Muscle weakness (generalized)

Demyelinating disorders (Guillain-Barré, chronic inflammatory demyelinating polyneuropathy [CIDP]).
Myasthenia gravis.
Infectious (poliomyelitis, diphtheria).
Toxic (botulism, tick paralysis, paralytic shellfish toxin, puffer fish, newts).

Metabolic (acquired or familial hypokalemia, hypophosphatemia, hypermagnesemia).
Metal poisoning (arsenic, thallium).
Porphyria.

WEAKNESS, GRADUAL ONSET

ICD-10CM #	M62.81	Muscle weakness (generalized)

Depression.
Malingering.
Anemia.
Hypothyroidism.
Medications (e.g., sedatives, antidepressants, narcotics).
CHF.
Renal failure.
Liver failure.
Respiratory insufficiency.
Alcoholism.
Nutritional deficiencies.
Disorders of motor unit.
Basal ganglia disorders.
Upper motor neuron lesions.

WEAKNESS, NONNEUROMUSCULAR CAUSES

ICD-10CM #	G93.3	Postviral fatigue syndrome
	R53.1	Weakness
	R53.81	Other malaise
	R53.83	Other fatigue

Anxiety disorder.
Infectious process.
Anemia.
Renal insufficiency.
Hyperventilation.
Malignancy.
Hypothyroidism.
Hypotension.
Hypercapnia.
Hypoglycemia.
Cardiac arrhythmias.
Hepatic insufficiency.
Electrolyte imbalance.
Malnutrition.
Cerebrovascular insufficiency.

WEIGHT GAIN

ICD-10CM #	R63.5	Abnormal weight gain
	E66.9	Obesity, unspecified

Sedentary lifestyle.
Fluid overload.
Discontinuation of tobacco abuse.
Endocrine disorders (hypothyroidism, hyperinsulinism associated with maturity-onset DM, Cushing's syndrome, hypogonadism, insulinoma, hyperprolactinemia, acromegaly).
Medications (nutritional supplements, oral contraceptives, glucocorticoids, etc.).
Anxiety disorders with compulsive eating.
Laurence-Moon-Biedl syndrome, Prader-Willi syndrome, other congenital diseases.
Hypothalamic injury (rare; <100 cases reported in medical literature).

WEIGHT LOSS

ICD-10CM #	R63.4	Abnormal weight loss

Malignancy.
Psychiatric disorders (depression, anorexia nervosa).
New-onset DM.
Malabsorption.
COPD.
AIDS.
Uremia, liver disease.
Thyrotoxicosis, pheochromocytoma, carcinoid syndrome.
Addison disease.
Intestinal parasites.
Peptic ulcer disease.
Inflammatory bowel disease.
Food faddism.
Postgastrectomy syndrome.

WHEEZING

ICD-10CM #	R06.2	Wheezing

Asthma.
COPD.
Interstitial lung disease.
Infections (pneumonia, bronchitis, bronchiolitis, epiglottitis).
Cardiac asthma.
GERD with aspiration.
Foreign body aspiration.
Pulmonary embolism.
Anaphylaxis.
Obstruction of airway (neoplasm, goiter, edema or hemorrhage from trauma, aneurysm, congenital abnormalities, strictures, spasm).
Carcinoid syndrome.

WHEEZING, PEDIATRIC AGE[9]

ICD-10CM #	R06.2	Wheezing

Reactive airways disease.
Atopic asthma.
Infection-associated airway reactivity.
Exercise-induced asthma.
Salicylate-induced asthma and nasal polyposis.
Asthmatic bronchitis.
Other hypersensitivity reactions:
- Hypersensitivity pneumonitis.
- Tropical eosinophilia.
- Visceral larva migrans.
- Allergic bronchopulmonary aspergillosis.

Aspiration:
- Foreign body.
- Food, saliva, gastric contents.
- Laryngotracheoesophageal cleft.
- Tracheoesophageal fistula, H-type.
- Pharyngeal incoordination or neuromuscular weakness.

Cystic fibrosis.
Primary ciliary dyskinesia.
Cardiac failure.
Bronchiolitis obliterans.
Extrinsic compression of airways:
- Vascular ring.
- Enlarged lymph node.
- Mediastinal tumor.
- Lung cysts.

Tracheobronchomalacia.
Endobronchial masses.
Gastroesophageal reflux.
Pulmonary hemosiderosis.
Sequelae of bronchopulmonary dysplasia.
"Hysterical" glottic closure.
Cigarette smoke, other environmental insults.

WRIST AND HAND PAIN, IN DIFFERENT AGE GROUPS[18]

ICD-10CM #	S69.80XA	Other specified injuries of unspecified wrist, hand and finger(s), initial encounter
	S69.90XA	Unspecified injury of unspecified wrist, hand and finger(s), initial encounter

Differential Diagnosis II

COMMON CAUSES OF WRIST AND HAND PAIN IN DIFFERENT AGE GROUPS

Childhood (2-10 yr)
Intraarticular
Infection.
Periarticular
Fracture.
Osteomyelitis.
Adolescence (10-18 yr)
Intraarticular
Infection.
Periarticular
Trauma.
Osteomyelitis.
Tumors.
Ganglion.
Idiopathic wrist pain.
Early Adulthood (18-30 yr)
Intraarticular
Inflammatory arthritis.
Infection.
Osteoarthritis.
Periarticular
Peripheral nerve entrapment.
Tendonitis.
Referred
Cervical.
Adulthood (30-50 yr)
Intraarticular
Inflammatory arthritis.
Infection.
Osteoarthritis.
Periarticular
Peripheral nerve entrapment.
Tendonitis.
Referred
Cervical.
Chest.
Cardiac.
Old age (>50 yr)
Intraarticular
Inflammatory arthritis.

Osteoarthritis.
Periarticular
Peripheral nerve entrapment.
Tendonitis.
Referred
Cervical.
Chest.
Cardiac.

WRIST PAIN

ICD-10CM #		
	S69.80XA	Other specified injuries of unspecified wrist, hand, and finger(s), initial encounter
	S69.90XA	Unspecified injury of unspecified wrist, hand, and finger(s), initial encounter

MECHANICAL

Osteoarthritis.
Ligament tear.
Fracture.
Ganglion.
De Quervain tenosynovitis.
Avascular necrosis (scaphoid, lunate).
Nonunion of scaphoid or lunate.
Neoplasm.

METABOLIC

Pregnancy.
Diabetes.
Gout.
Pseudogout.
Paget disease.
Acromegaly.
Hypothyroidism.
Hyperparathyroidism.

INFECTIOUS

Osteomyelitis.
Septic arthritis.
Cat-scratch disease.
Tick bite (Lyme disease, babesiosis).
Tuberculosis.

NEUROLOGIC

Peripheral neuropathy.
Nerve injury (median, ulnar, radial nerve).
Thoracic outlet compression syndrome.
Distal posterior interosseous nerve syndrome.

RHEUMATOLOGIC

Psoriasis.
RA.
SLE, mixed connective tissue disorder (MCTD).
Scleroderma.

MISCELLANEOUS

Granulomatous (sarcoidosis).
Amyloidosis.
Multiple myeloma.
Leukemia.

XEROPHTHALMIA[61]

ICD-10CM #		
	H11.149	Conjunctival xerosis, unspecified, unspecified eye

MEDICATIONS

Tricyclic antidepressants: amitriptyline, doxepin.
Antihistamines: diphenhydramine, chlorpheniramine, promethazine, and many cold and decongestant preparations.
Anticholinergic agents: antiemetics such as scopolamine, antispasmodic agents such as oxybutynin chloride.

ABNORMALITIES OF EYELID FUNCTION

Neuromuscular disorders.
Aging.
Thyrotoxicosis.

ABNORMALITIES OF TEAR PRODUCTION

Hypovitaminosis A.
Stevens-Johnson syndrome.
Familial diseases affecting sebaceous secretions.

ABNORMALITIES OF CORNEAL SURFACES

Scarring from past injuries and herpes simplex infection.

XEROSTOMIA[61]

ICD-10CM #		
	K11.7	Disturbances of salivary secretion
	R68.2	Dry mouth, unspecified

MEDICATIONS

Tricyclic antidepressants: amitriptyline, doxepin.
Antihistamines: diphenhydramine, chlorpheniramine, promethazine, and many cold and decongestant preparations.
Anticholinergic agents: antiemetics such as scopolamine, antispasmodic agents such as oxybutynin chloride.

DEHYDRATION

Debility.
Fever.

POLYURIA

Alcohol intake.
Arrhythmia.
Diabetes.

PREVIOUS HEAD AND NECK IRRADIATION SYSTEMIC DISEASES

Sjögren syndrome.
Sarcoidosis.
Amyloidosis.
HIV infection.
Graft-versus-host disease.

YELLOW URINE

ICD-10CM #		
	R82	Other abnormal findings in urine

Normal coloration.
Concentrated urine.
Use of multivitamin supplements.
Diet rich in carrots.
Use of Cascara.
Urinary tract infection

REFERENCES

1. Adams JG, et al.: *Emergency medicine, clinical essentials*, ed 2, Philadelphia, Elsevier.
2. Adkinson NF, et al.: *Middleton's allergy principles and practice*, ed 8, Philadelphia, 2014, Saunders.
3. Andreoli TE: *Cecil essentials of medicine*, ed 5, Philadelphia, Saunders.
4. Auerbach P: *Wilderness medicine*, Philadelphia, Saunders.
5. Bain BJ, Bates I, Laffan MA: *Dacie and Lewis practical haematology*, ed 12, Philadelphia, 2017, Elsevier.
6. Ballinger A: *Kumar & Clark's essentials of clinical medicine*, ed 6, Edinburgh, Saunders.
7. Barkin RM, Rosen P: *Emergency pediatrics: a guide to ambulatory care*, ed 5, St Louis, Mosby.
8. Baude AI: *Infectious diseases and medical microbiology*, ed 2, Philadelphia, Saunders.
9. Behrman RE: *Nelson textbook of pediatrics*, ed 16, Philadelphia, Saunders.
10. Bennett JE, Dolin R, Blaser MJ: *Mandell, Douglas, and Bennett's principles and practice of infectious diseases*, ed 8, Philadelphia, 2015, Saunders.
11. Bonow RO et al: *Braunwauld's heart disease*, ed 9, Philadelphia, Elsevier.
12. Bowling B: *Kanski's clinical ophthalmology*, ed 8, Philadelphia, 2016, Elsevier.
13. Boyer KM: Nonbacterial pneumonia. In Feigin RD, Cherry JD, editors: *Textbook of pediatric infectious diseases*, ed 4, Philadelphia, 1998, WB Saunders, pp 260–273.
14. Callen JP: *Color atlas of dermatology*, ed 2, Philadelphia, WB Saunders.
15. Cameron JL, Cameron AM: *Current surgical therapy*, ed 10, Philadelphia, Saunders.
16. Canoso J: *Rheumatology in primary care*, Philadelphia, Saunders.
17. Carlson KJ: *Primary care of women*, ed 2, St Louis, Mosby.
18. Carr A, Hamilton W: *Orthopedics in primary care*, ed 2, Philadelphia, Saunders.
19. Cherry JD: *Feigin and Cherry's pediatric infectious diseases*, ed 8, Philadelphia, 2019, Elsevier.
20. Conn R: *Current diagnosis*, ed 9, Philadelphia, Saunders.
21. Copeland LJ: *Textbook of gynecology*, ed 2, Philadelphia, Saunders.
22. Crum CP: *Diagnostic gynecologic and obstetric pathology*, ed 3, Philadelphia, 2018, Elsevier.
23. Custer JW, Rau RE: *The Harriet Lane handbook*, ed 18, St Louis, Mosby.
24. Danakas G: *Practical guide to the care of the gynecologic/obstetric patient*, St Louis, Mosby.
25. Eberlein M: A fall in Ghana, *Am J Med* 122:1091, 2009.

26. Feldman M, Friedman LS, Brandt LJ: *Sleisenger and Fordtran's gastrointestinal and liver disease*, ed 10, Philadelphia, 2016, Elsevier.
27. Firestein GS, Budd RC, Gabriel SE, et al.: *Kelly's textbook of rheumatology*, ed 9, Philadelphia, Saunders.
28. Floege J, et al.: *Comprehensive clinical nephrology*, ed 4, Philadelphia, Saunders.
29. Fuhrman BP, et al.: *Pediatric critical care*, ed 4, Philadelphia, Saunders.
30. Gabbe SG: *Obstetrics*, ed 6, Philadelphia, Saunders.
31. Goldberg RJ: *The care of the psychiatric patient*, ed 3, St Louis, Mosby.
32. Goldman L, Ausiello D: *Cecil textbook of medicine*, ed 21, Philadelphia, Saunders.
33. Goldman L, Braunwald E: *Braunwauld Primary cardiology*, Philadelphia, Saunders.
34. Goldman L, Schafer AI: *Goldman's Cecil medicine*, ed 24, Philadelphia, Saunders.
35. Gorbach SL: *Infectious diseases*, ed 2, Philadelphia, Saunders.
36. Grainger RG, Allison D: *Grainger & Allison's diagnostic radiology, a textbook of medical imaging*, ed 4, London, Churchill Livingstone.
37. Habif TP: *Clinical dermatology*, ed 6, Philadelphia, 2016, Elsevier.
38. Harrington J: *Consultation in internal medicine*, ed 2, St Louis, Mosby.
39. Henry JB: *Clinical diagnosis and management by laboratory methods*, ed 20, Philadelphia, Saunders.
40. Hochberg MC, et al.: *Rheumatology*, ed 5, Mosby: St. Louis.
41. Hoekelman R: *Primary pediatric care*, ed 3, St Louis, Mosby.
42. Hoffman R: *Hematology, basic principles and practice*, ed 6, Philadelphia, Saunders.
43. Hoffmann R, et al.: *Hematology: basic principles and practice*, ed 5, Philadelphia, Churchill Livingstone.
44. Hoffman R: *Hematology, basic principles and practice*, ed 7, Philadelphia, 2018, Elsevier.
45. James WD: *Andrews' diseases of the skin*, ed 12, Philadelphia, 2016, Saunders.
46. Kanski JJ, Bowling B: *Clinical ophthalmology, a systematic approach*, ed 7, Philadelphia, Saunders.
47. Kassirer J: *Current therapy in adult medicine*, ed 4, St Louis, Mosby.
48. Kassirer J: *Practical rheumatology*, London, Mosby.
49. Kaufman DM, Geyer HL, Milstein MJ: *Kaufman's clinical neurology for psychiatrists*, ed 8, Philadelphia, 2017, Elsevier.
50. Khan MG: *Rapid ECG interpretation, Philadelphia, Saunders.*
51. Kliegman RM, et al.: *Nelson textbook of pediatrics*, ed 19, Philadelphia, Saunders.
52. Kliegman RM: *Practical strategies in pediatric diagnosis and therapy*, Philadelphia, Saunders.
53. Lipshultz LI, Khera M, Atwal DT: *Urology and the primary care practitioner*, ed 3, Philadelphia, Elsevier.
54. Mahanty S, Nutman TB: Eosinophilia and eosinophil-related disorders. In Middleton EJ, Reed CE, Ellis EF et al editors: *Allergy: principles and practice*, ed 4, Mosby-Year Book: St Louis, p. 1077.
55. Mandell GL: *Mandell, Douglas, and Bennett's principles and practice of infectious diseases*, ed 6, New York, Churchill Livingstone.
56. Mann DL, Zipes DP, Libby P, Bonow RO: *Braunwald's heart disease*, ed 10, Philadelphia, 2015, Elsevier.
57. Marx JA: *Rosen's emergency medicine*, ed 8, Philadelphia, 2014, Saunders.
58. Mason RJ: *Murray & Nadel's textbook of respiratory medicine*, ed 5, Philadelphia, Saunders.
59. Melmed S, Polonsky KS, Larsen PR, Kronenberg HM: *Williams textbook of endocrinology*, ed 12, Philadelphia, Saunders.
60. Moore WT, Eastman RC: *Diagnostic endocrinology*, ed 2, St Louis, Mosby.
61. Noble J: *Primary care medicine*, ed 3, St Louis, Mosby.
62. Nseyo UO: *Urology for primary care physicians*, Philadelphia, Saunders.
63. Palay D: *Ophthalmology for the primary care physician*, St Louis, Mosby.
64. Park MK: *Park's Pediatric cardiology for practitioners*, ed 6, Philadelphia, 2014, Saunders.
65. Parrillo JE, Dellinger RP: *Critical care medicine, principles of diagnosis and management in the adult*, ed 4, Philadelphia, 2014, Elsevier.
66. Pope TL, Bloem HL, Beltran J, Morrison WB, Wilson DJ: *Musculoskeletal imaging*, ed 2, Philadelphia, 2014, Saunders.
67. Rakel RE: *Principles of family practice*, ed 6, Philadelphia, Saunders.
68. Ronco C: *Critical care nephrology*, ed 3, Philadelphia, 2019, Elsevier.
69. Rumack CM: *Diagnostic ultrasound*, ed 4, Philadelphia, 2011, Elsevier.
70. Schwarz MI: *Interstitial lung disease*, ed 2, St Louis, Mosby.
71. Seller RH: *Differential diagnosis of common complaints*, ed 4, Philadelphia, Saunders.
72. Sellke FW, del Nido PJ, Swanson SJ: *Sabiston & Spencer surgery of the chest*, ed 9, Philadelphia, 2016, Elsevier.
73. Siedel HM: *Mosby's guide to physical examination*, ed 4, St Louis, Mosby.
74. Skorecki K: *Brenner & Rector's the kidney*, ed 10, Philadelphia, 2016, Elsevier.
75. Souhami RL, Moxham J: *Textbook of medicine*, ed 4, London, Churchill Livingstone.
76. Specht N: *Practical guide to diagnostic imaging*, St Louis, Mosby.
77. Stein JH: *Internal medicine*, ed 5, St Louis, Mosby.
78. Stern TA: *Massachusetts General Hospital handbook of general hospital psychiatry*, ed 7, Philadelphia, 2018, Elsevier.
79. Swaiman KF: *Swaiman's pediatric neurology, principles and practice*, ed 6, Philadelphia, 2017, Elsevier.
80. Swain R, Snodgrass JG: Managing groin pain, *Phys Sportmed* 23(56), 1995.
81. Talley NJ, Martin CJ: *Clinical gastroenterology*, ed 2, Sydney, Churchill Livingstone.
82. Tschudy MM, Arcara KM: *The Harriet Lane handbook*, ed 19, Philadelphia, Mosby.
83. Vincent JL, et al.: *Textbook of critical care*, ed 6, Philadelphia, Saunders.
84. Webb WR, Brant WE, Major NM: *Fundamentals of body CT*, ed 4, Philadelphia, 2015, Saunders.
85. Wein AJ: *Campbell-Walsh urology*, ed 11, Philadelphia, 2016, Elsevier.
86. Weinberg SE, et al.: *Principles of pulmonary medicine*, ed 5, Philadelphia, Saunders.
87. Wiederholt WC: *Neurology for non-neurologists*, ed 4, Philadelphia, Saunders.
88. Wilson JD: *Williams textbook of endocrinology*, ed 9, Philadelphia, Saunders.

Clinical Algorithms

PLEASE NOTE: These algorithms are designed to assist clinicians in the evaluation and treatment of patients. They may not apply to all patients with a particular disorder and are not intended to replace the clinician's individual judgment.

Additional algorithms content available at ExpertConsult.com

Alveolar Hemorrhage (Figs. E19 and E20, Box E2)
Ambiguous Genitalia (Figs. E21, E22, Box E3)
Azoospermia (Figs. E29, E30)
Convulsive Disorder, Suspected, Pediatric Patient (Fig. E47)
Diarrhea, Watery (Fig. E53)
Dilated Pupil (Fig. E54)
Dyspepsia (Fig. E55)
Esophageal Foreign Body (Figs. E60 and E61, Tables E18 and E19)
Fever and Infection in High-Risk Hematology Patient without Obvious Source (Fig. E66)
Fever and Neutropenia, Pediatric Patient (Fig. E68)
Pruritus, Pregnant Patient (Fig. E115)
Pseudohermaphroditism (Fig. E116)
Purpura (Fig. E120)
Red Eye (Fig. E124-E128)
Renal Trauma (Fig. E132, Table E49)
Short Stature (Fig. E141)
Shoulder Pain (Fig. E142)
Skin Blisters (Fig. E145, Table E53)
Tachycardia, Diagnostic Approach (Table E57)
Tachycardia, Pediatric Patient (Fig. E157)
Thrombotic Microangiopathies, Differential Diagnosis (Fig. E161)
Traumatic Aortic Injury (Fig. E164, Box E14)

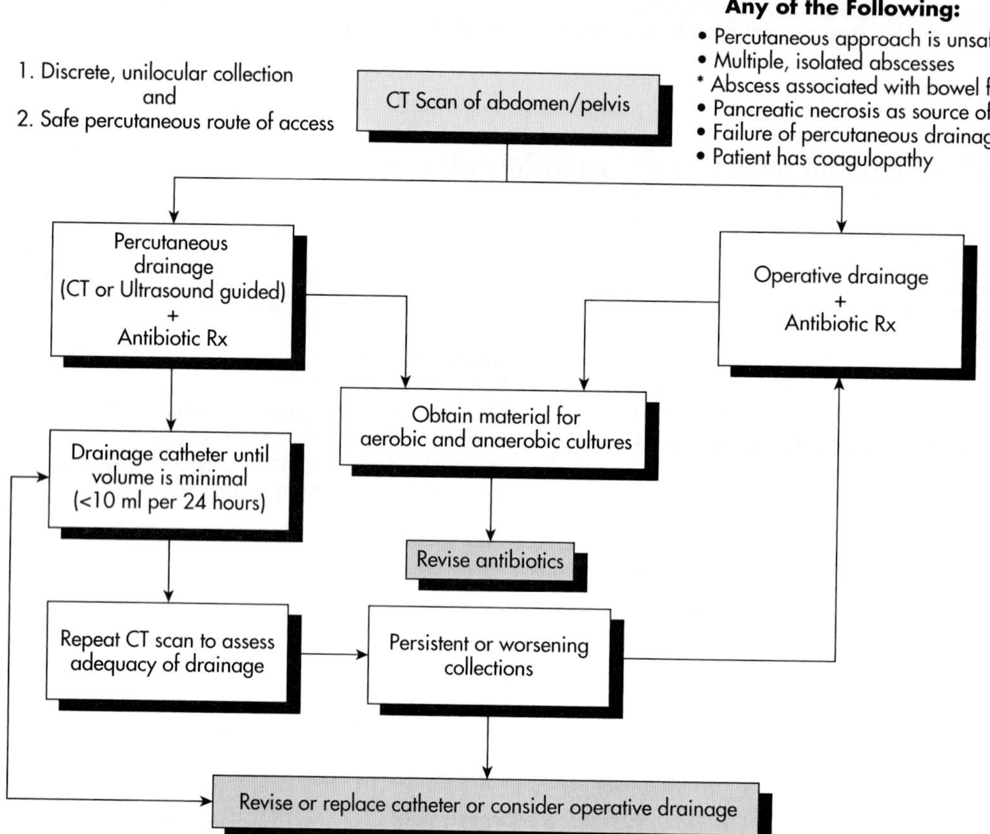
Any of the Following:
• Percutaneous approach is unsafe
• Multiple, isolated abscesses
* Abscess associated with bowel fistula
• Pancreatic necrosis as source of abscess
• Failure of percutaneous drainage
• Patient has coagulopathy
1. Discrete, unilocular collection
and
2. Safe percutaneous route of access
CT Scan of abdomen/pelvis
Percutaneous drainage (CT or Ultrasound guided) + Antibiotic Rx
Operative drainage + Antibiotic Rx
Obtain material for aerobic and anaerobic cultures
Drainage catheter until volume is minimal (<10 ml per 24 hours)
Revise antibiotics
Repeat CT scan to assess adequacy of drainage
Persistent or worsening collections
Revise or replace catheter or consider operative drainage

FIG. 1 Approach to management of intraabdominal abscesses including indications for consideration of percutaneous versus operative drainage. *CT,* computed tomography. (From Parrillo JE, Dellinger RP: *Critical care medicine, principles of diagnosis and management in the adult,* ed 4, 2014, Elsevier.)

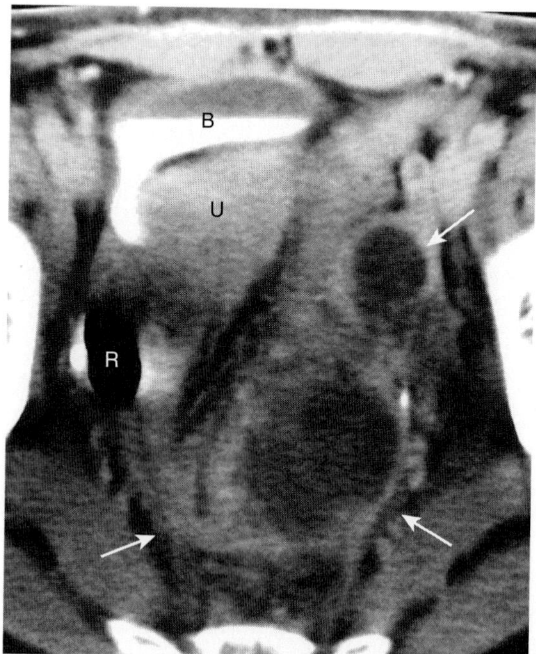
B
U
R

FIG. 2 Tuboovarian abscess. A poorly marginated cystic and solid inflammatory mass (between *arrows*) displaces the rectum (*R*), uterus (*U*), and bladder (*B*) anteriorly and rightward. The left ovary and dilated left fallopian tube are incorporated within the mass but are not definitively identified. The patient was suffering from sepsis and had acute pelvic pain. (From Webb WR, Brandt WE, Major NM: *Fundamentals of body CT,* ed 4, Philadelphia, 2015, Elsevier.)

TABLE 1 Comparison of Common Causes of Acute Abdominal Pain

Cause	Onset	Location	Character	Descriptor	Radiation	Intensity
Appendicitis	Gradual	Periumbilical area early; RLQ late	Diffuse early; localized later	Aching	None	++
Cholecystitis	Acute	RUQ	Localized	Constricting	Scapula	++
Pancreatitis	Acute	Epigastrium, back	Localized	Boring	Midback	++ to +++
Diverticulitis	Gradual	LLQ	Localized	Aching	None	++ to +++
Perforated peptic ulcer	Sudden	Epigastrium	Localized early, diffuse later	Burning	None	+++
Small bowel obstruction	Gradual	Periumbilical area	Diffuse	Cramping	None	++
Mesenteric ischemia, infarction	Sudden	Periumbilical area	Diffuse	Agonizing	None	+++
Ruptured abdominal aortic aneurysm	Sudden	Abdomen, back, flank	Diffuse	Tearing	None	+++
Gastroenteritis	Gradual	Periumbilical area	Diffuse	Spasmodic	None	+ to ++
Pelvic inflammatory disease	Gradual	Either LQ, pelvis	Localized	Aching	Upper thigh	++
Ruptured ectopic pregnancy	Sudden	Either LQ, pelvis	Localized	Sharp	None	++

+, mild; ++, moderate; +++, severe; *LLQ*, left lower quadrant; *LQ*, lower quadrant; *RLQ*, right lower quadrant; *RUQ*, right upper quadrant.
From Feldman M, Friedman LS, Brandt LJ: *Sleisenger and Fortran's gastrointestinal and liver disease*, ed 10, 2016, Elsevier.

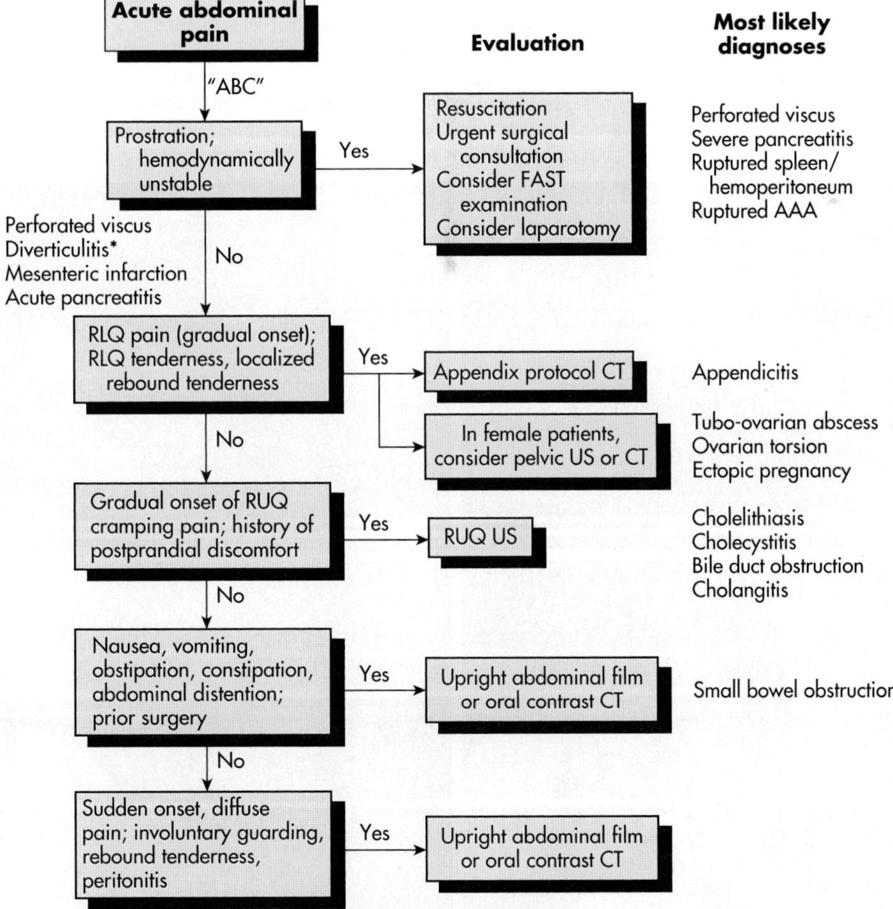

FIG. 3 An approach to the urgent evaluation of abdominal pain. Specific complaints and physical examination findings are coupled with appropriate radiologic imaging. *For left lower quadrant pain, the most likely diagnosis is diverticulitis. *AAA*, abdominal aortic aneurysm; *ABC*, airway, breathing, circulation; *CT*, computed tomography; *FAST*, focused abdominal sonogram for trauma; *RLQ*, right lower quadrant; *RUQ*, right upper quadrant. (From Feldman M, Friedman LS, Brandt LJ: *Sleisenger and Fortran's gastrointestinal and liver disease*, ed 10, 2016, Elsevier.)

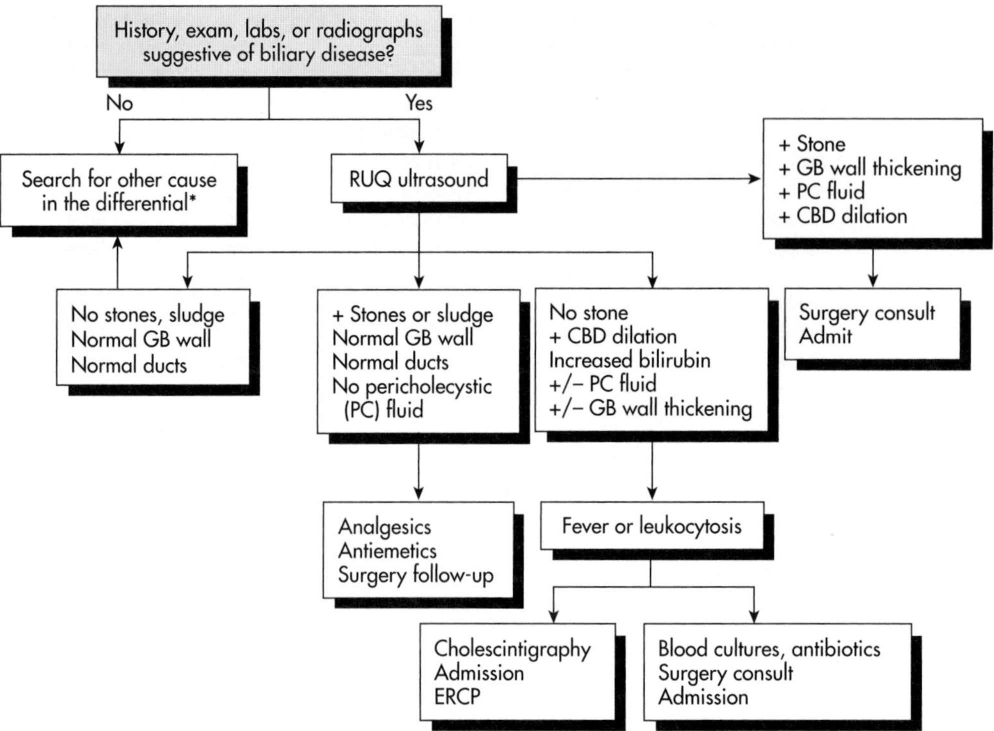

FIG. 4 Treatment algorithm for right upper quadrant (RUQ) pain. *Refer to Section II, Differential Diagnosis, Abdominal Pain Right Upper Quadrant. *CBD*, Common bile duct; *ERCP*, endoscopic retrograde cholangiopancreatography; *GB*, gallbladder; *RUQ*, right upper quadrant; +, with; −, without; ±, with or without. (From Adams JG et al: *Emergency medicine, clinical essentials*, ed 2, Philadelphia, 2013, Elsevier.)

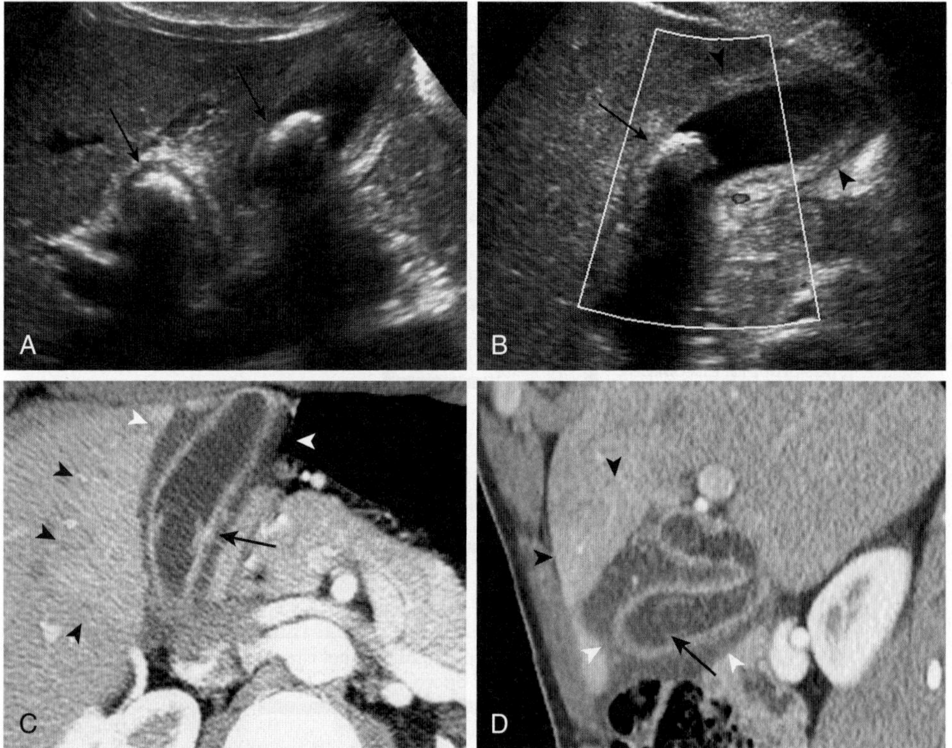

FIG. 5 A 43-year-old man with acute cholecystitis. Ultrasound images **(A** and **B)** demonstrate echogenic, shadowing gallstones *(arrows)* with gallbladder wall thickening *(arrowheads)* in a patient in whom a sonographic Murphy's sign was elicited. Axial **(C)** and sagittal **(D)** portal venous phase computed tomography images reveal a gallstone *(arrows)*, as well as a thickened gallbladder wall *(white arrowheads)*. Although not acquired in the arterial phase of contrast, hepatic hyperenhancement consistent with secondary inflammation is nevertheless seen *(black arrowheads)*. These findings are specific for this life-threatening complication and should be recognized and treated urgently. (From Soto JA, Lucey BC: *Emergency radiology, the requisites*, ed 2, 2017, Elsevier.)

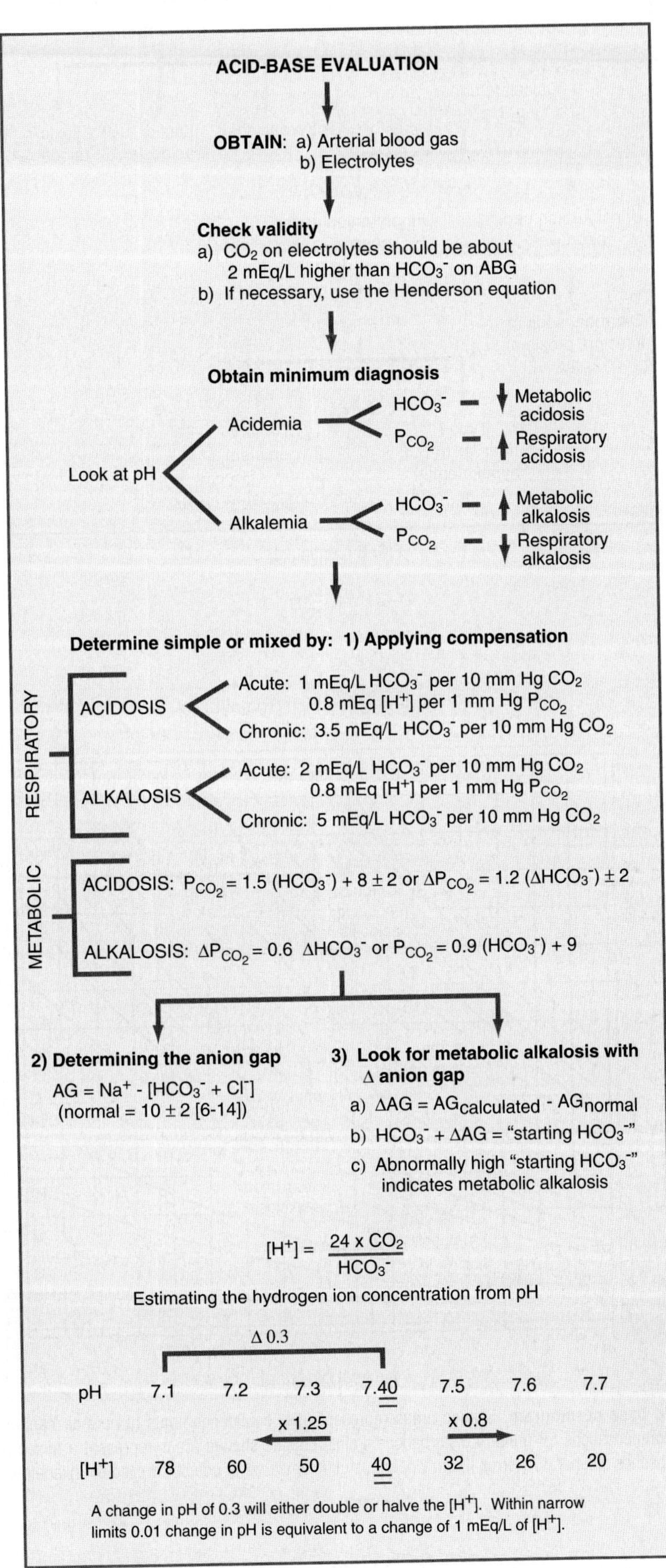

FIG. 6 Scheme for assessing acid-base homeostasis. (Modified from Andreoli TE [ed]: *Cecil essentials of medicine*, ed 7, Philadelphia, 2008, Saunders.)

Continued on next page

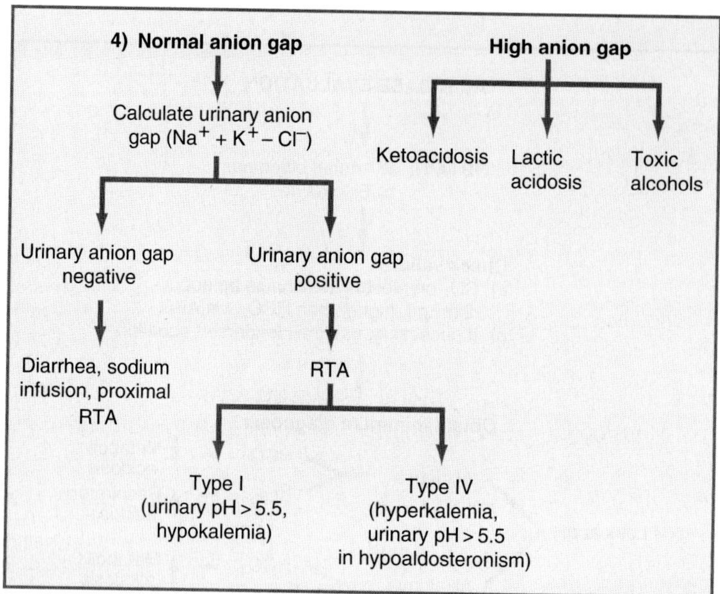

FIG. 6 (Continued)

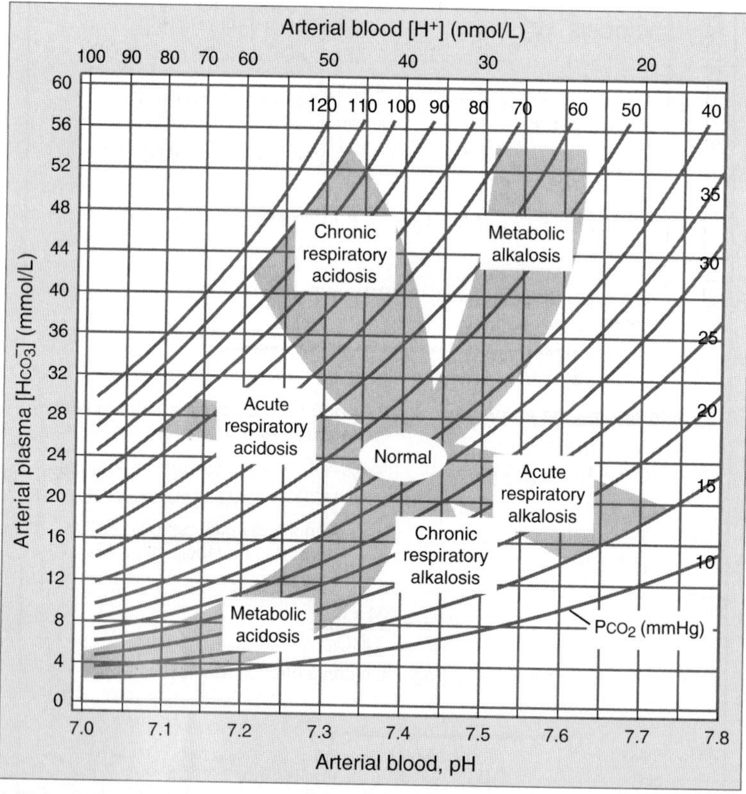

FIG. 7 Acid base normogram. Shaded areas represent 95% confidence limits of normal respiratory and metabolic compensations for primary disturbances. Points outside shaded areas represent a mixed disorder, assuming absence of laboratory error. (From Vincent JL et al: *Textbook of critical care*, ed 6, Philadelphia, 2011, Saunders.)

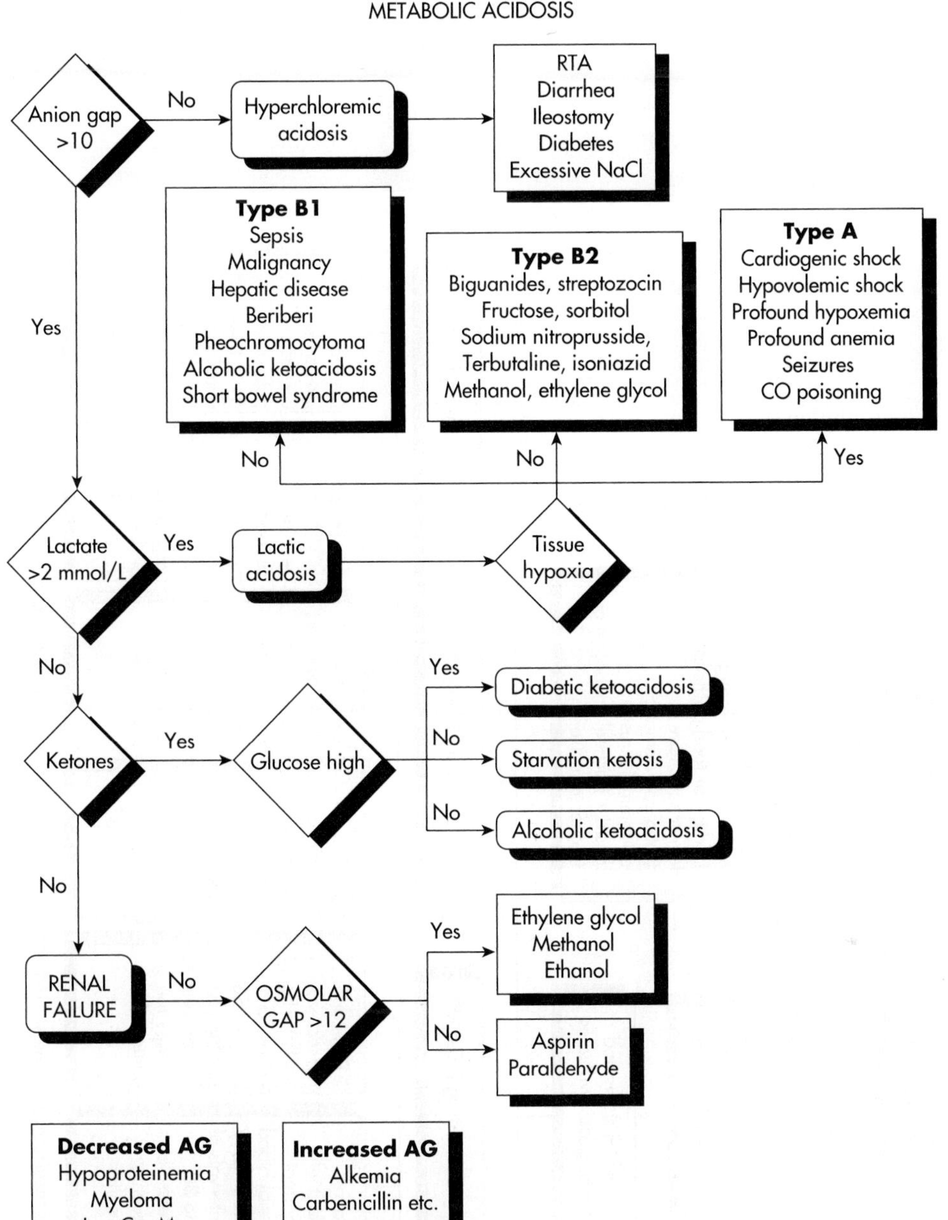

FIG. 8 Diagnostic approach to metabolic acidosis. *CO,* carbon monoxide; *RTA,* renal tubular acidosis. (From Vincent JL et al: *Textbook of critical care,* ed 7, Philadelphia, 2017, Elsevier.)

ICD-10CM # E87.2 Acidosis

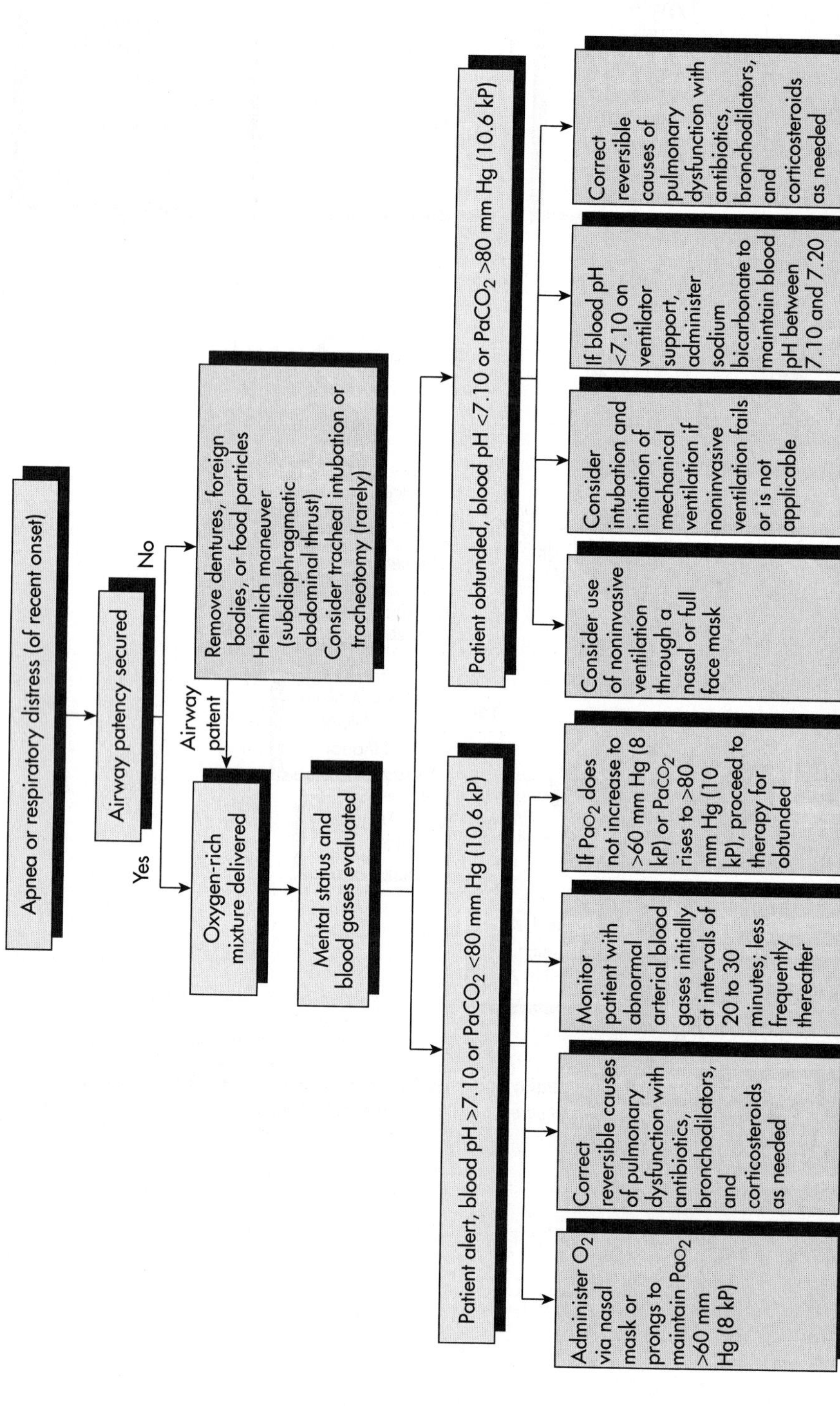

FIG. 9 Algorithm for management of acute respiratory acidosis. (From Johnson R et al: *Comprehensive clinical nephrology,* ed 5, Philadelphia, 2015, Saunders.)

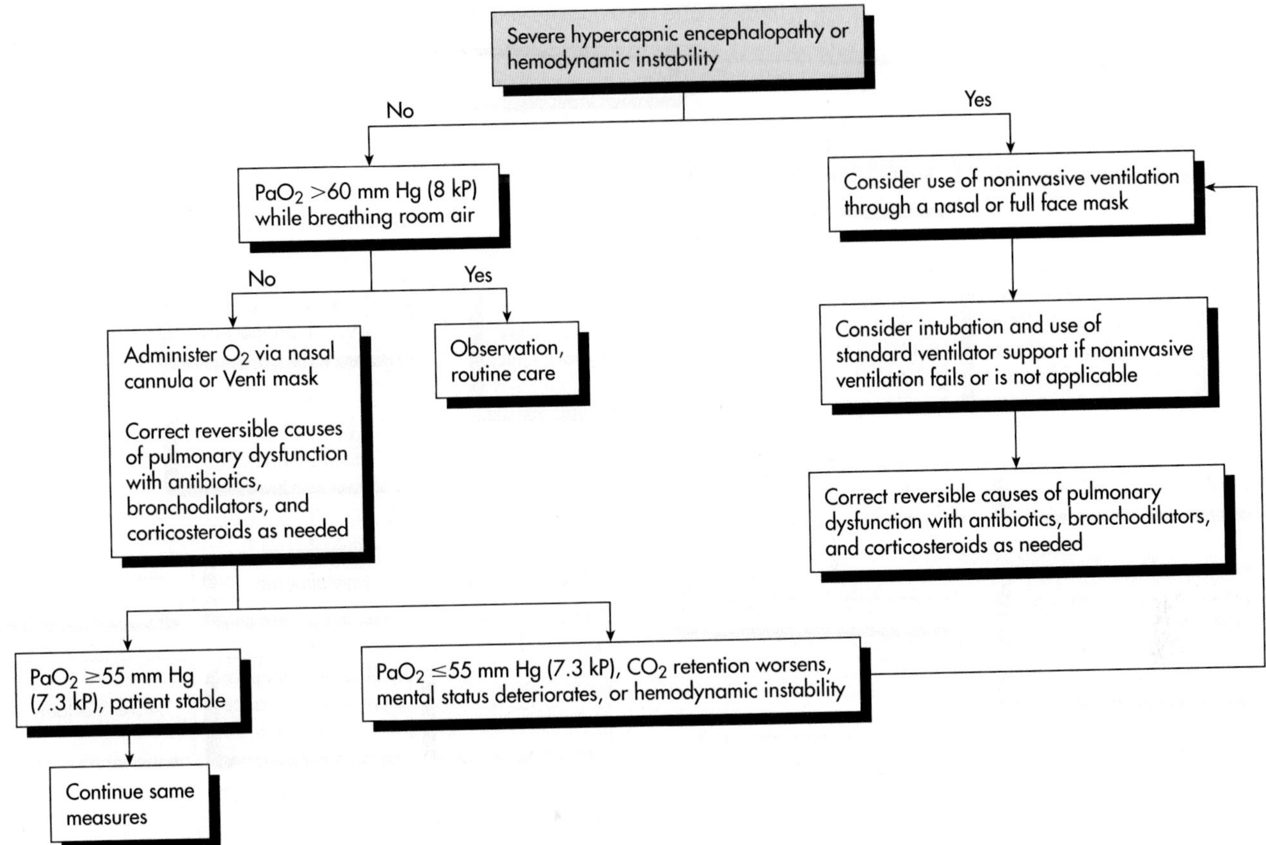

FIG. 10 Algorithm for management of chronic respiratory acidosis. *PaO_2*, partial pressure of oxygen. (From Johnson R et al: *Comprehensive clinical nephrology*, ed 5, Philadelphia, 2015, Saunders.)

TABLE 2 Causes of Chronic Alveolar Hypoventilation/Respiratory Acidosis

	Site of Defect	Condition
Defects in respiratory drive	Central and peripheral chemoreceptors	Brainstem lesions Primary alveolar hypoventilation syndrome (Ondine's curse), extreme obesity (Pickwickian syndrome)
Neuromuscular defects	Neuromuscular	Spinal cord lesions *Motor neuron disease:* critical illness polyneuropathy, multiple sclerosis, amyotrophic lateral sclerosis
	Muscular disease	Myasthenia gravis, critical illness myopathy
Defects in respiratory mechanics and gas exchange	Lung	*Increased dead space:* chronic obstructive pulmonary disease, chronic pulmonary embolism *Increased lung elastance*: pulmonary fibrosis *Increased chest wall elastance:* extreme obesity, fibrothorax, kyphoscoliosis *Increased respiratory resistance*: airway stenosis, chronic obstructive pulmonary disease

From Ronco C: *Critical care nephrology*, ed 3, Philadelphia, 2019, Elsevier.

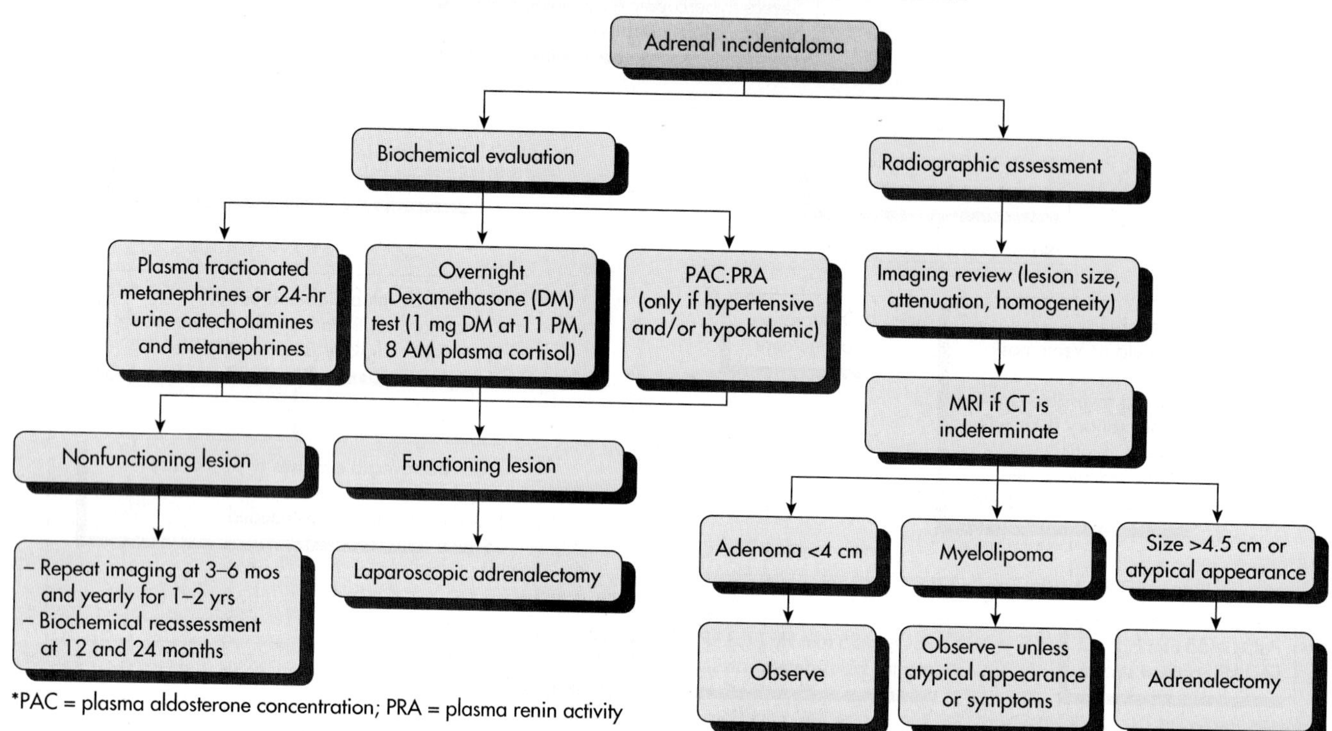

FIG. 11 Diagnostic and management algorithm for adrenal incidentaloma. *CT,* computed tomography. (From Cameron JL, Cameron AM: *Surgical therapy,* ed 12, Philadelphia, 2017, Elsevier.)

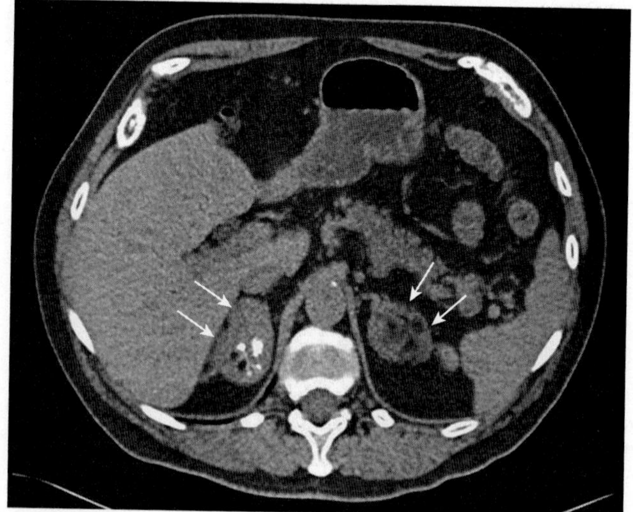

FIG. 12 Computed tomography scan of bilateral adrenal myelolipomas (*arrows*). Note the areas of macroscopic fat (hypodense areas) that are typical for this lesion. (From Cameron JL, Cameron AM: *Surgical therapy,* ed 12, Philadelphia, 2017, Elsevier.)

BOX 1 Differential Diagnosis for Adrenal Incidentaloma

Functional Tumors
Pheochromocytoma
Cortisol-producing adenoma/subclinical Cushing's syndrome
Aldosteronoma
Primary adrenal hyperplasia

Nonfunctional Lesions
Nonfunctioning cortical adenoma
Myelolipoma
Adrenal hemorrhage
Adrenal cyst
Ganglioneuroma

Malignant
Adrenocortical carcinoma
Metastases to the adrenal gland

From Cameron JL, Cameron AM: *Surgical therapy,* ed 12, Philadelphia, 2017, Elsevier.

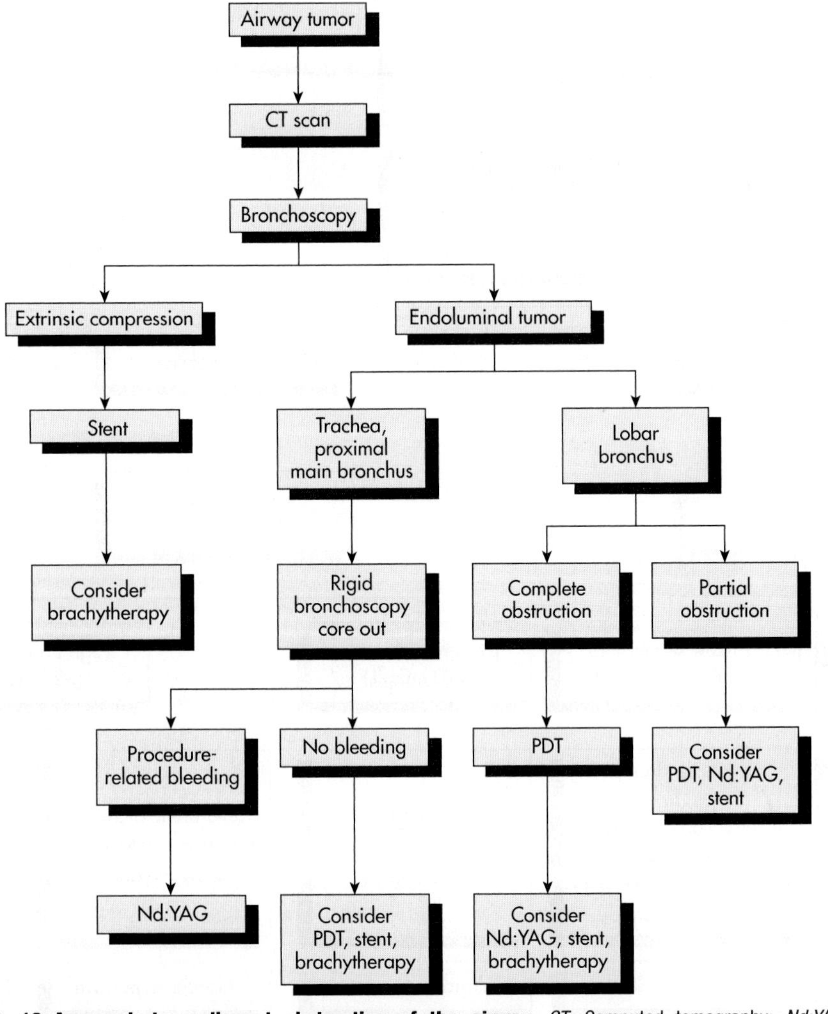

FIG. 13 Approach to malignant obstruction of the airway. *CT*, Computed tomography; *Nd:YAG*, neodymium:yttrium-aluminum-garnet; *PDT*, photodynamic therapy. (From Sellke FW, del Nido PJ, Swanson SJ: *Sabiston & Spencer surgery of the chest*, ed 9, 2016, Elsevier.)

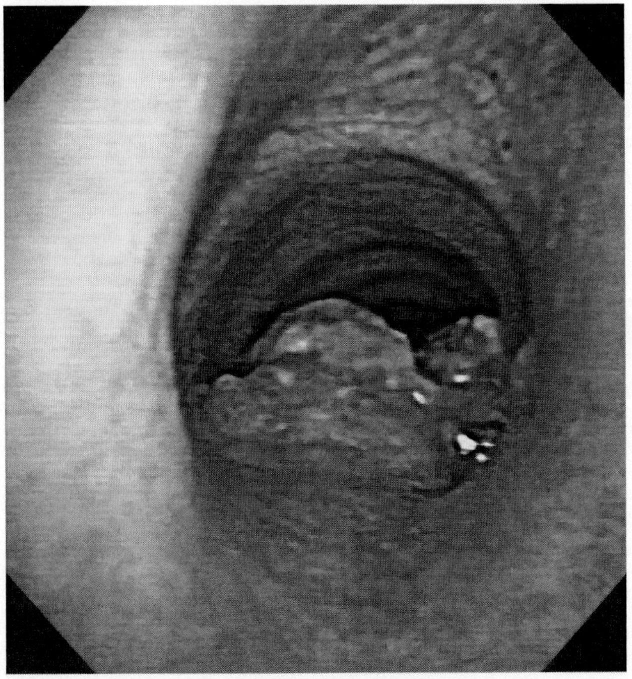

FIG. 14 An exophytic squamous cell carcinoma of the trachea. (From Sellke FW, del Nido PJ, Swanson SJ: *Sabiston & Spencer surgery of the chest*, ed 9, 2016, Elsevier.)

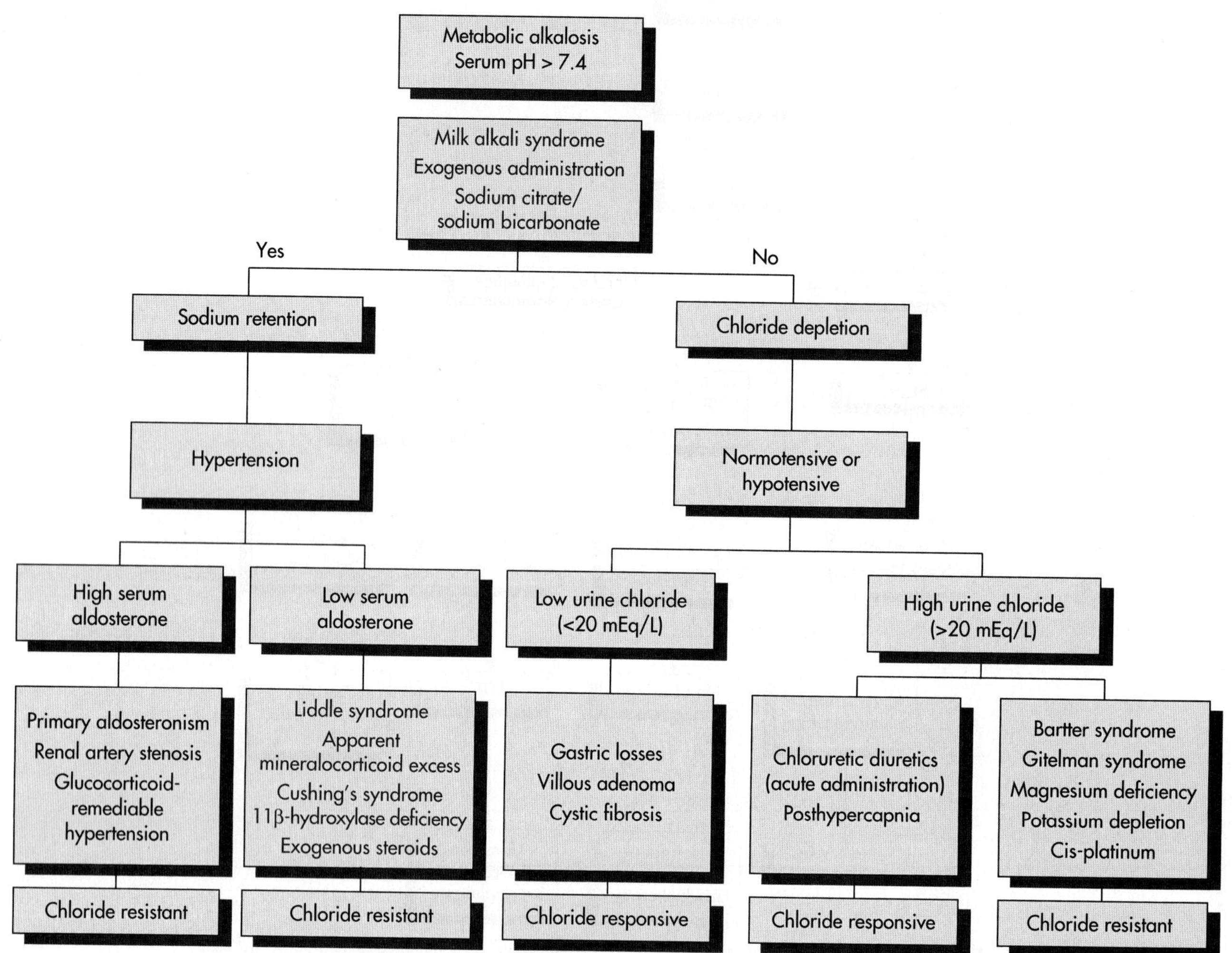

FIG. 15 Differential diagnosis of metabolic alkalosis. (From Ronco C: *Critical care nephrology,* ed 3, Philadelphia, 2019, Elsevier.)

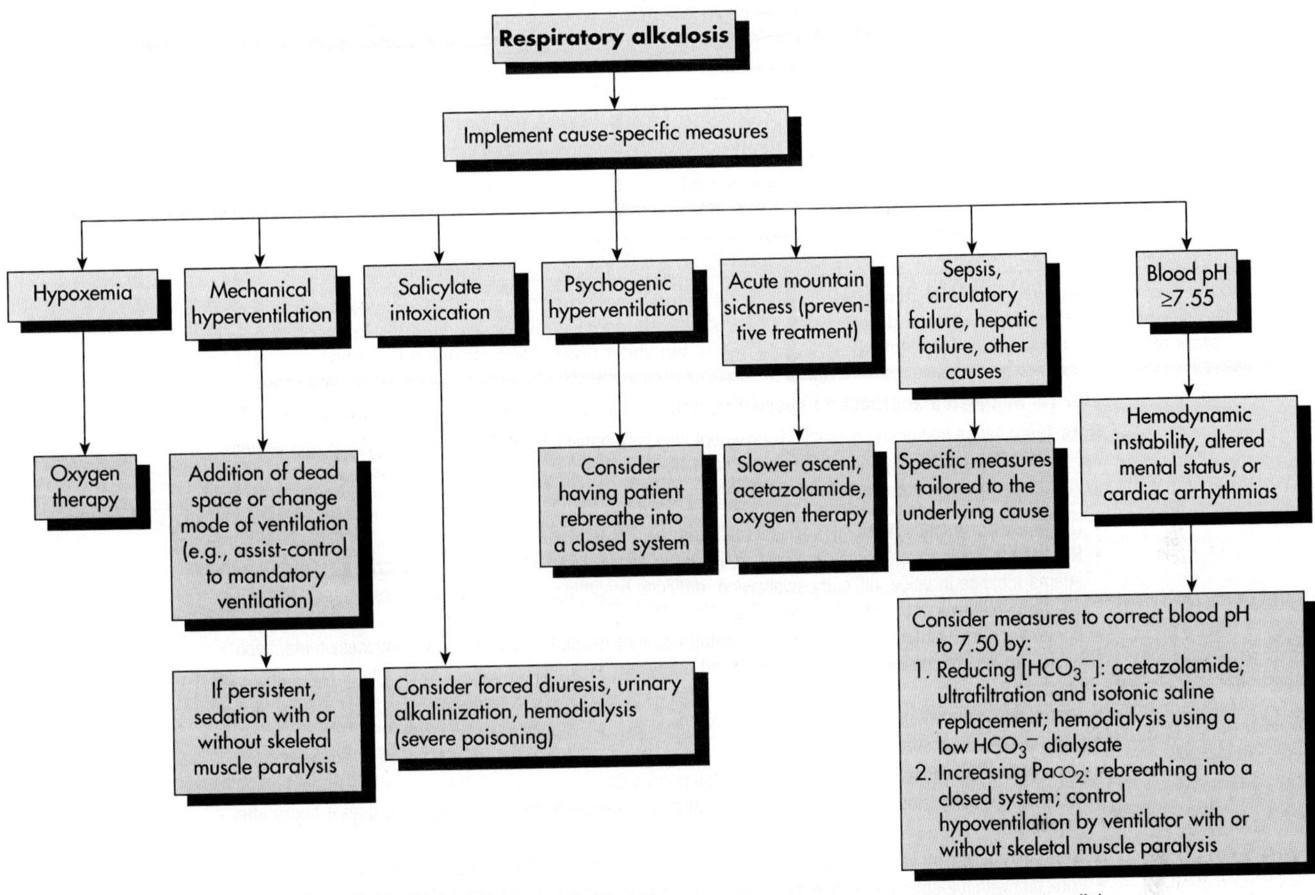

FIG. 16 Recommended treatment of respiratory alkalosis. (From Johnson R et al: *Comprehensive clinical nephrology*, ed 5, Philadelphia, 2015, Saunders.)

Clinical Algorithms III

TABLE 3 Causes of Alveolar Hyperventilation/Respiratory Alkalosis

	Site of Defect	Condition
Defects in respiratory drive	Central chemoreceptors	*Voluntary hyperventilation Psychogenic:* pain, panic attack *Central neurogenic hyperventilation:* brainstem injuries, brain tumors *Hormonal:* increased progesterone levels in pregnancy and liver cirrhosis *Infectious:* meningitis, encephalitis *Thermal hyperpnea:* fever, hyperthermia *Intoxication:* salicylate, topiramate *Therapeutic:* doxapram
	Peripheral chemoreceptors	*Increased activity of peripheral chemoreceptors:* hypoxic pulmonary disease, high altitude *Increased activity of lung receptors*, e.g., pulmonary edema, pneumonia, pulmonary embolism, interstitial fibrosis
Iatrogenic		*Mechanical ventilation:* excessive mechanical ventilation (accidental, or therapeutic for traumatic brain injury) *Extracorporeal gas exchange:* excessive extracorporeal CO2 removal

From Ronco C: *Critical care nephrology*, ed 3, Philadelphia, 2019, Elsevier.

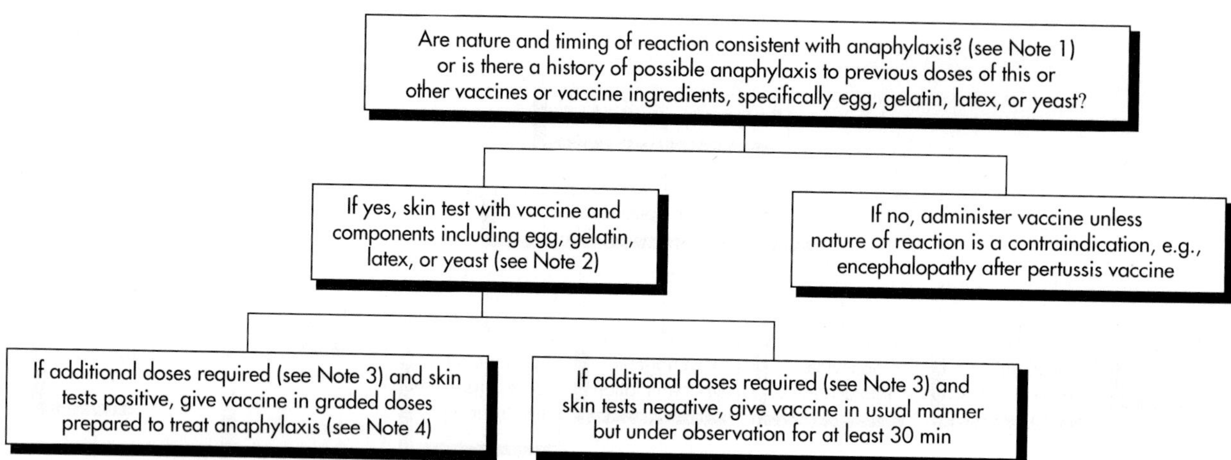

FIG. 17 Suggested approach to suspected immediate-type allergic reactions to vaccines.

Note 1. Are nature and timing of reaction consistent with a systemic IgE-mediated reaction? *Probable systemic IgE-mediated reaction:* reaction occurring within 4 hours of vaccine administration to include signs and/or symptoms from more than one of the following systems:

- Dermatologic: urticaria, flushing, angioedema, pruritis.
- Respiratory: rhinoconjunctivitis (red, watery, itchy eyes; stuffy, runny, itchy nose; sneezing), upper airway edema (change in voice, difficulty swallowing, difficulty breathing, stridor), bronchospasm/asthma (cough, wheeze, shortness of breath, chest tightness).
- Cardiovascular: hypotension, tachycardia, palpitations, light-headedness, loss of consciousness (note: hypotension or loss of consciousness with pallor and bradycardia is much more likely to be due to a vasovagal reaction).
- Gastrointestinal: cramping, nausea, vomiting, diarrhea.

Possible systemic IgE-mediated reaction:

- Signs and/or symptoms from only one system (as previously).
- Signs and/or symptoms from more than one system (as previously) but occurring more than 4 hours after vaccination.

Note 2. Skin tests with vaccine and components including egg, gelatin, latex, or yeast. *Vaccine skin tests:*

- Prick test with full-strength vaccine; consider 1:10 dilution if patient has a history of life-threatening reaction.
- If results of prick test with full-strength vaccine are negative, perform intradermal testing with 0.02 mL of vaccine at 1:100 dilution.
- Vaccine skin tests may cause false (or clinically irrelevant) positive reactions. Thus, if skin testing gives a positive reaction, also perform on normal control subjects.

Vaccine component skin tests:

- Prick tests with commercial extracts of egg (influenza and yellow fever vaccines) or Saccharomyces cerevisiae yeast (hepatitis B and quadrivalent human papillomavirus vaccines).
- Prick test with sugared gelatin (e.g., Jell-O): dissolve 1 teaspoon of gelatin powder in 5 mL of normal saline.
- Vaccines that contain gelatin: influenza (some brands), measles, mumps, rabies (some brands), rubella, typhoid (capsule), varicella, yellow fever, zoster.
- Prick test with latex: soak 2 fingers of latex glove or a toy balloon in 5 mL of normal saline. Vaccines that contain latex in packaging: available at http://www.cdc.gov/vaccines/pubs/pinkbook/downloads/appendices/B/latex-table.pdf.
- In vitro assays for specific IgE antibody to egg, gelatin, latex, and yeast are also commercially available as an alternative or complement to skin testing

Note 3. If fewer than the recommended number of doses are received, consider measuring level of IgG antibodies to immunizing agent. If the measured level is associated with protection from disease, consider withholding additional doses, although magnitude and duration of immunity may be less than if all doses received.

Note 4. Vaccine administration in graded doses:

- With a vaccine for which the usual dose is 0.5 mL, administer graded doses of vaccine at 15-minute intervals: 0.05 mL of 1:10 dilution, 0.05 mL of full strength, 0.10 mL of full strength, 0.15 mL of full strength, 0.20 mL of full strength. (From Adkinson NF et al: *Middleton's allergy principles and practice*, ed 8, Philadelphia, 2014, Saunders.)

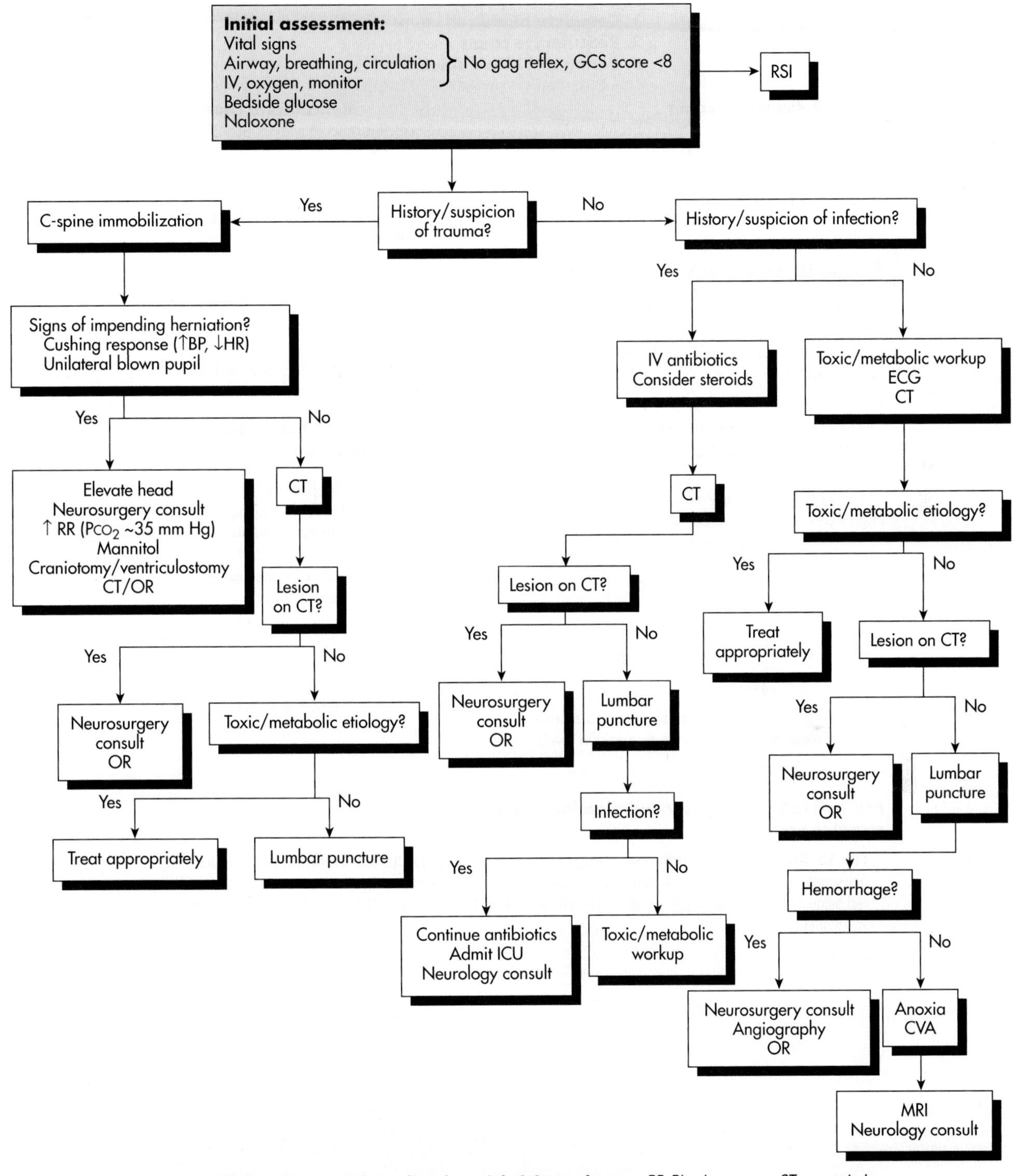

FIG. 18 Diagnostic approach to altered mental status and coma. *BP*, Blood pressure; *CT*, computed tomography; *CVA*, cerebrovascular accident; *ECG*, electrocardiography; *GCS*, Glasgow Coma Scale; *HR*, heart rate; *ICU*, intensive care unit; *MRI*, magnetic resonance imaging; *OR*, operating room; *RR*, respiratory rate; *RSI*, rapid-sequence intubation. (From Adams JG et al: *Emergency medicine, clinical essentials,* ed 2, Philadelphia, 2013, Elsevier.)

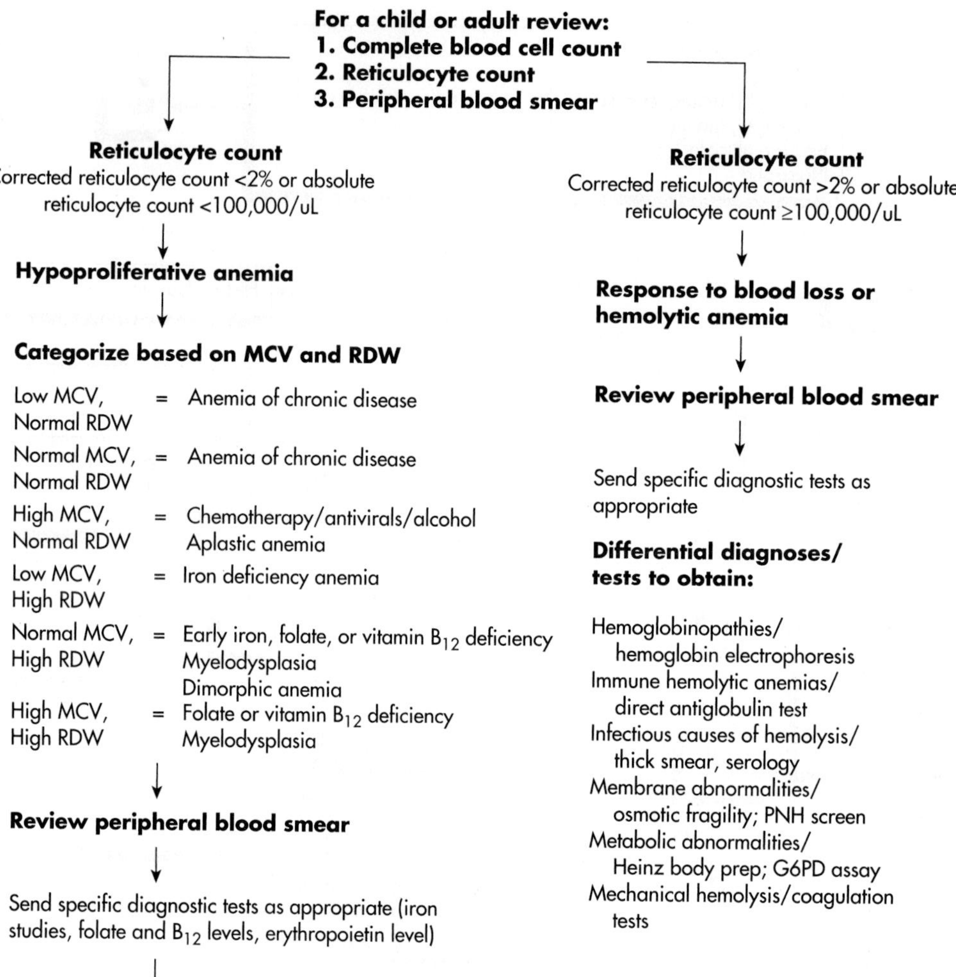
For a child or adult review:
1. Complete blood cell count
2. Reticulocyte count
3. Peripheral blood smear
Reticulocyte count
Corrected reticulocyte count <2% or absolute reticulocyte count <100,000/uL
Hypoproliferative anemia
Categorize based on MCV and RDW
Low MCV, Normal RDW = Anemia of chronic disease
Normal MCV, Normal RDW = Anemia of chronic disease
High MCV, Normal RDW = Chemotherapy/antivirals/alcohol Aplastic anemia
Low MCV, High RDW = Iron deficiency anemia
Normal MCV, High RDW = Early iron, folate, or vitamin B_{12} deficiency Myelodysplasia Dimorphic anemia
High MCV, High RDW = Folate or vitamin B_{12} deficiency Myelodysplasia
Review peripheral blood smear
Send specific diagnostic tests as appropriate (iron studies, folate and B_{12} levels, erythropoietin level)
Proceed to bone marrow examination if diagnosis remains unclear
Reticulocyte count
Corrected reticulocyte count >2% or absolute reticulocyte count ≥100,000/uL
Response to blood loss or hemolytic anemia
Review peripheral blood smear
Send specific diagnostic tests as appropriate
Differential diagnoses/ tests to obtain:
Hemoglobinopathies/ hemoglobin electrophoresis
Immune hemolytic anemias/ direct antiglobulin test
Infectious causes of hemolysis/ thick smear, serology
Membrane abnormalities/ osmotic fragility; PNH screen
Metabolic abnormalities/ Heinz body prep; G6PD assay
Mechanical hemolysis/coagulation tests

FIG. 23 Approach to the differential diagnosis of anemia in adults and children. *G6PD,* Glucose-6-phosphate dehydrogenase; *MCV,* mean corpuscular volume; *PNH,* paroxysmal nocturnal hemoglobinuria; *RDW,* red blood cell distribution width. (From Hoffman R: *Hematology, basic principles and practice,* ed 7, Philadelphia, 2018, Elsevier.)

ANEMIA, MACROCYTIC

ICD-10CM # D50.9 Microcytic (hypochromic) anemia

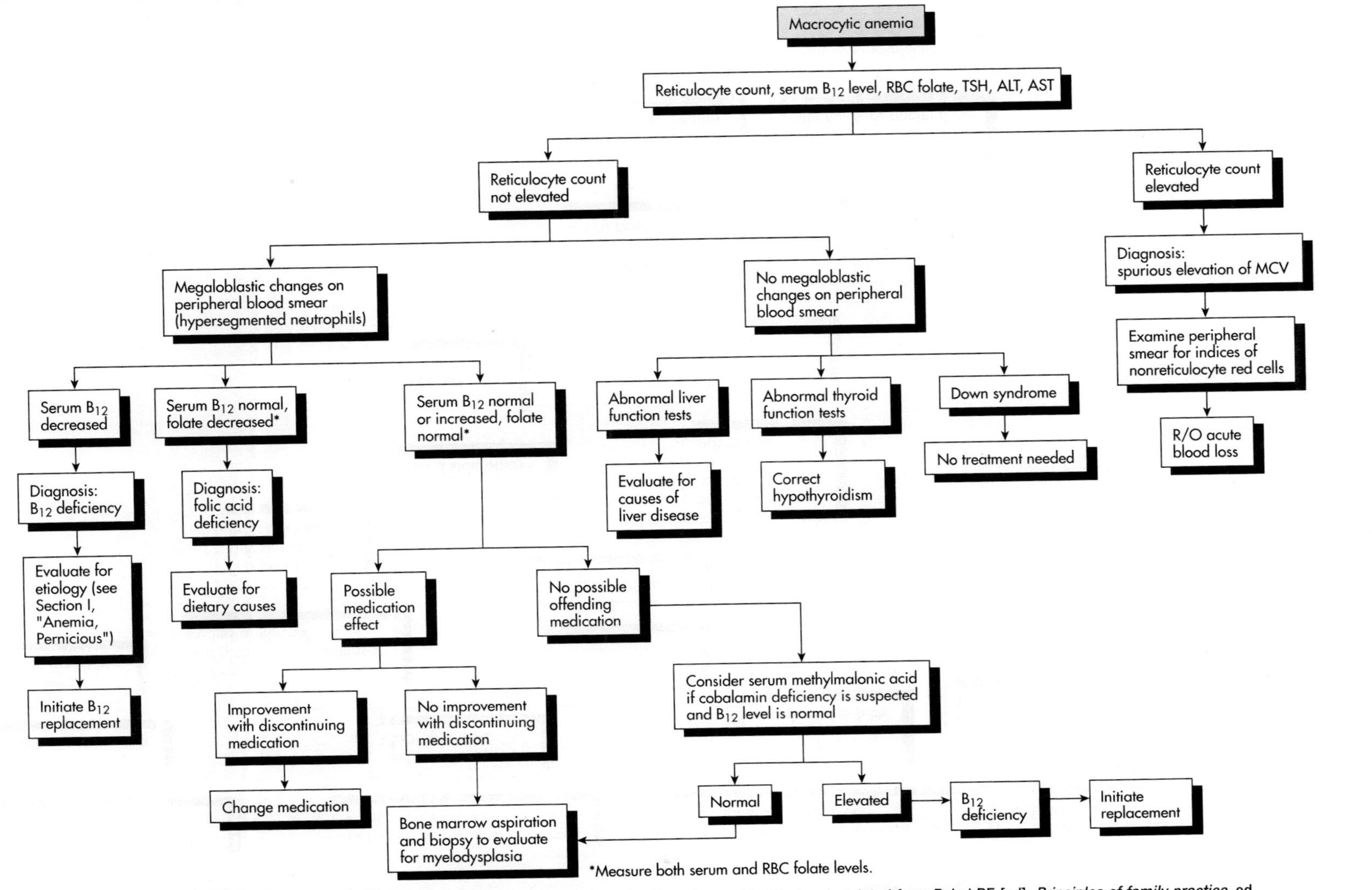

FIG. 24 Differential diagnosis of macrocytic anemia. *MCV,* Mean corpuscular volume. (Modified and updated from Rakel RE [ed]: *Principles of family practice*, ed 7, Philadelphia, 2007, Saunders.)

ICD-10CM # D50.9 Microcytic (hypochromic) anemia

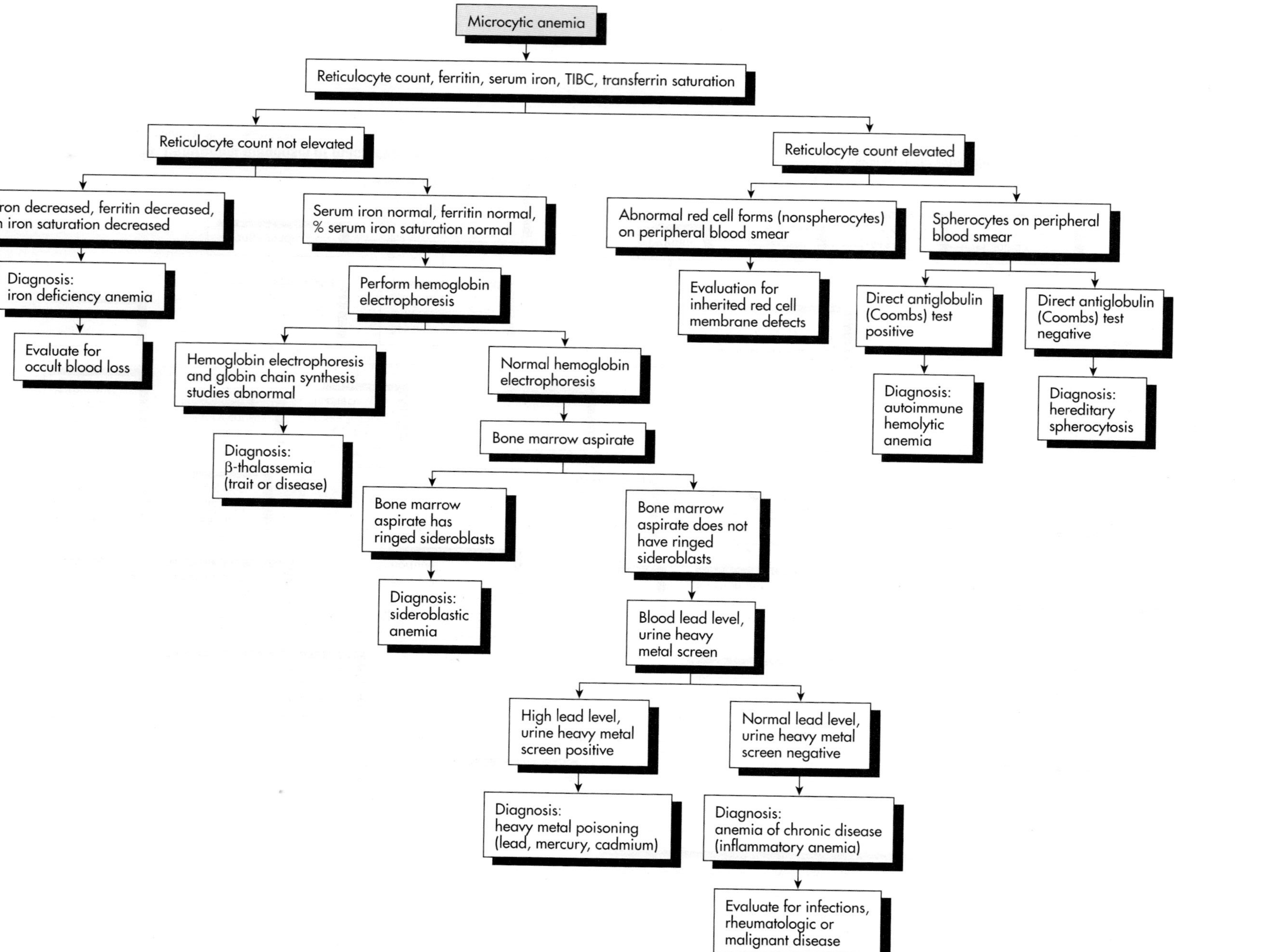

FIG. 25 Differential diagnosis of microcytic anemia. *TIBC*, Total iron binding capacity. (Modified and updated from Rakel RE [ed]: *Principles of family practice*, ed 7, Philadelphia, 2007, Saunders.)

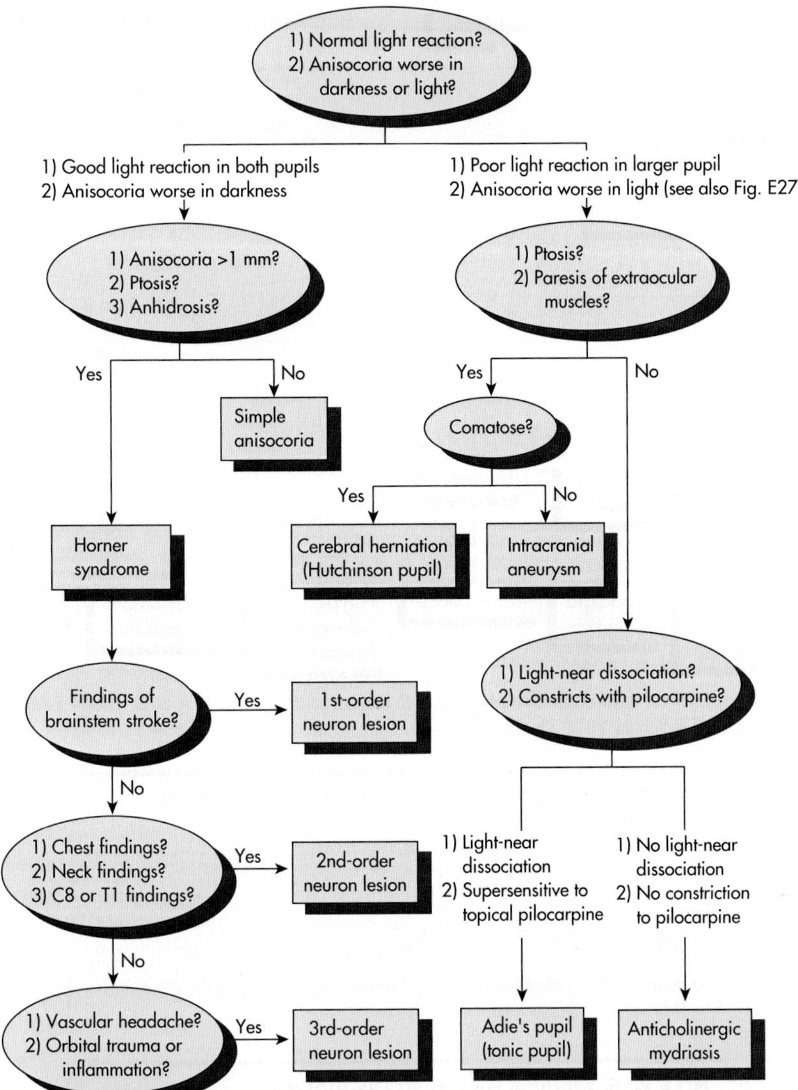

FIG. 26 Summary of approach to anisocoria. The first two questions (Is there a normal light reaction? and Is anisocoria worse in darkness or light?) distinguish problems with the pupillary dilator muscle (i.e., Horner syndrome, simple anisocoria; *left side* of the figure) from problems with the pupillary constrictor muscle (i.e., third cranial nerve, iris; *right side* of the figure). Two other tests distinguish Horner syndrome from simple anisocoria: the cocaine or apraclonidine eyedrop tests and pupillary dilator lag (i.e., the pupil dilates slowly in darkness, as documented by photographs). (From McGee S: *Evidence-based physical diagnosis,* ed 4, Philadelphia, 2018, Elsevier.)

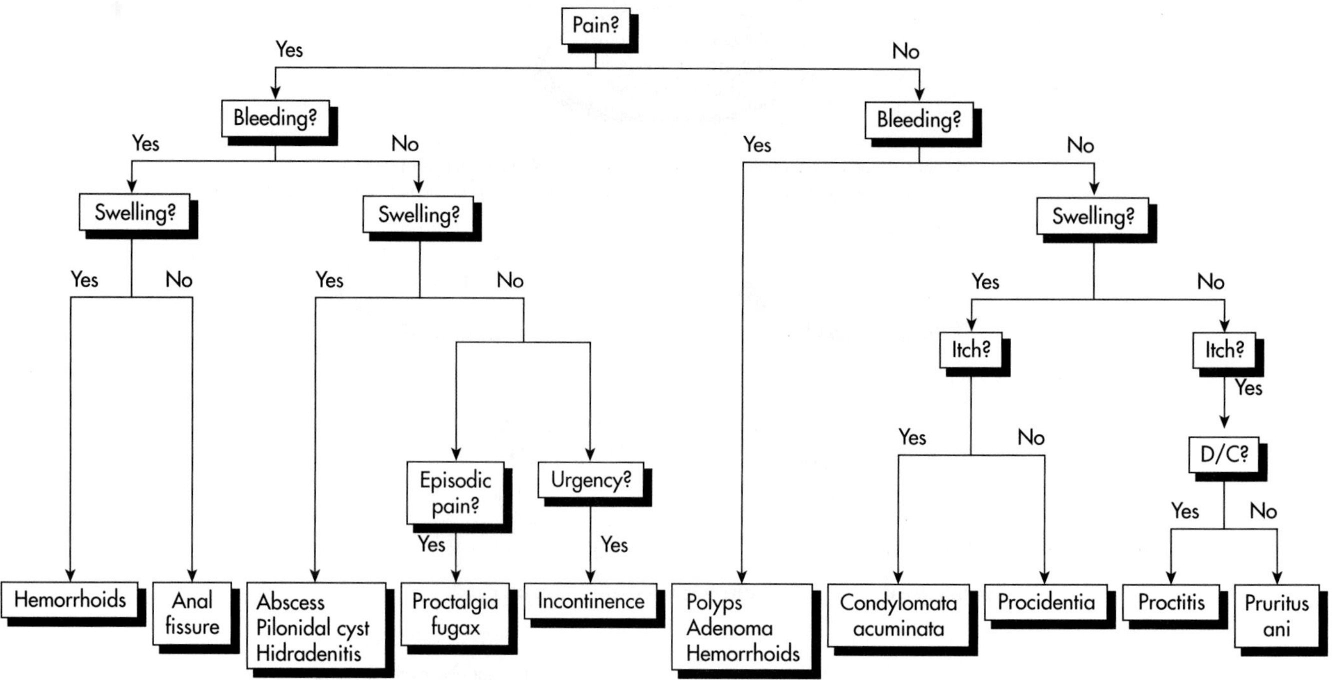

FIG. 28 Algorithm for anorectal complaints. *D/C,* discharge. (From Marx JA et al: *Rosen's emergency medicine*, ed 8, Philadelphia, 2014, Saunders.)

BOX 4, A The WASH Regimen for Management of Hemorrhoids

- *W*arm water
- *A*nalgesic agents
- *S*tool softeners
- *H*igh-fiber diet

From Marx JA et al: *Rosen's emergency medicine*, ed 8, Philadelphia, 2014, Saunders.

BOX 4, B Medical History in Diagnosis of Anorectal Disorders

Anorectal History
- Pain
- Bleeding
- Swelling
- Itching
- Discharge
- Urgency

Gastrointestinal History
- Change in bowel habits (straining, flatus, color, consistency, frequency)
- Nausea or vomiting
- Incontinence of stool
- Underlying GI disease (Crohn's disease, cancer, polyps)

Systemic Disease History
- Diabetes mellitus
- Coagulopathy
- Cancer
- HIV infection

Sexual History of the Anus
- Penetration
- Known STDs
- Assault

GI, Gastrointestinal; *HIV,* human immunodeficiency virus; *STD,* sexually transmitted disease.
From Marx JA et al: *Rosen's emergency medicine,* ed 8, Philadelphia, 2014, Saunders.

BACK PAIN

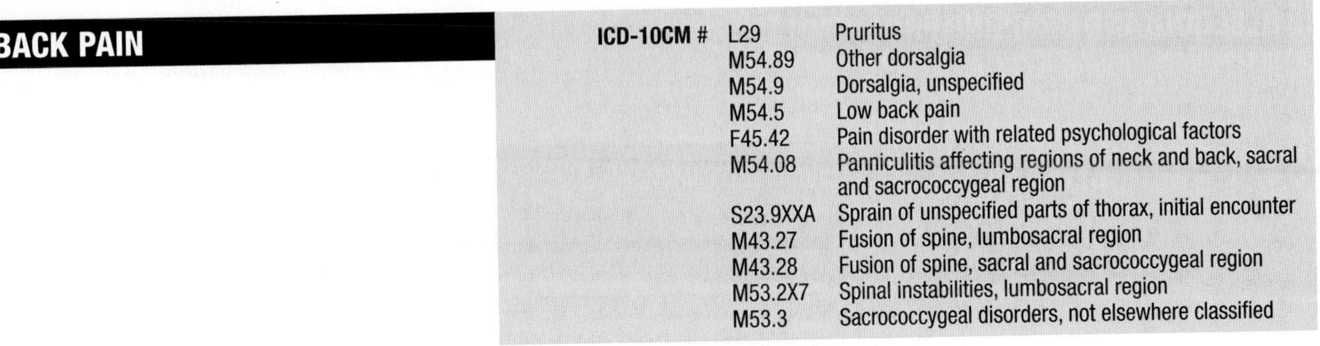

ICD-10CM #		
	L29	Pruritus
	M54.89	Other dorsalgia
	M54.9	Dorsalgia, unspecified
	M54.5	Low back pain
	F45.42	Pain disorder with related psychological factors
	M54.08	Panniculitis affecting regions of neck and back, sacral and sacrococcygeal region
	S23.9XXA	Sprain of unspecified parts of thorax, initial encounter
	M43.27	Fusion of spine, lumbosacral region
	M43.28	Fusion of spine, sacral and sacrococcygeal region
	M53.2X7	Spinal instabilities, lumbosacral region
	M53.3	Sacrococcygeal disorders, not elsewhere classified

Low back pain

Focused history and physical examination to categorize patients

Patients with "red flags" that indicate risk of systemic disease (infection, malignancy, spondyloarthritis) or vertebral compression fracture

Patients with neurologic signs and symptoms

Patients with nonspecific/ mechanical LBP

- Plain radiography
- ESR
- Consider MRI if abnormal or high index of suspicion

- Cauda equina syndrome suspected
- Presence of serious or progressive neurologic deficit

Radiculopathy without serious or progressive neurologic deficit

Spinal stenosis suspected

Conservative care

Systemic disease confirmed

No systemic disease

MRI and urgent surgical consultation

Plain radiography, ESR if concern for osteomyelitis

Serious or progressive neurologic deficit

No serious neurologic deficit

If not improved plain radiography and ESR to exclude systemic disease

Specific treatment

Conservative care

Conservative care for 4-6 weeks

MRI and surgical consultation

Conservative care

Continue conservative care if symptoms manageable

Consider interdisciplinary rehabilitation with cognitive behavioral therapy for severe disabling chronic LBP

MRI if no improvement Consider surgical consultation especially with neurologic progression

MRI and surgical consultation for development of disabling neurogenic claudication

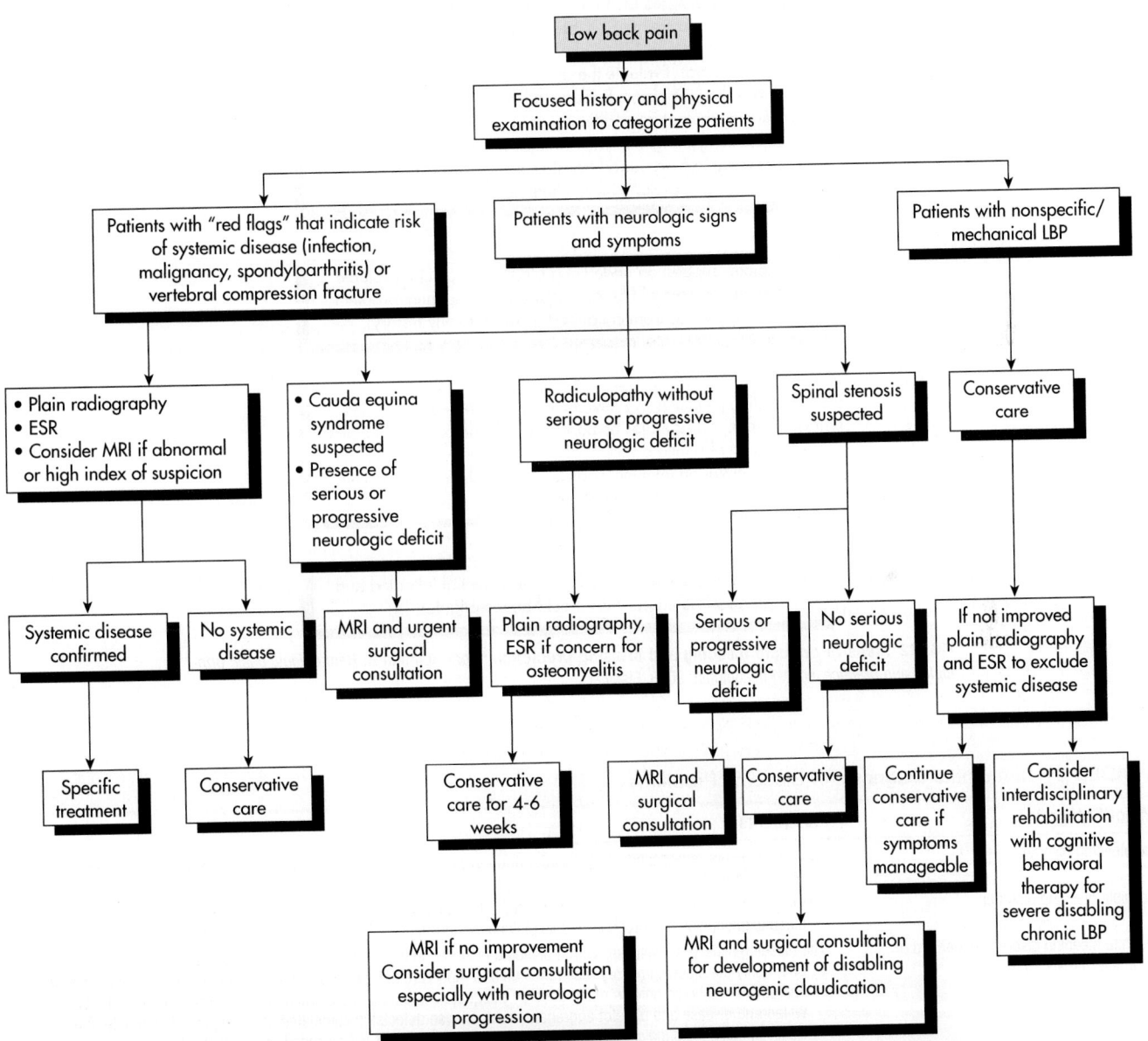

FIG. 31 Algorithm for the differential diagnosis and treatment of low back pain. *ESR*, erythrocyte sedimentation rate; *LBP*, low back pain; *MRI*, magnetic resonance imaging. (From Firestein GS, Budd RC, Gabriel SE et al: *Kelley and Firestein's textbook of rheumatology*, ed 10, Philadelphia, 2017, Elsevier.)

TABLE 4 Red Flags for Potentially Serious Conditions

Possible Fracture	Possible Tumor or Infection	Possible Cauda Equina Syndrome
From Medical History		
Major trauma, such as vehicle accident or fall from height Minor trauma or even strenuous lifting (in older or potentially osteoporotic patient)	Age over 50 or under 20 yr History of cancer Constitutional symptoms, such as recent fever or chills or unexplained weight loss Risk factors for spinal infection: recent bacterial infection (e.g., urinary tract infection), intravenous drug abuse, or immune suppression (from steroids, transplant, or human immunodeficiency virus) Pain that worsens when supine; severe nighttime pain	Saddle anesthesia Recent onset of bladder dysfunction, such as urinary retention, increased frequency, or overflow incontinence Severe or progressive neurologic deficit in the lower extremity

ICD-10CM # D68.9 Coagulation defect, unspecified
D68.8 Other specified coagulation defects

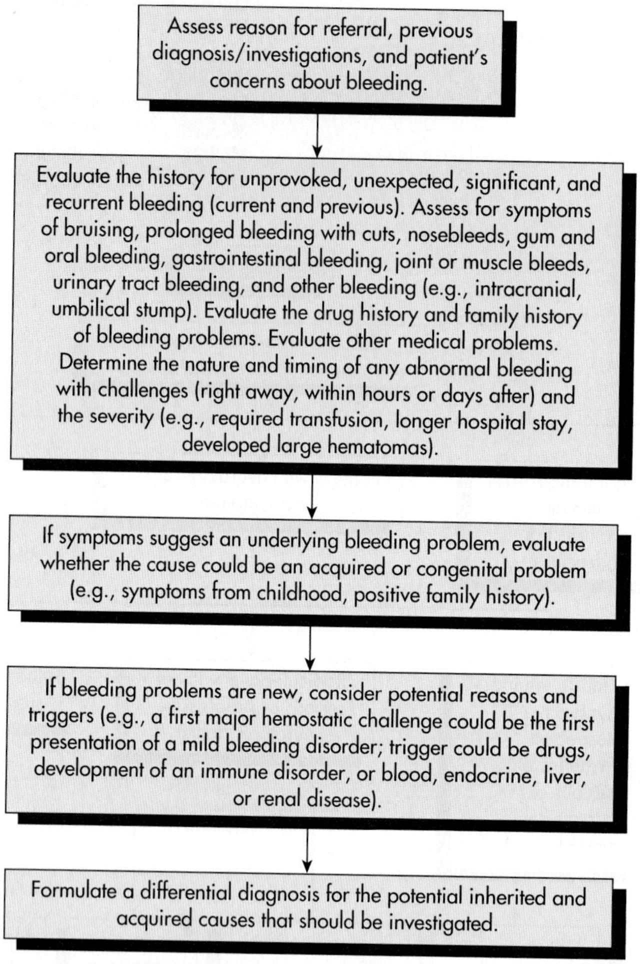

Assess reason for referral, previous diagnosis/investigations, and patient's concerns about bleeding.

↓

Evaluate the history for unprovoked, unexpected, significant, and recurrent bleeding (current and previous). Assess for symptoms of bruising, prolonged bleeding with cuts, nosebleeds, gum and oral bleeding, gastrointestinal bleeding, joint or muscle bleeds, urinary tract bleeding, and other bleeding (e.g., intracranial, umbilical stump). Evaluate the drug history and family history of bleeding problems. Evaluate other medical problems. Determine the nature and timing of any abnormal bleeding with challenges (right away, within hours or days after) and the severity (e.g., required transfusion, longer hospital stay, developed large hematomas).

↓

If symptoms suggest an underlying bleeding problem, evaluate whether the cause could be an acquired or congenital problem (e.g., symptoms from childhood, positive family history).

↓

If bleeding problems are new, consider potential reasons and triggers (e.g., a first major hemostatic challenge could be the first presentation of a mild bleeding disorder; trigger could be drugs, development of an immune disorder, or blood, endocrine, liver, or renal disease).

↓

Formulate a differential diagnosis for the potential inherited and acquired causes that should be investigated.

FIG. 32 Steps to evaluate bleeding and bruising problems. (From Hoffman R: *Hematology, basic principles and practice*, ed 7, Philadelphia, 2018, Elsevier.)

TABLE 5 Differential Diagnosis of Bleeding Problems

Major Categories	Comments
No bleeding disorder	Symptoms do not reflect a bleeding disorder and have another explanation (e.g., a surgical bleed, not caused by a bleeding disorder).
Possible bleeding disorder	The laboratory findings are nondiagnostic, and the bleeding history is considered equivocal (e.g., unexplained serious bleed with one surgical procedure; unexplained menorrhagia without other bleeding problems).
Definite bleeding disorder, undefined or indeterminate type	The bleeding history is consistent with a bleeding disorder; however, the laboratory findings are nondiagnostic. Commonly the bleeding history resembles mild to moderate defects in platelet function or von Willebrand factor. The diagnosis should only be made once an adequate evaluation for common bleeding disorders (e.g., for von Willebrand disease and platelet aggregation and release defects) is completed. If testing is not complete, the classification should indicate the types of conditions excluded or not excluded, for example: mild mucocutaneous bleeding problem, von Willebrand disease excluded, mild mucocutaneous bleeding problem, platelet release defects not yet excluded.
Definite bleeding disorder with cause	The symptoms and laboratory findings are considered diagnostic of a bleeding disorder. Tables 6 and 7 summarize many of a define the potential inherited and acquired causes.

From Hoffman R: *Hematology, basic principles and practice*, ed 7, Philadelphia, 2018, Elsevier.

Table 6 Differential Diagnosis of Congenital Bleeding Disorders

Disorder	Comments
Fibrinogen deficiency or dysfunction	Deficiencies can be mild-moderate hypofibrinogenemia or severe afibrinogenemia. Fibrinogen function is abnormal in dysfibrinogenemias, which can present with bleeding, thrombosis, or both. Fibrinogen levels can be reduced in some dysfibrinogenemias.
X-linked coagulation factor deficiencies—hemophilia	Presentation is influenced by the degree of deficiency. Factor VIII deficiency is more common than factor IX deficiency. If factor VIII is low, von Willebrand disease needs to be excluded as the cause.
Rarer, coagulation factor deficiencies	Deficiencies can affect factors XI, V, II, VII, or X, and the presentation is dependent on the severity of the deficiency. Hereditary deficiencies of multiple coagulation factors are rare (e.g., of factors V and VIII, or multiple vitamin K–dependent coagulation factors for congenital defects impairing γ-carboxylation) and can easily be excluded by measuring multiple factors.
Fibrinolytic defects	Causes include disorders caused by loss of function, such as α2-antiplasmin or PAI-1 deficiency, and by gain-of-function defects, such as Quebec platelet disorder (overexpression of urokinase plasminogen activator in megakaryocytes).
von Willebrand's disease	Causes include quantitative (partial type 1 to severe type 3) and qualitative defects (loss of function in type 2M and 2A, gain of function in type 2B and platelet-type). Type 1 von Willebrand disease can be confused with low von Willebrand factor levels (e.g., because of blood group O).
Platelet disorders	These conditions can affect platelet number, function, or both. The most common type of platelet function disorder is a platelet secretion defect, which may or may not also impair aggregation responses. Disorders of platelet function are commonly subclassified by the nature of the defect, such as the following: 1. Defects of membrane receptors for adhesive proteins (e.g., Glanzmann thrombasthenia and Bernard-Soulier syndrome) or agonists (e.g., $P2Y_{12}$ deficiency) 2. Defects of signaling or secretion (the largest subcategory) 3. Cytoskeletal defects (e.g., MYH9-related disorders) 4. Storage pool disorders (e.g., gray platelet syndrome, dense granule deficiency, $\alpha\gamma$-storage pool deficiency, Quebec platelet disorder) 5. Defects of procoagulant function (e.g., Scott syndrome)
Vascular disorders	Congenital vascular malformation, including hereditary hemorrhagic telangiectasia, Ehlers-Danlos syndrome

MYH9, Myosin heavy polypeptide 9; *PAI-1,* plasminogen activator inhibitor 1.
From Hoffman R: *Hematology, basic principles and practice,* ed 7, Philadelphia, 2018, Elsevier.

ICD-10CM # D68.9 Coagulation defect, unspecified
D68.8 Other specified coagulation defects

Table 7 Differential Diagnosis of Acquired Bleeding Problems

Disorder	Comments
Drug induced	Aspirin, NSAIDs, other platelet function inhibitors (e.g., $P2Y_{12}$ and $\alpha_{IIb}\beta_3$ inhibitors), anticoagulants, fibrinolytic drugs, and antidepressants are common causes.
Acquired factor deficiencies	The causes can be immune (e.g., acquired factor VIII deficiency, acquired factor V deficiency) or nonimmune. Reductions in multiple factors can result from vitamin K deficiency, treatment with vitamin K antagonists, liver disease, hemodilution, and rarely snakebites. Severe acquired hypofibrinogenemia is commonly caused by a postpartum coagulopathy or severe liver disease. Prothrombin deficiency occurs with some lupus anticoagulants. Amyloidosis can cause an acquired factor X deficiency, which may be associated with reductions in other coagulation factors synthesized in the liver if the liver is involved.
Disseminated intravascular coagulation	The manifestations can include thrombocytopenia, consumption of coagulation factors, including fibrinogen, and impairment of hemostatic mechanisms from the fibrin/fibrinogen degradation products. Causes are wide ranging and include postpartum consumptive states, prostate and other cancers, and snakebites.
Acquired von Willebrand disease	The cause can be immune (often in association with an IgG paraprotein) or nonimmune (e.g., increased proteolysis of von Willebrand factor with stenotic aortic valvular disease).
Immune thrombocytopenia	Bleeding is usually influenced by the extent of the thrombocytopenia. Some autoantibodies interfere with platelet membrane receptor function, causing bleeding disproportionate to the thrombocytopenia.
Non–drug-induced, acquired platelet function disorders	The cause can be immune (see earlier) or nonimmune, typically from bone marrow disorders, although secretion defects can be secondary to Cushing syndrome or hypothyroidism.
Liver disease	Liver disease can cause thrombocytopenia, deficiencies of coagulation factors, hypofibrinogenemia and dysfibrinogenemia, and increased fibrinolysis. In mild liver disease, factor VII and sometimes factors XI and XII are low. Fibrinogen is often increased in early liver disease, and if low, the finding suggests severe liver disease.
Renal disease	Anemia is an important predictor of uremic bleeding. Uremic bleeding is typically associated with severe renal impairment.
Hypothyroidism	Hypothyroidism can cause an acquired von Willebrand disease and acquired defects in platelet function.
Cushing's syndrome	This syndrome should be suspected when there are symptoms and findings suggestive of Cushing syndrome or treatment with systemic or topical glucocorticoids.
Surgical bleeding	This is often a diagnosis of exclusion, although the procedural notes sometimes document that a technical problem was encountered that led to abnormal bleeding.
Vitamin K deficiency	Newborns are at risk, as are individuals with malabsorption and/or receiving broad-spectrum antibiotics that reduce vitamin K production by reducing gut bacteria. Older adults are also at greater risk for developing vitamin K deficiency because of reduced stores from poorer intake of vitamin K. If the patient does not respond to parenteral vitamin K, other causes should be considered.
Vitamin C deficiency (scurvy)	This diagnosis should be considered when there is lethargy with skin and gum bleeding (perifollicular hemorrhages, gum bleeding with swelling). The condition is rare in developed countries. The cause is usually a very poor diet or malabsorption.

IgG, Immunoglobulin G; *NSAID,* nonsteroidal antiinflammatory drug.
From Hoffman R: *Hematology, basic principles and practice,* ed 7, Philadelphia, 2018, Elsevier.

BOX 5 The Laboratory Manifestations of Bleeding Disorders

The laboratory manifestations of bleeding disorders can include abnormalities from the following:
1. The underlying hemostatic defect
2. Bleeding complications (e.g., anemia, iron deficiency, coagulopathy secondary to hemodilution after resuscitation for a massive bleed, development of red cell antibodies after transfusion)
3. False-positive abnormalities (e.g., prolonged aPTT caused by incidental mild factor XII deficiency, which is found in about 1 of 200 patients, or a lupus anticoagulant, which can be a transient finding in about 5% of hospitalized patients)
4. Extremes of normal variation (e.g., mildly low von Willebrand factor levels in an individual who is blood group O, absent secondary aggregation with epinephrine in adjusted platelet rich–plasma aggregation studies).

From Hoffman R: *Hematology, basic principles and practice,* ed 7, Philadelphia, 2018, Elsevier.

BOX 6 Influences on Presenting Problems

When evaluating a bleeding history, it is important to recognize that the presenting problems are influenced by the following factors:

1. The nature and severity of the defect, and the presence of single or multiple risk factors for bleeding
2. Whether the bleeding problem is congenital or acquired
3. Antecedent exposure to hemostatic challenges (such as surgery, dental extraction, menses, and childbirth) and the risk for bleeding with each of these challenges
4. The presence of other medical problems (e.g., renal, hepatic, or thyroid disease), including anemia
5. Variability in the bleeding symptoms experienced by individuals without bleeding disorders (e.g., nosebleeds, bruising) and by individuals with known bleeding disorders, even within families with the same defect
6. Local factors (e.g., sun-damage to the skin, vascular lesions, diverticular disease, or cancerous lesions in the gastrointestinal tract) and the possibility of nonaccidental trauma
7. Treatments that increase the risk for bleeding (e.g., antiplatelet drugs, such as aspirin and nonsteroidal antiinflammatory drugs used for pain control, anticoagulant therapy, etc.)
8. Whether treatments were used to prevent or control bleeding
9. Whether treatments prescribed for other reasons may have reduced bleeding (e.g., reduced menstrual bleeding while on oral contraceptives to prevent pregnancy)

From Hoffman R: *Hematology, basic principles and practice,* ed 7, Philadelphia, 2018, Elsevier.

BOX 7 Case 1: Illustration of a Mild, Inherited Bleeding Problem

A 77-year-old man who is starting treatment for multiple myeloma was discovered to have a prolonged activated partial thromboplastin time. Review of his records indicated that the abnormality was present on a previous admission for spinal cord compression, which was treated with surgery. He required 4 units of packed red blood cells several days after this surgery because of delayed postoperative bleeding. There was no other bleeding history. He was found to have mild factor IX deficiency, unrelated to the myeloma, and his daughter proved to be a carrier of this defect.

From Hoffman R: *Hematology, basic principles and practice,* ed 7, Philadelphia, 2018, Elsevier.

BOX 8 Case 2: Illustration of the Importance of Assessing Both Personal and Familial Bleeding Problems

A 22-year-old woman was referred for evaluation of a possible platelet disorder. She had a history of menorrhagia (4 days out of 7 days of menstrual flow were heavy when not on treatment), prolonged nosebleeds in childhood, and hematuria with urinary tract infections. She did not have thrombocytopenia, and she had no exposure to major hemostatic challenges. Her father, uncle, and grandfather had a striking bleeding history, and two of them had thrombocytopenia. The bleeding in her relatives included joint bleeds with trauma and severe, delayed-onset bleeding after trauma and surgery (usually more than a day later), which continued for weeks despite platelet transfusions. One of these relatives reported no bleeding when he had a tooth extracted while receiving fibrinolytic inhibitor therapy. Although menorrhagia is not specific to any one type of bleeding disorder, the delayed bleeding in affected relatives suggests a possible autosomal dominant disorder and either a fibrinolytic defect of a factor defect or deficiency (e.g., affected relatives). Because of the family history of thrombocytopenia, joint bleeds, and delayed bleeding, which did not respond well to platelet transfusions, testing was done for the Quebec platelet disorder. Genetic testing for duplication mutation of the urokinase plasminogen activator gene confirmed this diagnosis in the patient and her relatives. The case illustrates the importance of evaluating both the personal and family bleeding history and highlights the fact that bleeding-symptom severity can vary among affected family members, in part because of their different exposures to challenges and treatments.

From Hoffman R: *Hematology, basic principles and practice,* ed 7, Philadelphia, 2018, Elsevier.

BOX 9 Case 3: Illustration of the Importance of Assessing Bleeding Problems Over Time

A 72-year-old man was referred for evaluation of a severe bleed after receiving a single dose of low-molecular-weight heparin for unconfirmed deep vein thrombosis. He had a history of a similar bleeding episode several years previously while on warfarin treatment for atrial fibrillation. There was no other bleeding history, and the patient subsequently developed a spontaneous iliopsoas bleed. He had undergone numerous surgeries earlier in life without any bleeding problems, and there was no family history of bleeding. The bleeding history suggested the possibility of an acquired bleeding problem, possibly acquired von Willebrand disease or an acquired factor XIII deficiency. Diagnostic testing indicated that he had acquired factor XIII deficiency. This case illustrates the fact that there may be more than one risk factor for bleeding: in this case, several exposures to anticoagulants triggered bleeding in a patient with an acquired factor deficiency. On initial treatment of his iliopsoas bleed with factor XIII concentrate, there was partial neutralization of the infused factor followed by accelerated clearance, consistent with acquired factor XIII deficiency secondary to an autoantibody.

From Hoffman R: *Hematology, basic principles and practice,* ed 7, Philadelphia, 2018, Elsevier.

ICD-10CM # D68.8 Other specified coagulation defects
D68.9 Coagulation defect, unspecified

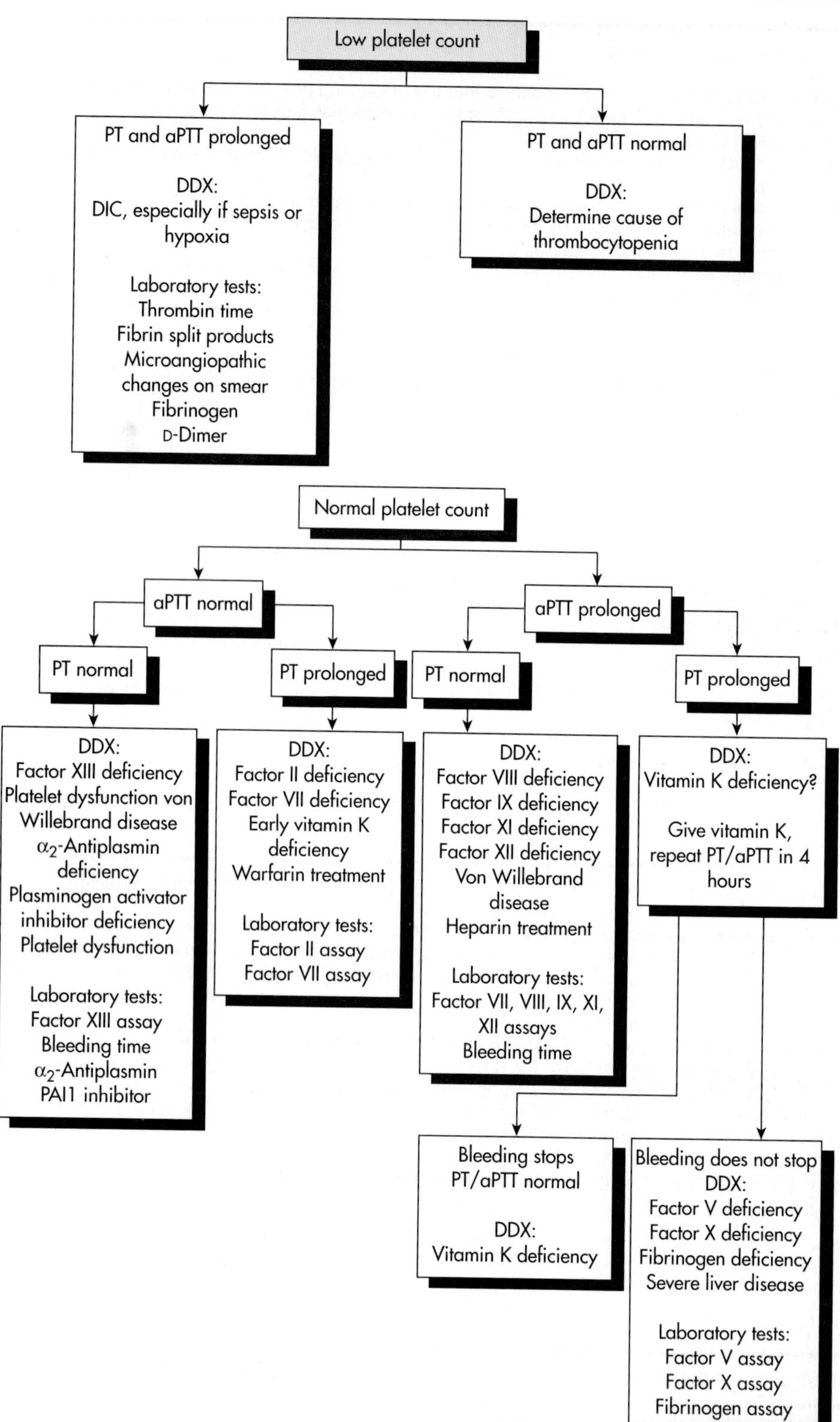

FIG. 33 Differential diagnosis (DDx) of bleeding disorders. (From Hughes HK, Kahl LK: *The Harriet Lane handbook*, ed 21, St Louis, 2018, Mosby.)

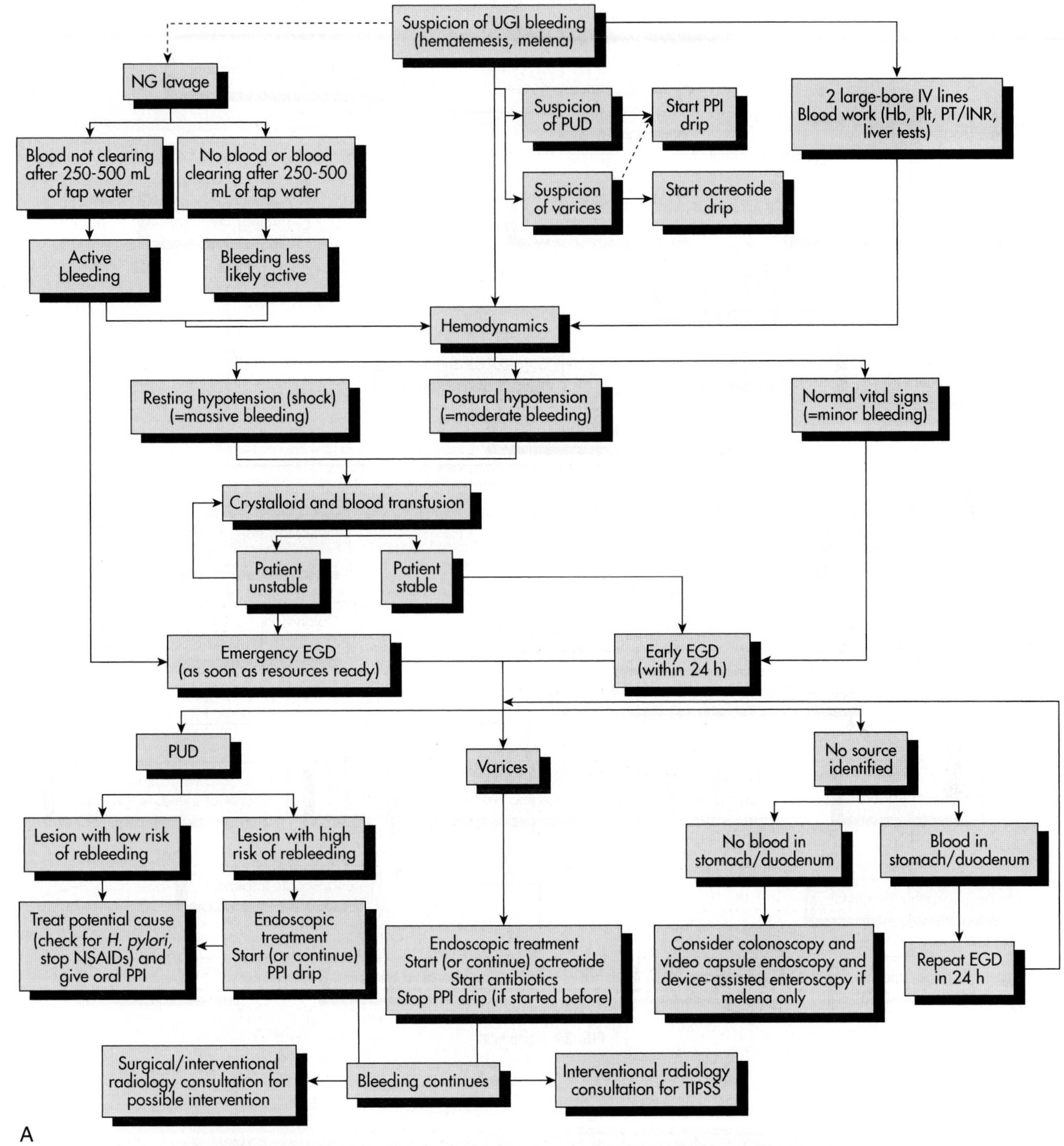

Suspicion of UGI bleeding (hematemesis, melena)

NG lavage

Blood not clearing after 250-500 mL of tap water

No blood or blood clearing after 250-500 mL of tap water

Active bleeding

Bleeding less likely active

Suspicion of PUD

Start PPI drip

Suspicion of varices

Start octreotide drip

2 large-bore IV lines Blood work (Hb, Plt, PT/INR, liver tests)

Hemodynamics

Resting hypotension (shock) (=massive bleeding)

Postural hypotension (=moderate bleeding)

Normal vital signs (=minor bleeding)

Crystalloid and blood transfusion

Patient unstable

Patient stable

Emergency EGD (as soon as resources ready)

Early EGD (within 24 h)

PUD

Varices

No source identified

Lesion with low risk of rebleeding

Lesion with high risk of rebleeding

No blood in stomach/duodenum

Blood in stomach/duodenum

Treat potential cause (check for *H. pylori*, stop NSAIDs) and give oral PPI

Endoscopic treatment Start (or continue) PPI drip

Endoscopic treatment Start (or continue) octreotide Start antibiotics Stop PPI drip (if started before)

Consider colonoscopy and video capsule endoscopy and device-assisted enteroscopy if melena only

Repeat EGD in 24 h

Surgical/interventional radiology consultation for possible intervention

Bleeding continues

Interventional radiology consultation for TIPSS

A

FIG. 34 A, Approach to managing upper gastrointestinal bleeding in critical care patients. **B,** Approach to managing lower gastrointestinal bleeding in critical care patients. *AVM*, arteriovenous malformation; *EGD*, esophagogastroduodenoscopy; *Hb*, hemoglobin; *INR*, international normalized ratio; *LGI*, lower gastrointestinal; *NG*, nasogastric; *NSAIDs*, nonsteroidal antiinflammatory drugs; *Plt*, platelets; *PPI*, proton pump inhibitor; *PT*, prothrombin time; *PUD*, peptic ulcer disease; *RBC*, red blood cell; *TIPSS*, transjugular intrahepatic portosystemic stent shunt; *UGI*, upper gastrointestinal. (From Parrillo JE, Dellinger RP: *Critical care medicine, principles of diagnosis and management in the adult*, ed 4, 2014, Elsevier.)

Continued on next page

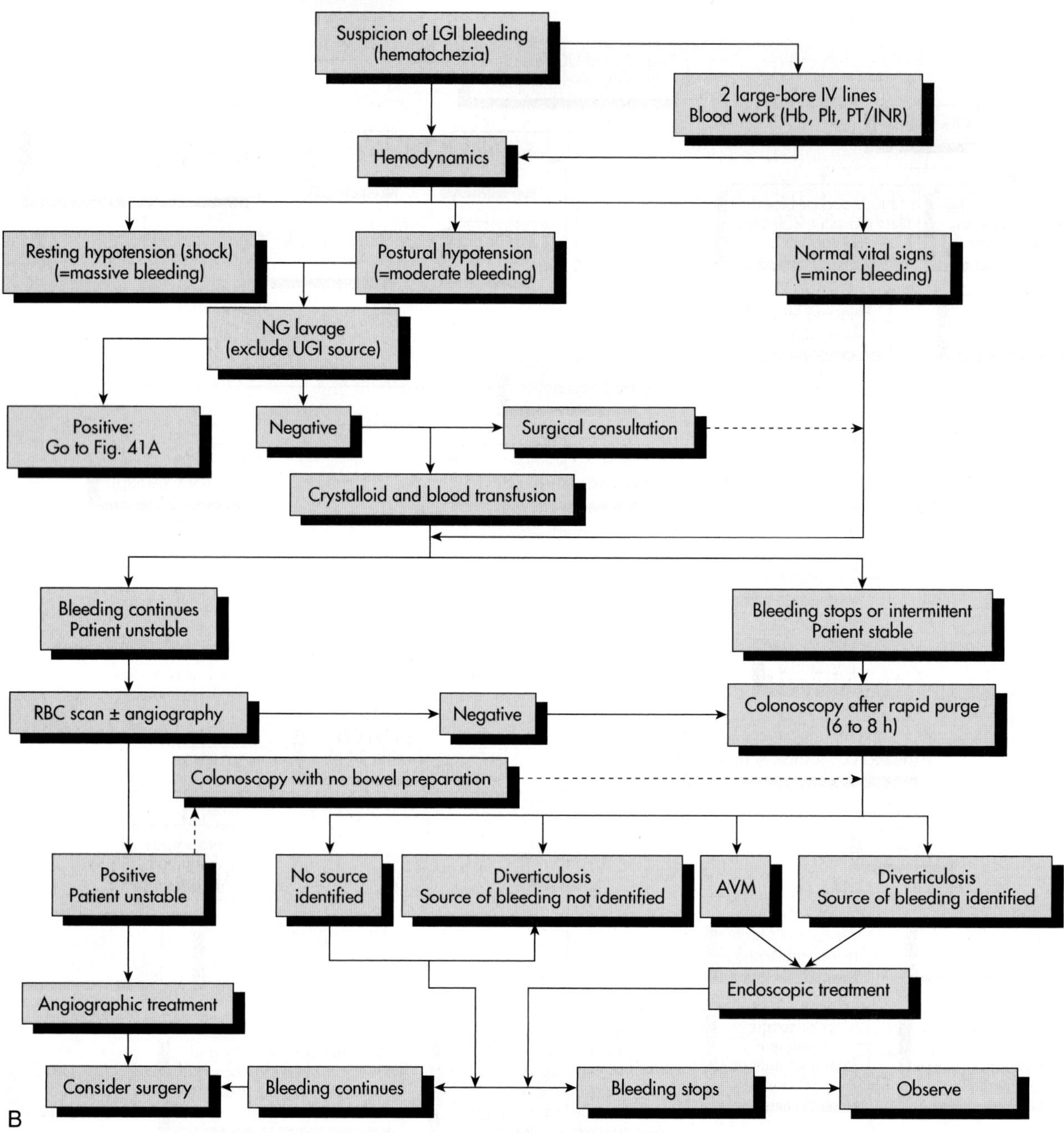

FIG. 34 (Continued)

Monitoring	Rhythm	Therapy
Unresponsive, apneic, and pulseless		CPR[a]
ECG by pads, quick look paddles, or limb leads	VF/VT	Defibrillate[b]
	PEA	• CPR • Diagnose and treat underlying cause[c] • Differentiate EMD vs. pseudo-EMD (vascular Doppler, echocardiography, arterial line)
	Asystole	• CPR • Diagnosis and treat underlying cause
$PETco_2$[h]	All rhythms	• Continue CPR • Advanced airway[d] confirm tube placement and ventilate • Intravenous access • Titrate chest compressions $PETco_2$ >10 mm Hg
	All rhythms	• Continue CPR • Vasopressor therapy[e]
	VF/VT	• Antidysrhythmic agent simultaneous to epinephrine[f] • Defibrillate every 2 min or 200 compressions
	PEA	• Atropine if heart rate <60 bpm[g]
Arterial line to monitor arterial diastolic (relaxation) pressure, use $Scvo_2$ catheter[i] if already in place	All rhythms	• Continue CPR and titrate therapy to: • AoDP >40 mm Hg • $Scvo_2$ >40 mm Hg • If CPR inadequate consider emergent extracorporeal circulation (ECMO) if available
	All rhythms	• Continue CPR and vasopressor therapy[e]
	VF/VT	• Additional antidysrhythmic agents[f] • Defibrillate every 2 min or 200 compressions

End resuscitative efforts when cardiopulmonary arrest is refractory to optimized therapy and reversible causes have been corrected.

FIG. 35 Emergency treatment algorithm for treatment of cardiac arrest. [a]If arrest is witnessed and known to be of short duration, immediate rhythm assessment and defibrillation or ventricular fibrillation/ventricular tachycardia (VF/VT) precede cardiopulmonary resuscitation (CPR). In cases of prolonged untreated VF/VT, 1 to 2 minutes of CPR before defibrillation may enhance the ability to achieve return of spontaneous circulation. *EMD,* Electromechanical dissociation; *PEA,* pulseless electrical activity. [b]Biphasic defibrillation should use manufacturer-recommended energy versus monophasic defibrillation (360 J). [c]See Section I, Pulseless Electrical Activity. [d]Endotracheal intubation or supraglottic airway when feasible with minimal interruption in chest compressions. [e]Epinephrine, initial dose of 1 mg intravenously (IV) or intraosseously (IO), or 2.5 mg by endotracheal tube (ETT). Repeat every 3 to 5 minutes. Subsequent doses may be increased up to 0.1 mg/kg. An alternative to epinephrine is vasopressin, 40 U via IV push. Vasopressin is potentially more effective if the presenting rhythm is asystolic. The dose (40 U) can be repeated once in 3 minutes, followed by administration of epinephrine every 3 to 5 minutes. [f]Amiodarone, 300 mg via IV push, followed by 150 mg every 30 minutes. Lidocaine is an alternative antidysrhythmic if amiodarone is not available. Magnesium sulfate, 1 to 2 g via IV push in torsades de pointes or known hypomagnesemia. [g]Atropine, 1 mg via IV push or 2.5 mg by ETT. Repeat dose every 3 to 5 minutes to a total dose of 0.04 mg/kg. *AoDP,* Aortic diastolic pressure; *ECG,* electrocardiogram; *$Scvo_2$,* central venous oxygen saturation. [h]Changes in the partial pressure of end-tidal carbon dioxide ($PETco_2$) may not be predictive of myocardial blood flow in the setting of high-dose vasopressor therapy. [i]Invasive monitoring should be performed only if adequate personnel are available and if it would not delay therapeutic interventions. (From Marx JA et al: *Rosen's emergency medicine,* ed 8, Philadelphia, 2014, Saunders.)

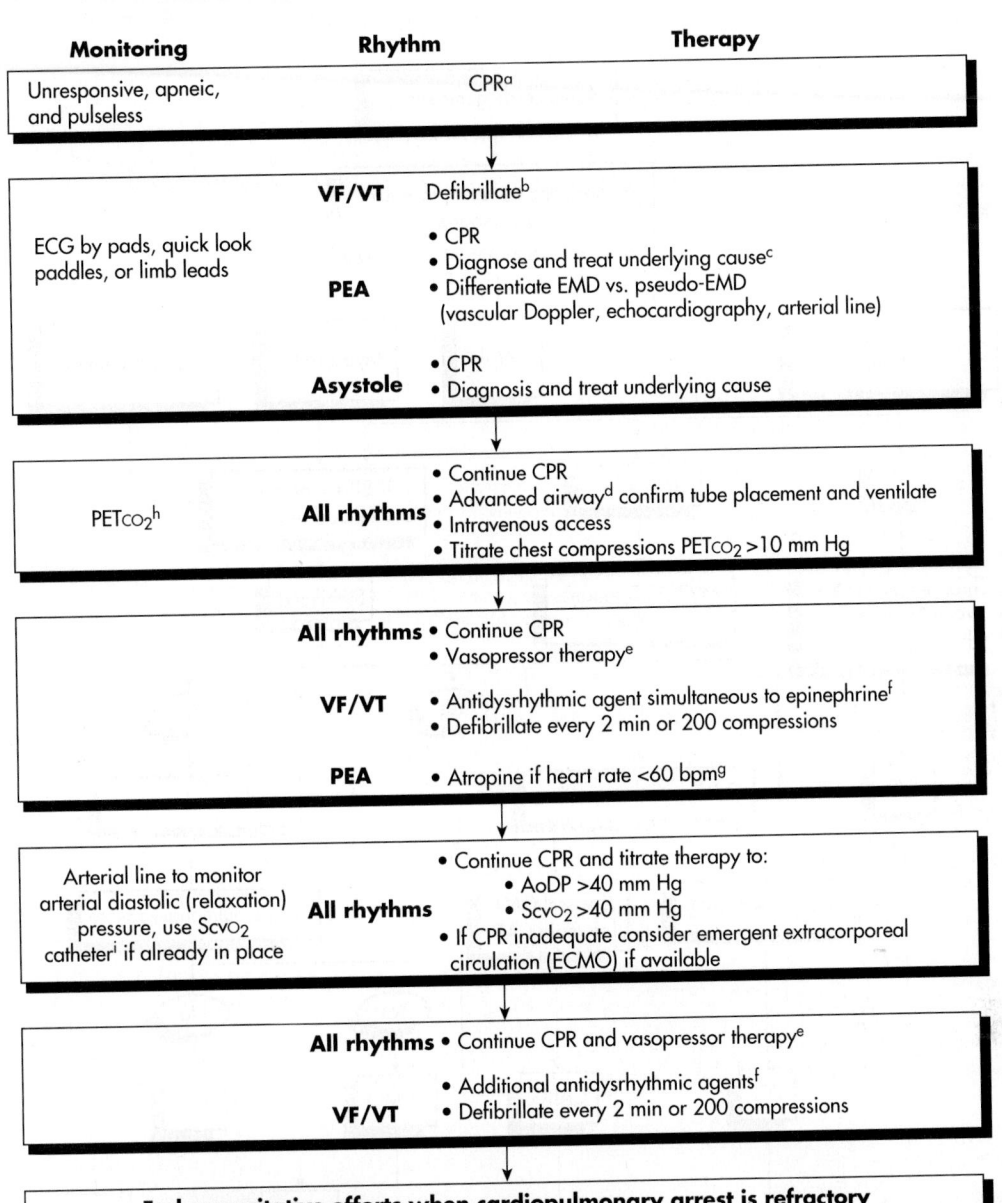

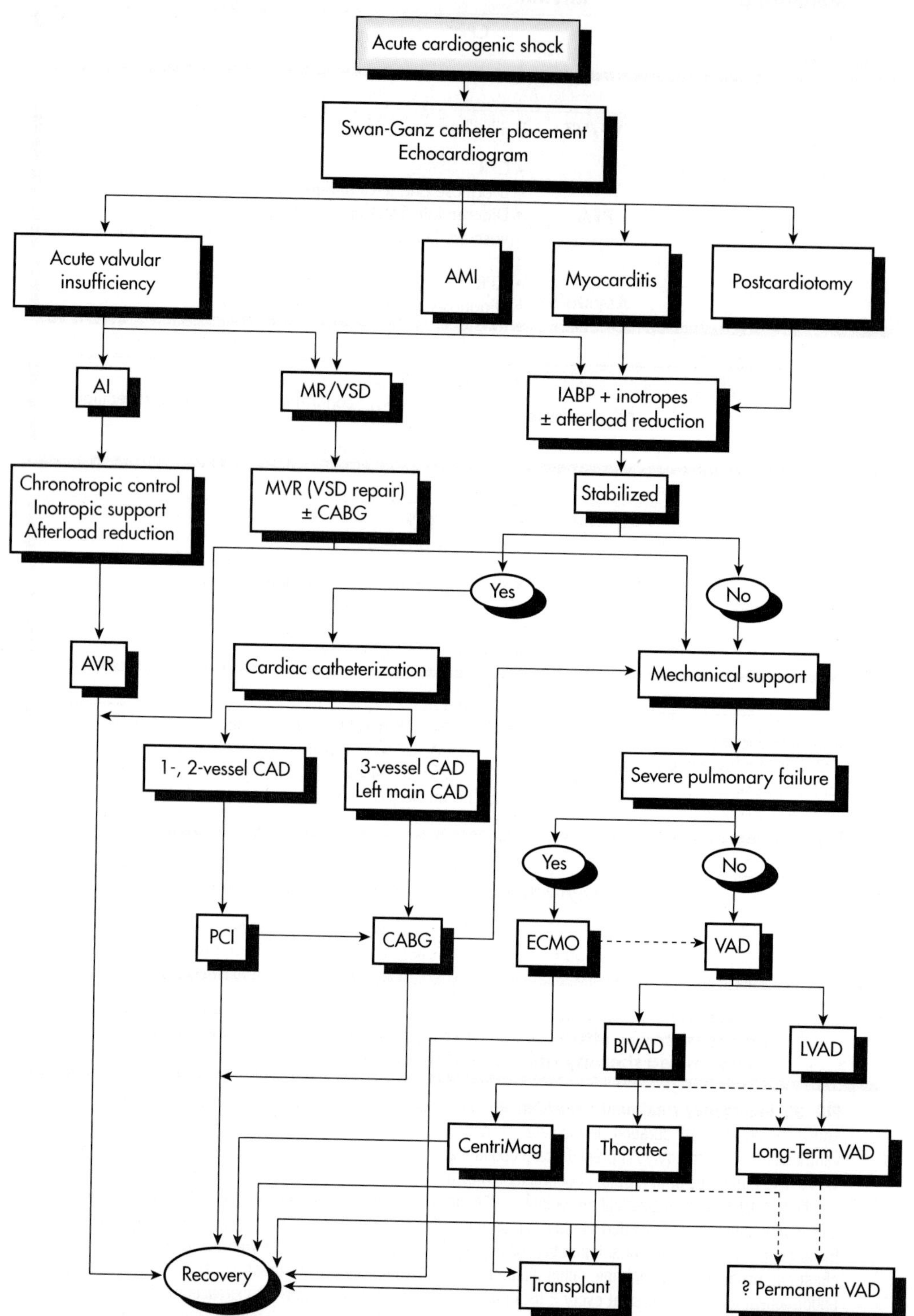

FIG. 36 Algorithm for the management of acute cardiogenic shock. *AI*, Aortic insufficiency; *AMI*, acute myocardial infarction; *AVR*, Acute valvular regurgitation; *BIVAD*, biventricular assist device; *CABG*, coronary artery bypass grafting; *CAD*, coronary artery disease; *ECMO*, extracorporeal membrane oxygenation; *IABP*, intraaortic balloon pump; *LVAD*, left ventricular assist device; *MR*, mitral regurgitation; *VAD*, ventricular assist device; *VSD*, ventricular septal defect. (From Vincent JL et al: *Textbook of critical case*, ed 7, Philadelphia, 2017, Elsevier.)

CARDIOMEGALY ON CHEST X-RAY

ICD-10CM #		
	I51.7	Cardiomegaly
	Q24.8	Other specified congenital malformations of heart
	I11.9	Hypertensive heart disease without heart failure
	I11.0	Hypertensive heart disease with heart failure
	Q23.8	Other congenital malformations of aortic and mitral valves

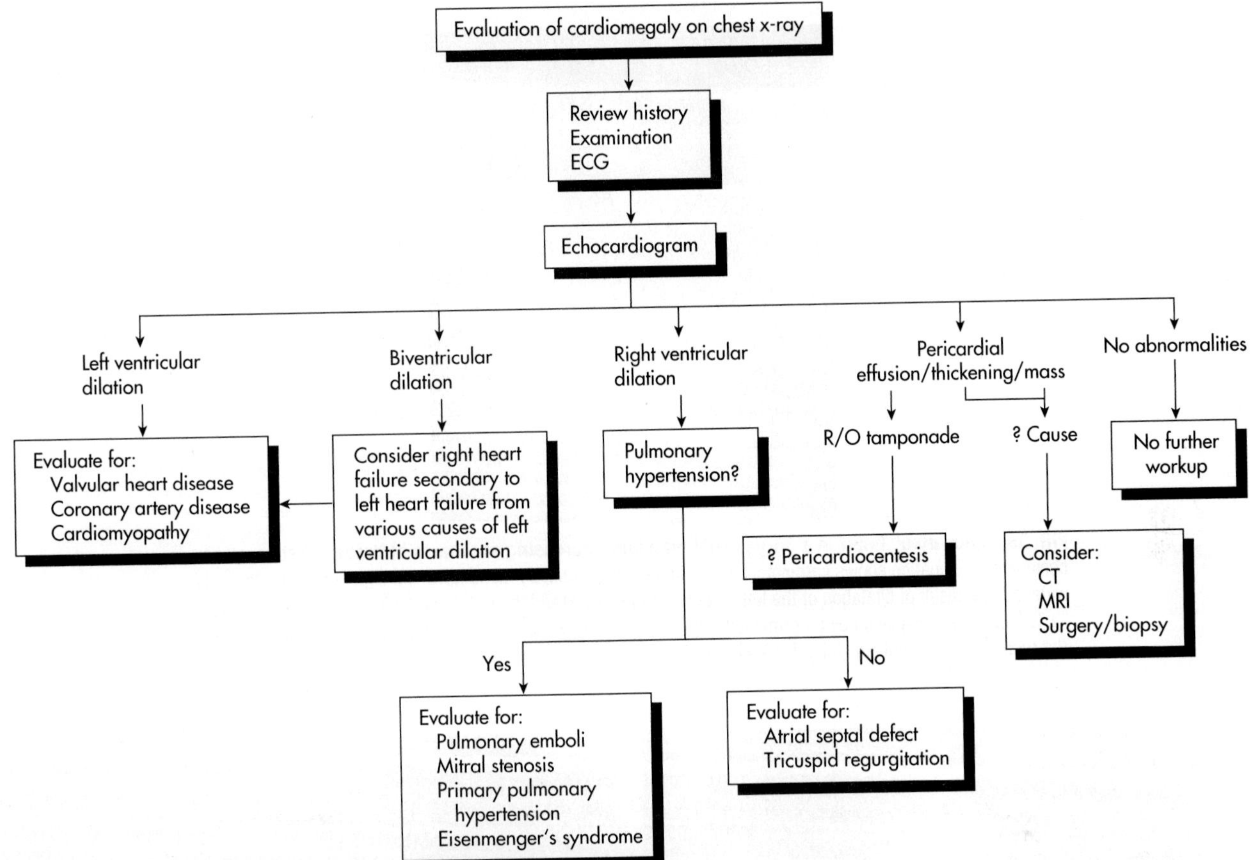

FIG. 37 Approach to the patient with cardiomegaly. When cardiomegaly is found on the chest radiograph, the history and physical examination should be reviewed and an electrocardiogram *(ECG)* performed before obtaining a two-dimensional Doppler echocardiographic study. Cardiomegaly may be explained by left ventricular dilation, biventricular dilation, right ventricular dilation, or pericardial abnormalities, or it may be found to be spurious on the echocardiogram. Rarely, isolated abnormalities of the atrium, particularly the left atrium, may cause abnormalities on the chest radiograph but will not cause true cardiomegaly. Depending on the echocardiographic findings, further tests can help elucidate the cause of echocardiographically confirmed cardiomegaly. *CT*, Computed tomography; *MRI*, magnetic resonance imaging; *R/O*, rule out. (From Goldman L, Braunwald E [eds]: *Primary cardiology*, ed 2, Philadelphia, 2003, Saunders.)

ICD-10CM #		
	I51.7	Cardiomegaly
	Q24.8	Other specified congenital malformations of heart
	I11.9	Hypertensive heart disease without heart failure
	I11.0	Hypertensive heart disease with heart failure
	Q23.8	Other congenital malformations of aortic and mitral valves

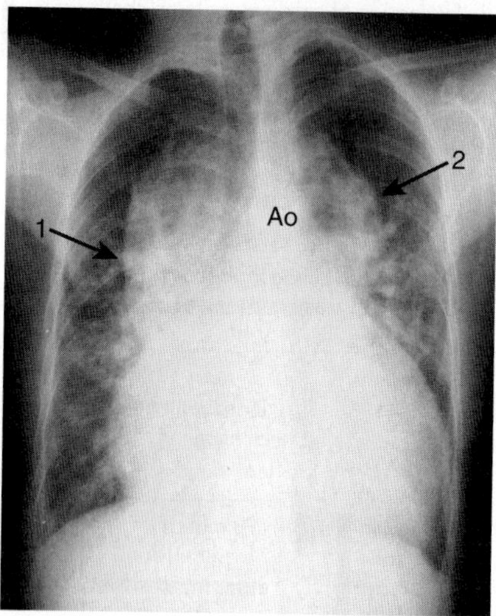

FIG. 38 "Snowman" heart in a 36-year-old man with increasing shortness of breath. Posteroanterior chest film examination shows cardiomegaly and increased pulmonary blood flow. The superior mediastinum is widened, the result of dilatation of the left vertical vein *(arrow 2)* and the right-sided superior vena cava *(arrow 1)*. The trachea is displaced by a normal left-sided aortic arch (Ao). (From Boxt LM, Abbara S: *Cardiac imaging: the requisites,* ed 4, Philadelphia, 2016, Elsevier.)

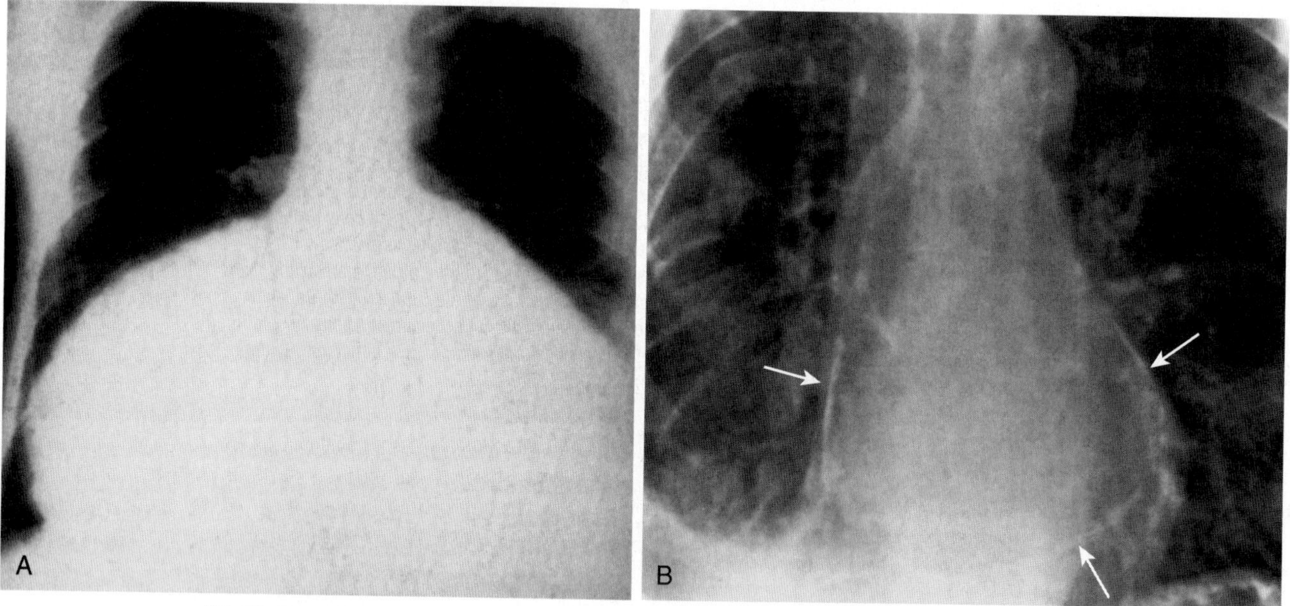

FIG. 39 Chest radiographs in a patient with a very large pericardial effusion. A, "Water bottle" sign. **B,** A patient with constrictive pericarditis and pericardial calcifications (*white arrows*). (From Vincent JL et al: *Textbook of critical care*, ed 7, Philadelphia, 2017, Elsevier.)

ICD-10CM # I51.7 Cardiomegaly
Q24.8 Other specified congenital malformations of heart
I11.9 Hypertensive heart disease without heart failure
I11.0 Hypertensive heart disease with heart failure
Q23.8 Other congenital malformations of aortic and mitral valves

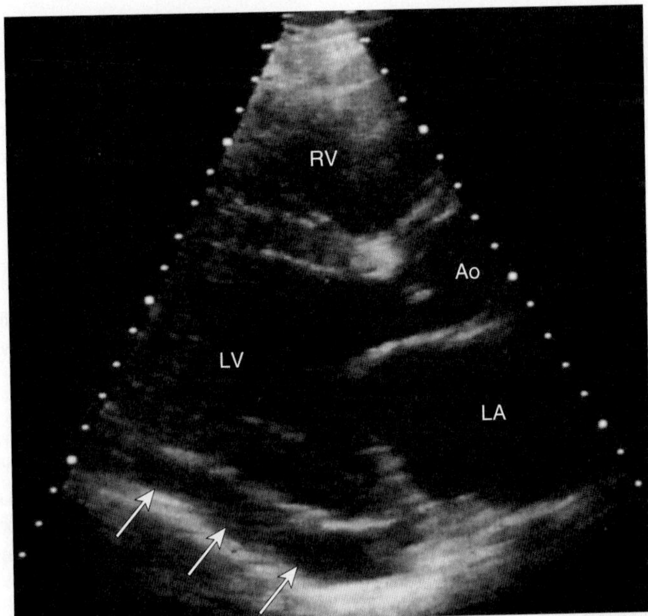

FIG. 40 Echocardiographic findings in a small to moderate pericardial effusion (*white arrows*). *Ao*, aortic root; *LA*, left atrium; *LV*, left ventricle; *RV*, right ventricle. (From Vincent JL et al: *Textbook of critical care*, ed 7, Philadelphia, 2017, Elsevier.)

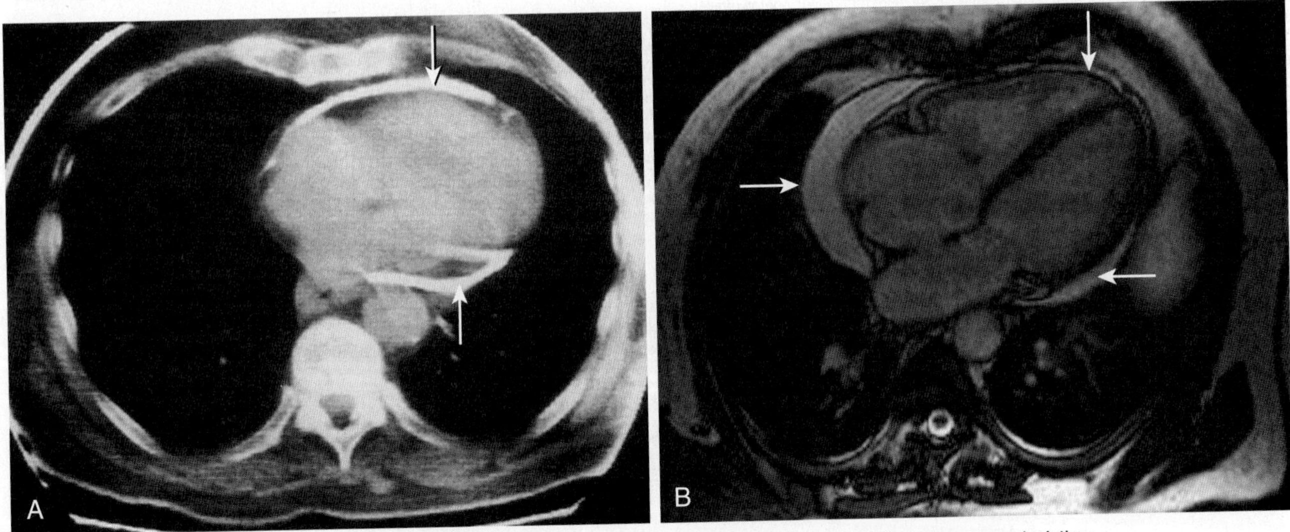

FIG. 41 A, Computed tomography findings in constrictive pericarditis. White vertical arrows are depicting thickened pericardium and pericardial calcification. **B,** The magnetic resonance imaging results of a patient with effusive-constrictive pericarditis are shown in the right image. Horizontal arrows show a loculated pericardial effusion, and the vertical arrow shows thickened pericardium. (From Vincent JL et al: *Textbook of critical care*, ed 7, Philadelphia, 2017, Elsevier.)

ICD-10CM #
I51.7 Cardiomegaly
Q24.8 Other specified congenital malformations of heart
I11.9 Hypertensive heart disease without heart failure
I11.0 Hypertensive heart disease with heart failure
Q23.8 Other congenital malformations of aortic and mitral valves

TABLE 8 Diagnosis of Cardiac Tamponade

Clinical presentation	Elevated systemic venous pressure,* hypotension,† pulsus paradoxus,‡ tachycardia,§ dyspnea, or tachypnea with clear lungs
Precipitating factors	Drugs (cyclosporine, anticoagulants, thrombolytics), recent cardiac surgery, indwelling instrumentation, blunt chest trauma, malignancies, connective tissue disease, renal failure, septicemia‖
ECG	Can be normal or nonspecifically changed (ST-T wave), electrical alternans (QRS, rarely T), bradycardia (end stage), electromechanical dissociation (agonal phase)
Chest radiograph	Enlarged cardiac silhouette with clear lungs
M-mode/two-dimensional echocardiogram	Diastolic collapse of the anterior RV free wall,¶ RA collapse, LA and rarely LV collapse, increased LV diastolic wall thickness "pseudohypertrophy," IVC dilatation (no collapse in inspiration), "swinging heart"
Doppler	Tricuspid flow increases and mitral flow decreases during inspiration (reverse in expiration)
	Systolic and diastolic flows are reduced in systemic veins in expiration and reverse flow with atrial contraction is increased
M-mode color Doppler	Large respiratory fluctuations in mitral/tricuspid flows
Cardiac catheterization	Confirmation of the diagnosis and quantification of the hemodynamic compromise
	RA pressure is elevated (preserved systolic × descent and absent or diminished diastolic y descent)
	Intrapericardial pressure is also elevated and virtually identical to RA pressure (both pressures fall in inspiration)
	RV mid-diastolic pressure is elevated and equal to the RA and pericardial pressures (no dip-and-plateau configuration)
	Pulmonary artery diastolic pressure is slightly elevated and may correspond to the RV pressure
	Pulmonary capillary wedge pressure is also elevated and nearly equal to intrapericardial and right atrial pressure
	LV systolic and aortic pressures may be normal or reduced
	Documenting that pericardial aspiration is followed by hemodynamic improvement**
	Detection of coexisting hemodynamic abnormalities (LV failure, constriction, pulmonary hypertension)
	Detection of associated cardiovascular diseases (cardiomyopathy, coronary artery disease)
RV/LV angiography	Atrial collapse and small hyperactive ventricular chambers
Coronary angiography	Coronary compression in diastole

IVC, Inferior vena cava; *LA*, left atrium; *LV*, left ventricle; *RA*, right atrium; *RV*, right ventricle.

*Jugular venous distention is less notable in hypovolemic patients or in "surgical tamponade." An inspiratory increase or lack of fall of pressure in the neck veins (Kussmaul sign), when verified by tamponade or after pericardial drainage, indicates effusive-constrictive disease.

†Heart rate is usually greater than 100 beats per minute but may be lower in patients with hypothyroidism or uremia.

‡Pulsus paradoxus is defined as a drop in systolic blood pressure greater than 10 mm Hg during inspiration, while diastolic blood pressure remains unchanged. It is easily detected by simply feeling the pulse, which diminishes significantly during inspiration. Clinically significant pulsus paradoxus is apparent when the patient is breathing normally. When this sign is present only in deep inspiration, it should be interpreted with caution. The magnitude of pulsus paradoxus is evaluated by sphygmomanometry. If pulsus paradoxus is present, the first Korotkoff sound is not heard equally well throughout the respiratory cycle but only during expiration at a given blood pressure. The blood pressure cuff is therefore inflated above the patient's systolic pressure. Then it is slowly deflated, while the clinician observes the phase of respiration. During deflation, the first Korotkoff sound is intermittent. Correlation with the patient's respiratory cycle identifies a point at which the sound is audible during expiration but disappears when the patient breathes in. As the cuff pressure drops further, another point is reached when the first blood pressure sound is audible throughout the respiratory cycle. The difference in systolic pressure between these two points is the clinical measure of pulsus paradoxus. Pulsus paradoxus is absent in tamponade complicating an atrial septal defect and in patients with significant aortic regurgitation.

§Occasional patients are hypertensive, especially if they have preexisting hypertension.

‖Febrile tamponade may be misdiagnosed as septic shock.

¶Right ventricular collapse can be absent in elevated right ventricular pressure and right ventricular hypertrophy or in right ventricular infarction.

**If after drainage of the pericardial effusion, the intrapericardial pressure does not fall below atrial pressure, effusive-constrictive disease should be considered.

From Vincent JL et al: *Textbook of critical care,* ed 7, Philadelphia, 2017, Elsevier.

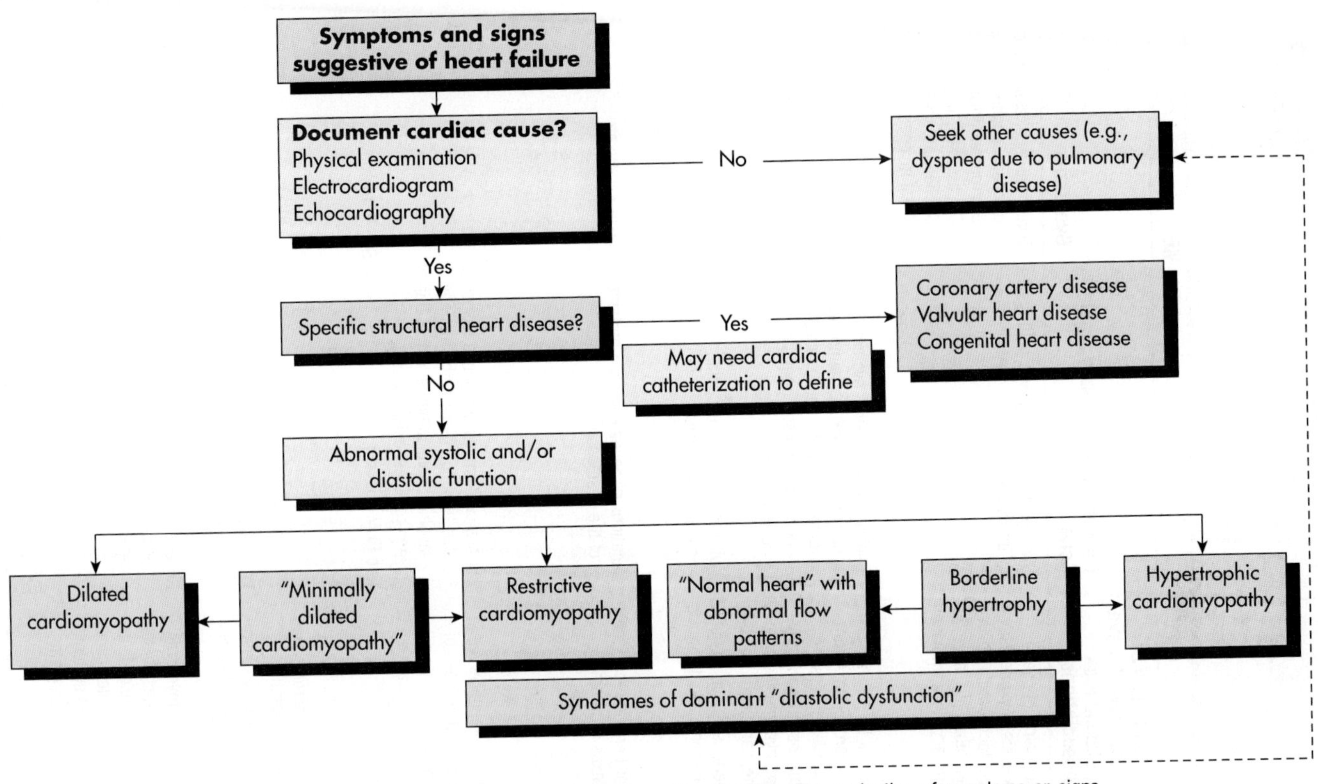

FIG. 42 Initial approach to classification of cardiomyopathy. The evaluation of symptoms or signs consistent with heart failure first includes confirmation that they can be attributed to a cardiac cause. Although this conclusion is often apparent from routine physical examination and electrocardiography, echocardiography serves to confirm cardiac disease and provides clues to the presence of other cardiac diseases, such as focal abnormalities suggesting primary valve disease or congenital heart disease. Having excluded these conditions, cardiomyopathy is generally considered to be dilated, restrictive, or hypertrophic, as shown in the figure. Patients with apparently normal cardiac structure and contraction are occasionally found to demonstrate abnormal intracardiac flow patterns consistent with diastolic dysfunction but should also be evaluated carefully for other causes of their symptoms. Most patients with so-called diastolic dysfunction also demonstrate at least borderline criteria for left ventricular hypertrophy, frequently in the setting of chronic hypertension and diabetes. A moderately decreased ejection fraction without marked dilation or a pattern of restrictive cardiomyopathy is sometimes referred to as minimally dilated cardiomyopathy, which may represent either a distinct entity or a transition between acute and chronic disease. (From Goldman L, Schafer AI: *Goldman Cecil medicine,* ed 25, Philadelphia, 2016, Saunders.)

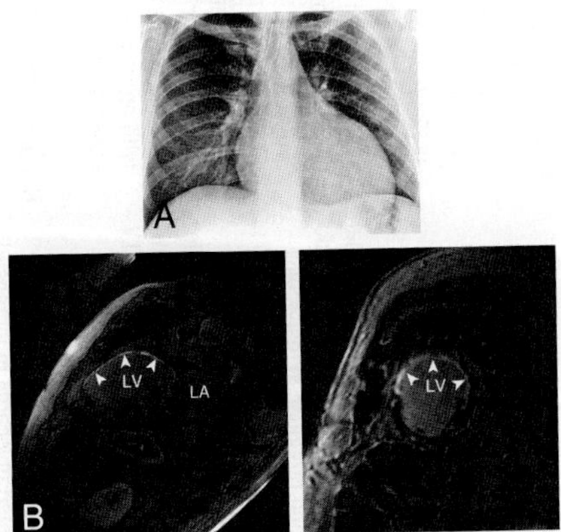

FIG. 43 Dilated cardiomyopathy. A, The heart shows enlargement of all four chambers. The azygos vein and superior vena cava are slightly dilated, reflecting high central venous pressure. **B,** Delayed enhanced magnetic resonance images demonstrate ischemic dilated cardiomyopathy. Extensive subendocardial delayed hyperenhancement *(arrowheads)* demonstrates features of old myocardial infarction: it follows a vascular territory (the left anterior descending), it is based on the subendocardium, and there is thinning of the affected myocardium. *LA,* Left atrium; *LV,* left ventricle. (Boxt LM, Abbara S: *Cardiac imaging: the requisites,* ed 4, Philadelphia, 2016, Elsevier.)

CARDIOMYOPATHY—cont'd

ICD-10CM # I42.5 Other restrictive cardiomyopathy
I42.8 Other cardiomyopathies

TABLE 9 Classification of the Cardiomyopathies by Phenome and Genome

	PHENOME				GENOME	
Type	**Morphology**	**Physiology**	**Pathology**	**Systemic Conditions or Diseases, Clinically Relevant Features, Classic Risk Factors, Associations**	**Nonsyndromic, Usually Single Gene**	**Syndromic**
Dilated (DCM)	LV/RV dilation with minimal or no wall thickening	Reduced contractility is the primary defect; variable degree of diastolic dysfunction	Myocyte hypertrophy; scattered fibrosis	Hypertension; alcohol use; thyrotoxicosis, myxedema; persistent tachycardia; toxins, e.g., chemotherapy, especially anthracyclines; radiation; pregnancy	Diverse gene ontology with >30 genes implicated	Diverse array of associated conditions, especially muscular dystrophies (MDs): Emery-Dreifuss MD, limb-girdle MD, Duchenne/Becker MD; Laing distal myopathy; Barth syndrome; Kearns-Sayre; others
Restrictive (RCM)	Usually normal chamber sizes; minimal wall thickening	Contractility normal or near-normal with a marked increase in end-diastolic filling pressure	Specific to type, diagnosis: amyloid, iron, glycogen storage disease, others	Endomyocardial fibrosis, amyloid, sarcoid, scleroderma, Churg-Strauss syndrome, cystinosis, lymphoma, pseudoxanthoma elasticum, hypereosinophilic syndrome, carcinoid	If not associated with a systemic genetic disease (e.g., hemochromatosis), genetic cause found most commonly to result from sarcomeric gene mutations	Gaucher disease, hemochromatosis, Fabry disease, familial amyloidosis. Mucopolysaccharidoses, Noonan syndrome
Hypertrophic (HCM)	Usually normal or reduced internal chamber dimension; wall thickening pronounced, especially septal hypertrophy	Systolic function increased or normal	Myocyte hypertrophy, classically with disarray	Severe hypertension can confound clinical, morphologic diagnosis	Mutations of genes encoding sarcomeric proteins	Noonan/Leopard, Danon, Fabry, WPW, Friedrich ataxia, MERRF, MELAS
Arrhythmogenic cardiomyopathy (ACM)	Scattered fibrofatty infiltration, classically of the right ventricle but also commonly involving the left ventricle; RV dilation, LV dilation, or both are common although not universal	Ventricular arrhythmias (VT, VF) early or late, reduced contractility with progressive disease; can mimic DCM	Islands of fatty replacement; fibrosis	Palmoplantar keratoderma, wooly hair in Naxos syndrome	Mutations of genes encoding proteins of the desmosome	Naxos syndrome
Left ventricular noncompaction (LVNC)	Ratio of noncompacted to compacted myocardium increased; normal chamber dimensions varying to a DCM phenotype	Normal to reduced systolic function	Myocardium normal and ranging to findings consistent with other coexisting cardiomyopathy	Phenotype has been observed in the setting of other types of cardiomyopathy	Various cardiomyopathy genes associated but uncertain whether genetic cause or developmental defect during organogenesis; see text	
Infiltrative	Usually thickened walls; occasional dilation	Restrictive physiology; systolic function usually mildly reduced	Specific to type, diagnosis: amyloid, iron, glycogen storage disease, others		See RCM above	See RCM above
Inflammatory	Normal or dilated without hypertrophy	Reduced systolic function	Inflammatory infiltrates	Hypereosinophilic syndrome (see text), acute myocarditis		
Ischemic	Normal or dilated without hypertrophy	Reduced systolic function	Areas of infarcted myocardium	Hypercholesterolemia, hypertension, diabetes, cigarette smoking, family history	Familial hypercholesterolemia; other heritable lipid disorders	Familial hypercholesterolemia
Infectious	Normal or dilated without hypertrophy	Reduced systolic function	Specific to infection	Viral (especially acute myocarditis); protozoal (e.g., Chagas); bacterial, direct infection (e.g., Lyme disease), or from acute cellular toxicity as a result of systemic toxins (*Streptococcus*, gram-negatives, etc.)	Genetic predisposition to infection and/or variable response to infective agent	

LV, left ventricle; *MELAS,* mitochondrial encephalopathy, lactic acidosis, and stroke-like symptoms; *MERRF,* myocyclonic epilepsy associated with ragged red fibers; *RV,* right ventricle; *VF,* ventricular fibrillation; *VT,* ventricular tachycardia.
From Mann DL, Zipes DP, Libby P, Bonow RO: *Braunwald's heart disease,* ed 10, Philadelphia, 2015, Elsevier.

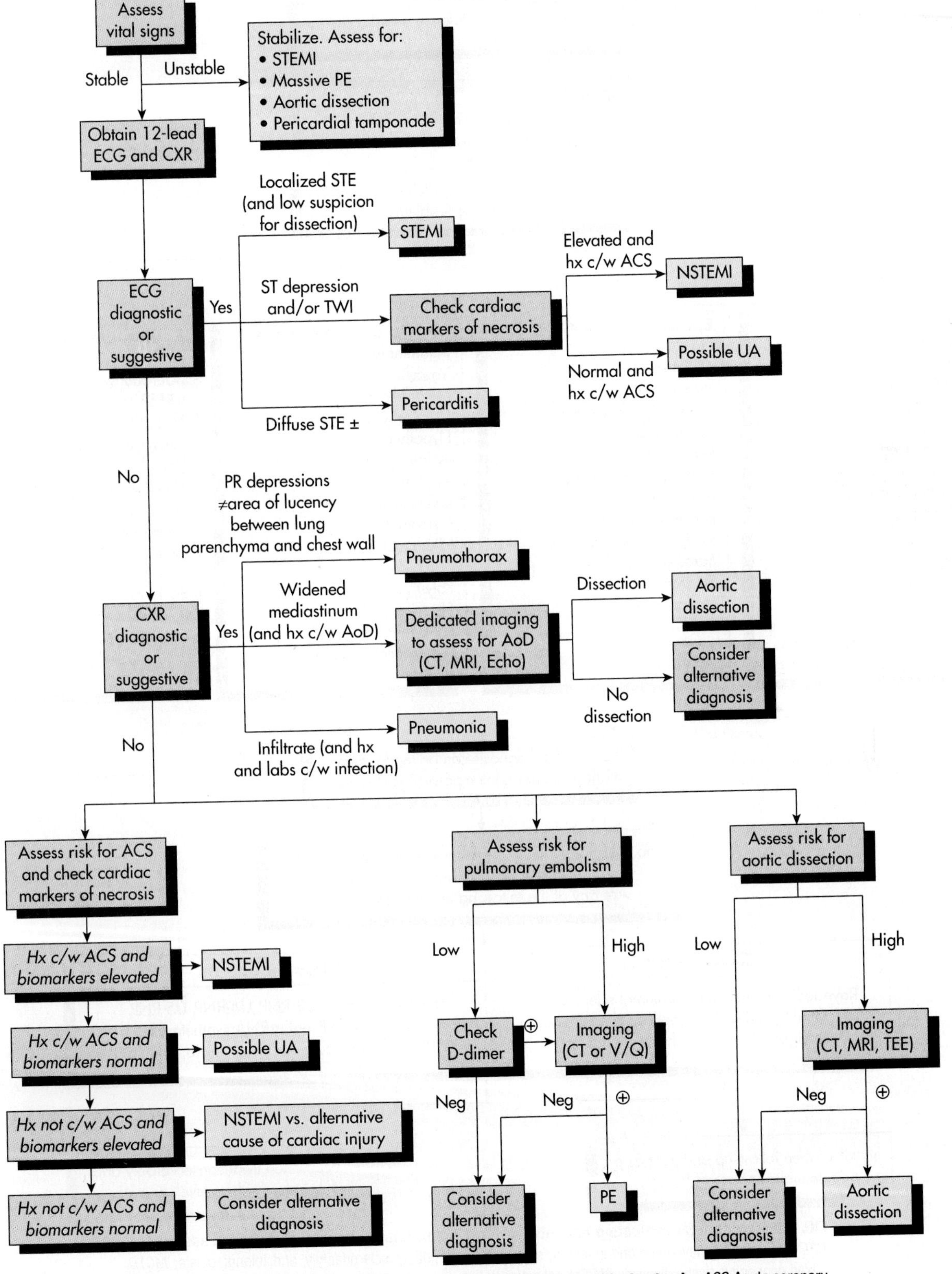

FIG. 44 Algorithm for the initial diagnostic approach to a patient with chest pain. *ACS*, Acute coronary syndrome; *AoD*, aortic dissection; *c/w*, consistent with; *CXR*, chest x-ray; *hx*, history; *NSTEMI*, non–ST-segment myocardial infarction; *PE*, pulmonary embolism; *STE*, ST elevation; *STEMI*, ST-segment myocardial infarction; *TEE*, transesophageal echocardiography; *TWI*, t-wave inversion; *UA*, unstable angina; *V/Q*, ventilation-perfusion scan. (Mann DL, Zipes DP, Libby P, Bonow RO: *Braunwald's heart disease*, ed 10, Philadelphia, 2015, Elsevier.)

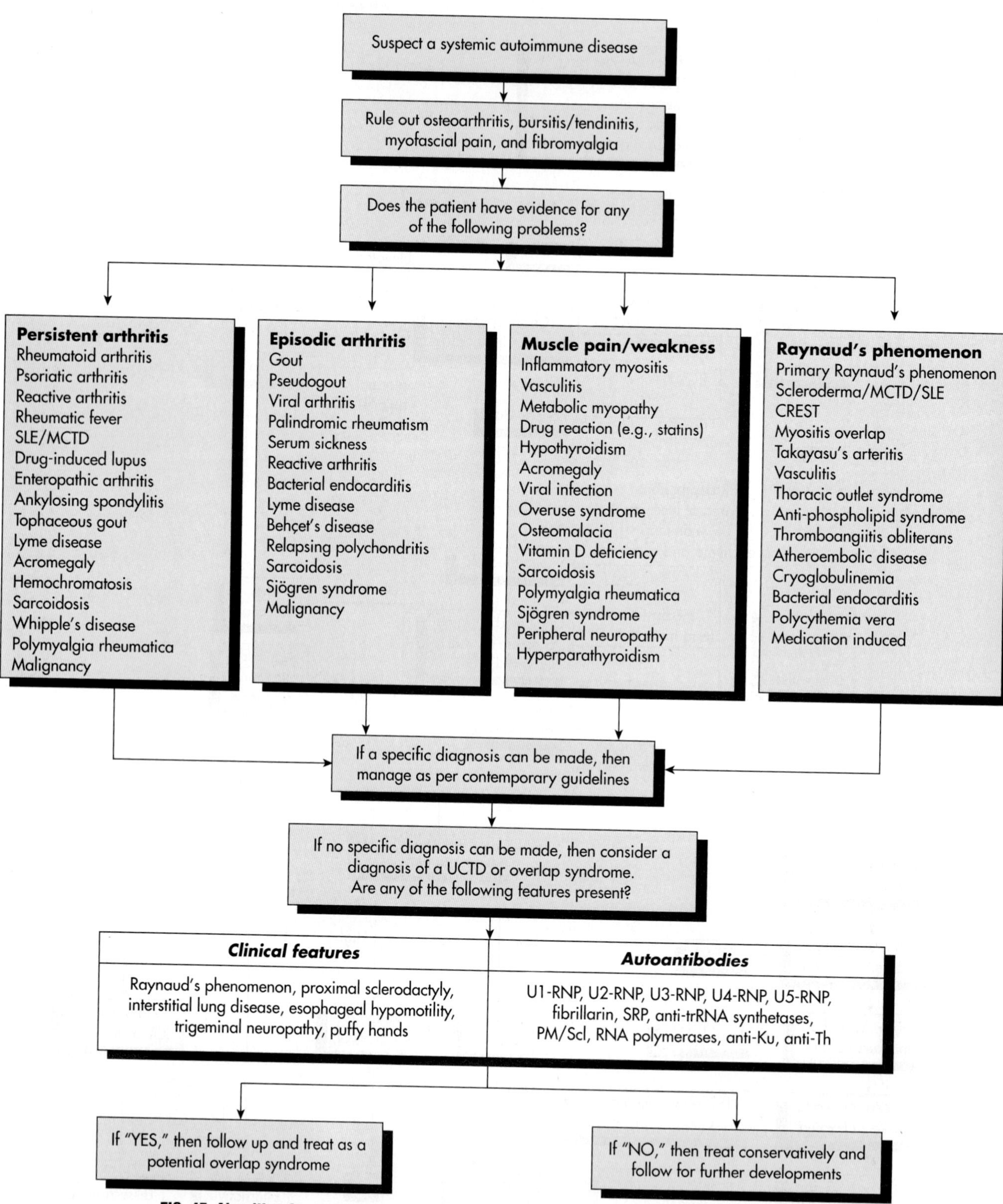

FIG. 45 Algorithm for evaluating patients with undifferentiated connective tissue disease (UCTD). *CREST,* Calcinosis, Raynaud's phenomenon, esophageal dysmotility, sclerodactyly, and telangiectasia; *MCTD,* mixed connective tissue disease; *PM/Scl,* polymyositis/scleroderma; *SLE,* systemic lupus erythematosus; *SRP,* signal recognition particle. (From Firestein GS, Budd RC, Gabriel SE et al: *Kelley and Firestein's textbook of rheumatology,* ed 10, Philadelphia, 2017, Elsevier.)

CONNECTIVE TISSUE LABORATORY TESTS

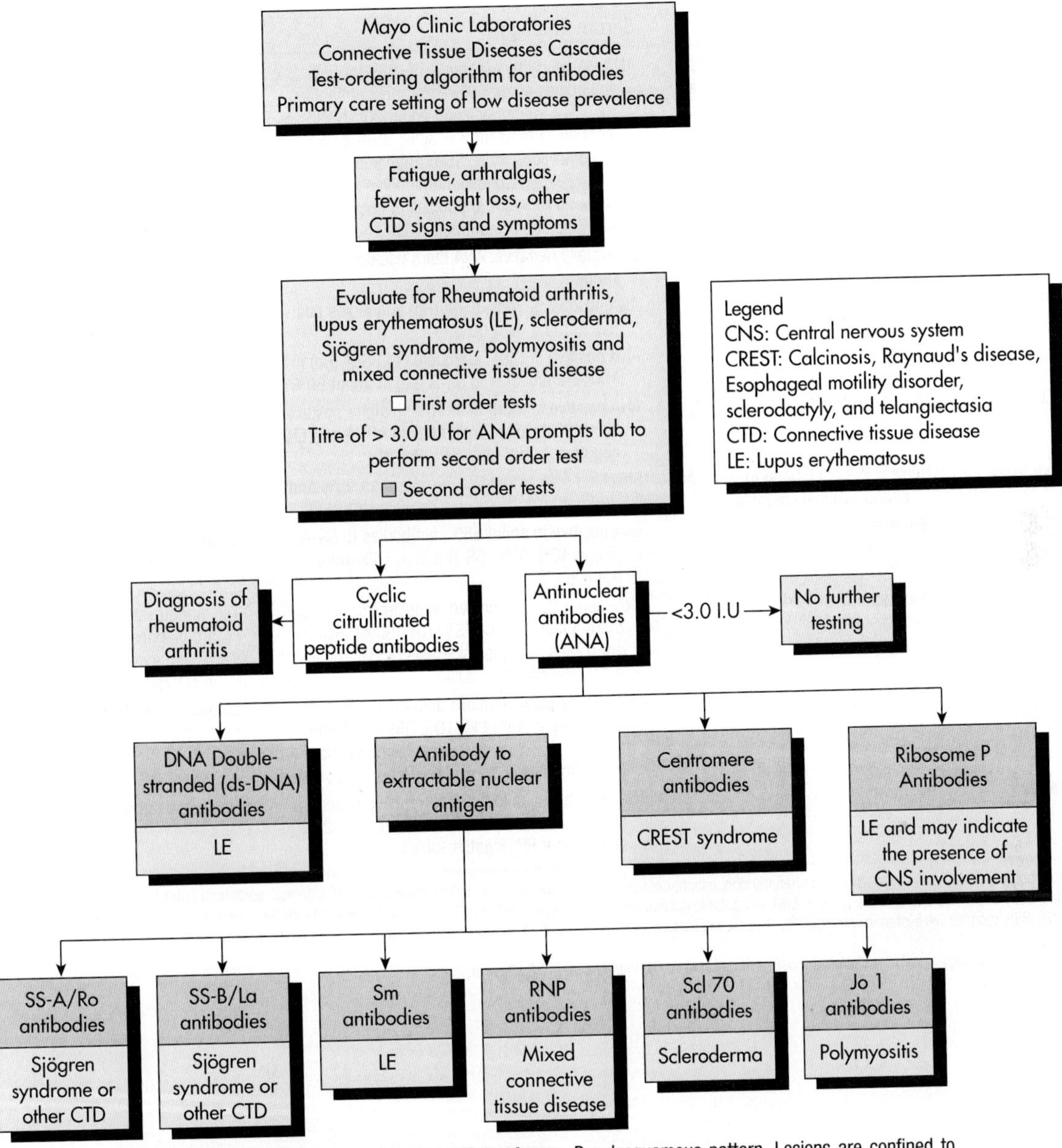

FIG. 46 Subacute cutaneous lupus erythematosus. Papulosquamous pattern. Lesions are confined to exposed areas on the upper half of the body. (From Habif TP: *Clinical dermatology, a color guide to diagnosis and therapy*, ed 6, Philadelphia, 2016, Elsevier.)

TABLE 10 Autoantibody Tests for Connective Tissue Diseases

Antibody	Clinical significance
Antinuclear antibodies	Screening for SLE and PSS
Centromere antibodies	Marker for CREST
Histone antibodies	To exclude drug-induced LE
ENA: Sm antibodies	Marker for SLE
RNP antibodies	SLE, MCTD, scleroderma
SS-A (Ro)/SS-B (La) antibodies	SLE, Sjögren syndrome, SCLE, and others
Scl-70 antibodies	Marker for scleroderma
Jo-1 antibodies	Marker for polymyositis
Ku (Ki) antibodies	Polymyositis/scleroderma overlap, SLE
Phospholipid antibodies (lupus anticoagulant)	Marker for SLE subset with thrombosis: frequent aborters

CREST, Calcinosis, Raynaud phenomenon, esophageal dysmotility, sclerodactyly, and telangiectasia; *ENA,* extractable nuclear antigen; *LE,* lupus erythematosus; *MCTD,* mixed connective tissue disease; *PSS,* progressive systemic sclerosis; *RNP,* ribonucleoprotein; *SCLE,* subacute cutaneous lupus erythematosus; *SLE,* systemic lupus erythematosus.
From Habif TP: *Clinical dermatology, a color guide to diagnosis and therapy*, ed 6, Philadelphia, 2016, Elsevier.

TABLE 11 Diagnostic Significance of Immunologic Findings in Serum and Skin Biopsies in Connective Tissue Diseases

Disease	Biopsy findings: Direct immunofluorescence	Serum findings	Relevance
Systemic LE	LE band (granular immune deposits, IgG, and/or IgM) IgA, C3 at DEJ in lesional and/or normal skin (over 90% in sun-exposed skin)	ANA elevated titers (about 95%-99%); nDNA antibodies about 50%-75%; DNP antibodies <50%; Sm antibodies in about 20%; RNP antibodies in about 5%-30%; SS-A antibodies in about 30%-40%; SS-B antibodies in about 1%-15%; phospholipid antibodies in about 30%-50%; PCNA antibodies in about 2%-10%; Ku(Ki) antibodies in about 10%	DIF, ANA, and ENA usually diagnostic; nDNA and Sm antibodies are diagnostic markers
Discoid LE	LE band, mostly IgG and C in lesion ONLY	Essentially negative; ANA titers usually in normal range	LE band highly characteristic
Subacute, cutaneous LE	LE band in lesion	ANA positive in 70%; SS-A (Ro) antibodies positive in more than 60%	DIF and anti–SS-A (Ro) highly characteristic
Neonatal LE	LE band in lesion (about 50%)	ANA positive in 30%; antibodies to SS-A (Ro) in 100%; antibodies to SS-B (La) in about 60%	DIF and anti–SS-A (Ro) highly characteristic
Drug-induced LE	LE band in lesion (rare)	ANA positive in more than 90%; histone positive about 90%; other antibodies to nDNA and ENA negative	DIF and histone antibodies in absence of other nuclear antibodies highly characteristic
Mixed connective tissue disease	Nuclear IgG or LE band in normal and/or lesional epidermis	Speckled ANA antibodies in more than 95% and RNP antibodies in more than 90%	Serology and/or DIF of nuclei diagnostic for MCTD, SLE, or PSS
Sjögren syndrome	Negative	ANA positive in about 55%; antibodies to SS-A (Ro) in 43%-88%; SS-B (La) in 14%-60%; RF positive	Positive serum results support diagnosis
Progressive systemic sclerosis (scleroderma)	Nucleolar IgG in epidermis in few cases; most negative	ANA (about 85%) speckled or nucleolar; centromere antibody in CREST (70%-90%); Scl-70 antibodies in diffuse sclerosis (45%) and in acrosclerosis (15%-20%)	DIF limited value; centromere antibodies are diagnostic marker in CREST; Scl-70 antibodies are diagnostic marker in scleroderma
Polymyositis/ dermatomyositis	Negative	ANA usually positive (more than 80%); Jo-1 antibodies in 30% PM, 10% DM; SS-A (Ro) antibodies in 55% PM/scleroderma overlap; Ku (Ki) antibodies in 10% PM/scleroderma overlap	Limited value, but positive serum results support diagnosis
Rheumatoid arthritis	Negative	ANA usually negative or low titer; RF positive in about 90%; RNA positive in about 70%-90% and 95% of RF-negative cases	Positive serum results support diagnosis

ANA, Antinuclear antibodies; *CREST,* calcinosis, Raynaud phenomenon, esophageal dysmotility, sclerodactyly, and telangiectasia; *DEJ,* dermal-epidermal junction; *DIF,* direct immunofluorescence; *DM,* dermatomyositis; *DNP,* deoxyribonucleoprotein protein; *ENA,* extractable nuclear antigen; *LE,* lupus erythematosus; *MCTD,* mixed connective tissue disease; *PCNA,* proliferating cell nuclear antigen; *PM,* polymyositis; *PSS,* progressive systemic sclerosis; *RF,* rheumatoid factor; *RNA,* antibodies to rheumatoid arthritis–associated nuclear antigen; *RNP,* ribonucleoprotein; *SLE,* systemic lupus erythematosus.

From Habif TP: *Clinical dermatology, a color guide to diagnosis and therapy,* ed 6, Philadelphia, 2016, Elsevier.

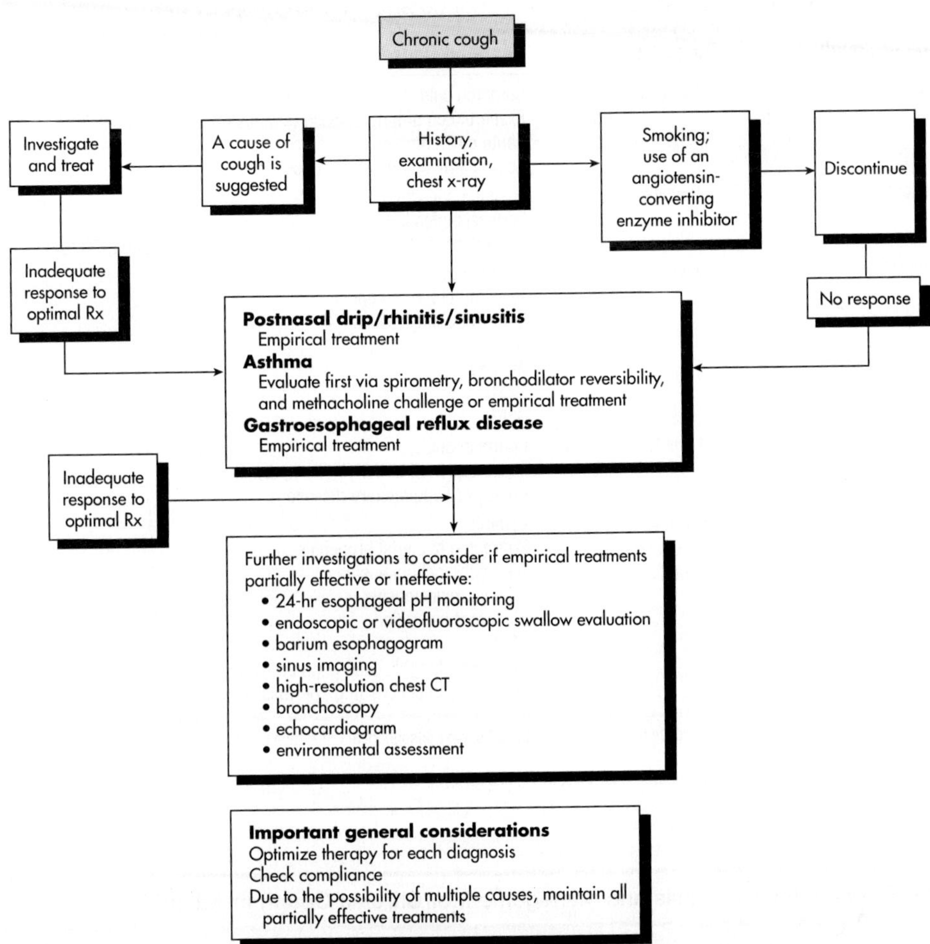

FIG. 48 Algorithm for the management of chronic cough lasting >8 weeks. *CT,* Computed tomography; *Rx,* prescription. (From Goldman L, Schafer AI: *Goldman's Cecil medicine,* ed 24, Philadelphia, 2012, Saunders.)

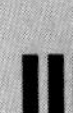

TABLE 12 Testing Characteristics of Diagnostic Protocol for Evaluation of Chronic Cough

Tests	Diagnosis	Positive Predictive Value (%)	Negative Predictive Value (%)
Sinus radiograph	Sinusitis	57-81	95-100
Methacholine inhalation challenge	Asthma	60-82	100
Modified barium esophagography	GERD, esophageal stricture	38-63	63-93
Esophageal pH*	GERD	89-100	>100
Bronchoscopy	Endobronchial mass/lesion	50-89	100

*24-Hour esophageal pH monitoring. *GERD,* Gastroesophageal reflux disease.
From Goldman L, Schafer AI [eds]: *Goldman's Cecil medicine,* ed 24, Philadelphia, 2012, Saunders.

TABLE 13 Definitions and Common Causes of Cough in Adults and Children

Age Group	Type of Cough	Duration	Common Causes
Adults	Acute	<3 weeks	Common cold Exacerbation of lung disease (e.g., asthma) Acute environmental exposure Acute cardiopulmonary disease
	Subacute	3-8 weeks	Postinfectious cough Pertussis infection Exacerbation of underlying lung disease (e.g., asthma, COPD, bronchiectasis)
	Chronic	>8 weeks	ACEI therapy Smoking/chronic bronchitis Underlying lung disease UACS Asthma NAEB GERD
Children	Acute	<4 weeks	Common cold Exacerbation of underlying lung disease Acute cardiopulmonary disease
	Chronic	>4 weeks	Asthma Protracted bacterial bronchitis Tracheobronchomalacia Chronic rhinosinusitis Recurrent aspiration GERD Underlying lung disease (e.g., bronchiectasis) Pulmonary infections (e.g., pertussis)

ACEI, Angiotensin-converting enzyme inhibitor; *COPD,* chronic obstructive pulmonary disease; *GERD,* gastroesophageal reflux disease; *NAEB,* nonasthmatic eosinophilic bronchitis; *UACS,* upper airway cough syndrome.
From Adkinson NF et al: *Middleton's allergy principles and practice*, ed 8, Philadelphia, 2014, Saunders.

BOX 10 Pitfalls and Errors in the Diagnosis and Management of Chronic Cough in Adults

General Considerations

- Failing to consider that UACS, asthma/NAEB, and/or GERD are likely when the chest radiograph is normal or near-normal in appearance and the patient is a nonsmoker and is not taking an ACEI
- Failing to include UACS, asthma/NAEB, and/or GERD in the differential diagnosis because clinical or radiographic evidence confirms the presence of an "obvious" cause of the patient's cough (e.g., solitary pulmonary nodule, idiopathic pulmonary fibrosis)
- Not recognizing multiple simultaneous causes of cough
- Failing to continue treatment trials long enough to accurately assess their effectiveness
- Prematurely diagnosing "unexplained" cough before a bronchoscopy has been performed to assess for unsuspected airway disease
- Mistakenly diagnosing "unexplained" cough or diagnosing psychogenic cough before a complete evaluation for cough has been performed

Upper Airway Cough Syndrome

- Failing to realize that UACS can manifest as cough productive of phlegm
- Not recognizing that chronic cough can be the sole manifestation of UACS in at least 20% of the cases
- Failing to consider sinusitis as a cause of UACS
- Mistakenly assuming that selective histamine H_1 receptor antagonists are effective in treating nonallergic causes of UACS
- Missing allergic rhinitis because symptoms are perennial
- Missing aspirin-exacerbated disease in a patient with nasal polyps

Asthma/NAEB

- Failing to realize that these conditions can sometimes manifest as cough productive of phlegm
- Not recognizing that chronic cough can sometimes be the sole manifestation of asthma (so-called cough variant asthma)
- Mistakenly assuming that a positive result on bronchial challenge (e.g., methacholine challenge) is diagnostic of asthma when it is merely *consistent* with the diagnosis
- Failing to consider NAEB when the bronchial challenge test yields a negative result
- Not recognizing that inhaled medications can sometimes provoke cough
- Failing to consider occupational and environmental causes of asthma/NAEB

Gastroesophageal Reflux Disease

- Failing to realize that GERD can sometimes manifest as cough productive of phlegm
- Not recognizing that chronic cough can sometimes be the sole manifestation of GERD (so-called silent GERD)
- Mistakenly concluding that cough cannot be due to GERD simply because cough does not resolve with relief of gastrointestinal symptoms
- Not considering nonacid reflux and mistakenly assuming that cough will always respond to acid suppression
- Failing to assess the adequacy of GERD treatment by using 24-hour monitoring of esophageal pH and impedance
- Not recognizing coexisting diseases (e.g., sleep apnea) and medications (e.g., nitrates, progesterone) that may impair the effectiveness of GERD treatment
- Failing to recognize that surgery may help when intensive medical therapy has failed

Angiotensin-Converting Enzyme Inhibitor

- Failing to consider ACEI therapy as a cause of chronic cough simply because the cough predated initiation of the ACEI
- Mistakenly concluding that ACEI therapy is not the cause of chronic cough because the cough did not resolve within 1 to 3 weeks of stopping the ACEI

ACEI, Angiotensin-converting enzyme inhibitor; *GERD,* gastroesophageal reflux disease; *NAEB,* nonasthmatic eosinophilic bronchitis; *UACS,* upper airway cough syndrome.
From Adkinson NF et al: *Middleton's allergy principles and practice*, ed 8, Philadelphia, 2014, Saunders.

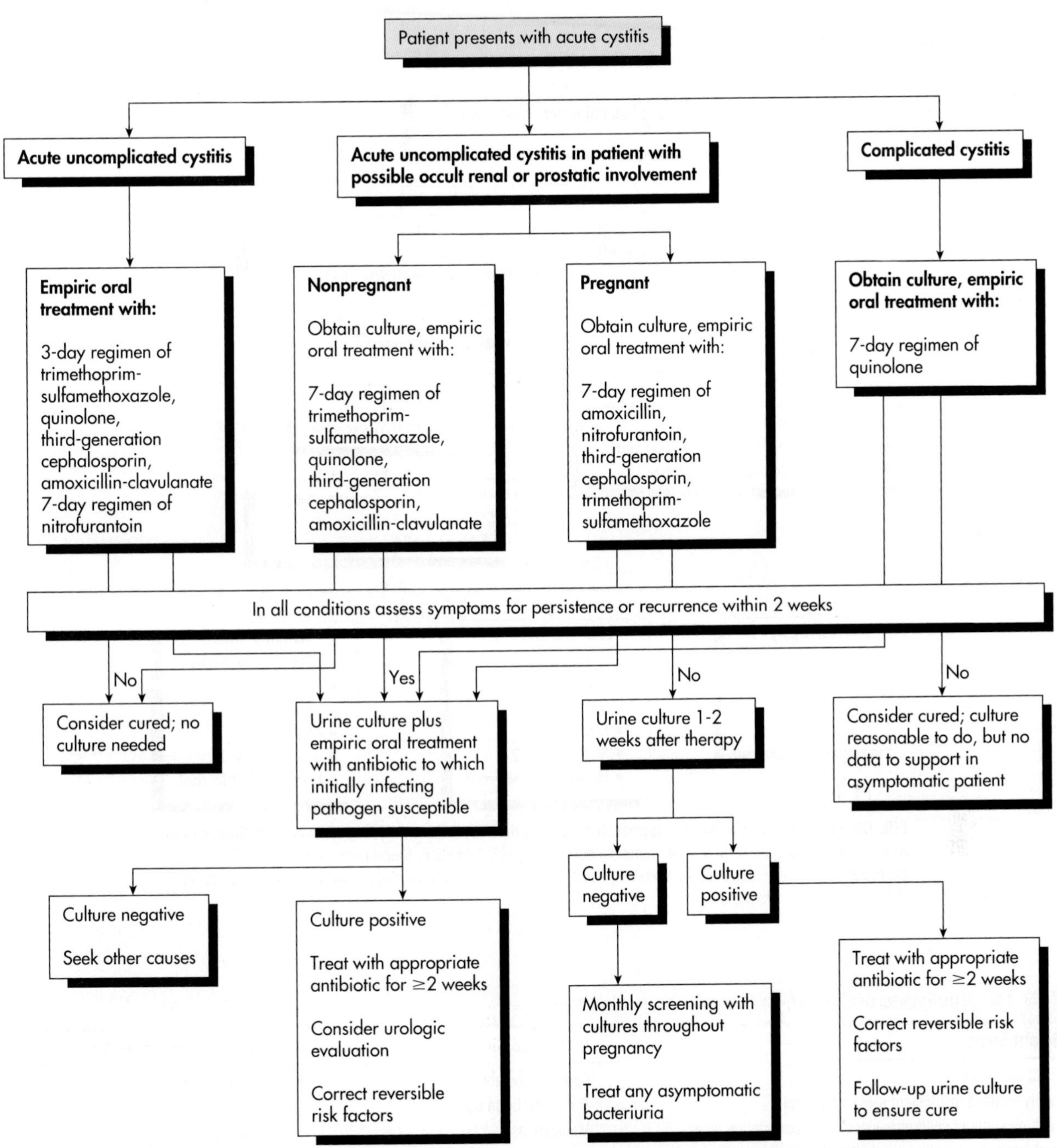

FIG. 49 Algorithm for management of acute cystitis based on severity and complicating factors. (From Johnson R et al: *Comprehensive clinical nephrology*, ed 5, Philadelphia, 2015, Saunders.)

DAYTIME SLEEPINESS, PEDIATRIC PATIENT

ICD-10CM # R40.0 Somnolence
G47.19 Other hypersomnia

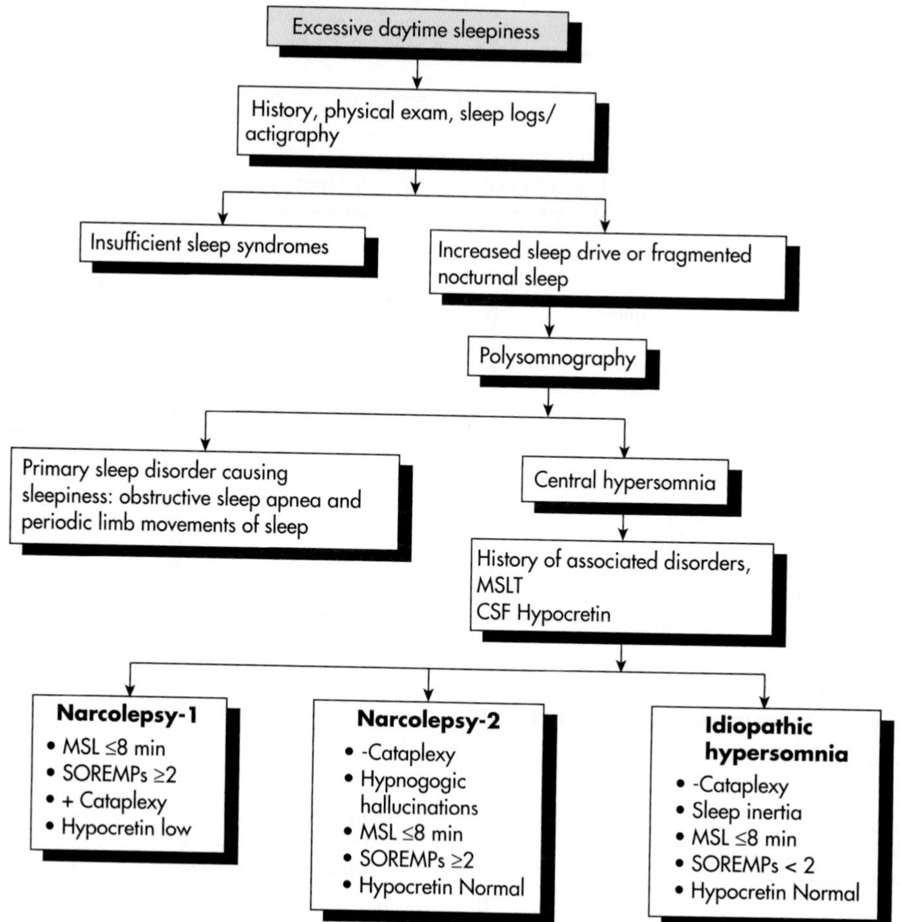

FIG. 50 Algorithm showing the approach in evaluation of children with excessive daytime sleepiness. *CSF*, Cerebrospinal fluid; *MSL*, mean sleep latency; *MSLT*, Multiple Sleep Latency Test; *SOREMPs*, sleep-onset rapid eye movement. (From Swaiman KF: *Swaiman's pediatric neurology, principles and practice,* ed 6, Philadelphia, 2017, Elsevier.)

TABLE 14 Etiologies of Excessive Sleepiness in Children

Insufficient Sleep	Increased Sleep Drive	Fragmented Nocturnal Sleep
Paradoxical insomnia	Central hypersomnias	Primary sleep disorder
Behaviorally induced insufficient sleep syndrome	Traumatic brain injury	GERD
Behavioral insomnia of children—sleep onset association type	Medications	Allergy, eczema
Behavioral insomnia of children—limit setting type	Infections	Asthma
Circadian rhythm sleep disorders	Metabolic disorders	Other medical disorders
Psychophysiological insomnia		Medications
Idiopathic insomnia		Illicit drugs, alcohol

GERD, Gastroesophageal reflux disease.
From Swaiman KF: *Swaiman's pediatric neurology, principles and practice*, ed 6, Philadelphia, 2017, Elsevier.

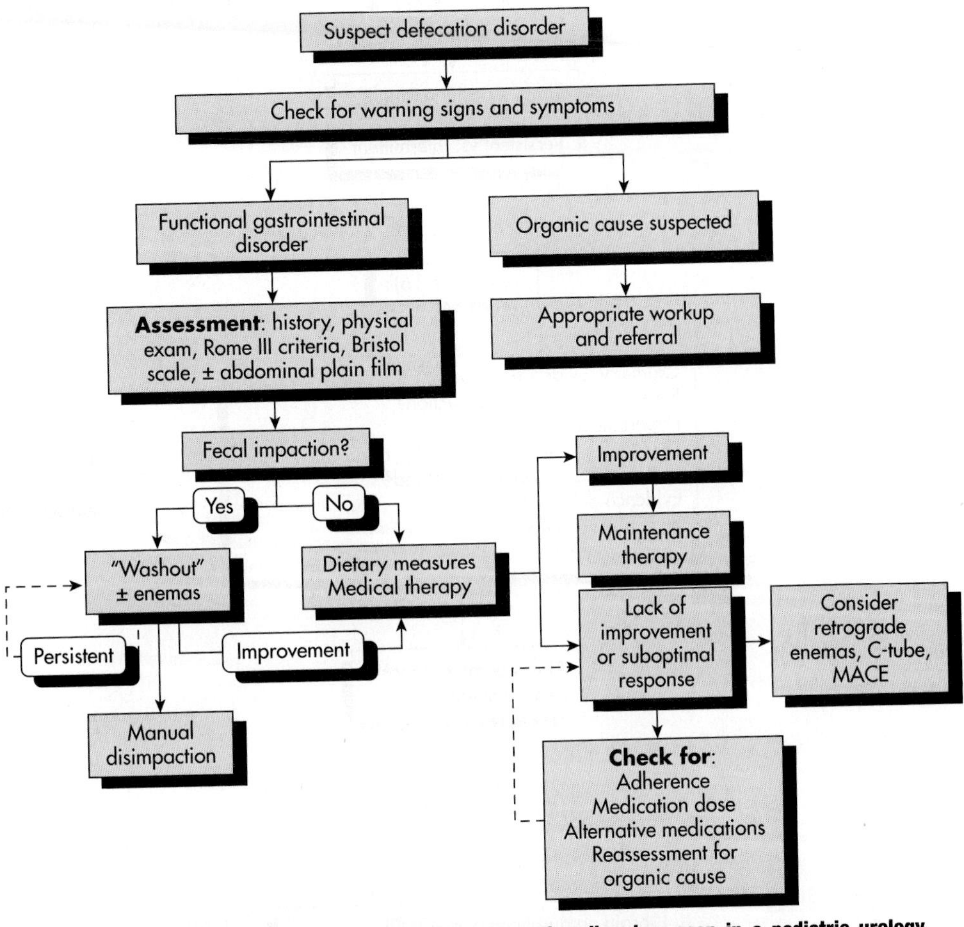

FIG. 51 Management algorithm for childhood defecation disorders seen in a pediatric urology practice. Lack of improvement or intractable constipation should be diagnosed based on worsening response, absence of response, or suboptimal response to adequate medical treatment for at least 3 months. *C-tube*, cecostomy tube; *MACE*, Malone antegrade continence enema procedure. (From Wein AJ, Kavoussi LR, Partin AW, Peters CA: *Campbell-Walsh urology*, ed 11, Philadelphia, 2016, Elsevier.)

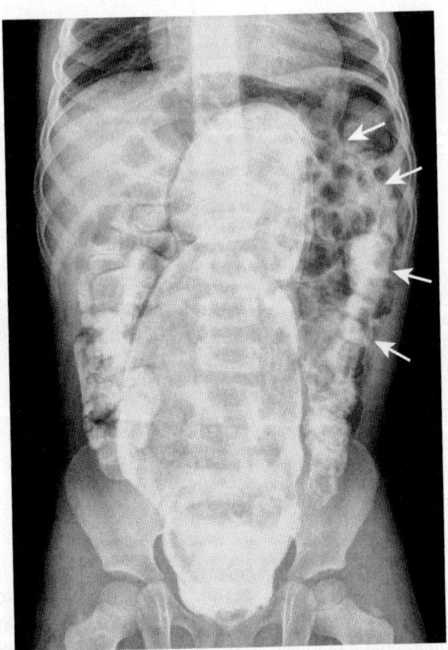

FIG. 52 Soluble contrast enema for evaluation of child with defecation problems since birth. Findings suggestive of Hirschsprung disease, including massively distended colon and rectum that can progress toward more normal-appearing large bowel *(arrows)*. This child was subsequently assessed with a rectal biopsy to confirm the diagnosis. (From Wein AJ, Kavoussi LR, Partin AW, Peters CA: Campbell-Walsh Urology, ed 11, Philadelphia, 2016, Elsevier.)

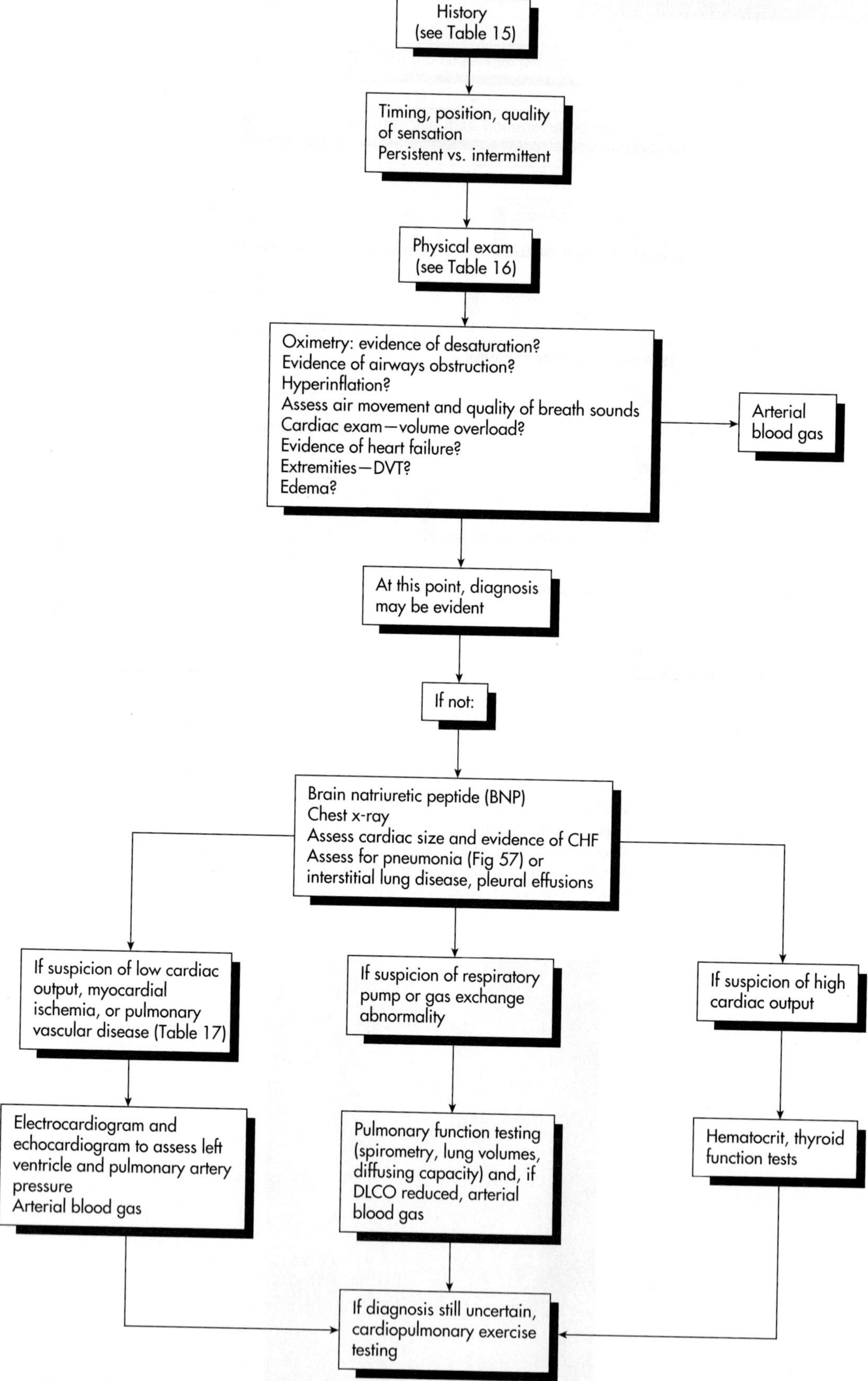

FIG. 56 Algorithm for the evaluation of the patient with dyspnea. The pace and completeness with which one approaches this framework depends on the intensity and acuity of the patient's symptoms. In a patient with severe, acute dyspnea, for example, an arterial blood gas measurement may be one of the first laboratory evaluations, whereas this measurement might not be obtained until much later in the workup in a patient with chronic breathlessness of unclear cause. A therapeutic trial of a medication, for example, a bronchodilator, may be instituted at any point if one is fairly confident of the diagnosis based on the data available at that time. *CHF,* Congestive heart failure; *DLCO,* diffusing capacity of the lung for carbon monoxide; *DVT,* deep venous thrombosis. (Modified from Schwartzstein RM, Feller-Kopman D: Approach to the patient with dyspnea. In Braunwald E, Goldman L [eds]: *Primary cardiology,* ed 2, Philadelphia, 2003, Saunders.)

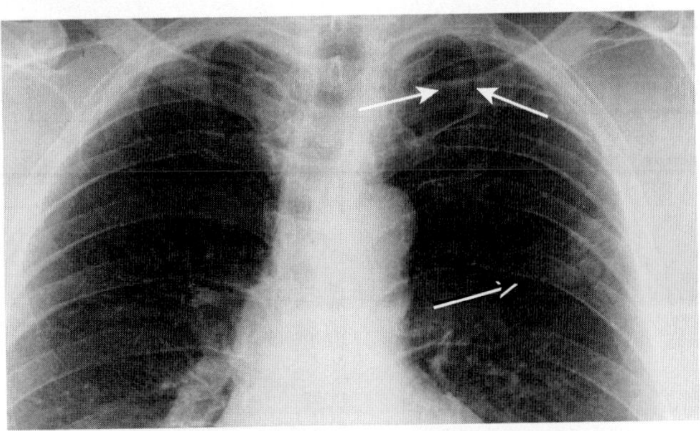

FIG. 57 Chest radiograph of a patient presenting with cough and fever. A faint area of opacification within the left midlung proved to be pneumonia *(black arrow)*. Additionally, a small left apical carcinoma was detected *(white arrows)*. Because of multiple overlying structures, including the first ribs and the clavicles, the pulmonary apices are a "danger" area in terms of risk of missed findings on chest radiographs. Close inspection of the apices is warranted on every chest radiograph. (Soto JA, Lucey BC: *Emergency radiology: the requisites,* ed 2, Philadelphia, 2017, Elsevier.)

TABLE 15 Differential Diagnoses for Acute Dyspnea

Organ System	Critical Diagnoses	Emergent Diagnoses	Nonemergent Diagnoses
Pulmonary	Airway obstruction Pulmonary embolus Noncardiogenic edema Anaphylaxis Ventilatory failure	Spontaneous pneumothorax Asthma Cor pulmonale Aspiration Pneumonia (CAP score >70)	Pleural effusion Neoplasm Pneumonia (CAP score ≤70) COPD
Cardiac	Pulmonary edema Myocardial infarction Cardiac tamponade	Pericarditis	Congenital heart disease Valvular heart disease Cardiomyopathy
Primarily Associated with Normal or Increased Respiratory Effort			
Abdominal		Mechanical interference Hypotension, sepsis from ruptured viscus, bowel obstruction, inflammatory or infectious process	Pregnancy Ascites obesity
Psychogenic			Hyperventilation syndrome Somatization disorder Panic attack
Metabolic or endocrine	Toxic ingestion DKA	Renal failure Electrolyte abnormalities Metabolic acidosis	Fever Thyroid disease
Infectious	Epiglottitis	Pneumonia (CAP score >70)	Pneumonia (CAP score ≤70)
Traumatic	Tension pneumothorax Cardiac tamponade Flail chest	Simple pneumothorax, hemothorax Diaphragmatic rupture	Rib fractures
Hematologic	Carbon monoxide poisoning Acute chest syndrome	Anemia	
Primarily Associated with Decreased Respiratory Effort			
Neuromuscular	CVA, intracranial insult Organophosphate poisoning	Multiple sclerosis Guillain-Barré syndrome Tick paralysis	ALS Polymyositis Porphyria

ALS, Amyotrophic lateral sclerosis; *CAP,* community-acquired pneumonia; *COPD,* chronic obstructive pulmonary disease; *CVA,* cerebrovascular accident; *DKA,* diabetic ketoacidosis.
From Marx JA et al: *Rosen's Emergency Medicine*, ed 8, Philadelphia, 2014, Saunders.

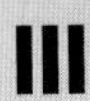

TABLE 16 Pivotal Findings in Physical Examination

Sign	Physical Finding	Diagnoses to Consider
Vital signs	Tachypnea	Pneumonia, pneumothorax
	Hypopnea	Intracranial insult, drug or toxin ingestion
	Tachycardia	PE, traumatic chest injury
	Hypotension	Tension pneumothorax
	Fever	Pneumonia, PE
General appearance	Cachexia, weight loss	Malignancy, acquired immune disorder, mycobacterial infection
	Obesity	Hypoventilation, sleep apnea, PE
	Pregnancy	PE
	Barrel chest	COPD
	"Sniffing" position	Epiglottitis
	"Tripoding" position	COPD or asthma with severe distress
	Traumatic injury	Pneumothorax (simple, tension), rib fractures, flail chest, hemothorax, pulmonary contusion
Skin and nails	Tobacco stains or odor	COPD, malignancy, infection
	Clubbing	Chronic hypoxia, intracardiac shunts, or pulmonary vascular anomalies
	Pallid skin or conjunctivae	Anemia
	Muscle wasting	Neuromuscular disease
	Bruising	Chest wall: rib fractures, pneumothorax
		Diffuse: thrombocytopenia, chronic steroid use, anticoagulation
	Subcutaneous emphysema	Rib fractures, pneumothorax, tracheobronchial disruption
	Hives, rash	Allergic reaction, infection, tick-borne illness
Neck	Stridor	Upper airway edema or infection, foreign body, traumatic injury, anaphylaxis
	JVD	Tension pneumothorax, COPD or asthma exacerbation, fluid overload or CHF, PE
Lung examination	Wheezes	CHF, anaphylaxis
		Bronchospasm
	Rales	CHF, pneumonia, PE
	Unilateral decrease	Pneumothorax, pleural effusion, consolidation, rib fractures or contusion, pulmonary contusion
	Hemoptysis	Malignancy, infection, bleeding disorder, CHF
	Sputum production	Infection (viral, bacterial)
	Friction rub	Pleurisy
	Abnormal respiratory pattern (e.g., Cheyne-Stokes)	Intracranial insult
Chest examination	Crepitance or pain on palpation	Rib or sternal fractures
	Subcutaneous emphysema	Pneumothorax, tracheobronchial rupture
	Thoracoabdominal desynchrony	Diaphragmatic injury with herniation; cervical spinal cord trauma
	Flail segment	Flail chest, pulmonary contusion
Cardiac examination	Murmur	PE
	S_3 or S_4 gallop	PE
	S_2 accentuation	PE
	Muffled heart sounds	Cardiac tamponade
Extremities	Calf tenderness, Homans' sign	PE
	Edema	CHF
Neurologic examination	Focal deficits (motor, sensory, cognitive)	Stroke, intracranial hemorrhage causing central abnormal respiratory drive; if long-standing, risk of aspiration pneumonia
	Symmetrical deficits	Neuromuscular disease
	Diffuse weakness	Metabolic or electrolyte abnormality (hypocalcemia, hypomagnesemia, hypophosphatemia), anemia
	Hyporeflexia	Hypermagnesemia
	Ascending weakness	Guillain-Barré syndrome

CHF, Congestive heart failure; *COPD,* chronic obstructive pulmonary disease; *JVD,* jugular venous distention; *PE,* pulmonary embolism.
From Marx JA et al: *Rosen's Emergency Medicine*, ed 8, Philadelphia, 2014, Saunders.

TABLE 17 Diagnostic Table: Patterns of Diseases Often Resulting in Dyspnea

Disease	History (Dyspnea)	Associated Symptoms	Signs and Physical Findings	Tests
Pulmonary embolism	• HPI: abrupt onset, pleuritic pain, immobility (travel, recent surgery) • PMH: malignancy, DVT, PE, hypercoagulability, oral contraception, obesity	Diaphoresis, exertional dyspnea	Tachycardia, tachypnea, low-grade fever	• Pulse oximetry, ABG (A-a gradient), D-dimer • ECG (dysrhythmia, right-sided heart strain) • CXR (Westermark sign, Hampton's hump), spiral CT, MRV • Pulmonary angiogram • Ultrasound positive for DVT
Pneumonia	Fever, productive cough, chest pain	Anorexia, chills, nausea, vomiting, exertional dyspnea, cough	Fever, tachycardia, tachypnea, rales or decreased breath sounds	CXR, CBC, sputum and blood cultures
Bacterial	SH: tobacco use			Pulse oximetry Waveform capnography if altered mental status, ABG if capnography unavailable and acid-base derangement or hypercarbia suspected
Viral	Exposure (e.g., influenza, varicella)			
Opportunistic	Immune disorder, chemotherapy			
Fungal or parasitic	Exposure (e.g., birds), indolent onset	Episodic fever, nonproductive cough		
Pneumothorax	Abrupt onset: trauma, chest pain, thin males more likely to have spontaneous pneumothorax	Localized chest pain	Decreased breath sounds, subcutaneous emphysema, chest wall wounds or instability	• CXR: pneumothorax, rib fractures, hemothorax • Ultrasound: pneumothorax, pleural effusion
Simple				Ultrasound positive for pneumothorax
Tension	Decompensation of simple pneumothorax	Diaphoresis	JVD, tracheal deviation, muffled heart sounds, cardiovascular collapse	Clinical diagnosis: requires immediate decompression. May verify via bedside ultrasound
COPD or asthma	Tobacco use, medication noncompliance, URI symptoms, sudden weather change	Air hunger, diaphoresis	• Retractions, accessory muscle use, tripoding, cyanosis • "Shark fin" capnograph	• CXR: rule out infiltrate, pneumothorax, atelectasis (mucus plug) • Ultrasound: distinguish from heart failure
	PMH: environmental allergies FH: asthma			Waveform capnography
Malignancy	Weight loss, tobacco, or other occupational exposure	Dysphagia	Hemoptysis	CXR, chest CT: mass, hilar adenopathy, focal atelectasis
Fluid overload	• Gradual onset, dietary indiscretion or medication noncompliance, chest pain • PMH: recent MI, diabetes, CHF	Worsening orthopnea, PND	JVD, peripheral edema, S_3 or S_4 gallop, new cardiac dysrhythmia, hepatojugular reflux	• CXR and/or ultrasound: pleural effusion, interstitial edema, Kerley B lines, cardiomegaly • ECG: ischemia, dysrhythmia • NT-proBNP
Anaphylaxis	Abrupt onset, exposure to allergen	Dysphagia	Oral swelling, stridor, wheezing, hives	

A-a, Alveolar-arterial; *ABG,* arterial blood gas; *CBC,* complete blood count; *CHF,* congestive heart failure; *CT,* computed tomography; *CXR,* chest x-ray examination; *DVT,* deep vein thrombosis; *ECG,* electrocardiogram; *FH,* family history; *HPI,* history of present illness; *JVD,* jugular venous distention; *MI,* myocardial infarction; *MRV,* magnetic resonance venography; *NT-proBNP,* amino-terminal pro-B–type natriuretic peptide; *PE,* pulmonary embolism; *PMH,* past medical history; *PND,* paroxysmal nocturnal dyspnea; *SH,* social history; *URI,* upper respiratory infection.

From Marx JA et al: *Rosen's emergency medicine,* ed 8, Philadelphia, 2014, Saunders.

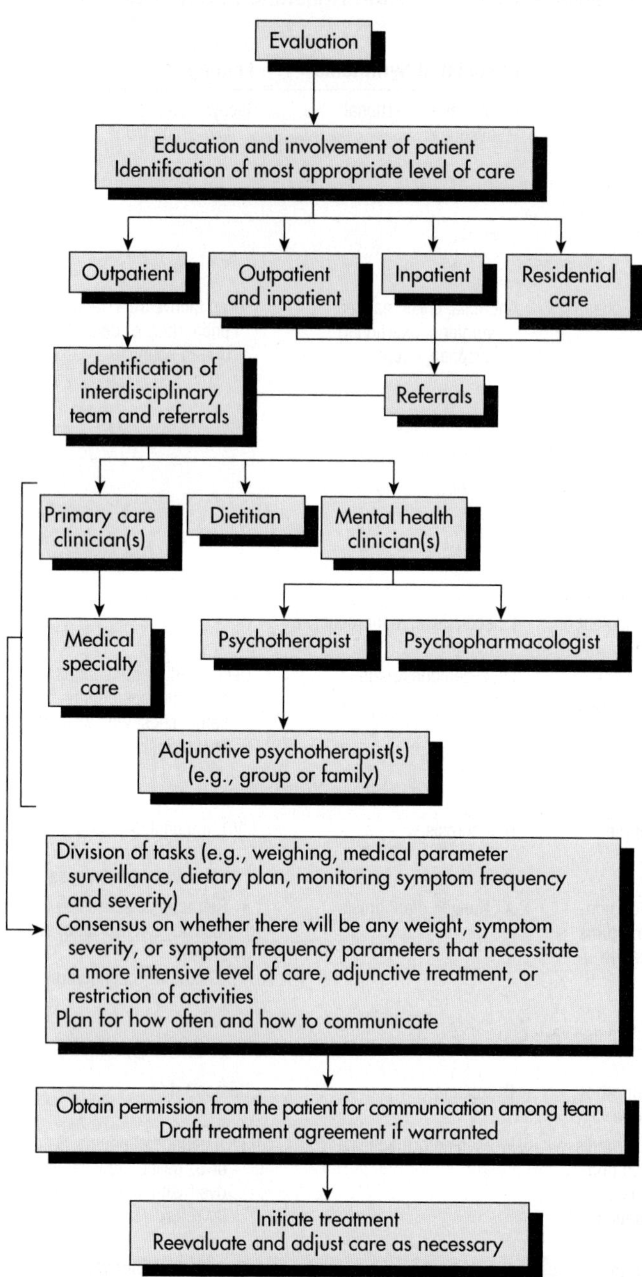

FIG. 58 Algorithm for team management of adult patients with an eating disorder. (Feldman M, Friedman LS, Brandt LJ: *Sleisenger and Fortran's gastrointestinal and liver disease,* ed 10, Philadelphia, 2016, Elsevier.)

ERYTHROCYTOSIS, ACQUIRED

ICD-10CM #		
	D75.1	Secondary polycythemia
	D75.0	Familial erythrocytosis
	D45	Polycythemia vera
	P61.1	Polycythemia neonatorum

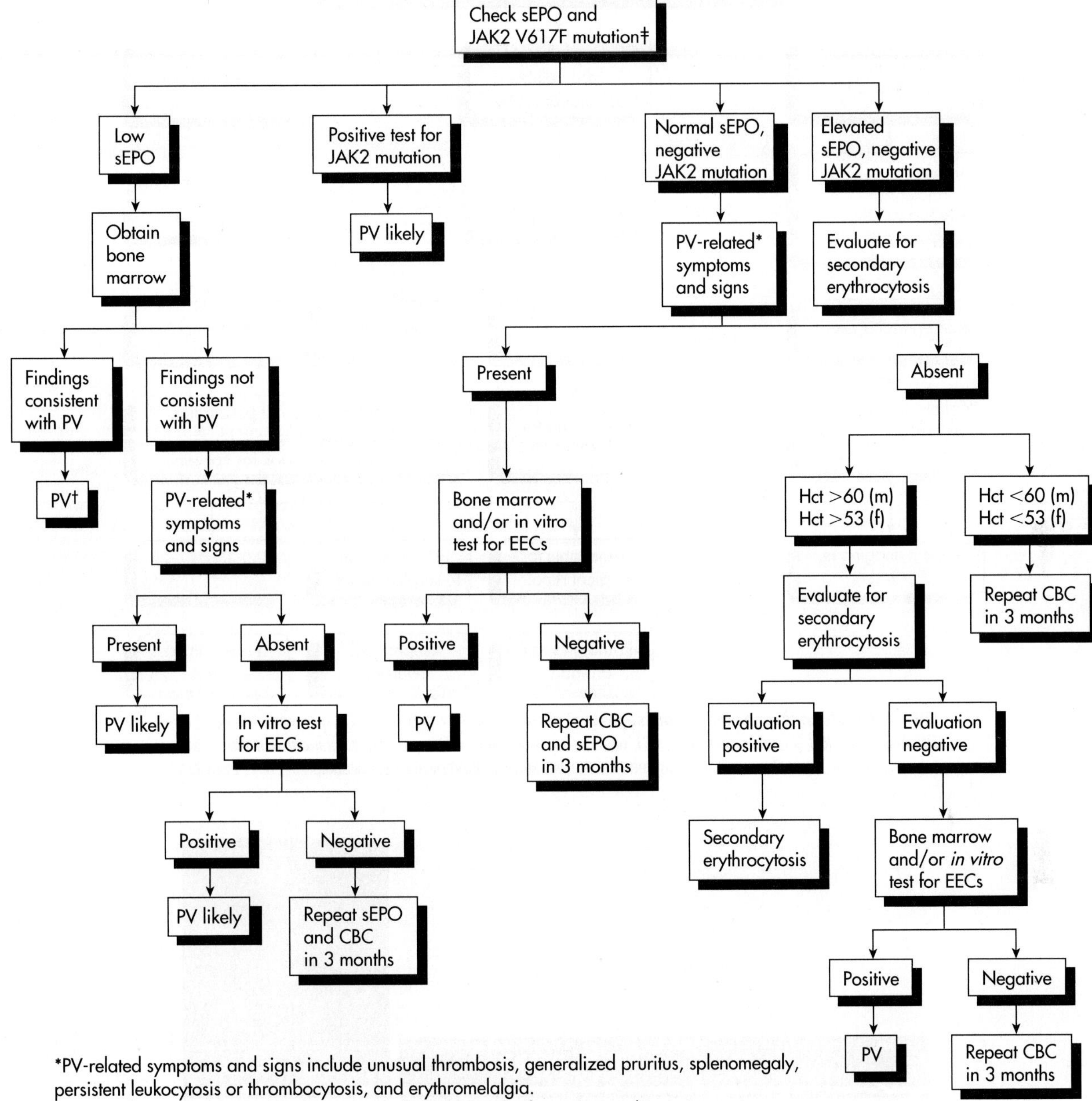

*PV-related symptoms and signs include unusual thrombosis, generalized pruritus, splenomegaly, persistent leukocytosis or thrombocytosis, and erythromelalgia.
†Note: Refer to Section I, Polycythemia Vera, for additional information on this topic.
‡The JAK2 mutation is found in >95% of patients with PV and can be used for diagnostic purposes.

FIG. 59 A diagnostic approach to acquired erythrocytosis. *CBC,* Complete blood cell count; *EEC,* endogenous (spontaneous) erythroid colonies; *f,* female; *Hct,* hematocrit; *m,* male; *PV,* polycythemia vera; *sEPO,* serum erythropoietin level. (Modified from Goldman L, Schafer AL [eds]: *Cecil textbook of medicine,* ed 24, Philadelphia, 2012, Saunders.)

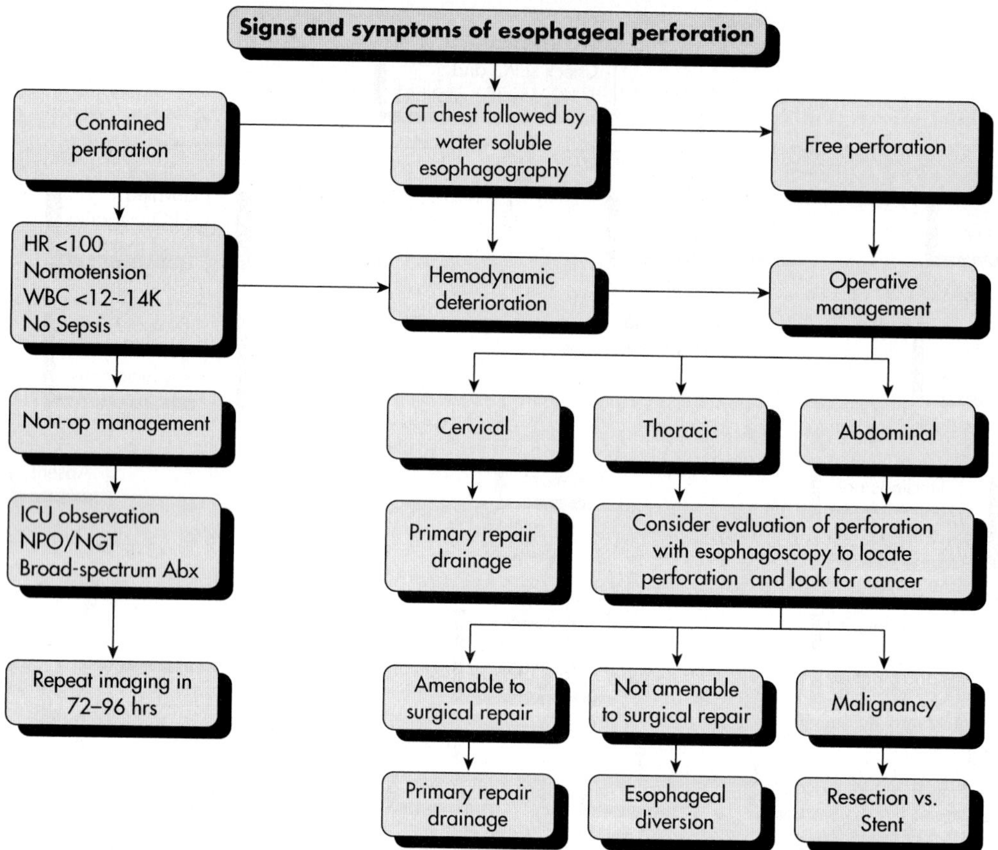

FIG. 62 Algorithm of management of esophageal perforation. *Abx,* Antibiotics; *CT,* computed tomography; *HR,* heart rate; *ICU,* intensive care unit; *NGT,* nasogastric tube; *NPO,* nothing by mouth *(nil per os)*; *WBC,* white blood cell count. (From Cameron JL, Cameron AM: *Current surgical therapy,* ed 12, Philadelphia, 2017, Elsevier.)

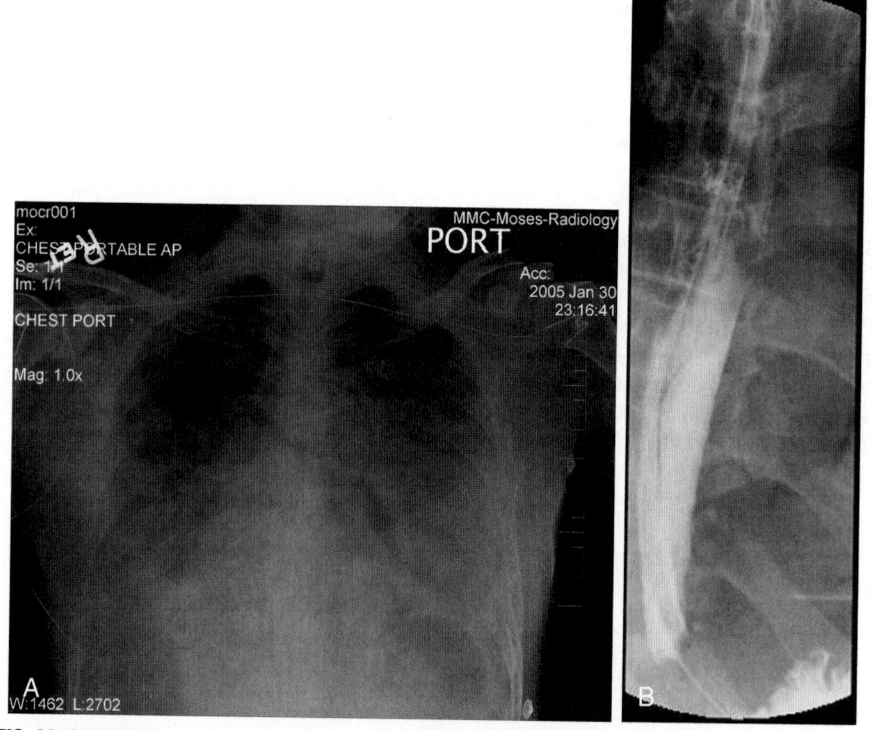

FIG. 63 A and **B,** Chest radiographs demonstrating pneumomediastinum and bilateral pleural effusions. (From Adams JG, Barton ED et al [eds]: *Emergency medicine: clinical essentials,* ed 2, Philadelphia, 2013, Saunders.)

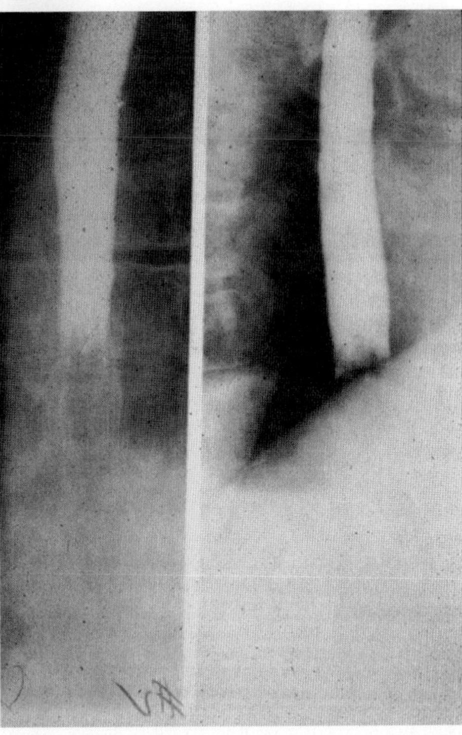

FIG. 64 Fluoroscopic swallow study showing extravasation of contrast agent (as seen from the left side of the film). (From Adams JG, Barton ED et al [eds]: *Emergency medicine: clinical essentials,* ed 2, Philadelphia, 2013, Saunders.)

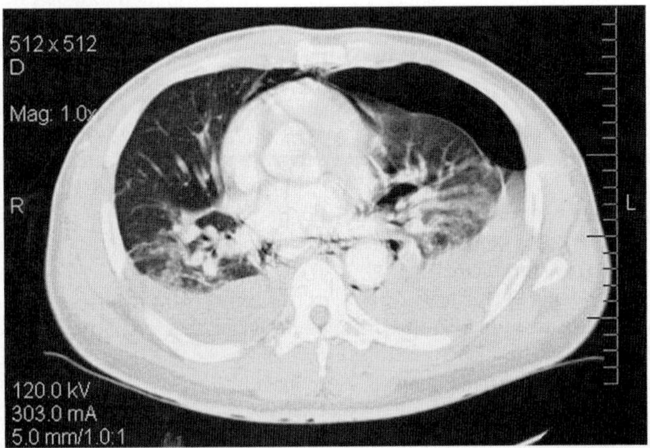

FIG. 65 Esophageal computed tomography scan demonstrating typical fluid collections in the setting of perforation. (From Adams JG, Barton ED et al [eds]: *Emergency medicine: clinical essentials,* ed 2, Philadelphia, 2013, Saunders.)

ICD-10CM # R50.9 Fever, unspecified
D70.3 Neutropenia due to infection

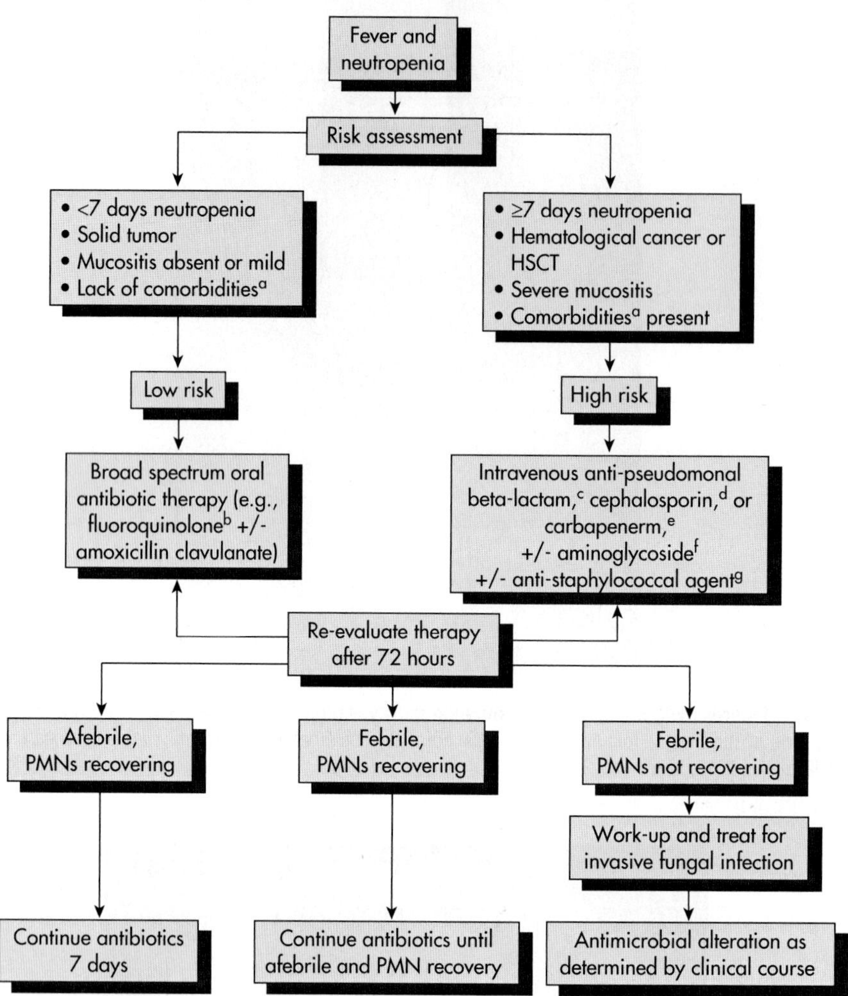

a Hypotension, altered mental status, neurologic changes, respiratory failure, abdominal pain, hemorrhage, cardiac compromise or new arrhythmia, catheter tunnel infection, extensive cellulitis, acute renal or liver failure
b Institution sensitivity dependent, ciprofloxacin, levofloxacin, moxifloxacin
c Drug selection and dosing institution-specific: piperacillin tazobactam, ticarcillin/clavulanate
d Drug selection and dosing institution-specific: ceftazidime
e imipenem, cefepime/cilastatin, meropenem, doripenem
f Gentamicin, tobramycin, or amikacin
g Drug selection and institution institution-specific: vancomycin, linezolid, daptomycin, ceftaroline

FIG. 67 Approach to patient with fever and neutropenia. *HSCT,* Hematopoietic stem cell transplant; *PMN,* polymorphonuclear neutrophil. (From Hoffman R: *Hematology: basic principles and practice,* ed 7, Philadelphia, 2018, Elsevier.)

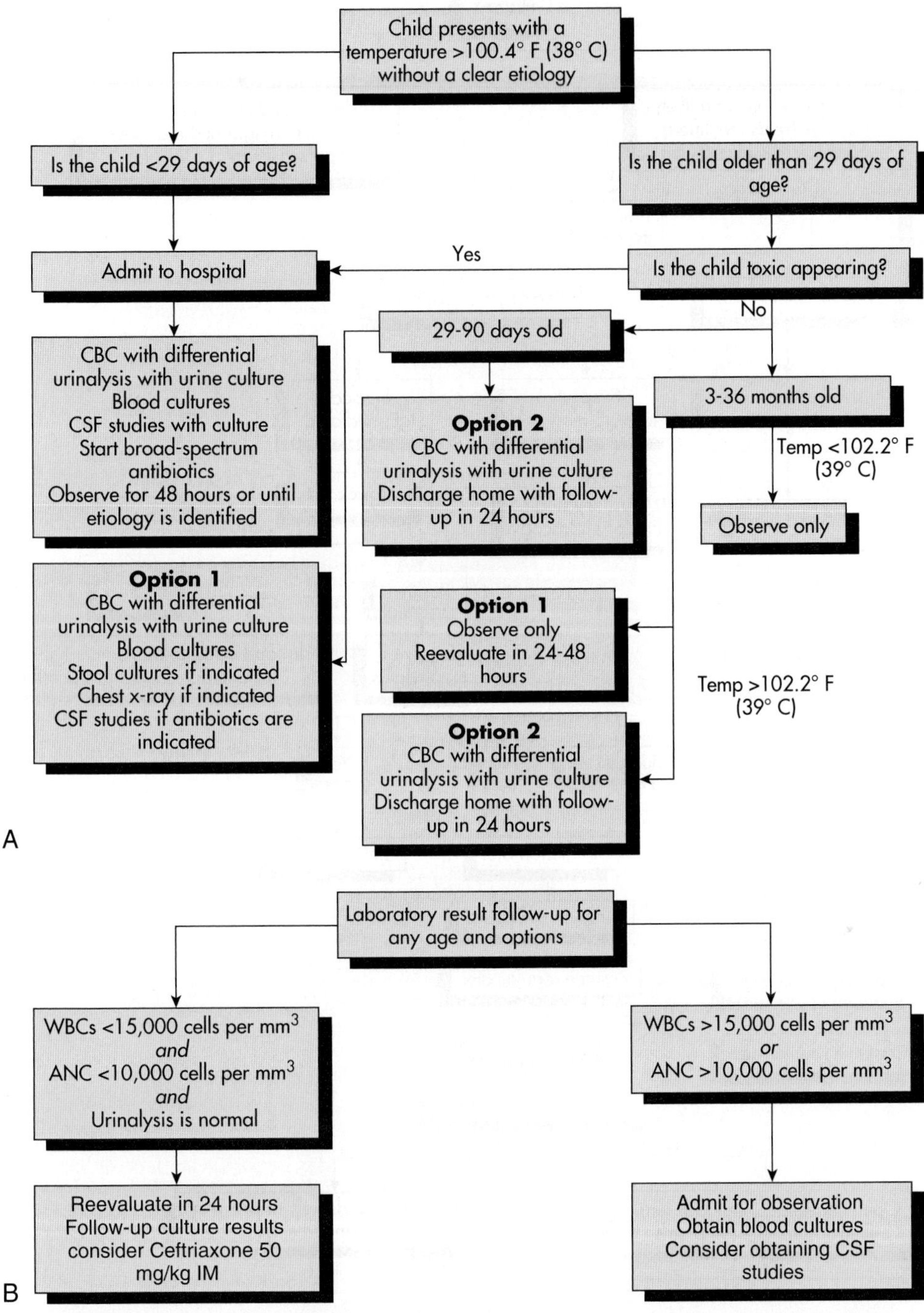

FIG. 69 **A,** Algorithm for the treatment of a child aged 0 to 36 months with a fever higher than 100.4° F (38° C) with no etiology for the fever. **B,** Continued considerations for the treatment of a child aged 0 to 36 months with a fever higher than 100.4° F (38° C) with no etiology for the fever. *ANC*, absolute neutrophil count; *CBC*, complete blood count; *CSF*, cerebrospinal fluid; *IM*, intramuscular; *WBCs*, white blood cells. (From Wein AJ, Kavoussi LR, Partin AW, Peters CA: *Campbell-Walsh urology,* ed 11, Philadelphia, 2016, Elsevier.)

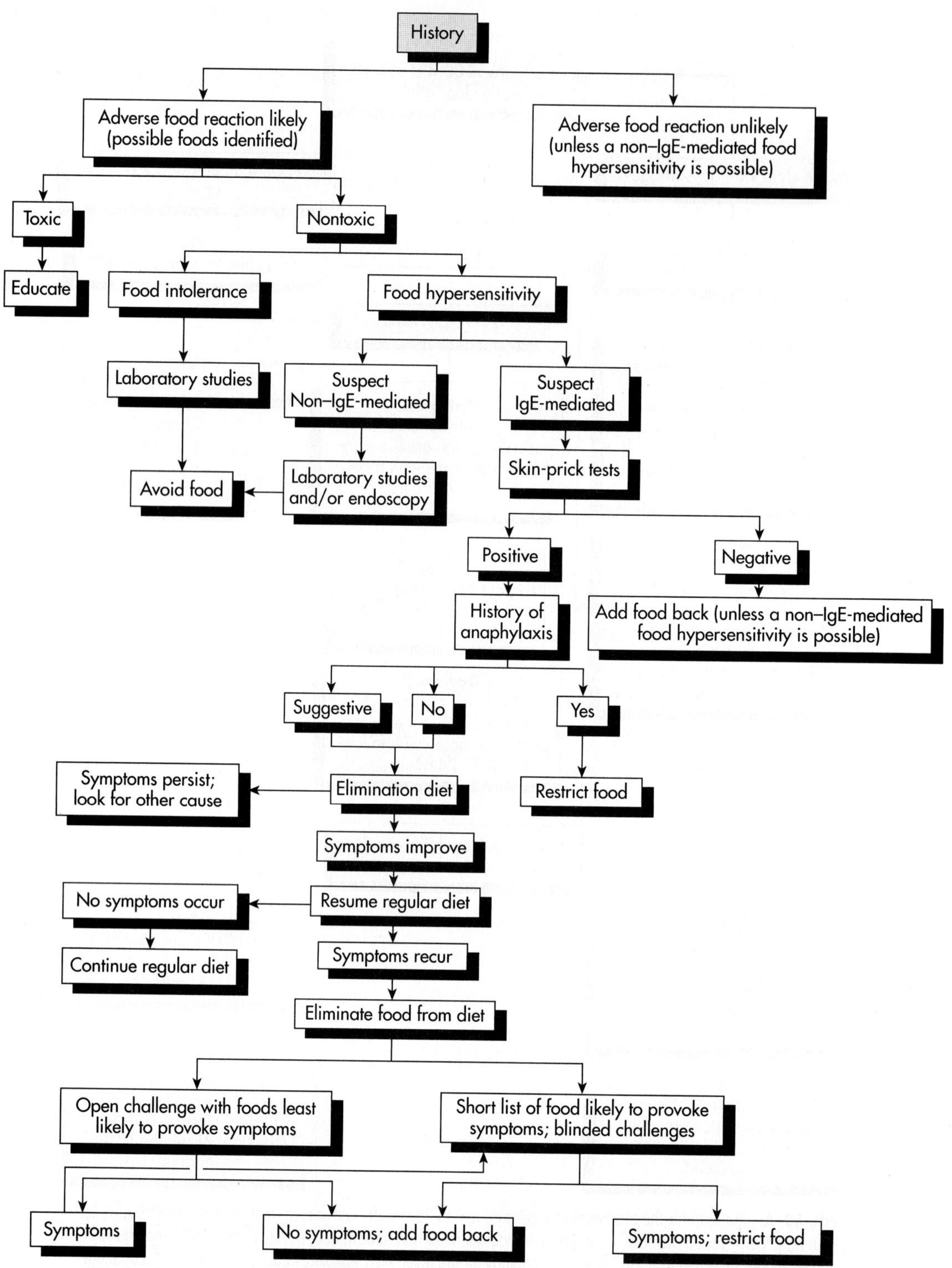

FIG. 70 Algorithm for the evaluation and management of adverse food reactions. (Feldman M, Friedman LS, Brandt LJ: *Sleisenger and Fortran's gastrointestinal and liver disease*, ed 10, Philadelphia, 2016, Elsevier.)

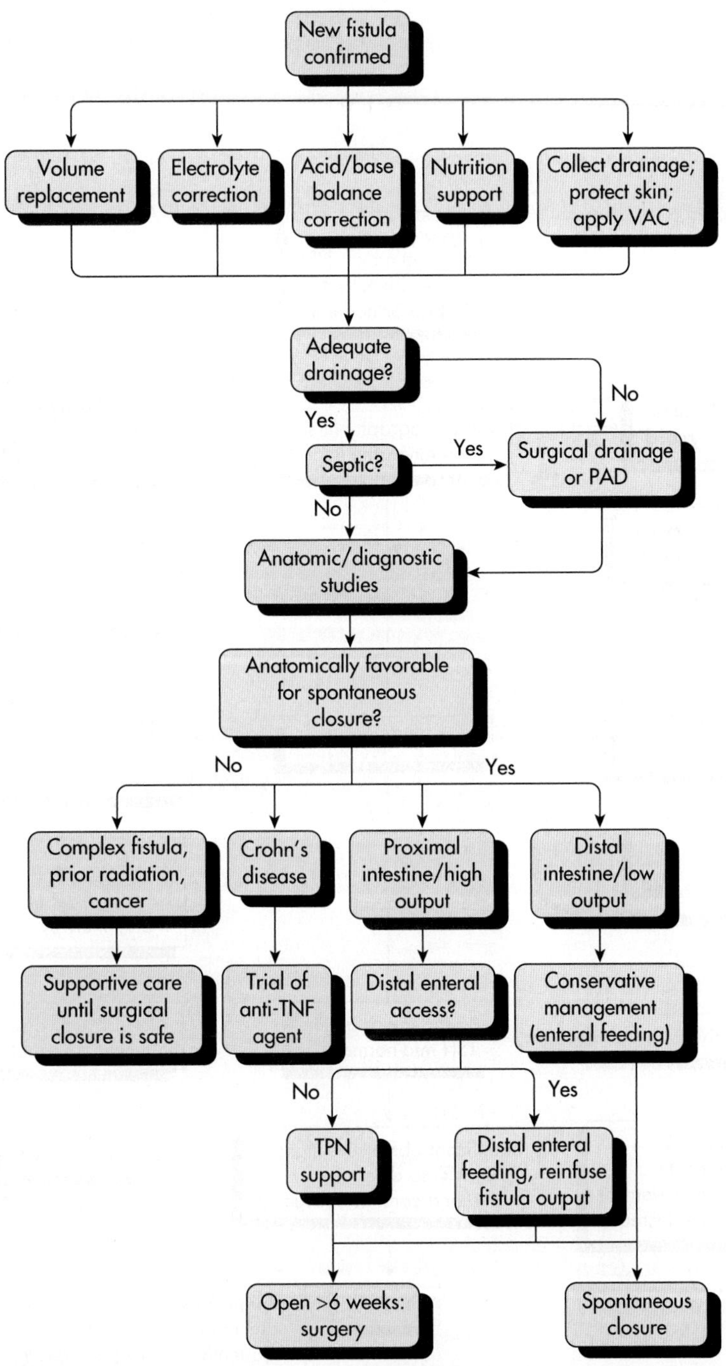

FIG. 71 Algorithm for the management of gastrointestinal fistulas. *PAD,* percutaneous abscess drainage; *TNF,* tumor necrosis factor; *TPN,* total parenteral nutrition; *VAC,* vacuum-assisted closure. (From Feldman M, Friedman LS, Brandt LJ: *Sleisenger and Fortran's gastrointestinal and liver disease,* ed 10, Philadelphia, 2016, Elsevier.)

GOITER EVALUATION AND MANAGEMENT

ICD-10CM #		
	E04.9	Nontoxic goiter, unspecified
	E01.2	Iodine-deficiency related (endemic) goiter, unspecified
	E04.0	Nontoxic diffuse goiter
	E05.10	Thyrotoxicosis with toxic single thyroid nodule without thyrotoxic crisis or storm
	E05.20	Thyrotoxicosis with toxic multinodular goiter without thyrotoxic crisis or storm
	E07.1	Dyshormogenetic goiter

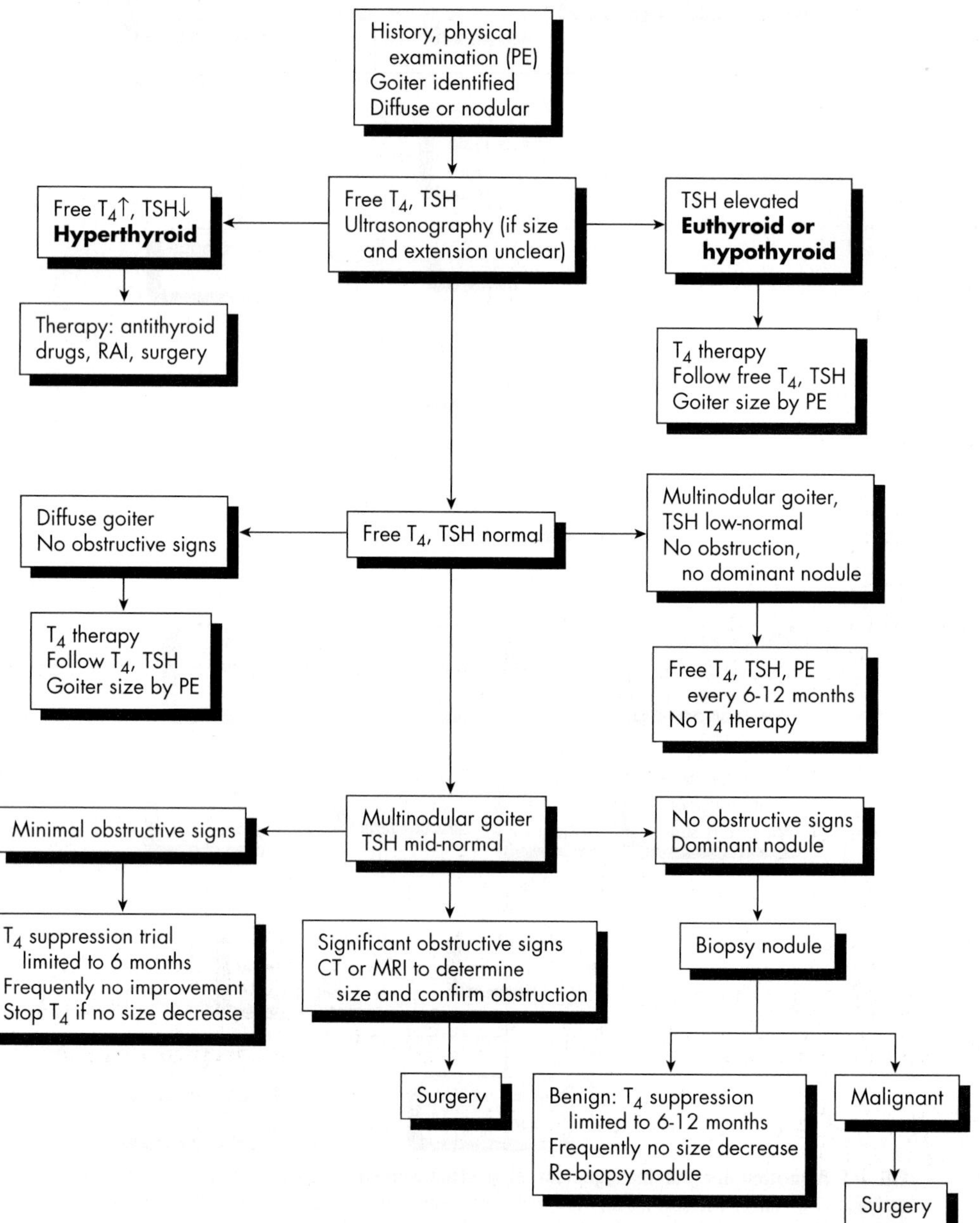

FIG. 72 Evaluation and management of patients with nontoxic diffuse and nodular goiter and undetermined thyroid status. *CT,* Computed tomography; *MRI,* magnetic resonance imaging; *RAI,* radioactive iodine; *TSH,* thyroid-stimulating hormone. (From Goldman L, Schafer AL [eds]: *Cecil textbook of medicine,* ed 24, Philadelphia, 2012, Saunders.)

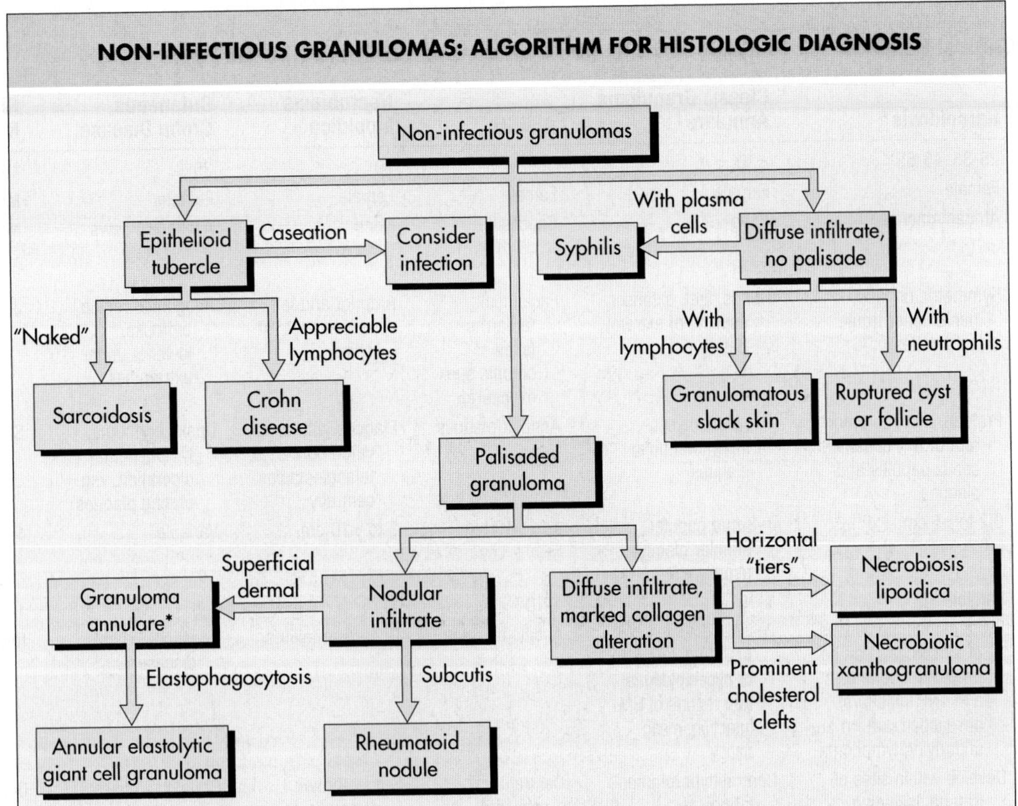

FIG. 73 Noninfectious granulomas: algorithm for histologic diagnosis. Interstitial granulomatous dermatitis and palisaded neutrophilic and granulomatous dermatitis may represent an additional diagnostic consideration. *May also have a patchy dermal interstitial pattern without palisades, or subcutaneous palisades with more mucin than rheumatoid nodules. (From Bolognia J: *Dermatology,* ed 4, Philadelphia, 2018, Elsevier.)

TABLE 20 Clinical Features of the Major Noninfectious Granulomatous Dermatitides

	Sarcoidosis*	Classic Granuloma Annulare†	AEGCG	Necrobiosis Lipoidica	Cutaneous Crohn Disease	Rheumatoid Nodule
Average age (y)	25-35, 45-65	<30	50-70	30	35	40-50
Sex predilection	Female	Female	Female	Female	Female	Male‡
Racial/ethnic predilection in US	African American	None	Caucasian	None	Ashkenazi Jews	None
Sites	Symmetric on face, neck, upper trunk, extremities	Hands, feet, extensor aspects of extremities	Face, neck, forearms (sites of chronic sun exposure)	Anterior and lateral aspects of shins	Anogenital region, buttocks, lower > upper extremities	Juxta-articular areas, especially elbows and hands
Appearance	Protean; most commonly red–brown or violaceous papules and plaques	Papules coalescing into annular plaques	Annular plaques	Plaques with elevated borders, telangiectasias centrally	Dusky erythema, lymphedema, ulceration, vegetating plaques	Skin-colored, firm, mobile subcutaneous nodules
Size of lesions	0.2 to >5 cm	1-3 mm papules, annular plaques usually <6 cm	2 to >10 cm	3 to >10 cm	Variable	1-3 cm
No. of lesions	Variable	1-10	1-10	1-10	1-5	1-10
Associations	Systemic manifestations of sarcoidosis can be drug-induced (e.g., IFN, TNF inhibitors) or reaction pattern to underlying lymphoma	Possible diabetes mellitus, thyroid disease, or hyperlipidemia; rare reports of HIV infection, malignancy	Actinic damage	Diabetes mellitus	Intestinal Crohn's disease	Rheumatoid arthritis
Special clinical characteristics	Develop within sites of trauma, including scars and tattoos	Central hyperpigmentation	Central atrophy and hypopigmentation	Yellow–brown atrophic centers, ulceration	Draining sinuses and fistulas	Occasional ulceration, especially at sites of trauma

*Clinical variants include lupus pernio and subcutaneous (Darier–Roussy), psoriasiform, ichthyosiform, angiolupoid, and ulcerative sarcoidosis.
†Clinical variants include generalized/disseminated, micropapular, nodular, perforating, subcutaneous, and patch granuloma annulare.
‡Although rheumatoid arthritis has a female:male ratio of 2-3:1.
IFN, Interferons, *TNF,* tumor necrosis factor.
Modified from Bolognia J: *Dermatology,* ed 4, Philadelphia, 2018, Elsevier.

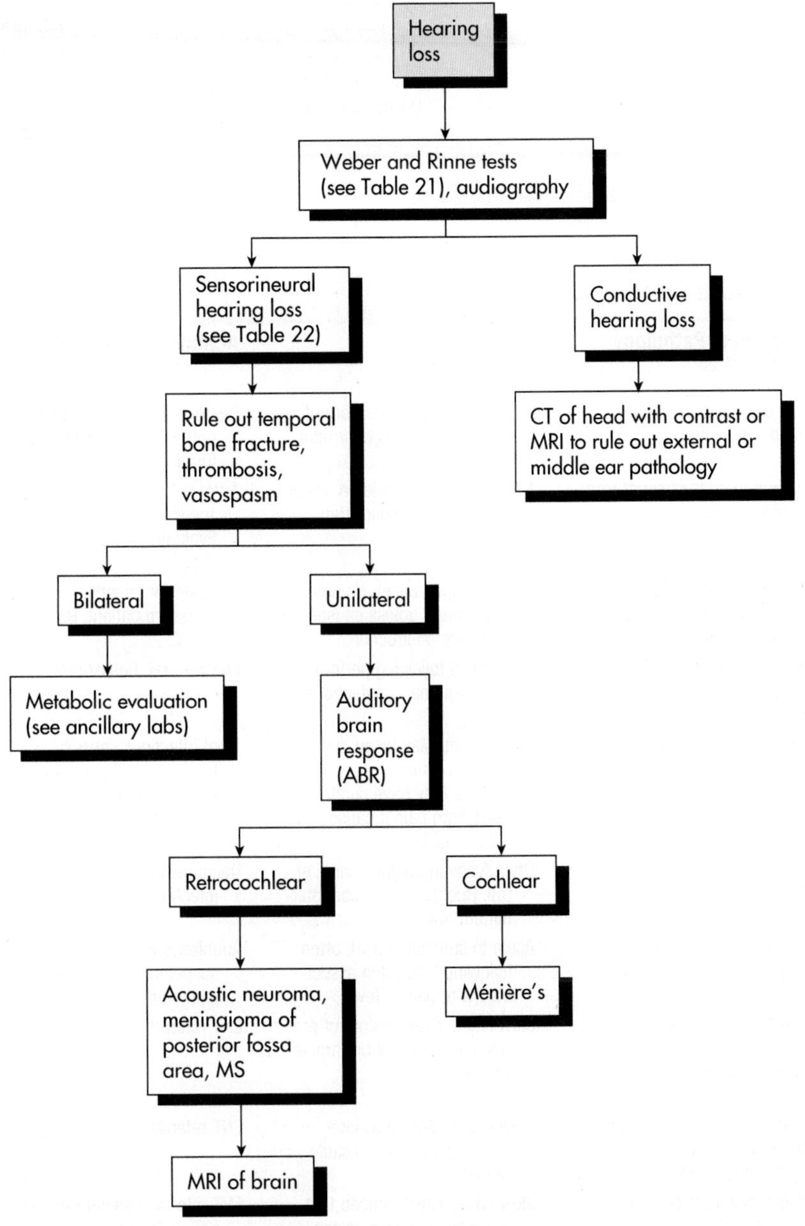

FIG. 74 Evaluation of hearing loss. *CT,* Computed tomography; *MRI,* magnetic resonance imaging; *MS,* multiple sclerosis. (From Ferri FF: *Ferri's best test: a practical guide to clinical laboratory medicine and diagnostic imaging,* ed 4, Philadelphia, 2018, Mosby.)

BOX 11 Hearing Loss

Diagnostic imaging	Lab evaluation
Best test	***Best test***
None	None
Ancillary tests	***Ancillary tests***
CT of head with contrast or MRI with contrast	CBC
CT of temporal bone without contrast	ALT, AST
	ANA, VDRL
	TSH

ALT, Alanine aminotransferase; *ANA,* antibody to nuclear antigens; *AST,* angiotensin sensitivity test; *CBC,* complete blood count; *CT,* computed tomography; *TSH,* thyroid-stimulating hormone; *VDRL,* Venereal Disease Research Laboratory.
From Ferri FF: *Ferri's best test: a practical guide to clinical laboratory medicine and diagnostic imaging,* ed 4, Philadelphia, 2018, Mosby.

TABLE 21 Interpretation of the Weber and Rinne Tests

	Weber without Lateralization	Weber Lateralizes Right	Weber Lateralizes Left
Rinne both ears: AC >BC	Normal	S/N loss in the left ear	S/N loss in the right ear
Rinne left ear: BC >AC	–	Combined loss: conduction and S/N loss in the left ear	Conduction loss in the left ear
Rinne right ear: BC >AC	–	Conduction loss in the right ear	Combined loss: conduction and S/N loss in the right ear

AC, Air conduction; *BC*, bone conduction; *S/N*, sensorineural.
From Adams JG et al: *Emergency medicine, clinical essentials*, ed 2, Philadelphia, 2013, Elsevier.

TABLE 22 Lesions That Cause Hearing Loss

	Description of Pathology	Onset/Course	Actions or Treatment	Prognosis
Conductive Lesion				
Foreign body	Mass in external canal blocks sound conduction	Acute onset associated or not with pain, drainage, or odor	Removal. Evaluate for infection. Evaluate for TM perforation	Excellent
Otitis externa	Edema and detritus obstruct external canal	Rapid onset. Pain, edema, swelling. Drainage, odor often present	Aural toilet to remove debris. Topical (±oral) antibiotics. Evaluate for necrotizing otitis	Excellent if treated appropriately
Exostosis	Bony growths obstruct canal. Often seen with prolonged exposure to cold water (divers)	Slow insidious onset. No pain or drainage unless causes complete obstruction	Evaluate for infection. Reassure patient. Refer to ENT	Good
Tympanosclerosis	TM scarring from perforations or infections. Decreased mobility impairs sound conduction	Slow onset following perforations, trauma, or infections	ENT referral. Reassurance	Variable
Perforated TM	Disruption of TM integrity results in impaired transmission of sound to ossicle	Acute onset. May follow direct trauma or sudden barotrauma. May have sudden relief from pain if caused by otitis media	Treat infectious causes. Counsel on importance of keeping water out of ear canal. ENT referral	Good
Sterile effusion (barotrauma)	Fluid in middle ear dampens conduction through ossicles	Often following flight, diving, or URI. Bubbles can cause intermittent pain	Decongestants. Evaluate for infection. Follow-up	Excellent
Acute otitis media	Pus (or fluid) in middle ear dampens conduction through ossicles	Acute to subacute onset, often following URI. Often associated with pain ± fever	Antibiotics (unless viral cause suspected), decongestants, pain control	Excellent if treated appropriately
Cholesteatoma	Trapped stratified squamous epithelial mass in middle ear. Interferes with ossicle conduction	Slow onset. Often history of previous perforations or chronic infections	ENT referral	Variable. May destroy ossicles or erode into surrounding structures
Glomus tumor	Vascular tumor occupies middle ear space. Interferes with ossicle conduction	Slow onset. May be associated with rushing pulsatile sensation	ENT referral	Variable
Cancer	Squamous cell most common. Obstructs external canal	Slow onset. Often noticed first by others. Painless unless occlusion causes otitis externa	ENT referral. Evaluate for secondary infection	Variable
Sensorineural Lesion				
Perilymph fistula (inner ear barotrauma)	Disruption of round or oval window allows leakage of perilymph into middle ear	Sudden onset of hearing loss often with tinnitus and vertigo. Frequently follows straining or abrupt change in pressure. Turning in direction of fistula exacerbates symptoms	Complete bed rest. Elevate head of bed and avoid increases in CSF pressure. Severe symptoms or noncompliance may require hospitalization. ENT consultation for possible oval or round window patch	Variable
Viral cochleitis	Cochlear inflammation. Often following URI	Rapid onset. Often following URI	Steroids often used (no good data)	Variable
Presbycusis	Age-related hearing loss. May be related to previous chronic noise exposure	Slow onset. Usually symmetric. High frequencies most affected. Tinnitus may occur	Hearing aid may help with both hearing loss and tinnitus	Variable

Continued

TABLE 22 Lesions That Cause Hearing Loss—cont'd

	Description of Pathology	Onset/Course	Actions or Treatment	Prognosis
Acoustic neuroma	Benign schwannoma of 8th cranial nerve	Slow onset. Usually unilateral. May exhibit tinnitus, vertigo. May exhibit facial hyperesthesias or twitching	May require surgical excision if symptoms debilitating	Variable
Ototoxic agents	Direct toxicity to inner ear structures	Variable onset. High frequency most affected. Exposure to ototoxic drugs. May have associated tinnitus	Stop use of offending agent	Variable. Hearing loss at time of stopping offending agent is usually permanent
Multiple sclerosis	Multiple demyelinating lesions interfere with nerve conduction	Often other associated neurologic findings. May wax and wane	Standard multiple sclerosis treatment (steroids, cytotoxic agents)	Variable
Stroke/CVA	Focal ischemic lesion of auditory nerve or auditory cortex	Sudden onset. Often associated with other neurologic deficits	Treat CVA risk factors (ASA, anticoagulants, glycemic control, BP control)	Variable
Meningitis	Infection enters inner ear through CNS-perilymph connection. Damages organ of Corti	Follows clinical picture of meningitis	Treat infection. Steroids may limit inflammation and damage	Variable
Ménière's disease (endolymphatic hydrops)	Abnormal homeostasis of inner ear fluids (clinical diagnosis; definitive diagnosis made histologically)	Episodic spells of vertigo. Associated sensation of fullness, tinnitus, and SNHL or auditory distortion. Low-frequency ranges most affected	Reduce salt, caffeine, nicotine (vasoconstrictors) intake. Consider diuretics, antihistamines, anticholinergics. ENT referral	Variable
Chronic noise exposure	Direct mechanical damage to cochlear structures and hair cells	Slow onset. Usually high frequency most affected	Prevention measures (earplugs). Stop exposure	Usually permanent
Skull trauma	Interruption of cranial nerve VIII, ossicle disruption, or shearing effects on organ of Corti	Sudden onset after trauma	ENT consultation for possible surgical repair	Variable: ossicle disruption has better prognosis than nerve or organ of Corti damage
Autoimmune causes	Vascular or neuronal inflammatory changes	Bilateral asymmetric SNHL. May be fluctuating or progressive. Often other systemic autoimmune findings	Outpatient autoimmune evaluation. Steroids and cytotoxic agents may slow progression	Variable

ASA, Acetylsalicylic acid; *BP*, blood pressure; CNS, central nervous system; *CSF*, cerebrospinal fluid; *CVA*, cerebrovascular accident; *ENT*, ear, nose, and throat; SNHL, sensorineural hearing loss; *TM*, tympanic membrane; *URI*, upper respiratory infection.

From Adams JG et al: *Emergency medicine, clinical essentials*, ed 2, Philadelphia, 2013, Elsevier.

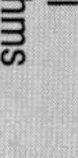

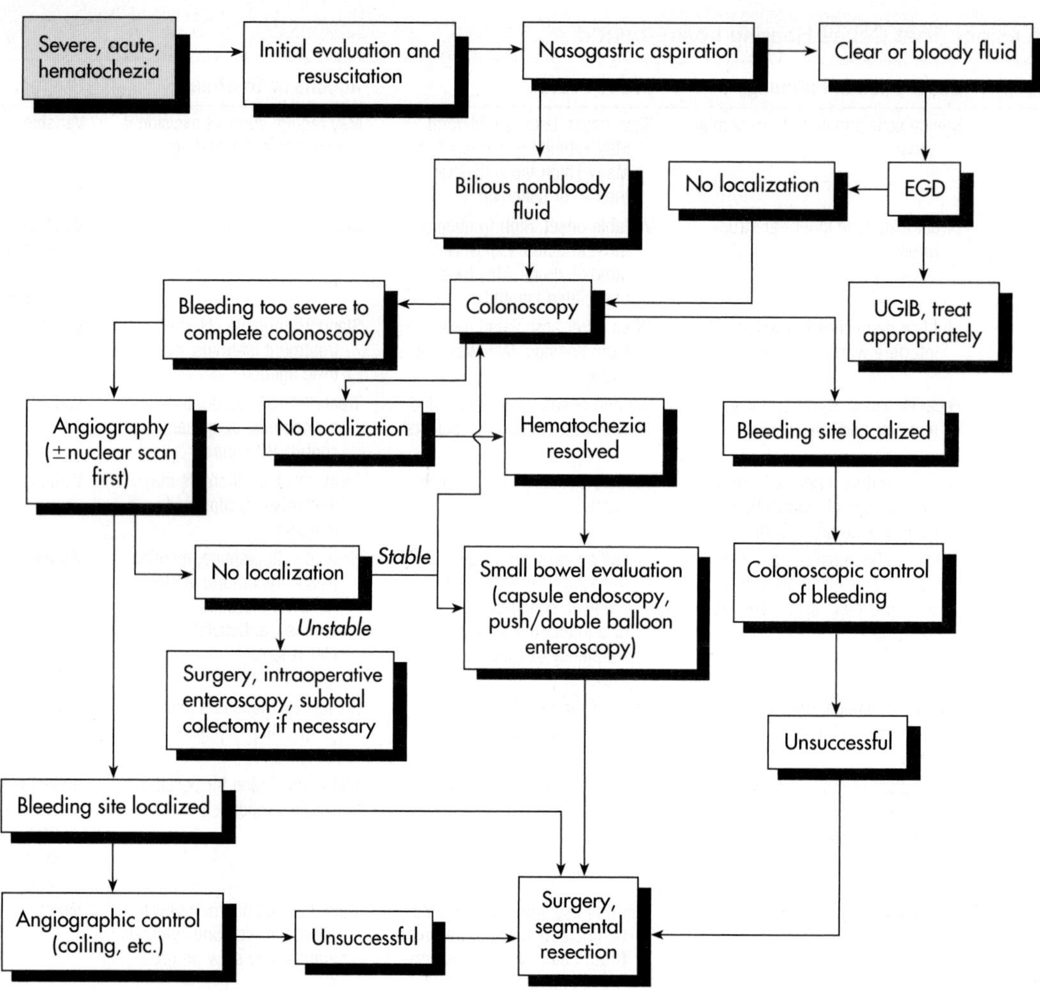

FIG. 75 Management algorithm for hematochezia. *EGD,* Esophagogastroduodenoscopy; *UGIB,* upper gastrointestinal biopsy. (From Cameron JL, Cameron AM: *Current surgical therapy,* ed 10, Philadelphia, 2011, Saunders.)

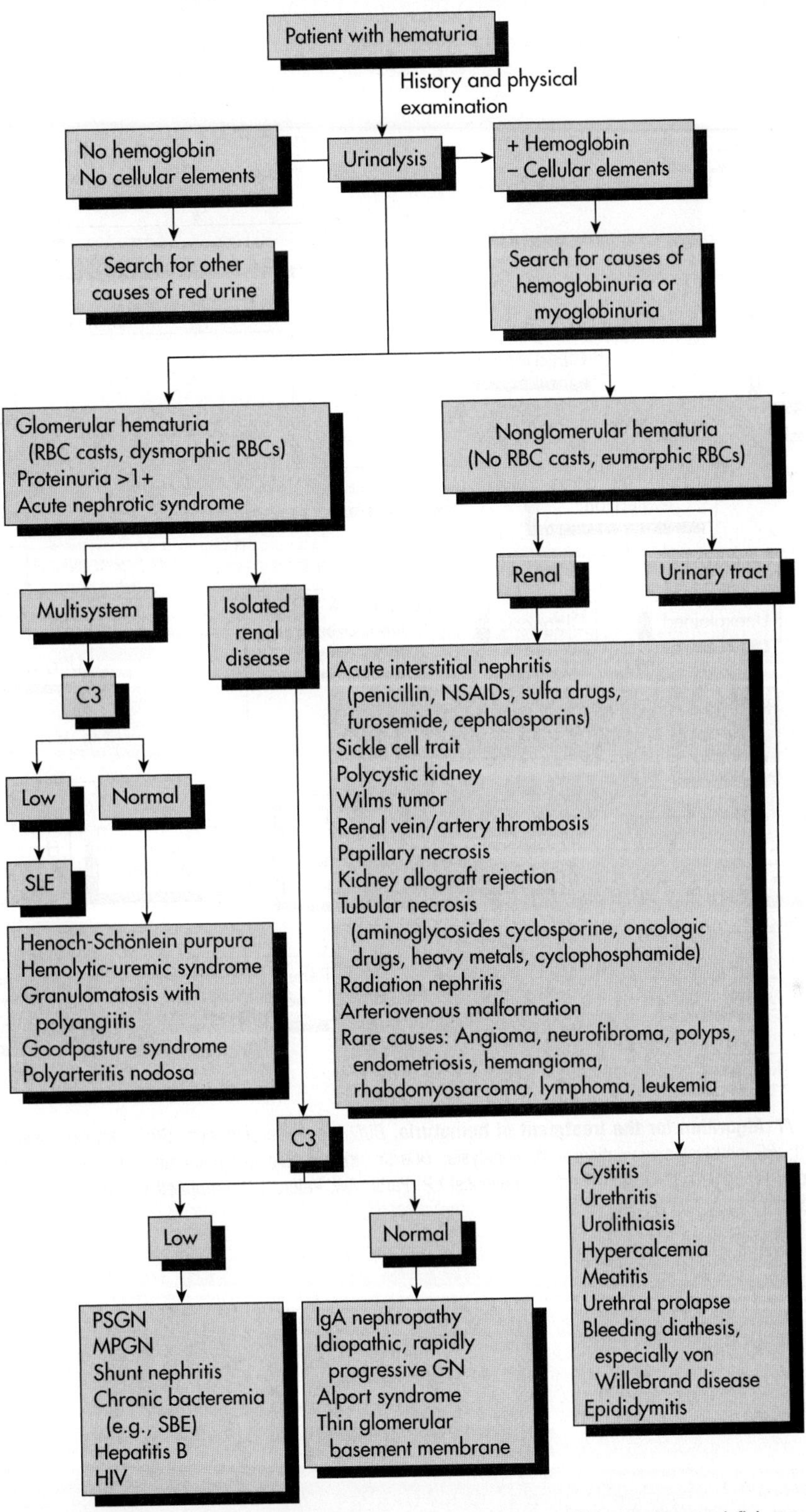

FIG. 76 Diagnostic strategy for hematuria. *GN,* glomerulonephritis; *HIV,* human immunodeficiency virus; *MPGN,* membranoproliferative glomerulonephritis; *NSAIDs,* nonsteroidal antiinflammatory drugs; *PSGN,* post-streptococcal glomerulonephritis; *RBC,* red blood cell; *SBE,* subacute bacterial endocarditis; *SLE,* systemic lupus erythematosus. (From The Johns Hopkins Hospital, Hughes HK, Kalh, LK: *The Harriet Lane handbook,* ed 21, St Louis, 2018, Elsevier.)

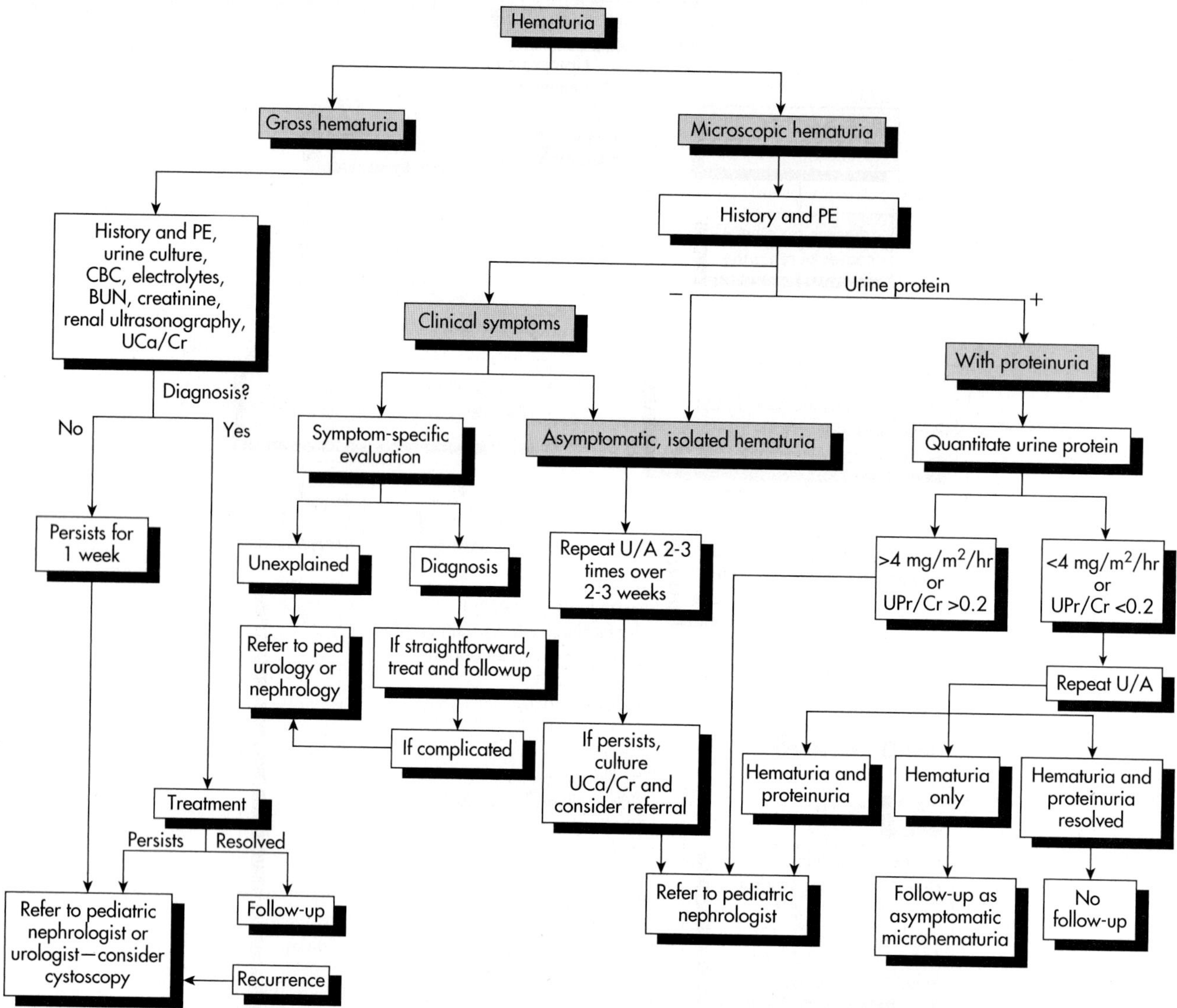

FIG. 77 Algorithm for the treatment of hematuria. *BUN*, blood urea nitrogen; *CBC*, complete blood cell count; *PE*, physical examination; *U/A*, urinalysis; *UCa/Cr*, urinary calcium/creatinine ratio; *UPr/Cr*, urinary protein/creatinine ratio. (From Wein AJ, Kavoussi LR, Partin AW, Peters CA: *Campbell-Walsh urology,* ed 11, Philadelphia, 2016, Elsevier.)

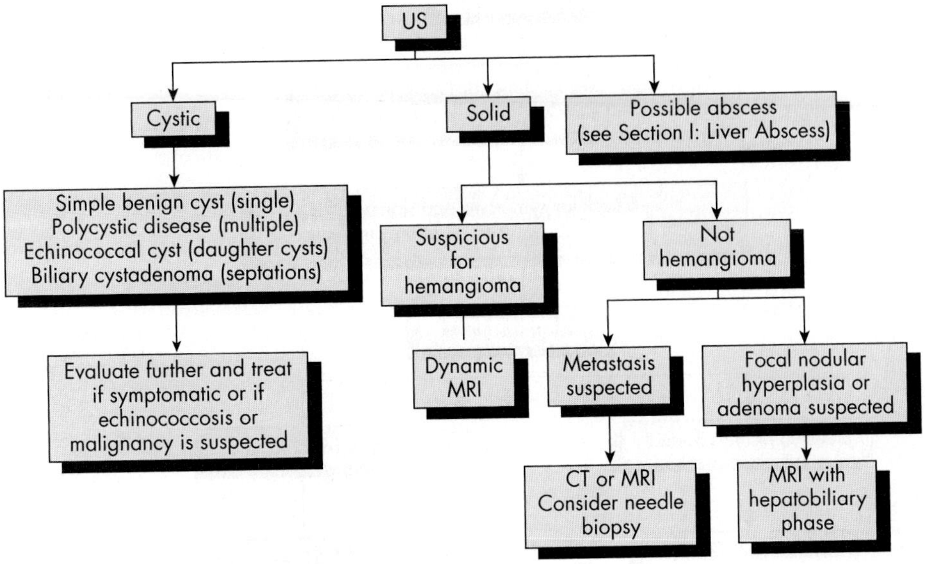

FIG. 78 A, Algorithm for the approach to the management of a patient, not known to have cirrhosis, with a hepatic mass (often incidental, possibly symptomatic). **B,** Algorithm for the approach to the management of a patient with known or suspected cirrhosis and a hepatic mass (found on routine surveillance, because of symptoms, or because of an increasing alpha-fetoprotein level). *Perform imaging modality not previously performed. *HCC*, hepatocellular carcinoma. (From Feldman M, Friedman LS, Brandt LJ: *Sleisenger and Fortran's gastrointestinal and liver disease,* ed 10, Philadelphia, 2016, Elsevier.)

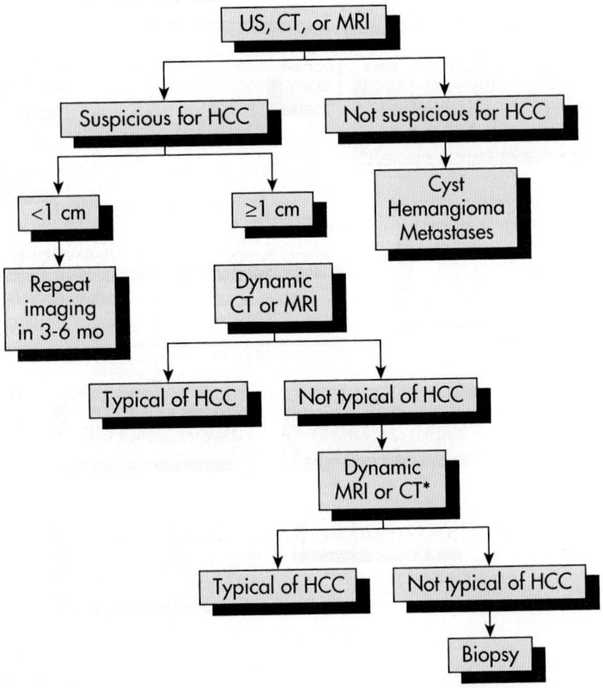

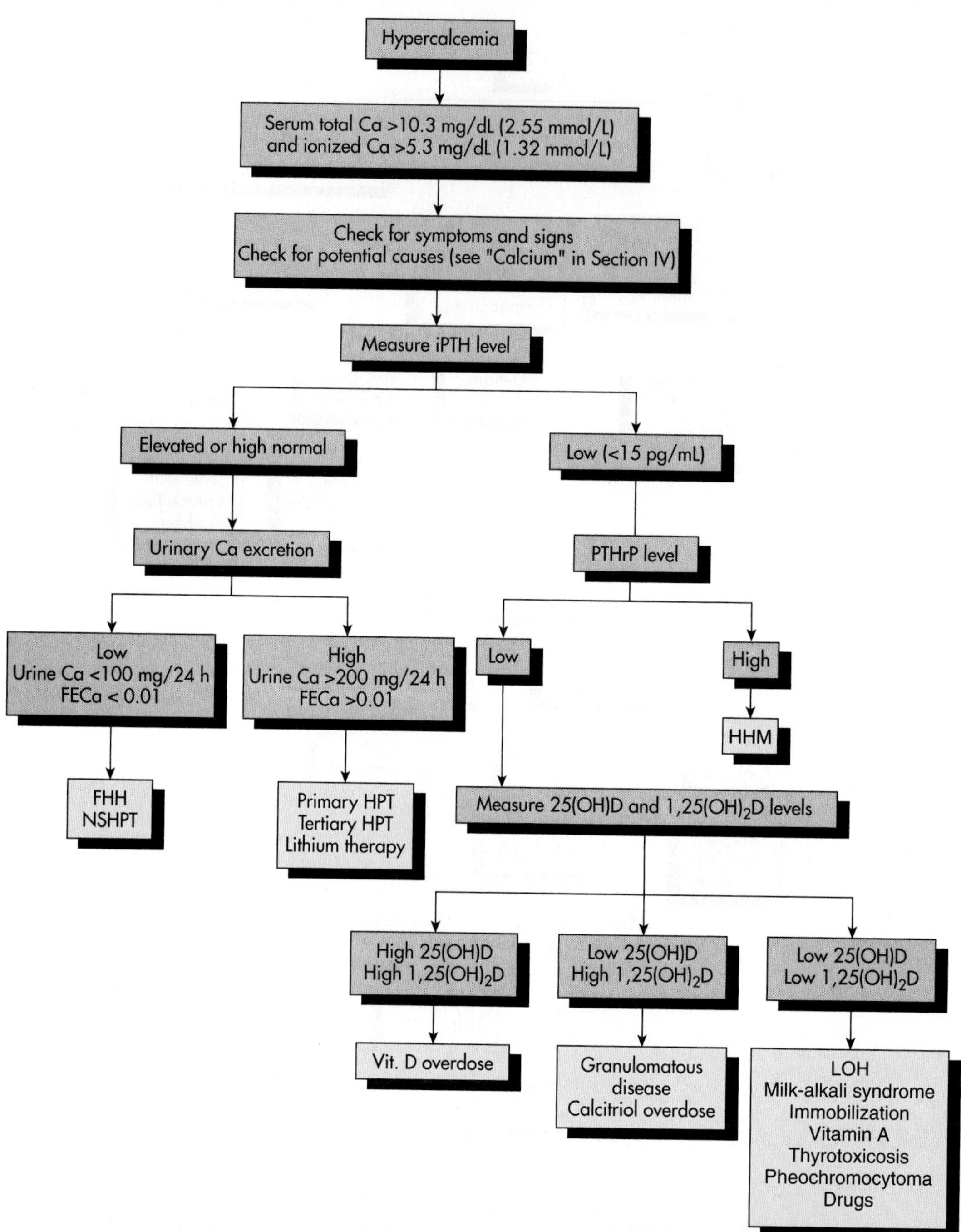

FIG. 79 Algorithm for evaluation of hypercalcemia. *FECa*, Fractional excretion of calcium; *FHH*, familial hypocalciuric hypercalcemia; *HHM*, humoral hypercalcemia of malignancy; *HPT*, hyperparathyroidism; *iPTH*, intact parathyroid hormone; *LOH*, localized osteolytic hypercalcemia; *NSHPT*, neonatal severe hyperparathyroidism; *PTHrP*, parathyroid hormone–related peptide. (Skorecki K, Chertow GM, Marsden PA, Taal MW, Yu ASL, Wasser WG: *Brenner & Rector's the kidney,* ed 10, Philadelphia, 2016, Elsevier.)

Diagnostic Imaging

Best Test(s)

None

Ancillary Tests

Radiograph of painful bones (r/o bone neoplasm, multiple myeloma)
Tc-99m parathyroid scan (r/o parathyroid adenoma)
Ultrasound of parathyroid glands
Ultrasound of kidneys (r/o renal cell carcinoma)

Lab Evaluation

Best Test(s)

Serum calcium level
PTH level

Ancillary Tests

Serum phosphate, magnesium, alkaline phosphatase, albumin
Electrolytes, BUN, creatinine
24-hour urine collection for calcium
Urinary cyclic AMP
PSA (if prostate carcinoma is suspected)
Serum and urine protein immunoelectrophoresis (if multiple myeloma suspected)

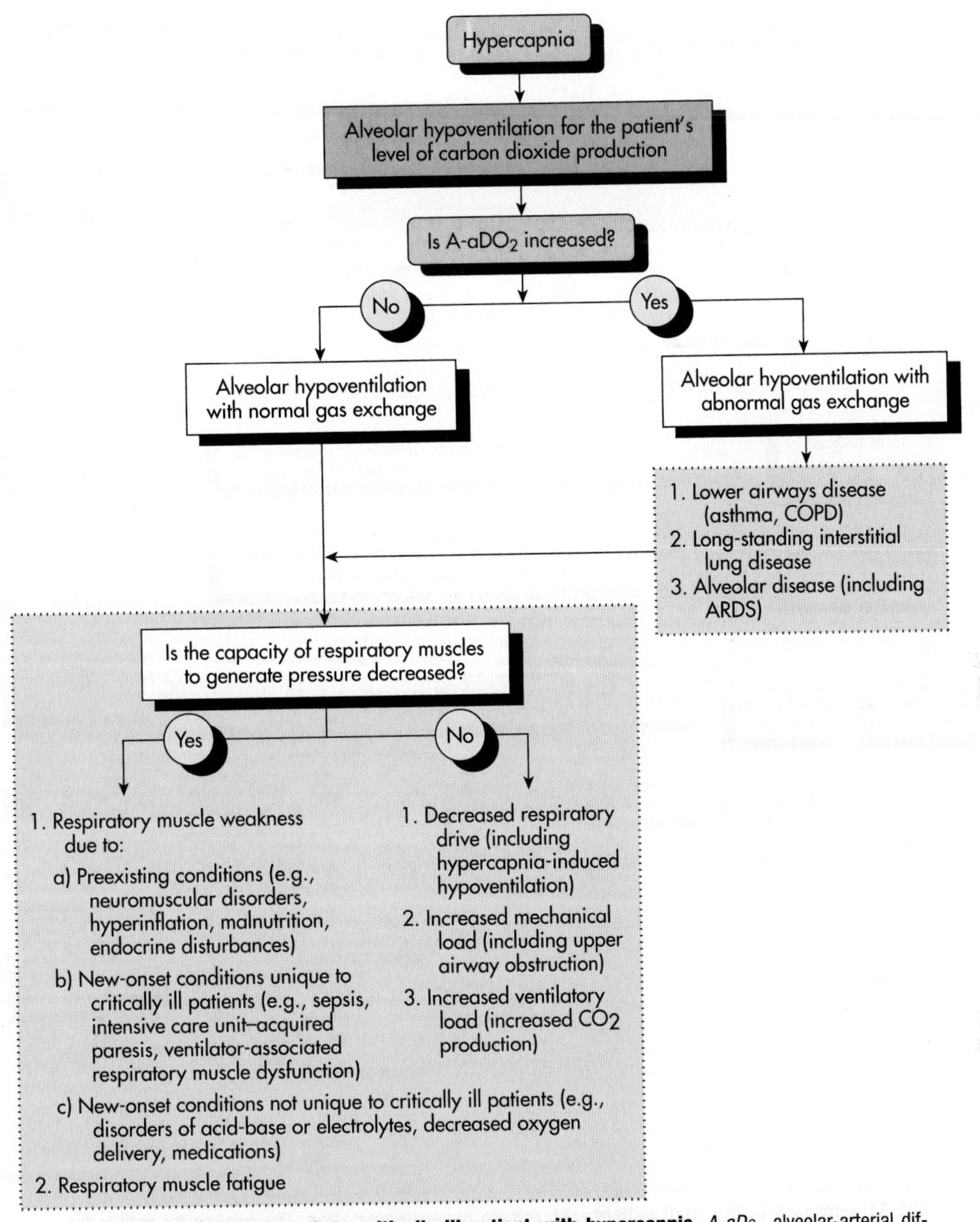

FIG. 80 Diagnostic approach to critically ill patient with hypercapnia. *A-aDo₂*, alveolar-arterial difference in partial pressure of oxygen; *ARDS*, acute respiratory distress syndrome; *COPD*, chronic obstructive pulmonary disease. (From Parrillo JE, Dellinger RP: *Critical care medicine: principles of diagnosis and management in the adult,* ed 4, Philadelphia, 2014, Elsevier.)

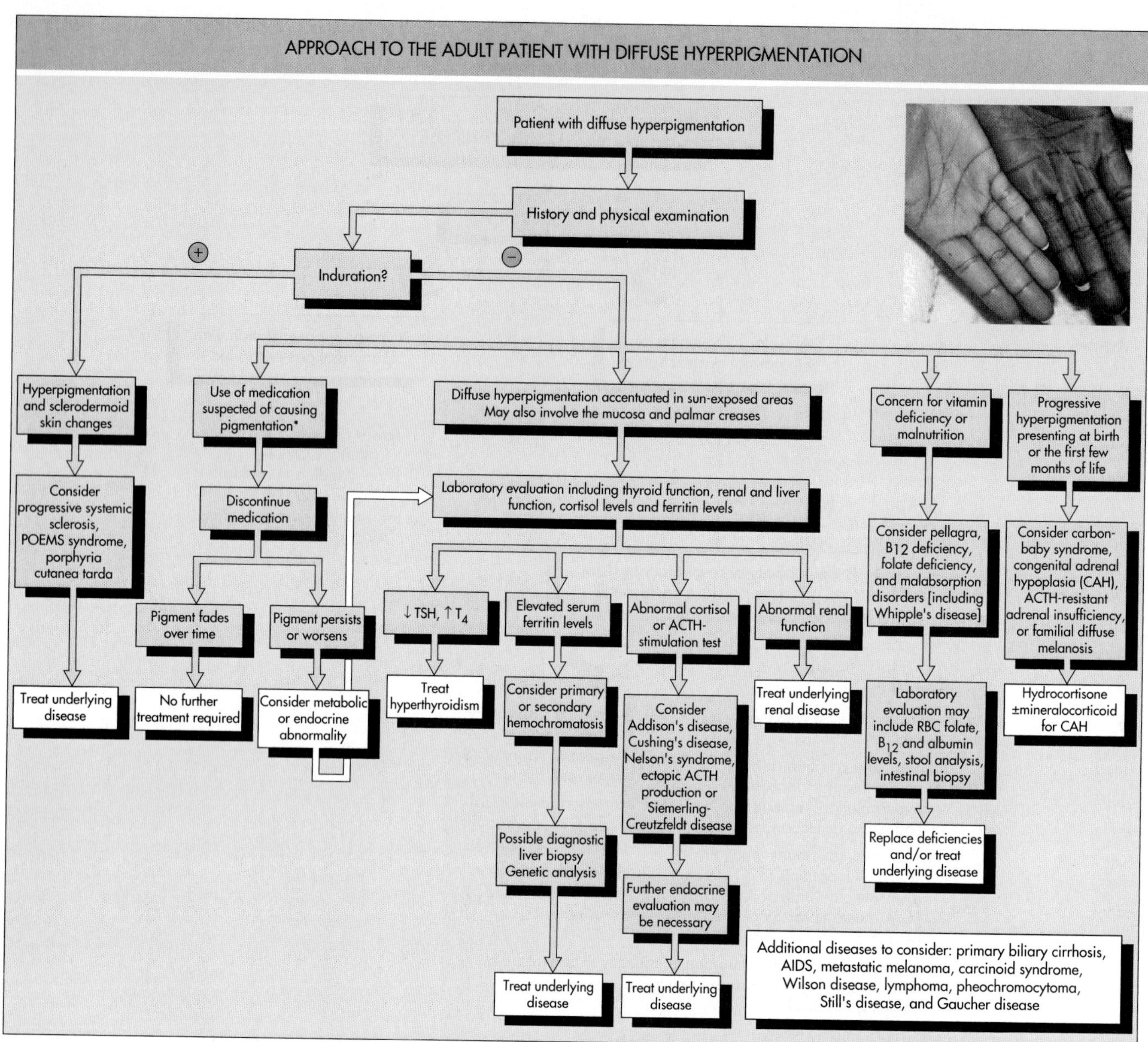

FIG. 81 Approach to the adult patient with diffuse hyperpigmentation. The palm on the right in the inset photograph shows diffuse hyperpigmentation in a patient with POEMS syndrome (*p*olyneuropathy, *o*rganomegaly, *e*ndocrinopathy, *m*onoclonal gammopathy and *s*kin lesions). *ACTH,* adrenocorticotropic hormone; T_4, thyroxine; *TSH,* thyroid-stimulating hormone. *See Table 23 for a list of drugs and chemicals associated with diffuse hyperpigmentation. (From Bolognia JL, Jorizzo JL, Schaffer JV: *Dermatology,* ed 3, St Louis, 2012, Elsevier.)

TABLE 23 Drugs and Chemicals Associated with Hyperpigmentation

Drug or Chemical	Clinical Features	Histopathology/Comment
Cancer Chemotherapeutic Agents		
BCNU (Topical)	• Hyperpigmentation at site of application (no reaction seen with parenteral administration)	• Hyperplasia of basal melanocytes consistent with postinflammatory hyperpigmentation
Bleomycin	• Linear, flagellate bands, associated with minor trauma • Nails may be involved • Hyperpigmentation overlying joints	• Increased epidermal melanin • Little dermal pigment incontinence • No increase in epidermal melanocytes
Busulfan	• Generalized hyperpigmentation resembling Addison's disease; sometimes seen in association with drug-induced pulmonary fibrosis	• Increased melanin in basal keratinocytes and in dermal macrophages
Cyclophosphamide	• Diffuse hyperpigmentation of the skin and mucous membranes • Localized pigment of the nails (transverse or longitudinal bands), palms and soles, or teeth	• Pigmentation usually regresses within 6 to 12 months after therapy is discontinued
Dactinomycin	• Generalized hyperpigmentation, most prominent on the face	• Pigmentation fades after treatment discontinued
Daunorubicin	• Hyperpigmentation of light-exposed areas • Transverse brown-black nail bands	• Structurally similar to doxorubicin
Doxorubicin	• Pigmentation of the nails; hyperpigmentation of the palmar creases, palms, soles, buccal mucosa, dorsae of the knuckles and tongue	• Increased epidermal melanin • Increased number of melanocytes
5-Fluorouracil	• Hyperpigmentation in sun-exposed areas • Increased pigmentation of skin overlying veins used for infusion, dorsae of the hands and trunk	• Synergistic hyperpigmentation of irradiation portal sites
Hydroxyurea	• Reversible hyperpigmentation over pressure points and the back • Nails may be involved	• Lichenoid eruption with secondary hyperpigmentation
Mechlorethamine (nitrogen mustard)	• Topical use for cutaneous lymphoma may result in generalized hyperpigmentation • More intense in lesional skin	• Disaggregation of melanosomes within keratinocytes • Increased number of melanocytes
Methotrexate	• Uniform hyperpigmentation in sun-exposed areas	• Uncommon • May be postinflammatory hyperpigmentation secondary to photosensitivity reaction
Antimalarials		
Amino quinolones (chloroquine, hydroxychloroquine, amodiaquine)	• Yellow-brown or gray to blue-black pigment, usually in pretibial areas; face, hard palate, and subungual areas may be involved	• Dyspigmentation in up to 25% of patients • Dermal deposition of melanin-drug complexes; hemosiderin around capillaries • May fade, but rarely resolves, upon discontinuation of drug
Heavy Metals		
Arsenic	• Areas of bronze hyperpigmentation ± superimposed raindrops • Keratoses on the palms and soles associated with pigmentation	• May appear 1-20 yr after exposure • Dermal and epidermal deposition of arsenic • Increased epidermal melanin synthesis
Bismuth	• Generalized blue-gray discoloration of face, neck, dorsal hands • Oral mucosa and gingivae may be involved	• Bismuth granules in the papillary and reticular dermis
Gold	• Permanent blue-gray discoloration in sun-exposed areas, mostly around the eyes (chrysiasis)	• Gold particles within macrophage lysosomes in the dermis
Iron	• Permanent brown pigment at injection or application sites	• Pigment coats collagen fibers and is deposited in dermal macrophages
Lead	• "Lead line" in gingival margin • Nail pigmentation	• Lead line is due to subepithelial deposition of lead granules
Mercury	• Slate-gray pigmentation, particularly in skin folds	• Brown-black granules free in dermis, in association with elastic fibers, and within macrophages
Silver	• Generalized slate-gray pigmentation, increased in sun-exposed areas • Nails and sclerae may also be involved • Localized at sites of application	• Silver granules in the basement membrane and on the membrana propria of eccrine glands
Hormones		
Oral contraceptives	• Melasma; increased pigment of nipples and nevi	• Increased melanocytes and increased melanin synthesis
ACTH/MSH	• Diffuse brown or bronze pigmentation; seen in Addison's disease and Cushing's syndrome	• Increased melanin synthesis
Miscellaneous Compounds		
Amiodarone	• Slate-gray to violaceous discoloration of sun-exposed skin	• Yellow-brown granules in dermis, mostly perivascular • Lysosomal inclusions with a lipid-like substance
Azidothymidine (zidovudine, AZT)	• Nail and mucocutaneous hyperpigmentation	• Skin biopsy shows increased epidermal and dermal melanin
Clofazimine	• Diffuse red to red-brown discoloration of skin • Violet-brown to bluish discoloration, especially lesional skin	• Redness secondary to drug in fat • Phagolysosomes with lipofuscin material

TABLE 23 Drugs and Chemicals Associated with Hyperpigmentation—cont'd

Drug or Chemical	Clinical Features	Histopathology/Comment
Dioxins	• Chloracne most common skin finding • Hyperpigmentation may occur in sun-exposed areas	• Rare, except in accidental exposure
Hydroquinone	• Hyperpigmentation in areas of application due to exogenous ochronosis	• Yellow-brown banana-shaped fibers in papillary dermis
Minocycline	• Blue-black discoloration in old acne scars or sites of inflammation as well as lower extremities • May also involve nails, sclerae, oral mucosa, bones, and teeth • Generalized "muddy brown" pigmentation pattern in some patients	• Iron-containing granules and/or increased melanin, depending on clinical type
Psoralens	• Increased pigmentation after exposure to UVA light (PUVA)	• Proliferation of follicular melanocytes • Increased synthesis and transfer of melanin
Psychotropic drugs (phenothiazine, chlorpromazine, imipramine, desipramine)	• Slate-gray discoloration in sun-exposed areas	• Golden-brown granules in the upper dermis • Electron-dense inclusion bodies

ACTH, Adrenocorticotropic hormone; *AZT,* azidothymidine, now renamed zidovudine; *MSH,* melanocyte-stimulating hormone.
From Bolognia JL et al [eds]: *Dermatology,* ed 2, St Louis, 2008, Mosby.

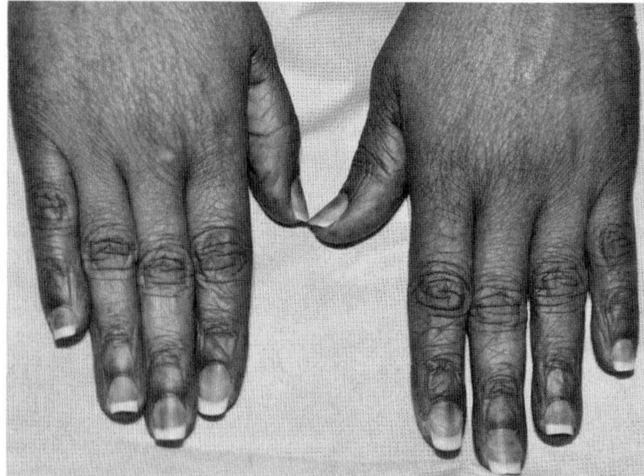

FIG. 82 Hyperpigmentation of the nails in a 61-year-old woman receiving paclitaxel for breast cancer. (From Callen JP, Jorizzo JL et al: *Dermatologic signs of systemic disease,* ed 5, 2017, Elsevier.)

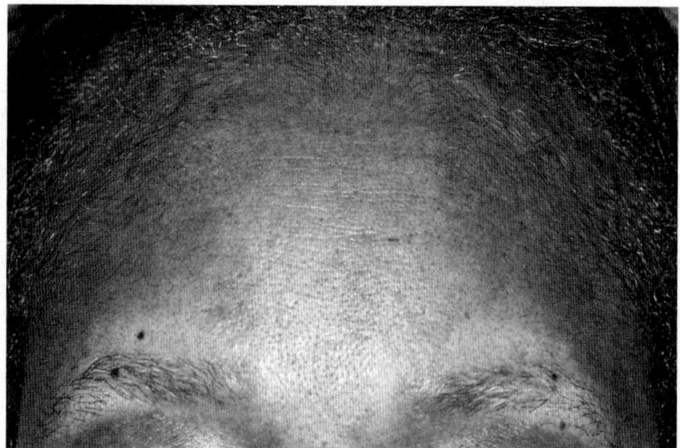

FIG. 83 Grade 1 skin (facial) hyperpigmentation in a 62-year-old woman, during treatment with imatinib for a gastrointestinal stromal tumor. (From Callen JP, Jorizzo JL et al: *Dermatologic signs of systemic disease,* ed 5, 2017, Elsevier.)

HYPOGONADISM

ICD-10CM # E28.310 Symptomatic premature menopause
E29.1 Testicular hypofunction
E28.39 Other primary ovarian failure
E23.6 Other disorders of pituitary gland

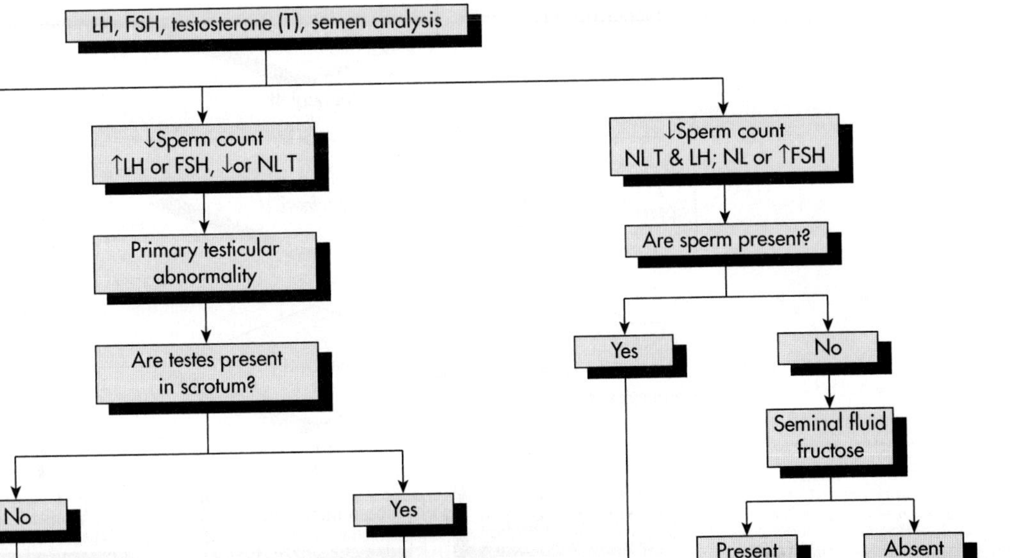

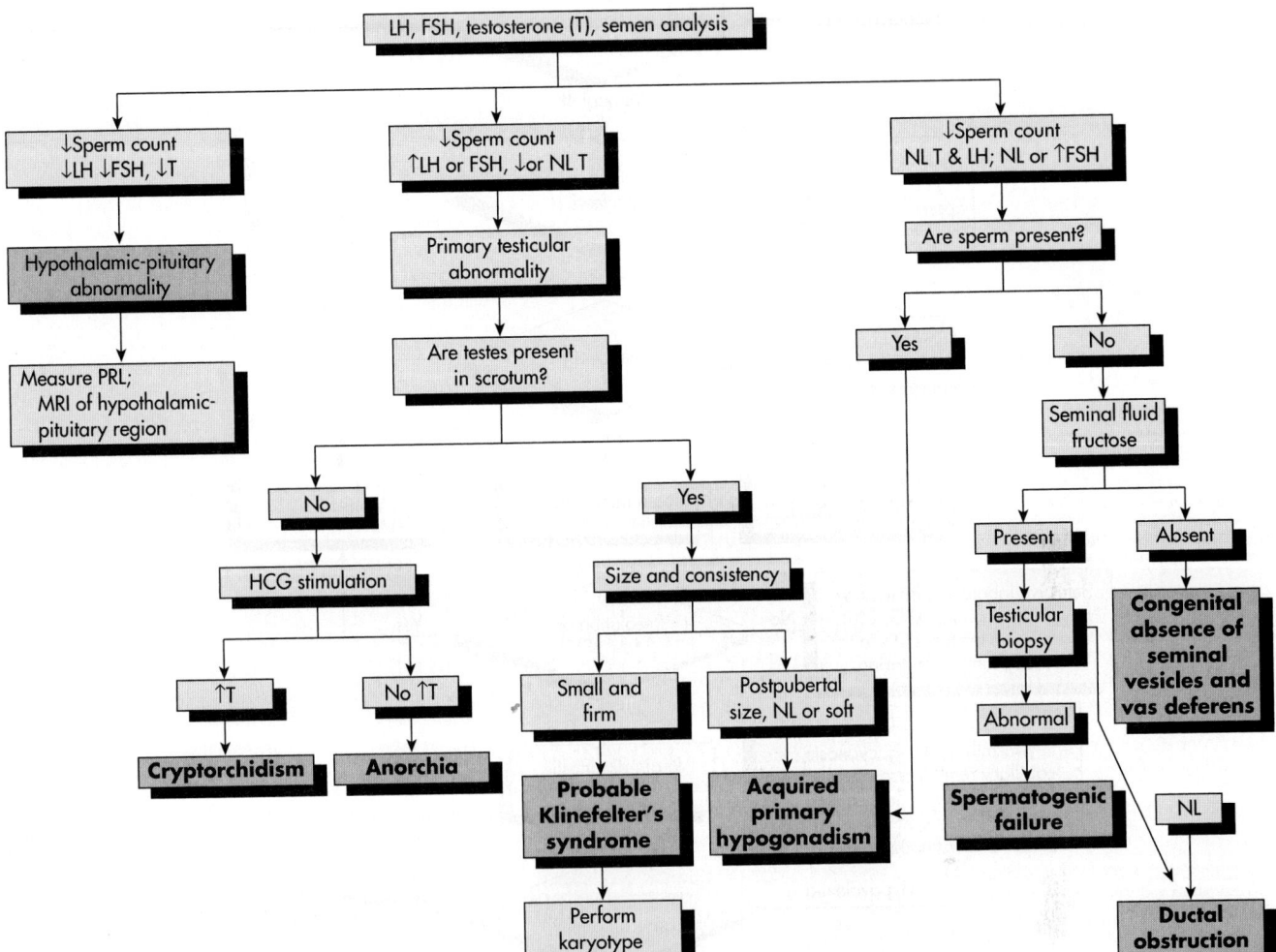

FIG. 84 Laboratory evaluation of hypogonadism. ↑, Elevated; ↓, decreased or low; *FSH*, follicle-stimulating hormone; *HCG*, human chorionic gonadotropin; *LH*, luteinizing hormone; *MRI*, magnetic resonance imaging; *NL*, normal; *PRL*, prolactin. (From Benjamin I et al: *Andreoli and Carpenter's Cecil essentials of medicine*, ed 9, Philadelphia, 2016, Saunders.)

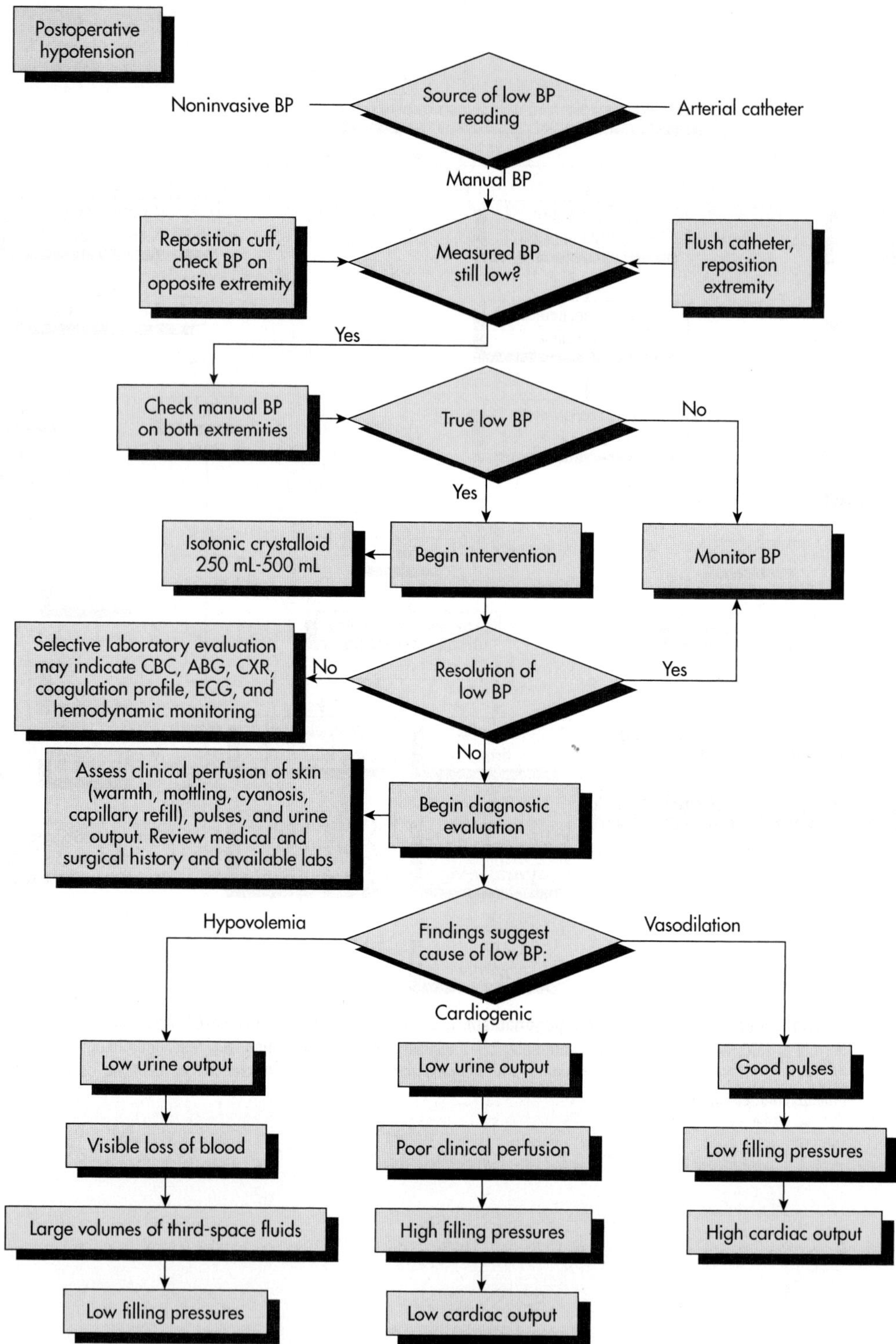

FIG. 85 Approach to managing postoperative hypotension. *ABG*, arterial blood gases; *BP*, blood pressure; *CBC*, complete blood count; *CXR*, chest x-ray study; *ECG*, electrocardiogram. (From Parrillo JE, Dellinger RP: *Critical care medicine: principles of diagnosis and management in the adult,* ed 4, Philadelphia, 2014, Elsevier.)

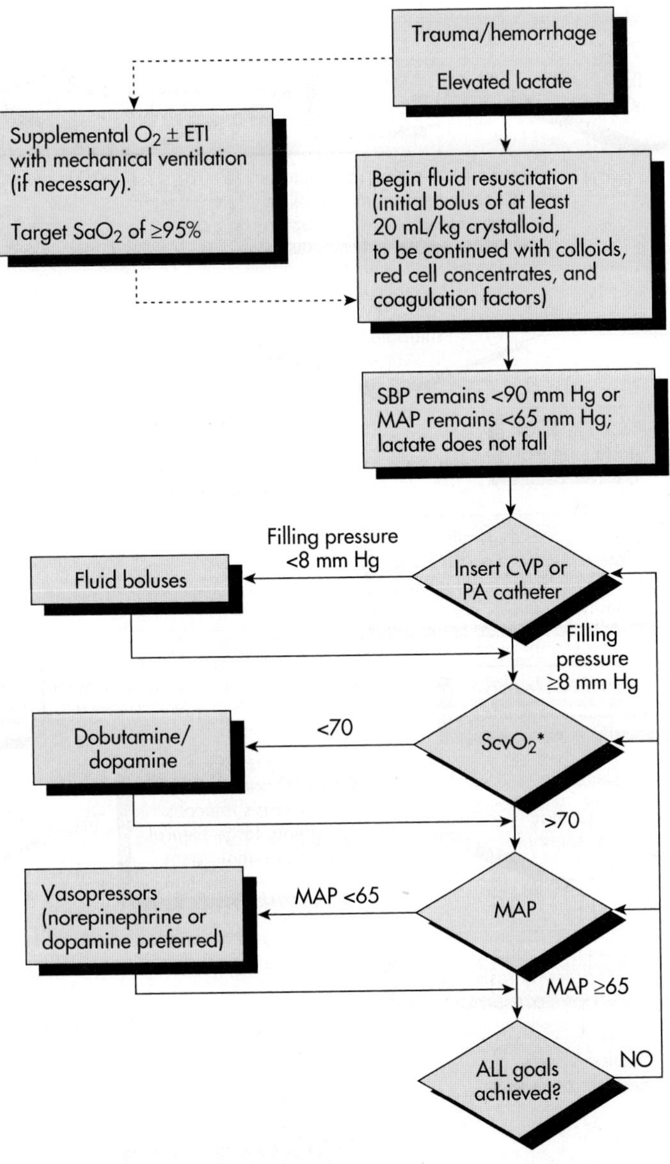

FIG. 86 Hypovolemic shock management protocol. *CVP*, central venous pressure; *ETI*, endotracheal intubation; *MAP*, mean arterial pressure; *PA*, pulmonary artery; *Sa_{O_2}*, oxygen saturation; *SBP*, systolic blood pressure; *Scv_{O_2}*, central venous oxygen saturation. (From Parrillo JE, Dellinger RP: *Critical care medicine: principles of diagnosis and management in the adult,* ed 4, Philadelphia, 2014, Elsevier.)

TABLE 24 Clinical Classification of Severity of Posthemorrhagic Hypovolemic Shock

Feature	Class I	Class II	Class III	Class IV
Blood loss				
mL	<750	750-1500	>1500-2000	>2000
%	<15	15-30	>30-40	>40
Heart rate (beats/min)	<100	>100	>120	>140
Blood pressure	Normal	Normal	Decreased	Decreased
Pulse pressure	Normal	Decreased	Decreased	Decreased
Respiratory rate	14-20	20-30	30-40	>40
Urinary output (mL/h)	>30	20-30	5-15	Negligible
Mental status	Slightly anxious	Mildly anxious	Anxious, confused	Confused, lethargic
Fluid replacement (mL/h)	Crystalloid	Crystalloid/colloid	Crystalloid and blood	Crystalloid and blood

From Parrillo JE, Dellinger RP: *Critical care medicine: principles of diagnosis and management in the adult,* ed 4, Philadelphia, 2014, Elsevier.

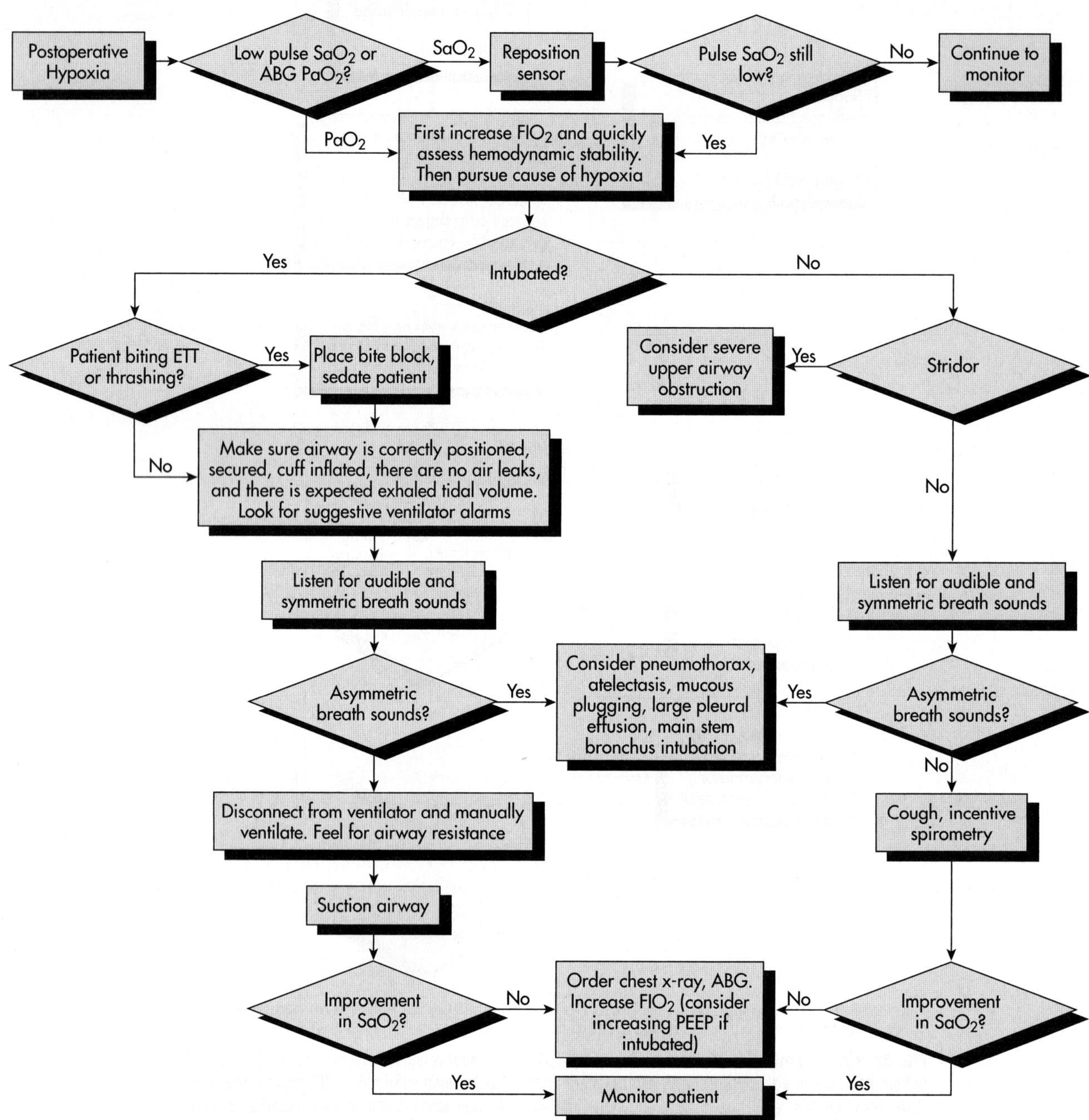

FIG. 87 Approach to managing postoperative hypoxemia. *ABG*, arterial blood gas; *ETT*, endotracheal tube; *FiO_2*, fraction of inspired oxygen; *PaO_2*, arterial oxygen tension; *PEEP*, positive end-expiratory pressure; *SaO_2*, arterial oxygen saturation. (From Parrillo JE, Dellinger RP: *Critical care medicine: principles of diagnosis and management in the adult,* ed 4, Philadelphia, 2014, Elsevier.)

INFECTIONS OF SOFT TISSUE, JOINTS, AND BONE

ICD-10CM # M00.9 Pyogenic arthritis, unspecified
M86.9 Osteomyelitis unspecified
T84.3 Infection and inflammatory reaction
M79.9 Soft tissue disorder, unspecified

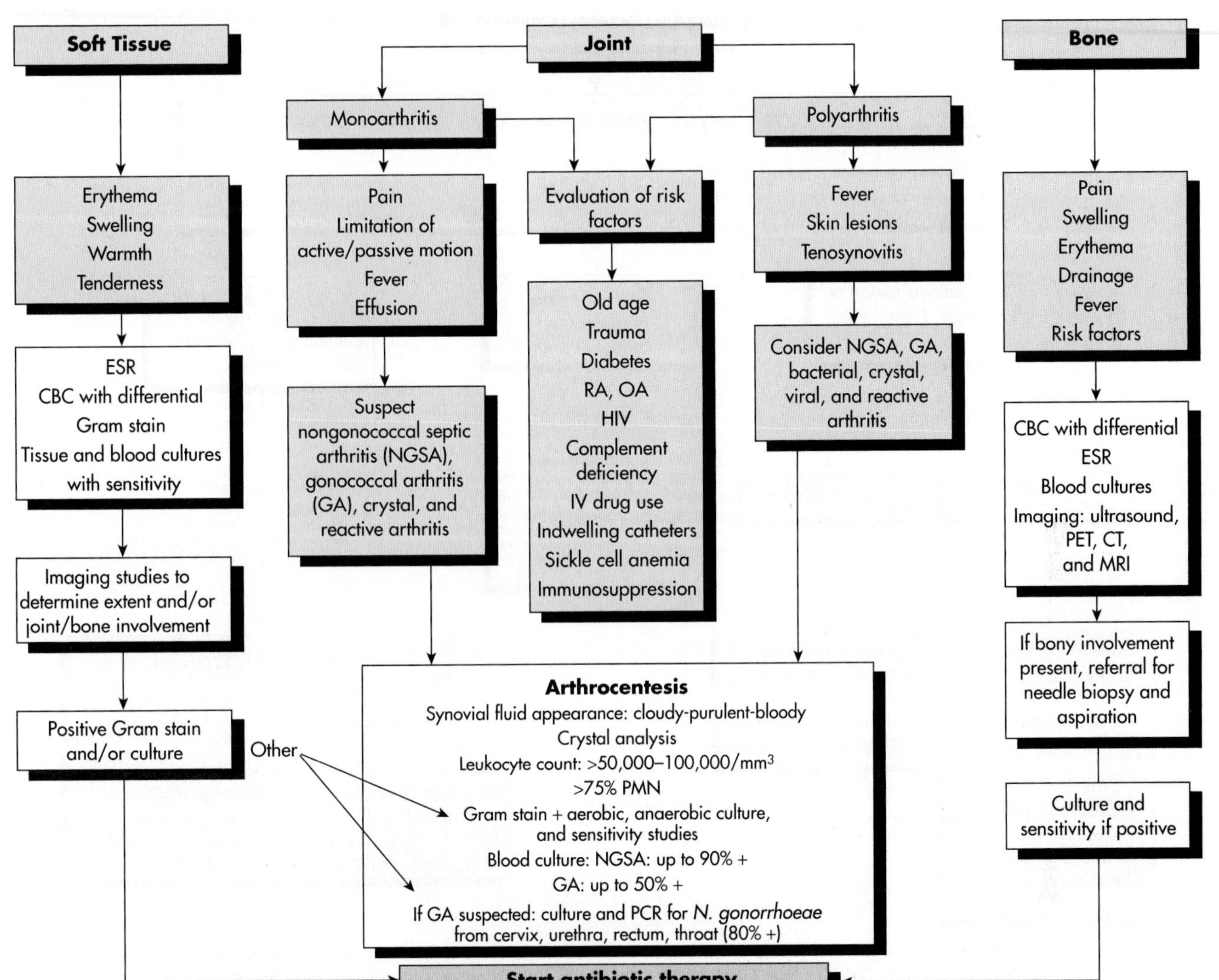

FIG. 88 Clinical evaluation of infections of soft tissues, joints, and bone. *CBC,* Complete blood count; *CT,* computed tomography; *ESR,* erythrocyte sedimentation rate; *GA,* gonococcal arthritis; *HIV,* human immunodeficiency virus; *IV,* intravenous; *MRI,* magnetic resonance imaging; *NGSA,* nongonococcal septic arthritis; *OA,* osteoarthritis; *PCR,* polymerase chain reaction; *PET,* positron emission tomography; *PMN,* polymorphonuclear leukocyte; *RA,* rheumatoid arthritis. (From Goldman L, Schafer AI: *Goldman Cecil medicine,* ed 25, Philadelphia, 2016, Saunders.)

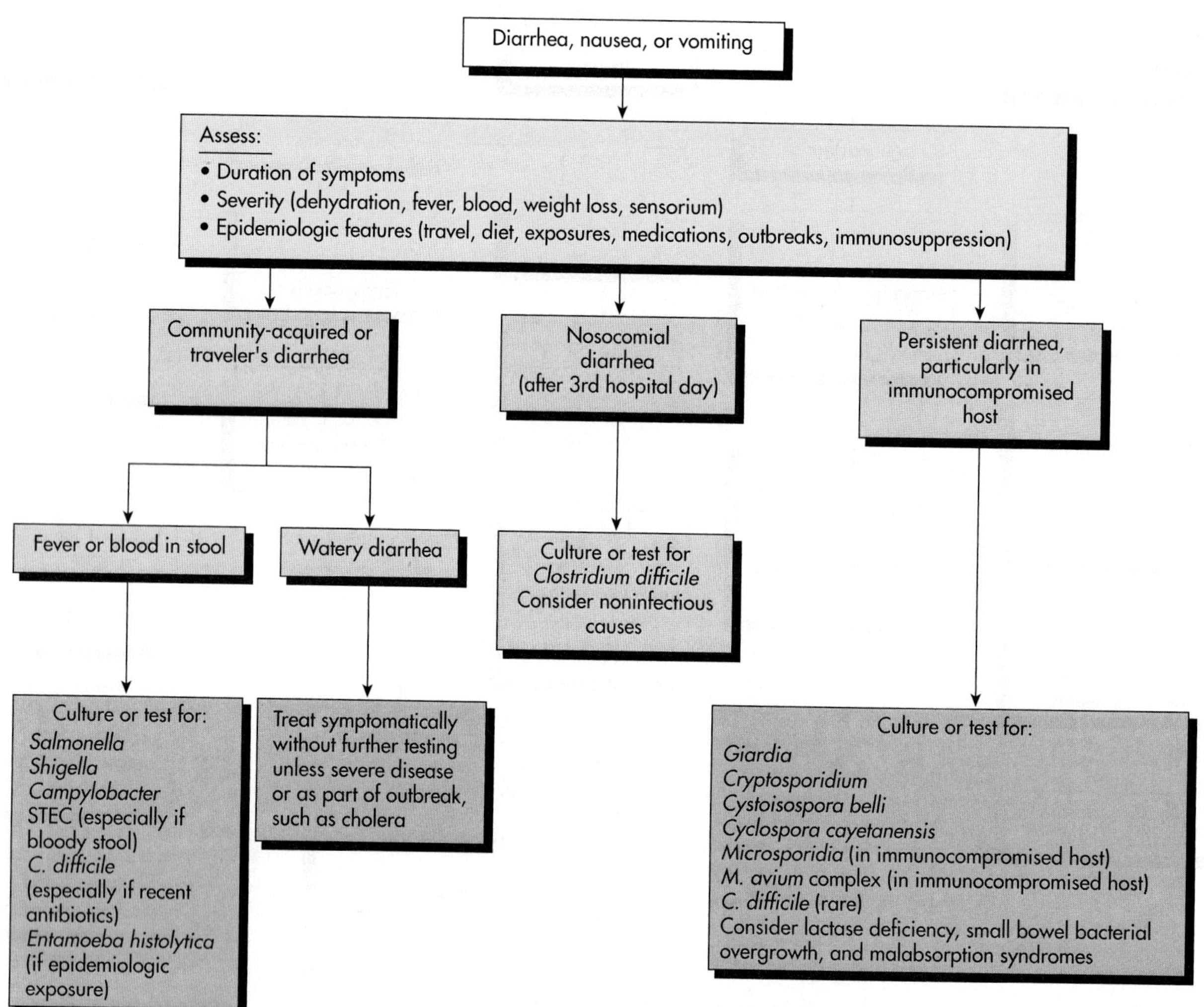

FIG. 89 Approach to diagnosis of infectious diarrhea. *STEC*, Shiga toxin–producing *Escherichia coli.* (From Bennett JE, Dolin R, Blaser MJ: *Mandell, Douglas, and Bennett's principles and practice of infectious diseases*, ed 8, Philadelphia, 2015, Saunders.)

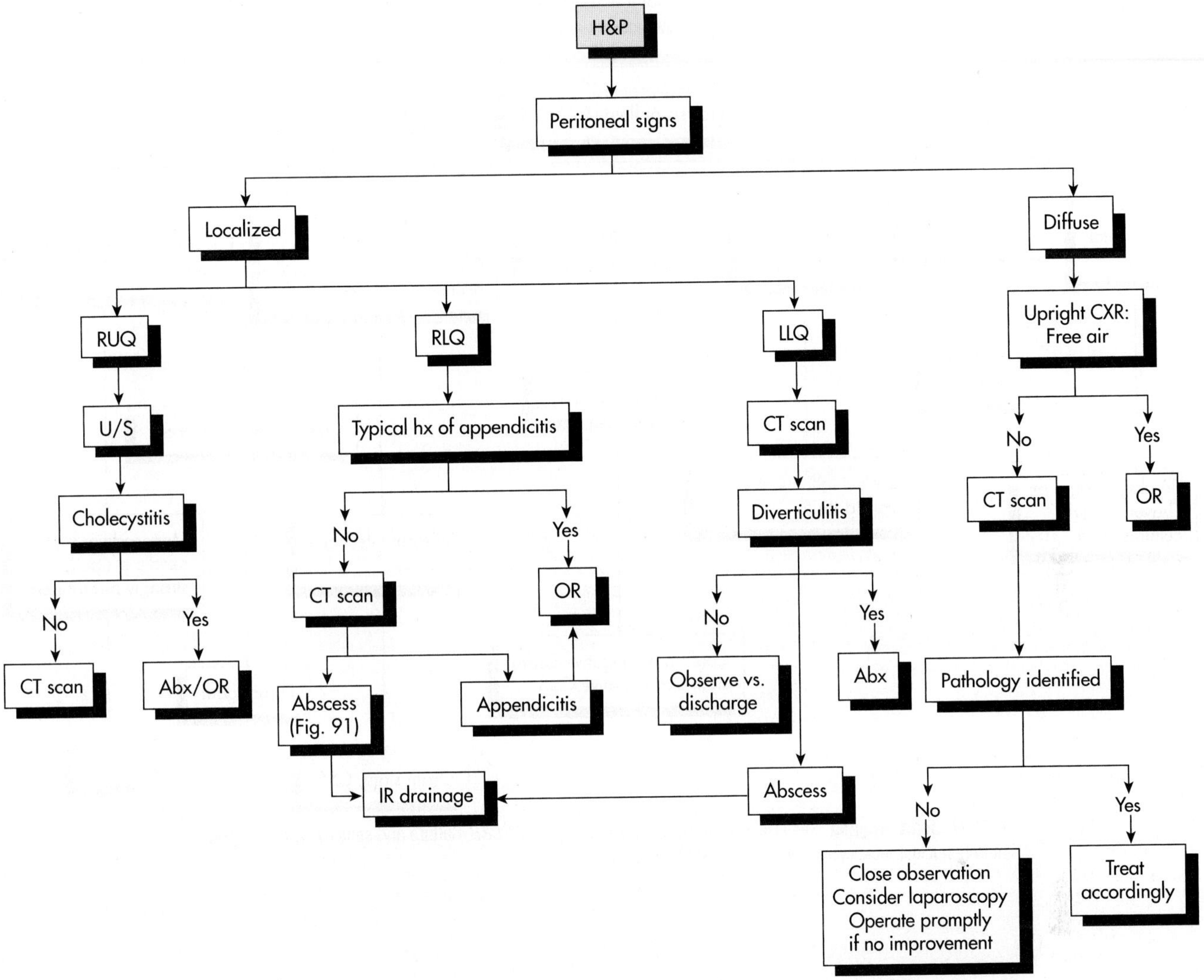

INTRAABDOMINAL INFECTION, SUSPECTED

- H&P
  - Peritoneal signs
    - Localized
      - RUQ
        - U/S
          - Cholecystitis
            - No → CT scan
            - Yes → Abx/OR
      - RLQ
        - Typical hx of appendicitis
          - No → CT scan
            - Abscess (Fig. 91) → IR drainage
            - Appendicitis → OR
          - Yes → OR
      - LLQ
        - CT scan
          - Diverticulitis
            - No → Observe vs. discharge
            - Yes → Abx
            - Abscess → IR drainage
    - Diffuse
      - Upright CXR: Free air
        - No → CT scan
          - Pathology identified
            - No → Close observation / Consider laparoscopy / Operate promptly if no improvement
            - Yes → Treat accordingly
        - Yes → OR

FIG. 90 Algorithm for the diagnosis and management of patients with suspected intraabdominal infection. *Abx,* antibiotics; *CT,* computed tomography; *CXR,* chest radiograph; *H&P,* History and physical exam; *hx,* history; *IR,* interventional radiology; *LLQ,* left lower quadrant; *RLQ,* right lower quadrant; *RUQ,* right upper quadrant; *U/S,* ultrasound. (From Cameron JL, Cameron AM: *Current surgical therapy,* ed 10, Philadelphia, 2011, Saunders.)

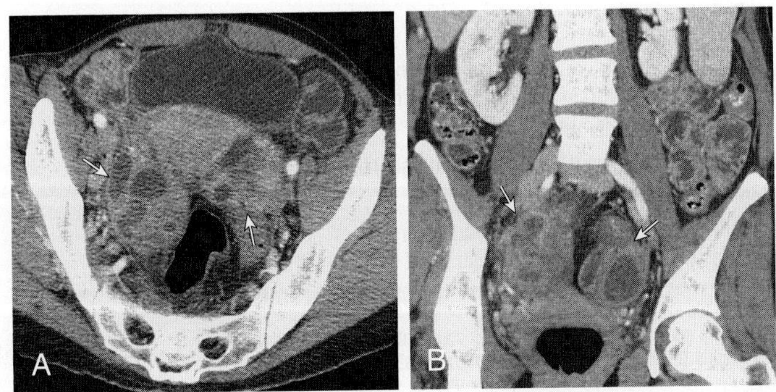

FIG. 91 Axial (A) and coronal (B) postcontrast computed tomographic images showing bilateral tuboovarian abscesses *(arrows)*. (Fielding JR et al: *Gynecologic imaging,* Philadelphia, 2011, Saunders.)

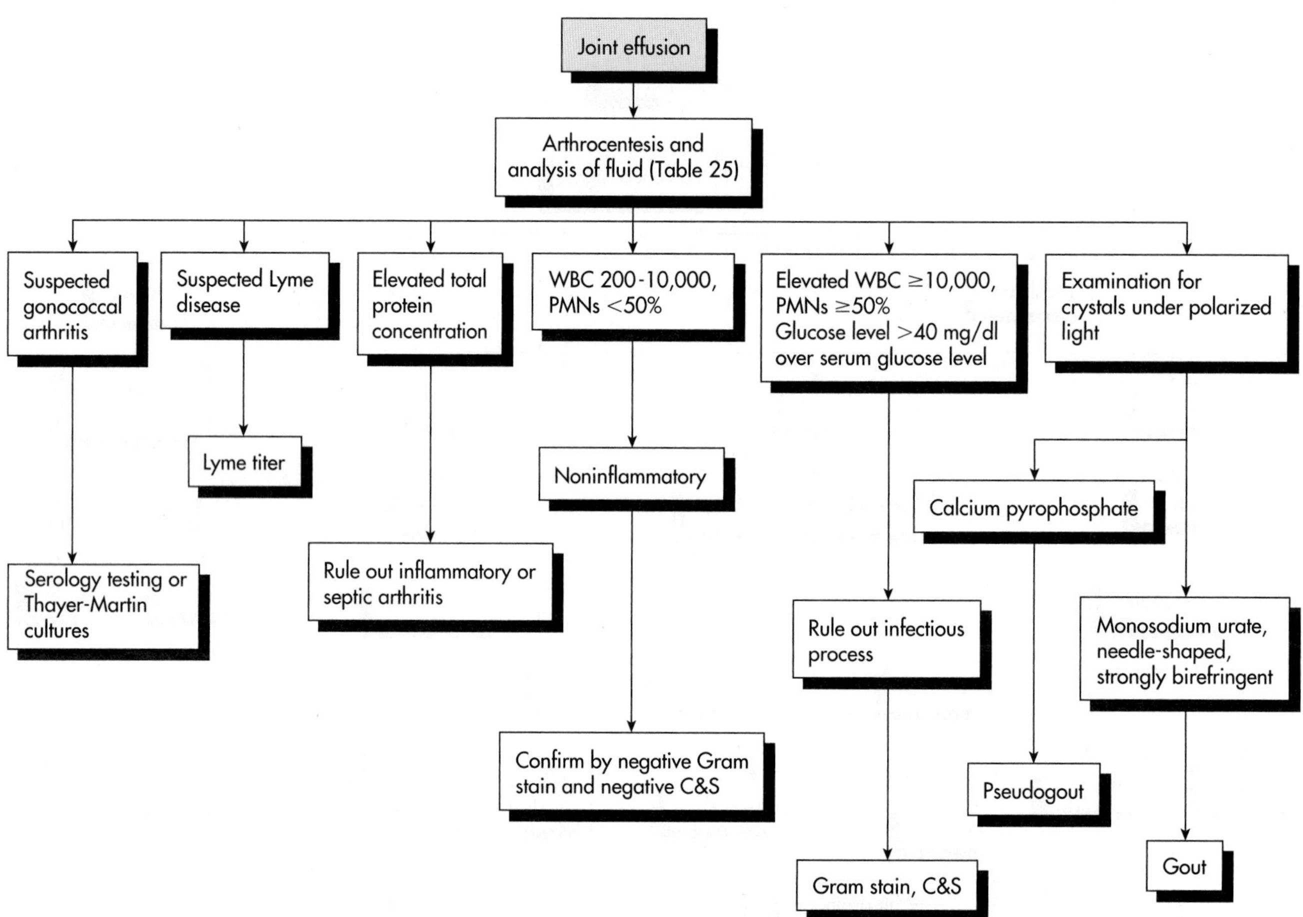

FIG. 92 Joint effusion. See also Section IV, "Arthrocentesis Fluid." *C&S,* Culture and sensitivity; *PMNs,* polymorphonuclear leukocytes; *WBC,* white blood cell count.

TABLE 25 Indications for Arthrocentesis

Undiagnosed Arthritis with Effusion

Characterize type of arthritis

- Noninflammatory (WBC <2000/mm^3)
- Inflammatory (WBC >2000/mm^3)
- Septic (WBC >50,000/mm^3)
- Definitive diagnosis
- Gout (urate crystals)
- Pseudogout (calcium pyrophosphate dihydrate crystals)
- Septic arthritis (Gram stain [rare] or culture)

Undiagnosed Arthritis without Effusion

May be definitive in gout (knee, first metatarsophalangeal joint)

Patient with Known Diagnosis

Septic arthritis (repeated taps for adequate drainage)
Other types of arthritis for symptomatic relief (with or without injection)*

WBC, white blood cells.
*Most studies show improved effect if fluid is aspirated before injection.
From Firestein GS et al: *Kelley's textbook of rheumatology,* ed 9, Philadelphia, 2013, Saunders.

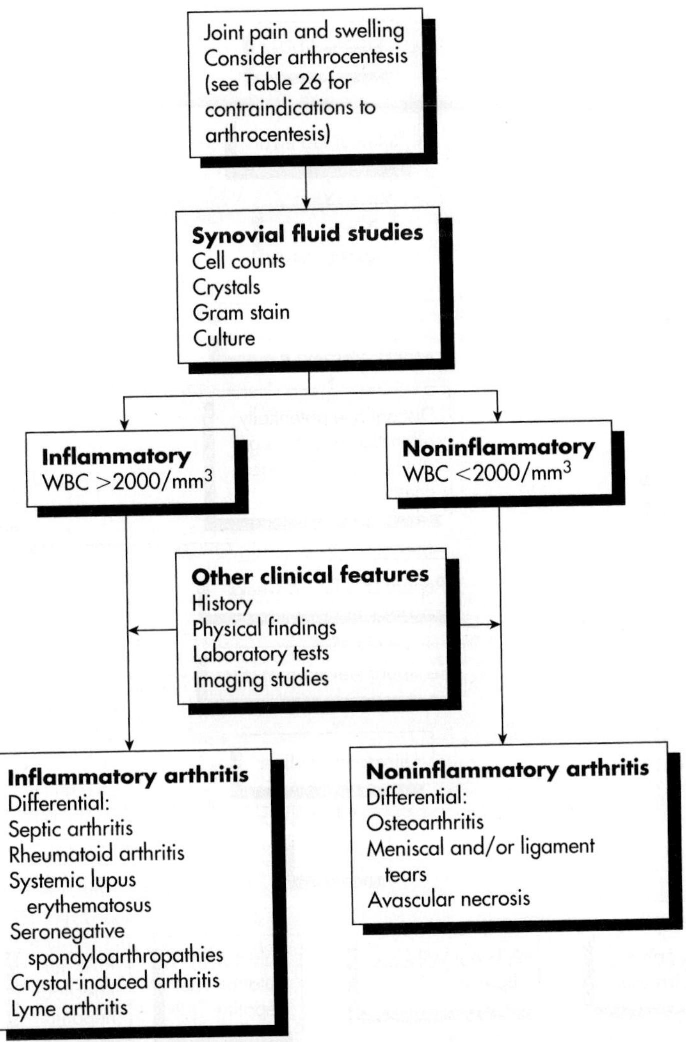

FIG. 93 Diagnostic approach for swollen joints. *WBC,* White blood cell count. (From Goldman L, Schafer AL [eds]: *Cecil textbook of medicine,* ed 24, Philadelphia, 2012, Saunders.)

TABLE 26 Contraindications to Arthrocentesis and Joint Injection

Contraindication	Comment
Established infection in nearby structures (e.g., cellulitis, septic bursitis)	Sometimes gout mimics cellulitis, creating a confusing picture
Septicemia (theoretic risk of introducing organism into joint)	Need to tap suspected septic joints in septic patients
Disrupted skin barrier (e.g., psoriasis)	Do not tap through lesions
Bleeding disorder (not absolute, but use more care)	Risk of bleeding very low, even in patients taking warfarin
Septic joint	Steroid injection contraindicated
Prior lack of response	Relative contraindication
Difficult-to-access joint	Relative contraindication without imaging aid

From Firestein GS et al: *Kelley's textbook of rheumatology,* ed 9, Philadelphia, 2013, Saunders

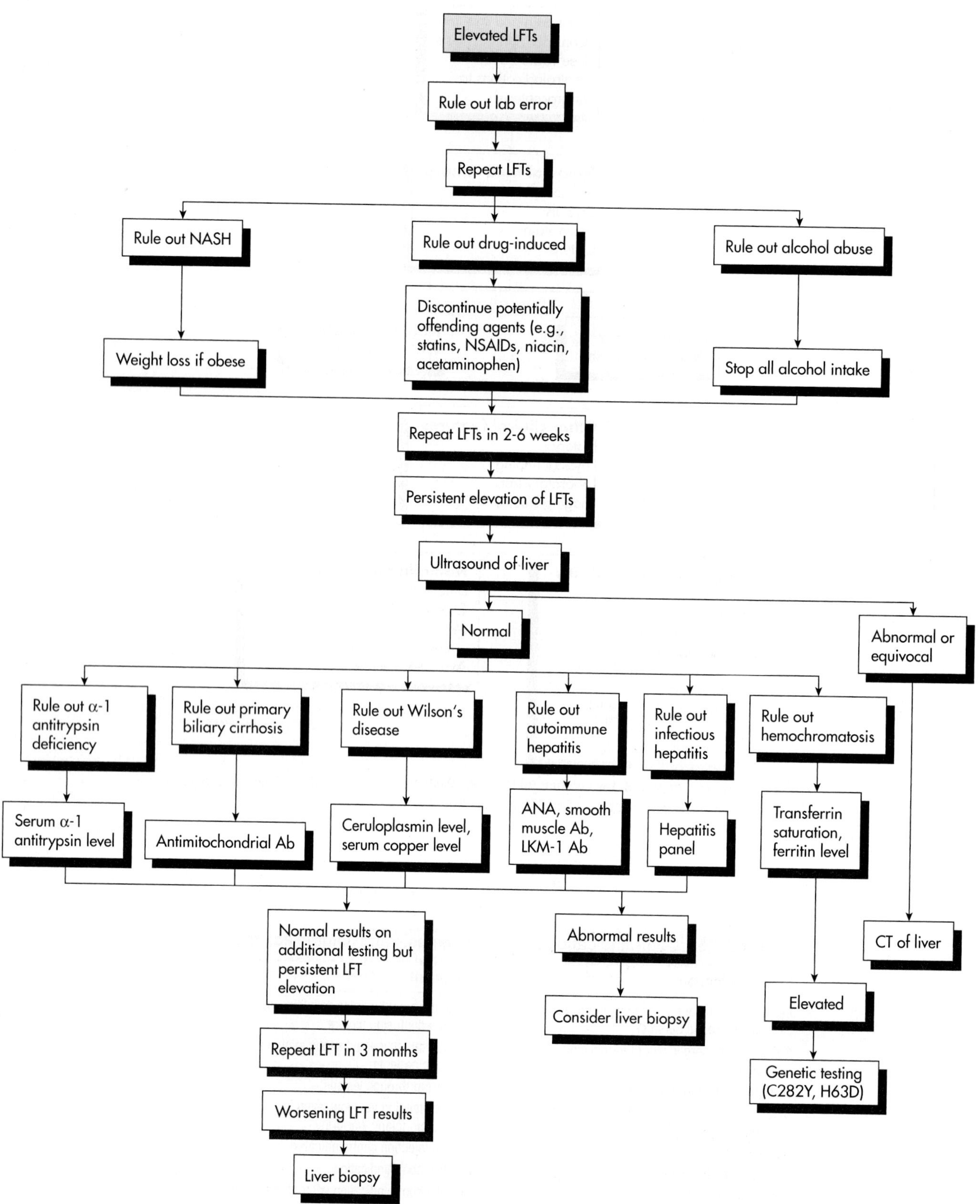

FIG. 94 Liver function test elevations. *Ab,* Antibody; *ANA,* antibody to nuclear antigens; *CT,* computed tomography; *LFTs,* liver function tests; *LKM,* liver-kidney microsome; *NASH,* nonalcoholic steatohepatitis; *NSAIDs,* nonsteroidal antiinflammatory drugs.

MENTAL STATUS CHANGE, ELDERLY PATIENT

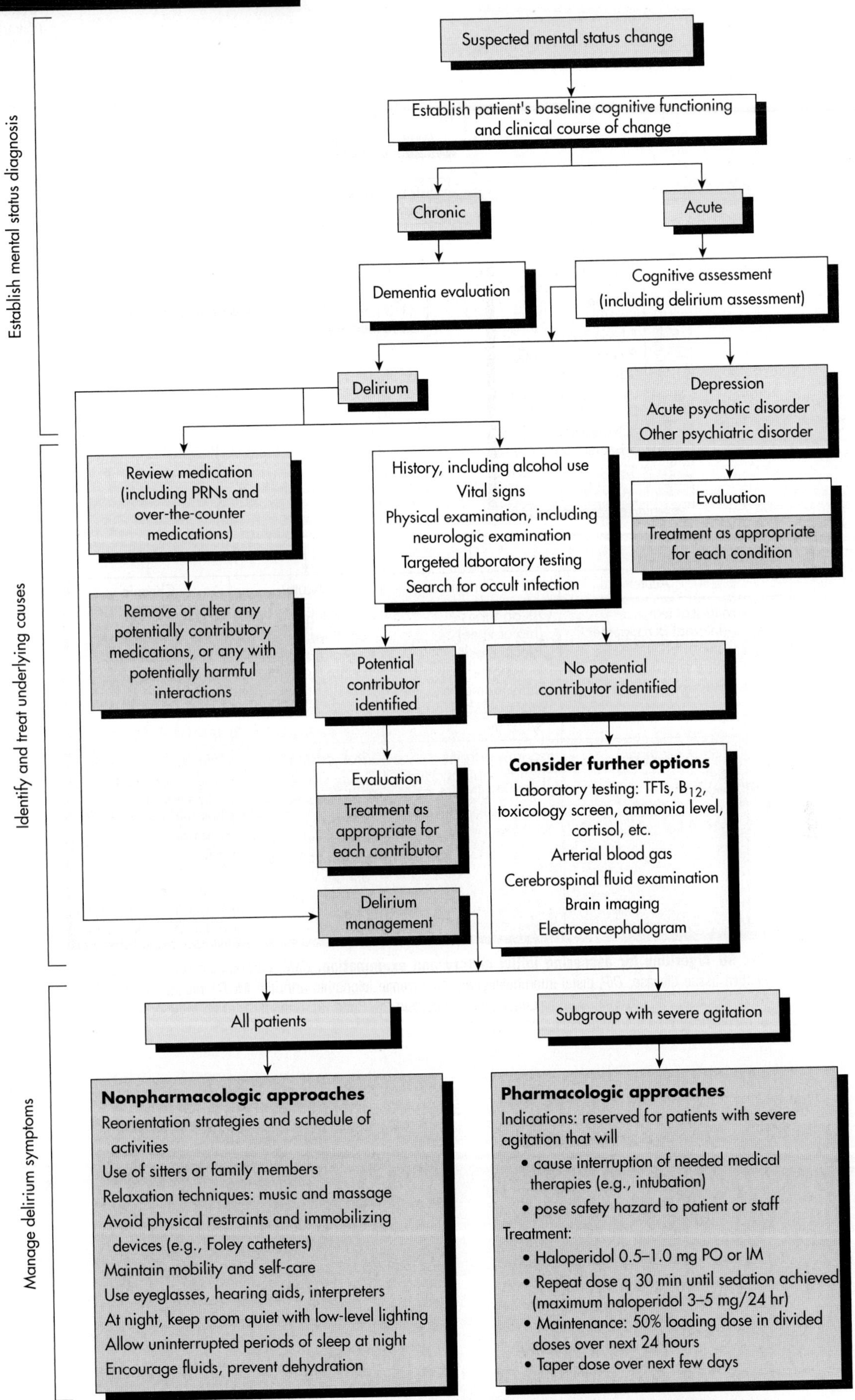

FIG. 95 Algorithm for the evaluation of suspected mental status change in older patients. *PRN*, As needed; *TFTs*, thyroid function tests. (From Goldman L, Schafer AI: *Goldman Cecil medicine*, ed 25, Philadelphia, 2016, Saunders.)

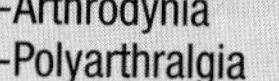

ICD-10CM # M25.50 -Pain(s) joint
-Arthralgia (allergic)
-Arthrodynia
-Polyarthralgia

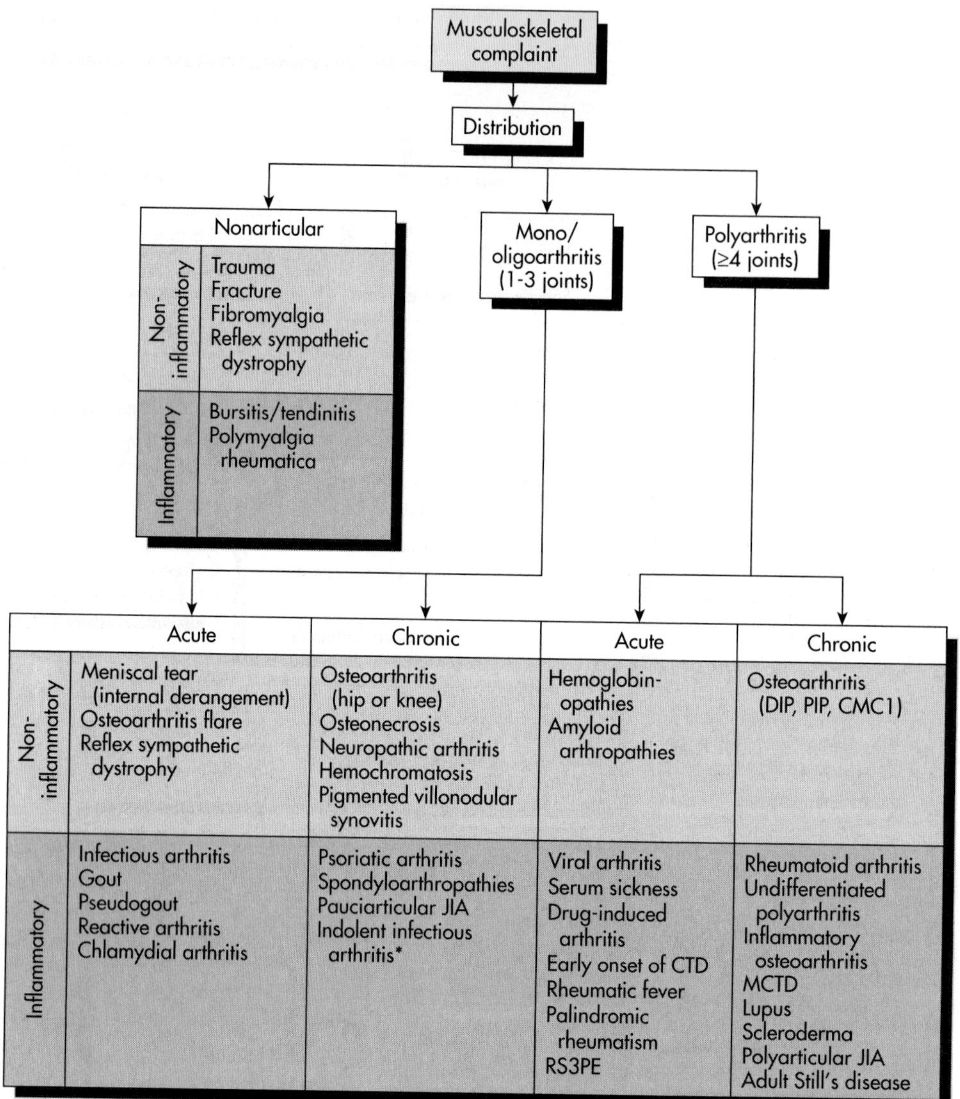

FIG. 96 Algorithm for assessing initial history and examination. *CMC*, Carpometacarpal; *CTD*, connective tissue disease; *DIP*, distal interphalangeal; *JIA*, juvenile idiopathic arthritis; *MCTD*, mixed connective tissue disease; *PIP*, proximal interphalangeal. (From Firestein GS, Budd RC, Gabriel SE et al: *Kelley's textbook of rheumatology*, ed 9, Philadelphia, 2013, Saunders.)

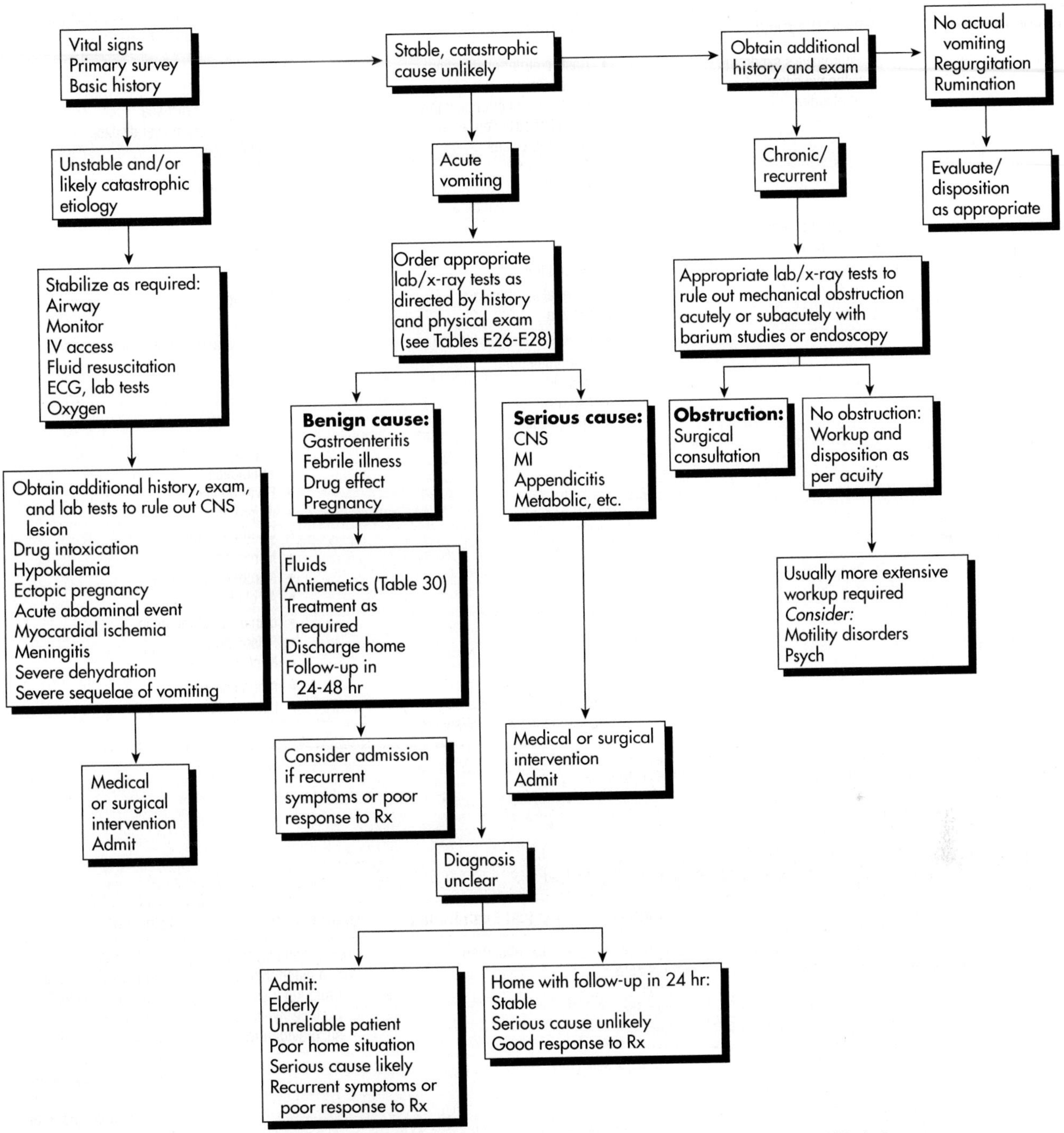

Vital signs
Primary survey
Basic history

Unstable and/or likely catastrophic etiology

Stabilize as required:
Airway
Monitor
IV access
Fluid resuscitation
ECG, lab tests
Oxygen

Obtain additional history, exam, and lab tests to rule out CNS lesion
Drug intoxication
Hypokalemia
Ectopic pregnancy
Acute abdominal event
Myocardial ischemia
Meningitis
Severe dehydration
Severe sequelae of vomiting

Medical or surgical intervention
Admit

Stable, catastrophic cause unlikely

Acute vomiting

Order appropriate lab/x-ray tests as directed by history and physical exam (see Tables E26-E28)

Benign cause:
Gastroenteritis
Febrile illness
Drug effect
Pregnancy

Fluids
Antiemetics (Table 30)
Treatment as required
Discharge home
Follow-up in 24-48 hr

Consider admission if recurrent symptoms or poor response to Rx

Serious cause:
CNS
MI
Appendicitis
Metabolic, etc.

Medical or surgical intervention
Admit

Diagnosis unclear

Admit:
Elderly
Unreliable patient
Poor home situation
Serious cause likely
Recurrent symptoms or poor response to Rx

Home with follow-up in 24 hr:
Stable
Serious cause unlikely
Good response to Rx

Obtain additional history and exam

No actual vomiting
Regurgitation
Rumination

Evaluate/disposition as appropriate

Chronic/recurrent

Appropriate lab/x-ray tests to rule out mechanical obstruction acutely or subacutely with barium studies or endoscopy

Obstruction:
Surgical consultation

No obstruction:
Workup and disposition as per acuity

Usually more extensive workup required
Consider:
Motility disorders
Psych

FIG. 97 Approach to the patient with nausea and vomiting. *CNS,* Central nervous system; *ECG,* electrocardiogram; *IV,* intravenous; *MI,* myocardial infarction; *Psych,* psychogenic; *Rx,* treatment. (From Marx JA et al: *Rosen's emergency medicine,* ed 8, Philadelphia, 2014, Saunders.)

TABLE 27 Differential Diagnosis of Nausea and Vomiting

Etiologic Category	Critical Diagnoses	Emergent Diagnoses	Nonemergent Diagnoses
Gastrointestinal (GI)	• Boerhaave's syndrome • Ischemic bowel • GI bleeding	• Gastric outlet obstruction • Pancreatitis • Cholecystitis or cholangitis • Bowel obstruction or ileus • Ruptured viscus • Appendicitis • Peritonitis • Spontaneous bacterial peritonitis	• Gastritis • Gastroparesis • Peptic ulcer disease • Inflammatory bowel disease • Biliary colic • Hepatitis • Gastroenteritis
Neurologic	• Intracerebral bleed • Meningitis	• Migraine • CNS tumor • Raised ICP	
Endocrine	• DKA	• Adrenal insufficiency • Uremia	• Thyroid
Pregnancy		• Hyperemesis gravidarum	• Nausea and vomiting of pregnancy
Drug toxicity		• Acetaminophen • Digoxin • Aspirin • Theophylline	
Therapeutic drug use			• Aspirin • Antibiotics • Erythromycin • Ibuprofen • Chemotherapy
Drugs of abuse			• Narcotics • Narcotic withdrawal • Alcohol
Genitourinary		• Gonadal torsion	• Urinary tract infection • Poisoning • Nephrolithiasis
Miscellaneous	• Myocardial infarctionSepsis	• Carbon monoxide • Electrolyte disorders • Organophosphate poisoning	• Motion sickness • Labyrinthitis

CNS, Central nervous system; *DKA,* diabetic ketoacidosis; *ICP,* intracranial pressure.
From Marx JA et al: *Rosen's emergency medicine,* ed 8, Philadelphia, 2014, Saunders.

TABLE 28 Disorders Commonly Associated with Vomiting

Disorder	History	Prevalence	Physical Examination	Useful Tests	Comments
Nausea and vomiting of pregnancy (NVP)	Vomiting occurs predominantly in the morning. Associated breast tenderness. NVP typically starts in weeks 4-7, peaks in weeks 10-16, and disappears by week 20. Vomiting that begins after week 12 or continues past week 20 should prompt a search for another cause.	Very common Affects 75% of all pregnancies	Benign abdomen	Urine pregnancy test Serum electrolytes, urine ketones to exclude hyperemesis gravidarum	Consider NVP in all females of childbearing age. Prognosis for mother and infant is excellent. NVP is associated with a decreased risk of miscarriage, fetal growth retardation, and fetal mortality.
Hyperemesis gravidarum	Severe, protracted form of NVP. No universally accepted definition of the disease. Generally accepted hallmarks include 5% weight loss, ketonuria, and electrolyte disturbance. Hyperemesis is associated with multiple gestation, molar pregnancy, and nulliparity.	Uncommon Affects <1% of pregnancies	Signs of dehydration Benign abdomen	β-hCG Urinalysis for ketones Serum electrolytes Ultrasound examination to exclude molar pregnancy or multiple gestation	Most studies have found no adverse outcomes for the fetus. A few studies, however, have shown a correlation with fetal growth retardation.
Gastroenteritis	Fever, diarrhea, and crampy abdominal pain. Vomiting and pain occur early, usually followed by diarrhea within 24 hr.	Very common	Benign abdomen	Usually not necessary	Early gastroenteritis, when only vomiting and periumbilical pain are present, may be confused with early appendicitis. Diarrhea is usually in the diagnosis of gastroenteritis.

Continued

TABLE 28 Disorders Commonly Associated with Vomiting—cont'd

Disorder	History	Prevalence	Physical Examination	Useful Tests	Comments
Gastritis	Epigastric pain, belching, bloating, fullness, heartburn, and food intolerance. Use of NSAIDs or ETOH common.	Very common	Mild epigastric tenderness may be present.	Lipase and pregnancy test may be necessary to exclude other diagnoses.	Removal of inciting agent along with antacid therapy will resolve symptoms in most patients.
Peptic ulcer disease (PUD)	Epigastric pain present in 90% of cases. Classically, duodenal ulcer pain is relieved by food whereas gastric ulcer pain is made worse. Presence of severe pain should raise suspicion of perforation.	Very common	Mild epigastric tenderness	Hemoglobin if bleeding is suspected Heme-positive stool Upright abdominal film if perforation is suspected	Three major causes of PUD are NSAIDs, *Helicobacter pylori* infection, and hypersecretory states.
Biliary disease	Abdominal pain may be midepigastric or right upper quadrant (RUQ). Onset frequently after a fatty meal. May have history of similar episodes in the past.	Very common	RUQ tenderness present in most cases. If instructed to breathe deeply during palpation in the RUQ, the patient experiences heightened tenderness and inspiratory arrest (Murphy's sign).	WBCs Lipase Serum bilirubin Alkaline phosphatase RUQ ultrasound examination ERCP	Normal temperature, WBCs, and spontaneous resolution of symptoms suggest biliary colic. Fever, Murphy's sign, elevated WBCs, and suggestive ultrasound indicate cholecystitis.
Myocardial infarction (MI)	Patients typically have substernal chest pain that may radiate to left arm or jaw. Often associated with dyspnea, diaphoresis, or dizziness.	Common	Patients often are anxious and in distress from pain. No diagnostic examination findings.	ECG (new Q waves, ST segment changes, or T wave inversions) troponin	Not all patients have chest pain. A subset of patients, particularly diabetics and elders, may have only nausea, vomiting, and epigastric discomfort.
Diabetic ketoacidosis (DKA)	Polydipsia and polyuria occur early. Without treatment, altered mental status and coma may develop. In patients with long-standing diabetes, DKA may be triggered by infection, trauma, MI, or surgery.	Common	"Fruity" breath odor results from serum acetone. Tachypnea occurs with attempts to "blow off" carbon dioxide to compensate for metabolic acidosis. Signs of dehydration may be present. Severe cases often manifest with altered mental status or coma.	Serum glucose, urine ketones, ABGs	DKA may be the first manifestation of diabetes in some patients. These patients often do not recognize the importance of polydipsia and polyuria. They often report only nausea, vomiting, and epigastric pain.
Pancreatitis	Presenting symptom is epigastric pain, which often radiates to the back. Most cases are caused by gallstones or alcoholism. Other causes include hypercalcemia, hyperlipidemia, drugs (sulfas and thiazides), ERCP.	Common	Epigastric tenderness is present. Associated paralytic ileus may cause abdominal distention and decreased bowel sounds. Frank shock may be present in severe cases.	Lipase WBCs, serum glucose, LDH, AST Hematocrit, BUN, calcium, ABGs	Criteria correlating with higher mortality: *At admission*—age >55 yr, WBCs >16,000/mm^3, glucose >200 dL, base deficit >4, LDH >350 IU/L, AST >250 U/L *Within 48 hours*—Hct drop of 10%, BUN >2 mg/dL, P_{O_2} <60 mm Hg, calcium <8 mg, fluid sequestration >4 L
Appendicitis	Abdominal pain classically begins in periumbilical region and later moves to right lower quadrant. Anorexia is common.	Common	Localized tenderness over right lower quadrant. Low-grade fever may be present.	WBCs Ultrasound Abdominal CT	Early appendicitis can be a difficult diagnosis to make. It is still frequently missed on the first physician encounter.
Bowel obstruction	Classically, abdominal pain consists of intermittent cramps occurring at regular intervals. The frequency of the cramps varies with the level of the obstruction; the higher the level, the more frequent the cramps. The location of the pain also varies with the level of the obstruction; high obstruction causes epigastric pain, midlevel obstruction causes periumbilical pain, colonic obstruction causes hypogastric pain.	Common	Abdominal distention, mild diffuse tenderness, and high-pitched "tinkling" bowel sounds may be present. Thorough search for hernias should be performed.	Supine and upright plain abdominal films Abdominal CT	Adhesions, hernias, and tumors account for 90% of bowel obstructions. Other causes include intussusception, volvulus, foreign bodies, gallstone ileus, inflammatory bowel disease, stricture, cystic fibrosis, and hematoma.
Carbon monoxide (CO) poisoning	Headache is usually present. CO poisoning often occurs during winter months when furnaces are turned on. Family members may have similar symptoms if they also have been exposed.	Uncommon	No reliable signs of early CO poisoning	CO level	Because CO is a tasteless, odorless gas, patients may not realize they have been exposed. It is important to keep a high index of suspicion during the cold months.

TABLE 28 Disorders Commonly Associated with Vomiting—cont'd

Disorder	History	Prevalence	Physical Examination	Useful Tests	Comments
Boerhaave's syndrome	Patients may have neck, chest, or epigastric pain. Forceful, protracted vomiting usually causes the tear. Most cases follow a bout of heavy eating and drinking. Other reported causes include childbirth, defecation, seizures, and heavy lifting.	Uncommon	Tachypnea, tachycardia, and hypotension may be present. Escaped air from the esophagus may produce subcutaneous emphysema. Air in the mediastinum produces a "crunching" sound as the heart beats (Hamman's sign).	CXR may show pleural effusion, widened mediastinum, pneumothorax, or pneumomediastinum. Esophagogram with water-soluble contrast is definitive.	The classic presentation includes forceful vomiting, severe chest pain, subcutaneous emphysema, and multiple CXR findings. There is a growing body of evidence that most cases do not have this "classic" picture. In more subtle presentations, the diagnosis can be difficult to make.

ABGs, arterial blood gases; *AST,* aspartate aminotransferase; *β-hCG,* β-human chorionic gonadotropin; *BUN,* blood urea nitrogen; *CT,* computed tomography; *CXR,* chest radiography; *ECG,* electrocardiogram; *ERCP,* endoscopic retrograde cholangiopancreatography; *ETOH,* ethyl alcohol; *Hct,* hematocrit; *LDH,* lactate dehydrogenase; *NSAID,* nonsteroidal antiinflammatory drug; *Po_2,* partial pressure of oxygen; *WBC,* white blood cell.

From Marx JA et al: *Rosen's emergency medicine,* ed 8, Philadelphia, 2014, Saunders.

TABLE 29 Etiology of Nausea and Vomiting in Pediatric Age Groups

Etiologic Category	Newborn	Infant	Child	Adolescent
Infectious	Sepsis, meningitis, UTI, thrush	Pneumonia, otitis media, thrush	Gastroenteritis	Gastroenteritis, URI
Anatomic	Atresia and webs, malrotation, stenosis, meconium ileus, Hirschsprung's disease	Pyloric stenosis, intussusception, Hirschsprung's disease	Bezoars, chronic granulomatous disease	PUD, superior mesenteric syndrome
Gastrointestinal	Reflux, overfeeding, gastric outlet obstruction, volvulus	Reflux, gastritis, milk intolerance	Appendicitis, pancreatic, hepatitis, other food intolerance	Achalasia, hepatitis
Neurologic	Subdural hematoma, hydrocephalus	Subdural hematoma	Neoplasia, migraine, Reye's syndrome, motion sickness, hypertension	Neoplasia, migraine, motion sickness, hypertension
Metabolic	Organic or amino acidemias, urea cycle defects, galactosemia, hypercalcemia, phenylketonuria, kernicterus	Hereditary fructose intolerance, disorders of fatty acid metabolism, uremia, adrenal hyperplasia, kernicterus	Diabetes, vitamin A excess	Diabetes, pregnancy, acute intermittent porphyria
Other	Idiopathic, cardiac failure	Rumination, cardiac failure	Cyclic vomiting syndrome, toxins, food poisoning, Munchausen syndrome by proxy	Psychogenic, anorexia

PUD, peptic ulcer disease; *URI,* upper respiratory infection; *UTI,* urinary tract infection.

Adapted from Li HK, Sunku BK: Vomiting and nausea. In Wyllie R, Hyams JS, editors: *Pediatric gastrointestinal and liver disease: pathophysiology, diagnosis, management.* Philadelphia: WB Saunders; 2005:127-149.

From Marx JA et al: *Rosen's emergency medicine,* ed 8, Philadelphia, 2014, Saunders.

TABLE 30 Commonly Used Medications for the Treatment of Nausea and Vomiting

Medication	Dose	Comments
Promethazine (Phenergan)	*Adult:* 12.5-25 mg IV, IM, PO, or by rectum *Pediatric:* 0.25-1 mg/kg/dose q4-6h prn IV, IM, PO, or by rectum; max 25 mg/dose	May be repeated every 4-6 hr until cessation of vomiting. May cause dry mouth, dizziness, blurred vision. Boxed warning for use under 2 yr old.
Prochlorperazine (Compazine)	*Adult:* 5-10 mg IM or PO; 2.5-10 mg IV; 25 mg by rectum *Pediatric:* 0.4 mg/kg/24 hr tid-qid PO or by rectum; 0.1-0.15 mg/kg/dose tid-qid IM; max 40 mg/24 hr	May be repeated every 4 hr IV or IM or every 12 hr by rectum until cessation of vomiting. May cause lethargy, hypotension, extrapyramidal effects.
Metoclopramide (Reglan)	*Adult:* 10 mg IM or IV, may repeat q6h *Pediatric:* 1-2 mg/kg/dose q2-6h IV q2-3h	May cause dystonic reactions, tardive dyskinesia, neuroleptic malignant syndrome.
Ondansetron (Zofran)	*Adult:* 4 mg IV single dose *Pediatric:* up to 40 kg: 0.1 mg/kg; >40 kg: 4 mg/dose IV single dose	May cause headache, dizziness, and musculoskeletal pain.

IM, intramuscularly; *IV,* intravenously; *PO,* orally; *prn,* as needed.

From Marx JA et al: *Rosen's emergency medicine,* ed 8, Philadelphia, 2014, Saunders

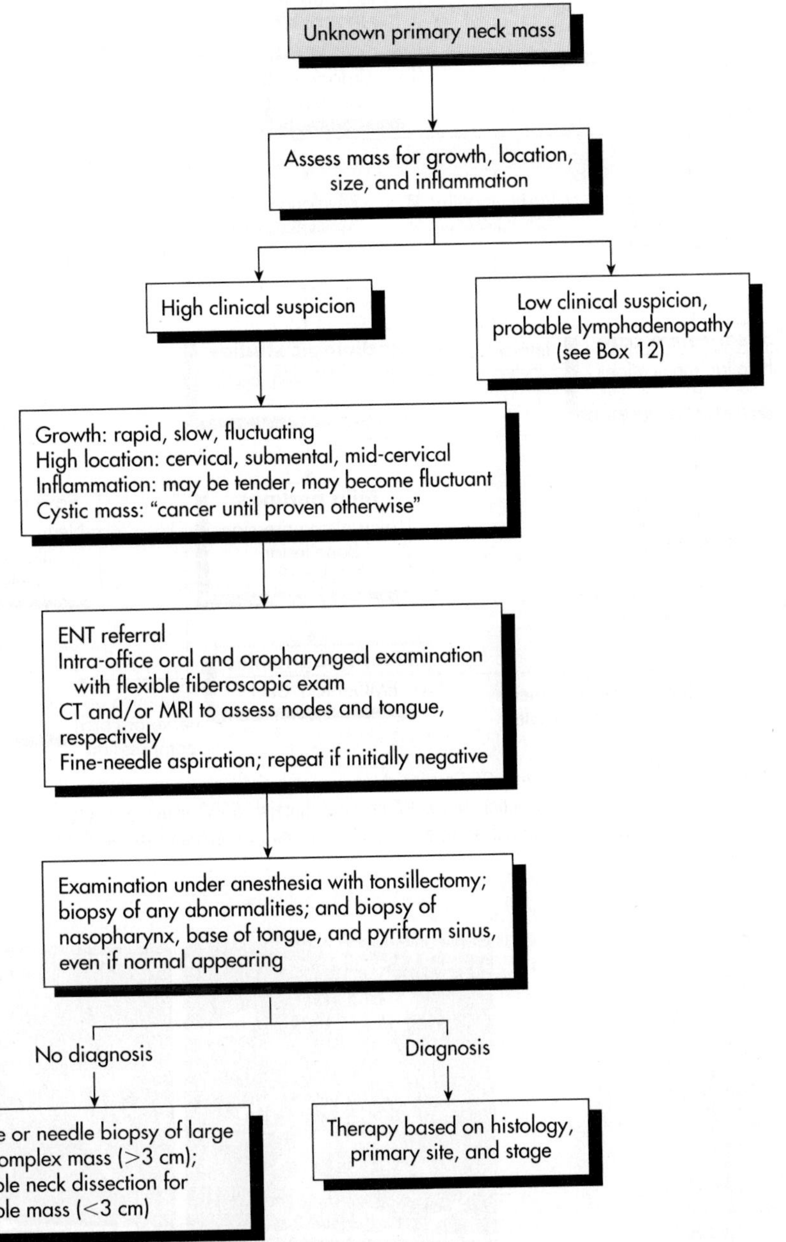

FIG. 98 Evaluation of an unknown primary neck mass. *CT,* Computed tomography; *ENT,* ear, nose, and throat; *MRI,* magnetic resonance imaging. (From Goldman L, Schafer AL [eds]: *Cecil textbook of medicine,* ed 24, Philadelphia, 2012, Saunders.)

BOX 12 An Approach to the Patient with Lymphadenopathy

- Does the patient have a known illness that causes lymphadenopathy? Treat and monitor for resolution.
- Is there an obvious infection to explain the lymphadenopathy (e.g., infectious mononucleosis)? Treat and monitor for resolution.
- Are the nodes very large and/or very firm and thus suggestive of malignancy? Perform a biopsy.
- Is the patient very concerned about malignancy and unable to be reassured that malignancy is unlikely? Perform a biopsy.
- If none of the preceding are true, perform a complete blood cell count and if it is unrevealing, monitor for a predetermined period (usually 2 to 6 weeks). If the nodes do not regress or if they increase in size, perform a biopsy.

From Goldman L, Ausiello D (eds): *Cecil textbook of medicine,* ed 23, Philadelphia, 2008, Saunders.

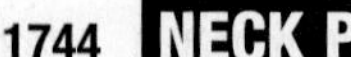

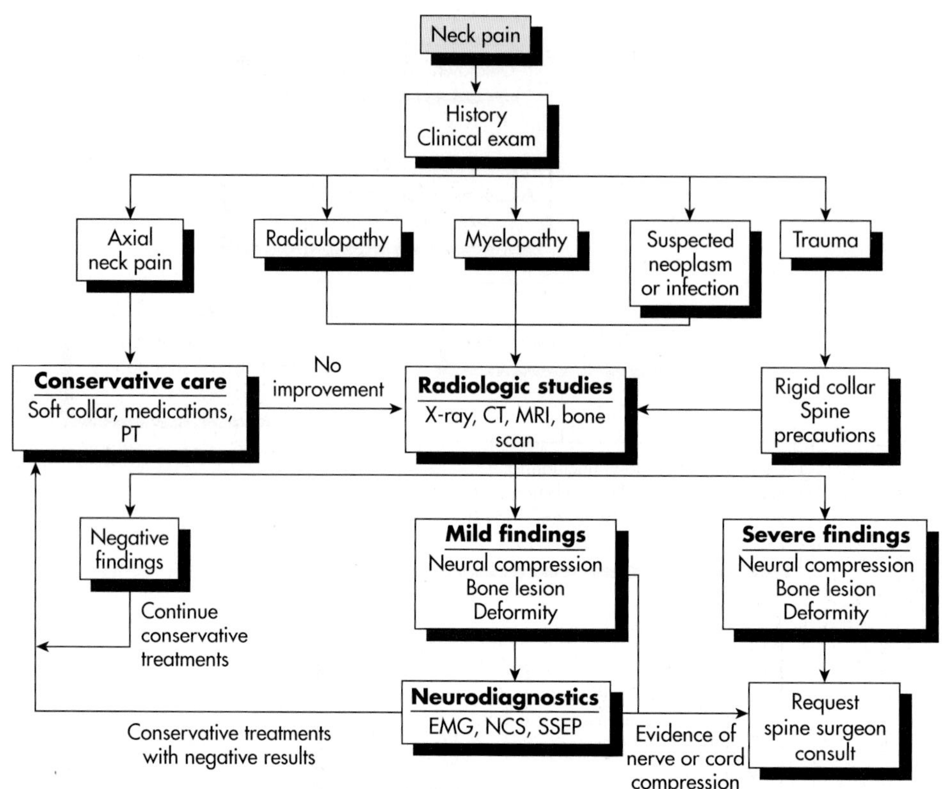

FIG. 99 Algorithm of neck pain. *CT,* Computed tomography; *EMG,* electromyogram; *MRI,* magnetic resonance imaging; *NCS,* nerve conduction study; *PT,* physical therapy; *SSEP,* somatosensory evoked potentials. (From Firestein GS, Budd RC, Gabriel SE et al: *Kelley's textbook of rheumatology,* ed 9, Philadelphia, 2013, Saunders.)

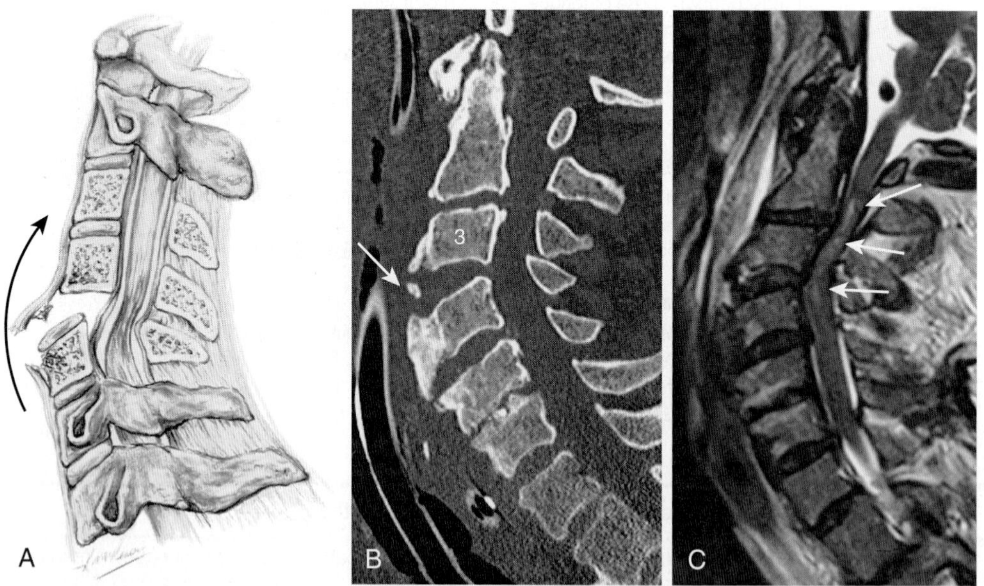

FIG. 100 Extension injury. A, Drawing shows mechanism and injury. There is a small avulsion from the anterosuperior margin of the vertebra immediately below the affected level. Note the wide disk space and retrolisthesis, hallmarks of this injury. The spinal cord is frequently injured in this setting. **B,** Sagittal reconstructed CT image shows widening of the C3 disk space with an avulsed fragment of bone *(arrow)* and retrolisthesis. **C,** T2-weighted MR image shows cord hemorrhage *(arrows).* The patient is quadriplegic. (From Pope TL, Bloem HL et al: *Musculoskeletal imaging,* ed 2, Philadelphia, 2015, Elsevier.)

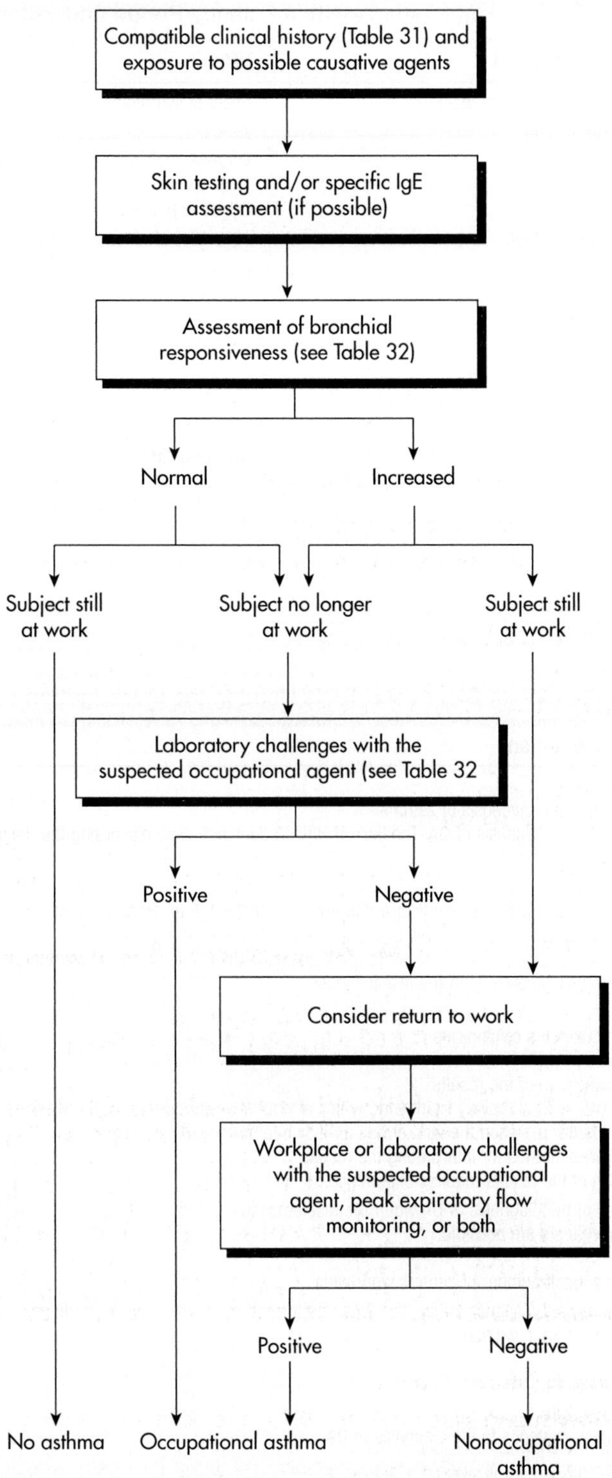

FIG. 101 Algorithm for the investigation of occupational asthma. *IgE,* Immunoglobulin E. (From Adkinson NF et al: *Middleton's allergy principles and practice*, ed 8, Philadelphia, 2014, Saunders.)

TABLE 31 Differences between Occupational Asthma with a Latency Period and Irritant-Induced Asthma

	OA With a Latency Period	IrIA
Latency period	Variable but at least a matter of weeks	Onset of symptoms within minutes or hours
Mechanisms	Immunologic sensitization	?
Physiopathology	Like common asthma	Massive epithelial desquamation with early deposition of collagen. No role of eosinophils. Oxidative process
Frequency	85%-90% of all cases of OA	10%-15% of all cases of OA
Symptoms	Wheeze predominant	Cough predominant
Function	The degree of airway hyperresponsiveness to methacholine reflects severity	Severity not reflected by the degree of responsiveness to methacholine
Response to bronchodilator	+++	++
Response to inhaled steroids	+++	++
Improvement with time	Good in general	Moderate, little, or absent

IrIA, irritant-induced asthma; *OA*, occupational asthma.
From Mason RJ, Broaddus CV et al: *Murray & Nadel's textbook of respiratory medicine,* ed 5, Philadelphia, 2010, Saunders.

TABLE 32 Advantages and Limitations of Diagnostic Tests Used in the Investigation of Occupational Asthma (OA)

Diagnostic Test(s)	Advantages/Limitations
Assessment of bronchial responsiveness	• Simple, low cost • Allow to confirm the diagnosis of asthma • Low specificity for diagnosis of OA. The lack of NSBHR does not allow discarding the diagnosis of OA in subjects who have been removed from the workplace.
Immunologic tests	• Easy to perform, low cost • Commercial extracts are available (skin-prick tests or specific IgE for HMW agents). • Lack of standardization for a majority of occupational allergens except latex • Measure of specific IgE available for some LMW agents (anhydrides, acids, isocyanates, aldehydes), but low sensitivity • Identify the sensitization but not the disease itself
PEF monitoring	• Low cost • Requires the worker's collaboration • Low adherence (<60%) • Possible falsification of the results • Requires 2 weeks at and away from work, which are not always possible for the workers • Impossible to perform when the worker has already been removed from exposure • No standardized method for interpreting the results • Interpretation of the results requires experience.
Specific inhalation challenges in the laboratory	• Confirmation of the diagnosis of OA when the test is positive • False-negative tests are possible • Costly • Available in a small number of centers worldwide
Specific inhalation challenges at the workplace	• Exclude diagnosis if response is negative when performed in the usual work conditions • Requires usual work condition • Costly
Noninvasive measures of airway inflammation	Sputum cell counts • Impossible to falsify • Bring additional evidence to the diagnosis of OA • Costly • Not widely available • Does not allow to confirm or discard the diagnosis of OA by itself Exhaled NO measurement • Easy to perform • Inconsistent results • Difficult to interpret • Affected by many different factors

HMW, High-molecular-weight; *IgE,* immunoglobulin E; *LMW,* low-molecular-weight; *NO,* nitric oxide; *NSBHR,* nonspecific bronchial hyperresponsiveness; *PEF,* peak expiratory flow.
From Adkinson NF et al: *Middleton's allergy principles and practice*, ed 8, Philadelphia, 2014, Saunders.

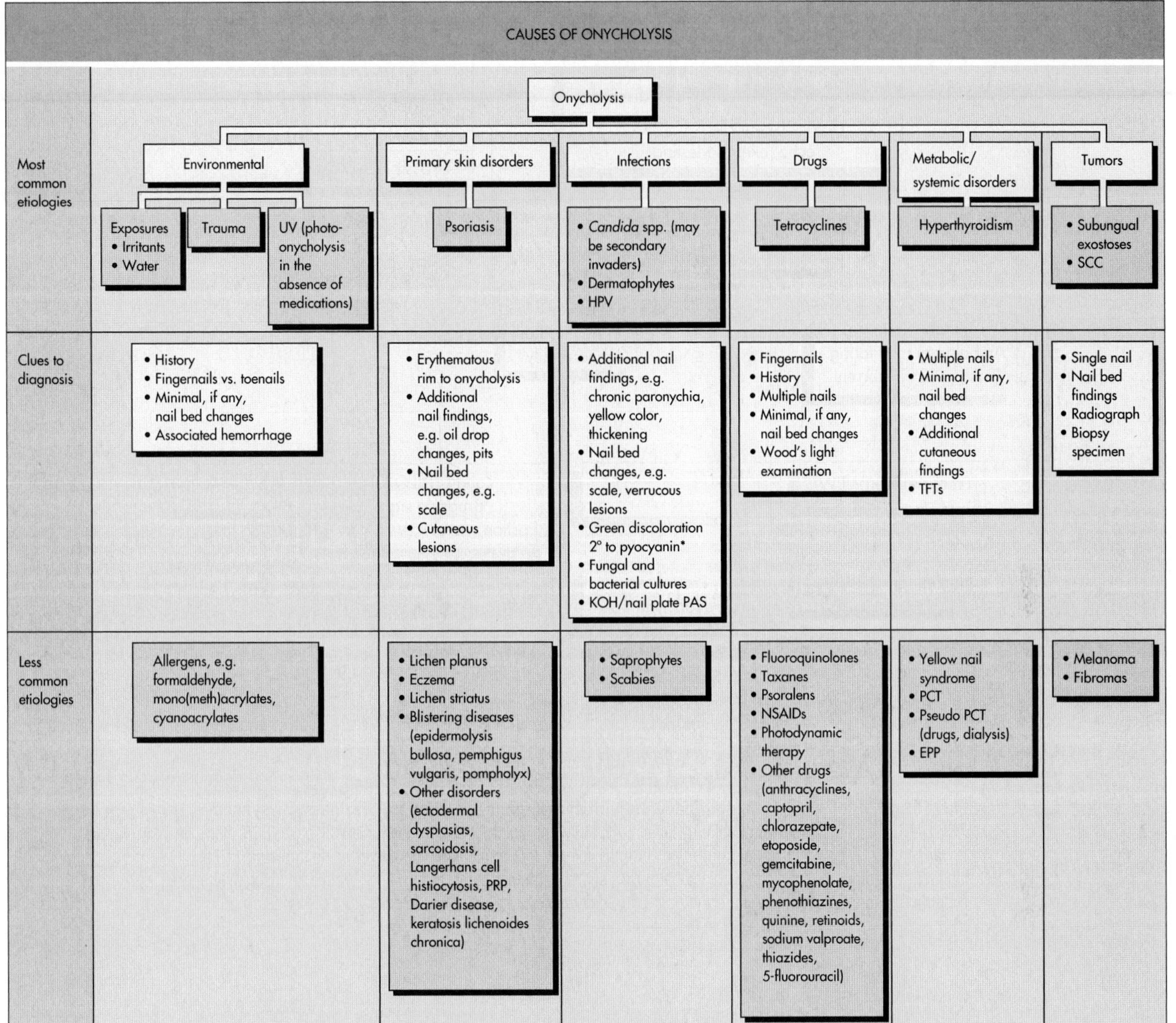

FIG. 102 Causes of onycholysis. *Due to secondary colonization with *Pseudomonas aeruginosa*. *EPP*, erythropoietic protoporphyria; *HPV*, human papillomavirus infection; *NSAIDs*, nonsteroidal antiinflammatory drugs; *PAS*, periodic acid-Schiff; *PCT*, porphyria cutanea tarda; *PRP*, pityriasis rubra pilaris; *SCC*, squamous cell carcinoma; *TFTs*, thyroid function tests. (From Bolognia JL, Jorizzo JL, Schaffer JV: *Dermatology*, ed 3, St Louis, 2012, Elsevier.)

ICD-10CM # R42 Dizziness and giddiness
R55 Syncope and collapse

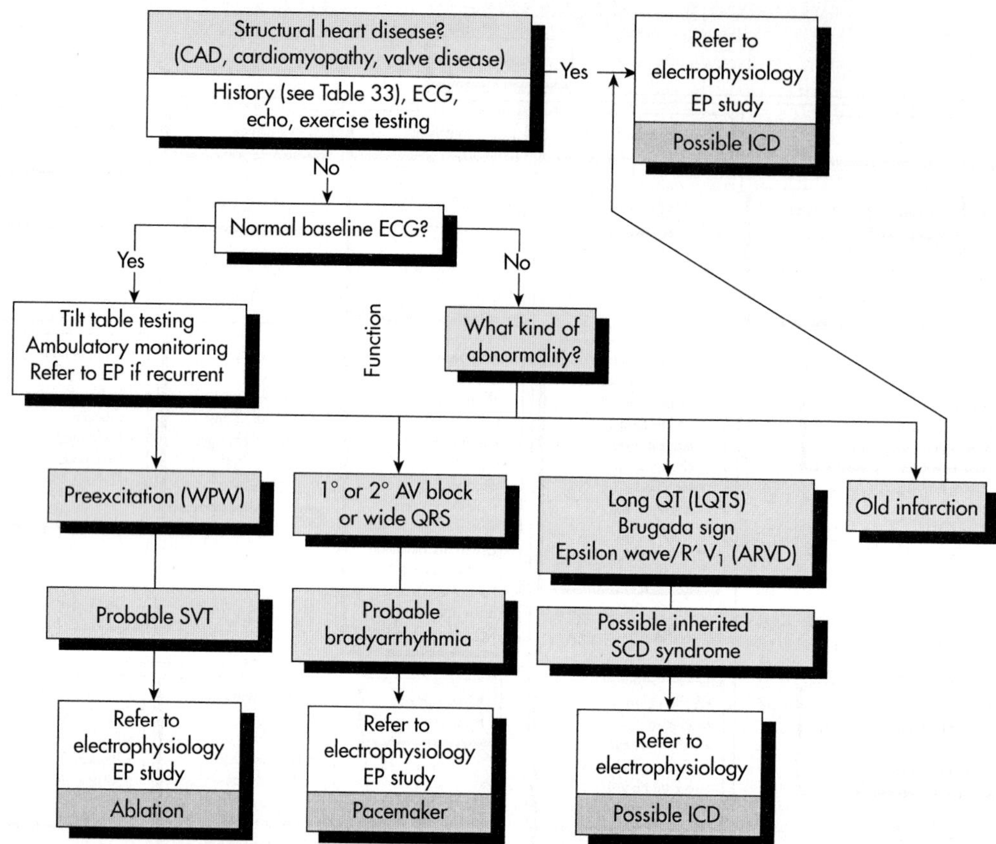

FIG. 103 Algorithm for evaluating patients with symptoms of palpitation, dizziness, or syncope. *ARVD*, arrhythmogenic right ventricular dysplasia; *AV*, atrioventricular; *CAD*, coronary artery disease; *ECG*, electrocardiogram; *echo*, echocardiogram; *EP*, electrophysiology; *ICD*, implantable cardioverter-defibrillator; *LQTS*, long QT syndrome; *SCD*, sudden cardiac death; *SVT*, supraventricular tachycardia; *WPW*, Wolff-Parkinson-White syndrome. (From Goldman L, Schafer AI: *Goldman Cecil medicine,* ed 25, Philadelphia, 2016, Saunders.)

TABLE 33 Items to Be Covered in History of Patient with Palpitation

Does the Palpitation Occur:	If So, Suspect:
As isolated "jumps" or "skips"?	Extrasystoles
In attacks known to be of abrupt beginning, with a heart rate of 120 beats/min or over, with regular or irregular rhythm?	Paroxysmal rapid heart action
Independent of exercise or excitement adequate to account for the symptom?	Atrial fibrillation, atrial flutter, thyrotoxicosis, anemia, febrile states, hypoglycemia, anxiety state
In attacks developing rapidly though not absolutely abruptly, unrelated to exertion or excitement?	Hemorrhage, hypoglycemia, tumor of the adrenal medulla
In conjunction with the taking of drugs?	Tobacco, coffee, tea, alcohol, epinephrine, ephedrine, aminophylline, atropine, thyroid extract, monoamine oxidase inhibitors
On standing?	Postural hypotension
In middle-aged women, in conjunction with flushes and sweats?	Menopausal syndrome
When the rate is known to be normal and the rhythm regular?	Anxiety state

From Goldman L, Braunwald E: Chest discomfort and palpitation. In Isselbacher KJ, Braunwald E et al [eds]: *Harrison's principles of internal medicine,* ed 13, New York, 1994, McGraw-Hill.

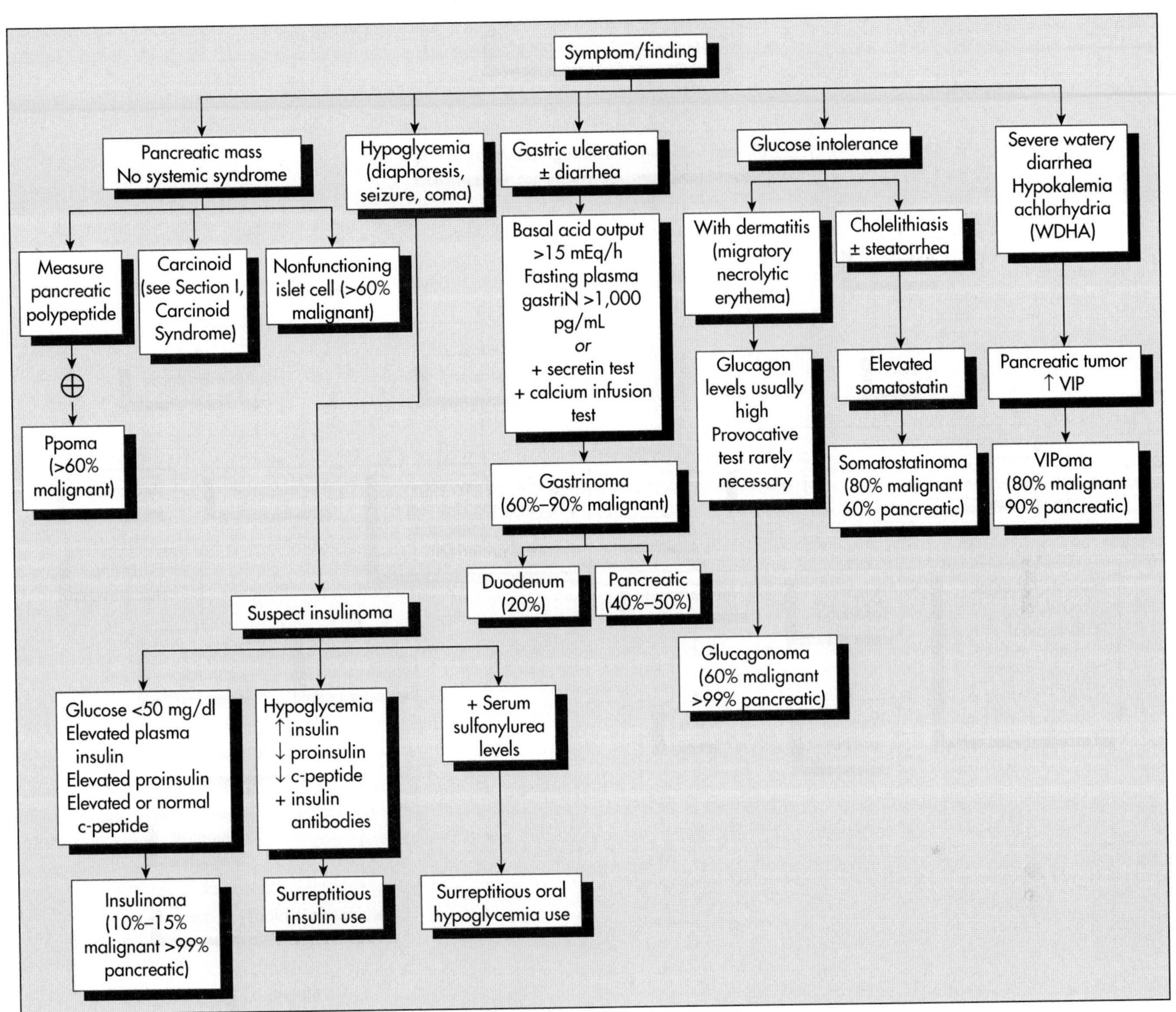

FIG. 104 Diagnosis of pancreatic islet cell tumors. *Ppoma,* Pancreatic polypeptide-secreting tumor; *VIP,* vasoactive intestinal peptide; *VIPoma,* vasoactive intestinal peptide secreted by a pancreatic islet tumor. (From Niederhuber JE, Armitage JO, Doroshow JH et al: *Abeloff's clinical oncology,* ed 5, Philadelphia, 2014, Saunders.)

ICD-10CM # C25.3 Malignant neoplasm of pancreatic duct
R19.06 Epigastric swelling, mass or lump

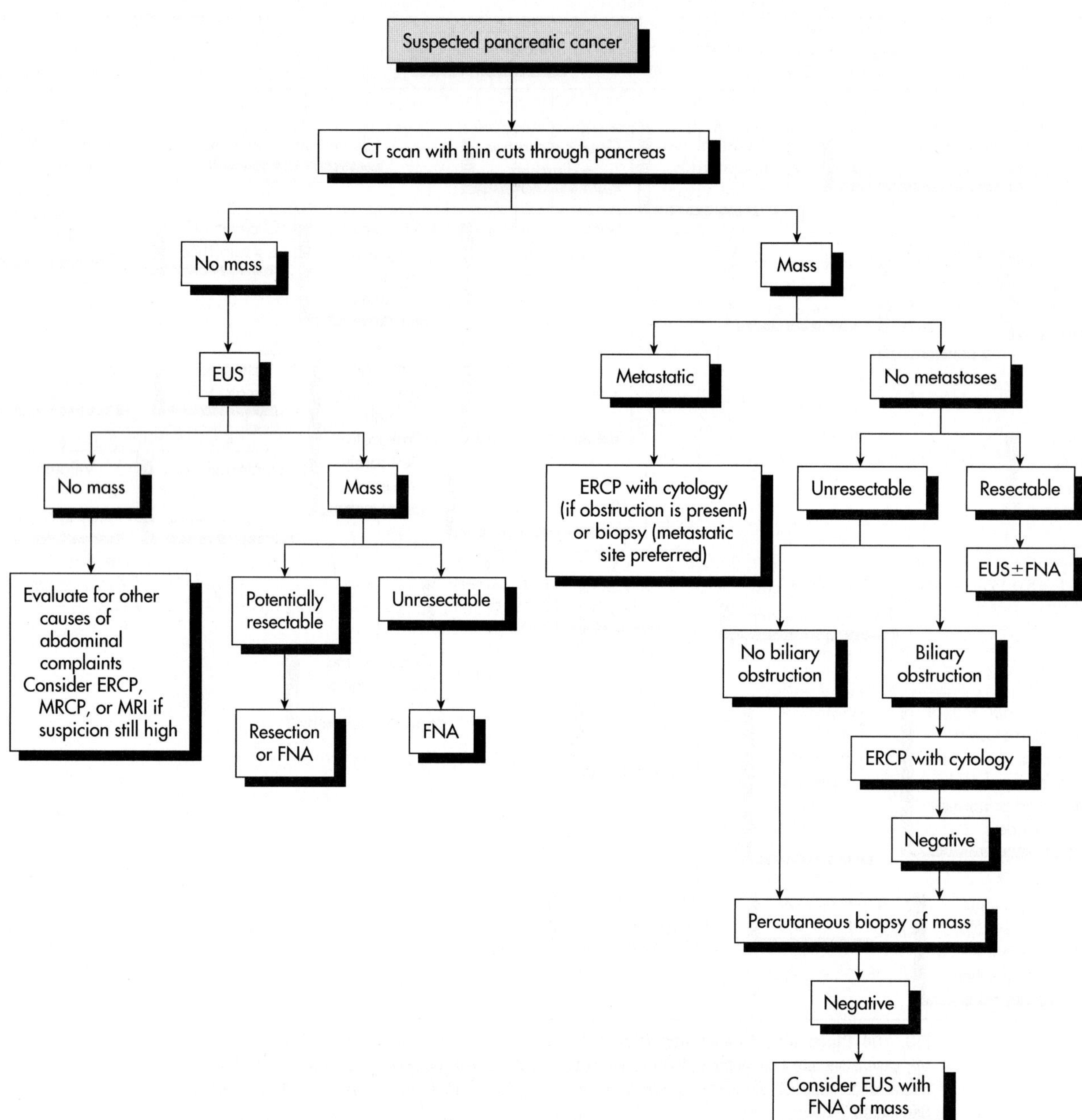

FIG. 105 Diagnostic algorithm for pancreatic cancer. Intraoperative fine-needle aspiration (FNA) if found inoperable during surgery. *CT,* Computed tomography; *ERCP,* endoscopic retrograde cholangiopancreatography; *EUS,* endoscopic ultrasonography; *MRCP,* magnetic resonance cholangiopancreatography; *MRI,* magnetic resonance imaging. (From Goldman L, Schafer AL [eds]: *Cecil textbook of medicine,* ed 24, Philadelphia, 2012, Saunders.)

PELVIC PAIN, WOMEN, DIAGNOSTIC EVALUATION

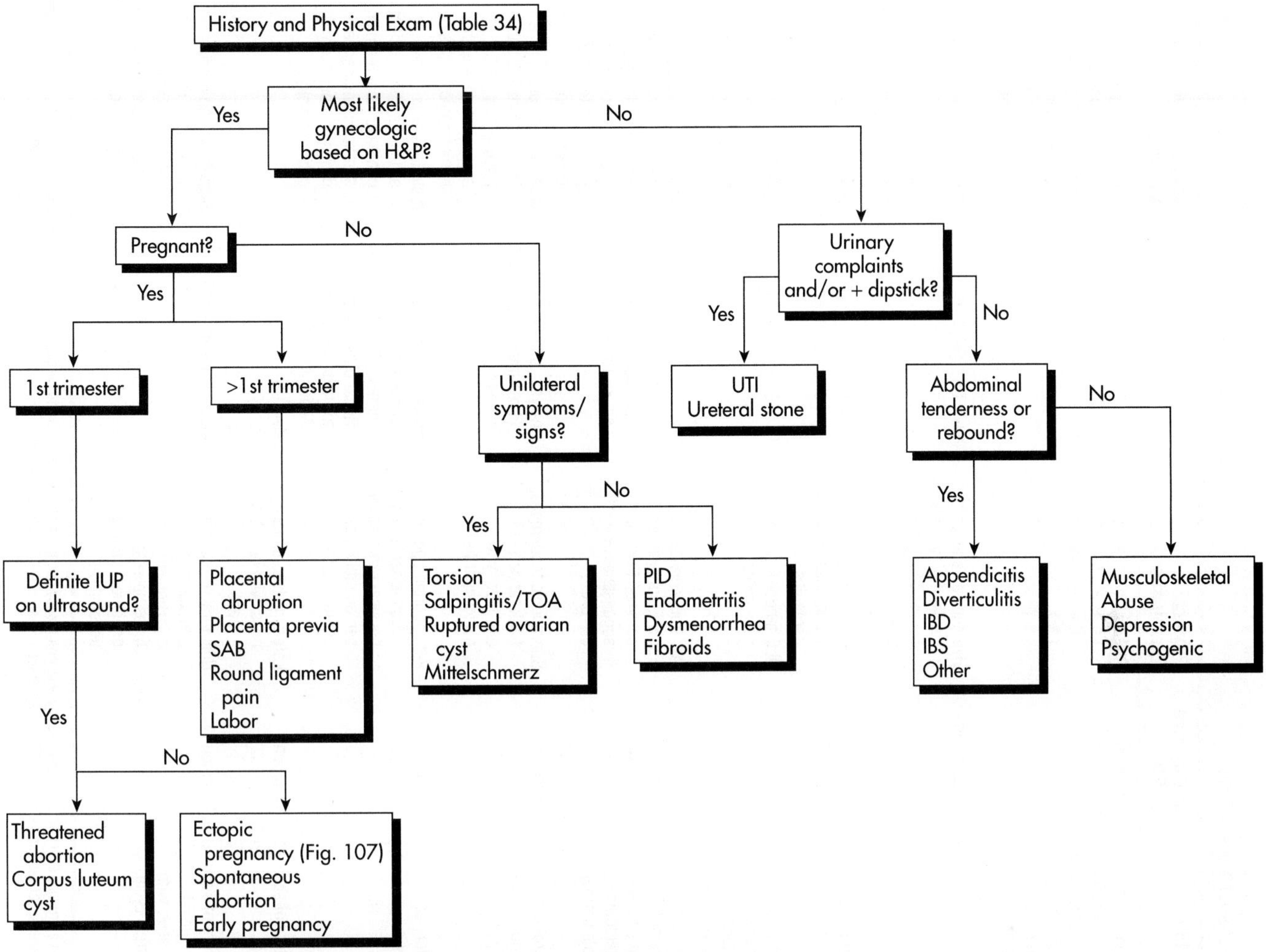

- History and Physical Exam (Table 34)
  - Most likely gynecologic based on H&P?
    - Yes → Pregnant?
      - Yes →
        - 1st trimester → Definite IUP on ultrasound?
          - Yes → Threatened abortion; Corpus luteum cyst
          - No → Ectopic pregnancy (Fig. 107); Spontaneous abortion; Early pregnancy
        - >1st trimester → Placental abruption; Placenta previa; SAB; Round ligament pain; Labor
      - No → Unilateral symptoms/signs?
        - Yes → Torsion; Salpingitis/TOA; Ruptured ovarian cyst; Mittelschmerz
        - No → PID; Endometritis; Dysmenorrhea; Fibroids
    - No → Urinary complaints and/or + dipstick?
      - Yes → UTI; Ureteral stone
      - No → Abdominal tenderness or rebound?
        - Yes → Appendicitis; Diverticulitis; IBD; IBS; Other
        - No → Musculoskeletal; Abuse; Depression; Psychogenic

FIG. 106 Diagnostic algorithm for acute pelvic pain. *H&P,* History and physical; *IBD,* inflammatory bowel disease; *IBS,* irritable bowel syndrome; *IUP,* intrauterine pregnancy; *PID,* pelvic inflammatory disease; *SAB,* spontaneous abortion; *TOA,* tubo-ovarian abscess; *UTI,* urinary tract infection. (From Marx JA et al: *Rosen's emergency medicine*, ed 8, Philadelphia, 2014, Saunders.)

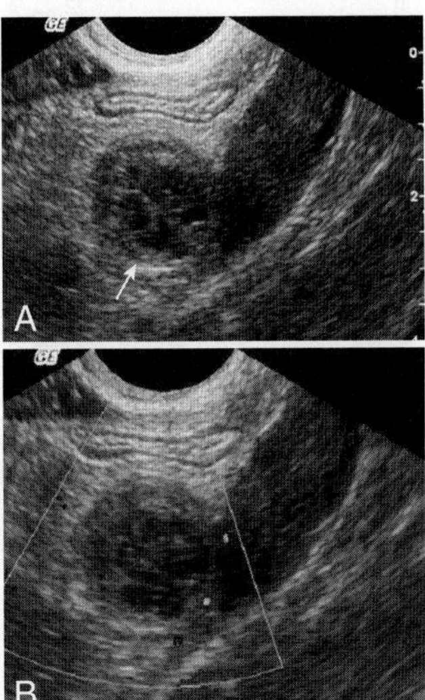

FIG. 107 Ectopic pregnancy seen as mixed-echogenicity mass. A 30-year-old woman presented with left lower quadrant pain at 7 weeks' gestation and β-hCG of 500 mIU/mL and falling over a 3-day period. **A,** In the left adnexa, medial to the left ovary, there was a 2-cm mass *(arrow)* with mixed echogenicity, and **B,** only minimal peripheral vascularity. A left ectopic pregnancy was confirmed and, based on a falling β-hCG, was treated expectantly and resolved without complication. (Rumack CM, Wilson SR, Charboneau JW, Levine D: *Diagnostic ultrasound,* ed 4, Philadelphia, 2011, Elsevier.)

TABLE 34 Differentiation of Common or Potentially Catastrophic Causes of Pelvic Pain

Causative Disorder or Condition	Pain History	Associated Symptoms	Supporting History	Prevalence in ED	Physical Examination	Useful Tests	Atypical or Additional Aspects
Ectopic pregnancy (critical if ruptured)	Classically severe, sharp, lateral pelvic pain, but severity, location, and quality highly variable.	Vaginal bleeding (often mild, can be absent).	Missed period; history of previous ectopic pregnancy, infertility, pelvic surgery, PID, or IUD use.	Common	Classically unilateral adnexal tenderness, adnexal mass, and CMT.	Pelvic US, quantitative β-hCG, T&C, laparoscopy.	Cannot reliably exclude diagnosis based on history and physical examination. Severe pain, hypotension, or peritonitis suggests rupture.
Ruptured ovarian cyst (emergent—critical with significant hemorrhage; otherwise, urgent)	Abrupt moderate to severe lateral pain.	Light-headedness if bleeding is severe; rectal pain arises from fluid in cul-de-sac.		Uncommon	Hypotension and tachycardia if blood loss is significant; possible peritonitis.	Pelvic US, CBC, T&C.	Physical examination findings often do not correlate with volume of blood in pelvis at US.
Ovarian torsion (emergent)	Acute onset of moderate to severe lateral pain.	Nausea and vomiting.	History of ovarian mass or cyst.	Uncommon	Adnexal mass and tenderness, possible peritonitis.	US with Doppler flow studies, laparoscopy.	Torsion can be intermittent.
Appendicitis (emergent)	Duration often <48 hr, generalized followed by localized RLQ pain.	Low-grade fever, nausea, anorexia.	Migration of pain to RLQ from center, abdominal pain before vomiting.	Common	RLQ tenderness, possible peritonitis.	US or CT in unclear cases.	Early in course, tenderness may be minimal or poorly localized.
PID, TOA (TOA: emergent; PID: urgent-emergent)	Without TOA, pain usually bilateral. May manifest acutely within 48 hr or subacutely with up to 3 wk of pain.	Fever, vaginal discharge.	Vaginal discharge, history of PID, history of unprotected intercourse or multiple partners.	PID: common TOA: uncommon	Pus from cervical os, CMT, adnexal tenderness. Peritonitis suggests severe PID or TOA.	CBC, ESR, CRP, pelvic US, laparoscopy, cervical cultures, cervical smear for WBCs.	History and physical examination may be inaccurate for diagnosis, particularly in patients with subacute presentation.
UTI (urgent)	Pain with urination. Patient may have flank pain from associated pyelonephritis.	Urinary urgency and frequency; fever and vomiting if patient has associated pyelonephritis.	Recent urologic procedure, prior history of UTI.	Common	Suprapubic tenderness, flank tenderness and fever with pyelonephritis.	Urinalysis, urine culture (if recurrent or complicated).	WBCs can be present in urine with PID and appendicitis. RBCs present in urine with hemorrhagic cystitis.
Ureteral colic (urgent)	Acute onset, manifests within hours. Pain is lateral, usually moderate to severe. Often radiates into the groin or costovertebral angle or flank.	Nausea and vomiting.	Prior history of stones.	Common	Patient often appears uncomfortable, but physical examination can be otherwise unremarkable.	Urinalysis: hematuria present in approximately 80% of cases. Renal ultrasound for hydronephrosis. Abdominal CT.	If stone is at ureterovesicular junction, patient can have localized pain that can mimic appendicitis or other acute pelvic pathology.
Unruptured ovarian cyst or tumor	Lateral ache, gradual onset.	Often minimal.	Prior history of similar pain.	Common	Lateral pelvic tenderness, with or without a mass.	Pelvic US.	
Endometriosis	Unilateral or bilateral pelvic pain, often recurrent.	Dysmenorrhea, dyspareunia.	Prior history of same type of pain in association with menstrual cycle.	Common	Unilateral or bilateral adnexal tenderness, occasionally pelvic mass present, peritoneal findings uncommon.	Pelvic US, laparoscopy.	Symptoms can mimic other types of pelvic pathology; laparoscopy often is needed for confirmation.

β-*hCG*, β-Human chorionic gonadotropin; *CBC*, complete blood count; *CMT*, cervical motion tenderness; *CRP*, C-reactive protein; *CT*, computed tomography; *ED*, emergency department; *ESR*, erythrocyte sedimentation rate; *IUD*, intrauterine device; *PID*, pelvic inflammatory disease; *RBC*, red blood cell; *RLQ*, right lower quadrant; *T&C*, type and crossmatch; *TOA*, tubo-ovarian abscess; *US*, ultrasonography; *UTI*, urinary tract infection; *WBC*, white blood cell.

From Marx JA et al: *Rosen's emergency medicine*, ed 8, Philadelphia, 2014, Saunders.

PELVIC PAIN, WOMEN, MANAGEMENT

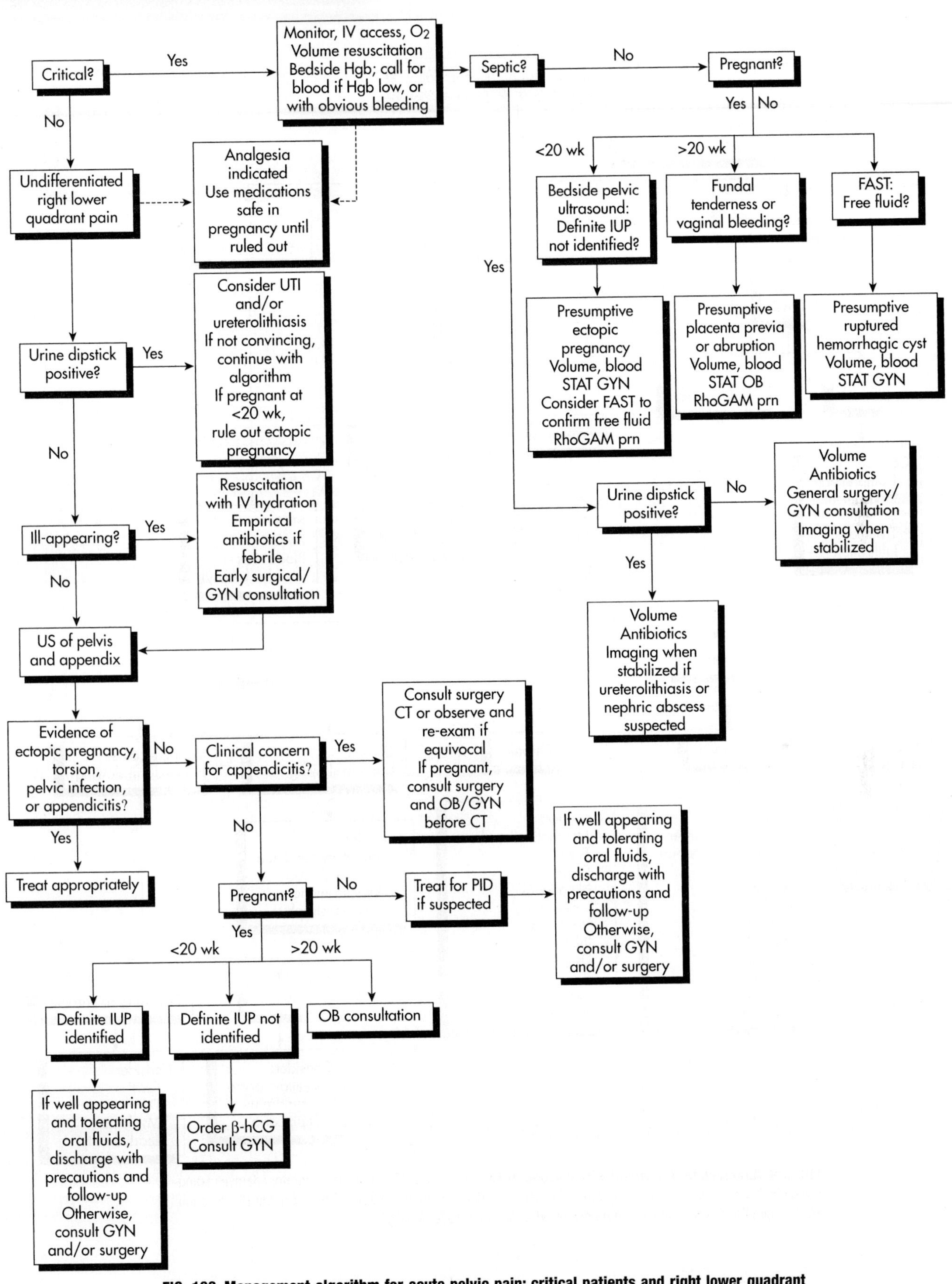

FIG. 108 Management algorithm for acute pelvic pain: critical patients and right lower quadrant pain presentations. *β-hCG*, β-Human chorionic gonadotropin; *CT*, computed tomography; *FAST*, focused assessment with sonography for trauma; *GYN*, gynecology; *Hgb*, hemoglobin; *IUP*, intrauterine pregnancy; *IV*, intravenous; *OB*, obstetrics; *PID*, pelvic inflammatory disease; *STAT*, immediately; *US*, ultrasound; *UTI*, urinary tract infection. (From Marx JA et al: *Rosen's emergency medicine*, ed 8, Philadelphia, 2014, Saunders.)

PERIPHERAL NEUROPATHY

ICD-10CM # G60.9 Hereditary and idiopathic neuropathy, unspecified
G57.10 Meralgia paresthetica, unspecified lower limb
G90.09 Other idiopathic peripheral autonomic neuropathy

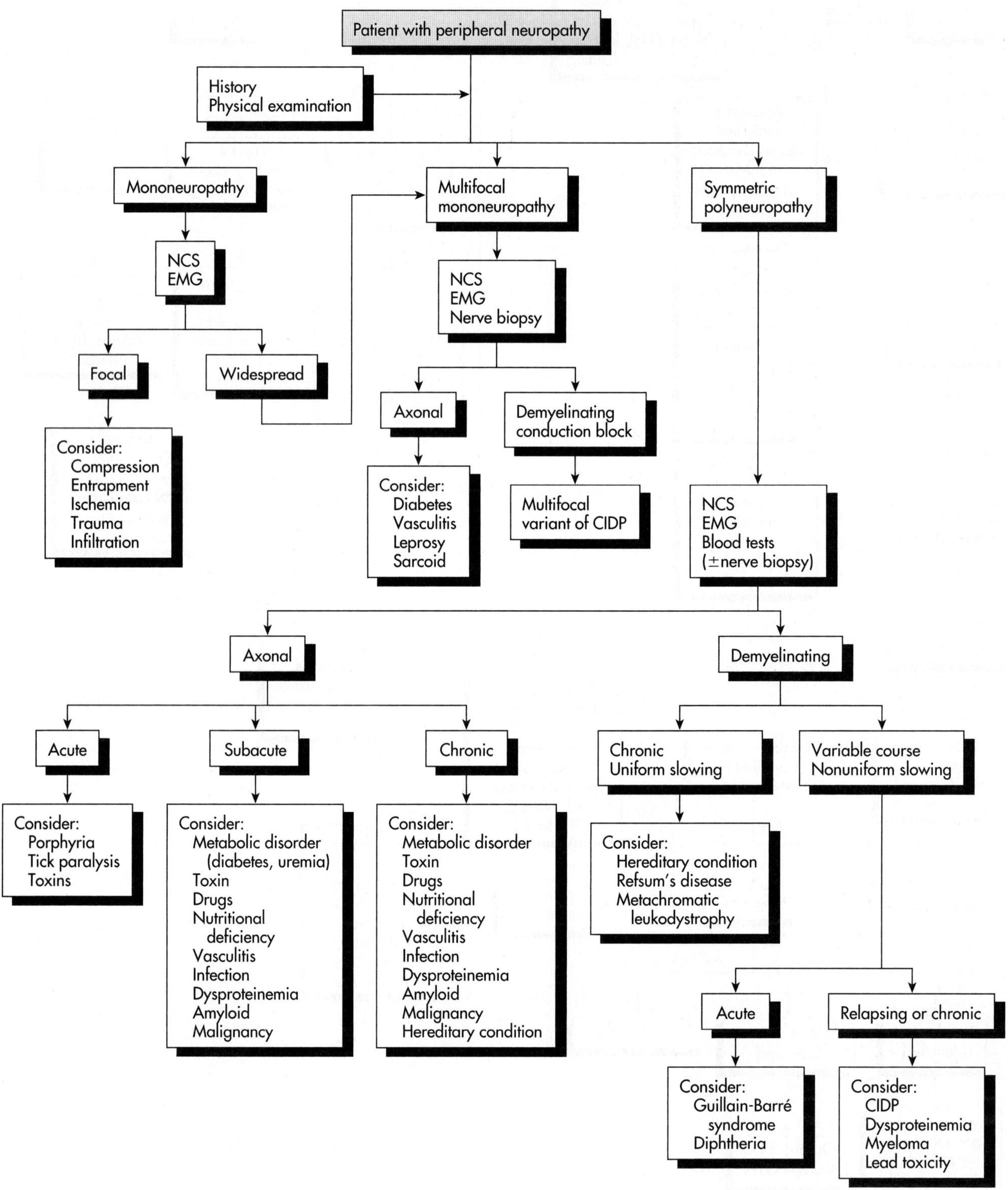

FIG. 109 Approach to the patient with peripheral neuropathy. *CIDP,* Chronic inflammatory demyelinating polyradiculopathy; *EMG,* electromyogram; *NCS,* nerve conduction studies. (Modified from Greene HL, Johnson WP, Lemcke DL: *Decision making in medicine*, ed 2, St Louis, 1988, Mosby.)

PHOTOSENSITIVITY

ICD-10CM # L56.0 Drug phototoxic response
L56.1 Drug photoallergic response
L56.2 Photocontact dermatitis [berloque dermatitis]

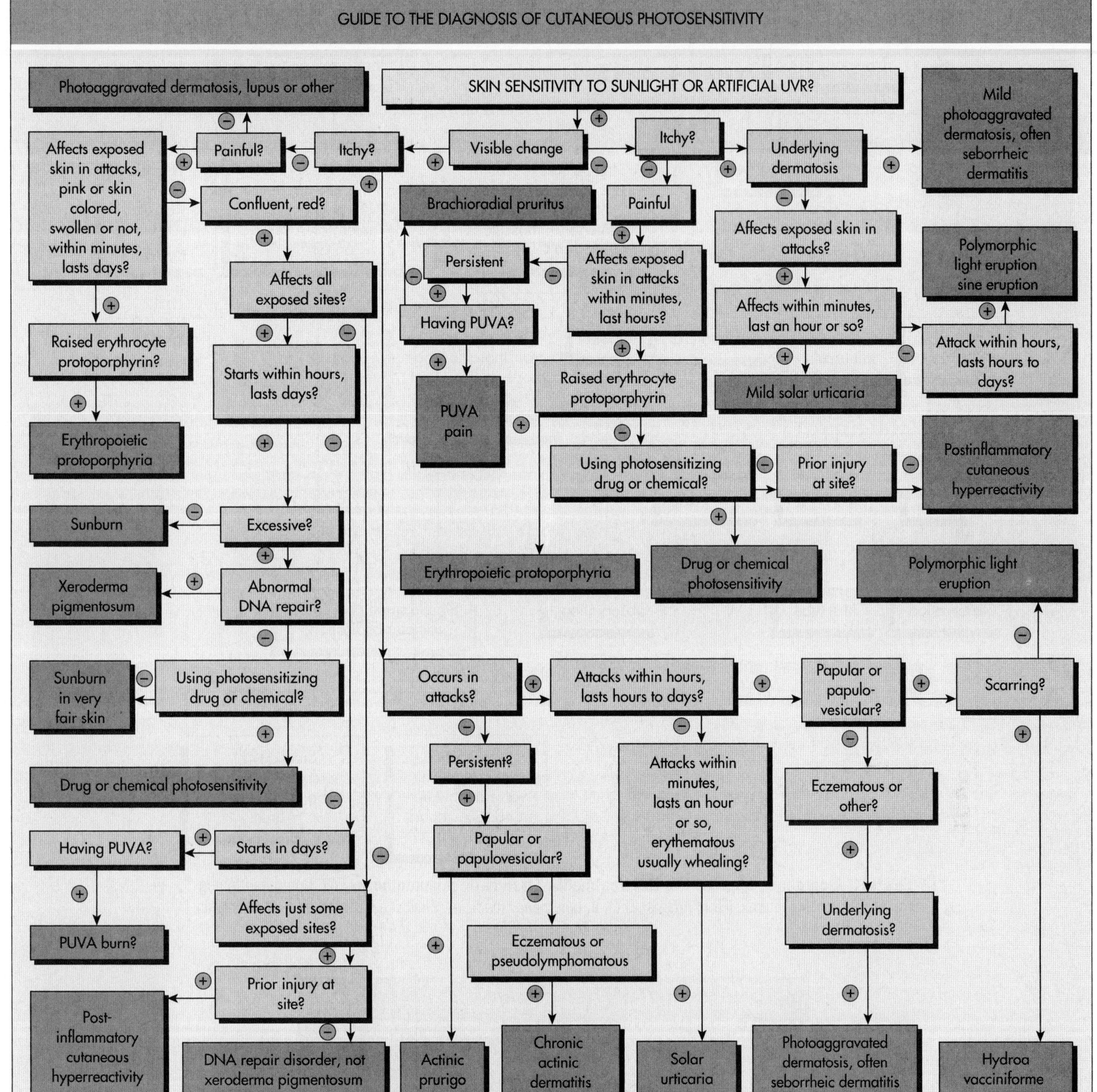

FIG. 110 Guide to the diagnosis of cutaneous photosensitivity. The diagnosis can generally be made from patient history and clinical findings, provided the titers of antinuclear antibodies and other LE-associated antibodies are normal. *PUVA*, Psoralen and ultraviolet A. (From Bolognia JL, Jorizzo JL, Schaffer JV: *Dermatology,* ed 3, St Louis, 2012, Elsevier.)

Clinical Algorithms III

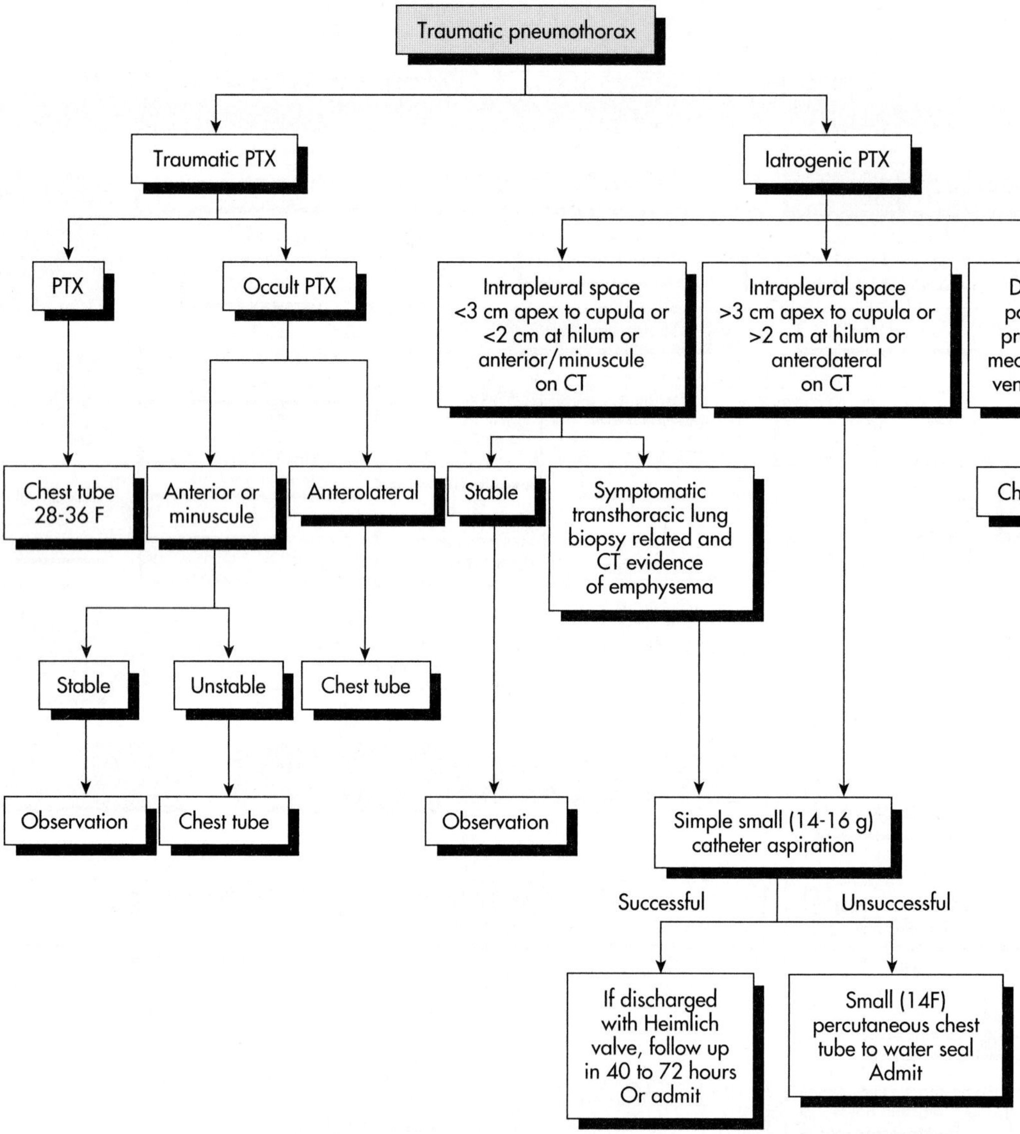

- Traumatic pneumothorax
  - Traumatic PTX
    - PTX
      - Chest tube 28-36 F
    - Occult PTX
      - Anterior or minuscule
        - Stable
          - Observation
        - Unstable
          - Chest tube
      - Anterolateral
        - Chest tube
  - Iatrogenic PTX
    - Intrapleural space <3 cm apex to cupula or <2 cm at hilum or anterior/minuscule on CT
      - Stable
        - Observation
      - Symptomatic transthoracic lung biopsy related and CT evidence of emphysema
        - Simple small (14-16 g) catheter aspiration
    - Intrapleural space >3 cm apex to cupula or >2 cm at hilum or anterolateral on CT
      - Simple small (14-16 g) catheter aspiration
        - Successful: If discharged with Heimlich valve, follow up in 40 to 72 hours Or admit
        - Unsuccessful: Small (14F) percutaneous chest tube to water seal Admit
    - Due to positive pressure mechanical ventilation
      - Chest tube

FIG. 111 Algorithmic approach to the treatment of traumatic pneumothorax. *CT*, Computed tomography; *PTX*, pneumothorax. (From Adams JG et al: *Emergency medicine: clinical essentials*, ed 2, Philadelphia, 2013, Elsevier.)

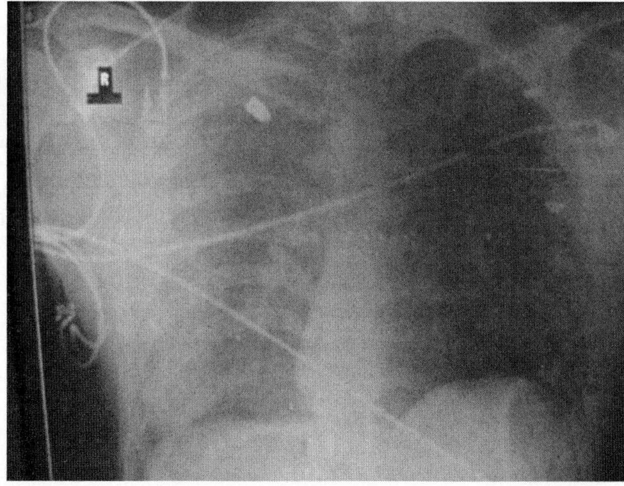

FIG. 112 Hemothorax secondary to gunshot wound. Note haziness over right hemithorax with bullet seen in right upper lobe. (From Marx JA et al: *Rosen's emergency medicine*, ed 8, Philadelphia, 2014, Saunders.)

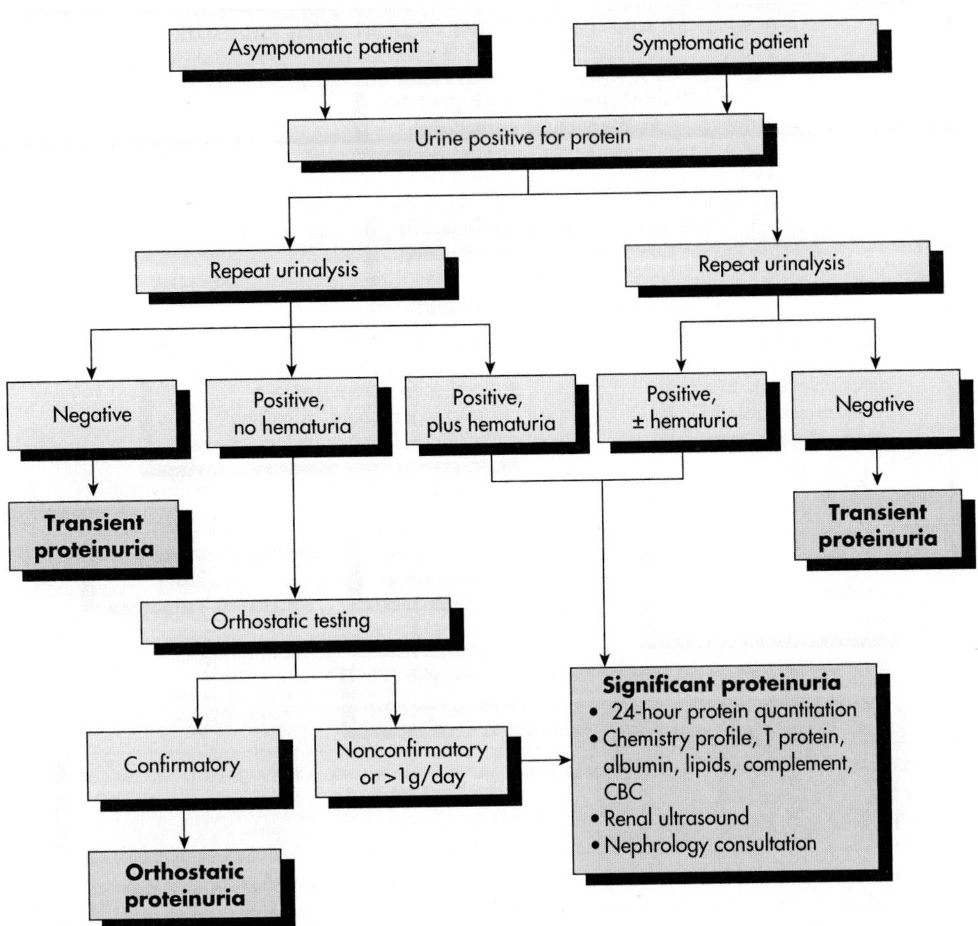

FIG. 113 Evaluation of children with proteinuria. *CBC*, complete blood cell count. (From Wein AJ et al: *Campbell-Walsh urology*, ed 11, Philadelphia, 2016, Elsevier.)

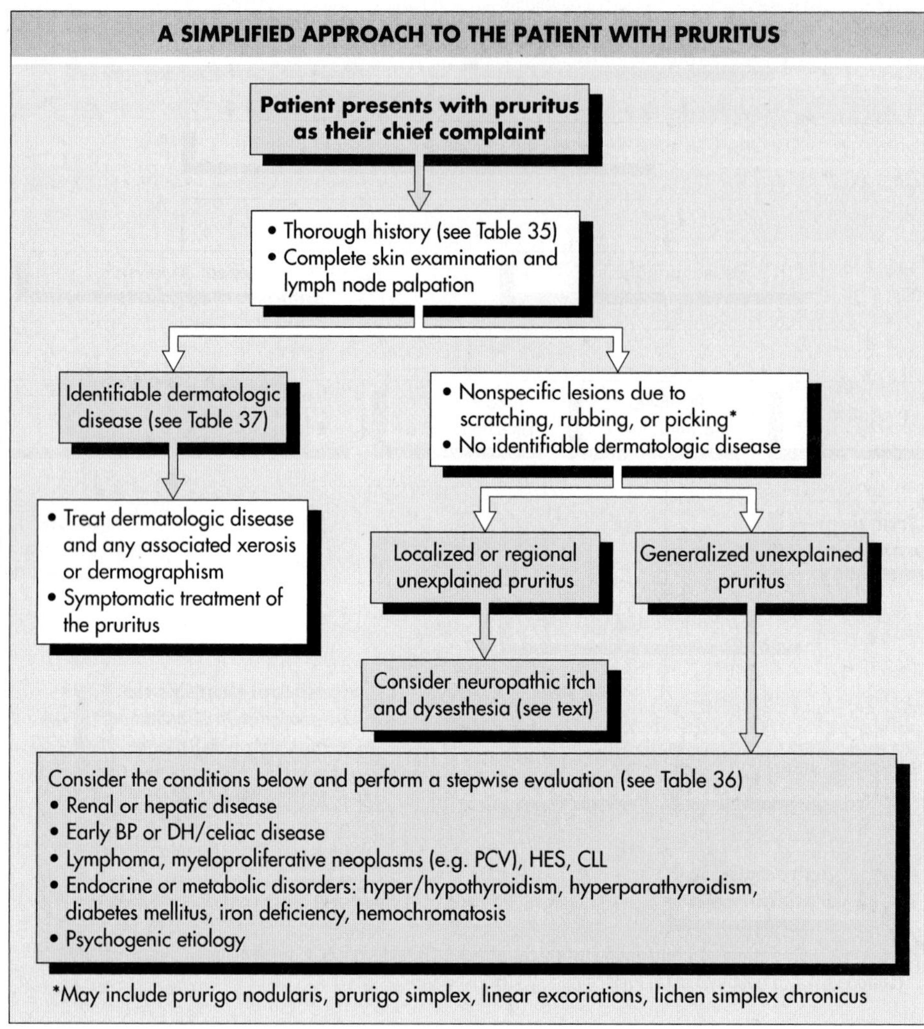
A SIMPLIFIED APPROACH TO THE PATIENT WITH PRURITUS
Patient presents with pruritus as their chief complaint
• Thorough history (see Table 35)
• Complete skin examination and lymph node palpation
Identifiable dermatologic disease (see Table 37)
• Nonspecific lesions due to scratching, rubbing, or picking*
• No identifiable dermatologic disease
• Treat dermatologic disease and any associated xerosis or dermographism
• Symptomatic treatment of the pruritus
Localized or regional unexplained pruritus
Generalized unexplained pruritus
Consider neuropathic itch and dysesthesia (see text)
Consider the conditions below and perform a stepwise evaluation (see Table 36)
• Renal or hepatic disease
• Early BP or DH/celiac disease
• Lymphoma, myeloproliferative neoplasms (e.g. PCV), HES, CLL
• Endocrine or metabolic disorders: hyper/hypothyroidism, hyperparathyroidism, diabetes mellitus, iron deficiency, hemochromatosis
• Psychogenic etiology
*May include prurigo nodularis, prurigo simplex, linear excoriations, lichen simplex chronicus

FIG. 114 A simplified approach to the patient with pruritus. *BP,* Bullous pemphigoid; *CLL,* chronic lymphocytic leukemia; *DH,* dermatitis herpetiformis; *HES,* hypereosinophilic syndromes; *PCV,* polycythemia vera. (From Bolognia J: *Dermatology,* ed 4, Philadelphia, 2018, Elsevier.)

TABLE 35 Descriptive Features of the Pruritus and Additional Patient History

Questions to Ask Regarding the Pruritus

- WHEN did it start? *Duration:* days, weeks, months, years
- WHERE did it start? WHERE is it now? *Location:* localized or generalized, unilateral or bilateral
- HOW did it start? *Onset:* abrupt, gradual, prior history of pruritic episodes
- HOW does it feel? *Nature:* prickling, crawling, burning, stinging
- HOW intense is it? *Severity:* mild, moderate, severe; interference with normal activities or sleep
- HOW often do you feel it? *Time course:* intermittent, continuous, cyclical, nocturnal
- WHAT makes it worse? *Provoking/aggravating factors:* heat, cold, water, air, exercise, occupation, hobbies
- WHAT makes it better? *Itch relief:* cold, heat, scratching/rubbing/hurting, cool/hot showering
- WHAT do you think is the cause? *Patient's theory of pruritus etiology*

Additional patient history

- Skin care, bathing habits, exposure to irritants
- Medications (including topical agents): prescribed, over-the-counter; duration of use and relationship to onset of pruritus
- Use of nicotine, alcohol, and recreational/illicit drugs
- Allergies (known and suspected): drugs, airborne, food, contact
- Atopic history: atopic dermatitis, allergic rhinoconjunctivitis, asthma
- Past and present medical history: thyroid, liver, or renal dysfunction; other systemic diseases; psychological disease; surgeries or accidents
- Family history: atopy, skin disease, similar pruritic conditions
- Occupation, hobbies, personal stress
- Household and personal contacts; pets and their care
- Dietary habits
- Sexual history
- Travel history
- Prior diagnoses made by physician or patient

From Bolognia J: *Dermatology,* ed 4, Philadelphia, 2018, Elsevier.

TABLE 36 Laboratory and Radiographic Evaluation in Patients with Pruritus of Unknown Etiology

Basic Initial Evaluation

- Complete blood cell count (CBC) with differential and platelet count
- Erythrocyte sedimentation rate (ESR) and C-reactive protein (CRP)
- Creatinine, blood urea nitrogen, electrolytes
- Liver transaminases, alkaline phosphatase, bilirubin
- Lactate dehydrogenase (LDH)
- Fasting glucose
- Thyroid stimulating hormone (TSH) ± free thyroxine

Possible Additional Evaluation

Skin biopsy

- Routine histology (if skin lesions are present)
- Direct immunofluorescence studies*

Other laboratory tests

- Serum total and/or allergen-specific IgE
- Serum ferritin, iron, total iron binding capacity
- Hemoglobin A1c
- Parathyroid function (calcium, phosphate, and parathyroid hormone levels)
- Stool for ova/parasites and/or occult blood
- Viral hepatitis panel (including hepatitis B and C viruses)
- HIV testing
- Anti-tissue transglutaminase ± epidermal transglutaminase IgA antibodies**
- Anti-BP180 and anti-BP230 bullous pemphigoid IgG antibodies
- Anti-mitochondrial and anti-smooth muscle antibodies
- Serum tryptase, histamine, and/or chromogranin-A levels
- Urinalysis with sediment evaluation
- 24-Hour urine collection for 5-hydroxyindoleacetic acid (5-HIAA; a serotonin metabolite) and porphyrins
- Serum protein electrophoresis, serum immunofixation electrophoresis

Radiographic studies

- Chest x-ray or CT scan
- Abdominal and pelvic ultrasonography or CT scan
- Lymph node ultrasonography
- Spinal x-ray or MRI (for regional pruritus)

Other investigations

- Patch testing
- Prick testing for major atopy and relevant occupational allergens
- Age-appropriate cancer screening (in conjunction with primary care physician)
- If hydroxyethyl starch (HES)-induced pruritus is suspected, electron microscopy of a biopsy sample from normal-appearing skin

*Biopsy perilesional skin or normal-appearing skin (in vicinity of lesions if present) to assess for bullous pemphigoid and dermatitis herpetiformis, respectively.

**Often performed in conjunction with serum total IgA; in patients with IgA deficiency, anti-tissue transglutaminase IgG antibodies should be assessed.

A1c, Glycated hemoglobin; *CT,* computed tomography; *IgA,* immunoglobin A; *IgE,* immunoglobin E, *IgG,* immunoglobin G; *MRI,* magnetic resonance imaging.

From Bolognia J: *Dermatology,* ed 4, Philadelphia, 2018, Elsevier.

TABLE 37 Primary Dermatologic Conditions Associated with Pruritus

Cause	Dermatologic Disease
Inflammation	• Atopic dermatitis • Allergic or irritant contact dermatitis • Seborrheic dermatitis, especially of the scalp • Stasis dermatitis • Psoriasis • Parapsoriasis • Pityriasis rubra pilaris • Lichen planus • Urticaria, dermographism • Mastocytosis • Papular urticaria, urticarial dermatitis • Drug eruptions, e.g., morbilliform • Polymorphous light eruption, actinic prurigo, chronic actinic dermatitis • Bullous diseases, e.g., DH, BP • Polymorphic eruption of pregnancy (PEP) • Eosinophilic folliculitis • Dermatomyositis • Prurigo pigmentosa • Lichen sclerosus • Graft-versus-host disease
Infestation/ bites & stings	• Scabies • Pediculosis • Arthropod bites
Infections	• Bacterial infections, e.g., folliculitis • Viral infections, e.g., varicella • Fungal infections, e.g., inflammatory tinea • Parasitic infections, e.g., schistosomal cercarial dermatitis
Neoplastic	• Cutaneous T-cell lymphoma, e.g., mycosis fungoides, Sézary syndrome
Genetic/nevoid	• Darier disease and Hailey–Hailey disease • Ichthyoses, e.g., Netherton, Sjögren–Larsson, and peeling skin syndromes • Pruriginosa subtype of dominant dystrophic EB • Porphyrias, e.g., porphyria cutanea tarda and erythropoietic protoporphyria • Inflammatory linear verrucous epidermal nevus (ILVEN) • Large/giant congenital melanocytic nevi, occasionally, especially in bulky lesions with neural differentiation
Other	• Xerosis, eczema craquelé • Primary cutaneous amyloidosis (macular, lichenoid) • Postburn pruritus • Scar-associated pruritus • Fiberglass dermatitis

BP, Bullous pemphigoid; *DH,* dermatitis herpetiformis; *EB,* epidermolysis bullosa.

From Bolognia J: *Dermatology,* ed 4, Philadelphia, 2018, Elsevier.

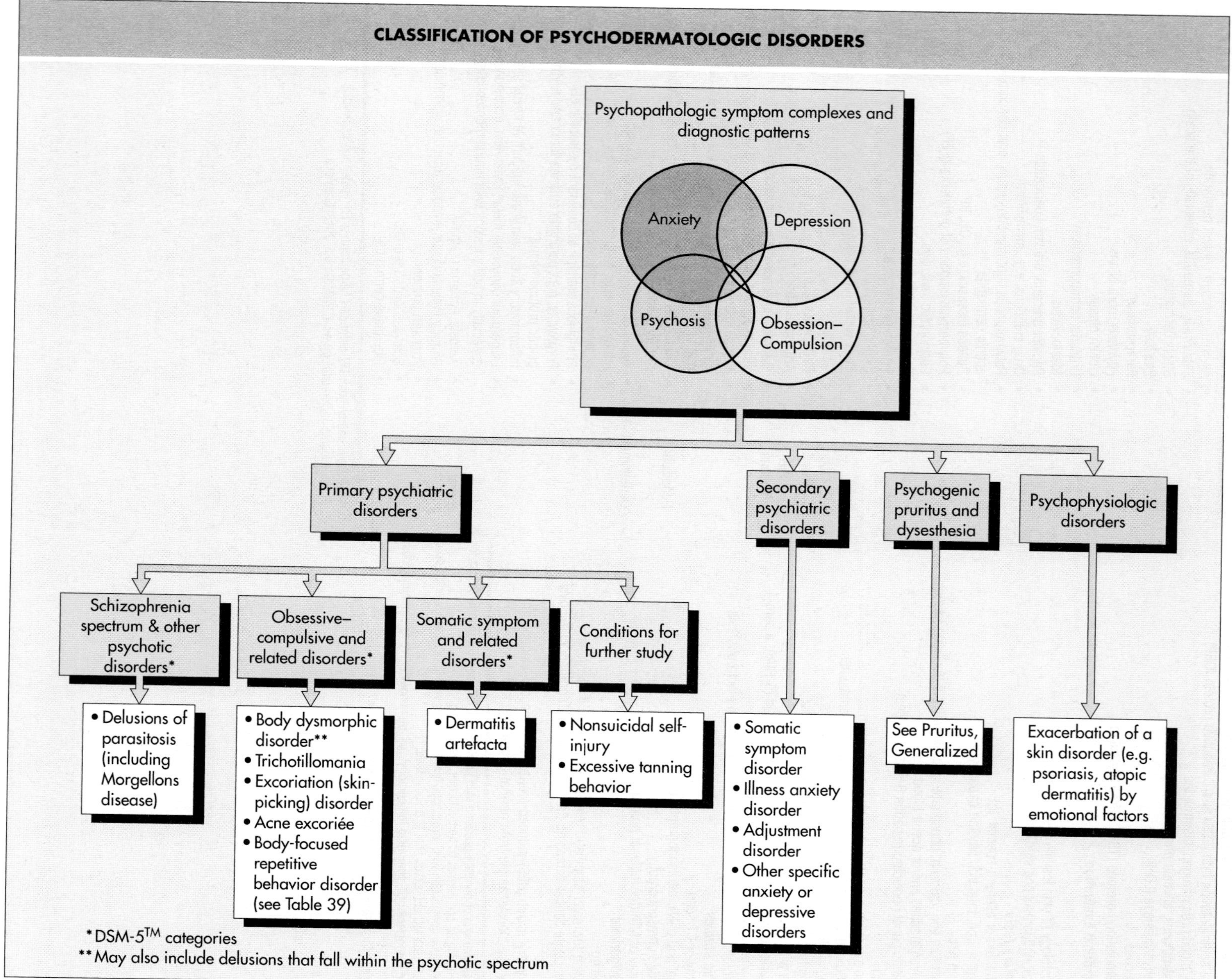

FIG.117 Classification of psychodermatologic disorders. Psychocutaneous disorders can be conceptualized by (1) the specific psychodermatologic condition and its classification, and (2) the presenting symptom complex of the underlying psychopathology. Primary psychiatric disorders are those in which the patient has no primary skin disease and all of the cutaneous findings are self-induced. Secondary psychiatric disorders involve the development of psychological problems as a result of a skin disease. *Psychophysiologic disorders* are those in which a primary skin condition, such as psoriasis, is exacerbated by emotional factors. A particular patient with a psychodermatologic disorder can have a presenting symptom complex with features from one or more of the four major psychopathologic patterns of anxiety, depression, psychosis, and obsessions/compulsions. (From Bolognia J: *Dermatology,* ed 4, Philadelphia, 2018, Elsevier.)

TABLE 38 Psychopathic Patterns and Psychotropic Medications Used in Dermatology

Underlying Psychopathology and Symptom Complex	Possible Pharmacologic Treatment	Comments and Precautions
Anxiety		
• Excessive anxiety and worry • Restlessness; feeling "keyed up" or "on edge" • Irritability • Fatigability • Difficulty concentrating or mind going blank • Muscle tension or feeling "shaky" • Sleep disturbance • Somatic symptoms, e.g., dizziness, sweating, palpitations, abdominal complaints	**Acute anxiety: Benzodiazepines** • Clonazepam (0.5-2 mg once or twice daily, as needed) • Lorazepam (0.5-2 mg every 6-8 hours, as needed)	• Treatment not to exceed 4 weeks because of dependency/addiction risk • May cause sedation • Taper dosage to avoid withdrawal symptoms

	Chronic anxiety: Nonbenzodiazepines—start low and titrate slowly
	• *Azapirone anxiolytic*
	  • Buspirone (15 mg/day, divided into 3 doses; increase daily dose by 5 mg every 2-3 days, up to a maximum of 60 mg/day if needed)
	• Selective serotonin reuptake inhibitors (*SSRIs*; see "Depression" below)
	• *Tricyclic antidepressants* (e.g., doxepin; see "Depression" below)
	• *Serotonin–norepinephrine reuptake inhibitor*
	  • Venlafaxine, extended release (37.5-75 mg/day, up to 225 mg/day)
		• Onset of action often delayed 2-4 weeks
		• Do not cause dependency/addiction

Depression		

• Depressed mood
• Anhedonia
• Unexplained weight loss/gain or appetite change
• Insomnia or hypersomnia
• Psychomotor agitation or retardation
• Fatigue, lack of energy
• Feelings of hopelessness, worthlessness
• Excessive guilt
• Difficulty with concentration, indecisiveness
• Suicidal ideation/plan
• Crying spells
• Preoccupation with physical concerns
	• *SSRIs*—start at minimal effective dose and increase every week or every other week as tolerated; if no response at 6-8 weeks, then change to a different class of antidepressants
	  • Fluoxetine (10-20 mg/day, up to 40 mg/day)
	  • Paroxetine (10-20 mg/day, up to 40 mg/day)
	  • Sertraline (25-50 mg/day, up to 200 mg/day)
	  • Escitalopram (5-10 mg/day, up to 30 mg/day)
	  • Citalopram (10-20 mg/day, up to 40 mg/day)
		• SSRIs have a slow onset of action, with full therapeutic response not seen until 6-8 weeks
		• SSRIs may cause gastrointestinal disturbances, sexual dysfunction
		• Avoid abrupt discontinuation of SSRIs, as may cause dysphoria, dizziness, gastrointestinal distress
		• Citalopram and escitalopram can cause dose-dependent QT prolongation

	• *Tricyclic antidepressants (TCAs)* • Doxepin (dosage for pruritus is typically 10-25 mg at bedtime; for depression, typically start at 10-25 mg at bedtime and increase every 1-2 weeks to a therapeutic dose of 25-150 mg at bedtime or up to 300 mg in divided doses, depending on tolerance and disease severity)	• TCAs can lead to weight gain, cardiac conduction abnormalities, orthostatic hypotension, and anticholinergic side effects • Doxepin often causes sedation, especially in the elderly and smaller individuals; should be started at low doses (e.g., 10 mg/day) in these individuals
Psychosis		
• Delusions are the most common feature that presents to dermatologists • Fixed false belief that the patient is convinced is true • Delusion is usually encapsulated (narrow focus)	• *Pimozide* (starting dose is 1 mg/day; increase by 1 mg every 1-2 weeks until optimal response is reached, typically at 4-6 mg/day)	• Must taper dosage of pimozide and not discontinue abruptly to avoid withdrawal symptoms such as dyskinetic movements • Pimozide is associated with QT prolongation, cardiac toxicity, extrapyramidal side effects (e.g., tardive dyskinesia), and drug interactions (avoid if taking macrolides, protease inhibitors, azole antifungals, grapefruit juice) • Baseline ECG often recommended when starting pimozide

	• *Atypical (second-generation) antipsychotics*
	  • Risperidone (1-2 mg/day, up to 4 mg/day)
	  • Olanzapine (5-10 mg/day, up to 20 mg/day)
	  • Aripiprazole (10-15 mg/day)
		• Weight gain, metabolic effects, and other side effects of atypical antipsychotics
		• Increasingly being used for delusions of parasitosis because of lower risk of tardive dyskinesia and QT prolongation compared to pimozide.

Continued

TABLE 38 Psychopathic Patterns and Psychotropic Medications Used in Dermatology—cont'd

Underlying Psychopathology and Symptom Complex	Possible Pharmacologic Treatment	Comments and Precautions
Obsessive–compulsive disorder (OCD)		

• Presence of intrusive obsessions and/or compulsions (see text)
• Varying degrees of insight
	• *SSRIs* (start at low dose and increase every week or every other week until reach therapeutic range)
	  • Fluoxetine (20 mg/day, up to 40-80 mg/day)
	  • Paroxetine (20 mg/day, up to 40-60 mg/day)
	  • Sertraline (50 mg/day, up to 200 mg/day)
	  • Fluvoxamine (50 mg/day, up to 200-300 mg/day)
	  • Escitalopram (10 mg/day, up to 20-40 mg/day)
	  • Citalopram (20 mg/day, up to 40 mg/day)
		• OCD often requires higher doses of SSRIs, and patients may take longer to respond (e.g., 10-12 weeks)
		• Once a therapeutic response is achieved, continue treatment for 1-2 yrs, followed by gradual tapering of the dosage

	• Tricyclic antidepressants • Clomipramine (50 mg/day, up to 100-250 mg/day)	• Clomipramine has a less tolerable side-effect profile than SSRIs, including cardiac toxicity and arrhythmias; check blood levels when the dose is ≥150 mg/day
	• Serotonin–norepinephrine reuptake inhibitor • Venlafaxine (75 mg/day, up to 225-350 mg/day)	• Venlafaxine may cause hypertension and an increased risk of gastrointestinal bleeding

Modified from Bolognia J: *Dermatology*, ed 4, Philadelphia, 2018, Elsevier.

TABLE 39 Body-Focused Repetitive Behaviors and Associated Mucocutaneous Findings

Body-Focused Repetitive Behavior	Associated Mucocutaneous Findings
Lip licking	Irritant contact dermatitis, secondary bacterial or yeast infections
Lip picking or biting	Multiple erosions or ulcerations, recurrent HSV
Cheek chewing or biting	Bite fibroma, morsicatio buccarum
Cuticle pulling, picking, or biting	Paronychia, nail surface irregularities
Nail biting (onychophagia)	Paronychia, nail dystrophy, subungual hemorrhages
Nail picking or pulling (onychotillomania)	
Habit-tic deformity of the thumbnail	Multiple midline Beau's lines with prominent longitudinal central depression
Thumb or finger sucking	Skin maceration, dermatitis, secondary bacterial or yeast infections
Nose picking (rhinotillexomania)	Erosions, secondary bacterial infections
Trichotillomania	
Excoriation (skin-picking) disorder	

HSV, Herpes simplex virus.

Body-focused repetitive behaviors occur on a chronic basis and present with characteristic mucocutaneous findings, depending on the body site and behavior type. These behaviors exist along a spectrum, with habits at one end and body-focused repetitive behavioral disorders at the other end. The latter disorders continue despite repeated attempts to stop and lead to impaired functioning (e.g., social, occupational) or to distress manifesting as feelings of loss of control, embarrassment, or shame.

Modified from Bolognia J: *Dermatology*, ed 4, Philadelphia, 2018, Elsevier.

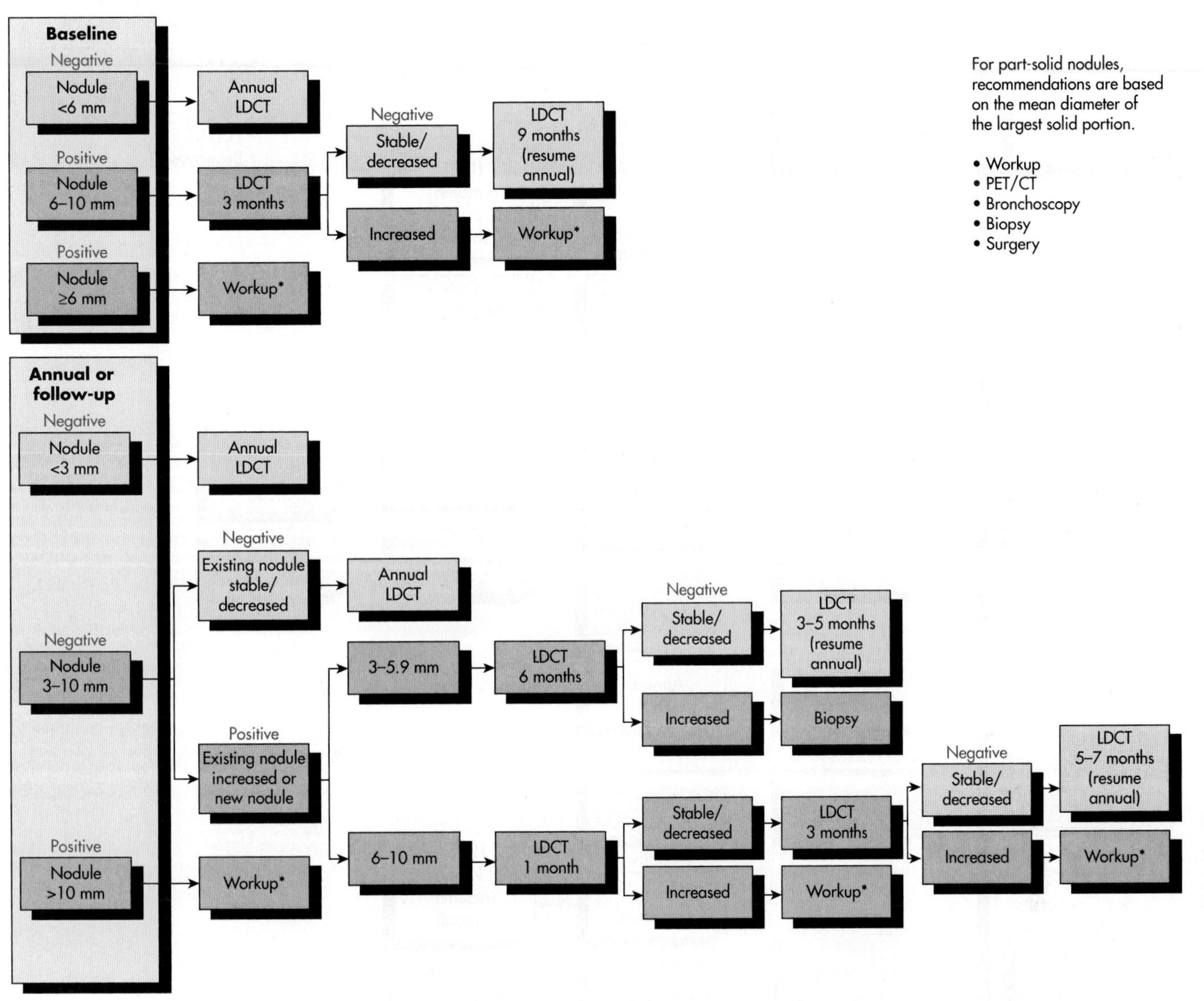

FIG. 118 The diagnostic algorithm for (A) solid or part-solid nodules and (B) nonsolid nodules. This algorithm was created through discussion by a multidisciplinary group composed of thoracic surgeons, radiologists, pulmonologists, oncologists, and pathologists. *Workup is at the discretion of the treating physicians but typically consists of a PET/CT and tissue diagnosis, either by bronchoscopy, CT-guided biopsy, or for highly suspicious nodules, minimally invasive surgery. *CT,* Computed tomography; *LDCT,* low-dose computed tomography; *PET,* positron emission tomography. (From Sellke FW, del Nido PJ, Swanson SJ: *Sabiston & Spencer surgery of the chest,* ed 9, Philadelphia, 2016, Elsevier. The Fleishner Society recommendations for computed tomography follow-up of pulmonary nodules are summarized in Tables 40–42.)

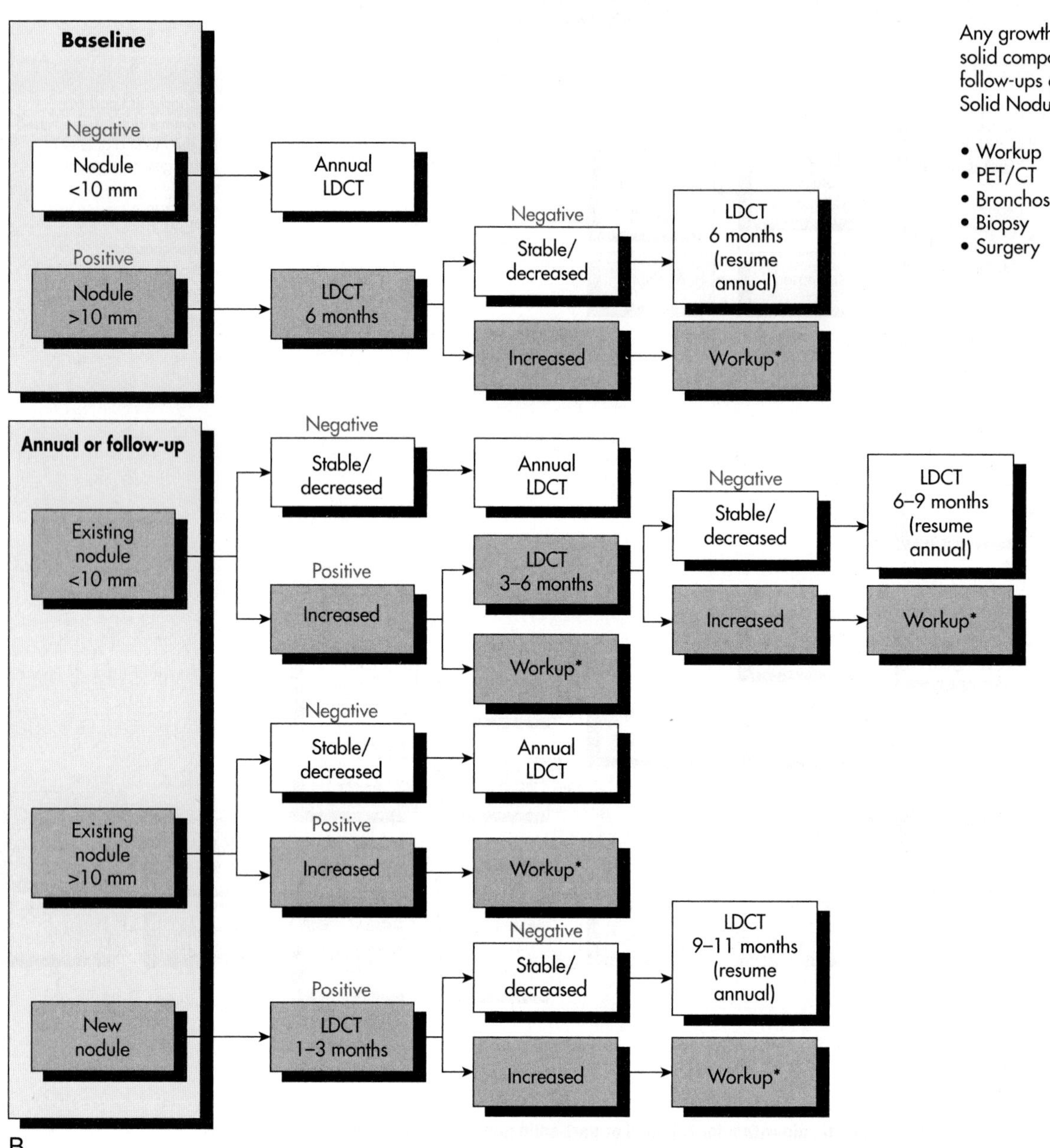

FIG. 118 (Continued)

TABLE 40 Fleischner Society Recommendations for Computed Tomography (CT) Follow-up (FU) of Solid Nodules*

Nodule Size	Low-Risk Patient	High-Risk patient
≤4 mm	No FU CT needed (FU is optional)	FU CT at 12 months; if unchanged, no further FU
>4-6 mm	FU CT at 12 months; if unchanged, no further FU	FU CT at 6-12 months, then at 18-24 months if no change
>6-8 mm	FU CT at 6-12 months, then at 18-24 months if no change	FU CT at 3-6 months, then at 9-12 and 24 months if no change
>8 mm	Options: FU CT at 3, 9, and 24 months; positron emission tomography; biopsy; video-assisted thoracic surgery	

*Nodule size is average of length and width. Low-risk patient, minimal or absent history of smoking or other known risk factors; high-risk patient, history of smoking or other known risk factors.
From Webb WR, Brant WE, Major NM: *Fundamentals of body CT*, ed 4, Philadelphia, 2015, Saunders.

TABLE 41 Fleischner Society Recommendations for Computed Tomography (CT) Follow-up (FU) of Solitary Ground-Glass Opacity (GGO) or Part-GGO Nodules

Nodule Type	Recommendation	Additional Remarks
Solitary pure GGO ≤5 mm	No FU CT required	Use 1-mm slices to confirm nodule is pure GGO
Solitary pure GGO >5 mm	FU CT at 3 months; if persistent, yearly FU for at least 3 yrs	Positron emission tomography of limited value and not recommended
Solitary part-solid nodules	FU CT at 3 months; if persistent and solid component <5 mm, yearly FU for at least 3 yrs; if persistent and solid component ≥5 mm, then biopsy or resection	Consider positron emission tomography if nodule >1 cm

From Webb WR, Brant WE, Major NM: *Fundamentals of body CT*, ed 4, Philadelphia, 2015, Saunders.

TABLE 42 Fleischner Society Recommendations for Computed Tomography (CT) Follow-up (FU) of Multiple Ground-Glass Opacity (GGO) or Part-GGO Nodules

Nodule Type	Recommendation	Additional Remarks
Multiple pure GGO ≤5 mm	FU CT at 2 and 4 yrs	Consider alternate cause for GGO nodules
Multiple pure GGO >5 mm; no dominant lesion	FU CT at 3 months; if persistent, yearly FU for at least 3 yrs	Positron emission tomography of limited value and not recommended
Dominant part-solid nodule(s)	FU CT at 3 months; if persistent, then biopsy or resection, particularly if solid component ≥ 5 mm	Consider lung-sparing surgery in patients with a dominant lesion suspicious for lung cancer

From Webb WR, Brant WE, Major NM: *Fundamentals of body CT*, ed 4, Philadelphia, 2015, Saunders.

ICD-10CM # D69.2 Other nonthrombocytopenic purpura
D69.0 Allergic purpura
D69.49 Other primary thrombocytopenia
M31.1 Thrombotic microangiopathy

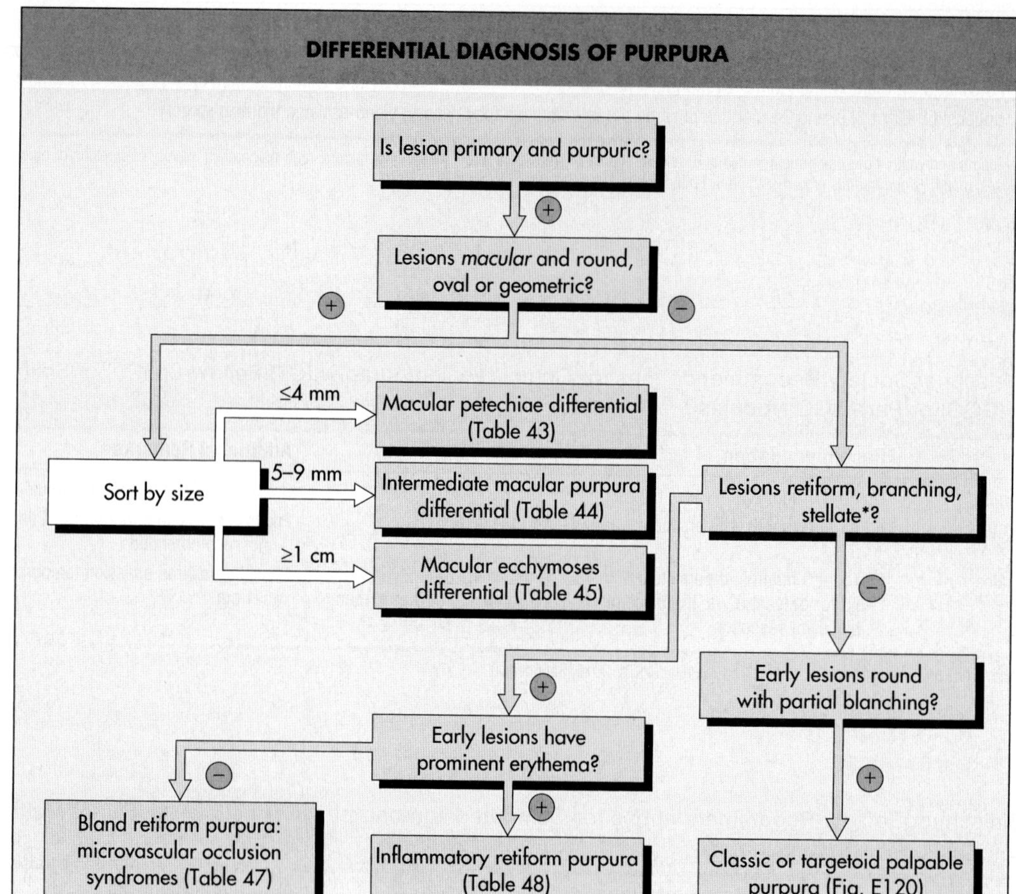

FIG. 119 Differential diagnosis of purpura. *Very few lesions are truly stellate, that is, characterized by a central area of necrosis or hemorrhage with radiating extensions, but some authors continue to use this term to describe these lesions. (From Bolognia J: *Dermatology,* ed 4, Philadelphia, 2018, Elsevier.)

TABLE 43 Differential Diagnosis of Macular Petechiae (≤4 mm in diameter)

Hemostatically Relevant Thrombocytopenia (<10, 000-20, 000/mm3)*

Major etiologies†

- Idiopathic thrombocytopenic purpura
- Thrombotic thrombocytopenic purpura
- Other acquired thrombocytopenias, including drug-related
  - Peripheral destruction (e.g., quinine, quinidine)
  - Drug-induced decreased production, idiosyncratic or dose-related (e.g., chemotherapy)
  - Bone marrow infiltration, fibrosis, or failure
- Disseminated intravascular coagulation (early sign)

Abnormal Platelet Function

Major etiologies†

- Congenital or hereditary platelet function defects
- Acquired platelet function defects
  - Aspirin, NSAIDs
  - Renal insufficiency
  - Monoclonal gammopathy (uncommon)
- Thrombocytosis secondary to myeloproliferative disorders (often >1,000,000/mm^3)

Nonplatelet Etiologies

Major etiologies†

- Spiking elevations of intravascular venous pressure (Valsalva maneuver-like, e.g., repetitive vomiting, childbirth, paroxysmal coughing, seizure)
- Fixed increased pressure (e.g., stasis, ligatures) or intermittent pressure (e.g., blood pressure cuff [Rumpel–Leede sign])
- Trauma (often linear)
- Perifollicular (vitamin C deficiency)
- Mildly inflammatory conditions
  - Pigmented purpuric eruptions
  - Hypergammaglobulinemic purpura of Waldenström

*Platelets provide factors necessary for hemostasis of endothelial cell junctions. When counts fall below 10,000-20,000/mm^3, inadequate platelet support leads to degradation of junction function, increased permeability, and hemorrhage.[3]

†Partial list.

From Bolognia J: *Dermatology,* ed 4, Philadelphia, 2018, Elsevier.

TABLE 44 Differential Diagnosis of Intermediate Macular Purpura (5-9 mm)

Major Etiologies*

- Hypergammaglobulinemic purpura of Waldenström
- Infection/inflammation in patients with thrombocytopenia
- Rarely, minimally inflamed cutaneous small vessel vasculitis (usually dependent distribution)

*Partial list.

From Bolognia J: *Dermatology,* ed 4, Philadelphia, 2018, Elsevier.

TABLE 45 Differential Diagnosis of Macular Ecchymoses (≥1 cm)

Procoagulant Defect Plus Minor Trauma

Major etiologies*

- Anticoagulant use
- Hepatic insufficiency with poor procoagulant synthesis
- Vitamin K deficiency
- Disseminated intravascular coagulation (some)

Poor dermal support of vessels plus minor trauma

Major etiologies*

- Solar (actinic, senile) purpura
- Corticosteroid therapy, topical or systemic
- Vitamin C deficiency (scurvy)
- Systemic amyloidosis (light chain-related, transthyretin-related
- Ehlers–Danlos syndrome

Platelet Disorders Plus Minor Trauma

Major etiologies*

- Platelet function defects, including von Willebrand disease and those induced by medications and metabolic diseases
- Acquired or congenital thrombocytopenia

Miscellaneous

- Papular purpuric gloves and socks syndrome

*Partial list.

From Bolognia J: *Dermatology,* ed 4, Philadelphia, 2018, Elsevier.

TABLE 46 Palpable Purpura: Inflammatory Purpura with Prominent Early Erythema

Leukocytoclastic Vasculitis due to Immune Complex Disease

Small vessels only

- Idiopathic, infection- or drug-associated IgG or IgM complexes
- Idiopathic IgA complexes (HSP), or IgA complexes associated with drugs or infection
- Hypergammaglobulinemic purpura of Waldenström
- Urticarial vasculitis: often minimally purpuric
- Pustular vasculitis (e.g. bowel bypass syndrome)

Small- and medium-sized (macroscopic) vessels may be involved

- Mixed cryoglobulinemia
- Rheumatic vasculitides (LE, RA, Sjögren syndrome)

Pauci-immune leukocytoclastic vasculitis

ANCA-associated

- Granulomatosis with polyangiitis
- Microscopic polyangiitis
- Eosinophilic granulomatosis with polyangiitis (Churg–Strauss syndrome)

Other

- Erythema elevatum diutinum
- Sweet syndrome (vasculitis unusual)

***Not* leukocytoclastic vasculitis**

Small vessels only

- Erythema multiforme
- Pityriasis lichenoides et varioliformis acuta (PLEVA)
- Pigmented purpuric eruptions
- Hypergammaglobulinemic purpura of Waldenström (although some lesions have histologic evidence of leukocytoclastic vasculitis)

Classic target lesion—usually erythema multiforme, but can be small vessel vasculitis, especially IgA-associated

AgG, Antigen G; *IgG,* immunoglobin G; *IgM,* immunoglobin M; *HSP,* Henoch–Schönlein purpura; *LE,* lupus erythematosus; *RA,* rheumatoid arthritis.

Modified from Bolognia J: *Dermatology,* ed 4, Philadelphia, 2018, Elsevier.

ICD-10CM # D69.2 Other nonthrombocytopenic purpura
D69.0 Allergic purpura
D69.49 Other primary thrombocytopenia
M31.1 Thrombotic microangiopathy

TABLE 47 Differential Diagnosis of Noninflammatory Retiform Purpura

Occlusion Primarily due to Platelet-Related Thrombopathy

Major etiologies*

- Heparin-induced thrombocytopenia syndrome (HITS)
- Thrombocytosis secondary to myeloproliferative disorders
- Paroxysmal nocturnal hemoglobinuria
- Thrombotic thrombocytopenic purpura (though platelet plugs form primarily in visceral vessels, and skin hemorrhage is due more often to thrombocytopenia)

Cold-related precipitation or agglutination

Major etiologies*

- Cryoglobulinemia, usually monoclonal (early lesions of mixed cryoglobulinemia are more often inflammatory and leukocytoclastic due to immune complex deposition)
- Cryofibrinogenemia (though most cryofibrinogens are incidental findings in hospitalized patients)
- Cold agglutinins (rarely cause occlusion; usually cause hemolysis or are asymptomatic)

Occlusion due to organisms growing in vessels

Major etiologies*

- Vessel-invasive fungi (e.g., *Mucor* spp., *Aspergillus* spp.; usually in immunocompromised patients)
- Ecthyma gangrenosum (often *Pseudomonas* spp. or other gram-negative bacilli proliferating in adventitia of subcutaneous arterioles)
- Disseminated strongyloidiasis
- Lucio phenomenon of Hansen disease
- Rocky Mountain spotted fever, other rickettsial spotted fevers

Systemic alteration in control of coagulation

Major etiologies*

- Protein C- and S-related
  - Homozygous protein C or protein S deficiency
  - Acquired protein C deficiency (some patients with sepsis-associated DIC)
  - Warfarin necrosis** (protein C dysfunction)
  - Postinfectious purpura fulminans (protein S dysfunction)
- Antiphospholipid antibody, lupus anticoagulant
- Levamisole-adulterated cocaine^

Vascular coagulopathy

- Livedoid vasculopathy/atrophie blanche (may also have a systemic prothrombotic component)
- Malignant atrophic papulosis/Degos disease (antiphospholipid antibody syndrome can mimic this disease)
- Sneddon syndrome (can be related to antiphospholipid antibody syndrome)
- Deficiency of adenosine deaminase 2 (ADA2)

Embolization or crystal deposition

Major etiologies*

- Cholesterol emboli
- Oxalate crystal deposition (rare)
- Marantic endocarditis, atrial myxoma, crystal globulins, hypereosinophilic syndrome (all rare)

Reticulocyte, red blood cell occlusion

- Sickle cell disease
- Severe malaria (usually *Plasmodium falciparum*)

Miscellaneous

- Cutaneous calciphylaxis
- Brown recluse (*Loxosceles*) spider bite reaction
- Intravascular B-cell lymphoma
- Hydroxyurea (rare)

DIC, Disseminated intravascular coagulation.
*Partial list.
**Also referred to as Coumadin® necrosis.
^Early lesions primarily thrombotic, but vasculitis can also occur.
From Bolognia J: *Dermatology,* ed 4, Philadelphia, 2018, Elsevier.

TABLE 48 Differential Diagnosis of Inflammatory Retiform Purpura

Vasculitis

Primarily dermal vessels

- IgA vasculitis

Dermal and Subcutaneous Vessels Usually Involved

- Mixed cryoglobulinemia
- Rheumatic vasculitides (LE, RA)
- Polyarteritis nodosa
- Microscopic polyangiitis
- Granulomatosis with polyangiitis
- Eosinophilic granulomatosis with polyangiitis (Churg–Strauss syndrome)

Dermal Vessel Inflammation/Occlusion/Constriction

- Livedoid vasculopathy
- Septic vasculitis
- Chilblains (pernio)
- Pyoderma gangrenosum

IgA, Immunoglobin A; *LE,* Lupus erythematosus; *RA,* rheumatoid arthritis.
From Bolognia J: *Dermatology,* ed 4, Philadelphia, 2018, Elsevier.

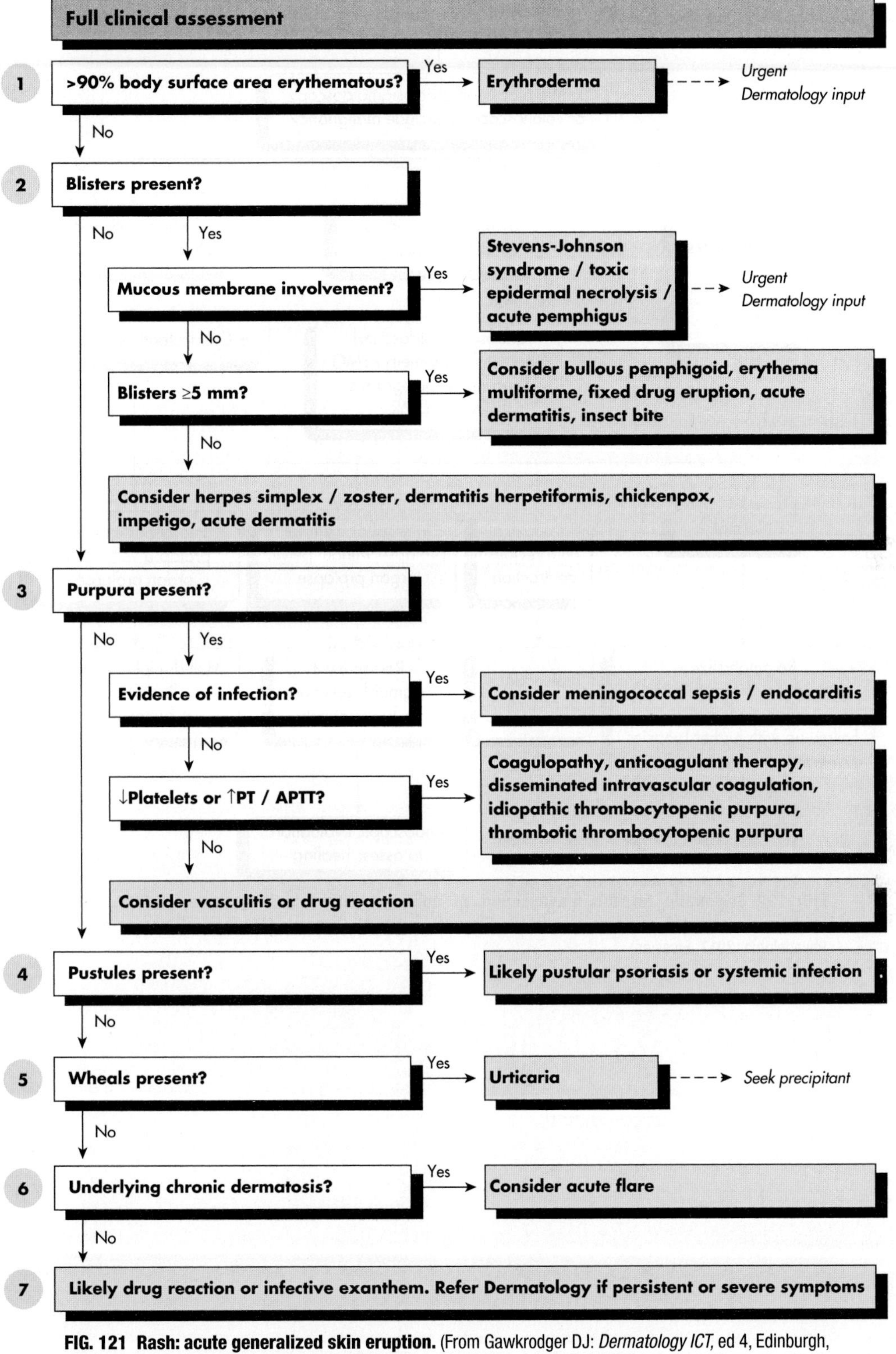

FIG. 121 Rash: acute generalized skin eruption. (From Gawkrodger DJ: *Dermatology ICT,* ed 4, Edinburgh, 2008, Churchill Livingstone; Japp AG, Robertson C: *Macleod's clinical diagnosis,* ed 2, Philadelphia, 2018, Elsevier.)

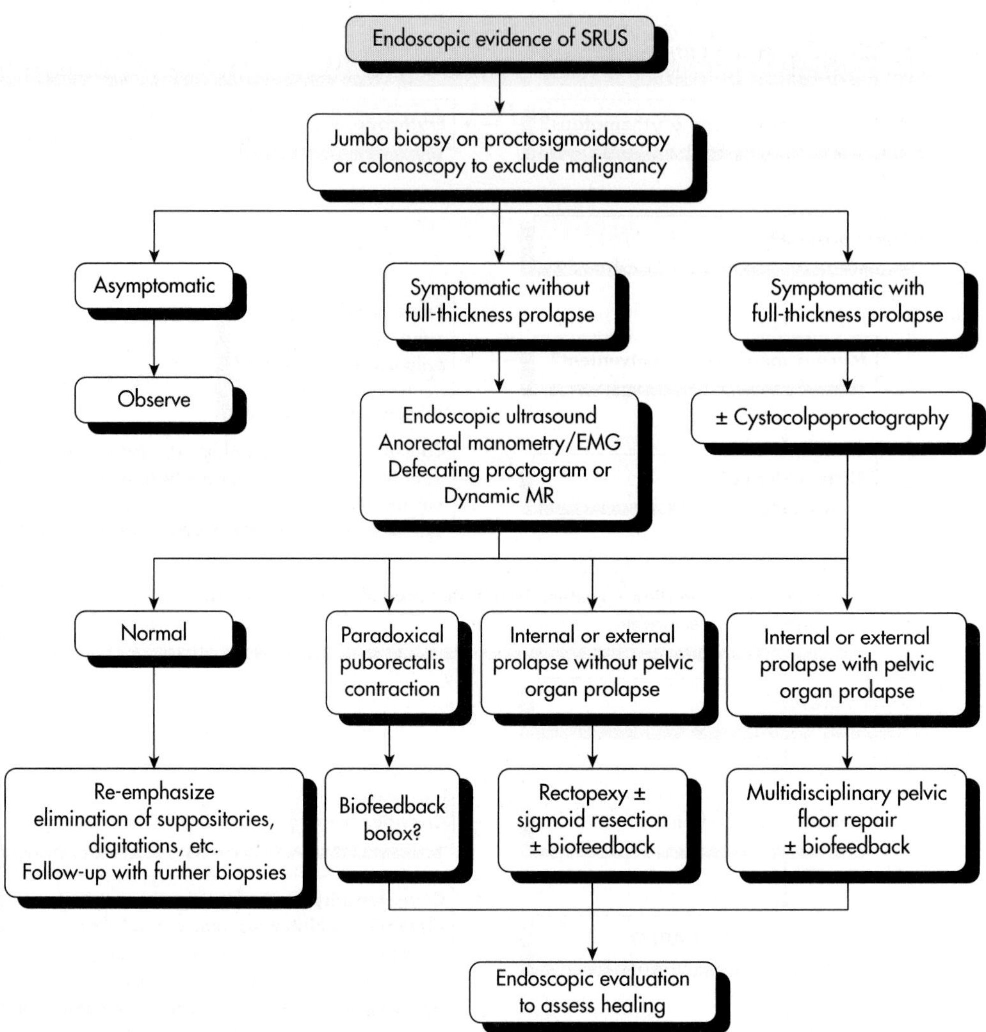

FIG. 122 Schematic for the management of solitary rectal ulcer syndrome (SRUS). *EMG*, Electromyography; *MR*, magnetic resonance. (From Cameron JL, Cameron AM: *Surgical therapy,* ed 12, Philadelphia, 2017, Elsevier.)

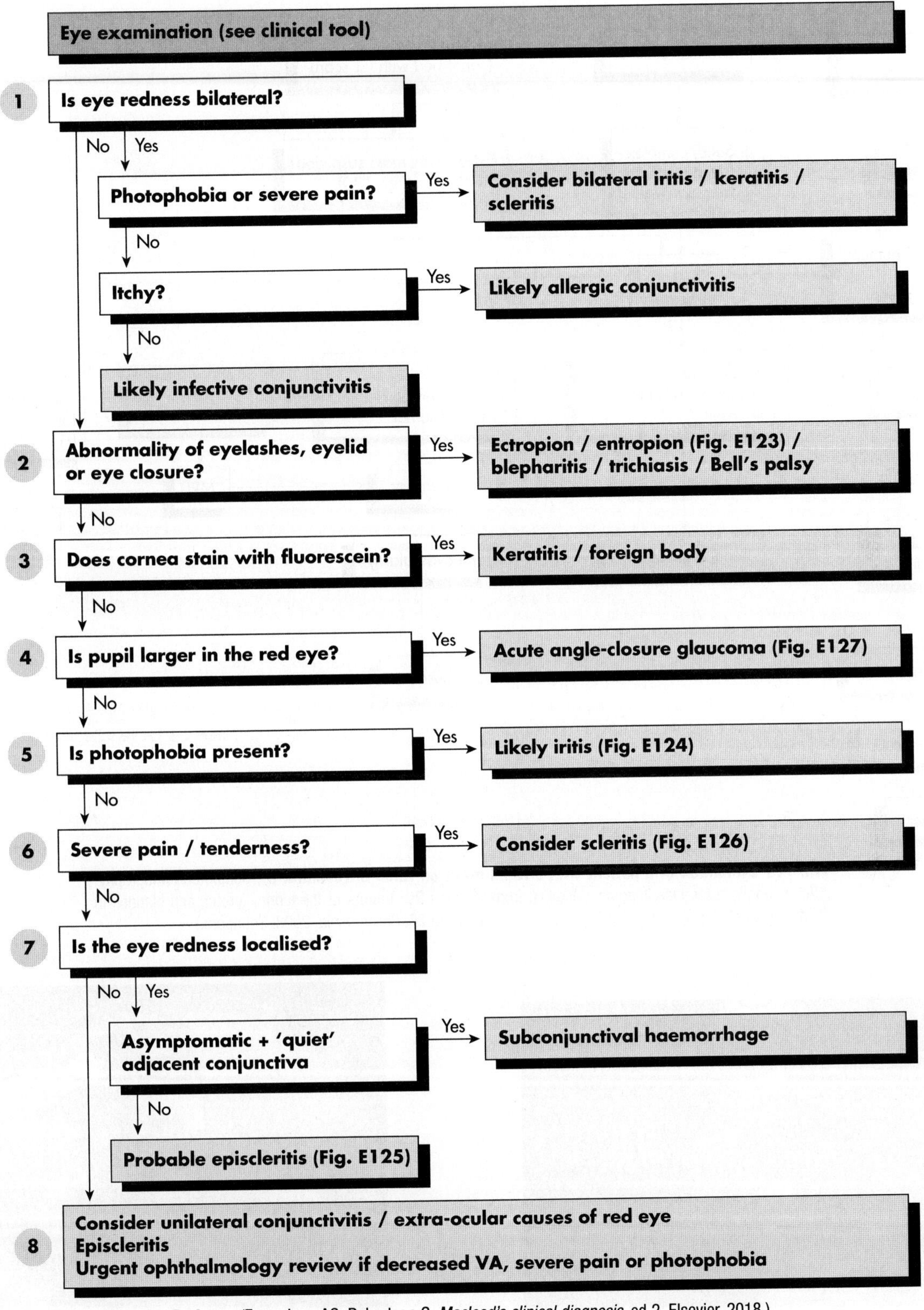

FIG. 128 Red eye. (From Japp AG, Robertson C: *Macleod's clinical diagnosis*, ed 2, Elsevier, 2018.)

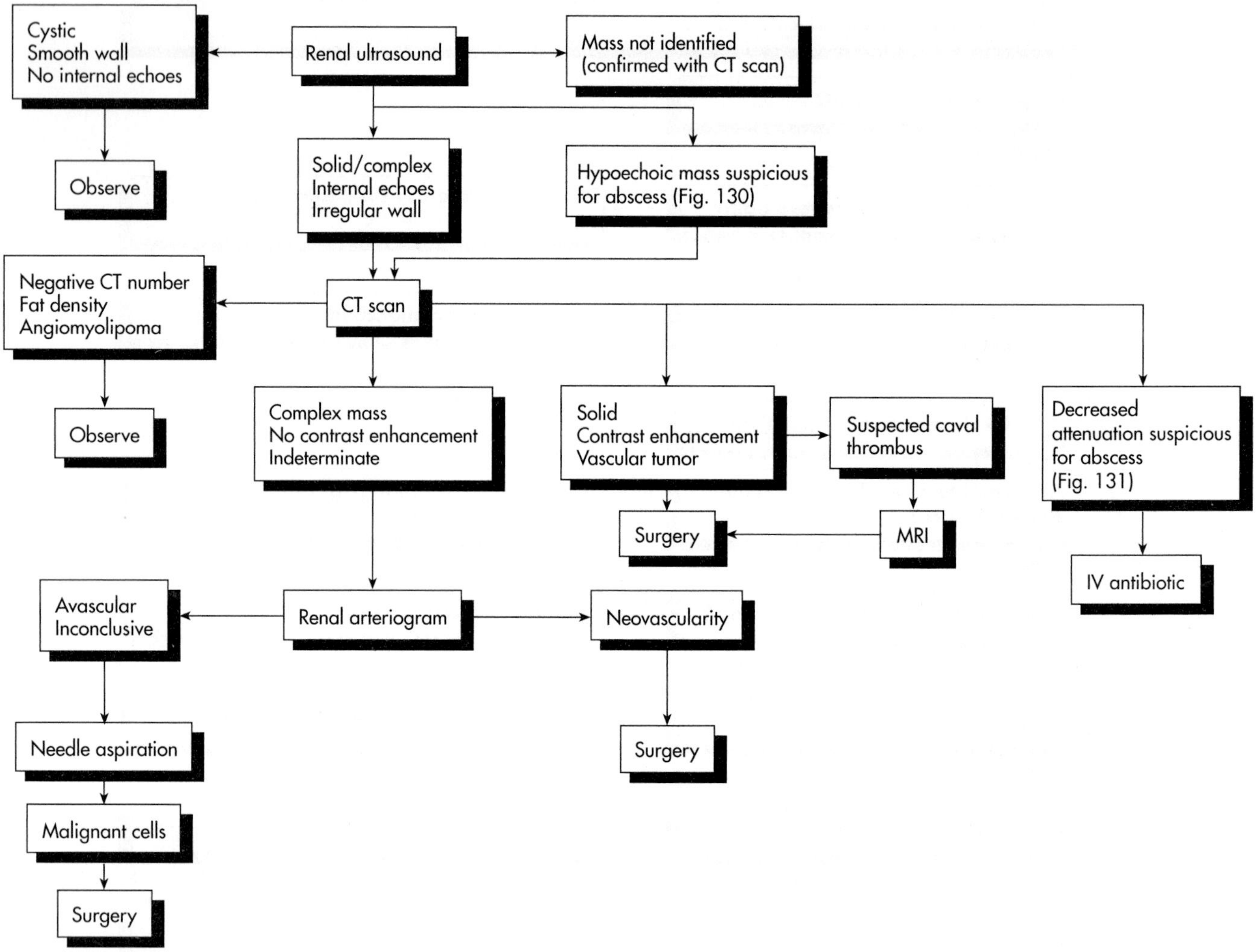

ICD-10CM # D41.10 Neoplasm of uncertain behavior of unspecified renal pelvis

Renal ultrasound
- → Cystic / Smooth wall / No internal echoes → Observe
- → Mass not identified (confirmed with CT scan)
- → Solid/complex / Internal echoes / Irregular wall → CT scan
- → Hypoechoic mass suspicious for abscess (Fig. 130) → CT scan

CT scan
- → Negative CT number / Fat density / Angiomyolipoma → Observe
- → Complex mass / No contrast enhancement / Indeterminate → Renal arteriogram
  - → Avascular / Inconclusive → Needle aspiration → Malignant cells → Surgery
  - → Neovascularity → Surgery
- → Solid / Contrast enhancement / Vascular tumor → Surgery
  - → Suspected caval thrombus → MRI → Surgery
- → Decreased attenuation suspicious for abscess (Fig. 131) → IV antibiotic

FIG. 129 Evaluation of a patient with a renal mass on renal ultrasound. *CT,* Computed tomography; *MRI,* magnetic resonance imaging. (Modified from Williams RD: Tumors of the kidney, ureter, and bladder. In Goldman L, Schafer AL [eds]: *Cecil textbook of medicine,* ed 23, Philadelphia, 2008, Saunders.)

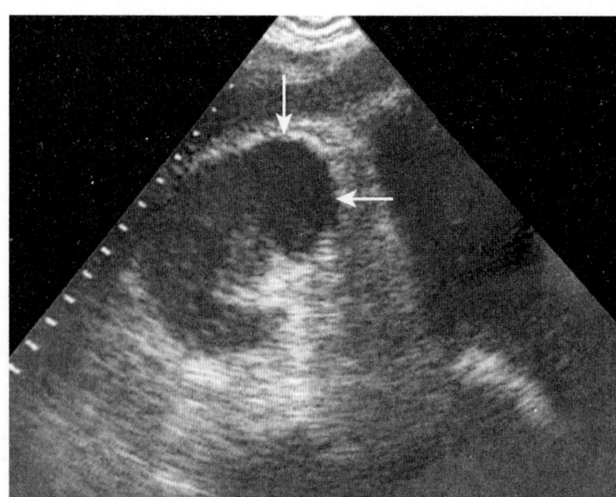

FIG. 130 Acute renal abscess. Transverse ultrasound image of the right kidney demonstrates a poorly marginated rounded focal hypoechoic mass *(arrows)* in the anterior portion of the kidney. *CT,* computed tomography. (From Wein AJ, Kavoussi LR, Partin AW, Peters CA: *Campbell-Walsh urology,* ed 11, Philadelphia, 2016, Elsevier.)

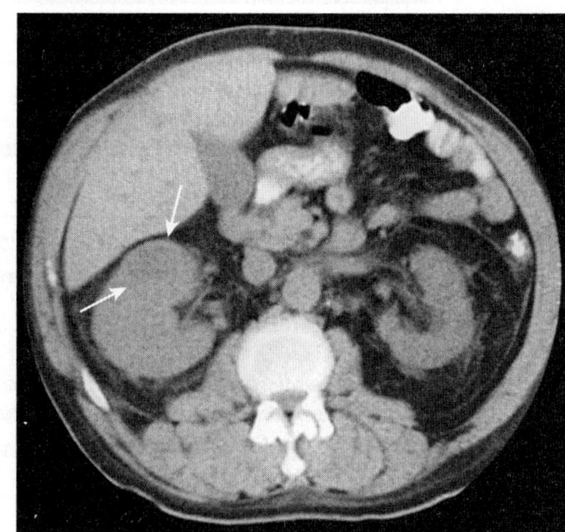

FIG. 131 Acute renal abscess. Nonenhanced computed tomography scan through the mid-pole of the right kidney demonstrates right renal enlargement and an area of decreased attenuation *(arrows).* After antimicrobial therapy, a follow-up scan showed complete regression of these findings. (From Wein AJ, Kavoussi LR, Partin AW, Peters CA: *Campbell-Walsh urology,* ed 11, Philadelphia, 2016, Elsevier.)

SCROTAL MASS

ICD-10CM # N44.2 Benign cyst of testis
N44.8 Other noninflammatory disorders of the testis
N50.3 Cyst of epididymis
N50.8 Other specified disorders of male genital organs

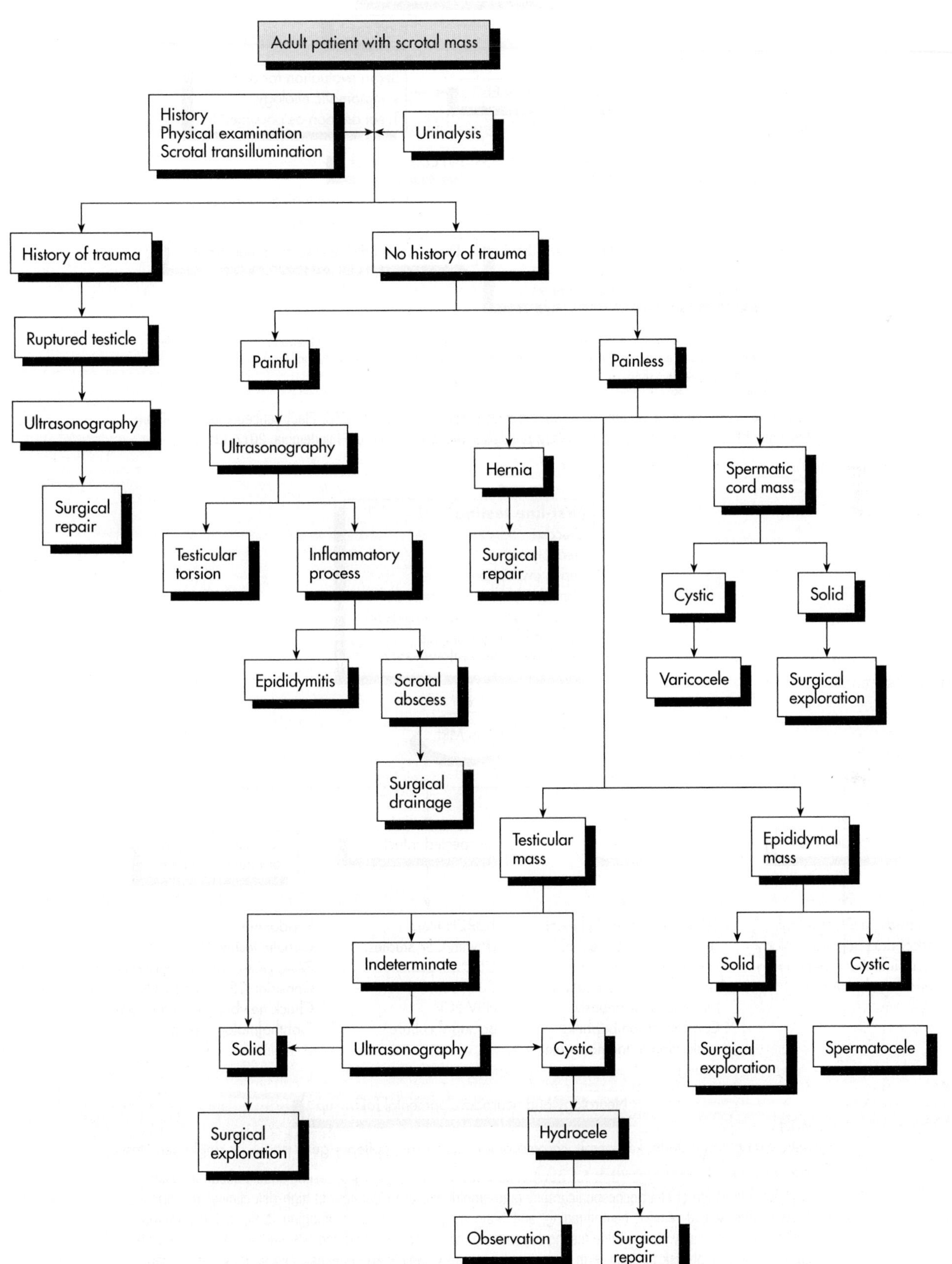

FIG. 133 Evaluation of scrotal mass. (Modified from Greene HL, Johnson WP, Lemcke DL [eds]: *Decision making in medicine*, ed 2, St Louis, 1998, Mosby.)

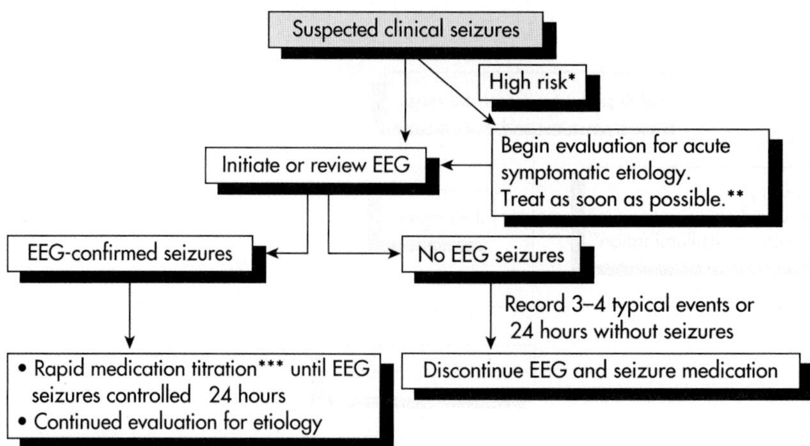

* High-risk scenarios: known or suspected acute brain injury, encephalopathy, previous EEG seizures, first 72 hours of life
** Reverse glucose or electrolyte abnormalities, and/or administer lorazepam 0.1 mg/kg IV, and/or administer phenobarbital loading dose.
*** Refer to Figure 136

FIG. 134 Assessment algorithm for newborns with suspected seizures. *EEG,* Electroencephalogram. (From Swaiman KF: *Swaiman's pediatric neurology, principles and practice,* ed 6, Philadelphia, 2017, Elsevier.)

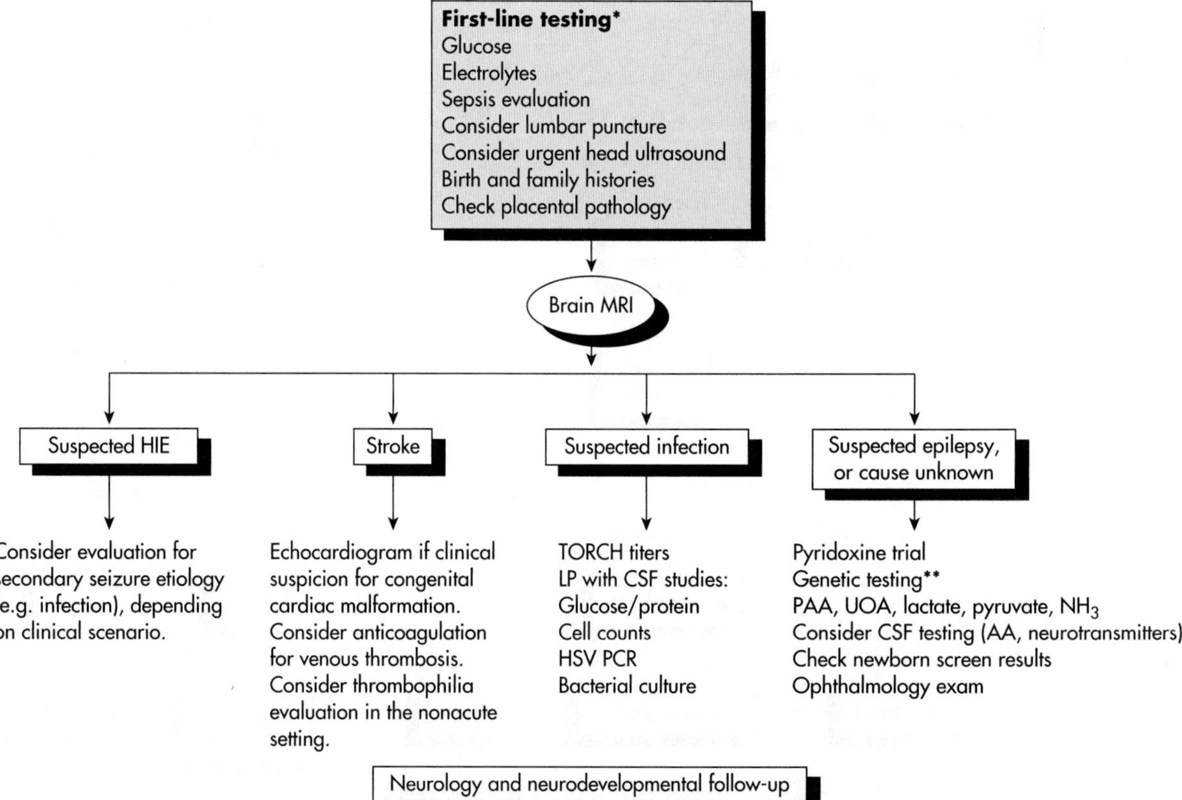

**Genetic testing can include: karyotype, chromosomal microarray, epilepsy gene panel, or single gene testing.

FIG. 135 Assessment algorithm for newborns with seizures. First-line testing should occur simultaneously with initiation of electroencephalography (and empiric seizure treatment in high-risk clinical scenarios). Most infants should receive neuroimaging, and brain magnetic resonance imaging (MRI) is the preferred neuroimaging modality. Second-line testing depends on the clinical scenario and MRI findings. Newborns with seizures are at high risk for long-term neurodevelopmental disability and epilepsy, and so they require careful follow-up by appropriate clinicians. *CSF,* Cerebrospinal fluid; *HIE,* hypoxic ischemic encephalopathy; *HSV,* herpes simplex virus; *LP,* lumbar puncture; *PCR,* polymerase chain reaction; *TORCH,* Toxoplasma gondii, other viruses, rubella, cytomegalovirus, and herpes simplex. (From Swaiman KF: *Swaiman's pediatric neurology: principles and practice,* ed 6, Philadelphia, 2017, Elsevier.)

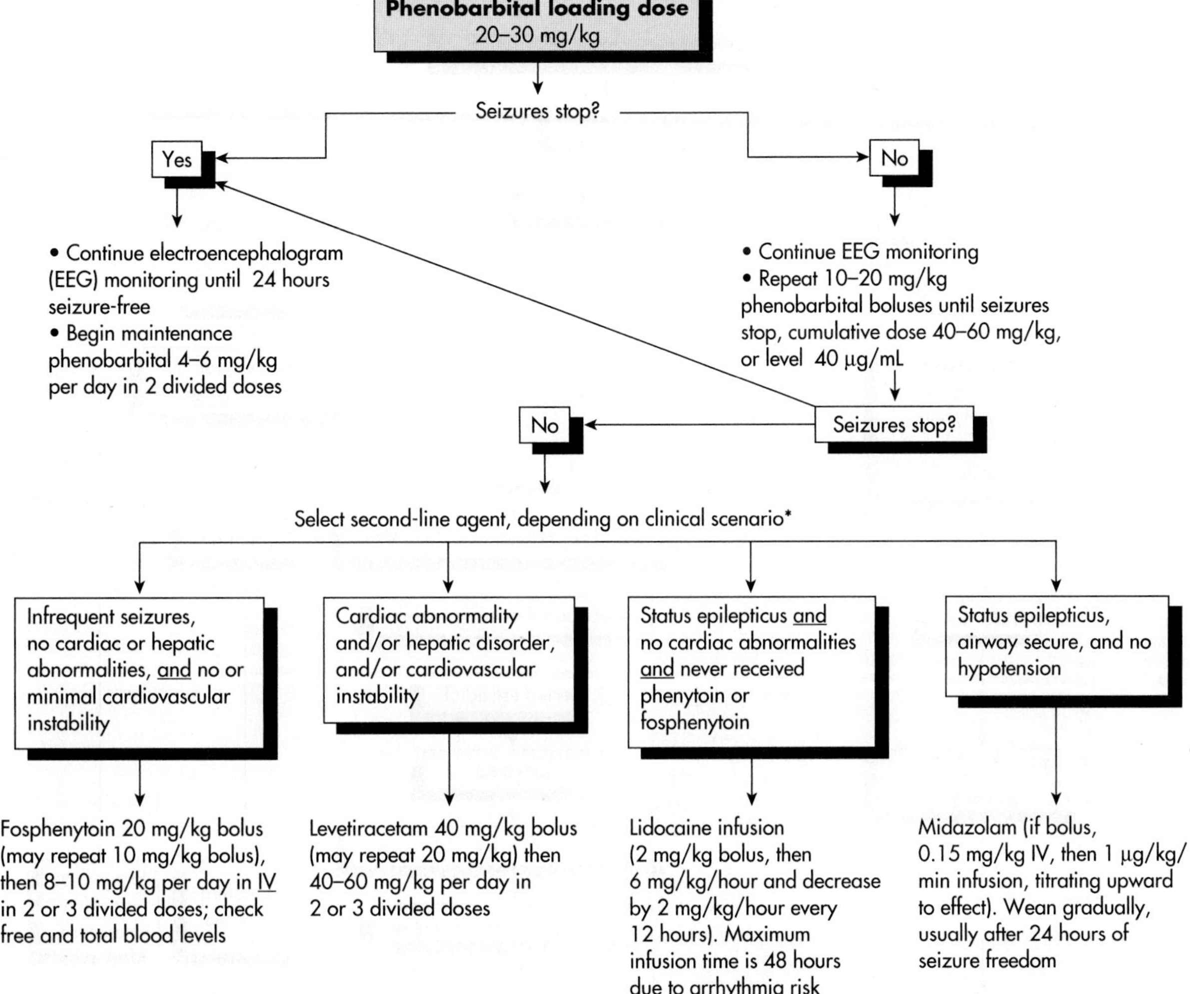

FIG. 136 Suggested treatment algorithm for neonatal seizures. The rapidity of medication administration will depend on local guidelines and resources. Frequent assessment of treatment response is recommended. (From Swaiman KF: *Swaiman's pediatric neurology: principles and practice*, ed 6, Philadelphia, 2017, Elsevier.)

SEXUAL PRECOCITY, FEMALE BREAST DEVELOPMENT

ICD-10CM # E30.1 Precocious puberty
E30.8 Other disorders of puberty

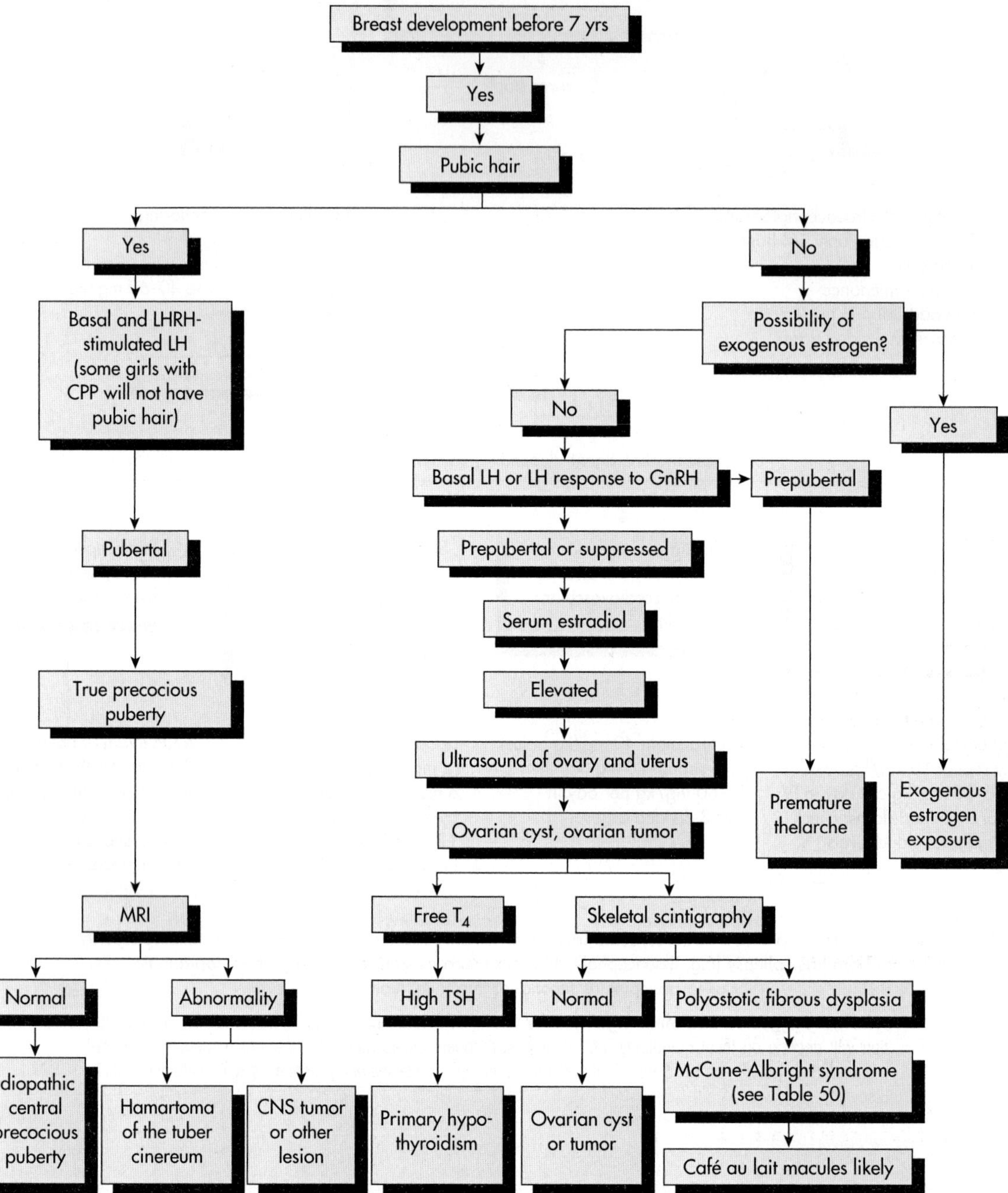

Note: See Section I, "Precocious Puberty," for more information on this topic

FIG. 137 Flow chart for diagnosing sexual precocity in girls. *CNS*, central nervous system; *CPP*, central precocious puberty; *FSH*, follicle-stimulating hormone; *GnRH*, gonadotropin-releasing hormone; *LH*, luteinizing hormone; *LHRH*, LH-releasing hormone; *MRI*, magnetic resonance imaging; *T_4*, thyroxine; *TSH*, thyroid-stimulating hormone. (From Melmed S, Polonsky KS, Larsen P et al: *Williams textbook of endocrinology*, ed 13, Philadelphia, 2016, Elsevier.)

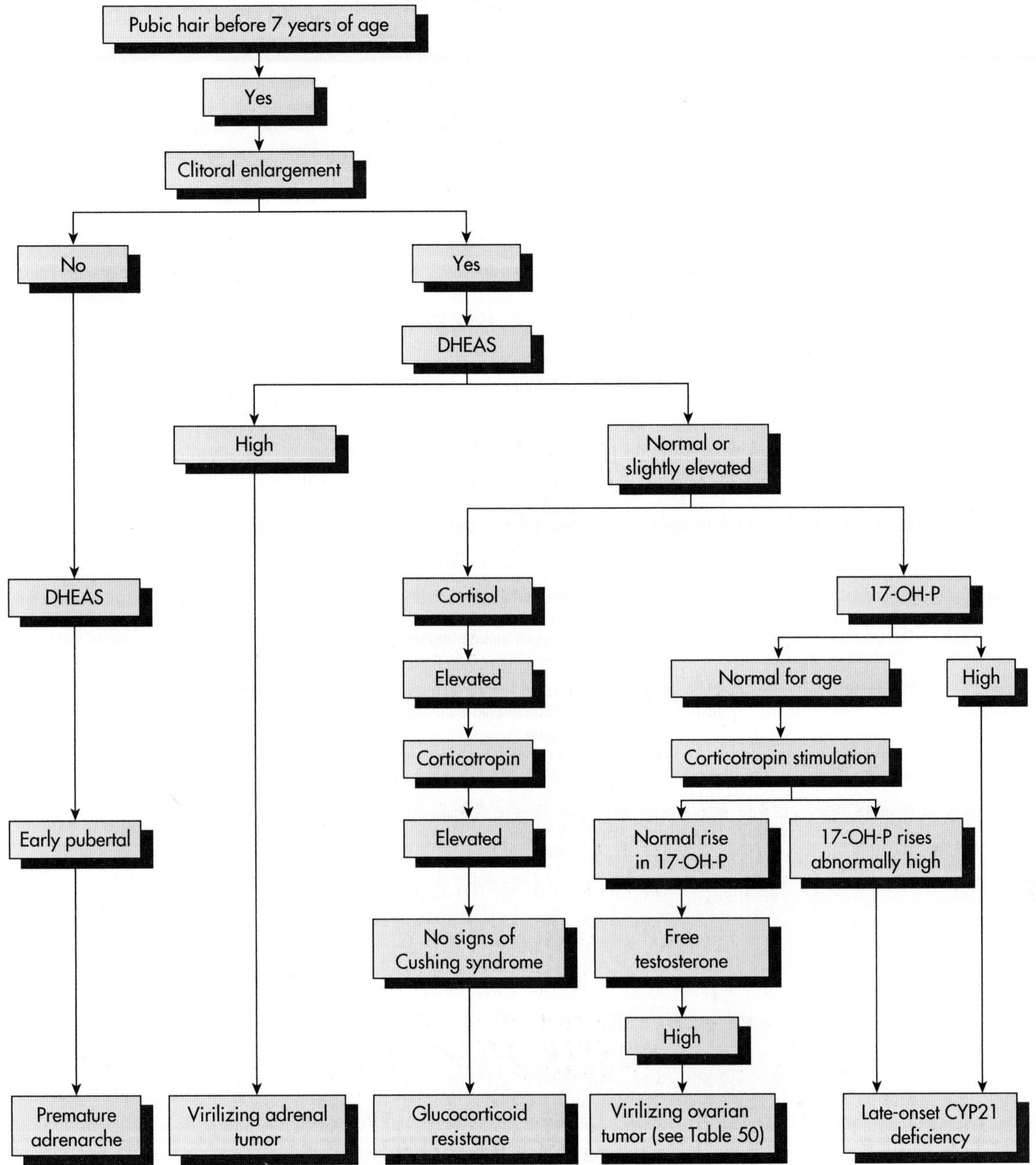

Note: See Section I, "Precocious Puberty," for more information on this topic.

FIG. 138 Flow chart for the evaluation of pubic hair in normal phenotypic girls before 7 years. *DHEAS*, dehydroepiandrosterone sulfate; 17-OH-P, 17-hydroxyprogesterone. (From Melmed S, Polonsky KS, Larsen P et al: *Williams textbook of endocrinology,* ed 13, Philadelphia, 2016, Elsevier.)

TABLE 50 Differential Diagnosis of Sexual Precocity

	Plasma Gonadotropins	LH Response to LHRH	Serum Sex Steroid Concentration	Gonadal Size	Miscellaneous
In Both Sexes					
McCune-Albright syndrome	Suppressed	Suppressed	Sex steroids pubertal or higher	Ovarian (on ultrasound); slight testicular enlargement	Skeletal survey for polyostotic fibrous dysplasia and skin examination for café-au-lait spots
Primary hypothyroidism	LH prepubertal; FSH may be slightly elevated	Prepubertal FSH may be increased	Estradiol may be pubertal	Testicular enlargement; ovaries cystic	TSH and prolactin elevated; T_4 low
Females					
Granulosa cell tumor (follicular cysts may present similarly)	Suppressed	Prepubertal LH response	Very high estradiol	Ovarian enlargement on physical examination, CT, or ultrasonography	Tumor often palpable on abdominal examination
Follicular cyst	Suppressed	Prepubertal LH response	Prepubertal to very high estradiol	Ovarian enlargement on physical examination, CT, or ultrasonography	Single or recurrent episodes of menses and/or breast development; exclude McCune-Albright syndrome
Feminizing adrenal tumor	Suppressed	Prepubertal LH response	High estradiol and DHEAS values	Ovaries prepubertal	Unilateral adrenal mass
Premature thelarche	Prepubertal	Prepubertal LH, pubertal estradiol response	Prepubertal or early	Ovaries prepubertal	Onset usually before 3 yrs of age
Premature adrenarche	Prepubertal	Prepubertal LH response	Prepubertal estradiol; DHEAS or urinary 17-ketosteroid values appropriate for pubic hair stage 2	Ovaries prepubertal	Onset usually after 6 yrs of age; more frequent in brain-injured children
Late-onset virilizing congenital adrenal hyperplasia	Prepubertal	Prepubertal LH response	Elevated 17-OHP in basal or corticotropin-stimulated state	Ovaries prepubertal	Autosomal recessive

CNS, Central nervous system; *CT,* computed tomography; *DHEAS,* dehydroepiandrosterone sulfate; *FSH,* follicle-stimulating hormone; *LH,* luteinizing hormone; 1 *7-OHP,* 17-hydroxy progesterone; T_4, thyroxine; *TSH,* thyrotropin.

From Larsen PR, Kronenberg HM, Melmed S, Polansky KS [eds]: *Williams textbook of endocrinology,* ed 11, Philadelphia, 2008, Saunders.

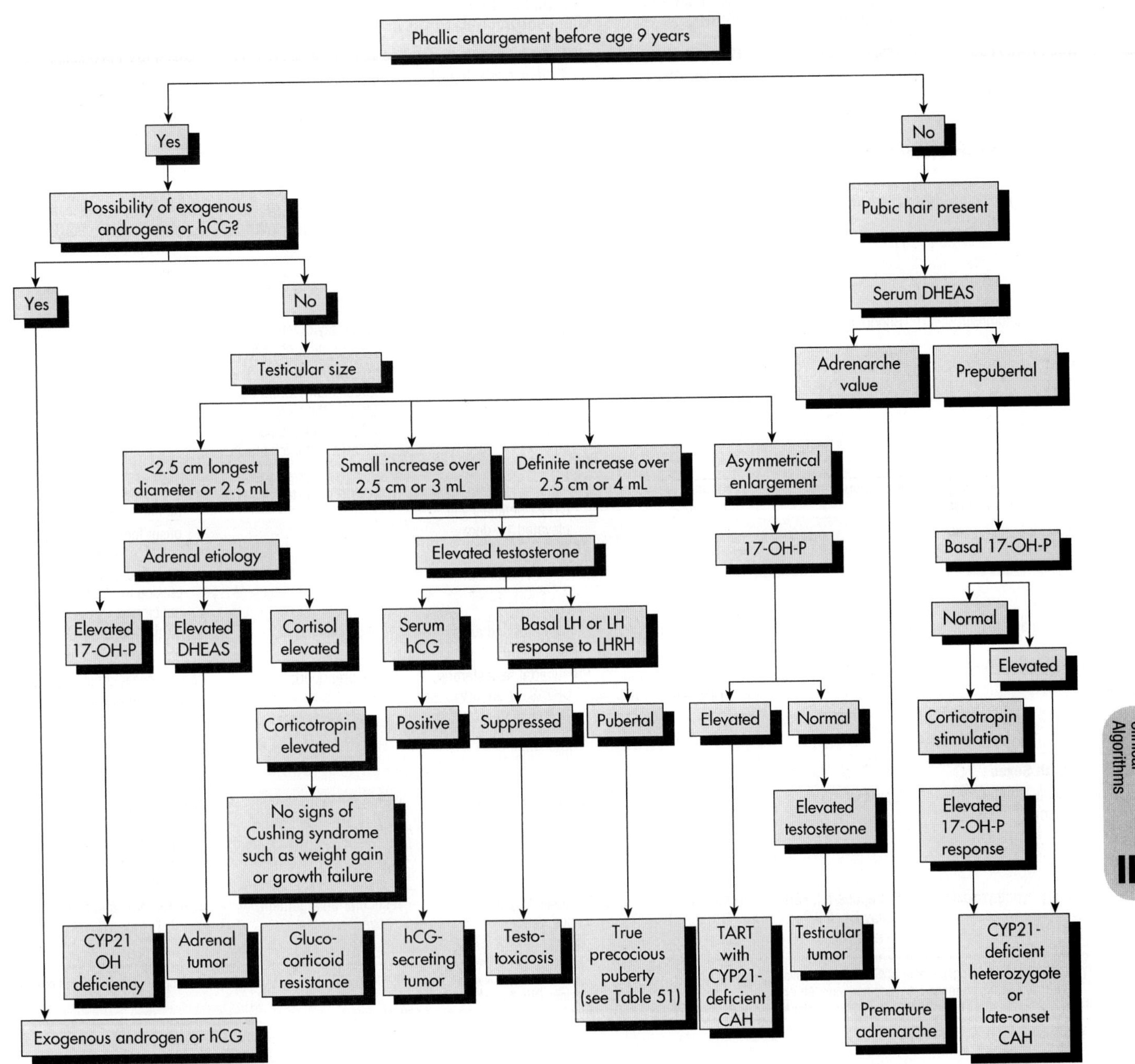

Note: See Section I, "Precocious Puberty," for more information on this topic.

FIG. 139 Flow chart for diagnosing sexual precocity in a phenotypic male. *CAH*, congenital adrenal hyperplasia; *DHEAS*, dehydroepiandrosterone sulfate; *hCG*, human chorionic gonadotropin; *LH*, luteinizing hormone; *LHRH*, LH-releasing hormone; *17-OH-P*, 17-hydroxyprogesterone; *TART*, testicular adrenal rest tissue. (From Melmed S, Polonsky KS, Larsen P et al: *Williams textbook of endocrinology,* ed 13, Philadelphia, 2016, Elsevier.)

ICD-10CM # E30.1 Precocious puberty
E30.8 Other disorders of puberty

TABLE 51 Causes of Male Sexual Precocity

	Plasma Gonadotropins	LH Response to LHRH	Serum Sex Steroid Concentration	Gonadal Size	Miscellaneous
True Precocious Puberty (premature reactivation of LHRH pulse generator)	Prominent LH pulses, initially during sleep	Pubertal LH response	Pubertal values of testosterone or estradiol	Normal pubertal testicular enlargement or ovarian and uterine enlargement (by ultrasonography)	MRI of brain to rule out CNS tumor or other abnormality; skeletal survey for McCune-Albright syndrome
Incomplete Sexual Precocity (pituitary gonadotropin-independent)					
Males					
Chorionic gonadotropin-secreting tumor in males	High hCG, low LH	Prepubertal LH response	Pubertal value of testosterone	Slight to moderate uniform enlargement of testes	Hepatomegaly suggests hepatoblastoma; CT scan of brain if chorionic gonadotropin-secreting CNS tumor suspected
Leydig cell tumor in males	Suppressed	No LH response	Very high testosterone	Irregular asymmetrical enlargement of testes	
Familial testotoxicosis	Suppressed	No LH response	Pubertal values of testosterone	Testes symmetrical and larger than 2.5 cm but smaller than expected for pubertal development; spermatogenesis occurs	Familial; probably sex-limited, autosomal dominant trait
Virilizing congenital adrenal hyperplasia	Prepubertal	Prepubertal LH response	Elevated 17-OHP in CYP21 deficiency or elevated 11-deoxycortisol in CYP11B1 deficiency	Testes prepubertal	Autosomal recessive, may be congenital or late-onset form, may have salt loss in CYP21 deficiency or hypertension in CYP11B1 deficiency
Virilizing adrenal tumor	Prepubertal	Prepubertal LH response	High DHEAS and androstenedione values	Testes prepubertal	CT, MRI, or ultrasonography of abdomen
Premature adrenarche	Prepubertal	Prepubertal LH response	Prepubertal testosterone, DHEAS, or urinary 17-ketosteroid values appropriate for pubic hair stage 2	Testes prepubertal	Onset usually after 6 yrs of age; more frequent in CNS-injured children
In Both Sexes					
McCune-Albright syndrome	Suppressed	Suppressed	Sex steroids pubertal or higher	Ovarian (on ultrasound); slight testicular enlargement	Skeletal survey for polyostotic fibrous dysplasia and skin examination for café-au-lait spots
Primary hypothyroidism	LH prepubertal; FSH may be slightly elevated	Prepubertal FSH may be increased	Estradiol may be pubertal	Testicular enlargement; ovaries cystic	TSH and prolactin elevated; T_4 low

17-OHP, 17-Hydroxyprogesterone; *CNS,* central nervous system; *CT,* computed tomography; *DHEAS,* dehydroepiandrosterone sulfate; *hCG,* human chorionic gonadotropin; *LH,* luteinizing hormone; *LHRH,* luteinizing hormone-releasing hormone; *MRI,* magnetic resonance imaging; T_4, thyroxine; *TSH,* thyrotropin.

From Larsen PR, Kronenberg HM, Melmed S, Polansky, KS [eds]: *Williams textbook of endocrinology,* ed 11, Philadelphia, 2008, Saunders.

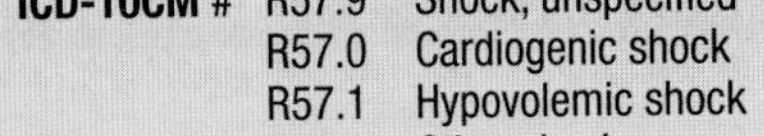

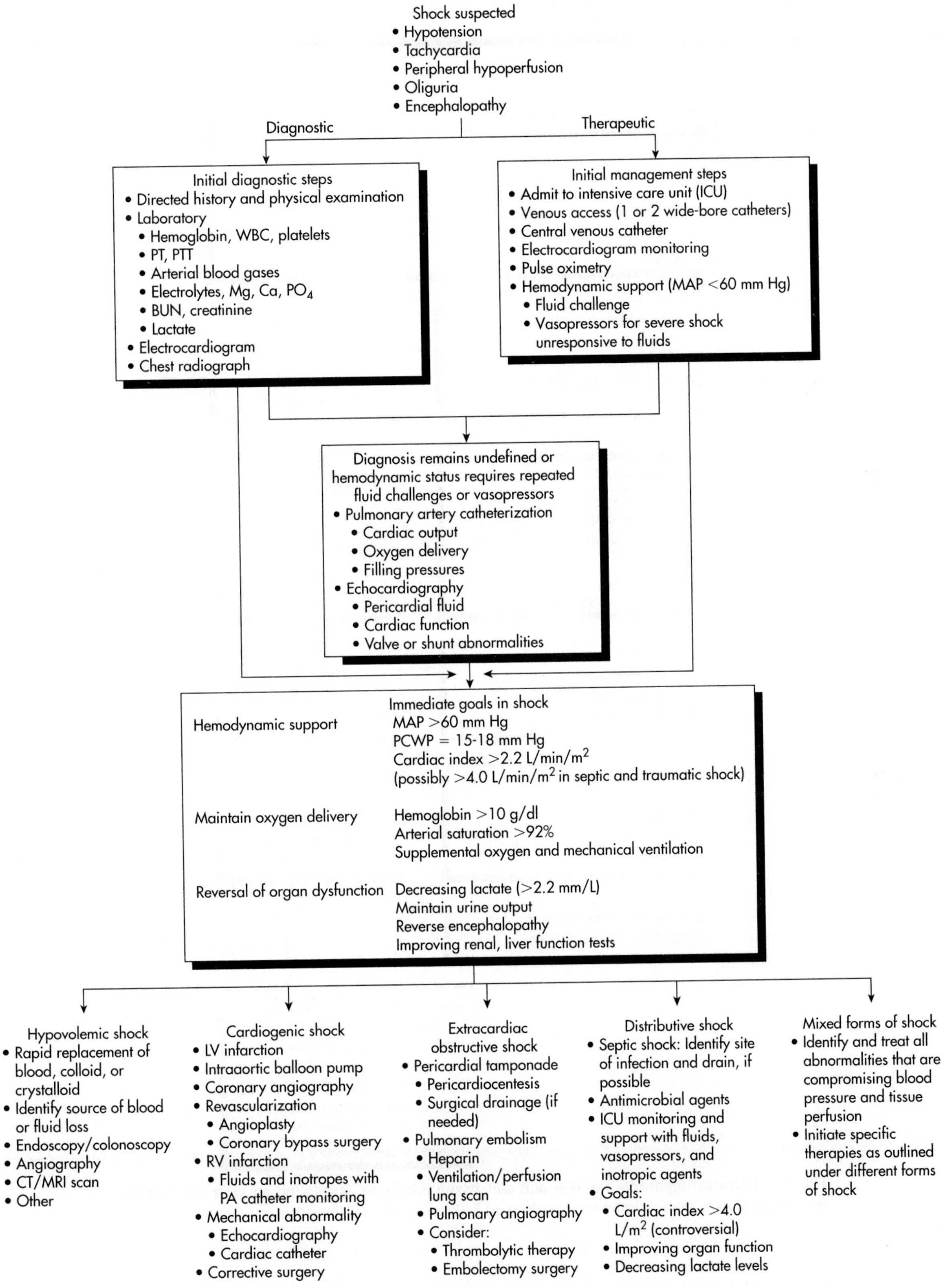

ICD-10CM # R57.9 Shock, unspecified
R57.0 Cardiogenic shock
R57.1 Hypovolemic shock
R57.8 Other shock

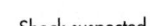

Shock suspected
- Hypotension
- Tachycardia
- Peripheral hypoperfusion
- Oliguria
- Encephalopathy

Diagnostic

Initial diagnostic steps
- Directed history and physical examination
- Laboratory
  - Hemoglobin, WBC, platelets
  - PT, PTT
  - Arterial blood gases
  - Electrolytes, Mg, Ca, PO_4
  - BUN, creatinine
  - Lactate
- Electrocardiogram
- Chest radiograph

Therapeutic

Initial management steps
- Admit to intensive care unit (ICU)
- Venous access (1 or 2 wide-bore catheters)
- Central venous catheter
- Electrocardiogram monitoring
- Pulse oximetry
- Hemodynamic support (MAP <60 mm Hg)
  - Fluid challenge
  - Vasopressors for severe shock unresponsive to fluids

Diagnosis remains undefined or hemodynamic status requires repeated fluid challenges or vasopressors
- Pulmonary artery catheterization
  - Cardiac output
  - Oxygen delivery
  - Filling pressures
- Echocardiography
  - Pericardial fluid
  - Cardiac function
  - Valve or shunt abnormalities

Immediate goals in shock

Hemodynamic support	MAP >60 mm Hg PCWP = 15-18 mm Hg Cardiac index >2.2 L/min/m^2 (possibly >4.0 L/min/m^2 in septic and traumatic shock)
Maintain oxygen delivery	Hemoglobin >10 g/dl Arterial saturation >92% Supplemental oxygen and mechanical ventilation
Reversal of organ dysfunction	Decreasing lactate (>2.2 mm/L) Maintain urine output Reverse encephalopathy Improving renal, liver function tests

Hypovolemic shock
- Rapid replacement of blood, colloid, or crystalloid
- Identify source of blood or fluid loss
- Endoscopy/colonoscopy
- Angiography
- CT/MRI scan
- Other

Cardiogenic shock
- LV infarction
- Intraaortic balloon pump
- Coronary angiography
- Revascularization
  - Angioplasty
  - Coronary bypass surgery
- RV infarction
  - Fluids and inotropes with PA catheter monitoring
- Mechanical abnormality
  - Echocardiography
  - Cardiac catheter
- Corrective surgery

Extracardiac obstructive shock
- Pericardial tamponade
  - Pericardiocentesis
  - Surgical drainage (if needed)
- Pulmonary embolism
  - Heparin
  - Ventilation/perfusion lung scan
  - Pulmonary angiography
  - Consider:
    - Thrombolytic therapy
    - Embolectomy surgery

Distributive shock
- Septic shock: Identify site of infection and drain, if possible
- Antimicrobial agents
- ICU monitoring and support with fluids, vasopressors, and inotropic agents
- Goals:
  - Cardiac index >4.0 L/m^2 (controversial)
  - Improving organ function
  - Decreasing lactate levels

Mixed forms of shock
- Identify and treat all abnormalities that are compromising blood pressure and tissue perfusion
- Initiate specific therapies as outlined under different forms of shock

FIG. 140 An approach to the diagnosis and treatment of shock. *BUN,* Blood urea nitrogen; *CT,* computed tomography; *LV,* left ventricular; *MAP,* mean arterial pressure; *MRI,* magnetic resonance imaging; *PA,* pulmonary arterial; *PCWP,* pulmonary capillary wedge pressure; *PT,* prothrombin time; *PTT,* partial thromboplastin time; *RV,* right ventricular; *WBC,* white blood cell count. (From Goldman L, Ausiello D [eds]: *Cecil textbook of medicine,* ed 24, Philadelphia, 2012, Saunders.)

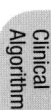

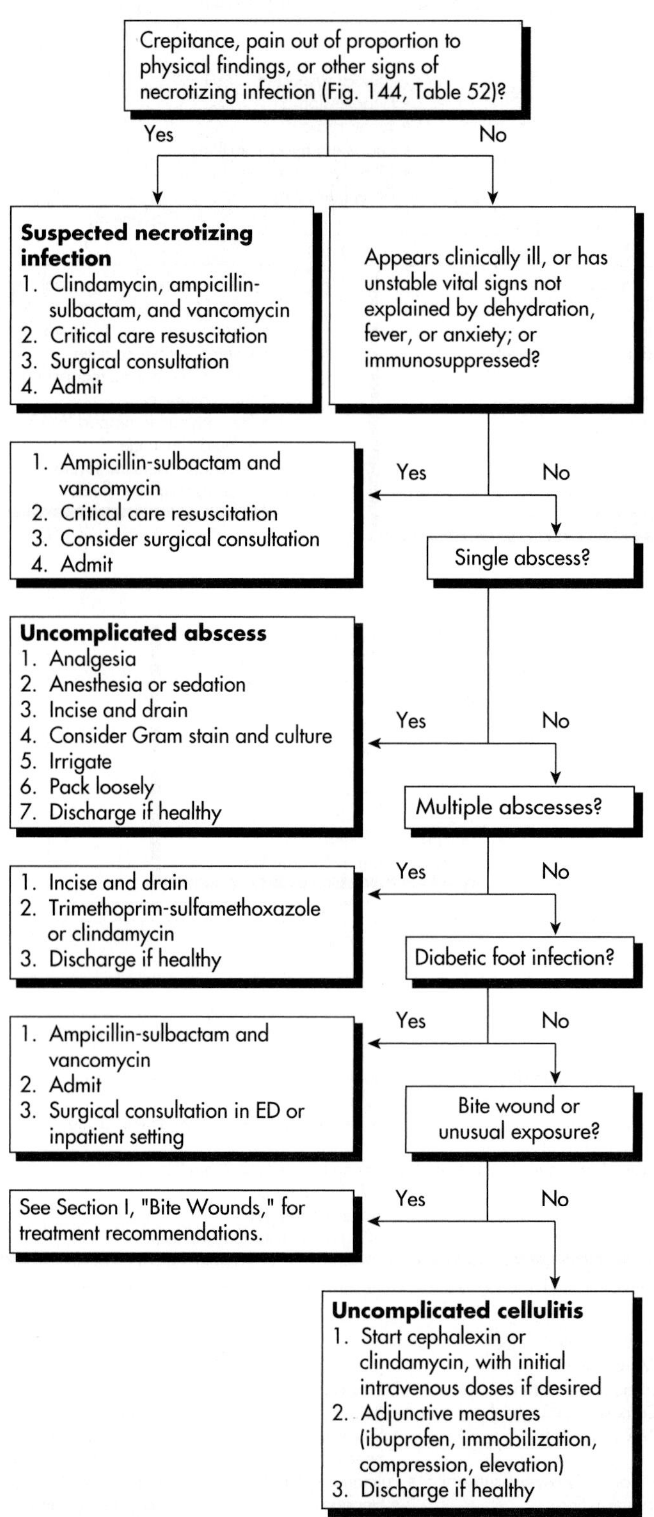

FIG. 143 Universal algorithm for skin and soft tissue infections (assuming no prior treatment). (From Marx JA et al: *Rosen's emergency medicine*, ed 8, Philadelphia, 2014, Saunders.)

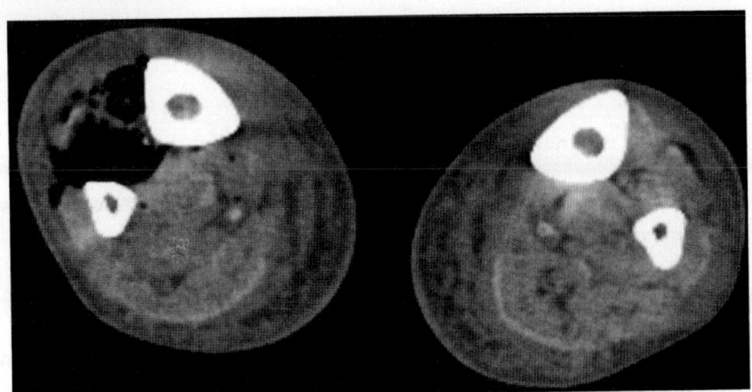

FIG. 144 Necrotizing fasciitis. Axial computed tomography through the lower extremities demonstrates gas in the anterior soft tissues. Necrotizing fasciitis is a clinical diagnosis. Imaging may lead to a delay in treatment. (From Webb WR, Brandt WE, Major NM: *Fundamentals of body CT,* ed 4, Philadelphia, 2015, Elsevier.)

TABLE 52 Differentiating Features of Necrotizing Skin and Soft Tissue Infections

Feature	Progressive Bacterial Synergistic Gangrene	Nonclostridial Anaerobic Cellulitis	Clostridial Myonecrosis (Gas Gangrene)	Necrotizing Fasciitis Type 1	Necrotizing Fasciitis Type 2
Risk factors	Surgery, ileostomy, colostomy, chronic ulceration	Diabetes mellitus	Trauma, surgery	Diabetes mellitus, surgery, perineal infection	Trauma, surgery, none
Microbiology	Microaerophilic streptococci plus *Staphylococcus aureus*	Non–spore-forming anaerobes ± coliforms, streptococci, *S. aureus*	*Clostridium* spp.	Polymicrobial (Enterobacteriaceae plus anaerobes)	Group A streptococci
Course	Slow	Slow or rapid	Very rapid	Rapid	Very rapid
Pain	++++	++/+++	++++	+++/++++	++++
Gas formation	–	++++	++	++	–
Appearance	Central necrotic ulcer, erythematous periphery	Erythematous skin necrosis	Bullae, necrosis	Bullae, skin	Bullae, necrotic skin and tissue
Drainage	Purulent if present	Purulent	Serosanguineous	"Dishwater," seropurulent	Serous if present
Depth of involvement	Skin, soft tissue	Skin, soft tissue	Muscle	Fascia	Fascia
Systemic toxicity	±	+++/++++	++++	+++/++++	++++

–, absent; ±, occasionally present; +, minimal; ++, mild; +++, moderate; ++++, marked or severe.
From Parrillo JE, Dellinger RP: *Critical care medicine: principles of diagnosis and management in the adult,* ed 4, Philadelphia, 2014, Elsevier.

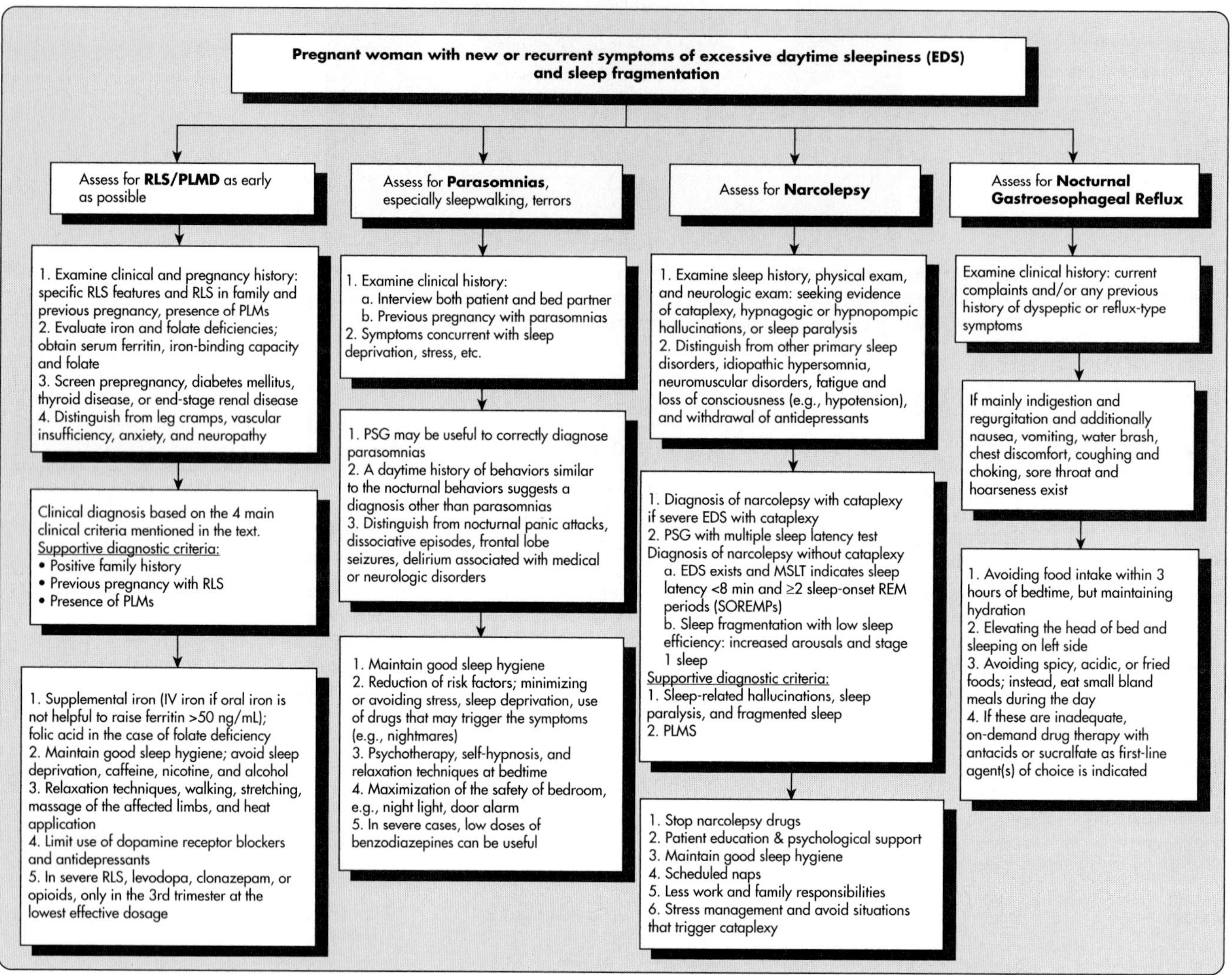

FIG. 146 Management and treatment of sleep-related disorders. *IV*, Intravenous; *MSLT*, Multiple Sleep Latency Test; *PLMs*, periodic leg movements; *PLMD*, periodic leg movement disorder; *PSG*, polysomnography; *REM*, rapid eye movement; *RLS*, restless legs syndrome; *SOREMP*, sleep-onset rapid eye movement sleep period. (Kryger M, Roth T, Dement WC: *Principles and practice of sleep medicine*, ed 6, Philadelphia, 2017, Elsevier.)

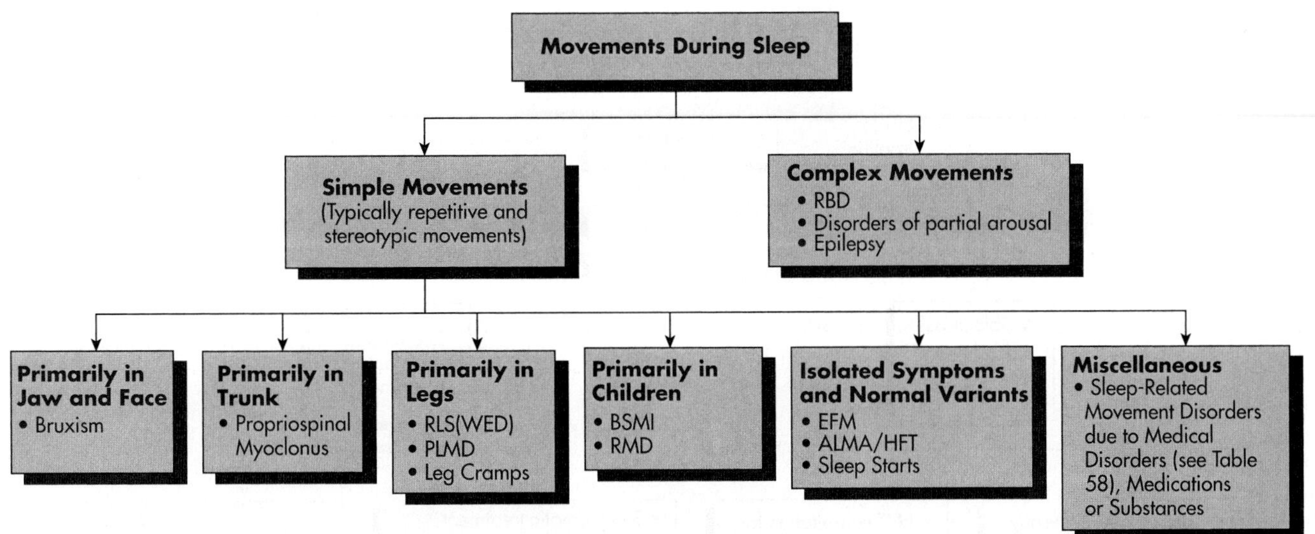

FIG. 147 Flow chart for the approach to the differential diagnosis of sleep-related movement disorders. *ALMA*, Alternating leg muscle activation; *BSMI*, benign sleep myoclonus of infancy; *EFM*, excessive fragmentary myoclonus; *HFT*, hypnagogic foot tremor; *PLMD*, periodic limb movement disorder; *RBD*, rapid eye movement (REM) sleep behavior disorder; *RLS (WED)*, restless legs syndrome (Willis-Ekbom disease); *RMD*, rhythmic movement disorder. (Kryger M, Roth T, Dement WC: *Principles and practice of sleep medicine,* ed 6, Philadelphia, 2017, Elsevier.)

TABLE 54 Distinguishing Features of Nocturnal Events

Feature	Disorders of Arousal	Sleep-Related Eating Disorder	REM Behavior Disorder	Recurrent Isolated Sleep Paralysis	Exploding Head Syndrome	Psychogenic Events	Nocturnal Seizures
Behavior	Confused; semi-purposeful movement with eyes open	Eating typically high-calorie foods; eyes open	Sometimes combative with eyes closed	Episodes of inability to move	Painless sensation of explosion inside the head	Variable	Dependent on the portion of brain involved
Age of onset	Childhood and adolescence	Variable	Older adult	Variable	Adult	Adolescence to adulthood	Variable
Time of occurrence	First third of night	First half of night	During REM	Typically on awakening	Usually near sleep onset but can be variable	Anytime	Anytime
Frequency of events	Less than one per night	Variable	Multiple per night	Variable less than weekly	Rare	Variable	Frontal seizures—multiple per night
Duration	Minutes	Minutes	Seconds to minute	Seconds to minutes	Seconds	Variable minutes or longer	Usually under 3 minutes
Memory of event	Usually none	Usually none or limited	Dream recall	Yes	Yes	None	Usually none
Stereotypical movements	No	No	No	No	Similar sensation	No	Yes
Polysomnogram findings	Arousals from slow wave sleep	Arousal from NREM sleep	Excessive electromyogram tone during REM sleep	Arousal from REM sleep	Usually occurs in light sleep	Occur from awake state	Potentially epileptiform activity

REM, Rapid eye movement; *NREM*, non-rapid eye movement.
From Kryger M, Roth T, Dement WC: *Principles and practice of sleep medicine,* ed 6, Philadelphia, 2017, Elsevier.

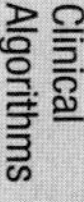

ICD-10CM # J02.9 Acute pharyngitis, unspecified
J31.2 Chronic pharyngitis
J02.0 Streptococcal pharyngitis

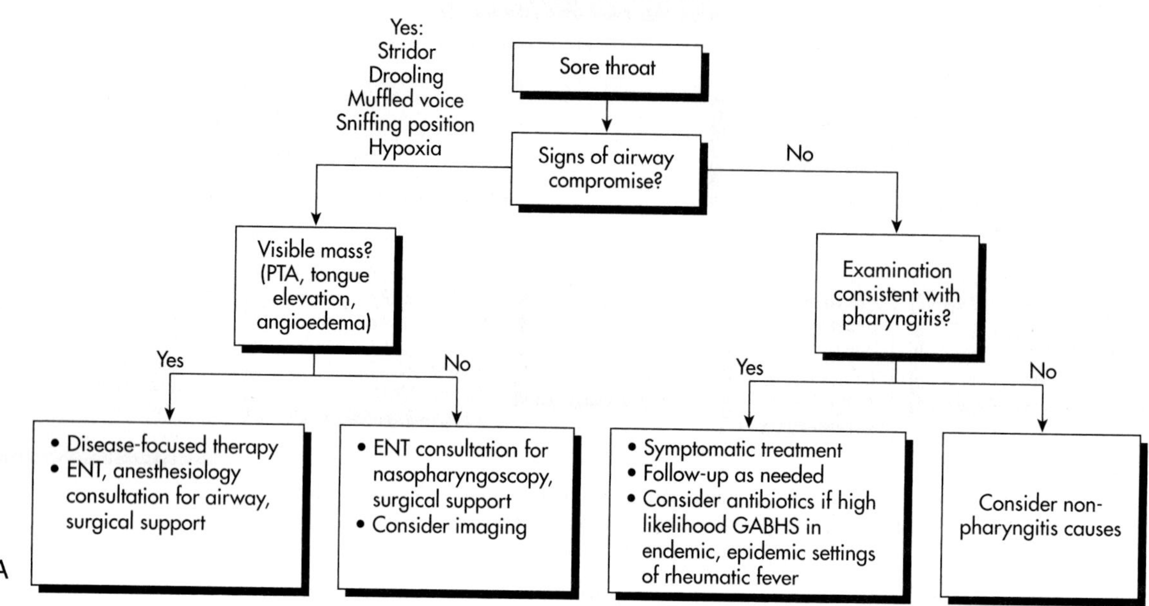

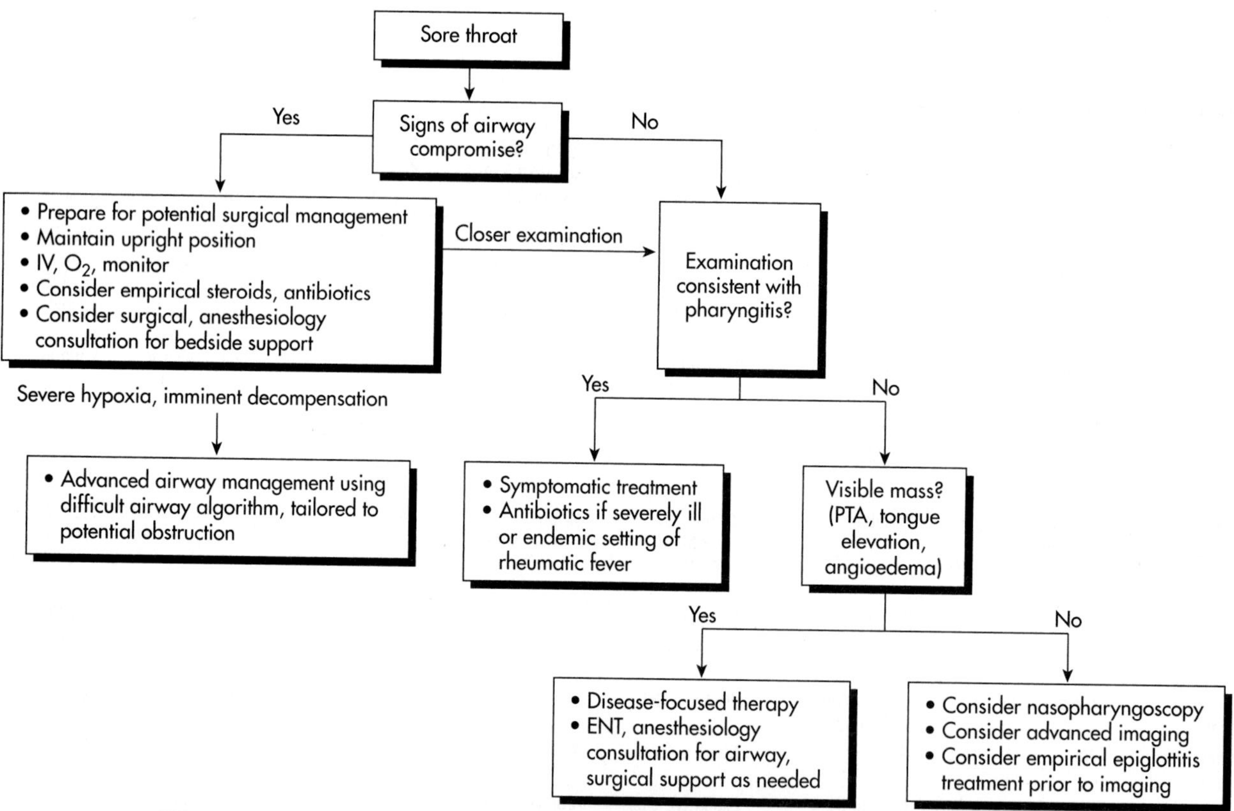

FIG. 148 Clinical approach to the patient with sore throat—diagnosis (A) and management (B). Refer to Section I, "Pharyngitis/Tonsillitis and Epiglottitis," for additional information on this matter. *ENT,* Ear-nose-throat; *GABHS,* group A beta-hemolytic streptococcus; *IV,* intravenous; *PTA,* peritonsillar abscess. (From Marx JA et al: *Rosen's emergency medicine,* ed 8, Philadelphia, 2014, Saunders.)

TABLE 55 Differential Diagnosis of Sore Throat

Type of Pharyngitis	Nature of Patient	Nature of Symptoms	Predisposing Factors	Physical Findings	Diagnostic Studies
Without Pharyngeal Ulcers					
Viral	All ages	Pain in throat Rapid onset Systemic symptoms	—	Exudate less likely than with streptococcal infections	—
Infectious mononucleosis	Adolescents and young adults Uncommon in elderly	Gradual onset	—	Low-grade temperature Occasional exudate Posterior cervical adenopathy Hepatosplenomegaly	Monospot test
Streptococcal pharyngitis	Patients younger than 25 yrs, especially age 6–12 yrs	Pain in throat Rapid onset Few systemic symptoms	Fall and winter Streptococcal infection in family Diabetes	Marked erythema and throat swelling Temperature >101°F Tender anterior cervical nodes Scarlatiniform rash Tonsillar exudate more likely than with viral infection	Culture Rapid streptococcal antigen screening Increased antistreptolysin O titer
Gonococcal pharyngitis	Most common in male homosexuals and people with anogenital gonorrhea	Often no symptoms	Orogenital sex	—	Culture
Sinusitis with postnasal drip	Adults	Mild throat soreness Symptoms often worse with recumbency	—	Evidence of sinusitis Postnasal drip	CT/flexible rhinoscopy (in recalcitrant cases)
Allergic pharyngitis	—	—	Seasonal allergies	No fever Intermittent postnasal drip Swollen pharynx with minimal injection	Allergy testing
With Pharyngeal Ulcers					
Herpangina	More common in children	Painful ulcers on tonsils, pillars, or uvula	Immunosuppression Summer and autumn	Vesicles 1-2-mm ulcers	Serologic tests
Fusospirochetal infection (Vincent's angina)	Children and people with poor oral hygiene	Painful ulcers Bleeding gums Foul breath	—	No vesicles Ulcerative gingivitis Gray, necrotic ulcers 2–30-mm ulcers Pseudomembrane	Gram stain: spirochetes
Candidiasis	Children Immunosuppressed patients Those taking antibiotics	—	Immunosuppression Antibiotics Inhaled steroids	3–11-mm ulcers No vesicles	KOH smear: *Candida* culture
Herpes simplex	Most common in children	Not usually a cause of sore throat	Immunosuppression	1–2-mm painful ulcers Vesicles present on lips, gingivae, buccal mucosa, or tongue	Tzanck smear (not very sensitive) viral culture, PCR, herpes simplex virus antibody assay

CT, Computed tomography; *PCR,* polymerase chain reaction.
Modified from Seller RH, Symons AB: *Differential diagnosis of common complaints,* ed 7, Philadelphia, 2018, Elsevier.

ICD-10CM # S36.00XA Unspecified injury of spleen, initial encounter
S35.32 Injury of splenic vein
S35.3 Injury of portal or splenic vein and branches

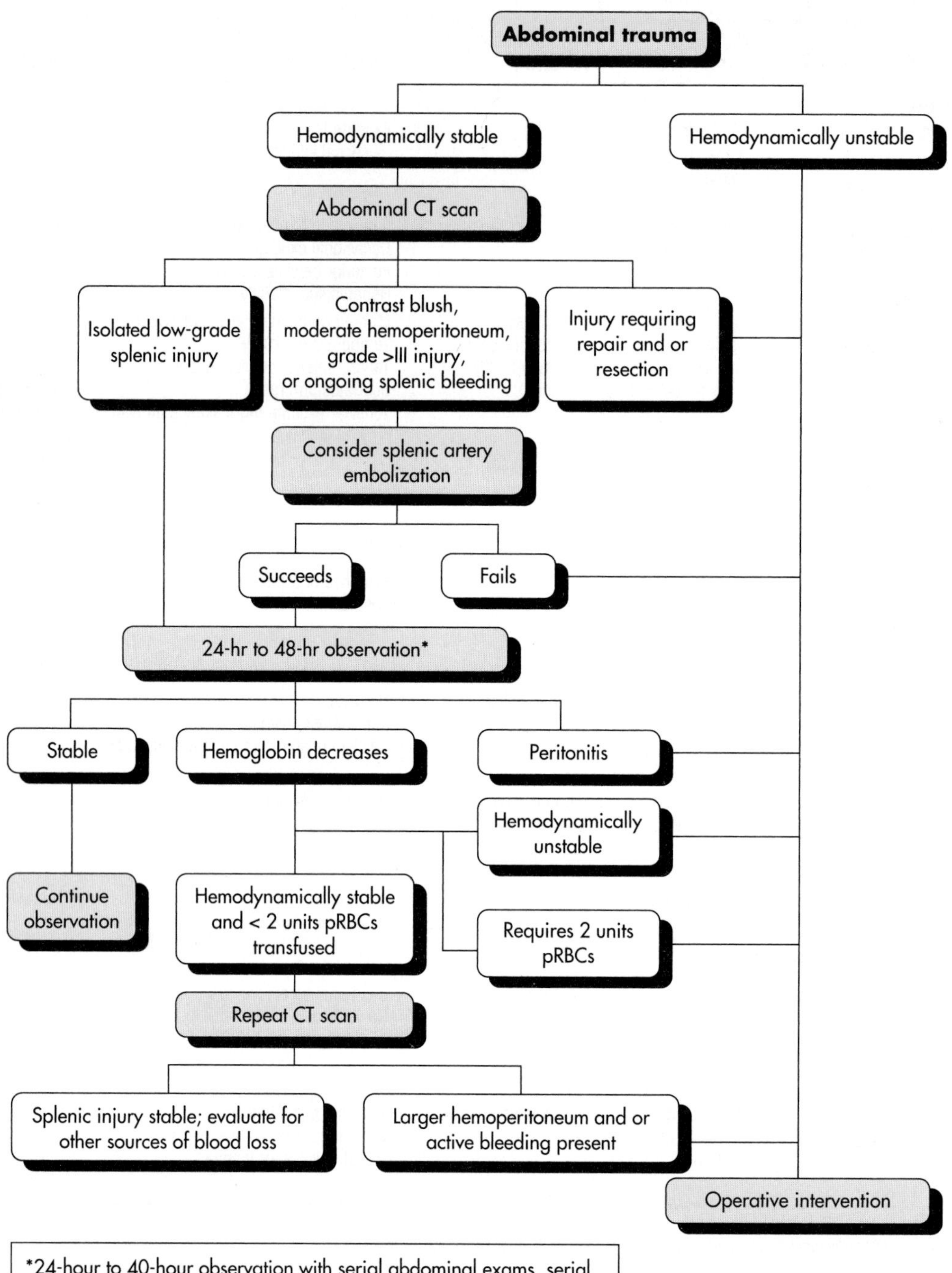

FIG. 149 Algorithmic approach to the management of traumatic splenic injury. *CT*, Computed tomography; *pRBC*, packed red blood cell. (From Cameron JL, Cameron AM: *Current surgical therapy,* ed 12, Philadelphia, 2017, Elsevier.)

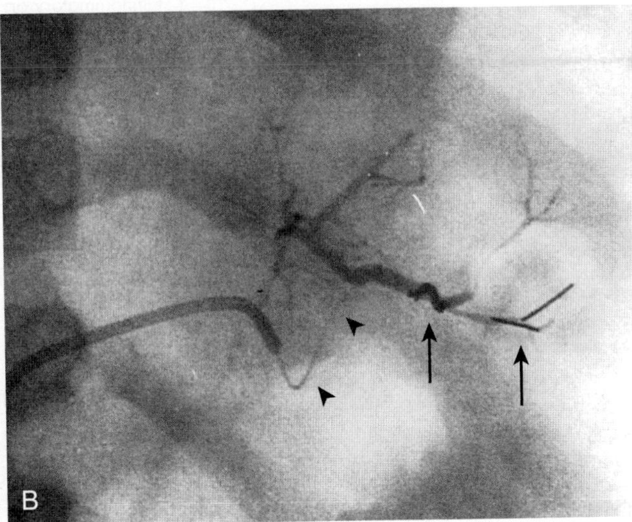

FIG. 150 A, Splenic pseudoaneurysm (*arrowheads*) indicate contrast with the pseudoaneurysm) after non-operative treatment of blunt splenic injury. **B,** Successful angiographic embolization (*arrows* show occlusion of ruptured vessels). (From Cameron JL, Cameron AM: *Current surgical therapy,* ed 12, Philadelphia, 2017, Elsevier.)

TABLE 56 Organ Injury Scale for the Spleen by the American Association for the Surgery of Trauma

Grade	Injury Type	Description of Injury
I	Hematoma	Subcapsular, nonexpanding, <10% surface area
	Laceration	Capsular tear, nonbleeding, <1 cm parenchymal depth
II	Hematoma	Subcapsular, nonexpanding, 10%–50% surface area; intraparenchymal, <5 cm in depth
	Laceration	Capsular tear, active bleeding, 1–3 cm parenchymal depth that does not involve a trabecular vessel
III	Hematoma	Subcapsular, >50% surface area or expanding; ruptured subcapsular or parenchymal hematoma with active bleeding; intraparenchymal hematoma ≥5 cm or expanding
	Laceration	>3 cm parenchymal depth or involving trabecular vessels
IV	Laceration	Laceration involving segmental or hilar vessels producing major devascularization (>25% of spleen)
V	Laceration	Completely shattered spleen
	Vascular	Hilar vascular injury with devascularized spleen

From Cameron JL, Cameron AM: *Current surgical therapy,* ed 12, Philadelphia, 2017, Elsevier.

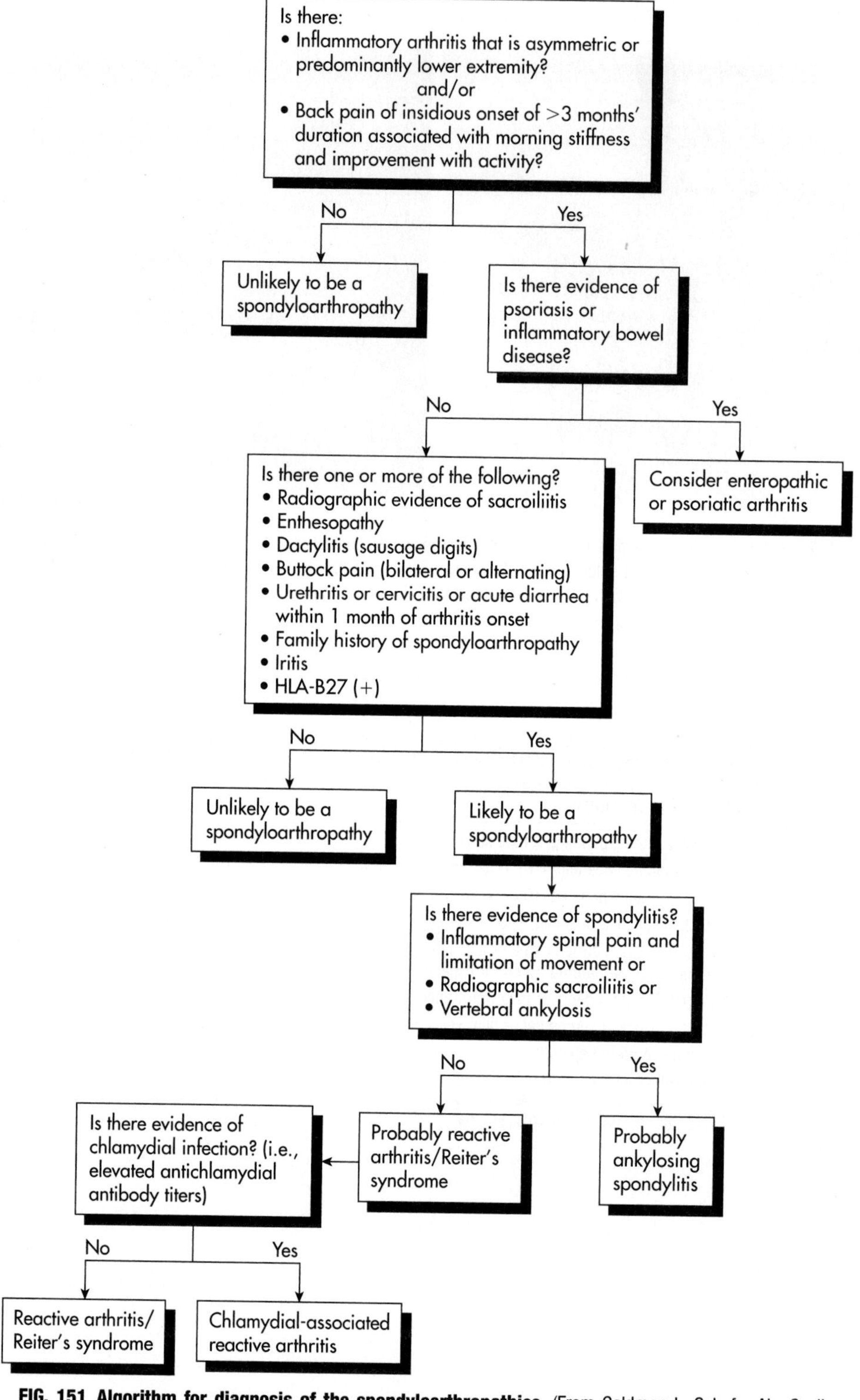

FIG. 151 Algorithm for diagnosis of the spondyloarthropathies. (From Goldman L, Schafer AL: *Cecil textbook of medicine,* ed 24, Philadelphia, 2012, Saunders.)

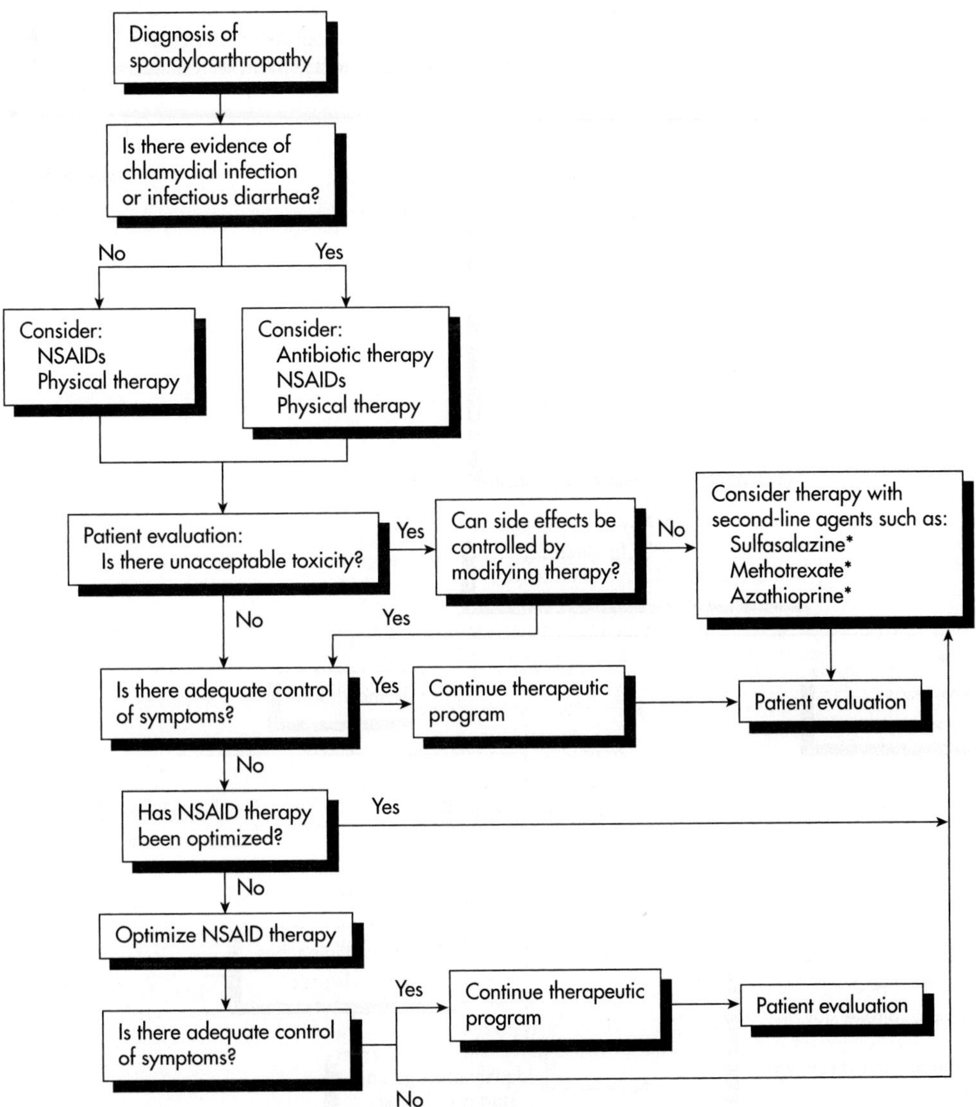

*Not approved by the FDA for treatment of spondyloarthropathies.

FIG. 152 Treatment algorithm for patients with a spondyloarthropathy. *FDA,* Food and Drug Administration; *NSAID,* nonsteroidal antiinflammatory drug. (From Goldman L, Schafer AL: *Cecil textbook of medicine,* ed 24, Philadelphia, 2012, Saunders.)

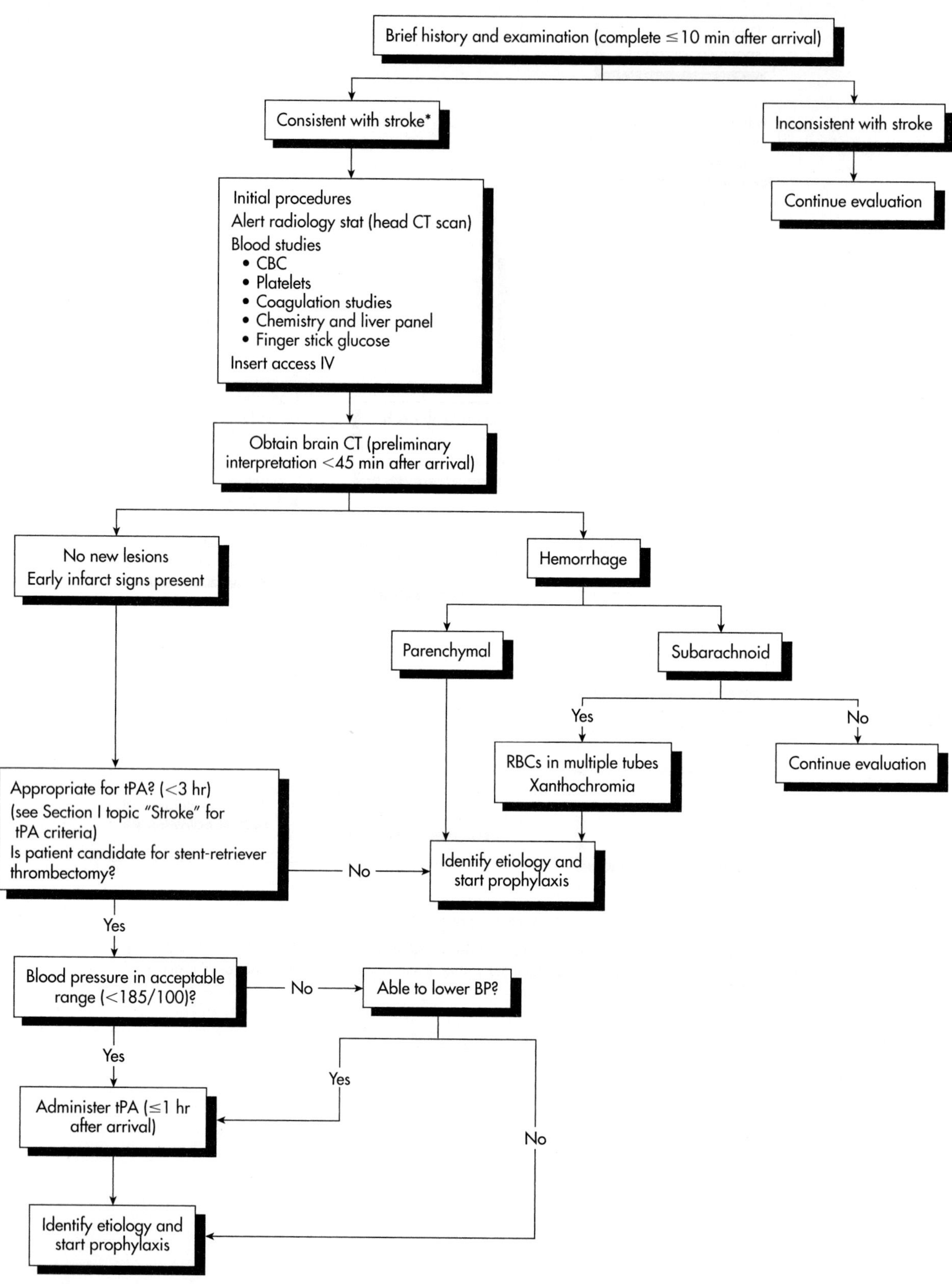

*Note: Refer to Section I for additional information on this topic.

FIG. 153 Algorithm for the emergency evaluation of a patient with suspected stroke. *BP,* Blood pressure; *CBC,* complete blood count; *CT,* computed tomography; *RBCs,* red blood cells; *tPA,* tissue plasminogen activator. (From Goldman L, Schafer AL [eds]: *Cecil textbook of medicine,* ed 24, Philadelphia, 2012, Saunders.)

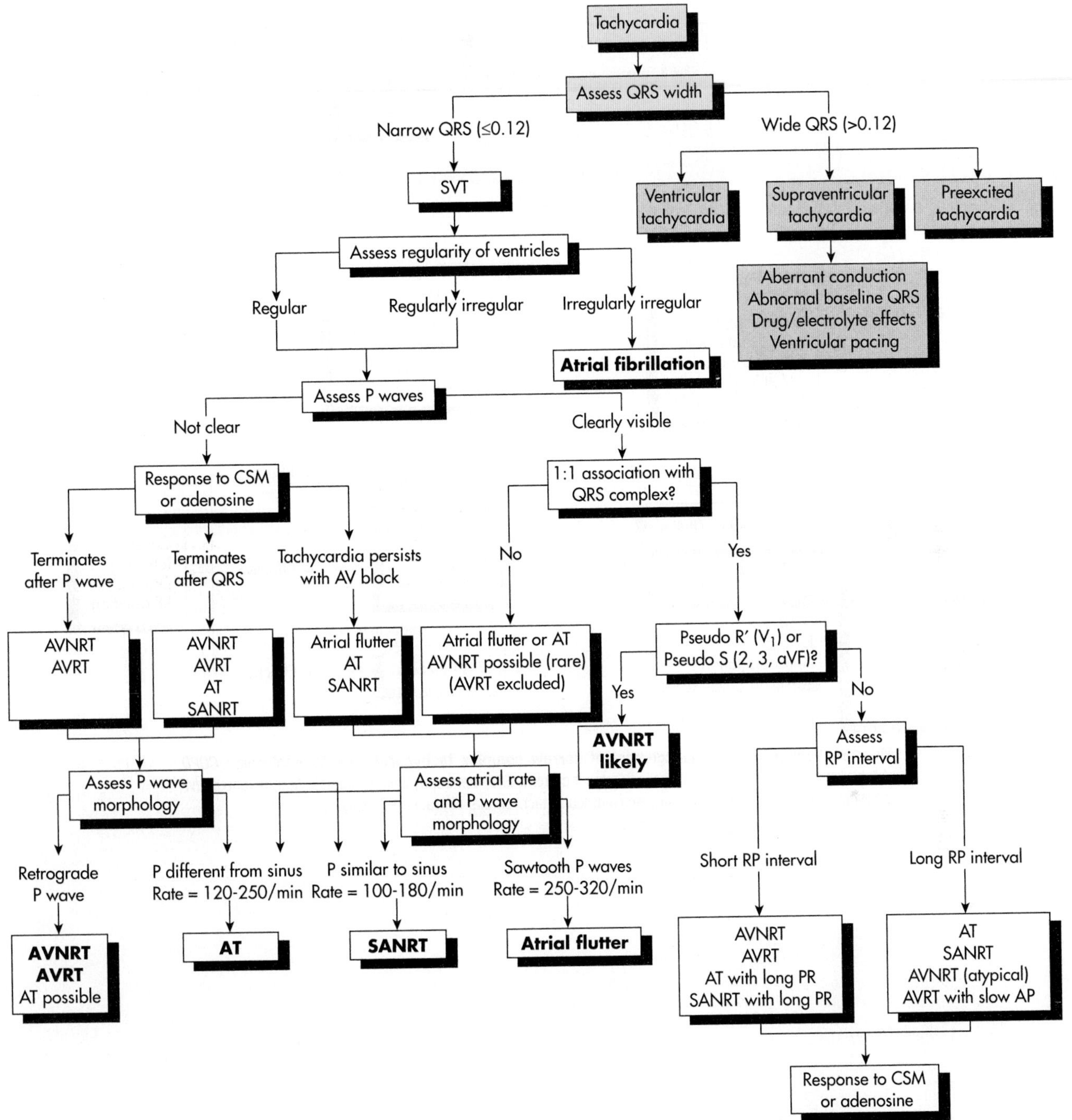

FIG. 154 Stepwise approach to diagnosis of the type of tachycardia based on a 12-lead echocardiogram during the episode. The initial step is to determine whether the tachycardia has a wide or narrow QRS complex (see Fig. 155). *AP*, accessory pathway; *AT*, atrial tachycardia; *AV*, atrioventricular; *AVNRT*, atrioventricular nodal reentrant tachycardia; *AVRT*, atrioventricular reciprocating tachycardia; *CSM*, carotid sinus massage; *SANRT*, sinoatrial nodal reentry tachycardia; *SVT*, supraventricular tachycardia. (From Mann DL, Zipes DP, Libby P et al: *Braunwald's heart disease*, ed 10, Philadelphia, 2015, Saunders.)

ICD-10CM # I49.02 Ventricular flutter
I49.8 Other specified cardiac arrhythmias
R00.1 Bradycardia, unspecified

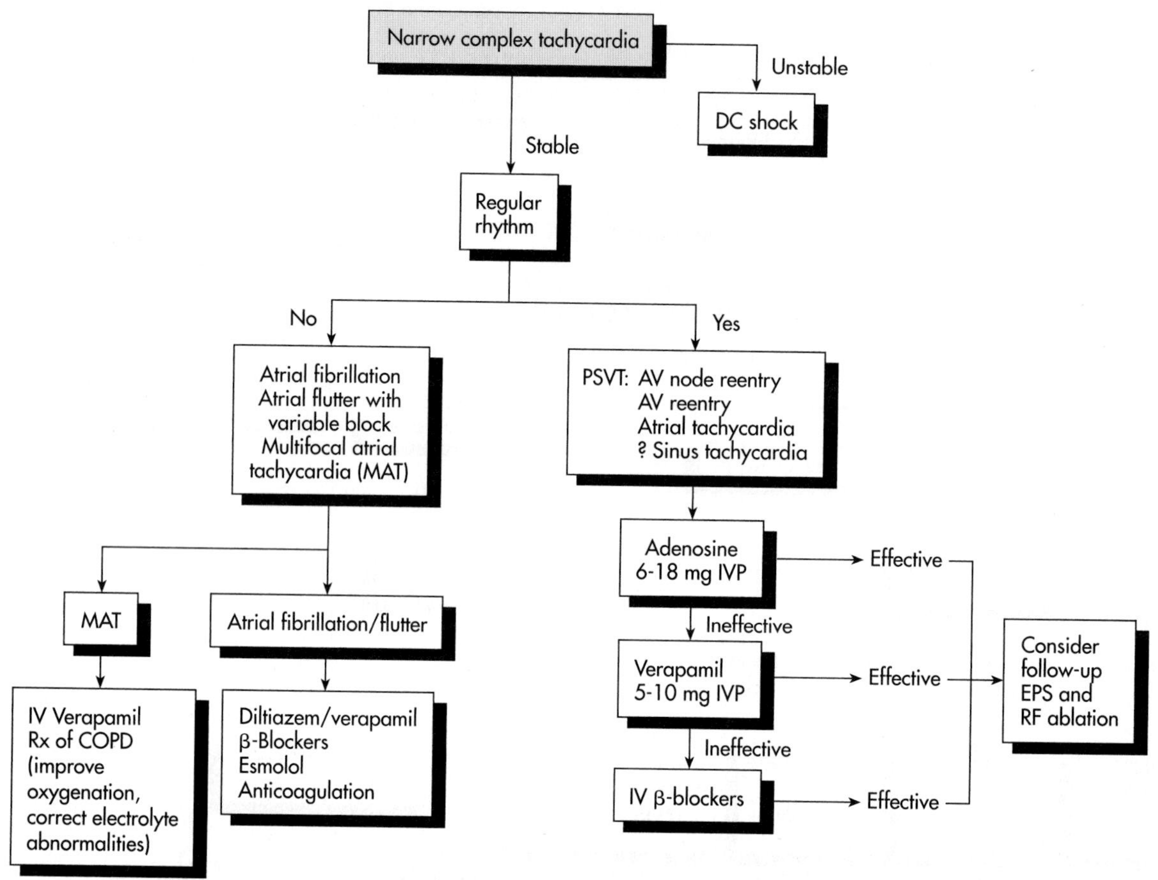

FIG. 155 Evaluation and management of narrow complex tachycardia. *AV,* Atrioventricular; *COPD,* chronic obstructive pulmonary disease; *DC,* direct current; *EPS,* electrophysiologic studies; *IV,* intravenous; *IVP,* intravenous push; *PSVT,* paroxysmal supraventricular tachycardia; *RF,* radiofrequency.

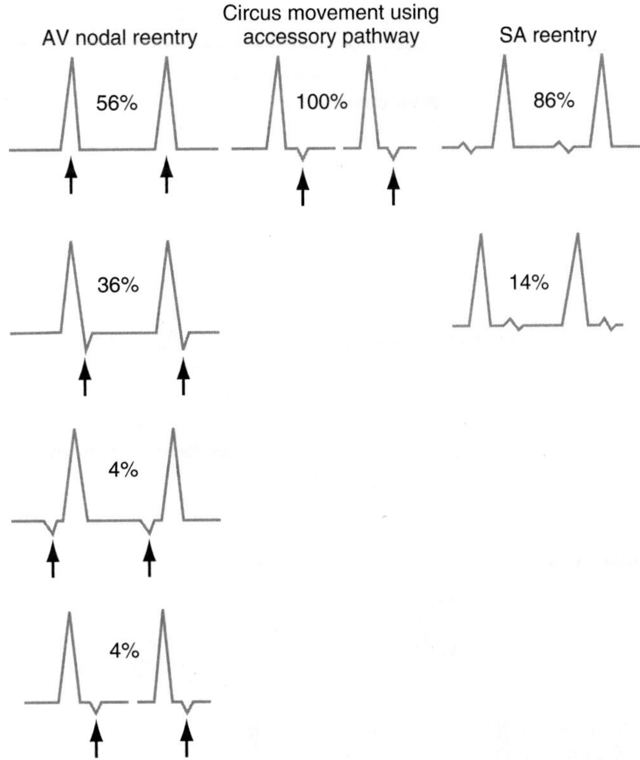

FIG. 156 Location of P waves in common causes of regular narrow-complex tachycardia. *AV,* atrioventricular; *SA,* sinoatrial. (From Marriott HJL, Conover MB: *Advanced concepts in dysrhythmias,* 2nd ed. St Louis, Mosby, 1989.) (Marx JA et al: *Rosen's emergency medicine,* ed 8, Philadelphia, 2014, Saunders.)

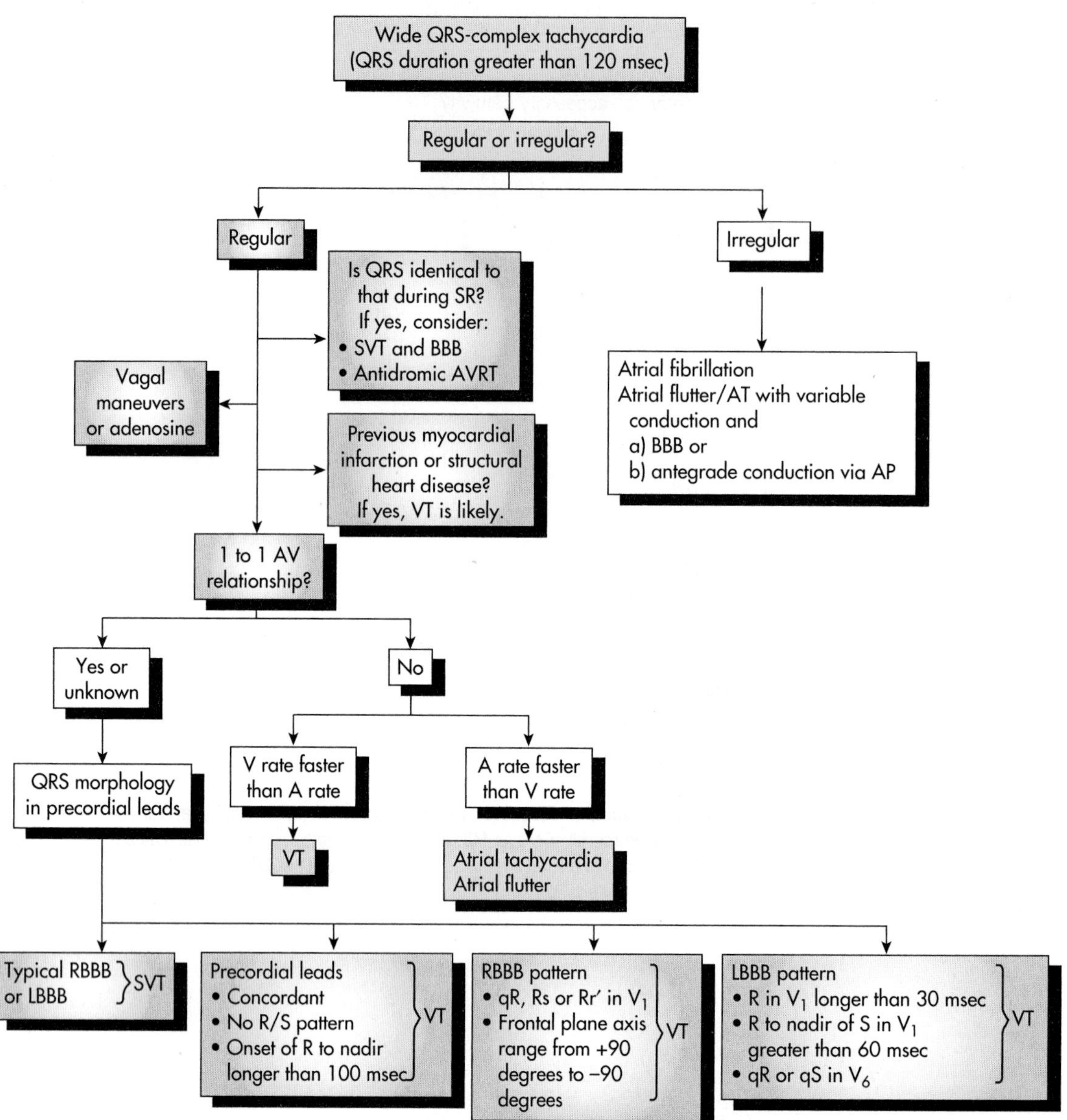

FIG. 158 Algorithm for diagnosis of wide-QRS tachycardia. *AP,* Accessory pathway; *AT,* atrial tachycardia; *AV,* atrioventricular; *AVRT,* AV reentrant tachycardia; *LBBB,* left bundle branch block; *RBBB,* right bundle branch block; *SVT,* supraventricular tachycardia; *VT,* ventricular tachycardia. (From Bloomstrom-Lundqvist C, Scheinman MM, Aliot EM, el al: ACC/AHA/ESC guidelines for the management of patients with supraventricular arrhythmias—executive summary: a report of the American College of Cardiology/American Heart Association Task Force on Practice Guidelines and the European Society of Cardiology Committee for Practice Guidelines [Writing Committee to Develop Guidelines for the Management of Patients with Supraventricular Arrhythmias]. *Circulation* 108:1871, 2003; Mann DL, Zipes DP, Libby P, Bonow RO: *Braunwald's heart disease*, ed 10, Philadelphia, 2015, Elsevier.)

TABLE 58 Stepwise Criteria Favoring Ventricular Tachycardia Patients with Wide-Complex Tachycardias Using Different Algorithms

ACC/AHA/ESC Algorithm*	Kindwall Criteria†	Wellens Criteria‡	Brugada Criteria§	Miller criteria§
See Figure 158	R >30 ms in V_1 or V_2 → VT	AV dissociation → VT	Absence of RS complex in all precordial leads → VT	Initial R wave in aVR → VT
	Any Q in V_6 → VT	QRS width >140 ms → VT	Longest R/S interval >100 ms in any precordial lead → VT	aVR with initial r or q >40 sec in duration → VT
	>60 ms to S wave nadir in V_1 or V_2 → VT	Left axis deviation > −30° → VT	AV dissociation → VT	aVR with a notch on the descending limb of a negative-onset and predominantly negative QRS in aVR → VT
	Notched downstroke S wave in V_1 or V_2 → VT	If RBBB morphology, monophasic or biphasic QRS in V_1 → SVT or R-to-S ratio of <1 in V_6 → VT If LBBB morphology, S in V_1-V_2 → VT	If RBBB morphology, monophasic R or qR in V_1 → VT R taller than R′ → VT rS in V_6 → VT If LBBB morphology, initial R >40 ms in duration → VT Slurred or notched S in V_1 or V_2 → VT Beginning Q or QS in V_6 → VT	In aVR, mV of initial 40 msec divided by terminal 40 msec ($v/v_t \le 1$) → VT

ACC, American College of Cardiology; *AHA,* American Heart Association; *ESC,* European Society of Cardiology; *LBBB,* Left bundle branch block; *RBBB,* right bundle branch block.

*Blomström-Lundqvist C, Scheinman MM, Aliot EM et al: ACC/AHA/ESC guidelines for the management of patients with supraventricular arrhythmias—executive summary: a report of the American College of Cardiology/American Heart Association Task Force on Practice Guidelines and the European Society of Cardiology Committee for Practice Guidelines (Writing Committee to Develop Guidelines for the Management of Patients With Supraventricular Arrhythmias). *Circulation* 108:1871, 2003.

†Kindwall KE, Brown J, Josephson ME: Electrocardiographic criteria for ventricular tachycardia in wide complex left bundle branch block morphology tachycardias. *Am J Cardiol* 61:1279, 1988.

‡Wellens HJ, Bär FW, Lie KI: The value of the electrocardiogram in the differential diagnosis of a tachycardia with a widened QRS complex. *Am J Med* 64:27, 1978.

§Brugada P, Brugada J, Mont L et al: A new approach to the differential diagnosis of a regular tachycardia with a wide QRS complex. *Circulation* 83:1649, 1991.

‖Vereckei A, Duray G, Szénási G et al: New algorithm using only lead aVR for differential diagnosis of wide QRS complex tachycardia. *Heart Rhythm* 5:89, 2008.

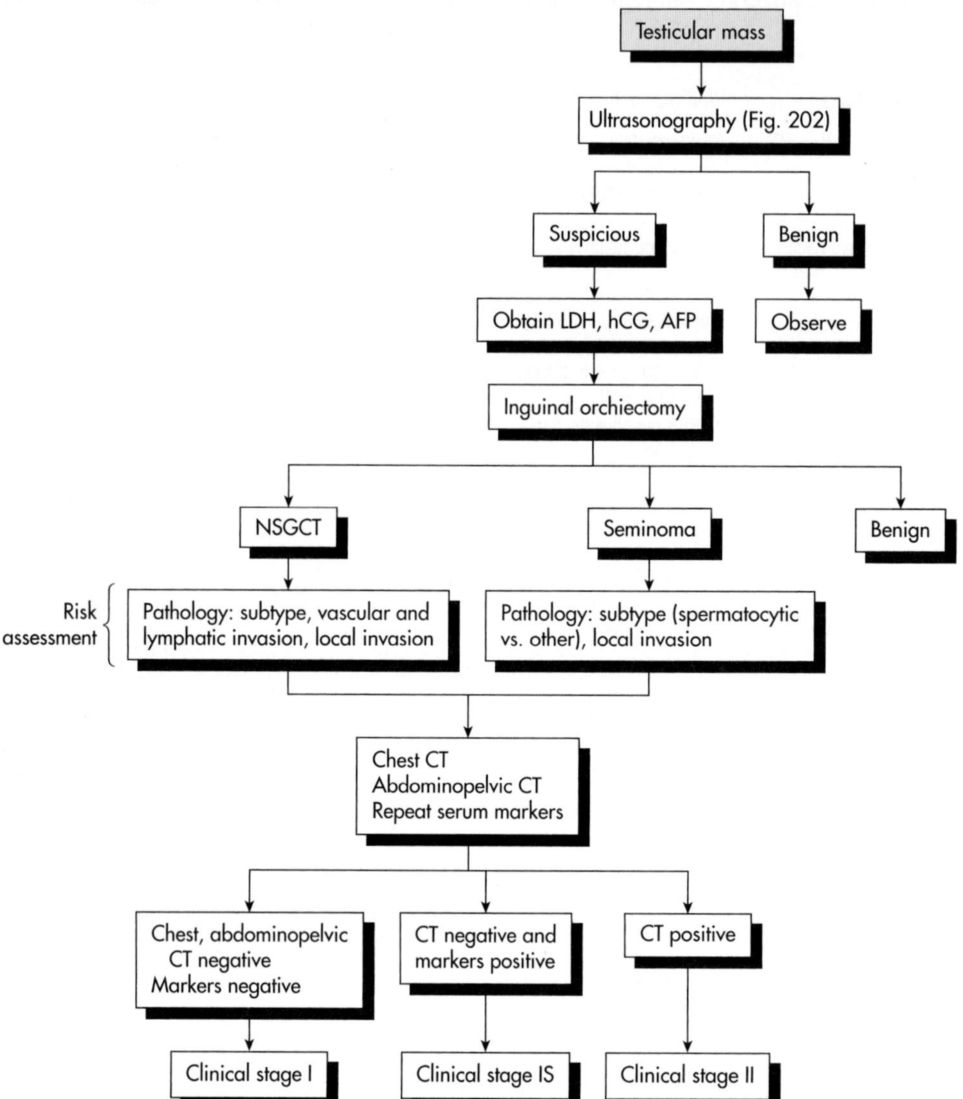

FIG. 159 Diagnosis, staging, and risk assessment of patients with testicular germ cell tumor. See Section I, "Testicular Cancer," for additional information. *AFP,* α-Fetoprotein; *CT,* computed tomography; *hCG,* human chorionic gonadotropin; *LDH,* lactic dehydrogenase; *NSGCT,* nonseminoma germ cell tumor. (From Abeloff MD: *Clinical oncology,* ed 4, New York, 2007, Churchill Livingstone.)

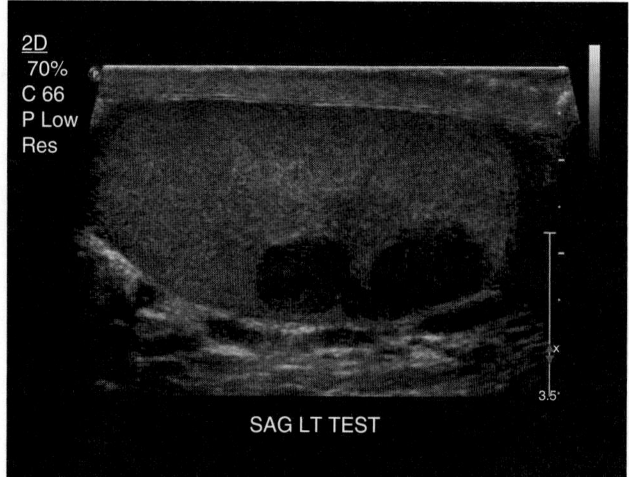

FIG. 160 Sagittal view of ultrasound of left testis showing multinodular hypoechoic intratesticular lesion confirmed to be pure seminoma at orchiectomy. (From Wein AJ, Kavoussi LR, Partin AW, Peters CA: *Campbell-Walsh urology,* ed 11, Philadelphia, 2016, Elsevier.)

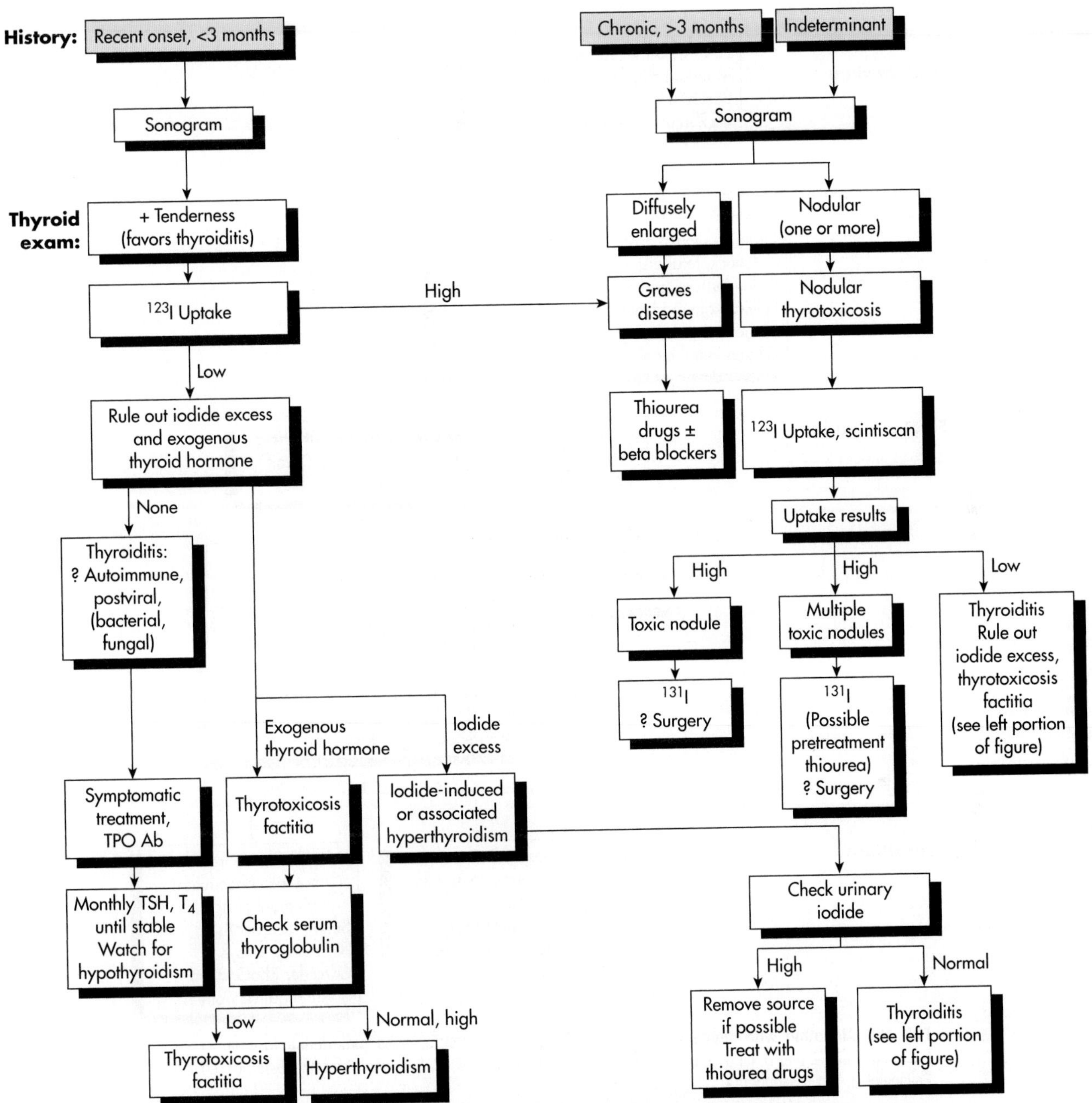

FIG. 162 Algorithm for determining the cause of thyrotropin-independent thyrotoxicosis. Additional information on thyrotoxicosis is available in Section I topics "Hyperthyroidism," "Thyroid Nodule", "Thyroiditis", "Thyroid Storm", and "Graves Disease". T_3, triiodothyronine; T_4, thyroxine; *TPO Ab*, thyroid peroxidase antibody; *TSH*, thyroid-stimulating hormone (thyrotropin). (From Melmed S, Polonsky KS, Larsen P et al: *Williams textbook of endocrinology*, ed 13, Philadelphia, 2016, Elsevier.)

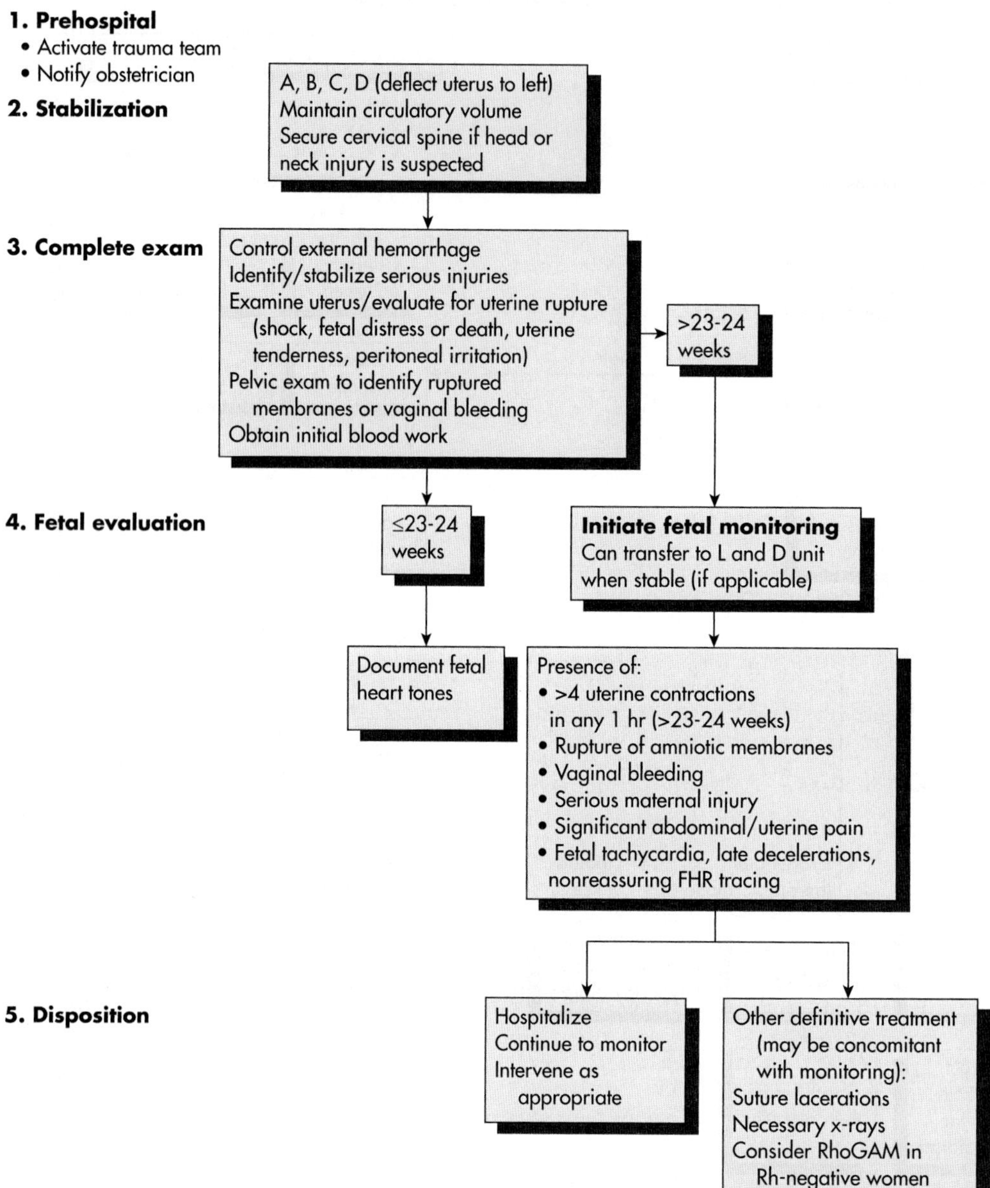
EMERGENCY DEPARTMENT MANAGEMENT: TRAUMA IN PREGNANCY
1. Prehospital
• Activate trauma team
• Notify obstetrician
2. Stabilization
A, B, C, D (deflect uterus to left)
Maintain circulatory volume
Secure cervical spine if head or neck injury is suspected
3. Complete exam
Control external hemorrhage
Identify/stabilize serious injuries
Examine uterus/evaluate for uterine rupture (shock, fetal distress or death, uterine tenderness, peritoneal irritation)
Pelvic exam to identify ruptured membranes or vaginal bleeding
Obtain initial blood work
>23-24 weeks
4. Fetal evaluation
≤23-24 weeks
Initiate fetal monitoring
Can transfer to L and D unit when stable (if applicable)
Document fetal heart tones
Presence of:
• >4 uterine contractions in any 1 hr (>23-24 weeks)
• Rupture of amniotic membranes
• Vaginal bleeding
• Serious maternal injury
• Significant abdominal/uterine pain
• Fetal tachycardia, late decelerations, nonreassuring FHR tracing
5. Disposition
Hospitalize
Continue to monitor
Intervene as appropriate
Other definitive treatment (may be concomitant with monitoring):
Suture lacerations
Necessary x-rays
Consider RhoGAM in Rh-negative women

FIG. 163 Algorithm with suggested care plan for pregnant women who experience trauma. *FHR*, fetal heart rate; *L and D*, labor and delivery. (From Gabbe SG, Niebyl JR, Simpson JL et al: *Obstetrics*, ed 7, Philadelphia, 2017, Saunders.)

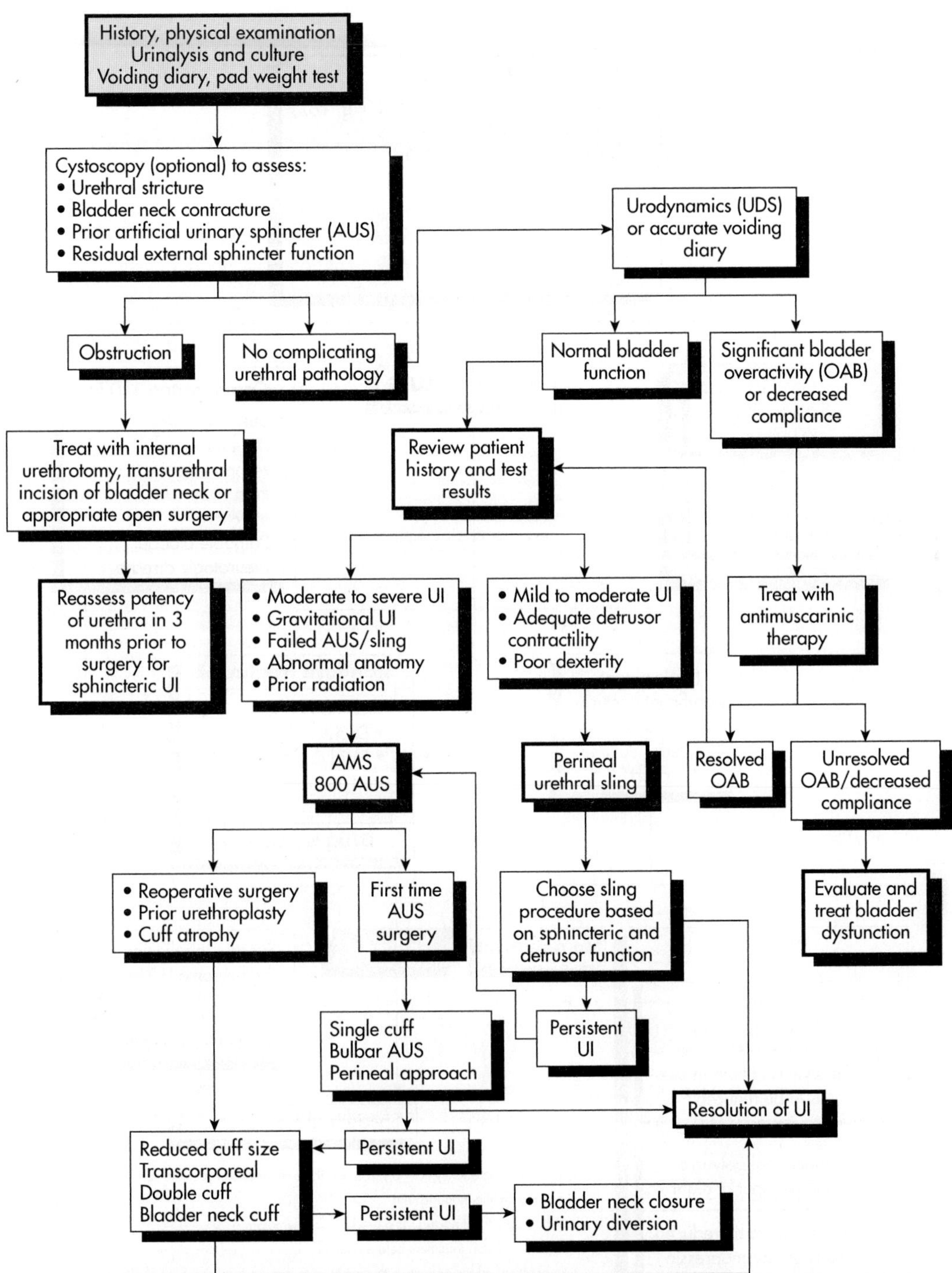

FIG. 165 Algorithm for the evaluation and management of sphincteric urinary incontinence. (From Wein AJ, Kavoussi LR, Partin AW, Peters CA: *Campbell-Walsh urology,* ed 11, Philadelphia, 2016, Elsevier.)

URINARY SYMPTOMS, LOWER URINARY TRACT

ICD-10CM # R33.9 Retention of urine, unspecified
N21.8 Other lower urinary tract calculus
R32 Unspecified urinary incontinence

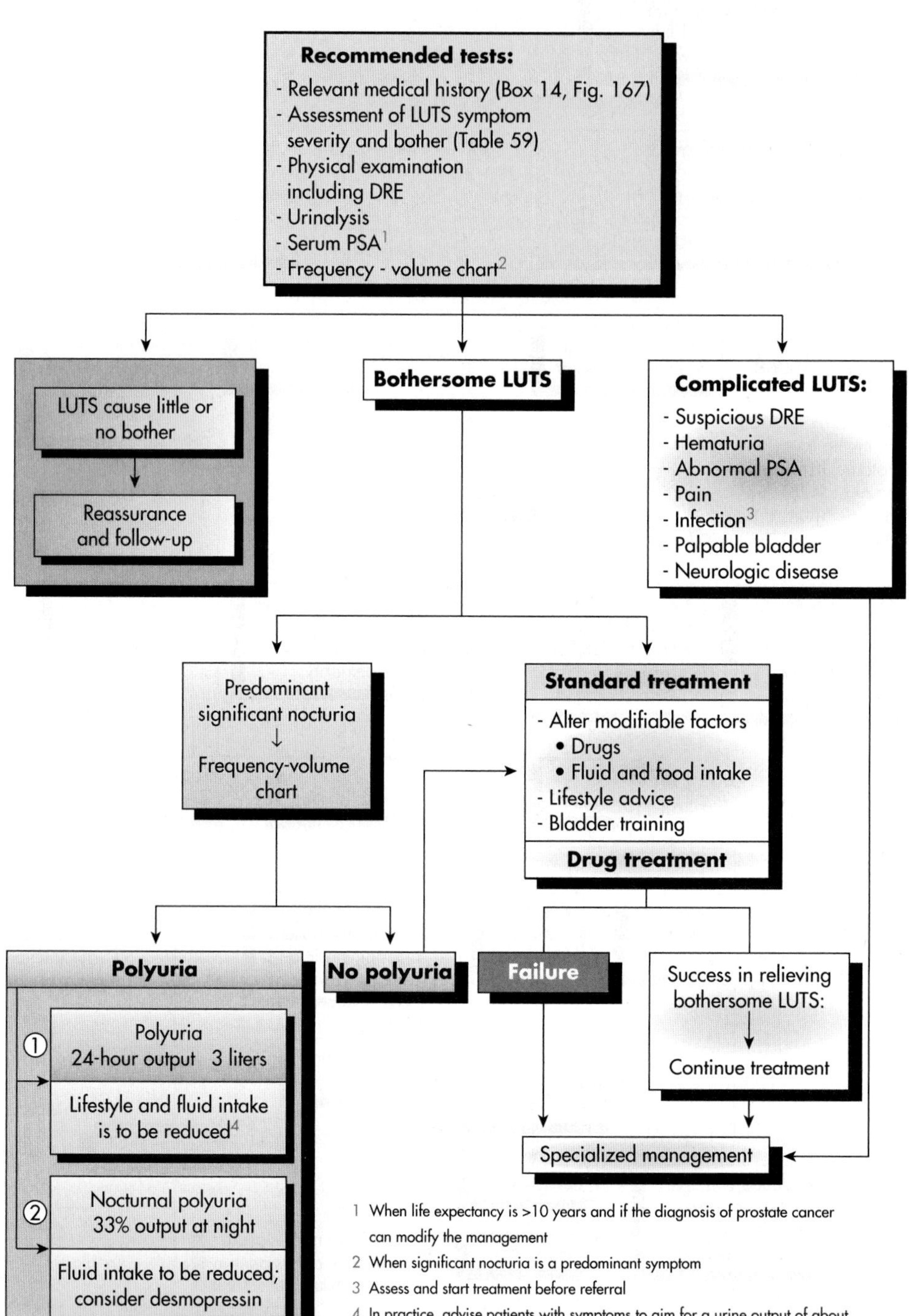

FIG. 166 Basic management of lower urinary tract symptoms (LUTS) in men. *DRE,* Digital rectal examination; *LUTS,* lower urinary tract symptoms; *PSA,* prostate-specific antigen. (From Fillit HM: *Brocklehurst's textbook of geriatric medicine and gerontology,* ed 8, Philadelphia, 2017, Elsevier.)

BOX 14 Causes of Male Lower Urinary Tract Symptoms

Benign prostatic enlargement (secondary to benign prostatic hyperplasia)
Urinary tract infection
Prostatitis
Overactive bladder
Neurogenic bladder dysfunction
Urethral stricture
Bladder neck contracture
Phimosis
Urinary tract stones
Bladder tumor
Advanced prostate cancer
Foreign body in the bladder
Medications, illicit drugs, and dietary factors (including caffeine, alcohol, ketamine, and decongestants)
Diabetes mellitus

From Fillit HM: *Brocklehurst's textbook of geriatric medicine and gerontology*, ed 8, Philadelphia, 2017, Elsevier.

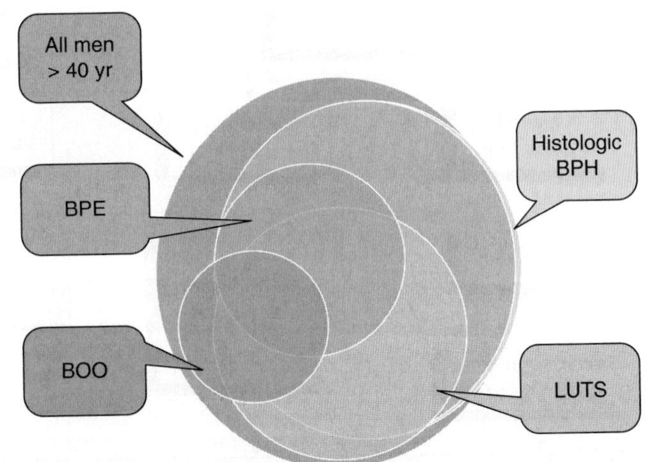

FIG. 167 Occurrence of LUTS with and without BOO, BPE, or BPH. *BOO*, Bladder outflow obstruction; *BPH*, benign prostate hyperplasia; *BPE*, benign prostate enlargement; *LUTS*, lower urinary tract symptoms. (From Fillit HM: Brocklehurst's textbook of geriatric medicine and gerontology, ed 8, Philadelphia, 2017, Elsevier.)

TABLE 59 International Continence Society Definitions of Lower Urinary Tract Symptoms

Voiding symptoms	• *Hesitancy* is difficulty in initiating micturition, resulting in a delay in the onset of voiding after being ready to pass urine. • *Slow stream* is the perception of reduced urine flow, usually compared to previous performance or in comparison to others. • *Splitting or spraying* of the urine stream. • *Intermittent stream* (intermittency) is the term used to describe urine flow that stops and starts, on one or more occasions, during micturition. • *Straining* to void describes the muscular effort used to initiate, maintain, or improve the urinary stream. • *Terminal dribble* is the term used to describe a prolonged final part of micturition, when the flow has slowed to a trickle or dribble.
Storage symptoms	• *Increased daytime frequency* is the complaint by the patient who considers that he voids too often during the day. • *Nocturia* is the complaint that the man has to wake at night one or more times to void. • *Urgency* is the complaint of a sudden compelling desire to pass urine that is difficult to defer. • *Urinary incontinence* is the complaint of any involuntary leakage of urine.
Postmicturition symptoms	• *Feeling of incomplete emptying* is a self-explanatory term for a feeling experienced by the individual after passing urine. • *Postmicturition dribble* is the term used to describe the involuntary loss of urine immediately after finishing passing urine, usually after leaving the toilet.

From Fillit HM: *Brocklehurst's textbook of geriatric medicine and gerontology*, ed 8, Philadelphia, 2017, Elsevier.

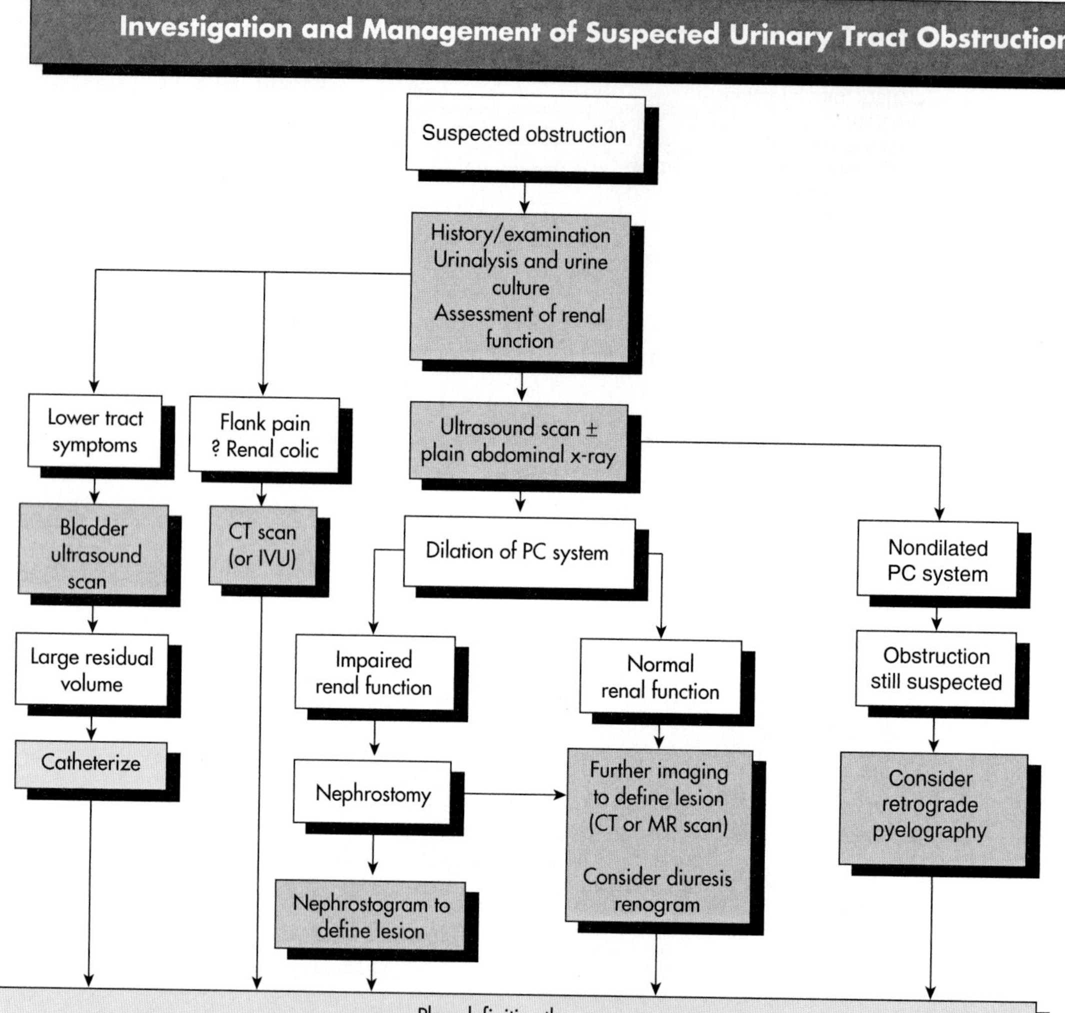

FIG. 168 Investigation and management of suspected urinary tract obstruction. A full history should be taken and a thorough examination performed, together with urinalysis, urine microscopy and culture, and measurement of renal function and serum electrolytes. Ultrasound is a useful first-line investigation for any patient with suspected urinary tract obstruction. Computed tomography *(CT)* is now the preferred imaging technique when renal calculi are suspected. Either CT or magnetic resonance *(MR)* urography can accurately diagnose both the site and cause of obstruction in most cases. If there is renal impairment, a nephrostomy allows the effective relief of the obstruction and time for renal function to recover while definitive therapy is planned. *IVU,* Intravenous urography; *PC,* pelvicalyceal. (From Johnson R, Feehally J, Floege J: *Comprehensive clinical nephrology*, ed 5, Philadelphia, 2015, Saunders.)

BOX 15 Diagnostic Tests Used in Obstructive Uropathy

Upper Urinary Tract Obstruction
- Sonography (ultrasound)
- Plain films of the abdomen (KUB)
- Excretory or intravenous pyelography (very rarely needed)
- Retrograde pyelography
- Isotopic renography
- Computed tomography (helical CT)
- Magnetic resonance imaging
- Pressure flow studies (the Whitaker test)

Lower Urinary Tract Obstruction
- Some of the tests listed at left
- Cystoscopy
- Voiding cystourethrogram
- Retrograde urethrography
- Urodynamic tests
- Debimetry
- Cystometrography
- Electromyography
- Urethral pressure profile

KUB, Kidneys, ureter, bladder.

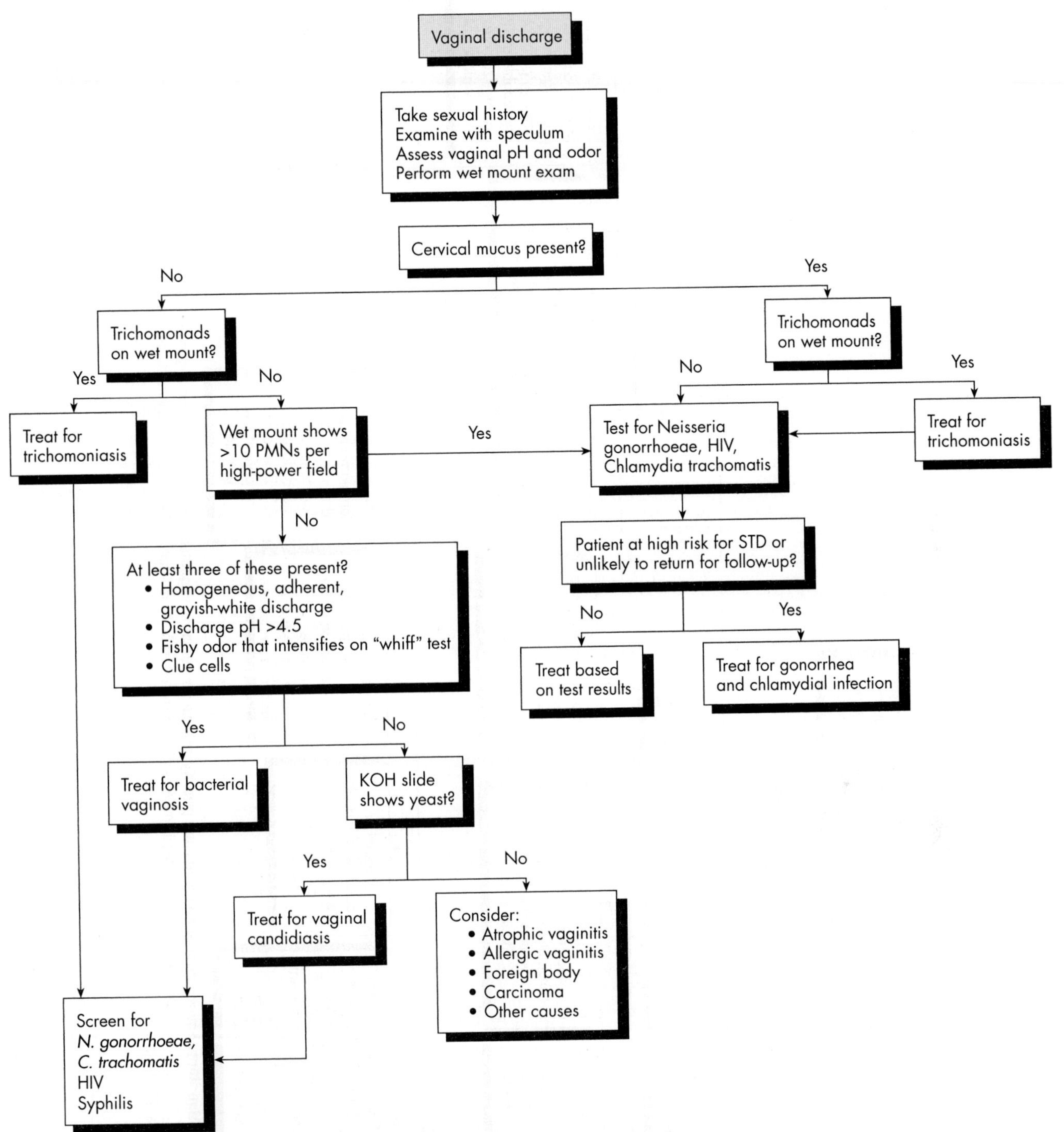
Vaginal discharge
Take sexual history
Examine with speculum
Assess vaginal pH and odor
Perform wet mount exam
Cervical mucus present?
No
Yes
Trichomonads on wet mount?
Yes
No
Treat for trichomoniasis
Wet mount shows >10 PMNs per high-power field
Yes
No
At least three of these present?
• Homogeneous, adherent, grayish-white discharge
• Discharge pH >4.5
• Fishy odor that intensifies on "whiff" test
• Clue cells
Yes
No
Treat for bacterial vaginosis
KOH slide shows yeast?
Yes
No
Treat for vaginal candidiasis
Consider:
• Atrophic vaginitis
• Allergic vaginitis
• Foreign body
• Carcinoma
• Other causes
Screen for
N. gonorrhoeae,
C. trachomatis
HIV
Syphilis
Trichomonads on wet mount?
No
Yes
Test for Neisseria gonorrhoeae, HIV, Chlamydia trachomatis
Treat for trichomoniasis
Patient at high risk for STD or unlikely to return for follow-up?
No
Yes
Treat based on test results
Treat for gonorrhea and chlamydial infection

FIG. 169 Evaluation of vaginal discharge. See Section I, "Vaginitis, Fungal, and Vaginitis Trichomonas" for additional information on vaginal discharge evaluation. *HIV,* Human immunodeficiency virus; *KOH,* potassium hydroxide; *PMN,* polymorphonuclear leukocyte; *STD,* sexually transmitted disease.

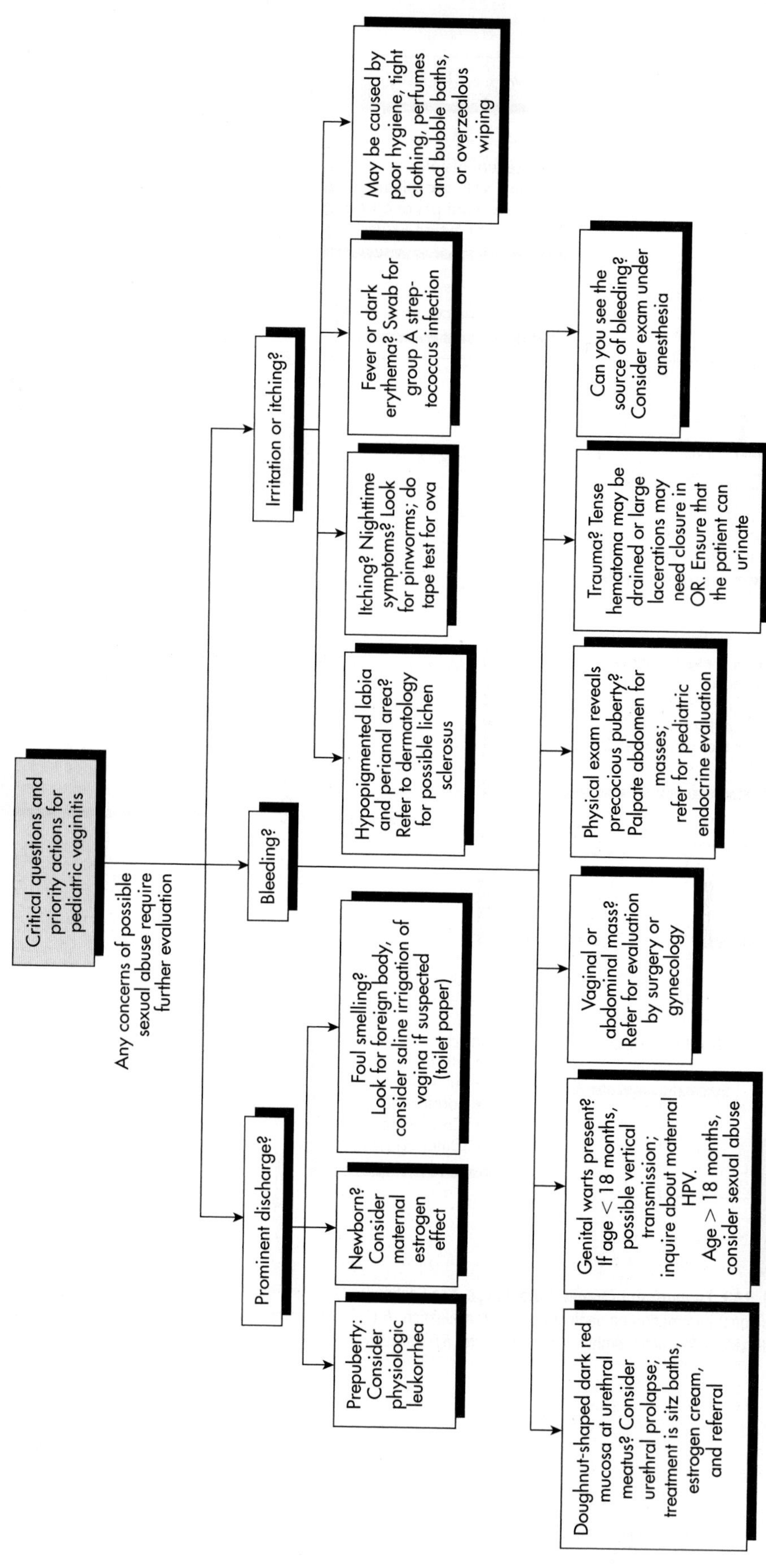
Critical questions and priority actions for pediatric vaginitis
Any concerns of possible sexual abuse require further evaluation
Prominent discharge?
Bleeding?
Irritation or itching?
Prepuberty: Consider physiologic leukorrhea
Newborn? Consider maternal estrogen effect
Foul smelling? Look for foreign body, consider saline irrigation of vagina if suspected (toilet paper)
Hypopigmented labia and perianal area? Refer to dermatology for possible lichen sclerosus
Itching? Nighttime symptoms? Look for pinworms; do tape test for ova
Fever or dark erythema? Swab for group A streptococcus infection
May be caused by poor hygiene, tight clothing, perfumes and bubble baths, or overzealous wiping
Doughnut-shaped dark red mucosa at urethral meatus? Consider urethral prolapse; treatment is sitz baths, estrogen cream, and referral
Genital warts present? If age < 18 months, possible vertical transmission; inquire about maternal HPV. Age > 18 months, consider sexual abuse
Vaginal or abdominal mass? Refer for evaluation by surgery or gynecology
Physical exam reveals precocious puberty? Palpate abdomen for masses; refer for pediatric endocrine evaluation
Trauma? Tense hematoma may be drained or large lacerations may need closure in OR. Ensure that the patient can urinate
Can you see the source of bleeding? Consider exam under anesthesia

FIG. 170 Algorithm showing critical questions and priority actions for pediatric vaginitis. Additional information on pediatric vaginitis is available in Section I, Vaginitis, Prepubescent. *HPV*, Human papillomavirus; *OR*, operating room. (From Adams JG et al: *Emergency medicine: clinical essentials*, ed 2, Philadelphia, 2013, Elsevier.)

VENTILATOR-ASSOCIATED PNEUMONIA

ICD-10CM # J15.9 Unspecified bacterial pneumonia
J15.1 Pneumonia due to pseudomonas
J15.6 Pneumonia due to other aerobic gram-negative bacteria
J15.212 Pneumonia due to methicillin-resistant Staphylococcus aureus

Patient has a baseline period of stability or improvement on the ventilator, defined by ≥2 calendar days of stable or decreasing daily minimum* FiO_2 or PEEP values. The baseline period is defined as the 2 calendar days immediately preceding the first day of increased daily minimum PEEP or FiO_2.
*Daily minimum defined by lowest value of FiO_2 or PEEP during a calendar day that is maintained for at least 1 hour.

↓

After a period of stability or improvement on the ventilator, the patient has at least one of the following indicators of worsening oxygenation:
1) Increase in daily minimum* FiO_2 of ≥0.20 (20 points) over the daily minimum FiO_2 in the baseline period, sustained for ≥2 calendar days.
2) Increase in daily minimum* PEEP values of ≥3 cm H_2O over the daily minimum PEEP in the baseline period,† sustained for ≥2 calendar days.
*Daily minimum defined by lowest value of FiO_2 or PEEP during a calendar day that is maintained for at least 1 hour.
†Daily minimum PEEP values of 0–5 cm H_2O are considered equivalent for the purposes of VAE surveillance.

↓

Ventilator-Associated Condition (VAC)

↓

On or after calendar day 3 of mechanical ventilation and within 2 calendar days before or after the onset of worsening oxygenation, the patient meets *both* of the following criteria:

1) Temperature >38° C or <36° C, **OR** white blood cell count ≥12,000 cells/mm^3 or ≤4,000 cells/mm^3.
AND
2) A new antimicrobial agent(s) is started, and is continued for ≥4 calendar days.

↓

Infection-related Ventilator-Associated Complication (IVAC)

↓

On or after calendar day 3 of mechanical ventilation and within 2 calendar days before or after the onset of worsening oxygenation, ONE of the following criteria is met (**taking into account organism exclusions specified in the protocol**):

1) Criterion 1: Positive culture of one of the following specimens, meeting quantitative or semiquantitative thresholds as outlined in protocol, *without* requirement for purulent respiratory secretions:
    - Endotracheal aspirate, ≥10^5 CFU/mL or corresponding semiquantitative result
    - Bronchoalveolar lavage, ≥10^4 CFU/mL or corresponding semiquantitative result
    - Lung tissue, ≥10^4 CFU/g or corresponding semiquantitative result
    - Protected specimen brush, ≥10^3 CFU/mL or corresponding semiquantitative result
2) Criterion 2: Purulent respiratory secretions (defined as secretions from the lungs, bronchi, or trachea that contain ≥25 neutrophils and ≤10 squamous epithelial cells per low power field [lpf, 100])† *plus* a positive culture of one of the following specimens (qualitative culture, or quantitative/semiquantitative culture without sufficient growth to meet criterion #1):
    - Sputum
    - Endotracheal aspirate
    - Bronchoalveolar lavage
    - Lung tissue
    - Protected specimen brush

    † If the laboratory reports semiquantitative results, those results must correspond to the above quantitative thresholds. See additional instructions for using the purulent respiratory secretions criterion in the VAE Protocol.
3) Criterion 3: One of the following positive tests:
    - Pleural fluid culture (where specimen was obtained during thoracentesis or initial placement of chest tube and NOT from an indwelling chest tube)
    - Lung histopathology, defined as: 1) abscess formation or foci of consolidation with intense neutrophil accumulation in bronchioles and alveoli; 2) evidence of lung parenchyma invasion by fungi (hyphae, pseudohyphae, or yeast forms); 3) evidence of infection with the viral pathogens listed below based on results of immunohistochemical assays, cytology, or microscopy performed on lung tissue
    - Diagnostic test for *Legionella* species
    - Diagnostic test on respiratory secretions for influenza virus, respiratory syncytial virus, adenovirus, parainfluenza virus, rhinovirus human metapneumovirus coronavirus

↓

Possible Ventilator-Associated Pneumonia (PVAP)

FIG. 171 Ventilator-associated events surveillance algorithm. *FiO_2*, Fraction of inspired oxygen; *PEEP*, positive end-expiratory pressure. (From The Centers for Disease Control and Prevention: Ventilator-associated event [VAE], device-associated module. *NHSN Patient Safety Component Manual*, pp 10-1–10-46, January 2015 [modified April 2015]. Available at http://www.cdc.gov/nhsn/pdfs/pscmanual/pcsmanual_current.pdf. Accessed October 15 2018.)

VENTRICULAR FIBRILLATION OR PULSELESS VENTRICULAR TACHYCARDIA

ICD-10CM # I49.01 Ventricular fibrillation

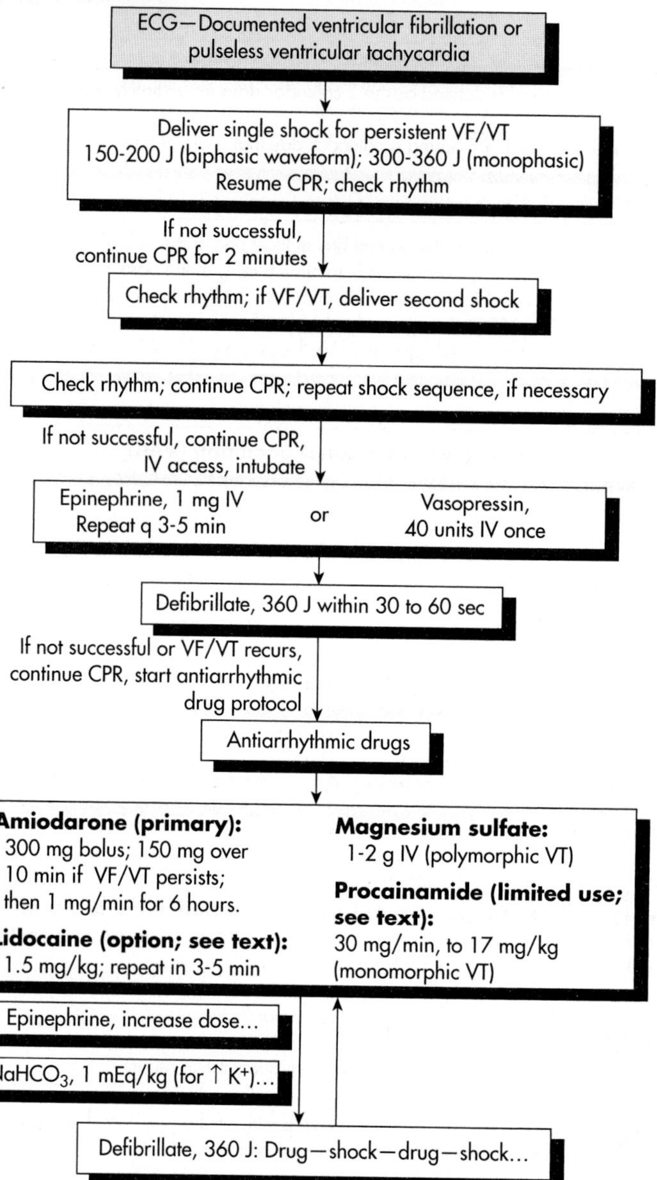
ECG—Documented ventricular fibrillation or pulseless ventricular tachycardia
Deliver single shock for persistent VF/VT
150-200 J (biphasic waveform); 300-360 J (monophasic)
Resume CPR; check rhythm
If not successful, continue CPR for 2 minutes
Check rhythm; if VF/VT, deliver second shock
Check rhythm; continue CPR; repeat shock sequence, if necessary
If not successful, continue CPR, IV access, intubate
Epinephrine, 1 mg IV
Repeat q 3-5 min
or
Vasopressin,
40 units IV once
Defibrillate, 360 J within 30 to 60 sec
If not successful or VF/VT recurs, continue CPR, start antiarrhythmic drug protocol
Antiarrhythmic drugs
Amiodarone (primary):
300 mg bolus; 150 mg over 10 min if VF/VT persists; then 1 mg/min for 6 hours.
Lidocaine (option; see text):
1.5 mg/kg; repeat in 3-5 min
Magnesium sulfate:
1-2 g IV (polymorphic VT)
Procainamide (limited use; see text):
30 mg/min, to 17 mg/kg (monomorphic VT)
Epinephrine, increase dose...
NaHCO3, 1 mEq/kg (for ↑ K+)...
Defibrillate, 360 J: Drug—shock—drug—shock...

FIG. 172 General algorithm for advanced cardiac life support (ACLS) response to ventricular fibrillation (VF) or pulseless ventricular tachycardia (VT). NOTE: In a 2008 advisory, 200 compression-only sequences were suggested as an alternative to standard CPR cycles between shocks, and this approach is under consideration for future guidelines. *CPR*, cardiopulmonary resuscitation; *ECG*, electrocardiogram. (From Goldman L, Schafer AI: *Goldman Cecil medicine*, ed 25, Philadelphia, 2016, Saunders.)

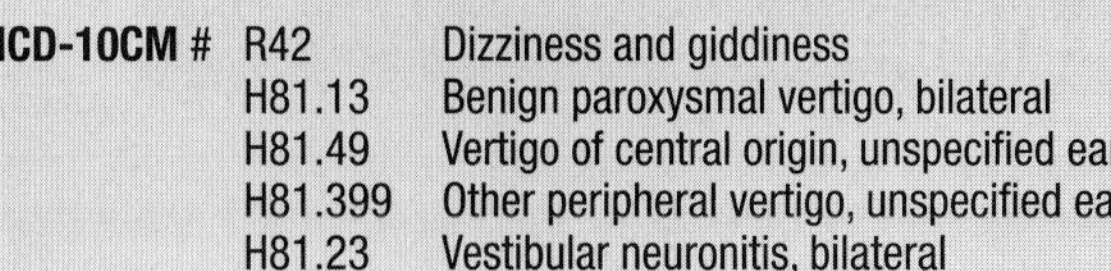

ICD-10CM #		
	R42	Dizziness and giddiness
	H81.13	Benign paroxysmal vertigo, bilateral
	H81.49	Vertigo of central origin, unspecified ear
	H81.399	Other peripheral vertigo, unspecified ear
	H81.23	Vestibular neuronitis, bilateral

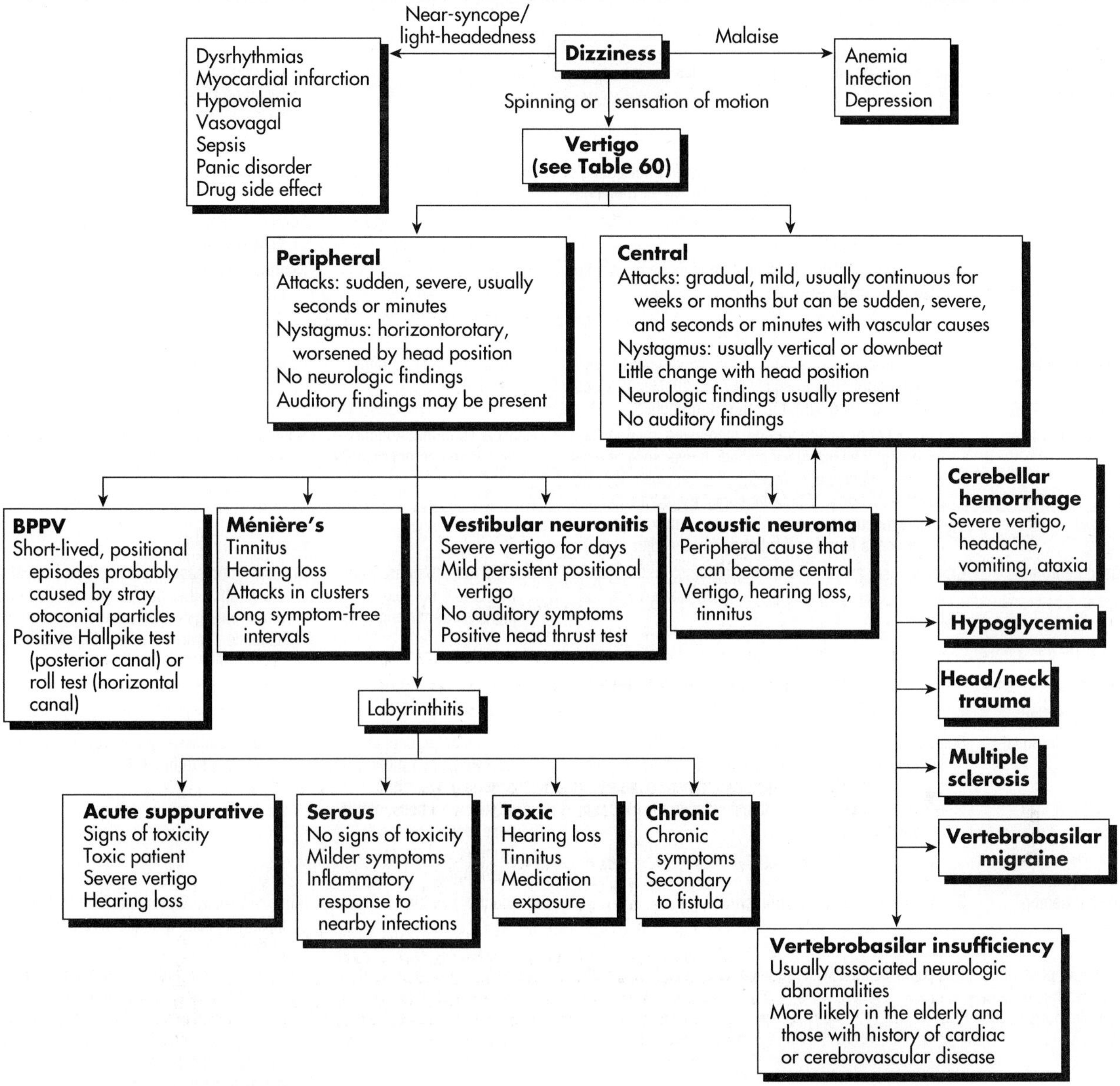

Dizziness

- Near-syncope/light-headedness → Dysrhythmias; Myocardial infarction; Hypovolemia; Vasovagal; Sepsis; Panic disorder; Drug side effect
- Malaise → Anemia; Infection; Depression
- Spinning or sensation of motion → **Vertigo (see Table 60)**

Vertigo

Peripheral
Attacks: sudden, severe, usually seconds or minutes
Nystagmus: horizontorotary, worsened by head position
No neurologic findings
Auditory findings may be present

Central
Attacks: gradual, mild, usually continuous for weeks or months but can be sudden, severe, and seconds or minutes with vascular causes
Nystagmus: usually vertical or downbeat
Little change with head position
Neurologic findings usually present
No auditory findings

Peripheral →

BPPV
Short-lived, positional episodes probably caused by stray otoconial particles
Positive Hallpike test (posterior canal) or roll test (horizontal canal)

Ménière's
Tinnitus
Hearing loss
Attacks in clusters
Long symptom-free intervals

Vestibular neuronitis
Severe vertigo for days
Mild persistent positional vertigo
No auditory symptoms
Positive head thrust test

Acoustic neuroma (→ Central)
Peripheral cause that can become central
Vertigo, hearing loss, tinnitus

Labyrinthitis →

Acute suppurative
Signs of toxicity
Toxic patient
Severe vertigo
Hearing loss

Serous
No signs of toxicity
Milder symptoms
Inflammatory response to nearby infections

Toxic
Hearing loss
Tinnitus
Medication exposure

Chronic
Chronic symptoms
Secondary to fistula

Central →

Cerebellar hemorrhage
Severe vertigo, headache, vomiting, ataxia

Hypoglycemia

Head/neck trauma

Multiple sclerosis

Vertebrobasilar migraine

Vertebrobasilar insufficiency
Usually associated neurologic abnormalities
More likely in the elderly and those with history of cardiac or cerebrovascular disease

FIG. 173 Diagnostic algorithm for dizziness and vertigo. Additional topics "Vestibular Neuronitis," "Acoustic Neuroma," "Labyrinthitis," "Ménière's Disease," and "Benign Paroxysmal Positional Vertigo" are available in Section I. *BPPV,* Benign paroxysmal positional vertigo. (From Marx JA et al: *Rosen's emergency medicine*, ed 8, Philadelphia, 2014, Saunders.)

ICD-10CM #		
	R42	Dizziness and giddiness
	H81.13	Benign paroxysmal vertigo, bilateral
	H81.49	Vertigo of central origin, unspecified ear
	H81.399	Other peripheral vertigo, unspecified ear
	H81.23	Vestibular neuronitis, bilateral

TABLE 60 Differential Diagnosis of Patients with True Vertigo

Cause	History	Associated Symptoms	Physical
Peripheral			
1. Benign paroxysmal positional vertigo	Short-lived, positional, fatigable episodes	Nausea, vomiting	Single position can precipitate vertigo. Positive result on Hallpike test (posterior semicircular canal) or Roll test (horizontal canal).
2. Labyrinthitis			
A. Serous	Mild to severe positional symptoms. Usually coexisting or antecedent infection of ear, nose, throat, or meninges.	Mild to severe hearing loss can occur	Usually nontoxic patient with minimal fever elevation
B. Acute suppurative	Coexisting acute exudative infection of the inner ear. Severe symptoms.	Usually severe hearing loss, nausea, vomiting	Febrile patient showing signs of toxicity. Acute otitis media.
C. Toxic	Gradually progressive symptoms: Patients on medication causing toxicity.	Hearing loss that may become rapid and severe, nausea and vomiting	Hearing loss. Ataxia common feature in chronic phase.
3. Ménière disease	Recurrent episodes of severe rotational vertigo usually lasting hours. Onset usually abrupt. Attacks may occur in clusters. Long symptom-free remissions.	Nausea, vomiting, tinnitus, hearing loss	Positional nystagmus not present
4. Vestibular neuritis	Sudden onset of severe vertigo, increasing in intensity for hours, then gradually subsiding over several days but can last weeks to months. Can be worsened with positional change. Sometimes history of infection or toxic exposure that precedes initial attack. Highest incidence is found in third and fifth decades.	Nausea, vomiting. Auditory symptoms do not occur.	Spontaneous nystagmus toward the involved ear may be present.
5. Acoustic neuroma	Gradual onset and increase in symptoms. Neurologic signs in later stages. Most occur in women aged 30 to 60.	Hearing loss, tinnitus. True ataxia and neurologic signs as tumor enlarges.	Unilateral decreased hearing. True truncal ataxia and other neurologic signs when tumor enlarges. May have diminution or absence of corneal reflex. Eighth cranial nerve deficit may be present.
Central			
1. Vascular disorders			
A. Vertebrobasilar insufficiency	Should be considered in any patient of advanced age with isolated new-onset vertigo without an obvious cause. More likely with history of atherosclerosis. Can occur with neck trauma. Initial episode usually lasts seconds to minutes.	Often headache. Usually neurologic symptoms including dysarthria, ataxia, weakness, numbness, double vision. Tinnitus and deafness uncommon.	Neurologic deficits usually present, but initially neurologic examination can be normal
B. Cerebellar hemorrhage	Sudden onset of severe symptoms	Headache, vomiting, ataxia	Signs of toxicity. Dysmetria, true ataxia. Ipsilateral sixth cranial nerve palsy may be present.
C. Occlusion of posterior inferior cerebellar artery (Wallenberg's syndrome)	Vertigo associated with significant neurologic complaints	Nausea, vomiting, loss of pain and temperature sensation, ataxia, hoarseness	Loss of pain and temperature sensation on the side of the face ipsilateral to the lesion and on the opposite side of the body, paralysis of the palate, pharynx, and larynx. Horner syndrome (ipsilateral ptosis, miosis, and decreased facial sweating).
2. Head trauma	Symptoms begin with or shortly after head trauma. Positional symptoms most common type after trauma. Self-limited symptoms that can persist weeks to months.	Usually mild nausea	Occasionally, basilar skull fracture
3. Vertebrobasilar migraine	Vertigo almost always followed by headache. Patient has usually had similar episodes in past. Most patients have a family history of migraine. Syndrome usually begins in adolescence.	Dysarthria, ataxia, visual disturbances, or paresthesias usually precede headache	No residual neurologic or otologic signs are present after attack
4. Multiple sclerosis	Vertigo presenting symptom in 7%-10% and appears in the course of the disease in a third. Onset may be severe and suggest labyrinth disease. Disease onset usually between ages 20 and 40. Often history of other attacks with varying neurologic signs or symptoms.	Nausea and vomiting, which may be severe	May have horizontal, rotary, or vertical nystagmus. Nystagmus may persist after the vertiginous symptoms have subsided. Bilateral internuclear ophthalmoplegia and ataxic eye movements suggest multiple sclerosis.
5. Temporal lobe epilepsy	Can be initial or prominent symptom in some patients with the disorder	Memory impairment, hallucinations, trancelike states, seizures	May have aphasia or convulsions
6. Hypoglycemia	Should be considered in diabetics and any other patient with unexplained symptoms	Sweating, anxiety	Tachycardia, mental status change may be present

From Marx JA et al: *Rosen's emergency medicine*, ed 8, Philadelphia, 2014, Saunders.

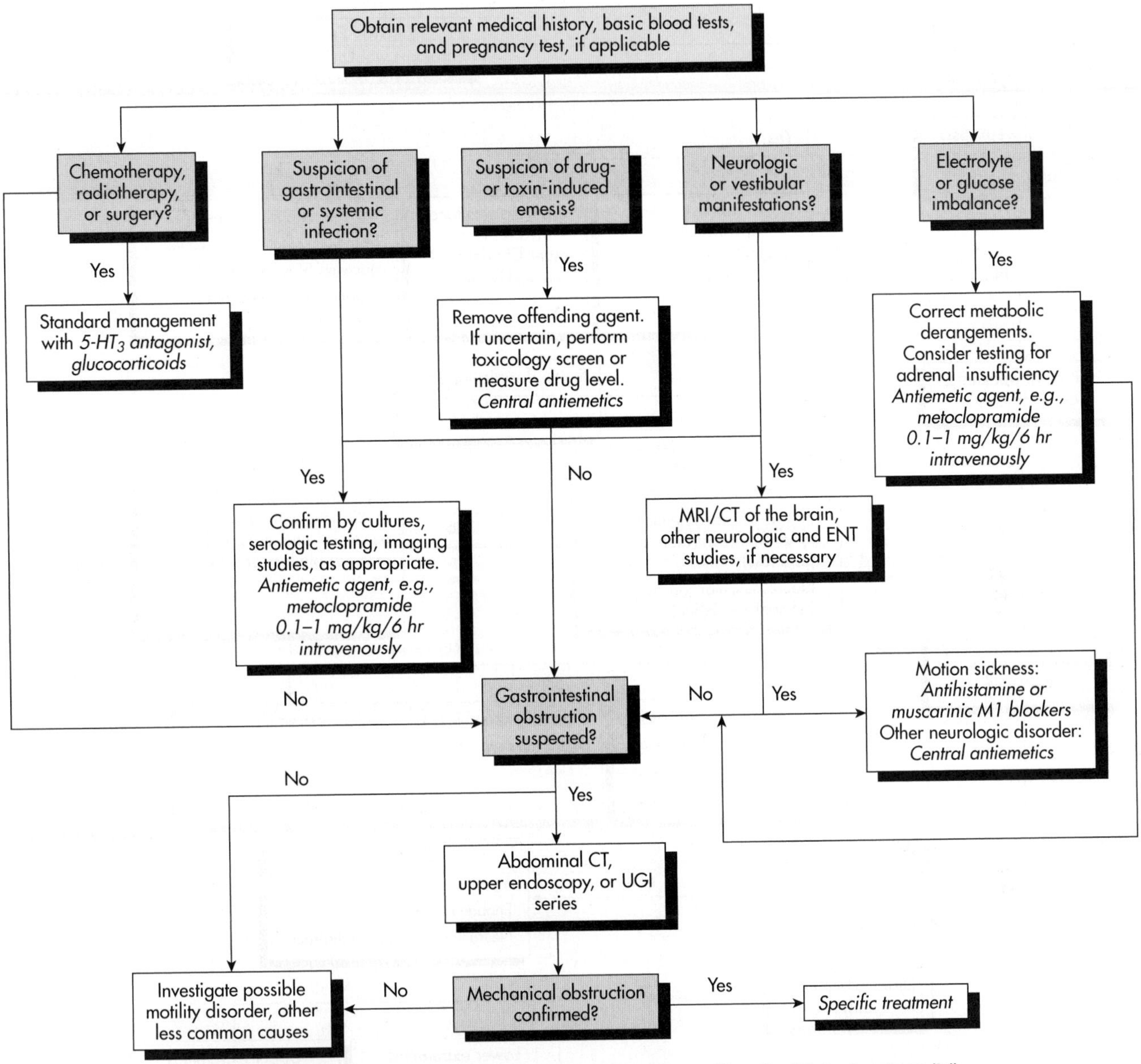

VOMITING, ACUTE, MANAGEMENT

ICD-10CM # R11.10 Vomiting, unspecified

Obtain relevant medical history, basic blood tests, and pregnancy test, if applicable

Chemotherapy, radiotherapy, or surgery?

Suspicion of gastrointestinal or systemic infection?

Suspicion of drug- or toxin-induced emesis?

Neurologic or vestibular manifestations?

Electrolyte or glucose imbalance?

Yes

Standard management with *5-HT$_3$ antagonist, glucocorticoids*

Yes

Remove offending agent. If uncertain, perform toxicology screen or measure drug level. *Central antiemetics*

Yes

Correct metabolic derangements. Consider testing for adrenal insufficiency *Antiemetic agent, e.g., metoclopramide 0.1–1 mg/kg/6 hr intravenously*

Yes

No

Yes

Confirm by cultures, serologic testing, imaging studies, as appropriate. *Antiemetic agent, e.g., metoclopramide 0.1–1 mg/kg/6 hr intravenously*

MRI/CT of the brain, other neurologic and ENT studies, if necessary

No

Gastrointestinal obstruction suspected?

No

Yes

Motion sickness: *Antihistamine or muscarinic M1 blockers* Other neurologic disorder: *Central antiemetics*

No

Yes

Abdominal CT, upper endoscopy, or UGI series

Investigate possible motility disorder, other less common causes

No

Mechanical obstruction confirmed?

Yes

Specific treatment

FIG. 174 Algorithm for management of a patient with acute vomiting. Possible treatments are italicized. *ENT*, ear, nose, and throat; *5-HT*, 5-hydroxytryptamine; *UGI*, upper GI. Potential treatments are shown in italics. (Feldman M, Friedman LS, Brandt LJ: *Sleisenger and Fortran's gastrointestinal and liver disease*, ed 10, Philadelphia, 2016, Elsevier.)

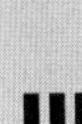

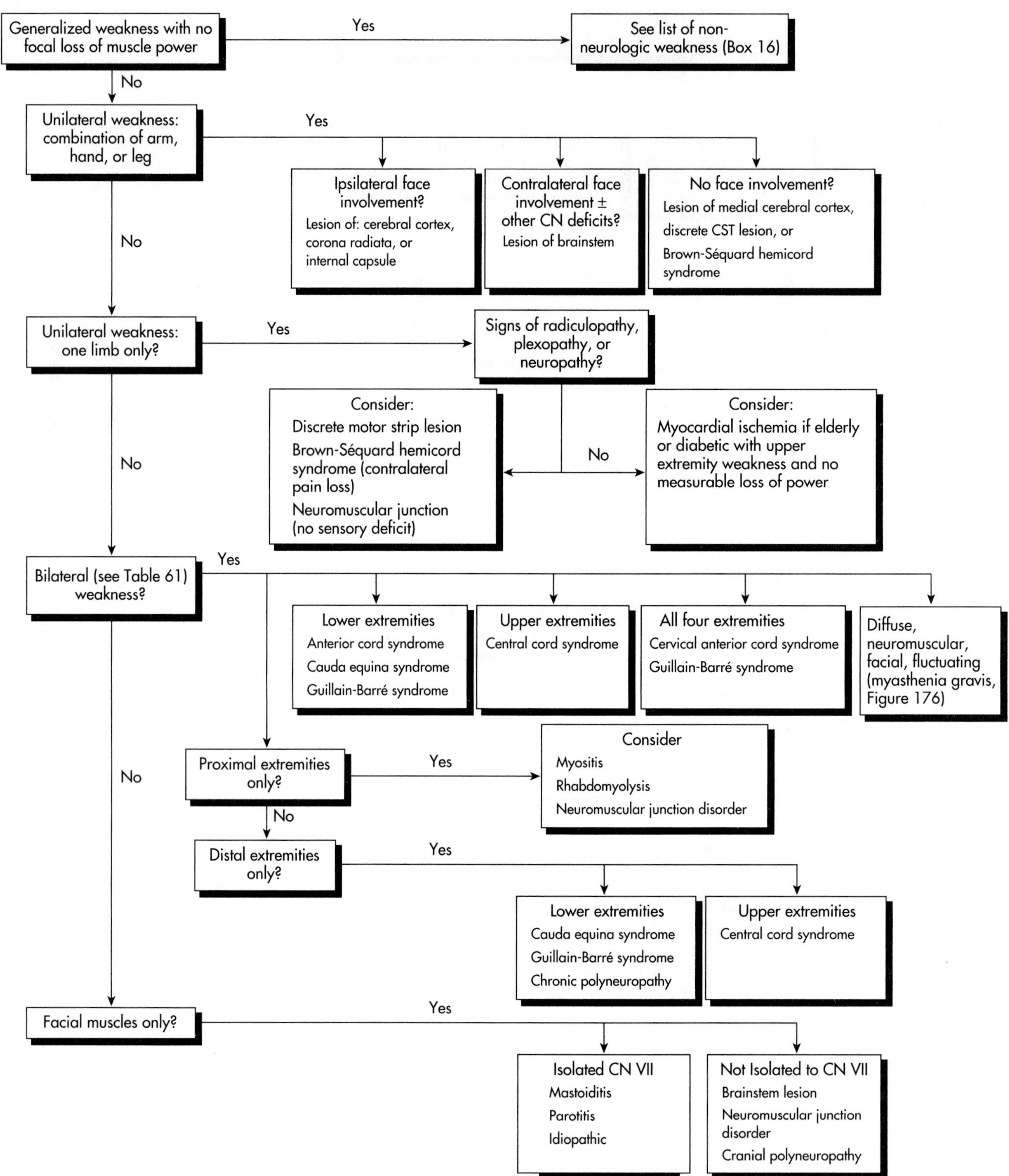

FIG. 175 Common clinical patterns of weakness, classified and assessed. *CN,* Cranial nerve; *CST,* corticospinal tract. (Modified from Marx JA et al: *Rosen's emergency medicine*, ed 8, Philadelphia, 2014, Saunders.)

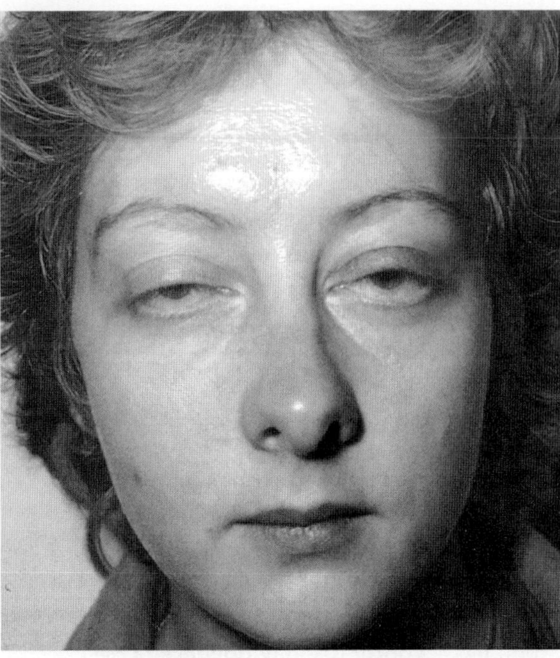

FIG. 176 Myopathic facies in myasthenia gravis. (From Bowling B: *Kanski's clinical ophthalmology, a systemic approach,* ed 8, 2106, Elsevier.)

TABLE 61 Critical and Emergent Causes of Neuromuscular Weakness

Critical Diagnoses	
Cerebral cortex or subcortical	Ischemic or hemorrhagic cerebrovascular accident (CVA)
Brainstem	Ischemic or hemorrhagic CVA
Spinal cord	Ischemia, compression (disk, abscess, or hematoma)
Peripheral nerve	Acute demyelination (Guillain-Barré syndrome)
Neuromuscular junction	Myasthenic or cholinergic crisis Botulism Tick paralysis Organophosphate poisoning
Muscle	Rhabdomyolysis
Emergent Diagnoses	
Cerebral cortex or subcortical	Tumor, abscess, demyelination
Brainstem	Demyelination
Spinal cord	Demyelination (transverse myelitis) Compression (disk, spondylosis)
Peripheral nerve	Compressive plexopathy (hematoma, aneurysm) Paraneoplastic vasculitis uremia
Muscle	Inflammatory myositis

From Marx JA et al: *Rosen's emergency medicine*, ed 8, Philadelphia, 2014, Saunders.

Clinical Algorithms III

BOX 16 Nonneurologic Weakness

- Alterations in plasma volume (dehydration)
- Alterations in plasma composition (glucose, electrolytes)
- Derangement in circulating red blood cells (anemia or polycythemia)
- Decrement in cardiac pump function (myocardial ischemia)
- Drop in systemic vascular resistance (vasodilatory shock from any cause)
- Increased metabolic demand (local or systemic infection, endocrinopathy, toxin)
- Mitochondrial dysfunction (severe sepsis or toxin-mediated)
- Global depression of the central nervous system (sedatives, stimulant withdrawal)

From Marx JA et al: *Rosen's emergency medicine*, ed 8, Philadelphia, 2014, Saunders.

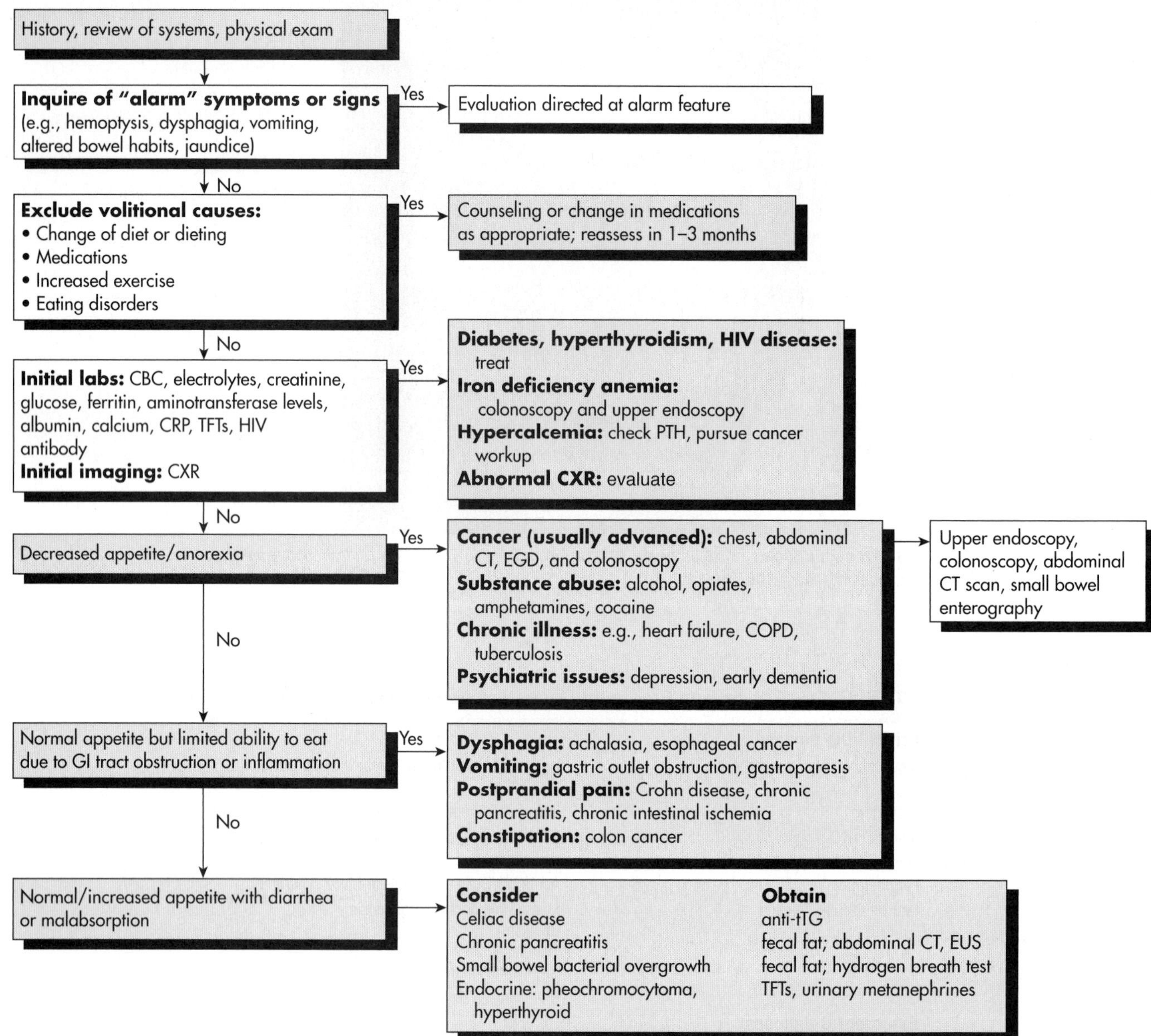

FIG. 177 Approach to the patient with unintentional weight loss of more than 5%. *CBC*, complete blood count; *COPD*, chronic obstructive pulmonary disease; *CRP*, C-reactive protein; *CT*, computed tomography; *CXR*, chest radiograph; *EGD*, esophagogastroduodenoscopy; *EUS*, endoscopic ultrasound; *GI*, gastrointestinal; *HIV*, human immunodeficiency virus; *PTH*, parathyroid hormone; *TFTs*, thyroid function tests; *tTG*, tissue transglutaminase. (From Goldman L, Schafer AI: *Goldman Cecil medicine*, ed 25, Philadelphia, 2016, Saunders.)

Laboratory Tests and Interpretation of Results

INTRODUCTION

This section contains over 300 commonly performed laboratory tests. In general, the tests are discussed in the following format:

1. Laboratory test.
2. Normal range in adult patients. Normal values are given using the present (traditional) reference interval, followed by the Système Internationale (SI) reference interval, the conversion factor (CF), and the suggested minimum increment (SMI).
3. Common abnormalities, such as positive test, increased, or decreased value.
4. Causes of abnormal result.

The normal ranges may differ slightly, depending on the laboratory. The reader should be aware of the "normal range" of the particular laboratory performing the test. Every attempt has been made to present current laboratory test data with emphasis on practical considerations.

ACE LEVEL

See ANGIOTENSIN-CONVERTING ENZYME

ACETONE (serum or plasma)

Normal: Negative
Elevated in: DKA, starvation, isopropanol ingestion

ACETYLCHOLINE RECEPTOR (AChR) ANTIBODY

Normal: <0.03 nmol/L
Elevated in: Myasthenia gravis. Changes in AChR concentration correlate with the clinical severity of myasthenia gravis following therapy and during therapy with prednisone and immunosuppressants. False-positive AChR antibody results may be found in patients with Eaton-Lambert syndrome.

ACID-BASE REFERENCE VALUES

See Tables 1, 2, and 3.

ACID PHOSPHATASE (serum)

Normal range: 0-5.5 U/L (0-90 nkat/L [CF: 16.67; SMI:2 nkat/L])
Elevated in: Carcinoma of prostate, other neoplasms (breast, bone), Paget disease, osteogenesis imperfecta, malignant invasion of bone, Gaucher disease, multiple myeloma, myeloproliferative disorders, benign prostatic hypertrophy, prostatic palpation or surgery, hyperparathyroidism, liver disease, chronic renal failure, idiopathic thrombocytopenic purpura, bronchitis

ACID SERUM TEST

See HAM TEST

ACTIVATED CLOTTING TIME (ACT)

Normal: This test is used to determine the dose of protamine sulfate to reverse the effect of heparin as an anticoagulant during angioplasty, cardiac surgery, and hemodialysis. The accepted goal during cardiopulmonary bypass surgery is usually 400-500 sec.

ACTIVATED PARTIAL THROMBOPLASTIN TIME (APTT, aPTT)

See PARTIAL THROMBOPLASTIN TIME

ADRENOCORTICOTROPIC HORMONE

Normal: 9-52 pg/ml. Table 4 describes patterns of serum levels of ACTH and cortisol in different adrenal gland disorders.
Elevated in: Addison's disease, ectopic ACTH-producing tumors, congenital adrenal hyperplasia, Nelson syndrome, pituitary-dependent Cushing's disease
Decreased in: Secondary adrenocortical insufficiency, hypopituitarism, adrenal adenoma or adrenal carcinoma

ALANINE AMINOPEPTIDASE

Normal:
Male: 1.11-1.71 mcg/ml
Female: 0.96-1.52 mcg/ml
Elevated in: Liver or pancreatic disease, ethanol use, oral contraceptives use, malignancy, tobacco use, pregnancy
Decreased in: Abortion

ALANINE AMINOTRANSFERASE (ALT, SGPT)

See Fig. 1, an algorithm for evaluation of elevated ALT. Table 5 describes patterns of liver function tests in liver disorders.
Normal range: 0-35 U/L (0.058 μkat/L [CF: 0.02 μkat/L])
Elevated in: Liver disease (hepatitis, cirrhosis, Reye syndrome), hepatic congestion, infectious mononucleosis, myocardial infarction, myocarditis, severe muscle trauma, dermatomyositis/polymyositis, muscular dystrophy, drugs (antibiotics, narcotics, antihypertensive agents, heparin, labetalol, statins, NSAIDs, amiodarone, chlorpromazine, phenytoin), malignancy, renal and pulmonary infarction, seizures, eclampsia, shock liver

TABLE 1 Commonly Used Acid-Base Reference Values for Arterial and Venous Plasma or Serum (Averaged from Various Sources)

	ARTERIAL		VENOUS	
	Conventional Units	SI Units*	Conventional Units	SI Units*
pH	7.40 (7.35-7.45)	7.40 (7.35-7.45)	7.37 (7.32-7.42)	7.37 (7.32-7.42)
Pco_2	40 mm Hg (35-45)	5.33 kPa (4.67-6.10)	45 mm Hg (45-50)	6.10 kPa (5.33-6.67)
Po_2	80-100 mm Hg	10.66-13.33 kPa	40 mm Hg (37-43)	5.33 kPa (4.93-5.73)
HCO_3 (CO_2 combining power)	24 mEq/L (20-28)	24 mmol/L (20-28)	26 mEq/L (22-30)	26 mmol/L (22-30)
CO_2 content	25 mEq/L (22-28)	25 mmol/L (22-28)	27 mEq/L (24-30)	27 mmol/L(24-30)

*International system.
From Ravel R: *Clinical laboratory medicine*, ed 6, St Louis, 1995, Mosby.

TABLE 2 Summary of Laboratory Findings in Primary Uncomplicated Respiratory and Metabolic Acid-Base Disorders*

Disorder	Pco_2	pH	Base Excess
Acute primary respiratory hypoactivity (respiratory acidosis)	Increase	Decrease	Normal/positive
Acute primary respiratory hyperactivity (respiratory alkalosis)	Decrease	Increase	Normal/negative
Uncompensated metabolic acidosis	Normal	Decrease	Negative
Uncompensated metabolic alkalosis	Normal	Increase	Positive
Partially compensated metabolic acidosis	Decrease	Decrease	Negative
Partially compensated metabolic alkalosis	Increase	Increase	Positive
Chronic primary respiratory hypoactivity (compensated respiratory acidosis)	Increase	Normal	Positive
Fully compensated metabolic alkalosis	Increase	Normal	Positive
Chronic primary respiratory hyperactivity (compensated respiratory alkalosis)	Decrease	Normal	Negative
Fully compensated metabolic acidosis	Decrease	Normal	Negative

*Base excess results refer to negative (–) values more than 22 and positive (+) values more than 12.
From Ravel R: *Clinical laboratory medicine*, ed 6, St Louis, 1995, Mosby.

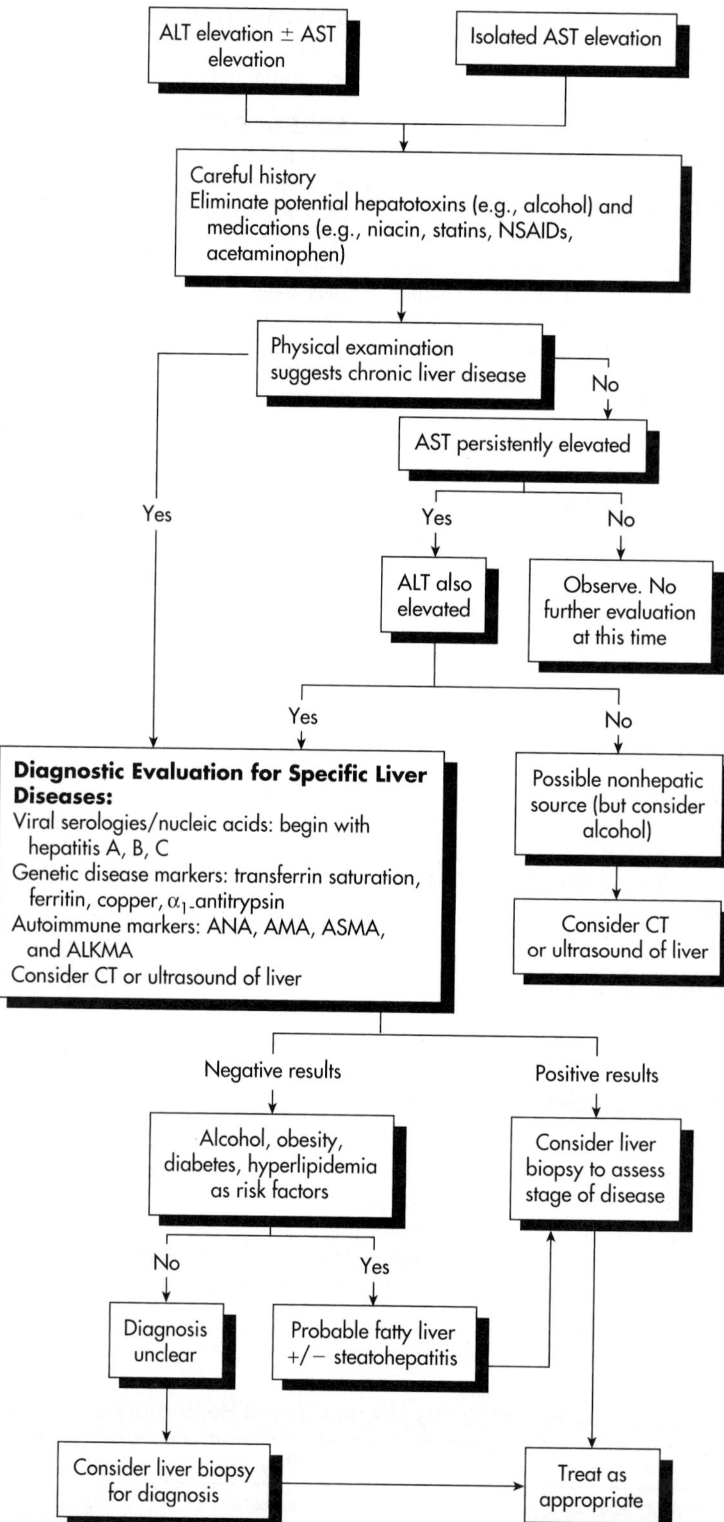

FIG. 1 Approach to the evaluation of isolated elevated levels of serum alanine aminotransferase *(ALT)* and/or aspartate aminotransferase *(AST)* in the asymptomatic patient. *ALKMA,* Anti–liver/kidney microsomal antibody; *AMA,* antimitochondrial antibody; *ANA,* antinuclear antibody; *ASMA,* anti–smooth muscle antibody; *NSAIDs,* nonsteroidal antiinflammatory drugs. (Modified from Goldman L, Ausiello D [eds]: *Cecil textbook of medicine,* ed 24, Philadelphia, 2012, Saunders.)

ALBUMIN (serum)

Normal range: 4-6 g/dl (40-60 g/L [CF:10; SMI: 1 g/L])
Elevated in: Dehydration (relative increase)
Decreased in: Liver disease, nephrotic syndrome, poor nutritional status, rapid IV hydration, protein-losing enteropathies (e.g., inflammatory bowel disease), severe burns, neoplasia, chronic inflammatory diseases, pregnancy, oral contraceptives, prolonged immobilization, lymphomas, hypervitaminosis A, chronic glomerulonephritis

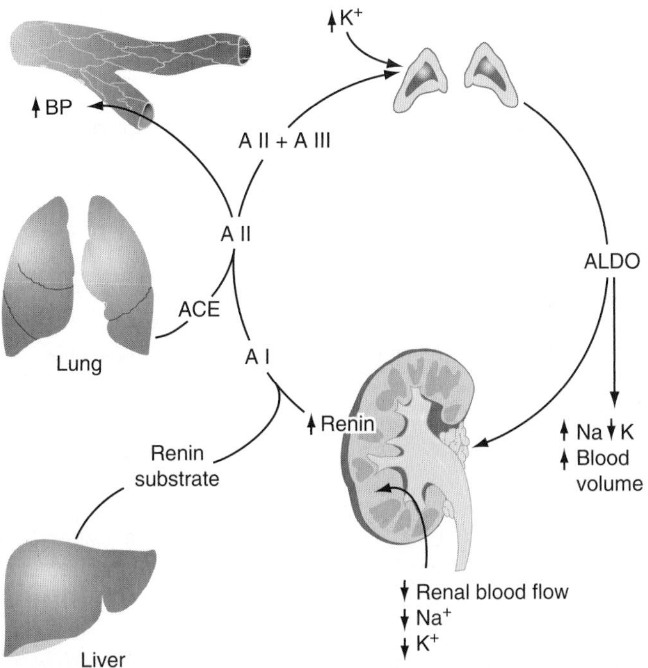

FIG. 2 The normal renin-angiotensin-aldosterone axis. Renin, secreted by the kidney, cleaves angiotensin I from renin substrate (angiotensinogen) produced by the liver. Angiotensin I is converted to angiotensin II by angiotensin-converting enzyme *(ACE)* mainly in the lung. Angiotensin II increases peripheral vascular resistance and, together with angiotensin III, stimulates aldosterone *(ALDO)* secretion, which results in sodium retention and increased plasma volume.
(Adapted from Stewart PM: The adrenal cortex. In Larsen PR, Kronenberg HM, Melmed S et al [eds]: *Williams textbook of endocrinology,* ed 10, Philadelphia, 2003, Saunders, p 499.
McPherson RA, Pincus MR: *Henry's clinical diagnosis and management by laboratory methods*, ed 23, St Louis, 2017, Elsevier.)

ALCOHOL DEHYDROGENASE

Normal: 0-7 U/L
Elevated in: Drug-induced hepatocellular damage, obstructive jaundice, malignancy, inflammation, infection

ALDOLASE (serum)

Normal range: 0-6 U/L (0-100 nkat/L [CF: 16.67; SMI: 20 nkat/L])
Elevated in: Muscular dystrophy, rhabdomyolysis, dermatomyositis/polymyositis, trichinosis, acute hepatitis and other liver diseases, myocardial infarction, prostatic carcinoma, hemorrhagic pancreatitis, gangrene, delirium tremens, burns
Decreased in: Loss of muscle mass, late stages of muscular dystrophy

ALDOSTERONE

Normal range:
Recumbent: 50-150 ng/L
Upright: 150-300 ng/L
(Highest levels in neonates, decreasing over time to adult levels). The normal renin-angiotensin-aldosterone axis is illustrated in Fig. 2.
Elevated in: Primary aldosteronism, secondary aldosteronism, pseudoprimary aldosteronism. Table 6 differentiates the various causes of hyperaldosteronism.
Decreased in
Patient with hypertension: diabetes mellitus, Turner syndrome, acute alcohol intoxication, excess secretion of deoxycorticosterone, corticosterone, and 18-hydroxycorticosterone
Patient without hypertension: Addison disease, hypoaldosteronism resulting from renin deficiency, isolated aldosterone deficiency. Table 7 differentiates the various causes of hypoaldosteronism.

ALKALINE PHOSPHATASE (ALP) (serum)

See Fig. 3 for investigating a raised ALP in general practice.
See Fig. E4 for approach to elevated ALP.
Normal range: 30-120 U/L (0.5-2 μkat/L [CF:0.01667; SMI: 0.1 μkat/L])
Elevated in
LIVER AND BILIARY TRACT ORIGIN
Extrahepatic bile duct obstruction
Intrahepatic biliary obstruction
Liver cell acute injury
Liver passive congestion
Drug-induced liver cell dysfunction
Space-occupying lesions
Primary biliary cirrhosis
Sepsis
BONE ORIGIN (OSTEOBLAST HYPERACTIVITY)
Physiologic (rapid) bone growth (childhood and adolescence)
Metastatic tumor with osteoblastic reaction
Fracture healing
Paget's disease of bone

TABLE 3 Acid-Base Abnormalities and Appropriate Compensatory Responses for Simple Disorders

Primary Acid-Base Disorders	Primary Defect	Effect on pH	Compensatory Response	Expected Range of Compensation	Limits of Compensation
Respiratory acidosis	Alveolar hypoventilation (↑ P_{CO_2})	↓	↑ Renal HCO_3- reabsorption (HCO_3- ↑)	Acute: $\Delta[HCO_3-] = +1$ mEq/L for each ↑ ΔP_{CO_2} of 10 mm Hg	$[HCO_3-] = 38$ mEq/L
				Chronic: $\Delta[HCO_3-] = +4$ mEq/L for each ↑ ΔP_{CO_2} of 10 mm Hg	$[HCO_3-] = 45$ mEq/L
Respiratory alkalosis	Alveolar hyperventilation (↓ P_{CO_2})	↑	↓ Renal HCO_3- reabsorption (HCO_3- ↓)	Acute: $\Delta[HCO_3-] = -2$ mEq/L for each ↓ ΔP_{CO_2} of 10 mm Hg	$[HCO_3-] = 18$ mEq/L
				Chronic: $\Delta[HCO_3-] = -5$ mEq/L for each ↓ ΔP_{CO_2} of 10 mm Hg	$[HCO_3-] = 15$ mEq/L
Metabolic acidosis	Loss of HCO_3- or gain of H^+ (↓ HCO_3-)	↓	Alveolar hyperventilation to ↑ pulmonary CO_2 excretion (↓P_{CO_2})	$P_{CO_2} = 1.5[HCO_3-] + 8 \pm 2$ P_{CO_2} = last 2 digits of pH × 100 $P_{CO_2} = 15 + [HCO_3-]$	$P_{CO_2} = 15$ mm Hg
Metabolic alkalosis	Gain of HCO_3- or loss of H^+ (↑ HCO_3-)	↑	Alveolar hypoventilation to ↓ pulmonary CO_2 excretion (↑ P_{CO_2})	$P_{CO_2} = +0.6$ mm Hg for $\Delta[HCO_3-]$ of 1 mEq/L. $P_{CO_2} = 15 + [HCO_3-]$	$P_{CO_2} = 55$ mm Hg

From Vincent JL, Abraham E, Moore FA et al: *Textbook of critical care*, ed 7, Philadelphia, 2017, Elsevier. Adapted and updated from Bidani A, Tauzon DM, Heming TA. Regulation of whole body acid-base balance. In DuBose TD, Hamm LL (eds). *Acid base and electrolytes disorders: a companion to Brenner and Rector's the kidney.* Philadelphia: Saunders; 2002, p. 1–21.

TABLE 4 Patterns of Serum Levels of Adrenocorticotropic Hormone (ACTH) and Cortisol in Different Adrenal Gland Conditions

Condition	Cortisol	ACTH	Dexamethasone Suppression, Low Dose	Dexamethasone Suppression, High Dose	Site of Disease
Normal adrenal	Normal	Normal	N/A	N/A	None
Primary hypoadrenalism	Low	High	N/A	N/A	Adrenal gland
Secondary hypoadrenalism	Low	Low	N/A	N/A	Pituitary
Primary hyperadrenalism—high cortisol, low ACTH	High	Low	N/A	N/A	Adrenal
Primary hyperadrenalism—high cortisol, borderline low ACTH	High	Borderline low	Positive	N/A	Adrenal
Primary hyperadrenalism due to adrenal hyperplasia—high cortisol, borderline low ACTH	High	Borderline low	Negative	Positive	Adrenal
Primary hyperadrenalism due to adrenal adenoma/carcinoma—high cortisol, borderline low ACTH	High	Borderline low	Negative	Negative	Adrenal
Secondary hyperadrenalism	High	High	N/A	N/A	Pituitary

McPherson RA, Pincus MR: *Henry's clinical diagnosis and management by laboratory methods*, ed 23, St Louis, 2017, Elsevier.

TABLE 5 Six Fundamental Patterns of Liver Function Tests

Condition	AST	ALT	LD	AP	TP	Albumin	Bilirubin	Ammonia
1. Hepatitis	H	H	H	H	N	N	H	N
2. Cirrhosis	N	N	N	N–sl H	L	L	H	H
3. Biliary obstruction	N	N	N	H	N	N	H	N
4. Space-occupying lesion	N or H	N or H	H	H	N	N	N–H	N
5. Passive congestion	Sl H	sl H	sl H	N–sl H	N	N	N–sl H	N
6. Fulminant failure	Very H	H	H	H	L	L	H	H

H, High; *N*, normal; *L*, low; *sl*, slightly; *AST*, aspartate aminotransferase; *ALT*, alanine aminotransferase; *LD*, lactate dehydrogenase; *AP*, alkaline phosphatase; *TP*, total protein.
McPherson RA, Pincus MR: *Henry's clinical diagnosis and management by laboratory methods*, ed 23, St Louis, 2017, Elsevier.

TABLE 6 Differentiating the Various Causes of Hyperaldosteronism

Disorder	Aldosterone	Renin	Serum K+
Primary hyperaldosteronism	↑	↓	↓
Renin-secreting tumor	↑	↑	↓—N
Dexamethasone-suppressible hyperaldosteronism	↑	↓	↓
Renovascular hypertension	N—↑	N—↑	↓—N
Bartter's syndrome	↑	↑	↓
Diuretics, congestive heart failure, cirrhosis, nephrotic syndrome	↑	↑	N—↓

N, Normal.
From McPherson RA, Pincus MR: *Henry's clinical diagnosis and management by laboratory methods*, ed 23, St Louis, 2017, Elsevier.

TABLE 7 Differentiating the Various Causes of Hypoaldosteronism

Disorder	Aldosterone	Renin	Serum K+
Addison's disease	↓	↑	↑
Cushing's syndrome	↓	↓	N or ↓
Liddle's syndrome	↓	↓	↓
Hyporeninemic hypoaldosteronism	↓	↓	↑
Apparent mineralocorticoid excess	↓	↓	↓
Isolated hypoaldosteronism	↓	↑	↑

N, Normal.
From McPherson RA, Pincus MR: *Henry's clinical diagnosis and management by laboratory methods*, ed 23, St Louis, 2017, Elsevier.

CAPILLARY ENDOTHELIAL ORIGIN
Granulation tissue formation (active)
PLACENTAL ORIGIN
Pregnancy
Some parenteral albumin preparations
OTHER
Thyrotoxicosis
Benign transient hyperphosphatasemia
Primary hyperparathyroidism
Decreased in: Hypothyroidism, pernicious anemia, hypophosphatemia, hypervitaminosis D, malnutrition

ALPHA-1-ANTITRYPSIN (serum)

Normal range: 110-140 mg/dl
Decreased in: Homozygous or heterozygous deficiency

ALPHA-1-FETOPROTEIN (serum)

See α-1 FETOPROTEIN

ALT

See ALANINE AMINOTRANSFERASE

ALUMINUM (serum)

Normal range: 0-6 ng/ml
Elevated in: Chronic renal failure on dialysis, parenteral nutrition, industrial exposure

AMA

See ANTIMITOCHONDRIAL ANTIBODY

AMEBIASIS SEROLOGIC TEST

Test description: Test is used to support diagnosis of amebiasis caused by *Entamoeba histolytica*. Serum acute and convalescent titers are drawn 1-3 weeks apart. A fourfold increase in titer is the most indicative result.

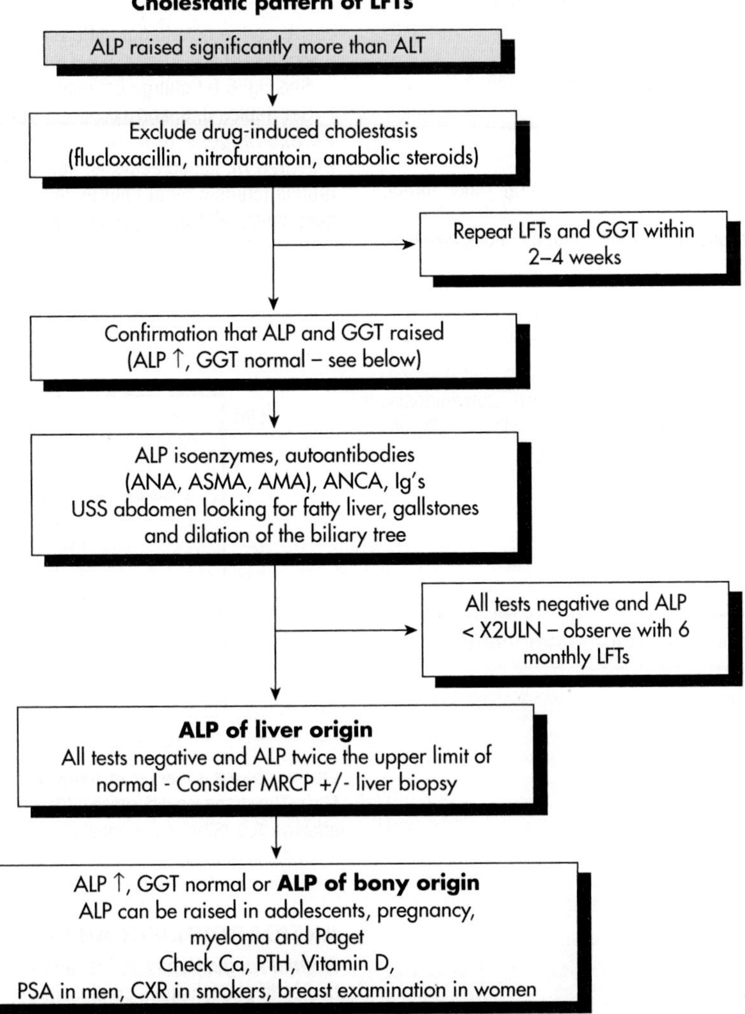

FIG. 3 Investigating a raised ALP in general practice. *ALP,* Alkaline phosphatase; *ALT,* alanine transaminase; *AMA,* antimitochondrial antibody; *ANA,* antinuclear antibody; *ANCA,* antineutrophil cytoplasmic antibody; *ASMA,* anti–smooth muscle antibody; *Ca,* calcium; *CXR,* chest x-ray; *GGT,* γ-glutamyl transpeptidase; *LFT,* liver function test; *MRCP,* magnetic resonance cholangiopancreatography; *PSA,* prostate-specific antigen; *PTH,* parathyroid hormone; *ULN,* upper limit of normal. (From Fillit HM: *Brocklehurst's textbook of geriatric medicine and gerontology*, ed 8, Philadelphia, 2017, Elsevier.)

AMINOLEVULINIC ACID (δ-ALA) (24-hr urine collection)

Normal: 1.5-7.5 mg/day
Elevated in: Acute porphyrias, lead poisoning, DKA, pregnancy, anticonvulsant drugs, hereditary tyrosinemia
Decreased in: Alcoholic liver disease

AMMONIA (serum)

See Box 1 for differential diagnosis of hyperammonemia.

See Fig. E5 for approach to hyperammonemia in pediatric patients.

Normal range: 10-80 μg/dl (5-50 μmol/L [CF: 0.5872; SMI:5 μmol/L])
Elevated in: Hepatic failure, hepatic encephalopathy, Reye syndrome, portacaval shunt, drugs (diuretics, polymyxin B, methicillin)
Decreased in: Drugs (neomycin, lactulose, tetracycline), renal failure

AMYLASE (serum)

Normal range: 0-130 U/L (0-2.17 μkat/L [CF: 0.01667; SMI: 0.01 μkat/L])
Elevated in: Acute pancreatitis, pancreatic neoplasm, abscess, pseudocyst, ascites, macroamylasemia, perforated peptic ulcer, intestinal obstruction, intestinal infarction, acute cholecystitis, appendicitis, ruptured ectopic pregnancy, salivary gland inflammation, peritonitis, burns, diabetic ketoacidosis, renal insufficiency, drugs (morphine), carcinomatosis (of lung, esophagus, ovary), acute ethanol ingestion, mumps, prostate tumors, post-endoscopic retrograde cholangiopancreatography, bulimia, anorexia nervosa
Decreased in: Advanced chronic pancreatitis, hepatic necrosis, cystic fibrosis

AMYLASE, URINE

See URINE AMYLASE

AMYLOID A PROTEIN (serum)

Normal: <10 mcg/ml
Elevated in: Inflammatory disorders (acute phase–reacting protein), infections, acute coronary syndrome, malignancies

ANA

See ANTINUCLEAR ANTIBODY

ANCA

See ANTINEUTROPHIL CYTOPLASMIC ANTIBODY

ANDROSTENEDIONE (serum)

Normal:
Male: 75-205 ng/dl
Female: 85-275 ng/dl

Elevated in: Congenital adrenal hyperplasia, polycystic ovary syndrome, ectopic ACTH-producing tumor, Cushing's syndrome, hirsutism, hyperplasia of ovarian stroma, ovarian neoplasm
Decreased in: Ovarian failure, adrenal failure, sickle cell anemia

ANGIOTENSIN II

Normal: 10-60 pg/ml
Elevated in: Hypertension, CHF, cirrhosis, renin-secreting renal tumor, volume depletion
Decreased in: ACE inhibitor drugs, ARB drugs, primary aldosteronism, Cushing's syndrome

ANGIOTENSIN-CONVERTING ENZYME (ACE level)

Normal range: <40 nmol/ml/min (<670 nkat/L [CF: 16.67; SMI: 10 nkat/L])
Elevated in: Sarcoidosis, primary biliary cirrhosis, alcoholic liver disease, hyperthyroidism, hyperparathyroidism, diabetes mellitus, amyloidosis, multiple myeloma, lung disease (asbestosis, silicosis, berylliosis, allergic alveolitis, coccidioidomycosis), Gaucher disease, leprosy

ANH

See ATRIAL NATRIURETIC HORMONE

BOX 1 Differential Diagnosis of Hyperammonemia

- Acute liver failure
- Chronic kidney disease
- Cigarette smoking
- Cirrhosis
- GI bleeding
- Inborn errors of metabolism
  - Proline metabolism disorders
  - Urea cycle defects (e.g., carbamoyl phosphate synthetase I deficiency, ornithine transcarbamylase deficiency, argininosuccinate lyase deficiency, *N*-acetylglutamate synthetase deficiency)
- Medications/toxins
  - Alcohol
  - Diuretics (e.g., acetazolamide)
  - Narcotics
  - Valproic acid
- Muscle exertion and ischemia
- Portosystemic shunts
- Technique and conditions of blood sampling
  - High body temperature
  - High-protein diet
- Tourniquet use

From Feldman M, Friedman LS, Brandt LJ: *Sleisenger and Fortran's gastrointestinal and liver disease*, ed 10, Philadelphia, 2016, Elsevier.

ANION GAP

The AG is the net change difference between the cations Na^+, K^+, and the anions Cl^- and HCO_3^-

See Fig. 6 for charge balance in blood plasma.

See Tables 8, 9, and 10.

Normal range: 9-14 mEq/L
Elevated in: Lactic acidosis, ketoacidosis (diabetes, alcoholic starvation), uremia (chronic renal failure), ingestion of toxins (paraldehyde, methanol, salicylates, ethylene glycol), hyperosmolar nonketotic coma, antibiotics (carbenicillin)
Decreased in: Hypoalbuminemia, severe hypermagnesemia, IgG myeloma, lithium toxicity, laboratory error (falsely decreased sodium or overestimation of bicarbonate or chloride), hypercalcemia of parathyroid origin, antibiotics (e.g., polymyxin)

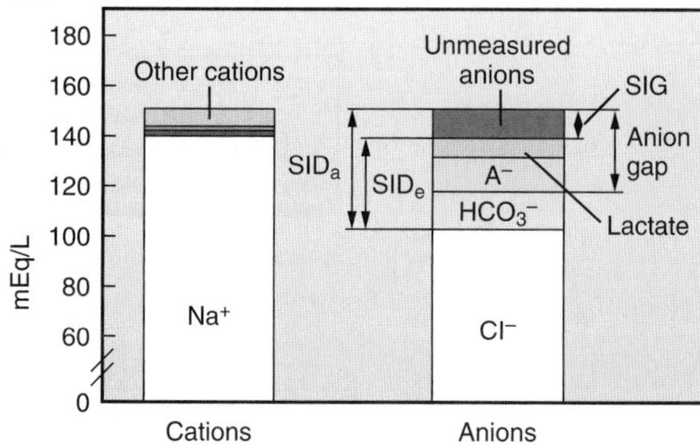

FIG. 6 Charge balance in blood plasma. "Other cations" include Ca^{2+} and Mg^{2+}. The strong ion difference (SID) is always positive (in plasma) and SID minus effective SID (SIDe) must equal 0. Any difference between SID apparent (SIDa) and SIDe is the strong ion gap (SIG) and must represent unmeasured anions. A^-, Concentration of dissociated weak acids; HCO_3^-, bicarbonate.

ANTICARDIOLIPIN ANTIBODY (ACA)

Normal range: Negative. Test includes detection of IgG, IgM, and IgA antibodies to phospholipid, cardiolipin
Present in: Antiphospholipid antibody syndrome, chronic hepatitis C

ANTICOAGULANT

See CIRCULATING ANTICOAGULANT

ANTIDIURETIC HORMONE

Normal range: mOsm/kg 295-300 (4-12 pg/ml)
Elevated in: SIADH, antipsychotic medications, ectopic ADH from systemic neoplasm, Guillain-Barré syndrome, CNS infections, brain tumors, nephrogenic diabetes insipidus

Table 8 Equations Used to Estimate the Quantity of Unmeasured Ions

Anion gap (AG)	$(Na^+ + K^+) - (Cl^- + HCO^-_3)$	Normal values: 12 ± mEq/L (with K^+) 8 ± 4 mEq/L (without K^+)
Connected anion gap (cAG)	$(Na^+ + K^+) - (Cl^- + HCO^-_3$ + 2[*albumin g/dL*] + 0.5[*phosphate mg/dL*] + *lactate*) SI (all units mEq/L): $(Na^+ + K^+) - (Cl^- + HCO^-_3$ + 0.2[*albumin g/L*] + 1.5[*phosphate mmol/L*] + *lactate*)	Normal values: 0 ± 5 mEq/L
Apparent strong ion different (SID_a)	$(Na^+ + K^+ + Ca^{2+} + Mg^{2+}) - (Cl^- + lactate)$	The difference between measured strong cations and anions. Concentrations should be expressed in mEq/L (Ca^{2+} and Mg^{2+} multiplied by 2 from mmol/L).
Effective strong ion difference (SID_e)	$(HCO^-_3$ + [albumin g/dL] × (0.123 × *pH* − 0.631) + $[PO^{2-}_4]$ × (0.39 × *pH* − 0.469)	
Strong ion gap (SIG)	$SID_a - SID_e$	Should theoretically approach 0, but is normally 5 (±5) in critically ill patients
$\Delta AG/\Delta HCO^-_3$ (delta ratio)	$(cAG - cAG_{normal})/(24 - HCO^-_3)$	Normal values 0.8 to 1.6
Osmolar gap	*measured osmolality* − ([1.86 × Na^+] + *glucose mg/dL*/18 + *BUN mg/dL*/2.8 + *ethanol mg/dL*/4.6) SI (all units mmol/L): *measured osmolality* − ([1.86 × Na^+] + *glucose* + *urea* + 1.25 × *ethanol*)	Normally ≤ 19 mmol/L

Ronco C et al: *Critical care nephrology*, ed 3, Philadelphia, 2019, Elsevier.

Decreased in: Central diabetes insipidus, nephritic syndrome, psychogenic polydipsias, demeclocycline, lithium, phenytoin, alcohol. Table 11 describes the water deprivation test used for diagnosing and classifying diabetes insipidus. Table 12 summarizes tests in the differential diagnosis of water homeostasis. Causes of polyuria due to water diuresis are described in Box 2.

TABLE 9 Causes of Increased Anion Gap or Strong Ion Gap

Common causes	Lactic acidosis*
	L-lactate (hypoxic and nonhypoxic)
	D-lactate (in short bowel syndrome)
	Renal failure
	Ketoacidosis
	Diabetic
	Alcoholic
	Starvation
	Metabolic errors
	Toxins
	Methanol
	Ethylene and propylene glycol
	Salicylates
	5-oxoproline (pyroglutamic acid)
	Sepsis
Rare causes	Severe liver disease
	Sodium salts
	Sodium lactate
	Sodium citrate
	Sodium acetate
	Sodium penicillin (>50 million units/day)
	Carbenicillin (>30 g/day)
	Decreased unmeasured cations
	Hypomagnesemia
	Hypocalcemia
	Massive rhabdomyolysis
	Alkalemia

*Lactate, Mg^{2+}, and Ca^{2+} are accounted for in the strong ion gap. From Ronco C: *Critical care nephrology*, ed 3, Philadelphia, 2019, Elsevier.

TABLE 10 Causes of Normal Anion Gap or Strong Ion Gap Acidosis

Nonrenal causes: urine SID (Na + K − Cl) < 0	Low SID infusions (e.g., normal saline)
	Strong cation (or HCO_3^-) losses though diarrhea
	Ureteral diversions
	Biliary or pancreatic fistulas
Renal causes: urine SID (Na + K − Cl) >0	Type 1 (distal) RTA
	Type 2 (proximal) RTA
	Type 4 (hypoaldosteronism) RTA

RTA, Renal tubular acidosis; *SID,* strong ion difference.
From Ronco C: *Critical care nephrology*, ed 3, Philadelphia, 2019, Elsevier.

ANTI-DNA

Normal range: Absent
Present in: Systemic lupus erythematosus, chronic active hepatitis, infectious mononucleosis, biliary cirrhosis

ANTI-DS DNA

Normal: <25 U
Elevated in: Systemic lupus erythematosus

ANTIGLOBULIN TEST

See COOMBS TEST

ANTIGLOMERULAR BASEMENT ANTIBODY

See GLOMERULAR BASEMENT MEMBRANE ANTIBODY

ANTIHISTONE

Normal: <1 U
Elevated in: Drug-induced lupus erythematosus

ANTIMITOCHONDRIAL ANTIBODY (AMA, Mitochondrial antibody)

Normal range: <1:20 titer
Elevated in: Primary biliary cirrhosis (85%-95%), chronic active hepatitis (25%-30%), cryptogenic cirrhosis (25%-30%)

TABLE 11 Water Deprivation Test for Diagnosing and Classifying Diabetes Insipidus

Patients with mild polyuria may be instructed to withhold all fluid intake from 10 PM onward. For those with more severe polyuria (8 to 10 L/day), water deprivation should be started early in the morning under close observation.

1. During testing, the patient is forbidden to take in anything by mouth.
2. Obtain the following baseline parameters: urine volume (Uvol) and urinary osmolality (Uosm), plasma osmolality (Posm), and plasma sodium (PNa). Also record the weight and blood pressure (BP)/pulse (P) seated and standing.
3. Urine and plasma are collected hourly for Uvol, Uosm, and Posm. Weight, BP, and P are also recorded. Record requests for fluid.
4. When the Uosm has plateaued (e.g., hourly increase <30 mOsm/kg for 3 consecutive hours), or when body weight has decreased by 3% to 5%, or the patient develops a >20-mm Hg drop in systolic BP, obtain samples for Uvol, Uosm, Posm, PNa, and AVP (plasma).
5. Administer 1 mcg of desmopressin IV or IM, or 5 mcg of AVP SC Uosm; urine output and Posm are recorded at 30, 60, and 120 minutes after the injection. The highest Uosm value is used to evaluate the patient's response to AVP.

Precautions

When possible, discontinue any medications that can influence ADH secretion. Observe for hypotension and nausea, which may stimulate ADH secretion. The patient should not be permitted to smoke during the test.

Interpretation

Normal	Final Uosm before AVP challenge is higher than Posm. Following AVP challenge, the Uosm is less than 10% higher than the maximal Uosm achieved with water restriction alone.
Neurogenic DI	Final Uosm before AVP challenge is less than Posm. Following AVP administration, there is a greater than 50% increase in Uosm.
Nephrogenic DI	Final Uosm before AVP challenge is less than Posm. Following AVP administration, there is a less than 10% increase in Uosm.
Partial central DI	Uosm may be higher than Posm following dehydration; however, there is only a 10% to 50% increase in Uosm following administration of AVP.
Partial nephrogenic DI	Uosm may be higher than Posm following dehydration; however, there is a greater than 10% increase in Uosm following administration of AVP.

Plotting basal and postdehydration Uosm and plasma ADH on the nomograms from Zerbe and Robertson will permit further distinction between partial nephrogenic DI, partial central DI, and primary polydipsia

ADH, Antidiuretic hormone; *AVP,* arginine vasopressin; *DI,* diabetes insipidus; *IM,* intramuscular; *IV,* intravenous; *SC,* subcutaneous.
From McPherson RA, Pincus MR: *Henry's clinical diagnosis and management by laboratory methods*, ed 23, St Louis, 2017, Elsevier.

TABLE 12 Tests in the Differential Diagnosis of Disorders of Water Homeostasis

	BASELINE			AFTER 12-HOUR FLUID RESTRICTION			
Disorder	**Serum Na+ and Osmolality**	**Urine Na+ and Osmolality**	**Serum ADH**	**Serum Na+ and Osmolality**	**Urine Na+ and Osmolality**	**Serum ADH**	**Urine Osmolality Post-AVP Challenge**
Normal control	N	N	N	N	High	High	Same
SIADH	Low	N-High	High	Low-N	High	High	—
Neurogenic DI	N-High	Low	Low	High	Low-N	Low	Increased
Nephrogenic DI	N-High	Low	N-High	High	Low-N	High	Same
Psychogenic polydipsia	Low–N	Low	Low	N	N-High	N-High	Same

ADH, Antidiuretic hormone; *AVP,* arginine vasopressin; *DI,* diabetes insipidus; *N,* normal; *SIADH,* syndrome of inappropriate secretion of ADH.
McPherson RA, Pincus MR: *Henry's clinical diagnosis and management by laboratory methods,* ed 23, St Louis, 2017, Elsevier.

BOX 2 Causes of Polyuria Due to Water Diuresis

Lack of ADH
Central diabetes insipidus (DI): congenital or acquired (idiopathic cell degeneration, tumors and granulomas, surgery, trauma, infarction, and infection of the pituitary gland or hypothalamus)
Dipsogenic: psychogenic, organic brain disease, iatrogenic
Gestational DI: Excess vasopressinase

Failure of the Kidney to Respond to ADH (Nephrogenic DI)
Congenital nephrogenic DI: a defect in ADH receptor, a defect in aquaporin expression.
Chronic renal failure.
Acquired nephrogenic DI: lithium toxicity, demeclocycline toxicity, methoxyflurane toxicity, amyloidosis, light chain nephropathy, hypercalcemia, hypokalemia, obstructive uropathy

From McPherson RA, Pincus MR: *Henry's clinical diagnosis and management by laboratory methods*, ed 23, St Louis, 2017, Elsevier.

ANTINEUTROPHIL CYTOPLASMIC ANTIBODY (ANCA)

Positive test: Cytoplasmic pattern (cANCA): positive in granulomatosis with polyangiitis (see Fig. E7 and Table E13 for approach to patient with positive c-ANCA)

Perinuclear pattern (pANCA): Positive in inflammatory bowel disease, primary biliary cirrhosis, primary sclerosing cholangitis, autoimmune chronic active hepatitis, crescentic glomerulonephritis (see Table E13 for approach to patient with positive P-ANCA)

ANTINUCLEAR ANTIBODY (ANA)

Fig. E8 describes an algorithm for the use of antinuclear antibodies in the diagnosis of connective tissue disorders. See Fig. E9 for approach to positive ANA pattern
Normal range: <1:20 titer
Positive test: Systemic lupus erythematosus (more significant if titer >1:160), drugs (phenytoin, ethosuximide, primidone, methyldopa, hydralazine, carbamazepine, penicillin, procainamide, chlorpromazine, griseofulvin, thiazides), chronic active hepatitis, autoimmune thyroid disease (positive ANA is found in up to 45% of patients), idiopathic thrombocytopenic purpura, multiple sclerosis, rheumatoid arthritis, scleroderma, mixed connective tissue disease, necrotizing vasculitis, Sjögren syndrome, tuberculosis, pulmonary interstitial fibrosis. Positive ANA results are nonspecific and can be found in healthy individuals (13.8% of the adult general population). Table 14 describes diseases associated with ANA subtypes. Fig. 10 illustrates various fluorescent ANA test patterns.

ANTI-RNP ANTIBODY

See EXTRACTABLE NUCLEAR ANTIGEN

ANTI-SCL-70

Normal: Absent
Elevated in: Scleroderma

ANTI-SM (anti-Smith) ANTIBODY

See EXTRACTABLE NUCLEAR ANTIGEN

ANTI-SMOOTH MUSCLE ANTIBODY

See SMOOTH MUSCLE ANTIBODY

ANTISTREPTOLYSIN O TITER (Streptozyme, ASLO titer)

Normal range for adults: <160 Todd units
Elevated in: Streptococcal upper airway infection, acute rheumatic fever, acute glomerulonephritis, increased levels of β-lipoprotein
NOTE: A fourfold increase in titer between acute and convalescent specimens is diagnostic of streptococcal upper airway infection regardless of the initial titer.

ANTITHROMBIN III

See Table 15.
Normal range: 81%-120% of normal activity; 17-30 mg/dl
Decreased in: Hereditary deficiency of antithrombin III, disseminated intravascular coagulation, pulmonary embolism, cirrhosis, thrombolytic therapy, chronic liver failure, postsurgery, third trimester of pregnancy, oral contraceptives, nephrotic syndrome, IV heparin >3 days, sepsis, acute leukemia, carcinoma, thrombophlebitis
Elevated in: Warfarin drugs, post-myocardial infarction

APOLIPOPROTEIN A-1 (Apo A-1)

Normal: Desirable >120 mg/dl
Elevated in: Familial hyperalphalipoproteinemia, statins, niacin, estrogens, weight loss, familial cholesteryl ester transfer protein (CETP) deficiency
Decreased in: Familial hypoalphalipoproteinemia, Tangier disease, diuretics, androgens, cigarette smoking, hepatocellular disorders, chronic renal failure, nephritic syndrome, coronary heart disease, cholestasis

APOLIPOPROTEIN B (Apo B)

Normal: Desirable <100 mg/dl; high risk >120 mg/dl
Elevated in: High saturated fat diet, high-cholesterol diet, hyperapobetalipoproteinemia, familial combined hyperlipidemia, anabolic steroids, diuretics, beta-blockers, corticosteroids, progestins, diabetes, hypothyroidism, chronic renal failure, liver disease, Cushing's syndrome, coronary heart disease
Decreased in: Statins, niacin, low-cholesterol diet, malnutrition, abetalipoproteinemia, hypobetalipoproteinemia, hyperthyroidism

ARTERIAL BLOOD GASES

Normal range:
Po_2: 75-100 mm Hg
Pco_2: 35-45 mm Hg
HCO_3: 24-28 mEq/L
pH: 7.35-7.45
Abnormal values: Acid-base disturbances (see the following)
METABOLIC ACIDOSIS
Causes of metabolic acidosis by net acid excretion are summarized in Box 3.
Metabolic acidosis with increased AG (AG acidosis)

TABLE 14 Disease-Associated Anti-Nuclear Antibody Subtypes

Nuclear Location	Disease(s)
"Native" DNA (dsDNA, or dsDNA/ssDNA complex)	SLE (60%-70%; range, 35%-75%) Also PSS (5%-55%), MCTD (11%-25%), RA (5%-40%), DM (5%-25%), SS (5%)
sNP	SLE (50%) Also other collagen diseases
DNP (DNA-histone complex)	SLE (52%) Also MCTD (8%), RA (3%)
Histones	Drug-induced SLE (95%) Also SLE (30%), RA (15%-24%)
ENA Sm	SLE (30%-40%; range, 28%-40%) Also MCTD (0%-8%); RNP (U1-RNP) MCTD (in high titer without any other ANA subtype present: 95%-100%) Also SLE (26%-50%), PSS (11%-22%), RA (10%), SS (3%)
SS-A (Ro)*	SS without RA (60%-70%) Also SLE (26%-50%), neonatal SLE (over 95%), PSS (30%), MCTD (50%), SS with RA (9%), PBC (15%-19%)
SS-B (La)	SS without RA (40%-60%) Also SLE (5%-15%), SS with RA (5%)
Scl-70*	PSS (15%-43%)
Centromere*	CREST syndrome (70%-90%; range, 57%-96%) Also PSS (4%-20%), PBC (12%)
Nucleolar	PSS (scleroderma) (54%-90%) Also SLE (25%-26%), RA (9%)
RAP (RANA)	SS with RA (60%-76%) Also SS without RA (5%)
Jo-1	Polymyositis (30%)
PM-1	Polymyositis or PMS/PSS overlap syndrome (60%-90%) Also DM (17%)
ssDNA	SLE (60%-70%) Also CAH, infectious mononucleosis, RA, chronic GN, chronic infections, PBC
Cytoplasmic Location	Disease(s)
Mitochondrial	PBC (90%-100%)Also CAH (7%-30%), cryptogenic cirrhosis (30%), acute hepatitis, viral hepatitis (3%), other liver diseases (0%-20%), SLE (5%), SS and PSS (8%)
Microsomal†	Chronic active hepatitis (60%-80%), Hashimoto thyroiditis (97%)
Ribosomal	SLE (5%-12%)
Smooth muscle‡	Chronic active hepatitis (60%-91%)

CAH, Chronic active hepatitis; *DM,* dermatomyositis; *GN,* glomerulonephritis; *MS,* multiple sclerosis; *PBC,* primary biliary cirrhosis; *SS,* Sjögren syndrome.
*Not detected using rat or mouse liver or kidney tissue method.
†Not detected by cultured cell method.
‡Detected by cultured cells but better with rat or mouse tissue.
From Ravel R: *Clinical laboratory medicine*, ed 6, St Louis, 1995, Mosby.

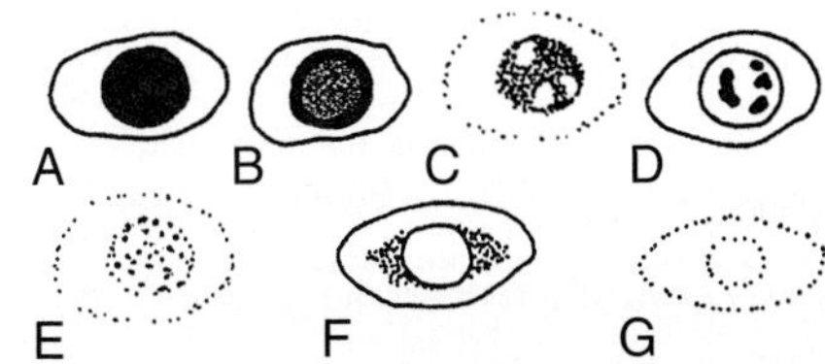

FIG. 10 Fluorescent antinuclear antibody test patterns (HEP-2 cells). **A,** Solid (homogeneous). **B,** Peripheral (rim). **C,** Speckled. **D,** Nucleolar. **E,** Anticentromere. **F,** Antimitochondrial. **G,** Normal (nonreactive). (From Ravel R [ed]: *Clinical laboratory medicine*, ed 6, St Louis, 1995, Mosby.)

Lactic acidosis (see Box 4)
Ketoacidosis (diabetes mellitus, alcoholic ketoacidosis)
Uremia (chronic renal failure)
Ingestion of toxins (paraldehyde, methanol, salicylate, ethylene glycol)
High-fat diet (mild acidosis)

Metabolic acidosis with normal AG (hyperchloremic acidosis)
Renal tubular acidosis (including acidosis of aldosterone deficiency)
Intestinal loss of HCO_3^- (diarrhea, pancreatic fistula)
Carbonic anhydrase inhibitors (e.g., acetazolamide)
Dilutional acidosis (as a result of rapid infusion of bicarbonate-free isotonic saline)
Ingestion of exogenous acids (ammonium chloride, methionine, cystine, calcium chloride)

TABLE 15 Assay Measurements in Heterozygous Antithrombin (ATIII) Deficiency for Diagnosis

	ACTIVITY		
Type	Antigen	Heparin Cofactor	Progressive ATIII
I	Low	Low	Low
II			
Active site defect	Normal	Low	Low
Heparin-binding site defect	Normal	Low	Normal

From Hoffman R et al: *Hematology: basic principles and practice,* ed 5, Philadelphia, 2009, Churchill Livingstone.

BOX 3 Causes of Metabolic Acidosis by Net Acid Excretion

Renal Acidosis: Absolute or Relative Reduction in Net Acid Excretion
Uremic acidosis
Renal tubular acidosis
- Distal renal tubular acidosis (type I)
- Proximal renal tubular acidosis (type II)
- Aldosterone deficiency or unresponsiveness (type IV)

Extrarenal Acidosis: Increase in Net Acid Excretion
Gastrointestinal loss of bicarbonate
Ingestion of acids or acid precursors: ammonium chloride, sulfur-containing compounds
Acid precursors or toxins: salicylate, ethylene glycol, methanol, toluene, acetaminophen, paraldehyde
Organic acidosis
- L-lactic acidosis
- D-lactic acidosis
- Ketoacidosis
- Pyroglutamic acidosis

From McPherson RA, Pincus MR: *Henry's clinical diagnosis and management by laboratory methods*, ed 23, St Louis, 2017, Elsevier.

BOX 4 Causes of L-Lactic Acidosis

Type A Lactic Acidosis Due to Tissue Hypoxia
Circulatory shock
Severe hypoxemia
Heart failure
Severe anemia
Grand mal seizure

Type B Lactic Acidosis, No Tissue Hypoxia
Acute alcoholism
Drugs and toxins (e.g., metformin, antiretroviral drugs, salicylate intoxication)
Diabetes mellitus
Leukemia
Deficiency of thiamin or riboflavin
Idiopathic

From McPherson RA, Pincus MR: *Henry's clinical diagnosis and management by laboratory methods,* ed 23, St Louis, 2017, Elsevier.

Ileostomy
Ureterosigmoidostomy
Drugs: amiloride, triamterene, spironolactone, β-blockers
RESPIRATORY ACIDOSIS
Pulmonary disease (COPD, severe pneumonia, pulmonary edema, interstitial fibrosis)
Airway obstruction (foreign body, severe bronchospasm, laryngospasm)
Thoracic cage disorders (pneumothorax, flail chest, kyphoscoliosis)
Defects in muscles of respiration (myasthenia gravis, hypokalemia, muscular dystrophy)
Defects in peripheral nervous system (amyotrophic lateral sclerosis, poliomyelitis, Guillain-Barré syndrome, botulism, tetanus, organophosphate poisoning, spinal cord injury)
Depression of respiratory center (anesthesia, narcotics, sedatives, vertebral artery embolism or thrombosis, increased intracranial pressure)
Failure of mechanical ventilator
METABOLIC ALKALOSIS. Divided into chloride-responsive (urinary chloride <15 meq/l) and chloride-resistant forms (urinary chloride level >15 meq/l)
Chloride-responsive
Vomiting
Nasogastric (NG) suction
Diuretics
Posthypercapnic alkalosis
Stool losses (laxative abuse, cystic fibrosis, villous adenoma)
Massive blood transfusion
Exogenous alkali administration
Chloride-resistant
Hyperadrenocorticoid states (Cushing's syndrome, primary hyperaldosteronism, secondary mineralocorticoidism [licorice, chewing tobacco])
Hypomagnesemia
Hypokalemia
Bartter's syndrome
RESPIRATORY ALKALOSIS
Hypoxemia (pneumonia, pulmonary embolism, atelectasis, high-altitude living)
Drugs (salicylates, xanthines, progesterone, epinephrine, thyroxine, nicotine)
Central nervous system (CNS) disorders (tumor, cerebrovascular accident [CVA], trauma, infections)
Psychogenic hyperventilation (anxiety, hysteria)
Hepatic encephalopathy
Gram-negative sepsis
Hyponatremia
Sudden recovery from metabolic acidosis
Assisted ventilation

ARTHROCENTESIS FLUID

Reference intervals for synovial fluid constituents are described in Table 16.

Interpretation of results:

1. **Color:** Normally it is clear or pale yellow; cloudiness indicates inflammatory process or presence of crystals, cell debris, fibrin, or triglycerides.
2. **Viscosity:** Normally it has a high viscosity because of hyaluronate; when fluid is placed on a slide, it can be stretched to a string >2 cm in length before separating (low viscosity indicates breakdown of hyaluronate [lysosomal enzymes from leukocytes] or the presence of edema fluid).
3. **Mucin clot:** Add 1 ml of fluid to 5 ml of a 5% acetic acid solution and allow 1 minute for the clot to form; a firm clot (does not fragment on shaking) is normal and indicates the presence of large molecules of hyaluronic acid (this test is nonspecific and infrequently done).
4. **Glucose:** Normally it approximately equals serum glucose level; a difference of more than 40 mg/dl is suggestive of infection.
5. **Protein:** Total protein concentration is <2.5 g/dl in the normal synovial fluid; it is elevated in inflammatory and septic arthritis.

TABLE 16 Reference Intervals for Synovial Fluid Constituents

Constituent	Synovial Fluid	Plasma
Total protein	1-3 g/dL	6-8 g/dL
Albumin	55%-70%	50%-65%
α1-Globulin	6%-8%	3%-5%
α2-Globulin	5%-7%	7%-13%
β-Globulin	8%-10%	8%-14%
γ-Globulin	10%-14%	12%-22%
Hyaluronic acid	0.3-0.4 g/dL	
Glucose	70-110 mg/dL	70-110 mg/dL
Uric acid	2-8 mg/dL	2-8 mg/dL
Lactate	9-29 mg/dL	9-29 mg/dL

Modified from Kjeldsberg CR, Knight JA: *Body fluids: laboratory examination of amniotic, cerebrospinal, seminal, serous and synovial fluids,* ed 3, Chicago, 1993, © American Society for Clinical Pathology, with permission.
McPherson RA, Pincus MR: *Henry's clinical diagnosis and management by laboratory methods,* ed 23, 2017, Elsevier

6. Microscopic examination for crystals
   a. **Gout:** Monosodium urate crystals
   b. **Pseudogout:** Calcium pyrophosphate dihydrate crystals

ASLO TITER

See ANTISTREPTOLYSIN O TITER

ASPARTATE AMINOTRANSFERASE (AST, SGOT)

Normal range: 0-35 U/L (0-0.58 μkat/L [CF: 0.01667, SMI: 0.01 μkat/L])
Elevated in:
HEART
Acute myocardial infarction
Pericarditis (active: some cases)
LIVER
Hepatitis virus, Epstein-Barr, or cytomegalovirus infection
Active cirrhosis
Liver passive congestion or hypoxia
Alcohol- or drug-induced liver dysfunction
Space-occupying lesions (active)
Fatty liver (severe)
Extrahepatic biliary obstruction (early)
Drug-induced
SKELETAL MUSCLE
Acute skeletal muscle injury
Muscle inflammation (infectious or noninfectious)
Muscular dystrophy (active)
Recent surgery
Delirium tremens
KIDNEY
Acute injury or damage
Renal infarct
OTHER
Intestinal infarction
Shock
Cholecystitis
Acute pancreatitis
Hypothyroidism
Heparin therapy (60%-80% of cases)
Fig. 1 describes an approach to the evaluation of AST elevation.
Box 5 describes causes of elevated serum aminotransferase levels.

ATRIAL NATRIURETIC HORMONE (ANH)

Normal: 20-77 pg/ml
Elevated in: CHF, volume overload, cardiovascular disease with high filling pressure
Decreased with: Prazosin and other alpha blockers

BOX 5 Causes of Elevated Serum Aminotransferase Levels*

Chronic, Mild Elevations, ALT > AST (<150 U/L or 5 × normal)

Hepatic Causes
α_1-Antitrypsin deficiency
Autoimmune hepatitis
Chronic viral hepatitis (B, C, and D)
Hemochromatosis
Medications and toxins
Steatosis and steatohepatitis
Wilson disease

Nonhepatic Causes
Celiac disease
Hyperthyroidism

Severe, Acute Elevations, ALT > AST (>1000 U/L or >20-25 × normal)

Hepatic Causes
Acute bile duct obstruction
Acute Budd-Chiari syndrome
Acute viral hepatitis
Autoimmune hepatitis
Drugs and toxins
Hepatic artery ligation
Ischemic hepatitis
Wilson disease

Severe, Acute Elevations, AST > ALT (>1000 U/L or >20-25 × normal)

Hepatic Cause
Medications or toxins in a patient with underlying alcoholic liver injury

Nonhepatic Cause
Acute rhabdomyolysis

Chronic, Mild Elevations, AST > ALT (<150 U/L, <5 × normal)

Hepatic Causes
Alcohol-related liver injury (AST/ALT > 2:1, AST nearly always <300 U/L)
Cirrhosis

Nonhepatic Causes
Hypothyroidism
Macro-AST
Myopathy
Strenuous exercise

*Virtually any liver disease can cause moderate aminotransferase elevations (5-15 × normal).
From Feldman M, Friedman LS, Brandt LJ: *Sleisenger and Fortran's gastrointestinal and liver disease*, ed 10, Philadelphia, 2016, Elsevier.

B-TYPE NATRIURETIC PEPTIDE (BNP)

Normal range: up to 100 mcg/L. Natriuretic peptides are secreted to regulate fluid volume, blood pressure, and electrolyte balance. They have activity in both the central and peripheral nervous systems. In humans the main source of circulatory BNP is the heart ventricles.
Elevated in: Heart failure. This test is useful to differentiate heart failure patients from those with chronic obstructive pulmonary disease presenting with dyspnea. Levels are also increased in asymptomatic left ventricular dysfunction, arterial and pulmonary hypertension, cardiac hypertrophy, valvular heart disease, arrhythmia, and acute coronary syndrome. See Fig. 11.

BASOPHIL COUNT

Normal range:
a. 0.4%-1% of total WBC; 40-100/mm^3
Elevated in: Leukemia, inflammatory processes, polycythemia vera, Hodgkin's lymphoma, hemolytic anemia, after splenectomy, myeloid metaplasia, myxedema
Decreased in: Stress, hypersensitivity reaction, steroids, pregnancy, hyperthyroidism, postirradiation

BICARBONATE

Normal:
- Arterial: 21-28 mEq/L
- Venous: 22-29 mEq/L

Elevated in: Metabolic alkalosis, compensated respiratory acidosis, diuretics, corticosteroids, laxative abuse
Decreased in: Metabolic acidosis, compensated respiratory alkalosis, acetazolamide, cyclosporine, cholestyramine, methanol or ethylene glycol poisoning

BILE, URINE

See URINE BILE

BILIRUBIN, DIRECT (conjugated bilirubin)

Normal range: 0-0.2 mg/dl (0-4 μmol/L [CF: 17.10; SMI: 2 μmol/L])
Elevated in: Hepatocellular disease, biliary obstruction, drug-induced cholestasis, hereditary disorders (Dubin-Johnson syndrome, Rotor syndrome)

BILIRUBIN, INDIRECT (unconjugated bilirubin)

Normal range:
0-1.0 mg/dl (2-18 μmol/L [CF: 17.10; SMI: 2 μmol/L])
Elevated in:
Increased bilirubin production (if normal liver, serum unconjugated bilirubin is usually less than 4 mg/100 ml)
- Hemolytic anemia
  - Acquired
  - Congenital
- Resorption from extravascular sources
  - Hematomas
  - Pulmonary infarcts
- Excessive ineffective erythropoiesis
  - Congenital (congenital dyserythropoietic anemias)
  - Acquired (pernicious anemia, severe lead poisoning; if present, bilirubinemia is usually mild)

Defective hepatic unconjugated bilirubin clearance (defective uptake or conjugation)
- Severe liver disease
- Gilbert syndrome
- Crigler-Najjar type I or II
- Drug-induced inhibition
- Portacaval shunt
- Congestive heart failure
- Hyperthyroidism (uncommon)

BILIRUBIN, TOTAL

See Fig. 12 and Table 17, for evaluation of hyperbilirubinemia and liver disease.
Normal range:
0-1.0 mg/dl (2-18 μmol/L [CF: 17.10, SMI: 2 μmol/L])
Elevated in: Liver disease (hepatitis, cirrhosis, cholangitis, neoplasm, biliary obstruction, infectious mononucleosis), hereditary disorders (Gilbert disease, Dubin-Johnson syndrome), drugs (steroids, statins, niacin, acetaminophen, diphenylhydantoin, phenothiazines, penicillin, erythromycin, clindamycin, captopril, amphotericin B, sulfonamides, azathioprine, isoniazid, 5-aminosalicylic acid, allopurinol, methyldopa, indomethacin, halothane, oral contraceptives, procainamide, tolbutamide, labetalol), hemolysis, pulmonary embolism or infarct, hepatic congestion secondary to congestive heart failure

BILIRUBIN, URINE

See URINE BILE

BLADDER TUMOR ASSOCIATED ANTIGEN

Normal:
≤14 U/ml. Test is used to detect bladder cancer recurrence. Sensitivity 57%-83% and specificity 68%-72%.
Elevated in: Bladder cancer, renal stones, nephritis, UTI, hematuria, renal cancer, cystitis, recent bladder or urinary tract trauma

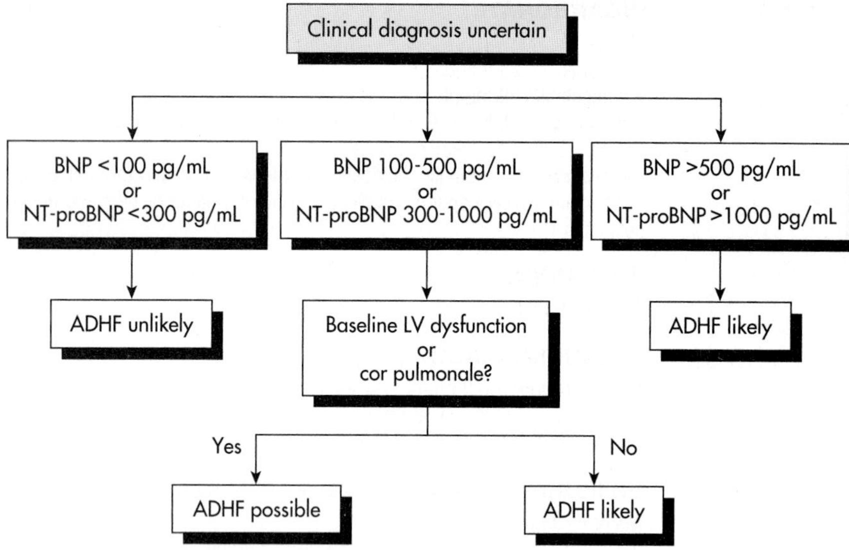

FIG. 11 Interpretation of natriuretic peptide levels. *ADHF,* Acute decompensated heart failure; *BNP,* B-type natriuretic peptide; *NT-proBNP,* inactive N-terminal fragment of BNP. (From Adams JG et al: *Emergency medicine, clinical essentials,* ed 2, Philadelphia, 2013, Elsevier.)

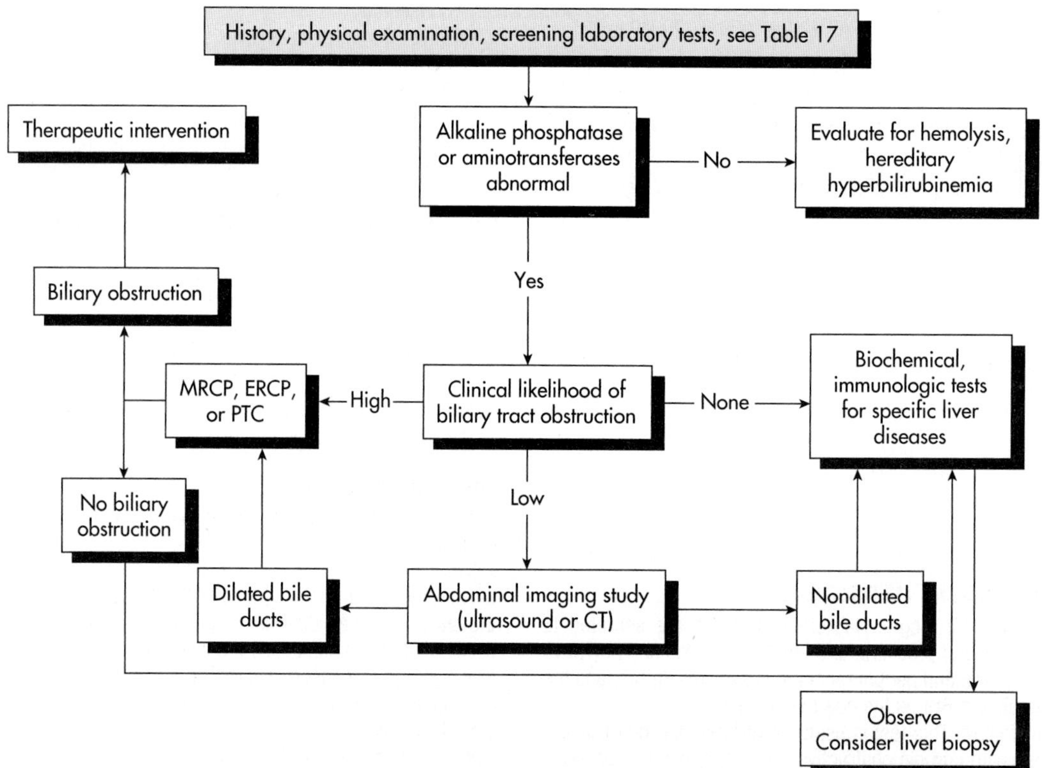

FIG. 12 Diagnosis algorithm for the evaluation of hyperbilirubinemia and other liver test abnormalities and/or signs and symptoms suggestive of liver disease. *CT,* Computed tomography; *ERCP,* endoscopic retrograde cholangiopancreatography; *MRCP,* magnetic resonance cholangiopancreatography; *PTC,* percutaneous cholangiogram. (From Goldman L, Ausiello D [eds]: *Cecil textbook of medicine,* ed 24, Philadelphia, 2012, Saunders. Modified and updated from Lidofsky SD, Scharschmidt BF: Jaundice. In Feldman M, Scharschmidt BF, Sleisenger MH [eds]: *Gastrointestinal and liver disease,* ed 6, Philadelphia, 1998, Saunders.)

TABLE 17 Obstructive Jaundice versus Cholestatic Liver Disease

Feature	Suggests Obstructive Jaundice	Suggests Parenchymal Liver Disease
History	Abdominal pain; fever, rigors; prior biliary surgery; older age; acholic stools	Anorexia, malaise, myalgias, suggestive of viral prodrome; known infectious exposure; receipt of blood products, use of intravenous drugs; exposure to known hepatotoxin; family history of jaundice
Physical examination	High fever; abdominal tenderness; palpable abdominal mass; abdominal scar	Ascites; other stigmata of liver disease (e.g., prominent abdominal veins, gynecomastia, spider angiomata, asterixis, encephalopathy, Kayser-Fleischer rings)
Laboratory studies	Predominant elevation of serum bilirubin and alkaline phosphatase; prothrombin time that is normal or normalizes with vitamin K administration; elevated serum amylase	Predominant elevation of serum aminotransferases; prolonged prothrombin time that does not correct with vitamin K administration; blood tests indicative of specific liver disease

From Goldman L, Ausiello D (eds): *Cecil textbook of medicine,* ed 24, Philadelphia, 2012, Saunders.

BLEEDING TIME (modified Ivy method)

See Fig. E13 for evaluation of patients with prolonged bleeding time.
Normal range: 2 to 9.5 min
Elevated in: Thrombocytopenia, capillary wall abnormalities, platelet abnormalities (Bernard-Soulier disease, Glanzmann disease), drugs (aspirin, warfarin, antiinflammatory medications, streptokinase, urokinase, dextran, β-lactam antibiotics, moxalactam), disseminated intravascular coagulation, cirrhosis, uremia, myeloproliferative disorders, von Willebrand's disease.

Bleeding time tests are no longer performed at many hospitals and have been replaced by the platelet function analyzer (PFA-100) assay.

BLOOD VOLUME, TOTAL

Normal: 60-80 ml/kg
Elevated in: Polycythemia vera, pulmonary disease, CHF, renal insufficiency, pregnancy, acidosis, thyrotoxicosis
Decreased in: Anemia, hemorrhage, vomiting, diarrhea, dehydration, burns, starvation

BNP

See B-TYPE NATRIURETIC PEPTIDE

BORDETELLA PERTUSSIS SEROLOGY

Test description: PCR of nasopharyngeal aspirates or secretions is used to identify *Bordetella pertussis,* the organism responsible for whooping cough.

BRCA ANALYSIS

DESCRIPTION OF ANALYSIS

Comprehensive BRCA analysis:

BRCA1: Full sequence determination in both forward and reverse directions of approximately 5500 base pairs comprising 22 coding exons and one noncoding exon (exon 4) and approximately 800 adjacent base pairs in the noncoding intervening sequence (intron). Exon 1, which is noncoding, is not analyzed. The wild-type *BRCA1* gene encodes a protein comprising 1863 amino acids.

BRCA2: Full sequence determination in both forward and reverse directions of approximately 10,200 base pairs comprising 26 coding exons and approximately 900 adjacent base pairs in the noncoding intervening sequence (intron). Exon 1, which is noncoding, is not analyzed. The wild-type *BRCA2* gene encodes a protein comprising 3418 amino acids.

The noncoding intronic regions of *BRCA1* and *BRCA2* that are analyzed do not extend more than 20 base pairs proximal to the 5' end and 10 base pairs distal to the 3' end of each exon.

Single-site BRCA analysis: DNA sequence analysis for a specified mutation in *BRCA1* and/or *BRCA2.*

Multisite 3 BRCA analysis: DNA sequence analysis of specific portions of *BRCA1* exon 2, *BRCA1* exon 20, and *BRCA2* exon 11 designed to detect only mutations 187delAG and 5385insC in *BRCA1* and 6174delT in *BRCA2.*

Interpretive Criteria:

"Positive for a deleterious mutation": Includes all mutations (nonsense, insertions, deletions) that prematurely terminate ("truncate") the protein product of *BRCA1* at least 10 amino acids from the C-terminus, or the protein product of *BRCA2* at least 110 amino acids from the C-terminus (based on documentation of deleterious mutations in *BRCA1* and *BRCA2*).

In addition, specific missense mutations and noncoding intervening sequence (IVS) mutations are recognized as deleterious on the basis of data derived from linkage analysis of high-risk families, functional assays, biochemical evidence, and/or demonstration of abnormal mRNA transcript processing.

"Genetic variant, suspected deleterious": Includes genetic variants for which the available evidence indicates a likelihood, but not proof, that the mutation is deleterious. The specific evidence supporting such an interpretation will be summarized for individual variants on each such report.

"Genetic variant, favor polymorphism": Includes genetic variants for which available evidence indicates that the variant is highly unlikely to contribute substantially to cancer risk. The specific evidence supporting such an interpretation will be summarized for individual variants on each such report.

"Genetic variant of uncertain significance": Includes missense mutations and mutations that occur in analyzed intronic regions whose clinical significance has not yet been determined, as well as chain-terminating mutations that truncate *BRCA1* and *BRCA2* distal to amino acid positions 1853 and 3308, respectively.

"No deleterious mutation detected": Includes nontruncating genetic variants observed at an allele frequency of approximately 1% of a suitable control population (providing that no data suggest clinical significance), as well as all genetic variants for which published data demonstrate absence of substantial clinical significance. Also includes mutations in the protein-coding region that neither alter the amino acid sequence nor are predicted to significantly affect exon splicing, and base pair alterations in noncoding portions of the gene that have been demonstrated to have no deleterious effect on the length or stability of the mRNA transcript.

There may be uncommon genetic abnormalities in *BRCA1* and *BRCA2* that will not be detected by *BRCA* analysis. This analysis, however, is believed to rule out the majority of abnormalities in these genes, which are believed responsible for most hereditary susceptibility to breast and ovarian cancer.

"Specific variant/mutation not identified": Specific and designated deleterious mutations or variants of uncertain clinical significance are not present in the individual being tested. If one (or rarely two) specific deleterious mutations have been identified in a family member, a negative analysis for the specific mutation(s) indicates that the tested individual is at the general population risk of developing breast or ovarian cancer.

BREATH HYDROGEN TEST (hydrogen breath test)

Normal: This test is for bacterial overgrowth. H_2 excretion fasting: 4.6 ± 5.1, after lactulose, early increase <12. Lactulose usually results in a colonic response >30 min after ingestion.
Elevated in: A high fasting breath H_2 level and an increase of at least 12 ppm within 30 min after lactulose challenge are indicative of bacterial overgrowth in the small intestine. The increase must precede the colonic response.

False positives in: Accelerated gastric emptying, laxative use
False negatives in: Use of antibiotics and patients who are nonhydrogen producers

BUN

See UREA NITROGEN, BLOOD

C282Y AND H63D MUTATION ANALYSIS

Procedure: Detection of the C282Y and H63D mutations is accomplished by amplification of exons 2 and 4 of the *HFE* gene on chromosome 6 by polymerase chain reaction (PCR) followed by allele-specific hybridization and chemiluminescent detection of hybridized probes. H63D is viewed by some as a polymorphism rather than a mutation because of its prevalence in the population, because 15% of the individuals affected with hereditary hemochromatosis (HH) are compound heterozygotes for C282Y and H63D and about 1% of patients are H63D homozygotes, which suggests that H63D may be causative in the development of the disorder at reduced penetrance.
Interpretation: Homozygosity for the C282Y mutation has been associated with an increased risk of being affected with HH compared with the general population. The genotype is observed in 60%-90% of individuals affected with HH and occurs in less than 1% of the general population. However, approximately 25% of asymptomatic individuals with this genotype do not develop the disorder.

C3

See COMPLEMENT

C4

See COMPLEMENT

CALCITONIN (serum)

Normal range: <100 pg/ml (<100 ng/L [CF: 1; SMI: 10 ng/L])
Elevated in: Medullary carcinoma of the thyroid (particularly if level >1500 pg/ml), carcinoma of the breast, apudomas, carcinoids, renal failure, thyroiditis

CALCIUM (serum)

See Figs. 14 and 15.

Normal range: 8.8-10.3 mg/dl (2.2-2.58 μmol/L [CF: 0.2495; SMI: 0.02 μmol/L])
ELEVATED
Relatively common:
Neoplasia
Bone primary
Myeloma
Acute leukemia
Nonbone solid tumors
Breast
Lung
Squamous nonpulmonary
Kidney
Neoplasm secretion of parathyroid hormone-related protein (PTHrP, "ectopic PTH")
Primary hyperparathyroidism
Thiazide diuretics
Tertiary (renal) hyperparathyroidism
Idiopathic
Spurious (artifactual) hypercalcemia
Dehydration
Serum protein elevation
Laboratory technical problem (lab error)
Relatively uncommon:
Sarcoidosis
Hyperthyroidism
Immobilization (mostly seen in children and adolescents)
Diuretic phase of acute renal tubular necrosis
Vitamin D intoxication
Milk-alkali syndrome
Addison's disease
Lithium therapy
Idiopathic hypercalcemia of infancy
Acromegaly
Theophylline toxicity

Table 18 describes the laboratory differential diagnosis of hypercalcemia.

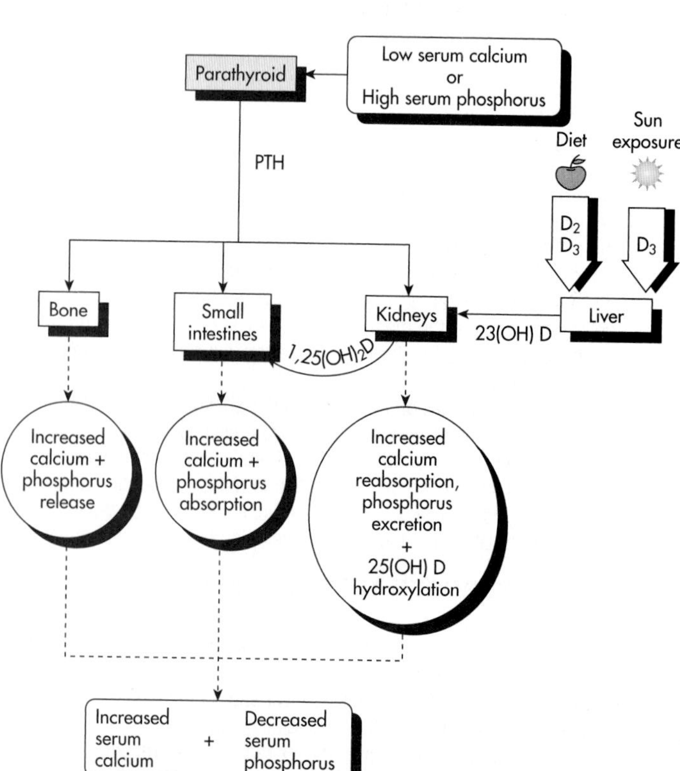

FIG. 14 Calcium homeostasis. Parathyroid hormone (PTH) is released from the parathyroid glands in response to hypocalcemia and hyperphosphatemia. PTH acts on bone, the small intestines, and the kidneys to effect a rise in serum calcium and a net decrease in serum phosphorus. Hydroxylation of inactive forms of vitamin D occurs in the liver and kidneys. 1,25(OH)2D facilitates intestinal absorption of calcium and phosphorus. *1,25(OH)2D*, 1,25-Dihydroxyvitamin D; *25(OH) D*, 25-hydroxyvitamin D; *D2*, vitamin D2; *D3*, vitamin D3. (From Adams JG et al: *Emergency medicine, clinical essentials*, ed 2, Philadelphia, 2013, Elsevier.)

Hypocalcemia
Repeat serum calcium level, check serum albumin level
Low serum calcium, normal albumin
Low serum calcium, low albumin
Serum PTH, phosphate magnesium levels
Hypocalcemia due to low albumin level
Check ionized calcium
Low magnesium
Low PTH
Appropriately elevated PTH
Hypomagnesemia
r/o drug-induced hypocalcemia (e.g., phenytoin, colchicine)
r/o pseudohypoparathyroidism
r/o hypovitaminosis D
Elevated phosphate
Hypoparathyroidism; hypomagnesemia, postparathyroidectomy
Hyperphosphatemia
Normal phosphate
Low serum phosphate
Vitamin D Level 25(OH)D Level
Chronic kidney disease
Rhabdomyolysis
Hyperalimentation
Malabsorption
Malnutrition
Anticonvulsants
Low
Normal
Vitamin D deficiency
1,25(OH)2D Level
Normal
High
Pseudohypoparathyroidism, vitamin D-resistant rickets
Vitamin D-resistant rickets

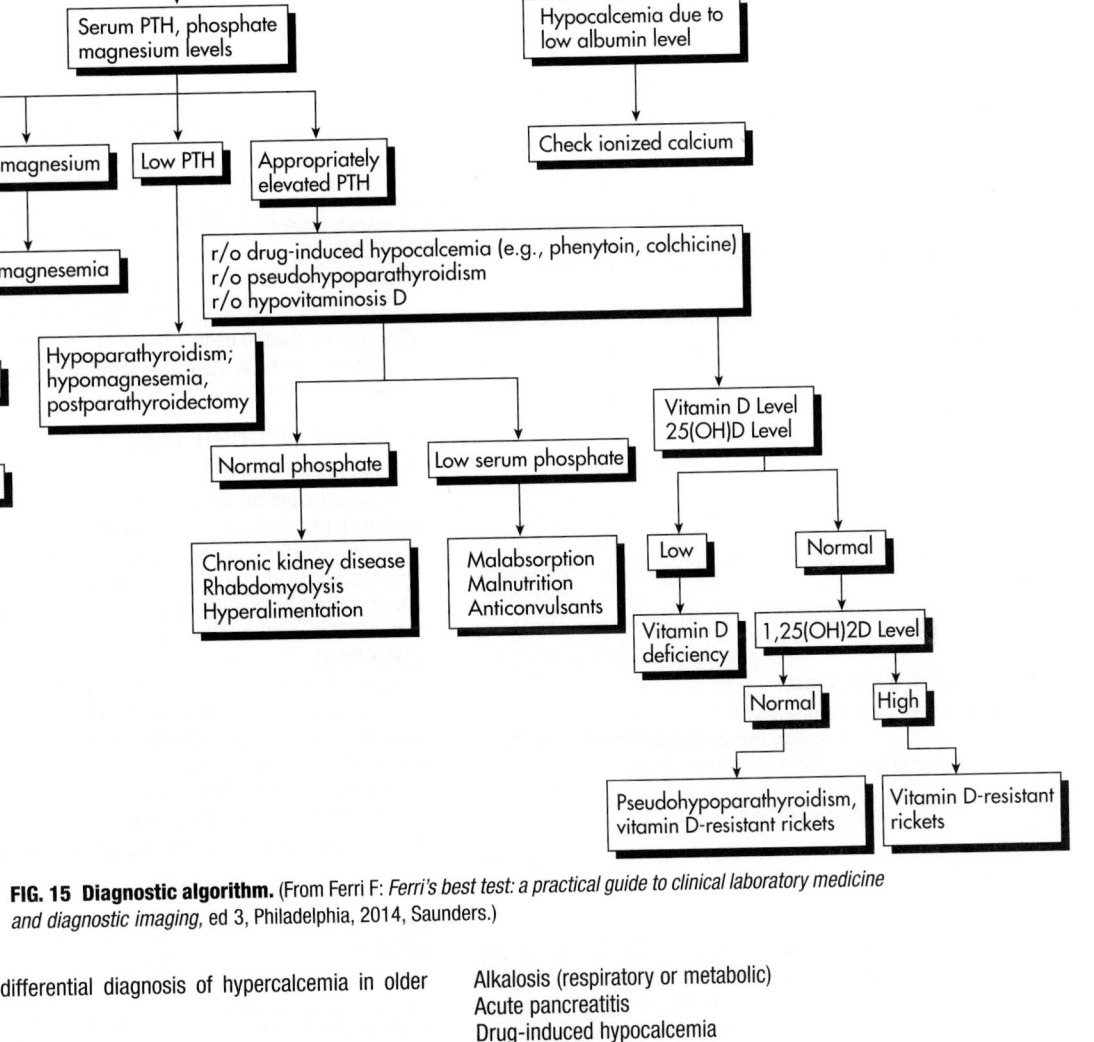

FIG. 15 Diagnostic algorithm. (From Ferri F: *Ferri's best test: a practical guide to clinical laboratory medicine and diagnostic imaging,* ed 3, Philadelphia, 2014, Saunders.)

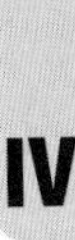

Box 6 describes the differential diagnosis of hypercalcemia in older adults.

DECREASED
Artifactual
Hypoalbuminemia
Hemodilution
Primary hypoparathyroidism
Pseudohypoparathyroidism
Vitamin D related
Vitamin D deficiency
Malabsorption
Renal failure
Magnesium deficiency
Sepsis
Chronic alcoholism
Tumor lysis syndrome
Rhabdomyolysis
Alkalosis (respiratory or metabolic)
Acute pancreatitis
Drug-induced hypocalcemia
Large doses of magnesium sulfate
Anticonvulsants
Mithramycin
Gentamicin
Cimetidine

Table 19 describes the laboratory differential diagnosis of hypocalcemia.

CALCIUM, URINE

See URINE CALCIUM

CANCER ANTIGEN 15-3 (CA 15-3)

Normal: <30 U/ml
Elevated in: Approximately 80% of women with metastatic breast cancer. Clinical sensitivity is 0.60, specificity 0.87, positive predictive value 0.91.

TABLE 18 Laboratory Differential Diagnosis of Hypercalcemia

Diagnosis	PLASMA TESTS					URINE TESTS			Comments
	Ca	PO_4	PTH	25(OH)D	$1,25(OH)_2D$	cAMP	TmP/GFR	Ca	
Primary hyperparathyroidism	↑	N/↓	↑	N	N/↑	↑	↓	↑	Parathyroid adenoma most common
MEN I									Parathyroid hyperplasia; also includes pituitary and pancreatic neoplasms
MEN IIa									Parathyroid hyperplasia; also includes medullary thyroid carcinoma and pheochromocytoma
MEN IIb									Parathyroid disease uncommon, primarily medullary thyroid carcinoma and pheochromocytoma
FHH	↑	N	N/↑	N	N	N/↑	N/↓	↓↓	Autosomal dominant inheritance; hypercalcemia present within first decade; benign
Malignancy									
Solid tumor, humoral	↑	N/↓	↓	N	N	↑	↓	↑↑	Primarily epidermoid tumors; PTH-related protein(s) is mediator
Solid tumor, osteolytic	↑	N/↑	↓	N	N	↓	↑	↑↑	
Lymphoma	↑	N/↑	↓	N/↓	↑	↓	↑	↑↑	
Granulomatous disease	↑	N/↑	↓	N/↓	↑↑	↓	↑	↑↑	Sarcoid most common etiology
Vitamin D intoxication	↑	N/↑	↓	↑↑	N	↓	↑	↑↑	
Hyperthyroidism	↑	N	↓	N	N	N	N	↑↑	Plasma concentrations of T_4 and/or T_3 are elevated

Ca, Calcium; *cAMP,* cyclic adenosine monophosphate; *FHH,* familial hypocalciuric hypercalcemia; *GFR,* glomerular filtration rate; *MEN,* multiple endocrine neoplasia; *25(OH)D,* 25 hydroxyvitamin D; *PO_4,* phosphate; *PTH,* parathyroid hormone; *T_3,* triiodothyronine; *T_4,* thyroxine; *TmP,* renal threshold for phosphorus.
From Moore WT, Eastman RC: *Diagnostic endocrinology*, ed 2, St Louis, 1996, Mosby.

BOX 6 Differential Diagnosis of Hypercalcemia in Older Adults

Primary hyperparathyroidism
Malignancy
Renal failure
Addison disease
Hyperthyroidism
Immobilization
Medications: thiazide diuretics, calcium supplements, lithium
Milk alkali syndrome
Paget disease (when immobilized)
Sarcoidosis
Tuberculosis
Vitamin D or vitamin A intoxication

Symptoms of Acute Hypercalcemia
Neurologic: drowsiness, confusion, irritability hypotonia, coma
Gastrointestinal: anorexia, nausea, vomiting, acute pancreatitis
Cardiovascular: arrhythmias
Renal: polyuria, polydipsia, dehydration

From Fillit HM: *Brocklehurst's textbook of geriatric medicine and gerontology*, ed 8, Philadelphia, 2017, Elsevier.

This test is generally used to predict recurrence of breast cancer and evaluate response to therapy. May also be elevated in liver cancer, pancreatic cancer, ovarian cancer, colorectal cancer. Elevations can also occur with benign breast and liver disease.

CANCER ANTIGEN 27-29 (CA 27-29)

Normal: <38 U/ml
Elevated in: Approximately 75% of women with metastatic breast cancer. Clinical sensitivity is 0.57, specificity 0.97, positive predictive value 0.83, negative predictive value 0.92. This test is generally used to predict recurrence of breast cancer and evaluate response to therapy. May also be elevated in liver cancer, pancreatic cancer, ovarian cancer, colorectal cancer. Elevations can also occur with benign breast and liver disease.

CANCER ANTIGEN 72-4 (CA 72-4)

Normal: <4.0 ng/ml
Elevated in: Gastric cancer (elevated in >50% of patients). Often used in combination with CA 72-4, CA 19-9, and CEA to monitor gastric cancer after treatment.

CANCER ANTIGEN 125 (CA 125)

Normal range: <1.4%
This test uses an antibody against antigen from tissue culture of an ovarian tumor cell line. Various published evaluations report sensitivity of about 75%-80% in patients with ovarian carcinoma. There is also an appreciable incidence of elevated values in nonovarian malignancies and in certain benign conditions (see below). Test values may transiently increase during chemotherapy.

MALIGNANT
Epithelial ovarian carcinoma, 75%-80% (range, 25%-92%; better in serous than mucinous cystadenocarcinoma)
Endometrial carcinoma, 25%-48% (2%-90%)
Pancreatic carcinoma, 59%
Colorectal carcinoma, 20% (15%-56%)
Endocervical adenocarcinoma, 83%
Squamous cervical or vaginal carcinoma, 7%-14%
Lung carcinoma, 32%
Breast carcinoma, 12%-40%
Lymphoma, 35%

BENIGN
Cirrhosis, 40%-80%
Acute pancreatitis, 38%
Acute peritonitis, 75%
Endometriosis, 88%
Acute pelvic inflammatory disease, 33%
Pregnancy first trimester, 2%-24%
During menstruation (occasionally)
Renal failure (?frequency)
Normal persons, 0.6%-1.4%

CAPTOPRIL STIMULATION TEST

Normal: Test performed by giving 25 mg captopril orally after overnight fast. Patient should be seated during test. After captopril, aldosterone <15 ng/dl, renin >2 ng angiotensin L/ml/hr.
Interpretation: In patients with primary aldosteronism, plasma aldosterone remains high and plasma renin activity remains low after captopril.

TABLE 19 Laboratory Differential Diagnosis of Hypocalcemia

Diagnosis	PLASMA TESTS					URINE TESTS					Comments
	Ca	PO_4	PTH	25(OH)D	1,25$(OH)_2$D	cAMP	cAMP after PTH	TmP/GFR	TmP/GFR after PTH	Ca	
Hypoparathyroidism	↓	↑	N/↓	N	↓	↓	↑↑	↑	↓↓	N/↓	Deficiency of PTH
Pseudohypoparathyroidism											
Type I	↓	↑	↑↑	N	↓	↓	NC	↑	↑	N/↓	Resistance to PTH; patients may have Albright's hereditary osteodystrophy and resistance to multiple hormones
Type II	↓	N	↑↑	N	↓	↓	↑	↑	↑	N/↓	Renal resistance to cAMP
Vitamin D deficiency	↓	N/↓	↑↑	↓↓	N/↓	↑	↑	↓	↓	↓↓	Deficient supply (e.g., nutrition) or absorption (e.g., pancreatic insufficiency) of vitamin D
Vitamin D–dependent Rickets											
Type I	↓	N/↓	↑↑	N	↓	↑↑		↓		↓↓	Deficient activity of renal 25(OH) D-1α-hydroxylase
Type II	↓	N/↓	↑↑	N	↑↑	↑		↓		↓↓	Resistance to 1,25$(OH)_2$D

Ca, Calcium; *cAMP,* cyclic adenosine monophosphate; *FHH,* familial hypocalciuric hypercalcemia; *GFR,* glomerular filtration rate; *MEN,* multiple endocrine neoplasia; *NC,* no change or small increase; *(OH)D,* hydroxycalciferol D; *PO_4,* phosphate; *PTH,* parathyroid hormone; *T_3,* triiodothyronine; *T_4,* thyroxine; *TmP,* renal threshold for phosphorus.
From Moore WT, Eastman RC: *Diagnostic endocrinology,* ed 2, St Louis, 1996, Mosby.

CARBAMAZEPINE (Tegretol)

Normal therapeutic range: 4-12 mcg/ml

CARBOHYDRATE ANTIGEN 19-9

Normal: <37.0 U/ml
Elevated in: GI cancer, most frequently pancreatic cancer. Amount of elevation has no relation to tumor mass. Elevations can also occur with cirrhosis, cholangitis, and chronic or acute pancreatitis.

CARBON DIOXIDE, PARTIAL PRESSURE

Normal:
Male: 35-48 mm Hg
Female: 32-45 mm Hg
Elevated in: Respiratory acidosis
Decreased in: Respiratory alkalosis

CARBON MONOXIDE

See CARBOXYHEMOGLOBIN

CARBOXYHEMOGLOBIN

Normal range: Saturation of hemoglobin <2%; smokers <9%
Elevated in: Smoking, exposure to smoking, exposure to automobile exhaust fumes, malfunctioning gas-burning appliances

CARCINOEMBRYONIC ANTIGEN (CEA)

Normal range:
Nonsmokers: 0-2.5 ng/ml (0-2.5 μg/L [CF: 1; SMI: 0.1 μg/L])
Smokers: 0-5 ng/ml (0-5 μg/L [CF: 1; SMI: 0.1 μg/L])
Elevated in:
Colorectal carcinomas*, pancreatic carcinomas, and metastatic disease (usually produce higher elevations: >20 ng/ml)
Carcinomas of the esophagus, stomach, small intestine, liver, breast, ovary, lung, and thyroid (usually produce lesser elevations)
Benign conditions (smoking, inflammatory bowel disease, hypothyroidism, cirrhosis, pancreatitis, infections) (usually produce levels <10 ng/ml)

CAROTENE (serum)

Normal range: 50-250 μg/dl (0.9-4.6 μmol/L [CF: 0.01863; SMI: 0.1 μmol/L])
Elevated in: Carotenemia, chronic nephritis, diabetes mellitus, hypothyroidism, nephrotic syndrome, hyperlipidemia
Decreased in: Fat malabsorption, steatorrhea, pancreatic insufficiency, lack of carotenoids in diet, high fever, liver disease

CATECHOLAMINES, URINE

See URINE CATECHOLAMINES

CBC

See COMPLETE BLOOD COUNT

CD40 LIGAND

Normal: <5 mcg/L. CD40 ligand is a soluble protein that is shed from activated leukocytes and platelets and used in risk stratification for acute coronary syndrome.
Elevated in: Acute coronary syndrome. Increased CD40 ligand is associated with higher incidence of death or nonfatal MI.

CD4+ T-LYMPHOCYTE COUNT (CD4+ T-cells)

Calculated as total WBC × % lymphocytes × % lymphocytes stained with CD4.

This test is used primarily to evaluate immune dysfunction in HIV infection. It is useful as a prognostic indicator and as a criterion for initiating prophylaxis for several opportunistic infections that are sequelae of HIV infection. Progressive depletion of CD4+ T-lymphocytes is associated with an increased likelihood of clinical complications (Table 20).

CEA

See CARCINOEMBRYONIC ANTIGEN

CEREBROSPINAL FLUID (CSF)

Interpretation of results:
Appearance of the fluid
Clear: normal.
Yellow color (xanthochromia) in the supernatant of centrifuged CSF within 1 hour or less after collection is usually the result of previous bleeding (subarachnoid hemorrhage); it may also be caused by increased CSF protein, melanin from meningeal melanosarcomas, or carotenoids.
Pinkish color is usually the result of a bloody tap; the color generally clears progressively from tubes 1 to 4 (the supernatant is usually crystal clear in traumatic taps).
Turbidity usually indicates the presence of leukocytes (bleeding introduces approximately 1 WBC/500 RBCs into the CSF).
CSF pressure: elevated pressure can be seen with meningitis, meningoencephalitis, pseudotumor cerebri, mass lesions, and intracerebral bleeding.

*To detect colorectal cancer, the sensitivity of CEA ranges from 68% for a threshold of 10 mcg/L to 82% for a threshold of 2.5 mcg/L, and the specificity ranges from 97% for a threshold of 10 mcg/L to 80% for a threshold of 2.6 mcg/L.

TABLE 22 Cerebrospinal Fluid Findings in Infectious and Inflammatory Diseases of the Central Nervous System

Condition	Pressure (mm H_2O)	Leukocytes/μL	Protein (mg/dL)	Sugar (mg/dL)	Specific Findings
Acute bacterial meningitis	Usually elevated; average 300	Several hundred to >10,000; usually a few thousand; occasionally <100 (especially meningococcal or early in disease); PMLs predominate	Usually 100–500, occasionally >1000	<40 in more than half the cases	Organism usually seen on smear or recovered on culture in >90% of cases
Subdural empyema	Usually elevated; average 300	<100 to a few thousand; PMLs predominate	Usually 100–500	Normal	No organisms on smear or by culture unless concurrent meningitis
Brain abscess	Usually elevated	Usually 10–200; fluid rarely is acellular; lymphocytes predominate	Usually 75–400	Normal	No organisms on smear or by culture
Ventricular empyema (rupture of brain abscess)	Elevated	Several thousand to 100,000; usually >90% PMLs	Usually several hundred	Usually <40	Organisms may be seen on smear or cultured
Cerebral epidural abscess	Slight to modest elevation	Few to several hundred or more cells; lymphocytes predominate	Usually 50–200	Normal	No organisms on smear or by culture
Spinal epidural abscess	Usually reduced with spinal block	Usually 10–100; lymphocytes predominate	Usually several hundred	Normal	No organisms on smear or by culture
Thrombophlebitis (often associated with subdural empyema)	Often elevated	Few to several hundred; PMLs and lymphocytes	Slightly to moderately elevated	Normal	No organisms on smear or by culture
Bacterial endocarditis (with embolism)	Normal or slightly elevated	Few to <100; lymphocytes and PMLs	Slightly elevated	Normal	No organisms on smear or by culture
Acute hemorrhagic encephalitis	Usually elevated	Few to >1000; PMLs predominate	Moderately elevated	Normal	No organisms on smear or by culture
Tuberculous infection	Usually elevated	Usually 25–100, rarely >500; lymphocytes predominate except in early stages when PMLs may account for 80% of cells	Nearly always elevated; usually 100–200; may be much higher if block in CSF flow	Usually reduced; <50 in 75% of cases	Acid-fast organisms may be seen on smear of protein coagulum (pellicle) or recovered from inoculated guinea pig or by culture
Cryptococcal infection	Usually elevated	Average 50 (0–800); lymphocytes predominate	Average 100; usually 20–500	Reduced in more than half of cases; often higher in patients with concomitant diabetes mellitus	Organisms may be seen in India ink preparation and on culture (Sabouraud medium); usually grow on blood agar; may produce alcohol in CSF from fermentation of glucose
Syphilis (acute)	Usually elevated	Average 500; usually lymphocytes; rarely PMLs	Average, 100; γ-globulin often high, with abnormal colloidal gold curve	Normal (rarely reduced)	Positive reagin test result for syphilis; spirochete not demonstrable by usual techniques of smear or by culture
Sarcoidosis	Normal to considerably elevated	0 to <100 mononuclear cells	Slight to moderate elevation	Normal	No specific findings

CSF, Cerebrospinal fluid; *PMLs,* polymorphonuclear leukocytes.
From Cherry JD: *Feigin and Cherry's pediatric infectious diseases*, ed 8, Philadelphia, 2019, Elsevier.

TABLE 20 Relation of CD4 Lymphocyte Counts to the Onset of Certain HIV-Associated Infections and Neoplasms in North America

CD4 Count (Cells/mm³)*	Opportunistic Infection or Neoplasm	Frequency (%)†
>500	Herpes zoster, polydermatomal	5-10
200-500	*Mycobacterium tuberculosis* infection, pulmonary and extrapulmonary	2-20
	Oral hairy leukoplakia	40-70
	Candida pharyngitis (thrush)	40-70
	Recurrent *Candida* vaginitis	15-30 (F)
	Kaposi sarcoma, mucocutaneous	15-30 (M)
	Bacterial pneumonia, recurrent	15-20
	Cervical neoplasia	1-2 (F)
100-200	*Pneumocystis carinii* pneumonia	15-60
	Herpes simplex, chronic, ulcerative	5-10
	Histoplasma capsulatum infection, disseminated	0-20
	Kaposi's sarcoma, visceral	3-8 (M)
	Progressive multifocal leukoencephalopathy	2-3
	Lymphoma, non-Hodgkin's	2-5
<100	*Candida* esophagitis	15-20
	Mycobacterium avium-intracellulare, disseminated	25-40
	Toxoplasma gondii encephalitis	5-25
	Cryptosporidium enteritis	2-10
	CMV retinitis	20-35
	Cryptococcus neoformans encephalitis	2-5
	CMV esophagitis or colitis	6-12
	Lymphoma, central nervous system	4-8

CMV, Cytomegalovirus; *F*, exclusively in women; *HIV*, human immunodeficiency virus; *M*, almost exclusively in men.
*Table indicates CD4 count at which specific infections or neoplasms generally begin to appear. Each infection may recur or progress during the subsequent course of HIV disease.
†Even within the United States, great regional differences in the incidence of specific opportunistic infections are apparent. For example, disseminated histoplasmosis is common in the Mississippi River drainage area but very rare in individuals who have lived exclusively on the East or West Coast.
From Andreoli TE (ed): *Cecil essentials of medicine*, ed 5, Philadelphia, 2000, Saunders.

Cell count: in the adult the CSF is normally free of cells (although up to 5 mononuclear cells/mm³ is considered normal); the presence of granulocytes is never normal.

Neutrophils: seen in bacterial meningitis, early viral meningoencephalitis, and early tuberculosis (TB) meningitis. Box 7 summarizes causes of increased CSF neutrophils.

Increased lymphocytes: TB meningitis, viral meningoencephalitis, syphilitic meningoencephalitis, fungal meningitis. Causes of CSF lymphocytosis are summarized in Box 8.

CSF plasmacytosis: Box 9 describes inflammatory and infectious causes of CSF plasmacytosis.

CSF eosinophilia: Causes of CSF eosinophilic pleocytosis are summarized in Box 10.

Protein: serum proteins are generally too large to cross the normal blood–CSF barrier; however, increased CSF protein is seen with meningeal inflammation, traumatic tap, increased CNS synthesis, tissue degeneration, obstruction to CSF circulation, and Guillain-Barré syndrome. Mean concentrations of plasma and CSF proteins are summarized in Table 21. Conditions associated with increased CSF total protein are summarized in Box 11.

Glucose

Decreased glucose is seen with bacterial meningitis, TB meningitis, fungal meningitis, subarachnoid hemorrhage, and some cases of viral meningitis.

BOX 7 Causes of Increased CSF Neutrophils

- Meningitis
  - Bacterial meningitis
  - Early viral meningoencephalitis
  - Early tuberculous meningitis
  - Early mycotic meningitis
  - Amebic encephalomyelitis
- Other infections
  - Cerebral abscess
  - Subdural empyema
  - AIDS-related CMV radiculopathy
- Following seizures
- Following CNS hemorrhage
  - Subarachnoid
  - Intracerebral
- Following CNS infarct
- Reaction to repeated lumbar punctures
- Injection of foreign material in subarachnoid space (e.g., methotrexate, contrast media)
- Metastatic tumor in contact with CSF

AIDS, Acquired immunodeficiency syndrome; *CMV*, cytomegalovirus; *CNS*, central nervous system; *CSF*, cerebrospinal fluid.
From McPherson RA, Pincus MR: *Henry's clinical diagnosis and management by laboratory methods*, ed 23, St Louis, 2017, Elsevier.

BOX 8 Causes of CSF Lymphocytosis

Meningitis
- Viral meningitis
- Tuberculous meningitis
- Fungal meningitis
- Syphilitic meningoencephalitis
- Leptospiral meningitis
- Bacterial due to uncommon organisms
- Early bacterial meningitis where leukocyte counts are relatively low
- Parasitic infestations (e.g., cysticercosis, trichinosis, toxoplasmosis)
- Aseptic meningitis due to septic focus adjacent to meninges

Degenerative Disorders
- Subacute sclerosing panencephalitis
- Multiple sclerosis
- Drug abuse encephalopathy
- Guillain-Barré syndrome
- Acute disseminated encephalomyelitis

Other Inflammatory Disorders
- Handl syndrome (headache with neurologic deficits and CSF lymphocytosis)
- Sarcoidosis
- Polyneuritis
- CNS periarteritis

CNS, Central nervous system; *CSF*, cerebrospinal fluid.
From McPherson RA, Pincus MR: *Henry's clinical diagnosis and management by laboratory methods*, ed 23, St Louis, 2017, Elsevier.

A mild increase in CSF glucose can be seen in patients with very elevated serum glucose levels.

Table 22 describes CSF findings in infectious and inflammatory diseases of the central nervous system and meninges.

Causes of xanthochromia are summarized in Table 23.

CERULOPLASMIN (serum)

Normal range: 20-35 mg/dl (200-350 mg/L [CF: 10; SMI: 10 mg/L])
Elevated in: Pregnancy, estrogens, oral contraceptives, neoplastic diseases (leukemias, Hodgkin's lymphoma, carcinomas), inflammatory states, systemic lupus erythematosus, primary biliary cirrhosis, rheumatoid arthritis
Decreased in: Wilson disease (values often <10 mg/dl), nephrotic syndrome, advanced liver disease, malabsorption, total parenteral nutrition, Menkes syndrome

BOX 9 Inflammatory and Infectious Causes of CSF Plasmacytosis

Acute viral infections
Guillain-Barré syndrome
Multiple sclerosis
Parasitic CNS infestations
Sarcoidosis
Subacute sclerosing panencephalitis
Syphilitic meningoencephalitis
Tuberculous meningitis

CNS, Central nervous system; *CSF,* cerebrospinal fluid.
(From McPherson RA, Pincus MR: *Henry's clinical diagnosis and management by laboratory methods*, ed 23, St Louis, 2017, Elsevier.)

BOX 10 Causes of CSF Eosinophilic Pleocytosis

Commonly associated with
- Acute polyneuritis
- CNS reaction to foreign material (drugs, shunts)
- Fungal infections
- Idiopathic eosinophilic meningitis
- Idiopathic hypereosinophilic syndrome
- Parasitic infections

Infrequently associated with
- Bacterial meningitis
- Leukemia/lymphoma
- Myeloproliferative disorders
- Neurosarcoidosis
- Primary brain tumors
- Tuberculous meningoencephalitis
- Viral meningitis

CNS, Central nervous system; *CSF,* cerebrospinal fluid.
Modified from Kjeldsberg CR, Knight JA: *Body fluids: laboratory examination of amniotic, cerebrospinal, seminal, serous and synovial fluids*, ed 3, Chicago, 1993, © American Society for Clinical Pathology, with permission. In McPherson RA, Pincus MR: *Henry's clinical diagnosis and management by laboratory methods*, ed 23, St Louis, 2017, Elsevier.

TABLE 21 Mean Concentrations of Plasma and CSF Proteins

Protein	CSF, mg/L	Plasma/CSF Ratio
Prealbumin	17.3	14
Albumin	155.0	236
Transferrin	14.4	142
Ceruloplasmin	1.0	366
Immunoglobulin (Ig)G	12.3	802
IgA	1.3	1346
α_2-Microglobulin	2.0	1111
Fibrinogen	0.6	4940
IgM	0.6	1167
β-Lipoprotein	0.6	6213

CSF, Cerebrospinal fluid.
Adapted and updated from Felgenhauer K: Protein size and cerebrospinal fluid composition, *Klin Wochenschr* 52:1158, 1974, with permission.
(McPherson RA, Pincus MR: *Henry's clinical diagnosis and management by laboratory methods,* ed 23, St Louis, 2017, Elsevier.)

CHLAMYDIA GROUP ANTIBODY SEROLOGIC TEST

Test description: Acute and convalescent sera is drawn 2-4 weeks apart. A fourfold increase in titer between acute and convalescent sera is necessary for confirmation. A single titer ≥1:64 is considered indicative of psittacosis or LGV.

BOX 11 Conditions Associated with Increased CSF Total Protein

Traumatic Spinal Puncture
Increased Blood-CSF Permeability
Arachnoiditis (e.g., following methotrexate therapy)
Meningitis (bacterial, viral, fungal, tuberculous)
Hemorrhage (subarachnoid, intracerebral)
Endocrine/metabolic disorders
- Milk-alkali syndrome with hypercalcemia
- Diabetic neuropathy
- Hereditary neuropathies and myelopathies
- Decreased endocrine function (thyroid, parathyroid)
- Other disorders (uremia, dehydration)

Drug Toxicity
Ethanol, phenothiazines, phenytoin

CSF Circulation Defects
Mechanical obstruction (tumor, abscess, herniated disk)
Loculated CSF effusion

Increased Immunoglobulin (Ig)G Synthesis
Multiple sclerosis

Neurosyphilis
Subacute sclerosing panencephalitis

Increased IgG Synthesis and Blood-CSF Permeability
Guillain-Barré syndrome
Collagen vascular diseases (e.g., lupus, periarteritis)
Chronic inflammatory demyelinating polyradiculopathy

CSF, Cerebrospinal fluid.
From McPherson RA, Pincus MR: *Henry's clinical diagnosis and management by laboratory methods*, ed 23, St Louis, 2017, Elsevier.

CHLAMYDIA TRACHOMATIS PCR

Test description: Test is performed on endocervical swab, urine, and intraurethral swab (see Table 24)
Normal: Negative

CHLORIDE (serum)

Normal range: 95-105 mEq/L (95-105 mmol/L [CF: 1; SMI: 1 mmol/L])
Elevated in: Dehydration, excessive infusion of normal saline solution, cystic fibrosis (sweat test), hyperparathyroidism, renal tubular disease, metabolic acidosis, prolonged diarrhea, drugs (ammonium chloride administration, acetazolamide, boric acid, triamterene)
Decreased in: Congestive heart failure, syndrome of inappropriate antidiuretic hormone secretion, Addison disease, vomiting, gastric suction, salt-losing nephritis, continuous infusion of D_5W, thiazide diuretic administration, diaphoresis, diarrhea, burns, diabetic ketoacidosis

CHLORIDE (sweat)

Normal: 0-40 mmol/L
Borderline/indeterminate: 41-60 mmol/L
Consistent with cystic fibrosis: >60 mmol/L

False low results can occur with edema, excessive sweating, and hypoproteinemia.

CHLORIDE, URINE

See URINE CHLORIDE

CHOLECYSTOKININ-PANCREOZYMIN (CCK, CCK-PZ)

Normal: <80 pg/ml
Elevated in: Pancreatic disease, celiac disease, gastric ulcer, postgastrectomy, IBS, fatty food intolerance

CHOLESTEROL, HIGH-DENSITY LIPOPROTEIN

See HIGH-DENSITY LIPOPROTEIN CHOLESTEROL

CHOLESTEROL, LOW-DENSITY LIPOPROTEIN

See LOW-DENSITY LIPOPROTEIN CHOLESTEROL

TABLE 23 Xanthochromia and Associated Diseases/Disorders

CSF Supernatant Color	Associated Diseases/Disorders
Pink	RBC lysis/hemoglobin breakdown products
Yellow	RBC lysis/hemoglobin breakdown products Hyperbilirubinemia CSF protein >150 mg/dL (1.5 g/L)
Orange	RBC lysis/hemoglobin breakdown products Hypervitaminosis A (carotenoids)
Yellow-green	Hyperbilirubinemia (biliverdin)
Brown	Meningeal metastatic melanoma

CSF, Cerebrospinal fluid; *RBC,* red blood cell.
McPherson RA, Pincus MR: *Henry's clinical diagnosis and management by laboratory methods,* ed 23, St Louis, 2017, Elsevier.

TABLE 24 Specimens for Detection of *Chlamydia trachomatis**

Disease	Specimen
Mucopurulent cervicitis	Endocervical swab, urine
Acute urethral syndrome (women)	Urethral swab, urine
Acute endometritis	Endometrial aspirate
Acute salpingitis	Fallopian tube biopsy
Nongonococcal urethritis (men)	Urethral swab, urine
Inclusion conjunctivitis	Conjunctival scrapings/swab
Trachoma	Conjunctival scrapings/swab
Lymphogranuloma venereum	Lymph node aspirate, biopsy of ulcerated lesion, serum
Pneumonitis (infants)	Serum, tracheobronchial aspirate, nasopharyngeal swab

*Urine is acceptable for some enzyme-linked immunoassays and for the commercial nucleic acid amplification tests.
McPherson RA, Pincus MR: *Henry's clinical diagnosis and management by laboratory methods,* ed 23, St Louis, 2017, Elsevier.

CHOLESTEROL, TOTAL

Normal range: Varies with age

Generally <200 mg/dl (<5.20 mmol/L [CF: 0.02586; SMI: 0.05 mmol/L])

Elevated in: Primary hypercholesterolemia, biliary obstruction, diabetes mellitus, nephrotic syndrome, hypothyroidism, primary biliary cirrhosis, high-cholesterol diet, pregnancy third trimester, myocardial infarction, drugs (steroids, phenothiazines, oral contraceptives). Classic hyperlipidemia phenotypes are summarized in Table 25.

Decreased in: Medications (statins, niacin), starvation, malabsorption, sideroblastic anemia, thalassemia, abetalipoproteinemia, hyperthyroidism, Cushing's syndrome, hepatic failure, multiple myeloma, polycythemia vera, chronic myelocytic leukemia, myeloid metaplasia, Waldenström's macroglobulinemia, myelofibrosis

CHORIONIC GONADOTROPINS, HUMAN (serum) (HCG)

Normal range, serum:

Female, premenopausal: <0.8 IU/L; postmenopausal <3.3 IU/L

Male: <0.7 IU/L

Elevated in:

Pregnancy, choriocarcinoma, gestational trophoblastic neoplasia (including molar gestations), placental site trophoblastic tumors; human antimouse antibodies (HAMA) can produce false serum assay for hCG.

The principal use of this test is to diagnose pregnancy. The concentration of hCG increases significantly during the initial 6 weeks of pregnancy.

Normal range: Varies with gestational stage:

1 wk: 5-50 mU/ml 1-2 wk: 50-550 mU/ml

2-3 wk: up to 5000 mU/ml

3-4 wk: up to 10,000 mU/ml

4-5 wk: up to 50,000 mU/ml

2-3 mo: 10,000-100,000 mU/ml

Peak values approaching 100,000 IU/L occur 60-70 days following implantation.

hCG levels generally double every 1-3 days. In patients with concentration <2000 IU/L, an increase of serum hCG <66% after 2 days is suggestive of spontaneous abortion or ruptured ectopic gestation.

CHYMOTRYPSIN

Normal: <10 mcg/L

TABLE 25 Classic Hyperlipidemia Phenotypes

WHO ICD and OMIM Numbers	Type	Particle	Triglycerides	Cholesterol	Comments
E78.3 238600	1 (familial chylomicronemia or LPL deficiency)	CM	High	Normal	Low cardiac risk; hereditary, found mostly in pediatric patients and young adults; autosomal recessive mutation in *LPL* or *APOC2; APOA5, LMF-1,* and *GPIHBP1* mutations are linked to this phenotype.
E78.0 143890	2A (heterozygous and homozygous familial hypercholesterolemia)	LDL	Normal	High	High cardiac risk; mostly polygenic disease; about 10% are monogenic; heterozygous form is due to mutations in *LDLR, APOB,* or *PCSK9*; homozygous form is due to mutations in *LDLR* or *LDLRAP1* (ARH).
E78.4 144250	2B (combined hyperlipoproteinemia)	VLDL, LDL	High	High	High cardiac risk; polygenic disease; links to mutations in *USF1, APOB,* and *LPL*
E78.2 107741	3 (dysbetalipoproteinemia)	IDL	High	High	High cardiac risk; mutations in *APOE* gene or homozygous for E2 allele of *APOE*
E78.1 144600, 145750	4 (primary hypertriglyceridemia)	VLDL	High	Normal	Lower cardiac risk than type 2 or 3; polygenic disease
E78.3 144650	5 (mixed hyperlipidemia)	VLDL, CM	High	High	Low cardiac risk; polygenic disease; 10% of patients have mutations in *LPL, APOC2,* and *APOA5*; mutations in *APOE, TRIB1, CHREBP, GALNT2, GCKR,* and *ANGPTL3* are thought to contribute to this disease.

ANGPTL3, Angiopoietin-like 3; *APOA5,* apolipoprotein A-V; *APOB,* apolipoprotein B; *APOC2,* apolipoprotein C-II; *APOE,* apolipoprotein E; *CHREBP,* carbohydrate response element binding protein (or *MLXIPL*); *CM,* chylomicron; *GALNT2,* UDP-N′-acetyl-alpha-D-galactosamine-polypeptide *N*-acetylgalactosaminyltransferase 2; *GCKR,* glucokinase regulator; *ICD,* International Classification of Diseases; *IDL,* intermediate-density lipoprotein; *LDL,* low-density lipoprotein; *LDLRAP1,* LDLR adaptor protein 1 (also known as ARH); *OMIM,* Online Mendelian Inheritance in Man; *TRIB1,* tribbles homologue 1; *USF1,* upstream transcription factor 1; *VLDL,* very-low-density lipoprotein; *WHO,* World Health Organization.
McPherson RA, Pincus MR: *Henry's clinical diagnosis and management by laboratory methods,* ed 23, St Louis, 2017, Elsevier.

TABLE 26 Characteristics of Coagulation Factors

Factor	Descriptive Name	Source	Approximate Half-Life (hr)	Function
I	Fibrinogen	Liver	120	Substrate for fibrin clot (CP)
II	Prothrombin	Liver (VKD)	60	Serine protease (CP)
V	Proaccelerin, labile factor	Liver	12-36	Cofactor (CP)
VII	Serum prothrombin conversion accelerator, proconvertin	Liver (VKD)	6	(?) Serine protease (EP)
VIII	Antihemophilic factor or globulin	Endothelial cells and (?) elsewhere	12	Cofactor (IP)
IX	Plasma thromboplastin component, Christmas factor	Liver (VKD)	24	Serine protease (IP)
X	Stuart-Prower factor	Liver (VKD)	36	Serine protease (CP)
XI	Plasma thromboplastin antecedent	(?) Liver	40-84	Serine protease (IP)
XII	Hageman factor	(?) Liver	50	Serine protease contact activation (IP)
XIII	Fibrin-stabilizing factor	(?) Liver	96-180	Transglutaminase (CP)
Prekallikrein	Fletcher factor	(?) Liver	?	Serine protease contact activation (IP)
High-molecular-weight kininogen	Fitzgerald factor, Flaujeac or Williams factor	(?) Liver	?	Cofactor, contact activation (IP)

CP, Common pathway; *EP*, extrinsic pathway; *IP*, intrinsic pathway; *VKD*, vitamin K dependent.
From Noble J (ed): *Primary care medicine*, ed 3, St Louis, 2001, Mosby.

Elevated in: Acute pancreatitis, chronic renal failure, oral enzyme preparations, gastric cancer, pancreatic cancer
Decreased in: Chronic pancreatitis, late cystic fibrosis

CIRCULATING ANTICOAGULANT (lupus anticoagulant)

Normal: Negative
Detected in: Systemic lupus erythematosus, drug-induced lupus, long-term phenothiazine therapy, multiple myeloma, ulcerative colitis, rheumatoid arthritis, postpartum, hemophilia, neoplasms, chronic inflammatory states, AIDS, nephrotic syndrome

NOTE: The name is a misnomer because these patients are prone to hypercoagulability and thrombosis.

CK

See CREATINE KINASE

CLONIDINE SUPPRESSION TEST

Interpretation: Clonidine inhibits neurogenic catecholamine release and will cause a decrease in plasma norepinephrine into the reference interval in hypertensive subjects without pheochromocytoma. Test is performed by giving 4.3 mcg clonidine/kg orally after overnight fast. Norepinephrine is measured at 3 hr. Result should be within established reference range and decrease to <50% of baseline concentration. Lack of decrease in norepinephrine is suggestive of pheochromocytoma.

CLOSTRIDIUM DIFFICILE TOXIN ASSAY (stool)

Normal: Negative
Detected in: Antibiotic-associated diarrhea and pseudomembranous colitis

CO

See CARBOXYHEMOGLOBIN

COAGULATION FACTORS

See Table 26 for characteristics of coagulation factors.

See Table 27 for differential diagnosis of low factor VIII.

Factor reference ranges:

a. V: >10%
b. VII: >10%
c. VIII: 50%-170%
d. IX: 60%-136%
e. X: >10%
f. XI: 50%-150%
g. XII: >30%

Table 28 describes screening laboratory results in coagulation factor deficiencies. Characterization of coagulation factors and their deficiencies is summarized in Table 29.

TABLE 27 Differential Diagnosis of a Low Factor VIII Level

1. FVIII <10%
   1. Severe or moderately severe hemophilia A
   2. Severe type 1 vWD
   3. Type 3 vWD
   4. Type 2N vWD
   5. Acquired hemophilia A
   6. Acquired vWD
2. FVIII: 10% to 50%
   1. Mild hemophilia A
   2. Type 1 vWD
   3. Type 2N vWD
   4. Combined FVIII and FV deficiency

FV, Factor V; *FVIII*, factor VIII; *VWD*, von Willebrand's disease.
From Hoffman R: *Hematology: basic principles and practice*, ed 6, Philadelphia, Saunders, 2013.

TABLE 28 Screening Laboratory Results in Coagulation Factor Deficiencies

Deficient Factor	Frequency	PT	PTT	TT
I (fibrinogen)	Rare	↑	↑	↑
II (prothrombin)	Very rare	↑	↑	↑
V 1:1,000,000	↑	↑	NL	
VII	1:500,000	↑	NL	NL
VIII	1:5000 (male)	NL	↑	NL
IX	1:30,000 (male)	NL	↑	NL
X 1:500,000	↑	↑	NL	
XI	Rare*	NL	↑	NL
XII or HMWK or PK†	Rare	NL	↑	NL
XIII	Rare	NL	NL	↑

↑Increased over normal range; *HMWK*, high-molecular-weight kininogen; *NL*, normal; *PK*, prekallikrein; *PT*, prothrombin time; *PTT*, partial thromboplastin time; *TT*, thrombin time.
*Except in those of Ashkenazi Jewish descent (approximately 4% are heterozygous for factor XI deficiency).
†Not associated with clinical bleeding.
From Andreoli TE (ed): *Cecil essentials of medicine*, ed 5, Philadelphia, 2001, Saunders.

TABLE 29 Characterization of Coagulation Factors and Their Deficiencies

Factor	Molecular Weight, kDa	Gene Location	Normal Circulating Half-Life	Incidence	Inheritance	Bleeding Severity
Fibrinogen	330	4q31.3-q32.1	2-4 days	1:1 million	Recessive	Mild–severe*
II	72	11p11.2	3-4 days	Very rare	Recessive	Mild–moderate
V	330	1q24.2	36 hours	1:1 million	Recessive	Moderate
V and VIII combined	—	LMAN1:18q21.32 MCFD2:2p21	36 hours for FV; 10-14 hours for FVIII	1:2 million	Recessive	Mild–moderate
VII	50	13q34	3-6 hours	1:500,000	Recessive	Mild–severe
VIII	330	Xq28	10-14 hours	1:10,000	Sex-linked	Mild–severe
IX	56	Xq27	18-24 hours	1:30,000	Sex-linked	Mild–severe
X	58	13q34	40-60 hours	1:500,000	Recessive	Mild–severe
XI	160	4q35.2	40-70 hours	Rare†	Recessive	Mild–moderate
XII	80	5q33-qter	50-70 days	Rare	Recessive	No bleeding
PK	88	4q33-q35	Not known	Very rare	Recessive	No bleeding
HK	120	3q27	9-10 hours	Extremely rare	Recessive	No bleeding
XIII	320	A:6p25.1 B:1q31.3	11-14 days	<1:1 million	Recessive	Moderate–severe

HK, High molecular weight kininogen; *PK*, prekallikrein.
*May be associated with thrombosis.
†Rare except in those of Ashkenazi Jewish descent.
McPherson RA, Pincus MR: *Henry's clinical diagnosis and management by laboratory methods*, ed 23, St Louis, 2017, Elsevier.

COBALAMIN, SERUM

See VITAMIN B_{12}

COLD AGGLUTININS TITER

Normal range: <1:32
Elevated in:
Primary atypical pneumonia (*Mycoplasma* pneumonia), infectious mononucleosis, CMV infection
Others: hepatic cirrhosis, acquired hemolytic anemia, frostbite, multiple myeloma, lymphoma, malaria

COMPLEMENT

Normal range:
C3: 70-160 mg/dl (0.7-1.6 g/L [CF: 0.01; SMI: 0.1 g/L])
C4: 20-40 mg/dl (0.2-0.4 g/L [CF: 0.01; SMI: 0.1 g/L])
Abnormal values:
Decreased C3: Active SLE, immune complex disease, acute glomerulonephritis, inborn C3 deficiency, membranoproliferative glomerulonephritis, infective endocarditis, serum sickness, autoimmune/chronic active hepatitis
Decreased C4: Immune complex disease, active SLE, infective endocarditis, inborn C4 deficiency, hereditary angioedema, hypergammaglobulinemic states, cryoglobulinemic vasculitis. NOTE: The complement system has daunting nomenclature; accordingly, some basic definitions are given in Box 12.

BOX 12 Definitions

Classical pathway: C1, C4, C2, C3, and the terminal components.
Alternative pathway: Factor B, factor D, properdin, and the terminal components.
Lectin activation pathway: MBL, MASP1, MASP2, C3, and the terminal components.
Anaphylatoxins: C3a, C4a, C5a. These are mediators of smooth muscle contraction, degranulation of mast cells, enhanced neutrophil aggregation, increased vascular permeability.
Opsonization: Renders a particle more easily phagocytosed.
C3 tickover: This term occasionally is used to describe spontaneous C3 hydrolysis.
Membrane attack complex (terminal components): C5, C6, C7, C8, C9.
CH50: Used to define the dilution of serum capable of lysing 50% of sensitized sheep red cells. This assay measures the intactness of the classical pathway through the terminal components.
AH50: Used to define the dilution of serum capable of lysing 50% of nonsensitized rabbit red cells. This assay measures the intactness of the alternative pathway through the terminal components.

From Adkinson NF et al: *Middleton's allergy principles and practice*, ed 8, Philadelphia, 2014, Saunders.

COMPLEMENT DEFICIENCY

Table 30 describes complement deficiency states.

COMPLETE BLOOD COUNT (CBC)

See Fig. 16, which describes an algorithm for the evaluation of patients with neutropenia.
White blood cells 3200-9800/mm^3 (3.2-9.8 × 10^9/L [CF: 0.001; SMI: 0.1 × 10^9/L])
Red blood cells
Male: 4.3-5.9 × 10^6/mm^3 (4.3-5.9 × 10^{12}/L [CF: 0.001; SMI: 0.1 × 10^{12}/L])
Female: 3.5-5 × 10^6/mm^3 (3.5-5 × 10^{12}/L [CF: 0.001; SMI: 0.1 × 10^{12}/L])
Hemoglobin
Male: 13.6-17.7 g/dl (136-172 g/L [CF: 10; SMI: 1 g/L])
Female: 12-15 g/dl (120-150 g/L [CF: 10; SMI: 1 g/L])
Hematocrit
Male: 39%-49% (0.39-0.49 [CF: 0.01; SMI: 0.01])
Female: 33%-43% (0.33-0.43 [CF: 0.01; SMI: 0.01])
Mean corpuscular volume (MCV): 76-100 μm^3 (76-100 fL [CF: 1; SMI: 1 fL])
Mean corpuscular hemoglobin (MCH): 27-33 pg (27-33 pg [CF: 1; SMI: 1 pg])
Mean corpuscular hemoglobin concentration (MCHC): 33-37 g/dl (330-370 g/L [CF: 10; SMI: 10 g/L])
Red blood cell distribution width index (RDW): 11.5%-14.5%
Platelet count: 130-400 × 10^3/mm^3 (130-400 × 10^9/L [CF: 1; SMI: 5 × 10^9/L])
Differential:
2-6 stabs (bands, early mature neutrophils)
60-70 segs (mature neutrophils)
1-4 eosinophils
0-1 basophils
2-8 monocytes
25-40 lymphocytes

CONJUGATED BILIRUBIN

See BILIRUBIN, DIRECT

COPPER (serum)

Normal range: 70-140 μg/dl (11-22 μmol/L [CF: 0.1574, SMI: 0.2 μmol/L])
Decreased in: Wilson disease, Menkes syndrome, malabsorption, malnutrition, nephrosis, total parenteral nutrition, acute leukemia in remission

TABLE 30 Complement Deficiency States

Component	No. of Reported Patients	Mode of Inheritance	Functional Defects	Disease Associations
Classic Pathway				
C1qrs	31	ACD	Impaired IC handling, delayed C' activation, impaired immune response	CVD, 48%; infection (encapsulated bacteria), 22%; both, 18%; healthy, 12%
C4	21	ACD	Impaired C' activation in absence of specific antibody	Infection (meningococcal), 74%; healthy, 26%
C2	109	ACD		
Alternative Pathway				
D	3	ACD	Impaired IC handling, opson/phag; granulocytosis, CTX, immune response and absent SBA	CVD, 79%; recurrent infection (encapsulated bacteria), 71%
P	70	XL		
Junction of Classic and Alternative Pathways				
C3	19	ACD	Impaired CTX; absent SBA	Infection (*Neisseria,* primarily meningococcal), 58%; CVD, 4%
Terminal Components				
C5	27	ACD	Absent SBA	Both, 1%
C6	77	ACD		Healthy, 25%
C7	73	ACD		
C8	73	ACD		
C9	165	ACD	Impaired SBA	Healthy, 91%; infection, 9%
Plasma Proteins Regulating C' Activation				
C1-INH	Many	AD	Uncontrolled generation of an inflammatory mediator on C' activation	Hereditary angioedema
H	13	Acq	Uncontrolled AP activation → low C3	CVD, 40%; CVD plus infection (encapsulated bacteria), 40%; healthy, 20%
I	14	ACD	Uncontrolled AP activation → low C3	Infection (encapsulated bacteria), 100%
Membrane proteins regulating C' activation	Many	Acq	Impaired regulation of C3b and C8 deposited on host RBCs; PMN, platelets → cell lysis	Paroxysmal nocturnal hemoglobinuria
Decay-accelerating factor				
Homologous restriction factor				
CD59	>20	ACD	Impaired PMN adhesive functions (i.e., margination), CTX, C3bi-mediated opson/phag	Infection (*Staphylococcus aureus, Pseudomonas* spp.), 100%
CR3 autoantibodies				
C3 nephritic factors	>59	Acq	Stabilize AP, convertase → low C3	MPGN, 41%; PLD, 25%; infection (encapsulated bacteria), 16%; MPGN plus PLD, 10%; PLD plus infection, 5%; MPGN plus PLD plus infection, 3%; MPGN plus infection, 2%
C4 nephritic factor		Acq	Stabilize CP, C3 convertase → low C3	Glomerulonephritis, 50%; CVD, 50%

ACD, Autosomal codominant; *Acq,* acquired; *AD,* autosomal dominant; *AP,* alternative pathway; *C',* complement; *CP,* classic pathway; *CTX,* chemotaxis; *CVD,* collagen-vascular disease; *IC,* immune complex, *MPGN,* membranoproliferative glomerulonephritis; *PLD,* partial lipodystrophy; *PMN,* polymorphonuclear neutrophil; *RBCs,* red blood cells; *SBA,* serum bactericidal activity; *XL,* X-linked.
From Mandell GL: *Mandell, Douglas, and Bennett's principles and practice of infectious diseases,* ed 6, New York, 2005, Churchill Livingstone.

Elevated in: Aplastic anemia, biliary cirrhosis, systemic lupus erythematosus, hemochromatosis, hyperthyroidism, hypothyroidism, infection, iron deficiency anemia, leukemia, lymphoma, oral contraceptives, pernicious anemia, rheumatoid arthritis

COPPER, URINE

See URINE COPPER

CORTICOTROPIN RELEASING HORMONE (CRH) STIMULATION TEST

Normal: A dose of 0.5 mg of dexamethasone is given every 6 hours for 2 days; 2 hours after last dose 1 mcg/kg CRH is given IV. Samples are drawn after 15 min. Normally there is a twofold to fourfold increase in mean baseline concentration of ACTH or cortisol. Cortisol >1.4 mcg/L is virtually 100% specific and 100% diagnostic.

Interpretation:

Normal or exaggerated response: Pituitary Cushing's disease

No response: Ectopic ACTH-secreting tumor

A positive response to CRH or a suppressed response to high-dose dexamethasone has a 97% positive predictive value for Cushing's disease. However, a lack of response to either test excludes Cushing's disease in only 64%-78% of patients. When the tests are considered together, negative responses from both have a 100% predictive value for ectopic ACTH secretion.

CORTISOL, PLASMA

Normal range:

Varies with time of collection (circadian variation):

8 AM: 4-19 μg/dl (110-520 nmol/L [CF: 27.59; SMI: 10 nmol/L])

4 PM: 2-15 μg/dl (50-410 nmol/L [CF: 27.59; SMI: 10 nmol/L])

Elevated in: Ectopic adrenocorticotropic hormone production (i.e., oat cell carcinoma of lung), loss of normal diurnal variation, pregnancy, chronic renal failure, iatrogenic, stress, adrenal or pituitary hyperplasia, or adenomas

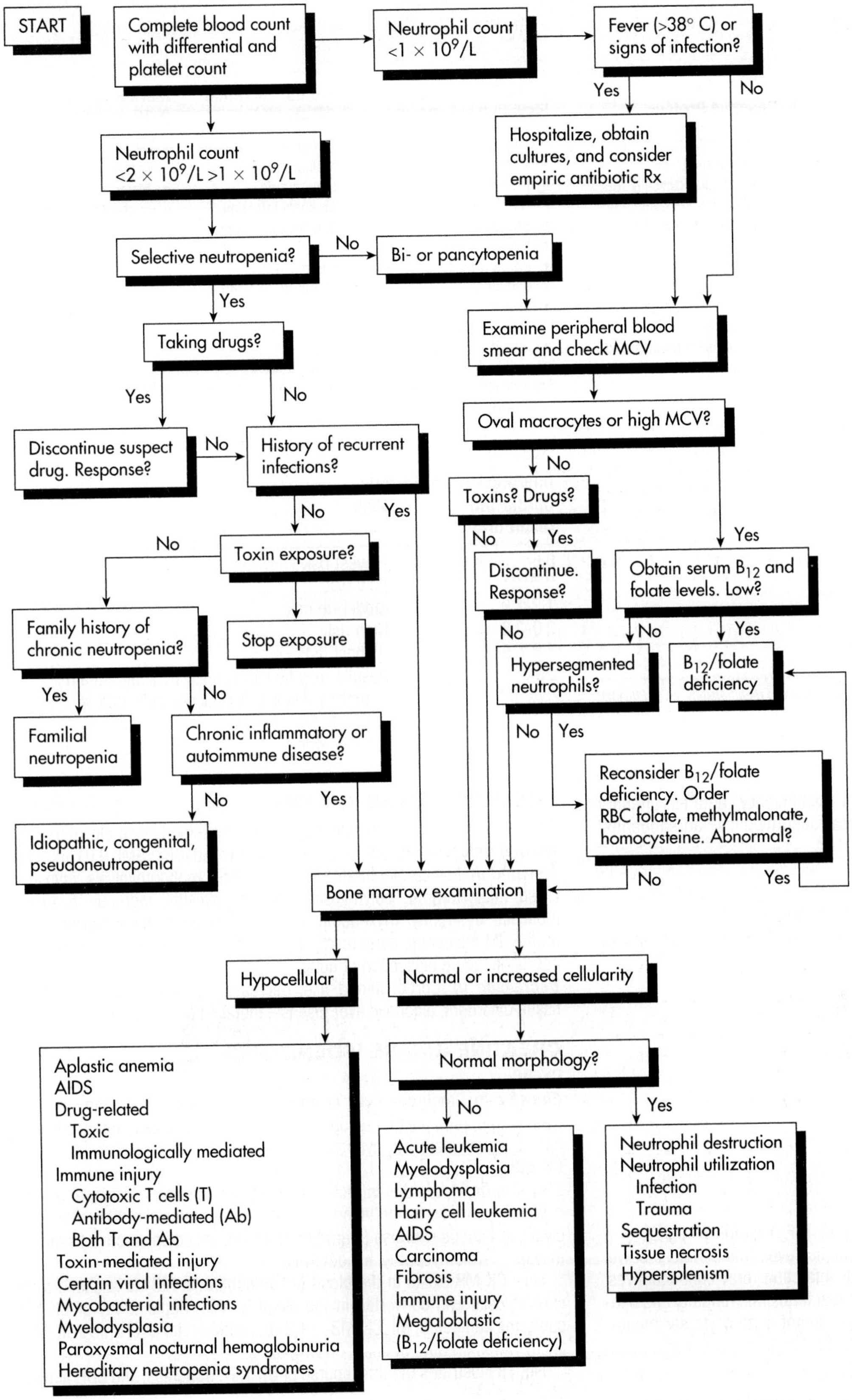

START

Complete blood count with differential and platelet count

→ Neutrophil count <1 × 10^9/L → Fever (>38° C) or signs of infection?
- Yes → Hospitalize, obtain cultures, and consider empiric antibiotic Rx → Examine peripheral blood smear and check MCV
- No → Examine peripheral blood smear and check MCV

→ Neutrophil count <2 × 10^9/L >1 × 10^9/L

Selective neutropenia?
- No → Bi- or pancytopenia → Examine peripheral blood smear and check MCV
- Yes → Taking drugs?
  - Yes → Discontinue suspect drug. Response?
    - No → History of recurrent infections?
  - No → History of recurrent infections?
    - Yes → Bone marrow examination
    - No → Toxin exposure?
      - Yes → Stop exposure
      - No → Family history of chronic neutropenia?
        - Yes → Familial neutropenia
        - No → Chronic inflammatory or autoimmune disease?
          - Yes → Bone marrow examination
          - No → Idiopathic, congenital, pseudoneutropenia

Examine peripheral blood smear and check MCV → Oval macrocytes or high MCV?
- No → Toxins? Drugs?
  - No → Bone marrow examination
  - Yes → Discontinue. Response?
    - No → Bone marrow examination
- Yes → Obtain serum B_{12} and folate levels. Low?
  - Yes → B_{12}/folate deficiency
  - No → Hypersegmented neutrophils?
    - No → Bone marrow examination
    - Yes → Reconsider B_{12}/folate deficiency. Order RBC folate, methylmalonate, homocysteine. Abnormal?
      - No → Bone marrow examination
      - Yes → B_{12}/folate deficiency

Bone marrow examination
- Hypocellular →
  - Aplastic anemia
  - AIDS
  - Drug-related
    - Toxic
    - Immunologically mediated
  - Immune injury
    - Cytotoxic T cells (T)
    - Antibody-mediated (Ab)
    - Both T and Ab
  - Toxin-mediated injury
  - Certain viral infections
  - Mycobacterial infections
  - Myelodysplasia
  - Paroxysmal nocturnal hemoglobinuria
  - Hereditary neutropenia syndromes
- Normal or increased cellularity → Normal morphology?
  - No →
    - Acute leukemia
    - Myelodysplasia
    - Lymphoma
    - Hairy cell leukemia
    - AIDS
    - Carcinoma
    - Fibrosis
    - Immune injury
    - Megaloblastic (B_{12}/folate deficiency)
  - Yes →
    - Neutrophil destruction
    - Neutrophil utilization
      - Infection
      - Trauma
    - Sequestration
    - Tissue necrosis
    - Hypersplenism

FIG. 16 A practical algorithm for the evaluation of patients with neutropenia. The fundamental diagnostic principle is that for patients with severe neutropenia or for those with bicytopenia or pancytopenia, bone marrow examination will likely be necessary unless the following diagnoses are made: (1) a nutritional (folate or vitamin B_{12}) deficiency or (2) drug- or toxin-induced neutropenia in a patient whose neutropenia resolves after discontinuation of the offending agent. *AIDS,* Acquired immunodeficiency syndrome; *MCV,* mean corpuscular volume; *RBC,* red blood cell. (From Goldman L, Ausiello D [eds]: *Cecil textbook of medicine,* ed 24, Philadelphia, 2012, Saunders.)

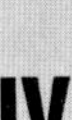

TABLE 31 Comparison of Erythrocyte Sedimentation Rate and C-Reactive Protein

	Erythrocyte Sedimentation Rate	C-Reactive Protein
Advantages	• Much clinical information in the literature • May reflect overall health status	• Rapid response to inflammatory stimuli • Wide range of clinically relevant values are detectable • Unaffected by age and gender • Reflects value of a single acute phase protein • Can be measured on stored sera • Quantitation is precise and reproducible
Disadvantages	• Affected by age and gender • Affected by red blood cell morphology • Affected by anemia and polycythemia • Reflects levels of many plasma proteins, not all of which are acute phase proteins • Responds slowly to inflammatory stimuli • Requires fresh sample • May be affected by drugs	• None

From Firestein GS, Budd RC, Gabriel SE et al: *Kelley's textbook of rheumatology*, ed 9, Philadelphia, 2013, Saunders.

TABLE 32 Conditions Associated with Elevated C-Reactive Protein Levels

Normal or Minor Elevation (<1 mg/dL)	Moderate Elevation (1-10 mg/dL)	Marked Elevation (>10 mg/dL)
• Vigorous exercise • Common cold • Pregnancy • Gingivitis • Seizures • Depression • Insulin resistance and diabetes • Several genetic polymorphisms • Obesity	• Myocardial infarction • Malignancies • Pancreatitis • Mucosal infection (bronchitis, cystitis) • Most connective tissue diseases • Rheumatoid arthritis	• Acute bacterial infection (80%-85%) • Major trauma • Systemic vasculitis

From Firestein GS, Budd RC, Gabriel SE et al: *Kelley's textbook of rheumatology*, ed 9, Philadelphia, 2013, Saunders.

Decreased in: Primary adrenocortical insufficiency, anterior pituitary hypofunction, secondary adrenocortical insufficiency, adrenogenital syndromes

C-PEPTIDE

Elevated in: Insulinoma, sulfonylurea administration
Decreased in: Insulin-dependent diabetes mellitus, factitious insulin administration

COOMBS DIRECT

See DIRECT ANTIGLOBULIN

COOMBS INDIRECT

See INDIRECT ANTIGLOBULIN

CPK

See CREATINE KINASE

C-REACTIVE PROTEIN

Normal range: 6.8-820 µg/dl (68-8200 µg/L [CF: 10; SMI: 10 µg/L])
Elevated in: Rheumatoid arthritis, rheumatic fever, inflammatory bowel disease, bacterial infections, myocardial infarction, oral contraceptives, third trimester of pregnancy (acute phase reactant), inflammatory and neoplastic diseases. Table 31 shows a comparison of erythrocyte sedimentation rate and C-reactive protein, and Table 32 shows conditions associated with elevated C-reactive protein levels.

C-REACTIVE PROTEIN, HIGH SENSITIVITY (hs-CRP, cardio-CRP)

This is a cardiac risk marker. It is increased in patients with silent atherosclerosis years before a cardiovascular event and is independent of cholesterol level and other lipoproteins. It can be used to help stratify cardiac risk.

Interpretation of Results

Cardio-CRP result (mg/L)	Risk
0.6	Lowest risk
0.7-1.1	Low risk
1.2-1.9	Moderate risk
2.0-3.8	High risk
3.9-4.9	Highest risk
≥5.0	Results may be confounded by acute inflammatory disease. If clinically indicated, a repeat test should be performed in 2 or more weeks.

CREATINE KINASE (CK, CPK)

Fig. E17 describes a diagnostic approach to creatine kinase elevation.
Normal range: 0-130 U/L (0-2.16 µkat/L [CF: 0.01667; SMI: 0.01 µkat/L])
Elevated in: Myocardial infarction, myocarditis, rhabdomyolysis, myositis, crush injury/trauma, polymyositis, dermatomyositis, vigorous exercise, muscular dystrophy, myxedema, seizures, malignant hyperthermia syndrome, IM injections, cerebrovascular accident, pulmonary embolism and infarction, acute dissection of aorta
Decreased in: Corticosteroid use, decreased muscle mass, connective tissue disorders, alcoholic liver disease, metastatic neoplasms

CREATINE KINASE ISOENZYMES

CK-BB
Elevated In: Cerebrovascular accident, subarachnoid hemorrhage, neoplasms (prostate, gastrointestinal tract, brain, ovary, breast, lung), severe shock, bowel infarction, hypothermia, meningitis
CK-MB
Elevated In: Myocardial infarction (MI), myocarditis, pericarditis, muscular dystrophy, cardiac defibrillation, cardiac surgery, extensive rhabdomyolysis, strenuous exercise (marathon runners), mixed connective tissue disease, cardiomyopathy, hypothermia

NOTE: CK-MB exists in the blood in two subforms. MB_2 is released from cardiac cells and converted in the blood to MB_1. Rapid assay of CK-MB subforms can detect MI (CK-MB_2 ≥1.0 U/L, with a ratio of CK-MB_2/CK-MB_1 ≥1.5) within 6 hours of onset of symptoms.

Fig. 18 illustrates the time course of CK, AST, troponins, and LDH activity after acute MI.

CK-MM
Elevated In: Crush injury, seizures, malignant hyperthermia syndrome, rhabdomyolysis, myositis, polymyositis, dermatomyositis, vigorous exercise, muscular dystrophy, IM injections, acute dissection of aorta

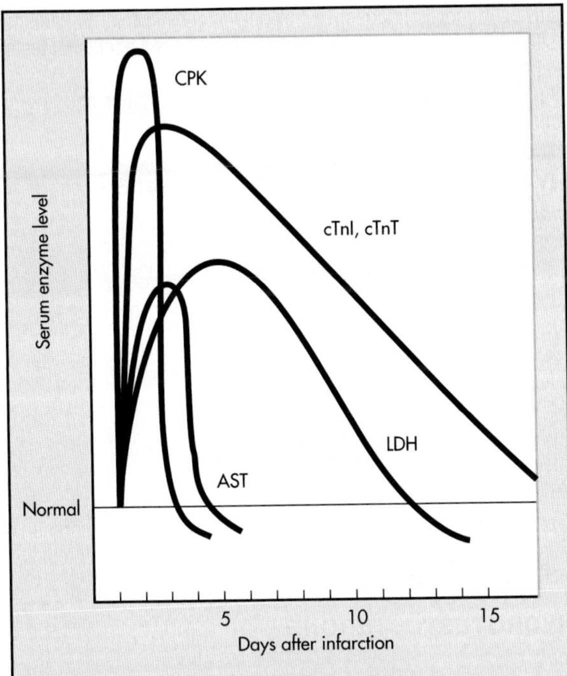

FIG. 18 Enzyme levels post-myocardial infarction. *AST,* Aspartate aminotransferase; *CPK,* creatine kinase; *cTnI,* cardiac troponin I; *cTnT,* cardiac troponin T; *LDH,* lactate dehydrogenase. (From Greene HL, Johnson WP, Lemcke D [eds]: *Decision making in medicine,* ed 2, St Louis, 1998, Mosby.)

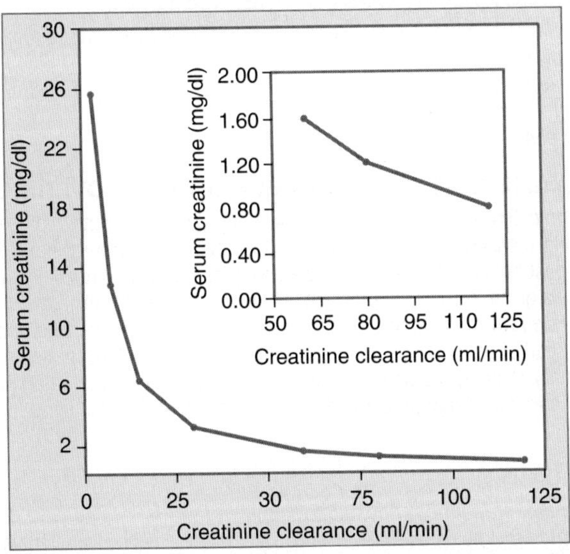

FIG. 19 Relationship between creatinine clearance and serum creatinine. In steady state, serum creatinine should increase twofold for each 50% reduction in creatinine clearance. *Inset* represents enlarged view of changes in serum creatinine as creatinine clearance decreases from 120 to 60 ml/min. If serum creatinine is 0.8 mg/dl when creatinine clearance is 120 ml/min, creatinine clearance can decrease by 33% such that increased serum creatinine is still within normal range. (From Vincent JL et al: *Textbook of critical care,* ed 6, Philadelphia, 2011, Saunders.)

CREATININE (serum)

Normal range: 0.6-1.2 mg/dl (50-110 μmol/L [CF: 88.4; SMI: 10 μmol/L]). Fig. 19 illustrates the relationship between creatinine clearance and serum creatinine. Factors that may alter serum creatinine level are described in Box 13.

Elevated in: Renal insufficiency (acute and chronic), decreased renal perfusion (hypotension, dehydration, congestive heart failure), urinary tract infection, rhabdomyolysis, ketonemia

Drugs (antibiotics [aminoglycosides, cephalosporins], hydantoin, diuretics, methyldopa)

BOX 13 Factors That May Alter Serum Creatinine (Cr) Level

Endogenous
- Reduced muscle mass: ↓
- Hyperbilirubinemia: ↓

Exogenous
- Medications inhibiting tubular secretion (trimethoprim, cimetidine): ↑

Medications Interfering with Laboratory Assays*
- Flucytosine and cefoxitin: ↑
- Catecholamines: ↓

*Varies by assay type used.
From Parrillo JE, Dellinger RP: *Critical care medicine, principles of diagnosis and management in the adult*, ed 4, Philadelphia, 2014, Elsevier.

TABLE 33 RIFLE Criteria for Acute Kidney Injury

	GFR and Serum Creatinine Changes	Urine Volume Changes
R (Risk)	Increase in SCreat >1.5×	Urine volume <0.5 mL/kg/hr >6 hr
	Decrease in GFR >25%	
I (Injury)	Increase in SCreat >2×	Urine volume <0.5 mL/kg/hr >12 hr
	Decrease in GFR >50%	
F (Failure)	Increase in SCreat >3×	Urine volume <0.3 mL/kg/hr >24 hr
	Decrease in GFR >75%	Anuria >12 hr
	SCreat >4 mg/dL	
L (Loss)	Complete loss of kidney function >4 weeks	
E (ESRD)	End-stage kidney disease >3 months	

SCreat, Serum creatinine.
McPherson RA, Pincus MR: *Henry's clinical diagnosis and management by laboratory methods,* ed 23, St Louis, 2017, Elsevier.

TABLE 34 New Classification for Acute Kidney Injury (AKI) Criteria

Stage	Serum Creatinine Criteria	Urine Output Criteria
1	>0.3 mg/dL (26.4 μmol/L) or >150% to 200%	<0.5 mL/kg for >6 hr
2	>200% to 300%	<0.5 mL/kg for >12 hr
3	>300%, 4 mg/dL (354 μmol/L) or acute increase of >0.5 mg/dL	<0.3 mL/kg for >24 hr or anuria >12 hr

McPherson RA, Pincus MR: *Henry's clinical diagnosis and management by laboratory methods,* ed 23, St Louis, 2017, Elsevier.

The RIFLE criteria for acute kidney injury is summarized in Table 33. A classification of acute kidney injury (AKI) is described in Table 34.

Falsely elevated in: Diabetic ketoacidosis, administration of some cephalosporins (e.g., cefoxitin, cephalothin)

Decreased in: Decreased muscle mass (including amputees and older persons), pregnancy, prolonged debilitation

CREATININE CLEARANCE

Normal range:
75-124 ml/min (1.24-2.08 ml/sec [CF: 0.01667; SMI: 0.02 ml/sec])
Box 14 describes a formula for calculation of creatinine clearance.
The Cockcroft-Gault formula to calculate creatinine clearance is described in Box 15.

Elevated in:
Pregnancy, exercise

Decreased in:
Renal insufficiency, drugs (cimetidine, procainamide, antibiotics, quinidine)

BOX 14 Calculation of Creatinine Clearance

$C_{cr} = U_{cr} \times V/P_{cr}$
where C_{cr} = clearance of creatinine (ml/min)
U_{cr} = urine creatinine (mg/dl)
V = volume of urine (ml/min) (for 24-hr volume: divide by 1440)
P_{cr} = plasma creatinine (mg/dl)
Normal range: 95 to 105 ml/min/1.75m^2

BOX 15 Cockcroft-Gault Formula to Calculate Creatinine Clearance (C_{cr})

$$C_{cr} = \frac{(140 - \text{age in year}) \times (\text{lean body weight in kg})}{S_{cr} \text{ in mg/dl} - 72}$$

CREATININE, URINE

See URINE CREATININE

CRYOGLOBULINS (serum)

Normal range: Not detectable
Present in: Collagen vascular diseases, chronic lymphocytic leukemia, hemolytic anemias, multiple myeloma, Waldenström's macroglobulinemia, chronic active hepatitis, Hodgkin's disease

CRYPTOSPORIDIUM ANTIGEN BY EIA (stool)

Normal range: Not detected
Present in: Cryptosporidiosis

CSF

See CEREBROSPINAL FLUID

CYSTATIN C

Normal: Cystatin C is a cysteine protease inhibitor that is produced at a constant rate by all nucleated cells. It is freely filtered by the glomerulus and reabsorbed (but not secreted) by the renal tubules with no extrarenal excretion. Its concentration is not affected by diet, muscle mass, or acute inflammation. Normal range when measured by particle-enhanced nephelometric immunoassay (PENIA) is <0.28 mg/L.
Elevated in: Renal disorders. Good predictor of the severity of acute tubular necrosis. Cystatin C increases more rapidly than creatinine in the early stages of GFR impairment. The cystatin C concentration is an independent risk factor for heart failure in older adults and appears to provide a better measure of risk assessment than the serum creatinine concentration.

CYSTIC FIBROSIS PCR

Test description: Test can be performed on whole blood or tissue. Common mutations in the cystic fibrosis transmembrane regulator (CFTR) gene can be used to detect 75%-80% of mutant alleles.

CYTOMEGALOVIRUS BY PCR

Test description: Test can be performed on whole blood, plasma, or tissue. Qualitative PCR is highly sensitive but may not be able to differentiate between latent and active infection.

D-DIMER

Normal range: <0.5 mcg/ml
Elevated in:
DVT, pulmonary embolism, high levels of rheumatoid factor, activation of coagulation and fibrolytic system from any cause
D-dimer assay by ELISA assists in the diagnosis of DVT and pulmonary embolism. This test has significant limitations because it can be elevated whenever the coagulation and fibrinolytic systems are activated and can also be falsely elevated with high rheumatoid factor levels.
A positive d-dimer is suggestive but not diagnostic for PE. Patients with positive d-dimer and clinical suspicion for PE need additional tests such as chest CT to confirm diagnosis.
PE might be ruled out in patients with negative d-dimer and low pretest probability for PE.

DEHYDROEPIANDROSTERONE SULFATE

Normal:
Males:

Ages 19-30:	125-619 mcg/dl
31-50:	59-452 mcg/dl
51-60:	20-413 mcg/dl
61-83:	10-285 mcg/dl
Females:	
Ages 19-30:	29-781 mcg/dl
31-50:	12-379 mcg/dl
Postmenopausal:	30-260 mcg/dl

Elevated in: Hirsutism, congenital adrenal hyperplasia, adrenal carcinomas, adrenal adenomas, polycystic ovary syndrome, ectopic ACTH-producing tumors, Cushing's disease, spironolactone

DEHYDROTESTOSTERONE (serum, urine)

Normal:
Serum: Males: 30-85 ng/dl; females: 4-22 ng/dl
Urine, 24 h: Males: 20-50 mcg/day; females: <8 mcg/day
Elevated in: Hirsutism
Decreased in: 5-α-reductase deficiency, hypogonadism

DEOXYCORTICOSTERONE (11-DEOXYCORTICOSTERONE, DOC) (serum)

Normal: 2-19 ng/dl. Normal secretion depends on ACTH and is suppressible by dexamethasone.
Elevated in: Adrenogenital syndromes due to 17- and 11-hydroxylase deficiencies, pregnancy
Decreased in: Preeclampsia

DEXAMETHASONE SUPPRESSION TEST, OVERNIGHT

Normal: Test is performed by giving 1 mg dexamethasone orally at 11 PM and measuring serum cortisol at 8 AM the following morning. Normal response is cortisol suppression to <3 mcg/dl; if dose of 4 mg dexamethasone is given, cortisol suppression will be to <50% of baseline.
Interpretation: Cushing's syndrome (<10 mcg/dl), endogenous depression (half of patients suppress test values <5 mcg/dl). Most patients with pituitary Cushing's disease demonstrate suppression, whereas patients with adrenal adenoma, carcinoma, and ectopic ACTH-producing tumors do not.

DIGOXIN

Normal therapeutic range: 0.5-2 ng/ml
Elevated in: Impaired renal function, excessive dosing, concomitant use of quinidine, amiodarone, verapamil, fluoxetine, nifedipine. Toxicity may occur at a lower blood concentration in the presence of hypokalemia, hypomagnesemia, and hypercalcemia. See Table 35.

DILANTIN

See PHENYTOIN

DIRECT ANTIGLOBULIN (Coombs Direct)

Normal: Negative
Positive: Autoimmune hemolytic anemia, erythroblastosis fetalis, transfusion reactions, drugs (α-methyldopa, penicillins, tetracycline, sulfonamides, levodopa, cephalosporins, quinidine, insulin)
False-positive: May be seen with cold agglutinins

DISACCHARIDE ABSORPTION TESTS

Normal: Test is used to diagnose malabsorption due to disaccharide deficiency. It is performed by giving disaccharide orally 1 g/kg body weight

TABLE 35 Applications for Direct and Indirect Antiglobulin Techniques

	Applications	Purpose	What Is Detected
Direct antiglobulin test (DAT)	Investigation of HTR	To detect circulating donor red cells that are sensitized with recipient antibody. A positive DAT is the first immunohematologic evidence of a hemolytic reaction after transfusion	DAT positive owing to IgG and/or C3d depending on the antibodies responsible
	Diagnosis of HDFN	To detect maternal antibodies that have crossed the placenta to sensitize fetal red cells	DAT almost always positive as a result of IgG; occasionally C3d if ABO antibodies involved
	Diagnosis of AIHA	To detect autoantibody sensitizing a patient's own red cells	Warm autoantibodies: DAT almost always positive owing to IgG Cold autoantibodies: DAT may be due to C3d only
	Investigation of drug-induced hemolysis	To detect antidrug/red cell antibodies and/or subsequent activation of the complement system	DAT may be positive owing to IgG, C3d, or both, depending on the mechanism involved (see under Investigation of Autoimmune Hemolytic Anemia section) Indirect antiglobulin test
	Antibody detection (or antibody screen)	To detect clinically significant IgG alloantibodies in the recipient	Recipient IgG antibodies bound to reagent screening cells*
	Antibody identification	To specifically identify those antibodies detected by reagent screening cells or by donor red cells	Recipient IgG antibodies bound to reagent cells from a panel of 10-12 donors*
	Crossmatching	To detect antibodies that may have been missed by the antibody screen because of absence of the corresponding antigen or presence of a dosing antibody	Recipient IgG antibodies bound to donor red cells*
	Red cell antigen typing	To type patient or donor red cells for antigens that can be detected by IgG antisera reactive only by the AGT. A common example of this would be the weak D test	Specific binding of reagent IgG antibodies to red cells positive for the corresponding antigen

AGT, Antihuman globulin test; *AIHA,* autoimmune hemolytic anemia; *HDFN,* hemolytic disease of the fetus and newborn; *HTR,* hemolytic transfusion reaction; *Ig,* immunoglobulin.
*If complement is fixed in vitro, it may be detected if polyspecific antiglobulin is used.
McPherson RA, Pincus MR: Henry's clinical diagnosis and management by laboratory methods, ed 23, St Louis, 2017, Elsevier.

to a total of 25 g. Blood is drawn at 0, 30, 60, 90, and 120 min. Normal response is a change in glucose from fasting value >30 mg/dl, inconclusive when increase is 20-30 mg/dl, abnormal when increase is >20 mg/dl. Test can also be performed by measuring air at 0, 30, 60, 90, and 120 min. Normal is H_2 >20 ppm above baseline level before a colonic response.
Decreased in: Disaccharide deficiency (lactose, fructose, sorbitol), celiac disease, sprue, acute gastroenteritis

DOC

See DEOXYCORTICOSTERONE

DONATH-LANDSTEINER (D-L) TEST FOR PAROXYSMAL COLD HEMOGLOBINURIA

Normal: No hemolysis
Interpretation: Hemolysis indicates presence of bithermic cold hemolysins or Donath-Landsteiner antibodies (D-L Ab)

DOPAMINE

Normal range: 175 pg/ml
Elevated in: Pheochromocytomas, neuroblastomas, stress, vigorous exercise, certain foods (bananas, chocolate, coffee, tea, vanilla)

D-XYLOSE ABSORPTION

Normal range: 21%-31% excreted in 5 hours
Decreased in: Malabsorption syndrome

D-XYLOSE ABSORPTION TEST

Normal range:
URINE: ≥4 g/5 hours (5-hour urine collection in adults >12 years [25-g dose])
SERUM: ≥25 mg/dl (adult, 1 hour, 25-g dose, normal renal function)
Normal results: In patients with malabsorption, normal results suggest pancreatic disease as an etiology of the malabsorption.
Abnormal results: Celiac disease, Crohn disease, tropical sprue, surgical bowel resection, AIDS. False-positives can occur with decreased renal function, dehydration/hypovolemia, surgical blind loops, decreased gastric emptying, vomiting.

ELECTROPHORESIS, HEMOGLOBIN

See HEMOGLOBIN ELECTROPHORESIS

ELECTROPHORESIS, PROTEIN

See PROTEIN ELECTROPHORESIS

ENA COMPLEX

See EXTRACTABLE NUCLEAR ANTIGEN

ENDOMYSIAL ANTIBODIES

Normal: Not detected
Present in: Celiac disease, dermatitis herpetiformis

EOSINOPHIL COUNT

Normal range:
1%-4% eosinophils (0-440/mm^3)
Elevated in
HELMINTHIC PARASITE
Ascaris lumbricoides (invasive larval stage)
Hookworms (invasive larval stage)
Strongyloides stercoralis (initial infection and autoinfection)
Trichinosis
Filariasis
Echinococcus granulosus and *E. multilocularis*
Toxocara species
Animal hookworms
Angiostrongylus cantonensis and *A. costaricensis*
Schistosomiasis
Liver flukes
Fasciolopsis buski
Anisakiasis
Capillaria philippinensis
Paragonimus westermani
"Tropical eosinophilia" (unidentified microfilariae)
NOTE: Table 36 describes an approach to investigation of eosinophilia in returning travelers.

TABLE 36 Eosinophilia Investigation in Returning Travelers

History	Allergies Drugs and vitamins (L-tryptophan) Regions, localities, and duration of exposure
Physical examination	Skin, subcutaneous tissues Liver/spleen Signs of other systemic disease
Initial investigations	Full blood count and differential white blood cell count Stool examination for ova and parasites (×3) Urine analysis Examination of midday urine for ova and parasites (×3) (in those who have traveled to Africa or the Middle East)
Further investigations as suggested by travel and exposure from history	*Strongyloides* culture and serologic testing Duodenal aspirate (strongyloidiasis, hookworm) Serologic testing (schistosomiasis, filariasis) Day/night blood films (filariasis)
Further studies if suggested by history and physical examination	Skin snips (onchocerciasis) Chest x-ray examination (hydatid cyst, tropical pulmonary eosinophilia, paragonimiasis) Soft tissue x-ray examination (cysticercosis) Sputum examination for ova and parasites (paragonimiasis) Abdominal ultrasound examination (hydatid cyst) Cystoscopy with or without biopsy (schistosomiasis) Rectal snips (schistosomiasis)

From Hoffman R: *Hematology: basic principles and practice*, ed 6, Philadelphia, Saunders, 2013.

OTHER INFECTIONS/INFESTATIONS
Pulmonary aspergillosis
Severe scabies
ALLERGIES
Asthma
Hay fever
Drug reactions
Atopic dermatitis
AUTOIMMUNE AND RELATED DISORDERS
Polyarteritis nodosa
Necrotizing vasculitis
Eosinophilic fasciitis
Pemphigus
NEOPLASTIC DISEASES
Hodgkin's disease
Mycosis fungoides
Chronic myelocytic leukemia
Eosinophilic leukemia
Polycythemia vera
Mucin-secreting adenocarcinomas
IMMUNODEFICIENCY STATES
Hyperimmunoglobulin E with recurrent infection
Wiskott-Aldrich syndrome
OTHER
Addison disease
Inflammatory bowel disease
Dermatitis herpetiformis
Toxic/chemical syndrome
Eosinophilic myalgia syndrome, tryptophan, toxic oil syndrome
Hypereosinophilic syndrome (unknown etiology)

Fig. 20 describes an algorithm for patients with eosinophil disorders.

Table 37 describes hematopoietic neoplasms accompanied by eosinophilia.

EPINEPHRINE, PLASMA

Normal range: 0-90 pg/ml
Elevated in: Pheochromocytomas, neuroblastomas, stress, vigorous exercise, certain foods (bananas, chocolate, coffee, tea, vanilla), hypoglycemia

EPSTEIN-BARR VIRUS SEROLOGY (Box 16)

Normal range: IgG anti-VCA <1:10 or negative>
Abnormal:
IgG anti-VCA >1:10 or positive indicates either current or previous infection
IgM anti-VCA >1:10 or positive indicates current or recent infection
Anti-EBNA ≥1.5 or positive indicates previous infection

Table 38 and Fig. 21 describe test interpretation.

ERYTHROCYTE SEDIMENTATION RATE (ESR, sed rate, sedimentation rate)

See Table 39 for erythrocyte sedimentation rate ranges in health.
Normal range:
Male: 0-15 mm/hr
Female: 0-20 mm/hr
Elevated in: Collagen vascular diseases, infections, myocardial infarction, neoplasms, inflammatory states (acute phase reactant), hyperthyroidism, hypothyroidism, rouleaux formation
Decreased in: Sickle cell disease, polycythemia, corticosteroids, spherocytosis, anisocytosis, hypofibrinogenemia, increased serum viscosity

ERYTHROPOIETIN (EP)

Normal: 3.7-16.0 IU/L by radioimmunoassay

Erythropoietin is a glycoprotein secreted by the kidneys that stimulates RBC production by acting on erythroid-committed stem cells.

Increased in:
Extremely high: Generally seen in patients with severe anemia (Hct, <25; Hb<7) such as in cases of aplastic anemia, severe hemolytic anemia, hematologic cancers
Very high: Patients with mild to moderate anemia (Hct, 25-35; Hb, 7-10)
High: Patients with mild anemia (e.g., AIDS, myelodysplasia)

Erythropoietin can be inappropriately elevated in patients with malignant neoplasms, renal cysts, postrenal transplant, meningioma, hemangioblastoma, and leiomyoma.

Decreased in: Renal failure, polycythemia vera, autonomic neuropathy

ESTRADIOL (serum)

Normal range:
Female, premenopausal: 30-400 pg/ml, depending on phase of menstrual cycle
Female, postmenopausal: 0-30 pg/ml
Male, adult: 10-50 pg/ml
Decreased in: Ovarian failure
Elevated in: Tumors of ovary, testis, adrenal, or nonendocrine sites (rare)

ESTROGEN

Normal range (serum):

Males:	20-80 pg/ml
Females:	
Follicular:	60-200 pg/ml
Luteal:	160-400 pg/ml
Postmenopausal:	<130 pg/ml

Normal Range (urine):

Males:	4-23 μg/g creatinine
Females:	
Follicular:	7-65 μg/g creatinine
Midcycle:	32-104 μg/g creatinine
Luteal:	8-135 μg/g creatinine

Elevated in: Hyperplasia of adrenal cortex, ovarian tumors producing estrogen, granulosa and thecal cell tumors, testicular tumors
Decreased in: Menopause, hypopituitarism, primary ovarian malfunction, anorexia nervosa, hypofunction of adrenal cortex, ovarian agenesis, psychogenic stress, gonadotropin-releasing hormone deficiency

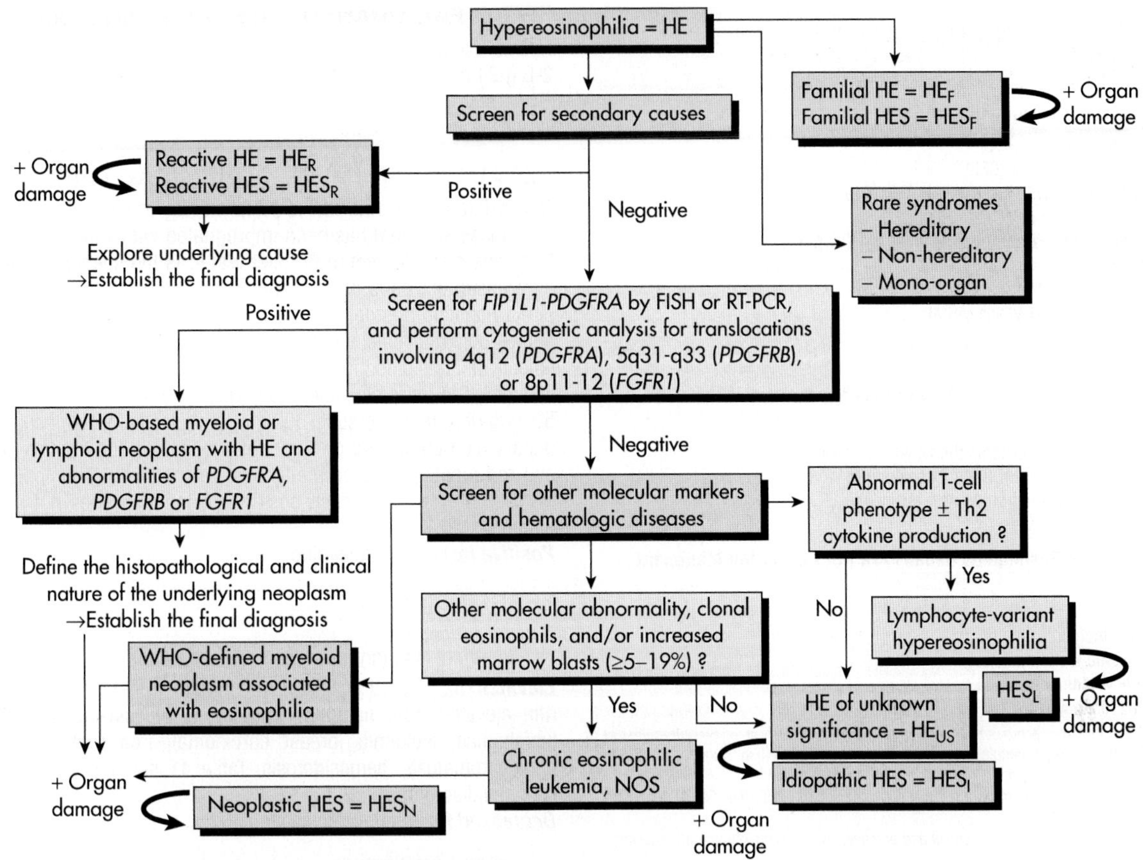

FIG. 20 Diagnostic algorithm for patients with eosinophil disorders. The first important step in the algorithm is to confirm the presence of HE, defined by a persistent (>4 weeks) increase in eosinophils above 1500/μL blood. The next important question is whether HE is reactive (HE_R) or neoplastic (clonal = HE_N) in nature. In patients with HE_N, WHO criteria should be applied in order to define the underlying molecular lesion. In addition, morphologic and histopathologic criteria are used to arrive at a final diagnosis regarding the underlying disease. In patients with HE_R, an underlying disease must also be defined. In both groups of patients, the next important question is whether (or not) HE-related organ damage is present. If such organopathy is found, it is appropriate to diagnose the (additional) presence of HES. According to the underlying etiology (disease), HES is classified again into HES_R and HES_N. In some patients with HES, a clonal T-cell population, but no lymphoproliferative disease, is detected. In these patients, the HES_L variant is diagnosed. If no clonal T cells and no underlying reactive or neoplastic condition is detected in a patient with HES, the (provisional) diagnosis of an HES_I is established. If no underlying disease and no HES are detected, the patient has HE_{US} by definition. Familial cases of HE or HES are very rare, and the same holds true for hereditary syndromes and mono-organ syndromes accompanied by HE. *HE,* Hypereosinophilia; *HES,* hypereosinophilic syndrome; *HES_F,* familial HES; *HES_I,* idiopathic HES; *HES_L,* lymphoid variant of HES; *HES_N,* primary (neoplastic) HES; *HES_R,* reactive HES; *HE_{US},* HE of undermined (unknown) significance; *WHO,* World Health Organisation. (From Hoffman R: *Hematology, basic principles and practice*, ed 7, Philadelphia, 2018, Elsevier.)

ETHANOL (blood)

Normal range:

Negative (values <10 mg/dl are considered negative)

Ethanol is metabolized at 10-25 mg/dl/hr. Levels ≥80 mg/dl are considered evidence of impairment for driving. Fatal blood concentration is considered to be >400 mg/dl. Table 40 summarizes the influence of acute ethanol ingestion on ethanol levels and behavior.

EXTRACTABLE NUCLEAR ANTIGEN (ENA COMPLEX, ANTI-RNP ANTIBODY, ANTI-SM, ANTI-SMITH)

Normal: Negative

Present in:

Systemic lupus erythematosus, rheumatoid arthritis, Sjögren syndrome, mixed connective tissue disease

FACTOR V LEIDEN

Test description: PCR test performed on whole blood or tissue. This single mutation, found in 2%-8% of the general Caucasian population, is the single most common cause of hereditary thrombophilia.

FASTING BLOOD SUGAR

See GLUCOSE, FASTING

FBS

See GLUCOSE, FASTING

FDP

See FIBRIN DEGRADATION PRODUCT

TABLE 37 Hematopoietic Neoplasms Accompanied by Eosinophilia

Neoplasms in Which Eosinophils Are Likely to Be Clonal Cells

Acute eosinophilic leukemia (AEL)
Chronic eosinophilic leukemia (CEL)
Acute myeloid leukemia with inv(16) (FAB AML M4eo)
Chronic myeloid leukemia (CML – *BCR-ABL1*⁺)
Myeloid neoplasms with *PDGFR* abnormalities (WHO types)
Hematopoietic neoplasms with *FGFR1* abnormalities (WHO types)
Smoldering systemic mastocytosis
Aggressive systemic mastocytosis (ASM)
Mast cell leukemia (MCL)
SM-AHN (SM-CEL)

Neoplasms in Which Eosinophils May or May Not Be Part of the Malignant Clone

Other myeloproliferative neoplasms (MPN) with eosinophilia[a]
Myelodysplastic syndromes (MDS) with eosinophilia
Other MDS/MPN overlap syndromes with eosinophilia[a]
Indolent systemic mastocytosis

Neoplasms in Which Eosinophils Usually Are Not Part of the Malignant Clone

Hodgkin's disease
B- or T-cell non-Hodgkin's lymphoma
Acute lymphoblastic leukemia (ALL)
Chronic lymphocytic leukemia (CLL)
Langerhans cell histiocytosis

AHN, Associated hematologic neoplasm; *FAB,* French–American–British Cooperative Study Group; *SM,* systemic mastocytosis; *WHO,* World Health Organisation.
[a]Other MPN or MPN/MDS: neoplasms where no abnormalities in the *PDGFR* or *FGFR1* genes are detectable.
From Hoffman R: *Hematology, basic principles and practice*, ed 7, Philadelphia, 2018, Elsevier.

BOX 16 Epstein-Barr Virus–Associated Malignancies

Malignancy	Epstein-Barr Virus Frequency
Hodgkin's disease	≈40%
Non-Hodgkin's lymphomas	
Burkitt lymphoma	20%-95%
Diffuse large B-cell lymphoma and CD30⁺ Ki-1⁺ anaplastic large cell lymphoma	10%-35%
Lymphomatoid granulomatosis	80%-95%
T cell–rich B-cell lymphoma	20%
Angioimmunoblastic lymphoma	>80%
T-cell, NK cell, and T/NK-cell lymphomas	30%-90%
Nasopharyngeal carcinoma	>95%
Gastric adenocarcinoma	5%-10%
Pyothorax-associated lymphoma	>95%
Leiomyosarcoma in immunocompromised patients	>95%

From Hoffman R: *Hematology: basic principles and practice*, ed 6, Philadelphia, Saunders, 2013.

FECAL FAT, QUANTITATIVE (72-hr collection)

Normal range:
2-6 g/24 hr (7-21 mmol/dl [CF: 3.515; SMI: 1 mmol/dl])
Elevated in:
Malabsorption syndrome

FECAL GLOBIN IMMUNOCHEMICAL TEST

Normal: Negative. This test is performed by immunochromatography on a cellulose strip that has been impregnated with various antibodies. The test uses a small amount of toilet water as the specimen and is placed onto absorbent pads of card similar to traditional OB card. There is no direct handling of stool. This test is specific for the globin portion of the hemoglobin molecule, which confers lower GI bleeding specificity. It specifically detects blood from the lower GI tract; guaic tests are not lower GI specific. It is more sensitive than typical Hemoccult test (detection limit 50 mcg Hb/g feces versus >500 mcg Hb/g feces for Hemoccult). It has no dietary restrictions and gives no false-positives due to plant peroxidases and red meats. It has no medication restrictions. Iron supplements and NSAIDs do not cause false-positives. Vitamin C does not cause false-negatives.
Positive in: Lower GI bleeding

FERRITIN (serum)

Normal range:
18-300 ng/ml (18-300 μg/L [CF: 1; SMI: 10 μg/L])
Elevated in: Hyperthyroidism, inflammatory states, liver disease (ferritin elevated from necrotic hepatocytes), neoplasms (neuroblastomas, lymphomas, leukemia, breast carcinoma), iron replacement therapy, hemochromatosis, hemosiderosis. Table 41 summarizes hereditary iron overload disorders.
Decreased in: Iron deficiency anemia

α-1 FETOPROTEIN

Normal range
0-20 ng/ml (0-20 μg/L [CF: 1; SMI: 1 μg/L])
Elevated in: Hepatocellular carcinoma (usually values >1000 ng/ml), germinal neoplasms (testis, ovary, mediastinum, retroperitoneum), liver

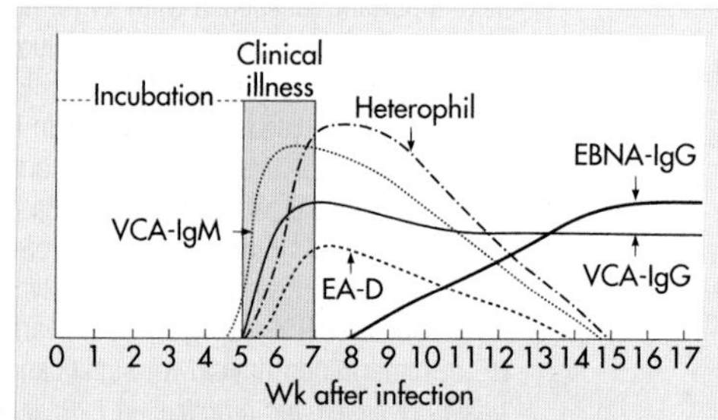

FIG. 21 Tests in Epstein-Barr viral infection. See Table 38 for abbreviations. (From Ravel R [ed]: *Clinical laboratory medicine,* ed 6, St Louis, 1995, Mosby.)

TABLE 38 Antibody Tests in Epstein-Barr Viral Infection

	Appearance	Peak	Disappears
Heterophil Ab	3-5 days after onset of Sx (range, 0-21 days)	During second wk after onset of Sx (1-4 wk)	2-3 mo after onset of Sx (still found at 1 yr in 20% of cases)
VCA-IgM	Beginning of Sx (1 wk before to 1 wk after Sx begin)	During first wk after onset of Sx (0-21 days)	2-3 mo after onset of Sx (1-6 mo)
VCA-IgG	3 days after onset of Sx (0-2 wk)	During second wk after onset of Sx (1-3 wk)	Decline to lower level, then persists for life
EBNA-IgG	3 wk after onset of Sx (1-4 wk)	8 mo after appearance (3-12 mo)	Lifelong
EA-D	5 days after onset of Sx (during first 1-2 wk after onset of Sx)	14-21 days after onset of Sx (1-4 wk)	9 wk after appearance (2-6 mo)
EBNA-IgM	Same as VCA-IgM	Same as VCA-IgM	Same as VCA-IgM

Ab, Antibody; *EA,* early antigen; *EBNA,* Epstein-Barr virus nuclear antigen; *Sx,* symptoms; *VCA,* viral capsid antigen.
From Ravel R: *Clinical laboratory medicine,* ed 6, St Louis, 1995, Mosby.

TABLE 39 Erythrocyte sedimentation ranges in health

Age Range (Years)	ESR Mean (mm in 1 h)
10–19	8
20–29	10.8
30–39	10.4
40–49	13.6
50–59	14.2
60–69	16
70–79	16.5
80–91	15.8
Pregnancy	
Early gestation	48 (62 if anaemic)
Later gestation	70 (95 if anaemic)

From Bain BJ, Bates I, Laffan MA: *Dacie and Lewis practical haematology*, ed 12, Philadelphia, 2017, Elsevier.

TABLE 40 Influence of Acute Ethanol Ingestion on Ethanol Levels and Behavior

Ounces	Blood Concentration	Influence
1-2	10-50 mg/dL (2.2-10.9 mmol/L)	1. None to mild euphoria
a. 3-4	50-100 mg/dL (10.9-21.7 mmol/L or greater)	Mild influence on stereoscopic vision and dark adaptation
	100 mg/dL (21.7 mmol/L)	Legally intoxicated
4-6	100-150 mg/dL (21.7-32.6 mmol/L)	1. Euphoria; disappearance of inhibition; prolonged reaction time
6-7	150-200 mg/dL (32.6-43.4 mmol/L)	Moderately severe poisoning; reaction time greatly prolonged; loss of inhibition and slight disturbances in equilibrium and coordination
8-9	200-250 mg/dL (43.4-54.3 mmol/L)	Severe degree of poisoning; disturbances of equilibrium and coordination; retardation of the thought processes and clouding of consciousness
10-15	250-400 mg/dL (54.3-86.8 mmol/L)	Deep, possibly fatal, coma

McPherson RA, Pincus MR: *Henry's clinical diagnosis and management by laboratory methods*, ed 23, St Louis, 2017, Elsevier.

TABLE 41 Hereditary Iron Overload Disorders

Disorder	Gene, Chromosome Location	Inheritance	Plasma Transferrin Saturation	Plasma Ferritin	Iron Deposition Sites	Clinical Manifestations
Hereditary hemochromatosis, *HFE*-associated (type 1; OMIM 235200)	*HFE*, 6p21	Autosomal recessive	Early increase; >45%	Later increase after third decade	Parenchymal iron overload affecting hepatocytes, heart, pancreas, other organs	Liver and heart disease, diabetes, gonadal failure, arthritis, skin pigmentation
Hereditary hemochromatosis, TfR2-associated (type 3; OMIM 604250)	*TFR2*, 7q22	Autosomal recessive	Early increase; >45%	Later increase after third decade	Parenchymal iron overload affecting hepatocytes, heart, pancreas, other organs	Liver and heart disease, diabetes, gonadal failure, arthritis, skin pigmentation
Juvenile hemochromatosis, hemojuvelin-associated (type 2A; OMIM 602390)	*HJV*, 1q21	Autosomal recessive	Early increase; >45%	Increased by second decade	Parenchymal iron overload affecting hepatocytes, heart, pancreas, other organs	As for hereditary hemochromatosis, but liver involvement less prominent
Juvenile hemochromatosis, hepcidin-associated (type 2B; OMIM 613313)	*HAMP*, 19q13	Autosomal recessive	Early increase; >45%	Increased by second decade	Parenchymal iron overload affecting hepatocytes, heart, pancreas, other organs	As for hereditary hemochromatosis, but liver involvement less prominent
Hemochromatosis, DMT1-associated (OMIM 206100)	*SCL11A2*, 12q13	Autosomal recessive	Early increase; >45%	Normal to moderately elevated	Hepatic iron overload, predominantly in hepatocytes	Severe microcytic anemia, liver dysfunction
Atransferrinemia (OMIM 209300)	*TF*, 3q22	Autosomal recessive	No plasma transferrin	Increased	Parenchymal iron overload affecting hepatocytes, heart, pancreas; no iron in bone marrow or spleen	Transfusion-dependent iron deficiency anemia, growth retardation, poor survival
Aceruloplasminemia (OMIM 604290)	*CP*, 3q24-q25	Autosomal recessive	Decreased	Increased	Marked iron accumulation in basal ganglia, liver, pancreas	Diabetes, progressive neurologic disease, retinal degeneration
Hemochromatosis, ferroportin-associated, with impaired iron export (type 4A; OMIM 606069)	*SLC40A1*, 2q32	Autosomal dominant	Remains normal or low	Early increase	Predominantly macrophage iron deposition	None
Hemochromatosis, ferroportin-associated, with hepcidin resistance (type 4B; OMIM 606069)	*SLC40A1*, 2q32	Autosomal dominant	Early increase; >45%	Early increase	Parenchymal iron overload affecting hepatocytes, heart, pancreas, other organs	Similar to HFE-associated hemochromatosis

From Hoffman R et al: *Hematology, basic principles and practice*, ed 6, Philadelphia, 2013, Saunders.

disease (alcoholic cirrhosis, acute hepatitis, chronic active hepatitis), fetal anencephaly, spina bifida, basal cell carcinoma, breast carcinoma, pancreatic carcinoma, gastric carcinoma, retinoblastoma, esophageal atresia

FIBRIN DEGRADATION PRODUCT (FDP)

Normal range:
<10 μg/ml
Elevated in: Disseminated intravascular coagulation, primary fibrinolysis, pulmonary embolism, severe liver disease

NOTE: The presence of rheumatoid factor may cause falsely elevated FDP.

FIBRINOGEN

Normal range:
200-400 mg/dl (2-4 g/L [CF: 0.01; SMI: 0.1 g/L])
Elevated in: Tissue inflammation or damage (acute phase protein reactant), oral contraceptives, pregnancy, acute infection, myocardial infarction
Decreased in: Disseminated intravascular coagulation, hereditary afibrinogenemia, liver disease, primary or secondary fibrinolysis, cachexia

FOLATE (folic acid)

Normal range:
Plasma: 2-10 ng/ml (4-22 nmol/L [CF: 2.266; SMI: 2 nmol/L])
Red blood cells: 140-960 ng/ml (550-2200 nmol/L [CF: 2.266; SMI: 10 nmol/L])
Decreased in: Folic acid deficiency (inadequate intake, malabsorption), alcoholism, drugs (methotrexate, trimethoprim, phenytoin, oral contraceptives, Azulfidine), vitamin B_{12} deficiency (defective red cell folate absorption), hemolytic anemia. Box 17 summarizes an etiophysiologic classification of folate deficiency.
Elevated in: Folic acid therapy

BOX 17 Etiopathophysiologic Classification of Folate Deficiency

Nutritional causes
- Decreased dietary intake—poverty and famine, institutionalized individuals (psychiatric/nursing homes)/chronic debilitating disease, prolonged feeding of infants with goat's milk, special slimming diets or food fads (folate-rich foods not consumed), cultural/ethnic cooking techniques (food folate destroyed)
- Decreased diet and increased requirements
  - Physiologic—pregnancy and lactation, prematurity, hyperemesis gravidarum, infancy
  - Pathologic
  - Intrinsic hematologic diseases involving hemolysis with compensatory erythropoiesis, abnormal hematopoiesis, or bone marrow infiltration with malignant disease
  - Dermatologic disease—psoriasis
- Folate malabsorption
- With normal intestinal mucosa
- Drugs—sulfasalazine, pyrimethamine, proton pump inhibitors (via inhibition of proton-coupled folate transporter [PCFT])
- Hereditary folate malabsorption (mutations in PCFTs) (rare)
- With mucosal abnormalities—tropical and nontropical sprue, regional enteritis

Defective cerebral spinal fluid folate transport—cerebral folate deficiency (mutation or autoantibodies to folate receptors) (rare)

Inadequate cellular utilization
- Folate antagonists (methotrexate)
- Hereditary enzyme deficiencies involving folate

Drugs (multiple effects on folate metabolism)—alcohol, sulfasalazine, triamterene, pyrimethamine, trimethoprim-sulfamethoxazole, diphenylhydantoin, barbiturates

From Hoffman R: *Hematology: basic principles and practice,* ed 6, Philadelphia, Saunders, 2013.

FOLLICLE-STIMULATING HORMONE (FSH)

Normal range:
5-20 mIU/ml
Elevated in: Menopause, primary gonadal failure, alcoholism, castration, Klinefelter's syndrome, gonadotropin-secreting pituitary hormones
Decreased in: Pregnancy, polycystic ovary disease, anorexia nervosa, anterior pituitary hypofunction

FREE T4

See T_4, FREE

FREE THYROXINE INDEX

Normal range:
1.1-4.3

INCREASED THYROXINE OR FREE THYROXINE VALUES

Laboratory error
Primary hyperthyroidism (T4/T3 type)
Severe thyroxine-binding globulin elevation
Excess therapy of hypothyroidism
Excessive dose of levothyroxine
Active thyroiditis (subacute, painless, early active Hashimoto disease)
Familial dysalbuminemic hyperthyroxinemia (some FT4 kits, especially analog types)
Peripheral resistance to T4 syndrome
Amiodarone or propranolol
Postpartum transient toxicosis
Factitious hyperthyroidism
Jod-Basedow (iodine-induced) hyperthyroidism
Severe nonthyroid illness
Acute psychosis (especially paranoid schizophrenia)
T4 sample drawn 2-4 hr after levothyroxine dose
Struma ovarii
Pituitary thyroid-stimulating hormone–secreting tumor
Certain x-ray contrast media (Telepaque and Oragrafin)
Acute porphyria
Heparin effect (some T4 and FT4 kits)
Amphetamine, heroin, methadone, and phencyclidine abuse
Perphenazine or 5-fluorouracil
Antithyroid or anti-IgG heterophil (HAMA) autoantibodies
"T4" hyperthyroidism
Hyperemesis gravidarum; about 50% of patients
High altitudes

DECREASED THYROXINE OR FREE THYROXINE VALUES

Laboratory error
Primary hypothyroidism
Severe nonthyroid illness
Lithium therapy
Severe thyroxine-binding globulin decrease (congenital, disease, or drug-induced) or severe albumin decrease
Dilantin, Depakene, or high-dose salicylate drugs
Pituitary insufficiency
Large doses of inorganic iodide (e.g., saturated solution of potassium iodide)
Moderate or severe iodine deficiency
Cushing's syndrome
High-dose glucocorticoid drugs
Pregnancy, third trimester (low normal or small decrease)
Addison disease; some patients (30%)
Heparin effect (a few FT4 kits)
Desipramine or amiodarone drugs
Acute psychiatric illness

FTA-ABS (serum)

Normal:
Nonreactive
Reactive in:
Syphilis, other treponemal diseases (yaws, pinta, bejel), SLE, pregnancy

FUROSEMIDE STIMULATION TEST

Normal: Test is performed by giving 60 mg furosemide orally after overnight fast. Patient should be on a normal diet without medications the week before the test. Normal results: renin 1-6 ng angiotensin L/ml/hr.
Elevated in: Renovascular hypertension, Bartter syndrome, high-renin essential hypertension, pheochromocytoma
No response in:
Primary aldosteronism, low-renin essential hypertension, hyporeninemic hypoaldosteronism

GAMMA-GLUTAMYL TRANSFERASE (GGT)

See γ-GLUTAMYL TRANSFERASE

GASTRIN (serum)

Normal range: 0-180 pg/ml (0-180 ng/L [CF: 1; SMI: 10 ng/L])
Elevated in: Zollinger-Ellison syndrome (gastrinoma), pernicious anemia, hyperparathyroidism, retained gastric antrum, chronic renal failure, gastric ulcer, chronic atrophic gastritis, pyloric obstruction, malignant neoplasms of the stomach, H_2-blockers, omeprazole, calcium therapy, ulcerative colitis, rheumatoid arthritis

GASTRIN STIMULATION TEST

Normal: Gastrin stimulation test after calcium infusion is performed by giving a calcium infusion (15 mg/kg in 500 ml normal saline over 4 hours). Serum is drawn in fasting state before infusion and at 1, 2, 3, and 4 hr. Normal response is little or no increase over baseline gastrin level.
Elevated in: Gastrinoma (gastrin >400 pg/ml), duodenal ulcer (gastrin level increase <400 ng/L)
Decreased in: Pernicious anemia, atrophic gastritis

GLIADIN ANTIBODIES, IGA AND IGG

Normal: <25 U, equivocal 20-25 U, positive >25 U. Test is useful to monitor compliance with gluten-free diet in patients with celiac disease.
Elevated in: Celiac disease with dietary noncompliance

GLOMERULAR BASEMENT MEMBRANE (GBM) ANTIBODY

Normal: Negative
Present in: Goodpasture syndrome

GLOMERULAR FILTRATION RATE

See Box 18 for a summary of common equations for calculating GFR or creatinine clearance. Chronic kidney disease stages based on GFR are summarized in Table 42.

Normal:

Ages 20-29	116 ml/min/1.73 m^2
Ages 30-39	107 ml/min/1.73 m^2
Ages 40-49	99 ml/min/1.73 m^2
Ages 50-59	93 ml/min/1.73 m^2
Ages 60-69	85 ml/min/1.73 m^2
Ages >75	75 ml/min/1.73 m^2

Decreased in: Renal insufficiency, decreased renal blood flow

GLUCAGON

Normal: 20-100 pg/ml
Elevated in: Glucagonoma (900-7800 pg/ml), chronic renal failure, diabetes mellitus, glucocorticoids, insulin, nifedipine, danazol, sympathomimetic amines
Decreased in: Hyperlipoproteinemia (types III, IV), beta-blockers, secretin

GLUCOSE, FASTING (FBS, fasting blood sugar)

Fig. E22 describes the approach to hypoglycemia. An algorithm for evaluation of hypoglycemia in children is described in Fig. E23.
Normal range: 60-99 mg/dl (3.8-6.0 mmol/L [CF: 0.05551; SMI: 0.1 mmol/L])
Elevated in: Diabetes mellitus, stress, infections, myocardial infarction, cerebrovascular accident, Cushing's syndrome, acromegaly, acute pancreatitis, glucagonoma, hemochromatosis, drugs (glucocorticoids, diuretics [thiazides, loop diuretics]), glucose intolerance, impaired fasting glucose

BOX 18 Common Equations for Estimating Glomerular Filtration Rate or Creatinine Clearance

Cockcroft-Gault (C_{Cr} · BSA/1.73 m^2)
For men: $C_{Cr} = [(140 - age) \cdot weight (kg)]/S_{Cr} \cdot 72$
For women: $C_{Cr} = ([(140 - age) \cdot weight (kg)]/S_{Cr} \cdot 72) \cdot 0.85$

MDRD (1)
$GFR = 170 \cdot [S_{Cr}]^{-0.999} \cdot [age]^{-0.176} \cdot$ [0.762 if patient is female] · [1.18 if patient is black] · $[BUN]^{-0170} \cdot [Alb]^{0.318}$

MDRD (2)
$GFR = 186 \cdot [S_{Cr.}]^{-1.154} \cdot [age]^{-0.203} \cdot$ [0.742 if patient is female] · [1.212 if patient is black]

Jellife (1) (C_{Cr} · BSA/1.73 m^2)
For men: $(98 - [0.8 \cdot (age - 20)])/S_{Cr}$
For women: $(98 - [0.8 \cdot (age - 20)])S_{Cr} \cdot 0.90$

Jellife (2)
For men: $(100/S_{Cr})^{-12}$
For women: $(80/S_{Cr})^{-7}$

Mawer
For men: weight · [29.3 − (0.203 · age)] · [1 − (0.03 · SCr)]
For women: weight · [25.3 − (0.175 · age)] · [1 − (0.03 · SC_r)]

Bjornsson
For men: $[27 - (0.173 \cdot age)] \cdot weight \cdot 0/S_{Cr}$
For women: $[25 - (0.175 \cdot age)] \cdot weight \cdot 0.07/S_{Cr}$

Gates
For men: $(89.4 \cdot S_{Cr}^{-1.2}) + (55 - age) \cdot (0.447 \cdot S_{Cr}^{-1.1})$
For women: $(89.4 \cdot S_{Cr}^{-1.2}) + (55 - age) \cdot (0.447 \cdot S_{Cr}^{-1.1})$

Salazar-Corcoran
For men: $[137 - age] \cdot [(0.285 \cdot weight) + (12.1 \cdot height^2)]/(51 \cdot S_{Cr})$
For women: $[146 - age] \cdot [(0.287 \cdot weight) + (9.74 \cdot height^2)]/(60 \cdot S_{Cr})$

From Vincent JL et al: *Textbook of critical care,* ed 6, Philadelphia, 2011, Saunders.

TABLE 42 Chronic Kidney Disease Stages

Stage	eGFR (mL/min/1.73 m^2)	Urinalysis Findings
1	≥90	Hematuria, proteinuria, or imaging abnormalities at >3 months
2	60-89	Hematuria, proteinuria, or imaging abnormalities at >3 months
3	30-59	↑ or normal
4	15-29	↑ or normal
5	0-14	↑ or normal

eGFR, estimated glomerular filtration rate.
Parrillo JE, Dellinger RP: *Critical care medicine, principles of diagnosis and management in the adult,* ed 4, Philadelphia, 2014, Elsevier.

Decreased in: Sulfonylurea therapy, insulin therapy, reactive hypoglycemia (e.g., subtotal gastrectomy), starvation, insulinoma, glycogen storage disorders, severe liver disease or renal disease, ethanol-induced hypoglycemia, mesenchymal tumors that secrete insulin-like hormones

GLUCOSE, POSTPRANDIAL

Normal range: <140 mg/dl (<7.8 mmol/L [CF: 0.05551; SMI: 0.1 mmol/L])
Elevated in: Diabetes mellitus, glucose intolerance
Decreased in: Post-gastrointestinal resection, reactive hypoglycemia, hereditary fructose intolerance, galactosemia, leucine sensitivity

GLUCOSE TOLERANCE TEST

Normal values above fasting:
30 min: 30-60 mg/dl (1.65-3.3 mmol/L [CF: 0.05551; SMI: 0.1 mmol/L])
60 min: 20-50 mg/dl (1.1-2.75 mmol/L [CF: 0.05551; SMI: 0.1 mmol/L])
120 min: 5-15 mg/dl (0.28-0.83 mmol/L [CF: 0.05551; SMI: 0.1 mmol/L])
180 min: fasting level or below
Abnormal in: Glucose intolerance, diabetes mellitus, Cushing's syndrome, acromegaly, pheochromocytoma, gestational diabetes

TABLE 43 Glycemic Goals in Adults*

		PREPRANDIAL GLUCOSE		POSTPRANDIAL GLUCOSE**	
	Hemoglobin A_{1c} (%)	mg/dL	mmol/L	mg/dL	mmol/L
ADA†: Adults	<7.0‡	80-130	4.4-7.2	<180	<10.0
Pregnant adults	<6.0	60-99	3.3-5.5	100-129	5.6-7.2
Older adults:					
Healthy	<7.5	90-130	5.0-7.2	90-150	5.0-8.3
Intermediate	<8.0	90-150	5.0-8.3	100-180	5.6-10.0
Poor health	<8.5	100-180	5.6-10.0	110-200	6.1-11.1
AACE§,¶	≤6.5	≤110	≤6.1	≤140	<7.8

*Youth <18 years of age: goal hemoglobin A_{1c} <7.5%.
**1 to 2 hours after beginning a meal for adults, except bedtime for older adults.
†American Diabetes Association (2015); Chiang et al (2014).
‡Lower goals may be appropriate for selected individuals if this can be accomplished safely (without significant hypoglycemia). Higher goals may be appropriate in some individuals (e.g., with a history of severe hypoglycemia, limited life expectancy, advanced complications, extensive comorbid conditions, or long-standing diabetes in whom the goal is difficult to achieve with appropriate education, monitoring, and therapies, including insulin).
§AACE, American Association of Clinical Endocrinologists, 2015.
¶For patients without concurrent serious illness and at low hypoglycemia risk.
From McPherson RA, Pincus MR: *Henry's clinical diagnosis and management by laboratory methods*, ed 23, St Louis, 2017, Elsevier.

GLUCOSE-6-PHOSPHATE DEHYDROGENASE (G6PD) SCREEN (blood)

Normal: G6PD enzyme activity detected
Abnormal: If a deficiency is detected, quantitation of G6PD is necessary; a G6PD screen may be falsely interpreted as "normal" after an episode of hemolysis because most G6PD-deficient cells have been destroyed.

γ-GLUTAMYL TRANSFERASE (GGT)

Normal range: 0-30 U/L (0.050 μkat/L [CF: 0.01667; SMI: 0.01 μkat/L])
Elevated in: Chronic alcoholic liver disease, neoplasms (hepatoma, metastatic disease to the liver, carcinoma of the pancreas), systemic lupus erythematosus, congestive heart failure, trauma, nephrotic syndrome, sepsis, cholestasis, drugs (phenytoin, barbiturates)

GLYCOHEMOGLOBIN (glycated glycosylated] hemoglobin), (HbA1c)

Normal range: 4.0%-5.9%. Glycemic goals in adults are summarized in Table 43.
Elevated in: Uncontrolled diabetes mellitus (glycated hemoglobin levels reflect the level of glucose control over the preceding 120 days), lead toxicity, alcoholism, iron deficiency anemia, hypertriglyceridemia
Decreased in: Hemolytic anemias, decreased red blood cell survival, pregnancy, acute or chronic blood loss, chronic renal failure, insulinoma, congenital spherocytosis, hemoglobin S, C, and D diseases

GROWTH HORMONE

Normal: Male: 1-9 ng/ml; female: 1-16 ng/ml
Elevated in: Pituitary gigantism, acromegaly, ectopic GH secretion, cirrhosis, renal failure, anorexia nervosa, stress, exercise, prolonged fasting, amphetamines, beta-blockers, insulin, levodopa, metoclopramide, clonidine, vasopressin, human growth hormone (HGH) supplementation
Decreased in: Hypopituitarism, pituitary dwarfism, adrenocortical hyperfunction, bromocriptine, corticosteroids, glucose

GROWTH HORMONE RELEASING HORMONE (GHRH)

Normal: <50 pg/ml
Elevated in: Acromegaly caused by GHRH secretion by neoplasms

GROWTH HORMONE SUPPRESSION TEST (after glucose)

Normal: Test is done by giving 1.75 g glucose/kg orally after overnight fast. Blood is drawn at baseline, after 60 min, and after 120 min of glucose load. Normal response is growth hormone suppression to <2 ng/ml or undetectable levels.
Abnormal: There is no or incomplete suppression from the high basal level in gigantism or acromegaly.

HAM TEST (acid serum test)

Normal: Negative
Positive in: Paroxysmal nocturnal hemoglobinuria
False-positive in: Hereditary or acquired spherocytosis, recent transfusion with aged red blood cells, aplastic anemia, myeloproliferative syndromes, leukemia, hereditary dyserythropoietic anemia type II

HAPTOGLOBIN (serum)

Normal range: 50-220 mg/dl (0.50-2.2 g/L [CF: 0.01; SMI: 0.01 g/L])
Elevated in: Inflammation (acute phase reactant), collagen vascular diseases, infections (acute phase reactant), drugs (androgens), obstructive liver disease
Decreased in: Hemolysis (intravascular more than extravascular), megaloblastic anemia, severe liver disease, large tissue hematomas, infectious mononucleosis, drugs (oral contraceptives)

HBA$_{1C}$

See GLYCOHEMOGLOBIN

HDL

See HIGH-DENSITY LIPOPROTEIN CHOLESTEROL

HELICOBACTER PYLORI (serology, stool antigen)

Normal range: Not detected
Detected in: *H. pylori* infection. Positive serology can indicate current or past infection. Positive stool antigen test indicates acute infection (sensitivity and specificity >90%). Stool testing should be delayed at least 4 weeks after eradication therapy.

HEMATOCRIT

Normal range:
Male: 39%-49% (0.39-0.49 [CF: 0.01; SMI: 0.01])
Female: 33%-43% (0.33-0.43 [CF: 0.01; SMI: 0.01])
Elevated in: Polycythemia vera, smoking, chronic obstructive pulmonary disease, high altitudes, dehydration, hypovolemia
Decreased in: Blood loss (gastrointestinal, genitourinary) anemia

HEMOGLOBIN

Normal range:
Male: 13.6-17.7 g/dl (136-172 g/L [CF: 10; SMI: 1 g/L])
Female: 12.0-15.0 g/dl (120-150 g/L [CF: 10; SMI: 1 g/L])
Elevated in: Hemoconcentration, dehydration, polycythemia vera, chronic obstructive pulmonary disease, high altitudes, false elevations (hyperlipemic plasma, white blood cells >50,000/mm^3), stress
Decreased in: Hemorrhagic (gastrointestinal, genitourinary) anemia

HEMOGLOBIN A_{1C}

See GLYCOHEMOGLOBIN

HEMOGLOBIN ELECTROPHORESIS

Table 44 describes neonatal hemoglobin electrophoresis patterns, Table 45 summarizes types of hemoglobin, and Table 46 describes classifications of hemoglobinopathies.

TABLE 44 Neonatal Hemoglobin (Hb) Electrophoresis Patterns*

FA	Fetal Hb and adult normal Hb; the normal newborn pattern.
FAV	Indicates the presence of both HbF and HbA. However, an anomalous band (V) is present, which does not appear to be any of the common Hb variants.
FAS	Indicates fetal Hb, adult normal HbA, and HbS, consistent with benign sickle cell trait.
FS	Fetal and sickle HbS without detectable adult normal HbA. Consistent with clinically significant homozygous sickle Hb genotype (S/S) or sickle β-thalassemia, with manifestations of sickle cell anemia during childhood.
FC†	Designates the presence of HbC without adult normal HbA. Consistent with clinically significant homozygous HbC genotype (C/C), resulting in a mild hematologic disorder presenting during childhood.
FSC	HbS and HbC present. This heterozygous condition could lead to the manifestations of sickle cell disease during childhood.
FAC	HbC and adult normal HbA present, consistent with benign HbC trait.
FSA	Heterozygous HbS/β-thalassemia, a clinically significant sickling disorder.
F†	Fetal HbF is present without adult normal HbA. Although this may indicate a delayed appearance of HbA, it is also consistent with homozygous β-thalassemia major, or homozygous hereditary persistence of fetal HbF.
FV†	Fetal HbF and an anomalous Hb variant (V) are present.
AF	May indicate prior blood transfusion. Submit another filter paper blood specimen when the infant is 4 mo of age, at which time the transfused blood cells should have been cleared.

NOTE: HbA: $\alpha 2\beta 2$; HbF: $\alpha 2\gamma 2$; HbA2: $\alpha 2\delta 2$.
*Hemoglobin variants are reported in order of decreasing abundance; for example, FA indicates more fetal than adult hemoglobin.
†Repeat blood specimen should be submitted to confirm the original interpretation.
From Tschudy MM, Arcara KM: *The Harriet Lane handbook,* ed 19, Philadelphia, 2012, Mosby.

TABLE 45 Types of Hemoglobin

	Hemoglobin	Structure	Comment
Normal	A	$\alpha_2\beta_2$	97% of adult hemoglobin
	A_2	$\alpha_2\delta_2$	2% of adult Hb; elevated in β-thalassemia
	F	$\alpha_2\gamma_2$	Normal Hb in fetus from 3rd to 9th month; increased in β-thalassemia
Abnormal chain production	H	β_4	Found in α-thalassemia, biologically useless
	Barts	γ_4	Found in α-thalassemia, biologically useless
Abnormal chain structure	S	$\alpha_2\beta_2$	Substitution of valine for glutamic acid in position 6 of β chain
	C	$\alpha_2\beta_2$	Substitution of lysine for glutamic acid in position 6 of β chain

From Ballinger A: *Kumar & Clark's essentials of clinical medicine,* ed 6, Edinburgh, 2012, Saunders.

Normal range:
HbA_1: 95%-98%
HbA_2: 1.5%-3.5%
HbF: <2%
HbC: absent
HbS: absent

HEMOGLOBIN, GLYCATED

See GLYCOHEMOGLOBIN

HEMOGLOBIN, GLYCOSYLATED

See GLYCOHEMOGLOBIN

HEMOGLOBIN H

See Table 45.
Normal: Negative
Present in: Hemoglobin H disease, alpha-thalassemia trait, unstable hemoglobin disorders

HEMOGLOBIN, URINE

See URINE HEMOGLOBIN, FREE

HEMOSIDERIN, URINE

See URINE HEMOGLOBIN, FREE

HEPARIN-INDUCED THROMBOCYTOPENIA ANTIBODIES

Normal: Antigen assay: Negative, <0.45; weak, 0.45-1.0; strong, >1.0
Elevated in: Heparin-induced thrombocytopenia

TABLE 46 Classification of Hemoglobinopathies

Structural hemoglobinopathies—hemoglobins with altered amino acid sequences that result in deranged function or altered physical or chemical properties
Abnormal hemoglobin polymerization—HBS
Altered oxygen affinity
High affinity—polycythemia
Low affinity—cyanosis, pseudoanemia
Hemoglobins that oxidize readily
Unstable hemoglobins, hemolytic anemia, jaundice
M hemoglobins—methemoglobinemia, cyanosis
Thalassemias—defective production of globin chains
α-Thalassemias
β-Thalassemias
δβ-, γδβ-, αβ-Thalassemias
Structural hemoglobinopathies—structurally abnormal Hb associated with coinherited thalassemia phenotype
HbE
Hb constant spring
Hb lepore
Hereditary persistence of fetal hemoglobin—persistence of high levels of HbF into adult life
Pancellular—all red blood cells contain elevated HbF levels
Nondeletion forms
Deletion forms
Hb Kenya
Heterocellular—only specific subpopulation of red blood cells contain elevated levels of HbF
Acquired hemoglobinopathies
Methemoglobin due to toxic exposures
Sulfhemoglobin due to toxic exposures
Carboxyhemoglobin
HbH in erythroleukemia
Elevated HbF in states of erythroid stress and bone marrow dysplasia, usually heterocellular

Hb, Hemoglobin.
From Hoffman R: *Hematology: basic principles and practice,* ed 6, Philadelphia, 2013, Saunders.

HEPATITIS A ANTIBODY

Normal: Negative

Present in: Viral hepatitis A; can be IgM or IgG (if IgM, acute hepatitis A; if IgG, previous infection with hepatitis A)

See Fig. 24 for serologic tests in HAV infection.

See Table 47 for serologic and virologic tests for hepatitis viruses.

HAV-IGM ANTIBODY

Appearance: About the same time as clinical symptoms (3-4 weeks after exposure; range, 14-60 days), or just before beginning of AST/ALT elevation (range, 10 days before to 7 days after)

Peak: About 3-4 weeks after onset of symptoms (1-6 weeks)

Becomes nondetectable: 3-4 months after onset of symptoms (1-6 months). In a few cases HAV-IgM antibody can persist as long as 12-14 months.

HAV TOTAL ANTIBODY

Appearance: About 3 weeks after IgM becomes detectable (therefore about the middle of clinical symptom period to early convalescence)

Peak: About 1-2 months after onset

Becomes nondetectable: Remains elevated for life but can somewhat slowly fall

HEPATITIS A VIRAL INFECTION

Best all-purpose test(s) to diagnose acute HAV infection = HAV-Ab (IgM)

Best all-purpose test(s) to demonstrate past HAV infection/immunity = HAV-Ab (total)

HEPATITIS B SURFACE ANTIGEN (HBsAg)

Normal: Not detected

Detected in: Acute viral hepatitis type B, chronic hepatitis B

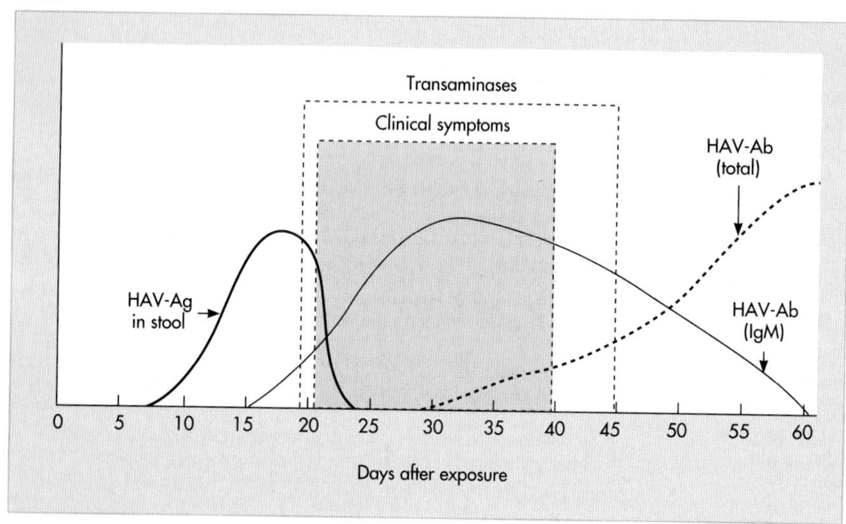

FIG. 24 Serologic tests in hepatitis A viral infection. (From Ravel R [ed]: *Clinical laboratory medicine,* ed 6, St Louis, 1995, Mosby.)

TABLE 47 Serologic and Virologic Tests for Hepatitis Viruses

IgM Anti-HAV	IgG Anti-HAV	HBsAg	Anti-HBs	IgM Anti-HBVc	HBeAg	Anti-HBe	HBV DNA	Anti-HCV Screen	HCV RNA	Anti-HDV	Anti-HEV
HAV:											
Acute	+	+									
Remote	+	+									
HBV:											
Early			+	−	+	+	−	+			
Window			−	−	+	−	−	+			
Resolving			−/+	+	−	−/+	+	−/+			
Chronic			+	−/+	−	+	+/−	+			
TX monitoring								+			
Remote			−	+	−	−/+	+/−	−/+			
HCV:											
Screen									+	+	
Acute									+/−	+	
Chronic									+	+	
TX monitoring										+	
Remote									+	−/+	
HDV:											
Superinfection			+	−	+/−	+	−/+	+/−			+
HEV											+

HAV, Hepatitis A virus; *HBe,* hepatitis E; *HBeAg,* hepatitis E antigen; *HBs,* hepatitis B surface; *HBsAg,* hepatitis B surface antigen; *HBV,* hepatitis B virus; *HCV,* hepatitis C virus; *HDV,* hepatitis D virus; *HEV,* hepatitis E virus; *IgM,* immunoglobulin M; +, positive; −, negative.

Data from CDC: Surveillance for acute hepatitis, United States, 2007, *MMWR* 58(SS-3), 2009.

From McPherson RA, Pincus MR: *Henry's clinical diagnosis and management by laboratory methods,* ed 23, Philadelphia, 2017, Elsevier.

Appearance: 2-6 weeks after exposure (range, 6 days to 6 months); 5%-15% of patients are negative at onset of jaundice
Peak: 1-2 weeks before to 1-2 weeks after onset of symptoms
Becomes nondetectable: 1-3 months after peak (range, 1 week to 5 months)

HEPATITIS B VIRAL INFECTION

See Table 48

Figs. 25, 26, and 27 illustrate antigens and antibodies in hepatitis B infection.

HB_S

-Ag

HB_SAg: shows current active HBV infection.
Persistence over 6 months indicates carrier/chronic HBV infection.
HBV nucleic acid probe: present before and longer than HB_SAg.
More reliable marker for increased infectivity than HB_SAg and/or HB_eAg.

TABLE 48 Serologic Markers of Hepatitis B Infection

	HBsAg	anti-HBc	anti-HBs	IgM anti-HBc
Susceptible to infection	Negative	Negative	Negative	Negative
Immune due to natural infection	Negative	Positive	Positive	Negative
Immune due to hepatitis B vaccination	Negative	Negative	Positive	Negative
Acutely infected	Positive	Positive	Negative	Positive
Chronically infected	Positive	Positive	Negative	Negative

From Ballinger A: *Kumar & Clark's essentials of clinical medicine,* ed 6, Edinburgh, 2012, Saunders.

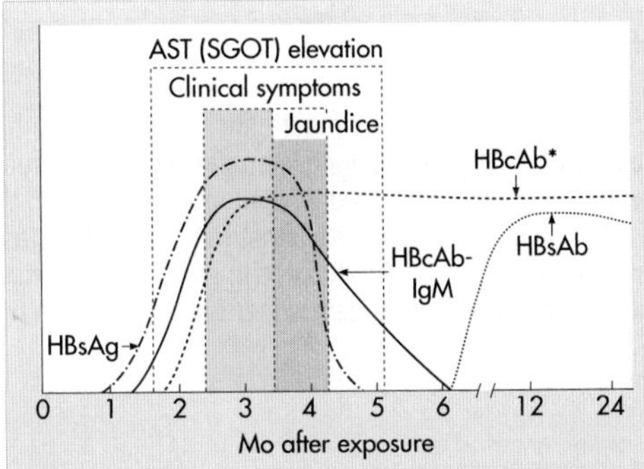

FIG. 25 Hepatitis B virus surface antigen-antibody and core antibodies. Note "core window." *$HB_CAb = HB_CAb$-IgM + HBCAb-IgG (combined). (From Ravel R [ed]: *Clinical laboratory medicine,* ed 6, St Louis, 1995, Mosby.)

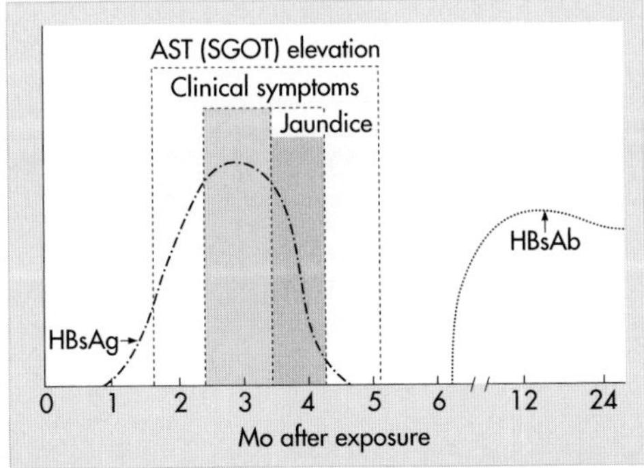

FIG. 26 Hepatitis B virus surface antigen and antibody (HB_SAg and HB_SAb-total). (From Ravel R [ed]: *Clinical laboratory medicine,* ed 6, St Louis, 1995, Mosby.)

-Ab

HB_SAb-total: shows previous healed HBV infection and evidence of immunity.

HB_C

-Ab

HB_CAb-IgM: shows either acute or very recent infection by HBV.
In convalescent phase of acute HBV, may be elevated when HB_SAg has disappeared (core window).
Negative HB_CAb-IgM with positive HB_SAg suggests either very early acute HBV or carrier/chronic HBV.
HB_CAb-total: only useful to show past HBV infection if HB_SAg and HB_cAb-IgM are both negative.

HB_E

-Ag

HB_e-AbAg: when present, especially without HB_eAb, suggests increased patient infectivity.
HB_eAb-total: when present, suggests less patient infectivity.

- HB_SAg positive, HB_CAb negative
  - About 5% (range, 0%-17%) of patients with early-stage HBV acute infection (HB_CAb rises later)
- HB_SAg positive, HB_CAb positive, HB_SAb negative
  - Most of the clinical symptom stage
  - Chronic HBV carriers without evidence of liver disease ("asymptomatic carriers")
  - Chronic HBV hepatitis (chronic persistent type or chronic active type)
- HB_SAg negative, HB_CAb positive,* HB_SAb negative
  - Late clinical symptom stage or early convalescence stage (core window)
  - Chronic HBV infection with HB_SAg below detection levels with current tests
  - Old previous HBV infection
- HB_SAg negative, HB_CAb positive, HB_SAb positive
  - Late convalescence to complete recovery
  - Old infection

HEPATITIS C VIRAL INFECTION

Fig. 28 illustrates antigens and antibodies in hepatitis C infection. Table 49 summarizes interpretation of patterns of HCV markers.

HEPATITIS C RNA

Normal: Negative
Elevated in: Hepatitis C. Detection of hepatitis C-RNA is used to confirm current infection and to monitor treatment. Quantitative assays (viral load) are needed before treatment to assess response (<2 log decrease after 12-week treatment indicates lack of response).

HCV

-Ag

HCV nucleic acid probe: shows current infection by HCV (especially with PCR amplification).

-Ab

HCV-Ab (IgG): current, convalescent, or old HCV infection.

HAV

-Ag

HAV-Ag by EM: shows presence of virus in stool early in infection.

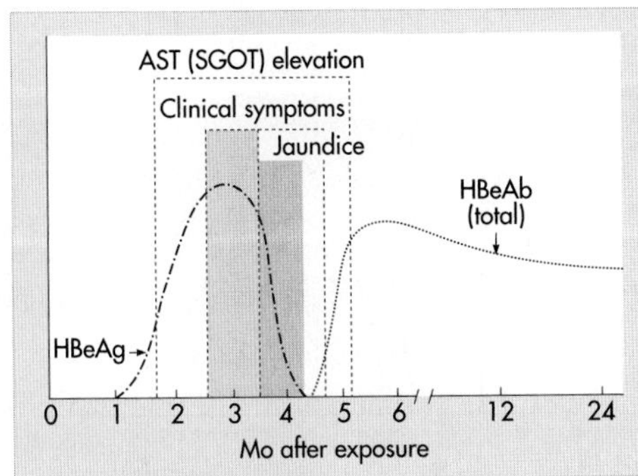

FIG. 27 HBVe antigen and antibody. (From Ravel R [ed]: *Clinical laboratory medicine,* ed 6, St Louis, 1995, Mosby.)

-Ab
HAV-Ab (IgM): current or recent HAV infection.
HAV-Ab (total): convalescent or old HAV infection.

HEPATITIS D VIRAL INFECTION

Fig. 29 illustrates antigens and antibodies in hepatitis D infection.
Best current all-purpose screening test = HDV-Ab (total)
Best test to differentiate acute from chronic infection = HDV-Ab (IgM)

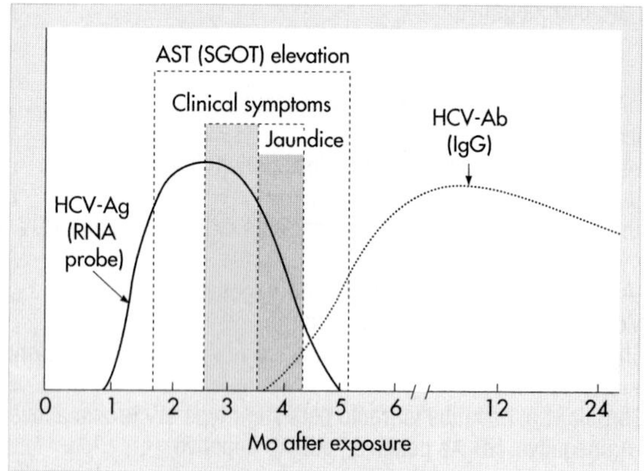

FIG. 28 Hepatitis C virus antigen and antibody. (From Ravel R [ed]: *Clinical laboratory medicine,* ed 6, St Louis, 1995, Mosby.)

TABLE 49 Interpretation of Patterns of HCV Markers

Interpretation	Anti-HCV	RIBA	HCV RNA
Acute HCV infection	–	–	+
Active HCV infection	+	+	+
Possible HCV clearance	+	+	–
False-positive HCV test	+	–	–
Requires further study	+	Indeterminate*	–

HCV, Hepatitis C; *RIBA,* recombinant immunoassay.
*Indeterminate result: only one band positive, or more than one band and nonspecific reactivity.
From McPherson RA, Pincus MR: *Henry's clinical diagnosis and management by laboratory methods,* ed 23, St Louis, 2017, Elsevier.

DELTA HEPATITIS COINFECTION (acute HDV1 acute HBV) **OR SUPERINFECTION** (acute HDV1 chronic HBV)

HDV

-Ag
HDV-Ag: shows current infection (acute or chronic) by HDV.
HDV nucleic acid probe: detects antigen before and longer than HDV-Ag by EIA.

-Ab
HDV-Ab (IgM): high elevation in acute HDV; does not persist.
Low or moderate elevation in convalescent HDV; does not persist.
Low to high persistent elevation in chronic HDV (depends on degree of cell injury and sensitivity of the assay).
HDV-Ab (total): high elevation in acute HDV; does not persist.
High persistent elevation in chronic HDV.

HDV-AG

Detected by DNA probe, less often by immunoassay
Appearance: Prodromal stage (before symptoms); just at or after initial rise in ALT (about a week after appearance of HB_SAg and about the time HB_CAb-IgM level begins to rise)
Peak: 2-3 days after onset
Becomes nondetectable: 1-4 days (may persist until shortly after symptoms appear)

HDV-AB (IgM)

Appearance: About 10 days after symptoms begin (range, 1-28 days)
Peak: About 2 weeks after first detection
Becomes nondetectable: About 35 days (range, 10-80 days) after first detection (most other IgM antibodies take 3-6 months to become nondetectable)

HDV-AB (total)

Appearance: About 50 days after symptoms begin (range, 14-80 days); about 5 weeks after HDV-Ag (range, 3-11 weeks)
Peak: About 2 weeks after first detection
Becomes nondetectable: About 7 months after first detection (range, 4-14 months)

HER-2/*NEU*

Normal: Negative
Present in: 25%-30% of primary breast cancers. It can also be found in other epithelial tumors, including lung, hepatocellular, pancreatic, colon, stomach, ovarian, cervical, and bladder cancer. Trastuzumab (Herceptin) is a humanized monoclonal antibody against Her-2/*neu.* This test is useful to identify patients with metastatic; recurrent; and/or treatment-refractory, unresectable, locally advanced breast cancer for trastuzumab treatment.

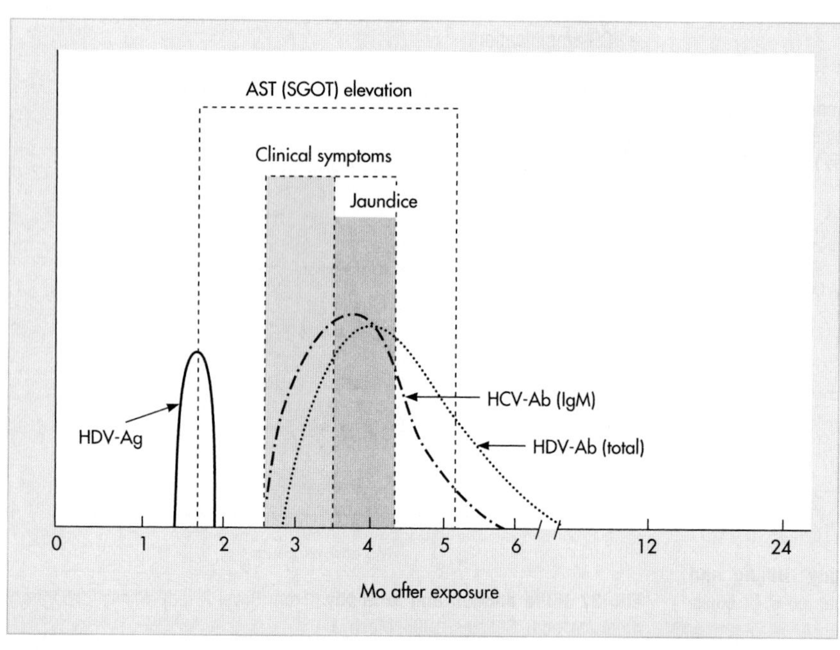

FIG. 29 Hepatitis D virus antigen and antibodies. (From Ravel R [ed]: *Clinical laboratory medicine,* ed 6, St Louis, 1995, Mosby.)

HERPES SIMPLEX VIRUS (HSV)

Test description: The PCR test can be performed on serum biopsy samples, CSF, vitreous humor.

HFE SCREEN FOR HEREDITARY HEMOCHROMATOSIS

Test description: PCR test can be performed on whole blood or tissue. One mutation (C282Y) and two polymorphisms (H63D, S65C) account for the majority of alleles associated with this disease.

HETEROPHIL ANTIBODY

Normal: Negative
Positive in: Infectious mononucleosis

HIGH-DENSITY LIPOPROTEIN (HDL) CHOLESTEROL

Normal range
Male: 40-70 mg/dl (0.8-1.8 mmol/L [CF: 0.02586; SMI: 0.05 mmol/L])
Female: 50-90 mg/dl (1.1-2.35 mmol/L [CF: 0.02586; SMI: 0.05 mmol/L])
Increased in: Use of gemfibrozil, statins, fenofibrate, nicotinic acid, estrogens, regular aerobic exercise, small (1 oz) daily alcohol intake
Decreased in: Deficiency of apoproteins, liver disease, probucol ingestion, Tangier disease

NOTE: A cholesterol/HDL ratio >4.0 is associated with increased risk of coronary artery disease. Table 50 summarizes significant human apolipoproteins.

HLA ANTIGENS

Associated disorders: see Table 51

HOMOCYSTEINE (plasma)

Normal range

0-30 years: 4.6-8.1 mcmol/L
30-59 years: 6.3-11.2 mcmol/L (males), 4.5-7.9 mcmol/L (females)
>59 years: 5.8-11.9 mcmol/L

Increased: Thrombophilic states, B_6, B_{12}, folic acid, riboflavin deficiency, pregnancy, homocystinuria

NOTE: An increased homocysteine level is an independent risk factor for atherosclerosis.

HUMAN CHORIONIC GONADOTROPIN (hCG)

Normal range: Varies with gestational stage:

1 wk: 5-50 mU/ml
1-2 wk: 50-550 mU/ml
2-3 wk: up to 5000 mU/ml
3-4 wk: up to 10,000 mU/ml
4-5 wk: up to 50,000 mU/ml
2-3 mo: 10,000-100,000 mU/ml

TABLE 50 Significant Human Apolipoproteins

					PLASMA CONCENTRATION	
Apolipoprotein	**Major Lipoproteins**	**Mr* (kDa)**	**Amino Acids**	**Chromosome**	**mmol/L**	**mg/dL**
A-I	HDL	29	243-245	11	32-46	90-130
A-II	HDL	17.4	154	1	18-29	30-50
A-IV	HDL, LDL	44.5	396	11		
(a)	Lp(a)	350-700	Variable	6		
B-100	VLDL, IDL, LDL	512.7	4536	2	1.5-1.8	80-100
B-48	CM	240.8	2152	2	<0.2	<5
C-I	CM, LDL	6.6	57	19	6.1-10.8	4-7
C-II	CM, LDL	8.9	78 or 79	19	3.4-9.1	3-8
C-III	CM	8.8	79	11	9.1-17.1	8-15
D	HDL	19	169	3		
E	CM, LDL, IDL	34.1	299	19	0.8-1.6	3-6
F	HDL, LDL, VLDL	29	162	12		8.35
H	VLDL	50	326	17		20
J	HDL	80	449	8		
L	HDL	39-42	383	22	Not present in plasma	
M	HDL, LDL, VLDL, CM	26	188	6		2-15
0	HDL, LDL, VLDL	22.3	198	X		

CM, Chylomicron; *HDL,* high-density lipoprotein; *IDL,* intermediate-density lipoprotein; *LDL,* low-density lipoprotein; *Lp(a),* lipoprotein A; *VLDL,* very-low-density lipoprotein.
*Relative molecular mass.
From McPherson RA, Pincus MR: *Henry's clinical diagnosis and management by laboratory methods*, ed 23, St Louis, 2017, Elsevier.

Laboratory Tests

IV

TABLE 51 HLA Antigens Associated with Specific Diseases

Antigen	**Condition**	**Antigen**	**Condition**
HLA-B27	Ankylosing spondylitis	HLA-B8, Dw3	Celiac disease
	Reiter's syndrome	HLA-B8, Dw3	Dermatitis herpetiformis
	Psoriatic arthritis	HLA-B8	Myasthenia gravis
HLA-A10, B18, Dw2	C2 deficiency	HLA-B8	Chronic active hepatitis in children
HLA-A2, B40, Cw3	C4 deficiency	HLA-Drw4	Active chronic hepatitis in adults
HLA-B7, Dw2	Multiple sclerosis	HLA-B13, Bw17	Psoriasis
HLA-A3	Hemochromatosis		

HLA, Human leukocyte antigen.
From Cerra FB: *Manual of critical care,* St Louis, 1987, Mosby.

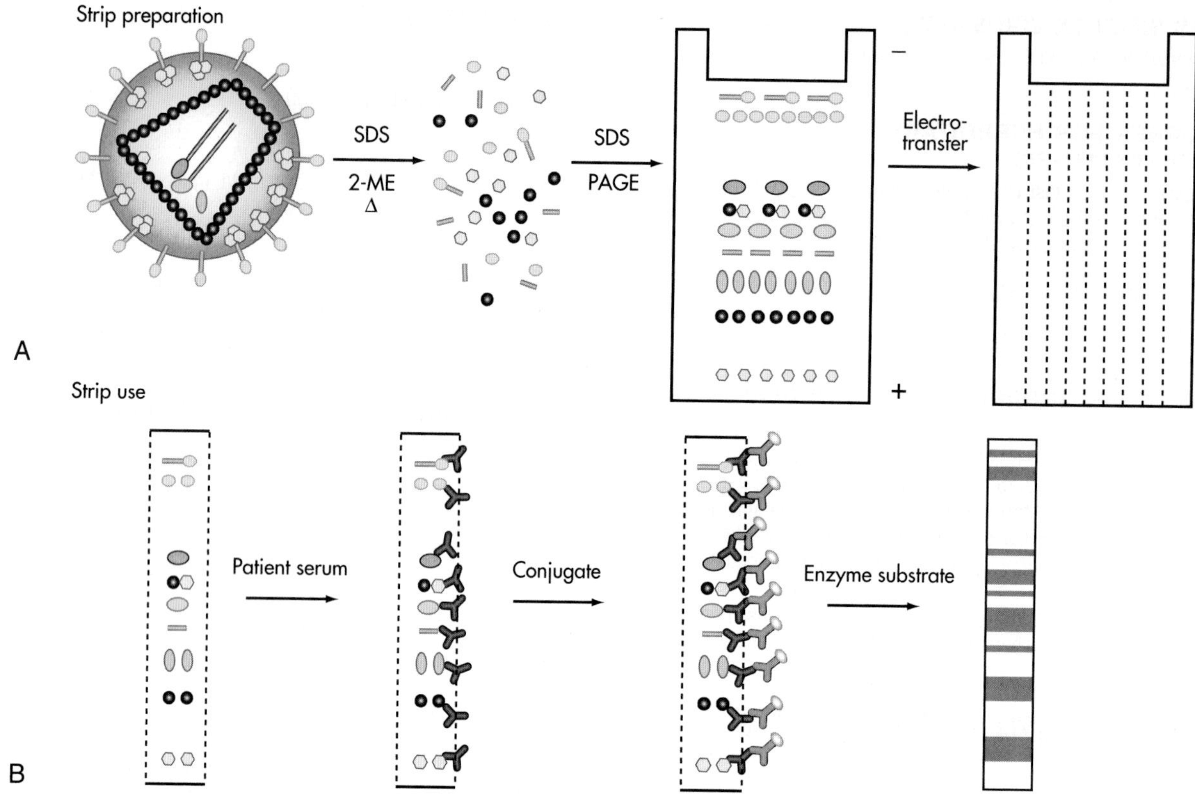

FIG. 30 Human immunodeficiency virus (HIV) Western blot. A, Western blot strips are prepared with purified HIV virions that are disrupted with ionic detergent and reducing agent, subjected to sodium dodecyl sulfate–polyacrylamide gel electrophoresis (SDS-PAGE), and electrotransferred to solid strips, typically of nitrocellulose. **B,** Strips are sequentially incubated with patient sample (serum, plasma, saliva, or urine); enzyme-conjugated antihuman IgG; and enzyme substrate. The positions of enzymes bound identify the presence of antibody to individual HIV proteins. (From Bennett JE, Dolin R, Blaser MJ: *Mandell, Douglas, and Bennett's principles and practice of infectious diseases,* ed 8, Philadelphia, 2015, Saunders.)

Elevated in: Normal pregnancy, hydatidiform mole, choriocarcinoma, germ cell tumors of testicle, some nontrophoblastic neoplasms (e.g., neoplasms of cervix, gastrointestinal tract, ovary, lung, breast)

HUMAN HERPES VIRUS 8 (HHV8)

Test description: PCR test can be performed on whole blood, tissue, bone marrow, and urine. HHV8 is found in all forms of Kaposi's sarcoma.

HUMAN IMMUNODEFICIENCY VIRUS ANTIBODY, TYPE 1 (HIV-1)

Normal range: Not detected

Abnormal result: HIV antibodies usually appear in the blood 1-4 months after infection.

Testing sequence

ELISA is the recommended initial screening test. Sensitivity and specificity are >99%. False-positive ELISA may occur with autoimmune disorders, administration of immune globulin manufactured before 1985, within 6 weeks of testing, in the presence of rheumatoid factor, in the presence of DLA-DR antibodies in multigravida female, with administration of influenza vaccine within 3 months of testing, with hemodialysis, with positive plasma reagin test, and with certain medical disorders (hemophilia, hypergammaglobulinemia, alcoholic hepatitis).

A positive ELISA is confirmed with Western blot (Fig. 30). False-positive Western blot may result from connective tissue disorders, human leukocyte antigen antibodies, polyclonal gammopathies, hyperbilirubinemia, presence of antibody to another human retrovirus, or cross-reaction with other non–virus-derived proteins in healthy persons. Undetermined Western blot may occur in AIDS patients with advanced immunodeficiency (caused by loss of antibodies) and in recent HIV infections.

PCR is used to confirm indeterminate Western blot results or negative results in persons with suspected HIV infection.

Fig. 31 describes tests in HIV infection; indications for plasma HIV RNA testing are described in Table 52.

HUMAN IMMUNODEFICIENCY VIRUS TYPE 1 (HIV-1) Antigen (p24), Qualitative (p24 antigen)

Normal range: Negative. This test detects uncomplexed HIV-1 p24 antigen. The core protein p24 is the first detectable protein encoded by the group-specific antigen *(gag)* gene. This protein is a marker for viremia. This test should not be used in place of HIV-1 antibody testing as a screen for HIV-1 infection. HIV-1 p24 may be detectable in the first month of acute HIV-1 infection and generally falls to undetectable levels during the asymptomatic stage of HIV-1 infection. A negative result does not exclude the possibility of infection or exposure to HIV-1. It is recommended that a negative result be followed with repeat testing at least 8 weeks after the original test. This test is used primarily for screening of donated blood and plasma and as an aid for the prognosis of HIV-1 infection.

HUMAN IMMUNODEFICIENCY VIRUS TYPE 1 (HIV-1) VIRAL LOAD

Normal range: HIV-1 RNA, quant. bDNA 3: less than 50 copies/ml or less than 1.7 log copies/ml

This test should be used only in individuals with documented HIV-1 infection for monitoring the progression of infection, response to antiretroviral therapy, and disease prognosis. It is not indicated for diagnosis of HIV infection.

HUMAN PAPILLOMA VIRUS (HPV)

Test description: PCR test can be performed on cervical smears, biopsies, scrapings, liquid cytology specimen, and anogenital tissues.

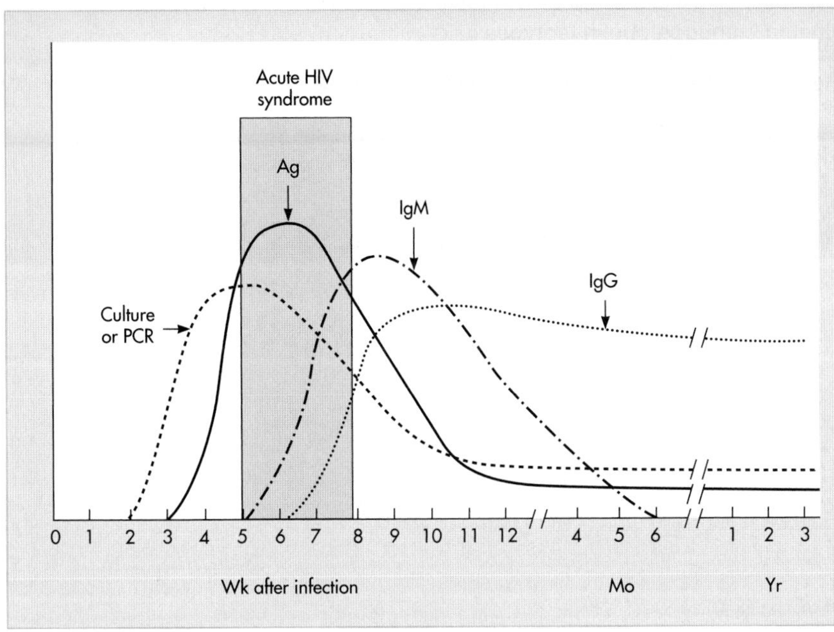

FIG. 31 Tests in human immunodeficiency virus infection (HIV)-1 infection. (From Ravel R [ed]: *Clinical laboratory medicine,* ed 6, St Louis, 1995, Mosby.)

TABLE 52 Indications for Plasma HIV RNA Testing*

Clinical Indication	Information	Use
Syndrome consistent with acute HIV infection	Establishes diagnosis when HIV antibody test is negative or indeterminate	Diagnosis†
Initial evaluation of newly diagnosed HIV infection	Baseline viral load set point	Decision to start or defer therapy
Every 3-4 mo in patients not on therapy	Changes in viral load	Decision to start therapy
4-8 wk after initiation of antiretroviral therapy	Initial assessment of drug efficacy	Decision to continue or change therapy
3-4 mo after start of therapy	Maximal effect of therapy	Decision to continue or change therapy
Every 3-4 mo in patients on therapy	Durability of antiretroviral effect	Decision to continue or change therapy
Clinical event or significant decline in CD4+ T cells	Association with changing or stable	Decision to continue, initiate, or change

*Acute illness (e.g., bacterial pneumonia, tuberculosis, HSV, PCP) and immunizations can cause increase in plasma HIV RNA for 2-4 wk; viral load testing should not be performed during this time. Plasma HIV RNA results should usually be verified with a repeat determination before starting or making changes in therapy. HIV RNA should be measured using the same laboratory and the same assay.

†Diagnosis of HIV infection determined by HIV RNA testing should be confirmed by standard methods (e.g., Western blot serology) performed 2-4 mo after the initial indeterminate or negative test.

From Report of the NIH Panel to Define Principles of Therapy of HIV Infection, *MMWR Recomm Rep* 47(RR-5):1-41, 1998.

HUNTINGTON'S DISEASE PCR

Test description: PCR can be performed on whole blood. Huntington's disease is caused by the expansion of the trinucleotide repeat CAG within IT 15 (huntingtin). Pre- and post-test counseling should be performed when ordering this test.

HYDROGEN BREATH TEST

See BREATH HYDROGEN TEST

5-HYDROXYINDOLE-ACETIC ACID, URINE

See URINE 5-HYDROXYINDOLE-ACETIC ACID

IMMUNE COMPLEX ASSAY

Normal: Negative

Detected in: Collagen vascular disorders, glomerulonephritis, neoplastic diseases, malaria, primary biliary cirrhosis, chronic acute hepatitis, bacterial endocarditis, vasculitis

IMMUNOGLOBULINS

Normal range:

IgA:	50-350 mg/dl (0.5-3.5 g/L [CF: 0.01; SMI: 0.01 g/L])
IgD:	<6 mg/dl (<60 mg/L [CF: 0.01; SMI: 0.01 g/L])
IgE:	<25 μg/dl (<0.00025 g/L [CF: 0.01; SMI: 0.01 g/L])
IgG:	800-1500 mg/dl (8-15 g/L [CF: 0.01; SMI: 0.01 g/L])
IgM:	45-150 mg/dl (0.45-1.5 g/L [CF: 0.01; SMI: 0.01 g/L])

Table 53 summarizes biologic properties of human immunoglobulin isotopes. Box 19 summarizes selected conditions associated with monoclonal immunoglobulins. Disease states associated with polyclonal hyperimmunoglobulinemia are described in Table 54.

Elevated in:

IgA: Lymphoproliferative disorders, Berger's nephropathy, chronic infections, autoimmune disorders, liver disease

IgE: Allergic disorders, parasitic infections, immunologic disorders, IgE myeloma (see Box 20 for summary of nonallergic diseases associated with high levels of IgE. Box 21 summarizes conditions with very high IgE levels)

IgG: Chronic granulomatous infections, infectious diseases, inflammation, myeloma, liver disease

IgM: Primary biliary cirrhosis, infectious diseases (brucellosis, malaria), Waldenström's macroglobulinemia, liver disease

Decreased in:

IgA: Nephrotic syndrome, protein-losing enteropathy, congenital deficiency, lymphocytic leukemia, ataxia-telangiectasia, chronic sinopulmonary disease

IgE: Hypogammaglobulinemia, neoplasms (breast, bronchial, cervical), ataxia-telangiectasia, primary biliary cirrhosis (see Box 20)

IgG: Congenital or acquired deficiency, lymphocytic leukemia, phenytoin, methylprednisolone, nephrotic syndrome, protein-losing enteropathy

IgM: Congenital deficiency, lymphocytic leukemia, nephrotic syndrome

INDIRECT ANTIGLOBULIN (Coombs Indirect)

Normal: Negative

Positive: Acquired hemolytic anemia, incompatible cross-matched blood, anti-Rh antibodies, drugs (methyldopa, mefenamic acid, levodopa)

Fig. 32 illustrates the mechanism of Coombs test.

TABLE 53 Selected Biologic Properties of Human Immunoglobulin Isotypes

Characteristics	IgG1	IgG2	IgG3	IgG4	IgM	IgA1	IgA2	IgD	IgE
Physical Properties									
Molecular weight (kD)	146	146	165	146	970*	160	160	170	190
Serum half-life (days)	29	27	7	16	5	6	6	–	2
Anatomic Distribution									
Mean serum level (mg/mL)	5-12	2-6	0.5-1.0	0.2-1.0	0.5-1.5	0.5-2.0	0-0.2	0-0.4	0-0.002
Transport across placenta	+++	+	++	±	–	–	–	–	–
Transport across epithelium	–	–	–	–	+	+++†	+++†	–	–
Extravascular diffusion	+++	+++	+++	+++	±	++‡	++‡	+	+
Functional Activity									
Antigen neutralization	++	++	++	++	++	++	++	–	–
Complement fixation	++	+	++	–	+++	+	+	–	–
ADCC	+	+	+	±	–	–	–	–	+
Immediate hypersensitivity	–	–	–	–	–	–	–	–	+++

ADCC, Antibody-dependent cellular cytotoxicity; –, no effect; ±, no effect or negligible degree; +, small degree; ++, moderate degree; +++, large degree.
*Pentameric IgM plus J chain.
†Dimer.
‡Monomer.
From Adkinson NF et al: *Middleton's allergy principles and practice*, ed 8, Philadelphia, 2014, Saunders.

BOX 19 Selected Conditions Associated with Monoclonal Immunoglobulins

- Multiple myeloma
- Macroglobulinemia of Waldenström
- Chronic lymphocytic leukemia
- Other leukemias
- Lymphomas
- "Benign" monoclonal gammopathy
- Systemic capillary leak syndrome
- Amyloidosis
- Chronic liver disease such as chronic active hepatitis, primary biliary cirrhosis
- Autoimmune disorders, including rheumatoid arthritis, systemic lupus erythematosus, thyroiditis, pernicious anemia, polyarteritis nodosa, Sjögren syndrome
- Gaucher disease
- Malignancies of various types
- Hereditary spherocytosis
- HIV infection, including AIDS

AIDS, Acquired immune deficiency syndrome; *HIV*, human immunodeficiency virus.
From McPherson RA, Pincus MR: *Henry's clinical diagnosis and management by laboratory methods*, ed 23, St Louis, 2017, Elsevier.

INFLUENZA A AND B TESTS

Test description: PCR can be performed on nasopharyngeal swab, wash, or aspirate
Normal: Negative

INSULIN AUTOANTIBODIES

Normal: Negative
Present in: Exogenous insulin from insulin therapy. The presence of islet cell antibodies indicates ongoing beta cell destruction. This test is useful in the early diagnosis of type 1a diabetes mellitus and in the identification of patients at high risk for type 1a diabetes.

INSULIN, FREE

Normal: <17 mcU/ml
Elevated in: Insulin overdose, insulin resistance syndromes, endogenous hyperinsulinemia
Decreased in: Inadequately treated type 1 diabetes mellitus

INSULIN-LIKE GROWTH FACTOR-1 (IGF-1) (Serum)

Normal range:

Ages 16-24:	182-780 ng/ml
Ages 25-39:	114-492 ng/ml
Ages 40-54:	90-360 ng/ml
Ages >55:	71-290 ng/ml

Elevated in: Adolescence, acromegaly, pregnancy, precocious puberty, obesity
Decreased in: Malnutrition, delayed puberty, diabetes mellitus, hypopituitarism, cirrhosis, old age

INSULIN-LIKE GROWTH FACTOR-II

Normal range: 288-736 ng/ml
Elevated in: Hypoglycemia associated with non–islet cell tumors, hepatoma, and Wilms tumor
Decreased in: Growth hormone deficiency

INTERNATIONAL NORMALIZED RATIO (INR)

The INR is a comparative rating of prothrombin time (PT) ratios. The INR represents the observed PT ratio adjusted by the International Reference Thromboplastin. It provides a universal result indicative of what the patient's PT result would have been if measured using the primary World Health Organization International Reference reagent. For proper interpretation of INR values, the patient should be on stable anticoagulant therapy.

RECOMMENDED INR RANGES

Proximal deep vein thrombosis:	2-3
Pulmonary embolism:	2-3
Transient ischemic attacks:	2-3
Atrial fibrillation:	2-3
Mechanical prosthetic valves:	2.5-3.5
Recurrent venous thromboembolic disease:	2.5-3.5

INTRINSIC FACTOR ANTIBODIES

Normal: Negative
Present in: Pernicious anemia (>50% of patients). Cyanocobalamin may give false-positive results.

IRON (Serum)

Normal: Male: 65-175 mcg/dl; female: 50-1170 mcg/dl

TABLE 54 Polyclonal Hyperimmunoglobulinemias: Some Associated Disease States

Condition	Immunoglobulin (Ig) Classes
Immunodeficiency Diseases	
Hyperimmunoglobulin E and recurrent infections	IgE
Wiskott-Aldrich syndrome	IgA, IgE
"Dysgammaglobulinemia type I"	IgM
Hyperimmunoglobulin A and recurrent infections	IgA
Acquired immune deficiency syndrome (AIDS)	All classes
Infections	
Congenital infections (syphilis, toxoplasmosis, rubella, cytomegalovirus)	IgM
Infectious mononucleosis	IgM or all
Trypanosomiasis	IgM or all
Intestinal parasitism	All classes
Several helminthic infections	IgE
Visceral larva migrans	All classes
Chronic granulomatous disease of childhood	All classes
Leprosy	All classes
Chronic infection in general	All classes, with a preference for IgG
Liver Diseases	
Chronic active hepatitis	IgG predominates
Acute hepatitis	IgG predominates
Biliary cirrhosis	IgM predominates
Lupoid hepatitis	All classes
Pulmonary Disorders	
Pulmonary hypersensitivity syndrome	All classes
Sarcoidosis	All classes
Berylliosis	All classes
"Autoimmune" Disorders	
Systemic lupus erythematosus	All classes
Rheumatoid arthritis	IgA or all
Many "autoimmune" states such as thyroiditis	All classes
Scleroderma	All classes
Cold agglutinin disease	IgM
Anaphylactoid purpura	IgA
Miscellaneous	
Down syndrome	All classes
Amyloidosis	All classes
Narcotic addiction	IgM
Renal tubular disease	All classes

McPherson RA, Pincus MR: *Henry's clinical diagnosis and management by laboratory methods*, ed 23, St Louis, 2017, Elsevier.

Elevated in: Hemochromatosis, excessive iron therapy, repeated transfusions, lead poisoning, hemolytic anemia, aplastic anemia, pernicious anemia

Decreased in: Iron deficiency anemia, hypothyroidism, chronic infection

IRON-BINDING CAPACITY, TOTAL (TIBC)

Normal range: 250-460 μg/dl (45-82 μmol/L [CF: 0.1791; SMI: 1 μmol/L])

Elevated in: Iron deficiency anemia, pregnancy, polycythemia, hepatitis, weight loss

Decreased in: Anemia of chronic disease, hemochromatosis, chronic liver disease, hemolytic anemias, malnutrition (protein depletion)

Table 55 describes TIBC and serum iron abnormalities.

BOX 20 Nonallergic Diseases Associated with Altered Total Serum Immunoglobulin E Levels

Increased Levels (≥500 IU/ml)

Parasitic Diseases
Ascariasis
Visceral larva migrans
Capillariasis
Paragonimiasis
Fascioliasis
Schistosomiasis
Hookworm
Trichinosis
Filariasis
Strongyloidiasis
Echinococcosis
Onchocerciasis
Malaria

Infections
Allergic bronchopulmonary mycosis
Systemic candidiasis
Coccidioidomycosis
Leprosy
Epstein-Barr virus mononucleosis
Cytomegalovirus mononucleosis
Viral respiratory infections
Human immunodeficiency virus (HIV) type 1 infections
Pertussis

Cutaneous Diseases
Alopecia areata
Bullous pemphigoid
Chronic acral dermatitis
Streptococcal erythema nodosum

Other Diseases and Disorders
Nephrotic syndrome
Drug-induced interstitial nephritis
Liver disease
Cystic fibrosis
Kawasaki disease
Infantile polyarteritis nodosa
Primary pulmonary hemosiderosis
Guillain-Barré syndrome
Burns
Rheumatoid arthritis
Bone marrow transplantation
Cigarette smoking
Alcoholism

Neoplastic Diseases
Hodgkin's disease
Immunoglobulin E (IgE) myeloma
Bronchial carcinoma

Immunodeficiency Diseases
Wiskott-Aldrich syndrome
Hyper-IgE syndrome
Thymic hypoplasia (DiGeorge syndrome)
Cellular immunodeficiency with immunoglobulins (Nezelof syndrome)
Selective IgA deficiency

Medications
Enfuvirtide
Pholcodine

Decreased Levels (<5 IU/ml)
Familial IgE deficiency and recurrent sinopulmonary infections
Human T cell lymphotropic virus type 1 infections
Primary biliary cirrhosis

From Adkinson NF et al: *Middleton's allergy principles and practice*, ed 8, Philadelphia, 2014, Saunders.

BOX 21 Conditions Associated with Unusually High Serum Immunoglobulin E Concentrations (≥500 IU/ml)

- Allergic bronchopulmonary mycosis
- Allergic fungal sinusitis
- Atopic dermatitis
- Human immunodeficiency virus (HIV) infection
- Hyperimmunoglobulin E (hyper-IgE) syndrome
- Immunoglobulin E myeloma
- Kimura disease
- Lymphoma
- Netherton syndrome
- Systemic helminthic parasitosis
- Tuberculosis

From Adkinson NF et al: *Middleton's allergy principles and practice*, ed 8, Philadelphia, 2014, Saunders.

TABLE 55 Serum Iron and Total Iron-Binding Capacity Patterns

SI↓	TIBC↓	Chronic diseases; uremia
SI↓	TIBC↑	Chronic iron deficiency anemia; pregnancy in third trimester
SI↑	TIBC↓	Hemochromatosis iron therapy overload (TIBC may be normal); hemolytic anemia; thalassemia; lead poisoning; megaloblastic anemia; aplastic, pyridoxine deficiency, or other sideroblastic anemias
SI↑	TIBC↑	Oral contraceptives; acute hepatitis (some report TIBC is low normal); chronic hepatitis (some patients)
SI↑	TIBCNL	B_{12} or folate deficiency
SI↓	TIBCNL	Chronic iron deficiency (some patients); acute infection, surgery, tissue damage
SI NL	TIBC↑	B_{12}/folate deficiency plus iron deficiency

NL, Normal; *SI,* serum iron; *TIBC,* total iron-binding capacity.
From Ravel R: *Clinical laboratory medicine*, ed 6, St Louis, 1995, Mosby.

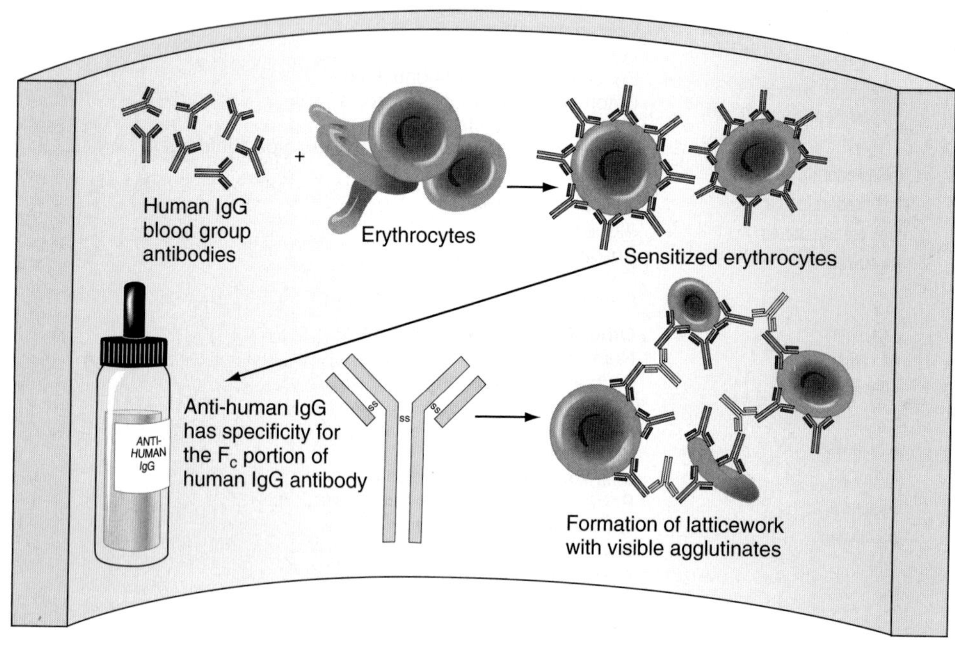

FIG. 32 Antihuman globulin antibodies form a bridge between adjacent erythrocytes sensitized with human immunoglobulin (Ig)G or complement components. (From McPherson RA, Pincus MR: *Henry's clinical diagnosis and management by laboratory methods*, ed 23, St Louis, 2017, Elsevier.)

IRON SATURATION (% Transferrin Saturation)

Normal:
Male: 20%-50%
Female: 15%-50%

Elevated in: Hemochromatosis, excessive iron intake, aplastic anemia, thalassemia, vitamin B_6 deficiency

Decreased in: Hypochromic anemias, GI malignancy

LACTATE (blood)

Normal range: 0.5-2.0 mEq/L

Elevated in: Tissue hypoxia (shock, respiratory failure, severe CHF, severe anemia, carbon monoxide or cyanide poisoning), systemic disorders (liver or renal failure, seizures), abnormal intestinal flora (d-lactic acidosis), drugs or toxins (salicylates, ethanol, methanol, ethylene glycol), G6PD deficiency

LACTATE DEHYDROGENASE (LDH)

Normal range: 50-150 U/L (0.82-2.66 μkat/L [CF: 0.01667; SMI: 0.02 μkat/L])

Elevated in:
Infarction of myocardium, lung, kidney
Diseases of cardiopulmonary system, liver, collagen, central nervous system
Hemolytic anemias, megaloblastic anemias, transfusions, seizures, muscle trauma, muscular dystrophy, acute pancreatitis, hypotension, shock, infectious mononucleosis, inflammation, neoplasia, intestinal obstruction, hypothyroidism

LACTATE DEHYDROGENASE ISOENZYMES

Normal range:

LDH_1:	22%-36% (cardiac, red blood cell) (0.22-0.36 [CF: 0.01, SMI: 0.01])
LDH_2:	35%-46% (cardiac, red blood cell) (0.35-0.46)
LDH_3:	13%-26% (pulmonary) (0.15-0.26)
LDH_4:	3%-10% (striated muscle, liver) (0.03-0.1)
LDH_5:	2%-9% (striated muscle, liver) (0.02-0.09)

Normal ratios:
$LDH_1 < LDH_2$
$LDH_5 < LDH_4$

Abnormal values:
LDH1 >LDH2: Myocardial infarction (can also be seen with hemolytic anemias, pernicious anemia, folate deficiency, renal infarct)
LDH5 >LDH4: Liver disease (cirrhosis, hepatitis, hepatic congestion)

TABLE 56 Laboratory Tests in the Differential Diagnosis of Diarrhea

Test	Method	Use
Initial Screening Tests		
Fecal leukocytes	Wright's stain or methylene blue	Identify inflammatory diarrhea
Fecal occult blood test	Immunochemical	Detect blood
Fecal osmotic gap	290 – 2 × (fecal Na^+ + K^+)	Distinguish secretory vs. osmotic diarrhea
Stool alkalinization	Color change after adding NaOH to stool/urine	Phenolphthalein laxative ingestion
Infectious Causes		
Stool bacterial culture	Routine culture and sensitivity	Identify *Shigella, Salmonella*
Stool special culture	Specialized culture and serotyping	Identify *E. coli* 0157:H7, *Yersinia, Campylobacter*
Stool *C. difficile* toxin assay	EIA for toxins A and B	Pseudomembranous colitis
HIV serology	EIA, Western blot	HIV enteritis
Stool rotavirus screen	EIA for antigen	Rotavirus enteritis
Stool ova and parasites	Concentration and stains	Enteric parasitic infection
Stool mycobacteria	Acid-fast stain, culture and sensitivity, PCR	*Mycobacterium*, antibiotic selection
Stool *E. histolytica* Ag	EIA for antigen	*Entamoeba histolytica*
Stool *Giardia* Ag	EIA for antigen	*Giardia lamblia*
Stool *Cryptosporidium* Ag	EIA for antigen	*Cryptosporidium parvum*
Endocrine Causes		
Urine 5-HIAA or blood serotonin	HPLC	Carcinoid syndrome
Serum VIP	RIA	VIPoma
Serum TSH, free T4	Immunoassay	Hyperthyroidism
Serum gastrin	RIA	Zollinger-Ellison syndrome
Serum calcitonin	RIA	Hypocalcemia-related diarrhea
Serum somatostatin	RIA	Somatostatinoma
Malabsorption		
Lactose tolerance test	See text	Lactase deficiency
Stool reducing sugars	Clinitest tablets	Carbohydrate intolerance
Sweat chloride	See text	Cystic fibrosis
D-Xylose absorption test	See text	Evaluate pancreatic and jejunal function
Fecal fat stain	Fat stain	Lipid malabsorption
Serum carotene	Spectrophotometry	Lipid malabsorption
^{14}C-glyceryl trioleate test malabsorption	See text	Lipid malabsorption
Serum IgA	Nephelometry	Rule out IgA deficiency
Antitissue transglutaminase antibody	EIA	Celiac disease
Hydrogen breath test	Electrochemical hydrogen monitorinomatography g	Carbohydrate malabsorption
Bacterial colony count	Small bowel aspirate and quantitative culture	Bacterial overgrowth
Other		
Serum ionized calcium	Ion-specific electrode	Hypocalcemia-related diarrhea
Serum protein and albumin	Nephelometry, photometry	IBD, protein-losing enteropathy
Stool alpha-1-antitrypsin	Nephelometry	Protein-losing enteropathy
Quantitative immunoglobulins	Nephelometry	Agammaglobulinemia
7α-Hydroxy-4-cholestin-3-one	HPLC	Bile salt malabsorption
Fecal elastase or pancreolauryl test	EIA	Pancreatic insufficiency
Intestinal biopsy	Endoscopic or open biopsy	Whipple disease, MAI, abetalipoproteinemia, neoplasia, lymphoma, amyloidosis, eosinophilic gastroenteritis, agammaglobulinemia, intestinal lymphangiectasia, Crohn disease, tuberculosis, graft-versus-host disease, *Giardia*, other parasitic infections, collagenous colitis, microscopic colitis
Extraintestinal causes	See text	Hyperthyroidism, diabetes, hypoparathyroidism, adrenal cortical insufficiency, hormone-secreting tumors

5-HIAA, 5-Hydroxyindoleacetic acid; *Ab*, antibody; *Ag*, amtigen; *EIA*, enzyme immunoassay; *HIV*, human immunodeficiency virus; *HPLC*, high-performance liquid chromatography; *IBD*, inflammatory bowel disease; *MAI*, *Mycobacterium avium-intracellulare*; *PCR*, polymerase chain reaction; *RIA*, radioimmunoassay; *TSH*, thyroid-stimulating hormone; *VIP*, vasoactive intestinal peptide.
From McPherson RA, Pincus MR: *Henry's clinical diagnosis and management by laboratory methods*, ed 23, St Louis, 2017, Elsevier.

LACTOSE TOLERANCE TEST (serum)

Normal: Test is performed by giving 2 g/kg body weight lactose orally and drawing glucose level at 0, 30, 45, 60, and 90 min. Normal response is change in glucose from fasting value to >30 mg/dl. Inconclusive response is increase of 20-30 mg/dl, abnormal response is increase <20 mg/dl. Table 56 summarizes laboratory tests in the differential diagnosis of diarrhea.

Abnormal in: Lactase deficiency

LAP SCORE

See LEUKOCYTE ALKALINE PHOSPHATASE

Laboratory Tests IV

LEAD

Normal: Child, <10 mcg/dl; adult, <25 mcg/dl; acceptable for industrial exposure, <50 mcg/dl
Elevated in: Lead exposure, lead poisoning

LDH

See LACTATE DEHYDROGENASE

LDL

See LOW-DENSITY LIPOPROTEIN CHOLESTEROL

LEGIONELLA PNEUMOPHILA PCR

Test description: PCR can be performed on lung tissue, water sputum, bronchoalveolar lavage, and other respiratory fluids.

LEGIONELLA TITER

Normal: Negative
Positive in: Legionnaires' disease (presumptive: ≥1:256 titer; definitive: fourfold titer increase to ≥1:128)

LEUKOCYTE ALKALINE PHOSPHATASE (LAP)

Normal range: 13-100 (33-188 U)
Elevated in: Leukemoid reactions, neutrophilia secondary to infections (except in sickle cell crisis—no significant increase in LAP score), Hodgkin's disease, polycythemia vera, hairy cell leukemia, aplastic anemia, Down syndrome, myelofibrosis
Decreased in: Acute and chronic granulocytic leukemia, thrombocytopenic purpura, paroxysmal nocturnal hemoglobinuria, hypophosphatemia, collagen disorders

LEUKOCYTE COUNT

See COMPLETE BLOOD COUNT

LIPASE

Normal range: 0-160 U/L (0-2.66 μkat/L [CF: 0.01667; SMI: 0.02 μkat/L])
Elevated in: Acute pancreatitis, perforated peptic ulcer, carcinoma of pancreas (early stage), pancreatic duct obstruction, bowel infarction, intestinal obstruction

LIPOPROTEIN(a)

Normal: Male: 1.35-19.6 mg/dl; female: 1.24-20.1 mg/dl. Fig. 33 illustrates lipoprotein structure. Table 57 summarizes the major classes of human plasma lipoproteins. The chemical composition of major classes of plasma lipoproteins is described in Table 58.
Elevated in: Coronary artery disease, uncontrolled diabetes, hypothyroidism, chronic renal failure, pregnancy, tobacco use, infections, nephritic syndrome
Decreased in: Niacin, omega-3 fatty acids, estrogens, tamoxifen, statins

LIPOPROTEIN CHOLESTEROL, HIGH-DENSITY

See HIGH-DENSITY LIPOPROTEIN CHOLESTEROL

LIPOPROTEIN CHOLESTEROL, LOW-DENSITY

See LOW-DENSITY LIPOPROTEIN CHOLESTEROL

LIVER KIDNEY MICROSOME TYPE 1 ANTIBODIES (LKM1)

Normal: <20 U
Elevated in: Autoimmune hepatitis type 2

LKM1

See Liver Kidney Microsome Type 1 Antibodies

LOW-DENSITY LIPOPROTEIN (LDL) CHOLESTEROL

Normal range: 50-130 mg/dl (1.30-1.68 mmol/L [CF: 0.02586; SMI: 0.05 mmol/L]). Fig. 34 illustrates the LDL receptor pathway and regulation of cholesterol metabolism.

<70	Optimal in diabetics, prior MI, and patients with cardiac risk factors
100-129	Near or above optimal
130-159	Borderline high
160-189	High
≥190	Very high

LUPUS ANTICOAGULANT

See CIRCULATING ANTICOAGULANT

LUTEINIZING HORMONE

Normal range: 5-25 mIU/ml
Elevated in: Postmenopause, pituitary adenoma, primary gonadal dysfunction, polycystic ovary syndrome

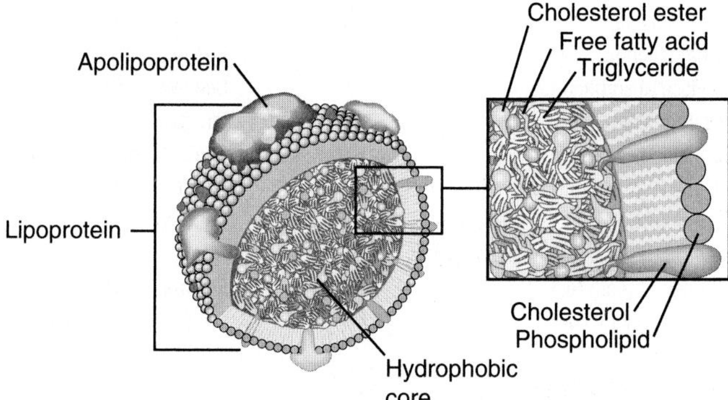

FIG. 33 Lipoprotein structure. Lipoproteins are spherical particles with a hydrophobic core and an amphiphilic surface. The surface consists of a single layer of phospholipids. This surface layer also contains proteins and free cholesterol. The hydrophobic core mainly contains triglycerides and cholesterol esters. (From McPherson RA, Pincus MR: *Henry's clinical diagnosis and management by laboratory methods*, ed 23, St Louis, 2017, Elsevier.)

TABLE 57 Major Classes of Human Plasma Lipoproteins: Physicochemical Characteristics

Particle	Electrophoretic Mobility*	Major Apolipoproteins	Diameter (Å)	Density (kg/L)	Sf†
Chylomicrons	Origin	ApoA-I, A-IV, B-48, C-I, C-II, C-III, E	750-12,000	<0.95	>400
VLDL	Pre-β	ApoB-100, C-I, C-II, C-III, E	300-700	0.95-1.006	20-400
IDL	β or pre-β	ApoB-100, E1.006–1.019	12-20		
LDL	B	ApoB-100	180-300	1.019-1.063	0-12
HDL_2	A	ApoA-I, A-II, E	50-120	1.063-1.125	
HDL_3	A	ApoA-II, A-I, E	50-120	1.125-1.210	
Lp(a)	Pre-β	ApoB-100, Apo(a)		1.045-1.080	

HDL_2, Ultracentrifugation subclass of high-density lipoprotein; *HDL_3*, ultracentrifugation subclass of high-density lipoprotein; *IDL*, intermediate-density lipoprotein; *LDL*, low-density lipoprotein; *Lp(a)*, lipoprotein A; *VLDL*, very-low-density lipoprotein.
*Agarose gel electrophoresis.
†Svedberg flotation rate.
McPherson RA, Pincus MR: *Henry's clinical diagnosis and management by laboratory methods*, ed 23, St Louis, 2017, Elsevier.

TABLE 58 Chemical Composition of Major Classes of Plasma Lipoproteins

	Protein (%)*	Free Cholesterol (%)	Cholesterol Esters (%)	Triglyceride (%)	Phospholipid (%)
Chylomicrons	1-2	1-3	2-4	80-95	3-6
VLDL	6-10	4-8	16-22	45-65	15-20
IDL	Intermediate between VLDL and LDL				
LDL	18-22	6-8	45-50	4-8	18-24
HDL	45-55	3-5	15-20	2-7	26-32

Data from Albers (1974), Gaubatz et al (1983), Fless et al (1984), Gotto et al (1986), Gries et al (1988), and Hegele (2009).
HDL, High-density lipoprotein; *IDL,* intermediate-density lipoprotein; *LDL,* low-density lipoprotein; *VLDL,* very-low-density lipoprotein.
*Percentage of dry weight.
McPherson RA, Pincus MR: *Henry's clinical diagnosis and management by laboratory methods,* ed 23, St Louis, 2017, Elsevier.

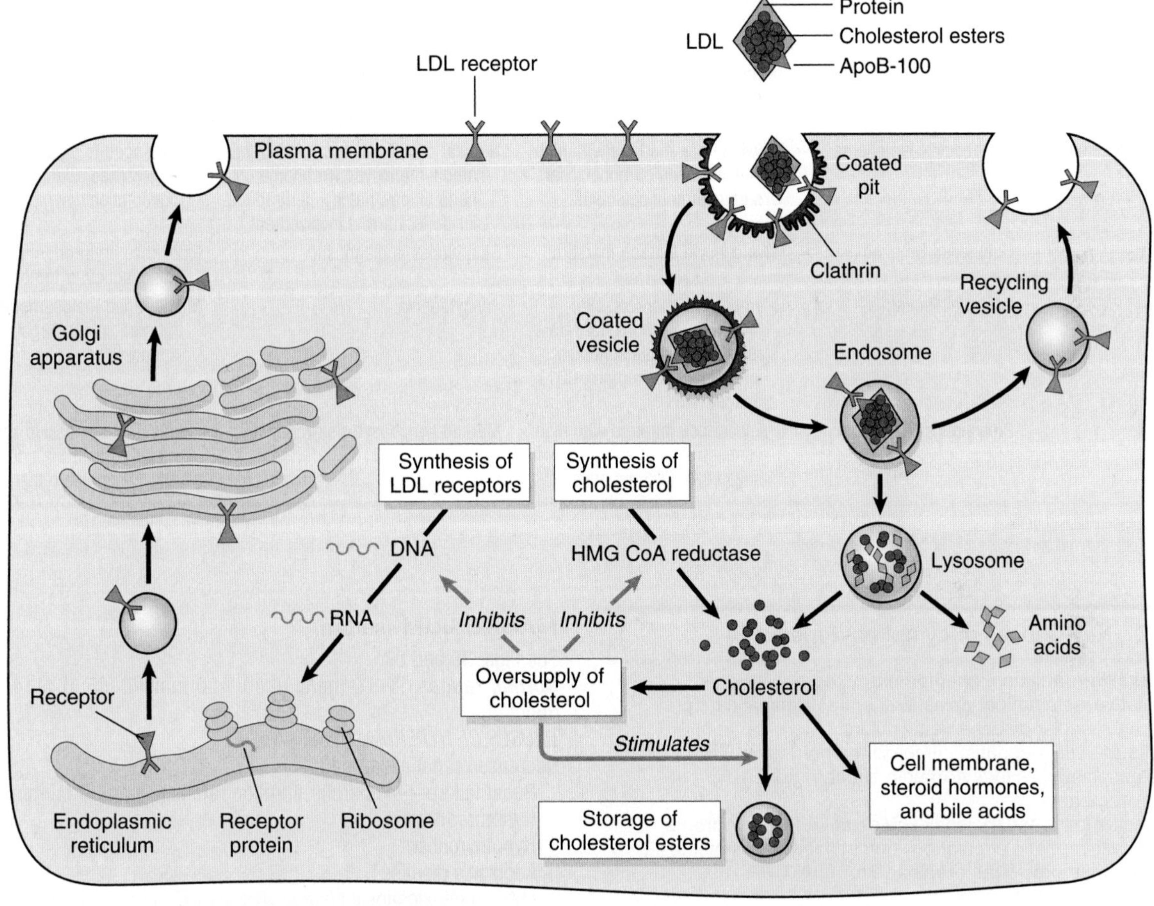

FIG. 34 The low-density lipoprotein (LDL) receptor pathway and regulation of cholesterol metabolism. (From McPherson RA, Pincus MR: *Henry's clinical diagnosis and management by laboratory methods,* ed 23, St Louis, 2017, Elsevier.)

Decreased in: Severe illness, anorexia nervosa, malnutrition, pituitary or hypothalamic impairment, severe stress

LYME DISEASE ANTIBODY TITER

Normal range: Negative
Positive result: Fig. 35 illustrates the usual serologic response in Lyme disease.

A serologic test is not necessary or helpful for several days after a tick bite because it is only 40%-50% sensitive in this stage, and a negative test does not rule out the diagnosis.

LYMPHOCYTES

Normal range:
15%-40%
Total lymphocyte count = 800-2600/mm3
Total T lymphocyte = 800-2200/mm3

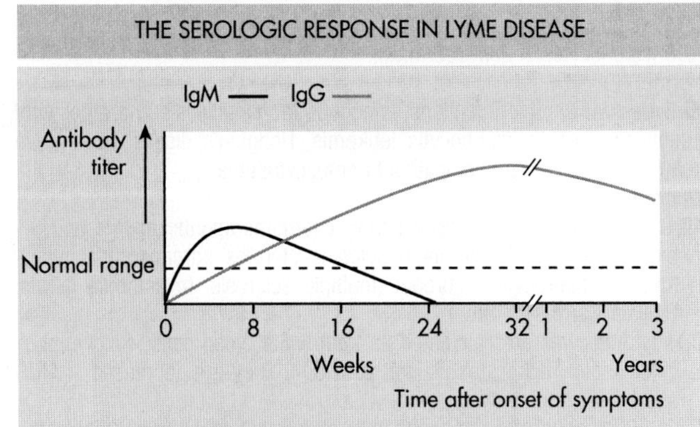

FIG. 35 IgM and IgG responses in Lyme disease.

TABLE 59 Differential Diagnosis of Abnormal Lymphocytes in Peripheral Blood

Lymphocyte Type	Usual Disease Association	Cytologic Features	Laboratory Features	Clinical Features
Small lymphocyte	Chronic lymphocytic leukemia	B-cell surface markers with low concentration of surface immunoglobulin, CD5 antigen	Hypogammaglobulinemia in 50%; positive direct Coombs test in 15%; on node biopsy, diffuse, well-differentiated lymphocytic infiltrate	Elderly adults; presentation runs gamut from asymptomatic with lymphocytosis only to bulky disease with adenopathy, splenomegaly, and "packed" bone marrow
Atypical lymphocyte	Infectious mononucleosis, other viral illnesses	Suppressor T-cell markers	Heterophil agglutinin; positive serology for Epstein-Barr virus, cytomegalovirus, toxoplasma, HBsAg	Pharyngitis, fever, adenopathy, rash, splenomegaly, palatal petechiae, jaundice
Plasmacytoid lymphocyte	Waldenström's macroglobulin anemia	Cytoplasmic IgM, periodic acid-Schiff positivity	IgM paraprotein, rouleaux, cryoglobulins	Adenopathy, splenomegaly, absence of bone lesions, hyperviscosity syndrome, cryopathic phenomena
Lymphoblast	ALL	Terminal transferase positivity, common ALL antigen, B- or T-precursor markers	Anemia, granulocytopenia, thrombocytopenia, hyperuricemia, diffuse bone marrow infiltration	Peak incidence in childhood, acute onset, bone pain frequent
Lymphosarcoma cell	Lymphocytic lymphoma	B-cell surface markers with high concentration of monoclonal surface immunoglobulin	Nodular or diffuse, poorly differentiated lymphocytic lymphoma on node biopsy, patchy, peritrabecular bone marrow involvement	Middle-aged to older adults, generalized adenopathy, constitutional symptoms
Sézary cell	Cutaneous lymphomas	T-lymphocyte surface markers	Skin biopsy is diagnostic	Exfoliative erythroderma, cutaneous plaques or tumors
Hairy cell	Hairy cell leukemia	B-lymphocyte markers, cytoplasmic projections, tartrate-resistant acid phosphatase, interleukin-2 receptors, CD11 antigen	Pancytopenia	Middle-aged males, moderate to marked splenomegaly without adenopathy
Prolymphocyte	Prolymphocytic leukemia	B-cell surface markers with high concentration of surface immunoglobulin, CD5 negative	Marked lymphocytosis (frequently $>100 \times 10^9$/L)	Elderly adults, massive splenomegaly, minimum adenopathy, poor response to therapy

ALL, Acute lymphoblastic leukemia.
From Stein JH (ed): *Internal medicine,* ed 5, St Louis, 1998, Mosby.

BOX 22 Key Causes of Lymphocytopenia

- Destructive—radiation, chemotherapy, corticosteroids
- Debilitative—starvation, aplastic anemia, terminal cancer, collagen vascular disease, renal failure
- Infectious—viral hepatitis, influenza, typhoid fever, TB
- AIDS-associated—HIV cytopathic effect, nutritional imbalance, drug effect
- Congenital immunodeficiency—Wiskott-Aldrich syndrome
- Abnormal lymphatic circulation—intestinal lymphangiectasia, obstruction, thoracic duct drainage/rupture, CHF

AIDS, Acquired immunodeficiency syndrome; *CHF,* congestive heart failure; *HIV,* human immunodeficiency virus; *TB,* tuberculosis.
From McPherson RA, Pincus MR: *Henry's clinical diagnosis and management by laboratory methods*, ed 23, St Louis, 2017, Elsevier.

CD4 lymphocytes = ≥ 400/mm3
CD8 lymphocytes = 200-800/mm3
Normal CD4/CD8 ratio is 2.0.

Elevated in: Chronic infections, infectious mononucleosis and other viral infections, chronic lymphocytic leukemia, Hodgkin's disease, ulcerative colitis, hypoadrenalism, idiopathic thrombocytopenia

Decreased in:
AIDS, bone marrow suppression from chemotherapeutic agents or chemotherapy, aplastic anemia, neoplasms, steroids, adrenocortical hyperfunction, neurologic disorders (multiple sclerosis, myasthenia gravis, Guillain-Barré syndrome)
CD4 lymphocytes are calculated as total white blood cells × % lymphocytes × % lymphocytes stained with CD4. They are decreased in AIDS and other immune dysfunction.
Table 59 describes various lymphocyte abnormalities in peripheral blood. Box 22 summarizes key causes of lymphocytopenia.

MAGNESIUM (serum)

See Figs. 36 and 37.

Normal range: 1.8-3.0 mg/dl (0.80-1.20 mmol/L [CF: 0.4114; SMI: 0.02 mmol/L])

CAUSES OF HYPERMAGNESEMIA
Decreased renal excretion
  Renal failure—glomerular filtration rate less than 30 ml/min
  Hyperparathyroidism
  Hypothyroidism
  Addison's disease
  Lithium intoxication
  Familial hypocalciuric hypercalcemia
Other causes: usually in association with decrease in glomerular filtration rate
  Endogenous loads
    Diabetic ketoacidosis
    Severe tissue injury—burns
  Exogenous loads
    Gastrointestinal
      Magnesium-containing laxatives and antacids
      High-dose vitamin D analogs
Parenteral: management of toxemia of pregnancy

CAUSES OF HYPOMAGNESEMIA
Alcoholic abuse
Diuretic use
Renal losses
Acute and chronic renal failure
Postobstructive diuresis
Acute tubular necrosis
Chronic glomerulonephritis
Chronic pyelonephritis

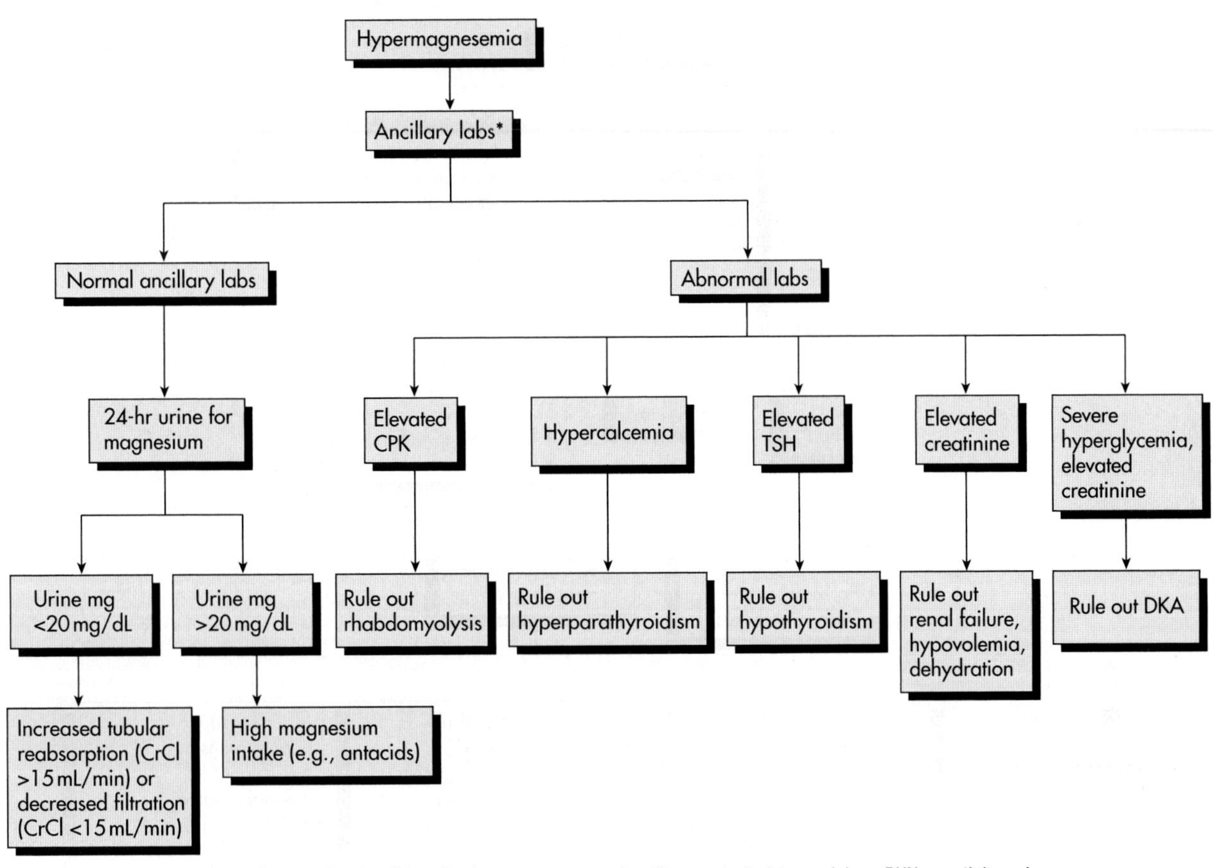

FIG. 36 Diagnostic algorithm for hypermagnesemia. *Serum electrolytes, calcium, BUN, creatinine, glucose, TSH, CPK. (From Ferri, F: *Ferri's best test: a practical guide to clinical laboratory medicine and diagnostic imaging,* ed 3, Philadelphia, 2014, Saunders.)

Interstitial nephropathy
Renal transplantation
Gastrointestinal losses
Chronic diarrhea
Nasogastric suctioning
Short bowel syndrome
Protein-calorie malnutrition
Bowel fistula
Total parenteral nutrition
Acute pancreatitis
Endocrine
Diabetes mellitus
Hyperaldosteronism
Hyperthyroidism
Hyperparathyroidism
Acute intermittent porphyria
Pregnancy
Drugs
Aminoglycosides
Amphotericin
β-agonists
Cisplatin
Cyclosporine
Diuretics
Foscarnet
Pentamidine
Theophylline
Congenital disorders
Familial hypomagnesemia
Maternal diabetes
Maternal hypothyroidism
Maternal hyperparathyroidism

MEAN CORPUSCULAR VOLUME (MCV)

Normal range: 76-100 μm^3 (76-100 fL) (76-100 fL [CF: 1; SMI: 1 fL])

Table 60 summarizes clinical conditions not to be confused with megaloblastosis. See Tables 61, 62, and 63 for descriptions of MCV abnormalities. Table 64 describes the usefulness of the MCV and RBC distribution width in the diagnosis of anemia. Table 65 describes peripheral blood film evaluation in a patient with red cell membrane disorder.

METANEPHRINES, URINE

See URINE METANEPHRINES

METHYLMALONIC ACID (Serum)

Normal: <0.2 mcmol/L
Elevated in: Vitamin B_{12} deficiency, pregnancy, methylmalonic acidemia

MITOCHONDRIAL ANTIBODY (AMA)

Normal: Negative
Present in: Primary biliary cirrhosis (>90% of patients)

MONOCYTE COUNT

Normal range: 2%-8%
Elevated in: Viral diseases, parasites, infections, neoplasms, inflammatory bowel disease, monocytic leukemia, lymphomas, myeloma, sarcoidosis

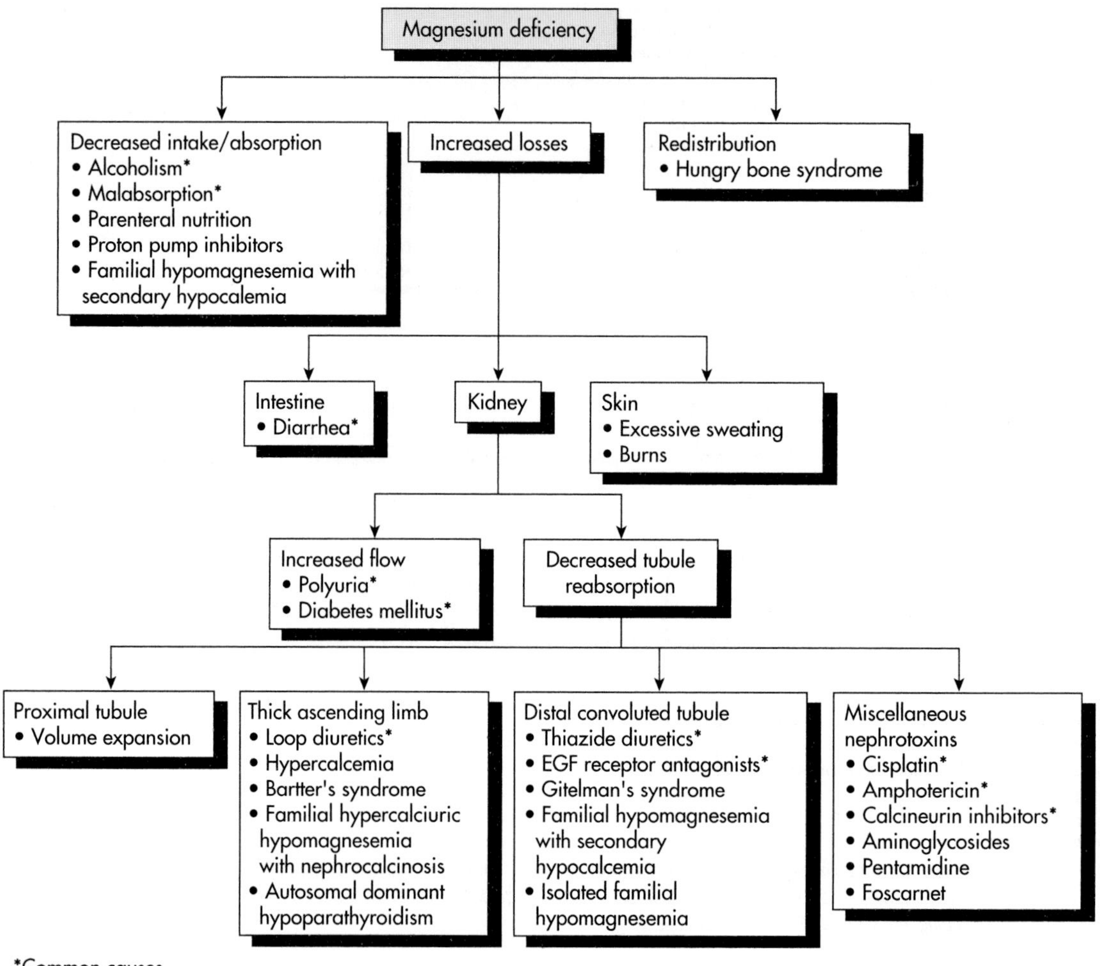

FIG. 37 Causes of magnesium deficiency. (From Skorecki K, Chertow GM, Marsden PA et al: *Brenner & Rector's the kidney*, ed 10, Philadelphia, 2016, Elsevier.)

TABLE 60 Clinical Conditions Not to Be Confused with Megaloblastosis

Macrocytosis* without Megaloblastosis†
Reticulocytosis
Liver disease
Aplastic anemia
Myelodysplastic syndromes (especially 5q-)
Multiple myeloma
Hypoxemia
Smokers
Spurious Increases in MCV without Macro-Ovalocytosis‡
Cold agglutinin disease
Marked hyperglycemia
Leukocytosis
Older individuals

MCV, Mean corpuscular volume.
*The central pallor that normally occupies about one third of the normal red blood cell is decreased in macro-ovalocytes. This contrasts with the finding of thin macrocytes, in which the central pallor is increased.
†Although megaloblastosis implies that a bone marrow test has been performed, with the addition of highly sensitive tests for the specific diagnosis of cobalamin and folate deficiency, the need for a bone marrow test is often dictated by the urgency to make the diagnosis.
‡When the Coulter counter readings of a high MCV are not confirmed by looking at the peripheral smear.
From Hoffman R: *Hematology: basic principles and practice,* ed 6, Philadelphia, 2013, Saunders.

Decreased in: Aplastic anemia, lymphocytic leukemia, glucocorticoid administration
See Table 66 for changes in monocyte number.

MYCOPLASMA PNEUMONIAE PCR

Test description: PCR can be performed on sputum, bronchoalveolar lavage, nasopharyngeal and throat swabs, other respiratory fluids, and lung tissue

MYELIN BASIC PROTEIN, CEREBROSPINAL FLUID

Normal: <2.5 ng/ml
Elevated in: Multiple sclerosis, CNS trauma, stroke, encephalitis

MYOGLOBIN, URINE

See URINE MYOGLOBIN

TABLE 61 Some Causes of Increased Mean Corpuscular Volume (Macrocytosis)

Causes	% of all Macrocytosis Patients*	% of Macrocytosis in Each Disease†
Common		
Folate or B_{12} deficiency	20-30 (5-50)‡	80-90 (4-100)
Chronic liver disease	15-20 (6-28)	25-30 (8-65)
Chronic alcoholism	10-12 (3-15)	60 (26-90)
Cytotoxic chemotherapy	10-15 (2-20)	30-40 (13-82)
Cardiorespiratory abnormality	8 (7-9.5)	?
Reticulocytosis	6-7 (0-15)	Depends on severity
Myelodysplastic syndromes	Frequent over age 40 yr	>60 in RAEB and RARS
Unexplained	25 (22.5-27)	—
Normal newborn		
Less Common	**<4%**	
Noncytotoxic drugs		
> Zidovudine		
Phenytoin		30 (14-50)
Azathioprine		
Hypothyroidism		20-30 (8-55)
Chronic leukemia/ myelofibrosis		
Radiotherapy for malignancy		
Chronic renal disease (occasional patients)		
Distance-runner macrocytosis (some persons)		
Down syndrome		
Artifactual (e.g., cold agglutinins)		

RAEB, Refractory anemia with excessive blasts; *RARS,* refractory anemia with ring sideroblasts (formerly called "IASA," or idiopathic acquired sideroblastic anemia).
*Percentage of all patients with macrocytosis.
†Percentage of patients with each condition listed who have macrocytosis.
‡Numbers in parentheses are literature range.
From Ravel R: *Clinical laboratory medicine,* ed 6, St Louis, 1995, Mosby.

TABLE 62 Some Causes of Decreased Mean Corpuscular Volume (Microcytosis)

Common	Less Common
Chronic iron deficiency	Some cases of polycythemia
α- or β-thalassemia (minor)	Some cases of lead poisoning
Anemia of chronic disease	Some cases of congenital spherocytosis
	Some cases of sideroblastic anemia
	Certain abnormal hemoglobins (HbE, Hb Lepore)

From Ravel R: *Clinical laboratory medicine,* ed 6, St Louis, 1995, Mosby.

TABLE 63 Differential Diagnosis of Microcytic Hypochromic Anemia

Decreased Body Iron Stores
Iron-deficiency anemia
Normal or increased body iron stores
Anemia of chronic disease
Defective absorption, transport, or use of iron
Iron-refractory, iron-deficiency anemia after parenteral iron
Atransferrinemia
Aceruloplasminemia
Divalent metal transporter 1 (DMT1 or SLC11A2) deficiency
Ferroportin-associated hemochromatosis with impaired iron export (type 4A)
Heme oxygenase 1 deficiency
Disorders of globin synthesis
Thalassemia
Other microcytic hemoglobinopathies
Disorders of heme synthesis: sideroblastic anemias
Hereditary
Acquired

From Hoffman R et al: *Hematology, basic principles and practice,* ed 6, Philadelphia, 2013, Saunders.

TABLE 64 Usefulness of the Mean Corpuscular Value and Red Blood Cell Distribution Width in the Diagnosis of Anemia

	Low MCV (<80 fL)	Normal MCV (80–99 fL)	High MCV (≥100 fL)
Normal RDW	Anemia of chronic disease α- or β-Thalassemia trait Hemoglobin E trait	Acute blood loss Anemia of chronic disease Anemia of renal disease	Aplastic anemia Chronic liver disease Chemotherapy, antivirals, or alcohol
Elevated RDW	Iron deficiency Sickle cell-β–thalassemia	Early iron, folate, or vitamin B_{12} deficiency Dimorphic anemia (for example, iron + folate deficiency) Sickle cell anemia Sickle cell disease Chronic liver disease Myelodysplasia	Folate or vitamin B_{12} deficiency Immune hemolytic anemia Cytotoxic chemotherapy Chronic liver disease Myelodysplasia Hereditary spherocytosis, hereditary elliptocytosis, congenital hemoglobinopathies, and RBC enzymopathies

MCV, Mean corpuscular value; *RDW,* red blood cell distribution width.
From Hoffman R: *Hematology, basic principles and practice,* ed 7, Philadelphia, 2018, Elsevier.

TABLE 65 Peripheral Blood Film Evaluation in a Patient with Red Cell Membrane Disorder

Shape	Pathobiology	Diagnosis
Microspherocytes	Loss of membrane lipids leading to a reduction of surface area resulting from deficiencies of spectrin, ankyrin, or band 3 and protein 4.2 Removal of membrane material from antibody-coated red cells by macrophages Removal of membrane-associated Heinz bodies, with the adjacent membrane lipids, by the spleen	HS Immunohemolytic anemias Heinz body hemolytic anemias
Elliptocytes	Permanent red cell deformation resulting from a weakening of skeletal protein interactions (such as the spectrin dimer-dimer contact). This facilitates disruption of existing protein contacts during shear-stress-induced elliptical deformation. Subsequently, new protein contacts are formed that stabilize elliptical shape Unknown	Mild common HE Iron deficiency, megaloblastic anemias, myelofibrosis, myelophthisic anemias, myelodysplastic syndrome, thalassemias
Poikilocytes/ fragments	Weakening of skeletal protein contacts resulting from skeletal protein mutations Unknown	Hemolytic HE/HPP Iron deficiency, megaloblastic anemias, myelofibrosis, myelophthisic anemias, myelodysplastic syndrome, thalassemias
Schistocytes, fragmented red cells	Red cells "torn" by mechanic trauma (fibrin strands, turbulent flow)	"Microangiopathic" hemolytic anemia associated with disseminated intravascular coagulation, thrombotic thrombocytopenic purpura, vasculitis, heart valve prostheses
Acanthocytes	Uptake of cholesterol and its preferential accumulation in the outer leaflet of the lipid bilayer Selective accumulation of sphingomyelin in the outer lipid leaflet Unknown	Spur cell hemolytic anemia in severe liver disease Abetalipoproteinemia Chorea-acanthocytosis syndrome, malnutrition, hypothyroidism, McLeod phenotype
Echinocytes	Expansion of the surface area of the outer hemileaflet of lipid bilayer relative to the inner hemileaflet Unknown	Hemolytic anemia associated with hypomagnesemia and hypophosphatemia in malnourished patients, pyruvate kinase deficiency; in vitro artifact of low blood storage (ATP depletion), contact with glass or elevated pH Hemolysis in long-distance runners, renal failure
Stomatocytes	Expansion of the surface area of the inner hemileaflet of the bilayer relative to the outer leaflet Unknown	Exposure of red cells to cationic anesthetics in vitro; in vivo the drug concentrations may not be sufficient to produce similar effect Alcoholism, inherited disorders of membrane permeability (hereditary stomatocytosis)
Target cells	Absolute excess of membrane lipids (both cholesterol and phospholipids: "symmetric" lipid gain), followed by an increase of cell surface area Relative excess of surface area because of a decrease in cell volume	Obstructive jaundice, liver disease with intrahepatic cholestasis Thalassemias and some hemoglobinopathies (C, D, E)

ATP, Adenosine triphosphate; *HE,* hereditary elliptocytosis; *HPP,* hereditary pyropoikilocytosis; *HS,* hereditary spherocytosis.
From Hoffman R: *Hematology, basic principles and practice*, ed 7, Philadelphia, 2018, Elsevier.

TABLE 66 Changes in Monocyte Number

Monocytosis
Infections: tuberculosis, granulomatous infection, brucellosis, subacute bacterial endocarditis
Connective tissue disorder
Recovery from myelosuppression
Hematologic malignancies
  MDS, MPD, MDS–MPD overlap, CMML
  Acute and chronic monocytic leukemia, myelomonocytic leukemia
  Hodgkin's and non-Hodgkin's lymphomas
Monocytopenia
Hairy cell leukemia
MonoMAC syndrome
Aplastic anemia
Drugs: chemotherapy, IFN-α, glucocorticoids (transient)
Radiation therapy

CMML, Chronic myelomonocytic leukemia; *IFN,* interferon; *MDS,* myelodysplastic syndrome; *monoMAC,* monocytopenia and mycobacterium avium complex syndrome; *MPD,* myeloproliferative disorder.
From Hoffman R: *Hematology, basic principles and practice*, ed 6, Philadelphia, 2013, Saunders.

NEISSERIA GONORRHOEAE PCR

Test description: Test can be performed on endocervical swab, urine, and intraurethral swab
Normal: Negative

NEUTROPHIL COUNT

Normal range: 50%-70%
Subsets:
l. Stabs (bands, early mature neutrophils): 2%-6%
m. Segs (mature neutrophils): 60%-70%
Elevated in: Acute bacterial infections, acute myocardial infarction, stress, neoplasms, myelocytic leukemia
Decreased in: Viral infections, aplastic anemias, immunosuppressive drugs, radiation therapy to bone marrow, agranulocytosis, drugs (antibiotics, antithyroidals, clopidogrel), lymphocytic and monocytic leukemias

Box 23 describes various drugs that can cause neutropenia. Table 67 describes miscellaneous inherited neutropenia disorders. Classification of neutropenia is covered in Table 68. Table 69 lists drugs associated with agranulocytosis. Table 70 describes causes of neutrophilia.

TABLE 67 Miscellaneous Inherited Neutropenia Disorders

Diagnosis	Genetics	Mapping	Mutant Gene	Additional Features
Hyper IgM syndrome, type 1	X-L	Xq26	*CD40L*	↓IgG, IgA, IgE, autoimmune cytopenias
Hermansky-Pudlak syndrome, type 2	AR	5q14.1	*AP3B1*	↓IgG, partial albinism, platelet dysfunction
Griscelli syndrome, type 1	AR	15q21	*MYO5A*	Neurologic dysfunction, partial albinism
Griscelli syndrome, type 2	AR	15q21	*RAB27A*	Same as type 1 plus hemophagocytosis
Chédiak-Higashi syndrome	AR	1q42.1-q42.2	*LYST (CHSI)*	Immunodeficiency, partial albinism
Poikiloderma with neutropenia	AR	16q13	*C160RF57*	Rash, short stature, dystrophic nails
P14 deficiency	AR	1q22	*MAPBPIP*	Immunodeficiency, hypopigmentation
Cohen syndrome	AR	8q22-q23	*VPS13B/COH1*	Retinopathy, retardation, skeletal anomalies
Charcot-Marie-Tooth syndrome, type 2	AD	19p13.2	*DMN2*	Axonal demyelinating neuropathy

AD, Autosomal dominant; *AR,* autosomal recessive; *Ig,* immunoglobulin; *X-L,* X-linked recessive.
Data compiled from Online Mendelian Inheritance in Man (http://ncbi.nlm.nih.gov/omim); From Hoffman R: *Hematology: basic principles and practice,* ed 6, Philadelphia, 2013, Saunders.

BOX 23 Drugs That Cause Neutropenia

Antiarrhythmics: tocainide, procainamide, propranolol, quinidine
Antibiotics: chloramphenicol, penicillins, sulfonamides, *p*-aminosalicylic acid (PAS), rifampin, vancomycin, isoniazid, nitrofurantoin
Antimalarials: dapsone, quinine, pyrimethamine
Anticonvulsants: phenytoin, mephenytoin, trimethadione, ethosuximide, carbamazepine
Hypoglycemic agents: tolbutamide, chlorpropamide
Antihistamines: cimetidine, brompheniramine, tripelennamine
Antihypertensives: methyldopa, captopril
Antiinflammatory agents: aminopyrine, phenylbutazone, gold salts, ibuprofen, indomethacin
Antithyroid agents: propylthiouracil, methimazole, thiouracil
Diuretics: acetazolamide, hydrochlorothiazide, chlorthalidone
Phenothiazines: chlorpromazine, promazine, prochlorperazine
Immunosuppressive agents: antimetabolites
Cytotoxic agents: alkylating agents, antimetabolites, anthracyclines, *Vinca* alkaloids, cisplatin, hydroxyurea, dactinomycin
Other agents: recombinant interferons, allopurinol, ethanol, levamisole, penicillamine, zidovudine, streptokinase, carbamazepine, clopidogrel, ticlopidine

Modified and updated from Goldman L, Ausiello D (eds): *Cecil textbook of medicine,* ed 22, Philadelphia, 2004, Saunders.

NOREPINEPHRINE

Normal range: 0-600 pg/ml
Elevated in: Pheochromocytomas, neuroblastomas, stress, vigorous exercise, certain foods (bananas, chocolate, coffee, tea, vanilla)

5′-NUCLEOTIDASE

Normal range: 2-16 IU/L (3-27 $\times$ 10^8 kat/L [CF: 1.67 $\times$ 10^8; SMI: 1 $\times$ 10^8 kat/L])
Elevated in: Biliary obstruction, metastatic neoplasms to liver, primary biliary cirrhosis, renal failure, pancreatic carcinoma, chronic active hepatitis

TABLE 68 Classification of Neutropenia

Congenital

Primary
- Autoimmune neutropenia
- Pure white cell aplasia
- Idiopathic
- Thymoma
- Hematologic malignancies (e.g., T-LGL leukemia)
- Infections/postinfectious
- Viral
  - Measles, mumps, roseola, rubella, RSV, influenza
  - Hepatitis A, B, and C
  - CMV, EBV, HIV
  - Parvovirus
- Bacterial
  - Tuberculosis
  - Brucellosis
  - Tularemia
  - Typhoid fever
- Rickettsial
  - Rocky Mountain spotted fever
  - Ehrlichiosis
- Fungal
  - Histoplasmosis
- Parasitic
  - Malaria, leishmaniasis
- Autoimmune conditions (e.g., SLE, RA)
- Drugs and chemicals
- Neutropenia associated with immunodeficiency
- Severe nutritional deficiencies
- Neutropenia caused by increased margination
- Iatrogenic (e.g., hemodialysis)

CMV, Cytomegalovirus; *EBV,* Epstein-Barr virus; *HIV,* human immunodeficiency virus; *RA,* refractory anemia; *RSV,* respiratory syncytial virus; *SLE,* systemic lupus erythematosus; *T-LGL,* T-cell large granular lymphocyte.
Modified from Hoffman R: *Hematology, basic principles and practice,* ed 7, Philadelphia, 2018, Elsevier.

TABLE 69 Drugs Associated with Agranulocytosis

	ETIOLOGIC FRACTION	
	Agranulocytosis (%)	Aplastic Anemia (%)
Overall	64	62
IAAAS	12	27
United States	72	17
Thailand	70	2

Drugs associated with agranulocytosis (IAAAS and other drugs of interest)

- Acetyldigoxin
- ACE inhibitors
- Allopurinol
- Amodiaquine
- Benzafibrate
- β-Blockers
- β-Lactam antibiotics
- Carbamazepine
- Cinepazide
- Corticosteroids
- Cotrimoxazole, other sulfonamides
- Dipyridamole
- Deferasirox (Exjade)
- Dypirone
- Histamine-2 receptor antagonist
- Indomethacin
- Isoniazid
- Macrolides
- Mefloquine
- Nifedipine
- Phenytoin
- Procainamide
- Salicylates
- Sulfasalazine
- Sulfonylureas
- Tetracyclines
- Thenalidine
- Thyrostatics
- Troxerutine

ACE, Angiotensin-converting enzyme; *IAAAS,* International Agranulocytosis and Aplastic Anemia Study.
Modified from Hoffman R: *Hematology, basic principles and practice,* ed 7, Philadelphia, 2018, Elsevier.

TABLE 70 Causes of Neutrophilia

- Hematologic malignancy (CML, CNL, CMML)
- Infection
- Inflammation, physiologic stress, hemorrhage, hemolysis
- Hereditary or congenital neutrophilias
- Smoking
- Drugs: colony-stimulating factors, glucocorticoids, epinephrine, lithium
- Nonhematologic malignancy
- Asplenia
- Obesity
- Recovery from neutropenia

CML, Chronic myeloid leukemia; *CMML,* chronic myelomonocytic leukemia; *CNL,* chronic neutrophilic leukemia.
From Hoffman R: *Hematology, basic principles and practice,* ed 7, Philadelphia, 2018, Elsevier.

OSMOLALITY (serum)

Normal range: 280-300 mOsm/kg (280-300 mmol/kg [CF: 1; SMI: 1 mmol/kg])

It can also be estimated by the following formula:

$$2\,([\text{Na}] + [\text{K}] + \text{glucose}/18 + \text{BUN}/2.8)$$

The relationship between plasma osmolality and plasma arginine vasopressin is illustrated in Fig. 38.

The relationships between plasma and urine osmolality are illustrated in Fig. 39.

Elevated in: Dehydration, hypernatremia, diabetes insipidus, uremia, hyperglycemia, mannitol therapy, ingestion of toxins (ethylene glycol, methanol, ethanol), hypercalcemia, diuretics

Decreased in: Syndrome of inappropriate diuretic hormone secretion, hyponatremia, overhydration, Addison's disease, hypothyroidism

OSMOLALITY, URINE

Normal range: 50-1200 mOsm/kg (50-1200 mmol/kg [CF: 1; SMI: 1 mmol/kg])

Elevated in: Syndrome of inappropriate antidiuretic hormone secretion, dehydration, glycosuria, adrenal insufficiency, high-protein diet

Decreased in: Diabetes insipidus, excessive water intake, IV hydration with D_5W, acute renal insufficiency, glomerulonephritis

The relationship between plasma urine osmolality and plasma arginine vasopressin in patients with polyuria is illustrated in Fig. 40. Box 24 describes urine osmolality variances in common clinical situations.

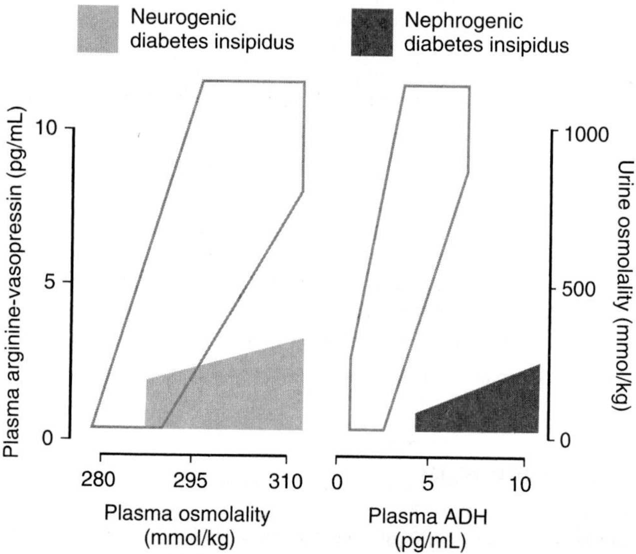

FIG. 38 *Left,* Relationship between plasma arginine vasopressin (AVP/ADH) and plasma osmolality during the infusion of hypertonic saline. Patients with primary polydipsia and nephrogenic diabetes insipidus (DI) have values within the normal range *(open area),* in contrast to patients with neurogenic DI, who show a subnormal plasma ADH response to a rise in osmolality *(pink). Right,* Relationship between urine osmolality and plasma ADH during dehydration and water loading. Patients with primary polydipsia and neurogenic DI have values within the normal range *(open area),* in contrast to patients with nephrogenic DI, who have hypotonic urine despite high plasma ADH *(green).*

(Redrawn from Bichet DG: Diabetes insipidus and vasopressin. In Moore TW, Eastman RC [eds]: *Diagnostic endocrinology,* ed 2, St Louis, 1996, Mosby, p. 168, with permission.)

(McPherson RA, Pincus MR: *Henry's clinical diagnosis and management by laboratory methods,* ed 23, St Louis, 2017, Elsevier.)

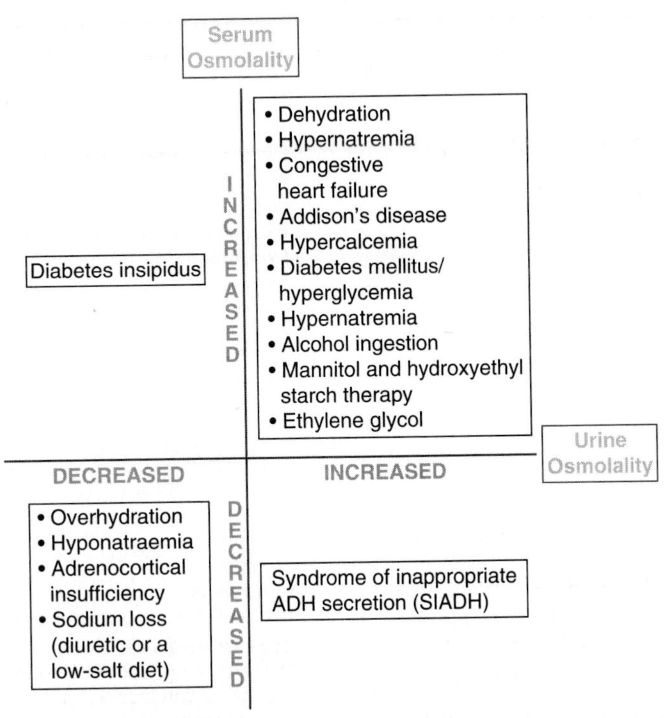

FIG. 39 Relationships between plasma and urine osmolality. (From Vincent JL, Abraham E, Moore FA et al: *Textbook of critical care*, ed 7, Philadelphia, 2017, Elsevier.)

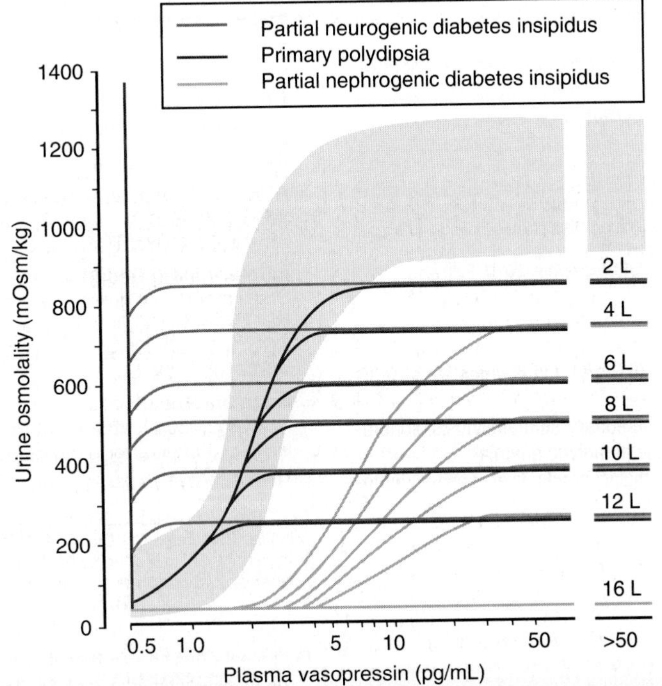

FIG. 40 The relationship between urine osmolality (Uosm) and plasma arginine vasopressin (AVP/ADH) in patients with polyuria of diverse causes and severity. Each of the three categories of polyuria is described by its own family of sigmoid curves of differing heights. Differences in height within a family reflect differences in maximum concentrating capacity caused by "washout" of the medullary concentration gradient. They are proportional to the severity of the polyuria (indicated in liters per day at the right end of each plateau). The normal response is depicted in yellow. The three categories of polyuria differ principally in the ascending portion of the dose-response curve. In patients with partial neurogenic diabetes insipidus (DI), the curve lies to the left of normal, reflecting increased sensitivity to the antidiuretic effects of very low concentrations of plasma ADH. In contrast, in patients with partial nephrogenic DI, the curve lies to the right of normal, reflecting decreased sensitivity to ADH. In primary polydipsia, the relationship of Uosm to ADH remains relatively normal.
(Redrawn from Bichet DG: Diabetes insipidus and vasopressin. In Moore WT, Eastman RC [eds]: *Diagnostic endocrinology*, ed 2, St Louis, 1996, Mosby, p 158, with permission.)
(McPherson RA, Pincus MR: *Henry's clinical diagnosis and management by laboratory methods*, ed 23, St Louis, 2017, Elsevier.)

BOX 24 Urine Osmolality in Common Clinical Situations

High Urine Osmolality
AKI or when assessing effective circulating volume
Prerenal states
Volume depletion (GI losses, renal losses, skin losses, third spacing)
Heart failure
Cirrhosis
Hypoalbuminemia
Hyponatremia
Prerenal states
Volume depletion (GI losses, renal losses, skin losses, third spacing)
Heart failure
Cirrhosis
Hypoalbuminemia
Syndrome of inappropriate ADH secretion
Hypernatremia
GI losses (vomiting, diarrhea, nasogastric tube, fistula)
Skin losses (fever, exercise, ventilation)
Sodium overload (received excess normal saline or sodium bicarbonate)
Mineralocorticoid excess
Seizures (↑ intracellular osmoles → water shifts → transient increase in serum Na)

Low Urine Osmolality
AKI or when assessing effective circulating volume
Euvolemic or hypervolemic
Established AKI
Chronic kidney disease
Hyponatremia
In process of correcting hyponatremia
Primary polydipsia
Extremely low solute intake (tea and toast diet or beer potomonia)
Hypernatremia
Osmotic diuresis (glucose, mannitol, urea)
Loop diuretics
Nephrogenic DI
Central DI

ADH, Antidiuretic hormone; *AKI,* acute kidney injury; *DI,* diabetes insipidus; *GI,* gastrointestinal.
From Ronco C: *Critical care nephrology*, ed 3, Philadelphia, 2019, Elsevier.

OSMOTIC FRAGILITY TEST

Normal: Hemolysis begins at 0.50, w/v [5.0 g/L] and is complete at 0.30, w/v [3.0 g/L] NaCl.
Elevated in: Hereditary spherocytosis, hereditary stomatocytosis, spherocytosis associated with acquired immune hemolytic anemia
Decreased in: Iron deficiency anemia, thalassemias, liver disease, leptocytosis associated with asplenia

PARACENTESIS FLUID

Testing and evaluation of results:
Process the fluid as follows:
Tube 1: LDH, glucose, albumin
Tube 2: protein, specific gravity
Tube 3: cell count and differential
Tube 4: save until further notice
Draw serum LDH, protein, albumin.
Gram stain, AFB stain, bacterial and fungal cultures, amylase, and triglycerides should be ordered only when clearly indicated; bedside inoculation of blood-culture bottles with ascitic fluid improves sensitivity in detecting bacterial growth.
If malignant ascites is suspected, consider a carcinoembryonic antigen level on the paracentesis fluid and cytologic evaluation.
In suspected spontaneous bacterial peritonitis (SBP) the incidence of positive cultures can be increased by injecting 10 to 20 ml of ascitic fluid into blood culture bottles.

BOX 25 Causes of Peritoneal Effusions

Transudates: Increased Hydrostatic Pressure or Decreased Plasma Oncotic Pressure
Congestive heart failure
Hepatic cirrhosis
Hypoproteinemia (e.g., nephrotic syndrome)

Exudates: Increased Capillary Permeability or Decreased Lymphatic Resorption
Infections
- Primary bacterial peritonitis
- Secondary bacterial peritonitis (e.g., appendicitis, bowel rupture)
- Tuberculosis

Neoplasms
- Hepatoma
- Lymphoma
- Mesothelioma
- Metastatic carcinoma
- Ovarian carcinoma
- Prostate cancer

Trauma
Pancreatitis
Bile peritonitis (e.g., ruptured gallbladder)

Chylous Effusion
Damage to or obstruction of thoracic duct (e.g., trauma, lymphoma, carcinoma, tuberculosis and other granulomas [e.g., sarcoidosis, histoplasmosis], parasitic infestation)

From McPherson RA, Pincus MR: *Henry's clinical diagnosis and management by laboratory methods*, ed 23, St Louis, 2017, Elsevier.

BOX 26 Criteria for Evaluation of Peritoneal Lavage

Positive Result
Aspiration of >15 mL gross blood on catheter placement
Grossly bloody lavage fluid
RBC >100,000/μL after blunt trauma
RBC >50,000/μL after penetrating trauma
WBC >500/μL
Amylase >110 U/dL

Indeterminate Result
Small amount of gross blood on catheter placement
RBC 50,000-100,000/μL after blunt trauma
RBC 1000-50,000/μL after penetrating trauma
WBC 100-500/μL

Negative Result
RBC <50,000/μL after blunt trauma
RBC <1000/μL after penetrating trauma
WBC <100/μL

RBC, Red blood cells; *WBC,* white blood cells.
Modified from Feied CF: Diagnostic peritoneal lavage, *Postgrad Med* 85:40, 1989, with permission. In McPherson RA, Pincus MR: *Henry's clinical diagnosis and management by laboratory methods*, ed 23, St Louis, 2017, Elsevier.

Peritoneal effusion can be subdivided as exudative or transudative based on its characteristics (see Section II).
The serum-ascites albumin gradient (serum albumin level–ascitic fluid albumin level [SAAG]) correlates directly with portal pressure and can also be used to classify ascites. Patients with gradients ≥1.1 g/dl have portal hypertension, and those with gradients ≤1.1 g/dl do not; the accuracy of this method is >95%.
For the differential diagnosis of ascites, refer to Section II.
An ascitic fluid polymorphonuclear leukocyte count >500/μl is suggestive of SBP.
A blood-ascitic fluid albumin gradient. Box 25 summarizes causes of peritoneal effusions. Useful criteria for evaluation of peritoneal lavage is summarized in Box 26. Recommended tests in peritoneal effusions are summarized in Box 27.

BOX 27 Recommended Tests in Peritoneal Effusions

Useful in Most Patients
Gross examination
Cytology
Stains and culture for microorganisms
Serum-ascites albumin concentration gradient

Useful in Selected Disorders
Total leukocyte and differential cell counts
RBC count (lavage)
Bilirubin
Creatinine/urea nitrogen
Enzymes (ADA, ALP, amylase, LD, telomerase)
Lactate
Cholesterol (malignant ascites)
Fibronectin
Tumor markers (CEA, PSA, CA 19-9, CA 15-3, CA-125)
Immunocytology/flow cytometry
Tuberculostearic acid

ADA, Adenosine deaminase; *ALP,* alkaline phosphatase; *CEA,* carcinoembryonic antigen; *LD,* lactate dehydrogenase; *PSA,* prostate-specific antigen; *RBC,* red blood cell.
Modified from Kjeldsberg CR, Knight JA: *Body fluids: Laboratory examination of amniotic, cerebrospinal, seminal, serous and synovial fluids*, ed 3, Chicago, 1993, © American Society for Clinical Pathology, with permission. In McPherson RA, Pincus MR: *Henry's clinical diagnosis and management by laboratory methods*, ed 23, St Louis, 2017, Elsevier.

TABLE 71 Clinical Peculiarities of Coagulation Protein Screening Tests

Long aPTT, normal or long PT, no bleeding	Normal aPTT, PT, *with bleeding*
Long aPTT Only	
Factor XII deficiency	Factor XIII deficiency or inhibitor
Prekallikrein deficiency	α_2-Antiplasmin deficiency or defect
High-molecular-weight kininogen	Plasminogen activator inhibitor deficiency or defect
Lupus anticoagulant	α_1-Antitrypsin Pittsburgh defect
Long aPTT and PT	
Dysfibrinogenemia with fibrinopeptide B release	
Lupus anticoagulant	

From Hoffman R et al: *Hematology: basic principles and practice*, ed 5, Philadelphia, 2009, Churchill Livingstone.

PARATHYROID HORMONE (PTH)

Normal:
Serum, intact molecule 10-65 pg/ml
Plasma 1.0-5.0 pmol/L
Elevated in:
Hyperparathyroidism (primary or secondary), pseudohypoparathyroidism, anticonvulsants, corticosteroids, lithium, INH, rifampin, phosphates, Zollinger-Ellison syndrome, hereditary vitamin D deficiency
Decreased in: Hypoparathyroidism, sarcoidosis, cimetidine, beta-blockers, hyperthyroidism, hypomagnesemia

PARIETAL CELL ANTIBODIES

Normal: Negative
Present in: Pernicious anemia (>90%), atrophic gastritis (up to 50%), thyroiditis (30%), Addison's disease, myasthenia gravis, Sjögren syndrome, type 1 DM

PARTIAL THROMBOPLASTIN TIME (PTT), ACTIVATED PARTIAL THROMBOPLASTIN TIME (APTT)

See Table 71 for interpretation of coagulation protein screening tests.

Normal range: 25-41 sec
Elevated in: Heparin therapy, coagulation factor deficiency (I, II, V, VIII, IX, X, XI, XII), liver disease, vitamin K deficiency, disseminated intravascular coagulation, circulating anticoagulant, warfarin therapy, specific factor inhibition (PCN reaction, rheumatoid arthritis), thrombolytic therapy, nephrotic syndrome
NOTE: Useful to evaluate the intrinsic coagulation system.

PEPSINOGEN I

Normal: 124-142 ng/ml
Elevated in: ZE syndrome, duodenal ulcer, acute gastritis
Decreased in: Atrophic gastritis, gastric carcinoma, myxedema, pernicious anemia, Addison's disease

PH, BLOOD

Normal values:
Arterial: 7.35-7.45
Venous: 7.32-7.42
For abnormal values, refer to ARTERIAL BLOOD GASES.

PH, URINE

See URINE pH

PHENOBARBITAL

Normal therapeutic range: 15-30 mc g/ml for epilepsy control

PHENYTOIN (Dilantin)

Normal therapeutic range: 10-20 mcg/ml

PHOSPHATASE, ACID

See ACID PHOSPHATASE

PHOSPHATASE, ALKALINE

See ALKALINE PHOSPHATASE

PHOSPHATE (serum)

Normal range: 2.5-5 mg/dl (0.8-1.6 mmol/L [CF: 0.3229; SMI: 0.05 mmol/L])
DECREASED
Parenteral hyperalimentation
Diabetic acidosis
Alcohol withdrawal
Severe metabolic or respiratory alkalosis
Antacids that bind phosphorus
Malnutrition with refeeding using low-phosphorus nutrients
Renal tubule failure to reabsorb phosphate (Fanconi's syndrome; congenital disorder; vitamin D deficiency)
Glucose administration
Nasogastric suction
Malabsorption
Gram-negative sepsis
Primary hyperthyroidism
Chlorothiazide diuretics
Therapy of acute severe asthma
Acute respiratory failure with mechanical ventilation
INCREASED
Renal failure
Severe muscle injury
Phosphate-containing antacids
Hypoparathyroidism
Tumor lysis syndrome
For a diagnostic algorithm of hyperphosphatemia, see Fig. 41.
For a diagnostic algorithm for hypophosphatemia, see Fig. 42.
For causes and treatment of hypophosphatemia see Tables 72 and 73.

PLASMINOGEN

Normal: Immunoassay (antigen): <20 mg/dl
Elevated in: Infection, trauma, neoplasm, myocardial infarction (acute phase reactant), pregnancy, bilirubinemia

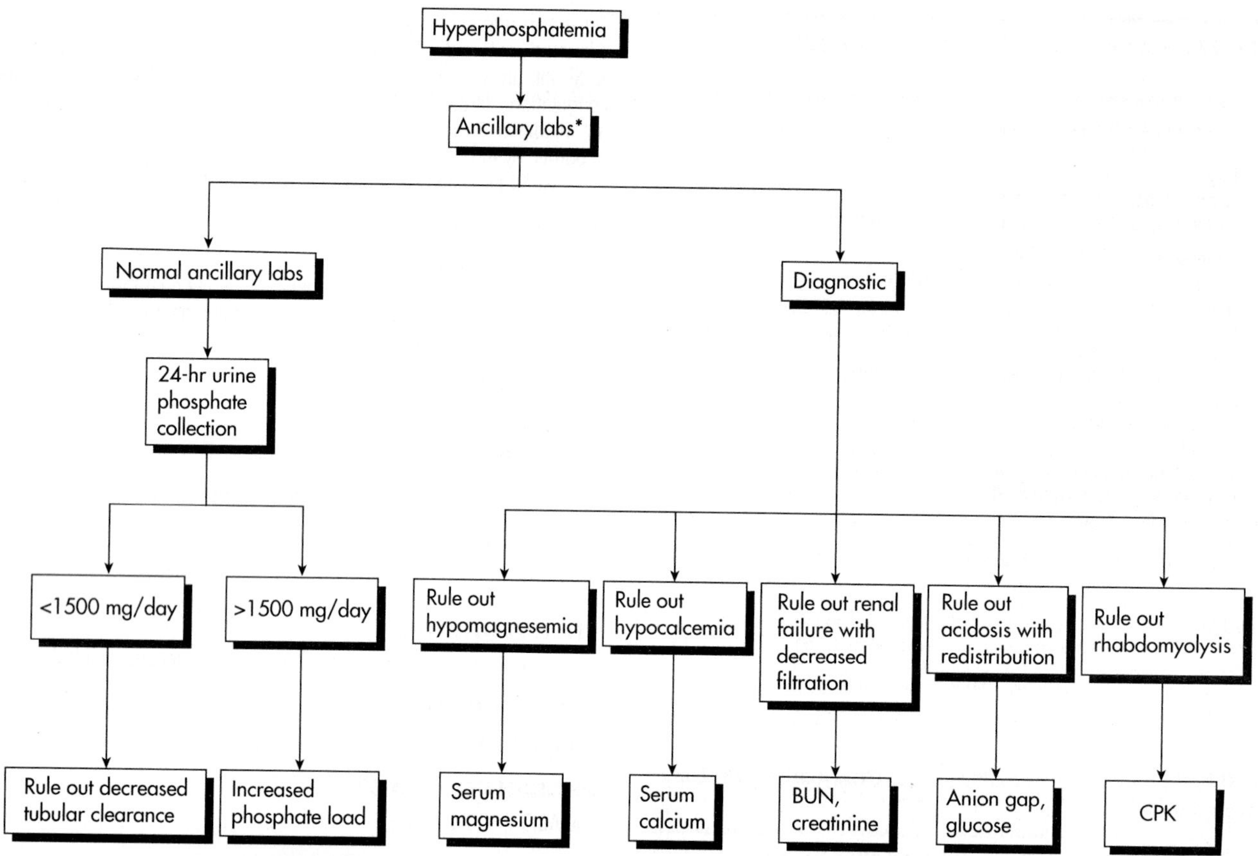

FIG. 41 Diagnostic algorithm for hyperphosphatemia. *Serum calcium, electrolytes, creatinine, glucose, ABGs, urinalysis, CPK, magnesium. (From Ferri, F: *Ferri's best test: a practical guide to clinical laboratory medicine and diagnostic imaging*, ed 4, Philadelphia, 2017, Saunders.)

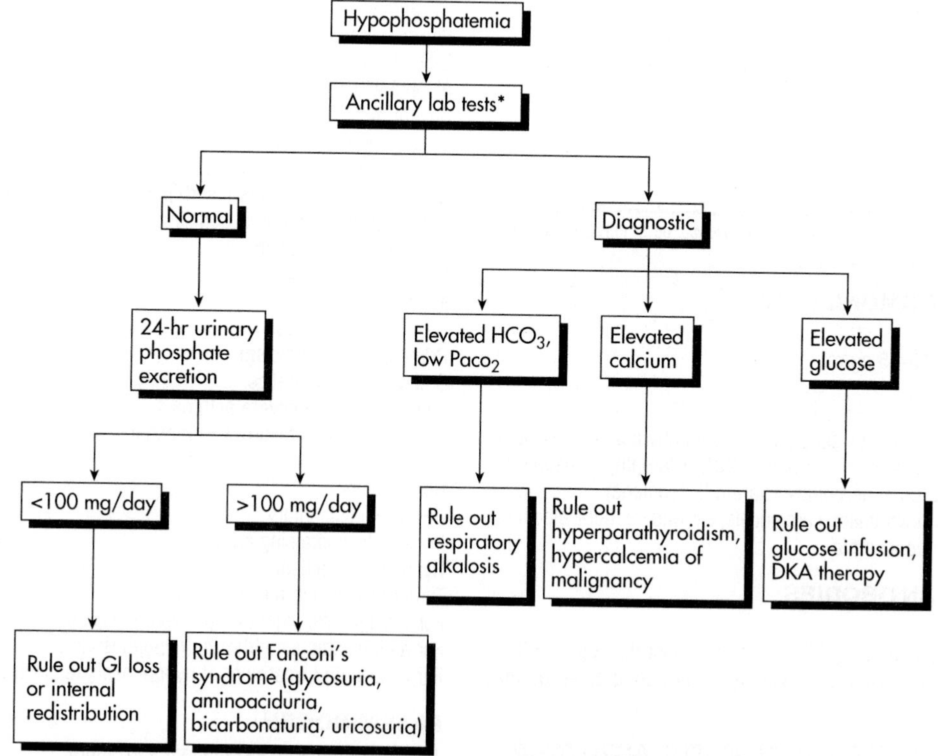

FIG. 42 Diagnostic algorithm for hypophosphatemia. *Serum creatinine, BUN, electrolytes, magnesium, calcium, glucose, urinalysis, CPK. (From Ferri, F: *Ferri's best test: a practical guide to clinical laboratory medicine and diagnostic imaging*, ed 4, Philadelphia, 2017, Saunders.)

TABLE 72 Causes of Hypophosphatemia

Decreased Phosphate Intake

- Starvation, inadequate phosphate intake, chronic diarrhea, chronic alcoholism
- Total parenteral nutrition with insufficient phosphate content

Increased Loss of Phosphate

- Increased renal phosphate excretion
  - Primary hyperparathyroidism
  - Secondary hyperparathyroidism: vitamin D deficiency or resistance (including 1α-hydroxylase deficiency, VDR mutations, VDDR); imatinib
  - Excess FGF-23 or phosphatonins: X-linked hypophosphatemia, AD hypophosphatemic rickets, tumor-induced osteomalacia, epidermal nevus, McCune-Albright syndrome
  - Fanconi's syndrome, cystinosis, Wilson disease, Dent disease, Lowe syndrome, multiple myeloma, amyloidosis, heavy-metal toxicity, rewarming of hyperthermia, Na/Pi-IIa and Na/Pi-IIc mutation (HHRH)
  - PTHrP-dependent hypercalcemia of malignancy
  - Hypomagnesemia
- Decreased intestinal absorption
  - Vitamin D deficiency or resistance (VDDR I and II)
  - Malabsorption
- Increased intestinal loss
  - Phosphate binding antacids used in treating peptic ulcers
- Increased loss from other routes
  - Skin: severe burns
  - Vomiting

Phosphate Shifting from Extracellular Compartment to Cells and Bones

- Diabetic ketoacidosis
- Alcohol intoxication
- Acute respiratory alkalosis, salicylate intoxication, gram-negative sepsis, toxic shock syndrome, acute gout
- Refeeding syndromes from starvation, anorexia nervosa, hepatic failure: acute intravenous glucose, fructose, glycerol
- Rapid cellular proliferation: intensive erythropoietin therapy, GM-CSF therapy, leukemic blast crisis
- Recovery from hypothermia
- Heat stroke
- Post parathyroidectomy; "hungry bone" disease: osteoblastic metastases, antiresorptive treatment of severe Paget disease
- Catecholamine (albuterol, dopamine, terbutaline, epinephrine)
- Thyrotoxic periodic paralysis
- Hypocalcemic periodic paralysis

Miscellaneous

Hyperaldosteronism

- Oncogenic hypophosphatemia
- Post kidney transplantation
- Post partial hepatectomy
- High-dose corticosteroids, estrogens
- Medications: ifosfamide; toluene; calcitonin; bisphosphonate; tenofovir; paraquat, cisplatin; acetazolamide and other diuretics
- Post obstructive diuresis

AD, Autosomal dominant; *FGF-23,* fibroblast growth factor 23; *GM-CSF,* granulocyte-macrophage colony-stimulating factor; *HHRH,* hereditary hypophosphatemic rickets with hypercalciuria; *Na/Pi-II,* type II sodium-dependent phosphate cotransporter; *PTHrP,* parathyroid hormone–related peptide; *VDR,* vitamin D receptor; *VDDR,* vitamin D–dependent rickets.
From Skorecki K, Chertow GM, Marsden PA et al: *Brenner & Rector's the kidney,* ed 10, Philadelphia, 2016, Elsevier.

TABLE 73 Treatment of Hypophosphatemia

Therapy	Dosage	Administration
Mild and Moderate Hypophosphatemia		
	Low-fat milk	Phosphate 0.9 mg/mL
	Buffered Na phosphate (Fleet enema)	1-3 g/day in 4 divided doses
	Neutra-Phos (250 mg elemental phosphorus per capsule)	1-3 g/day in 4 divided doses
	Calcitriol	30-70 ng/kg body weight per day
Asymptomatic Severe Hypophosphatemia		
Elemental phosphate	2.5 mg/kg body weight	IV over 6 hr
Symptomatic Severe Hypophosphatemia		
Elemental phosphate	5 mg/kg body weight	IV over 6 hr

IV, Intravenously.
From Skorecki K, Chertow GM, Marsden PA et al: *Brenner & Rector's the kidney,* ed 10, Philadelphia, 2016, Elsevier.

TABLE 74 Differential Diagnosis of Thrombocytopenia in Suspected Disseminated Intravascular Coagulation

Differential Diagnosis	Additional Diagnostic Clues
DIC	Prolonged aPTT and PT, increased FDP, low levels of AT or protein C
Sepsis without DIC	Positive (blood) cultures, positive sepsis criteria, hematophagocytosis in BM aspirate
Massive blood loss	Major bleeding, low hemoglobin, prolonged aPTT and PT
Thrombotic microangiopathy	Schistocytes in blood smear, Coombs-negative hemolysis, fever, neurologic symptoms, renal insufficiency, coagulation test results usually normal, ADAMTS13 levels decreased
Heparin-induced thrombocytopenia	Use of heparin, venous or arterial thrombosis, positive HIT test (usually immunoassay for heparin-platelet factor 4 antibodies), increase in platelet count after cessation of heparin; coagulation tests usually normal
Immune thrombocytopenia	Antiplatelet antibodies, normal or increased number of megakaryocytes in BM aspirate, TPO decreased; coagulation tests usually normal
Drug-induced thrombocytopenia	Decreased number of megakaryocytes in BM aspirate or detection of drug-induced antiplatelet antibodies, increase in platelet count after cessation of drug; coagulation test results usually normal

ADAMTS13, A disintegrin and metalloproteinase with a thrombospondin type 1 motif, member 13; *aPTT,* activated partial thromboplastin time; *AT,* antithrombin; *BM,* bone marrow; *DIC,* disseminated intravascular coagulation; *FDP,* fibrin degradation product; *HIT,* heparin-induced thrombocytopenia; *PT,* prothrombin time; TPO, thrombopoietin.
From Souoffman R: *Hematology, basic principles and practice,* ed 6, Philadelphia, Saunders, 2013.

Decreased in: DIC, severe liver disease, thrombolytic therapy with streptokinase or urokinase, alteplase

PLATELET AGGREGATION

Normal: Full aggregation (generally >60%) in response to epinephrine, thrombin, ristocetin, ADP, collagen
Elevated in: Heparin, hemolysis, lipemia, nicotine, hereditary and acquired disorders of platelet adhesion, activation, and aggregation
Decreased in: Aspirin, some penicillins, chloroquine, chlorpromazine, clofibrate, captopril, Glanzmann thrombasthenia, Bernard-Soulier syndrome, Wiskott-Aldrich syndrome, cyclooxygenase deficiency. In von Willebrand's disease there is normal aggregation with ADP, collagen, and epinephrine but abnormal agglutination with ristocetin.

PLATELET ANTIBODIES

Normal: Absent
Present in: ITP (>90% of patients with chronic ITP). Patients with nonimmune thrombocytopenias may have false-positive results.

PLATELET COUNT

See Fig. E43 for evaluation of thrombocytosis. Box E28 describes testing for thrombocytopenia. See Table 74 for differential diagnosis. Table 75 describes antibody-mediated thrombocytopenic disorders caused by autoantibodies, alloantibodies, or potentially both. Tables 76 and 77

TABLE 75 Antibody-Mediated Thrombocytopenic Disorders Caused by Autoantibodies (Immune Thrombocytopenia), Alloantibodies (Neonatal Alloimmune Thrombocytopenia), or Potentially Both (Posttransfusion Purpura)

	Immune Thrombocytopenia	Neonatal Alloimmune Thrombocytopenia	Posttransfusion Purpura
Immune reaction	Autoimmune	Alloimmune	Features of both allo- and autoimmunity
Incidence	5 per 100,000 population	40 per 100,000 births (or 1 per 2500)	1 per 100,000 blood transfusions
Principal antigenic target	GPIIb/IIIa	HPA-1a	HPA-1a plus autoantigens
Nature of the antibody	Intermittent	Persistent (past 1 year)	Persistent often at high titers
Mode of sensitization	Autoantibody	Alloantibody	Features of allo- and autoantibodies
Sensitizing event	Mostly unknown; some viral illnesses, chronic infection	Exposure to fetal platelet antigens early in first pregnancy	Blood transfusion (RBCs or platelets) 5–10 days earlier
Bleeding frequency	Uncommon	Common	Very common
Epidemiology	Higher incidence in children and elderly adults; female predominance in early adulthood	Majority affects fetus or newborn carrying the HPA-1a antigen	Almost all are HPA-1bb women sensitized by previous transfusion or pregnancy

GP, Glycoprotein; *HPA,* human platelet antigen; *RBC,* red blood cell.
From Hoffman R: *Hematology, basic principles and practice*, ed 7, Philadelphia, 2018, Elsevier.

TABLE 76 Differential Diagnosis of Thrombocytopenia in Newborns

Perinatal Hypoxemia
Placental Insufficiency
Congenital Infection
- Sepsis
- Toxoplasmosis
- Rubella
- Cytomegalovirus

Autoimmune
- Maternal immune thrombocytopenia
- Maternal systemic lupus erythematosus

Disseminated Intravascular Coagulation
Maternal Drug Exposure
Congenital Heart Disease
Hereditary Thrombocytopenia
- MYH9 macrothrombocytopenia (including May-Hegglin anomaly)
- Thrombocytopenia absent radii syndrome
- Amegakaryocytic thrombocytopenia
- Wiskott-Aldrich syndrome
- Fanconi anemia

Hemangioma with Thrombocytopenia
- Kasabach-Merritt syndrome

Bone Marrow Infiltration
- Congenital leukemia

From Hoffman R: *Hematology, basic principles and practice*, ed 7, Philadelphia, 2018, Elsevier.

TABLE 77 Differential Diagnosis of Thrombocytopenia in Pregnancy

Incidental thrombocytopenia of pregnancy (gestational thrombocytopenia)
Preeclampsia or eclampsia[a]
DIC secondary to:
- Abruptio placentae
- Endometritis
- Amniotic fluid embolism
- Retained fetus
- Preeclampsia or eclampsia[a]

Peripartum or postpartum thrombotic microangiopathy
- TTP
- HssUS

DIC, Disseminated intravascular coagulation; *HUS,* hemolytic uremic syndrome; *TTP,* thrombotic thrombocytopenic purpura.
[a]Preeclampsia or eclampsia usually is not associated with overt DIC.
From Hoffman R: *Hematology, basic principles and practice*, ed 7, Philadelphia, 2018, Elsevier.

indicate differential diagnosis of thrombocytopenia in newborns and differential diagnosis of thrombocytopenia in pregnancy, respectively. Table 78 describes laboratory tests used to investigate a patient with thrombocytopenia.

Normal range: 130-400 × 103/mm3 (130-400 × 109/L [CF: 1; SMI: 5 × 109/L])

Elevated in

REACTIVE THROMBOCYTOSIS
Infections or inflammatory states: vasculitis, allergic reactions, etc.
Surgery and tissue damage: myocardial infarction, pancreatitis, etc.
Postsplenectomy state
Malignancy: solid tumors, lymphoma
Iron deficiency anemia, hemolytic anemia, acute blood loss
Uncertain etiology
Rebound effect after chemotherapy or immune thrombocytopenia
Renal disorders: renal failure, nephrotic syndrome

MYELOPROLIFERATIVE DISORDERS
Chronic myeloid leukemia
Primary thrombocythemia
Polycythemia vera
Idiopathic myelofibrosis

Decreased:

Increased destruction (see Table 79)
- Immunologic
  - Drugs: quinine, quinidine, digitalis, procainamide, thiazide diuretics, sulfonamides, phenytoin, aspirin, penicillin, heparin, gold, meprobamate, sulfa drugs, phenylbutazone, NSAIDs, methyldopa, cimetidine, furosemide, INH, cephalosporins, chlorpropamide, organic arsenicals, chloroquine
  - Idiopathic thrombocytopenic purpura
  - Transfusion reaction: transfusion of platelets with platelet antigen HPA-1a (PL^{A1}) in recipients without PL^{A1}
  - Fetal/maternal incompatibility
  - Vasculitis (e.g., systemic lupus erythematosus)
  - Autoimmune hemolytic anemia
  - Lymphoreticular disorders (e.g., chronic lymphocytic leukemia)
- Nonimmunologic
  - Prosthetic heart valves
  - Thrombotic thrombocytopenic purpura
  - Sepsis
  - Disseminated intravascular coagulation
  - Hemolytic-uremic syndrome
  - Giant cavernous hemangioma

Decreased production
- Abnormal marrow

TABLE 78 Laboratory Tests Used to Investigate a Patient with Thrombocytopenia

Test	Rationale
Common Tests	
CBC	Isolated thrombocytopenia usually is caused by platelet destruction, but involvement of all cell lines suggests underproduction or sequestration
Examination of the blood film	Pseudothrombocytopenia (platelet clumps)
	Toxic changes and granulocyte "left shift" suggest septicemia
	Atypical lymphocytes suggest viral infection
	RBC fragments suggest TTP or HUS
	Parasites (e.g., in malaria)
	White cell inclusions suggest hereditary macrothrombocytopenia
Blood cultures	Bacteremia, fungemia
ANA test	Systemic lupus erythematosus
Direct antiglobulin test	Exclude immune hemolysis accompanying ITP (Evans syndrome)
Coagulation Assays	
aPTT, PT (INR), thrombin time, fibrinogen, D-dimer assay	DIC
LA assay (nonspecific inhibitor), anticardiolipin and anti-β_2-glycoprotein I assays	aPL antibody syndrome
Serum protein electrophoresis; IgG, IgM, IgA levels	ITP associated with lymphoproliferative disorder (monoclonal); hypersplenism associated with chronic hepatitis (polyclonal)
HIV serologic studies	HIV-associated thrombocytopenia
BM aspiration, biopsy	Assess megakaryocyte numbers and morphology; exclude primary BM disorder
Specialized Tests	
GP-specific platelet antibody assays (e.g., MAIPA)	Relatively specific assay for primary and secondary ITP
Drug-dependent increase in platelet-associated IgG	Specific assay for D-ITP
Drug-dependent platelet activation test (e.g., platelet serotonin release assay) or PF4–heparin (or PF4-polyanion) ELISA	HIT
Radionuclide platelet life span study with imaging (e.g., ^{111}In platelet survival study)	Define the mechanism of thrombocytopenia; identify an "accessory" spleen postsplenectomy

ANA, Antinuclear antibody; *aPL,* antiphospholipid; *aPTT,* activated partial thromboplastin time; *BM,* bone marrow; *CBC,* complete blood count; *DIC,* disseminated intravascular coagulation; *D-ITP,* drug-induced immune thrombocytopenia; *ELISA,* enzyme-linked immunosorbent assay; *GP,* glycoprotein; *HIT,* heparin-induced thrombocytopenia; *HIV,* human immunodeficiency virus; *HUS,* hemolytic uremic syndrome; *IgG,* immunoglobulin G; *INR,* international normalized ratio; *ITP,* idiopathic (immune) thrombocytopenic purpura; *LA,* lupus anticoagulant; *MAIPA,* monoclonal antibody immobilization of platelet antigens; *PF4,* platelet factor 4; *PT,* prothrombin time; *RBC,* red blood cell; *TTP,* thrombotic thrombocytopenic purpura.
From Hoffman R: *Hematology, basic principles and practice,* ed 7, Philadelphia, 2018, Elsevier.

TABLE 79 Mechanisms of Platelet Destruction

Type of Thrombocytopenia	Specific Example(s)
Immune Mediated	
Autoantibody-mediated platelet destruction by reticuloendothelial system (RES)	Primary immune thrombocytopenic purpura; secondary immune thrombocytopenia associated with lymphoproliferative disease; collagen vascular disease; infections such as infectious mononucleosis; human immunodeficiency virus syndrome
Alloantibody-mediated platelet destruction by RES	Neonatal alloimmune thrombocytopenia; posttransfusion purpura; passive alloimmune thrombocytopenia; alloimmune platelet transfusion refractoriness
Drug-dependent, antibody-mediated platelet destruction by RES	Drug-induced immune thrombocytopenic purpura (e.g., quinine)
Platelet activation by binding of immunoglobulin G (IgG) Fc of drug-dependent IgG to platelet FcγIIa receptors	Heparin-induced thrombocytopenia
Non–Immune Mediated	
Platelet activation by thrombin or proinflammatory cytokines	Disseminated intravascular coagulation; septicemia/systemic inflammatory response syndromes
Platelet destruction via ingestion by macrophages (hemophagocytosis)	Infections; certain malignant lymphoproliferative disorders
Platelet destruction through platelet interactions with altered von Willebrand factor	Thrombotic thrombocytopenic purpura; hemolytic-uremic syndrome; aortic stenosis
Platelet losses on artificial surfaces	Cardiopulmonary bypass surgery; use of intravascular catheters
Decreased platelet survival associated with cardiovascular disease	Congenital and acquired heart disease; cardiomyopathy; pulmonary embolism

Modified with permission from Warkentin TE, Kelton JG: Thrombocytopenia due to platelet destruction and hypersplenism. In Hoffman R, Benz EJ Jr, Shattil SJ et al (eds): *Hematology: basic principles and practice.* Philadelphia, 2005, Elsevier Churchill Livingstone, pp 2305–2325.
McPherson RA, Pincus MR: *Henry's clinical diagnosis and management by laboratory methods,* ed 23, St Louis, 2017, Elsevier.

TABLE 80 Classification of Inherited Thrombocytopenias by Platelet Size

Small Platelets (MPV <7 fL)	Normal-Sized Platelets (MPV 7-11 fL)	Large Platelets (MPV >11 fL)
Wiskott-Aldrich syndrome	Congenital amegakaryocytic thrombocytopenia	*MYH9*-related disorders
X-linked thrombocytopenia	Thrombocytopenia absent radius syndrome	Bernard-Soulier syndrome
	Radioulnar synostosis with amegakaryocytic thrombocytopenia	Gray platelet syndrome
	RUNX1 mutations (FPD/AML)	Velocardiofacial syndrome
	ANKRD26-related thrombocytopenia	*GATA*-1 mutations
	CYCS-related thrombocytopenia	Type 2B von Willebrand's disease
		Platelet-type von Willebrand's disease
		Paris-Trousseau (Jacobsen) syndrome
		TUBB1-related macrothrombocytopenia
		Thrombocytopenia associated with sitosterolemia

Modified with permission from Kumar R, Kahr WHA: Congenital thrombocytopenia: Clinical manifestations, laboratory abnormalities, and molecular defects of a heterogeneous group of conditions. In Rao AK (ed): *Hematology/oncology clinics of North America: disorders of the platelets,* vol 27, Philadelphia, 2013, Elsevier, pp 465–494.
In McPherson RA, Pincus MR: *Henry's clinical diagnosis and management by laboratory methods*, ed 23, St Louis, 2017, Elsevier.

Marrow infiltration (e.g., leukemia, lymphoma, fibrosis)
Marrow suppression (e.g., chemotherapy, alcohol, radiation)
Hereditary disorders (see Table 80)
Wiskott-Aldrich syndrome: X-linked disorder characterized by thrombocytopenia, eczema, and repeated infections
May-Hegglin anomaly: increased megakaryocytes but ineffective thrombopoiesis
Vitamin deficiencies (e.g., vitamin B_{12}, folic acid)
Splenic sequestration, hypersplenism
Dilutional, secondary to massive transfusion

PLATELET FUNCTION ANALYSIS 100 ASSAY (PFA)

Normal: This test is a two-component assay where blood is aspirated through two capillary tubes, one of which is coated with collagen and ADP (COL/ADP) and the other with collagen and epinephrine (COL/EPI). The test measures the ability of platelets to occlude an aperture in a biologically active membrane treated with COL/ADP and COL/EPI. During the test, the platelets adhere to the surface of the tube and cause blood flow to cease. The closing time refers to the cessation of blood flow and is reported in conjunction with the hematocrit and platelet count. Hematocrit count must be >25% and platelet count >50 K/microliter for the test to be performed.
COL/ADP: 70-120 sec
COL/EPI: 75-120 sec
Elevated in: Acquired platelet dysfunction, von Willebrand's disease, anemia, thrombocytopenia, use of aspirin and NSAIDs

PLEURAL FLUID

Testing and evaluation of results

Pleural effusion fluid should be differentiated in exudate or transudate.
The initial laboratory studies should be aimed only at distinguishing an exudate from a transudate.
Tube 1: protein, LDH, albumin.
Tubes 2, 3, 4: save the fluid until further notice. In selected patients with suspected empyema, a pH level may be useful (generally ≤7.0). See following for proper procedure to obtain a pH level from pleural fluid.
A serum/effusion albumin gradient of ≤1.2 g/dl is indicative of exudative effusions, especially in patients with congestive heart failure (CHF) treated with diuretics.
Note the appearance of the fluid:
A grossly hemorrhagic effusion can be a result of a traumatic tap, neoplasm, or an embolus with infarction.
A milky appearance indicates either of the following:
Chylous effusion: caused by trauma or tumor invasion of the thoracic duct; lipoprotein electrophoresis of the effusion reveals chylomicrons and triglyceride levels >115 mg/dl.
Pseudochylous effusion: often seen with chronic inflammation of the pleural space (e.g., TB, connective tissue diseases).
If transudate, consider CHF, cirrhosis, chronic renal failure, and other hypoproteinemic states and perform subsequent workup accordingly.
If exudate, consider ordering these tests on the pleural fluid:
Cytologic examination for malignant cells (for suspected neoplasm).
Gram stain, cultures (aerobic and anaerobic), and sensitivities (for suspected infectious process).
AFB stain and cultures (for suspected TB).
pH: a value <7.0 suggests parapneumonic effusion or empyema; a pleural fluid pH must be drawn anaerobically and iced immediately; the syringe should be prerinsed with 0.2 ml of 1:1000 heparin.
Glucose: a low glucose level suggests parapneumonic effusions and rheumatoid arthritis.
Amylase: a high amylase level suggests pancreatitis or ruptured esophagus.
Perplexing pleural effusions are often a result of malignancy (e.g., lymphoma, malignant mesothelioma, ovarian carcinoma), TB, subdiaphragmatic processes, prior asbestos exposure, and postcardiac injury syndrome.
Box 29 Describes a cellular differential of pleural effusions. Features differentiating exudative from transudative pleural effusion are summarized in Table 81.

BOX 29 Cellular Differential of Pleural Effusions

Neutrophilia (>50%)
Bacterial pneumonia (parapneumonic effusion)
Pulmonary infarction
Pancreatitis
Subphrenic abscess
Early tuberculosis
Transudates (>10%)

Lymphocytosis (>50%)
Tuberculosis
Viral infection
Malignancy (lymphoma, other neoplasms)
True chylothorax
Rheumatoid pleuritis
Systemic lupus erythematosus
Uremic effusions
Transudates (≈30%)

Eosinophilia (>10%)
Pneumothorax (air in pleural space)
Trauma
Pulmonary infarction
Congestive heart failure
Infection (especially parasitic, fungal)
Hypersensitivity syndromes
Drug reaction
Rheumatologic diseases
Hodgkin's disease
Idiopathic

From McPherson RA, Pincus MR: *Henry's clinical diagnosis and management by laboratory methods*, ed 23, St Louis, 2017, Elsevier.

TABLE 81 Features Differentiating Exudative from Transudative Pleural Effusion

Feature	Transudate	Exudate
Appearance	Serous	Cloudy
Leukocyte count	<10,000/mm³	>50,000/mm³
pH	>7.2	<7.2
Protein	<3.0 g/dL	>3.0 g/dL
Ratio of pleural fluid protein to serum	<0.5	>0.5
Lactate dehydrogenase (LDH)	<200 IU/L	>200 IU/L
Ratio of pleural fluid LDH to serum	<0.6	>0.6
Glucose	≥60 mg/dL	<60 mg/dL

From Bennett JE, Dolin R, Blaser MJ: *Mandell, Douglas, and Bennett's principles and practice of infectious diseases*, ed 8, Philadelphia, 2015, Saunders.

POTASSIUM (serum)

Normal range: 3.5-5 mEq/L (3.5-5 mmol/L [CF: 1; SMI: 0.1 mmol/L])

CAUSES OF HYPERKALEMIA

See Fig. E44 for evaluation and treatment of hyperkalemia, and Fig. E45 for electrocardiographic changes in hyperkalemia.

Pseudohyperkalemia
- Hemolysis of sample
- Thrombocytosis
- Leukocytosis
- Laboratory error

Increased potassium intake and absorption
- Potassium supplements (oral and parenteral)
- Dietary: salt substitutes
- Stored blood
- Potassium-containing medications

Impaired renal excretion
- Acute renal failure
- Chronic renal failure
- Tubular defect in potassium secretion
  1. Renal allograft
  2. Analgesic nephropathy
  3. Sickle cell disease
  4. Obstructive uropathy
- Hypoaldosteronism
  - Primary (Addison disease)
  - Secondary
    - Hyporeninemic hypoaldosteronism (type IV RTA)
    - Congenital adrenal hyperplasia
    - Drug-induced
      - NSAIDs
      - ACE inhibitors
      - Heparin
      - Cyclosporine
- Transcellular shifts
  - Acidosis
  - Hypertonicity
  - Insulin deficiency
  - Drugs
    - β-blockers
    - Digitalis toxicity
    - Succinylcholine
  - Exercise
  - Hyperkalemic periodic paralysis
- Cellular injury
  - Rhabdomyolysis
  - Severe intravascular hemolysis
  - Acute tumor lysis syndrome
  - Burns and crush injuries

CAUSES OF HYPOKALEMIA

For the clinical approach to hypokalemia, see Fig. 46.

- Decreased intake
  - Decreased dietary potassium
  - Impaired absorption of potassium
  - Clay ingestion
  - Kayexalate
- Increased loss
  - Renal
    - Hyperaldosteronism
      - Primary
        - (1) Conn syndrome
        - (2) Adrenal hyperplasia
      - Secondary
        - (1) Congestive heart failure
        - (2) Cirrhosis
        - (3) Nephrotic syndrome
        - (4) Dehydration
      - Bartter syndrome
    - Glycyrrhizic acid (licorice, chewing tobacco)
    - Excessive adrenal corticosteroids
      - a. Cushing's syndrome
      - b. Steroid therapy
      - c. Adrenogenital syndrome
    - Renal tubular defects
      - a. Renal tubular acidosis
      - b. Obstructive uropathy
      - c. Salt-wasting nephropathy
  - Drugs
    - a. Diuretics
    - b. Aminoglycosides
    - c. Mannitol
    - d. Amphotericin
    - e. Cisplatin
    - f. Carbenicillin
  - Gastrointestinal
    1. Vomiting
    2. Nasogastric suction
    3. Diarrhea
    4. Malabsorption
    5. Ileostomy
    6. Villous adenoma
    7. Laxative abuse
  - Increased losses from the skin
    1. Excessive sweating
    2. Burns
  - Transcellular shifts
    - A. Alkalosis
      1. Vomiting
      2. Diuretics
      3. Hyperventilation
      4. Bicarbonate therapy
    - B. Insulin
      1. Exogenous
      2. Endogenous response to glucose
    - C. β_2-Agonists (albuterol, terbutaline, epinephrine)
    - D. Hypokalemia periodic paralysis
      1. Familial
      2. Thyrotoxic
- Miscellaneous
  - A. Anabolic state
  - B. Intravenous hyperalimentation
  - C. Treatment of megaloblastic anemia
  - D. Acute mountain sickness

POTASSIUM, URINE

See URINE POTASSIUM

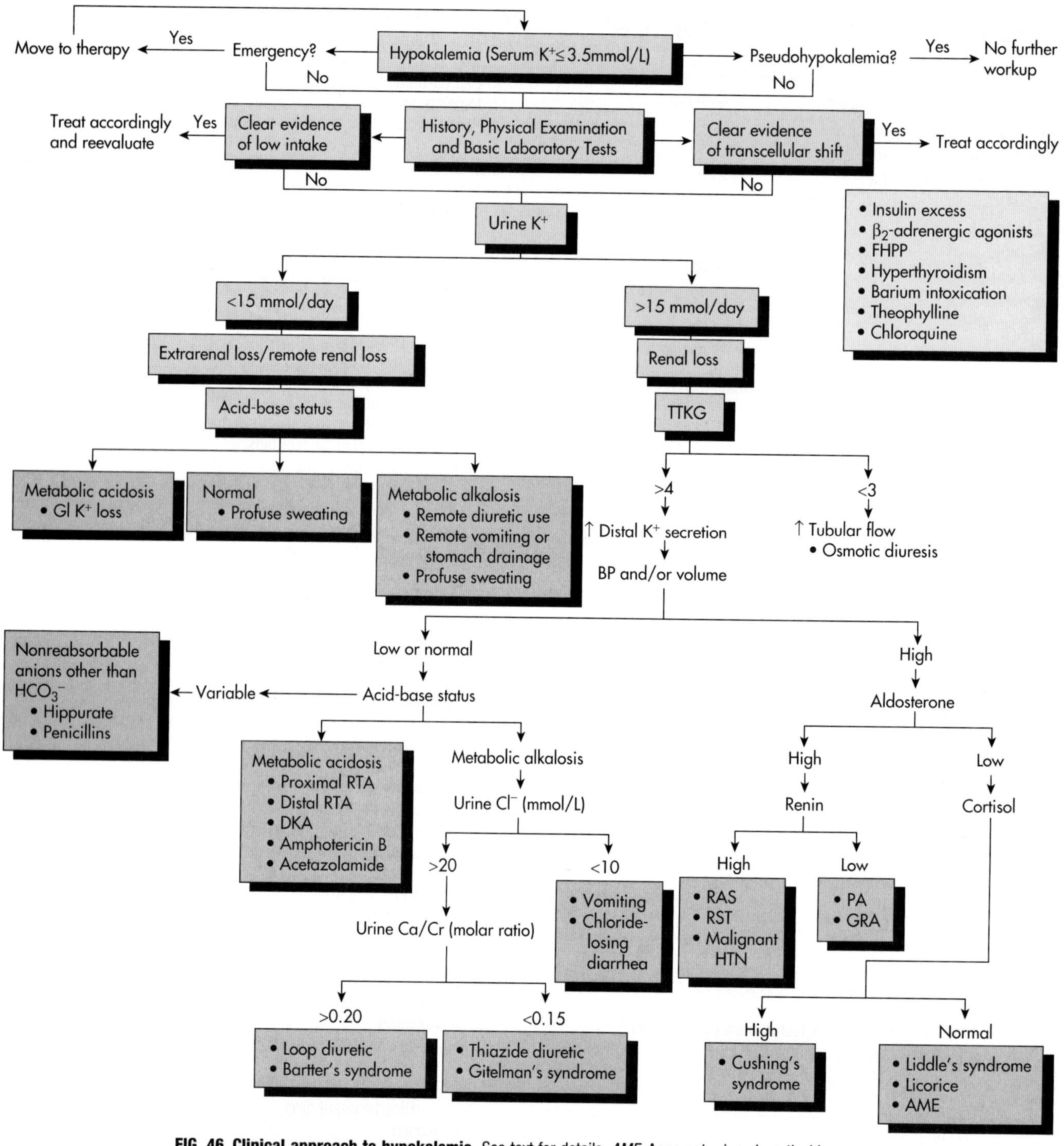

Move to therapy
Yes
Emergency?
No
Hypokalemia (Serum K⁺≤3.5mmol/L)
Pseudohypokalemia?
Yes
No further workup
No
Treat accordingly and reevaluate
Yes
Clear evidence of low intake
History, Physical Examination and Basic Laboratory Tests
Clear evidence of transcellular shift
Yes
Treat accordingly
No
No
- Insulin excess
- β_2-adrenergic agonists
- FHPP
- Hyperthyroidism
- Barium intoxication
- Theophylline
- Chloroquine

Urine K^+
<15 mmol/day
Extrarenal loss/remote renal loss
Acid-base status
Metabolic acidosis
- GI K^+ loss

Normal
- Profuse sweating

Metabolic alkalosis
- Remote diuretic use
- Remote vomiting or stomach drainage
- Profuse sweating

>15 mmol/day
Renal loss
TTKG
>4
↑ Distal K^+ secretion
BP and/or volume
<3
↑ Tubular flow
- Osmotic diuresis

Low or normal
Acid-base status
Variable
Nonreabsorbable anions other than HCO_3^-
- Hippurate
- Penicillins

Metabolic acidosis
- Proximal RTA
- Distal RTA
- DKA
- Amphotericin B
- Acetazolamide

Metabolic alkalosis
Urine Cl^- (mmol/L)
>20
Urine Ca/Cr (molar ratio)
>0.20
- Loop diuretic
- Bartter's syndrome

<0.15
- Thiazide diuretic
- Gitelman's syndrome

<10
- Vomiting
- Chloride-losing diarrhea

High
Aldosterone
High
Renin
High
- RAS
- RST
- Malignant HTN

Low
- PA
- GRA

Low
Cortisol
High
- Cushing's syndrome

Normal
- Liddle's syndrome
- Licorice
- AME

FIG. 46 Clinical approach to hypokalemia. See text for details. *AME*, Apparent mineralocorticoid excess; *BP*, blood pressure; *CCD*, cortical collecting duct; *DKA*, diabetic ketoacidosis; *FHPP*, familial hypokalemic periodic paralysis; *GI*, gastrointestinal; *GRA*, glucocorticoid-remediable aldosteronism; *HTN*, hypertension; *PA*, primary aldosteronism; *RAS*, renal artery stenosis; *RST*, renin-secreting tumor; *RTA*, renal tubular acidosis; *TTKG*, transtubular potassium gradient. (From Skorecki K, Chertow GM, Marsden PA et al: *Brenner & Rector's the kidney*, ed 10, Philadelphia, 2016, Elsevier.)

PROCAINAMIDE

Normal therapeutic range: 4-10 mcg/ml

PROGESTERONE (serum)

Normal:

Female: Follicular phase: 15-70 ng/dl
Luteal phase: 200-2500 ng/dl
Male: 15-70 ng/dl

Elevated in: Congenital adrenal hyperplasia, clomiphene, corticosterone, 11-deoxycortisol, dihydroprogesterone, molar pregnancy, lipoid ovarian tumor
Decreased in: Primary or secondary hypogonadism, oral contraceptives, ampicillin, threatened abortion

PROLACTIN

See Fig. E47 for the evaluation of hyperprolactinemia.
Normal range: <20 ng/ml (<20 μg/L [CF: 1; SMI: 1 μg/L])

Elevated in: Prolactinomas (level >200 micrograms/L highly suggestive), drugs (phenothiazines, cimetidine, tricyclic antidepressants, metoclopramide, estrogens, antihypertensives [methyldopa], verapamil, haloperidol), postpartum, stress, hypoglycemia, hypothyroidism, chronic liver disease, end-stage renal disease, brain radiation therapy, polycystic ovary syndrome, seizures, exercise, coitus, lactation. Mild hyperprolactinemia (<100 micrograms/L) can also be caused by large sellar masses, including nonfunctioning pituitary adenoma.

PROSTATE-SPECIFIC ANTIGEN (PSA)

Normal range: 0-4 ng/ml

Table 82 describes age-specific reference ranges for PSA.

Elevated in: Benign prostatic hypertrophy, carcinoma of prostate, prostatitis, postrectal examination, prostate trauma.

Factors affecting serum PSA are described in Table 83.

NOTE: Measurement of free PSA is useful to assess the probability of prostate cancer in patients with normal digital rectal examination and total PSA between 4 and 10 ng/ml. In these patients, the global risk of prostate cancer is 25%; however, if the free PSA is >25%, the risk of prostate cancer decreases to 8%, whereas if the free PSA is <10%, the risk of cancer increases to 56%. Free PSA is also useful to evaluate the aggressiveness of prostate cancer. A low free PSA percentage generally indicates a high-grade cancer, whereas a high free PSA percentage is generally associated with a slower-growing tumor.

Decreased in: 5-α reductase inhibitors (finasteride, dutasteride), saw palmetto use, antiandrogens

PROSTATIC ACID PHOSPHATASE

Normal: 0-0.8 U/L

Elevated in: Prostate cancer (especially in metastatic prostate cancer), BPH, prostatitis, post-prostate surgery or manipulation, hemolysis, androgens, clofibrate

Decreased in: Ketoconazole

TABLE 82 Age-Specific Reference Ranges for PSA

	SERUM PSA (NG/ML)		
Age (yr)	**Whites**	**Japanese**	**African Americans**
40-49	0-2.5	0-2.0	0-2.0
50-59	0-3.5	0-3.0	0-4.0
60-69	0-4.5	0-4.0	0-4.5
70-79	0-6.5	0-5.0	0-5.5

PSA, Prostate-specific antigen.
From Nseyo UO (ed): *Urology for primary care physicians,* Philadelphia, 1999, Saunders.

TABLE 83 Factors Affecting Serum PSA

Factors Affecting Serum PSA	Duration of Effect
Prostate cell number	NA
Prostate size	NA
Recent ejaculation	6-48 hours
Prostate manipulation	
Vigorous massage	1 week
Cystoscopy	1 week
Prostate biopsy	4-6 weeks
Prostatitis	
Acute	3-6 months
Chronic	Unknown
Prostate cancer	NA
Drugs: finasteride*	3-6 months

NA, Not applicable; *PSA,* prostate-specific antigen.
*Lowers PSA for as long as patient is on the medication.
From Nseyo UO (ed): *Urology for primary care physicians,* Philadelphia, 1999, Saunders.

PROTEIN (serum)

Normal range: 6-8 g/dl (60-80 g/L [CF: 10; SMI: 1 g/L])

Elevated in: Dehydration, multiple myeloma, Waldenström's macroglobulinemia, sarcoidosis, collagen vascular diseases

Decreased in: Malnutrition, low-protein diet, overhydration, malabsorption, pregnancy, severe burns, neoplasms, chronic diseases, cirrhosis, nephrosis

PROTEIN C ASSAY

See Table 84.

Normal: 70%-140%

Elevated in: Oral contraceptives, stanozolol

Decreased in: Congenital protein C deficiency, warfarin therapy, Vitamin K deficiency, renal insufficiency, consumptive coagulopathies

PROTEIN ELECTROPHORESIS (serum)

Normal range:

Albumin: 60%-75% (0.6-0.75 [CF: 0.01; SMI: 0.01])
- α-1: 1.7%-5% (0.02-0.05)
- α-2: 6.7%-12.5% (0.07-0.13)
- β: 8.3%-16.3% (0.08-0.16)
- γ: 10.7%-20% (0.11-0.2)

Albumin: 3.6-5.2 g/dl (36-52 g/L [CF: 0.01; SMI: 1 g/L])
- α-1: 0.1-0.4 g/dl (1-4 g/L)
- α-2: 0.4-1 g/dl (4-10 g/L)
- β: 0.5-1.2 g/dl (5-12 g/L)
- γ: 0.6-1.6 g/dl (6-16 g/L)

Elevated in:

Albumin: dehydration
α-1: neoplastic diseases, inflammation
α-2: neoplasms, inflammation, infection, nephrotic syndrome
β: hypothyroidism, biliary cirrhosis, diabetes mellitus
γ: See IMMUNOGLOBULINS

Decreased in:

Albumin: malnutrition, chronic liver disease, malabsorption, nephrotic syndrome, burns, systemic lupus erythematosus
α-1: emphysema (α-1 antitrypsin deficiency), nephrosis
α-2: hemolytic anemias (decreased haptoglobin), severe hepatocellular damage
β: hypocholesterolemia, nephrosis
γ: See IMMUNOGLOBULINS

Fig. 48 describes serum protein electrophoretic patterns.

PROTEIN S ASSAY

See Table 85.

Normal: 65%-140%

Elevated in: Presence of lupus anticoagulant

Decreased in: Hereditary deficiency, acute thrombotic events, DIC, surgery, oral contraceptives, pregnancy, hormone replacement therapy, l-asparaginase treatment

PROTHROMBIN TIME (PT)

See Table 86.

Normal range: 10-12 sec

Elevated in: Liver disease, oral anticoagulants (warfarin), heparin, factor deficiency (I, II, V, VII, X), disseminated intravascular coagula-

TABLE 84 Assay Measurement in Heterozygote Protein C Deficiency

	ACTIVITY		
Type	**Antigen**	**Amidolytic**	**Coagulant**
I	Low	Low	Low
II	Normal	Low	Low
	Normal	Normal	Low

From Hoffman R et al: *Hematology: basic principles and practice,* ed 5, Philadelphia, 2009, Churchill Livingstone.

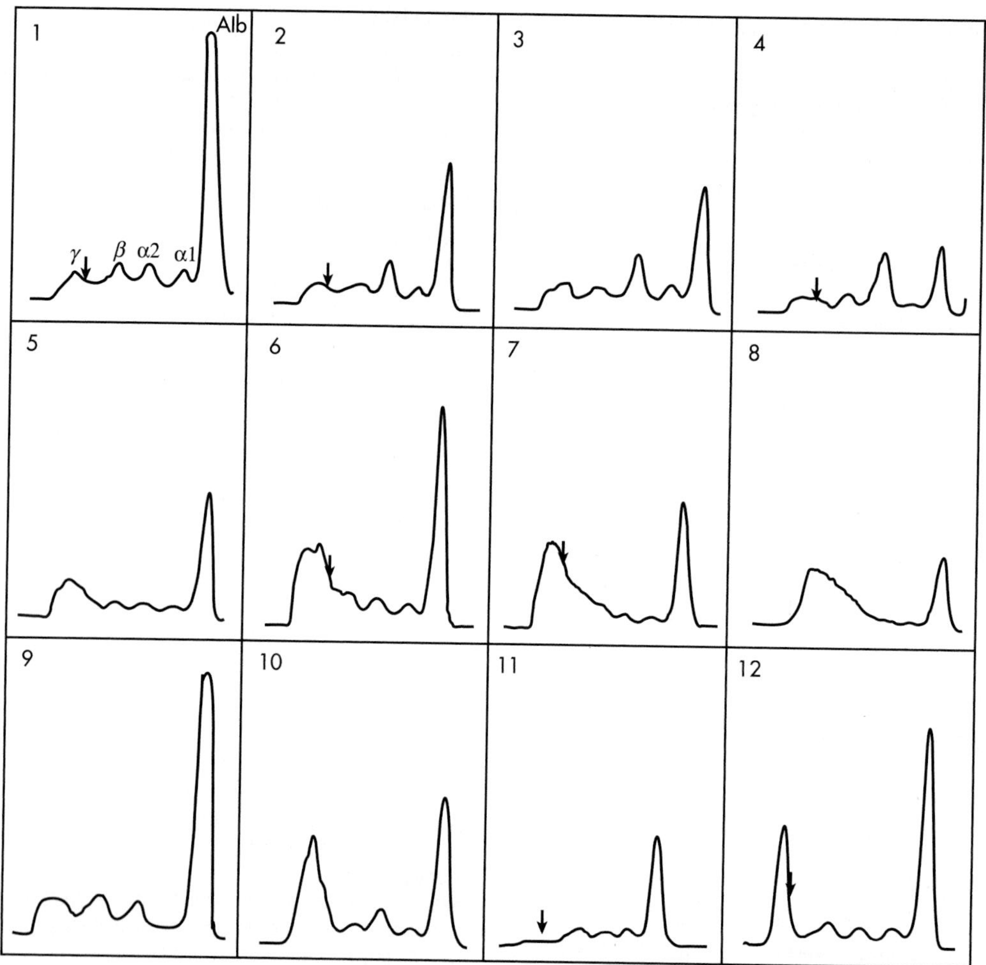

FIG. 48 Typical serum protein electrophoretic patterns. ***1,*** Normal (*arrow* near γ region indicates serum application point). ***2,*** Acute reaction pattern. ***3,*** Acute reaction or nephrotic syndrome. ***4,*** Nephrotic syndrome. ***5,*** Chronic inflammation, cirrhosis, granulomatous diseases, rheumatoid-collagen group. ***6,*** Same as 5, but γ elevation is more pronounced. There is also partial (but not complete) β-γ fusion. ***7,*** Suggestive of cirrhosis but could be found in the granulomatous diseases or the rheumatoid-collagen group. ***8,*** Characteristic pattern of cirrhosis. ***9,*** α-1 Antitrypsin deficiency with mild γ elevation suggesting concurrent chronic disease. ***10,*** Same as 5, but the γ elevation is marked. The configuration of the γ peak superficially mimics that of myeloma, but is more broad-based. There are superimposed acute reaction changes. ***11,*** Hypogammaglobulinemia or light-chain myeloma. ***12,*** Myeloma, Waldenström's macroglobulinemia, idiopathic or secondary monoclonal gammopathy. (From Ravel R [ed]: *Clinical laboratory medicine,* ed 6, St Louis, 1995, Mosby.)

TABLE 85 Assay Measurements in Heterozygote Protein S Deficiency

	ACTIVITY		
Type	**Protein S Total Antigen**	**Protein S Free Antigen**	**Protein S Activity**
I (classic)	Low	Low	Low
II	Normal	Normal	Low
III	Normal	Low	Low

From Hoffman R et al: *Hematology: basic principles and practice,* ed 5, Philadelphia, 2009, Churchill Livingstone.

tion, vitamin K deficiency, afibrinogenemia, dysfibrinogenemia, drugs (salicylate, chloral hydrate, diphenylhydantoin, estrogens, antacids, phenylbutazone, quinidine, antibiotics, allopurinol, anabolic steroids). Table 87 describes a differential diagnosis of abnormal coagulation screening tests.

Decreased in: Vitamin K supplementation, thrombophlebitis, drugs (glutethimide, estrogens, griseofulvin, diphenhydramine)

PROTOPORPHYRIN (Free erythrocyte)

Normal range: 16-36 μg/dl of red blood cells (0.28-0.64 μmol/L [CF: 0.0177; SMI: 0.02 μmol/L])
Elevated in: Iron deficiency, lead poisoning, sideroblastic anemias, anemia of chronic disease, hemolytic anemias, erythropoietic protoporphyria

PSA

See PROSTATE-SPECIFIC ANTIGEN

PT

See PROTHROMBIN TIME

PTH

See PARATHYROID HORMONE

PTT

See PARTIAL THROMBOPLASTIN TIME

TABLE 86 Causes of Increased Prothrombin Time/International Normalized Ratio (PT/INR) and/or Activated Partial Prothrombin Time (APTT)

Increased PT/INR—Defect in Extrinsic Pathway

Deficiency or inhibitor of factor VII

Early warfarin (Coumadin) therapy

Early liver disease

Increased APTT—Defect in Intrinsic Pathway

Deficiency or inhibitor of factors XII, XI, IX, or VIII

Heparin (though usually affects PT as well)

Liver disease (though usually affects PT as well)

Lupus anticoagulant (may affect PT as well)

Increased PT/INR and APTT—Defect in Common Pathway or Combined Defect in Extrinsic and Intrinsic Pathways

Heparin (all serine proteases affected, especially II and X)

Disseminated intravascular coagulation (all factors, including pro- and anticoagulants, affected)

Liver disease (all factors except VIII affected)

Warfarin (factors II, VII, IX, and X affected)

Vitamin K deficiency (factors II, VII, IX, and X affected)

Direct thrombin inhibitors

Lupus anticoagulant

Modified from: Rizoli S, Aird WC. Coagulopathy. In Vincent JL, Abraham E, Moore FA et al (eds): *Textbook of critical care*. ed 6, Philadelphia, 2011, Elsevier.

TABLE 87 Differential Diagnosis of Abnormal Coagulation Screening Tests

Abnormal Activated Partial Thromboplastin Time (APTT) Alone

Associated with bleeding: VIII, IX, and XI defects

Not associated with bleeding: XII, prekallikrein (PK), high molecular weight kininogen, lupus anticoagulants

Abnormal Prothrombin Time (PT) Alone

Factor VII defects

Combined Abnormal APTT and PT

Medical conditions: Anticoagulants, disseminated intravascular coagulation (DIC), liver disease, vitamin K deficiency, massive transfusion

Rarely dysfibrinogenemia; factor X, V, and II defects

From McPherson RA, Pincus MR: *Henry's clinical diagnosis and management by laboratory methods*, ed 23, St Louis, 2017, Elsevier.

RAPID PLASMA REAGIN (RPR)

Description: Non-treponemal test traditionally used as a screening test for syphilis. It is a quantitative test and antibody titers can be monitored to assess treatment response.
Normal: Negative
Positive: Syphilis. False-positive results may occur with pregnancy, autoimmune diseases, tuberculosis, and other inflammatory conditions. Positive results should be confirmed with treponemal serologic tests (e.g., T-pallidum enzyme immunoassay [TP-EIA])

RDW

See RED BLOOD CELL DISTRIBUTION WIDTH

RED BLOOD CELL (RBC) COUNT

Normal range:
Male: 4.3-5.9 × 10^6/mm^3 (4.3-5.9 × 10^{12}/L [CF: 1; SMI: 0.1 × 10^{12}/L])
Female: 3.5-5 × 10^6/mm^3 (3.5-5 × 10^{12}/L [CF: 1; SMI: 0.1 × 10^{12}/L])

TABLE 88 Combining the Reticulocyte Count and Red Blood Cell Parameters for Diagnosis

MCV, RDW	Reticulocyte Count <100,000/µL	Reticulocyte Count ≥100,000/µL
Low, normal	Anemia of chronic disease	
Normal, normal	Anemia of chronic disease	
High, normal	Chemotherapy, antivirals, or alcohol Aplastic anemia	Chronic liver disease
Low, high	Iron-deficiency anemia	Sickle cell-β–thalassemia
Normal, high	Early iron, folate, vitamin B_{12} deficiency Myelodysplasia	Sickle cell anemia, sickle cell disease
High, high	Folate or vitamin B_{12} deficiency	Immune hemolytic anemia
	Myelodysplasia	Chronic liver disease

MCV, Mean corpuscular volume; *RDW,* red blood cell distribution width.
From Hoffman R: *Hematology, basic principles and practice*, ed 7, Philadelphia, 2018, Elsevier.

Elevated in: Polycythemia vera, smokers, high altitude, cardiovascular disease, renal cell carcinoma and other erythropoietin-producing neoplasms, stress, hemoconcentration/dehydration
Decreased in: Anemias, hemolysis, chronic renal failure, hemorrhage, failure of marrow production

RED BLOOD CELL DISTRIBUTION WIDTH (RDW)

Measures variability of red cell size (anisocytosis)
Normal range: 11.5-14.5
Normal RDW and elevated mean corpuscular volume (MCV): Aplastic anemia, preleukemia
Normal MCV: Normal, anemia of chronic disease, acute blood loss or hemolysis, chronic lymphocytic leukemia (CLL), chronic myelocytic leukemia, nonanemic enzymopathy or hemoglobinopathy
Decreased MCV: Anemia of chronic disease, heterozygous thalassemia
Elevated RDW and elevated MCV: Vitamin B_{12} deficiency, folate deficiency, immune hemolytic anemia, cold agglutinins, CLL with high count, liver disease
Normal MCV: Early iron deficiency, early vitamin B_{12} deficiency, early folate deficiency, anemic globinopathy
Decreased MCV: Iron deficiency, red blood cell fragmentation, HbH disease, thalassemia intermedia

See Table 88 for combining the reticulocyte count and RBC parameters for diagnosis.

RED BLOOD CELL FOLATE

See FOLATE

RED BLOOD CELL MASS (volume)

Normal range:
Male: 20-36 ml/kg body weight (1.15-1.21 L/m^2 body surface area)
Female: 19-31 ml/kg body weight (0.95-1.00 L/m^2 body surface area)
Elevated in: Polycythemia vera, hypoxia (smokers, high altitude, cardiovascular disease), hemoglobinopathies with high oxygen affinity, erythropoietin-producing tumors (renal cell carcinoma)
Decreased in: Hemorrhage, chronic disease, failure of marrow production, anemias, hemolysis

RED BLOOD CELL MORPHOLOGY

Table 89 describes features of the peripheral blood smear. Table 90 summarizes peripheral blood film evaluation in a patient with red cell membrane disorder. See Fig. 49 for useful peripheral blood and RBC features in the evaluation of anemia.

RENIN (serum)

Elevated in: Drugs (thiazides, estrogen, minoxidil), chronic renal failure, Bartter syndrome, pregnancy (normal), pheochromocytoma, renal hypertension, reduced plasma volume, secondary aldosteronism

TABLE 89 Features of the Peripheral Blood Smear

Red Blood Cell Morphology	Definition	Interpretation
Polychromasia	Large, bluish RBCs lacking normal central pallor on peripheral blood smear; bluish stain is the result of residual ribonucleic acid	Rapid production and release of RBCs from BM; elevated reticulocyte count; most commonly seen in any hemolytic anemia and states of increased RBC turnover
Basophilic stippling	Many small bluish dots in portion of erythrocytes; comes from staining of clustered polyribosomes in young circulating RBCs	Seen in a variety of erythropoietic disorders, including acquired (e.g., myelodysplasia) and congenital hemolytic anemias and occasionally in lead poisoning
Pappenheimer bodies	Several grayish, irregularly shaped inclusions in a portion of erythrocytes visible on peripheral smear; composed of aggregates of ribosomes, ferritin, and mitochondria	Erythropoietic malfunction in congenital anemias such as hemoglobinopathies, particularly with splenic hypofunction or acquired anemias such as megaloblastic anemia
Heinz bodies	Several grayish, round inclusions visible after supravital staining with methyl crystal violet of the peripheral blood smear, often in the context of bite cells; represent aggregates of denatured hemoglobin	Indicative of oxidative injury to the erythrocyte, such as occurs in G6PD deficiency and other RBC enzymopathies or unstable hemoglobins
Howell-Jolly bodies	Usually one or at most a few purplish inclusions in the erythrocyte visible on the routine peripheral blood smear; represent residual fragments of nuclei containing chromatin	Associated with states of splenic hypofunction, splenic atrophy, splenic thrombosis, or after splenectomy
Schistocytes	RBCs that are fragmented into a variety of shapes and sizes, including helmet-shaped cells; indicative of shearing of the erythrocyte within the circulation	Associated with microangiopathic hemolytic anemias, including DIC, TTP, HUS, or aHUS, as well as other mechanical causes of hemolysis, such as prosthetic heart valves or severe cardiac valvular stenosis
Spherocytes	RBCs that have lost their central pallor and appear spherical; indicative of loss of cytoskeletal integrity from internal or external causes	Associated with hereditary spherocytosis, autoimmune hemolytic anemia; may also be observed in addition to schistocytes in the presence of microangiopathic hemolytic anemia
Teardrop cells	Pear-shaped erythrocytes visible on peripheral blood smear; indicative of mechanical stress on the RBC during release from the BM or passage through the spleen	Seen in a variety of conditions along with other poikilocytes, including severe iron deficiency anemia, congenital anemias such as thalassemias, hemoglobinopathies, and acquired disorders such as megaloblastic anemia. As isolated poikilocyte, teardrop RBCs may be initial changes of myelophthisis (BM replacement or infiltration), e.g., myelodysplastic syndrome or myelofibrosis.
Burr cells (echinocytes)	RBCs that have smooth undulations present on the surface circumferentially; pathogenesis unknown	Indicative of uremia when present on a properly made peripheral blood smear
Spur cells (acanthocytes)	RBCs that have spiny points present on the surface circumferentially; reflective of abnormal lipid composition of RBC membrane	Most commonly indicative of hemolytic anemia of advanced liver disease when present in significant numbers; also seen in abetalipoproteinemia and in RBCs lacking the Kell blood group antigen

aHUS, Atypical hemolytic uremic syndrome; *BM,* bone marrow; *DIC,* disseminated intravascular coagulation; *G6PD,* glucose-6-phosphate dehydrogenase; *HUS,* hemolytic uremic syndrome; *RBC,* red blood cell; *TTP,* thrombotic thrombocytopenic purpura.
From Hoffman R: *Hematology, basic principles and practice,* ed 7, Philadelphia, 2018, Elsevier.

TABLE 90 Peripheral Blood Film Evaluation in a Patient with Red Cell Membrane Disorder

Shape	Pathobiology	Diagnosis
Microspherocytes	Loss of membrane lipids leading to a reduction of surface area resulting from deficiencies of spectrin, ankyrin, or band 3 and protein 4.2; removal of membrane material from antibody-coated red cells by macrophages; removal of membrane-associated Heinz bodies, with the adjacent membrane lipids, by the spleen	HS Immunohemolytic anemias; Heinz body hemolytic anemias
Elliptocytes	Permanent red cell deformation resulting from a weakening of skeletal protein interactions (such as the spectrin dimer-dimer contact). This facilitates disruption of existing protein contacts during shear stress–induced elliptical deformation. Subsequently, new protein contacts are formed that stabilize elliptical shape; unknown	Mild common HE; iron deficiency, megaloblastic anemias, myelofibrosis, myelophthisic anemias, myelodysplastic syndrome, thalassemias
Poikilocytes/ Fragments	Weakening of skeletal protein contacts resulting from skeletal protein mutations; unknown	Hemolytic HE/HPP; iron deficiency, megaloblastic anemias, myelofibrosis, myelophthisic anemias, myelodysplastic syndrome, thalassemias
Schistocytes, fragmented red cells	Red cells "torn" by mechanical trauma (fibrin strands, turbulent flow)	"Microangiopathic" hemolytic anemia associated with disseminated intravascular coagulation, thrombotic thrombocytopenic purpura, vasculitis, heart valve prostheses
Acanthocytes	Uptake of cholesterol and its preferential accumulation in the outer leaflet of the lipid bilayer; selective accumulation of sphingomyelin in the outer lipid leaflet; unknown	Spur cell hemolytic anemia in severe liver disease; abetalipoproteinemia; chorea-acanthocytosis syndrome, malnutrition, hypothyroidism; McLeod phenotype
Echinocytes	Expansion of the surface area of the outer hemileaflet of lipid bilayer relative to the inner hemileaflet; unknown	Hemolytic anemia associated with hypomagnesemia and hypophosphatemia in malnourished patients, pyruvate kinase deficiency; in vitro artifact of low blood storage (ATP depletion), contact with glass or elevated pH Hemolysis in long-distance runners, renal failure
Stomatocytes	Expansion of the surface area of the inner hemileaflet of the bilayer relative to the outer leaflet; unknown	Exposure of red cells to cationic anesthetics in vitro; in vivo the drug concentrations may not be sufficient to produce similar effect; alcoholism, inherited disorders of membrane permeability (hereditary stomatocytosis)
Target cells	Absolute excess of membrane lipids (both cholesterol and phospholipids: "symmetric" lipid gain), followed by an increase of cell surface area; relative excess of surface area because of a decrease in cell volume	Obstructive jaundice, liver disease with intrahepatic cholestasis; thalassemias and some hemoglobinopathies (C, D, E)

ATP, Adenosine triphosphate; *HE,* hereditary elliptocytosis; *HPP,* hereditary pyropoikilocytosis; *HS,* hereditary spherocytosis.
From Hoffman R et al: *Hematology, basic principles and practice,* ed 7, Philadelphia, 2018, Saunders.

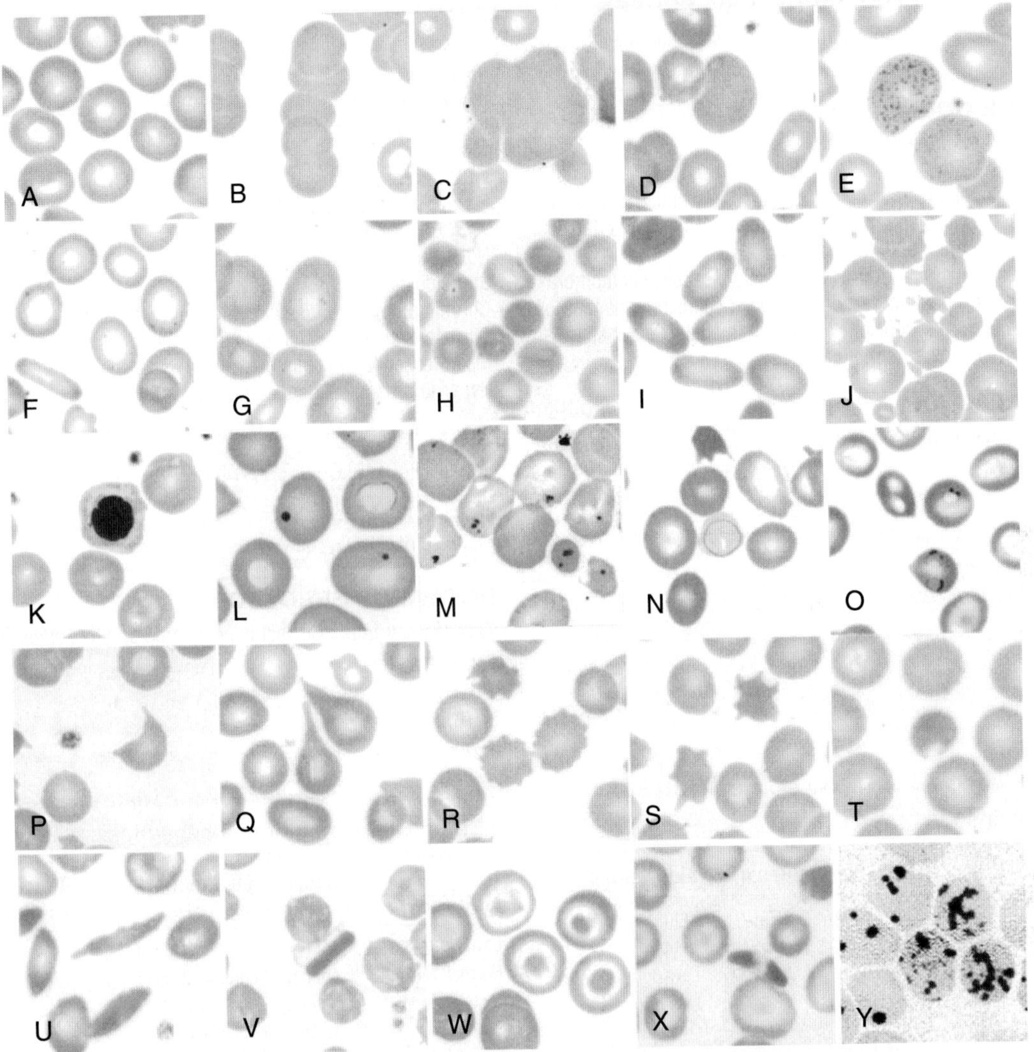

FIG. 49 Useful peripheral blood and red blood cell features in the evaluation of anemia. A, Normal red blood cells (RBCs). Note that the central pallor is one-third the diameter of the entire cell. **B,** Rouleaux formation is indicative of increased plasma protein. **C,** Agglutination indicates an antibody-mediated process such as cold agglutinin disease. **D,** Polychromatophilic cell. The gray-blue color is attributable to RNA and the cell is equivalent to a reticulocyte, which must be identified with a reticulocyte stain. **E,** Basophilic stippling. This also is attributable to increased RNA caused either by a left shift in erythroid cells or lead toxicity. **F,** Hypochromic microcytic cells typical of iron-deficiency anemia. Note the widened central pallor and the "pencil" cell in the *lower left.* **G,** Macroovalocyte as can be seen in either megaloblastic anemia or myelodysplastic syndrome. **H,** Microspherocytes typical of hereditary spherocytosis. **I,** Elliptocytes (ovalocytes) from a patient with hereditary elliptocytosis. **J,** RBC fragments from thermal injury (burn patient). **K,** Nucleated RBC. **L,** Howell-Jolly bodies indicative of splenic dysfunction or absence. **M,** Pappenheimer bodies from a patient with sideroblastic anemia. **N,** Cabot ring, as can be seen in megaloblastic anemia or MDS. **O,** Malarial parasites *(Plasmodium falciparum).* **P,** Schistocyte typical of a microangiopathic hemolytic anemia. **Q,** Tear-drop form indicates marrow fibrosis and extramedullary hematopoiesis. **R,** Echinocyte (Burr cell) with rounded edges. **S,** Acanthocyte (spur cell) with more irregular pointed ends. This was from a patient with neuroacanthocytosis. They can also be seen in patients with liver disease and lipid abnormalities. **T,** "Bite" cell from a patient with glucose-6-phosphate dehydrogenase (G6PD) deficiency. **U,** Sickle cell, from a patient with homozygous sickle cell disease. **V,** Hemoglobin C crystal. **W,** Target cells. **X,** Hemoglobin C disease. Note that the RBC in center has condensed hemoglobin at each pole. **Y,** Heinz body preparation (supravital stain) from a patient with G6PD deficiency. Note that the cells to the right have increased precipitated hemoglobin. From Hoffman R: *Hematology, basic principles and practice*, ed 7, Philadelphia, 2018, Elsevier.

Decreased in: Adrenocortical hypertension, increased plasma volume, primary aldosteronism, drugs (propranolol, reserpine, clonidine)

Table 91 describes typical renin-aldosterone patterns in various conditions.

RESPIRATORY SYNCYTIAL VIRUS (RSV) SCREEN

Test description: PCR test can be performed on nasopharyngeal swab, wash, or aspirate

RETICULOCYTE COUNT

See Fig. E50, Fig. 51, and Table 92.

Normal range: 0.5%-1.5%

Elevated in: Hemolytic anemia (sickle cell crisis, thalassemia major, autoimmune hemolysis), hemorrhage, postanemia therapy (folic acid, ferrous sulfate, vitamin B_{12}), chronic renal failure

Decreased in: Aplastic anemia, marrow suppression (sepsis, chemotherapeutic agents, radiation), hepatic cirrhosis, blood transfusion, anemias of disordered maturation (iron deficiency anemia, megaloblastic anemia, sideroblastic anemia, anemia of chronic disease)

RHEUMATOID FACTOR

Normal: Negative. Present in titer >1:20

RHEUMATIC DISEASES

Rheumatoid arthritis
Sjögren syndrome
Systemic lupus erythematosus
Polymyositis/dermatomyositis
Mixed connective tissue disease
Scleroderma

INFECTIOUS DISEASES

Subacute bacterial endocarditis
Tuberculosis
Infectious mononucleosis
Hepatitis
Syphilis
Leprosy
Influenza

MALIGNANCIES

Lymphoma
Multiple myeloma
Waldenström's macroglobulinemia
Postradiation or postchemotherapy

MISCELLANEOUS

Normal adults, especially the elderly
Sarcoidosis
Chronic pulmonary disease (interstitial fibrosis)
Chronic liver disease (chronic active hepatitis, cirrhosis)
Mixed essential cryoglobulinemia
Hypergammaglobulinemic purpura

RNP

See EXTRACTABLE NUCLEAR ANTIGEN

RPR

See RAPID PLASMA REAGIN

ROTAVIRUS SEROLOGY

Test description: PCR test is performed on stool specimen

Normal: Negative

TABLE 91 Typical Renin-Aldosterone Patterns in Various Conditions

	Plasma Renin	Aldosterone
Primary aldosteronism	Low	High
"Low-renin" essential hypertension	Low	Normal
Cushing's syndrome	Low	Low-normal
Licorice ingestion syndrome	Low	Low
High-salt diet	Low	Low
Oral contraceptives	High	Normal
Cirrhosis	High	High
Malignant hypertension	High	High
Unilateral renal disease	High	High
"High-renin" essential hypertension	High	High
Pregnancy	High	High
Diuretic overuse	High	High
Juxtaglomerular tumor (Bartter's syndrome)	High	High
Low-salt diet	High	High
Addison's disease	High	Low
Hypokalemia	High	Low

From Ravel R (ed): *Clinical laboratory medicine,* ed 6, St Louis, 1995, Mosby.

TABLE 92 Combining the Reticulocyte Count and Red Blood Cell Parameters for Diagnosis

MCV, RDW	Reticulocyte Count <75,000/μL	Reticulocyte Count >100,000/μL
Low, Normal	Anemia of chronic disease	
Normal, Normal	Anemia of chronic disease	
High, Normal	Chemotherapy/antivirals/ alcohol Aplastic anemia	Chronic liver disease
Low, High	Iron deficiency anemia	Sickle cell-β-thalassemia
Normal, High	Early iron, folate, vitamin B_{12} deficiency Myelodysplasia	Sickle cell anemia, sickle cell disease
High, High	Folate or vitamin B_{12} deficiency Myelodysplasia	Immune hemolytic anemia Chronic liver disease

MCV, Mean corpuscular volume; *RDW,* red blood cell distribution width.

From Hoffman R et al: *Hematology: basic principles and practice,* ed 5, Philadelphia, 2009, Churchill Livingstone.

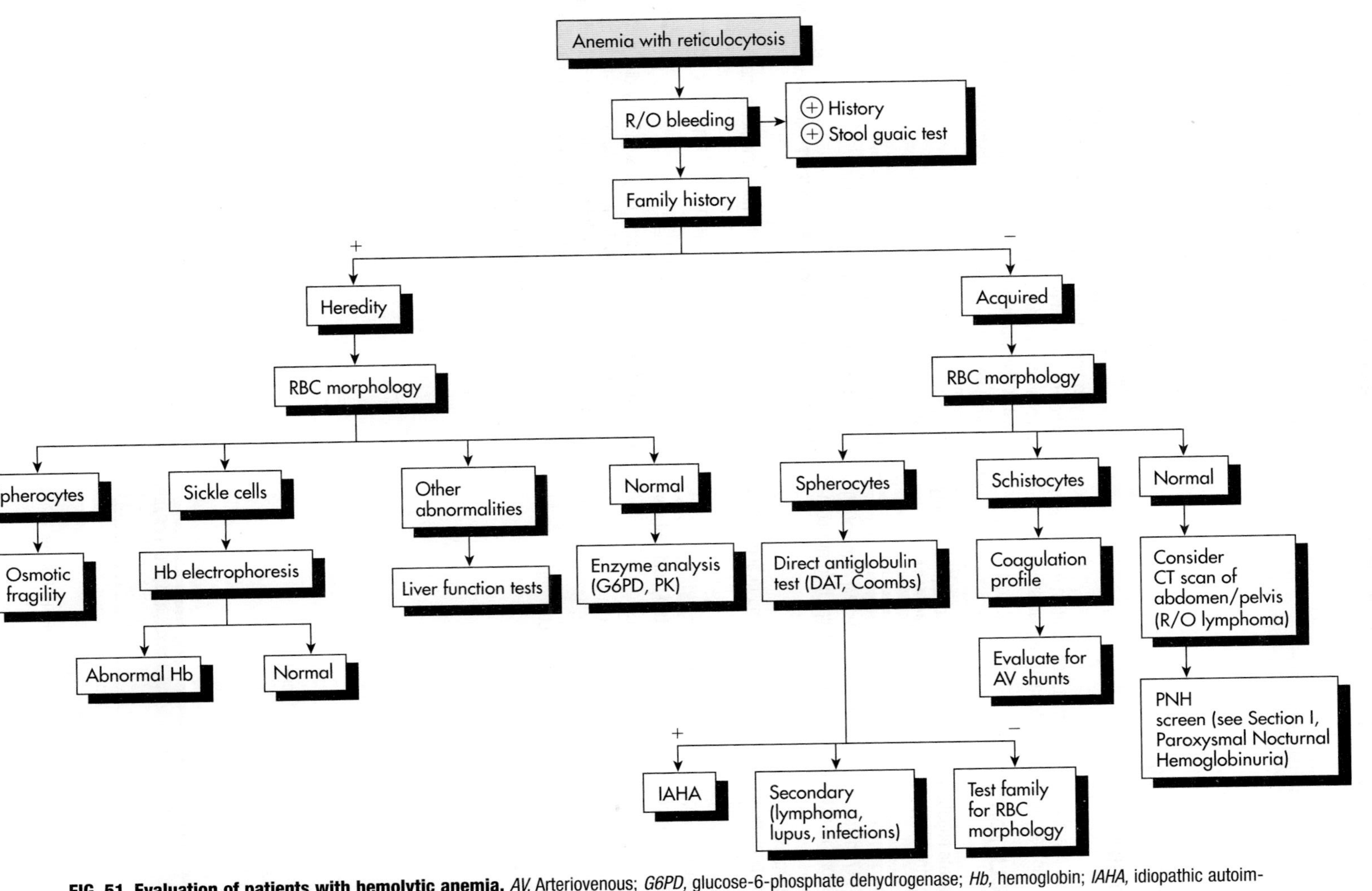

FIG. 51 Evaluation of patients with hemolytic anemia. *AV,* Arteriovenous; *G6PD,* glucose-6-phosphate dehydrogenase; *Hb,* hemoglobin; *IAHA,* idiopathic autoimmune hemolytic anemia; *LS,* liver spleen; *PK,* pyruvate kinase; *PNH,* paroxysmal nocturnal hemoglobinuria; *RBC,* red blood cell; *R/O,* rule out.

SED RATE

See ERYTHROCYTE SEDIMENTATION RATE

SEDIMENTATION RATE

See ERYTHROCYTE SEDIMENTATION RATE

SEMEN ANALYSIS

Table 93 describes semen analysis reference ranges.

SGOT

See ASPARTATE AMINOTRANSFERASE

SGPT

See ASPARTATE AMINOTRANSFERASE

SICKLE CELL TEST

Normal: Negative
Positive in: Sickle cell anemia, sickle cell trait, combination of *Hb S* gene with other disorders such as alpha-thalassemia, beta-thalassemia.

SMOOTH MUSCLE ANTIBODY

Normal: Negative
Present in: Chronic acute hepatitis, primary sclerosing cholangitis, primary biliary cirrhosis, autoimmune hepatitis, infectious mononucleosis

SODIUM (serum)

Normal range: 135-147 mEq/L (135-147 mmol/L [CF: 1; SMI: 1 mmol/L]). Electrolyte concentrations in extracellular and intracellular fluid are summarized in Table 94.

HYPONATREMIA See Fig. 52.

Common causes of hyponatremia and electrolyte patterns in serum and urine with normal renal function are described in Table 95. Table E96 describes drugs associated with hyponatremia.

Sodium and water depletion (deficit hyponatremia)
- Loss of gastrointestinal secretions with replacement of fluid but not electrolytes
  - Vomiting
  - Diarrhea
  - Tube drainage
- Loss from skin with replacement of fluids but not electrolytes
  - Excessive sweating
  - Extensive burns
- Loss from kidney
  - Diuretics
  - Chronic renal insufficiency (uremia) with acidosis
- Metabolic loss
  - Starvation with acidosis
  - Diabetic acidosis
- Endocrine loss
  - Addison's disease
  - Sudden withdrawal of long-term steroid therapy
- Iatrogenic loss from serous cavities
  - Paracentesis or thoracentesis

TABLE 93 Semen Analysis Reference Ranges

Color	Grayish white
pH	7.3-7.8 (literature range, 7.0-7.8)
Volume	2.0-5.0 ml (literature range, 1.5-6.0 ml)
Sperm count	20-250 million/ml (literature range for upper limit varies from 100-250 million/ml)
Motility	>60% motile <3 hours after specimen is obtained (literature range, >40% to >70%)
% Normal sperm	>60% (literature range, >60% to >70%)
Viscosity	Can be poured from a pipet in droplets rather than a thick strand

From Ravel R (ed): *Clinical laboratory medicine,* ed 6, St Louis, 1995, Mosby.

Excessive water (dilution hyponatremia)
- Excessive water administration
- Congestive heart failure
- Cirrhosis
- Nephrotic syndrome
- Hypoalbuminemia (severe)
- Acute renal failure with oliguria

Inappropriate antidiuretic hormone (IADH) syndrome
Intracellular loss (reset osmostat syndrome)
False hyponatremia (actually a dilutional effect)
- Marked hypertriglyceridemia
- Marked hyperproteinemia
- Severe hyperglycemia

HYPERNATREMIA See Fig. 53.

Common causes of hypernatremia and electrolyte patterns in serum and urine with normal renal function are summarized in Table 97.
Dehydration is the most frequent overall clinical finding in hypernatremia.
Deficient water intake (either orally or intravenously)
Excess kidney water output (diabetes insipidus, osmotic diuresis)
Excess skin water output (excess sweating, loss from burns)
Excess gastrointestinal tract output (severe protracted vomiting or diarrhea without fluid therapy)
Accidental sodium overdose
High-protein tube feedings

STREPTOZYME

See ANTISTREPTOLYSIN O TITER

SUCROSE HEMOLYSIS TEST (sugar water test)

Normal: Absence of hemolysis
Positive in: Paroxysmal nocturnal hemoglobinuria
False-positive: autoimmune hemolytic anemia, megaloblastic anemias
False-negative: may occur with use of heparin or EDTA

SUDAN III STAIN (qualitative screening for fecal fat)

Normal: Negative. Test should be preceded by diet containing 100-150 g of dietary fat/day for 1 week, avoidance of high-fiber diet, and avoidance of suppositories or oily material before specimen collection.
Positive in: Steatorrhea, use of castor oil or mineral oil droplets

SYNOVIAL FLUID ANALYSIS

Table 98 describes the classification and interpretation of synovial fluid analysis. An algorithm for analysis of joint fluid is illustrated in Fig. 54.

TABLE 94 Electrolyte Concentrations in Extracellular and Intracellular Fluids

	PLASMA		INTERSTITIAL FLUID		PLASMA WATER		CELL WATER (MUSCLE)	
	(mmol/L)	(mmol/L)	(mmol/L)	(mmol/L)	(mmol/L)	(mmol/L)	(mmol/L)	(mmol/L)
Na^+	140	140	145.3	145.3	149.8	149.8	13	13
K^+	4.5	4.5	4.7	4.7	4.8	4.8	140	140
Ca^{++}	5.0	2.5	2.8	1.4	5.3	5.3	10^{-7}	0.5×10^{-7}
Mg^{++}	1.7	0.85	1.0	0.5	1.8	0.9	7.0	3.5
Cl^-	104	104	114.7	114.7	111.4	111.4	3	3
HCO_3^-	24	24	26.5	26.5	25.7	25.7	10	10
SO_4^{2-}	1.0	0.5	1.2	0.6	1.1	0.55	–	–
P	2.1	1.2^+	2.1^{++}	1.2^+	2.2	1.25^+	107	57^{+++}
Protein	15	1	8	0.5	16	1	40	2.5*
Organic anion	5	5	5.6	5.6	5.3	5.3	–	–

+The calculation is based on the assumption that the pH of the extracellular fluid is 7.4 and the pK of inorganic $H_2PO_4^-$ is 6.8.
++The concentration of P in the interstitial fluid would be increased by the Donnan effect, but reduced by the lower protein-bound phosphate, and these two opposing effects keep interstitial phosphate concentration about equal to that of plasma.
+++The intracellular molal concentration of phosphate is calculated with the assumption that the pK of organic phosphates in the cell is 6.1 and the intracellular pH 7.0.
*The calculation is based on the assumption that each mmol of intracellular protein has an average of 15 mEq.
(From McPherson RA, Pincus MR: *Henry's clinical diagnosis and management by laboratory methods*, ed 23, St Louis, 2017, Elsevier.)

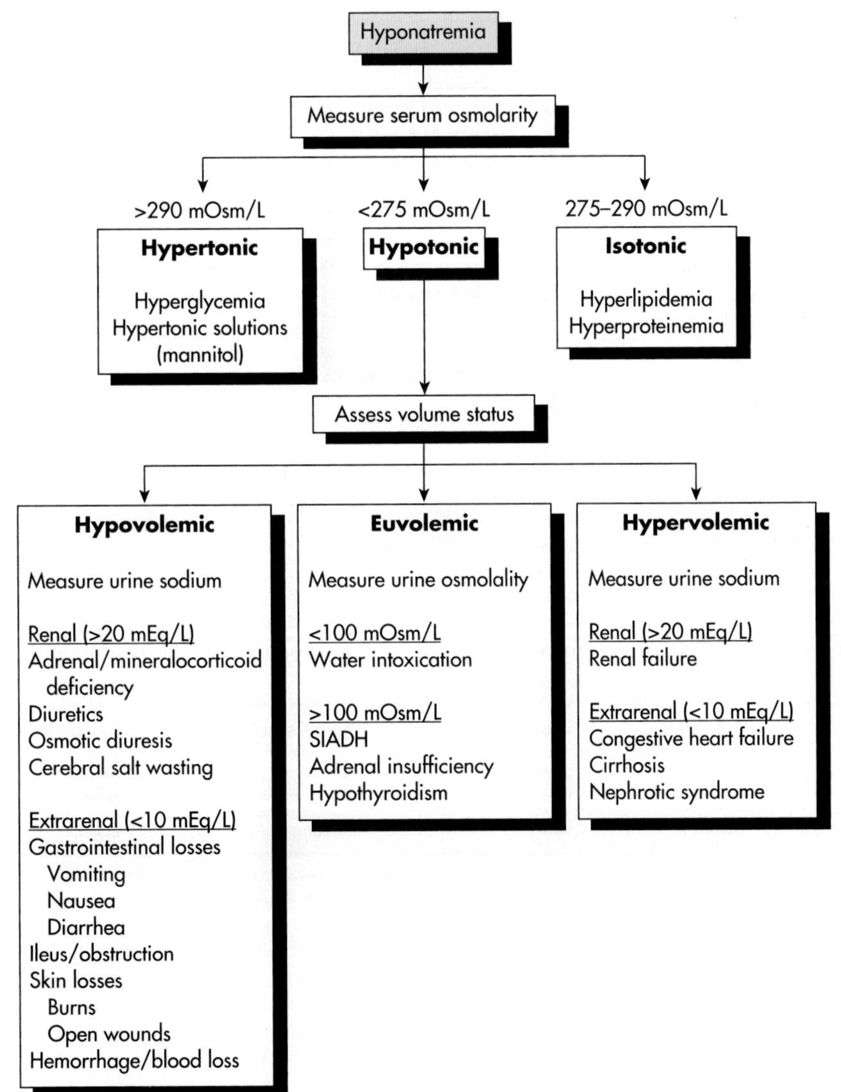

FIG. 52 Algorithm for diagnosis and treatment of hyponatremia. *SIADH*, Syndrome of inappropriate antidiuretic hormone. (From Cameron JL, Cameron AM: *Electrolyte disorders: current surgical therapy*, ed 10, Philadelphia, 2011, Saunders.)

TABLE 95 Common Causes of Hyponatremia and Electrolyte Patterns in Serum and Urine with Normal Renal Function*

Cause	Serum Na	Urine Na (UNa)	Urine Osmolality	Serum K	24-Hour UNa
1. Overhydration	Low	Low	Low	Normal or low	Low
2. Diuretics	Low	Low	Low	Low	High
3. SIADH†	Low	High	High	Normal or low	High
4. Adrenal failure	Low	Mildly elevated	Normal	High	High
5. Bartter syndrome	Low	Low	Low	Low	High
6. Diabetic hyperosmolarity‡	Low	Normal	Normal	High	Normal

*All Na and K values are concentrations, except for 24-hour UNa, which is the total number of milliequivalents of Na excreted in 24 hours in the urine.
†Secretion of inappropriate levels of antidiuretic hormone.
‡In this condition, serum glucose is markedly elevated.
(From McPherson RA, Pincus MR: *Henry's clinical diagnosis and management by laboratory methods*, ed 23, St Louis, 2017, Elsevier.)

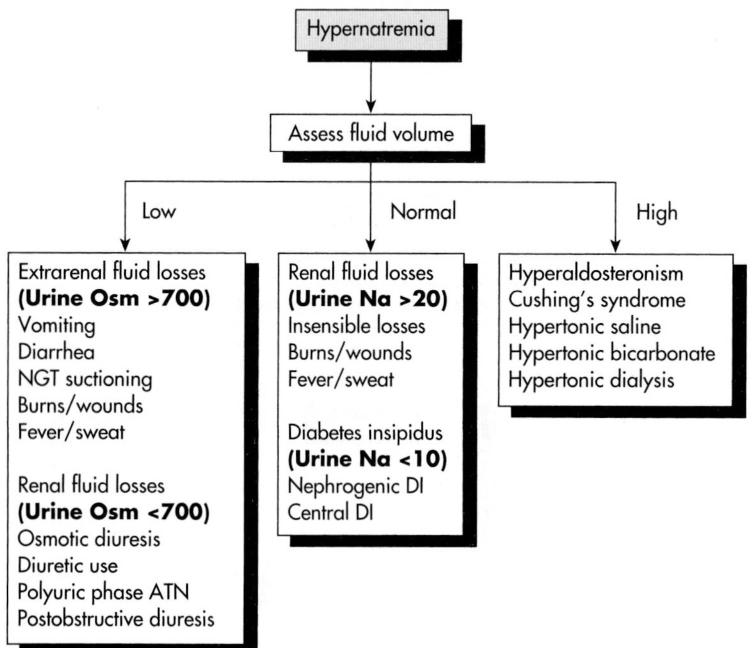

FIG. 53 Algorithm for evaluation of hypernatremia. (From Cameron JL, Cameron AM: *Electrolyte disorders: current surgical therapy*, ed 10, Philadelphia, 2011, Saunders.)

TABLE 97 Common Causes of Hypernatremia and Electrolyte Patterns in Serum and Urine with Normal Renal Function*

Cause	Serum Na	Urine Na (UNa)	Urine Osmolality	Serum K	24-Hour UNa
1. Dehydration	High	High	High	Normal	Varies
2. Diabetes insipidus	High	Low	Low	Normal	Low
3. Cushing's disease or syndrome	High	Low	Normal	Low	Low

*All Na and K values are concentrations, except for 24-hour UNa, which is the total number of milliequivalents of Na excreted in 24 hours in the urine.
(From McPherson RA, Pincus MR: *Henry's clinical diagnosis and management by laboratory methods*, ed 23, St Louis, 2017, Elsevier.)

TABLE 98 Classification and Interpretation of Synovial Fluid Analysis

Group	Diseases	Appearance	Viscosity	Mucin Clot	WBC/mm³	% PMN	Glucose (mg/dl) (Blood-Synovial Fluid)	Protein (g/dl)
Normal	—	Clear	↑	Firm	<200	<25	<10	<2.5
I (noninflammatory)	Osteoarthritis, aseptic necrosis, traumatic arthritis, erythema nodosum, osteochondritis dissecans	Clear, yellow (may be xanthochromic if traumatic arthritis)	↑	Firm	↑ Up to 10,000	<25	<10	<2.5
II (inflammatory)	Crystal-induced arthritis, rheumatoid arthritis, Reiter's syndrome, collagen vascular disease, psoriatic arthritis, serum sickness, rheumatic fever	Clear, yellow, turbid	↓	Friable	↑↑ Up to 100,000	40-90	<40	<2.5
III (septic)	Bacterial (staphylococcal, gonococcal, tuberculosis)	Turbid	↓/↑	Friable	↑↑↑ Up to 5 million	40-100	20-100	>2.5

↑, Elevated; ↑↑ >markedly high; ↓, decreased; *PMN,* polymorphonuclear leukocytes. Note that there is considerable overlap in the numbers listed above.

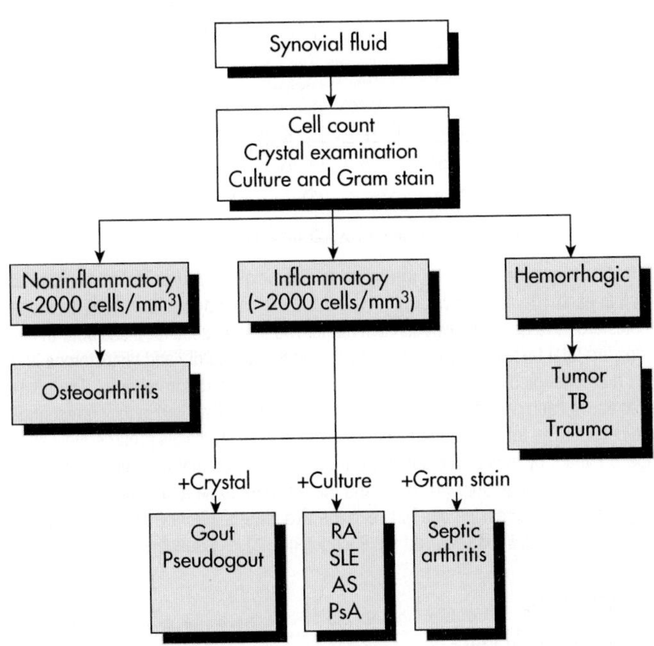

FIG. 54 Algorithm for analysis of joint fluid. Examples of inflammatory arthritis are indicated, although many conditions can produce these findings. *AS,* ankylosing spondylitis; *PsA,* psoriatic arthritis; *RA,* rheumatoid arthritis; *SLE,* systemic lupus erythematosus; *TB,* tuberculosis. (From Goldman L, Schafer AI: *Goldman's Cecil medicine,* ed 24, Philadelphia, 2012, Saunders.)

T_3 (triiodothyronine)

See Table 99 for T_3 abnormalities.

Normal range: 75-220 ng/dl (1.2-3.4 nmol/L [CF: 0.01536; SMI: 0.1 nmol/L])

Abnormal values:

Elevated in hyperthyroidism (usually earlier and to a greater extent than serum T_4).

Useful in diagnosing:

- T_3 hyperthyroidism (thyrotoxicosis): increased T_3, normal FTI.
- Toxic nodular goiter: increased T_3, normal or increased T_4.
- Iodine deficiency: normal T_3, possibly decreased T_4.
- Thyroid replacement therapy with liothyronine (Cytomel): normal T_4, increased T_3 if patient is symptomatically hyperthyroid.

TABLE 99 Findings in Thyroid Function Tests in Various Clinical Conditions

Condition	T_4	FT_4I	T_3	FT_3I	TSH	TSI	TRH Stimulation
Hyperthyroidism							
Graves disease	↑	↑	↑	↑	↓	+	↓
Toxic nodular goiter	↑	↑	↑	↑	↓	–	↓
Pituitary TSH-secreting tumors	↑	↑	↑	↑	↑	–	↓
T_3 thyrotoxicosis	N	N	↑	↑	↓	+, –	↓
T_4 thyrotoxicosis	↑	↑	N	N	↓	+, –	↓
Hypothyroidism							
Primary	↓	↓	↓	↓	↑	+, –	↑
Secondary	↓	↓	↓	↓	↓N	–	↓
Tertiary	↓	↓	↓	↓	↓, N	–	N
Peripheral unresponsiveness	↑, N	↑, N	↑, N	↑	↑, N	–	N,↑

↑, Increased; ↓, decreased; +, – variable; *N,* normal.
From Tilton RC, Barrows A: *Clinical laboratory medicine,* St Louis, 1992, Mosby.

Not ordered routinely but indicated when hyperthyroidism is suspected and serum-free T_4 or FTI inconclusive.

T_3 RESIN UPTAKE (T_3RU)

Normal range: 25%-35%

Abnormal values: Increased in hyperthyroidism. T_3 resin uptake (T_3RU or RT_3U) measures the percentage of free T_4 (not bound to protein); it does not measure serum T_3 concentration; T_3RU and other tests that reflect thyroid hormone binding to plasma protein are also known as *thyroid hormone-binding ratios* (THBR).

T_4, FREE (Free thyroxine)

Normal range: 0.8-2.8 ng/dl

Elevated in:

Graves disease, toxic multinodular goiter, toxic adenoma, iatrogenic and factitious causes, transient hyperthyroidism

Serum-free T_4 directly measures unbound thyroxine. Free T_4 can be measured by equilibrium dialysis (gold standard of free T_4 assays) or by

TABLE 100 Effects of Pregnancy on Thyroid Physiology

Physiologic Change	Thyroid-Related Consequences
↑ Serum thyroxine-binding globulin	↑ Total T_4 and T_3; ↑ T_4 production
↑ Plasma volume	↑ T_4 and T_3 pool size; ↑ T_4 production; ↑ cardiac output
D3 expression in placenta and (?) uterus	↑ T_4 production
First-trimester ↑ in hCG	↑ Free T_4; ↓ basal thyrotropin; ↑ T_4 production
↑ Renal I– clearance	↑ Iodine requirements
↑ T_4 production; fetal T_4 synthesis during second and third trimesters	
↑ Oxygen consumption by fetoplacental unit, gravid uterus, and mother	↑ Basal metabolic rate; ↑ cardiac output

D3, type 3 iodothyronine deiodinase; *I–*, plasma iodide; *hCG*, human chorionic gonadotropin; T_3, triiodothyronine; T_4, thyroxine.
From Melmed S, Polonsky KS, Larsen PR, Kronenberg HM: *Williams textbook of endocrinology*, ed 12, Philadelphia, 2011, Saunders.

immunometric techniques (influenced by serum levels of lipids, proteins, and certain drugs). The free thyroxine index (FTI) can also be easily calculated by multiplying T_4 times T_3RU and dividing the result by 100; the FTI corrects for any abnormal T_4 values secondary to protein binding: $FTI = T_4 \times T_3RU/100$.
Normal values equal 1.1 to 4.3.

T_4, SERUM T_4

Normal range: 0.8-2.8 ng/dl (10-36 pmol/L [CF: 12.87; SMI: 1 pmol/L])
Abnormal values: Serum thyroxine (T_4)
Elevated in:
Graves disease
Toxic multinodular goiter
Toxic adenoma
Iatrogenic and factitious
Transient hyperthyroidism
- Subacute thyroiditis
- Hashimoto's thyroiditis
- Silent thyroiditis

Rare causes: hypersecretion of TSH (e.g., pituitary neoplasms), struma ovarii, ingestion of large amounts of iodine in a patient with preexisting thyroid hyperplasia or adenoma (Jod-Basedow phenomenon), hydatidiform mole, carcinoma of thyroid, amiodarone therapy of arrhythmias.
Serum thyroxine test measures both circulating thyroxine bound to protein (represents >99% of circulating T_4) and unbound (free) thyroxine. Values vary with protein binding; changes in the concentration of T_4 secondary to changes in thyroxine-binding globulin (TBG) can be caused by the following:

Increased TBG (↑T4)	Decreased TBG (↓T4)
Pregnancy	Androgens, glucocorticoids
Estrogens	Nephrotic syndrome, cirrhosis
Acute infectious hepatitis	Acromegaly
Oral contraceptives	Hypoproteinemia
Familial	Familial
Fluorouracil, clofibrate	Phenytoin, ASA and other NSAIDs, heroin, methadone, high-dose penicillin, asparaginase, chronic debilitating illness

To eliminate the suspected influence of protein binding on thyroxine values, two additional tests are available: T_3 resin uptake and serum free thyroxine. Table 100 summarizes the effects of pregnancy on thyroid physiology, and Table 101 describes changes in thyroid hormone levels during illness.

TABLE 101 Changes in Thyroid Hormone Levels during Illness

Severity of Illness	Free T_3	Free T_4	Reverse T_3	TSH	Probable Cause
Mild	↓	N	↑	N	↓ D2, D1
Moderate	↓↓	N, ↑↓	↑↑	N, ↓	↓↓ D2, D1,?↑ D3
Severe	↓↓↓	↓	↑	↓↓	↓↓ D2, D1, ↑D3
Recovery	↓	↓	↑	↑	?

D1 through *D3*, iodothyronine deiodinases; *N*, no change; T_3, triiodothyronine; T_4, thyroxine; *TSH*, thyroid-stimulating hormone.
From Melmed S, Polonsky KS, Larsen PR, Kronenberg HM: *Williams textbook of endocrinology*, ed 12, Philadelphia, 2011, Saunders.

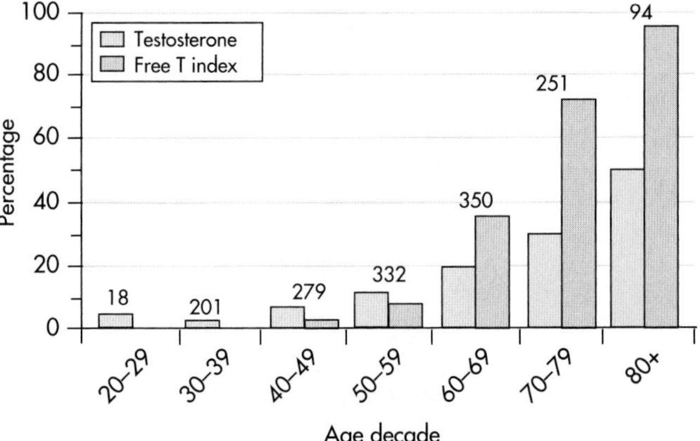

FIG. 55 Hypogonadism in aging men. Bar height indicates the percentage of men in each 10-year interval, from the third to the ninth decades, with at least one testosterone value in the hypogonadal range. The criteria used for these determinations are total testosterone less than 11.3 nmol/L (325 ng/dL) and testosterone and sex hormone–binding globulin (free T index) less than 0.153 nmol/nmol. The numbers above each pair of bars indicate the number of men studied in the corresponding decade. The fraction of men who are hypogonadal increases progressively after age 50 years by either criterion. More men are hypogonadal by free T index than by total testosterone after 50 years, and there seems to be a progressively greater difference with increasing age between the two criteria. (From Goldman L, Schafer AI: *Goldman's Cecil medicine*, ed 24, Philadelphia, 2012, Saunders.)

TEGRETOL

See CARBAMAZEPINE.

TESTOSTERONE (total testosterone)

Normal range: Variable with age and sex. Testosterone circulates in plasma mostly bound to plasma proteins and sex hormone–binding globulin (SHBG). Approximately 2% of testosterone circulates in free form (biologically active form). Low testosterone levels in obese patients may be due to reduced levels of SHBG; therefore, it is essential to measure free testosterone when evaluating androgen deficiency in obese patients.

Serum/plasma
Males: 280-1100 ng/dl Females: 15-70 ng/dl
Urine
Males: 50-135 μg/day Females: 2-12 μg/day

Elevated in: Testicular tumors, ovarian masculinizing tumors, testosterone replacement therapy
Decreased in: Hypogonadism, obesity, insulin resistance, sleep apnea. Fig. 55 illustrates testosterone level changes with age. The diagnosis of androgen deficiency should be based on at least 2 morning testosterone measurements (collected on separate days) in a symptomatic patient.

THEOPHYLLINE

Normal therapeutic range: 10-20 mcg/ml

THORACENTESIS FLUID

See PLEURAL FLUID

THROMBIN TIME (TT), THROMBIN CLOTTING TIME (TCT)

Normal range: 11.3-18.5 sec
Elevated in: Thrombolytic and heparin therapy, disseminated intravascular coagulation, hypofibrinogenemia, dysfibrinogenemia

See Table 102 for synthesizing results of PT, APTT, and TCT.

TABLE 102 Synthesizing Results of PT, APTT, and TCT

TEST			
PT	**APTT**	**TCT**	**Possible Diagnoses**
Normal	Normal	Normal	Normal hemostasis, disorder of platelet function, factor XIII deficiency, disorder of vascular hemostasis, mild coagulation protein deficiency, mild vWD, disorder of fibrinolysis (α_2-antiplasmin deficiency/defect, plasminogen activator inhibitor-1 deficiency/defect)
Prolonged	Normal	Normal	Factor VII deficiency; early oral anticoagulation; lupus anticoagulant; mild factor II, V, or X deficiency; specific factor inhibitor
Normal	Prolonged	Normal	Factor VIII, IX, XI, XI, prekallikrein, or HMWK deficiency; lupus anticoagulant; amyloid-adsorbed factor IX; specific factor inhibitor
Prolonged	Prolonged	Normal	Multiple factor deficiency (e.g., liver failure, vitamin K deficiency, oral anticoagulants); factor V, X, or II deficiency; amyloid-adsorbed factor X; specific factor inhibitor
Prolonged	Prolonged	Prolonged	Anticoagulants, DIC, dilutional coagulopathy, liver disease, fibrinogen deficiency/disorder, inhibition of fibrin polymerization, hyperfibrinolysis

APTT, Activated partial thromboplastin time; *DIC,* disseminated intravascular coagulation; *HMWK,* high-molecular-weight kininogen; *PT,* prothrombin time; *TCT,* thrombin clotting time; *vWD,* von Willebrand's disease.
(From Hoffman R: *Hematology, basic principles and practice,* ed 7, Philadelphia, 2018, Elsevier.)

THYROGLOBULIN

Normal: 3-40 ng/ml. Thyroglobulin is a tumor marker for monitoring the status of patients with papillary or follicular thyroid cancer following resection.
Elevated in: Papillary or follicular thyroid cancer, Hashimoto thyroiditis, Graves disease, subacute thyroiditis

THYROID MICROSOMAL ANTIBODIES

Normal: Undetectable. Low titers may be present in 5%-10% of normal individuals
Elevated in: Hashimoto disease, thyroid carcinoma, early hypothyroidism, pernicious anemia

THYROID-STIMULATING HORMONE (TSH)

See Fig. 56 for an algorithmic approach to thyroid testing.
Normal range: 2-11 μU/ml (2-11 mU/L [CF: 1; SMI: 1 mU/L])

CONDITIONS THAT INCREASE SERUM THYROID-STIMULATING HORMONE VALUES

Laboratory error
Primary hypothyroidism
Synthroid therapy with insufficient dose
Lithium or amiodarone; some patients
Hashimoto thyroiditis in later stage
Large doses of inorganic iodide (e.g., SSKI)
Severe nonthyroid illness in recovery phase
Iodine deficiency (moderate or severe)
Addison disease
TSH specimen drawn in evening (peak of diurnal variation)
Pituitary TSH-secreting tumor
Therapy of hypothyroidism (3-6 wk after beginning therapy [range, 1-8 wk]; sometimes longer when pretherapy TSH is over 100 μU/ml)
Acute psychiatric illness
Peripheral resistance to T_4 syndrome
Antibodies (e.g., HAMA) interfering with monoclonal sandwich method of TSH assay
Telepaque (iopanoic acid) and Oragrafin (ipodate) x-ray contrast media
Amphetamines
High altitudes

CONDITIONS THAT DECREASE SERUM THYROID-STIMULATING HORMONE VALUES

Laboratory error
T_4/T_3 toxicosis (diffuse or nodular etiology)
Excessive therapy for hypothyroidism
Active thyroiditis (subacute, painless, or early active Hashimoto disease)
Multinodular goiter containing areas of autonomy
Severe nonthyroid illness (especially acute trauma, dopamine, or glucocorticoid)
T_3 toxicosis
Pituitary insufficiency
Cushing's syndrome (and some patients on high-dose glucocorticoid)
Jod-Basedow (iodine-induced) hyperthyroidism
Thyroid-stimulating hormone drawn 2-4 hr after levothyroxine dose
Postpartum transient toxicosis
Factitious hyperthyroidism
Struma ovarii
Radioimmunoassay, surgery, or antithyroid drug therapy for hyperthyroidism 4-6 weeks (range, 2 wk to 2 yr) after the treatment
Interleukin-2 drugs (3%-6% of cases) or α-interferon therapy (1% of cases)
Hyperemesis gravidarum
Amiodarone therapy.
See Table 101 for changes in thyroid hormone levels during illness.

THYROTROPIN (TSH) RECEPTOR ANTIBODIES

Normal: <130% of basal activity
Elevated in: Values between 1.3 and 2.0 are found in 10% of patients with thyroid disease other than Graves disease. Values >2.8 have been found only in patients with Graves disease.

THYROTROPIN-RELEASING HORMONE (TRH) STIMULATION TEST

Normal: Baseline TSH <11 microU/ml; Stimulated TSH: more than double the baseline.

In primary hypothyroidism the TSH increase is 2× to 3× the normal result. In secondary hypothyroidism no TSH response occurs. In tertiary hypothyroidism (hypothalamic failure) there is a delayed rise in the TSH level.

THYROXINE (T_4)

Normal range: 4-11 μg/dl (51-142 nmol/L [CF: 12.87; SMI: 1 nmol/L])
Elevated: Hyperthyroidism (see Fig. 56)

TIBC

See IRON-BINDING CAPACITY, TOTAL

TISSUE TRANSGLUTAMINASE ANTIBODY

Normal: Negative
Present in: Celiac disease (specificity; 94%-97%, sensitivity, 90%-98%), dermatitis herpetiformis

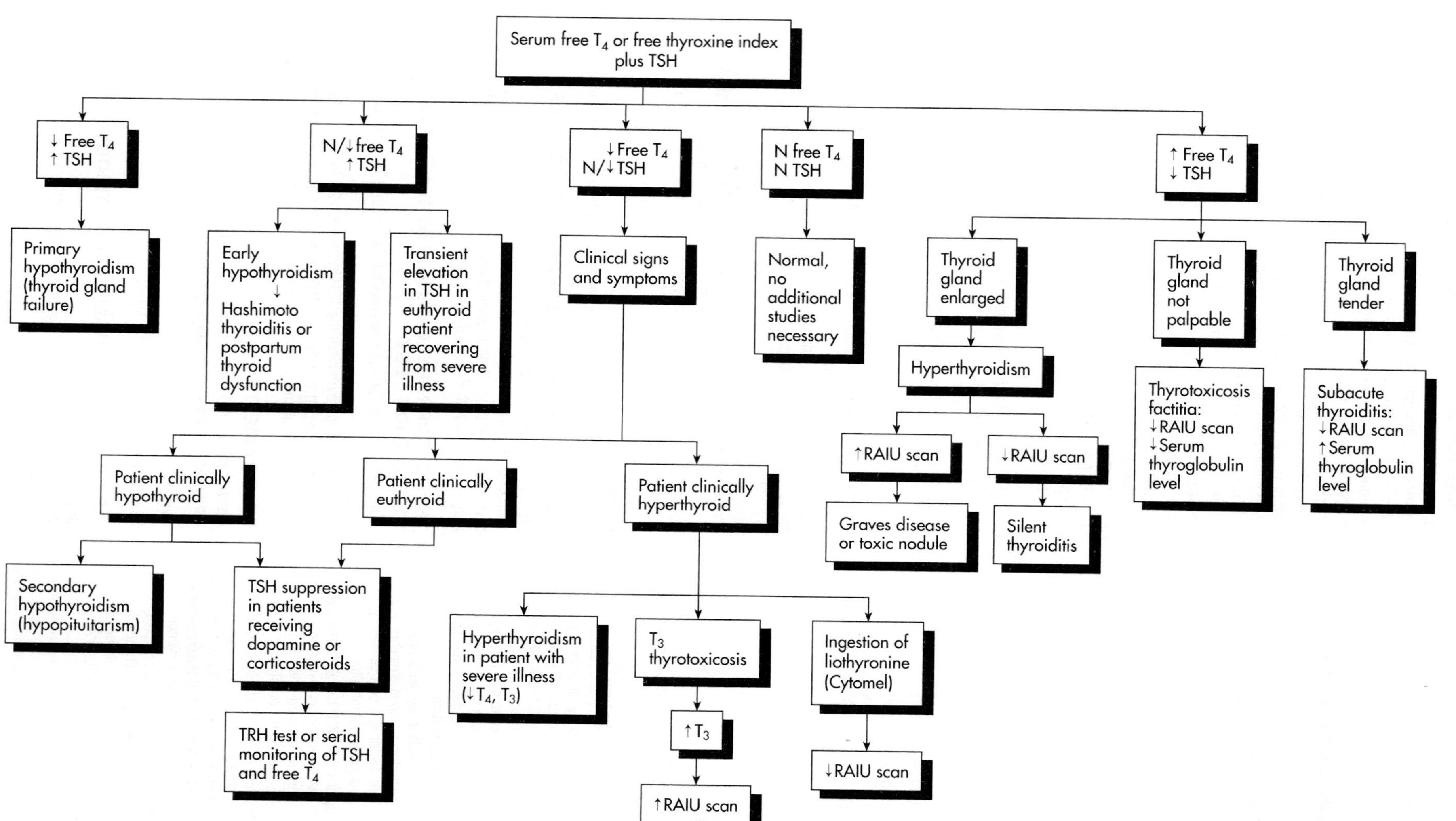

FIG. 56 Diagnostic approach to thyroid testing. *N,* Normal; *RAIU,* radioactive iodine uptake; *TRH,* thyrotropin-releasing hormone; *TSH,* thyroid-stimulating hormone. (From Ferri FF: *Practical guide to the care of the medical patient*, ed 8, St Louis, 2011, Mosby.)

BOX 30 Causes of Serum Troponin T and I Elevations, Including Both Acute Coronary Syndromes, Noncoronary Cardiac Events, and Noncardiac Ailments

Acute coronary syndrome/acute myocardial infarction
Shock of any form (cardiogenic, obstructive, distributive)
Myocarditis and myopericarditis
Cardiomyopathies
Acute congestive heart failure (pulmonary edema)
Sepsis
Pulmonary embolism
Renal failure
Sympathomimetic ingestions
Polytrauma
Burns
Acute CNS event
Rhabdomyolysis
Cardiac neoplasm, inflammatory syndromes, and infiltrative diseases
Congenital coronary anomalies
Extreme physical exertion

From Vincent JL et al: *Textbook of critical care,* ed 6, Philadelphia, 2011, Saunders.

TRANSFERRIN

Normal range: 170-370 mg/dl (1.7-3.7 g/L [CF: 0.01; SMI: 0.01 g/L])
Elevated in: Iron deficiency anemia, oral contraceptive administration, viral hepatitis, late pregnancy
Decreased in: Nephrotic syndrome, liver disease, hereditary deficiency, protein malnutrition, neoplasms, chronic inflammatory states, chronic illness, thalassemia, hemochromatosis, hemolytic anemia

TRIGLYCERIDES

Normal range: <150 mg/dl (<1.80 mmol/L [CF: 0.01129; SMI: 0.02 mmol/L])
Elevated in: Hyperlipoproteinemias (types I, IIb, III, IV, V), hypothyroidism, pregnancy, estrogens, acute myocardial infarction, pancreatitis, alcohol intake, nephrotic syndrome, diabetes mellitus, glycogen storage disease
Decreased in: Malnutrition, congenital abetalipoproteinemias, drugs (e.g., gemfibrozil, fenofibrate, nicotinic acid, clofibrate)

TRIIODOTHYRONINE

See T_3

TROPONINS (serum)

See Box 30 for causes of troponin elevations.
Normal range: 0-0.4 ng/ml (negative). If there is clinical suspicion of evolving acute MI or ischemic episode, repeat testing in 5-6 hours is recommended.
Indeterminate: 0.05-0.49 ng/ml. Suggest further tests. In a patient with unstable angina and this troponin I level, there is an increased risk of a cardiac event in the near future.
Strong probability of acute MI: ≥0.05 ng/ml
Cardiac troponin T (cTnT) is a highly sensitive marker for myocardial injury for the first 48 hours after MI and for up to 5-7 days (see Fig. 19, under "Creatine Kinase Isoenzymes"). It may also be elevated in renal failure, chronic muscle disease, and trauma.
Cardiac troponin I (cTnI) is highly sensitive and specific for myocardial injury (≥CK-MB) in the initial 8 hours, peaks within 24 hours and lasts up to 7 days. With progressively higher levels of cTnI, the risk of mortality increases because the amount of necrosis increases.

TSH

See THYROID-STIMULATING HORMONE

TT

See THROMBIN TIME

BOX 31 PPD Reaction Size Considered "Positive" (Intracutaneous 5 TU Mantoux Test at 48 hr)

5 mm or More
HIV infection or risk factors for HIV
Close recent contact with active TB case
Persons with chest x-ray consistent with healed TB

10 mm or More
Foreign-born persons from countries with high TB prevalence in Asia, Africa, and Latin America
IV drug users
Medically underserved low-income population groups (including Native Americans, Hispanics, and blacks)
Residents of long-term care facilities (nursing homes, mental institutions)
Medical conditions that increase risk for TB (silicosis, gastrectomy, undernourishment, diabetes mellitus, high-dose corticosteroids or immunosuppression Rx, leukemia or lymphoma, other malignancies)
Employees of long-term care facilities, schools, child care facilities, health care facilities

15 mm or More
All others not already listed

TB, Tuberculosis; *TU,* tuberculin units.

BOX 32 Factors Associated with False-Negative Tuberculin Tests

Technical Errors
Improper administration
Inaccurate reading
Loss of potency of antigen

Patient-Related Factors (Anergy)
Age (elderly)
Nutritional status
Medications: corticosteroids, immunosuppressive agents
Severe tuberculosis
Coexisting diseases
- HIV infection
- Viral illness or vaccination
- Lymphoreticular malignancies
- Sarcoidosis
- Solid tumors
- Lepromatous leprosy
- Sjögren syndrome
- Ataxia telangiectasia
- Uremia
- Primary biliary cirrhosis
- Systemic lupus erythematosus

Severe systemic disease of any etiology

From Stein JH (ed): *Internal medicine,* ed 4, St Louis, 1994, Mosby.

TUBERCULIN TEST (PPD)

Abnormal results: see Box 31. Box 32 describes factors associated with false-negative tuberculin tests.

UNCONJUGATED BILIRUBIN

See BILIRUBIN, DIRECT

UREA NITROGEN, BLOOD (BUN)

Normal range: 8-18 mg/dl (3-6.5 mmol/L [CF: 0.357; SMI: 0.5 mmol/L])

Box 33 describes factors affecting BUN level independent of renal function.

Elevated in: Dehydration, drugs (aminoglycosides and other antibiotics, diuretics, lithium, corticosteroids), gastrointestinal bleeding, decreased renal blood flow (shock, congestive heart failure, myocardial infarction), renal disease (glomerulonephritis, pyelonephritis, diabetic nephropathy), urinary tract obstruction (prostatic hypertrophy)

Decreased in: Liver disease, malnutrition, third trimester of pregnancy, overhydration, acromegaly, celiac disease

URIC ACID (serum)

Normal range: 2-7 mg/dl

Elevated in: Renal failure, gout, excessive cell lysis (chemotherapeutic agents, radiation therapy, leukemia, lymphoma, hemolytic anemia), hereditary enzyme deficiency (hypoxanthine-guanine-phosphoribosyl transferase), acidosis, myeloproliferative disorders, diet high in purines or protein, drugs (diuretics, low doses of ASA, ethambutol, nicotinic acid), lead poisoning, hypothyroidism, Addison disease, nephrogenic diabetes insipidus, active psoriasis, polycystic kidneys

Decreased in: Drugs (allopurinol, febuxostat, high doses of ASA, probenecid, warfarin, corticosteroid), deficiency of xanthine oxidase, syndrome of inappropriate antidiuretic hormone secretion, renal tubular deficits (Fanconi syndrome), alcoholism, liver disease, diet deficient in protein or purines, Wilson disease, hemochromatosis

URINALYSIS

Normal range:

Color: light straw
Appearance: clear
Ketones: absent
pH: 4.5-8 (average, 6)
Protein: absent
Glucose: absent
Specific gravity: 1.005-1.030
Occult blood absent
Microscopic examination:
- Red blood cells: 0-5 (high-power field)
- White blood cells: 0-5 (high-power field)
- Bacteria (spun specimen): absent
- Casts: 0-4 hyaline (low-power field)

Abnormalities in the microscopic examination of urine are described in Table 103. Causes of abnormal appearance and color of urine are described in Table 104. Urine color changes with commonly used drugs are summarized in Table 105.

BOX 33 Factors Affecting Blood Urea Nitrogen Level Independent of Renal Function

Disproportionate Increase in Blood Urea Nitrogen
Volume depletion ("prerenal azotemia")
Gastrointestinal hemorrhage
Corticosteroid or cytotoxic agents
High-protein diet
Obstructive uropathy
Sepsis
Catabolic states, tissue breakdown

Disproportionate Decrease in Blood Urea Nitrogen
Low-protein diet
Liver disease

From Andreoli TE (ed): *Cecil essentials of medicine,* ed 5, Philadelphia, 2001, Saunders.

URINE AMYLASE

Normal range: 35-260 U Somogyi/hr (6.5-48.1 U/hr [CF: 0.185; SMI: 1 U/hr])

Elevated in: Pancreatitis, carcinoma of the pancreas

URINE BILE

Normal: Absent

Abnormal:

Urine bilirubin: hepatitis (viral, toxic, drug-induced), biliary obstruction

Urine urobilinogen: hepatitis (viral, toxic, drug-induced), hemolytic jaundice, liver cell dysfunction (cirrhosis, infection, metastases)

URINE CALCIUM

Normal range: <250 mg/24 hr (<6.2 mmol/dl [CF: 0.02495; SMI: 0.1 mmol/dl])

Elevated in: Primary hyperparathyroidism, hypervitaminosis D, bone metastases, multiple myeloma, increased calcium intake, steroids, prolonged immobilization, sarcoidosis, Paget disease, idiopathic hypercalciuria, renal tubular acidosis

Decreased in: Hypoparathyroidism, pseudohypoparathyroidism, vitamin D deficiency, vitamin D–resistant rickets, diet low in calcium, drugs (thiazide diuretics, oral contraceptives), familial hypocalciuric hypercalcemia, renal osteodystrophy, potassium citrate therapy

URINE CAMP

Elevated in: Hypercalciuria, familial hypocalciuric hypercalcemia, primary hyperparathyroidism, pseudohypoparathyroidism, rickets

Decreased in: Vitamin D intoxication, sarcoidosis

URINE CATECHOLAMINES

Normal range:

Norepinephrine: <100 μg/24 hr (<590 nmol/day [CF: 5.911; SMI: 10 nmol/day])

Epinephrine: <10 μg/24 hr (55 nmol/day [CF: 5.458; SMI: 5 nmol/day])

Elevated in: Pheochromocytoma, neuroblastoma, severe stress

TABLE 103 Microscopic Examination of the Urine

Finding	Associations
Casts	
Red blood cell	Glomerulonephritis, vasculitis
White blood cell	Interstitial nephritis, pyelonephritis
Epithelial cell	Acute tubular necrosis, interstitial nephritis, glomerulonephritis
Granular	Renal parenchymal disease (nonspecific)
Waxy, broad	Advanced renal failure
Hyaline	Normal finding in concentrated urine
Fatty	Heavy proteinuria
Cells	
Red blood cell	Urinary tract infection, urinary tract inflammation
White blood cell	Urinary tract infection, urinary tract inflammation
Eosinophil	Acute interstitial nephritis
(Squamous) epithelial cell	Contaminants
Crystals	
Uric acid	Acid urine, acute uric acid nephropathy, hyperuricosuria
Calcium phosphate	Alkaline urine
Calcium oxalate	Acid urine, hyperoxaluria, ethylene glycol poisoning
Cystine	Cystinuria
Sulfur	Sulfa-containing antibiotics

From Andreoli TE (ed): *Cecil essentials of medicine,* ed 5, Philadelphia, 2001, Saunders.

TABLE 104 Appearance and Color of Urine

Appearance	Cause	Remarks
Colorless Cloudy	Very dilute urine	Polyuria, diabetes insipidus
	Phosphates, carbonates	Soluble in dilute acetic acid
	Urates, uric acid	Dissolve at 60° C and in alkali
	Leukocytes	Insoluble in dilute acetic acid
	Red blood cells ("smoky")	Lyse in dilute acetic acid
	Bacteria, yeasts	Insoluble in dilute acetic acid
	Spermatozoa	Insoluble in dilute acetic acid
	Prostatic fluid	May be flocculent
	Mucin, mucous threads	Phosphates, oxalates
	Calculi, "gravel"	Rectovesical fistula
	Clumps, pus, tissue	In acid urine
	Fecal contamination	
	Radiographic dye	
Milky	Many neutrophils (pyuria)	Insoluble in dilute acetic acid
	Fat	Nephrosis, crush injury – soluble in ether
	Lipiduria, opalescent	Lymphatic obstruction-soluble in ether
	Chyluria, milky	Vaginal creams
	Emulsified paraffin	
Yellow	Acriflavine	Green fluorescence
Yellow-orange	Concentrated urine	Dehydration, fever
	Urobilin in excess	No yellow foam
	Bilirubin	Yellow foam if sufficient bilirubin
Yellow-green	Bilirubin-biliverdin	Yellow foam
Yellow-brown	Bilirubin-biliverdin	"Beer" brown, yellow foam
Red	Hemoglobin	Positive
	Erythrocytes	Positive } Reagent strip for blood
	Myoglobin	Positive
	Porphyrin	May be colorless
	Fuscin, aniline dye	Foods, candy
	Beets	Yellow alkaline, genetic
	Menstrual contamination	Clots, mucus
Red-purple	Porphyrins	May be colorless
Red-brown	Erythrocytes	Acid pH
	Hemoglobin on standing	Muscle injury
	Methemoglobin	Result of unstable hemoglobin
	Myoglobin	
	Bilifuscin (dipyrrole)	
Brown-black	Methemoglobin	Blood, acid pH
	Homogentisic acid	On standing, alkaline; alkaptonuria
	Melanin	On standing, rare
Blue-green	Indicans	Small intestine infections
	Pseudomonas infections	Mouth deodorants
	Chlorophyll	

From McPherson RA, Pincus MR: *Henry's clinical diagnosis and management by laboratory methods*, ed 23, St Louis, 2017, Elsevier.

URINE CHLORIDE

Normal range: 110-250 mEq/day (110-250 mmol/day [CF: 1; SMI: 1 mmol/day])
Elevated in: Corticosteroids, Bartter syndrome, diuretics, metabolic acidosis, severe hypokalemia
Decreased in: Chloride depletion (vomiting), colonic villous adenoma, chronic renal failure, renal tubular acidosis

URINE COPPER

Normal range: <40 μg/24 hr (<0.6 μmol/day [CF: 0.01574; SMI: 0.2 μmol/day])

URINE CORTISOL, FREE

Normal range: 10-110 μg/24 hr (30-300 nmol/day [CF: 2.759; SMI: 10 nmol/day])

TABLE 105 Urine Color Changes with Commonly Used Drugs*

Drug	Color
Alcohol, ethyl	Pale, diuresis
Anthraquinone laxatives (senna, cascara)	Reddish, alkaline; yellow-brown, acid
Chlorzoxazone (Paraflex) (muscle relaxant)	Red
Deferoxamine mesylate (Desferal) (chelates iron)	Red
Ethoxazene (Serenium) (urinary analgesic)	Orange, red
Fluorescein sodium (given IV)	Yellow
Furazolidone (Furoxone) (Tricofuron) (an antibacterial, antiprotozoal nitrofuran)	Brown
Indigo carmine dye (renal function, cystoscopy)	Blue
Iron sorbitol (Jectofer) (possibly other iron compounds forming iron sulfide in urine)	Brown on standing
Levodopa (L-dopa) (for parkinsonism)	Red then brown, alkaline
Mepacrine (Atabrine) (antimalarial) (intestinal worms, *Giardia)*	Yellow
Methocarbamol (Robaxin) (muscle relaxant)	Green-brown
Methyldopa (Aldomet) (antihypertensive)	Darkens; if oxidizing agents present, red to brown
Methylene blue (used to delineate fistulas)	Blue, blue-green
Metronidazole (Flagyl) (for *Trichomonas* infection, amebiasis, *Giardia*)	Darkening, reddish brown
Nitrofurantoin (Furadantin) (antibacterial)	Brown-yellow
Phenazopyridine (Pyridium) (urinary analgesic), also compounded with sulfonamides (e.g., Azo Gantrisin)	Orange-red, acid pH
Phenindione (Hedulin) (anticoagulant) (important to distinguish from hematuria)	Orange, alkaline; color disappears on acidifying
Phenol poisoning	Brown; oxidized to quinones (green)
Phenolphthalein (purgative)	Red-purple, alkaline pH
Phenolsulfonphthalein (also sulfobromophthalein)	Pink-red, alkaline pH
Rifampin (Rifadin, Rimactane) (tuberculosis therapy)	Bright orange-red
Riboflavin (multivitamins)	Bright yellow
Sulfasalazine (Azulfidine) (for ulcerative colitis)	Orange-yellow, alkaline pH

*Other commonly used drugs have been noted to produce color change once or occasionally: amitriptyline (Elavil)—blue-green; phenothiazines—red; triamterene (Dyrenium)—pale blue (blue fluorescence in acid urine).
From McPherson RA, Pincus MR: *Henry's clinical diagnosis and management by laboratory methods*, ed 23, St Louis, 2017, Elsevier.

Elevated: See CORTISOL, PLASMA

URINE CREATININE (24 hr)

Normal range:
Male: 0.8-1.8 g/day (7-16 mmol/day [CF: 8.840; SMI: 0.1 mmol/day])
Female: 0.6-1.6 g/day (5.3-14 mmol/day)
NOTE: Useful test as an indicator of completeness of 24-hr urine collection.

URINE CRYSTALS

Uric acid: acid urine, hyperuricosuria, uric acid nephropathy
Sulfur: antibiotics containing sulfa
Calcium oxalate: ethylene glycol poisoning, acid urine, hyperoxaluria
Calcium phosphate: alkaline urine
Cystine: cystinuria

URINE EOSINOPHILS

Normal: Absent

TABLE 106 Factors That Interfere with Determination of Urinary 5-HIAA

Foods	Drugs
Factors That Produce False-Positive Results	
Avocado	Acetaminophen
Banana	Acetanilid
Chocolate	Caffeine
Coffee	Fluorouracil
Eggplant	Guaifenesin
Pecan	l-Dopa
Pineapple	Melphalan
Plum	Mephenesin
Tea	Methamphetamine
Walnuts	Methocarbamol
	Methysergide maleate
	Phenmetrazine
	Reserpine
	Salicylates
Factors That Cause False-Negative Results	
None	Corticotropin
	p-Chlorophenylalanine
	Chlorpromazine
	Heparin
	Imipramine
	Isoniazid
	Methenamine mandelate
	Methyldopa
	Monoamine oxidase inhibitors
	Phenothiazine
	Promethazine

5-HIAA, 5-hydroxyindoleacetic acid.
From Melmed S, Polonsky KS, Larsen PR, Kronenberg HM: *Williams textbook of endocrinology*, ed 12, Philadelphia, 2011, Saunders.

Present in: Interstitial nephritis, acute tubular necrosis, urinary tract infection, kidney transplant rejection, hepatorenal syndrome

URINE GLUCOSE (qualitative)

Normal: Absent
Present in: Diabetes mellitus, renal glycosuria (decreased renal threshold for glucose), glucose intolerance

URINE HEMOGLOBIN, FREE

Normal: Absent
Present in: Hemolysis (with saturation of serum haptoglobin binding capacity and renal threshold for tubular absorption of hemoglobin)

URINE HEMOSIDERIN

Normal: Absent
Present in: Paroxysmal nocturnal hemoglobinuria, chronic hemolytic anemia, hemochromatosis, blood transfusion, thalassemias

URINE 5-HYDROXYINDOLE-ACETIC ACID (urine 5-HIAA)

Normal range: 2-8 mg/24 hr (10-40 μmol/day [CF: 5.23; SMI: 5 μmol/day])
Elevated in: Carcinoid tumors, after ingestion of certain foods (bananas, plums, tomatoes, avocados, pineapples, eggplant, walnuts), drugs (monoamine oxidase inhibitors, phenacetin, methyldopa, glycerol guaiacolate, acetaminophen, salicylates, phenothiazines, imipramine, methocarbamol, reserpine, methamphetamine). See Table 106.

URINE INDICAN

Normal: Absent
Present in: Malabsorption secondary to intestinal bacterial overgrowth

TABLE 107 Medications That May Increase Measured Levels of Fractionated Catecholamines and Metanephrines

Tricyclic antidepressants (including cyclobenzaprine)
Levodopa
Drugs containing adrenergic receptor agonists (e.g., decongestants)
Amphetamines
Buspirone and antipsychotic agents
Prochlorperazine
Reserpine
Withdrawal from clonidine and other drugs (e.g., illicit drugs)
Illicit drugs (e.g., cocaine, heroin)
Ethanol

From Melmed S, Polonsky KS, Larsen PR, Kronenberg HM: *Williams textbook of endocrinology*, ed 12, Philadelphia, 2011, Saunders.

TABLE 108 Differentiation of Hematuria, Hemoglobinuria, and Myoglobinuria

Condition	Plasma Findings	Urine Findings
Hematuria	Color—normal	Color—normal, smoky, pink, red, brown
		Erythrocytes—many
		Renal—red blood cell casts
		Protein—marked increase
		Lower urinary tract—no casts
		Protein—present or absent
Hemoglobinuria	Color—pink (early)	Color—pink, red, brown
	Haptoglobin—low	Erythrocytes—occasional
		Pigment casts—occasional
		Protein—present or absent
		Hemosiderin—late
Myoglobinuria	Color—normal	Color—red, brown
	Haptoglobin—normal	Erythrocytes—occasional
	Creatine kinase—marked increase	Dense brown casts—occasional
	Aldolase—increased	Protein—present or absent

From McPherson RA, Pincus MR: *Henry's clinical diagnosis and management by laboratory methods*, ed 23, St Louis, 2017, Elsevier.

URINE KETONES (semiquantitative)

Normal: Absent
Present in: Diabetic ketoacidosis, alcoholic ketoacidosis, starvation, isopropanol ingestion

URINE METANEPHRINES

Normal range: 0-2.0 mg/24 hr (0-11.0 μmol/day [CF: 5.458; SMI: 0.5 μmol/day])
Elevated in: Pheochromocytoma, neuroblastoma, drugs (caffeine, phenothiazines, monoamine oxidase inhibitors), stress. Table 107 summarizes medications that may increase metanephrine levels.

URINE MYOGLOBIN

Normal: Absent
Present in: Severe trauma, hyperthermia, polymyositis/dermatomyositis, carbon monoxide poisoning, drugs (narcotic and amphetamine toxicity), hypothyroidism, muscle ischemia

Table 108 differentiates hematuria and hemoglobinuria from myoglobinuria.

URINE NITRITE

Normal: Absent
Present in: Urinary tract infections

URINE OCCULT BLOOD

Normal: Negative
Positive in: Trauma to urinary tract, renal disease (glomerulonephritis, pyelonephritis), renal or ureteral calculi, bladder lesions (carcinoma, cystitis), prostatitis, prostatic carcinoma, menstrual contamination, hematopoietic disorders (hemophilia, thrombocytopenia), anticoagulants, ASA

URINE OSMOLALITY

See OSMOLALITY, URINE

URINE PH

Normal range: 4.6-8 (average, 6)
Elevated in: Bacteriuria, vegetarian diet, renal failure with inability to form ammonia, drugs (antibiotics, sodium bicarbonate, acetazolamide)
Decreased in: Acidosis (metabolic, respiratory), drugs (ammonium chloride, methenamine mandelate), diabetes mellitus, starvation, diarrhea

URINE PHOSPHATE

Normal range: 0.8-2.0 g/24 hr
Elevated in: Acute tubular necrosis (diuretic phase), chronic renal disease, uncontrolled diabetes mellitus, hyperparathyroidism, hypomagnesemia, metabolic acidosis, metabolic alkalosis, neurofibromatosis, adult-onset vitamin D–resistant hypophosphatemic osteomalacia
Decreased in: Acromegaly, acute renal failure, decreased dietary intake, hypoparathyroidism, respiratory acidosis

URINE POTASSIUM

Normal range: 25-100 mEq/24 hr (25-100 mmol/day [CF: 1; SMI: 1 mmol/day])
Elevated in: Aldosteronism (primary, secondary), glucocorticoids, alkalosis, renal tubular acidosis, excessive dietary potassium intake
Decreased in: Acute renal failure, potassium-sparing diuretics, diarrhea, hypokalemia
Box 34 describes urine potassium in hypokalemia.

BOX 34 Urine Potassium in Hypokalemia

Low 24-hour urinary potassium (<25 mEq/day) or low spot urine potassium (<15 mEq/L) or low potassium-to-creatinine ratio (<1.5 mEq/mmol)
GI losses: vomiting, diarrhea, nasogastric tube
Sweat losses: extreme heat, cystic fibrosis
Low intake

High 24-hour urinary potassium (>25 mEq/day) or high spot urine potassium (>40 mEq/L) or high potassium-to-creatinine ratio (>1.5 mEq/mmol)
Renal potassium wasting
- Diuretics, amphotericin B
- Increased mineralocorticoid activity
- Excretion of bicarbonate (vomiting, RTA)
- Excretion of other nonreabsorbable anion (hippurate, beta-hydroxybutyrate, penicillin derivative)

Transcellular shifts
Hypomagnesemia
Bartter, Gitelman, Liddle syndromes

High 24-hour urinary potassium (>25 mEq/day) and high potassium-to-creatinine ratio (>1.5 mEq/mmol) but low spot urine potassium (<15 mEq/L)
Established AKI (tubular dysfunction ± dilutional)
Primary polydipsia (dilutional)
Other polyuric states (osmotic and water diuresis)

From Ronco C: *Critical care nephrology*, ed 3, Philadelphia, 2019, Elsevier.
AKI, Acute kidney injury; *RTA,* renal tubular acidosis.

URINE PROTEIN (quantitative)

Normal range: <150 mg/24 hr (<0.15 g/day [CF: 0.001; SMI: 0.01 g/day])
Elevated in:
Nephrotic syndrome as a result of primary renal diseases
Malignant hypertension
Malignancies: multiple myeloma, leukemias, Hodgkin's disease
Congestive heart failure
Diabetes mellitus
Systemic lupus erythematosus, rheumatoid arthritis
Sickle cell disease
Goodpasture's syndrome
Malaria
Amyloidosis, sarcoidosis
Tubular lesions: cystinosis
Functional (after heavy exercise)
Pyelonephritis
Pregnancy
Constrictive pericarditis
Renal vein thrombosis
Toxic nephropathies: heavy metals, drugs
Radiation nephritis
Orthostatic (postural) proteinuria
Benign proteinuria: fever, heat or cold exposure

URINE SEDIMENT

See Fig. 57 for visual evaluation of common abnormalities. Table 109 summarizes characteristics of amorphous and crystalline urinary sediments.

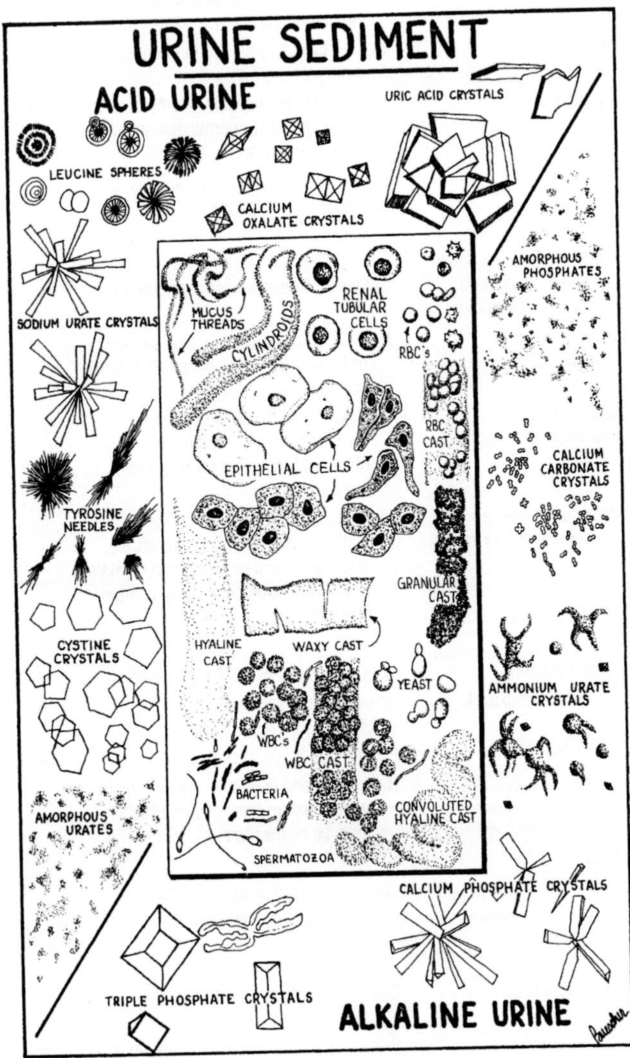

FIG. 57 Microscopic examination of urinary sediment. From Grigorian Greene M: *The Harriet Lane handbook: a manual for pediatric house officers,* ed 17, St Louis, 2007, Mosby.

TABLE 109 Characteristics of Amorphous and Crystalline Urinary Sediments

Substance	Description	URINE PH WHERE FOUND Acid	Neutral	Alkaline	Solubility Characteristics and Comments
Ampicillin	Uncommon—from high dose; colorless; long prisms that form clusters, sheaves	+	–	–	
Bilirubin	Reddish brown; amorphous needles, rhombic plates, or cubes; may color uric acid crystals	+	–	–	Soluble in alkali, acid, acetone, and chloroform
Cholesterol	Rare; colorless; flat plate with corner notch; accompanies fatty casts and oval fat bodies	+	+	–	Very soluble in chloroform, ether, and hot alcohol
Calcium carbonate	Colorless; small granules in pairs, fours; spheres; rarely needles	–	+	+	Soluble in acetic acid with effervescence
Calcium oxalate	Dihydrate—common; colorless; small refractile octahedron Monohydrate—uncommon; dumbbell and ovoid rectangle	+	+	–	Soluble in dilute HCl
Cystine	Colorless; hexagonal plates, often laminated; rapidly destroyed by bacteria; may be confused with uric acid, but cystine is soluble in dilute hydrochloric acid	+	–	–	Soluble in alkali (especially ammonia) and dilute HCl; insoluble in boiling water, acetic acid, alcohol, ether; apply cyanide-nitroprusside reaction
Hematin	Small, biconvex "whetstone" seen with hemoglobinuria	+	–	–	
Hemosiderin	Golden brown; granules in clumps, in cells, casts	+	+	–	Blue with Prussian blue
Hippuric acid	Rare; colorless, needles, rhombic plates and four-sided prisms; distinguish from phosphates	+	+	+	Soluble with hot water and alkali; insoluble in acetic acid
Indigotin	Rare; blue; amorphous or small crystals; colors other crystals	+	+	+	Very soluble in chloroform; soluble in ether; insoluble in acetone
Phosphates					
Amorphous phosphate (magnesium, calcium)	Colorless; fine, granular precipitate	–	+	+	Insoluble with heat; soluble with acetic acid, dilute HCl
Calcium hydrogen phosphate	Less common; colorless, star-shaped or long, thin prisms or needles; form rosettes	sl	+	sl	Slightly soluble in dilute acetic acid, soluble in dilute HCl
Triple phosphate (ammonium, magnesium)	Common form: colorless; three- to six-sided prisms, "coffin lids" Less often: Flat, fern leaf form, sheets, flakes	–	+	+	Soluble in dilute acetic acid
Radiographic media (meglumine diatrizoate)	Intravenous: Colorless; thin, rhombic plates, some with notch, resemble cholesterol plates; elongated crystals Retrograde: Colorless; long, pointed crystals	+	–	–	Soluble in 10% NaOH: Insoluble in ether and chloroform; high specific gravity in urine: polarizes with interference colors
Sulfonamides					
Acetylsulfadiazine	Wheat sheaves with eccentric binding	+	–	–	
Acetylsulfamethoxazole	Brown; dense spheres or irregular divided spheres	+	–	–	
Sulfadiazine	Brown; dense globules	+	–	–	Soluble in acetone
Tyrosine	Rare; colorless or yellow, appears black with focusing; fine silky needles in sheaves or rosettes	+	–	–	Soluble in alkali, dilute mineral acid, relatively heat soluble; insoluble in alcohol, ether
Urates					
Amorphous (calcium, magnesium, sodium, potassium)	Common; colorless to yellow-brown; amorphous, granular precipitate	+	+	–	Soluble in dilute alkali; soluble at 60 °C or lower; change to uric acid crystal with concentrated HCl or acetic acid
Monosodium urate	Colorless; needles or amorphous precipitate	+	–	–	
Urates (sodium, potassium, ammonium)	Brown; small, spherical; clusters resemble biurates	sl	+	–	Soluble at 60 °C; change to uric acid with glacial acetic acid

continued

TABLE 109 Characteristics of Amorphous and Crystalline Urinary Sediments—cont'd

Substance	Description	URINE PH WHERE FOUND Acid	Neutral	Alkaline	Solubility Characteristics and Comments
Ammonium biurate	Common in "old" urine; dark yellow or brown; spheres or "thorn apples" (spheres with horns)	–	+	+	Soluble at 60° C with acetic acid; soluble strong alkali; change to uric acid with concentrated hydrochloric or acetic acid
Uric acid	Common; yellow, red-brown, brown; large variety of shapes—rhombic, four-sided plates, rosettes, "whetstones" lemon shapes; rarely, colorless hexagonals	+	–	–	Soluble in alkali: Insoluble in alcohol and acids; polarizes with interference colors
Xanthine	Rare; colorless; small, rhombic plates	+	+	–	Soluble in alkali; soluble with heat; insoluble in acetic acid

sl, Slight.
From McPherson RA, Pincus MR: *Henry's clinical diagnosis and management by laboratory methods*, ed 23, St Louis, 2017, Elsevier.

TABLE 110 Urine Electrolytes* in the Differential Diagnosis of Hypokalemia

Condition	URINE ELECTROLYTE Na^+	Cl–
Vomiting		
Recent	High†	Low‡
Remote	Low	Low
Diuretics		
Recent	High	High
Remote	Low	Low
Diarrhea or Laxative Abuse	Low	High
Bartter or Gitelman Syndrome	High	High

*Do not use the urine electrolytes in this fashion during polyuric states.
†High = urine concentration >15 mmol/L.
‡Low = urine concentration <15 mmol/L.
From Vincent JL et al: *Textbook of critical care*, ed 6, Philadelphia, 2011, Saunders.

TABLE 111 Urinalysis Findings in Acute Kidney Injury (AKI)

Etiologic Disorder	Urine Chemistry	Urine Sediment
Prerenal	U_{Na} <20 mmol/L FE_{Na} <1% FE_{urea} <35%	Normal or nearly normal (hyaline casts and rare granular casts)
Acute tubular necrosis	U_{Na} >40 mmol/L FE_{Na} >2% FE_{urea} >60%	Renal tubular epithelial cells, epithelial cell casts, coarse pigmented (muddy brown) casts
Acute interstitial nephritis	Variable; U_{Na} may be >40 mmol/L, FE_{Na} may be >2%	Red blood cells, white blood cells, white blood cell casts, eosinophils
Acute glomerulonephritis	Variable; U_{Na} may be <20 mmol/L, FE_{Na} may be <1%	Red blood cells (dysmorphic), red blood cell casts
Acute vascular disease	Variable; U_{Na} may be <20 mmol/L, FE_{Na} may be <1%	Red blood cells, red blood cell casts in HUS/TTP, eosinophils in atheroembolic disease
Crystal-associated AKI	Variable	Crystalluria Uric acid crystals in tumor lysis syndrome Calcium oxalate crystals in ethylene glycol ingestion Drug crystals (acyclovir, methotrexate, indinavir, triamterene, sulfadiazine)
Obstructive	Variable; early U_{Na} may be <20 mmol/L, FE_{Na} may be <1%; late U_{Na} may be >40 mmol/L, FE_{Na} may be >2%	Normal or red blood cells, white blood cells and crystals

FE_{Na}, fractional excretion of sodium; *FE_{urea},* fractional excretion of urea; *HUS,* hemolytic-uremic syndrome; *TTP,* thrombotic thrombocytopenic purpura; *U_{Na},* urine sodium concentration.
From Parrillo JE, Dellinger RP: *Critical care medicine, principles of diagnosis and management in the adult,* ed 4, Philadelphia, 2014, Elsevier.

URINE SODIUM (quantitative)

See Table 110 for use of urine electrolytes in the differential diagnosis of hypokalemia. Table 111 describes urine sodium findings in acute kidney injury (AKI).

Normal range: 40-220 mEq/day (40-220 mmol/day [CF: 1; SMI: 1 mmol/day])

Elevated in: Diuretic administration, high sodium intake, salt-losing nephritis, acute tubular necrosis, vomiting, Addison disease, syndrome of inappropriate antidiuretic hormone secretion, hypothyroidism, congestive heart failure, hepatic failure, chronic renal failure, Bartter syndrome, glucocorticoid deficiency, interstitial nephritis caused by analgesic abuse, mannitol, dextran, or glycerol therapy, milk-alkali syndrome, decreased renin secretion, postobstructive diuresis

Decreased In: Increased aldosterone, glucocorticoid excess, hyponatremia, prerenal azotemia, decreased salt intake

URINE SPECIFIC GRAVITY

Normal range: 1.005-1.030

Elevated in: Dehydration, excessive fluid losses (vomiting, diarrhea, fever), x-ray contrast media, diabetes mellitus, congestive heart failure, syndrome of inappropriate antidiuretic hormone secretion, adrenal insufficiency, decreased fluid intake

Decreased in: Diabetes insipidus, renal disease (glomerulonephritis, pyelonephritis), excessive fluid intake or IV hydration

URINE VANILLYLMANDELIC ACID (VMA)

Normal range: <6.8 mg/24 hr (<35 μmol/day [CF: 5.046; SMI: 1 μmol/day])

Elevated in: Pheochromocytoma, neuroblastoma, ganglioblastoma, drugs (isoproterenol, methocarbamol, levodopa, sulfonamides, chlorpromazine), severe stress, after ingestion of bananas, chocolate, vanilla, tea, coffee

Decreased in: Drugs (monoamine oxidase inhibitors, reserpine, guanethidine, methyldopa)

VARICELLA-ZOSTER VIRUS (VZV) SEROLOGY

Test description: Test can be performed on whole blood, tissue, skin lesions, and CSF

VASOACTIVE INTESTINAL PEPTIDE (VIP)

Normal: <50 pg/ml
Elevated in: Pancreatic VIP-omas, neuroblastoma, pancreatic islet cell hyperplasia, liver disease, MEN I, ganglioneuroma, ganglioneuroblastoma

VDRL

Normal range: Negative
Positive test: Syphilis, other treponemal diseases (yaws, pinta, bejel)

NOTE: A false-positive test may be seen in patients with systemic lupus erythematosus and other autoimmune diseases, infectious mononucleosis, HIV, atypical pneumonia, malaria, leprosy, typhus fever, rat-bite fever, relapsing fever.

NOTE: See Table 112 for interpretation of serologic tests for syphilis.

VISCOSITY (serum)

Normal range: 1.4-1.8 relative to water (1.10-1.22 centipoise)
Elevated in: Monoclonal gammopathies (Waldenström's macroglobulinemia, multiple myeloma), hyperfibrinogenemia, systemic lupus erythematosus, rheumatoid arthritis, polycythemia, leukemia

VITAMIN B_{12} (cobalamin)

See Box 35 for etiopathophysiologic classification of cobalamin deficiency. Causes of false-positive and false-negative serum cobalamin levels are summarized in Table 113. Table 114 describes causes of megaloblastosis not responding to therapy with cobalamin or folate. Table 115 summarizes indications for prophylaxis with cobalamin or folate.

Normal:
190-900 ng/ml

Causes of vitamin B_{12} deficiency:

a. Pernicious anemia (antibodies against intrinsic factor and gastric parietal cells)
b. Dietary (strict lacto-ovo vegetarians, food faddists)
c. Malabsorption (achlorhydria, gastrectomy, ileal resection, pancreatic insufficiency, drugs [omeprazole, cholestyramine])

Falsely low levels occur in patients with severe folate deficiency, in patients using high doses of ascorbic acid, and when cobalamin levels are measured after nuclear medicine studies (radioactivity interferes with cobalamin radioimmunoassay).

Falsely high or normal levels in patients with cobalamin deficiency can occur in severe liver disease and chronic granulocytic leukemia.

The absence of anemia or macrocytosis does not exclude the diagnosis of cobalamin deficiency.

VITAMIN D, 1,25 DIHYDROXY CALCIFEROL

Normal: 16-65 pg/ml
Elevated in: Tumor calcinosis, primary hyperparathyroidism, sarcoidosis, tuberculosis, idiopathic hypercalciuria
Decreased in: Nutritional deficiency, postmenopausal osteoporosis, chronic renal failure, hypoparathyroidism, tumor-induced osteomalacia, rickets, elevated blood lead levels. Table 116 compares vitamin D levels in various disorders. Fig. 59 illustrates vitamin D physiology.

VITAMIN K

Normal: 0.10-2.20 ng/ml
Decreased in: Primary biliary cirrhosis, anticoagulants, antibiotics, cholestyramine, GI disease, pancreatic disease, cystic fibrosis, obstructive jaundice, hypoprothrombinemia, hemorrhagic disease of the newborn

VON WILLEBRAND FACTOR

Normal: Levels vary according to blood type; blood type O: 50-150 U/dl; blood type non-O: 90-200 U/dl
Decreased in: von Willebrand's disease (however, in type II von Willebrand's disease the antigen may be normal but the function is impaired)

TABLE 112 Interpretation of Serologic Tests for Syphilis*

Nontreponemal Tests	Treponemal Tests	Interpretation of Finding: Is Syphilis Present?*
Nonreactive	Nonreactive	Early primary syphilis is not ruled out by negative serologic tests. Early syphilis is present in 13%-30% of patients who have a negative microhemagglutination *Treponema pallidum* test; in about 30% of patients who present with chancre but have a nonreactive reagin test; and in about 10% of patients who have a negative FTA-ABS test. Late syphilis is present in a very small fraction of patients. Adequately treated syphilis in remote past may produce these results, but treponemal tests usually remain reactive.
	Reactive	Observed in about 10% of patients with chancre. The treponemal tests may turn positive shortly before the reagin tests. Reagin tests repeated after several days are generally positive. In adequately treated early syphilis, the reagin test may return to nonreactive within 1-2 yr, whereas the treponemal tests generally do not. Late syphilis is not ruled out by a negative reagin test. The sensitivity of the reagin tests is lower than that of treponemal tests in untreated late syphilis. In secondary syphilis, rarely, a highly reactive serum appears negative when tested undiluted with a reagin test because flocculation is inhibited by relative antibody excess. Not reported to occur with treponemal tests. Quantitative reagin tests are positive. False-positive treponemal tests occur in 40% of patients with Lyme disease.
Reactive	Nonreactive borderline (FTA-ABS)	Finding is not diagnostic of syphilis but constitutes a classic biologic false-positive reaction. Not diagnostic of syphilis; most patients (90%) with this pattern do not develop clinical or serologic evidence of syphilis. Repeat test is indicated. Chronic borderline results are associated with a variety of conditions other than syphilis.
	Beaded (FTA-ABS)	Not diagnostic of syphilis. Seen with collagen vascular disease.
	Reactive	Findings diagnostic of syphilis or other treponemal disease. In adequately treated syphilis, one would expect (1) a sustained fourfold drop in titer of reagin test, although reagin test may remain positive after adequate therapy; (2) treponemal tests remain positive after adequate therapy. Concurrent false-positive results on both nontreponemal and treponemal tests could occur in rare instances. It may be impossible to rule out syphilis in an individual with this test profile.

FTA-ABS, Fluorescent treponemal antibody, absorbed.
*Serologic data must always be interpreted in the light of a total clinical evaluation. Diagnosis based on serologic criteria alone is fraught with error. Serologic tests apparently in conflict with clinical diagnosis should be confirmed by repetition or possibly referral to a reference laboratory.
From Stein JH (ed): *Internal medicine,* ed 4, St Louis, 1994, Mosby.

BOX 35 Etiopathophysiologic Classification of Cobalamin Deficiency

- Nutritional cobalamin deficiency (insufficient cobalamin intake)—vegetarians, poverty-imposed near-vegetarians, breastfed infants of mothers with pernicious anemia
- Abnormal intragastric events (inadequate proteolysis of food cobalamin)—atrophic gastritis, hypochlorhydria, proton pump inhibitors, H_2 blockers
- Loss/atrophy of gastric oxyntic mucosa (deficient intrinsic factor [IF] molecules)—total or partial gastrectomy, adult and juvenile pernicious anemia, caustic destruction (lye)
- Abnormal events in the small bowel lumen
  - Inadequate pancreatic protease (R factor–cobalamin not degraded, cobalamin not transferred to IF)
  - Insufficient pancreatic protease—pancreatic insufficiency
  - Inactivation of pancreatic protease—Zollinger-Ellison syndrome
  - Usurping of luminal cobalamin (inadequate binding of cobalamin to IF)
  - By bacteria-stasis syndromes (blind loops, pouches of diverticulosis, strictures, fistulas, anastomosis), impaired bowel motility (scleroderma), hypogammaglobulinemia
  - By *Diphyllobothrium latum* (fish tapeworm)
- Disorders of ileal mucosa/IF-cobalamin receptors (IF-cobalamin not bound to IF-cobalamin receptors [cubam receptors])
  - Diminished or absent cubam receptors—ileal bypass/resection/fistula
  - Abnormal mucosal architecture/function—tropical/nontropical sprue, Crohn disease, tuberculous ileitis, amyloidosis
  - Cubam receptor defects—Imerslund-Gräsbeck syndrome
  - Drug-effects—metformin, cholestyramine, colchicine, neomycin
- Disorders of plasma cobalamin transport (transcobalamin [TCII]-cobalamin not delivered to TCII receptors)—congenital TCII deficiency, defective binding of TCII-cobalamin to TCII receptors (rare)
  - Metabolic disorders (cobalamin not used by cell)
  - Inborn enzyme errors—cblA to cblG disorders
  - Acquired disorders (cobalamin inactivated by irreversible oxidation)—nitrous oxide

From Hoffman R: *Hematology: basic principles and practice,* ed 6, Philadelphia, Saunders, 2013.

TABLE 113 Serum Cobalamin: False-Positive and False-Negative Test Results

Falsely Low Serum Cobalamin in the Absence of True Cobalamin Deficiency
Folate deficiency (one-third of patients)
Multiple myeloma
TCI deficiency
Megadose vitamin C therapy
Falsely Raised Cobalamin Levels in the Presence of True Deficiency*
Cobalamin binders (TCI and II) increased (e.g., myeloproliferative states, hepatomas, and fibrolamellar hepatic tumors)
TCII-producing macrophages are activated (e.g., autoimmune diseases, monoblastic leukemias and lymphomas)
Release of cobalamin from hepatocytes (e.g., active liver disease)
High serum anti-IF antibody titer

IF, Intrinsic factor; *TC,* transcobalamin.

*Although a low serum cobalamin level is not synonymous with cobalamin deficiency, 5% of patients with true cobalamin deficiency have low-normal cobalamin levels, a potentially serious problem because the patient's underlying cobalamin deficiency will progress if uncorrected.

From Hoffman R et al: *Hematology, basic principles and practice,* ed 6, Philadelphia, 2013, Saunders.

TABLE 114 Causes of Megaloblastosis Not Responding to Therapy with Cobalamin or Folate

Wrong Diagnosis
Combined folate and cobalamin deficiencies being treated with only one vitamin
Associated iron deficiency
Associated hemoglobinopathy (e.g., sickle cell disease, thalassemia)
Associated anemia of chronic disease
Associated hypothyroidism

From Hoffman R: *Hematology, basic principles and practice,* ed 7, Philadelphia, 2018, Elsevier.

TABLE 115 Indications for Prophylaxis with Cobalamin or Folate

Prophylaxis with Cobalamin
Infants on specialized diets[a]
Premature infants
Infants of mothers with pernicious anemia[a]
Infants and children of mothers with nutritional cobalamin deficiency
Vegetarianism and poverty-imposed near-vegetarianism[a]
Total gastrectomy[b]
Prophylaxis with Folic Acid[c]
All women contemplating pregnancy (at least 400 μg/day)[d]
Pregnancy and lactation, premature infants
Mothers at risk for delivery of infants with neural tube defects[e,f]
Hemolytic anemias/hyperproliferative hematologic states
Patients with rheumatoid arthritis or psoriasis on therapy with methotrexate[g]
Patients on antiepileptic drugs
Patients with ulcerative colitis

[a]For vegetarians, prophylaxis with cobalamin (5- to 10-μg tablet/day) orally should suffice. In all other conditions involving any abnormality of cobalamin absorption, cobalamin tablets of 1000 μg/day should be administered orally to ensure that cobalamin transport by passive diffusion across the intestine is sufficient to meet daily needs.

[b]Consider late development of cobalamin deficiency and iron malabsorption (prophylaxis with oral cobalamin and iron).

[c]Ensure that the patient does not have a cobalamin deficiency before initiating long-term folate prophylaxis.

[d]For prevention of first occurrence of neural tube defects.

[e]Previous delivery of a child with neural tube defects (e.g., anencephaly, spina bifida, meningocele) imparts a 10-fold greater risk for subsequent delivery of infant with neural tube defects.

[f]Folic acid (4 mg/day) administered periconceptionally and throughout the first trimester.

[g]To reduce toxicity of the antifolate.

From Hoffman R: *Hematology, basic principles and practice,* ed 7, Philadelphia, 2018, Elsevier.

TABLE 116 Serum Calcium, Phosphate, and Vitamin D Levels in Various Disorders

Disorder	Calcium	25(OH)D	1,25(OH)D	Phosphate
25(OH)D intoxication	High	High	Low, normal	Normal, high
Primary hyperparathyroidism	High	Normal	Normal, high	Low
Secondary hyperparathyroidism	Low	Low, normal, high	Low, normal, high	Low, normal, high
Tertiary hyperparathyroidism	Normal, high*	Low, normal, high	Low, normal, high	Low, normal, high
Malignancy	High	Normal	Low, normal	Low
Vitamin D deficiency	Low	Low	Low, normal, high	Low
Renal failure	Low	Normal	Low	High
Hyperphosphatemia	Low	Normal	Low	High
Vitamin D rickets type I, II	Low	Normal, high	Low, normal, high	Low
Granulomatous diseases (sarcoid/TB)	High	Low, normal, high	High	Normal, high
Postmenopausal osteoporosis	Normal	Normal	Normal	Normal
Senile osteoporosis	Normal	Normal	Normal	Normal
Osteomalacia	Low, normal	Low, normal	Low	Low, normal, high

*Calcium may be normal in the setting of concurrent 1,25$(OH)_2D_3$ deficiency.
From McPherson RA, Pincus MR: *Henry's clinical diagnosis and management by laboratory methods*, ed 23, St Louis, 2017, Elsevier.

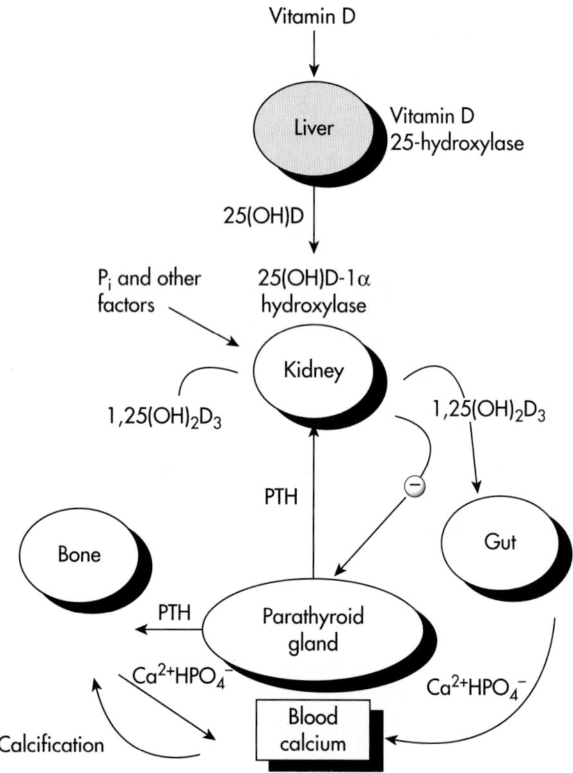

FIG. 59 Vitamin D physiology. *P_i*, Inorganic phosphate; *PTH,* parathyroid hormone. (From Ronco C: *Critical care nephrology*, ed 3, Philadelphia, 2019, Elsevier.)

Clinical Practice Guidelines

Childhood and Adolescent Immunizations

TABLE 1 Recommended Immunization Schedule for Children and Adolescents Aged 18 Years or Younger—United States, 2019. (For those who fall behind or start late, see that catch-up schedule [Table 2])

These recommendations must be read with the footnotes that follow. For those who fall behind or start late, provide catch-up vaccination at the earliest opportunity as indicated by the divided bars. To determine minimum intervals between doses, see the catch-up schedule (Table 2). School entry and adolescent vaccine age groups are shaded in gray.

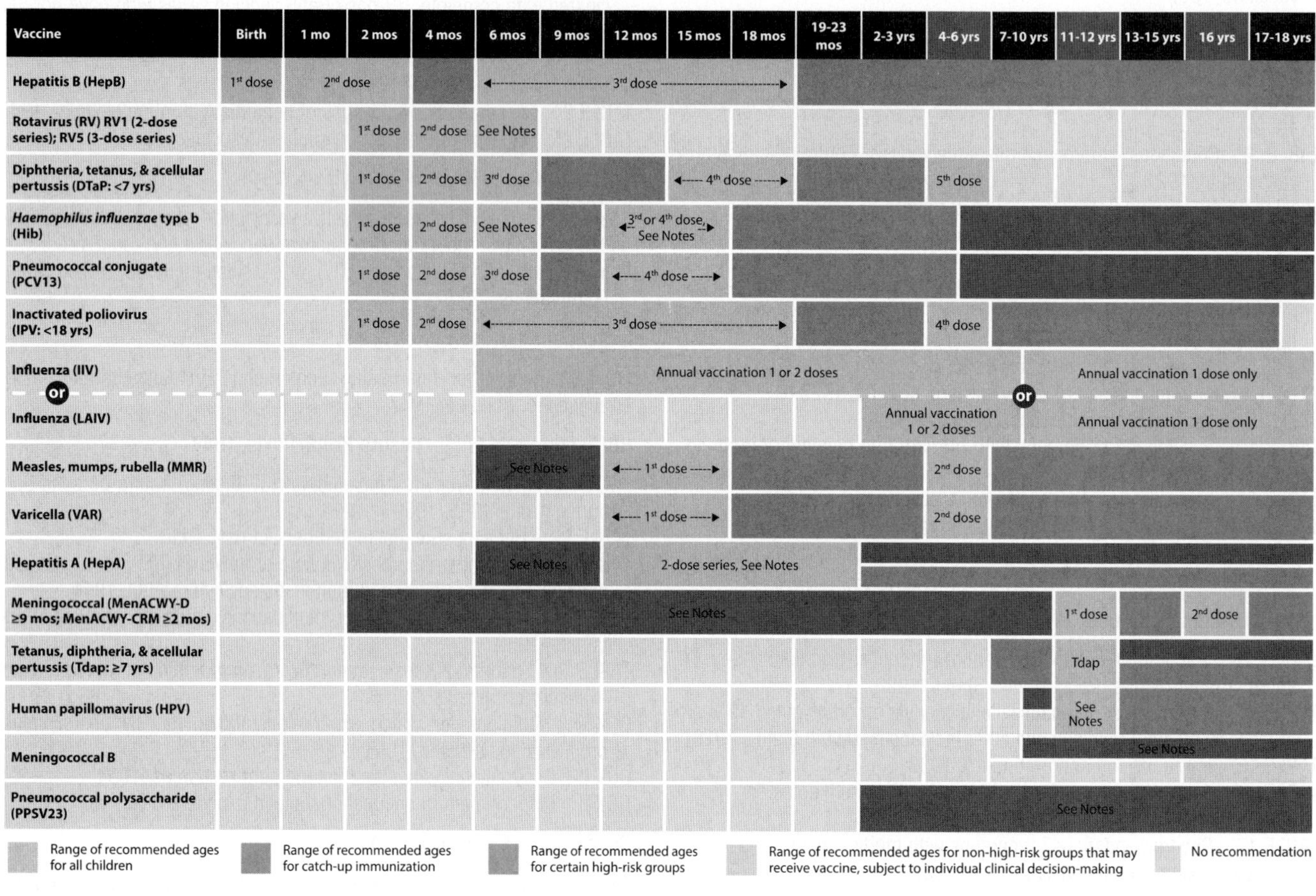

Vaccine	Birth	1 mo	2 mos	4 mos	6 mos	9 mos	12 mos	15 mos	18 mos	19-23 mos	2-3 yrs	4-6 yrs	7-10 yrs	11-12 yrs	13-15 yrs	16 yrs	17-18 yrs
Hepatitis B (HepB)	1st dose	2nd dose			←3rd dose→												
Rotavirus (RV) RV1 (2-dose series); RV5 (3-dose series)			1st dose	2nd dose	See Notes												
Diphtheria, tetanus, & acellular pertussis (DTaP: <7 yrs)			1st dose	2nd dose	3rd dose			←4th dose→				5th dose					
Haemophilus influenzae type b (Hib)			1st dose	2nd dose	See Notes		←3rd or 4th dose, See Notes→										
Pneumococcal conjugate (PCV13)			1st dose	2nd dose	3rd dose		←4th dose→										
Inactivated poliovirus (IPV: <18 yrs)			1st dose	2nd dose	←3rd dose→							4th dose					
Influenza (IIV)					Annual vaccination 1 or 2 doses									Annual vaccination 1 dose only			
or														or			
Influenza (LAIV)											Annual vaccination 1 or 2 doses			Annual vaccination 1 dose only			
Measles, mumps, rubella (MMR)					See Notes		←1st dose→					2nd dose					
Varicella (VAR)							←1st dose→					2nd dose					
Hepatitis A (HepA)					See Notes		2-dose series, See Notes										
Meningococcal (MenACWY-D ≥9 mos; MenACWY-CRM ≥2 mos)			See Notes											1st dose		2nd dose	
Tetanus, diphtheria, & acellular pertussis (Tdap: ≥7 yrs)														Tdap			
Human papillomavirus (HPV)														See Notes			
Meningococcal B														See Notes			
Pneumococcal polysaccharide (PPSV23)											See Notes						

Range of recommended ages for all children | Range of recommended ages for catch-up immunization | Range of recommended ages for certain high-risk groups | Range of recommended ages for non-high-risk groups that may receive vaccine, subject to individual clinical decision-making | No recommendation

TABLE 2 Catch-up Immunization Schedule for Persons Aged 4 Months Through 18 Years Who Start Late or Who Are More Than 1 Month Behind—United States, 2019

The table below provides catch-up schedules and minimum intervals between doses for children whose vaccinations have been delayed. A vaccine series does not need to be restarted, regardless of the time that has elapsed between doses. Use the section appropriate for the child's age. Always use this table in conjunction with Table 1 and the footnotes that follow.

Vaccine	Minimum Age for Dose 1	Minimum Interval Between Doses			
		Dose 1 to Dose 2	Dose 2 to Dose 3	Dose 3 to Dose 4	Dose 4 to Dose 5
Children age 4 months through 6 years					
Hepatitis B	Birth	**4 weeks**	**8 weeks *and* at least 16 weeks after first dose.** Minimum age for the final dose is 24 weeks.		
Rotavirus	6 weeks Maximum age for first dose is 14 weeks, 6 days	**4 weeks**	**4 weeks** Maximum age for final dose is 8 months, 0 days.		
Diphtheria, tetanus, and acellular pertussis	6 weeks	**4 weeks**	**4 weeks**	**6 months**	**6 months**
Haemophilus influenzae type b	6 weeks	**No further doses needed** if first dose was administered at age 15 months or older. **4 weeks** if first dose was administered before the 1st birthday. **8 weeks (as final dose)** if first dose was administered at age 12 through 14 months.	**No further doses needed** if previous dose was administered at age 15 months or older. **4 weeks** if current age is younger than 12 months ***and*** first dose was administered at younger than age 7 months, ***and*** at least 1 previous dose was PRP-T (ActHib, Pentacel, Hiberix) or unknown. **8 weeks *and* age 12 through 59 months (as final dose)** if current age is younger than 12 months ***and*** first dose was administered at age 7 through 11 months; OR if current age is 12 through 59 months ***and*** first dose was administered before the 1st birthday, ***and*** second dose administered at younger than 15 months; OR if both doses were PRP-OMP (PedvaxHIB; Comvax) ***and*** were administered before the 1st birthday.	**8 weeks (as final dose)** This dose only necessary for children age 12 through 59 months who received 3 doses before the 1st birthday.	
Pneumococcal conjugate	6 weeks	**No further doses needed** for healthy children if first dose was administered at age 24 months or older. **4 weeks** if first dose administered before the 1st birthday. **8 weeks (as final dose for healthy children)** if first dose was administered at the 1st birthday or after.	**No further doses needed** for healthy children if previous dose administered at age 24 months or older. **4 weeks** if current age is younger than 12 months and previous dose given at <7 months old. **8 weeks (as final dose for healthy children)** if previous dose given between 7-11 months (wait until at least 12 months old); OR if current age is 12 months or older and at least 1 dose was given before age 12 months.	**8 weeks (as final dose)** This **dose** only necessary for children age 12 through 59 months who received 3 doses before age 12 months or for children at high risk who received 3 doses at any age.	
Inactivated poliovirus	6 weeks	**4 weeks**	4 weeks if current age is < 4 years. 6 months (as final dose) if current age is 4 years or older.	**6 months** (minimum age 4 years for final dose).	
Measles, mumps, rubella	12 months	**4 weeks**			
Varicella	12 months	**3 months**			
Hepatitis A	12 months	**6 months**			
Meningococcal	2 months MenACWY-CRM 9 months MenACWY-D	**8 weeks**	See Notes	See Notes	
Children and adolescents age 7 through 18 years					
Meningococcal	Not Applicable (N/A)	**8 weeks**			
Tetanus, diphtheria; tetanus, diphtheria, and acellular pertussis	7 years	**4 weeks**	**4 weeks** if first dose of DTaP/DT was administered before the 1st birthday. **6 months (as final dose)** if first dose of DTaP/DT or Tdap/Td was administered at or after the 1st birthday.	**6 months** if first dose of DTaP/DT was administered before the 1st birthday.	
Human papillomavirus	9 years	**Routine dosing intervals are recommended.**			
Hepatitis A	N/A	**6 months**			
Hepatitis B	N/A	**4 weeks**	**8 weeks *and*** at least 16 weeks after first dose.		
Inactivated poliovirus	N/A	**4 weeks**	**6 months** A fourth dose is not necessary if the third dose was administered at age 4 years or older and at least 6 months after the previous dose.	A fourth dose of IPV is indicated if all previous doses were administered at <4 years or if the third dose was administered <6 months after the second dose.	
Measles, mumps, rubella	N/A	**4 weeks**			
Varicella	N/A	**3 months** if younger than age 13 years. **4 weeks** if age 13 years or older.			

Footnotes — Recommended Child and Adolescent Immunization Schedule for ages 18 years or younger, United States, 2019

For vaccine recommendations for persons 19 years of age and older, see the Recommended Adult Immunization Schedule.

Additional information

- Consult relevant ACIP statements for detailed recommendations at www.cdc.gov/vaccines/hcp/acip-recs/index.html.
- For information on contraindications and precautions for the use of a vaccine, consult the General Best Practice Guidelines for Immunization and relevant ACIP statements at www.cdc.gov/vaccines/hcp/acip-recs/index.html.
- For calculating intervals between doses, 4 weeks = 28 days. Intervals of ≥4 months are determined by calendar months.
- Within a number range (e.g., 12–18), a dash (–) should be read as "through."
- Vaccine doses administered ≤4 days before the minimum age or interval are considered valid. Doses of any vaccine administered ≥5 days earlier than the minimum age or minimum interval should not be counted as valid and should be repeated as age-appropriate. The repeat dose should be spaced after the invalid dose by the recommended minimum interval. For further details, see Table 3-1, Recommended and minimum ages and intervals between vaccine doses, in General Best Practice Guidelines for Immunization at www.cdc.gov/vaccines/hcp/acip-recs/general-recs/timing.html.
- Information on travel vaccine requirements and recommendations is available at wwwnc.cdc.gov/travel/.
- For vaccination of persons with immunodeficiencies, see Table 8-1, Vaccination of persons with primary and secondary immunodeficiencies, in General Best Practice Guidelines for Immunization at www.cdc.gov/vaccines/hcp/acip-recs/general-recs/immunocompetence.html, and Immunization in Special Clinical Circumstances (In: Kimberlin DW, Brady MT, Jackson MA, Long SS, eds. *Red Book: 2018 Report of the Committee on Infectious Diseases*. 31st ed. Itasca, IL: American Academy of Pediatrics; 2018:67–111).
- For information regarding vaccination in the setting of a vaccine-preventable disease outbreak, contact your state or local health department.
- The National Vaccine Injury Compensation Program (VICP) is a no-fault alternative to the traditional legal system for resolving vaccine injury claims. All routine child and adolescent vaccines are covered by VICP except for pneumococcal polysaccharide vaccine (PPSV23). For more information, see www.hrsa.gov/vaccinecompensation/index.html.

1. Diphtheria, tetanus, and pertussis (DTaP) vaccination (minimum age: 6 weeks [4 years for Kinrix or Quadracel])

Routine vaccination
- 5-dose series at 2, 4, 6, 15–18 months, 4–6 years
  - **Prospectively:** Dose 4 may be given as early as age 12 months if at least 6 months have elapsed since dose 3.
  - **Retrospectively:** A 4th dose that was inadvertently given as early as 12 months may be counted if at least 4 months have elapsed since dose 3.

Catch-up vaccination
- Dose 5 is not necessary if dose 4 was administered at age 4 years or older.
- For other catch-up guidance, see Table 2.

2. *Haemophilus influenzae* type b vaccination (minimum age: 6 weeks)

Routine vaccination
- **ActHIB, Hiberix, or Pentacel:** 4-dose series at 2, 4, 6, 12–15 months
- **PedvaxHIB:** 3-dose series at 2, 4, 12–15 months

Catch-up vaccination
- **Dose 1 at 7–11 months:** Administer dose 2 at least 4 weeks later and dose 3 (final dose) at 12–15 months or 8 weeks after dose 2 (whichever is later).
- **Dose 1 at 12–14 months:** Administer dose 2 (final dose) at least 8 weeks after dose 1.
- **Dose 1 before 12 months and dose 2 before 15 months:** Administer dose 3 (final dose) 8 weeks after dose 2.
- **2 doses of PedvaxHIB before 12 months:** Administer dose 3 (final dose) at 12–59 months and at least 8 weeks after dose 2.
- **Unvaccinated at 15–59 months:** 1 dose
- For other catch-up guidance, see Table 2.

Special situations
- **Chemotherapy or radiation treatment:**
  12–59 months
  - Unvaccinated or only 1 dose before age 12 months: 2 doses, 8 weeks apart
  - 2 or more doses before age 12 months: 1 dose at least 8 weeks after previous dose

  Doses administered within 14 days of starting therapy or during therapy should be repeated at least 3 months after therapy completion.
- **Hematopoietic stem cell transplant (HSCT):**
  - 3-dose series 4 weeks apart starting 6 to 12 months after successful transplant regardless of Hib vaccination history
- **Anatomic or functional asplenia (including sickle cell disease):**
  12–59 months
  - Unvaccinated or only 1 dose before 12 months: 2 doses, 8 weeks apart
  - 2 or more doses before 12 months:1 dose at least 8 weeks after previous dose

  Unvaccinated persons age 5 years or older*
  - 1 dose
- **Elective splenectomy:**
  Unvaccinated persons age 15 months or older*
  - 1 dose (preferably at least 14 days before procedure)
- **HIV infection:**
  12–59 months
  - Unvaccinated or only 1 dose before age 12 months: 2 doses, 8 weeks apart
  - 2 or more doses before age 12 months: 1 dose at least 8 weeks after previous dose

  Unvaccinated persons age 5–18 years*
  - 1 dose
- **Immunoglobulin deficiency, early component complement deficiency:**
  12–59 months
  - Unvaccinated or only 1 dose before age 12 months: 2 doses, 8 weeks apart
  - 2 or more doses before age 12 months: 1 dose at least 8 weeks after previous dose

**Unvaccinated* = Less than routine series (through 14 months) OR no doses (14 months or older)

3. Hepatitis A vaccination (minimum age: 12 months for routine vaccination)

Routine vaccination
- 2-dose series (**Havrix** 6–12 months apart or **Vaqta** 6–18 months apart, minimum interval 6 months); a series begun before the 2nd birthday should be completed even if the child turns 2 before the second dose is administered.

Catch-up vaccination
- Anyone 2 years of age or older may receive HepA vaccine if desired. Minimum interval between doses: 6 months
- Adolescents 18 years and older may receive the combined HepA and HepB vaccine, **Twinrix**, as a 3-dose series (0, 1, and 6 months) or 4-dose series (0, 7, and 21–30 days, followed by a dose at 12 months).

International travel
- Persons traveling to or working in countries with high or intermediate endemic hepatitis A (wwwnc.cdc.gov/travel/):
  - **Infants age 6–11 months:** 1 dose before departure; revaccinate with 2 doses, separated by 6–18 months, between 12 to 23 months of age.
  - **Unvaccinated age 12 months and older:** 1st dose as soon as travel considered

Special situations

At risk for hepatitis A infection: 2-dose series as above
- **Chronic liver disease**
- **Clotting factor disorders**
- **Men who have sex with men**
- **Injection or non-injection drug use**
- **Homelessness**
- **Work with hepatitis A virus** in research laboratory or nonhuman primates with hepatitis A infection

- **Travel** in countries with high or intermediate endemic hepatitis A
- **Close, personal contact with international adoptee** (e.g., household or regular babysitting) in first 60 days after arrival from country with high or intermediate endemic hepatitis A (administer dose 1 as soon as adoption is planned, at least 2 weeks before adoptee's arrival)

4. **Hepatitis B vaccination**
(minimum age: birth)

Birth dose (monovalent HepB vaccine only)

- **Mother is HBsAg-negative:** 1 dose within 24 hours of birth for **all** medically stable infants ≥2,000 grams. Infants <2,000 grams: administer 1 dose at chronological age 1 month or hospital discharge.
- **Mother is HBsAg-positive:**
  - Administer **HepB vaccine** and **0.5 mL of hepatitis B immune globulin (HBIG)** (at separate anatomic sites) within 12 hours of birth, regardless of birth weight. For infants <2,000 grams, administer 3 additional doses of vaccine (total of 4 doses) beginning at age 1 month.
  - Test for HBsAg and anti-HBs at age 9–12 months. If HepB series is delayed, test 1–2 months after final dose.
- **Mother's HBsAg status is unknown:**
  - Administer **HepB vaccine** within 12 hours of birth, regardless of birth weight.
  - For infants <2,000 grams, administer **0.5 mL of HBIG** in addition to HepB vaccine within 12 hours of birth. Administer 3 additional doses of vaccine (total of 4 doses) beginning at age 1 month.
  - Determine mother's HBsAg status as soon as possible. If mother is HBsAg-positive, administer **0.5 mL of HBIG** to infants ≥2,000 grams as soon as possible, but no later than 7 days of age.

Routine series

- 3-dose series at 0, 1–2, 6–18 months (use monovalent HepB vaccine for doses administered before age 6 weeks)
- Infants who did not receive a birth dose should begin the series as soon as feasible (see Table 2).
- Administration of **4 doses** is permitted when a combination vaccine containing HepB is used after the birth dose.
- **Minimum age** for the final (3rd or 4th) dose: 24 weeks
- **Minimum intervals:** dose 1 to dose 2: 4 weeks / dose 2 to dose 3: 8 weeks / dose 1 to dose 3: 16 weeks (when 4 doses are administered, substitute "dose 4" for "dose 3" in these calculations)

Catch-up vaccination

- Unvaccinated persons should complete a 3-dose series at 0, 1–2, 6 months.
- Adolescents age 11–15 years may use an alternative 2-dose schedule with at least 4 months between doses (adult formulation **Recombivax HB** only).
- Adolescents 18 years and older may receive a 2-dose series of HepB **(Heplisav-B)** at least 4 weeks apart.
- Adolescents 18 years and older may receive the combined HepA and HepB vaccine, **Twinrix**, as a 3-dose series (0, 1, and 6 months) or 4-dose series (0, 7, and 21–30 days, followed by a dose at 12 months).
- For other catch-up guidance, see Table 2.

5. **Human papillomavirus vaccination**
(minimum age: 9 years)

Routine and catch-up vaccination

- HPV vaccination routinely recommended for all adolescents **age 11–12 years (can start at age 9 years)** and through age 18 years if not previously adequately vaccinated
- 2- or 3-dose series depending on age at initial vaccination:
  - **Age 9 through 14 years at initial vaccination:** 2-dose series at 0, 6–12 months (minimum interval: 5 months; repeat dose if administered too soon)
  - **Age 15 years or older at initial vaccination:** 3-dose series at 0, 1–2 months, 6 months (minimum intervals: dose 1 to dose 2: 4 weeks / dose 2 to dose 3: 12 weeks / dose 1 to dose 3: 5 months; repeat dose if administered too soon)
- If completed valid vaccination series with any HPV vaccine, no additional doses needed

Special situations

- **Immunocompromising conditions, including HIV infection:** 3-dose series as above
- **History of sexual abuse or assault**: Start at age 9 years
- **Pregnancy:** HPV vaccination not recommended until after pregnancy; no intervention needed if vaccinated while pregnant; pregnancy testing not needed before vaccination

6. **Inactivated poliovirus vaccination**
(minimum age: 6 weeks)

Routine vaccination

- 4-dose series at ages 2, 4, 6–18 months, 4–6 years; administer the final dose on or after the 4th birthday and at least 6 months after the previous dose.
- 4 or more doses of IPV can be administered before the 4th birthday when a combination vaccine containing IPV is used. However, a dose is still recommended after the 4th birthday and at least 6 months after the previous dose.

Catch-up vaccination

- In the first 6 months of life, use minimum ages and intervals only for travel to a polio-endemic region or during an outbreak.
- IPV is not routinely recommended for U.S. residents 18 years and older.

Series containing oral polio vaccine (OPV), either mixed OPVIPV or OPV-only series:

- Total number of doses needed to complete the series is the same as that recommended for the U.S. IPV schedule. See www.cdc.gov/mmwr/volumes/66/wr/mm6601a6.htm?s_cid=mm6601a6_w.
- Only trivalent OPV (tOPV) counts toward the U.S. vaccination requirements. For guidance to assess doses documented as "OPV," see www.cdc.gov/mmwr/volumes/66/wr/mm6606a7.htm?s_cid=mm6606a7_w.
- For other catch-up guidance, see Table 2.

7. **Influenza vaccination**
(minimum age: 6 months [IIV], 2 years [LAIV], 18 years [RIV])

Routine vaccination

- 1 dose any influenza vaccine appropriate for age and health status annually (2 doses separated by at least 4 weeks for **children 6 months–8 years** who did not receive at least 2 doses of influenza vaccine before July 1, 2018)

Special situations

- **Egg allergy, hives only:** Any influenza vaccine appropriate for age and health status annually
- **Egg allergy more severe than hives** (e.g., angioedema, respiratory distress): Any influenza vaccine appropriate for age and health status annually in medical setting under supervision of health care provider who can recognize and manage severe allergic conditions
- **LAIV should not be used** for those with a history of severe allergic reaction to any component of the vaccine (excluding egg) or to a previous dose of any influenza vaccine, children and adolescents receiving concomitant aspirin or salicylate-containing medications, children age 2 through 4 years with a history of asthma or wheezing, those who are immunocompromised due to any cause (including immunosuppression caused by medications and HIV infection), anatomic and functional asplenia, cochlear implants, cerebrospinal fluid-oropharyngeal communication, close contacts and caregivers of severely immunosuppressed persons who require a protected environment, pregnancy, and persons who have received influenza antiviral medications within the previous 48 hours.

8. **Measles, mumps, and rubella vaccination**
(minimum age: 12 months for routine vaccination)

Routine vaccination

- 2-dose series at 12–15 months, 4–6 years
- Dose 2 may be administered as early as 4 weeks after dose 1.

Catch-up vaccination

- Unvaccinated children and adolescents: 2 doses at least 4 weeks apart
- The maximum age for use of *MMRV* is 12 years.

Continued

Special situations

International travel

- **Infants age 6–11 months:** 1 dose before departure; revaccinate with 2 doses at 12–15 months (12 months for children in high-risk areas) and dose 2 as early as 4 weeks later.
- **Unvaccinated children age 12 months and older:** 2-dose series at least 4 weeks apart before departure

9. **Meningococcal serogroup A,C,W,Y vaccination** (minimum age: 2 months [MenACWY-CRM, Menveo], 9 months [MenACWY-D, Menactra])

Routine vaccination

- 2-dose series: 11–12 years, 16 years

Catch-up vaccination

- Age 13–15 years: 1 dose now and booster at age 16–18 years (minimum interval: 8 weeks)
- Age 16–18 years: 1 dose

Special situations

Anatomic or functional asplenia (including sickle cell disease), HIV infection, persistent complement component deficiency, eculizumab use:

- **Menveo**
  - Dose 1 at age 8 weeks: 4-dose series at 2, 4, 6, 12 months
  - Dose 1 at age 7–23 months: 2-dose series (dose 2 at least 12 weeks after dose 1 and after the 1st birthday)
  - Dose 1 at age 24 months or older: 2-dose series at least 8 weeks apart
- **Menactra**
  - **Persistent complement component deficiency:**
    - Age 9–23 months: 2 doses at least 12 weeks apart
    - Age 24 months or older: 2 doses at least 8 weeks apart
  - **Anatomic or functional asplenia, sickle cell disease, or HIV infection:**
    - **Age 9–23 months:** Not recommended
    - **24 months or older:** 2 doses at least 8 weeks apart
    - **Menactra** must be administered at least 4 weeks after completion of PCV13 series.

Travel in countries with hyperendemic or epidemic meningococcal disease, including countries in the African meningitis belt or during the Hajj (wwwnc.cdc.gov/travel/):

- Children age less than 24 months:
  - **Menveo (age 2–23 months):**
    - Dose 1 at 8 weeks: 4-dose series at 2, 4, 6, 12 months
    - Dose 1 at 7–23 months: 2-dose series (dose 2 at least 12 weeks after dose 1 and after the 1st birthday)
  - **Menactra (age 9–23 months):**
    - 2-dose series (dose 2 at least 12 weeks after dose 1; dose 2 may be administered as early as 8 weeks after dose 1 in travelers)
- Children age 2 years or older: 1 dose **Menveo** or **Menactra**

First-year college students who live in residential housing (if not previously vaccinated at age 16 years or older) or military recruits:

- 1 dose **Menveo** or **Menactra**

Note: Menactra should be administered either before or at the same time as DTaP. For MenACWY booster dose recommendations for groups listed under "Special situations" above and additional meningococcal vaccination information, see meningococcal *MMWR* publications at www.cdc.gov/vaccines/hcp/acip-recs/vacc-specific/mening.html.

10. **Meningococcal serogroup B vaccination** (minimum age: 10 years [MenB-4C, Bexsero; MenB-FHbp, Trumenba])

Clinical discretion

- MenB vaccine may be administered based on individual clinical decision to **adolescents not at increased risk** age 16–23 years (preferred age 16–18 years):
- **Bexsero:** 2-dose series at least 1 month apart
- **Trumenba:** 2-dose series at least 6 months apart; if dose 2 is administered earlier than 6 months, administer a 3rd dose at least 4 months after dose 2.

Special situations

Anatomic or functional asplenia (including sickle cell disease), persistent complement component deficiency, eculizumab use:

- **Bexsero:** 2-dose series at least 1 month apart
- **Trumenba:** 3-dose series at 0, 1–2, 6 months

Bexsero and **Trumenba** are not interchangeable; the same product should be used for all doses in a series. For additional meningococcal vaccination information, see meningococcal *MMWR* publications at www.cdc.gov/vaccines/hcp/acip-recs/vacc-specific/mening.html.

11. **Pneumococcal vaccination** (minimum age: 6 weeks [PCV13], 2 years [PPSV23])

Routine vaccination with PCV13

- 4-dose series at 2, 4, 6, 12–15 months

Catch-up vaccination with PCV13

- 1 dose for healthy children age 24–59 months with any incomplete* PCV13 series
- For other catch-up guidance, see Table 2.

Special situations

High-risk conditions below: When both PCV13 and PPSV23 are indicated, administer PCV13 first. PCV13 and PPSV23 should not be administered during same visit.

Chronic heart disease (particularly cyanotic congenital heart disease and cardiac failure); chronic lung disease (including asthma treated with high-dose, oral corticosteroids); diabetes mellitus:

<u>Age 2–5 years</u>

- Any incomplete* series with:
  - 3 PCV13 doses: 1 dose PCV13 (at least 8 weeks after any prior PCV13 dose)
  - Less than 3 PCV13 doses: 2 doses PCV13 (8 weeks after the most recent dose and administered 8 weeks apart)
- No history of PPSV23: 1 dose PPSV23 (at least 8 weeks afterany prior PCV13 dose)

<u>Age 6–18 years</u>

- No history of PPSV23: 1 dose PPSV23 (at least 8 weeks after any prior PCV13 dose)

Cerebrospinal fluid leak, cochlear implant:

<u>Age 2–5 years</u>

- Any incomplete* series with:
  - 3 PCV13 doses: 1 dose PCV13 (at least 8 weeks after any prior PCV13 dose)
  - Less than 3 PCV13 doses: 2 doses PCV13, 8 weeks after the most recent dose and administered 8 weeks apart
- No history of PPSV23: 1 dose PPSV23 (at least 8 weeks after any prior PCV13 dose)

<u>Age 6–18 years</u>

- No history of either PCV13 or PPSV23: 1 dose PCV13, 1 dose PPSV23 at least 8 weeks later
- Any PCV13 but no PPSV23: 1 dose PPSV23 at least 8 weeks after the most recent dose of PCV13
- PPSV23 but no PCV13: 1 dose PCV13 at least 8 weeks after the most recent dose of PPSV23

Sickle cell disease and other hemoglobinopathies; anatomic or functional asplenia; congenital or acquired immunodeficiency; HIV infection; chronic renal failure; nephrotic syndrome; malignant neoplasms, leukemias, lymphomas, Hodgkin disease, and other diseases associated with treatment with immunosuppressive drugs or radiation therapy; solid organ transplantation; multiple myeloma:

<u>Age 2–5 years</u>

- Any incomplete* series with:
  - 3 PCV13 doses: 1 dose PCV13 (at least 8 weeks after any prior PCV13 dose)
  - Less than 3 PCV13 doses: 2 doses PCV13 (8 weeks after the most recent dose and administered 8 weeks apart)
- No history of PPSV23: 1 dose PPSV23 (at least 8 weeks after any prior PCV13 dose) and a 2nd dose of PPSV23 5 years later

Age 6–18 years

- No history of either PCV13 or PPSV23: 1 dose PCV13, 2 doses PPSV23 (dose 1 of PPSV23 administered 8 weeks after PCV13 and dose 2 of PPSV23 administered at least 5 years after dose 1 of PPSV23)
- Any PCV13 but no PPSV23: 2 doses PPSV23 (dose 1 of PPSV23 administered 8 weeks after the most recent dose of PCV13 and dose 2 of PPSV23 administered at least 5 years after dose 1 of PPSV23)
- PPSV23 but no PCV13: 1 dose PCV13 at least 8 weeks after the most recent PPSV23 dose and a 2nd dose of PPSV23 administered 5 years after dose 1 of PPSV23 and at least 8 weeks after a dose of PCV13

Chronic liver disease, alcoholism:

Age 6–18 years

- No history of PPSV23: 1 dose PPSV23 (at least 8 weeks after any prior PCV13 dose)

*An incomplete series is defined as not having received all doses in either the recommended series or an ageappropriate catch-up series. See Tables 8, 9, and 11 in the ACIP pneumococcal vaccine recommendations (www.cdc.gov/mmwr/pdf/rr/rr5911.pdf) for complete schedule details.

12. **Rotavirus vaccination**
(minimum age: 6 weeks)
Routine vaccination
- **Rotarix:** 2-dose series at 2 and 4 months.
- **RotaTeq:** 3-dose series at 2, 4, and 6 months.

If any dose in the series is either **RotaTeq** or unknown, default to 3-dose series.
Catch-up vaccination
- Do not start the series on or after age 15 weeks, 0 days.
- The maximum age for the final dose is 8 months, 0 days.
- For other catch-up guidance, see Figure 2.

13. **Tetanus, diphtheria, and pertussis (Tdap) vaccination**
(minimum age: 11 years for routine vaccination, 7 years for catch-up vaccination)
Routine vaccination
- **Adolescents age 11–12 years:** 1 dose Tdap
- **Pregnancy:** 1 dose Tdap during each pregnancy, preferably in early part of gestational weeks 27–36
- Tdap may be administered regardless of the interval since the last tetanus- and diphtheria-toxoid-containing vaccine

Catch-up vaccination
- **Adolescents age 13–18 years who have not received Tdap:** 1 dose Tdap, then Td booster every 10 years
- **Persons age 7–18 years not fully immunized with DTaP:** 1 dose Tdap as part of the catch-up series (preferably the first dose); if additional doses are needed, use Td.
- **Children age 7–10 years** who receive Tdap inadvertently or as part of the catch-up series should receive the routine Tdap dose at 11–12 years.
- **DTaP inadvertently given after the 7th birthday:**
  - **Child age 7–10 years:** DTaP may count as part of catch-up series. Routine Tdap dose at 11–12 should be administered.
  - **Adolescent age 11–18 years:** Count dose of DTaP as the adolescent Tdap booster.
- For other catch-up guidance, see Table 2.
- For information on use of Tdap or Td as tetanus prophylaxis in wound management, see www.cdc.gov/mmwr/volumes/67/rr/rr6702a1.htm.

14. **Varicella vaccination**
(minimum age: 12 months)
Routine vaccination
- 2-dose series: 12–15 months, 4–6 years
- Dose 2 may be administered as early as 3 months after dose 1 (a dose administered after a 4-week interval may be counted).

Catch-up vaccination
- Ensure persons age 7–18 years without evidence of immunity (see *MMWR* at www.cdc.gov/mmwr/pdf/rr/rr5604.pdf) have 2-dose series:
  - **Ages 7–12 years:** routine interval: 3 months (minimum interval: 4 weeks)
  - **Ages 13 years and older:** routine interval: 4–8 weeks (minimum interval: 4 weeks).
  - The maximum age for use of *MMRV* is 12 years.

General Recommendations on Immunization

TABLE 3 Recommended and Minimum Ages and Intervals between Vaccine Doses[*†]

Vaccine and Dose Number	Recommended Age for this Dose	Minimum Age for this Dose	Recommended Interval to Next Dose	Minimum Interval to Next Dose
HepB-1[§]	Birth	Birth	1-4 months	4 weeks
HepB-2	1-2 months	4 weeks	2-17 months	8 weeks
HepB-3[¶]	6-18 months	24 weeks	—	—
DTaP-1[§]	2 months	6 weeks	2 months	4 weeks
DTaP-2	4 months	10 weeks[***]	2 months	4 weeks
DTaP-3	6 months	14 weeks	6-12 months	6 months[**††]
DTaP-4	15-18 months	12 months	3 years	6 months[**]
DTaP-5	4-6 years	4 years	—	—
Hib-1[§§§]	2 months	6 weeks	2 months	4 weeks
Hib-2	4 months	10 weeks	2 months	4 weeks
Hib-3[¶¶]	6 months	14 weeks	6-9 months	8 weeks
Hib-4	12-15 months	12 months	—	—
IPV-1[§]	2 months	6 weeks	2 months	4 weeks
IPV-2	4 months	10 weeks	2-14 months	4 weeks
IPV-3	6-18 months	14 weeks	3-5 years	6 months
IPV-4[***]	4-6 years	4 years	—	—
PCV-1[§§]	2 months	6 weeks	8 weeks	4 weeks
PCV-2	4 months	10 weeks	8 weeks	4 weeks
PCV-3	6 months	14 weeks	6 months	8 weeks
PCV-4	12-15 months	12 months	—	—
MMR-1[†††]	12-15 months	12 months	3-5 years	4 weeks
MMR-2[†††]	4-6 years	13 months	—	—
Varicella-1[†††]	12-15 months	12 months	3-5 years	12 weeks[§§§]
Varicella-2[†††]	4-6 years	15 months	—	—
HepA-1	12-23 months	12 months	6-18 months[**]	6 months[**]
HepA-2	≥18 months	18 months	—	—
Influenza inactivated[¶¶¶]	≥6 months	6 months[****]	1 month	4 weeks
LAIV (intranasal)[¶¶¶]	2-49 years	2 years	1 month	4 weeks
MCV4-1[††††]	11-12 years	2 years	5 years	8 weeks
MCV4-2	16 years	11 years (+8 weeks)	—	—
MPSV4-1[††††]	—	2 years	5 years	5 years
MPSV4-2	—	7 years	—	—
Td	11-12 years	7 years	10 years	5 years
Tdap[§§§§]	≥11 years	7 years	—	—
PPSV-1	—	2 years	5 years	5 years
PPSV-2[¶¶¶¶]	—	7 years	—	—
HPV-1[*****]	11-12 years	9 years	2 months	4 weeks
HPV-2	11-12 years (+2 months)	9 years (+4 weeks)	4 months	12 weeks[†††††]
HPV-3[†††††]	11-12 years (+6 months)	9 years (+24 weeks)	—	—
Rotavirus-1[§§§§§]	2 months	6 weeks	2 months	4 weeks
Rotavirus-2	4 months	10 weeks	2 months	4 weeks
Rotavirus-3[¶¶¶¶¶]	6 months	14 weeks	—	—
Herpes zoster[******]	≥60 years	60 years	—	—
Pneumococcal vaccine[††††††]	—	—	—	—

DTaP, Diphtheria and tetanus toxoids and acellular pertussis; *HepA,* hepatitis A; *HepB,* hepatitis B; *Hib, Haemophilus influenzae* type b; *HPV,* human papillomavirus; *IPV,* inactivated poliovirus; *LAIV,* live, attenuated influenza vaccine; *MCV4,* quadrivalent meningococcal conjugate vaccine; *MMR,* measles, mumps, and rubella; *MMRV,* measles, mumps, rubella, and varicella; *MPSV4,* quadrivalent meningococcal polysaccharide vaccine; *PCV,* pneumococcal conjugate vaccine; *PPSV,* pneumococcal polysaccharide vaccine; *PRP-OMB,* polyribosylribitol phosphate-meningococcal outer membrane protein conjugate; *Td,* tetanus and diphtheria toxoids; *Tdap,* tetanus toxoid, reduced diphtheria toxoid, and acellular pertussis.

*Combination vaccines are available. Use of licensed combination vaccines is generally preferred to separate injections of their equivalent component vaccines. When administering combination vaccines, the minimum age for administration is the oldest age for any of the individual components; the minimum interval between doses is equal to the greatest interval of any of the individual components.

†Information on travel vaccines, including typhoid, Japanese encephalitis, and yellow fever, is available at www.cdc.gov/travel. Information on other vaccines that are licensed in the United States but not distributed, including anthrax and smallpox, is available at https://www.cdc.gov/vaccines/hcp/vis/current-vis.html.

§Combination vaccines containing the hepatitis B component are available. These vaccines should not be administered to infants aged <6 weeks because of the other components (i.e., Hib, DTaP, HepA, and IPV).

¶HepB-3 should be administered at least 8 weeks after HepB-2 and at least 16 weeks after HepB-1 and should not be administered before age 24 weeks.

**Calendar months.

††The minimum recommended interval between DTaP-3 and DTaP-4 is 6 months. However, DTaP-4 need not be repeated if administered at least 4 months after DTaP-3.

§§For Hib and PCV, children receiving the first dose of vaccine at age ≥7 months require fewer doses to complete the series.

TABLE 3 Recommended and Minimum Ages and Intervals between Vaccine Doses*†—cont'd

¶¶If PRP-OMP (Pedvax-Hib, Merck Vaccine Division) was administered at ages 2 and 4 months, a dose at age 6 months is not necessary.
***A fourth dose is not needed if the third dose was administered at ≥4 years and at least 6 months after the previous dose.
†††Combination MMRV vaccine can be used for children aged 12 months to 12 years.
§§§The minimum interval from Varicella-1 to Varicella-2 for persons beginning the series at age ≥13 years is 4 weeks.
¶¶¶One dose of influenza vaccine per season is recommended for most persons. Children aged <9 years who are receiving influenza vaccine for the first time or who received only 1 dose the previous season (if it was their first vaccination season) should receive 2 doses this season.
****The minimum age for inactivated influenza vaccine varies by vaccine manufacturer. See package insert for vaccine-specific minimum ages.
††††Revaccination with meningococcal vaccine is recommended for previously vaccinated persons who remain at high risk for meningococcal disease. (Source: CDC. Updated recommendations from the Advisory Committee on Immunization Practices (ACIP) for revaccination of persons at prolonged increased risk for meningococcal disease. *MMWR* 2009;58:[1042-3]).
§§§§Only 1 dose of Tdap is recommended. Subsequent doses should be given as Td. For one brand of Tdap, the minimum age is 11 years. For management of a tetanus-prone wound in persons who have received a primary series of tetanus-toxoid–containing vaccine, the minimum interval after a previous dose of any tetanus-containing vaccine is 5 years.
¶¶¶¶A second dose of PPSV 5 years after the first dose is recommended for persons aged ≤65 years at highest risk for serious pneumococcal infection and those who are likely to have a rapid decline in pneumococcal antibody concentration. (Source: CDC. Prevention of pneumococcal disease: recommendations of the Advisory Committee on Immunization Practices [ACIP]. *MMWR* 1997;46[No. RR-8].)
*****Bivalent HPV vaccine is approved for females aged 10-25 years. Quadrivalent HPV vaccine is approved for males and females aged 9-26 years.
†††††The minimum age for HPV-3 is based on the baseline minimum age for the first dose (i.e., 108 months) and the minimum interval of 24 weeks between the first and third dose. Dose 3 need not be repeated if it is administered at least 16 weeks after the first dose.
§§§§§The first dose of rotavirus must be administered at age 6 weeks through 14 weeks and 6 days. The vaccine series should not be started for infants aged ≥15 weeks, 0 days. Rotavirus should not be administered to children older than 8 months, 0 days of age regardless of the number of doses received between 6 weeks and 8 months, 0 days of age.
¶¶¶¶¶If 2 doses of Rotarix (GlaxoSmithKline) are administered as age appropriate, a third dose is not necessary.
******Herpes zoster vaccine is recommended as a single dose for persons aged ≥60 years.

TABLE 4 Guidelines for Spacing of Live and Inactivated Antigens

Antigen Combination	Recommended Minimum Interval between Doses
Two or more inactivated*	May be administered simultaneously or at any interval between doses
Inactivated and live	May be administered simultaneously or at any interval between doses
Two or more live intranasal or injectable†	28 days minimum interval, if not administered simultaneously

*Certain experts suggest a 28-day interval between tetanus toxoid, reduced diphtheria toxoid, and acellular pertussis (Tdap) vaccine and tetravalent meningococcal conjugate vaccine if they are not administered simultaneously.
†Live oral vaccines (e.g., Ty21a typhoid vaccine and rotavirus vaccine) may be administered simultaneously or at any interval before or after inactivated or live injectable vaccines.
From Centers for Disease Control and Prevention: General recommendations on immunization: recommendations of the Advisory Committee on Immunization Practices (ACIP), *MMWR* 60(2):38, 2011.

TABLE 5 Guidelines for Administering Antibody-Containing Products* and Vaccines

Type of Administration	Products Administered		Recommended Minimum Interval Between Doses
Simultaneous (during the same office visit)	Antibody-containing products and inactivated antigen		Can be administered simultaneously at different anatomic sites or at any time interval between doses
	Antibody-containing products and live antigen		Should not be administered simultaneously.† If simultaneous administration of measles-containing vaccine or varicella vaccine is unavoidable, administer at different sites and revaccinate or test for seroconversion after the recommended interval
Nonsimultaneous	**Administered First**	**Administered Second**	
	Antibody-containing products	Inactivated antigen	No interval necessary
	Inactivated antigen	Antibody-containing products	No interval necessary
	Antibody-containing products	Live antigen	Dose related†‡
	Live antigen	Antibody-containing products	2 weeks†

*Blood products containing substantial amounts of immune globulin include intramuscular and intravenous immune globulin, specific hyperimmune globulin (e.g., hepatitis B immune globulin, tetanus immune globulin, varicella zoster immune globulin, and rabies immune globulin), whole blood, packed red blood cells, plasma, and platelet products.
†Yellow fever vaccine; rotavirus vaccine; oral Ty21a typhoid vaccine; live, attenuated influenza vaccine; and zoster vaccine are exceptions to these recommendations. These live, attenuated vaccines can be administered at any time before or after or simultaneously with an antibody-containing product.
‡The duration of interference of antibody-containing products with the immune response to the measles component of measles-containing vaccine, and possibly varicella vaccine, is dose related.
From Centers for Disease Control and Prevention: General recommendations on immunization: recommendations of the Advisory Committee on Immunization Practices (ACIP), *MMWR* 60:(RR-2), 2011.

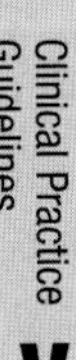

TABLE 6 Recommended Intervals between Administration of Antibody-Containing Products and Measles- or Varicella-Containing Vaccine, by Product and Indication for Vaccination

Product/Indication	Dose (mg IgG/kg) and Route*	Recommended Interval before Measles- or Varicella-Containing Vaccine† Administration (months)
Tetanus IG	250 units (10 mg IgG/kg) IM	3
Hepatitis A IG		
Contact prophylaxis	0.02 ml/kg (33 mg IgG/kg) IM	3
International travel	0.06 ml/kg (10 mg IgG/kg) IM	3
Hepatitis B IG	0.06 ml/kg (10 mg IgG/kg) IM	3
Rabies IG	20 IU/kg (22 mg IgG/kg) IM	4
Varicella IG	125 units/10 kg (60–200 mg IgG/kg) IM, maximum 625 units	5
Measles prophylaxis IG		
Standard (i.e., nonimmunocompromised) contact	0.25 ml/kg (40 mg IgG/kg) IM	5
Immunocompromised contact	0.50 ml/kg (80 mg IgG/kg) IM	6
Blood transfusion		
RBCs, washed	10 ml/kg negligible IgG/kg IV	None
RBCs, adenine-saline added	10 ml/kg (10 mg IgG/kg) IV	3
Packed RBCs (hematocrit 65%)§	10 ml/kg (60 mg IgG/kg) IV	6
Whole blood (hematocrit 35%-50%)§	10 ml/kg (80-100 mg IgG/kg) IV	6
Plasma/platelet products	10 ml/kg (160 mg IgG/kg) IV	7
Cytomegalovirus IGIV	150 mg/kg maximum	6
IGIV		
Replacement therapy for immune deficiencies¶	300-400 mg/kg IV¶	8
Immune thrombocytopenic purpura treatment	400 mg/kg IV	8
Postexposure varicella prophylaxis**	400 mg/kg IV	8
Immune thrombocytopenic purpura treatment	1000 mg/kg IV	10
Kawasaki disease	2 g/kg IV	11
Monoclonal antibody to respiratory syncytial virus F protein (Synagis [MedImmune])††	15 mg/kg IM	None

HIV, human immunodeficiency virus; *IG,* immune globulin; *IgG,* immune globulin G; *IGIV,* intravenous immune globulin; *mg IgG/kg,* milligrams of immune globulin G per kilogram of body weight; *IM,* intramuscular; *IV,* intravenous; *RBCs,* red blood cells.

*This table is not intended for determining the correct indications and dosages for using antibody-containing products. Unvaccinated persons might not be protected fully against measles during the entire recommended interval, and additional doses of IG or measles vaccine might be indicated after measles exposure. Concentrations of measles antibody in an IG preparation can vary by manufacturer's lot. Rates of antibody clearance after receipt of an IG preparation also might vary. Recommended intervals are extrapolated from an estimated half-life of 30 days for passively acquired antibody and an observed interference with the immune response to measles vaccine for 5 months after a dose of 80 mg IgG/kg.

†Does not include zoster vaccine. Zoster vaccine may be given with antibody-containing blood products.

§Assumes a serum IgG concentration of 16 mg/ml.

¶Measles and varicella vaccinations are recommended for children with asymptomatic or mildly symptomatic HIV infection but are contraindicated for persons with severe immunosuppression from HIV or any other immunosuppressive disorder.

**The investigational VariZIG, similar to licensed varicella-zoster IG (VZIG), is a purified human IG preparation made from plasma containing high levels of antivaricella antibodies (IgG). The interval between VariZIG and varicella vaccine (Var or MMRV) is 5 months.

††Contains antibody only to respiratory syncytial virus.

From Centers for Disease Control and Prevention: General recommendations on immunization: recommendations of the Advisory Committee on Immunization Practices (ACIP), *MMWR* 60:(RR-2), 2011.

TABLE 7 Contraindications and Precautions* to Commonly Used Vaccines

Vaccine	Contraindications	Precautions
DTaP	Severe allergic reaction (e.g., anaphylaxis) after a previous dose or to a vaccine component Encephalopathy (e.g., coma, decreased level of consciousness, or prolonged seizures), not attributable to another identifiable cause, within 7 days of administration of previous dose of DTP or DTaP	Progressive neurologic disorder, including infantile spasms, uncontrolled epilepsy, progressive encephalopathy; defer DTaP until neurologic status clarified and stabilized Temperature of ≥105° F (≥40° C) within 48 hours after vaccination with a previous dose of DTP or DTaP Collapse or shock-like state (i.e., hypotonic hyporesponsive episode) within 48 hours after receiving a previous dose of DTP/DTaP Seizure ≤3 days after receiving a previous dose of DTP/DTaP Persistent, inconsolable crying lasting ≥3 hours within 48 hours after receiving a previous dose of DTP/DTaP GBS <6 weeks after previous dose of tetanus toxoid-containing vaccine History of Arthus-type hypersensitivity reactions after a previous dose of tetanus toxoid-containing vaccine; defer vaccination until at least 10 years have elapsed since the last tetanus-toxoid–containing vaccine Moderate or severe acute illness with or without fever
DT, Td	Severe allergic reaction (e.g., anaphylaxis) after a previous dose or to a vaccine component	GBS <6 weeks after previous dose of tetanus toxoid-containing vaccine History of Arthus-type hypersensitivity reactions after a previous dose of tetanus toxoid-containing vaccine; defer vaccination until at least 10 years have elapsed since the last tetanus-toxoid–containing vaccine Moderate or severe acute illness with or without fever
Tdap	Severe allergic reaction (e.g., anaphylaxis) after a previous dose or to a vaccine component Encephalopathy (e.g., coma, decreased level of consciousness, or prolonged seizures), not attributable to another identifiable cause, within 7 days of administration of previous dose of DTP, DTaP, or Tdap	GBS <6 weeks after a previous dose of tetanus toxoid-containing vaccine Progressive or unstable neurologic disorder, uncontrolled seizures, or progressive encephalopathy until a treatment regimen has been established and the condition has stabilized History of Arthus-type hypersensitivity reactions after a previous dose of tetanus toxoid-containing vaccine; defer vaccination until at least 10 years have elapsed since the last tetanus toxoid-containing vaccine Moderate or severe acute illness with or without fever
IPV	Severe allergic reaction (e.g., anaphylaxis) after a previous dose or to a vaccine component	Pregnancy Moderate or severe acute illness with or without fever
MMR[†§]	Severe allergic reaction (e.g., anaphylaxis) after a previous dose or to a vaccine component Pregnancy: Known severe immunodeficiency (e.g., from hematologic and solid tumors, receipt of chemotherapy, congenital immunodeficiency, or long-term immunosuppressive therapy[¶] or patients with HIV infection who are severely immunocompromised)[§]	Recent (≤11 months) receipt of antibody-containing blood product (specific interval depends on product) History of thrombocytopenia or thrombocytopenic purpura Need for tuberculin skin testing[††] Moderate or severe acute illness with or without fever
Hib	Severe allergic reaction (e.g., anaphylaxis) after a previous dose or to a vaccine component Age <6 weeks	Moderate or severe acute illness with or without fever
Hepatitis B	Severe allergic reaction (e.g., anaphylaxis) after a previous dose or to a vaccine component	Infant weight <2000 g[§§] Moderate or severe acute illness with or without fever
Hepatitis A	Severe allergic reaction (e.g., anaphylaxis) after a previous dose or to a vaccine component	Pregnancy: Moderate or severe acute illness with or without fever
Varicella	Severe allergic reaction (e.g., anaphylaxis) after a previous dose or to a vaccine component Known severe immunodeficiency (e.g., from hematologic and solid tumors, receipt of chemotherapy, congenital immunodeficiency, or long-term immunosuppressive therapy[¶] or patients with HIV infection who are severely immunocompromised)[§] Pregnancy	Recent (≤11 months) receipt of antibody-containing blood product (specific interval depends on product)[¶¶] Moderate or severe acute illness with or without fever
PCV	Severe allergic reaction (e.g., anaphylaxis) after a previous dose (of PCV7, PCV13, or any diphtheria toxoid-containing vaccine) or to a component of a vaccine (PCV7, PCV13, or any diphtheria toxoid-containing vaccine)	Moderate or severe acute illness with or without fever
TIV	Severe allergic reaction (e.g., anaphylaxis) after a previous dose or to vaccine component, including egg protein	GBS <6 weeks after a previous dose of influenza vaccine Moderate or severe acute illness with or without fever
LAIV	Severe allergic reaction (e.g., anaphylaxis) after a previous dose or to vaccine component, including egg protein Pregnancy Immunosuppression Certain chronic medical conditions***	GBS <6 weeks after a previous dose of influenza vaccine Moderate or severe acute illness with or without fever
PPSV	Severe allergic reaction (e.g., anaphylaxis) after a previous dose or to a vaccine component	Moderate or severe acute illness with or without fever
MCV4	Severe allergic reaction (e.g., anaphylaxis) after a previous dose or to a vaccine component	Moderate or severe acute illness with or without fever
MPSV4	Severe allergic reaction (e.g., anaphylaxis) after a previous dose or to a vaccine component	Moderate or severe acute illness with or without fever
HPV	Severe allergic reaction (e.g., anaphylaxis) after a previous dose or to a vaccine component	Pregnancy: Moderate or severe acute illness with or without fever

Continued

TABLE 7 Contraindications and Precautions* to Commonly Used Vaccines—cont'd

Vaccine	Contraindications	Precautions
Rotavirus	Severe allergic reaction (e.g., anaphylaxis) after a previous dose or to a vaccine component SCID	Altered immunocompetence other than SCID: History of intussusception Chronic gastrointestinal disease††† Spina bifida or bladder exstrophy††† Moderate or severe acute illness with or without fever
Zoster	Severe allergic reaction (e.g., anaphylaxis) after a previous dose or to a vaccine component Substantial suppression of cellular immunity Pregnancy	Moderate or severe acute illness with or without fever

DT, diphtheria and tetanus toxoids; *DTaP,* diphtheria and tetanus toxoids and acellular pertussis; *GBS,* Guillain-Barré syndrome; *HBsAg,* hepatitis B surface antigen; *Hib, Haemophilus influenzae* type b; *HIV,* human immunodeficiency virus; *HPV,* human papillomavirus; *IPV,* inactivated poliovirus; *LAIV,* live, attenuated influenza vaccine; *MCV4,* quadrivalent meningococcal conjugate vaccine; *MMRV* measles, mumps, rubella; *MPSV4,* quadrivalent meningococcal polysaccharide vaccine; *PCV,* pneumococcal conjugate vaccine; *PPSV,* pneumococcal polysaccharide vaccine; *SCID,* severe combined immunodeficiency; *Td,* tetanus and diphtheria toxoids; *Tdap,* tetanus toxoid, reduced diphtheria toxoid, and acellular pertussis; *TIV,* trivalent inactivated influenza vaccine.

*Events or conditions listed as precautions should be reviewed carefully. Benefits of and risks for administering a specific vaccine to a person under these circumstances should be considered. If the risk from the vaccine is believed to outweigh the benefit, the vaccine should not be administered. If the benefit of vaccination is believed to outweigh the risk, the vaccine should be administered. Whether and when to administer DTaP to children with proven or suspected underlying neurologic disorders should be decided on a case-by-case basis.

†HIV-infected children may receive varicella and measles vaccine if CD4+ T-lymphocyte count is <15%. (Source: Adapted from American Academy of Pediatrics. Passive immunization. In: Pickering LK, ed. *Red book: 2009 report of the committee on infectious diseases.* 28th ed. Elk Grove Village. IL: American Academy of Pediatrics: 2009.)

§MMR and varicella vaccines can be administered on the same day. If not administered on the same day, these vaccines should be separated by at least 28 days.

¶Substantially immunosuppressive steroid dose is considered to be ≥2 weeks of daily receipt of 20 mg or 2 mg/kg body weight of prednisone or equivalent.

††Measles vaccination might suppress tuberculin reactivity temporarily. Measles-containing vaccine can be administered on the same day as tuberculin skin testing. If testing cannot be performed until after the day of MMR vaccination, the test should be postponed for ≥4 weeks after the vaccination. If an urgent need exists to skin test, do so with the understanding that reactivity might be reduced by the vaccine.

§§Hepatitis B vaccination should be deferred for infants weighing <2000 g if the mother is documented to be HBsAg-negative at the time of the infant's birth. Vaccination can commence at chronological age 1 month or at hospital discharge. For infants born to HBsAg-positive women, hepatitis B immune globulin and hepatitis B vaccine should be administered within 12 hours after birth, regardless of weight.

¶¶Vaccine should be deferred for the appropriate interval if replacement immune globulin products are being administered.

***Source: CDC. Prevention and control of seasonal influenza with vaccines: recommendations of the Advisory Committee on Immunization Practices (ACIP), 2010. *MMWR* 2010;59(No. RR-8).

†††For details see CDC. Prevention of rotavirus gastroenteritis among infants and children: recommendations of the Advisory Committee on Immunization Practices. *MMWR* 2009;58(No. RR-2).

From Centers for Disease Control and Prevention: General recommendations on immunization: recommendations of the Advisory Committee on Immunization Practices (ACIP), *MMWR* 60:(RR-2), 2011.

TABLE 8 Conditions Commonly Misperceived as Contraindications to Vaccination

Vaccine	Conditions Commonly Misperceived as Contraindications (i.e., Vaccination May be Administered under These Conditions)
General for all vaccines, including DTaP, pediatric DT, adult Td, adolescent-adult Tdap, IPV, MMR, Hib, hepatitis A, hepatitis B, varicella, rotavirus, PCV, TIV, LAIV, PPSV, MCV4, MPSV4, HPV, and herpes zoster	Mild acute illness with or without fever Mild-to-moderate local reaction (i.e., swelling, redness, soreness); low-grade or moderate fever after previous dose Lack of previous physical examination in well-appearing person Current antimicrobial therapy* Convalescent phase of illness Preterm birth (hepatitis B vaccine is an exception in certain circumstances)[†] Recent exposure to an infectious disease History of penicillin allergy, other nonvaccine allergies, relatives with allergies, or receiving allergen extract immunotherapy
DTaP	Fever of <105° F (<40° C), fussiness or mild drowsiness after a previous dose of DTP/DTaP Family history of seizures Family history of sudden infant death syndrome Family history of an adverse event after DTP or DTaP administration Stable neurologic conditions (e.g., cerebral palsy, well-controlled seizures, or developmental delay)
Tdap	Fever of ≥105° F (≥40° C) for <48 hours after vaccination with a previous dose of DTP or DTaP Collapse or shock-like state (i.e., hypotonic hyporesponsive episode) within 48 hours after receiving a previous dose of DTaP Seizure <3 days after receiving a previous dose of DTP/DTaP Persistent, inconsolable crying lasting <3 hours within 48 hours after receiving a previous dose of DTP/DTaP History of extensive limb swelling after DTP/DTaP/Td that is not an Arthus-type reaction Stable neurologic disorder History of brachial neuritis Latex allergy that is not anaphylactic Breastfeeding Immunosuppression
IPV	Previous receipt of ≥1 dose of oral polio vaccine
MMR[§,¶]	Positive tuberculin skin test Simultaneous tuberculin skin testing** Breastfeeding Pregnancy of recipient's mother or other close or household contact Recipient is female of childbearing age Immunodeficient family member or household contact Asymptomatic or mildly symptomatic HIV infection Allergy to eggs
Hepatitis B	Pregnancy Autoimmune disease (e.g., systemic lupus erythematosus or rheumatoid arthritis)
Varicella	Pregnancy of recipient's mother or other close or household contact Immunodeficient family member or household contact[††] Asymptomatic or mildly symptomatic HIV infection Humoral immunodeficiency (e.g., agammaglobulinemia)
TIV	Nonsevere (e.g., contact) allergy to latex, thimerosal, or egg Concurrent administration of Coumadin or aminophylline
LAIV	Health care providers that see patients with chronic diseases or altered immunocompetence (an exception is providers for severely immunocompromised patients requiring care in a protected environment) Breastfeeding Contacts of persons with chronic disease or altered immunocompetence (an exception is contacts of severely immunocompromised patients requiring care in a protected environment)
PPSV	History of invasive pneumococcal disease or pneumonia
HPV	Immunosuppression Previous equivocal or abnormal Papanicolaou test Known HPV infection Breastfeeding History of genital warts
Rotavirus	Prematurity Immunosuppressed household contacts Pregnant household contacts
Zoster	Therapy with low-dose methotrexate (≤0.4 mg/kg/week), azathioprine (≤3.0 mg/kg/day), or 6-mercaptopurine (≤1.5 mg/kg/day) for treatment of rheumatoid arthritis, psoriasis, polymyositis, sarcoidosis, inflammatory bowel disease, or other conditions Health care providers of patients with chronic diseases or altered immunocompetence Contacts of patients with chronic diseases or altered immunocompetence Unknown or uncertain history of varicella in a U.S.-born person

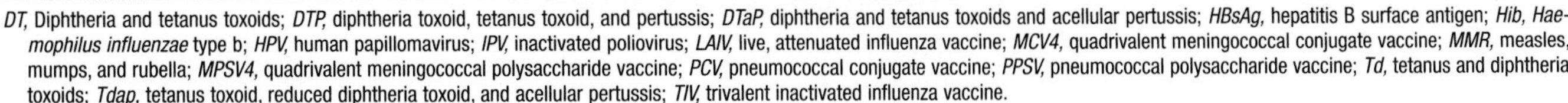

DT, Diphtheria and tetanus toxoids; *DTP,* diphtheria toxoid, tetanus toxoid, and pertussis; *DTaP,* diphtheria and tetanus toxoids and acellular pertussis; *HBsAg,* hepatitis B surface antigen; *Hib, Haemophilus influenzae* type b; *HPV,* human papillomavirus; *IPV,* inactivated poliovirus; *LAIV,* live, attenuated influenza vaccine; *MCV4,* quadrivalent meningococcal conjugate vaccine; *MMR,* measles, mumps, and rubella; *MPSV4,* quadrivalent meningococcal polysaccharide vaccine; *PCV,* pneumococcal conjugate vaccine; *PPSV,* pneumococcal polysaccharide vaccine; *Td,* tetanus and diphtheria toxoids; *Tdap,* tetanus toxoid, reduced diphtheria toxoid, and acellular pertussis; *TIV,* trivalent inactivated influenza vaccine.

Continued

TABLE 8 Conditions Commonly Misperceived as Contraindications to Vaccination—cont'd

*Antibacterial drugs might interfere with Ty21a oral typhoid vaccine, and certain antiviral drugs might interfere with varicella-containing vaccines and LAIV.

†Hepatitis B vaccination should be deferred for infants weighing <2000 g if the mother is documented to be HBsAg-negative at the time of the infant's birth. Vaccination can commence at chronologic age 1 month or at hospital discharge. For infants born to HBsAg-positive women, hepatitis B immune globulin and hepatitis B vaccine should be administered within 12 hours after birth, regardless of weight.

§MMR and varicella vaccines can be administered on the same day. If not administered on the same day, these vaccines should be separated by at least 28 days.

¶HIV-infected children should receive immune globulin after exposure to measles. HIV-infected children can receive varicella and measles vaccine if $CD4^+$ T-lymphocyte count is >15%. (Source: Adapted from American Academy of Pediatrics. Passive immunization. In: Pickering LK, ed. *Red book: 2009 report of the Committee on Infectious Diseases,* 28th ed. Elk Grove Village, IL: American Academy of Pediatrics; 2009.)

**Measles vaccination might suppress tuberculin reactivity temporarily. Measles-containing vaccine can be administered on the same day as tuberculin skin testing. If testing cannot be performed until after the day of MMR vaccination, the test should be postponed for at least 4 weeks after the vaccination. If an urgent need exists to skin test, do so with the understanding that reactivity might be reduced by the vaccine.

††If a vaccinee experiences a presumed vaccine-related rash 7-25 days after vaccination, the person should avoid direct contact with immunocompromised persons for the duration of the rash.

From Centers for Disease Control and Prevention: General recommendations on immunization: recommendations of the Advisory Committee on Immunization Practices (ACIP), *MMWR* 60:(RR-2), 2011.

VACCINE ADMINISTRATION*

INFECTION CONTROL AND STERILE TECHNIQUE

Persons administering vaccines should follow appropriate precautions to minimize risk for spread of disease. Hands should be cleansed with an alcohol-based, waterless antiseptic hand rub or washed with soap and water between each patient contact. Occupational Safety and Health Administration (OSHA) regulations do not require that gloves be worn when administering vaccinations unless persons administering vaccinations are likely to come into contact with potentially infectious body fluids or have open lesions on their hands. Needles used for injections must be sterile and disposable to minimize the risk for contamination. A separate needle and syringe should be used for each injection. Changing needles between drawing vaccine from a vial and injecting it into a recipient is not necessary. Different vaccines should never be mixed in the same syringe unless specifically licensed for such use, and no attempt should be made to transfer between syringes.

For all intramuscular injections, the needle should be long enough to reach the muscle mass and prevent vaccine from seeping into subcutaneous tissue, but not so long as to involve underlying nerves, blood vessels, or bone. Vaccinators should be familiar with the anatomy of the area where they are injecting vaccine. Intramuscular injections are administered at a 90-degree angle to the skin, preferably into the anterolateral aspect of the thigh or the deltoid muscle of the upper arm depending on the age of the patient.

Decision on needle size and site of injection must be made for each person on the basis of the size of the muscle, the thickness of adipose tissue at the injection site, the volume of the material to be administered, injection technique, and the depth below the muscle surface into which the material is to be injected (Fig. E1). Aspiration before injection of vaccines or toxoids (i.e., pulling back on the syringe plunger after needle insertion before injection) is not required because no large blood vessel exists at the recommended injection sites.

INFANTS (AGED <12 MONTHS)

For the majority of infants, the anterolateral aspect of the thigh is the recommended site for injection because it provides a large muscle mass (Fig. E2). The muscles of the buttock have not been used for administration of vaccines in infants and children because of concern about potential injury to the sciatic nerve, which is well documented after injection of antimicrobial agents into the buttock. If the gluteal muscle must be used, care should be taken to define the anatomic landmarks.† Injection technique is the most important parameter to ensure efficient intramuscular vaccine delivery. If the subcutaneous and muscle tissue are bunched to minimize the chance of striking bone, a 1-inch needle is required to ensure intramuscular administration in infants. For the majority of infants, a 1-inch, 22- to 25-gauge needle is sufficient to penetrate muscle in an infant's thigh. For newborn (first 28 days of life) and premature infants, a 5/8-inch-long needle usually is adequate if the skin is stretched flat between thumb and forefinger and the needle inserted at a 90-degree angle to the skin.

TODDLERS AND OLDER CHILDREN (AGED 12 MONTHS TO 10 YEARS)

The deltoid muscle should be used if the muscle mass is adequate. The needle size for deltoid site injections can range from 22 to 25 gauge and from 5/8 to 1 inch on the basis of the size of the muscle and the thickness of adipose tissue at the injection site (Fig. E3). A 5/8-inch needle is adequate only for the deltoid muscle and only if the skin is stretched flat between the thumb and forefinger and the needle inserted at a 90-degree angle to the skin. For toddlers, the anterolateral thigh can be used, but the needle should be at least 1 inch in length.

ADOLESCENTS AND ADULTS (AGED >11 YEARS)

For adults and adolescents, the deltoid muscle is recommended for routine intramuscular vaccinations. The anterolateral thigh also can be used. For men and women weighing <130 lb (<60 kg) a 5/8- to 1-inch needle is sufficient to ensure intramuscular injection. For women weighing 130 to 200 lb (60 to 90 kg) and men 130 to 260 lb (60 to 118 kg), a 1- to 1½-inch needle is needed. For women weighing >200 lb (>90 kg) or men weighing >260 lb (>118 kg), a 1½-inch needle is required.

SUBCUTANEOUS INJECTIONS

Subcutaneous injections are administered at a 45-degree angle, usually into the thigh for infants younger than 12 months and in the upper-outer triceps area of persons aged 12 months and older. Subcutaneous injections can be administered into the upper-outer triceps area of an infant if necessary. A 5/8-inch, 23- to 25-gauge needle should be inserted into the subcutaneous tissue (Figs. E4 and E5).

TABLE 9 Treatment of Anaphylaxis in Children and Adults with Drugs Administered Intramuscularly or Orally

Drug	Dosage
Children	
Primary Regimen	
Epinephrine 1:1000 (aqueous) (1 mg/ml)*	0.01 mg/kg up to 0.5 mg (administer 0.01 ml/kg/dose up to 0.5 mL) IM repeated every 10-20 minutes up to 3 doses
Secondary Regimen	
Diphenhydramine	1-2 mg/kg oral, IM, or IV, every 4-6 hours (100 mg, maximum single dose)
Hydroxyzine	0.5-1 mg/kg oral, IM, every 4-6 hours (100 mg, maximum single dose)
Prednisone	1.5-2 mg/kg oral (60 mg, maximum single dose); use corticosteroids as long as needed
Adults	
Primary Regimen	
Epinephrine 1:1000 (aqueous)*	0.01 mg/kg up to 0.5 mg (administer 0.01 ml/kg/dose up to 0.5 ml) IM repeated every 10-20 minutes up to 3 doses
Secondary Regimen	
Diphenhydramine	1-2 mg/kg up to l00 mg IM or oral, every 4-6 hours

IM, Intramuscular; *IV*, intravenous.

*If the agent causing the anaphylactic reaction was administered by injection, epinephrine may be injected into the same site to slow absorption.

From Centers for Disease Control and Prevention: General recommendations on immunization: recommendations of the Advisory Committee on Immunization Practices (ACIP), *MMWR* 60:(RR-2), 2011. Adapted from American Academy of Pediatrics. Passive immunization. In: Pickering LK, Baker CJ, Kimberlin DW, Long SS, eds: *Red book: 2009 report of the Committee on Infectious Diseases,* 28th ed. Elk Grove Village, IL: American Academy of Pediatrics, 2009:66-7; Immunization Action Coalition. Medical management of vaccine reactions in adult patients (available at www.immunize.org/catg.d/p3082.pdf); and *Mosby's drug consult,* St Louis, 2005, Mosby.

TABLE 10 Vaccination of Persons with Primary and Secondary Immunodeficiencies

Primary	Specific Immunodeficiency	Contraindicated Vaccines*	Risk-Specific Recommended Vaccines*	Effectiveness and Comments
B-lymphocyte (humoral)	Severe antibody deficiencies (e.g., X-linked agammaglobulinemia and common variable immunodeficiency)	OPV† Smallpox LAIV BCG Ty21a (live typhoid) Yellow fever	Pneumococcal Consider measles and varicella vaccination	The effectiveness of any vaccine is uncertain if it depends only on the humoral response (e.g., PPSV or MPSV4). IVIG interferes with the immune response to measles vaccine and possibly varicella vaccine.
	Less severe antibody deficiencies (e.g., selective IgA deficiency and IgG subclass deficiency)	OPV† BCG Yellow fever Other live vaccines appear to be safe.	Pneumococcal	All vaccines likely effective; immune response might be attenuated.
T-lymphocyte (cell-mediated and humoral)	Complete deficits (e.g., severe combined immunodeficiency [SCID] disease, complete DiGeorge syndrome)	All live vaccines§,¶,**	Pneumococcal	Vaccines might be ineffective.
	Partial defects (e.g., most patients with DiGeorge syndrome, Wiskott-Aldrich syndrome, ataxia-telangiectasia)	All live vaccines§,¶,**	Pneumococcal Meningococcal Hib (if not administered in infancy)	Effectiveness of any vaccine depends on degree of immune suppression.
Complement	Persistent complement, properdin, or factor B deficiency	None	Pneumococcal Meningococcal	All routine vaccines likely effective.
Phagocytic function	Chronic granulomatous disease, leukocyte adhesion defect, and myeloperoxidase deficiency	Live bacterial vaccines§	Pneumococcal††	All inactivated vaccines safe and likely effective. Live viral vaccines likely safe and effective.
Secondary	HIV/AIDS	OPV† Smallpox BCG LAIV Withhold MMR and varicella in severely immunocompromised persons. Yellow fever vaccine might have a contraindication or a precaution depending on clinical parameters of immune function***	Pneumococcal Consider Hib (if not administered in infancy) and meningococcal vaccination.	MMR, varicella, rotavirus, and all inactivated vaccines, including inactivated influenza, might be effective.§§
	Malignant neoplasm, transplantation, immunosuppressive or radiation therapy	Live viral and bacterial, depending on immune status§,¶	Pneumococcal	Effectiveness of any vaccine depends on degree of immune suppression.
	Asplenia	None	Pneumococcal Meningococcal Hib (if not administered in infancy)	All routine vaccines likely effective.
	Chronic renal disease	LAIV	Pneumococcal Hepatitis B¶¶	All routine vaccines likely effective.

AIDS, acquired immunodeficiency syndrome; *BCG,* bacille Calmette-Guérin; *Hib, Haemophilus influenzae* type b; *HIV,* human immunodeficiency virus; *Ig,* immunoglobulin; *IGIV,* immune globulin intravenous; *LAIV,* live, attenuated influenza vaccine; *MMR,* measles, mumps, and rubella; *MPSV4,* quadrivalent meningococcal polysaccharide vaccine; *OPV,* oral poliovirus polysaccharide vaccine; *PPSV,* pneumococcal polysaccharide vaccine.

*Other vaccines that are universally or routinely recommended should be given if not contraindicated.

†OPV is no longer available in the United States.

§Live bacterial vaccines: BCG and oral Ty21a *Salmonella typhi* vaccine.

¶Live viral vaccines: MMR, MMRV, OPV, LAIV, yellow fever, zoster, rotavirus, varicella, and vaccinia (smallpox). Smallpox vaccine is not recommended for children or the general public.

**Regarding T-lymphocyte immunodeficiency as a contraindication for rotavirus vaccine, data exist only for severe combined immunodeficiency.

††Pneumococcal vaccine is not indicated for children with chronic granulomatous disease beyond age-based universal recommendations for PCV. Children with chronic granulomatous disease are not at increased risk for pneumococcal disease.

§§HIV-infected children should receive IG after exposure to measles and may receive varicella and measles vaccine if CD4+ T-lymphocyte count is ≥15%.

¶¶Indicated based on the risk from dialysis-based bloodborne transmission.

***Symptomatic HIV infection or CD4+ T-lymphocyte count of <200/mm^3 or <15% of total lymphocytes for children aged <6 years is a contraindication to yellow fever vaccine administration. Asymptomatic HIV infection with CD4+ T-lymphocyte count of 200–499/mm^3 for persons aged ≥6 years or 15%–24% of total lymphocytes for children aged <6 years is a precaution for yellow fever vaccine administration. Details of yellow fever vaccine recommendations are available from CDC. (CDC. Yellow fever vaccine recommendations of the Advisory Committee on Immunization Practices [ACIP]. *MMWR* 2010;59[No. RR-7].)

From Centers for Disease Control and Prevention: General recommendations on immunization: recommendations of the Advisory Committee on Immunization Practices (ACIP), *MMWR* 60:(RR-2), 2011. Adapted from American Academy of Pediatrics. Passive immunization. In: Pickering LK, Baker CJ, Kimberlin DW, Long SS, eds: *Red book: 2009 report of the Committee on Infectious Diseases,* 28th ed. Elk Grove Village, IL: American Academy of Pediatrics; 2009:74–5.

TABLE 11 Immunizations for Pediatric Oncology Patients

Vaccine	Indications and Comments
DTaP	Indicated for incompletely immunized children <7 yr, even during active chemotherapy
Td	Indicated 1 yr after completion of therapy in children 7 yr
Hib	Indicated for incompletely immunized children if <7 yr
HBV	Indicated for incompletely immunized children
23PS	Indicated for asplenic patients
PCV13	Indicated for incompletely immunized children <5 yr
Meningococcus	Consider in asplenic patients
IPV	Indicated for incompletely immunized children; also recommended for all household contacts requiring immunization to reduce the risk of vaccine-associated polio
MMR	Contraindicated until child is in remission and finished with all chemotherapy for 3-6 mo; may need to reimmunize after chemotherapy if titers have fallen below protective levels
Influenza	Defer in active chemotherapy; may give as early as 3-4 wk after remission and off chemotherapy if during influenza season; peripheral granulocyte and lymphocyte counts should be >1000/µL; should also be given to household contact of children with cancer
Varicella	Consider immunizing children who have remained in remission and have finished chemotherapy for >1 yr; with absolute lymphocyte count of >700/µl and platelet count of >100,000/µL within 24 hr of immunization; check titers of previously immunized children to verify protective levels of antibodies

DTaP, Diphtheria, tetanus, and pertussis; *HBV,* hepatitis B virus; *Hib, Haemophilus influenzae* type b; *IPV,* inactivated polio vaccine; *MMR,* measles, mumps, rubella; *PCV13,* pneumococcal conjugate vaccine; *Td,* tetanus, diphtheria; *23PS,* 23-valent pneumococcal polysaccharide vaccine.
From *MMWR* 49(RR-10):1-147, 2000.

TABLE 12 Approaches to the Evaluation and Vaccination of Persons Vaccinated Outside the United States Who Have No (or Questionable) Vaccination Records

Vaccine	Recommended Approach	Alternative Approach*
MMR	Revaccination with MMR	Serologic testing for IgG antibodies to measles, mumps, and rubella
Hib	Age-appropriate revaccination	—
Hepatitis A	Age-appropriate revaccination	Serologic testing for IgG antibodies to hepatitis A
Hepatitis B	Age-appropriate revaccination and serologic testing for HBsAg†	—
Poliovirus	Revaccinate with inactivated poliovirus vaccine	Serologic testing for neutralizing antibody to poliovirus types 1, 2, and 3 (limited availability)
DTaP	Revaccination with DTaP, with serologic testing for specific IgG antibody to tetanus and diphtheria toxins in the event of a severe local reaction	Persons whose records indicate receipt of ≥3 doses: serologic testing for specific IgG antibody to diphtheria and tetanus toxins before administering additional doses, or administer a single booster dose of DTaP, followed by serologic testing after 1 month for specific IgG antibody to diphtheria and tetanus toxins with revaccination as appropriate
Tdap	Age-appropriate vaccination of persons who are candidates for Tdap vaccine on the basis of time since last diphtheria and tetanus-toxoid–containing vaccines.	—
Varicella	Age-appropriate vaccination of persons who lack evidence of varicella immunity	—
Pneumococcal conjugate	Age-appropriate vaccination	—
Rotavirus	Age-appropriate vaccination	—
HPV	Age-appropriate vaccination	—
Zoster	Age-appropriate vaccination	—

DTaP, Diphtheria and tetanus toxoids and acellular pertussis; *HBsAg,* hepatitis B surface antigen; *Hib, Haemophilus influenzae* type b; *HPV,* human papillomavirus; *IgG,* immune globulin G; *MMR,* measles, mumps, and rubella; *Tdap,* tetanus toxoid, reduced diphtheria toxoid, and acellular pertussis.

*There is a recommended approach for all vaccines and an alternative approach for some vaccines.

†In rare instances, hepatitis B vaccine can give a false-positive HBsAg result up to 18 days after vaccination; therefore, blood should be drawn to test for HBsAg before vaccinating. (Source: CDC. A comprehensive immunization strategy to eliminate transmission of hepatitis B virus infection in the United States: recommendations of the Advisory Committee on Immunization Practices [ACIP]; Part I: Immunization in infants, children, and adolescents, *MMWR* 2005;54(No. RR-16.)

From Centers for Disease Control and Prevention: General recommendations on immunization: recommendations of the Advisory Committee on Immunization Practices (ACIP), *MMWR* 60:(RR-2), 2011.

Immunizations for Adults

RECOMMENDED IMMUNIZATION SCHEDULE FOR ADULTS AGED 19 YEARS OR OLDER, UNITED STATES, 2017

In February 2017, the *Recommended Immunization Schedule for Adults Aged 19 Years or Older, United States, 2017* became effective, as recommended by the Advisory Committee on Immunization Practices (ACIP) and approved by the Centers for Disease Control and Prevention (CDC). The 2017 adult immunization schedule was also reviewed and approved by the following professional medical organizations:

- American College of Physicians (www.acponline.org)
- American Academy of Family Physicians (www.aafp.org)
- American College of Obstetricians and Gynecologists (www.acog.org)
- American College of Nurse-Midwives (www.midwife.org)

CDC announced the availability of the 2017 adult immunization schedule at https://www.cdc.gov/vaccines/schedules/easy-to-read/adult.html in the *Morbidity and Mortality Weekly Report (MMWR)*.[1] The schedule is published in its entirety in the *Annals of Internal Medicine*.[2]

The adult immunization schedule describes the age groups and medical conditions and other indications for which licensed vaccines are recommended. The 2017 adult immunization schedule consists of:

- Table 13. Recommended immunization schedule for adults by age group
- Table 14. Recommended immunization schedule for adults by medical condition and other indications
- Footnotes that accompany each vaccine containing important general information and considerations for special populations

Consider the following information when reviewing the adult immunization schedule:

- The tables in the adult immunization schedule should be read with the footnotes that contain important general information and information about vaccination of special populations.
- When indicated, administer recommended vaccines to adults whose vaccination history is incomplete or unknown.
- Increased interval between doses of a multi-dose vaccine does not diminish vaccine effectiveness; therefore, it is not necessary to restart the vaccine series or add doses to the series because of an extended interval between doses.
- Adults with immunocompromising conditions should generally avoid live vaccines, e.g., measles, mumps, and rubella vaccine. Inactivated vaccines, e.g., pneumococcal or inactivated influenza vaccines, are generally acceptable.
- Combination vaccines may be used when any component of the combination is indicated and when the other components of the combination vaccine are not contraindicated.
- The use of trade names in the adult immunization schedule is for identification purposes only and does not imply endorsement by the ACIP or CDC.

Details on vaccines recommended for adults and complete ACIP statements are available at www.cdc.gov/vaccines/hcp/acip-recs/index.html. Additional CDC resources include:

- A summary of information on vaccination recommendations, vaccination of persons with immunodeficiencies, preventing and managing adverse reactions, vaccination contraindications and precautions, and other information can be found in *General Recommendations on Immunization* at www.cdc.gov/mmwr/preview/mmwrhtml/rr6002a1.htm.
- Vaccine Information Statements that explain benefits and risks of vaccines are available at https://www.cdc.gov/vaccinesafety/Concerns/Index.html
- Information and resources regarding vaccination of pregnant women are available at https://www.cdc.gov/vaccines/pregnancy/pregnant-women/index.html
- Information on travel vaccine requirements and recommendations is available at www.cdc.gov/travel/destinations/list.
- *CDC Vaccine Schedules App* for clinicians and other immunization service providers to download is available at https://www.cdc.gov/vaccines/schedules/
- *Recommended Immunization Schedule for Children and Adolescents Aged 18 Years or Younger* is available at https://www.cdc.gov/vaccines/schedules/hcp/child-adolescent.html#schedule

Report suspected cases of reportable vaccine-preventable diseases to the local or state health department.

Report all clinically significant post-vaccination reactions to the Vaccine Adverse Event Reporting System at www.vaers.hhs.gov or by telephone, 800-822-7967. All vaccines included in the 2017 adult immunization schedule except herpes zoster and 23-valent pneumococcal polysaccharide vaccines are covered by the Vaccine Injury Compensation Program. Information on how to file a vaccine injury claim is available at www.hrsa.gov/vaccinecompensation or by telephone, 800-338-2382.

Submit questions and comments regarding the 2017 adult immunization schedule to CDC through www.cdc.gov/cdc-info or by telephone, 800-CDC-INFO (800-232-4636), in English and Spanish, 8:00am–8:00pm ET, Monday–Friday, excluding holidays.

The following acronyms are used for vaccines recommended for adults:

HepA	hepatitis A vaccine
HepA-HepB	hepatitis A and hepatitis B vaccines
HepB	hepatitis B vaccine
Hib	*Haemophilus influenzae* type b conjugate vaccine
HPV vaccine	human papillomavirus vaccine
HZV	herpes zoster vaccine
IIV	inactivated influenza vaccine
LAIV	live attenuated influenza vaccine
MenACWY	serogroups A, C, W, and Y meningococcal conjugate vaccine
MenB	serogroup B meningococcal vaccine
MMR	measles, mumps, and rubella vaccine
MPSV4	serogroups A, C, W, and Y meningococcal polysaccharide vaccine
PCV13	13-valent pneumococcal conjugate vaccine
PPSV23	23-valent pneumococcal polysaccharide vaccine
RIV	recombinant influenza vaccine
Td	tetanus and diphtheria toxoids
Tdap	tetanus toxoid, reduced diphtheria toxoid, and acellular pertussis vaccine
VAR	varicella vaccine

[1] MMWR Morb Mortal Wkly Rep. 2017;66(5). Available at www.cdc.gov/mmwr/volumes/66/wr/mm6605e2.htm?s_cid=mm6605e2_w.

[2] Ann Intern Med. 2017;166:209-218. Available at annals.org/aim/article/doi/10.7326/M16-2936.

TABLE 13 Recommended Immunization Schedule for Adults Aged 19 Years or Older by Age Group, United States, 2019

These recommendations must be read with the footnotes that follow.

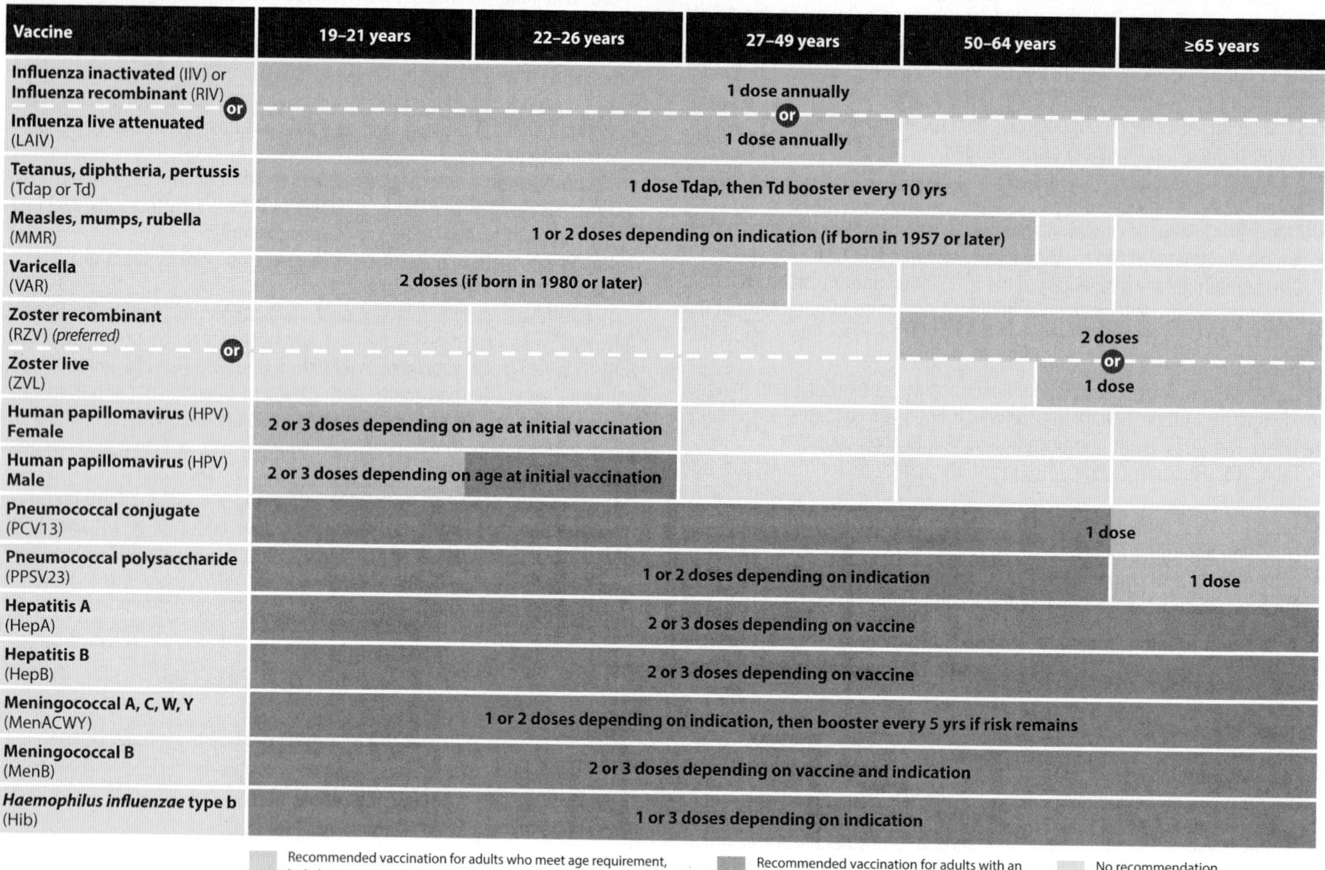

Vaccine	19–21 years	22–26 years	27–49 years	50–64 years	≥65 years
Influenza inactivated (IIV) or **Influenza recombinant** (RIV)	1 dose annually				
or					
Influenza live attenuated (LAIV)	1 dose annually				
Tetanus, diphtheria, pertussis (Tdap or Td)	1 dose Tdap, then Td booster every 10 yrs				
Measles, mumps, rubella (MMR)	1 or 2 doses depending on indication (if born in 1957 or later)				
Varicella (VAR)	2 doses (if born in 1980 or later)				
Zoster recombinant (RZV) *(preferred)*				2 doses	
or					
Zoster live (ZVL)					1 dose
Human papillomavirus (HPV) **Female**	2 or 3 doses depending on age at initial vaccination				
Human papillomavirus (HPV) **Male**	2 or 3 doses depending on age at initial vaccination				
Pneumococcal conjugate (PCV13)					1 dose
Pneumococcal polysaccharide (PPSV23)	1 or 2 doses depending on indication				1 dose
Hepatitis A (HepA)	2 or 3 doses depending on vaccine				
Hepatitis B (HepB)	2 or 3 doses depending on vaccine				
Meningococcal A, C, W, Y (MenACWY)	1 or 2 doses depending on indication, then booster every 5 yrs if risk remains				
Meningococcal B (MenB)	2 or 3 doses depending on vaccine and indication				
***Haemophilus influenzae* type b** (Hib)	1 or 3 doses depending on indication				

Recommended vaccination for adults who meet age requirement, lack documentation of vaccination, or lack evidence of past infection

Recommended vaccination for adults with an additional risk factor or another indication

No recommendation

TABLE 14 Recommended Immunization Schedule for Adults Aged 19 Years or Older by Medical Condition and Other Indications, United States, 2019

These recommendations must be read with the footnotes that follow.

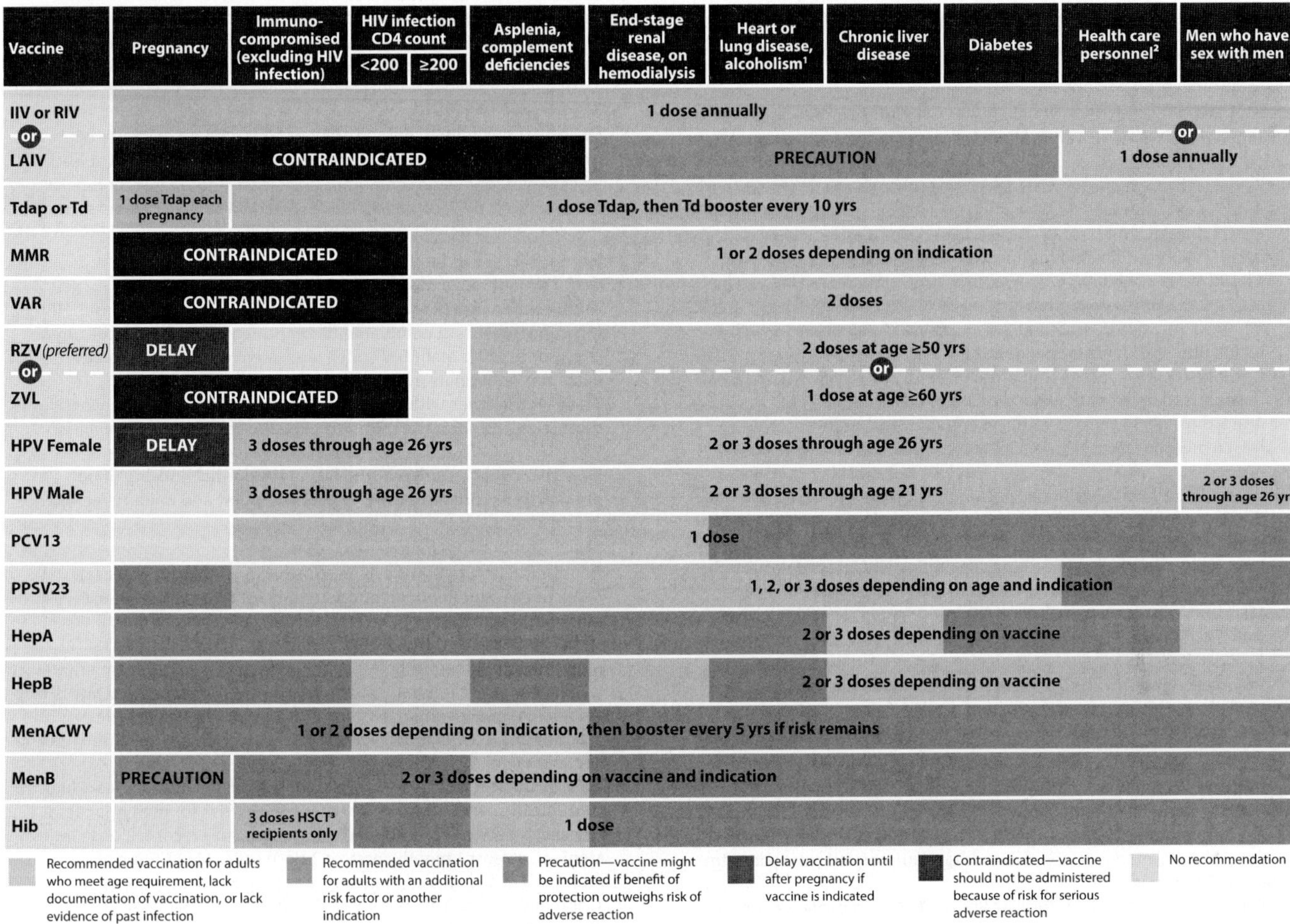

Vaccine	Pregnancy	Immuno-compromised (excluding HIV infection)	HIV infection CD4 count <200	HIV infection CD4 count ≥200	Asplenia, complement deficiencies	End-stage renal disease, on hemodialysis	Heart or lung disease, alcoholism[1]	Chronic liver disease	Diabetes	Health care personnel[2]	Men who have sex with men
IIV or RIV	1 dose annually										
or LAIV	CONTRAINDICATED					PRECAUTION				1 dose annually	
Tdap or Td	1 dose Tdap each pregnancy	1 dose Tdap, then Td booster every 10 yrs									
MMR	CONTRAINDICATED			1 or 2 doses depending on indication							
VAR	CONTRAINDICATED			2 doses							
RZV (preferred)	DELAY				2 doses at age ≥50 yrs						
or ZVL	CONTRAINDICATED				1 dose at age ≥60 yrs						
HPV Female	DELAY	3 doses through age 26 yrs			2 or 3 doses through age 26 yrs						
HPV Male		3 doses through age 26 yrs			2 or 3 doses through age 21 yrs						2 or 3 doses through age 26 yrs
PCV13		1 dose									
PPSV23		1, 2, or 3 doses depending on age and indication									
HepA	2 or 3 doses depending on vaccine										
HepB	2 or 3 doses depending on vaccine										
MenACWY	1 or 2 doses depending on indication, then booster every 5 yrs if risk remains										
MenB	PRECAUTION	2 or 3 doses depending on vaccine and indication									
Hib		3 doses HSCT[3] recipients only	1 dose								

Recommended vaccination for adults who meet age requirement, lack documentation of vaccination, or lack evidence of past infection

Recommended vaccination for adults with an additional risk factor or another indication

Precaution—vaccine might be indicated if benefit of protection outweighs risk of adverse reaction

Delay vaccination until after pregnancy if vaccine is indicated

Contraindicated—vaccine should not be administered because of risk for serious adverse reaction

No recommendation

1. Precaution for LAIV does not apply to alcoholism. **2.** See notes for influenza; hepatitis B; measles, mumps, and rubella; and varicella vaccinations. **3.** Hematopoietic stem cell transplant.

Footnotes. Recommended Adult Immunization Schedule United States, 2019

1. ***Haemophilus influenzae*** **type b vaccination**
   Special situations
   - **Anatomical or functional asplenia (including sickle cell disease):** 1 dose Hib if previously did not receive Hib; if elective splenectomy, 1 dose Hib, preferably at least 14 days before splenectomy
   - **Hematopoietic stem cell transplant** (HSCT): 3-dose series Hib 4 weeks apart starting 6–12 months after successful transplant, regardless of Hib vaccination history
2. **Hepatitis A vaccination**
   Routine vaccination
   - **Not at risk but want protection from hepatitis A** (identification of risk factor not required): 2-dose series HepA (Havrix 6–12 months apart or Vaqta 6–18 months apart [minimum interval: 6 months]) or 3-dose series HepA-HepB (Twinrix at 0, 1, 6 months [minimum intervals: 4 weeks between doses 1 and 2, 5 months between doses 2 and 3])

   Special situations
   - **At risk for hepatitis A virus infection:** 2-dose series HepA or 3-dose series HepA-HepB as above
     - **Chronic liver disease**
     - **Clotting factor disorders**
     - **Men who have sex with men**
     - **Injection or non-injection drug use**
     - **Homelessness**
     - **Work with hepatitis A virus** in research laboratory or nonhuman primates with hepatitis A virus infection
     - **Travel in countries with high or intermediate endemic hepatitis A**
     - **Close personal contact with international adoptee** (e.g., household, regular babysitting) in first 60 days after arrival from country with high or intermediate endemic hepatitis A (administer dose 1 as soon as adoption is planned, at least 2 weeks before adoptee's arrival)
3. **Hepatitis B vaccination**
   Routine vaccination
   - **Not at risk but want protection from hepatitis B** (identification of risk factor not required): 2- or 3-dose series HepB (2-dose series Heplisav-B at least 4 weeks apart [2-dose series HepB only applies when 2 doses of Heplisav-B are used at least 4 weeks apart] or 3-dose series Engerix-B or Recombivax HB at 0, 1, 6 months [minimum intervals: 4 weeks between doses 1 and 2, 8 weeks between doses 2 and 3, 16 weeks between doses 1 and 3]) or 3-dose series HepA-HepB (Twinrix at 0, 1, 6 months [minimum intervals: 4 weeks between doses 1 and 2, 5 months between doses 2 and 3])

   Special situations
   - **At risk for hepatitis B virus infection:** 2-dose (Heplisav-B) or 3-dose (Engerix-B, Recombivax HB) series HepB, or 3-dose series HepA-HepB as above
     - **Hepatitis C virus infection**
     - **Chronic liver disease** (e.g., cirrhosis, fatty liver disease, alcoholic liver disease, autoimmune hepatitis, alanine aminotransferase [ALT] or aspartate aminotransferase [AST] level greater than twice upper limit of normal)
     - **HIV infection**
     - **Sexual exposure risk** (e.g., sex partners of hepatitis B surface antigen (HBsAg)-positive persons; sexually active persons not in mutually monogamous relationships, persons seeking evaluation or treatment for a sexually transmitted infection, men who have sex with men)
     - **Current or recent injection drug use**
     - **Percutaneous or mucosal risk for exposure to blood** (e.g., household contacts of HBsAg-positive persons; residents and staff of facilities for developmentally disabled persons; health care and public safety personnel with reasonably anticipated risk for exposure

to blood or blood-contaminated body fluids; hemodialysis, peritoneal dialysis, home dialysis, and predialysis patients; persons with diabetes mellitus age younger than 60 years and, at discretion of treating clinician, those age 60 years or older)
  - **Incarcerated persons**
  - **Travel in countries with high or intermediate endemic hepatitis B**

4. **Human papillomavirus vaccination**
   Routine vaccination
   - **Females through age 26 years and males through age 21 years:** 2- or 3-dose series HPV vaccine depending on age at initial vaccination; males age 22 through 26 years may be vaccinated based on individual clinical decision (HPV vaccination routinely recommended at age 11–12 years)
   - **Age 15 years or older at initial vaccination:** 3-dose series HPV vaccine at 0, 1–2, 6 months (minimum intervals: 4 weeks between doses 1 and 2, 12 weeks between doses 2 and 3, 5 months between doses 1 and 3; repeat dose if administered too soon)
   - **Age 9 through 14 years at initial vaccination and received 1 dose, or 2 doses less than 5 months apart:** 1 dose HPV vaccine
   - **Age 9 through 14 years at initial vaccination and received 2 doses at least 5 months apart:** HPV vaccination complete, no additional dose needed
   - If completed valid vaccination series with any HPV vaccine, no additional doses needed

   Special situations
   - **Immunocompromising conditions (including HIV infection) through age 26 years:** 3-dose series HPV vaccine at 0, 1–2, 6 months as above
   - **Men who have sex with men and transgender persons through age 26 years:** 2- or 3-dose series HPV vaccine depending on age at initial vaccination as above
   - **Pregnancy through age 26 years:** HPV vaccination not recommended until after pregnancy; no intervention needed if vaccinated while pregnant; pregnancy testing not needed before vaccination

5. **Influenza vaccination**
   Routine vaccination
   - **Persons age 6 months or older:** 1 dose IIV, RIV, or LAIV appropriate for age and health status annually
     For additional guidance, see www.cdc.gov/flu/professionals/index.htm

   Special situations
   - **Egg allergy, hives only:** 1 dose IIV, RIV, or LAIV appropriate for age and health status annually
   - **Egg allergy more severe than hives** (e.g., angioedema, respiratory distress): 1 dose IIV, RIV, or LAIV appropriate for age and health status annually in medical setting under supervision of health care provider who can recognize and manage severe allergic conditions
   - **Immunocompromising conditions (including HIV infection), anatomical or functional asplenia, pregnant women, close contacts and caregivers of severely immunocompromised persons in protected environment, use of influenza antiviral medications in previous 48 hours, with cerebrospinal fluid leak or cochlear implant:** 1 dose IIV or RIV annually (LAIV not recommended)
   - **History of Guillain-Barré syndrome within 6 weeks of previous dose of influenza vaccine:** Generally should not be vaccinated

6. **Measles, mumps, and rubella vaccination**
   Routine vaccination
   - **No evidence of immunity to measles, mumps, or rubella:** 1 dose MMR
     - Evidence of immunity: Born before 1957 (except health care personnel [see below]), documentation of receipt of MMR, laboratory evidence of immunity or disease (diagnosis of disease without laboratory confirmation is not evidence of immunity)

   Special situations
   - **Pregnancy with no evidence of immunity to rubella:** MMR contraindicated during pregnancy; after pregnancy (before discharge from health care facility), 1 dose MMR
   - **Non-pregnant women of childbearing age with no evidence of immunity to rubella:** 1 dose MMR
   - **HIV infection with CD4 count ≥200 cells/μL for at least 6 months and no evidence of immunity to measles, mumps, or rubella:** 2-dose series MMR at least 4 weeks apart; MMR contraindicated in HIV infection with CD4 count <200 cells/μL
   - **Severe immunocompromising conditions:** MMR contraindicated
   - **Students in postsecondary educational institutions, international travelers, and household or close personal contacts of immunocompromised persons with no evidence of immunity to measles, mumps, or rubella:** 1 dose MMR if previously received 1 dose MMR, or 2-dose series MMR at least 4 weeks apart if previously did not receive any MMR
   - **Health care personnel born in 1957 or later with no evidence of immunity to measles, mumps, or rubella:** 2-dose series MMR at least 4 weeks apart for measles or mumps, or at least 1 dose MMR for rubella; if born before 1957, consider 2-dose series MMR at least 4 weeks apart for measles or mumps, or 1 dose MMR for rubella

7. **Meningococcal vaccination**
   Special situations for MenACWY
   - **Anatomical or functional asplenia (including sickle cell disease), HIV infection, persistent complement component deficiency, eculizumab use:** 2-dose series MenACWY (Menactra, Menveo) at least 8 weeks apart and revaccinate every 5 years if risk remains
   - **Travel in countries with hyperendemic or epidemic meningococcal disease, microbiologists routinely exposed to *Neisseria meningitidis*:** 1 dose MenACWY and revaccinate every 5 years if risk remains
   - **First-year college students who live in residential housing (if not previously vaccinated at age 16 years or older) and military recruits:** 1 dose MenACWY

   Special situations for MenB
   - **Anatomical or functional asplenia (including sickle cell disease), persistent complement component deficiency, eculizumab use, microbiologists routinely exposed to *Neisseria meningitidis*:** 2-dose series MenB-4C (Bexsero) at least 1 month apart, or 3-dose series MenB-FHbp (Trumenba) at 0, 1–2, 6 months (if dose 2 was administered at least 6 months after dose 1, dose 3 not needed); MenB-4C and MenBFHbp are not interchangeable (use same product for all doses in series)
   - **Pregnancy:** Delay MenB until after pregnancy unless at increased risk and vaccination benefit outweighs potential risks
   - **Healthy adolescents and young adults age 16 through 23 years (age 16 through 18 years preferred) not at increased risk for meningococcal disease:** Based on individual clinical decision, may receive 2-dose series MenB-4C at least 1 month apart, or 2-dose series MenB-FHbp at 0, 6 months (if dose 2 was administered less than 6 months after dose 1, administer dose 3 at least 4 months after dose 2); MenB-4C and MenB-FHbp are not interchangeable (use same product for all doses in series)

8. **Pneumococcal vaccination**
   Routine vaccination
   - **Age 65 years or older** (immunocompetent): 1 dose PCV13 if previously did not receive PCV13, followed by 1 dose PPSV23 at least 1 year after PCV13 and at least 5 years after last dose PPSV23
     - Previously received PPSV23 but not PCV13 at age 65 years or older: 1 dose PCV13 at least 1 year after PPSV23
     - When both PCV13 and PPSV23 are indicated, administer PCV13 first (PCV13 and PPSV23 should not be administered during same visit)

   Special situations
   - **Age 19 through 64 years with chronic medical conditions (chronic heart [excluding hypertension], lung, or liver disease; diabetes), alcoholism, or cigarette smoking:** 1 dose PPSV23
   - **Age 19 years or older with immunocompromising conditions (congenital or acquired immunodeficiency [including B- and T-lymphocyte deficiency, complement deficiencies, phagocytic disorders, HIV infection], chronic renal failure, nephrotic syndrome, leukemia, lymphoma, Hodgkin disease, generalized malignancy, iatrogenic immunosuppression [e.g., drug or radiation therapy], solid organ transplant, multiple myeloma) or anatomical or functional asplenia (including sickle cell disease and other hemoglobinopathies):** 1 dose PCV13 followed by 1 dose PPSV23 at least 8 weeks later, then another dose PPSV23 at least 5 years after previous PPSV23; at age 65 years or older, administer 1 dose PPSV23 at least 5 years after most recent PPSV23 (note: only 1 dose PPSV23 recommended at age 65 years or older)
   - **Age 19 years or older with cerebrospinal fluid leak or cochlear implant:** 1 dose PCV13 followed by 1 dose PPSV23 at least 8 weeks later; at age 65 years or older, administer another dose PPSV23 at least 5 years after PPSV23 (note: only 1 dose PPSV23 recommended at age 65 years or older)

9. **Tetanus, diphtheria, and pertussis vaccination**
   Routine vaccination
   - **Previously did not receive Tdap at or after age 11 years:** 1 dose Tdap, then Td booster every 10 years

   Special situations
   - **Previously did not receive primary vaccination series for tetanus, diphtheria, and pertussis:** 1 dose Tdap followed by 1 dose Td at least 4 weeks after Tdap, and another dose Td 6–12 months after last Td (Tdap can be substituted for any Td dose, but preferred as first dose); Td booster every 10 years thereafter
   - **Pregnancy:** 1 dose Tdap during each pregnancy, preferably in early part of gestational weeks 27–36
   - For information on use of Tdap or Td as tetanus prophylaxis in wound management, see www.cdc.gov/mmwr/volumes/67/rr/rr6702a1.htm

10. **Varicella vaccination**
    Routine vaccination
    - **No evidence of immunity to varicella:** 2-dose series VAR 4–8 weeks apart if previously did not receive varicella-containing vaccine (VAR or MMRV [measlesmumps-rubella-varicella vaccine] for children); if previously received 1 dose varicella-containing vaccine: 1 dose VAR at least 4 weeks after first dose
      - Evidence of immunity: U.S.-born before 1980 (except for pregnant women and health care personnel [see below]), documentation of 2 doses varicellacontaining vaccine at least 4 weeks apart, diagnosis or verification of history of varicella or herpes zoster by a health care provider, laboratory evidence of immunity or disease

    Special situations
    - **Pregnancy with no evidence of immunity to varicella:** VAR contraindicated during pregnancy; after pregnancy (before discharge from health care facility), 1 dose VAR if previously received 1 dose varicellacontaining vaccine, or dose 1 of 2-dose series VAR (dose 2: 4–8 weeks later) if previously did not receive any varicella-containing vaccine, regardless of whether U.S.-born before 1980
    - **Health care personnel with no evidence of immunity to varicella:** 1 dose VAR if previously received 1 dose varicella-containing vaccine, or 2-dose series VAR 4–8 weeks apart if previously did not receive any varicella-containing vaccine, regardless of whether U.S.-born before 1980
    - **HIV infection with CD4 count ≥200 cells/μL with no evidence of immunity:** Consider 2-dose series VAR 3 months apart based on individual clinical decision; VAR contraindicated in HIV infection with CD4 count <200 cells/μL
    - **Severe immunocompromising conditions:** VAR contraindicated

11. **Zoster vaccination**
    Routine vaccination
    - **Age 50 years or older:** 2-dose series RZV 2–6 months apart (minimum interval: 4 weeks; repeat dose if administered too soon) regardless of previous herpes zoster or previously received ZVL (administer RZV at least 2 months after ZVL)
    - **Age 60 years or older:** 2-dose series RZV 2–6 months apart (minimum interval: 4 weeks; repeat dose if administered too soon) or 1 dose ZVL if not previously vaccinated (if previously received ZVL, administer RZV at least 2 months after ZVL); RZV preferred over ZVL

    Special situations
    - **Pregnancy:** ZVL contraindicated; consider delaying RZV until after pregnancy if RZV is otherwise indicated
    - **Severe immunocompromising conditions (including HIV infection with CD4 count <200 cells/μL):** ZVL contraindicated; recommended use of RZV under review

The Advisory Committee on Immunization Practices (ACIP) recommendations and package inserts for vaccines provide information on contraindications and precautions related to vaccines. Contraindications are conditions that increase chances of a serious adverse reaction in vaccine recipients and the vaccine should not be administered when a contraindication is present. Precautions should be reviewed for potential risks and benefits for vaccine recipient. For a person with a severe allergy to latex, e.g., anaphylaxis, vaccines supplied in vials or syringes that contain natural rubber latex should not be administered unless the benefit of vaccination clearly outweighs the risk for a potential allergic reaction. For latex allergies other than anaphylaxis, vaccines supplied in vials or syringes that contain dry, natural rubber or natural rubber latex may be administered.

TABLE 15 Immunization and Pregnancy

Vaccine	Before Pregnancy	During Pregnancy	After Pregnancy	Type of Vaccine	Route
Hepatitis A	If at high risk for disease	If at high risk for disease	If at high risk for disease	Inactivated	IM
Hepatitis B	Yes, if at risk	Yes, if at risk	Yes, if at risk	Inactivated	IM
Human papillomavirus (HPV)	Yes, if 9 to 26 years of age	No, under study	Yes, if 9 to 26 years of age	Inactivated	IM
Influenza TIV	Yes	Yes	Yes	Inactivated	IM
Influenza LAIV	Yes, if <50 years and healthy; avoid conception for 4 weeks	No	Yes, if <50 years and healthy; avoid conception for 4 weeks	Live	Nasal spray
MMR	Yes, avoid conception for 4 weeks	No	Yes, give immediately postpartum if susceptible to rubella	Live	SC
Meningococcal	If indicated	If indicated	If indicated		
Polysaccharide				Inactivated	SC
Conjugate				Inactivated	IM
Pneumococcal polysaccharide	If indicated	If indicated	If indicated	Inactivated	IM or SC
Tetanus/diphtheria Td	Yes, Tdap preferred	If indicated	Yes, Tdap preferred	Toxoid	IM
Tdap, one dose only	Yes, preferred	If high risk of pertussis; otherwise, Td preferred	Yes, preferred	Toxoid/inactivated	IM
Varicella	Yes, avoid conception for 4 weeks	No	Yes, give immediately postpartum if susceptible	Live	SC

IM, Intramuscular; *LAIV,* live, attenuated influenza vaccine; *SC,* subcutaneous; *Tdap,* tetanus and diphtheria toxoids and acellular pertussis; *TIV,* trivalent inactivated influenza vaccine.

TABLE 16 Immunizing Agents and Immunization Schedules for Health Care Workers (HCWs)*

Generic Name	Primary Schedule and Booster(s)	Indications	Major Precautions and Contraindications	Special Considerations
Immunizing Agents Strongly Recommended for Health Care Workers				
Hepatitis B (HB) recombinant vaccine	Two doses IM 4 wk apart; third dose 5 mo after second; booster doses not necessary	**Preexposure:** HCWs at risk for exposure to blood or body fluids	Based on limited data no risk of adverse effects to developing fetuses is apparent. Pregnancy should *not* be considered a contraindication to vaccination of women. Previous anaphylactic reaction to common baker's yeast is a contraindication to vaccination.	The vaccine produces neither therapeutic nor adverse effects on HB-infected persons. Prevaccination serologic screening is not indicated for persons being vaccinated because of occupational risk. HCWs who have contact with patients or blood should be tested 1-2 mo after vaccination to determine serologic response.
Hepatitis B immune globulin (HBIG)	0.06 ml/kg IM as soon as possible after exposure. A second dose of HBIG should be administered 1 mo later if the HB vaccine series has not been started.	**Postexposure prophylaxis:** For persons exposed to blood or body fluids containing HBsAg and who are not immune to HBV infection—0.06 ml/kg IM as soon as possible (but no later than 7 days after exposure)		
Influenza vaccine (inactivated whole-virus and split-virus vaccines)	Annual vaccination with current vaccine Administered IM	HCWs who have contact with patients at high risk for influenza or its complications; HCWs who work in long-term care facilities; HCWs with high-risk medical conditions or who are aged ≥65 yr	History of anaphylactic hypersensitivity to egg ingestion	No evidence exists of risk to mother or fetus when the vaccine is administered to a pregnant woman with an underlying high-risk condition. Influenza vaccination is recommended during second and third trimesters of pregnancy because of increased risk for hospitalization.
Measles live-virus vaccine	One dose SC; second dose at least 1 mo later	HCWs† born during or after 1957 who do not have documentation of having received two doses of live vaccine on or after the first birthday **or** a history of physician-diagnosed measles or serologic evidence of immunity. Vaccination should be considered for all HCWs who lack proof of immunity, including those born before 1957.	Pregnancy; immunocompromised persons,‡ including HIV-infected persons who have evidence of severe immunosuppression; anaphylaxis after gelatin ingestion or administration of neomycin; recent administration of immune globulin	MMR is the vaccine of choice if recipients are likely to be susceptible to rubella and/or mumps as well as measles. Persons vaccinated between 1963 and 1967 with a killed measles vaccine alone, killed vaccine followed by live vaccine, or with a vaccine of unknown type should be revaccinated with two doses of live measles virus vaccine.
Mumps live-virus vaccine	One dose SC; second dose at least 1 mo later	HCWs† believed to be susceptible can be vaccinated. Adults born before 1957 can be considered immune.	Pregnancy; immunocompromised persons,‡ history of anaphylactic reaction after gelatin ingestion or administration of neomycin	MMR is the vaccine of choice if recipients are likely to be susceptible to measles and rubella, as well as mumps.
Hepatitis A virus (HAV) vaccine	Two doses of vaccine either 6-12 mo apart (HAVRIX), or 6 mo apart (VAQTA)	Not routinely indicated for HCWs in the United States. Persons who work with HAV-infected primates or with HAV in a research laboratory setting should be vaccinated.	History of anaphylactic hypersensitivity to alum or, for HAVRIX, the preservative 2-phenoxyethanol. The safety of the vaccine in pregnant women has not been determined; the risk associated with vaccination should be weighed against the risk for hepatitis A in women who may be at high risk for exposure to HAV.	

TABLE 16 Immunizing Agents and Immunization Schedules for Health Care Workers (HCWs)*—cont'd

Generic Name	Primary Schedule and Booster(s)	Indications	Major Precautions and Contraindications	Special Considerations
Meningococcal vaccine	One dose in volume and by route specified by manufacturer; single booster for adults 19 to 21 years of age if the first dose was given before age 16	Laboratory personnel and others with exposure risk.	The safety of the vaccine in pregnant women has not been evaluated; it should not be administered during pregnancy unless the risk for infection is high.	
Typhoid vaccine, IM, SC, and oral	IM vaccine: One 0.5-ml/dose, booster 0.5 ml every 2 yr SC vaccine: Two 0.5-ml doses, ≥4 wk apart, booster 0.5 ml SC or 0.1 ID every 3 yr if exposure continues Oral vaccine: Four doses on alternate days. The manufacturer recommends revaccination with the entire 4-dose series every 5 yr	Workers in microbiology laboratories who frequently work with *Salmonella typhi*	Severe local or systemic reaction to a previous dose. Ty21a (oral) vaccine should not be administered to immunocompromised persons† or to persons receiving antimicrobial agents.	Vaccination should not be considered an alternative to the use of proper procedures when handling specimens and cultures in the laboratory.
Vaccinia vaccine (smallpox)	One dose administered with a bifurcated needle; boosters administered every 10 yr	Laboratory workers who directly handle cultures with vaccinia, recombinant vaccinia viruses, or orthopox viruses that infect human beings	The vaccine is contraindicated in pregnancy, in persons with eczema or a history of eczema, and in immunocompromised persons† and their household contacts.	Vaccination may be considered for HCWs who have direct contact with contaminated dressings or other infectious material from volunteers in clinical studies involving recombinant vaccinia virus.
Other Vaccine-Preventable Diseases				
Tetanus and diphtheria and pertussis (Tdap)	Two IM doses 4 wk apart or tetanus and diphtheria toxoid for adults with uncertain or incomplete primary vaccination; third dose 6-12 mo after second dose; booster every 10 yr. Substitute a one-time dose of Tdap for one of the doses of Td, either in the primary series or for the routine booster, whichever comes first.	All adults	Except in the first trimester, pregnancy is not a precaution. History of a neurologic reaction or immediate hypersensitivity reaction after a previous dose. History of severe local (Arthus-type) reaction after a previous dose. Such persons should not receive further routine or emergency doses of Td for 10 yr.	Tetanus prophylaxis in wound management‡
Pneumococcal polysaccharide vaccine (23 valent)	One dose, 0.5 ml, IM or SC; revaccination recommended for those at highest risk ≥5 yr after the first dose	Adults who are at increased risk of pneumococcal disease and its complications because of underlying health conditions; older adults, especially those age ≥65 who are healthy	The safety of vaccine in pregnant women has not been evaluated; it should not be administered during pregnancy unless the risk for infection is high. Previous recipients of any type of pneumococcal polysaccharide vaccine who are at highest risk for fatal infection or antibody loss may be revaccinated ≥5 yr after the first dose.	
Rubella live-virus vaccine	One dose SC; second dose at least 1 mo later	Indicated for HCWs,† both men and women, who do not have documentation of having received live vaccine on or after their first birthday **or** laboratory evidence of immunity. Adults born before 1957, **except women who can become pregnant,** can be considered immune.	Pregnancy; immunocompromised persons†; history of anaphylactic reaction after administration of neomycin	The risk for rubella vaccine–associated malformations in the offspring of women pregnant when vaccinated or who become pregnant within 3 mo after vaccination is negligible. Such women should be counseled regarding the theoretic basis of concern for the fetus. MMR is the vaccine of choice if recipients are likely to be susceptible to measles or mumps as well as rubella.

Continued

TABLE 16 Immunizing Agents and Immunization Schedules for Health Care Workers (HCWs)*—cont'd

Generic Name	Primary Schedule and Booster(s)	Indications	Major Precautions and Contraindications	Special Considerations
Varicella-zoster live-virus vaccine	Two 0.5-ml doses SC 4-8 wk apart if ≥13 yr	Indicated for HCWs† who do not have either a reliable history of varicella or serologic evidence of immunity	Pregnancy, immunocompromised persons,‡ history of anaphylactic reaction after receipt of neomycin or gelatin. Avoid salicylate use for 6 wk after vaccination.	Vaccine is available from the manufacturer for certain patients with acute lymphocytic leukemia in remission. Because 71%-93% of persons without a history of varicella are immune, serologic testing before vaccination is likely to be cost effective.
Varicella-zoster immune globulin (VZIG)	Persons <50 kg: 125 µg/10 kg IM; persons ≥50 kg: 625 µg§	Persons known or likely to be susceptible (particularly those at high risk for complications, e.g., pregnant women) who have close and prolonged exposure to a contact case or to an infectious hospital staff worker or patient		Serologic testing may help in assessing whether to administer VZIG. If use of VZIG prevents varicella disease, patient should be vaccinated subsequently.
BCG Vaccination				
Bacille Calmette-Guérin (BCG) vaccine (TB)	One percutaneous dose of 0.3 ml; no booster dose recommended	Should be considered only for HCWs in areas where multidrug TB is prevalent, a strong likelihood of infection exists, and where comprehensive infection control precautions have failed to prevent TB transmission to HCWs	Should not be administered to immunocompromised persons,‡ pregnant women	In the United States TB-control efforts are directed toward early identification, treatment of cases, and preventive therapy with isoniazid.
Other Immunobiologics That Are or May Be Indicated for HCWs				
Immune globulin (hepatitis A)	**Postexposure**—One IM dose of 0.02 ml/kg administered ≤2 wk after exposure	Indicated for HCWs exposed to feces of infectious patients	Contraindicated in persons with IgA deficiency; do not administer within 2 wk after MMR vaccine or 3 wk after varicella vaccine. Delay administration of MMR vaccine for ≥3 mo and varicella vaccine ≥5 mo after administration of immune globulin	Administer in large muscle mass (deltoid, gluteal).

HBsAg, Hepatitis B surface antigen; *HBV,* hepatitis B virus; *HIV,* human immunodeficiency virus; *IM,* intramuscular; *MMR,* measles, mumps, rubella vaccine; *SC,* subcutaneous; *TB,* tuberculosis.

*Persons who provide health care to patients or work in institutions that provide patient care (e.g., physicians, nurses, emergency medical personnel, dental professionals and students, medical and nursing students, laboratory technicians, hospital volunteers, and administrative and support staff in health care institutions).

†All HCWs (i.e., medical or nonmedical, paid or volunteer, full time or part time, student or nonstudent, with or without patient-care responsibilities) who work in health care institutions (e.g., inpatient and outpatient, public and private) should be immune to measles, rubella, and varicella.

‡Persons immunocompromised because of immune deficiency diseases, HIV infection, leukemia, lymphoma or generalized malignancy, or immunosuppressed as a result of therapy with corticosteroids, alkylating drugs, antimetabolites, or radiation.

§Some experts recommend 125 µg/10 kg regardless of total body weight.

Modified from *MMWR* 46(RR-18), 1998.

TABLE 17 Recommendations for Persons with Medical Conditions Requiring Special Vaccination Considerations

Condition	Tdap	MMR	Varicella	HBV	HAV	Pneumovax[a]	Influenza[b]	HbCV	Meningococcal	IPV	Other Live Vaccines[c]	Other Killed Vaccines[d]
HIV infection	Rou	Rou/Contr[e]	Contr[f]	Rou[g]	Rou	Rec	Rec	Cons	Rou	Rou	Contr	Rou
Severe immunocompromise[h]	Rou	Contr	Contr[f]	Rou[g]	Rou	Rec	Rec	Rou[i]	Rou	Rou	Contr	Rou
Renal failure	Rou	Rou	Rou	Rec[g]	Rou	Rec	Rec	Rou	Rou	Rou	Rou	Rou
Diabetes	Rou	Rou	Rou	Rou	Rou	Rec	Rec	Rou	Rou	Rou	Rou	Rou
Chronic liver disease	Rou	Rou	Rou	Rou	Rec	Rec	Rec	Rou	Rou	Rou	Rou	Rou
Cardiac disease	Rou	Rou	Rou	Rou	Rou	Rec	Rec	Rou	Rou	Rou	Rou	Rou
Pulmonary disease	Rou	Rou	Rou	Rou	Rou	Rec	Rec	Rou	Rou	Rou	Rou	Rou
Alcoholism	Rou	Rou	Rou	Rou	Rou	Rec	Rec	Rou	Rou	Rou	Rou	Rou
Functional/anatomic asplenia	Rou	Rou	Rou	Rou	Rou	Rec[j]	Rec	Rec[j]	Rec[j]	Rou	Rou	Rou
Terminal complement deficiency	Rou	Rou	Rou	Rou	Rou	Rou	Rou	Rou	Rec	Rou	Rou	
Clotting factor disorders	Rou	Rou	Rou	Rec	Rec	Rou	Rou	Rou	Rou	Rou	Rou	Rou

Cons, Consider vaccination; *Contr,* contraindicated; *HAV,* hepatitis A virus; *HbCV, Haemophilus influenzae* conjugate vaccine; *HBV,* hepatitis B virus; *IPV,* inactivated poliomyelitis vaccine; *MMR,* measles-mumps-rubella; *Rec,* recommended; *Rou,* routine as outlined for all adults; *Tdap,* tetanus and diphtheria toxoids and acellular pertussis.

[a]Pneumovax should be repeated in 5 yr for patients in whom vaccine is recommended. Asthma without chronic obstructive pulmonary disease is not an indication for the vaccine.

[b]Influenza vaccine should also be given to caregivers and household members.

[c]Includes bacille Calmette-Guérin, vaccinia, oral typhoid, yellow fever (if exposure cannot be avoided, persons with HIV can be given yellow fever vaccine; see text).

[d]Includes rabies (check postvaccination titers in HIV or severely immunocompromised persons), Lyme disease, inactivated typhoid, cholera, plague, and anthrax.

[e]For asymptomatic, nonseverely immunocompromised persons with HIV, MMR can be used; it is contraindicated in severely immunocompromised persons. MMR can be considered in symptomatic HIV patients without severe immunocompromise.

[f]Varicella can be given to household members and caregivers, but if varicella-like rash develops after vaccination, contact should be avoided.

[g]Recommended for persons with severe chronic renal failure approaching or already receiving dialysis, and higher doses should be given. Antibody titers should be measured after vaccination in these patients and in those with HIV or severe immunocompromise (who may require higher doses) to ensure adequate response. Yearly titers should be measured in dialysis patients.

[h]Severe immunocompromise can result from congenital immunodeficiency, leukemia, lymphoma, malignancy, organ transplant, chemotherapy, radiation therapy, or high-dose corticosteroids.

[i]Only for persons with Hodgkin's disease.

[j]Give at least 2 wk in advance of elective splenectomy.

Modified and updated from *MMWR* 42(RR-4):16, 1993.

Vaccinations for International Travel

TABLE 18 Recommended Immunizations for Travelers to Developing Countries

	LENGTH OF TRAVEL		
Immunizations	**Brief (<2 wk)**	**Intermediate (2 wk–3 mo)**	**Long-Term Residential (>3 mo)**
Review and complete age-appropriate childhood schedule	+	+	+
DTaP, poliovirus, pneumococcal, and *Haemophilus influenzae* type B vaccines may be given at 4-week intervals if necessary to complete the recommended schedule before departure. Rotavirus vaccine has maximum ages for the first and last doses; consideration should be given to the timing of an infant's travel so that the infant will be able to receive the vaccine series.			
Measles: Infants 6–11 mo of age should receive 1 dose of MMR vaccine before departure. Two additional doses are given if younger than 12 mo of age at first dose.			
Varicella			
Hepatitis A*			
Hepatitis B†			
Vaccines against the following diseases should be considered depending on the geographic area and circumstances of the visit:			
Japanese encephalitis‡	±	±	+
Meningococcal disease§	±	±	±
Rabies¶	±	+	+
Typhoid fever**	±	+	+
Yellow fever††	+	+	+

DTaP, Diphtheria–tetanus–acellular pertussis.
*Indicated for travelers to areas with intermediate or high endemic rates of hepatitis A virus infection.
†If insufficient time to complete 6-month primary series, an accelerated series can be given.
‡For regions with endemic infection. For high-risk activities in areas experiencing outbreaks, vaccine is recommended, even for brief travel.
§Recommended for regions of Africa with endemic infection and during local epidemics and required for travel to Saudi Arabia for the Hajj.
¶Indicated for persons at high risk for animal exposure (especially dogs) and for travelers to countries with endemic infection.
**Indicated for travelers who will consume food and liquids in areas of poor sanitation.
††For regions with endemic infection.
From Cherry JD: *Feigin and Cherry's pediatric infectious diseases*, ed 8, Elsevier, 2019. (Modified from American Academy of Pediatrics. Immunizations in special clinical circumstances. In: Kimberlin DW, Brady MT, Jackson MA, Long SS, eds. *Red book: 2015 report of the Committee on Infectious Diseases,* ed 30. Elk Grove Village, IL: American Academy of Pediatrics, 2015, 101–107; Centers for Disease Control and Prevention. Health information for international travel, 2016: international travel with infants and young children. Available at http://wwwnc.cdc.gov/travel/yellowbook/2016/international-travel-with-infants-children/vaccine-recommendations-for-infants-children.)

Prevention of Hepatitis B Virus Infection in the United States: Recommendations of the Advisory Committee on Immunization Practices

TABLE 19 Recommended Doses of Hepatitis B Vaccine, by Group and Vaccine Type

	SINGLE-ANTIGEN VACCINE				COMBINATION VACCINE			
	RECOMBIVAX		ENGERIX		PEDIARIX*		TWINRIX†	
Age Group (y)	**Dose (μg)**	**Vol (mL)**	**Dose (μg)**	**Vol (mL)**	**Dose (μg)**	**Vol (mL)**	**DOSE (MG)**	**Vol (mL)**
Birth–10	5	0.5	10	0.5	10*	0.5	N/A	N/A
11–15	10§	1	N/A	N/A	N/A	N/A	N/A	N/A
16–19	5	0.5	10	0.5	N/A	N/A	N/A	N/A
≥20	10	1	20	1	N/A	N/A	20†	1
Hemodialysis Patients and Other Immune-Compromised Persons								
<20	5	0.5	10	0.5	N/A	N/A	N/A	N/A
≥20	40	1	40	2	N/A	N/A	N/A	N/A

N/A, Not applicable.
*Pediarix is approved for use in persons aged 6 weeks through 6 years (before the 7th birthday).
†Twinrix is approved for use in persons aged ≥18 years.
§Adult formulation administered on a 2-dose schedule.
From Schillie S, Vellozzi C, Reingold A, et al. Prevention of hepatitis B virus infection in the United States: recommendations of the Advisory Committee on Immunization Practices. *MMWR Recomm Rep* 67(No. RR-1):1–31, 2018.

TABLE 20 Hepatitis B Vaccine Schedules for Infants, by Infant Birthweight and Maternal HBsAg Status

		SINGLE-ANTIGEN VACCINE		SINGLE-ANTIGEN + COMBINATION VACCINE†	
Birthweight	**Maternal HBsAg Status**	**Dose**	**Age**	**Dose**	**Age**
≥2000 g	Positive	1	Birth (≤12 hr)	1	Birth (≤12 hr)
		HBIG§	Birth (≤12 hr)	HBIG	Birth (≤12 hr)
		2	1–2 mo	2	2 mo
		3	6 mo¶	3	4 mo
				4	6 mo¶
	Unknown*	1	Birth (≤12 hr)	1	Birth (≤12 hr)
		2	1–2 mo	2	2 mo
		3	6 mo¶	3	4 mo
				4	6 mo¶
	Negative	1	Birth (≤24 hr)	1	Birth (≤24 hr)
		2	1–2 mo	2	2 mo
		3	6–18 mo¶	3	4 mo
				4	6 mo¶
<2000 g	Positive	1	Birth (≤12 hr)	1	Birth (≤12 hr)
		HBIG	Birth (≤12 hr)	HBIG	Birth (≤12 hr)
		2	1 mo	2	2 mo
		3	2–3 mo	3	4 mo
		4	6 mo¶	4	6 mo¶
	Unknown	1	Birth (≤12 hr)	1	Birth (≤12 hr)
		HBIG	Birth (≤12 hr)	HBIG	Birth (≤12 hr)
		2	1 mo	2	2 mo
		3	2–3 mo	3	4 mo
		4	6 mo¶	4	6 mo¶
	Negative	1	Hospital discharge or age 1 mo	1	Hospital discharge or age 1 mo
		2	2 mo	2	2 mo
		3	6–18 mo¶	3	4 mo
				4	6 mo¶

HBIG, Hepatitis B immune globulin; *HBsAg,* hepatitis B surface antigen.
*Mothers should have blood drawn and tested for HBsAg as soon as possible after admission for delivery; if the mother is found to be HBsAg positive, the infant should receive HBIG as soon as possible but no later than age 7 days.
†Pediarix should not be administered before age 6 weeks.
§HBIG should be administered at a separate anatomical site from vaccine.
¶The final dose in the vaccine series should not be administered before age 24 weeks (164 days).
From Schillie S, Vellozzi C, Reingold A, et al. Prevention of hepatitis B virus infection in the United States: recommendations of the Advisory Committee on Immunization Practices. *MMWR Recomm Rep* 67(No. RR-1):1–31, 2018.

TABLE 21 Hepatitis B Vaccine Schedules for Children, Adolescents, and Adults

Age Group	Schedule* (Interval Represents Time in Months from First Dose)
Children (1–10 y)	0, 1, and 6 mo
	0, 1, 2, and 12 mo
Adolescents (11–19 y)	0, 1, and 6 mo
	0, 12, and 24 mo
	0 and 4–6 mo†
	0, 1, 2, and 12 mo
	0, 7 d, 21–30 d, 12 mo§
Adults (≥20 y)	0, 1, and 6 mo
	0, 1, 2, and 12 mo
	0, 1, 2, and 6 mo¶
	0, 7 d, 21–30 d, 12 mo§

*Refer to package inserts for further information. For all ages, when the HepB vaccine schedule is interrupted, the vaccine series does not need to be restarted. If the series is interrupted after the first dose, the second dose should be administered as soon as possible, and the second and third doses should be separated by an interval of at least 8 weeks. If only the third dose has been delayed, it should be administered as soon as possible. The final dose of vaccine must be administered at least 8 weeks after the second dose and should follow the first dose by at least 16 weeks; the minimum interval between the first and second doses is 4 weeks. Inadequate doses of hepatitis B vaccine or doses received after a shorter-than-recommended dosing interval should be readministered, using the correct dosage or schedule. Vaccine doses administered ≤4 days before the minimum interval or age are considered valid. Because of the unique accelerated schedule for Twinrix, the 4-day guideline does not apply to the first three doses of this vaccine when administered on a 0-day, 7-day, 21–30-day, and 12-month schedule (new recommendation).
†A 2-dose schedule of Recombivax adult formulation (10 μg) is licensed for adolescents aged 11–15 years. When scheduled to receive the second dose, adolescents aged >15 years should be switched to a 3-dose series, with doses 2 and 3 consisting of the pediatric formulation administered on an appropriate schedule.
§Twinrix is approved for use in persons aged ≥18 years and is available on an accelerated schedule with doses administered at 0, 7, and 21–30 days and 12 months.
¶A 4-dose schedule of Engerix administered in two 1 mL doses (40 μg) on a 0-, 1-, 2-, and 6-month schedule is recommended for adult hemodialysis patients.
From Schillie S, Vellozzi C, Reingold A, et al. Prevention of hepatitis B virus infection in the United States: recommendations of the Advisory Committee on Immunization Practices. *MMWR Recomm Rep* 67(No. RR-1):1–31, 2018.

TABLE 22 Postexposure Management of Health Care Personnel After Occupational Percutaneous or Mucosal Exposure to Blood or Body Fluids, by Health Care Personnel HepB Vaccination and Response Status

	POSTEXPOSURE TESTING		POSTEXPOSURE PROPHYLAXIS		
HCP Status	**Source Patient (HBsAg)**	**HCP Testing (Anti-HBs)**	**HBIG**	**Vaccination**	**Postvaccination Serologic Testing**
Documented responder after complete series			No action needed		
Documented nonresponder after two complete series	Positive/unknown	–*	HBIG ×2 separated by 1 month	—	N/A
	Negative			No action needed	
Response unknown after complete series	Positive/unknown	<10 mIU/mL	HBIG ×1	Initiate revaccination	Yes
	Negative	<10 mIU/mL	None	Initiate revaccination	Yes
	Any result	≥10 mIU/mL		No action needed	
Unvaccinated/incompletely vaccinated or vaccine refusers	Positive/unknown	—	HBIG ×1	Complete vaccination	Yes
	Negative	—	None	Complete vaccination	Yes

Anti-HBs, Antibody to hepatitis B surface antigen; *HBIG,* hepatitis B immune globulin; *HBsAg,* hepatitis B surface antigen; *HCP,* health care personnel; *N/A,* not applicable.
*Not indicated.
From Schillie S, Vellozzi C, Reingold A, et al. Prevention of hepatitis B virus infection in the United States: recommendations of the Advisory Committee on Immunization Practices. *MMWR Recomm Rep* 67(No. RR-1):1–31, 2018.

TABLE 23 Postexposure Management After Distinct Nonoccupational Percutaneous or Mucosal Exposure to Blood or Body Fluids

	MANAGEMENT	
Exposure*	**Unvaccinated Person**	**Previously Vaccinated Person**
HBsAg-positive source	HepB vaccine series and HBIG	HepB vaccine dose
HBsAg status unknown for source	Hep B vaccine series	No management

HBIG, Hepatitis B immune globulin; *HBsAg,* hepatitis B surface antigen; *HepB,* hepatitis B.
*Exposures include percutaneous (e.g., bite or needlestick) or mucosal exposure to blood or body fluids, sex or needle-sharing contact, or victim of sexual assault/abuse.
From Schillie S, Vellozzi C, Reingold A, et al. Prevention of hepatitis B virus infection in the United States: recommendations of the Advisory Committee on Immunization Practices. *MMWR Recomm Rep* 67(No. RR-1):1–31, 2018.

BOX 1 Persons Recommended to Receive Hepatitis B Vaccination

- All infants
- Unvaccinated children aged <19 years
- Persons at risk for infection by sexual exposure
  - Sex partners of hepatitis B surface antigen (HBsAg)–positive persons
  - Sexually active persons who are not in a long-term, mutually monogamous relationship (e.g., persons with more than one sex partner during the previous 6 months)
  - Persons seeking evaluation or treatment for a sexually transmitted infection
  - Men who have sex with men
- Persons at risk for infection by percutaneous or mucosal exposure to blood
  - Current or recent injection-drug users
  - Household contacts of HBsAg-positive persons
  - Residents and staff of facilities for developmentally disabled persons
  - Health care and public safety personnel with reasonably anticipated risk for exposure to blood or blood-contaminated body fluids
  - Hemodialysis patients and predialysis, peritoneal dialysis, and home dialysis patients
  - Persons with diabetes aged 19–59 years; persons with diabetes aged ≥60 years at the discretion of the treating clinician
- Others
  - International travelers to countries with high or intermediate levels of endemic hepatitis B virus (HBV) infection (HBsAg prevalence of ≥2%)
  - Persons with hepatitis C virus infection
  - Persons with chronic liver disease (including persons with cirrhosis, fatty liver disease, alcoholic liver disease, autoimmune hepatitis, and an alanine aminotransferase [ALT] or aspartate aminotransferase [AST] level greater than twice the upper limit of normal)
  - Persons with HIV infection
  - Incarcerated persons
- All other persons seeking protection from HBV infection

From Schillie S, Vellozzi C, Reingold A, et al. Prevention of hepatitis B virus infection in the United States: recommendations of the Advisory Committee on Immunization Practices. *MMWR Recomm Rep* 67(No. RR-1):1–31, 2018.

BOX 2 Testing Anti-HBs for Health Care Personnel (HCP) Vaccinated in the Past

The issue: An increasing number of HCP have received routine hepatitis B (HepB) vaccination during childhood. No postvaccination serologic testing is recommended after routine infant or adolescent HepB vaccination. Because vaccine-induced antibody to hepatitis B surface antigen (anti-HBs) wanes over time, testing HCP for anti-HBs years after vaccination might not distinguish vaccine nonresponders from responders.

Guidance for health care institutions: Health care institutions may measure anti-HBs upon hire or matriculation for HCP who have documentation of a complete HepB vaccine series in the past (e.g., as part of routine infant or adolescent vaccination). HCP with anti-HBs <10 mIU/mL should receive one or more additional doses of HepB vaccine and retesting (see Fig. 6). Institutions that decide to not measure anti-HBs upon hire or matriculation for HCP who have documentation of a complete HepB vaccine series in the past should ensure timely assessment and postexposure prophylaxis following an exposure (see Table 22).

Considerations: The risk for occupational HBV infection for vaccinated HCP might be low enough in certain settings so that assessment of anti-HBs status and appropriate follow-up should be done at the time of exposure to potentially infectious blood or body fluids. This approach relies on HCP recognizing and reporting blood and body fluid exposures and therefore may be applied on the basis of documented low risk, implementation, and cost considerations. Certain HCP occupations have lower risk for occupational blood and body fluid exposures (e.g., occupations involving counseling versus performing procedures), and nontrainees have lower risks for blood and body fluid exposures than trainees. Some settings also will have a lower prevalence of HBV infection in the patient population served than in other settings, which will influence the risk for HCP exposure to HBsAg-positive blood and body fluids.

From Schillie S, Vellozzi C, Reingold A, et al. Prevention of hepatitis B virus infection in the United States: recommendations of the Advisory Committee on Immunization Practices. *MMWR Recomm Rep* 67(No. RR-1):1–31, 2018.

BOX 3 Persons Recommended to Receive Serologic Testing Before Vaccination*

- Household, sexual, or needle contacts of hepatitis B surface antigen (HBsAg)–positive persons†
- HIV-positive persons†
- Persons with elevated alanine aminotransferase/aspartate aminotransferase of unknown etiology†
- Hemodialysis patients†
- Men who have sex with men†
- Past or current persons who inject drugs†
- Persons born in countries of high and intermediate hepatitis B virus (HBV) endemicity (HBsAg prevalence ≥2%)
- U.S.-born persons not vaccinated as infants whose parents were born in countries with high HBV endemicity (≥8%)
- Persons needing immunosuppressive therapy, including chemotherapy, immunosuppression related to organ transplantation, and immunosuppression for rheumatologic or gastroenterologic disorders
- Donors of blood, plasma, organs, tissues, or semen

*Serologic testing comprises testing for hepatitis B surface antigen (HBsAg), antibody to HBsAg, and antibody to hepatitis B core antigen.
†Denotes persons also recommended for hepatitis B vaccination. Serologic testing should occur before vaccination. Serologic testing should not be a barrier to vaccination of susceptible persons. The first dose of vaccine should typically be administered immediately after collection of the blood for serologic testing.
From Schillie S, Vellozzi C, Reingold A, et al. Prevention of hepatitis B virus infection in the United States: recommendations of the Advisory Committee on Immunization Practices. *MMWR Recomm Rep* 67(No. RR-1):1–31, 2018.

BOX 4 Persons Recommended to Receive Postvaccination Serologic Testing* After a Complete Series of Hepatitis B Vaccination

- Infants born to hepatitis B surface antigen (HBsAg)–positive mothers or mothers whose HBsAg status remains unknown (e.g., when a parent or person with lawful custody safely surrenders an infant confidentially shortly after birth infants safely surrendered at or shortly after birth)†
- Health care personnel and public safety workers
- Hemodialysis patients and others who might require outpatient hemodialysis (e.g., predialysis, peritoneal dialysis, and home dialysis)
- HIV-infected persons
- Other immunocompromised persons (e.g., hematopoietic stem-cell transplant recipients or persons receiving chemotherapy)
- Sex partners of HBsAg-positive persons

*Postvaccination serologic testing for persons other than infants born to HBsAg-positive (or HBsAg-unknown) mothers consists of anti-HBs.
†Postvaccination serologic testing for infants born to HBsAg-positive (or HBsAg-unknown) mothers consists of anti-HBs and HBsAg. Persons with anti-HBs <10 mIU/mL after the primary vaccine series should be revaccinated. Infants born to HBsAg-positive mothers or mothers with an unknown HBsAg status should be revaccinated with a single dose of HepB vaccine and receive postvaccination serologic testing 1–2 months later. Infants whose anti-HBs remains <10 mIU/mL after single dose revaccination should receive two additional doses of HepB vaccine, followed by postvaccination serologic testing 1–2 months after the final dose. Based on clinical circumstances or family preference, HBsAg-negative infants with anti-HBs <10 mIU/mL may instead be revaccinated with a second, complete 3-dose series, followed by postvaccination serologic testing performed 1–2 months after the final dose of vaccine. For others with anti-HBs <10 mIU/mL after the primary series, administration of 3 additional HepB vaccine doses on an appropriate schedule, followed by anti-HBs testing 1–2 months after the final dose, is usually more practical than serologic testing after ≥1 dose of vaccine.
From Schillie S, Vellozzi C, Reingold A, et al. Prevention of hepatitis B virus infection in the United States: recommendations of the Advisory Committee on Immunization Practices. *MMWR Recomm Rep* 67(No. RR-1):1–31, 2018.

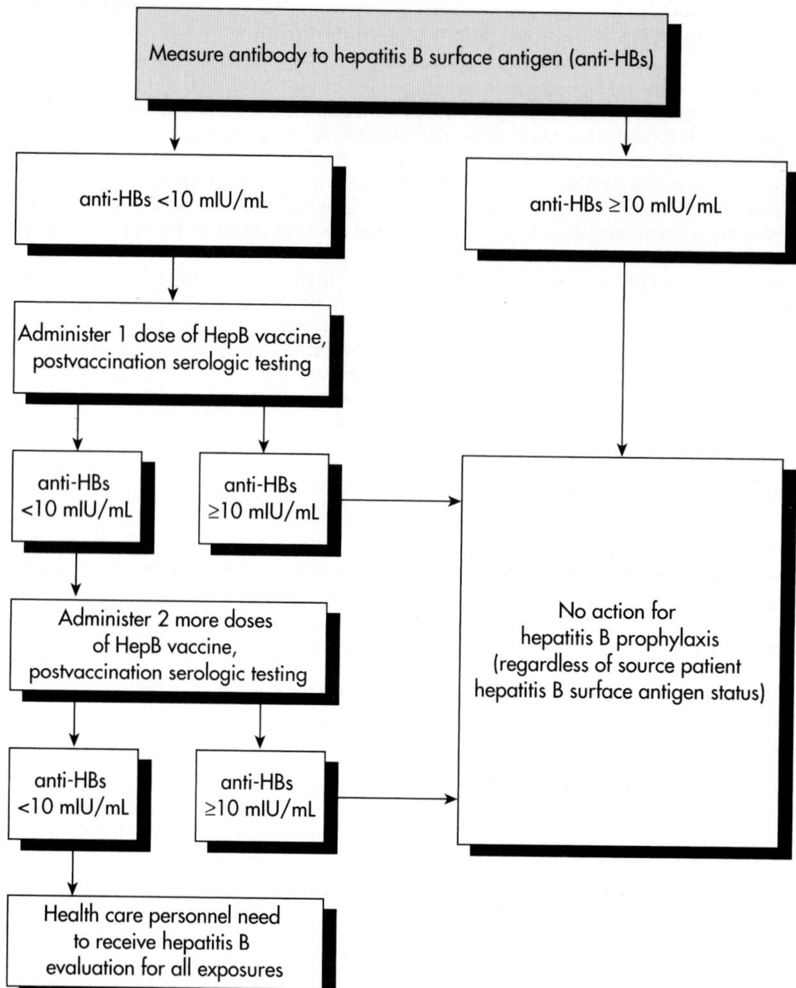

FIG. 6 Pre-exposure evaluation for health care personnel previously vaccinated with complete, ≥3-dose HepB vaccine series who have not had postvaccination serologic testing.* Source: Adapted from CDC: A comprehensive immunization strategy to eliminate transmission of hepatitis B virus infection in the United States: recommendations of the Advisory Committee on Immunization Practices (ACIP). Part II: immunization of adults. *MMWR* 55(No. RR-16), 2006.

*Should be performed 1–2 months after the last dose of vaccine using a quantitative method that allows detection of the protective concentration of anti-HBs (≥10 mIU/mL) (e.g., enzyme-linked immunosorbent assay [ELISA]). From Schillie S, Vellozzi C, Reingold A, et al. Prevention of hepatitis B virus infection in the United States: recommendations of the Advisory Committee on Immunization Practices. *MMWR Recomm Rep* 67(No. RR-1):1–31, 2018.

Hepatitis A Prophylaxis

TABLE 24 Recommended Dosages of Hepatitis A Immune Globulin

Setting	Duration of Coverage	Dose
Preexposure prophylaxis	Short term (<3 mo) Long term (3-5 mo)*	0.02 ml/kg 0.06 ml/kg
Postexposure prophylaxis	—	0.02 ml/kg

NOTE: Immune globulin should be administered intramuscularly into the deltoid or gluteal muscle in children younger than 24 mo; it may be administered in the anterolateral thigh muscle.
*Repeat every 5 mo if continued exposure to hepatitis A virus occurs.
Modified from Centers for Disease Control and Prevention: Prevention of hepatitis A through active or passive immunization: recommendations of the Advisory Committee on Immunization Practices (ACIP), *MMWR* 55(RR-07):9, 2006.

TABLE 25 Licensed Dosages of Hepatitis A Vaccines

Vaccine	Patient's Age	Dose	Volume (ml)	Number of Doses	Schedule (mo)*
Hepatitis A vaccine, inactivated (Havrix)	12 mo to 18 yr ≥19 yr	720 EL.U. 1440 EL.U.	0.5 1.0	2 2	0, 6-12 0, 6-12
Hepatitis A vaccine, inactivated (Vaqta)	12 mo to 18 yr ≥19 yr	25 U 50 U	0.5 1.0	2 2	0, 6-18 0, 6-18
Combined hepatitis A and hepatitis B vaccine (Twinrix)	≥18 yr	720 EL.U. of hepatitis A antigen and 20 mcg of hepatitis B surface antigen protein	1.0	3	0, 1, and 6

*Zero represents the timing of the initial dose; subsequent numbers represent months after the initial dose.
Modified from Centers for Disease Control and Prevention: Prevention of hepatitis A through active or passive immunization: recommendations of the Advisory Committee on Immunization Practices (ACIP), *MMWR* 55(RR-07):10, 2006.

Influenza Treatment and Prophylaxis

BOX 5 Summary of Seasonal Influenza Vaccination Recommendations

Children	Adults
All children aged 6 months to 18 years should be vaccinated annually. Children and adolescents at higher risk for influenza complications should continue to be a focus for vaccination efforts as providers and programs transition to routinely vaccinating all children and adolescents, including those who: • are aged 6 months to 4 years (59 months) • have chronic pulmonary (including asthma), cardiovascular (except hypertension), renal, hepatic, cognitive, neurologic/neuromuscular, hematologic, or metabolic disorders (including diabetes mellitus) • are immunosuppressed (including immunosuppression caused by medications or by human immunodeficiency virus) • are receiving long-term aspirin therapy and therefore might be at risk for experiencing Reye's syndrome after influenza virus infection • are residents of long-term care facilities • will be pregnant during the influenza season **Note:** Children aged <6 months cannot receive influenza vaccination. Household and other close contacts (e.g., day-care providers) of children aged <6 months, including older children and adolescents, should be vaccinated.	Annual vaccination against influenza is recommended for any adult who wants to reduce the risk of becoming ill with influenza or of transmitting it to others. Vaccination is recommended for all adults without contraindications in the following groups, because these persons either are at higher risk for influenza complications, or are close contacts of the persons at higher risk: • persons aged ≥50 years • women who will be pregnant during the influenza season • persons who have chronic pulmonary (including asthma), cardiovascular (except hypertension), renal, hepatic, cognitive, neurologic/neuromuscular, hematologic, or metabolic disorders (including diabetes mellitus) • persons who have immunosuppression (including immunosuppression caused by medications or by human immunodeficiency virus) • residents of nursing homes and other long-term care facilities • health care personnel • household contacts and caregivers of children aged <5 years and adults aged ≥50 years, with particular emphasis on vaccinating contacts of children aged <6 months • household contacts and caregivers of persons with medical conditions that put them at higher risk for severe complications from influenza

Modified from *MMWR* 58:(RR-8), 2009.

TABLE 26 Live, Attenuated Influenza Vaccine (LAIV) Compared with Inactivated Influenza Vaccine (TIV) for Seasonal Influenza, U.S. Formulations

Factor	LAIV	TIV
Route of administration	Intranasal spray	Intramuscular injection
Type of vaccine	Live virus	Noninfectious virus (i.e., inactivated)
Number of included virus strains	3 (2 influenza A, 1 influenza B)	3 (2 influenza A, 1 influenza B)
Vaccine virus strains updated	Annually	Annually
Frequency of administration	Annually*	Annually*
Approved age	Persons aged 2-49 yr	Persons aged ≥6 mo
Interval between 2 doses recommended for children aged ≥6 mo to 8 yr who are receiving influenza vaccine for the first time	4 wk	4 wk
Can be administered to persons with medical risk factors for influenza-related complications†	No	Yes
Can be administered to children with asthma or children aged 2-4 yr with wheezing during the preceding year§	No	Yes
Can be administered to family members or close contacts of immunosuppressed persons not requiring a protected environment	Yes	Yes
Can be administered to family members or close contacts of immunosuppressed persons requiring a protected environment (e.g., hematopoietic stem cell transplant recipient)	No	Yes
Can be administered to family members or close contacts of persons at high risk but not severely immunosuppressed	Yes	Yes
Can be simultaneously administered with other vaccines	Yes¶	Yes**
If not simultaneously administered, can be administered within 4 wk of another live vaccine	Prudent to space 4 wk apart	Yes
If not simultaneously administered, can be administered within 4 wk of an inactivated vaccine	Yes	Yes

*Children aged 6 months to 8 years who have never received influenza vaccine before should receive 2 doses. Those who only receive 1 dose in their first year of vaccination should receive 2 doses in the following year, spaced 4 weeks apart.

†Persons at higher risk for complications of influenza infection because of underlying medical conditions should not receive LAIV. Persons at higher risk for complications of influenza infection because of underlying medical conditions include adults and children with chronic disorders of the pulmonary or cardiovascular systems; adults and children with chronic metabolic diseases (including diabetes mellitus), renal dysfunction, hemoglobinopathies, or immunosuppression; children and adolescents receiving long-term aspirin therapy (at risk for developing Reye's syndrome after wild-type influenza infection); persons who have any condition (e.g., cognitive dysfunction, spinal cord injuries, seizure disorders, or other neuromuscular disorders) that can compromise respiratory function or the handling of respiratory secretions or that can increase the risk for aspiration; pregnant women; and residents of nursing homes and other chronic-care facilities that house persons with chronic medical conditions.

§Clinicians and immunization programs should screen for possible reactive airways diseases when considering use of LAIV for children aged 2-4 years and should avoid use of this vaccine in children with asthma or a recent wheezing episode. Health care providers should consult the medical record, when available, to identify children aged 2-4 years with asthma or recurrent wheezing that might indicate asthma. In addition, to identify children who might be at greater risk for asthma and possibly at increased risk for wheezing after receiving LAIV, parents or caregivers of children aged 2-4 years should be asked: "In the past 12 months, has a health care provider ever told you that your child had wheezing or asthma?" Children whose parents or caregivers answer "yes" to this question and children who have asthma or who had a wheezing episode noted in the medical record during the preceding 12 months should not receive LAIV.

¶LAIV coadministration has been evaluated systematically only among children aged 12-15 months who received measles, mumps, and rubella vaccine or varicella vaccine.

**TIV coadministration has been evaluated systematically only among adults who received pneumococcal polysaccharide or zoster vaccine.

Modified from *MMWR* 56(RR-6), 2007.

INDICATIONS FOR USE OF ANTIVIRALS

PERSONS FOR WHOM ANTIVIRAL TREATMENT SHOULD BE CONSIDERED

If possible, antiviral treatment should be started within 48 hours of influenza illness onset. The effectiveness of initiating antiviral treatment more than 48 hours after illness onset has not been established. Persons for whom antiviral treatment should be considered include:

- Persons hospitalized with laboratory-confirmed influenza (limited data suggest benefit even for persons whose antiviral treatment is initiated more than 48 hours after illness onset)
- Persons with laboratory-confirmed influenza pneumonia
- Persons with laboratory-confirmed influenza and bacterial coinfection
- Persons with laboratory-confirmed influenza infection who are at higher risk for influenza complications
- Persons presenting to medical care with laboratory-confirmed influenza within 48 hours of influenza illness onset who want to decrease the duration or severity of their symptoms and transmission of influenza to others at higher risk for complications

PERSONS FOR WHOM ANTIVIRAL CHEMOPROPHYLAXIS SHOULD BE CONSIDERED DURING PERIODS OF INCREASED INFLUENZA ACTIVITY IN THE COMMUNITY

- Persons at high risk during the 2 weeks after influenza vaccination (after the second dose for children younger than 9 years who have not previously been vaccinated) if influenza viruses are circulating in the community
- Persons at high risk for whom influenza vaccine is contraindicated
- Family members or health care providers who are unvaccinated and are likely to have ongoing, close exposure to persons at high risk or unvaccinated persons or infants younger than 6 months
- Persons and their family members and close contacts and health care workers when circulating strains of influenza virus in the community are not matched with vaccine strains
- Persons with immune deficiencies or those who might not respond to vaccination (e.g., persons infected with HIV or other immunosuppressed conditions or who are receiving immunosuppressive medications)
- Unvaccinated staff and persons during response to an outbreak in a closed institutional setting with residents at high risk (e.g., extended-care facilities)

Modified from *MMWR* 57(RR-7), 2008.

NOTE: Recommended antiviral medications (neuraminidase inhibitors) are not licensed for chemoprophylaxis of children younger than 1 year (oseltamivir) or younger than 5 years (zanamivir). Updates or supplements to these recommendations (e.g., expanded age or risk group indications for licensed vaccines) might be required. Health care providers should be alert to announcements of recommendation updates and should check the CDC influenza website periodically for additional information (www.cdc.gov/flu).

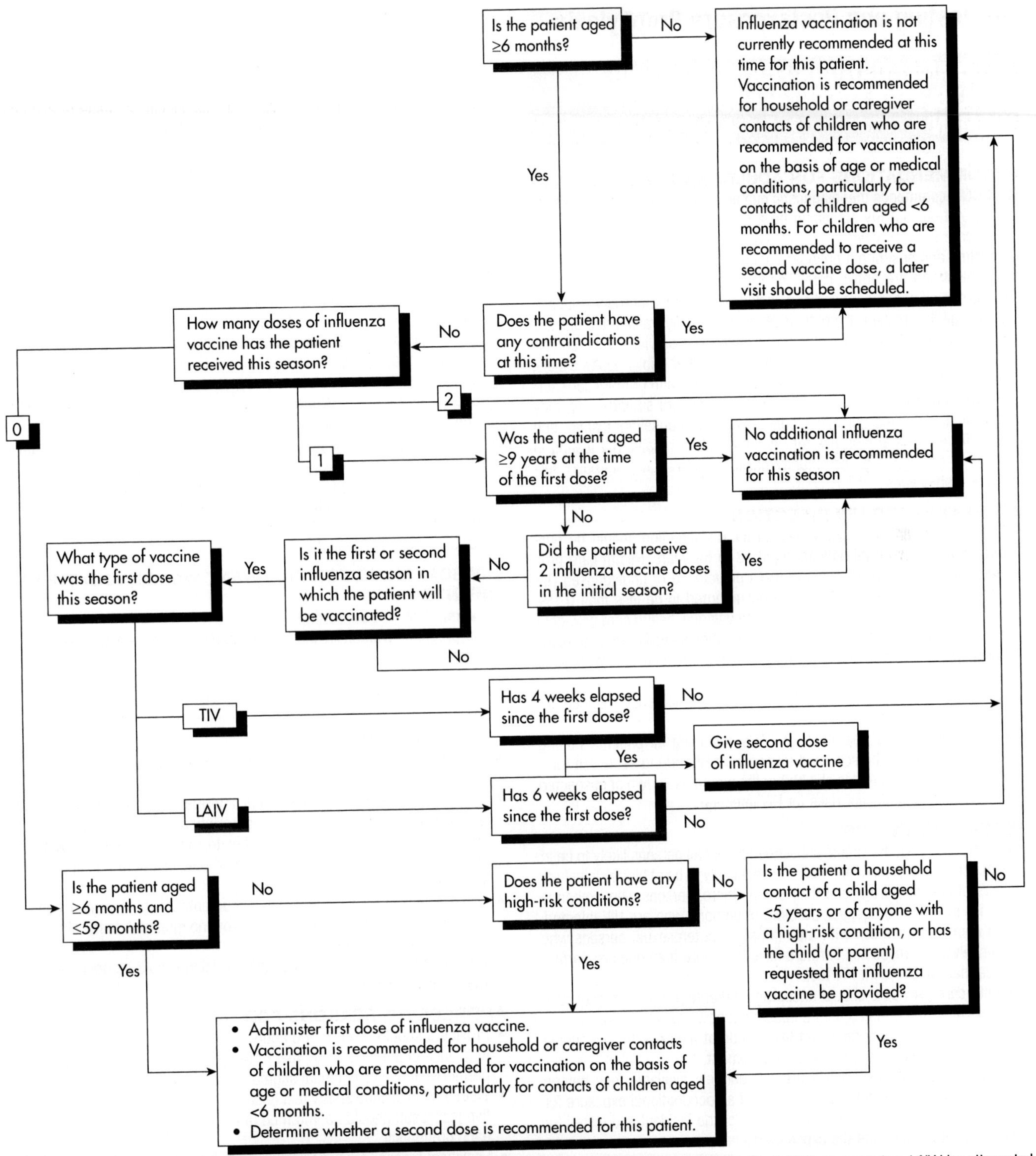

Is the patient aged ≥6 months?

No → Influenza vaccination is not currently recommended at this time for this patient. Vaccination is recommended for household or caregiver contacts of children who are recommended for vaccination on the basis of age or medical conditions, particularly for contacts of children aged <6 months. For children who are recommended to receive a second vaccine dose, a later visit should be scheduled.

Yes → Does the patient have any contraindications at this time?

Yes → (Influenza vaccination is not currently recommended at this time for this patient.)

No → How many doses of influenza vaccine has the patient received this season?

2 → No additional influenza vaccination is recommended for this season

1 → Was the patient aged ≥9 years at the time of the first dose?

Yes → No additional influenza vaccination is recommended for this season

No → Did the patient receive 2 influenza vaccine doses in the initial season?

Yes → No additional influenza vaccination is recommended for this season

No → Is it the first or second influenza season in which the patient will be vaccinated?

No → No additional influenza vaccination is recommended for this season

Yes → What type of vaccine was the first dose this season?

TIV → Has 4 weeks elapsed since the first dose?

LAIV → Has 6 weeks elapsed since the first dose?

Yes → Give second dose of influenza vaccine

No → (Influenza vaccination is not currently recommended at this time for this patient.)

0 → Is the patient aged ≥6 months and ≤59 months?

No → Does the patient have any high-risk conditions?

No → Is the patient a household contact of a child aged <5 years or of anyone with a high-risk condition, or has the child (or parent) requested that influenza vaccine be provided?

No → (Influenza vaccination is not currently recommended at this time for this patient.)

Yes →

- Administer first dose of influenza vaccine.
- Vaccination is recommended for household or caregiver contacts of children who are recommended for vaccination on the basis of age or medical conditions, particularly for contacts of children aged <6 months.
- Determine whether a second dose is recommended for this patient.

FIG. 7 Algorithm for determining recommended influenza immunization actions for children. *TIV,* Trivalent inactivated influenza vaccine; *LAIV,* Live attenuated influenza vaccine. Modified with permission from the American Academy of Pediatrics' Committee on Infectious Diseases: Prevention of influenza: recommendations for influenza immunization of children, 2006-2007, *Pediatrics* 119:846-51, 2007.

HIV Testing and Postexposure Prophylaxis

RECOMMENDATIONS FOR HIV TESTING OF ADULTS, ADOLESCENTS, AND PREGNANT WOMEN

RECOMMENDATIONS FOR ADULTS AND ADOLESCENTS

The CDC recommends that diagnostic human immunodeficiency virus (HIV) testing and opt-out HIV screening be a part of routine clinical care in all health care settings while also preserving the patient's option to decline HIV testing and ensuring a provider-patient relationship conducive to optimal clinical and preventive care. The recommendations are intended for providers in all health care settings, including hospital emergency departments, urgent-care clinics, inpatient services, sexually transmitted disease (STD) clinics or other venues offering clinical STD services, tuberculosis (TB) clinics, substance abuse treatment clinics, other public health clinics, community clinics, correctional health care facilities, and primary care settings. The guidelines address HIV testing in health care settings only; they do not modify existing guidelines concerning HIV counseling, testing, and referral for persons at high risk for HIV who seek or receive HIV testing in nonclinical settings (e.g., community-based organizations, outreach settings, or mobile vans).[3]

SCREENING FOR HIV INFECTION

- In all health care settings, screening for HIV infection should be performed routinely for all patients aged 13 to 64 years. Health care providers should initiate screening unless prevalence of undiagnosed HIV infection in their patients has been documented to be less than 0.1%. In the absence of existing data for HIV prevalence, health care providers should initiate voluntary HIV screening until they establish that the diagnostic yield is less than 1 per 1000 patients screened, at which point such screening is no longer warranted.
- All patients initiating treatment for TB should be screened routinely for HIV infection.
- All patients seeking treatment for STDs, including all patients visiting STD clinics, should be screened routinely for HIV during each visit for a new complaint, regardless of whether the patient is known or suspected to have specific behavior risks for HIV infection.

REPEAT SCREENING

- Health care providers should subsequently test all persons likely to be at high risk for HIV at least annually. Persons likely to be at high risk include users of injection drugs and their sex partners, persons who exchange sex for money or drugs, sex partners of persons who are HIV infected, and men who have sex with men (MSM) or heterosexual persons who themselves or whose sex partners have had more than one sex partner since their most recent HIV test.
- Health care providers should encourage patients and their prospective sex partners to be tested before initiating a new sexual relationship.
- Repeat screening of persons not likely to be at high risk for HIV should be performed on the basis of clinical judgment.
- Unless recent HIV test results are immediately available, any person whose blood or body fluid is the source of an occupational exposure for a health care provider should be informed of the incident and tested for HIV infection at the time the exposure occurs.

CONSENT AND PRETEST INFORMATION

- Screening should be voluntary and undertaken only with the patient's knowledge and understanding that HIV testing is planned.
- Patients should be informed orally or in writing that HIV testing will be performed unless they decline (opt-out screening). Oral or written information should include an explanation of HIV infection and the meanings of positive and negative test results, and the patient should be offered an opportunity to ask questions and decline testing. With such notification, consent for HIV screening should be incorporated into the patient's general informed consent for medical care on the same basis as are other screening or diagnostic tests; a separate consent form for HIV testing is not recommended.
- Easily understood informational materials should be made available in the languages of the commonly encountered populations within the service area. The competence of interpreters and bilingual staff to provide language assistance to patients with limited English proficiency must be ensured.
- If a patient declines an HIV test, this decision should be documented in the medical record.

DIAGNOSTIC TESTING FOR HIV INFECTION

- All patients with signs or symptoms consistent with HIV infection or an opportunistic illness characteristic of acquired immunodeficiency syndrome (AIDS) should be tested for HIV.
- Clinicians should maintain a high level of suspicion for acute HIV infection in all patients who have a compatible clinical syndrome and who report recent high-risk behavior. When acute retroviral syndrome is a possibility, a plasma RNA test should be used in conjunction with an HIV antibody test to diagnose acute HIV infection.
- Patients or persons responsible for the patient's care should be notified orally that testing is planned, advised of the indication for testing and the implications of positive and negative test results, and offered an opportunity to ask questions and decline testing. With such notification, the patient's general consent for medical care is considered sufficient for diagnostic HIV testing.

HIV SCREENING FOR PREGNANT WOMEN AND THEIR INFANTS*

Universal Opt-Out Screening

- All pregnant women in the United States should be screened for HIV infection.
- Screening should occur after a woman is notified that HIV screening is recommended for all pregnant patients and that she will receive an HIV test as part of the routine panel of prenatal tests unless she declines (opt-out screening).
- HIV testing must be voluntary and free from coercion. No woman should be tested without her knowledge.
- Pregnant women should receive oral or written information that includes an explanation of HIV infection, a description of interventions that can reduce HIV transmission from mother to infant, and the meanings of positive and negative test results. They should be offered an opportunity to ask questions and decline testing.
- No additional process or written documentation of informed consent beyond what is required for other routine prenatal tests should be required for HIV testing.
- If a patient declines an HIV test, this decision should be documented in the medical record.

ADDRESSING REASONS FOR DECLINING TESTING

- Providers should discuss and address reasons for declining an HIV test (e.g., lack of perceived risk, fear of the disease, and concerns regarding partner violence or potential stigma or discrimination).
- Women who decline an HIV test because they have had a previous negative test result should be informed of the importance of retesting during each pregnancy.
- Logistical reasons for not testing (e.g., scheduling) should be resolved.
- Certain women who initially decline an HIV test might accept at a later date, especially if their concerns are discussed. Certain women will continue to decline testing, and their decisions should be respected and documented in the medical record.

Timing of HIV Testing

- To promote informed and timely therapeutic decisions, health care providers should test women for HIV as early as possible during each pregnancy. Women who decline the test early in prenatal care should be encouraged to be tested at a subsequent visit.
- A second HIV test during the third trimester, preferably less than 36 weeks of gestation, is cost effective even in areas of low HIV prevalence and may be considered for all pregnant women. A second HIV test during

---

[3] Data from *MMWR* 57(RR-10), 2008.

the third trimester is recommended for women who meet one or more of the following criteria:

1. Women who receive health care in jurisdictions with elevated incidence of HIV or AIDS among women aged 15 to 45 years. In 2004, these jurisdictions included Alabama, Connecticut, Delaware, the District of Columbia, Florida, Georgia, Illinois, Louisiana, Maryland, Massachusetts, Mississippi, Nevada, New Jersey, New York, North Carolina, Pennsylvania, Puerto Rico, Rhode Island, South Carolina, Tennessee, Texas, and Virginia.[4]
2. Women who receive health care in facilities in which prenatal screening identifies at least one pregnant woman who is infected with HIV per 1000 women screened.
3. Women who are known to be at high risk for acquiring HIV (e.g., users of injection drugs and their sex partners, women who exchange sex for money or drugs, women who are sex partners of persons who are infected with HIV, and women who have had a new or more than one sex partner during this pregnancy).
4. Women who have signs or symptoms consistent with acute HIV infection. When acute retroviral syndrome is a possibility, a plasma RNA test should be used in conjunction with an HIV antibody test to diagnose acute HIV infection.

Rapid Testing During Labor

- Any woman with undocumented HIV status at the time of labor should be screened with a rapid HIV test unless she declines (opt-out screening).
- Reasons for declining a rapid test should be explored (see "Addressing Reasons for Declining Testing").
- Immediate initiation of appropriate antiretroviral prophylaxis should be recommended to women on the basis of a reactive rapid test result without waiting for the result of a confirmatory test.

Postpartum/Newborn Testing

- When a woman's HIV status is still unknown at the time of delivery, she should be screened immediately postpartum with a rapid HIV test unless she declines (opt-out screening).
- When the mother's HIV status is unknown postpartum, rapid testing of the newborn as soon as possible after birth is recommended so that antiretroviral prophylaxis can be offered to infants exposed to HIV. Women should be informed that identifying HIV antibodies in the newborn indicates that the mother is infected.
- For infants whose HIV exposure status is unknown and who are in foster care, the person legally authorized to provide consent should be informed that rapid HIV testing is recommended for infants whose biologic mothers have not been tested.
- The benefits of neonatal antiretroviral prophylaxis are best realized when it is initiated within 12 hours after birth.

Confirmatory Testing

- Whenever possible, uncertainties regarding laboratory test results indicating HIV infection status should be resolved before final decisions are made regarding reproductive options, antiretroviral therapy, cesarean delivery, or other interventions.
- If the confirmatory test result is not available before delivery, immediate initiation of appropriate antiretroviral prophylaxis should be recommended to any pregnant patient whose HIV screening test result is reactive to reduce the risk for perinatal transmission.

[4] A second HIV test in the third trimester is as cost effective as other common health interventions when HIV incidence among women of childbearing age is =17 HIV cases per 100,000 person-years. In 2004, in jurisdictions with available data on HIV case rates, a rate of 17 new HIV diagnoses per year per 100,000 women aged 15 to 45 years was associated with an AIDS case rate of at least nine AIDS diagnoses per year per 100,000 women aged 15 to 45 years (CDC, unpublished data, 2005). As of 2004, the jurisdictions listed above exceeded these thresholds. The list of specific jurisdictions where a second test in the third trimester is recommended will be updated periodically based on surveillance data.

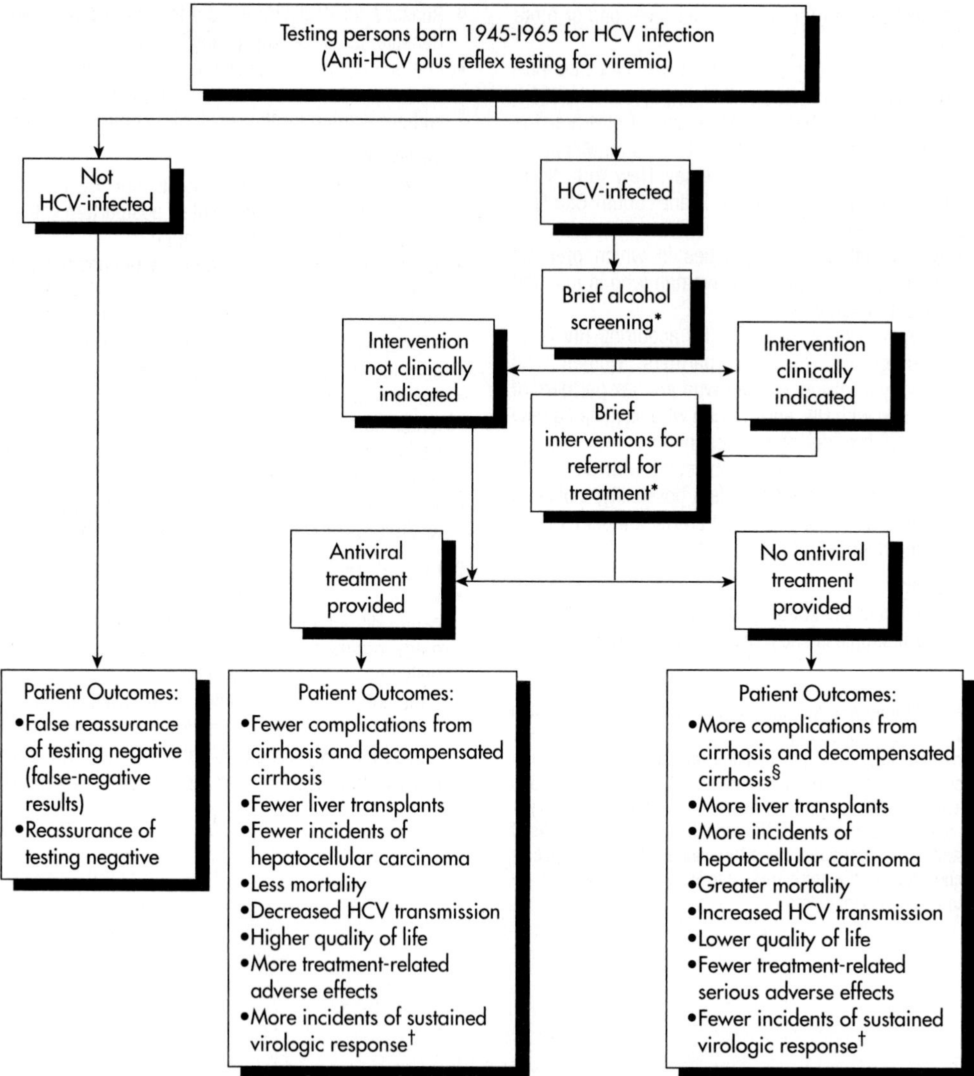

FIG. 8 Analytic Framework for Guiding HCV Testing Among Persons Born During 1945-1965. *Together, these interventions are known as alcohol screening and brief interventions (SBI) for referral for treatment. †Viral eradication after treatment completion. §Cirrhosis with the diagnosis of at least one of the following: ascites, variceal bleeding, encephalopathy, or impaired hepatitis synthetic function. From Centers for Disease Control and Prevention: Recommendations for the identification of chronic hepatitis C virus infection among persons born during 1945-1965. *MMWR* 2012:61(4).

TABLE 27 HIV Exposure, Estimated Per-Act Risk

Exposure Route	Risk per 10,000 Exposures to an Infected Source
Blood transfusion	9000
Needle-sharing injection drug use	67
Receptive anal intercourse	50
Percutaneous needle stick	30
Receptive penile-vaginal intercourse	10
Insertive anal intercourse	6.5
Insertive penile-vaginal intercourse	5
Receptive oral intercourse	1
Insertive oral intercourse	0.5

NOTE: Estimates of risk for transmission from sexual exposures assume no condom use. Source refers to oral intercourse performed on a man.

TABLE 28 Recommended Postexposure Prophylaxis (PEP) for All Occupational Exposures to Human Immunodeficiency Virus (HIV)

PREFERRED HIV PEP REGIMEN	
Raltegravir (Isentress) 400 mg PO (by mouth) twice daily *plus* Tenofovir DF (Viread) 300 mg + emtricitabine (Emtriva) 200 mg; available as Truvada, PO once daily	
ALTERNATIVE REGIMENS	
May combine one drug or drug pair from the left column with one pair of nucleoside/nucleotide reverse transcriptase inhibitors from the right column	
Dolutegravir (Tivicay)	Tenofovir DF (Viread) + emtricitabine (Emtriva); available as Truvada
Raltegravir (Isentress)	Tenofovir DF (Viread) + emtricitabine (Emtriva); available as Truvada
Darunavir (Prezista) + ritonavir (Norvir)	Tenofovir DF (Viread) + lamivudine (Epivir)
Etravirine (Intelence)	Zidovudine (Retrovir) + lamivudine (Epivir); available as Combivir
Rilpivirine (Edurant)	Zidovudine (Retrovir) + emtricitabine (Emtriva)
Atazanavir (Reyataz) + ritonavir (Norvir)	
Lopinavir/ritonavir (Kaletra)	
Stribild (elvitegravir, cobicistat, tenofovir DF, emtricitabine); a complete fixed-dose combination regimen with no additional antiretrovirals needed	
ALTERNATIVE ANTIRETROVIRAL AGENTS FOR USE AS PEP *ONLY* WITH EXPERT CONSULTATION	
Abacavir (Ziagen)	
Efavirenz (Sustiva)	
Enfuvirtide (Fuzeon)	
Fosamprenavir (Lexiva)	
Maraviroc (Selzentry)	
Saquinavir (Invirase)	
Stavudine (Zerit)	
ANTIRETROVIRAL AGENTS GENERALLY NOT RECOMMENDED FOR USE AS PEP	
Didanosine (Videx EC)	
Nelfinavir (Viracept)	
Tipranavir (Aptivus)	
ANTIRETROVIRAL AGENTS CONTRAINDICATED AS PEP	
Nevirapine (Viramune)	

Adapted from Kuhar DT, Henderson DK, Struble KA, et al. Panlilio AL, Heneine W, Thomas V, Cheever LW, Gomaa A. Updated U.S. Public Health Service guidelines for the management of occupational exposures to HIV and recommendations for postexposure prophylaxis. *Infect Control Hosp Epidemiol.* 2013; 34:875-892. In Cameron JL, Cameron AM: *Current surgical therapy*, ed 12, Philadelphia, 2017, Elsevier.

TABLE 29 Antiretroviral Therapy Medications, Adult Dosage, and Side Effects

Medication	Adult Dosage*	Side Effects and Toxicities
Combination Tablets		
Lopinavir/ritonavir (Kaletra)‡	3 tablets twice daily 400 mg lopinavir/100 mg ritonavir	Diarrhea, nausea, vomiting; asthenia; elevated transaminases; hyperglycemia; fat redistribution; lipid abnormalities; possible increased bleeding in persons with hemophilia; pancreatitis
Zidovudine/lamivudine (Combivir)	1 tablet twice daily 300 mg zidovudine/150 mg lamivudine	See following individual medications
Zidovudine/lamivudine/abacavir (Trizivir)	1 tablet twice daily 300 mg zidovudine/150 mg lamivudine/300 mg abacavir	See following individual medications
Lamivudine/abacavir (Epzicom)	1 tablet once daily 300 mg lamivudine/600 mg abacavir	See following individual medications
Emtricitabine/tenofovir (Truvada)	1 tablet once daily 200 mg emtricitabine/300 mg tenofovir	See following individual medications
Single Agents		
Nucleoside and nucleotide reverse transcriptase inhibitors (side effects as a class: lactic acidosis, severe hepatomegaly with steatosis, including some fatal cases)		
Abacavir (Ziagen, ABC)‡	300 mg twice daily or 600 mg once daily	Severe hypersensitivity reaction (can be fatal); nausea; vomiting
Didanosine (Videx, ddI)‡	>60 kg (132 lb) body weight: 200 mg twice daily or 400 mg daily; if with tenofovir, 250 mg/daily <60 kg (132 lb): 125 mg twice daily or 250 mg daily; if with tenofovir, dose not established Do not use with stavudine (d4T, Zerit) during pregnancy; avoid ddI/d4T combination in general because of increased risk for adverse events (e.g., neuropathy, pancreatitis, and hyperlactatemia)	Pancreatitis; nausea, diarrhea; peripheral neuropathy
Emtricitabine (Emtriva, FTC)	200 mg once daily	Minimal toxicity; lactic acidosis and hepatic steatosis a rare but possibly life-threatening event
Lamivudine (Epivir, 3TC)‡	150 mg twice daily or 300 mg once daily	Minimal toxicity; lactic acidosis and hepatic steatosis a rare but possibly life-threatening event
Stavudine (Zerit, d4T)‡	>60 kg (132 lb) body weight: 40 mg twice daily <60 kg (132 lb) body weight: 30 mg twice daily Do not use with didanosine (ddI, Videx) during pregnancy; avoid ddI/d4T combination in general because of increased risk of adverse events (e.g., neuropathy, pancreatitis, and hyperlactatemia)	Pancreatitis; peripheral neuropathy; rapidly progressive ascending neuromuscular weakness (rare)
Tenofovir (Viread)	300 mg daily	Nausea, vomiting, diarrhea; headache; asthenia; flatulence; renal impairment
Zidovudine (Retrovir, AZT)‡	200 mg three times daily or 300 mg twice daily	Bone marrow suppression (anemia, neutropenia); gastrointestinal intolerance; headache; insomnia; asthenia; and myopathy
Nonnucleoside reverse transcriptase inhibitors (side effects as a class: Stevens-Johnson syndrome)		
Efavirenz (Sustiva)	600 mg daily at bedtime	Rash; central nervous system symptoms (e.g., dizziness, impaired concentration, insomnia, and abnormal dreams); transaminase elevation; false-positive cannabinoid test
Protease inhibitors (side effects as a class: gastrointestinal intolerance, hyperlipidemia, hyperglycemia, diabetes, fat redistribution, and possible increased bleeding in hemophiliacs; do not use during known or possible pregnancy)		
Atazanavir (Reyataz)	400 mg once daily; if administered with tenofovir plus ritonavir, 300 mg once daily	Indirect hyperbilirubinemia; prolonged PR interval (use caution in patients with underlying cardiac conduction defects or on concomitant medications that can cause PR prolongation)
Fosamprenavir (Lexiva)‡	1400 mg twice daily	Gastrointestinal intolerance, nausea, vomiting, diarrhea; rash; elevated transaminases; headache
Indinavir (Crixivan)	800 mg q8h With ritonavir (might increase risk for renal adverse events): 800 mg indinavir and 100 mg ritonavir q12h or 800 mg indinavir and 200 mg ritonavir every q12h	Gastrointestinal intolerance, nausea; nephrolithiasis; headache; asthenia; blurred vision; metallic taste; thrombocytopenia; hemolytic anemia; indirect hyperbilirubinemia (inconsequential)
Nelfinavir (Viracept)‡	750 mg three times daily or one 250 mg twice daily	Diarrhea; elevated transaminases
Ritonavir (Norvir)‡	See doses used in combination with other specific protease inhibitors	Gastrointestinal intolerance; nausea, vomiting, diarrhea; paresthesias; hepatitis; pancreatitis; asthenia; taste perversion; many drug interactions
Saquinavir (hard-gel capsule) (Invirase)	With ritonavir: 400 mg saquinavir and 400 mg ritonavir twice daily or 1000 mg saquinavir and 100 mg ritonavir twice daily	Gastrointestinal intolerance; nausea, diarrhea; headache; elevated transaminases
Saquinavir (soft-gel capsule) (Fortovase)	With ritonavir: 400 mg saquinavir and 400 mg ritonavir twice daily or 1000 mg saquinavir and 100 mg ritonavir twice daily	Gastrointestinal intolerance; nausea, diarrhea; abdominal pain; dyspepsia; headache; elevated transaminases

*For pediatric dosing information, see *Guidelines for use of antiretroviral agents in pediatric HIV infection.* Available at https://aidsinfo.nih.gov/guidelines/html/2/pediatric-arv/108/role-of-therapeutic-drug-monitoring-in-management-of-pediatric-hiv-infection.

‡Pediatric formulation available.

Sources: Modified from U.S. Department of Health and Human Services and the Henry J. Kaiser Family Foundation: *Guidelines for the use of antiretroviral agents in HIV-infected adults and adolescents.* Available at https://aidsinfo.nih.gov/guidelines/html/1/adult-and-adolescent-arv/0 (refer to website for updated versions); Bartlett JG, Finkbeiner AK: HIV drugs: the guide to living with HIV infection, 2001. Available at http://www.thebody.com/content/art32314.html

TABLE 30 Laboratory Tests Generally Recommended for Persons after Exposure to HIV*

	RECOMMENDED DURING TREATMENT		RECOMMENDED AT FOLLOW-UP		
Test	**Baseline**	**Symptom-Directed†**	**4-6 wk**	**12 wk**	**24 wk**
ELISA for HIV antibodies	Yes	Yes	Yes	Yes	Yes
Creatinine, liver function, and complete blood count with differential count	Yes	Yes	No	No	No
HIV viral load	No	Yes	No	No	No
Anti-HBs antibodies	Yes‡	No	No	No	No
HBsAg	Yes‡§	No	No	No	No
HCV antibodies	Yes	No	Yes	Yes	Yes
HCV RNA‖	No	Yes	Yes	Yes	Yes
Screening, including rapid plasma reagin test, for other sexually transmitted infections¶	Yes	Yes	No	Yes	No

Anti-HBs antibodies, Hepatitis B virus surface antibodies; *ELISA,* enzyme-linked immunosorbent assay; *HBsAg,* hepatitis B surface antigen; *HCV,* hepatitis C virus.

*Patients who receive zidovudine plus lamivudine–based regimens should have a complete blood count and measurement of liver-enzyme levels at 2 weeks of treatment, irrespective of the presence or absence of clinical symptoms. Tenofovir plus emtricitabine–based regimens generally involve few side effects, and symptom-directed assessment of serum creatinine or liver-enzyme levels should be considered. The addition of a ritonavir-boosted protease inhibitor should be followed by symptom-directed assessment of liver-enzyme levels, serum glucose levels, or both.

†Symptom-directed tests are for signs or symptoms of toxic effects (rash, nausea, vomiting, or abdominal pain) or HIV seroconversion (fever, fatigue, lymphadenopathy, rash, or oral or genital ulcers).

‡If tests for anti-HBs antibodies and HBsAg are both negative, a vaccination series against HBV infection should be initiated and completed.

§If the patient is HBsAg-positive, he or she should have monthly follow-up of liver function tests after discontinuation of postexposure prophylactic regimens containing tenofovir, lamivudine, or emtricitabine; referral to a specialist in viral hepatitis should be considered.

‖HCV RNA testing may identify early HCV seroconversion; early detection and treatment during acute HCV infection may avert or ameliorate chronic disease. Data are from Dienstag and McHutchison.

¶Rapid plasma reagin testing and testing of urethral-swab and rectal-swab specimens for gonorrhea and chlamydia and of pharyngeal-swab specimens for gonorrhea should be performed as appropriate, according to the patient's sexual risk-taking behaviors and the type of exposure to HIV.

From Landovitz RJ, Currier JS: Postexposure prophylaxis for HIV infection, *N Engl J Med* 361:1768-1775, 2009.

BOX 6 Situations for Which Expert Consultation for HIV Postexposure Prophylaxis Is Advised[5]

- Delayed (i.e., later than 24-36 hours) exposure report
  1. The interval after which there is no benefit from postexposure prophylaxis (PEP) is undefined
- Unknown source (e.g., needle in sharps disposal container or laundry)
  1. Decide use of PEP on a case-by-case basis
  2. Consider the severity of the exposure and the epidemiologic likelihood of HIV exposure
  3. Do not test needles or other sharp instruments for HIV
- Known or suspected pregnancy in the exposed person
  1. Does not preclude the use of optimal PEP regimens
  2. Do not deny PEP solely on the basis of pregnancy
- Resistance of the source virus to antiretroviral agents
  1. Influence of drug resistance on transmission risk is unknown
  2. Selection of drugs to which the source person's virus is unlikely to be resistant is recommended if the source person's virus is known or suspected to be resistant to one or more of the drugs considered for the PEP regimen
  3. Resistance testing of the source person's virus at the time of the exposure is not recommended
- Toxicity of the initial PEP regimen
  1. Adverse symptoms such as nausea and diarrhea are common with PEP
  2. Symptoms often can be managed without changing the PEP regimen by prescribing antimotility and/or antiemetic agents
  3. Modification of dose intervals (i.e., administering a lower dose of drug more frequently throughout the day, as recommended by the manufacturer) in other situations might help alleviate symptoms

[5]Local experts and/or the National Clinicians' Postexposure Prophylaxis Hotline (PEPline [888-448-4911]).

BOX 7 Occupational Exposure Management Resources

National Clinicians' Postexposure Prophylaxis Hotline (PEPline) Run by University of California–San Francisco/San Francisco General Hospital staff; supported by the Health Resources and Services Administration, Ryan White CARE Act, HIV/AIDS Bureau, AIDS Education and Training Centers, and CDC	Phone: 888-448-4911 Internet: http://nccc.ucsf.edu/clinician-consultation/pep-post-exposure-prophylaxis/
Hepatitis Hotline	Phone: 888-443-7232 Internet: www.cdc.gov/ncidod/diseases/hepatitis/index.htm
Reporting to CDC: Occupationally acquired HIV infections and failures of PEP	Phone: 800-893-0485
HIV Antiretroviral Pregnancy Registry	Phone: 800-258-4263 Fax: 800-800-1052 Address: 1410 Commonwealth Dr., Suite 215, Wilmington, NC 28405 Internet: http://www.apregistry.com/
Food and Drug Administration Report unusual or severe toxicity to antiretroviral agents	Phone: 800-332-1088 Address: MedWatch, HF-2, FDA, 5600 Fishers Lane, Rockville, MD 20857 Internet: www.fda.gov/medwatch
HIV/AIDS Treatment Information Service	Internet: www.hivatis.org

BOX 8 Management of Occupational Blood Exposures

Provide Immediate Care to the Exposure Site
- Wash wounds and skin with soap and water
- Flush mucous membranes with water

Determine Risk Associated with Exposure
- Type of fluid (e.g., blood, visibly bloody fluid, other potentially infectious fluid or tissue, and concentrated virus)
- Type of exposure (e.g., percutaneous injury, mucous membrane or nonintact skin exposure, and bites resulting in blood exposure)

Evaluate Exposure Source
- Assess the risk of infection using available information
- Test known sources for HBsAg, anti-HCV, and HIV antibodies (consider using rapid testing)
- For unknown sources, assess risk of exposure to HBV, HCV, or HIV infection
- Do not test discarded needles or syringes for virus contamination

Evaluate the Exposed Person
- Assess immune status for HBV infection (i.e., by history of hepatitis B vaccination and vaccine response)

Give PEP for Exposures Posing Risk of Infection Transmission
- HBV: See Table 5
- HCV: PEP not recommended
- HIV: See Tables 28, 29, and 30 and Fig. 8
  1. Initiate PEP as soon as possible, preferably within hours of exposure
  2. Offer pregnancy testing to all women of childbearing age not known to be pregnant
  3. Seek expert consultation if viral resistance is suspected
  4. Administer PEP for 4 weeks if tolerated

Perform Follow-up Testing and Provide Counseling
- Advise exposed persons to seek medical evaluation for any acute illness occurring during follow-up

HBV Exposures
- Perform follow-up anti-HBs testing in persons who receive hepatitis B vaccine
  1. Test for anti-HBs 1 to 2 months after last dose of vaccine
  2. Anti-HBs response to vaccine cannot be ascertained if HBIG was received in the previous 3 to 4 months

HCV Exposures
- Perform baseline and follow-up testing for anti-HCV and alanine aminotransferase 4 to 6 months after exposure
- Perform HCV RNA at 4 to 6 weeks if earlier diagnosis of HCV infection desired
- Confirm repeatedly reactive anti-HCV enzyme immunoassays with supplemental tests

HIV Exposures
- Perform HIV-antibody testing for at least 6 months after exposure (e.g., at baseline, 6 weeks, 3 months, and 6 months)
- Perform HIV-antibody testing if illness compatible with an acute retroviral syndrome occurs
- Advise exposed persons to use precautions to prevent secondary transmission during the follow-up period
- Evaluate exposed persons taking PEP within 72 hr after exposure and monitor for drug toxicity for at least 2 weeks

HBIG, Hepatitis B immune globulin; *HBsAg,* hepatitis B surface antigen; *HBV,* hepatitis B virus; *HCV,* hepatitis C virus; *HIV,* human immunodeficiency virus; *PEP,* postexposure prophylaxis; *RNA,* ribonucleic acid.

Endocarditis Prophylaxis[6]

TABLE 31 Cardiac Conditions Associated with the Highest Risk of Adverse Outcome from Endocarditis for Which Prophylaxis with Dental Procedures Is Recommended

Prosthetic cardiac valve

Previous infective endocarditis

CHD*

Unrepaired cyanotic CHD, including palliative shunts and conduits

Completely repaired congenital heart defect with prosthetic material or device, whether placed by surgery or by catheter intervention, during the first 6 mo after the procedure†

Repaired CHD with residual defects at the site or adjacent to the site of a prosthetic patch or prosthetic device (that inhibit endothelialization)

Cardiac transplant recipients who develop cardiac valvulopathy

CHD, Congenital heart disease.
*Except for the conditions listed above, antibiotic prophylaxis is no longer recommended for any other form of CHD.
†Prophylaxis is recommended because endothelialization of prosthetic material occurs within 6 mo after the procedure.

TABLE 32 Dental Procedures for Which Endocarditis Prophylaxis Is Recommended for Patients in Table 31

All dental procedures that involve manipulation of gingival tissue or the periapical region of teeth or perforation of the oral mucosa*

*The following procedures and events do not need prophylaxis: routine anesthetic injections through noninfected tissue, taking dental radiographs, placement of removable prosthodontic or orthodontic appliances, adjustment of orthodontic appliances, placement of orthodontic brackets, shedding of deciduous teeth, and bleeding from trauma to the lips or oral mucosa.

TABLE 33 Regimens for a Dental Procedure

	REGIMEN: SINGLE DOSE 30-60 MIN BEFORE PROCEDURE		
Situation	**Agent**	**Adults**	**Children**
Oral	Amoxicillin	2 g	50 mg/kg
Unable to take oral medication	Ampicillin	2 g IM or IV	50 mg/kg IM or IV
	OR		
	Cefazolin or ceftriaxone*	1 g IM or IV	50 mg/kg IM or IV
Allergic to penicillins or ampicillin, oral	Cephalexin*†	2 g	50 mg/kg
	OR		
	Clindamycin	600 mg	20 mg/kg
	OR		
	Azithromycin or clarithromycin	500 mg	15 mg/kg
Allergic to penicillins or ampicillin and unable to take oral medicine	Cefazolin or ceftriaxone†	1 g IM or IV	50 mg/kg IM or IV
	OR		
	Clindamycin	600 mg IM or IV	20 mg/kg IM or IV

IM, Intramuscular; *IV,* intravenous.
*Or other first-generation or second-generation oral cephalosporin in equivalent adult or pediatric dosage.
†Cephalosporins should not be used in an individual with a history of anaphylaxis, angioedema, or urticaria with penicillins or ampicillin.

[6]From Prevention of infective endocarditis. A guideline from the American Heart Association Rheumatic Fever, Endocarditis, and Kawasaki Disease Committee, Council on Cardiovascular Disease in the Young, and the Council on Clinical Cardiology, Council on Cardiovascular Surgery and Anesthesia, and the Quality of Care and Outcomes Research Interdisciplinary Working Group. Circulation published online Apr 19, 2007, DOI: 10.1161/CIRCULATIONAHA.106.183095. Print ISSN: 0009-7322. Online ISSN: 1524-4539.

TABLE 34 Summary of Major Changes in Updated Recommendations

We concluded that bacteremia resulting from daily activities is much more likely to cause IE than bacteremia associated with a dental procedure.
We concluded that only an extremely small number of cases of IE might be prevented by antibiotic prophylaxis even if prophylaxis is 100% effective.
Antibiotic prophylaxis is not recommended based solely on an increased lifetime risk of acquisition of IE.
Limit recommendations for IE prophylaxis only to those conditions listed in Table 31.
Antibiotic prophylaxis is no longer recommended for any other form of CHD, except for the conditions listed in Table 31.
Antibiotic prophylaxis is recommended for all dental procedures that involve manipulation of gingival tissues or periapical region of teeth or perforation of oral mucosa only for patients with underlying cardiac conditions associated with the highest risk of adverse outcome from IE (see Table 31).
Antibiotic prophylaxis is recommended for procedures on respiratory tract or infected skin, skin structures, or musculoskeletal tissue only for patients with underlying cardiac conditions associated with the highest risk of adverse outcome from IE (see Table 31).
Antibiotic prophylaxis solely to prevent IE is not recommended for GU or GI tract procedures.
The writing group reaffirms the procedures noted in the 1997 prophylaxis guidelines for which endocarditis prophylaxis is not recommended and extends this to other common procedures, including ear and body piercing, tattooing, and vaginal delivery and hysterectomy.

NOTE: A guide to the clinical preventive services described is available online at www.ahrq.gov/clinic/pocketgd07/. *CHD,* Congenital heart disease; *GI,* gastrointestinal; *GU,* genitourinary; *IE,* infective endocarditis.

Hepatitis C Testing (See Fig. 8)

BOX 9 Recommendations for Prevention and Control of Hepatitis C Virus (HCV) Infection and HCV-Related Chronic Diseases

Recommendations for the Identification of Chronic Hepatitis C Virus Infection Among Persons Born During 1945–1965[7]

- Adults born during 1945-1965 should receive one-time testing for HCV without prior ascertainment of HCV risk.
- All persons with identified HCV infection should receive a brief alcohol screening and intervention as clinically indicated, followed by referral to appropriate care and treatment services for HCV infection and related conditions.[8,9]

Guidelines for Prevention and Treatment of Opportunistic Infections in HIV-Infected Adults and Adolescents[8,9]

- HIV-infected patients should be tested routinely for evidence of chronic HCV infection. Initial testing for HCV should be performed using the most sensitive immunoassays licensed for detection of antibody to HCV (anti-HCV) in blood.

Recommendations for Prevention and Control of Hepatitis C Virus (HCV) Infection and HCV-Related Chronic Disease
Routine HCV testing is recommended for

- Persons who ever injected illegal drugs, including those who injected once or a few times many years ago and do not consider themselves drug users.
- Persons with selected medical conditions, including:
  1. persons who received clotting factor concentrates produced before 1987;
  2. persons who were ever on chronic (long-term) hemodialysis;
  3. persons with persistently abnormal alanine aminotransferase levels.
- Prior recipients of transfusions or organ transplants, including:
  1. persons who were notified that they received blood from a donor who later tested positive for HCV infection;
  2. persons who received a transfusion of blood or blood components before July 1992; and
  3. persons who received an organ transplant before July 1992.

Routine HCV testing is recommended for persons with recognized exposures, including

- Health care, emergency medical, and public safety workers after needle sticks, sharps, or mucosal exposures to HCV-positive blood.
- Children born to HCV-positive women.

[7]Source: Centers for Disease Control and Prevention: Recommendations for the identification of chronic hepatitis C virus infection among persons born during 1945–1965. *MMWR* 2012;61(No. RR–4).
[8]Source: Centers for Disease Control and Prevention: Recommendations for prevention and control of hepatitis C virus (HCV) infection and HCV-related chronic disease. *MMWR* 1998;47(No. RR–19).
[9]Source: Centers for Disease Control and Prevention: Guidelines for prevention and treatment of opportunitistic infections in HIV-infected adults and adolescents: Recommendations from CDC, the National Institutes of Health, and the HIV Medicine Association of the Infectious Diseases Society of America. *MMWR* 2009;58(No. RR–4).
From Centers for Disease Control and Prevention: Recommendations for the identification of chronic hepatitis C virus infection among persons born during 1945-1965. *MMWR* 2012:61(4).

Recommendations for Meningococcal Vaccination

TABLE 35 Recommendations for Meningococcal Vaccination of Children at Increased Risk for Meningococcal Disease

Vaccine	Age of Primary Vaccination	Booster Doses	Indicated for Infants	Not Indicated for Infants
MenACWY-CRM (Menveo)	2, 4, 6, and 12 mo	1st booster 3 yr after primary series Additional boosters every 5 yr	Complement component deficiencies Functional or anatomic asplenia The risk groups for an outbreak for which vaccination is recommended Traveling to or residing in epidemic or hyperendemic regions	
MenACWY-D (Menactra)	9 and 12 mo	1st booster 3 yr after primary series Additional boosters every 5 yr	Complement component deficiencies The risk groups for an outbreak for which vaccination is recommended Traveling to or residing in epidemic or hyperendemic regions	Functional or anatomic asplenia
Hib-MenCY-TT (MenHibrix)	2, 4, 6, and 12–15 mo	1st booster (using MenACWY-CRM or MenACWY-D) 3 y after primary series	1st booster 3 yr after primary series	Traveling to or residing in epidemic or hyperendemic regions
MenB-FHbp (Trumenba)	3-dose series, with 2nd and 3rd doses after 2 and 6 mo after 1st dose; 2nd dose 6 mo after 1st dose is an option	None	≥10 yr at increased risk for serogroup B disease (complement component deficiencies, functional or anatomic asplenia, the risk groups for an outbreak for which vaccination is recommended)	Children aged <10 yr Traveling to or residing in epidemic or hyperendemic regions
MenB-4C (Bexsero)	2-dose series, with doses at least 1 mo apart	None	≥10 yr at increased risk for serogroup B disease (complement component deficiencies, functional or anatomic asplenia, the risk groups for an outbreak for which vaccination is recommended)	Children aged <10 yr Traveling to or residing in epidemic or hyperendemic regions

From Cherry JD: *Feigin and Cherry's pediatric infectious diseases*, ed 8, Elsevier, 2019.

I. Complementary and Alternative Medicine

II. Nutrition

III. Acute Poisoning

IV. Impairment and Disability Issues

V. Protection of Travelers

VI. Physician Quality Reporting System (PQRS) Measures (available online)

VII. Patient Teaching Guides (available online)

Definitions of Complementary and Alternative Medicine Terms

Acupuncture Thin needles are inserted superficially on the skin at locations throughout the body. These points are located along "channels" of energy. Heat can be applied by burning (moxibustion), electric current (electroacupuncture), or pressure (acupressure). Healing is proposed by the restoration of a balance of energy flow called *Qi.* Another explanation suggests that, possibly, the stimulation activates endorphin receptors.

Alexander Technique A bodywork technique in which rebalancing of "postural sets" (i.e., physical alignment) is taught by mentally focusing on the way correct alignments should look and feel and through verbal and tactile guidance by the practitioner.

Applied Kinesiology A form of treatment that uses nutrition, physical manipulation, vitamins, diets, and exercise to restore and energize the body. Weak muscles are proposed as a source of dysfunctional health.

Aromatherapy A form of complementary medicine that uses various plant oils such as those from lavender. Route of administration can be through absorption in the skin or inhalation. The aromatic biochemical structures of certain plants are thought to act in areas of the brain related to past experiences and emotions (e.g., limbic system).

Ayurveda A major health system that originated in India and incorporates the body, mind, and spirit to prevent and treat disease. Includes special types of diets, herbs, and minerals.

Biofeedback A mind-body therapy procedure in which sensors are placed on the body to measure muscle tension, heart rate, and sweat responses or neural activity. Information is provided by visual, auditory, or body-muscle cell activation so as to teach either to increase or decrease physiologic activity, which, when reconstituted, is proposed to improve health problems (e.g., pain, anxiety, or high blood pressure). In some cases, relaxation exercises complement this procedure.

Chelation Therapy Involves the removal—through intravenous infusion of a chelating agent (synthetic amino acid ethylenediamine tetraacetic acid [EDTA])—of heavy metals, including lead, nickel, and cadmium, as a way to treat certain diseases. Ancillary treatments include the use of vitamins, changes in diet, and exercise.

Cognitive Therapy Psychological therapy in which the major focus is altering and changing irrational beliefs through a type of Socratic dialogue and self-evaluation of certain illogical thoughts. Conditioning and learning are important components of this therapy.

Craniosacral Therapy A form of gentle manual manipulation used for diagnosis and for making corrections in a system made up of cerebrospinal fluid, cranial and dural membranes, cranial bones, and sacrum. This system is proposed to be dynamic, with its own physiologic frequency. Through touch and pressure, tension is proposed to be reduced and cranial rhythms normalized, leading to improvement in health and disease.

Modified and updated from Spencer JW: *Complementary/alternative medicine: an evidence-based approach*, St. Louis, 1999, Mosby.

Diathermy The use of high-frequency electrical currents as a form of physical therapy and in surgical procedures. The term *diathermy,* derived from the Greek words *dia* and *therma,* literally means "heating through." The three forms of diathermy used by physical therapists are short wave, ultrasound, and microwave.

Eye Movement Desensitization and Reprocessing (EMDR) A technique that proposes to remove painful memories by behavioral techniques. Rhythmic, multisaccadic eye movements are produced by allowing the patient to track and follow a moving object while imagining a stressful memory or event. By using deconditioning, including verbal interaction with the therapist, the painful memory is extinguished and health improved.

Feldenkrais Method A bodywork technique that integrates physics, judo, and yoga. The practitioner directs sequences of movement using verbal or hands-on techniques or teaches a system of self-directed exercise to treat physical impairments through the learning of new movement patterns.

Hatha Yoga The branch of yoga practice that involves physical exercise, breathing practices, and movement. These exercises are designed to have a salutary effect on posture, flexibility, and strength and are intended ultimately to prepare the body to remain still for long periods of meditation.

Hellerwork A bodywork technique that treats and improves proper body alignment through the development of a more complete awareness of the physical body. The goal is to realign fascia for improvement of standing, sitting, and breathing using "body energy," verbal feedback, and changing emotions and attitudes.

Homeopathy A form of treatment in which substances (minerals, plant extracts, chemicals, or disease-producing germs), which in sufficient doses would produce a set of illness symptoms in healthy individuals, are given in microdoses to produce a "cure" of those same symptoms. The *symptom* is not thought to be part of the illness but part of a curative process.

Hyperbaric Oxygen A therapy in which 100% oxygen is given at or above atmospheric pressure. An increase in oxygen in the tissue is proposed to increase blood circulation and improve healing and health and influence the course of disease.

Jin Shin Jyutsu An ancient bodywork technique to harmonize body, mind, and spirit by gentle touch that uses specific "healing points" at the body surface. The points are proposed to overlie flowing energy (Qi). The therapist's fingers are used to "redirect, balance, and provide a more efficient energy flow" to and throughout the body.

Light Therapy Natural light or light of specified wavelengths is used to treat disease. This may include ultraviolet light, colored light, or low-intensity laser light. Generally, the eye is the initial entry point for the light because of its direct connection to the brain.

Magnetic Therapy Magnets are placed directly on the skin, theoretically stimulating living cells and increasing blood flow by ionic currents that are created from polarities on the magnets.

Mediterranean Diet A diet that includes 50% to 60% carbohydrates, 30% fats, and 10% proteins. The diet is derived from the eating habits of people in the Mediterranean area, who were shown to have reduced rates of cardiovascular disease. Clinical trial evidence has indicated that it may reduce the risk of cardiovascular disease in people at high risk for CVD.

Mind-Body Therapies A group of therapies that emphasize using the mind or brain in conjunction with the body to assist healing. Mind-body therapies can involve varying degrees of levels of consciousness, including *hypnosis,* in which selective attention is used to induce a specific altered state (trance) for memory retrieval, relaxation, or suggestion; *visual imagery,* in which the focus is on a target visual stimulus; *yoga,* which involves integration of posture and controlled breathing, relaxation, and/or meditation; *relaxation,* which includes lighter levels of altered states of consciousness through indirect or direct focus; and *meditation,* in which there is an intentional use of posture, concentration, contemplation, and visualization.

Muscle Energy Technique A manual therapy in osteopathic medicine that includes both passive mobilization and muscle reeducation. Diagnosis of somatic dysfunction is performed by the practitioner, after which the patient is guided to provide corrective muscle contraction.

Music Therapy The use of music in an either active or passive mode. Used mainly to reduce stress, anxiety, and pain, especially in the palliative care setting

Naturopathy A major health system that includes practices that emphasize diet, nutrition, homeopathy, acupuncture, herbal medicine, manipulation, and various mind-body therapies. Focal points include self-healing and treatment through changes in lifestyle and emphasis on health prevention.

Ornish Diet A life-choice program based on eating a vegetarian diet containing less than 10% fat. The diet is high in complex carbohydrates and fiber. Meat and fish are generally avoided.

Oslo Diet An eating plan that emphasizes increased intake of fish and reduced total fat intake. Diet is combined with regular endurance exercise.

Pilates An educational and exercise approach using the proper body mechanics, movements, truncal and pelvic stabilization, coordinated breathing, and muscle contractions to promote strengthening. Attention is paid to the entire musculoskeletal system.

Prayer The use of prayer(s) that are offered to "some higher being" or authority to heal and/or arrest disease. May be practiced by the individual patient, by groups, or by other(s) with or without the patient's knowledge (e.g., intercessory).

Pritikin Diet A weight management plan that is based on a vegetarian framework. Meals are low in fat, high in fiber, and high in complex carbohydrates.

Qi Gong A form of Chinese exercise-stimulation therapy that proposes to improve health by redirecting mental focus, breathing, coordination, and relaxation. The goal is to "rebalance" the body's own healing capacities by activating proposed electrical or energetic currents that flow along meridians located throughout the body. These meridians, however, do not follow conventional nerve or muscle pathways. In Chinese medical training and practice this therapy includes "external Qi," which is energy transmitted from one person to another so as to heal.

Raja Yoga Yoga practice that includes all of the other forms of yoga. The practitioner is instructed to follow moral directives, physical exercises, breathing exercises, meditation, devotion, and service to others to facilitate religious awakening.

Reflexology A bodywork technique that uses reflex points on the hands and feet. Pressure is applied at points that correspond to various body parts, to eliminate blockages thought to produce pain or disease.

Reiki Comes from the Japanese word meaning "universal life force energy." The practitioner serves as a conduit for healing energy directed into the body or energy field of the recipient without physical contact with the body.

Rolfing A bodywork technique that involves the myofascia. The body is realigned by using the hands to apply deep pressure and friction that allow more sufficient posture, movement, and the "release" of emotions from the body.

Shiatsu A Japanese bodywork technique involving finger pressure at specific points on the body mainly to balance "energy" in the body. The major focus is on prevention by keeping the body healthy. The therapy uses more than 600 points on the skin that are proposed to be connected to pathways through which energy flows.

T'ai Chi A technique that uses slow, purposeful motor-physical movements of the body to control and achieve a more balanced physiologic and psychological state.

Therapeutic Touch A body energy field technique in which hands are passed over the body without actually touching to recreate and change proposed "energy imbalances" for restoring innate healing forces. Verbal interaction between patient and therapist helps maximize effects.

Traditional Chinese Medicine An ancient form of medicine that focuses on prevention and secondarily treats disease with an emphasis on maintaining balance through the body by stimulating a constant, smooth-flowing Qi energy. Herbs, acupuncture, massage, diet, and exercise are also used.

Trager Psychophysical Integration A bodywork technique in which the practitioner enters a meditative state and guides the client through gentle, light, rhythmic, nonintrusive movements. "Mentastics" exercises using self-healing movements are taught to the clients.

AUTHOR: **ANNE L. HUME, PHARM.D.**

Relaxation Techniques

Relaxation Techniques

Relaxation Technique	Summary	Further Resources
Breathing exercise	This is the foundation of most relaxation techniques. Have patients place one hand on the chest and the other on the abdomen. Instruct them to take a slow, deep breath, as if they were sucking in all the air in the room. While doing this, the hand on the abdomen should rise higher than the hand on the chest. This promotes diaphragmatic breathing that increases alveolar expansion in the bases of the lungs. Have them hold the breath for a count of 7 and then exhale. Exhalation should take twice as long as inhalation. Repeat this for a total of five breaths, and encourage patients to do this three times a day.	*Conscious Breathing* by Gay Hendricks is one of many good resources on using breathing for relaxation and health.
Meditation		
Transcendental/The relaxation response	To prevent distracting thoughts, the subject repeats a mantra (a word or sound) over and over again while sitting in a comfortable position. If a distracting thought comes to mind, it is accepted and let go, with the mind focusing again on the mantra.	*The Relaxation Response* by Herbert Benson; www.tm.org for information on transcendental meditation.
Mindful meditation	This represents the philosophy of living in the present or in the moment. The *body scan* is one technique where the subject uses breathing to obtain a relaxed state while lying or sitting. The mind progressively focuses on different parts of the body, where it feels any and all sensations intentionally but nonjudgmentally before moving on to another part of the body. A patient with back pain may focus on the quality and characteristics of the pain as if to better understand it and bring it under control.	*Full Catastrophe Living* by Jon Kabat-Zinn describes this technique in full and the program for stress reduction at the University of Massachusetts Medical Center.
Centering prayer	This is a form similar to transcendental meditation that has a more religious foundation. The subject repeats a "sacred word" similar to a mantra. As thoughts come to mind, they are accepted and let go, clearing the mind to become more centered on the spirit within, as if the mind's preoccupied thoughts are the layers of an onion that are peeled away, allowing better understanding of the spirit at the core.	www.centeringprayer.com; look under "method of centering prayer" for a nondenominational discussion.
Progressive muscle relaxation (PMR)	A form of relaxation in which the subject is attuned to the difference in feeling when the muscles are tensed and then relaxed. In a comfortable position, start by tensing the whole body from head to toe. While doing this, notice the feelings of tightness. Take a deep breath in and as you let it out, let the tension release and the muscles relax. This is then followed by progressive tension and relaxation throughout the body. One may start by clenching the fists and then tensing the arms, shoulders, chest, abdomen, hips, legs, and so on, with each step followed by relaxation.	*You Must Relax* is a book by the founder of this technique, Edmund Jacobson. Anxiety Canada: www.anxietycanada.com/adults/how-do-progressive-muscle-relaxation Mayo Clinic: http://www.mayoclinic.org/healthy-lifestyle/stress-management/in-depth/relaxation-technique/art-20045368 Oncology Nursing Society: www.ons.org/intervention/progressive-muscle-relaxation-pmr
Visualization/Self-hypnosis	The subject uses visualization to recruit images that create a relaxed state. For example, if a person is anxious, visualizing images of a place and a time that were peaceful and comforting would help induce relaxation. This is best used in conjunction with a breathing exercise.	There are many CDs, MP3s, and DVDs that can guide people through a visualization "script" that can result in relaxation. Emmett Miller is one well-known author.
Autogenic training	This induces a physiologic response by using simple phrases. For example, "My legs are heavy and warm" is meant to increase the blood flow to this area, resulting in relaxation. This is done progressively from head to toe with the use of deep breathing and repetition of the phrase. After completing this, focus attention on any body part that may still be tense, and then focus the breath and phrase to that area until the whole body is relaxed.	The British Autogenic Society at www.autogenic-therapy.org.uk/ is a good resource for more information.

Continued on following page

Relaxation Techniques—cont'd

Relaxation Technique	Summary	Further Resources
Exercise/Movement		
Aerobic	While performing an aerobic exercise, focus attention on a phrase, sound, word, or prayer and passively disregard other thoughts that may enter the mind. Some may focus on their breathing, saying to themselves, "In" with inhalation and "Out" with exhalation, or repeating "one-two, one-two" with each step they take with jogging. Doing this will help the mind focus, preventing other thoughts that may cause tension.	*Beyond the Relaxation Response* by Herbert Benson includes discussion of his research on inducing the relaxation response while exercising.
Yoga	This has been practiced for thousands of years in India. In America, it has been divided into three aspects: breathing (pranayama yoga), bodily postures or asanas (hatha yoga), and meditation to maintain balance and health. Regular practice induces relaxation.	For Yoga, t'ai chi, and qi gong therapies, it is best to encourage patients to take a class at a local community center or gym and to pick up an introductory book at a library or bookstore.
T'ai chi	An ancient Chinese martial art that uses slow, graceful movements combined with inner mindfulness and breathing techniques to help bring balance between the mind and body.	See above.
Qi gong	A traditional Chinese practice that uses movement, meditation, and controlled breathing to balance the body's vital energy force, Qi.	See above.

Updated from Rakel RE (ed): *Principles of family practice*, ed 6, Philadelphia, 2002, Saunders.

Overview of Selected Natural Products

This table includes a few of the common uses and side effects of selected natural products. The evidence supporting the uses and side effects of these products varies considerably and may be based on anecdotal information or theoretical concerns with the natural products.

Natural Products	Common Use(s)	Adverse Effects/Potential Concerns
African plum (Pygeum)	Benign prostatic hyperplasia	Nausea and abdominal pain have been reported, but pygeum is generally well tolerated. Pygeum does not decrease prostate size or influence PSA concentrations.
Black cohosh	Management of hot flashes in peri- and postmenopausal women	Dyspepsia, rash, weight gain, headache, and cramping have been reported. Concern exists that black cohosh causes liver toxicity, although the botanical was part of a multi-ingredient blend. The potential development of mild estrogen-like adverse effects, especially endometrial hyperplasia, is of concern.
Butterbur	Prevention of migraine headaches and supported by 2012 American Academy of Neurology; allergic rhinitis	Diarrhea, stomach upset, fatigue, belching, headache, and drowsiness may occur. Due to concern about hepatotoxicity, butterbur products should be free of pyrrolizidine alkaloids. Products should be standardized to 15% petasin and isopetasin.
Chamomile (German)	Motion sickness, anxiety, insomnia; gastrointestinal spasms; mucositis	Allergic reactions occur on rare occasion. Patients with a ragweed allergy should use chamomile with caution.
Chasteberry	Premenstrual dysphoric disorder, premenstrual syndrome, menopausal symptoms, female infertility, mastalgia	Gastrointestinal upset, headache, rash, acne, weight gain, and menstrual bleeding have been reported.
Chitosan	Weight loss, Crohn's disease, hypercholesterolemia, anemia	Gastrointestinal upset, nausea, flatulence, and constipation have been reported. Patients with a shellfish allergy should avoid the use of chitosan.
Chondroitin sulfate	Osteoarthritis, osteoporosis, hyperlipidemia	Gastrointestinal upset, nausea, diarrhea, constipation, and alopecia. Concern exists that chondroitin may have anticoagulant activity due to its structural similarity to part of heparin.
Cinnamon	Type 2 diabetes mellitus, flatulence, gastrointestinal spasms, anorexia, menopausal symptoms, impotence	Cassia cinnamon is one of three types of cinnamon in commercial food products; this is the only type that may have minor effects to improve blood glucose concentrations.
Coenzyme Q10	Chronic heart failure, angina, dilated cardiomyopathy, statin-induced myopathy, Parkinson's disease	Nausea, vomiting, diarrhea, anorexia, heartburn, and rash have been reported. Coenzyme Q10 is structurally similar to vitamin K; concern exists about potential interaction with warfarin.
Cranberry	Prevention and treatment of urinary tract infections; type 2 diabetes mellitus; chronic fatigue syndrome; pleurisy	Gastrointestinal upset and diarrhea have been reported with large doses of cranberry. Uric acid kidney stone formation is also possible with large doses of cranberry over prolonged periods of time.
Dehydroepiandrosterone (DHEA)	Slow or reverse aging, weight loss, metabolic syndrome, erectile dysfunction, immune stimulant, osteoporosis, systemic lupus erythematosus, multiple sclerosis, depression, schizophrenia	Acne and other androgenic effects commonly occur in women. Alopecia, insulin resistance, hepatic dysfunction, and hypertension have been reported. Ingested wild yam and soy cannot be converted into DHEA by humans.
Devil's claw	Osteoarthritis, atherosclerosis, gout, myalgias, fever, migraines	Diarrhea, nausea, and vomiting, as well as allergic reactions, have been reported.
Echinacea	Prevention and treatment of viral respiratory infections; urinary tract infections; chronic fatigue syndrome; attention deficit hyperactivity disorder	Nausea, vomiting, diarrhea, heartburn, headaches, dizziness, arthralgias, and allergic reactions have been reported with echinacea. Patients with a ragweed allergy should avoid use of echinacea.
Eleuthero (Siberian ginseng)	Maintenance of a normal blood pressure; atherosclerosis; Alzheimer's disease; chronic fatigue syndrome; diabetes; herpes simplex infections	Drowsiness, anxiety, and irritability have been reported.

Continued on following page

Overview of Selected Natural Products

Natural Products	Common Use(s)	Adverse Effects/Potential Concerns
Evening primrose oil (EPO)	Premenstrual syndrome, mastalgia, osteoporosis, asthma, menopausal symptoms, eczema, chronic fatigue syndrome	EPO is well tolerated.
Fenugreek	Type 2 diabetes mellitus, anorexia, atherosclerosis; also used as galactogogue	Gastrointestinal upset, flatulence, and hypoglycemia are possible side effects. Patients with a peanut allergy (and an allergy to related plants) should use fenugreek with caution. Nursing mothers who use fenugreek may notice a "maple syrup" smell in their sweat and in the urine of their infants. This may be mistaken to be maple syrup urine disease in the infant.
Feverfew	Prevention of migraines; fever; menstrual-related problems; arthritis; infertility; asthma	Gastrointestinal side effects are the most common with feverfew. A "post-feverfew syndrome" has been reported in individuals who have taken feverfew for prolonged periods of time and then have abruptly stopped the herbal.
Fish oil	Hypertriglyceridemia, coronary heart disease, hypertension, asthma, depression, rheumatoid arthritis, osteoporosis, psoriasis	Heartburn, nausea, rash, and a "fishy" aftertaste can occur. Contamination with pesticides (as well as with mercury and other heavy metals) is a potential concern, although this is unlikely.
Garlic	Hyperlipidemia, hypertension, peripheral arterial disease, type 2 diabetes mellitus	Nausea, vomiting, heartburn, and body odor are most common. "Deodorized" garlic products may lack the active ingredient, allicin.
Ginger	Nausea and vomiting secondary to pregnancy, chemotherapy, motion sickness, surgery	Heartburn, belching, and dermatitis have been reported. In overdoses, ginger has been associated with central nervous system depression and arrhythmias. Efficacy for hyperemesis gravidarum is unknown, and use is not recommended.
Ginkgo	Alzheimer's disease, vascular dementias, tinnitus, acute mountain sickness, intermittent claudication	Gastrointestinal side effects, headaches, dizziness, and allergic skin reactions. Seizures have been reported in several case reports. Products should contain 24% ginkgo flavone glycosides and 6% terpenoids.
Ginseng (Panax)	Increased resistance to stress and improved well-being; increased physical stamina; depression; diabetes; erectile dysfunction	Insomnia has been reported with ginseng. Vaginal bleeding, mastalgia, and amenorrhea have also been reported.
Glucosamine sulfate	Osteoarthritis	Nausea, heartburn, skin reactions, and headache have been reported. Increased glucose concentrations have been a concern but have not been documented. Patients with a shellfish allergy should use glucosamine with caution.
Green tea	Improve cognitive performance; prevention of breast, prostate, and colon cancer; hyperlipidemia; Parkinson's disease; obesity; diabetes; cardiovascular disease	Nausea, vomiting, dyspepsia, dizziness, insomnia, and nervousness have been reported. Side effects may be a result of the large amount of caffeine in green tea products. Hepatotoxicity has been a potential concern with green tea.
Hawthorn	Mild heart failure, angina, arrhythmias, hypertension	Mild gastrointestinal effects, dizziness, rash, palpitations, and nervousness have been reported.
Hoodia	Obesity	Side effects have not been reported. Many products have been adulterated and lack the actual ingredient.
Horse chestnut	Chronic venous insufficiency, including varicose veins; benign prostate hyperplasia; diarrhea	Mild nausea, vomiting, dizziness, headache, and itching. Products are standardized to 16%–20% aescin.
Huperzine	Alzheimer's disease, increased alertness and energy, myasthenia gravis, memory enhancement	Nausea, vomiting, diarrhea, sweating, and blurred vision as a result of the cholinergic effects of huperzine have been reported.
Kava	Anxiety, insomnia, restlessness, seizure disorders, depression, chronic fatigue syndrome	Gastrointestinal upset, headache, dizziness, "kava" dermopathy, and allergic skin reactions. Hepatotoxicity is the primary concern with kava; some countries have banned the use of kava.
Melatonin	Jet lag, insomnia, migraine, chronic fatigue syndrome, breast cancer, gastritis/PUD, osteoporosis; also used for insomnia in children with ADHD	Daytime drowsiness, headache, and dizziness have been reported. Vaginal bleeding has occurred in perimenopausal women. Melatonin from animal sources should be avoided.
Melissa	Cold sores (topically), anxiety, insomnia, Alzheimer's disease, hypertension, dyspepsia	Nausea, vomiting, dizziness, and wheezing have occurred with oral melissa.
Methylsulfonylmethane (MSM)	Chronic pain, arthritis, diabetes, osteoporosis, allergies, obesity, premenstrual syndrome	Nausea, bloating, diarrhea, fatigue, and insomnia have been associated with MSM. This substance is used frequently in combination with glucosamine and chondroitin.
Milk thistle	Protective agent against liver damage due to alcohol, acetaminophen, and carbon tetrachloride; hepatitis C	Nausea, abdominal fullness, diarrhea, and allergic reactions. Patients with a ragweed allergy should use milk thistle with caution.
Peppermint	Irritable bowel syndrome, sinusitis, morning sickness, dysmenorrhea	Heartburn has been reported, as well as laryngeal and bronchial spasm in infants and children.
Policosanol	Hyperlipidemia, intermittent claudication, atherosclerosis	Migraines, insomnia, dizziness, skin rash, and bleeding have been reported with policosanol. The product has antiplatelet effects.
Probiotics	Treatment and prevention of diarrhea including antibiotic-associated diarrhea; irritable bowel syndrome; atopic dermatitis; Crohn's disease	Theoretically, probiotic products may increase risk of infections in immunocompromised individuals.
Red clover phytoestrogens	Menopausal symptoms, premenstrual syndrome, asthma	Rash, myalgias, headaches, and vaginal bleeding have been reported. Theoretically, endometrial hyperplasia is an adverse effect from the use of these compounds.
Red yeast rice	Hyperlipidemia, indigestion, diarrhea, circulatory conditions	Gastrointestinal upset and dizziness may occur. Red yeast rice may contain lovastatin-like compounds and potentially cause rhabdomyolysis.

Natural Products	Common Use(s)	Adverse Effects/Potential Concerns
S-adenosylmethionine (SAM-e)	Depression, anxiety, dementia, osteoarthritis, heart disease	Nausea, vomiting, diarrhea, headache, and nervousness have been reported. Concern exists that SAM-e raises homocysteine levels.
St. John's wort	Depression, anxiety, chronic fatigue syndrome, HIV/AIDS	Anxiety, gastrointestinal upset, vaginal bleeding, neuropathy, and rash can occur. Hypomania has been induced by St. John's wort.
Tea tree oil	Topical use for acne, fungal infections, lice, scabies	Local inflammation and contact dermatitis may occur.
Valerian	Insomnia, depression, chronic fatigue syndrome, menstrual cramps	Headaches, gastrointestinal upset, and drowsiness can occur. Hepatotoxicity is a potential concern with valerian.

AIDS, Acquired immune deficiency syndrome; *HIV*, human immunodeficiency virus.

AUTHOR: **ANNE L. HUME, PHARM.D.**

Natural Products and Drug Interactions

This table lists interactions between selected natural products and prescription and nonprescription drugs. Many of the listed interactions are theoretical in nature and have not been documented to occur in humans. However, interactions with St. John's wort are potentially life threatening in nature. Other interactions are based on small studies of healthy volunteers and use pharmaceutical-quality natural products that may or may not be commercially available.

Natural Products	Drugs	Interactions
Black cohosh	Hepatotoxic drugs	Concern exists that the risk of hepatotoxicity with black cohosh is increased in the presence of hepatotoxic drugs.
	Cisplatin	Animal studies suggest that the efficacy of cisplatin against breast cancer cells may be decreased by black cohosh.
	CYP2D6 substrates	Black cohosh may modestly inhibit CYP2D6 enzyme activity to result in higher drug concentrations.
Butterbur	CYP3A4 inducers (rifampin, carbamazepine, etc.)	Drugs that induce the activity of CYP3A4 increase the risk of the formation of hepatotoxic metabolites from pyrrolizidine alkaloids from some butterbur products.
Chamomile	CNS depressants	Chamomile may have additive CNS depressant effects.
	CYP1A2 substrates	Chamomile may inhibit CYP1A2 enzyme activity to result in higher drug concentrations.
	CYP3A4 substrates	Chamomile may inhibit CYP3A4 enzyme activity to result in higher drug concentrations.
	Estrogens	Chamomile may compete for estrogen receptors.
	Tamoxifen	Chamomile may interfere with the effects of tamoxifen because of its estrogenic effects.
Chaste tree berry	Antipsychotic agents	Chaste tree berry may antagonize the effects of antipsychotic agents through its dopaminergic activity.
	Metoclopramide	Chaste tree berry may antagonize the effects of metoclopramide through its dopaminergic activity.
	Dopamine agonists	Chaste tree berry may possess additive effects to drugs such as levodopa through its dopaminergic activity.
	Oral contraceptives/estrogens	Chaste tree berry may possess additive hormonal effects.
Chondroitin	Warfarin	High-dose chondroitin has structural similarity to a heparinoid and may possess weak anticoagulant effects.
Cinnamon	Hypoglycemic agents	Cinnamon may possess additive effects on blood glucose to those of hypoglycemic agents.
Coenzyme Q10	Antihypertensive agents	Coenzyme Q10 may possess additive effects on blood pressure to those of antihypertensive agents.
	Warfarin	Coenzyme Q10 may lessen the anticoagulant effects of warfarin because of its structural similarity to vitamin K.
	Chemotherapy	The antioxidant effects of coenzyme Q10 may blunt the efficacy of chemotherapeutic agents that depend on the formation of free radicals.
Cranberry	CYP2C9 substrates (warfarin)	Cranberry may inhibit CYP2C9 enzyme activity to result in higher drug concentrations, although evidence with warfarin is contradictory.
Dehydroepiandrosterone (DHEA)	Tamoxifen and aromatase inhibitors such as anastrozole.	DHEA may interfere with the antiestrogenic effects of these drugs.
	CYP3A4 substrates	DHEA may slightly inhibit CYP3A4 enzyme activity to result in higher drug concentrations.

Natural Products	Drugs	Interactions
Devil's claw	Antihypertensive agents	Devil's claw may possess additive effects on blood pressure to those of antihypertensive agents.
	Hypoglycemic agents	Devil's claw may possess additive effects on blood glucose to those of hypoglycemic agents.
	H_2 antagonists and PPIs	Devil's claw may raise gastric pH and blunt the efficacy of H_2 antagonists and PPIs.
	CYP3A4 substrates	Devil's claw may inhibit CYP3A4 enzyme activity to result in higher drug concentrations.
	CYP2C9 substrates	Devil's claw may inhibit CYP2C9 enzyme activity to result in higher drug concentrations.
	CYP2C19 substrates	Devil's claw may inhibit CYP2C19 enzyme activity to result in higher drug concentrations.
	Warfarin	Devil's claw may inhibit CYP2C9 enzyme activity to result in higher concentrations of warfarin; purpura has been reported.
Echinacea	Immune suppressants	Echinacea may stimulate immune function, potentially decreasing the effectiveness of drugs such as cyclosporine and prednisone.
	CYP3A4 substrates	Echinacea may modestly induce hepatic CYP3A4 enzyme activity to result in lower drug concentrations.
	CYP1A2 substrates	Echinacea may inhibit CYP1A2 enzyme activity to result in higher drug concentrations.
Eleuthero (Siberian ginseng)	CNS depressants	Eleuthero may have additive CNS depressant effects.
	Antiplatelet and anticoagulant agents	Eleuthero may have antiplatelet activity, potentially increasing the risk of bleeding.
	CYP3A4 substrates	Eleuthero may inhibit CYP3A4 enzyme activity to result in higher drug concentrations.
	CYP1A2 substrates	Eleuthero may modestly inhibit CYP1A2 enzyme activity to result in higher drug concentrations.
	CYP2C9 substrates	Eleuthero may modestly inhibit CYP2C9 enzyme activity to result in higher drug concentrations.
	CYP2D6 substrates	Eleuthero may inhibit CYP2D6 enzyme activity to result in higher drug concentrations.
	Digoxin	Concentration of digoxin has been reported to increase but without evidence of toxicity.
Evening primrose oil (EPO)	Antiplatelet and anticoagulant agents	EPO may have anticoagulant activity, potentially increasing the risk of bleeding.
Fenugreek	Antiplatelet and anticoagulant agents	Fenugreek may have antiplatelet activity, potentially increasing the risk of bleeding.
	Hypoglycemic agents	Fenugreek may potentially lower blood glucose concentrations and have additive effects with hypoglycemic agents.
Feverfew	Antiplatelet and anticoagulant agents	Feverfew may have antiplatelet activity, potentially increasing the risk of bleeding.
	CYP3A4 substrates	Feverfew may inhibit CYP3A4 enzyme activity to result in higher drug concentrations.
	CYP1A2 substrates	Feverfew may inhibit CYP1A2 enzyme activity to result in higher drug concentrations.
	CYP2C9 substrates	Feverfew may inhibit CYP2C9 enzyme activity to result in higher drug concentrations.
	CYP2C19 substrates	Feverfew may inhibit CYP2C19 enzyme activity to result in higher drug concentrations.
Fish oils (omega-3 fatty acids)	Antiplatelet and anticoagulant agents	Fish oils may have antiplatelet activity, potentially increasing the risk of bleeding, although this has not been documented in humans.
	Antihypertensive agents	Fish oils may possess additive effects on blood pressure to those of antihypertensive agents.
	Oral contraceptives	Oral contraceptives may potentially interfere with the triglyceride-lowering effects of fish oil.
Garlic	Antiplatelet and anticoagulant agents	Garlic may have antiplatelet activity, potentially increasing the risk of bleeding.
	CYP3A4 substrates	Garlic may potentially induce CYP3A4 enzyme activity to result in lower drug concentrations; evidence is contradictory.
	CYP2E1 substrates	Garlic may modestly inhibit CYP2E1 enzyme activity to result in higher drug concentrations.
Ginger	Antiplatelet and anticoagulant agents	Ginger may have antiplatelet activity, potentially increasing the risk of bleeding.
	Hypoglycemic agents	Ginger may potentially lower blood glucose concentrations and have additive effects with hypoglycemic agents.
Ginkgo	Antiplatelet and anticoagulant agents	Ginkgo may have antiplatelet activity, potentially increasing the risk of bleeding.
	CYP2C19 substrates	Ginkgo may induce CYP2C19 enzyme activity to result in lower drug concentrations.
	CYP1A2 substrates	Ginkgo may modestly inhibit CYP1A2 enzyme activity to result in higher drug levels.
	CYP2C9 substrates	Ginkgo may modestly inhibit CYP2C9 enzyme activity to result in higher drug concentrations.
	CYP2D6 substrates	Ginkgo may inhibit CYP2D6 enzyme activity to result in higher drug concentrations.
Ginseng (Panax)	Antiplatelet and anticoagulant agents	Panax ginseng may have antiplatelet properties; American ginseng may decrease the effectiveness (international normalized ratio [INR]) of warfarin.
	CYP2D6 substrates	Panax ginseng may modestly inhibit CYP2D6 enzyme activity to result in higher drug concentrations.
	Immune suppressants	Panax ginseng may stimulate immune function, potentially decreasing the effectiveness of drugs such as cyclosporine and prednisone.
	Hypoglycemic agents	Panax ginseng may potentially lower blood glucose levels and have additive effects with hypoglycemic agents.
Glucosamine	Warfarin	High-dose glucosamine (along with high-dose chondroitin) may have additive effects to those of warfarin because of structural similarity to heparin. Evidence is lacking.

Continued on following page

Natural Products	Drugs	Interactions
Green tea extract	Antiplatelet agents	Green tea possesses compounds that may have antiplatelet activity, potentially increasing the risk of bleeding.
	Amphetamines	Caffeine in green tea may increase the risk of CNS toxicity.
	Cocaine	Caffeine in green tea may increase the risk of CNS toxicity.
	Oral contraceptives	Oral contraceptives may decrease the clearance of caffeine in green tea.
	Warfarin	Small amounts of vitamin K have been reported to be present in green tea, potentially decreasing the effectiveness of warfarin.
	Theophylline	Caffeine potentially decreases theophylline clearance.
	Verapamil	Verapamil decreases caffeine clearance, resulting in increased concentrations.
	Quinolone antibiotics	Some quinolone antibiotics decrease the clearance of caffeine.
	Hepatotoxic drugs	Concern exists that the risk of hepatotoxicity with green tea is increased in the presence of hepatotoxic drugs.
Hawthorn	β-Blockers	Hawthorn and β-blockers may have additive effects on blood pressure and heart rate.
	CCBs, nitrates	Hawthorn and CCBs (or nitrates) may have additive effects due to coronary vasodilation.
	Digoxin	Hawthorn may have additive effects to those of digoxin.
	Phosphodiesterase inhibitors	Hawthorn may have additive vasodilatory and hypotensive effects with these drugs.
Horse chestnut seed extract (HCSE)	Antiplatelet and anticoagulant agents	HCSE may have antiplatelet activity, potentially increasing the risk of bleeding.
	Hypoglycemic agents	HCSE may potentially lower blood glucose concentrations and have additive effects with hypoglycemic agents.
Huperzine	AChE inhibitors (donepezil, etc.)	Huperzine may have additive effects when combined with AChE inhibitors.
	Anticholinergic drugs	The effectiveness of huperzine and/or the anticholinergic drug may be decreased by their concomitant administration.
	Cholinergic drugs (bethanechol, etc.)	Huperzine may have additive effects when combined with cholinergic drugs.
Kava	CYP3A4 substrates	Kava may inhibit CYP3A4 enzyme activity to result in higher drug concentrations.
	CYP1A2 substrates	Kava may inhibit CYP1A2 enzyme activity to result in higher drug concentrations.
	CYP2C9 substrates, CYP2C19 substrates	Kava may inhibit CYP2C9 and CYP2C19 enzyme activity to result in higher drug concentrations.
	CYP2D6 substrates	Kava may inhibit CYP2D6 enzyme activity to result in higher drug concentrations.
	P-glycoprotein substrates (digoxin; itraconazole; diltiazem, verapamil; and many other drugs)	Kava may inhibit P-glycoprotein transporter systems.
	Hepatotoxic drugs	Concern exists that the risk of hepatotoxicity from kava is increased in the presence of hepatotoxic drugs.
Melatonin	Antiplatelet and anticoagulant agents	Melatonin may potentiate the effects of antiplatelets and anticoagulants, although the mechanism is unknown.
	CNS depressants	Melatonin may have additive CNS depressant effects.
	Fluvoxamine	Fluvoxamine may increase levels of melatonin.
	Immune suppressants	Melatonin may stimulate immune function, potentially decreasing the effectiveness of drugs such as cyclosporine and prednisone.
	Hypoglycemic agents	Melatonin may impair glucose utilization and may decrease the efficacy of hypoglycemic agents.
Milk thistle	Estrogens (and other drugs that undergo glucuronidation)	Silymarin may increase the clearance of estrogens.
	CYP2C9 substrates	Milk thistle may modestly inhibit CYP2C9 enzyme activity to result in higher drug concentrations.
Peppermint oil	H_2 antagonists and proton pump inhibitors	Peppermint oil may raise gastric pH and blunt efficacy of H_2 antagonists and PPIs.
	CYP3A4 substrates	Peppermint oil may modestly inhibit CYP3A4 enzyme activity to result in higher drug concentrations.
	CYP1A2 substrates	Peppermint oil may modestly inhibit CYP1A2 enzyme activity to result in higher drug concentrations.
	CYP2C9 substrates, CYP2C19 substrates	Peppermint oil may modestly inhibit CYP2C9 and CYP2C19 enzyme activity to result in higher drug concentrations.
Policosanol	Antiplatelet and anticoagulant agents	Policosanol may have antiplatelet activity, potentially increasing the risk of bleeding.
Probiotics	Antibiotics	Antibiotics may kill the live organisms in different probiotic preparations.
	Immune suppressants	Theoretically, probiotics may cause bacterial or fungal infections in patients who are taking immune suppressants chronically.
Red clover phytoestrogens	Antiplatelet and anticoagulant agents	Theoretically, red clover may possess coumarins, which increase the risk of bleeding with antiplatelet and anticoagulants. Evidence is lacking.
	CYP3A4 substrates	Red clover may inhibit CYP3A4 enzyme activity to result in higher drug concentrations.
	CYP2C9 substrates, CYP2C19 substrates	Red clover may inhibit CYP2C9 and CYP2C19 enzyme activity to result in higher drug concentrations.
	CYP1A2 substrates	Red clover may inhibit CYP1A2 enzyme activity to result in higher drug concentrations.

Natural Products	Drugs	Interactions
Red yeast rice	CYP3A4 inhibitors	Drugs that inhibit CYP3A4 may decrease the metabolism of lovastatin in red yeast rice.
	Statins	Red yeast rice contains lovastatin and increases the risk of myopathy.
	Fibrates and niacin	Fibrates and niacin may increase concentrations of lovastatin in red yeast rice.
S-adenosylmethionine (SAM-e)	Antidepressants (including MAOIs)	Additive effects are possible, and there is potential for toxicity.
	Serotonergic drugs (triptans, SSRIs, tramadol, dextromethorphan, etc.)	SAM-e may increase the risk of development of serotonin syndrome when used concomitantly.
Soy phytoestrogens	Estrogens	Soy potentially may inhibit the effects of estrogen.
	Tamoxifen/aromatase inhibitors	Soy's estrogenic effects may antagonize the antitumor effects of tamoxifen/aromatase inhibitors.
	MAOIs	Fermented soy products may contain tyramine.
St. John's wort	CYP3A4 substrates	St. John's wort strongly induces CYP3A4 enzyme activity to result in lower drug concentrations.
	CYP1A2 substrates	St. John's wort modestly induces CYP1A2 enzyme activity to result in lower drug levels.
	CYP2C9 substrates	St. John's wort induces CYP2C9 enzyme activity to result in lower drug concentrations.
	P-glycoprotein substrates (digoxin; itraconazole; diltiazem, verapamil; and many other drugs)	St. John's wort induces P-glycoprotein transporter systems.
	Serotonergic drugs (triptans, SSRIs, tramadol, dextromethorphan, etc.)	St. John's wort may increase the risk of development of serotonin syndrome when used concomitantly.
Valerian	CNS depressants	Valerian may increase the sedative effects of CNS depressants.
	CYP3A4 substrates	Valerian may modestly inhibit the CYP3A4 enzyme activity.

AChE, Acetylcholinesterase; *CCBs,* calcium channel blockers; *CNS,* central nervous system; *MAOIs,* monoamine oxidase inhibitor; *PPIs,* proton pump inhibitors; *SSRIs,* selective serotonin reuptake inhibitors.

EXAMPLES OF DRUGS METABOLIZED BY CYP ENZYMES

The following are examples of drugs that are metabolized through the different cytochrome P450 isoenzymes:

CYP1A2 substrates: theophylline, imipramine, clozapine, naproxen

CYP2C9 substrates: warfarin, tamoxifen, irbesartan, ibuprofen, glipizide

CYP2C19 substrates: omeprazole and other proton pump inhibitors, phenytoin, phenobarbital, cyclophosphamide

CYP2D6 substrates: S-metoprolol, propafenone, paroxetine, risperidone, tramadol

CYP2E1 substrates: acetaminophen, alcohol

CYP3A4 substrates: most statins, indinavir, amlodipine, verapamil, alprazolam, buspirone

AUTHOR: **ANNE L. HUME, PHARM.D.**

Appendix Ie

Commonly Ingested Plants with Significant Toxic Potential

Plant	Symptoms	Management
Autumn crocus *(Colchicum autumnale)*	Vomiting Diarrhea Initial leukocytosis followed by bone marrow failure Multisystem organ failure	Activated charcoal decontamination Aggressive fluid resuscitation and supportive care
Belladonna alkaloids: jimson weed *(Datura stramonium)* Belladonna ("deadly nightshade"; *Atropa belladonna*)	Anticholinergic toxidrome Seizures	Supportive care, benzodiazepines Consider physostigmine if patient is a threat to self or others; only use if no conduction delays on ECG
Cardiac glycoside–containing plants (foxglove, lily of the valley, oleander, yellow oleander, etc.)	Nausea Vomiting Bradycardia Dysrhythmias (AV block, ventricular ectopy) Hyperkalemia	Digoxin-specific Fab fragments
Jequirity bean and other abrin-containing species (e.g., rosary pea, precatory bean)	Oral pain Vomiting Diarrhea Shock Hemolysis Renal failure	Supportive care, including aggressive volume resuscitation and correction of electrolyte abnormalities
Monkshood (*Aconitum* species)	Numbness and tingling of lips/tongue Vomiting Bradycardia	Atropine for bradycardia Supportive care
Oxalate-containing plants: *Philodendron, Dieffenbachia, Colocasia* ("elephant ear")	Local tissue injury Oral pain Vomiting	Supportive care, pain control
Poison hemlock *(Conium maculatum)*	Vomiting Agitation followed by CNS depression Paralysis Respiratory failure	Supportive care
Pokeweed	Hemorrhagic gastroenteritis Burning of mouth and throat	Supportive care
Rhododendron	Vomiting Diarrhea Bradycardia	Atropine for symptomatic bradycardia Supportive care
Tobacco	Vomiting Agitation Diaphoresis Fasciculations Seizures	Supportive care
Water hemlock (*Cicuta* species)	Abdominal pain Vomiting Delirium Seizures	Supportive care, including benzodiazepines for seizures
Yew (*Taxus* species)	GI symptoms QRS widening Hypotension CV collapse	Supportive care Atropine for bradycardia Sodium bicarbonate does not appear to be effective

AV, atrioventricular; *CNS,* central nervous system; *CV,* cardiovascular; *ECG,* electrocardiogram; *Fab,* fragment, antigen binding; *GI,* gastrointestinal.
From Kliegman RM et al: *Nelson textbook of pediatrics,* ed 20, Philadelphia, 2016, Saunders.

Herbs Associated with Toxicity

Herbal Product	Toxic Chemicals	Toxic Effects
Aconite (*Aconitum* spp.)	Aconitine alkaloids	Nausea, vomiting, paresthesia, weakness, hypotension, asystole, arrhythmia, bradycardia
Chamomile *(Matricaria chamomilla, Anthemis nobilis)*	Allergens	Anaphylaxis, contact dermatitis
Chapparal *(Larrea divaricata, Larrea tridentata)*	Nordihydroguaiaretic acid	Nausea, vomiting, lethargy, hepatitis
Cinnamon oil *(Cinnamomum)*	Cinnamaldehyde	Dermatitis, abuse syndrome
Coltsfoot *(Tussilago farfara)*	Pyrrolizidines	HVOD
Comfrey *(Symphytum officinale)*	Pyrrolizidines	HVOD
Crotalaria spp.	Pyrrolizidines	HVOD
Echinacea (*Echinacea angustifolia, Compositae* spp.)	Polysaccharides	Asthma, atopy, angioedema, anaphylaxis, urticaria
Eucalyptus *(Eucalyptus globulus)*	1,8-cineole	Drowsiness, ataxia, nausea, vomiting, seizure, coma, respiratory failure
Garlic *(Allium sativum)*	Allicin	Dermatitis, chemical burn, oxidant
Germander *(Teucrium chamaedrys)*		Hepatotoxicity
Ginseng *(Panax ginseng)*	Ginsenoside	Ginseng abuse, diarrhea, anxiety, insomnia, hypertension
Glycerated asafetida	Oxidants	Methemoglobinemia
Grousel *(Senecio longilobus)*	Pyrrolizidines	HVOD
Heliotrope, turnsole *(Crotalaria fulva, Heliotropium, Cynoglossum officinale)*	Pyrrolizidines	HVOD
Jin bu huan (*Stephania* spp., *Corydalis* spp.)	l-Tetrahydropalmatine	Hepatitis, lethargy, coma
Kava-kava *(Piper methysticum)*	Kavain, methysticin	Hepatic failure, "kavaism" neurotoxicity
Kelp	Iodine	Thyroid dysfunction
Laetrile	Cyanide	Coma, seizure, death
Licorice *(Glycyrrhiza glabra)*	Glycyrrhetic acid	Hypertension, arrhythmia, hypokalemia
Ma huang *(Ephedra sinica)*	Ephedrine	Arrhythmia, seizure, stroke, hypertension
Monkshood *(Aconitum napellus, A. columbianum)*	Aconite	Arrhythmia, weakness, coma, shock, paresthesia, vomiting, seizure
Nutmeg *(Myristica fragrans)*	Myristicin, eugenol	Hallucination, emesis, headache
Nux vomica	Strychnine	Seizure, abdominal pain, respiratory arrest
Pennyroyal (*Mentha pulegium* or *Hedeoma* spp.)	Pulegone	Centrilobular liver necrosis, fetotoxicity, seizure, shock
Ragwort (golden) *(Senecio aureus, Echium)*	Pyrrolizidines	HVOD
Wormwood (*Artemisia* spp.)	Thujone	Seizure, dementia, tremor, headache

HVOD, hepatic veno-occlusive disease.
Modified from Committee on Injuries & Poison Prevention: *Children's environmental health,* ed 3. Elk Grove Village, IL, 2009, American Academy of Pediatrics. In Fuhrman BP et al: *Pediatric critical care,* ed 5, Philadelphia, 2017, Elsevier.

Websites Providing Data on Herbal Therapy Hazards

Web Address	Website
www.fda.gov	On the U.S. Food and Drug Administration website under the title "MedWatch," some herb warnings can be found ("special adverse event monitoring system" link)
www.faseb.org/aspet/H&MIG3.htm#top	ASPET Herbal and Medicinal Plant Interest Group: a site for an herb discussion group with pharmacologists
www.nnlm.nlm.nih.gov/pnr/uwmhg/	University of Washington Medicinal Herb Garden
www.abc.herbalgram.org	American Botanical Council
http://nccih.nih.gov/	The National Center for Complementary and Integrative Health is 1 of 27 institutes and centers that make up the U.S. National Institutes of Health; their mission is to define, through rigorous scientific investigation, the usefulness and safety of complementary and integrative health interventions and their roles in improving health and health care
http://toxnet.nlm.nih.gov/	A cluster of databases on toxicology, hazardous chemicals, and related areas

Modified from Floege J et al: *Comprehensive clinical nephrology,* ed 4, Philadelphia, 2010, Saunders.

Dietary Supplements: What Every Primary Care Provider Should Know

Primary care providers must be knowledgeable regarding the safety, efficacy, and drug interactions associated with common dietary supplements because of the following:

- An estimated 33.2% of adults ages 18 years and older reported the use of at least one form of complementary health approach, according to the National Health Interview Survey in 2012.
- 18% of adults specifically reported the use of dietary supplements, with fish oil, glucosamine, chondroitin, melatonin, and pre/probiotics the most frequently used nonvitamin, nonmineral supplement.
- In a 2010 AARP telephone survey of older adults, almost one-third reported the use of herbal and other supplements, and almost half of those individuals using supplements did not tell their health care provider. https://nccih.nih.gov/research/statistics/2010

COMMON TERMINOLOGY

- A *dietary supplement* is defined as an oral product containing vitamins, minerals, herbs, or other botanicals; amino acids; dietary substances used to supplement the diet by increasing the total dietary intake; or a concentrate, metabolite, constituent, extract, or combination.
- *CAM* refers to the broad domain of healing practices that include diverse health systems, modalities, and practices and their accompanying theories and beliefs (see glossary of terms in Appendix Ia).
- *Complementary therapies* are those that are used *in addition to* conventional therapies, whereas *alternative therapies* are those that are used *instead of* conventional therapies. Integrative therapy is generally defined as the use of complementary medicine with conventional Western medicine in a coordinated manner. https://nccih.nih.gov/health/integrative-health#integrative

LEGISLATION

The U.S. Food and Drug Administration (FDA) is frequently criticized for not closely regulating dietary supplements and monitoring their safety. However, although the agency regulates prescription drugs and over-the-counter (OTC) products, the FDA has limited regulatory authority over dietary supplements. This is because the Dietary Supplement and Health Education Act (DSHEA) of 1994 and its resulting regulations limit the FDA's authority. As a result of DSHEA, the FDA is able to act only when a dietary supplement has been documented to contain a prescription drug, such as sildenafil and related compounds in supplements for erectile dysfunction or sibutramine in a weight-loss preparation. In addition, the FDA can act when safety issues related to a product have been clearly documented, although these cases are frequently challenged in the courts.

HEALTH CLAIMS

Dietary supplements generally are marketed under three types of health claims. The first category is the "nutrient content" claim, in which the product is identified as an excellent source of, typically, a mineral such as calcium, based on recommended daily values. The second type is the "significant scientific agreement" claim; these claims are used when some evidence of the product's efficacy exists (e.g., fish oil supplements). The third and most common type of health claim is called a "structure/function" claim; these claims state that the product has some effect on health—for example, "helps to maintain a healthy heart." However, dietary supplements are not permitted to carry claims stating that they are effective in preventing, treating, or curing diseases.

INFORMATION RESOURCES

Appendix Ic provides a brief overview of common dietary supplements. In the past, few evidence-based resources on dietary supplements were available. Clinical studies and systematic reviews on dietary supplements are now widely available through PubMed, EMBASE, and the Cochrane Database of Systematic Reviews. Although more information is available, references on specific products vary in their interpretation of the available evidence and may exhibit an unintentional bias, either pro or con, regarding the safety and efficacy of dietary supplements.

"Gold standard" evidence-based databases on dietary supplements (subscription required) include the following:

- Natural Medicines Professional Database (https://naturalmedicines.therapeuticresearch.com/) contains multiple databases including one listing many dietary supplements. Monographs include the different common and scientific names; uses and likely effectiveness for different uses; chemical constituents; interactions with drugs, diseases, foods, and laboratory tests; adverse effects; and cautions. The information is extensively referenced and is updated on a daily basis.
- Consumerlabs.com has a subscription-based database containing common popular dietary supplements as well as almost daily updates related to supplements in the news on its website (www.consumerlab.com/). This organization is not affiliated with Consumer Reports and primarily conducts independent tests of the content of commercially available supplements.

Evidence-based free websites on dietary supplements include the following:

- National Center for Complementary and Integrative Health (NCCIH) https://nccih.nih.gov/health/providers
- Memorial Sloan-Kettering Cancer Center www.mskcc.org/cancer-care/diagnosis-treatment/symptom-management/integrative-medicine/herbs

DRUG INTERACTIONS

Clinically significant interactions have been documented between dietary supplements and prescription or OTC drugs. The challenge for primary care providers is to identify real, clinically relevant interactions versus potential or theoretical interactions. Data on interactions with dietary supplements are usually based on isolated case reports or on studies enrolling healthy volunteers. As with drug-drug interactions, the likelihood of an interaction and its severity are influenced especially by concomitant medical conditions, such as heart failure and presence or absence of impaired kidney and liver function. Data also has suggested that the individual's genetic profile may influence the potential for drug-botanical supplement interactions.

Appendix Id lists interactions between selected dietary supplements and prescription and nonprescription drugs. The following two broad interactions are particularly important in primary care practice:

- St. John's wort, commonly used for depression, is a potent inducer of cytochrome P450 3A4 isoenzymes and has been documented to increase the clearance of many drugs that are metabolized through this and other pathways. In addition, St. John's wort may induce P-glycoprotein transporter systems that are important for digoxin and some chemotherapeutic agents. St. John's wort has also been associated with the development of serotonin syndrome when used with drugs that have significant serotonergic activity.
- Dietary supplements such as garlic, ginkgo, and feverfew, as well as many others, have been purported to either have antiplatelet activity or have effects on the clotting cascade. This may be important for adults also taking aspirin and other platelet-active agents, as well as warfarin and the direct acting oral anticoagulants (DOACs).

COUNSELING POINTS

The single most important counseling point related to dietary supplements is to ask patients about their use of these products and to do so in an open, nonjudgmental manner. The approach should emphasize that many consumers have been interested in vitamins, minerals, herbs, teas, and so on, to maintain their health or to treat illness. If the clinician is unaware of the safety, efficacy, and interactions of a specific product, several websites are available to quickly scan for information. Also, access to drug information centers at colleges of pharmacy is frequently available, and some hospitals now offer programs in integrative medicine.

Patients should be asked about their goals in using the product, as well as how long they have taken it and in what dosage. Allergies to plants should be documented because cross-allergies are common. Clinicians should appreciate that individuals who use dietary supplements may be interested in making lifestyle changes and potentially decreasing their use of prescription drugs. In addition, if an individual is also consulting an alternative medicine practitioner, clinicians should recognize that some alternative health systems discourage the use of established therapies such as vaccines.

Although problems with safety and efficacy have been identified, many dietary supplements are benign except for their cost. Some patients are at higher risk for adverse outcomes from the use of dietary supplements (e.g., those with chronic kidney and liver disease). Patients should be counseled specifically to avoid purchasing dietary supplements over the Internet.

RESEARCH ISSUES

Many clinical and observational studies of dietary supplements have been published. In the past, clinicians frequently stated either that published studies of dietary supplements did not exist or that only a few were available. The reason for this finding was that in the past the National Library of Medicine did not abstract from the peer-reviewed alternative medicine literature. As with all research, the more rigorous the study methodology, the less likely the dietary supplement is to demonstrate clinical benefit.

In evaluating published studies of dietary supplements, the following should be considered:

- Has the correct plant and part of the plant (root, stem, leaf) been used? This critical information may not be known to many clinicians. Consulting a resource such as the National Medicines database can usually provide the needed information to judge this component of the study.
- Has the content of active ingredients been verified throughout the study? In a review of 81 major randomized controlled trials of herbal products, only 12 (15%) reported performing tests to quantify actual contents, and 3 (4%) provided adequate data to compare actual with expected content values of at least one chemical constituent.
- Is the severity of the disease appropriate for study? Negative studies with dietary supplements sometimes inappropriately enroll participants who have moderate-to-severe disease (e.g., those with depression or benign prostatic hyperplasia) when only mild disease would be appropriate.
- Is the duration of the study appropriate? Early studies comparing glucosamine and nonsteroidal antiinflammatory agents (NSAIAs) demonstrated greater efficacy with the NSAIAs because of an inadequate study duration for glucosamine to show any benefit.
- Is a placebo group included? Recent studies with dietary supplements for menopausal symptoms and osteoarthritis have demonstrated placebo responses over 40% to 50%.
- Was the blinding maintained throughout the study? Some dietary supplements, such as saw palmetto, have distinctive odors and tastes that are not easily masked.
- Is the preparation commercially available? Most important, when a study with dietary supplements does show benefit, it frequently is difficult to use the product in practice because the specific formulation studied is not commercially available.

AUTHOR: **ANNE L. HUME, PHARM.D.**

Vitamins and Their Functions

	Biochemistry and Physiology	Deficiency [RDA*]	Toxicity [TUL†]	Assessment of Status
Fat-Soluble Vitamins				
Vitamin A	A family of the retinoid compounds, each member having biologic activity qualitatively similar to retinol. Carotenoids are structurally related to retinoids. Some carotenoids, most notably β-carotene, are metabolized into compounds with vitamin A activity and are therefore considered to be provitamin A compounds. Vitamin A is an integral component of rhodopsin and iodopsins, light-sensitive proteins in rod and cone cells in the retina. *Additional functions:* induction and maintenance of cellular differentiation in certain tissues; signal for appropriate morphogenesis in the developing embryo; maintenance of cell-mediated immunity. 1 μg of retinol = 3.33 IU of vitamin A.	Follicular hyperkeratosis and night blindness are early indicators. Conjunctival xerosis, degeneration of the cornea (keratomalacia), and dedifferentiation of rapidly proliferating epithelia are later indications of deficiency. *Bitot spots* (focal areas of the conjunctiva or cornea with foamy appearance) are an indication of xerosis. Blindness, due to corneal destruction and retinal dysfunction, ensues if left uncorrected. Increased susceptibility to infection is also a consequence. [F: 700 μg; M: 900 μg]	In adults, >150,000 μg may cause *acute* toxicity: fatal intracranial hypertension, skin exfoliation, and hepatocellular necrosis. *Chronic* toxicity may occur with habitual daily intake of >10,000 μg: alopecia, ataxia, bone and muscle pain, dermatitis, cheilitis, conjunctivitis, pseudotumor cerebri, hepatocellular necrosis, hyperlipidemia, and hyperostosis are common. Single, large doses of vitamin A (30,000 μg) or habitual intake of >4500 μg/day in early pregnancy can be teratogenic. Excessive intake of carotenoids causes a benign condition characterized by yellowish discoloration of the skin. Habitually large doses of canthaxanthin, a carotenoid, have the additional capability of inducing a retinopathy. [3000 μg]	Retinol concentration in the plasma and vitamin A concentrations in the milk and tears are reasonably accurate measures of adequate status. Toxicity is best assessed by elevated levels of retinyl esters in plasma. A quantitative measure of dark adaptation for night vision and electroretinography are useful functional tests.
Vitamin D	A group of sterol compounds whose parent structure is cholecalciferol (vitamin D_3). Cholecalciferol is formed in the skin from 7-dehydrocholesterol (provitamin D_3) by exposure to UVB radiation. A plant sterol, ergocalciferol (provitamin D_2), can be similarly converted into vitamin D_2 and has similar vitamin D activity. The vitamin undergoes sequential hydroxylations in the liver and kidney at the 25 and 1 positions, respectively, producing the most bioactive form of the vitamin, 1,25-dihydroxy vitamin D. Vitamin D maintains intracellular and extracellular concentrations of calcium and phosphate by enhancing intestinal absorption of the two ions and, in conjunction with PTH, promoting their mobilization from bone mineral. It retards proliferation and promotes differentiation in certain epithelia. Purported actions of vitamin D as an anti-diabetes, antiinflammatory, and cancer preventive agent remain controversial and are under investigation. 1 μg = 40 IU.	Deficiency results in decreased mineralization of newly formed bone called *rickets* in childhood and *osteomalacia* in adults. Expansion of the epiphyseal growth plates and replacement of normal bone with unmineralized bone matrix are the cardinal features of rickets; the latter feature also characterizes osteomalacia. Deformity of bone and pathologic fractures occur. Decreased serum concentrations of calcium and phosphate may occur. [15 μg, ages 19-70 yr; 20 μg, age >70 yr]	Excess amounts result in abnormally high concentrations of calcium and phosphate in the serum; metastatic calcifications, renal damage, and altered mentation may occur. [100 μg for ages ≥9 yr]	The serum concentration of the major circulating metabolite, 25-hydroxyvitamin D, is the best indicator of systemic status except in advanced kidney disease (stages 4 and 5), in which the impairment of renal 1-hydroxylation results in disassociation of the mono- and dihydroxyvitamin concentrations. Measurement of the serum concentration of 1,25-dihydroxyvitamin D is then necessary.

Continued on following page

	Biochemistry and Physiology	Deficiency [RDA*]	Toxicity [TUL†]	Assessment of Status
Vitamin E	A group of at least 8 naturally occurring compounds, some of which are tocopherols and some of which are tocotrienols. At present, the only dietary form that is thought to be biologically active in humans is α-tocopherol. Vitamin E acts as an antioxidant and free radical scavenger in lipophilic environments, most notably in cell membranes. It acts in conjunction with other antioxidants, such as selenium.	Deficiency due to dietary inadequacy is rare. It is usually seen in premature infants, individuals with fat malabsorption, and individuals with abetalipoproteinemia. Red blood cell fragility occurs and can produce a hemolytic anemia. Neuronal degeneration produces peripheral neuropathies, ophthalmoplegia, and destruction of posterior columns of spinal cord. Neurologic disease is frequently irreversible if deficiency is not corrected early enough. May contribute to the hemolytic anemia and retrolental fibroplasia seen in premature infants. Reported to suppress cell-mediated immunity. [15 mg]	Depressed levels of vitamin K–dependent procoagulants and potentiation of oral anticoagulants have been reported, as has impaired WBC function. Doses of 800 mg/day have been reported to increase slightly the incidence of hemorrhagic stroke. [1000 mg]	Plasma or serum concentration of α-tocopherol is most commonly used. Additional accuracy is obtained by expressing this value per milligram of total plasma lipid. RBC peroxide hemolysis test is not entirely specific but is a useful functional measure of the antioxidant potential of cell membranes.
Vitamin K	A family of naphthoquinone compounds with similar biologic activity. Phylloquinone (vitamin K_1) is derived from plants; a variety of menaquinones (vitamin K_2) are derived from bacterial and animal sources. Vitamin K serves as an essential cofactor in the post-translational γ-carboxylation of glutamic acid residues in many proteins. These proteins include several circulating procoagulants and anticoagulants as well as proteins in a variety of tissues.	Deficiency syndrome is uncommon except in breast-fed newborns, in whom it may cause "hemorrhagic disease of the newborn"; in adults with fat malabsorption or who are taking drugs that interfere with vitamin K metabolism (e.g., coumarin, phenytoin, broad-spectrum antibiotics); and in individuals taking large doses of vitamin E and anticoagulant drugs. Excessive hemorrhage is the usual manifestation. [F: 90 µg; M: 120 µg]	Rapid intravenous infusion of K_1 has been rarely associated with dyspnea, flushing, and cardiovascular collapse; this is likely related to the dispersing agents in the solution. Supplementation may interfere with coumarin-based anticoagulation. Pregnant women taking large amounts of the provitamin menadione may deliver infants with hemolytic anemia, hyperbilirubinemia, and kernicterus. [no TUL established]	Prothrombin time is typically used as a measure of functional K status; it is neither sensitive nor specific for vitamin K deficiency. Determination of fasting plasma vitamin K is an accurate indicator of status. Undercarboxylated plasma prothrombin is also an accurate metric, but only for detecting the deficient state, and is less widely available than plasma vitamin K.
Water-Soluble Vitamins				
Thiamin (vitamin B_1)	A water-soluble compound containing substituted pyrimidine and thiazole rings and a hydroxyethyl side chain. The coenzyme form is thiamin pyrophosphate (TPP). Thiamin serves as a coenzyme in many α-ketoacid decarboxylation and transketolation reactions. Inadequate thiamin availability leads to impairments of these reactions, resulting in inadequate adenosine triphosphate synthesis and abnormal carbohydrate metabolism, respectively. It may have an additional role in neuronal conduction independent of the aforementioned actions.	Classic deficiency syndrome (beriberi) is described in Asian populations consuming a polished rice diet. Alcoholism, chronic renal dialysis, and persistent nausea and vomiting after bariatric surgery are also common precipitants. High carbohydrate intake increases need for B_1. *Mild deficiency*: irritability, fatigue, and headaches *More severe deficiency*: combinations of peripheral neuropathy, cardiovascular dysfunction, and cerebral dysfunction. Cardiovascular involvement (wet beriberi): congestive heart failure and low peripheral vascular resistance. Cerebral disease: nystagmus, ophthalmoplegia, and ataxia (Wernicke's encephalopathy); hallucinations, impaired short-term memory, and confabulation (Korsakoff's psychosis) Deficiency syndrome responds within 24 hr to parenteral thiamin but is partially or wholly irreversible after a certain stage. [F: 1.1 mg; M: 1.2 mg]	Excess intake is largely excreted in the urine, although parenteral doses of >400 mg/day are reported to cause lethargy, ataxia, and reduced tone of the gastrointestinal tract. [TUL not established]	The most effective measure of B_1 status is the erythrocyte transketolase activity coefficient, which measures enzyme activity before and after addition of exogenous TPP; RBCs from a deficient individual express a substantial increase in enzyme activity with addition of TPP. Thiamin concentrations in blood or urine are also used.
Riboflavin (vitamin B_2)	Consists of a substituted isoalloxazine ring with a ribitol side chain. Riboflavin serves as a coenzyme for a diverse array of biochemical reactions. The primary coenzymatic forms are flavin mononucleotide and flavin adenine dinucleotide. Riboflavin holoenzymes participate in oxidation-reduction reactions in myriad metabolic pathways.	Deficiency is usually seen in conjunction with deficiencies of other B vitamins. Isolated deficiency of riboflavin produces hyperemia and edema of nasopharyngeal mucosa, cheilosis, angular stomatitis, glossitis, seborrheic dermatitis, and a normochromic, normocytic anemia. [F: 1.1; M: 1.3]	Toxicity is not reported in humans. [TUL not established]	The most common method of assessment is to determine the activity coefficient of glutathione reductase in RBCs (the test is invalid for individuals with glucose-6-phosphate dehydrogenase deficiency). Measurements of blood and urine concentrations are less desirable methods.

	Biochemistry and Physiology	Deficiency [RDA*]	Toxicity [TUL†]	Assessment of Status
Niacin (vitamin B_3)	Refers to nicotinic acid and the corresponding amide, nicotinamide The active coenzymatic forms are composed of nicotinamide affixed to adenine dinucleotide, forming NAD or NADP. More than 200 apoenzymes use these compounds as electron acceptors or hydrogen donors, either as a coenzyme or as a co-substrate. The essential amino acid tryptophan is a precursor of niacin; 60 mg of dietary tryptophan yields approximately 1 mg of niacin. Dietary requirements thus depend partly on tryptophan intake. Requirement is often determined on basis of calorie intake (i.e., niacin equivalents/1000 kcal). Large doses of nicotinic acid (1.5-3 g/day) effectively lower low-density lipoprotein cholesterol and elevate high-density lipoprotein cholesterol.	*Pellagra* is the classic deficiency syndrome and is often seen in populations in which corn is the major source of energy; it is still endemic in parts of China, Africa, and India. Diarrhea, dementia (or associated symptoms of anxiety or insomnia), and a pigmented dermatitis that develops in sun-exposed areas are typical features. Glossitis, stomatitis, vaginitis, vertigo, and burning dysesthesias are early signs. It is reported occasionally to occur in carcinoid syndrome because tryptophan is diverted to other synthetic pathways. [F: 14 mg; M: 16 mg]	Human toxicity is known largely through studies examining hypolipidemic effects. Includes vasomotor phenomenon (flushing), hyperglycemia, parenchymal liver damage, and hyperuricemia. [35 mg]	Assessment of status is problematic; blood levels of the vitamin are not reliable. Measurement of urinary excretion of the niacin metabolites *N*-methylnicotinamide and 2-pyridone is thought to be the most effective means of assessment at present.
Vitamin B_6	Refers to several derivatives of pyridine, including pyridoxine, pyridoxal, and pyridoxamine, which are interconvertible in the body. The coenzymatic forms are pyridoxal-5-phosphate (PLP) and pyridoxamine-5-phosphate. As a coenzyme, B_6 is involved in many transamination reactions (and thereby in gluconeogenesis), in the synthesis of niacin from tryptophan, in the synthesis of several neurotransmitters, and in the synthesis of δ-aminolevulinic acid (and therefore in heme synthesis). It also has functions unrelated to coenzymatic activity: pyridoxal and PLP bind to hemoglobin and alter oxygen affinity; PLP also binds to steroid receptors, inhibiting receptor affinity to DNA and thereby modulating steroid activity.	Deficiency is usually seen in conjunction with other water-soluble vitamin deficiencies. Stomatitis, angular cheilosis, glossitis, irritability, depression, and confusion occur in moderate to severe depletion; normochromic, normocytic anemia has been reported in severe deficiency. Abnormalities on electroencephalography and, in infants, convulsions have also been observed. Some sideroblastic anemias respond to B_6 administration. Isoniazid, cycloserine, penicillamine, ethanol, and theophylline can inhibit B_6 metabolism. [Ages 19-50 yr: 1.3 mg; >50 yr: 1.5 mg for women, 1.7 mg for men]	Long-term use with doses exceeding 200 mg/day (in adults) may cause peripheral neuropathies and photosensitivity. [100 mg]	Many useful laboratory methods of assessment exist. The plasma or erythrocyte PLP levels are most common. Urinary excretion of xanthurenic acid after an oral tryptophan load and activity indices of RBC alanine or aspartate transaminase are functional measures of B_6-dependent enzyme activity.
Folate	A group of related pterin compounds More than 35 forms of the vitamin are found naturally. The fully oxidized form, folic acid, is not found in nature but is the pharmacologic form of the vitamin. All folate functions relate to its ability to transfer one-carbon groups. It is essential in the de novo synthesis of nucleotides and in the metabolism of several amino acids; it is an integral component for the regeneration of the "universal" methyl donor, *S*-adenosylmethionine. Inhibition of bacterial and cancer cell folate metabolism is the basis for the sulfonamide antibiotics and chemotherapeutic agents, such as methotrexate and 5-fluorouracil, respectively.	Women of childbearing age are most likely to be deficient. *Classic deficiency syndrome*: megaloblastic anemia, diarrhea. The hematopoietic cells in bone marrow become enlarged and have immature nuclei, reflecting ineffective DNA synthesis. The peripheral blood smear demonstrates macro-ovalocytes and polymorphonuclear leukocytes with an average of more than 3.5 nuclear lobes. Megaloblastic changes also occur in other epithelia that proliferate rapidly (e.g., oral mucosa and gastrointestinal tract, producing glossitis and diarrhea, respectively). Sulfasalazine and diphenytoin inhibit absorption and predispose to deficiency. [400 µg of dietary folate equivalents (DFE); 1 DFE = 1 µg food folate = 0.6 µg folic acid]	Doses >1000 µg/day may partially correct the anemia of B_{12} deficiency and may therefore mask (and perhaps exacerbate) the associated neuropathy. Large doses are also reported to lower seizure threshold in individuals prone to seizures. Parenteral administration is rarely reported to cause allergic phenomena, which is probably due to dispersion agents. [1000 µg]	Serum folate measures short-term folate balance, whereas RBC folate is a better reflection of tissue status. Serum homocysteine rises early in deficiency but is nonspecific because B_{12} or B_6 deficiency, renal insufficiency, and older age may also cause elevations.

Continued on following page

	Biochemistry and Physiology	Deficiency [RDA*]	Toxicity [TUL†]	Assessment of Status
Vitamin C (ascorbic and dehydroascorbic acid)	Ascorbic acid readily oxidizes to dehydroascorbic acid in aqueous solution. Dehydroascorbic acid can be reduced in vivo, so it possesses vitamin C activity. Total vitamin C is therefore the sum of ascorbic and dehydroascorbic acid content. Vitamin C serves primarily as a biologic antioxidant in aqueous environments. Biosyntheses of collagen, carnitine, bile acids, and norepinephrine as well as proper functioning of the hepatic mixed-function oxygenase system depend on this property. Vitamin C in foodstuffs increases the intestinal absorption of nonheme iron.	Overt deficiency is uncommon in developed countries. The classic deficiency syndrome is *scurvy:* fatigue, depression, and widespread abnormalities in connective tissues, such as inflamed gingivae, petechiae, perifollicular hemorrhages, impaired wound healing, coiled hairs, hyperkeratosis, and bleeding into body cavities. In infants, defects in ossification and bone growth may occur. Tobacco smoking lowers plasma and leukocyte vitamin C levels. [F: 75 mg; M: 90 mg; increase requirement for cigarette smokers by 35 mg/day]	≥500 mg/day (in adults) may cause nausea and diarrhea. >1 g/day modestly increases risk for oxalate kidney stones. Supplementation may interfere with laboratory tests based on redox potential (e.g., fecal occult blood testing, serum cholesterol, and glucose). Withdrawal from chronic ingestion of high doses of vitamin C supplements should be done gradually because accommodation appears to occur, raising a concern of "rebound scurvy." [2 g]	Plasma ascorbic acid concentration reflects recent dietary intake, whereas WBC levels more closely reflect tissue stores. Women's plasma levels are approximately 20% higher than men's for any given dietary intake.
Vitamin B_{12}	A group of closely related cobalamin compounds composed of a corrin ring (with a cobalt atom in its center) connected to a ribonucleotide through an aminopropanol bridge. Microorganisms are the ultimate source of all naturally occurring B_{12}. The two active coenzyme forms are deoxyadenosylcobalamin and methylcobalamin. These coenzymes are needed for the synthesis of succinyl CoA, which is essential in lipid and carbohydrate metabolism, and for the synthesis of methionine. The synthesis of methionine is essential for amino acid metabolism, for purine and pyrimidine synthesis, for many methylation reactions, and for the intracellular retention of folates.	Dietary inadequacy is a rare cause of deficiency except in strict vegetarians. Most deficiencies arise from loss of intestinal absorption, which may occur with pernicious anemia, pancreatic insufficiency, atrophic gastritis, small bowel bacterial overgrowth, or ileal disease. Megaloblastic anemia and megaloblastic changes in other epithelia (see Folate) are the result of sustained depletion. Demyelination of peripheral nerves, posterior and lateral columns of spinal cord, and nerves within the brain may occur. Altered mentation, depression, and psychoses occur. Hematologic and neurologic complications may occur independently. Folate supplementation, in doses of 1000 µg/day, may partly correct the anemia, thereby masking (or perhaps exacerbating) the neuropathic complication. [2.4 µg]	A few allergic reactions have been reported to crystalline B_{12} preparations and are probably due to impurities, not the vitamin. [TUL not established]	Serum or plasma concentrations are generally accurate. Subtle deficiency with neurologic complications, as described in the Deficiency column, can best be established by concurrently measuring the concentration of plasma B_{12} and serum methylmalonic acid, which is a sensitive indicator of cellular deficiency.
Biotin	A bi-cyclic compound consisting of a ureido ring fused to a substituted tetrahydrothiophene ring. Endogenous synthesis by intestinal flora may contribute significantly to biotin nutriture. Most dietary biotin is linked to lysine, a compound called biotinyl lysine, or biocytin. The lysine must be hydrolyzed by an intestinal enzyme called biotinidase before intestinal absorption occurs. Biotin acts primarily as a coenzyme for several carboxylases; each holoenzyme catalyzes an adenosine triphosphate–dependent carbon dioxide transfer. The carboxylases are critical enzymes in carbohydrate and lipid metabolism.	Isolated deficiency is rare. Deficiency in humans has been produced by prolonged total parenteral nutrition lacking the vitamin and by ingestion of large quantities of raw egg white, which contains avidin, a protein that binds biotin with such high affinity that it renders it bioun-available. Alterations in mental status, myalgias, hyperesthesias, and anorexia occur. Later, a seborrheic dermatitis and alopecia develop. Deficiency is usually accompanied by lactic acidosis and organic aciduria. [30 µg]	Toxicity has not been reported in humans with doses as high as 60 mg/day in children. [TUL not established]	Plasma and urine concentrations of biotin are diminished in the deficient state. Elevated urine concentrations of methyl citrate, 3-methylcrotonylglycine, and 3-hydroxyisovalerate are also observed in deficiency.

	Biochemistry and Physiology	Deficiency [RDA*]	Toxicity [TUL†]	Assessment of Status
Pantothenic acid	Consists of pantoic acid linked to β-alanine through an amide bond Pantothenic acid is an essential component of CoA and phosphopantetheine, which are essential for synthesis and β-oxidation of fatty acids as well as for synthesis of cholesterol, steroid hormones, vitamins A and D, and other isoprenoid derivatives. CoA is also involved in the synthesis of several amino acids and δ-aminolevulinic acid, a precursor for the corrin ring of vitamin B_{12}, the porphyrin ring of heme, and of cytochromes. CoA is also necessary for the acetylation and fatty acid acylation of a variety of proteins.	Deficiency is rare; it has been reported only as a result of feeding of semisynthetic diets or an antagonist to the vitamin. Experimental, isolated deficiency in humans produces fatigue, abdominal pain, vomiting, insomnia, and paresthesias of the extremities. [5 mg]	In doses of 10 g/day, diarrhea is reported to occur. [TUL not established]	Whole blood and urine concentrations of pantothenate are indicators of status; serum levels are not thought to be accurate.

CoA, coenzyme A; *NAD,* nicotinamide adenine dinucleotide; *NADP,* nicotinamide adenine dinucleotide phosphate; *PTH,* parathyroid hormone; *RBC,* red blood cell; *UVB,* ultraviolet B; *WBC,* white blood cell.

*Recommended daily allowance (RDA) established for female (F) and male (M) adults by the U.S. Food and Nutrition Board, 1999-2001. In some instances, insufficient data exist to establish an RDA, in which case the adequate intake (AI) established by the board is listed.

†Tolerable upper limit (TUL) established for adults by the U.S. Food and Nutrition Board, 1999-2001.

From Goldman L, Schafer AI: *Goldman-Cecil medicine,* ed 25, Philadelphia, 2016, Elsevier.

Nutritional Trace Elements and Their Clinical Implications

	Biochemistry and Physiology	Deficiency [RDA*]	Toxicity [TUL†]	Assessment of Status
Chromium	Dietary chromium consists of both inorganic and organic forms. Its primary function in humans is to potentiate insulin action. It accomplishes this function as a circulating complex called *glucose tolerance factor*, thereby affecting carbohydrate, fat, and protein metabolism.	Deficiency in humans has been described only in long-term total parenteral nutrition (TPN) patients receiving insufficient chromium. Hyperglycemia or impaired glucose tolerance occurs. Elevated plasma free fatty acid concentrations, neuropathy, encephalopathy, and abnormalities in nitrogen metabolism are also reported. Whether supplemental chromium may improve glucose tolerance in glucose-intolerant individuals remains controversial. [F: 25 μg; M: 35 μg]	Toxicity after oral ingestion is uncommon and seems confined to gastric irritation. Airborne exposure may cause contact dermatitis, eczema, skin ulcers, and bronchogenic carcinoma. [TUL not established]	Plasma or serum concentration of chromium is a crude indicator of chromium status; it appears to be meaningful when the value is markedly above or below the normal range.
Copper	Copper is absorbed by a specific intestinal transport mechanism. It is carried to the liver, where it is bound to ceruloplasmin, which circulates systemically and delivers copper to target tissues in the body. Excretion of copper is largely through bile and then into the feces. Absorptive and excretory processes vary with the levels of dietary copper, providing a means of copper homeostasis. Copper serves as a component of many enzymes, including amine oxidases, ferroxidases, cytochrome *c* oxidase, dopamine β-hydroxylase, superoxide dismutase, and tyrosinase.	Dietary deficiency is rare; it has been observed in premature and low-birthweight infants fed exclusively a cow's milk diet and in individuals on long-term TPN lacking copper. It has also been described after gastric bypass surgery and with chronic zinc supplementation. Clinical manifestations include depigmentation of skin and hair, myelopathy and other neurologic lesions, leukopenia, anemia, and skeletal abnormalities. Anemia arises from impaired utilization of iron and therefore often is manifested as a sideroblastic anemia. The peripheral smear and bone marrow may mimic myelodysplasia. A deficiency syndrome is also observed in Menkes' disease, a rare inherited condition associated with impaired copper utilization. [900 μg]	Acute copper toxicity has been described after excessive oral intake and with absorption of copper salts applied to burned skin. Milder manifestations include nausea, vomiting, epigastric pain, and diarrhea; coma and hepatic necrosis may ensue in severe cases. Toxicity may be seen with doses as low as 70 μg/kg/day. Chronic toxicity is also described. Wilson's disease is a rare, inherited disease associated with abnormally low ceruloplasmin levels and accumulation of copper in the liver and brain, eventually leading to damage to these two organs. [10 mg]	Practical methods to detect marginal deficiency are not available. Marked deficiency is reliably detected by diminished serum copper and ceruloplasmin concentrations as well as by low red blood cell superoxide dismutase activity.
Fluorine	Known more commonly by its ionic form, fluoride. Fluorine is incorporated into the crystalline structure of bone, thereby altering its physical characteristics.	Intake of <0.1 mg/day in infants and <0.5 mg/day in children is associated with an increased incidence of dental caries. Optimal intake in adults is between 1.5 and 4 mg/day. [F: 3 mg; M: 4 mg]	Acute ingestion of >30 mg/kg body weight is likely to cause death. Excessive chronic intake (0.1 mg/kg/day) leads to mottling of teeth (dental fluorosis), calcification of tendons and ligaments, and exostoses and may increase the brittleness of bones. [10 mg]	Estimates of intake and clinical assessment are used because no good laboratory test exists.

	Biochemistry and Physiology	Deficiency [RDA*]	Toxicity [TUL†]	Assessment of Status
Iodine	Iodine is readily absorbed from the diet, concentrated in the thyroid, and integrated into the thyroid hormones thyroxine and triiodothyronine. These hormones circulate largely bound to thyroxine-binding globulin. They modulate resting energy expenditure and, in the developing human, growth and development.	In the absence of supplementation, populations relying primarily on food from soils with low iodine content have endemic iodine deficiency. Maternal iodine deficiency leads to fetal deficiency, which produces spontaneous abortions, stillbirths, hypothyroidism, cretinism, and dwarfism. Permanent cognitive deficits may result from iodine deficiency during the first 2 years of life. In the adult, compensatory hypertrophy of the thyroid (goiter) occurs along with varying degrees of hypothyroidism. [150 μg]	Large doses (>2 mg/day in adults) may induce hypothyroidism by blocking thyroid hormone synthesis. Supplementation with >100 mg/day to an individual who was formerly deficient occasionally induces hyperthyroidism. [1.1 mg]	Iodine status of a population can be estimated by the prevalence of goiter. Urinary excretion of iodine is an effective laboratory means of assessment. Thyroid-stimulating hormone blood level is an indirect and therefore not entirely specific means of assessment.
Iron	Conveys the capacity to participate in redox reactions to a number of metalloproteins, such as hemoglobin, myoglobin, cytochrome enzymes, and many oxidases and oxygenases. The primary storage form of iron is ferritin and, to a lesser degree, hemosiderin. Intestinal absorption is 15-20% for "heme" iron and 1-8% for iron contained in vegetables. Absorption of the latter form is enhanced by the ascorbic acid in foodstuffs; by poultry, fish, or beef; and by an iron-deficient state. It is decreased by phytate and tannins.	Iron deficiency is the most common micronutrient deficiency in the world. Women of childbearing age are the group at highest risk because of menstrual blood losses, pregnancy, and lactation. The classic deficiency syndrome is hypochromic, microcytic anemia. Glossitis and koilonychia ("spoon" nails) are also observed. Easy fatigability often is an early symptom, before anemia appears. In children, mild deficiency of insufficient severity to cause anemia is associated with behavioral disturbances and poor school performance. [postmenopausal F and M: 8 mg; premenopausal F: 18 mg]	Iron overload typically occurs when habitual dietary intake is extremely high, intestinal absorption is excessive, repeated parenteral administration occurs, or a combination of these factors exists. Excessive iron stores usually accumulate in the reticuloendothelial tissues and cause little damage (hemosiderosis). If overload continues, iron eventually begins to accumulate in tissues such as the hepatic parenchyma, pancreas, heart, and synovium, causing hemochromatosis Hereditary hemochromatosis results from homozygosity of a common recessive trait. Excessive intestinal absorption of iron is seen in homozygotes. [45 mg]	Negative iron balance initially leads to depletion of iron stores in the bone marrow; a bone marrow biopsy and the concentration of serum ferritin are accurate indicators of early depletion. As the severity of deficiency proceeds, serum iron (SI) decreases and total iron-binding capacity (TIBC) increases; an iron saturation (SI/TIBC) of <16% suggests iron deficiency. Microcytosis, hypochromia, and anemia ensue. Elevated levels of serum ferritin or an iron saturation of >60% suggests iron overload, although systemic inflammation elevates serum ferritin regardless of iron status.
Manganese	A component of several metalloenzymes. Most manganese is in mitochondria, where it is a component of manganese superoxide dismutase.	Manganese deficiency in the human has not been conclusively demonstrated. It is said to cause hypocholesterolemia, weight loss, hair and nail changes, dermatitis, and impaired synthesis of vitamin K–dependent proteins. [F: 1.8 mg; M: 2.3 mg]	Toxicity by oral ingestion is unknown in humans. Toxic inhalation causes hallucinations, other alterations in mentation, and extrapyramidal movement disorders. [11 mg]	Until the deficiency syndrome is better defined, an appropriate measure of status will be difficult to develop.
Molybdenum	A cofactor in several enzymes, most prominently xanthine oxidase and sulfite oxidase	A probable case of human deficiency is described as being secondary to parenteral administration of sulfite and resulted in hyperoxypurinemia, hypouricemia, and low sulfate excretion. [45 μg]	Toxicity not well described in humans, although it may interfere with copper metabolism at high doses. [2 mg]	Laboratory means of assessment are not meaningful until the deficiency syndrome is better described.

Continued on following page

	Biochemistry and Physiology	Deficiency [RDA*]	Toxicity [TUL†]	Assessment of Status
Selenium	Most dietary selenium is in the form of an amino acid complex. Nearly complete absorption of such forms occurs. Homeostasis is largely performed by the kidney, which regulates urinary excretion as a function of selenium status. Selenium is a component of several enzymes, most notably glutathione peroxidase and superoxide dismutase. These enzymes protect against oxidative and free radical damage of various cell structures. The antioxidant protection conveyed by selenium apparently operates in conjunction with vitamin E because deficiency of one seems to potentiate damage induced by a deficiency of the other. Selenium also participates in the enzymatic conversion of thyroxine to its more active metabolite, triiodothyronine.	Deficiency is rare in North America but has been observed in individuals on long-term TPN lacking selenium. Such individuals have myalgias or cardiomyopathies. Populations in some regions of the world, most notably some parts of China, have marginal intake of selenium. In these regions *Keshan's disease*, a condition characterized by cardiomyopathy, is endemic; it can be prevented (but not treated) by selenium supplementation. [55 μg]	Toxicity is associated with nausea, diarrhea, alterations in mental status, peripheral neuropathy, and loss of hair and nails; such symptoms were observed in adults who inadvertently consumed 27-2400 mg. [400 μg]	Erythrocyte glutathione peroxidase activity and plasma or whole blood selenium concentrations are the most commonly used methods of assessment. They are moderately accurate indicators of status.
Zinc	Intestinal absorption occurs by a specific process that is enhanced by pregnancy and corticosteroids and diminished by coingestion of phytates, phosphates, iron, copper, lead, or calcium. Diminished intake of zinc leads to an increased efficiency of absorption and decreased fecal excretion, providing a means of zinc homeostasis. Zinc is a component of more than 100 enzymes, among which are DNA polymerase, RNA polymerase, and transfer RNA synthetase.	Zinc deficiency has its most profound effect on rapidly proliferating tissues. *Mild deficiency:* growth retardation in children. *More severe deficiency:* growth arrest, teratogenicity, hypogonadism and infertility, dysgeusia, poor wound healing, diarrhea, dermatitis on the extremities and around orifices, glossitis, alopecia, corneal clouding, loss of dark adaptation, and behavioral changes. Impaired cellular immunity is observed. Excessive loss of gastrointestinal secretions through chronic diarrhea and fistulas may precipitate deficiency. *Acrodermatitis enteropathica* is a rare, recessively inherited disease in which intestinal absorption of zinc is impaired. [F: 8 mg; M: 11 mg]	Acute zinc toxicity can usually be induced by ingestion of >200 mg of zinc in a single day (in adults). It is manifested by epigastric pain, nausea, vomiting, and diarrhea. Hyperpnea, diaphoresis, and weakness may follow inhalation of zinc fumes. Copper and zinc compete for intestinal absorption: long-term ingestion of >25 mg/day of zinc may lead to copper deficiency. Long-term ingestion of >150 mg/day has been reported to cause gastric erosions, low high-density lipoprotein cholesterol levels, and impaired cellular immunity. [40 mg]	No accurate indicators of zinc status exist for routine clinical use. Plasma, red blood cell, and hair zinc concentrations are often misleading. Acute illness, in particular, is known to diminish plasma zinc levels, in part by inducing a shift of zinc out of the plasma compartment and into the liver. Functional tests that determine dark adaptation, taste acuity, and rate of wound healing lack specificity.

*Recommended daily allowance (RDA) established for female (F) and male (M) adults by the U.S. Food and Nutrition Board, 1999–2001. In some instances, insufficient data exist to establish an RDA, in which case the adequate intake (AI) established by the board is listed.

†Tolerable upper limit (TUL) established for adults by the U.S. Food and Nutrition Board, 1999–2001.

From Goldman L, Schafer AI: *Goldman-Cecil medicine,* ed 25, Philadelphia, 2016, Elsevier.

Summary of Vitamin and Mineral Deficiencies

Vitamin and Mineral Deficiencies	Neurologic Syndrome or Syndromes	Supporting Tests	Treatment	Causes (Other Than Malnutrition)
A (retinol)	Blindness from retinal or corneal damage	Visual fields, visual acuity Serum level <30-65 μg/dl	30,000 IU vitamin A daily × 1 wk	Hypothyroidism, diabetes, renal or liver failure
B_1 (thiamine)	Wernicke's encephalopathy: ataxia, nystagmus, ophthalmoparesis, confusion, delirium Korsakoff's syndrome: amnesia, confabulation Beriberi: axonal neuropathy	MRI: symmetric lesions of midbrain (periaqueductal area), pons, hypothalamus, thalamus, cerebellum MRI: necrosis of mammillary bodies, dorsomedial and anterior thalamus Nerve conduction tests: decreased amplitude Serum thiamine level <20 ng/dl Erythrocyte transketolase	Prevent by 100 mg PO daily before and 1 year after bariatric surgery, 100 mg IV before glucose administration or refeeding Treat Wernicke's encephalopathy with 5 days of thiamine, 100-500 mg IV or IM daily, then PO 100 mg daily Antioxidants (*N*-acetylcysteine)	Alcoholism, bariatric or other major GI surgery, prolonged vomiting, hemodialysis, diuretic treatment of heart failure, cachexia, 5-fluorouracil, other blockers of thiamine phosphate production
B_3 (niacin)	Pellagra: confusion, dementia, weakness, ataxia, spasticity, myoclonus, glossitis, dermatitis, photosensitivity	Erythrocyte NAD, plasma niacin, urinary N_1-methylnicotinamide	Nicotinic acid, 50 mg PO tid or 25 mg IV tid; nicotinamide, 50-100 mg IM or PO tid	Alcoholism, corn- or cereal-based diet, Hartnup's syndrome, carcinoid syndrome
B_5 (pantothenic acid)	Dysesthesias, foot paresthesias	Deficient coenzyme A	5 mg PO daily	Severe malnutrition
B_6 (pyridoxine)	Neuropathy, sensory ataxia, depression Infantile pyridoxine-deficient epilepsy	Plasma PLP <27 nmol/L; urinary 4-pyridoxic acid, <3 nmol ↑ Homocysteine after methionine loading challenge ↑ α-AASA in urine, plasma, CSF	50-100 mg PO daily for neuropathy (preventive use if taking B_6 antagonist) 100-200 mg daily for adult epilepsy	Diverticulosis, isoniazid, cycloserine, other antagonists Genetic defects in antiquitin (aldehyde dehydrogenase), pyridoxal synthesis
B_{12} (cobalamin)	Myelopathy with spastic paraparesis and sensory ataxia, peripheral neuropathy, optic neuropathy, memory loss, dementia; indirect contributor to stroke	Blood level <200 pg/ml ↑ Methylmalonic acid >145 nmol/L Intrinsic factor antibodies Schilling test, megaloblastic anemia Delayed somatosensory evoked potentials ↑ Homocysteine, total >12.5 μmol/L	IM B_{12}, 1000 μg daily for 1 week, then weekly for 1 month, then monthly or oral B_{12}, 1000 μg daily, or nasal B_{12}, 500 μg weekly for lifetime if abnormal absorption, 50-100 μg daily if normal absorption	Achlorhydria, gastric or ileal resection, blind loop syndrome, sprue, HIV infection, nitrous oxide anesthesia (especially abuse), fish tapeworm, vegan diet
D (calciferol)	Proximal myopathy, often painful; cognitive impairment Secondary compression of spinal cord, plexus, or peripheral nerves from rickets or osteomalacia	25-(OH) vitamin D_3 level <10 ng/ml in urine Serum calcium ↑ PTH >54 pg/ml Osteopenia/porosis on bone densitometry	Daily supplementation with 400 IU, >50,000 IU 3 times per wk if malabsorption; use blood level or urine calcium excretion to guide (should be >100 mg/day)	Lack of exposure to sunlight, including sunblock protection; chronic antiepileptic drug use

Continued on following page

Summary of Vitamin and Mineral Deficiencies

Vitamin and Mineral Deficiencies	Neurologic Syndrome or Syndromes	Supporting Tests	Treatment	Causes (Other Than Malnutrition)
E (tocopherol)	Spinal and cerebellar ataxia, Babinski's sign, ophthalmoplegia, peripheral neuropathy, retinitis pigmentosa	Vitamin E level <2.5 mg/L (normal, 6-15 with normal lipid level) ↑ A-β-lipoprotein levels, antigliadin antibodies Genetic analysis to rule out other spinocerebellar ataxias such as Friedreich's ataxia	Supplement with 6-800 IU, 5-10 mg/kg twice daily, for ataxia of genetic causes, water-soluble 200 mg/kg/day or IM α-tocopherol for malabsorption	Biliary atresia, celiac sprue, Genetic: ↓ α-tocopherol transport protein (8q13), microsomal triglyceride transfer protein
Folate	Dementia, B_{12} deficiency, stroke	↑ Homocysteine, plasma level <2.5 μg/L	1 mg 3 times per day until normal level, then maintenance of 1 mg/day Pregnancy: additional 0.4 mg/day if taking a folate antagonist	Malabsorption or use of antagonist (methotrexate) or antiepileptic medication
K (phytonadione)	Intracranial hemorrhage	INR or PT elevation	IM phytonadione at birth, maternal vitamin K for last month of pregnancy	Medication use that increases metabolism, such as phenytoin
Copper	Myelopathy, neuropathy	Serum Cu <75 μg/dl, ↓ urinary Cu, ceruloplasmin <23 mg/dl MRI: ↑ T_2 signal in cervical cord, dorsal column Mutation in ATP7A gene (Menkes' disease)	Elemental Cu, 8 mg/day PO week 1, 6 mg/day week 2, 4 mg/day week 3, 2 mg/day ongoing malabsorption Menkes' disease: 250 mg SC bid	Wilson's disease, Menkes' disease, alcoholism, malabsorption, gastric bypass, zinc toxicity
Magnesium	Seizures, encephalopathy	Serum magnesium <1.5 mg/ dl, correct for low albumin	Magnesium sulfate IV or PO Avoid magnesium-wasting drugs	Alcoholism, especially beer
Potassium	Muscle weakness, chronic, acute	Serum potassium <3.5 mEq/L, ECG	IV or PO KCl until normalized	Diuretic use, bulimia

AASA, Aminoadipic semialdehyde; *CSF,* cerebrospinal fluid; *ECG,* electrocardiography; *GI,* gastrointestinal; *HIV,* human immunodeficiency virus; *IM,* intramuscularly; *INR,* international normalized ratio; *IU,* international units; *IV,* intravenously; *MRI,* magnetic resonance imaging; *NAD,* nicotinamide adenine dinucleotide; *PLP,* pyridoxal-5-phosphate (active coenzyme of pyridoxine); *PO,* by mouth; *PT,* prothrombin time; *PTH,* parathyroid hormone; *tid,* three times a day.

From Goldman L, Schafer AI: *Goldman's Cecil medicine,* ed 24, Philadelphia, 2012, Saunders.

Historical and Physical Findings in Poisoning

Sign	Toxin
Odor	
Bitter almonds	Cyanide
Acetone	Isopropyl alcohol, methanol, paraldehyde, salicylates
Alcohol	Ethanol
Wintergreen	Methyl salicylate
Garlic	Arsenic, thallium, organophosphates, selenium
Ocular Signs	
Miosis	Opioids (except propoxyphene, meperidine, and pentazocine), organophosphates and other cholinergics, clonidine, phenothiazines, sedative-hypnotics, olanzapine
Mydriasis	Atropine, cocaine, amphetamines, antihistamines, TCAs, carbamazepine, serotonin syndrome, PCP, LSD, postanoxic encephalopathy
Nystagmus	Phenytoin, barbiturates, sedative-hypnotics, alcohols, carbamazepine, PCP, ketamine, dextromethorphan
Lacrimation	Organophosphates, irritant gas or vapors
Retinal hyperemia	Methanol
Cutaneous Signs	
Diaphoresis	Organophosphates, salicylates, cocaine and other sympathomimetics, serotonin syndrome, withdrawal syndromes
Alopecia	Thallium, arsenic
Erythema	Boric acid, elemental mercury, cyanide, carbon monoxide, disulfiram, scombroid, anticholinergics
Cyanosis (unresponsive to oxygen)	Methemoglobinemia (e.g., benzocaine, dapsone, nitrites, phenazopyridine), amiodarone, silver
Oral Signs	
Salivation	Organophosphates, salicylates, corrosives, ketamine, PCP, strychnine
Oral burns	Corrosives, oxalate-containing plants
Gum lines	Lead, mercury, arsenic, bismuth
Gastrointestinal Signs	
Diarrhea	Antimicrobials, arsenic, iron, boric acid, cholinergics, colchicine, withdrawal
Hematemesis	Arsenic, iron, caustics, NSAIDs, salicylates
Cardiac Signs	
Tachycardia	Sympathomimetics (e.g., amphetamines, cocaine), anticholinergics, antidepressants, theophylline, caffeine, antipsychotics, atropine, salicylates, cellular asphyxiants (cyanide, carbon monoxide, hydrogen sulfide), withdrawal
Bradycardia	β-blockers, calcium channel blockers, digoxin, clonidine and other central α_2 agonists, organophosphates, opioids, sedative-hypnotics
Hypertension	Sympathomimetics (amphetamines, cocaine, LSD), anticholinergics, clonidine (early), monoamine oxidase inhibitors
Hypotension	β-blockers, calcium channel blockers, cyclic antidepressants, iron, phenothiazines, barbiturates, clonidine, theophylline, opioids, arsenic, amatoxin mushrooms, cellular asphyxiants (cyanide, carbon monoxide, hydrogen sulfide), snake envenomation
Respiratory Signs	
Depressed respirations	Opioids, sedative-hypnotics, alcohol, clonidine, barbiturates
Tachypnea	Salicylates, amphetamines, caffeine, metabolic acidosis (ethylene glycol, methanol, cyanide), carbon monoxide, hydrocarbons

Continued on following page

Historical and Physical Findings in Poisoning

Sign	Toxin
Central Nervous System Signs	
Ataxia	Alcohol, anticonvulsants, benzodiazepines, barbiturates, lithium, dextromethorphan, carbon monoxide, inhalants
Coma	Opioids, sedative-hypnotics, anticonvulsants, cyclic antidepressants, antipsychotics, ethanol, anticholinergics, clonidine, GHB, alcohols, salicylates, barbiturates
Seizures	Sympathomimetics, anticholinergics, antidepressants (especially TCAs, bupropion, venlafaxine), isoniazid, camphor, lindane, salicylates, lead, organophosphates, carbamazepine, tramadol, lithium, ginkgo seeds, water hemlock, withdrawal
Delirium/psychosis	Sympathomimetics, anticholinergics, LSD, PCP, hallucinogens, lithium, dextromethorphan, steroids, withdrawal
Peripheral neuropathy	Lead, arsenic, mercury, organophosphates

GHB, Gamma hydroxybutyrate; *LSD,* lysergic acid diethylamide; *NSAID,* nonsteroidal antiinflammatory drug; *PCP,* phencyclidine; *TCA,* tricyclic antidepressant.
From Goldman L, Schafer AI: *Goldman's Cecil medicine,* ed 24, Philadelphia, 2012, Saunders.

Recognizable Poison Syndromes ("Toxidromes")

Toxidrome	SIGNS: Vital signs	Mental status	Pupils	Skin	Bowel sounds	Other	Possible toxins
Sympathomimetic	Hypertension, tachycardia, hyperthermia	Agitation, psychosis, delirium, violence	Dilated	Diaphoretic	Normal to increased		Amphetamines, cocaine, PCP, bath salts (cathinones), ADHD medication
Anticholinergic	Hypertension, tachycardia, hyperthermia	Agitated, delirium, coma, seizure	Dilated	Dry, hot	Diminished	Ileus urinary retention	Antihistamines, tricyclic antidepressants, atropine, jimson weed
Cholinergic	Bradycardia BP and temp typically normal	Confusion, coma, fasciculations	Small	Diaphoretic	Hyperactive	Diarrhea, urination, bronchorrhea, bronchospasm, emesis, lacrimation, salivation	Organophosphates (insecticides, nerve agents), carbamates (physostigmine, neostigmine, pyridostigmine) Alzheimer medications, myasthenia treatments
Opioids	Respiratory depression bradycardia, hypotension, hypothermia	Depression, coma, euphoria	Pinpoint	Normal	Normal to decreased		Methadone, buprenorphine, morphine, oxycodone, heroin, etc.
Sedative–hypnotics	Respiratory depression, HR normal to decreased, BP normal to decreased, temp normal to decreased	Somnolence, coma	Small or normal	Normal	Normal		Barbiturates, benzodiazepines, ethanol
Serotonin syndrome (similar findings with neuroleptic malignant syndrome)	Hyperthermia, tachycardia, hypertension or hypotension (autonomic instability)	Agitation, confusion, coma	Dilated	Diaphoretic	Increased	Neuromuscular hyperexcitability: clonus, hyperreflexia (lower extremities > upper extremities)	SSRIs, lithium, MAOIs, linezolid, tramadol, meperidine, dextromethorphan
Salicylates	Tachypnea, hyperpnea, tachycardia, hyperthermia	Agitation, confusion, coma	Normal	Diaphoretic	Normal	Nausea, vomiting, tinnitus, ABG with primary respiratory alkalosis and primary metabolic acidosis; tinnitus or difficulty hearing	Aspirin and aspirin-containing products, methyl-salicylate
Withdrawal (sedative–hypnotic)	Tachycardia, tachypnea, hyperthermia	Agitation, tremor, seizure, hallucinosis, delirium tremens	Dilated	Diaphoretic	Increased		Lack of access to ethanol, benzodiazepines, barbiturates, GHB, or excessive use of flumazenil
Withdrawal (opioid)	Tachycardia	Restlessness, anxiety	Dilated	Diaphoretic	Hyperactive	Nausea, vomiting, diarrhea	Lack of access to opioids or excessive use of naloxone

ABG, Arterial blood gas; *ADHD*, attention-deficit/hyperactivity disorder; *BP*, blood pressure; *GHB*, γ-hydroxybutyrate; *HR*, heart rate; *MAOI*, monoamine oxidase inhibitor; *PCP*, phencyclidine; *SSRI*, selective serotonin reuptake inhibitor; *temp*, temperature.

From Kliegman RM et al: *Nelson textbook of pediatrics*, ed 20, Philadelphia, 2016, Elsevier.

Antidotes and Indications for Use

Antidote	Indication for Use	Dose*	Treatment End Point	Comments
Antivenom, *Crotalidae* (Fab)[†]	Crotaline snake (e.g., rattlesnakes, copperhead)	4-6 vials; repeat for persistent or worsening clinical condition; repeated doses of 2 vials at 6, 12, and 18 hr after initial antivenom dose are recommended	Halt in progression of circumferential and proximal swelling Resolving systemic effects	Better safety profile than historical equine-derived antivenom Repetitive dosing indicated for recurrent soft tissue swelling Less effective at correcting hematologic (i.e., coagulation and platelet) disorders
Antivenom, *Latrodectus* (equine)[†]	Black widow spider (*Latrodectus* sp)	1 vial diluted in 50-100 mL NS, infused during 1 hr; can repeat	Resolution of symptoms, vital signs normal	Dilution and slow infusion rate are *critical* to avoid anaphylactoid reaction Indications include severe pain unresponsive to opioids and severe hypertension Serum sickness can occur IV calcium is ineffective
Atropine	Carbamates Nerve agents Organophosphorus compounds	2 mg IV; double the dose every 5 min to achieve atropinization and hemodynamic stability; then start continuous infusion of 10-20% of total stabilizing dose per hour	Cessation of excessive oral and pulmonary secretions, >80 beats/min, systolic blood pressure >80 mm Hg	Doubling of the dose every 5 min (e.g., 2, 4, 8, and 16 mg) estimated to achieve atropinization within 30 min Stop infusion when patient develops concerning signs or symptoms of anticholinergic toxidrome (see Table 110-1); restart infusion at lower rate when signs or symptoms abate
Calcium salt[‡]	Calcium-channel antagonists	Calcium chloride 10%, 10 mL (1 g) during 10 min; can be given in 1 min if critically ill Calcium gluconate 10%, 30 mL (3 g) during 10 min; can be given in 1 min if critically ill	Reversal of hypotension; may not reverse bradycardia	*All indications:* Monitor ionized calcium levels IV extravasation causes tissue necrosis, especially with calcium chloride Can administer at faster than stated rates for immediate life-threatening conditions (i.e., in 1 min) Calcium chloride contains three times more elemental calcium than calcium gluconate does
	Hydrofluoric acid	Systemic toxicity: calcium gluconate 10%, 1-3 g (10-30 mL) per dose IV during 10-min period; repeat as needed every 5-10 min	Reversal of life-threatening manifestations of hypocalcemia and hyperkalemia	Can dilute and give intra-arterially or IV with a Bier block for extremity exposures and burns
	Hyperkalemia (except cardiac glycosides)	Calcium gluconate 10%, 1 g (10 mL) per dose IV during 10-min period; repeat as needed every 5-10 min	Reversal of myocardial depression and conduction delays	May precipitate ventricular arrhythmias
	Hypermagnesemia	Calcium gluconate 10%, 1-2 g (10-20 mL) per dose IV during 10-min period; repeat as needed every 5-10 min	Reversal of respiratory depression, hypotension, and cardiac conduction blocks	Simultaneous therapies to increase magnesium elimination should be instituted
	Hypocalcemia (e.g., ethylene glycol)	Calcium gluconate 10%, 0.5-1.0 g (5-10 mL) per dose during 10-min period; repeat as needed every 10 min	Reversal of tetany	Correct symptomatic hypocalcemia; avoid excessive administration that may increase production of calcium oxalate crystals in ethylene glycol poisoning
L-Carnitine	Valproate-induced hyperammonemia or hepatotoxicity	100 mg/kg (maximum 6 g) IV during 30 min, then 15 mg/kg IV during 30-min period q4h (maximum 6 g/day)	Treat until clinical improvement occurs	Levocarnitine is active form Adjust dose for end-stage renal disease

Antidote	Indication for Use	Dose*	Treatment End Point	Comments
Cyanide antidote kit Amyl nitrite Sodium nitrite Sodium thiosulfate [Hydroxocobalamin is preferred if available, see below]	Cyanide	Amyl nitrite: 0.3-mL pearls, crush and inhale during 30-sec period Sodium nitrite 3%: 10 mL IV during 10-min period Sodium thiosulfate 25%: 50 mL (12.5 g) IV during 10-min period	Resolution of lactic acidosis and moderate to severe clinical signs and symptoms: seizures, coma, dyspnea, apnea, hypotension, bradycardia	Coordinate amyl nitrite with continued oxygenation and give only until sodium nitrite infusion is begun; nitrites may produce hypotension and excess methemoglobinemia Sodium nitrite dose must be adjusted if patient has hemoglobin <12 g/dL Sodium thiosulfate dosing can be repeated
Deferoxamine	Iron	Initiate at 5 mg/kg/hr, titrate to 15 mg/kg/hr IV (maximum 8 g/day) Mild to moderate: administer for 6-12 hr Severe toxicity: administer 24 hr	Resolution of clinical signs and symptoms Do not use urine color, which is an unreliable marker for iron clearance Laboratory testing is unreliable while antidote is being received	Indications: symptomatic patients with lethargy, severe abdominal pain, hypovolemia, acidosis, shock; any symptomatic patient with peak serum iron level >350 g/dL Prolonged therapy can cause pulmonary toxicity
Digoxin-specific antibody fragments (Fab)	Digoxin Digitalis and related plants (e.g., oleander, lily of the valley) Other cardiac glycosides (e.g., bufadienolides [Bufo toads])	Unknown digoxin dose or serum level, or for plant or toad source: acute toxicity—10-20 vials; chronic toxicity—3-6 vials Digoxin dose known: number of vials = (mg ingested × 0.8) ÷ 0.5 Digoxin serum level known: number of vials = [serum level (ng/mL) × weight (kg)] ÷ 100 Infuse dose during 30 min	Resolution of hyperkalemia, symptomatic bradydysrhythmias, ventricular arrhythmias, Mobitz II or third-degree heart block	Each vial binds 0.5 mg of digoxin or digitoxin Monitor ECG and potassium levels Digoxin serum levels unreliable after antidote administered unless test is specific for free serum digoxin
Dimercaprol (BAL)	Arsenic Lead Mercury, elemental and inorganic salts	Arsenic: 3-5 mg/kg IM q4h Lead: 75 mg/m^2 (4 mg/kg) IM q4h for 5 days Inorganic mercury: 5 mg/kg IM, then 2.5 mg/kg IM q12h for 10 days or until patient is clinically improved	Arsenic: 24-hr urinary arsenic <50 µg/L Lead: encephalopathy resolved, blood lead level <100 µg/dL, and succimer therapy can be started Mercury, elemental and inorganic: 24-hr urinary mercury <20 µg/L	Formulated in peanut oil; painful IM injection and caution with allergy Maximum adult dose is 3 g/day BAL started 4 hr before initiation of concomitant $CaNa_2$ EDTA for lead encephalopathy Dosing not well established for arsenic and elemental or inorganic mercury toxicity; not used for organic mercury poisoning Adverse effects: painful injections, fever, diaphoresis, agitation, headache, salivation, nausea and vomiting, hemolysis in G6PD-deficient patients, chelation of essential metals Check essential metal levels if chelation is prolonged Succimer is replacing BAL for many indications except lead encephalopathy Treatment end points for arsenic and mercury include improving clinical condition
Edetate calcium disodium ($CaNa_2$ EDTA)	Lead	1500 mg/m^2/24 hr (maximum 3 g) by continuous infusion	Treat for 5 days, followed by 2-day hiatus; repeat until encephalopathy resolved, lead level <100 µg/dL, and succimer therapy can be started	Use in patients with lead encephalopathy or lead level >100 g/dL Administer BAL 4 hr before initiating $CaNa_2$ EDTA Hydrate patient and establish good urinary output before starting therapy Avoid thrombophlebitis by diluting in NS or D_5W to a concentration ≤0.5% Substitution of Na_2 EDTA can cause fatal hypocalcemia
Flumazenil	Benzodiazepines	0.1 mg/min IV to a total dose of 1 mg	Reversal of coma	Limit use to reversal of inadequate ventilation in benzodiazepine-toxic patients Acute benzodiazepine withdrawal may occur in patients dependent on benzodiazepines Increases intracranial pressure and risk for seizures in presence of underlying seizure disorder or ingestion of seizure-producing toxicants Monitor for resedation up to 2 hr after last dose

Continued on following page

Antidote	Indication for Use	Dose*	Treatment End Point	Comments
Folinic acid (tetrahydrofolic acid [leucovorin])	Methanol Methotrexate	Methanol: 50 mg IV q4h Methotrexate: 100 mg/m^2 IV during 15-30 min q3-6h; dosing lower when used as "rescue" in chemotherapy	Methanol: methanol undetectable, metabolic acidosis cleared Methotrexate: serum level $<1 \times 10^{-8}$ mol/L	Essential therapy for both toxicants Little concern with excessive dosing when used for methotrexate overdose Methotrexate: large overdoses may require increased dose Glucarpidase administered 2-4 hr before or after folinic acid
Fomepizole	Ethylene glycol Methanol	Dose 1: 15 mg/kg IV Doses during next 48 hr: 10 mg/kg IV All subsequent doses: 15 mg/kg IV Administer q12h, except when HD performed: HD initiation: next dose if >6 hr since last dose HD ongoing: q4h End of HD (based on time of last dose): <1 hr, no dose; 1-3 hr, next dose; >3 hr, next dose	For both: serum level <25 mg/dL and metabolic acidosis resolved	Start immediately if toxic alcohol suspected, without waiting for confirmatory levels Dose amount is not affected by interval timing of doses
Glucagon	β-Adrenergic receptor antagonists Calcium-channel antagonists	Bolus of 3-5 mg IV; can repeat to achieve clinical effect, then infusion of 2-10 mg/hr	Reversal of hypotension and bradycardia; taper infusion	Can precipitate vomiting; be prepared to protect airway Mild hyperglycemia occurs Maximum dosing amounts unknown; bolus doses up to 30 mg reported Duration of effect is 15 min; thus infusion must be started immediately
Hydroxocobalamin	Cyanide	Initial: 5 g IV during 15-min period Second dose: 5 g IV during 15 min to 2 hr; maximum total dose is 10 g Follow each hydroxocobalamin dose with sodium thiosulfate 25%: 50 mL (12.5 g) IV during 10-min period	Resolution of lactic acidosis and moderate to severe clinical signs and symptoms: seizures, coma, dyspnea, apnea, hypotension, bradycardia	Can be administered IV push if patient is in cardiac arrest Do not give hydroxocobalamin and sodium thiosulfate through the same IV line Adverse effects: red discoloration of plasma, urine, mucous membranes, skin; transient hypertension Interference with laboratory colorimetric assays: Levels increased: bilirubin; creatinine; glucose; hemoglobin; magnesium; co-oximetry total Hb, COHb%, MetHb% Levels decreased: AST, ALT, creatinine, co-oximetry O_2 Hb%
Hyperbaric oxygen (HBO)	Carbon monoxide Experimental: carbon tetrachloride, cyanide, hydrogen sulfide	3.0 atm pressure for 60 min (25 min O_2, 5 min air, 25 min O_2, 5 min air), then 2.0 atm for 65 min (30 min O_2, 5 min air, 30 min O_2), then "surface" to 1.0 atm	One treatment Repeated treatment controversial	Carbon monoxide: treatment protocols may vary HBO indicated for loss of consciousness; seizures; cerebellar dysfunction; impaired cognition; headache, nausea/vomiting persisting after 4 hr of O_2 therapy regardless of carboxyhemoglobin level
Insulin-glucose	Calcium-channel antagonists β-Adrenergic receptor antagonists	Regular insulin, 1 U/kg bolus, followed by 0.5-1 U/kg/hr Titrate 50% dextrose IV to avoid hypoglycemia	Reversal of myocardial depression	Initiate early to reverse myocardial depression Monitor glucose and potassium; hypoglycemia can occur during and after therapy Hyperglycemia results from calcium-channel antagonist–induced insulin resistance, and initial dextrose requirements may be less than anticipated Recovery may be heralded by normalization of glucose levels, with increased dextrose required to avoid hypoglycemia
Lipid emulsion	Cardiac toxicity from local anesthetics (e.g., bupivacaine, ropivacaine) Experimental: verapamil, diltiazem, tricyclic antidepressants, bupropion, propranolol, and other lipophilic toxicants	Use 20% formulation Initial bolus: 1.5 mL/kg IV during 1 min, followed immediately by infusion of 0.25 mL/kg/min for 30-60 min Can repeat bolus for asystole	Return of hemodynamic stability	Use for other than bupivacaine based on animal experiments and human case reports; numerous dosing regimens have been used Use if advanced life support measures fail; continue CPR as needed during drug administration

Antidote	Indication for Use	Dose*	Treatment End Point	Comments
Methylene blue	Methemoglobin-producing agents	1-2 mg/kg body weight (0.1-0.2 mL/kg of 1%) methylene blue during 5-min period; repeat dose for persistent or recurrent symptoms or signs	Resolution of dyspnea and altered mental status	Use if patient is symptomatic (i.e., dyspneic, altered mental status) Maximum dose should not exceed 7 mg/kg (0.7 mL/kg) Contraindicated in G6PD-deficient patients; may cause hemolysis Some toxicants (e.g., dapsone) may require prolonged therapy
N-Acetylcysteine (NAC)[7]	Acetaminophen Experimental: carbon tetrachloride, chloroform, pennyroyal oil	Oral (total 72 hr) Load: 140 mg/kg Maintenance (starting 4 hr after load): 70 mg/kg q4h × 17 doses IV (total 21 hr) Load: 150 mg/kg during 1-hr period Maintenance infusion: 12.5 mg/kg/hr during 4-hr period, then 6.25 mg/kg/hr over 16 hr as continuous infusion	At the end of therapy, repeat AST and APAP levels: if AST normal and APAP not detected, treatment complete; if AST normal and APAP detected, continue NAC; if AST elevated, continue NAC After patient has received full course of NAC therapy, if INR ≥2.0 or severe hepatotoxicity present (AST >1000 U/L), continue NAC until INR <2.0 and aminotransferases normalize	Most effective if initiated within 8 hr after ingestion; may be started any time after ingestion and is beneficial in severe hepatotoxic states Longer duration of treatment may be required in patients with hepatotoxicity Treatment end points simplified for ease of use INR result not valid indicator if FFP recently administered
Naloxone	Opioids	Opioid dependence possible: 40-50 μg (0.04-0.05 mg) IV titrated upward to reversal, while avoiding withdrawal if concerns for opioid dependence Opioid dependence not likely: 0.4 mg by any route and titrate up to 10 mg Continuous infusion: establish bolus dose required to reverse respiratory depression; begin infusing two thirds of reversal dose every hour and titrate to maintain adequate respirations; repeated bolus with half of reversal dose 15 min after reversal of respiratory depression	Initial: reversal of respiratory depression with resolution of hypoxia and hypercapnia Final: resolution of CNS and respiratory depression	Pre-ventilate patients with respiratory depression by bag-valve-mask or intubation before administration Use smaller doses in opioid-dependent patients Some opioids (e.g., buprenorphine) may require larger doses of naloxone Use continuous infusion for recurrent symptoms and prolonged action of some formulations (e.g., sustained-release morphine, methadone) Re-sedation can occur Do not use naltrexone to reverse acute toxicity
Octreotide	Sulfonylurea-induced hypoglycemia	50 mg SC q6h	Resolution of hypoglycemia and dextrose not required	Maintain dextrose infusion as needed Not for insulin-induced hypoglycemia
Physostigmine	Anticholinergic agents (e.g., diphenhydramine, jimsonweed [*Datura* sp], scopolamine)	1-2 mg IV during 5-min period; can repeat in 5 min if no effect and cholinergic effects do not occur	Reversal of anticholinergic effects	Duration of effect is 60-90 min Benzodiazepine used for subsequent treatment of agitation and seizures; additional physostigmine used rarely (e.g., refractory seizures or agitation) Adverse effects include seizures, excessive oral secretions, bradyarrhythmias; contraindicated in cyclic antidepressant toxicity
Pralidoxime chloride	Organophosphorus compounds Nerve agents: sarin, VX	30 mg/kg IV bolus (maximum 2 g) during 30 min, followed by continuous infusion of 8-10 mg/kg/hr (maximum 650 mg/hr)	Resolution of signs and symptoms, atropine no longer required	Can give initial dose during 2-min period for life-threatening clinical effects Administer early when diagnosis known or strongly suspected Efficacy variable, depending on the organophosphate Fat-soluble organophosphates may require prolonged treatment

Continued on following page

Antidote	Indication for Use	Dose*	Treatment End Point	Comments
Pyridoxine	Ethylene glycol Isoniazid Monomethylhydrazine (*Gyromitra esculenta* mushrooms)	100 mg IV 5 g IV, repeat for refractory seizures	One dose Resolution of seizures	Efficacy theoretical for ethylene glycol to enhance elimination of toxic metabolites Pyridoxine may be required even with benzodiazepines to stop seizures, but patient can remain comatose (isoniazid, *Gyromitra* mushrooms) Excessive dosing can cause neuropathy
Sodium bicarbonate ($NaHCO_3$)	Reversal of myocardial sodium-channel blockers (e.g., cyclic antidepressants, cocaine, sodium-channel–blocking antiarrhythmics with $\tau_{recovery}$ >1 sec, piperidine phenothiazines (thioridazine, mesoridazine)	1-2 mEq $NaHCO_3$/kg by intermittent bolus; repeat as needed	Narrowing of prolonged QRS, resolution of ventricular arrhythmias, reversal of hypotension	Monitor blood pH (optimal pH approximately 7.50); avoid pH >7.55
	Altered tissue distribution or enhanced elimination of salicylates; may be used for chlorophenoxy herbicides, formic acid, methotrexate, phenobarbital	1-2 mEq $NaHCO_3$/kg, followed by 3 ampules (150 mL) $NaHCO_3$(44 mEq per 50 mL) in 850 mL of D_5W, infused at 2-3 times normal maintenance fluid rate	Serum salicylate <30 mg/dL and patient clinically stable	Target blood pH: 7.50-7.55 Monitor urinary pH hourly; adjust infusion to maintain urine pH of 7.5-8.0 (avoid blood pH >7.55) Monitor ABGs Maintain normokalemia
Succimer (DMSA)	Arsenic Lead Mercury, all forms	10 mg/kg/dose q8h for 5 days, followed by q12h for 14 days Drug holiday for 2 weeks; repeat if treatment end point not reached	Arsenic: 24-hr urinary arsenic <50 μg/L Lead: resolution of encephalopathy, gastrointestinal symptoms, neuropathy, nephropathy, arthralgias, myalgias, and blood lead level <70 μg/dL Mercury, elemental and inorganic: 24-hr urinary mercury <20 μg/L Mercury, organic: end point not well established	Oral chelator; adverse effects include rash, transient AST and alkaline phosphatase elevations, and gastrointestinal distress; minimal chelation of essential metals occurs Dosing for arsenic and mercury not well established Therapeutic end point for organic mercury not established; neurotoxicity not responsive to chelation therapy; suggest chelation until blood mercury level within normal-value range for reference laboratory
Vitamin K	Vitamin K antagonist anticoagulants (e.g., warfarin, long-acting anticoagulant rodenticides [LAARs]) [note that this is not for normalizing a supratherapeutic INR in patients prescribed warfarin]	Subcutaneous: AquaMEPHYTON (K_1), 10-25 mg, repeat every 6-12 hr until oral vitamin K_1 started Oral: 25-50 mg q6h; larger doses may be required	INR is normal 48-72 hr after stopping vitamin K_1 therapy Can also monitor factor VII activity	Anaphylactoid reaction can occur with rapid IV administration Severe bleeding may also require FFP, prothrombin protein concentrate (off label), or factor concentrates Base decision to treat on finding of elevated INR; do not administer prophylactic vitamin K_1 Oral therapy may be required for months with LAAR poisoning because of lipophilicity of toxicant, with slow body clearance

ABGs, Arterial blood gases; *ALT*, alanine aminotransferase; *APAP*, acetyl-*p*-aminophenol (acetaminophen); *AST*, aspartate aminotransferase; *BAL*, British antilewisite; *CNS*, central nervous system; *COHb%*, percentage carboxyhemoglobin; *CPR*, cardiopulmonary resuscitation; D_5W, 5% dextrose in water; *DMSA*, 2,3-dimercaptosuccinic acid; *ECG*, electrocardiogram; *FFP*, fresh-frozen plasma; *G6PD*, glucose-6-phosphate dehydrogenase; *Hb*, hemoglobin; *HD*, hemodialysis; *INR*, international normalized ratio; *MetHb%*, percentage methemoglobinemia; *NS*, normal saline; $O_2Hb\%$, percentage oxyhemoglobin; $\tau_{recovery}$, drug blockade recovery rate.

*Dose concentrations and infusion times are not given. Drug dosages may require adjustment in patients with renal or hepatic failure.

†Administer antivenom in a monitored setting; antivenom must be reconstituted and then diluted; initially infuse at a rate of 2-5 mL/hr, and double the infusion rate every 5 min as tolerated to administer antivenom during a 1-hr period.

‡Ten percent calcium chloride solution = 100 mg/mL (27.2 mg/mL elemental calcium); 10% calcium gluconate solution = 100 mg/mL (9 mg/mL elemental calcium).

From Goldman L, Schafer AI: *Goldman-Cecil medicine*, ed 25, Philadelphia, 2016, Elsevier.

Management of Acute Poisoning

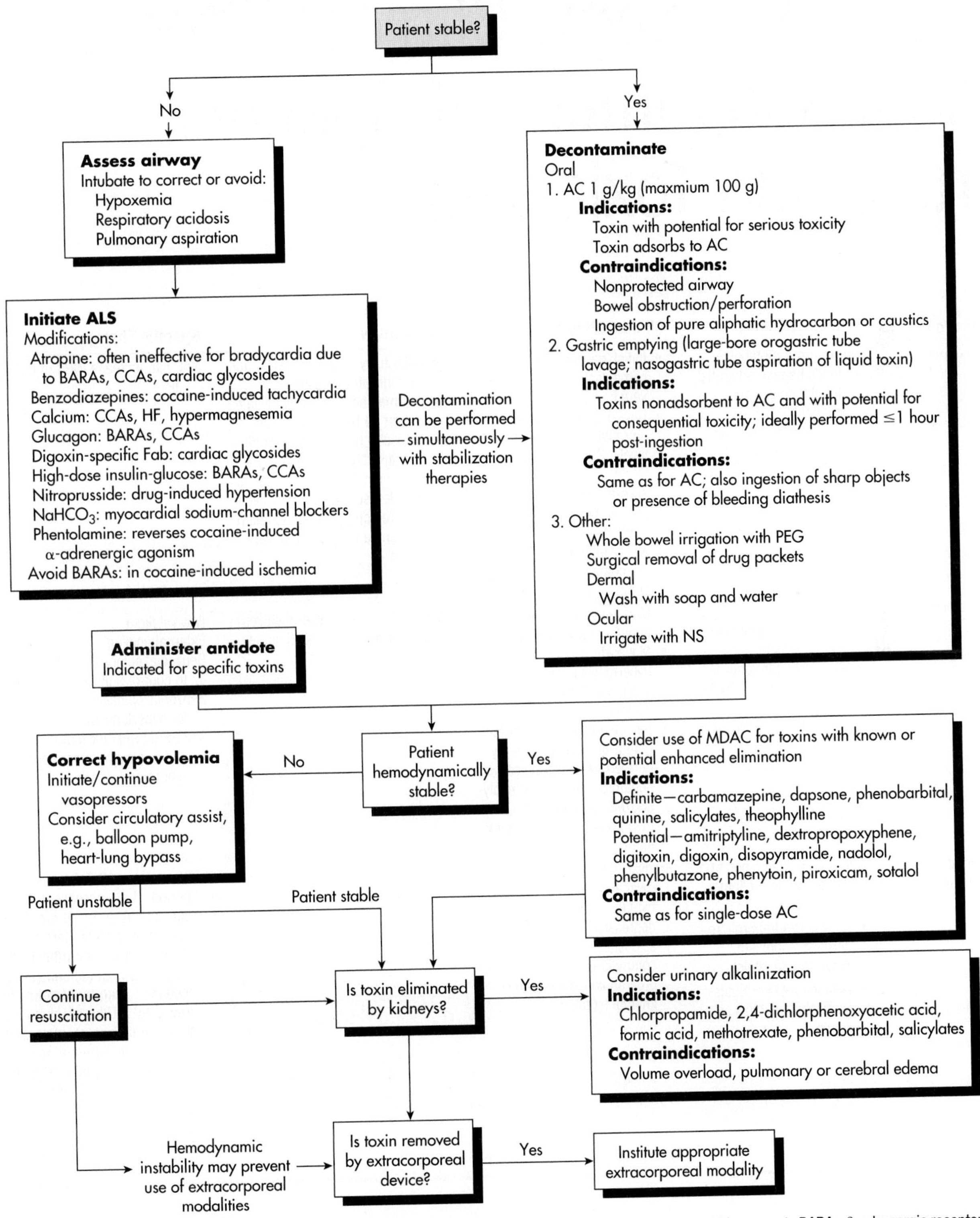

Algorithm for the management of acute poisoning. See also Appendix IIIe. *AC*, Activated charcoal; *ALS*, advanced life support; *BARAs*, β-adrenergic receptor antagonists; *CCAs*, L-type calcium-channel antagonists; *HF*, hydrofluoric acid; *MDAC*, multidose activated charcoal; *NS*, 0.9% saline solution; *PEG*, nonabsorbable polyethylene glycol solution. (Modified from Goldman L, Schafer AI: *Goldman-Cecil medicine*, ed 25, Philadelphia, 2016, Elsevier.)

Pathophysiology, Clinical Effects, and Management of Specific Drugs and Toxicants

Drug or Toxicant	Pathophysiology	Clinical Effects	Laboratory	Specific Therapy
Acetaminophen	NAPQI (toxic metabolite) binds hepatic and renal tubular cells; acetaminophen itself induces transient decrease in functional factor VII	• Initial: nausea, vomiting, coma, lactic acidosis in severe cases • Days 1-3: elevated INR, aminotransferase, and bilirubin levels; RUQ tenderness; increased creatinine level in severe cases • Days 4-14: gradual recovery or continued increase in INR and creatinine, lactic acidosis, coma, cerebral edema, death	• Potentially toxic level ≥150 μg/ml 4 hr after ingestion* • INR may be transiently elevated in first 24 hr because of decrease in functional factor VII; further increases indicate hepatic necrosis; elevated aminotransferase and bilirubin levels not predictive of hepatic failure • Creatinine elevated in severe cases	NAC can increase INR but not aPTT†
Amphetamines	• Increased release of presynaptic norepinephrine and dopamine • Increased serotonin release (especially MDMA, PMA, DOB, other synthetic amphetamines)	• Mild: euphoria, decreased appetite, repetitive behavior • Moderate: vomiting, agitation, hypertension, tachycardia, mydriasis, bruxism, diaphoresis • Severe: hypertension or hypotension, arrhythmias, hyperthermia, seizures, coma, hepatotoxicity, rhabdomyolysis, DIC, hyponatremia (SIADH), renal failure, cerebral infarction or hemorrhage	Not helpful; many false-positives and false-negatives on screening tests	IV crystalloid External cooling Benzodiazepines or barbiturates to control agitation or seizure Benzodiazepines or nitroprusside for hypertension See SSRIs/SRIs for features and treatment of serotonin syndrome
β-Adrenergic receptor antagonists	Blocks catecholamines from β-adrenergic receptors • α- and β-adrenergic receptor antagonism: carvedilol, labetalol • Delayed rectifier potassium-channel blockade: sotalol	Bradyarrhythmias, decreased myocardial contractility, hypotension, respiratory depression, decreased consciousness with seizures or coma (lipophilic agents, e.g., propranolol), prolonged QT interval (sotalol)	• ECG • No specific tests	• IV glucagon, 3.5-5 mg over 2-min period; if no increase in BP or HR, can repeat up to 10 mg; if effective, immediately start continuous infusion at 2-10 mg/hr; if still unstable, options include (1) regular insulin, 1 U/kg by IV bolus, followed by 1 U/kg/hr, plus dextrose to maintain euglycemia; (2) norepinephrine or dobutamine infusion titrated to desirable BP and HR; (3) IV milrinone, 50 μg/kg over 10-min period, then 0.375-0.75 μg/kg/min based on hemodynamic status‡ • Electrical pacing and IABP in refractory cases

Drug or Toxicant	Pathophysiology	Clinical Effects	Laboratory	Specific Therapy
L-type calcium-channel antagonists	• Blocks L-type voltage-sensitive calcium channels, thereby decreasing calcium entry into myocardial and vascular smooth muscle cells • Decreases pancreatic insulin release and increases insulin resistance	Bradyarrhythmias (verapamil, diltiazem), hypotension, hyperglycemia	• ECG • No specific tests	• IV 10% calcium chloride, 10-20 mg/kg (0.1-0.2 ml/kg); can repeat once; if BP improves, continuous infusion at 0.2-0.5 ml/kg/hr (20-50 mg/kg/hr) • Ionized Ca^{2+} levels should not exceed 2× normal (severe cases will be refractory to calcium therapy) • Glucagon, high-dose insulin and dextrose, catecholamines, and milrinone (as for β-adrenergic antagonists)
Cardiac glycosides, including digoxin, bufadienolides (toxic toad venom), or cardenolides (e.g., oleander, lily of the valley, dogbane)	• Inhibits Na^+, K^+-ATPase • Decreased CNS sympathetic output • Decreased baroreceptor sensitivity • Increased vagal acetylcholine discharge	Bradyarrhythmias, including second- and third-degree AV block and asystole Ventricular ectopy, tachycardia, fibrillation Junctional tachycardia, paroxysmal atrial tachycardia with block Weakness, visual disturbances, nausea, vomiting	Serum digoxin level Serum potassium (hyperkalemia occurs in acute poisoning; hypokalemia may be present in chronic poisoning), magnesium, and creatinine levels	Correct hypokalemia and hypomagnesemia; do not give calcium Digoxin-specific antibody fragments (Fab) indicated if patient has hemodynamically significant arrhythmias, serum potassium ≥5 mg/L, Mobitz II or third-degree AV block, ingestion of bufadienolide- or cardenolide-containing agents, or renal insufficiency Empirical dose Chronic: 2-5 vial Acute: 10-20 vial Calculated dose Chronic: number of vials = 2 × serum digoxin level (ng/ml) × 5.6 × weight (kg)/1000 Acute: number of vials = 2 × oral digoxin dose (mg) × 0.8
Cyclic antidepressants	Myocardial sodium- and potassium-channel blockade Blockade of α-adrenergic and cholinergic muscarinic receptor Inhibition of norepinephrine reuptake	• Decreased level of consciousness (can develop rapidly), myoclonus, seizures, coma • Anticholinergic toxidrome • Sinus tachycardia, ventricular conduction delays, ventricular arrhythmias, asystole • Hypotension	Serum levels not helpful in management	• Intermittent IV boluses of $NaHCO_3$ (1 mEq/kg) to maintain arterial pH at 7.5 because acidemia can worsen cardiovascular complications • Intubation and neuroparalytic drugs may be useful to ameliorate acidemia from muscular hyperactivity while seizures are being treated • Contraindicated drugs: types IA and IC antiarrhythmic agents; physostigmine, flumazenil
Ethylene glycol, methanol (e.g., antifreeze, window cleaners, camping stove fuels)	• Ethylene glycol: toxic metabolites produce cytotoxicity in CNS, kidneys, lungs, heart, liver, muscles; metabolic acidosis is due to glycolate accumulation; oxalate complexes with calcium, so hypocalcemia can develop • Methanol: metabolized to formic acid, which is responsible for metabolic acidosis and inhibition of cytochrome aa3; target organs include retina, optic nerve, CNS	• Ethylene glycol: CNS depression, cerebral edema, seizures, anion gap metabolic acidosis, renal failure with acute tubular necrosis, pulmonary edema, myositis • Methanol: nausea, vomiting; cerebral edema, hemorrhage, infarcts; necrosis of thalamus and putamen; anion gap metabolic acidosis; visual disturbances, papilledema, hyperemic optic disc, nonreactive pupils	• Serum ethylene glycol and methanol levels; levels may be low or undetectable if significant metabolism has occurred • Ethylene glycol: serum calcium, creatinine, BUN levels; examine urine for calcium oxalate crystals; false hyperlactatemia occurs with certain analyzers using l-lactate oxidase, which cross-reacts with glycolic and glyoxylic acids	• For both: fomepizole (which inhibits alcohol dehydrogenase and blocks formation of toxic metabolites), 15 mg/kg IV loading dose, then 10 mg/kg IV for 4 doses during the next 48 hr, then 15 mg/kg for subsequent doses; interval dosing is q12h (q4h during hemodialysis, with dosing interval adjustments at start and finish); continue until ethylene glycol or methanol is no longer detectable • Use of ethanol is no longer recommended • Hemodialysis: initiate if level is ≥50 mg/dl or metabolic acidosis with end-organ toxicity; continue until acidosis resolves and serum level of ethylene glycol or methanol is undetectable • Monitor for cerebral edema with possible herniation • Ethylene glycol: IV calcium for symptomatic hypocalcemia • Methanol: folinic acid, 50 mg IV q4h until methanol not detectable and acidosis cleared

Continued on following page

Drug or Toxicant	Pathophysiology	Clinical Effects	Laboratory	Specific Therapy
γ-Hydroxybutyrate (GHB) and its precursors (γ-butyrolactone and 1,4-butanediol [1,4-BD])	Agonist effect on CNS GHB receptors; indirect action with opioid receptors (may increase proenkephalins); metabolized to GABA, interacts with $GABA_B$ receptors; decreases dopamine release	• CNS: rapid loss of consciousness, with recovery typical within 2-4 hr; myoclonus (possible seizures) • Respiratory depression; bradycardia; nausea, vomiting	No specific tests	• Supportive care, including respiratory support as needed • Withdrawal resembles sedative-hypnotic withdrawal and can be treated with benzodiazepines or pentobarbital
Lithium	Decreases brain inositol; alters CNS serotonin, dopamine, and norepinephrine; inhibits adenylate cyclases, including those that mediate vasopressin-induced renal concentration and thyroid function	• Chronic toxicity usually more severe than acute toxicity: tremor, hyperreflexia, drowsiness, incoordination, clonus, confusion, ataxia; in severe cases, seizures, coma, death; recovery may take weeks, and CNS deficits may persist • Sinus node dysfunction, QT prolongation, T wave abnormalities, U waves • Nephrogenic diabetes insipidus, hypothyroidism, hyperthyroidism, hypercalcemia, pseudotumor cerebri • Acute toxicity: nausea, vomiting, diarrhea, and milder neurologic findings	• Peak serum levels: • Normal dose 2-3 hr; up to 5 hr for sustained-release lithium • Acute overdose: peak may be delayed ≥4-12 hr	• Replenish intravascular volume, maintain urinary output at 1-2 ml/kg/hr • Consider GI decontamination with oral polyethylene glycol electrolyte solution within 1-2 hr after acute overdose of sustained-release drug • Hemodialysis[§] in patients with altered mental status, ataxia, seizures, or coma or in patients with mild symptoms in the setting of acute overdose or renal insufficiency • Ineffective or contraindicated therapies include oral activated charcoal, diuretics, and aminophylline
Opioids (e.g., heroin, morphine, oxycodone, fentanyl)	Agonist effect at CNS μ, κ, and δ opioid receptors; result is cell hyperpolarization and decreased neurotransmitter release	• CNS depression, respiratory depression, miosis • Dextromethorphan increases CNS serotonin and inhibits NMDA receptors, which causes hallucinations • Propoxyphene and its metabolite norpropoxyphene block sodium channels and can cause seizures and wide-complex arrhythmias similar to cyclic antidepressants; $NaHCO_3$ treats arrhythmias • Seizure risk with tramadol, meperidine, propoxyphene • Rapid, powerful heroin-like effect when sustained-release oxycodone is crushed before ingestion, snorting, or smoking • QTc prolongation and torsades de pointes with methadone	Rapid urine drug screens detect morphine and codeine but may not detect semisynthetic and synthetic opioids; some interferents/irrelevants	• IV naloxone, 0.4-2 mg; can repeat up to 10 mg if no response • Continuous infusion for recurrent symptoms or sustained-release opioid ingestion; give 50% of dose that produces desired effect 15 min after initial effect is obtained, then infuse two thirds of this dose every hr; infusion rate can be increased or decreased to maintain normal respiration and avoid withdrawal symptoms • Contraindicated therapies: nalmefene and naltrexone should not be used for acute opioid reversal
Organo-phosphorus compounds and carbamates (e.g., diazinon, mevinphos, fenthion, aldicarb)	Inhibits acetylcholinesterase, resulting in excessive acetylcholine stimulation of nicotinic and muscarinic receptors in autonomic and somatic motor nervous systems and CNS	• Nicotinic-mediated effects: tachycardia, mydriasis, hypertension, delirium, coma, seizures, muscle weakness, fasciculations • Muscarinic-mediated effects: salivation, lacrimation, urination, vomiting, defecation, miosis, bronchorrhea, bronchospasm, bradycardia	• Serum (butyrylcholinesterase) or RBC (acetylcholinesterase) activity <50% of normal • Clinical recovery occurs before serum cholinesterase levels normalize	• Atropine, 1-2 mg by initial IV bolus; double the dose every 5 min (2 mg, 4 mg, 8 mg, 16 mg, etc.) until drying of bronchial secretions, adequate oxygenation, pulse >80 bpm, systolic blood pressure >80 mm Hg achieved; continuous infusion at 10%-20% of total stabilizing dose per hr; stop infusion if patient develops any signs or symptoms of anticholinergic toxidrome; restart infusion at lower rate when signs or symptoms abate • Pralidoxime‖ chloride 30 mg/kg (maximum 2 g) IV bolus over 30 min, then 8-10 mg/kg/hr (maximum 650 mg/hr) continuous infusion; administer as soon as possible after poisoning; continue 12-24 hr after atropine no longer required and symptoms resolve

Drug or Toxicant	Pathophysiology	Clinical Effects	Laboratory	Specific Therapy
Salicylates	Inhibits cyclooxygenase; decreases formation of prostaglandins and thromboxane A_2; stimulates CNS medullary respiratory receptor and chemoreceptor trigger zone; impairs platelet function; disrupts carbohydrate metabolism; uncouples oxidative phosphorylation; increases vascular permeability	• Acute toxicity • Mild: nausea, vomiting, diaphoresis, tinnitus, decreased hearing, hyperpnea, tachypnea • Moderate–severe: confusion, delirium, coma, seizures, hyperthermia, ALI; death can occur within hours of overdose • Chronic toxicity: same as acute, but may not have diaphoresis or vomiting • Consider diagnosis in patients with new-onset confusion, anion gap metabolic acidosis, or ALI	• Serum salicylate level: toxic ≥30 mg/dl; level ≥100 mg/dL indicates life-threatening toxicity with possible sudden, rapid clinical deterioration; in chronic toxicity, levels may be minimally elevated (>30 mg/dl), and clinical evaluation is more reliable for gauging degree of toxicity • Arterial blood gases: respiratory alkalosis with metabolic acidosis • Anion gap metabolic acidosis • Prolonged PT and PTT, ketonuria, ketonemia	Multidose activated charcoal q2-3h in acute overdose with progressive symptoms or rising salicylate level
SSRIs/SRIs	• Inhibits reuptake of serotonin • SRIs have additional effects (e.g., duloxetine inhibits norepinephrine reuptake, nefazodone inhibits serotonergic 5-HT2 receptors, trazodone inhibits peripheral α-adrenergic receptors, venlafaxine inhibits norepinephrine and dopamine reuptake)	• Vomiting, blurred vision, CNS depression, tachycardia • Seizures and coma rare • Torsades de pointes reported with citalopram • Serotonin syndrome: clonus, agitation, tremor, diaphoresis, hyperreflexia; hyperthermia and hypertonicity in severe cases	• No specific tests • If serotonin syndrome suspected: electrolytes, BUN, glucose, liver enzymes, coagulation panel, blood gases, chest radiograph	• Respiratory support as needed • Benzodiazepines for agitation or seizures • Serotonin syndrome: consider cyproheptadine, 12 mg PO initial dose then 2 mg PO q2h (to a maximum of 32 mg/day) until symptoms resolve • Critical care therapies for hyperthermia, rhabdomyolysis, DIC, ARDS, renal and hepatic dysfunction, torsades de pointes

ALI, Acute lung injury; *aPTT,* activated partial thromboplastin time; *ARDS,* acute respiratory distress syndrome; *AV,* atrioventricular; *BP,* blood pressure; *bpm,* beats per minute; *BUN,* blood urea nitrogen; *CNS,* central nervous system; *DIC,* disseminated intravascular coagulation; *DOB,* 4-bromo-2,5-dimethoxyamphetamine; *ECG,* electrocardiogram; *GABA,* α-aminobutyric acid; *GI,* gastrointestinal; *HR,* heart rate; *IABP,* intra-aortic balloon counterpulsation; *INR,* international normalized ratio; *IV,* intravenous; *MDMA,* 3,4-methylenedioxymethamphetamine; *Na^1,K^1-ATPase,* sodium, potassium adenosine triphosphatase; *NAC,* N-acetylcysteine; *NAPQI,* N-acetyl-p-benzoquinone imine; *NMDA,* N-methyl-D-aspartate; *PMA,* paramethoxyamphetamine; *PT,* prothrombin time; *PTT,* partial thromboplastin time; *RBC,* red blood cell; *RUQ,* upper right quadrant (abdomen); *SIADH,* syndrome of inappropriate antidiuretic secretion; *SRI,* serotonin reuptake inhibitor; *SSRI,* selective serotonin reuptake inhibitor.

*A nomogram to evaluate the potential toxicity of levels drawn more than 4 hours after ingestion is provided in Fig. 7, from Rumack BH, Matthew H: Acetaminophen poisoning and toxicity, *Pediatrics* 1975(55):871-876. The nomogram is valid only for levels drawn after a single acute ingestion.

†NAC can be discontinued in patients with uncomplicated disease after a loading dose plus six maintenance doses if hepatic aminotransferase levels are normal and acetaminophen is not detected; otherwise, the full regimen should be administered.

‡Adjust infusion for reduced renal function.

§Continue hemodialysis until the serum lithium level is less than 1 mEq/L. Recheck the level 8 hr after dialysis, and restart hemodialysis if the level is higher than 1 mEq/L. Repeat this cycle until the serum lithium level remains lower than 1 mEq/L.

ǁA double-blind, randomized, placebo-controlled trial of pralidoxime in acute organophosphorus poisoning found no significant difference in mortality rates or need for intubation.

From Goldman L, Schafer AI: *Goldman's Cecil medicine,* ed 24, Philadelphia, 2012, Elsevier.

Accidental Poisoning by an Exposure to Other Drugs Acting on the Autonomic Nervous System

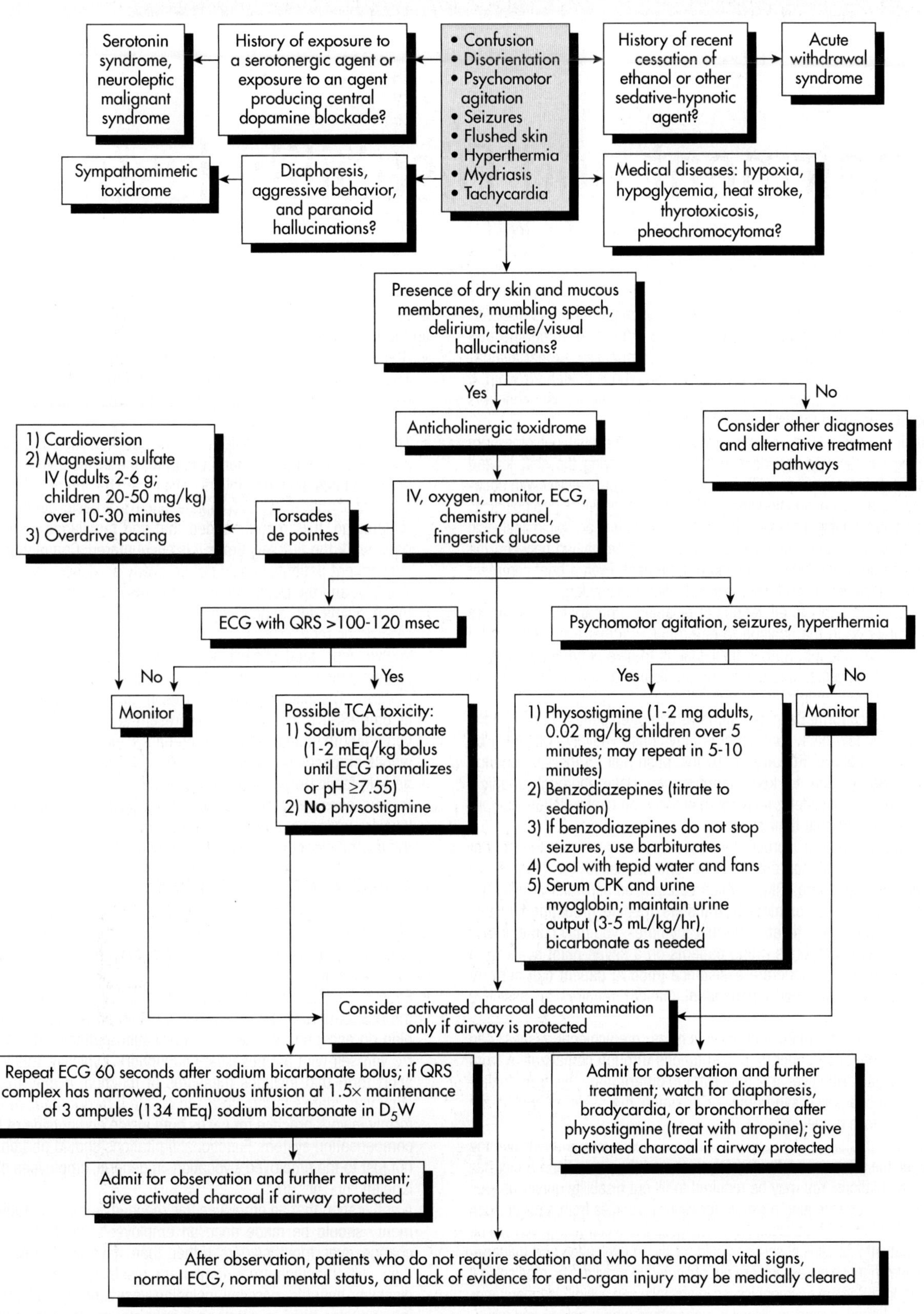

Algorithm for the recognition and treatment of anticholinergic toxicity. *CPK*, Creatine phosphokinase; *D_5W*, 5% dextrose in water; *ECG*, electrocardiogram; *IV*, intravenous line; *TCA*, tricyclic antidepressant. (From Adams JG et al: *Emergency medicine: clinical essentials*, ed 2, Philadelphia, 2013, Elsevier.)

Appendix IV

Impairment and Disability Issues

Impairment describes harm to anatomy and physiology, whereas *disability* denotes the difficulty a person has performing a function. Reporting disability for different sectors of society has its own nuances. Proper evaluation of impairment/disability starts with knowing who is asking for what. It is an area of practice in which an understanding of some basic concepts can make it rewarding rather than distressing.

- Ultimately, disability is a measure of function. Functional outcomes are becoming increasingly important in medicine, mirroring the shift toward patient-centeredness. All practitioners should have some facility with documenting the effects of an intervention on a patient's physical, psychological, and social functioning. For example, the continuation of an opioid analgesic should be predicated on meeting functional goals negotiated between the patient and physician before initiation of treatment. Even a brief comment on walking distance or work tolerance is better than nothing.
- Some concepts apply to all venues of disability. Primary care providers should rarely be in the position to determine whether a patient can be on or off a specific job. Rather, their task is to give general parameters about which physical exertions are medically dangerous. Try to be specific and use objective criteria where appropriate, but don't be intimidated by a form. Ballpark estimates can often suffice. For example, many chronic low back pain patients may conservatively and safely be described as able to lift/carry up 10 lbs, push/pull 25 lbs, and change positions as needed to keep comfortable. Have thorough medical records and be consistent; lawyers may focus on contradictions in your documentation to help their clients.
- Rehabilitation centers across the country are required to monitor function using a standardized set of criteria called the "Functional Independence Measure (FIM)," which categorizes activities of daily living into divisions such as mobility, transfers, feeding, grooming/hygiene, dressing, bathing, and toileting. In therapy notes, you may come across scores in these categories rating patients on a seven-point scale from totally dependent to moderate-assistance (mod A; patient can perform 50% of task) to modified-independent (patient requires an assistive device) to independent.
- Psychosocial contributing factors such as medicolegal issues can profoundly influence patients' presentations through somatization from secondary gain. However, it is important to differentiate this from malingering, Munchausen's syndrome, or "gaming the system," which are remarkably less prevalent.
- The number of stakeholders expands in the disability system to include the employer, the government, the legal system, and the payer. Each sector has its own regulations. You may be required to fill out disability questionnaires as a condition of accepting payment for clinical services from a payer, such as in the workers' compensation system. Much more commonly, you will be seeing patients for clinical services paid for by an evaluation and management code. In these cases, you are not obligated to provide free medicolegal assessments. Settling payment issues in advance can avoid misunderstanding. Again, before assessing disability, understand who is asking and why.

GOVERNMENT-ADMINISTERED DISABILITY

State Temporary Disability Insurance (TDI) programs, the Family Medical Leave Act of 1993 (FMLA), the Social Security Administration (SSA), and the Department of Veterans Affairs offer disability benefits through the state and federal government.

- State TDI forms must be filled out for the patient to receive any income. They are generally very basic and just engage the social support network for a patient. This may not be the best venue to stipulate partial disability.
- The FMLA provides unpaid leave for qualified medical and family reasons. Because it is a federal program, the forms involved are standard across states and employers. They can be intimidating at first, but are reasonably easy to complete once the basic definitions used are understood. It is recommended that you familiarize yourself with this paperwork the first few times it is encountered. Completing the form for subsequent patients should not be overly burdensome.
- The SSA and the Department of Veterans Affairs have their own internal mechanisms for quantifying disability, but they may subpoena your records or request a summary narrative as part of their processes. If you've kept good clinical notes, your existing documentation should satisfy their requirements. Many patients choose to apply for Social Security Disability Insurance (SSDI) and/or Supplemental Security Income (SSI) through a legal representative. These lawyers may send you a lengthy questionnaire to prepare their case. There are physicians whose practices perform these services and who can be hired by attorneys to facilitate patients' applications. If this nonclinical work appeals to you, consider affiliating with the SSA or contracting your time to lawyers under separate indenture. If not, you may want to recommend the law office contact a suitable practice.

WORKERS' COMPENSATION

In workers' compensation, the payer and employer join the provider in trying to rehabilitate the injured worker. Confidentiality issues are handled differently because these stakeholders may have a right to protected health information.

- Each state has their own laws regarding reporting requirements, and the U.S. Department of Labor governs injured federal employees. If you plan on accepting workers' compensation patients, you must familiarize yourself with the necessary paperwork. Typically, this is a standard, short form that includes measures of function. It may make sense to copy your state's parameters and create a "work note" to be used uniformly in your practice for cases both inside and outside of the workers' compensation system. Functional limitations should pertain to any task, not just to the employee's vocation. In general, employees should not be labeled "on" or "off."
- A notification that an employee has reached "maximal medical improvement" should be made once an employee's condition is expected to change over months/years rather than days/weeks. At this juncture they will transition from temporary disability benefits to permanent disability benefits, possibly including vocational rehabilitation. If ongoing sequelae exist, a permanent impairment rating may be needed to resolve an employee's claim and allow them to progress to the next stage of their life. These are more sophisticated determinations, usually directed by the American Medical Association's (AMA) *Guides to the Evaluation of Permanent Impairment*, now in its sixth edition. Analysis of

permanent impairment, causation, and apportionment generally fall outside of workers' compensation reporting requirements. Someone with appropriate training may be best suited to complete this task. Consider providing these more detailed services under a separate indenture, such as a consultation arrangement with the employee's attorney. Your state workers' compensation board may have specific guidelines governing these reports. In any case, the work should be done under a clear written agreement, not based on a verbal request by the employee. Very complex cases may also require a formal functional capacity evaluation through an appropriate rehabilitation resource.

PERSONAL INJURY

Patients hurt in car accidents or other personal injuries often are involved in legal cases covering medical care, personal damages, and pain and suffering. Most commonly, you will be helping these patients with their clinical issues under their regular medical insurance, although some providers agree to provide services under a legal lien on the claim. Regardless of your role in a personal injury case, it is helpful to document objective details about the injury and functional parameters. If you are asked to keep someone out of work, try to delineate functional limitations as you would in a workers' compensation employee.

- Similar to the workers' compensation system, it is helpful to state when a patient has reached maximal medical improvement. Personal injury claims can take longer to resolve than in the workers' compensation system, as the employer and insurance company are strongly incentivized to reach a resolution in those cases. In general, an ongoing legal case may hinder a patient from achieving a healthful balance of wellness. It is in the patient's best interest to move the claim toward completion.
- Quantifying permanent disability is a key component of resolving these cases. If a clinician is providing services under a legal lien, there may be a conflict of interest in having that provider quantify the permanent impairment. There may be financial implications to the degree of disability awarded, and this may influence whether or not the clinician will receive payment on their lien. These cases are almost always contentious, and may be best handled by providers with special training, such as an independent medical examiner. Again, the determination typically follows the AMA's *Guides to the Evaluation of Permanent Impairment.* A clinician's role is to manage the patient's injuries, not to negotiate medicolegal issues. If you are not appropriately trained, consider deferring questions regarding disability to someone who is.

PRIVATE DISABILITY

Some patients purchase private insurance plans to provide income in addition to that offered through the government in the case of long-term disability. These forms vary by insurance carrier and change over time. They may need to be filled out periodically to maintain benefits. Many providers opt to charge a separate fee for the completion of this type of paperwork.

CONCLUSION

In summary, impairment and disability are measures of function and should be followed by all good doctors as part of patient-centered care. Providers can be most effective interacting with the various disability systems if they know when they are acting as clinicians and when they are acting as legal consultants. Understanding the principles involved with the different sectors will help you avoid confusion between obligations and opportunities when doing this work.

SUGGESTED READINGS

American Academy of Physical Medicine and Rehabilitation: Disability evaluation. Available at http://now.aapmr.org/rehab-essentials/special-assessment-mgmt-strategy/Pages/Disability-evaluation.aspx. Accessed March 7, 2014.

Holmes EB: Impairment rating and disability determination. Available at http://emedicine.medscape.com/article/314195-overview#a1. Accessed March 7, 2014.

Rondinelli RD: *Guides to the evaluation of permanent impairment*, ed 6, Arlington, 2009, American Medical Association.

AUTHOR: **MATTHEW J. SMITH, M.D.**

Protection of Travelers

TABLE 1 Structured Approach to the Pretravel Office Visit with a Traveler to the Developing World

Perform Risk Assessment

The following must always be ascertained to determine appropriate preventive medical recommendations. Preprinted medical record forms may be used to record these.

Exact itinerary, including regions within each country to be visited
Dates of travel to assess risk of seasonal diseases
Age
Past vaccination history
Underlying illness(es)
Current medications
Pregnancy status
Allergies
Purpose of trip
Risk exposures—blood, body fluids, adventure or extensive outdoor exposures
Urban versus rural travel
Type of accommodations
Level of aversion to risk
Financial limitations that may necessitate prioritization of interventions

Administer Immunizations

Administer routine vaccinations that are not up-to-date.
Administer indicated travel vaccines.
Provide to patient legally mandated Vaccine Information Statements from the Centers for Disease Control and Prevention (http://www.cdc.gov/vaccines/pubs/vis/).
Provide printed checklist to patient, listing vaccines administered.
Record in the clinic record vaccines administered, lot number, and date.
Document vaccines offered to but declined by patient, as well as nonrecommended vaccines administered at the patient's request.

Provide Malaria Prevention (If Indicated)

Determine whether malaria risk exists for the destination country. If yes:
Does the patient's itinerary within that country put him or her at risk? If yes:
Recommend malaria chemoprophylaxis. Several equally effective drugs of choice may be indicated. Ascertain which is best suited to the individual patient and itinerary.
Educate on personal protection against arthropods.

Educate on Traveler's Diarrhea

Recommend food and water precautions.
Prescribe and educate on standby therapy with a quinolone antibiotic or azithromycin and advise on use of loperamide and oral hydration if needed.

Teach Essential Preventive Behaviors

Most travel-related health problems, including vaccine-preventable diseases, can be avoided through simple behaviors initiated by the traveler.
Educate on appropriate strategies in the following categories (some topics are not applicable to all destinations): blood-borne and sexually transmitted diseases, safety and crime avoidance, injury prevention, swimming safety, rabies, skin/wound care, tuberculosis, packing for healthy travel, obtaining health care abroad.

Discuss Other Applicable Heath Issues

Advise and prescribe for altitude illness, motion sickness, or jet lag.
Discuss prevention of specific travel-related infections that are of some risk to the traveler and have a possible preventive strategy not included in the strategies above.
Discuss any minimal-risk conditions (e.g., hemorrhagic fevers) that are a frequent cause of patient anxiety.

From Bennett JE, Dolin R, Blaser MJ: *Mandell, Douglas, and Bennett's principles and practice of infectious diseases*, ed 8, Philadelphia, 2015, Elsevier.

TABLE 2 In-Depth Information Resources for Travel Medicine

Authoritative Websites Updated Constantly with Epidemiologic and Outbreak Information

Centers for Disease Control and Prevention (CDC) Travelers Health http://www.cdc.gov/travel
World Health Organization (WHO) Travelers Health http://www.who.int/ith
Public Health Agency of Canada. Committee to Advise on Tropical Medicine and Travel (CATMAT) http://www.phac-aspc.gc.ca/tmp-pmv/catmat-ccmtmv/index-eng.php
WHO Disease Outbreak News http://www.who.int/csr/don/en/
WHO Weekly Epidemiological Record http://www.who.int/wer
CDC Morbidity and Mortality Weekly Report http://www.cdc.gov/mmwr
WHO Disease by Disease Health Topics http://www.who.int/health-topics/

In-Depth References on Specialized Topics

Centers for Disease Control and Prevention. Health Information for International Travel 2018 (The "CDC Yellow Book"). U.S. Public Health Service. Atlanta. Full text and hard copy order information available at https://wwwnc.cdc.gov/travel/page/yellowbook-home
World Health Organization. International Travel and Health (WHO "Green" Book). Published annually. Available from authorized WHO book agents. Full text online at http://www.who.int/ith/en/
Keystone JS, Kozarsky P, Connor B, et al, eds: *Travel medicine,* ed 4, Philadelphia, 2019, Elsevier (ISBN: 9780323546966)
Plotkin SA, Orenstein WA, Offit P, Edwards K: *Plotkin's vaccines,* ed 7, Philadelphia, 2017, Elsevier (ISBN: 9780323393010)
Auerbach PS, Cushing TA, Harris NS: *Wilderness medicine,* ed 7, St Louis, 2016, Elsevier (ISBN: 9780323359429)

Updated from Bennett JE, Dolin R, Blaser MJ: *Mandell, Douglas, and Bennett's principles and practice of infectious diseases,* ed 8, Philadelphia, 2015, Elsevier.

Japanese encephalitis, countries or areas at risk, 2011

Countries or areas at risk

Yellow fever vaccination recommendations in the Americas, 2011

Vaccination recommended

Vaccination generally not recommended*

Vaccination not recommended

Yellow fever vaccination recommendations in Africa, 2011

Vaccination recommended

Vaccination generally not recommended*

Vaccination not recommended

Hepatitis A, countries or areas at risk

Countries or areas with moderate to high risk

Hepatitis B, countries or areas at risk

Countries or areas with moderate to high risk

Rabies, countries or areas at risk

High risk

Medium risk

Low risk

No risk

Dengue, countries or areas at risk, 2011

Countries or areas where dengue has been reported

Polio-infected countries for which WHO recommends polio immunization or boosting to travelers, as of 01 Feb 2013

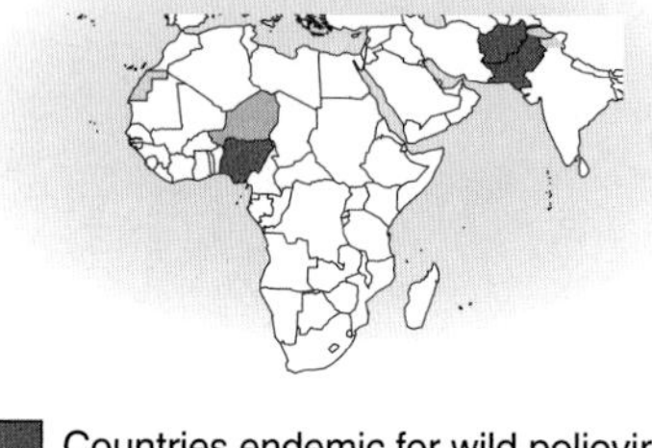

Countries endemic for wild poliovirus

Countries with reestablished virus transmission or recently reporting imported wild poliovirus

Meningococcal meningitis, countries or areas at high rsik, 2011

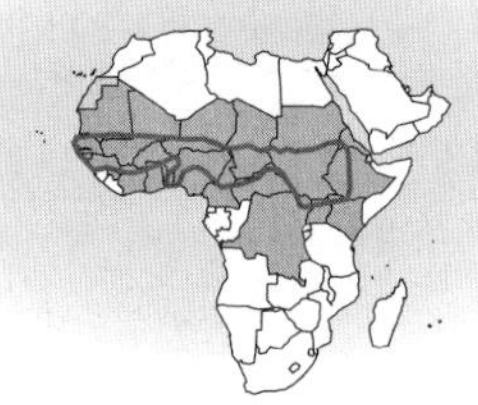

Countries at high epidemic risk

Meningitis belt, areas at high epidemic risk

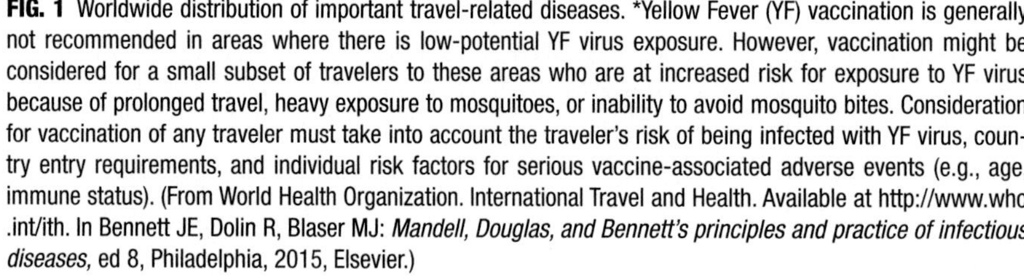

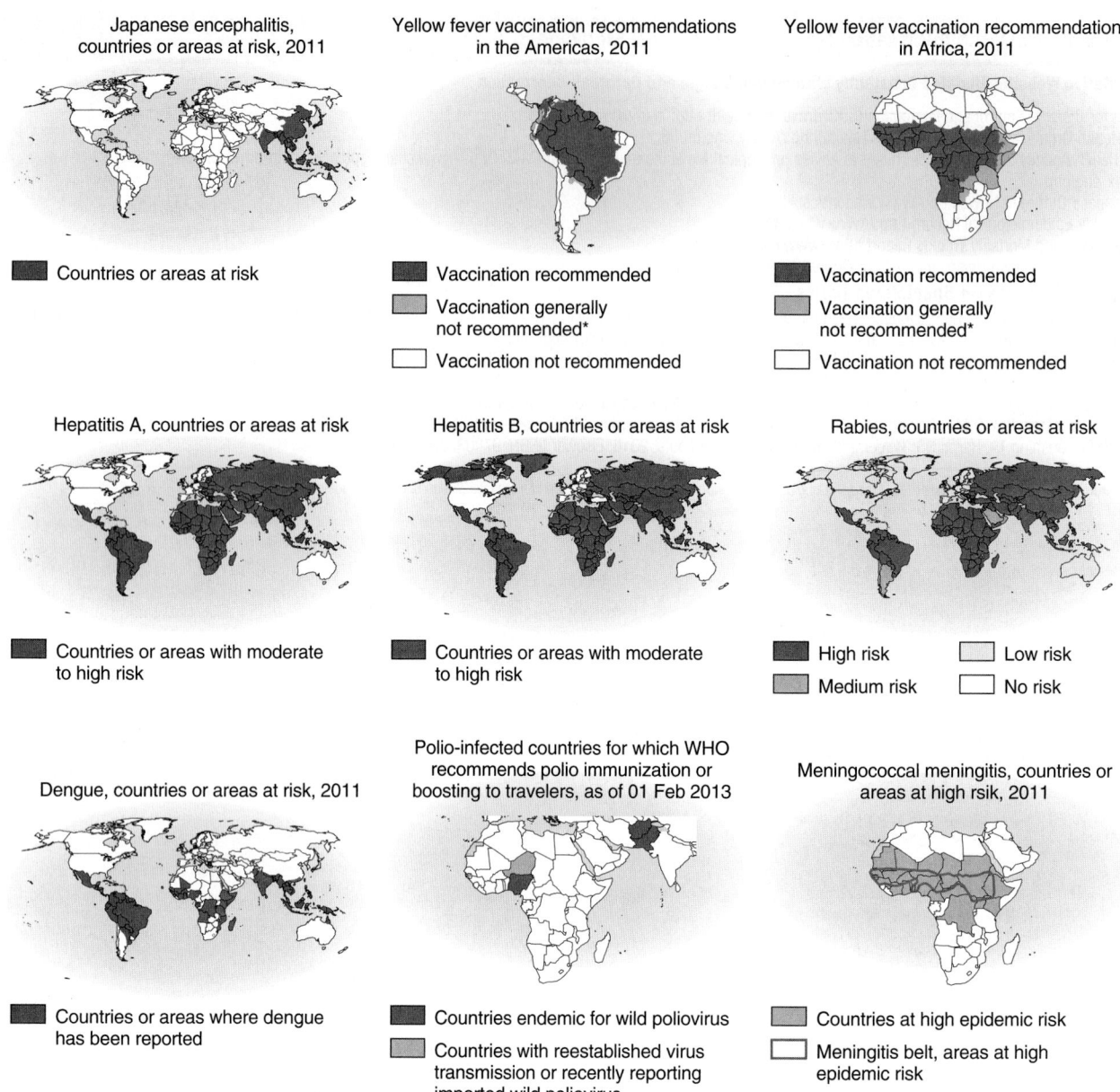

FIG. 1 Worldwide distribution of important travel-related diseases. *Yellow Fever (YF) vaccination is generally not recommended in areas where there is low-potential YF virus exposure. However, vaccination might be considered for a small subset of travelers to these areas who are at increased risk for exposure to YF virus because of prolonged travel, heavy exposure to mosquitoes, or inability to avoid mosquito bites. Consideration for vaccination of any traveler must take into account the traveler's risk of being infected with YF virus, country entry requirements, and individual risk factors for serious vaccine-associated adverse events (e.g., age, immune status). (From World Health Organization. International Travel and Health. Available at http://www.who.int/ith. In Bennett JE, Dolin R, Blaser MJ: *Mandell, Douglas, and Bennett's principles and practice of infectious diseases,* ed 8, Philadelphia, 2015, Elsevier.)

TABLE 3 Travel-Related Vaccines of Adults

DISEASE	VACCINE	PRIMARY COURSE	ROUTE	FURTHER BOOSTERS
Vaccines to Consider for All Destinations				
Hepatitis A	Killed virus	0, 6-18mo[a]	IM	None
Hepatitis B	Recombinant viral antigen	0, 1, 6mo	IM	None
		A: 0, 1, 2, and 12mo	IM	None
		A: 0, 1, 3wk and 12mo[b]	IM	
Hepatitis A/B	Combination of monovalent preparations	0, 1, 6mo	IM	None
		A: 0, 1, 3wk and 12mo	IM	None
Typhoid	Capsular Vi polysaccharide	Single dose	IM	2-3yr
	Live-attenuated Ty21a bacteria	0, 2, 4, 6 days	Oral	5yr
Influenza	Inactivated viral	Single dose	IM	Annual
	Live-attenuated virus	Single dose	Nasal	Annual
Varicella	Live-attenuated virus	0, 4-8wk	SC	None
Vaccines for Selected Destinations				
Yellow fever	Live-attenuated 17D virus	Single dose	SC	Lifetime protection[c]
Meningococcus	Quadrivalent conjugated polysaccharide (A, C, Y, W135)	Single dose	IM	5yr
Rabies	Inactivated cell culture viral	0, 7, 21-28 days	IM[d]	None routinely but two doses after each exposure
Japanese encephalitis (Vero cell)	Inactivated viral	0, 28 days	IM	1yr if at continued risk. No data on subsequent doses
Polio[e]	Inactivated viral	Single dose if adequate childhood series	SC; IM acceptable	None
Cholera	Killed bacteria + recombinant B toxin subunit[f,g]	0, 1wk	Oral	2yr for cholera; 3mo for ETEC
Tick-borne encephalitis[h]	Inactivated viral	0, 1-3mo, 9-12mo	IM	3yr

[a]Second dose may be delayed up to 8 years without diminished efficacy.
[b]Regimen not approved by the U.S. Food and Drug Administration for monovalent hepatitis B vaccine but approved for combination hepatitis A/B vaccine containing the same quantity of hepatitis B antigen.
[c]Until 2016, some countries that have mandatory entry requirements may require vaccination every 10 years.
[d]Intradermal rabies preexposure vaccine is no longer produced, and the intramuscular 1.0-mL vials are not licensed for intradermal use in a 0.1-mL dose.
[e]Oral polio vaccine is no longer produced in the United States.
[f]Not available in the United States but available in Canada and most European countries. No cholera vaccine of any kind is currently available in the United States.
[g]Also licensed in some countries for traveler's diarrhea because of enterotoxigenic *Escherichia coli.*
[h]Not available in United States but available in endemic areas and in Canada and the United Kingdom by special release.
A, accelerated regimen to be used for imminent departures; *ETEC,* enterotoxigenic *E. coli; IM,* intramuscular; *SC,* subcutaneous.
From Bennett JE, Dolin R, Blaser MJ: *Mandell, Douglas, and Bennett's principles and practice of infectious diseases,* ed 8, Philadelphia, 2015, Elsevier.

A

Page numbers followed by "f" indicate figures, "t" indicate tables and "b" indicate boxes.

C

D

G

H

J

K

L

O

Q

R

T

U

V

W

X

Y

Z

PULMONARY DISEASE

RHEUMATOLOGY

SURGERY, GENERAL

UROLOGY